NELSON Textbook of
PEDIATRICS

NELSON Textbook of PEDIATRICS

THIRTEENTH EDITION

RICHARD E. BEHRMAN, M.D.

Dean, School of Medicine and
Professor, Department of Pediatrics,
Case Western Reserve University School of Medicine;
Attending Physician, Rainbow Babies and Childrens Hospital,
Cleveland, Ohio

VICTOR C. VAUGHAN, III, M.D.

Professor of Pediatrics,
Temple University School of Medicine;
Attending Physician, St. Christopher's Hospital for Children;
Senior Medical Evaluation Officer, National Board of Medical Examiners,
Philadelphia, Pennsylvania

Senior Editor
WALDO E. NELSON, M.D.

Professor of Pediatrics, Medical College of Pennsylvania and
Temple University School of Medicine;
Attending Physician, St. Christopher's Hospital for Children,
Philadelphia, Pennsylvania

1987
W. B. SAUNDERS COMPANY
Harcourt Brace Jovanovich, Inc.
Philadelphia ■ London ■ Toronto ■ Montreal ■ Sydney ■ Tokyo

W. B. SAUNDERS COMPANY
Harcourt Brace Jovanovich, Inc.

West Washington Square
Philadelphia, PA 19105

Library of Congress Cataloging-in-Publication Data

Textbook of pediatrics.

Nelson textbook of pediatrics.

Includes bibliographies and index.

1. Pediatrics.   I. Behrman, Richard E., 1931–   .
II. Vaughan, Victor C., 1919–   .   III. Nelson, Waldo E.
(Waldo Emerson), 1898–   . [DNLM: 1. Pediatrics.
WS 100 N4321]

RJ45.T43 1987   618.92   86–17727

ISBN 0-03-011442-X

Listed here are the latest translated editions of this book together with the language of the translation and the publisher.

French—Vol. I (*10th Edition*)—Doin Editeurs, S.A., Paris, France

French—Vol. II (*10th Edition*)—Doin Editeurs, S.A., Paris, France

Russian (*12th Edition*)—Meditsina Publishing House, Moscow, U.S.S.R.

Editor: Darlene Cooke
Developmental Editor: David Kilmer
Designer: W. B. Saunders Staff
Production Manager: Bob Butler
Manuscript Editor: Mark Coyle
Illustration Coordinator: Peg Shaw
Indexer: Julie Schwager

Nelson Textbook of Pediatrics   ISBN 0-03-011442-X

Last digit is the print number: 9   8   7   6   5   4   3

To the generations of pediatricians, house officers, and medical students, whose personal commitment to their own continuing education is the foundation of quality care for children.

PREFACE

The Thirteenth Edition of the Nelson Textbook of Pediatrics has been produced and published during an almost unprecedented surge of progress in biomedical science and technology, which is rapidly advancing the knowledge and techniques of caring for children. This comprehensive and concise one-volume edition devoted to the welfare of children has tried to meld this progress with the art of pediatrics to meet the needs of practitioners, house staff, and medical students.

This edition includes many essentially new sections as well as many substantially modified and expanded sections, all of which have been produced in the light of the new knowledge and concerns. Our review of the field of pediatrics has left practically no area of the book untouched, and, we hope, no section unimproved. We greatly appreciate the efforts of our contributors in achieving the completeness, relevance, and conciseness the book displays. We have all been committed to producing an edition that will continue to be helpful to those caring for children or wishing to know more about them.

Since the last edition, we have lost three contributors through death. The participation of Henry W. Baird, Harry A. Feldman, and C. Henry Kempe is much missed.

In this edition we have had the invaluable assistance of the faculty of the Department of Pediatrics at Case Western Reserve University. We are especially indebted to Suzanne Hazan, who, as editorial assistant, has played a vital role in the quality of the final written text. Victor H. Auerbach, Ph.D., and J. Richard Hamilton, M.D., have served as associate editors for the sections on Inborn Errors of Metabolism and Gastroenterology, respectively.

The preparation of this Thirteenth Edition has also required the help and cooperation of many other persons. To each of them we acknowledge our debt of gratitude. We especially wish to express our heartfelt thanks to Ann Behrman and Deborah Vaughan. Without their understanding, forbearance, and help this textbook would not have been possible.

RICHARD E. BEHRMAN
VICTOR C. VAUGHAN, III

NOTICE

Extraordinary efforts have been made by the authors, the editors, and the publisher of this book to ensure that dosage recommendations are precise and in agreement with standards officially accepted at the time of publication.

It does happen, however, that dosage schedules are changed from time to time in the light of accumulating clinical experience and continuing laboratory studies. This is most likely to occur in the case of recently introduced products.

It is urged, therefore, that you check the manufacturer's recommendations for dosage, *especially if the drug to be administered or prescribed is one that you use only infrequently or have not used for some time.*

THE PUBLISHER

CONTRIBUTORS

TARO AKABANE, M.D., Ph.D.
Chairman and Professor of Pediatrics, Shinshu University
School of Medicine; Attending Physician, Shinshu University
Hospital, Japan

ARTHUR J. AMMANN, M.D.
Director, Collaborative Medical Research Program, Genentech, Inc.; Adjunct Professor of Immunology/Rheumatology, University of California, San Francisco, San Francisco, California

DOROTHY M. ARAM, Ph.D.
Associate Professor, Department of Pediatrics, Case Western Reserve University School of Medicine; Attending Physician, Rainbow Babies and Childrens Hospital, Cleveland, Ohio

STEPHEN C. ARONOFF, M.D.
Assistant Professor, Department of Pediatrics, Case Western Reserve University School of Medicine, Cleveland, Ohio

VICTOR H. AUERBACH, Ph.D.
Senior Research Professor in Pediatrics (Biochemistry), Temple University School of Medicine; Formerly Director of Laboratories, St. Christopher's Hospital for Children, Philadelphia, Pennsylvania

WILLIAM F. BALISTRERI, M.D.
Professor of Pediatrics and Medicine, University of Cincinnati College of Medicine; Director, Division of Pediatric Gastroenterology and Nutrition, Children's Hospital Medical Center, Cincinnati, Ohio

GIULIO J. BARBERO, M.D.
Professor and Chairman, Department of Child Health, University of Missouri School of Medicine; Chief of Pediatric Service, University of Missouri Hospital, Columbia, Missouri

LEWIS A. BARNESS, M.D.
Professor and Chairman, Department of Pediatrics, University of South Florida College of Medicine; Attending Physician, Tampa General Hospital, Tampa, Florida

JOHN B. BARTRAM, M.D.
Professor Emeritus of Pediatrics, Temple University School of Medicine; Honorary Attending Pediatrician, St. Christopher's Hospital for Children, Philadelphia, Pennsylvania

RICHARD E. BEHRMAN, M.D.
Dean, School of Medicine, and Professor, Department of Pediatrics, Case Western Reserve University School of Medicine; Attending Physician, Rainbow Babies and Childrens Hospital, Cleveland, Ohio

JERRY MICHAEL BERGSTEIN, M.D.
Professor, Department of Pediatrics, Indiana University School of Medicine; Director, Section of Nephrology, James Whitcomb Riley Hospital for Children, Indianapolis, Indiana

ROBERT J. BERKOWITZ
Associate Professor and Director, Division of Preventive Dentistry, School of Dental and Oral Surgery, Columbia University; Attending Staff, Presbyterian Hospital, New York, New York

JAMES B. BESUNDER, D.O.
Fellow, Department of Pediatrics, Case Western Reserve University School of Medicine, Cleveland, Ohio

CHARLES D. BLUESTONE, M.D.
Professor, Department of Otolaryngology, University of Pittsburgh School of Medicine; Director, Department of Pediatric Otolaryngology, Children's Hospital of Pittsburgh, Pittsburgh, Pennsylvania

THOMAS F. BOAT, M.D.
Professor and Chairman, Department of Pediatrics, University of North Carolina School of Medicine; Director of Pediatrics, North Carolina Memorial Hospital, Chapel Hill, North Carolina

PHILIP A. BRUNELL, M.D.
Professor, Department of Pediatrics, University of Texas Health Science Center at San Antonio; Attending Physician, Medical Center Hospital and Santa Rosa Children's Hospital, San Antonio, Texas

THOMAS M. BUCHANAN, M.D.
Professor of Medicine, University of Washington School of Medicine; Attending Physician, Pacific Medical Center and Harborview Medical Center; Chief, Immunology Research Laboratory, Pacific Medical Center, Seattle, Washington

HUGO F. CARVAJAL, M.D.
Professor of Pediatrics and Surgery, and Director, Division of Pediatric Critical Care, Department of Pediatrics, University of Texas Medical School at Houston, Houston, Texas

JAMES D. CHERRY, M.D., M.Sc.
Professor of Pediatrics and Chief, Division of Pediatric Infectious Diseases, Center for the Health Sciences, UCLA School of Medicine; Attending Physician, UCLA Medical Center, Los Angeles, California

RUSSELL W. CHESNEY, M.D.
Professor and Vice Chairman, Department of Pediatrics, and Director, Pediatric Nephrology, University of California—Davis Medical Center, Sacramento, California

J. JULIAN CHISOLM, Jr., M.D.
Associate Professor of Pediatrics, Johns Hopkins University School of Medicine; Director, Childhood Lead Poisoning Prevention Program, Kennedy Institute for Handicapped Children; Senior Staff Pediatrician, Francis Scott Key Medical Center, Baltimore, Maryland

DAVID F. CLYDE, M.D., Ph.D., D.T.M.& H.
Adjunct Professor, Johns Hopkins University School of Medicine; Research Professor of Medicine, University of Maryland School of Medicine, Baltimore, Maryland

PAUL M. COATES, Ph.D.
Research Associate Professor, Department of Pediatrics, University of Pennsylvania School of Medicine; Associate Director, Lipid–Heart Research Center, Children's Hospital of Philadelphia, Philadelphia, Pennsylvania

SANFORD N. COHEN, M.D.
Senior Vice President for Academic Affairs, Provost, and Professor of Pediatrics, Wayne State University School of Medicine; Attending Physician, Children's Hospital of Michigan, Detroit, Michigan

A. W. CONN, M.D., B.Sc.(Med.), F.A.C.A., F.R.C.P.(C), F.A.A.P.
Professor of Anaesthesia, University of Toronto; Director Emeritus, Intensive Care Unit, Hospital for Sick Children, Toronto, Ontario, Canada

JEAN A. CORTNER, M.D.
Professor, Department of Pediatrics, University of Pennsylvania School of Medicine; Director, Lipid–Heart Research Center, and Senior Physician, Children's Hospital of Philadelphia, Philadelphia, Pennsylvania

FRANKLIN L. DeBUSK, M.D.
Professor of Pediatrics, University of Florida College of Medicine; Active Staff, Shands Hospital, Gainesville, Florida

FLOYD W. DENNY, M.D.
Professor of Pediatrics, University of North Carolina School of Medicine; Attending Pediatrician, North Carolina Memorial Hospital, Chapel Hill, North Carolina

ANGELO M. DiGEORGE, M.D.
Professor of Pediatrics, Temple University School of Medicine; Chief, Endocrine and Metabolic Disease Section, St. Christopher's Hospital for Children, Philadelphia, Pennsylvania

CARL F. DOERSHUK, M.D.
Professor of Pediatrics, Case Western Reserve University School of Medicine; Associate Pediatrician, Rainbow Babies and Childrens Hospital, Cleveland, Ohio

JOHN J. DOWNES, M.D.
Professor of Anesthesia and Pediatrics, University of Pennsylvania School of Medicine; Anesthesiologist-in-Chief and Director, Department of Anesthesia and Critical Care, Children's Hospital of Philadelphia, Philadelphia, Pennsylvania

JOHN M. DUNN, M.D.
Former Clinical Associate Professor, Temple University School of Medicine, Philadelphia, Pennsylvania; Staff Child Psychiatrist, Grandview Hospital, Sellersville, Pennsylvania

ELLIOT F. ELLIS, M.D.
Professor of Pediatrics, State University of New York at Buffalo; Director, Allergy/Clinical Immunology Division, The Children's Hospital of Buffalo, Buffalo, New York

NANCY B. ESTERLY, M.D.
Professor of Pediatrics and Dermatology, Northwestern University Medical School; Head, Division of Dermatology, Children's Memorial Hospital, Chicago, Illinois

JAMES C. FALLIS, M.D., F.R.C.S.(C)
Assistant Professor in Surgery and in Pediatrics, University of Toronto; Active Staff, Departments of Surgery and Pediatrics, and Director, Emergency Services, Hospital for Sick Children, Toronto, Ontario, Canada

RALPH D. FEIGIN, M.D.
J.S. Abercrombie Professor of Pediatrics and Chairman of the Department of Pediatrics, Baylor College of Medicine; Physician-in-Chief, Texas Children's Hospital; Physician-in-Chief, Pediatric Service, Harris County Hospital District; Chief, Pediatric Service, The Methodist Hospital, Houston, Texas

THE LATE HARRY A. FELDMAN, M.D.
Formerly Professor and Chairman, Department of Preventive Medicine, State University of New York, Upstate Medical Center; Attending Physician, State University Hospital, Syracuse, New York

MARC A. FORMAN, M.D.
Professor of Psychiatry, Clinical Professor in Pediatrics, and Director, Division of Child Psychiatry, Tulane University School of Medicine; Clinical Professor of Psychiatry, Louisiana State University School of Medicine; Consultant, Children's Hospital of New Orleans and New Orleans Adolescent Hospital, New Orleans, Louisiana

GORDON FORSTNER, M.D., F.R.C.P.(C)
Professor of Pediatrics, University of Toronto; Chief, Division of Gastroenterology, Hospital for Sick Children, Toronto, Ontario, Canada

WELTON M. GERSONY, M.D.
Professor of Pediatrics, College of Physicians and Surgeons of Columbia University; Director, Division of Pediatric Cardiology, Columbia-Presbyterian Medical Center, New York, New York

ELI GOLD, M.D.
Clinical Professor of Pediatrics, University of Washington; Emeritus Professor of Pediatrics, University of California, Davis; Attending Pediatrician, Children's Hospital and Medical Center, Seattle, Washington

RICARDO GONZALEZ, M.D.
Professor, Director of Pediatric Urology, Department of Urologic Surgery, University of Minnesota; Attending Urologist, University of Minnesota Hospital; Active Staff, Minneapolis Children's Medical Center, Minneapolis, Minnesota

I. BRUCE GORDON, M.D.
Associate Professor of Pediatrics and Vice Chairman, Department of Pediatrics, Case Western Reserve University School of Medicine; Director, Department of Pediatrics, Cleveland Metropolitan General Hospital, Cleveland, Ohio

N. THORNE GRISCOM
Professor of Radiology, Harvard Medical School; Radiologist, Children's Hospital, Boston, and Brigham and Women's Hospital, Boston, Massachusetts

GABRIEL G. HADDAD, M.D.
Associate Professor of Pediatrics, Columbia University College of Physicians and Surgeons; Attending Physician, Babies Hospital/Presbyterian Hospital, New York, New York

SCOTT B. HALSTEAD, M.D.
Associate Director, Health Sciences Division, Rockefeller Foundation, New York, New York

J. RICHARD HAMILTON, M.D., F.R.C.P.(C)
Professor and Chairman, Department of Pediatrics, McGill University; Physician-in-Chief, Montreal Children's Hospital, Montreal, Quebec, Canada

JAMES BARRY HANSHAW, M.D.
Professor of Pediatrics, Dean, and Provost, University of Massachusetts Medical School; Lecturer, Department of Pediatrics, Harvard Medical School; Consultant, University of Massachusetts Hospital, St. Vincent Hospital, and Worcester Memorial Hospital, Worcester, Massachusetts

HAROLD E. HARRISON
Professor Emeritus in Pediatrics, Johns Hopkins University School of Medicine; Pediatrician, Johns Hopkins Hospital, Baltimore, Maryland

ALFRED D. HEGGIE, M.D.
Associate Professor of Pediatrics and Pathology, Case Western Reserve University School of Medicine; Attending Pediatrician, Rainbow Babies and Childrens Hospital; Associate Director, Virology Laboratory, University Hospitals of Cleveland, Cleveland, Ohio

WERNER HENLE, M.D.
Professor Emeritus of Virology, University of Pennsylvania; Director, Division of Research Virology, Joseph Stokes Jr. Research Institute, Children's Hospital of Philadelphia, Philadelphia, Pennsylvania

JOHN J. HERBST, M.D.
Professor and Chairman, Department of Pediatrics, Louisiana State University School of Medicine at Shreveport; Attending Physician, University Hospital, Louisiana State University Medical Center, Shreveport, Louisiana

WILLIAM HETZNECKER, M.D.
Clinical Professor of Psychiatry, Clinical Professor in Pediatrics, Temple University School of Medicine; Attending Physician, St. Christopher's Hospital for Children and Temple University Hospital, Philadelphia, Pennsylvania

KURT HIRSCHHORN, M.D.
Herbert H. Lehman Professor and Chairman, Mount Sinai School of Medicine; Pediatrician-in-Chief, Mount Sinai Hospital, New York, New York

LEWIS B. HOLMES, M.D.
Associate Professor of Pediatrics, Harvard Medical School; Pediatrician and Chief, Embryology-Teratology Unit, Massachusetts General Hospital, Boston, Massachusetts

RICHARD HONG, M.D.
Professor of Pediatrics, University of Wisconsin Clinical Science Center; Attending Physician, University Hospitals, Madison, Wisconsin

HAROLD W. HOROWITZ, M.D.
Research Associate in Geographic Medicine, Clinical Fellow in Infectious Diseases, Tufts University School of Medicine, Boston, Massachusetts

R. RODNEY HOWELL, M.D.
David R. Park Professor and Chairman, Department of Pediatrics, University of Texas Medical School at Houston; Pediatrician in Chief, University Children's Hospital at Hermann; Consultant in Pediatrics, M.D. Anderson Hospital and Tumor Institute and Shriners Hospital for Crippled Children, Houston, Texas

GEORGE HUG, M.D.
Professor of Pediatrics, University of Cincinnati College of Medicine; Attending Pediatrician and Director, Divisions of Enzymology and the Clinical Research Center, Children's Hospital Medical Center, Cincinnati, Ohio

PETER R. HUTTENLOCHER, M.D.
Professor of Pediatrics and Neurology, University of Chicago School of Medicine; Chief, Pediatric Neurology Section, Wyler Children's Hospital, Chicago, Illinois

DAVID C. JOHNSEN, D.D.S., M.S.
Professor and Chairman, Department of Pediatric Dentistry, School of Dentistry, Case Western Reserve University, Cleveland, Ohio

RICHARD B. JOHNSTON, JR., M.D.
William H. Bennett Professor and Chairman, Department of Pediatrics, University of Pennsylvania School of Medicine; Physician-in-Chief, Children's Hospital of Philadelphia, Philadelphia, Pennsylvania

KENNETH LYONS JONES, M.D.
Associate Professor, Department of Pediatrics, University of California, San Diego, La Jolla, California; Attending Physician, University Hospital, San Diego, California

BARBARA S. KAPLAN, M.D.
Clinical Intructor, Case Western Reserve University School of Medicine; Attending Physician, Mt. Sinai Medical Center, Cleveland, Ohio

SHELDON L. KAPLAN, M.D.
Associate Professor, Department of Pediatrics, Baylor College of Medicine; Chief, Infectious Disease Service, Texas Children's Hospital; Attending Pediatrician, Ben Taub General Hospital, Houston, Texas

RALPH E. KAUFFMAN, M.D.
Professor of Pediatrics and Pharmacology, Wayne State University School of Medicine; Attending Physician and Director, Division of Clinical Pharmacology/Toxicology, Children's Hospital of Michigan, Detroit, Michigan

JAMES W. KAZURA, M.D.
Associate Professor of Medicine, Case Western Reserve University School of Medicine; Attending Physician, University Hospitals of Cleveland, Cleveland, Ohio

WESLEY E. KERSCHBAUM, M.D.
Instructor in Psychiatry (Child), Temple University School of Medicine; Child Psychiatrist, St. Christopher's Hospital for Children, Philadelphia, Pennsylvania

JOHN A. KIRKPATRICK, Jr., M.D.
Professor of Radiology, Harvard Medical School; Radiologist-in-Chief, Children's Hospital, Boston; Radiologist (Pediatric), Brigham and Women's Hospital, Boston, Massachusetts

ROBERT M. KLIEGMAN, M.D.
Associate Professor, Case Western Reserve University School of Medicine; Vice Chairman, Department of Pediatrics, Rainbow Babies and Children's Hospital, Cleveland, Ohio

RICHARD D. KRUGMAN, M.D.
Associate Professor and Vice Chairman, Department of Pediatrics, University of Colorado School of Medicine; Director, C. Henry Kempe National Center for the Prevention and Treatment of Child Abuse and Neglect; Attending Physician, University Hospital, Denver, Colorado

BRIGID G. LEVENTHAL, M.D.
Associate Professor, Oncology and Pediatrics, Johns Hopkins Medical Institutions; Director, Clinical Research Administration, Johns Hopkins Oncology Center, Johns Hopkins Hospital, Baltimore, Maryland

MELVIN D. LEVINE, M.D., F.A.A.P.
Professor of Pediatrics, University of North Carolina School of Medicine; Director, Clinical Center for the Study of Development and Learning, University of North Carolina, Chapel Hill, North Carolina

IRIS F. LITT, M.D.
Associate Professor of Pediatrics, Stanford University School of Medicine; Director, Division of Adolescent Medicine, Stanford University Hospital and The Children's Hospital at Stanford, Stanford, California

C. CHARLTON MABRY, M.D.
Professor of Pediatrics, University of Kentucky; Attending Pediatrician, University Hospital, Lexington, Kentucky

ADEL A. F. MAHMOUD, M.D., Ph.D.
Professor of Medicine, Professor of Molecular Biology and Microbiology, Case Western Reserve University School of Medicine; Attending Physician, Department of Medicine, and Chief, Division of Geographic Medicine, University Hospitals of Cleveland, Cleveland, Ohio

MILTON MARKOWITZ, M.D.
Professor of Pediatrics and Associate Dean, Student Affairs, University of Connecticut School of Medicine, Farmington, Connecticut

RICHARD J. MARTIN, M.D.
Associate Professor of Pediatrics, Case Western Reserve University School of Medicine; Co-Director of Neonatology, Rainbow Babies and Childrens Hospital, Cleveland, Ohio

LOIS J. MARTYN, M.D.
Associate Professor of Ophthalmology and Associate Professor in Pediatrics, Temple University School of Medicine; Pediatric Ophthalmologist, St. Christopher's Hospital for Children, Philadelphia, Pennsylvania

REUBEN MATALON, M.D., Ph.D.
Professor of Pediatrics and Genetics, Head, Division of Genetics and Metabolism; and Director, PKU Clinic, University of Illinois at Chicago College of Medicine, Chicago, Illinois

KENNETH McINTOSH, M.D.
Professor of Pediatrics, Harvard Medical School; Clinical Chief, Division of Infectious Diseases, Children's Hospital, Boston, Massachusetts

R. JAMES McKAY, M.D.
Professor of Pediatrics, University of Vermont College of Medicine; Attending Pediatrician, Medical Center Hospital of Vermont, Burlington, Vermont

ROBERT B. MELLINS, M.D.
Professor of Pediatrics, Columbia University College of Physicians and Surgeons; Attending Physician, Babies Hospital/Presbyterian Hospital, New York, New York

MICHAEL H. MERSON, M.D.
Director, Diarrheal Diseases Control Programme, World Health Organization, Geneva, Switzerland

ALFRED F. MICHAEL, M.D.
Regents' Professor, Department of Pediatrics and Department of Laboratory Medicine and Pathology, University of Minnesota Medical School; Attending Physician, University of Minnesota Hospital, Minneapolis, Minnesota

ALBERT MILLER, B.S., M.S., Ph.D.
(Retired) Associate Professor of Parasitology, Tulane University School of Public Health and Tropical Medicine, New Orleans, Louisiana

RICHARD A. MILLER, M.D.
Assistant Professor of Medicine, Division of Infectious Diseases, University of Washington; Attending Physician, Division of Infectious Diseases, Pacific Medical Center, Seattle, Washington

ROBERT W. MILLER, M.D., Dr.P.H.
Chief, Clinical Epidemiology Branch, National Cancer Institute, Bethesda, Maryland

THOMAS P. MONATH, M.D.
Director, Division of Vector-Borne Viral Diseases, Center for Infectious Diseases, Centers for Disease Control, Fort Collins, Colorado

E. A. MORTIMER, M.D.
Elisabeth Severance Prentiss Professor of Epidemiology and Pediatrics, and Vice Chairman, Department of Epidemiology and Biostatistics, Case Western Reserve University School of Medicine; Associate Pediatrician, University Hospitals of Cleveland and Cleveland Metropolitan General Hospital, Cleveland, Ohio

NADIA NOGUEIRA, M.D., Ph.D.
Associate Professor, Department of Medical and Molecular Parasitology and Department of Medicine, New York University Medical Center, New York, New York

MICHAEL E. NORMAN, M.D.
Professor and Associate Chairman, Department of Pediatrics, Jefferson Medical College of Thomas Jefferson University, Philadelphia, Pennsylvania; Director of Pediatrics, The Medical Center of Delaware, Inc., Newark, Delaware

JAMES C. OVERALL, Jr., M.D.
Professor of Pediatrics and Pathology; Chief, Pediatric Infectious Diseases, Department of Pediatrics; Associate Director, Diagnostic Virology Laboratory, Department of Pathology; Center for Infectious Diseases, Diagnostic Microbiology, and Immunology; University of Utah School of Medicine; Consultant in Infectious Diseases, Primary Children's Medical Center, Salt Lake City, Utah

DEMOSTHENES PAPPAGIANIS, M.D., Ph.D.
Professor, Department of Medical Microbiology and Immunology, University of California, Davis, School of Medicine, Davis, California

ROBERT H. PARROTT, M.D.
Professor, George Washington University School of Medicine and Health Sciences; Director Emeritus, Children's Hospital National Medical Center, Washington, D.C.

JEROME A. PAULSON, M.D.
Assistant Professor of Pediatrics, Case Western Reserve University School of Medicine; Assistant Pediatrician, Rainbow Babies and Childrens Hospital; Assistant Visiting Pediatrician, Cleveland Metropolitan General Hospital, Cleveland, Ohio

HOWARD A. PEARSON, M.D.
Professor of Pediatrics, Yale University School of Medicine; Attending Physician, Yale–New Haven Hospital, New Haven, Connecticut

CAROL F. PHILLIPS, M.D.
Professor and Chairman, Department of Pediatrics, University of Vermont College of Medicine; Chief of Pediatric Service, Medical Center Hospital of Vermont, Burlington, Vermont

STANLEY A. PLOTKIN, M.D.
Professor of Pediatrics and Microbiology, University of Pennsylvania School of Medicine; Associate Chairman, Department of Pediatrics, Division of Infectious Diseases, Children's Hospital of Philadelphia, Philadelphia, Pennsylvania

ALBERT W. PRUITT, M.D.
Ellington Charles Hawes Professor and Chairman, Department of Pediatrics, Medical College of Georgia; Chief of Pediatrics, Medical College of Georgia Hospital and Clinics, Augusta, Georgia

PAUL G. QUIE, M.D.
Professor of Pediatrics, Microbiology, and Laboratory Medicine and Pathology, University of Minnesota School of Medicine; Attending Physician, University of Minnesota Hospital and Clinics, Minneapolis, Minnesota

RUSSELL C. RAPHAELY, M.D.
Associate Professor of Anesthesia and Pediatrics, University of Pennsylvania School of Medicine; Director, Pediatric Critical Care Complex, Children's Hospital of Philadelphia, Philadelphia, Pennsylvania

JACK S. REMINGTON, M.D.
Chairman, Department of Immunology and Infectious Diseases, Research Institute, Palo Alto Medical Foundation, Palo Alto, California; Professor of Medicine, Stanford University Medical Center, Department of Medicine, Division of Infectious Diseases, Stanford, California

IRAJ REZVANI, M.D.
Professor of Pediatrics, Temple University School of Medicine; Attending Physician, Section of Pediatric Endocrinology and Metabolism, Department of Pediatrics, St. Christopher's Hospital for Children, Philadelphia, Pennsylvania

THOMAS A. RIEMENSCHNEIDER, M.D., M.B.A.
Professor of Pediatrics, Epidemiology, and Biostatistics, and Associate Dean, Case Western Reserve University School of Medicine; Associate Pediatrician, Division of Pediatric Cardiology, Rainbow Babies and Childrens Hospital, Cleveland, Ohio

ALAN M. ROBSON, M.D., F.R.C.P.
Professor of Pediatrics, Washington University School of Medicine; Director, Division of Pediatric Nephrology, St. Louis Children's Hospital, St. Louis, Missouri

BARRY H. RUMACK, M.D.
Professor of Pediatrics, University of Colorado School of Medicine; Director, Rocky Mountain Poison and Drug Center; Attending Physician, Denver General Hospital, Denver, Colorado

JANE GREEN SCHALLER, M.D.
Professor and Chairman, Tufts University School of Medicine; Pediatrician-in-Chief, Floating Hospital for Infants and Children, New England Medical Center Hospitals, Boston, Massachusetts

BARTON D. SCHMITT, M.D.
Associate Professor of Pediatrics, University of Colorado School of Medicine; Director of Consultative Services, Children's Hospital of Denver, Denver, Colorado

ROBERT SCHWARTZ, M.D.
Professor of Pediatrics and of Medical Science, Program in Medicine, Division of Biology and Medicine, Brown University; Director of Pediatric Metabolism and Nutrition, Rhode Island Hospital, Providence, Rhode Island

BARRY SHANDLING, M.B., Ch.B., F.R.C.S.(Eng.), F.R.C.S.(C), F.A.C.S.
Associate Professor, Department of Surgery, University of Toronto; Senior Staff Surgeon, Hospital for Sick Children; Director, Bowel Clinic, Hugh McMillan Medical Centre; Consultant Surgeon, Sunnybrook Hospital and North York General Hospital, Toronto, Ontario, Canada

DAVID O. SILLENCE, M.D., B.S., F.R.A.C.P., F.R.C.P.A.
Professor of Medical Genetics, University of Sydney, Sydney, Australia; Head, Medical Genetics Unit and Bone Dysplasia Clinic, Children's Hospital, Camperdown, Australia

JOSEPH SIMON, M.D.
Director, Emergency Services, Scottish Rite Children's Hospital, Atlanta, Georgia

WILLIAM T. SPECK, M.D.
Gertrude Lee Chandler Tucker Professor and Chairman, Department of Pediatrics, Case Western Reserve University School of Medicine; Director, Department of Pediatrics, Rainbow Babies and Childrens Hospital, Cleveland, Ohio

MARK A. SPERLING, M.D.
Professor of Pediatrics and Associate Professor of Medicine, University of Cincinnati College of Medicine; Director, Division of Endocrinology/Diabetes, Children's Hospital Medical Center, Cincinnati, Ohio

ROBERT C. STERN, M.D.
Professor of Pediatrics, Case Western Reserve University School of Medicine; Associate Pediatrician, Rainbow Babies and Childrens Hospital, Cleveland, Ohio

MARSHALL L. STOLLER, M.D.
Attending Physician, University of California at San Francisco Affiliated Hospitals, San Francisco, California

LEON STREBEL, M.D.
Hoffmann–La Roche, Inc., Basel, Switzerland

FREDERICK J. SUCHY, M.D.
Associate Professor of Pediatrics, University of Cincinnati College of Medicine; Attending Gastroenterologist, Children's Hospital Medical Center; Attending Physician, University Hospital, Cincinnati, Ohio

LAWRENCE T. TAFT, M.D.
Professor and Chairman, Department of Pediatrics, University of Medicine and Dentistry of New Jersey—Robert Wood Johnson Medical School; Chief of Pediatrics, Robert Wood Johnson University Hospital; Consultant in Pediatric Neurology, St. Peter's Medical Center, Hunterdon Medical Center, and Somerset Medical Center; Consultant, Jersey Shore Medical Center, Muhlenberg Hospital, and Morristown Memorial Hospital, New Brunswick, New Jersey

PHILIP TOLTZIS, M.D.
Instructor, Department of Pediatrics, Harvard University School of Medicine; Assistant in Medicine, Children's Hospital, Boston, Massachusetts

VICTOR C. VAUGHAN, III, M.D.
Professor in Pediatrics, Temple University School of Medicine; Adjunct Professor of Pediatrics, University of Pennsylvania School of Medicine; Senior Medical Evaluation Officer, National Board of Medical Examiners; Attending Pediatrician, St. Christopher's Hospital for Children, Philadelphia, Pennsylvania

HUGH G. WATTS, M.D.
Clinical Professor of Orthopedics, King Saud University; Consultant Pediatric Orthopedist, King Faisal Specialist Hospital and Research Center, Riyadh, Saudi Arabia

RALPH J. WEDGWOOD, M.D.
Professor and Head, Division of Immunology and Rheumatology, Department of Pediatrics, University of Washington; Chief, Rheumatology Service, and Attending Physician, Children's Hospital and Medical Center, Seattle, Washington

DAVID WENGER, Ph.D.
Professor of Medicine and Biochemistry, Jefferson Medical College of Thomas Jefferson University, Philadelphia, Pennsylvania

ROBERT E. WOOD, M.D., Ph.D.
Associate Professor of Pediatrics and Chief, Pediatric Pulmonary Medicine, University of North Carolina School of Medicine, Chapel Hill, North Carolina

DAVID J. WYLER, M.D., F.A.C.P.
Professor of Medicine, Tufts University School of Medicine; Physician, New England Medical Center Hospitals, Boston, Massachusetts

CONTENTS

4. PREVENTIVE PEDIATRICS AND EPIDEMIOLOGY 155

5. GENERAL CONSIDERATIONS IN THE CARE OF SICK CHILDREN.. 169

6. PRENATAL DISTURBANCES... 242

7. INBORN ERRORS OF METABOLISM 277

8. THE FETUS AND THE NEONATAL INFANT 358

12. THE DIGESTIVE SYSTEM 756

13. THE RESPIRATORY SYSTEM 854

14. THE CARDIOVASCULAR SYSTEM 943

15. DISEASES OF THE BLOOD 1033

16. NEOPLASMS AND NEOPLASM-LIKE STRUCTURES 1079

20. METABOLIC DISORDERS 1248

21. THE NERVOUS SYSTEM... 1274

22. NEUROMUSCULAR DISEASES 1331

23. THE BONES AND JOINTS 1343

24. THE SKIN 1385

25. PEDIATRIC OPHTHALMOLOGY 1447

26. UNCLASSIFIED DISEASES 1480

NELSON Textbook of
PEDIATRICS

COLOR PLATES

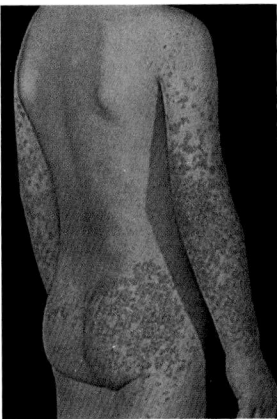

Figure 10–20. Schönlein-Henoch purpura (anaphylactoid purpura). (From Korting GW: Hautkrankheiten bei Kindern und Jugendlichen. Stuttgart, Germany, FK Schattauer Verlag, 1969.)

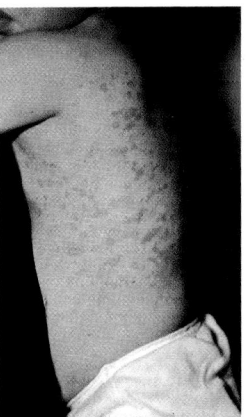

Figure 10–14. Rash of rheumatoid arthritis.

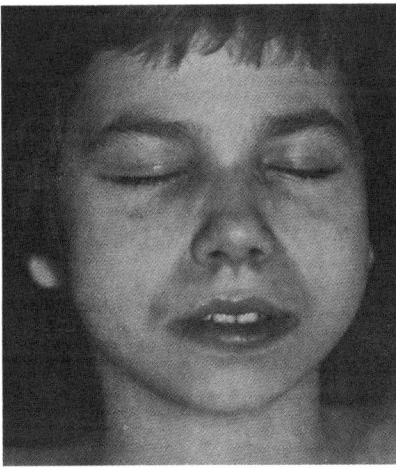

Figure 10–21. The facial rash of dermatomyositis. Note the faint erythema over the bridge of the nose and malar areas, and the heliotrope discoloration of the upper eyelids.

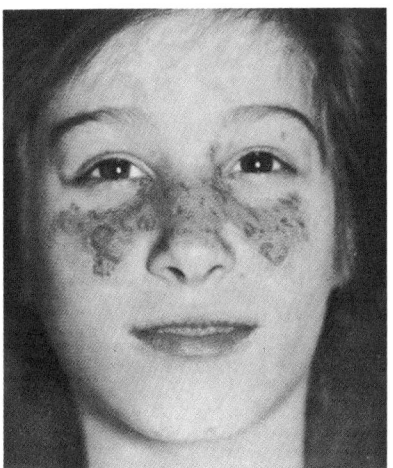

Figure 10–19. The butterfly rash of systemic lupus erythematosus.

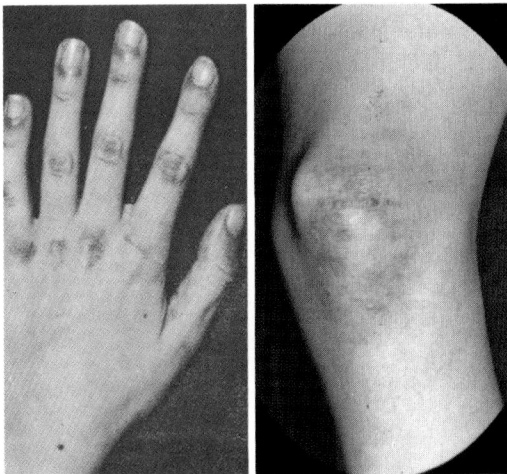

Figure 10–22. Rash of dermatomyositis. Skin changes over the knuckles (left) and over the knee (right).

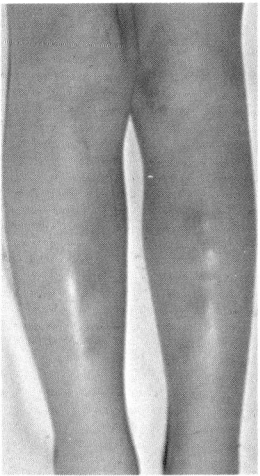

Figure 10–24. Erythema nodosum.

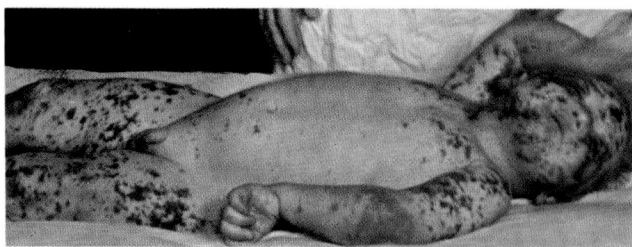

Figure 11–1. Fulminating meningococcemia in child 2½ yr of age. Onset 36 hr before admission, with vomiting and fever; 18 hr before admission, extensive purpuric eruption began; death 8 hr after admission. Blood culture positive for meningococcus type II. Nasal and cerebrospinal fluid cultures negative. One sibling had meningitis; another was found to be a carrier.

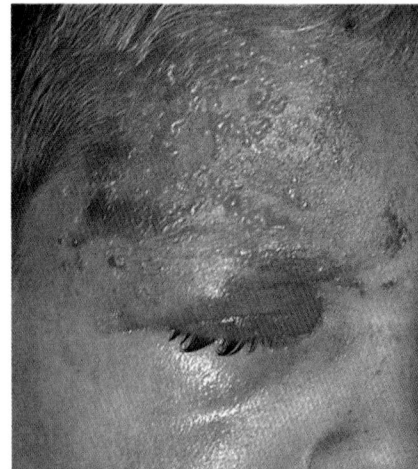

Figure 11–19. Herpes zoster ophthalmicus. (From Korting GW: Hautkrankheiten bei Kindern und Jugendlichen. Stuttgart, Germany, FK Schattauer Verlag, 1969.)

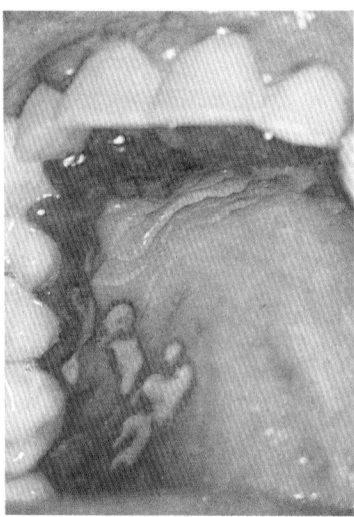

Figure 11–28. Herpangina. (From Korting GW: Hautkrankheiten bei Kindern und Jugendlichen. Stuttgart, Germany, FK Schattauer Verlag, 1969.)

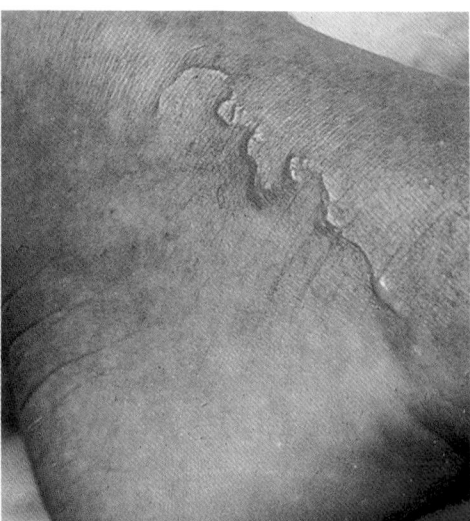

Figure 11–36. Creeping eruption of cutaneous larva migrans. (From Korting GW: Hautkrankheiten bei Kindern und Jugendlichen. Stuttgart, Germany, FK Schattauer Verlag, 1969.)

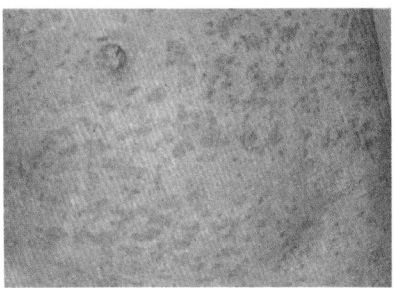

Figure 11–10. Maculopapular rash of measles. (From Korting GW: Hautkrankheiten bei Kindern und Jugendlichen. Stuttgart, Germany, FK Schattauer Verlag, 1969.)

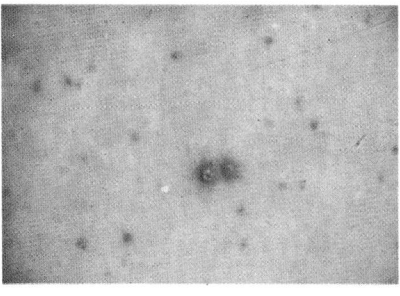

Figure 11–17. Skin lesions of chickenpox. Note the varying stages of development (macules, papules, and vesicles) present at the same time. (Courtesy of Dr. P. F. Lucchesi.)

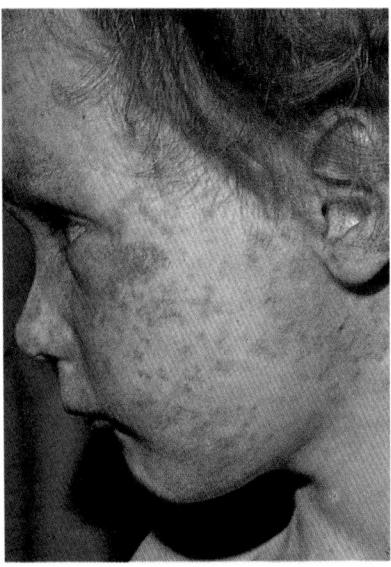

Figure 11–12. Rash of rubella (German measles). (From Korting GW: Hautkrankheiten bei Kindern und Jugendlichen. Stuttgart, Germany, FK Schattauer Verlag, 1969.)

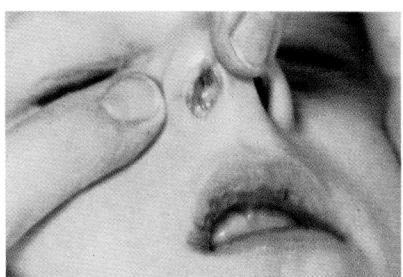

Figure 11–2. Nasal diphtheria. (Courtesy of Dr. Robert A. Lyon.)

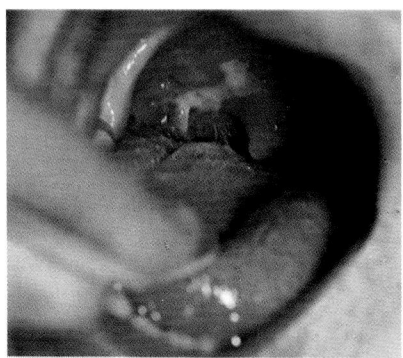

Figure 11–3. Pharyngotonsillar membrane of diphtheria. (Courtesy of Dr. Robert A. Lyon.)

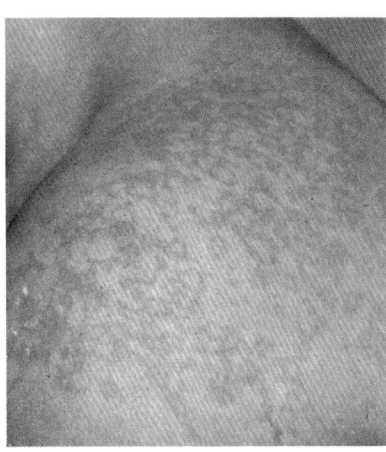

Figure 11–13. Erythema infectiosum. (From Korting GW: Hautkrankheiten bei Kindern und Jugendlichen. Stuttgart, Germany, FK Schattauer Verlag, 1969.)

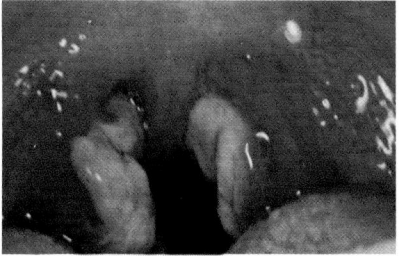

Figure 11–20. Tonsillitis with membrane formation in infectious mononucleosis. (Courtesy of Dr. Alex J. Steigman.)

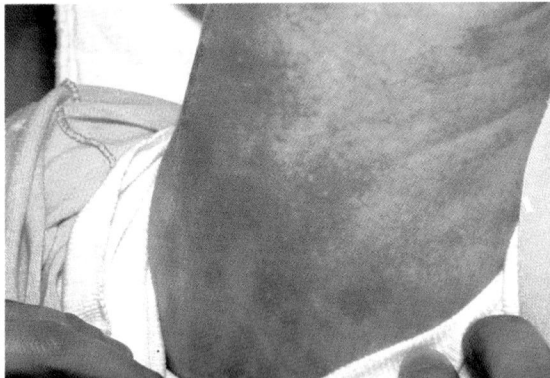

Figure 24–1. Erythema toxicum on the trunk of a newborn infant.

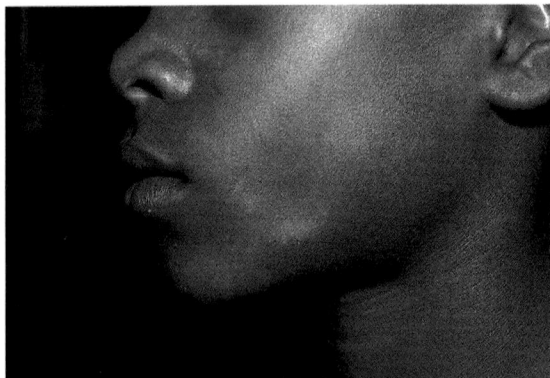

Figure 24–22. Patchy hypopigmented lesions with diffuse borders characteristic of pityriasis alba.

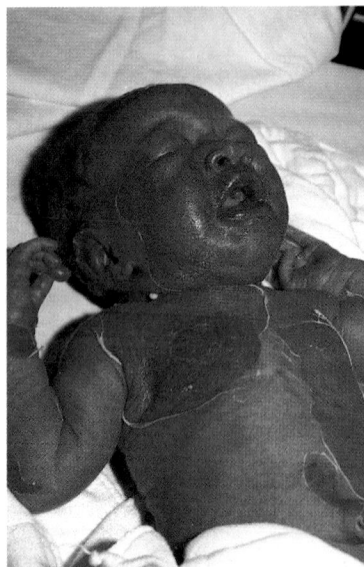

Figure 24–40. Infant with staphylococcal scalded skin syndrome.

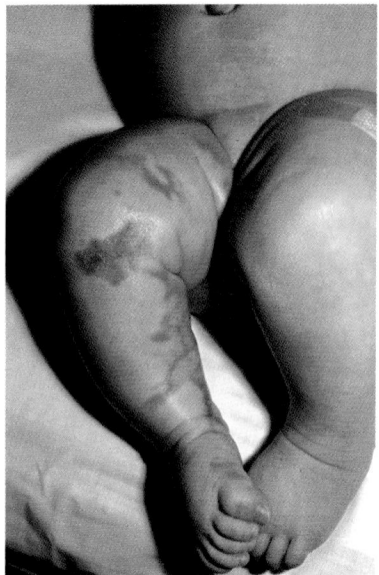

Figure 24–7. Marbled pattern of cutis marmorata telangiectatica congenita on the right leg.

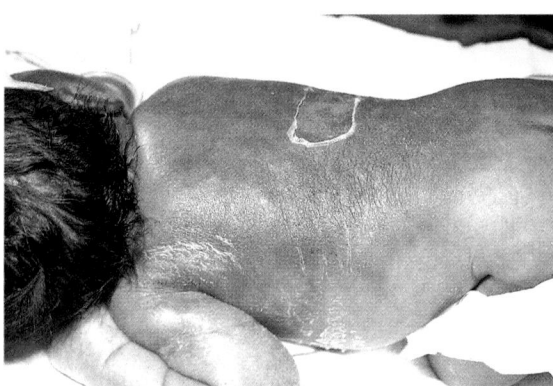

Figure 24–36. Red purple nodular infiltration of skin of back and upper arms due to subcutaneous fat necrosis.

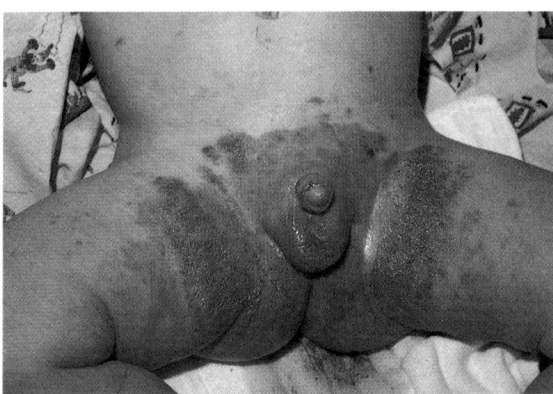

Figure 24–45. Erythematous confluent plaque with satellite pustules due to candidal infection.

NELSON Textbook of
PEDIATRICS

1

THE FIELD OF PEDIATRICS

Unlike medical specialties that deal primarily with particular organ systems or biologic processes, pediatrics is concerned with any disturbances of the health or the orderly growth and development of the child. The pediatrician's commitment is to secure for all children the opportunity to achieve their full native potential. As guardians of children's physical, mental, and emotional progress from conception to maturity, pediatricians are in the vanguard of social concern for children and their families. The caring qualities of any society may best be measured by the concerns it manifests for its aged, its disadvantaged (the dependent, handicapped, retarded, or incarcerated, for example), and its young. The young are often among the most disadvantaged.

THE SCOPE AND HISTORY OF PEDIATRICS

Pediatrics emerged as a medical specialty over a century ago in response to a growing appreciation that the health problems of children are different from those of adults and that the child's reaction to them varies with age. The focus and scope of pediatrics are being continually revised.

The health problems of children vary widely among the nations of the world in accordance with many factors, which include (1) the prevalence and ecology of infectious agents and their hosts; (2) climate and geography; (3) agricultural resources and practices; (4) educational, economic, and sociocultural considerations; and (5), in many instances, the gene frequencies for some disorders. These factors are often interrelated.

Not only do problems differ in various parts of the world, but priorities do also, since they must reflect local concerns, resources, and needs. The assessment of the state of health of any community must begin with epidemiologic and other studies that describe the incidence of illness and must continue with studies that show the changes that occur with time and in response to programs of prevention, case finding, therapy, and adequate surveillance. As contemporary problems in any community yield to study and to improved management, new problems become the foci of attention and efforts of pediatric clinicians and research workers. Accordingly, with time, there may be major changes in the relative importance of the various causes of childhood morbidity and mortality.

In the late 19th century in the United States, of every 1000 children born alive 200 might be expected to die before the age of 1 yr of such conditions as dysentery, pneumonia, measles, diphtheria, whooping cough, and the like. The efforts of pediatricians, combined with those of immunologists and pioneers in public health, have led to such better understanding of the origin and management of many problems of infants that in the past half century the infant mortality in the United States has fallen from around 75/1000 live births in 1925 to about 10.9 in 1983. Figure 8–1 shows that both neonatal (1st mo) and postneonatal (1–11 mo) mortality have had major reductions. Figure 1–1 shows that the great majority (about 75%) of deaths of infants under 1 yr of age occur within the first 28 days of life, most of these within the first 7 days; moreover, more than half of those within the first 7

days occur within the 1st day (about 40% of all deaths in the 1st yr). Table 1–1 shows the disproportionately high death rate within the 1st yr, as compared with the remainder of childhood.

Early in the 20th century efforts at control of infectious disease began to be complemented by better understanding of nutrition. New and continuing discoveries in these areas led to establishment of well child clinics. Along with acute infections and the chronic disturbances associated with deficits of calories, vitamins, minerals, or proteins, the acute nutritional and metabolic disturbances that accompany acute diarrhea also received attention.

In the middle years of the 20th century, a profound revolution in child health was brought about by the introduction of antibacterial chemicals and antibiotic agents. With improved control of infectious disease through both prevention and treatment and with other scientific and technical advances, pediatric medicine turned its attention increasingly to conditions affecting relatively small numbers of children. These included both potentially lethal conditions and temporarily or permanently handicapping conditions; among these disorders were leukemia, cystic fibrosis, diseases of the newborn infant, congenital heart disease, mental retardation, genetic defects, rheumatic diseases, renal diseases, and metabolic and endocrine disorders.

More recently, increasing attention has been given behavioral and social aspects of child health, ranging from a reexamination of child-rearing practices to the creation of major programs aimed at prevention and management of abuse and neglect of infants and children. Developmental psychologists,

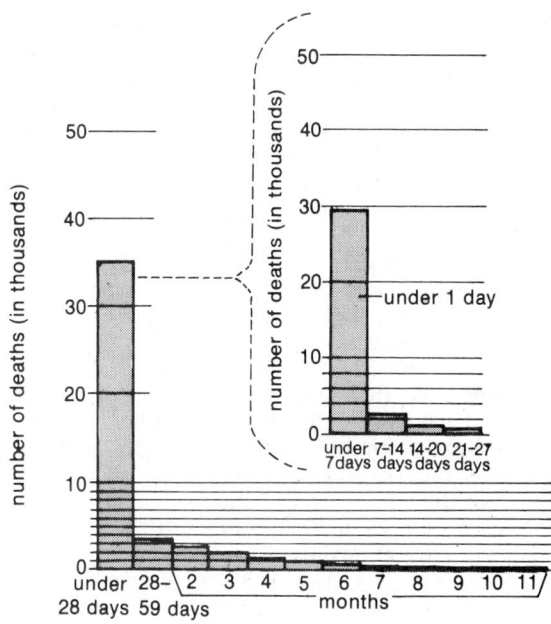

Figure 1–1. Infant mortality by age, United States, 1976. (United States Department of Health and Human Services; data from National Center for Health Statistics.)

1

Table 1–1. **Death Rates* for All Causes, According to Sex, Race, and Age: United States, Selected Years, 1959–1984**

	1950		1960		1970		1980		1984	
	White	Black	White	Black	White	Black	White	Black	White	Black
Male										
<1 yr	3401 ⎫		2694	5307	2113	4299	1230	2587	997	2222
1–4 yr	136 ⎬	1413	105	209	84	151	66	111	52	84
5–14 yr	67	95	53	75	48	67	35	47	28	44
15–24 yr	152	290	144	212	171	321	167	209	142	163
Female										
<1 yr	2567 ⎫		2008	4162	1614	3369	963	2124	827	1841
1–4 yr	112 ⎬	1139	85	173	66	129	49	84	39	68
5–14 yr	45		35	54	30	44	23	31	19	25
15–24	72	73 / 213	55	108	62	112	56	71	50	57

*Death rates per 100,000 population.
Adapted from Table 10, Health, United States, 1985. DHHS (PHS) Pub. No. 86–1232, pp. 38–39. Hyattsville, MD, National Center for Health Statistics, 1985.

child psychiatrists, sociologists, anthropologists, ethnologists, and others have brought us new insights into human potential, including new views of the importance of the circumstances surrounding birth and the early hours together of infants and parents (Sec. 2.3, 2.5, and 2.23).

Table 1–2 shows the 10 leading causes of death in various age groups in 1978. Tables 1–3, 1–4, 4–1, 4–2, and 4–3 show how certain of these problems of children have changed in the United States over a generation. Tables 1–2 and 4–3 highlight the impact of violent deaths upon mortality in older children, adolescents, and young adults.

Figure 8–1 shows that the nonwhite children of the United States have not fully benefited from the changes in infant mortality in this century owing to a variety of socioeconomic and other disadvantages that have resisted the efforts of many who have struggled to reduce this disparity, including many pediatricians. Similar disparities between races occur in several indices of health such as rates of diseases of the heart and homicides.

In 1981 a Select Panel for the Promotion of Child Health completed a comprehensive assessment of the health needs of children in the United States. The study found that existing programs for meeting child health problems are not available to all families in need, with gaps between eligibility for public support and ability to pay costs; that needed services are often either nonexistent or fragmented among programs, agencies, or policies; that programs are poorly coordinated; that data collection is inadequate; and that the resources available for maternal and child health care services are generally inadequate. These findings reflect a need, not just in the United States but in many other parts of the world as well, for continuing re-examination and revision of the system of health care.

The Select Panel reported that from 1970–1978 the percentage of mothers 25–30 yr old who were employed in the labor force had risen from 45% to 62% and that the children of working mothers had increased in numbers by 3.3 million between 1970–1977, 38% of them by 1977 under 6 yr old; these changes occurred even though the actual number of children under the age of 18 yr had fallen between the 1970 and 1980 censuses from about 70 million to 62 million. The study further reported that the number of children living in homes in which there was only 1 parent (usually the mother) had increased from 9% in 1960 to 19% in 1978. Many such 1-parent families live at poverty levels of income.

The above findings generated 3 sets of goals. The 1st set included that all families have access to adequate perinatal, preschool, and family-planning services; that governmental activities be effectively coordinated; that services be so orga-

Table 1–2. **Death Rates for the 10 Leading Causes of Death, by Specified Age Groups: United States, 1978 (Refers only to resident deaths occurring within the United States. Rates per 100,000 population)**

Rank Order in 1978	Cause of Death* and Age	Rate
	Under 1 Yr—All Causes	1378.4
1	Congenital anomalies	252.1
2	Immaturity, unqualified	110.3
3	Respiratory distress syndrome	99.7
4	Asphyxia of newborn, unspecified	88.7
5	Hyaline membrane disease	80.0
6	Birth injury without mention of cause	55.5
7	Influenza and pneumonia	46.0
8	Accidents	37.9
9	Septicemia	32.8
10	Conditions of placenta	23.0
—	All other causes	552.3
	1–4 Yr—All Causes	69.2
1	Accidents	28.8
—	Motor vehicle accidents	10.6
—	All other accidents	18.2
2	Congenital anomalies	8.4
3	Malignant neoplasms, including neoplasms of lymphatic and hematopoietic tissues	4.9
4	Influenza and pneumonia	2.9
5	Homicide	2.6
6	Diseases of heart	2.3
7	Meningitis	1.8
8	Meningococcal infections	0.9
9	Cerebrovascular diseases	0.8
10	Anemias	0.6
—	All other causes	15.1
	5–14 Yr—All Causes	33.9
1	Accidents	17.2
—	Motor vehicle accidents	8.8
—	All other accidents	8.4
2	Malignant neoplasms, including neoplasms of lymphatic and hematopoietic tissues	4.2
3	Congenital anomalies	1.8
4	Homicide	1.3
5	Diseases of heart	1.0
6	Influenza and pneumonia	0.9
7	Cerebrovascular diseases	0.6
8	Suicide	0.4
9	Anemias	0.2
10	Benign neoplasms and neoplasms of unspecified nature	0.2
—	All other causes	6.0

Table continued on opposite page

Table 1–2. Death Rates for the 10 Leading Causes of Death, by Specified Age Groups: United States, 1978 (Refers only to resident deaths occurring within the United States. Rates per 100,000 population) *Continued*

Rank Order in 1978	Cause of Death* and Age	Rate
	15–24 Yr—All Causes	117.5
1	Accidents	64.5
—	Motor vehicle accidents	46.4
—	All other accidents	18.1
2	Homicide	13.2
3	Suicide	12.4
4	Malignant neoplasms, including neoplasms of lymphatic and hematopoietic tissues	6.3
5	Diseases of heart	2.7
6	Congenital anomalies	1.6
7	Influenza and pneumonia	1.3
8	Cerebrovascular diseases	1.1
9	Diabetes mellitus	0.3
10	Benign neoplasms and neoplasms of unspecified nature	0.3
—	All other causes	13.8

Table adapted from Monthly Vital Statistics Report 28(13):23, 25, 1980.
*(Eighth Revision, International Classification of Diseases, Adapted, 1965)

nized that they reach populations at special risk; that there be no insurmountable or inequitable financial barriers to adequate care; that the health care of children have continuity from prenatal through adolescent age periods; and that ultimately every family have access to *all* needed services, including dental, genetic, and mental health services. A 2nd set of goals addressed the needs for reducing accidents and environmental risks, for meeting nutritional needs, and for health education aimed at fostering health-promoting life styles. A 3rd set of goals specified needs for research in biomedical and behavioral science, in fundamentals of bioscience and human biology, and in the particular problems of mothers and children.

The unfinished business in the quest for physical, mental, and social health in the community is impressively illustrated by the disparities with which deaths due to disease, to accidents, and to violence are distributed between white and nonwhite children. Homicide has become a major cause of adolescent deaths and has increased in rate also among the very young, among whom the increase may in part represent the more accurate identification of child abuse (Sec. 2.57); among adolescents it may reflect unresolved social tensions and an unhealthy preoccupation in our society with violence. Some of the issues underlying these problems are discussed in Sec. 2.20, 2.35, 2.44, 2.57, 9.1, and 9.3.

PATTERNS OF HEALTH CARE

In 1981 nearly 15% of all office visits for health care, including about half the visits of children under the age of 15 yr, were made to the offices of pediatricians. Private offices or clinics or group practices either of pediatricians or other medical practitioners served most of these children, with about 10% using the outpatient clinics or the emergency rooms of hospitals. Nonwhite children are about 4 times as likely as white children to use these hospital facilities for ambulatory care. About 25% of visits made to pediatricians' offices in 1975 involved health assessment or health maintenance activities; the remainder concerned problems of acute or chronic illness, most often (about 35%) involving the respiratory tract or ears.

Hospitals, particularly in urban areas, are sources of both routine and intensive child care, with medical and surgical services which may range from immunization and developmental counseling to open heart surgery or renal transplantation. Procedures involving hyperintensive care are likely to be clustered in university-affiliated centers serving as regional resources.

PLANNING A SYSTEM OF CARE

Physicians caring for children have been increasingly called upon to advise in the management of disturbed behavior or of relationships between child and parent, child and school, or child and community and are increasingly concerned with problems of mental, social, and societal health. There is also an increasing concern with disparities in how the benefits of what we know about child health reach various groups of children. Just as in many developing countries, so in the United States the health of children lags far behind what it could be if the means and will to apply current knowledge could be brought to bear. The medical problems of the children are often intimately related to problems of mental and social health. The children most at risk are disproportionately represented among ethnic minority groups. Pediatricians have a responsibility to address themselves aggressively to problems such as these.

Table 1–3. Death Rates* for Diseases of the Heart According to Sex, Race, and Age: United States, Selected Years, 1950–1983

	1950 White	1950 Black	1960 White	1960 Black	1970 White	1970 Black	1980 White	1980 Black	1983 White	1983 Black
Male										
<1 yr	4.1	} 4.8	6.9	13.9	12.0	33.5	22.5	42.8	24.1	54.5
1–4 yr	1.1		1.0	3.8	1.5	3.9	2.1	6.3	2.2	5.1
5–14 yr	1.7	6.4	1.1	3.0	0.8	1.4	0.9	1.3	0.9	1.5
15–24 yr	5.8	18.0	3.6	8.7	3.0	8.3	2.9	8.3	2.7	6.6
Female										
< 1 yr	2.7	} 3.9	4.3	12.0	7.0	31.3	15.7	43.6	19.3	45.6
1–4 yr	1.1		0.9	2.8	1.2	4.2	2.1	4.4	2.1	3.6
5–14 yr	1.9	8.8	0.9	3.0	0.7	1.8	0.8	1.7	0.8	1.1
15–24 yr	5.3	19.8	2.8	10.0	1.7	6.0	1.7	4.6	1.6	4.4

*Death rates per 100,000 population.
Adapted from Table 17, Health, United States, 1985. DHHS (PHS) Pub. No. 86–1232, pp. 48–49. Hyattsville, MD, National Center for Health Statistics, 1985.

Table 1–4. **Death Rates* for Malignant Neoplasms According to Sex, Race, and Age:**
United States, Selected Years, 1950–1983

	1950		1960		1970		1980		1983	
	White	Black	White	Black	White	Black	White	Black	White	Black
Male										
<1 yr	9.6	8.2	7.9	6.8	4.3	5.3	3.5	4.5	3.5	3.9
1–4 yr	13.1		13.1	7.9	8.5	7.6	5.4	5.1	5.3	4.7
5–14 yr	7.6	5.8	8.0	4.4	7.0	4.8	5.2	3.7	4.4	4.1
15–24 yr	9.9	7.9	10.3	9.7	10.6	9.4	7.8	8.1	6.7	5.6
Female										
<1 yr	7.8	7.0	6.8	6.7	5.4	3.3	2.7	3.0	3.5	3.3
1–4 yr	11.3		9.7	6.9	6.9	5.7	3.6	3.9	4.4	3.1
5–14 yr	5.3	3.9	6.2	4.8	5.4	4.0	3.6	3.4	3.4	3.6
15–24 yr	7.5	8.8	6.5	6.9	6.2	6.4	4.7	5.7	4.6	5.0

*Death rates per 100,000 population.
Adapted from Table 19, Health, United States, 1985. DHHS (PHS) Pub. No. 86–1232, pp. 52–53. Hyattsville, MD, National Center for Health Statistics, 1985.

Linked to these views of the broad scope of pediatric concern is the concept that access to health services is a right of every person, to be supported in aspects ranging from the molecular to the social by the commitment and effort of the community or society to which that person belongs. The failure of health services and health benefits to reach all who need them has led to re-examination of the design of health care systems in many countries; but unresolved problems remain in most health care systems, such as the maldistribution of physicians, institutional unresponsiveness to the perceived needs of the individual, failure of medical services to be adapted to the need and convenience of the patient, and deficiencies in health education. Efforts to make the delivery of health care more efficient and effective have led imaginative pediatricians to create new categories of health care providers, such as physicians' assistants or pediatric nurse practitioners or associates, who can multiply the effectiveness of the individual physician.

New insights into the needs of children have reshaped the child care system in other ways. Growing understanding of the need of the infant for certain qualities of stimulation and care has led to restudy and revision of the care of the newborn infant (Sec. 2.3 and 2.23) and of procedures leading to adoption or to foster care (Sec. 2.31 and 2.32). It seems likely that for handicapped children the massive centralized institutions of past years will be replaced by community-centered arrangements offering a better opportunity for these children to achieve their maximal potential. Pediatricians have been involved in shaping these institutions, and their insights and active contributions will continue to be needed.

COSTS OF HEALTH CARE

The growth of high technology, the redesign of health institutions (particularly with respect to the needs for and the uses of personnel), and the manner in which the costs of health care are paid (by public or private insurance programs based on fee-for-service) have driven the costs of health care in the United States up to a point at which health care has become a dominant industry. Efforts currently under way to contain these costs have led to revisions of the way in which funds are to be used for payment of physicians or hospitals. Limits have been set on the fees for some services, capitated prepayment systems flourish, and a program of reimbursement (diagnosis-related groups, or DRG's) based on the diagnosis rather than on the particular services rendered to the individual patient has been developed. It remains to be seen what the impact of these will be; they will in any case force difficult decisions upon those responsible for allocation of health resources (Sec. 2.72).

EVALUATION OF HEALTH CARE

The shaping of health care systems to the meeting of actual needs will require accurate statistical data and difficult decisions in the setting of priorities. Along with growing concerns with the design and cost of health care systems and their ability to distribute creative child care has come more intense preoccupation with the quality of health care and with both its efficiency and its effectiveness. There is increasing public and political pressure for explicit, continuing evaluation of care in terms of what actually takes place rather than what modern medical knowledge has made possible. Methods of record-keeping and peer review have been developed that can expose problems in the quality of care and point the way toward their resolution.

GROWTH OF SPECIALIZATION

The amount of information relevant to child health care doubles about every 8–10 yr now, and no person can make herself or himself master of it all. Physicians are increasingly dependent upon one another for the highest quality of care for their patients; group practices in pediatrics are on the rise, each member developing some special knowledge and skills. The vast majority of pediatricians are generalists, but as many as 25% claim an "area of special interest."

The growth of specialization within pediatrics has taken a number of different forms: interests in problems of *age groups* of children have created neonatology and adolescent medicine; interests in *organ systems* have created pediatric cardiology, allergy, hematology, nephrology, gastroenterology, pulmonology, endocrinology, and specialization in metabolism and genetics; interests in *the health care system* have created pediatricians devoted to ambulatory care on the one hand, or to intensive care on the other; and finally, multidisciplinary subspecialties have grown up around the problems of *handicapped children*, to which pediatrics, neurology, psychiatry, psychology, nursing, physical and occupational therapy, special education, speech therapy, audiology, and nutrition all make essential contributions. This growth of specialization has been most conspicuous in university-affiliated departments of pediatrics and medical centers for children. The development of such areas of special interest among private practitioners is particularly likely among those pediatricians who practice in groups.

THE NEED FOR CONTINUING SELF-EDUCATION

The explosion of information has also created a need for continuing education, which was much less keenly felt in earlier years, when the new information in any field of medicine was easily accessible through a relatively small number of journals, texts, or monographs. Now, relevant information is so widely scattered among the many journals published that elaborate electronic data systems are necessary to make it accessible. New auditory and visual aids to learning abound as well as postgraduate courses through which the participating physician can be brought up to date on various aspects of child health care. The American Board of Pediatrics and the American Academy of Pediatrics have arranged for the close linkage of continuing education of the pediatrician to recertification in pediatrics.

There is no touchstone through which physicians can assure that the process of their own continuing education will keep them abreast of advancing knowledge in the field, but they must find a way if they are to discharge their responsibility to their patients. An essential element of this process may be for the physician to take an *active* role. The passive role of simply reading or listening or watching is far less effective than an active one in which the physician translates what is read, seen, or heard into some action of his or her own. Efforts in continuing self-education will be fostered, for example, if the physician can use these efforts to teach, particularly if they are relevant to problems actually encountered in practice. Each clinical problem can be made a stimulus for a review of standard literature, alone or in consultation with an appropriate colleague or consultant. This continuing review will do much to identify those inconsistencies or contradictions which will indicate, in the ultimate best interest of the patient, that things are not what they seem or have been said to be. Physicians still learn most from their patients, but not if they fall into the easy habit of accepting their patients' problems casually or at face value because they appear to be simple.

The tools which the physician must use in dealing with the problems of children and their families fall into three main categories: *cognitive* (up-to-date factual information regarding diagnostic and therapeutic issues, available on recall or easily found in readily accessible sources); *interpersonal or manual* (the ability to carry out a productive interview, execute a reliable physical examination, perform a deft venipuncture, or manage cardiac arrest or the resuscitation of a depressed newborn infant, for example); and *attitudinal* (the physician's commitment to fullest possible implementation of knowledge and skills on behalf of children and their families in a climate of empathetic sensitivity and concern).

The workaday needs of professional persons for knowledge and skills in care of children will vary widely. The primary care physician needs depth in developmental concepts and in the ability to organize an effective system for achieving quality and continuity in assessing and planning for health care during the entire period of growth. There may often be little

or no need for immediate recall of esoterica. On the other hand, the consultant or subspecialist not only needs a comfortable grasp of esoterica within his or her field and perhaps within related fields, but must be able also to cope with controversial issues, with flexibility which will permit adaptation of a variety of points of view to the best interest of his or her unique patient.

At whatever level of care (primary, secondary, or tertiary), or in whatever role (as student, as pediatric nurse practitioner, as resident pediatrician, as a practitioner of pediatrics or of family medicine, or as a pediatric or other subspecialist), professional persons dealing with children must be able to identify their roles of the moment and their levels of engagement with a child's problem; each must determine whether his or her experience and other resources at hand are adequate to deal with this problem and must be ready to seek other help when they are not. Among the needed resources will be general textbooks, more detailed monographs in subspecialty areas, selected journals, audiovisual materials, and above all, colleagues with exceptional or complementary experience and expertise. The intercommunication of all these levels of engagement with medical and health problems of children offers the best hope that subsequent generations will progressively bring us closer to the goal of providing the opportunity for all children to achieve their maximum potential.

VICTOR C. VAUGHAN, III

Access to Ambulatory Health Care: United States, 1974. Advance Data, No 17, February 23, 1978.

Ambulatory Medical Care Rendered in Physicians' Offices. Advance Data, No 12, October 12, 1977.

Ambulatory Medical Care Rendered in Pediatricians' Offices. Advance Data, No 13, October 13, 1977.

Better Health for Our Children: A National Strategy. The Report of the Select Panel for the Promotion of Child Health (in 3 vols). DHHS (PHS) Publication No. 79–55071. Washington, DC, U.S. Government Printing Office, 1981. (For sale by the Superintendent of Documents.)

Foundations for Evaluating the Competency of Pediatricians. Chicago, American Board of Pediatrics, Inc., 1974.

Healthy People: The Surgeon General's Report on Health Promotion and Disease Prevention. The Report and Background Papers. DHEW (PHS) Publications No. 79–55071 and 79–55071A. Washington, DC, U.S. Government Printing Office 1979. (For sale by Superintendent of Documents.)

Health—United States. 1984. DHHS Publication No. 85–1232. Hyattsville, MD. National Center for Health Statistics, 1985.

Morley D: Paediatric Priorities in the Developing World. London, Butterworths, 1973.

Program for Recertification in Pediatrics. Chapel Hill, NC, American Board of Pediatrics, 1981.

Promoting Health/Preventing Disease: Objectives for the Nation. Department of Health and Human Services. Public Health Service. Office of the Assistant Secretary for Health and Surgeon General (JB Richmond, M.D.). Washington, DC, U.S. Government Printing Office, 1980.

Inquiries regarding the publications of the National Center for Health Statistics (NCHS) can be made to National Center for Health Statistics. Center Building, Room 1–57, 3700 East-West Highway, Hyattsville, MD, 20782. Telephone: (301) 436–8500.

2

DEVELOPMENTAL PEDIATRICS

GROWTH AND DEVELOPMENT

2.1 INTRODUCTION

The basic science of pediatrics is growth and development. All health personnel having responsibility for the care of children should be sufficiently familiar with the normal patterns and milestones so that they can recognize overt deviations from the normal ranges as early as possible, in order for underlying disorders to be identified and given appropriate attention.

The term *growth and development* refers to the process by which the fertilized ovum eventually attains adult status. *Growth* principally implies changes in size of the body as a whole or of its separate parts; *development* embraces other aspects of differentiation of form, but principally involves changes of function, including those largely shaped by interaction with the structural, emotional, or social environment.

The degree to which, and the process through which, a person achieves biologic potential are the consequences of many interrelated factors. *Genetic* factors are sometimes thought of as establishing final limits to biologic potential, but these are intimately interwoven with the environment. *Physical trauma* may affect growth and development; it may be prenatal or postnatal, nutritional, chemical, residual from infection, or immunologic. *Nutritional* factors may reflect primarily *socioeconomic* realities. *Social and emotional* factors affecting growth potential include the position of the child in the family, the quality of interaction of the infant or child with siblings, parents, and others, the personal concerns and needs of the parents, and the child-rearing patterns of the parents

or of the community. *Cultural considerations* may either limit or expand the range of behavior of children by establishing conventional expectations, and may conspicuously alter the schedule for acquisition of skills, such as sitting or walking, which were once regarded as depending almost entirely upon maturation. *Politics* and culture are closely related, inasmuch as the political life of any community provides the arena in which public priorities are set, including those which may have profound effects upon children.

Manifestations of *physical growth and development* range from those at the molecular level, such as the activation of enzymes in the course of differentiation, to the complex interplay of metabolic and physical changes associated with puberty and adolescence.

In early infancy the elements of *cognitive growth and development* may be difficult to differentiate from neurologic and behavioral maturation. In later infancy and childhood cognitive and intellectual functions are increasingly measured by communicative skills and by the ability to handle abstract and symbolic material.

The experience of each child is unique, and the patterns of development may be profoundly different for individual children within the broad limits that designate "normality." Indeed, patterns of growth and development have such variability that they can often be expressed only in statistical terms. The appropriate statistical principles and terms are discussed later (Sec. 2.10). Following below is a description of children generally within the normal range of development at each age, with some indication of what that range may be.

GROWTH AND DEVELOPMENT OF FETUS, INFANT, AND CHILD

2.2 THE FETUS

Intrauterine life comprises two principal phases: *embryonic* and *fetal*. The embryonic period is usually considered to be the first 8 wk of growth, during which the ovum differentiates rapidly into an organism having most of the gross anatomic features of the human form. Organogenesis continues beyond 8 wk in some systems, so that some prefer to designate the embryonic period as the 1st trimester of pregnancy, or the first 12 wk. The period between the 12th and the 40th wk of gestation is marked by rapid growth and elaboration of function. Not until the 24th–26th wk, however, is the fetus generally considered *viable*.

Physical. The 1st wk of embryonic life is *germinal*, consisting of active cellular division. During the 2nd wk the tissues differentiate into two layers (ectoderm and entoderm); during the 3rd wk mesoderm is added. During the 4th wk, the growing organism elaborates the somites, and between the 4th and 8th wk undergoes rapid differentiation into an essentially human form. At 8 wk of age the fetus weighs about 1 g and is about 2.5 cm in length; at 12 wk it weighs about 14 g

and is about 7.5 cm long. By the end of the 1st trimester the sex of the fetus can be distinguished on external examination. By the end of the 2nd trimester (28 wk) the fetus weighs about 100 g and is about 35 cm (14 in) in length. During the *3rd trimester* the further increase in size of the now viable fetus involves primarily subcutaneous tissue and muscle mass.

During the *2nd trimester* there is rapid acquisition of new functions. The *circulatory* system of the fetus attains its final form between the 8th and 12th wk of gestation. The details of its structure and the changes that occur with birth are discussed in Chapters 8 and 14.

Respiratory movements of the fetus may be seen as early as the 18th wk of gestation, but the development of the alveolar structures will usually not be sufficient to permit survival until the 24th–26th wk. The development of pulmonary surfactant is under way by 20 wk of gestation, but may not be adequate until late in the 3rd trimester (Sec. 8.32). The tidal flow of amniotic fluid into and out of the developing lung may contribute to pulmonary arborization. Late in pregnancy, when amniotic fluid contains more cells and may contain meconium and other debris, aspiration may deposit these materials in the alveoli and lead to respiratory difficulties following delivery.

The hemoglobin of the fetus is predominantly fetal in type (Hgb F). At a given oxygen tension, Hgb F carries more oxygen than adult hemoglobin (Hgb A) does. Hgb A is produced in late fetal life and represents about 30% of the hemoglobin in the mature newborn infant. (See also Sec. 15.2.)

Bile begins to be formed by about 12 wk of gestation, and *digestive* enzymes soon thereafter. Meconium, the distinctive intestinal content of the fetus, is present by 16 wk; it consists of desquamated intestinal cells and intestinal juices, and of squamous cells and lanugo hair swallowed by the fetus in amniotic fluid.

The fetus makes swallowing movements as early as the 14th wk of gestation; at 17 wk it may protrude the upper lip on stimulation in the oral area, and by the 20th wk it may protrude both lips on stimulation. At 22 wk the lips are pursed upon stimulation, and by 26–28 wk the fetus may actively suck in attempting to gain nourishment.

The *placenta* is the chief route of metabolic exchange between mother and fetus. Its most urgent function is to provide for gas exchange; for this, adequate perfusion is needed on both the fetal and the maternal sides. The placenta elaborates hormones and enzymes that participate in the regulation of pregnancy, and it effects the selective transfer of nutrients and metabolites between mother and infant. Maternal hormones and drugs may also be transferred to the infant. Placental permeability is selective even for such closely related substances as the antibodies against viruses and those against bacteria; the former (as IgG) are more readily transmitted than the latter (as IgM). Much of the transfer of calcium, iron, and IgG to the infant occurs in the last trimester, with the result that the infant born prematurely may have greater need than the fullterm infant for calcium and iron and may be more susceptible to infection (Sec. 8.58).

Neurodevelopmental. Neurologic activity in the fetus is first manifest by about 8 wk of gestation, when isolated muscular contractions may be seen in response to local stimulation. By 9 wk contralateral flexion may be followed by ipsilateral flexion, and some spontaneous movements occur. By 9 wk of gestation the palms and soles have also become reflexogenic; by 13–14 wk graceful flowing movements may be produced by stimulation of all areas except the back, the back of the head, and the vertex. At this time the movements of the fetus may first be felt by the mother. The grasp reflex is evident by 17 wk and is generally well developed by 27 wk. Respiratory movements may occur in the fetus delivered at 18 wk; at 22 wk there may be weak phonation. By 25 wk the earliest signs of the Moro response can be elicited. The fetus is capable in late pregnancy of *habituation* to certain sensory stimuli; e.g., fetal movement and acceleration of the fetal pulse in response to noise transmitted through the mother's abdomen are blunted on repetition of the noise (see *orienting response* in Sec. 2.3).

Fetuses differ in levels of activity, and there is evidence that fetal activity may be responsive to maternal emotions, possibly as a result of placental transfer of epinephrine or other substances. Little is known about how the activity of newborn infants or the quality of the infant's demands during the first few weeks of life may reflect aspects of gestation that are dependent upon maternal emotional states. The comfort that some newborn infants receive from rhythmic motion or rhythmic sound may stem from similar sensations imparted by maternal motion, breathing, or heart sounds.

Problems of Embryonic and Fetal Life. The mortality of the *embryonic* period is probably higher than at any other time of life. Causes include abnormalities of genes and chromosomes and alterations in maternal health. These may be interrelated; advanced maternal age, for example, disposes to certain chromosomal abnormalities. Maternal infection or the administration of certain drugs to the mother during the 1st trimester may alter the differentiation of the fetus and result in congenital anomalies. Intrauterine environmental factors responsible for defects in differentiation exert their effects principally within the 1st trimester (Sec. 8.7).

Morbidity during the *fetal period* may result from a variety of intrauterine factors. These include interference with oxygenation secondary to disturbances of the placenta or umbilical cord; infections of bacterial, viral, or protozoan origin; injury by radiation, trauma, or noxious chemicals; immunologic disorders due to maternal immunization and transfer of isoantibodies; and maternal nutritional disturbances.

The effects of *intrauterine malnutrition* upon cerebral structure or function in later life are not fully understood. The rate of increase in the number of neurons is high during gestation, and their number probably continues to increase at a decreasing rate until about 18 mo of postnatal age. In this postnatal period there is also an increase in the number and complexity of dendritic connections, in the number of neuroglial cells, in the size of neurons and glial cells, and in myelinization. The effects on the central nervous system of malnutrition that occurs after this time can be much more readily reversed than those that result from undernutrition during periods of rapid cellular proliferation.

2.3 THE NEWBORN INFANT

Physical. An average newborn infant weighs about 3.4 kg (7½ lb); boys are slightly heavier than girls. About 95% of fullterm newborn infants weigh 2.5–4.6 kg (5½–10 lb). Length averages about 50 cm (20 in); approximately 95% of infants are within the range of 45–55 cm (18–22 in). Head circumference averages about 35 cm (14 in), with a range of 32.6–37.2 cm between the 5th and 95th percentiles.

Body proportions of newborn infants differentiate them sharply from older infants, children, and adults (Fig. 2–1). The head is relatively larger, the face rounder, and the mandible smaller than in older children or adults. The chest tends to be rounded rather than flattened anteroposteriorly; the abdomen is relatively prominent, and the extremities relatively short. The midpoint of stature of the newborn infant is near the level of the umbilicus, whereas in the adult it is at the symphysis pubis.

At birth minor traumatic effects of labor may be apparent, such as edema of the vertex or overriding of cranial bones, and infrequently there may be more severe injuries. There may be other minor anatomic variants of little or no significance. Normal anatomic features differentiating the newborn from the older child include external auditory canals that are relatively short and straight, with thicker drums that are placed more obliquely to the canal. The middle ear contains a mucoid substance that may be mistaken for an exudate of infection. The eustachian tube is short and broad. There is usually a single mastoid cell in the antrum; maxillary and ethmoid sinuses are small, and the frontal and sphenoidal ones undeveloped. The liver and spleen are commonly felt at or just below the costal margins, and the kidneys are often palpable.

The posture of the newborn infant tends to be one of partial flexion, simulating the fetal position. The latter can often be determined by "folding" the infant into its most comfortable position, in which a more or less ovoid shape is created. Sometimes minor and occasionally major orthopedic abnormalities of the infant will reflect the effect of intrauterine posture and pressure on the growing fetus.

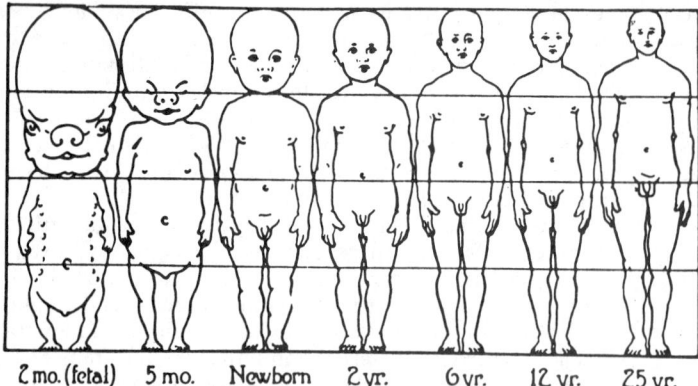

Figure 2–1. Changes in body proportions from 2nd fetal mo to adulthood. (From Robbins et al.: Growth. New Haven, Yale University Press. By permission of publisher.)

2 mo.(fetal)   5 mo.   Newborn   2 yr.   6 yr.   12 yr.   25 yr.

Physiologic. The prime need of the newborn infant is to establish adequate respirations for the exchange of gases. The rate of established respirations ranges generally from 35 to 50/min; brief excursions well outside this range are relatively common.

Cardiac adjustments of the neonatal period are often associated with transient murmurs. The heart rate ranges from 120 to 160/min. The heart of the newborn infant seems large in proportion to the thorax when assessed by adult standards.

Activity of newborn infants addressed toward the meeting of nutritional needs includes crying when hungry, and a tendency when hungry to turn the head toward and to "root" about for the nipple or another stimulus placed close to the oral area (rooting reflex) (Sec. 3.10). Sucking, gagging, and swallowing reflexes are active. The newborn infant may experience nausea and vomiting.

The infant initially expresses hunger at irregular intervals, but by the end of the 1st wk will usually be reasonably comfortably feeding at intervals ranging from 2 to 5 hr. No schedule of feedings will meet the demands or needs of all infants; if infant and mother are close to each other during the immediate postnatal period, as in a rooming-in arrangement, the opportunities for comfortably finding the baby's patterns of sleeping, awakening, and feeding will be as favorable as can be expected.

The first stools will generally be passed within 24 hr and will consist of meconium. When milk feedings are established, these will begin to be replaced on the 3rd–4th day by *transitional* stools, which are greenish brown and may contain milk curds. The typical milk stool of the older infant follows after an interval of 3–4 days. The frequency of stools in the newborn infant seems closely related to the frequency of feeding and to the amount of food obtained, averaging 3–5/day by the end of the 1st wk. On any given day during the 1st wk about 1 infant in 50 will have no stool at all; it is not unusual for a healthy infant to have as many as 6–7 stools/day after the 2nd day, particularly if breast fed.

At delivery the body temperatures of mother and infant are virtually the same. The infant's temperature falls quickly but transiently; it is usually restored within 4–8 hr. The caloric requirement of the newborn infant for maintenance of body heat and basal activity is usually about 55 kcal/kg/24 hr. By the end of the 1st wk the caloric needs will be approximately 110 kcal/kg/24 hr, of which 50% supplies basal metabolic needs, 40% is invested in growth and in activity, 5% is for the specific dynamic action of protein, and 5% is lost in feces and urine.

In the newborn infant the extracellular fluid compartment may constitute up to 35% of body weight. During the first few days there is loss of fluid which, in the absence of unusual oral intake, generally averages about 6% of body weight and may occasionally exceed 10%. When this loss is excessive, there may be dehydration or inanition fever on the 3rd–4th day. After the 1st wk the need for water will range between 120 and 150 mL/kg/24 hr. About half of this will be devoted to formation of urine and the rest to insensible loss by lungs and by skin and to other losses. Insensible loss is in a relatively fixed relationship to the calories metabolized by the infant (about 40 mL/100 kcal). Losses in stool are variable, those in sweat minimal.

Metabolism in newborn infants favors the anaerobic or glycolytic pathway, so that they are more tolerant of periods of hypoxia than older infants, children, or adults. This tolerance for anoxia is only relative, however. If oxygenation of the newborn infant is not quickly established, there may be a rapidly progressive metabolic and respiratory acidosis (from accumulation of lactic acid and carbon dioxide) and hypoxic tissue injury.

Glomerular filtration rate (GFR) and urine output are low in the first days of life and increase rapidly in the first 2 weeks. The GFR does not approach adult standards until the end of the first year. During the 1st wk proteinuria is common, and the urine may contain an abundance of urates, which may give the diaper a pink stain. Urea clearance is low, and the ability to concentrate urine is limited. Production of ammonium ion also is limited, and phosphate clearance is low. The blood urea nitrogen level may rise transiently.

The hemoglobin level of the newborn infant ranges around 17–19 g/dL, and mild reticulocytosis and normoblastemia may be observed for the first day or two of life (see Table 15–3). Leukocytes number about 10,000/μL at birth and generally increase in number for the first 24 hr, with a relative neutrophilia. Counts as high as 25,000 to 35,000 may be encountered. After the 1st wk the total white cell count is likely to be below 14,000, with the characteristic relative lymphocytosis of infancy and early childhood. Stressful situations in the newborn infant, including overwhelming infections, may be associated with little or no leukocytosis and even with leukopenia.

There is little or no transfer of certain clotting factors from mother to infant. Establishment of normal hemostatic mechanisms depends on the acquisition of normal intestinal flora and elaboration of vitamin K (Sec. 15.45).

Placental transfer of maternal hormones produces temporary changes in the breasts and genitalia of the newborn infant (Sec. 8.3) and possibly in other tissues; and the withdrawal of maternal hormones or other metabolites may contribute to temporary hypofunction of the parathyroid. Maternal hyperglycemia may dispose the infant to hyperinsulinemia and hypoglycemia (Sec. 8.56 and 8.57). Blood levels of sugar and of calcium are normally relatively low in the newborn infant, and further decreases (below about 20 mg/dL of sugar or about 7.5 mg/dL of calcium) may cause convulsions.

The gamma globulin level of the newborn infant (almost entirely maternal IgG) is slightly higher than that of the mother, owing to an active transport mechanism. The IgG affords protection against many viral and some bacterial diseases. On the other hand, IgM antibodies, like isohemag-glutinins, do not cross the placenta in substantial amounts. The IgM fraction of maternal immune globulins contains antibodies against certain antigens of gram-negative entero-bacteria; infants denied these are, accordingly, at increased risk of gram-negative bacillary infection. IgM antibodies may be formed by the fetus, however, in response to intrauterine infection. IgA antibodies and IgE do not generally cross the placenta. T lymphocyte functions are somewhat reduced in newborn infants.

The gamma globulin level of the infant falls to a low level by about 3 mo of age, as maternal antibody disappears; a rise then occurs, as the infant produces his or her own immuno-globulins to the levels that characterize older children and adults. Responses to artificial immunizations are relatively sluggish in term newborn infants and markedly so in pre-mature infants. Antibodies of the major blood group system (ABO) usually appear by the 2nd mo of life.

The digestive enzymes are usually adequate for the diet of the newborn infant, though fat is handled somewhat less well than protein or carbohydrate. At the cellular level, however, a number of deficiencies may have important clinical conse-quences. The red blood cells of the newborn infant have relatively low levels of reduced glutathione, which may con-tribute to increased hemolysis under a variety of circum-stances. A deficiency in capacity of the liver to conjugate bilirubin with glucuronic acid leads to hyperbilirubinemia, often with no evidence of hemolysis. A diminished capacity for the metabolism of certain drugs may place the newborn infant at increased risk when drug therapy is needed.

Neurodevelopmental. Many of the behavioral features and neurologic responses of the newborn infant are described in Sec. 8.3, 8.17, and 21.3. As indicated there and in Sec. 2.4, responses will depend upon the level of maturity of the infant. Beyond the conventional neurologic or reflex behavior of the newborn infant, however, lies a capacity for interaction with the environment which was unappreciated until recently, and which gives evidence of a complex neurologic organiza-tion.

It has been shown that the quality of the behavior that can be elicited from the newborn infant is highly dependent upon the *behavioral state* or the level of arousal of the infant. Six levels of arousal have been defined: deep sleep; sleep with rapid eye movements (REM); a drowsy state; a quiet, alert state; an awake and active state; and a state of active, intense crying. It is in the quiet and alert state that newborn infants are capable of their most responsive and complex interactions with the environment.

Within 1–2 hr after normal delivery of an unanesthetized and unsedated infant, the infant will commonly spend a good deal of time in the quiet, alert state. From the moment of birth the infant is quite capable of visual fixation on objects and of following the movements of these objects; he or she is capable of visual scanning of simple geometric figures; and among somewhat similar and rather complex figures will give preferential attention to figures that resemble the human face. Within the next few days the amount of time spent by the baby in this state will constitute about 10% of the day, and then increases with age. Sleep patterns of newborn infants begin to change as early as the 2nd day from the predomi-nantly REM type sleep of the older fetus toward the patterns of older infants and children.

Through complex mechanisms infants hold fixation of faces or of points of contrast, movement, or changing intensity of light within their visual fields. During the 1st wk they are able to maintain these fixations against passive movements of their bodies (doll's eye reflex); subsequently, responses orig-inally partly vestibular become increasingly oculomotor alone.

Certain behaviors of infants in response to environmental change have been called the *orienting response*. As a new stimulus is received in the auditory and/or visual or other sensory field, the infant becomes more alert, with a suppres-sion of spontaneous movement, with a likely turning of the head toward the stimulus, and with physiologic changes, such as changes in heart rate. There is a tendency for the heart rate to decelerate when the baby orients to a more or less familiar stimulus, whereas acceleration occurs when a totally unfamiliar or noxious stimulus is received. When a substantially unchanging new stimulus becomes repetitive, the orienting response rapidly habituates; there is less startle reaction or cardiac acceleration, and as the stimulus becomes familiar, cardiac deceleration may supervene.

Brazelton has brought together a number of observations of neonatal behavior to form a behavioral scale that may provide a more precise and predictive assessment of the newborn infant than a traditional neurologic examination. The scale assesses the behavior of the infant in four dimen-sions: *interactive* processes (orientation; alertness; consolabil-ity; cuddliness); *motor* processes (muscular tone; motor ma-turity; defensive reactions; hand-to-mouth activity; general activity level; and reflex behavior); *control of physiologic state* (habituation to a bright light, a rattle, a bell, and a pinprick; self-quieting behavior); and *response to stress* (tremulousness; lability of skin color; and startle reaction). This Neonatal Behavioral Assessment Scale has been used to identify deficits in neurobehavioral function, to describe the level and quality of normal behavior, to assess the impact on behavior of injury, drugs, or other interventions, and to attempt prediction of future development and function. In this last function, the results of the Brazelton evaluation may during the first week or two give a more accurate prognosis than the Apgar score at 1 and 5 min; and as late as 1 wk after delivery the use of this examination has detected changes in the infant's behavior due to drugs given to the mother (such as phenobarbital). The demonstration to parents of some of the items in the scale may foster healthy attachment as they reveal the infant's complexity and early evidence of the infant's personality and individuality (Sec. 2.17).

Psychosocial. The infant is born into a social milieu in which he or she has already for some time been an important participant, represented in the hopes and fears of parents, and particularly in the mother's experiences during preg-nancy. To these earlier experiences are added the events surrounding the mother's labor and the delivery of the child. These experiences have the effect of *bonding* the parents in greater or lesser degree to the child. Bonding consists of those emotional ties and commitments that characterize the rela-tionship between each parent or other participant in this social event and the infant who becomes the central figure. During the next hours, days, weeks, and months the infant reciprocates this bonding with his or her *attachment* to the significant persons in the environment to whom he or she will turn in the future for protection, nurturance, and love. Analogues of bonding and attachment have been studied in animals and their newborn, under the designation of *imprint-ing*; and such studies have greatly enriched the study of socialization in human infants.

The equipment that the infant brings to bonding and attachment is striking in its complexity, beginning with the observation that the infant in the first minutes of life responds visually preferentially to figures that resemble the human face. Such behavior may be important in facilitating or eliciting those interactions leading to the formation of social bonds. For example, the steady gaze of the newborn infant into her eyes is often experienced by the mother as a powerful stimulus to her emotional attachment. Moreover, newborn infants give attention preferentially to high pitched or female voices, and can be shown within the 1st wk of life to turn their heads more readily toward the sounds of their own mothers' voices than to voices not previously heard, and even to be able to distinguish a familiar sound in that voice. Further, the motor behavior of infants is responsive to the cadences of speech of a person engaging them in a social relationship. This responsiveness to vocal stimulation may have importance for social bonding, and its lack may give a mother her first clue that her infant is abnormal, without either her or her physician knowing at first that the infant is deaf.

The attraction of the newborn infant for the human face may have a basis in some predetermined and poorly understood preprogramming of a genetic nature. It has been shown that the infant may somehow carry a preregistration of what he or she may see, as evidenced by the fact that the infant will imitatively stick out the tongue to someone who sticks out a tongue at him or her. Other evidence of intersensory organization in the infant is that the infant will at the moment of birth turn the eyes with more than random likelihood toward a sound heard at one side of the head, as if knowing that to hear a sound from that source means that there is something to be seen there.

Infants are capable within the 1st wk of life of differentiating breast pads containing the odor of the milk and breast of their own mothers. Other sensory modalities have been less well studied for their social implications. Prenatal and postnatal experiences involve kinesthetic, somesthetic, thermal, olfactory, and proprioceptive stimuli. Some of these may reflect the intrauterine experience. The baby is exposed in utero to the regular rhythm and rate of the maternal heartbeat and respiration, for example, and it has been shown that sounds having the quality, rhythm, and rate of a normal heartbeat can sometimes comfort fretful infants.

The 1st or 2nd hr after birth, when the infant is in the quiet, alert state, may offer a particularly favorable opportunity for facilitating bonding and attachment (Sec. 8.6). Events at this time may influence not only the quality of relationship established between mother and infant, but also, to a degree, between the infant and other persons sharing the experience, even if only as onlookers (say, as godparents). It is not known whether there exist for bonding and attachment in humans *critical periods* comparable to those for imprinting in animals. It seems unlikely given the resilience with which many infants, parents, and families surmount neonatal experiences that might have had devastating effects. On the other hand, for some fragile infants or parents the loss of some opportunities for harmonious interaction may be irretrievable within a few hours or days. These lost opportunities may be in some instances a first step in the development in later life of emotional disorders, child abuse and neglect, or failure to achieve potential levels of intellectual or social development. In any case, such effects are perhaps more likely to represent trauma to or changes in the relationship between parent and infant than to reflect the loss of any physiologic "now or never" period.

Growing appreciation of the importance of childbirth as a social rather than a medical event has led to substantial revision of traditional practices. Mothers and fathers have both become involved in prenatal programs oriented to education for childbirth and for child-rearing, to further encouragement of family-centered activities for pregnancy and childbirth, to greater restraint in the use of analgesic and anesthetic medication in labor, to further encouragement of breast feeding, and to rooming-in arrangements in the neonatal period that will optimize the opportunities for newborn infants, their mothers, and their families to get to know each other within the first hours and days of life.

2.4 THE INFANT BORN PREMATURELY

The fetus born prematurely begins to have a substantial chance of survival at about 26–28 wk of gestation. The physical features of infants ranging between gestational ages of 26 and 40 wk are described in detail in Sec. 8.17. Their behavioral characteristics also evolve with their increasing gestational ages.

Neurodevelopmental. Infants whose birth weights are 1000–1500 g tend to be predominantly atonic and to lie in a tonic neck attitude, often with little motion of the extremities. Vocalization is weak, as are the grasp and Moro responses. Sucking responses may also be weak, and these infants may show little hunger on deprivation of food. It is difficult to tell whether they are awake or asleep, though they can be stimulated to greater alertness.

Infants weighing 1500–2000 g have good muscle tone when stimulated, more vigorous grasp, and complete Moro responses. A sleep pattern is easily discernible, and they are able visually to fixate some objects in their environment. The more vigorous of these babies are able to manage breast feeding.

Infants weighing 2000–2500 g at birth generally have the appearance of small fullterm infants, from which they cannot usually be differentiated by developmental examination. They have good cry and sustained muscle tone.

Although a small premature infant, by the time he or she reaches the expected date of delivery, may seem more alert and active than a fullterm baby born on that day, the actual developmental level reached within a few weeks will generally be lower than that indicated by chronologic age. The deficit in level tends to correspond to the level of prematurity. These differences will generally have disappeared by the end of the 2nd year of life, so long as no complicating factors occur.

Problems. The premature infant faces difficulties from failure of adequate maturation of enzymatic, respiratory, renal, metabolic, hematologic, and immunologic mechanisms (Chapter 8). Developmental defects are more common in premature infants than in fullterm infants and often include impairments of motor or intellectual function. The latter are commonly due to residual damage from anoxia or infection.

The premature infant is particularly vulnerable to the effects of sensory or social deprivation in the neonatal period, owing to the restrictions imposed by necessities of care and by the sometimes prolonged period of relative isolation. Recent studies emphasize the importance of involving the mothers of even the smallest babies in some aspects of their care as early as possible in order to enhance the opportunities for mutual emotional bonding and attachment (Sec. 2.3 and 8.6).

2.5 THE FIRST YEAR

Physical. Most fullterm infants regain their birth weights by the age of 10 days. The fullterm infant will generally double birth weight by 5 mo and triple it by 1 yr (Table 2–1). The premature infant is likely to gain about 6–7 kg (13–15 lb) in the 1st yr, which is about the average gain for fullterm infants. The length of the normal infant increases during the 1st yr by 25–30 cm (10–12 in). An increase in subcutaneous tissue in the early mo of life reaches its peak at about 9 mo.

The anterior fontanel may increase in size after birth, but generally diminishes after 6 mo and may become effectively closed between 9 and 18 mo. The posterior fontanel is usually closed to palpation by 4 mo.

Head circumference (normally 34–35 cm [13.4–13.8 in] at birth) increases to approximately 44 cm by 6 mo and to 47 cm by 1 yr (Table 2–2). The head circumference is slightly larger than that of the chest at birth, but the two become equal by the end of the 1st yr.

The first deciduous teeth erupt in most children between 5 and 9 mo. The first to appear are the lower central incisors, followed by the upper central and then the upper lateral incisors. The lower lateral incisors, the 1st deciduous molars,

Table 2–1. **Formulas for Approximate Average Height and Weight of Normal Infants and Children (After Weech)**

Weight	Kilograms	(Pounds)
(a) at birth	3.25	(7)
(b) 3–12 mo	$\dfrac{age(mo) + 9}{2}$	(age(mo) + 11)
(c) 1–6 yr	age(yr) × 2 + 8	(age(yr) × 5 + 17)
(d) 7–12 yr	$\dfrac{age(yr) \times 7 - 5}{2}$	(age(yr) × 7 + 5)

Height	Centimeters	(Inches)
(e) at birth	50	(20)
(f) at 1 yr	75	(30)
(g) 2–12 yr	age(yr) × 6 + 77	(age(yr) × 2½ + 30)

cuspids (canines), and 2nd deciduous molars follow in that order. By the age of 1 yr most children have 6–8 teeth. Occasionally an infant has as few as 2 teeth at 1 yr without other evidence of any growth disturbance.

THE FIRST THREE MONTHS
(Table 2–3)

Neurodevelopmental. The newborn infant placed upon a firm surface is able to avoid suffocation by turning the face from side to side; by 4 wk of age the head is lifted above the surface as it is turned. By then a rather symmetrical flexed posture has become more relaxed, and the infant is likely to lie, when supine, in a tonic neck posture (head turned to one side, with the extremities extended on that side).

When the infant within the first 4–8 wk of life is pulled from a supine to a sitting position, the head lags, and with the infant in the upright position head control is absent. By 12 wk there is some control of the head as the infant is drawn to sitting position, but the head is tilted a little forward on the upright body; irregular head control results in a bobbing motion.

When held in ventral suspension (i.e., lifted from the prone position by a hand held under the trunk), the newborn infant will be in a posture of flexion of head and extremities around the supporting hand (Landau response). By 1 mo of age the infant will raise the head momentarily to the plane of the body, and by 2 mo will be able to sustain the head in that plane. By 3 mo the head will be raised above the plane of the body and the legs will be extended as well.

In the first days of life infants visually fixate best those objects that are placed close to or moved through their line of vision. Depending upon their level of interest, they may maintain fixation with movement of the eyes and head to nearly 90° to either side of the midline. By 2 mo of age a supine infant will be able to follow an object presented 90° from the midline through an arc of 180°.

Reflex grasp persists until the age of about 8 wk, after which, with growing eye and hand coordination, an active grasp becomes more evident. Reaching and grasping evolve out of earlier coordinate but incomplete motions of the arms and hands in response to the sight of objects in motion nearby ("larval reach"); by 12 wk the infant attempts to make contact with an offered object and will hold it briefly if appropriate contact is made. The coordination of eye and hand implicit in this activity seems to have been facilitated in some measure by the tonic neck attitude.

The infant begins at about 4 wk to make small throaty noises; some vowel sounds will be produced at 8 wk, and these will be uttered with evident pleasure on social contact by 12 wk.

Psychosocial. With neonatal experiences fostering bonding and attachment, and with continuing social interaction, infants soon show that they differentiate persons and objects in their environments. As early as 2–6 wk they are clearly more comfortable with familiar persons than with strangers.

Newborn and even prematurely born infants often display fragmentary smiles, usually in response to internal stimuli of uncertain nature during REM sleep or moments of drowsiness. A fully developed social smile becomes manifest usually between 3 and 5 wk of age. There is evidence that the smile of the very young infant may be elicited primarily by the infant's discovery that he or she has control over some

Table 2–2. **Median Head Circumferences of Infants and Children**

BOYS				Age	GIRLS			
Median	Percentiles (5th–95th)	Median	Percentiles (5th–95th)		Median	Percentiles (5th–95th)	Median	Percentiles (5th–95th)
Centimeters		(Inches)			Centimeters		(Inches)	
34.8	32.6–37.2	(13.7)	(12.8–14.7)	Birth	34.3	32.1–35.9	(13.5)	(12.6–14.1)
37.2	34.9–39.6	(14.7)	(13.7–15.6)	1 mo	36.4	34.2–38.3	(14.3)	(13.5–15.1)
40.6	38.4–43.1	(16.0)	(15.1–17.0)	3 mo	39.5	37.3–41.7	(15.6)	(14.7–16.4)
43.8	41.5–46.2	(17.2)	(16.3–18.2)	6 mo	42.4	40.3–44.6	(16.7)	(15.9–17.6)
45.8	43.5–48.1	(18.0)	(17.1–18.9)	9 mo	44.3	42.3–46.4	(17.4)	(16.7–18.3)
47.0	44.8–49.3	(18.5)	(17.6–19.4)	1 yr	45.6	43.5–47.6	(18.0)	(17.1–18.7)
48.4	46.3–50.6	(19.1)	(18.2–19.9)	1.5 yr	47.1	45.0–49.1	(18.5)	(17.7–19.3)
49.2	47.3–51.4	(19.4)	(18.6–20.2)	2 yr	48.1	46.1–50.1	(18.9)	(18.2–19.7)
49.9	48.0–52.2	(19.7)	(18.9–20.6)	2.5 yr	48.8	47.0–50.8	(19.2)	(18.5–20.0)
50.5	48.6–52.8	(19.9)	(19.1–20.8)	3 yr	49.3	47.6–51.4	(19.4)	(18.8–20.2)

From Health Survey of National Center for Health Statistics, 1976 (see footnote to Table 2–8).

Estimating Formula (First Year Only):	Boys and Girls Combined	Centimeters	(Inches)
Normal range of head circumference (5th–95th percentile) = $\left[\dfrac{Length\ (cm)}{2} + 9.5\right] \pm 2.5$	Median head circumference at 4 yr \ at 5 yr	50.4 \ 50.8	(19.8) \ (20.0)
	From Studies of Harvard School of Public Health (see text).		

After Dine et al, 1981.

Table 2–3. **Length, Weight and Head Circumference by Age**
Boys and Girls: Birth to 36 Months

	Boys: Percentiles								Girls: Percentiles						
	5th	*10th*	*25th*	*50th*	*75th*	*90th*	*95th*	Measurement	*5th*	*10th*	*25th*	*50th*	*75th*	*90th*	*95th*
BIRTH	46.4 (18¼)	47.5 (18¾)	49.0 (19¼)	50.5 (20)	51.8 (20½)	53.5 (21)	54.4 (21½)	Length-mm (in)	45.4 (17¾)	46.5 (18¼)	48.2 (19)	49.9 (19¾)	51.0 (20)	52.0 (20½)	52.9 (20¾)
	2.54 (5½)	2.78 (6¼)	3.00 (6½)	3.27 (7¼)	3.64 (8)	3.82 (8½)	4.15 (9¼)	Weight-kg (lb)	2.36 (5¼)	2.58 (5¾)	2.93 (6½)	3.23 (7)	3.52 (7¾)	3.64 (8)	3.81 (8½)
	32.6 (12¾)	33.0 (13)	33.9 (13¼)	34.8 (13¾)	35.6 (14)	36.6 (14½)	37.2 (14¾)	Head C-cm (in)	32.1 (12¾)	32.9 (13)	33.5 (13¼)	34.3 (13½)	34.8 (13¾)	35.5 (14)	35.9 (14¼)
1 month	50.4 (19¾)	51.3 (20¼)	53.0 (20¾)	54.6 (21½)	56.2 (22¼)	57.7 (22¾)	58.6 (23)	Length-cm (in)	49.2 (19¼)	50.2 (19¾)	51.9 (20½)	53.5 (21)	54.9 (21½)	56.1 (22)	56.9 (22½)
	3.16 (7)	3.43 (7½)	3.82 (8½)	4.29 (9½)	4.75 (10½)	5.14 (11¼)	5.38 (11¾)	Weight-kg (lb)	2.97 (6½)	3.22 (7)	3.59 (8)	3.98 (8¾)	4.36 (9½)	4.65 (10¼)	4.92 (10¾)
	34.9 (13¾)	35.4 (14)	36.2 (14¼)	37.2 (14¾)	38.1 (15)	39.0 (15¼)	39.6 (15½)	Head C-cm (in)	34.2 (13½)	34.8 (13¾)	35.6 (14)	36.4 (14¼)	37.1 (14½)	37.8 (15)	38.3 (15)
3 months	56.7 (22¼)	57.7 (22¾)	59.4 (23½)	61.1 (24)	63.0 (24¾)	64.5 (25½)	65.4 (25¾)	Length-cm (in)	55.4 (21¾)	56.2 (22¼)	57.8 (22¾)	59.5 (23½)	61.2 (24)	62.7 (24¾)	63.4 (25)
	4.43 (9¾)	4.78 (10½)	5.32 (11¾)	5.98 (13¼)	6.56 (14½)	7.14 (15¾)	7.37 (16¼)	Weight-kg (lb)	4.18 (9¼)	4.47 (9¾)	4.88 (10¾)	5.40 (12)	5.90 (13)	6.39 (14)	6.74 (14¾)
	38.4 (15)	38.9 (15¼)	39.7 (15¾)	40.6 (16)	41.7 (16½)	42.5 (16¾)	43.1 (17)	Head C-cm (in)	37.3 (14¾)	37.8 (15)	38.7 (15¼)	39.5 (15½)	40.4 (16)	41.2 (16¼)	41.7 (16½)
6 months	63.4 (25)	64.4 (25¼)	66.1 (26)	67.8 (26¾)	69.7 (27½)	71.3 (28)	72.3 (28½)	Length-cm (in)	61.8 (24¼)	62.6 (24¾)	64.2 (25¼)	65.9 (26)	67.8 (26¾)	69.4 (27¼)	70.2 (27¾)
	6.20 (13¾)	6.61 (14½)	7.20 (15¾)	7.85 (17¼)	8.49 (18¾)	9.10 (20)	9.46 (20¾)	Weight-kg (lb)	5.79 (12¾)	6.12 (13½)	6.60 (14½)	7.21 (16)	7.83 (17¼)	8.38 (18½)	8.73 (19¼)
	41.5 (16¼)	42.0 (16½)	42.8 (16¾)	43.8 (17¼)	44.7 (17½)	45.6 (18)	46.2 (18¼)	Head C-cm (in)	40.3 (15¾)	40.9 (16)	41.6 (16½)	42.4 (16¾)	43.3 (17)	44.1 (17¼)	44.6 (17½)
9 months	68.0 (26¾)	69.1 (27¼)	70.6 (27¾)	72.3 (28½)	74.0 (29¼)	75.9 (30)	77.1 (30¼)	Length-cm (in)	66.1 (26)	67.0 (26½)	68.7 (27)	70.4 (27¾)	72.4 (28½)	74.0 (29¼)	75.0 (29½)
	7.52 (16½)	7.95 (17½)	8.56 (18¾)	9.18 (20¼)	9.88 (21¾)	10.49 (23¼)	10.93 (24)	Weight-kg (lb)	7.00 (15½)	7.34 (16¼)	7.89 (17½)	8.56 (18¾)	9.24 (20¼)	9.83 (21¾)	10.17 (22½)
	43.5 (17¼)	44.0 (17¼)	44.8 (17¾)	45.8 (18)	46.6 (18¼)	47.5 (18¾)	48.1 (19)	Head C-cm (in)	42.3 (16¾)	42.8 (16¾)	43.5 (17¼)	44.3 (17½)	45.1 (17¾)	46.0 (18)	46.4 (18¼)
12 months	71.7 (28¼)	72.8 (28¾)	74.3 (29¼)	76.1 (30)	77.7 (30½)	79.8 (31½)	81.2 (32)	Length-cm (in)	69.8 (27½)	70.8 (27¾)	72.4 (28½)	74.3 (29¼)	76.3 (30)	78.0 (30¾)	79.1 (31¼)
	8.43 (18½)	8.84 (19½)	9.49 (21)	10.15 (22½)	10.91 (24)	11.54 (25½)	11.99 (26½)	Weight-kg (lb)	7.84 (17¼)	8.19 (18)	8.81 (19½)	9.53 (21)	10.23 (22½)	10.87 (24)	11.24 (24¾)
	44.8 (17¾)	45.3 (17¾)	46.1 (18¼)	47.0 (18½)	47.9 (18¾)	48.8 (19¼)	49.3 (19½)	Head C-cm (in)	43.5 (17¼)	44.1 (17¼)	44.8 (17¾)	45.6 (18)	46.4 (18¼)	47.2 (18½)	47.6 (18¾)
18 months	77.5 (30½)	78.7 (31)	80.5 (31¾)	82.4 (32½)	84.3 (33¼)	86.6 (34)	88.1 (34¾)	Length-cm (in)	76.0 (30)	77.2 (30½)	78.8 (31)	80.9 (31¾)	83.0 (32¾)	85.0 (33½)	86.1 (34)
	9.59 (21¼)	9.92 (21¾)	10.67 (23½)	11.47 (25¼)	12.31 (27¼)	13.05 (28¾)	13.44 (29½)	Weight-kg (lb)	8.92 (19¾)	9.30 (20½)	10.04 (22¼)	10.82 (23¾)	11.55 (25½)	12.30 (27)	12.76 (28¼)
	46.3 (18¼)	46.7 (18½)	47.4 (18¾)	48.4 (19)	49.3 (19½)	50.1 (19¾)	50.6 (20)	Head C-cm (in)	45.0 (17¾)	45.6 (18)	46.3 (18¼)	47.1 (18½)	47.9 (18¾)	48.6 (19¼)	49.1 (19¼)
24 months	82.3 (32½)	83.5 (32¾)	85.6 (33¾)	87.6 (34½)	89.9 (35½)	92.2 (36¼)	93.8 (37)	Length-cm (in)	81.3 (32)	82.5 (32½)	84.2 (33¼)	86.5 (34)	88.7 (35)	90.8 (35¾)	92.0 (36¼)
	10.54 (23¼)	10.85 (24)	11.65 (25¾)	12.59 (27¾)	13.44 (29¾)	14.29 (31½)	14.70 (32½)	Weight-kg (lb)	9.87 (21¾)	10.26 (22½)	11.10 (24½)	11.90 (26¼)	12.74 (28)	13.57 (30)	14.08 (31)
	47.3 (18½)	47.7 (18¾)	48.3 (19)	49.2 (19¼)	50.2 (19¾)	51.0 (20)	51.4 (20¼)	Head C-cm (in)	46.1 (18¼)	46.5 (18¼)	47.3 (18½)	48.1 (19)	48.8 (19¼)	49.6 (19½)	50.1 (19¾)
30 months	87.0 (34¼)	88.2 (34¾)	90.1 (35½)	92.3 (36¼)	94.6 (37¼)	97.0 (38¼)	98.7 (38¾)	Length-cm (in)	86.0 (33¾)	87.0 (34¼)	88.9 (35)	91.3 (36)	93.7 (37)	95.6 (37¾)	96.9 (38¼)
	11.44 (25¼)	11.80 (26)	12.63 (27¾)	13.67 (30¼)	14.51 (32)	15.47 (34)	15.97 (35¼)	Weight-kg (lb)	10.78 (23¾)	11.21 (24¾)	12.11 (26¾)	12.93 (28½)	13.93 (30¾)	14.81 (32¾)	15.35 (33¾)
	48.0 (19)	48.4 (19)	49.1 (19¼)	49.9 (19¾)	51.0 (20)	51.7 (20¼)	52.2 (20½)	Head C-cm (in)	47.0 (18½)	47.3 (18½)	48.0 (19)	48.8 (19¼)	49.4 (19½)	50.3 (19¾)	50.8 (20)
36 months	91.2 (36)	92.4 (36½)	94.2 (37)	96.5 (38)	98.9 (39)	101.4 (40)	103.1 (40½)	Length-cm (in)	90.0 (35½)	91.0 (35¾)	93.1 (36¾)	95.6 (37¾)	98.1 (38½)	100.0 (39¼)	101.5 (40)
	12.26 (27)	12.69 (28)	13.58 (30)	14.69 (32½)	15.59 (34½)	16.66 (36¾)	17.28 (38)	Weight-kg (lb)	11.60 (25½)	12.07 (26½)	12.99 (28¾)	13.93 (30¾)	15.03 (33¼)	15.97 (35¼)	16.54 (36½)
	48.6 (19¼)	49.0 (19¼)	49.7 (19½)	50.5 (20)	51.5 (20¼)	52.3 (20½)	52.8 (20¾)	Head C-cm (in)	47.6 (18¾)	47.9 (18¾)	48.5 (19)	49.3 (19½)	50.0 (19¾)	50.8 (20)	51.4 (20¼)

These data are those of the National Center for Health Statistics (NCHS), Health Resources Administration, DHEW. They were based on studies of The Fels Research Institute, Yellow Springs, Ohio. Metric data have been smoothed by a least-squares cubic spline technique. For details see Hamill PVV, et al: NCHS Growth Charts, 1976. Monthly Vital Statistics Report 25(3):1, 1976. These data and those in Tables 2–4 and 2–5 were first made available to us with the help of William M. Moore, M.D., of Ross Laboratories, who supplied the conversion from metric measurements to approximate inches and pounds. This help is gratefully acknowledged.

contingencies in the environment, such as securing care or attention from mother or another caretaker, or from being able to control the behavior of inanimate objects. The infant who does not have a social smile by the age of 8–12 wk should be regarded as possibly seriously deviant with respect to developmental potential or to quality of environmental experience.

The earliest days and weeks of life find the infant attaining control of reflex and homeostatic mechanisms, and entering into interactions with the personal and inanimate environment. Patterns or rhythms of feeding and sleeping are found, and the ability to control his or her own state through self-stimulation, as by finger- or thumb-sucking. A major part of the interaction between mother and infant in the first weeks of life is initiated by the infant, not simply as changes of state indicating distress or immediate need, but as part of a growing and complex system of signals between infant and mother (or other caretakers). Through these communicative exchanges emotional attachments are formed; the infant learns to sort out his or her own internal states for their meaning and to convey information regarding them; and the mother learns to read and respond appropriately to the infant's signals, with activities that have the capacity to comfort, to reassure, or at times to make tolerable the appropriate or necessary frustration or postponement of gratification.

There is reason to feel that during this period the sense of security of the infant will be optimally fostered when care is given by the mother or mother-figure in a prompt, loving, and confident manner. Both consistency and promptness seem important in the responses of the caretakers to the behavior of the infant. In instances of defective mothering the infant's normal or appropriate behavior may not be consistently or reliably rewarded by reduction of tension, or an effective maternal response may come so late and after so much anxiety or tension that the infant cannot associate any specific action of his or her own with relief of that tension. Such infants may come to feel that they have no way to affect their environments through their own actions. Long-term retreat, anxiety, or hostility may be the consequences.

THREE TO SIX MONTHS
(Table 2–3)

Neurodevelopmental. By the age of 3 mo infants in the prone position on a firm surface are generally able to raise head and chest with their arms extended. From the same position, by 4 mo they are able to raise the head to a vertical axis and turn it easily from side to side.

When the infant of 4 mo is pulled to a sitting position, the head is brought up without lag; in the upright position the head tilts a little forward, but is held steady without bobbing. The head will be maintained erect and steady by 5 mo of age.

At 5–6 mo of age the infant begins purposefully to roll over, at first from the prone to the supine position and then in the reverse direction.

Between 3 and 4 mo of age the infant gradually abandons the tonic neck attitude as the predominant posture, and the head becomes generally maintained in the midline, with the arms and legs in more or less symmetric positions, and the hands often brought together in the midline or at the mouth (*symmetrotonic posture*). In this position the 4–6 mo old infant often develops a bald spot over the occiput.

By 4–5 mo the infant will enjoy being supported in an upright posture and becomes increasingly attracted to objects presented on a plane surface. By 6 mo he or she will be able to change the orientation of the entire body to reach toward a desired object.

By 4 mo the infant becomes more adept in making contact with objects brought within reach and will often bring them to the midline and to the mouth for oral exploration. Whereas at 4 mo the infant will be able to grasp an object of moderate size, he or she will have only limited interest in a small object, such as a pellet. By 7 mo the pellet is promptly seen and may be vigorously pursued by raking motions of the fingers, but the infant is not apt to be able to pick it up. After 6 mo the functions of the hands are increasingly lodged in the structures on the radial side, the thumb being used in conjunction with the palm. By 6–6.5 mo most infants can grasp a large object, such as a rattle, and transfer it from hand to hand.

With growing skills in manipulation of arms and hands, infants discover the rest of their body, face at first, then head, trunk, lower extremities, and genitalia. Their discovery that the genitalia can be handled with pleasure may engender anxiety in parents.

At 5–6 mo infants can often be pulled from a sitting to a standing position and will support their weight upon extended legs. At 6–6.5 mo in this same position they will often flex the knees momentarily and return to a standing posture. A 6–6.5 mo infants are often able to sit alone, leaning forward upon their hands, or with slight support of the pelvis; they will not yet have developed a lumbar lordosis, and the spine will have a gentle kyphotic curve from cervical region to sacrum.

Psychosocial. As infants become more intricately related to objects and persons in the environment, their smiles continue as catalysts of social exchange. By 4 mo they begin to laugh aloud at pleasurable social contacts. They may also, on interruption of a pleasant social contact, show displeasure by changes of expression, fussing, or crying. Between 4 and 7 mo of age infants become increasingly responsive to the emotional tone of social contacts, and by 7 mo will respond to changes in the facial expressions of those having close rapport with them. By the end of the 6th mo normal infants will have developed clear preferences for social contact with the persons giving them the most care, and will, particularly when in the mother's arms, begin to show anxiety at the approach of strangers. By contrast, in a setting where they are alone with a stranger, new social contacts may be accepted without protest. Development of separation anxieties and fear of strangers may depend in some measure on the depth to which infants have developed comfortable patterns of communication and emotional exchange with primary caretakers.

SIX TO TWELVE MONTHS
(Table 2–3)

Neurodevelopmental. By 7 mo the infant in the prone position is able to *pivot* in pursuit of an object, but if it is not within reach, may be unable to attain it. By 9–10 mo most infants have learned to *creep* or to *crawl*.

Supine infants are able by 6 mo or so to lift their heads and become increasingly interested in their legs and feet. By 8–9 mo they are able to assume a sitting position without help and are soon able to maintain it with the back straight. They are often able at 8 mo to stand steadily for a short time so long as the hands are held, and by 9 mo may be able to take some steps with both hands held.

Between 6 and 9 mo the radial-palmar grasp becomes clearly elaborated into movements involving thumb and forefinger. The index finger is used to poke at objects by 9 mo, and at this time the thumb and forefinger can be brought into sufficiently accurate apposition to permit a pellet to be picked up with a pincer motion. This movement is apt to be made with the ulnar surface of the hand supported on the same surface upon which the pellet lies. By 12 mo the pincer will be executed without this ulnar support.

Between 6 and 12 mo the infant's behavior becomes more imitative. At 6 mo the infant may crudely imitate the tapping

Table 2–4A. **Weight by Length*** **Boys and Girls Less Than 4 Years**

Recumbent Length	Boys: Weight Percentiles, kg and (lb)							Girls: Weight Percentiles, kg and (lb)						
	5th	*10th*	*25th*	*50th*	*75th*	*90th*	*95th*	*5th*	*10th*	*25th*	*50th*	*75th*	*90th*	*95th*
48–50 cm (19–19¾ in)			2.86 (6¼)	3.15 (7)	3.50 (7¾)					3.02 (6¾)	3.29 (7¼)	3.59 (8)		
50–52 cm (19¾–20½ in)			3.16 (70)	3.48 (7¾)	3.86 (8½)					3.25 (7¼)	3.55 (7¾)	3.89 (8½)		
52–54 cm (20½–21¼ in)			3.52 (7¾)	3.88 (8½)	4.28 (9½)					3.56 (7¾)	3.89 (8½)	4.26 (9½)		
54–56 cm (21¼–22 in)	3.49 (7¼)	3.65 (8)	3.95 (8¾)	4.34 (9½)	4.76 (10½)	5.13 (11¼)	5.33 (11¾)	3.54 (7¾)	3.64 (8)	3.93 (8¾)	4.29 (9½)	4.70 (10¼)	5.02 (11)	5.21 (11½)
56–58 cm (22–22¾ in)	3.90 (8½)	4.09 (9)	4.43 (9¾)	4.84 (10¾)	5.29 (11¾)	5.69 (12½)	5.88 (13)	3.93 (8¾)	4.05 (9)	4.37 (9¾)	4.76 (10½)	5.20 (11½)	5.55 (12¼)	5.77 (12¾)
58–60 cm (22¾–23½ in)	4.37 (9¾)	4.58 (10)	4.94 (11)	5.38 (11¾)	5.84 (12¾)	6.28 (13¾)	6.47 (14¼)	4.38 (9¾)	4.50 (10)	4.85 (10¾)	5.27 (11½)	5.73 (12¾)	6.12 (13½)	6.36 (14)
60–62 cm (23½–24½ in)	4.88 (10¾)	5.10 (11¼)	5.49 (12)	5.94 (13)	6.42 (14¼)	6.88 (15¼)	7.08 (15½)	4.85 (10¾)	4.99 (11)	5.37 (11¾)	5.82 (12¾)	6.30 (14)	6.70 (14¾)	6.95 (15¼)
62–64 cm (24½–25¼ in)	5.43 (12)	5.65 (12½)	6.05 (13¼)	6.52 (14¼)	7.02 (15½)	7.50 (16½)	7.72 (17)	5.35 (11¾)	5.50 (12)	5.91 (13)	6.39 (14)	6.89 (15¼)	7.30 (16)	7.55 (16¾)
64–66 cm (25¼–26 in)	5.99 (13¼)	6.20 (13¾)	6.62 (14½)	7.11 (15¾)	7.63 (16¾)	8.13 (18)	8.36 (8½)	5.87 (13)	6.03 (13¼)	6.47 (14¼)	6.97 (15¼)	7.48 (16½)	7.90 (17½)	8.15 (18)
66–68 cm (26–26¾ in)	6.55 (14½)	6.76 (15)	7.19 (15¾)	7.70 (17)	8.23 (18¼)	8.75 (19¼)	8.99 (19¾)	6.38 (14)	6.56 (14½)	7.02 (15½)	7.55 (16¾)	8.07 (17¾)	8.50 (18¾)	8.75 (19¼)
68–70 cm (26¾–27½ in)	7.10 (15¾)	7.31 (16)	7.75 (17)	8.27 (18¼)	8.82 (19½)	9.35 (20½)	9.62 (21¼)	6.89 (15¼)	7.08 (15½)	7.56 (16¾)	8.11 (17¾)	8.64 (19)	9.08 (20)	9.33 (20½)
70–72 cm (27½–28¼ in)	7.63 (16¾)	7.84 (17¼)	8.28 (18¼)	8.82 (19½)	9.39 (20¾)	9.93 (22)	10.21 (22½)	7.37 (16¼)	7.58 (16¾)	8.08 (17¾)	8.64 (19)	9.18 (20¼)	9.63 (21¼)	9.88 (21¾)
72–74 cm (28¼–29¼ in)	8.13 (18)	8.33 (18¼)	8.78 (19¼)	9.33 (20½)	9.92 (21¾)	10.48 (23)	10.77 (23¾)	7.82 (17¼)	8.05 (17¾)	8.56 (18¾)	9.14 (20¼)	9.68 (21¼)	10.15 (22½)	10.41 (23)
74–76 cm (29¼–30 in)	8.58 (19)	8.78 (19¼)	9.24 (20¼)	9.81 (21¾)	10.43 (23)	10.99 (24¼)	11.29 (25)	8.24 (18¼)	8.49 (18¾)	9.00 (19¾)	9.59 (21¼)	10.14 (22¼)	10.63 (23½)	10.91 (24)
76–78 cm (30–30¾ in)	9.00 (19¾)	9.21 (20¼)	9.68 (21¼)	10.27 (22¾)	10.91 (24)	11.48 (25¼)	11.78 (26)	8.62 (19)	8.90 (19½)	9.42 (20¾)	10.02 (22)	10.57 (23¼)	11.08 (24½)	11.39 (25)
78–80 cm (30¾–31½ in)	9.40 (20¾)	9.62 (21¼)	10.09 (22¼)	10.70 (23½)	11.36 (25)	11.94 (26¼)	12.25 (27)	8.99 (19¾)	9.29 (20½)	9.81 (21¾)	10.41 (23)	10.97 (24¼)	11.51 (25¼)	11.85 (26)
80–82 cm (31½–32¼ in)	9.77 (21½)	10.01 (22)	10.49 (23¼)	11.12 (24½)	11.80 (26)	12.39 (27¼)	12.69 (28)	9.34 (20½)	9.67 (21¼)	10.19 (22½)	10.80 (23¾)	11.37 (25)	11.93 (26¼)	12.29 (27)
82–84 cm (32¼–33 in)	10.14 (22¼)	10.39 (23)	10.88 (24)	11.53 (25½)	12.23 (27)	12.83 (28¼)	13.13 (29)	9.68 (21¼)	10.04 (22¼)	10.57 (23¼)	11.18 (24¾)	11.75 (26)	12.35 (27¼)	12.72 (28)
84–86 cm (33–33¾ in)	10.49 (23¼)	10.76 (23¾)	11.27 (24¾)	11.93 (26¼)	12.65 (28)	13.26 (29¼)	13.56 (30)	10.03 (22)	10.41 (23)	10.94 (24)	11.56 (25½)	12.15 (26¾)	12.76 (28¼)	13.15 (29)
86–88 cm (33¾–34¾ in)	10.85 (24)	11.14 (24½)	11.67 (25¾)	12.34 (27¼)	13.07 (28¾)	13.69 (30¼)	14.00 (30¾)	10.39 (23)	10.78 (23¾)	11.33 (25)	11.95 (26¼)	12.55 (27¾)	13.19 (29)	13.57 (30)
88–90 cm (34¾–35½ in)	11.22 (24¾)	11.53 (25½)	12.08 (26¾)	12.76 (28¼)	13.50 (29¾)	14.13 (31¼)	14.44 (31¾)	10.76 (23¾)	11.17 (24½)	11.74 (26)	12.36 (27¼)	12.98 (28½)	13.63 (30)	14.01 (31)
90–92 cm (35½–36¼ in)	11.60 (25½)	11.94 (26¼)	12.52 (27½)	13.20 (29)	13.94 (30¾)	14.58 (32¼)	14.90 (32¾)	11.16 (24½)	11.58 (25½)	12.17 (26¾)	12.80 (28¼)	13.45 (29¾)	14.10 (31)	14.45 (31¾)
92–94 cm (36¼–37 in)	12.00 (26½)	12.37 (27¼)	12.97 (28½)	13.65 (30)	14.40 (31¾)	15.05 (33¼)	15.39 (34)	11.59 (25½)	12.02 (26½)	12.63 (27¾)	13.27 (29¼)	13.95 (30¾)	14.61 (32¼)	14.92 (33)
94–96 cm (37–37¾ in)	12.42 (27½)	12.81 (28¼)	13.45 (29¾)	14.14 (31¼)	14.88 (32¾)	15.54 (34¼)	15.90 (35)	12.05 (26½)	12.48 (27½)	13.12 (29)	13.77 (30¼)	14.48 (32)	15.14 (33½)	15.42 (34)
96–98 cm (37¾–38½ in)	12.88 (28½)	13.28 (29¼)	13.96 (30¾)	14.66 (32¼)	15.39 (34)	16.06 (35½)	16.43 (36¼)	12.55 (27¾)	12.98 (28½)	13.64 (30)	14.31 (31½)	15.04 (33¼)	15.71 (34¾)	15.99 (35¼)
98–100 cm (38½–39¼ in)	13.37 (29½)	13.78 (30½)	14.50 (32)	15.21 (33½)	15.94 (35¼)	16.62 (36¾)	17.00 (37½)	13.10 (29)	13.51 (29¾)	14.19 (31¼)	14.87 (32¾)	15.63 (34½)	16.32 (36)	16.64 (36¾)
100–102 cm (39¼–49¼ in)	13.90 (30¾)	14.30 (31½)	15.06 (33¼)	15.81 (34¾)	16.54 (36½)	17.22 (38)	17.60 (38¾)	13.68 (30¼)	14.08 (31)	14.77 (32½)	15.46 (34)	16.25 (35¾)	16.96 (37½)	17.39 (38¼)
102–104 cm (40¼–41 in)	14.48 (32)	14.85 (32¾)	15.65 (34½)	16.45 (36¼)	17.18 (37¾)	17.87 (39½)	18.24 (40¼)							

*Data in Tables 2–4A and 2–4B are those of the National Center for Health Statistics (NCHS), Health Resources Administration, DHEW. Data of Table 2–4A are based on studies of The Fels Research Institute, Yellow Springs, Ohio; those of Table 2–4B are based on the Health Examination Surveys of the NCHS. For details see footnote to Table 2–3.

Table 2–4B. Weight by Stature*
Boys and Girls: Prepubescent

Stature	Boys: Weight Percentiles, kg and (lb)							Girls: Weight Percentiles, kg and (lb)						
	5th	10th	25th	50th	75th	90th	95th	5th	10th	25th	50th	75th	90th	95th
90–92 cm (35½–36¼ in)	11.70 (25¾)	11.97 (26½)	12.59 (27¾)	13.41 (29½)	14.35 (31¾)	15.25 (33½)	15.72 (34¾)	11.45 (25¼)	11.67 (25¾)	12.28 (27)	13.14 (29)	14.11 (31)	14.98 (33)	15.74 (34¾)
92–94 cm (36¼–37 in)	12.07 (26½)	12.36 (27¼)	13.03 (28¾)	13.89 (30½)	14.84 (32¾)	15.87 (35)	16.41 (36¼)	11.86 (26¼)	12.10 (26¾)	12.74 (28)	13.63 (30)	14.63 (32¼)	15.57 (34¼)	16.42 (36¼)
94–96 cm (37–37¾ in)	12.46 (27½)	12.77 (28¼)	13.49 (29¾)	14.38 (31¾)	15.34 (33¾)	16.45 (36¼)	17.06 (37½)	12.26 (27)	12.53 (27½)	13.21 (29)	14.12 (31¼)	15.14 (33½)	16.13 (35½)	17.05 (37½)
96–98 cm (37¾–38½ in)	12.87 (28¼)	13.21 (29)	13.98 (30¾)	14.89 (32¾)	15.87 (35)	17.01 (37½)	17.69 (39)	12.66 (28)	12.97 (28½)	13.70 (30¼)	14.62 (32¼)	15.66 (34½)	16.69 (36¾)	17.65 (39)
98–100 cm (38½–39¼ in)	13.31 (29¼)	13.67 (30¼)	14.48 (32)	15.43 (34)	16.41 (36¼)	17.56 (38¾)	18.29 (40¼)	13.06 (28¾)	13.42 (29½)	14.19 (31¼)	15.13 (33¼)	16.19 (35¾)	17.24 (38)	18.23 (40¼)
100–102 cm (39¼–40¼ in)	13.77 (30¼)	14.15 (31¼)	15.00 (33)	15.98 (35¼)	16.98 (37½)	18.11 (40)	18.89 (41¾)	13.48 (29¾)	13.88 (30½)	14.69 (32½)	15.65 (34½)	16.73 (37)	17.80 (39¼)	18.80 (41½)
102–104 cm (40¼–41 in)	14.25 (31½)	14.65 (32¼)	15.54 (34¼)	16.65 (36½)	17.57 (38¾)	18.67 (41¼)	19.50 (43)	13.91 (30¾)	14.36 (31¾)	15.21 (33½)	16.20 (35¾)	17.28 (38)	18.38 (40½)	19.38 (42¾)
104–106 cm (41–41¾ in)	14.76 (32½)	15.18 (33½)	16.10 (35½)	17.13 (37¾)	18.18 (40)	19.25 (42½)	20.12 (44¼)	14.36 (31¾)	14.85 (32¾)	15.75 (34¾)	16.75 (37)	17.86 (39¼)	18.98 (41¾)	19.98 (44)
106–108 cm (41¾–42½ in)	15.30 (33¾)	15.73 (34¾)	16.68 (36¾)	17.74 (39)	18.82 (41½)	19.86 (43¾)	20.76 (45¾)	14.84 (32¾)	15.37 (34)	16.30 (36)	17.33 (38¼)	18.46 (40¾)	19.62 (43¼)	20.61 (45½)
108–110 cm (42½–43¼ in)	15.85 (35)	16.31 (36)	17.28 (38)	18.37 (40½)	19.49 (43)	20.51 (45¼)	21.45 (47¼)	15.35 (33¾)	15.91 (35)	16.87 (37¼)	17.94 (39½)	19.09 (42)	20.30 (44¾)	21.29 (47)
110–112 cm (43¼–44 in)	16.43 (36¼)	16.91 (37¼)	17.90 (39½)	19.02 (42)	20.18 (44½)	21.22 (46¾)	22.18 (49)	15.90 (35)	16.48 (36¼)	17.47 (38½)	18.56 (41)	19.76 (43½)	21.03 (46¼)	22.03 (48½)
112–114 cm (44–45 in)	17.04 (37½)	17.53 (38¾)	18.54 (40¾)	19.70 (43½)	20.91 (46)	21.98 (48½)	22.98 (50¾)	16.48 (36¼)	17.09 (37¾)	18.08 (39¾)	19.22 (42¼)	20.47 (45¼)	21.81 (48)	22.84 (50¼)
114–116 cm (45–45¾ in)	17.66 (39)	18.18 (40)	19.20 (42¼)	20.39 (45)	21.66 (47¾)	22.82 (50¼)	23.85 (52½)	17.11 (37¾)	17.72 (39)	18.72 (41¼)	19.91 (44)	21.23 (46¾)	22.67 (50)	23.73 (52¼)
116–118 cm (45¾–46½ in)	18.32 (40½)	18.85 (41½)	19.89 (43¾)	21.11 (46½)	22.45 (49½)	23.73 (52¼)	24.80 (54¾)	17.77 (39¼)	18.40 (40½)	19.40 (42¾)	20.64 (45½)	22.04 (48½)	23.60 (52)	24.71 (54½)
118–120 cm (46½–47¼ in)	18.99 (41¾)	19.55 (43)	20.60 (45½)	21.85 (48¼)	23.28 (51¼)	24.73 (54½)	25.83 (57)	18.48 (40¾)	19.11 (42¼)	20.11 (44¼)	21.42 (47¼)	22.92 (50½)	24.62 (54¼)	25.81 (57)
120–122 cm (47¼–48 in)	19.70 (43½)	20.28 (44¾)	21.34 (47)	22.63 (50)	24.15 (53¼)	25.80 (57)	26.96 (59½)	19.22 (42¼)	19.85 (43¾)	20.87 (46)	22.25 (49)	23.88 (52¾)	25.73 (56¾)	27.03 (59½)
122–124 cm (48–48¾ in)	20.43 (45)	21.03 (46¼)	22.11 (48¾)	23.45 (51¾)	25.07 (55¼)	26.96 (59½)	28.18 (62¼)	19.99 (44)	20.64 (45½)	21.68 (47¾)	23.13 (51)	24.91 (55)	26.95 (59½)	28.37 (62½)
124–126 cm (48¾–49½ in)	21.20 (46¾)	21.82 (48)	22.92 (50½)	24.32 (53½)	26.05 (57½)	28.18 (62¼)	29.50 (65)	20.80 (45¾)	21.47 (47¼)	22.54 (49¾)	24.09 (53)	26.05 (57½)	28.27 (62¼)	29.87 (65¾)
126–128 cm (49½–50½ in)	21.99 (48½)	22.64 (50)	23.77 (52½)	25.24 (55¾)	27.10 (59¾)	29.48 (65)	30.92 (68¼)	21.65 (47¾)	22.34 (49¼)	23.47 (51¾)	25.11 (55¼)	27.28 (60¼)	29.71 (65½)	31.51 (69½)
128–130 cm (50½–51¾ in)	22.82 (50¼)	23.50 (51¾)	24.67 (54½)	26.22 (57¾)	28.21 (62¼)	30.86 (68)	32.44 (71½)	22.53 (49¾)	23.25 (51¼)	24.46 (54)	26.22 (57¾)	28.63 (63)	31.28 (69)	33.33 (73½)
130–132 cm (51¼–52 in)	23.69 (52¼)	24.59 (53¾)	25.62 (56½)	27.26 (60)	29.41 (64¾)	32.31 (71¼)	34.07 (75)	23.44 (51¾)	24.22 (53½)	25.52 (56¼)	27.40 (60½)	30.09 (66¼)	32.99 (72¾)	35.33 (78)
132–134 cm (52–53¾ in)	24.59 (54¼)	25.32 (55¾)	26.62 (58¾)	28.38 (62½)	30.68 (67¾)	33.82 (74½)	35.81 (79)	24.38 (53¾)	25.22 (55½)	26.66 (58¾)	28.68 (63¼)	31.68 (69¾)	34.84 (76¾)	37.53 (82¾)
134–136 cm (52¾–53½ in)	25.53 (56¼)	26.30 (58)	27.68 (61)	29.58 (65¼)	32.05 (70¾)	35.40 (78)	37.67 (83)	25.35 (56)	26.28 (58)	27.88 (61½)	30.06 (66¼)	33.41 (73¾)	36.84 (81¼)	39.93 (88)
136–138 cm (53½–54¼ in)	26.51 (58½)	27.32 (60¼)	28.80 (63½)	30.86 (68)	33.51 (74)	37.05 (81¾)	39.65 (87½)	26.34 (58)	27.39 (60½)	29.19 (64¼)	31.54 (69½)	35.29 (77¾)	39.01 (86)	42.54 (93¾)
138–140 cm (54½–55 in)	27.53 (60¾)	28.38 (62½)	29.99 (66)	32.23 (71)	35.08 (77¼)	38.77 (85½)	41.74 (92)							
140–142 cm (55–56 in)	28.59 (63)	29.48 (65)	31.25 (69)	33.70 (74¼)	36.75 (81)	40.55 (89½)	43.97 (97)							
142–144 cm (56–56¾ in)	29.70 (65½)	30.64 (67½)	32.58 (71¾)	35.27 (77¾)	38.54 (85)	42.39 (93½)	46.32 (102)							
144–146 cm (56¾–57½ in)	30.86 (68)	31.85 (70¼)	34.00 (75)	36.95 (81½)	40.45 (89¼)	44.29 (97¾)	48.80 (107½)							

*See footnote to Table 2–4A.

of a pencil upon a table. At 9 mo the infant will wave bye-bye or bring the hands together imitatively; at 12 mo a child may enter into very simple games with a toy such as a ball.

At 9 mo an infant may be able to release an object upon request, if the object is grasped as the request is made. By 1 yr most infants will extend the object and release it into an offered hand.

Language. The infant is able to make repetitive vowel sounds by 6.5 mo and by 8 mo is likely to produce repetitive consonant sounds, such as ba-ba, ma-ma, and da-da, though not necessarily associating these sounds with objects. Children of 8–9 mo become attentive to the sounds of their own names. They may knowingly use a few words besides ma-ma or da-da by the age of 1 yr, and may show by their behavior that they know the names of some objects.

Psychosocial. The preference for their mothers that was manifested at 6 mo often evolves into separation anxiety between the ages of 6 and 8 mo. About this same time a mother may experience difficulty in putting to sleep a baby who always went willingly before. Sometimes a mother whose child is fretful when she leaves the room can comfort him or her by maintaining vocal contact. By 9–10 mo infants begin to be less dependent upon the physical presence of their mothers, partly because with creeping or crawling they are increasingly able to follow her around. Also at this time, if an object that has attracted attention is covered with a cloth before the infant has an opportunity to grasp it, he or she will be able to uncover it and grasp it, with apparent knowledge that its being out of sight does not mean that it is not available. Peek-a-boo often becomes a pleasant game about this time, and gives the infant an opportunity to test and retest his or her ability to recreate the absent parent.

At the end of the first year, with a secure interactive system between infant and mother and other caretakers, including fathers and sometimes siblings, and with the development of locomotion, the infant is ready to move from a position of dependency towards more independent activities, and to explore a larger world.

2.6 THE SECOND YEAR

Physical. During the 2nd yr of life there is a further deceleration in the rate of growth; the average child will gain about 2.5 kg (5–6 lb) and about 12 cm (5 in) (Tables 2–3 and 2–4A and B). After 10 mo of age there is often a decrease in appetite extending well into the 2nd year. The result is a loss during the 2nd yr of some of the subcutaneous tissue which reached its maximal development around 9 mo; the plump infant begins to change gradually into the lean and muscular child. With the upright posture, the mild lordosis and protuberant abdomen appear that are characteristic of the 2nd and 3rd yr of life.

The growth of the brain also decelerates during the 2nd yr; head circumference, which increased approximately 12 cm during the 1st yr, will increase only 2 cm during the 2nd. By the end of the 1st yr the brain has reached approximately two thirds, and at the end of the 2nd yr four fifths, of its adult size.

During the 2nd yr 8 more teeth erupt, making a total of 14–16, including the first deciduous molars and the cuspids (canines). The order of eruption may be irregular; the cuspids commonly appear after the 1st molars have erupted.

Neurodevelopmental. During the 2nd yr the infant moves from an awkward upright stance in which he or she could walk with support to a high degree of locomotor control. By 15 mo infants are generally able to walk alone and by 18 mo to run stiffly.

At 18 mo the infant can climb stairs, if one hand is held, going one step at a time; by 20 mo he or she is able to go downstairs, one hand held, and may be able to climb stairs holding to the stair railing. By 24 mo children normally enter the "run about" age. They are able to move quickly from a safe environment into danger and will need constant surveillance.

The child who at 12 mo was able to release a pellet into the hand of a person requesting it will at 15 mo generally be able to put the pellet into a small bottle. He or she may attempt to remove the pellet from the bottle by inserting a finger, and by 18 mo will be able to dump it from the bottle.

By 15 mo the child is able to put a 1 inch cube on top of another in response to a demonstration; by 18 mo he or she is able to make a tower of 3 cubes and by 24 mo a tower of 6 cubes. Imitative and conceptual behavior continue to evolve, with spontaneous scribbling and with imitation of vertical lines at 18 mo; by 24 mo the child imitates circular strokes and can make a horizontal line.

Language. The child normally has a vocabulary of 10 words by 18 mo. There is wide variation in the times at which words begin to flow readily; it is not unusual for a normal child to have few or no sounds conveying definite meaning until 18 mo or later. Some children with delay in development of recognizable speech have a rich jargon before communicative sounds appear; this jargon often has many of the intonations and punctuations of speech, but otherwise conveys no meaning. In those normal children in whom speech is delayed to 18–20 mo, there is often rapid acquisition of words and meanings after this time, with the result that most normal children by their 2nd birthday are able to put 3 words together.

Psychosocial. With the advent of their 2nd yr, children enter a period when they will vigorously and imitatively exploit the objects in their environment. They can empty wastebaskets, drawers, and shelves and may try to examine everything within reach. *Household poisons, drugs, and chemicals must be kept in places inaccessible to them.*

During the 2nd yr imitative behavior extends to persons other than the mother, including siblings and playmates. Until the end of the 2nd yr, however, play is generally solitary and consists in active manipulation of available objects. During the 3rd yr of life children move increasingly into play activities in which other children are involved. By the end of the 4th year the child is increasingly engaged in activity with other children in which the group begins to enact imaginative roles and activities. This tendency to role-playing will increase in the school years.

By 18–24 mo most children are able to verbalize their toilet needs and can be helped at this time to follow acceptable social patterns in meeting them. Whenever the young child has comfortable and adequate models, toilet training need not become the focus either of emotion-laden educational activity or of disciplinary concern.

The expectation that children at this time will submit to increasing control of their bodies and of their environments in accordance with social and cultural pressures often produces frustration and anger. Temper tantrums, breath-holding spells, and less dramatic outbursts are common. These episodes respond best to management by firm and loving parents who are able to set the necessary limits for the child (Sec. 2.20 and 2.45).

2.7 THE PRESCHOOL YEARS

Physical. During the 3rd, 4th, and 5th yr of life gains in weight and height are relatively steady at approximately 2.0 kg (4.5 lb) and about 6–8 cm (2.5–3.5 in)/yr, respectively (Tables 2–3 and 2–5A and B). Most children are lean relative to their earlier body configuration. The lordosis and protuberant abdomen of late infancy tend to disappear by the 4th yr, as do the pads of fat that earlier camouflage the normal arches of the feet.

By 2.5 yr the 20 deciduous teeth have usually erupted. During the rest of the preschool period the face tends to grow proportionately more than the cranial cavity and the jaw to widen preparatory to the eruption of permanent teeth.

Neurodevelopmental. Refinement of motor skills includes alternation of feet in ascending stairs by 3 yr and alternation in descending stairs by 4 yr. By 3 yr most children can stand for a short period on one foot; by 5 yr they are generally able to hop on one foot and soon to skip.

By 3 yr a child may be able to imitate crudely the drawing of a cross. By 4 yr the cross figure may be copied without prior demonstration, by some as a four-element figure. By 4–5 yr the child can make correctly proportionate copies of the figures and for the first time becomes able to copy figures with slanting lines, such as triangles. A diamond-shaped figure may not be accurately and proportionately reproduced until the 6th yr.

By the age of 6 yr the child begins to develop the ability to translate abstract conceptions into figures and structures (e.g., the sound of T into the letter T, the idea of two into the figure 2).

Psychosocial. By 3 yr most children can state their ages and whether they are boys or girls. With increasing awareness that they are destined to become larger children and adults, children in the later preschool period begin to seek adequate models from whom to learn. The most accessible models are, of course, the parents and other members of the immediate family. The child's imperfect perception of the realities of the future often engenders conflicting pressures and anxieties. A child of 4, 5, or 6 yr assumes those habits of thought, feeling, and action that represent his or her growing perception or fantasy as to the future. Inside the home the child's fantasies about the future roles include playing the part of the parent of the same sex, and there may be increasing curiosity and concern as to what the realities of these roles may be.

Outside the home, concerns and fantasies about future roles are likely to be expressed in dramatic play. The interest of children of this age in sex differences, which often appears as questions inside the home, may commonly appear in the form of sex play among children of each sex, which is to be expected.

Changing patterns of parent-child interaction and of other relationships in and out of the home often leave elements of anxiety, hostility, or aggression in the child's behavior, thoughts, or fantasies. Anxieties may be expressed as nightmares or as fears of separation, death, or bodily injury. Children with serious problems may resume or continue bedwetting or thumb-sucking, show speech or learning difficulties, be unable to enter into a comfortable sharing relationship, or display temper tantrums or other behavior appropriate to earlier years.

2.8 THE EARLY SCHOOL YEARS

Physical. The early school years are a period of relatively steady growth ending in a preadolescent growth spurt by about the age of 10 yr in girls and about 12 in boys. The average gain in weight during these years is about 3–3.5 kg (7 lb)/yr, and in height about 6 cm (2.5 in)/yr. Growth in head circumference is slowed, the circumference increasing from about 51 cm (20 in) to 53–54 cm (21 in) between the ages of 5–12 yr. At the end of this period the brain has reached virtually adult size.

The development of the facial bones is active during the school years, particularly with enlargement of the nasal accessory sinuses. The frontal sinus has usually made its appearance by the 7th yr.

The 1st permanent teeth, the 1st molars, most often erupt during the 7th yr of life. With these so-called 6 yr molars in place, the shedding of deciduous teeth begins; it follows approximately the same sequence as their acquisition. They are replaced at a rate of about 4 teeth/yr over the next 5 yr. The 2nd permanent molars commonly erupt by the 14th yr; the 3rd molars may not appear until the early 20's. See also Sec. 12.1.

The school years are a time of vigorous physical activity. The spine becomes straighter, but the child's body is supple, and postures may be assumed that are disturbing to parents and to teachers. Mild degrees of knock-knee or flatfoot that may have been apparent in the late preschool years tend to correct themselves during the first year or two of the school years. The motor activities of the earlier years, such as running and climbing, become increasingly directed to more specialized activities and games requiring particular motor and muscular skills.

Lymphatic tissues are at the peak of their development during these years and generally exceed the amount of such tissue in the normal adult. The abundance of lymphoid tissue during this time of life bears some relationship to the frequency with which tonsillectomy and adenoidectomy are incorrectly recommended. Respiratory infections are common during these years, and the response of the child to infection begins to be more like that of the adult than of the infant or young child. The usual number of respiratory infections during the school years is high; as many as 6–7 illnesses/yr are not uncommon.

Psychosocial. With the transfer of a large portion of the child's life from the home to the school environment, children begin increasingly to live independently and to look outside the home for goals and for standards of behavior. This shifting of interests is often anxiety-provoking for parents, and if earlier problems between parent and child have not been adequately resolved, adjustments to forces outside the home are apt to be difficult.

A major task of the school years is the creation in the child of the senses of duty, of responsibility, and of realistic accomplishment. There is a possibility of great frustration for parents and children when the child's achievement does not measure up to parental hopes. The child unable to meet expected standards may learn for the first time the sense of *failure* and may react with anxiety, depression, or hostility. Antisocial behavior may develop through which the child attempts to gain recognition that he or she cannot attain otherwise (Sec. 2.20, 2.29, and 2.45).

VICTOR C. VAUGHAN, III
IRIS F. LITT

Bower TGR: Development in Infancy. San Francisco, WH Freeman, 1974.

Bower TGR: A Primer of Infant Development. San Francisco, WH Freeman, 1977.

Bower TGR: The Perceptual World of the Child. Cambridge, Harvard University Press, 1977.

Brazelton TB: Neonatal Behavior Assessment Scale. Clin Dev Med Ser No 50. London, William Heinemann, 1973.

Brazelton TB, Parker WB, Zuckerman B: Importance of assessment of the neonate. Curr Prob Pediatr 7:1, 1976.

Brazelton TB, Vaughan VC III (eds): The Family: Setting Priorities. New York, Science & Medicine Publishing Co, 1979.

Condon WS, Sander L: Neonatal movement is synchronized with adult speech: Interactional participation and language acquisition. Science 183:99, 1974.

Erikson EH: Childhood and Society. 2nd ed. New York, WW Norton, 1963.

Klaus MH, Kennell JH: Parent-Infant Bonding. 2nd ed. St. Louis, CV Mosby, 1982.

McKay HE, McKay A, Sinisterra L: Behavioral intervention studies with malnourished children: A review of experiences. *In*: Kallen DJ: Nutrition,

Table 2–5A. **Stature and Weight by Age*** **Boys: 2 to 18 Years**

{ **Stature:** centimeters and (inches)
{ **Weight:** kilograms and (pounds)

Age years	Boys: Percentiles 5th	10th	25th	50th	75th	90th	95th
2.0†	82.5 (32½) 10.49 (23¼)	83.5 (32¾) 10.96 (24¼)	85.3 (33½) 11.55 (25½)	86.8 (34¼) 12.34 (27¼)	89.2 (35) 13.36 (29½)	92.0 (36¼) 14.38 (31¾)	94.4 (37¼) 15.50 (34¼)
2.5†	85.4 (33½) 11.27 (24¾)	86.5 (34) 11.77 (26)	88.5 (34¾) 12.55 (27¾)	90.4 (35½) 13.52 (29¾)	92.9 (36½) 14.61 (32¼)	95.6 (37¾) 15.71 (34¾)	97.8 (38½) 16.61 (36½)
3.0	89.0 (35) 12.05 (26½)	90.3 (35½) 12.58 (27¾)	92.6 (36½) 13.12 (29¾)	94.9 (37¼) 14.62 (32¼)	97.5 (38½) 15.78 (34¾)	100.1 (39½) 16.95 (37¼)	102.0 (40¼) 17.77 (39¼)
3.5	92.5 (36½) 12.84 (28¼)	93.9 (37) 13.41 (29½)	96.4 (38) 14.46 (32)	99.1 (39) 15.68 (34½)	101.7 (40) 16.90 (37¼)	104.3 (41¼) 18.15 (40)	106.1 (41¾) 18.98 (41¾)
4.0	95.8 (37¾) 13.64 (30)	97.3 (38¼) 14.24 (31½)	100.0 (39¼) 15.39 (34)	102.9 (40½) 16.69 (36¾)	105.7 (41½) 17.99 (39¾)	108.2 (42½) 19.32 (42½)	109.9 (43¼) 20.27 (44¾)
4.5	98.9 (39) 14.45 (31¾)	100.6 (39½) 15.10 (33¼)	103.4 (40¾) 16.30 (36)	106.6 (42) 17.69 (39)	109.4 (43) 19.06 (42)	111.9 (44) 20.50 (45¼)	113.5 (44¾) 21.63 (47¾)
5.0	102.0 (40¼) 15.27 (33¾)	103.7 (40¾) 15.96 (35¼)	106.5 (42) 17.22 (38)	109.9 (43¼) 18.67 (41¼)	112.8 (44½) 20.14 (44½)	115.4 (45½) 21.70 (47¾)	117.0 (46) 23.09 (51)
5.5	104.9 (41¼) 16.09 (35½)	106.7 (42) 16.83 (37)	109.6 (43¼) 18.14 (40)	113.1 (44½) 19.67 (43¼)	116.1 (45¾) 21.25 (46¾)	118.7 (46¾) 22.96 (50½)	120.3 (47¼) 24.66 (54¼)
6.0	107.7 (42½) 16.93 (37¼)	109.6 (43¼) 17.72 (39)	112.5 (44¼) 19.07 (42)	116.1 (45¾) 20.69 (45½)	119.2 (47) 22.40 (49½)	121.9 (48) 24.31 (53½)	123.5 (48½) 26.34 (58)
6.5	110.4 (43½) 17.78 (39¼)	112.3 (44¼) 18.62 (41)	115.3 (45½) 20.02 (44¼)	119.0 (46¾) 21.74 (48)	122.2 (48) 23.62 (52)	124.9 (49¼) 25.76 (56¾)	126.6 (49¾) 28.16 (62)
7.0	113.0 (44½) 18.64 (41)	115.0 (45¼) 19.53 (43)	118.0 (46½) 21.00 (46¼)	121.7 (48) 22.85 (50¼)	125.0 (49¼) 24.94 (55)	127.9 (50¼) 27.36 (60¼)	129.7 (51) 30.12 (66½)
7.5	115.6 (45½) 19.52 (43)	117.6 (46¼) 20.45 (45	120.6 (47½) 22.02 (48½)	124.4 (49) 24.03 (53)	127.8 (50¼) 26.36 (58)	130.8 (51½) 29.11 (64¼)	132.7 (52¼) 32.73 (72¼)
8.0	118.1 (46½) 20.40 (45)	120.2 (47¼) 21.39 (47¼)	123.2 (48½) 22.09 (51)	127.0 (50) 25.30 (55¾)	130.5 (51½) 27.91 (61½)	133.6 (52½) 31.06 (68½)	135.7 (53½) 34.51 (76)
8.5	120.5 (47½) 21.31 (47)	122.7 (48¼) 22.34 (49¼)	125.7 (49½) 24.21 (53¼)	129.6 (51) 26.66 (58¾)	133.2 (52½) 29.61 (65¼)	136.5 (53¾) 33.22 (73¼)	138.8 (54¾) 36.96 (81½)
9.0	122.9 (48½) 22.25 (49)	125.2 (49¼) 23.33 (51½)	128.2 (50½) 25.40 (56)	132.2 (52) 28.13 (62)	136.0 (53½) 31.46 (69¼)	139.4 (55) 35.57 (78½)	141.8 (55¾) 39.58 (87¾)
9.5	125.3 (49¼) 23.25 (51¼)	127.6 (50¼) 24.38 (53¾)	130.8 (51½) 26.88 (58¾)	134.8 (53) 29.73 (65½)	138.8 (54¾) 33.46 (73¾)	142.4 (56) 38.11 (84)	144.9 (57) 42.35 (93¼)
10.0	127.7 (50¼) 24.33 (53¾)	130.1 (51¼) 25.52 (56¼)	133.4 (52½) 28.07 (62)	137.5 (54¼) 31.44 (69¼)	141.6 (55¾) 35.61 (78½)	145.5 (57¼) 40.80 (90)	148.1 (58¼) 45.27 (99¾)
10.5	130.1 (51¼) 25.51 (56¼)	132.6 (52¼) 26.78 (59)	136.0 (53½) 29.59 (65¼)	140.3 (55¼) 33.30 (73½)	144.6 (57) 37.92 (83½)	148.7 (58½) 43.63 (96¼)	151.5 (59¾) 48.31 (106½)
11.0	132.6 (52¼) 26.80 (59)	135.1 (53¼) 28.17 (62)	138.7 (54½) 31.25 (69)	143.33 (56½) 35.30 (77¾)	147.8 (58¼) 40.38 (89)	152.1 (60) 46.57 (102¾)	154.9 (61) 51.47 (113½)
11.5	135.0 (53¼) 28.24 (62¼)	137.7 (54½) 29.72 (65½)	141.5 (55¾) 33.08 (73)	146.4 (57¾) 37.46 (82½)	151.1 (59½) 43.00 (94¾)	155.6 (61¼) 49.61 (109¼)	158.5 (62½) 54.73 (120¾)
12.0	137.6 (54¼) 29.85 (65¾)	140.3 (55¼) 31.46 (69¼)	144.4 (56¾) 35.09 (77¼)	149.7 (59) 39.78 (87¾)	154.6 (60¾) 45.77 (101)	159.4 (62¾) 52.73 (116¼)	162.3 (64) 58.09 (128)
12.5	140.2 (55¼) 31.64 (69¾)	143.0 (56¼) 33.41 (73¾)	147.4 (58) 37.31 (82¼)	153.0 (60¼) 42.27 (93¼)	158.2 (62¼) 48.70 (107¼)	163.2 (64¼) 55.91 (123¼)	166.1 (65½) 61.52 (135¾)
13.0	142.9 (56¼) 33.64 (74¼)	145.8 (57½) 35.60 (78½)	150.5 (59¼) 39.74 (87½)	156.5 (61½) 44.95 (99)	161.8 (63¾) 51.79 (114¼)	167.0 (65¾) 59.12 (130¼)	169.8 (66¾) 65.02 (143¼)
13.5	145.7 (57¼) 35.85 (79)	148.7 (58½) 38.03 (83¾)	153.6 (60½) 42.40 (93½)	159.9 (63) 47.81 (105½)	165.3 (65) 55.02 (121¼)	170.5 (67¼) 62.35 (137½)	173.4 (68¼) 68.51 (151)
14.0	148.8 (58½) 38.22 (84¼)	151.8 (59¾) 40.64 (89½)	156.9 (61¾) 45.21 (99¾)	63.1 (64¼) 50.77 (112)	168.5 (66¼) 58.31 (128½)	173.8 (68½) 65.57 (144½)	176.7 (69½) 72.13 (159)
14.5	152.0 (59¾) 40.66 (89¾)	155.0 (61) 43.34 (95½)	160.1 (63) 48.08 (106)	166.2 (65½) 53.76 (118½)	171.5 (67½) 61.58 (135¾)	176.6 (69½) 68.76 (151½)	179.5 (70½) 75.66 (166¾)
15.0	155.2 (61) 43.11 (95)	158.2 (62¼) 46.06 (101½)	163.3 (64¼) 50.92 (112¼)	169.0 (66½) 56.71 (125)	174.1 (68½) 64.72 (142¾)	178.9 (70½) 71.91 (158½)	181.9 (71½) 79.12 (174½)
15.5	158.3 (62¼) 45.50 (100¼)	161.2 (63½) 48.69 (107¼)	166.2 (65½) 53.64 (118¼)	171.5 (67½) 59.51 (131¼)	176.3 (69½) 67.64 (149)	180.8 (71¼) 74.98 (165¼)	183.9 (72½) 82.45 (181¾)
16.0	161.1 (63½) 47.74 (105¼)	163.9 (64½) 51.16 (112¾)	168.7 (66½) 56.16 (123¾)	173.5 (68¼) 62.10 (137)	178.1 (70) 70.26 (155)	182.4 (71¾) 77.97 (172)	185.4 (73) 85.62 (188¾)
16.5	163.4 (64¼) 49.76 (109¾)	166.1 (65½) 53.39 (117¾)	170.6 (67¼) 58.38 (128¾)	175.2 (69) 64.39 (142)	179.5 (70¾) 72.46 (159¾)	183.6 (72¼) 80.84 (178¼)	186.6 (73½) 88.59 (195¼)
17.0	164.9 (65) 51.50 (113½)	167.7 (66) 55.28 (121¾)	171.9 (67¾) 60.22 (132¾)	176.2 (69¼) 66.31 (146¼)	180.5 (71) 74.17 (163½)	184.4 (72½) 83.58 (184¼)	187.3 (73¾) 91.31 (201¼)
17.5	165.6 (65¼) 52.89 (116½)	168.5 (66¼) 56.78 (125¼)	172.4 (67¾) 61.61 (135¾)	176.7 (69½) 67.78 (149½)	181.0 (71¼) 75.32 (166)	185.0 (72¾) 86.14 (190)	187.6 (73¾) 93.73 (206¾)
18.0	165.7 (65¼) 53.97 (119)	168.7 (66½) 57.89 (127½)	172.3 (67¾) 62.61 (138)	176.8 (69½) 68.88 (151¾)	181.2 (71¼) 76.0 (167¾)	185.3 (73) 88.41 (195)	187.6 (73¾) 95.76 (211)

*Data in Tables 2–5A and 2–5B are those of the National Center for Health Statistics, Health Resources Administration, DHEW, collected in its Health Examination Surveys. Metric data have been smoothed by the least-squares cubic spline technique. For details see footnote to Table 2–3.

†Stature data for 2.0 to 3.0 years include some recumbent length measurements, which make values slightly higher than if all measurements had been of stature.

Table 2–5B. **Stature and Weight by Age* Girls: 2 to 18 Years**

Stature: centimeters and (inches)
Weight: kilograms and (pounds)

Age years	Girls: Percentiles 5th	10th	25th	50th	75th	90th	95th
2.0	81.6 (32¼)	82.1 (32¼)	84.0 (33)	86.8 (34¼)	89.3 (35¼)	92.0 (36¼)	93.6 (36¾)
	9.95 (22)	10.32 (22¾)	10.96 (24¼)	11.80 (26)	12.73 (28)	13.58 (30)	14.15 (31¼)
2.5	84.6 (33¼)	85.3 (33½)	87.3 (34½)	90.0 (35½)	92.5 (36½)	95.0 (37½)	96.6 (38)
	10.80 (23¾)	11.35 (25)	12.11 (26¾)	13.03 (28¾)	14.23 (31¼)	15.16 (33½)	15.76 (34¾)
3.0	88.3 (34¾)	89.3 (35¼)	91.4 (36)	94.1 (37)	96.6 (38)	99.0 (39)	100.6 (39½)
	11.61 (25½)	12.26 (27)	13.11 (29)	14.10 (31)	15.50 (34¼)	16.54 (36½)	17.22 (38)
3.5	91.7 (36)	93.0 (36½)	95.2 (37½)	97.9 (38½)	100.5 (39½)	102.8 (40½)	104.5 (41¼)
	12.37 (27¼)	13.08 (28¾)	14.00 (30¾)	15.07 (33¼)	16.59 (36½)	17.77 (39¼)	18.59 (41)
4.0	95.0 (37½)	96.4 (38)	98.8 (39)	101.6 (40)	104.3 (41)	106.6 (42)	108.3 (42¾)
	13.11 (29)	13.84 (30½)	14.80 (32¾)	15.96 (35¼)	17.56 (38¾)	18.93 (41¾)	19.91 (44)
4.5	98.1 (38½)	99.7 (39¼)	102.2 (40¼)	105.0 (41¼)	107.9 (42½)	110.2 (43½)	112.0 (44)
	13.83 (30½)	14.56 (32)	15.55 (34¼)	16.81 (37)	18.48 (40¾)	20.06 (44¼)	21.24 (46¾)
5.0	101.1 (39¾)	102.7 (40½)	105.4 (41½)	108.4 (42¾)	111.4 (43¾)	113.8 (44¾)	115.6 (45½)
	14.55 (32)	15.26 (33¾)	16.29 (36)	17.66 (39)	19.39 (42¾)	21.23 (46¾)	22.62 (49¾)
5.5	103.9 (41)	105.6 (41½)	108.4 (42¾)	111.6 (44)	114.8 (45¼)	117.4 (46¼)	119.2 (47)
	15.29 (33¾)	15.97 (35¼)	17.05 (37½)	18.56 (41)	20.36 (45)	22.48 (49½)	24.11 (53¼)
6.0	106.6 (42)	108.4 (42¾)	111.3 (43¾)	114.6 (45)	118.1 (46½)	120.8 (47½)	122.7 (48¼)
	16.05 (35½)	16.72 (36¾)	17.86 (39¼)	19.52 (43)	21.44 (47¼)	23.89 (52¾)	25.75 (56¾)
6.5	109.2 (43)	111.0 (43¾)	114.1 (45)	117.6 (46¼)	121.3 (47¾)	124.2 (49)	126.1 (49¾)
	16.85 (37¼)	17.51 (38½)	18.76 (41¼)	20.61 (45½)	22.68 (50)	25.50 (56¼)	27.59 (60¾)
7.0	111.8 (44)	113.6 (44¾)	116.8 (46)	120.6 (47½)	124.4 (49)	127.6 (50¼)	129.5 (51)
	17.71 (39)	18.39 (40½)	19.78 (43½)	21.84 (48¼)	24.16 (53¼)	27.39 (60½)	29.68 (65½)
7.5	114.4 (45)	116.2 (45¾)	119.5 (47)	123.5 (48½)	127.5 (50¼)	130.9 (51½)	132.9 (52¼)
	18.62 (41)	19.37 (42¾)	20.95 (46¼)	23.26 (51¼)	25.90 (57)	29.57 (65¼)	32.07 (70¾)
8.0	116.9 (46)	118.7 (46¾)	122.2 (48)	126.4 (49¾)	130.6 (51½)	134.2 (52¾)	136.2 (53½)
	19.62 (43¼)	20.45 (45)	22.26 (49)	24.84 (54¾)	27.88 (61½)	32.04 (70¾)	34.71 (76½)
8.5	119.5 (47)	121.3 (47¾)	124.9 (49¼)	129.3 (51)	133.6 (52½)	137.4 (54)	139.6 (55)
	20.68 (45½)	21.64 (47¾)	23.70 (52¼)	26.58 (58½)	30.08 (66¼)	34.73 (76½)	37.58 (82¾)
9.0	122.1 (48)	123.9 (48¾)	127.7 (50¼)	132.2 (52)	136.7 (53¾)	140.7 (55½)	142.9 (56¼)
	21.82 (48)	22.92 (50½)	25.27 (55¾)	28.46 (62¾)	32.44 (71½)	37.60 (83)	40.64 (89½)
9.5	124.8 (49¼)	126.6 (49¾)	130.6 (51½)	135.2 (53¼)	139.8 (55)	143.9 (56¾)	146.2 (57½)
	23.05 (50¾)	24.29 (53½)	26.94 (59½)	30.45 (67¼)	34.94 (77)	40.61 (89½)	43.85 (96¾)
10.0	127.5 (50¼)	129.5 (51)	133.6 (52½)	138.3 (54½)	142.9 (56¼)	147.2 (58)	149.5 (58¾)
	24.36 (53¾)	25.76 (56¾)	28.71 (63¼)	32.55 (71¾)	37.53 (82¾)	43.70 (96¼)	47.17 (104)
10.5	130.4 (51¼)	132.5 (52¼)	136.7 (53¾)	141.5 (55¾)	146.1 (57½)	150.4 (59¼)	152.8 (60¼)
	25.75 (56¾)	27.32 (60¼)	30.57 (67½)	34.72 (76½)	40.17 (88½)	46.84 (103¼)	50.57 (111½)
11.0	133.5 (52½)	135.6 (53½)	140.0 (55)	144.8 (57)	149.3 (58¾)	153.7 (60½)	56.2 (61½)
	27.24 (60)	28.97 (63¾)	32.49 (71¾)	36.95 (81½)	42.84 (94½)	49.96 (110¼)	54.00 (119)
11.5	136.6 (53¾)	139.0 (54¾)	143.5 (56½)	148.2 (58¼)	152.6 (60)	156.9 (61¾)	159.5 (62¾)
	28.83 (63½)	30.71 (67¾)	34.48 (76)	39.23 (86½)	45.48 (100¼	53.03 (117)	57.42 (126½)
12.0	139.8 (55)	142.3 (56)	147.0 (57¾)	151.5 (59¾)	155.8 (61¼)	160.0 (63)	162.7 (64)
	30.52 (67¼)	32.53 (71¼)	36.52 (80½)	41.53 (91½)	48.07 (106)	55.99 (123½)	60.81 (134)
12.5	142.7 (56¼)	145.4 (57¼)	150.1 (59)	154.6 (60¾)	158.8 (62½)	162.9 (64½)	165.6 (65¼)
	32.30 (71¾)	34.42 (76)	38.59 (85)	43.84 (96¾)	50.56 (111½)	58.81 (129¾)	64.12 (141¼)
13.0	145.2 (57¼)	148.0 (58¼)	152.8 (60¼)	157.1 (61¾)	161.3 (63½)	165.3 (65)	168.1 (66¼)
	34.14 (75¼)	36.35 (80¼)	40.55 (89½)	46.10 (101¾)	52.91 (116¾)	61.45 (135½)	67.30 (148¼)
13.5	147.2 (58)	150.0 (59)	154.7 (61)	159.0 (62½)	163.2 (64¼)	167.3 (65¾)	170.0 (67)
	35.98 (79¼)	38.26 (84¼)	42.65 (94)	48.26 (106½)	55.11 (121½)	63.87 (140¾)	70.30 (155)
14.0	148.7 (58½)	151.5 (59¾)	155.9 (61½)	160.4 (63¼)	164.6 (64¾)	168.7 (66½)	171.3 (67½)
	37.76 (83¼)	40.11 (88½)	44.54 (98¼)	50.28 (110¾)	57.09 (125¾)	66.04 (145½)	73.08 (161)
14.5	149.7 (59)	152.5 (60)	158.8 (61¾)	161.2 (63½)	165.6 (65¼)	169.8 (66¾)	172.2 (67¾)
	39.45 (87)	41.83 (92¼)	46.28 (102)	52.10 (114¾)	58.84 (129¾)	67.95 (149¾)	75.59 (166¾)
15.0	150.5 (59¼)	153.2 (60¼)	157.2 (62)	161.8 (63¾)	166.3 (65¼)	170.5 (67¼)	172.8 (68)
	40.99 (90¼)	43.38 (95¾)	47.82 (105½)	53.68 (118¼)	60.32 (133)	69.54 (153¼)	77.78 (171½)
15.5	151.1 (59½)	153.6 (60½)	157.5 (62)	162.1 (63¾)	166.7 (65¾)	170.9 (67¼)	173.1 (68¼)
	42.32 (93¼)	44.72 (98½)	49.10 (108¼)	54.96 (121¼)	61.48 (135½)	70.79 (156)	79.59 (176½)
16.0	151.6 (59¾)	154.1 (60¾)	157.8 (62¼)	162.4 (64)	166.9 (65¾)	171.1 (67¼)	173.3 (68¼)
	43.41 (95¾)	45.78 (101)	50.09 (110½)	55.89 (123¼)	62.29 (137¼)	71.68 (158)	80.99 (178½)
16.5	152.2 (60)	154.6 (60¾)	158.2 (62¼)	162.7 (64)	167.1 (65¾)	171.2 (67½)	173.4 (68¼)
	44.20 (97½)	46.54 (102½)	50.75 (112)	56.44 (124½)	62.75 (138¼)	72.18 (159¼)	81.93 (180½)
17.0	152.7 (60)	155.1 (61)	158.7 (62½)	163.1 (64¼)	167.3 (65¾)	171.2 (67½)	173.5 (68¼)
	44.74 (98¾)	47.04 (103¾)	51.14 (112¾)	56.69 (125)	62.91 (138¾)	72.38 (159½)	82.46 (181¾)
17.5	153.2 (60¼)	155.6 (61¼)	159.1 (62¾)	163.4 (64¼)	167.5 (66)	171.1 (67¼)	173.5 (68¼)
	45.08 (99½)	47.33 (104¼)	51.33 (113¼)	56.71 (125)	62.89 (138¾)	72.37 (159½)	82.62 (182¼)
18.0	153.6 (60½)	156.0 (61½)	159.6 (62¾)	163.7 (64½)	167.6 (66)	171.0 (67¼)	173.6 (68¼)
	45.26 (99¾)	47.47 (104¾)	51.39 (113¼)	56.62 (124¾)	62.78 (138½)	72.25 (159¼)	82.47 (181¾)

*See footnotes to Table 2–5A.

Development, and Social Behavior. Washington DC, DHEW Publication No 73–242.

Prechtl H, Beintema D: The Neurological Examination of the Full Term Newborn Infant. Clin Dev Med Ser No 12. Philadelphia, JB Lippincott, 1975. Repr of 1965 ed.

Vaughan VC III, Brazelton TB (eds): The Family—Can It Be Saved? Chicago, Year Book Publishers, 1976.

2.9 GROWTH AND DEVELOPMENT DURING ADOLESCENCE

The most important organizing event of adolescence is puberty, and because puberty occurs and progresses across a wide range of chronologic ages and differs between the sexes, attempts at chronologic categorization are fraught with boundary problems. Accordingly, it is reasonable to define *early, middle,* and *late* adolescence in terms of *stages of pubertal development,* since these follow a consistent pattern for individuals regardless of chronologic age.

Unfortunately, many of the physiologic and other data about adolescence have been derived in accordance with age criteria that limit their potential usefulness. That notwithstanding, we will attempt to reorganize existing information into the model of physical development whenever possible, so as to present a developmentally integrated picture of the adolescent at each stage.

Many of the features of adolescent development have been shown to be more closely related to the stage of pubertal development, or *sex maturity rating (SMR),* than to chronologic age. The schema of Tanner is the most widely used for assignment of SMR. SMRs 1 and 2 belong to early adolescence, SMRs 3 and 4 to middle adolescence, and SMR 5 to late adolescence and full sex maturity. The criteria are shown in Tables 2–6 for girls and in Table 2–7 for boys. The corresponding clinical features for each stage are seen in Figures 2–2 and 2–3, and their interrelationships are shown diagrammatically in Figures 2–4 and 2–5. Within each developmental category, physical development, psychologic development, and social development will be described, and those areas of particular interest to the health professional will be emphasized. Tools and methods of assessment will also be described when appropriate.

Early adolescence (SMR 2) generally has its onset between the ages of 10 and 13 yr and lasts for 6 mo to 1 yr in girls. In boys, its onset is between 10.5 and 15, lasting from 6 mo to 2 yr. Middle adolescence (SMR 3–4) occurs anywhere from 11 to 14 yr in girls, lasting between 2 and 3 yr on average. In boys, middle adolescence typically begins between the ages of 12 and 15.5 yr and lasts 6 mo to 3 yr. Late adolescence (SMR 5) is reached by the average girl between the ages of 13 and 17 yr and by the average boy between 14 and 16 yr.

GROWTH AND DEVELOPMENT DURING THE EARLY ADOLESCENT YEARS

Physical. During the early stages of pubertal maturation (SMRs 1 and 2), gains in weight and in height differ little

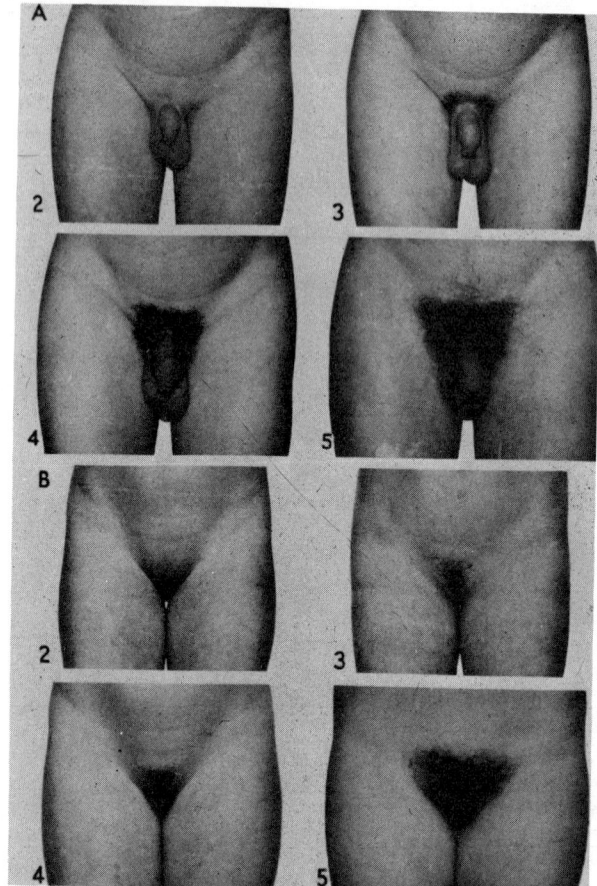

Figure 2–2. Sex maturity ratings of pubic hair changes in adolescent boys and girls. (Courtesy JM Tanner, M.D., Institute of Child Health, Department of Growth and Development, University of London, London, England.)

from those in the preceding years, approximating 2 kg and 6–8 cm each year. This apparent continuity with earlier years belies the changes of body composition that occur with the onset of puberty.

In females, increase in fatness is associated with each successive stage of pubertal development. Subscapular skin-fold thickness, a measure of adiposity, increases an average of about a third in the transition from SMR 1 to SMR 2, about a quarter from SMR 2 to 4, and about another half from SMR 4 to 5.

Between SMR 1 and SMR 5, the total fat content of the female body increases from approximately 10 to 20%. Males become more muscular, rather than fatter, during adolescence, but there is little increase in muscle tissue between SMR 1 and 2. Body fat content has been shown to decrease in males reaching SMR 2 (genital).

Development of secondary sex characteristics forms the definitional basis for puberty. The earliest stage of puberty,

Table 2–6. **Classification of Sex Maturity Stages in Girls**

SMR Stage	Pubic Hair	Breasts
1	Preadolescent	Preadolescent
2	Sparse, lightly pigmented, straight, medial border of labia	Breast and papilla elevated as small mound; areolar diameter increased
3	Darker, beginning to curl, increased amount	Breast and areola enlarged, no contour separation
4	Coarse, curly, abundant but amount less than in adult	Areola and papilla form secondary mound
5	Adult feminine triangle, spread to medial surface of thighs	Mature; nipple projects, areola part of general breast contour

Adapted from Tanner JM: Growth at Adolescence. Ed 2. Oxford, Blackwell Scientific Publications, 1962.

Table 2–7. **Classification of Sex Maturity Stages in Boys**

SMR Stage	Pubic Hair	Penis	Testes
1	None	Preadolescent	Preadolescent
2	Scanty, long, slightly pigmented	Slight enlargement	Enlarged scrotum, pink texture altered
3	Darker, starts to curl, small amount	Longer	Larger
4	Resembles adult type, but less in quantity; coarse, curly	Larger; glans and breadth increase in size	Larger, scrotum dark
5	Adult distribution, spread to medial surface of thighs	Adult size	Adult size

Adapted from Tanner JM: Growth at Adolescence. Ed 2. Oxford, Blackwell Scientific Publications, 1962.

SMR 2, occurs as a result of sleep-augmented secretion of pituitary gonadotropins and growth hormone. There is some recent evidence that these well-documented phenomena are preceded by falling levels of melatonin from the 7th yr on. In females, breast buds first appear in SMR 2, whereas in 30 to 50% of males this occurrence (gynecomastia) is variable and inconsistent in its timing during the pubertal period.

In females breast development results from stimulation by ovarian secretion of estrogens in response to follicle-stimulating hormone (FSH). The predominant effect of FSH is to stimulate growth of the ovaries, a process that begins approximately 1 yr before the stage of breast budding (SMR 2). Further evidence of estrogen production by the ovaries includes thickening of the vaginal mucosa, increased pigmentation, vascularization, and eroticization of the labia majora, and slight enlargement of the clitoris, as well as enlargement of the uterus, which is at this stage equally divided between

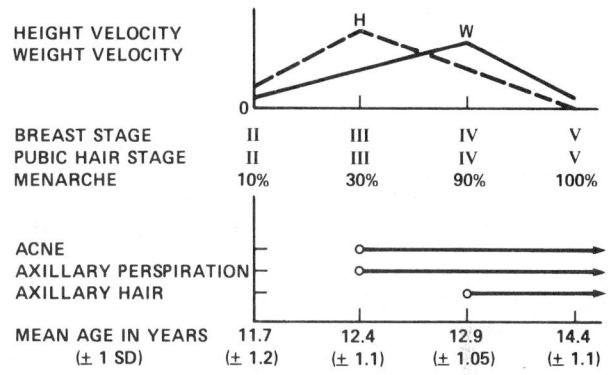

Figure 2–4. Sequence of maturational events in females. (Adapted from Marshall WA, Tanner JM: Arch Dis Child 44:291, 1969.)

corpus and cervix. Endometrial thickening and differentiation begin, while the myometrium begins to increase the cellular content of actomyosin, creatine kinase (CK), and adenosine triphosphate (ATP), presumably in preparation for menses and childbirth. Increased depositon of glycogen within the cells of the vaginal mucosa, another effect of estrogen, favors the growth of Doederlein's lactic acid–forming bacteria and results in a change to an acid pH, as well as in increased susceptibility to yeast infections.

In males SMR 2 consists of enlargement of the testes due to increased size of seminiferous tubules and increased numbers of Leydig and Sertoli cells; secretion of testosterone is responsible for the changes that follow. Enlargement of the

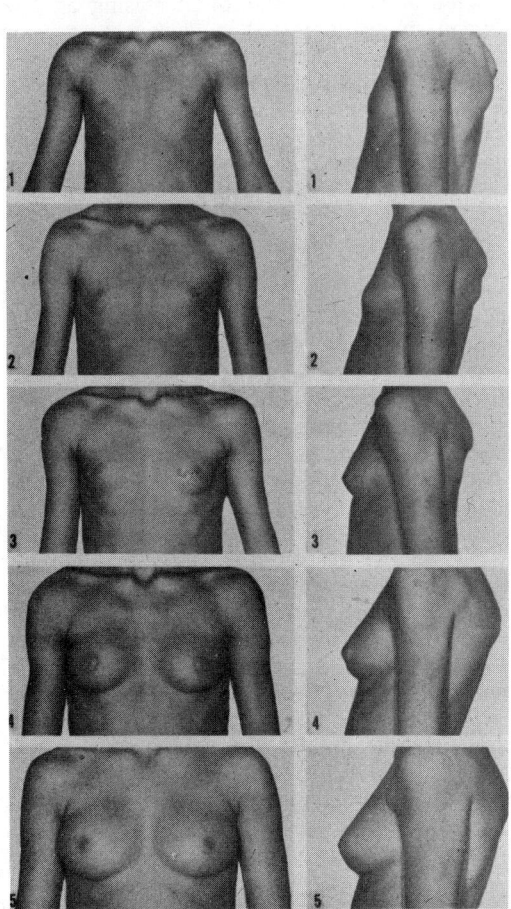

Figure 2–3. Sex maturity ratings of breast changes in adolescent girls. (Courtesy JM Tanner, M.D., Institute of Child Health, Department of Growth and Development, University of London, London, England.)

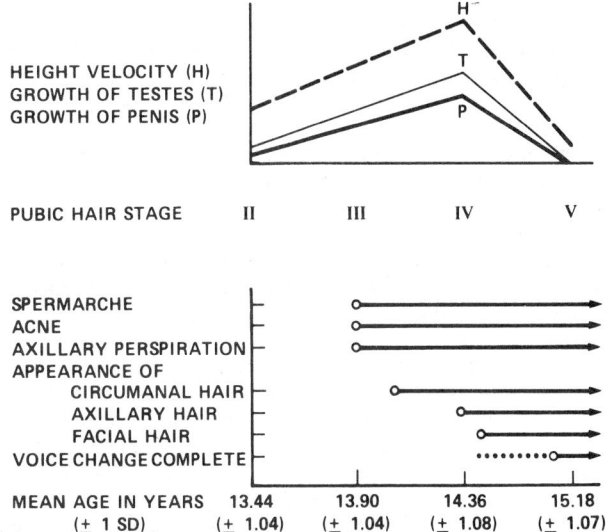

Figure 2–5. Sequence of maturational events in males. (Adapted from Marshall WA, Tanner JM: Arch Dis Child 44:291, 1969.)

epididymis, seminal vesicles, and prostate begins. The epididymis grows less than the testes, coincident with thinning and hypervascularity of the scrotum. The latter assumes the adult configuration, with a narrower proximal portion and the left testis lower than the right. Enlargement of the penis begins shortly thereafter. The penis remains thinner in proportion to its length until later puberty, when acceleration of the growth of the corpora cavernosa penis over that of the urethra eventuates in the adult width.

In addition to secretion of testosterone in males, increased concentrations of adrenal androgens occur in both sexes and are responsible in both for initiation of development of pubic and axillary hair. The consistency and distribution of pubic hair follows a predictable pattern in both sexes, and consequently is a reliable index of pubertal progression, in conjunction with breast development in females and development of the genitalia in males. The relationships among these events are diagrammed in Figures 2–4 and 2–5. At SMR 2, pubic hair is fine and silky and appears in the midline of the labia in females and surrounding the base of the penis in males. Another effect of androgen is to increase both the size and secretions of the sebaceous follicles. These effects are the forerunners of acne, which may thus also be considered a secondary sex characteristic (Sec. 24.31).

There are dramatic functional as well as structural changes in the male genitalia during puberty. Ejaculation, usually initially in response to masturbation, occurs approximately 1 year following the onset of testicular growth, at the time of appearance of pubic hair.

The cuspids (canines) and first molars of the primary dentition are shed by *early* adolescence; the permanent cuspids, 1st and 2nd premolars, and molars erupt during this period. There is close correlation between the times of eruption of the second permanent molar and of the menarche (r = 0.62).

Neurodevelopmental. Although no gross changes in brain morphology are apparent, electroencephalographic studies demonstrate continuing neurodevelopmental maturation during adolescence, which is characterized by an increase in alpha$_2$ wave activity that parallels a decrease in theta and that is most dramatic in girls during *early* adolescence. By *early* adolescence, an individual should manifest a "mature" response on all items of a standardized neurodevelopmental assessment. The last of the items to mature do so by the age of 12 yr and include the ability to identify correctly stimulated fingers in a finger localization task and to distinguish left and right starting from new bases, such as those in marching commands, and the ability to separate the 3rd and 4th fingers without "overflow" movement to other fingers.

Cognitive. Until recently, cognitive development has been described largely in relation to chronologic age. Accordingly, the relationship between stages of pubertal development and cognitive development remains unclear. Carey, in studies of face recognition, concluded that the onset of puberty has a disruptive effect on cognition in girls, whereas Peterson, using different measures of cognition, failed to document the hypothesized disruption.

Since SMR 2 in females spans the ages from 10 to 13 yr (mean ± one standard deviation) and that for males is broader, from 10.5 to 14.5 yr, it is apparent that in the piagetian sequence some at each age will be at the stage of concrete operations and some at the stage of formal operations. At the stage of formal operational thinking, the individual is capable of generating hypotheses to be tested before action is initiated, can think abstractly, can entertain multiple contingencies simultaneously, and can generalize and consider possible consequences of behavior in a logical manner without actually experiencing them first. There are potential implications of attainment of the level of formal operations

for health. As health behaviors are influenced by the patient's ability to understand consequences of proposed therapy (or the risk of pregnancy, for example), an individual may not be in a position to enter into a mature, confidential relationship with the physician until he or she has reached the stage of formal operations. Achievement of this stage is often associated with development of interests in the occult or in mysticism, as well as in religion.

Piagetian theory has in recent years dominated the thinking about the development of cognition, but more recently his description of clear-cut, discrete stages has been challenged. The present approach emphasizes "developmental trends" that evolve during childhood and adolescence and involve more overlap and variation than previously described. These trends include:

1. *Information-processing capacity.* Adolescents appear superior to younger children in their *functional* information-processing capacities, but it is not yet known whether this reflects any increase in "hard-wired *structural* capacity" with age.

2. *Domain-specific knowledge.* As a child ages, he or she accumulates more and more organized knowledge in different, specific domains, allowing for problem-solving by memory processes unavailable to the younger child.

3. *Concrete and formal operations.* The piagetian notions are viewed as trends, rather than specific stages, such that the younger child's approach is viewed as more "empirico-deductive," whereas that of the adolescent is more "hypothetico-deductive."

4. *Quantitative thinking.* Adolescents tend to approach problems with a "more quantitative, measurement-oriented set" than younger children as a result of acquisition "of the concept of a unit measure."

5. *"A sense of the game."* With increasing age, children become increasingly interested in *thinking* as a competitive game and are challenged by it.

6. *Metacognition.* This concept refers to thinking about thinking and is divided by Flavell into metacognitive knowledge and metacognitive experiences. The first "refers to accumulated declarative and procedural knowledge concerning cognitive matters," and the second to affective experiences of the "Eureka!" or, conversely, the "This doesn't make sense to me" variety. Metacognition develops considerably between childhood and adolescence.

7. *Improving existing competencies.* The maturation of competencies once acquired is a continuing process during development. Sex differences appear to emerge during *early* adolescence, with boys performing better in areas of spatial ability and mathematics, and girls excelling in verbal ability.

Closely related to cognitive development is that of moral thought, an area explored by Kohlberg (Sec. 2.21). At the time of entry into formal operations in the piagetian schema, the individual should be at the postconventional level of moral development in the Kohlberg classification. This level is "characterized by a major thrust toward autonomous moral principles which have validity and application apart from authority of the groups or persons who hold them and apart from the individual's identification with those persons or groups."

Psychosocial. The *early* adolescent must function in three arenas: the family, peer group, and school. In each arena there exists a complex interplay of determinants of successful function.

The major developmental task of early adolescence is that of initiating independence from the family, and it is at this time that earlier familial relationships may be most visibly disrupted. Often at the same time, the onset of pubertal development signals a wish for privacy, and often for increased distance from a physically affectionate parent of the opposite sex. The adolescent's unspoken wish for parents to set limits is in conflict with his or her need for autonomy, and unresolved parental needs are often reawakened by these stresses. As a result, the adolescent tends to turn toward a same-sex peer group.

Friendships at this early adolescent stage of development are typically with members of the same sex and tend to center more on the joint activity "than on the interaction itself," according to Douvan and Adelson, who describe the friendships of early adolescence as relatively devoid of depth or mutuality. Costanzo and Shaw have found the highest degree of conformity to exist in the peer groups of early adolescence, with little difference between those of males and females in this age group.

Function in the school setting appears at this age to be multifactorially determined. Synchrony of pubertal development with that of the peer group has been found by a number of investigators to be an important factor in adjustment. Gross and Duke found that boys who were late maturers performed less well in school and had lower educational expectations and aspirations than the early-maturing males. Simmonds and associates found that early-maturing girls in a middle school setting had poor self-image and lower grade point averages than their later-maturing peers or those who were still in an elementary school (8th grade or less) setting. The emergence of sex differences in cognition in early adolescence as described above may contribute to changes in school performance.

GROWTH AND DEVELOPMENT IN THE MIDDLE ADOLESCENT YEARS

Middle adolescence refers to the period corresponding to SMR 3 and 4 and spans roughly the chronologic ages from 12 to 14 years in females and from 12.5 to 15 years in males. It is the period of the most dramatic growth and change. There is at this time acceleration in weight and linear growth, as well as further development of secondary sex characteristics. Middle adolescence is the time of the peak of the weight velocity curve, which follows the peak of the height velocity curve by approximately 6 months. It is during this phase that the bulk of fat tissue is deposited in females and of muscle mass in males (with a 4–fold greater increase in number of muscle cells in males than in females). In males the peak of grip strength occurs about 14 months following the peak of the height velocity curve.

During the growth spurt of middle adolescence, females average an increment in height of 8 cm/yr at a mean age of 12 years, whereas the later growth spurt of males (at a mean age of 14 years) averages 10 cm/yr. There is an orderly pattern of progression of skeletal growth from distal to proximal parts of the body, beginning with growth of the feet. This is followed approximately 6 months later by that of the lower leg, and then of the thigh. A similar pattern is found for the upper extremity, the resultant disproportionately large hands and feet contributing to the apparent clumsiness of adolescents. The peak acceleration of leg length is followed approximately 4 months later by that of width of chest and hips. Elongation of the trunk and increase in the anteroposterior diameter of the chest are the last manifestations of the pubertal growth spurt.

Just as sex differences arise in soft tissue growth during middle adolescence, there are also sex differences in patterns of skeletal growth. The greater biacromial width of males is androgen-determined, while the estrogen-determined wider bitrochanteric diameter contributes to the adult female contour. The longer arms and legs of males, relative to total body length, result from the later onset of their growth spurt. The carrying angle of the male arm is less than that of the female as a result of differential growth of cartilage of the lateral humeral epicondyle during puberty.

In middle adolescence development of secondary sex characteristics involves enlargement of the female breast and areola, and, in about 75% of girls (in SMR 4), the demarcation of the contours of breast and areola by an elevation of the latter. Pubic hair darkens, coarsens, curls, and extends proximally and laterally to cover the mons. In the male, the penis elongates and widens, testes enlarge, and the scrotum becomes more pigmented. The most dramatic event of puberty for the female is the menarche; it occurs at a mean age of 12.5 years in our culture. Its timing is closely linked to other pubertal events: it occurs at SMR 2 in 10%, SMR 3 in 20%, SMR 4 in 60%, and SMR 5 in 10% of girls, and is, accordingly, largely an event of middle adolescence. The timing of menarche is closely related to the peak of the weight velocity curve and to the deceleration phase of the height velocity curve. The timing is determined by a number of factors, the most important of which is undoubtedly genetic. There is close concordance between mothers' and daughters' ages at menarche, and even closer correlation between those of siblings. Other factors, such as nutritional status, are also important; obese girls have their menarche earlier than those who are lean. The very lean, and particularly athletes, are delayed in their menarche when compared with nonathletic controls. Any chronic illness that adversely affects nutritional status or tissue oxygenation will also delay pubertal maturation and ultimately the timing of menarche.

Much more variable in timing of appearance is growth of circumanal hair, which tends to antedate axillary and facial hair; the latter two appear about the time when pubic hair reaches SMR 4. In males facial hair first appears at the corners of the upper lip and spreads medially. Coincident with the appearance of axillary hair is that of body odor, which results from androgenic stimulation of apocrine sweat glands and is often a source of concern to the already self-conscious adolescent.

It is also typically during middle adolescence that many males manifest gynecomastia, which may be bi- or unilateral and can persist up to 18 months after onset. Although common and nonpathologic, it often causes great consternation to the young man who develops it. Reassurance that this is normal is required of the physician even in the absence of inquiry by the patient.

Neurodevelopmental. Neurodevelopmental maturity appears to be reached before or during early adolescence. Nothing of which we are aware distinguishes middle adolescence from the neurodevelopmental perspective. On the other hand, although no apparent growth of the central nervous system occurs during middle adolescence, sleep studies suggest that physiologic changes do occur. As an individual moves from SMR 3 to SMR 4, there is a decrease in sleep latency time and an increase in daytime sleepiness. Parents may misinterpret these normal events as signs of laziness.

Cognitive Development. The trends in cognitive development described in the section on early adolescence continue.

Psychosocial Development. The contexts of adolescents' behavior with family, school, and peer group during this middle adolescent stage remain similar to those of early adolescence; school and peer group gain in importance, and now sex differences in peer relationships become apparent. According to Savin-Williams, "The developmental tasks during adolescence for boys are dominated by needs for achievement and independence, best worked through in a group; for girls, developing interpersonal skills and love, which are best achieved in dyadic relationships." Loyalty and commitment and intimacy of shared information are more valued in female than in male friendships.

During middle adolescence, social groups may extend to include members of the opposite sex, and paired dating may begin. A developmental progression in dating behavior has been described: stage 1 consists of dating without physical contact; stage 2 of kissing, with touching of clothed breasts; stage 3 of touching of unclothed breasts or genital apposition; stage 4 of sexual intercourse with a single partner; and stage 5 of intercourse with multiple partners. Although there is a great deal of variability among subgroups of adolescents, it appears that the majority of teenagers in the middle adolescent years do not progress to stage 4. For those who do, however, the risk of unintended pregnancy and sexually transmitted disease is quite high, making prevention an important agenda item for the care of those in this age group (Chapter 9).

During middle adolescence vocational and educational decisions are often made. As indicated earlier, synchrony with the peer group in timing of physical maturation can influence school performance, as well as aspirations for educational achievement. The physical effects of pubertal development become incorporated into one's self-image during these years, often with profound consequences. When the increased adiposity of pubertal development is viewed negatively by a young woman, a chain of events culminating in anorexia nervosa may ensue (Sec. 9.6). Asymmetric breast development may cause an adolescent to view herself as abnormal. Poor self-image is a common problem during this time, particularly for females and those with chronic illness. Development of self-image during middle adolescence also involves "trying on" or experimenting with different social roles. In the eriksonian categorization of life crises, it is the time for self-definition or development of an identity. It is also the time when sexual identity becomes solidified and a sense of sexual adequacy is developed.

GROWTH AND DEVELOPMENT DURING LATE ADOLESCENCE

Physical. It is during this phase of development that the body approximates its young adult proportions and size. Little additional linear growth is achieved after the growth spurt of middle adolescence has passed. Remaining epiphyses, such as those of the femur, humerus, and sternoclavicular junction, become fused, sometimes as late as in the early 20's. Development of secondary sex characteristics is completed with spread of pubic hair to the medial aspects of the thighs in both sexes, attainment of adult genitalia and full reproductive capacity in the male, and attainment of adult breast configuration in the female. In the male facial hair spreads to the chin, and chest hair appears as the last event in the progression of hair growth. The deepening of voice is completed as testosterone stimulates growth of the thyroid and cricoid cartilages and of laryngeal muscles. In the female the adult relationship of larger uterine fundus to smaller cervix is attained.

Neurodevelopmental. Neurophysiologic structures and functions appear to be completely developed by the end of middle adolescence. No further developmental processes are known. On the other hand, cognitive, social, and moral development may continue through the rest of life.

Psychosocial. In late adolescence issues of career decisions are usually firmly and sometimes finally faced, and the rebelliousness of earlier stages, if manifest, is often replaced by a gradual return to the family, albeit on a new footing. Although still often moralistic and absolute in their thinking, adolescents of this stage are often more able to engage in a dialogue with parents. The ability to engage in an empathetic, intimate relationship with another person begins, and the sometimes exploitative, narcissistic sexual relationships of earlier stages are supplanted. By the age of 19 years, approximately 60% of females and 80% of males in the United States have had sexual intercourse. Even in same-sex relationships, differences emerge in late adolescence such that loyalty, trust, and support in an emotional crisis are characteristics most valued in friendships of 17 yr olds, whereas 13 yr olds stress good moral character and "niceness" in their friendships. (See also Sec. 2.30.)

If the psychosocial crisis of earlier adolescence was, in Erikson's schema, that of identity, then that of late adolescence is the need to develop the capacity for intimacy. Once the individual has a self to give, he or she is capable of giving it.

IRIS F. LITT
VICTOR C. VAUGHAN, III

Bazan MT: Anomalous dental development with medical and genetic implications. Pediatr Ann 14:108, 1985.

Chess S, Thomas A, Cameron M: Sexual attitudes and behavior patterns in a middle-class adolescent population. Am J Orthopsychiatry 4:46, 1976.

Costanzo PR, Shaw ME: Conformity as a function of age level. Child Develop 37:967, 1966.

Diamond R, Carey S, Back KJ: Genetic influences on the development of spatial skills during early adolescence. Cognition 13:167, 1983.

Douvan E, Adelson J: The Adolescent Experience. New York, John Wiley & Sons, 1966.

Flavell J: Cognitive Development. 2nd ed. Englewood Cliffs, NJ, Prentice Hall, 1985.

Gross RT, Duke PM: The effect of early versus late physical maturation on adolescent behavior. Pediatr Clin North Am 27:71, 1980.

Katchadourian HA: Biology of Adolescence. San Francisco, WH Freeman, 1977.

Kohlberg L, Gilligan C: The adolescent as a philosopher: the discovery of the self in a post conventional world. In: Kagan J, Coles R (eds): 12 to 16. Early Adolescence. New York, WW Norton, 1972.

Levine MD: Developmental assessment. In: Levine MD, Carey W, Crocker A, et al (eds): Developmental-Behavioral Pediatrics. Philadelphia, WB Saunders, 1983.

Peterson AC: Pubertal change and cognition. In: Brooks-Gunn J, Peterson AC (eds): Girls at Puberty. New York, Plenum Press, 1983.

Savin-Williams R: Dominance hierarchies in groups of early adolescents. Child Develop 50:923, 1979.

Schofeld M: The Sexual Behavior of Young People. Boston, Little, Brown, 1965.

Simmonds RG, Blyth DA, McKinney KL: The social and psychological effects of puberty on white females. In: Brooks-Gunn J, Peterson AC (eds): Girls at Puberty. New York, Plenum Press, 1983.

Tanner JM: Growth at Adolescence. 2nd ed. Oxford, Blackwell Scientific Publications, 1962.

2.10 ASSESSMENT OF GROWTH AND DEVELOPMENT

The accurate assessment of developmental status is critical to health care of the infant, child, or adolescent. Many structural and functional details of growth and development are inconspicuous in the broad patterns of growth outlined above, but take on significance when they are factors in the evaluation of clinical problems. The physician who monitors the growth and development of the child will need to know or have access to information regarding the limits of normal variability in these details, not only quantitatively and qualitatively, but also with respect to their interrelationships. The wide variation in patterns of growth often requires that some elements be examined in statistical rather than absolute terms (see also Sec. 4.3).

When biologic data vary over a range of normal values, the largest number of measurements tend to cluster about an *average* or *mean* value. When such data are plotted on a graph, the result is often a close approximation of the ideal gaussian (bell-shaped) curve that describes the distribution of continuously variable values about a population mean. Statistical treatment of such data may generate a number of useful

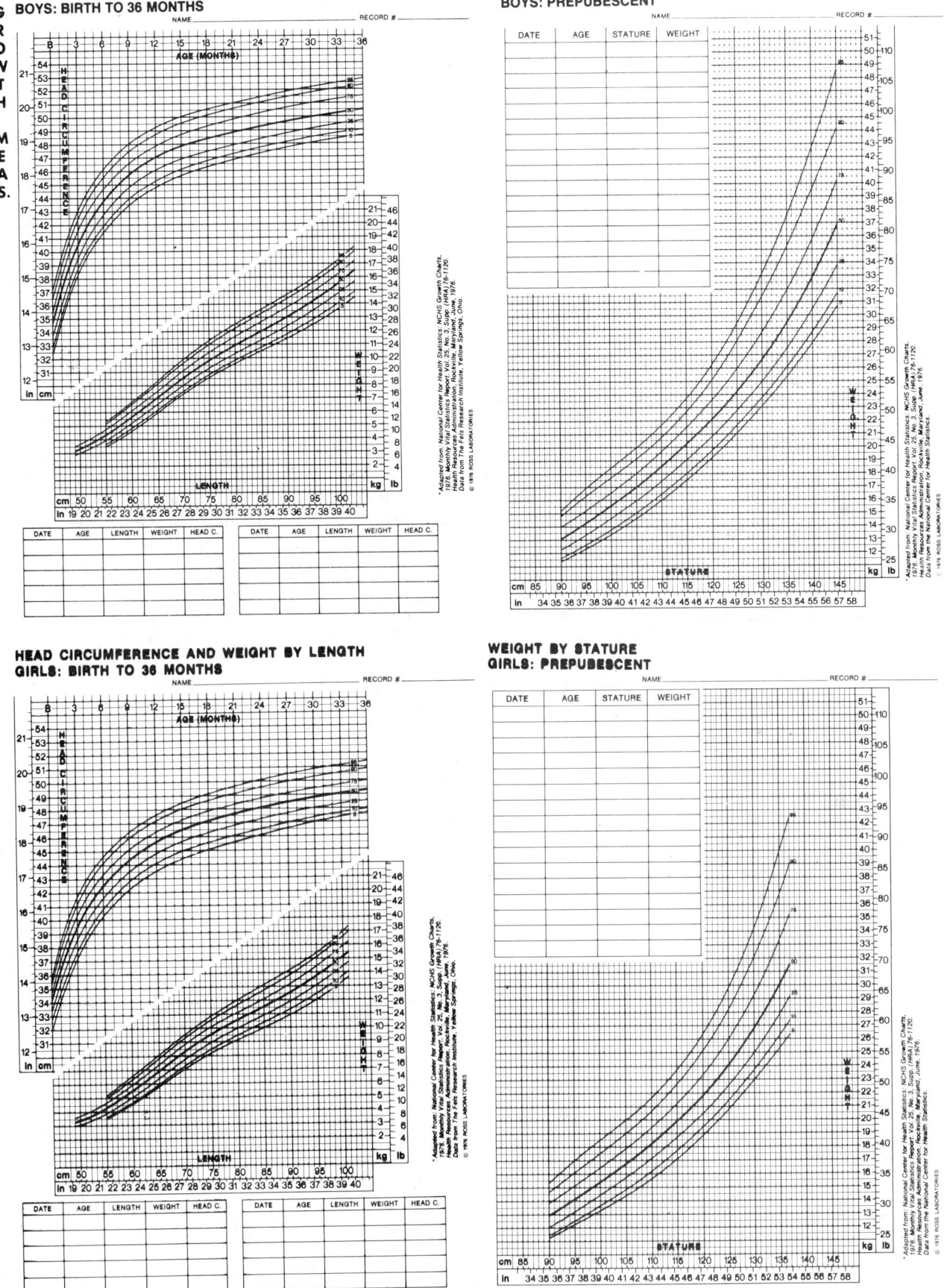

Figure 2–6. Charts for BOYS (Fig. 2–6*A*, above), and for GIRLS (Fig. 2–6*B*, below) of *weight by length [or stature],* for infants and young children (left) and for older [prepubertal] children (right). *Head circumference by age* is given for infants and young children (upper left). These charts are based upon the data in Tables 2–3 and 2–4, and have been adapted from NCHS Growth Charts by Ross Laboratories. Permission to use them is gratefully acknowledged.

observations, the most important of which are the mean or average value and the *standard deviation of the mean.*

In a theoretically perfect distribution of random values the average value will be the one most commonly found (i.e., the mode or norm) within the population under study. If, on the other hand, a distribution includes a disproportionately larger number of high values than low, or vice versa, the average value may not be the most representative (modal) for the population being investigated. Asymmetric curves are generated, which are said to be *skewed* or to show *kurtosis.* Under these circumstances the *median* or central value (see below) may be more representative of the population.

When a bimodal curve is found, it may generally be inferred that not one but two populations are being measured, which have some feature differentiating them from each other. When two different samples or populations differ with respect to average values for some biologic trait, it is often difficult to evaluate this difference unless the distribution or dispersion of values in each sample is known. When the standard deviations of the two samples are known, the likelihood can be calculated that an observed difference between them could have occurred by chance alone, or is likely to be a significant differential factor.

The standard deviation (SD) measures the degree of dispersion of observed values as they deviate from the mean value. The values lying between the points 1 SD below and 1 SD above the mean value will include about 68% of all values in a theoretic (gaussian) distribution about this mean. The range, *mean plus or minus 2 SD*, will include about 95% of values distributed about this mean, and the range, *mean plus or minus 3 SD*, will include about 99.7% of such values.

The above measures of dispersion are commonly used to locate an individual member of a population with respect to the average member. The growth charts in common use for following the course of physical development of children make this location easy by showing developmental lines at a number of different positions corresponding to deviations from average values, either about or below the mean. These deviations are often expressed not in terms of SD, but as *percentile* location in the distribution pattern.

When quantitative data are arranged in order of ascending or descending magnitude, a value, the *median*, can be found, on either side of which lie half of the observations. In the distribution described by the symmetrical normal curve, the median, the mean, and the mode fall at the same point. Values may also be designated which divide the data into two groups at the first *quartile* point, below which will lie one quarter of the values, at the second quartile point (the median), and at the third quartile point, below which lie three quarters of the observed values. The *percentile* points in a distribution of ordered data have similar meaning, one tenth of observations falling below the 10th percentile, three tenths below the 30th percentile, nine tenths below the 90th percentile, and so on.

Appraisal of growth and development has its greatest usefulness only when the data obtained are accurate, and

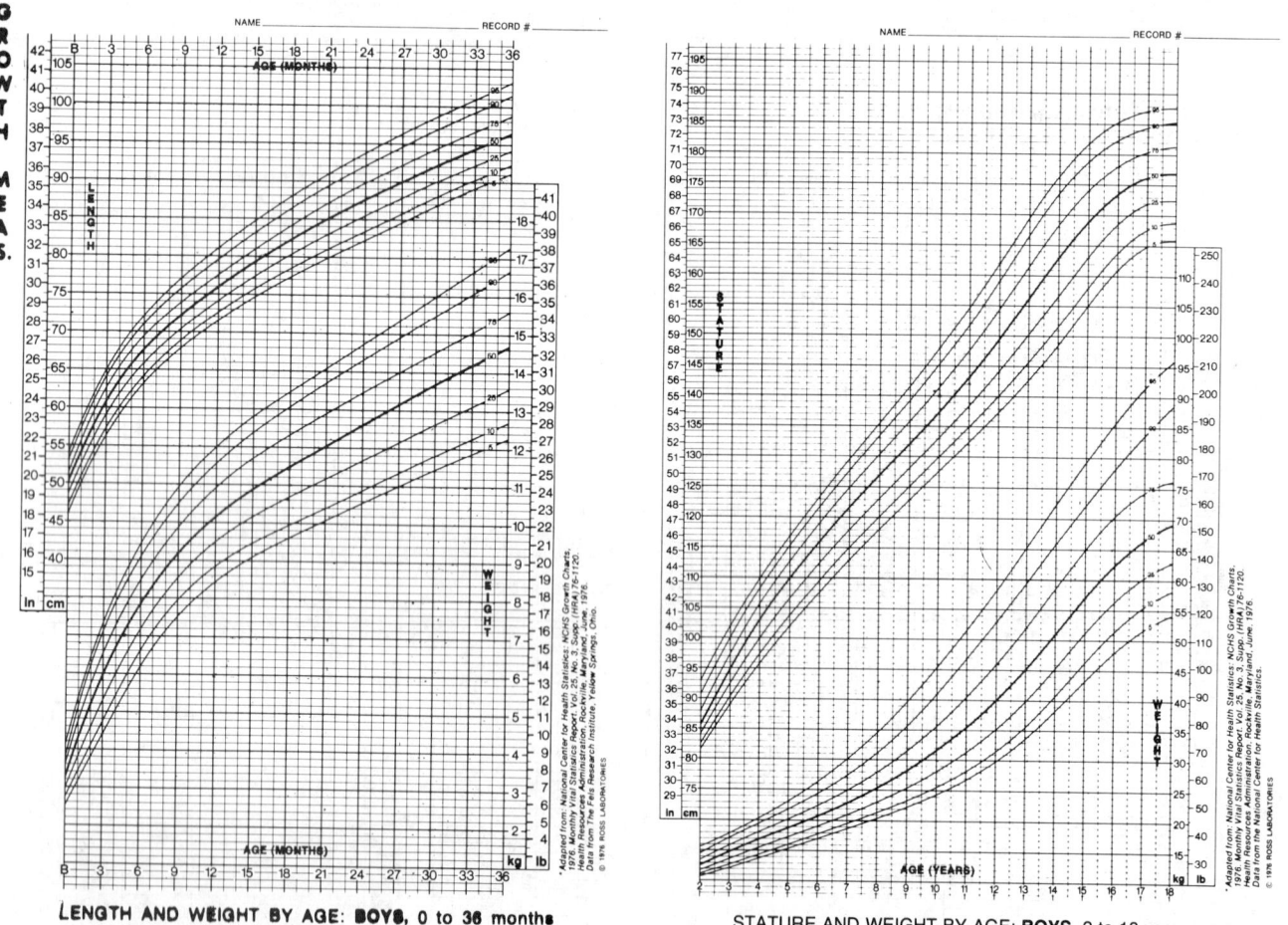

LENGTH AND WEIGHT BY AGE: BOYS, 0 to 36 months

STATURE AND WEIGHT BY AGE: BOYS, 2 to 18 years

Figure 2–7. *A* (above) and *B* (opposite), Charts for BOYS and GIRLS of *length [or stature] by age* (upper curves) and *weight by age* (lower curves), each curve corresponding to the indicated percentile level. These charts are based upon the data in Tables 2–3 and 2–5 and have been adapted from NCHS Growth Charts by Ross Laboratories. Permission to use them is gratefully acknowledged.

usually when the data are obtained through serial measurements over periods of months or years.

ASSESSMENT OF PHYSICAL GROWTH AND DEVELOPMENT

In the infant the most useful routine physical measurements are head circumference, length, and weight (Figs. 2–6 and 2–7 and Tables 2–2 to 2–5). These are supplemented by observation of the nutritional state, dentition, and size or patency of the fontanels. In older children measurements of stature and weight may be supplemented by measurements of lengths of body segments (extremities, span, and sitting height). Interpretation of the growth status of adolescents requires, in addition to height and weight, assessments of sex maturity rating, height velocity, and body fat content. Measurements of skinfold thickness and arm or leg circumference may be useful in the estimation of muscle mass or of body fat content.

Charts depicting patterns of normal growth, with indications of its variability, were developed more than 50 yr ago. Among them were the Harvard and Iowa charts, data for which were derived from Caucasian children predominantly of middle class origin, and the Wetzel grid, which drew from a wide assortment of sources. Such charts may not now reflect the characteristics of growth patterns of contemporary ethnic, genetic, or socioeconomic groups. Inasmuch as there is evidence that ethnic differences depend in largest measure upon differences in prevalence of malnutrition and infectious disease in various parts of the world, there can be no universal standard.

The National Center for Health Statistics (NCHS) has conducted a large survey of characteristics of the growth of children in the United States, from which the data were developed that are shown in Tables 2–2 to 2–5 and in Figures 2–6 and 2–7. The children studied represented a cross-section of ethnic and economic groups; accordingly, some genetic, ethnic, and socioeconomic differences are embedded in the data. The data and the derived charts are best regarded, therefore, as *reference standards* rather than as descriptive of any particular group of children. As such standards, they have some justification: (1) they are reasonably up to date; (2) they reflect the status of generally well-nourished children whose health has been about as good as is likely to be achieved in an industrially developed country; and (3) they appear to indicate conditions close to asymptotic for the secular trend of increasing growth in height that has been evident for several centuries. In these respects their usefulness as reference standards may be relatively long-standing.

Tables 2–3 and 2–5A and B and Fig. 2–7 present data regarding the relationship of distributions of length (or stature) and weight to age. Table 2–4A and B and Fig. 2–6, on the other hand, present data with respect to the distributions of relationships between weight and length (or stature) irrespective of age. In conjunction with data relating height to age, the latter data may be particularly informative. For example, children with low heights for age who have acceptable weight for height may have experienced nutritional or growth failure in the past, whereas if both height for age and weight for height are strikingly low, then both past and current nutritional or growth failure may be suspected. By contrast, children with normal height for age who have

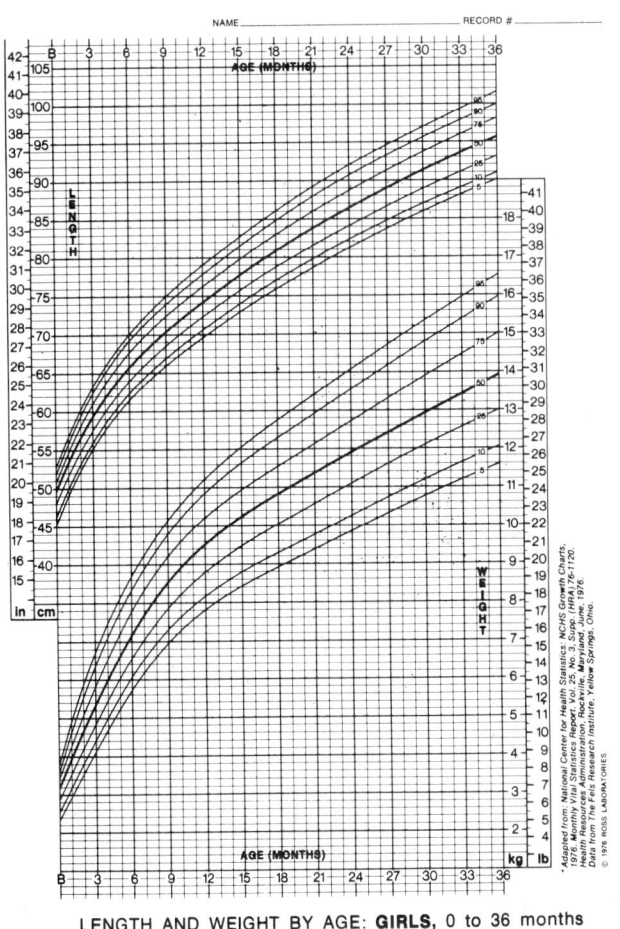

LENGTH AND WEIGHT BY AGE: **GIRLS**, 0 to 36 months

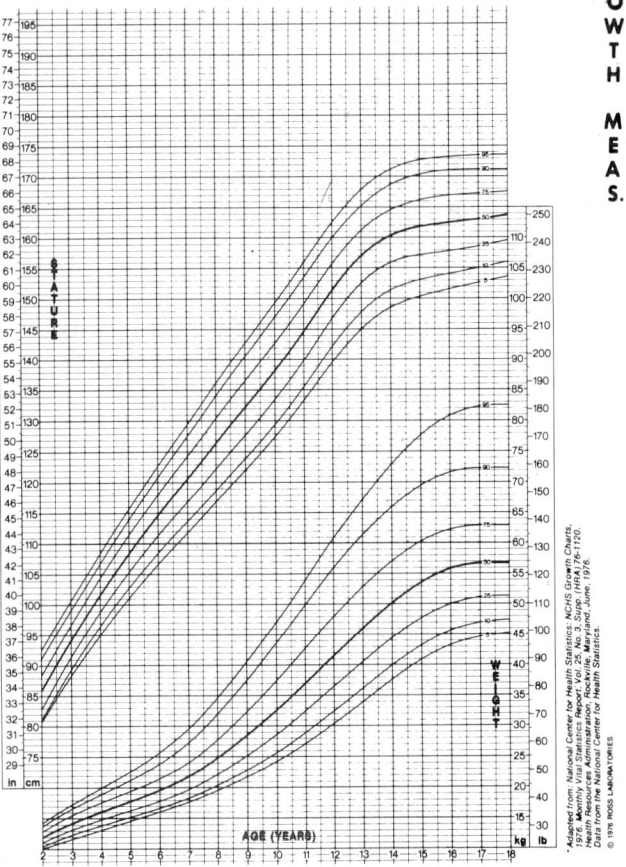

STATURE AND WEIGHT BY AGE: **GIRLS**, 2 to 18 years

Figure 2–7B. See legend on opposite page.

conspicuously low weight for height are likely to have either relatively acute nutritional or growth problems or variant physiques. Children whose weights are at less than the 5th or over the 95th percentile for their actual heights should be evaluated. A physical assessment, in conjunction with a review of history of illness, of dietary habits, of family patterns of growth, and of the psychosocial circumstances of the family, will suggest whether more extensive studies are indicated.

Measurements of weight, height, and head circumference at any given time will indicate the status of a child with respect to other children of the same age, but only sequential measurements will indicate the quality of the process through which each child is achieving his or her growth potential. A child below the 10th percentile in weight for age may be suspected of being undernourished, but 10% of normal children are found to be below this level. If such children manifest regular sequential growth in height and weight along a percentile curve above the 3rd or 5th percentile, they may often be manifesting normal physical growth. On the other hand, other children whose height and weight are at higher percentiles for their ages may be found to be significantly below their own ideal levels when sequential measurements are evaluated; alternatively, some children with obesity or illness may be found to have height or weight above that expected for age.

The growth curves of each healthy child at his or her appropriate percentile point in the normal distribution are sufficiently smooth so that any substantial perturbations of the growth line are likely to reflect physical illness, nutritional disturbances, or psychosocial difficulties. The early recognition of such disturbances may depend heavily upon the care with which regular and accurate measurements are made.

It will be useful in assessing children's height to take into account family patterns. Tanner and coworkers have developed for children between the ages of 2 and 9 yr standards for height appropriately adjusted for parental height. Wingert and coworkers also have indicated how an appraisal of the preadolescent child's height can take parental height into account.

Inasmuch as the NCHS data relating height and weight to age represent averages of the population at each age, the data obscure differences that distinguish early- from late-maturing adolescents. For these two groups the curves that relate *growth velocity* to age will be markedly different, and it is unlikely that any adolescent will follow precisely the standard curve. Reliable estimates of growth velocity require accurate measurements at relatively frequent intervals (3–6 mo).

Variability in Body Proportions

Besides the usual changes in body proportions from fetal to adult life (Fig. 2–1), there are individual differences that express innate growth potential and environmental influences. These variations in body forms of normal persons may be expressed by differences in *physique*. *Somatotype* connotes loosely the potentialities at the time of birth for the development of a particular physique: ectomorphic, mesomorphic, or endomorphic. The ectomorph is characterized by relative linearity, light bone structure, and small mass in respect to

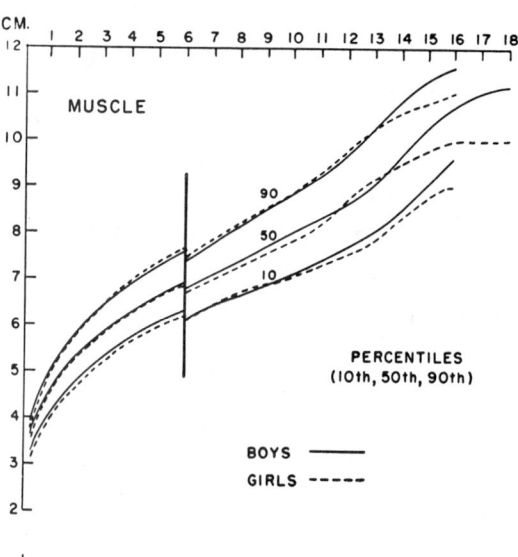

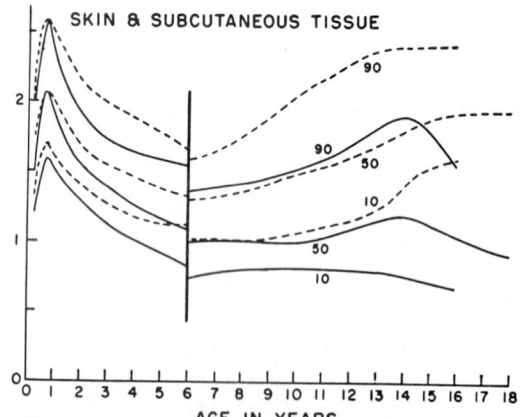

Figure 2–9. Breadths of muscle and of double layers of skin and subcutaneous tissue at greatest width of calf by age and sex from 3 mo to 18 yr of age. The graphs reveal the close similarity in pattern of the curves for muscle to those of general growth, but a unique pattern of increase and decrease and a sex difference in the skin and subcutaneous tissue. (For details, see Stuart and Sobel: J Pediatr 28:637, 1946, and Lombard: Child Dev, Vol 21, 1950. For distribution of subcutaneous fat in childhood and adolescence, see Reynolds: Monographs Soc Res Child Dev, Vol 15, 1950.)

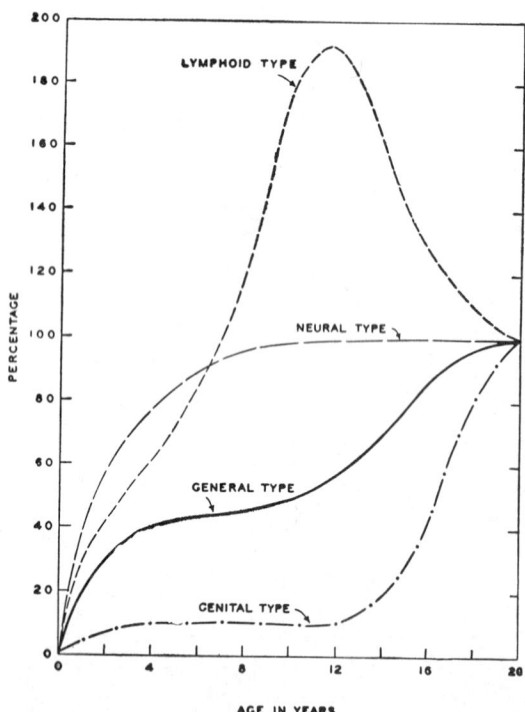

Figure 2–8. Main types of postnatal growth of the various parts and organs of the body. (After Scammon: The measurement of the body in childhood. *In* Harris et al.: The Measurement of Man. Minneapolis, University of Minnesota Press, 1930.)

body length. The endomorph is characterized by relatively stocky build, with large amounts of soft tissue. The physique of the mesomorph is in between, often relatively muscular. Some functional attributes, including some psychologic ones, may be loosely related to somatotype.

Somatotype may be evident in early childhood or become clear only with the termination of the growth period. Somatotype does not seem closely related to the ultimate height or weight achieved, but the endomorph appears to mature earlier than the ectomorph. As a result of this early maturation the endomorphic child may have a tendency to be taller than the ectomorphic one in late childhood, with the differences being reduced as the ectomorph completes growth.

Other variations in body proportions depend on the different rates of growth of body parts. The size of the brain and cranial cavity approaches adult levels much more rapidly than the size of the face or the length of the legs. This relative preponderance of growth at the cranial end of the body (with corresponding early elaboration of function) has been termed the cephalocaudad progression.

Alterations in proportionate sizes of trunk, extremities, and head are characteristic of certain growth disturbances and may give insight into the underlying pathophysiologic processes. Helpful measurements include sitting and standing heights, span, body weight, and head circumference. Normally, sitting height represents about 70% of length in the newborn infant, 57% at 3 yr, and about 52% at the time of menarche (Tanner Stage 3) in girls and at about Tanner Stage 4 in boys. There is then a slight increase of 1–2 percentage points, as the trunk has some growth after the limbs have ceased growing.

Figure 2–8 illustrates the proportionate rates of growth for several body systems, and shows distinctive variations in patterns, which are often closely correlated with function. Standards for weights of organs at various ages show certain organ-specific patterns; these may be designated as lymphoid, neural, general, and genital. There may be variations within patterns: whereas ovary and testis follow the designated genital pattern, the uterus and adrenals are relatively large at birth, and show involution in the early weeks of life. The

Table 2–8. Time of Appearance in Roentgenograms of Centers of Ossification in Infancy and Childhood

Boys—Age at Appearance Mean ± Std. Deviation*	Bones and Epiphyseal Centers	Girls—Age at Appearance Mean ± Std. Deviation*
3 wk	*Humerus*, head	3 wk
	Carpal bones	
2 mo ± 2 mo	Capitate	2 mo ± 2 mo
3 mo ± 2 mo	Hamate	2 mo ± 2 mo
(30 mo ± 16 mo)	(Triangular)†	(21 mo ± 14 mo)
(42 mo ± 19 mo)	(Lunate)†	(34 mo ± 13 mo)
(67 mo ± 19 mo)	(Trapezium)†	(47 mo ± 14 mo)
(69 mo ± 15 mo)	(Trapezoid)†	(49 mo ± 12 mo)
(66 mo ± 15 mo)	(Scaphoid)†	(51 mo ± 12 mo)
(no standards available)	(Pisiform)†	(no standards available)
	Metacarpal bones	
18 mo ± 5 mo	II	12 mo ± 3 mo
20 mo ± 5 mo	III	13 mo ± 3 mo
23 mo ± 6 mo	IV	15 mo ± 4 mo
26 mo ± 7 mo	V	16 mo ± 5 mo
32 mo ± 9 mo	I	18 mo ± 5 mo
	Fingers (epiphyses)	
16 mo ± 4 mo	Proximal phalanx, 3rd finger	10 mo ± 3 mo
16 mo ± 4 mo	Proximal phalanx, 2nd finger	11 mo ± 3 mo
17 mo ± 5 mo	Proximal phalanx, 4th finger	11 mo ± 3 mo
19 mo ± 7 mo	Distal phalanx, 1st finger	12 mo ± 4 mo
21 mo ± 5 mo	Proximal phalanx, 5th finger	14 mo ± 4 mo
24 mo ± 6 mo	Middle phalanx, 3rd finger	15 mo ± 5 mo
24 mo ± 6 mo	Middle phalanx, 4th finger	15 mo ± 5 mo
26 mo ± 6 mo	Middle phalanx, 2nd finger	16 mo ± 5 mo
28 mo ± 6 mo	Distal phalanx, 3rd finger	18 mo ± 4 mo
28 mo ± 6 mo	Distal phalanx, 4th finger	18 mo ± 5 mo
32 mo ± 7 mo	Proximal phalanx, 1st finger	20 mo ± 5 mo
37 mo ± 9 mo	Distal phalanx, 5th finger	23 mo ± 6 mo
37 mo ± 8 mo	Distal phalanx, 2nd finger	23 mo ± 6 mo
39 mo ± 10 mo	Middle phalanx, 5th finger	22 mo ± 7 mo
152 mo ± 18 mo	Sesamoid (adductor pollicis)	121 mo ± 13 mo
	Hip and knee	
Usually present at birth	Femur, distal	Usually present at birth
Usually present at birth	Tibia, proximal	Usually present at birth
4 mo ± 2 mo	Femur, head	4 mo ± 2 mo
46 mo ± 11 mo	Patella	29 mo ± 7 mo
	Foot and ankle‡	

*To nearest month.

†Except for the capitate and hamate bones, the variability of carpal centers is too great to make them very useful clinically.

‡Standards for the foot are available, but normal variation is wide, including some familial variants, so that this area is of little clinical use.

The norms in Tables 2–8 and 2–9 present a composite of published data from the Fels Research Institute, Yellow Springs, Ohio (Pyle SI, Sontag L. Am J Roentgenol Vol 49, 1943), and unpublished data from the Brush Foundation, Case Western Reserve University, Cleveland, Ohio, and the Harvard School of Public Health, Boston, Massachusetts. Compiled by Lieb, Buehl, and Pyle.

Table 2–9. **Modal Age at Onset and Completion of Fusion in Skeletal Areas in Adolescence**

Boys—Modal Age Between	Area	Girls—Modal Age Between
	Elbow	
13.0–13.5 yr	Onset in humerus	11.0–11.5 yr
15.0–15.5	Complete in ulna	12.5–13.0
	Foot and ankle	
14.0–14.5	Onset in great toe	12.5–13.0
15.5–16	Complete in tibia, fibula	14.0–14.5
	Hand and wrist	
15.0–15.5	Onset in distal phalanges	13.0–13.5
17.5–18.0	Complete in radius	16.0–16.5
	Knee	
15.0–15.5	Onset in tibial tuberosity	13.5–14.0
17.5–18.0	Complete in fibula	16.0–16.5
	Hip and pelvis	
15.5–16.0	Onset in greater trochanter	14.0–14.5
after 18.0	Complete in symphysis	17.5–18.0
	Shoulder and clavicle	
15.5–16.0	Onset in greater tubercle of humerus	14.0–14.5
after 18.0	Complete in clavicle	17.5–18.0

See footnote to Table 2–8.

absolute amount of lymphoid tissue in the school-age child may exceed that in the normal adult; involution is evident at puberty. The weight of the thymus is labile in childhood, decreasing rapidly during illness. It tends to follow the general pattern of growth during the first 5 yr of life, with involution at adolescence. The spleen appears to follow the lymphoid pattern, and the liver the general one. Skeletal muscle follows the general pattern, but is slow to achieve its ultimate mass. Cardiac muscle is initially proportionately large to body size; after the neonatal period it follows the general growth curve.

The proportionate mass of subcutaneous tissue is greatest at about 9 mo; it decreases steadily to about 6 yr, when the increase begins that presages the "fat spurt" of preadolescence, at which time sex differences become apparent (Fig. 2–9). The usefulness of skinfold thickness (SFT) as a measure

of fat content diminishes somewhat during adolescence. The ratio of total body water to body weight may be a more accurate measurement of body fat, correlating at about 0.62 with SFT. In office practice, however, measurements of triceps and subscapular SFT will generally suffice, and can be referred to standards such as those prepared by Tanner and coworkers.

Evaluation of Osseous Maturation

Ossification of the fetal skeleton begins at about the 5th mo and makes increasing demands upon the maternal supply of bone-forming substances. Ossification appears first in the clavicles and membranous bones of the skull, and follows rapidly in long bones and spine. The distal femoral and proximal tibial epiphyses are usually ossified in the normal

Table 2–10. **Chronology of Human Dentition**
Primary or Deciduous Teeth

	Calcification		Eruption		Shedding	
	Begins at	Complete at	Maxillary	Mandibular	Maxillary	Mandibular
Central incisors	5th fetal mo	18–24 mo	6–8 mo	5–7 mo	7–8 yr	6–7 yr
Lateral incisors	5th fetal mo	18–24 mo	8–11 mo	7–10 mo	8–9 yr	7–8 yr
Cuspids (canines)	6th fetal mo	30–36 mo	16–20 mo	16–20 mo	11–12 yr	9–11 yr
First molars	5th fetal mo	24–30 mo	10–16 mo	10–16 mo	10–11 yr	10–12 yr
Second molars	6th fetal mo	36 mo	20–30 mo	20–30 mo	10–12 yr	11–13 yr

Secondary or Permanent Teeth

	Calcification		Eruption	
	Begins at	Complete at	Maxillary	Mandibular
Central incisors	3–4 mo	9–10 yr	7–8 yr	6–7 yr
Lateral incisors	Max., 10–12 mo Mand., 3–4 mo	10–11 yr	8–9 yr	7–8 yr
Cuspids (canines)	4–5 mo	12–15 yr	11–12 yr	9–11 yr
First premolars (bicuspids)	18–21 mo	12–13 yr	10–11 yr	10–12 yr
Second premolars (bicuspids)	24–30 mo	12–14 yr	10–12 yr	11–13 yr
First molars	Birth	9–10 yr	6–7 yr	6–7 yr
Second molars	30–36 mo	14–16 yr	12–13 yr	12–13 yr
Third molars	Max., 7–9 yr Mand., 8–10 yr	18–25 yr	17–22 yr	17–22 yr

Adapted from chart prepared by PK Losch, Harvard School of Dental Medicine, who provided the data for this chart.

fullterm infant. The fusion of the humeral capitellum with the shaft is said to mark the end of the period of most rapid growth in girls and to predict menarche within a year.

A general index of growth status is given by the bone age, as determined from roentgenograms. Bone age is based on (1) the number and size of epiphyseal centers, (2) the size, shape, density, and sharpness of outline of the ends of bones, and (3) the distance separating the epiphyseal center from the zone of provisional calcification or the degree of fusion between these two elements. Examination of hand and wrist is useful at all ages; useful information can also be derived from the leg, especially in early infancy.

Tables 2–8 and 2–9 show expected times of appearance and fusion of various ossification centers, with their normal variation. Since girls are more advanced than boys in skeletal development at all ages, separate standards are necessary. Variability is less for girls than for boys, especially in later childhood. In boys the standard deviation of bone age in relation to chronologic age is about 2 mo in the 1st yr of life, and increases to 4 mo during the 2nd yr, to 6 mo during the 3rd yr, and to 10 mo by the 7th yr. Thereafter, for the rest of the growth period, the standard deviation is about 12–15 mo. Larger standard deviations during adolescence reflect the different rates of pubertal maturation; bone age corresponds more closely to sex maturity rating than to chronologic age.

Evaluation of Dental Development

See also Chapter 12.

Calcification of teeth begins in about the 7th month of fetal life; it involves deciduous teeth until shortly before term, when calcification begins in those permanent teeth that will be the first to erupt.

Table 2–10 lists the times of eruption of the deciduous and permanent teeth. Delay in eruption of deciduous teeth occurs in hypothyroidism and in other nutritional and growth disturbances, but the normal variability in dental eruption prevents such delay from being useful as an indicator of a disorder of growth. In some families the children have conspicuously early or late dentition without other signs of retardation or acceleration of growth.

The first permanent teeth to erupt are the 6 yr molars; they may be mistaken for deciduous teeth. It is important to know that the first permanent molars stabilize the dental arch and have a great deal to do with the ultimate shape of the jaw and the orderly arrangement of teeth. Caries or other defects in them should receive prompt attention; their extraction should be avoided.

Nutritional disorders or prolonged illness, or use of certain drugs (such as tetracyclines) in infancy or childhood may interfere with calcification of deciduous and permanent teeth. Such disturbances, if temporary, may leave defects in the enamel ranging from a line of small pits across the tooth to a broader band of hypoplasia. It is possible at times to date a nutritional disturbance by these pits or bands.

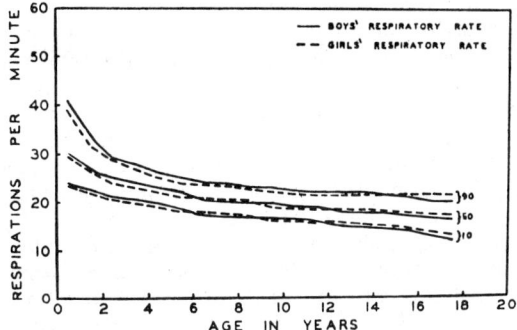

Figure 2–10. Respiratory rates in infants and children.

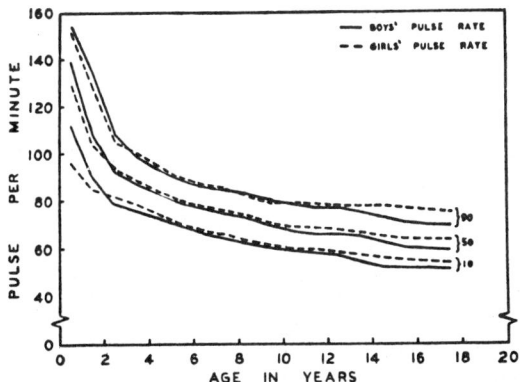

Figure 2–11. Pulse rates in infants and children.

The formation of healthy tooth structure is fostered by a diet adequate in protein, calcium, phosphate, and vitamins, especially C and D, and depends further upon an adequate supply of thyroid hormone. Resistance to dental caries is increased when the diet contains optimal amounts of fluoride.

Special Features of Growth in the Respiratory Tract

The status of the sinuses in the newborn infant is described in Sec. 2.3. The sphenoidal sinuses appear by about the age of 3 yr, and the frontal sinuses between 3 and 7 yr of age. Figure 2–10 shows the changes in respiratory rate with age, with 10th and 90th percentile lines, and shows how the rates differ for boys and girls, with the distinctive changes at adolescence. (See also Sec. 13.1–13.4.)

Special Features of Growth in the Cardiovascular System

The heart is relatively large at birth, and there is a pubertal growth spurt in heart size that parallels the general growth spurt. As a result, there may need to be different standards for radiologic interpretation of cardiac diameter in adolescents. Figure 2–11 shows how the pulse rate varies with age, and Figures 14–1 and 14–2 show the changes in blood pressure with age. It is seen that the mean systolic pressure for boys continues to advance with age after that of girls has begun to reach an asymptote. The levels of serum urate increase and those of high density lipoprotein (HDL) cholesterol decrease with advancing age in male adolescents. (See Sec. 7.39–7.47.)

Special Aspects of Metabolism and Nutrition

Caloric needs increase with growth in size but bear a relatively constant relationship to body surface area, which appears to be as closely correlated with the body's mass of metabolically active tissue as any other simple measurement. Measurements of body surface that correspond to given heights and weights are available; estimates can be obtained

Table 2–11. **Approximation of Surface Area (m²) to Weight (kg)**

Weight Range	Approximate Surface Area
1 to 5 kg	m² = (0.05 × kg) + 0.05
6 to 10 kg	m² = (0.04 × kg) + 0.10
11 to 20 kg	m² = (0.03 × kg) + 0.20
21 to 40 kg	m² = (0.02 × kg) + 0.40

(The figures 5, 10, 20, and 40 are given in italics to indicate a simple mnemonic. The formula m² = (0.02 × kg) + 40 is reasonably accurate from 21 to 70 kg.)

from nomograms (see Chapter 29). Cruder estimates from weight alone can be made for children whose physique is normal; Lowe's formula is:

$$\text{Surface area (m}^2\text{)} = \sqrt[3]{Wt^2 \text{ (kg)}} \times 0.1$$

Other crude estimates for children of average physique are given by the simple formulas in Table 2–11.

In reference to body surface, basal caloric needs appear to be somewhat lower in premature infants than in fullterm ones. These caloric needs increase during the 1st yr of life from about 30 kcal/m²/hr to about 50 by the 2nd yr, with a subsequent fall to adult levels of 35–40 kcal/m²/hr. The rate of decline is slowed or may be reversed during prepubertal or adolescent years by the need for additional energy to support the increase in growth rate that occurs at this time. This increased need for calories is matched by increased need for other nutritional factors, including iron for both sexes (for muscular development in males and to replace menstrual blood loss in postmenarchal females).

Needs for water and electrolytes remain roughly constant in their proportion to body surface through most of the growing period; the inevitable variations in intake are met by the capacity of homeostatic mechanisms to adjust to varying conditions of supply and demand.

Adolescent growth is particularly susceptible to impairment by dietary fads or by behaviors that deprive the youngster of essential calories or other nutritional substances. Drugs also may impair adolescent growth; among these are certain of the stimulants given for attention deficit disorder or learning disabilities (methylphenidate or dextroamphetamines).

A variety of metabolic changes in adolescence are reflected in changes in normal values for levels of components of serum. The activity of alkaline phosphatase increases during the period of increase in height velocity. Changes in levels of somatomedins, hematocrit, HDL cholesterol, serum iron, and other measurements correlate more closely with sex maturity rating than with chronologic age. An increase in creatinine level is correlated with increasing muscle mass in males.

Developmental Aspects of Drug Metabolism

Changes in metabolic activity with age may significantly alter the response to drugs, and require adjustments of dosage. This is particularly evident with respect to administration of drugs to newborn infants (Sec. 5.51). Some variability in rates of metabolism reflects the rapidity with which the infant or child acquires a normal capacity to metabolize drugs for which the metabolic pathways are incomplete or incompletely activated at birth. Normal activities of glucuronidase, phenylalanine transaminase, and other enzymes may be achieved only after days, weeks, or months, sometimes with clinical consequences.

During puberty, changes in body composition, such as increased adipose tissue in females and decreased total body water in both sexes, will affect patterns of drug distribution. Competition for enzymes that metabolize drugs may result from increased levels of sex steroids as well. In male adolescents high levels of androgens increase the binding capacity of the cytochrome P_{450} system. Hein and coworkers have shown that the rate of elimination of theophylline is more closely related to sex maturity than to age. A similar relationship can be expected for other drugs.

Genetic variability also may determine the rate of metabolism or the pharmacologic effect of some substances. Acetylation, methylation, demethylation, sulfation, and other processes may be involved. For example, the rapidity of acetylation and excretion of such drugs as isoniazid, hydralazine, and some sulfonamides is genetically set by autosomal recessive genes. Persons who are fast acetylators may need larger doses of drugs and respond poorly to them, whereas slow acetyla-

tors are at higher risk of toxic effects associated with elevated levels.

Other developmental aspects of pharmacology that are not well understood include the paradoxic reactions of some children to some drugs; excitement as a response to phenobarbital and abatement of hyperkinesis with amphetamine are examples. Moreover, children appear to have increased sensitivity or reactivity to the effects of some drugs under other conditions; children with deficiencies of glucose-6–phosphate dehydrogenase (G-6-PD) have, for example, generally more severe reactions from ingestion of the offending drugs than do susceptible adults.

Techniques of Physical Measurements

Accuracy of measurement is essential to the reliable interpretation of growth data; slight variations in technique may result in significantly large errors in the placement of children according to percentile rank.

Height. *Recumbent length* can be more accurately measured than standing height in children under the age of 5 yr, after which measurement of standing height is generally more convenient. Recumbent length is measured as the child lies on a firm table that has a measuring stick at least 125 cm or 50 inches long fastened along one edge. The soles of the feet are held firmly against a fixed upright placed at the zero mark. A movable upright crosses the table above the head and is brought firmly against the vertex. If recumbent length is used after 5 yr of age, the value obtained may be reduced by 1 cm from that for standing height.

Standing height is measured as the child stands erect, with heels, buttocks, upper part of the back, and occiput against a vertical upright; the heels should be close together, and the arms should hang naturally at the sides. (The external auditory meatus and the lower border of the orbit should be in a plane parallel with the floor.) A wooden headpiece having two faces at right angles may be placed firmly on the head against a 2-meter or 6-foot measuring scale attached to the vertical surface against which the child is positioned.

During adolescence serial measurements of height should be plotted on a *height velocity* chart, in order that the acceleration of growth that should occur at this time may be documented. Moreover, the interpretation of findings should take into account the sex maturity rating of the patient in order to determine whether the velocity curve is consistent with that expected for the developmental stage. Standards have been prepared by Tanner and coworkers.

Body Composition. Measurement of skinfold thickness (SFT) provides a rough estimate of body composition. Triceps SFT is measured over the posterior surface of the triceps of the left arm by calipers placed at a point halfway between the acromion and the olecranon as the arm hangs vertically in a relaxed fashion at the patient's side. Subscapular SFT is measured below the angle of the left scapula. Values obtained may be converted to estimates of body fat using standard conversion tables. SFT and arm circumference together give crude information regarding muscle mass.

Sex Maturity Rating (SMR). Inspection of the patient is generally adequate to establish his or her SMR, which is based on examination of the breasts and pubic hair in girls, and on examination of the testes, penis, and pubic hair in boys. Tables 2–6 and 2–7 give the criteria for determining SMR. Staging of testicular size is aided by use of an orchiometer.

Head Circumference. This measurement is particularly valuable in infants; it need not be taken routinely after 3 yr of age. The tape is applied firmly over the glabella and supraorbital ridges anteriorly and that part of the occiput that gives the maximal circumference. Difficulties will sometimes arise when the head has an unusual or abnormal shape, as in hydrocephalus. Under these circumstances serial measurements of the changing size of the head may best be made by positioning the tape over whatever points on the forehead and occiput give *maximal* circumference. If cloth tapes are used, they may stretch with aging and should be checked frequently against wooden or steel standards.

Chest Circumference. Measurement is made in midrespiration at the level of the xiphoid cartilage or substernal notch. Measurement is made with the child recumbent up to age 5 yr, and standing thereafter.

Abdominal Circumference. This measurement is taken to 3 yr only and will be of value principally in recognizing and following the course of chronic intestinal disturbances. Meas-

urement is made in the plane of the umbilicus when the infant is recumbent.

2.11 NEURODEVELOPMENTAL ASSESSMENT

See also Sec. 2.36, 21.2, and 21.3.

An informal assessment of the neurodevelopmental status of infants and children should be a routine part of each clinical encounter. Only with such an assessment can the physician be adequately sensitive to deviations indicating slight impairment or retardation, and be able to inform parents, respond

Table 2–12. **Emerging Patterns of Behavior During the First Year of Life***

	Neonatal Period (First 4 Weeks)
Prone:	Lies in flexed attitude; turns head from side to side; head sags on ventral suspension
Supine:	Generally flexed and a little stiff
Visual:	May fixate face or light in line of vision; "doll's-eye" movement of eyes on turning of the body
Reflex:	Moro response active; stepping and placing reflexes; grasp reflex active
Social:	Visual preference for human face

	At 4 Weeks
Prone:	Legs more extended; holds chin up; turns head; head lifted momentarily to plane of body on ventral suspension
Supine:	Tonic neck posture predominates; supple and relaxed; head lags on pull to sitting position
Visual:	Watches person; follows moving object
Social:	Body movements in cadence with voice of other in social contact; beginning to smile

	At 8 Weeks
Prone:	Raises head slightly farther; head sustained in plane of body on ventral suspension
Supine:	Tonic neck posture predominates; head lags on pull to sitting position
Visual:	Follows moving object 180 degrees
Social:	Smiles on social contact; listens to voice and coos

	At 12 Weeks
Prone:	Lifts head and chest, arms extended; head above plane of body on ventral suspension
Supine:	Tonic neck posture predominates; reaches toward and misses objects; waves at toy
Sitting:	Head lag partially compensated on pull to sitting position; early head control with bobbing motion; back rounded
Reflex:	Typical Moro response has not persisted; makes defense movements or selective withdrawal reactions
Social:	Sustained social contact; listens to music; says "aah, ngah"

	At 16 Weeks
Prone:	Lifts head and chest, head in approximately vertical axis; legs extended
Supine:	Symmetrical posture predominates, hands in midline; reaches and grasps objects and brings them to mouth
Sitting:	No head lag on pull to sitting position; head steady, held forward; enjoys sitting with full truncal support
Standing:	When held erect, pushes with feet
Adaptive:	Sees pellet, but makes no move to it
Social:	Laughs out loud; may show displeasure if social contact is broken; excited at sight of food

	At 28 Weeks
Prone:	Rolls over; may pivot
Supine:	Lifts head; rolls over; squirming movements
Sitting:	Sits briefly, with support of pelvis; leans forward on hands; back rounded
Standing:	May support most of weight; bounces actively
Adaptive:	Reaches out for and grasps large object; *transfers* objects from hand to hand; grasp uses radial palm; rakes at pellet
Language:	Polysyllabic vowel sounds formed
Social:	Prefers mother; babbles; enjoys mirror; responds to changes in emotional content of social contact

	At 40 Weeks
Sitting:	Sits up alone and indefinitely without support, back straight
Standing:	Pulls to standing position
Motor:	Creeps or crawls
Adaptive:	Grasps objects with *thumb and forefinger*; pokes at things with forefinger; picks up pellet with assisted pincer movement; uncovers hidden toy; attempts to retrieve dropped object; releases object grasped by other person
Language:	Repetitive consonant sounds (mama, dada)
Social:	Responds to sound of name; plays peek-a-boo or pat-a-cake; waves bye-bye

	At 52 Weeks (1 Year)
Motor:	Walks with one hand held; "cruises" or walks holding on to furniture
Adaptive:	Picks up pellet with unassisted pincer movement of forefinger and thumb; releases object to other person on request or gesture
Language:	A few words besides mama, dada
Social:	Plays simple ball game; makes postural adjustment to dressing

*Data are derived from those of Gesell, Shirley, Provence, Wolf, Bailey, and others.

Table 2–13. **Emerging Patterns of Behavior from 1 to 5 Years of Age***

	15 Months
Motor:	Walks alone; crawls up stairs
Adaptive:	Makes tower of 2 cubes; makes a line with crayon; inserts pellet in bottle
Language:	Jargon; follows simple commands; may name a familiar object (ball)
Social:	Indicates some desires or needs by pointing; hugs parents

	18 Months
Motor:	Runs stiffly; sits on small chair; walks up stairs with one hand held; explores drawers and waste baskets
Adaptive:	Piles 3 cubes; imitates scribbling; imitates vertical stroke; dumps pellet from bottle
Language:	10 words (average); names pictures; identifies one or more parts of body
Social:	Feeds self; seeks help when in trouble; may complain when wet or soiled; kisses parent with pucker

	24 Months
Motor:	Runs well; walks up and down stairs, one step at a time; opens doors; climbs on furniture
Adaptive:	Tower of 6 cubes; circular scribbling; imitates horizontal stroke; folds paper once imitatively
Language:	Puts 3 words together (subject, verb, object)
Social:	Handles spoon well; often tells immediate experiences; helps to undress; listens to stories with pictures

	30 Months
Motor:	Jumps
Adaptive:	Tower of 8 cubes; makes vertical and horizontal strokes, but generally will not join them to make a cross; imitates circular stroke, forming closed figure
Language:	Refers to self by pronoun "I"; knows full name
Social:	Helps put things away; pretends in play

	36 Months
Motor:	Goes up stairs alternating feet; rides tricycle; stands momentarily on one foot
Adaptive:	Tower of 9 cubes; imitates construction of "bridge" of 3 cubes; copies a circle; imitates a cross
Language:	Knows age and sex; counts 3 objects correctly; repeats 3 numbers or a sentence of 6 syllables
Social:	Plays simple games (in "parallel" with other children); helps in dressing (unbuttons clothing and puts on shoes); washes hands

	48 Months
Motor:	Hops on one foot; throws ball overhand; uses scissors to cut out pictures; climbs well
Adaptive:	Copies bridge from model; imitates construction of "gate" of 5 cubes; copies cross and square; draws a man with 2 to 4 parts besides head; names longer of 2 lines
Language:	Counts 4 pennies accurately; tells a story
Social:	Plays with several children with beginning of social interaction and role-playing; goes to toilet alone

	60 Months
Motor:	Skips
Adaptive:	Draws triangle from copy; names heavier of 2 weights
Language:	Names 4 colors; repeats sentence of 10 syllables; counts 10 pennies correctly
Social:	Dresses and undresses; asks questions about meaning of words; domestic role-playing

*Data are derived from those of Gesell, Shirley, Provence, Wolf, Bailey, and others. After 5 years the Stanford-Binet, Wechsler-Bellevue and other scales offer the most precise estimates of developmental level. In order to have their greatest value, they should be administered only by an experienced and qualified person.

to their questions, or make appropriate recommendations for further study.

Tables 2–12 and 2–13 list expected behaviors of infants and children at various ages. In evaluating these behaviors the examiner will often use materials (such as readily available toys or other materials) that have not been standardized but that will often reveal whether a standardized screening test or a formal psychologic evaluation is indicated.

The casual examination should be interpreted with caution, particularly when an infant or child who is irritable, hungry, or ill does not perform at his or her expected level. For such patients a future examination should be scheduled. For the infant born prematurely, the observed developmental level should be adjusted in relation to chronologic age during the first 2 yr of life.

Procedure. Examination of young infants may begin with observation in the prone and supine positions, note being made of spontaneous behavior, and then of the manner in which the infant adjusts to being pulled from a supine to a sitting position and to being held in ventral suspension (Landau response). The reaction to moving persons or objects within the visual field or line of sight or within reach can be observed, both for relatively large objects, such as a rattle or

stethoscope, and for small objects such as a raisin or pellet. Behavior when standing with support should also be observed.

After 6 mo of age the infant may be given blocks (1 inch cubes), and after 12 mo blocks and crayon and paper, observation being made of the ability to imitate or copy patterns of construction with blocks or the drawings of simple figures, as demonstrated by the examiner. After 2½ yr the child can be asked to draw a person, to draw geometric figures, and to count pennies or raisins.

Standardized Screening Tests. A number of relatively simple tests permit the physician or his or her assistant to make helpful assessments of the developmental or cognitive levels of older children as a part of normal office practice. Some of these are in the form of questionnaires for parents, and others are administered directly, with use of standardized materials. Such tests include the Quick Test, the Raven Matrices, the Thorpe Developmental Inventory, the Denver Developmental Screening Test (DDST), and the Revised Developmental Screening Inventory (based on Gesell, by Knobloch). In using these or other tools for evaluation of performance the tester should become thoroughly familiar with the procedures, the rules for their administration, and their limitations.

2.12 PSYCHOSOCIAL ASSESSMENT

The assessment of psychosocial problems and their management are discussed in Sec. 2.13 et seq.

VICTOR C. VAUGHAN, III
IRIS F. LITT

Bayer LM, Bayley N: Growth Diagnosis. Chicago, University of Chicago Press, 1959.

Dine, MS, Gartside PS, Glueck CJ, et al: Relationship of head circumference to length in the first 400 days of life: A mnemonic. Pediatrics 67:506, 1981.

Frankenburg WK, Goldstein AD, Camp BW: The Revised Denver Developmental Screening Test: Its accuracy as a screening instrument. J Pediatr 79:988, 1971.

Frankenburg WK, Thornton SM, Cohrs ME: Pediatric Developmental Diagnosis. New York, Thieme-Stratton Inc., 1981.

Greulich WW, Pyle SI: Radiographic Atlas of Skeletal Development of the Hand and Wrist. Stanford, CA, Stanford University Press, 1950; 2nd ed, 1959.

Iliff A, Lee VA: Pulse rate, respiratory rate, and body temperature of children between two months and eighteen years of age. Child Develop 23:237, 1952.

Knobloch H, Pasamanick B (eds): Gesell and Amatruda's Developmental Diagnosis. 3rd ed. Hagerstown, MD, Harper & Row, 1974.

Knobloch H, Stevens F, Malone AF: Manual of Developmental Diagnosis. Hagerstown, MD, Harper & Row, 1980.

Pyle SI, Reed RB, Stuart HC: Patterns of skeletal development in the hand. Pediatrics 24:886, 1959.

Reynolds EL, Asakawa T: Skeletal development in infancy: Standards for clinical use. Am J Roentgenol Radium Ther 65:403, 1951.

Tanner, JM, Goldstein H, Whitehouse RH: Standards for children's height at 2–9 years allowing for height of parents. Arch Dis Child 45:755, 1970.

Todd TW: Atlas of Skeletal Maturation (Hand). St. Louis, CV Mosby, 1937.

Vogt EC, Vickers VS: Osseous growth and development. Radiology 31:441, 1938.

Weech AA: Signposts on highway of growth. Am J Dis Child 88:452, 1954.

Wingert J, Solomon IL, Schoen EJ: Parent-specific height standards for preadolescent children of three racial groups, with method for rapid determination. Pediatrics 52:555, 1973.

PSYCHOSOCIAL DIMENSIONS OF PEDIATRICS

2.13 INTRODUCTION

The term *psychosocial* recognizes that the activities, functions, and behaviors of a child include two dimensions: *psychic* or *internal*, which consists of feelings, attitudes, thoughts, fantasies, memory, judgment, values, and self-image; and *social, external,* or *interactional,* encompassing relationships with the environment, people, and circumstances within which the child lives. The psychosocial orientation in no way neglects the biologic or organic aspects of development. Biologic (physiologic or pathologic) facts significant to psychosocial development or disturbances will be identified.

The psychosocial viewpoint considers the child's emotional and social development and its deviations and disturbances in terms of *interaction* between fetus, infant, or child and the environment. For example, to state that an infant's cry indicates hunger is to infer a physiologic or biologic state. The inference seems justified when the cry subsides after feeding. But the process of feeding has had, besides its nutritional significance, emotional and social aspects for both infant and mother. Holding, cuddling, crooning to, or talking to the infant expresses emotional and social states of the mother, and the infant perceives and feels ("ingests") and responds to these aspects of the feeding relationship as surely as to the food itself.

Maturation involves those intrinsic processes that are genetically or otherwise organically programmed; but even maturational features of development depend for their healthy achievement upon environmental factors.

Development refers to the progressive differentiation, refinement, and specialization of the organism and its constituent parts. Development is interactional and depends upon both general and specific internal and environmental conditions. The major intrapsychic dimensions of psychosocial development include the *cognitive* and the *affective*. Cognitive processes underlie perceptual reasoning, judgment, and memory—generally, the intellectual features of intrapsychic function. Affective states include anxiety, depression, fear, anger, sadness, joy, elation, jealousy, calmness, and placidity (the dimensions of feeling or emotion).

Most activities of the child integrate both affective and cognitive processes. The risk for most clinicians is that attention to affective distress may be neglected until it is blatant. The affective component in a child's temper tantrum is unmistakable; but a child's poor performance in school may be too easily construed as primarily a cognitive or perceptual difficulty, with little attention given to strong feelings of guilt, discouragement, fear of failure, and displaced anger.

The formation of *conscience* and its exercise are psychic processes with important cognitive and affective features.

Anxiety and the desire for approval are early affective precursors. Identifying and remembering approved and disapproved actions, and choosing among behavioral alternatives are cognitive aspects of the formation and function of conscience.

BASIC PRINCIPLES

1. All human experiences have psychosocial as well as biologic or organic contexts.

2. The biologic equipment with which the child is born is modifiable. Its function can be facilitated or impaired, sometimes irreversibly, in both the physical and the psychosocial domains.

3. All behavior has meaning. This meaning can be known to both the actor and the observer; or this meaning may be obscure to both. Meanings may frequently be given one label by a child, and other labels by parents, peers, teachers, physicians, or others.

4. Everyone has theories that explain his or her own behavior and the behaviors of others. The clinician will choose among various theories in attempting to comprehend the development and the behavior of children. Conceptual models such as those described below may give meaning to aspects of children's behavior by providing useful frameworks of assumptions, hypotheses, and empirical data.

FREQUENTLY OVERLOOKED ISSUES

1. Both acute and chronic illnesses frequently produce in children lassitude and affective dullness bordering on depression. Even common viral illnesses often leave residual depression and irritability for days or weeks after other signs and symptoms have disappeared. Emotional, social, and academic behavior may be slow to return to pre-illness levels of function. Patience is required of parents and teachers, and parents may need reassurance from the clinician.

2. Events such as a household move, illness of a family member, a substitute classroom teacher, separation from a friend, or death of a pet always have some and may have major psychosocial impact on the child. Even when the child's overt reaction is minimal, it is important to explore the meaning of these events. How a child handles separation and loss, whether temporary or permanent, provides important information about his or her psychosocial style and adaptability.

The child who has little or no reaction to a major event is not displaying optimal adaptability. Relationships should be important to children, and they should learn to invest emotions freely in them, and be able to show their feelings when significant relationships are interrupted or terminated. Children unable to make emotional investments or who have to protect themselves from open reactions to losses may have significant developmental disturbances.

3. The specific ways in which affection is given and received among family members are important determinants of the manner and comfort with which children will express positive regard for others. To label a parent "cold" or "aloof" is less useful than finding out whether and under what conditions he or she can or cannot express physical, verbal, or emotional affection. Such data will help both in assessment and in planning appropriate intervention in support of family relationships.

2.14 SOME CONCEPTUAL MODELS OF CHILD DEVELOPMENT

No single psychosocial theory accounts adequately for all aspects of the development or behavior of children, whether normal or disturbed. On the other hand, the clinician needs to be familiar with the general outlines of the major theories, as a set of perspectives within which to understand children and with respect to which he or she can make clear and explicit his or her own theoretic stance. Common sense is not an adequate basis for intervention into either organic or psychosocial aspects of health or disease; unfortunately, many physicians well informed of the physiologic and pathologic aspects of physical illness have only primitive knowledge of the data and theories of psychosocial health and illness.

Children and the societies in which they live present complex interrelationships. *Systems theory* attempts to improve understanding of these relationships by describing hierarchies of interrelated systems. Any conceptual model usually deals with only one or a few of the many systems within which the child lives. The following conceptual models for the development of children are listed from "inside out."

The first model is generally (but narrowly) called the *medical* or *physiologic* model. Consider this analogy: the liver has at different ages differing metabolic capacities, and the child can be understood, for certain purposes, in terms of liver function and age; and in illness or in health this physiologic system has very direct communication with the intrapsychic system through nervous and hormonal subsystems. The psychosocial impact upon the child of asthma, heart disease, central nervous system disorders, and a host of other conditions can sometimes be best understood or dealt with in such a physiologic perspective.

Sigmund Freud and Erikson, among others, have contributed to the development of the *psychoanalytic* or *psychosocial* models of development, in which the child is seen as motivated by basic sexual and aggressive drives and as passing through successive and critical stages of development, influenced at first primarily by parents and then by an enlarging group of social experiences. For instance, the oral stage (psychoanalytic) of the first half of the first year of life is seen as a stage during which basic trust (psychosocial) is learned, so long as both the child's physical apparatus and the environment are intact and supportive. Anna Freud added a longitudinal concept to the same model in describing *developmental lines*. For instance, the only child of articulate parents might seem quite advanced in the language line over his or her peers, owing to the preponderance of time spent with adults. On the other hand, the emotional line might be found lagging with respect to tolerance for independence, creating a disparate psychosocial assessment along these two lines.

A more circumscribed conceptual model is the *cognitive*, to which Piaget has contributed through his studies of the step-by-step acquisition of knowledge. His observations help in understanding how a 5 yr old and a 15 yr old differ in their capacities to know or to think about concepts such as sex, the future, or death.

The *behavioral* model of child development is less concerned with what goes on in the mind or body than with predictable patterns in the child's overt response to external stimuli at different age levels. This model is based on learning theories, and emphasizes that most of the behavior of children is learned. Appropriate behavior may be positively reinforced by pleasant, rewarding experiences. Similarly, inappropriate behavior may be diminished or eliminated not by reinforcing it, but by ignoring it. Use of this model helps physicians to counsel parents how to *teach* children (for example, to go to bed without undue delay). The model helps parents to see how their own behavior determines the responses of their children. Some parents do not know that unwanted behaviors are just as learned as wanted ones. The child who finds that screaming is the only stimulus that gets a response from mother will use that behavior when the need for mother overrides the consideration that her attention may be aversive. The behavioral model can help plan strategies aimed at changing such specific behaviors as enuresis, avoidance due to phobias, and others.

The physician should be familiar with the *family system* as a conceptual model. The child develops within a complex set of interpersonal systems that include relationships with parents or parent-surrogates and other members of the family or household, as well as their relationships with each other. The child models his or her behavior on that of the parents, at first by unconsciously imitating, and then by identifying with, their styles, attitudes, behavior, and values. The standards of parents and others have a heavy impact upon the child's life. It is the parent who monitors the child's health and brings him or her to the physician; and a hyperkinetic child whose parents are opposed to drug therapy will not get the benefits of that treatment, no matter how important the physician may feel it to be. The parents and the family and their relationships and expectations *acculturate* the child. Their rules and ways of functioning are the basic standards that the child ultimately makes his or her own. Children often incorporate into their own repertoires of feeling and behavior the manners in which their parents become ill or respond to illness. An anxious parent, for example, can magnify a child's minor pain into a frightening experience for both.

The *social* or *cultural* model recognizes that children at any age are part of a larger community or society. The broader the scope of the notion of society or culture, however, the less certain we can be about what this means to a given child. At one level, a variety of socioeconomic and sociocultural considerations increase the chances of prematurity, lead poisoning, rat bites, malnutrition, child abuse, and sudden infant death; at another level, the child-rearing practices of any community have profound effects upon how children view themselves and their future.

One of the most influential social systems outside the family is the school, which is perhaps the most age-structured system the child will experience. School provides the setting and framework within which the child is measured and in turn measures himself or herself academically, emotionally, socially, and physically. Though parents may have adapted to a child's immature speech, he or she will face on entering school a need to re-evaluate and change modes of speech. A pediatrician who points out this potential problem early may be able to initiate changes that prevent a major confrontation when school begins. Such early intervention is more successful than that which is deferred to the time of imperative need.

The physician, too, is part of the child's social system, playing a part ascribed by the family and its subculture. Physicians may play this part comfortably or uncomfortably, depending upon their level of familiarity and comfort with that culture and upon their capacity for adjustment.

THE ROLE OF PARENTS IN CHILD DEVELOPMENT

2.15 FAMILY PLANNING

Unfortunately, the first encounters of pediatricians with the families of their patients generally occur after the birth of the first child. The timing of the birth of the first child has heavy influence upon parental relationships and sets the pattern for the spacing and number of future children. The pediatrician has an important role in examining with parents the questions and issues in family planning. Central to family planning is the notion of *choice*. The National Association for Social Work has made the following statement: "Potential parents should be free to decide for themselves without duress, and according to their personal beliefs and convictions, whether they want to become parents, how many children they are willing and able to nurture, and the opportune time for them to have children." Pediatricians should encourage parents to discuss family planning, but must approach sensitive areas of personal beliefs and values with caution and concern. Variations in the birth rate, the tendency of some prospective parents to wish to influence or control the sex of their unborn child, and the diagnostic role of amniocentesis in cases of genetic risk all reflect a growing personal and technologic sophistication in family planning.

Perhaps the most common question on family planning asked of pediatricians is: what is the optimal interval between the births of siblings? This is a matter ultimately for parents to decide. They may be guided, however, by the consideration that an interval of approximately 2.5 yr allows time for maternal replenishment from the first pregnancy, time for comfortable reciprocal attachment between parents and the first child, time for the older child to master locomotion, toilet training, and other self-care that will free the mother for care of the new infant, and opportunity for a reasonably close-in-age relationship between the siblings.

2.16 PARENTAL ATTITUDES AND EXPECTATIONS

All adults bring to parenthood certain attitudes toward the roles of mother and father and certain expectations of and attitudes about children. These ideas are strongly influenced by childhood experiences and by the notions, models, and beliefs that each culture holds about children. Our society has a variety of views about children, and these views are frequently incongruent. For example, the young infant is seen as both innocent and uncivilized, or as a tabula rasa and as largely genetically predetermined. These attitudes about childhood have deep historic, philosophic, religious, and, more recently, scientific roots. And when mother and father hold conflicting attitudes about children and child-rearing, areas of compromise must be found so that they may develop an effective partnership as parents.

At the first encounter with each family the physician should elicit the parents' attitudes toward children and toward their own child by inquiring into *expectations*. Among the most common and abrasive sources of distress within and between human beings are the gaps between expectations and achievement, or between incompatible expectations. Even with regard to the infant in utero parents have attitudes and expectations. The content and quality depend on many factors, including the adequacy of the marriage, the couple's feelings about each other, the economic circumstances of the family, and the unmet emotional needs of the parents as individuals. The unborn child may be viewed as a "mistake" or as a "savior," or may represent an unconscious or deliberate attempt to hold a shaky marriage together or a compensatory

substitute for an ungratifying partner. In more normal circumstances, parents tend to view children as extensions of themselves, and to see in children their genetic legacy and certain aspects of their own personalities. Such a perspective can become pathologic if children are expected to fulfill the unrealized dreams and ambitions of their parents, rather than to lead their own lives. The child who is planned as a replacement for one who has recently died is at particular risk, and may be treated as fragile, with overindulgence, and as though vulnerable to the same fate that befell the previous child. The first child to be born after one or more miscarriages may be viewed similarly. Anticipatory exploration of feelings by the physician, with guidance and counseling, can be of considerable benefit in these instances.

Parents of children who are chronically ill, emotionally disturbed, mentally retarded, or severely handicapped are at risk of development of unhealthy and destructive attitudes toward their children, society, or themselves. Such children may provide little gratification and represent serious disappointment. The pediatrician must help such parents recognize and express their feelings and must guard against conveying unprofessional negative or condemning attitudes toward them. Physicians need to be sure of their own systems of beliefs and values with regard to parental roles, child rearing, and children; but they must be careful lest they impose their own idiosyncratic values on the children and families they seek to help (Sec. 2.72).

2.17 TEMPERAMENT IN PARENT-CHILD RELATIONSHIPS

The notion of *temperament* embraces the individual's particular pattern of physiologic organization, probably genetically determined, through which a uniquely personal way of thinking, feeling, and acting is predictably and more or less continually effected. Temperament is the core of the personality; personality may in turn be shaped by the environment, which can mellow or muffle temperament but never eradicate it. For example, the reaction times of newborn infants to certain stimuli and the adaptabilities of infants to change appear to be among the first signs of temperament, and may predict the activity level of older children or adults. For the most part the temperaments of parents and the complex superstructures of their personalities will permit them to interact comfortably and effectively with the possibly differing temperaments of their children, but the interpersonal experiences of parents sometimes differ so much with different children that parents have a sense of awe at the degree to which their children are not alike. Policies of child management successful for one child may not at all suit another. Thomas and Chess refer to "goodness of fit" or "consonance between the individual and the environment" as predisposing to optimal development. In cases of uncomfortable interaction with a given child, parents may develop unrealistic guilt. If such guilt leads them to anxiety or withdrawal, the child may become irritable or withdraw in turn. Parents may turn to anger as a defense against frustration or guilt.

The physician is in a favorable position to evaluate the temperaments of infants and of mothers and fathers. The mother who says she has a "good" baby generally means that their temperaments are in a complementary and happy relationship. On the other hand, a hyperactive ("good") infant and a placid, slow-moving mother may not engage each other sufficiently in growth-promoting interactions. The physician can encourage or train such mothers to provide more sensory stimulation or exchanges for such children. Such mother-infant pairs may need, for example, to have the times of picking up and rocking structured for them, rather than depending for interaction on their own low levels of exchange of cues. In the opposite case, an intrusive mother with a highly reactive child may need help in damping stimuli to the child, to prevent undue irritability. For the measurement of infant temperament, Carey and McDevitt have developed a 95-item questionnaire that yields ratings in 9 categories: activity, rhythmicity, adaptability, approach, sensory threshold, intensity, mood, distractibility, and persistence. Scales and questionnaires are also available for the assessment of temperament in toddlers (Fullard, McDevitt, and Carey), 3–7 yr old children (McDevitt and Carey), and 8–12 yr old children (Hegvik, McDevitt, and Carey).

Mothers and fathers often differ in temperament, and either can sometimes provide relief to the other or to the child when one of the parent-child relationships is in trouble. A more active, expressive, or creative parent can, for example, give special attention to the child in activities contributing to adaptive learning, whereas a more placid and relaxed parent can take over child care when a period of quiet is needed to consolidate and assimilate new experiences. The physician can help both parents to coordinate their different temperaments and personalities in action for the child's benefit, in this way preventing parental blocking or *stasis*. Stasis occurs when each parent sees the other's temperament as being "bad" for the child. If the label can be changed from "bad" to "different and complementary," the parents can conceptualize their joint efforts as mutually effective and supportive rather than destructive. The same considerations apply to parent-surrogates, such as grandparents, and at times even to siblings. All family members can be encouraged to contribute something of their own to the child, so long as these contributions are orchestrated positively and comfortably by the primary caregiver, rather than being offered in a chaotic or oppositional way.

Both temperamental differences and the child's developmental stages become more or less effectively enmeshed with the temperaments and personalities of parents. A mother who has always found it exciting to deal with new challenges finds her child's adolescence a stimulating and positive experience. A nurturant, stable, hyporeactive father may, on the other hand, find that he is more effective with the preschool toddler than with the inquisitive 10 yr old.

2.18 PARENTS AS TEACHERS

The parent is the child's first and most important teacher. Most parents do not view themselves as educators of their children, but they present in direct and indirect ways an essential and far-reaching curriculum. The parents "teach" the infant how to trust, rely on, and depend on people and circumstances—the basis for the child's future view of interpersonal relationships. Parents not only teach a son or daughter how to throw a ball, but also impart notions of sportsmanship and fair play. Parents who read to their children motivate reading. Parents who explain to and inform children foster language development, serve as models of a communicative style, and provide the ingredients for mastery of problem-solving techniques. Parents who display aggressive and temperamental outbursts in response to minor frustrations model a style of behavior which may find ready imitators. In all of these educative ventures, parents not only offer content, information, and advice, but also transmit the values of their families and of their cultures. Children as "students" may be willing, unwitting, or resistant.

Parents tend to be unaware of or to undervalue their educative role, deferring to school teachers as professionals who "know more" or can "teach better." In recent years, however, the community mental health movement and programs of compensatory education have re-emphasized the importance of the teaching skills of parents, both in their natural affective roles and in the cognitive domain. With appropriate training and support, parents have learned to use their talents as teachers of language development in infant stimulation programs, as therapists in behavior modification with children who have maladaptive behavior patterns, as classroom aides, and in a variety of other endeavors with their own and other children.

For these complex educative roles as well as for the nurturant and economic roles of parenthood, most prospective parents receive little or no preparation. Most persons "learn" how to be parents primarily from their relationships with their own parents and from caretaking responsibilities they may have had for younger siblings. But sociocultural changes and urbanization have increasingly limited these experiences for many children. Furthermore, maladaptive and conflictive patterns, as well as positive ones, may be learned from parents and passed on to succeeding generations; children of child abusers, for example, tend to be child abusers. Courses on parenthood have been introduced into the curricula of some high schools, but it would be more useful if throughout the school years children had organized experiences in relating to and in helping to take care of younger children.

2.19 DEPENDENCE VERSUS AUTONOMY

Psychologically, children become independent beings during the phase of development that Mahler has called *separation* and *individuation*. It extends between 6 and 30 mo of age and does not evolve as a steady movement toward separation and individuation; rather, both psychologically and literally the child departs from and returns to the mother in a predictable pattern. The end of this process finds 3–4 yr old children in a stage of autonomy, wanting to do things themselves, but, within the parents' view of reality, still needing a great deal of support.

At adolescence the child goes through a second and more definitive emergence as a person separate from his or her parents, as he or she strives for an identity as an independent adult. The adolescent has many advantages over the 4 yr old, including the capacity for abstract reason, the physical equipment of a young adult, and a great deal more knowledge and experience; but periodic regressions again reflect the underlying tension between needs for dependence and for autonomy. The 19–22 yr old finally pulls up roots and establishes himself or herself apart. But the pendulum between dependence and autonomy never rests, even in successive stages of adult life. The more success parents have in helping children to be comfortable with both autonomy and dependence, the more successfully will the children live as adults.

Infants appear totally dependent upon their mothers or caregivers, but their strivings for new sights, sounds, movements, and other growth-promoting experiences must be unhindered, within the bounds of safety, if learning is to occur. On the other hand, when 15 yr olds learn and test independent behavior by staying out at night and taking unreasonable chances, parents may need to show concern and provide limits which help the adolescent to consolidate gains before moving out again into new experiences.

All new learning represents a striving for autonomy, but it can be successful and its effect positive only if the child feels secure. Overly dependent children may feel that their nurturant base is threatened by illness in their mothers or fathers or by parental conflicts, so that they cling to home all the harder. Parents may themselves view the world as a dangerous and untrustworthy place and foster similar feelings in their children. Physical illness increases dependency; this dependency is counterproductive if, after physiologic systems are back to normal, parents do not expect the child to resume appropriate autonomy.

Some children are forced into premature independence by loss of a parent. A 12 yr old who, because of his or her mother's death or separation, has to take over the care of a household or of a younger sibling may be able to assume this responsibility and independence without regression. But sometimes the apparently successful child will have trouble in dealing later with the dependent needs of his or her own children or of others, basically feeling cheated and resentful.

There are periods when the striving of children for more independent behavior creates crises for their parents. The physician can be an important neutral consultant or arbitrator, who can help parents to decide whether it is more realistic to yield some independence or to hold their children to certain limits. This is a particularly difficult issue for handicapped children, who require more care and restrictions. Helping such children achieve an inner sense of independence calls for creativity from both parents and physicians.

Finally, children learn about independence by observing their parents and grandparents and older siblings. A mother who becomes overly involved in her own mother's waning years provides both a model and a dependency conflict for her 12 yr old daughter, who may both want and not want to be closer to her own mother.

2.20 SOCIALIZATION, DISCIPLINE, AND PUNISHMENT

Socialization. Socialization is primarily an interactional process between the developing child and his or her parents and other significant adults. Socialization involves the knowledge, skills, and techniques that accomplish an adaptive fit between the child and the social environment. These are acquired both formally and informally, in conscious and unconscious ways, and by precept and example. Although successful socialization continues into adulthood, and is a lifelong process, the time from birth to late adolescence is generally considered the period of establishment of primary adaptive social attitudes and behaviors.

Discipline. Discipline has been defined as training in proper conduct and action. It has mental and moral aspects. As a verb, *discipline* means to educate, to train, and especially to bring under control. The term also carries notions of protection, prevention, and punishment. In the early life of the child discipline emerges from the relationship with parents, involving conformity to their expectations and obedience to their commands; it becomes generalized as the child grows older, shaping responsiveness to persons in authority generally, and contributing to notions of personal autonomy, authority, and integrity that are later codified in rules, regulations, laws, morals, and religious and ethical principles.

The child begins at about 18 mo to experience discipline when he or she is faced with growing numbers of rules, regulations, and expectations within the family. As children mature physically, cognitively, emotionally, and socially, they progressively internalize these standards and develop those internal controls of behavior that are termed self-discipline. The purpose of discipline is to provide children with incentives, reasons, values, and the instrumental means to achieve self-discipline. Discipline is too often seen only in terms of punishment, whereas at its healthiest it is a complex set of attitudes, behaviors, formal and informal instruction, rewards, and punishments that serve not to inhibit, restrict, subjugate, or repress children but to help them internalize appropriate cognitive processes, ideals, and values. With these they will be able ultimately to exercise their own judgments and choose their own behaviors in ways best adapted to their situations.

Social and cultural factors strongly influence the kinds and effectiveness of discipline. In some relatively homogeneous communities, strong and commonly held traditions of national, ethnic, philosophic, or religious values give strong support to the socializing and disciplinary actions of parents toward their children. In such communities discipline may seem easier, both in the congruence of views among adults who support each other's parental behaviors and in the common experience of the children. But when families move from their communities of origin, kinship ties are often nonexistent or attenuated over long distances. Many married couples, moreover, may have come together from competing or contradictory traditions and values, the marriage transcending differences in religion, ethnic origin, or ties of community or class.

It is important that parents be secure and explicit in their attitudes and values regarding child rearing, especially as they concern discipline. Difficulties in control or in adaptive socialization in children often stem from contradictions and conflicts between parents over the systems of expectations, rewards, and punishments that will be appropriate to the disciplining of children.

Certain principles can be stated with regard to parental approaches to discipline:

1. Parents must help children appreciate the value of learning from the results of their behaviors; parents help children to do this when they recognize and reward approved behavior and let their disapproval of unacceptable behavior be known.

2. Parents need to understand clearly the differences between hurting and retaliation, and teaching through discipline and punishment; they need to examine how to resist exerting either power or authority for its own sake, rather than as a tool for the edification and education of the child.

3. Parents need to recognize and resist the tendency to demean or to humiliate those who oppose their will.

4. Parents need to review and understand their own childhood experiences with parental discipline and to recognize attitudes or behaviors of their own that are unreasonable residua; these can include overdemanding expectations, overreliance on authoritarian and power-oriented discipline, a tendency to respond impulsively or angrily or cruelly, the use of discipline to humiliate or demean, or a tendency to be so vacillating or inappropriately oversympathetic with a child that discipline lacks firmness and consistency.

Chess and Thomas have described a group of basically normal but "difficult" children, whose temperamental characteristics include a high level of intensity, some degree of impulsivity, a low tolerance for frustration, negative mood, and a tendency to recoil from new experiences. Parents of many such children regard them as having disciplinary problems. On the other hand, the stubborn or difficult child may have qualities that the parents admire and want preserved or developed, such as that they have "a mind of their own," or are "not easily led." Such children may become rather independent and creative thinkers or leaders, but these qualities may emerge only in late adolescence or early adulthood; during childhood such children may be regarded as unpleasantly stubborn, defiant, and resistant.

Punishment. Punishment is an aspect of discipline; it includes a variety of techniques for fostering approved and discouraging disapproved behavior. Punishment is related to the general area of conscience formation, which depends upon attitudes, values, motivation, effects of adult models, and visibility of legal, social, and cultural expectations, rewards, and sanctions. Punishment, whether it be construed as physical or psychologic, may have a relatively limited role in the formation of a mature, autonomous conscience. Studies of animals and of preschool and early school-age children have identified some of the variables determining the effectiveness of punishment. Some conclusions of these studies are as follows:

Timing. Most studies agree that the shorter the delay between an act of transgression and the punishment for it, the more effective the punishment will be in preventing repetition of the prohibited behavior. The implication for parents is that punishment should be effected as soon as possible after a transgression is observed or known. Warning or admonishing the child who appears about to perform a forbidden act is frequently effective in preventing transgressions.

Intensity. Studies of animals indicate that the higher the intensity of punishment, the more effective will be the prohibition. This relationship is not so clear for children since it is unacceptable to use a high intensity of physical punishment. It has been further shown that punishment of high intensity is likely to interfere with learning when the child must make relatively complex discriminations in order to comply with expectations. Two principal recommendations emerge: first, the intensity of punishment should be high enough so that a mild to moderate amount of anxiety is generated in the younger child, but not so high that the child is frightened, panicked, or terror-stricken (by physical punishment) or made so angry (by either physical or emotional punishment) that he or she cannot learn the lesson; second, for the preschool child the rules and the discriminations surrounding expected behaviors should be simple. The more complicated the discrimination needed, the less intense should be any punishment that follows transgression.

Emotional Context of Punishment. Both clinical and experimental studies indicate that punishment is most effective when it takes place in the context of a warm, affectionate, and generally accepting relationship between parent and child. In naturalistic studies of child-rearing, relatively cold and aloof parents who used spanking as a means of physical punishment found it less effective than other parents who also used spanking frequently, but who were temperamentally warm and affectionate toward their children. Retrospective studies of delinquent boys indicate that often their fathers have been cruel, harsh, and punitive, with little love, respect, or affection. Parents should understand that being affectionate and kind toward their children and praising them is not in conflict with the need from time to time to punish them.

Another aspect of punishment, involving the relationship between child and parent, is termed the temporary withdrawal of nurturance or of love. The more children desire the approval of their parents and care about their parents' positive regard for them, the more sensitive they are to shame and to indications of their parents' diminished respect. This does not mean that for a parent to reject the child or to declare that he or she no longer loves the child is a good method of punishment. Rather, it indicates that a moderate amount of disapproval can help to promote prescribed behaviors in the context of a relationship in which the child values the parents' approval and affection. The flow of nurturance and warmth from fathers to sons is particularly important, and the development of these harmonious relationships is important in itself, as well as contributing to the increased effectiveness of paternal discipline. Parents who are particularly sensitive to threats to their own power or authority may be unduly punitive and harsh in the discipline of their children, and may be less likely to be warm and affectionate in their overall relationships with them. They may need particular help in finding comfortable ground in this area.

Association of Punishment with Cognitive Methods: Reasoning. Reasoning and physical punishment are more effective together than physical punishment alone in bringing about the incorporation of approved behaviors in children; moreover, combinations of reasoning with nonphysical forms of punishment, such as deprivation of privileges, or withdrawal of nurturance, are more effective than any one alone. On the other hand, reasoning alone is more effective than any punishment alone. And even when punishment is delayed after the transgression, its effectiveness is increased if the child is provided reasons for the punishment. Studies of effects of reasoning indicate the importance of explanation and of careful labeling of proscribed behaviors. Internalization of standards (the acquisition of self-discipline) requires a cognitively oriented training procedure. The cognitive elements include the careful *labeling* of the prohibited behaviors, a careful *description* and *reconstruction* with the child of the nature of any transgression, a parental *demonstration* of the deviant act before punishment, and an indication as to what *consequences* or *results* of the deviant action are to be avoided. The efficacy of reasoning increases, of course, as the growing child can better understand a cognitive approach.

The following recommendations may be used in guiding parents. For the child between 12 and 30 mo old techniques that are direct, clear, and immediate, and that produce a moderate amount of anxiety without unduly frightening or angering the child, seem to be the most effective in producing inhibition of transgressions. With increasing understanding of language, by 20–24 mo, clear and simple explanations of the reasons for punishment should be given, without elaboration. In older children techniques of punishment seem most effective that diminish anxiety and emphasize the verbal control of behavior through attention to general rules, appeals to reason and common sense, and other cognitively oriented techniques. For children of any age a moderate amount of disapproval or of shaming may be useful in promoting the child's self-control, so long as it is used in the context of a positive, supportive, and respectful relationship.

Consistency. Studies of delinquent children and of the child-rearing practices of parents of normal children, as well as experimental studies, indicate that parental *consistency* is an important factor in promoting approved behavior in children. Erratic disciplinary procedures, including punitiveness and laxity, are highly correlated with increased delinquency. Consistency is relative; no individual, still less two parents, can be totally consistent in child-rearing. It is important, however, that parents establish a generally consistent style in terms of what, when, how, and to what degree punishment is appropriate to each transgression. The pediatrician should encourage parents who are attempting to establish new disciplinary procedures or alter previously unsuccessful ones to be patient and persistent. Parents usually feel that a few trials at a changed pattern of discipline ought to produce immediate results in the child. This is quite unrealistic, both for themselves and for their children, since their current patterns of behavior probably took months or years to develop. Moreover, studies indicate that inconsistent discipline builds resistance to changes in response to later, more consistent behavior. The physician must instruct and encourage parents in maintaining reasonable and appropriate disciplinary procedures, even if favorable results are not immediately forthcoming.

Undesirable Consequences of Punishment. A clearly undesirable consequence of punishment is the modeling of aggressive behavior, best illustrated by the father or mother who in correcting a child for a temper tantrum becomes angry and physically cruel. The angrier the parent, the more likely he or she is to lose control and to punish too severely. Such parents can look foolish to their children and feel so themselves, which may increase the parent's anger so that the child may be held accountable in such terms as "he's trying to make a fool of me." Such parents may feel involved in struggles with their children for control.

Loss of control tends to diminish the positive effects and increase the negative effects of punishment. It arouses anxiety and anger in children, which turn them against their parents and against their parents' desires. Severe and demeaning disapproval can make the child feel small, helpless, and inadequate. Feelings of resentment, fantasies of retaliation, or a sense of worthlessness may arise. Such feelings reduce the effectiveness of punishment as a positive learning experience.

As children get older, physical punishment becomes much less effective and its negative effects increase. At any age slapping or whipping a child can be cruel and abusive and lead to the results cited above, and to alienation of the child from the family. Even moderate degrees of spanking in school-age or older children can make them feel humiliated and resentful. The intended lesson is lost. Some children may begin to use repetition of the specific transgressions for which they were punished as a means of retaliation against punitive, cruel, or humiliating parents. Others, when escape is impossible and retaliation too dangerous, react by passivity and withdrawal, and instead of becoming angry, develop passive-aggressive or passive-withdrawal personalities that may inhibit development.

Reinforcement of Approved Behavior. This method of discipline involves essentially the encouragement of positive behavior. The parent generally ignores or musters a mild reproof for undesirable behavior, while encouraging cooperation, helpfulness, and sympathetic, prosocial behavior. Encouragement by helpful and kind words has been shown to reduce aggressive behavior both in college students and in 8–12 yr old children. With this positive approach to discipline many of the unwanted side effects of punishment are avoided. This approach can often be incorporated as an element of discipline, and although it takes more time initially it may save time in the end.

Modeling. Studies by Bandura, Walters, and others of aggressive behavior in children indicate that adult models significantly influence children's learning. Bandura contends that modeling can produce learning on a single trial, in contrast to the learning with multiple trials that is posited by theories of classical and operant conditioning. Modeling is equivalent to the phrase "good example." Parents repeatedly demonstrate the power of deeds over words in their behavior toward each other, as well as in the behaviors they manifest toward their children. In displays of affection, of anger and its control, of respect, honesty, and openness of communication, parents model behavior that children identify with and *imitate*. Modeling also involves *identification*, the process by which one feels he or she is like another person. Both verbal and nonverbal aspects of behavior, such as tone of voice, facial expressions, gestures, and expressions of physical affection or aggression, are sources of imitation and identification that may be powerful influences on children.

2.21 CONSCIENCE FORMATION

Theories of conscience formation have sought to identify factors that cause children to learn approved behavior and to resist temptations to transgress against rules, first of parents and later of society. Psychoanalytic theory has postulated that the psychologic structure has three functional aspects: ego, superego, and id. The *superego* has the functions of conscience, with both conscious and unconscious aspects. The superego is primarily a negative governor (or inhibitor), incorporating the do's and don't's of parents and of society; the latter reach the child through parents, peers, teachers, and laws. The concept of *ego ideal* represents positive aspects and goals of living toward which one strives. The strong affective component of the superego is *guilt*. Guilt serves as an internal punishment for transgression, and the avoidance of the pain of guilt is the major deterrent to contemplated aggression.

The wish or desire to transgress can mobilize defense mechanisms aimed at avoidance of the awareness of guilt. Such mechanisms include repression, denial, displacement, and projection. Psychoanalytic theory suggests that a healthy, stable, and mature superego requires appropriate resolution of the oedipal complex, which occurs around the 6th or 7th yr of life. In repressing both sexual feelings for the parent of the opposite sex and hostility toward the parent of the same sex, the young child establishes a firm gender identity and internalizes the values, attitudes, beliefs, and standards of the parents, particularly the parent of the same sex.

Erikson has broadened psychoanalytic theory by giving attention to important social and cultural factors. To the concept of the oedipal complex he adds notions of the influence of social rules upon children at this critical stage. Socialization is for Erikson a matter of learning roles by observation, imitation, and rehearsal and has cognitive, affective, and behavioral components. In the young child much thought is carried out as an internal monologue, often uttered aloud but intended for the child alone. Language is also a major tool for socialization. The voices of parents and others become internalized, often concretely as voices at first, then as statements, and rather later as thoughts. Children also internalize the behaviors and attitudes that they have seen, rehearsing and adapting them through imitation and fantasy in play. Children's consciences are built from the superegos and sociocultural traditions of their parents. Erikson holds that the superego can be construed as the child becoming "parent"—a carrier of tradition. Children internalize not just what their parents teach but what they are as persons. In Erikson's view the ego has an active role in formation of conscience, and the child's superego is as individual as the ego.

Other theories of the development of conscience can be called "cognitive developmental." Piaget, Kohlberg, and Aronfreed have studied both the reactions of children to temptation in various experimental situations and how children have attempted to explain their behaviors in reaction to moral dilemmas. Kohlberg's theory has outlined stages in development of conscience; they have no timetable, but the order is invariable. Some adults never reach the final, most mature stage, owing to constitutional, temperamental, or environmental factors, or to psychologic or social disturbances of the developing conscience. Kohlberg has posited 3 major levels of conscience development, with 2 stages within each level. In general, the stages move from a primary emphasis on the self or parents as referents for moral judgments and actions to more remote referents such as law or universal principles.

Level I: Preconventional. Moral reasoning is determined by the consequences of behavior: punishment, reward, exchange of favors, or the physical power of people in authority, particularly parents.

Stage 1: Behavior is determined primarily by efforts to avoid punishment or to seek pleasure of rewards. Obedience to the power embodied in adults is more or less automatic.

Stage 2: Behavior is based upon a desire to satisfy one's own needs and at times those of others. The child's view of reciprocity is concrete: "You scratch my back and I'll scratch yours." There is some consideration of feelings of others but only as a matter of secondary convenience. Notions of loyalty and justice are not strong at this stage.

Level II: Conventional. The child's moral reasoning at this level has the dual focus of the interests of others and of the desire to maintain the respect and support of others. There is also an aspect of reasoning that involves justifying the existing social order.

Stage 3: For the first time behavior is judged not only by its outcome but by its intention, which becomes important. Many moral decisions are now based upon a desire to please others, to help them, and in turn to receive their approval and aid.

Stage 4: The notion of duty now emerges. Right behavior is seen as doing one's duty or meeting one's obligations. A desire develops to ally one's self with the existing authority, rules, and social order, particularly as they are embodied in custom and law.

Level III: Postconventional. This level is not attained until adulthood, if at all. Here the individual begins to develop a set of moral principles and to use them in solving rather complicated problems of moral and ethical behavior. These principles become more or less universal in concept, extending beyond the immediate family, the community, or even the national mores as these last may be codified in rules, laws, or customs.

Stage 5: The notion of social contract which embodies personal rights and responsibilities within a society becomes important. An emphasis on the legal aspect of morality includes the possibility of changing laws or customs so that they may be more equitable or reasonable, or may deal more effectively with moral wrongs.

Stage 6: Morality is conceived now in universal terms or principles, such as justice, equality, reciprocity, and respect for the individual. These universal concepts are seen as applying to all humankind, regardless of status, nationality, class, race, sex, and the like.

Children of 2–3 yr of age do modulate behavior to avoid pain and to seek approval and reward. Available data indicate that Kohlberg's stages 1 and 2 are typically found in elementary school children. Stages 3 and 4 emerge in adolescence and early adulthood; stage 5 occurs in some adults; stage 6 may occur in only a few.

The value of Kohlberg's work lies in its assessment of the role of reasoning in the development of moral judgments. There is clearly no precise relationship between a person's capacity for reasoning and his or her actions; moreover, the individual may reason at one moral level in some situations and at higher or lower levels in others.

2.22 COMPETENCE AND MASTERY

Learning theory sees the infant, child, adolescent, and adult as reactive primarily to external stimuli, whereas psychoanalytic and motivational theories hold that defense operations are involved in maintaining a steady or homeostatic state through reduction of drives. These theories tend to deny, neglect, or give cursory attention to the possibility that the infant may have inherent mechanisms for developing competence in manipulating or mastering the environment. Notions of competence and mastery, emphasizing the proactive rather than the reactive aspect of the infant and child, first gained wide attention through the work of R. W. White, who gave the name *effectance* to such intrinsic motivation and pointed out that traditional theories neglected the importance of the feedback that the child obtains as a result of his or her actions.

Piaget emphasized that infants and children play active roles in building "schemata," which are cognitive behavioral structures. The process involves "assimilation" of new experiences and "accommodation" of the prestimulus states to the features of the new experience that are not familiar. For example, during the sensorimotor period (birth to about 15–18 mo) the infant constructs schemata from such activities as touching, crawling, reaching, grasping, and bringing closer for detailed examination by looking, tasting, smelling, and so on. Grasping a rattle establishes an additional sensory reality for the external object and conveys the ability to affect it by moving it, turning it for a new look, or putting it in the mouth. In such ways the infant gains power over the world of objects as growing cognitive structures help formulate the separateness of self and the external world. Piaget held that the infant or child manipulates the environment to learn about it, developing concurrently the cognitive strengths that lead to further competence and mastery.

Stimulating interactions with impersonal as well as personal elements in the environment are also important for perceptual cognitive development. The interactions with persons and with inanimate objects support each other; for example, 1 yr old infants explore a controlled environment more actively in the presence of their mothers than with strangers. Infants appear to need and thrive on informational input as if it were analogous to a nutritional requirement. In an unchanging environment, lacking in a flow of new information, the infant may become apathetic, and ultimately retarded in cognitive and social development. A balanced and sensible approach is needed, however; too many mobiles or a constant barrage of music may overstimulate, and some varieties of stimuli may be ineffective or irrelevant before 2–3 mo of age. Parents should be advised that the infant first needs adequate interpersonal stimulation, and that perceptual or sensory stimulation should be secondary and complementary. Parents should learn to judge what is interesting or pleasing for each child, how much becomes too exhausting, or what is too complex, beyond the child's capacity to exploit and enjoy.

SPECIFIC DEVELOPMENTAL ISSUES

2.23 ATTACHMENT BEHAVIOR

See Sec. 2.3 and 8.6.

The continuing support of a nurturant family is vital for children in all stages of their development; when serious social and emotional deprivation occur, especially within the first 2 yr of life, there may be psychologic and cognitive sequelae. Some deleterious effects may be reversible, but some children may experience lasting damage to social development, especially when deprivation occurs within the context of major familial conflict, psychotic illness in one or both parents, prolonged separation, or abandonment. "Failure to thrive" in infants is commonly a subacute manifestation of maternal depression and reflects the inability of the mother to give her child adequate psychologic warmth and care (Sec. 2.60). Effective treatment requires that the mother must be helped to emerge from her withdrawn or depressive state into more active involvement with her child. Chronic social deprivation has been shown to contribute to intellectual retardation and to major emotional disturbances. On the other hand, minor variants of feeding practices, mother-child contact, and mother-child interaction in the first few days or months of life do not predict later problems in social or cognitive development.

When mothers working outside the home have arranged for adequate day care for their children and see them daily, there appears to be little risk of serious harm to the children. Caldwell et al found no significant differences in maternal attachment at the age of 30 mo between children in day care and children reared at home. The former may, however, be more aggressive and less cooperative when they later enter nursery school. Some children raised in depriving circumstances or by depressed mothers may benefit from the intellectual and social stimulation that good day care offers. Essentially nothing is known about the effects of "informal" day care, in which children are entrusted to untrained caretakers while their parents work. A national commitment to day care must provide a large pool of competent and dedicated personnel.

A mother who is to be separated from her child for a prolonged period of time should find a single consistent and stable surrogate, rather than a series of caretakers. Hospitalization of children under the age of 5–6 yr should, wherever possible, involve the rooming-in of the mother, in order to minimize the child's anxiety and to prevent subsequent maladaptive emotional responses (Sec. 2.54). Normal children show separation anxiety at the age of 7–9 mo, the onset of this phenomenon reflecting an important step in the evolution of attachment behavior between mother and infant. The child becomes fretful when the mother leaves the room and fearful when persons outside the family attempt to remove him or her from the mother's arms. Parents can be reassured that such children have simply begun to recognize their separateness from and dependence upon the mother, and that after a few more months they will have a better understanding of her permanence, and separation anxiety will diminish.

Maternal care during the first 2 yr should be sufficiently reliable, predictable, and warm to give the child a sense of basic trust about the world, but should not be overindulgent. The infant's learning that he or she can survive and tolerate some frustrations, as well as inevitable or appropriate delays in the satisfaction of wishes, probably contributes positively to the quality of social development and to the strength and health of mother-child attachment.

Parents of infants handicapped by physical abnormalities may, owing to feelings of depression or shame, maintain an emotional distance from the children and create a situation of relative deprivation. Blind, deaf, and physically disabled infants and children require considerable interaction and stimulation to reach their full potential; a diminution of parental contact compounds their difficulties.

The role of the mother is vital in early infant-parent attachment. Less is known of the role of fathers, which may be quite variable; there is little doubt, however, that the participation of fathers and siblings in the care and stimulation of infants may be of paramount importance in their emotional development.

2.24 GENDER IDENTITY AND ROLE

The establishment of gender identity and appropriate gender role behavior is a complex process; it begins before the birth of the child on at least 2 levels. At the biologic level, the sex chromosomes predetermine the development of male or female gonads and sex organs. At another level, the gender of the unborn baby is involved in the wishes, hopes, anxieties, expectations, and projections of the parents, whose degrees of satisfaction in their own gender identities and roles and whose previous experiences as parents of boys or girls will establish certain expectations or wishes, both positive and negative.

The terms that refer to aspects of the development of sexual identity and role should be clearly understood. *Chromosomal sex* is the sex assignment determined by karyotype. *Somatotype* is the sex assigned at birth, in accord with the appearance of the external genitalia. Genitals and chromosomal sex are generally congruent. (Exceptions are discussed in Sec. 19.40.) *Gender identity* is the *subjectively* felt conviction that one is male or female. *Gender role* or *sex role* consists of the personal and social expectations and behaviors through which the individual gives expression to being male or female.

Biologic Factors. Neither gender identity nor gender role is determined finally by chromosomal sex. Individuals with ambiguous genitalia who have been assigned at birth to somatotypes inappropriate to their chromosomal sex have generally adopted gender identities, gender roles, and sex roles in accordance with the somatotype assigned. On the other hand, transsexuals, whose external genitalia and sex chromosomes are in accord, have a subjectively felt gender identity that is incongruent. Neither the true sex of the gonads, nor the influence of adrenal or other hormones, nor the form of the external genitalia determines finally what gender identity or role will be adopted. On the other hand, prenatal exposure to steroids of the progesterone type may influence certain stereotypic gender role behaviors; for example, masculine behavior has been found more evident in girls exposed prenatally to synthetic progestins, and study of boys and girls exposed prenatally to progestins found them to score higher than their siblings on scales of independence and self-sufficient behaviors.

Psychosocial Aspects. It is the *social* determinants of gender identity and gender role that are critical in sexual typing.

These arise from within the family and from the larger social environment. Money et al indicate that by 18 mo of age the child may have an irreversibly firm grip on his or her gender role. Others feel that the final identification of sexual self occurs between 2.5 and 3 yr. Two thirds of 3 yr olds and almost all 4 yr olds are able to identify their own gender correctly.

Among the factors determining gender identity and role behaviors are those standards, expectations, and behaviors of parents, other adults, and siblings, which have sexual implications for the child. If parents and other important persons in the environment of children label, raise, and treat them consistently as belonging to one sex, it is that gender identity they will internalize. Sexual standards, which are beliefs about the behaviors or attitudes appropriate to gender roles, serve as an internal guide to what is male and what is female. Standards arise from identification with important models of gender roles, parents especially, and out of growing expectations that certain behaviors or attitudes will be approved, and others not. By the age of 7 yr the child's notion of sex roles as dichotomous has been established. Physical attributes perceived by the child as identifying sex roles are fairly clear and direct. Young children's drawings distinguish gender on the basis of hair, clothing, jewelry, occasionally breasts, and only rarely by external genitalia.

Traditional Western cultural standards rate aggressive, assertive, and instrumental behavior as masculine, whereas dependent, socially compliant, more emotionally expressive behavior is regarded as typically feminine. These cultural stereotypes present boys as more dominant in interpersonal relationships, more interested in mechanical things, more interested and active in sports, developing greater skill in the use of large muscles, and more independent, whereas girls are typified as more expressive emotionally, more concerned and skilled in interpersonal relationships, and more nurturant, with athletic prowess limited to certain sports. These cultural stereotypes, however, are undergoing significant changes.

Preschool children choose their parents of the same sex as models for sex roles. Boys are usually required by cultural standards and expectations to make sex role preferences and a clear definition earlier, more consistently, and more stringently than girls. For example, parents will frequently be unnecessarily anxious if their 3–4 yr old boy is still interested in dolls or in "girls' activities and games," but girls seem to have more latitude in terms of "tomboy" behaviors. In traditional families, girls show a strong feminine preference in preschool years which seems to diminish as they get older, whereas the preference of boys for the male role increases steadily throughout the elementary years.

The most obvious behavioral differences between boys and girls in the preschool years lie in the greater assertiveness and aggressiveness of boys, which become manifest between 2 and 2.5 yr of age, along with their identification of their own sex. This may be the result of constitutional and temperamental differences between boys and girls that presumably exert their influence from birth or may reflect parental and cultural attitudes and expectations incorporated from the earliest weeks of life.

Gender identity, the belief about one's own sexual traits, involves a very emotionally laden set of feelings. There is never perfect correspondence between sexual standards and sexual identity, but some congruity is necessary to the emotional health and successful adaptation of the child. Seeing one's self as similar to the parent of the same sex and different in certain critical ways from the other parent is important in achieving a secure gender identity. Children with weak or vague gender-related traits may have unusual difficulty in identifying themselves as female or male. Upon entry into school, the child's basis for comparison broadens in the world of peers; this may either strengthen or threaten the depth or nature of convictions about his or her own gender.

Academic achievement is not specifically sex typed, but our culture tends to stress academic success for boys, particularly in adolescence and in pursuit of vocational success. Girls in the elementary school years generally perform better than boys academically, except in mathematics, and are more fluent verbally, although boys may actually know more words. Learning disabilities are 3–6 times more frequent in boys than in girls. By adolescence, boys have generally caught up with and at times surpassed girls in many areas of academic achievement. Differential rates of maturation and development may influence these differences; other possibilities include the fact that striving for intellectual achievements may be viewed by girls or by their adult models as aggressive or assertive behavior in conflict with traditional female sex roles. An achievement-oriented girl will likely engage in behavior that puts her into competition with boys, and she may feel that the possibility of her being loved and cherished is threatened. Such attitudes reflect a cultural prescription designed to maintain psychologic and economic domination of women by men and to make the female attractive as a marital candidate. This attitude also supports the traditional notion that the female role is to be loved and provided for, and protected in her future role fulfillment as a mother, and it assumes that her economic security will come from her husband's efforts to maintain her and her children.

The women's liberation movement has challenged the cultural stereotypes of gender roles both for adults and for children. Its supporters have questioned the child rearing techniques and sex role standards that may mold girls into passive, nonassertive, noncompetitive adults, emphasizing exclusively the nurturant or emotionally expressive sides of personality development. The movement challenges the assumption that the principal task of little girls is to prepare for the role of wife and mother and contends that cultural concerns with the security of the male ego and with protection of the dominant socioeconomic position of men both wittingly and unwittingly support traditional sex role standards and behaviors.

Pediatricians can expect some problems of child behavior and child-rearing to reflect these new attitudes toward the behaviors, games, interests, and activities heretofore assigned to one gender or the other. Moreover, the way in which parents serve as sexual role models may undergo some marked shifts. All this may proceed smoothly and agreeably in any given family or be marked with conflict and strife. For a generation or more among some middle class couples gender roles have been blurred in respect to many household activities, but the persons primarily responsible for day to day care of children have continued to be mothers or their female helpers (grandmothers, baby sitters, and so on). There is now greater pressure on the husband and father to share more directly in child rearing responsibilities, and conflict may occur over whether and how this is done. Although studies are in progress, neither the immediate nor the long-term effect of these new life styles is as yet known.

The physician who is consulted regarding appropriate gender roles or who finds children caught in the struggle between such roles can help parents to see that they are engaged in a renegotiation of their family relationships (or social contract). The physician can promote an atmosphere for this negotiation in which each party states his or her terms and expectations and can then decide which conflicting areas or issues can be compromised or traded off. Physicians must help parents to avoid generating conflicting loyalties in the children and possibly confusing them about their own gender identities. Children are very vulnerable when caught in struggles between their parents for their loyalty and affection. A typical response of such children is to develop symptoms—physical, behavioral, or emotional.

Sex Activity. Boys may develop erections from the time of birth. Girls can produce lubrication of their vaginas also from birth. During the first year, all children explore their bodies and identify various areas or zones as particularly sensitive. Boys identify the penis as sensitive to both pleasurable and painful stimuli. One third of the mothers of 1 yr old infants have reported some sort of genital manipulation. Boys were noted mostly to simply pull at their penises, girls to rub or otherwise stimulate the genital area. Between 2 and 5 yr approximately one half of boys and one third of girls are observed to be involved in some sort of genital handling. Girls engage in friction of the thighs together as well as in direct genital rubbing.

Very young children frequently touch their mothers' breasts, brothers' or fathers' penises, or buttocks of both parents, principally out of curiosity and interest. Preschool children often engage in thinly veiled sexual games such as playing "mother and father," "doctor and nurse," or other games that involve dressing and undressing. Such games allow for visual and at times manual exploration of each other's bodies, including the genitals of both sexes. Children at this age are curious about the sexual differences in their parents and will often intrude upon parents in the bathroom or when they are getting dressed.

These behaviors are to be viewed as a normal part of the curiosity that children have about themselves and the world they live in. Parents are well advised not to show shock, repugnance, anger, or shaming behavior toward children found in these various curiosity-generated and harmless pleasure-seeking activities. Parents need not engage in exposure or nudity that they are not comfortable with, albeit some boys first urinate in a standing position only after their fathers model this behavior. Children should not share a bed with parents nor sleep in the same room when this can be avoided. Such affectionate displays as kissing, hugging, and a certain amount of sensual exchange between parents are healthy for children to see and be aware of, but parents should not engage in erotic and explicit sexual behavior in the presence of their children, not even in the hope of providing an enlightened household or encouraging their acceptance of sexuality as normal and good. If a child accidentally or intentionally happens upon parents involved in sexual activities, the parents should be neither embarrassed nor ashamed, still less enraged. If the incident is handled calmly and casually, with the child requested to leave or return to his or her bedroom, it is likely that the incident will be treated quite naturally by the child. If the child asks, he or she should be provided with a simple, direct, and calm explanation of what has been seen, and the statement that this is one of the ways that parents show their love and affection for each other.

By 5–7 yr of age many children develop an increasing sense of modesty about their own dressing and undressing, toileting, and bathing behaviors, and this sense of privacy often increases toward puberty.

Prepubertal children used to be thought to exhibit little sexual activity. This "latency period" of psychoanalytic theory is now known to contain considerable sexual activity and concern. One study found masturbation in 10% of 7 yr old boys and 80% of 13 yr olds. Heterosexual interests may include a boy's identifying a specific girlfriend, sharing activities with her and exchanges of affection, and at times experiences of erotic nature. A study has found that 5% of 5 yr olds, 33% of 8 yr olds, and two thirds of 13 yr olds can acknowledge heterosexual interests or curiosities, with the last group claiming a fair amount of experience. Most 10–12 yr old girls or boys said that they had a boy- or girlfriend;

two thirds of 10 yr olds and 85% of 12 yr olds stated that they had kissed their girl- or boyfriend. Sexual interests of girls and boys move from the notion of wanting to get married in a general way to wanting to marry a particular boy or girl, to actually having a boyfriend or girlfriend, and then to some social and heterosexual activities with the friend.

2.25 PHYSICAL ACTIVITY

Mobile exploration is a vital step in acquiring knowledge and a sense of initiative, but parental supervision is necessary to minimize the risk of accidents. Stairways must be barred, poisonous substances placed out of reach, electrical outlets plugged, and the handles of gas burners out of reach or removed. Physicians should see that parents receive careful instruction on safety measures; they also must encourage parents to allow the child considerable freedom to move about in safe places.

Data indicate that restraint of the child's mobility by surgical and medical procedures involving splints or casts, oxygen or mist tents, prolonged intravenous feedings, dressings for burns, and the like may contribute to the development of subsequent emotional or personality problems or to speech or learning difficulties. When restraint of the child's locomotor function is necessary, it should be done with considerable emotional support, with rooming-in of parents and close contact with medical and other staff, and with diversions such as appropriate games, television, and so on.

Excessive motor activity in the toddler may be an early sign of the attention deficit disorder, *hyperactivity syndrome* (Sec. 2.46). Involved children may be reported to have many accidents, "to get into things," to wander away from home, "not to understand the meaning of the word *NO*," and to be "always on the go." However, except where there is evidence of constitutional hyperactivity, difficulties in managing the active toddler mostly reflect inconsistent discipline by the parents. This period can be a difficult one, the toddler "feeling his oats," exercising newly developed skills, and testing limits. Occasionally the setting is complicated by the birth of a new sibling. Effective discipline requires that parents know what they want, mean what they say, use a firm approach, and follow through in a consistent fashion (Sec. 2.20). Usually parental reproach, sometimes repeated, and removal of the child from an undesired activity will suffice. Temper tantrums are common, with peak incidence around 2.5 yr of age. Parents should generally accept these excellent attention-getting devices as understandable expressions of the child's frustration at having no power to change the rules; when tantrums prove useless, the child tends to give them up (Sec. 2.45).

2.26 TOILET TRAINING

The impact of conflicts around toilet training on the child's emotional development has been exaggerated. There is little to indicate that the experiences involved in the toilet training of most children are of major psychologic consequence. Only when toilet training becomes a battlefield between the child and overdemanding parents or is pursued overzealously or unrealistically early would one expect conflict over toilet training to have any effect on personality development.

Parents may wish to start toilet training when the child is old enough to verbalize needs for care after wetting or soiling, and when he or she can appreciate a simple reward system. The substitution of training pants for diapers is an important step in the toilet training process, though it is to be expected that accidents will occur. If resistance is significant, parents should not make toileting a battleground but merely postpone further efforts for several weeks or months. Though it may be disappointing, annoying, or irritating to parents, it is neither uncommon nor harmful for toilet training to be achieved as late as the 3rd yr. Many children, by tuning in on the parents' implicit or gently expressed wishes, appear to train themselves; some are trained by the encouragement of siblings.

2.27 SIBLING RELATIONSHIPS

The impact of a new sibling upon a young child can be felt very early. As soon as she knows she is pregnant the mother may alter her attitudes toward her other children and sometimes begin to intensify her concern with activities such as feeding, toilet training, and so on, which she wants to have under a different level of control by the time the new baby is born. The physician should explore such areas of family dynamics, and may well caution mothers against letting the deadline of the date of expected delivery provoke conflict in these areas. With the birth of a new sibling, the older child may show responses ranging from denial of the sibling's birth through regressive behavior, such as wetting or soiling, to happy acceptance of the event. The older child requires such preparation for the sibling's birth as will impart the reassurance that he or she remains loved and will have some caretaking responsibilities, even if minor, for the new sibling. Questions regarding babies, hospitals, and birth should be answered as factually and comfortably as possible.

The ordinal position of siblings has no proven effect on their development of personality. Firstborn children are not necessarily more neurotic or more gifted, and there is little evidence that they are reared essentially differently from subsequent children. Ordinal position may be used to rationalize other problems to which it bears no relationship.

Bickering and competition among siblings are normal and help to develop interpersonal skills. Rough and tumble play is probably beneficial to such growth. Severe problems in sibling relationship, however, frequently reflect marital difficulties or inadequacies in parental management. Sometimes one of several siblings may be unconsciously assigned a role by one or both parents that involves him or her in a conflict between them, and such a child may be implicitly encouraged by one parent to be an ally against the other. Similarly, a sibling may serve as a scapegoat for other family psychopathology, owing to the timing of birth, a birth defect, or his or her temperament, sex, or resemblance to or identification with a parent or grandparent. At times a child may unconsciously fall into or choose the role of scapegoat in order to maintain a balance in family psychopathology so that a more serious or threatening disintegration in family interaction is held off.

Parents frequently complain about sibling jealousies as one of the problems in raising more than one child, but older siblings are important in the education, socialization, and support of younger ones, and siblings may be the closest of friends.

2.28 NORMAL FEARS OF CHILDREN

Fears are normal and perhaps a necessary part of psychologic development. To be realistically afraid of real danger and to take steps to avoid it or to minimize its effects are necessary for adaptation and survival. Fear is the perception of an external threat, real or possible. Anxiety implies the feelings associated with fear in the absence of any immediate perception of external threat. It may be the result of fantasies reflecting internal conflicts. Though the object of fear or anxiety may be imaginary or fictitious, the sensation itself, of course, is real and has familiar physiologic components. The distinction between fear and phobia is essentially that between normal and pathologic—phobias involving certain mechanisms of defense, such as repression, projection, or displacement.

The things children are likely to fear change with age, becoming more specific to their environment and experience as they grow older. The younger child's fears are centered on basic conditions or situations such as darkness, or being left alone or abandoned, or upon cultural stereotypes of fear-inducing objects, such as animals, monsters, ghosts, and goblins. Preverbal and even school-age children do not necessarily have fears that correspond to the concerns adults may have for them or may try to inculcate. They may not, for example, be concerned about fire, traffic, or the friendly stranger who may spirit them away. As they become older, their fears become more oriented toward specific culturally appropriate threats in the environment and toward specific past experiences of their own. They may generalize isolated experiences of their own that were threatening or fear-inducing, sometimes appropriately, sometimes not.

Children's fears may readily reflect those of their parents, and these fears may be transmitted from parents to child explicitly, or more often implicitly. Among the common fears of preschool and young school-age children are those of thunder and lightning, punishment, pain, hospitals, and such people as physicians or dentists. Parents also may be feared. Even when parents are not punitive, cruel, or harsh, most children are afraid of them under some situations. The anger of a parent is particularly frightening for the child, even when the parent refrains from physical contact with the child.

Children manifest their fears in various ways, depending upon age and sophistication and upon ability to verbalize and willingness to do so. The preverbal child may cling, cry, scream, and try to escape from situations that frighten, and it may be very difficult to identify the fear-provoking stimulus. The older child may be hesitant to discuss or even name what he or she is afraid of, because of fantasy and fear that talking about it will make it come true, the words being given magical powers.

The physician can help parents to be patient with children's fears. Even intense fears are not necessarily a sign of emotional disturbance, still less of cowardice. For the preverbal and young verbal child, the parents can be encouraged to give support through hugging, holding, and physical comforting, conveying reassurance through their availability and presence that the feared object or condition has no power actually to hurt. For such young children who are anxious and excited, logical explanation is incomprehensible.

For the child of school age and older, verbal reassurance should supplement physical and emotional support, for the child can respond to it in terms both of its tone and of its realism. Simple, direct explanations often require repetition each time the feared situation or object is encountered; the child may gain strength and support even as the logical and reasonable explanation is repeated in the same way each time. After a while the child may internalize the formula and be heard saying it to himself or herself or to younger brothers and sisters when they show concern with the same object or situation. The child becomes able to distinguish the feeling of fear from the fact that the feared situation, object, or condition has no real power to do harm. Parents should be advised neither to shame nor to demean fearful children, nor to try to force them into feared situations hoping that, in surviving them without support or in crying it out, they will overcome fear. This procedure may induce terror and complicate subsequent management of fears.

The unrealistically feared situation needs eventually to be faced by the child, and parents may need advice in devising appropriate ways to help children to master specific fears. Children afraid to be separated from their parents at night may be allowed to stay outside their bedroom sleeping on the hall floor, to be moved into their own bedrooms or into the bedrooms of siblings as they become more secure. It helps if they can be given some power over the situation, such as being able to turn on or keep a light on if they are afraid of the dark, to reach their parents by telephone when they have been left for an evening, or to have contact with a nonthreatening puppy or kitten if fears center on dogs or cats. Each time a child masters even in a slight way the fearful situation, he or she should be given praise and encouragement. Whatever is done, the parents' own capacities to be calm, reassuring,·encouraging, and supportive are essential.

Parents whose own fears of the dark, of being alone, of thunder or lightning, or of dentist or doctor provide models for their children's fears have the responsibility to underplay those situations. If their children ask them if they are afraid, it is important that parents be able to acknowledge their own fears, since to deny those fears is to deny the child's accurate perception, and this denial could be confusing. Parents do not have to be fearless nor to appear so to the child. Parents should be able to say, "Yes, I have the same fear and I know it is not sensible, but I have learned to live with it." They may then be able to give their children some advice about how to handle fears and may encourage them to feel that they do not have to be burdened with the fears of their parents. With this approach children may learn to cope with fears with more success than their parents.

When fears last an inordinately long time, when one set of fears is replaced by another, or when fears become increasingly incapacitating to the child or to parental or family function, a more definitive psychologic and psychiatric evaluation will be needed.

2.29 PRESCHOOL AND SCHOOL

Preschool experiences can be of value to the young child, enhancing socialization, peer group interaction, and perhaps even cognitive learning. Four year olds and, in selected instances, 3 yr olds who appear to be mature enough to spend a half day away from home should be enrolled in nursery school. Even at 18 mo of age some children may benefit from a half day or more each week in a supervised setting where they may interact with other children (Sec. 2.23).

The refusal to go to school (school phobia) is not uncommon in kindergarten or first or second grade children. The children involved are generally good students with obsessive traits, who often have had earlier problems in separating from parents or from home. Somatic complaints may accompany the refusal to attend school. The physician should first help parents to insist upon the young child's prompt return to school and continued attendance, and then try to determine and alleviate the cause. Otherwise, early and transient school refusal may evolve into an ingrained and chronic difficulty. In preadolescence and adolescence, though, an episode of school refusal may indicate rather serious psychopathology, and it is wise not to insist on a return to school until psychiatric assessment finds that appropriate.

Poor school performance in an intellectually able child may be the result of emotional problems, sensory deficits, other physical illness, or inadequate teaching. Boys may be less ready developmentally than girls to assume the passive role of student, and the normally exuberant activity of young grade school boys may present problems for teachers in the early school years. As a general principle, it may be wise not to have boys begin their first grade experience before the age of 6, or at times closer to 7 yr. Despite some dangers of inaccurate diagnoses and mislabeling, the early school years provide a good setting for identifying such health, psychologic or educational problems as mental retardation, reading disorders, hyperkinesis, sensory deficits, and emotional difficulties. Identification is of value, however, only if appropriate remedial programs are available. In recent years schools have been experimenting with new educational techniques, including "open classrooms," programmed learning, "family" groupings, and operant conditioning; these may be more useful for some children than for others. For example, a withdrawn and inhibited child may function quite well in an open setting; an overactive child may require a more structured educational program. Most children, however, do well in school, and schools do well by most children. Wherever possible, those interested in children should work closely with schools, both around individual children with problems and in collaborative efforts that will strengthen the ability of schools to foster children's emotional development. The development of disadvantaged children, in particular, can be favored by good educational experiences.

2.30 PUBERTY AND ADOLESCENCE

See Sec. 2.9 and Chapter 9.

Adolescence is a physical and psychosocial process of long duration, lasting in Western society from an onset at 10–13 yr to the late teens or early 20's. Assignment of an end point to adolescence depends upon whether one is measuring it by relatively internalized psychologic processes or by more social benchmarks such as economic and social emancipation from the parental family.

Adolescent "Turmoil." Psychoanalytic theory has held that adolescence is normally a period of "turmoil," marked by a desire for independence and a quest for sexual identity and maturity, and by a casting off of parental images and values in order to solidify one's own personality structure. Turmoil was once regarded as an inevitable, necessary part of growth. This view held, further, that if turmoil does not occur in adolescence, the individual will pay the cost later in inhibition, constriction of personality, or dependency.

More recent studies of adolescents, comparisons of patients and controls, and examinations of large populations of boys and girls suggest less conflict. Rutter et al found in a review of normative studies that "most adolescents are not particularly critical of their parents, and very few reject them." Parents and adolescents may have disagreements, and most adolescents would prefer their parents to be less restrictive; but the great majority of adolescents tend to admire their parents, get along quite well with them, and are generally satisfied and happy at home. Contrary to popular belief, they are more worried about parental disapproval than about the disapproval of friends. They are not particularly alienated unless they have psychologic disturbances, and there is no evidence that the increase in sexual activity, including intercourse, is correlated with psychiatric disturbances (see below). Normal adolescents experience anxiety and depression as inherent in growing up, but do not experience major turmoil, confusion, or withdrawal.

An adolescent who is clearly unhappy or whose recurrent crises suggest serious conflict requires careful evaluation. Among signs requiring attention are sudden declines in scholastic achievement, choices of new companions with whom parents are uncomfortable or of whom they disapprove, or evidence of a preference almost exclusively for activities outside the home, especially when there appears to be a breakdown in a communication within the home. When such signs appear, the family physician or pediatrician should suspect such illness as may warrant psychiatric referral. A disturbed adolescent should not be dismissed as a normal variant with a necessary and transient disturbance. Such an adolescent was likely disturbed earlier as a child, and will be a disturbed adult unless intervention occurs.

Sexual Behavior. (See also Sec. 9.7.) In recent years traditional standards of sexual conduct have changed, with adolescents becoming more experienced sexually. This change is real and marked. In 1971, 30% of unmarried female teenagers in the age group 15–19 residing in metropolitan areas had experienced sexual intercourse; this increased to 43% by 1976 and to 50% by 1979. In 1976, more adolescents were using birth control, especially the pill, but more than a third were "unprotected" at the time of last intercourse. By 1979 contraceptive use had increased but there had also been an increase in ineffective measures, such as withdrawal, and 13% of unmarried teenagers had been pregnant. Sorenson's 1973 study found that 59% of American adolescent boys and 45% of adolescent girls had had sexual intercourse. The adolescents indicated that they saw sexual activity as occurring in the context of a relationship, as a means of communication, as a part of self-realization, and as an aspect of love. About half of the boys and 62% of the girls 16–19 yr old had used contraception during their most recent intercourse. Many adolescents who did not use birth control relied on the possibility of abortion or of having and keeping a baby without getting married.

The physician who deals with adolescents, even those who may be sexually active, should not assume that their theoretical knowledge, particularly in the area of contraception, is measured by their experience. Many sexually active adolescents find it difficult to admit ignorance about sexual matters; for them, bravado, airs of sophistication, and face-saving are often highly invested coping styles. Accordingly, the physician must often take the initiative in providing instruction and guidance.

The failure of some adolescents to use contraceptives involves motivational factors as well as ignorance (Sec. 9.7). Obtaining and using contraceptives makes the intention to have intercourse explicit. By not being prepared, the adolescent attempts to avoid guilt through the fiction that intercourse resulted from overwhelming passion or a miscalculation. For some girls pregnancy fulfills conscious or unconscious needs; it can boost self-esteem, provide reassurance of femininity, become an act of defiance or of self-denigration, or be used as a weapon against family, boyfriend, or self. For some boys, impregnating their girlfriends serves as proof of virility.

Guidance. In guiding the adolescent, the physician must take into account the relationships between adolescents and parents, and those between adolescents and their peers. The young adolescent may vacillate between attempts at extreme independence and sudden reversions to overt or camouflaged dependence. The adolescent is testing new ideas and new relationships and trying to renegotiate the old relationship with parents to win somewhat new and different terms. Adolescence in Western society can be viewed as a time of rehearsal for a variety of adult roles, and it is natural that early attempts at adult performance may be clumsy, exaggerated, and not satisfactory either to the adolescent or to others. One of the most important roles of the physician is to point out to adolescents, and particularly to parents, that they are entering upon a new phase of relationship. Both parents and adolescents must get used to the idea that they are in a process of separating from each other, reaching the final stage of a process that began with birth. Anxiety and depression are to be expected at times, on the part either of the child or of the parent, as they modify their earlier closer bond. The parental attitudes most threatening to the adolescent may be either premature total emancipation on the one hand or a resort to inappropriately severe restrictions on the other. Parental indifference might be equally threatening. Adolescents also fear and do their best to avoid loss of face, the appearance of being fools to themselves or to their peers, siblings, or parents. The physician can be most helpful to parents if, as a semi-objective outsider, he or she can help them to avoid power struggles in which the loss of face by child or parent is a frequent outcome.

In treating *drug-related problems*, physicians must know such things as types of drugs; frequency of use; among which age groups the drugs are used; whether the use is distinctive by social class, by school, or by local community; and what parental, school, and other community resources are doing about drug problems. Only adequately informed physicians can help adolescents or their families who face problems of drug abuse (Sec. 9.4).

The *choice of career*, whether it follows immediately upon high school or after college and postgraduate work, is an important preoccupation of adolescents. The physician can be helpful in knowing what resources are available for vocational training and in offering advice regarding choice of colleges or the kind of preparation needed for a career in which the adolescent is interested. Adolescents frequently need to discuss with experienced adults their concerns about their future.

Adolescents in the United States are today under great pressure to succeed both academically and vocationally. They are likely to expect too much of themselves, to become discouraged and give up, or to strive inordinately hard, paying a high price emotionally and socially, and sometimes with health. Suicide attempts are at peak incidence in the age group between 15 and 25 yr (Sec. 2.44).

Piaget and other investigators have indicated that in the adolescent period the final stage is reached in development of abstract reasoning and facility with logic, along with increased sophistication in moral reasoning (Sec. 2.21). The physician can help adolescents and their parents by providing developmental interpretations of behavior. Discussion and arguments around such issues as religion, philosophy, politics, social concerns, and ethical questions are one way in which some adolescents develop and test their new cognitive and logical skills.

The typical adolescent is subject to anxiety and to episodes of depression. Fairly effective strategies for dealing with stress and avoiding too much self-preoccupation include development of goal-directed academic or extracurricular or social activities. Discussions with their peers support adolescents in coping with the stresses and strains of everyday life. Humor is a major coping strategy, the targets of which may be parents and adult-dominated institutions, but also the adolescents themselves, and often each other.

SOCIAL ISSUES

2.31 ADOPTION

Most adopted children and their families handle the matter with considerable common sense and sensitivity, but some issues concerning adoption require comment.

Adoptions accomplished through approved agencies are preferred to independent adoptions, since they tend to more adequately assess the psychosocial setting of the prospective adoptive family and perhaps provide better safeguards for the physical condition of the infant. Adoptive placement should be made as soon after birth as possible in order to foster attachment and bonding between infant and adoptive mother (Sec. 2.23). Adoptions of older children, or across religious and ethnic lines, or by single parents are, in appropriate instances, reasonable alternatives to having adoptable children languish in institutions or temporary foster homes, but adoptions of older children present some risks. For example, a family seeking to rescue a 4–5 yr old child with a history of severe emotional deprivation and multiple foster home placements may find that the child has been severely traumatized and will later display major psychologic disturbances, even in the best of adoptive homes.

Adopted children should be told of their adoption as soon as they have achieved reasonably good verbal facility and comprehension, by the age of 3 or at the latest 4 yr. The explanation can be repeated when circumstances are appropriate, such as during a family discussion about the birth of a neighbor's baby, but should not become ritual. Children's books on adoption can be read to young children; later they can read them themselves.

Controversy continues as to whether adopted children are at increased risk for development of emotional problems. If they are, it is likely to reflect problems of parental management. Since the adopted child generally arrives in the context of marital infertility, he or she may be treated with considerable overindulgence as a "special child." Adoption need not be perceived by the child as a threat to self-esteem, but in the case of individual and family problems, the child's adoptive status may reinforce otherwise existing doubts about his or her competence and worth. Not infrequently a natural child is born following an adoption to previously "infertile" parents. For the adopted child the event may initiate a competitive struggle requiring both understanding and firmness on the part of the parents.

Occasionally, foster parents wish to adopt a child who has been in their care for a number of years, but who has not been legally relinquished by the natural parents. Historically, the courts have upheld the claim of biologic parents for the child, even in those instances in which the natural parents abandoned the child and the foster parents have been essentially the child's only long-standing, nurturant, and consistent (psychologic) parents. Such legal decisions reinforce the notion that children are to be treated as property, rather than having their own needs and rights. Recent decisions to the contrary, however, show the courts' growing appreciation of the child's need for continuity of care.

In some states, adopted persons who have attained their majority are entitled to access to their adoption records and to information about their biologic parents. On the whole, this is a commendable development; this right-to-know must be weighed, however, against the rights of biologic parents to privacy, if they desire it.

2.32 FOSTER CARE

Placement in foster care is typically provided by local welfare authorities for abandoned, severely neglected, or abused children. For many children, foster care offers a lifesaving environment that gives them the opportunity to be physically replenished, to grow, and to develop innate potential. For others, however, foster care represents yet another episode in a lifelong history of deprivation. Unfortunately, we have yet to develop in the United States a comprehensive and well-supervised system of foster care that provides integrated services for children already at risk. Undermanned and underbudgeted departments of public welfare are often unable adequately to prepare, supervise, and support foster parents who may have to deal with difficult, traumatized children. Children are transferred from one foster home to another because foster parents move, the child doesn't "adjust," or unsupervised foster parents are deemed to be inadequate. Some children move in and out of placement according to the whims of natural parents who can neither care for them nor let them go permanently. For some children multiple foster care placements have disastrous effects on abilities to learn, trust, and relate to others. Such children, already made vulnerable by the circumstances that led to their placement, are placed at further risk by the vagaries of foster care. Serious retardation in reading, antisocial behavior, apathetic states, and defects in socialization have all been compellingly described by Eisenberg as the sequelae of such experiences. This situation will not change until the needs of children receive high priority in social planning and legislation. Only recently have trends in state and federal legislation been aimed at "permanency planning," with the use of adoptive placement or permanent foster care, and with earlier relinquishment or termination of the rights of parents who are unwilling or unable to care for their own children.

2.33 EFFECTS OF A MOBILE SOCIETY

For the first 30 yr after World War II approximately 20% of the population of the United States changed residence each year; there has been a slight decline in mobility in recent years.

The effects of this movement on children and families are frequently overlooked. For children the move is essentially involuntary; they move because a parent has obtained employment elsewhere, because the birth of a sibling has made a larger home desirable, or for other reasons. When such changes in family structure as divorce or death precipitate moves, children face the stresses created by both the precipitating events and moving itself. When parents are sad because of the circumstances surrounding the move, this unhappiness will be transmitted to their children. Children who move lose their old friends, lose the comfort of a familiar bedroom and house, and lose their ties to school and community. Not only must they sever old relationships, but they are faced with developing new ones in new neighborhoods and new schools. Because movement upward in social standing often accompanies a geographic move, children may enter neighborhoods with new and different customs and values. And since academic standards and curricula vary from community to community, children who have performed well in one school may find themselves struggling in a new one. Frequent moves during the school years are likely to have adverse consequences on social and academic performance.

Parents should prepare children well in advance of any move, and allow them to express any unhappy feelings or misgivings. Parents should acknowledge their own mixed feelings and agree that they will miss their old home while looking forward to a new one. Visits to the new home in advance are often useful preludes to the actual move. Transient periods of regressive behavior may be noted in preschool children after moving, and these should be understood and accepted. Parents should assist the entry of their children into the new community, and exchanges of letters with old friends and visits, whenever possible, should be encouraged.

2.34 SEPARATION AND DEATH

The younger the child, the more likely it is that the response to the loss of a parent through separation or death will be characteristic of age. In older children the reactions are more individualized and reflect differential characteristics of their own experiences. Relatively brief separations and reunions usually produce rather transient effects, in response either to the separation or to the reunion. The potential impact of each event must be considered in the light of the age and stage of development of the child and the particular relationship with the absent person, as well as the nature of the separation. It is more frightening for children to be separated from a parent at a hospital than within the familiar surroundings of home (Sec. 2.54).

In young children the initial reaction to separation may involve crying, either of a tantrum-like, protesting type or of a quieter, sadder type. After a few hours or a day or so of separation, the child may appear more subdued, withdrawn, and quiet or irritable, fussy, moody, and resistant to authority. Disturbance of appetite may occur, and there may be special difficulties at bedtime, such as reluctance in going to bed and problems in getting to sleep, with a resurgence of old fears, and in younger children perhaps such regressive behavior as bed wetting. Children may repeatedly ask where the absent parent is and when he or she will return home; some children may not refer to parental absence at all. The child may go to the window or door or out into the neighborhood looking for the absent parent; a few may even leave home or their places of temporary placement to try to find where their parents are. This last rather unusual response needs to be considered when a child cannot be found for a while shortly after the separation or departure of a parent.

The child's response to reunion may surprise or alarm the parent who is not prepared. The parent who joyfully returns to the family may be met by wary or cautious children, who, after a brief interchange of affection, may move away from the parent and seem indifferent to his or her return. The interpretation of this response will depend on the child and his or her style; it may indicate anger at being left and wariness that the event will happen again, or since children tend to personalize, the child may have felt he or she caused the parent's departure. For instance, if the mother who frequently says, "Stop it, or you'll give me a headache," is hospitalized, the child may unrealistically feel at fault and guilty. As a result of these feelings children may seem to be more closely attached to the other parent than the absent one, or even to the grandparent or babysitter who cared for them during their parent's absence. Immediately after the reunion or after a few days, some children, particularly younger ones, may become more clinging and dependent than they were prior to separation, while continuing any regressive behavior that had occurred during separation. Such behavior may engage the returned parent more closely and help to re-establish the bond that the child felt was broken. Usually such reactions are transient; within a week or two the child will have recovered usual behavior and equilibrium. Recurrent separations may tend to make the child more wary and guarded about re-establishing the relationship with the repeatedly absent parent, and these traits may affect other personal relationships. Parents should not try to ameliorate a child's behavior by threatening to leave.

Experiences of loss such as divorce or placement in foster care can give rise to the same kinds of reactions listed above, but more intense and possibly more lasting. School-age children may respond with evident depression, seem indifferent, or be markedly angry. Other children appear to deny or avoid the issue, behaviorally or verbally. Most children may cling to the hope or fantasy that the actual placement or separation is not real. Guilt may be generated by the child's feeling that this loss, separation, or placement represents rejection and perhaps punishment for misbehavior. The child may protect the parents at his or her own expense, believing and asserting that one's own badness caused the parent to depart or to place him or her with relatives or strangers, rather than that the parent has been bad or irresponsible. Besides having their own feelings of guilt, children cannot blame their parents because they sense it may be fairly risky. The parent who discovers that the child harbors resentment might punish further for these thoughts or feelings. Children who feel that their misbehavior caused their parents to separate or become divorced have the fantasy that their own trivial or recurrent behavioral patterns have caused their parents to become angry with each other. Some children develop behavioral or psychosomatic symptoms and unwittingly adopt a "sick" role as a strategy for reuniting the parents.

In response to separation and divorce of parents older children and adolescents commonly show more intense anger.

Almost all children cling to the magical belief that their parents will reunite. Wallerstein and Kelly found that 5 yr after the breakup more than 30% of the children were "consciously and intensely unhappy and dissatisfied with their life in the post-divorce family." Moderate to severe depression was common in this group. On the other hand, many children stabilize within 2–5 years after the parental separation. Their good adjustment seems related to ongoing involvement with two psychologically healthy parents and the support system offered by siblings. Joint custody arrangements appear to reduce ongoing parental conflict, but a recent study by Steinman revealed that one third of children in joint custody "felt overburdened by the demands and requirements of maintaining a strong presence in 2 homes."

As to the ultimate separation—death of a parent—most preadolescent children do not seem to go through a typical mourning process as psychoanalytically defined. The child's mourning may be masked by behavior not typically seen in adults. Among school-age to adolescent children who had lost a parent through death, Wolfenstein found that immediately after the loss sad feelings were not markedly evident, nor was there much crying. Children continued in everyday activities, the major mechanism in dealing with catastrophe being denial, both overt and unconscious, and maintained by the magical wish and hope for reunion and reappearance. Any depressed moods that occurred were not connected with thoughts of the parent's death; this could be acknowledged intellectually as a fact but was isolated in the emotionally nurtured expectation of return. Some children seemed to maintain remarkably good moods; some were more active than usual. Wolfenstein saw these good moods as an effective accompaniment of denial: "If one does not feel bad, then nothing bad has happened." Some children show hostile and angry feelings toward the surviving parent and tend to identify with and idealize the lost parent, sometimes with reunion fantasies accompanying denial. Guilt may be present, reflecting the child's egocentric tendency. An orphan of the Hiroshima bomb said, "We did nothing bad—and still our parents died."

Children under the age of 5 yr view death as reversible, possibly with belief in the dead coming back to life and in ghosts. In the next stage, up to 8–9 yr, death is personified, e.g., as the "grim reaper" who punishes and avenges. Only after this age does the child realistically understand death as a universal and final biologic process.

The physician can help children and surviving caretakers through a period of separation or adjustment to death of parent or sibling, first by helping them recognize that the adults themselves are going through a period of grief and mourning. It is not unhealthy for children to see their surviving or remaining parent mourn the loss of a mate or grieve for a divorced or separated spouse. In the case of a dead parent the child needs the support and reassurance of having the remaining parent or other important caretakers available. Close physical contact and emotional exchange, with verbal explanations and reassurance for those children who can understand, are important aspects of support. Children

should not be expected or forced to discuss all their feelings or to put into words their reactions to a parent's death. They should not be expected to interrupt usual social or recreational activities for weeks or months after death of a parent, either out of respect for that parent or in recognition of the remaining parent's sorrow or grief. Continuance of usual activities should not be interpreted by adults or older children as callousness or indifference, but rather as the child's way of dealing at his or her stage of development with what is as much a catastrophe for him or her as it is for the adult. Further, the child should not be expected to serve as a primary support to the remaining parent or others in their grief.

In most cases it seems helpful for the child to participate appropriately in the rituals that generally surround the death and burial of a parent. A young child can attend a funeral, viewing, or wake so long as there is no morbid preoccupation or demand that the child remain a long time or be involved in prolonged religious ceremonies. To keep the young child away from some participation in the burial rituals, whatever they are, will be a misguided effort to protect and ultimately will be more confusing and isolating than helpful.

2.35 IMPACT OF TELEVISION

It is estimated that American children watch television for an average of 30–40 hr/wk. This is more time than they spend in school, and for many it is their major scheduled activity. Television places children in passive roles and offers them entertainment generally requiring little engagement or imagination. It entices them away from important activities such as reading, hobbies, physical exercise, and relationships with peers and with other family members.

Educational programs aimed at preschool children through television may enhance cognitive development in reading readiness and acquisition of vocabulary. At best, however, such programs can only supplement rather than substitute for the activities of parents in conveying knowledge, skills, and information, and in motivating learning (Sec. 2.18). Television may inform older children of current events, politics, history, and science; it more commonly, however, displays scenes of violence that serve as models for aggressive behavior. Exposure to violence in films increases interpersonal aggressiveness among children. Optimists may hope that most children will be able to separate themselves from the steady diet of violence they witness on television; but children readily imitate all types of models, and the effects of television violence on children may be considerably more pervasive than we now know. It is certain that some children already emotionally disturbed may act out aggressively as the direct result of crime or horror programs, and that the action may follow the models presented.

All parents should know what their children are watching on television, should decide whether certain programs are appropriate, and should feel in no way reluctant to meet their own standards in imposing restrictions on the time and content of television viewing.

2.36 ASSESSMENT AND INTERVIEWING

THE CLINICAL INTERVIEW (HISTORY)

The clinical interview is the most common procedure in medicine, but the nature of the process is often poorly defined. The interview is not simply history taking; still less is it a cross-examination of the patient that attempts to fulfill the requirements of a review of systems. It is basically a working alliance between the patient and the physician, aimed

at the orderly exchange of any and all clinically relevant information between them (also see Sec. 5.3). The patient is seeking reassurance or help, and the physician possesses knowledge, skills, and the social sanction to be helpful. *The most useful perspective in which to view the clinical interview is as a major means of engaging the patient in the active management of his or her own care.*

One well-practiced aspect of the clinical interview in most

pediatric and general medical settings is the simple collection of those historical medical data that disclose and review the signs and symptoms of a presenting illness, the nature and course of past medical illnesses, the family history, and a review of systems. Other aspects of the patient's life, such as the psychosocial, often get less or scant attention in interviewing. Physicians need to find ways to use clinical interviews to assess the emotional states of their patients, their usual reactions to stress, their levels of self-concept, their systems of values, the natures of their personal relationships, something of their personalities, the quality of their coping abilities, and clues that might point to psychosocial distress or disturbance.

To become an effective interviewer requires motivation, skill, and continuous attentive practice. The skills required develop throughout the course of one's professional life. They are frequently overlooked in medical school, or poorly taught, or seen as related only to psychiatric patients, or taken for granted once medical school is completed. The development of effective interviewing skills is facilitated when the student has the opportunity to practice with simulated patients, to make and hear recordings of his or her work with simulators or with actual patients, and to have these activities supervised by competent teachers or consultants.

Time. An interview that attempts comprehensively to explore both psychosocial and biomedical aspects of the condition of a stranger who has just become a new patient needs at least 30–40 min for significant exchange of the most basic relevant information. Physician and patient must have time to become comfortable with each other and to establish the rapport that facilitates the exploration of psychologic and social information. When patient and physician have had an adequate earlier initial interview, and the physician therefore knows some of the major aspects of the patient's psychosocial status, it is possible to focus on particular issues in periods as brief as 10 min, but an initial interview of 10 min is ineffective and it may communicate to the family a lack of respect for the sensitivity and importance of material given such casual attention.

Setting. Privacy is essential, but unfortunately it is often difficult to maintain in children's hospitals or in busy outpatient clinics. The need for privacy is most likely to be overlooked with children, who are frequently managed with less respect and sensitivity than is given adults. It is difficult to carry on an interview in a relatively unsheltered cubicle in an outpatient department or at bedside, even with curtains drawn to shield the child or family from visual intrusion or distractions. If possible, it is often more productive to seat the hospitalized child in a chair next to the bed rather than to converse with the child while he or she lies in bed. Adverse physical conditions negatively affect the quality and the effectiveness of the clinical interview. Though it may be difficult, it is worth considerable effort to find a private place; in hospitals this may be a treatment room, an empty conference room, or even an unoccupied office or patient's room. Privacy is more easily arranged in the office of the practicing physician, where closed doors and reasonable comfort are ordinarily routine.

Goals. The most common deficiency within an interview is the failure of the clinician to define clearly the goals of that particular encounter. No single interview can accomplish everything that needs to be done to complete a clinical assessment. *The clinician must set, define, and state priorities.* These will depend upon the nature of the patient's condition, whether the interview is an initial visit or a follow-up one, or whether the physician has to elicit sensitive material or to transmit unpleasant or unhappy diagnostic or prognostic information to patient or family. Physicians must become sufficiently familiar with their own styles and learn enough

from past experiences to be able to judge accurately what can be accomplished in each interview. For example, if the work of the first interview is to establish a working alliance with a child and family and to identify the primary problems or concerns, then it may be a mistake to attempt a total developmental, family, or school survey on such an occasion.

Communication. The major purpose and process of the clinical interview is the exchange of information. When the patients are children, this exchange occurs between parents and physician, between child and parents, and between parents, as well as between child and physician. In any social interaction communication has two major features: one is the *content* or *message;* the other is the *process,* or the manner in which content is exchanged within the relationship.

The notion of *content* refers to the literal meaning of the words exchanged between communicating parties; content is the message or the *what* of communication. The notion of *process* refers to the relational or nonverbal aspects of communication. The tone of voice, the rate of speech, the inflection of words and phrases, facial expressions, head movements, hand gestures, and body postures and movement all communicate meaning, often more accurately than the words exchanged. The words usually capture the major conscious attention, but the process may frequently determine the success of the venture. The nonverbal features of communication are continually monitored by each sender and receiver, often preconsciously or subconsciously. The nonverbal conveys the cognitive, emotional, social, or rather global state of the sender with respect to what he or she is saying, and indicates to the receiver *how the content is to be interpreted.*

Children attend to and interpret nonverbal communication before they understand the meanings of words. Reciprocal communication of basic feelings and emotions between parent and infant takes place through sounds, gestures, and body contacts long before the infant or the toddler can identify feelings or know what words appropriately express them. Physicians should be aware of how their own facial expressions, tones of voice, or gestures influence children's reactions and determine how messages are interpreted; this knowledge contributes greatly to skill in interviewing. The complementary skill required of the physician is to recognize and correctly interpret the child's emotional state through careful observation of facial expression, tone and inflection of voice, body posture, gestures, and other responses. Children may be unresponsive to questions because they are upset by the loudness of the physician's voice, by the suddenness with which he or she initiates an examination, or even by the closeness of the physician's body. Some children have temperamental characteristics predisposing them to anxiety in new or unfamiliar situations and the physician has the responsibility for recognizing the signs and knowing how anxiety may be dealt with. Many children are frightened of unfamiliar office or hospital settings, of physical pain, of separation, of uncertainty, of persons or figures to whom they may attribute awesome authority and power, and of all else that goes with the word "doctor."

Children need continually to know what is happening and what is going to happen to them in the immediate future. Their anxiety will be significantly reduced when physicians take time to explain what they are doing and what they are going to do, and when they engage the child as an active participant as much as the clinical situation and good judgment will allow. Making life predictable, within the framework of a short or even a 50 min encounter in office or hospital can have a profound effect on the likelihood of obtaining the cooperation of children.

Some children as young as 3–4 yr and most children by the age of 8 can participate verbally as well as physically in their own health care. All too frequently, conversation involves only the clinician and the parent, with the interaction between clinician and child being limited to the physical examination and some pleasantries. Children can and will respond relevantly to seriously posed questions about themselves.

By the age of 13 yr the young person is to be considered the primary informant and should be dealt with directly in his or her own right. If parents are at hand, they may be interviewed with the adolescent or separately; but at this age all explanations of diagnostic and treatment procedures should be directed first to the young person rather than to the parents. This procedure does not imply that the patient has veto power over the recommendations of the physician. The patient is still dependent on his or her parents, and the parents are still the major decision makers. Physical examinations of adolescents should be conducted with their parents not present, unless the patient requests otherwise.

Script. The distinction between content and process as aspects of communication requires further discussion of the content or message aspect. The use of words to convey messages has an aspect called *script.*

Script is the specific set of words used to convey a message. The impact of nonverbal communication upon the meaning of messages has been stressed above. The notion of script recognizes that the specific word content of the message may also convey subtleties of meaning, quite apart from nonverbal cues. Certain words or phrases, in accordance with their connotation or their usual reception, will inhibit or impede communication, whereas other words or phrases conveying substantially the same message will facilitate or promote effective communication and elicit relevant responses.

An example may clarify this. A mother might ask her 6 yr old child, "Why did you do that?" Alternatively, she might have said, "What reason did you have in mind when you did that?" or "What made you decide to do that?" If the mother's purpose is really to know *why,* then the first question is semantically adequate; on the other hand, the pejorative context in which such a question is usually phrased renders it much less likely to be effective in opening and revealing communication than the alternatives, both of which ask the same question in words that invite a more creative or process-oriented dialogue.

The first form of the above question belongs to a rather large set of stock phrases which, we learned as children, have various meanings hidden behind the words. We use these same stock phrases or questions as adults in communicating with a new generation of children. These phrases may have one or more of several characteristics:

1. Some phrases are likely to put a respondent on the defensive, such as: Why? What on earth makes you think that?

2. Some phrases subtly or blatantly impugn the veracity of the respondent, such as: You really don't believe that! Everyone knows that. That's just an old wives' tale.

3. Some phrases can express moral reproach about feelings or opinions of the respondent, such as: A good boy doesn't feel that way about his mother (father, etc.). I can't imagine anyone feeling that way. That kind of behavior never bothers *me.*

4. Some such phrases state or imply that the speaker enjoys a position of particular wisdom or virtue which the respondent could adopt to his or her benefit if only he or she could come to think, feel, or act in the same way as the speaker. For example: If I were you . . . Why don't you . . . ? It just takes patience (or understanding, or love, or firmness) to. . .

5. Many such phrases convey the patronizing, formalistic, condescending flavor of the sloganeer: Stop worrying. Take it easy. Learn to relax.

On the whole, such stock phrases emphasize the power side of a relationship. The speaker is frequently in a role of traditional power—doctor, parent, or teacher, or an adult engaged with a child. These words and phrases are accompanied by congruent tones of voice, gestures, facial expressions, and body postures. They are intended to admonish or to convince the hearer to admit error or wrong-doing or stupidity, and to change feelings, thoughts, or behaviors in directions indicated by the speaker, but the effect is to inhibit, reduce, or close off communication, with the respondent feeling wounded, hurt, rejected, helpless, depressed, exhausted, irritated, angry, or (rarely) amused or entertained.

Physicians must identify and evaluate their own stock phrases and substitute others that will facilitate communication. In a sense, a new script is substituted for a set of habitual questions and responses. The new script may have surprising and gratifying results.

1. I'd like to understand your reasons for that (idea, feeling, behavior). Can you explain them?

2. Disliking (hating) your daughter (mother, husband) must be a very unpleasant feeling. How does it affect you?

3. Not everyone looks at a stuffy nose in the same way. What do you think it means?

4. There are a lot of conflicting opinions about hyperactivity (toilet training, sex education), and it's often hard for parents to sort out which one is going to be the most useful. Here is an approach some people have found successful. You may not find it exactly right for you, but you can try it.

5. I strongly recommend that you . . . (NOTE: there is nothing at all wrong with a physician taking a strong stand in making professional recommendations to parents regarding the health of their children, but the proper way is clearly and simply to state that position without contaminating it with demeaning or pejorative phrases or with such nonverbal communication as scowls, raised voices, bombast, finger pointing, or other inappropriate gestures.)

6. I know it's hard to take your mind off your child's leukemia. What have you found that sometimes helps?

7. Try to ignore his constant pestering. If you find you can't, then let's figure out some other strategies.

The alternatives to stock phrases are usually longer and more tentative, allow the other person more autonomy and leeway in terms of possible choices, and promote an alliance rather than the dominance of one party over the other. Successful alternatives help the hearer feel that his or her position and integrity are respected, even when these alternatives convey the message that there is an area of disagreement.

Many physicians find that tape recordings of their interviews will help them to identify the phrases, as well as the tones of voice and inflections that they may wish to change or modify. They should practice saying aloud the alternative phrases that they propose, to see how they sound to others as well as to themselves. The procedure and effort may seem awkward and artificial at first, the experience sometimes resembling learning to play a musical instrument correctly after using incorrect techniques for years; but the awkwardness gives way to a much improved performance.

Talking with Children. Professional conversations with children have certain rules:

1. Don't talk to children in a condescending way, but as a physician talks with any patient.

2. Don't convey to the child your thought that his or her feelings, concerns, or ideas are "childish."

3. Don't laugh at what a child says unless you are quite sure the child intends to be humorous.

4. Don't try always to be funny or amusing to children. Such efforts are best saved for few occasions only, and for children you know and who know you very well. Children know the difference between doctors and funny people.

5. Never tease a child unless you know him or her *very*

well and the child knows he or she has permission to tease you in return.

6. Initial or casual encounters with young children are often made easier when introduced in a whisper, which young children may find more personal, private, and reassuring than jollity; they commonly whisper in response.

7. When children are old enough, at 3–4 yr, form the habit of discussing with them their symptoms, diagnoses, and treatments in terms they can understand.

8. Never discuss the illness or treatment of a hospitalized child who has acquired receptive language functions in the child's presence unless you are discussing it with him or her as well.

9. When a child fails to cooperate in his or her care in office or hospital, the first assumption should be that negativism or struggling means that he or she is frightened and reacting to fear in a customary personal manner; such behavior is often erroneously perceived as immature and irritating, embarrassing, provocative, or frightening by parents and other adults.

In the last context it can be noted that one can always ultimately overpower a child, verbally or physically or both. Sometimes, though rarely, that may be necessary, but there is always a cost to the child, to the physician, and to the relationship. Physicians frequently delegate the task of enforcing control of children to parents, nurses, students, or aides, or to drugs. This may give the physician a sense of distance from the regrettable or unpleasant necessity, but he or she is ultimately responsible. Calling upon naked power, whether it be verbal or physical, has at least three undesirable results: it increases the patient's sense of helplessness and powerlessness; it models the technique for students, residents, and other health care staff; and it narrows and restricts the clinician's own rapport, sometimes dulling sensibility to the feelings of others as well as to his or her own.

Other Aspects of the Interview. Certain signs indicate that the progress of an interview or examination should be assessed or reassessed for the effectiveness of communication.

1. When parents do not appear readily reassured by the diagnostic and treatment procedures, look for hidden anxiety from unanswered questions that they may have difficulty recognizing or stating. Latent anger may have the same result. The physician should make it comfortable and easy for parents to ask "stupid" questions or to admit "shameful" thoughts or "ungrateful" or angry feelings.

2. When a child is giving evidence of feeling pain, it is a psychologic impossibility that nothing hurts. When parents scold a child with "That doesn't hurt," they must be helped to understand that pain is a purely subjective experience and needs to be respected. Their acceptance of this may help greatly to clear the air.

3. Parents will sometimes be heard denigrating or shaming a child by using such terms as "baby," which is almost as bad as being intentionally cruel or frightening. Such behavior should be dealt with by the physician promptly and its inappropriateness discussed, with as much empathy for the parents' position as possible. "I can see that it's upsetting to you to have your child behaving this way, but I don't think that this approach is going to help us. Let's look at it from her (his) point of view . . ."

4. Exhortation and other emotional appeals to reason will be frequently heard used by parents and are among the weakest methods of attempting to alter behavior or attitudes. Again, ". . . Let's look at it from the child's point of view . . ."

5. When only one parent accompanies the child, it is almost always the mother. In many families, including those with working mothers, issues of health care are viewed as maternal responsibilities. Physicians should feel increasingly uncomfortable as time passes and they have not yet met the fathers of children for whom they have assumed the responsibility of continuing care. Many fathers will be found eager to see a physician who extends a specific invitation, has clearly stated expectations, and will accommodate his time and schedules.

6. The physician will often, if he or she adequately explores the matter, find that parents have not complied with recommendations made for the care of their children. Compliance is not simply a matter of hearing, understanding, and doing what the doctor says; nor is noncompliance to be explained simply as ignorance, neglect, or a personality clash. The parent who fails to comply with recommendations may do so for a number of reasons, and these must be accurately identified.

Did the parent really understand what was prescribed or recommended? Does noncompliance express the parent's reservations as to the appropriateness of the recommendations or were the recommendations beyond the capacity of these parents to execute them, for technical, emotional, or financial reasons? Had the parents enough opportunity to ask questions and to discuss the details and ramifications of the child's condition and treatment? Is a noncompliant parent being influenced or torn by information or advice contrary to that of the physician, which may come from the other parent, a grandmother, a friend, a newspaper or magazine article, or TV programs?

Does the parent or do the parents have personal or marital problems which so upset and distract them that they cannot be effective; or does the child's illness itself have them so emotionally upset that they cannot accept the initiative and responsibility that has been thrust upon them? Depressed mothers can be so psychologically depleted as to be unavailable to the child even though they may consciously want or intend to carry out recommendations. Is the parent expressing anger at the physician through noncompliance? Is the parent of an anxious and resistant child unable to execute a prescribed regimen that may be difficult or uncomfortable because he or she fears that the child may become hurt, resentful, or angry if the required firmness is exercised?

OTHER SOURCES FOR ASSESSMENT

Institutions or Agencies. Besides the clinical interview, other data can greatly help in psychosocial assessment. Birth records, for example, may help in questions of injury during pregnancy or at birth. Such records are often deficient, but they may provide the only objective view of events of the patient's birth and early days. Other health records, including those from other physicians or agencies who have cared for the patient, may provide essential information concerning acute or chronic illness, show a pattern of unusually frequent visits to the physician's office for relatively minor problems, or reveal an obsessive focus on certain areas of the body.

School reports are important to the psychosocial assessment, especially if they include both an academic assessment and a description of the child's relationships with schoolmates and teachers. Requests for school reports should be made only with the written permission of the child's parents or legal guardians.

Reports from child care agencies may also be helpful, especially in the case of adopted children or children in foster care. Such agencies often have extensive background material and may have reports of earlier psychologic examinations.

Psychologic Testing. Relatively simple screening tests such as the Peabody Picture Vocabulary Test, the Denver Developmental Screening Test (Sec. 2.11), the Thorpe Developmental Inventory, and others may be administered by the trained pediatrician or by his or her assistant. They may indicate areas of possible or patent intellectual or perceptual dysfunction that need further study. The major danger of these tests is that they may be relied upon too heavily as giving definitive assessments, whereas they should be regarded purely as screening tests.

Some psychologic tests should be administered and interpreted only by or under the supervision of trained psychologists; others can be used by trained school personnel. They are generally of four types. The first type is concerned with *perceptual-motor* integrity. This type is felt to be especially sensitive to "organicity," or to reflect structural or physiologic abnormalities in the central nervous system. The Bender-Gestalt test is probably the best known in this category. The second category is that of *intelligence* tests such as the Stanford-Binet or the Wechsler Intelligence Scale for Children (WISC). The WISC is a 10-category test that gives both verbal and performance IQ scores. The third type of test includes the *achievement* tests that are usually administered in schools. Tests such as the Wide Range Achievement Test (WRAT) report the grade level of achievement in such subject areas as reading, spelling, and mathematics. The fourth type includes the *projective* tests such as the Rorschach test (ink blot) or the Thematic Apperception Test (TAT). These give some indication of the fantasy life of the child as well as the reality testing and personality characteristics. When tests have already been done by the school, the results should be examined before new tests that may prove redundant or unnecessary are requested.

The tests to be used should be chosen by the psychologist after physician and psychologist have discussed the nature of the problem and the reason for consultation. As much as possible, tests should be chosen to assess specific problems, rather than as an exhaustive battery, some of which may have only vague relationships to any clearly defined problems or goals. When the physician is at all uncertain of the nature of the tests or the implications conveyed in their interpretation, a joint meeting should be arranged with the psychologist and parents for an interpretive review; otherwise, costly tests may be ordered, the results of which are never fully exploited.

Occasionally, genetic, endocrine, or neurologic studies will be required to determine whether organic problems may contribute to or be responsible for psychologic disorders.

Psychiatric Consultation. A psychiatric consultation may be a valuable part of the assessment of children in whom vague or unexplained physical symptoms may have substantial psychogenic determinants; it will often be most acceptable and useful when the child has been hospitalized for study. Other indications include the evaluation of depression in children with major acute or chronic illness, of chronic neurotic problems, of underachievement, and of serious aggressive difficulties. The physician should inform both parent and child of the reasons for the psychiatric consultation, obtain their consent, and prepare them for what to expect.

Correlation of Data. The physician must avoid early diagnostic closure even when the parents' initial description of their problem gives a reasonably clear idea of what is going on. So long as the physician remains a receptive and perceptive listener, new and important information will emerge, as parents and perhaps patient begin to feel more trusting, and as they are educated by the physician's questions. Furthermore, the weighing of data must be done in the context of the family's sociocultural pattern. It is important that the physician not use his or her personal value system or style of living as a yardstick against which to measure the family's behavior or their success or failure in coping with their life situation. Their own feelings of anger, frustration, anxiety, failure, or depression are more valid indicators of where they need help.

It is important that the principal item of concern be accurately identified. Parents may present as the prime concern, for example, a problem such as bedwetting of many years duration. Why then have they come for help now? It is important to determine whether there may, in fact, be more important hidden issues the parents do not recognize or acknowledge, or cannot face. By the same token it must be understood that the parents' assessment of the problem is critical for the child. Sometimes a physician, having collected and assessed appropriate data, can conclude only that a child presented by his or her parents as having a problem is functioning within normal limits. In such a case it must be determined what personal, familial, social, or cultural considerations compel the parents to see the child's behavior as a major problem. It must then be determined what re-education they may need in order to feel reassured and not be left with the impression that their anxiety has been casually dismissed.

Referral. When problems have not been internalized by the child it may be sufficient simply to counsel the parents or school personnel, or both. If this has been done and a maladaptive child or situation continues to present problems, the child and family will probably require more intensive or extensive help and should be referred to a child psychiatrist or to a psychiatric clinic. It is important that physicians avoid the position that psychiatric referral is a last resort. The need for a psychiatric consultation or referral can perhaps best be expressed in terms of the joint need of the family and physician for help in areas where the psychiatrist has special expertise, with the understanding that the collaboration of physician and family in management of the other health needs of the child remains intact.

2.37 PSYCHOSOCIAL PROBLEMS

A psychosocial disorder in a child may become manifest as a disturbance in feelings (e.g., depression, anxiety), in bodily functions (psychosomatic disorders), in behavior (e.g., conduct disturbances, passive-aggressive behavior), or in performance (learning problems). Dysfunction may involve any or all of these areas. Psychosocial problems may be produced by such physical or emotional stresses as birth defects, physical injury, inconsistent and contradictory child-rearing practices, marital conflict, child abuse and neglect, overindulgence, chronic illness, and so on. Particular agents do not, however, produce specific symptoms or disorders; rather, children's psychosocial problems are multifactorial in origin, their expression depending on many variables, including temperament, developmental level, the nature and duration of stress, past experiences, and the coping and adaptive abilities of the family. In general, chronic stresses, or a series of stressful events, are much more difficult for child and family to manage than a single acute stressful episode. Children may react immediately to traumatic events, or may keep their feelings dormant until maladaptive reactions become apparent during later periods of vulnerability.

Anticipatory guidance during periods of stress may considerably help children and their families to achieve more positive outcomes. Parents should be encouraged to prepare their children in advance for potentially traumatic events that can be anticipated (e.g., elective surgery, separation, or divorce). Children should be allowed or encouraged to express their feelings of dismay, fear, or anger, rather than being told to be a "good girl" or "brave boy."

Infants and toddlers tend to react to stressful situations

with impairment of physiologic functions, such as disturbances of feeding and sleep, with relatively global expressions of anger or fear, as in temper tantrums, or with withdrawal and avoidance behavior. School-age children demonstrate their difficulties through altered interpersonal relationships with peers and family members, through impairment of school performance, by the development of specific psychologic syndromes, such as phobias or psychosomatic disorders, or by "regressing" to earlier, more "childish" modes of functioning.

Parents are frequently concerned whether the particular behaviors of their children are "normal" or whether they represent problems that require intervention. Some "symptomatic" actions of children may be part of normal development. For example, a temper tantrum may express the normal negativism of a toddler; on the other hand, temper tantrums on slight provocation in a 6 yr old may indicate psychosocial disturbance. Whether behavior is judged to be a developmental variation or evidence of a more serious problem depends upon the age of the child, upon the frequency, intensity, and number of symptoms, and especially upon the degree of functional impairment. The decision of parents to seek help is determined, in turn, by the characteristics of their children's behavior, by the amount of distress it causes the children, parents, teachers, and others, and by their past experiences in discussing psychosocial matters with their physicians.

2.38 PSYCHIATRIC CONSIDERATIONS OF CENTRAL NERVOUS SYSTEM INJURY

Psychiatric difficulties may follow infection, injury, or intoxication, or genetic, metabolic, or idiopathic illness involving the central nervous system. These are not to be confused with the manifestations of "minimal cerebral dysfunction" (also known as minimal brain dysfunction, dysfunctional child, attention deficit disorder, or, in behavioral terms, the hyperactive or hyperkinetic child. For the last condition see Sec. 2.46).

Brain injury increases the risk both for intellectual impairment and for psychiatric disorder, especially when the injury is severe. Social disinhibition appears to be a specific sequela of brain injury, but no typical psychiatric syndrome is associated. The particular expression of disturbance depends more on the child's developmental level, past history, temperament, and family relationships than on the nature of the insult. Psychosis is not a typical result of brain injury or illness in childhood. Chess has reported an autism-like syndrome in children who have had congenital rubella, but autistic psychosis is probably the result primarily of unspecified genetic, physiologic, and organic factors (Sec. 2.52).

Psychiatric disorder accompanies or follows brain injury or illness or epilepsy in a significant percentage of affected children. The epidemiologic survey of the Isle of Wight found brain-injured or epileptic children 5–15 yr old to have 5 times the normal risk of psychiatric disorders. Mentally retarded children also are at increased risk of psychiatric disorders.

Prenatal factors have long been suspected of causing brain damage and psychiatric or behavioral disorders. Prematurity and neonatal complications involving hypoxia have been seen as causing such conditions as hyperactivity, impulsivity, difficulties in socialization, and poor control of emotions, especially anger. On the other hand, Graham's study of 350 children at the age of 3.5 yr who had suffered neonatal asphyxia found no more behavioral or emotional disturbances than were found in a control group matched for social class and family factors.

Children under the age of 3 yr who survive encephalitis or meningitis seem to show more lasting effects on personality and behavior than those who have these illnesses later. The result contradicts the notion that the brain might in the earlier years have greater potential for recovery without significant residual dysfunction.

Children with hydrocephalus and motor deficits have a 7 times greater than average incidence of psychiatric disorder. The additional findings of low IQ, language disorder, or bilaterality of the motor handicap increase the incidence of psychiatric disturbance significantly, but again there is no specificity in the type of disturbance encountered.

When children with brain damage or injury have problems with impulse or anger control, aggressiveness, hyperactivity, or other emotional reactions, these do not differ in quality from those of children with intact nervous systems who have the same disturbances.

The most significant factor in the child's adjustment to a chronic handicapping organic condition is the capacity of his parents to adjust and cope.

In some affected children stimulant drugs improve the ability to perform in school, smooth out emotional reactivity, and facilitate social interactions with peers and adults. Such medication taken for extended periods may produce growth retardation, which must be weighed against possible beneficial effects. Tranquilizers may lessen anxiety and improve emotional control and behavior, but they tend also to produce obtundation and somnolence, which may interfere with learning.

Most children with psychologic disturbances related to central nervous system injuries, and their families, benefit from understanding psychosocial support. A frequently beneficial approach is to help the child to identify his or her ineffective reaction patterns, along with more successful patterns. The approach combines "coaching" and education, with an opportunity to discuss depression, isolation, and anger and those feelings of being different, rejected, or exploited that so much affect self-esteem. The parents will have their own needs and will need advice, counseling, and emotional support in dealing with their child's emotional and behavioral problems, both in family matters and in his or her life at school and with friends. Fair, firm discipline is always useful. Behavior modification techniques can help children in whom specific target behaviors can be identified; the technique may be used at home or at school. Both aberrant psychosocial behaviors and learning difficulties may respond (Sec. 2.66).

2.39 PSYCHOSOMATIC DISORDERS

Psychologic conflict may lead to alterations in somatic function or so-called "psychosomatic disorders." Contrary to earlier views, particular types of feeling or conflict do not produce specific kinds of psychosomatic illness; rather, any kind of emotional distress may be associated with any type of psychosomatic disorder in a child. There appear to be both innate constitutional vulnerabilities and environmental factors, none of which are well understood, that determine why one organ or system becomes dysfunctional rather than another. Psychosomatic illnesses are of two types: conversion ("hysterical") reactions, and psychophysiologic disorders.

Conversion reactions are sudden in onset, and can usually be traced to a precipitating environmental event. Voluntary musculature and organs of special sense are the most frequent target sites for the "hysterical" expressions of psychologic conflict. Such reactions may take many forms, including hysterical blindness, paralysis, diplopia, gait disturbances, and the like. Physical examination often fails to reveal objective abnormalities. Deep tendon reflexes can be elicited in a paralyzed leg, and pupillary responses to light are noted in hysterical blindness. Affected children and their families tend to be rather dramatic and hypochondriacal and often give a past history of previous conversion episodes.

La belle indifférence, or "beautiful indifference" to symptoms, supposedly characteristic of hysterical patients, is an inconsistent and unreliable finding. The benefit of secondary gain does not distinguish the hysteric from the patient with organic illness, as both may unconsciously use disability as a method of obtaining relief from stressful life experiences.

Psychophysiologic disorders have a more insidious onset. Chronic anxiety produces functional abnormalities within the autonomic nervous system that lead to structural changes within organ systems. Eczema, bronchial asthma, ulcerative colitis, and peptic ulcer are considered to be psychophysiologic disorders or at least to have significant psychophysiologic components in some children. Children with psychophysiologic disorders have been reported to be obsessive and inhibited, but there is no compelling evidence for specific personality characteristics.

Several general principles guide management of children with psychosomatic disorders:

1. The symptoms of affected children are not within their conscious control; they are not "acting" or malingering; their pain and their problems are real.

2. It is essential that a psychiatric assessment be arranged early in the management of these disorders; otherwise, after elaborate and expensive tests have been done, the child and family will often be convinced that he or she has a very serious illness for which a "real" cause exists that cannot be found.

3. An explanation of the role of the emotions in the genesis of these disorders must be accepted by the parents before truly effective intervention can be accomplished.

4. Psychotherapy for the child and counseling for the family are often indicated, as well as pediatric management; psychiatrist and pediatrician must be in close communication with each other in a therapeutic alliance; modest amounts of minor tranquilizing medication may be a useful adjunct.

5. Child and family should be encouraged and helped to live as normally as possible to avoid crippling psychologic invalidism, with stress put on early return to school after acute illness, upon participation in recreational activities, and upon normal peer interactions. Parents should know that some children unconsciously use their symptoms to maintain dependency, and that firm, gentle insistence upon the fullest possible range of activities for the child is indicated.

6. The physician should be alert for indications of psychosomatic or physical illness in parents, with which children may unconsciously identify; successful treatment of parental illness may be necessary for a favorable outcome in the child.

The diagnosis of conversion reaction should not be based solely on normal physical findings, but should be supported by the positive psychologic findings noted above. Up to 30% of patients originally thought to have conversion reactions may subsequently be proved to have organic illness.

2.40 DISORDERS RELATED TO VEGETATIVE FUNCTIONS

Obesity. Sec. 3.20.

Anorexia Nervosa and Bulimia. Sec. 9.6.

Pica. Pica is a habit disorder involving repeated or chronic ingestion of non-nutrient substances, which may include plaster, charcoal, clay, wool, ashes, paint, and earth. The tasting or mouthing of objects is normal in infants and toddlers, but pica after the 2nd yr of life needs investigation. Pica is most often a symptom of family disorganization, poor supervision, and affectional neglect. It appears to be more prevalent in lower socioeconomic classes and may be related to poor nutrition. Pica may also be seen in severely retarded

children, as part of their tendency to mouth objects indiscriminately. Children with pica are at increased risk for lead poisoning (Sec. 28.15) and parasitic infections (Sec. 11.100).

Enuresis. Enuresis, the involuntary discharge of urine after the age by which bladder control should usually have been established, is one of the most common and perplexing problems brought to the attention of the pediatrician. Because of wide variation in the age of achievement of bladder mastery, children are not generally labeled "enuretic" unless the symptom persists beyond the age of 5 yr. Nocturnal enuresis occurs once a month or more in 8% of school-age children. Persistent diurnal enuresis is much less common, usually represents a more serious problem, and, especially in girls, may be associated with infection.

Bedwetting occurs more frequently in boys than girls and becomes less common as the child approaches puberty. It will often have been present in one of the parents. Bedwetting may be divided into the *persistent* (or *primary*) type, in which the child has never been dry at night, and the *regressive* type, in which a previously continent child begins to wet the bed again. Persistent nocturnal enuresis is often the result of inadequate or inappropriate toilet training. Parents who demand coercively that the child become toilet trained promptly may mobilize an angry response, the child unconsciously defying them by wetting the bed. On the other hand, parents who are not sufficiently close to the needs of the child to support toilet training may undermine his or her attempts at bladder mastery. Chronic psychologic stress unrelated to toilet training experiences but occurring during the toddler period can also impair the child's ability to achieve bladder control.

The regressive type of bedwetting is precipitated by stressful environmental events, such as a move to a new home, marital conflict, birth of a sibling, or death in the family. Such bedwetting is often intermittent and transitory; prognosis is better and management less difficult than in children with primary enuresis.

In both types of bedwetting, organic pathology can be found in only a very small number of cases. Physical examination and urinalysis are indicated, but more strenuous procedures such as urography and cystoscopy are usually not warranted, and should not be pursued unless there is some indication of an organic lesion (Sec. 17.39–17.43).

Treatment of the child with enuresis depends on an understanding of the possible specific causative factors suggested by an adequate psychosocial inventory and physical examination; for example, a child can be helped to deal with feelings about a new younger sibling, or the parents may be helped to establish proper attitudes and climate for a child's success in toilet training. Some general suggestions are:

1. It is important to enlist the cooperation of and to motivate the child to deal with the problem. Rewarding the child for being dry at night is a useful step. Child or parent can chart the dry nights, and with one or two dry nights a small token or reward can be given, with more substantial rewards with increasing success.

2. Older children should be expected to launder their own soiled bedclothes and pajamas.

3. Children should be given no liquids after dinnertime.

4. The child should void before retiring.

5. Waking the child repeatedly to take him or her to the bathroom is useful in only a few children and may further mobilize or aggravate anger in child or parent.

6. Punishment or humiliation of the child by parents or others should be strongly discouraged.

The use of conditioning devices (such as an alarm that rings when the child wets a special sheet) is usually not necessary, and should be reserved for persistent and refractory cases in which the child's self-esteem has been seriously eroded, and only with the consent of the child. Imipramine (Tofranil) (see

Table 2–14) is generally only briefly effective, and drug tolerance is common. This medication has a variety of side effects (hypotension, hypertension, tachycardia, restlessness, nightmares, dry mouth, rarely blood dyscrasia), and its use is not without risk.

Encopresis. Encopresis is the involuntary passage of feces at an age by which bowel control should have been established. By the age of 4–5 yr it is viewed as a symptom, rather than a developmental variation. As in the case of enuresis, organic defects are rarely found. Encopresis is much less common than enuresis (though the two may coexist), and it indicates a more serious emotional disturbance. Chronic soiling may persist from infancy onward, or may appear as a regressive phenomenon. Encopresis is often associated with chronic constipation, fecal impaction, and overflow incontinence, and may progress to psychogenic megacolon. This symptom usually represents unconscious anger and defiance in the child, and the parents may respond with retaliatory, punitive measures. School performance and attendance may be affected, as the child becomes the target of scorn and derision from schoolmates because of the offensive odor. Chronic use of enemas and laxatives should be avoided; they are usually of no benefit, call further attention to the symptom, and make the child more defiant. Measures similar to those used in the supportive treatment of enuresis may be useful with encopretic children, but the fixed and disabling nature of the symptom frequently requires psychotherapeutic intervention with child and family. See Sec. 12.13.

Sleep Disorders. Sleep disorders are common in childhood, and may be temporary, intermittent, or chronic in nature. Infants who show difficulty in establishing regular nighttime sleep patterns may also show general fussiness and irritability as a temperamental characteristic. Sleep disorders in infancy may also be a result of parental anxiety or strife. Older children may experience transient nighttime fears of burglars, noises, thunder and lightning, being kidnapped, and so on, and this anxiety will interfere with their sleep. Children may express their fears overtly, or they may disguise them, often by invoking tactics designed to delay bedtime. The fearful child may also seek to sleep in the parents' bedroom or may attempt to come into their bedroom after they are asleep.

Separation anxiety is often a causative factor. Children may unconsciously and symbolically view sleep as a time when they are removed from parental love and concern. If there is conflict within the family, or if separation or divorce has occurred, such anxiety will be naturally exacerbated. Bedtime fears often relate to such normal separations as occur with the child's first attendance in nursery school or kindergarten. As growing children become more aware of death, they may be unwilling to go to sleep at night for fear that they may die. This fear will be heightened if a family member has recently died. Finally, anxiety related to any other areas of the child's life—family, peers, school performance—may be expressed as a sleep disorder.

Parental support, reassurance, and encouragement are vital for alleviating sleep disorders. Angry threats and punitive measures are to be avoided. Parents should adopt calm, understanding, but firm attitudes. Bedtime should be set for a regular and stated time, variations being kept to a minimum. The parents should discourage the child from sleeping in their room, but may temporarily allow a fearful child to sleep in a sibling's room. A night light and allowing the child to leave the door open are often reassuring. The interval before bedtime should be quiet and restful; stimulating television programs should be avoided. A warm bath, a light snack, and a quiet affectionate moment with parents are conducive to sleep. Some children may become drowsy if allowed to read a favorite book for a few minutes after they are settled in bed. Diphenhydramine may serve as a mild sedative.

Nightmares in children are of two types: the more common anxiety dream or "bad" dream, and the rarer "night terror." The anxiety dream occurs during REM sleep; the child awakens, becomes lucid quickly, and usually remembers the content of the dream. He or she can be reassured and comforted by being held and by soothing words. *Night terrors* usually have their onset in the preschool years and occur with arousal from stage 4 (non-REM) sleep; the child is confused and disoriented, shows signs of intense autonomic activity (labored breathing, dilated pupils, sweating, tachypnea, tachycardia), may complain of peculiar visual phenomena, and appears to be very frightened. A period of somnambulism (sleepwalking) may follow, during which the child may be at risk of injury. Some minutes may pass before the child seems to be oriented. Usually he or she cannot recall dream content causing the night terror. Night terrors are often self-limited and may be related to a specific developmental conflict or to a precipitating traumatic event.

Persistent nightmares reflect chronic underlying anxiety and warrant a comprehensive evaluation of the child, including psychologic status. Diazepam (5–10 mg at bedtime) has been reported to be of benefit in the treatment of night terrors and somnambulism.

For sleep disorders in adolescence, see Sec. 9.5.

2.41 HABIT DISORDERS

Habit disorders include many tension-discharging phenomena, such as head banging, body rocking, thumb sucking, nail biting, hair pulling, and teeth grinding. Tics, which involve the involuntary movement of various muscle groups of the body, are included. Stuttering and masturbation will be discussed with the habit disorders, though the latter is not usually considered a disorder.

All children show at various developmental levels repetitive patterns of movement that can be described as habits. Whether they come to be considered disorders depends on the degree to which they interfere with the child's functioning—physically, emotionally, or socially. Some habit patterns may be learned by imitation of adults. Many begin as a purposeful movement that for some reason becomes repetitive, the habit losing its original significance and becoming a means of discharge of tension. For example, a child with an eye irritation or one attempting not to shed tears might try closing his or her eyelids several times in rapid succession. This activity might become repetitive, and incorporated into the child's behavior as an outlet for tension. Such symptoms are often reinforced by attention from parents or others. Other movements, such as rhythmic head banging and rocking in early life, can persist without parental reinforcement, occurring when the child is put to bed or is alone; they seem to provide a kind of sensory solace to the child feeling otherwise uncared for and understimulated by human touch or interaction. These movements represent in this sense a kind of internal stroking. Such patterns are often seen in the mentally retarded or in children suffering from maternal or emotional deprivation. Equivalent movements are evident in children who twist their hair or touch or play with parts of their bodies in repetitive ways. These rhythmic movements are often most prominent just before sleep or as the child passes from wakefulness into sleep, and they seem to help the child cope with anxieties. As involved children become older, they learn to inhibit some of their rhythmic habit patterns, particularly in social situations; but in the more seriously disturbed the rhythmic habit patterns may persist.

Teeth grinding (bruxism) seems to result from tension originating in unexpressed anger or resentment. It may create problems in dental occlusion. Helping the child to find other ways to express resentment may relieve the teeth grinding.

Bedtime can be made more enjoyable and relaxed, with reading or talking with the child permitting re-experience and review of some of the fears or angers of the day. Praise and other emotional support for the child are useful at these times.

Thumb sucking is normal in early infancy. In the older child it has the unfortunate effects of making the child appear immature, and of interfering with the normal alignment of teeth. Like other rhythmic patterns it can be seen as a way in which the child secures extra self-nurturance. Providing the child with evidence of concern and with other forms of satisfaction is generally the best strategy for dealing with thumb sucking. Parents should ignore the symptom if possible, while they give attention to more positive aspects of the child's behavior. The child actively trying to restrain thumb sucking should be given praise and encouragement.

Tics involve repetitive movements of muscle groups, but have no apparent function. They may have been first intentional, sometimes becoming nonintentional very quickly. Parts of the body most frequently involved are muscles of the face, neck, shoulders, trunk, and hands. There may be lip smacking, grimacing, tongue thrusting, eye blinking, throat clearing, and so on. Tics appear to represent discharges of tension originating in emotional states which involve the muscular system. It is very difficult for the person with a tic to inhibit it. Tics can be distinguished from variants of minor seizures in that the child does not experience a transient loss of consciousness or amnesia. Tics occasionally accompany other psychiatric syndromes or follow encephalitis. Most cases seem to have had no physical antecedents and are transient. Undue parental attention can reinforce tics, whereas ignoring them may diminish their occurrence.

Gilles de la Tourette syndrome (also called Tourette syndrome) is a rare condition seen in children, some of whom have severe psychopathology; it is characterized by tics, compulsive barking, or the shouting of obscene words. It can be helped to some extent by counseling the child and parents. Haloperidol (a potent dopaminergic inhibitor) has been found to lessen the frequency and intensity of the tics and to reduce anxiety (see Table 2–14).

Masturbation is manipulation of the genitals for sexual pleasure. There may be movements or contractions of the musculature of the thighs, with copulatory movements. Younger children unaware of cultural taboos against masturbation may be observed by their parents in this activity, but most children sense parental disapproval, and the activity is carried out in privacy. Open masturbation by the older child suggests poor awareness of social reality or a lack of parental censorship. It is important for parents to understand that masturbation may be normal at any age and is virtually universal among children and adolescents. It presents a self-gratification analogous to thumb sucking. In the older child or adolescent it serves the purpose of exploring and experimenting with newly developing sexual feelings and capacities. It also serves to discharge sexual tensions, and may aid in gaining control over sexual urges. Masturbation is most common at bedtime, when anxiety is increased owing to separation or to fear of loss of control over sexual or aggressive impulses. Children are most likely to masturbate when alone and feeling lonely, or when they are having sexual fantasies. Beyond normal release of sexual tension, masturbation can be done in a repetitious and compulsive way as a reassurance against fear of injury to the genitalia. Excessive masturbation suggests some problem or deficiency in the child's or adolescent's ability to relate to others.

It is appropriate for parents to discourage open masturbation and to be concerned about excessive masturbation. On the other hand, it is important that masturbation be accepted as a normal aspect of the child's sexual life, and that guilt or anxiety relative to it be avoided. By the time of puberty, children should be given explanations of its normality. This can be done in conjunction with explanations of ejaculation, orgasm, and menstruation, so that children can understand them, too, as normal bodily functions.

Stuttering is not generally regarded as a tension-releasing activity but it can become so in a secondary fashion. Most theorists of stuttering agree that primary stuttering comes about as an atypical development during the learning of speech. As it becomes more fixed, secondary compulsive and repetitive movements of various muscle systems come into play as the child attempts to "force" out the words and release the build-up of tension. The physician can help parents accept the child's early patterns of dysfluent speech; the less emphasis paid to these early patterns, the better the outcome. The child can be made to feel successful and cared for in other areas. If the pattern persists, a speech therapist should be consulted. Approaches to treatment include breath control exercises or the use of a miniaturized metronome that "paces" the rhythm of speech (Sec. 2.68).

EMOTIONAL DISORDERS

2.42 NEUROSES

According to psychoanalytic theory, psychoneuroses arise from intrapsychic conflict between one's wishes for expression of sexual and aggressive drives and the prohibitions of the conscience against these expressions. This internalized conflict is outside conscious awareness, but the symptoms of anxiety become apparent. Anxiety can be expressed as irritability or whimpering, or as worry in older children. It can also appear as a phobia, such as fear of the dark or of going outside. Sometimes anxiety is converted into a somatic symptom, i.e., a conversion reaction, such as paralysis of a limb or inability to see clearly. The neurotic conflict may express itself also in obsessive-compulsive rituals.

Psychoneurotic conflict does not reach awareness because of *repression*, a defense mechanism that may intermittently or generally keep the conflict from consciousness; when repression fails, neurotic symptoms appear. Specific neuroses usually do not appear by themselves in children; rather, intermittently there may be multiple neuroses, or neurotic traits. Neurotic traits may be interwoven with underlying personality disorders. The essence of neurotic symptoms is that affected patients are aware of them, will admit to them, and find them unpleasant. The prognosis for most childhood neurosis is relatively good.

The overanxious child is upset beyond apparent reason. There may be excessive shyness, shaking, frequent crying, insomnia, tics, and so on. One form of overanxiety is seen in the so-called *school phobia* (Sec. 2.29). Affected children have a problem of separation, rather than a true phobia. Besides showing anxiety in the morning, affected children become excessively anxious at night, when the gradual diminution of sensory input leaves them relatively more aware of their fearful fantasies. The physician should help the parents look for hidden sources of anxiety that can be dealt with openly by child and parents.

Children with *phobias* have organized their anxieties into focused and projected mental patterns. Instead of feeling generally anxious, they are anxious only under specific conditions: in the presence of a dog, in the dark, on high places, outside the home, at the sight of men with beards, and so on. The choice of object to be feared is in some unconscious way related to the origins of the anxiety; for example, aggressive or murderous thoughts unacceptable to the conscience are repressed, and projected into fears of the robber or of the monster lurking in the dark. Phobic neuroses may resolve spontaneously if they are not reinforced by new sources of anxiety. It appears also that children can be desensitized to their phobias by the techniques of behavior modification, the phobias becoming attenuated and disappearing without their underlying sources necessarily having been revealed or dealt with. Whether these unresolved unconscious conflicts affect the future mental or emotional life of the patient is uncertain.

The parents of a phobic child should remain calm in the face of the child's anxiety or panic. If they become upset, the child will conclude that there is in fact something to fear. Calm acceptance provides a useful model for the child in dealing with the normal and unavoidable anxieties of growing up. The most powerful therapeutic tools physicians can use in these conditions are their listening, their understanding, and their own calmness.

The child with an *obsessive-compulsive* neurosis has further elaborated anxiety and conflict into a system of apparently pointless rituals. For example, a boy in conflict over sexual urges may become hyperalert to the genital area. He may next project the thought that others can see his penis, which may also represent a repressed exhibitionistic wish. He may begin looking down each time he enters a room to make sure that his pants are buttoned or zipped, or he may check his belt every few minutes to make sure that everything is in place. Obsessive-compulsive rituals are not always seen as pathologic. When they become so intense and persistent, however, as to interfere with comfortable function, they require psychiatric help. Obsessive-compulsive neuroses are generally harder to treat than phobias, and some theorists feel that there may be an inborn element to their formation. A past history of depressive disorder may be found. Affected children tend to be very serious, "grown up," rigid, and finicky, and to find it hard to reach out to others with positive affect. On the other hand, within limits some obsessive-compulsive traits may be healthy manifestations of self-discipline, may help children to stay organized, and may contribute to their success in various activities and to their self-esteem. A good student striving for scholastic achievement, who puts off immediate gratification in order eventually to become a professional person, may have obsessive-compulsive traits working to his or her advantage.

Children with *hysterical neuroses* are able to achieve massive repression of certain ego states without overt evidence of anxiety (equivalent to forgetting). In the *dissociated state* a child may at times feel that he or she is someone else. In a more organized rendition of this, the *fugue state*, the child may act out a complicated series of behaviors, return to his or her usual ego state, and have no memory of the period of fugue. This is not the same as sleepwalking (Sec. 2.40), but more akin to the phenomenon of multiple personalities. Parents of many children report that their children have transient marked changes in personality, but these variant behaviors are almost always under the control of markedly divergent moods, rather than true fugues or dissociations. Temporal lobe epilepsy may produce strange behavioral sequences, but these rarely last more than a few minutes; they are unremembered, as in fugue states, but unlike the latter are followed by postictal sleepiness. Electroencephalography may be of help in differential diagnosis.

A more common hysterical neurosis is the *conversion neurosis*, which is a somatization of a repressed psychic conflict and often, if not always, follows a model in the child's experience (Sec. 2.39). For example, a child with bronchitis may overcome the infection, but maintain or reintroduce later a chronic hysterical cough. The symptom appears to be an attempt to recreate an ego state that at the time of bronchitis served the purpose of conflict resolution, permitting the receipt of dependency gratifications without guilt. For another example, a young child with a crippled grandmother might get a twinge in the knee at times when he or she wishes to withdraw from stressful situations, these factors correlating with ego states in which the child pictures himself or herself at a certain level as an invalid, and acts out this internalized picture. Conversion symptoms often have a bizarre "unmedical" quality. They represent the unsophisticated notions of how it is to be paralyzed, blind, voiceless, in pain, and so on. Affected children are not pretending or malingering, and should not be so charged. They consciously believe in their condition, and their parents often join them in this belief. Referrals to psychiatric consultants can be difficult, since such referral challenges the integrity of the perceptions of the children or parents, or both. Referral is best accomplished by presenting the need for consultation as part of an adequate investigation (Sec. 2.55). Probably most conversion symptoms will disappear with positive suggestion by the physician. The most important diagnostic and therapeutic considerations involve identifying the secondary gain achieved by the symptom (e.g., absence from school, dependency). If this can be reduced or eliminated, the symptom will often abate.

2.43 DEPRESSION

It was formerly widely believed that children do not become depressed, but disorders of affect can occur in children of any age, including early infancy.

Anaclitic depression was first described by Spitz as a devastating effect of disruption of the mother-child relationship in early infancy. Spitz observed the condition in infants of mothers who were separated by imprisonment from their months- to year-old infants. The infants were then cared for in a clean, hygienic, and well-run babies' home. The staff, however, were able to provide only minimal routine care, rather than the close, affectionate, and stimulating relationship of the usual mother-child dyad. The infants showed profound disturbances in health and in motor, social, and language development. Some died.

There is a characteristic pattern to the anaclitic depression of infancy. By 6 mo of age infants have normally formed a strong attachment to a mothering figure (Sec. 8.6). Separation for a significant period at this time leads to a profound reaction in many infants, especially in those who have had the warmest and most satisfying relationships. The initial reaction is protest: crying, searching, almost panic behavior, with a good deal of motor activity in both arms and legs. Later, when an adult who is not the mother or usual caretaker approaches, the infant will first search anxiously to see if the mother has returned and then turn away from the approaching figure. The final phase of reaction is a period of apathy, in which the infant is hypotonic and inactive, with a sad facial expression. Affected infants cry silently and stare into space. When picked up, they search again for the familiar face; they will cling to a stranger and cry, but are not consoled.

Depressive conditions exist from preschool age through adolescence. Estimates of their frequency vary widely, from 2 to 50%, depending upon the population studied. Depressive *symptoms* may occur in 4-8% of preschool children, but whether distinctive depressive *syndromes* occur remains to be elucidated. In school-age children, however, syndromes do emerge; one study found 4-5% of 9 yr old children to have a depressive syndrome. The incidence of depressive illness in adolescence is uncertain, but many teenagers experience symptoms of depression, and the full range of adulthood affective syndromes occurs in adolescence. Girls are more likely than boys to report feeling depressed.

Depressive conditions in childhood are probably not homogeneous, but the finer distinctions in types and subtypes identified in adult disorders have not been elaborated for children. The diagnostic criteria set forth in the Diagnostic and Statistical Manual of the American Psychiatric Association (DSM–III) have been increasingly applied to childhood depressive disorders, and specialized diagnostic inventories and instruments have been developed.

Depressed children present a variety of symptoms. General features include a sad or downcast face, easy tears, irritability, withdrawal from some usual activities and interests, and loss of pleasure in such things as friendships, sports, games, and family outings. The depressed child may spend more time than usual alone, often watching television. School performance may be impaired. Depending on his or her personality style, the child may become more clinging and dependent; more aloof, withdrawn, and seclusive; or more disruptive, aggressive, and defiant. Conflicts may often arise in relationships with family and friends; they may add to the child's negative feelings as well as provoke anger, criticism, and rejection from others. Depressed children may at times show some of the psychomotor retardation, slouched posture, and decreased activity characteristic of adult depression. When asked how they feel, they will frequently say that they are bored, that they don't like anything, or that nothing is fun any more, rather than describing their state as depressed. Their capacity to look forward to pleasurable events is impaired or absent. They may express feelings of hopelessness or helplessness in terms appropriate to their age and verbal ability. They often communicate a sense of being unattractive and unloved, and complain that others in the family are favored or that everyone else is having a good time while they are not. Sleep disturbances are probably more common than is realized, because children do not report them unless asked.

In the more severe depressive conditions, such as *major depressive disorder* and *dysthymic disorder*, key symptoms are a generalized, persistent dysphoria, combined with a loss or impairment of pleasure derived from enjoyable experiences (anhedonia). In *major depressive disorder*, the dysphoric mood is unrelenting during the depressive episode, and the anhedonia is marked, pervasive, and persistent. Loss of appetite is common in adult depression, but more difficult to assess in children, given their fluctuating food preferences and the normal variations in amounts eaten between meals; one sign of appetite disturbance is failure to attain an age-appropriate weight. Sleep disturbances (insomnia in its various patterns, or hypersomnia), increase or decrease in motor activity, loss of energy and easy fatigability, decreased ability to concentrate, and slowed thinking are experienced. The child may feel worthless or inappropriately guilty. There may be recurrent thoughts of death, calamity, or suicide; occasionally, depressed children attempt to harm themselves. Associated findings in major depressive disorder include hallucinations with a depressive content (mood-congruent); these are more likely in prepubertal children. Mood-congruent delusions, if they occur, are more common in adolescents. Separation anxiety is very common in major depressive disorder and may lead to refusal to attend school. Somatic complaints (headaches, abdominal or chest pain, etc.) or a preoccupation with physical health may be found. Substance abuse becomes a risk during adolescence.

In *dysthymic disorder*, the dysphoria is generally more intermittent, with periods of normal mood lasting several days to several weeks. The dysphoria is less intense, but more chronic, lasting up to several years. With the exception of hallucinations and delusions, the other symptoms of major depression may be present. Concomitant disorders may include attention deficit disorder, conduct disorder, mental retardation, or personality disorder.

The course and form of childhood depression vary, but can be conveniently divided into acute depressive *reactions* and chronic depressive *disorders*. Acute depressive reactions are almost invariably preceded by some precipitating event such as an illness requiring hospitalization; loss of a parent through separation, divorce, or death; loss of a significant relationship with a friend or a pet; or a move of the family from one residence or city to another. As children enter the preadolescent period, experiences that damage self-esteem can precipitate acute depressive responses. Included are such events as failures in school, social exclusion, the disruption of an intense friendship or early romantic relationship, or even the growing awareness that childhood is over and that significant responsibilities and concerns of adolescence are approaching.

Acute depressive responses may last only a few days or weeks and often resolve spontaneously. When physicians, parents, or teachers become aware of these changes in children, their solicitous concern, their recognition of feelings, their allowing the children to talk about it if they are able, and the emotional support given by verbal and physical expressions of affection can help depressed children to regain feelings of self-worth. When a clear-cut event has precipitated a depression, parents can discuss the matter with the depressed child, helping the child understand both the event and his or her feelings about it. Medication is rarely indicated.

Chronic depressive disorders are not as common as acute reactions. There is usually no clear-cut precipitating event. Some of the affected children may represent a "depressive-reactive" style of personality. Such children have for some time had frequent disruptions in important relationships, often from early infancy onward. There is usually, moreover, a history of depressive illness in one or both parents, and usually during the child's lifetime. Affected children often show marginal emotional and social adjustment throughout their lives. Sometimes they present a picture of helpless, passive, clinging, dependent, and lonely children. At other times they relate to others in a more hardened, negativistic, aloof, or almost cynical manner. Having experienced many disappointments in interpersonal relationships, they expect further disappointment from adults and others. They are reluctant to invest emotion or trust in relationships, and frequently develop rather manipulative or expedient approaches to human affairs. They may engage in potentially self-destructive behavior, risking physical danger or exposing themselves to socially dangerous situations in which they can be harmed or exploited by adults. They are less likely than acutely depressed children to show episodes of crying, and they attempt to hide their depressive affect. They are often very wary and guarded in discussing anything that has to do with their personal feelings, thoughts, or attitudes.

Children with serious depressive disorders, such as dysthymic disorder or major depressive disorder, experience problems in school achievement and in their relationships with family and peers. They are at risk for conduct disorders or substance abuse. With effective treatment, school performance and separation anxiety respond rapidly, with improvement in depression, whereas problems in interpersonal relationships change more slowly.

The initial episode of major depressive disorder has a considerably shorter duration, about 32 wk, than the presenting episode of dysthymic disorder, which averages 3 yr. For both disorders, an earlier age of onset is associated with a more protracted course. Within 2 yr of their first episode, 40% of children with major depressive disorder experienced a relapse. One study found that 69% of children diagnosed as having dysthymic disorder developed a first episode of major depressive disorder within 5 yr of the onset of the dysthymic disorder.

As many as 20% of teenagers with major depressive disorders hospitalized for major depression may develop a manic episode of bipolar manic-depressive illness within 3–4 yr. Three predictors of such an outcome are (1) a depressive symptom cluster characterized by rapid onset, psychomotor retardation, and mood-congruent psychotic features; (2) a family history of either bipolar illness or "loading" for affective illness; and (3) induction of hypomania by antidepressant medication.

Several etiologic models attempt to account for childhood depression. The biochemical model examines variations in the production, utilization, or degradation of monoamine neurotransmitters. The finding of biologic markers or evidence of genetic transmission is consistent with this model. To date, the conditions that show such evidence are major depressive disorder and bipolar manic-depressive disorder. In major depressive disorder, especially, characteristics of the electroencephalogram during sleep and certain biochemical correlates have been noted. These findings have not yet been incorporated into clinical practice. Both major depressive disorder and manic-depressive disorder tend to have strong family histories of affective illness. Other models for depression include the learned helplessness model, the life stress model, the cognitive distortion model, and the behavioral reinforcement and sociologic models. Attempts are being made to examine each of these, with appropriate modification, in studies of children.

Children with chronic and serious depressive illness usually require psychotherapeutic help and are best referred to consultants or mental health facilities for diagnosis and management. A long-term supportive and therapeutic relationship with the family is often necessary.

For serious depressive disorders in prepubertal children, tricyclic antidepressants have been used. Imipramine is effective in ameliorating the symptoms of major depressive disorder in preadolescents. Its usefulness in adolescents is less clear-cut, possibly owing to the teenager's changing hormonal status. The side effects of tricyclics, especially the cardiotoxic ones, require careful monitoring. In any case, the use of a psychopharmacologic agent in treatment of a child's or adolescent's psychiatric disorder should be only one aspect of a comprehensive program that includes appropriate psychotherapy for the child and family, with attention to educational, social, and recreational needs. In certain unusually severe depressions or those in which the environment is unresponsive, intolerable, or very stressful, the depressed child may require a period of hospitalization.

For special features of depression in adolescence, see Sec. 9.2.

2.44 SUICIDAL BEHAVIOR

Our cultural myths deny that before the age of adolescence children are sexually interested and active, that they become depressed, or that they may at times have murderous wishes or behavior; we have also been slow to accept that young children have suicidal thoughts, and that with measurable frequency they act on suicidal thoughts and impulses.

Among children and adolescents predisposed to suicidal behavior there is no consistent clinical picture. Depression is quite common, but anger, jealousy, anxiety, feelings of rejection, and loneliness may all contribute to the suicidal thoughts and behaviors generated by the pressure to reduce intense stress. An involved child may have tried many other means to reduce this stress. Suicidal threats or behavior may be directed both at the environment and at the self, a significant motive often being to cause people in the environment to react, either with a rescue attempt or with feelings of guilt, remorse, or sorrow. There is some skepticism as to whether young children with inadequate concepts of death can really intend suicide, but studies in depth have revealed that many children perceive death as having life-like qualities, including the ability to fulfill their needs and provide them with love.

The incidence of suicide in children under the age of 15 yr is low, but is rising. For boys, the suicide rate tripled between 1950 and 1977, reaching a peak of 1.6/100,000 deaths; the rate then declined to 1.1/100,000 by 1979. The rate for girls has steadily increased, and by 1979 had reached 0.5/100,000—five times the incidence in 1950. Studies of clinically distressed children indicate that both thoughts of and attempts at suicide are much more common than earlier believed. A study of randomly selected children in a school setting found almost 12% to have had suicidal thoughts, threats, or attempts.

Older adolescents (15 to 19 yr old) have shown a 3-fold increase in their suicide rate between 1950 and 1979. Four times as many males (13.4/100,000) as females (3.2/100,000) in this age group commit suicide, making it second only to accidents as a cause of death. The higher incidence of suicide in specific age groups is especially significant since the higher rate within such groups persists as the group progresses in age, including during adulthood—a "cohort effect."

The methods of suicide vary with age. Among preadolescents, jumping from heights is the most common, followed by self-poisoning, hanging, stabbing, and running into traffic. The likelihood that self-administration of a poison is a suicidal gesture or attempt increases with the age of the child. Episodes of self-poisoning that occur after the age of 6 yr are less likely to be accidental and should be treated as if the behavior had suicidal potential or as a possible instance of child abuse or neglect. Of the estimated 100,000 self-poisoning episodes per year in children aged 5–14 yr and the 150,000/yr for the 15–24 yr old age group, about 46% are severe enough to produce symptoms and 24% require hospitalization. Estimates of the ratio of suicidal gestures to completed suicide in adolescents have ranged from 16:1 to 200:1.

While boys are more likely to commit suicide, girls are 2–3 times more likely to attempt it. Suicide attempts tend to be most common in the 15–19 yr age group. In children hospitalized for suicidal behavior, major depressive disorder, adjustment disorder, and specific developmental disabilities have been associated with increased risk, whereas schizophrenia and mental retardation correlated negatively with suicidal behavior.

Studies in England and the U.S. have identified significant dynamic and family factors in children who attempt and in those who succeed at suicide. Of intrapsychic factors, the most prominent and important is depression, both recent and past. This may derive from a number of causes. The loss of a loved person (or, less often, animal) may produce acute or prolonged grief, loneliness, or despair. Sometimes death is viewed as a means of reunion. Concern over failure at school may also be a prominent feature in some children. Guilty and self-deprecating children often used the attempt or threat of suicide as a cry for help directed outside the immediate family, which was seen as unresponsive or hostile. A child who has recently been aggressive may harm himself in fearful anticipation of harsh retribution. Abused children often internalize self-hate and have been found to be at high risk for self-harming behavior. In some adolescents who attempt suicide and in at least half of those who succeed, the notion of revenge or hostility is prominent, directed either outwardly or against the self. Suicidal behavior may be an attempt to gain evidence of parental love or involvement, sometimes in reaction to a self-perception of being "in the way" or expendable. A small percentage of suicide attempts are felt to result from playing a "suicide game."

Familial influences hold particular importance in suicidal behavior. Family dissolution through parental separation, divorce, or death is a major factor. A family history of illness, either medical or emotional, is also common. Fathers of suicidal youngsters have been more often noted to be depressed themselves and to have low self-esteem, whereas mothers have experienced greater anxiety or suicidal ideation. Both parents have tended to consume more alcohol than usual. Drug use is a common family problem. Suicidal children should be questioned about physical or sexual abuse, since they are more likely to have been victimized.

Many suicidal children have shown for a month or more prior to a suicide attempt some outward signs of distress, including signs of depression, as noted by teachers, family, or friends; others have had difficulties in adjustment for several months to a year or more. Especially prominent are a preoccupation with death and dying, a wish to die, and feelings of hopelessness or worthlessness. In children under 12 yr old, boys were more severely depressed than girls and were at continuing risk for suicidal behavior. At least half of the children who succeeded at suicide had personalities that were seen as irritable, easily hurt or aroused to anger, or impulsive. Successful suicides occurred in children who had higher IQ's, and were more likely to be relatively advanced in physical development. In a third of childhood suicide cases, a parent, sibling, or other first degree relative had shown some sort of overt suicidal behavior.

For special aspects of suicide in adolescents, see Sec. 9.3.

Of possible importance is the familiarity that a child with problems may have with the idea or experience of suicide. Parents may have served as models of thinking about, talking about, or actually attempting suicide, sometimes with signs of clinical depression. Some children hear threats or discussion of suicide by peers, or in movies, television, or books; many know of the actual suicides of cultural idols in the entertainment world. These models and this familiarity make suicide seem a possible solution to intolerable stress, conflict, loss of self-esteem, or intense hostility, particularly in the early or middle adolescent years.

Recidivism in suicidal attempts is primarily related either to the adolescent's inability to change his or her life situation (which may involve depression, entrapment related to poverty, alcoholism in a parent, chronic illness, unwanted pregnancy, homosexual guilt, thought disorders, or acting out) or to inability to respond to changes that have occurred in the environment. Hospitalization or institutionalization has not been very helpful. Finding of a thought disorder bodes a poor prognosis. The most important risk factors for recurrence are severe depression, thought disorder, and deteriorating home environment.

Management of Suicidal Behavior in Children and Adolescents. Threats of or attempts at suicide should be seen as acts communicating desperation, and all such threats or attempts should be taken seriously. Physicians, parents, and others must scrupulously avoid sarcasm or kidding, daring, or belittling them. If the physician labels such behavior "manipulative," power or control becomes the major issue influencing his or her response. Such a position reduces the psychologic flexibility required to deal effectively with child and family at a time of great stress.

The physician assessing suicidal behavior in a child or adolescent should carefully explore, with scrupulous attention to details, the child's life for the 48–72 hr prior to either the threat or the event of a suicide attempt. The physician must identify any precipitating events, as well as any possible hints or early warnings of a suicidal attempt that had been missed or ignored by family members, teachers, or friends. It is crucial to assess the degree of premeditation or impulsivity, whether the patient intended to be stopped or discovered by the timing of the action, and whether the behavior prior to or subsequent to the attempt would promote or impede the patient's being discovered in the attempt. The physician needs to judge the margin of error allowed by the patient in terms of the method used or proposed, the closeness or remoteness of available help, whether the patient actually called for help

immediately after the attempt if it was not immediately discovered, and whether the patient calculated correctly whether the family would return in time to discover him or her or planned it so that he or she would not be discovered. *The most significant factor in assessing intended lethality is the possibility and probability of rescue as foreseen by the child or adolescent.*

When the patient is able or willing, the physician should investigate the child's frame of mind, the degree of hopelessness, helplessness, or overwhelming shame or guilt, and the presence or absence of anger, and whether directed against others or self. The degree of depression should be carefully evaluated both in terms of the seriousness of the attempt and whether or not the patient presents a continued risk. It is also important to determine whether or not the child acted out of a psychotic delusion or paranoid ideation, or as the result of such hallucinatory experiences as might produce intolerable anxiety or panic—all of which are very high risk factors. Some psychotic and some young children have feelings of magical omnipotence that nothing can hurt or kill them; it is important to assess this possibility.

After the patient has recovered from the effects of attempted suicide, it is important to assess the frame of mind, to determine whether the intent to suicide persists or whether there is now a more optimistic sense of being able to solve or to seek help for problems in a manner other than through suicide. It is important to know whether the patient has some sense of what the immediate future may hold or feels that the future may not be totally hopeless or bleak.

When suicidal patients have been seen in the physician's office or in an emergency room, it is often best to admit them for a day or more to the hospital, so that a more adequate evaluation can be made of the patient's frame of mind and of the circumstances of the family or environment. Such admissions usually require only 2 or 3 days, unless medical needs require a longer stay or unless serious psychiatric disorders are found, such as severe depression or psychosis. If social services and psychiatric assessment are adequate and arrangements for appropriate follow-up care can be made, disposition can be fairly rapidly made. The physician must give careful attention to how family and friends have responded to the patient's act. A hostile and angry family, such as is frequently found, will indicate a different disposition or resolution than a family that is supportive, sympathetic, and understanding. Some families may deny completely the seriousness of the behavior; this can be quite discouraging or provocative to a patient whose act has been a desperate attempt to get a different response. It is important that family members examine their roles in the interactions that preceded an attempted suicide, without being made overly guilty. Judgments about the supportiveness of the family are essential to deciding whether a patient can return home immediately or not.

In planning care of patients after suicidal threats or attempts, the physician must consider the following:

1. Has the patient been restored physiologically? For example, have the effects of drugs cleared? What is the state of consciousness, orientation, memory, attention, concentration, and so on? Many drugs produce an acute brain syndrome or delirium that persists after the coma or stupor has lifted.

2. Is the patient less depressed, or has the depression simply become submerged? This may be difficult to determine quickly, and may require a psychiatric consultant who is familiar with children. The family may sometimes help determine if or when the patient seems to be more like his or her usual self.

3. Does the patient appreciate the seriousness of what he or she tried to do, and did he or she want to die? Does the wish to die persist? Answers to these questions may indicate

that the patient needs a psychiatric hospitalization or an immediate referral to a psychiatric facility before any final decision about a return to home and community can be made.

4. Are the precipitating events or other reasons that provoked the suicidal behavior still actively influential? The answer requires assessment of the family and of the environment by physician, social worker, nurse, or mental health professional.

5. Have the family, friends, teachers, or other persons significant to the patient responded in a relatively positive manner? It is important to determine whether parents or other significant adults have recovered from their anger or excessive guilt, since the child will need their functional support when he or she returns home. Have parents and child been able to identify for themselves some changes that they can make in order to improve relationships in the home, at school, or in the neighborhood?

6. Does the child show evidence of a future orientation? Has the child something to look forward to when he or she returns home? This may be as simple as going out with friends, attending a sports event, or an outing with the family.

7. Have the child's anger and disappointment, shame, guilt, depression, grief, and other strong feelings moderated or remitted to the point that he or she feels in better control and less at the mercy of impulses and feelings? It is particularly important to assess whether hopelessness and helplessness have declined and whether a sense of control over one's life or one's situation has reappeared.

Whenever possible, every suicidal attempt or threat should initiate a psychiatric or mental health consultation at the time of the event, or shortly thereafter. This may be in the emergency room or hospital, or by immediate referral to a local mental health practitioner or facility. The motivation and willingness of the family may be crucial to the success of referral, since the child is frequently unable to accept this on his or her own. Usually it is best for the physician to make personal contact with the referral resource, in addition to encouraging and enabling the family to do so. Follow-up care should be arranged.

2.45 CONDUCT DISTURBANCES IN EARLY CHILDHOOD

Around the ages of 2–3 yr children begin to develop a need for some autonomy, a sense of wanting and being able to do things their own way. They do not, however, have the full range of motor or social skills to be successful. Frustration and much anger may result. Common manifestations of anger are crying and screaming, breath-holding spells, temper tantrums, and physical aggression against objects or people.

Breath-holding is fairly common in the first 2 yr of life. Parents are best advised to leave the room when a child makes such attempts to control parental behavior; this leaves the child without reinforcement for the behavior, which soon disappears. A few children hold their breath until they lose consciousness for a few seconds. Such children have no increased risk of seizure disorders later on.

Defiance, oppositional behavior, and *temper tantrums* are all related to the child's learning how to express aggression. A child should learn that expression of anger in appropriate ways is an acceptable and important part of his or her life. Children can be frightened by the strength of their own angry feelings, or by the intensity of angry feelings that they arouse in their parents. It is not often apparent, though it is true, that children are as concerned as their parents about learning to control their own anger. When children successfully control themselves, they should be praised. And it is also of prime importance that parents provide those models in control of their own anger and aggressive feelings that they wish their children to follow. Many parents who are horrified at their children's loss of control of anger are unable to see that they have often lost control themselves; they are not, therefore, helping their children to internalize controls. Physicians must learn from the parents how they handle anger before making recommendations about how the child's problems are to be helped.

Defiant and oppositional behavior is to some extent normal in the older toddler, as an effort to achieve a sense of autonomy or individuality. This oppositional behavior should be accepted by parents so long as it does not go beyond the parents' own limits. The child at this age needs to know that his or her parents are going to be reassuring in a calm and firm way. A technique for dealing with children who have strong oppositional feelings is to provide them with choices, both or all choices being ones that the parents can accept. This gives the child a feeling that he or she has some options, with the knowledge also that the parents are still in the background, able to keep things from getting out of control. If a child becomes irrational and extremely angry, parents may have the child go to his or her room, or leave the child and become busy in some other part of the house. Children sometimes substitute a younger brother or sister as the object for anger, when parents are too threatening to confront.

A distinction is to be made between *temper outbursts* and full-blown *temper tantrums*. In the former the child is angry, but still has some control over feelings and can at times respond to a calm approach on the part of parents who accept the anger. When the stage of temper tantrum is reached, the child no longer has either control or an observing ego, except that he or she remains aware that the frustrating parent is still within scope. In this latter case, no form of verbalization will control the child's behavior. It is then important for the parent to separate physically from the child. Parents can sometimes divert their children to other activities before they reach the point of loss of control, or help them to isolate themselves voluntarily until they feel better. It is important not to demean the child or make fun of his or her angry state. Such behavior tends to send confusing messages to children; they may develop the notion that their behavior is desired by parents who seem to be getting perverse pleasure from it. Children need to know that angry feelings are normal, but that the control of excessive anger is an important part of growing up and being mature.

Stealing can sometimes be an expression of anger or of revenge for real or imagined frustration by parents. It is also evidence that the child's internalization of controls has not reached a level where temptation can be resisted. Stealing is sometimes learned from parents. Parents, for instance, who boast of outwitting tax laws or of exceeding speed limits or getting away with other illegal practices are telling their children that these are acceptable forms of behavior. Another formulation that leads children to steal is their sense of the lack or loss of something, perhaps on an emotional level, such as a feeling of not being cared for. Stealing in these cases is a concrete effort to replace the loss. Finally, it appears that in many instances of children's stealing there is a strong element of the child's wanting to be caught, almost as if the theft were arranged so that a confrontation with the parents could serve the child's need for an "emotional reward." Children may find, in effect, that this is one way in which they can compel parents to show an intense feeling toward them, and this gives them a power over their parents that they cannot resist using.

Whatever the cause of stealing, it is important that parents help the child to undo the theft by returning the stolen articles, or by rendering their equivalent either in money that the child can earn or in services. When it is apparent that children are not able to control temptation, money and valuable objects should not be left in their paths to increase the chances of stealing. Almost all children steal something at some time during their childhood. It is important to respond to the event appropriately. It is also important that the act not be overemphasized, lest the behavior or the response to it become so exciting that it is reproduced in future periods of discontent.

Lying is another conduct problem commonly brought to the attention of physicians by concerned parents. It is important first to determine whether a lying child is developmentally capable of understanding what he or she has said or whether the parents may be misinterpreting statements that sound untruthful to them but may not be so intended by the child. In one sense, lying is a form of fantasy for the child, who is describing things as they are wished rather than as they are. For instance, a child who has not done something that a parent wanted done may say that it has been done in order to avoid an unpleasant confrontation. The child's sense of time does not permit the realization that this only postpones an even angrier confrontation. Some children lie because they seem to enjoy masochistically the response of their upset parents. Most often, lying seems to represent children's not wanting to accept the pain of a relative loss of self-esteem. That is, most lying is an effort to cover up something that the child does not want to accept in his or her behavior. The lie is invented, therefore, to achieve temporary good feeling. Finally, lying, like stealing, can be the result of parental modeling, in which case the child's interpretations of reality are often conflicting, confusing, or unclear. For instance, when mothers and fathers accuse each other frequently of lying, the child may become hopelessly unsure of how the word lying is to be interpreted; moreover, a loyalty conflict is added to the already distorted process of reality testing.

For the child who presents a history of repeated accidents or of *accident-prone behavior,* a complete assessment of physical, psychologic, and developmental status should be made, together with a careful evaluation of family and especially parental interactions. The child's impulsivity and self-harm may be related to problems of marital discord, or the withdrawal or depression of a parent. The preoccupations of parents with their own needs and interests can markedly reduce their investment in activities as parents. Unresolved parental anger, resentment, or ambivalence toward the child can also result in neglect of normal considerations of safety. As children get older, their risky, careless behaviors may become intended or unconscious ways of getting parental attention, or such behavior may reflect the child's own perception of not being wanted. Children thus internalize negative views of themselves and behave as though they do not care about their safety.

When a physician judges that accident proneness does not primarily depend on a parental or marital disturbance, he or she can rely on careful instructions to the parents to protect the child and to decrease hazards and risk to health and safety. On the other hand, if accident proneness is judged to be a sign of emotional disturbance in the child or to reflect a parental or family disturbance, then the physician should refer the family to a family service or children's service agency or to a mental health clinic or consultant.

2.46 ATTENTION DEFICIT DISORDER
(Hyperactive Syndrome)

The term *attention deficit disorder* (ADD) designates the central disturbances of a group of children heretofore labeled as suffering from hyperactivity, hyperkinesis, minimal brain damage, or minimal cerebral dysfunction. Subgroups of chil-

dren with attention deficit disorder include those *with* hyperactivity, those *without* hyperactivity, and a residual type. Criteria for diagnosis of each of these types are detailed in the DSM–III Manual of the American Psychiatric Association. Hyperactivity, once thought to be the core symptom of this syndrome, is not always present, and tends to improve or disappear as the child becomes older. Difficulty in maintaining attention, and impulsivity, are more consistent problems. The overlap of these symptoms with other problem behaviors is enormous: it is estimated that in children showing aggressiveness and/or hyperactivity, only 17% were exclusively hyperactive and 18% exclusively aggressive—65% showed a combination of the two traits. This finding supports mounting evidence that conduct disorder and attention deficit often coexist, and perhaps represent a spectrum of, rather than discrete, conditions. Since learning disorders are common in both ADD and conduct disorders, it is quite possible that these diagnostic categories are expressions of a common underlying condition or group of conditions.

Etiology. Opinions vary as to the origin and features of this disorder. Some believe the disorder results from disturbances in the neurochemistry or neurophysiology of the central nervous system, with metabolites of brain catecholamines (norepinephrine and dopamine) receiving particular attention. Phenylethylamine (PEA) excretion has shown promise as a biological marker for ADD. The syndrome has been attributed to a number of gestational or noxious factors, including lead poisoning, birth complications (prematurity, trauma, or anoxia), temperament, child-rearing practices, and allergic reactions. Recent studies have emphasized a genetic component.

Incidence. Depending on its definition, an attention deficit disorder with hyperactivity is estimated to occur in 5–10% of school-age children. Specific learning disabilities overlap with hyperactivity. The incidence of hyperactivity in boys is 4–6 times that in girls.

Clinical Manifestations. About twice as many children with an attention deficit have motor overactivity as do not. Evidence suggests that these two conditions have significant differences: Hyperactive children have been found to demonstrate aggressive behavior with little expression of guilt, to have poor school performance, and to be very unpopular with peers. Nonhyperactive children with ADD were anxious and socially withdrawn and, in addition to poor academic performance, had difficulty in sports. In general, children with ADD have short attention spans, are distractable and impulsive, and tend to act without considering or reflecting upon the consequences. They have a low tolerance for frustration and are emotionally labile and excitable. Their moods tend to be neutral or oppositional; they are frequently gregarious, but socially clumsy. Some are hostile and negative, but these traits are often secondary to the psychosocial problems they experience (Sec. 2.37 and 2.61). Some are excessively dependent; others are so independent as to be foolhardy.

Emotional and behavioral difficulties are common, and are related to the negative social impact of the behavior. Affected children receive criticism and punishment from parents and teachers, and social ostracism from peers. They fail chronically at academic tasks, and many are not well enough coordinated or self-controlled to be successful at sports. They have a poor self-image and low self-esteem, and frequently suffer from depression. There is a high incidence of learning disabilities in reading, mathematics, spelling, and handwriting. Academic performances may lag by 2 yr or more, and lower than would be expected based on measured intelligence.

Past and Developmental History. Probably the most important tools in evaluation are the developmental history and the teacher's report of academic problems and behavior in the classroom. The history is often diagnostic: typically, the mother remembers the baby as alert, active, and demanding, with intense emotional responses, with feeding and sleeping difficulties in the early months; usually the baby was difficult to get quiet at bedtime and slow to establish diurnal rhythms. Colic is rather commonly reported. Developmental milestones are usually normal; some children stand, walk, and run quite early. As toddlers, these children are "into everything," constantly intrusive and demanding, and their mothers learn that they need constant supervision to keep out of mischief or danger.

Diagnosis. It is difficult among 2–4 yr old children to identify those who will develop hyperactivity from those who are simply active, boisterous, and gregarious. The latter learn during the preschool period to master motor output, to maintain attention and concentration, and to modulate social behavior in preparation for school. The pediatrician should be alert to the possibility of nascent hyperactive syndrome in toddlers or preschool children as part of normal longitudinal assessment. Mothers who describe their children as hyperactive should not be told they "will outgrow it," nor should stimulant or other medication be given without adequate study (see below).

To assess accurately the term "hyperactive" the physician needs descriptions of behavior; these will clarify the expectations of parents and reveal their levels of tolerance for motor activity such as running, playing, shouting, and so on. Parents who value physical and emotional control may judge a normally active boy or girl as hyperactive or "bad." The physician must assess the psychosocial structure within which judgments of "normal," "hyperactive," "deviant," or "stubborn" are made.

The initial identification of children as "hyperactive" commonly occurs as they enter nursery or elementary school. Their teachers report that they are uncontrollable, can't sit still, intrude into the space and activities of other children, are boisterous and inattentive, won't concentrate, or won't follow instructions. They are often said to provoke others to anger, not to seem to hear instructions, not to learn from mistakes, and not to respond to the usual disciplinary actions. Parents may report many of the same traits, their prior management perhaps reflecting their range of tolerance or their experience with other children. Some children with attention deficit syndrome are clumsy, but others are well coordinated, meeting the physical requirements of sports or games but having difficulty with social requirements, with keeping to the rules, paying attention, and concentrating. They may be particularly disabled in activities requiring cooperation.

Affected children are frequently unable to sit still, even for television. They may quietly watch a television program they like but be disruptive and intrusive when they have little interest. The dinner table is an arena of frustration and conflict.

Clinical Evaluation. Children with attention deficits not uncommonly maintain good control in the physician's examining room, sitting quietly, paying attention, and responding to directions. The physician should not be misled; these children may be suppressing characteristic behavior in this structured situation free of the distractions and demands of home or school. The most useful information is often obtained from adult observers—parents and teachers. Behavior rating scales can help describe and quantify behavior (Conners).

Physical examination does not generally contribute to the diagnosis. Children with attention deficits are generally believed to show increased numbers of neurologic "soft signs." The diagnostic precision of these findings is debatable, since they occur in learning disabled children as well as in Gilles de la Tourette syndrome. They include mixed hand preference, impaired balance, astereognosis, dysdiadochokinesia,

and choreiform movements. A recent study found that impairments of short-term memory, fine motor performance, synkinesis and awareness of laterality were more specifically related to ADD.

Laboratory and Other Studies. No laboratory studies establish the diagnosis of attention deficit disorder. Children with hyperactivity are reported to have increased content of slow waves in the electroencephalogram without evidence of progressive neurologic disease or epilepsy, but this finding has doubtful significance. EEG spectra and event-related potentials have been analyzed by computer to diagnose children with learning problems, but these techniques are not widely available. For children whose history suggests the possibility of lead poisoning, the blood lead level should be measured.

Psychologic and Psychoeducational Testing. It is uncertain whether hyperactive children with attention deficit syndrome have significantly lower IQ scores than children appropriately matched for age, school grade level, socioeconomic status, and the like who do not have this syndrome. Some hyperactive children have verbal scores more than 10 points higher than performance scores on the Wechsler Intelligence Scale for Children (WISC) and lower scores on the attention/concentration subset. Educational levels, as measured on the Peabody Individual Achievement Test (PIAT), Woodcock-Johnson Psychoeducational Battery, or Wide Range Achievement Test (WRAT) may be lower than expected for age or IQ in one or several areas. More specific tests for learning disabilities, such as the Woodcock Reading Mastery Test or the Key Math Diagnostic Test, can then be administered to pinpoint areas of difficulty. The Vineland Adaptive Behavior Scale can be used to gauge a child's socialization skills. Projective tests such as the Thematic Apperception Test (TAT) and Rorschach are not helpful in diagnosis of attention deficit disorder, though they may provide information on psychodynamics and on emotional strengths and weaknesses.

Differential Diagnosis. Sensory impairment, particularly auditory, should be investigated in children who present with difficulty concentrating. Hyperactivity and learning disabilities often occur together; the child suspected of having one should be evaluated for the other. Children with problems in sustaining attention may also have problems in learning, but such problems are not called a "learning disability." The latter term refers to those problems which arise out of perceptual-motor difficulties, such as those described in Sec. 2.63, and affect achievement in reading and/or mathematics. Convulsive disorders, particularly petit mal, may produce apparent lack of concentration or attention, but children with petit mal do not have an attention deficit disorder unless these disorders coexist. Certain medications, including anticonvulsants such as phenobarbital, have been implicated in producing hyperactivity and attention problems in at least some children. Children whose activity, boisterousness, and aggressiveness are at the upper extreme of normal usually respond to appropriate techniques of socialization and discipline, and rapidly learn to maintain the attention, concentration, and impulse control required in a structured environment. Children suffering from depressive disorders (Sec. 2.43) may show increased activity and social disturbances, but they do not have the characteristic history of excessive activity and impulsivity in early life. Conduct disorders and Gilles de la Tourette syndrome may coexist with ADD.

Treatment. Treatment of children with attention deficit disorders is directed at the social environment of the home and classroom and at the child's personal academic and psychosocial needs, with judicious use of medication. A clear explanation of the child's condition must be given both to the parents and to the child.

A program that will give structure to the child's environment will decrease the effects of the handicap and help in academic and social learning. The children should have a regular daily routine, which they are expected to follow promptly and for which they are rewarded with praise. Rules should be simple, clear, and as few as possible, and coupled with firm limits, enforced fairly and sympathetically through restrictions or deprivations for transgressions. Overstimulation and excessive fatigue should be avoided. The child will need time for relaxation after play, particularly after vigorous physical activity. The period before bedtime should be quiet, with avoidance of exciting television programs and rough and tumble games. It is probably best that young children with attention deficit syndrome who are hyperactive not be taken on long trips by automobile or on extensive shopping trips. The confined space of the car and the excessive stimulation in large stores may intensify the child's symptoms. The home should be arranged so that all valuable, dangerous, or breakable objects are out of the reach of the young child. Parents should reward even partially successful efforts at control of behavior or academic responsibilities with recognition, affection, and regular praise. Often helpful are more formal operant conditioning techniques that reward the child with stars or tokens (exchangeable for toys and activities), contingent upon improved behavior.

Medication. Medication is often an integral part of the treatment of attention deficit disorder. A variety of medications are used, the most common and safe being the stimulants. Dextroamphetamine and magnesium pemoline are members of this class, but the stimulant most widely used and with the fewest side effects is methylphenidate. These drugs probably modify fundamental disturbances in attention span, concentration, and impulsivity. Since the response to medication is difficult to predict, a clinical trial is usually required; 2–3 wk of daily medication may be needed, with adjustments in dosage, to determine whether a beneficial effect will occur. To know the effect of stimulant medications, the physician should obtain reports from teachers and parents every 5–7 days; a standardized scale, such as that developed by Conners, can be used for this purpose.

The daily dosage range for methylphenidate is 0.3–1.0 mg/kg, and for dextroamphetamine is 0.2–0.5 mg/kg (see Table 2–14). Although dextroamphetamine tablets and sustained release preparations have a longer half-life than methylphenidate, the therapeutic effect of amphetamine preparations is reported to be no longer than 4 hr. Methylphenidate tablets generally have an effect over a period of 2–4 hr; the sustained release form, available only in 20 mg tablets, may last longer, but has not been well studied to date. Initial work with plasma levels of methylphenidate suggested that there may be a differential response of target symptoms to dosage levels, with attention improving optimally at 0.3 mg/kg, but behavior ameliorating at 1.0 mg/kg. A more recent study indicates a linear improvement in both target symptoms as dosage increases from 0.3 to 0.8 mg/kg.

The effect of magnesium pemoline on hyperactivity develops more slowly and lasts about 12 hr. Initial doses of 18.75 mg (half of the 37.5 mg tablet) have been suggested, to be increased by a half tablet/wk (see Table 2–14). Three to 4 wk are required to determine its efficacy. About 1–2% of children treated with magnesium pemoline may show changes in liver function; accordingly, pre-treatment studies and the monitoring of liver function are required. Side effects include increased nervousness and jitteriness.

Dextroamphetamine and methylphenidate can be given with or after meals to minimize appetite suppression. They should not be given after 3–4 PM to avoid insomnia. The response to both medications, if they are at a therapeutic level, is noticeable soon after medication is started. The child should be less fidgety and hyperactive, less impulsive, and better able to concentrate. Children who do not respond show little or no change in behavior with increasing doses. Parents or teachers may report that the child is worse. Before a child is judged to be unresponsive, a full therapeutic trial should be undertaken, so long as side effects are not serious.

With onset of treatment some children become tearful and sensitive to criticism, whereas they may have earlier seemed impervious to correction, criticism, or punishment. The reaction should subside after 1–2 wk; if it persists, reduction of dosage or a change of medication should be considered. Other short-term side effects include drowsiness, headaches, tics, and nail biting. With chronic medication some children develop a pale, sallow, drawn, glassy-eyed appearance; it is not thought to represent a significant disturbance, but can be distressing to child and parents. If these effects do not abate with decreases in dose, another medication may be tried.

Major short-term side effects include anorexia, upper abdominal pain, and difficulty in going to sleep. Upper abdominal pain is usually without nausea or vomiting and usually responds to a decrease in dose; suspension of medication is rarely required. It is best to avoid the use of sedative drugs to treat the sleep disturbance.

Long-term effects include increased heart rate and growth suppression. The implications of increased heart rate are not clear; there may be a chronic increase in the workload of the heart. The issue of growth suppression is controversial. Kalachnik et al found no suppression at dosages of methylphenidate as high as 0.8 mg/kg/day, even after 3 yr. By contrast, Mattes and Gittelman reported a drop in height of 2 percentile points in children who had taken an average of 40 mg/day for 2–4 yr. Moreover, the effect seemed directly related to cumulative dosage. It is certainly wise to monitor the growth of children receiving stimulants and to employ drug-free holidays (weekends, holidays, summer vacation) when practical. Stopping the medication each summer permits parents and the child to reassess the need for continued medication. A drug-free period of 2–3 wk a year should routinely be tried for this purpose.

The age range benefiting from stimulant medication is longer than once thought, embracing adolescents and even adults with attention deficits. Stimulants are not approved by the FDA for children under the age of 6 yr. There is no evidence that children treated with stimulant drugs are at increased risk of becoming abusers of such drugs in adolescence. Quite commonly an overemphasis on medication develops, involving both the child and important adults in the child's life. The child may receive anxious inquiries each morning, or in every case of an emotional outburst, as to whether he or she has taken the medication, rather than more appropriate and helpful attempts at intervention. More importantly, improvements in the child's behavior and performance are attributed to the medication alone, creating the illusion of a "chemical conscience," whereas a more beneficial practice would be to praise the child for making progress. These pitfalls should be avoided since they deny the child the discipline and positive reinforcement needed in order to gain a sense of self-mastery and self-esteem.

Other medications have been used to treat attention deficit disorder. Some studies report tricyclic antidepressants to be very effective in ameliorating symptoms of ADD, but they have more side effects (Sec. 2.56 and Table 2.14). They should be used if stimulants are not effective. Phenothiazines, and particularly thioridazine, may moderate the child's motor behavior. They are less attractive than stimulant medication because of their side effects: somnolence, irritability, and dysphoria. The more obtunded child will probably have no improvement in attention or concentration at school. The combination of a phenothiazine and a stimulant may be effective in children who are not helped by either type of drug given alone. The use of stimulants for children with tics or a family history of tics is controversial, since there is evidence that Gilles de la Tourette syndrome may be precipitated. Some children unresponsive to stimulant medication may derive benefit from the mildly tranquilizing effects of diphenhydramine or hydroxyzine. Diphenhydramine has been used in children under 6 yr of age; fairly high doses are required.

The benefits and disadvantages of medication must be weighed carefully by the physician, with full disclosure to parents, and to the child as well, within the limits of his or her understanding. Informed consent is a necessary condition for effective treatment, since adequate management of the hyperactive child with the attention deficit syndrome requires parents and child to sustain a regimen that may last for many years. The trust and confidence established in an initial working alliance between parents, child, and physician are of paramount importance. An important strategy is to engage the hyperactive child increasingly in responsibility for his or her own management to the degree permitted by age, understanding, and emotional stability. This assumption of responsibility involves not only medication but social and academic behaviors.

School. The child with the attention deficit syndrome with hyperactivity often has a learning disability, and may need any of the special educational approaches prescribed for learning disabilities. Some children may be maintained in regular class placement with additional tutoring. Special classes frequently use contingency or operant conditioning for behavior modification; when carefully planned and carried out by teachers well grounded in theory and practice, such approaches can help these children. In fact, behavior therapy can be more efficacious than medication for treating certain problems, especially aggression. It is essential that physician and school personnel maintain close communication about the child's progress. Decisions about medication or about referral to a mental health facility may well depend foremost upon the information obtained from a cooperative and perceptive teacher.

Psychotherapy. When severe psychosocial difficulties have produced serious family distress and parents are ineffective in carrying out a prescribed regimen, referral to a mental health professional or an appropriate mental health clinic is indicated. There is no conclusive evidence that psychotherapy is primarily beneficial in the attention deficit syndrome, but individual and family therapy is indicated when ADD is complicated by depression, social withdrawal or negativism, eroded self-esteem, or chronic family conflict.

Other Therapies. Few conditions have generated as many controversial approaches as has ADD. There is little evidence to support the use of dietary treatment. No evidence exists for a positive effect of diets utilizing megavitamins, restricting sugar, or supplementing trace minerals. A small percentage of affected children (5–10%) may respond to diets low in food additives or coloring; even for those children, it is not clear that such treatment is superior to more conventional approaches. When a physician chooses one of these therapies, owing to personal preference or to parental pressure, certain untoward effects should be kept in mind. Megavitamin treatment carries a risk of toxicity due to overdosage. For diets having many restrictions, the child is likely to experience a sense of deprivation and of being punished that will exacerbate the negative feelings and self-perceptions that have already resulted.

Prognosis. The attention deficit syndrome may last through childhood and adolescence, and also into adulthood. The random motor movements and social intrusiveness may diminish, but learning disabilities and behavioral and psychosocial problems may become even more intense and handicapping in late childhood and adolescence. An optimistic prognosis can be made if the child can succeed sufficiently at learning to make progress through school approximately with his or her age group, and if the secondary psychosocial effects can be ameliorated by a supportive family.

2.47 AGGRESSIVE BEHAVIOR AND AGGRESSIVE DISORDERS

Aggression is a problem both of normal development and of psychosocial disturbance. There is no totally satisfactory theory of the nature and causes of human aggressive behavior, though various disciplines have contributed to partial understanding of its nature and control. Some believe that aggression is primarily innate or instinctual; studies of aggression in fish, birds and lower mammals, subhuman primates, and man reveal certain similarities. A common finding is that certain configurations of stimuli give rise to aggressive responses, especially those involving territory, mating, food, protection of the nest and young, and social hierarchy. A striking observation of many studies is that intraspecies aggression is rarely fatal, particularly in subhuman primates.

In the development of psychoanalytic theory Freud named aggression as one of the two basic drives, conceiving of it as a death instinct in contrast to a life instinct. Later theorists have paired an aggressive instinct with the sexual instinct as two basic drives. In accounting for the perpetuation of aggressive behaviors, learning theories stress conditioning and contingency theories stress positive reinforcement. Social theorists suggest that modern crowding, the breakdown in commonly shared values, the demise of traditional family patterns of child-rearing in kinship systems, and social alienation both in individuals and in large groups are leading to increased aggression in children, adolescents, and adults. Aggression in children has also been correlated with familial unemployment, discord, criminality, and psychiatric disorders.

There are individual constitutional differences within species. For example, boys are almost universally reported more aggressive than girls. In many animals, giving male sex hormones to females produces more aggressive behavior. Larger children are often more aggressive than smaller ones. More active and intrusive children are perceived as more aggressive. Other dimensions of temperament also influence aggressive activity (Sec. 2.17).

Aggressive behavior that results in some kind of injury may be distinguished from initiative behavior that intrudes upon the environment for the sake of learning, mastering, or achieving. Many hyperactive, clumsy children are termed aggressive because of the accidental results of their behavior, their intentions being benign. Intentional aggression may be primarily *instrumental*, to achieve an end, or primarily *hostile*, part of the motivation of the latter being to inflict physical or psychologic pain. Clinically, it is important to attempt to differentiate among these motives. Other factors needing attention in assessment include the developmental level and circumstances of the child, the social acceptance accorded the child, the models the child may have for aggression, the possibility of emotional disturbances, and familial, social or subcultural patterns of behavior.

The child of 2–5 yr may show aggressive outbursts ranging from temper tantrums and screaming to hurting others or destroying toys and furniture. In these situations aggressive behavior frequently arises out of particular frustrations. Usually such aggressive behavior in 2–3 yr olds is directed toward the parents in response to demands for performance or compliance, or as a response to frustration of the wishes or intent of the child. By the age of 4–5 yr such behavior is more likely to be directed at siblings or peers, owing to the greater social interaction at these ages. Verbal aggression increases between the ages of 2 and 4 yr, and after the age of 3 yr revenge and retaliation become more prominent as determinants of aggression.

Aggressive behavior in boys is relatively stable from the preschool period through adolescence; a boy with a high level of aggressive behavior in the period between 3 and 6 yr of age has a high probability of carrying this behavior into adolescence. On the other hand, a study reveals that girls under 6 yr old who were aggressive toward their peers did not continue to be aggressive at older ages, nor did this earlier aggression correlate with adult competitiveness. This is probably because aggressive girls suffer anxiety in the conflict between competitiveness and development of the traditional gender role.

Aggressive children have also been noted to have an increased incidence of underlying reading disorder; incarcerated youths have been shown to have a high incidence of neuropsychological impairment and psychiatric illness.

Frustration is commonly viewed as the response to those conditions that bar an individual from achieving goals important to self-esteem or that create internal conflicts between incompatible responses. Frustration and aggression are closely associated: the frustrated individual responds with aggressive behavior to a degree depending on his or her personality. If a child learns that reacting aggressively against sources of frustration removes them, this experience reinforces the aggressive behavior, and may cause it to be perpetuated. But in making judgments about aggressive behavior one should take into account the age of the child, the stage of development, the nature of the environment, and whether what is termed aggression is a misplaced attempt to persevere in the face of obstacles or to engage in appropriate problem solving. It is important not to attribute malice to the child whose aggression is really self-assertion in response to anxieties or feelings of incompetence or low self-esteem.

Children exposed to aggressive models on television or in play, whether these models be other children, adults, or cartoon figures, will display increased aggressive behavior when compared with children not exposed to these models. Parents also must understand that their anger and aggressive or harsh punishment will model behavior that children may imitate when they themselves have been physically or psychologically hurt.

Our culture provides universal support for violence and aggressive behavior through literature, films, and television, and the influence is significant. As nations attempt to solve problems by aggression, so adults attempt to satisfy their needs or to right wrongs through aggressive and violent behaviors ranging from personal assault, murder, and rape to terrorist activities against individuals or social institutions. Societies, in turn, respond with aggressive counterbehavior in dealing with suspected or actual perpetrators of crime. Reports of police brutality, of the violence of parents or teachers against children, and of riots and confrontations all create a climate in which, unfortunately, violence is seen as a legitimate and even valued means of solving human problems or of dealing with human conflict.

2.48 PASSIVE-AGGRESSIVE BEHAVIOR

The *passive-aggressive* child expresses hostility indirectly, as procrastination, "forgetting," dawdling, stubbornness, resistance, or "willful" behavior. Parents often complain that such children don't hear them and that they fail to respond to repeated requests. Academic underachievement is common. Their early histories may reveal excessive negativism during the infancy and toddler periods, feeding disturbances, and problems in bladder and bowel training.

Children may unconsciously adopt passive-aggressive strategies for a variety of motives: to gain independence while maintaining dependency; to counter underlying low self-esteem; to maintain control and autonomy when threatened by anxiety; and to get revenge. Children using these strategies are essentially fearful of direct expression of aggression and hostility; consequently, anger is disguised through passive-aggressive maneuvers. The child-rearing styles of their parents are often intimidating, critical, and authoritarian, or on the other hand indulgent and permissive. Both children and parents may find it difficult to deal directly and overtly with anger, and neither may be able to acknowledge the anger that contributes to and is generated by the passive-aggressive behavior. Physicians should encourage parents to handle passive-aggressive behavior by setting firm limits and expectations for the child. The parents and the child should reach agreement upon what they will consider his or her most important tasks and responsibilities. Deficiencies in lesser or minor areas should be temporarily overlooked so that confrontations over unimportant issues are avoided. Age-appropriate assertiveness and independence should be promoted and rewarded. The more refractory cases require psychiatric intervention to reveal and modify the underlying psychodynamics.

2.49 DEPENDENCY

The *dependent child* is inhibited in self-expression, shy, and fearful in social situations, often described as "sensitive" and "easily hurt." Dependent children tend to cling to parents and to avoid taking initiatives, unconsciously wishing and arranging that others take care of them. Recreational activities and peer group interactions may be shunned because of fear of competition and injury. Dependent children have frequently been overprotected and overindulged by parents, and their development of normal independence and autonomy has been hindered. The child is often viewed by the parents as sickly and fragile, even when any physical illnesses have been minor.

Successful management depends on the parents' willingness to encourage the child to take the normal risks of growing up. The pediatrician should support and reassure parents, as they assist the child in meeting new situations in small, calibrated steps. Nursery school for the preschool child and organized recreational activities for the older child are helpful initial steps in aiding the child's psychologic separation from parents. Any small change toward more independent and autonomous function should be praised and rewarded. Expectations should not be raised too high too quickly. If supportive advice and direction are unavailing, psychiatric intervention should be considered.

2.50 THE SCHIZOID CHILD

The *schizoid child* is characterized not only by limited socialization skills but also by seeming not to desire any. Schizoid children are not out of touch with reality, delusional, or having hallucinations, but they resemble in some ways adults with simple schizophrenia. Their interests seem shallow, their energies limited. The schizoid child can often become obsessed with some limited activity and appear quite content. Since such children generate few demands on their parents or teachers, their illness can remain undetected. They are not mentally retarded but emotionally and socially immature.

They may appear neither to have nor to want substantial friendships, whereas shy or withdrawn children want to be involved with others but are too fearful. The latter children may be quite animated and friendly in their family groups but not at school.

The schizoid child may have some inborn neurophysiologic disorder, but this is not proved. Schizoid children are at risk for more serious disorders in late adolescence and young adulthood unless they are well protected and their lives structured for them. Under stress they may become frankly psychotic or adopt antisocial behavior. As the child gets older, there may be deterioration in intellectual abilities; the child may come to resemble a person with organic brain damage.

Parents of schizoid children need long-term guidance and help in providing socialization experiences for their children. They will have to be firm in supporting and implementing activities that enhance ego growth, even though the child is reluctant. Medication is of little or no help. Diagnostic assessment should be made as early in the child's life as the above pattern can be recognized. Evaluation can be made through a child psychiatrist or a mental health clinic.

2.51 VARIATIONS IN SEXUAL BEHAVIOR

Children are naturally curious—about the world around them, about other people, and about themselves. Their bodies are of particular interest, following the discovery of body parts in the first year of life. The 2 yr old child can and ought to be told the proper names for the parts of his or her body, including the genital parts. It is to be hoped that the child's exploration, manipulation, and enjoyment of his or her own body, including the genitals, will be met with calm understanding on the part of the parents, rather than with anxiety or anger.

Young boys and girls commonly undress together and engage in looking and touching behavior involving the genitalia. In preschool children hugging, kissing, and perhaps lying on top of each other may be the extent of the physical contact, genital behavior being usually confined to mutual touching and stroking. Preschool children who engage in more explicit sexual behavior, such as oral contacts, attempts at simulated intercourse, or anal stimulation, have probably learned such behavior by watching or being involved in such activities by older children or adults. The majority of sexual abuses against young children are perpetrated by adolescents or adults well known to the child, often by family members, and sometimes with the tacit approval of or in default of supervision on the part of other responsible adults (Sec. 2.57 and 18.6).

Children can be advised that questions about sexual matters are natural and can be answered by their parents, by their doctor, or by books. There are many well designed, factual, and sensitive sex education materials, some distributed through such organizations as Planned Parenthood, religious groups, sex education societies, and other organizations, as well as through medical societies and public health organizations. Parents can be advised to explain to each child that his or her own body is private and personal, and that the same consideration applies to the bodies of other children.

Sexual interests and activities have had negative sanctions in Western culture, and still evoke strong emotions in adults. All adults, and physicians above all, should be extremely cautious in inferring meaning for the current or future sexual development of children from any isolated act or even a series of sexual acts. This is especially true for preschool children, though gender identity and gender role development are well advanced in preschool children (Sec. 2.24).

Transvestism may occur transiently as a part of normal development or it may be a chronic manifestation of a disturbance in gender identity or gender role. Preschool boys may frequently dress up in clothing of their mothers or sisters and strut around, sometimes to the delight and sometimes to the consternation of others. Parents rarely remark on "cross-dressing" in girls; in fact it is almost impossible to define the condition, since girls are permitted to wear "boys' clothing" from early childhood through adulthood. Neither fathers nor mothers should become angry, accusatory, or anxious about transient cross-dressing in little boys; nor should they be entertained by or encourage it. Ignoring the behavior or firmly but calmly discouraging it is probably the best means of handling it. At the same time, physicians and parents should understand that the transient behavior may be a sign of a more fundamental anxiety or concern on the part of the young boy, having to do with his discomfort with what he believes to be the masculine role.

Parental concern is warranted when transient cross-dressing becomes chronic and recurrent, or furtive, and when the boy dresses in girls' or women's underwear, pays a great deal of attention to jewelry and cosmetics, and seems uncomfortable with the usual activities of boys of his age. The physician should then investigate other areas of gender identification. Does the child verbalize a preference to be the opposite sex? Is the child preoccupied with the stereotypical activities and dress of the opposite sex (a characteristic harder to assess in girls than in boys)? Does the child deny or disparage his or her own sexual anatomy, or assert that he or she will develop the anatomical structures of the opposite sex? When these behaviors recur regularly and persistently despite parental disapproval, the possibility of a disturbance in gender role or sex identity needs to be considered, especially if the child is more than 5–6 yr old.

The pediatrician should not label the child as a transvestite, but merely note that he is showing episodes of cross-dressing behavior. Neither should it be inferred immediately by parents or clinician that the child is becoming or will become a homosexual. Transvestism usually appears after masculine identity has been established. The adult transvestite man does not question his being male, though he may be at times uncomfortable with his masculinity and manifest this discomfort by feminine behavior and cross-dressing. An essential characteristic of adult transvestite behavior is the man's knowledge that he has a penis. He may frequently become sexually aroused during periods of cross-dressing or develop fetishistic attachments to certain articles of women's clothing in order to obtain genital arousal and/or orgasm. The older pubertal child who persists in transvestite behavior may have the same experiences.

Transsexualism is the psychologic conviction in a person biologically (chromosomally, gonadally, hormonally, and genitally) belonging to one sex that he or she is a member of the other sex. Transsexualism is differentiated from homosexuality, transvestism, and effeminacy. In adults this has become a medically important entity, since hormonal and surgical treatment can accomplish a change of sex for both male and female transsexuals. The results of surgery, however, are controversial with respect to improvement in personal, social, or work adjustment. The true incidence of this disturbance among adults is unknown. In children the condition is rare; it has been reported, however, in male children ranging in age from 3 yr to puberty.

Transsexualism manifests itself in cross-dressing of an elaborate, persistent, and intransigent nature. It almost always arises from a psychologic conviction in the male child that he is or will become a woman. Studies of psychologic roots and early attitudes of transsexuals have found that evidence may have been apparent as early as within the first 18 mo of life.

By all measures currently known there are no biologic determinants, nor does it seem due to genetically inherited behaviors or dispositions. Affected boys adopt gestures, postures, gaits, voices, mannerisms, games, and interests that are feminine. They prefer to play almost exclusively with girls and willingly adopt female roles in various fantasy games.

Affected children are not psychotic; rather, they may be pleasant, creative, socially attractive to both peers and adults, intelligent, and articulate. Their behavior is not primarily characterized by overt erotic or sexual interaction with peers. Rather it is gender role behavior that belongs to the gender identity assumed, which may be encouraged and supported by the family dynamics. Stoller reports that the mothers of affected boys are uncertain about their own sexuality and not particularly active sexually, but not evidently homosexual. Their lives have frequently had a sense of emptiness, with no close interpersonal relationships. Their relationships with their own mothers seemed problematic and unrewarding. The fathers of these boys have been psychologically and physically absent, both to their children and to their wives. Stoller reports that the mothers of affected boys lavish physical attention upon them, not only as infants but through the preschool years. They are held, cuddled, petted, and allowed to be close to mother in bed, during bathing, and in dressing, as if there were no psychologic or physical boundary or social distance between mother and son. Mothers of affected boys characteristically gratify them completely, seeing their life's mission as giving these boys pleasure and rewarding their every whim and wish.

Exploring and counseling with parents regarding questions of gender role dysfunction requires great sensitivity and tact. Clinicians must be aware of their own anxiety in dealing with problems in this area, which may be expressed as punitiveness, disgust, brusque referral, or denial and avoidance. A successful referral to a mental health practitioner or agency may be crucial to helping parents and child in understanding the possible sources and meaning of the behavior. Such a referral may also help the child adapt with less distress to the conflict between somatic sex assignment and psychosocial role behaviors.

HOMOSEXUAL BEHAVIOR

Developmental same-sex (homosexual) behavior. Sexual behavior between members of the same sex is not uncommon in children; its incidence in relation to age and sex is not known. The impression that it is more common between boys is biased by a cultural sensitivity and anxiety about male homosexual behavior, as well as by the cultural stereotype that boys are intrinsically more interested and active sexually than girls. In addition, adult male homosexuality has been more publicly recognized. The physician should not infer that sexual relations between boys or between girls is likely to be a sign either of a basic homosexual identity or of serious psychiatric disturbance. The important questions are similar to those addressed to any other behavior. What are the ranges of normal expectation as they relate to age, developmental level, the gender of the individual, and the circumstances under which the behavior occurred? Other judgments relate to whether or not the behavior is adaptive; its frequency and duration; whether it interferes with normal function; and whether it is an aspect of more generally disturbed psychosocial function. Sexual behavior is likely to be given the center of the emotional stage. The physician must be able to maintain his or her own perspective and help others to consider sexual behavior as only one aspect of the child's global development, interpersonal functioning, and personal adaptation.

If the physician judges that same-sex behavior reported by a parent in a child is normal developmental behavior or transient and circumstantial, he or she can adopt the following management: parents will need reassurance and some advice as to how to handle any recurrence of such behavior; the physician will need to help the parents control their anxiety, anger, disgust, guilt, or feelings that the child is destined to develop a deviant sexual orientation. Reassurance and guidance are crucial in helping the parents to achieve the attitudes and emotional control that will permit them to be helpful and supportive to their child.

The first task of physicians or parents is to help younger children feel safe and less guilty. Parents should avoid suspicious, scolding, threatening, shaming, or guilt-inducing attitudes or behaviors toward the child. The physician can serve as a model for the parent through his or her own calm, sensitive, careful and supportive exploration of feelings and behavior with the child. The physician should expect denials on the part of the child, and avoidance of and embarrassment with the subject, but discussion will help the child to understand that sexual behavior is comprehensible, and that sexual feelings and curiosity are normal. It is important to know whether the child's information and understanding of sexual matters are appropriate to his or her age. If the same-sex behavior involves another child in the family, he or she should be treated in the same manner. If an older child is the initiator or seducer, he or she should be told clearly and firmly that such behavior will not be tolerated and that he or she will be expected to act with responsibility and control. The older child should talk with a physician or mental health professional, and if there are concerns about emotional or social adjustment, referral for psychiatric evaluation is indicated.

The physician must not let his or her own negative feelings aggravate the disgust, anger, or punitive feelings that parents may have for an older child seen as perpetrator, especially if the older child is not a member of the younger child's family. The physician may need to help parents of exploited children refrain from ill-considered acts of revenge against offenders. If, on the other hand, there has been physical violence or psychologic coercion, both psychiatric and legal intervention are indicated.

Parents can be advised that it is appropriate to make a careful inventory of their children's activities and friends. Vigilance over the child may be increased, but it should not become punitive, suspicious, or guilt-inducing.

Circumstantial same-sex behavior occurs in situations where there are not opportunities for heterosocial or heterosexual behavior, especially among adolescents. Same-sex detention centers and prisons for youth, residential treatment centers, and group-living situations provide occasions for circumstantial homosexuality. In these settings, many involved in such behavior are not homosexual in psychologic orientation. Such circumstances may, however, bring latent homosexual orientations or desires to overt expression. Sexual exploitation and sadistic behavior, including rape, may occur in these situations. Most homosexual experimentation in adolescence is developmental or circumstantial and not premonitory of a later fixed homosexual orientation.

HOMOSEXUALITY

True homosexual orientation is a complex phenomenon, different from merely developmental or circumstantial same-sex behavior. It is essentially a psychologic orientation through which the individual has sexual desires toward or attraction to and gratification from sexual and sensuous contact with members of the same sex. The true homosexual orientation is not exclusively or even primarily genital, but rather a global psychosocial involvement. Only a minority of homosexual persons demonstrate such discordant gender role behavior as effeminacy in men or masculine behavior in women.

The cause of homosexual orientation is uncertain; there are

probably various pathways to it. Theories have proposed genetic, biochemical, neurohumoral, and psychologic factors. It does not appear that homosexual parents produce homosexual children. Two studies have found no appreciable difference between children of lesbian mothers and the general population in social and emotional adaptation or in gender identification. Homosexual orientation is probably not fixed until middle or late adolescence. Various forms of therapy (psychoanalytic, behavioral, group) have produced heterosexual orientations in some homosexual persons who have sought this goal.

Historically, acceptance of homosexuality has waxed and waned within societies. The view is currently held by some that homosexuality is best regarded as an alternative life style. The American Psychiatric Association no longer lists homosexuality among mental disorders.

Homosexuality in Boys. Factors seen as influential in the development of homosexual orientation in boys have included lack of adequate male role models and of support from parents, peers, and subculture for male behavior.

The potentially damaging father is psychologically distant, demeaning, or punitive, especially if such attitudes are aimed at his son's attempts at gender role behaviors. For example, a father who criticizes his son's interest in volleyball as "sissy" and is openly disappointed or angry at the boy's lack of interest in or skill at sports demanding physical contact may produce in the boy feelings of failure, inadequacy, and loss of self-esteem, with doubts about meeting the gender role expectations so vehemently valued within the family. Some fathers with intense, eroticized feelings toward their sons may inadvertently provoke anxiety-producing homosexual feelings.

The mother may, on the other hand, be overprotective and indulgent. She may also be intentionally or unintentionally seductive in her behavior, stimulating intense sensuous and sexual feelings that the boy finds intolerable, and that may reach consciousness only in the form of anxiety, placing the child in a situation of irreconcilable conflict. The boy who wants to be close to his mother and enjoy the rewards of her interest and affection is made very uncomfortable by the overt and covert erotic aspects of the relationship. This may compel him to avoid her or to develop an irritable, angry facade that keeps her at a distance and alleviates his own anxiety. The boy may then generalize this pattern of interaction to his relationship with girls. At adolescence this conflict may become so intensified that the boy orients himself to male company as a way of avoiding the anxiety generated by his eroticized relationship with his mother.

Homosexual feelings in adolescents and young men may often also arise from excessive dependency, and other feelings of ineffectiveness or incompetency in male role behaviors; these feelings may produce an unconscious desire for a passive-dependent relationship with a strong man.

Some cautions are indicated. The intrafamilial dynamics just described, which correspond in a general way to the psychoanalytic theory of inadequate resolution of the oedipal conflict, do not necessarily lead to homosexual orientation in boys. It is important that physicians not accuse mothers or fathers of sexually seductive attitudes or behavior toward their children. Such accusations are extremely harmful. They impugn the intentions and integrity of parents, and even when only implied, could make parents extremely guilty (or angry). Parents are then likely to reject further counsel from the physician and avoid further contact, reacting toward the child with increased psychologic distance owing to their anxiety, guilt, or self-disgust. The child suffers the attenuation of the relationship with parents and is in turn confused and guilty. The erotic aspects of parent-child relationships can usually be discussed only with professionals with special training and experience.

A physician who is concerned about the possibility of such an abnormal relationship between parents and child can approach the need for change by discussing the adverse effects of excessive dependency and the need to help the young boy become more grown up and autonomous. Suggestions about modesty in the home and about the privacy of adult sexual behavior can be given in the form of general counseling without the parents feeling accused of negligence or of seductive actions. It is important that both parents be involved in counseling around such issues, so that they can both understand what has been said and be supportive to each other, and so that the physician can assess the father's role in promotion or maintenance of the excessive closeness of mother and son, or assess the degree to which the father's relationship with his son is defective.

Some young boys who may be able to handle social contacts with girls become anxious or guilty or feel incompetent when the relationship begins to become sexualized. Such boys may also experience impotence in their early attempts at sexual activity with girls. The accompanying shame or feeling of failure may be augmented by the girl's reaction of disappointment or teasing. The boy may compare himself unfavorably with his peers' reports of sexual exploits. Such boys may turn to homosexual behavior as less anxiety-provoking than to risk further social or sexual failure with girls—a homosexual orientation by default.

Such boys and young men need professional help and referral to a mental health facility. Their parents need to be advised that such a referral is not a luxury, nor should they expect such boys simply to "outgrow" their shyness. Such referrals should at least promote opportunities for the adolescent to feel free to explore heterosexual orientation. He may otherwise be excluded from such options owing to paralyzing anxiety or to intermittent depression accompanying loss of self-esteem.

Boys of elementary school age who display effeminate traits (see below), who lack interest in boys as friends, or who have excessive attachment to their mothers and predominant interest in the activities of girls and women deserve an adequate psychiatric evaluation, and treatment if indicated.

Homosexuality in Girls. Knowledge of the development of homosexuality in girls and young women is more tenuous than for males. Women who as young adolescents become homosexually oriented often give a history of a very unsatisfying, non-nurturant relationship with their mothers, persistent from early childhood. Their mothers may have been aloof and distant, punitive and rejecting, or so involved elsewhere that the young girl felt a sense of rejection and abandonment. If mother or father shows an excessive interest in male siblings, the girl feels ashamed of or questions the value of her own sexual role. As she becomes older, she may become attracted to other girls for the opportunity they afford for nurturance, dependency, gratification, and attention.

Many girls go through a normal developmental stage marked by "crushes" on other girls. These positive emotional feelings can also involve inseparable social companionship and such physical contacts as hand holding. Such behavior is culturally more accepted in girls than in boys, girls being generally allowed much more latitude in physical interaction with other girls than boys are allowed with other boys. For some girls neither "crush" relationships nor such socially acceptable activites as dancing together or slumber parties provide any sexual or erotic stimulation. For others they may provide occasions for more deeply felt and strongly desired physical, erotic, or sexual contact with other girls. The eroticization of these relationships may both be exciting and fulfill needs for closeness and affection.

Some homosexual girls may be extremely masculine in behavior, with hair cut short, and wearing such masculine clothes as leather jackets and heavy boots. They often quite explicitly reject all things feminine and female, but it is not necessarily correct to infer that they are homosexual in genital orientation. Some are asexual and have adopted the masculine façade as a way of avoiding any sexual or even social contact with boys owing to anxieties in this area. Such girls may have felt that male roles in their families were especially or excessively valued by parents, or may regard the male role in society as valued and prized over the female, and as perhaps essential to various social, academic, and economic rewards. They may also have underlying fears about passivity and dependency for which they compensate by adoption of the masculine gender role in behavior and dress, often in an exaggerated way. Some have had distant, unsatisfying relationships with their mothers and perhaps too close, affectionate, and eroticized relationships with their fathers. Anxiety arising from the sexual aspects of this relationship may have forced them to deny and abandon feminine sexuality as a way of denying incestuous wishes toward their fathers or competition with their mothers.

Management. There is probably a wide range of intrafamilial, interpersonal, and cultural dynamics besides the above that may give rise to homosexual orientation in girls or boys. It is important that the physician not conclude from apparent gender role of behavior that a masculinized girl or an effeminate boy has an underlying homosexual orientation. Children displaying these behaviors merit careful evaluation by a competent mental health professional. Their parents should be advised that punishment, castigation, shaming, or rejection will not support their children's attempts to struggle with whatever intrapsychic, interpersonal, or cultural conflicts they may have. Parents also need reassurance that they did not wish or intend for such behavior to develop. Homosexual orientation in their children is very threatening to parents, in terms both of their possible responsibility and of underlying uncertainties and fears about their own sexual identities. Some children act out the underlying unconscious or unfulfilled wishes of their parents, and this principle might extend to homosexual orientations; but such possibilities are not to be explored in the usual relationship between physician and family. They require the evaluation and counsel of a fully trained and specifically qualified mental health professional.

EFFEMINACY IN BOYS

Effeminacy in boys may be noted by a physician or brought to his or her attention by an anxious parent. In either case, a full profile of the child's behavior should be reviewed before reassurance is given to the parent or a referral made to a psychiatrist. The attitudes and behaviors of parents are crucial to evaluation of the significance of this symptom. Newman distinguishes two categories of cross-sex behaviors: the first category includes cross-dressing, a verbal wish on a boy's part to be a girl, taking feminine roles in games and fantasies, and the imitation of the gestures of girls; the second category includes dislike of rough or competitive games, disinterest in mechanical toys, preference for artistic activities, enjoyment of girls as playmates, gracefulness in body movements, and being teased as a "sissy." Newman believes that the behaviors in the second category do not themselves constitute serious effeminacy, but that the combination of any first category behavior with one or more second category behaviors requires careful psychiatric evaluation and possible treatment. He found that for boys who wished to be girls the prognosis is good for reversal of the wish when therapy for child and parents is begun in early childhood, whereas after puberty, the prognosis for change is poor. Young boys exhibiting feminine behavior have a higher than normal incidence of serious problems of gender identity in adult life. The two parental factors that seem most commonly related to effeminacy in boys are a distant, disinterested father and a mother who covertly or overtly encourages the boy's identification with her, as revealed, for example, by her enjoying her son's dressing in feminine apparel.

INCESTUOUS BEHAVIOR

Most *incestuous behavior* involves sexual relations between a father and pubertal or teenage daughter. Incest is a form of child abuse and is required by law to be reported by physicians to local child welfare authorities (Sec. 2.59 and 18.6). Unfortunately, mothers are often reluctant to face consciously what they fear is taking place, and the daughter feels fearful and guilty. The fathers involved are manifesting arrested psychosexual development. A recent study found that fathers of incest victims usually had a history of violence, and mothers were often chronically ill, battered, depressed, or alcoholic. The family needs not only to have the problem exposed and faced but to have the continuing support of the physician, since the revelation of incest can lead to the father's imprisonment, the mother's becoming dependent on public welfare, and the daughter's suffering great guilt and shame. Referral to a family counseling center is imperative, as incest is usually not a single event but part of a pattern of inappropriate sexual behavior between parent and child.

When younger children have been or are alleged to have been sexually molested by family members, the physician should try not to identify with the anger of a parent or both parents at the alleged molester; such parental anger may be a defensive reaction against feelings of guilt for not having prevented the event. The molested child may feel anger both at the molester and at the parents who failed to protect him or her. Fear and guilt are inevitable. The role of the physician is not simply to seek justice; that is left to public authorities. The physician can help alleviate unnecessary fear, conflict, and guilt by protecting the child from insistent or inappropriate questioning as well as preventing the child from developing an unhealthy attention-getting device. It is also helpful to point out to the parents that the child's understanding of the situation is different from their own and that with adequate evaluation and counseling or other therapy, lasting adverse effects can generally be avoided.

EXHIBITIONISM

Exhibitionistic and voyeuristic activities (including undressing games, such as the "doctor" game) are common among preschool children. Exhibitionism diminishes through the early grade school years; intermittent episodes of voyeurism may occur as the child attempts to gain more knowledge about sexual activities, especially when parents have been unwilling or unable to impart sexual information.

Compulsive male exhibitionism may occur as a symptom of disturbance during adolescence. The adolescent exhibitionist is not only "seeking attention." He may be seeking reassurance as to his genital equipment and sexual identity, albeit in perverse fashion; but the underlying motive is frequently aggressive—the exhibitionist shocks and frightens his victims. The exhibitionist may also be reacting to covert seductive behavior or overly repressive sexual attitudes by parents. Unconscious guilt compels him into situations in which he will inevitably be caught and punished. Persistent exhibitionism generally indicates serious psychologic disturbance, and psychiatric intervention for both the adolescent and his family is essential. Overt sexual exhibitionism is seen less commonly in adolescent girls.

2.52 PSYCHOSES IN CHILDHOOD

Psychoses are rare but important disorders in children. They may be divided into those of early onset (infancy and preschool) and those of late onset (preadolescence and adolescence).

PSYCHOSES OF EARLY ONSET

Autism. Early infantile autism is characterized by profound impairment of the child's ability to relate to people, including parents. Autism affects 0.7–4.5/10,000 children. Typically, autistic children come to the attention of the physician because the emergence of speech is delayed. Historical review may reveal that the autistic child did not appear to be "cuddly" as an infant, that social smiling was delayed or absent, and that the child did not assume anticipatory postures prior to being picked up.

The autistic child is withdrawn and may spend hours in solitary play, favorite toys and activities being preferred to human contact. Ritualistic behavior prevails and reflects the child's need to maintain a constant environment. The child has compulsive routines (e.g., the touching of objects in a prescribed sequence); disruption of routines may provoke tantrum-like rage reactions. Eye contact with others is minimal or absent, and the child is indifferent to the attempts of others to engage him or her in play. Head banging, teeth grinding, whirling, and rocking may be noted. These activities may lead to self-mutilation of such degree that the child's life is in danger. Visual scanning of hand and finger movements, mouthing of objects, and rubbing of surfaces may indicate a heightened awareness and sensitivity to some stimuli, whereas diminished responses to pain and lack of startle responses to sudden loud noises reflect a lowered sensitivity to other stimuli. If speech is present, echolalia, pronominal reversal ("he" to refer to self, for example), nonsense rhyming, and other idiosyncratic language forms may predominate. IQ by conventional psychologic testing usually falls in the functionally retarded range, but deficits in language and socialization make it difficult to obtain an accurate estimate of the autistic child's intellectual potential. Some autistic children perform adequately in nonverbal tests, and those with developed speech may demonstrate adequate intellectual capacity. Occasionally, an autistic child may have an isolated, remarkable talent, analogous to that of the adult "idiot savant."

The cause of autism is speculative. Theories have centered on a variety of agents, including brain injury, constitutional vulnerability, developmental aphasia, and deficits in the reticular activating system. Recent evidence appears to indicate that autism is neurophysiologic in origin. Contrary to notions in vogue two decades ago, autism is not induced by parents.

Many different therapies have been attempted with autistic children, but success has been quite limited. Some gains in acquisition of speech have been reported with approaches utilizing behavior therapy and operant conditioning. Behavior modification has also been useful in controlling destructive, self-mutilating, and nonfunctional perseverative behavior. Intensive psychotherapy has been of limited value. Tranquilizing medication is generally useful in controlling aggressive and self-mutilating outbursts. There is evidence that lower-dose antipsychotic drugs (haloperidol, and piperazine phenothiazines such as trifluoperazine) may bring improvement in stereotypic behavior, social withdrawal, and ability to learn. Treatment in a therapeutic residential setting may be indicated, especially when parents feel unable to manage the child at home.

The prognosis for autistic children is guarded. Some, especially those with speech, may grow up to live marginal, self-sufficient, albeit isolated, lives in the community; but for most, chronic placement in institutions is the ultimate outcome. The relationship between autism and schizophrenia is uncertain. Instances in which autistic children have later developed schizophrenic symptoms are rare.

Symbiotic Psychosis. Symbiotic psychosis is not so well defined as autism, and there is controversy as to whether it exists as a separate entity. The disorder, as originally described by Mahler in 1952, has its onset between the ages of 2 and 5 yr. Early development is often described as normal, though traces of temperamental "oversensitivity" may have been noted in infancy. A precipitating event, such as the birth of a sibling, causes acute, sudden, panic-like anxiety, together with severe regression in social behavior and intellectual functioning. The symbiotic child clings intensely to his or her mother, but may also show marked dependent attachment to others in an indiscriminate manner. Speech, which may have been present prior to onset, becomes jargonistic and idiosyncratic, losing its communicative value. Regression may lead to a state of "secondary autism," which is chronic and persistent, and resembles early infantile autism. Some of the same etiologic factors already described for autism have been imputed for the symbiotic psychosis, but the cause remains unknown. The prognosis is perhaps slightly more favorable than that of autism.

PSYCHOSES OF LATE ONSET

Psychotic reactions in older children tend more closely to resemble the psychoses of adulthood, and the same diagnostic criteria apply. Affective psychoses have been described earlier (Sec. 2.43). In childhood schizophrenia, prominent symptoms include thought disorder, delusions, and hallucinations. In contrast to the psychoses of early onset, psychoses occurring later in childhood occur in families with a higher than expected rate of schizophrenia. As opposed to schizophrenics, autistic children tend to have different symptoms (notably they lack hallucinations and delusions), much earlier onset, lower IQ scores, and more perinatal complications.

For schizophrenia, chemotherapy, behavior therapy, family supportive therapy, and individual therapy are useful interventions. Hospitalization may be indicated during periods of acute crisis, and prolonged residential treatment for severely affected individuals. Prognosis, while more favorable than that of early-onset psychosis, is poor. There may be periods of remission, but a 20 yr follow-up of childhood schizophrenics found that they had retained their original symptomatology and were similar in presentation to adults with simple schizophrenia.

2.53 PREVENTION OF PSYCHOLOGIC DISORDERS IN THE SICK CHILD

Whenever an illness alters children's functions or changes the way in which their parents or others feel about them, there may be psychologic disturbances. These effects can be minimized and psychogenic problems may be prevented through anticipatory guidance. The psychologic impact of illness may derive from discomfort, anxiety, and changes of sensorium (clouding of consciousness, hallucinations, delusions, and disorientation) and may be manifested as withdrawal, depression, irritability, and regression. Regression is normal for ill children and for ill adults as well. The caretaking process reinforces regression and can lead to prolongation of illness if excessive and inappropriate. The sick child withdraws interest from the outside world and invests it in self and his or her hurt. This is normal for a while, but parents should be advised to increase their expectations of the patient as clinical signs of illness subside.

2.54 PSYCHOSOMATIC INTERPLAY

Psychosocial factors modify responses to experiences, including illnesses. Every clinical phenomenon has reverberations at all organizational levels: molecular, anatomic, physiologic, intrapsychic, interpersonal, familial, and social. This has three important implications for the physician:

1. He or she must maintain an open attitude toward the cause of the patient's discomfort, rather than a position that symptoms are *either* organic *or* psychologically determined.

2. The psychosocial aspects of illness should from the outset be examined along with the physiologic aspects.

3. The physician can act as a model for the parents and the child by showing interest in the child's feelings and demonstrating that it is possible and appropriate to communicate discomfort in verbal, symbolic language, and not just in somatic language. A good opening question is "How are you feeling?" rather than "Where does it hurt?"

For the young child who is hospitalized, potential challenges include coping with separation (Sec. 2.34), adapting to a new environment, adjusting to multiple caretakers, often associating with very sick children, and sometimes experiencing being submitted to machines in an intensive care unit, to anesthesia, or to surgery. The most intense fears for the infant or the young child are created by separation from the parents, often felt as loss of love and/or abandonment. Bowlby has described the following sequence of reactions in hospitalized young children: angry protest with panic-like anxiety; depression and despair; eventual apathy and detachment. Older children may be more concerned with painful procedures, some of which carry the threat of bodily mutilation, and with the loss of control implicit in the use of anesthesia. Repeated hospital admissions are significantly associated with disturbance in later childhood. All of these reactions may be reduced through preventive measures that ease adaptation to the hospital and lessen psychologic and behavioral consequences (Sec. 5.47).

For the child whose future admission to the hospital is arranged, an earlier visit is very important: to see where he or she will be, to meet the people who will be caring for him or her, and to receive answers to questions as to what will happen. For the child under the age of 5–6 yr, the rooming-in of the parent is basic, if it is at all feasible. Creative and active recreational or socialization programs, with liberal or open visiting hours (including visits from siblings), and chances to act out feared procedures in play with dolls or mannequins are all helpful. The hospital staff should maintain sensitive, sympathetic, and accepting attitudes toward child and parent. Some nurses or physicians find themselves at times at odds with parents toward whom they take condescending or critical attitudes, overtly or unconsciously. Such nurses or physicians may feel, for example, that they are better able to meet the child's needs than parents who appear to be anxious or distraught or, alternatively, less concerned than circumstances seem to warrant. At these times, such nurses or physicians may convey to the parents an "I can be a better parent than you" feeling which may greatly impair the adjustment of the parents and child to hospitalization. Parents often already, albeit irrationally, feel guilty enough that their child became ill; they may react in a hostile manner to compensate for their feelings of guilt, or they may not be able to ask crucial questions for fear of "sounding stupid." The physician, nurse, and other professional persons all need to help to establish and to maintain effective communication and a climate of interest and affection for the child and family.

Ambulatory care presents particular problems in clinics in which patients receive discontinuous care from a series of physicians whose intercommunication is often negligible. Differences of language and culture may raise additional barriers to communication. Parents are often unable to verbalize major concerns about their children. Recommendations for care may become inappropriate or irrelevant, and compliance with advice or directions becomes poor. At the end of any initial diagnostic or management activity, the physician should habitually inquire whether there are other things parents or children may wish to ask or talk about during this visit. In the busy emergency rooms of hospitals in urban centers, conflicting expectations exist between how professional staff expect the emergency room to be used (for trauma or for acute and serious illness of recent onset) and what the patients actually need (a local medical agency offering the services of a family-oriented physician). When these different expectations are critically examined, ways may be found to deal more effectively with the patterns of use of emergency services. Employment in emergency rooms of ombudsmen to whom patients and parents can turn for help has been shown often to clarify and resolve individual, social, and cultural differences and conflicts.

The *chronically or fatally ill child* presents special problems to the physician, some of which are discussed in Sec. 2.71. Here we shall touch on certain preventive measures that can lessen the psychologic discomfort of child and parents during illness and prevent psychologic problems for surviving parents and siblings.

Every symptom experienced by children is vaguely or perhaps unconsciously perceived by them and by their parents as a threat to their physical integrity and, when carried to its extreme, as a threat to life and a reminder of their mortality. The more serious the clinical state, the greater the intensity of emotions aroused. The young child feels this primarily as discomfort, and perhaps as an anxiety that reflects parental anxiety. By the age of 9 yr, however, children begin to conceive of death as meaning more than just going away. By adolescence they can think of death in philosophic terms much like adults, albeit with limited experience.

In chronic illnesses that shorten life, such as cystic fibrosis, parents need the physician's early support in developing a relatively guilt-free understanding of the disease and how to help ameliorate it. They need guidance also in answering comfortably the child's questions about the disease. The young child will take most cues from the parent. With the older child, and especially the adolescent, parents must be prepared for the anger of the child at his or her fate. This anger will be lessened and easier to accept if the child has been given at each phase of illness such relatively consistent, accurate, and simple information as is needed and can be assimilated. The child needs both the parents' psychologic strengths and resources and the physician's availability and objectivity.

The role of the physician is difficult. He or she must stand for hope and for relief of discomfort, ready to help parents and child avoid emotionally crippling psychologic handicaps. For example, parents must be encouraged to meet their own needs, even when this requires temporary and perhaps recurrent separation from the child; at times this might help the child learn to tolerate frustration. Parents of chronically or fatally ill children may creatively support each other in groups meeting under the professional guidance of physician, psychologist, or social worker (Sec. 2.71).

In more potentially fulminant lethal processes, the intensity of parental anxiety, guilt, and despair may be greater than in more chronic illnesses. With most children over 9–10 yr of age it has been found most supportive to treat fatal illnesses such as leukemia factually with the child, so far as diagnosis and prognosis are concerned, but always offering realistic hope. Children do not usually ask the physician if or when they are going to die, though they may reveal their fears to others in the hospital. Young children primarily want to be reassured that their parents will not desert them and that they are loved. Both in and outside the hospital the team representing medical, nursing, psychologic, and social work disciplines, and perhaps others, should provide support. The primary physician also needs to stay involved and close to the child and to the clinical situation; he or she often knows the child and family best and can be most supportive. The hospital team needs frequent conferences for their own mutual support in the difficult situation of losing a patient. If objectivity is lost, physicians who feel they have failed may themselves become anxious or depressed and lose their ability to support patient and family.

After the death of a child the parents will need opportunities to talk out their feelings with the physician, one of whose goals should be to help them avoid psychologically encapsulating the lost child in an unmourned state (Sec. 2.71). Many parents can be helped and comforted by being with and holding the dying infant or child or seeing and touching him or her after death.

Organ transplant in children has most often involved the kidney. Hemodialysis may precede renal transplant for varying lengths of time and begins in the hospital, but parents are often expected to learn to carry out this procedure at home. They may be ambivalent about being given control of a life-threatening process. The child receiving dialysis becomes psychologically dependent and often withdrawn. Bone marrow transplant also involves many psychologic considerations, such as donor relationships and the stress of isolation.

Family problems multiply with the question of who will donate an organ. If relatives are available as donors, there may be tension about who should "make the sacrifice." In some cases guilt may be relieved if the physician arbitrarily (but thoughtfully) makes this decision. A medical support team of carefully chosen staff is essential to decision-making and continuing care. There is a high suicide rate among adults on hemodialysis, but it appears to be less traumatic to children, probably owing to the child's greater capacities for denial and acceptance of a support system. Adolescents are concerned with distortions of body image, which they cannot always express verbally. The physician needs the patience to listen (both to the stated and to the implied questions and misconceptions), to interpret, to set appropriate limits, and to help families and patients with technical details and with decision-making.

2.55 MANAGEMENT OF ESTABLISHED PSYCHOLOGIC DISORDERS

Planning Psychotherapy. When it has been determined that psychopathology exists in a child or within a family that requires intervention, the physician may develop and implement the therapeutic plan, or may refer to a more specialized level of care. Referral should not, however, end the role of the primary physician as the ongoing medical caretaker; there will be a need to assess the psychiatric intervention being offered and what the child or family appear to gain from it.

When referral for psychotherapy is considered, the resources in the community may include not only private practitioners in child psychiatry, social work, or psychology, but also child guidance agencies, child welfare and family service agencies, and children's psychiatric wards or hospitals. Some school districts have both psychologic evaluative and treatment services, as well as special classes. In justifying referral to child or parent, the simplest statement is the best, one that conveys the physician's confidence that it is necessary. The choice of treatment should be left to the consultant, with the referring physician reassuring the family and patient that close communication with the consultant will be maintained. The referring physician should ordinarily plan actively for the continuing medical care of the patient, including episodic illnesses. The child or parents should not be left with the feeling that "there is nothing more" the physician can do.

Treatment Methods Used by the Psychiatrist. In classic psychotherapy, the therapist works directly with the child in the task of resolving intrapsychic conflict. If intensive, it is called child psychoanalysis; if less intensive, it is termed child psychotherapy. Efforts may range from specific suggestions to the child for alteration of behavior to interpretive therapy aimed at giving the child an opportunity to change his or her intrapsychic structure and coping behavior. Some allegiance to the therapeutic effort is required on the part of the child.

Parents may be involved in concurrent casework, or may be seen by the child's therapist in parental counseling on a frequent or occasional basis. The *psychodynamic* approach stresses the importance of having child and parents come to understand how past patterns of behavior have influenced current feelings and function. The *behavior modification* approach stresses a complete analysis of the behavior of the child, in terms of the current behavior's immediate antecedents and consequences. Desirable behavioral changes are then brought about by changing the reinforcement system.

A second approach involves working with the family as a group, in part or in whole, giving most attention to relationships between family members, rather than to the inner emotional life of each individual. There is heavy stress on mending communication difficulties between family members and upon having each member learn what his or her healthy role is, accept it, gain acceptance for it, and function effectively within it.

A third approach involves group therapy for children, which is particularly useful for the child who has problems in development of social skills. Group therapy for preadolescent children tends to emphasize physical and other structured activities through which therapist and children alike can discover how they relate to each other and find ways to change.

Psychotherapy by the Nonpsychiatric Physician. Barriers to the involvement of the generalist or pediatrician in psychotherapeutic activities with children include presumed lack of time and lack of adequate conceptual background. The experience of successfully grappling with some of these problems will give many physicians the confidence that they *can* treat many of them.

The first therapeutic impact is conveyed by interest, in listening thoughtfully and in asking questions that evoke new thoughts in parents or children that help them to gain more objective views of their lives as a family. This process is helped if parents are given from time to time the opportunity to state at their level of understanding how *they* see a problem. When well-established and trusting relationships exist between physician and family, it may be appropriate to convey directly and simply some diagnostic impressions and suggestions for management. The physician may recommend that parents and children talk about their feelings about the problem and feel freer to express them.

Adolescents should usually be included in discussions that formulate the problem and suggest changes. Some supportive therapy of this kind can be viewed as representing a contract between physician, parents, and child, which indicates the actions to be taken by each party with respect to a focal point of concern. Progress toward solution of a problem is reviewed at successive visits with questions on how well or whether goals have been met and what new problems may have come up. If little or no improvement occurs, the primary physician may wish to seek the advice of a psychiatrist or refer the patient for more intensive study or therapy.

Psychotherapy by the nonpsychiatric physician emphasizes listening and interviewing, conceptualization of the problem (first to self and then to parents), exploration of problem-solving techniques with parents in one or more conferences, a willingness to stay involved as long as needed, and a readiness to accept limitations and to make referrals when these are appropriate.

Hospitalization. At times hospitalization of the disturbed or emotionally ill child in a general or pediatric hospital will be helpful or necessary, and may serve a number of functions. In the case of many psychosomatic disorders or of a suicidal or drugged adolescent, indications may be medical as well as psychiatric. If treatment of a child in a psychiatric hospital is thought to be necessary, consulting with a psychiatrist or a social agency is necessary in decision-making and planning. Admission to residential treatment reflects the family's decompensation as often as the child's.

2.56 PSYCHOPHARMACOLOGY

Using drugs to modify children's behavior is controversial. The specific ways in which commonly used psychopharmaceutic agents act upon the central nervous system are generally unclear. Their effects on behavior are influenced by the

Table 2–14. **Psychopharmacologic Agents**

Medication Class	Indications	Dosage	Side Effects/Toxicity/Cautions
I. Antipsychotics 　A. Low potency/high dosage: 　　Thioridazine 　　　(Mellaril) 　　Chlorpromazine 　　　(Thorazine) 　B. Mid-potency/mid-dosage: 　　Mesoridazine 　　　(Serentil) 　C. High potency/low dosage: 　　Trifluoperazine 　　　(Stelazine) 　　Thiothixene 　　　(Navane) 　　Haloperidol 　　　(Haldol)	*All Classes:* Severe anxiety, agitation; childhood and adolescent schizophrenia; emotional lability, aggressivity, and/or hyperactivity associated with severe conduct disorder; pervasive developmental disorder; mania; stereotypic and withdrawal symptoms of pervasive developmental disorder and autism; self-abuse, pica, and aggressivity in mental retardation *High Potency Class:* Gilles de la Tourette syndrome, other tic disorders (haloperidol)	A. Low potency: 30–150 mg/24 hr in divided doses; available in concentrated form B. Mid potency: 10–75 mg/24 hr in divided doses C. High Potency: 1–6 mg/24 hr in divided doses	*All Classes:* Sedation, weight gain; anticholinergic effects (dry mouth, blurred vision, constipation); hypersensitivity reactions (hepatic, skin); blood dyscrasias; parkinsonism Long term effects: Risk of tardive dyskinesia and "withdrawal-emergent" syndrome (see text)
II. Stimulants (6 yr and older) 　Methylphenidate (Ritalin)	Attention deficit disorder	0.3–1.0 mg/kg/24 hr	Insomnia, decreased appetite, possible weight loss, irritability and tearfulness; abdominal pain, headache; elevated systolic blood pressure. A long-term effect may be height and weight reduction (Sec. 2.56). *Pemoline* is associated with hypersensitivity reactions, especially hepatic. .
Dextroamphetamine (Dexedrine)	Attention deficit disorder	0.2–0.5 mg/kg/24 hr	
Pemoline (Cylert)	Attention deficit disorder	37.5–112.5 mg/24 hr	
III. Antidepressants 　Imipramine (Tofranil)	Major depressive disorder; separation anxiety; attention deficit disorder unresponsive to stimulants (12 yr and older); enuresis (6 yr and older)	For major depressive disorder and separation anxiety: 2–3 mg/kg/24 hr in divided doses. For enuresis, 25–50 mg/24 hr	EKG and blood pressure should be monitored for hypertension, orthostatic hypotension, cardiac arrhythmia or lengthening of PR or QRS interval. Side effects: anticholinergic (dry mouth, blurred vision, constipation); rarely parkinsonian symptoms. Possible withdrawal reactions (Sec. 2.56). Monitor plasma levels for therapeutic range.
Desipramine (Norpramin)	Major depressive disorder (12 yr and older)	25–100 mg/24 hr	
IV. Miscellaneous 　Diphenhydramine (Benadryl)	Hyperactivity, anxiety, sleep disorders	For hyperactivity, 25–150 mg/24 hr, in divided doses; sleep disorders, 25–50 mg at bedtime; can be given as elixir	Dry mucous membranes, rash

*Also see Table 29–1B.

maturity of the central nervous system, by intrapsychic and psychosocial factors, by the personality or charisma of the physician prescribing them, by the problem itself, and by the milieu (patient, parents, time of day given, etc.).

Table 2–14 lists the psychopharmaceutic agents most commonly used outside of hospitals for treating behavioral disorders in ambulatory patients, together with appropriate dosage schedules, indications, and adverse reactions. The medications are of three general types: stimulants, antipsychotic medications, and antidepressants.

The uses of dextroamphetamine and methylphenidate for the child with attention deficit disorder are discussed in Sec. 2.46 and 2.66.

Indications for the use of antipsychotic medications in children are not well established, especially in young children. In disturbed adolescents, these drugs may be used in much the same manner as they are in young adults. The antipsychotic medications most commonly used in child psychiatry are the aliphatic phenothiazines (thioridazine and chlorpromazine) and haloperidol. The use of antipsychotic medications should generally be reserved for children with serious disorders, characterized by excessive agitation, aggressiveness, anxiety, or psychosis. When the decision is made to discontinue antipsychotic medication, the physician should be alert to the possibility of "withdrawal-emergent" syndrome, whose symptoms include nausea, vomiting, diaphoresis, ataxia, oral dyskinesia, and dystonic movements of the limbs, trunk, and head. Symptoms tend to have a spontaneous remission 8–12 wk after discontinuation. *Tardive dyskinesia*, an involuntary movement disorder characterized by choreoathetoid movements of trunk, limbs, and facial musculature, has been reported in children and adolescents treated with antipsychotic agents. It can occur not only with high-dose, long-term treatment, but with low doses of antipsychotics over a span of several months, and may be irreversible.

Antidepressant medication may have to be discontinued in a slowly tapering regimen for children to prevent withdrawal symptoms (abdominal pain, nausea, vomiting, drowsiness, decreased appetite, tearfulness, and agitation). The process may extend over several weeks.

Since bipolar disorder is very unusual in the pediatric age group, lithium is rarely used in children. It has been employed for bipolar illness in adolescents, using the same dosage guidelines and blood levels as in adults.

Prior to treatment with antipsychotic medication, with pemoline, with lithium, or with antidepressants, baseline laboratory studies should be obtained, and blood studies repeated about every 6 mo. Appropriate studies include a complete blood count with differential and platelet count, and a liver function profile. Thyroid and renal function studies are necessary for patients taking lithium. Monitoring of EKG and blood pressure are indicated for patients receiving imipramine or on high doses of aliphatic phenothiazines. Therapeutic plasma levels have been established for various drugs, and dosages and levels should be monitored.

As the biologic basis of psychiatric disorders becomes better understood, additional psychoactive medications and therapeutic indications undoubtedly will be discovered. Lithium and haloperidol have both been found useful in decreasing excessively aggressive behavior. Clonidine has shown success in children with attention deficit disorder, as well as in children who have a personal or family history of tics (including Gilles de la Tourette syndrome). Pimozide, still an experimental drug in the United States, seems to be effective in the treatment of Tourette syndrome.

The increasing experience with and sophistication of chemotherapy must not create overconfidence in or overdependence on medication as a therapeutic tool. Since some parents are adamantly opposed to the use of psychotropic drugs, the physician contemplating their use must make sure of the parental attitudes. If drugs are to be used, it should be for as short a period as possible. As in any clinical disorder, the physician should avoid using multiple medications and should not shift back and forth from one medication to another when no immediate response occurs. Since psychotropic medications have significant biochemical effects on the developing child, it is important that the physician give an appropriate explanation to the parents and child as to the rationale for medication. Even for disorders in which chemotherapy has a definite place, medication is rarely, if ever, the sole treatment indicated. The complexity of emotional conditions demands an integrated approach involving various therapies: psychodynamic (individual, family, or group); behavioral; milieu; chemotherapeutic; and use of resources in the family, school, and community. These factors must be knowledgeably selected, judiciously coordinated, and skillfully applied to ensure the maximal benefit for the child.

MARC A. FORMAN
WESLEY E. KERSCHBAUM
WILLIAM H. HETZNECKER
JOHN M. DUNN

General

Chess S, Hassibi M: Principles and Practice of Child Psychiatry. New York, Plenum Press, 1978.
Erikson EH: Childhood and Society. Ed 2. New York, WW Norton, 1963.
Flavell JH: The Developmental Psychology of Jean Piaget. Princeton, NJ, Von Nostrand, 1963.
Freud A: Normality and Pathology in Childhood. New York, International Universities Press, 1965.
Hetznecker W, Forman MA: On Behalf of Children. New York, Grune & Stratton, 1974.
Kagan J.: The Nature of the Child. New York, Basic Books, 1984.
Rutter M (ed): Scientific Foundations of Developmental Psychiatry. London, William Heinemann Medical Books Ltd, 1980.
Rutter M, Tizard J, Whitmore K: Education, Health and Behavior. New York, John Wiley & Sons, 1970.

Role of Parents in Child Development

Becker W: Parents Are Teachers. Urbana, IL, Research Press, 1971.
Carey WB: The importance of temperament-environment interaction for child health and development. *In*: Lewis M, Rosenblum L (eds): The Uncommon Child. New York, Plenum Press, 1981.
Carey WB, McDevitt SC: Revision of the infant temperament questionnaire. Pediatrics 61:735, 1978.
Deur JL, Parke RD: The effects of inconsistent punishment on aggression in children. Dev Psychobiol 2:403, 1970.
Dodson F: How to Parent. Los Angeles, Nash Publishing Corp, 1970.
Fullard W, McDevitt SC, Carey WB: Assessing temperament in one to three year old children. J Pediatr Psychol 9:205, 1984.
Haselkorn F (ed): Family Planning: A Source Book and Case Material for Social Work Education. New York, Council on Social Work Education, 1971.
Hegvik RL, McDevitt SC, Carey WB: The middle childhood temperament questionnaire. J Dev Behav Pediatr 3:197, 1982.
Kohlberg L: Stages of moral development as the basis for moral education. *In*: Beck C, Sullivan E, Crittendon D (eds): Moral Education. Toronto, University of Toronto Press, 1971.
Maccoby EE: The development of moral values and behavior in childhood. *In*: Clausen JA (ed): Socialization and Society. Boston, Little, Brown, 1968.
McDevitt SC, Carey WB: The measurement of temperament in 3–7 year old children. J Child Psychol Psychiatry 19:245, 1978.
Parke RD: The role of punishment in the socialization process. *In*: Hoppe RA, Milton GA, Simmel EC (eds): Early Experience and the Process of Socialization. New York, Academic Press, 1970.
Siegel E: The biological effects of family planning—preventive pediatrics: The potential of family planning. J Med Educ 44:74, 1969.
Smith BM: Competence and socialization. *In*: Clausen JA (ed): Socialization and Society. Boston, Little, Brown, 1968.
Thomas A, Chess S: Genesis and evolution of behavioral disorders: From infancy to early adult life. Am J Psychiatry 141:1,1984.
White RW: Motivation reconsidered: The concept of competence. Psychol Rev 66:297, 1959.

Specific Developmental Issues

Aronfreed J: Conduct and Conscience: The Socialization of Internalized Control over Behavior. New York, Academic Press, 1968.
Bakeman R, Brown JV: Early interaction: Consequences for social and mental development at three years. Child Development 51:437, 1980.

Bowlby J: Attachment. New York, Basic Books, 1969.

Bowlby J: Attachment and Loss. Vol II, Separation. New York, Basic Books, 1973.

Brown GW, Harris T: Social Origins of Depression. London, Tavistock Publications, 1978.

Caldwell BM, Wright CM, Honig AS, et al: Infant day care and attachment. Am J Orthopsychiatry 40:397, 1970.

Chess S, Thomas A: Infant bonding: Mystique and reality. Am J Orthopsychiatry 52:213, 1982.

Douvan E, Adelson Y: The Adolescent Experience. New York, John Wiley & Sons, 1966.

Egeland B, Vaughn B: Failure of "bond formation" as a cause of abuse, neglect and maltreatment. Am J Orthopsychiatry 51:78, 1981.

Ehrhardt AA, Money J: Progestin-induced hermaphroditism; IQ and psychosexual identity in a study of ten girls. J Sex Res 3:83, 1967.

Green R, Money J (eds): Transsexualism and Sex Reassignment. Baltimore, Johns Hopkins Press, 1969.

Green R: Sexual identity of 37 children raised by homosexual and transsexual parents. Am J Psychiatr 135:692, 1978.

Hutt C: Biological bases of psychological sex differences. Am J Dis Child 132:170, 1978.

Kagan J: Acquisition and significance of sex typing and sex role identity. In: Hoffman ML, Hoffman LW (eds): Review of Child Development Research. Vol I. New York, Russell Sage Foundation, 1964.

Masterson JF: The psychiatric significance of adolescent turmoil. Am J Psychiatry 124:107, 1968.

Money J: Psychosexual differentiation. In: Money J (ed): Sex Research; New Developments. New York, Holt, Rinehart and Winston, 1965.

Ounstead C, Taylor DC (eds): Gender Differences: Their Ontogeny and Significance. Edinburgh, Churchill Livingstone, 1972.

Reinisch JM, Karow WG: Prenatal exposure to synthetic progestins and estrogens: Effects on human development. Arch Sex Behav 6:257, 1977.

Rutter M: Social-emotional consequences of day care for preschool children. Am J Orthopsychiatry 51:4, 1981.

Rutter M, Chadwick OFD, Yule W: Adolescent turmoil: Fact or fiction? J Child Psychol Psychiatry 17:35, 1976.

Schofield M: The Sexual Behavior of Young People. Boston, Little, Brown, 1965.

Schooler C: Birth order effects: Not here, not now. Psychol Bull 78(3):161, 1972.

Schwartz J, Strickland RG, Krolick G: Infant day care: Behavioral effects at preschool age. Dev Psychol 10:502, 1974.

Sibinga MS, Friedman CJ: Restraint and speech. Pediatrics 48:116, 1971.

Sorensen RC: Adolescent Sexuality in Contemporary America. New York, World Publishing, 1972.

Zelnik M, Kantner JF: Sexual activity, contraceptive use and pregnancy among metropolitan-area teenagers: 1971–1979. Family Planning Perspect 12:230, 1980.

Social Issues

Anthony S: The Discovery of Death in Childhood and After. New York, Basic Books, 1971.

Eisenberg L: The sins of the fathers: Urban decay and social pathology. Am J Orthopsychiatry 32:5, 1962.

Gardner RA: The Boys' and Girls' Book About Divorce. New York, Science House, 1970.

Ilfield F, Ilfield H, Alexander JR: Does joint custody work? A first look at outcome data of relitigation. Am J Psychiatry 139:62, 1982.

Maluccio A, Fein E, Hamilton J, et al: Beyond permanency planning. Child Welfare 59:515, 1980.

Nagy M: The child's meaning of death. In: Feifel H (ed): The Meaning of Death. New York, McGraw-Hill, 1959.

Rothenberg MB: The role of television in shaping the attitudes of children. J Am Acad Child Psychiatry 22:86, 1983.

Steinman S: The experience of children in a joint custody arrangement: A report of a study. Am J Orthopsychiatry 51:403, 1981.

Wallerstein JS, Kelly JB: Surviving the Breakup: How Children Actually Cope with Divorce. New York, Basic Books, 1980.

Wolfenstein M: How is mourning possible? In The Psychoanalytic Study of the Child. New York, International Universities Press, 1966.

Assessment and Interviewing

Beiser HR: Psychiatric diagnostic interviews with children. Am Acad Child Psychiatry 1:656, 1962.

Rich J: Interviewing Children and Adolescents. London, Macmillan, 1968.

Schulman JL: Management of Emotional Disorders in Pediatric Practice. Chicago, Year Book Medical Publishers, 1967.

Simmons JE: Psychiatric Examination of Children. 3rd ed. Philadelphia, Lea & Febiger, 1981.

Wood DJ: Talking to young children. Dev Med Child Neurol 24:856, 1982.

Psychosocial Problems

Abikoff, H, Gittleman R: Does behavior therapy normalize the classroom behavior of hyperactive children? Arch Gen Psychiatry 41:449, 1984.

Adams RM, Kocsis JJ, Estes RE: Soft neurological signs in learning-disabled children and controls. Am J Dis Child 128:614, 1974.

American Psychiatric Association: Diagnostic and Statistical Manual of Mental Disorders. 3rd ed. DSM-III, Washington, 1980.

Bandura A: Aggression: A Social Learning Analysis. Englewood Cliffs, NJ, Prentice-Hall, 1973.

Berg I: Day wetting in children. J Child Psychol Psychiatry 16:289, 1975.

Camp BW, Blom GE, Herbert F, et al: "Think aloud": A program for developing self-control in young aggressive boys. J Abnorm Child Psychol 5:157, 1977.

Chess S: Autism in children with congenital rubella. J Autism Child Schizophrenia 1:33, 1971.

Cohen DJ, Nathanson JA, Young MG, et al: Clonidine in Tourette's syndrome. Lancet 2:551, 1979.

Conners CK: A teacher rating scale for use in drug studies with children. Am J Psychiatry 126:884, 1969.

Earls F: The epidemiology of depression in children and adolescents. Pediatr Ann 13:23, 1984.

Eastgate, J, Gilmour L: Long term outcome of depressed children: A follow-up study. Dev Med Child Neurol 26:68, 1984.

Eisenberg L: The epidemiology of suicide in adolescents. Pediatr Ann 13:47, 1984.

Eron L, Walden L, Lefkowitz M: Learning of Aggression in Children. Boston, Little, Brown, 1971.

Garfinkel BD, Froese A, Hood J: Suicide attempts in children and adolescents. Am J Psychiatry 139:1257, 1982.

Golden GS: Controversial therapies. Pediatr Clin North Am 31:459, 1984.

Golombok S, Spencer A, Rutter M: Children in lesbian and single-parent households: psychosexual and psychiatric appraisal. J Child Psychol Psychiatry 24:551, 1983.

Goodyer I: Hysterical conversion reactions in childhood. J Child Psychol Psychiatry 22:179, 1981.

Graham FK, Ernhardt CB, Thurston CB, et al: Development three years after perinatal anoxia and other potentially damaging newborn experiences. Psychol Monographs 76:1, 1962.

Guilleminault C, Anders JF: Sleep disorders in children. In: Schulman I (ed): Advances in Pediatrics, Vol 22. Chicago, Year Book Medical Publishers, 1976.

Hansen CR, Cohen D: Multimodality approaches in the treatment of attention deficit children. Pediatr Clin North Am 31:499, 1984.

Herman J, Hirschman L: Families at risk for father-daughter incest. Am J Psychiatry 138:967, 1981.

Hetznecker W, Forman MA: Developmental issues and psychosocial problems in children: I. Normal development and minor behavioral problems. II. More serious behavioral and performance disorders. In: Smith DW (ed): Introduction to Clinical Pediatrics. 2nd ed. Philadelphia, WB Saunders, 1977.

Hoare P: The development of psychiatric disorder among school children with epilepsy. Dev Med Child Neurol 26:3, 1984.

Kalachnik JE, Sprague RL, Sleator EK, et al: Effect of methylphenidate hydrochloride on stature of hyperactive children. Dev Med Child Neurol 24:586, 1982.

Kandel DB, Davies M: Epidemiology of depressive mood in adolescents. Arch Gen Psychiatry 39:1205, 1982.

Kashani JH, Husain A, Shekim WO, et al: Current perspectives on childhood depression: An overview. Am J Psychiatry 138:143, 1981.

Kashani JH, McGee RO, Clarkson SE, et al: Depression in a sample of nine-year-old children. Arch Gen Psychiatry 40:1217, 1983.

Keith PR: Night terrors. J Am Acad Child Psychiatry 14:477, 1975.

Kirkpatrick M, Smith C, Roy R: Lesbian mothers and their children: A comparative study. Am J Orthopsychiatry 51:545, 1981.

Kovacs M, Feinberg TL, Crouse-Novak MA, et al: Depressive disorders in childhood: I. A longitudinal prospective study of characteristics and recovery. Arch Gen Psychiatry 41:229, 1984.

Kovacs M, Feinberg TL, Crouse-Novak MA, et al: Depressive disorders in childhood. II. A longitudinal study of the risk for a subsequent major depression. Arch Gen Psychiatry 41:643, 1984.

Lahey B, Schaughency E, Strauss C, et al: Are attention deficit disorder with and without hyperactivity similar or dissimilar disorders? J Am Acad Child Psychiatry 23:302, 1984.

Lapouse R, Monk MA: An epidemiologic study of behavioral characteristics in children. Am J Pub Health 48:1134, 1958.

Lazare A: Current concepts in psychiatry: Conversion symptoms. N Engl J Med 305:745, 1981.

Lebovitz P: Feminine behavior in boys: Aspects of outcome. Am J Psychiatry 128:10, 1972.

Lewis D, Balla DA: Delinquency and Psychopathology. New York, Grune and Stratton, 1976.

MacKeith R, Sandler J (eds): Psychosomatic Aspects of Paediatrics. London, Pergamon Press, 1961.

Maloney MJ, Klykylo WM: An overview of anorexia nervosa, bulimia, and obesity in children and adolescents. J Am Acad Child Psychiatry 22:99, 1983.

Mattes J, Gittleman R: Effects of artificial food colorings in children with hyperactive symptoms. Arch Gen Psychiatry 38:714, 1981.

Mattes J, Gittleman R: Growth of hyperactive children on maintenance regimen of methylphenidate. Arch Gen Psychiatry 40:317, 1983.

McGhee R, Silva PA, Williams S: Behavior problems in a population of seven year old children: Prevalence, stability and types of disorder—A research report. J Child Psychol Psychiatry 25:251, 1984.

McIntire MS, Angle CR (eds): Suicide Attempts in Children and Youth. Hagerstown, MD, Harper & Row, 1980.

Minuchin S: Families and Family Therapy. Cambridge, Harvard University Press, 1974.

Newman LE: Treatment for the parents of feminine boys. Am J Psychiatry 133:683, 1976.

Petti TA, Law W: Imipramine treatment of depressed children: A double-blind pilot study. J Clin Psychopharm 2:107, 1982.

Pfeffer C: Clinical aspects of childhood suicidal behavior. Pediatr Ann 13:56, 1984.

Puig-Antich J: Clinical and treatment aspects of depression in childhood and adolescence. Pediatr Ann 13:37, 1984.

Rapoport J, Elkins R, Langer DH, et al: Childhood obsessive-compulsive disorder. Am J Psychiatry 138:1545, 1981.

Raskin L, Shaywitz S, Shaywitz B, et al: Neurochemical correlates of attention deficit disorder. Pediatr Clin North Am 31:387, 1984.

Rutter M: Family, area and school influences in the genesis of conduct disorders. In: Hersov LA, Berger M, Shaffer D (eds): Aggression and Antisocial Behavior in Childhood and Adolescence. Oxford, Pergamon Press, 1978.

Rutter M: Psychological sequelae of brain damage in children. Am J Psychiatry 138:1533, 1981.

Safer DJ, Allen RP, Barr E: Growth rebound after termination of stimulant drugs. J Pediatr 86:113, 1975.

Schachar R, Rutter M, Smith A: The characteristics of situationally and pervasively hyperactive children: implications for syndrome definition. J Child Psychol Psychiatry 22:375, 1981.

Scott JP: Biology and human aggression. Am J Orthopsychiatry 40:568, 1970.

Shaffer D: Suicide in childhood and early adolescence. J Child Psychol Psychiatry 15:275, 1974.

Shaywitz S, Shaywitz B: Diagnosis and management of attention deficit disorder: A pediatric perspective. Pediatr Clin North Am 31:429, 1984.

Spitz R: Anaclitic depression. In: Eissler RS (ed): Psychoanalytic Study of the Child. Vol II. New York, International Universities Press, 1946.

Stoller RJ: Male child transsexualism. J Am Acad Child Psychiatry 7:193, 1968.

Strober M, Carlson G: Bipolar illness in adolescents with major depression. Arch Gen Psychiat 39:549, 1982.

Tishler CL, McKenry PC: Parental negative self and adolescent suicide attempts. J Am Acad Child Psychiatry 21:404, 1982.

Varley C: Diet and the behavior of children with attention deficit disorder. J Am Acad Child Psychiatry 23:182, 1984.

Weiss G, Hechtman L: The hyperactive child syndrome. Science 205:1348, 1979.

Weizman A, Weitz R, Szekely G, et al: Combination of neuroleptic and stimulant treatment in attention deficit disorder with hyperactivity. J Am Acad Child Psychiatry 23:295, 1984.

Wender PH: Minimal Brain Dysfunction in Children. New York, Wiley Interscience, 1971.

Whalen C, Henker B: Hyperactivity and the attention deficit disorders: Expanding frontiers. Pediatr Clin North Am 31:397, 1984.

West DJ: Homosexuality. 3rd ed. London, Duckworth, 1968.

Zucker KJ: Childhood gender disturbance: Diagnostic issues. J Am Acad Child Psychiatry 21:274, 1982.

Childhood Psychoses

Green WH, Campbell M, Hardesty AS, et al: A comparison of schizophrenic and autistic children. J Am Acad Child Psychiatry 23:399, 1984.

Howells JG, Giurguis W: Childhood schizophrenia 20 years later. Arch Gen Psychiatry 41:123, 1984.

Kanner L: Early infantile autism. Am J Orthopsychiatry 19:416, 1949.

Kolvin I: Psychoses in childhood. In: Rutter M (ed): Infantile Autism—Concepts, Characteristics, and Treatment. London, Churchill, 1971.

Mahler MS, Furer M, Settlage CF: Severe emotional disturbances in childhood psychoses. In: Arieti S (ed): American Handbook of Psychiatry. Vol 1. New York, Basic Books, 1959.

Ornitz EM, Ritvo ER: The syndrome of autism: A critical review. Am J Psychiatry 133:609, 1976.

Petty L, Ornitz E, Michelman EG, et al: Autistic children who became schizophrenic. Arch Gen Psychiatry 41:129, 1984.

Prevention of Psychologic Disorders in the Sick Child

Bergman T: Children in the Hospital. New York, International Universities Press, 1966.

Brunnquell D, Hall MD: Issues in the psychological care of pediatric oncology patients. Am J Orthopsychiatry 52:32, 1982.

Douglas JWB: Early hospital admissions and later disturbances of behavior and learning. Dev Med Child Neurol 17:456, 1975.

Lansky SB: Childhood leukemia. J Am Acad Child Psychiatry 13:499, 1974.

Prugh DG: Toward an understanding of psychosomatic concepts in relation to illness in children. In: Solnit AJ, Provence SA (eds): Modern Perspectives in Child Development; in Honor of Milton JE Senn. New York, International Universities Press, 1963.

Quinton D, Rutter M: Early hospital admissions and later disturbances of behavior: An attempted replication of Douglas' findings. Dev Med Child Neurol 18:447, 1976.

Robertson J: Young Children in Hospitals. New York, Basic Books, 1958.

Sampson TF: The child in renal failure: Emotional impact of treatment on the child and his family. J Am Acad Child Psychiatry 14:462, 1975.

Solnit AJ, Green M: Psychologic considerations in the management of deaths on pediatric hospital services. I. The doctor and the child's family. Pediatrics 24(1):106, 1959.

Tisza VB, Dorsett P, Morse J: Psychological implications of renal transplantation. J Am Acad Child Psychiatry 15:709, 1976.

Wallinga J: Human ecology: Primary prevention in pediatrics. Am J Orthopsychiatry 52:141, 1982.

Film: You See, I Had a Life. The Eccentric Circle Cinema Workshop, PO Box 1981, Evanston, IL, 60204.

Management of Established Psychologic Disorders

Balint M: The Doctor, His Patient and the Illness. New York, International Universities Press, 1957.

Denckla MB, Bemporad JR, Mackay MC: Tics following methylphenidate adminstration. JAMA 235:1349, 1976.

Gualtieri CT, Guimond M: Tardive dyskinesia and the behavioral consequences of chronic neuroleptic treatment. Dev Med Child Neurol 23:255, 1981.

Werry J: An overview of pediatric psychopharmacology. J Am Acad Child Psychiatry 21:3, 1982.

Wiener JM: Psychopharmacology in childhood disorders. Psychiatr Clin North Am 7:831, 1984.

ABUSE AND NEGLECT OF CHILDREN

Child abuse is any maltreatment of children or adolescents by their parents, guardians, or other caretakers. Physicians must be able to recognize abused children and confirm the diagnosis; recognition is especially important in the first 6 mo of life because if the diagnosis is missed at this age, risk of fatality is high. Physicians have three main responsibilities toward abused children: detection, reporting, and prevention. In all 50 states the laws require physicians to report suspected cases of child abuse or neglect to a local child protective agency; laws protect physicians from liability should their suspicions prove unfounded.

2.57 THE SPECTRUM OF CHILD ABUSE AND NEGLECT

The types of child abuse and neglect seen by physicians are approximately 70% physical abuse, 25% sexual abuse, and 5% failure to thrive due to underfeeding. *Physical abuse* or nonaccidental trauma inflicted by a caretaker may include bruises, burns, head injuries, fractures, and the like; their severity can range from minor bruises to fatal subdural hematomas. Corporal punishment that causes bruises or leads to an injury that requires medical treatment is outside the range of normal disciplinary action; reckless and dangerous punishment (e.g., kicking a child in the abdomen) is absolutely unacceptable, even if injuries do not occur. *Nutritional neglect* or deliberate underfeeding is the most common cause of underweight in infancy and may account for over half of the cases of failure to thrive. *Sexual abuse* usually occurs within the family (incest) and is the most often overlooked type of child abuse.

Intentional drugging or poisoning includes giving children medications that are harmful or are not intended for children, or sharing illegal drugs with them. Barbiturates and tranquilizers are the drugs most frequently given. Occasionally, the parent has lethal intent. *Neglect of medical care* recommended for a child with chronic disease may lead to deterioration in the condition and require court-enforced supervision or placement in foster care. Court orders to hospitalize and treat are also needed when an emergency exists for the child that parents will not acknowledge or not permit to be treated. Accidents to children from *neglect of safety* constitute child neglect if there is gross lack of supervision, especially if the child involved is under 3 yr of age. Rare types of child abuse include hypernatremic dehydration due to water deprivation, hyponatremia from forcing water, hypothermia due to cold water punishment, near drowning following forced immersion, intentional suffocation, deprivational dwarfism, and kwashiorkor due to cult diets.

The term *Münchausen syndrome by proxy* describes instances in which children are victims of illnesses fabricated or induced by parents. The children are usually under 6 yr old and too young to reveal the deception. The induced symptoms and signs lead to unnecessary medical investigations, hospital admissions, and treatment. Occasionally a child dies, as when the parent induces apnea. The involved parent often is a nurse or has an illness with features similar to those being induced in the child. Factitious symptoms often include bleeding from various sites. If specimens are requested, the parent adds his or her own blood to them. Factitious signs include recurrent sepsis from injecting contaminated fluids, chronic diarrhea from laxatives, false renal stones from pebbles, fever from rubbing or heating thermometers, or rashes from rubbing the skin or applying caustic substances. All such cases should be reported to child protective services and the police in order to prevent the child's being taken to a different hospital or fatal treatment of the child by the parent when confronted with the evidence.

Emotional abuse is the continual rejection or scapegoating of a child by caretakers; severe verbal abuse is usually part of this picture. Emotional abuse is difficult to prove. The diagnostic criteria include severe psychopathology in the child, as determined by a psychiatrist, with the persistent refusal by the parents of treatment for the child. Psychologic terrorism (e.g., locking a child in a dark cellar or threats of mutilation) may also occur.

2.58 PHYSICAL ABUSE

Epidemiology. Each year in the United States approximately 1% of children are reported to be abused or neglected. Substantiated new cases of physical abuse are 1200/million population/yr. About 10% of injuries to children under 5 yr of age seen in hospital emergency rooms are due to abuse. The mortality is about 3% or 4000 deaths/yr. The ages of victims of physical abuse are estimated to be one third under 1 yr, one third from 1–6 yr of age, and one third over 6 yr. Premature infants are at a 3-fold greater risk of abuse.

Etiology. The abuser is a related caretaker in 90% of cases, a male friend of the mother in 5%, an unrelated babysitter in 4%, and a sibling in 1%. Parents who abuse their children exist in all ethnic, geographic, religious, educational, occupational, and socioeconomic groups. Groups living in poverty may have an increased incidence of child abuse because of the increased number of crises in their lives (e.g., unemployment or overcrowding) and because they have limited access to economic or social resources. An increased incidence of child physical abuse has been noted on military bases. The presence of spouse abuse doubles the likelihood of child abuse. Women are more likely to be involved in abuse than are men, but this is not usually the case in families in which the fathers are home, unemployed.

Over 90% of abusing parents have neither psychotic nor criminal personalities; they tend to be lonely, unhappy, angry adults under heavy stress. They injure their children in anger after being provoked by some misbehavior, and often themselves have experienced physical abuse as children. They usually believe that all misbehavior is deliberate and that severe punishment is necessary in teaching children to respect authority. If parents do not fit this description, suspicion of abuse should turn to babysitters and other parties.

The occurrence of physical abuse requires not only the particular parent but also a specific child and occasion. The child often has characteristics that make him or her provocative, such as negativism or a difficult temperament; some of the more offensive misbehaviors are intractable crying, wetting, soiling, and spilling. The occasion initiating the abuse is usually a family crisis; the most common include loss of a job or home, marital strife or upheavals, birth of a sibling, or physical exhaustion.

Clinical Manifestations. Many cases of physical abuse are first suspected because the injury is unexplained. More commonly an explanation is offered, but it is implausible. Inconsistencies are common between the history offered of a minor accident and the physical findings of a major injury, or between the history and the child's developmental level. Normal parents usually know to the moment when and where their children were hurt, and bring their children immediately for examination. In the case of abused children, there is often delay in seeking medical help, sometimes for several days.

Bruises, welts, lacerations, and scars identify physical abuse. The most common sites of accidental bruises are over the forehead, anterior tibia, and other bony prominences; however, bruises confined to the buttocks and lower back are almost always related to punishment. Finger and thumb prints may be found on the arms where a child has been forcefully grabbed. A slap leaves a bruise on the cheek with 2 or 3 parallel lines running through it. Attempts to silence a screaming child with impatient, forced attempts at feeding may bruise the upper lip and frenulum. Human bite marks are distinctive, paired, crescent-shaped bruises facing each other. When a blunt instrument is used in punishment, a bruise or welt will often resemble it in shape. Loop marks or scars on the skin are secondary to a doubled-over cord or rope. Lash marks are seen after beating with a belt, tree branch, or hard-edged ruler. Choke marks may be seen on the neck, or circumferential marks of ropes tied around the ankles or wrists. Traumatic alopecia may occur when the hair is yanked; the scalp has a normal appearance and the damaged hairs are broken off at varying lengths. A subgaleal hematoma may form under the site. Bruises and scars may be found at various stages of healing. Petechiae of the face and shoulders may follow intense retching, coughing, or crying. A mongolian spot may be mistaken for a bruise, but the color of the spot is solely blue-gray without any red hue.

Approximately 10% of cases of physical abuse involve burns. Hot solid burns are easiest to diagnose. These are usually 2nd-degree burns without blister formation and involve only one surface of the body. The shape of the burn is pathognomonic if the child is held against a heating grate or electric hot plate. Cigarette burns produce circular, punched-out lesions of uniform size. These are often found on the hands or feet and may be confused with bullous impetigo.

Hot water burns are the most common type of inflicted burn; blisters are usually present. A dunking burn occurs when a parent holds the thighs against the abdomen and places the buttocks and perineum in scalding water as punishment for enuresis or resistance to toilet training. This results in a circular type of burn restricted to the buttocks. With deeper, forced immersions, the scald extends to a clear-cut water level on the thighs and waist. The hands and feet are spared, which is incompatible with falling into a tub or turning on the hot water while in the bathtub. Forcible immersion of a hand or foot as punishment can be suspected when a burn goes well above the wrist or ankle. Toxic epidermal necrolysis can be confused with scalds.

Subdural hematoma is the most dangerous inflicted injury, often causing death or serious sequelae. Over 95% of serious intracranial injuries during the first year of life are the result of abuse. Affected infants often present with coma, convulsions, and increased intracranial pressure. Subdural hematomas may be associated with skull fractures secondary to a direct blow to the head, but over one half of the cases involve no skull fracture or bruises. These cases are the result of violent, whiplash-type, shaking injuries; the rapid acceleration and deceleration of the head as it bobs about may lead to tearing of the bridging cerebral veins with bleeding into the subdural space, usually bilaterally. Retinal hemorrhages are nearly always present, and there may be grab mark bruises of the upper extremities, shoulders, or chest.

Intra-abdominal injuries are the second most common cause of death in battered children. Affected children may present with recurrent vomiting, abdominal distention, absent bowel sounds, localized tenderness, or shock. Because the abdominal wall is flexible, the force of the blow is usually absorbed by the internal organs and the overlying skin is free of bruises. The most common finding is a ruptured liver or spleen. Much rarer are tears or other injuries of the small intestine at sites of ligamental support such as the duodenum and proximal jejunum. Intramural hematomas at these sites can lead to temporary obstruction. Chylous ascites and pseudocyst of the pancreas have been reported.

Laboratory Data. Screening tests for a bleeding diathesis should be obtained if medically indicated or if the parents deny the possibility of inflicted injury and give a history of easy bruisability.

When physical abuse is suspected in a child under 2 yr of age, a roentgenologic bone survey consisting of films of skull, thorax, and long bones should be made; pelvis and spine films may be indicated if any of the preceding films are positive. These films are of great diagnostic value since the clinical findings of fracture often disappear in 6–7 days even without orthopedic care. For most children 2–5 yr of age, a bone survey is indicated unless the child has very minor injuries or has been in a supervised setting (e.g., preschool). For children over the age of 5 yr roentgenograms need be obtained only if there is bone tenderness or a limited range of motion on physical examination. If films of a tender site are initially negative, they should be repeated in 2 wk to detect any calcification of subperiosteal bleeding or nondisplaced epiphyseal separations that may have occurred. Bone trauma is found in 10–20% of physically abused children.

Most inflicted fractures are due to wrenching or pulling injuries that damage the metaphysis, and the classic early finding is a chip fracture in which a corner of the metaphysis of a long bone is torn off, along with the epiphysis and periosteum. Ten to 14 days later calcification of subperiosteal bleeding becomes visible at the periphery. By 4–6 wk after the injury the subperiosteal calcification will be solid and start to smooth out and remodel. Inflicted fractures of the shaft are usually spiral rather than transverse, and spiral fractures of the femur prior to the age of walking are usually inflicted. Fractures of the ribs, scapula, or sternum should arouse suspicion of nonaccidental trauma. Cardiopulmonary resuscitation (CPR) rarely if ever causes rib fractures in children.

Diagnosis. A tentative diagnosis of physical abuse should be made if an injury is inadequately explained. Often a child over the age of 3 yr will be able to tell a sensitive and skillful interviewer that a particular adult hurt him or her. Certain bruises, burns, and scars are pathognomonic, and subdural hematomas do not occur spontaneously. Roentgenographic findings of chip fractures or multiple bony injuries at different stages of healing, implying repeated assaults, are also diagnostic.

Rare bone diseases such as scurvy and syphilis may resemble nonaccidental bone trauma, but the bony changes in these diseases are often symmetrical. Children with osteogenesis imperfecta, severe osteomalacia, or sensory deficits (e.g., myelomeningocele or paraplegia) have an increased incidence of pathologic fractures, but not of the metaphysis.

Treatment. A child suspected of being abused or neglected should usually be hospitalized, regardless of the extent of injuries, in order to protect the child until evaluation of the family with respect to the safety of the home is complete. If parents refuse hospitalization, a police or court order should be obtained. Some cases of child abuse can be safely evaluated without hospitalization when the child can be placed in an emergency receiving home or when the person inflicting the trauma no longer has access to the child. Children over the age of 6 yr with mild injuries may be evaluated in the home under certain circumstances.

Once the child is in the hospital, the medical and surgical problems should receive appropriate care. The parents should be told by the physician that inflicted injury is suspected, the reasons for this concern, and that the physician is legally obligated to report it. It should be emphasized that this problem is treatable, that a child welfare agency will be involved (not usually the police), and that everyone's goal is not to punish but to help the parents find better ways of dealing with their child's needs. The protective service agency should then be contacted immediately by telephone; required written reports should be sent subsequently. Siblings should have full examinations within 12 hr of the report of child abuse in the family. Approximately 20% of them will also have signs of physical abuse.

Feeling angry with abusing parents is natural, but expressing the anger damages rapport, making the cooperation of parents less likely. Repeated interrogations, confrontations, and accusations must be avoided. The parents should be encouraged to visit their children, and the hospital staff must do their best to be courteous and helpful. The primary physician should see the parents or telephone them daily. An evaluation by hospital social services should be obtained to determine the nature of problems in the family and environment and the safety of the home. A psychiatric evaluation may be appropriate in some instances.

Every hospital caring for children should designate a group of professionals responsive to the needs of abused or neglected children and their families. The group should include a pediatric consultant, a hospital social worker, a pediatric nurse, a psychologist or psychiatrist, and a coordinator. There should be clearly defined liaisons with public agencies and the courts, and legal consultants should be available. Within 1 wk of admitting any child for abuse or neglect, evaluations should be completed and the team should meet with the child's physician and nurse, the child protective service representative, and, as appropriate, the police or any other community agencies involved with the family, to decide on the best immediate and long-range plans.

The pediatrician can coordinate the health care of the abused child, who needs more intensive surveillance and well-child care than the average child. Child welfare agencies are primarily responsible for coordinating and making home visits and for evaluating the therapy of the entire family. Because of the number of difficulties experienced by most abusive families, usually no single agency or discipline can provide all the needed services. Innovative types of therapy that have been successful when designed for individual families include Lay Therapists or Parent Aides, Homemakers,

Parents Anonymous groups, telephone hotlines, environmental crisis therapy, and child-rearing counseling. Traditional psychotherapy is often ineffective.

Prevention. Parents at high risk for being unable adequately to love and care for their offspring can be identified early if attention is given to such things as abuse of a previous child, drug addiction or serious psychiatric illness in a new mother, negative parental comments about the newborn infant, lack of evidence of maternal attachment, infrequent visits to a new baby whose discharge is delayed because of prematurity or illness, the spanking of a young infant, or the severe neglect of infant hygiene. Abuse and serious neglect may be prevented when such families receive an intensive form of well baby care, including prenatal classes, contact between mother and baby in the delivery room, rooming-in, increased parental contact with premature infants, extra help with calming the crying infant, more frequent office visits, ongoing counseling regarding discipline, visits of public health nurses, nurseries to which infants and young children can be admitted for short-term respite care at the times of family crises, close follow-up of acute illnesses, telephone lifelines, arrangement for day care, and assistance in family planning.

Prognosis. With comprehensive, intensive treatment of the entire family, 80–90% of families involved in child abuse or neglect can be rehabilitated to provide adequate care for their children. Approximately 10–15% of such families can only be stabilized, and will require an indefinite continuation of supporting services until their children are old enough to leave home. Termination of parental rights or continued foster placement is required in 2–3% of cases.

Of abused children returned to their parents without any intervention, about 5% will be killed and 25% seriously injured. Children with repeated injuries to the central nervous system may develop mental retardation, organic brain syndrome, seizures, hydrocephalus, or ataxia. Common emotional traits of abused children are fearfulness, aggression, and hyperactivity. Further, untreated families tend to produce children who become the juvenile delinquents and violent members of our society and the next generation of child abusers.

2.59 INCEST
(Family-Related Sexual Abuse)

See also Sec. 2.51 and 18.6.

Incest refers to any sexual activity between persons too closely related to marry; most legal codes include adopted and/or stepchildren in the definition. Sexual mistreatment of children by family members is the most common type, and by friends and acquaintances of the child or family is the next most common. Least common is sexual abuse by strangers. This section will not deal with extrafamilial child sexual abuse, although the steps in medical evaluation of both types are similar. Intrafamilial sexual abuse is more difficult to manage because the child must be protected from additional abuse at the same time that one tries to preserve the family unit.

Three types of incest are molestation, sexual intercourse, and rape. Child molestation includes touching or fondling the genitals of the child or asking the child to fondle the adult's genitals; forced exposure to sexual acts or pornography is also part of this definition. Sexual intercourse includes vaginal, oral, or rectal penetration (or attempted penetration) on a nonassaultive basis. Without detection and intervention molestation almost always progresses to full sexual intercourse. Less than 10% of incest is assaultive, forced intercourse (family-related rape).

Epidemiology. At least 0.2–0.3% of children have been involved in persistent incestuous relationships for an average

period of 5 yr. Brief sexual encounters occur more frequently. The victims of incest are 90% female and 10% male. (In cases of third party molestation in child care centers, which are being recognized with increasing frequency, the sex ratio is more nearly equal.) No age of child is exempt. Approximately one third are less than 6 yr of age, one third 6–12, and one third 12–18. Incest is often repeated with successive daughters. The offenders are 99% male. The incidence among stepfathers is about 5 times higher than among natural fathers. Incest cuts across socioeconomic lines to a greater degree than physical abuse.

Etiology. Most incest involves fathers and daughters. Sexual relationships usually begin gradually and without any violence. The father brings to this relationship a need for sexual gratification, and the daughter brings a need for tender affection and nurturance. The father is usually rigid, patriarchal, and emotionally immature. He is unlikely to engage in extramarital relationships, but he may have a tendency to alcoholism. Mothers are usually chronically depressed, unavailable to their husbands because of work or illness, and often themselves the childhood victims of sexual abuse. The child victim tends to be pseudomature and has taken on many of the housekeeping tasks. The families are often closely knit and socially isolated. In cases of violent family-related rape, the father is usually a sociopath, and his sexual abuse extends outside the family circle.

Clinical Manifestations. Victims of family-related rape are usually brought to an emergency room in acute distress. The child may disclose the incestuous relationship to her mother and be brought to a physician at that time. If the mother does not believe the child, the child may later tell a girlfriend, friend's mother, or school counselor. Some adolescents will disclose their secret to a physician in a private interview. At other times the physician must elicit the history of incest on suspicion, e.g., when the prepubertal child presents with vaginal bleeding, other unexplained genital symptoms, recurrent urinary tract infections, enuresis, or encopresis. The main cause of venereal disease in the prepubertal child is sexual transmission from adults. Nonsexual contamination from an older female with gonorrhea occasionally occurs in children under 4 yr of age. In the case of a pregnant adolescent who is not dating and who offers no information regarding the baby's father, incest should be suspected.

Investigation of the possibility of incest requires sensitive and thorough history-taking because less than half of the victims have any abnormal physical or laboratory findings. A detailed explicit account of sexual experiences by a prepubertal child should be considered hard evidence in these cases. Physical findings are usually absent because of the long delay before the victim feels safe in telling someone about his or her plight. Interviewing should proceed gently and at the child's pace. Pictures or dolls should be used to clarify body parts; the child's vocabulary should be learned from the parent. If a social worker has carried out the initial interview, the physician can review this material and need not repeat the interview.

Female victims usually prefer that a female physician examine them, but this is not mandatory. An examination of the skin should be carried out for any signs of trauma, especially bite marks. The abdominal examination should assess the possibility of pregnancy. The mouth should be examined for signs of trauma such as redness, abrasions, or purpura. The rectum should be examined for signs of trauma or laxity. The external genitals should be examined for signs of trauma, laxity, or discharge. In prepubertal girls, a hymenal opening of 5 mm or greater is probably abnormal. A speculum examination of the vagina is indicated when the victim is postpubertal or when nonmenstrual vaginal bleeding or major trauma of the external genitals is present.

Laboratory Data. The amount of laboratory evidence sought depends on the history. Molestation victims usually receive only a vulvar washing for sperm. Sexual intercourse victims should have routine tests for sperm, acid phosphatase, and gonorrhea. In the vagina, motile sperm can be found for 6 hr and nonmotile for 72 hr or longer. Acid phosphatase is present for 24 hr. Sperm and semen may also be recovered from the mouth and rectum. While the presence of semen substantiates the victim's history, the absence of semen does not contradict the history of vaginal intercourse. Cultures should be taken from the mouth, vagina, and rectum; occasionally they are positive at sites initially denied by the child because of embarrassment. Less than 5% of the victims have positive cultures for gonorrhea. Symptomatic victims should also have tests for syphilis and *Chlamydia*. Additional materials that may help to identify the perpetrator in third-party cases include pubic hair, scalp hair, fingernail scrapings, blood samples, and sperm. The specimens are usually transferred to the police laboratory in sealed, signed, and dated envelopes.

Diagnosis. The diagnosis of child molestation and most instances of sexual intercourse rests on the graphic history offered by the victim. False accusations are rare except in cases involving psychotic patients, sexually active adolescents who are angry at their father or stepfather, and some custody disputes. If sexual intercourse has occurred within the previous 72 hr, laboratory evidence of acid phosphatase or sperm helps to confirm the diagnosis. The presence of a nonvirginal hymen suggests penetration, but the victim must clarify whether this was caused by a penis, finger, or other object. In family-related rape cases, the diagnosis is readily confirmed by evidence of recent trauma as well as positive laboratory findings. Normal physical and laboratory examinations, however, are compatible with most types of sexual abuse.

Treatment. Evaluation and management of sexual abuse is similar to but more complex than that of physical abuse. All victims of sexual abuse require psychologic support. Often both parents deny the girl's accusation and rebuke or punish her for reporting the incident. Victims of a single nonviolent episode of molestation may need only reassurance and a chance to express their feelings about the event on one or two occasions. Usually they are less distressed by the incident than are their parents. In a single, violent episode of family-related rape the patient is usually in serious emotional distress and requires the services of a child psychiatrist and/or rape victim advocate. Most such patients make a good adjustment after several sessions in age-appropriate psychotherapy. The victims of multiple episodes of sexual abuse almost always need long-term psychotherapy. The victim may be able to return home if the perpetrator is out of the home or has confessed and is in therapy. The child should be placed in foster care if this is his or her desire, if the mother doesn't believe the child's story, if family life is chaotic, or if collection of evidence is not yet complete. Medication to prevent pregnancy may be given to postmenarcheal girls in mid-cycle, who have experienced vaginal intercourse within the previous 72 hr. At a minimum all victims should revisit their physicians within 2 wk to evaluate their psychologic functioning and to assess the services that have been implemented.

Many incest offenders are treatable. The offending parent requires a psychiatric evaluation, and the spouse should be evaluated by a social worker. Offenders are always investigated by the police, and criminal prosecution commonly occurs. Sentencing is usually deferred if the father becomes honestly involved in therapy. Both parents usually need psychotherapy and marital therapy. The offender in family-related rape cases is usually placed in jail, and criminal prosecution and sentencing do occur. The sociopaths are usually untreatable. Offenders with alcoholism may be helped by Alcoholics Anonymous groups.

Prevention. The primary prevention of sexual abuse includes encouraging children to "not keep secrets," "say no," and to "tell someone." Over one hundred books, plays, cartoons, films and mime shows on sexual abuse are currently available in the United States. Such programs may bring out declarations by children already sexually abused, but whether they will protect others from seductive or predatory adults is not clear. At present, the best protection for children is alert adults who will not leave them in high-risk situations (e.g., day care centers that prohibit visiting) and who will listen to them and recognize their symptoms of stress.

Prognosis. With intervention most incest victims can lead normal adult lives. Without intervention many of them run away from home and become adolescent prostitutes and drug addicts; those who stay at home manifest depression, suicidal gestures, and conversion reactions; as adults most of them have difficulties with close relationships and need psychiatric help.

2.60 NONORGANIC FAILURE TO THRIVE

See also Sec. 5.36.

Failure to thrive (FTT) has several causes. Approximately 70% of cases are nonorganic and 30% are organic. The nonorganic group is composed of 50% neglectful or psychologic FTT and 20% accidental, e.g., errors in formula preparation or errors in feeding techniques. Here we will consider neglectful failure to thrive, which rarely occurs after 2 yr of age because older children can obtain food for themselves. Under bizarre circumstances an older child can lose weight or gain poorly because he is confined to a room or deliberately starved. The main cause of FTT in infancy is that the baby is not fed enough. The mother may neglect feeding because she is busy with external problems (e.g., overwhelmed with work), preoccupied with inner problems, or doesn't like the baby. Emotional deprivation is inevitably concurrent with nutritional deprivation. Most of the involved mothers feel deprived and unloved themselves; many are acutely or chronically depressed. The baby is usually unplanned and unwanted. Multiple and continuing crises, frequently compounded by the physical absence of the father, may overwhelm the mother, who reacts by neglecting her infant.

Clinical Manifestations. The dietary history in infants with nutritional neglect is usually not helpful because the parent reports that the baby is receiving adequate calories. In some cases, the mother's report that the baby has vomiting and diarrhea is not confirmed by the baby's hospital course. The parents have not usually sought medical care for their baby and immunizations are not up-to-date. By contrast, the feeding history is extremely helpful in accidental FTT because the parents are open about their feeding errors and misunderstandings.

The infant with FTT usually exhibits thin extremities, a narrow face, prominent ribs, and wasted buttocks. Neglect of hygiene is often evidenced by rampant diaper rash, unwashed skin, untreated impetigo, uncut fingernails, or filthy clothing. A flattened occiput points to being left unattended for undue hours. Delays in social and speech development are common but are rarely detected before 4 mo of age. Findings include an avoidance of eye contact, an expressionless face, and the absence of a cuddling response. The amount of time the mother spends holding, playing with, and talking to her baby is usually reduced or inappropriate. A rejecting mother will often feed her baby with anger and unnecessary force.

Laboratory Data. Investigation of the etiology of failure to thrive is discussed in Sec. 5.36. Extensive laboratory evaluation should usually be delayed until dietary management has

expressive language; selective attention and activity; and increasingly higher orders of conceptualization. These functions are supported by the somewhat more general or pervasive apparatuses of memory (auditory, visual, sequential, short-term, and long-term) and of motor output. All of these elements serve the child in a psychosocial context shaped by past experiences and acquired values, by learned skills and coping styles, and by the child's emotional health and feelings of self-esteem.

The dysfunctions of youngsters with mental deficiency or multiple handicaps have similar elements. The retarded may often differ from the subtly handicapped only in the severity or multiplicity of their deficits.

2.62 CAUSES OF DEVELOPMENTAL DYSFUNCTION

The search for specific etiology of developmental dysfunction in school-age children has rarely been fruitful. One can often identify certain "risk factors" or predispositions in early medical and developmental history, such as premature birth, small size for gestational age, or traumatic delivery; however, one can rarely be certain that such associations are, in fact, causes of the child's current difficulties, since statistical associations between perinatal stresses and later development are weak and inconsistent. Many children born of difficult pregnancies and deliveries, with stormy neonatal courses, function normally during the school years.

Certain families have a high incidence of reading problems with no ready environmental explanation. Some children with attention deficits have parents whose behavior was similar during childhood; in such cases, it may be difficult to separate genetic effects from modeling. Some genetic syndromes have specific processing problems; girls with Turner syndrome, for example, have difficulties with visual-spatial organization.

Infections of the central nervous system and encephalopathies such as lead poisoning may also produce developmental dysfunctions.

2.63 THE ELEMENTS OF DEVELOPMENTAL FUNCTION

VISUAL-SPATIAL ORIENTATION

Normal Function. From birth infants begin to be aware of spatial relationships through integrating visual imagery with somesthetic input through tactile, kinesthetic, and proprioceptive senses and reflexes. Piaget called the developmental period, during which infants first and principally employ sensory cues to construct a world of objects, the *stage of sensorimotor intelligence*. This stage of development is clearly dependent upon the adequacy of *visual perception* and in turn on the capacity for *visual-motor integration*.

Perception is the process whereby the central nervous system organizes sensory data. Visual-perceptual function permits recognition and discrimination among patterns and their relationships in space. This is *visual-spatial orientation*. It entails the appreciation of details, relative position, size, contour, and distinctions between background and foreground. The ability to differentiate visually among symbols and letters is critical for reading and ultimately for writing, and is closely linked to the ability to perceive an overall pattern, in contradistinction to the limited ability to identify only the separate items or portions of a figure or a structure.

Visual-motor integration is essential in praxis (i.e., the planning and execution of complex motor movements). Catching a ball, tying shoelaces, copying designs, and buttoning a shirt are acts requiring such integration.

Dysfunction. Delays in development of visual-perceptual and visual-motor functions may be difficult to identify in infancy and in the preschool years. Initial manifestations may include difficulties in learning to tie shoelaces, in discrimination between left and right, in confusion and anxiety over recognition of letters or delay in acquiring skills in drawing or copying. Ultimately, a child with visual-spatial disorientation may encounter problems in learning to read (Sec. 2.64), to write, and to arrange words and sentences on a page. There has been a tendency to attribute most reading problems to inadequacies in visual perception, but recent observations have not supported this assumption. Some investigators now suggest that difficulties in matching or associating specific visual images with the sound and meaning of their verbal equivalents may be responsible for many of the delays in acquiring reading skills. Such a difference might reflect a disorder of associative memory, or perhaps generally poor linguistic skills. Inadequacies in visual perception do, however, appear to be related to inefficiencies in spelling, writing, and other eye-hand coordination activities. Some children develop compensatory strategies, independently or with help, and may overcome visual processing handicaps to varying degrees.

Some, but not all, children with visual-perceptual disorders experience delays in the development of some functions; on the other hand, not all children with delays in their motor development have evidence of visual-spatial disorganization.

Assessment. The diagnosis of deficits in visual perception can be difficult. Most commonly, children are asked to copy specific forms standardized for age (Fig. 2–12). Such tests, however, depend upon fine motor function, as well as upon visual-motor integration; moreover, a child who is reflective is likely to reproduce such forms more accurately than an impulsive youngster. The skill may also be dependent on previous experience. For these reasons, one must interpret such assessments cautiously. Delay in acquiring skill in form-copying does not prove the existence of a visual-perceptual problem, but might be taken as evidence of such a deficit. More discriminatory evidence may come from some of the subtests on the Wechsler Intelligence Scale for Children (WISC) (in particular, object assembly, picture completion, and block design); other standardized tests such as Frostig's Developmental Test of Visual Perception and Raven's Pro-

FORMS TO COPY FOR THE SCREENING OF VISUAL-PERCEPTUAL-MOTOR FUNCTION

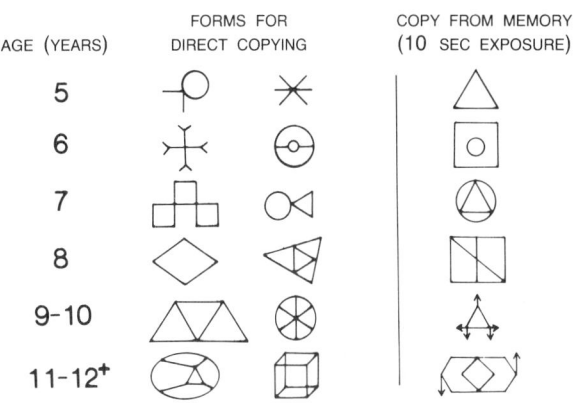

Figure 2–12. Examples of forms standardized for age. These forms can be utilized by pediatricians as screening devices for visual-perceptual-motor deficits. Impaired performance on such a task might also be due to other problems, such as inattention, inexperience, fine motor difficulties, or problems with conceptualization. These forms should never be used as the ultimate diagnostic indicator; instead, they might indicate the need for further evaluation of a visual-perceptual-motor problem.

gressive Matrices are more direct measures of visual perception.

TEMPORAL-SEQUENTIAL ORGANIZATION

Normal Function. Just as children develop visual-spatial orientation, so do they acquire concepts of time and sequence. This function is localized to a large extent in the left hemisphere of the brain, whereas appreciation of overall form and pattern is thought to be a function mainly of the right hemisphere (in right-handed persons).

Much of a child's information gathering and daily activity depends upon sequence. Watches, calendars, schedules, and routines testify to the importance given time and sequence in our society. Young children acquire an appreciation of sequence as they master the routine order of meals, days, months, and years, and learn such concepts as *before* and *after*, *today* and *tomorrow*, and *now* and *later*. Sequential organization is closely related to memory. Its capacity and range expand with age.

Dysfunction. Children with deficits in sequential organization may have serious problems with short-term memory. Parents and teachers may complain that they seldom follow instructions, seem unable to retain what has just been said, or get "overloaded" or bewildered by a series of directions. They may have difficulty with story telling or reporting, may show confusion over temporal prepositions, and may be delayed in learning to tell time. Sequencing difficulties may be primarily auditory or mainly visual or motor; some involve many or all areas. Affected children may show maladaptive classroom behaviors, as protective strategies or as evidence of frustration and anxiety.

Difficulties in temporal-sequential organization often follow a fairly typical pattern. The earliest manifestations (such as problems in telling time or in following multistep directions) may be slowly mastered, only to be followed by scholastic difficulties, such as problems in remembering the multiplication tables. Ultimately, these too improve, but may be replaced in adolescence by problems in organization of study habits, with long-range projects, and with the completion of multistep proofs in geometry.

Assessment. There are several methods of screening for temporal-sequential organization. The *digit span* tests immediate recall of a sequence of spoken numbers, as a test of auditory-sequential memory; but performance may be influenced by the strength of the child's number concept as well as by anxiety or inattention. In the *object span* test the child is asked to tap or point to a series of objects in an order demonstrated by the examiner. The *block tapping* exercise is done the same way, except that a series of similar squares is tapped instead of different objects. These tests of visual-sequential memory are influenced by a child's attentional strength. *Serial commands* involve a sequence of oral instructions. Motor sequencing involves imitation of a sequence of motor activities, as demonstrated by the examiner. These tests for sequential organization are summarized in Table 2–15.

Standardized tests of visual-sequential and auditory-sequential memory form part of the Illinois Test of Psycholinguistic Abilities. The Digit Span and Picture Arrangement subtests of the WISC may also offer indications of sequencing problems.

MEMORY

The quality of memory depends upon the strength of attention, the extent of motivation, the adequacy of processing of the information to be stored, the frequency of exposure, and the techniques used to register and to retrieve data. There is no single brain center that houses all of memory; rather, the capacity for retention is widely distributed over the many associative areas of the brain. The ability to store and retrieve *specific kinds* of data varies considerably from person to person.

Neurophysiologists distinguish between short- and long-term memory. The former is limited in its capacity, whereas the latter seems to have nearly inexhaustible storage space. Short-term memory is influenced by the strength of attention and by the quality of information processing. Adequacy of long-term memory is enhanced by frequent retrieval and elaboration, by strong cognitive and affective associations of stored information, and by the relevance of the information to the memorizer.

A critical aspect of memory has to do with *access* to stored data. The two most commonly cited processes are recognition and retrieval. The capacity to recognize as familiar something

Table 2–15. **Tasks for the Assessment of Temporal-Sequential Organization**

Age	Digit Span — Series of spoken numbers (1–9), given one per second, to be repeated by child	Object Span — Series of objects tapped in random order; child imitates in same order	Block Tapping — Series of squares tapped in random order; child then imitates in same order	Serial Commands — Series of simple commands; child performs in correct order	Motor Sequence — Child performs act after examiner
5–6 yr	4 forward digits	4 objects	4 squares	3-step series	Simultaneously open and close both hands, arms extended
6–7 yr	4–5 forward digits	4 objects	4 squares	4-step series	Imitative finger tapping (both hands, 3–4 steps)
7–8 yr	5 forward digits	5 objects	5 squares	5-step series	Imitative mixed finger-foot tapping (4–5 steps)
9–10 yr	6 forward digits 4 reverse digits	5 objects	5 squares	5-step series	Alternate left and right open and close fists, arms extended
11–12 + yr	6 forward digits 5 reverse digits	6 objects	6 squares	6-step series	Imitate edge of hand on knee, then palm on knee, then clenched fist (4 cycles)

one has encountered before is relatively simple. Much more complex is the ability to recall sets of related information, such as someone's name on sight or the spelling of a word during writing.

It appears that by the 1st grade youngsters have developed about the same degree of proficiency in recognition memory as have 6th grade students. During these elementary school years, however, there is a distinct increase in the ability to retrieve stored knowledge. As children progress toward junior high school, they have a critical need that retrieval capacity become highly developed in order that large areas of their knowledge can be readily accessed without much effort. This enables the student to recall certain information or skills while performing another act. In this way, for example, a youngster can form letters with his or her pen and recall spelling and some needed facts all at the same time.

Most youngsters become increasingly adept in employing *memory strategies*, so that by 6th grade the more apt students can be expected to employ mnemonic strategies that include imaging, developing rich associations with new data, subvocalizing, classifying, and other techniques. Many youngsters with learning disorders lack these strategies, and fail to develop "metamemory," a conscious understanding of how one's own memory operates best.

Dysfunction. Evidence suggests that many children with learning problems have related memory deficits. Some of these memory disorders may be related to other conceptual problems; for example, a youngster with visual-perceptual problems may also have a difficulty with visual memory that aggravates writing and spelling deficiencies. One with poor language processing may have difficulties with auditory memory. Students who lag in temporal-sequential organization are prone to sequential memory deficiencies. Those with attentional problems commonly develop rather bizarre and unpredictable patterns of memory. Some students have trouble in holding one process in mind while performing a related action. Consequently, they may forget what they are doing in the middle of a task. For example, during the performance of mental arithmetic, they may become confused and lose track of various substeps of a problem. It is not unusual for such youngsters to develop test-taking anxiety in anticipation of memory failure during examinations. The anxiety itself further compromises memory.

A careful clinical history may provide anecdotal clues regarding memory deficiencies. For example, some children have difficulty in retaining instructions in the classroom or at home, and others in recalling skills or information following a school vacation. Weakness in such academic skills as spelling, multiplication tables, and foreign languages may be evidence of poor memory ability. The detection of specific deficits requires both time and considerable experience in conducting and evaluating the various tests and measurements now available; accordingly, the diagnostic survey should generally be carried out by a clinical psychologist experienced in the educational field.

RECEPTIVE LANGUAGE AND CENTRAL AUDITORY PROCESSING

Normal Function. Acquisition of the ability to decode words and sentences greatly facilitates children's understanding and assimilation of their surroundings, their perception of themselves, their interactions with others, and their ultimate academic skills. Learning the rules of syntax or grammar gives words meaning in context.

Language skills are presumed when the child enters school. During elementary school years, there is surprisingly little growth in vocabulary, but conspicuous progress in complex and sophisticated grammatical constructions, in drawing in-ferences from abstract figures of speech, and in perception of irony, paradox, and humor. In the early grades, the language and ideational content of a reading passage is well below what the child may be expected to grasp in conversation. As the student approaches and enters secondary school, the verbal sophistication of texts surpasses that of conversation, usually during 8th grade. Youngsters who have subtle difficulties with receptive language may ultimately display serious impairments of reading comprehension.

Good language processing in one's native tongue is critical to mastery of a second language. Some children in their high school years show impairment in their ability to acquire competence in a foreign language. In some cases, this may reflect subclinical disabilities in the native language that have not surfaced earlier owing to the preponderance of verbal activity in early life.

Receptive language function involves interpretation of auditory stimuli and extraction of meaning from words and sentences. The first step is selective attention to speech sounds. Auditory discrimination, which is a differentiation of similar sounds, follows. Basic units of sound are then identified as words with meanings, which can then be given syntactic relationships.

Dysfunction. Auditory perceptual difficulties may involve both difficulty with recognition of discrete units of sound or with auditory figure-sound relationships and difficulty in association of meanings with words or understanding the significance of grammatical structures. Affected children may be restless and inattentive in verbal environments.

Children with impaired language reception may have trouble analyzing words phonetically. Delays in reading, spelling, and written output can result from relatively subtle receptive weaknesses. Secondary inattention, emotional difficulties, and social maladjustment are common. Young children with these problems can become confused and anxious or panic-stricken, as they perceive the classroom experience as through a bad telephone connection or a badly tuned radio.

Assessment. Screening for speech and language disabilities begins with a careful history and with informed interaction with the child. No single speech and language screening test serves all ages. Such tests as the Preschool Language Scale (Zimmerman, Steiner, and Evatt) or the Screening Test for Preschool Children (Fluharty) are useful for children until the age of 5 yr.

An expressive language disorder (see below) may be accompanied by difficulty with receptive processing. Children with difficulties in articulation, word finding, and narration may also have underlying auditory-perceptual deficits, weaknesses of auditory memory, or other language deficiencies. Physicians must be alert for perceptive language problems, and not assume that conventional psychologic testing will reliably detect language disabilities interfering with school performance.

Adequate hearing acuity is basic to receptive language function and to speech development in infancy, and to adequate function at any older age. For further discussion of hearing, speech, and language see Sec. 2.67 and 2.68.

EXPRESSIVE LANGUAGE

Normal Function. Useful language depends on the capacity to call up relevant words, the arrangement of them in phrases or sentences that conform to linguistic rules, and the development of ideas in a meaningful sequence. During the school years, written and spoken language occupies the center stage in education, in self-monitoring, in controlling social interaction, in dealing with and understanding one's own feelings, and in demonstrating competence.

Dysfunction. Disorders of expressive language include:

1. Deficits of resonance: abnormal oral-nasal sound balance, usually heard as hypernasality or hyponasality.

2. Voice disorders: deviations in quality, pitch, or loudness of physiologic or psychologic origin.

3. Fluency disorders: disruption in the natural flow of connected speech, most commonly as stuttering.

4. Articulation disorders: a major group of problems in which the production of speech sounds is imprecise.

5. Language disorders: problems in comprehension and manipulation of the symbol systems of language.

Disorders of resonance and voice are common and ordinarily require the assistance of a speech therapist (Sec. 2.68). During the normal development of language, all children show some evidence of nonfluent speech between 1 and 4 yr of age. These may consist of pauses, repetitions of sounds, revisions of sentences, lapses in responding, or prolongation of sounds. *Stuttering* is felt by some to be due often to inappropriate response by a listener to this normal developmental dysfluency; the resulting feelings of inadequacy by the child aggravate the nonfluency. The majority of stuttering children are identified between the ages of 3 and 4 yr. Stuttering may appear later, with the first school experience or with the approach of adolescence. In all likelihood, stuttering is a symptom with multiple causes. Its association with wider neurologic dysfunction is unusual. It may occur in families, but it is not generally regarded as genetic or learned by imitation. The attitude of the family toward normal nonfluency and other expectations may explain its occurrence in siblings. Some children may derive secondary gains from stuttering. Stuttering children need early, careful psychologic assessments and evaluations of speech and language. Most should be referred to a speech pathologist.

Disorders of articulation are the most commonly encountered speech problems in children, and involve three types of errors: *substitutions*, replacement of one sound with another (e.g., wight for light); *omissions*, failure to produce certain speech sounds (e.g., boo for book); and *distortions*, inappropriate sounds replacing the correct ones. Wide variability is observed in the number of consonants and vowels that are misarticulated. Errors may range from a few misarticulated sounds to speech that is sometimes unintelligible. Poor articulation may be caused by anatomic abnormalities within the oral cavity (including dental irregularities, or abnormal shape or structure of the hard palate), paralysis or weakness of the tongue, or occasionally hearing loss. Articulation deficits may be associated with developmental language disabilities. Environmental and psychologic factors may also predispose to poor speech sound production.

Evidence suggests that many children or adults with articulation disabilities have difficulty in using sensory information from the mouth (buccal somesthetic and kinesthetic feedback). Such an articulation disorder may be analogous to other perceptual-motor problems.

Disabilities of expressive language create a variety of problems; one is an inability to use syntax in a manner commensurate with developmental age. Affected youngsters are often shy; commonly, they rely on gestures and on communication through single words or phrases, appearing at times to speak in telegraphic style. There may be a history of delay in achievement of language milestones. Children with deficits in expressive language must be evaluated for generalized developmental delay, auditory sensory loss, emotional disturbance, autism, and elective mutism.

Some children able to express themselves in appropriate syntax require excessive time and effort; they have difficulty keeping pace in conversations and become reluctant to use narrative. Some such children are afraid of being called upon during class discussions. Although they have good ideas, they are ashamed of their hesitancy and impaired quality of expression. Such students may be helped by teachers who will ask them questions that can be answered "yes" or "no."

Word-finding disorders, as expressive language handicaps, are more common than has been recognized. Parents of an affected child may report that "he can't say what he wants," or "it's as if it's just at the tip of her tongue." The child is momentarily unable to recall the name of an object or event for which previous knowledge exists, may be slow to name pictures or objects, or may attempt to use gestures or pantomimes that conform closely to the object. Some children will speak in definitions or approximations rather than specific words; others will label things by association (e.g., rain for umbrella, or tobacco for pipe). Sometimes a word is substituted that sounds like the word sought (e.g., slow for low). Word-finding deficits often occur with other language handicaps, such as difficulties with syntax and auditory memory.

Disorders of narrative may take several forms, such as an inability to comment on content, or reduced story-telling skills. Affected youngsters may speak only in the most concrete way about events. Many cannot organize a narrative, but ramble and build incoherent structures.

Deficits of word-finding and of narrative organization may not be detected by parents or teachers. An affected child may even be verbose; but careful study will show the content of expressive language to be developmentally delayed, the words used relatively simple and below the child's developmental level in other areas, and sentence structure relatively primitive.

Language impairments may disrupt the development of social relationships within the family, or with peer groups, and behavioral disorganization or regression may be observed. Many children with expressive language problems have difficulties in reading. Their plight intensifies when they are required to produce high volumes of written material (Sec. 2.64). Early detection and intervention are particularly urgent.

Assessment. The evaluation of expressive language requires assessment of the child's ability to formulate sentences, to name, and to narrate. A history of recurrent otitis media, of delayed acquisition of intelligible speech, or of persistent articulation problems may point to dysfunction in this area.

In addition to assessing the intelligibility of speech, one should judge the child's voice quality, pitch, and resonance. Pediatricians should be on the alert for youngsters with problems in articulation, for school-age children who overuse short declarative sentences, for sparseness of vocabulary, for frequent hesitations or circumlocutions, or for unusual reluctance in verbal expression. Picture-naming tests are used to uncover possible problems with word-finding. When there are doubts about any of these, a full-scale evaluation of speech and language should be undertaken (Sec. 2.68).

VOLUNTARY MOTOR OUTPUT

Normal Function. Gross and fine motor control reflect the constant feedback of visual and somesthetic cues, which contribute to a sense of body position, to control over movement quality, to the maintenance of posture, and to decisions as to whether to continue, to modify, or to complete motor acts. Motor function involves also the facilitation and inhibition of muscle groups, the planning (praxis), execution, and monitoring of actions. Fine motor function, such as dexterity with the hands, critical for writing skills, depends upon afferent stimuli involving visual, proprioceptive, and kinesthetic feedback and various aspects of memory. Effective gross motor control offers obvious dividends in the enhancement of self-image through sports and other recreations. Some claim that motor therapy can improve learning, but there is little evidence of such a relationship.

Dysfunction. Specific types of fine motor dysfunction may compromise writing or drawing, or delay acquisition of such self-help skills as the tying of shoelaces. Some affected youngsters show deficiencies of eye-hand coordination, and others have difficulty with proprioceptive-kinesthetic feedback. Failure of finger localization (*finger agnosia*) can result in slow and awkward written output. Such youngsters, in particular, may adopt awkward pencil grasps, and may be overwhelmed by lengthy writing assignments or by tests taken under timed conditions.

Children with another kind of fine motor dysfunction (dyspraxia) have difficulty with motor implementation or muscular coordination. Dyspractic writers know what they want to do but cannot execute the appropriate sequence of motor movements. Many of the children with fine motor dyspraxia also have problems in speech articulation.

Some children have difficulties with *motor memory*. Most commonly one encounters fluctuating patterns of motor recall. A student momentarily "forgets" how to form letters while in the process of doing so, and tends to form the same letter in different ways in the same sentence. During writing there are frequent hesitations, retracings, and crossing out. Illegibility is common.

Children with gross motor delays may develop profound feelings of inadequacy, avoiding interaction with their peers for fear of such humiliation as always being picked last for teams. Some degree of social ostracism may result from their visible awkwardness or clumsiness.

Assessment. In evaluating fine motor function, children should be observed performing some tasks that entail use of a pencil and some that do not. Eye-hand coordination can be assessed by watching the rate and precision with which a child picks up matchsticks or pennies, or the rate at which a child puts a string through a series of eye hooks that follow a circuitous pathway in a board. Pencil control can be evaluated as a child draws a line through a maze, connects dots, or copies designs. The latter may also be used to assess motor planning.

Knowledge of a child's orientation toward graphic arts, fixing things, and craft activities may suggest strengths in certain aspects of fine motor output. Historical data regarding the acquisition of writing skills are critical. Children who are resistant and/or delayed in mastering cursive writing frequently have underlying deficiencies of motor memory. The ANSER System Questionnaires, commonly used in the evaluation of children with learning problems, contain specific questions to detect such developmental problems.

The examination of a child's gross motor control involves presenting developmentally appropriate tasks. Table 2–16 lists examples of such activities as rough guidelines. Motor performance is poorly standardized for older children, however, owing to the effects of cultural differences and experience. The quality of performance may be more important than simply whether or not the child can perform a given task. For gross movement, one should observe coordination, balance, visual-motor integration, and motor-sequential organization.

In the school-age child, a history of skills and interest in specific sports may provide insights into a child's gross motor proficiency. Athletic pursuits differ in the demands made upon gross motor output. For example, baseball requires an ability to program gross motor activity within a visual-spatial context, whereas skiing and swimming emphasize body positioning and kinesthetic sense. For children with possible gross motor delays the Lincoln-Oseretsky Test offers developmentally appropriate tests of gross motor function.

SELECTIVE ATTENTION AND ACTIVITY

See also Sec. 2.46.

Normal Function. Attention is a continuing and self-reinforcing process of selection. At any instant, a host of internal and external stimuli compete for attention; these include immediate auditory or visual sensations, data stored in long- or short-term memory, impulses originating in viscera, muscles, and joints, or fantasies, feelings, or associations. By a process of selection, one or a few of these inputs take priority, while the others are relegated to the background.

The process of selective attention allows children to focus purposefully and for appropriate lengths of time on incoming data that will lead to productive activities or to learning. When the process is operating optimally, the resistance to distraction and the degrees of reflection and persistence are adequate for tasks involving comprehension and problem solving. Choice of action is also dependent upon selectivity.

Dysfunction. Chronic inattention and poorly controlled activity are frequent concomitants of academic and social failure in the school-age child. Not all affected children are "hyperkinetic" or "overactive," nor are learning disabilities necessarily associated. Children in whom extreme activity is purposeful and effective should not be considered dysfunctional.

Symptoms commonly encountered in children with attention deficits include distractibility, impersistence at tasks, impulsivity, insatiability, restlessness, difficulty in delaying gratification, extreme inconsistency of performance, sleep problems, and poor self-monitoring. These traits compromise not only academic performance but also behavioral adjustment and social interaction.

Four categories of disorders of activity and attention can be defined: *primary disorders of attention; secondary disorders of attention* related to handicaps in one or more areas of information processing or emotional difficulties; *situational inattention* in children who have no functional difficulty but rather an environmental problem; and *mixed types* of attention deficit. A full discussion of the effects, assessment, and treatment of attention deficit disorder (hyperactivity) is presented in Sec. 2.46.

NEUROLOGIC MATURATION

Normal Function. With the maturation of structure and function within the central nervous system and the cumulative

Table 2–16 Tasks for the Assessment of Gross Motor Function

Age	Gross Motor
5–6 years	Skip Walk on heels Tandem gait forward Hop in place
6–7 years	Tandem gait backward Stand on one foot, eyes open (10 sec)
7–8 years	Crouch on tiptoes, eyes closed (10 sec) Hop twice in place on each foot in succession (3 cycles) Stand in tandem gait position (heel-toe), eyes closed (10 sec)
9–10 years	Tandem gait sideways Catch tennis ball in air, one hand Throw tennis ball at target
10–12 years	Balance on tiptoes, eyes closed (15 sec) Jump in air, clap heels together Jump in air, clap hands three times

effects of experience, normal children achieve increasing efficiency and adaptability in their behavior as they mature.

Dysfunction and Assessment. The degree of organization and maturation of the central nervous system has commonly been assessed through examination of "soft neurologic signs." Some of these signs are normally encountered in many preschool children, but rarely in older ones. Accordingly, disappearance of these signs has been linked to central nervous system maturation. Many of them reappear during senescence. The persistence of such signs beyond the ages at which they usually disappear has been associated with learning disorders, behavior problems, and other manifestations of developmental dysfunction. A single such sign in isolation may not have much meaning. Some very successful children may show one or more of these indicators, while others with significant developmental dysfunctions may have no such evidence of neuromaturational delay. Clusters of these signs may be more accurate discriminators than any one alone.

The examination of the child for "soft signs" most commonly focuses attention upon:

1. Mirror (synkinetic) movements, in which one side of the body mimics an activity of the other side (e.g., a child asked to oppose the right thumb and forefinger repeatedly carries out the action in both hands). Mirror movements are rare beyond the age of 8 yr.

2. Other unnecessary or inefficient movements (e.g., mouth movements, head bobbing, or foot tapping) in conjunction with some unrelated activity.

3. Diadochokinesis, rapidly repeated alternating movements such as pronation and supination of the hands. Dysdiadochokinesis involves awkward performance in the hands, or flailings of the arms owing to poor control of the proximal musculature of the arms.

4. Finger agnosia, inability to know or state the position of the fingers without visual clues (e.g., the examiner asks how many fingers or which are being touched or held between two of the examiner's fingers). Reduced awareness of fingers may indicate some degree of unreadiness for educational activities.

5. Stimulus extinction, a tendency of the young child to lose the perception of one of two stimuli presented simultaneously (e.g., in two-point discrimination or when touched repeatedly on hand and face; in the latter instance, only the face may be reported after a few trials [rostral dominance]). This is not normally found after 7 yr of age.

6. Choreiform movements, involuntary arrhythmic or rotatory movements in outstretched fingers or tongue when the child is asked to close the eyes, protrude the tongue, extend arms and hands, spread the fingers, and hold the position for 30 sec.

7. Motor impersistence, an inability to sustain for 30 sec the position described in item 6 above (e.g., arms fall, tongue darts in and out, eyes open).

8. Lateral dominance, the preference for use of one side of the body to initiate action. Hand dominance is usually established by 4–6 yr (and usually for the right side), eye dominance by 2 yr. The significance of mixed dominance (e.g., to be right-eyed and left-handed) is less certain than it has seemed in the past.

9. Left-right discrimination, a sense of laterality (not just ability to name right and left, but to refer these to one's own body—e.g., "Show me your right hand" [by 6 yr] or "Touch your left ear with your right hand" [by 8 yr] or refer the same to the body of another person [by 9 yr]). Children with visual-spatial dysfunction often have delays in left-right discrimination.

The above signs of neuromaturational delay do not have direct implications for intervention, but they may suggest the degree of deficit. In some cases, delays in neuromaturation are accompanied by other forms of maturational lag: in skeletal age, stature, dentition, onset of puberty, emotional maturity, or social insight.

"HIGHER-ORDER" PROCESSING AND INTEGRATION

Normal Function. The higher levels of cognitive processes include:

1. Reasoning on an abstract or symbolic level.

2. Developing and applying generalizations, classifications, or rules that facilitate further behavior and learning.

3. Agility of mental movement between the concrete and the abstract-symbolic.

4. Capacity to put concrete and/or abstract materials into new juxtapositions (i.e., creativity and imagination).

5. Ability to identify discrepancies and consistencies within complex materials.

6. Skill at inferential reasoning.

7. Mobilization of effective problem-solving strategies.

In young children, one can study the pace and the order of development of the above functions. Specific stages are dominated by the emergence of particular components of intelligence, which have implications both for learning and for behavior and moral development (Sec. 2.20–2.22).

Dysfunction. Many children with difficulty in higher-order conceptualization, abstraction, and so on, also have other developmental dysfunctions. Their difficulties with higher-order processing may prevent them from developing strategies to deal with their other handicaps. On the other hand, some children with perceptual problems or other cognitive deficits may have relative strengths in such higher-order processes as reasoning, creativity, and generalization, which may help them to compensate and to develop effective learning and behavioral styles.

Assessment. The similarities and block design subtests of the WISC have been thought to measure conceptualization in verbal and nonverbal areas, respectively. Other assessments of higher order conceptual abilities have been based on the work of Piaget, but these have not yet been proved useful in the evaluation of children with learning disorders. Careful observation of children with learning problems at home and at school by parents and teachers can sometimes identify cognitive styles and strengths.

The results of intelligence tests in children with developmental dysfunctions must be interpreted with care (Sec. 2.61). Youngsters with attention deficits may show low test-retest reliability. Moreover, a child's calculated IQ may largely reflect a deficit in a single relatively narrow area of function. There are few tests that assess children's capacities to develop problem-solving strategies, to overcome adversity, to be creative, or to use imagination.

MOTIVATION

The learning and working achievements of school children depend heavily on motivation, which is dependent in turn upon a multitude of factors. Reduced motivation may be the result of a learning problem as well as contribute to its severity. Role models in the family or among peers can fortify or dissipate motivation. Certain youngsters are inclined to be attracted to some discrete subject areas but not others. Other driving factors include the quality of teaching, the likelihood of success, and the child's own self-esteem. It is important that youngsters with learning disabilities not have more demanded of them than they have a reasonable chance of achieving, and that their successes receive appropriate recognition and praise.

2.64 AREAS OF PERFORMANCE

Systematic observation and analysis of a child's academic performance can identify various functional components, including degree of reflectivity, persistence, reactions to frustration, responses to positive reinforcement, preferred styles or modalities of learning, and areas of processing deficit. Analysis of the components of a task and observation of the nature of a child's success or failure at it will permit the diagnosis or the description of developmental dysfunction as well as areas of strength. Many of the tests for language and learning disabilities lack standards for older children and adolescents. The direct observation of performance is especially important, therefore, in diagnostic evaluation of adolescents.

READING

During the early school years a serious impediment in reading may sow the seeds of later inhibitions or negative attitudes toward learning. It is important, therefore, that reading difficulties receive early diagnosis and prompt intervention.

Delays in learning to read may result from a variety of cognitive, psychologic, and social influences. In assessment of a child's reading performance, the following should be evaluated:

1. Reading level or grade equivalent.
2. Reading rate.
3. Sight vocabulary (the ability to recognize words almost instantly).
4. Word analysis skill (the capacity to sound out or analyze phonetically a word not remembered or previously encountered).
5. Tracking (the ability to keep one's place).
6. Level of comprehension.
7. Ability to recall and retell.

Deficits may be indicated by excessive use of finger pointing (a possible indication of a visual tracking problem); over-reliance on context; sequencing errors (incorrect juxtaposition of letters within a word or words within a sentence); deficits in visual discrimination (e.g., substituting *b's* for *d's* or mis-reading words for those of similar overall configuration); poorly established sound-symbol association; disregard of punctuation; word-by-word reading or monotony of tone; and word substitutions or omissions. Some professionals classify as dyslexic children who misinterpret visual symbols during reading, but who have adequate peripheral sensory mechanisms. By observing the types of errors and stylistic tendencies, a diagnostician or teacher may identify certain patterns consistent with specific neurodevelopmental deficits. Appropriate strategies for educational intervention may follow.

The health care team, but more likely the school, can easily administer such standardized tests as the Wide Range Achievement Test, the Stanford Reading Achievement Tests, the Woodcock-Johnson Reading Battery, and the Gray Oral Reading Paragraphs. When these are supplemented by developmental tests, specific themes of dysfunction may become discernible.

SPELLING

As with reading, careful analysis of the tasks and performances involved in spelling can yield valuable data descriptive of a child's learning style or handicaps. Difficulty with spelling (dysorthographia) may not in itself constitute a significant obstacle to success in life, but in combination with other areas of dysfunction, it may contribute to emotional anguish and to poor performance.

The manner in which a grade level for spelling achievement is measured is critical. Some youngsters who have great difficulty in spelling words from dictation will be highly accurate in selecting a correctly spelled word from a list of incorrect ones. Some students spell a dictated word list accurately, but reveal considerable inaccuracy when spelling within a paragraph.

A child's errors can be revealing: some children produce spellings that are correct phonetically but inaccurate visually (e.g., lite for light); others mistake similar configurations (e.g., laugh for light), or persistently commit errors of sequencing

(e.g., lihgt for light); still others show mixed errors. It may be useful to have a child read a list of words that are well ingrained in his or her sight vocabulary, and immediately thereafter try to spell them from dictation. Some youngsters have great difficulty with the revisualization of words, even those they have just seen.

Disorders of visual memory, sequencing, and receptive language are common in children with poor spelling, but in many cases problems with spelling appear to be isolated deficits without other developmental or psychologic correlates.

Spelling can be assessed using the Stanford or Wide Range Achievement Tests. The Boder Spelling Lists can be used to assess revisualization.

WRITING

In the middle and upper elementary school grades, earlier emphasis on relatively passive skills in recognition and discrimination gives way to increasing stress on written work. Most school-age children respond to this transition effectively and welcome the opportunity to express themselves, but some children have difficulty with written compositions, one of the highest forms of language and the last to be learned. It is not unusual for children at the late elementary or early junior high school level to become discouraged with their writing. Some children with disorders of writing have multiple deficits; others have isolated or discrete problems. The common disturbances are:

1. Weakness of fine motor control: difficulty with eye-hand coordination, defective or inefficient pencil grasp, or problems executing or recalling automatically the motor patterns needed to form letters, numbers, or words.
2. Disorders of visual-motor integration: problems perceiving visual configurations and converting them into a blueprint from which written words or sentences can be drawn. Affected children may be able to narrate and read with fluency, but still encounter obstacles in writing.
3. Problems with visual memory or revisualization: inability to retain visual images of letters, words, or shapes to permit their reproduction from memory (even in some children who can copy them well). Affected children would have difficulty writing or spelling from dictation.
4. Dysnomia: slowness in finding words in either written or oral expression.
5. Deficiencies in composition, organization, and syntax: inability to arrange thoughts in an organized way in writing and at times in speech.
6. Spatial disorganization: difficulty in orderly arrangement of letters, words, or sentences.
7. Diminished rate of processing: difficulty with accomplishing the task at an appropriate rate. Affected children become discouraged with the slow, laborious nature of writing effort, avoid writing when possible, and obtain less practice.

Three other factors need consideration in evaluating writing failure:

1. Because poor writing can be a permanent exhibit of a child's inadequacies, some children may be embarrassed and reluctant to write, especially when perfection is demanded too soon.
2. Children with little opportunity to write are unlikely to write well.
3. Writing is under strong cultural influence, there being low incentive for writing in families with little stress on the written word.

Children with developmental disorders of written language are frequently branded as unmotivated, lazy, disinterested, or depressed. They may become anxious or emotionally disturbed because of their limited productivity, with further inhibition of written output.

In evaluating a child with writing difficulties, a writing sample may be sufficient. It is useful to have the child perform on at least three levels: first, copying some sentences or words; second, writing from dictation; and third, writing a paragraph on a particular subject. Observations can be made on grasp of pencil and on fine motor control, word finding, organizational skills, direct visualization and revisualization, sophistication of language, and visual-motor integration.

MATHEMATICS

Dyscalculia, or disability in mathematics, subsumes a group of common but poorly understood disorders. Visual processing problems may impair visual recognition of numbers; visual-spatial problems present obstacles to arranging numbers or columns of numbers systematically on a page, or difficulties with the geometric aspects of mathematics.

Some children with sequencing problems have particular difficulty learning the multiplication tables, performing geometric proofs, and/or integrating basic number concepts; some with language disabilities have difficulty relating the symbolism of arithmetic operations to everyday situations, and may be greatly confused in dealing with word problems. Attentional difficulties and excessive impulsivity may impair ability to organize details of written numerical problems. Some youngsters with fine motor problems have difficulty aligning numbers for addition, subtraction, or multiplication.

Higher-order conceptualizations are critical in arithmetic. Children with dyscalculia may have difficulties with the notion of conservation of quantity (e.g., 1 dime equals 2 nickels), with formulating and applying principles for problem solving, with associating auditory with visual symbols, with ideas of one-to-one correspondence (e.g., 4 people need 4 spoons to consume their soup), or with counting (as opposed to rote repetition of numbers in sequence).

Some youngsters with disabilities in mathematics have problems with *active working memory*. They forget critical aspects of what they are doing or what numbers they are using *while* engaged in computation. They have trouble particularly with mental arithmetic. Such students often report that after prodigious study for an examination they seem to forget during the test.

Assessment of arithmetic skill should consider the child's computational skill, rate of problem solving, computational accuracy, and ability to tackle word problems. Analysis of errors can be helpful. The Wide Range Achievement Test and the KayMath Test of Arithmetic Abilities cover a broad range of mathematical operations.

SOCIAL COMPETENCE

Success in social interactions depends on appropriate experience, on emotional health, and on many other social and cultural factors. Some children may lack the capacity or sensitivity to read facial expressions of approval or disapproval, to perceive and respond to the needs of others, or to comprehend basic social skills such as sharing or offering support to another individual; or they may be persistently egocentric and insatiable.

Children with gross motor delays may have difficulty establishing gratifying social interactions in a milieu that accords a high value to athletic competence. Impulsive and inattentive children are often rejected by their peers and may experience isolation as early as the preschool years. Children with receptive or expressive language difficulties may have problems in building relationships, as may those with stuttering or other articulation problems. Failure often leads to a sense of inadequacy and a retreat from peers. Such youngsters may prefer the company of younger children or of the opposite sex. Some

such young children may feel most comfortable in the company of adults. Others feel alienated from the adult world owing to their failure to meet its expectations.

For children with developmental dysfunction, knowing the patterns of social interaction at home, in school, and in the neighborhood is important to understanding their needs. This can often be obtained from the child, and supplemented by the insights of parents and teachers. The child's interactions with the physician may *not* offer a valid sample of social performance.

2.65 DIAGNOSIS OF DEVELOPMENTAL DYSFUNCTIONS

Children with developmental dysfunction present complex and sometimes baffling diagnostic challenges. Their problems are not easily classified, each discipline tending to perceive problems in the context of its own subject matter.

The health care team can play a critical role in diagnostic evaluation and follow-up, through cooperation with educators, psychologists, and other specialists. Schools may seek medical help in identifying emotional and neurologic factors predisposing to failure. Parents may ask for assistance in obtaining evaluations free of distortions inherent in some school-based evaluations, in which personalities, budgets, and space may at times bias diagnosis and management.

The individual physician or nurse may collect the data leading to a plan for appropriate services, but in many cases a multi-professional team evaluation will be the most appropriate.

An initial evaluation should include:

1. A review of pregnancy and the perinatal period, early temperament, early development (motor, language, and social), health record, and family background, with particular attention to early life events that are frequently associated with developmental dysfunction. One should attempt to evaluate the degree of stimulation or deprivation in the child's life, and the quality of interaction between parents and child. Standardized questionnaires for parents and teachers (such as the ANSER System, a group of questionnaires) are designed for this purpose. Data so obtained can be elucidated or supplemented during an interview.

2. A description of the child's present home and school settings. The structure, living arrangements, and style of the family should be noted so far as possible, with a sense of the child's activities, supports, and interactions at home, in the neighborhood, and in the classroom. There should be an analysis of the curriculum and of any extra help the child is receiving.

3. A physical examination. Careful evaluation of vision and hearing and a traditional neurologic examination are required. Note should be given to evidence of maturation delay; growth retardation; malnutrition; deprivation; and medical conditions that might interfere with attention and learning, such as allergies, sinus infections, or chronic serous otitis.

4. A clear description of present function. Rating systems which measure a child's activity and attentional strength include the Conners Scales, the Weery Scales, and the ANSER System. Parents can fill these out prior to the child's visit. Behavioral inventories can record positive or maladaptive behaviors that may be associated with the child's dysfunction; other instruments elicit ratings by teachers of academic performance, attention, activity, and associated behaviors.

5. A mental health assessment. Parents and child should be interviewed separately by the mental health member of the team. The child should be evaluated as to self-esteem, personality, affect, mood, relatedness, and evidence of organicity. A child's drawing of his or her family may be helpful.

6. A neurodevelopmental screening assessment. This should screen for neuromaturational delay and for the specific deficits outlined earlier. The health care team can work with the psychoeducational specialist in direct observations of performance.

7. Psychoeducational testing. This should include assessments of intelligence and academic achievement and, as indicated, of specific

developmental areas, such as language, memory, or visual-spatial processing.

The diagnostic process should be able to describe a child on five levels:

1. *Neurodevelopmental*, with an analysis of constitutional, maturational, and developmental factors interfering with function and underlying strengths.

2. *Psychosocial*, elucidating factors in the environment, in the family, and in the past experience or present emotional health of the child that either enhance or compromise current performance.

3. *Secondary psychological*, with an account of the emotional effects of failure and the present level and stability of self-esteem.

4. *Supportive*, with a description of how the family, the school, and the community understand and are attempting to cope with the child's dysfunction.

5. *Strategic*, with an analysis of the child's strategies for dealing with failure.

2.66 MANAGEMENT OF DEVELOPMENTAL DYSFUNCTIONS

In the United States Public Law 94–142 established that children with developmental disabilities and other sources of learning difficulty have a right to a multidisciplinary assessment in school, leading to an Individualized Educational Plan (IEP) to meet their specific educational, developmental, and counseling needs.

The roles of pediatricians or other child health providers in this planning vary from state to state. Schools or parents seeking an outside opinion commonly involve physicians in "independent evaluations." The health team and the school should collaborate in developing an IEP that includes specific recommendations for counseling parents and child and, when necessary, for further study or consultation. A plan for follow-up and accountability should be instituted.

EDUCATIONAL PLANS

Health care personnel and educators are increasingly working together in planning for children with developmental dysfunction. The selection and utilization of curricular materials and classroom activities are functions primarily of educators. Health professionals need to know more about educational systems and alternatives, and educators must become more familiar with the medical and developmental aspects of school failure.

IEP's may involve:

Alteration of classroom structure. Some children with chronic inattention or poor activity control may function far more effectively in smaller classrooms with higher teacher:pupil ratios and in highly structured programs. On the other hand, recommendations need to be based on knowledge of the specific settings and options available and objective information about their educational relevance.

Modification of teacher-student interaction. Teachers aware of a child's developmental dysfunctions can apply specific educational strategies. Problems with sequencing require presentation of materials in small units, and instructions given one step at a time. The child may need to confirm receipt of multiple-step instructions by repeating them. Children with visual distractibility may benefit from a somewhat isolated carrel or a workspace; those with auditory distractibility, from sitting near the front of the room or having an opportunity to do some work in relatively quiet settings each day. Teachers need to discover whether a given child learns best through visual or auditory channels.

Children with output problems may require more time or reduced assignments. Youngsters chronically deprived of mastery will profit if their teachers can regularly assign tasks in which success is assured.

Additional specialized help. Many youngsters may require specialized assistance outside of regular classrooms. There is a growing movement in this country not to segregate children with educational problems into "special" classes. This trend is referred to as "mainstreaming." Students in need can leave the regular classroom for portions of the day for specialized help in special settings ("learning centers," "resource rooms"). There each child can receive individualized assistance from such professionals as learning disabilities teachers, speech and language pathologists, and reading specialists, whose efforts are aimed both at strengthening basic skills and at overcoming specific dysfunctions, through specific exercises directed at visual-perceptual motor function, sequencing, fine motor problems, or language disabilities.

Some children with attentional problems may learn best in a one-to-one relationship. Appropriate feedback and reinforcement, an emphasis on reflective behavior, and the elimination of distractions and peer pressure may dramatically facilitate performance and learning in such youngsters.

For some children a multisensorial approach to learning is based on the assumption that a weak modality can be compensated for by input through several channels. For example, a youngster with a visual-perceptual problem might learn to recognize letters by combining auditory, visual, tactile, and kinesthetic input, a child with difficulty in visual learning might be taught through the use of tape recordings, or a child whose fine motor problems impair writing might use a typewriter.

Remedial help in performance areas. As children grow older, more emphasis is placed on direct tutorial help in subject areas, with less emphasis on readiness skills. Such intervention may be very beneficial to a child whose slow rate of processing creates difficulty with the tempo of a regular classroom.

Curriculum modifications and substitutions. The selection of curriculum and teaching methods should be directed by an understanding of the child's developmental status and learning style. There are differing, valid approaches to the learning of basic skills, and specific curricula may accommodate individual styles.

Modifications in course content may help dysfunctional children. For example, those with gross motor lags who are intimidated by physical education classes may flourish in other areas after being excused from regular gym classes or being enrolled in an adaptive physical education program.

Other curricular issues, such as the introduction of foreign languages, the special demands of the sciences, and the provision of specific vocational training, need to be considered as children with learning problems enter the upper grades. Whenever possible, highly motivating educational experiences need to be included.

Many educational interventions have not been adequately evaluated and are espoused on the basis of anecdotal reports and uncontrolled trials. Investigations need to allow for wide individual variations, for the inevitable effects of maturation, and for the tendency of all helping gestures to produce nonspecific gains.

COUNSELING PARENTS AND CHILDREN

Physicians and health care professionals can play major roles in the counseling of children with developmental dysfunction and of their parents, through a continuing relationship with the family. The interaction should focus upon the specific deficits and manifestations, upon the child's strengths, upon the social milieu, and upon associated issues, including coping with day-to-day situations. The physician or nurse can also interpret biomedical, developmental, and educational findings, helping to "demystify" the child's problem.

Health care professionals should avoid excessive reassurance. Such assertions as "she'll outgrow it," or "I was the same way when I was his age," are inappropriate. Reassurance can be beneficial, but its overuse can prevent a child from receiving appropriate services or impede further evaluation.

Children should be included in discussions about their learning difficulties; they are likely otherwise to fantasize uncomfortably about secret conversations between professionals and their parents. Many students with developmental dysfunctions fear that they are pervasively "dumb" or defective. They need to hear or overhear that their learning problems are discrete and embedded in assets.

Provision should be made for counseling directly with children by a physician, nurse, guidance counselor, or other professional. Counseling should aim in part at elucidating for the children their specific problems and strengths in understandable language with encouragement to talk about such problems and to report how they are coping.

Professionals and parents can together seek to identify areas of creative talent in which children can achieve a sense of mastery or triumph. Parents should be encouraged to balance criticism with praise, and to be reasonable and consistent in their expectations.

Health care professionals, parents, and teachers should be careful not to moralize about a child's learning problem. Such terms as "bad," "lazy," and "poorly motivated" never motivate, probably intensify negative self-images, and may act as self-fulfilling prophecies.

Psychotherapy may be indicated in instances of family disorganization and conflict, or when significant psychopathology is evident in the child. When referral is necessary, the physician, child, and family may need to meet several times to plan the use of mental health services to increase the likelihood of a successful referral (Sec. 2.55).

MEDICAL MANAGEMENT

The first responsibility of the health care team is to ensure that any medical problems interfering with function, such as sensory deficits, neurologic problems, seizures, or chronic medical problems, receive appropriate care. Children with allergies, for example, may have learning difficulties aggravated by serous otitis, chronic nasal congestion, or excessive fatigue. Antihistamines may produce chronic fatigue and inattention in the classroom. If teachers are aware of medication being taken, their observations may lead to helpful alterations of dosages or schedules.

Many children with developmental dysfunctions have associated symptoms, such as abdominal pain, enuresis, encopresis, headaches, or other complaints. Alleviation of these can improve function in other areas.

PHARMACOTHERAPY

Drugs used for children with problems in learning and attention have included cerebral stimulants, tranquilizers, antidepressants, and anticonvulsants. Their efficacy has been a matter of controversy; ethical concerns have been expressed regarding "behavioral control" of children, though dramatic improvements in learning and life style occur in some children receiving such therapy (Sec. 2.46 and 2.56). The most commonly used stimulant drugs are dextroamphetamine (Dexedrine), methylphenidate (Ritalin), and pemoline (Cylert).

Their use, side effects, and contraindications are discussed in Sec. 2.46.

Stimulants should not be given without a comprehensive evaluation both of specific learning deficits and of psychopathology. The hasty offering of these drugs may delay other much needed help.

THERAPEUTIC CAUTIONS

Other therapeutic offerings of poorly substantiated quality and validity have included use of special diets, megavitamin therapy, allergic hyposensitization, optometric exercises, the use of thyroid medication and insulin, motor patterning exercises, self-hypnosis, anti–motion sickness drugs, and transcendental meditation.

It has been suggested that food additives may have a deleterious effect on the learning and behavior of certain children. The question is being studied, but data are still inconclusive. It is unlikely that an additive-free diet will benefit the usual child with learning problems. If a trial of diet is made, close supervision will be important.

Others have suggested that high levels of dietary carbohydrate impair learning and behavior in many young children. Use of a high protein, low carbohydrate diet has, however, meager data to support it. Dietary manipulation may produce nutritional deficiencies, elevate hopes unrealistically, or delay the child's receiving appropriate educational and counseling services. Advocates of special biochemical and orthomolecular approaches to learning disorders, or of optometric, motor, and other interventions, have yet to present adequately controlled studies. In some cases, schools themselves have endorsed questionably valid treatment programs.

As advocates for parents and children, pediatricians can help to minimize their susceptibility to irresponsible claims. Many parents seek help elsewhere when they feel abandoned by the health and educational systems. Adequate continuing support and appropriate intervention with families will lessen their need to seek "miraculous cures."

PROGNOSIS

Children with developmental dysfunctions leading to mild physiologic impairments may be helped to compensate quite adequately by support of family, by early cognitive experiences, by cultural values, and by emotional factors. Longitudinal studies of children with perinatal complications and of others with malnutrition in infancy have shown that behavior and achievement are influenced by socioeconomic class as well as by the antecedent risk factors; a poor outcome for the child is surer when biologic insult and lower socioeconomic class occur together.

A child's particular strengths may compensate for weaknesses, allowing some resiliency. If dysfunctions are severe enough or sufficiently maladaptive, however, even strong environmental support may be inadequate to prevent failure.

Resiliency in development may continue into adult life, but adult performance and life style may be influenced adversely by the experience of failure in early life. Outcomes are sometimes tragic: alcoholism, drug abuse, unemployment, serious automobile accidents, and crime have been linked to developmental dysfunctions. The comprehensive early evaluation and treatment of such dysfunctions may be essential to a future stable and productive adulthood.

Increasing attention is being paid to the temperamental characteristics of infants as predictors of later developmental function, and neurologic examinations such as the Brazelton Neonatal Assessment Scale have revised the assessment of behavior and neurologic organization in the newborn. Insatiability, irritability, and unpredictability have been described as intrinsic traits of some infants who later develop behavioral disorganization and problems with learning. The predictive validity of observations of temperament or of the Brazelton Scale has yet to be established for children of school age.

Developmental assessments in infancy are useful in the detection of severely handicapped children, but their ability to predict handicaps of low severity appears limited. In the preschool years, early detection may become increasingly feasible with use of educational readiness examinations that examine perceptual-motor, language, and memory functions more closely than do traditional developmental assessments.

PREVENTION

During the first years of life the earliest screening for developmental dysfunction is a responsibility of the primary health care team, which has a critical role in recognizing risk factors or in uncovering physical indicators of evolving handicaps.

A variety of preventive programs have been proposed to minimize the effects of both blatant and subtle handicaps and to foster the nurturance of the developing child. Some have assumed responsibility for optimizing the early health, development, and education of children. Demonstration models, such as the Brookline Early Education Project, have "enrolled" children in public school programs before they were born. The ultimate gains engendered by such programs and their cost-benefit ratios are highly encouraging.

COMMUNITY ACTION

Where resources for children with developmental dysfunction are lacking, physicians, nurses, and educators can lead the way to changes in public policy that will generate needed help. Where school systems lack the personnel and facilities for special educational treatment and evaluation, the health care team can help document the need. Where multidisciplinary diagnostic programs do not exist, health providers can take the initiative in creating appropriate team efforts. Physicians, nurses, and other professionals can also educate the community about the nature of developmental dysfunctions, the predicament experienced by failing children and their families, and the ultimate high cost to society and the individual of neglect of inadequacy in early life.

MELVIN D. LEVINE

Kenniston AH, Flarell JH: A developmental study of intelligent retrieval. Child Development 50:1144, 1979.
Levine MD: Developmental Variation and Learning Disorders. Cambridge, MA, Educators Publishing Service, 1987.
Levine MD, Brooks R, and Shonkoff J: A Pediatric Approach to Learning Disorders. New York, John Wiley & Sons, 1980.
Levine MD, Busch B, Aufeeser C: The dimension of inattention in children with school problems. Pediatrics 70:387, 1982.
Levine MD, Carey W, Crocker A, et al: Developmental-Behavioral Pediatrics. Philadelphia, WB Saunders, 1983.
Levine MD, Melmed RD: The unhappy wanderers: Children with attention deficits. Pediatr Clin North Am 29:105, 1982.
Levine MD, Oberklaid F, Meltzer L: Developmental output failure: A study of low productivity in school-aged children. Pediatrics 67:18, 1981.
Levine MD, Satz P: Middle Childhood: Development and Dysfunction. Baltimore, University Park Press, 1984.
Levine MD, Zallen B: The learning disorders of adolescents: Organic and nonorganic failure to strive. Pediatr Clin North Am 31:345, 1984.
Luria A: Higher Cortical Function in Man. New York, Basic Books, 1980.
Ross DM, Ross SA: Hyperactivity: Current Issues, Research, and Theory. New York, Wiley Interscience, 1982.
Rubin KH, et al: Symposium: Social competence and peer status. Child Development 54:1383, 1983.
Rutter M (ed): Developmental Neuropsychiatry. New York, Guilford Press, 1983.
Torgesen JK: The role of non-specific factors in the task performance of learning disabled children: A theoretical assessment. J Learning Disabilities 10:27, 1977.
Vellutino FR: Dyslexia: Theory and Research. Cambridge, MA, MIT Press, 1979.
Wallach GP, Butler KG: Language Learning Disabilities in School-Age Children. Baltimore, Williams & Wilkins, 1984.

DISORDERS OF HEARING, SPEECH, AND LANGUAGE

2.67 HEARING DISORDERS

Significance and Prevalence. Hearing is the primary sensory modality for acquisition of speech and language, providing a fundamental basis for social adjustment and academic and vocational achievement. Even mild or unilateral hearing loss during childhood has been shown to have a negative impact on language and learning. More severe hearing loss presents a major handicap for speech, language, academic, and vocational attainment and requires intensive special education.

The prevalence of hearing loss varies with the criteria for hearing loss used, the technique for detection employed, and the population studied. Among groups of neonates at high risk the incidence of severe bilateral hearing loss ranges from 1.7% to greater than 5%. The National Center for Health Statistics (1982) estimated a prevalence of 0.63% among children less than 5 years of age and 1.63% among children 5 to 14 years.

Of children under 5 yr of age, 4% have bilateral losses greater than 15 dB, and an additional 8–10% have unilateral losses greater than 15 dB.

Types and Causes. Four types of hearing loss are present in infants and children:

Conductive hearing loss involves interference with the reception of sound by the external ear or with the transmission of sound from the external to the inner ear. If the inner ear is unimpaired, only sound conducted by air is diminished, whereas normal reception is given to sound conducted through the skull and temporal bones. Total occlusion of the air-conduction pathways (such as occurs in atresia of the auditory canal, absence of the oval window, complete stapes fixation, or ossicular malformation), may produce a maximal loss of 60 dB in air-conduction hearing. Lesser degrees of hearing loss occur from partial disruptions of transmission, including structural abnormalities or growths and middle ear effusions. Primary among conditions contributing to conductive hearing loss among pediatric patients are congenital or acquired structural abnormalities of the external ear, the canal, the ossicles, or eardrum; stenosis of the ear canal, or collapsed ear canals; the presence of foreign bodies, cerumen, and growths; inflammatory conditions such as otitis media; and the presence of middle ear effusion. Many craniofacial conditions and syndromes have associated deformities of the external and middle ear or carry an increased incidence of middle ear pathology. Conductive hearing loss often may be treated successfully through medical or surgical means.

Sensorineural hearing loss results from abnormalities of the cochlear hair cells or the auditory nerve; hearing losses are comparable for air-conducted and bone-conducted stimuli. More than 50% of severe to profound congenital sensorineural hearing losses are hereditary; about 40% are autosomal recessive, 10% dominant, and 3% sex-linked. Other major causes of sensorineural hearing losses include hypoxia, trauma, hyperbilirubinemia, ototoxicity of drugs, intrauterine infections, and bacterial infections of the pharynx. Less frequent or suspected causes include viral infections, such as measles, mumps, or chicken pox.

Sensorineural hearing losses are generally irreversible and do not respond to medical or surgical management, though the use of cochlear implants is being explored with increasingly younger patients who have severe to profound hearing losses. Depending on the severity and configuration of the hearing loss, hearing aid amplification and special education are the usual modes of habilitation. Early prescription and use of a hearing aid offers the single most important habilitative tool for infants and young children.

Mixed hearing loss occurs when both a conductive and a sensorineural hearing loss are present (such as when a child with moderately severe hereditary sensorineural loss has a superimposed mild conductive hearing loss as a result of middle ear effusion). Hearing loss may be severe. Medical or surgical management of both the conductive component and the sensorineural component is typically required.

Central auditory disorders arise from dysfunction of the central auditory nervous system (CANS), the complex system of interconnecting afferent and efferent neural pathways between the cochlea and cerebral cortex. These neural structures are felt to be responsible for the analysis of frequency, intensity, and temporal components of auditory stimuli as well as complex auditory tasks such as sound localization, binaural synthesis and separation, and identification of figure-ground stimuli. Disorders of the CANS may arise from a variety of pre-, peri-, and postnatal factors. While thresholds for sound are often normal for children with central auditory disorders they have difficulty attending to, discriminating, retaining and analyzing auditory information.

Identification of Hearing Loss. Early identification of hearing loss is fundamental to its effective management in infants and young children. Audiologists working with children who are very young or difficult to test require special training in working with such children. The types of hearing tests used may be broadly grouped as follows:

Infant Hearing Screening Programs. If hearing loss present during the neonatal period is not detected before discharge from the hospital, its subsequent detection and confirmation is typically delayed many months, with treatment often not beginning before 18 to 24 mo, when stages have passed that are critical for early language and learning. Recognition of such delays has led to the practice of screening infants at risk for hearing loss prior to their hospital discharge. The Joint Committee on Newborn Hearing has recommended that the hearing of infants in high risk categories be screened during the newborn period or no later than 6 mo of age. The definitions of high risk are summarized in Table 2–17 (the High Risk Register).

Infants identified through the use of the High Risk Register are screened for hearing loss through one or more of three means: observation of behavioral responses to calibrated noisemakers; auditory brain stem evoked responses (ABER); or automatized infant hearing screening devices. Observation of the infant's behavioral responses to soundmakers of known intensity and frequency is most cost-effective but least reliable. ABER yields the lowest rate of false negative findings but the highest false positive, owing in part to the dependence of brain stem responses on the maturational level of the newborn. ABER is the most costly and time-consuming means of

Table 2–17. **High Risk Registry Criteria**

A. *Neonatal asphyxia* (including infants with Apgar scores of 0–3, those who fail to exhibit spontaneous respiration by 10 minutes, and those with hypotonia persisting to 2 hours of age).

B. *Bacterial meningitis* (including *H. influenzae*, streptococcal, and neisserial infections).

C. *Congenital* or *perinatal infections* (including cytomegalovirus infection, rubella, herpes, toxoplasmosis, or syphilis).

D. *Defects* of head or neck (e.g., craniofacial syndromes, overt or submucous cleft palate, morphologic abnormalities of the pinna).

E. *Serum bilirubin* levels exceeding indications for exchange transfusion.

F. *Family history* of hearing impairment in childhood.

G. *Birthweight less than 1.5 kg.*

Adapted from Gerkin KP: The high risk register for deafness. ASHA 26(4):17, 1984.

infant hearing screening. For these reasons ABER generally is not advocated for hearing screening of large numbers of infants. Use of automated hearing screening devices, such as the Crib-O-Gram and the Auditory Response Cradle, is efficient in reducing time and cost and provides objective readings with acceptable false positive rates and very low false negative rates. Through use of motion-sensitive transducers these automated devices establish a baseline activity level against which the activity levels following repeated presentations of an 85 or 90 dB stimulus are recorded. These microprocessor-based units are fully automated, both performing the test and interpreting the results. It must be noted that infant screening procedures are effective in identifying moderate to severe hearing losses but are not sensitive to mild losses, unilateral losses, or progressive losses of later onset.

Whenever a hearing loss has been suspected during the newborn period, follow-up hearing evaluation to confirm its presence is essential, typically between 3 and 6 mo of age.

Clinical Audiologic Tests. Clinical audiologic tests rely principally on measuring a child's response to auditory stimuli of known intensity and frequency and are conducted in a sound-proof booth. The testing paradigms vary with the age and ability level of the child. From birth to 12 mo of age, systematic observations are made of reflexive responses to auditory stimuli (such as startle patterns, localization movements, increased or decreased body movement, and eye blinks). By 1 yr of age, or at times younger, infants and young children can be taught to associate a visual stimulus with a test tone through classical conditioning techniques, ultimately responding to the auditory tone in anticipation of presentation of the visual stimulus. By 2½ yr of age, if reinforcement is provided, most children can be taught to respond with voluntary motor action to perception of sound, for example, by placing pegs in a pegboard. By 5 yr of age, most children can respond reliably by raising their hand in response to test tones, which is the principal method of response used in testing older children and adults.

Except in instances in which a child will not tolerate earphones, auditory stimuli are presented through earphones, which allow control over the ear tested, as well as over the intensity and frequency of the tone presented. In pure-tone threshold testing, both air and bone conduction thresholds for responses are obtained, in order to differentiate conductive from sensorineural hearing loss and to determine the configuration of either. In addition to pure-tone testing, tests of hearing thresholds to speech, and of the ability to discriminate speech sounds are done. When a central auditory disorder is suspected, special batteries of tests are administered; such tests have not yet been developed for clinical use in children under 6 yr of age.

Electrophysiologic Hearing Tests. Among the several electrophysiologic tests available for assessing the physiologic integrity of the hearing and vestibular mechanisms, impedance audiometry and auditory evoked responses have the most widespread use with pediatric patients. Impedance audiometry includes tympanometry and measurement of static compliance and of the acoustic reflex threshold. *Tympanometry* charts objectively the movement of the tympanic membrane as the air pressure in the external auditory canal is varied. This technique has been useful in measuring middle ear pressure, detecting inadequate eustachian tube functioning, identifying perforations of the tympanic membrane, and confirming the patency of pressure equalization tubes. A *static compliance measure* of the ossicles and middle ear muscles also can be obtained which aids in differentiating among middle ear disorders. Finally, the *acoustic reflex threshold* measures the intensity level at which the stapedial muscle contracts; this provides an objective means for determining the presence of cochlear pathology and is useful in differential diagnosis of conductive and sensorineural hearing loss.

Auditory evoked response audiometry, of which auditory brain stem evoked responses (ABER) is one form, provides a computer-generated average of the brain's electrical response latency to auditory stimuli. ABER provides a record of the wave-form latencies considered to correspond to stages of brain stem reception of auditory stimuli. ABER provides a record of the wave-form latencies considered to correspond to stages of brain stem reception of auditory stimuli. ABER provides information regarding the degree of hearing loss to air-conducted stimuli and may identify the brain stem as the site of a lesion, but interpretation of these data is not fully understood. The limitations of ABER as a screening procedure for neonates have been noted, but it is useful in providing objective measurements of sensorineural hearing status in children who are difficult to test. ABER typically requires sedation in infants and young children; accordingly, this technique is usually reserved for children who cannot be tested reliably through behavioral techniques.

Severity of Hearing Loss and the Effect on Language and Learning. The severity of a hearing impairment is determined by the degree of hearing loss present and the range of frequencies affected. Responses to pure-tone stimuli at controlled frequencies and intensities are charted for each ear by air and bone conduction on an audiogram similar to that given in Figure 2–13. Figure 2–13 shows moderately severe bilateral conductive loss in which bone conduction thresholds are bilaterally within normal limits (at 10 dB) across the frequency range tested, but air conduction thresholds are elevated to between 40 and 60 dB. This audiogram suggests significant middle ear pathology with normal sensorineural hearing, possibly secondary to ossicular discontinuity.

The features of normal hearing vary with age and stimulus; the level of responsivity improves from infancy to 2 years of age. The greatest concentration of acoustic energy for speech falls between 500 and 2000 Hz, yet frequencies as low as 125 Hz and up to at least 8000 Hz are important for learning and discriminating some speech sounds. The handicapping effect of a hearing loss depends both on the frequencies involved and on the degree of loss at each frequency. In addition to its dependency on the severity of the hearing loss, the prognosis for language, learning, and educational achievement depends on the age of onset of the hearing loss, on how early the loss was identified, on the age at which amplification and remediation were instituted, on the quality of parental support, and on any associated anomalies. Table 2–18 summarizes the levels of disability likely to correspond to the degree of hearing loss, the degree of handicap likely if

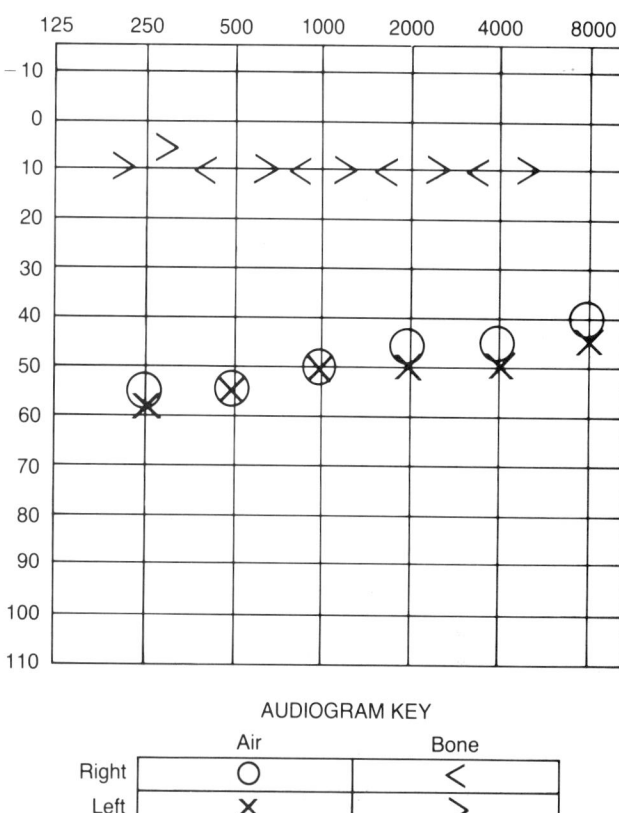

PURE-TONE AUDIOGRAM
Frequency in cycles per second

AUDIOGRAM KEY

	Air	Bone
Right	O	<
Left	×	>

Figure 2–13. Audiogram demonstrating a bilateral conductive hearing loss.

the condition is not recognized and treated in the first year of life, and the probable special educational needs.

Treatment of Hearing Loss. Treatments available for children with hearing impairments include medical and surgical interventions, amplification of residual hearing, and special education programs. Medical management of conductive hearing loss includes pharmacologic treatment of otitis media, middle ear effusions, and other middle ear diseases. Surgical measures include correction of congenital or other structural malformations of the outer and middle ear and insertion of pressure equalization tubes for recurrent or chronic middle ear effusion.

Amplification of residual hearing is accomplished through monaural or binaural hearing aids and classroom amplification systems. Since even mild or unilateral hearing loss may impede development of speech and language and impair academic achievement, some form of remedial education is usually required for all children with hearing loss. For less severe problems this may be confined to speech and language therapy, possibly coupled with scholastic tutoring. Children with more significant losses typically require special educational programs throughout the preschool and school years. From infancy to 3 yr, parent-infant programs teach parents to capitalize on the child's residual hearing and provide a visual language through sign or lipreading. In most communities intensive classroom instruction in language, speech, and learning for hearing-impaired children is available by 3 years of age and is mandated by Public Law 94–142 for school-age children. The primary emphasis of these programs, especially in the early years, is on teaching language and speech through visual and tactile modalities and on developing whatever

Table 2–18. **Hearing Handicap as a Function of Average Hearing Threshold Level of the Better Ear**

Average Threshold Level at 500–2000 Hz (ANSI)*	Description	Common Causes	What Can Be Heard without Amplification	Degree of Handicap (if not treated in 1st year of life)	Probable Needs
0–15 dB	Normal range		All speech sounds	None	None
16–25 dB	Slight hearing loss	Serous otitis, perforation, monomeric membrane, sensorineural loss, tympanosclerosis	Vowel wounds heard clearly, may miss unvoiced consonant sounds	Possible mild or transitory auditory dysfunction Difficulty in perceiving some speech sounds	Consideration of need for hearing aid Lip reading Auditory training Speech therapy Preferential seating Appropriate surgery
26–40 dB	Mild	Serous otitis, perforation, tympanosclerosis, monomeric membrane, sensorineural loss	Hears only some of speech sounds; the louder voiced sounds	Auditory learning dysfunction Mild language retardation Mild speech problems Inattention	Hearing aid Lip reading Auditory training Speech therapy Appropriate surgery
41–65 dB	Moderate hearing loss	Chronic otitis, middle ear anomaly, sensorineural loss	Misses most speech sounds at normal conversational level	Speech problems Language retardation Learning dysfunction Inattention	All of the above, plus consideration of special classroom situation
66–95 dB	Severe hearing loss	Sensorineural loss or mixed loss due to sensorineural loss plus middle ear disease	Hears no speech sound of normal conversations	Severe speech problems Language retardation Learning dysfunction Inattention	All of the above; probable assignment to special classes
96 + dB	Profound hearing loss	Sensorineural loss or mixed	Hears no speech or other sounds	Severe speech problems Language retardation Learning dysfunction Inattention	All of the above; probable assignment to special classes

*ANSI = American National Standards Institute.
From Northern JL, Downs MP: Hearing in Children. 3rd ed. Baltimore, Williams & Wilkins, 1984.

residual hearing remains. School-age hearing-impaired children who are functioning well in aural-verbal language may receive part or all of their educational programs in classrooms shared with normally hearing children. Alternatively, they may be educated in self-contained programs for the hearing-impaired. There has been controversy among educators of the hearing-impaired as to how dependent these programs should be on aurally received and verbally expressed language, as opposed to sign language. Considerable evidence now suggests that a *total communication* approach, in which language information is encouraged in all modalities, may be the most effective approach for developing language in young children with hearing impairment.

2.68 SPEECH AND LANGUAGE DISORDERS

Speech and language provide an early and primary form of communication for children and adults. Acquisition of language represents one of the first learning tasks presented to young children. Failure to learn language normally and speak correctly has been found to be negatively correlated with later academic and vocational achievement and may foreshadow later learning problems. Prevalence figures for disordered speech and language vary with the definitions and measures for detection used in various studies. The National Center for Health Statistics reported a prevalence for speech impairment of 0.92% for children under 5 yr old and 1.94% for those 5 to 14 yr old in a study based on parental report and excluding hearing-impaired children and those with cleft palate. Direct

evaluations of school-age children have reported prevalence rates as high as 3.8 times those found by interview only. Such findings suggest that speech and language impairment may involve as many as 4–5% of children.

TYPES OF SPEECH AND LANGUAGE FUNCTION

Language Functions. The term *language* refers to a system of symbolic representations that may be accessed and expressed through various modalities including listening, reading, writing, and speaking. Language is made up of at least four components that, although interrelated, may be differentially disrupted in various types of language disorders. These include: (1) *phonology*, the sound system of a language and the linguistic rules that govern the permissible sound sequences (for example, the vowels and consonants of a language and the combinations in which they occur); (2) *syntax*, the linguistic rules governing word order and the use of grammatic marker endings such as plurality and verb tense (for example, the distinctions between "the car hits the train" and "the train hits the car," and between "the cat plays" and "the cats play"); (3) *semantics*, the cognitive-linguistic knowledge needed to interpret meanings of words and word relationships; and (4) *pragmatics*, the sociolinguistic system that indicates the social appropriateness of language (for example, the differences in language usage in informal and formal contexts).

Language disorders in children represent a failure to comprehend or express one or more of these four components of language. To date, there is no widely agreed upon classification system for developmental language disorders, although several have been proposed. Most speech-language pathologists distinguish between disorders of language comprehension and language expression; and the relative strengths or deficits in phonology, syntax, semantics, and pragmatics are usually described and contrasted among subgroups of language disorders in children.

Speech Functions. The term *speech* concerns the physical production of verbal language through execution of the movements involved in producing, modifying, and articulating sound. The three types of speech disorders are those of voice, articulation, and fluency. *Voice disorders* include abnormal vocal tone produced by the breathing and laryngeal mechanisms or abnormal resonance due to irregularities of the normal coupling of the pharyngeal, nasal, and oral cavities. An *articulation disorder* is deviant production of speech sounds arising principally from abnormalities in lip, tongue, and palatal movements secondary to physical limitations or habituation of incorrectly learned patterns. A *fluency disorder*, often referred to as stuttering, is characterized by impaired rate and rhythm of the flow of speech often accompanied by struggle behavior. Fluency disorders may occur on a genetic basis, be a symptom of neurological dysfunction, or have a psychosocial basis.

NORMAL SPEECH AND LANGUAGE DEVELOPMENT

Active acquisition of speech and the various components of language begins during the first year of life, for example in the initial practice of sounds and babbling and interpersonal interactions with the caretaker. Rapid development occurs in all aspects of speech and language during the preschool years, and refinement extends well into the school-age years. Table 2–19 summarizes some early language milestones that may serve as a broad guide for judging the normalcy of a child's language development.

REQUISITES FOR SPEECH AND LANGUAGE

For a child to develop normal speech and language, four systems must be intact. Disruptions in any of these systems may cause a speech or language disorder.

1. The *social environment* provides the interpersonal interactions basic to all communication and presents the language model to be emulated. Environmental deprivation may be reflected in a child's speech and language.

2. The *input system* concerns primarily the reception and perception of auditorily received speech, but also includes the visual and tactile-kinesthetic integrity of the child. The importance of the auditory system for learning speech and language has been detailed above. Language patterns are characteristically altered in children with severe visual limitations, and certain articulation disorders have been linked to subtle tactile deficits.

3. The *central speech and language system* is dependent on the physical integrity of those aspects of the central nervous system felt to be responsible for the comprehension, interpretation, formulation, and planning of language as well as for the intellectual activity and ability of the child. The neurologic basis of language processing among children is not fully understood; it is felt to be principally a function of left hemisphere activity, with contributions from the right hemisphere and subcortical structures. A central nervous system dysfunction interfering with language comprehension or expression is typically referred to as producing childhood dysphasia. The child's cognitive-intellectual development determines the level of language attainment possible. The presence of a language disorder is typically determined in reference to more generalized cognitive abilities, especially performance on nonverbal cognitive tasks. An intellectually limited child may have language abilities commensurate with his performance on nonverbal cognitive tasks, in which case the child would not be considered to present a language disorder, but rather a more generalized retardation. Other children with some degree of more generalized retardation may present even more pronounced deficits in language areas, in which case the retarded child would be considered also to have a language disorder.

4. The *production system* comprises the laryngeal, pharyngeal, nasal, and oral structural and neuromuscular mechanisms involved in modifying breathing for speech, generating laryngeal sound, shaping that sound into articulate speech through altering the shape of and airflow through the pharyngeal, laryngeal, and oral cavities. Any disruption of the breathing mechanism may interfere with the breath support required for speech and contribute to a voice disorder, seen most dramatically in children sustaining tracheostomies for prolonged periods but also evident in many neuromuscular disorders affecting children. Laryngeal pathology, such as vocal fold paresis or vocal nodules, will produce abnormal voice quality as well as resonance abnormalities governed by the coupling of the pharyngeal, nasal, and oral cavities. Disruption of normal velar valving of the nasal cavity will produce hypernasality, as seen in children with clefts of the hard and soft palate or velar-pharyngeal incompetence. The velum also has a crucial role in articulation of speech sounds. When it is lowered, the nasal sounds /m/, /n/, and /ng/ are produced, and its effective seal of the nasal port permits buildup of intraoral pressure required for production of stop-plosive sounds (p, b, t, d, k, g) and fricatives (f, v, s, z, sh, zh, ch). Lip movements are involved in normal production of several consonants and vowels (oo, b, p, m, f, v), although effective compensations often can be made for inadequate lip mobility. Precise, rapid movements of the tongue, however, are required for acceptable articulation of many speech sounds, and any limitation in tongue mobility or sensitivity may contribute to an articulation disorder.

SCREENING FOR SPEECH AND LANGUAGE DISORDERS

During the preschool years, the pediatrician often is responsible for initial identification of speech and language disorders. Often alerted by parental concerns, the pediatrician can assess the need for further evaluation by comparing the child's observed or reported speech and language ability to normative data, such as those presented in Tables 2–19 and 2–20. Several tools for screening speech and language are commercially available (such as the *Receptive-Expressive Emergent Language Scale* and the *Early Language Milestone Scale*). Many speech-language pathologists advise that a child be referred for additional evaluation if he or she does not say single words at 18 mo, use word combinations at 2 yr, or utter simple, intelligible sentences at 3 yr. After 3 yr of age, failure to sustain conversation, abbreviated attention to language, or notably deviant articulation of speech sounds warrants further investigation. Lack of responsivity to sound, failure to comprehend language as expected, speech production requiring increased effort, or an abnormal voice quality warrants referral at any age (Table 2–21).

REFERRAL FOR SPEECH AND LANGUAGE SERVICES

When a speech or language disorder is suspected, referral to a qualified speech-language pathologist for further evaluation is indicated. Speech-language pathologists are certified

Table 2–19. **Speech and Language Development**

Age	Phonology (Sound System)	Syntax (Grammar)/Semantics (Meaning)	Pragmatics (Use of Language)

6–12 months	Babbling—labial consonants dominant (p,b,m)
	Sound play
	Begins learning intonation patterns
	Imitates:
	  First sounds that can be made spontaneously
	  Later attempts to imitate new sounds not yet made spontaneously
			Vocalizations have a range of functions/intentions: e.g., responding, greeting, protesting, attention getting
			Verbal and nonverbal turn-taking
			Shared eye contact (attends to object other looks at)
			Communication games

12–18 months	Consonant-vowel (e.g., ma) or consonant-vowel-consonant-vowel reduplicated (e.g., mama)
	Early consonants: nasals (m,n); front consonants (t, b, d); followed by back consonants (k)
	May not distinguish between voiced and voiceless consonants (t/d)
	Vowels—ah, ee, oo
	May use deferred imitation of words heard earlier
		Begins using single words meaningfully
		Holophrastic words (one word = whole sentence)
		Uses a few function words (there, no, all gone); names (mama, pet); object labels (cup, doggie)
		Undergeneralizations—uses words more narrowly
		Overgeneralization of referents
		Gesture and words
		About 50 words by 18 months
			Intentions expressed:
			  request for object or attention
			  reject
			  comment
			  routine

18–24 months	18–48 months—simplification of adult syllable structures, e.g.:
	  1. Final consonants deleted
	  2. Delete unstressed syllables
	  3. Repeat syllable: byebye, mama, dada
	  4. Reduction of consonant clusters
	  5. Assimilation in which production of one sound is influenced by second sound in the word
	  6. Substitution of sounds, e.g.: front/back consonants (t/k), stop/fricative (d/s)
		Sudden increase in vocabulary
		Onset of 2-word combinations
		Noun phrase, may include modifiers
		Verbs do not include inflectional ending except occasional -ing
		No or *not* used to negate entire phrase;
		Encode semantic relations such as: recurrence (more milk), cessation (no milk), disappearance (no doggie), possession (mommie juice)
			Symbolic play emerges
			Onset of verbal dialogue
			Answers speech with speech

24–36 months	Develops voiced-voiceless distinction (e.g., t/d, p/b, k/g) Begins using consonants in final position of word	3–4 word "telegraphic" sentences Can name and tell use of common objects Noun phrases are elaborated to include modifiers, demonstratives, articles, and possessives Verb phrases used: -ing, regular past -ed, auxiliaries can, will, be emerge Yes/no questions marked by rising intonation Simple *what* and *where* questions asked; *Why, who* and *how* questions infrequent Negatives placed between noun and verb phrases; may include *can't, don't* and *won't*	Revises language secondary to listener's response Can put 2–3 sentences together to hold brief conversation Rapid topic change
36–48 months	By 3 years, all vowels acquired 3 years: p, m, h, n, w* Uses final consonants in words	Grammatically complete simple sentences Noun phrases elaborated to include adjectives Verbs: *be-ing* appears; begin use of modals: *could, would, should, must, might* Present tense contracted or uncontracted forms of *can* (e.g., can't, cannot), *will, do, be* Begins to move auxiliary for yes-no questions *When* questions emerge	Sustains topic Systematic changes in speech depending on listener

48 months and beyond	By 4 years: intelligible to strangers
	4 years: b, k, g, d, f, y; early consonant clusters: sm, sn, sp, st, sk;*
	6 years: t, ng, r, l*
	7 years: ch, sh, j, voiceless th;*
	8 years: s, z, v, voiced th;*
	8 years +: zh;*
	—Perfects consonant clusters
	—Develops accurate pronunciation of multi-syllabic, complex words (e.g., electrician, electricity, electrically)
	—Sophistication in use of stress, pitch changes and intonation patterns
		Verb system completed
		Negation system completed
		Complex sentence structures, e.g.:
		  Relative clauses (She sees the girl who's on the bike)
		  Verb complements (Jaime thinks that John's stupid)
		Coordinates sentences by:
		  Conjunctions (I went to the store and I bought some cookies)
		  Embeddings (I went to the store to buy juice and cookies)
		Achieves full semantic contrast of word pairs such as *more-less, before-after*
		Continues to develop vocabulary and meaning of words into adulthood
			Develops metalinguistic awareness (ability to think about language)
			Perfects social appropriateness of language use
			Develops ability to role-play and assume another perspective

*Customarily used by 90% of children studied. (Sander, 1972.)

Table 2–20. **Development of Speech and Language**

Age at Which Behavior Should Be Established (Months)	Receptive Language Behavior	Expressive Language Behavior
1	Random activity arrested by sound	Random vocalization; primarily vowel sounds
2	Appears to listen to speaker; may smile at speaker	Vocal signs of pleasure; social smile
3	Looks in direction of speaker	Cooing and gurgling; smile in response to speech
4	Responds differentially to angry vs. pleasant voice	Responds vocally to social stimuli
5	Responds to own name (see also Sec. 2.5)	Begins to mimic sounds
6	Recognizes words like "bye-bye," "Mamma," "Daddy"	Protests vocally; squeals with delight
7	Responds with gestures to words such as "up," "come," "bye-bye"	Begins to use wordlike sounds, some jargon
8	Stops activity when own name is called	Imitates sound sequences
9	Stops activity in response to "no"	Imitates intonation pattern of speech
10	Accurately imitates pitch variations	First words appear
11	Responds to simple questions ("where is the dog?") by looking or pointing	Jargon well established
12	Responds with gestures to a variety of verbal requests	Announces awareness of familiar objects by name
15	Recognizes names of various parts of body	True words heard embedded in jargon, often with gestures
18	Identifies pictures of familiar objects when they are named	Uses words more than gestures to express desires
21	Follows two consecutive, related directions ("pick up your hat and put it on the chair")	Begins combining words ("Daddy car," "Mamma up")
24	Understands more complex sentences ("after we get in the car we'll go to the store")	Refers to self by name

by the American Speech-Language and Hearing Association. They may maintain private practices or may be affiliated with school systems or with various health care agencies. A speech and language evaluation typically describes the nature and severity of the disorder, identifies the possible contributing causes, and outlines a treatment program if indicated. Assessment or treatment may involve referral to other professionals, such as neurologists, otolaryngologists, psychiatrists, or psychologists. There may be a need for enrollment in preschool or special school programs, or the institution of direct speech and language therapy. Language therapy aims to teach language rules, facilitate more rapid language development, and when necessary provide alternative forms of communication, such as sign language or communication boards. The goals of speech therapy are to correct deviant speech or teach compensatory strategies for more acceptable speech production.

DOROTHY M. ARAM

Table 2–21. **Signs of Problems in Language and Speech Development in Preschool Children**

1. At 6 mo of age does not turn eyes and head to sound coming from behind or to side
2. At 10 mo does not make some kind of response to his or her name
3. At 15 mo does not understand and respond to "no-no," "bye-bye," and "bottle"
4. At 18 mo is not saying up to 10 single words
5. At 21 mo does not respond to directions (e.g., "sit down," "come here," "stand up")
6. After 24 mo has excessive, inappropriate jargon or echoing
7. At 24 mo does not on request point to body parts (e.g., mouth, nose, eyes, ears)
8. At 24 mo has no z-word phrases
9. At 30 mo has speech that is not intelligible to family members
10. At 36 mo uses no simple sentences
11. At 36 mo has not begun to ask simple questions
12. At 36 mo has speech that is not intelligible to strangers
13. At 3.5 yr of age consistently fails to produce the final consonant (e.g., "ca" for *cat*, "bo" for *bone*, etc.)
14. After 4 yr of age is noticeably dysfluent (stutters)
15. After 7 yr of age has any speech sound errors
16. At any age has noticeable hypernasality or hyponasality, or has a voice that is a monotone, of inappropriate pitch, unduly loud, inaudible, or consistently hoarse

Andrews G, Craig A, Foyer AM, et al: Stuttering: A review of research findings and theories circa 1982. J Speech Hear Disord 48:226, 1983.
Aram DM, Nation JE: Child Language Disorders. St. Louis, CV Mosby, 1982.
Bzoch K, League R: Assessing Language Skills in Infancy. Gainesville, FL, Tree of Life Press, 1971.
Capute AJ, Accardo PJ: Linguistic and auditory milestones during the first two years of life. Clin Pediatr 17:847, 1978.
Coplan J: The Early Language Milestone Scale. Tulsa, OK, Modern Education Corporation, 1983.
Gerkin KP: The high risk register for deafness. ASHA 26(4):17, 1984.
Lass NJ, McReynolds LV, Northern JL, et al (eds): Speech, Language and Hearing. Vol I–III. Philadelphia, WB Saunders, 1982.
Miller JF: Assessing Language in Children. Baltimore, University Park Press, 1981.
Northern JL, Downs MP: Hearing in Children. 3rd ed. Baltimore, Williams & Wilkins, 1984.
Prutting CA: Process \prä | ses\n: The action of moving forward progressively from one point to another on the way to completion. J Speech Hear Disord 44:3, 1979.
Reilly AP (ed): The Communication Game: Perspectives on the Development of Speech, Language and Nonverbal Communication Skills. Johnson & Johnson Pediatric Round Table Series, 1980.
Sander EK: When are speech sounds learned? J Speech Hearing Dis 37:55, 1972.

OTHER DEVELOPMENTAL ISSUES
2.69 MENTAL RETARDATION

Mental retardation is a symptom found in many disorders of known and unknown etiologies. It is often difficult to define or to grade as to its severity. The diagnosis should be made only when evidence has made its presence certain; otherwise, the stigmatizing effect of the label can itself be seriously handicapping.

Mental retardation should be considered in any child who performs more than 2 standard deviations below the mean for his or her age on a standard psychometric test measuring intelligence. The intelligence quotient, or IQ, is the ratio of mental age to chronologic age, multiplied by 100. It is important to recognize that almost 3% of any "normal" population falls 2 standard deviations below the mean on any "intelligence" test. Pitfalls of intelligence tests are discussed elsewhere. They generally measure several brain functions, including auditory memory, visual-spatial capability, and expressive and receptive language. The calculated IQ is an average of these measurements and does not indicate specific strengths and weaknesses. Binet, who designed the first IQ test, did not intend it as a measure of innate cognitive ability but simply as a tool to predict school performance, for which the IQ proves after the age of 3 yr to be a rather reliable predictor, but far from perfect. The IQ may not reflect the optimal cerebral function or potential of the individual. It is in some respects insensitive to the adverse effects of cultural and environmental factors on achievement of the fullest potential.

The limitations of the IQ as a criterion for diagnosis of mental retardation have led to development of scales that assess the ability to adapt successfully to environmental and societal demands. For example, adaptation may be measured in terms of a child's ability to care for personal needs such as dressing and feeding as compared to that of children of similar chronologic age. Social skills may be assessed, as well as the ability to adapt to general educational demands in a normal school setting. Focus may center on the degree to which, as an adult, the individual can be expected to be personally independent, socially accepted, and vocationally competitive.

The reported incidence of mental retardation varies with age (Fig. 2–14), owing principally to the need to adapt to changing environmental circumstances. The number of children recognized as "retarded" rises during the school years, for it is at this time that the social setting results in comparisons among large numbers of children of the same age. The incidence decreases in late adolescence when scholastic demands are no longer an obstacle to functional adequacy. Many young adults with mild mental retardation make satisfactory adaptations in the community, both vocationally and socially. They function independently and competitively, though their intellectual handicap has added to their difficulties in reaching this goal. It is estimated that 30–70% of adults with IQ's of 60–80 make adequate adjustment to community life without the assistance of health, social, or correctional agencies.

None of the many adaptive scales proposed have been universally accepted as devices for classification. Accordingly, in spite of its limitations the IQ remains the principal diagnostic criterion used by the health professions and agencies that deal with the mentally retarded. Table 2–22 gives the classification of retardation currently in general use. It is estimated that over 90% of retarded persons are in the mild or borderline range. Only 5% are severely or profoundly retarded.

Etiology. Table 2–23 classifies the principal causes of mental retardation. In the majority of patients whose mental retardation is mild to borderline, comprehensive medical evaluations have not found evidence of a defective brain. The majority of these mildly retarded individuals are at the lower end of the socioeconomic scale; accordingly, one is led to the hypothesis that their poor adaptive function is likely to be secondary to adverse sociocultural influences, including the lack of a stimulating environment. This theory is in keeping with the observation that children of lower socioeconomic groups have gradual declines in IQ's with maturation. On the other hand, it is possible that the defective brain function may not be detected by present neuroinvestigative techniques or that polygenic or mutifactorial determinants of intelligence may be playing a role. Moreover, there may be prevalent in the lower socioeconomic environment subtly detrimental "organic" effects that are not readily apparent. For example, blood lead levels are often higher in inner-city, economically deprived children than in suburban children from affluent families. Subclinical lead intoxication, acting over a prolonged period of time, can impair cognitive abilities. Cytomegalovirus infection is also more frequently noted among mothers of lower socioeconomic status, and their infants are more frequently found to excrete the virus than infants from more affluent families. The likelihood of nutritional deficiency also correlates with socioeconomic status. Malnutrition, smoking, and deficiencies in prenatal care are all more common among socioeconomically disadvantaged mothers and are known to have detrimental effects on fetal brain development.

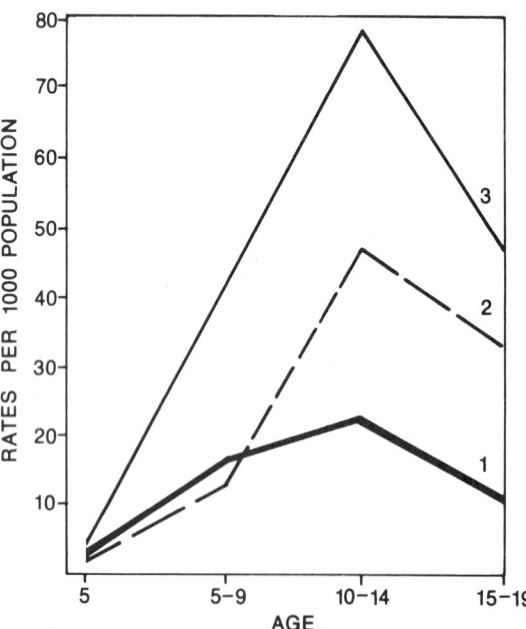

Figure 2–14. Incidence of mental retardation in different age groups as reported from three different surveys. 1. Report of the Mental Deficiency Commission, London, His Majesty's Stationery Office, 1929, Pts 1, 2, 3, and 4. 2. Lemkau P, et al.: Mental Hygiene Problems in an Urban District. 3. New York State Department of Mental Hygiene, Mental Health Research Unit: A Special Census of Suspected Referred Mental Retardation, Onondaga County, N.Y. Syracuse, N.Y., 1955, p 84.

Table 2–22. Levels of Mental Retardation and Associated Features

Borderline (IQ 68–83)	Children with IQ's above 69 are not retarded, strictly speaking, but are vulnerable to educational problems. They are usually able to function adequately in slow sections of regular classes. Most achieve independent social and vocational adjustment.
Mild (IQ 52–67)	This group includes 90% of children formally classified as retarded. Most need special class placement, and some can achieve 4th–6th grade reading levels. Those who are well adjusted may be able to function independently as adults.
Moderate (IQ 36–51)	Children in this group will usually function in classes for the trainable retarded, with emphasis on gaining maximal self-care and perhaps some academic skills. Those who are well adjusted may be able to function semi-independently in supervised living and sheltered workshop settings.
Severe (IQ 20–35)	Children in this group can learn minimal self-care skills and simple conversational skills. They need much supervision and are often institutionalized.
Profound (IQ below 20)	Children in this group need total supervision. Very minimal self-care skills are possible. Some may be toilet trained. Language development will be minimal.

Diagnosis and Clinical Manifestations. The assessment of a child who is functioning in the mentally retarded range must first answer the following questions:

1. Does the brain dysfunction have an organic basis?
2. If so, is the organic deficit due to a static or progressive lesion?
3. Is the condition treatable?
4. Is there evidence of a familial or hereditary disorder?

A comprehensive history can be the best aid to diagnosis. Certain high risk factors (prenatal, perinatal, or postnatal) increase the likelihood of brain damage (Table 2–24), but the finding of one or more of these factors offers only circumstantial evidence that cerebral injury has resulted. It is not unusual to find in an infant at high risk who performs poorly on standard developmental testing that findings on medical, neurologic, and comprehensive laboratory examinations are normal. In such cases, to conclude that there is no relationship between the high risk factor and evidence of brain injury may be unjustifiable. Clinical judgment is required in assessing the relationship between high-risk events and later neurologic status.

A variety of findings on physical examination may give clues as to etiology or organicity. It is important to determine whether certain congenital stigmata are present (Table 2–25). Various patterns of stigmata indicate specific syndromes. Some are secondary to chromosomal abnormalities or teratogenic effects; others may be of unknown cause. Identification of syndromes has been made easier through compendia that index stigmata to known syndromes. One is often unable to identify a syndrome even though the prevalence of stigmata

clearly suggests that the central nervous system anomaly may have the same origin as the external abnormalities. On the other hand, each of these stigmata occurs in normal persons, albeit with much lower frequency than among the mentally retarded.

Head circumference may be of diagnostic significance if it is more than 2 standard deviations below or above the normal mean or if head circumference and height are significantly discrepant though both are within normal limits. Clues to progressive degenerative diseases of the brain or to metabolic diseases include choreoretinitis, optic atrophy, pigmentary degeneration of the retina, cataracts, uveitis, skin lesions (vitiligo, café-au-lait spots, port-wine stains, hemangiomas, incontinentia pigmenti, nevus unius lateris, and adenoma sebaceum), organomegaly, abnormal genitalia, excessively short or tall stature, abnormal body proportions, unusual smell to urine or skin, light hair color, and sparse or friable

Table 2–23. Causes of Mental Retardation

Nonorganic—environmentally determined
  Sociocultural factors
  Emotional disturbances

Organic
  Static encephalopathies
    Prenatal origin
      Cerebral malformation—1st trimester
        Chromosomal aberrations
        Intrauterine infections (e.g., TORCHES infections*)
        Teratogens
        Placental dysfunction
        Unknown causes
      Cerebral deformation—2nd and 3rd trimesters
        Intrauterine infection (e.g., TORCHES infections*)
        Teratogens
        Maternal diabetes mellitus
        Maternal toxemia of pregnancy
        Placental dysfunction
        Maternal urinary tract infection (?)
        Maternal malnutrition
    Perinatal origin
      Complications of prematurity
      Asphyxia and/or ischemia neonatorum
      Birth trauma
      Meningitis
      Cerebrovascular accidents
    Postnatal origin
      Head and central nervous system trauma
      Cerebrovascular accident
      Neurotoxins (e.g., lead)
      Intracranial infections
      Anoxic episodes (e.g., near-drowning)

  Progressive encephalopathies
    Metabolic
      Aminoacidurias (e.g., PKU)
      Carbohydrate disorders (e.g., galactosemia)
      Mucopolysaccharidoses (e.g., Hurler syndrome)
      Cerebral lipidoses (e.g., Tay-Sachs disease); with hepatomegaly (Gaucher disease)
      Leukodystrophies (e.g., metachromatic leukodystrophy)
      Uric acid disturbance (e.g., Lesch-Nyhan syndrome)
      Hormonal imbalance (e.g., hypothyroid, pseudohypoparathyroid)
      Nutritional deficiencies
      Neuroectodermal dysplasia (e.g., tuberous sclerosis)
      Other degenerative diseases (e.g., Alper disease, muscular dystrophy [occasionally], myotonic dystrophy [occasionally])
    Infectious
      Kuru
      Subacute sclerosing panencephalitis

*TORCHES infections are toxoplasmosis, rubella, cytomegalovirus infection, herpesvirus infection, and syphilis.

Table 2–24. **Factors indicating Increased Risk of Infants or Children for Mental Retardation**

Prenatal
Toxemia
Placenta previa
Abruptio placentae
Exposure to ionizing radiation during 1st trimester
Syphilis
TORCHES infections
Ingestion of teratogens
Multiple pregnancy
Previous miscarriage
Family history of cerebral dysfunction, speech and language dysfunction, hearing impairment
Maternal malnutrition
Vaginal bleeding in the 2nd or 3rd trimesters
Maternal age less than 16 yr or over 40 yr
Consanguinity of parents

Perinatal
Prematurity
Small birth weight for gestational age
Birth anoxia or hypoxia
Birth trauma
Apgar scores—under 4 at 1 min and/or under 6 at 5 min
Neonatal seizures
Abnormal neonatal neurobehavioral examination
Early difficulty in sucking
Hypoglycemia

Postnatal
Delayed language development
Delayed motor development
Delayed adaptive behavior
Disadvantaged socioeconomic environment
Intracranial infection
Significant head trauma
Encephalitis
Meningitis
Ingestion or inhalation of neurotoxins (e.g., lead)
Cerebral hypoxia (e.g., secondary to near-drowning or carbon monoxide poisoning)
Cerebrovascular accident
Severe malnutrition

hair. A formal neurologic examination should evaluate the status of the entire neuraxis and peripheral nervous system, including assessment of cranial nerves; muscular strength, tone, and coordination; deep tendon and primitive reflexes; and cortical sensory function. Examination is also made for the presence of "soft" neurologic signs (Table 2–26).

The laboratory investigations necessary to assess the patient with mental retardation should vary with the clinical findings. Table 2–27 lists laboratory tests that should be considered in the context of historical events and findings on physical and neurologic examination.

Treatment. The primary goal of management of the mentally retarded is that each affected person reach his or her optimal developmental potential and be able to cope as effectively as possible with the handicap. In helping to achieve this, the physician must assist the family as a whole in developing strategies that will allow each member to make a rapid and optimal adaptation to the stress of living with a handicapped person.

Treatment begins as soon as diagnosis is suspected. It is important that the physician be scrupulously honest regarding the diagnosis and prognosis and also be willing to share uncertainty or ignorance on certain points. This truthful approach must be tempered by compassion. Parents who are told for the first time that their child is mentally retarded will not infrequently deny that the problem exists. Denial may be accompanied by anger toward the physician and by a search for contrary medical opinions. These parental reactions are normal. A defensive or angry response on the part of the physician whose diagnosis and advice are thus rejected or disbelieved will further alienate the parents and complicate future contacts. The physician will usually need to reassure parents that they are not themselves responsible for the child's handicap. Such reassurance is particularly important when the etiology is not known.

When a diagnosis conveying the probability or certainty of mental retardation is evident during the neonatal period, the physician should meet with both parents and explain his or her concern about the baby, avoiding a tendency to focus only upon abnormal findings or probable weaknesses. Attention of the parents should also be directed to normal features and positive attributes the baby may have, such as vitality, muscular strength, nice appearance, or alertness. Such observations may help parents to accept the infant as a person and foster the healthy bonding important to the infant's later development. Parents who learn that they have a retarded child rather than the fantasized ideal extension of themselves may go into a period of mourning as though they had lost a family member (Sec. 2.34).

Retarded infants should be referred early to infant stimulation programs. These programs may be based either in centers or in the home. They have two primary functions: (1) to help the infant develop optimally by helping the parents to understand their baby's developmental problem, strengths, and limitations; and (2) to offer a curriculum of multisensory stimulation aimed at facilitation of cognitive, physical, and emotional development. A third function is to support parents and other family members through individual and/or group counseling. Infant stimulation programs vary in strategies aimed toward sensorimotor development. Although their effectiveness has not been convincingly demonstrated, many clinicians believe that they have value in immediate supportive and educational counseling of parents, which may decrease their need to "shop" for other opinions and may shorten the time necessary for them to adapt to the experience of having and living with a handicapped offspring. The sapping of emotional energy and financial resources through searching for contrary opinions can adversely affect maternal-infant bonding and impair or frustrate the nurturance needed by the handicapped infant.

Since 1975, Federal legislation (PL 94–142) has established that all retarded children in the United States, irrespective of the severity of their functional deficits, have the legal right to an education from 3 to 21 yr of age. The educational services are to be in school settings, either in regular classes with the help of extra resources ("mainstreaming") or in special classes geared to the handicapped child's educational, social, and behavioral needs. Education does not necessarily mean studying academic subjects, but can mean learning self-care activities and social skills.

Physicians should encourage parents to enroll their handicapped children in school programs and, with parents' permission, should exchange information with the school about educationally relevant medical and physical findings. They should participate in the formulation of the child's educational needs. To be effective in securing an appropriate educational program for any child with a learning disability, the physician must become familiar enough with his or her own local school system to understand and cope with the administrative and political issues that may interfere with provision of the appropriate individualized educational program to which the child is entitled. The physician who accepts and meets the challenge of bringing about communication among various professional persons involved in services to children with disabilities and to their families can be particularly helpful because of his or her understanding of human development.

Table 2–25. Stigmata Associated with Mental Retardation

Head
  Maximal occipitofrontal circumference less than 3rd percentile or over 97th percentile
  Plagiocephaly

Hair
  Double whorl; sparse or absent hair
  Fine, friable, prematurely gray or white locks

Eyes
  Microphthalmia
  Hypertelorism
  Hypotelorism
  Upward-and-outward or downward-and-outward slant
  Inner or outer epicanthal folds
  Coloboma of iris or retina
  Brushfield spots
  Eccentrically placed pupil
  Nystagmus
  Telangiectasia

Ears
  Low-set ears
  Simple or abnormal helix formation

Nose
  Flattened bridge
  Small size
  Upturned nares

Face
  Increased length of philtrum
  Hypoplasia of maxilla and/or mandible

Mouth
  Inverted "V" shape of upper lip
  Wide or high-arched palate

Teeth
  Evidence of abnormal enamelogenesis
  Abnormal odontogenesis

Neck
  Short neck
  Lack of full mobility
  Webbing

Extremities
  Unusually short or long limbs
  Increased carrying angle at elbows

Hands
  Short 4th or 5th metacarpals
  Short stubby fingers
  Long, thin tapered fingers
  Broad thumbs
  Clinodactyly
  Abnormal dermatoglyphics (e.g., distal triradius)
  Simian line
  Abnormal nails

Feet
  Overlap of toes
  Short stubby toes
  Broad, large big toes
  Deep crease leading from angle of 1st and 2nd toes
  Abnormal dermatoglyphics
  Short 4th or 5th metatarsals

Abdomen
  Protuberant abdomen
  Umbilical hernia

Genitalia
  Ambiguous genitalia
  Micropenis
  Abnormal placement of urethral meatus
  Undescended testicles
  Large testicles

Chest
  Pectus excavatum or carinatum
  Supernumerary nipples

Skin
  Café-au-lait spots
  Depigmented nevi
  Adenoma sebaceum
  Malar flush
  Eczema
  Linear nevus unius lateris

Unfortunately, many retarded persons are not befriended by their normally functioning age-mates or classmates. Social and recreational activities must be planned for them. Organized activities for retarded persons are often available, and parents should become familiar with them. Attendance at summer camps for the retarded should be encouraged. Such programs help the retarded to acquire comfortable social interactions and to achieve more independent function.

Many communities have sheltered workshops for retarded adults who are capable of simple repetitive tasks but unable to compete in the labor market. For severely retarded individuals who cannot function in sheltered workshops, community-based activity centers offer a chance for socialization and recreation.

Table 2–26. Soft Neurologic Signs

Poor fine and/or gross coordination
Strabismus
Verbal dyspraxia
Motor dyspraxia
Motor impersistence (positive Prechtl sign)
Immature overflow patterns (mirror movements)
Immature sequencing (motor, auditory, visual)
Graphomotor difficulties
Constructional dyspraxia
Dysdiadochokinesia

The United States is moving toward "normalizing" as much as possible the lives of retarded individuals. Foster care or placement in small group homes is becoming available as an alternative to large residential institutions for children or adults who need to be cared for away from their own homes. Group homes are usually situated within the community where the retarded person's family lives, and in such homes "house parents" are responsible for care of a small number of compatible handicapped individuals; this care is coordinated with other resources of the community, such as public schools, recreational facilities, and sheltered workshops. Early residential placement of retarded children or adults outside the home should not be casually advised by the physician, but the possibility can be mentioned as an option when it becomes evident that a particular family is finding it difficult to cope with the situation and/or when the particular child's behavior is deteriorating. The physician should discuss all options without passing moral judgments as to what the family should or should not do. When parents make decisions in accord with *their* needs and resources, all options considered, the physician should be supportive.

Every retarded child needs someone to take the responsibility for monitoring progress, for assisting with educational placement and obtaining social and recreational experiences, and for supporting and advising parents and siblings during periods of crisis. This individual should also inform the family about the programmatic and financial assistance to which

Table 2–27. Diagnostic Strategy for Infant or Child with Mental Retardation

Chromosomal *karyotyping* indicated in children with
  Unusual number and/or character of physical stigmata
  History of maternal exposure to a teratogen
  Abnormal genitalia
Examination for *aminoaciduria* indicated in children with
  Unexplained seizures — neonatal period
  Unusual smell to urine or skin
  Unusually light-colored hair
  Microcephaly
  Family history
  Dermatitis
Examination of urine for *mucopolysaccharides* indicated in children with
  Coarse features
  Kyphosis
  Short extremities
  Short trunk
  Cloudy cornea
  Impaired hearing
  Dwarfism
  Stiff joints
Examination of urine for *reducing substances* indicated in children with
  Cataracts
  Hepatomegaly
  Seizures
Examination of *serum ammonia level* indicated in children with
  Episodic vomiting and metabolic acidosis
Examination of urine for *ketoacids* indicated in children with
  Seizures
  Short friable hair
Examination of *blood lead level* indicated in children with
  History of pica
  Anemia
  Unexplained mental retardation in inner-city child
Examination of *serum zinc level* indicated in children with
  Acrodermatitis
Examination of *skull roentgenograms* indicated in children with
  Microcephaly
  Macrocephaly
  Plagiocephaly
  Suspected intracerebral mass
Examination of *serum copper and ceruloplasmin levels* indicated in children with
  Involuntary movements
  Cirrhosis
  Kayser-Fleischer rings
Examination of *serum neuroenzyme activities* and/or *skin biopsy* indicated in children with
  Loss of milestones or functions in motor and/or cognitive areas
  Optic atrophy
  Retinal degeneration
  Recurrent cerebellar ataxia
  Myoclonus
  Hepatosplenomegaly
  Coarse loose skin
  Seizures
  Enlarged head beginning after 1 yr of age
Examination of *VMA levels* indicated in children with
  Episodic vomiting
  Poor suck
  Symptoms of autonomic dysfunction
Examination of *serum uric acid levels* indicated in children with
  Self-mutilation
  Rage attacks
  Gout
  Choreoathetosis
Computed tomography (CT scan) of head indicated in children with
  Progressive enlargement of head
  Tuberous sclerosis
  Suspected gross malformation of brain
  Focal seizures
  Suspected intracranial mass

they may be entitled. A concerned pediatrician can discharge this function particularly well; at routine health visits for preventive care more global issues can be explored with the family. Pediatricians who do not feel that they can provide these services should suggest that help be sought at a local chapter of the Association for Retarded Citizens or through the responsible governmental agency (generally, the Crippled Children's Program).

Parents of handicapped children are often excessively devoted to the care of their handicapped child, leaving no time for themselves. Many communities have respite centers in foster care or residential settings where parents can leave their children temporarily with responsible caretakers while they have relief for a weekend or longer from the continuing demands of the care of the handicapped child. The physician should suggest such arrangements to parents and help them not to feel guilty about their need for periodic relief or vacation.

The sexual drives of mild or moderately retarded persons do not differ from those of persons of normal intelligence. On the other hand, their levels of comprehension of socially acceptable sexual behavior may present a problem, depending on their particular levels of intellectual functioning. Many retarded persons will need family-planning services adjusted to their levels of understanding and function. In some instances, sterilization may warrant consideration as a form of contraception, though ethical and legal issues surround its use. Sterilization of retardates for eugenic purposes is not acceptable in the United States.

Prognosis. If a mildly retarded adult is to have a chance of functioning independently within the community, he or she must have socially acceptable behavior. This achievement is not easy, given the environmental burden mentally handicapped children must cope with. They are frequently frustrated by their inability to attain academic or social success and feel the effects of parental unhappiness or dissatisfaction at their slow progress. The result is loss of self-esteem and decreased motivation to achieve. Some retarded persons feel that they can achieve recognition only by aggressive or acting-out behavior, which further alienates them from peers and family. Retarded persons with cosmetic difficulties have additional experiences of rejection.

Mildly retarded persons usually require placement in special educational programs, though a few succeed in regular classes. Many can achieve a 5th grade level in reading or in mathematics. Usually, they can find employment only in unskilled jobs. Not infrequently, mildly retarded persons marry and raise children in a responsible fashion. Assuming responsibility for a family can be a risky venture, however, especially for retarded persons with poor judgment who must compete in an increasingly technologic society.

Moderately, severely, and profoundly retarded children cannot be expected to acquire academic skills. They can, however, learn self-care activities and social competencies. They will always require supervisory care, either by a guardian in a home setting or in residential placement. Some may be able to participate in a sheltered workshop or an activity center.

LAWRENCE T. TAFT

Alford CA: Prenatal infections and psychosocial development in children born into lower socioeconomic settings. *In:* Mittler P (ed): Research to Practice in Mental Retardation and Biomedical Aspects. Vol III. Baltimore, University Park Press, 1977.
Birch HG: Functional effect of malnutrition. *In:* Chess S, Thomas A (eds): Annual Progress in Child Psychiatry and Child Development. New York, Brunner/Hazel, 1972.
Brooks-Gunn J, Hearn RP: Early intervention and developmental dysfunction: Implications for pediatrics. Adv Pediatr 29:497, 1982.
Cruickshank W: The relation of physical disability to fear and guilt feelings. Child Dev 22:291, 1951.

Denhoff E: Status of infant stimulation or enrichment programs for children with developmental disabilities. Pediatrics 67:32, 1981.

Diagnostic and Statistical Manual of Mental Disorder III. Washington DC, American Psychiatric Association, 1979.

Dobbing J, Hopewell JW, Lynch A: Vulnerability of developing brain. VII. Permanent deficits of neurons in cerebral and cerebellar cortex following early mild malnutrition. Exp Neur 32:439, 1971.

Green M: The management of children with chronic disease. In: Green AM, Haggerty RJ (eds): Ambulatory Pediatrics II. Philadelphia, WB Saunders, 1977.

Haggerty RJ (ed): Chronic disease in children. Pediatr Clin North Am 31 (No 1), 1984.

Mattson A: Long-term physical illness in childhood: A challenge to psychosocial adaptation. Pediatrics 50:801, 1972.

Meier JH: Screening, assessment and intervention for young children at developmental risk. In: Tjossem TD (ed): Intervention Strategies for High Risk Infants and Young Children. Baltimore, University Park Press, 1976, p 251.

Rosen M, Clark GR, Kivitz MO (eds): The History of Mental Retardation. Baltimore, University Park Press, 1976.

Schneider AP, Hanshaw JB, Simeoussou RH, et al: The study of children with congenital cytomegalovirus infection. In: Mittler P (ed): Research to Practice in Mental Retardation and Biomedical Aspects. Vol III. Baltimore, University Park Press, 1977.

Solnit AJ, Stark MH: Mourning and the birth of a defective child. Psychoanal Study Child 16:523, 1961.

Sparrow S, Zigler E: Evaluation of a patterning treatment for retarded children. Pediatrics 63:137, 1978.

Turnbull AP, Turnbull HR III: Parents Speak Out, Views from the Other Side of the Two-Way Mirror. Columbus, OH, Charles E Merrill Publishing Co, 1978.

Wright GF: The pediatrician's role in Public Law 94–142. Pediatr Rev 4:191, 1982.

Zigler E: Dealing with retardation. (Review of The Mentally Retarded and Society, by MJ Begab and SA Richardson). Science 196:1192, 1977.

2.70 CARE OF THE CHILD WITH A PERMANENT HANDICAP

Permanent handicaps of children include a wide variety of disorders that limit the activity or developmental potential of children in various ways. The most salient features of the handicapping condition may include mental retardation; limitations of physical activity; sensory, learning, and communicative difficulties; conspicuous physical deformities; needs for special arrangements to achieve such normal functions as toileting, mobility, feeding, and the like; evidences of chronic illness or its treatment; and so on. Whatever the particulars, the handicapped child must live in a social world that is perceived as being somewhat apart. And, ultimately, the successful management of children who have chronic and perhaps permanent disabilities depends as often on the social, academic, and home adjustments that can be achieved as it does on purely technical and medical procedures. The parents and family have the major responsibility in caring for and nurturing their children, including the child with the handicap; but the physician should play a direct and supportive role, with others, in helping the family to meet their responsibilities for identifying, finding, and providing those things needed for optimal development.

The Physician. Some physicians are not suited by temperament or training to manage the handicapped child and the family. The comprehensive care required is time-consuming, and many of the children as well as their parents appear at times uncooperative, unappreciative, and even negative. Much time must be spent with parents whose emotional reactions frequently demand more attention than the condition of the child. The physician who extends his or her responsibility beyond the treatment of the "chief complaint," however, will find it rewarding to help young handicapped patients and their families live more comfortably and effectively.

Physicians may feel inadequate because the problems appear complex or insoluble or beyond the means at immediate command. They must be aware of their own possible negative attitudes, prejudices, and limitations and must, above all, be able to utilize other professional persons or disciplines, to make appropriate referrals, and to use other resources in the community while they maintain the role of primary physician.

The physician may feel inadequate if a specific diagnosis cannot be made or if the evaluation cannot be completed at one visit. The physician to handicapped children and their families must be a patient, unthreatening listener, satisfied with small gains and able to understand the child's and the parents' positions sufficiently to offer intelligent support when cure or recovery is not possible. It is important not to cling to outmoded concepts or be unaware of either the possibilities or the limitations of habilitation. The physician must communicate and work effectively with others in the community in providing adequate general pediatric care for the child and support for an acceptable role for parents. Physicians who are uncomfortable in these roles should arrange for care of the child and family by others prepared and willing to assume these responsibilities. When such a transfer of care is arranged, it should not be implied that the reason for it is any shortcoming of the family.

Management of the Child. Management begins at the first meeting with the family, with a functional appraisal of the child and a simple explanation to the parents. Further management should include the same comprehensive health services given to all children. Through continuing contacts and interest in the child and family the physician can help in developing and periodically revising a realistic plan. The ultimate goal is for the child to make use of his or her abilities as effectively as possible and to become as socially acceptable and self-sufficient as limitations permit. Immediate goals should be sufficiently realistic that success is possible and likely since failure discourages further effort, whereas success and praise of effort encourage and motivate.

Children with single or multiple handicaps often have limited opportunities for the experiences upon which normal learning and development depend; accordingly, particular effort must be made to arrange appropriate experiences at each developmental level. Opportunities for learning, for social and group experiences, and for the achievement of self-discipline should be provided. A variety of sensory stimuli and of close, warm, and stimulating parent-child interactions are essential from birth for optimal child development. It is especially important that the parents of infants and children whose avenues to learning may be blocked be reminded to create adequate opportunities for early social and environmental stimulation and interaction. A balance between overprotection and overstimulation must be sought. Misguided protection or indulgence may deprive the child of normal experiences, such as being held to normal limits of acceptable behavior and discipline through self-control. Every effort should be made to minimize secondary handicaps in personality development, which may otherwise become more serious than the primary defect.

The physician should above all else try to help the child lead a happy life. Every effort should be made to involve the child as well as the parents in understanding the problem, in planning, and in decision making. The wise and understanding physician takes time to explain to the child at the child's level of comprehension why he or she is different, what is planned, what is to be done, and why. The physician must interpret the child's condition and behavior to those who are in regular or occasional contact with him or her.

The Family's Problems. The environment and emotional climate of the home of the handicapped child are often more crucial than medical care for the child's eventual adjustment; accordingly, the family must be helped to understand their own feelings and to fulfill their own needs. They should always be given something constructive to do. Parents' reactions to a child with a defect depend on the extent to which they feel that their competency, social standing, and anticipated way of life are threatened. Most parents attempt initially to deny the reality of the defect, particularly if it is not apparent physically. Denial is usually followed by frustration, disorganization, self-accusation, and questioning; fears and anxieties about the future may become overwhelming. Simple explanation, support, and guidance for the family are particularly necessary at this time. As parents' defenses become organized further, denial, hostility, and attempts to assign responsibility develop. A physician who is not aware that the parents' feelings of guilt may be projected as anger toward him or her will be unprepared to react with the necessary understanding and patience and may emerge with a bruised ego. If communication and counseling are not effective, the "no one ever told me" reaction sets in and "shopping around" ensues. Frequently, introduction of the family to group discussions with other parents will prove helpful through providing opportunities for sharing of feelings or for education about the condition itself.

The physician's ability to communicate a genuine professional concern for the child and for the family's feelings often spells the difference between the family's active involvement and their rejection of help. Depending upon their maturity and emotional resources, the family can be helped to plan realistically and constructively for the long-term needs of the child. Parents and other family members should join in assessment and re-evaluation of the child's progress and actively participate in developing and carrying out recommendations. If the family cannot approve or accept recommendations, even ideal ones, or if recommended community services are not available, substitutes should be found. Group or individual counseling about problems of management may be appropriate. The support that the church can give to families in time of stress should not be overlooked.

The problems are as varied as the people involved. Most parents, regardless of their backgrounds, have feelings of guilt which must be resolved lest attitudes of self-sacrifice, excessive protection, or rejection of the child develop. Most families have ambivalent feelings varying from overt hostility to gross overindulgence. The handicapped child may frequently be the precipitating factor in marital difficulties not basically related to him or her.

As the child grows older, the parents have to make adaptations that would otherwise not be necessary, because of the child's prolonged dependency upon them. Problems of social isolation, schooling, sexual development, and sometimes unpleasant behavior become increasingly important.

In some circumstances the principles of behavior modification should be discussed with the family and help given in establishing and maintaining an appropriate program of conditioning for acceptable behavior. Parents should be given support and suitable materials for ongoing health and sex education for their children.

Family Therapy. Parents often complain in retrospect that the status of the child was not made clear to them, that the diagnosis was based on an incomplete examination or hasty judgment, that a poor prognosis was not justified, or that their part in helping the child was not explained. It must be remembered that many parents hear, retain, and comprehend only in part and that interpretations and suggestions must be given *and repeated* in an acceptable and understandable way to all those concerned. Reinforcement of information given the family may be made by other members of the physician's staff or by members of various other disciplines if consultation services are available.

The initial explanation of the facts about a child with a handicap should be made to the parents *together* as simply as possible. A statement as to what is wrong and what will be done about it is less confusing than a technical explanation. Emphasis should be placed on normalities and similarities to other children rather than on deficiencies and differences. Long-term prognosis and planning should be left for later interviews; attention should be focused on management of immediate problems and symptoms. If necessary, for example, simple techniques could be demonstrated: how to handle an infant who arches the back; how to help an infant in sucking, swallowing, or chewing or in the use of a spoon or cup; how to choose appropriate toys or activities to encourage language development.

Questions should be answered simply and reassurance given to minimize guilt feelings. The physician should also stress the need for patience because it will take time to clarify the child's developmental potential. Attention cannot be given too early to the need to avoid secondary emotional problems in the child and family. The practical problems of carrying out a reasonable program can be best appreciated by a visit to the home. Grandparents and other relatives who may be involved in family affairs should be brought into explanations and planning so that the parents' efforts with the child will be supported.

The parents need clear, simple, valid explanations and interpretations of what the referring physician and consultants have observed and recommended in the form of statements as to what has been found, along with copies of reports and consultations. Such reports should be factual, should contain relevant positive and negative observations about the child and his or her developmental progress, and should make appropriate recommendations. They should not become complex scientific treatises but efficient working papers.

Care should be taken to assure siblings an equal share of parents' time, attention, and interest. With inadvertent or intentional neglect their problems may become greater than those of the affected child. Their questions about the abnormal child should be answered simply and honestly. The experience of living with a seriously handicapped brother or sister may be used constructively to teach tolerance, patience, and understanding of others. If parents openly accept the child as an individual despite limitations, and if they accept failures as gracefully as they do more limited successes, a good example is set for others.

The question of the probable outcome of future pregnancies is frequently raised by parents. If the cause of the disability is clearly an accidental one, it is easy to be reassuring. If it is known to be genetically determined or to arise as a result of circumstances that might recur, the physician should explain the facts as simply and clearly as possible and help the parents to make their own decision based on available evidence and their own circumstances.

Institutional Care. When a seriously handicapped child will always be completely or partially dependent on others for care, the question of suitability of institutional placement arises. The physician should objectively discuss with the family the advantages and disadvantages of such care. Infants and young children have a better developmental future if they live with a consistent mothering figure in an emotionally sound home environment. Moreover, parents generally feel more comfortable about later placement if they have gradually gained full understanding and acceptance of the child's limitations by fulfilling their normal roles as parents. Premature placement may lead to doubts and greater feelings of guilt. Before advising the use of supportive or educational facilities away from home, as opposed to what may be available in the community, the physician should assess their appropriateness, their cost, and their availability. In any case, the decision is the family's and not the physician's, though the physician, if convinced that such a solution would be beneficial to all, may diplomatically initiate the discussion when the family appears reluctant to open the question.

Temporary care away from home is indicated when the child can profit by greater opportunities in a different environment, or for a short term when inevitable family emergencies arise, or when a vacation is needed by all.

Use of Community Resources. The physician is in a unique position to interpret to others in the school, the church, and the community the special problems presented by children with handicaps, and the physician should help to develop and make effective use of community resources. Needs may include medical facilities for early diagnosis, evaluation, and treatment; social case work; genetic counseling; psychologic evaluation and counseling; home care by nurses; "homemaker" services, babysitting, or temporary boarding home care; day care; special educational and recreational facilities; occupational and vocational placement; sheltered workshops; and smaller, local residential programs for respite care.

The physician should support current trends to centralize and coordinate diagnostic and treatment services for children with related handicaps in order to avoid discontinuity, waste of professional effort, frustration of parents, fragmentation of services for the child, and general administrative inefficiency. The "developmental disability" approach is an example of such an effort to bring together programs involving several categorical disorders.

Mainstreaming is an educational movement to channel children with major special needs into regular classes in the schools in the hope of providing a more normal environment and of avoiding the stigma associated with special programs which label such children as different. This has had limited success in comparison with classes offering special education of good quality, structured to meet pupils' individual learning needs. Mainstreaming may become more effective as teachers are better prepared, as more adequate resources and supports are provided in the classrooms, as teachers are able to communicate more effectively with parents and with other concerned professionals, and as the attitudes and expectations of all concerned become more tolerant and realistic. In the shift from placement of retarded or severely handicapped children in relatively large isolated institutions toward care in the home or in smaller, neighborhood facilities, many of the anticipated benefits have been delayed because of deficiencies of local services and in clarifying administrative responsibility. Still to be clarified also are the ideal size of the group, the best physical environment, the kinds of disabilities that can be dealt with appropriately in smaller units, and the ages at which affected children can best be served. The smaller units seem, however, to be providing a stimulus for more appropriate individualized programs and for better social behavior.

Parents' Organizations. Parents' organizations and groups of handicapped persons themselves have been outstandingly successful in providing those with common problems opportunities to share their anxieties, to gain strength and hope through identification with a group, and to bring about effective changes in legislation, in community health and educational programs, and in support of legal and civil rights of the handicapped. These and other efforts in behalf of community education, support of research, voluntary participation in a variety of services, and public recognition are psychologically important to the families of children with handicaps and are constructively helpful to the community.

JOHN B. BARTRAM

Gordon S: Facts about Sex for Exceptional Youth. New Jersey Association for Brain Injured Children, 61 Lincoln Street, East Orange, NJ 07017.
Kempton W, et al: Guide for Parents: Love, Sex and Birth Control for Mentally Retarded. Planned Parenthood Association of Southeastern Pennsylvania, 1402 Spruce Street, Philadelphia, Pa 19102.
Lobato D: Siblings of handicapped children: A review. J Autism Dev Disord 13:347, 1983.
Pattullo A: Puberty in the Girl Who Is Retarded. National Association for Retarded Citizens, 2709 Avenue E East, Arlington, Tex 76010.
White B: First Three Years of Life. Englewood Cliffs, NJ, Prentice-Hall, 1975.

2.71 CARE OF THE CHILD WITH A FATAL ILLNESS

From time to time every physician has the painful duty of caring for a child with a fatal illness. It is then his or her responsibility to help the family cope with *their* pain and grief in such ways that the experience may become growth-promoting rather than destructive of family integrity or of the emotional well-being of the family members. When physicians accept these goals as realistic and commit professional skills to them, their efforts will help to blunt their sense of frustration, grief, or professional inadequacy. (See also Sec. 2.34).

CARE OF PARENTS

When the physician is certain of a fatal outcome, there should ordinarily be no equivocation in conveying the diagnosis to the family in a direct and empathetic way. If both parents are available, the fact that their child has an illness from which recovery is not expected should be conveyed to them when they are together. The words chosen and the manner of the physician should be gentle and honest, and he or she should be prepared to meet the parents' anguish or disbelief with answers to their questions and with information as to what measures will be taken to try to forestall what seems to be inevitable (Sec 2.54).

The place in which this conversation occurs should be carefully chosen. It should be apart from the other activities of the hospital or office and should be available for an adequate, uninterrupted time. The privacy of this time should be carefully protected. It needs to be understood that much of the conversation at this time will not be fully registered or accurately remembered by the parents of the sick child, and the physician should plan another session later in the day or on the next day when the information given can be reviewed and new or recurring questions answered.

Ordinarily the physician should avoid taking the position that nothing can be done but should emphasize the positive steps that the physician and parents together can take to surmount the difficulties ahead. Physicians should generally avoid detailed predictions of the course or duration of the illness, emphasizing that in such situations one generally lives from day to day and that it is usually possible to avoid undue suffering or pain. When the illness may endure for months or years, it may not be inappropriate to hold out hope that medical research may provide methods of control that are not currently available.

Parents are often reluctant to ask whether some other physician or the resources of some other medical center may offer more hope, or even whether the diagnosis may be in doubt. They will need help in expressing these concerns and should be encouraged and helped to seek additional medical opinions if they wish. These matters should be discussed in such a way that the family should feel no embarrassment, and they should know that they are causing none. They can be told that medical communication is generally good enough to provide prompt dissemination of any real breakthrough in the management of the otherwise fatal illness of their child. It is also reasonable to advise them that they may do the ill child and the rest of the family a disservice if they dissipate the family's emotional and other resources in a frantic search for something that is not available.

It is natural and inevitable that parents will ask themselves whether the fatal illness of their child was not somehow avoidable. Some will seek causes in inadequate medical care, in incompetent physicians, or in other environmental circumstances; others will assume a burden of guilt at their own failure to recognize the symptoms of illness or to take action quickly enough so that a cure could have been effected. Each of these reactions may be irrational. When these feelings are implicit in questions or responses of parents, the physician should make them explicit, point out the inevitability of such feelings, and, when it can be honestly done, reassure the parents that there are no grounds for their shouldering blame for a situation which no one could say might have been averted. The feeling of guilt or of punishment may be particularly strong in genetic disorders. Here it may be helpful to encourage the family to regard genetic mutations as tragic accidents, almost always beyond the ability of man to avoid.

In the management of the affected child parents should be encouraged to handle the life situation of the child as normally as possible. This may be difficult for guilt-ridden or grieving parents who may think that their usual disciplinary activities may make the child's pain or illness worse. The parents should be encouraged to maintain the child in the normal place in the family hierarchy. Special arrangements, such as the celebration of Christmas in the summertime or public dramatizations of the child's illness, should be discouraged; they may be more anxiety-provoking for the child than fulfilling of any need. As much as possible, the parents should be encouraged to participate in the care of the child in the hospital as long as their responsibilities to other children at home are adequately met. They may also need encouragement to take adequate respite from the care of the ill child.

As the physician follows the evolution of a fatal illness in a child, the manner in which the parents are coping with the situation should be observed. For example, some parents may increasingly turn their attention to other sick children in the hospital. This is a healthy sign if it is not premature; if it comes too early, it may represent the parents' unresolved burden of guilt or their pain in facing the ill child. This turning away to help other children is healthy as long as the parents still have adequate resources and strength for the needs of their own child.

At times the guilt of parents is intensified by a wish that the illness were over or by an unexpected sense of relief or release at the terminal event itself. The considerate and skillful physician will be on the watch for signs of these reactions and find the right words of reassurance or encouragement that such feelings are normal and that the parents have given everything that could have been expected of them in a situation that they have found very trying and toward which they will forever have sensitive and tender feelings.

CARE OF THE CHILD

What to tell the child who has a fatal illness about the future will vary with the condition and circumstances. Most young children do not ask whether they are going to die.

They can often be told that they have an illness that may last for some time and has ups and downs, and that it is important for them to get adequate rest and to be active when they feel up to it. Unrealistic reassurances that they look well and are doing fine will be less helpful than the frank recognition of the child's feeling that being ill is no fun and that having it going on so long is discouraging. If the child is in a stage of illness requiring temporary hospitalization, he or she needs assurance that school and normal activity will begin again as soon as possible. Meanwhile it is supportive, when appropriate, for the child to receive attention from schoolteachers and play therapists in the hospital, who will help blunt the sense of inevitability of worsening illness.

In the case of preadolescent or adolescent children with chronic and fatal illness, the plan for care may often include sharing the diagnosis with the child and examining with parents and child together the implications of diagnosis and prognosis, answering their questions, and laying out with them a program of action and support that will have as its goal keeping the patient as comfortable as possible and forestalling any conclusion to the effort as long as possible. In this atmosphere of frankness, trust, and cooperation, free of secrets or evasions, many families and patients will find an unexpectedly healthy climate for the expression of tenderness and love toward each other, and the physician may find his or her own work easier. As a chronic illness becomes terminal, this climate makes it easier to meet the needs of the patient for a sense of not being abandoned, for assurances of the continuing love and affection of those around, and for reasonably prompt responses to needs for care. The decision as to when or how the diagnosis of a potentially fatal illness is to be shared with the child must have the full understanding, consent, and cooperation of parents, and the parents will need to have given some thought to how the news of the child's illness is to be handled with siblings, relatives, and neighbors.

OTHER RESOURCES

In dealing with the problems of patient and family around a fatal illness, the physician will often call upon other professional persons for help. The family minister or other spiritual advisor can be of immense comfort. When family problems can be ameliorated by use of community resources, the help of a social worker may be important. When the family is not intact, owing to the death or previous separation of a parent, the likelihood of emotional difficulties complicating the management of the illness is sufficiently great that social service resources should probably be involved from the time the diagnosis is known.

The fatal chronic illnesses of children tend to cluster around certain diseases, such as leukemia or other malignancy, cystic fibrosis, and metabolic or degenerative disorders (such as Tay-Sachs disease). When groups of families who share a common problem can be brought together to discuss aspects of the care of their children under the guidance of a knowledgeable and skillful professional person (physician, social worker, or nurse), they can often help one another in the management of the illness as well as in coping with the feelings that go with the inevitability of ultimate loss.

TERMINAL CARE

In the management of terminal illness physicians should not leave decisions about what is to be done for the child to parents but should give positive advice as to what they plan to do. The physician should be responsive, however, to the suggestions of parents when these represent helpful and realistic appraisals of their children's needs.

When death is imminent, the patient should be kept comfortable and the parents, as much as possible, should be close at hand. The physician should be available both to parents and to the patient. The physician's control of his or her own feelings is important; if the physician's personal distress is allowed to increase the distance from or decrease involvement with the patient, the anger of the child or parents with what may be perceived as abandonment of them may make terminal care much more difficult. The continued interest and concern of the physician are important in preventing the emotional situation from deteriorating at this time.

As the moment of death approaches, the child should be in a room where he or she can be alone with parents or loved ones at the bedside or nearby. The sensitive physician will see that the occasion is accorded appropriate dignity and not rendered more frustrating or agonizing by efforts to prolong vital functions in a climate of fruitless hyperactivity.

When death has occurred, the patient, bed, and room should be made neat, and the paraphernalia of illness removed. If the parents are not at hand, they should be asked to come to the hospital and be informed of the circumstances. Parents should be given the opportunity to be with the child a little while in the relatively peaceful and uncluttered setting that has been created. A brief and tender parting may help the parents in the adjustments they must ultimately make.

After an infant or child has died, the opportunity for groups of parents with similar experiences to share them may be as important and as supportive as before the death of the child, as long as professional guidance is adequate. Members of such groups can help each other with the process of mourning and can foster the reassurance that comes with sharing such common and otherwise frightening experiences as the guilt felt at the sense of relief that the illness is over or the fear of losing touch with reality that comes with having set a place at the table for the dead child or with finding oneself listening for his or her footstep or voice. Regardless of whether such parent programs exist, physicians should plan for a number of visits with the parents in the weeks after a child's death in order to review such matters with them, to answer their continuing questions, and to assess their status.

DEATH OF THE NEWBORN INFANT

Acute fatal illnesses have a major cluster in the neonatal period, and neonatal nurseries and intensive care units must be responsive to the needs of parents who have had no preparation for a catastrophic loss. Mother and infant are usually apart at the moment of death. The body of the newborn infant can often be taken to the mother or to both parents at her bedside or at some other point in the hospital where the chance to hold and examine the baby may be the mother's only opportunity to establish for herself the reality of the birth and death of her infant and to adjust toward

reality her current or future fantasies as to what the baby might *really* have been like or what might *really* have happened. For the mother of the malformed infant this may be even more important than for the mother of the otherwise intact infant. The defects can be examined by her in reality rather than in fantasy and their implications gently discussed, with the observation perhaps that the baby was in every other way perfectly formed. Mothers whose infants have died are in critical need of help in mourning; they should be as involved as they may wish or as circumstances permit in decisions occasioned by the death, including such ceremonial leave-taking as funerals or memorial services.

Neonatal intensive care units find it helpful to maintain small discussion groups for mothers who have lost infants, within which they can share their experiences with others during the first few weeks of mourning. The quality of professional guidance of such groups is crucial to their success.

Physicians should make sure that parents understand that the mourning process for a dead infant or older child ought to be reasonably complete and a stable state reached before they decide to have another child. This generally requires 9 mo to a year or more. A new infant conceived too soon is likely to be too closely identified with the dead child and to be surrounded by inordinate anxiety or inappropriate expectations.

POST MORTEM EXAMINATION

A request for post mortem examination should be made by the responsible physician who knows the family best, often not the house officer but the attending or referring physician. The need for post mortem examination should be urged as strongly as conviction permits. Parents can be assured that such examinations are always helpful, that information is gathered and saved which may be useful in years to come in solving similar problems of other children or in providing definitive answers to questions of other children in the family or of their relatives or descendants concerning the patient's illness. Later the physician should describe the important and relevant findings of the gross post mortem examination for the parents in simple terms, and they should have a chance to discuss them as freely as they desire.

Bluebond-Langner M: The Private Worlds of Dying Children. Princeton NJ, Princeton University Press, 1978.
Davidson GW: Death of the wished-for child: A case study. Death Educ 1:265, 1977.
Howell DA: A child dies. J Pediatr Surg 1:2, 1966.
Kübler-Ross E: On Death and Dying. New York, Macmillan, 1969. (Available also in paperback.)
Schulman JL, Kupst MJ: The Child with Cancer: Clinical Approaches to Psychosocial Care—Research in Psychosocial Aspects. Springfield, IL, Charles C Thomas, 1980.

2.72 ETHICAL DECISIONS IN PEDIATRICS

Among the more difficult decisions faced by the physician caring for children and their families are those which involve a variety of ethical or moral judgments with respect to which the community has no uniformity of feeling or of standards. Among these are informed consent for surgery or other procedures or for the enlistment of a child in an experimental procedure; decisions regarding organ transplantation; genetic counseling; amniocentesis; abortion or other interruption of pregnancy; euthanasia; judgments about the quality of life; and determination of the point at which the potential has been passed for vital processes to be restored and the patient who still has a beating heart is effectively dead.

The increasing attention given these decisions reflects increased public and professional concern that they be made only after adequate study of the issues involved and that they meet certain standards of objectivity and accountability.

Among the factors that may influence or ultimately determine the responses of physicians to such problems are such considerations as the educational level, culture, and religion of the involved families; the larger social issues of eugenics, overpopulation, or other interests of the community; and, in many instances, legal constraints. In some cases the rights of parents and the rights of their children may appear to be in conflict. There is a growing feeling in the United States that the child deserves his or her own advocacy before the law. The rights of adolescents to receive medical care without the consent or knowledge of their parents have been recognized in a number of states through legislation aimed particularly at helping the adolescent in difficulties with sexual problems or with drug abuse.

Physicians faced with difficult decisions involving moral or ethical judgment will generally assume positions they regard as appropriate and rational, sometimes with the support of notions borrowed from the physiologic or psychologic disciplines of medicine. But they must accept that their own logical, scientific, and intellectual positions or attitudes may not at all be so construed by others. The investment of emotions in some issues may be great, with intense feelings of fear, guilt, anger, and anxiety.

In dealing with these matters, an overriding principle ought to be that the issues must be examined in the context of the value system of the *patient* and of the *patient's family*, not only that of the physician. The goal is to help the family find the acceptable solution to their problem with which they can live most comfortably. With an assessment of the needs and resources of patients and their families, the physician serves as a catalyst through which the most satisfying or least damaging solutions of difficult problems may be found.

Some decisions, such as those which may have as their result the shortening or the termination of life or the prolongation of a life of limited potential, are of such nature that to require parents to choose between alternatives is to lay upon them a devastating burden. Sometimes, decisions of such difficulty must be made by the physician on behalf of the family, but he or she must be as sure as circumstances permit that the decision is one the family can accept in terms of *their* system of values, not his or her own. When all the issues have been examined and when the physician has formed a reasonable judgment as to what decision will be most growth-promoting or least destructive, then the physician should move toward this decision in discussions with the family, subject to re-examination at any point. The aim will be to arrive jointly with the family at the best or least bad plan, which may sometimes be appropriately regarded as the lesser of two tragedies.

Bioethical decision-making is no longer the exclusive domain of the physician, the patient, and the patient's family. A growing public concern with ethical issues in health care has led to the formation of ethics committees in many hospitals, the role of which is to assist in bioethical decision-making. Such committees are multidisciplinary, with representation not only from the health professions but also from law, the clergy, the public, and the field of ethics itself. The roles of such committees may include consultation, policy formation, education, multidisciplinary discussion, resource allocation, formulating institutional commitments, and providing emotional support for patients and their families.

The question is still unresolved as to whether ethics committees are to be regarded primarily as advisory or as final arbiters when ethical questions arise. Committees are ordinarily likely to be consultative and advisory, their concern being that due process (adequate presentation and consideration of all points of view, with acceptable resolution of questions) has been followed in arriving at decisions regarding patients around whose care ethical issues appear to have developed. On the other hand, committees may alternate between these roles; when questions that cannot be easily resolved through decisions arrived at jointly by physician, patient, and family are brought before them, the committees function as appeals boards.

The other possible roles for ethics committees besides consultation have not been widely or fully developed. Institutional policies may be set with regard to some ethical issues, with impact upon the definition of the institutional commitment and upon allocation of resources. The educational role of such committees may be to see that the nature of ethical issues be brought before the staff, and that they attend or participate in discussions, not necessarily to decide about a particular patient but as a consciousness-raising exercise for the institution as a whole.

Thomasma has pointed out that ethical disagreements involve the clash of cherished values, and that one role of the ethics committee may be to offer a forum in which, when irreconcilable differences of opinion arise, these differences can be accepted on both sides as deeply held convictions, and to foster a climate of mutual forgiveness when parties cannot agree.

When decisions have been made that it can be anticipated will cause periods of continuing grief or requestioning, the physicians who have participated in these decisions must be available to the concerned families and ready to satisfy their continuing needs for information, understanding, and support.

If a physician becomes involved in moral or ethical issues concerning which the family cannot accept his or her judgment, then it should be made clear to the family that they should feel free to seek advice from another consultant.

It is tempting to provide guidelines and examples of how specific problems ought to be handled. But there are often no specific guidelines, and each occasion must be evaluated on its own merits. The skills most useful to the physician will be in the psychotherapeutic realm and will involve skillful listening, gentle and sensitive probing, and compassionate help in decision-making.

VICTOR C. VAUGHAN, III

American Academy of Pediatrics: Guidelines for infant bioethics committees. Bioethics Reporter 3:940, 1984.
Reiser SJ, Dyck AJ, Curran WJ (eds): Ethics in Medicine: Historical Perspectives and Contemporary Concerns. Cambridge, MA, MIT Press, 1977.
Summing Up: The Ethical and Legal Problems in Medicine and Biomedical and Behavioral Research. Report of President's Commission for the Study of Ethical Problems in Medicine and Biomedical and Behavioral Research. Washington, DC, U.S. Government Printing Office, 1983.
Thomasma, DG. Hospital Ethics Committees and Hospital Policy. QRB 11:204, 1985.

3

NUTRITION AND NUTRITIONAL DISORDERS

NUTRITIONAL REQUIREMENTS

Individual nutritional requirements vary with genetic and metabolic differences. For infants and children, however, the basic goals are satisfactory growth and the avoidance of deficiency states. Good nutrition helps to prevent acute and chronic illness and to develop physical and mental potential; it should also provide reserves for stress.

The Food and Nutrition Board (NAS–NRC, 1980) has identified appropriate dietary allowances for a number of substances that prevent deficiency states in most persons (Table 3–1). Because some essential substances remain unidentifiable, a varied diet may be the only prudent way of providing them after early infancy. Only human milk appears to supply all essentials for a prolonged time. While some essential foods should be included in the daily diet, others are stored by the body and may be supplied periodically.

Although any diet producing good nutrition varies considerably, mild excesses of nutrients or calories may be as undesirable as mild deficiencies. Since dietary influence on aspects of the aging process, for example, atherosclerosis and longevity, remains incompletely understood, avoiding excessive caloric intake appears to be wise at all ages.

3.1 WATER

Water is essential for existence; lack of it results in death in a matter of days. The water content of infants is relatively higher (70–75% of the body weight) than that of adults (60–65%). Assuming that water constitutes 70% of the body weight, 7% is blood plasma, 18% is interstitial fluid, and 45% is intracellular fluid. Although fluids provide the principal source of water, some is obtained from the oxidation of foods (mixed diets yield about 12 g H_2O/100 kcal) and body tissues.

Human needs for water are related to caloric consumption, to insensible loss, and to the specific gravity of the urine. The infant must consume much larger amounts of water per unit of body weight than the adult, but when calculated per unit of caloric intake, the amounts required are nearly identical (Tables 3–2 and 3–3). The daily consumption of fluid by the healthy infant is equivalent to 10–15% of body weight, compared to 2–4% in the adult. The usual food of infants and children is high in water content; most of the solid food in the child's diet contains 60–70% water, and many of the fruits and vegetables contain 90%.

Water is absorbed throughout the intestinal tract. The quantity of water in the interstitial compartment is readily changed to maintain homeostatic balance between the intracellular and vascular compartments. The interchange of water among these compartments depends on their respective protein and electrolyte concentrations. Depending upon the rate of growth, about 0.5–3% of the fluid intake will be retained. Retention of water is in the range of 9–13 mL/24 hr for the "male reference infant" in the first year of life.

Water balance depends on variables such as fluid intake, protein and mineral content of diet, solute load presented for renal excretion, metabolic and respiratory rates, and body temperature. Water requirements for low birthweight infants are estimated at 85–170 mL/kg/24 hr. Fecal losses are small (3–10% of intake). Evaporation from lungs and skin accounts for 40–50% of intake (sometimes more) and renal excretion for 40–50% or more. The kidney preserves the fluid and electrolyte equilibrium of the body by varying the osmolar content and volume of urine. Urine usually has a greater osmotic pressure (300–1000 mosm/L) than the internal environment (293 mosm/L); maximum normal urinary concentration is approximately 600–700 mosm/L.

3.2 CALORIES

The unit of heat in metabolism is the large calorie or kilocalorie (1 Cal = 1 kcal); it is used to refer to the energy content of food. A kilocalorie is defined as the amount of heat necessary to raise the temperature of 1 kg of water from 14.5° to 15.5° C. The production of heat varies in the oxidation of different foods, so that measuring the amount of oxygen consumed or measuring the end products of oxidation, carbon dioxide, and water approximates the values obtained by direct calorimetry.

Energy needs of children at different ages and under various conditions (Fig. 3–1) vary greatly. The approximate average expenditures of energy by the child 6–12 yr of age are basal metabolism, 50%; growth, 12%; physical activity, 25%; and fecal loss, about 8%, mainly as unabsorbed fat.

Basal metabolism is measured at room temperature (20° C) 10–14 hr after a meal, with the patient physically and emotionally quiet. For each centigrade degree of fever, basal metabolism increases approximately 10%. The basal requirement in infants is about 55 kcal/kg/24 hr; it decreases to 25–30 kcal/kg/24 hr at maturity. The term *specific dynamic action* (SDA) refers to the increase in metabolism over the basal rate by the ingestion and assimilation of food. Protein digestion may increase metabolism as much as 30% above the basal level, except when it is being deposited in tissues, whereas fat and carbohydrate, which have a "sparing" effect on the specific dynamic action of protein and upon each other, cause increases of only 4 and 6%, respectively. In infants, about 7–8% of the total caloric intake goes to specific dynamic action, whereas in older children on an ordinary mixed diet it is unlikely to constitute more than about 5% of total intake. The estimated energy necessary to build body tissue (*growth*) is the difference between the calories ingested and those expended for other purposes. The average requirement for *physical activity* is 15–25 kcal/kg/24 hr, with peak utilizations as high as 50–80 kcal/kg/24 hr for short periods of time. The amount of energy-producing food lost in the stools, except when absorption is impaired, is not more than 10% of the intake.

Although caloric requirements can best be predicted from the surface area rather than from age or weight, the final

Table 3–1. Food and Nutrition Board, National Academy of Sciences—National Research Council Recommended Daily Dietary Allowances,* Revised 1980

Designed for the maintenance of good nutrition of practically all healthy people in the U.S.A.

	Age (Years)	Weight (kg)	Weight (lb)	Height (cm)	Height (in)	Protein (g)	Fat-Soluble Vitamins — Vitamin A (RE)†	Fat-Soluble Vitamins — Vitamin D (µg)‡	Fat-Soluble Vitamins — Vitamin E (α-TE)§	Water-Soluble Vitamins — Vitamin C (mg)	Thiamine (mg)	Riboflavin (mg)	Niacin (mg NE)¶	Vitamin B_6 (mg)	Folacin** (µg)	Vitamin B_{12} (µg)	Minerals — Calcium (mg)	Phosphorus (mg)	Magnesium (mg)	Iron (mg)	Zinc (mg)	Iodine (µg)	Energy Needs (kcal)
Infants	0.0–0.5	6	13	60	24	kg × 2.2	420	10	3	35	0.3	0.4	6	0.3	30	0.5††	360	240	50	10	3	40	kg × 115
	0.5–1.0	9	20	71	28	kg × 2.0	400	10	4	35	0.5	0.6	8	0.6	45	1.5	540	360	70	15	5	50	kg × 105
Children	1–3	13	29	90	35	23	400	10	5	45	0.7	0.8	9	0.9	100	2.0	800	800	150	15	10	70	1300
	4–6	20	44	112	44	30	500	10	6	45	0.9	1.0	11	1.3	200	2.5	800	800	200	10	10	90	1700
	7–10	28	62	132	52	34	700	10	7	45	1.2	1.4	16	1.6	300	3.0	800	800	250	10	10	120	2400
Males	11–14	45	99	157	62	45	1000	10	8	50	1.4	1.6	18	1.8	400	3.0	1200	1200	350	18	15	150	2700
	15–18	66	145	176	69	56	1000	10	10	60	1.4	1.7	18	2.0	400	3.0	1200	1200	400	18	15	150	2800
	19–22	70	154	177	70	56	1000	7.5	10	60	1.5	1.7	19	2.2	400	3.0	800	800	350	10	15	150	2900
	23–50	70	154	178	70	56	1000	5	10	60	1.4	1.6	18	2.2	400	3.0	800	800	350	10	15	150	2700
	51+	70	154	178	70	56	1000	5	10	60	1.2	1.4	16	2.2	400	3.0	800	800	350	10	15	150	2400
Females	11–14	46	101	157	62	46	800	10	8	50	1.1	1.3	15	1.8	400	3.0	1200	1200	300	18	15	150	2200
	15–18	55	120	163	64	46	800	10	8	60	1.1	1.3	14	2.0	400	3.0	1200	1200	300	18	15	150	2100
	19–22	55	120	163	64	44	800	7.5	8	60	1.1	1.3	14	2.0	400	3.0	800	800	300	18	15	150	2100
	23–50	55	120	163	64	44	800	5	8	60	1.0	1.2	13	2.0	400	3.0	800	800	300	18	15	150	2000
	51+	55	120	163	64	44	800	5	8	60	1.0	1.2	13	2.0	400	3.0	800	800	300	10	15	150	1800
Pregnant						+30	+200	+5	+2	+20	+0.4	+0.3	+2	+0.6	+400	+1.0	+400	+400	+150	‡‡	+5	+25	+300
Lactating						+20	+400	+5	+3	+40	+0.5	+0.5	+5	+0.5	+100	+1.0	+400	+400	+150	‡‡	+10	+50	+500

*The allowances are intended to provide for individual variations among most normal persons as they live in the United States under usual environmental stresses. Diets should be based on a variety of common foods in order to provide other nutrients for which human requirements have been less well defined.

†Retinol equivalents. 1 retinol equivalent = 1 µg retinol or 6 µg β carotene = 3.3 IU vitamin A.

‡As cholecalciferol. 10 µg cholecalciferol = 400 IU of vitamin D.

§α-tocopherol equivalents. 1 mg d-α tocopherol = 1 α-TE.

¶1 NE (niacin equivalent) is equal to 1 mg of niacin or 60 mg of dietary tryptophan.

**The folacin allowances refer to dietary sources as determined by Lactobacillus casei assay after treatment with enzymes (conjugases) to make polyglutamyl forms of the vitamin available to the test organism.

††The recommended dietary allowance for vitamin B_{12} in infants is based on average concentration of the vitamin in human milk. The allowances after weaning are based on energy intake (as recommended by the American Academy of Pediatrics) and consideration of other factors, such as intestinal absorption; see text.

‡‡The increased requirement during pregnancy cannot be met by the iron content of habitual American diets or by the existing iron stores of many women; therefore the use of 30–60 mg of supplemental iron is recommended. Iron needs during lactation are not substantially different from those of nonpregnant women, but continued supplementation of the mother for 2–3 months after parturition is advisable in order to replenish stores depleted by pregnancy.

Table 3–2. **Water Requirements**

Urine Specific Gravity	Infant—3 kg 300 Calories* Intake			Adult—70 kg 3000 Calories* Intake		
	Water Intake			Water Intake		
	mL	g/100 kcal	g/ kg	mL	g/100 kcal	g/ kg
1.005	650	217	220	6300	210	90
1.015	339	113	116	3180	106	45
1.020	300	100	100	2790	93	40
1.030	264	88	91	2430	81	35

*In this sense Calorie = large calorie = 1 kcal = 1 Cal (see text).

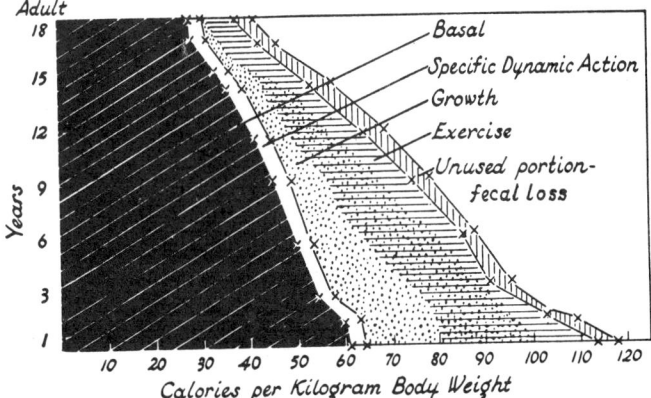

Figure 3–1. Total daily expenditure of calories with approximate distribution among individual factors in relation to age and weight (Calorie = large calorie = 1 kcal = 1 Cal).

criteria for evaluating the child's needs depend upon the growth pattern, the sense of well-being, and satiety. The daily requirement is approximately 80–120 kcal/kg for the first year of life, with subsequent decreases of about 10 kcal/kg for each succeeding 3 yr period. Periods of rapid growth and development near puberty require increased caloric consumption. The distribution of calories in human milk, in most formulas, and in a well balanced diet is similar. Approximately 9–15% of the calories are derived from protein, 45–55% from carbohydrate, and 35–45% from fat.

Each gram of ingested protein or carbohydrate provides 4 kcal. One gram of short-chain fatty acids provides 5.3 kcal; medium-chain, 8.3 kcal; and long-chain, 9 kcal. A continued caloric intake greater or less than the body expenditure will increase or decrease body fat. In general, a consistent caloric imbalance of 500 kcal/24 hr changes body weight by about 450 g (1 pound)/wk.

3.3 PROTEINS

Protein constitutes about 20% of adult body weight. Its amino acids are essential nutrients in forming cell protoplasm. The kind, number, and arrangement of amino acids in a protein molecule determine its characteristics. Twenty-four amino acids have been identified; nine were found to be essential for infants (threonine, valine, leucine, isoleucine, lysine, tryptophan, phenylalanine, methionine, and histidine). Arginine, cystine, and, perhaps, taurine are essential for low birthweight infants. Nonessential amino acids can be

Table 3–3. **Range of Average Water Requirements of Children at Different Ages Under Ordinary Conditions**

Age	Average Body Weight in kg	Total Water in 24 Hours, mL	Water per kg Body wt in 24 Hours, mL
3 days	3.0	250–300	80–100
10 days	3.2	400–500	125–150
3 mo	5.4	750–850	140–160
6 mo	7.3	950–1100	130–155
9 mo	8.6	1100–1250	125–145
1 yr	9.5	1150–1300	120–135
2 yr	11.8	1350–1500	115–125
4 yr	16.2	1600–1800	100–110
6 yr	20.0	1800–2000	90–100
10 yr	28.7	2000–2500	70–85
14 yr	45.0	2200–2700	50–60
18 yr	54.0	2200–2700	40–50

synthesized and need not be supplied in the diet. New tissue cannot be formed without all of the essential amino acids simultaneously present in the diet; the absence or deficiency of only one essential amino acid results in a negative nitrogen balance.

Proteins are broken down in the digestive process to oligopeptides and α-amino acids. The hydrochloric acid of the stomach provides the optimal pH for peptide cleavage by pepsin. Rennin changes casein of milk to paracasein, which pepsin hydrolyzes along with other proteins. The various proteases show preference for splitting specific peptide linkages; some cleave linkages in the interior of the peptide chain, and others act at more terminal junctures. In the alkaline medium of the intestine, trypsin, chymotrypsin, and carboxypeptidase from the pancreas hydrolyze these proteins and peptones to peptides and to some amino acids; other peptidases from the intestinal juices carry digestion to the amino acid stage.

Minute amounts of certain proteins may be absorbed unchanged, as evidenced by immunologic reactions, but the hydrolytic products, the amino acids and some peptides, are normally absorbed through the intestinal mucosa. Large oligopeptides may be absorbed in the first few months of life or after episodes of gastroenteritis. The amino acids are carried to the liver by the portal circulation and from there are distributed to other tissues. Amino acids are reconstituted to functional human proteins, e.g., albumin, hemoglobin, hormones. Excess amino acids undergo deamination, and the nitrogenous portions are converted to urea in the liver and excreted by the kidneys. The carbon from amino acids is oxidized much like that of carbohydrate or fat; some amino acids are glycogenic, others ketogenic. Proteins cannot be effectively stored. In protein depletion states, proteins from muscle may be broken down to supply amino acids for more essential sites such as brain and enzymes.

Aberrations in the metabolism of protein and the amino acids constitute a significant portion of the disease entities known as inborn errors of metabolism (Chapter 7).

Protein requirements at various ages are listed in Table 3–1. "Biologic value" of proteins indicates effectiveness of utilization; proteins of high biologic value have the quantity and distribution of essential amino acids appropriate for resynthesis of body tissues and provide little waste, as determined by nitrogen balance studies (Table 3–4). Abundant protein is available for children in the United States, but the supply in many countries is so limited that it is the greatest need of children throughout the world.

Table 3–4. Functions, Effects of Deficiency and Excess, Requirements, and Sources of Water, Proteins, Carbohydrates, and Fats

Foodstuffs	Functions	Effects of Deficiency	Effects of Excess	Requirements	Sources
Water	Structure of cells; solvent for cellular changes; medium for ions; transport of nutrients and waste products; regulation of body temperature	Thirst, dryness of tongue, dehydration, anhydremia, high sp. gr. of urine, loss of kidney function (acidosis, oliguria, uremia, death)	Abdominal discomfort, headache, cramps (water without salt), intoxication, convulsions, edema, and circulatory failure	See Tables 3–2 and 3–3 Related to calories consumed; greater in hot weather	Water as such All foods
Proteins	Supply amino acids for growth and repair of tissue cells; sols for osmotic equilibrium; ions in acid-base balance. With prosthetic groups to form hemoglobin, nucleoproteins, glycoprotein, and lipoproteins. Enzymes, hormones, cellular respiratory substance, antibodies. Protective structures (nails and hair). Source of energy	Lassitude, abdominal enlargement, edema; depletion of plasma proteins, negative nitrogen balance (no clinical syndrome due to lack of specific amino acid); kwashiorkor (protein malnutrition); marasmus (protein-calorie malnutrition)	Prolonged high protein intake probably not harmful. Important in certain anomalies involving amino acid and protein metabolism	See Table 3–1	Milk, eggs, meat, fish, poultry, cheese, soybeans, peas, beans, cereals, nuts, lentils
Carbo-hydrates	Readily available source of energy, antiketogenic, structure of cells, antibodies, source of stored calories (glycogen and fat), conversion to fat, resynthesis of amino acids, roughage	Ketosis if intake is less than 15% of calories or in starvation; underweight if total calories are low	Overweight if total calories are high. Various syndromes due to inborn errors of sugar metabolism	To supply 25–55% of calories	Milk, cereals, fruits, sucrose, syrups, starches, vegetables
Fats	Concentrated source of energy; physical protection for vessels, nerves, organs; insulation against changes in temperature; structure of body tissues, cell membranes, and nuclei; vehicle for absorption of vitamins (A, D, E, and K); appetite appeal; aids satiety (delays emptying time of stomach); avoids necessity of ingestion of large bulk of foods; spares protein, vitamin A, and thiamine; supplies linoleic acid	Lack of satiety (craving for fat); underweight; skin changes with intakes very low in linoleic acid	Overweight; abdominal symptoms in familial hyperlipidemia; high cholesterol intakes may be harmful to selected populations	Minimal not known; usually supplies 35% of calories; probably 1–2% of calories as linoleic acid	Milk, butter, egg yolk, lard, bacon, meat, fish, cheese, nuts, vegetable oils Breast milk usually supplies 4–5% of calories as linoleic acid; vegetable oils vary greatly, safflower, corn, soy, and others being especially rich

3.4 CARBOHYDRATES

Carbohydrates, while supplying the necessary bulk of the diet, also supply most of the body's energy needs. In its absence the body uses proteins and fats for energy. Stored chiefly as glycogen in the liver and muscles, carbohydrates probably constitute no more than 1% of the body weight. Since the size of the infant's liver is 10% of the adult's and the muscle mass 2%, the infant's glycogen reserve is a fraction (about 3.5%) of the adult's.

Carbohydrates are oxidized as glucose (dextrose) but are consumed in various forms: the monosaccharides (glucose, fructose, galactose), the disaccharides (lactose, sucrose, maltose, isomaltose), and the polysaccharides (starches, dextrins, glycogen, gums, cellulose). Pentoses are poorly absorbed.

Through a series of enzymatic and chemical reactions in the digestive tract, complex carbohydrates are split into simpler structures. Salivary and pancreatic amylases are principally involved in the breakdown of starch to oligosaccharides (dextrins) and disaccharides (primarily maltose). Intestinal amylase may be decreased during the first 4 mo of life. The

disaccharides are absorbed intact into the intestinal brush border cells, where the various disaccharidases in the membrane fraction of the microvilli complete the hydrolysis to the monosaccharides: 1 molecule of maltose to 2 of glucose; sucrose to glucose and fructose; lactose to glucose and galactose. The monosaccharides are rapidly absorbed; glucose and galactose are actively taken up against concentration gradients, whereas fructose absorption is passive. During absorption, phosphoric acid "carrier" radicals combine with hexose sugars in the intestinal mucosa for transport across the cell membrane. Sodium must be present for absorption to continue when the intraintestinal sugar concentration is low. These hexose-phosphates separate again into their component parts, permitting the sugar to diffuse into the portal blood stream.

Some glucose may be oxidized directly, as in the brain and heart. Most of the absorbed sugar is converted to glycogen in the liver, though glycogenesis also occurs in other tissues. Up to 15% of the weight of the liver and 3% of the muscle may be glycogen; small amounts are also found in practically all other organs. Glycogenolysis in the liver yields glucose as the chief product, whereas glycogen breakdown in the muscle yields lactic acid. The overall oxidation of glucose has two phases, the anaerobic (glycolysis) and the aerobic (tricarboxylic acid cycle). In the former, glucose is broken down to pyruvic acid; in the aerobic cycle pyruvic acid is completely oxidized to carbon dioxide and water. Insulin and the pituitary and adrenal hormones are involved in these processes, and nicotinic acid, thiamine, riboflavin, and pantothenic acid take part in the enzymatic reactions. Carbohydrate that is not oxidized or stored as glycogen is converted to fat.

The principal carbohydrate metabolic disorders are diabetes mellitus, glycogen storage disease, galactosemia, fructose intolerance, and glucose intolerance; deficiencies of sugar-splitting enzymes in the intestines (lactase, sucrase, maltase) are associated with diarrhea and malabsorption resulting from the osmotic effect of the unabsorbed sugar and from fermentation of the carbohydrate by intestinal bacteria.

3.5 FATS

Fats or their metabolic products form an integral part of cellular membranes and are efficient stores of energy. They impart palatability to food and serve as vehicles for fat-soluble vitamins A, D, E, and K. Approximately 98% of natural fats are triglycerides, 3 fatty acids combined with glycerol. The remaining 2% include free fatty acids, monoglycerides, diglycerides, cholesterol, and phospholipids (including lecithin, cephalin, sphingomyelin, and cerebrosides).

Naturally occurring fats contain straight-chain fatty acids, both saturated and unsaturated, varying in length from 4 to 24 carbon atoms. The degree of absorption generally varies with the melting point, the degree of unsaturation, and the positions of the fatty acids on the glycerol molecule.

Ingested triglycerides are partially hydrolyzed by lingual lipase and emulsified in the stomach. In the duodenum pancreatic lipase hydrolyzes the triglycerides to monoglycerides and fatty acids; intraluminal solubility is greatly enhanced by the presence of bile salts. The remaining unsplit diglycerides and triglycerides are insoluble even in the presence of bile salts. Low birthweight infants have decreased amounts of bile and decreased absorption of fat.

Long-chain fatty acids and monoglycerides (those with more than 10 carbon atoms) are presumably absorbed into the mucosal cell by diffusion. Transport across the cell involves re-esterification of these fatty acids and monoglycerides to triglycerides, which are then "coated" with lipoprotein to form the chylomicron, in which the fat is transported in the lymph system to the venous circulation via the thoracic duct. Transport proteins include very low density (VLDL), low density (LDL), and high density (HDL) lipoproteins synthesized in the liver.

Short- and medium-chain triglycerides are handled differently; they are readily hydrolyzed by pancreatic lipase to free fatty acids which are transported through the cell. Even when intraluminal hydrolysis is inadequate because of deficiency of pancreatic lipase or of bile salts, these fats will be absorbed and hydrolyzed to free fatty acids within the cell by mucosal lipase. With neither esterification to triglycerides nor subsequent chylomicron formation, these free fatty acids directly enter the intestinal veins and pass to the liver via the portal system. This alternate pathway for short- and medium-chain triglycerides is utilized in nutritional formulations for children with severe absorptive problems.

Linoleic and Arachidonic Acids. Humans do not synthesize linoleic acid, an 18-carbon atom chain with 2 double bonds (dienoic acid); hence, it must be supplied in the diet. Linolenic (3 double bonds) and arachidonic (4 double bonds) acids also may be essential to infants. Unsaturated fatty acids are nec-essary for growth, skin and hair integrity, regulation of cholesterol metabolism, lipotropic activity, synthesis of the prostaglandins, decreased platelet adhesiveness, and reproduction. Diets containing less than 1–2% of the calories as linoleic acid require greater caloric consumption for comparable growth. In children with essential fatty acid deficiency, serum levels of trienoic acid increase relative to tetraenoic acids. Excess linoleic acids increase peroxidation and may cause membrane destruction. Rapidly growing young infants maintained on diets very low in linoleic acid develop intertrigo and dryness, thickening, and desquamation of the skin.

The relation of dietary fat intake to intimal fat streaking in the major arterial vessels in early life and atheromatous changes in adults remains to be clarified (Sec. 7.39–7.47).

3.6 MINERALS

The physiologic roles and dietary sources of the principal minerals with nutritional significance are summarized in Table 3–5. Requirements are shown in Table 3–1, except for several of the trace elements.

The ash content of the fetus is about 3% of the body weight at birth. It increases continuously throughout childhood, both absolutely and relatively. Adult ash content is 4.35% of body weight; 83% is in the skeleton and 10% in the muscle. For each gram of protein retained, 0.3 g of mineral matter is deposited. The principal cations are calcium, magnesium, potassium, and sodium; the comparable anions are phosphorus, sulfur, and chloride. Iron, iodine, and cobalt appear in important organic complexes. The trace elements fluorine, copper, zinc, chromium, and manganese have known metabolic roles; selenium, silicon, boron, nickel, aluminum, arsenic, bromine, molybdenum, and strontium are present in the diet and in the body.

3.7 VITAMINS

The word "vitamin" refers to organic compounds required in minute amounts to catalyze cellular metabolism essential for growth or maintenance of the organism. Vitamin requirements for infants and children are listed in Table 3–1. For vitamin functions and disorders, see Table 3–6 and Sec. 3.21–3.33.

MISCELLANEOUS FACTORS

Roughage. The quantity of indigestible vegetable fiber in acceptable diets may be as much as 170–300 mg/kg/24 hr. Most children who receive well balanced diets obtain sufficient amounts of roughage. Highly refined foods contain little fiber and may be associated with increased incidence of constipation, appendicitis, diverticulitis, and other intestinal disorders. High fiber intake may result in decreased absorption of zinc and other essential nutrients.

Digestibility. The relative amount of a given nutrient available for assimilation is high in most of the common food classes: carbohydrate, 97%; fat, 95%; protein, 92%. Cooking is a factor in digestibility. For example, the boiling of milk reduces the size of the curd and renders it more digestible; on the other hand, heating destroys activity of vitamin C.

Satiety. The ingestion of a meal should provide a sense of well-being. Whole milk, cream, eggs, and fatty foods have high satiety values; sugar increases the flow of gastric juice and delays emptying of the stomach, thus increasing satiety. Bread and potatoes have relatively low satiety values, as do lean meat, fish, vegetables, and many fruits.

Table 3–5. **Physiology and Sources of Nutritionally Important Minerals**

Mineral	Function and Metabolism	Effects of Deficiency	Effects of Excess	Sources
Calcium	Structure of bone and teeth, muscle contraction, nerve irritability, coagulation of blood, cardiac action, production of milk Absorbed from upper small intestine: aided by vitamin D, ascorbic acid, lactose, acid reaction; hindered by excesses of dietary oxalic acid, phytic acid, fat, fiber, phosphate. Deposited in bone trabeculae and maintained in dynamic equilibrium with body tissues through action of parathyroid hormone and thyrocalcitonin About 70% excreted in feces, 10% in urine; 15–25% retained, depending on growth rate. Serum level 9–11 mg/dL, 60% ionized	Poor mineralization of bones and teeth; osteomalacia; osteoporosis; tetany; rickets; impairment of growth	Unknown (dietary) Heart block and renal stones (parenteral)	Milk, cheese, green leafy vegetables, canned salmon, clams, oysters
Chloride	Osmotic pressure; acid-base balance; HCl in gastric juice Readily absorbed; about 92% of intake is excreted, mainly in the urine, some in feces and sweat; comprises about 2/3 of the blood plasma anions; blood serum level, 99–106 mEq/L; in intracellular and extracellular fluids; parallels sodium intake and output	Hypochloremic alkalosis may occur with prolonged vomiting or excessive sweating, with parenteral administration of glucose without saline, with excessive ACTH therapy, and with congenital alkalosis	Unknown	Table salt, meat, milk, eggs
Chromium	Glycemia regulation and insulin metabolism	Diabetes in animals	None known	Yeast
Cobalt	Component of vitamin B_{12} (cobalamin) molecule and of erythropoietin Not utilized for synthesis of cobalamin by man; readily absorbed and excreted	None known ?Hypothyroidism	Cardiomyopathy; medicinally it may be goitrogenic or may produce cardiomyopathy	Widely distributed
Copper	Essential for production of red blood cells; catalyst in hemoglobin formation; absorption of iron. Associated with activities of tyrosinase, catalase, uricase, cytochrome C oxidase, delta-aminolevulinic acid dehydrase, lysyl oxidase. Absorbed with sulfur-rich proteins: transported in plasma bound to plasma proteins and in ceruloplasmin; present in erythrocytes in a labile form and the more stable hemocuprein; highest concentration in liver and central nervous system (cerebrocuprein); excreted mainly via the intestinal wall and bile; deranged metabolism in Wilson disease (hepatolenticular degeneration), and Menkes syndrome.	May be cause of refractory anemia, osteoporosis, neutropenia, depigmentation and ataxia Increased serum cholesterol.	?Cirrhosis	Liver, oysters, meats, fish, whole grains, nuts, legumes
Fluorine	Tooth and bone structure Retained when intake is above 0.6 mg/day; excreted in urine and sweat; deposited in bones as fluorapatite (dynamic equilibrium)	Tendency to dental caries	Fluorosis: mottling of teeth with intake of more than 4–8 mg/24 hr	Water, sea foods, plant and animal foods (dependent upon content in soil and water)
Iodine	Constituent of thyroxine (T_4) and triiodothyronine (T_3) Readily absorbed from intestine; circulates as inorganic and organic iodide; selectively concentrated about 25:1 in the thyroid gland, quickly iodized and incorporated into a complex known as thyroglobulin; proteolytic enzymes release thyroxine and triiodothyronine into the blood. Excretion mainly in urine. Antithyroid compounds interfere with iodine metabolism: goitrins and brassicae; certain drugs	Simple goiter, endemic cretinism	Not harmful (less than 1 mg/24 hr); medicinally may cause goiter	Iodized salt, sea food, food grown in nongoitrous areas

Table continued on opposite page

Table 3–5. **Physiology and Sources of Nutritionally Important Minerals** *Continued*

Mineral	Function and Metabolism	Effects of Deficiency	Effects of Excess	Sources
Iron	Structure of hemoglobin and myoglobin for O_2 and CO_2 transport; oxidative enzymes: cytochrome C and catalase Absorbed in ferrous form according to body need, aided by gastric juice and ascorbic acid; hindered by fiber, phytic acid, steatorrhea Transported in plasma in ferric state bound to transferrin (a beta globulin); stored in liver, spleen, bone marrow, and kidney as ferritin and hemosiderin; carefully conserved and reused; minimal losses in urine and sweat; about 90% of intake excreted in the stool	Anemia: hypochromic, microcytic	Hemosiderosis in Bantu people of Africa due to low phosphorus and high iron contents of diet Poisoning by medicinal iron	Liver, meat, egg yolk, green vegetables, whole grains, legumes, nuts
Magnesium	Structure of bones and teeth; activation of enzymes in carbohydrate metabolism; muscle and nerve irritability. Important intracellular cation, essential to metabolic processes Principal cation of soft tissue; absorption from small intestine varies with intake; some urinary excretion, but excellent renal conservation; antagonist to calcium action	Occurs in malabsorption and deficiency states; may be expressed clinically as tetany; associated frequently with hypocalcemia, hypokalemia	None (dietary); toxicity from intravenous medication	Cereals, legumes, nuts, meat, milk
Manganese	Enzyme activation, especially superoxide dismutase; normal bone structure, carbohydrate metabolism Poor absorption from intestine; transported in plasma; particularly high turnover rate in mitochondria; excretion mainly via the intestine in bile; competes with iron	Not known	None (dietary); toxicity from chronic inhalation (encephalopathy)	Legumes, nuts, whole grain cereals, green leafy vegetables
Molybdenum	Component of enzymes: xanthine oxidase for conversion to uric acid and mobilization of ferritin iron in liver, liver aldehyde oxidase Readily absorbed from intestine; excreted chiefly in urine, some in bile	Not observed in man	Not established	Legumes, grains, dark green leafy vegetables, animal organs
Phosphorus	Constituent of bones and teeth; structure of nucleus and cytoplasm of all cells; acid-base balance; key position in energy transformations and transmission of nerve impulses; metabolism of carbohydrate, protein, and fat About 70% of intake absorbed as free phosphates from intestine; vitamin D and parathormone implicated in intestinal absorption and kidney retention; excreted in urine and feces; occurs in blood as phospholipids, organic esters, and inorganic phosphates; inorganic phosphates in blood serum of infants and children, 4–7 mg/dL; ratio of inorganic to organic phosphates in whole blood is about 1:20	Rickets may develop in rapidly growing, very low birthweight babies with low intakes of both P and Ca; muscle weakness	Possibility of tetany during recovery from rickets or in newborn on formula with low Ca:P (1:1) ratio	Milk, milk products, egg yolk, fresh foods, legumes, nuts, whole grains
Potassium	Muscle contraction; nerve impulse conduction; intracellular osmotic pressure and fluid balance; heart rhythm Primarily intracellular; absorption via intestine; excretion 80% in urine—some in sweat and feces; about 8% retained by growing child; blood serum level 4.0–5.6 mEq/L	In starvation or in such pathologic conditions as diarrhea, diabetic acidosis, ACTH excess: muscle weakness, anorexia, nausea, abdominal distention, nervous irritability, drowsiness, confusion, tachycardia; deficiency exaggerates effects of sodium	Heart block at serum levels of 10 mEq/L; important in Addison disease, renal failure, or administration of K-containing salts	All foods
Selenium	Cofactor for glutathione peroxidase in tissue respiration	Muscle diseases in animals. Kashan cardiomyopathy, ?arthritis	Toxicity observed in animals	Vegetables, meats

Table continued on following page

Table 3–5. **Physiology and Sources of Nutritionally Important Minerals** Continued

Mineral	Function and Metabolism	Effects of Deficiency	Effects of Excess	Sources
Sodium	Osmostic pressure; acid-base balance; water balance; muscle and nerve irritability Readily absorbed from intestine; excreted chiefly in urine (98%); parallels chloride intake; renal excretion controlled by adrenal cortical hormone; extracellular cation, but small amount in muscle and cartilage; blood serum level, 135–145 mEq/L	Nausea; diarrhea, muscle cramps, dehydration	Edema if inadequate excretion or excessive parenteral fluids	Table salt, flesh foods, milk, eggs, sodium compounds as baking soda and powder, glutamate, seasonings, and preservatives
Sulfur	Constituent of all cellular protein; cocarboxylase; melanin; mucopolysaccharides of mucous secretions, vitreous humor, synovial fluid, connective tissues, cartilage, heparin; insulin; metabolism of nerve tissue; detoxification mechanisms; tissue metabolism as SH group in coenzyme A, cystathionine, and glutathione Only sources utilized are cystine and methionine; inorganic forms unavailable to body; excreted as inorganic sulfate or ethereal sulfate via urine and bile	Not known; growth failure from protein deficiency may be due in part to deficiency of S-containing amino acids	Not harmful; excreted in urine as sulfates	Protein foods contain about 1%
Zinc	Constituent of several enzymes: carbonic anhydrase (in erythrocytes) essential for CO_2 exchange; carboxypeptidase of intestine for hydrolysis of protein; dehydrogenase of liver Found in liver and organs, muscles, bones, red and white cells; higher tissue concentration in young subjects; excreted chiefly from intestine, competes with copper	Dwarfism, iron deficiency anemia, hepatosplenomegaly, hyperpigmentation and hypogonadism, acrodermatitis enteropathica, depression of immunocompetence, poor wound healing	Gastrointestinal upsets (from galvanized iron cooking utensils); copper deficiency; decreased high density lipoprotein	Meat, grain, nuts, cheese

Table 3–6. **Physical and Metabolic Properties and Food Sources of the Vitamins**

Name and Synonyms	Characteristics	Biochemical Action	Effects of Deficiency	Effects of Excess	Sources
Vitamin A: Retinol (vitamin A_1) is an alcohol of high molecular weight *Provitamin A:* The plant pigments, alpha-, beta-, and gamma-carotenes and cryptoxanthin	Fat-soluble; heat-stable; destroyed by oxidation, drying; bile necessary for absorption; stored in liver; protected by vitamin E	Component of retinal pigments, rhodopsin and iodopsin, for vision in dim light; bone and tooth development; formation and maturation of epithelia	Nyctalopia, photophobia, xerophthalmia, conjunctivitis, keratomalacia leading to blindness; faulty epiphyseal bone formation; defective tooth enamel; keratinization of mucous membranes and skin; retarded growth	Excessive carotene intake may produce carotenemia with xanthosis cutis. Individual variation in sensitivity includes anorexia, slow growth, drying and cracking of skin, enlargement of liver and spleen, swelling and pain of long bones, bone fragility, increased intracranial pressure	Liver, fish-liver oils, whole milk, milk fat products, egg yolk, fortified margarines. Carotenoids from plants—green vegetables, yellow fruits and vegetables
Vitamin B Complex: *Thiamine:* Vitamin B_1; antiberiberi vitamin; aneurin	Water- and alcohol-soluble; fat-insoluble; stable in slightly acid solution; labile to heat, alkali, sulfites	Component of thiamine pyrophosphate carboxylases, which act in various oxidative decarboxylations, including that of pyruvic acid	Beriberi—fatigue, irritability, anorexia, constipation, headache, insomnia, tachycardia, polyneuritis, cardiac failure, edema; elevated pyruvic acid in the blood	None from oral intake	Liver, meat, especially pork, milk, whole grain or enriched cereals, wheat germ, legumes, nuts
Riboflavin: Vitamin B_2	Sparingly soluble in water; sensitive to light and alkali; stable to heat, oxidation, acid	Constituent of flavoprotein enzymes important in hydrogen transfer reactions: amino acid, fatty acid, and carbohydrate metabolism and cellular respiration. Retinal pigment for light adaptation	Ariboflavinosis; photophobia, blurred vision, burning and itching of eyes, corneal vascularization, poor growth	Not harmful	Milk, cheese, liver and other organs, meat, eggs, fish, green leafy vegetables, whole or enriched grains

Table continued on opposite page

Table 3–6. **Physical and Metabolic Properties and Food Sources of the Vitamins** *Continued*

Name and Synonyms	Characteristics	Biochemical Action	Effects of Deficiency	Effects of Excess	Sources
Niacin: Nicotinamide; nicotinic acid; antipellagra vitamin	Water- and alcohol-soluble; stable to acid, alkali, light, heat, oxidation	Constituent of coenzymes I and II, cofactors in a number of dehydrogenase systems	Pellagra: multiple B-vitamin deficiency syndrome	Nicotinic acid (not the amide) is vasodilator; skin flushing and itching, may induce hepatopathy	Meat, fish, poultry, liver, whole grain and enriched cereals, green vegetables, peanuts
Folacin: Group of related compounds containing pteridine ring, para-amino benzoic acid, and glutamic acid. Pteroylglutamic acid (PGA)	Slightly soluble in water; labile to heat, light, acid	Concerned with formation and metabolism of one-carbon units; participates in synthesis of purines, pyrimidines, nucleoproteins, and methyl groups	Megaloblastic anemia (infancy, pregnancy); usually is secondary to malabsorption disease	Unknown	Liver, green vegetables, nuts, cereals, cheese
Vitamin B_6: 3 active forms: pyridoxine, pyridoxal, pyridoxamine	Water-soluble; destroyed by ultraviolet light and by heat	Constituent of coenzymes for decarboxylation, transamination, transsulfuration; fatty acid metabolism	Irritability, convulsions, hypochromic anemia; peripheral neuritis in patients receiving isoniazid	Sensory neuropathy	Meat, liver, kidney, whole grains, peanuts, soybeans
Cobalamin: Vitamin B_{12}	Slightly soluble in water; stable to heat in neutral solution; labile in acid or alkaline ones; destroyed by light. Castle intrinsic factor of the stomach required for absorption	Transfer of one-carbon units in purine and labile-methyl group metabolism; essential for maturation of red blood cells in bone marrow; metabolism of nervous tissue	Juvenile pernicious anemia, due to defect in absorption rather than to dietary lack; also secondary to gastrectomy, celiac disease, inflammatory lesions of small bowel, long term drug therapy (PAS, neomycin)	Unknown	Muscle and organ meats, fish, eggs, milk, cheese
Biotin	Crystallized from yeast; soluble in water	Coenzyme of acetyl coenzyme A carboxylase; involved in CO_2 transfer	Dermatitis, seborrhea; inactivated by avidin in raw egg white	None known	Yeast, animal products; synthesized in intestine
Vitamin C: Ascorbic acid: Vitamin C; antiscorbutic vitamin	Water-soluble; easily oxidized, accelerated by heat, light, alkali, oxidative enzymes, traces of copper or iron	Integrity and maintenance of intercellular material in all tissues; facilitates absorption of iron and conversion of folic acid to folinic acid; metabolism of tyrosine and phenylalanine; contributes to activity of succinic dehydrogenase and serum phosphatase in infants, not in adults	Scurvy and poor wound healing	Oxaluria	Citrus fruits, tomatoes, berries, cantaloupe, cabbage, green vegetables. Cooking has destructive effect
Vitamin D: Group of sterols having similar physiologic activity. D_2-calciferol is activated ergosterol. D_3 is activated 7-dehydrocholesterol	Fat-soluble; stable to heat, acid, alkali, and oxidation; bile necessary for absorption	Regulates absorption and deposition of calcium and phosphorus, presumably by affecting permeability of intestinal membrane; regulates level of serum alkaline phosphatase, which is believed to be concerned with calcium phosphate deposition in bones and teeth	Rickets (high serum phosphatase level appears before bone deformities); infantile tetany, poor growth, osteomalacia	Wide variation in tolerance; in general over 500 μg/24 hr toxic when continued for weeks; prolonged administration of 45 μg/24 hr may be toxic (see Sec. 3.31); manifestations are nausea, diarrhea, weight loss, polyuria, nocturia, calcification of soft tissues, including heart, renal tubules, blood vessels, bronchi, stomach	Vitamin D–fortified milk and margarine, fish-liver oils, exposure to sunlight or other ultraviolet sources

Table continued on following page

Table 3–6. **Physical and Metabolic Properties and Food Sources of the Vitamins** *Continued*

Name and Synonyms	Characteristics	Biochemical Action	Effects of Deficiency	Effects of Excess	Sources
Vitamin E: Group of related chemical compounds—tocopherols—with similar biologic activities	Fat-soluble; unstable to ultraviolet light, alkali; readily oxidized by oxygen, iron, rancid fats. Antioxidant; bile necessary for absorption	Minimizes oxidation of carotene, vitamin A, and linoleic acid in the intestine	Requirements related to polyunsaturated fat intake; red blood cell hemolysis in premature infants; loss of neural integrity	Unknown	Germ oils of various seeds, green leafy vegetables, nuts, legumes
Vitamin K: Group of naphthoquinones with similar biologic activities; K_1 is phytoquinone	Natural compounds are fat-soluble; water-soluble products have been developed (menadione); Stable to heat and reducing agents; labile to oxidizing agents, strong acids, alkali, light; bile salts necessary for intestinal absorption of fat-soluble forms	Prothrombin formation, coagulation factors II, VII, IX, X and osteocalcin are K-dependent	Hemorrhagic manifestations; bone metabolism	Not established; medicinally may produce hyperbilirubinemia in premature infants	Green leafy vegetables, pork liver. Widely distributed

Availability. Poverty, ignorance, and lack of practical education in buying and preparing food are the main causes of malnutrition in children. Diets of lower-income families are often deficient in milk, fruits, fresh vegetables, and meats. A suggested method for planning low cost meals is to divide the money available for food into fifths: one fifth each for vegetables and fruits; for milk and cheese; for meats, fish, and eggs; for bread and cereals; and for fats, sugar, and other food adjuncts.

Geographic location may influence the availability of foods, especially among low socioeconomic populations. An effect of geographic factors on deficiency diseases is evidenced by the relation of dental caries to lack of fluoride in communal water supplies.

Bacterial Synthesis of Vitamins. Certain vitamins are synthesized in the human gastrointestinal tract; however, the extent to which they can meet the body's needs is uncertain. Once the bacterial flora of the intestinal tract has been established, vitamin K is produced and is available to the body. Pantothenic acid and biotin, essential to human metabolism, can be supplied by bacterial synthesis alone. Thiamine, riboflavin, niacin, vitamin B_6, vitamin B_{12}, and folic acid are synthesized in some species, but synthesis is limited or does not exist in humans. The kind of food or the nature of intestinal flora may affect vitamin production or availability. For instance, 3% of the population in Kobe, Japan, harbored intestinal bacteria that split thiamine; evidence of beriberi appeared in these persons.

Antimicrobial Factors. Administration of antimicrobial agents may affect nutritional status. Appetite is sometimes impaired or bacterial flora producing vitamin K are sufficiently altered to precipitate borderline deficiency. Several antibiotics are known to produce steatorrhea. Neomycin may produce malabsorption. Orally administered broad-spectrum antibiotics decrease nitrogen balance. Isoniazid combines with pyridoxal phosphate and may produce symptoms of vitamin B_6 deficiency. Antimicrobial compounds may be transmitted in breast milk or in foods from animals fed these compounds.

Endocrine Factors. Antithyroid substances that increase the requirement for iodine (goitrogens) have been found in turnips, rutabagas, cabbage, soybeans, cobalt-containing foods, food additives, and medications. Administering ACTH or corticosteroids necessitates an increase in protein and calcium and a decrease in sodium intake. Transient hypoparathyroid-

ism with tetany has been observed in the neonatal period after excessive intake of vitamin D or of phosphates.

Radioactivity. Apparently, little danger results from carbon-14 because of its low activity. Iodine-131 is removed from milk by aeration or storage. Cesium-137, which may be found in meat and milk products, can be counteracted by a high potassium intake or by acetazolamide. Only 10% of strontium-90 ingested by the cow is found in cow's milk.

Emotional Factors. Along with increased knowledge of the significance of various nutrients, excessive parental and professional concern has developed over the food the individual infant or child eats. The mother, developing a sense of fear or guilt about her child's eating habits, may create a battle of wits between her and her child which may have far-reaching effects. The physician must know the nutritional fundamentals in order to recognize and manage emotional behavioral problems arising from undesirable food habits or eating problems.

3.8 EVALUATION OF DIET

The pediatrician should know the basic properties of various foods in order to take and evaluate a dietary history, to know which laboratory tests are valuable for diagnosis, and to interpret therapeutic responses. (See Tables 3–7 and 29–9 and 29–10 of the Appendix.)

The recall interview for determining children's food habits is usually satisfactory, but for a more accurate accounting the mother should observe and record the actual food intake in terms of the standard measuring cup or tablespoon, weight, or size of pieces, which can then be converted to "servings" appropriate to the child's age (Table 3–7). It is important to include items that may not be consumed daily.

The dietary guide according to food groups provides flexibility for cultural, religious, and personal preferences and seasonal, regional, and economic availability. A food intake record can indicate possible nutritional imbalances. An excessive intake of foods of one group may result in a high caloric level producing an overweight child while at the same time leading to a dangerously low intake of some essential nutrients, e.g., the overconsumption of milk and the underconsumption of meat and eggs, the resultant danger of which is iron deficiency anemia. When key foods, such as milk, eggs,

Table 3–7. Recommended Food Intake for Good Nutrition According to Food Groups and the Average Size of Servings at Different Age Levels

Food Group	Servings per Day	Average Size of Servings					
		1 year	2–3 years	4–5 years	6–9 years	10–12 years	13–15 years
Milk and cheese (1.5 oz cheese = 1 C* milk)	4	½ C*	½–¾ C	½–¾ C	½–1 C	½–1 C	½–1 C
Meat group (protein foods) Egg	3 or more	1	1	1	1	1	1 or more
Lean meat, fish, poultry (liver once a week)		2 Tbsp†	2 Tbsp	4 Tbsp	2–3 oz (4–6 Tbsp)	3–4 oz	4 oz or more
Peanut butter			1 Tbsp	2 Tbsp	2–3 Tbsp	3 Tbsp	3 Tbsp
Fruits and vegetables Vitamin C source (citrus fruits, berries, tomato, cabbage, cantaloupe)	At least 4, including: 1 or more (twice as much tomato as citrus)	⅓ C (citrus)	½ C	½ C	1 medium orange	1 medium orange	1 medium orange
Vitamin A source (green or yellow fruits and vegetables)	1 or more	2 Tbsp	3 Tbsp	4 Tbsp (¼ C)	¼ C	⅓ C	½ C
Other vegetables (potato and legumes, etc.) *or*	2	2 Tbsp	3 Tbsp	4 Tbsp (¼ C)	⅓ C	½ C	¾ C
Other fruits (apple, banana, etc.)		¼ C	⅓ C	½ C	1 medium	1 medium	1 medium
Cereals (whole-grain or enriched) Bread	At least 4	½ slice	1 slice	1½ slices	1–2 slices	2 slices	2 slices
Ready-to-eat cereals		½ oz	¾ oz	1 oz	1 oz	1 oz	1 oz
Cooked cereal (including macaroni, spaghetti, rice, etc.)		¼ C	⅓ C	½ C	½ C	¾ C	1 C or more
Fats and carbohydrates Butter, margarine, mayonnaise, oils: 1 Tbsp = 100 Calories (kcal)	To meet caloric needs	1 Tbsp	1 Tbsp	1 Tbsp	2 Tbsp	2 Tbsp	2–4 Tbsp
Desserts and sweets: 100-Calorie portions as follows: ⅓ C pudding or ice cream, 2 3″ cookies, 1 oz cake, 1⅓ oz pie, 2 tbsp jelly, jam, honey, sugar		1 portion	1½ portions	1½ portions	3 portions	3 portions	3–6 portions

*C = 1 cup or 8 oz or 240 mL.
†Tbsp = Tablespoon (1 Tbsp = ca. 15 mL = ca. ½ oz).
Modified with Mildred J. Bennett, Ph.D., from "Four Food Groups of the Daily Food Guide," Institute of Home Economics, U.S.D.A., and Publication #30, Children's Bureau of the United States Department of Health, Education, and Welfare.

and citrus fruits, are eliminated for personal or medical reasons, the deficiencies may be compensated for by judicious substitutions. Following is a list of the principal food groups' nutrients:

Milk: high quality protein, calcium, and phosphorus; riboflavin; vitamin A; vitamin D (if fortified)
Meat and eggs: high quality protein, iron, B vitamins; vitamin A from liver and eggs
Fruits and vegetables: vitamin C; provitamin A from green and yellow ones; trace elements; fiber

Cereals: less expensive and supplementary amounts of protein, minerals, fiber, B vitamins

Suspected dietary insufficiencies may be corroborated by appropriate laboratory tests and clinical evaluation. When malnutrition, either as dietary deficiency or excess, or failure to thrive exists in spite of an apparently satisfactory food intake, the infant or child's family relationships must be evaluated, not only for organic causes but especially for psychosocial ones (Sec. 2.60).
(References follow next section.)

3.9 FEEDING OF INFANTS

Successful infant feeding requires cooperation between the mother and her baby, beginning with the initial feeding experience and continuing throughout the child's period of dependency. Promptly establishing comfortable, satisfying feeding practices contributes greatly to the infant's and mother's emotional well-being (Sec 8.5–8.6). Feeding time should be pleasurable for both mother and child. Since maternal feelings are readily transmitted to the baby and largely determine the emotional setting in which feeding takes place, tense, anxious, irritable, easily upset, or emotionally labile mothers are more likely to experience a difficult feeding relationship, but they frequently become more comfortable and confident with appropriate guidance and support from an empathetic and experienced relative, friend, or physician.

As soon after birth as an infant can safely tolerate enteral nutrition, as judged by normal activity, alertness, suck, and cry, feedings should be initiated to maintain normal metabolism and growth during the transition from fetal to extrauterine life, to promote maternal-infant bonding and to decrease the risks of hypoglycemia, hyperkalemia, hyperbilirubinemia, and azotemia. Mistakes are made by feeding the infant too much or too little. Inadequate fluid intake, particularly in hot weather, may result in "dehydration fever." Most infants may start feeding by 6 hr of life. When any question about the tolerance of feeding arises because of physical or neurologic status, feeding should be withheld and parenteral fluids substituted. The schedule of initial feeding in a hospital is less important than the principle of the unhurried beginning and patient assistance and support for the mother. Mothers wishing to initiate breast feeding in the delivery room and continue on a demand basis thereafter should be supported. However, since the hospital must maintain a general feeding schedule when rooming-in is unavailable or not desired and demand feeding is impractical, the infant can be taken to the mother for the first feeding at 10 A.M. or 6 P.M., whichever is nearer the end of a 6 hr postpartum rest. Subsequent formula or breast feedings are given every 3–4 hr/day and night by the mother, except for the first night, when the 2 A.M. feeding is given by the nursing staff. Artificially fed infants should receive sterile water for the first feeding, since regurgitation and aspiration of this liquid are less likely to cause significant irritation of the respiratory tract.

The feeding of infants requires practical interpretation of specific nutritional needs and of the widely varying limits of the normal baby's appetite and behavior regarding food. The time it takes the infant's stomach to empty may vary from 1 to 4 hr or more; thus, considerable difference in the infant's desire for food is expected at different times of the day. Ideally, the feeding schedule should be based on this reasonable "self-regulation." Variation in the time between feedings and in the amount taken per feeding is to be expected in the first few weeks during the establishment of the self-regulation plan. By the end of the first month more than 90% of infants will have established a suitable and reasonably regular schedule.

Most healthy, bottle-fed infants will want 6–9 feedings/24 hr by the end of the first week of life. Some will take enough at one feeding to satisfy themselves for approximately 4 hr; others who are smaller or whose gastric emptying time is more rapid will want milk about every 2–3 hr; breast-fed infants often prefer shorter intervals. Most term infants will rapidly increase their intake from 30 mL to 80–90 mL every 3–4 hr at 4–5 days of life. Feeding should be considered as having progressed satisfactorily if the infant is no longer losing weight by 5–7 days and is gaining weight by 12–14 days. Some infants will not awaken for a middle-of-the-night feeding after 3–6 wk of age; some may never want it. Many will not want a late evening feeding between 4 and 8 mo of age and will be satisfied with 3 meals a day by 9–12 mo.

It is important to appreciate that babies cry for other reasons besides hunger, and *they need not be fed every time they cry*; some infants are placid, some unusually active, some irritable. Sick infants are often uninterested in food. Babies who awaken and cry consistently at short intervals may not be receiving enough milk at each feeding or may have discomfort from some cause other than hunger, e.g., too much clothing; soiled, wet, or uncomfortable diapers and clothing; colic; swallowed air ("gas"); uncomfortably hot or cold environment; or illness. Some babies cry to gain sufficient or additional attention, whereas others deprived of adequate mothering become indifferent. Some infants simply need to be held. Those who stop crying when they are picked up or held do not usually need food, but those who continue to cry when held and when food is offered should be carefully evaluated for other causes of distress. The habit of offering frequent, small feedings or of holding and feeding to pacify all crying should not be cultivated.

However, the advantages in satisfying the infant's true hunger needs as they are expressed are several: physiologic requirements are met promptly; the infant does not learn to associate prolonged crying and discomfort with feeding; and the infant is less likely to develop poor eating practices such as gulping the feedings or taking small amounts too frequently. Infants soon establish a regular schedule which permits the family to resume normal function. If this does not occur, individual feedings or the whole day's schedule can be moved ahead or delayed sufficiently to avoid conflicts with necessary family activities.

Some mothers will not understand the goals of infant "self-regulation"; some will misinterpret the physician's instructions, and others may be unable to adjust themselves to the regimen of the infant. *The orderly, overanxious, and compulsive parent will do better with a more specific outline for the infant's activities.*

The postpartum period is often a time of great anxiety and insecurity for the first-time mother, who may be temporarily overwhelmed by the responsibilities of motherhood. The hospital setting and the attitude of the hospital personnel should be comforting and supporting while the mother finds and develops confidence in her maternal abilities. *Time should be set aside to consider the questions of inexperienced or uncertain mothers at the hospital or in the home.* Fathers and other household members should be included by physicians in these anticipatory guidance sessions. Knowing the personalities and expectations of both parents is invaluable in helping to avert physical and psychologic problems centered on feeding. Parental misconceptions and confusion about the dietary and satiety needs of infants and children are often the bases for abnormal parent-child relations which can be avoided by appropriate counseling.

3.10 BREAST FEEDING

Breast feeding continues to have practical and psychologic advantages that should be considered when the mother selects the method for feeding. Human milk is the most appropriate of all available milks for the human infant since it is uniquely adapted to his or her needs.

Advantages of Breast Feeding. *Breast milk is the natural food for full-term infants during the first months of life.* It is always readily available at the proper temperature and needs no time for preparation. The milk is fresh and free of contaminating bacteria, which lessens the chances of gastrointestinal disturbances. Although little if any difference exists in mortality rates in formula-fed and breast-fed infants receiving good care, among the lower socioeconomic groups and those living in unsanitary conditions, the breast-fed infant is much more likely to survive.

Allergy and intolerance to cow's milk create significant disturbances and feeding difficulties not seen in breast-fed infants. The symptoms include diarrhea, intestinal bleeding, and occult melena. "Spitting up," colic, and atopic eczema are less common in infants receiving human milk. (See also Sec. 13.81.)

Human milk contains bacterial and viral antibodies, including relatively high concentrations of secretory IgA antibodies, which prevent micro-organisms from adhering to the intestinal mucosa. Breast-fed infants of mothers with high anti-poliomyelitis titers are relatively resistant to infection by the attenuated live poliomyelitis vaccine viruses, an effect that may be pronounced in the neonatal period but does not seem to interfere with active immunization at 2, 4, and 6 mo of age. Growth of the mumps, influenza, vaccinia, and Japanese B encephalitis viruses can be inhibited by substances in human milk. These ingested antibodies from human colostrum and milk may afford local gastrointestinal immunity against organisms entering the body via this route.

Macrophages normally present in human colostrum and milk may be able to synthesize complement, lysozyme, and lactoferrin. Breast milk is also a source of lactoferrin, the iron-binding whey protein which is normally about one third saturated with iron, which has an inhibitory effect on the growth of E. coli in the intestine. The stool of the breast-fed infant has a pH lower than that of the infant fed cow's milk, and its bacterial content is predominantly of the lactobacillus group in contrast to a preponderance of the coliform group in artificially fed infants. Human milk contains a "growth factor" which facilitates intestinal colonization by Lactobacillus bifidus. The intestinal flora of infants fed human milk may protect them against infections caused by some species of E. coli. Bile salt–stimulated lipase kills Giardia lamblia and Entamoeba histolytica.

Milk from the mother whose diet is sufficient and properly balanced will supply the necessary nutrients, except, perhaps, fluoride and, after several months, Vitamin D (Sec. 3.29). Iron stores are sufficient for the first 6–9 mo in term infants. Human milk iron is well absorbed by the infant; breast-fed infants may not require supplemental iron during the first year, but their diets should be supplemented after 6 mo of age by the addition of cereal and meat or by administration of one of the ferrous iron preparations. Human milk contains sufficient vitamin C for the infant's needs, provided the mother's intake is adequate.

The psychologic advantages of breast feeding for both mother and infant are well recognized, and successful breast feeding is a satisfying experience for both. The mother is personally involved in the nurturing of her baby, gaining both a feeling of being essential and a sense of accomplishment. The infant is afforded a close and comfortable physical relationship with the mother. Breast feeding offers increased opportunity for close sensual contact between mother and infant; studies suggest that early and intimate tactile and visual contact are important in determining the quality of attachment and mothering which is provided the infant (Sec. 8.6).

The mother who is unable or does not wish to nurse her infant, however, need have no less sense of accomplishment or of affection for her baby. The quality of attachment and mothering and the degree of security and affection provided can be identical.

Contraindications to Breast Feeding. For the average, healthy, full-term infant there are no disadvantages to breast feeding, provided the mother's milk supply is ample and her diet contains sufficient amounts of protein and vitamins. Infrequently, allergens to which the infant is sensitized may be conveyed in the milk. In such instances an attempt should be made to find the specific allergen and to remove it from the mother's diet; its presence rarely is a valid reason for weaning the baby.

From the mother's standpoint there are few contraindications to breast feeding. Markedly inverted nipples may be troublesome. Fissuring or cracking of the nipples can usually be avoided if engorgement is prevented. Mastitis may be alleviated by continued and frequent nursing on the affected breast to keep it from becoming engorged, local heat applications, and antibiotics. Acute infection in the mother may

contraindicate breast feeding if the infant does not have the same infection; otherwise there is no need to stop nursing unless the condition of either necessitates it. When the infant is unaffected and the mother's condition permits, the breast may be emptied and the milk given to the infant. Septicemia, nephritis, eclampsia, profuse hemorrhage, active tuberculosis, typhoid fever, and malaria are permanent contraindications to nursing, as are chronic poor nutrition, debility, severe neuroses, and postpartum psychoses.

The resumption of menstruation should not deter continued nursing, although temporary behavior changes of mother or baby may call for reassurance. Pregnancy does not necessitate immediate cessation of nursing, but the combined demands of supplying milk to the infant and nutrients to the fetus are formidable and require special attention to maternal nutrition.

Prematurely born infants weighing 2000 g (4½ pounds) or more usually thrive on breast milk. Infants of lesser birth-weights, however, may have such rapid rates of growth that human milk alone may not supply sufficient essential nutrients for normal growth (Sec. 8.17). Low birthweight infants too weak to suck or those tiring before ingesting an adequate volume may be given human milk by gavage. Many such infants have thrived.

The low vitamin K content of human milk may contribute to hemorrhagic disease of the newborn. *Administration of 1 mg of vitamin K_1 parenterally at birth is recommended for all infants, especially for those who will be breast-fed.*

Unconjugated hyperbilirubinemia in breast-fed infants is discussed in Sec. 8.44.

Hemolytic disease of the newborn (erythroblastosis fetalis) is not a contraindication to breast feeding if the infant's general condition warrants it, since antibodies in the mother's milk are inactivated in the intestinal tract and do not contribute to further hemolysis of the infant's blood cells.

Preparation of the Prospective Mother. Most women are physically capable of breast feeding, provided they receive sufficient encouragement and are protected from discouraging experiences and comments while the secretion of breast milk is becoming established. The physician interested in aiding the prospective mother to breast feed should discuss its advantages during the midtrimester of pregnancy or whenever the mother begins planning for her baby. Many mothers ambivalent toward breast feeding will be able to nurse successfully if they are reassured and supported. If the mother rejects the suggestion that she nurse her infant, overpersuasion may be detrimental to mother-infant relationships.

Physical factors conducive to a good breast feeding experience include establishing and maintaining a state of good health, proper balance of rest and exercise, freedom from worry, early and sufficient treatment of any intercurrent disease, and adequate nutrition.

Retracted nipples usually benefit from daily manual breast pump traction during the latter weeks of pregnancy; truly inverted nipples may be helped by the use of milk cups, starting as early as the 3rd mo of pregnancy.

The mother may be confidently told that she need not gain or lose weight if her diet is adequate. She should be reassured that breast tone will be preserved by the use of a properly fitted brassiere to support the breasts, especially before delivery and during the nursing period. During the latter part of pregnancy, the mother gains weight and stores fat which is utilized in lactation. Nutritional requirements for lactation are listed in Table 3–1.

ESTABLISHING AND MAINTAINING THE MILK SUPPLY

The most satisfactory stimulus to the secretion of human milk is regular and complete emptying of the breasts; milk production is reduced when the secreted milk is not drained. Once lactation is well established, mothers are capable of producing more milk than their infants need. There are many reasons for incomplete nursing, but the principal ones are unsupportive hospital practices, weakness of the infant, and failure to initiate the natural hunger cycle. Efforts should be directed toward the early establishment of normal, vigorous nursing by letting the infant empty the breast frequently during the time when only colostrum is being formed. The infant should be allowed to nurse when hungry, whether or not there appears to be any milk.

Breast feeding should be begun as soon after delivery as the condition of the mother and of the baby permits, preferably within several hours. Infants who cannot be fed on demand should be brought to the mother for feeding about every 3 hr during the day and every 4 hr during the night. Many infants are hungry within 2 hr of a satisfying nursing episode, and about 75% of the breast's milk has been replenished by this time.

Appropriate care for tender or sore nipples should be instituted before severe pain from abrasions and cracking develops. Exposing the nipples to air; applying pure lanolin; avoiding soap, alcohol, and tincture of benzoin; frequently changing disposable nursing pads lining the brassiere cups; nursing more frequently; manually expressing milk; nursing in different positions; and keeping the breast dry between feedings are recommended. When the tenderness causes the mother apprehension the *milk ejection reflex* may be delayed, leading to frustration in the infant and to increasingly vigorous nursing, which further injures the nipple and areolar area. Occasionally, nipple shields may be of help.

The first 2 wk of the neonatal period are crucial for establishing breast feeding. Lactogenic hormones are ineffective in stimulating human breast secretion. Daily weight gains are overly emphasized, and early supplemental bottle feedings given to achieve this goal compromise attempts at breast feeding. The infant usually finds that it is easier to get milk from a bottle than from a breast and becomes satiated. The difference between breast and bottle nipples may also confuse the infant, leading to disruption of the feeding pattern and/or injury of the mother's nipples.

On the day the mother is discharged from the hospital lactation may not be well established, and the excitement of going home may impede an initially successful nursing experience there. A wise physician anticipates this experience and discusses it with the mother. In some instances, providing her with enough isocaloric formula for 1–2 complementary feedings may prevent discouragement which might prejudice further nursing.

Psychologic Factors. No factor is more important than a happy, relaxed state of mind. Worry and unhappiness are the most effective means for decreasing or abolishing breast secretions.

Mothers may worry that their babies are abnormal when they cry, are drowsy, sneeze, or regurgitate milk. Mothers are upset by any suggestion that their milk may be lacking in quantity or quality. They may be disturbed at the scanty supply of colostrum, at tenderness of the nipples, and at the fullness of the breast on the 4th or 5th day. Many mothers do not feel comfortable when trying to nurse in an open ward or with another person in the room. Mothers may worry about what is going on at home while they are in the hospital or about what is going to happen when they arrive home. An alert physician realizes these worries, particularly if the baby is a first born, and by tactful reassurance and explanation can help prevent or minimize worry, thus contributing to successful breast feeding.

Fatigue. Avoiding fatigue is important, but the mother should exercise sufficiently to promote her sense of physical well-being.

Hygiene. Once a day the breasts should be washed. If soap is drying to the nipple and areolar area, it should be discontinued. The nipple area should be kept dry. *Boric acid must not be used.* Care should be taken to prevent irritation and infection of the nipples caused by prolonged initial nursing, maceration from wetness of the nipple, or rubbing of clothing.

Some mothers may be more comfortable if they wear a properly fitted brassiere day and night. Plastic liners should be removed. An absorbent pad (commercially available) or a clean cloth or handkerchief may be placed inside the brassiere to absorb any milk that leaks out.

Diet. The diet should contain enough calories to compensate for those secreted in the milk as well as for those required to produce it. The nursing mother needs a varied diet, sufficient to maintain her weight and high in fluid, vitamins, and minerals. She should avoid weight-reducing diets. Milk is important but should not replace other essential foods. If the mother is allergic to or dislikes milk, 1 g of calcium may be added to her daily diet. The fluid intake should approximate 3 quarts daily; urinary output is a good measure of the adequacy of fluid in the daily diet.

The idea that substances such as milk, beer, oatmeal, and tea are galactogenic is mistaken. Singular foods in the mother's diet seldom disturb the breast-fed infant. Occasionally, however, eating certain berries, tomatoes, onions, members of the cabbage family, chocolate, spices, and condiments may cause gastric distress or loose stools in the infant. No food need be withheld from the mother unless it causes distress to the infant. Whenever possible, nursing mothers should not take drugs since many preparations are harmful to the neonate and many have not been evaluated (Table 8–4). Antithyroid medications, lithium, anticancer agents, isoniazid, and phenindione are contraindicated. Temporary cessation of nursing is recommended if the mother requires diagnostic radiopharmaceuticals, chloramphenicol, metronidazole, sulfonamides, or anthroquinone-derivative laxatives. Lactating women should not eat sport fish from waters contaminated with polychlorinated biphenyls (PCB's). It is better to control maternal constipation by inclusion in her diet of raw and cooked fruits and vegatables, whole wheat bread, and an adequate amount of water than by use of laxatives. Smoking cigarettes and drinking alcoholic beverages are discouraged. Substances such as arsenicals, barbiturates, bromides, iodides, lead, mercurials, salicylates, opium, atropine, most antimicrobial agents, and cascara may be transmitted through the milk and exert an effect on the infant.

TECHNIQUE OF BREAST FEEDING

The technical aspects of breast feeding require careful consideration. Breast feeding sometimes becomes impossible simply because the attending physician fails to recognize that the difficulties are in the feeding technique.

At feeding time the infant should be hungry, dry, neither too cold nor too warm, and held in a comfortable, semisitting position for his or her enjoyment and for ease of eructation without vomiting. The mother, too, must be comfortable and completely at ease. When she is able to be out of bed, a moderately low chair with armrest is preferable, and a low stool is advantageous for resting her foot and raising her knee on the nursing side. The baby is supported comfortably with the face held close to the mother's breast by one arm and hand while the other hand supports the breast so that the nipple is easily accessible to the infant's mouth and yet does not obstruct the infant's nasal breathing. The baby's lips should be expected to engage considerable areola as well as nipple.

Success in infant feeding depends greatly upon the adjustments made during the first few days of life. Difficulties often result from attempts to adapt the infant to a nursing procedure rather than designing a procedure that satisfies the infant's natural desires. Rigidly adhering to clock schedules and the "assembly line" manner in which babies are handled in many nurseries may make adjustment at home more difficult. Most problems can be avoided by conforming to the infant's spontaneous pattern. If the infant is breast fed when he or she normally cries in hunger and feeding ends when the baby's appetite is satisfied, the fundamental requirements are met.

At birth the normal infant is equipped with several reflexes, or behavior patterns, that facilitate breast feeding. These reflexes are concerned with the actual getting of food—rooting, sucking, swallowing, and satiety reflexes. The *rooting reflex* is the first to come into play. When babies smell milk they move their heads around, attempting to find its source. If their cheek is touched by a smooth object, they will turn toward that object, opening their mouths in anticipation of grasping the nipple. This suggests how milk should be given to babies: applying their cheek to the mother's breast will start them rooting with their mouths for the nipple.

The infant's rooting reflex brings the entire areolar area into the mouth; the contact of the nipple against the palate and posterior tongue elicits sucking or "milking," and the buccal fat pads help keep the nipple in place. This *sucking reflex* is a process of squeezing the sinuses of the areola rather than simply suction on the nipple. The infant's sucking results in afferent impulses to the mother's hypothalamus and then to both anterior and posterior pituitary. Prolactin from the anterior pituitary stimulates milk secretion in the cuboidal cells in the acini or alveoli of the breast. Finally, milk in the infant's mouth triggers the *swallowing reflex*. In contrast, bottle feeding requires the infant to compress the nipple to avoid choking.

Mothers should know that if the infant is not hungry, he or she will not search for the nipple or suck. Infants are usually sleepy for several days and most, initially, are not avid suckers. On the 3rd day, when there has been some weight loss, mothers become anxious about infants who seem uninterested in nursing. It reassures them to learn that most healthy babies "wake up" and become good nursers on the 4th day. Infants whose mothers received obstetric sedation during labor suck at lower rates and pressures and consume less milk than comparable infants of mothers given no sedation.

Some infants will empty a breast in 5 min; others nurse more leisurely for 20 min. Most of the milk is obtained early in the feeding: 50% in the first 2 min and 80–90% in the first 4 min. The baby should be permitted to suck until satisfied unless the mother has sore nipples. If the baby does not "unlatch" from the breast, a finger inserted into the corner of the baby's mouth decreases suction and facilitates removal. The baby should not be pulled from the breast. Waking a sleepy baby to nurse by slapping feet, pinching, or shaking is usually unsuccessful.

At the end of the nursing period the infant should be held erect over the mother's shoulder or on her lap with or without gently rubbing or patting the back to assist in expelling swallowed air; often this "burping" procedure is necessary one or more times during the feeding as well as 5–10 min after the infant has been put into the crib. It is an essential procedure during the early months but should not be overdone. When nursing is completed, the infant should be placed in the crib on the abdomen or on the right side to facilitate emptying of the stomach into the intestines and to lessen the chances of regurgitation or aspiration.

One or Both Breasts Per Feeding. The infant should empty at least one breast at each feeding; otherwise it will not be stimulated to refill. Both breasts should be used at each feeding in the early weeks to encourage maximal production of milk. After the milk supply has been established, the breasts may be alternated at successive feedings, and the

baby will usually be satisfied with the amount obtained from one. If the secretion of milk becomes too great, both breasts may again be offered at each feeding and incompletely emptied with the intent of securing a partial decrease in lactation.

Determining Adequacy of Milk Supply. If the infant is satisfied after each nursing period, sleeps 2–4 hr, and gains weight adequately, the milk supply is probably sufficient. Infants who are "light sleepers" require a lot of body contact with the mother during the first months. Mothers of these wakeful and alert infants should not be thought to have a poor milk supply. However, if the infant nurses avidly and completely empties both breasts but appears unsatisfied afterwards, does not go to sleep, or sleeps fitfully and awakens after 1–2 hr, and fails to gain weight satisfactorily, the milk supply is probably inadequate. The program of La Leche League,* which establishes close relationships between successful nursing mothers and mothers needing assistance, is often helpful in such circumstances.

The "let-down" or *milk-ejection reflex* in the mother is an important sign of successful nursing. Sucking or psychologic stimuli associated with nursing lead to secretion of oxytocin by the posterior pituitary. As a result, the myoepithelial cells surrounding the alveoli deep in the breast contract, squeezing milk into the larger ducts, where it is more easily available to the sucking infant. When this reflex functions well, milk flows from the opposite breast as the baby begins to nurse. This reflex is frequently absent or erratic during periods of pain, fatigue, or emotional distress, and its malfunction is thought to be responsible for milk retention in women unsuccessful in breast feeding.

In general, a mother's weighing her baby before and after nursing is neither necessary nor desirable in judging milk supply adequacy. The amount of milk an infant takes at a time is usually unimportant (the amount ingested at each feeding ranges from one to several oz throughout a 24 hr period), and the results obtained are readily misinterpreted. Small gains may worry the mother, and in turn may diminish her milk supply. She may give the baby a bottle to assure herself that the infant is getting enough to eat. The better result with the "test bottle" may be so discouraging that subsequent breast feeding becomes impossible, even when she has an adequate supply of milk. Before assuming that the mother produces insufficient milk, three possibilities should be excluded: (1) errors in feeding technique responsible for the infant's inadequate progress; (2) remediable maternal factors related to diet, rest, or emotional distresss; or (3) physical disturbances in the infant that interfere with eating or with gain in weight. Infrequently infants who seem to be nursing well may not thrive because of insufficiency of milk; increased frequency of feeding may be indicated. Nursing more than every 2 hr may inhibit prolactin secretion of the anterior pituitary, decreasing production; this is usually corrected by delaying feedings to 2½ hr intervals. Other aids include stimulation of prolactin secretion by administering small doses of chlorpromazine for a few days or by devices such as the Lact-aid which supplement the infant's intake.

Manual Expression of Breast Milk. This is achieved by two movements. First, the whole breast is compressed between the hands, starting at the base and continuing toward the areola. Firm pressure maintained throughout the movement, which is repeated several times, impels milk to the lacteal sinuses. The second movement empties the sinuses: the breast is supported with one hand while the tissue just behind the areola is repeatedly compressed between the thumb and first

*La Leche League International, 9616 Minneapolis Avenue, Franklin Park, Illinois 60131, has many local affiliates composed of successfully nursing mothers willing to assist other mothers desiring to nurse.

finger of the other hand. The force is directed backward toward the center of the breast rather than toward the nipple. The fingers remain in this initial position, and the skin over the breast tissue is never rubbed. The procedure should not be painful, even if the nipples are sore and cracked.

Mechanical Expression of Breast Milk. Hand pumps are often ineffectual and may increase the irritation and pain in congested breast and nipple tissues. Many mothers prefer electric breast pumps.

Supplementary Feedings. An occasional replacement feeding, after the first 6 wk when nursing has been adequately established, permits the mother greater freedom in her activities. For the normal, healthy infant who is getting insufficient breast milk, artificial feeding may be offered either immediately after or in place of one or more breast feedings. An attempt should first be made to increase the supply of breast milk. Any of the milk formulas described in Sec. 3.11 may be offered to the infant in sufficiently satisfying amounts. If formula is to be given after the infant has completed a breast feeding, the warmed bottle should be handy so it can be offered immediately after the infant has been burped. The holes in the nipples should not be so large that the infant gets this portion of food without any effort, or the infant will quickly abandon any efforts to suck adequately at the mother's breast.

Weaning. Most infants gradually reduce the volume of and frequency of their demand for breast feedings at 6–12 mo of age, and they become accustomed to increasing amounts of solid foods and of liquids by bottle and cup. As they demand less breast milk, the mother's supply will gradually diminish, causing the mother no discomfort from engorgement. Weaning should be initiated by substituting whole cow's milk by bottle or cup for part of a breast feeding, and subsequently for all of a breast feeding. Over several days, one of the breast feedings is replaced and then subsequently another, and so on, until the infant is weaned completely. Occasionally, the baby takes the cup as readily as the bottle, avoiding the intermediate transfer from bottle to cup. These changes should be made gradually for they should provide a pleasant experience, not a conflict, for mother and infant. Praise, loving attention, and cuddling are vital to successful weaning.

When cessation of nursing is necessary at an earlier age because of maternal illness or prolonged illness or death of the infant, a tight breast binder may be used and ice bags applied for a day or so to decrease milk production. Restriction of the mother's fluid intake is also helpful. Hormones, such as small doses of estrogen for 1–2 days, also may help decrease milk production at the termination of nursing.

3.11 FORMULA FEEDING

Whole cow's milk or its modified form is the basis for most formulas, although other milks and milk substitutes are available for infants who cannot tolerate it. Sterilization and refrigeration of the formula greatly reduces morbidity and mortality from gastrointestinal infections. Milk processing (ranging from simple home boiling to commercial pasteurization, homogenization, and evaporation) alters the casein so that small and readily digestible curds form in the stomach, eliminating the principal cause for indigestibility of cow's milk protein.

Though breast feeding is considered superior to formula feeding for normal infants, many infants receive formula from birth. Changing social and cultural patterns have increased formula feeding. Because they are employed outside the home, many mothers are reluctant to nurse their infants. Others fear that nursing will limit their activities. Some refuse to nurse because they fear failure at nursing. Others regard weight gain and loss of breast tone as unattractive, and some

consider breast feeding as socially unacceptable. Whatever the reasons, the present popularity of artificial feeding could not have been reached without prior improvements in the safety and quality of the substitute milks.

Objective nutritional studies of growing infants (rate of growth in weight and length, normality of various constituents in blood, performance in metabolic studies, body composition, etc.) show relatively small differences between infants fed human milk and those fed cow's milk. Although such techniques may not record small but important variations, these investigations attest to the normal infant's ability to thrive by making satisfactory physiologic adjustments to wide ranges of ingested protein, fat, carbohydrate, and minerals.

Conventional formulas of whole and evaporated cow's milk provide approximately 3–4 g of protein/kg/24 hr ("high protein" intake largely exceeding the basic need), whereas breast milk and many commercially prepared feedings simulating the composition of breast milk supply 1.5–2.5 g/kg/24 hr ("low protein" intake supplying a smaller degree of excess).

Fomon has calculated the rate of increase in total body protein mass in the "male reference" term infant to average approximately 3.5 g/24 hr in the first 4 mo of life. Assuming 0.5 g/24 hr nitrogen loss from the skin, total protein need is estimated to be about 4.0 g/24 hr during the first 4 mo and slightly less during the remainder of the first year.

Commercial formulas are modified from a cow's milk base, and their protein and ash levels are reduced nearer to those of human milk, thus decreasing osmolality and renal excretory load. The saturated fat of cow's milk is replaced with some unsaturated vegetable fatty acids, and vitamins are added. The concentration of lactose is lower in cow's milk than in human milk. Some formulas include higher lactoproteins and lower casein as in breast milk. Low birthweight infants in particular may benefit from the increased cystine of lactoproteins. Until more information is available, breast feeding for all infants appears prudent, but if this is impossible, then a formula as compositionally close to breast milk as possible is desirable.

TECHNIQUE OF ARTIFICIAL FEEDING

The setting should be similar to that for breast feeding, with the mother and infant in a comfortable position, unhurried, and free from distractions. The infant should be hungry, fully awake, warm, and dry and be held as though being breast fed. The bottle should be held so that milk, not air, channels through the nipple. Bottle propping, even with a "safe" holder, should be avoided, since it not only deprives the infant of the physical contact, comfort, and security of being held but may also be dangerous to small infants, who may aspirate if unattended. Otitis media is more common in babies fed with the propped bottle.

The bottle of milk is customarily warmed to body temperature, though no harmful effects have been demonstrated from feedings at room temperature or cooler. The temperature may be tested by dropping milk onto the wrist. The nipple holes should be of the size so that milk will drop slowly.

Especially during the first 6–7 mo of life, the eructation of air swallowed during feeding is important for avoiding regurgitation and abdominal discomfort. This technique is similar to that described after breast feeding. A few infants relieve themselves best after being replaced in the crib. All infants will, at times, regurgitate or "spit up" a small amount of milk after feeding, a fact that the mother should know. Spitting up occurs more often in the artificially fed than in the breast-fed infant.

A feeding may last from 5 to 25 min, depending on the vigor and the age of the infant. Since the appetite varies from feeding to feeding, each bottle should contain more than the average amount taken per feeding. In no instance should the infant be urged to take more than desired, and excess milk should be discarded.

COMPARISON OF HUMAN MILK AND COW'S MILK

Average values for the various constituents of human milk and whole fresh cow's milk are listed in Table 3–8. Both differ during the various stages of lactation and among individuals, although the differences in human milk from women with adequate diets are insignificant. Milk late in pregnancy and early after birth contains more protein, calcium, and other minerals than later during lactation.

Colostrum. The secretion of the breasts during the latter part of pregnancy and for the 2–4 days after delivery is termed "colostrum." It has a deep lemon yellow color, its reaction is alkaline, and its specific gravity is 1.040–1.060, in contrast to the average specific gravity of 1.030 for mature breast milk. The total amount of colostrum secreted daily is 10–40 mL. Human or cow colostrum contains several times the protein of mature breast milk, more minerals, but less carbohydrate and fat. Human colostrum also contains some unique immunologic factors. After the first few days of lactation, colostrum is replaced by secretion of a transitional form of milk which gradually assumes the characteristics of mature breast milk by the 3rd or 4th wk.

Water. The relative amounts of water and solids in human and cow's milks are about the same.

Calories. The energy value of each milk may vary slightly and is about 20 kcal/oz or 0.67 kcal/mL.

Protein. There are quantitative differences between the proteins of the 2 milks. Human milk contains only 1.0–1.5% protein in contrast to about 3.3% in cow's milk. The increased protein of cow's milk results almost entirely from its 6-fold higher content of casein. Human milk protein consists of approximately 60% whey proteins, largely lactalbumins and lactoglobulins, and 40% casein; the cow's milk ratio is reversed, to 18:82.

Carbohydrate. The sugars of the 2 milks differ only quantitatively; both contain lactose. Human milk contains 6.5–7.0% and cow's milk about 4.5%.

Fat. The fat content of milks varies more than any of their other constituents; the average content is about 3.5%. In human milk fat content varies somewhat with maternal diet; during a single nursing it is higher in the latter portion of the feeding, which may help satiate the infant at the conclusion of nursing.

The milks of different breeds of cattle vary in fat content. Most market milk in urban areas, however, is pooled, and the fat content is adjusted to a standard level, generally from 3.25–4%.

Qualitative differences exist in the fats of human and of cow's milks. The fats of each are composed principally of the triglycerides olein, palmitin, and stearin, but human milk contains twice as much of the more absorbable olein. The volatile fatty acids (butyric, capric, caproic, and caprylic) comprise only about 1.3% of human milk fat, but about 9% of cow's milk fat. Usually the small amount of linoleic acid in cow's milk is sufficient to prevent deficiency. The premature or debilitated infant may have steatorrhea after ingesting cow's milk fat. For such infants it is wise to substitute a more readily assimilated vegetable fat or human milk.

Minerals. Cow's milk contains much more of all the minerals except iron and copper than human milk; total mineral content of cow's milk is 0.7–0.75%; that of human milk is 0.15–0.25%. Cow's milk contains inadequate iron; breast milk iron, while low, may be sufficient for the infant because it is better absorbed, and during the first 4 mo or so of life iron stored during fetal life compensates for the milk's deficiency.

Table 3–8. **Approximate Composition of Colostrum, Human Milk, and Cow's Milk***

Constituent g/100 g	Human Milk	Human Colostrum	Cow's Milk
Water	88	87	88
Protein	0.9	2.7	3.3
Casein	0.4	1.2	2.7
Lactalbumin	0.4		0.4
Lactoglobulin	0.2	1.5	0.2
Fat	3.8	2.9	3.8
% polyunsaturated	8.0	7.0	2.0
Lactose	7.0	5.3	4.8
Ash	0.2	0.5	0.8
Calcium mg/100 g	34	30	117
Phosphorus mg/100 g	15	15	92
Sodium mEq/L	7	48	22
Potassium mEq/L	13	74	35
Chloride mEq/L	11	80	29
Magnesium mg/100 g	4	4	12
Sulfur mg/100 g	14	22	30
Chromium μg/L			10
Manganese μg/L	10	tr	30
Copper μg/L	400	600	300
Zinc mg/L	4	6	4
Iodine μg/L	30	120	47
Selenium μg/L	30		30
Iron mg/L	0.5	0.1	0.5
Amino acids (mg/100 mL)			
Histidine	22		95
Leucine	68		228
Isoleucine	100		350
Lysine	73		277
Methionine	25		88
Phenylalanine	48		172
Threonine	50		164
Tryptophan	18		49
Valine	70		245
Arginine	45		129
Alanine	35		75
Aspartic acid	116		166
Cystine	22		32
Glutamic acid	230		680
Glycine	0		11
Proline	80		250
Serine	69		160
Tyrosine	61		179
Vitamins (liter)			
Vitamin A (IU)	1898		1025
Thiamine (μg)	160		440
Riboflavin (μg)	360		1750
Niacin (μg)	1470		940
Pyridoxine (μg)	100		640
Pantothenate (mg)	2		3
Folacin (μg)	52		55
B_{12} (μg)	0.3		4
Vitamin C (mg)	43		11
Vitamin D (IU)	22		14
Vitamin E (mg)	2		0.4
Vitamin K (μg)	15		60

*Collated largely from Fomon SJ: Infant Nutrition. Ed 2. Philadelphia, WB Saunders Co, 1974, pp 360 ff, and Macy IG, Kelly HJ, Sloan RE: The Composition of Milks, NAS-NRC Publ. 254, 1953.

Although the need for calcium and phosphorus is great during periods of rapid growth, adequate balances are maintained on breast milk despite its low content of these minerals.

Vitamins. The vitamin content of each milk varies with the maternal intake, although each has large amounts of vitamin A. Cow's milk is low in vitamins C and D. Breast milk usually contains adequate vitamin C if the mother eats appropriate foods, and adequate vitamin D unless she is insufficiently exposed to sunlight or is darkly pigmented. Cow's milk contains more thiamine and riboflavin than human milk, and about an equal amount of niacin. Both milks seem to contain adequate amounts of vitamin A and the B-complex vitamins for the nutritional needs of infants in the first months of life.

Bacterial Content. Although human milk is essentially uncontaminated by bacteria, pathogenic organisms in significant numbers may enter the milk from mastitis. Tubercle and typhoid bacilli and herpes, hepatitis B, rubella, mumps, and cytomegaloviruses may be found at times in the milk of women infected with these organisms. Cow's milk is regularly contaminated, but in most instances by bacteria that are not harmful to man. Milk, however, is a good culture medium for pathogenic bacteria, and many infections are milk-borne, including streptococcal diseases, diphtheria, typhoid fever, salmonellosis, tuberculosis, and brucellosis. Furthermore, certain bacteria that may not affect older children or adults may cause diarrhea in infants. In most cities, however, pasteurization of all marketed whole milk is required. In addition, terminal sterilization or boiling the milk immediately before mixing the infant's formula is advisable.

Digestibility. The stomach empties more rapidly after human than after whole cow's milk; however, no appreciable difference in gastrointestinal passage time exists between human milk and processed milk formulas during the first 45 days of life. The curd of cow's milk is reduced in size by boiling; it is made considerably less tough and much smaller by the heating required in evaporation, by the addition of acid or alkali, and by homogenization. In contrast, the curd of breast milk is fine and flocculent and readily broken down in the stomach. The fat of cow's milk is less readily digested than that of breast milk.

MILK USED IN FORMULAS

Raw Milk. This is not advised for infant feeding; it forms large curds in the stomach, is slowly digested, and is easily contaminated with pathogenic organisms. Its sale is forbidden in most urban communities in the United States.

Pasteurized Milk. Pasteurization destroys pathogenic bacteria and modifies casein so that smaller, less tough curds are produced in the stomach. Raw milk is pasteurized by holding heated milk at a specified temperature for a specific length of time, e.g., at 145° F (63° C) for 30 min or, more commonly, at 161° F (72° C) for 15 sec, then rapidly cooling it to 148° F (65° C) or lower (60° C). Standards for the bacterial content of pasteurized milk vary in different cities, tolerable counts ranging as high as 50,000 nonpathogenic bacteria/mL; average counts in many cities, however, are as low as 5000–10,000. Pasteurized milk should be boiled when used for infant feeding. If it is allowed to stand in the refrigerator for as long as 48 hr, its bacterial count may significantly increase.

Homogenized Milk. During the process of homogenization, the fat globules are broken into minute particles and remain dispersed. The principal advantage of homogenized milk is the smaller, less tough curd produced in the stomach.

Evaporated Milk. This milk has many advantages, including almost universal availability. The unopened can will keep for months without refrigeration. The casein curd produced in the stomach is softer and smaller than that of boiled whole milk; homogenization of the fat also contributes to smaller curd formation. The lactalbumin appears to be less allergenic than that of fresh milk. The sugar is unchanged. When necessary, evaporated milk can be fed in higher concentrations than whole milk formulas. The standard can contains 13 fluid oz* (384 mL). Each fluid oz equals about 44 kcal; in

practice the value is generally considered to be 40 kcal. Vitamin D is usually added in the processing so that each reconstituted quart contains 400 IU.

Prepared Milks. Many commercially prepared modified milks requiring only the addition of water in a 1:1 proportion are widely used in infant feeding (Tables 3–9 and 3–10). Most are derived from cow's milk, and many are available in both liquid and powder forms. The composition of the majority simulates breast milk in various ways. All are fortified with vitamin D; many contain other vitamins, and some have added iron.

These milks are nutritionally adequate for normal infants, simple to prepare, and convenient to use. They cost somewhat more than evaporated milk–water formulas.

Other prepared milks that may have virtue for special circumstances are now available. Those with very low electrolyte content (mineral content similar to that in human milk) may be helpful for infants with congestive heart failure, nephrogenic diabetes insipidus, or marginal renal function. A low sodium milk, containing about 1 mEq of sodium per reconstituted quart, is commercially available for managing infants with congestive heart failure, but should be used with caution. Milks low in phenylalanine content are useful in managing infants and children with phenylketonuria.

Condensed Milk. About 45% cane sugar has been added in sweetened condensed milk, making the carbohydrate content approximately 60% in the evaporated form before dilution. The usual dilutions (1:10–14) are disproportionately high in sugar and low in fat and protein. Although readily digestible, it has no use in infant feeding for more than short periods when a high calorie diet is desired.

Dried Whole Milk. The fat content of fluid milk is adjusted to 3.5%, and the milk is rapidly evaporated to powder form by spray-, freeze-, or roller-drying. Reconstituted dried milk has most of the advantages of evaporated milk but does not keep well when exposed to air.

Dried Skim Milk. Both nonfat skim milk (fat content 0.5%) and half-skim milk (fat content 1.5%) are available. The use of these milks is limited to infants with fat intolerance. Skim milk should not be used in the first year of life for reducing weight. Its high protein and mineral content in proportion to calories may cause severe dehydration. Many of these products do not contain added vitamin D.

Acid and Fermented Milk. So-called acid milks are prepared by adding acid to previously boiled and cooled cow's milk formulas, or are fermented by adding lactic acid–producing organisms. These milks require less hydrochloric acid for gastric digestion. The casein is altered so that smaller, less tough curds form in the stomach. Acidified milks are now rarely used in infant feedings, as they are prone to cause acidosis.

Goat's Milk. In many countries goat's milk is used extensively for infant feeding; in the United States its use is limited to managing cow's milk allergies. Because of inconsistent, antigenic cross-reaction between cow's and goat's milks, the latter is less popular than the soy "milks" or formulas derived from lamb and beef and from casein hydrolysis.

Although similar in composition to cow's milk, goat's milk contains less sodium, more potassium and chloride, and more of the essential linoleic and arachidonic acids. Its fat may be more digestible and its curd tension lower than that found in cow's milk. It is low in Vitamin D, iron, and folic acid; infants fed exclusively on goat's milk are prone to megaloblastic anemia due to folate deficiency. Since the goat is especially susceptible to brucellosis, its milk should be boiled before use. It is commercially available in evaporated and powdered forms.

Milk Protein. Powdered protein is used chiefly for increasing protein content of some formulas fed to premature or

---

*One fluid oz is equivalent to approximately 29.57 mL.

Table 3–9. Natural Milks, Prepared Milks, and Milk Substitutes Used in Infant Feeding

| | Normal Dilution kcal/oz* | Approximate Percentage Composition in Normal Dilution (g per 100 mL) | | | | | Approximate Electrolyte Composition in Normal Dilution (Milliequivalents per Liter) | | | Milligrams per Liter | | |
		Protein	Carbo-hydrate	Fat	PUFA	Minerals	Na	K	Cl	Ca	P	Fe
Human milk, mature, average	22	1.1	7.0	3.8	—	0.21	7	14	12	340	150	1.5
Cow's milk, market, average	20	3.3	4.8	3.7	—	0.72	25	35	29	1170	920	1.0
Cow's milk, evaporated	22	3.8	5.4	4.0	—	0.8	28	39	32	1300	1100	1.0
Prepared formulas, cow's milk based												
Aptamil Milupa	20	1.5	7.2	3.6	—	0.3	10.4	12.2	10	580	368	10
Bebelac No. 1, Lijemph	—	1.8	8.6	3.0	—	0.4	—	—	—	950	540	0.4
Dumex Baby Food, Dumex	22	2.0	7.3	3.2	—	0.42	9.0	15	13	594	396	7.9
Dutch Baby Food, Friesland	20	1.9	6.6	3.0	0.33	—	5.8	13.7	11.5	408	274	0.4
Enfamil, Mead Johnson	20	1.5	6.9	3.8	1.11	0.3	9	18	12.0	460	320	1.0
Frisolac, Friesland	20	1.4	7.4	3.4	0.60	—	5.5	12.8	10.3	455	274	0.4
Lactalac V, Friesland	20	3.5	4.9	3.7	0.10	—	23.0	45.0	32.1	1340	1145	0.1
Lactogen, Nestlē	20	1.9	7.1	3.1	0.40	0.41	11.7	21.0	17.7	670	520	8.0
Lactogen FP, Nestlē	20	3.1	7.5	2.7	0.35	0.69	20.0	35.0	29.2	1110	860	12.0
Mamex, Dumex	22	1.6	7.3	3.5	—	0.26	6.0	14	10	500	333	7.7
Nan, Nestlē	20	1.6	7.4	3.4	0.44	0.30	7.4	19.2	14.4	530	300	8.0
Nativa, Nestlē	20	1.8	6.9	3.6	0.36	0.31	9.1	16.7	11	580	380	8.0
Perlargon, Nestlē	20	1.9	7.7	3.1	0.39	0.43	12.6	22.3	18.3	690	540	8.0
Similac, Ross (also 13, 24, 27 kcal/oz)	20	1.5	7.2	3.6	1.4	0.33	10	21	14	510	390	1.5
Similac Advance, Ross	16	2.0	5.5	2.7	1.5	0.35	10	23	15	510	390	12
Similac PM 60/40, Ross	20	1.5	6.9	3.8	1.2	0.22	7	15	11	400	200	1.5
Similac with Whey + Iron, Ross	20	1.5	7.2	3.6	1.4	0.34	10	19	12	400	300	12
SMA, Wyeth (also 13, 24, 27 kcal/oz)	20	1.5	7.2	3.6	0.49	0.25	6.5	14	11	443	330	12.7
Hypoallergenic products, soy based												
Alsoy, Nestlē	20	1.9	7.4	3.3	0.8	0.35	10.0	20.5	13.8	600	430	8.0
Isomil (soy), Ross	20	1.8	6.8	3.7	1.4	—	13	18	15	700	500	12
Meat base (beef heart), Gerber	20	2.8	6.2	3.3	—	0.4	7.8	9.5	6	980	650	13.7
Nursoy (soy), Wyeth	20	2.1	6.9	3.6	0.49	0.35	8.7	18.9	10.6	634	443	12.7
Nutramigen (casein hydrolysate), Mead Johnson	20	2.2	8.8	2.6	0.3	0.5	14	18	13	630	480	12.7
ProSobee (soy), Mead Johnson	20	2.0	6.9	3.6	1.0	0.4	13	20	16	630	500	12.7
Soyalac (soy), Loma Linda	20	2.1	6.7	3.8	—	0.4	14.3	18.7	—	600	500	15.0
Specialty products												
Advance, Ross	16	2.0	5.5	2.7	1.5	0.35	10	23	15	510	390	12.0
Alfare, Nestlē	20	2.2	7.0	3.3	0.38	0.42	16.9	21.0	19.1	540	340	8
Casec, Mead Johnson, 100 g powder	†	88	—	2	0.03	4.5	6.5	0.26	0.28	1600	800	—
Citrotein, Doyle, egg	20	2.3	7.0	0.5	0.1	—	17.3	10	15.1	600	600	21
Compleat B, Doyle, meat, vegetables	31	4.3	12.8	4.3	1.6	—	55.3	35	24.5	670	1340	12
Criticare HN, Mead Johnson	30	3.8	22.2	0.3	0.23	0.7	27.0	34	30	530	530	9.5
Electrodialysed whey, Wyeth/100 g	—	35	56	3	1.1	—	15	43	45	700	419	0.2
Enfamil human milk fortifier (per 4 packets)	14	0.7	2.7	0.04	0.01	0.19	7	15.6	17.7	60	33	—

Table continued on following page

Table 3–9. **Natural Milks, Prepared Milks, and Milk Substitutes Used in Infant Feeding** Continued

	Normal Dilution kcal/oz*	Approximate Percentage Composition in Normal Dilution (g per 100 mL)					Approximate Electrolyte Composition in Normal Dilution (Milliequivalents per Liter)			Milligrams per Liter		
		Protein	Carbohydrate	Fat	PUFA	Minerals	Na	K	Cl	Ca	P	Fe
Ensure Plus, Ross, casein, soy	44	5.5	20.0	5.3	4.3	0.22	50	60	57	630	630	14
Isocal, Mead Johnson, casein, soy oil, MCT oil	30	3.4	13.3	4.4	2.3	0.6	23	34	30	630	530	9.5
Lactalac MCT, Friesland	20	3.5	5.2	2.1	0.01	—	29	56.9	41.5	1675	1445	0.1
Lofenalac, Mead Johnson	20	2.2	8.8	2.7	1.6	0.5	14	19	15	630	480	13
Lonalac, Mead Johnson, low sodium	20	3.5	5.0	3.7	0.7	0.6	1.1	31.0	15	1195	1060	0.1
MSUD Powder, Mead Johnson, AA (corn oil)	20	1.2	8.8	2.8	—	0.5	12	18	15	700	382	13
Phenyl-free, Mead Johnson, AA	25	4.3	14	1.4	0.58	0.8	37	74	55	1060	1060	25
PKU-1 Milupa (also Hist-1, Hom-1, Lys-1, Tyr, MSUD 051)	20	3.7	1.3	—	—	—	3.4	4.3	3.4	176	136	—
Portagen, Mead Johnson	20	2.4	7.8	3.2	0.39	0.5	14	22	16	630	480	12.7
Precision, Doyle, egg	31	3.0	15.0	3.1	0.48	—	34.7	25.0	29.8	666	666	1.2
Precision LR, Doyle, egg	38	3.0	28.0	1.8	0.15	—	34.7	25.0	29.8	666	666	1.2
Pregestimil, Mead Johnson	20	1.9	9.1	2.7	0.97	0.5	14	19	16	630	420	12.7
Protein Free, Mead Johnson, 100 g powder (contains corn oil)		0	71.8	22.5	—	2.7	3.1	8.7	3.8	540	300	11
RCF, Ross	12	2.0	0	3.6	1.4	0.38	14	20	17	700	500	1.5
S-14, Wyeth	20	1.1	7.1	3.7	0.5	0.28	6.9	12.1	10.1	423	317	12.8
S-29, Wyeth, low solute	20	1.7	10.1	2.3	0.3	0.13	0.4	8.1	0.3	138	169	12.8
S-44, Wyeth, no vitamins	20	1.7	10.1	2.3	0.3	0.13	0.4	8.1	0.3	138	169	12.8
Vital, Ross	30	4.2	18.5	10.8	0.5	0.53	21	34	26	670	670	12
Vivonex, Norwich Eaton, elemental	32	2.1	24.6	0.15	—	—	37.4	29.9	51.8	555	555	10
Vivonex, HN, Norwich Eaton, elemental	32	4.2	22.6	0.10	—	—	33.5	17.9	52.4	333	333	6
3200 AB, Mead Johnson, low phenylalanine/tyrosine	20	2.2	8.8	2.7	—	0.5	14	18	14	630	480	12
3200 K, Mead Johnson, soy, low methionine	20	2.1	6.7	3.7	—	0.4	11.3	14.8	12.2	580	420	13
3232A, Mead Johnson, mono- & disaccharide free‡	20	1.9	9.1	2.8	—	0.5	12.7	19	16.9	636	424	13
Formulas for low birthweight infants												
Alprem, Nestlé	21	2.0	8.0	3.4	0.31	0.31	10	18.5	11.3	550	300	8
Enfamil, Premature Formula, Mead Johnson	24	2.4	8.9	4.1	1.0	0.5	14	23	19.4	950	480	1.3
Similac 24 LBW, Ross	24	2.2	8.5	4.5	0.6	0.5	16	31	26	730	560	3
Similac Special Care, Ross	24	2.2	8.6	4.4	0.8	0.5	17	29	20	1440	720	3
SMA Preemie, Wyeth	24	2.0	8.6	4.4	0.6	0.4	13.9	19	15	750	400	3

kcal = kilocalories = Cal.
†Casec is a protein supplement; it does not have a "normal dilution."
‡When total recommended carbohydrate has been added.

Table 3–10. Recommended Ranges of Nutrient Levels in Infant Formulas

Nutrient (per 100 kcal)	Adequate		Not to Exceed	
Protein (g)	1.8*		4.5	
Fat (g)	3.3	(30% of Cal)	6	(54% of Cal)
Including essential fatty acid (linoleate) (mg)	300	(2.7% of Cal)		
Vitamins				
A (IU)	250	(75 µg)†	750	(225 µg)†
D (µg cholecalciferol)‡	1		2.5	
K (µg)	4		—	
E (tocopherol equivalents)§	0.5	(at least 0.5/g linoleic acid)		
C (ascorbic acid) (mg)	8		—	
B₁ (thiamine) (µg)	40		—	
B₂ (riboflavin) (µg)	60		—	
B₆ (pyridoxine) (µg)	20 µg/g protein		—	
B₁₂ (µg)	0.15			
Niacin (µg)	250	(or 0.8 niacin equivalent)	—	
Folic acid (µg)	4		—	
Pantothenic acid (µg)	300		—	
Biotin (µg)	1.5		—	
Choline (mg)	7¶		—	
Inositol (mg)	4¶			
Minerals‖				
Calcium (mg)	60**		—	
Phosphorus (mg)	30**		—	
Magnesium (mg)	6		—	
Iron (mg)	0.15		2.5††	
Iodine (µg)	5		25	
Zinc (mg)	0.5		—	
Copper (µg)	60		—	
Manganese (µg)	5		100	
Selenium (µg)	3		—	
Sodium (mg)	20	(5.8 mEq/L)	60	(17.5 mEq/L)
Potassium (mg)	80	(13.7 mEq/L)	200	(34.3 mEq/L)
Chloride (mg)	55	(10.4 mEq/L)	150	(28.3 mEq/L)

AAP Committee on Nutrition, 1976 Recommendations with 1982 Modifications

*Nutritionally equivalent to casein. For use of other proteins refer to the Commentary on Breast Feeding and Infant Formulas, including Proposed Standards for Formulas. Pediatrics 57:278, 1976.

†Retinol equivalents.

‡1 µg cholecalciferol = 40 IU vitamin D.

§1.49 IU = 1 mg d-α-tocopherol equivalent. The β and γ isomers have less activity.

¶Average present in milk-base formulas; should be included in this amount in other formulas.

**Calcium to phosphorus ratio should not be less than 1.1 or more than 2.

††Prudence indicates there should be an upper limit for iron. If formula is labeled "infant formula with iron" it must not contain less than 1 mg/100 kcal.

‖Formula should be made with water low in fluoride and in all cases contain less than 45 µg/100 kcal. For explanation see Statement on Fluoride Supplementation: Revised Dosage Schedule. Pediatrics 63:150, 1979.

debilitated infants or to infants with diarrhea. Because of the increased metabolic products and the easy conversion from a balanced to an unbalanced diet, such products should be used carefully and for short durations.

Milk Substitutes and Hypoallergenic Milks. A number of milks and milk substitutes are available for infants allergic to cow's milk. These include evaporated goat's milk, a preparation in which nutrient nitrogen is supplied as an amino acid

mixture (casein hydrolysate), nonmilk foods in which the protein is derived from soybeans, and meat-base formulas (beef and lamb sources). All appear to be nutritionally satisfactory and have a place in the management of infants who cannot tolerate cow's milk; those not containing lactose are useful for infants with galactosemia. Powdered casein (Casec) and medium-chain triglycerides (MCT oil) are available for special purposes.

Filled and Imitation Milks. Imitation milk products and nondairy "white" beverages in which vegetable fat is substituted for cow (butter) fat are being developed and tested for use in countries where milk and other high quality protein sources are in short supply. Many of these products lack the full nutritional benefits of fluid milk; they are not intended as formula for infants or as a substitute for breast milk. When they are used for older children, the physician should be aware of the composition and limitations of the product.

Elemental Dietary Substitutes for Milk. A number of specialty products have been developed to meet complicated dietary and nutritional problems in children and adults with malabsorption due to primary disease or extensive surgical resection of the small bowel. These include diets prepared with known quantities of purified chemical elements (free glucose, amino acids, and essential fatty acids). All are low residue, chemically defined, and nutritionally adequate, at least for short-term use. They have been most useful in treating severely ill infants with intractable diarrhea, in reducing stooling and/or "resting" the colon in inflammatory bowel disease, in making maximum use of short bowel segments after surgery, and in maintaining very ill patients in positive nitrogen balance while decreasing the bulk and bacterial content of the colon prior to and after major bowel surgery. (See Table 3–9.)

MILK FORMULAS

The formulas combine milk, sugar, and water, and some modification for a more desirable, smaller curd formation. They should contain about 20 kcal/oz.

Caloric Requirements (Sec. 3.4). The average caloric requirements of fullterm infants are about 45–55 kcal/lb or 80–120 kcal/kg during the first few months of life and about 45 kcal/lb or 100 kcal/kg by 1 yr of age; individual variations are significant, and for many infants intakes of this order exceed caloric need.

Fluid Requirements (Table 3–3). Fluid requirements are high during infancy. During the first 6 mo of life they range from 2 to 3 oz/lb/24 hr, or 130 to 190 ml/kg/24 hr and may increase during hot weather. As a rule, the infant regulates his or her own fluid intake, provided adequate amounts are offered. Most of the fluid required is in the formula, but some is supplied in orange juice and other foods and by water between feedings.

Number of Feedings Daily. The number of feedings required per day decreases throughout the first year; by 1 yr of age most infants are satisfied with 3 meals a day (Table 3–11). The interval between feedings differs considerably among

Table 3–11. Average Number of Feedings per 24 Hours

Age	Average Number of Feedings in 24 Hours
Birth–1 wk	6–10
1 wk–1 mo	6–8
1–3 mo	5–6
3–7 mo	4–5
4–9 mo	3–4
8–12 mo	3

Table 3–12. Average Quantity of Feedings

Age	Average Quantity Taken in Individual Feedings
1st and 2nd wk	2–3 oz (60–90 mL)
3 wk–2 mo	4–5 oz (120–150 mL)
2–3 mo	5–6 oz (150–180 mL)
3–4 mo	6–7 oz (180–210 mL)
5–12 mo	7–8 oz (210–240 mL)

infants but, in general, ranges from 3–5 hr during the first year of life, averaging 4 hr for fullterm, healthy infants. Small and/or weak infants may prefer feedings at 2–3 hr intervals. For the first month or two, feedings are taken throughout the 24 hr period, but thereafter, as the quantity of milk consumed at each feeding increases and the infant adjusts his or her demand to the family pattern of daytime activity, the infant will usually sleep for longer periods of time at night. As the infant develops psychologically and the loving relationship between parent and infant evolves, demand feeding should gradually progress to a comfortable, regular feeding regimen that accounts for the needs of both infant and parents.

Quantity of Formula. Although the quantity taken at a feeding will vary with different infants of the same age and with the same infant at different feedings, it is important to know the average amounts taken at various ages.

Each infant must be primarily responsible for determining the quantity of intake (Table 3–12). Rarely will an infant want to take more than 7–8 oz of milk at one feeding, if caloric and nutritional needs are adequately supplemented by other foods. The relative requirement for milk is somewhat less in the first 2 wk than in the succeeding 5–6 mo. After this time milk, though still of great value, has diminishing importance in meeting total nutritional requirements.

It is rarely necessary to use more than 1 can (13 fluid oz) of evaporated milk or 1 quart of whole milk/day. By the time the infant is taking these quantities, other foods will be added to the diet in increasing amounts. Ingesting more milk has no advantage, but the disadvantage is that other essential foods may be displaced. Some of the milk may be incorporated in the cereal and in the preparation of foods such as custards, soups, and sauces.

During the first few months the high quantity of protein and minerals in undiluted cow's milk makes such unmodified milk unsuitable for most infants. Diluting the milk supplies free water, and adding carbohydrate increases the caloric content (Table 3–13).

While lactose is the milk sugar of most mammals, it is expensive and other carbohydrates are usually used in home-prepared formulas. Cane sugar, dextrin-maltose preparations, or other easily digestible sugars can be added. Ingested lactose

Table 3–13. Household Measures of Some Commonly Used Sugars*

	Tablespoonfuls per Ounce
Lactose	3
Sucrose (cane)	2
Dextrin-maltose preparations:	
Mead's Dextri-Maltose	4
Karo	2
Cartose	2
Dexin	6
Polycose fluid	2

*Caloric value of each is 120 Calories per ounce, except Dexin, 115, and polycose, 60.

produces a lower pH in the intestine than formulas containing other sugars. The acid pH improves calcium absorption.

Representative evaporated or whole milk formulas for the first 10 days of life are given in Table 3–14. These formulas are satisfactory for an initial prescription. Subsequent adjustments of milk and water should be made in accordance with the infant's satiety and the growth curve.

Preparation of Formula. Several more bottles than the number required for feedings are needed for holding water and orange juice. Bottles should be made of heat-resistant glass, be smooth inside, and be marked in ounces. A wide-mouthed bottle is preferable because it is more easily cleaned, and those with an adequate cover for the nipple are preferable if the baby is to be fed away from home. There should be several more nipples than the number required for feedings. Alternatively, disposable bottles are now widely used in some communities. Other useful utensils include a graduate made of heat-resistant glass and marked in ounces, a saucepan for heating and mixing the formula, a container for nipples, a glass funnel if narrowmouthed bottles are used, a large kettle or special bottle sterilizer, a measuring spoon, a can opener, a knife, a standard tablespoon, and a strainer.

All utensils required for the mixing and storing of the formula should be sterilized by boiling for 5–10 min. The rubber nipples and caps should not be boiled more than 5 min. After each feeding the bottle and nipple should be thoroughly flushed and the bottle filled with water until washed with water and a detergent.

The hands should be thoroughly scrubbed and the sterilized bottles and utensils arranged on a clean table. If whole milk is used, the bottle is shaken so that its contents are mixed, and the top is washed with hot water before the cap is removed. The water for the formula (it is necessary to allow for a slight loss in boiling) is brought to the boiling point in a saucepan; the amount of whole milk ordered is added; and the mixture is boiled for 5 min. Constant stirring is necessary. The sugar is added while the milk is still warm.

If evaporated milk is used, the top of the can is washed with soap and hot water and rinsed with hot water; 2 holes are punctured in it. The water for the formula is boiled for 5 min, and the evaporated milk and sugar are added to it. No further boiling is necessary.

The freshly prepared and sterile formula is poured in appropriate amounts into sterilized nursing bottles. The bottles are capped by aseptic technique and stored in the refrigerator until time for the feedings.

Terminal Heating. This method is most commonly used today; it has practical advantages and does not require pre-sterilization of bottles or utensils. The formula is poured into clean nursing bottles, and the nipples are applied. The nipples are then loosely covered with glass, metal, or paper caps and

Table 3–14. Representative Formulas

	1–3 Days	Cal	4–10 Days	Cal	10 Days	Cal
Evaporated milk	6 oz	240	7 oz	280	13 oz	520
Sugar	1 tbsp	60	1 tbsp	60	3 tbsp	180
Water	14 oz		14 oz		17 oz	
	20 oz	300	21 oz	340	30 oz	700
Cal/oz		14		16		22
Cal/100 mL		47		56		70
Whole milk	12 oz	240	14 oz	280	26 oz	520
Sugar	1 tbsp	60	1 tbsp	60	3 tbsp	180
Water	8 oz		7 oz		6 oz	
	20 oz	300	21 oz	340	32 oz	700

Total volume is divided into 6 bottles, and the total intake is regulated by the infant.

the bottles placed in a rack in a container tall enough to prevent the bottles from touching the lid. The container is filled with water to about the midpoint of the bottles, covered, and placed over a moderate flame. The water is allowed to boil gently for 25 min. The bottles are then removed with tongs and placed in a container of cold water for 10 min. The caps are then tightened and the bottles stored in a refrigerator.

3.12 OTHER FOODS

Vitamins. Most marketed whole and artificial milks are fortified with 400 IU of vitamin D per reconstituted quart, and commercially prepared milks vary in the content of other vitamins. Therefore, knowing the vitamin content of the milk is essential before prescribing additional vitamins for the bottle-fed baby.

Orange and other citrus fruit juices are natural sources of *vitamin C*, but since many young infants do not seem to tolerate them in amounts large enough to supply an adequate vitamin intake, it is preferable to give 50 mg of ascorbic acid. When at least 2 oz of fresh, frozen, or canned orange juice (or equivalent amounts of other sources of vitamin C) is taken daily, the ascorbic acid may be discontinued.

Vitamin D should be started early in the neonatal period with a daily intake of approximately 400 IU only if the infant is taking a formula which does not contain vitamin D or is receiving an insufficient volume of milk to meet the daily requirement. Low birthweight infants require supplementation (Sec. 8.17). Vitamin D supplement is not necessary during the first few months of breast feeding of white infants but may be for black infants and those not exposed to adequate sunlight. Concentrates in water-miscible vehicles are desirable to avoid aspiration of oil.

Iron. Foods rich in iron tend to be limited in the diet of the less affluent of the population. The most effective way to prevent iron deficiency is to provide iron supplementation in the form of an iron-fortified milk formula or medicinal iron (2 mg/kg up to a total of 15 mg/24 hr) beginning at 6 wk of age. It is doubtful that iron-supplemented cereals can provide sufficient supplementation for infants with reduced iron stores.

"Solid" Foods. The caloric contents of the various prepared baby foods differ widely (Table 29–10). Egg yolk, cereals with added milk, meats, and puddings have greater caloric density than milk, whereas vegetables and fruits have an energy value similar to or lower than milk. Without appropriate advice, many mothers do not know how to select foods for their infants. Among their errors is the tendency to select foods with high caloric values that result in obesity. Little evidence exists for claiming that adding solid foods to the diet before 4–6 mo of age contributes significantly to the health of the normal infant.

Any new food should be initially offered once a day in small amounts (1–2 teaspoonfuls). Any small spoon that easily fits the baby's mouth may be used. New foods are generally best accepted if fairly thin or dilute. Food is frequently pushed out by the tongue rather than back because the baby cannot yet swallow efficiently. This should be mentioned to the mother, who might otherwise interpret the "spitting out" of new foods as dislike. It is usually wise to offer the same food daily until the baby becomes accustomed to it and not to introduce new foods more often than every 1–2 wk.

The feeding at which these foods are offered is not particularly important. They should be given when the baby's hunger is no longer satisfied by milk alone and when they fit into the daily schedule. There is no reason for persisting with or forcing a particular food that is definitely disliked. The family's dislikes and prejudices for particular foods are con-

tagious and should not be displayed before the infant. The physician should avoid prescribing a definite amount of a given food lest the mother interpret the suggestion too literally. *Many infants are overfed by overzealous parents who mistake acceptance of food for appetite.* The infant's appetite is the best index of the proper amount, and respect for the infant's wishes will avoid many problems.

Cereal. The various precooked cereals on the market provide in a convenient form a variety of grains excellent for infants. Most contain iron and factors of the vitamin B complex.

Fruits. Strained or puréed cooked fruits furnish minerals and some water-soluble vitamins and usually have a mildly laxative effect. Raw ripe mashed banana is readily digested and enjoyed by most babies. Many infants who are slow in accepting new foods seem to prefer fruits.

Vegetables. Vegetables are moderately good sources of iron and other minerals and of the vitamins of the B complex. They should be freshly cooked and strained or commercially prepared. Vegetables are usually added to the infant's diet by about 7 mo of age.

Meats, Eggs, and Starchy Foods. Eggs and starchy foods are usually introduced during the second 6 mo of life, although some physicians offer egg yolk at an earlier age. The yolk of the egg is used initially and is preferably hard-cooked. As with all new foods, a small amount is offered at first, with gradual increases up to a whole yolk 1–3 times a week. Egg white should be introduced with equal caution to minimize any possible allergic manifestations.

Potatoes, rice, spaghetti, bread, and similar starchy foods have principally a caloric value. As a rule, they are not included in the infant's diet until the more essential foods mentioned above are being taken regularly. Zwieback, toast, or graham crackers may be offered to the infant when he or she shows an interest in "gumming" on coarser foods (usually 6–8 mo of age). It is with such foods that infants learn to chew and to feed themselves.

Meat is an excellent source of protein as well as of iron and vitamins. Ground fresh beef or liver or the strained canned meats may be used initially by about 6 mo of age. Meats may be more readily accepted when mixed with another food.

The commercial soups and meat and vegetable mixtures are relatively high in carbohydrate and are not considered optimal sources of iron or protein. Many home-prepared soups are bulky out of proportion to their food value, and much of the vitamin content is lost by overcooking.

Desserts. Puddings, junkets, and custard are good foods for older infants, particularly if they temporarily prefer milk in that form. If, however, such foods are given as a bribe or reward or only after other foods have been finished, poor eating habits are apt to be established. Sweet foods should be offered as casually as the rest of the meal and at any place in the meal that the child desires.

Salt Intake. To increase their palatability, particularly for the parent, excessive salt used to be added to baby foods. Recently this practice has been discontinued. The significance of large intakes of sodium, which are in the ranges seen in populations with a high incidence of hypertension, is not clear, but the possibility that they might contribute to the development of hypertension later in life cannot be ignored.

Food Additives. Naturally occurring chemicals and food additives, particularly the artificial flavors and colors, have been implicated in health problems. It has been estimated that more than 3000 flavors are currently being used, and few children are spared exposure to them in their daily diet. Artificial flavors and colors have been associated with respiratory allergic disorders, with urticaria and angioedema, with lesions of the tongue and buccal mucosa, with digestive disturbances, with arthralgia and hydrarthroses, and with headache and behavioral disturbances, including hyperkinesis in childhood.

3.13 FIRST-YEAR FEEDING PROBLEMS

Underfeeding. Underfeeding is suggested by restlessness and crying and by failure to gain weight adequately, despite complete emptying of the breast or bottle. Underfeeding may also result from the infant's failure to take a sufficient quantity of food even when offered. In these instances the frequency of feedings, the mechanics of feeding, the size of the holes in the nipple, the adequacy of eructation of air, the possibility of abnormal mother-infant "bonding," and possible systemic disease in the baby should be investigated (Sec. 5.36). The extent and duration of underfeeding determine the clinical manifestations. Constipation, failure to sleep, irritability, and excessive crying are to be expected. There may be poor gain in weight or an actual loss. In the latter instance the skin becomes dry and wrinkled, subcutaneous tissue disappears, and the infant assumes the appearance of an "old man." Deficiencies of vitamins A, B, C, and D and of iron and protein may be responsible for characteristic clinical manifestations.

Treatment consists of increasing the fluid and caloric intake, correcting deficiencies in vitamin and mineral intake, and instructing the mother in the art of infant feeding. If some underlying systemic disease or psychologic problem is responsible, specific management of these disorders will be necessary.

Overfeeding. Overfeeding may be quantitative or qualitative. Regurgitation and vomiting are frequent symptoms of overfeeding. As a rule, infants can be depended upon not to take excessive quantities, but occasionally an infant who has postprandial discomfort from eating too much may nonetheless gain weight excessively. Diets too high in fat delay gastric emptying, cause distention and abdominal discomfort, and may cause excessive gain in weight. Diets too high in carbohydrate are likely to cause undue fermentation in the intestine, resulting in distention and flatulence and in too rapid gain in weight. Such diets may be deficient in essential protein, vitamins, and minerals. Formulas too high in caloric content in the first 1–2 wk of life are likely to result in loose or diarrheal stools. Obesity is undesirable at any time in life; often the excessively fed infant becomes the obese child and adult.

Regurgitation and Vomiting. The return of small amounts of swallowed food during or shortly after eating is termed "regurgitation" or "spitting up." More complete emptying of the stomach, especially occurring some time after feeding, is termed "vomiting." Within limits, regurgitation is a natural occurrence, especially during the first 6 mo or so of life. It can be reduced to a negligible amount, however, by adequate eructation of swallowed air during and after eating, by gentle handling, by avoiding emotional conflicts, and by placing the infant on the right side or abdomen for a nap immediately after eating. The head should not be lower than the rest of the body during the rest period, since gastroesophageal reflux is common during the first 4–6 mo.

Vomiting, one of the most common symptoms in infancy, may be associated with a variety of disturbances, both trivial and serious. It should be distinguished from rumination; its cause should always be investigated (Sec. 12.13, 12.15, and 12.16).

Loose or Diarrheal Stools. Acute infectious diarrhea and chronic diarrheal conditions are discussed in Sec. 11.8 and 12.40; only mild disturbances of dietary origin will be considered here.

The stool of the breast-fed infant is naturally softer than that of the infant fed cow's milk. From about the 4th to the 6th day of life the stools go through a transitional stage in which they are rather loose and greenish yellow and contain mucus; within a few days the typical "milk stool" appears. Subsequently, the use of laxatives or the ingestion of certain foods by the mother may be temporarily responsible for an infant's loose stools. Excessive intake of breast milk may also increase the frequency and the water content of the stool. Actual diarrhea in a breast-fed infant is unusual and should be considered infectious until proved otherwise.

Though the stools of artificially fed infants tend to be firmer than those of breast-fed infants, under certain circumstances loose stools may result from artificial feeding. In the first 2 wk or so of life, overfeeding is likely to cause loose, frequent stools. Later, formulas too concentrated or too high in sugar content, especially in lactose, may produce loose, frequent stools. Many temporary diarrhea disturbances in artificially fed infants result from food contaminations that would not disturb an older child and are not serious enough to cause prolonged difficulty for the infant. The ease with which artificially fed infants acquire diarrheal disturbances and their potential seriousness are strong arguments for extreme care in providing food free of pathogenic bacteria.

Mild diarrheal disturbances due to overfeeding respond quickly to temporary decrease or cessation of feeding. Withholding all solid food and one or several milk feedings, substituting boiled water or 5% glucose in water or in a balanced electrolyte solution, is usually all that is required.

Constipation (Sec. 12.13). Constipation is practically unknown in breast-fed infants receiving an adequate amount of milk, and is rare in artificially fed infants receiving an adequate diet. The nature of the stool, not its frequency, is the mark of constipation. Although most infants have one or more stools daily, an occasional infant will have a stool of normal consistency only at intervals of 36–48 hr. Whenever constipation or obstipation is present from birth or shortly thereafter, a rectal examination should be performed. Tight or spastic anal sphincters may occasionally be responsible for obstipation, and correction usually follows finger dilatation. Anal fissures or cracks may also cause constipation. If irritation is alleviated, healing usually occurs quickly. Aganglionic megacolon may be manifested by constipation in early infancy; the absence of stool in the rectum on digital examination suggests this possibility.

Constipation in the artificially fed infant may be due to an insufficient amount of food or fluid. In other instances it may result from diets too high in fat or protein or deficient in bulk. Simply increasing the amount of fluid or sugar in the formula may be corrective in the first few months of life. After this age better results are obtained by adding or increasing the amounts of cereal, vegetables, and fruits. Prune juice (½–1 oz) may be given as a temporary measure, but it is better to add foods with some bulk. Enemas and suppositories should never be more than temporary measures. Milk of magnesia may be given in doses of 1–2 teaspoonfuls but should be reserved for unresponsive or severe constipation.

Colic. The term "colic" describes a frequent symptom complex of paroxysmal abdominal pain, presumably of intestinal origin, and of severe crying. It usually occurs in infants under 3 mo of age.

The clinical pattern is characteristic: the attack usually begins suddenly; the cry is loud and more or less continuous; so-called paroxysms may persist for several hours; the face may be flushed, or there may be circumoral pallor; the abdomen is distended and tense; the legs are drawn up on the abdomen, though they may be momentarily extended; the feet are often cold; the hands are clenched. The attack may terminate only when the infant is completely exhausted, but often there is apparent relief with the passage of feces or flatus.

Certain infants seem to be peculiarly susceptible to colic. The cause of recurrent attacks is usually not apparent, though they may be associated with hunger and with swallowed air which has passed into the intestine. Overfeeding may also cause discomfort and distention. Certain foods, especially those of high carbohydrate content, may be responsible for excessive fermentation in the intestines, but a change in diet only occasionally prevents further colic attacks. Crying from intestinal discomfort is seen in infants with intestinal allergy, but colic is not limited to this group. Intestinal obstruction or peritoneal infection may mimic an attack of colic. Recurrent attacks commonly occur late in the afternoon or evening, suggesting that events in the household routine may possibly cause them. Worry, fear, anger, or excitement may cause vomiting in an older child and may cause colic in an infant. No single factor consistently accounts for colic, nor does any treatment consistently provide satisfactory relief. Careful physical examination is important to eliminate the possibility of intussusception, strangulated hernia, hair in eye, otitis, pyelonephritis, or other disorders.

Holding the baby upright or permitting the baby to lie prone across the lap or on a hot water bottle or heating pad occasionally helps. Passage of flatus or fecal material spontaneously or with expulsion of a suppository or enema sometimes affords relief. Carminatives before feedings are ineffective in preventing the attacks. Sedation is occasionally indicated for a prolonged attack and is sometimes given to parent or child for a period of time if other measures fail. Temporary hospitalization of the infant, often without more than a change in the infant's feeding routine and providing a period of rest for the mother, may help in extreme cases. Prevention of attacks should be sought by improving feeding techniques, including burping, providing a stable emotional environment, identifying possibly allergenic foods in the infant's or nursing mother's diet, and avoiding underfeeding or overfeeding. Colic rarely persists after 3 mo of age. A supportive, sympathetic physician is important in successfully resolving the problem.

3.14 FEEDING DURING THE SECOND YEAR OF LIFE

Most infants naturally adapt themselves to a schedule of three meals a day by about the end of the 1st yr of life. Though considerable latitude in the diet of each infant should be permitted to allow for personal idiosyncrasies and family habits, the mother should be given an outline of the daily basic dietary needs (Table 3–7).

Reduced Caloric Intake. Toward the end of the 1st yr of life and during the 2nd yr, because of the constantly decelerating rate of growth, there is a gradual reduction in the infant's caloric intake per unit of body weight. In addition, it is not unusual to have temporary periods of lack of interest in certain foods or even in food in general. Failure to recognize these features, especially the decreasing caloric needs, results in attempts to force feed. The child naturally rebels and feeding problems ensue. Since preventing problems is more effective than correcting them, the changing pattern of the infant's food habits during the 2nd yr of life should be explained to the mother before it appears.

Self-Selection of Diet. Children's strong likes or dislikes of particular foods should be respected whenever possible and practicable. Spinach is an example of a nonessential food whose virtues have been overemphasized. When consistently rejected foods include basic staples such as milk and eggs, food allergy should be considered.

Children, including infants, tend to select diets which, over several days, assume a balanced nature. Thus, the child may be permitted a wide choice of foods, as long as he or she eats adequately over the longer period. Normally, the child determines the quantity to be eaten of a given food and of the entire meal. At this age eating habits may be strongly influenced by older children in the family, particularly in respect to food likes and dislikes. Eating patterns and habits developed in the first 2 yr of life usually persist for several years.

Self-Feeding by Infants. Before 1 yr of age the infant should be permitted to participate in the act of feeding. By 6 mo or so the infant can hold a bottle; within another 2–3 mo, a cup. Zwieback, graham crackers, or other hand-held foods can be introduced by the age of 7–8 mo. A spoon may be used as soon as it can be held and directed to the mouth, possibly by 10–12 mo of age. Mothers often inhibit this learning process because they object to its messiness.

Acquiring the ability to feed oneself is an important step in developing self-reliance and responsibility. By the end of the second year of life, infants should be largely responsible for feeding themselves.

Permitting infants and children to go to sleep while sucking intermittently from a bottle of formula, whole milk, sweetened fruit juice, or water should be discouraged. Pedodontists stress the correlation between this habit and enamel erosion in deciduous teeth, terming it the "baby bottle syndrome."

Although nutritional requirements per unit of body weight constantly decrease with increasing age (110 kcal/kg in infancy; 50 kcal/kg at 15 yr), the need for calories as well as for protein, vitamins, and minerals is relatively greater in children than it is in adults.

Daily Basic Diet. Parents should be given a daily basic diet for the child from which the family menu can be prepared. Daily selection from each of the food groups provides a balanced diet with sufficient macro- and micronutrients. The quantity of intake after the basic requirements have been met can usually be determined by the healthy growing child. The child's history of dietary habits is essential for evaluating the nutritive intake, but such histories are often unreliable unless an accurate dietary diary is kept for several days. From such information, correcting the diet may be more effective. The recommended daily dietary intake is shown in Table 3–7.

The older child should learn the content of a basic diet and its importance to proper growth and good health, but this information should never be presented as a threat to enforce rigid feeding practices.

Eating Habits. Eating habits formed in the first year or two of life distinctly affect those of the subsequent years. Feeding difficulties between the ages of 2 and 5 yr frequently result from excessive parental insistence on eating and subsequent anxiety when the child does not conform to some arbitrary standard. The child's negative reactions naturally result from undue mealtime stress, and correction requires improvement in parent-child relations. Other factors that disturb eating are too much confusion at mealtime, insufficient time for eating, either on the part of the adult or of the child, food dislikes of other members of the family, and poorly prepared and unattractively served food. A comfortable chair of proper height with a foot-rest is important for a child's ease at the table. Mealtimes should be happy and the conversation should be on subjects of interest to the entire family. The child's appetite should be respected; if his or her desire for food at times is below average, there should be no persuasion to eat more. Adults should realize that eating habits are taught better by example than by formal explanation.

Snacks Between Meals. During the second year and even for several years thereafter, orange juice or other fruit juice or fruit, together with a cracker, may be given in either or both of the between-meal periods. Snacks served in nursery schools and kindergartens should be nutritious. Older children should avoid between-meal snacking if it reduces their appetite for the next meal. After-school snacks, especially of fruit, should be encouraged if they produce greater enthusiasm and energy for play and do not reduce the appetite for the evening meal.

VEGETARIAN DIET

All-vegetable diets supply all needed nutrients when vegetables are selected from different classes. Vegetables are high in fiber content, vitamins, and minerals. Vegetarians usually have faster gastrointestinal transit time, bulkier stools, and low serum cholesterol levels and are said to have less diverticulitis and appendicitis than meat eaters. Those who consume eggs are ovovegetarians. Those who consume milk are lactovegetarians. Those who consume neither are vegans. Vegans may develop vitamin B_{12} deficiency and, because of high fiber intake, may develop trace mineral deficiency. Nursing vegan mothers must be given added vitamin B_{12} to prevent methylmalonic acidemia in their infants. Vegetarian infants may not grow as rapidly as omnivores in the first 2 yr.

DIET FOR ATHLETIC ACTIVITIES

Adequate caloric intake is necessary for growth and activity. A varied diet supplies all necessary nutrients. Special food supplements are unnecessary and may be harmful. Water intake should be scheduled regularly before and during athletic events.

Aldrich CA: Ancient processes in scientific age: Feeding aspects. Am J Dis Child 64:714, 1942.
Am. Soc. for Parenteral and Enteral Nutrition, Inc.: Product Resource Manual, 2nd ed, 1982.
Bahna SL, Heiner DC: Cows' milk allergy. Adv Pediatr 25:1, 1978.
Committee on Nutrition, AAP: Composition of milks. Pediatrics 26:1039, 1960.
Committee on Nutrition, AAP: Vitamin K supplementation for infants receiving milk substitute infant formulas and for those with fat malabsorption. Pediatrics 48:483, 1971.
Committee on Nutrition, AAP: Filled milks, imitation milks, and coffee whiteners. Pediatrics 49:770, 1972.
Committee on Nutrition, AAP: Pediatric Nutrition Handbook. Chicago, 1979.
Committee on Nutrition, AAP: On the feeding of supplemental foods to infants. Pediatrics 65:1178, 1980.
Committee on Nutrition, AAP: Nutritional Aspects of Obesity in Childhood. Pediatrics 68:880, 1981.
Committee on Nutrition, AAP: Toward a prudent diet for children. Pediatrics 71:78, 1983.
Committee on Nutrition, AAP: Soy protein formulas? Recommendations for use in infant feeding. Pediatrics 72:359, 1983.
Cunningham AS: Morbidity in breast-fed and artificially fed infants. J Pediatr 90:726, 1977.
Feingold BF: Food additives and child development. Hosp Pract (No 10) 8:11, 1973.

Fomon SJ: Body composition of the male reference infant. Pediatrics 40:863, 1967.
Fomon, SJ: Infant Nutrition. 2nd ed. Philadelphia, WB Saunders, 1974.
Food and Nutrition Board: Recommended Dietary Allowances. 9th ed. National Academy of Sciences, 1980.
Friedman Z, Danon A, Stahlman MT, et al: Rapid onset of essential fatty acid deficiency in the newborn. Pediatrics 58:640, 1976.
Garonger JD, Brown MS, Laster L: The columnar epithelial cell of the small intestine: Digestion and transport. N Engl J Med 283:1196, 1264, 1317, 1970.
Gartner LM, Arias IM: Studies of prolonged neonatal jaundice in the breast-fed infant. J Pediatr 68:54, 1966.
Goldfarb J, Tibbetts E: Breast-feeding Handbook. Hillside, NJ, Enslow Publ, 1980.
Goldman AS, Pong AJH, Goldblum RM: Host defenses: Development and maternal contributions. Adv Ped 33:71, 1985.
Gryboski J: Gastrointestinal Problems in the Infant. Philadelphia, WB Saunders, 1975.
Hambreus L: Proprietary milk versus human breast milk in infant feeding. Pediatr Clin North Am 24:17, 1977.
Hansen AE, Stewart RA, Hughes G, et al: The relation of linoleic acid to infant feeding: A review. Acta Pediatr 51:Suppl, 1982.
Holt, LE Jr, Snyderman SE: The amino acid requirements of infants. JAMA 175:100, 1961.
Howald H, Poortmans, JR: Metabolic adaptation to prolonged physical exercise. Proc 2nd International Symposium on Biochemistry of Exercise, Magglingen, 1973. Basel, 1975.
Kagan BM, Stanincova V, Felix NS, et al: Body composition of premature infants: Relation to nutrition. Am J Clin Nutr 25:1153, 1973.
Klaus MH, Jerauld R, Kreger NC, et al: Maternal attachment: Importance of the first postpartum days. N Engl J Med 286:460, 1972.
La Leche League International. The Womanly Art of Breast Feeding. Franklin Park, IL, 1976.
Lebenthal E (ed): Textbook of Gastroenterology and Nutrition in Infants. New York, Raven Press, 1981.
Macy IG, Kelly HJ, Sloan RE: The composition of milks. A compilation of the comparative composition and properties of human, cow and goat milk, colostrum and transitional milk. Washington, DC, Publication 254, National Academy of Science–National Research Council, 1953.
McMillan JA, Landaw SA, Oski FA: Iron insufficiency in breast-fed infants and the availability of iron from human milk. Pediatrics 58:686, 1976.
Neville MC: Methodologies in human lactation: Report of a workshop. J Pediatr Gastroenterol Nutr 3:268, 1984.
Powers GF: Infant feeding: Historical background and modern practice. JAMA 105:753, 1935.
Prasad AS (ed): Trace Elements in Human Health and Diseases. Vol 1. Zinc and Copper, New York, Academic Press, 1976.
Raiha NCR, Heinonen K, Rassin DK, et al: Milk protein quantity and quality in low birth weight infants. I. Metabolic responses and effects on growth. Pediatrics 57:659, 1976.
Reeves JD, Vichinsky E, Addiego J, et al: Iron deficiency in health and disease. Adv Pediatr 30:281, 1983.
Reina D: Infant nutrition. Clin Perinatol 2:373, 1975.
Roy RN, Sinclair JC: Hydration of the low birth weight infant. Clin Perinatol 2:393, 1975.
Spock B: Baby and Child Care. New York, Pocket Books, 1962.
Suskind RM (ed): Textbook of Pediatric Nutrition. New York, Raven Press, 1981.
Watkins JB: Mechanisms of fat absorption and the development of gastrointestinal function. Pediatr Clin North Am 22:721, 1975.

NUTRITIONAL DISORDERS

3.15 MALNUTRITION

Worldwide, malnutrition is one of the leading causes of morbidity and mortality in childhood (Sec. 4.4).

Malnutrition may be due to improper and/or inadequate food intake or may result from inadequate absorption of food. Insufficient food supply, poor dietary habits, food faddism, and emotional factors may limit intake. Certain metabolic abnormalities may also cause malnutrition. Requirements for essential nutrients may be increased during stress and disease and during the administration of antibiotics or of catabolic or anabolic drugs. Malnutrition may be acute or chronic, reversible or irreversible.

Precise evaluation of nutritional status is difficult. Severe disturbances are readily apparent, but mild disturbances may be overlooked, even after careful physical and laboratory examinations. The diagnosis of malnutrition rests on an accurate dietary history; upon evaluation of present deviations from average height, weight, head circumference, and past rates of growth; upon comparative measurements of midarm circumference and skinfold thickness; and upon chemical and other tests. Decreased skinfold thickness suggests protein-calorie malnutrition; excessive thickness indicates obesity. Muscle mass is calculated by subtracting skinfold measurements from arm circumference. For older children and adults midarm muscle circumference (cm) = arm circumference (cm) − (skinfold thickness [cm] × 3.14). Lean body mass can be estimated from 24 hr creatinine excretion. Deficiencies of some nutrients may be revealed by finding low blood levels of them or their metabolites, by observing biochemical or clinical effects of administration of the nutrients or their products, or by giving the patient substantial amounts of appropriate nutrients and noting the rate at which they are excreted. Protein reserves are assessed from serum albumin, transferrin, hemoglobin, prealbumin, or retinol-binding protein. Serum levels of essential amino acids may be lower than those of nonessential amino acids. Excretion of hydroxyproline is decreased and of 3-methylhistidine increased, and hair is easily plucked out in the severely malnourished child.

The most acute nutritional disturbances are those which involve water and electrolytes, especially sodium, potassium, chloride, and hydrogen ions (Chapter 5). Chronic malnutrition usually involves deficits of more than a single nutrient. Immunologic insufficiency is common in malnutrition and is demonstrated by total lymphocyte counts less than 1500/mm³ and anergy to skin test antigens, e.g., streptokinase-streptodornase, *Candida*, mumps, or tuberculin in exposed persons (Sec. 10.22 and 10.27).

3.16 MARASMUS
(Infantile Atrophy, Inanition, Athrepsia)

Severe malnutrition in infants is common in areas with insufficient food, inadequate knowledge of feeding techniques, or poor hygiene. The synonyms of marasmus listed above apply to patterns of clinical illness emphasizing one or more features of protein and calorie deficiency.

Etiology. The clinical picture of marasmus stems from an inadequate caloric intake due to insufficient diet, to improper feeding habits such as those of disturbed parent-child relations, or to metabolic abnormalities or congenital malformations. Severe impairment of any body system may result in malnutrition.

Clinical Manifestations. Initially, there is failure to gain weight, followed by loss of weight until emaciation results, with loss of turgor in skin which becomes wrinkled and loose as subcutaneous fat disappears. Because fat is lost last from the sucking pads of the cheeks, the face may retain a relatively normal appearance for some time before becoming shrunken and wizened. The abdomen may be distended or flat, and the intestinal pattern may be readily visible. Atrophy of muscles occurs, with resultant hypotonia. Edema may be present.

The temperature is usually subnormal, the pulse may be slow, and the basal metabolic rate tends to be reduced. At first the infant may be fretful but later becomes listless, and the appetite diminishes. The infant is usually constipated, but the so-called starvation type of diarrhea may appear, with frequent, small stools containing mucus.

3.17 PROTEIN MALNUTRITION
(PCM, Protein-Calorie Malnutrition, Kwashiorkor)

Because they are growing, children must consume enough nitrogenous food to maintain a positive nitrogen balance, whereas adults need only maintain nitrogen equilibrium.

Etiology. Although deficiencies of calories and other nutrients complicate the clinical and chemical patterns, the principal symptoms of protein malnutrition are due to insufficient intake of protein of good biologic value. There may also be impaired absorption of protein, as in chronic diarrheal states, abnormal losses of protein in proteinuria (nephrosis), infection, hemorrhage or burns, and failure of protein synthesis, as in chronic liver disease.

Kwashiorkor is a clinical syndrome that results from a severe deficiency of protein and an inadequate caloric intake. It is the most serious and prevalent form of malnutrition in the world today, especially in industrially underdeveloped areas.

Kwashiorkor means "deposed child," i.e., the child no longer suckled; it may become evident from early infancy to about 5 yr of age, usually after weaning from the breast.

Although gains in height and weight are accelerated with treatment, these measurements never equal those of consistently well-nourished children.

Clinical Manifestations (Fig. 3-2). Early clinical evidence of protein malnutrition is vague, but does include lethargy, apathy, or irritability. When well advanced, it results in inadequate growth, lack of stamina, loss of muscular tissue, increased susceptibility to infections, and edema. Secondary immunodeficiency is one of the most serious and constant manifestations. For example, measles, a relatively benign disease of the well nourished, can be devastating and fatal in malnourished children. The child may develop anorexia, flabbiness of subcutaneous tissues, and loss of muscle tone. The liver may enlarge early or late; fatty infiltration is common. Edema usually develops early; failure to gain weight may be masked by edema, which is often present in internal organs before it can be recognized in the face and limbs. Renal plasma flow, glomerular filtration rate, and renal tubular function are decreased. The heart may be small in the early stages of the disease but is usually enlarged later.

Dermatitis is common. Darkening of the skin appears in irritated areas but not in those exposed to sunlight, a contrast to the situation in pellagra (Sec. 3.25). Dyspigmentation may occur in these areas after desquamation or may be generalized. The hair is often sparse and thin and loses its elasticity. In dark-haired children, dyspigmentation may result in streaky red or gray hair color (hypochromotrichia). Hair texture becomes coarse in chronic disease.

Infections and parasitic infestations are common, as are anorexia, vomiting, and continued diarrhea. The muscles are weak, thin, and atrophic, but occasionally there may be an excess of subcutaneous fat. Mental changes, especially irritability and apathy, are common. Stupor, coma, and death may follow.

Laboratory Data. Decrease in the concentration of serum albumin is the most characteristic change. Ketonuria is common in the early stage of inanition but frequently disappears in the later stages. Blood glucose values are low, but glucose tolerance curves may be diabetic in type. Urinary excretion of hydroxyproline relative to creatinine may be decreased. Plasma values of essential amino acids may be decreased relative to nonessential ones, and there may be increased aminoaciduria. Potassium and magnesium deficiencies are frequent. The serum cholesterol level is low, but it returns to normal after a few days of treatment. The serum values of amylase, esterase, cholinesterase, transaminase, lipase, and alkaline phosphatase are decreased. There is diminished activity of the pancreatic enzymes and of xanthine oxidase, but these values return to normal shortly after the onset of treatment. Anemia may be normocytic, microcytic, or macrocytic. Other nutritional deficiencies, as of vitamins and minerals, are usually evident. Bone growth is usually delayed. Growth hormone secretion may be increased.

Differential Diagnosis. Differential diagnosis of protein deprivation includes chronic infections, diseases in which there is an excessive loss of protein through urine or stools, and conditions with a metabolic inability to synthesize protein.

Prevention. This requires a diet containing an adequate quantity of protein of good biologic quality. Since kwashiorkor has not only a serious and often fatal course but often permanent and devastating aftereffects in recovered children and their offspring, adequate dietary instruction and food distribution are urgently needed in endemic areas.

Treatment. Immediate management of any acute problems such as those of severe diarrhea, renal failure, and shock (Sec. 5.41) and, ultimately, the replacement of missing nutrients is essential. Moderate or severe dehydration, manifest or suspected infection, eye signs of severe vitamin A deficiency,

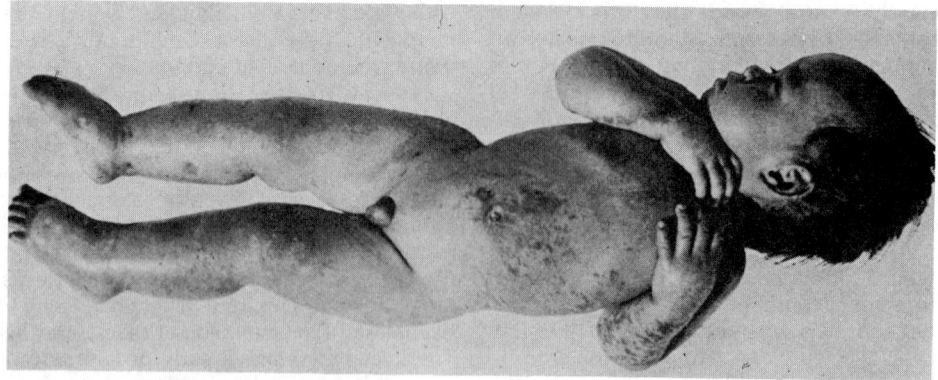

A

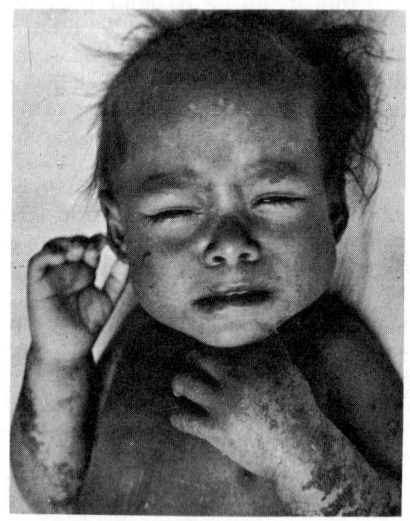

B

Figure 3–2. *A*, Kwashiorkor in a 2 yr old boy. Note the generalized edema, the typical skin lesions, and the state of prostration. *B*, Close-up of the same child showing the hair changes and psychic alterations (apathy and misery); the edema of the face and the skin lesions can be seen more clearly. (Photographs made available by the Institute of Nutrition of Central America and Panama [INCAP], Guatemala, through the courtesy of Dr. Moisés Béhar.)

severe anemia, hypoglycemia, continuing or recurrent diarrhea, skin and mucous membrane lesions, anorexia, and hypothermia all must be treated. For mild to moderate dehydration fluids are administered orally or by nasogastric tube (Sec. 5.24). A breast-fed infant should be nursed as often as he or she wants. For severe dehydration, intravenous fluids are necessary (Sec. 5.22). If intravenous fluids cannot be given, a rapid intraperitoneal infusion of 70 mL/kg of half-strength Ringer lactate solution may be lifesaving. Procaine benzylpenicillin and ampicillin should be given intramuscularly for 5–10 days.

When dehydration is corrected, oral feeding starts with small, frequent feeds of dilute milk; strength and volume are gradually increased and frequency decreased over the next 5 days. By day 6–8, the child should receive 150 mL/kg/day in 6 feeds. Cow's milk, or yogurt for the lactose-intolerant, should be made with 50 g sugar/L. Special feeds are available from UNICEF. In the recovery period high energy feeds made with milk, oil, and sugar are needed. Skim milk, casein hydrolysates, or synthetic amino acid mixtures may be used to supplement the basic fluid and nutritional regimen.

When high calorie and high protein diets are given too early and rapidly, the liver may become enlarged, the abdomen becomes markedly distended, and the child improves more slowly. Vegetable fat is better absorbed than cow's milk fat. Impaired glucose tolerance may be improved in some affected children by the daily administration of 250 μg of chromium chloride. Vitamins and minerals, especially vitamin A, potassium, and magnesium, are necessary from the outset of treatment. Iron and folic acid will usually correct the anemia.

Bacterial infections must be treated concomitantly with the dietary therapy, whereas treatment of parasitic infestations, if not severe, may be postponed until recovery is under way.

After treatment has been initiated, the patient may lose weight for a few weeks, due to loss of apparent or inapparent edema. Serum and intestinal enzymes return to normal, and intestinal absorption of fat and protein improves.

If growth and development has been extensively impaired, mental and physical retardation may be permanent. Apparently, the younger the infant at the time of deprivation, the more devastating are the long-term effects. Deficits in perceptual and abstract abilities are especially long-lasting.

3.18 MALNUTRITION IN CHILDREN BEYOND INFANCY

Etiology. Malnutrition in children may be a continuation of an undernourished state begun in infancy, or it may stem from factors that become operative during childhood. In general, the causes are the same as those responsible for malnutrition in infants. The problem may be complex. Poor dietary habits may be associated with a generally poor hygienic situation, with chronic disease, with finicky eating habits of other members of the family, or with disturbed parent-child relations (Sec. 5.36).

Poor eating habits in children under the age of 5 or 6 yr can often be traced directly to parental factors, of which overconcern about the quantity or quality of the diet is a common one. In children of all ages, insufficient sleep and too much emotional excitement, such as that associated with the movies and television, are important factors. School-age children often develop irregular or inappropriate eating habits, especially at breakfast and lunch, because sufficient time is not allotted or because the meals may be inadequate. During adolescence girls frequently restrict their dietary intake for cosmetic reasons. Eating between meals, especially of such items as candy and snack foods, usually reduces the mealtime appetite.

Clinical Manifestations. Malnutrition does not invariably result in underweight. Fatigue, lassitude, restlessness, and irritability are frequent manifestations. Restlessness and overactivity are frequently misinterpreted by parents as evidences of lack of fatigue. Anorexia, easily induced digestive disturbances, and constipation are common complaints, and even in older children the starvation type of mucoid diarrheal stool may be observed. Malnourished children often have a limited span of attention and do poorly in school. They have increased susceptibility to infections. Muscular development is inadequate, and the flabby muscles result in a posture of fatigue, with rounded shoulders, flat chest, and protuberant abdomen. Such children often look tired; the face is pale, the complexion is "muddy," and the eyes lack luster. Hypochromic anemia is common. In protracted cases there may be delayed epiphyseal development, irregularities in dentition, and delayed puberty.

Evaluation should always include a careful history of dietary habits, psychosocial maladjustments, physical hygiene, and illness; a thorough physical examination; and appropriate laboratory examinations.

Treatment. There is a great need for individualized treatment aimed at correcting underlying psychologic and physical disturbances. An adequate diet (Sec. 3.14) should be outlined; vitamin concentrates may be added and continued for a time after the dietary intake has become adequate. When anorexia is a problem, the essential items of the diet should be provided in as concentrated a form as possible, and the fat content should be low. Between-meal snacks need not be prohibited if they do not interfere with the appetite for the next meal; milk or candy should not be given at such times; fruit or fruit juices are appropriate. Re-educating of the entire family about eating habits may be necessary (Sec. 5.36).

Cupoli JM, Hallock JA, Barness LA: Failure to thrive. Current Probl Pediatr No. 11, Sept, 1980.

Hegsted DM: Protein-calorie malnutrition. Am Scientist 66:61, 1978.

Katz M, Stiehm ER: Host defense in malnutrition. Pediatrics 59:490, 1977.

Robinson H, Picou D: A comparison of fasting plasma insulin and growth hormone concentrations in marasmic, kwashiorkor, marasmic-kwashiorkor and underweight children. Pediatr Res 11:637, 1977.

Sleisenger MH, Kim YS: Protein digestion and absorption. N Engl J Med 300:659, 1979.

Zain BK, Haquani AH, Qureshi N, et al: Studies on the significance of hair root protein and DNA in protein calorie malnutrition. Am J Clin Nutr 30:1094, 1977.

3.19 PROTEIN EXCESS

Excessive protein intake, especially in the absence of sufficient water, may lead to signs of dehydration—protein fever. Signs of protein excess are rare, but premature infants fed a high protein diet may have an increased morbidity. Marasmic infants fed high protein diets during the recovery phase may develop hyperammonemia; protein intoxication has also been noted in children with other liver disease. Some weight reducing diets with high protein content may be responsible for protein intoxication.

Barness LA, Omans WB, Rose CS, et al: Progress of premature infants fed a formula containing demineralized whey. Pediatrics 32:52, 1963.

3.20 OBESITY

No exact line separates good nutrition and overnutrition; practically, the diagnosis is made from the child's appearance rather than from an arbitrary weight excess. Stocky children may have relatively large skeletal frames and more than the average amount of muscular tissue so that their weight and height as well as their "bigness" exceed those of the average child of their age, but they are not to be considered obese. Obesity or overnutrition is a generalized, excessive accumulation of fat in subcutaneous and other tissues that can be quantitated by measuring skinfold thickness with calipers.

Etiology. Obesity is usually due to an excessive intake of food. Appetite may be influenced by a variety of factors that include psychologic disturbances; hypothalamic, pituitary, or other brain lesions; and hyperinsulinism. Genetic predisposition to obesity occurs in certain animals and may occur in man. In a study of adults, obesity was found to be seven times more common in the lowest than in the highest socioeconomic class. Lack of activity may be responsible for obesity even though intake of food may not be unusual. Illnesses that keep a child in bed for prolonged periods of time may also result in obesity. Some inherited syndromes such as the Laurence-Moon-Biedl, Prader-Willi, and Cushing usually include obesity, on either an endocrine or inactivity basis.

Obesity may result from increases in numbers or in size of fat cells, adipocytes. Adipocytes appear to increase in number when caloric intake is increased, especially in the gestational months and during the first year of life. This stimulus to increase in number continues, though at a reduced rate, throughout puberty, so that during periods of adolescent weight reduction, the size but not the number of adipocytes decreases.

The obese may become resistant to insulin, resulting in an increase in levels of circulating insulin. Insulin decreases lipolysis and increases fat synthesis and uptake. The obese respond to a carbohydrate meal with increased insulin and a decreased utilization of free fatty acids. During weight reduction regimens, the obese deliver less food to their cells than the lean, owing to decreased mobilization of free fatty acids. In starvation after obesity, fat is mobilized as serum insulin decreases. Protein conservation is facilitated as the brain utilizes ketones for energy. During starvation, serum alanine levels decrease and glycine levels rise.

Purified sugars as well as high protein diet may cause greater secretion of insulin than do complex carbohydrates.

The chronic and uncritical offering of a bottle as a means of dealing with a fretful or crying infant may establish a habit that leads the infant to expect or seek food whenever experiencing frustration. If obesity is initiated early, it is likely to persist. Similarly, the uncritical early introduction of high calorie solid foods may lead to rapid weight gain and to obesity.

Clinical Manifestations. Obesity may become evident at any age, but it appears most frequently in the first year of life, at 5–6 yr of age, and during adolescence. The child whose obesity is due to excessively high caloric intake is usually not only heavier than others in his or her cohort but also taller, and bone age is advanced. The facial features often appear disproportionately fine. The adiposity in the mammary regions of boys is often suggestive of breast development and therefore an embarrassing feature. The abdomen tends to be pendulous, and white or purple striae are often present. The external genitalia of boys appear disproportionately small but actually are most often of average size; the penis is often imbedded in the pubic fat. Puberty may occur early, with the result that the ultimate height of the obese may be less than that of their slower maturing peers. The development of the external genitalia is normal in the majority of girls, and menarche is usually not delayed. The obesity of the extremities is usually greater in the upper arm and thigh and is at times limited to them. The hands may be relatively small and the fingers tapering. Genu valgum is common.

Psychologic disturbances are common in obese children.

Even in the apparently well adjusted child adequate psychologic evaluation often discloses significant underlying emotional problems. These may have initially contributed to the causes of obesity and usually are an additive factor in its maintenance.

Prevention and Treatment. Because obesity may be self-perpetuating for psychologic or physiologic reasons, children of obese parents or those with obese siblings should be encouraged to adhere to a systematic program of energetic exercise and a balanced low calorie diet. Idealized weight is desirable not only for esthetic reasons but also to prevent such complications of obesity as diabetes, shortness of breath, and early death. Untreated overweight infants almost always remain overweight as adults. Treatment of the obese child usually fails unless the child is motivated to lose weight. Modifying behavior to include increased activity is helpful.

In planning the diet, the basic nutritional needs must be met. All the essential dietary needs may be included in an 1100- to 1300-calorie diet for children 10–14 yr of age for several months (Table 3–15). Some children avoid excessive eating after they have been allowed to return to a free choice of diet. The diet should contain as much bulk as possible. At times greater cooperation is secured if small portions of the diet are permitted between meals, especially in the afternoon. If there is doubt that the daily vitamin intake is adequate, vitamin concentrates may be prescribed. Vitamin D should be included, as for all growing children. Rapid decreases in weight should not be attempted, and medical supervision should be maintained. During the growing years, maintenance of weight while the child increases in height is often a sufficient goal. At best there is a limited place for drug therapy. Psychologic support is often an essential element in management, and both dietary and psychologic treatment should involve the entire family.

The *pickwickian syndrome* (for the fat boy, Joe, in Dickens' *Pickwick Papers*) is a rare complication of extreme exogenous obesity, in which there is severe cardiorespiratory distress. The extreme obesity causes alveolar hypoventilation, with a decrease in pulmonary, tidal, and expiratory reserve volumes. The manifestations include polycythemia, hypoxemia, cyanosis, cardiac enlargement, congestive cardiac failure, and

Table 3–15. **1100-1300-Calorie Diet**

Breakfast

1 orange, ½ grapefruit, or 1 cup of tomato juice
1 egg
1 slice of whole-wheat bread or 1 serving of cereal without sugar
1 teaspoonful of butter
6 oz of whole milk

Lunch

2 ounces of lean meat, 1 egg, or ½ cup of cottage cheese
1 serving of raw vegetable as salad—no dressing
1 slice of whole-wheat bread
1 teaspoonful of butter
1 serving of fresh or unsweetened fruit
6 oz of whole milk

Dinner

2 ounces of lean meat (liver once a week), poultry, or fish
2 servings of green, yellow, or red vegetables*
1 serving of fresh or unsweetened fruit
6 oz of whole milk
    (Part or all of bread and butter from one of the other meals
    may be included here)
A 1000-Calorie diet may be obtained by eliminating the butter or cream from milk. In this case it becomes especially important to add vitamin A to the daily diet.

*Does not include Irish or sweet potatoes, parsnips, dried peas or beans, lima beans, or corn.

somnolence. High concentrations of oxygen may be dangerous in treating the cyanosis since respiration may depend solely on the stimulatory effect of hypoxia. Weight reduction is extremely important and should be accomplished as rapidly as feasible.

American Academy of Pediatrics Committee on Nutrition: Obesity in infancy and childhood. Pediatrics 68:880, 1981.
Bistrian BR, Blackburn GL, Stanbury JB: Metabolic aspects of a protein-sparing modified fast in the dietary management of Prader-Willi obesity. N Engl J Med 296:774, 1977.
Felig P, Wahren J: Fuel homeostasis in exercise. N Engl J Med 293:1078, 1975.
Striker EM: Hyperphagia. N Engl J Med 298:1010, 1978.

VITAMINS

Vitamins are essential nutrients that must be supplied exogenously. Functions of vitamins are summarized in Table 3–6, and recommended daily allowances in Table 3–1. Toxicity is more commonly seen with excesses of the fat-soluble vitamins A and D than with the water-soluble vitamins. The vitamin-dependent states are summarized in Table 3–16.

3.21 VITAMIN A DEFICIENCY

The term vitamin A is a generic label for all β-ionone derivatives other than provitamin A carotenoids. Retinol signifies vitamin A alcohol retinyl ester, vitamin A ester; retinal, vitamin A aldehyde; and retinoic acid, vitamin A acid.

"Provitamin A carotenoids" is the generic term for all carotenoids that have the biologic activity of β-carotene. They or their derivatives with vitamin A activity are required in the diets of infants and children.

Beta-carotene is partly absorbed by the intestinal lymphatics; the remainder is cleaved into two molecules of retinol. Dietary retinyl ester is hydrolyzed to retinol in the intestine. Retinol is esterified inside the mucosal cell with palmitic acid and is stored in the liver as retinyl palmitate; this in turn is hydrolyzed to free retinol for transport to its site of action. Zinc is required for this mobilization. Normal plasma values of retinol in infants are 20–50 μg/dL; in children and adults, 30–225 μg/dL.

Heavy ingestion of carotenoids may result in large amounts of carotene in the blood and in yellow discoloration of the skin but not of the sclera. This disorder, carotenemia, is especially apt to occur in children with liver disease, diabetes mellitus, or hypothyroidism and in those who have congenital absence of enzymes that convert provitamin A carotenoids.

Etiology. The liver at birth has a low vitamin A content which is rapidly augmented since colostrum and breast milk furnish large amounts of the vitamin. Breast milk and whole cow's milk are satisfactory sources of vitamin A. Other foods (vegetables, fruits, eggs, butter, liver) or vitamin supplements also provide vitamin A. Loss of it in cooking, canning, and freezing of foodstuffs is small; oxidizing agents, however, destroy it.

The risk of vitamin A deficiency is small in healthy children with balanced diets. Deficient diets commonly cause disease by 2–3 yr of age. Vitamin A deficiency also results from inadequate intestinal absorption, as, for example, with chronic intestinal disorders, celiac disease, hepatic and pancreatic diseases, iron deficiency anemia, chronic infectious diseases, or chronic ingestion of mineral oil. Low intake of dietary fat results in low vitamin A absorption. Vitamin A excretion is increased in cancer, urinary tract disease, and chronic infectious diseases. Low protein intake results in deficient carrier protein and in decreases in plasma concentration of vitamin A.

Pathology. The human retina contains two distinct photoreceptor systems: the rods are sensitive to light of low inten-

Table 3–16. **Vitamin Dependency States**

Vitamin	Disease	Untreated State	Daily Dosage
A	Darier	Hyperkeratosis follicularis	25,000 IU
B₁	Leigh—pyruvic-lactic acidosis	Ataxia, retardation	600 mg
	Thiamine-responsive anemia	Megaloblastic anemia	20 mg
	Maple syrup urine disease	Hypotonia, seizures	10 mg
Riboflavin	Pyruvate kinase deficiency	Hemolysis	10 mg
Niacin	Hartnup	Ataxia, eczema	200 mg
B₆	Cystathioninuria	No symptoms	200 mg
	Homocystinuria	Retardation	200 mg
	B₆-anemia	Hypochromic microcytic anemia	10 mg
	B₆-seizures	Seizures	25 mg
	Xanthurenic aciduria	Retardation	10 mg
	Gyrate atrophy of choroid	Blindness	100 mg
	Oxaluria	Oxalate crystals	100 mg
Folic acid	Formiminotransferase deficiency	Retardation	5 mg
	Folate reductase deficiency	Megaloblastic anemia	5 mg
	Homocystinuria	Retardation	10 mg
B₁₂	Methylmalonic acidemia	Retardation	1 mg
Biotin	Propionic acidemia	Retardation	10 mg
	β-Methylcrotonyl glycinuria	Coma	10 mg
C	Chédiak-Higashi	Infections	50 mg
D	Dependency	Rickets	4000 IU
	Familial hypophosphatemia	Rickets	100,000 IU

sity, the cones to colors and to light of high intensity. Retinal is the prosthetic group of the photosensitive pigment in both rods and cones. The major difference between the visual pigments in rods (rhodopsin) and in cones (iodopsin) is the nature of the protein bound to retinal. All-*trans* retinal isomerizes in the dark to 11-*cis* form. This combines with opsin to form rhodopsin. Energy from light quanta reconverts 11-*cis* retinal back to the all-*trans* form; this energy exchange, transmitted via the optic nerves to the brain, results in visual sensation. Beta-carotene has been effective in ameliorating photosensitivity in patients with erythropoietic protoporphyria. It has also been suggested that retinitis pigmentosa may be related to a defect in retinol-binding protein.

Vitamin A is apparently necessary for membrane stability. Both excess and deficiency of vitamin A lead to rupture of lysosomal membranes with release of hydrolases.

The vitamin plays a role in keratinization, cornification, bone metabolism, placental development, growth, spermatogenesis, and mucus formation. Characteristic changes in epithelium include proliferation of basal cells, hyperkeratosis, and the formation of stratified, cornified, squamous epithelium. Epithelial changes in the respiratory system may result in bronchiolar obstruction. Squamous metaplasia of the renal pelves, ureters, urinary bladder, enamel organs, and pancreatic and salivary ducts may lead to an increase in infections in these areas.

Clinical Manifestations. Ocular lesions develop insidiously. Initially, the posterior segment of the eye is affected, with impairment of dark adaptation resulting in night blindness. Later, drying of the conjunctiva (xerosis conjunctivae) and of the cornea (xerosis corneae) is followed by wrinkling and cloudiness of the cornea (keratomalacia) (Fig. 3–3). Dry, silver-gray plaques may appear on the bulbar conjunctiva (Bitot spots), with follicular hyperkeratosis and photophobia.

Vitamin A deficiency may result in retardation of mental and physical growth and in apathy. Anemia with or without hepatosplenomegaly is usually present.

The skin is dry and scaly, and at times follicular hyperker-

atosis may be found on the shoulders, buttocks, and extensor surfaces of the extremities. The vaginal epithelium may become cornified, and epithelial metaplasia of the urinary tract may contribute to pyuria and hematuria. Increased intracranial pressure with wide separation of cranial bones at the sutures may occur. Hydrocephalus, with or without paralyses of the cranial nerves, is an infrequent manifestation.

Diagnosis. Dark adaptation tests may be helpful. Xerosis conjunctivae can be detected by biomicroscopic examination of the conjunctiva. Examination of the scrapings from the eye

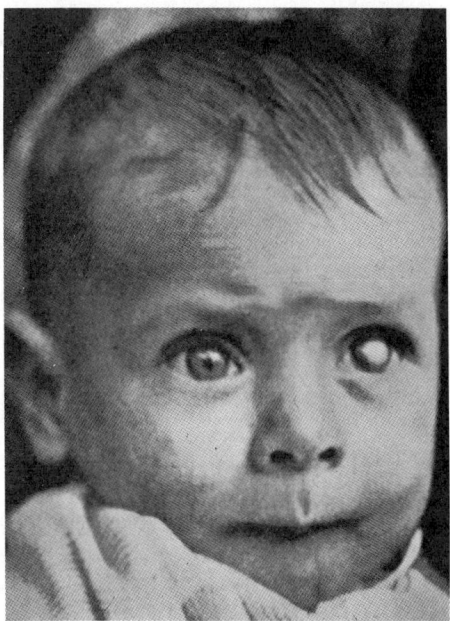

Figure 3–3. Recovery from xerophthalmia, showing permanent eye lesion. (From Bloch: Am J Dis Child, Vol 27.)

and vagina is recommended as a diagnostic aid. The plasma carotene concentration falls quickly, but that of vitamin A decreases more slowly. A standard absorption test for vitamin A is available. Low absorption curves are obtained in children with cystic fibrosis, celiac disease, obliteration of the bile ducts, and cretinism (Sec. 12.49).

Prevention. Infants should receive at least 500 μg* daily; older children and adults, 600–1500 μg of vitamin A or carotene. The average diets of infants and children in this country supply enough vitamin A to prevent symptoms of deficiency.

For therapeutic reasons low fat diets should be supplemented with vitamin A. In disorders with poor absorption of fat or increased excretion of vitamin A, water-miscible preparations of vitamin A should be administered in amounts several times the usual daily requirement. Premature infants, who absorb fats and vitamin A less efficiently than do full-term infants, should also receive water-miscible preparations. In areas of the world where vitamin A deficiency occurs, 100,000 IU of vitamin A should be given orally in a water-miscible base 4 times yearly; the same dose should be given postpartum to the mothers of breast-fed infants in these regions.

Treatment. In cases of latent vitamin A deficiency, a daily supplement of 5000 IU of vitamin A is sufficient. For xerophthalmia, 5000 IU/kg/24 hr is given orally for 5 days and then continued with intramuscular injection of 25,000 IU of vitamin A in oil daily until recovery occurs.

Hypervitaminosis A. Acute hypervitaminosis A may occur in infants after ingesting 300,000 IU or more. The symptoms are nausea, vomiting, drowsiness, and bulging of the fontanel. Diplopia, papilledema, cranial nerve palsies, and other symptoms suggestive of brain tumor (*pseudotumor cerebri*) may also occur.

Chronic hypervitaminosis A appears after ingestion of excessive doses for several weeks or months. The child has anorexia, pruritus, and a lack of weight gain. There is increasing irritability, limitation of motion, and tender swelling of the bones. Alopecia, seborrheic cutaneous lesions, fissuring of the corners of the mouth, increased intracranial pressure, and hepatomegaly may develop. Craniotabes and desquamation of the palms and soles are common. Roentgenograms reveal hyperostosis affecting several long bones; it is most notable at the middle of the shafts (Fig. 3–4).

Severe congenital malformations may occur in infants of mothers consuming large amounts of oral retinoids used in treating acne.

A history of excessive ingestion of vitamin A helps to differentiate it from cortical hyperostosis (Sec. 23.42). Besides a history of excess, the serum vitamin A level is elevated and hypercalcemia or liver cirrhosis occasionally occurs.

DeLuca HF: Retinoic acid metabolism. Fed Proc 38:2519, 1979.
Fisher KD, Carr CJ, Huff JE, et al: Dark adaptation and night vision. Fed Proc 29:1605, 1970.
Goodman DS: Vitamin A metabolism. Fed Proc 39:2716, 1980.
Gouras P, Chauder G: Retinitis pigmentosa and retinol-binding protein. Invest Ophthalmol 13:239, 1974.
Mahoney CP, Margolis T, Knauss TA, et al: Chronic vitamin A intoxication in infants fed chicken liver. Pediatrics 65:893, 1980.
Mathews-Roth MM, Pathak MA, Fitzpatrick TB, et al: Beta-carotene as an oral protective agent in erythropoietic protoporphyria. JAMA 228:1004, 1974.
McLaren DS, Shirajain E, Tchallian M, et al: Xerophthalmia in Jordan. Am J Clin Nutr 17:117, 1965.
Peck GL: Prolonged remissions of cystic and conglobate acne with 13-cis-retinoic acid. N Engl J Med 300:299, 1979.
Sporn MB, Newton DL: Chemoprevention of cancer with retinoids. Fed Proc 38:2528, 1979.

*One international unit (IU) of vitamin A is equivalent to 0.3 μg of retinol (vitamin A alcohol).

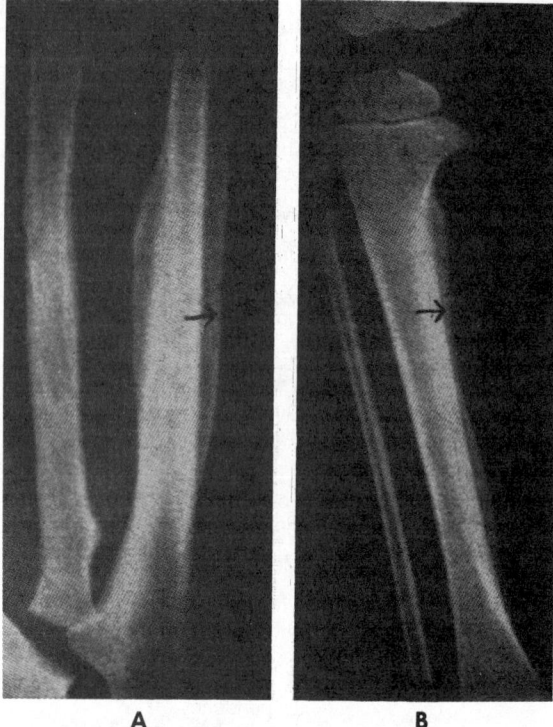

A   **B**

Figure 3–4. Hyperostosis of the ulna and the tibia in an infant 21 mo of age, resulting from vitamin A poisoning. *A*, Long, wavy cortical hyperostosis of ulna. *B*, Long, wavy cortical hyperostosis of right tibia; striking absence of metaphyseal changes. (From Caffey J: Pediatrics, Vol 5. Courtesy of Charles C Thomas, Publisher, Springfield, IL.)

3.22 VITAMIN B COMPLEX DEFICIENCY

Vitamin B complex includes several factors whose chemical composition and function vary widely (Table 3–6). All are important constituents of enzyme systems. Since many of these enzymes are closely related functionally, lack of a single factor can interrupt an entire chain of chemical processes, producing diverse clinical manifestations.

Diets deficient in any one factor of the B complex are frequently poor sources of other B vitamins. Since manifestations of several B deficiencies can usually be found in the same patient, it is generally practical to treat the patient with the entire B complex.

Factors such as pantothenic acid, choline, and inositol are important for the normal functioning of the human organism, but at present no specific deficiency syndromes can be ascribed to their lack in the diets of children.

3.23 THIAMINE DEFICIENCY
(Beriberi)

Etiology. Vitamin B_1 (thiamine) is water-soluble and, as thiamine pyrophosphate or cocarboxylase, functions as a coenzyme in carbohydrate metabolism. Thiamine is required for the synthesis of acetylcholine, and deficiency results in impaired nerve conduction. It is the coenzyme in transketolation and in decarboxylation of α-keto acids. Transketolase participates in the hexose monophosphate shunt which generates NADPH and pentose.

Breast milk or cow's milk, vegetables, cereals, fruits, and eggs are sources of thiamine. Infants whose source of food is the milk of thiamine-deficient mothers may develop beriberi. Older children whose diet contains good sources of thiamine such as meats and legumes do not require thiamine supplements.

Thiamine is easily destroyed by heat in neutral or alkaline media and is readily extracted from foodstuffs by cooking water. An enzyme factor destructive to thiamine is present in some fish. Since the covering of grains of cereals contains most of the vitamin, polishing reduces its availability.

Thiamine absorption decreases with gastrointestinal or liver disease. Requirements increase with fever, surgery, or stress. Thiamine dependency has been described in a child with megaloblastic anemia and in an infant with otherwise typical maple syrup urine disease. The urine of children with *Leigh encephalomyelopathy* and of their parents inhibits the formation of thiamine pyrophosphate. Large doses of thiamine improve some of the physical abnormalities associated with the disease.

Pathology. In fatal cases of beriberi, lesions are located principally in the heart, peripheral nerves, subcutaneous tissue, and serous cavities. The heart is dilated, and fatty degeneration of the myocardium is common. Generalized edema or edema of the legs, serous effusions, and venous engorgement may be present. The peripheral nerves undergo varying degrees of degeneration of myelin and axon cylinders, with wallerian degeneration, beginning in the distal locations. The nerves of the lower extremities are affected first. Lesions in the brain include vascular dilatation and hemorrhage.

Clinical Manifestations. Early manifestations of deficiency include fatigue, apathy, irritability, depression, drowsiness, poor mental concentration, anorexia, nausea, and abdominal discomfort. Signs of progression include peripheral neuritis with tingling, burning, and paresthesias of the toes and feet; decreased tendon reflexes; loss of vibration sense; tenderness and cramping of leg muscles; congestive heart failure; and psychic disturbances. There may be ptosis of the eyelids and atrophy of the optic nerve. Hoarseness due to paralysis of the laryngeal nerve is a characteristic sign. Muscle atrophy and tenderness of nerve trunks are followed by ataxia, loss of coordination, and loss of deep sensation. Paralytic symptoms are more common in adults than in children. Later, signs of increased intracranial pressure, meningismus, and coma occur.

In *dry* beriberi the child may appear plump but is pale, flabby, listless, and dyspneic; the heart rate is rapid and the liver enlarged. In *wet* beriberi the child is undernourished, pale, and edematous and has dyspnea, vomiting, and tachycardia. The skin appears waxy. The urine may contain albumin and casts.

The cardiac signs at first are slight cyanosis and dyspnea. Tachycardia, enlargement of the liver, loss of consciousness, and convulsions may develop rapidly. The heart is enlarged, especially to the right. The electrocardiogram shows increased Q-T interval, inversion of T waves, and low voltage, changes which rapidly revert to normal with treatment. Cardiac failure may lead to death in either chronic or acute beriberi.

Diagnosis. Since the early symptoms are encountered in many types of nutritional disturbances besides thiamine deficiency, demonstrations of lowered red cell transketolase and high blood or urinary glyoxylate values have been proposed as diagnostic tests. Excretion after an oral loading dose of thiamine or its metabolites, thiazole or pyrimidine, may help to identify the deficiency state. Clinical response to administration of thiamine remains the best test for thiamine deficiency.

Prevention. A maternal diet containing sufficient amounts of thiamine prevents this deficiency in breast-fed infants (Table 3–1). Thiamine requirements increase with a high carbohydrate content of the diet.

Treatment. If beriberi occurs in a breast-fed infant, both mother and child should be treated with thiamine. The daily dose for adults is 50 mg and for children 10 mg or more. Oral administration is effective unless gastrointestinal disturbances prevent absorption. Thiamine should be given intramuscularly or intravenously to children with cardiac failure. Such treatment is followed by dramatic improvement, though complete cure requires several weeks. The heart is not permanently damaged. Since beriberi patients often suffer from other B complex deficiencies, all other vitamins of the B complex should be administered, in addition to large doses of thiamine chloride.

3.24 RIBOFLAVIN DEFICIENCY
(Ariboflavinosis)

Riboflavin deficiency without deficiencies of other members of the B complex is rare. Riboflavin, a yellow, fluorescent, water-soluble substance, is stable to heat and acids but destroyed by light and alkalis. The coenzymes flavin mononucleotide (FMN) and flavin adenine dinucleotide (FAD) are synthesized from riboflavin, forming the prosthetic groups of several enzymes important in electron transport. Riboflavin is essential for growth and tissue respiration; it may play a role in light adaptation and is required for conversion of pyridoxine to pyridoxal phosphate. Large amounts of riboflavin occur in liver, kidney, brewer's yeast, milk, cheese, eggs, and leafy vegetables; cow's milk contains about five times as much riboflavin as human milk.

Riboflavin deficiency is usually due to inadequate intake. Faulty absorption may contribute in patients with biliary atresia or hepatitis or in those receiving probenecid, phenothiazine, or oral contraceptives. Phototherapy destroys riboflavin.

Clinical Manifestations. Evidences of riboflavin deficiency include cheilosis (perlèche), glossitis, keratitis, conjunctivitis, photophobia, lacrimation, marked corneal vascularization, and seborrheic dermatitis. Cheilosis begins with pallor at the angles of the mouth, followed by thinning and maceration of the epithelium. Superficial fissures often covered by yellow crusts develop in the angles of the mouth and extend radially into the skin for distances of 1–2 cm. Cheilosis epidemics occur in institutions and in families whose diet is inadequate. With glossitis the tongue is smooth, and loss of papillary structure occurs. A normocytic, normochromic anemia with bone marrow hypoplasia is common.

Diagnosis. Urinary excretion of riboflavin below 30 μg/24 hr is abnormally low. Levels of erythrocyte glutathionine reductase, a flavoprotein requiring FAD, may reflect the stores of riboflavin. A patient with hemolysis due to pyruvate kinase deficiency and reduced erythrocyte glutathionine reductase had both enzyme activities restored to normal on administration of riboflavin.

Prevention. Recommended daily allowances are presented in Table 3–1. Riboflavin deficiency is usually prevented by a diet that contains adequate amounts of milk, eggs, leafy vegetables, and lean meats.

Treatment. Treatment consists in the oral administration of 3–10 mg of riboflavin daily. If no response occurs within a few days, intramuscular injections of 2 mg of riboflavin in saline solution may be made three times daily. The child should also be given a well balanced diet and, at least temporarily, more than the usual requirements of the B complex.

3.25 NIACIN DEFICIENCY
(Pellagra)

Etiology. Pellagra (*pellis*, skin; *agra*, rough), a deficiency disease due mainly to a lack of niacin (nicotinic acid), affects all tissues of the body. Niacin forms part of two enzymes important in electron transfer and glycolysis: nicotinamide adenine dinucleotide (NAD) and nicotinamide adenine dinucleotide phosphate (NADP). Although dietary tryptophan can partially substitute for niacin, other sources of niacin are necessary. Liver, lean pork, salmon, poultry, and red meat are good sources, but most cereals contain only small amounts of it. Pellagra occurs chiefly in countries where corn (maize), a poor source of tryptophan, is a basic foodstuff. Milk and eggs, which contain little niacin, are good pellagra-preventive foods because of their high content of tryptophan. Because niacin is a stable compound, there are only small losses in cooking.

Pathology. Histologically, edema and degeneration of the superficial collagen of the dermis occur. The papillary vessels are engorged, and there is perivascular lymphocytic infiltration in the dermis. The epidermis is hyperkeratotic and later becomes atrophic.

Changes comparable to those in the skin are present in the tongue, buccal mucous membranes, and vagina. These changes may be associated with secondary infection and ulceration. The walls of the colon are thickened and inflamed with patches of pseudomembrane; later the mucosa atrophies. Changes in the nervous system occur relatively late in the disease and consist of patchy areas of demyelinization and degeneration of ganglion cells; demyelinization in the spinal cord may involve the posterior and lateral columns.

Clinical Manifestations. The early symptoms of pellagra are vague. Anorexia, lassitude, weakness, burning sensations, numbness, and dizziness may be prodromal symptoms. After a long period of niacin deficiency the characteristic symptoms appear. The classic triad consists of dermatitis, diarrhea, and dementia. Manifestations in children who have parasites or chronic disorders may be especially severe.

The most characteristic manifestations are the cutaneous ones, which may develop suddenly or insidiously and may be elicited by irritants, particularly by intense sunlight. They first appear as symmetric erythema of the exposed surfaces that may resemble sunburn and in mild cases may escape recognition. The lesions are usually sharply demarcated from the healthy skin around them, and their distribution may change frequently. The lesions on the hands sometimes have the appearance of a glove (pellagrous glove) (Fig. 3–5), and similar demarcations are occasionally seen on the foot and leg (pellagrous boot) or around the neck (Casal necklace). In some instances vesicles and bullae develop (wet type), or there may

be suppuration beneath the scaly, crusted epidermis; in others the swelling disappears after a short time and desquamation begins. The healed parts of the skin may remain pigmented.

The cutaneous lesions are sometimes preceded by stomatitis, glossitis, vomiting, or diarrhea. Swelling and redness of the tip of the tongue and its lateral margins may be followed by intense redness of the entire tongue and of the papillae and even ulceration.

Nervous symptoms include depression, disorientation, insomnia, and delirium.

The classic symptoms of pellagra are usually not well developed in infants and children. Anorexia, irritability, anxiety, and apathy are common in "pellagra families." They may also have sore tongues and lips, and the skin is usually dry and scaly. Diarrhea and constipation may alternate and a moderate secondary anemia may occur. Children who have pellagra often have evidences of other nutritional deficiency diseases.

Diagnosis. Diagnosis is usually made from the physical signs of glossitis, gastrointestinal symptoms, and a symmetrical dermatitis. Rapid clinical response to niacin is an important confirming test. N-methylnicotinamide, a normal metabolite of niacin, is almost undetectable in urine during niacin deficiency.

Prevention. A well balanced diet containing meat, vegetables, eggs, and milk meets the recommended daily allowances (Table 3–1), so supplements of niacin are necessary only in breast-fed infants whose mothers have pellagra or in children on restricted diets.

Treatment. Children respond rapidly to antipellagral therapy. A liberal and well balanced diet should be supplemented with 50–300 mg of niacin daily; 100 mg may be given intravenously in severe cases or in cases of poor intestinal absorption. Administering large doses of niacin is often followed within a half hour by a sensation of increased local heat and flushing and burning of the skin, unpleasant effects that are not produced by niacinamide. But large doses of niacin may cause cholestatic jaundice or hepatotoxicity.

The diet should be supplemented with other vitamins, especially with other members of the B complex. Sun exposure should be avoided during the active phase; the skin lesions may be covered with soothing applications. A blood transfusion may be helpful when there is severe anemia; less severe hypochromic anemia should be treated with iron. The diet of the cured pellagrin should be continuously supervised to prevent recurrence.

Thiamine Deficiency

Brin M: Erythrocyte as a biopsy tissue for functional evaluation of thiamin adequacy. JAMA 187:762, 1964.
McCandless DW, Schenker S: Neurologic disorders of thiamine deficiency. Nutr Rev 27:213, 1969.

Riboflavin Deficiency

Rillotson JA, Baker EM: An enzymatic measurement of the riboflavin status in man. Am J Clin Nutr 25:425, 1972.
Rivlin RS: Hormones, drugs and riboflavin. Nutr Rev 37:241, 1979.
Staal GEJ, Van Berkel TJC, Nijessen JG, et al: Normalization of red blood cell pyruvate kinase in pyruvate kinase deficiency by riboflavin treatment. Clin Chim Acta 60:323, 1975.

Niacin Deficiency

Darby WJ, McNutt KW, Todhunter EN: Niacin. Nutr Rev 33:289, 1975.

3.26 PYRIDOXINE (VITAMIN B₆) DEFICIENCY

Vitamin B_6 includes pyridoxal, pyridoxine, and pyridoxamine. These are converted to pyridoxal-5-phosphate (or pyridoxamine-5-phosphate), which acts as a coenzyme in decarboxylation and transamination of amino acids, e.g., in

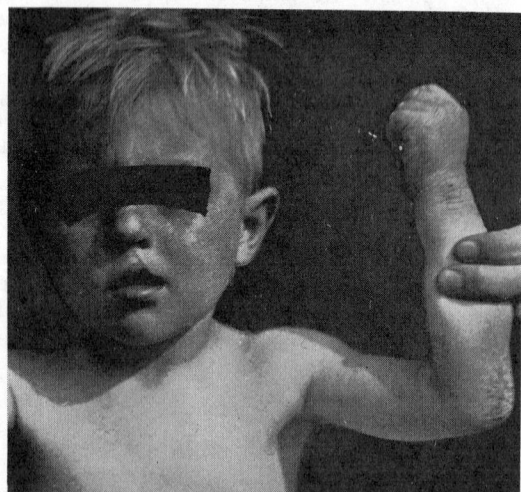

Figure 3–5. Pellagra in a boy 3 yr of age, showing lesions on the hand and elbow and an early lesion over the nose and malar eminences.

the decarboxylation of 5-hydroxytryptophan in the formation of serotonin, and in the metabolism of glycogen and fatty acids. Vitamin B_6 is also essential for the breakdown of kynurenine. When this does not occur, xanthurenic acid appears in the urine. Adequate functioning of the nervous system depends on pyridoxine, deficiency of which leads to seizures and to peripheral neuropathy. Pyridoxal phosphate is the coenzyme for both glutamic decarboxylase and γ-aminobutyric acid transaminase; each is necessary for normal brain metabolism. It participates in active transport of amino acids across cell membranes, chelates metals, and participates in the synthesis of arachidonic acid from linoleic acid. If it is lacking, glycine metabolism may lead to oxaluria. It is excreted largely as 4-pyridoxic acid.

Etiology. Pyridoxine is adequately available in human and cow's milk and in cereals, but prolonged heat processing of the latter two destroys it. Diseases with malabsorption, such as celiac syndrome, may contribute to vitamin B_6 deficiency.

There are several types of *vitamin B_6 dependency syndromes*, presumably the result of errors in enzyme structure or function, in which the patient responds to very large amounts of pyridoxine. These syndromes include B_6-dependent convulsions, a B_6-responsive anemia, xanthurenic aciduria, cystathioninuria, and homocystinuria.

Pyridoxine antagonists, such as isonicotinic acid hydrazide (isoniazid) used in the treatment of tuberculosis, increase the requirements for pyridoxine, as do pregnancy and drugs such as penicillamine, hydralazine, and the oral progesterone-estrogen contraceptives.

Clinical Manifestations. Deficiency symptoms are not as common in children as in adults. Four clinical disturbances due to vitamin B_6 deficiency have been described in man: convulsions in infants, peripheral neuritis, dermatitis, and anemia.

Infants fed a formula deficient in vitamin B_6 for 1–6 mo exhibit irritability and generalized seizures. Gastrointestinal distress and an aggravated startle response are common.

Peripheral neuropathy may occur during treatment of tuberculosis with isonicotinic acid hydrazide. The neuropathy responds to administration of pyridoxine or to a decrease in the dose of the drug. Administration of isonicotinic acid may also be followed by manifestations of pellagra.

Skin lesions include cheilosis, glossitis, and seborrhea around the eyes, nose, and mouth. Microcytic anemia, oxaluria, oxalic acid bladder stones, hyperglycinemia, lymphopenia, decreased antibody formation, and infections occur.

Convulsions from B_6 dependency may occur several hours to as long as 6 mo after birth. Seizures are typically myoclonic with hypsarrhythmic patterns on the electrocardiogram. In several instances the mother had received large doses of pyridoxine during pregnancy for control of emesis.

In *B_6-dependent anemia* the red cells are microcytic and hypochromic. There are increased serum iron concentrations, saturation of iron-binding protein, hemosiderin deposits in bone marrow and liver, and failure of iron utilization for hemoglobin synthesis.

Xanthurenic aciduria following tryptophan load tests is an apparently benign occurrence in some families. Xanthurenic acid excretion becomes normal following large doses of vitamin B_6. *Cystathioninuria* is similarly not accompanied by any clear clinical disturbance. Cystathioninase is vitamin B_6 dependent (Sec. 7.5).

In some patients with *homocystinuria*, serum levels of homocysteine will fall following B_6 administration. Cystathionine synthetase is B_6 dependent (Sec. 7.5).

Laboratory Data. Anemia is not common in affected infants. After administration of 100 mg/kg of tryptophan, large amounts of xanthurenic acid will be found in the urine of patients with pyridoxine deficiency; in normal persons none is detected. The result of this test may be normal in patients with "pyridoxine dependency."

Diagnosis. Infants with seizures should be suspected of having vitamin B_6 deficiency or dependency. If more common causes of infantile seizures, such as hypocalcemia, hypoglycemia, and infection, can be eliminated, 100 mg of pyridoxine should be injected. If the seizure stops, B_6 deficiency should be suspected, and a tryptophan loading test is indicated. Similarly, in older children with seizure disorders, 100 mg of pyridoxine may be injected intramuscularly while the electroencephalogram is being recorded; a favorable response of the EEG suggests pyridoxine deficiency.

Erythrocyte glutamic pyruvic transaminase is reduced in pyridoxine deficiency; its concentration may be used as an indicator of vitamin B_6 status.

Prevention. Balanced diets usually contain enough pyridoxine so that deficiency is rare. Children receiving high protein diets should have vitamin B_6 added. Infants whose mothers have received large doses of pyridoxine during pregnancy are at increased risk of seizures due to pyridoxine dependency. Any child receiving a pyridoxine antagonist such as isoniazid should be carefully observed for neurologic manifestations. If these develop, either pyridoxine should be administered or the dose of the antagonist decreased. Daily intake of 0.3–0.5 mg of pyridoxine in the infant, 0.5–1.5 mg in the child, or 1.5–2.0 mg in the adult prevents deficiency states.

Treatment. For convulsions possibly due to pyridoxine deficiency, 100 mg of the vitamin should be given intramuscularly. One dose should suffice if the diet is adequate. For "pyridoxine-dependent" children, 2–10 mg intramuscularly or 10–100 mg orally may be necessary daily.

Toxicity. Excessive intake may cause sensory neuropathy.

Aly HE, Donald EA, Simpson MHW: Oral contraceptives and vitamin B_6 metabolism. Am J Clin Nutr 22:97, 1971.

Cinnamon AD, Beaton JR: Biochemical assessment of vitamin B_6 status in man. Am J Clin Nutr 26:96, 1970.

Frimpter GW, Andelman RJ, George WF: Vitamin B_6-dependency syndromes. Am J Clin Nutr 22:794, 1959.

Hansson O, Hagberg B: Effect of pyridoxine treatment in children with epilepsy. Acta Soc Med Upsal 73:35, 1968.

Schaumburg H, Kaplan J Windebank A, et al: Sensory neuropathy from pyridoxine abuse. N Engl J Med. 309:445, 1983.

Scriver CR: Vitamin B_6 deficiency and dependency in man. Am J Dis Child 113:109, 1967.

3.27 BIOTIN

Biotin deficiency is rare. It is found in those consuming the biotin antagonist, avidin, found in raw egg white. Many microorganisms produce biotin.

Etiology. Biotin enzymes include carboxylases, transcarboxylases and decarboxylases. Avidin ingestion causes symptoms of deficiency. Deficiencies have appeared in those receiving all their nutrition parenterally and occasionally in infants whose mothers are biotin deficient.

Clinical Manifestations. Brawny dermatitis, somnolence, hallucinations and hyperesthesia with accumulation of organic acids are common. Other neurological signs and defective immunity may occur.

Diagnosis. Elevated organic aciduria, particularly propionic and hydroxy–short chain acids, with response to clinical and biochemical abnormalities following treatment, suggests biotin deficiency.

Prevention and Treatment. Parenteral solutions should contain biotin. Deficient patients respond to oral administration of 10 mg.

3.28 VITAMIN C (ASCORBIC ACID) DEFICIENCY
(Scurvy)

Ascorbic acid is essential for the normal formation of collagen; the defects in collagen structure stemming from deficiency of the vitamin produce many of the metabolic deviations and clinical manifestations of scurvy. Alterations in collagen formation are partly due to failure to incorporate hydroxyproline and proline.

Vitamin C is a potent reducing agent, easily oxidized and destroyed by heating. The adrenals and lenses have particularly high contents of vitamin C.

Ascorbic acid functions in a number of enzymatic activities (Table 3–6 and Sec. 7.3). Transient tyrosinemia in the neonatal period, relatively common among low birthweight infants and occasionally seen in fullterm ones fed high protein diets, is corrected by administering ascorbic acid (Sec. 7.3).

Ascorbic acid deficiency may also be a factor in some instances of megaloblastic anemia by interfering in the conversion of folic acid or other conjugates (Table 3–6 and Sec. 15.10).

Etiology. The infant is born with adequate stores of vitamin C if the mother's intake has been adequate; the vitamin C content of cord blood plasma is 2–4 times greater than that of maternal plasma. Under these circumstances breast milk contains about 4–7 mg/dL of ascorbic acid and is an adequate source of vitamin C. Deficiency of vitamin C in the mother's diet may result in scurvy in her breast-fed infant. Infants fed with formula must receive vitamin C supplements; such supplements will provide additional protection for the breast-fed infant.

The need for vitamin C is increased by febrile illnesses, particularly infectious and diarrheal diseases, and by iron deficiency, cold exposure, protein depletion, or smoking.

Pathology. During vitamin C deficiency formation of collagen and of chondroitin sulfate is impaired. The tendencies to hemorrhage, defective tooth dentin, and loosening of the teeth are due to deficient collagen. Since osteoblasts no longer form their normal intercellular substance (osteoid), endochondral bone formation ceases. The bony trabeculae that have been formed become brittle and fracture easily. The periosteum becomes loosened, and subperiosteal hemorrhages occur, especially at the ends of the femur and tibia. In severe scurvy there may be degeneration in skeletal muscles, cardiac hypertrophy, bone marrow depression, and adrenal atrophy.

Clinical Manifestations. Scurvy may occur at any age but is extremely rare in the newborn infant. The majority of cases occur in infants 6–24 mo of age. Clinical manifestations require time to develop; after a variable period of vitamin C depletion, vague symptoms of irritability, tachypnea, digestive disturbances, and loss of appetite appear. The irritability becomes progressively greater, and there is evidence of general tenderness, especially noticeable in the legs when the infant is picked up or when the diaper is changed. The pain results in pseudoparalysis, and the legs assume the typical "frog position" (Fig. 3–6), in which the hips and knees are semiflexed with the feet rotated outward. Edematous swelling along the shafts of the legs may be present, and in some cases a subperiosteal hemorrhage can be palpated at the end of the femur. The facial expression is apprehensive. Changes in the gums, most noticeable when the teeth are erupted, are characterized by bluish purple, spongy swellings of the mucous membrane, usually over the upper incisors. There may be a "rosary" at the costochondral junctions and a depression of the sternum. The angulation of the "scorbutic beads" is usually sharper than that of the rachitic rosary, since it is produced by a subluxation of the sternal plate at the costochondral junction (Fig. 3–6) rather than by widening of the softened epiphyses as occurs in rickets (Sec. 3.29).

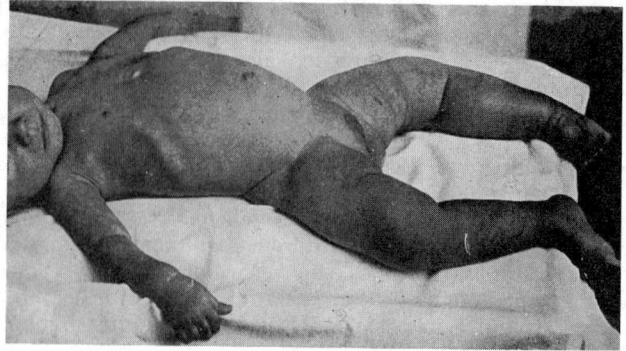

Figure 3–6. Scorbutic rosary, depression of sternum, and the so-called frog position.

Petechial hemorrhages may occur in the skin and mucous membranes. Hematuria, melena, and orbital or subdural hemorrhages may be found. Low-grade fever is usually present. Anemia may reflect inability to utilize iron or impaired folic acid metabolism (Sec. 15.10). Wound healing is delayed, and apparently healed wounds may break down. Swollen joints and follicular hyperkeratosis may develop, as well as the "sicca" syndrome of Sjögren, which is usually associated with collagen disorders and includes xerostomia, keratoconjunctivitis sicca, and enlargement of the salivary glands (Sec. 10.85).

Roentgenographic Manifestations. The diagnosis of scurvy is usually based on roentgenographic changes in the long bones, especially at their distal ends. Changes are greatest, as a rule, in the area of the knee. In the early stages the appearance resembles that of simple atrophy of bone. The trabeculae of the shaft cannot be discerned, and the bone assumes a "ground-glass" appearance. The cortex is reduced to "pencil-point thinness," and the epiphyseal ends are sharply outlined. The white line of Fraenkel, which represents the zone of well calcified cartilage, can be clearly discerned as an irregular but thickened white line at the metaphysis. The epiphyseal centers of ossification also have a ground-glass appearance and are surrounded by a white ring (Fig. 3–7).

At this stage scurvy cannot be diagnosed with certainty from the roentgenogram unless the zone of rarefaction under the white line at the metaphysis becomes apparent. The zone of rarefaction is a linear break in the bone proximal and parallel to the white line. Often it does not traverse the shaft in its entire width and may be seen only in its lateral parts as a triangular defect (Fig. 3–7B). A spur, as a lateral prolongation of the white line, may be present. Epiphyseal separation may occur along the line of destruction, with linear displacement or compression of the epiphysis against the shaft. Subperiosteal hemorrhages are not visible roentgenographically in active scurvy. During healing, however, the elevated periosteum becomes calcified, and the affected bone assumes a dumbbell or club shape.

Diagnosis. Diagnosis is based mainly on the characteristic clinical picture, the roentgenographic appearance of the long bones, and history of poor intake of vitamin C. Occasionally, a mother may have been boiling the infant's fruit juices.

Laboratory tests for scurvy are unsatisfactory. A fasting vitamin C level of the blood plasma of over 0.6 mg/dL aids in the exclusion of scurvy, but a lower vitamin C level does not prove its presence. Evidence of vitamin C deficiency is better furnished by the ascorbic acid concentration in the white cell–platelet layer (buffy layer) of centrifuged oxalated blood. A level of zero in this layer indicates latent scurvy, even in the absence of clinical signs of deficiency. The saturation of the tissues with vitamin C can be estimated from the amount of urinary excretion of the vitamin after a test dose of ascorbic acid. During the 3–5 hr after parenteral administration of the

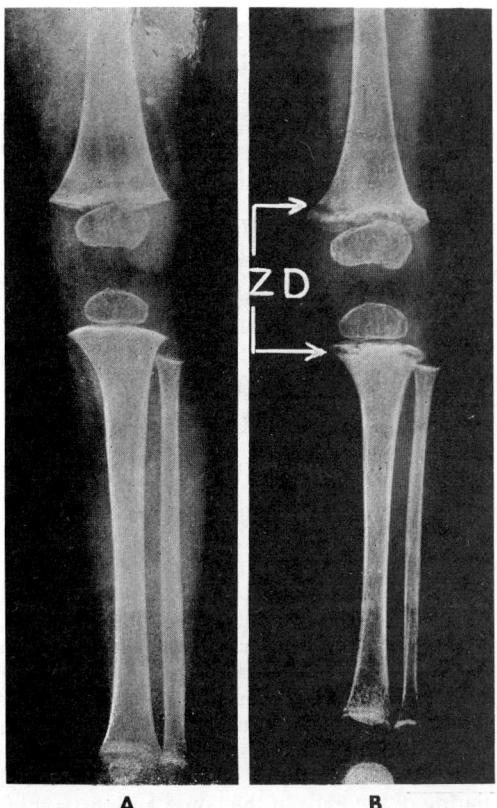

Figure 3–7. Roentgenograms of leg. *A*, Early scurvy: "white line" is visible on the ends of the shafts of the tibia and fibula; rings around epiphyses of femur and tibia. *B*, More advanced scorbutic changes; zones of destruction (ZD) in femur and tibia.

test dose, 80% of it can be found in the urine of normal children. A generalized, nonspecific aminoaciduria occurs in scurvy, while blood values of amino acids remain normal. After a tyrosine load the scorbutic infant excretes metabolites similar to those of the premature infant. Prothrombin time may be markedly increased.

Differential Diagnosis. The tenderness of the limbs and the pain elicited by movement have often led to a false diagnosis of arthritis or acrodynia. The patient's age aids in differentiating scurvy from rheumatic fever, since rheumatic fever is rare in children under 2 yr of age. Suppurative arthritis and osteomyelitis should be considered in the differential diagnosis. The pseudoparalysis of syphilis usually occurs at an earlier age than does that of scurvy and is often accompanied by other signs of syphilis; a roentgenogram may aid in the diagnosis. Poliomyelitis causes a true flaccid paralysis, and, in infants, the exquisite tenderness present in the limbs in scurvy is absent. Henoch-Schönlein purpura, thrombocytopenic purpura, leukemia, meningitis, or nephritis may be suspected.

Prognosis. With proper treatment recovery occurs rapidly in infants, but the swelling of subperiosteal hemorrhage may require months to disappear. Body growth usually is quickly resumed.

Prevention. Scurvy is prevented by a diet adequate in vitamin C; citrus fruits and juices are excellent sources. Formula-fed infants should receive 35 mg of ascorbic acid daily. Lactating mothers should take 100 mg; 45–60 mg daily is needed by children or adults (Table 3–1).

Treatment. The administration of 3–4 ounces of orange juice or tomato juice daily will quickly produce healing, but ascorbic acid is preferable. The daily therapeutic dose is 100–200 mg or more, orally or parenterally.

Irwin MI, Hutchins BK: A conspectus of research on vitamin C requirements in man. J Nutr 106:823, 1976.

3.29 RICKETS OF VITAMIN D DEFICIENCY*

Rickets is the term signifying a failure in mineralization of growing bone or osteoid tissue. The characteristic early changes are seen roentgenographically at the ends of long bones; evidence of demineralization also exists in the shafts. Subsequently, if healing is not initiated, clinical manifestations appear (see below). Failure of mature bone to mineralize is termed osteomalacia.

Etiology. During the first third of this century, the predominant cause of rickets was nutritional deficiency of vitamin D due either to inadequate direct exposure to ultraviolet rays in sunlight (296–310 nm; these rays do not pass through ordinary window glass) or to inadequate intake of vitamin D, or both. Vitamin D deficiency rickets has been nearly eliminated among infants and children in the industrialized countries by prophylactic means. Deficiency may occur in unsupplemented dark-skinned infants or in breast-fed infants of mothers unexposed to sunlight.

Currently in industrialized countries, it appears that conditions besides inadequate nutritional prophylaxis with vitamin D collectively produce most of the observed rachitic lesions (Sec. 23.46–23.52). These conditions include clinical entities that interfere with the metabolic conversion and activation of vitamin D, such as hepatic and renal lesions, or that disrupt calcium and phosphorus homeostasis in other ways.

Two forms of vitamin D are of practical importance. Vitamin D_2, or calciferol, available as irradiated ergosterol, largely replaced the fish liver oils (cod and percomorph) as a source of dietary and therapeutic vitamin D. Vitamin D_3, now available synthetically, is naturally present in human skin in the provitamin stage as 7-dehydrocholesterol. It is activated photochemically to cholecalciferol and transferred to the liver. Each of these irradiated sterols is hydroxylated in the liver to 25-OH-cholecalciferol and, subsequently, in the renal cortical cells to 1,25-dihydroxycholecalciferol, an end product considered a hormone. Its antirachitic functions include facilitation of intestinal absorption of calcium and phosphorus and of reabsorption of phosphorus in the kidney and a direct effect on mineral metabolism of bone (deposition and reabsorption). In conjunction with parathormone and calcitonin, it plays a major role in homeostasis of calcium and phosphorus in the body's fluids and tissues.

The diet of infants may contain only small amounts of vitamin D; cow's milk contains only 5–40 IU/quart.† Cereals, vegetables, and fruits contain only negligible amounts. Egg yolk contains 140–390 IU/g. Most marketed cow's milk is fortified with 400 IU of vitamin D per quart, and most commercially prepared milks for infant formulas are also fortified.

Besides lack of dietary vitamin D and the skin's lack of exposure to ultraviolet irradiation, several factors may predispose to vitamin D deficiency. Rickets or epiphyseal dysplasia is particularly apt to develop during rapid growth, such as in low birthweight infants and in adolescents. Black children are singularly susceptible to rickets, due to either the pigmentation of their skin or inadequate penetration of sunlight.

---

*For a review of the rachitic lesions reference should be made to Table 3–5 and Sec. 5.10 and 5.14 for calcium and phosphorus metabolism; Sec. 3.29 and 5.34 for hypocalcemic tetany; Sec. 19.17 for parathormone, vitamin D, and calcitonin activities; and to Table 3–6 and Sec. 23.46–23.52 for additional discussion of vitamin D metabolism and its activities.

†1 µg = 40 IU.

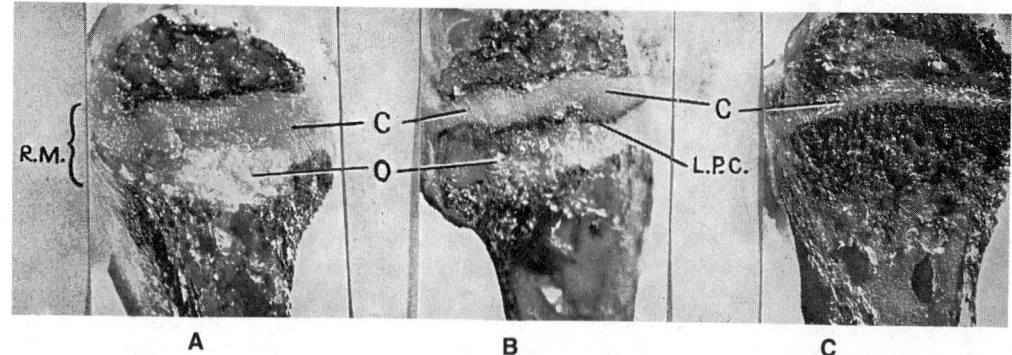

Figure 3–8. Line tests in rats (proximal end of tibia) (calcified tissue stained with silver appears black). *A,* Active rickets. The light broad zone between epiphysis and shaft represents the rachitic metaphysis (R.M.); C, cartilage; O, osteoid. *B,* Healing rickets. Line of preparatory calcification (L.P.C.) between zone of cartilage (C) and osteoid (O). *C,* Healed rickets. Cartilaginous disk (C) between epiphysis and normal shaft.

Children with disorders of absorption, such as celiac disease, steatorrhea, pancreatitis, or cystic fibrosis, may acquire rickets because of deficient absorption of vitamin D and calcium or of both. Anticonvulsant therapy, as for example with the phenytoins or with phenobarbital, may interfere in the metabolism of vitamin D; rickets has been seen with some frequency in institutionalized children receiving such therapy who also have inadequate exposure to sunlight (Sec. 23.50). Glucocorticoids appear to be antagonistic to vitamin D in calcium transport.

Pathology. New bone formation is initiated by the osteoblast, which is responsible for matrix deposition and its subsequent mineralization. Osteoblasts secrete collagen, and changes in polysaccharides, phospholipids, alkaline phosphatase, and pyrophosphatase follow until mineralization occurs in the presence of adequate calcium and phosphorus. Resorption of bone occurs when osteoclasts secrete enzymes on the bone surface, dissolving and removing matrix and mineral. Osteocytes covered by bone both resorb and redeposit bone. Factors affecting bone growth are poorly understood, but phosphorus, calcium, fluoride, and growth hormone all have some influence.

In rickets defective growth of bone results from retardation or suppression of normal growth of epiphyseal cartilage and of normal calcification. These changes are dependent upon a deficiency in serum of calcium and phosphorus salts for mineralization. Cartilage cells fail to complete their normal cycle of proliferation and degeneration, and subsequent failure of capillary penetration occurs in a patchy manner. The result is a frayed, irregular epiphyseal line at the end of the shaft. Failure of osseous and cartilaginous matrix to mineralize in the zone of preparatory calcification, followed by deposition of newly formed uncalcified osteoid results in a wide, irregular, frayed zone of nonrigid tissue (the rachitic metaphysis) (Fig. 3–8). This zone, responsible for many of the skeletal deformities, becomes compressed and bulges laterally, producing flaring of the ends of the bones and the rachitic rosary (Figs. 3–9 and 3–10).

Mineralization is also lacking in subperiosteal bone; pre-existing cortical bone is resorbed in a normal manner but is replaced by osteoid tissues over the entire shaft, which fails to mineralize. If this process continues, the shaft loses its rigidity, and the resulting softened and rarefied cortical bone is readily distorted by stress; deformities and fractures result (Fig. 3–10).

Healing Rickets. With healing, degeneration of cartilage cells occurs along the metaphyseal-diaphyseal border, capillary penetration of the resultant spaces is resumed, and calcification takes place in the zone of preparatory calcification. This calcification, occurring approximately at the line at

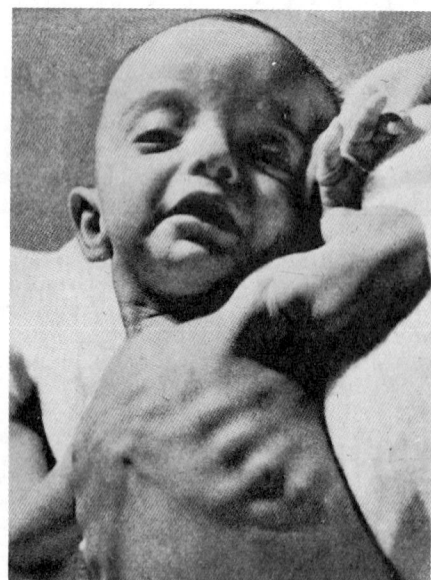

Figure 3–9. Rachitic rosary in a young infant. (From Lyons and Wallinger: Pediatrics and Pediatric Nursing.)

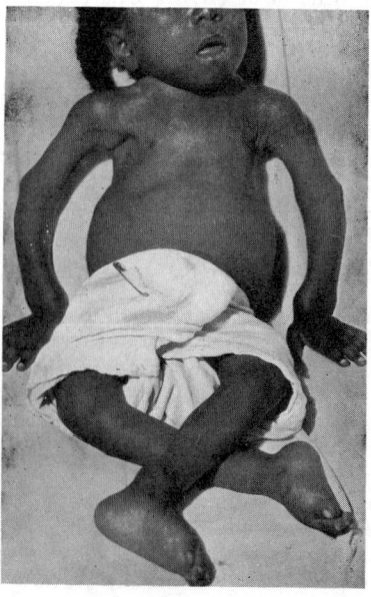

Figure 3–10. Curvature of arms, deformed "violin-shaped" chest, potbelly, enlarged epiphyses in a child with rickets, 3 yr of age.

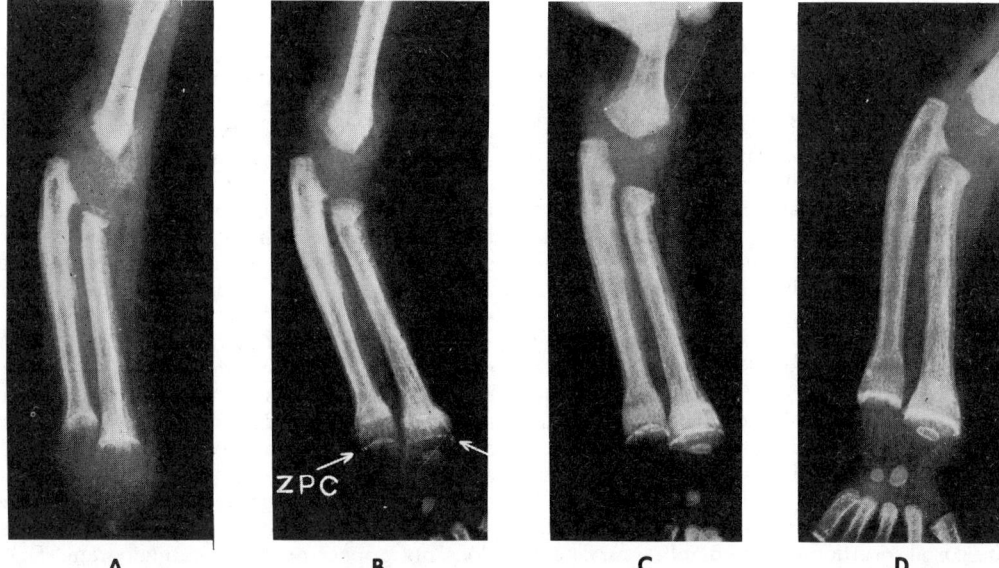

Figure 3–11. *A*, Active rickets; cupping and fraying of distal ends of radius and ulna; double contour along lateral outline of radius (periosteal osteoid). The 2 dense zones in the shaft of the ulna are calluses of greenstick fractures. *B*, Healing rickets after 12 days of treatment with vitamin D. Zones of preparatory calcification (ZPC); above them in the rachitic metaphyses there is beginning calcification. *C*, Healing rickets after 18 days of treatment. The zones of preparatory calcification are well defined, and the rachitic metaphyses appear well calcified. The epiphysis of the radius has become visible. *D*, Healing rickets after 29 days of treatment. Zones of preparatory calcification, rachitic metaphyses, and shafts have become united.

which normal calcification would have occurred had the rachitic process not supervened, produces a line clearly demonstrable in roentgenograms (Fig. 3–11*A* and *B*). As healing progresses, the osteoid tissue between this line of preparatory calcification and the diaphysis also becomes mineralized (Fig. 3–8). Osteoid tissue in the cortex and about the trabeculae in the shaft rapidly becomes mineralized. Months or years may be required to repair the deformities, and in extreme instances complete repair may be impossible.

Chemical Pathology. In healthy infants the inorganic serum phosphorus concentration is 4.5–6.5 mg/dL, whereas in rachitic infants it is usually reduced to 1.5–3.5 mg/dL. The serum calcium level is usually normal, but under certain conditions it too is reduced, and tetany may develop.

Vitamin D deficient rickets can be assumed to be the body's attempt to maintain normal serum calcium levels, presumably because calcium is necessary for normal function of nerve, muscle, and endocrine glands and for intercellular bridging. In the absence of vitamin D, less calcium is absorbed from the intestine. With slightly lowered serum calcium, parathormone is secreted, leading to mobilization of calcium and phosphorus from the bone. The serum calcium concentration is thus maintained, but secondary effects occur, including the changes of rickets in bone, the lowered serum phosphorus concentration (because parathormone decreases phosphorus reabsorption in the kidney), and elevated serum phosphatase (due to increased osteoblastic activity).

The alkaline phosphatase of serum, which in normal children is less than 200 IU/dL, is elevated in mild rickets to more than 500 IU/dL. As rickets heals, the phosphatase value returns slowly to the normal range. Serum alkaline phosphatase may be normal in infants with rickets who are protein and/or zinc depleted.

Calcium and phosphorus homeostasis depends on the intestinal absorption of dietary calcium and phosphorus. Maximum calcium absorption occurs in man when the ratio of calcium to phosphorus in the diet is about 2:1; increase in phosphate decreases absorption of calcium. Acidity of intes-

tinal contents increases absorption of calcium. An increase in calcium absorption also occurs when lactose is the dietary sugar. Chelating agents such as ethylenediaminetetraacetic acid (EDTA) or the phytates of cereals may decrease calcium absorption, and dietary iron may decrease absorption of phosphate. High dietary levels of stearic and palmitic acids, which are poorly absorbed, also decrease calcium absorption.

Calcium absorption is facilitated by 1,25-dihydroxycholecalciferol or similar hydroxylated forms of vitamin D. Calcium deficiency alone rarely leads to the failure of calcification as seen in rickets and osteomalacia; it results in a diminished amount of bone.

Vitamin D deficiency is also accompanied by generalized aminoaciduria, a decrease of citrate in bone and its increased urinary excretion, decreased ability of the kidneys to make an acid urine, phosphaturia, and, occasionally, mellituria. The parathyroid glands hypertrophy in rickets, and urinary cyclic AMP is increased.

Clinical Manifestations. Osseous changes of rickets can be recognized after several months of vitamin D deficiency. In breast-fed infants whose mothers have osteomalacia, rickets may develop within 2 mo. Florid rickets appears toward the end of the 1st and during the 2nd yr of life. Later in childhood manifest vitamin D deficient rickets is rare.

One of the early signs of rickets, craniotabes, is due to thinning of the outer table of the skull and detected by pressing firmly over the occiput or posterior parietal bones. A ping-pong ball sensation will be felt. Craniotabes near the suture lines is a normal variant. Low birthweight infants are particularly prone to early development of rickets and to craniotabes. Palpable enlargement of the costochondral junctions (the "rachitic rosary") (Fig. 3–9) and thickening of the wrists and ankles (Fig. 3–11) are other early evidences of osseous changes. Increased sweating, particularly around the head, may also be present.

Advanced Rickets. Signs of advanced rickets are easily recognized.

HEAD. Craniotabes may disappear before the end of the 1st

yr, though the rachitic process continues. The softness of the skull may result in flattening and, at times, permanent asymmetry of the head. The anterior fontanel is larger than normal; its closure may be delayed until after the 2nd yr of life. The central parts of the parietal and frontal bones are often thickened, forming prominences or bosses, which give the head a boxlike appearance (caput quadratum). The head may be larger than normal and may remain so throughout life. Eruption of the temporary teeth may be delayed, and there may be defects of the enamel and extensive caries. The permanent teeth that are calcifying may be affected; the permanent incisors, canines, and first molars usually show enamel defects.

THORAX. Enlargement of the costochondral junctions may become prominent; the beading of the ribs is not only palpable but also visible (Fig. 3–9). The sides of the thorax become flattened, and the longitudinal grooves develop posterior to the rosary. The sternum with its adjacent cartilages appears to be projected forward, producing the so-called pigeon breast deformity. Along the lower border of the chest develops a horizontal depression, Harrison groove (Fig. 3–12), which corresponds to the costal insertions of the diaphragm. There may be a variety of other thoracic deformities, including those of the shoulder girdle.

SPINAL COLUMN. Slight to moderate degrees of lateral curvature (scoliosis) are common, and a kyphosis may appear in the dorsolumbar region of rachitic children when sitting. Lordosis of the lumbar region may be seen in the erect position.

PELVIS. In children with lordosis there is frequently a concomitant deformity of the pelvis, which is also retarded in growth. The pelvic entrance is narrowed by a forward projection of the promontory; the exit, by a forward displacement of the caudal part of the sacrum and the coccyx. In the female these changes, if they become permanent, add to the hazards of childbirth and may necessitate cesarean section.

EXTREMITIES. As the rachitic process continues, the epiphyseal enlargement at the wrists and ankles becomes more noticeable. The enlarged epiphyses can be seen (Fig. 3–11) or palpated but are not distinct in roentgenograms since they consist of cartilage and uncalcified osteoid tissue. Bending of the softened shafts of the femur, tibia, and fibula results in bowlegs or knock knees; the femur and the tibia may also acquire an anterior convexity. Coxa vara is sometimes the result of rickets. Greenstick fractures occur in the long bones; often there are no clinical symptoms.

Deformities of the spine, pelvis, and legs result in reduced stature, rachitic dwarfism.

LIGAMENTS. Relaxation of ligaments helps to produce deformities and partly accounts for knock knees, overextension of the knee joints, weak ankles, kyphosis, and scoliosis.

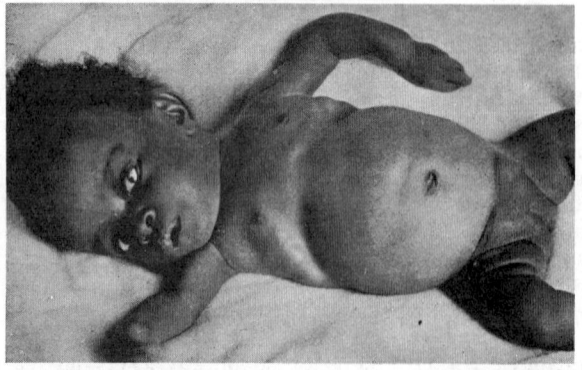

Figure 3–12. Deformities in rickets, showing curvature of the limbs, potbelly, and Harrison groove.

MUSCLES. The muscles are poorly developed and lack tone. As a result, children with moderately severe rickets are late in standing and walking. The common condition of potbelly (Figs. 3–10 and 3–12) depends to a large extent upon weakness of the abdominal muscles; weakness of the gastric and intestinal walls may contribute.

Diagnosis. The diagnosis of rickets is based on a history of inadequate intake of vitamin D and on clinical observation; it is confirmed chemically and by roentgenographic examination. The serum calcium level may be normal or low, the serum phosphorus level is below 4 mg/dL, and the serum alkaline phosphatase is elevated. Urinary cyclic AMP is elevated, and serum 25-hydroxycholecalciferol is decreased.

Roentgenographic Changes (Fig. 3–11). ACTIVE RICKETS. A roentgenogram of the wrist is best for early diagnosis, since characteristic changes of the ulna and radius occur at an early stage. The distal ends appear widened, concave (cupping), and frayed, in contrast to the normally sharply demarcated and slightly convex ends. The distance from the distal ends of the ulna and radius to the metacarpal bones is increased since the large rachitic metaphysis, which is not calcified, does not appear on the roentgenogram. The density of the shafts is decreased, but the trabeculae are unusually prominent.

HEALING RICKETS (Fig. 3–11). Initial healing is indicated by the appearance of the line of preparatory calcification. This line is separated from the distal end of the shaft by a zone of decreased calcification, the zone of the osteoid tissue. As healing progresses and the osteoid tissue becomes calcified, the shaft "grows" toward the line of preparatory calcification until it becomes united with it.

Differential Diagnosis. Nonrachitic craniotabes, at times present in the immediate postnatal period, tends to disappear before rachitic softening of the skull would become manifest (2nd–4th mo of life). Craniotabes also occurs in hydrocephalus and osteogenesis imperfecta, but it is not difficult to differentiate these conditions from rickets.

Enlargement of the costochondral junctions occurs in rickets, scurvy, and chondrodystrophy. The enlargements in rickets are rounded knobs, but in scurvy a ledgelike depression with the chondral or sternal portion is displaced below the osseous ribs. In chondrodystrophy there may be irregular, concave outlines of the distal ends of the bones, but no roentgenographic evidence of fraying. Other epiphyseal lesions that may require differentiation include congenital epiphyseal dysplasia, cytomegalic inclusion disease, syphilis, rubella, and copper deficiency. It is sometimes difficult to distinguish rachitic deformities of the chest from congenital ones. Bowlegs can be the result of rickets but may be a familial characteristic. Vitamin D resistant rickets and other metabolic disturbances with osseous lesions resembling rickets must also be differentiated (Sec. 23.45).

Complications. Respiratory infections such as bronchitis and bronchopneumonia are common in rachitic infants, and pulmonary atelectasis is frequently associated with severe deformities of the chest. Anemia due to iron deficiency or accompanying infections often develops in severe rickets.

Prognosis. If sufficient amounts of vitamin D are administered, healing begins within a few days and progresses slowly until the normal bony structure is restored. In many instances, the enlargement of the epiphyses of the long bones, including the ribs, and the deformities of the skull disappear only after months or years of treatment. Even rather severe bowing of the legs may disappear within several years without osteotomies. In advanced cases there may be permanent osseous alterations in the form of bowlegs, knock knees, curvature of the upper arms, deformities of the chest and spine, rachitic pelvis and coxa vara, and dwarfism.

Rickets in itself is not a fatal disease, but complications and intercurrent infections such as pneumonia, tuberculosis, and enteritis are more likely to cause death in rachitic than in normal children.

Prevention. Rickets can be prevented by exposure to ultraviolet light or by oral administration of vitamin D. Sunlight, as a prophylactic agent, may be effective in the temperate zones only during the summer months in haze-free areas.

The daily requirement of vitamin D is 10 µg or 400 IU. Much of the whole milk available in urban areas and evaporated milk are fortified with vitamin D concentrate so that 1 quart of fresh, whole milk or a can of evaporated milk contains this amount. Prematurely born infants or breast-fed infants whose mothers are not exposed to adequate sunlight should receive supplemental vitamin D daily.

Vitamin D should also be administered to pregnant and lactating mothers.

Treatment. Natural and artificial light are effective therapeutically, but oral administration of vitamin D is preferred. The daily administration of 50–150 µg of vitamin D_3 or 0.5–2 µg of 1,25-dihydroxycholecalciferol will produce healing demonstrable on roentgenograms within 2–4 wk except in the unusual cases of vitamin D refractory rickets.

Administering 15,000 µg of vitamin D in a single dose without further therapy for several months may be advantageous. More rapid healing will follow, possibly with earlier differential diagnosis from genetic vitamin D resistant rickets and less dependence on parents for daily administration of the vitamin. If no healing occurs, the rickets is probably resistant to vitamin D (Sec. 23.48). After healing is complete, the dose of vitamin D should be lowered to 10 µg daily.

DeLuca HF: Some new concepts emanating from a study of the metabolism and function of vitamin D. Nutr Rev 38:169, 1980.

Harrison HE, Harrison HC: Rickets then and now. J Pediatr 87:1144, 1975.

Raisz LG: Physiologic and pharmacologic regulations of bone resorption. N Engl J Med 282:909, 1970.

Rasmussen H: Cell communication, calcium ion, and cyclic adenosine monophosphate. Science 170:404, 1970.

Root AW, Harrison HE: Recent advances in calcium metabolism. I. Mechanisms of calcium homeostasis. II. Disorders of calcium homeostasis. J Pediatr 88:1, 177, 1976.

3.30 TETANY OF VITAMIN D DEFICIENCY
(Infantile Tetany)

See also Sec. 5.33.

Tetany due to deficiency of vitamin D occasionally accompanies rickets. Relatively common in former times, this type of tetany is rare today owing to the widespread prophylactic use of vitamin D. Occasionally, tetany is associated with celiac disease, probably as a result of deficient absorption of both vitamin D and calcium. Tetany of vitamin D deficiency occurs most frequently between the ages of 4 mo and 3 yr.

Chemical Pathology. When the serum calcium concentration falls below 7–7.5 mg/dL, muscular irritability occurs, apparently owing to the loss of the inhibitory control that serum ionized calcium exerts upon the neuromuscular junctions. It remains unclear why serum calcium is occasionally decreased in association with rickets; failure of the parathyroids to compensate for the low serum calcium level may be a factor.

Clinical Manifestations. The symptoms and signs of tetany are manifested, and rickets usually occurs concurrently. Vitamin D deficient tetany may exist in either a latent or a clinically manifest stage.

Latent Tetany. Symptoms are not evident, but they can be elicited by means of the Chvostek, Trousseau, and Erb procedures. The serum calcium level is less than 7–7.5 mg/dL.

Manifest Tetany. Spontaneous clinical manifestations include carpopedal spasm, laryngospasm, and convulsions. The serum calcium level is often well under 7 mg/dL.

Diagnosis. The diagnosis is based on the combined presence of rickets, low serum calcium level, and symptoms of tetany. The serum phosphorus level is usually low; the serum alkaline phosphatase level is increased. In the differential diagnosis causes of tetany such as hypoparathyroidism, hypomagnesemia, and ingestion of phenothiazine must be eliminated.

Prognosis. The prognosis is good unless treatment is delayed. Death rarely occurs, though it may result from laryngospasm and possibly from cardiac dilatation, so-called cardiac tetany.

Prevention. Prophylactic treatment is identical to that for rickets (Sec. 3.29).

Treatment. Active treatment raises the serum calcium above the tetany level. This level may be attained by administration of calcium chloride in 1–2% solution in milk. For the first 1–2 days, 4–6 g daily may be given in 1 g doses, the initial dose being 2–3 g; smaller doses of 1–3 g a day should then be continued for 1–2 wk. Calcium chloride in more concentrated solution may cause severe gastric ulceration, and large doses may cause acidosis. Calcium lactate may be added to milk in doses of 10–12 g a day for 10 days. When oral medication is impractical, calcium gluconate (5–10 mL of a 10% solution) can be administered intravenously but not subcutaneously or intramuscularly owing to the dangers of local necrosis.

Oxygen inhalation is indicated during convulsive seizures. When intravenously administered calcium gluconate does not quickly control the attacks, sodium phenobarbital may be given intramuscularly. Prolonged attacks of laryngospasm are usually controlled by sedation and by administering calcium salts. Intubation is only occasionally necessary. After the acute manifestations have been controlled, vitamin D in daily doses of 50–100 µg should be started and the oral administration of calcium continued (see above). When the rickets is healed, the dose of vitamin D should be decreased to the usual prophylactic one.

Fraser D, Kook SW, Scriver CR: Hyperparathyroidism as the cause of hyperaminoaciduria and phosphaturia in human vitamin D deficiency. Pediatr Res 1:425, 1967.

3.31 HYPERVITAMINOSIS D

Ingesting excessive amounts of vitamin D results in signs and symptoms similar to those of idiopathic hypercalcemia (Sec. 23.55), which may be due to hypersensitivity to vitamin D. Symptoms develop after 1–3 mo of large intakes of vitamin D; they include hypotonia, anorexia, irritability, constipation, polydipsia, polyuria, and pallor. Hypercalcemia and hypercalciuria are notable. Evidences of dehydration are usually present. Aortic valvular stenosis, vomiting, hypertension, retinopathy, and clouding of the cornea and conjunctiva may occur.

The urine may show proteinuria. With continued excessive intake, renal damage and metastatic calcification occur. Roentgenograms of the long bones reveal metastatic calcification and generalized osteoporosis.

Excessive intake of vitamin D may result from inadvertently substituting its concentrated form for one more dilute, from the parents' increasing their child's prescribed dose, and from inadequately controlling dosages for children receiving large amounts of vitamin D for chronic hyperphosphatemic states (Sec. 23.56).

Differential Diagnosis. Metastatic calcification occurs in chronic nephritis, hyperparathyroidism, and idiopathic hypercalcemia. The latter two are accompanied by hypercalcemia.

Prevention. Prevention requires careful evaluation of vitamin D dosage.

Treatment. This includes discontinuing vitamin D intake and decreasing intake of calcium. For severely involved infants, aluminum hydroxide by mouth, cortisone, or sodium versenate may be used.

Forbes GB, Cafarelli C, Manning J: Vitamin D and infantile hypercalcemia. Pediatrics 42:203, 1968.

3.32 VITAMIN E DEFICIENCY

The effects of vitamin E deficiency vary in different animal species. Vitamin E (α-tocopherol) is a fat-soluble antioxidant which may be involved in nucleic acid metabolism, but its precise biochemical action is unclear. Vitamin E is present in many foods (Table 3–6).

Deficiency may occur in malabsorption states such as cystic fibrosis and acanthocytosis. Diets high in unsaturated fatty acid increase the vitamin E requirement in premature infants who absorb vitamin E poorly. Excess iron administration exaggerates signs of vitamin E deficiency.

Some patients deficient in vitamin E have creatinuria, ceroid deposition in smooth muscle, focal necrosis of striated muscle, and muscle weakness. Some improvement may occur after administration of vitamin E. Vitamin E deficiency has been suggested as a causative factor in the anemia of kwashiorkor. Premature infants may have low serum levels of tocopherol, with development of a hemolytic anemia at 6–10 wk of age, correctable by administration of vitamin E. The role of vitamin E in retinopathy of prematurity is discussed in Sec. 8.17 and 25.13.

In deficiency states, platelet adhesiveness increases, as do blood platelet levels. Treatment of hemolysis in glucose-6-phosphate dehydrogenase deficiency, of sickle cell anemia, of leg cramps, or of coronary artery disease represents unsubstantiated use of vitamin E.

Diagnosis. If vitamin E has recently been administered, 3 days should elapse before determination of blood levels, since oral vitamin E may circulate for 1–2 days.

Prevention. Minimal daily requirements of vitamin E are not known; 0.7 mg/g of unsaturated fat in the diet appears adequate. Children with deficient fat absorption should take more. Premature infants may be given 15–25 IU/24 hr. Large oral or parenteral doses of vitamin E may prevent permanent neurologic abnormalities in children with biliary atresia or abetalipoproteinemia.

Gross S: Hemolytic anemia in premature infants: Relationship to vitamin E, selenium, glutathione peroxidase, and erythrocyte lipids. Sem Hemat 13:187, 1976.

3.33 VITAMIN K DEFICIENCY

Vitamin K is a naphthoquinone that participates in oxidative phosphorylation. Its absence or its failure to be absorbed from the intestinal tract results in hypoprothrombinemia and decreased hepatic synthesis of proconvertin. Prothrombin (factor II) and proconvertin (factor VII) are important to the 2nd stage of coagulation (Sec. 15.45). The 2nd stage of coagulation is studied by the 1-stage prothrombin time (Quick). Administering vitamin K to the newborn infant increases concentrations of prothrombin, proconvertin, plasma thromboplastin component (factor IX, PTC), and Stuart-Prower factor (factor X). Protein C is a vitamin K dependent factor that when activated inhibits coagulant function of factor VIII and factor V, and stimulates fibrinolysis. Vitamin K dependent calcium binding proteins such as osteocalcin promote phospholipid interactions in coagulation and in calcium metabolism.

Sources of Vitamin K. Naturally occurring vitamin K is fat soluble; it is found in high concentrations in hog's liver, soybeans, and alfalfa and in smaller amounts in some vegetables such as spinach, tomatoes, and kale. The natural vitamin (2-methyl-3-phytyl-1,4-naphthoquinone) has been labeled vitamin K_1 to distinguish it from synthetic naphthoquinones with vitamin K activity.

Many bacteria, including normal intestinal flora, are capable of synthesizing quinones with vitamin K activity. Suppression of intestinal bacteria by various antibiotics may be responsible for vitamin K deficiency, which results in diminution of prothrombin. Irradiated foods have produced vitamin K deficiency in animals. Cow's milk has more vitamin K than human milk.

Clinical Manifestations. Deficiency of vitamin K or hypoprothrombinemia should be considered in all patients with a hemorrhagic disturbance. The incidence of hemorrhagic disease of the newborn (Sec. 8.49) has been sharply decreased by the prophylactic administration of vitamin K. In childhood, the deficiency is usually due to factors affecting absorption or utilization of fat or to factors limiting its synthesis in the intestine, such as prolonged use of antibiotics. Diarrhea in infants, particularly breast-fed ones, may cause vitamin K deficiency. Diseases of the liver may lead to hypoprothrombinemia, which usually does not respond to administration of vitamin K.

Hypoprothrombinemia may also result from administering certain drugs. Dicumarol, obtained from spoiled sweet clover, is used specifically for the production of hypoprothrombinemia in the prevention and treatment of venous thrombosis. Bishydroxycoumarin (dicumarol) is thought to prevent the liver from utilizing vitamin K without exerting an effect on prothrombin. Blood prothrombin is continually destroyed in the body; since dicumarol prevents its replacement, a fall in prothrombin occurs. If a dangerously low level results, massive doses of vitamin K_1 may be necessary to restore prothrombin, and whole blood transfusions may also be necessary.

Salicylic acid, a degradation product of dicumarol, produces hypoprothrombinemia by similar action. The fall in prothrombin resulting from salicylates, however, is mild compared with that of dicumarol. The hemorrhagic manifestations in acute rheumatic fever may be due in some instances to large doses of salicylates; vitamin K is effective in neutralizing this action. Its use in children receiving large doses of salicylates would appear justified.

Treatment. Oral administration of vitamin K may correct mild prothrombin deficiency. One to 2 mg daily for an infant will usually suffice. If prothrombin deficiency is severe and hemorrhagic manifestations have appeared, 5 mg of vitamin K_1 daily should be given parenterally. Large doses of synthetic vitamin K analogues, but not of vitamin K_1, may result in hyperbilirubinemia and kernicterus in the glucose-6-phosphate dehydrogenase (G-6-PD)–deficient newborn and in the premature infant. In hypoprothrombinemia due to liver damage, vitamin K_1 may be given, but whole blood is usually also necessary.

LEWIS A. BARNESS

Corrigan JJ: The vitamin K dependent proteins. Adv Pediatr 28:57, 1981.

4

PREVENTIVE PEDIATRICS AND EPIDEMIOLOGY

Preventive pediatrics consists of efforts to avert rather than to cure disease and disability. It includes primary prevention, the attempts to avoid disease before it begins, such as tetanus immunization or chlorination of water supplies; secondary prevention, the recognizing and eliminating of the precursors of disease, such as screening programs for elevated blood lead levels and the Pap smear, and also efforts to identify and reverse disease in its early stages, such as a screening program for scoliosis in adolescents; and tertiary prevention, the measures for ameliorating or arresting the disabilities arising from established disease, such as physiotherapy to prevent contractures in patients with chronic neurologic disorders. Most successful primary preventive measures require understanding the cause, the pathogenesis, and the natural history of disease. For secondary or tertiary prevention, however, determining the cause is not essential.

Significant changes have occurred in child health in the United States during this century as a result of primary preventive medicine. Table 4–1 shows that in 1900, 53% of infant deaths were ascribed to infection; by 1984 this had decreased to 4%. Because of the striking diminution of deaths due to infections, other conditions loom proportionately larger in importance now than in the past. For example, although infant mortality rates from congenital anomalies declined by almost one half from 1900 to 1984, the proportion attributable to anomalies rose from 3% to 22% during those years. Similarly, although the frequency of sudden infant death syndrome has not increased in recent years, it is now responsible for one eighth of all infant deaths owing to the declining mortality from other conditions. Table 4–2 illustrates that in 1900 nearly 2% of all children 1–4 yr old died annually and 4 of 5 deaths were due to infection. By 1984 overall mortality in this age group was reduced by 97%, primarily owing to the reduction of death due to infections. Neoplastic diseases, congenital anomalies, and violence, all of which caused less than 5% of all deaths in this age group in 1900, were the primary cause in 63% in 1984 and thus now are proportionately more important, despite their actual reported decrease.

Table 4–1. **Certain Causes of Death for US Children Less Than 1 Yr of Age, 1900, 1950, and 1984***

Causes	1900	1950	1984
All	16,200	3,299	1079
Infection	8,586	543	43
Enteric	4,212	136	4
Anomalies	469	447	233
Perinatal	3,592	1,937	509
SIDS†	—	—	143
Accidents and violence	129	114	43
All others	3,424	258	108

*Deaths/100,000 children.
†Data not available until 1979.

Table 4–2. **Certain Causes of Death for US Children 1–4 Yr of Age, 1900, 1950, 1984***

Causes	1900	1950	1984
All	1980	141	52
Infection	1566	51	5
Respiratory	479	21	2
Enteric	311	6	<1
Neoplasms	8	13	4
Anomalies	9	11	7
Accidents and violence	74	37	22
All others	323	29	14

*Deaths/100,000 children.

These remarkable reductions in childhood mortality are attributable partly to medical advances such as immunization, anti-infective drugs, and various other diagnostic and therapeutic developments and partly to certain public health measures, such as filtration and chlorination of public water supplies, hygienic food handling (especially of milk), mosquito control, and isolation of infected persons. The indirect effects of social, economic, and educational advances have also played a role. However, many of the salutary changes in childhood mortality cannot be fully explained; for example, the annual crude mortality rates from measles declined 98% from 1900 to 1955 before the introduction of measles vaccine.

As a consequence of the decline in mortality, substantial changes in emphases in pediatric practice have occurred. Except for accident prevention, general pediatricians can do little to reduce the residual mortality from malignant neoplasms or congenital anomalies. Thus, increasing emphasis is placed on maintaining and enhancing the quality of the child's life and on ensuring that each child reaches adult life as physically, intellectually, and emotionally healthy as possible. Activities such as anticipatory guidance, developmental counseling, assisting families with children's school-related problems, sexual counseling, secondary prevention by screening for incipient disease, and attempting to ameliorate the precursors of adult disease have become integral parts of pediatric practice.

4.1 PRIMARY PREVENTION

Primary prevention occurs both within the community and in the pediatrician's office.

Community Primary Prevention. Several measures preventing disease at the community level have had enormous effects on childhood morbidity and mortality in the United States: sewage disposal and water sanitation, improved housing, hygienic control of food including pasteurization of milk, iodination of salt, and control of arthropod vectors of disease (such as mosquito control by swamp drainage in malarial areas). In areas of the world where these measures are still incompletely adopted, the spectrum of childhood mortality resembles that of the United States in 1900.

Many other public health programs of proven merit have not been universally adopted.

Fluoridation of public water supplies is efficacious in reducing dental caries. Its safety and its high benefit to cost ratio are well established. However, fluoridated water is currently available to only about half of all infants and children in the United States, since about 20% of the population live in areas without communal water supplies and 30% or more reside in communities where fluoridation, although feasible, has not been instituted for social, political, or economic reasons. Community fluoridation programs should be supported. In unfluoridated areas school programs should be established to provide fluoride tablets or rinses as alternative approaches. Additional measures include fluoride supplements from birth, and parental education about the importance of fluoridation.

Rat control is important in both rural and urban areas. By 1982 federally supported inner-city rat control programs resulted in the eradication of rats from neighborhoods in which 9.2 million people resided. These programs are directed primarily at environmental cleanup and sanitation and secondarily at extermination by baiting. They should be continued and expanded. Rural rat control is more difficult to achieve.

Pasteurization of milk prevents outbreaks of diarrheal disease caused by contaminating pathogenic bacteria. But the recent interest in the United States in "natural foods" has led to the increased consumption of raw milk under the fallacious assumption that it is nutritionally superior to pasteurized milk. Consequently, local outbreaks of diarrheal disease, which include fatalities, have occurred owing to the presence of strains of *Salmonella, Brucellosis, Campylobacter* and other gram-negative bacilli transmitted by milk. Pediatricians should educate parents and local authorities concerning the risks of raw milk (certified or not).

Accidents (Sec 5.37) and *homicide* (Chapter 1) result in 51% of all deaths in children 1–14 yr old; of these, 20% are due to automobile accidents (Table 4–3). Between 15 and 24 years of age, 86% of all deaths are due to external causes, and nearly half of these relate to the automobile; 40% of automobile fatalities in this age group are alcohol-related. Thus, external causes, including accidents, poisoning, homicide, and suicide are currently responsible for a major proportion of deaths of the United States' youth. Moreover, nonfatal injuries, including poisoning, account for much acute childhood morbidity (Table 4–4), and many of these injuries result in permanent disability.

Accident prevention is difficult because of the diversity of childhood injuries. Three approaches to primary prevention of childhood accidents have been used:

1. Public health education such as encouraging "childproofing" of the home.

2. Changes in children's environment, either mandated by law or voluntarily built in by manufacturers, such as flame-

Table 4–4. Childhood Morbidity From Acute Injury,* US, 1981†

	0–5 Yr	6–16 Yr
Injuries	36.7	40.3
Days of limited activity	21.6	38.4
Days of bed disability	12.1	29.1
School days lost	—	36.5

*Acute injury is defined as any injury, including poisoning, requiring medical attention or resulting in 1 or more days of restricted activity.
†Rate/100 children/yr.

resistant fabrics, childproof containers, paint of minimal lead content, window guards for apartment buildings, safe spacing of crib rails, and others. As of 1985, all but one state in the United States had passed an infant car seat law. These measures have been far more effective than public education.

3. One-on-one parent education by the child's physician. To provide effective parental guidance, the physician should know the household risk factors and the propensities of children at various ages for different types of accidents (Sec. 5.37). Particularly important are the medicine cabinet; areas where toxic household chemicals such as solvents, furniture polish, and the like are stored; the stove; matches; electrical wires and devices; and sharp objects such as glassware and knives. Outside the home the automobile and unprotected bodies of water endanger toddlers.

Accident prevention for older children and adolescents requires a proper balance between excessive restriction and undue permissiveness. Most sports, competitive or not, are associated with some jeopardy, though usually minor. Contact sports, such as football and hockey, present greater risk; proper equipment, supervision, and instruction minimize these risks. The trampoline is so potentially dangerous that it should not be available to children. Similarly, the excessive risks of boxing have caused both the American Medical Association and the American Academy of Pediatrics to advocate its discontinuation. Pediatricians should assume community responsibilities for certain aspects of accident prevention such as ensuring that playgrounds are reasonably safe and that sports programs are adequately supervised. Under some circumstances, developing and advocating mandatory regulations at the community or state level are indicated.

Poisoning has become a relatively more important child health problem as others have been ameliorated (Chapter 28). In Greater Cleveland during the years of 1971–1974, accidental poisoning was responsible for 3.1% of all hospital admissions and 2.2% of total hospital days for children 1–4 yr old. In the United States in 1979, 115 children 1–4 yr old died from accidental poisoning, which accounted for 1.0% of deaths in this age group. Pediatricians should work for primary prevention of poisoning not only from their offices but also in the community by supporting efforts at educating parents, childproofing containers, properly storing and disposing of toxic substances, and establishing poison control centers. During 1969–1979, toddler mortality from accidental poisoning declined by two-thirds largely because of Poison Control Center efforts.

Pediatricians should also participate in developing approaches to four major community problems for which satisfactory solutions have not yet been defined: homicide, adolescent pregnancy, suicide, and substance abuse.

Homicide statistics illustrated in Table 4–3 indicate that homicides accounted for 5% and 12% of deaths in 5–14 and 15–24 yr olds, respectively, in 1984; homicides among 15–19 yr olds accounted for more than a third of deaths. Homicide rates for young black males over the past 15 years have been distinctly greater than for other groups; in 1979 for white males it was 14.8 and for black males 78.9 per 100,000. More

Table 4–3. All Causes and External Causes of Death of US Persons 1–24 Yr of Age, 1984*

Causes	Age in Years		
	1–4	*5–14*	*15–24*
All	51.9	26.7	96.8
External	22.6	14.6	75.1
Motor vehicle	6.9	6.7	36.7
Suicide	—	0.7	12.5
Homicide	2.4	1.3	12.0

*Deaths/100,000 persons.

than 75% of these deaths were due to firearms and usually unrelated to criminal activities. The amount of permanent disability occurring to gunshot wound survivors can only be speculated. Suicide rates among the young increased about 40% during the 1970's; rates are higher for males, particularly white males. Most are carried out with firearms. The causes of homicide and suicide are undoubtedly multiple and include complex social and economic factors. Pediatricians should warn parents of the dangers of firearms and should participate in developing a public solution.

Adolescent Pregnancy. A problem involving all aspects of prevention is sexuality and consequent pregnancy in adolescents (Sec. 9.7). Teenage pregnancy causes major social, psychologic, educational, and financial burdens for the young parent(s). The infant of a teenage mother is at enhanced risk physically and developmentally, although, after adjustment for socioeconomic status and prenatal care, the only immediate consequences attributable to maternal youth are increases in pre-eclampsia and in low birthweight infants. In recent years rates of live births to teenage females have decreased slightly but absolute numbers of births to teenagers have not because of increases in the adolescent population. Fertility rates for girls under 15 yr, however, have changed very little since the mid-1970's, prior to which they had risen rapidly. In 1982, about 24,000 pregnancies occurred in girls less than 15 years old; of these about 60% were terminated by abortion, and nearly 10,000 were carried to term. At these rates 1 of 75 girls becomes pregnant between her 10th and 15th birthdays, and 1 in 180 delivers a live baby in this interval. Similarly, 1 in 6 females becomes pregnant between her 15th and 18th birthdays; 1 in 10 has a live born child. Rates in nonwhites are more than double those in whites.

The multiple and complex reasons for teenage pregnancies make control difficult to achieve; not all are accidental. Though precise data are not available, teenage sexual activity and pregnancy affect all population groups, but pregnancy appears to occur more frequently in lower socioeconomic groups.

The optimal solution to the problem would be the reduction or avoidance of sexual activity during adolescence. Because this goal is unrealistic, most efforts have been directed at encouraging and facilitating use of contraceptives by sexually active teenagers (Sec. 9.8). The key factors in successful programs directed at this problem have been outreach, nonjudgmental counseling to reduce ambivalent feelings about pregnancy and contraceptives, making contraceptives readily available and linking services with school health programs. For pregnant teenagers, counseling about options and encouraging regular prenatal care are important, as are helping to develop plans for care of the infant, continuing the mother's education, and preventing further pregnancies until maturity.

Substance abuse is discussed in Sec. 9.4.

Primary Prevention in the Pediatrician's Office. The purposes of routine child health care are to foster the smooth, normal development of the child from infancy to adulthood and to help ensure that each child achieves his or her full physical, intellectual, and emotional adult potential. In infancy, interaction between the pediatrician and the child is largely mediated by the parents; in later childhood and adolescence, a direct relationship between the physician and the child increasingly develops. Children's regularly scheduled health maintenance checkups are evaluative and preventive. Evaluations include the usual interval history and inquiries into any perceived problem, assessment of growth and development by history and examination, and screening for various abnormalities or their precursors. Preventive management includes efforts to correct or ameliorate any abnormalities, specific preventive measures such as immunization,

and anticipatory guidance. The following general recommendations derived from the American Academy of Pediatrics comprise general guidelines for the care of normal infants and children; the needs of individual children and their families may require modification. For example, an experienced family with a third child may require fewer visits than new anxious parents whose prior pregnancy terminated in death due to prematurity.

Prenatal Period. It is desirable, particularly with first pregnancies, for the parents to talk with their pediatrician sometime during the 3rd trimester about any of their problems or concerns. At this time they can review the pediatrician's role in the subsequent care of the child, which includes care in the newborn nursery, the proposed schedule of visits, planned immunizations, and the like. Financial arrangements may also be discussed. Other topics might include desirability of breast feeding, the pros and cons of circumcision, living arrangements for the baby, and what help may be available at home during the first week or two after birth. The pediatrician may also help to instill confidence in the parents by pointing out there is no single correct method of caring for the baby and that for the most part their own instincts in dealing with the infant from day to day should be followed.

Newborn Care. See also Sec. 8.4–8.6. Every infant should receive prophylaxis for ophthalmia neonatorum and a single intramuscular dose of a vitamin K preparation (0.1–0.2 mg menadione sodium bisulfite or 0.5 mg vitamin K_1). A test for PKU should be done and T_4 measured. Ten to 15 mL of cord blood should be collected at birth and saved in the refrigerator for 7 days for typing, Coombs testing, and other tests if needed.

Just prior to discharge it is important to sit down with the parents to review care at home, to reassure the parents of a normal infant, and, particularly, to encourage them to enjoy their baby. The parents also should be assured of the availability of the pediatrician by phone; a telephone conversation after the baby has been home 1–2 wk is desirable.

Follow-up. The optimal time for the first routine follow-up visit depends on the status of the infant and the experience of the parents. An office visit at 3–4 wk after birth ensures that feeding is going well, provides answers to questions that have arisen, identifies and solves minor problems, and reassures the parents. Table 4–5A and B suggests schedules for evaluation and preventive measures at specific ages.

Routine Immunization. The schedule for immunization is that recommended for routine protection of children by the Committee on Infectious Diseases of the American Academy of Pediatrics and the Advisory Committee on Immunization Practices (ACIP), U.S. Public Health Service. Pediatricians should understand the benefits and risks of children's vaccines and adequately inform parents about them.

Diphtheria and Tetanus Toxoids and Pertussis Vaccine (DTP). Immunization is ordinarily started at 8 wk of age; two additional doses are given at 2 mo intervals. A 4th dose is given at approximately 15–18 mo of age and a 5th dose at the time of school entry. DTP is not given after the 7th birthday. Instead, tetanus and diphtheria toxoids for adult use, combined (Td), containing a smaller amount of diphtheria toxoid are recommended at 10 yr intervals. DTP and Td should be given intramuscularly, preferably in the anterolateral thigh in young infants and either in the thigh or the deltoid in older children. Although the first of three doses of DTP may be given at 1 mo intervals with the initial dose at 4 wk of age if widespread pertussis is occurring, the 2 mo interval avoids unnecessary expense and inconvenience to parents.

There are three contraindications to administering DTP: (1) an acute febrile illness, since confusion may result as to the cause of subsequent symptoms (a minor respiratory infection

Table 4–5A. Evaluation at Specific Ages

Note: Interval history, dietary and sleep patterns, height, and weight should be included in each routine visit and are not listed on the table. Items not previously performed, as with an older child who is a new patient, should be carried out at the initial visit.

Procedure	Months							Years									
	2	4	6	9	12	15	18	2	3	4	5	6	8	10	12	14	16
Interview																	
Family history	+											+					+
Pregnancy and delivery	+																
Neonatal course	+																
Other past history	+																
Immunizations		+															
Developmental evaluation (see Chap. 2)																	
Body systems (for special attention)																	
Hearing, vision	+	+	+	+	+		+										
GI (defecation, etc.)	+			+			+	+	+	+							
Urinary	+							+									
Dental care									+	+	+	+	+	+	+	+	+
Drugs, alcohol, tobacco															+	+	+
Pica					+	+	+	+	+	+							
Sexual behavior														+	+	+	+
Physical examination (for special attention)																	
Head circumference	+	+	+	+	+												
Blood pressure									+	+	+	+	+	+	+	+	+
Vision																	
Fixed eyes	+																
Red reflex	+																
Fundus			+						+								
Strabismus			+														
Snellen chart									+		+			+			
Hearing																	
Gross	+			+													
Audiometer											+	+		+			
Speech					+			+	+								
Hip dislocation	+	+	+														
Gait						+	+	+									
Scoliosis													+	+	+	+	+
Pubertal development														+	+	+	+
Laboratory																	
Hgb or Hct				+				+					+				+
Urinalysis			+					+					+				+
Urine culture (girls)					+						+			+		+	
Tuberculin					+				+				+	+	+	+	+

Table 4–5B. Preventive Measures at Specific Ages

Measure	Months							Years									
	2	4	6	9	12	15	18	2	3	4	5	6	8	10	12	14	16
Immunizations																	
DTP	+	+	+			+*											
Td																+	
OPV	+	+	±	(optional)		+*	+				+						
MMR						+											
H. influenzae type b								+									
Influenza viral (high risk only)					+			Annually hereafter									
Pneumococcal (high risk only)								+									
Counseling (for special attention)																	
Diet	+	+	+	+	+	+	+	+	+					+	+	+	
Sleep	+	+	+		+		+	+	+			+		+	+	+	
Toilet training						+	+	+									
Accidents (see Sec. 5.37)																	
Day care									+								
School problems												+	+	+	+	+	+
Puberty and sexuality														+	+	+	+
Substance abuse													+	+	+	+	+

*The fourth dose of DTP and the third dose of OPV may be given simultaneously with the MMR at 15 mo, or DTP and OPV may be deferred until 18 mo.

is not a contraindication); (2) an evolving or suspected neurologic illness (for the same reason); and (3) a severe reaction to a prior dose of DTP.

DTP immunization of infants with underlying neurologic disorders, real or suspected, presents a special problem. Because DTP may precipitate or unmask manifestations of pre-existing neurologic problems and because temporal coincidence may result in confusion about causation, delaying initiation of DTP in such an infant for a few months until the situation is resolved is recommended. Detailed recommendations for immunizing these infants, published by the American Academy of Pediatrics and the U.S. Public Health Service, should be consulted.

Reactions that follow a DTP injection may be of three varieties. The first is minor, including local swelling and tenderness at the site of injection, slight fever, and irritability. A fever of greater than 105° F (40.5° C) is a contraindication to further doses of DTP. Second, reactions that are upsetting but without demonstrated sequelae include excessive somnolence beyond that attributable to a visit to the physician and disruption of daily schedule, protracted inconsolable crying that may last 4 hr or more, and an unusual shock-like syndrome that also may last for hours. The pathogenesis of these reactions is unknown. The shock-like syndrome is a contraindication to further injections of DTP. The degrees of excessive somnolence or inconsolable crying sufficient to warrant discontinuation of DTP are matters of judgment. Third, neurologic reactions contraindicating further DTP include occasional convulsions and, fortunately only rarely, frank encephalopathy, sometimes with brain damage or death. Because most of the reactivity of DTP is due to the pertussis component, the occurrence of one of these reactions does not contraindicate continuation of immunization against diphtheria and tetanus using diphtheria and tetanus toxoids for pediatric use (DT). Although local and febrile reactions to this preparation may occur, they are less severe than those to DTP and, except for extraordinarily rare anaphylactic reactions to tetanus toxoid, are not dangerous. Because no firm evidence exists that decreasing the dose of DTP significantly reduces the reactivity of the pertussis component, and because administering partial doses of DTP needs to be continuous until the full 12 units of pertussis vaccine (1.5 mL) are given, such divided doses are not warranted.

Polio Vaccines. Two types of vaccine are licensed in the United States: OPV, a live, attenuated trivalent polio vaccine (Sabin), and IPV, an inactivated (killed) trivalent polio vaccine (Salk). A full course of either vaccine protects the recipient against paralytic poliomyelitis almost without exception. Because rare cases of paralytic poliomyelitis occur in recipients of OPV or in their close contacts, some have advocated returning to IPV for routine immunization of children. Epidemiologic support for this recommendation comes from Sweden and other countries in which eradication of poliomyelitis has been achieved by IPV alone. The current IPV preparation, more potent than the earlier product, is presently being field tested in the United States. However, immunization advisory groups in the United States have continued to recommend OPV for routine immunization of children because of the virtual eradication of poliomyelitis from the United States by OPV and because of the belief that circulation of wild virus in the community is controlled better by the greater intestinal immunity afforded by OPV. Four doses of IPV are necessary for primary immunization: at 2, 4, and 6 mo, and 6–12 mo after the third dose.

The first dose of OPV should be given at approximately 2 mo of age and the second 2 mo later. Ninety-five percent of recipients are protected against all three strains of poliomyelitis by this regimen. In communities close to areas of high endemicity of poliomyelitis, such as the southwestern United States, a third dose at 6 mo of age is recommended. An additional dose is given to all children at approximately 15–18 mo of age and another prior to school entry. An interval of at least 2 mo between doses of OPV is required because intestinal carriage of vaccine virus may persist for up to 6 wk with consequent viral interference. The doses administered at 15–18 mo and prior to school entry are considered as "fillers" rather than boosters in case one of the original doses did not "take." The same schedule is recommended for IPV.

OPV should not be given to individuals proven or suspected to be immunocompromised, including those with congenital and acquired immunodeficiencies and those whose immune mechanisms are impaired by therapy. OPV also should not be given to household contacts of immunocompromised individuals or to subsequent siblings of a child with congenital immunodeficiency until the younger child is shown to be normal.

Unimmunized parents of infants scheduled for poliomyelitis immunization represent a special problem owing to their risk, albeit remote, of acquiring paralytic poliomyelitis from the vaccinated infant. In this situation two courses of action are acceptable. The first is administering OPV to the infant, regardless of the immune status of household contacts, the usual practice in the United States. The second is to give three consecutive monthly doses of IPV to the adult household contacts, administering the initial dose of OPV to the infant at the time of the third dose of IPV to the contacts. If the adult household contacts have been partially immunized with OPV or IPV, they should be given OPV or IPV, respectively, at the same time that the initial dose of OPV is administered to the infant. Adults and children traveling to areas where poliomyelitis is endemic should be fully immunized with polio vaccine (Sec. 4.4).

Measles-Mumps-Rubella Vaccine, Combined (MMR). Routine immunization with these live attenuated viruses should be administered at 15 mo of age. Because of persistent maternal antibody, vaccine failures, particularly with the measles component, occur when MMR is administered prior to this time; the younger the infant, the more likely is failure. However, when outbreaks of measles occur, the vaccine should be given as early as 9 mo of age but repeated some time after 15 mo. Teenagers who escaped natural rubella and measles in childhood and who were unimmunized should be identified and immunized. Currently these two diseases are more frequent in children over 10 yr than in better immunized younger children. Epidemics among college students have led to recommendations that these students be required to present documentation of immunity to measles and other vaccine-preventable diseases as a prerequisite to registration (Sec 11.61). MMR ensures seroconversion to all three antigens in 90–95% of recipients. Most vaccine failures, particularly to measles, are attributable to improper refrigeration, exposure to light, administration at too early an age, or the simultaneous use of immune serum globulin. There is no justification for the routine use of monovalent measles, mumps, or rubella vaccines in children.

Contraindications to MMR are pregnancy, immunodeficiency or therapeutic immunosuppression, or an acute febrile illness. Although the accumulated experience has not found any deleterious effects on the fetus when these vaccines were given in the first trimester, not giving MMR to pregnant women is prudent. Additionally, women of childbearing age given MMR should be cautioned to avoid pregnancy for the next 3 mo. As with any live virus vaccine, immunocompromised individuals should not be immunized. Immunization of individuals receiving immunosuppressive therapy should be delayed until at least 3 mo following discontinuation of therapy. The measles and mumps vaccines are grown in chick-embryo cell culture. Because allergic reactions to these vaccines have been reported in at least five children with prior anaphylaxis from egg ingestion, such children should not receive either vaccine. Other types of egg allergy are not contraindications. In contrast to OPV, transmission of measles, mumps, or rubella vaccine virus to susceptible contacts has not occurred. Therefore, the presence of a pregnant or immunocompromised household contact does not contraindicate immunization with MMR.

Adverse reactions to MMR attributable to the measles component include transient rashes and fever up to 103° F (39.4° C) occurring in a few individuals at 6–11 days after immunization. Subacute sclerosing panencephalitis (SSPE) has been attributed on rare occasions to measles vaccine. If it occurs, it does so at a much lower rate than that following natural measles. Additionally, because of the rubella component, transient arthralgia, rarely arthritis, and paresthetic pains may occur in 1–2% of children and a higher percentage of adults, especially females, 2–8 wk following immunization. These phenomena usually last only a few days; cases of rheumatoid arthritis in children occurring after rubella vaccine probably are coincidental, although this may not be the case in adults. Recognizable reactions to the mumps component have not occurred.

Delayed Immunization. Infants more than 2 mo but less than 14 mo of age without any immunization should be started on the same sequence of immunizations and intervals between doses as those recommended for young infants. Infants and children who previously received one or more doses of any vaccine at intervals longer than those routinely recommended do not require reinitiation of the series; completion of full immunization, counting the original doses, should be undertaken.

Children 14 mo–7 yr of age who have received no immunizations should receive DTP, OPV, and a tuberculin test at the first visit. To provide prompt protection against measles, MMR should be given 1 mo later, followed by DTP and OPV after an additional month. Approximately 2 mo after the second DTP and OPV (4 mo after the initial doses), the third dose of DTP and, in poliomyelitis-endemic areas, the third dose of OPV should be given. DTP and OPV should be repeated approximately 1 yr later. For a child more than 4 yr of age at completion of this regimen, further immunization prior to school entry is unnecessary; otherwise DTP and OPV should be given again between 5 and 7 yr of age. All children should receive a dose of Td in early adolescence.

When immunization is delayed, questions arise about simultaneously administering multiple antigens, such as DTP, OPV, and MMR at the initial visit. There is no interference between DTP and OPV (or IPV). Although one study suggested that DTP and MMR given at the same time resulted in reduced seroconversion rates to measles, others have shown no difference. MMR and the "filler" dose of OPV are effective when given simultaneously in the 2nd yr; whether giving MMR and the first dose of OPV at this time compromises immune response is not known. Likewise, it is not known whether giving initial doses of DTP and OPV with MMR to an unimmunized child 15 mo or older is fully effective. Nonetheless, when such an older unimmunized child is seen in whom the adequacy of follow-up is doubtful, simultaneously administering DTP, OPV and MMR is reasonable. An interval of at least 1 mo should always be allowed between doses of the same or different vaccines (2 mo between doses of OPV) when they are not given simultaneously.

Special Vaccines. Annual immunization against **viral influenza** diseases is inappropriate for normal children, but *should* be given to children at high risk from infections of the lower respiratory tract. Examples include children susceptible to: pulmonary infections from congenital or acquired heart disease (such as left to right shunts); disorders that compromise pulmonary function, including cystic fibrosis, severe asthma, neuromuscular and orthopedic conditions that distort or weaken the thoracic cage, and pulmonary dysplasia as a consequence of the neonatal respiratory distress syndrome; chronic azotemic renal disease or the nephrotic syndrome; diabetes mellitus; and chronic severe anemia such as thalassemia or sicklemia. Immunodeficient and immunocompromised children may also benefit. Since the constituents of influenza vaccine must be changed yearly owing to shifts in prevalent influenza viruses, annual recommendations of the U.S. Public Health Service, published in the *Morbidity and Mortality Weekly Report,* should be consulted for doses and schedules.

The 23 valent **pneumococcal vaccine** presently licensed in the United States is not recommended for routine use in children. As with other polysaccharide vaccines, its efficacy is minimal in children under 2 yr of age. Experience with children having sickle cell anemia indicates that the vaccine is useful in children older than 2 yr having functional or anatomic asplenia. The dose is 0.5 mL intramuscularly or subcutaneously; because antibodies persist and because reactivity is high even as long as 4 yr after the initial dose, reimmunization with pneumococcal vaccine is currently not indicated. The vaccine is probably ineffective in preventing otitis media.

The vaccine against *Haemophilus influenzae type b* is discussed in Sec. 11.20. The indications for the occasional use of other vaccines, such as meningococcal polysaccharide vaccine and typhoid vaccine, are discussed under those disease sections and in Sec. 4.5. Mixed respiratory vaccines and autogenous respiratory vaccines, oral or injected, are ineffective. Smallpox vaccine is discussed in Sec. 11.67.

Tuberculin Test. This should be performed early in the 2nd yr of life. It may be given before or, for convenience, at the time MMR is administered. Subsequent tuberculin testing is advisable prior to school entry and in early adolescence, but the physician should deviate from this schedule when circumstances, such as the local prevalence of tuberculosis, dictate.

Other Primary Preventions. In 1983 there were 2,010,000 deaths in the United States. Arteriosclerotic heart disease and stroke accounted for nearly 40% and cancer for 22% of these deaths. Because there is evidence that the factors responsible for degenerative vascular disease commence in childhood and that they may be somewhat controllable, considerable interest has developed in screening children for risk factors for premature degenerative cardiovascular disease and in attempting to change these risks. Risk factors include hyperlipidemia (Sec. 7.39–7.46), obesity, hypertension (Sec. 14.88), smoking, and, perhaps, sedentary habits. Although there are uncertainties about the role of these risk factors, their interactions, and the effects of intervention in the young, it seems prudent to discourage obesity and the initiation of smoking and to monitor blood pressure of all children. Children whose parent or grandparent had early coronary artery disease appear to be at highest risk and, therefore, should be screened for hyperlipidemia after 2 yr of age.

Reducing the likelihood of cancer in later life by childhood intervention is an even more difficult problem. Age-adjusted cancer mortality rates increased 10% between 1940 and 1983; this was almost entirely due to the more than 4-fold increase in mortality from respiratory cancer, which is largely attributable to cigarettes. Thus, preventing the initiation of smoking would produce enormous benefits. Other personal activities, including dietary habits, are variably associated epidemiologically with excessive rates of cancer at certain anatomic sites. For example, an apparent relationship between meat ingestion and bowel cancer suggests that perhaps a high fiber diet may reduce the risk of intestinal cancer; however, these data are not sufficiently firm to warrant major dietary changes in children. The effects of environmental pollution are even more uncertain. Although occupational exposure to some substances, such as arsenic, asbestos, and vinyl chloride, is known to be responsible for certain tumors (Sec. 16.1 and 28.16), the effect of general environmental pollution on cancer incidence or mortality is yet unclear. This uncertainty may be due to the long latent period between the exposure and the appearance of neoplasia and to the fact that the dramatic increase in exposure to chemicals began only 2–3 decades ago.

4.2 SECONDARY AND TERTIARY PREVENTION

Many facets of routine pediatric care (Table 4–5A and B) represent secondary preventive efforts. The family history, monitoring of development, sensory evaluation, blood pressure, and the like, are designed to identify the susceptibilities to, or antecedents of, later disease and thus are secondary preventive measures. Others include screening for tuberculosis, urinary tract infections, proteinuria, scoliosis, and early signs of congenital hip dysplasia. Care for the common, acute childhood illnesses also largely represents secondary prevention in that treatment for such illnesses in many cases prevents sequelae that would occur in very few. For example, streptococcal pharyngitis is treated to prevent rheumatic fever and suppurative complications, such as peritonsillar abscess. Further, acute bacterial otitis media will subside spontaneously in up to 95% of instances; the major benefit of antimicrobial therapy is the prevention of mastoiditis and/or chronic perforation of the drum.

Similarly, a great deal of care for chronic illness and disability in childhood represents tertiary prevention. Examples include many facets of care for children with cystic fibrosis, orthopedic measures for cerebral palsy and neural tube defects, anti-streptococcal prophylaxis for those having had rheumatic fever, and physiotherapy for children with rheumatoid arthritis. The pediatrician is additionally responsible for providing continuous support to the family while ameliorating as much as possible the social, psychologic, and financial effects of chronic illness on the child and other family members. Because such children often require the attention of subspecialists and various services such as physiotherapy, occupational therapy, and nutritional counseling, the pediatrician must coordinate these activities while providing regular child health care and treatment of intercurrent illness. The pediatrician must ensure that care proffered or recommended by other providers, including subspecialists and nonmedical health care professionals, is considered comprehensively, with respect to all aspects of the child and the family and to the probabilities that diagnostic and therapeutic benefits will outweigh the risks, untoward effects, and costs.

4.3 EPIDEMIOLOGY IN PEDIATRICS

Epidemiology is the scientific study of factors influencing health, disease, and the control of disease in populations rather than in individuals. Historically, epidemiology began with the search for clues to the causation of disease; more recently it has been employed in assessing preventive and therapeutic measures and in evaluating health services, including costs.

Physicians are constantly applying *clinical epidemiology* as a science of probabilities in making decisions. For example, whether to obtain a throat culture from a child with fever and an injected pharynx is a decision involving an assessment of the likelihood that group A streptococci will be recovered from the culture, which depends on a wide spectrum of variables, including age of the child, the season of the year, existing disease patterns in the community, the clinical features of the child's illness, and the chance of the child developing rheumatic fever if streptococcal pharyngitis is not recognized and treated because the throat was not cultured. These variables comprise a series of probabilities established by others' observations of large groups of children with and without streptococcal pharyngitis and by the physician's own experiences. These probabilities cannot always be precise but are subject to judgment; nonetheless they are useful in clinical decision making.

There are three types of epidemiologic studies. *Descriptive epidemiology* records the incidence and prevalence of death, disability, and disease of various types and causes. National, state, county, city, and local health departments and other agencies in the United States tabulate current information about health and disease. The National Center for Health Statistics and the Centers for Disease Control publish detailed morbidity and mortality data for the entire United States, for individual states, and, to a limited extent, for counties and metropolitan areas. *Causative (analytic) epidemiology* searches for clues to the causes of disease based on the fact that disease does not occur randomly in the population. Differences exist between those who incur a disease and those who do not, which may be due to inherent characteristics of the individuals themselves or due to the experiences of the individual. A given characteristic is said to be "associated" with a disease, e.g., it is found more often in those with the illness than in those without it. *Experimental epidemiology* uses clinical trials to compare responses to different therapies in groups of subjects.

There are three subtypes of *causative epidemiology* studies: cross-sectional, prospective, and retrospective. *Cross-sectional studies* are usually surveys that determine differences in prevalences of disease among various segments of the population at a particular time. A *prospective* study identifies a cohort of individuals who exhibit a particular characteristic, such as hypertension or exposure to an environmental pollutant, and follows them over time for the development of disease; a comparable cohort of persons without hypertension or exposure would also be similarly followed over time for the development of disease. The major advantage of such studies is that the actual rate of disease attributable to the factor in question can be determined because the numbers of those at risk, those not at risk, and those who develop disease in both groups are available. Disadvantages include that the investigator must suspect in advance which factor is associated with the disease, that an unrecognized causative factor may exist but not be considered, and that the disease must be reasonably frequent, since the cohorts of exposed and unexposed persons would otherwise be of unwieldy size. Sometimes conducting a prospective study by retrospection is possible by identifying cohorts of exposed and unexposed persons from prior records; an example is the study of gynecologic abnormalities in female offspring of women who did or did not receive DES during their pregnancies.

Retrospective (case-control) epidemiologic studies start with disease and search for past differences in exposure or other characteristics between groups of affected and nonaffected persons. This type of study is particularly useful in two situations: first, when few or no clues to causation exist; and second, when the causative agent is strongly suspected but the disorders in question are so rare that prospective studies are not feasible logistically and economically. An example of the first type is a study of Reye syndrome in which parents of patients and controls were asked about possible exposures to different types of medications and to various environmental substances; a strong association between salicylate use and subsequent Reye syndrome was observed.

Retrospective studies have certain disadvantages. The **absolute risk** of disease following exposure (the number of cases per 100,000 exposed persons) cannot be determined because the denominator of exposed individuals is unavailable. Only an estimate of **relative risk** (ratio of disease frequencies in exposed and unexposed persons) can be obtained. There is also considerable potential for bias in the selection of controls and in the differences of recall that exist between patients and controls.

Causative epidemiologic studies are frequently criticized because association does not prove causation. This is true; however, the strength of the association (i.e., the magnitude of the difference between cases and controls) and the lack of a plausible alternative for explaining the difference may be such that association is tantamount to causation even though the specific etiologic mechanism is unknown. Causation studies often require a judgmental decision, as with aspirin and Reye syndrome.

In *experimental epidemiology* or a clinical trial, the effect of a new preventive or therapeutic measure is compared with another form of treatment or to no treatment by randomly assigning comparable patients to each measure. Groups of patients are usually necessary for comparison purposes because the outcomes of most diseases are variable, which prevents drawing conclusions from only one or several individuals. Randomization within certain subgroups, such as by age or sex, is sometimes desirable and is called stratified randomization. In a double-blind study, both the experimenters and the subjects are unaware of treatment assignment. In a single-blind study, the experimenters but not the patients are aware of treatment assignment. In a triple-blind study, not only the experimenters and patients but also those conducting the analyses are unaware of assignment.

In comparative epidemiologic studies (causative and experimental epidemiology), there is always potential for three types of bias; selection, confounding, and observational. Selection bias is an inherent difference between the study and control groups that might influence the results. For example, in a clinical trial of a new drug or a new surgical procedure, if the control group is more seriously ill than the study group, the benefits might be mistakenly attributed to the new measure. Alternatively, if the study group comprised more severe cases, a beneficial effect of the new treatment might be obscured. Selection bias may occur also in causative epidemiology if the control group differs, in addition to the factor in question, in some other inherent characteristic or exposure related to the outcome. An example is the reported association between coffee consumption and cancer of the pancreas. Coffee consumption by patients and controls hospitalized with other diseases was determined by interview. Patients with alcohol and tobacco-related diseases were excluded from the control group, but because alcohol and tobacco use are associated with coffee consumption, it is possible that persons who drink little or no coffee were overly represented in the control group. Thus the association may be spurious.

Confounding bias occurs when another factor linked to the disease or issue in question is also associated with the characteristic under study. For example, one might conclude that chronic tonsillitis occurred more frequently in a suburban community than in the inner city because of the greater number of tonsillectomies performed in the suburbs. However, this conclusion is unjustified, because affluence is associated both with an increased tonsillectomy rate and with living in a suburb.

Observational bias occurs either when the study or the control group is observed more intensively than the other group, when there is greater interest in recalling past events by patients than by controls, or when there is a placebo effect. An example of observational bias due to the placebo effect is a study of a cold vaccine conducted on the University of Minnesota students prior to World War II. Students reporting undue susceptibility to colds received a vaccine and during the subsequent year noted a 70% reduction in colds. However, unknown to the students, about half of them received a saline placebo, and those students in this group experienced the same reduction.

Pediatricians are constantly exposed to new information intended to modify the way they practice medicine, and they have a responsibility to approach such information critically, using their basic medical knowledge and their knowledge of study design and analysis. They should examine the studies' methods, particularly for the possibility of bias. Because degrees of bias are inescapable in almost all studies, it is important to make a judgment based on medical knowledge about whether the bias is sufficient to negate the conclusions. If the results seem valid, pediatricians should then decide whether these apply to their patient populations and whether they should alter their own medical practices.

Biostatistics. This is the method used in clinical epidemiology to determine the likelihood that an observed difference between the groups studied is explained by chance. A p value of less than 0.05, for example, indicates that the probability that the difference between the groups due to chance is less than 5%; one is 95% sure that the difference is not due to chance. Three corollaries of this approach should be kept in mind. First, a p value indicates only the probability of a true difference but this does not mean that the true difference is exactly that which has been observed; it may turn out to be more or less if the study populations were expanded to include infinite numbers of subjects. Confidence limits are frequently provided to indicate the range of probabilities created by the use of a finite number of subjects. For example, a causative epidemiologic study might find that, compared with unexposed controls, exposure to a given chemical increases the likelihood of developing a particular cancer 12-fold (a relative risk of 12). But if the study was based on only 20 patients with the tumor, it would be reported as a relative risk of 12 (95% confidence limits 7.3 to 18.5), meaning that one can be 95% confident that exposure to the chemical increases the risk of that cancer between 7-fold and 18-fold.

Second, a p value of 0.05 means that one *expects* a difference as large as that observed to occur once in 20 times owing to chance. That is, if statistical tests are made of 100 variables in a study, one should not be surprised to find that five of the tests produced p values of 0.05; indeed one of them should reach the 0.01 level. For example, in repeatedly flipping a coin, the probability that heads will appear five times in a row is 0.03125 (p < 0.04). This also means that, if one flips a coin in repeated series of five tosses, all heads should occur once in every 32 series of five flips.

The third corollary is that biostatistical significance tests are not a substitute for critically assessing the study methods combined with medical judgment, which includes assessing the importance of the health problem in question.

There are multiple statistical tests, each applicable to special situations. Most commonly employed are tests for differences between proportions, such as the percentage of patients cured with one drug compared with those cured with another, e.g., the chi-square test. For comparisons of means, Student's t-test is employed. Reference texts should be consulted for further explanation of these and other methods of statistical and epidemiologic analysis.

General

Fulginiti VA, Bartlett VE, Book LS, et al: Pediatric patient education: Challenge for the '80s. Pediatrics (Suppl)74:913, 1984.

Roghmann KJ, Hoekelman RA, McInerny TK: The changing pattern of primary pediatric care: Update for one community. Pediatrics 73:363, 1984.

Morbidity and Mortality

National Center for Health Statistics: Advance report of final mortality statistics, 1982. Monthly Vital Statistics Report (Suppl)33:1, 1984.
National Center for Health Statistics: Current estimates from the national health interview survey: United States, 1981. Data from the national health survey. Series 10. No. 141. DHHS Publication No. (PHS)82–1569, 1982.
National Center for Health Statistics and its predecessors: Vital statistics of the United States, 1900–1978.
Wegman ME: Annual summary of vital statistics—1983. Pediatrics 74:981, 1984.

Public Health Measures

Centers for Disease Control: Urban rat control—United States, Second Quarter, Fiscal Year 1982. Morbid Mortal Weekly Rep 31:602, 1982.
Horowitz AM, Thomas HB (eds): Promoting the use of fluorides in communities: Past accomplishments and future perspectives. Horowitz AM, Thomas HB, eds. A symposium. Presented at the annual session of the American Association for Dental Research, March 20, 1980, Los Angeles. J Pub Health Dent 40:211, 1980.
Potter ME, Kaufman AF, Blake PA, et al: Unpasteurized milk: The hazards of a health fetish. JAMA 252:2048, 1984.

Accidents and Violence

Boyce WT, Sprunger LW, Sobolewski S, et al: Epidemiology of injuries in a large, urban school district. Pediatrics 74:342, 1984.
Centers for Disease Control: Temporal patterns of motor-vehicle-related fatalities associated with young drinking drivers—United States, 1983. Morbid Mortal Weekly Rep 33:699, 1984.
Centers for Disease Control: Violent deaths among persons 15–25 years of age—United States, 1970–1978. Morbid Mortal Weekly Rep 32:453, 1983.
Chafee-Bahamon C, Lovejoy FH Jr: Effectiveness of a regional poison center in reducing excess emergency room visits for children's poisonings. Pediatrics 72:164, 1983.
Committee on Accident and Poison Prevention, American Academy of Pediatrics: Automatic passenger protection systems. Pediatrics 74:146, 1984.
Decker MD, Dewey MJ, Hutcheson RH Jr, et al: The use and efficacy of child restraint devices. JAMA 252:2571, 1984.
Sudak HS, Ford AB, Rushforth NB: Suicide in the Young. Boston, John Wright–PSG Inc, 1984.
Torg J, Das M: Trampoline-related quadriplegia: Review of the literature and reflections on the American Academy of Pediatrics' position statement. Pediatrics 74:804, 1984.
Westman JS, Morrow G III: Moped injuries in children. Pediatrics 74:820, 1984.

Adolescent Pregnancy

Brann EA, Edwards L, Callicott T, et al: Strategies for the prevention of pregnancy in adolescents. Advances in Planned Parenthood 14:68, 1979.
National Center for Health Statistics: Advance report of final natality statistics, 1982. Monthly Vital Statistics Report (Suppl) 33:1, 1984.

Routine Child Health Maintenance

Committee on Psychosocial Aspects of Child and Family Health, American Academy of Pediatrics: The prenatal visit. Pediatrics 73:561, 1984.
Committee on Standards of Child Health Care. 3rd ed. American Academy of Pediatrics. Evanston, IL, 1977.
Recommendation of the Immunization Practices Advisory Committee (ACIP): Diphtheria, tetanus, and pertussis: Guidelines for vaccine prophylaxis and other preventive measures. Morbid Mortal Weekly Rep 34:405, 1985.
Recomendation of the Immunization Practices Advisory Committee (ACIP): Polysaccharide vaccine for prevention of *Haemophilus influenzae* type b disease. Morbid Mortal Weekl Rep 34:201, 1985.
Report of the Committee on Infectious Diseases. Ed 19. American Academy of Pediatrics, Evanston, IL, 1982.

Prevention of Disease in Later Life

American Heart Association. Inter-Society Commission for Heart Disease Resources: Special report: Optimal resources for primary prevention of atherosclerotic diseases. Circulation 70:153A, 1984.
Committee on Nutrition, American Academy of Pediatrics: Toward a prudent diet for children. Pediatrics 71:78, 1983.

Epidemiology

Cody CL, Baraff LJ, Cherry JD, et al: Nature and rates of adverse reactions associated with DTP and DT immunizations in infants and children. Pediatrics 68:650, 1981.
Diehl HS, Baker AB, Cowan DW: Cold vaccines. JAMA 111:1168, 1938.

Fletcher RH, Fletcher SW, Wagner EH: Clinical Epidemiology: The Essentials. 2nd ed. Baltimore, Williams & Wilkins, 1982.
Friedman GD: Primer of Epidemiology. 2nd ed. New York, McGraw-Hill, 1980.
Goldbloom R: Science and empiricism in pediatrics. Pediatrics 73:693, 1984.
Halpin TJ, Holtzhauer FJ, Campbell RJ, et al: Reye's syndrome and medication use. JAMA 248:687, 1982.
Haynes RB: How to read clinical journals: II. To learn about a diagnostic test. Can Med Assoc J 124:703, 1981.
MacMahon B, Yen S, Trichopoulos D, et al: Coffee and cancer of the pancreas. N Engl J Med 304:630, 1981.
Mausner JS, Kramer S: Epidemiology: An Introductory Text. Philadelphia, WB Saunders, 1985.
Miller DL, Ross EM, Alderslade R, et al: Pertussis immunisation and serious acute neurological illness in children. Br Med J 282:1595, 1981.
Sackett DL: How to read clinical journals: I. Why to read them and how to start reading them critically. Can Med Assoc J 124:555, 1981.
Sackett DL: How to read clinical journals: V. To distinguish useful from useless or even harmful therapy. Can Med Assoc J 124:1156, 1981.
Trout KS: How to read clinical journals: IV. To determine etiology or causation. Can Med Assoc J 124:985, 1981.
Tugwell PX: How to read clinical journals: III. To learn the clinical course and prognosis of disease. Can Med Assoc J 124:869, 1981.

4.4 CHILD HEALTH IN THE DEVELOPING WORLD

The health status of most children in the world is pathetically different from that in developed countries such as the United States. In the developing world about 15% of children born each year die before they reach 5 yr of age compared to 1.4% of such children in the United States. In areas such as Upper Volta (now Burkina Faso), Afghanistan, and Sierra Leone in 1981 this death rate was 23%, a rate similar to that in the United States in 1900. These enormous differences exist for many reasons, the most important of which are social, political, and economic, and access to the beneficial effects of modern medical science is in large part dependent on solutions to these underlying problems.

Immediate contributing medical causes of childhood death and morbidity in developing countries are the high prevalence of infants born at low birthweight, of children with inadequate nutrition, and of infants and children with serious infectious diseases, especially diarrhea, respiratory infections, and parasitic infestations (Sec. 11.100–11.128). It is estimated that of deaths occurring before 5 yr of age, one third (5 million) are due to measles, pertussis, and neonatal tetanus (Fig. 4–1). As of 1986, UNICEF and WHO have revised these estimates downward by including only those deaths which were directly attributable to specific vaccine-preventable diseases. Thirty to 50% are attributed to diarrhea and malnutrition, and the remainder to respiratory diseases and other causes.

Vital statistics on health in the developing world are imprecise and vary from country to country. Further, their interpretation is confounded by the interaction of malnutrition with infection, especially the debilitating cycle of diarrhea and malnutrition. For example, measles is clearly associated with higher mortality in young children of borderline nutritional status who experience enteritis shortly prior to or during measles. Conversely, episodes of enteritis soon after recovery from measles are more apt to be fatal. Moreover, measles may itself exacerbate chronic diarrheal states.

Comparison of patterns of childhood mortality in currently developing countries with those that existed in the now-developed countries at the turn of this century suggests certain similarities and differences. For example, in 1900 more than 60% of childhood deaths in the United States were attributed to infection, as they are in developing countries today. However, children in the developing world at present probably suffer somewhat more from malnutrition and have more parasitic diseases. It is also important to note that the decline in such mortality in the developed countries began prior to the application of preventive and therapeutic medical

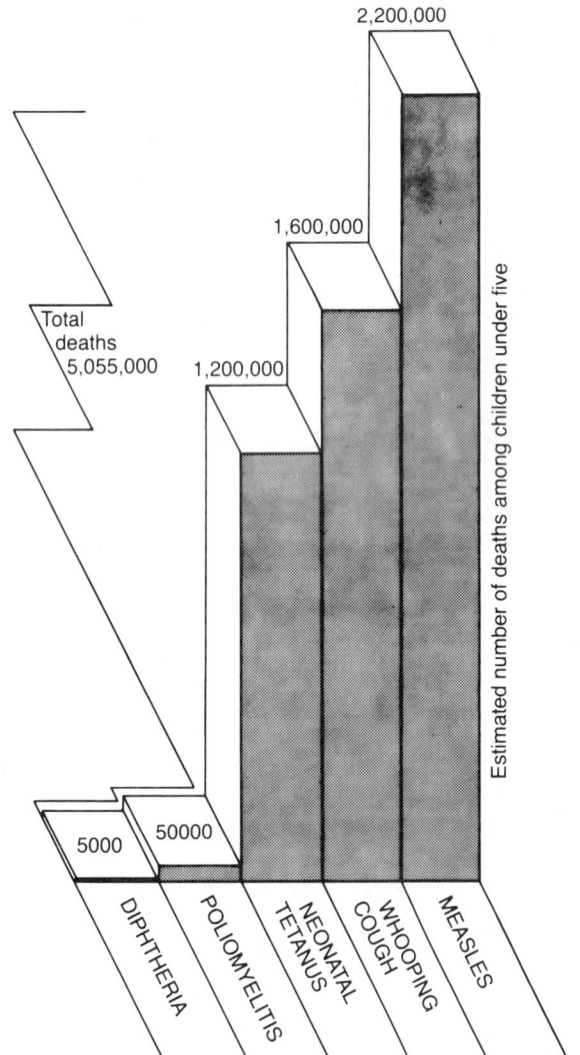

Figure 4–1. Total deaths of children less than 5 yr from immunization-preventable diseases, 1980. (Reprinted with permission of UNICEF from State of the World's Children 1984. New York, Oxford University Press, 1983. Data derived from WHO estimates.)

to childhood as well as result from inadequate food during pregnancy (food supplements for such pregnant women are associated with higher birthweights of their infants); (2) maternal infection, such as tuberculosis, malaria, and other parasitic diseases (this is mediated through aggravation of nutritional deficits as well as having an independent effect); and (3) short intervals between pregnancies. Encouragement of breast feeding, which interferes with conception, and family planning can reduce this problem.

Childhood Malnutrition (See Sec. 3.15–3.18). Inadequate nutrition is often initiated by low birthweight; these small infants are 3 to 4 times more likely to become malnourished children than are those of normal weight. Malnutrition in childhood is further aggravated by diarrhea and other infections. Countries with the highest infant mortality rates also have the highest death rates for children 1–4 yr old. In these countries the average caloric intake is 30% less than in those countries with the lowest mortality; in many the caloric deficits are greater, and within each of these countries there are populations with even greater deficits.

Morley thinks that the most important cause of childhood malnutrition is infection, including repeated diarrhea, parasitic diseases, measles, pertussis, and tuberculosis. These infections, whether acute or chronic, induce anorexia and divert nutrient energy from growth and development. He also points out that diets based largely on grain (such as gruel and pap) have such a low calorie content that the sheer bulk required for normal energy and growth requirements exceeds the ingestion capacity of many small children. This problem is uncommon in developed countries where high calorie fats and oils constitute a larger part of children's diets. Further, in some instances, adequate caloric intake but deficient protein

measures, such as immunizations and antimicrobial agents, suggesting that other factors, known and unknown, played major roles in reducing childhood mortality. Because of interactions among low birthweight, malnutrition, and infections, there is a need to address these problems concurrently. Further, because the severity of these child health problems parallels that of social, economic, educational, and political problems, and because these problems are sometimes complicated by unanticipated natural disasters, nonmedical problems should be addressed concomitantly with direct medical intervention to achieve optimum results.

Low Birthweight (See also Sec. 8.17). About 23 million of the 121 million infants born annually worldwide weigh less than 2500 g; increased mortality rates in surviving infants continue throughout the first few years of life, in part because low birthweight infants are more likely to become malnourished children. In countries with infant mortality rates exceeding 100/1000 live births, the proportion of low birthweight infants (less than 2500 g) averages 2½ times that in developed countries; in some countries it is up to 5-fold greater (Fig. 4–2). These low birthweight infants are 2 to 3 times as likely to die in infancy as are those of normal weight.

Three factors amenable to intervention contribute to low birthweight: (1) maternal malnutrition, which may date back

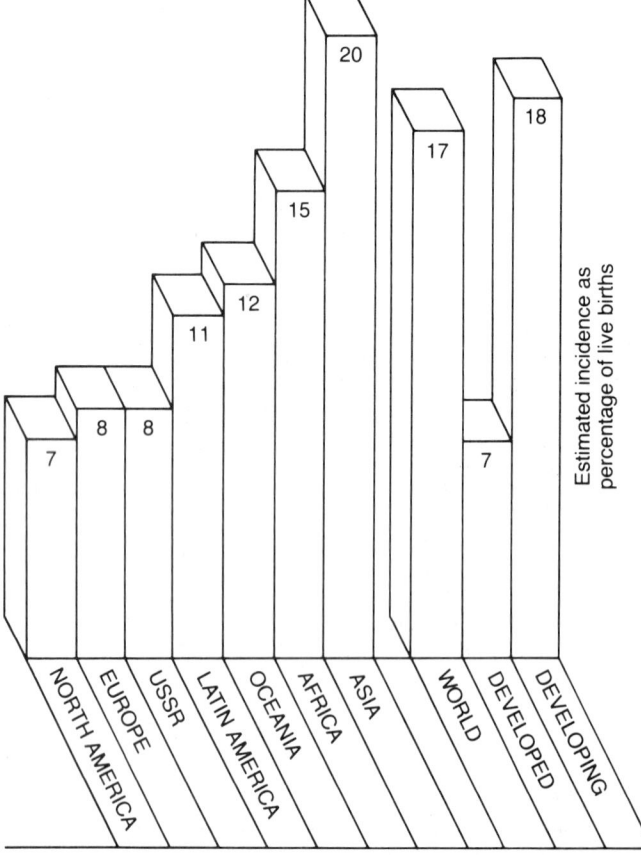

Figure 4–2. Global incidence of birthweights of 2.5 kg or less. (Source: WHO: The incidence of low birthweight: a critical review of available information. World Health Statistics Quarterly 33:No. 3, 1980.)

may contribute to protein malnutrition (Sec. 3.17). Lastly, Morley cites inadequate knowledge of elementary diet requirements as a major cause of malnutrition. As a corollary, mothers in deprived areas often do not recognize that their children are malnourished, because they look no different from other children they see.

These factors, in combination with each other and often initiated by low birthweight, constitute a debilitating complex of causation that is not easily overcome. Mortality is high, and in survivors growth is stunted and psychologic and emotional development is impaired. Further, the malnourished child has little energy available for normal childhood activities that contribute to normal development; the daily caloric expenditure of malnourished African children in play is about 40% that of their European counterparts. Amelioration of childhood malnutrition in the developing world requires attracting the attention of affected populations, especially the mothers, to the problem and educating them about its solutions. Morley advocates providing a simple chart, for the mother as well as for health care workers, that graphically indicates growth in height and weight and development. If the mothers are literate, messages about family planning, immunizations, available resources for health care, and other information may be included with the chart.

Diarrhea and Other Enteric Diseases. UNICEF and WHO estimate that worldwide one child dies of diarrhea every 6 seconds. Rates of enteric infection and consequent mortality are closely related to the lack of sanitary water supplies and to improper food handling. Safe public water is available to few in the developing world; refrigeration, food inspection, and other measures for control of enteric disease are usually lacking. For economic, political, logistic, and other reasons, these deficits are unlikely to be corrected in the near future. However, two interventions useful in ameliorating this problem are breast feeding and oral rehydration therapy (ORT).

Unfortunately, about 25 years ago a trend away from breast feeding and toward bottle feeding began in the developing world. But bottle feeding requires safe water, sterilization, and refrigeration, resources that are often unavailable. Further, powdered milk is costly and therefore may be overdiluted to save money, and illiterate parents may make errors in preparing formula. Often the result is contaminated formula, improperly diluted, leading to diarrhea and malnutrition. Recognizing that the widespread use of artificial infant feeding significantly contributes to morbidity and mortality from diarrhea in developing countries, the World Health Organization (WHO), United Nations Children's Fund (UNICEF), and various governments have instituted strong measures to encourage breast feeding and discourage artificial feeding. In 1981, the World Health Organization issued stringent guidelines (a Code) to limit the marketing of artificial milk substitutes by prohibiting or restricting various advertising and promotional practices. Governments were also urged vigorously to encourage breast feeding. Where these recommendations have been observed, sharp reductions in morbidity and mortality from infant diarrhea have occurred.

Oral rehydration therapy (ORT) is based on the observation that diarrheal dehydration rarely occurs if the affected infants can drink and retain adequate fluid containing small amounts of electrolyte and carbohydrate (Sec. 5.24). WHO and UNICEF, as well as certain countries, distribute nearly 100 million individual packets each year containing NaCl 3.5 g, NaHCO$_3$ 2.5 g, KCl 1.5 g, and glucose 20 g in dried form, to be dissolved in a liter of water. WHO and UNICEF estimate that more than 90% of diarrheal episodes in children can be treated inexpensively with ORT. In some communities in which ORT has been employed, childhood mortality from diarrhea has been reduced 50–60%. However, there are a billion or more episodes of childhood diarrhea worldwide with more than 5 million deaths from dehydration each year. The number of ORT packets produced annually is insufficient, and many children reside in areas too remote for supplies to be available. Therefore, in many countries indigenous health care workers and mothers are trained to substitute ingredients that are readily available locally for those in the packet. For example, in Bangladesh, mothers are instructed to mix a three-finger pinch of salt and a fistful of molasses in a "seer" (about a quart) of water: analyses of the electrolyte content of mixtures so prepared indicate that a safe and effective solution almost always results.

Immunization-Preventable Diseases. Since 1977, WHO and UNICEF have conducted vigorous efforts (the Expanded Programme on Immunization, EPI) to make immunization against six illnesses available to all children in the developing world. These diseases are diphtheria, pertussis, tetanus, measles, poliomyelitis, and tuberculosis, which are estimated to kill one child every 6 sec and to disable another child every 6 sec. As of 1983, WHO estimated that immunization was unavailable to 80% of the over 100 million children born annually in the developing world. The major problems in achieving a goal of universal immunization are societal and organizational.

The EPI plan was for WHO and UNICEF to encourage and assist individual countries in developing their own EPI's. Although many countries have done so and indeed are beginning to keep records of the incidence of these diseases and the numbers of children immunized, major problems in implementation have occurred. Senior and middle-level managers have been trained by EPI, but the subsequent recruitment, training, and supervision of the thousands of field workers who are ultimately responsible for the delivery of these vaccines to children have been impeded by lack of governmental commitment and delegation of authority, insufficient financial resources, and increasing ineffectiveness in the quality of training as it is passed from one level to the next. There are also major logistic problems in reaching children who live in poverty in cities and who live in remote areas.

Achieving compliance with the full immunization series is also extremely difficult: parents may not understand the importance, they may have other pressing responsibilities, and access to the field health center, although short in miles, may be limited owing to absence of roads, vehicles, and other means of transportation.

There are, of course, also technical problems, particularly in remote areas. Maintenance of the "cold chain" necessary for vaccine preservation may not be possible because of the absence of electricity. Attempts are being made to develop new means of refrigeration and new methods for determining whether a vaccine has been inactivated by breaks in the cold chain. There are also problems with sterilization; disposable syringes and needles are too expensive and impractical for many areas.

The health problems of children in the developing world require that immunization be combined with other primary health care services, including prenatal care and family planning for mothers, efforts to control enteric diseases, and nutritional services. These services depend on community involvement and interest, which in turn depend on social, political, economic, and geographic considerations.

The customs, mores, attitudes, and priorities as well as the political and organizational situations in developing countries usually differ from those in the developed world, as well as from each other. Sensitivity to these differences is critical to successful implementation of preventive health measures.

Finally, effects of the outcome of a given preventive program on other problems should be considered. A reduction of infant mortality by immunization and ORT in a community with inadequate nutritional resources to feed increased numbers of children requires family planning, greater food production, and other changes in order to achieve real benefits from the increased survival.

E. A. MORTIMER

Abed FH: Household teaching of ORT in rural Bangladesh. Case study. Assignment Children (UNICEF) 61/62:249, 1983.

Henderson R: Expanded immunization. In: UNICEF: State of the World's Children 1984. New York, Oxford University Press, 1983, p 82.

Kerr RA: Fifteen years of African drought. Science 227:1453, 1985.

McKeown T: The Role of Medicine. Dream, Mirage or Nemesis? Princeton, NJ, Princeton University Press, 1979.

Morley D: Growth monitoring: In: UNICEF: State of the World's Children 1984. New York, Oxford University Press, 1983, p 77.

Relucio-Clavano N: The promotion of breastfeeding. In: UNICEF: State of the World's Children 1984. New York, Oxford University Press, 1983, p 86.

Rohde JE: Oral rehydration therapy. In: UNICEF: State of the World's Children 1984. New York, Oxford University Press, 1983, p 72.

Shah KP: Food supplements. In: UNICEF: State of the World's Children 1984. New York, Oxford University Press, 1983, p 101.

UNICEF: State of the World's Children 1984. New York, Oxford University Press, 1983.

WHO/UNICEF: The management of diarrhea and use of oral rehydration therapy. A joint WHO/UNICEF statement. Assignment Children 61/62:77, 1983.

4.5 PROTECTION OF TRAVELING CHILDREN

Parents of children or adolescents who are planning to take them to live or to visit outside their country of residence should consult with public health authorities or physicians well in advance of their departure for a realistic assessment of risks, for immunizations and chemoprophylactic measures, and for advice on how to handle disease if it occurs. Up to date information is needed to assess the relative risk of acquiring one of the many infectious diseases that have specific geographic distribution or that are more common in the areas to be visited. Very young children are at a particular disadvantage when exposed to many of these infectious agents. Furthermore, knowledge of the general principles of prevention is necessary to avoid undue exposures. The major components of protection of traveling children are outlined below.

IMMUNIZATIONS

Childhood Vaccines. The risk of exposure to several of the common childhood infections increases when traveling in areas with less than optimal preventive and sanitary measures. Such children should have received the recommended schedule of immunizations against poliomyelitis, measles, mumps, rubella, diphtheria, tetanus, and pertussis (Sec. 4.1). Booster doses of polio, tetanus, diphtheria, and measles vaccines are recommended for adolescents before traveling.

Other Vaccines. Three additional immunizations are highly recommended to protect traveling children since they are particularly susceptible to these infections (Table 4–6). There are relatively few countries in the world where transmission of typhoid and rabies does not occur. Furthermore, the risk of hepatitis B is high in many areas including sub-Saharan Africa, Southeast Asia, and parts of the Caribbean and South Pacific. Assessment of the risk of acquiring any of these infections may be difficult since the availability of reliable prevalence data is poor. Pre-exposure vaccination against rabies (Sec. 11.78) using the human diploid cell vaccine is recommended for children who will be living for long periods of time in countries where the infection is known to exist. The vaccine is administered intramuscularly according to doses outlined in Table 4–6. Intradermal injection of human diploid cell rabies vaccine is currently being evaluated and

Table 4–6. **Additional Vaccines Recommended for Travelers to Areas with High Risk of Exposure**

Vaccine	Primary Series × No. of Injections	Interval	Booster
Rabies (human diploid cell)	1.0 mL intramuscularly × 3	1 wk and 2–3 wk	2 yr
Typhoid	<10 yr 0.25 mL subcutaneously × 2	4 wk	3 yr
	≥10 yr 0.5 mL subcutaneously × 2	4 wk	3 yr
Hepatitis B	<10 yr 0.5 mL intramuscularly × 3	1 mo and 6 mo	5 yr
	≥10 yr 1.0 mL intramuscularly × 3	1 mo and 6 mo	5 yr

may result in decreasing the necessary doses and cost of vaccination. Typhoid (Sec. 11.27) is also common in most countries in Asia, Africa, and Central and South America, and vaccination is, therefore, recommended for children who will remain in these areas for prolonged periods. Hepatitis B vaccine (Sec. 11.76) is recommended for children and adults traveling to areas with a high prevalence of carriers or who are likely to have direct contact with blood or secretions from infected individuals.

Required Vaccines. Under the WHO regulations certain countries may require International Certificate of Vaccination; currently only yellow fever and cholera are included.

Vaccination against yellow fever (Sec. 11.80) is recommended for all travelers to endemic areas (consult Health Information for International Travel, 1986). Infants under 6 mo should be vaccinated only if travel to high risk areas cannot be delayed. The vaccine preparation must have been approved by WHO and must be administered at a designated Yellow Fever Vaccination Center. The primary or booster dose of yellow fever vaccine for children older than 6 mo is 0.5 mL subcutaneously. The certificate is valid for 10 yr, beginning 10 days after the primary vaccination or on the date of revaccination if within 10 yr of the first injection. Yellow fever vaccine results in a high degree of immunity. In contrast, the efficacy of cholera vaccine (Sec. 11.29) is questionable; however, certain countries still require a valid vaccination certificate. The primary series of vaccination is two injections 1–4 wk apart. The dose is 0.2 mL (for 6 mo–4 yr), 0.3 mL (for 5–10 yr) and 0.5 mL (for >10 yr). Similar doses are recommended for booster injections every 6 mo. The WHO cholera vaccination certificate is valid for 6 mo beginning 6 days after one injection of the vaccine or on the date of revaccination if within 6 mo of first injection.

Passive Immunization. Protection against hepatitis A (Sec. 11.76) requires administering immune gamma globulin, which is recommended for travelers to most developing countries, particularly when planning to visit outside the major urban centers. For short-term visits (less than 3 mo) the intramuscular dose for children less than 23 kg is 0.5 mL, and for those 23–45 kg, 1.0 mL is recommended. These doses should be doubled for those planning to stay longer than 3 mo and should be repeated at 4–6 mo intervals.

MALARIA CHEMOPROPHYLAXIS

Malaria (Sec. 11.104) is becoming one of the most significant risks of international travel. Figure 4–3 illustrates the extent of its geographic distribution. Control of infection in most endemic areas is complicated by the emergence of drug resistance in the parasite and its mosquito vector.

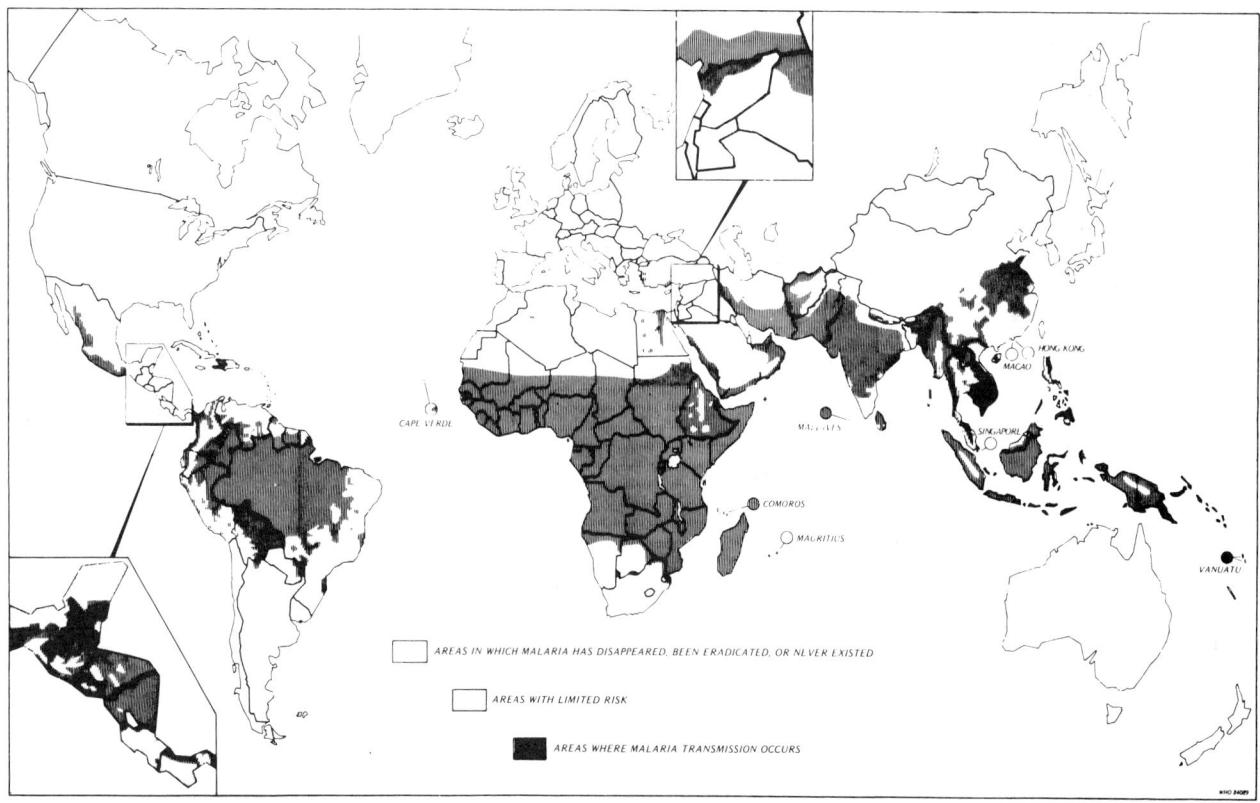

Figure 4–3. Geographic distribution of malaria. (From Health Information for International Travel, 1985. U.S. Department of Health and Human Services, Public Health Service, Centers for Disease Control, Atlanta, GA 30333. HHS Publication No. CDC 85–8280.)

Chloroquine, the major chemoprophylactic agent, should be administered as chloroquine phosphate, 8.5 mg salt/kg, once every week. It should be started 2 wk prior to traveling to a malaria endemic area and continued regularly during the visit and for 6 wk following departure. For young children and infants, liquid chloroquine preparations are available throughout the world but not in the United States. Chloroquine or any other malaria chemoprophylaxis will not prevent the acquisition of infection, but rather will prevent clinical manifestations while the drugs are being administered. Continuing the drug for 6 wk after departure from endemic areas ensures a high degree of protection against a clinical attack due to *Plasmodium falciparum* infection. Nevertheless, clinical malaria whether due to *P. falciparum* or other species can still occur after completion of the 6 wk of chloroquine. The chance decreases markedly after 3–6 mo for *P. falciparum* but the potential for a clinical attack from any of the three other human species may remain for years. Because of the latter possibilities, some recommend administering primaquine following a visit to areas known for high endemicity of *P. vivax*. However, this practice is not based on specific scientific information and should be discouraged because of the potential side effects of primaquine.

Chloroquine-resistant *P. falciparum* infection is spreading to many areas endemic for malaria. The geographic distribution of resistant parasites is depicted in Table 4–7. Furthermore, resistance to the alternative drug (pyrimethamine-sulfadoxine) is now reported from several endemic areas in Southeast Asia, East Africa, and Brazil; the use of this combination is also complicated by the risk of severe adverse reactions including death. Therefore, for those going to areas of risk for periods of less than 3 wk chloroquine is recommended. If these individuals are not known to have a previous history of

sulfonamide intolerance, they should also be supplied with a single treatment dose of pyrimethamine-sulfadoxine to be taken in the event of a febrile illness. This temporary measure should be followed by a medical consultation and should not be considered an alternative to continuing chloroquine prophylaxis. The presumptive therapeutic dose of pyrimethamine-sulfadoxine for children is: ¼ tablet for children aged 2–11 mo, ½ tablet for 1–3 yr, 1 tablet for 4–8 yr, 2 tablets for 9–14 yr, and the adult dose of 3 tablets for adolescents. For persons planning longer than 3 wk stay in areas where risk of exposure to chloroquine resistance is high, living conditions, availability of medical care, and the local patterns of malaria transmission should be taken into consideration.

Table 4–7. Countries with Malaria Caused by Chloroquine-Resistant *Plasmodium Falciparum* in 1985

General Area	Specific Countries
Western hemisphere	Bolivia, Brazil, Colombia, Ecuador, French Guiana, Guyana, Panama, Peru, Suriname, Venezuela
Asia	Bangladesh, Burma, China, India, Indonesia, Kampuchea, Laos, Malaysia, Pakistan, Papua New Guinea, Philippines, Solomon Islands, Sri Lanka, Thailand, Viet Nam
Africa	Angola, Burundi, Cameroon, Central African Republic, Comoros, Congo, Gabon, Kenya, Madagascar, Malawi, Mozambique, Namibia, Rwanda, South Africa, Sudan, Swaziland, Tanzania, Uganda, Zaire, Zambia, Zimbabwe

Combined prophylaxis using chloroquine and pyrimethamine-sulfadoxine may still be used as long as the individuals are aware of the possible side effects of the combination, which include skin and mucous membrane manifestations such as itching, rash, sore throat, or mucous membrane ulcers. The recommended pediatric dose is 0.5 mg/kg pyrimethamine and 10 mg/kg sulfadoxine once a week, administered according to the same schedule as for chloroquine.

Because drugs do not provide complete protection against malaria, it is important that up-to-date information be used in advising travelers and that in case of doubt physicians consult the Centers for Disease Control, Atlanta, GA. Other measures such as mosquito nets, insect repellents, and exercising reasonable precautions against insect bites are still highly recommended procedures.

GENERAL ADVICE

International travel entails changes in time zones, altitudes, quality of water and food, and exposure to other environmental hazards. Travelers should be advised on how to handle the risks associated with each of these hazards, what are the dangerous clinical symptoms, and how to seek further medical advice. *Traveler's diarrhea* is one of the most common hazards. No prophylactic chemotherapeutic agent is effective and safe, and none, therefore, is recommended. Individuals should be advised to investigate the quality of drinking water and to avoid eating fresh vegetables and fruits without properly washing them. Mild traveler's diarrhea is usually self limited. Considerable diarrhea, if associated with fever, severe abdominal cramps, or bloody stools, should alert the child or parent to consult immediately with a physician. Parents should be cautioned that children are particularly vulnerable to the effects of dehydration and electrolyte loss and advised to travel with several packets of the oral rehydration salts, which can be used for replacement therapy (Sec. 5.24 and 11.8). Two chemotherapeutic agents, trimethoprim-sulfamethoxazole (Bactrim) and doxycycline, are effective for treating many patients with travelers diarrhea, but their use should be closely monitored because of frequent side effects.

ADEL A. F. MAHMOUD

Health Information for International Travel, 1986. US Department of Health and Human Services, Public Health Service, Centers for Disease Control, Atlanta, GA, 30333. HHS Publication No. (CDC 86-8280).

Warren KS, Mahmoud AAF (eds): Tropical and Geographical Medicine. New York, McGraw-Hill, 1984.

Warren KS, Mahmoud AAF: Geographic Medicine for the Practitioner. 2nd ed. New York, Springer-Verlag, 1985.

5

GENERAL CONSIDERATIONS IN THE CARE OF SICK CHILDREN

5.1 CLINICAL EVALUATION OF INFANTS AND CHILDREN

The evaluation of the infant, child, or adolescent should be comprehensive and continuing and should embrace psychologic and environmental as well as somatic factors. A careful and complete history and physical examination are generally more informative than laboratory tests, which should be used (1) as screening procedures when direct observation is impossible or when specific and otherwise hidden conditions are being sought, (2) for confirmation or further definition of suspected conditions, (3) as guides to complex therapy, or (4) as a means of gathering research data.

Certain qualities in the physician are appreciated by all patients and will enhance effective gathering of data, ensure greater therapeutic compliance, and increase mutual satisfaction in the doctor-patient relationship. Among them are:

Gentleness. The physician's touch should be gentle, both literally and figuratively. Roughness, rudeness, or crudeness in manner, speech, or handling of the patient should be scrupulously avoided; they usually lead to conscious or unconscious resistance.

Respect. Self-respect is essential to mental health and a sense of well-being. The child's self-evaluation depends partly on the perception of how others treat his or her parents. Children gain self-respect when they see their parents valued.

A basic form of respect is to care enough to learn and use a person's name. The name the child prefers should be asked at the first encounter and consistently remembered and used thereafter. It is unfortunate that many physicians and other medical personnel address adults whom they feel to be socially, educationally, or intellectually inferior (including the aged) by their first names in the absence of previous first name familiarity; this is a sign of condescension. The common practice of addressing parents as "Mom" and "Dad" or referring to boys as "males" and girls as "females" also tends to depersonalize the child or parent and to create or widen gaps in communication or feeling.

Understanding. Children and parents may be unpleasant, uncooperative, and hostile. However, the physician should recognize that this behavior may be dictated by forces beyond their control. Efforts to understand why parents are angry, depressed, or withdrawn usually improve the doctor-patient relationship and the care of the child.

Sympathy. The warm expression of sympathy by word or touch relieves the uncomfortable child or troubled parent of feeling alone with pain or worry. It is greatly appreciated and adds to the rapport between physician and parent. Empathetic physicians can respond to negative attitudes and behavior with therapeutic rather than antagonistic or defensive behavior. Likewise, when physicians can share the feelings of patients and parents, they are better able to supply needed support and are less likely to view an unhappy encounter as one that should be terminated as quickly as possible.

Kindness. The physician who willingly seeks small ways of making the patient feel more comfortable in mind or body increases the patient's trust and is rewarded by the patient's appreciation.

5.2 INITIAL CONTACT

The physician should first identify himself or herself in a friendly manner to both parents and child, even if the latter is a small infant. In subsequent encounters a friendly greeting to both is always desirable. Establishing a relaxed and friendly atmosphere facilitates taking a history and performing a physical examination. Expressions of concern for the comfort of both parent and child increase confidence in the physician, since they indicate personal interest and sensitivity. The *infant* usually remains in the parent's arms during an interview. The *small child*, if ill, may do the same but should otherwise be provided with a box of toys or other distraction to prevent boredom. If sensitive areas of the child's own behavior and management are going to be discussed, it may be better to arrange to talk with the parent or parents alone. Serious prognoses should also be discussed out of the child's presence until some decision is reached on how to handle probable questions.

The child of *school age* can usually be expected to remain quiet during an interview and should be included from time to time in the questioning. Interviews with parents alone may alarm children of this age who are excluded from the conversation by implying that something serious is being kept from them. Opinions differ about the degree to which the older child should be included in the discussion of serious illness and prognosis; it is probably best to make individual judgments in this regard (Sec. 2.36). Speaking with parents alone is important when discussing behavior disorders; however, with parents' concurrence, the physician should frankly discuss with the child the subject, if not the content, of the earlier conversation with the parents.

The parents of *adolescents* often need opportunities to express their concerns about their children to the physician without the patient present, but the physician should always make it clear, both to them and to the adolescent, that the basic relationship exists between the physician and the adolescent. The interviewing procedures should be arranged accordingly.

5.3 HISTORY

The initial medical history is made up of the following components:

Chief Complaint (C.C.), i.e., the chief reason for the visit.
Present Illness (P.I.), i.e., all details bearing directly on the chief complaint.
Past History (P.H.), including previous illnesses, a review

169

of systems, and data concerning prophylactic or screening measures, such as immunizations and tuberculin tests.

Family History (F.H.), i.e., all medical conditions present in blood relatives that may by their presence or absence have a bearing on the health of the patient.

Social History (S.H.), i.e., environmental circumstances that may bear on the physical or emotional well-being of the patient.

The history obtained at subsequent contacts is usually limited to a C.C. and P.I.; new items of P.H., F.H., and S.H. are added as they arise and are appropriate.

In eliciting the medical history of a child, the physician should initially ask the reason for the visit or hospitalization. With acutely ill patients the reason may be obvious and may be better regarded as implicit. In other situations, simple questions such as "Would you tell me what the problem is from your point of view?" are appropriate for opening communication. The physician should listen carefully and respectfully to what follows and should not interrupt with questions. At the end of the parent's or the child's free recital, the physician should recapitulate what was understood from the story to make certain that all are in agreement on what has been said and what it means. Often a number of problems other than the chief complaint are touched upon. They should be noted as they emerge for later investigation (the "problem-oriented" approach). During the recital the observant physician may gain important clues from parent-child and parent-parent interactions, also from near-tearfulness, blushing, nail-biting, changes in tone of voice, and neuromuscular tension during the telling or discussion of specific items of the history.

Particular care should be taken to allow the informant to answer each question fully before going on to another. Failure to do so implies impatience or disrespect and carries the impression to the parent or child that the interviewer is not really interested in or listening to what is being related. It is important also to *avoid leading questions,* which may result in an inaccurate history. Sympathetic remarks (e.g., "All that activity must really tire you out at times") or oblique questions (e.g., "Does your husband's job often keep him away on weekends?") are frequently more effective than direct or blunt questions in eliciting data in sensitive areas. Material in such areas (family relations, sexual information, or behavior) may be withheld by parents until one or more visits have reassured them of the physician's interest, concern, empathy, and discretion.

At the conclusion of many interviews, the physician is well advised to formulate some question such as "I want to be sure that I have answered all your questions; can you tell me just what you expected or wanted to get from this visit?" Sometimes only in this way will the physician discover that the prime concern of the mother of a hypothyroid infant is constipation rather than the endocrine status; compliance in management of the latter may be obtained only after her concerns with the former are relieved.

See also Sec. 2.36 for a detailed discussion of interviewing as part of the clinical assessment.

5.4 PHYSICAL EXAMINATION

Setting. The room in which a child is examined contributes to the emotional climate. White is cold and buff impersonal to the small child; pastel walls achieve a cheerful and familiar effect, as do bright colors, comfortable furniture, and pictures. Glaring lights and unfamiliar equipment may be frightening. The latter should be introduced in familiar terms; the blood pressure cuff may be called a "special" or "funny" balloon, and the otoscope and ophthalmoscope "funny" or "special" flashlights. The warmth and texture of cotton flannel sheets instead of paper will make lying on the examining table more comfortable for the unclothed infant or child.

Approach. The approach to physical examination of the infant and child should be unhurried and not structured according to preconceived notions. The anxieties of even 6–8 wk old infants may be allayed and their cooperation obtained by getting them to smile in response to friendly voice sounds before beginning the examination. This is also reassuring to parents, whose anxiety at brusque manipulation may otherwise be transmitted to the infant by vocal or neuromuscular tension. Small children usually need to have a little time to get used to the examiner and to the place where they are to be examined, which is best accomplished by allowing the child freedom to explore while the history is being obtained. He or she should then be told ("I want you"), not asked ("Will you please?"), to remove all clothing, specifically excepting underpants since the latter seem to represent a last bastion of self-respect and protection against assault. At the end of the examination, when the child has confidence that the examiner does not intend to hurt him or her, the underpants can usually be lowered or removed without objection.

The physical examination may be performed on an examining table or on the parent's lap, whichever seems more opportune. Some children are very comfortable if examined standing. Small children are reassured if they are not required to be supine until the end of the examination when they have gained confidence in the examiner's gentleness and good intentions. The older child can be treated more as an adult; this implies no less gentleness, respect, and consideration for feelings of anxiety or the desire for privacy. The least threatening order of examination is usually inspection, palpation, percussion, auscultation, ophthalmoscopy (children 2½ or older will usually cooperate if not mentally retarded or emotionally disturbed), and otoscopy. Examining the pharynx is left for last with small children since it is usually the most uncomfortable. On the other hand, many children of 3 yr and older are quite comfortable standing, with an examination "to look you over from tip to toe" that begins with "shining a light in your ear" and moves easily to nose, mouth, teeth, pharynx, and so on to the soles.

Content. The content and order of recording the physical examination should be reasonably standardized for ease of review and should differ little from those used in adult medicine except for (1) the inclusion of head circumference as a standard measurement for children under 2 yr; (2) the use of a growth chart (see Figs. 2–6 and 2–7); (3) the inclusion of a developmental evaluation, especially for small children; and (4) an assessment of speech. The emphasis on developmental data is the major difference between the physical examinations of the child and of the adult and is essential to the interpretation of data in health and in disease, since many physical signs (e.g., blood pressure, pulse, heart sounds, breath sounds, organ size, neurologic signs) are influenced by the developmental process.

5.5 THE PROBLEM-ORIENTED MEDICAL RECORD

The problem-oriented medical record formalizes and structures some time-honored principles of medical record-keeping in a way that discourages oversight, simplifies audit of performance in regard to management of individual conditions, reinforces logical thought, makes explicit the process followed, and facilitates computerization of medical data. Problem-oriented record-keeping is the cornerstone of problem-oriented medical practice, which consists of (1) establishing and using a defined *data base*; (2) formulating and maintaining a *problem list*; (3) making a *plan* for managing each problem; (4) *educating* the patient in regard to items in the data base, problem list, plans, and their implementation; and (5) establishing and maintaining some form of continuing audit.

Data Base. The data base in the medical record is the recorded information pertinent to the patient and the problem(s). It may be general and comprehensive or limited to the problem of immediate concern. The *basic components* of the pediatric data base are the medical history, physical examination, growth charts, developmental flow sheet, screening tests, and baseline laboratory data. The content of the data base varies with the *age* of the patient, the *population* from which the patient is drawn, and the *reason* for any specific patient-physician encounter. Other factors affecting the content include the ability and willingness of the patient or others to pay for its development; the interests or concerns of individual physicians or health agencies initiating the collection of the data (these may reflect professional anxieties, confusions, or research interests); and changes in medical practice or knowledge.

Ideally, the standard or general data base should be completely defined and uniform; in practice it varies with the factors listed above. The additional data bases for individual patients, diseases, or circumstances (e.g., defined data base for a specific complaint such as diarrhea and vomiting) are added only as necessary. *Flow sheets* are a form of continuing data base which may be standard, as for health supervision or diabetes, or tailored to the needs of an individual with a rare disease or complication. The effort involved in developing a defined data base is usually more than repaid by professional satisfaction in knowing that nothing important has been overlooked and by the long-term saving of professional time.

The initial defined data base is often best obtained by using a questionnaire appropriate to the age and environment of the patient (see Margolis, 1978).

It is a convention of the problem-oriented record that all data are recorded under the headings of "*Subjective*" (related by the patient or other lay person) or "*Objective*" (observed directly by the physician or delegate or reported by another physician or a laboratory). Although these distinctions sometimes become blurred, they are generally useful, particularly in recording progress notes.

Once the initial data base is recorded, a *problem list* is developed and further data are recorded in relation to the specifically named and numbered problems on the list. The *number* of the problem is entered in the left-hand margin of the page or is circled for easy reference, and the *name* of the problem is the first part of the entry. A more detailed data base is obtained and recorded for each problem if all relevant data are not contained already in the initial data base. In many instances it is convenient to develop defined data bases, using check-off forms for specific illnesses or categories of illnesses.

Problem List. This list, which is developed from information contained in the data base, should include any medical, social, developmental, psychologic, economic, or environmental problems that have been identified, with each problem assigned a number and a name. Each subsequent entry in the record, including those on the hospital order sheet, is identified with the number and name of the problem to which it refers. This form of record-keeping makes it easier to locate all entries relating to a single problem, simplifies an *audit* of the record, and can be adapted to computerization, with easy ultimate retrieval of the data, notes, and orders referable to specific problems.

The *name of a problem* is customarily entered as (1) a diagnosis, (2) a physiologic or behavioral manifestation, (3) a symptom or physical finding, (4) an abnormal laboratory finding, (5) the history of a disease in the patient or the family, or (6) a social, environmental, or demographic circumstance that bears significantly on the patient, the illness, or management.

Each problem should be expressed only at a level of understanding or confidence that can be substantiated by objective evidence, including the course of the illness. This helps the formulator of the problem list keep an open mind about diagnostic possibilities and avoid jumping to potentially erroneous diagnostic conclusions. For example, the initial entry on the problem list of a child with suspected meningitis would be "Fever, vomiting, and stiff neck." If a spinal tap shows purulent fluid, an arrow is drawn and the problem updated to "meningitis." If the cerebrospinal fluid culture grows out *Haemophilus influenzae* 2 days later, the problem is again updated to the final diagnosis of "*H. influenzae* meningitis." Each time an arrow is drawn to update a problem, the date or time of the updating is indicated over the shaft of the arrow. The problem list thus encourages logical rather than intuitive thinking in clinical appraisal of the patient.

Generally, a problem is entered into the problem list and given a number when it requires specific and separate attention or action. Several conventions may be employed to keep the problem list from becoming unwieldy. For children, *health supervision* may be entered routinely as Problem No. 1 and all items relating to the observation of normal development, anticipatory guidance, and immunization referred to it. If a developmental abnormality of major or continuing importance (such as enuresis or mental retardation) becomes apparent, it is then listed as a separate problem with a separate number. Transient or minor complaints without sequelae are often entered as "Temporary Problems." These are listed separately with space to indicate the dates of recurrences; if the latter are frequent, transfer to the main problem list may be justified. Certain problems may be critical at the time they occur but of little long-term significance, which is particularly likely with problems leading to hospitalization. Consider, for example, the case of a child whose appendicitis is complicated by wound infection and dehiscence, bacteremia, penicillin reaction, water intoxication with convulsions, hypokalemia, and a near-fatal accidental overdose of morphine. Each of these is a major problem at some time, but only appendicitis, appendectomy, and penicillin allergy would be appropriate for inclusion in the permanent problem list. This situation may be handled either (1) by entering the associated problems as subproblems of appendectomy, e.g., wound infection, or (2) by listing each complication as a separate problem on a "single-admission problem list" and transcribing only "appendicitis → status postappendectomy" and "penicillin allergy" onto the permanent problem list, which remains separate from the single-admission problem list.

Ideally there should be only one problem list per patient, and it should be continuous from birth to death, but in practice this may be cumbersome. As a result, problem lists may have to be revised periodically. Moreover, other health professionals who see patients may need their own problem lists to guide them. In any event, the *primary physician* should be responsible for keeping a "permanent" or "master" problem list which is shared with patient or parent and which can serve as a guide to maintaining perspective and to ensuring that individual problems are not forgotten.

Although disagreements may arise as to what should be entered as separate problems, all perceived problems should be specifically identified and management efforts directed accordingly. The list should help the physician to deliver comprehensive and auditable care.

Assessment. Ordinarily, regular assessments should be made of each problem, including in each instance a direct or implied statement of the goal of the *plan* which is to be followed. For instance, if the assessment is "Probable febrile convulsion, r/o (rule out) meningitis," the implied goal of the initial plan is eliminating meningitis as a diagnostic possibility. Once that has been done, the fever may become a problem separate from the convulsion, each requiring its own assessment and plan (which may be merely that certain possibilities should be diagnostically eliminated). In each instance, the assessment should place in perspective a reasonable, explicit or implicit goal and a logical plan of action that will achieve that goal; accordingly, the assessment might be not to work up a problem at all, or it might define the extent of therapeutic effort to be expended.

Plan. Each plan should consist of four clearly stated components: (1) information related to diagnosis (Dx), (2) treatment (Rx), (3) patient or parent education (Ed), and (4) follow-up (FU). If no plan is made, its absence should be noted.

Progress Notes. These should be identified by the number and name of the problem to which they refer. Each note should contain four sections: (1) *subjective* data, usually supplied by the patient or parent; (2) *objective*, for directly ascertained data such as a new physical or laboratory finding; (3) *assessment*, for a statement of the significance of the data, including an explicit or implied goal for the following plan, and (4) *a plan* that follows logically from the content of (1), (2), and (3). The mnemonic **SOAP** is often used to designate the sections of the progress note.

Flow Sheets. Most good plans for continuing problems require flow sheets that list the appropriate variables to be followed, thus serving as both simplified progress notes and reminders that certain items should be or have been checked periodically. For example, on a flow sheet for health supervision the guidance items may be checked off on the sheet as they are carried out, and thus the physician has a handy record of what has and has not been done in this regard. The use of flow sheets increases the efficiency of the physician; once they have been prepared, most of the data can be gathered by an assistant for review and decision making by the physician.

Drug Lists. The use of an increasing number of drugs and an increasing knowledge of their interactions and adverse effects (Table 5–30) makes it important to maintain a drug list as well as a problem list, particularly for children with chronic diseases. The list should include all drugs taken, indicate the date each was started and stopped, and note any adverse effect. Future adverse reactions then may be foreseen or prevented or both.

Audit. Audit of the problem-oriented record consists of two phases: nonprofessional and professional. *Nonprofessional audit* can be done by a nonphysician through use of a checklist. It chiefly focuses on aspects of thoroughness, such as:

Was a data base obtained?
Are all the components of the data base contained in the record?
Are the components completed as defined?
Is there a problem list?
Are all entries in the progress notes referred to specific problems?
Were plans carried out?
Was patient education done?
Was planned follow-up carried out?

Professional audit is for quality of care; it includes (1) review of the nonprofessional audit, if that has been done; (2) review of the data base to see if all problems have been identified and entered on the problem list; and (3) general review of the record for thoroughness, efficiency, analytic sense, reliability, and professional knowledge and competence.

Disadvantages. The relatively rigid and detailed structure of the problem-oriented record can result, when improperly and overcompulsively used, in a greatly increased expenditure of time and paper. The emphasis on identification and management of each problem as a separate entity may lead not only to fragmentation of the record but to a loss of perspective; the neophyte, for instance, may be so intent on handling his or her patient's fever, vomiting, convulsions, and stiff neck as separate problems that the diagnosis of meningitis may be elusive or delayed. Problems encountered in its implementation and use are more easily handled if users recognize that arbitrary judgments must be made in the adaptation of any system to local conditions and that the user must remain the master; the system, the tool.

R. JAMES McKAY

Barness LA: Manual of Pediatric Physical Diagnosis. 5th ed. Chicago, Year Book Medical Publishers, 1980.
Korsch BM: The pediatrician's approach to his patient. Am J Dis Child 126:146, 1973.
Margolis CG: The Pediatric Problem-Oriented Record. A Manual for Implementation. Bedford Hills, NY, Redgrave Publishing Co., 1978.
Walker HK, Hurst JW, Woody MF (eds): Applying the Problem-Oriented System. New York, MEDCOM Press, 1973.

5.6 THE PATHOPHYSIOLOGY OF BODY FLUIDS

The physiology of body fluids should be considered from three perspectives:

1. *The total amounts of water and solutes in the body as a whole*, which result from carefully regulated balances between intake and output. Many controlling mechanisms, especially for substances having physiologic significance, are extremely complex. Those especially important to the clinician will be discussed in some detail.

2. *The distribution of water and solutes in the various compartments of the body*, which is critically important. Considerable energy is required to maintain steady state equilibrium for most substances.

3. *The concentration of the solutes within each compartment*, which depends on the relative amounts of both solute and solvent (water) in that compartment. Thus, concentration can be changed by altering the content of either or both.

Regulatory mechanisms appear to be designed for preventing large changes in solute concentrations, which can lead to profound functional alterations. Generally the rate and percentage of change in concentration of the various solutes are more physiologically and clinically significant than absolute change. For example, an alteration of 3 mEq/L from normal in the extracellular fluid concentration of potassium represents a change of approximately 70% and may result in profound physiologic effects, but an alteration of 3 mEq/L in the extracellular fluid sodium concentration represents a change of only 2%, is well tolerated, and is of little clinical significance.

Changes in volume are relatively well tolerated, although percentage and rate of change are again more critical than absolute change. Thus, the loss of 100 mL of blood in a few minutes produces a negligible disturbance in an adolescent but results in shock in a newborn infant; extended over several days, the same hemorrhage in the infant could be fairly well tolerated.

5.7 WATER

TOTAL BODY WATER

Water constitutes 78% of body weight at birth but drops to the adult level of approximately 60% by 1 yr of age (Fig. 5–1). A close linear relationship exists between total body water (TBW) and body weight (wt), described by the equation TBW (liters) = 0.611 wt (kg) + 0.251. Thus, estimates of TBW can be approximated from body weight alone. However, since fat is low in water content, TBW represents a smaller percentage of body weight in an obese than in a normal person. Because mature females have a higher body fat content than do mature males, their TBW is 55% of their body weight compared with 60% of the males'. A more exact estimate of TBW can be obtained from lean body mass (LBM) in which the relationship is TBW (liters) = 0.72 LBM (kg).

Fluid Compartments. Body water consists of intracellular and extracellular components (Fig. 5–2). In the fetus, *extracellular fluid* (ECF) volume is larger than the intracellular space, but the ratio of extracellular water to intracellular water falls to the adult level by 9 mo of postnatal life (Fig. 5–1). This relative loss of extracellular fluid presumably results from the increasing growth of cellular tissue and the decreasing rate of growth of collagen relative to muscle during the early months of life. Thereafter, extracellular fluid bears a fairly straight-line relation to weight (ECF = 0.239 wt [kg] + 0.325) and to total body water in normal infants and children. Under conditions of normal hydration in the older child (Fig. 5–2),

it constitutes 20–25% of body weight and is composed of plasma water (5% of body weight), interstitial water (15% of body weight), and transcellular water (1–3% of body weight).

The *transcellular water* compartment is composed primarily of gastrointestinal secretions plus cerebrospinal, intraocular, pleural, peritoneal, and synovial fluids. Transcellular fluid is usually considered a specialized fraction of extracellular fluid, although it is probably more accurate to consider the fluid in the gastrointestinal tract as extracorporeal. The volume of the transcellular compartment varies greatly, depending on the absorptive and secretory activities of the intestine; during the fasting state it represents about 1–3% of body weight.

Intracellular fluid (ICF) volume, the difference between total body water and extracellular water, approximates 30–40% of body weight. Although frequently considered a homogeneous phase, intracellular fluid represents the sum of fluids from cells in different locations with varying functions and differing intracellular compositions.

REGULATION OF BODY WATER

The plasma osmolality, the concentration of solute particles in plasma, remains almost constant at 285–295 mOsm/kg H_2O regardless of day-to-day fluctuations in solute and water intake. This is due largely to precise control of the amount of water in the body through a finely regulated feedback system involving osmoreceptors and volume receptors, the hypothalamus, the posterior pituitary, and the collecting ducts of the nephrons. To maintain a constant state, the amount of body water derived from intake and from oxidation of carbohydrate, fat, and protein of both exogenous and endogenous origin must equal losses from the kidneys, lungs, skin, and gastrointestinal tract. Water balance is controlled by regulating both intake and excretion, the latter being the more important regulatory mechanism.

Intake. Intake of water is normally stimulated by a sensation of *thirst*; this mechanism is a major defense against fluid depletion and hypertonicity. Thirst, regulated by a center in the midhypothalamus, occurs either when plasma osmolality increases by as little as 1–2% or when the volume of body fluids is significantly reduced, as occurs with hemorrhage or sodium depletion. The changes in osmolality are monitored by osmoreceptors (see below) located in the hypothalamus and possibly in the pancreas and hepatic portal vein. The

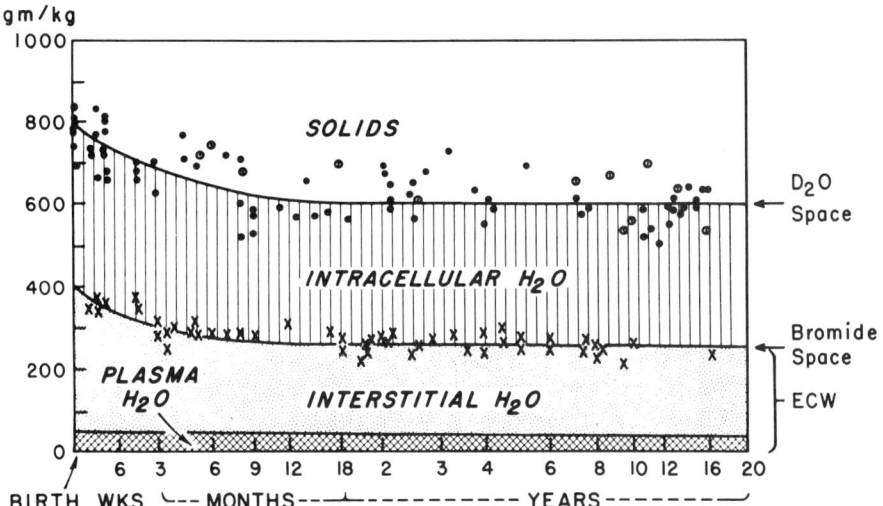

Figure 5–1. Body content and distribution of water at various ages. Deuterium oxide (D_2O) space represents total body water. (From Talbot NB, Richie RH, Crawford JD: Metabolic Homeostasis. Harvard University Press, 1959, p 3.)

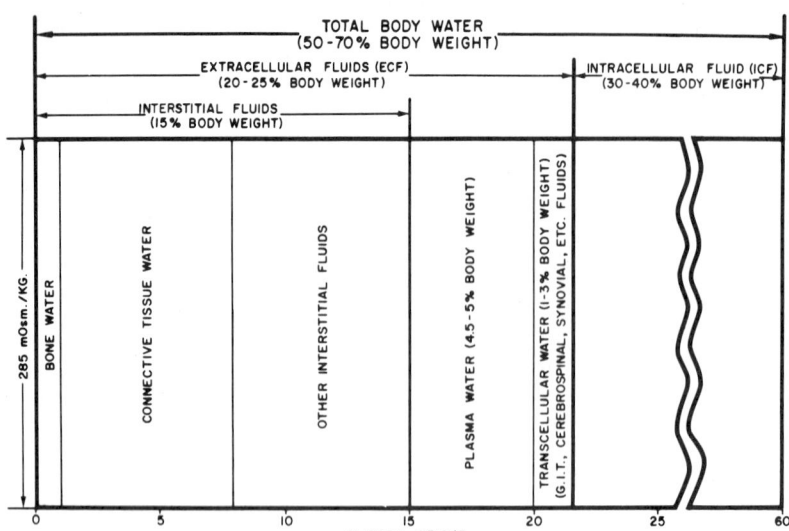

Figure 5–2. The distribution of water in the body of the older child. G.I.T. = gastrointestinal tract.

mechanisms by which volume depletion induces thirst are less well understood, but it may be monitored by baroreceptors in the atria and elsewhere in the vascular bed. Considerable circumstantial evidence suggests that elevated plasma levels of angiotensin II stimulate drinking and may mediate thirst in hypovolemic and hypotensive states. The kidney may also be involved in regulating water intake, possibly through the renin-angiotensin system.

In clinical situations, when conflicting stimuli such as hypotonicity and decreased intravascular volume occur together, the volume signal is dominant and thirst causes increased water intake, restoring volume at the expense of tonicity.

The thirst mechanism and the release of antidiuretic hormone (ADH) may be interrelated. However, at least some of the thirst centers are separated functionally and physically from those involved in release of ADH.

Disorders of the thirst mechanism may be seen in psychologic disorders associated with diseases of the central nervous system, in potassium deficiency, and in malnutrition. These may lead to increased drinking, even though the content of body water is greater than usual and osmolality decreased.

Absorption. Ingested water is absorbed in the gastrointestinal tract by passive diffusion in response to active transport of solute from intestinal lumen to interstitial fluid and plasma. The active transport of sodium is the chief process responsible for generating the osmotic gradient leading to water movement. Any inhibition of sodium transport or failure of reabsorption of solute, as in disaccharidase deficiency, can lead to the presence of large volumes of unabsorbed intestinal water, resulting in diarrhea.

Excretion. Loss of water occurs from the lungs, skin, gastrointestinal tract, and kidneys. The losses from the lungs and skin are evaporative and, in conjunction with that part of the urine volume necessary to excrete its solute load, are referred to as *obligatory losses*. These losses represent the minimum volume of fluid a person must ingest every day to maintain fluid balance.

Water excretion is regulated by varying the rate of urine flow. A fall in plasma osmolality, indicating relative excess of water, is corrected by the excretion of an increased volume of dilute urine which has an osmolality below that of plasma. This loss of free water restores plasma osmolality to normal. Conversely, when plasma osmolality rises above normal, the volume of urine falls and its osmolality rises above that of plasma. This regulation of urine volume and concentration depends principally on the neurohypophyseal-renal axis, the effector of which is ADH. However, since urine volume can

be reduced to only that necessary to excrete the solute load, it is influenced by diet. Other factors that influence urine flow include glomerular filtration rate (GFR), the state of the renal tubular epithelium, and plasma concentrations of adrenal steroids.

Unlike the excretion of water by the kidneys, which responds to the content of water in the body, evaporative water losses are regulated by factors generally independent of body water. They are proportionate to the surface area of the body and are influenced by body and environmental temperature, by the rate of respiration, and by the partial pressure of water vapor in the environment. Thus, evaporative water losses cannot be used to regulate water losses that occur owing to changes in the body's water content. The rate of sweating varies with the body temperature and is controlled in part by the autonomic nervous system. It may be reduced in heat stress, by *severe* deficits in volume of body fluids or by concentration of electrolytes, but still does not represent a major mechanism for regulating body water.

Antidiuretic Hormone (ADH). Human ADH (arginine vasopressin), a cyclic octapeptide, is synthesized in the supraoptic nuclei. This neurosecretory substance is transported down axons which descend through the infundibular stem to be stored in the terminal arborizations in the pars nervosa of the posterior pituitary. Release of ADH into the blood stream occurs by exocytosis in response to stimuli from the hypothalamus. Depletion of ADH in the posterior pituitary occurs in animals deprived of water; storage occurs when water loads are administered.

Secretion of ADH is regulated by the effective osmotic pressure of the extracellular fluid, i.e., that produced by solutes (primarily sodium and chloride) which do not readily penetrate cell membranes. This regulation is monitored by vesicles in the supraoptic nuclei which act as osmoreceptors: they swell when the osmolality of extracellular fluid is less than that of the intracellular fluid and shrink when the osmolality of extracellular fluid exceeds that of the intracellular fluid. Thus, administering urea, which readily diffuses across cell membranes to increase the osmolality of both extracellular and intracellular fluids, produces little shift of water between cells and interstitial fluid and does not evoke consistent antidiuresis. On the other hand, intravenous hypertonic saline solution evokes intense antidiuresis; the sodium remains predominantly in the extracellular fluid, increasing its osmolality in relation to that of intracellular fluid. Conversely, administering water inhibits the release of ADH.

Normally, the threshold for release of ADH is 280 mOsm/kg

H_2O. Release of vasopressin may be initiated or inhibited with changes in plasma osmolality of as little as 1–2%. Response is graded, permitting the urine volume and the osmolality of extracellular fluid to be continuously regulated, thus preventing the fluctuations in osmolality that would occur as a consequence of normal variations in intake of fluid and solutes. Levels of ADH also increase significantly after 8% or greater dehydration, the rise being exponential with more marked dehydration.

The primary action of ADH is to increase the permeability of the renal collecting ducts to water. Under conditions of antidiuresis, the interstitium of the renal medulla has an osmolality of up to 1200 mOsm/kg H_2O at the level of the papilla. This level of osmolality is achieved by the actions of the countercurrent multiplier (loops of Henle) and the exchange (medullary vasa recta blood vessels) systems. In the presence of ADH, luminal urine entering the collecting duct has an osmolality of about 285 mOsm/kg H_2O and becomes progressively more concentrated along the course of the collecting duct as water diffuses out of the urine into the hypertonic medullary interstitium by passive osmotic diffusion. By the time the urine enters the calyces, it has achieved the same concentration as the fluid in the hypertonic medullary papillae. If ADH is absent, continued reabsorption of sodium in the distal tubule and collecting duct leads to further dilution of the urine. Since, in the absence of ADH, these segments of the nephron are impermeable to water, diffusion into the hypertonic medulla does not occur and dilute urine is formed.

Influence of Disease States. Interruption of the supraoptic hypophyseal system causes diabetes insipidus. A failure of the renal collecting ducts to respond to ADH results in nephrogenic diabetes insipidus. Both are accompanied by an inability to concentrate the urine. Release of ADH may be stimulated or inhibited by emotional factors. Stressful stimuli such as pain or the mass discharge of peripheral receptors resulting from trauma, burns, or surgery increase ADH output and are important considerations in fluid therapy. Nicotine, prostaglandins, and cholinergic and beta-adrenergic drugs are potent stimulators of ADH output. Demerol, morphine, and barbiturates are probably antidiuretic in this way, although their reduction of GFR may contribute to their reduction of urine flow. Alcohol is a potent inhibitor of ADH release with a consistent dose-response relation. Diphenylhydantoin and possibly glucocorticoids also inhibit ADH release. Anesthesia reduces urinary flow, probably by altering renal hemodynamics. The presence of nonabsorbable, osmotically active solutes in the renal tubular lumen, e.g., glucose in diabetes mellitus, reduces the amount of water that can diffuse into the hypertonic medulla, thus limiting the ability of ADH to conserve water.

MECHANISMS FOR DISTRIBUTING FLUID WITHIN THE BODY

The distribution of water between intracellular and extracellular spaces is determined by physical factors. *Intracellular volume* is maintained relatively constant by osmotic forces operating across cell membranes freely permeable to water. The maintenance of these forces depends on active transport of potassium into and sodium out of cells by energy-requiring processes. No evidence exists for active transport or secretion of water per se. A rise in extracellular osmolality (e.g., with a sodium load) results in a fall in cell water. Conversely, water intoxication decreases extracellular osmolality and leads to an increase in cell volume. Disturbances in cellular function may also result in an increase in the fluid content of cells.

The volume of fluid in the *intravascular space* (plasma water) is maintained in a steady state by a balance between filtration and oncotic forces at the capillary level. Oncotic pressure (colloid osmotic pressure) represents only a small fraction of total osmotic pressure,* but its osmotic pressure is exerted by molecules, primarily albumin, which do not readily pass through the capillary pores. Thus, colloid osmotic pressure produces an effective osmotic gradient across capillary walls. At the arteriolar end of the capillaries the dominant effect of intracapillary hydrostatic pressure results in a net loss of plasma ultrafiltrate. Normally, at the venous end of the capillary, oncotic pressure causes the net return of an equivalent amount of fluid and electrolytes.

Decreases in protein concentration (as in the nephrotic syndrome) lead to reductions in plasma volume and equivalent increases in *interstitial volume*. These changes may compromise the intravascular volume enough to reduce the GFR and blood flow to other vital organs, but, since the volume of plasma is only one third that of interstitial fluid, plasma volume reduction by shifting of water into the interstitial space may not be observed clinically as *edema*. An increase in capillary permeability to protein, as in angioneurotic edema, produces a rise in protein concentration of the interstitial fluid. This rise reduces oncotic pressure, causing a net shift of fluid, which increases interstitial volume. The increase may be localized, appearing as a wheal or urticaria, or may be generalized. Interstitial fluid volume may also be increased by an increase in the hydrostatic pressure at the venous end of the capillary, as occurs with increased venous pressure associated with heart failure or with retention of sodium and resultant hypervolemia in glomerulonephritis.

The *transcellular fluid* space may increase markedly in inflammatory bowel disease, e.g., eosinophilic gastroenteropathy; in early severe diarrhea; or in ileus with multiple fluid levels.

OSMOLALITY OF BODY FLUIDS

Individual solute concentrations in the extracellular and intracellular fluids vary (Fig. 5–3). However, the osmolality in each compartment is comparable (Fig. 5–2); the chemical activity of water (i.e., the tendency of molecules to escape to another compartment) is the same in each compartment. Nevertheless, the water content of the different body fluids does differ considerably, and variations from normal in these values can be clinically significant. For example, when serum solids such as the proteins and lipids are elevated, as may occur in diabetic ketosis with hyperlipemia, the water content in the serum is markedly decreased (when expressed per liter of serum) because of volume displacement of water by lipids. Since electrolytes are dissolved in the aqueous phase of serum, electrolyte concentrations determined and expressed in the usual way (as mEq per liter of serum) will appear decreased even though their concentration per liter of serum water will be normal; spurious hyponatremia may be noted. Treatment of such *pseudohyponatremia* is unnecessary and may be detrimental to the patient. Its occurrence can be recognized by simultaneously measuring osmolality by freezing point depression, which measures solute concentration of the water fraction of serum. Thus it more accurately reflects sodium

---

*The principal colloids in the plasma are the plasma proteins, which exert an osmotic pressure of approximately 28 mm Hg compared with the 5100 mm Hg exerted by the plasma's crystalloidal solutes. However, the capillary walls are very permeable to the crystalloidal solutes, which, therefore, exert no osmotic force across the capillary walls. Albumin, the most abundant plasma protein and the one having the lowest molecular weight, is the principal solute responsible for colloid osmotic pressure and for regulating net water movement across capillary walls.

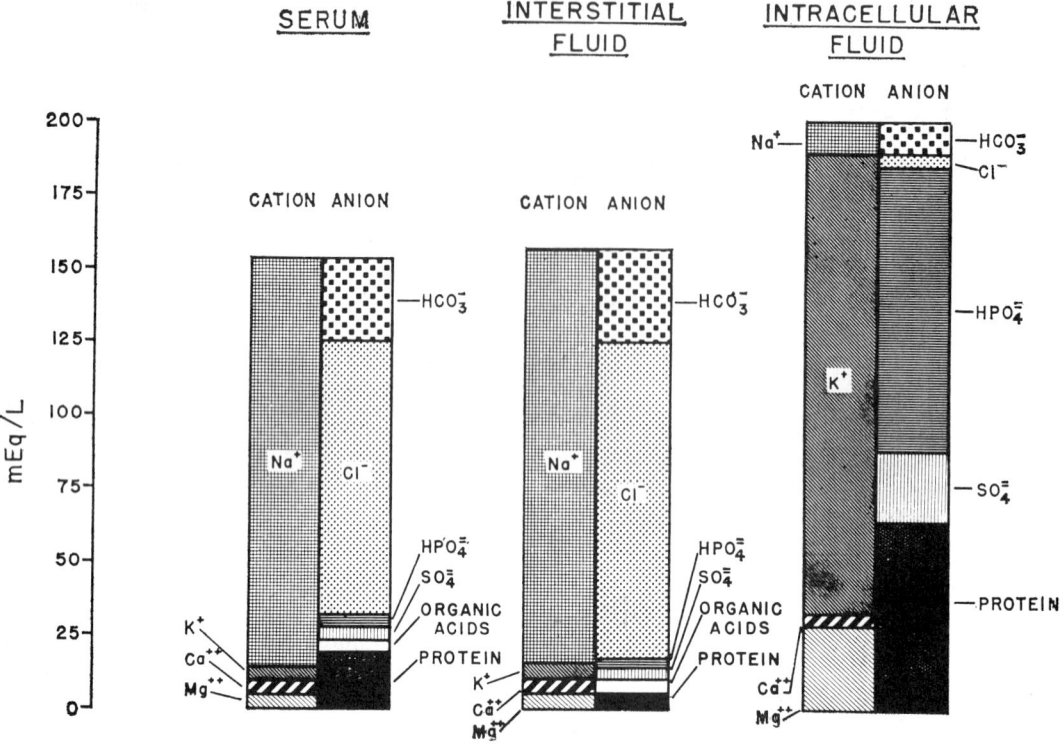

Figure 5–3. Differences in composition of intracellular and extracellular fluids.

concentration in the serum water. The problem of pseudo-hyponatremia is avoided by newer methods measuring sodium concentration with ion-specific electrodes.

5.8 SODIUM

BODY CONTENT OF SODIUM

Sodium, the bulk cation of the extracellular fluid, is the principal osmotically active solute responsible for the maintenance of intravascular and interstitial volumes. The quantity of sodium in the body approximates 58 mEq/kg, more than 30% of which is either nonexchangeable or only slowly exchangeable. Of total body sodium, 6.5 mEq/kg (11.2% of total) is present in the plasma sodium pool, 16.8 mEq/kg (29%) in the interstitial lymph fluid, and 1.4 mEq/kg (2.4%) in the intracellular fluid. About 25 mEq/kg (43.1%) is present in bone, but only one third of the sodium in bone is exchangeable. Dense connective tissue and cartilage sodium is 11.7%.

The *sodium content of the fetus* is relatively higher than that of the adult; exchangeable sodium averages approximately 85 mEq/kg compared with the adult value of 40 mEq/kg because the fetus has relatively large amounts of cartilage, connective tissue, and extracellular fluid (all of which contain considerable amounts of sodium) and a relatively small mass of muscle cells (which have a low sodium content).

REGULATION OF SODIUM

Intake. The amount of sodium in the body is determined by the balance between intake and excretion. When compared with the thirst mechanism for water, the regulatory mechanism of sodium *intake* is poorly developed but may respond to large changes; e.g., salt craving may occur in some patients with salt-wasting syndromes. However, sodium intake normally depends on cultural customs. In the United States the average adult usually takes in 100–170 mEq/day, equivalent

to 6–10 g of salt. Children take in less, proportionate to their smaller food intake. However, infants generally have a relatively high sodium intake because of the high sodium content of cow's milk.

Absorption. Occurring throughout the gastrointestinal tract, minimally in the stomach and maximally in the jejunum, absorption probably takes place by way of a sodium-potassium–activated adenosine triphosphatase (ATPase) system, a transport mechanism augmented by aldosterone or desoxycorticosterone acetate (DCA).

Excretion. This occurs in the urine, sweat, and feces, with the kidney the principal organ for the facultative regulation of sodium output. Normally, the concentration of sodium in sweat ranges from 5 to 40 mEq/L. Higher values are seen in cystic fibrosis and Addison disease, lower values in sodium depletion and hyperaldosteronism, but there is little evidence that changes in the level of sodium in sweat are part of the excretory mechanism for regulating the sodium content of the body. In the absence of diarrhea, fecal concentrations of sodium are low.

Renal regulation of sodium excretion depends on a balance between glomerular and tubular functions. Normally the amount of sodium filtered daily by the kidneys is more than 100 times that ingested and more than five times the total amount of sodium in the body. However, less than 1% of the filtered sodium is excreted in the urine; the remaining 99% is reabsorbed along the length of the renal tubule.

Under normal conditions changes in glomerular filtration rate (GFR) do not affect sodium homeostasis; changes in the filtered load of sodium produced by alterations in GFR are compensated for by appropriate changes in tubular reabsorption of sodium. Moreover, sodium balance can be achieved even when sodium intake varies and GFR remains stable. However, the reduction in GFR that occurs with severe depletion of the volume of extracellular fluid and the increase that accompanies volume expansion may facilitate sodium regulation. Even then it has been shown that experimentally induced changes in GFR, over a wide range, are accompanied by proportional changes in sodium reabsorption in the proximal tubule. Such glomerular-tubular balance reduces changes in the delivery of sodium to more distal segments of the nephron, even when the filtered load of sodium alters markedly, and presumably acts as a protective mechanism.

Approximately two thirds of the filtered sodium is reabsorbed by the *proximal convoluted tubule*. With contraction of extracellular fluid volume this fraction increases; with volume expansion, it decreases. The percentages of filtered sodium and water reabsorbed in the proximal tubule are proportional, so that the fluid remaining at the end of the proximal convoluted tubule has a sodium concentration comparable to that in the blood. Net movement of sodium out of the proximal tubule represents the balance between sodium reabsorbed from the luminal fluid and that returned through intercellular spaces. Since such a high flux of sodium enters the epithelial cells across the luminal membranes, the sodium flux is unlikely to occur by purely passive mechanisms. Reabsorbed sodium is actively transported out of the cells across their basolateral membranes, producing an osmotic gradient that causes the movement of an equivalent amount of water. The resulting hydrostatic force in the intercellular spaces and interstitial fluid, as well as the exertion of oncotic pressure by the plasma protein in the peritubular capillary, is responsible for returning the reabsorbed sodium and water into the vascular space. The balance between glomerular filtration rate and reabsorption of fluid from the proximal tubule (glomerulotubular balance) may be modulated through changes in the protein concentration in the blood at the level of the glomerular and peritubular capillaries.

Sodium reabsorption in the proximal tubules may be regulated by altering the amount of sodium returned to the lumen through the intercellular spaces and tight junctions. It may also be controlled by a natriuretic hormone secreted from the midbrain or hypothalamic region. Although considerable indirect evidence supports this hypothesis, such a hormone has yet to be isolated.

Significant sodium reabsorption occurs in the *loop of Henle* and is central to the countercurrent multiplier system essential for water balance and the concentration of urine (see above). Water reabsorption occurs in the descending limb of the loop of Henle, sodium reabsorption in the ascending limb. Sodium transport at this site may be secondary to the active transport of chloride rather than primary as it is at most other sites. Although the loop of Henle is important in the overall control

of sodium reabsorption, no precise regulating mechanism has yet been delineated, nor has a maximal rate for sodium transport at this site been demonstrated. When the load of sodium delivered to the loop is increased, by changes either in glomerular filtration rate or in sodium reabsorption in the proximal tubule, most of the excess load is reabsorbed in the loop, providing a further protective mechanism and limiting the magnitude of changes of sodium delivery to the distal convoluted tubule.

The fine regulation of sodium balance probably occurs throughout the distal nephron in both the *distal convoluted tubules* and the *collecting ducts*. Sodium reabsorption at these sites is stimulated by aldosterone, whose secretion is governed by the renin-angiotensin system, by some aspect of potassium balance (Fig. 5–4), and by a tropic hormone. The stimulus for release of renin may be a decrease in renal perfusion pressure or a change in sodium concentration (or delivery) in the distal tubule at the level of the macula densa; either system provides a "servo-mechanism" to prevent excessive changes in sodium balance. Throughout the distal tubule and collecting duct, sodium is reabsorbed against a large concentration gradient from lumen to plasma. However, in comparison with the proximal convoluted tubule and the loop of Henle, the total capacity for sodium reabsorption is more limited. Thus, if the load of sodium reaching the distal tubule increases significantly, reabsorption does not increase proportionately and the added load is excreted in the urine.

Additional mechanisms may be responsible for the renal regulation of sodium. Cortical nephrons, which have short loops of Henle, may be sodium-losing nephrons and the juxtamedullary nephrons with long loops of Henle, sodium-retaining nephrons. Sodium balance could be accomplished by altering the proportion of renal blood flow directed to these two populations of nephrons. Such a regulatory mechanism could be intrarenal and respond to local release of renin.

Granules in the cardiac atria have been found to contain peptides that are released into the circulation with volume loading. One of the most potent of these is a 24-amino-acid peptide referred to as atriopeptin III, which causes marked dilatation of blood vessels and induces a diuresis and natriuresis of an order of magnitude greater than that produced by diuretics. These peptides may represent one of the major regulators of sodium balance.

In health, less than 1% of filtered sodium is normally

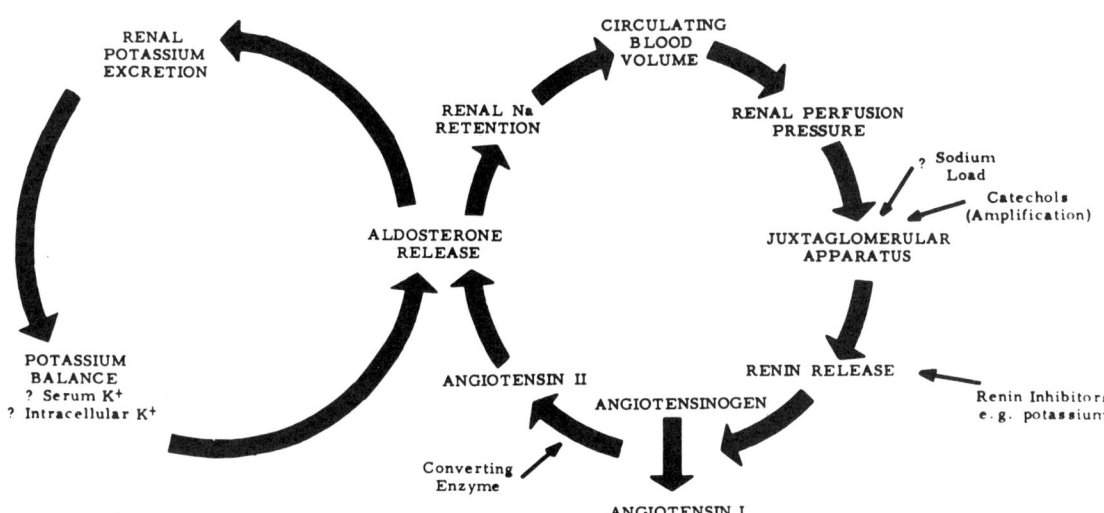

Figure 5–4. The interrelationship of the volume and potassium feedback loops with aldosterone secretion. Integration of signals from each loop determines the level of aldosterone secretion. (From Williams GH, Dluhy RG: Am J Med 53:595, 1972.)

excreted in the urine. However, to maintain sodium balance this figure may increase to 10% or higher with a high sodium intake and can decrease to very low levels in response to reduced dietary sodium. Thus, there is considerable flexibility which prevents a significantly positive or negative sodium balance when dietary sodium intake fluctuates. However, it takes about 3 days for a new steady state to be achieved after dietary intake of sodium has been markedly altered.

DISTRIBUTION OF BODY SODIUM

Although cell membranes are relatively permeable to it, sodium is predominantly extracellular in distribution. Intracellular concentrations are maintained at levels of approximately 10 mEq/L and extracellular concentrations at approximately 140 mEq/L. The low intracellular concentration is achieved by active extrusion of sodium from cells by the sodium-potassium–activated and magnesium-activated ATPase systems. No other cation can replace sodium stimulation of ATPase, but potassium can be replaced by ammonium, rubidium, cesium, and lithium. Calcium inhibits ATPase, as do ouabain and related cardiac glycosides.

Although intracellular concentrations of sodium are low and represent a small part of total body sodium, they may be critical in modifying certain intracellular enzyme activities. Thus, intracellular sodium content is usually relatively constant, and changes in total body sodium reflect mostly changes in extracellular sodium. However, redistribution of sodium between the intracellular and extracellular compartments may occur in the absence of significant changes in total body sodium. Such a change may be observed in the severely ill patient, in whom it usually is referred to as the "sick cell syndrome."

Because of the Donnan distribution of anionic proteins, the concentration of sodium in interstitial fluid is approximately 97% that of the serum sodium value; changes in concentration of sodium in the serum are reflected by proportional changes in the concentration of sodium in the interstitial fluid. Concentrations of sodium in transcellular fluids vary considerably because such fluids are not in simple diffusion equilibrium with plasma (Table 5–1). Unexpected changes in composition of these fluids may occur and may necessitate the changing of therapeutic regimens designed to replace their abnormal loss.

Table 5–1. Sodium, Potassium, and Chloride Concentrations in Transcellular Fluids

Fluid	Sodium (mEq/L)	Potassium (mEq/L)	Chloride (mEq/L)
Saliva	33.1 ± 13.4	19.5 ± 3.4	33.9 ± 10.2
Gastric juice	60.4 (9–116)	9.2 (0.5–32.5)	84.0 (7.8–154.5)
Ileal fluid	129.4 (105.4–143.7)	11.2 (5.9–29.3)	116.2 (90–136.4)
Cecal fluid	52.5	7.9	42.5
Pancreatic juice	141.1 (113–153)	4.6 (2.6–7.4)	76.6 (54.1–95.2)
Bile	148.9 (131–164)	4.98 (2.6–12)	100.6 (89–117.6)
Cerebrospinal fluid	140.0 (130–150)	3.3 (2.7–3.9)	126.8 (115.5–132.4)
Aqueous humor (rabbits)	143.0 (141.7–145.0)	4.7	107.9 (106.2–109.5)
Sweat	See Table 5–7		

From Edelman IS, Liebman J: Am J Med 27:256, 1959.

INFLUENCE OF DISEASE STATES

In many disease states the body loses its ability to regulate sodium normally. Such abnormalities usually result in changes in volume rather than in changes in sodium concentration. Retention of sodium is typically compensated for by a retention of an equivalent amount of water, so that edema develops. Sodium concentration remains in, or near, the normal range. Excessive losses of sodium may cause hyponatremia, but they are often paralleled by comparable losses of water, thus resulting in volume contraction with little change in sodium concentration.

Patients with *chronic renal disease* can usually modify their rate of sodium excretion, but both the upper and lower limits of sodium tolerance are characteristically limited. Some renal diseases, especially those affecting the tubules, are associated with a limited renal ability to conserve sodium. In such patients the unnecessary restriction of sodium will result in volume contraction and a further reduction in renal function. Conversely, exceeding the upper limit for sodium tolerance produces positive sodium balance and edema, a condition most often seen in patients with glomerular diseases. However, patients with chronic renal disease frequently do not develop positive sodium balance until their GFR falls to levels below 5–10% of normal or unless they have a nephrotic syndrome. Positive sodium balance may also be found in association with acute decreases in GFR such as that seen in acute glomerulonephritis and may also result from a decrease in the oncotic pressure of plasma (e.g., with the nephrotic syndrome), from a decrease in effective arterial volume (e.g., with congestive heart failure), or from the administration or increased secretion of steroids with mineralocorticoid effects.

In *diabetes mellitus* the high level of osmotically active solute in the tubular urine is due to the presence of glucose, which retards passive reabsorption of water and causes the limiting gradient for sodium transport to be attained inappropriately, thus reducing sodium transport. This osmotic effect, exerted principally beyond the proximal tubule, produces both natriuresis and diuresis and can cause negative sodium balance. Negative salt balance (with an inappropriate elevation of sodium in the urine) is also seen in Addison disease and in some patients with neurologic lesions. More commonly, it results from extrarenal losses of sodium, such as those that occur with severe or protracted diarrhea when urine sodium concentrations should be low.

Alterations in sodium concentration most often reflect an abnormality in the handling of water. *Hyponatremia* (serum sodium <135 mEq/L) indicates that there is relatively less sodium than water in the extracellular fluid (ECF) space. It can be due to ECF sodium depletion but often results from expansion of the ECF by water, which may arise from inappropriate reduction of water loss, e.g., with the inappropriate ADH syndrome, or from excessive water administration (Sec. 5.32). Mild degrees of hyponatremia result in remarkably few symptoms. With more severe decreases in sodium concentration the presenting symptom typically is confusion. When serum sodium concentrations fall to 120 mEq/L or less, they should be treated promptly since convulsions may occur as the osmotically induced movement of water into cerebral cells causes them to swell and produce seizures.

Hypernatremia (serum sodium >150 mEq/L) occurs when the amount of sodium in the ECF is increased in relation to the amount of water in this space. The content of sodium in the ECF may be increased but can be normal or even decreased if there have been major losses of water. Thus, as with hyponatremia, hypernatremia can result from derangements of sodium or water balance either alone or in combination. Examples include (1) sodium retention due to excess sodium administration either as saline or as salt tablets or with accidental substitution of salt for sugar in infant formulas and

(2) negative water balance due to inadequate replacement of either excessive losses (e.g., patients with central or nephrogenic diabetes insipidus) or normal losses (e.g., a comatose patient). (See Sec. 5.32.)

5.9 POTASSIUM

BODY CONTENT OF POTASSIUM

The body content of potassium, the major intracellular cation, correlates well with lean body mass. Because potassium is predominantly intracellular, the change in body potassium content that occurs with growth is an excellent index of cellular mass at different ages. In the adult, potassium approximates 53 mEq/kg body weight, 95% of which is exchangeable. Intracellular potassium amounts to 48 mEq/kg (89.6%); extracellular (plasma [0.4%], interstitial lymph [1.0%], dense connective tissue and cartilage [0.4%], and bone [7.6%]), only 5.5 mEq/kg (9.4%), of which 4 mEq/kg is in bone.

Intracellular concentrations of potassium approximate 150 mEq/L of cell water. Most is unbound and osmotically active, but sequestration by active transport in subcellular particles, such as mitochondria, is likely. Extracellular concentrations of potassium are maintained normally at 4–5 mEq/L.

REGULATION OF POTASSIUM

Potassium is present in remarkably constant quantities in almost all animal and vegetable tissues. A daily intake of 1–2 mEq/kg body weight is recommended, but intakes vary widely. Absorption of potassium is reasonably complete in the upper gastrointestinal tract. More distally, body potassium is exchanged for sodium present in the lumen of the lower bowel.

Chronic potassium balance is primarily regulated by the kidneys, which can adjust the amount of potassium excreted over a wide range. Normally the rate of potassium excretion in the urine approximates 10–15% of that filtered. With the administration of large amounts of potassium, urinary excretion may be more than twice the amount filtered at the glomerulus. Conversely, urinary concentrations can be reduced to very low levels if potassium conservation is required. Thus, in the adult, rates of urinary potassium excretion may range from less than 5 mEq to 1000 mEq/day.

Potassium is freely filtered in the glomerulus. Its concentration along the length of the proximal convoluted tubule is similar to that of plasma, indicating that reabsorption of potassium in this segment of the nephron is proportionate to that of water, with 60% or more of the filtered potassium being absorbed. Concentrations of potassium are increased in the loop of Henle. However, by the time tubular fluid reaches the early distal convoluted tubule, its potassium concentration is below that of plasma, so that the amount of potassium delivered to more distal segments of the nephron is less than 10% of the filtered load. Under states of maximal potassium conservation, continued reabsorption occurs in the distal tubule; when dietary intake is normal or when excretion is increased for other reasons, secretion of potassium takes place in the distal tubule and possibly in the collecting duct. Most of the potassium in the final urine probably results from tubular secretion rather than glomerular filtration.

The mechanisms responsible for the control of net secretion of potassium in the distal nephron are extremely complex and not fully understood. Potassium transfer across the luminal membrane is passive and depends on electrical and chemical gradients as well as on the membrane's potassium permeability. The electrical gradient generated by reabsorption of sodium from the fluid in the distal tubule represents a major driving force for this potassium secretion. The rate of potassium secretion, however, is always less than that of sodium reabsorption. Moreover, the variable ratio of the two rates indicates the processes are not tightly coupled. Furthermore, the hydrogen ion is also excreted into the distal tubule in exchange for sodium, and renal production of ammonia, a regulatory system for acid-base balance, is also intimately related to potassium homeostasis. These observations may explain the interrelation of hydrogen ion and potassium excretion and account for the effects of acid-base balance on urinary losses of potassium. For example, kaliuresis and hypokalemia frequently occur with systemic alkalosis.

The concentration gradient for potassium between the distal tubular fluid and the distal tubular cells also modifies the addition of potassium to the fluid in the distal nephron. This process may be regulated in large part by modulation of intracellular concentrations of potassium through the active transport of potassium at the contraluminal cell membrane. Such a scheme could account for the observation that potassium excretion frequently cannot be correlated with serum potassium levels but may be better correlated with intracellular concentrations of the cation. An increased flow rate of distal tubule fluid increases the concentration gradient as well as the rate of loss of potassium in the urine.

Active transport of potassium may also occur at the luminal membrane, from the tubular fluid back into the cells. It has been proposed that this process could represent the final regulating mechanism. In summary, factors affecting distal nephron potassium secretion include mineralocorticoid activity, dietary potassium, acid-base status, distal tubular flow rate, and sodium delivery to the distal tubule.

Aldosterone plays a major role in potassium regulation in the kidney as well as in other tissues. Injected intravenously into a patient with Addison disease, it reduces urinary excretion of sodium and increases that of potassium. It acts at the distal tubule by altering permeability of the luminal membrane to sodium, thus allowing increased exchange between luminal sodium and intracellular potassium. Aldosterone secretion appears to be affected by both sodium and potassium balance (Fig. 5–4).

Potassium is also lost in the feces and the sweat. The exchange of plasma potassium for sodium present in the colonic contents contributes to sodium conservation and permits the colon to participate in potassium homeostasis. However, even under conditions of chronic potassium loading, fecal potassium constitutes only a small percentage of the total amount of potassium excreted. The human colon responds to mineralocorticoids by decreasing sodium and increasing the potassium content of the stool. Glucocorticoids have a similar effect.

The potassium content of sweat, normally 10–25 mEq/L, is increased by mineralocorticoids and may be elevated in aldosteronism as well as in cystic fibrosis. Losses of potassium by this route, however, usually are insignificant even in disease states.

Acute potassium loads require well developed extrarenal mechanisms to prevent severe hyperkalemia and to avoid potassium toxicity. In the first 4–6 hr following a potassium load, only half of the potassium is excreted by the kidneys. Some is secreted into the intestinal tract. More than 40%, however, is translocated into cells, primarily in the liver and muscle. This process is an important protective mechanism and is regulated by both insulin and epinephrine, which enhance potassium uptake. The catecholamine effect appears to be mediated through β-receptors. Stimulation of α-adrenergic receptors impairs extrarenal disposal of an acute potassium load. Aldosterone plays a key role in the extrarenal handling of potassium. Its primary site of action may be the gastrointestinal tract, although it also affects muscle transport of potassium. Glucocorticoids may be important in extrarenal potassium homeostasis, too. Glucagon infusion causes a transient hyperkalemia, but its role in potassium regulation is not clear.

Acid-base balance affects intracellular shifts of potassium. Systemic acidosis results in movement of potassium out of cells; alkalosis produces the opposite effect. For every 0.1 unit change in blood pH, the plasma potassium concentration changes 0.3–1.3 mEq/L in the opposite direction. The changes depend on numerous factors; for example, the increase in serum potassium accompanying respiratory acidosis is much less than that with metabolic acidosis.

Potassium Depletion. Abnormally low amounts of total body potassium occur in a variety of disease states, such as muscular dystrophy, which are characterized by a decrease in muscle mass. These disorders are not necessarily accompanied by *hypokalemia*. A low serum potassium may result from a prolonged decreased intake, from increased renal excretion, or from increased extrarenal losses. Renal losses may be increased by the use of diuretics including osmotic diuretics and carbonic anhydrase inhibitors; by tubular defects such as renal tubular acidosis; by acid-base disturbances; in endocrinopathies such as Cushing syndrome, primary aldosteronism, and thyrotoxicosis; in diabetic ketoacidosis; in Bartter syndrome; and in magnesium deficiency. Extrarenal losses may occur from the bowel, e.g., with diarrhea, chronic catharsis, frequent enemas, protracted vomiting, biliary drainage, or enterocutaneous fistulas, or from the skin if there is profuse sweating. Movement of potassium into cells during correction of a metabolic acidosis, for example, may also result in hypokalemia, as may *familial hypokalemic periodic paralysis*, a rare disorder in which episodes of paralysis are usually accompanied by an abrupt and marked hypokalemia due to movement of potassium into an extravascular body compartment.

External losses of potassium result in a shift of potassium from the intracellular to the extracellular fluid. Intracellular potassium is replaced in part by sodium, hydrogen ions, and dibasic amino acids. If these changes become severe, intracellular acidosis in the renal tubular cells may result in excessive exchange of intracellular hydrogen for sodium in the distal tubular fluid leading to aciduria with the increased urinary excretion of ammonia and to systemic alkalosis.

The relation of extracellular to intracellular potassium concentration is vital to cell function. Membrane depolarization, the process responsible for initiating muscle contraction, requires the abrupt influx of sodium into cells and a comparable efflux of potassium out of them. The process is reversed with repolarization. With hypokalemia the ratio of intracellular to extracellular potassium concentrations is increased. The transmembrane electrical potential gradient increases so that a wider differential between the resting and excitation potentials exists, which interferes with impulse formation, propagation, and muscle contraction. Thus hypokalemia produces functional alterations in skeletal muscle, in smooth muscle, and in the heart. Although it is impossible to predict accurately the degree of potassium loss from the body by measuring serum potassium, a 1 mEq/L decrease in serum potassium concentration secondary to potassium loss generally corresponds to a loss of approximately 5–10% of body potassium. Many patients will tolerate this degree of loss without symptoms. Rate of change in potassium levels as well as magnitude of losses probably affects severity of symptoms. Weakness is an early manifestation typically noted first in limb muscles before trunk and respiratory muscles. Areflexia, paralysis, and death from respiratory muscle failure can develop. Paralytic ileus and gastric dilation reflect smooth muscle dysfunction. Electrocardiographic abnormalities, especially a low-

ered T-wave voltage and the appearance of a U wave, are characteristic. In the kidney, potassium deficiency results in vacuolar changes in the tubular epithelium. If sustained for a long time, it leads to nephrosclerosis and interstitial fibrosis, pathologic lesions indistinguishable from those of chronic pyelonephritis. The kidney has a reduced ability to concentrate or dilute the urine, with polyuria and polydipsia developing. An increase in bicarbonate reabsorption and hydrogen ion secretion results in systemic alkalosis. When the source of potassium loss is not apparent, measuring urinary potassium may help. A urine concentration of 15 mEq/L or less indicates renal conservation of potassium and suggests that the loss occurred from a nonrenal source.

Increases in Body Potassium. Increases comparable in magnitude to the deficits discussed have not been described; they probably would be lethal. Indeed, *hyperkalemia* with serum potassium levels of 5.5 mEq/L or greater may result from surprisingly small increases in total body potassium. Because the kidney has a large capacity to excrete excess potassium and to prevent hyperkalemia, this electrolyte abnormality is most often seen when renal excretory mechanisms are impaired. Thus it may occur in acute or chronic renal failure, in adrenal insufficiency, in hyporeninemic hypoaldosteronism, and with the use of potassium-sparing diuretics. Acute increases in potassium intake may also result in hyperkalemia, although it is typically transient in duration. Sources of such potassium include the use of potassium salts of penicillin (1.7 mEq/million units) and of salt substitutes by patients on a salt-restricted diet. Acute tissue breakdown, e.g., from trauma, major surgery, or burns, can also release sufficient potassium into the extracellular fluid to cause hyperkalemia. Finally, transcellular redistribution of potassium may cause an elevated serum potassium, seen typically in metabolic acidosis. It may also occur shortly before death or in severely ill patients. Certain drugs may increase the serum potassium by similar mechanisms. Succinylcholine inhibits membrane repolarization which requires cellular uptake of potassium. Severe digitalis overdose may cause severe hyperkalemia, presumably by inhibiting sodium-potassium exchange by cell membranes. Since intracellular levels of potassium are 30 times as high as those in the extracellular fluid, lysis of red cells during the collection or handling of a blood sample or release of potassium from platelets during clotting may result in pseudohyperkalemia, in which apparent elevations of serum potassium are recorded by the laboratory.

The major consequences of hyperkalemia are due to its neuromuscular effects. It reduces transmembrane potential toward threshold levels and therefore results in delayed depolarization, faster repolarization, and a slowing of conduction velocity. Paresthesias are followed by weakness and eventually by flaccid paralysis if treatment is not instituted. The heart is particularly vulnerable to hyperkalemia. The electrocardiogram typically shows peaking of the T waves. Lengthening of the P-R interval and widening of the QRS complex develop later and are particularly ominous, as they often herald the development of ventricular fibrillation. Since the sequence of cardiotoxic events often progresses rapidly, hyperkalemia should be treated as a medical emergency (Sec. 5.32).

5.10 CALCIUM

BODY CALCIUM

See also Sec. 3.6, 5.34, and 23.46.

At all ages 99% of the body's calcium is in bone. Since the bones of infants are less densely mineralized than are those of adults, the body contents of calcium in infants and adults are significantly different, i.e., about 400 and 950 mEq/kg of body weight, respectively.

In health the extracellular pool of calcium remains remarkably constant despite fairly free exchange with the enormous reservoir in bone. The calcium concentration in serum is also maintained within narrow limits, averaging 2.5 mM/L (10 mg/dL). Approximately 40% is protein-bound, of which 80–90% is bound to albumin. The remaining 60% is ultrafilterable or diffusible; about 14% is complexed with anions such as phosphate and citrate, and the remaining 46% (1.2 mM/L or 4.8 mg/dL) is present as free ionic calcium. The ionized calcium is of greatest physiologic importance.

REGULATION

Body calcium content is regulated primarily through the gastrointestinal tract. The recommended daily dietary intake is 360 mg in the first 6 mo of life, 540 mg in the second 6 mo, 800 mg from ages 1–10 yr, and 1200 mg from ages 11–18. Dairy products constitute the most important single source. Dietary calcium is absorbed along the small intestine, primarily in the duodenum and early jejunum by a process enhanced by 1,25-dihydroxy vitamin D_3. It is proposed that hypocalcemia stimulates release of parathyroid hormone (PTH) which, in turn, increases the renal conversion of 25-hydroxy vitamin D_3 to its 1,25 derivative.

The efficiency of intestinal absorption of dietary calcium is increased on a low calcium intake, in the growing child, in pregnancy, and during depletion of body calcium stores. The mechanisms responsible for this adaptation are unknown. Administering vitamin D and PTH also increases calcium absorption, the latter probably by its effect on vitamin D metabolism. Increases in absorption leading to hypercalcemia occur in sarcoidosis, carcinomatosis, and multiple myeloma. Decreased absorption of calcium results from the presence in the gastrointestinal tract of phytate, oxalate, and citrate (all of which complex the dietary calcium); from increased gastric motility; from reduction of bowel length; and from protein depletion, which may cause a deficiency of the calcium-binding protein in the intestinal mucosa. Some calcium is secreted into the intestinal lumen by the bowel, but this process probably does not represent a regulatory mechanism.

Excretion. Plasma non–protein-bound calcium (ultrafilterable calcium) is filtered at the glomerulus. Normally, about 99% of this filtered calcium is reabsorbed by the tubules, ionized calcium being transported more easily than the complexed form. Reabsorption occurs throughout the nephron. That which occurs in the proximal tubule (50–55%) and loop of Henle (20–30%) appears to parallel sodium reabsorption; factors influencing transport of one of these cations also affect the other. Calcium transport in the distal convoluted tubule (10–15%) and the collecting duct (2–8%) is independent of sodium transport; these sites probably represent the mechanisms that are specifically calciuric. Calcium reabsorption is stimulated specifically by 1,25-dihydroxy vitamin D_3 and inhibited by thyrocalcitonin. Parathyroid hormone increases reabsorption of calcium by the renal tubules, but this effect may be masked by the concomitant hypercalcemia and resultant increase in the glomerular filtered load of calcium seen in hyperparathyroidism. Urinary excretion of calcium is also increased by many nonspecific mechanisms. These include expansion of extracellular fluid volume; the administration of osmotic diuretics, furosemide, thiazides, growth hormone, thyroid hormone, or glucagon; metabolic acidosis; prolonged fasting; and an increase in serum phosphate.

There is a diurnal variation in the excretion of calcium, which peaks at the middle of the day. Alterations in dietary calcium result in only small changes in urinary excretion of calcium, probably reflecting adaptive changes in intestinal absorption of calcium. Physical inactivity is associated with

increased urinary excretion of calcium and, if prolonged, may result in formation of renal stones.

Influence of Disease States. The amount of ionized calcium is physiologically important in determining the significance of changes in plasma calcium concentration. Since some calcium is bound to protein, especially albumin, total calcium levels vary directly with the level of serum albumin. However, with hypoalbuminemia, a low total calcium level in the serum is rarely associated with symptoms or signs of hypocalcemia because the level of serum ionized calcium remains normal.

The balance between deposition and mobilization of calcium in bone largely determines the concentration of ionized calcium in the blood. PTH and 1,25-dihydroxy vitamin D_3 promote increased calcium resorption from bone and elevate the serum calcium. Thyrocalcitonin has the opposite effects. The amounts of calcium absorbed from the renal tubular fluid and from the bowel also affect concentrations of plasma-ionized calcium but to a lesser extent. Changes in hydrogen ion activity in the plasma modify the percentage of total calcium that is ionized; a pH change of 1.0 unit alters the concentration of ionized calcium by 10%. Acidosis increases and alkalosis decreases the proportion ionized so that symptomatic hypocalcemia may be seen during the rapid correction or overcorrection of acidosis. In addition, the serum concentrations of sodium and potassium may play some role in the balance between deposition and mobilization of bone calcium; thus, treating hypernatremia with fluids low in potassium content may result in hypocalcemia.

Symptomatic *hypocalcemia* due to a low concentration of ionized calcium results from vitamin D deficiency, which in turn is caused by nutritional deficiency, malabsorption, or abnormal metabolism of vitamin D. Hypocalcemia may also be due to hypoparathyroidism or pseudohypoparathyroidism, hyperphosphatemia, magnesium deficiency, and acute pancreatitis.

The neonate is particularly susceptible to hypocalcemia in association with hypoparathyroidism, abnormal vitamin D metabolism, a low calcium intake, or a high phosphate intake (Sec. 5.14, 5.34, 8.54, and 19.18). Bone mineralization is frequently inadequate in very low birthweight infants during the neonatal period, increasing the incidence of radiologic rickets and fractures. These lesions most likely result from an inadequate intake of calcium and phosphorus at the time of rapid postnatal growth and may not respond to vitamin D metabolites.

Causes of *hypercalcemia* include primary or tertiary hyperparathyroidism, hyperthyroidism, vitamin D intoxication, immobilization, malignancies (especially those which metastasize to bone), use of thiazide diuretics, milk-alkali syndrome, and sarcoidosis. An idiopathic form may occur in infancy associated with typical "elfin" facies and supravalvular aortic stenosis; this syndrome may be due to hypersensitivity to vitamin D. If their dietary intake of phosphorus is inadequate, low birthweight infants may develop hypercalcemia owing to resorption of both phosphorus and calcium from bone.

Calcium loading increases renal excretion of sodium and potassium and profoundly reduces the ability to concentrate the urine, an effect that may explain the polyuria and polydipsia seen clinically in patients with hypercalcemia due to hypervitaminosis D. Concentrated calcium solutions should always be administered cautiously, using electrocardiographic monitoring whenever possible to minimize cardiac arrhythmias (Sec. 14.70).

5.11 MAGNESIUM

Magnesium, the fourth most abundant cation in the body, plays a major role in cellular enzymatic activity, especially glycolysis and the stimulation of the ATPases.

Total body magnesium amounts to approximately 22 mEq/kg in the infant. It increases in adults to 28 mEq/kg. Sixty percent of body magnesium is in bone, of which about one third is freely exchangeable. Most of the remaining 40% is intracellular; more than 50% is in muscle and much of the remainder in liver. Only 20–30% of the intracellular magnesium is exchangeable, the remainder being bound to proteins, RNA, and ATP.

Extracellular magnesium accounts for only 1% of body magnesium. Although freely exchangeable with the large exchangeable pools in bone and cells, extracellular concentrations are maintained at low levels within a relatively narrow normal range. Serum magnesium normally ranges from 1.5–1.8 mEq/L, although wider normal ranges have been reported. Approximately 80% is ultrafilterable; this consists of 55% ionized and 25% complexed. The remaining 20% is protein bound.

The **intake** of magnesium in children ranges from 10 to 25 mEq/day, depending on age; the highest intakes are required during periods of rapid growth. Green vegetables and many other foods contain high concentrations of magnesium; the intake of most individuals exceeds the minimum requirement of 3.6 mg/kg/day (12 mg magnesium is equivalent to 1 mEq or 0.5 mM). Absorption of dietary magnesium occurs primarily in the upper gastrointestinal tract by mechanisms that are not fully delineated. Vitamin D, PTH, and increased sodium absorption enhance magnesium absorption; calcium, phosphorus, and increased intestinal motility decrease it. Absorption is far from complete; an amount of magnesium equal to about two thirds the intake is present in the feces. A small proportion of this magnesium is secreted by the bowel.

Maintenance of balance depends primarily on urinary excretion. Normally, less than 5% of the filtered load of magnesium appears in the urine. Twenty to 30% is reabsorbed in the proximal tubule and most of the remainder in the loop of Henle, especially the thick ascending limb. Regulation of magnesium absorption is incompletely understood. Under a variety of conditions magnesium reabsorption parallels that of calcium and sodium. There is competition between magnesium and calcium for transport. Urinary excretion of magnesium usually amounts to about one third of intake. It is increased by expansion of extracellular fluid volume; by osmotic, thiazide, mercurial, and loop diuretics; by glucagon; and by calcium loading. Conversely, volume contraction, magnesium deficiency, thyrocalcitonin, and PTH increase the renal reabsorption of magnesium.

The maintenance of magnesium balance and serum magnesium concentrations, however, requires a complex interaction of both renal and nonrenal factors. For example, a low magnesium diet results in reduced urinary magnesium. This reduction may be the consequence of modest reductions in the serum concentration of magnesium, which have been shown to increase the release of PTH. In turn, PTH release decreases urinary loss of magnesium and also causes the release of both magnesium and calcium into the extracellular fluid with increased concentrations of both cations. Tubular reabsorption of filtered magnesium can be almost complete. However, the gastrointestinal tract continues to secrete small amounts of magnesium, and depletion may result.

Influence of Disease States. The concentration of magnesium in serum depends not only on intake and output but also on mobilization of magnesium from both bone and soft tissue. It is not always a reliable indicator of magnesium balance but may remain normal even with marked *magnesium depletion*. Thus, in severe nutritional deficiency states such as kwashiorkor, serum levels of magnesium may be normal even though the content of magnesium in the muscle is decreased. Conversely, reduced levels may be seen in the absence of appreciable losses.

Hypomagnesemia occurs in a variety of clinical states, including malabsorption syndromes, hypoparathyroidism, diuretic therapy, hypercalcemia, renal tubular acidosis, primary aldosteronism, alcoholism, and prolonged intravenous fluid therapy with magnesium-free fluids. At special risk are infants who undergo surgery and receive such fluids for protracted periods of time. Infants with either early or late neonatal tetany often also have hypomagnesemia (Sec. 5.34, 8.54, and 19.18). When associated with early neonatal tetany, it tends to be mild and transient and may not require treatment with magnesium. In late neonatal tetany, hypocalcemia may fail to respond to treatment until magnesium levels have been returned to normal.

The symptoms of hypomagnesemia are primarily those of increased neuromuscular irritability and include tetany, severe seizures, and tremors. Personality changes, nausea, anorexia, abnormal cardiac rhythms, and electrocardiographic changes may also be seen. Symptoms do not always correlate with serum magnesium levels, perhaps because serum levels do not always reflect the body content of magnesium, a predominantly intracellular cation. Alternatively, the symptoms of hypomagnesemia may be minor compared with the symptoms of the primary disease causing the magnesium depletion. A third possibility is that symptoms may reflect whether hypomagnesemia is complicated by hypocalcemia. Severe hypomagnesemia interferes with release of PTH and induces skeletal resistance to the action of PTH. Thus, hypomagnesemia and hypocalcemia often coexist.

Hypermagnesemia, or an increase in body magnesium, rarely occurs in the absence of decreased renal function. Normally, the kidney prevents elevations of serum magnesium to dangerous levels even when large magnesium loads are administered. However, hypermagnesemia with serum levels exceeding 5 mEq/L can occur. The usual sources of a magnesium load include magnesium-containing laxatives, enemas, and intravenous fluids. Severe hypermagnesemia may be seen in neonates born of mothers who were treated with intramuscular injections of magnesium sulfate for the hypertension of pre-eclampsia. Neonates born prematurely with asphyxia and/or hypotonia are at special risk, although it remains to be determined whether the elevated magnesium is the cause or consequence of these abnormalities. Serum magnesium levels tend to spontaneously return to normal within 72 hr. There is also an increased incidence of hypermagnesemia in patients with Addison disease. Symptoms of hypermagnesemia occur when levels exceed 5 mg/dL. Hyporeflexia antedates respiratory depression, drowsiness, and coma. They are rapidly reversed by intravenous administration of calcium. Coma and death usually occur when the serum magnesium level increases above 15 mg/dL.

5.12 HYDROGEN ION
(Acid-Base Balance)

TERMINOLOGY

Acid-base balance has been complicated historically by a confusion of terminologies. The current approach emphasizes the *hydrogen ion*—or proton—which is a hydrogen atom with its neutralizing electron removed. *pH* is the negative logarithm of the concentration of free hydrogen ions. An *acid* is a proton (hydrogen ion) donor. Hydrochloric, sulfuric, phosphoric, and carbonic acids are conventional acids, each dissociating to liberate protons. A strong acid is one that is highly dissociated and, therefore, presents a high concentration of hydrogen ions; a weak acid is one that is poorly dissociated. A *base* is a hydrogen ion acceptor. Thus, bases bind free hydrogen ions, reducing their concentration. Examples include hydroxyl ions, ammonia, and the anions of weak acids. A *buffer* is defined as a substance that reduces the change in free hydrogen ion concentration of a solution upon the addition of an acid or base. The presence of a buffer in a solution increases the amount of acid or alkali that must be added to cause a change in pH. The addition of a strong acid to any of these buffer systems results in the production of a neutral salt and a weak acid. By generating a poorly dissociated acid, the buffer significantly reduces the increment in free hydrogen ion concentration when the reaction is compared to one that is not buffered. *Aprotes* are either cations such as sodium, potassium, calcium, and magnesium that carry one or more positive charges, depending on valence, or anions such as chloride and sulfate that carry negative charges. Since aprotes are able neither to donate nor to accept protons, they are not acids, bases, or buffers.

REGULATING MECHANISMS

The number of potential hydrogen ions in the body is huge. Most are buffered and, therefore, are not in free form. At the usual pH of 7.4 the concentration of free hydrogen ions in the blood is only 0.0000398 mEq/L or 3.98×10^{-8} Eq/L (often expressed as 40 nEq/L):

$$pH = -\log (H^+) = -\log (3.98 \times 10^{-8})$$
$$= -(0.60 - 8.0) = 7.4$$

Normally, the hydrogen ion concentrations of body fluids are maintained in relatively narrow ranges by the presence of buffers. Buffers represent the first line of defense against changes in pH, but they cannot maintain acid-base balance. Since, in the presence of disease states or abrupt alteration of hydrogen ion production, buffer systems may not be able to maintain a normal pH for a prolonged period, their action needs to be supplemented by compensatory and corrective physiologic changes in the lungs and the kidneys.

Compensation of a primary acid-base disorder is a slower process than buffering, but it is more effective in returning pH to normal. In a primary metabolic disorder the respiratory system provides the compensating mechanism; the kidneys compensate in a primary respiratory disorder. Compensation reduces pH changes but must be followed by *correction* which returns all acid-base measurements to normal. This occurs when the primary disorder is cured. The kidneys correct a metabolic disorder, the lungs a respiratory one. Although discussed separately, the buffering, pulmonary, and renal systems are interdependent and act in concert with one another.

Buffer Systems. The principal buffer in the extracellular fluid is the bicarbonate–carbonic acid system; intracellular buffers include various proteins and organic phosphates. In the urine, phosphate in its mono- and dihydrogen forms is the major buffer. Only the extracellular fluid buffer mechanisms will be considered in detail.

Hydrogen ions, when added to the plasma, are buffered in large part by bicarbonate with the generation of a neutral salt and carbonic acid.

$$HA + NaHCO_3 \rightarrow NaA + H_2CO_3$$

Carbonic acid is a weak acid with a relatively low solubility coefficient and is in equilibrium with dissolved carbon dioxide as follows:

$$[H^+] \cdot [HCO_3^-] \rightleftharpoons H_2CO_3 \rightleftharpoons CO_2 + H_2O$$

The addition of hydrogen ions drives this equation to the right, generating CO_2 and H_2O. Thus, despite the addition of hydrogen ions, the buffering mechanisms result in relatively little change in free hydrogen ion concentration and in pH. However, buffering is accomplished at the expense of a decrease in bicarbonate concentration (this decrease has been

referred to as representing *base deficit*) and an increase in carbon dioxide (pCO_2) levels. The Henderson-Hasselbalch equation indicates that these changes must result in some change in pH:

$$pH = pK + \log \frac{Base}{Acid}$$

In the bicarbonate–carbonic acid system, pK (a constant derived from the dissociation of the acid-base pair) is 6.1. Thus:

$$pH = 6.1 + \log \frac{Bicarbonate}{Carbonic\ acid}$$

Since carbonic acid is in equilibrium with dissolved carbon dioxide, measurement of the partial pressure of carbon dioxide (pCO_2) can be used as a clinical estimate of carbonic acid concentration. By decreasing bicarbonate concentration and increasing pCO_2, the addition of hydrogen ion to the plasma will still result in some decrease in pH despite the presence of buffers. However, the changes are of lesser magnitude than would occur in the absence of the buffering mechanism.

Pulmonary Mechanisms. The above equation indicates that pH depends not on absolute levels of bicarbonate and carbonic acid (pCO_2) but on the *ratio* of the two concentrations. A decrease or increase in concentration of bicarbonate will not modify pH if the pCO_2 is lowered or increased in proportion. Thus by altering the rate at which carbon dioxide is excreted, the lungs are able to regulate pCO_2 and modify pH. Although enormous quantities of carbon dioxide are produced from normal metabolic activity (Table 5–2), little change in pH results because of the unique properties of the bicarbonate–carbonic acid buffer system and a highly developed respiratory control mechanism. An increased respiratory rate, stimulated by increased levels of carbon dioxide, increases the excretion of carbon dioxide, decreases pCO_2, and thus increases pH. Conversely, a decreased respiratory rate will result in an increase in pCO_2 and a decrease in pH.

Even though the lungs can modify pH by changing pCO_2 and altering the ratio of carbonic acid to bicarbonate, this process cannot cause any loss (or gain) in hydrogen ions. The lungs are incapable of regenerating bicarbonate to replace that lost when hydrogen ion was buffered. The generation of new bicarbonate and, when required, the excretion of bicarbonate are the responsibilities of the kidneys.

Renal Mechanisms. The excretion of excess hydrogen ions with generation of new bicarbonate or the excretion of bicarbonate, occurs by regulation of two basic steps: (1) Reclamation of nearly all of the filtered bicarbonate occurs in the proximal tubule. No net hydrogen ion excretion results, but, in the adult, this process is responsible for reclaiming up to 5000 mEq of bicarbonate which is filtered through the glomeruli each day. If this bicarbonate were not reclaimed, its loss would be equivalent to the retention of an equal amount of hydrogen ions, which would result in severe systemic acidosis. (2) Generation of new bicarbonate occurs in more distal segments of the nephron and results in the net secretion of hydrogen ions needed to maintain hydrogen ion balance under most circumstances.

Table 5–2. Approximate Order of Magnitude of Certain Factors in Hydrogen Ion Metabolism in Standard Man of 1.73 M²

Total CO_2 turnover	24,000 mM/24 hr
Total hydrogen ion turnover	69 mEq/24 hr
Total buffer in body	2100 mEq
Total hydrogen ion in buffer (max. capacity)	700 mEq
Total hydrogen ion in buffer (normal amount)	105 mEq
Total free hydrogen ion in body fluids	0.0021 mEq

From Elkinton JR: Ann Intern Med 57:660, 1962.

The mechanisms for both of these steps are highly developed, energy-requiring, active transport processes, in contrast to the pulmonary excretion of carbon dioxide, which results from simple, passive diffusion. Both steps require the generation of hydrogen ions by the same basic reaction. Fig. 5–5 shows that the proximal renal tubular cells, under the influence of carbonic anhydrase, hydrolyze carbon dioxide to carbonic acid. This carbonic acid is then dissociated into hydrogen ion and bicarbonate. The hydrogen ions are transported into the proximal tubule and exchanged for filtered sodium, which is reabsorbed into the peritubular capillaries with the bicarbonate generated from the formation of hydrogen ion. In the lumen of the proximal tubule the hydrogen ion combines with filtered bicarbonate to form carbon dioxide and water. These mechanisms ensure that virtually no bicarbonate passes to more distal segments of the nephron and that an amount of sodium bicarbonate equal to the amount filtered is returned to the peritubular capillaries.

Hydrogen ions are generated in the distal tubular cells by the same process as that described for the proximal tubular

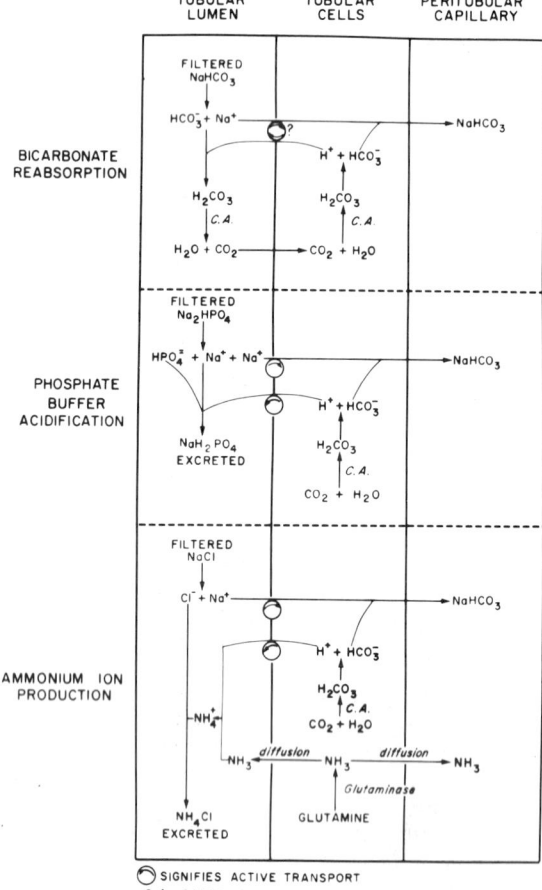

TUBULAR LUMEN   TUBULAR CELLS   PERITUBULAR CAPILLARY

BICARBONATE REABSORPTION

FILTERED $NaHCO_3$

$HCO_3^- + Na^+$ → $NaHCO_3$

$H^+ + HCO_3^-$

H_2CO_3 H_2CO_3
C.A.   C.A.
$H_2O + CO_2$ $CO_2 + H_2O$

PHOSPHATE BUFFER ACIDIFICATION

FILTERED Na_2HPO_4

$HPO_4^= + Na^+ + Na^+$ → $NaHCO_3$

$H^+ + HCO_3^-$

NaH_2PO_4 EXCRETED H_2CO_3
C.A.
$CO_2 + H_2O$

AMMONIUM ION PRODUCTION

FILTERED NaCl

$Cl^- + Na^+$ → $NaHCO_3$

$H^+ + HCO_3^-$
H_2CO_3
C.A.
$CO_2 + H_2O$

NH_4^+
NH_3 *diffusion* → NH_3 *diffusion* → NH_3
Glutaminase
NH_4Cl EXCRETED   GLUTAMINE

⊖ SIGNIFIES ACTIVE TRANSPORT
C.A. = CARBONIC ANHYDRASE

Figure 5–5. The renal mechanisms involved in acid-base homeostasis. Bicarbonate reabsorption normally occurs in the proximal tubule, where the presence of carbonic anhydrase on the luminal brush border facilitates the conversion of bicarbonate to carbon dioxide and water. This mechanism does not effect any net excretion of hydrogen ion from the body but results in the reclamation of bicarbonate in an amount equal to that lost from the plasma into the glomerular filtrate. Incomplete reabsorption of bicarbonate in the proximal tubule results in bicarbonate entering the distal nephron, where it decreases the amount of hydrogen ion available for producing ammonium and titrating phosphate to sodium dihydrogen phosphate, thus reducing net acid excretion. It is still uncertain whether the movement of sodium and hydrogen ions across the luminal border of the proximal tubular cell occurs by an active linked-transport mechanism.

cells. They are also excreted into the lumen in exchange for sodium, probably by an active process. The transport of hydrogen ions at this site appears to be gradient-limited, with the distal tubule able to generate a gradient for free hydrogen ion from tubular lumen to tubular cell of up to 1000:1. Transport is thus facilitated by the presence of buffers in the tubular fluid that decrease the concentration of free hydrogen ion and permit increased movement of hydrogen ion from cells into the tubular fluid. The principal buffers at this site are phosphate and ammonia.

Under most conditions large amounts of *phosphate* are present in the distal tubular fluid. In the presence of a high concentration of free hydrogen ions, the phosphate is converted from a monohydrogen to a dihydrogen form (Fig. 5–5), reducing the concentration of free hydrogen ion in the tubular fluid. The amount of hydrogen ion excreted in the urine in this form can be measured by determining the amount of alkali required to bring the urine to a neutral pH and is termed *titratable acidity.*

Ammonia, a hydrogen ion acceptor, is synthesized in tubular cells from the deamidation and deamination of glutamine in the presence of glutaminase; this reaction is stimulated by systemic acidosis. Ammonia diffuses through the lipid membrane of the cells into the tubular fluid, where it reacts with hydrogen ion to form ammonium ion, NH_4^+. This charged cation cannot readily diffuse back from luminal fluid.

These two processes, by reducing free hydrogen ion concentration in the tubular fluid, enable an increased rate of transport of hydrogen ions into the distal renal tubule fluid and allow the generation of new bicarbonate which can enter the plasma and replenish depleted levels of plasma bicarbonate (Fig. 5–5).

The absolute net rate of excretion of hydrogen ions by the kidney is calculated as the sum of the excretion rates in the urine of titratable acid and ammonium ion minus urine bicarbonate. Living on an average mixed diet, an adult in the United States must excrete about 70 mEq of hydrogen ions each day to maintain balance. Approximately one third is excreted as titratable acid, the remaining two thirds as ammonium.

A number of factors cause an increase in the rate of hydrogen ion secretion in the proximal tubules and lead to increased bicarbonate reabsorption with consequent elevation of serum bicarbonate. These include elevation of plasma pCO_2, hypokalemia, reduction in effective arterial blood volume (e.g., after vomiting or hemorrhage), and administration of mineralocorticoids. Conversely, hydrogen ion secretion, and thus bicarbonate reabsorption, is decreased by a decreased plasma pCO_2, by expansion of extracellular fluid volume, by inhibition of carbonic anhydrase (e.g., by drugs such as acetazolamide), and by mineralocorticoid deficiency. Reduction in plasma bicarbonate may occur in these situations. Similarly, disease states such as cystinosis or heavy metal poisoning associated with structural or functional damage to the proximal tubule may limit bicarbonate reabsorption at this site and result in systemic acidosis. The distal acidification mechanisms may be impaired by intrinsic defects in the tubule, which cause primary distal renal tubular acidosis, or by a variety of insults such as nephrocalcinosis, vitamin D intoxication, or amphotericin B administration, which produce secondary forms of distal renal tubular acidosis.

USUAL ACID-BASE BALANCE

Most mixed diets produce a net amount of hydrogen ions; true vegetarians ingest a neutral ash diet. Protein is the largest source of hydrogen ions; its metabolism accounts for approximately 65% of the total, generated primarily from the oxidation of sulfur-containing amino acids to yield sulfuric acid and from the oxidation and hydrolysis of phosphoproteins to yield phosphoric acid. The remainder of the hydrogen ions comes from the incomplete catabolism of carbohydrates, fats, and organic acids such as pyruvic, lactic, acetoacetic, and citric acids. Complete oxidation of these compounds does not produce excess hydrogen ions, since water and carbon dioxide are the final reaction products; incomplete metabolism results in the formation of organic acids and adds hydrogen ions. Thus, milk and meat diets generate about 70 mEq of hydrogen ions/day in the adult and require the kidney to daily excrete an equal amount to maintain a normal blood pH of 7.35–7.45. The infant and child must excrete proportionally similar amounts of hydrogen ion. In consequence the daily turnover of hydrogen ions is large, amounting to more than 50% of the hydrogen ions usually present in the body buffers and 10% of the maximum storage capacity of the buffers (Table 5-2). This hydrogen ion is initially buffered by the intra- and extracellular fluid buffers, and then there is respiratory compensation before the kidneys excrete the hydrogen ion to maintain balance.

DISTURBANCES OF ACID-BASE BALANCE

Systemic acidosis or alkalosis may result from either primary metabolic or respiratory abnormalities.

Metabolic Acidosis. Systemic acidosis may result from increased production or inadequate excretion of hydrogen ions or from excessive loss of bicarbonate in the urine or stools. Rapid expansion of the extracellular fluid space by a bicarbonate-free solution may also produce metabolic acidosis by diluting the bicarbonate in the extracellular fluid. The hydrogen ion load is buffered initially by bicarbonate in the extracellular fluid and by intracellular buffers such as hemoglobin and phosphate. Bone may be a further source of buffer. Serum bicarbonate and pH fall (but to a lesser extent than if no buffering mechanism were available) and pCO_2 rises. The resulting systemic acidosis and increased pCO_2 stimulate the respiratory center (and possibly peripheral chemoreceptors in the carotid artery and aorta) to increase the respiratory rate, thereby increasing the rate of excretion of carbon dioxide. Plasma pCO_2 and carbonic acid levels fall, partially or almost totally correcting the acidosis but at the expense of lowering both plasma bicarbonate and pCO_2. Thus blood pH is decreased but rarely drops as low as might be predicted from the low level of plasma bicarbonate.

The acidosis also stimulates the kidney to increase ammonia production and hydrogen ion excretion into the urine. As a result, there is an increased generation of new bicarbonate, returning plasma bicarbonate to normal if the primary disease process has been alleviated. In turn, the respiratory rate subsequently decreases, with the pCO_2 returning to normal. At this point the patient's acid-base status has returned to the normal state existing before the hydrogen ion load was administered.

The clinical picture of metabolic acidosis is usually dominated by its underlying cause and by the deep, rapid respirations (Kussmaul breathing) needed for respiratory compensation. However, severe acidosis itself may cause a decrease in peripheral vascular resistance and cardiac ventricular function, resulting in hypotension, pulmonary edema, and tissue hypoxia. The laboratory findings are decreased serum pH, bicarbonate, and pCO_2. For every 1 mEq/L fall from normal in plasma bicarbonate, arterial pCO_2 should decrease 1.0–1.5 mm Hg. If this does not occur, a mixed disturbance should be suspected (see below). When the acidosis is due to bicarbonate loss, the anion gap is normal and hyperchloremia is present. An increased anion gap usually signifies the increased production of hydrogen ion or its decreased excretion. A more detailed discussion of anion gap is presented in Sec. 5.13.

Renal causes of metabolic acidosis are numerous. Diseases involving the proximal tubules may limit the ability of this segment of the nephron to secrete hydrogen ions and cause incomplete bicarbonate reabsorption. Increased amounts of bicarbonate are presented to the distal tubular fluid, resulting in the proximal form of *renal tubular acidosis*. In distal renal tubular acidosis the distal tubule cannot maintain a normal hydrogen ion gradient so that urine pH remains relatively alkaline, rarely falling below 5.5. A reduction of titratable acid, decreased secretion of hydrogen ion, and systemic acidosis result. With *chronic renal insufficiency*, acidification mechanisms work normally or at supranormal rates. However, the reduced tubular mass limits the capacity of the kidney to generate sufficient ammonia and thus to excrete adequate amounts of hydrogen ions. A *low glomerular filtration rate*, as in the newborn, also limits the renal capacity to excrete hydrogen ion. In addition, the filtered load of phosphate is reduced, the bulk being reabsorbed in the proximal tubule; little is left for buffering of added hydrogen ion in the distal tubule. Hydrogen ion transport is thus reduced by rapid attainment of a maximal concentration gradient in the absence of buffer. Rarely, *reduction in ammonia synthesis*, as in the cerebro-oculo-renal syndrome of Lowe, limits the ability to excrete hydrogen ions.

Other Causes. Metabolic acidosis may also develop in *diabetic ketoacidosis* from incomplete metabolism of body lipids and catabolism of body protein, accompanied by the production of large amounts of acetoacetic, β-hydroxybutyric, phosphoric, and sulfuric acids. In *salicylism*, metabolic acidosis results not only from hydrogen ion derived from salicylic acid but also from the uncoupling of oxidative phosphorylation by salicylate. In severe *diarrhea* the increased losses of bicarbonate in diarrheal fluid and, possibly, the formation of organic acids from incomplete breakdown of carbohydrate in the stools result in metabolic acidosis. *Hyperalimentation, lactic acidosis, starvation*, and *poisoning with either methyl alcohol or ethylene glycol* cause systemic acidosis by increased production of various strong acids. Metabolic acidosis is seen also in certain *inherited aminoacidurias* (e.g., methylmalonicaciduria), in hypoxemia, and in shock.

Metabolic Alkalosis. This may result from three basic mechanisms: (1) excessive loss of hydrogen ion, as in prolonged gastric aspiration or persistent vomiting associated with pyloric stenosis; (2) increased addition of bicarbonate to the extracellular fluid, which may result from excessive administration by the parenteral route or by oral intake as in the milk-alkali syndrome, or from increased renal reabsorption of bicarbonate due to profound potassium depletion, primary hyperaldosteronism, Cushing syndrome, Bartter syndrome, or excessive intake of licorice; and (3) contraction of the extracellular fluid volume, which increases bicarbonate concentration in this fluid space and increases bicarbonate reclamation in the renal tubule.

The buffer systems minimize pH change, but both plasma bicarbonate and pH are increased. Respiration may be depressed with some increase in plasma pCO_2, but this response is limited by increasing hypoxia so that respiratory compensation is always incomplete and never restores pH to normal. The renal threshold for bicarbonate is exceeded, and bicarbonate appears in the urine, which may have a pH as high as 8.5–9.0. However, factors such as volume depletion and hypokalemia often coexist and they, along with the increased pCO_2 itself, tend to increase renal reabsorption of bicarbonate, maintaining the metabolic alkalosis. Metabolic alkalosis may be refractory to treatment in the presence of either hypokalemia or depletion of extracellular fluid volume and often can be corrected only after these deficiencies have been corrected.

The diagnosis of metabolic alkalosis should be considered in any patient with an appropriate history; there are no pathognomonic signs of this electrolyte disturbance. Patients may have cramps or feel weak and may have the signs of tetany if ionized calcium has been reduced by the alkalosis.

Characteristically, pH, plasma bicarbonate, and pCO_2 of arterial blood are elevated. Hypochloremia and hypokalemia are usually present, the latter principally due to increased urinary losses of potassium. Classically, the urine pH is alkaline, but in the presence of severe depletion of potassium, urinary potassium is low and paradoxic aciduria is present. In those patients with volume depletion who will be responsive to sodium chloride, urine chloride concentrations should be less than 10 mEq/L. In contrast, patients who have metabolic alkalosis due to excessive mineralocorticoid activity or potassium depletion have a urine chloride exceeding 20 mEq/L and are resistant to sodium chloride treatment.

Respiratory Acidosis. This disturbance results from inadequate pulmonary excretion of carbon dioxide in the presence of normal production of this gas. It may be seen acutely in neuromuscular disorders such as brain stem injury, Guillain-Barré syndrome, or sedative overdose; in airway obstruction such as that caused by a foreign body, severe bronchospasm, or laryngeal edema; in vascular diseases such as massive pulmonary embolism; and in other conditions such as pneumothorax, pulmonary edema, or severe pneumonia. Chronic respiratory acidosis may accompany the pickwickian syndrome, poliomyelitis, chronic obstructive airway disease, kyphoscoliosis, or chronic administration of sedatives.

In health, increased production of CO_2 stimulates its increased respiratory excretion so that a normal pCO_2 is maintained and acid-base status remains normal. In any of the disease states causing respiratory acidosis, the level of pCO_2 increases until it is elevated sufficiently to cause pulmonary excretion of carbon dioxide equal to its production. Although a new steady state is reached, the increase in pCO_2 (hypercapnia) causes a systemic acidosis by increasing serum concentrations of carbonic acid and, therefore, of hydrogen ions.

Since CO_2 is a major component of the principal buffer system of the extracellular fluid, the rise in pCO_2 must be buffered initially by the nonbicarbonate buffers, i.e., the proteins in the extracellular fluid and phosphate, hemoglobin, other proteins, and lactate in the cells. The acidosis and increased pCO_2 stimulate the kidney to increase hydrogen ion excretion as ammonium and titratable acid and to generate and reabsorb more bicarbonate; thus plasma bicarbonate levels may be increased somewhat above normal. At this stage the increase in plasma bicarbonate compensates for the primary increase in pCO_2 so that pH returns toward normal and the respiratory acidosis has been "compensated" by renal mechanisms. The only way to *correct* the abnormality is to reverse the primary disorder.

Causes of acute respiratory acidosis are often associated with hypoxemia, which usually dominates the clinical picture, along with the signs of respiratory distress. Hypercapnia results in vasodilatation, increases cerebral blood flow, and may be responsible for the headaches and raised intracranial pressure sometimes found in these patients. Severe hypercapnia may be a cerebral depressant; arterial pH is low, pCO_2 elevated, and plasma bicarbonate elevated moderately.

Respiratory Alkalosis. Excessive pulmonary losses of carbon dioxide in the presence of normal production results in a fall in pCO_2 and respiratory alkalosis. It may be observed with hyperventilation of psychogenic origin, with overventilation from mechanically assisted ventilation, and in the early stages of salicylate overdosage due to stimulation of the respiratory center by salicylate or to increased sensitivity of the respiratory center to pCO_2.

Plasma pCO_2 falls and pH rises. A rapid buffering of this pH change occurs, with hydrogen ions released from body buffers to decrease plasma bicarbonate. Approximately 99% of this hydrogen ion is released from intracellular buffers and the remaining 1% from extracellular buffers. The renal excretion of bicarbonate, slowly increasing by mechanisms that are incompletely understood, reduces plasma bicarbonate levels and compensates for the excessive loss of carbon dioxide, returning pH toward normal. However, correction cannot occur until the causative disorder is removed.

The clinical picture usually is that of the underlying disease process. However, acute hypercapnia may result in neuromuscular irritability and paresthesias in the extremities and periorally, due to a decrease in the concentration of ionized calcium. Arterial pH is elevated, pCO_2 and plasma bicarbonate decreased. Despite systemic alkalosis the urine usually remains acid.

Mixed Disorders. Under certain circumstances, mixed disturbances may occur in which more than a single primary cause is responsible for the abnormal acid-base balance. For example, in respiratory distress syndrome metabolic and respiratory acidoses often coexist. The respiratory disease prevents the compensatory fall in pCO_2, and the metabolic component limits the ability to increase plasma bicarbonate, which would normally buffer a respiratory acidosis. In such a situation the decrease in pH is often profound, of greater magnitude than that seen when only a single disturbance exists.

Other types of mixed disturbances may be seen. Patients with congestive heart failure and chronic respiratory acidosis may develop a component of metabolic alkalosis if they excessively use diuretics. Plasma bicarbonate and pH will be higher than in a simple chronic respiratory acidosis. Indeed, pH may be normal or even slightly elevated. Patients with hepatic failure may have both a metabolic acidosis and a respiratory alkalosis. Plasma bicarbonate and pCO_2 may be lower than expected with a simple disorder, whereas pH may be little changed from normal. Respiratory and metabolic alkaloses may also coexist under some circumstances.

CLINICAL ASSESSMENT OF ACID-BASE DISORDERS

For clinical purposes acid-base status is determined from serum pH, pCO_2, and bicarbonate levels. This approach has replaced measuring base excess or deficit and estimating buffer base as the sum of concentrations of the buffer anions of whole blood, i.e., bicarbonate, plasma proteins, and hemoglobin. Base excess was measured by titration of whole blood with a strong acid to pH 7.40 at a pCO_2 of 40 mm Hg at 37°C and base deficit, by titrating with base. Values were expressed as mEq/L.

Measurements. Blood pH can be measured accurately with small blood samples; normal values are from 7.35 to 7.45. The concentration of carbonic acid (H_2CO_3) in biologic fluids is quantitatively negligible compared with dissolved carbon dioxide. The latter is measured as the partial pressure of carbon dioxide (pCO_2) in a gas phase in equilibrium with the biologic fluid; the normal value approximates 40 mm Hg.

The concentration of bicarbonate ion in plasma can be measured directly, but the precision of this determination is not required for clinical purposes. It is customary to determine total carbon dioxide concentration of the serum as an estimate of bicarbonate level. This value is 1–2 mEq/L higher than that of true bicarbonate. It is obtained either by titration or by generation of carbon dioxide from serum with a strong acid. The carbon dioxide is derived principally from bicarbonate but also from dissolved carbon dioxide, carbonic acid, carbonate ion, and carbamino compounds. The normal value is 25–28 millimoles (mM)/L, except in the 1st yr of life when values are 20–23 mM/L, probably because of the low renal threshold for bicarbonate.

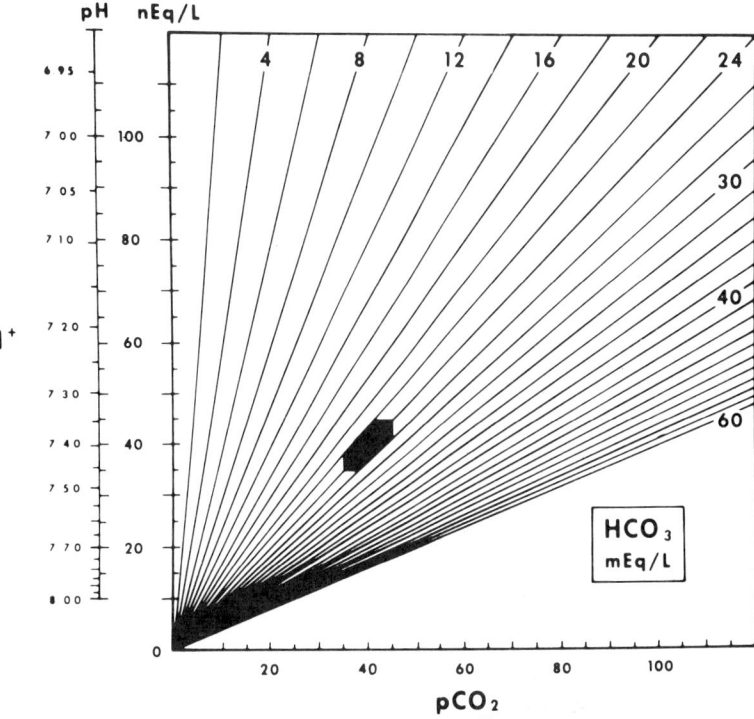

Figure 5–6. A nomogram permitting estimation of pH, pCO_2, or serum bicarbonate levels when only 2 of these measurements have been determined in the laboratory. The shaded area in the center of the plot represents the normal values. (From Cohen JJ: Ann Intern Med 66:159, 1967.)

If only two of these values are known, the third can be derived from one of the nomograms developed for this purpose (Fig. 5–6) or can be calculated by one of the several methods based on the Henderson-Hasselbalch equation.* If all three measurements have been made, the same formulas can be used to check the validity of the values.

Interpretation. It is relatively easy to correctly diagnose a simple acid-base disorder, given blood pH, pCO_2, and bicarbonate levels and using an acid-base nomogram such as that shown in Fig. 5–7 or the summary of laboratory findings shown in Fig. 5–8. Diagnosing a mixed disorder, however, is more difficult. In simple disorders pCO_2 and bicarbonate levels always change in the same direction. If any patient's values do not show this relationship, a mixed disorder should be considered. Similarly, results that plot outside any of the shaded areas shown in Fig. 5–7 indicate a 95% chance of a mixed disorder, which can be diagnosed from the clinical setting, as discussed, and from the information presented in Fig. 5–8.

INTRACELLULAR pH

Normal intracellular pH has been estimated to be 6.8; values as low as 6.0 have been obtained using microelectrodes. Mitochondrial pH may be even lower since intracellular pH is probably inhomogeneous.

---

*pCO_2 may be estimated from the equation

$$pCO_2 = \frac{[H^+] \times [\text{total } CO_2 \text{ content in mEq/L}]}{25}$$

$[H^+]$, expressed as nanoequivalents per liter (nEq/L), can easily be estimated from serum pH. At a pH of 7.40 $[H^+]$ is approximately 40 nEq/L (see Regulating Mechanisms). Each decrease in pH of 0.01 unit is associated with an increased $[H^+]$ of 1 nEq/L. Conversely, each increase in pH of 0.01 unit is associated with a decreased $[H^+]$ of 1 nEq/L. Thus, $[H^+]$ at a pH of 7.30 is 50 nEq/L and at 7.45 is 35 nEq/L. The maximum error in pCO_2 calculated by this simple formula is 7% for pH values from 7.10–7.50 and even less in the pH range of 7.28–7.45. (See N Engl J Med 272:1067, 1965.)

Carbon dioxide diffuses readily across cell membranes so that intracellular and extracellular values for pCO_2 are similar. Thus, intracellular changes in hydrogen ion concentration may occur as a result of primary respiratory disorders that cause either hypocapnia or hypercapnia. With *hypo*capnia, intracellular alkalosis is proportional to the degree of extracellular alkalosis. With *hyper*capnia, however, because intracellular bicarbonate concentrations cannot be adjusted as rapidly as those in the extracellular fluid, intracellular acidosis may be proportionally greater than that seen in the extracellular fluid. In contrast to the situation in respiratory acidosis, intracellular pH may be maintained in the face of severe metabolic acidosis until extracellular pH drops below 7.0.

The effects of extracellular acidosis and alkalosis on cellular functions are not fully understood. A low pH produces a slight change in the Donnan distribution across the capillary membrane; therefore some decrease in oncotic pressure results in a reduced plasma volume. Low pH also seems to reduce myocardial contractility and impair catecholamine action, and it increases the likelihood of arrhythmia, particularly with hypoxia. Moreover, if hydrogen ion concentration rises rapidly, it may inhibit further transport of the ion in the kidney. Metabolic disturbances also lead to an alteration in exchange of sodium and potassium for hydrogen ion; deficiency of potassium may result in a decrease in the intracellular pH at the same time that extracellular pH is elevated.

Changes in intracellular pH probably affect the activities of many enzymes. Decrease in carbohydrate tolerance has been observed in acidosis, and increase in neuromuscular irritability (latent or manifest tetany) occurs in alkalosis. Hypocapnia leads to an increase in blood lactic acid with a decrease in bicarbonate concentration and production of metabolic acidosis.

Cerebrospinal Fluid pH. Bicarbonate–carbonic acid represents virtually all the buffering capacity in this fluid. Carbon dioxide can diffuse freely between the blood and cerebrospinal fluid. Thus, increases or decreases in pCO_2 in the blood are reflected by similar changes in the cerebrospinal fluid, although this latter value is also modified by the rates of carbon dioxide production in the brain. In contrast, increases or

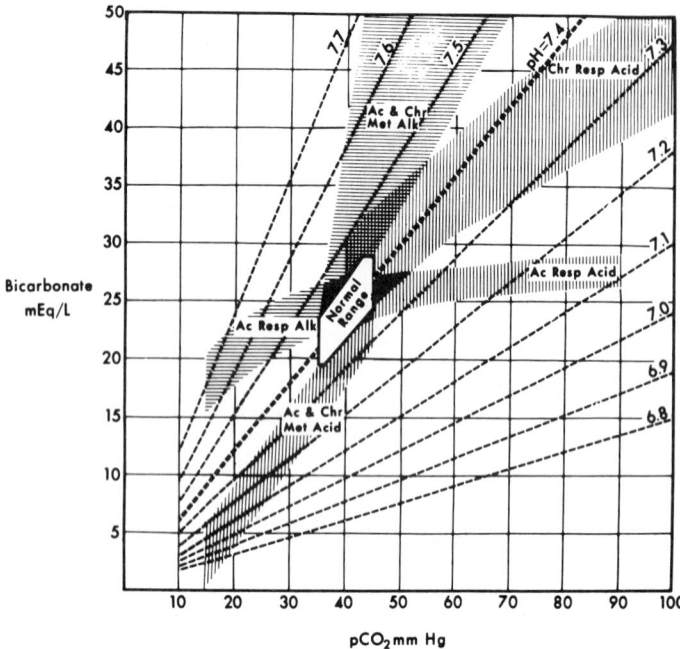

Figure 5–7. Determining simple acid-base disorders from measurements of pH, pCO_2, and serum bicarbonate. Ac, acute; Acid, acidosis; Alk, alkalosis; Chr, chronic; Met, metabolic; Resp, respiratory. (From Arbus GS: Can Med Assoc J *109*:291, 1973.)

decreases in concentration of bicarbonate in blood lead only slowly to small changes in bicarbonate in cerebrospinal fluid. Consequently, the concentration of hydrogen ion in the cerebrospinal fluid does not change instantaneously with changes in extracellular pH; the pHs of these fluids may differ significantly at times, especially if active respiratory compensation of a metabolic acidosis or alkalosis has occurred. Particular problems may be seen if a compensated metabolic acidosis is corrected too quickly. Correction results in an increase in both pCO_2 and bicarbonate levels in the extracellular fluid, but only the pCO_2 rises in the cerebrospinal fluid. The pH of the extracellular fluid returns to normal, but that of the cerebrospinal fluid falls even further. Thus, continuing neurologic symptoms and abnormalities in respiration may result.

5.13 CHLORIDE

Chloride is the major anion of extracellular fluid. Total body chloride amounts to 33 mEq/kg. Most of it is in the extracellular (plasma chloride, 13.6%; interstitial lymph, 37.3%; dense connective tissue and cartilage, 17%; bone, 15.2%) and transcellular (4.5%) fluids, with small quantities present intracellularly (12.4%). Exchangeable chloride remains relatively constant per unit of body weight at different ages.

The intake and output of chloride parallel those of sodium. Its transport is largely passive and travels down an electrochemical gradient created in part by sodium transport. However, chloride transport at several sites, including the thick ascending limb of the loop of Henle, may be active. The potency of furosemide as a diuretic may be due to the specific inhibition of this mechanism.

Under most clinical circumstances alterations in chloride concentration in the blood parallel those of sodium. Thus, hypo- and hyperchloremia are usually associated with comparable degrees of hypo- and hypernatremia, respectively, and are seen most often with dehydration secondary to diarrhea. Occasionally, however, changes in chloride concentration are not accompanied by equivalent changes in sodium concentration.

Chloride is not directly involved in regulating the concentration of free hydrogen ion. Nevertheless, as metabolic adjustments within the kidney are made and plasma levels of bicarbonate change secondary to secretion of hydrogen ions, reciprocal changes in the plasma concentration of chloride generally occur. Thus, *hypochloremia* is typically seen in metabolic alkalosis. It occurs also when chloride is lost from the body in excess of sodium losses. Examples include loss from the bowel with vomiting or gastric drainage or in chloride diarrhea, a rare congenital disorder in which there is a defect

		PH	PCO₂	BICARBONATE
Simple disorders				
	Metabolic acidosis	↓	↓	↓
	Metabolic alkalosis	↑	↑	↑
	Respiratory acidosis	↓	↑	↑
	Respiratory alkalosis	↑	↓	↓
Mixed disorders				
	Metabolic acidosis with respiratory acidosis	↓ ↓	↑,N,↓	↑,N,↓
	Metabolic alkalosis with respiratory acidosis	↑,N,↓	↑	↑
	Metabolic acidosis with respiratory alkalosis	↑,N,↓	↓	↓
	Metabolic alkalosis with respiratory alkalosis	↑ ↑	↑,N,↓	↑,N,↓

Figure 5–8. Typical serum findings in clinical disturbances of acid-base balance. In the simple disorders it has been assumed that the primary acid-base disturbance has been compensated (see text for details). ↑ = increased from normal, ↓ decreased from normal, N = normal.

in bowel transport of chloride. Urinary losses of chloride may exceed those of sodium during the correction of metabolic acidosis and in potassium deficiency. Indeed, with potassium deficiency both potassium and chloride must be given before the potassium deficits can be corrected. Similarly, administering chloride is necessary to correct most cases of metabolic alkalosis irrespective of whether or not it is associated with potassium deficiency. In patients with metabolic alkalosis, using either potassium or sodium chloride, as appropriate, results in the prompt excretion of bicarbonate into the urine and correction of the alkalosis. Hypochloremia will also result from a protracted inadequate intake of chloride. Thus, infants fed a chloride-deficient milk formula for several months developed chronic depletion of body chloride, severe hypochloremia (serum sodium levels usually remained normal), severe hypokalemic metabolic alkalosis, loss of appetite, failure to thrive, muscle weakness, and lethargy. Although adding chloride to the diet quickly reverses the electrolyte abnormalities, long-term sequelae may develop, including disturbed behavioral patterns.

Hyperchloremia may result when chloride is conserved by the kidney in excess of sodium and potassium. It occurs when alkaline urine is formed during the renal correction of alkalosis. An increased fractional reabsorption of chloride in the renal proximal tubule in distal renal tubular acidosis also results in hyperchloremia. Early amino acid solutions used in parenteral alimentation contained excessive amounts of chloride, and their administration resulted in hyperchloremic acidosis. Substituting acetate has largely solved this problem.

Measurements of serum chloride are necessary to determine a patient's **anion gap**. The concentration of the most abundant serum cation (sodium) is greater than the sum of the two most abundant serum anions (chloride and bicarbonate). The difference, referred to as the anion gap, is normally about 12 mEq/L (range 8–16 mEq/L). It is due to the combined concentrations of the unmeasured anions such as phosphate, sulfate, proteins, and organic acids, which exceed those of the unmeasured cations, primarily potassium, calcium, and magnesium. Calculating the anion gap permits the detection of an abnormal concentration of an unmeasured anion or cation. An increased anion gap in renal failure is due to increased concentrations of phosphate and sulfate; in diabetic ketoacidosis, to β-hydroxybutyrate and acetoacetate; in lactic acidosis, to lactate; in hyperglycemic nonketotic coma, to unidentified organic acids; and in disorders of amino acid metabolism, to a variety of organic acids. Increased anion gap also follows the administration of large amounts of penicillin. After ethylene glycol ingestion, it is caused by glycolate production; after methanol ingestion, by formate production; and after salicylate poisoning, by the salicylate anion and a variety of organic anions secondary to the uncoupling of oxidative phosphorylation.

A decreased anion gap occurs less frequently. It may be found in nephrotic syndrome, in which it is due to a decreased serum concentration of albumin which is anionic at pH 7.4; after lithium ingestion, lithium being an unmeasured cation; and in multiple myeloma, due to the presence of cationic proteins.

5.14 PHOSPHORUS

Confusion may exist in understanding the physiology of phosphorus, because the terms "phosphorus" and "phosphate" have frequently and erroneously been used interchangeably. Measurements of "phosphate" in biologic samples are usually performed as and expressed in terms of total elemental phosphorus concentration. Since the atomic weight of phosphorus is 30.98, a concentration of 3.1 mg/dL (31 mg/L) of phosphorus

is equivalent to 1 mM phosphorus/L. Most of the measured plasma phosphorus exists as both monovalent and divalent orthophosphate and thus behaves as though it has a valency of 1.8 at pH 7.40. Consequently, at pH 7.40, 1 mM of phosphate is equivalent to 1.8 mEq of phosphate (mM × valency = mEq).

Body Phosphorus. Infants retain phosphorus avidly. A 3 kg infant may retain 40–80 mg/day, which is more than 50% of usual intake. Consequently, total body phosphorus per unit of fat-free body weight (FFBW) increases throughout childhood; it doubles from birth to adulthood, at which time its value is approximately 12 gm/kg FFBW. This doubling is due primarily to an increase in skeletal phosphorus content; more than 80% of body phosphorus is in bone, and the remainder is distributed through all soft tissues.

In plasma, two thirds of phosphorus is present as phospholipids (Table 5–3). These compounds are insoluble in acid and are not measured in routine "plasma phosphorus" determinations. The measured portion of plasma phosphorus is acid soluble and is composed of inorganic phosphorus, primarily orthophosphate, 10% of which is bound to protein. The remaining 90% is ultrafilterable, 5% of which is complexed as calcium, magnesium, and sodium phosphates and 85% of which is present as "free phosphate." Of the latter, 80% is the divalent anion (HPO_4^{--}) and 20% the monovalent anion ($H_2PO_4^-$). Concentrations of phosphorus are low in interstitial fluids, but this fluid is not a simple ultrafiltrate of plasma. Each organ may have an interstitial fluid composition to meet its own needs.

Cellular phosphorus is present in cell membranes and subcellular organelles as organic phosphoglycerides and sphingolipids. Acid-soluble moeities of intracellular phosphorus include ATP and other nucleotides, various glucose-phosphate compounds, creatinine phosphate, and a small amount of cytosolic inorganic phosphate. Thus, intracellular phosphate plays an essential role in forming and releasing energy, as well as in intracellular enzyme activity. Inorganic phosphorus is the principal urinary buffer and plays a critical function in the regulation of free hydrogen ions (see above).

The principal sources of *dietary phosphorus* are milk, milk products, and meat. The recommended daily intake is 880 mg/day for ages 1–10 yr and 1200 mg for older children. Breast fed infants ingest 25–30 mg of phosphorus/kg/24 hr. Up to two thirds of the dietary phosphate is absorbed from the bowel, primarily in the jejunum. This absorption is stimulated by vitamin D and its metabolites as well as by parathyroid hormone (PTH); it is decreased by thyrocalcitonin, by the presence in the bowel of binders such as aluminum

Table 5–3. **Major Components of Plasma Phosphorus**

Total Plasma Phosphorus		3.9 mM/L
Acid insoluble	2.6 mM/L	
Organic (phospholipids)		
Acid soluble	1.3 mM/L	
Organic (esters)	0.1 mM/L	
Inorganic	1.2 mM/L	

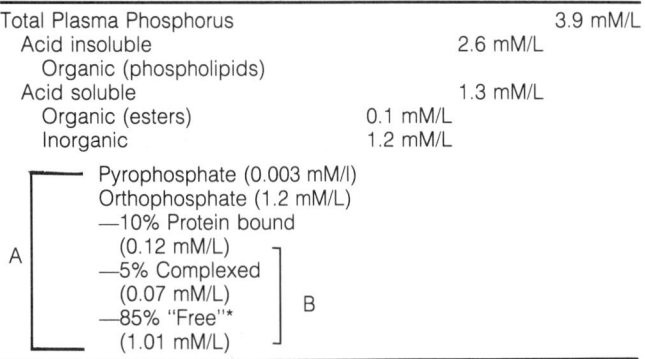

A = measured as plasma phosphorus
B = ultrafilterable phosphorus
*At pH 7.4: 17% as $H_2PO_4^-$ (0.20 mM/L), 68% as HPO_4^{--} (0.81 mM/L)

hydroxide and carbonate, and, at least in animals, by a high dietary calcium intake.

Even though phosphate is actively transported across the bowel wall, it is the kidney that plays a major role in regulating body phosphate. Renal handling of phosphate consists of glomerular filtration with facultative reabsorption by the tubule. Ultrafilterable phosphate is freely filtered at the glomerulus with an average of 90% of this filtered load normally being reabsorbed. Sixty to 70% of the reabsorption occurs in the proximal tubule and the remainder in more distal segments. Under certain circumstances phosphate may also be secreted by the distal tubules. Although a maximal rate for tubular reabsorption of phosphate (Tm phosphate) exists, it varies with filtration rate and is not attained under normal circumstances. Urinary excretion of phosphate shows a circadian rhythm—lowest in the morning and highest in early evening.

Tubular reabsorption of phosphate is regulated by *PTH*, the effects of which are mediated by the adenylate cyclase system. This hormone reduces tubular reabsorption of phosphorus and is associated with phosphaturia. Conversely, large doses of vitamin D stimulate reabsorption of phosphate in the proximal tubule, as does growth hormone. Under many circumstances renal tubular transport of phosphate parallels that of sodium. Thus, expansion of extracellular fluid results in phosphaturia, as does the administration of diuretics, especially those that inhibit carbonic anhydrase. Phosphate transport is also linked to that of glucose and to changes in pH; therefore, hyperglycemia results in phosphaturia and reduced Tm for phosphorus. Similarly, conditions that result in an alkaline urine also decrease reabsorption of phosphate.

Regulation of Plasma Phosphate. In addition to the factors already discussed, plasma phosphate concentration is affected by the continuous exchange of phosphate between the large stores in bone and those in the extracellular fluid. Net reabsorption of phosphate from bone is promoted by 1,25-dihydroxyvitamin D_3 and PTH but is opposed by thyrocalcitonin. Phosphate is also readily transported across all cell membranes. Administering glucose or insulin decreases plasma phosphate concentration, probably because of an intracellular flux of phosphate secondary to the phosphorylation of glucose. Hyperventilation, alkalosis, and administration of epinephrine also decrease plasma phosphate concentration. Marked, acute increases in plasma phosphate concentration result in hypocalcemia. Changes in calcium concentration, however, do not necessarily reciprocally alter plasma phosphate concentration.

Plasma phosphorus concentrations are high during infancy and childhood. Values at birth range from 1.4 to 2.8 mM/L and increase progressively in the first week of life to 2.0–3.3 mM/L before declining slowly during childhood. Levels fall to those of the adult (1.0–1.3 mM/L) upon completion of growth. Premature infants also have high plasma phosphorus values of 2.5–3.0 mM/L, provided their intake of phosphorus is adequate.

Hyperphosphatemia is characteristic of hypoparathyroidism but rarely occurs in the absence of renal insufficiency. Although small changes in glomerular filtration rate (GFR) have little effect on phosphate excretion in health, *reduction in GFR to below 25%* leads to an elevation of serum inorganic phosphate and to reciprocal changes in serum calcium, resulting in secondary hyperparathyroidism. This process begins with small decreases in GFR but usually does not clinically appear until GFR has fallen to low levels. *In the young infant* GFR is low in relation to active cell mass and the dietary phosphorus intake is high; consequently, serum inorganic phosphorus is high. Hence, reduction in GFR or relative hypoparathyroidism in infants rapidly leads to very high serum values of phosphate, with consequent depression of calcium concentration and latent or manifest tetany (Sec. 5.33, 5.34, 8.54, and 19.18).

Hyperphosphatemia may also result from the excessive administration of phosphate by the oral or intravenous routes or as phosphate-containing enemas. Using cytotoxic drugs to treat malignancies, especially lymphomas or leukemias, will result in cytolysis, with hyperphosphatemia due to release of phosphate into the circulation. The major clinical consequences of hyperphosphatemia are symptoms of the resulting hypocalcemia.

Hypophosphatemia may result from phosphate deficiency in association with, for example, starvation, protein-calorie malnutrition, and malabsorption syndromes. It may result from intracellular shifts of phosphate such as occur with respiratory or metabolic acidosis, during the treatment of diabetic ketoacidosis (typically during the first 24 hr), and following the administration of corticosteroids. Increased urinary losses of phosphate may be sufficiently severe to reduce plasma concentration; this reduction is observed in primary and tertiary hyperparathyroidism, in renal tubular defects, after ECF volume expansion, or after administration of diuretics. Often a combination of pathophysiologic mechanisms is responsible for the hypophosphatemia. Examples include vitamin D–deficient (Sec. 3.29) and vitamin D–resistant rickets (Sec. 23.46). The very low birthweight infant requires a high phosphorus intake at the time of rapid postnatal growth. Inadequate intake results in phosphorus depletion and hypophosphatemia. In addition, bone demineralization, hypercalcemia, and calciuria may occur, probably owing to mobilization of phosphorus and calcium from the bone.

In most instances, hypophosphatemia is mild or moderate in degree and is asymptomatic. Occasionally, plasma phosphate concentration may fall to very low levels (0.3 mM/L; 1.0 mg/dL or less). Such low levels have been observed with the *prolonged use of intravenous alimentation without phosphate supplements* and may result in a very severe, well-defined syndrome. Red cell concentrations of 2,3-diphosphoglycerate and ATP are decreased. The resulting decrease in release of oxygen by the red cells produces tissue anoxia. Increased hemolysis may also occur, as may leukocyte and platelet dysfunction. Some patients display the symptoms of a metabolic encephalopathy, including irritability, paresthesias, confusion, seizures, and coma, and some may develop abnormalities in the electroencephalogram. Hypercalcemia, thought to be due to increased release of calcium from bone, rhabdomyolysis, cardiomyopathy, and possibly hepatocellular dysfunction, has also been reported. Renal tubular defects may occur, and the kidney's ability to excrete hydrogen ions is impaired. Promptly recognizing and treating this syndrome, preferably by orally administering phosphate salts, is beneficial, but permanent defects may result. Thus, prevention of severe hypophosphatemia should always be the goal.

Ac Hoc Committee on Acid-Base Terminology: Report. Ann NY Acad Sci 133:25, 1966.

Bronner F, Coburn JW (eds): Disorders of Mineral Metabolism. Volume II: Calcium Physiology. Volume III: Pathophysiology of Calcium, Phosphorus and Magnesium. New York, Academic Press, 1981.

Cooke RE (ed): The Biologic Basis of Pediatric Practice. New York, McGraw-Hill, 1968.

Emmett M, Narins RG: Clinical use of the anion gap. Medicine 56:38, 1977.

Hellerstein S, Duggan E, Merveille O, et al: Follow up studies on children with severe dietary chloride deficiency during infancy. Pediatrics 75:1, 1985.

Hicks JM, Boeckx RL (eds): Pediatric Clinical Chemistry. Philadelphia, W B Saunders, 1984.

Klahr S (ed): The Kidney and Body Fluids in Health and Disease. 2nd ed. New York, Plenum Press, 1984.

Needleman P, Adams SP, Cole BR, et al: Atriopeptins as cardiac hormones. Hypertension 7:469, 1985.

Plum F, Price RW: Acid-base balance of cisternal and lumbar cerebrospinal fluid in hospital patients. N Engl J Med 289:1346, 1973.

Schrier RW (ed): Renal and Electrolyte Disorders. 2nd ed. Boston, Little, Brown & Company, 1980.

Winters RW (ed): Principles of Pediatric Fluid Therapy. 2nd ed. Boston, Little, Brown & Company, 1982.

5.15 PARENTERAL FLUID THERAPY

Infants and young children are especially susceptible to the consequences of illnesses that affect fluid balance. The infant's usual daily turnover of water is equal to almost 25% of total body water, compared with 6% in the adult. Thus, the effects of any disease that reduces fluid intake (e.g., vomiting) or increases fluid losses (e.g., diarrhea) appear much more rapidly in the infant than in the adult.

Calculation of Requirements. Fluid therapy can be considered in three phases. *Deficit therapy* is designed to replace losses of fluids and electrolytes resulting from an illness before the patient was brought for medical care. Its goal is to return volume and composition to normal. *Maintenance therapy* is designed to replace ongoing normal and abnormal losses of fluids and electrolytes. The purpose is to maintain patients in normal balance and to prevent deficits from developing. *Supplemental therapy* is used in certain diseases that require specific fluids and electrolytes in addition to those for repair of deficits and maintenance.

Total fluid and electrolyte needs are calculated as the sum of these individual phases of treatment. For example, after uncomplicated surgery a patient frequently only requires normal maintenance—the replacement of fluids and electrolytes usually lost from the body through the lungs and as urine, sweat, and feces. A postoperative patient with gastric drainage will require maintenance therapy to replace not only normal losses but also the increased losses of water and electrolytes in the gastric fluid. A dehydrated patient with severe diarrhea will require deficit therapy to replace the losses resulting from the diarrhea, and maintenance therapy to replace normal losses as well as the continuing abnormal stool losses for as long as the diarrhea persists. A patient with severe salicylate intoxication will require replacement of deficits that occurred prior to hospital admission; replacement of usual losses as well as the increased losses due to hyperventilation and fever; and supplemental treatment in which alkalinization of the urine and induction of diuresis are frequently employed to increase salicylate excretion in the urine.

Each of these phases of fluid therapy is considered separately. *As with potentially lethal drugs, amounts of fluids and electrolytes should preferably be calculated independently by at least two people, and the results should be reconciled before administration is begun.*

Monitoring of Patient. Regardless of the accuracy of planning a therapeutic regimen, a patient's response is not always predictable. Consequently, frequent assessment is required so that appropriate modifications of therapy can be instituted promptly if needed. Typically, such monitoring consists of frequent physical examinations to determine changes in body weight, and frequent review of intake and output charts. These clinical determinations may need to be supplemented by repeated laboratory determinations. Serial measurements of serum electrolytes, blood urea nitrogen, and serum creatinine may be essential; the interval between determinations depends on the patient's clinical status.

5.16 MAINTENANCE THERAPY

5.17 REPLACEMENT OF NORMAL LOSSES

A healthy person deprived of a normal oral intake will continue to lose basal amounts of fluids and electrolytes from the body as urine, sweat, and feces and will have additional losses of water from the lungs as evaporation in exhaled air. Water and electrolytes are required to replace these obligatory losses, or deficits will result. Protein and calories are also required, but complete parenteral replacement is difficult and

is not essential unless oral intake is restricted for a protracted period of time.

The amount and type of these losses may be modified by disease states. For example, pyrexia may be associated with increased sweating; renal disease may result in either oliguria or polyuria; both diarrhea and gastric suction will result in increased losses from the gastrointestinal tract. Less easily recognized but equally important losses are those that may result from sequestration of fluid in a body space; e.g., a patient with paralytic ileus may have pooling of fluid in the gastrointestinal tract. Even though total body fluid and electrolyte content may not be changed, this pooled fluid may not be in equilibrium with the vascular compartment and may cause a functional deficit. Failure to replace any of these losses will result in the development of fluid and electrolyte deficits. The influence of disease states on maintenance requirements will be discussed after normal maintenance needs have been analyzed.

Calculation of Normal Maintenance Therapy. I: Basic Method. Fluid and electrolyte requirements for purposes of maintenance are directly related to metabolic rate. An increase in metabolic rate requires an increase in catabolism of metabolic fuels and has three effects: (1) it increases the rate of endogenous water production from the oxidation of carbohydrate, fats, and protein; (2) it increases urinary solute excretion which, in turn, increases obligatory urine flow rates and urinary water losses; and (3) it increases heat production, which increases water loss as sweat and water loss through respiration. Similarly, the turnover rates of electrolytes are related to water loss and to metabolic rate. Therefore, if a patient's caloric expenditure can be estimated, his or her maintenance requirements of fluids and electrolytes can be calculated because the amounts of water, sodium, and potassium required for every 100 kcal metabolized are well established from numerous observations.

Calculation of Caloric Expenditure. Metabolic rate depends on age, body weight, degree of activity, and body temperature. *Basal metabolic rate* can be obtained from Table 5–4, which depicts the values for each sex at various body weights. To

Table 5–4. **Standard Basal Caloric Output**

Weight (kg)	Male	Kilocalories/24 hr Male and Female	Female
3		140	
5		270	
7		400	
9		500	
11		600	
13		650	
15		710	
17		780	
19		830	
21		880	
25	1020		960
29	1120		1040
33	1210		1120
37	1300		1190
41	1350		1260
45	1410		1320
49	1470		1380
53	1530		1440
57	1590		1500
61	1640		1560

Modified from Talbot.
Increments or decrements:
1. Add or subtract 12% of above for each degree C (8% for each degree F) above or below rectal temperature of 37.8° C (100° F).
2. Add 0 to 30% increments for activity.

calculate maintenance requirements from caloric expenditure, these basal values must be adjusted for the patient's activity, body temperature, and any pathologic state. *Adjustments for activity* are made from observing the patient. No increments are needed for patients in coma or under anesthesia. Usual activity in bed rarely increases basal expenditure by more than 30%. Caloric expenditure is increased by fever (12% per °C rise in body temperature) and by hypermetabolic states such as salicylism and hyperthyroidism (25–75%). It is decreased by hypothermia (12% per °C fall in body temperature) and by hypometabolic states such as hypothyroidism (10–25%).

These calculations permit a good estimate of caloric expenditure in all but the very young infant and the obese subject. In the neonate, activity during the first 3–5 days of life is low; total caloric expenditure does not usually exceed 50 kcal/kg of body weight per day; this figure should be used to calculate maintenance requirements during this period. In obese infants and children, "ideal" weight (50th percentile for age and height) should be used to calculate basal metabolic rate.

Translation of Caloric Expenditure to Water and Electrolyte Requirements. As shown in Table 5–5, the usual losses of water and electrolytes from lungs, skin, stool, and urine can be related to caloric expenditure (Table 5–4). For every 100 kcal metabolized the patient requires a total of approximately 125 mL of water, 3.2 mEq of sodium, and 2.4 mEq of potassium to replace normal losses. However, maintenance requirements for water have to be reduced by 10–15 mL/100 kcal metabolized to allow for the release of an equivalent volume of water during oxidation of endogenous and exogenous carbohydrate, fat, and protein. Thus, water, sodium, and potassium requirements for normal maintenance therapy are estimated at 115 mL, 3 mEq, and 2.5 mEq, respectively, for every 100 kcal metabolized. Bottle-fed infants require a higher fluid intake of 140 mL/100 kcal of food since their milk diet has a high protein content which increases the solute load to be excreted by the kidneys and the obligatory renal water loss.

These recommendations assume that the kidney can adjust rates of urine flow and electrolyte excretion over wide ranges. The maintenance requirements calculated above do not require maximal renal concentration or dilution of urine or exceed the solute load which can be excreted by the kidney or its ability to conserve electrolytes. The designated requirements thus provide some latitude in the amounts of fluids and electrolytes that can be administered safely. With renal damage, or in other disease states, this is frequently not the case, and maintenance requirements must be modified precisely, as outlined below.

Calculation of Normal Maintenance Therapy. II: Alternative Method. Several alternate methods have been developed to estimate caloric expenditure and to calculate fluid and electrolyte requirements. They are derived from the principles

Table 5–6. A Simplified Alternative Method for Calculating Caloric Expenditure from Body Weight

Body Weight (kg)	Caloric Expenditure/Day
Up to 10	100 kcal/kg
11–20	1000 kcal + 50 kcal/kg for each kg above 10 kg
Above 20	1500 kcal + 20 kcal/kg for each kg above 20 kg

Modified from Holliday and Segar. kcal = kilocalories = 1000 calories = 1000 Cal.

outlined but do not require the availability of reference tables. More simple to use, they relate maintenance requirements to either body weight or body surface.

One such method to estimate caloric expenditure is shown in Table 5–6. The values are for the average hospitalized patient and allow for usual activity in bed. Although values for caloric expenditure are slightly higher than those used in the basic system, the derived values for maintenance requirements are identical, since it is recommended that for every 100 kcal expended only 100 mL of fluid should be administered (compared with 115 mL with the basic system); this solution should contain 25 mEq of sodium and 20 mEq of potassium per liter, and 5% dextrose. Commercially prepared solutions with this composition are available (Table 29–8) which also provide magnesium (3 mEq/L), phosphate (3 mEq/L) and either lactate or acetate (23 mEq/L).

Comparison of Methods. Maintenance requirements calculated by the alternative method are virtually identical to those calculated by the basic method. For example, for an afebrile, previously healthy male child weighing 45 kg, basic caloric expenditure obtained from Table 5–4 would be 1410. Allowing a 20% increment for physical activity, the estimated caloric expenditure would be 1692 kcal. Daily water requirements would be $16.92 \times 115 = 1946$ mL; sodium requirements, $16.92 \times 3 = 51$ mEq (equivalent to 26 mEq/L of administered solution); and potassium requirements, $16.92 \times 2.5 = 42$ mEq (or 21 mEq/L of administered solution). The administered fluid should contain 5% dextrose. Using the alternative system (Table 5–6) caloric expenditure would be estimated as 2000 kcal, which would indicate the need to administer 2000 mL of the maintenance solution containing 5% dextrose, 25 mEq/L of sodium, and 20 mEq/L of potassium.

5.18 MODIFICATION OF MAINTENANCE REQUIREMENTS BY DISEASE STATES

Disease states may result in either markedly increased or decreased losses of water and/or electrolytes (Table 5–5). Maintenance therapy must be adjusted appropriately to maintain a patient's fluid and electrolyte balance.

Decreased Requirements. In *anuria* or extreme oliguria, urine output may be negligible, often less than 10 mL/100 kcal, compared with a normal 65 mL. Only stool and evaporative water losses occur, and the rate of fluid administered must be reduced accordingly. More than 45 mL of exogenous water is rarely required for each 100 kcal. It is preferable to underestimate rather than to overestimate fluid requirements in such cases, since it is easier to administer additional fluids later if needed than to remove excess fluid administered inappropriately. Administration of electrolytes should also be reduced in anuric patients. In the absence of complications such as diarrhea, sodium and potassium losses through the sweat and stools are usually negligible, and no electrolytes may be required for maintenance in these patients.

In some patients, particularly those with *meningitis*, excessive or inappropriate release of antidiuretic hormone may occur. The rate of flow of urine is markedly reduced, and

Table 5–5. Water and Electrolyte Losses/100 Kcal Metabolized Under Normal Conditions and in Disease States

Route of Loss	Usual Loss			Range Observed in Disease States		
	H_2O (mL)	Na (mEq)	K (mEq)	H_2O (mL)	Na (mEq)	K (mEq)
Evaporative						
Lungs	15	0	0	10–60	0	0
Skin	40	0.1	0.2	20–100	0.1–3.0	0.2–1.5
Stool	5	0.1	0.2	0–50	0.1–4.0	0.2–3.0
Urine	65	3.0	2.0	0–400	0–30.0	0–30.0
Total	125	3.2	2.4			

fluid intake should be reduced to reflect these decreased losses. *Patients in highly humidified atmospheres* (e.g., incubators or croup tents) also have reduced fluid requirements since the high humidity may reduce evaporative losses of water by 20–50%. In *congestive heart failure* restriction of sodium and water intake is indicated when planning parenteral as well as oral intake.

Increased Requirements. The amount and nature of abnormally increased losses of fluids and electrolytes depend on the underlying disease process and the site of loss. Considerable variation exists in the composition of abnormal *gastrointestinal losses* from patient to patient and from time to time in the same patient. An estimate of the composition of the more common fluid losses can be based on Table 5–7. These losses should be replaced as nearly as possible, volume for volume, as they occur to prevent physiologic readjustment that may further deplete the body of water and electrolytes. If such estimates are too imprecise, the electrolyte concentrations in the fluid being lost should be measured to exactly determine replacement needs.

In general, losses in gastric or intestinal drainage can be replaced satisfactorily by isotonic or somewhat hypotonic solutions which contain more chloride than sodium for gastric replacement and more sodium than chloride for intestinal replacement. Although gastric fluid contains relatively little potassium, the alkalosis that develops from the loss of significant quantities of hydrogen ion in the gastric juice usually results in increased urinary potassium loss; therefore, replacement fluid for a patient with gastric drainage should contain 10–20 mEq of potassium/L (provided renal function is well maintained).

Increased losses of sodium chloride in *sweat* usually are of little significance except in adrenal insufficiency and cystic fibrosis; heat stress should be avoided in such patients. In *hyperventilation* and *heat stress*, evaporative losses of water may increase as much as 90 and 120 mL/100 kcal, respectively.

When *renal* concentrating and diluting ability is lost, as in chronic renal disease, water requirements may rise to 150 mL/100 kcal and, as in diabetes insipidus of nephrogenic or hypothalamic origin, to as high as 400 mL/100 kcal.

Under most circumstances fluid losses are replaced volume-for-volume and electrolyte losses, milliequivalent-for-milliequivalent, but sometimes this is inappropriate. For example, the increased urine output seen in the diuretic phase of acute tubular necrosis may eliminate fluid retained during the oliguric phase of the disease. All of these increased losses are not replaced, since such therapy would only perpetuate the presence of edema. Sodium and water losses can be replaced rapidly. Potassium losses are replaced over a more protracted period of time, especially if administered parenterally.

ADMINISTRATION OF MAINTENANCE REQUIREMENTS

Losses should be replaced by mouth if possible, otherwise by intravenous route. Using subcutaneous injections of fluids is not recommended because of variable rates of absorption and other complications. However, if technical or other difficulties dictate that therapy be given by this route, glucose in water or in very dilute electrolyte solution should not be given because diffusion of sodium chloride into such an extravascular pool and the subsequent loss of fluid from the extracellular fluid may reduce plasma volume acutely and precipitate shock.

Precisely replacing large quantities of fluid may be difficult. In such instances, thirst, changes in body weight, and urinary output are usually more reliable indicators of the patient's needs than are the physician's estimates. Such patients should be re-evaluated every 8 hr, or more frequently, to ensure that the balance is maintained.

Caloric Intake

In a patient receiving maintenance fluids parenterally, matching caloric expenditure with adequate caloric intake is difficult and, fortunately, is unnecessary if maintenance therapy is needed for only short periods of time. However, administering maintenance electrolytes in a 5% dextrose solution is desirable as a routine measure to provide approximately 20% of the calories metabolized and to produce a decreased catabolism of endogenous protein and a decreased solute load to be excreted by the kidney. Concentrations of dextrose above 5% are not recommended, because when they are administered at infusion rates sufficient to meet water requirements, they frequently result in hyperglycemia. The consequent loss of dextrose in the urine may actually increase water requirements through an osmotic diuretic effect. At slower infusion rates, such as those used in the anuric patient or in the neonate, higher concentrations of dextrose may be used, but they increase the risk of intravenous thrombosis and infection.

Intravenous Alimentation

The foregoing regimens for replacing and maintaining fluid and electrolytes are calorically inadequate and will not sustain growth. They are suitable, therefore, for short periods of time only. In some infants and children, especially newborns undergoing major surgery and children with protracted diarrhea, parenteral nutrition for prolonged periods is necessary. Regimens developed to meet this need may effectively maintain positive nitrogen balance and growth for periods of 60 days or longer.

The standard infusate is prepared from a crystalline amino acid solution and contains 20% glucose and various electrolytes (Table 5–8). A multiple vitamin preparation is added to the solution, avoiding excess amounts of vitamin E; zinc, copper, chromium, and manganese are added in recommended trace amounts. The solution is infused into a central vein by means of a constant speed infusion pump through a catheter tunneled subcutaneously to reduce the risk of infection. Infused at rates of up to 135 mL/kg/24 hr, this solution provides approximately 120 cal/kg/24 hr and meets protein requirements estimated to be in the range of 2.0–3.0 g/kg/24 hr. Lipids may be given daily, but the more cost-effective intravenous transfusion of 20 mL/kg of lipids (containing linolenic and linoleic acids) every 10 days will provide adequate amounts of essential fatty acids.

In patients in whom it is impossible to use a central venous catheter and in neonates, parenteral nutrition may be given

Table 5–7. **Composition of External Abnormal Losses**

Fluid	Na	K	Cl	Protein g%
	mEq/L			
Gastric	20–80	5–20	100–150	—
Pancreatic	120–140	5–15	90–120	—
Small intestine	100–140	5–15	90–130	—
Bile	120–140	5–15	80–120	—
Ileostomy	45–135	3–15	20–115	—
Diarrheal	10–90	10–80	10–110	—
Sweat:*				
Normal	10–30	3–10	10–35	—
Cystic fibrosis	50–130	5–25	50–110	—
Burns	140	5	110	3–5

*Sweat sodium concentrations progressively increase with increasing sweat flow rates.

Table 5–8. **Composition of Typical Infusate Used in Intravenous Alimentation**

Constituent	Concentration (Per Liter)	Approximate** Infusion Rate (Per kg/day)
Amino acids* (g)	16	2.2
Glucose (g)	200	27
Sodium† (mEq)	32	4.3
Potassium† (mEq)	30	4.1
Chloride† (mEq)	30	4.1
Acetate (mEq)	32	4.1
Calcium‡ (mEq)	9	1.2
Magnesium (mEq)	8	1.1
Sulfate (mEq)	8	1.1
Phosphate (mM)	10	1.4
Total calories (kcal)	864	117
Osmolality (mOsm)	1462	209
pH	6.4	

*Derived from crystalline amino acid preparations such as FreAmine III or Trophamine (McGaw), Neoaminosol (Abbott Laboratories), or Travasol (Baxter Laboratories).
†May be adjusted to meet individual patient's needs.
**Based on an infusion rate of 135 mL/kg/day.
‡Some sources recommend a higher calcium concentration.

by peripheral vein. The glucose concentration in these infusates should be reduced to 10%. To compensate partially for the reduced caloric content of this infusate, the amino acid content is increased to 30 gm/L if an older child is to be treated. Since neonates do not tolerate this solution well, they should receive a solution containing the lower amino acid and glucose content even though it provides only 464 calories/L. The neonates should, however, receive lipids daily.

Complications of intravenous alimentation are common. They include sepsis; severe hyperglycemia, especially in the early stages of treatment of low birthweight infants; profound hypophosphatemia, which can be life threatening and can occur most often in the first week of the parenteral nutrition of malnourished patients; hyperammonemia, typically seen in small infants with bowel disease; severe metabolic acidosis; and other disturbances in electrolyte concentrations. To minimize complications, inserting catheters and changing lines should be performed only by persons trained in these techniques; the patient's clinical status and state of hydration should be monitored closely; urines should be regularly checked for glucosuria, especially in the first week of treatment; and serum electrolytes, phosphate, glucose, urea nitrogen, and hemoglobin should be measured before treatment is started and at weekly intervals thereafter. Serum calcium, ammonia, and albumin should be measured at less frequent intervals. Checking liver function and certain trace metal or vitamin levels may also be necessary should these studies be indicated on clinical grounds.

5.19 DEFICIT THERAPY

Deficits in body water and electrolytes may result from reduced intake with continuing normal losses, from excessive losses occurring with or without usual intake, or from a combination of these mechanisms. The *absolute deficits* of water and electrolytes observed in dehydration produced by different disease states are estimated in Table 5–9, which provides some representative values and illustrates the similarity in the magnitudes of deficits irrespective of the precipitating condition. This similarity is not surprising, since deficits reflect not only the results of direct losses but also the physiologic readjustments by the patient. As a consequence, *patients with deficits resulting from many different causes can be*

treated successfully in a similar manner. In most instances, management is dictated more by the severity and type of deficit than by its underlying cause. The *severity of the clinical disturbances* typically depends on the magnitude of the deficit in relation to body reserves and on the rate at which the deficit developed. The *type of deficit* depends on the relationship between the magnitude of loss of water and that of electrolytes, principally sodium.

SEVERITY OF DEFICIT

The magnitude or severity of a deficit can be gauged from change in body weight. Any loss of body weight in excess of 1%/day represents loss of body water. In young infants a weight loss of up to 5% is considered mild, 5–10% moderate, and 10–15% severe dehydration, the last of which is frequently associated with peripheral circulatory failure. Deficits in excess of 15% of body weight are rarely compatible with life.

In older children and adults total body water and extracellular fluid volume each represent a smaller percentage of body weight than in the infant. In these patients, any given percentage loss of body weight resulting from fluid and electrolyte deficits indicates more severe depletion than in infants. Thus, comparable figures for severity of the deficit in older patients are 3% (mild), 6% (moderate), and 9% (severe).

The rapidity with which a deficit develops is also important. A 10% weight loss occurring over 24 hr in an infant is severe. The same weight loss developing over several days is better tolerated, and its effects typically are only moderately severe.

5.20 TYPES OF DEHYDRATION

The serum sodium in dehydrated patients may be normal, low, or high, depending on the relative losses of water and electrolytes. Dehydration is classified on this basis, being termed *isonatremic* when serum sodium levels are 130–150 mEq/L, *hyponatremic* when serum sodium levels are less than 130 mEq/L, and *hypernatremic* when serum sodium levels are above 150 mEq/L. Since plasma osmolality in large part reflects sodium concentrations, these forms of dehydration are usually *isotonic, hypotonic,* and *hypertonic,* respectively. Changes in tonicity do not always correspond to changes in sodium concentration, however, so the two sets of terms cannot be used interchangeably. For example, in diabetic ketoacidosis or in uremia, serum sodium concentration may be low, but the plasma is hypertonic as a result of elevated plasma levels of glucose or urea, respectively.

Classifying dehydration into these three types, based on sodium concentrations, is of practical importance. Each form is associated with different relative losses of fluid from intracellular (ICF) and extracellular (ECF) compartments. In *isonatremic* dehydration the fluid and electrolyte loss is from the

Table 5–9. **Probable Deficits of Water and Electrolytes in Infants with Moderately Severe Dehydration**

Condition	H₂O (mL)	Na (mEq)	K* (mEq)	Cl (mEq)
		Per kg of Body Weight		
Fasting and thirsting	100–120	5–7	1–2	4–6
Diarrhea				
Isonatremic	100–120	8–10	8–10	8–10
Hypernatremic	100–120	2–4	0–4	−2−−6†
Hyponatremic	100–120	10–12	8–10	10–12
Pyloric stenosis	100–120	8–10	10–12	10–12
Diabetic acidosis	100–120	8–10	5–7	6–8

*Converted for breakdown of tissue cells: −1 g N = 3 mEq of K.
†Negative balance of chloride indicates excess at beginning of therapy.

extracellular fluid which remains isotonic. Since there is no osmotic gradient across cell walls, intracellular fluid volume remains virtually constant; the majority of fluid loss is borne by the extracellular compartment. In *hyponatremic* dehydration the hypotonicity of the extracellular fluid results in an osmotically induced movement of fluid from the extracellular compartment into cells, resulting in even further depletion of extracellular fluid and some increases in intracellular fluid. Conversely, in *hypernatremic* dehydration the increase in osmolality of the extracellular fluid results in movement of fluid out of the cells so that the intracellular fluid volume is depleted; depletion of extracellular fluid is less than expected. This analysis assumes that the plasma does not contain pathologic concentrations of other molecules which are osmotically effective across cell walls. As a consequence of these differences, the three forms of dehydration are characterized by variations in clinical presentation and in physical findings, each requiring appropriate modification in therapeutic approach.

5.21 ESTIMATION OF MAGNITUDE AND TYPE OF DEFICIT

This assessment should consist of a detailed history and a thorough physical examination, often augmented by appropriate laboratory studies.

History. Some important aspects are shown in Table 5–10. If a patient's preillness weight is known, the change from this value will provide an accurate estimate of the magnitude of fluid losses. Without such information, a detailed estimate of losses and the exact quantities and composition of the infant's feedings prior to being seen may permit a less exact assessment of the magnitude of the deficit and also indicate the type of dehydration. It is important to remember that body composition of dehydrated patients is influenced not only by losses but also by *concomitant intake*. The severity and type of dehydration are the result of the sum of intake and losses of both water and electrolytes. For example, a patient with severe diarrhea, losing fluid with a sodium concentration as low as 40 mEq/L, may continue to drink tap water containing virtually no sodium. Water losses will be partially compensated for by the water intake but sodium losses will not be replaced. Thus, despite the primary loss of excessive quantities of hyponatremic fluid (diarrhea), this patient may still present with hyponatremia. Conversely, the same patient treated with homemade electrolyte mixtures given by mouth may be hypernatremic, especially if the solution has been prepared with excessive amounts of salt or sodium bicarbonate, an all too common problem which has frequently been observed to result in severe hypernatremia.

The time and frequency of recent urinations, whether excessive or suppressed, may provide some appreciation of

Table 5–10. Historical Data Required in Estimating Magnitude and Types of Deficit and in Planning Deficit Therapy

Intake — during period of illness
  Quantity and how given
  Kind: water, electrolyte, protein, drugs
Output — during period of illness
  Quantity
  Kind: urine, vomiting, diarrhea, sweat, drainage
Balance
  Weight change
General medical
  Age
  Cardiovascular, respiratory, renal or central nervous system
    disease

the severity of dehydration or indicate its cause. Urine output characteristically is decreased with dehydration, except in some low birthweight infants. Continued frequent and excessive urination with dehydration suggests diabetes mellitus, diabetes insipidus, or nephrogenic diabetes insipidus. Output and usual amounts of urine without increased intake of water, in association with physical signs of dehydration, indicates a loss in the capacity of the kidneys to conserve water and suggests renal disease.

Physical Examination. Table 5–11 details the physical findings associated with dehydration of different degrees of severity. In general, these findings occur irrespective of the etiology of the volume of depletion. Table 5–12 summarizes how different types of dehydration modify the physical signs.

Most infants and children appear ill when dehydrated. Frequently, the eyes appear sunken and the skin around them dark. Intraocular pressure, elicited by lightly pressing on the closed eyes, is low. The mucous membranes of the mouth are usually dry, but prolonged mouth breathing or the tachypnea of acidosis may cause dry mucous membranes in the absence of dehydration. Tissue turgor may be reduced. Normally, when the skin and subcutaneous tissue are pinched between the thumb and first finger and then released, they return to position immediately. Delay in return (*tenting*) indicates dehydration. Skin and subcutaneous tissue must be tested together or laxity of skin may be misinterpreted as dehydration. Skin over the abdominal and chest walls and of the thigh should be tested. Testing the abdomen alone may cause this sign to be missed, since abdominal distention may mask loss of turgor at this site. Further, in the well-nourished infant or child, skin turgor may remain fairly normal in the presence of dehydration. Depression of the anterior fontanel in the infant is often an accurate indication of dehydration.

Physical examination may also help to determine the type of dehydration (Table 5–13). Patients with hyponatremic dehydration have increased losses of fluid from the extracellular compartment and are more likely to develop shock; conversely, evidence of depletion of intracellular fluid may be apparent in patients with hypernatremic dehydration and be reflected in a doughy or putty-like consistency of the skin and subcutaneous tissue on palpation.

Shock manifested by tachycardia, a thin and thready pulse, cyanosis, and low blood pressure may supervene with severe dehydration. Blood pressure is frequently hard to determine, but a useful estimate of systolic pressure only can often be obtained by palpation. The Doppler technique may enable an accurate measurement of blood pressure. The state of the peripheral circulation can be assessed by the warmth and color of the skin and by the rapidity of filling of the cutaneous capillary bed after pressure over the ear lobe, the nail bed, and the dorsum of the hand or the foot. However, peripheral circulation can be affected by local factors such as ambient temperature, and care must be taken when evaluating these signs.

Some disease states result in specific losses. For example, severe diarrhea is associated with marked losses of bicarbonate resulting in systemic acidosis. In pyloric stenosis, major losses of hydrogen and chloride cause a hypochloremic alkalosis. Chronic diarrhea may result in hypomagnesemia from continuing losses of magnesium. The findings on physical examination that may indicate such deficits are summarized in Table 5–13. Such signs are not infallible or uniform. For example, the characteristic signs of metabolic acidosis (relatively slow, regular breathing with increased depth and a prolonged expiratory phase, referred to as *Kussmaul breathing*) may be less marked in the presence of severe circulatory insufficiency. The compensatory diminution in breathing associated with alkalosis, though usually absent in adults, may be seen in infants with pyloric stenosis. Deficiencies of potas-

Table 5–11. **Clinical Assessment of Severity of Dehydration**

Signs and Symptoms	Mild Dehydration	Moderate Dehydration	Severe Dehydration
General appearance and condition:			
Infants and young children	Thirsty; alert; restless	Thirsty; restless or lethargic but irritable to touch or drowsy	Drowsy; limp, cold, sweaty, cyanotic extremities; may be comatose
Older children and adults	Thirsty; alert; restless	Thirsty; alert; postural hypotension	Usually conscious; apprehensive; cold, sweaty, cyanotic extremities; wrinkled skin of fingers and toes; muscle cramps
Radial pulse	Normal rate and strength	Rapid and weak	Rapid, feeble, sometimes impalpable
Respiration	Normal	Deep, maybe rapid	Deep and rapid
Anterior fontanel	Normal	Sunken	Very sunken
Systolic blood pressure	Normal	Normal or low	Less than 90 mm; may be unrecordable
Skin elasticity	Pinch retracts immediately	Pinch retracts slowly	Pinch retracts very slowly (>2 sec)
Eyes	Normal	Sunken (detectable)	Grossly sunken
Tears	Present	Absent	Absent
Mucous membranes	Moist	Dry	Very dry
Urine flow	Normal	Reduced amount and dark	None passed for several hours; empty bladder
% body weight loss	4–5%	6–9%	10% or more
Estimated fluid deficit	40–50 mL/kg	60–90 mL/kg	100–110 mL/kg

Modified from World Health Organization guide.

sium, calcium, or magnesium may exist without obvious physical findings. Hypokalemia may not always be present even when the cells are depleted of potassium so that such deficits may have to be inferred from history alone.

In summary, mild dehydration may be indicated only by the presence of thirst. If two or more signs of moderate dehydration (Table 5–11) are present, the patient should be considered to have moderate dehydration even if all the signs are not present. A similar guide should be used for severe dehydration. In the absence of known changes in body weight, examining the anterior fontanel, skin elasticity, and the eyes, as well as taking a history of the recent pattern of urination, helps to assess the degree of dehydration in an infant.

Laboratory Data. Admission laboratory values are helpful in characterizing the type of deficit and in planning therapy.

None is so essential, however, that adequate therapy cannot be initiated without it. Serial laboratory determinations are of greater importance. They permit the assessment of the results of treating deficits and guide subsequent maintenance therapy.

Hemoconcentration (increase in *hemoglobin*, *hematocrit*, and *plasma proteins*) may indicate the severity of dehydration. However, with pre-existing anemia, both hemoglobin and hematocrit may be normal even with severe dehydration. Similarly, the measurement of plasma proteins may have limited usefulness at the beginning of therapy, especially in the malnourished patient. Depite such limitations, these measurements, when correlated with physical findings, may be useful in planning therapy. Repeat measurements help to assess effectiveness of treatment.

Dehydration may result in a decrease in glomerular filtration

Table 5–12. **Effects of Type of Dehydration on Physical Signs**

	Isonatremic Dehydration (Proportionate Loss of Water and Sodium)	Hyponatremic Dehydration (Loss of Sodium in Excess of Water)	Hypernatremic Dehydration (Loss of Water in Excess of Sodium)
ECF Volume*	Markedly decreased	Severely decreased	Decreased
ICF Volume*	Maintained	Increased	Decreased
Physical Signs			
Skin			
Color†	Gray	Gray	Gray
Temperature	Cold	Cold	Cold or hot
Turgor‡	Poor	Very poor	Fair
Feel	Dry	Clammy	Thickened, doughy
Mucous membrane	Dry	Slightly moist	Parched§
Eyeball	Sunken and soft	Sunken and soft	Sunken
Fontanel	Sunken	Sunken	Sunken
Psyche	Lethargic	Coma	Hyperrritable
Pulse†	Rapid	Rapid	Moderately rapid
Blood pressure†	Low	Very low	Moderately low

*ECF = extracellular fluid; ICF = intracellular fluid.
†Signs of shock rather than of dehydration itself.
‡Reflects magnitude of fluid loss from ECF.
§Tongue often has shriveled appearance owing to loss of cellular fluid.

Table 5–13. Physical Signs of Variations in Concentration of Specific Ions

Acidosis (metabolic)
  Respiration: increased depth and rate
Alkalosis (metabolic)
  Respiration: decreased depth and rate
  Latent or manifest tetany
Hypopotassemia
  Heart: fast or slow, poor quality to heart sounds
  Skeletal muscle: weakness or paralyses, diminished reflexes
  Smooth muscle: abdominal distention, ileus
Hyperpotassemia
  Heart: slow or fast, poor quality to heart sounds
  Skeletal muscle: fibrillation, paralyses
Hypocalcemia
  Latent tetany (Sec. 5.33)
  Manifest tetany (Sec. 5.33)
Hypercalcemia
  Gastrointestinal: fecal masses
  Hypotonia
Hypomagnesemia
  Latent or manifest tetany
  Muscular twitching
Hypermagnesemia
  Decreased deep tendon reflexes
  Central nervous system depression

rate so that both *blood urea nitrogen* and *creatinine* levels will increase. Such elevations may also result from intrinsic renal disease. Measuring urine concentration can help to separate these two entities; *urinalysis* showing a specific gravity of less than 1.020 with dehydration indicates a defect in urinary concentrating mechanisms and suggests intrinsic renal disease. With dehydration there may be mild to moderate proteinuria, and the urine may contain hyaline and granular casts, white blood cells, and, occasionally, red blood cells. Such findings do not necessarily indicate intrinsic renal disease, but urinalysis should be repeated after recovery from the dehydration. Serial measurements of urinary output and specific gravity are of value in evaluating the effectiveness of therapy and in guiding it.

Serum or *plasma electrolyte values* are especially useful. Serum sodium concentration reflects the relative losses of water and electrolytes. *Total body sodium is typically depleted in all patients with dehydration, even in those with hypernatremia.* Serum potassium concentrations at the beginning of therapy are of limited value, because they do not help to determine body content of this cation. Values may be elevated because of anoxia, diminished renal function, or acidosis, even when significant cellular deficits exist. Serial electrocardiograms may provide clues to disturbances of intracellular potassium and calcium. *Serum bicarbonate* concentrations help to define whether the patient has acidemia or alkalemia. Values may have to be supplemented by determining blood pH and pCO_2. These determinations are particularly valuable as guides to the severity of metabolic disorders or of respiratory disorders, such as occur in patients receiving assisted or artificial respiration. Measuring *serum chloride* concentration permits calculation of anion gap (Sec. 5.13). Normally, the difference between the sum of measured cations (sodium and potassium) and that of measured anions (chloride and bicarbonate) is 15 ± 5 mEq/L. This value is increased in renal disease, as a result of retention of phosphate sulfate and other unmeasured anions, as well as in ketosis and lactic acidosis. The difference may also indicate the possibility of laboratory error in electrolyte determinations.

5.22 PRINCIPLES OF THERAPY

In some dehydrated patients, e.g., those in shock, administering fluids must be treated as a medical emergency. A complete evaluation of the patient can be undertaken after fluid therapy has begun and the patient's condition has been stabilized. However, most errors in fluid management occur in the initial stages of rehydration. When possible, it is preferable not to administer fluids until the patient's state of hydration has been assessed clinically and the type and amounts of fluids to be given for initial rehydration have been determined carefully. When planning this therapy for the dehydrated patient, the important considerations are the magnitude of the sodium and water deficits, the qualitative changes in body composition that have resulted from relative losses of electrolytes in relation to water, and the status of both potassium and hydrogen ion balances. *Similar basic therapeutic approaches with only minor modification may be used for patients having dehydration resulting from widely differing etiologies.*

Oral rehydration may be appropriate in patients with mild or moderate dehydration. Amounts of fluid and electrolytes adequate to correct the deficits often can be administered by mouth to such patients (Sec. 5.24). Parenteral administration is required for patients with more severe dehydration, for those who are vomiting, or for those having profound ongoing losses; for example, it is recommended for any patient with diarrhea of amounts greater than 100 mL/kg/hr. The intravenous route is preferred for parenterally replacing deficits, although replacement fluids have been given intraperitoneally and subcutaneously.

Parenteral rehydration therapy has three phases. *Initial therapy,* consisting of rapid re-expansion of extracellular fluid volume, is designed to improve circulatory dynamics and renal function, which are of primary importance in the morbidity and mortality of dehydration. *Subsequent therapy* is aimed at replacing the remaining intracellular and extracellular deficits of water and electrolytes but at a slower rate, with sodium replacement preceding potassium replacement. The *final phase,* consisting of the return of the patient's normal nutritional state, usually begins when the patient is able to return to oral feedings.

Initial Therapy. This phase is designed to treat or prevent shock by rapidly expanding the volume of extracellular fluid, especially the plasma. Ideally, the entire fluid used for initially treating dehydration should remain in the vascular space. Whole blood, however, is not the treatment of choice. Delays during typing and cross-matching the blood may occur, and thrombosis accompanying the administration of blood in the dehydrated patient is a risk. Similarly, the risk of hepatitis makes the use of pooled plasma undesirable. Instead, an electrolyte solution with a sodium concentration similar to that of blood is recommended. Glucose should be included in this fluid, since the sick infant is susceptible to hypoglycemia. Suitable preparations which fulfill these criteria are commercially available (Table 29–8). Isotonic saline (0.9%; Na and Cl both 154 mEq/L) containing glucose, 5 g/dL, is one alternative especially useful in dehydrated patients with metabolic alkalosis (e.g., from pyloric stenosis). Using this solution in a patient with acidosis is less optimal since it does not correct the acidosis unless renal perfusion is increased, permitting increased excretion of hydrogen ions by the kidneys, and since it might even aggravate the acidosis by further diluting the plasma bicarbonate. In an acidotic patient a solution containing some bicarbonate or a bicarbonate precursor is preferred, i.e., adding 28 mL of 7.5% sodium bicarbonate solution to 750 mL of 0.9% sodium chloride solution and increasing the final volume to 1 L with 5% dextrose in water. This solution contains 140 mEq of sodium, 115 mEq of chloride, and 25 mEq of bicarbonate/L. Similar commercial solutions containing lactate or acetate instead of bicarbonate are available but are disadvantageous in that the bicarbonate precursor may not be readily metabolized to bicarbonate in severely dehydrated patients with impaired circulation; thus therapy with these solutions may aggravate the existing acidosis.

The solution chosen for the initial phase of therapy can be started immediately even though serum electrolyte values are not known. The volume given should equal 20–30 mL/kg and be administered as rapidly as possible if there are signs of shock, or within 1 hr in less severely ill patients. If clinical signs of shock persist, a second and, rarely, a third infusion of 20–30 mL/kg may be necessary to restore circulation. Ordinarily, however, normal circulation is restored by the time 20 mL/kg has been administered, at which point the laboratory findings are usually available and one can proceed more slowly with logically planned subsequent therapy. If large volumes of fluid are administered, monitoring central venous pressure is desirable to minimize the danger of volume overload.

This therapy is equally appropriate in hypo-, iso-, and hypernatremic dehydration; the administered fluid tends to return the serum sodium toward normal in most cases. In some patients with hypernatremic dehydration, serum sodium may increase even further upon administering isotonic saline solution, the mechanism of which is unclear. However, this increase is usually 5 mEq/L or less and does not appear to affect the clinical course adversely.

Potassium should not be administered at this stage of therapy unless the patient is severely hypokalemic; it should be given only after establishing that the kidneys are functioning.

Occasionally, the therapy outlined above is inadequate to reverse shock, and blood (10 mL/kg) or other plasma volume expander is required.

Subsequent Therapy. Once circulation is restored, therapy during the remainder of the first 24 hr is aimed both at completely correcting the remaining sodium and water deficits and at replacing ongoing abnormal and normal obligatory losses. Replacement of potassium losses may be started but is not essential. Frequently, it is not attempted until after the first 24 hr. The exception is the presence of proven hypokalemia or a situation known to be associated with severe losses of potassium. Examples include the hypochloremic alkalosis of pyloric stenosis, prolonged diarrhea, or diabetes acidosis, when potassium may be administered even when pretreatment serum levels are normal or only mildly reduced. Even in such patients, however, potassium should not be administered until urine flow has been established.

By the time this phase of therapy is reached, the patient's serum electrolytes should be known and therapy can be modified, depending on the presenting serum sodium level.

Isonatremic Dehydration. In this disorder there are not only external losses of sodium from the extracellular fluid but also movement of sodium from extracellular into intracellular fluid to compensate for intracellular potassium losses. Therefore, administering sodium in an amount equal to the loss from the extracellular fluid would be excessive and would result in an increase in the patient's total body sodium; the increment of sodium in the intracellular fluid would later return to the extracellular fluid when potassium was administered, resulting in expansion of the latter compartment. To avoid this, only two thirds of the approximate losses of sodium and water from the extracellular fluid is replaced during the first 24 hr of treatment.

For example, in a patient with severe isonatremic dehydration and a 15% loss of body weight, the calculated fluid deficit would be 150 mL/kg (15% of body weight) and the sodium deficit 21 mEq/kg (assuming a serum sodium concentration of 140 mEq/L). In the first 24 hr only 100 mg/kg of water and 14 mEq/kg of sodium should be administered. Of this, 20–30 mL/kg of fluid and 3–4 mEq/kg of sodium (possibly more if the patient did not respond to this treatment) would be

administered in the first 2–3 hr as initial therapy to expand the extracellular fluid. The remaining 70–80 mL/kg of water and 10–11 mEq/kg of sodium would then be given during the ensuing 21–22 hr. The fluid used for this phase of therapy would be similar to that used in the first 2–3 hr, i.e., 0.9% saline or its equivalent, and treatment is aimed at replacing the bulk of the deficits of water and sodium.

In addition to replacing deficits, total fluid and electrolyte administration during this and subsequent phases of treatment must include replacement for both ongoing normal losses and any continuing abnormal losses such as those from diarrhea, intestinal suction, and so forth (Sec. 5.18). They are added to those needed to correct initial deficits, and thus an estimate of total requirements for the first 24 hr of treatment is obtained.

After the first 24 hr, the objective is to achieve complete replacement of sodium and water losses and to start replacing potassium losses. The sodium and water requirements at this point can be estimated by adding 25% to estimated normal maintenance requirements and by adding requirements for any ongoing abnormal losses. Potassium losses in dehydration may equal sodium losses, but potassium is lost almost exclusively from the intracellular fluid and has to be replaced by administration into the extracellular compartment. If potassium were replaced at a rate comparable to that used to replace sodium, severe hyperkalemia would almost certainly result. Thus, potassium losses are usually replaced over a 3–4 day period. Potassium should also not be administered if the serum potassium is elevated or until it is established that the kidneys are functioning. Moreover, in the presence of severe acidosis, it should be administered cautiously. Except under unusual circumstances, the concentration of potassium in the administered fluid should not exceed 40 mEq/L, and the rate of potassium administration should not exceed 3 mEq/kg/24 hr.

Hyponatremic Dehydration. This condition results from relatively greater losses of sodium than of water. The extra sodium loss can be calculated from the formula:

$$\text{Sodium deficit [mEq]} = (135 - S_{Na}) \times \text{total body water [in liters]}$$

where S_{Na} represents the serum sodium observed on admission (135 is a low normal value for serum sodium). Because the patient is dehydrated, total body water should be estimated at 50–55% of admission weight rather than as the usual value of 60%. Even though sodium is principally an extracellular cation, total body water is used for calculating sodium deficit. This allows for repletion of sodium lost from the extracellular fluid, for any expansion of the extracellular fluid that occurs with repletion, and for repletion of sodium lost from other pools of exchangeable sodium, such as that in bone.

Treatment of hyponatremic dehydration is similar to isonatremic dehydration, except that when calculating sodium administration, the extra losses of that ion should be taken into account. Administering the extra amounts of sodium needed to replace the additional losses can be spread over several days so that gradual correction of the hyponatremia is accomplished as volume is expanded. Sodium concentrations should not be abruptly elevated by administering hypertonic saline solutions unless symptoms of water intoxication, such as convulsions, are present. Symptoms rarely occur unless serum sodium levels fall below 120 mEq/L, and they are usually rapidly controlled by intravenously administering a 3% solution of sodium chloride at a rate of 1 mL/min to a maximum of 12 mL/kg of body weight. *Hypotonic solutions should be avoided, especially in the initial phase of treatment, because of the risk of inducing symptomatic hyponatremia.*

Hypernatremic Dehydration. This presents one of the more difficult problems in fluid therapy since severe hyperosmolality may result in cerebral damage, with widespread cerebral hemorrhages and thromboses or subdural effusions. This cerebral injury may result in permanent neurologic deficit. Even in the absence of such obvious pathologic lesions, seizures are common in patients with severe hypernatremia. The diagnosis of cerebral injury secondary to hypernatremia is assisted by finding an elevated protein level in the cerebrospinal fluid.

Frequently, seizures occur when the serum sodium is returning to normal owing to treatment. They may result from an increase in the sodium content of cerebral cells during the period of dehydration, which in turn results in an excessive movement of water into these cells during rehydration before excess sodium is extruded. Although the mechanism by which this water movement results in seizures is uncertain, the incidence may be reduced by correcting hypernatremia slowly over a period of days. Therefore, therapy is adjusted to return serum sodium levels toward normal by not more than 10 mEq/L/24 hr.

The sodium deficit in hypernatremic dehydration is relatively small and the extracellular fluid volume relatively well maintained so that the amounts of both sodium and water to be administered in this phase of therapy are reduced, compared with those in hypo- or isonatremic dehydration. A suitable regimen is to administer 60–75 mL/kg/24 hr of a 5% dextrose solution containing 25 mEq/L of sodium as a combination of the bicarbonate and chloride.

Amounts of maintenance fluid and sodium should be reduced by about 25% during this phase because the hypernatremic patient has high levels of antidiuretic hormone (ADH), resulting in a low volume of urine. Replacement of ongoing abnormal losses does not require modification.

If seizures do occur, they may often be controlled by intravenously administering 3–5 mL/kg of a 3% sodium chloride solution or by administering hypertonic mannitol.

Treatment of hypernatremic dehydration with large amounts of water, with or without salt, frequently results in expansion of the extracellular fluid volume before there is any notable excretion of chloride or correction of the acidosis. As a consequence, edema and cardiac failure may develop, necessitating digitalization. Hypocalcemia is also seen occasionally during treatment of hypernatremic dehydration; it may be prevented by administering appropriate amounts of potassium. Once developed, it may require intravenous administration of calcium. Another complication is renal tubular injury with azotemia and loss of concentrating ability, which may necessitate modification of the therapeutic regimen.

Although hypernatremic dehydration can be successfully treated, management is difficult and seizures frequently occur even with the best-designed regimens. It is better to emphasize prevention since this particul·rly dangerous form of dehydration is frequently iatrogenic in etiology (Sec. 5.24).

Correction of Nutritional Deficiencies. Although parenteral fluid therapy results in a caloric intake inadequate to meet the patient's needs, the inadequate calories are rarely a cause for concern because of the short periods of time usually involved. When the patient is able to return to a normal diet, any deficits in body fat and protein are soon corrected.

Should parenteral fluid therapy be required for prolonged periods (e.g., when patients are unable to eat or when they develop severe diarrhea as oral feeding is restarted), increased caloric and nutritional intake may be required to prevent the development of serious malnourishment. This intake is best given by the intravenous alimentation technique (Sec. 5.18).

Assessment of Response. Many factors modify the amounts and types of fluids to be administered. Thus, it is vitally important that the clinician monitor the response to therapy, which should include frequent clinical observation emphasizing the child's cry, degree of activity, skin turgor, and blood pressure. In addition, carefully charting intake and output, by recording stool and urine volumes separately, is valuable in assessing response to therapy, as is frequently measuring the body weight. Under certain circumstances, serially measuring serum and urine electrolytes, osmolality, and central venous pressure, as well as monitoring the electrocardiogram, may also be required. In the severely ill child, recording these serial determinations on a carefully maintained flow sheet and using them as a guide for adjusting therapy may be lifesaving. Unpredicted responses to therapy are not uncommon; hence, monitoring should be meticulous and, when indicated, appropriate modifications of the regimens should be instituted promptly.

SIMPLIFIED METHODS TO CALCULATE REQUIREMENTS

These alternative methods usually estimate deficit and maintenance needs together on the basis of the above principles. They are implemented once initial therapy for treating or preventing shock (Sec. 5.22) has been completed.

One method in widespread use expresses fluid and electrolyte requirements per unit of body surface—the *meter-squared system* (Table 5–14). The kidneys' ability to markedly regulate and to alter the excretion of water and electrolytes ensures that in health administering of fluid and electrolytes can be tolerated over wide ranges. As shown in the table, various disease states may reduce the maximum (ceiling) or increase the minimum (floor) amounts of water or electrolytes that can be tolerated. However, the average dehydrated child with functioning kidneys still has relatively large ranges of tolerance. If water and electrolytes are provided in adequate quantities within the limits of tolerance, the patients will cure themselves with renal function providing final regulation.

According to the meter-squared system, normal maintenance of water and electrolytes in older infants and children is provided by 1500 mL/m²/24 hr of a solution containing 5% dextrose, 25 mEq/L of sodium, and 20 mEq/L of potassium. This rate of administration may be increased 2- or 3-fold in dehydration or reduced in overhydration. With experience the clinician can determine fluid and electrolyte requirements using these guidelines and need not necessarily go through the several stages of calculations presented earlier. The important exceptions to this generalization are found in patients with marked renal insufficiency, craniopharyngioma, adrenal insufficiency, or other defects in the homeostatic mechanisms responsible for regulating water and sodium metabolism. In such patients severe impairment of renal or other regulatory mechanisms markedly limits the ranges of tolerance and requires that each component of fluid and electrolyte therapy be carefully calculated for the individual on a daily or even more frequent basis.

5.23 THERAPY IN SPECIFIC DISEASE STATES

5.24 DIARRHEA

See Sec. 11.8 and 12.40.

Acute. Diarrhea continues to be a serious problem in many areas of the world. It results in large losses of both water and electrolytes, especially sodium and potassium (Table 5–9), and frequently is complicated by severe systemic acidosis.

In approximately 70% of patients, the losses of water and sodium are proportionate, with *isonatremic dehydration* developing. *Hyponatremic dehydration* is seen in approximately 10%

Table 5–14. **Principles of Meter-Squared System for Determining Fluid and Electrolyte Therapy**

Substance	Range of Tolerance (in Health)	Ceiling Lowered	Floor Raised
Water	$1–13 \text{ L/m}^2/24 \text{ hr}$ (1–5 in first week of life)	General anesthesia Morphine and related drugs "Nephritis" Hypothalamic lesions Circulatory failure Neonatal period	Diabetes insipidus Nephrogenic diabetes insipidus Cellular K deficiency Na intoxication
Sodium	$5–250 \text{ mEq/m}^2/24 \text{ hr}$	Zero potassium intake Hypoalbuminemia Cardiac failure Severe stress Corticosteroid therapy Cushing syndrome Renal disease	Hypoadrenocorticism Abnormal loss of GI fluids Extensive burns Renal tubular disease (diuretic therapy)
Potassium	$10–250 \text{ mEq/m}^2/24 \text{ hr}$	Marked dehydration Circulatory failure Low Na intake Reduced GFR Hypoadrenocorticism Congenital adrenal hyperplasia	Diarrhea GI drainage High Na intake Corticosteroid therapy
Phosphorus	$0–4000 \text{ mg/m}^2/24 \text{ hr}$ (expressed as phosphorus)	Normal newborn Reduced GFR Hypoparathyroidism Pseudohypoparathyroidism Circulatory failure	Vitamin D intoxication Hyperparathyroidism
Chloride	$0–250 \text{ mEq/m}^2/24 \text{ hr}$		
Bicarbonate	$5–250 \text{ mEq/m}^2/24 \text{ hr}$		
Glucose	$50–300 \text{ g/m}^2/24 \text{ hr}$		

of all patients with diarrhea. It occurs when large amounts of electrolytes, especially sodium, are lost in the stool out of proportion to fluid losses. Thus, it is seen more frequently with bacillary dysentery or cholera. In these diseases, as opposed to diarrhea due to rotavirus, to other nonspecific (presumably virus) infections, and to many noninfectious causes, the concentration of sodium in the stool rises with increasing volume of stool. Hyponatremia may be accentuated or produced if, during the period of diarrhea, a considerable oral intake consisting of low electrolyte or electrolyte-free fluids is continued.

Disproportionately large net losses of water compared to electrolytes result in *hypernatremic dehydration*, which is seen in approximately 20% of patients with diarrhea and often results during the course of diarrhea from orally administering homemade electrolyte solutions with too high concentrations of salt. It may also occur in young infants with diarrhea if their renal ability to conserve water is limited, especially if the renal solute load is increased by feeding boiled skim milk. Such factors may be potentiated by fever, high environmental temperatures, or hyperventilation, each of which increases evaporative water loss significantly.

Using intravenous fluids for treating dehydration from severe diarrhea is discussed in Sec. 5.22. An important development in recent years has been the demonstration that dehydration from diarrhea of any etiology can be treated effectively, in a wide range of age groups, using a simple glucose-electrolyte solution given by mouth. Such oral rehydration is used in many countries and significantly reduces the mortality rate from acute diarrhea and lessens diarrhea-associated malnutrition. Patients in shock; those with severe dehydration or with uncontrollable vomiting; those with amounts of diarrhea exceeding 100 mL/kg/hr; those unable to drink because of extreme fatigue, stupor, or coma; or those with other serious complications such as severe gastric disten-

tion require intravenous therapy. However, oral rehydration can be attempted in the remainder, provided adequate supervision is available.

The composition of the oral rehydration solution (ORS) recommended by the Diarrhea Disease Control Program of the World Health Organization is shown in Table 5–15. The ingredients should be available in powder form in preweighed packages. Using teaspoons or other household items for measuring the amount of the solutes is inaccurate and not recommended. In the United States, a suitable preparation is available commercially (*Hydra-lyte*). Alternatively, an ORS with similar composition can be prepared from readily available solutions as follows: NaCl (0.9% saline solution) 390 mL; glucose (5% in water) 400 mL; KCl (2 mEq/mL) 10 mL; $NaHCO_3$ (1 mEq/mL) 30 mL; water to 1 L. Glucose is the

Table 5–15. **Comparison of Composition of Oral Solutions (mM/L)**

	WHO* (ORS)	Traditional† Solution	Reformulated†,** Solution
Sodium	90	30	50
Potassium	20	25	25
Chloride	80	25	45
Bicarbonate	30	36	30
Glucose	111	28‡	28‡

*World Health Organization oral rehydration solution composed of (g/L water): NaCl, 3.5; $NaHCO_3$, 2.5; KCl, 1.5; glucose 20.0.

†Bicarbonate usually present as a precursor such as citrate. Also contains (mEq/L): Ca, 4; Mg, 4; SO_4, 4; PO_4, 5.

**Lytren (Mead Johnson). Other solutions are similar except for sodium and chloride concentrations which range from 45 to 75 mEq/L.

‡Additional sugars provided as corn syrup to total carbohydrate content of 77 g/L.

preferred sugar for use in ORS, because its high concentration facilitates the transport of sodium across the bowel wall. Sucrose can be substituted but has a slightly lower success rate, possibly because it has to be hydrolyzed before being absorbed as glucose. The concentration of sucrose in g/L should be twice that of glucose in order to obtain the same osmolarity.

As a guideline for oral rehydration, 50 mL/kg of the ORS should be given within 4 hr to patients with mild dehydration and 100 mL/kg over 6 hr to those with moderate dehydration. The amounts and rates should be increased if the patient continues to have diarrhea or if rehydration does not appear complete; they should be decreased if the patient appears fully hydrated earlier than expected or develops periorbital edema. Breast feeding should be allowed ad libitum after treatment has been started in infants who are breast fed; in other patients, plain water should be offered. Vomiting may occur during the first 2 hr of administration of ORS but does not prevent successful oral rehydration. To reduce vomiting, the ORS should be given slowly, in small amounts at short intervals. If sustained severe vomiting occurs, intravenous therapy should be used. The patient's progress should be assessed frequently, and changes in body weight monitored, if possible, to determine the degree of rehydration.

When rehydration is complete, maintenance therapy can be started. Patients with mild diarrhea can be treated at home. Using 100 mL ORS/kg/24 hr until diarrhea stops is recommended. Breast feeds or supplemental water intake should be maintained. Those patients with more severe diarrhea require continued supervision. The volume of ORS ingested should equal the volume of stool losses. If stool volume cannot be measured, an intake of 10–15 mL ORS/kg/hr is appropriate.

This regimen has not been universally accepted. The sodium concentration of ORS (90 mM/L) is three times that of fluids (such as *Pedialyte* or *Lytren*; see Tables 5–15 and 29–8) which have traditionally been recommended for oral therapy in patients with diarrhea. These low sodium solutions were advocated because hypernatremia was seen frequently in the United States when oral electrolyte solutions with sodium concentrations of 50 mEq/L or more were used to treat infantile diarrhea. In contrast, extensive use of ORS in many developing countries has documented hypernatremia to be a rare complication, probably because ORS has been used primarily for rehydration (the major previous role for oral therapy was to prevent dehydration or for maintenance), because large amounts of water are ingested in addition to ORS, and because ORS has been administered under close supervision by trained personnel. More recently, oral rehydration has been found effective in treating acute diarrheal illnesses in well-nourished children in developed countries. Hypernatremia did not occur even when solutions containing sodium 90 mEq/L were used. Several commercially available electrolyte solutions for oral use have been reformulated with a sodium concentration increased to 50 mEq/L or higher (Table 5–15).

Occasionally, an infant receiving 2–3 liters of carbohydrate and electrolyte mixtures per day by mouth may have an apparently related increase in the volume of stools, but such instances are sufficiently rare that they do not contraindicate an initial trial of oral therapy.

It has been traditional to omit oral feedings initially when treating infants having more severe diarrhea. However, even during acute diarrhea, the small intestine can absorb a variety of nutrients and may absorb up to 60% of the food eaten. Since better weight gain has been documented in infants given a liberal dietary intake during diarrhea when compared to others on a more restricted intake, since fasting has been shown to further reduce the ability of the small intestine to absorb nutrients, and since no physiologic basis exists for giving the bowel a "rest" during acute diarrhea, regimens in developing countries for treating acute diarrhea have encouraged continuing the oral intake of nutrients. This approach may cause an increase in the volume of stool resulting in continuing large losses of fluid and electrolytes (Table 5–5), which must be replaced and may require instituting or extending parenteral therapy for several days. Despite this approach, studies have shown that rehydration occurs as rapidly with oral as with parenteral therapy in most patients.

Typically, frequency and volume of stools lessens within 48 hr in fasted patients treated with intravenous therapy. When stooling subsides, provided gastric distention and vomiting are absent, oral feeding of one of the carbohydrate and electrolyte mixtures may be initiated. As soon as oral feeding is tolerated without exacerbating the diarrhea, the caloric intake may be increased gradually by substituting mixtures that also contain fat and protein until the usual dietary intake is attained, which usually occurs within 7–8 days. Prematurely administering large quantities of calories in the form of milk may exacerbate diarrhea. In the young infant with a family history of allergy, a hypoallergenic feeding mixture is recommended for the recovery phase, since permeability of the gastrointestinal tract to whole protein may be increased during this time.

In addition to replacing the deficits of water and electrolytes, efforts should be made to obtain an etiologic diagnosis so that specific antimicrobial therapy may be given if indicated. Antibiotics are required in cases in which the diarrhea is due to cholera, shigella, amebic dysentery, or acute giardiasis. Such treatment does not modify fluid therapy. Drugs such as opiates which inhibit peristaltic activity of the bowel or absorbents such as kaolin or pectin have relatively little or no effect on the course of infantile diarrhea and are not recommended.

Diarrhea in Chronically Malnourished Children. Severe malnutrition complicated by diarrheal dehydration is common in tropical and subtropical countries and occurs occasionally in the temperate zones. Therapy should be adapted to meet the specific disturbances in body composition characteristic of the dehydrated *and* malnourished infant, in whom there appears to be an overexpansion of the intracellular space, accompanied by extracellular and presumably intracellular hypo-osmolality. Serum sodium, potassium, and magnesium levels tend to be low, and tetany may occasionally result from magnesium deficiency. Serum proteins are frequently below 3.6 gm/dL. The sodium content of muscle is high; potassium and magnesium contents are low. The electrocardiogram frequently shows tachycardia, low amplitude, and flat or inverted T waves. Cardiac reserve seems lowered, and heart failure is a common complication.

Despite clinical signs of dehydration and reduced body water, urinary osmolality may be low in the chronically malnourished child. This defect in renal concentration may result from the relative absence of urea to contribute to a hypertonic fluid in the renal papillae, a defect associated with a low dietary protein intake and resulting in a failure of tubular conservation of water. However, the GFR is low, resulting in a smaller loss of water than would otherwise be expected, and renal concentrating ability returns after several days of high-protein feedings.

Survival of the malnourished infant with diarrhea is limited by caloric deficit to a greater extent than by water and electrolyte deficit. Reparative calories can be given by slow drip through an indwelling nasogastric tube while electrolytes and water are given parenterally. If appetite is poor and vomiting and gastric distention are absent, feeding is begun early (30–40 Cal/kg/24 hr), given by slow intragastric drip. Increases to 50–100 Cal/kg/24 hr and 1–2 g of protein/kg/24 hr are made in a few days. Ad lib intake should be permitted in the succeeding weeks, up to 250-300 Cal/kg/24 hr and should include an adequate supply of iron and copper.

Initial parenteral therapy is designed to improve the circulation and to expand extracellular volume. The repair solutions recommended resemble those of hyponatremic dehydration. If edema is present, the quantity of fluid and rate of administration should be reduced from recommended levels to avoid pulmonary edema. Blood should be given if the patient is in shock, severely ill, or anemic. Potassium salts can be given early if urine output is good. Controlled trials suggest that survival can be improved by the intramuscular injection of 1.0–1.5 mL of a 50% solution of magnesium sulfate (4.0 mEq/mL) every 12 hr for 1–3 days. Clinical and electrocardiographic improvement may be more rapid with magnesium therapy, and seizures occurring during recovery from diarrhea complicating severe malnutrition may respond to magnesium.

Chronic Diarrhea. Parenteral alimentation (Sec. 5.18) may be required when diarrhea is severe and prolonged. Occasionally, this therapy must be supplemented by full oral feedings during chronic diarrhea, especially in severe malnutrition. Cow's milk protein allergy or specific disaccharidase deficiencies should be suspected in infants having persistent diarrhea. Acquired disaccharidase deficiency (especially for lactose) may develop as a complication of many chronic disorders of the gastrointestinal or other systems. Hypoallergenic feeding mixtures containing monosaccharides as the sole carbohydrate should be administered until the diarrhea ceases and nutrition improves. Specific tests of carbohydrate (disaccharide) splitting and absorption and of milk protein sensitivity can then be carried out but can be potentially dangerous, sometimes resulting in severe diarrhea with marked fluid and electrolyte losses.

Congenital Alkalosis of Gastrointestinal Origin. Rarely, chronic diarrhea may result from a congenital defect in the transport of chloride in both the small and large bowel. The watery stools of such patients have a high content of chloride, and alkalosis results from the ensuing volume depletion. Potassium is lost in the stools and in the urine, the latter losses being a consequence of the alkalosis. Treatment of fluid and electrolyte deficits is similar to that used in pyloric stenosis. Long-term therapy must provide an adequate dietary intake of potassium and chloride. A rare acute chloride-losing diarrhea may also occur.

5.25 PYLORIC STENOSIS

This condition exemplifies the correction of deficits associated with alkalosis. The therapy differs little from that for other causes of dehydration, except that potassium replacement should begin early, as soon as the child has urinated, and relatively more sodium and potassium should be given as the chloride salt than is usual in treating dehydration, partly because of the larger deficit of chloride seen in pyloric stenosis, and partly because this results in some correction of the alkalosis as volume is expanded. Correction of the hypochloremia and alkalosis by administering ammonium chloride without correcting the potassium deficit is not recommended because it results in continued dysfunction of renal tubular and other cells.

Severe depletion of intracellular potassium results in increased exchange of hydrogen ion for sodium in the distal tubules of the kidney. Thus, the paradoxic presence of an acid urine with systemic alkalosis should be interpreted as signifying a marked potassium deficit and a need to increase the amount of potassium used for repletion.

It is not uncommon for deficits to be replaced and serum levels of electrolytes returned to normal within 12 hr. However, except in the mildly ill infant without signs of dehydration, it is preferable to delay operation for at least 36–48 hr to achieve optimal readjustment of body functions. During this preparation period adequate fluid therapy prevents dehydration, and the stomach may be decompressed by gentle suction (Sec. 5.31 and 12.27).

5.26 FASTING AND THIRSTING

Parenteral fluid therapy is usually required in initially treating the infant or child who has taken little or no water and food for 1–5 days. Such infants are deficient not only in water, which has evaporated from the lungs and skin, but also in electrolytes, particularly sodium and chloride, which have been excreted in the urine (Table 5–9). Administering electrolyte-free solutions under such circumstances leads only to an increase in urine volume, with possible increased losses of electrolytes, and may actually increase the dehydration. If fasting and thirsting continue beyond 4–5 days, urinary output will fall to such low levels there will be no significant continued loss of electrolytes. Further severe deficiency of water alone will occur because of evaporative losses and will result in hypernatremia.

Therapy is begun with an isonatremic solution to produce rapid and safe expansion of extracellular volume and to improve renal function. Subsequent therapy is described in Sec. 5.22. Because relatively smaller extracellular reservoirs exist as age increases, children and adults should be given approximately one fourth to one third less water and sodium/kg than infants for a given degree of clinical dehydration. Potassium deficits are relatively the same in infants, children, and adults. Water, carbohydrate, and electrolytes may be administered to the mildly ill patient by mouth. Infants, however, often vomit when they are dehydrated, and for this reason initial therapy is usually given parenterally.

5.27 DIABETIC ACIDOSIS

See Sec. 20.1.

The deficit therapy of diabetic acidosis approximates that of other forms of dehydration. Initially, extracellular volume is expanded rapidly with Ringer lactate or 0.9% NaCl. The balance of the replacement therapy is carried out slowly over the remainder of the first 24 hr. The early administration of carbohydrate permits glycogenation of the liver after response to insulin and reduces the danger of hypoglycemia. During the early stages of treatment of children with severe ketoacidosis, serum electrolytes, pH, blood gases, and blood sugar may have to be monitored at regular 4 hr intervals.

5.28 BURNS

Maintenance requirements for water are diminished when a large area of burned skin is covered by wet dressings that limit evaporative losses from this site; evaporation from the lungs is normal or increased. Urinary output of water is probably limited by some antidiuresis resulting from massive stimulation of nerve receptors. Thus, the fluid therapy of burns is principally concerned with replacing abnormal losses. Some of these losses are external, such as oozing of plasma from the burned surface, but the largest part of the abnormal loss is *internal* in the form of plasma and plasma ultrafiltrate sequestered around the burn site. After 48 hr, the sequestered fluid may then return to the vascular compartment, producing acute pulmonary edema, particularly if there has been thermal injury to the lungs. See Sec. 5.44 for full discussion of treatment.

5.29 SALICYLATE POISONING

The treatment of salicylate intoxication exemplifies the importance of supplemental therapy in which water and electrolytes are given above the usual needs, even in the absence of specific deficits, to facilitate excretion of the drug. Also see Sec. 28.5.

Initially, high blood concentrations of salicylate sensitize the respiratory center to carbon dioxide. The resultant hyperventilation, with its characteristic marked prolongation of the expiratory phase of respiration, leads to increased evaporative losses of water and to respiratory alkalosis, for which the kidneys compensate by excreting large amounts of sodium and potassium bicarbonate. In addition, toxic levels of salicylate uncouple oxidative phosphorylation and may reduce hepatic glycogen, usually resulting in ketonemia and ketonuria. Hyperglycemia and glycosuria are common; hypoglycemia may be seen occasionally.

The loss of sodium and potassium in excess of chloride and the accumulation of acetoacetic and beta-hydroxybutyric acids eventually produce severe metabolic acidosis, which is aggravated by the release of two moles of free hydrogen ion from each mole of aspirin absorbed and hydrolyzed. Thus, a dose of salicylate of 200 mg/kg adds an acute hydrogen ion load of 2 mEq/kg. Transition from respiratory alkalosis to a mixed disturbance of acid-base balance with severe metabolic acidosis complicated by respiratory alkalosis may be relatively rapid; therefore, therapy must be followed by periodic monitoring of the serum carbon dioxide content and the pH of the blood and urine.

Except in poisoning due to repeated therapeutic administration of salicylates, the significance of an isolated blood salicylate level depends in part on the interval between the time the drug was ingested and the time the blood sample was obtained; a level of 35 mg/dL 36 hr after an acute ingestion or after the start of aspirin therapy may be more significant than a level of 60 mg/dL 2 hr after acute ingestion when peak levels may be expected. Fig. 5–9 can help determine the

severity of an acute overdose, given the serum salicylate level and the time since ingestion.

In chronic ingestion it should be remembered that even though a salicylate level of 35 mg/dL may be required to obtain therapeutic benefits in older children, fatal cases of salicylism have occurred in infants with lower blood levels; the need for active treatment depends only in part on blood levels of salicylate and on whether the overdose is acute or chronic. Clinical factors are equally important. Coma, convulsions, marked hyperventilation, oliguria, respiratory depression, severe azotemia, or marked reduction in the plasma level of bicarbonate or pCO_2 indicates the need for active therapeutic intervention.

Treatment is designed to prevent further absorption of salicylate, to correct deficits and replace ongoing losses of fluids and electrolytes (which are increased above normal), and to reduce tissue levels of salicylate by facilitating excretion of the drug.

The efficacy of attempting to empty the gastrointestinal tract of salicylate is controversial. However, in the absence of central nervous system depression, gastric emptying can be attempted for up to 10 hr following ingestion of the salicylate. Syrup of ipecac (dose in children over 1 yr of age: 1 tablespoon [15 mL] repeated after 20 min if vomiting does not occur) is probably still the most effective emetic, and a slurry of activated charcoal can be given later in an attempt to prevent further absorption of any remaining salicylate from the bowel. If the patient is in shock, an isonatremic solution is indicated to expand plasma volume; otherwise a hyponatremic solution can be used to replace fluid and electrolyte deficits.

The amount of fluid required ranges in individual patients from 2000 to 5500 mL/m²/24 hr. This fluid should contain sodium, 40–50 mEq/L, some of which should be sodium bicarbonate, and, if there is adequate renal function, potassium, to 40 mEq/L. Oral potassium salts may be used to supplement the intravenous therapy. Administering carbohydrate appears to improve prognosis; intravenous fluids should contain at least 5% glucose.

Treatment is designed to replace maintenance losses of fluids and electrolytes, which may be twice normal owing to increased evaporative losses, to replace deficits, and to maintain a diuresis to facilitate excretion of salicylate. A urine volume of at least 2000 mL/m²/24 hr with a specific gravity of less than 1.010 is a reasonable goal. The early administration of sodium bicarbonate to maintain an alkaline urine (pH higher than 7.5) facilitates excretion of salicylate by reducing its back-diffusion in ionized form from tubular urine through the lipid membranes of the renal tubular cells; the clearance of salicylate with a urine pH greater than 8.0 is 20 times that at a urine pH of 6.0. The dose of bicarbonate necessary to alkalinize the urine is approximately 2 mEq/kg, given over 1 hr. An additional 2 mEq/kg of sodium bicarbonate should be given if urine pH does not reach 7.0. The urinary pH should then be checked every 30 min. If the pH falls below 7.0, additional sodium bicarbonate should be given with appropriate amounts of potassium to avoid renal tubular potassium depletion and paradoxic aciduria.

Acetazolamide (5 mg/kg repeated 2–3 times in 24 hr) will also increase salicylate excretion; this therapy has not received general acceptance because of reported complications, including seizures, and an increased mortality in experimental animals. Peritoneal dialysis or hemodialysis should be considered for severely ill patients as a means for removing additional amounts of salicylate loosely bound to plasma proteins. Such patients include those with blood levels of salicylate above 100 mg/dL, those with an elevated pCO_2, those with severe acidosis, or those who have failed to respond adequately to alkalinization. The efficiency of dialysis is increased by the addition of albumin to the dialysis fluid. Exchange

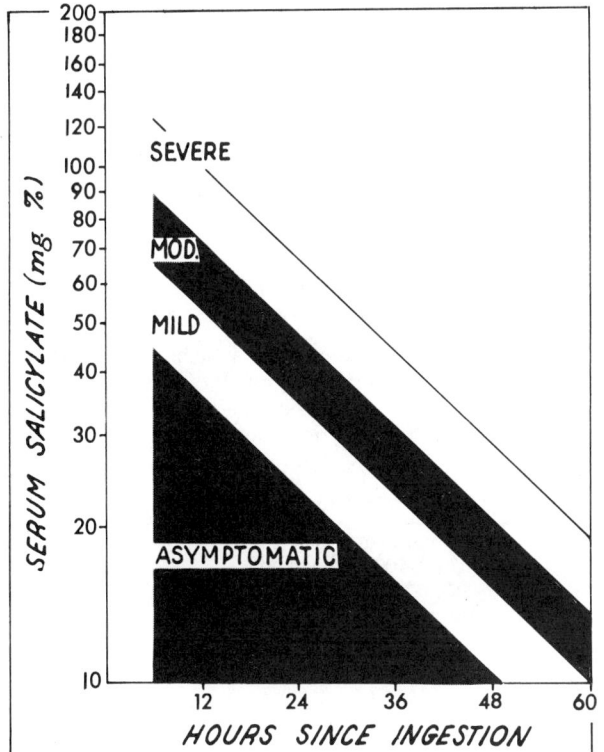

Figure 5–9. Nomogram relating serum salicylate concentration and expected severity of intoxication at varying intervals following the ingestion of a single dose of salicylate. (From Done AK: Pediatrics 26:800, 1960.)

transfusion is a relatively inefficient means of removing salicylate in the critically ill patient. If done, heparinized blood should be used because of the often lethal exacerbation of acidosis if citrated blood is used.

Vitamin K_1 oxide (Konakion) should be given intramuscularly to offset possible prothrombin deficiency.

5.30 ELECTROLYTE DISTURBANCES ASSOCIATED WITH CENTRAL NERVOUS SYSTEM DISORDERS

Diseases of the central nervous system are frequently associated with disturbances in sodium concentration. Three types of changes have been described:

1. Patients with diverse lesions, such as surgical or traumatic damage to the brain, encephalitis, bulbar poliomyelitis, cerebrovascular accidents, tumors of the 4th ventricle, and subdural hematomas, may lose large amounts of sodium in the urine. Dehydration, hypotension, and azotemia result unless large amounts of salt are administered and the intake of water is limited.

2. Patients with tuberculous meningitis who are severely ill and comatose are frequently hyponatremic but exhibit no symptoms that can be attributed to hyponatremia. This situation may be analogous to the asymptomatic hyponatremia of severe malnutrition or pulmonary disease. Relatively large amounts of salt may be lost in the urine when attempts are made to correct the hyponatremia by salt loading. Careful clinical and laboratory observations are essential to ensure that salt depletion and water intoxication do not occur. Potassium should be administered in amounts at least 50% greater than with usual maintenance therapy.

3. Patients with acute infections of the central nervous system occasionally have symptoms of acute water intoxication, with a rapid fall in serum sodium. These patients retain an excessive amount of water and have increased thirst. Convulsions are severe and resistant to drug therapy but respond to the intravenous administration of hypertonic saline solution and subsequent restriction of fluid.

These disorders may result from lesions involving the thirst center, osmoreceptors, or supraopticohypophyseal tract or from inappropriate secretion of ADH or other lesions.

Convulsions or other symptoms from cerebral edema may respond to hypertonic mannitol solution, although care in its administration should be taken in patients with impaired renal function.

5.31 PREOPERATIVE, INTRAOPERATIVE, AND POSTOPERATIVE FLUIDS

See Sec. 5.45–5.49.

Preoperatively preparing a patient having no pre-existing deficit or in whom the deficit has been repaired consists mainly in supplying carbohydrate to ensure adequate storage of glycogen in the liver. Usual maintenance requirements of water and electrolytes are appropriate. Small infants who are not vomiting should receive carbohydrate and sodium chloride mixtures by mouth until 3 hr before operation. Such fluids are readily absorbed from the gastrointestinal tract and will not produce aspiration pneumonitis if vomited and aspirated.

Preoperatively preparing the newborn involves certain unique hazards. Deficits of water and electrolytes from vomiting or from stasis owing to intestinal obstruction should be replaced before operating. If aspiration pneumonitis is suspected, it should be treated with antibiotics. Nasogastric suction may be inadequate. If so, *gastrostomy* should be performed to aid in decompression and in postoperative feeding. In intestinal obstruction conjugated bilirubin may be deglucuronidated by intestinal enzymes; an enterohepatic circulation of unconjugated bilirubin can then lead to high serum levels and kernicterus. Hypoprothrombinemia should be prevented by administering 1.0 mg of vitamin K_1 oxide.

The most common error in administering parenteral fluid during and after surgery is overadministration, particularly of dextrose in water. Table 5–16 lists maintenance water requirements during surgery. Additional amounts of blood, plasma, saline, or other volume expander must be given if blood loss or tissue trauma is significant. The magnitude of such losses is judged best by the experienced surgeon as he or she operates.

Under most circumstances no potassium should be administered during this time, since extensive tissue trauma or anoxia may result in the release of large amounts of intracellular potassium with the potential of causing hyperkalemia. Moreover, if shock occurs, it may be complicated by acute renal failure, making treatment of the hyperkalemia more difficult.

Postoperatively, intake should be limited for 24 hr. Thereafter, usual maintenance therapy is gradually resumed. The water intake should not exceed 85 mL/100 kcal metabolized because of antidiuresis resulting from trauma or circulatory readjustment unless renal capacity to concentrate the urine is limited (e.g., in sickle cell anemia). If the intake of water is not limited, whether given parenterally or by mouth, water intoxication may result. Maintenance sodium intake should also be low because of the low caloric expenditure during anesthesia and postoperatively.

5.32 THERAPY OF ISOLATED DISTURBANCES IN CONCENTRATIONS OF ELECTROLYTES

Acidosis. *Respiratory acidosis*, in which the pH may be markedly lowered, primarily as a result of retention of carbon dioxide, may be seen with severe respiratory insufficiency, with respiratory distress syndrome in the newborn infant,

Table 5–16. **Approximate Requirements of Water Without Electrolytes During Operation**

Weight (kg)	Basal kcal/24 Hr	Evap. Water mL/hr (90 mL/100 kcal/24 hr)*	Urine Water, mL/hr (30 mL/100 kcal/24 hr)†	Total‡ mL/hr
3	150	6	2	8
5	270	10	3	13
7	410	15	5	20
10	550	21	7	28
20	850	32	10	42
30	1100	41	14	55
40	1300	49	16	65

From Harned HS Jr, Cooke RE: Surg Gynecol Obstet *104*:543, 1957. By permission.
*This value is assumed to be high because of possible sweating and hyperventilation.
†This value is assumed to be low because of probable antidiuresis.
‡Does not include abnormal losses of fluid (hemorrhage, wound edema, suction) which must be replaced by appropriate electrolyte-containing fluids.

and in patients receiving assisted ventilation for any reason. Mild metabolic acidosis may also exist because hypoxia leads to the accumulation of lactic and other organic acids in the extracellular fluid. Measurements of blood pH and gases should guide correction of acidosis. The appropriate treatment is to improve ventilation by assisting respiration rather than by administering sodium bicarbonate, which may produce hyperosmolality and cardiac failure.

Metabolic acidosis, resulting, for example, from renal tubular acidosis or from accumulation of organic acids, may require the administration of alkali, especially if symptoms are evident. In lactic acidosis, in glycogen disorders, or in circulatory insufficiency and hypoxia, sodium lactate may not be adequately metabolized; in these situations sodium bicarbonate is the preferred agent. The usual initial dose is 1–2 mEq/kg. However, a more precise estimate of the dosage required is given by the general formula

$$(C_d - C_a) \times f_d \times \text{body weight in kg} = \text{mEq required}$$

where C_d and C_a represent, respectively, the serum bicarbonate concentration desired and the one actually present, expressed as mEq/L; and f_d represents that fraction of the total body weight in which the administered material is apparently (not actually) distributed (the value for f_d varies with the substance administered). The f_d for bicarbonate or potential bicarbonate approximates 0.5–0.6. Such calculations indicate that 0.5 mL/kg of a molar solution of sodium bicarbonate would raise the serum bicarbonate concentration approximately 1 mEq/L. However, responses to administered bicarbonate vary widely, since it may be sequestered in bone or muscle or lost in urine.

With glomerular insufficiency, acidosis must be corrected cautiously, because the sodium administered with bicarbonate may result in further expansion of the extracellular fluid volume. It is rarely necessary to attempt to increase serum bicarbonate levels above 15 mEq/L unless the patient continues to be markedly symptomatic from the acidosis. Overcorrecting acidosis also may be complicated by tetany. If hyperphosphatemia coexists with acidosis, it should be treated simultaneously with low phosphate diets and oral aluminum gels.

Treating with sodium bicarbonate should always be considered a temporizing measure; every attempt should be made to treat the underlying cause, e.g., using glucose and insulin in diabetic ketoacidosis, improving circulation in shock, or eliminating salicylates, methanol, or other toxins.

Alkalosis. Normally the kidney has an enormous capacity to excrete bicarbonate, and increased amounts of blood bicarbonate are promptly excreted. However, under certain circumstances, *metabolic alkalosis* may develop and be maintained. Typically, it is caused by the administration of excess amounts of alkali, by the loss of hydrogen ion, or by volume contraction with disproportionate losses of chloride. Severe hypokalemia can result in alkalosis, too, or may perpetuate it.

Plasma bicarbonate is elevated and respiratory compensation results in hypoventilation and an increase in pCO_2. Rarely, respiration may be so depressed in infants with severe hypochloremic alkalosis that blood oxygenation is diminished. Severe alkalotic tetany may also occur. In such instances, administering ammonium chloride may effect symptomatic improvement; the dose may be calculated from the general formula presented above, with the probable f_d being 0.2–0.3. Such therapy relieves only symptoms and should not be used in place of correcting the contracted volume of body fluids or administering potassium chloride to repair intracellular deficits.

Metabolic alkalosis associated with volume contraction responds to measures designed to expand volume and replace the chloride and potassium deficits. It occurs in patients with acid-base disorders due to vomiting, gastric suction, congenital chloride diarrhea, dietary chloride deficiency, or administration of diuretics. Their urinary chloride concentration is low (10 mM/L or less). A minority of patients are "chloride-resistant" with urinary chloride concentrations of 15 mM/L or greater owing to hyperadrenalism, Bartter syndrome, severe potassium depletion, or licorice ingestion. Potassium repletion and specific therapy directed to the underlying condition is indicated.

Respiratory alkalosis occurs in salicylate intoxication; in various central nervous system diseases such as trauma, infection, or tumors; with anxiety or fever; and in congestive heart failure, hepatic insufficiency, and gram-negative septicemia. Treatment should be directed at removing the underlying cause, although measures designed to return pCO_2 to normal may be indicated. Acidifying agents such as ammonium chloride are not indicated.

Hyponatremia. Serum sodium is most commonly reduced as a result of either sodium depletion or water "intoxication" or a combination of both (Table 5–17). A low serum sodium, thought to be due to redistribution of total body sodium, may also occur in association with severe illnesses or in the terminally ill patient. In addition, *apparent* hyponatremia may be observed as an artifact, e.g., in diabetic ketoacidosis when the water content of plasma is reduced by the presence of

Table 5–17. Clinical States Complicated by Hyponatremia

Expansion of extracellular space by water
  Excessive intake
    Parenteral fluid therapy — glucose in water
    Oral (with diminished output)
    Tap water enemas
    Allergy to cow's milk (very rare)
  Diminished output (usual intake)
    Renal
      Intrinsic: nephritis, nephrotic syndrome, tubular necrosis, prematurity
      Extrinsic
        Excess of antidiuretic hormone: acute and chronic central nervous system disease, vasopressin therapy, surgery, pulmonary disease
        Circulatory: heart failure, cardiovascular surgery, malnutrition
    Skin: premature infant in high humidity
Deficiency of extracellular sodium
  Inadequate intake
    Low salt diet
    Parenteral therapy with glucose in water
  Excessive losses
    Gastrointestinal: vomiting, salivary, gastric, biliary, pancreatic drainage, diarrhea, resin therapy, tap water enemas (especially in megacolon)
    Genitourinary
      Intrinsic renal disease: chronic nephritis, acute tubular necrosis (recovery phase), nephrotic syndrome (diuresis)
      Extrinsic influences: diuretics, acetazolamide, hypoadrenalism, central nervous system disease (rare), expanded volume (Pitressin, excessive water therapy)
    Skin
      Normal sweat
      Abnormal sweat: cystic fibrosis, adrenal insufficiency
      Burn therapy with silver nitrate (hypochloremia)
    Cerebrospinal fluid
      Draining myelomeningocele
      Arachnoureterostomy
      Continuous drainage of CSF, e.g., in lead encephalopathy
    Parenteral: thoracentesis, paracentesis, burns
  Redistribution
    Severe malnutrition
    Potassium deficiency
    Trauma

increased quantities of lipids. This error is avoided by laboratory methods that determine sodium activity rather than concentration.

Patients with a serum sodium below 120 mEq/L are usually symptomatic (i.e., convulsions, shock); those with lesser degrees of hyponatremia are frequently asymptomatic. Treatment of *asymptomatic hyponatremia* depends on its cause. With water overload, fluid restriction is the appropriate measure; serum sodium may return rapidly to normal if there is good renal function but may take several days or weeks with the inappropriate ADH syndrome. When sodium deficits are present, adding extra salt to the diet or increasing the sodium concentration of parenterally administered fluid often corrects the deficit. Measuring urine sodium concentration helps to determine the cause of hyponatremia. Typically with sodium depletion, urine sodium concentration is 10 mEq/L or less, although such low values are also found in nephrotic syndrome, congestive heart failure, or hepatic failure. Expansion of the extracellular fluid with water or renal tubular injury results in a higher urinary sodium concentration (around 50 mEq/L). The wrong treatment will not correct the defect and may be detrimental. For example, administering sodium to a patient with hyponatremia due to water excess, such as that seen with the chronic edema of heart failure, nephrotic syndrome, or cirrhosis, may result only in further expanding the extracellular fluid without correcting the serum sodium.

Treatment of *symptomatic hyponatremia* consists of administering a hypertonic saline solution, calculated according to the formula in the preceding section on acidosis, with C representing serum sodium rather than bicarbonate. Since there is osmotic equilibrium between cells and extracellular water, changes in osmolality are distributed over total body water so that the value for f_d should be 0.6–0.7. A dose of 12 mL/kg of body weight of 3% sodium chloride solution (6 mEq sodium/kg) usually raises the serum sodium approximately 10 mEq/L. Elevation of the sodium concentration should be effected in small increments (5–10 mEq/L) over 1–4 hr.

Hypernatremia. The treatment of hypernatremic dehydration was discussed in Sec. 5.22. It may also result from faulty preparation of infant formulas: using condensed instead of evaporated milk or using heaped or packed instead of level measures of milk powder. These errors increase the solute load to be excreted by the kidney relative to the amount of water provided and may result in an osmotic diuresis and negative water balance. The accidental ingestion of excessive amounts of sodium chloride *(salt poisoning)* also may result in hypernatremia with serious residuals. The accidental substitution of salt for cane sugar in private homes and institutions occurs with sufficient frequency to justify the routine use of liquid sugars in infant feeding. The excessive intake of sodium is accompanied by increases in total body sodium and in the volume of extracellular water. Severe acidosis results from a shift of organic acids and free hydrogen ions to extracellular fluid. With shift of water from brain cells, distention of cerebral vessels occurs, leading to subdural, subarachnoid, and intracerebral hemorrhage. The complications and residuals of salt poisoning are similar to, but may be more severe than, those seen with hypernatremic dehydration.

Treatment is directed toward the rapid removal of excess sodium from the body. Intravenous fluids should consist of glucose in water, potassium acetate, and calcium as needed. *Intermittent peritoneal dialysis* with glucose solutions can remove large quantities of sodium, correcting the hyperosmolality without the danger of pulmonary edema and heart failure. Approximately 45 mL/kg of a dialysis solution containing 4.25% glucose can be injected intraperitoneally for severe hypernatremia (serum sodium concentration more than 200 mEq/L) and withdrawn 1 hr later. As the concentration of sodium in the serum falls, subsequent dialysis may be carried out using a solution with 1.5% glucose so as not to remove too much water and dehydrate the patient. Exchange transfusion is not a substitute for dialysis, because enormous quantities of blood would be required to effect a change in osmolality of total body water. Phenobarbital should be administered to prevent or control seizures. Digitalization may be necessary to counteract heart failure.

Hypokalemia. Disturbances in the potassium concentration occurring without changes in volume of body fluids have been described in primary hyperaldosteronism and in Bartter syndrome. Large amounts of potassium are lost in the urine, resulting in low serum potassium and high serum bicarbonate concentrations. In congenital alkalosis of gastrointestinal origin, large amounts of potassium and chloride are lost in the stools. Using thiazide and loop diuretics (e.g., ethacrynic acid and furosemide) causes kaliuresis and natriuresis; prolonged use may result in significant potassium loss and hypokalemia.

Severe hypokalemia may result in weakness of skeletal muscles, decreased peristalsis, ileus, and an inability of the kidney to concentrate urine. Prolonged hypokalemia results in characteristic pathologic changes in the kidney and a decrease in function, which may persist even after potassium repletion.

Treatment consists of administration of large amounts of potassium (usually up to 3 mEq/kg/24 hr); in Bartter syndrome up to 10 mEq/kg may have to be given orally.

Hyperkalemia. Marked elevation of the serum potassium results in ventricular fibrillation and death. Levels above 6.5 mEq/L should be treated promptly. The possibility of orally or parenterally administering excessive amounts of potassium should be considered and all potassium intake discontinued. The rapid intravenous administration of sodium bicarbonate (up to 2 mEq/kg over a 5–10 min period) or glucose and insulin (0.5 g glucose/kg with 0.3 unit crystalline insulin/g of glucose, given over a 2 hr period) will result in the intracellular movement of potassium and will lower serum potassium. Intravenous calcium gluconate (up to 0.5 mL of a 10% solution/kg given over 2–4 min) will counter the cardiac toxicity of potassium, but the ECG should be monitored while it is being administered. None of these measures removes significant quantities of potassium from the patient; they are temporizing measures until negative potassium balance is established by the use of ion exchange resins (Kayexalate, 1 g/kg/24 hr, in divided oral doses twice daily or as a retention enema), by hemodialysis, or by peritoneal dialysis.

Hypocalcemia and **hypercalcemia** are discussed in Sec. 3.29, 5.10, 5.34, 8.54, and 19.18.

Hypomagnesemia. The importance of magnesium in intravenous therapy is reviewed in Sec. 5.11 and 5.24. The only definitive symptom complex associated with hypomagnesemia (serum magnesium less than 1.3 mEq/L) is that of latent or manifest tetany. Convulsions, muscular twitching, disorientation, athetoid movements, carpopedal spasm, and hyper-reactivity to mechanical and auditory stimulation have been observed. Lowered serum concentrations and whole body deficits of magnesium are found in chronic diarrhea or vomiting, sprue, celiac disease, prolonged parenteral fluid therapy, and hyperaldosteronism. Low serum magnesium levels have been observed in infantile tetany, presumably on the basis of transient hypoparathyroidism. The intramuscular injection of 0.1 mL of a 24% solution of $MgSO_4 \cdot 7H_2O$ (0.2 mEq/kg) repeated every 6 hr for three to four doses produces symptomatic and biochemical improvement. Adding 3 mEq/L of magnesium to maintenance fluids for patients requiring long-term therapy may decrease the chance of serious deficiency. See Sec. 8.54.

Hypermagnesemia. Levels of serum magnesium higher

than 10 mEq/L are accompanied by drowsiness and, occasionally, coma. Deep tendon reflexes may also be abolished, and respiratory depression may occur at higher concentrations. Disturbances in atrioventricular and intraventricular conduction may be detected at levels of 5 mEq/L. Acute renal failure and Addison disease are accompanied by significantly elevated serum magnesium. Iatrogenic poisoning can result from using magnesium in treating hypertension or toxemia of pregnancy; deaths have been reported from using magnesium sulfate enemas in megacolon and from orally administering it for purging.

Intravenously administering calcium gluconate rapidly reverses the depressant effects of hypermagnesemia as well as the associated cardiac abnormalities.

PARENTERAL SOLUTIONS

Table 29–8 lists some solutions commercially available for use in fluid therapy. The many carbohydrate and electrolyte mixtures available permit great flexibility and individualization of therapy.

ALAN M. ROBSON

Darrow DC, Pratt EL: Fluid therapy: Relation to tissue composition and expenditure of water and electrolyte. JAMA 154:365, 1950.
Feliciano DV, Telander RL: Total parenteral nutrition in infants and children. Mayo Clin Proc 51:647, 1976.
Fomon SJ (ed): Infant Nutrition. 2nd ed. Philadelphia, WB Saunders, 1974.
Harris F: Pediatric Fluid Therapy. Philadelphia, FA Davis, 1972.
Levine MM, Pizarro D: Advances in therapy of diarrheal dehydration: Oral rehydration. Adv Pediatr 31:207, 1984.
Nalin DR, Levine MM, Mata L, et al: Oral rehydration and maintenance of children with rotavirus and bacterial diarrheas. Bull WHO 57:453, 1979.
Santosham M, Daum RS, Dillman L, et al: Oral rehydration therapy of infantile diarrhea. N Engl J Med 306:1070, 1982.
Segar WE: Parenteral Fluid Therapy. Current Problems in Pediatrics. Chicago, Year Book Medical Publishers, 1972.
Weil WB: A unified guide to parenteral fluid therapy. J Pediatr 75:1, 1969.
WHO Treatment and prevention of dehydration in diarrheal diseases. Guide for use of primary health care personnel. Scientific Publication No. 336, 1977.
Winters RW (ed): Principles of Pediatric Fluid Therapy. 2nd ed. Boston, Little, Brown, and Co, 1982.
Wu PYK (ed): Fluid balance in the newborn infant. Clin Perinatol 9:645, 1982.

5.33 TETANY

Tetany, the state of hyperexcitability of the central and peripheral nervous systems, results from abnormal concentrations of ions in the fluid bathing nerve cells. These abnormalities may be decreases of H^+ (alkalosis), of Ca^{++}, or of Mg^{++}. Decrease of H^+ may precipitate tetany when concentrations of Ca^{++} or Mg^{++} may otherwise lie above the threshold for manifest tetany. A decrease of K^+ can prevent tetany despite low Ca^{++} concentrations, but a rising K^+ can precipitate tetany in a' patient with low Ca^{++}. Hypomagnesemic tetany, on the other hand, can occur despite reduction of K^+ concentration. Thus, a range of ionic concentrations exists at which tetany can be either latent or manifest.

The serum calcium, as usually measured, includes both Ca^{++} and undissociated calcium proteinate; albumin is the chief serum protein to form a complex with calcium. Ca^{++} can be measured, but the procedure is unavailable in most clinical laboratories. At normal concentrations of serum albumin about 40–50% of the total calcium is ionized, i.e., 4.0–5.2 mg/dL. When serum albumin is reduced, total serum calcium is decreased without a decrease in Ca^{++}; a rule of thumb states that with each decrease of 1 g/dL of albumin, a decrease of 0.8 mg/dL of calcium results. A nephrotic child with a serum albumin level of 1 g/dL might, therefore, be expected to have a total serum calcium concentration of 7.5–8.0 mg/dL without reduction of Ca^{++}.

At physiologic concentrations of H^+ and K^+, tetany may develop at Ca^{++} concentrations of less than 3.0 mg/dL and will almost always be manifest at Ca^{++} concentrations less than 2.5 mg/dL. At normal concentrations of serum albumin, these levels correspond to total serum calcium concentrations of approximately 7 mg/dL and 5 mg/dL, respectively.

The normal level of magnesium in serum ranges between 1.6 and 2.6 mg/dL, of which about 75% is Mg^{++}. Total serum magnesium reduced to less than 1.0 mg/dL may be associated with hyperexcitability of the nervous system.

Manifest Tetany. The classic signs of peripheral hyperexcitability of motor nerves are spasms of the muscles of the wrists and ankles (carpopedal spasm) and of the vocal cords (laryngospasm). In *carpopedal spasm* the wrists are flexed, the fingers extended, the thumbs adducted over the palms, the feet extended and adducted. These muscular spasms can be quite painful. *Laryngospasm* causes inspiratory obstruction accompanied by a high-pitched inspiratory crow; apnea may result. The sensory manifestations are paresthesias, particularly numbness and tingling of the hands and feet. Motor excitability of the central nervous system may be manifested by often brief but recurrent convulsions which are usually generalized but may be localized to one side of the body. Between seizures the patient may be apparently conscious, but after a prolonged series of convulsions a postictal state may result. In young infants convulsions are frequently the only evidence of the nervous system's hyperexcitability.

Latent Tetany. This is the condition in which ischemia or mechanical or electrical stimulation of motor nerves is required to produce the motor response characteristic of tetany. Carpopedal spasm may be induced in latent tetany through the production of ischemia of the motor nerves by reducing the arterial blood supply with a tourniquet (*Trousseau sign*); a blood pressure cuff on the arm is inflated above the systolic blood pressure for 3 min. Motor nerve impulses can be elicited by mechanical tapping, but under normal physiologic conditions this is not possible. The facial nerve can be stimulated by tapping anterior to the external auditory meatus. Contraction of the orbicularis oris occurs with a twitch of the upper lip or entire mouth (*Chvostek sign*). The peroneal nerve can be stimulated by tapping the place where it passes over the head of the fibula; a positive *peroneal sign* is dorsiflexion and abduction of the foot.

The motor nerves can also be stimulated electrically. *Erb sign* is a positive response of motor nerves to electrical stimulation by galvanic currents of amperage less than that required for their stimulation under normal physiologic conditions.

Another manifestation of reduced Ca^{++} concentrations is a prolonged Q-T interval for a given heart rate on the electrocardiogram.

Alkalotic Tetany. This is very rare in infants and young children. Tetany can be induced through spontaneous overventilation, producing respiratory alkalosis; such hyperventilation is most often of psychogenic origin. The treatment of alkalotic tetany due to spontaneous hyperventilation is to have the patient rebreathe into a bag or balloon to increase pCO_2. In patients with low Ca^{++} concentrations tetany may be precipitated by overventilation or by a metabolic alkalosis following administration of sodium bicarbonate, but the metabolic alkalosis resulting from loss of gastric juice owing to pyloric obstruction is rarely associated with tetany. Alkalotic tetany has occurred in patients with renal disease who have been protected by concurrent metabolic acidosis from the consequences of low Ca^{++} concentration; correcting the acidosis has caused tetany and convulsions.

5.34 HYPOCALCEMIC TETANY

Disorders of Parathyroid Function. The most common disorder of parathyroid function is transient physiologic hypoparathyroidism of the newborn infant, sometimes referred to as *neonatal hypocalcemia*. Clinically, these infants can be separated into two groups, one group with hypocalcemia during the first 36 hr of life, usually before achieving a significant oral intake of milk, and a second group with hypocalcemia due to high phosphate load, which develops only after receiving cow's milk for a number of days. The onset of symptoms in the second group occurs most commonly during the first 5–10 days of life; clinical manifestations have occasionally appeared as late as 6 wk of age. Both forms presumably result from physiologically inactive parathyroid glands that fail to respond normally to low Ca^{++} concentrations. Serum calcium values correlate directly with gestational age, and less mature infants have a greater chance of developing hypocalcemia.

Besides a relative lack of parathyroid hormone output in the newborn period, a partial refractoriness of the target cells to parathyroid hormone may exist. Moreover, excessive secretion of thyrocalcitonin may be a major contributing factor in persistent hypocalcemia of premature infants, particularly those stressed by anoxia. The low birthweight infant whose mother has had an inadequate intake of vitamin D and little exposure to sunshine also has a low plasma concentration of 25-hydroxy vitamin D_3, the deficiency of which is associated with relative refractoriness to parathyroid hormone.

The relative hypoparathyroidism of the newborn has been attributed to the increased serum calcium of the fetus, which reflects a calcium gradient across the placenta. In addition, this inhibition of the fetal parathyroids by calcium ion may be augmented by mild maternal hyperparathyroidism. Physiologic hyperparathyroidism, indicated by increased parathyroid hormone levels found during pregnancy, may occur more intensely in diabetic women. Occasional cases of infant transient hypoparathyroidism have been associated with maternal clinical hyperparathyroidism.

Early Hypocalcemia. The infants at greatest risk are low birthweight infants, especially those with intrauterine growth retardation; infants born of diabetic mothers; and infants who have been subjected to prolonged, difficult deliveries. Calcium intake may also be decreased owing to the infant's small size or to illness, and endogenous phosphate may be increased from catabolism. The incidence of hypocalcemia in prematurely born infants is extremely high, particularly in those with respiratory distress and those who have received intravenous sodium bicarbonate. Evaluating the role of hypocalcemia in the morbidity and mortality of such infants is difficult. Although hypocalcemia should be suspected as a possible cause of convulsions, it can be diagnosed only by determining serum calcium concentrations.

Asymptomatic hypocalcemia of premature infants usually resolves spontaneously. However, when possible, oral calcium gluconate should be given, since it usually obviates the subsequent need for intravenous therapy and its attendant complications.

Treatment requires the intravenous injection of 10% calcium gluconate in a dose of about 2 mL/kg (18 mg Ca/kg), which must be given slowly, while monitoring the cardiac rate for bradycardia; blood containing excessive calcium concentration that reaches the right auricle may inhibit the rhythmic electrical activity of the sinus node, causing cardiac arrest. Tissue necrosis and calcification may occur if this solution extrava-

sates or is given intramuscularly. The intravenous dose of calcium gluconate can be repeated at 6–8 hr intervals until calcium homeostasis becomes stable, or the calcium gluconate (75 mg elemental Ca/kg/24 hr) can be added to a constant intravenous infusion. Administering either 1,25-dihydroxy vitamin D_3 or 25-hydroxy vitamin D_3 in the first day of life to prematurely born infants at risk for hypocalcemia has successfully prevented or reduced the severity and duration of hypocalcemia, but neither is recommended for routine prevention. If hypomagnesemia is present, it usually also requires treatment before hypocalcemia responds to therapy. Calcium gluconate or calcium lactate also may be added to the feeding (see below) at the same time. There may be a gradual return to normal calcium levels after 1–3 days. Oral calcium should be continued for about 1 wk.

Late Hypocalcemia. Following the feeding of high phosphate milk, tetany can occur in both full-term and prematurely born infants and in infants whose clinical histories have been benign. The intake of a high phosphate food (cow's milk) in relatively large volume leads to an elevated serum phosphate owing to relatively high tubular reabsorption of phosphate and the physiologically low glomerular filtration rate of the newborn. The elevated serum phosphate depresses serum calcium through deposition of calcium in bone. The normal physiologic response would be an increased output of parathyroid hormone, which would increase both the solubilization of bone mineral and urine phosphate. This would restore the normal serum levels of both calcium and phosphate. If the infant's parathyroid glands are not yet able to respond with such an increase of parathyroid hormone, the level of serum calcium progressively falls and symptomatic hypocalcemia may result.

Clinical Manifestations. The most important presentation of hypocalcemia in infants is convulsions; carpopedal spasm is not usually seen and, because the Chvostek sign is common in newborn infants, it cannot be interpreted as a sign of tetany. Laryngospasm with cyanosis and apneic episodes may occur. Irritability, muscular twitchings, jitteriness, and tremors are frequent clinical manifestations in the newborn. Besides the characteristic signs from increased excitability of the nervous system, the nonspecific symptoms clinically suggestive of sepsis may also occur, such as poor feeding, vomiting, and lethargy rather than irritability. Serum calcium determinations and other diagnostic studies should be made in infants suspected of having sepsis. Bradycardia with heart block is rarely noted. A prolonged Q-T interval on the electrocardiogram suggests hypocalcemia. A serum calcium concentration below 7 mg/dL establishes the diagnosis; below 7.5 mg/dL is suggestive. The serum phosphate level is increased, sometimes to 10–12 mg/dL. The blood urea nitrogen is not elevated, distinguishing this condition from the hyperphosphatemia of severe renal dysfunction. Normal newborns fed cow's milk have serum phosphate concentrations of 6–8 mg/dL; normal premature infants may have concentrations even higher. Hypomagnesemia may also be present.

A favorable response to administering calcium is insufficient in itself to make the diagnosis, since calcium may act nonspecifically during seizures. Furthermore, symptoms such as irritability and tremors may subside spontaneously, and convulsions resulting from cerebral edema, anoxia, or injury may not be repeated during the neonatal period. Examination of the spinal fluid is indicated because of the possibility of a convulsion caused by infection or hemorrhage in the central nervous system.

Treatment. Initial treatment of the convulsing infant is intravenous injection of 10% calcium gluconate, 2 mL/kg, with the precautions given above. The response may be dramatic. After this, specific treatment aims at reducing the serum phosphate in late hypocalcemia. Since human milk is low in phosphorus, breast-fed infants rarely, if ever, develop hypocalcemia. "Humanized" infant foods prepared from dialyzed whey of cow's milk are considerably higher in phosphate than is human milk. Phosphate absorption from food can be suppressed, however, by adding to the formula a great excess of calcium, which precipitates as calcium phosphate in the lumen of the gut, e.g., adding calcium lactate or gluconate to the milk feeding to achieve a calcium to phosphorus ratio of 4:1. Calcium lactate powder is preferred, and its addition to milk produces no significant gastrointestinal disturbances. Since calcium lactate is 13% calcium, 770 mg of this salt provides 100 mg of calcium; calcium gluconate is 9% calcium, so that 1100 mg of it provides 100 mg of calcium. A soluble preparation of calcium gluconate (syrup of Neo-calglucon), containing 92 mg Ca/tsp, is a less desirable method of adding calcium since the required amounts have caused diarrhea. Calcium chloride may cause gastric irritation and hyperchloremic acidosis. Because the salt must dissolve in the milk, calcium lactate tablets should not be used, since compressed tablets are insoluble even if fragmented.

Sample calculation. An infant taking a volume of prepared infant feeding estimated to contain 300 mg of P and 450 mg of Ca can achieve a 4:1 ratio of Ca to P, by adding 750 mg of calcium for total calcium intake of 1200 mg. This requires addition of 6 g of calcium lactate powder to the total feeding or 1 g per feeding given every 4 hr.

As treatment decreases the serum phosphorus level, the serum calcium returns to normal, possibly even rising to hypercalcemic levels. At this point, the calcium supplement is reduced in steps, not stopped abruptly, since the serum phosphorus may rise precipitously and the calcium concentration fall again to tetanic levels. In most infants restoration of normal calcium homeostasis and presumably normal parathyroid responsiveness occurs in 1–2 wk.

Occasionally, a more prolonged calcium supplementation period is needed, in which case the treatment must be individualized by serial measurements of calcium and phosphate concentrations. If the infant responds poorly to treatment, the calculations should be checked to determine if sufficient calcium is being added, and the feeding should be examined to see if the calcium lactate or gluconate has been dissolving completely. If no errors are found and the therapeutic response is inadequate, the diagnosis of congenital hypoparathyroidism should be entertained, or, in older infants, vitamin D deficiency or an absorptive or metabolic abnormality of vitamin D.

The *prognosis* of early hypocalcemia with seizures depends on the primary disease; infants with late tetany have an excellent prognosis.

Congenital absence of the parathyroids can occur in association with aplasia of the thymus (*DiGeorge syndrome*), in combination with abnormalities of the great vessels of the heart, or as an isolated parathyroid aplasia. Such patients present the same symptoms as those in infants with transient physiologic hypoparathyroidism but respond incompletely to the simple treatment outlined above and have relapsing hypocalcemia which requires more definitive treatment. In total parathyroid deficiency, substituting pharmacologic amounts of vitamin D, vitamin D metabolites, or vitamin D analogues for parathyroid hormone is required. Dihydrotachysterol is preferable; at pharmacologic doses it is more potent than vitamin D in correcting hypocalcemia. Since it is also more rapidly inactivated in the body, it is not stored as is vitamin D and is not as cumulatively toxic. In the young infant 0.05–0.1 mg of dihydrotachysterol should be given daily, and the dose adjusted by determining serum calcium concentrations, which should be returned to levels of about 9–10 mg/dL. The highly active vitamin D metabolite, 1,25-dihydroxy vitamin D_3, is now available and in doses of 0.25–

0.5 μg/24 hr is effective in treating hypoparathyroidism. As the child grows, the dosage of either steroid must be increased, as indicated by serum calcium concentrations. Hypoparathyroidism in older children is discussed in Sec. 19.18.

Hypocalcemia and Tetany Due to Vitamin D Deficiency or Abnormalities of Vitamin D Metabolism. The onset of vitamin D deficiency tetany usually occurs at 3–6 mo of age, since depletion of the infant's vitamin D stores requires this amount of time. However, an infant born of a vitamin D–deficient mother may develop hypocalcemia from vitamin D deficiency within the first week of life. Tetany and nutritional vitamin D deficiency are now rare, but the latter occasionally develops in a breast-fed infant whose mother, unaware of human milk's vitamin D deficiency, does not provide supplementary vitamin D. See Sec. 3.29.

Hypocalcemia may also be due to failure of normal metabolism of vitamin D, which undergoes two hydroxylation steps, first in the liver and second in the kidney, before becoming the metabolically active 1,25-dehydroxy vitamin D_3. Infants with liver disease, such as neonatal hepatitis, cytomegalic inclusion disease, or atresia of the bile ducts, may show manifestations of vitamin D deficiency with hypocalcemia owing to failure of the liver to metabolize vitamin D. In atresia of the bile ducts, malabsorption of vitamin D may complicate the problem. In the genetic defect of vitamin D metabolism called vitamin D–dependent (pseudodeficient) rickets, the probable failure of the 1-hydroxylation step in the kidney affects infants who may also present with hypocalcemia. Vitamin D deficiency can also result from steatorrhea due to pancreatic lipase deficiency or to intrinsic intestinal mucosal disorders. In addition, rickets and osteomalacia are associated with the treatment of convulsive disorders by large doses of combined anticonvulsant drugs, principally phenobarbital, diphenylhydantoin, and primidone, which alter the liver's metabolism of vitamin D. Diphenylhydantoin also inhibits intestinal transport of calcium, and patients may present with hypocalcemia as well as skeletal changes. See Sec. 23.46–23.52.

Initially, patients with tetany resulting from vitamin D deficiency or failure of normal metabolism of vitamin D can be symptomatically relieved by intravenous injection of 10 mL of 10% calcium gluconate, with the usual precautionary monitoring of heart rate to prevent a too rapid injection. The definitive treatment is a highly concentrated vitamin D preparation which should be given in amounts adequate to achieve a rapid physiologic effect, e.g., vitamin D, 600,000 units, in a single dose or divided into several doses over a 24 hr period. The common solution of vitamin D in propylene glycol (Drisdol), 10,000 units/g, is unsuitable for this type of therapy, since the large volume of propylene glycol is depressant. An alternative therapy is 10,000 units of vitamin D daily for 3 wk. These large doses of vitamin D given orally will be effective in true vitamin D deficiency. If there is impaired vitamin D absorption or a defect in the metabolism of vitamin D, larger doses may be required. The active vitamin D metabolites, 25-hydroxy vitamin D_3 and 1,25-dihydroxy vitamin D_3, are now available for treatment. The hypocalcemia of hepatic disorders or of vitamin D–dependent rickets respond to large doses of vitamin D, but more precise treatment with 25-hydroxy vitamin D_3 or 1,25-dihydroxy vitamin D_3 is now possible. Treatment must be individualized and patients closely monitored to avoid vitamin D intoxication. (See also Sec. 3.31.)

5.35 HYPOMAGNESEMIC TETANY

Hypomagnesemia has reportedly caused tetany associated with either low or normal serum calcium concentrations. In transient physiologic hypoparathyroidism of the newborn, low serum magnesium concentrations may accompany the hyperphosphatemia and hypocalcemia. This hypomagnesemia usually responds to treatment directed at reducing the serum phosphate concentration. Occasionally, newborn infants with severe hypomagnesemia require specific magnesium therapy, which can be injected intramuscularly with 0.2 mL/kg of a 50% solution of $MgSO_4 \cdot 7H_2O$ (25% solution of $MgSO_4$). This treatment will raise serum Mg concentrations into the normal range within an hour and should maintain adequate concentrations for several hours. Often, no further therapy is needed. The mechanism of this transient hypomagnesemia is not understood. Hypomagnesemic tetany and convulsions seen beyond the newborn period may result from congenital disorders of magnesium transport, causing either failure of absorption of diet magnesium or failure of tubular reabsorption of magnesium with excessive urinary loss. In Bartter syndrome hypomagnesemia, hypokalemia, and tetany can occur secondary to a renal tubular dysfunction. Intestinal malabsorption of magnesium also results from acquired intestinal injury such as inflammatory bowel disease or resection of small intestine. Renal loss of magnesium may be secondary to nephropathy caused by aminoglycosides or cis-platinum. Magnesium depletion, whatever the pathogenesis, can be associated with hypocalcemia, since magnesium is needed for both secretion of parathyroid hormone and responsiveness of target tissues to the hormone. Treatment requires magnesium

administered either intramuscularly as above; intravenously, 2–10 mL/kg of 1% magnesium sulfate solution by slow infusion; or orally in the form of magnesium salts, such as the chloride or gluconate. See also Sec. 5.11.

HAROLD E. HARRISON

Bakwin H: Tetany in newborn infants. Am J Dis Child 54:1211, 1937.
Booth BE, Johanson A: Hypomagnesemia due to renal tubular defect in reabsorption of magnesium. J Pediatr 84:350, 1974.
Brown DR, Steranka BH, Taylor FH: Treatment of early-onset neonatal hypocalcemia. Am J Dis Child 135:24, 1981.
Callenbach JC, Sheehan MB, Anderson SJ, et al: Etiologic factors in rickets of very low-birth-weight infants. J Pediatr 98:800, 1981.
Changaris DG, Purohit DM, Balentine JD, et al: Brain calcification in severely stressed neonates receiving parenteral calcium. J Pediatr 104:941, 1984.
Colletti RP, Pan MW, Smith EWP, et al: Detection of hypocalcemia in susceptible neonates. The Q-oTc interval. N Engl J Med 290:931, 1974.
Gardner LI: Tetany and parathyroid hyperplasia in the newborn infant. Influence of dietary phosphate load. Pediatrics 9:534, 1962.
Harrison HE, Lifshitz F, Blizzard RM: Comparison between crystalline dihydrotachysterol and calciferol in patients requiring pharmacologic vitamin D therapy. N Engl J Med 276:894, 1967.
Harrison HE, Harrison HC: Disorders of Calcium and Phosphate Metabolism in Childhood and Adolescence. Philadelphia, WB Saunders, 1979.
Paunier L, Radde IC, Kooh SW, et al: Primary hypomagnesemia with secondary hypocalcemia in an infant. Pediatrics 41:385, 1968.
Richens A, Rowe DJF: Disturbance of calcium metabolism by anticonvulsant drugs. Br Med J 4:73, 1970.
Tsang RC, Light IJ, Sutherland JM, et al: Possible pathogenetic factors in neonatal hypocalcemia of prematurity. J Pediatr 82:423, 1973.

5.36 FAILURE TO THRIVE

Failure to thrive identifies infants and children who, without superficially evident cause, fail to gain weight and often lose weight. This problem occurs most often in infants but also is observed later in childhood. It can occur commonly among institutionalized children, especially those who are mentally retarded.

Etiology. Failure to thrive usually results from psychosocial circumstances, not always immediately apparent, that adversely affect the child's intake, absorption, or utilization of food. Emotional deprivation and neglect or abuse (Sec. 2.60), including the withholding of food (Sec. 2.57), are commonly associated with this condition. An increased incidence of failure to thrive, accompanied by malabsorption, has been reported among children with autism and adults with schizophrenia. Sometimes the physical or emotional deprivation of the child is related to a physical handicap, such as cerebral palsy or cleft palate, or to difficult behavior owing to temperament or other causes. The syndrome may also result from rare organic abnormalities as well as from easily discoverable diseases in which growth failure occurs. For many children who experience a period of failure to thrive with no ascertainable organic or environmental cause, retrospective analysis indicates the likelihood of psychosocial origin. Table 5–18 lists some of the psychosocial and organic conditions associated with failure to thrive.

Clinical Manifestations. Failure to gain weight or to grow at the expected rate may be the only sign. More characteristically, this is accompanied by signs of developmental retardation and of physical and emotional deprivation, such as apathy, poor hygiene, intense eye contact with people, withdrawing behavior; and disorders of oral intake, which may be manifested as anorexia, voracious appetite, or pica. Vomiting, regurgitation, diarrhea, and general neuromuscular spasticity or hypotonia may be concurrent.

Diagnosis and Differential Diagnosis. The diagnosis of failure to thrive is complex, because of the many factors that affect a child's growth. History may provide clarification of

whether inadequate intake, increased losses from vomiting or diarrhea, or disturbed food utilization is the mechanism leading to the growth failure. Frequently, the mechanism is unclear, but information gathered from other observers and through repeated interviews may reveal unsuspected adverse factors in the child's environment.

Constructing and studying both a growth chart and a developmental flow sheet may identify when the child began failing to thrive and may help uncover the environmental or physical factors responsible. If growth parallels the normal growth pattern but is below the expected level (e.g., usually below the 3rd percentile), constitutional short stature and endocrine, genetic, and other systemic disorders must be considered. A physical examination that reveals no abnormality except for growth and development is usually compatible with an environmental cause, although some organic etiologies may exhibit no gross physical findings.

Hospitalizing the child provides an opportunity for quantitating factors governing the net caloric intake (food intake, vomiting, stools) and for observing the child's interactions—especially during feeding and play—with parents, health personnel, and other children. Hospitalization frequently leads to dramatic improvement in weight gain and in social responses and thus provides evidence that environmental factors are causative, eliminating the need for searching further for underlying organic disease.

If the history or physical examination suggests disturbance in any organ system, appropriate diagnostic study is warranted, beginning with screening tests (i.e., routine blood counts and urinalyses) and proceeding further only if these are positive. Extensive study to rule out underlying organic lesions is justified only if the initial data base has failed to provide clues pointing to a specific environmental or organic etiology; failure of a favorable response to hospitalization should also be demonstrated.

Children chronically deprived of food may have stools consistent with malabsorption when an adequate dietary intake is initiated. They gain weight, however, and resume a normal stool pattern after some weeks or months.

Prevention. Failure to thrive arising from psychosocial factors is exceedingly difficult to prevent, since it frequently results from complex social or familial disruptions and intense stress. Preventive counseling involves the identification of families with a new infant having significant current life stresses, of problems during the pregnancy and perinatal period, and of poor relationships between parent and infant in the postnatal period. The family relationships may be characterized by violence and hostility, and members may have limited support systems. The involvement of a supporting network of community volunteers may facilitate the growth of parental capability and self-esteem.

Treatment. For necessary evaluation, a temporary change of environment, such as the hospital, may relieve transient tension among family members. When hospitalization is coupled with counseling and support from a physician, social worker, and family service agency, as appropriate, the family may be able to make adjustments needed to ensure adequate care of the child when he or she returns home. Temporary or permanent placement in a foster home may be necessary in some cases. Identified organic disease should be appropriately treated.

Prognosis. It is difficult to generalize about the prognosis of nonorganic failure to thrive because of the many variables involved in each patient. Children involved in a significant crisis affecting the family over a limited period may eventually achieve adequate physical growth and development. However, studies have shown that some may later exhibit neurotic or antisocial traits, reading problems, and poor verbal development. In some patients, inadequate rate of growth and development continues for a protracted time. A number of children with failure to thrive are also abused, and some may even die under suspicious circumstances. The personality of the child, the degree of deprivation, and the nature of the environmental experiences all are important variables in the ultimate outcome of this disturbance.

GIULIO J. BARBERO

Accardo PJ (ed): Failure to Thrive in Infancy and Early Childhood: A Multidisciplinary Team Approach. Baltimore, University Park Press, 1982.
Barbero GJ, Shaheen E: Environmental failure to thrive: A clinical view. J Pediatr 71:5, 1967.
Hufton IW, Oakes RK: Nonorganic failure to thrive: A long-term follow-up. Pediatrics 59:73, 1977.
Pollett E and Leibel R: Biological and social correlates of failure to thrive. In Greene LS, Johnston, FE (eds): Social and Biological Predictors of Nutritional Status, Physical Growth, and Neurological Development. New York, Academic Press, 1980, pp 173–200.
Smith CA, Berenberg W: The concept of failure to thrive. Pediatrics 46:661, 1970.

Table 5–18. Some Causes of Failure to Thrive and Screening Tests for Them

Cause	Screening Tests
Environmental and Psychosocial	
Inadequate caloric intake	History; observation in hospital
Emotional deprivation and disruptions	History; observation in hospital
Rumination; chronic diarrhea, gastroesophageal reflux	History; observation in hospital
Anorexia nervosa and bulimia	History; examination
Secondary to impact of organic disease	History and observation
Organic	
Central nervous system abnormalities, infection	Neurodevelopmental assessment; transillumination of skull; brain scan
Gastrointestinal system Malabsorption, cystic fibrosis, inflammatory bowel disease, parasites, aganglionic megacolon; liver disease; GE refux	Examination of stools: stool fat, sweat test, stool ova and parasites; liver function tests; barium swallow
Partial cleft palate	Physical examination; observation of feeding
Chronic heart failure	Physical examination; chest x-ray
Endocrine disorders	Growth chart; thyroid function; blood tests; bone age
Pulmonary disease Bronchopulmonary dysplasia; bronchiectasis	Physical examination; chest x-ray; tuberculin test
Renal disease Anomalies; infection; renal failure; renal tubular disorder	Urinalysis; BUN; ultrasound; urinary amino acid screen; urine pH
Chromosomal disorders Turner syndrome	Chromosomal analysis; identification of peculiar facies or multisystem defects
Other metabolic or inborn errors	Urine amino acid screen
Chronic infection Tuberculosis, mycotic, congenital; AIDS or AIDS-related complex	Tuberculin test; appropriate laboratory identification of infectious agent
Chronic inflammation Juvenile rheumatoid arthritis	Physical examination; sedimentation rate
Immunodeficiency disease DiGeorge syndrome; combined immunodeficiency	History of rash and diarrhea; thymus size; tonsil size; skin tests; CBC
Malignancies (kidney, adrenal, brain)	X-ray of abdomen, chest; ultrasound; brain scan
Congenital syndromes due to alcohol, dilantin, drugs, infection	Physical examination

5.37 ACCIDENTAL INJURIES

Accidents are a major cause of morbidity and mortality in children. Of children 1–14 yr of age, accidents cause more deaths in the United States than the next six most prevalent causes combined, about four times more deaths than cancer, the second highest cause. Of 15–24 yr olds, accidents cause more deaths than all combined causes, about four times the deaths from homicide, the second highest cause for this age group. The monetary cost of fatal accidents is staggering: the direct cost for individuals less than 24 yr old is estimated at $109 million per year.

SITES OF ACCIDENTAL INJURIES

Most accidental injuries and deaths of children occur on the streets, at home, and in school.

The Road. *Motor vehicle deaths* are the leading cause of accidental deaths and of all deaths for individuals 1–25 yr of age. Persons under age 20 account for 10% of the drivers but 18% of the auto fatalities. Although no controlled prospective studies of the efficacy of public school drivers' education programs have been performed, evidence suggests that the fatal accident rate for 16–17 yr old drivers with driver training is comparable to that of those without it.

Injuries can be reduced by improving motor vehicle design; developing collapsible steering wheels, padded dashboards, and improved car window glass has contributed to a decreased death rate. Improving roadside guardrails and signposts and lowering the national speed limit to 55 mph have also lessened the highway death toll.

Convincing people to use restraint devices, such as seat

belts or young children's seat restraints, for keeping themselves in place and for distributing deceleration forces to levels tolerable to the human body has been another major effort in automotive safety. However, most adults in the United States do not wear their seat belts, and, prior to the passage of seat restraint laws for children, over 90% of children were reportedly riding unrestrained. In Australia, after a law requiring the use of seat belts had been instituted, a 21% decrease in automobile mortality in metropolitan areas and a 10% decrease in rural areas occurred. Seat restraint laws have been passed in nearly all states. Tennessee has had a 50% decrease in mortality following passage of its mandatory seat belt law. Data from Washington state suggest that appropriately using seat belts or seat restraints could decrease infant deaths in automobile accidents by 91% and infant injury by 78%; corresponding decreases for older children would be 81% and 64%.

Children—even in utero—need to be restrained at all times when they travel in automobiles. The death of the mother is the largest single cause of fetal death in unrestrained automobile accidents. Pregnant women wearing seat belts sustain fewer injuries and deaths. Infants should be in a seat restraint on their first trip home from the hospital and during all other motor vehicle trips. Any child carried in an adult's arms is unsafe. The body of an 8 kg, 6 mo old infant attains a force equivalent to almost 350 kg during a collision at 30 miles/hr, the equivalent of a fall from a third story window. Children in the first 3 yr of life have a higher death rate in motor vehicle accidents than do older children up to adolescence. Therefore, the pediatrician should begin informing the new parent about seat restraints at their very first encounter. For children over 1 yr of age who can sit up adequately, seat belts provide an acceptable alternative to infant seat restraints.

Various passive restraints not requiring the automobile driver's or passenger's efforts in order to be effective may be installed in motor vehicles. Passive shoulder harnesses and a knee bar do not protect children less than 45 kg in weight and 104 cm in height. Air bags offer some protection for children of all ages and all sizes but to be most effective, they should be used in conjunction with a lap type seat belt, which can also be used with various infant seat restraint systems.

Motorcycles, motorscooters, motorbikes, and *mopeds* are increasingly used for transportation because of their low initial cost and relative fuel economy. Many of the riders of these vehicles are adolescents. Motorcycle accidents usually result in trauma to the musculoskeletal or central nervous systems; deaths are usually associated with trauma to the great vessels or to the central nervous system.

The number of motorcycles in the United States contributes disproportionately to the amount of accidental deaths. In 1983, there were 75 fatalities/100,000 registered motorcycles, over three times the rate for other registered motor vehicles. The death rate for all motor vehicles was 2.7 deaths/100,000,000 miles, but about 30 deaths/100,000,000 motorcycle miles. In 1983 motorcycles accounted for 3% of the registered motor vehicles and 9% of motor vehicle fatalities.

The use of helmets by riders of motorcycles and similar vehicles results in lower morbidity and mortality from accidents. In states that enacted laws requiring motorcycle riders to wear helmets, death rates declined markedly; where the laws were repealed, the death rate increased. The use of bright-colored paint and clothing and of the headlight at all times decreases accidents by making the rider and vehicle more visible.

Bicycle accidents result in relatively few deaths (approximately 1000/yr in the United States); however, they cause many injuries and are the most common cause of product-related injuries. In a study of all bicycle accidents reported to

police over a 2 yr period, there was one death; about 10% of the cyclists required hospitalization; 40% had a minor injury requiring medical care; and 20% had no injury. In another study of 3–12 yr old children, about two third of the injuries requiring medical treatment were abrasions, contusions, and lacerations. Of patients hospitalized after bicycle accidents, 67% had craniocerebral trauma, 18% had upper limb fractures and 7% had lower limb fractures.

The majority of bicycle-related injuries to infants occur when they are carried as passengers. Their feet and legs may get caught in the wheel of the bicycle, where spokes can cause a laceration and where the extremity can become squeezed between the wheel and the frame of the bicycle causing crush and shearing injuries. Children should be carried on a bicycle only in a special seat equipped with leg guards; parents also need to know that such infant carriers may make the bicycle more difficult to handle.

The majority of fatal bicycle accidents involve a motor vehicle, and the injury leading to death is usually craniocerebral trauma. The type of accident causing the greatest proportion of deaths (24.6%) is the motor vehicle overtaking the bicyclist from the rear.

Children under 13 account for 10% of bicycle traffic but 28% of bicycle injuries. One study showed that in 38% of the accidents, motorists received traffic citations with failure to yield the right-of-way as the most common charge. Bicyclists were in violation of traffic laws in 70% of the accidents; most of them were guilty of wrong-way riding (riding facing traffic), failure to yield the right-of-way, and turning violations. Young children may be unable to process their perceptions of road situations quickly enough to ride safety in traffic.

Separating bicycle from motor vehicle traffic, e.g., by providing a separate bicycle path, may be one way to decrease bicycle accidents. Bicyclists should also make their bicycles and themselves as visible as possible by wearing light colors, such as yellow, and by using adequate lights, especially at night. Bicyclists should also wear helmets.

Children are frequently involved in road accidents as *pedestrians.* Those under age 24 account for nearly 60% of all pedestrian fatalities. These children are most commonly 3–7 yr old; as in most other types of accidents, boys outnumber girls. Usually children are unsupervised by adults at the time of the accident and often dart out into the street. Frequently, prior to an accident, a child is hidden from the driver by parked cars, bushes, or other roadside objects. In addition, young children often do not see traffic signs or they misinterpret them.

To make children safer pedestrians, they should be dressed in brightly colored reflective clothing to be seen more easily. In addition, children should be separated from traffic by fences and closed streets, and under- or overpasses should be provided for crossing. Prohibiting parking and roadside obstructions near corners may allow drivers to see children sooner. Modifying motor vehicles by increasing external padding, decreasing external protuberances, and making bumper areas at more appropriate heights should decrease injuries.

Home. The home is frequently the site of both fatal and nonfatal accidents, and children in the 2–3 yr old age group are most commonly involved. The types of accidents that occur in the home are legion. See Sec. 5.44 for discussion of burns, Sec. 5.43 for discussion of drowning and near-drowning and Chapter 28 for discussion of poisoning.

School. Between the ages of 5 and 18, children spend up to 20% of their waking hours in school. For children in the primary grades, physical education and unorganized activities have the highest accident rates. For older children, accidents most commonly occur in physical education, the school building in general, interscholastic sports, and shops and laboratories. Overall, injuries occur at a rate of 49 injuries/1000 students; severe injuries, amputations, 3rd degree burns, concussions, crush injuries, fractures, and multiple injuries occur at a rate of about 9 injuries/1000 students. Adolescent males account for 30% of all injuries.

Playground equipment is frequently the source of product-related accidents. Approximately 118,000 children/yr have accidents related to playground equipment, with injuries severe enough to require an emergency room visit. Most of these injuries relate to falls from the equipment; approximately 50% of these falls result in injuries to the head and neck. The surface over which the playground equipment is installed may be a critical factor; many times this surface is concrete or asphalt rather than an energy-absorbing material such as loose sand, wood chips, or foam mats. A fall from a height of 1 foot onto concrete or asphalt can create forces sufficient to cause death if the child lands directly on his or her head. A fall from 3 feet onto packed dirt can also lead to death. But falls onto energy-asorbing material can be tolerated from a much greater height; all playground equipment should be installed over such surfaces. It also should be adequately maintained, e.g., checked for weakness due to rust, for sharp edges and protrusions, and for loose nuts and bolts.

The older the children, the more likely they are to be injured in physical education activities. Although these injuries are usually relatively minor, they are frequent—almost four injuries/100 participants/yr—and cause the loss of slightly more than one school day/injury.

The injury rate in interscholastic sports is higher in each succeeding level of school. It is highest for boys in high school football (2.3 accidents/100,000 student days) and highest for girls in high school basketball (0.23 accidents/100,000 student days). In one study, 92% of the injured athletes required physician services; however, 73% of those injured were able to return to their sport in fewer than 5 days. Two thirds of the injuries occurred during practice rather than during competition.

SPORTS INJURIES

Heat cramps, heat exhaustion, and **heat stroke** are serious athletic injuries. Heat cramps, which occur during or after physical exercise, involve the muscles used during the exercise and are associated with acute sodium loss. Heat exhaustion, the most common heat injury, is associated with a deficit of extracellular fluid, of total body water, or of sodium. Heat stroke is the most severe heat injury and is the second leading cause of death of athletes in the United States. It consists of marked hyperpyrexia (core temperatures greater than 41.1° C [106° F]), neurologic symptoms, and decreasing sweating or anhydrosis.

Heat injuries are preventable. Athletes should become acclimatized to warm ambient temperatures over several weeks. Sports practices and events should be scheduled for cooler parts of the day and should be canceled on hot, humid days. Large volumes of fluid should be provided before, during, and after the event. Salt tablets are not indicated.

Heat cramps can usually be treated with massage or oral or intravenous sodium replacement. Heat exhaustion can usually be managed by moving the patient to a cool environment and by providing several liters of fluid over several hours, either orally or intravenously.

Heat stroke is a medical emergency and should be treated aggressively. The airway must be protected and intravenous fluids administered to manage hypotension. The patient's core temperature should be monitored and cooling accomplished with a bath of cool water or ice or both. Short-acting anticonvulsants may be used for seizures. Some hypotension may be corrected by cooling alone. The patient also needs to be monitored for arrhythmias, evidence of rhabdomyolysis, renal failure, and disseminated intravascular coagulopathy.

The more common injuries sustained by high school athletes are usually less severe: **sprains** (30%), **strains** (29%), **contusions** (14%), **fractures** (6%), **inflammations** (5%), **lacerations** (2%), and other injuries (12%). Initial treatment of strains, sprains, contusions, and other inflammatory processes consists of *ice, compression,* and *elevation.* Such treatment can be started in the field prior to a detailed evaluation, and, if after evaluation no other definitive therapy is indicated, it should be continued for at least 24 hr.

The athlete should not return to activity as long as there is swelling or pain of the affected part. Overall fitness may be maintained by using forms of exercise that do not involve the injured area. Specific rehabilitation programs should be designed for the injured area after the swelling and pain have resolved.

See also Sec. 9.13 and 23.12 for orthopedic trauma, Sec. 12.8 for oral trauma, Sec. 17.46 for trauma to the genitourinary tract, and Sec. 25.17 for injuries to the eye.

REDUCING INJURY

Since "accident" connotes an unexpected, unavoidable, or unintentional event implying that nothing can be done to prevent such an occurrence, it is useful to consider this problem in terms of reducing injury in addition to preventing accidents.

Measures directed toward reducing injuries may attempt either to control the environment or to alter human behavior. The former usually requires the cooperation of relatively few individuals on few occasions but influences the lives of many. The latter requires the cooperation of many individuals on multiple occasions. Five steps that should be taken to reduce injury include (1) defining the frequency and severity of injuries that occur in a community and identifying high risk groups and/or situations; (2) determining what caused the injuries and, when possible, predicting situations that are likely to result in injuries in the future; (3) planning control measures; (4) implementing the control measures; and (5) evaluating the control measures for effectiveness.

Education is the most common approach to injury reduction, but it is often relatively ineffective; e.g., seat belts are unused and home hazards persist despite efforts to educate the population. In contrast, passive interventions have frequently resulted in decreased injury rates, e.g., prevention of poisoning through the use of childproof bottlecaps, changes in dashboard design of automobiles, and breakaway highway lamp posts.

THE ACCIDENT-PRONE CHILD

This term has been used to describe a child having a personality trait thought to predispose the child to having accidents. Such a personality trait does not exist. The child with repeated injuries should alert physicians to families with psychosocial problems; to a child with motor, attention, or temperament problems; and to the possibility of child abuse (Sec. 2.58).

JEROME A. PAULSON

General References

Munoz E: Economic costs of trauma. United States, 1982. J Trauma 24:237, 1984.
National Safety Council, Accident Facts, 1984 edition. Chicago, National Safety Council, 1984.

The Road Environment

Automobiles: Drivers and Passengers

Crosby W, Costiloe J: Safety of lap belt restraints for pregnant victims of automobile collisions. N Engl J Med 284:632, 1971.

Decker MD, Dewey MJ, Hutcheson RH, et al: The use and efficacy of child restraint devices. The Tennessee experience, 1982 and 1983. JAMA 252:2571, 1984.

Mohan D, Schneider LW: An evaluation of adult clasping strength for restraining lap held infants. Human Factors 21:635, 1979.

Robertson LS: Crash involvement of teenaged drivers when driver education is eliminated from high school. Am J Public Health 70:599, 1980.

Scherz R: Restraint systems for the prevention of injury to children in automobile accidents. Am J Public Health 66-451, 1976.

Motorcycles

Robertson LS: An instance of effective legal regulation: Motorcycle helmet and daytime head lamp laws. Law and Society Review 10:467, 1976.

Watson GS, Zador PL, Wilks A: A repeal of helmet use laws and increased motorcyclist mortality in the United States, 1975–1978. Am J Public Health 70:579, 1980.

Bicycles

Cross K, Fisher G: A Study of Bicycle/Motor Vehicle Accidents: Identification of Problem Types and Counter Measure Approaches, Vol I. Santa Barbara, Calif, Anacapa Sciences Inc., 1977.

Kravitz HL: Preventing injuries from bicycle spokes. Pediatr Ann 6:713, 1977.

Pedestrians

Sandels S: Young children in traffic. Br J Educ Psychol 40:111, 1970.

The School Environment

Boyce WT, Sprunger LW, Sobolewska S, et al: The epidemiology of injuries in large, urban school districts. Pediatrics 79:342, 1984.

Reichelderfer TE, Overback A, Greensher J: Unsafe playground. Pediatrics 56:526, 1979.

Heat Injuries

Anderson RJ, Reed G, Knochel J. Heatstroke. Adv Int Med 28:115, 1983.

O'Donnell TF. Management of heat stress injuries in the athlete. Orthop Clin North Am 11:841, 1980.

Reducing Injury

Haddon W: Energy damage and the ten counter measure strategies. J Trauma 13:21, 1973.

Schaplowsky A: Community injury control—a management approach. Am J Public Health 53:252, 1973.

Schlesinger ER, Dickenson DG, Westag J, et al: Study of health education in accident prevention. Am J Dis Child 111:490, 1966.

The Accident-Prone Child—The Abused Child

Husband P: The accident prone child. Practitioner 211:335, 1973.

References for Parents

American Academy of Pediatrics, 141 Northwest Point Rd, PO Box 927, Elk Grove Village, IL 60007.

Child Restraint Systems for Your Automobile, US Department of Transportation, National Highway Traffic Safety Administration, Washington DC 20590.

Don't Risk Your Child's Life! Physicians for Automotive Safety, PO Box 930, Armonk, NY 10504.

5.38 PEDIATRIC CRITICAL CARE

5.39 INTENSIVE CARE

The objective of intensive care is to provide maximal surveillance and care to patients with acute, temporary, life-threatening impairment of pulmonary, cardiovascular, renal, or nervous system functions. The major elements of intensive care are (1) physicians and nursing and paramedical personnel specially trained in the care of the critically ill; (2) monitoring and alarm systems for continuous assessment of vital functions; (3) respiratory therapy and resuscitation equipment and drugs; (4) immediately available physician specialists in anesthesiology, pediatrics, and surgery; and (5) 24 hr laboratory service for hematologic studies and rapid, precise determination of blood pH, gas tensions, and electrolytes on ultramicro samples.

Commercially available systems are adequate for continuous monitoring and have appropriate alarms for respiratory rate (impedance pneumograph), heart rate, arterial and central venous pressures, and body temperature (thermistor probes) in small infants and children. As in the operating room (Sec. 5.48), continuously measuring inspired oxygen concentration, arterial oxygen saturation, and end-tidal expired carbon dioxide concentration may be indicated to provide essential information about the effectiveness of gas exchange at negligible risk to the patient having cardiopulmonary failure. Cannulation of a peripheral artery permits continuous pressure monitoring and frequent blood sampling for pH and gas tensions in older infants and children.

Intravenous fluids can be precisely administered by using mechanical syringe pumps. Total or partial caloric requirements may be infused parenterally in infants able to tolerate a hyperosmolar infusion into a major vein.

Patients with existing or impending **respiratory failure** (Sec. 13.21) require intensive respiratory therapy. Respiratory failure exists if the impairment of ventilation poses an immediate threat to life. An acute rise in $paCO_2$ over 55 mm Hg or paO_2 under 100 mg Hg at an inspired oxygen concentration over 50% (except in cyanotic heart disease) indicates life-threatening impairment of ventilatory function. Successful therapy usually requires an artificial airway (nasotracheal intubation or tracheostomy, Table 5–19), mechanical ventilation, continuous humidification of inspired gases, and sterile tracheobronchial toilet at 1–3 hr intervals. Infants and children with severe acute lung disease, especially those with an artificial tracheal airway, also require chest percussion, vibration, and postural drainage for removing secretion and providing airway patency.

Approximately 3–5% of premature infants who develop severe respiratory distress syndrome or have major anomalies that affect cardiopulmonary function progress to bronchopulmonary dysplasia (Sec. 8.17) and chronic respiratory failure. Some of these infants, as well as those with severe myopathies or central nervous system disorders, will require tracheostomy and mechanical ventilation for months and even years; a few of those infants with myopathies or central nervous system disorders may need only negative pressure cuirass ventilation without a tracheostomy. Earlier experiences in some centers suggested a poor outcome for infants with chronic respiratory failure. However, if these patients are cared for in a well-coordinated, multidisciplinary program emphasizing nutrition, growth, and psychologic as well as physical development, the results can be very gratifying for the child and the family. This is especially likely for infants and children whose condition stabilizes enough to allow them to receive such care at home.

Diffuse alveolar injury, also called *adult respiratory distress syndrome* (Sec. 13.89), often can be the inevitable consequence of severe trauma, extensive cardiopulmonary surgery, septic shock, or severe pneumonitis. Decreased air-containing lung volume, increased work of breathing, and severe arterial hypoxemia result. The hypoxemia usually requires more aggressive therapy than merely increasing the inspired oxygen

Table 5–19. **Specifications for Pediatric Orotracheal Tubes***†

Age	Internal Diameter (ID in mm)	Length‡ (cm)	15 mm Male Connector Size (mm ID)
Newborn (<1.5 kg)	2.5	10	3
Newborn (≥1.5 kg)–3 mo	3.0	11	3
3–7 mo	3.5	11	4
7–15 mo	4.0	12	4
15–30 mo	4.5	13	5
2.5–4 yr	5.0	14	5
5–6 yr	5.5	16	6
7–8 yr	6.0	18	6
9–10 yr	6.0 cuffed§	20	6
11–12 yr	6.5 cuffed	22	7
13–15 yr	7.0 cuffed	24	7

*The ID size for age is based on the average size of tracheal tube in that age patient during general anesthesia which permitted an audible tracheal air leak at 20 to 25 cm H_2O peak inspiratory airway pressure. (Lee KW, et al: Selection of tracheal tube size in infants and children. Submitted for publication, 1982.) For age over 2 yr, the size formula:

$$ID (mm) = \frac{16 + age (yr)}{4}$$

†Clear polyvinyl-chloride tracheal tubes which satisfy the USP tissue implant test for inertness and the American National Standards Institute specifications will be labeled "Z-79" and are recommended. Connectors should have an ID equal to or greater than that of the tube and should be of lightweight plastic material.

‡Nasotracheal tubes should be 2 to 4 cm longer.

§High volume, low pressure cuffs inflated to permit an audible leak at 20 cm H_2O peak pressure are recommended.

concentration, which produces arterial gas tension compatible with intact recovery while avoiding toxic effects of oxygen on the lung. Fluid restriction and diuretics help reduce total body and intrapulmonary water; furosemide also may enhance pulmonary lymphatic flow. Positive end-expiratory airway pressure (PEEP) increases alveolar gas volume and helps maintain peripheral small airway patency, which causes better matching of ventilation with perfusion resulting in improved arterial oxygen tensions at lower inspired oxygen concentrations. Although high PEEP may increase the work of breathing, most patients accomplish adequate alveolar ventilation by spontaneous efforts and need only infrequent ventilator breaths (intermittent mechanical ventilation, IMV). The frequency of mechanical ventilator breaths (tidal volume 12–20 mL/kg) can be adjusted to achieve a normal arterial pH and $paCO_2$. The advantages of this technique over controlled mechanical ventilation with neuromuscular blockade or profound sedation include lower airway pressures with less risk of barotrauma; minimal interference with circulation; less need for sedation and neuromuscular blockade; and improved coordination of the patient with the ventilator, resulting in less work and better matching of alveolar gas with pulmonary blood flow.

Circulatory failure also can occur in patients with major trauma or sepsis and following complex cardiovascular operations (Sec. 5.41). Pediatric patients can benefit from precise control of intravascular volume, vasomotor tone, and blood flow by assessment of directly measured systemic arterial and right atrial (central venous) pressures; cardiac output; and blood oxygen content, pH, and gas tensions. In more complex conditions, introducing a quadralumen, flow-directed (Swan-Ganz) catheter into the pulmonary artery allows evaluation of pulmonary arterial and pulmonary occluded (wedge) pressures, which reflect right ventricular function as well as left atrial end-diastolic pressure. Treatment should be directed at the specific physiologic dysfunction by using the information obtained from monitoring to precisely adjust *blood volume* with diuretics or fluid infusions and *tissue perfusion* with selected catecholamines and vasodilators that alter myocardial contractility, heart rate, and vasomotor tone (Sec. 14.69).

Intracranial hypertension often occurs following severe head trauma and intracranial operations. Early recognition of increased intracranial pressure (ICP) and carefully monitored therapy can reduce the hyperemia and edema that impair cerebral perfusion, but the conditions may result in ischemia and permanent central nervous system damage. A hollow stainless steel threaded cannula (subdural bolt) inserted through a burr hole into the subarachnoid space provides a simple, safe, and usually reliable means of estimating ICP. The therapy for intracranial hypertension includes fluid restriction (one half to one third maintenance fluids), diuretics (furosemide 1 mg/kg intravenously) to reduce the cerebral edema, 30 degree head-up tilt with the head faced forward to enhance cerebral venous drainage and reduce intracranial blood volume, and dexamethasone (1.5 mg/kg initially, and 1.0 mL/kg/day for five days) for patients with cerebral swelling secondary to head trauma. Children whose ICP exceeds 15 mm Hg despite this therapy should undergo tracheal intubation, neuromuscular blockade, and mechanical hyperventilation to a $paCO_2$ range of 22–28 mm Hg; if this fails to control ICP, barbiturate coma and total body hypothermia to depress cerebral metabolic rate and reduce pressure may be effective in preserving central nervous system function; these are, however, exceedingly complex forms of therapy requiring specialized medical and nursing skills and extensive monitoring of pulmonary, cardiovascular, and renal function.

5.40 CARDIOPULMONARY RESUSCITATION

Cessation of *effective* ventilation or circulation requires immediate treatment. The cardinal signs of respiratory arrest are apnea and cyanosis. Absence of heart sounds and of carotid and femoral pulses indicates circulatory arrest. Respiratory arrest can be caused by airway obstruction, central nervous system depression, or neuromuscular paralysis. Circulatory arrest is due to asystole, ventricular fibrillation, and cardiovascular collapse associated with extreme arterial hypotension. If cardiopulmonary arrest is suspected, coordinated artificial ventilation and closed-chest cardiac massage is indicated.

Airway. The airway should be cleared immediately. Vomitus and secretions should be aspirated or removed with fingers and a hankerchief. Soft tissue obstruction can be overcome by extending the occipitoatlantal joint and displacing the mandible forward.

Ventilation. The lungs should be inflated with air or oxygen, which can be effectively accomplished by mouth-to-mouth or mouth-to-nose insufflation or by bag and mask devices. A good fit of the mask on the face with minimal or no leaks is essential. The hallmark of adequate lung inflation is synchronous thoracoabdominal motion. The lungs should be inflated rapidly, with a breath interposed between every four to five cardiac compressions.

During compression of the sternum preceding the intended interposition of a breath, positive pressure should be applied to the airway and maintained throughout the systolic and diastolic phases of the cardiac cycle. As pressure on the sternum is released (diastolic phase), gas will flow into the lungs without a pause in the rate and rhythm of cardiac compression, which promotes a higher cardiac output and improves perfusion of vital organs.

Table 5–20. **Drugs for Resuscitation**

Drug	Concentration	Intravenous Dose	Intracardiac Dose	Frequency Dose
Sodium bicarbonate*	1 mEq/mL	2–4 mEq/kg, up to 200 mEq	1/2 intravenous	5–10 min
Epinephrine	1:10,000 (0.1 mg/mL)	0.01 mg/kg, up to 0.5 mg	Same as intravenous	5–10 min
	µg/mL numerically equal to wt in kg	0.2–2.0 µg/kg/min	—	Continuous infusion
Isoproterenol	1:10,000 (0.1 mg/mL)	0.01 mg/kg, up to 0.5 mg	—	Single dose
	µg/mL numerically equal to wt in kg	0.2–2.0 µg/kg/min	—	Continuous infusion
Dopamine	µg/mL numerically equal to wt in kg × 10	2.0–20.0 µg/kg/min	—	Continuous infusion
Dobutamine	µg/mL numerically equal to wt in kg × 10	2.0–20.0 µg/kg/min	—	Continuous infusion
Atropine sulfate	400 µg/mL	10–20 µg/kg	—	30 min
Calcium chloride	10% (100 mg/mL)	20 mg/kg	—	10 min
Calcium gluconate	10% (100 mg/mL)	60 mg/kg	—	10 min
Lidocaine	20 mg/mL	1 mg/kg	—	Single dose

Defibrillation: 2–5 watt-seconds/kg (external)

*Obtain arterial sample for pH, pCO_2, base excess, as soon as possible to guide alkali therapy.

Circulation. An effective cardiac output in the newborn or small infant can be produced by applying maximum pressure with the tips of two fingers over the middle third of the sternum while the vertebral column is firmly supported. In larger infants and children the pressure is applied by the heel of one hand over the sternum opposite the 4th interspace. In large children the heel of the left hand is placed over the right hand to provide the strength of both arms and shoulders. If the maximum compression is held for a fraction of a second, a larger stroke volume will be ejected. The usual rate in infants is approximately 100/min, and 60/min in older patients.

When ventilation and massage are effective, carotid and femoral pulses become palpable, pupils constrict, and the color of the mucous membranes improves.

Open thoracotomy and direct cardiac massage are rarely indicated outside the operating room or intensive care unit.

Drugs. As soon as artificial ventilation and cardiac massage are effectively established, sodium bicarbonate and epinephrine should be administered (Table 5–20) either intravenously or directly into the heart. Sodium bicarbonate compensates for the extreme metabolic acidosis which develops rapidly after circulation ceases. Epinephrine, which increases myocardial contractile force without decreasing the systemic vascular resistance, should be given if artificial ventilation, cardiac

Table 5–21. **Recommended Contents for a Pediatric Resuscitation Cart**

Airway Equipment
1. Bag and masks (infant, child, adult) with nonrebreathing valve that has universal 15 mm female adapter for male 15 mm endotracheal tube connectors
2. Oropharyngeal airways (Guedel sizes 00, 0, 1, 2, 3, 4)
3. Orotracheal uncuffed tubes (complete sterile set of 2 of each size, 2.5 mm ID to 8.0 mm ID) with appropriate size straight 15 mm male connectors; cuffed tubes, 6.0 to 8.0 mm ID; all tubes cut to oral minimum length plus 2 cm
4. Laryngoscope:
   Adult handle, pediatric handle
   Blades: Miller—premature
          Wis-Hipple 1 and 1½
          Flagg—child
          Macintosh—adult (no. 3, 4)
   2 extra batteries
   1 extra light
   1 extra light for each blade
5. Aspiration equipment
   Metal tonsil aspirator (Yankauer)
   Disposable sterile plastic suction catheters, sizes (French) 5, 8, 10, 14
6. Magill forceps
7. Stylets (Teflon coated for tubes sized 2.5–8.0 mm ID)
8. EKG paper

Drugs
Sodium bicarbonate (1 mEq/mL)
Epinephrine (1.0 mg/mL)
Isoproterenol (0.2 mg/mL)
Calcium chloride (100 mg/mL)
Calcium gluconate (100 mg/mL)
Atropine sulfate (400 µg/mL)
Dopamine (0.2 µg/mL)

Dobutamine (0.2 µg/mL)
Dextrose (500 mg/mL)
Diazepam (5 mg/mL)
Mannitol (0.25 g/mL or 12.5 g/50 mL)
Lidocaine (20 mg/mL)
Saline (for dilution)

Defibrillator
Direct current with range of 20–400 watt-seconds
Saline-soaked 4 × 4 in gauze pads stored with external paddles
Pediatric (5 cm diameter) and adult (10 cm diameter) external paddles

Miscellaneous
Intracardiac needles: 20 and 22 gauge, 6–8 cm length
Plastic intravenous cannulas (16, 18, 20, and 22 gauge) and scalp vein sets
Sterile cutdown tray with pediatric instruments
Tongue blades   Scissors
Alcohol swabs   Syringes (plastic disposable)
Sterile hemostat   Needles
Sterile 4 × 4 gauze sponges   Lubricant, water-soluble, disposable single-use packets

massage, and sodium bicarbonate have not restored spontaneous, effective circulation within 3 min.

Defibrillation. An electrocardiogram should be obtained and run continuously as soon as possible after the diagnosis of circulatory arrest to detect ventricular fibrillation. External defibrillation can be achieved with an appropriate electric shock (2 watt-seconds/kg initially, 3–5 watt-seconds/kg up to total of 400 watt-seconds in subsequent shocks) applied through paddles of appropriate size to skin surfaces covered locally with a conductive electrode jelly or saline-soaked pads.

Postresuscitation Care. Subsequent care includes treatment of the cause of the collapse, plus monitoring and regulating the electrocardiogram, arterial pressure, and arterial pH and gas tensions. Cerebral edema may occur with increased intracranial pressure and may require specific treatment (Sec. 21.24 and 21.26).

Successful resuscitation cannot be achieved without careful preplanning, proper equipment (Table 5–21), and a coordinated team effort. One individual at a resuscitation should be designated the recorder, to note times and details of the entire resuscitation. A log of all resuscitations should be retained by a medical or nursing department of the hospital.

JOHN J. DOWNES
RUSSELL C. RAPHAELY

Downes JJ, Godinez RI: Upper airway obstruction in the child. American Society of Anesthesiologists Refresher Courses. Vol 8. Philadelphia, JB Lippincott, 1980, pp 29–48.

Downes JJ, Goldberg AI: Airway management, mechanical ventilation, and cardiopulmonary resuscitation. In: Scarpelli E, Auld PAM, Goldman HS (eds): Pulmonary Disease in the Fetus, Infant, and Child. Philadelphia, Lea and Febiger, 1978, pp 99–131.

Downes JJ, Schreiner MS, Kettrick RG, et al: Chronic respiratory failure in infancy—causes and survival. Crit Care Med 12:339, 1984.

Kettrick RG, Donar ME: The ventilator-dependent child: Medical and social care. In: Shoemaker WC (ed): Critical Care—State of the Art. Vol 6. Fullerton, CA, Society for Critical Care Medicine Publications, 1985, pp 31–38.

Mager T, Walker ML, Johnson DG, et al: Causes of morbidity and mortality in severe pediatric trauma. JAMA 245:719, 1981.

Phenninger J, Gerber A, Tschappeler H, et al: Adult respiratory distress syndrome in children. J Pediatr 101:352, 1982.

Raphaely RC: Shock. In: Fleisher G, Ludwig S (eds): Textbook of Pediatric Emergency Medicine. Baltimore, Williams and Wilkins, 1983, pp 31–42.

Raphaely RC: Respiratory support—ventilators. In: Welch KJ, Randolph JG, Ravitch MM, et al (eds): Pediatric Surgery. 4th ed. Chicago, Year Book Medical Publishers, 1986, pp 68–73.

Raphaely RC, Swedlow DB, Downes JJ, et al: Management of severe pediatric head trauma. Pediatr Clin North Am 27:715, 1980.

Shoemaker WC, Thompson WL, Holbrook PR (eds): Textbook of Critical Care. Philadelphia, WB Saunders, 1984.

Standards and Guidelines for Cardiopulmonary Resuscitation (CPR) and Emergency Cardiac Care (ECC): Part IV—Pediatric Basic Life Support. JAMA 255:2954, 1986.

5.41 SHOCK SYNDROMES

Shock is circulatory insufficiency. Its clinical presentation varies so greatly that shock can be best understood as a collection of syndromes unified by a common pathophysiology. Three factors influence its variation of clinical presentation:

1. Shock may be a complication of a diverse collection of illnesses, each with its own signs and symptoms.

2. The degrees of circulatory insufficiency experienced by major organ systems vary from patient to patient. For example, in one child central nervous system symptomatology may predominate; in another, signs of peripheral circulatory insufficiency may be most evident.

3. Since children have exceptionally effective cardiovascular compensatory mechanisms that blunt the effects of circulatory insufficiency on major organ systems, the symptoms of shock may be masked until it is far advanced.

Etiology. *Hypovolemia* secondary to dehydration or hemorrhage is the most common cause of shock in pediatric patients. *Septic (endotoxic) shock* is second in frequency, often occurring in children requiring immunosuppression. Although gram-negative enteric bacilli and the meningococcus have been the chief pathogens in septic shock, the gram-positive cocci, such as the group B streptococcus, the pneumococcus, and *Staphylococcus aureus* have assumed increasing importance. Occurring with increased frequency, *cardiogenic shock*, the failure of the pumping action of the myocardium, may follow open heart surgery or occur secondary to myocarditis, to life-threatening dysrhythmias, or to advanced septic shock. Sudden vascular collapse occurs infrequently secondary to hypersensitivity reactions or anaphylaxis, to central nervous system injuries, endocrine failure, such as adrenocortical insufficiency, and to mechanical obstruction of the circulation by cardiac compression, pericardial tamponade, or pulmonary embolism.

Pathophysiology. The basic defect in all shock states is inadequate blood supply to tissue. This may be produced by loss of blood or fluid, by myocardial depression with resultant pump failure, or by maldistribution of arterial flow and venous return to the heart, one of the major pathophysiologic factors in septic shock.

Despite the different mechanisms producing circulatory insufficiency, early cardiorespiratory adjustments commonly occur in most patients in shock. There is an outpouring of catecholamines which increase heart rate, myocardial contractility, myocardial oxygen consumption, peripheral vasoconstriction, and alveolar ventilation. This early phase may be undetected owing to minimal or absent hypotension. For example, in hypovolemic shock intense arteriolar and venular constriction will shift interstitial fluid into the circulatory volume. Provided the volume loss is not overwhelming, hypotension may be avoided and perfusion to vital organs may be preserved at the expense of skin and musculoskeletal perfusion. In cardiogenic shock, the myocardium cannot significantly improve its performance; thus the effect of sympathetic activity is usually intense vasoconstriction with an inadequate increase in the blood flow to major organ systems despite maintenance of a normal mean arterial blood pressure. The vasoconstriction may even be detrimental by increasing the workload of the myocardium. In contrast, during early septic shock, when the myocardium is normal and fluid loss is absent, there is enhanced peripheral perfusion and minimal catecholamine effect, often termed the "warm shock" syndrome.

The subsequent phase of shock is characterized by a redistribution of organ and microcirculatory blood flow; flow is preferentially diverted to the brain and heart at the expense of the kidney, gastrointestinal tract, liver, and skin. If ischemia occurs, there may be hypoxia, acidosis, and cellular injury; lactic acid and other metabolic products from injured tissue accumulate. Late in this stage, the precapillary blood vessels no longer respond to vasoconstriction and their fluid is lost from the plasma into the interstitial space.

In endotoxic shock it is probable that the polysaccharide component of endotoxin (a lipid-polysaccharide-peptide macromolecule found in the outer layers of the baterial cell) will activate the complement system, leading to the aggregation of leukocytes and platelets and to the release of vasoactive amines, including histamine, serotonin, and kinins. Blood pressure decreases secondary to diminished peripheral arterial resistance and to an increased venous tone, with a substantial portion of the total volume of fluid pooling in the venous capacitance vessels. Some capillary bed arteriovenous shunting is also promoted so that the capillary beds of many tissues are bypassed, reducing the "effective circulating blood volume."

During shock, the pulmonary capillary is particularly sensitive to injury, which results in leakage of water, electrolytes, and protein into the interstitium and alveolar space. A ventilation-perfusion abnormality follows, which further complicates shock by accentuating hypoxia, by reducing pulmonary compliance, and by increasing the work of breathing. This syndrome has been termed "shock lung" or **adult respiratory distress syndrome** (ARDS). The capillary leakage may also result from the action of endotoxin on the pulmonary capillary or from a series of reactions involving the complement cascade, neutrophil aggregation, the coagulation system, and lung prostaglandins in acute endothelial injury. Intense systemic vasoconstriction may cause capillary leakage by forcing volume into the pulmonary circulation. See also Sec. 13.89.

Diffuse intravascular coagulation (DIC) may also occur during shock, further reducing nutrient blood flow to tissues (Sec. 15.50).

The later stages of shock are a reflection of tissue ischemia and persistent anaerobic metabolism. Inadequate oxygenation eventually leads to irreversible damage of mitochondria and to disruption of cell membranes. Cardiac function, generally adequate early in hypovolemic and septic shock, becomes compromised as the acidosis and hypotension persist. Coronary circulation receives two thirds of its blood flow during diastole; tachycardia and prolonged hypotension reduce this diastolic flow. Myocardial ischemia may be severe enough to produce areas of endocardial infarction. Patients with cardiogenic shock generally tolerate little additional stress, deteriorating rapidly when acidosis begins to complicate their shock state.

Central nervous system blood flow is normally about 15% of the cardiac output. The brain tolerates any degree of hypoxia very poorly. Initially, the brain may reflexly preserve its blood flow despite a moderate reduction in cardiac output, but with persistent hypotension and diminished cardiac output, cerebral anoxia and death ensue.

Clinical Manifestations. Most patients with septic or cardiogenic shock have a history of significant antecedent illness or open heart surgery. In hypovolemic shock there is often a history of vomiting, diarrhea, gastrointestinal bleeding, or trauma.

There are signs of increased sympathetic activity such as cool, mottled, or moist skin, tachycardia, diaphoresis, and apprehension. Cold lower extremities suggest diminished perfusion. Toe temperature and the progression of skin temperature changes along the lower extremity can be used to monitor the progression of shock and its response to treatment. Blood pressure may be difficult to record because of intense vasoconstriction. In early shock, hypotension may be absent or minimal, espcially in patients who are septic. Fever, petechiae, and ecchymoses generally suggest bacteremia. Profound hypothermia may occur as a late manifestation of any form of shock. Patients with septic shock often have edema of the extremities in contrast to hypovolemic patients, who may have loss of skin turgor and dry mucous membranes. There may be signs of intra-abdominal hemorrhage, pulmonary edema, myocardial dysfunction, or abnormalities of the central nervous system.

Monitoring and Laboratory Data. The period from the onset of shock until death may be short; therefore, after a therapeutic decision has been made, it is essential to immediately assess the hemodynamic response. The ability to do so has been facilitated by thermodilution techniques that measure cardiac output and by flow-directed intravascular catheters that measure central venous, right atrial, pulmonary arterial, systolic, mean, and wedge pressures and allow calculation of pulmonary vascular resistance (Table 5–22). Such monitoring is recommended for children with cardiogenic shock and, frequently, for those with septic shock, because of probable associated myocardial compromise. For patients with hypo-

Table 5–22. **Direct Circulatory Measurements**

Parameter	Normal Values (mm Hg)
Aortic pressure	100/60
Mean arterial pressure (MAP)	75
Pulmonary arterial pressure:	
Systolic	20
Diastolic	10
Mean (MPAP)	15
Wedge (PAWP)	6–10
Left ventricular pressure:	
Systolic	100
End diastolic	8–10
Right ventricular pressure:	
Systolic	25
End diastolic	3–5
Right atrial pressure	3–5
Central venous pressure (CVP)	3–5

volemic shock, a prompt and sustained response to initial therapy may eliminate the need for invasive monitoring. In less stable cases of hypovolemic shock, such as with active gastrointestinal bleeding, central venous pressure (CVP) may need to be monitored.

The pulmonary artery wedge pressure is an excellent indication of left ventricular filling status and a useful guide to fluid and inotrope therapy. In contrast, the central venous or right atrial pressure may not reflect left ventricular (end-diastolic) filling pressure in patients with myocardial dysfunction.

A cannula should be inserted in the radial artery to monitor blood pressure and other parameters and to sample arterial blood gases.

Measurement of urine output is indicated and generally requires a urinary catheter. Urine production should be at least 1 mL/kg/hr and, if maintained at this level, indicates adequate renal perfusion and cardiac output. Red blood cells and casts in the urine indicate renal injury. The BUN may be elevated following gastrointestinal bleeding, but a urine/serum nitrogen ratio of less than 20:1 or a fractional excretion of sodium greater than 3% suggests acute renal injury.

Laboratory evaluation may be helpful. The serum potassium may increase with cellular damage or renal insufficiency, while the serum sodium decreases with loss of cell membrane integrity. Serum albumin leaks through damaged capillaries and should be kept at normal levels to maintain intravascular oncotic pressure and to retard further capillary losses. Serum calcium (ionized calcium in particular), often depressed in patients with shock, should be normalized to prevent further loss of cardiac contractility. Serum enzymes such as SGOT, SGPT, LDH, and amylase may be elevated owing to hepatic and pancreatic involvement. Stool blood may reflect primary intestinal lesions, and bleeding may occur secondary to intestinal ischemia. Serum glucose levels may be elevated early as a result of adrenergic activity but decrease as glycogen stores are depleted. An elevated arterial lactic acid level results from poor perfusion and anaerobic metabolism. Hemoglobin levels should be monitored to ensure adequate oxygen carrying capacity. The patient suspected of septic shock should have a complete bacteriologic workup. The CBC, platelet count, and clotting factors, such as prothrombin time, partial thromboplastin time, and fibrinogen level, should be evaluated for evidence of intravascular coagulation. The electrocardiogram is commonly employed to continuously monitor cardiac rhythm and electrical activity. The chest roentgenogram with evidence of pulmonary edema should suggest the presence of the shock lung syndrome or congestive heart failure.

Treatment. The principles of shock therapy are (1) identifying and treating the underlying disorders producing shock, (2) improving cardiac output, (3) improving the distribution of the patient's limited cardiac output, and (4) relieving respiratory insufficiency.

Identifying and treating underlying disorders is most difficult when shock is produced by more than one mechanism. For example, both cardiogenic and hypovolemic shock often complicate septic shock. Although aggressive invasive monitoring is often the only way to define precisely the mechanisms at work in a given patient, careful clinical evaluation plus the use of echocardiography in selected cases will supply enough data to guide initial treatment. For other patients a CVP line may be indicated. A few patients will require monitoring of cardiac output, systemic vascular resistance, and pulmonary vascular resistance.

The first priority of improving cardiac output is to provide adequate blood volume and to control hemorrhage or fluid loss. A fluid challenge of 10–20 mL/kg should be administered to any patient suspected of being volume depleted or, if such parameters are quickly available, to any patient displaying a CVP less than 5–8 mm Hg and a pulmonary arterial wedge pressure less than 10 mm Hg. If no significant increase in pressure occurs, additional fluids should be administered until the CVP is 10–12 mm Hg and the wedge pressure 16–18 mm Hg. Although these pressures are considered optimal ventricular filling conditions, each patient's response may vary depending on factors such as myocardial contractility, lung compliance, and level of respiratory support; serial cardiac output and blood pressure measurements performed during volume loading are necessary to determine the optimal cardiac filling pressures for each patient.

During early therapy, the administration of saline or Ringer lactate is acceptable to meet emergency volume needs. However, their effects are usually short-lived since fluid is quickly lost from the vascular into the intersitial space. This is especially true for patients with septic shock who have increased systemic and pulmonary capillary leakage; aggressive therapy with excess crystalloids may produce serious pulmonary sequelae. Blood, plasma, or albumin should be employed for volume expansion when available. These colloids improve mean arterial pressure, cardiac output, oxygen consumption, and left ventricular stroke work to a far greater degree than crystalloids, and the benefits are prolonged. In advanced shock, however, even colloids may leak from the vascular space.

The response to fluids may unmask the presence of decreased myocardial contractility. An elevation in filling pressures without an increase in cardiac output indicates that the myocardium is depressed and inotropic support may be needed. Sympathomimetic amines are most commonly employed because of their rapid onset, ease of accurate dosage, and ultra-short half-lives (Table 5–23). *Isoproterenol* stimulates the beta-adrenergic receptors to produce a cardiac inotropic and chronotropic effect as well as dilatation of skeletal muscle vascular beds; it involves the risk of increasing myocardial oxygen consumption, reducing coronary blood flow, and predisposing to myocardial ischemia and arrhythmias. *Epinephrine* has the advantage of being strongly inotropic with a dose-dependent dual vascular effect: at lower dosage, its effect is to reduce systemic vascular resistance, while at higher dosage, increased resistance occurs. *Dopamine* is a precursor of norepinephrine and also an activator of the sympathetic receptors in a dose-dependent fashion. At very low dosage, its principal effect is renal and splanchnic vasodilatation and a reduction of systemic vascular resistance. At moderate doses, the inotropic effects occur, along with vasodilatation, while at larger doses, there is inotropy with vasoconstriction. *Dobutamine* is synthesized from isoproterenol, and uniquely acts inotropicly with little peripheral vascular effect; it may be particularly helpful to patients with cardiogenic shock and an elevated peripheral vascular resistance. The high dose range of epinephrine and dopamine is recommended in patients with septic shock and decreased systemic vascular resistance and hypotension. The use of digitalis to increase inotropy of patients in shock should be discouraged because of its slow onset of action and long half-life and the unstable electrolyte status and renal function of these patients.

Acidosis depresses myocardial function and interferes with the circulatory response to sympathomimetic amines. The pH should be maintained above 7.25 with sodium bicarbonate to ensure adequate response to these vasoactive amines. Persistent metabolic acidosis, despite therapy, indicates continued inadequate tissue perfusion and a poor prognosis. If the serum ionized calcium is low, administering calcium chloride may produce a positive inotropic response with increased blood pressure.

Myocardial failure coexists with elevated systemic vascular resistance in most patients with cardiogenic shock and in many children in the later stages of septic shock. If the cardiac filling pressures are increased, with normal or elevated blood pressure and with depressed cardiac output, a vasodilator such as *sodium nitroprusside* should be employed for reducing systemic vascular resistance. Adequate cardiac filling, supplemented by inotropic agents and/or by afterload reduction, will improve cardiac performance unless irreversible myocardial damage has occurred.

Corticosteroids are reported to have improved cardiac output early in the course of shock. However, their effect on long-term survival is controversial. The recommended dosage is 30 mg/kg for methylprednisolone and 1.5–6.0 mg/kg for dexamethasone.

Redistributing cardiac output to improve renal and splanchnic blood flow may require low or moderated dose dopamine even after a relatively good response to volume loading. Another means of redistributing blood flow, until recently

Table 5–23. **Vasoactive Agents**

Medication	Dosage (μg/kg/min)	Action
Isoproterenol	0.1–3	Tachycardia, increased contractility, vasodilatation
Epinephrine	0.1–1	Increased contractility, mild vasodilatation
	1–3	Increased contractility, vasoconstriction
Dopamine	0.5–2	Increased renal and splanchnic flow, mild vasodilatation
	2–10	Mildly increased contractility, mild vasoconstriction, and increased renal blood flow
	10–20	Moderately increased contractility, tachycardia, vasoconstriction
	>20	As above, but further vasoconstriction
Dobutamine	2–20	Increased contractility, decreased systemic vascular resistance

used almost exclusively in the prehospital setting, is military antishock trousers (MAST). This tool is now being used by many emergency facilities to direct cardiac output away from the lower extremities and toward critical organ systems. Simple leg elevation is another means of promoting such a redistribution of blood flow.

Many patients with cardiogenic and septic shock require mechanical ventilation to relieve respiratory insufficiency. It is indicated if the paO$_2$ is less than 60–80 torr, despite an enrichment of the inspired oxygen. Controlled ventilation will alleviate the patients' respiratory distress and reduce oxygen consumption. If extravasation of fluid into the alveolus has occurred or if shock lung is present, levels of positive end-expiratory pressure (PEEP) of 10 cm H$_2$O or greater may be necessary. With very high PEEP levels (15 cm water or greater), the venous return may be impaired and cardiac output reduced. High levels require measuring cardiac output and filling pressures to ensure adequate cardiac performance.

JOSEPH SIMON

Hodes HL: Endotoxin shock. In: Smith CA (ed): The Critically Ill Child. Philadelphia, WB Saunders, 1977.
Joly RH, Weil MH: Temperature of the great toe as an indication of the severity of shock. Circulation 39:131, 1969.
Rinaldo JE, Rogers RM: Adult respiratory-distress syndrome: Changing concepts of lung injury and repair. N Engl J Med 306:900, 1982.
Shoemaker WC: Pathophysiology, monitoring, and therapy of shock syndromes. In: Shoemaker SC, Thompson WL (eds): Critical Care. Fullerton, CA, Society of Critical Care Medicine, 1980.
Siegel JH, Greenspan M, Del Guercio LRM: Abnormal vascular tone, defective oxygen transport and myocardial failure in human septic shock. Ann Surg 165:504, 1967.
Sprung CL, Caralis PV, Marcial EH: The effects of high-dose corticosteroids in patients with septic shock: A prospective, controlled study. N Engl J Med 311:1137, 1984.
Stiem RE, Rich K: Recognition and management of shock in pediatric patients. Current Problems in Pediatrics. Chicago, Year Book Medical Publishers, 1973.
The Organ in Shock. The proceedings of the second symposium on recent research developments and current clinical practice in shock. Thompson WL, Moderator. Kalamazoo, MI, Upjohn, 1977.
Wiel MH: Current understanding of mechanisms and treatment of circulatory shock caused by bacterial infections. Ann Clin Res 9:181, 1977.

5.42 HEMORRHAGIC SHOCK AND ENCEPHALOPATHY

This syndrome of unknown etiology characterized by profound circulatory collapse, signs of encephalopathy, fever, often disseminated intravascular coagulopathy, and variable signs of hepatic and renal dysfunction has recently been reported in infants. The onset of illness is sudden in previously well children usually less than 1 yr of age. Frequently it is preceded by 1–2 days of malaise and vomiting, but occasionally there is no prodrome. Clinical manifestations include signs of shock, often resistant to volume correction; seizures, coma, and hypotonia followed by decerebrate posturing, spasticity, and signs of increased intracranial pressure; hyperpyrexia; watery or bloody diarrhea; bleeding from the respiratory tract or venipuncture sites; and hepatomegaly. Laboratory studies reveal severe metabolic acidosis; markedly deranged clotting studies with subsequent thrombocytopenia and anemia; elevated blood urea, creatinine, transaminases, and bilirubin; and occasionally mild hypernatremia. Bacterial, viral, and toxicologic investigations have been negative. Mortality and central nervous system morbidity are high, despite intensive treatment of shock, elevated intracranial pressure, bleeding, and acidosis. At autopsy brains are edematous and soft to liquid in consistency, intestines have mucosal and submucosal hemorrhages and inflammatory infiltrates, and the liver has patchy swelling and degeneration of hepatocytes without fatty or other changes suggesting Reye syndrome. The differential diagnosis includes septicemia, viremia, Reye

syndrome, toxic shock and other toxin-induced diseases, heat stroke, viral hemorrhagic fevers, and poisonings.

RICHARD E. BEHRMAN

Leven M, Kay JDS, Gould JD, et al: Haemorrhagic shock and encephalopathy: A new syndrome with high mortality in young children. Lancet 2:64, 1983.
Whittington LK, Roscelli JD, Parry WH: Hemorrhagic shock and encephalopathy: Further description of a new syndrome. J Pediatr 106:599, 1985.

5.43 DROWNING AND NEAR-DROWNING

Drowning is death from suffocation by submersion in water, causing severe asphyxia from respiratory obstruction, with or without the aspiration of water. Death may be immediate or may follow unsuccessful resuscitation. Successful resuscitation, termed *near-drowning*, is the complete or temporary survival following a submersion incident. The victim may later die (termed *near-drowning with delayed death*) or may recover completely or partially. Fortunately, for each near-drowned child who later dies, there are four who survive, and most (92%) make a complete recovery.

Most drownings are accidental: infants drown in bathtubs; inadequately attended toddlers drown in swimming pools; small children fall into ponds, streams, and flooded excavations; accomplished swimmers overestimate their endurance; occupants of pleasure boats fall overboard without life jackets; and the incautious of all ages plunge through thin ice.

Incidence. Annually, approximately 140,000 people die worldwide from drowning. In the United States, there are about 7000 deaths/yr, with a higher proportion of males than females and of nonwhites than whites. Over half the victims are children, adolescents, and young adults (less than 25 yr old). The highest incidence occurs in the 1–4 yr age group. In children, the incidence of drowning varies with location: in Florida, it is the third most common cause of death for all children under 14; in Australia, drowning causes more deaths of children under 6 than motor vehicle accidents.

Creeks, rivers, and other bodies of water are the sites of about half the deaths of persons less than 25 yr of age; the bathtub is the site in almost 20% of the cases. Bathtub drownings most often occur to children unsupervised at the time of the accident, and particularly to those 10–12 mo old who are the youngest or next to youngest members of larger families. Swimming pools are the site of the highest death rates for children 1–3 yr of age, and in about three fourths of the drownings, the children were unsupervised in a pool having no fence around it. The incidence of drownings and near-drownings could be decreased, especially in this group, if all swimming pools were required to be enclosed on all four sides by a fence with a self-latching gate. In addition, parents need to be taught that young children should never swim or bathe unsupervised.

Pathophysiology. Drowning is characterized by increasing hypoxemia affecting all organs and tissues, the severity of which is determined by the *duration of submersion*, the presence of *pulmonary aspiration*, and by the *individual's responses*.

The duration of submersion is critical because arterial oxygen tension falls exponentially during asphyxia. It was believed that the maximum submersion period before irreversible damage occurred was 3–5 min. However, cases have been reported of prolonged submersion (10–40 min) with complete recovery, especially of children in cold water who developed acute hypothermia. Although full recovery is rare after more than 20 min submersion, resuscitation should always be attempted.

Pulmonary aspiration, which occurs in 80–90% of all cases,

may have profound effects. The near-drowned patient's subsequent course depends on the nature, composition, and amount of aspirate, which includes variables such as sea water or fresh water, cold water or warm water, pathogenic bacteria or fungi, toxic chemicals, mud and vegetable matter, gastric contents, and so forth. Aspirated sea water produces hypoxia by mechanisms that differ from those of fresh water. Because sea water is hypertonic (approximately 3% saline), body fluid is initially drawn into the alveoli, producing hypoxia. In contrast, aspirated hypotonic fresh water alters the surface tension properties of pulmonary surfactant, resulting in unstable alveoli, which become atelectatic, thus producing intrapulmonary shunting and hypoxemia. In both types, pulmonary insufficiency with intrapulmonary shunting and ventilation/perfusion mismatching occurs, lung compliance decreases, dead space to tidal volume ratio increases, and airway resistance increases.

Of greater immediate consequence than the nature of the aspirated water is its temperature and volume. In drowning animals, aspirated cold fresh water is rapidly absorbed and can produce significant "core" cooling (including cerebral hypothermia) prior to circulatory arrest. This process, "acute submersion hypothermia," may delay the onset of irreversible damage, making complete recovery possible despite prolonged submersion. Aspirated cold sea water is less likely to cause such profound central cooling, although the lung may function as a heat exchanger. Alternatively, humans who hyperventilate when submerged in icy water may have massive absorption and movement of cold water into their circulation; they may drown immediately from severe intravascular hemolysis with hyperkalemic circulatory arrest or from acute "core" hypothermia with unconsciousness or ventricular fibrillation. More commonly, aspiration of smaller volumes occurs and may produce mild hemolysis with hematuria and possible renal failure.

The volume of fresh water aspirated during a brief period of submerged respiration can exceed 100 mL/kg body weight, and Swann showed that the blood volume could increase up to 10 times in dogs submerged for 2–3 min.

The water load may be exacerbated by administering large volumes of fluid during resuscitation, producing excessive third-space fluid and late complications. Regardless of large fluid shifts during drowning, no clinically significant electrolyte changes are present within 15 min of successful resuscitation.

The acute aspiration of as little as 2.2 mL/kg of water produces a profound decrease in arterial oxygen tension, and after aspiration of 11 mL/kg of fresh water or sea water, the PaO_2 consistently drops to values of 30–40 torr and remains depressed for at least 72 hr in survivors. In the recovery phase, there may be hypoxia during room air breathing that was not evident during oxygen breathing, suggesting persistent areas of ventilation/perfusion mismatching. $paCO_2$ initially increases following aspiration in experimental animals but rapidly returns to normal as hyperventilation supervenes; measurements of $paCO_2$ in human near-drowning victims are variable. Carbon dioxide levels may be elevated by hypoventilation but rapidly return to normal with increased spontaneous or mechanical ventilation, indicating no barrier to the elimination of carbon dioxide. In the late recovery period, pulmonary function returns to normal and lung sequelae are rare.

Pulmonary damage may be exacerbated by inhaled irritating chemicals, virulent microorganisms, and mud or other vegetative material. In addition, near-drowned victims may swallow large volumes of fluid, develop gastric distention, and then regurgitate, which accounts for the water often seen issuing from the mouth after rescue. Stomach contents are aspirated in nearly 25% of cases, especially during cardiopulmonary resuscitation (CPR).

Approximately 12% of near-drowned victims do not aspirate, although they develop severe hypoxia and hypercarbia during submersion. If rescued and given artificial ventilation prior to circulatory arrest, they usually recover completely. The 10% of victims who drown without aspiration die acutely from breathholding or laryngospasm.

All body organ systems are affected by progressive hypoxemia and hypercarbia. However, the primary responses of the central nervous and cardiovascular systems while the victim is submerged are of greatest importance. Initially, panic and anxiety with breathholding occur, followed by swallowing and loss of consciousness. Subjective sensations are rarely reported, owing to retrograde amnesia in severe cases. Later, involuntary respiration usually occurs, followed by apnea from medullary depression. In animals, initially there is tachycardia followed after a minute or so by extreme hypertension (presumably the result of endogenous catecholamine release) with reflex bradycardia. Increasing cardiac irregularities follow, and within 3–5 min the circulation suddenly fails, secondary to myocardial hypoxia (producing "pulselessness"). The heart continues to beat briefly, but effective perfusion is absent, and successful resuscitation rapidly becomes impossible. In humans, without significant core hypothermia, a similar narrow margin exists between the onset of "pulselessness" and the inability to resuscitate. With cardiac arrest, total ischemia-anoxia supervenes and multiple organ failure results.

Pathology. Postmortem changes after drowning are nonspecific. Cutis anserina ("goose flesh"), water-wrinkling of the skin of the hands and feet, pale or sanguineous water foam from the nose and mouth, and vomitus and aquatic debris in the respiratory tract are common. The lungs may be irregularly congested and hyperinflated. Inhaled water interacts with mucus present in small airways to produce copious amounts of froth, which obstruct the exit of alveolar air. Microscopic sections show varying degrees of alveolar distention, edematous protein precipitate, infiltrates, and focal intraalveolar hemorrhage. In forensic medicine, the findings of diatoms, flagellates, or algae in the lung provide irrefutable proof of death by drowning.

The whole brain of drowning victims always looks swollen, but in delayed death after near-drowning its microscopic appearance varies with the degree of anoxia and duration of survival. With early death, edema and anoxic perivascular hemorrhages may be the only changes. In late death from near-drowning with prolonged and severe hypoxia, the changes may progress to cystic degeneration of the basal ganglia or midbrain. The heart usually appears normal, but some left ventricular dilation may occur. The liver, spleen, and kidneys appear congested, and the stomach may contain swallowed fluid.

Clinical Manifestations. Clinical death at the time of rescue does not always signify biologic death, especially in hypothermic children. Since such patients may have a good prognosis, great efforts to resuscitate are justified, despite the difficulties of restarting a cold, anoxic heart. After successful resuscitation, cardiac irregularities and low output are rare, unless severe hypoxia and metabolic acidosis persist owing to prolonged submersion. Pulmonary edema frequently occurs in the immediate postresuscitation period secondary to increased capillary permeability from anoxia, massive fluid overload, or myocardial failure. Severe pulmonary infection associated with aspiration is a common complication requiring vigorous respiratory care. Later, central nervous system dysfunction may become obvious as the result of cerebral hypoxia, ischemia, or both. Cerebral edema rarely develops; brain perfusion and cellular integrity may be further compromised by intracranial hypertension.

Treatment. Following rescue, immediate treatment is vital. If the patient is apneic, mouth-to-mouth ventilation should begin at once and be replaced as soon as possible with positive pressure ventilation. Closed chest massage should be added to ventilatory support if effective circulation is not present. CPR must be maintained continuously during transport to hospital (Sec. 5.40). If the patient was diving into water, near-drowning may be complicated by injury to the head or cervical spine, and care must be taken to maintain the neck in a neutral position. In the emergency room, routine resuscitative measures usuallly include intravenous administration of sodium bicarbonate, since severe metabolic acidosis is common. Measurement of core temperature and assessment for neurologic classification (Table 5–24) are valuable for prognostic purposes.

All patients with a history of significant submersion, even though asymptomatic, should be admitted to the hospital and observed for at least 24 hr, because they risk pulmonary insufficiency, infection, and neurologic depression.

Subsequent respiratory and circulatory support should be appropriate to the patient's condition. If the patient is alert and ventilating adequately to clear carbon dioxide, continuous positive airway pressure (CPAP) may be applied to the airway using a tight-fitting mask to increase functional residual capacity and to prevent alveoli from collapsing. A nasogastric tube should be inserted and the face observed for pressure points. CPAP should be titrated to the level at which the least intrapulmonary shunt occurs without harmful effects on cardiovascular function. If hypovolemia is present, CPAP, particularly at high levels, may decrease cardiac output and increase the need for circulatory support. Withdrawal from CPAP should be in decremental steps; sudden discontinuation of CPAP or of routine suctioning may result in significant deterioration of oxygenation. If the patient cannot maintain a normal $paCO_2$, if respirations are labored, or if paO_2 does not significantly improve, the trachea should be intubated and intermittent mandatory ventilation (IMV) should be provided at the rate determined by the arterial pH and pCO_2. If hypotension or low output exists or recurs, the use of inotropes and volume expanders is indicated.

If the patient is comatose, intensive care is required (Sec. 5.39). Intubation is necessary to protect the airway and to provide ventilatory support as indicated by the arterial blood gases. Maintaining a $paCO_2$ of less than 30 torr and a paO of greater than 55 torr may diminish the development of cerebral edema. The patient's inability to maintain an adequate arterial oxygen tension at inspired oxygen concentrations of less than 40% necessitates aggressive ventilatory therapy, which may include mechanical ventilation with positive end-expiratory pressure (PEEP) and respiratory paralysis.

Nebulized isoproterenol, racemic epinephrine, or intravenous aminophylline may be useful if bronchospasm is present. Occasionally, diuretics may also be beneficial in mobilizing interstitial pulmonary edema, but they must be used cautiously in the hypovolemic patient. Inotropic agents and plasma in large amounts may be necessary to maintain perfusion. Bronchoscopy is indicated only if food or solid material has been aspirated. Decompressing gastric dilatation with a nasogastric tube decreases the risk of regurgitation and aspiration and also may improve ventilation by decreasing intra-abdominal pressure. Prophylactic use of corticosteroids or antibiotics is not recommended.

Only after the circulation has remained stable for several hours following resuscitation should diuretics be given. Usually, maintenance fluid is decreased for several days. However, with sea water aspiration, large amounts of protein may be lost through the lungs, and colloid replacement may be indicated. Pulmonary edema after aspirating fresh or sea water may cause the loss of large volumes of fluid into the lung, which requires circulatory replacement. Pulmonary edema may also occur secondary to congestive heart failure and require fluid and pharmacologic management (Sec. 14.80 and 14.81), as well as PEEP. Significant electrolyte imbalances, coagulopathy, or anemia should be appropriately diagnosed and corrected.

Near-drowning may precipitate multiple organ system failure. Therefore, appropriate cardiopulmonary, renal, and central nervous system monitoring is required. The initial chest roentgenogram may be relatively clear even in the face of extreme hypoxia, particularly after aspiration of fresh water. Atelectasis, shock lung (Sec. 5.41 and 13.89), pneumothorax (Sec. 13.99), and pneumomediastinum (Sec. 13.100) may occur. Associated injuries, such as those of the spinal cord and intracranial bleeding, also should be ruled out.

Intracranial pressure monitoring and treatment with hyperventilation, muscle relaxants, diuretics, mannitol infusion, hypothermia, and barbiturates have been used to prevent subsequent anoxic and ischemic injury to the brain. The risks and benefits of these therapies are controversial, and they should not be used routinely.

Prognosis. The mortality rate for children admitted to the hospital following a near-drowning incident approximates 20%; most of the deaths occur in the first few days from cardiopulmonary failure. Among the survivors, the most serious sequela is neurologic damage, the reported incidence of which ranges from 0 to 21%. Although no prospective studies on the subject exist, retrospective studies suggest that those who are awake at the scene of rescue, or unconscious at the scene but fully awake on arrival at the emergency room (even after CPR) did not suffer serious neurologic sequelae (Table 5–24). The results seem similar for patients with a blunted level of consciousness, e.g., lethargic, semicomatose, agitated, confused, or combative on arrival at the hospital. In these groups, treatment consisted of cardiopulmonary support without aggressive cerebral resuscitation. In contrast, patients comatose on arrival at the hospital who required appropriate cardiopulmonary support were found to have nearly a 50% survival rate without brain damage, whether treated with only mild hyperventilation and steroids or with aggressive hyperventilation, fluid restriction, hyperoxia, steroids, muscle paralysis, and barbiturate coma. Aggressive treatment may decrease morbidity and mortality in those with decorticate or decerebrate signs, but, in general, severe anoxic injury occurs in the flaccid comatose patient, in those submerged for more than 6 min, in those requiring cardiopulmonary resuscitation in the emergency room, or in those needing continual mechanical ventilation. Rarely, following cold water drowning, hypothermic children who appeared clinically dead have recovered completely.

A. W. CONN

Conn AW, Barker GA: Fresh water drowning and near-drowning. Can Anaesth Soc J 31:S38–44, 1984.

Conn AW, Montes JE, Barker GA, et al: Cerebral salvage in near-drowning following neurological classification by triage. Can Anaesth Soc J 27:201, 1980.

Hoff BH: Multisystem failure: A review with special reference to drowning. Crit Care Med 7:210, 1979.

Table 5–24. Fresh Water Drowning and Near-Drowning (1970–1982), Hospital for Sick Children, Toronto

Neurologic Category	Total Cases	Results		
		Dead	Abnormal CNS	Normal
A (Awake)	56	0	0	56 (100%)
B (Blunted)	19	1 (5.5%)	0	18 (94.5%)
C (Comatose)	65	25 (38.5%)	9 (13.8%)	31 (47.7%)
Total cases	140	26 (18.6%)	9 (6.4%)	105 (75%)

Modell JH: The Pathophysiology and Treatment of Drowning and Near-Drowning. Springfield, IL, Charles C Thomas, 1971.

Modell JH, Graves SA, Kuck EJ: Near-drowning: Correlation of level of consciousness and survival. Can Anaesth Soc J 27:211, 1980.

Peterson B: Morbidity of childhood near-drowning. Pediatrics 29:364, 1977.

Swann HG, Spafford NR: Body salt and water changes during fresh and sea water drowning. Tex Rep Biol Med 9:356–382, 1981.

5.44 BURNS

Burns are the effects of thermal energy having made contact with skin and/or other tissues. Tissue damage begins when temperatures reach 40° C; the rate of injury increases logarithmically as the tissue temperature rises. Burns are classified according to the depth of tissue injured. *First degree burns*, such as sunburns, involve only the epithelium. *Second degree burns* destroy the epithelium and part of the corium but spare dermal appendages, from which re-epithelialization may occur. *Third degree burns* destroy the entire thickness of the dermis; consequently, re-epithelialization is restricted to the periphery of the lesions. Burns covering less than 10% of the body surface may be inconsequential unless they involve key areas such as the hands, face, or flexural regions. Morbidity and mortality increase with increasing extent and degree of burn.

Incidence. Approximately 2,000,000 people receive medical attention, 100,000 are hospitalized, and 7800 die each year in the United States because of burn injuries. Fires produce the second highest death rate in the world and the highest in industrial nations. Burns are the second leading cause of nonvehicular accidental death; 30% of these deaths occur in children under 15 yr of age. Among children aged 1–4 yr, burns are the leading cause of accidental death in the home and second only to vehicular injuries overall. Among 5–14 yr old children, burns are the third leading cause of accidental deaths.

Etiology. The young, the elderly, and the socioeconomically disadvantaged are at increased risk for burn injuries. Most children's burns occur in the home during waking hours. The major vectors of heat energy are hot liquids and solids, materials such as flammable fabrics, volatile flammable liquids, and domestic dwellings. Combustible materials are most commonly ignited by matches, poorly guarded space heaters, kitchen ranges, or water heaters. Scalds are the leading cause of burn injuries in the first 3 yr of life and are usually limited to small areas of the body. Chemical burns are rare and usually benign, except for those involving the esophagus. Burns due to the ignition of combustible materials are most common after infancy, and the resultant injuries are usually large and life-threatening.

Prevention. Preventing burns requires (1) educating the public about potential risks and ways to avoid them, (2) regulating product safety, and (3) attenuating the vectors of heat energy and their ignitors through technologic advances. Common strategies for preventing burns by controlling the sources and expenditure of energy are outlined in Table 5–25. Physicians have a major responsibility for educating parents and for encouraging appropriate legislative controls. For example, physicians strongly supported the federal regulation of flammability of children's sleepwear that reduced considerably the hazard of burn injury from flammable garments. Similar efforts are being made to regulate the maximum temperature of home water heaters and the ignition and burning power of cigarettes and matches.

Pathophysiology. Hemodynamic, autonomic, cardiopulmonary, renal, and metabolic disturbances develop rapidly following severe burns. Within seconds of the injury, cardiac output decreases, presumably because of exaggerated reflex responses and decreased venous return. Myocardial contrac-

Table 5–25. Prevention of Trauma, Adapted to Burn Injuries

General Principles	Examples of Application to Burns
Prevent marshaling of latent energy	Do not store gasoline in the home
Reduce the amount of marshaled energy	Reduce temperature of bath or shower water
Modify the rate at which energy can propagate	Use flame-retardant fabrics
Separate in time or space the energy from the susceptible structure	Locate water heaters away from flammable liquids
Separate by interposition of a barrier	Use safeguards for space heaters
Strengthen the structure that might be damaged by energy	Apply more stringent building and fireproofing codes
Detect the danger and counter its rapid continuation and extension	Use fire alarms, sprinkler systems, fire extinguishers

tility is not initially affected. A plasma factor that depresses myocardial contractility has been isolated from severely burned animals and humans during the latter stages of shock, but its significance is poorly understood.

Soon after the injury, the permeability of the vascular system may increase, accompanied by the loss of water, electrolytes, and proteins from the vascular compartment into the interstitium of injured and noninjured tissues. Animal studies suggest that this effect occurs at a maximum of 30 min after the burn and that capillary integrity is restored within 12 hr of the injury; however, only mild and transient leaks into noninjured tissues occurred in burns extending to as much as 40% of the body surface.

Within minutes following a substantial burn, renal plasma flow and glomerular filtration rate decreases. Oliguria develops, and tubular function is at least transiently compromised. Secretions of antidiuretic hormone (ADH) and aldosterone are increased, further contributing to reduced urine formation; tubular reabsorption of sodium is stimulated, excretion of potassium is enhanced, and the urine is maximally concentrated. This antidiuresis is most prominent during the first 12–24 hr after the burn, but it may persist for several days.

Destruction of red blood cells in the period immediately after a burn seldom exceeds 10% of circulating erythrocytes. Additional losses may occur subsequently, as partly damaged cells are lysed and blood is lost from granulation tissues. For these and other reasons, anemia is likely to develop within 4–7 days of major burn injuries.

Emergency Management of Severe Burns. It is imperative that care be administered in an orderly fashion (Table 5–26). First, the adequacy of the airway should be established, especially in a child with facial burns or one who has inhaled smoke. Then a rapid assessment is made, which includes (1) inspecting wounds, (2) evaluating the cardiorespiratory status, and (3) determining previously unrecognized injuries. An intravenous infusion of isotonic fluids is started, to expand the blood volume; lactated Ringer solution, isotonic saline, or plasma may be infused at a rate of 20 mL/kg/hr until more accurate estimates of fluid requirements are made.

The stomach is emptied with a nasogastric tube to prevent gastric dilatation or vomiting. Before the tube is withdrawn, a small quantity of antacid is instilled to retard the development of stress ulcers. A urinary catheter is then inserted so that output can be monitored.

Since the quantities of fluids and medications to be administered depend on the size of the patient and the extent of injury, the patient's weight and height should be carefully measured, and the total body surface area and the burned

Table 5–26. **Priorities of Medical Procedures in the Emergency Phase of Burn Injuries**

Procedure	Indication	Comment
Establish an adequate airway	Burns of the face Laryngeal edema Smoke inhalation	Avoid emergency tracheostomy
Examine for trauma to head, skeleton, or nervous system	Explosions	Remove clothing; radiologic examination helpful
Begin intravenous infusion	To prevent intravascular dehydration	Use isotonic fluids
Empty stomach through a nasogastric tube	To prevent gastric dilatation, vomiting, or aspiration	Antacids may be helpful
Insert an indwelling urinary catheter	To monitor hourly urine output	Use a closed drainage system
Examine the burn wound	To estimate depth and extent	Use burn charts corrected for age
Clean, debride, and dress the burn area	To minimize microbial colonization	Use topical antimicrobial therapy
Medications	To treat infections; to prevent tetanus; for sedation	Use intravenous route for sedation
Begin fluid, electrolyte, and protein replacement	To correct antecedent deficits and concurrent losses	Use appropriate formula to estimate requirements

surface area estimated. Weight should be measured both before and after dressings, bedclothing, or restraints are applied. The wounds should be cleansed and debrided, their depth assessed, and the extent of 2nd and 3rd degree burns estimated by using body surface charts corrected for age (Fig. 5–10). The wounds should then be covered with dressings saturated with an antimicrobial agent. In addition, circumferential 3rd degree burns should be identified and escharotomies performed to prevent ischemia of extremities or respiratory embarrassment from chest wall involvement.

Sedatives may be given, preferably via the intravenous route, if there are no injuries to the central nervous system. Respiratory depressants should be avoided. Tetanus toxoid and parenteral penicillin are indicated for tetanus and β-hemolytic streptococcal infections, respectively.

Fluid, Electrolyte, and Colloid Therapy During the First Day. The primary goal of administering fluid during the first 24 hr after a burn is to restore the patient's volume and osmotic homeostasis promptly, thereby preventing or minimizing organ dysfunction and edema formation. Restoring homeostasis is achieved by replacing antecedent and concurrent deficits of fluid, electrolytes, and proteins. In addition, therapy should anticipate and replace maintenance fluid and electrolyte requirements before significant deficits develop (Sec. 5.16).

The specific aim of fluid treatment is to attain and maintain a normal or near-normal state of hydration in all body fluid compartments; to correct acid-base imbalance; and to restore cardiovascular, pulmonary, and renal hemodynamics. Restoring and maintaining perfusion pressures leads to maximal

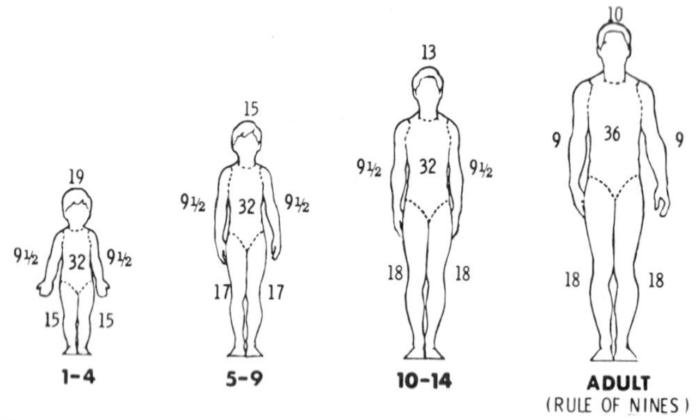

oxygenation of injured and noninjured tissues, which promotes spontaneous healing, prevents wound conversion, minimizes bacterial colonization, and prepares the injured areas for early grafting.

Errors in fluid therapy may have grave consequences. Underhydration can prolong a state of shock, worsen metabolic acidosis, and induce organ dysfunction; overhydration fosters edema formation and pulmonary congestion. Accurately predicting fluid requirements is especially difficult, since most formulas for fluid therapy of burn victims were designed for adults, whose fluid needs are estimated solely from body weight and percentage of body surface burned. Furthermore, current versions of these formulas do not include allowances for maintenance fluids and the fluid needed to replace burn related losses, the net result of which is a tendency to underhydrate small children and to overestimate the fluid requirements of the large or obese child. Similar errors also occur at the extremes of burn size. Therefore, using "single figure" formulas, such as the Parkland or the modified Brooke formula, is not recommended for hydration of burned children.

Compared with adults, children—and particularly infants—have high rates of heat exchange relative to size and weight, high rates of water exchange in relation to total body water, and significant differences in muscle water and electrolyte composition. Children also require relatively larger volumes of urine for excretion of waste products than do adults, and insensible water losses, when expressed in terms of body weight, are significantly greater than are those in adults. Therefore, calculating fluid and electrolyte requirements on the basis of body surface area offers greater accuracy, consistency, and simplicity.

When these concepts are applied to managing the burned child, the quantity of fluids to administer during the first 24 hr after the burn is estimated as follows:

2000 mL/m² of body surface/24 hr
plus
5000 mL/m² of body surface *burned*/24 hr

Half of this amount is administered during the first 8 hr and the other half during the subsequent 16 hr (Fig. 5–11). No upper limit for the area of body surface burned is used. Fluid received before arriving at a center for definitive care must be reviewed and appropriate adjustments made.

Example. A 4 yr old child having a body surface area of 0.68 m² sustained 3rd degree burns to approximately 40% of his body surface. Despite having received 200 mL of lactated Ringer solution during the first hour, he appeared dehydrated on admission.

Figure 5–10. Burn assessment chart. (Body proportions modified from Lund and Brower.) Numbers under the figures indicate age; the others indicate % of body surface.

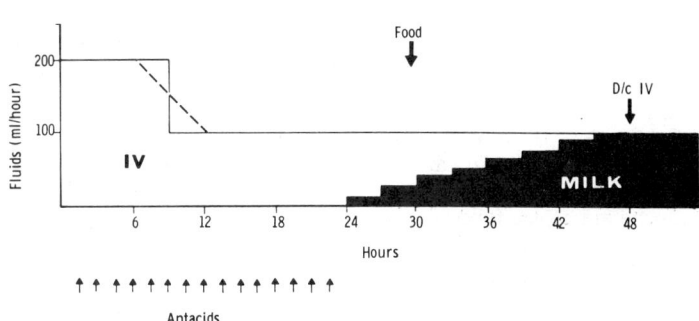

Figure 5–11. Rate of fluid administration. Half of the first day fluid estimate is administered intravenously during the first 8 hr after injury. The other half is given during the subsequent 16 hr. Homogenized milk by mouth and food are begun during the second day. Only antacids are given orally during the first day. (IV, intravenous; D/c, discontinue.)

Comments. (1) Fluids received during the initial evaluation period (lactated Ringer saline or plasma) need not be included in the calculation of requirements for the first 24 hr. These fluids may be given at a rate of approximately 20 mL/kg/hr for 1–2 hr.

(2) Calculation of the first 24 hr requirements: 2000 mL/m^2 of body surface/24 hr.

Example.

$$2000 \times 0.68 = 1360 \text{ mL/24 hr}$$
plus
$$5000 \text{ mL/m}^2 \text{ of body surface burned/24 hr}$$

Example.

$$5000 \times 0.68 \times 0.4 = 1360 \text{ mL/24 hr}$$

Total requirement for the first 24 hr (maintenance plus burn replacement) is 1360 mL + 1360 mL = 2720 mL.

(3) Half of the estimated amount is given during the first 8 hr and half during the subsequent 16 hr.

Example.

First 8 hr = 170 mL/hr
Second 8 hr = 85 mL/hr
Third 8 hr = 85 mL/hr

Although this method offers definite advantages in children, it still provides only reasonable estimates of the quantities of fluid needed for the first 24 hr. Successful fluid treatment of the burned child requires not only the use of an appropriate formula but also a clear understanding of the fluid therapy protocol as a whole, which includes:

1. Burn charts, properly corrected for age, to assess the extent of the injury (see Fig. 5–10).

2. Careful measurement of height and weight to calculate surface area from standard nomograms (see Figs. 29–1 and 29–2).

3. Accurate prediction of fluid requirements using the surface area formula.

4. An appropriate hydrating solution.

5. Well-defined guidelines to monitor the state of hydration.

Choice of Hydrating Solutions. The composition of the fluids administered is controversial, and various solutions such as plasma and saline, dextrose, lactated Ringer solution, and hypertonic saline have been proposed. The major issue is whether or not the initial use of crystalloid or colloid-containing solutions will improve the outcome of severe burns. Although this question remains unanswered, evidence now suggests that leakage of albumin from the intravascular to the interstitial spaces is a short-lived phenomenon, lasting 8–12 hr and of significance for only the first 6 hr after the burn; that the addition of albumin to resuscitation fluids reduces fluid requirements and, consequently, edema for-

mation; that the addition of 12.5 g of albumin to each liter of fluid given during the first 24 hr prevents the development of hypoalbuminemia and its consequences; and lastly that isotonic solutions containing 130–135 mEq of sodium/L and 20–30 mEq of bicarbonate or lactate/L maintain serum osmolality and electrolytes within normal limits and usually promptly correct any underlying metabolic acidosis. Thus, we recommend the use of lactate or bicarbonate isotonic salt solutions that contain albumin and adequate quantities of carbohydrate (e.g., 5% glucose) to provide a protein-sparing effect. This solution can be prepared by adding 12.5 g of human serum albumin (50 mL of 25% solution) to 950 mL of lactated Ringer solution in 5% dextrose. The final composition of the mixture is: Na—132 mEq/L; Cl—109 mEq/L; lactate—28 mEq/L; K—4 mEq/L; glucose—47.5 g/L; and albumin—1.25 g/dL.

For infants less than 1 yr of age the concentration of sodium in the hydrating fluids should be decreased to avoid hypernatremia. We recommend a solution prepared by mixing 930 mL of 5% dextrose in 0.3% sodium chloride solution, 20 mL of sodium bicarbonate (1 mEq/mL), and 50 mL of 25% human serum albumin. The final composition of this mixture is: Na—77 mEq/L; Cl—57 mEq/L; bicarbonate—20 mEq/L; glucose—46.5 gm/L; and albumin–1.25 g/dL. Potassium is not added during the first 24 hr, since large amounts of this ion are released from injured cells into the extracellular fluids. Acidosis and renal failure may also result in dangerous hyperkalemia. After the first day, depending on the blood urea nitrogen (BUN) level, urine output, and condition of the patient, 20–30 mEq of potassium phosphate may be added to each liter of intravenous fluid.

The advantages of using composite burn solutions are (1) only one type of solution is required; (2) fluid, electrolyte, and protein are administered simultaneously; and (3) only the rate of infusion needs adjustment. No oral fluids other than ice chips should be given for the first 24 hr; during this time, absorption of fluid and electrolytes from the gastrointestinal tract is unpredictable, and paralytic ileus and vomiting may develop. However, antacids (Maalox, 20 mL/m^2 of body surface/hr) should be administered hourly to decrease the incidence of stress ulcers (Fig. 5–11).

Monitoring Hydration Therapy. No single criterion suffices to guide fluid therapy. Since renal function and ADH secretion in burned patients are modified by factors other than blood volume, urine output may not adequately reflect the state of hydration. Significant oliguria, however, does not occur unless there is renal damage or severe dehydration. The urine output varies considerably from hour to hour, but when averaged over 4 to 8 hr intervals, 30 mL/hr/m^2 of body surface is the usual rate of urine production during the first 24 hr. Attempts to increase urine output beyond these limits usually cause increased peripheral and/or pulmonary edema. The state of hydration is better judged by frequent periodic assessment of the sensorium, pulse, blood pressure, venous capillary filling, body weight, hematocrit, BUN, and serum and urine electrolytes and osmolality rather than by urine output. Invasive techniques to measure other variables (e.g., cardiac output, central venous pressure) are usually unnecessary.

Calculation of Fluid Needs After the First 24 Hours. Fluid requirements for the 2nd and subsequent days usually average three fourths of the first day's allowance and may be estimated with the aid of the following formula:

$$1500 \text{ mL/m}^2 \text{ of body surface/24 hr}$$
plus
$$2750 \text{ mL/m}^2 \text{ of body surface } burned/24 \text{ hr}$$

From the 2nd day on, fluids are administered at a constant rate, and the hourly allowance should not be exceeded, regardless of whether the oral and/or intravenous route is used. By the end of the first 24 hr, antacids are discontinued and homogenized milk offered instead. Milk feedings should be started in small amounts and, if tolerated, progressively increased; intravenous fluids are reduced correspondingly (Fig. 5–11). A soft diet in small amounts is usually tolerated by the 2nd or 3rd day.

During the next several days (subacute phase), the child should be supported medically to facilitate the healing of 2nd degree burns and the autografting of 3rd degree burns. Management includes daily wound irrigation with antiseptic solutions, wound debridement, topical antimicrobial therapy, splinting of affected parts, and other indicated surgical procedures. Body weight, serum electrolytes, plasma proteins, colloid osmotic pressure, hematocrit, and hemoglobin should be monitored to detect any developing fluid or electrolyte disturbance, hypoalbuminemia, or anemia. Serum albumin levels should be maintained above 2 g/dL and oncotic pressure above 15 mm Hg to prevent edema and contraction of the intravascular volume. This may require infusing human serum albumin as a 5% solution over 12–24 hr. The usual quantity of human serum albumin needed to maintain the above serum level ranges from 100 to 150 mg/m² of burned body surface/wk in three divided doses. An equivalent amount of plasma can be used instead of albumin, but the risk of hepatitis or transfusion reactions or both must be taken into consideration.

Blood lost as the direct result of the injury or its complications should be replaced on the 2nd to 5th day after the burn, depending on the severity of anemia. Except for the patient with active bleeding or severe concomitant hypoproteinemia, transfusions of packed red blood cells are safer than whole blood and better tolerated. For most patients, 10 mg/kg of packed cells given over a 3–4 hr period is sufficient. Although transfusions may be needed at 3–4 day intervals, quantities of blood in excess of 15 mL/kg should not be given within a 24 hr period unless the patient is actively bleeding; larger quantities frequently result in cardiopulmonary congestion or hypertension or both.

Caloric Requirements. Hypermetabolism, increased glucose utilization, and severe protein and fat wasting are characteristic responses to major trauma and infection. This response is never as great as it is following thermal injury. Resting metabolic rate increases in curvilinear fashion with increasing burn size from near-normal for burns less than 10% total body surface area to 1.5 times normal for burns of 25% total body surface area, to a maximum of twice normal for burns in excess of 40% total body surface area.

The precise energy requirements needed to reach weight and nitrogen balance have been calculated in adults from linear regressive analysis of weight change versus predicted dietary intake: approximately 25 kilocalories/kg plus 40 kilocalories/% body surface area burned/24 hr are required. For children, maintenance caloric requirements should be estimated on the basis of 1800 kilocalories/m² of body surface/day,

and the calories required for the burn itself should be estimated on the basis of 2200 kilocalories/m² of body surface burned/day. Hildreth and Carvajal found that only 3 of 45 severely burned children having an average caloric intake equal to or in excess of that recommended by this formula lost weight; the others either gained or maintained their weight and clinically appeared well nourished.

In children, the increased caloric demands are usually met by oral feedings of milk or a lactose-free formula, plus a well-balanced diet containing 15% protein calories, 40% fat calories, and 45% carbohydrate calories. Most patients tolerate hourly feedings well and welcome the orally administered calories. In some cases, however, continuous nasogastric tube feeding may be preferable to promote normal sleeping habits or because of complications.

Lactose intolerance may lead to diarrhea severe enough to limit enteral alimentation. The use of lactose-free formulas from the onset or soon after the diagnosis of disaccharidase deficiency is suspected frequently decreases or completely eliminates diarrhea.

Complications. With appropriate fluid therapy, cardiac output usually returns to normal in 24–48 hr. The cause of persistent *cardiac dysfunction* in burns is unknown but may involve a circulating substance, presumably of pancreatic origin with a molecular weight of less than 1000, which has been reported in patients severely burned or with septic shock (Sec. 5.41). This myocardial depressant factor (MDF) decreases contractility and reduces cardiac output. Burned children are especially prone to congestive heart failure and pulmonary edema during septic shock or to renal failure. Treatment may require digitalis, diuretic agents (e.g., furosemide), and, in extreme cases, phlebotomy or peritoneal dialysis. The development of overt congestive failure in burned and septic children may be prevented by cautious hydration; we maintain our patients slightly underhydrated.

Respiratory problems are common, particularly with smoke inhalation or facial burns (Sec. 13.80); Phillips and Cope found that pulmonary lesions contributed to or were directly responsible for 80% of burn deaths. The most common respiratory problems are pulmonary edema, tracheobronchitis, bronchopneumonia, and the alveolar-capillary block syndrome. In addition, poisoning by inhalation of toxic gases, such as carbon monoxide, may occur in burns.

Severe oliguria during the immediate postburn period is most likely the result of ADH secretion and a reduction in glomerular filtration rate, but the possibility of *renal damage* should not be discarded until normal renal function is demonstrated. For example, in the presence of oliguria, the failure of the urine to become concentrated or to show conservation of sodium is indicative of renal dysfunction.

Renal failure may be transient, owing to acute hypovolemia or shock, or persistent; with persistent azotemia the patient may be oliguric. The prognosis for oliguric azotemia is extremely poor, but with adequate supportive therapy recovery may occur. Recognizing nonoliguric renal failure is important because an adequate urine output may mask the fact that the urine volume is fixed. Water and sodium retention, hypervolemia, and congestive heart failure may then develop. If, on the other hand, the condition is promptly recognized, appropriate restrictions of water, salt, and protein intake will usually sustain relatively normal fluid balance and allow for recovery of renal function. When renal failure, particularly the oliguric type, complicates burns, peritoneal dialysis or hemodialysis is often required.

Sepsis is a leading cause of death in burned children. Besides the loss of the protective skin barrier, additional defects in host resistance such as deficiencies in thymic-dependent lymphocytes, in phagocytic function, in complement, and in macrophage activation may predispose the patient to infection lasting for weeks. Serum levels of immunoglobulins fall in the first week owing to loss of plasma into the interstitium, but antibody formation is spared. The infecting organisms vary with exposure; the principal pathogens are *Staphylococcus aureus* and gram-negative bacteria such as *Pseudomonas aeruginosa*. The main portals of entry are the wound, the respiratory tract, the urinary tract, intravenous catheters, and possibly the gastrointestinal tract.

Successful treatment depends on early diagnosis and prompt use of parenteral antibiotic therapy. No clinical signs are pathognomonic of sepsis. The diagnosis must be suspected when there is (1) wound infection, (2) hyper- or hypothermia, (3) tachypnea, (4) gastrointestinal symptoms, (5) thrombocytopenia, (6) sudden change in sensorium, (7) oliguria, or (8) hypotension. With such findings, blood and other appropriate cultures should be obtained and antibiotic therapy begun. Although the bacteriologic history of the patient should be reviewed to choose the most appropriate antibiotic, in most cases a combination of tobramycin and a penicillinase-resistant penicillin (oxacillin, dicloxacillin, methicillin) is adequate. Both drugs should be administered in maximal therapeutic doses for a minimum of 2 wk. Whenever possible, therapy should be revised according to in vitro antibiotic sensitivity tests, serum antibiotic levels, and assessment of the minimal inhibitory concentrations of the administered antibiotics.

The condition of septic burned children is unstable, and vascular collapse may lead to death within a few hours. Fluctuating body temperature, profuse sweating, anxiety, clouded sensorium, changes in vital signs, hypotension, and decreased urine output should be considered incipient signs of septic shock (Sec. 5.41). If no improvement occurs following initial antibiotic therapy, ticarcillin and steroids should be added, e.g., prednisolone, 30 mg/kg as a single intravenous dose over 45 min.

Endotoxemia usually has multiple untoward effects on renal, respiratory, and cardiovascular functions. Therefore, fluid management should be conservative; a reasonable objective is to maintain the blood pressure just above shock levels and to achieve minimal urine output. Isotonic fluids containing albumin may be used initially, but as soon as the colloidosmotic pressure and arterial blood pressure stabilize, lower concentrations of sodium solutions without albumin should be administered. The cautious use of vasoactive drugs (isoproterenol, dopamine, dobutamine) and digitalis is recommended to maintain blood pressure and avoid administering excessive quantities of fluids.

Rehabilitation. Since the physical and psychologic effects of burns are potentially crippling, a vigorous rehabilitation program to counter these effects should be instituted as soon as possible. Residual deformities or loss of function may greatly impair the child's body image and self-esteem, and prolonged hospitalization may lead to a dependency reaction that extends beyond the period of confinement. The child or parents may harbor guilt feelings about the injury. In the parents, such feelings tend to interfere with their ability to cope with the illness of the child; early discussion of these issues with the child and family may ameliorate this problem. The services of a mental health professional and social worker may be required. Psychologic support should be closely coordinated with the medical, nursing, and surgical programs and other rehabilitative measures, including physical therapy, play therapy, and continuation of schoolwork.

Plans should be made to return the child to as normal a home life as possible. The parents and child should be instructed in home care procedures such as wound dressing, splints, pressure dressings, and physical therapy. These measures are particularly important in reducing hypertrophic scars. The child should return to school and other social activities as soon as possible; this is usually feasible within the first week after the end of hospitalization. The child's

continuing rehabilitation may involve the cooperative efforts of the family physician, physical therapist, mental health professional, and reconstructive surgeon. Procedures should be planned so that they will interfere as little as possible with the child's schoolwork and other normal social activities.

HUGO F. CARVAJAL

Arturson G: Pathophysiologic aspects of the burn syndrome with special reference to liver injury and alterations of capillary permeability. Acta Chir Scand (Suppl.) 274:1, 1961.

Artz CP, Moncrief JA: The Treatment of Burns. 2nd ed. Philadelphia, WB Saunders, 1969.

Baxter CR, Moncrief JA, Prager MH, et al: A circulating myocardial depressant factor in burn shock. *In*: Matter P, Barclay TL, Kowicfova S (eds): Research in Burns. Transactions of Third International Congress on Research in Burns, Prague. Bern, Hans Huber Publishers, 1971.

Baxter CR, Shires GT: Physiologic response to crystalloid resuscitation of severe burns. Ann NY Acad Sci 150:874, 1968.

Berman W Jr, Goldman AS, Reichelderfer T, et al: Childhood burn injuries and deaths. Pediatrics 51:1069, 1973.

Bernstein NR: Emotional Care of the Facially Burned and Disfigured. Boston, Little, Brown, 1976.

Brouhard BH, Carvajal HF, Linares, HA: Burn edema and protein leakage in the rat. I. Relationship to time of injury. Microvasc Res 15:221, 1978.

Carvajal HF: A physiologic approach to fluid therapy in severely burned children. Surg Gynecol Obstet 150:379, 1980.

Carvajal HF: Management of severely burned patients: Sorting out the controversies. Emerg Med Reports 6(12):89, 1985.

Carvajal HF, Feinstein R, Traber DL, et al: An objective method for early diagnosis of gram-negative septicemia in burned children. J Trauma 21:221, 1981.

Carvajal HF, Linares HA, Brouhard BH: Relationship of burn size to vascular permeability changes in rats. Surg Gynecol Obstet 149:193, 1979.

Carvajal HF, Parks D: Survival statistics in burned children. JBCR 3:81, 1982.

Carvajal HF, Reinhart JA, Traber DL: Renal and cardiovascular functional response to thermal injury in dogs subjected to sympathetic blockade. Cir Shock 3:287, 1976.

Clark AM: Burns in childhood. World J Surg 2:175, 1978.

Cope O, Moore FD: The redistribution of body water in the fluid therapy of the burned patient. Ann Surg 126:1010, 1947.

Dubois J: Water and electrolyte content of human skeletal muscle—variations with age. Rev Europ Etudes Clin Biol 17:505, 1972.

Durtschi MB, Kohler TR, Finley A, et al: Burn injury in infants and young children. Surg Gynecol Obstet 150:651, 1980.

Feller I: Prevention for one and two year olds. NBIE Newsletter 1(2), 1980.

Feller I: Trends in burn wound management. (Abstract.) Proceedings of ABA 13th Annual Meeting, Washington, DC, 1981, p. 13.

Granger ND, Gabel JC, Drake RE, et al: Physiologic basis for the clinical use of albumin solutions. Surg Gynecol Obstet 146:97, 1978.

Gump FE, Kinney JM: Energy balance and weight loss in burned patients. Arch Surg 103:442, 1971.

Haddon W Jr: On the escape of tigers: An ecologic note. Technology Review 72(7), 1970.

Hildreth M, Carvajal HF: Caloric requirements in burned children: A simple formula to estimate daily caloric requirements. JBCR 3:78, 1982.

Holleman JH, Gable JC, Hardy JD: Pulmonary effects of intravenous fluid therapy and burn resuscitation. Surg Gynecol Obstet 149:161, 1978.

Hutcher N, Hayes BW Jr: The Evans formula revisited. J Trauma 12:453, 1972.

Innes RL, Goldman AS, Schmitt R, et al: A study of the etiology and epidemiology of burn injuries in children. *In*: Matter P, Barclay TL, Kowicfova S (eds): Research in Burns. Transactions of the First International Congress on Research in Burns, Prague. Bern, Hans Huber Publishers, 1971.

Janzekovic Z: The burn wound from a surgical point of view. J Trauma 15:42, 1975.

Larson DL: Burns in childhood: Invited commentary. World J Surg 2:181, 1978.

Larson DL, Abston S, Willis B, et al: Contracture and scar formation in the burn patient. Clin Plast Surg 1:653, 1974.

Lloyd JR: Thermal trauma: Therapeutic achievements and investigative horizons. Surg Clin North Am 57:121, 1977.

Lund CL, Browder NC: The estimation of areas of burns. Surg Gynecol Obstet 79:352, 1944.

Monafo WW: The treatment of burn shock by the intravenous and oral administration of hypertonic lactated saline solution. J Trauma 10:575, 1970.

Moncrief JA: Burns. N Engl J Med 288:444, 1973.

Phillips AW, Cope O: The revelation of respiratory tract damage as a principal killer of the burned patient. Ann Surg 155:1, 1962.

Pruitt BA Jr: Advances in fluid therapy and the early care of the burn patient. World J Surg 2:139, 1978.

Shook CW, MacMillan BC, Altemeier WA: Pulmonary complications of the burned patient. Arch Surg 97:215, 1968.

Stoll AM, Chianta MA: Heat transfer through fabrics as related to thermal injury. Trans NY Acad Sci 33:649, 1971.

Stone, HH: The composite burn solution. *In*: Polk HC Jr, Stone HH (eds): Contemporary Burn Management. Boston, Little, Brown, 1971.

5.45 PREANESTHETIC AND POSTANESTHETIC CARE

Safe and effective anesthesia for infants and children requires a thorough comprehension of the basic principles of modern anesthetic practice and of the pharmacology of the drugs used. The anesthesiologist must understand (1) the ways in which pediatric patients differ from adults in anatomy, physiology, and response to drugs; (2) the emotional reactions to anesthesia and surgery by various pediatric age groups; and (3) the physical status of the patient, the nature of the surgical lesion, and the operation to be performed. These factors enable the anesthesiologist to make an appropriate preoperative evaluation, to produce the desired degree of preanesthetic sedation, to select the least hazardous anesthetic agents and techniques that will produce satisfactory operating conditions, to determine the appropriate modes of monitoring various vital functions, and to provide for maintenance of an adequate circulating blood volume as well as fluid, electrolyte, and acid-base equilibrium.

5.46 PREANESTHETIC EVALUATION

A careful history will enable the anesthesiologist to plan more effectively the management of anesthesia and the postanesthetic period. It should include specific information about the following:

The child's previous anesthetic and surgical procedures
Family history of major anesthetic complications
History of apnea, breathing irregularities or cyanosis (especially in infants under age 6 mo)
Recent upper respiratory tract infection
Exposure to exanthems
Previous laryngotracheitis (croup)
History of allergies, drug hypersensitivities, asthma, or wheezing during respiratory infections
Abnormal weight loss
Exercise tolerance
Bleeding tendencies
Blood transfusion reactions
Current medications
Prior administration of corticosteroids
Emotional reactions of the child to the proposed operation
When and what the child last ate (especially in emergency procedures)

A history of frequent croup will require special airway management during anesthesia; a familial history of abnormal response to muscle relaxants might indicate a genetically abnormal pseudocholinesterase, which the anesthesiologist must consider when selecting a muscle relaxant; infants and children receiving cortisone, antiepileptic or sedative drugs, or certain antibiotics may have altered responses to anesthetic and adjuvant agents; a patient with a full stomach risks aspiration during induction of anesthesia.

Following inhalation anesthesia, infants less than 6 mo of age born at a gestational age less than 36 wk may be prone to periodic breathing and apnea, with an increased risk of bradycardia and cardiac arrests. The mechanisms by which anesthetics affect the control of breathing in infants remain unclear. These infants are at even greater risk if they have a history of apneic or cyanotic episodes, if their postconceptual age is less than 1 yr, or if they present any of the risk factors associated with an increased susceptibility to the sudden infant death syndrome (SIDS) (Sec. 26.1). Regional or spinal anesthesia has limited application in small infants and each presents its own undesirable side effects. Because of these considerations, as well as the occasional unexplained post-

anesthetic death of a young infant born at term, we recommend delaying *purely elective* operations until after the age of 6 mo.

With the increased survival of severely premature infants (<1500 g birthweight) and their propensity to develop inguinal hernias, the risk of early operation must be weighed against the risks of delaying the hernia repair until after age 6 mo, which carries the possibility of developing an incarcerated or strangulated hernia and acute intestinal obstruction requiring an emergency herniorraphy at a time when the infant may be in less than optimal condition. If proceeding with the operation is decided, the infant should be observed with ECG and respiratory monitoring in the recovery room for at least 2 hr. If the infant also presents with one or more of the high risk factors associated with postanesthetic apnea with bradycardia cited above, in-hospital monitoring with close nursing surveillance for 24–48 hr is usually indicated.

The physical examination should emphasize the heart, lungs, and upper airways. The presence of heart murmurs, rales in the chest, or wheezing requires careful cardiac or pulmonary evaluation before proceeding. Small, narrow nares filled with secretions, loose teeth, tonsils and adenoids large enough to cause mouth-breathing, or a small, under-developed mandible with a protruding maxilla may contribute to upper airway obstruction after sedation or induction of anesthesia. Tracheal intubation may be difficult if the larynx lies anterior to its normal position.

Laboratory tests desirable before anesthesia include determination of hemoglobin or hematocrit, white cell count, and urinalysis. In patients with serious systemic disease or those about to undergo extensive surgery, a preoperative roentgenogram of the chest and measurement of arterial pH, paO_2 and $paCO_2$, serum electrolytes, and blood glucose or urea nitrogen may be indicated.

5.47 PREANESTHETIC PREPARATION AND SEDATION

Children are frightened on leaving the security and familiarity of home, especially those 1–4 yr of age, who are unable to understand the purpose of hospitalization. Terrifying experiences during induction of anesthesia or in the immediate postoperative period can produce disabling psychologic changes such as night terrors, enuresis, and temper tantrums. Certain steps will minimize the psychologic trauma: (1) For the child over 3 yr of age, parents should explain the purpose of the proposed operation in simple terms, telling of the probable sequence of events and discomfort involved. (2) Parents should be encouraged to display confidence and cheerfulness; their tension and anxiety are readily transmitted to the child. (3) The anesthesiologist should visit the child prior to operation, in the presence of the parents if possible, so that the child will regard the anesthesiologist as a sympathetic, caring friend. (4) Preanesthetic sedation should permit the child to be transported to the operating room lightly asleep, allow induction of anesthesia without awakening, and provide some analgesia during postanesthetic recovery.

Improvements in pediatric anesthesia over the past 20 yr permit children with no organic disturbances or some mild to moderate abnormalities to be admitted to a surgical facility, undergo general anesthesia and superficial, noncomplex operative procedures, recover, and return home on the same day. The requirements for safe "day surgery" include a history and physical examination, basic laboratory studies, and a visit with the anesthesiologist, preferably within 30 days prior to operation as well as a brief preanesthetic review by the anesthesiologist on the day of operation; and an extended recovery period to ensure that the child can retain oral liquids, has voided, is not vomiting, and has adequate relief of pain.

Elective anesthesia and operation in the healthy infant less than 6 mo of age carries an increased risk of certain serious, even potentially lethal complications. Infants, in contrast to older children and adults, experience more rapid uptake from the lungs and require higher blood levels to achieve effective anesthesia with halothane, the most widely used volatile anesthetic agent. Severe systemic arterial hypotension at an effective anesthetic dose occurs more frequently in the infant, indicating a narrow margin of safety. Unexplained apneic episodes in apparently recovered infants may occur after anesthesia, resulting in severe brain damage and death if undetected. Hemoglobin concentration may be at its nadir and limit oxygen content reserves in the blood. Delayed or partial recovery from muscle relaxants may also occur during this period, especially if the infant's body temperature falls below 36° C (96.8° F). All of these complications are rare, yet are more likely to occur in the infant born preterm who is less than 40 wk postconception. Appropriate use of halothane, muscle relaxants, and oxygen provides safe, reliable anesthesia in infants; however, extending postanesthetic observation and maintaining body temperature will help ensure the safety of anesthesia in this age group.

A wide variety of drugs are used for preanesthetic sedation. Table 5–27 lists appropriate oral and intramuscular drugs and dosages for various age groups. Atropine provides more effective abolition of vagal reflexes than does scopolamine and, therefore, is preferred in infants under 1 yr of age, in whom vagal reflexes tend to be more active. In children over 1 yr of age a small volume oral preanesthetic sedation in a fruit-flavored syrup containing meperidine, diazepam, and atropine given 2 hr prior to anesthetic induction is safe and effective. A barbiturate combined with an opiate and atropine given intramuscularly produces suitable preanesthetic sedation in most children requiring more profound sedation or in those about to undergo painful and extensive operative procedures.

Although the child's stomach should be free of solids prior to anesthesia, it is important not to interrupt fluid intake longer than necessary. No milk or solids should be given less than 12 hr prior to anesthesia. Clear fluids with glucose should be given up to 4 hr prior to inducing anesthesia in infants and up to 6–8 hr prior to induction in older children. Since this preoperative oral fluid regimen may not prevent mild dehydration, intravenous isotonic electrolyte solution with glucose is warranted for all but the shortest minor procedures. (See Sec. 5.31.)

Before proceeding with an operation the anesthesiologist should correct dehydration, decrease excessive fever, correct acidosis, and restore a depleted blood volume.

The febrile, dehydrated child who requires emergency surgery, such as appendectomy, should receive at least partial rehydration rapidly, along with correction of any concomitant metabolic acidosis by intravenous sodium bicarbonate (2–3 mEq/kg). General endotracheal anesthesia with neuromuscular blockade and controlled ventilation followed by surface cooling with water mattresses on the anterior and posterior body surfaces can then be instituted. Cooling should be continued until the colonic or esophageal temperature is under 38° C (100.4° F). The anterior water mattress can be removed when the body temperature is below 39° C (102.2° F), and the operation safely started.

Newborn infants who require immediate surgery and who have made little or no recovery from birth asphyxia or who have a body temperature below 35° C (95° F) require oxygen, intravenous sodium bicarbonate (2–3 mEq/kg), and elevation of body temperature toward 37° C (98.6° F). Analyzing blood for pH, $paCO_2$, paO_2, electrolytes, glucose, osmolality, and hematocrit is essential to initial monitoring and to evaluate the patient's ventilation and metabolic status.

5.48 INTRAOPERATIVE MANAGEMENT

All the common inhalation agents have been used in children, but during the past 20 yr halothane (Fluothane) and nitrous oxide with neuromuscular blockage have replaced flammable agents such as cyclopropane and diethyl ether. For induction, most anesthesiologists prefer gravity flow of nitrous oxide and halothane over the face, with application of a face mask only after the child has lost consciousness. Intravenous induction, using a 25–27 gauge scalp vein needle, may be achieved rapidly with intravenous thiopental (3–4 mg/kg); ketamine can also be used for intravenous induction in infants and young children, but is contraindicated in older children and adolescents because of the frequency of postanesthetic hallucinations in this age group. Newer inhalation agents such as enflurane (Ethrane) and isoflurane (Forane) also have been used for inhalation anesthesia in children and offer certain advantages over halothane in some patients. In equipotent dosage, isoflurane causes less arterial hypotension and enflurane fewer cardiac dysrrhythmias than halothane. Regional anesthesia has limited application in infants and small children because of their fears of the operating room.

Experience has shown that nondepolarizing muscle relaxants (metubine, d-tubocurarine, pancuronium, and the shorter-acting atracurium and vecuronium) can be used with effectiveness and safety even in the newborn infant. Tracheal intubation and controlled ventilation provide optimal gas exchange, and neostigmine preceded by atropine restores neuromuscular transmission at the conclusion of anesthesia.

Tracheal intubation is indicated in (1) operations about the head and neck, (2) intrathoracic and intraperitoneal procedures, (3) operations in the prone position, (4) most procedures in infants under 1 yr of age and (5) virtually all emergency procedures because there is uncertainty about the contents of the stomach. Ventilation should be controlled manually or mechanically in all intrathoracic procedures and intraperitoneal operations and in patients lying in the prone position.

Table 5–27. **Preanesthetic Medication**

	Age	Drug
Intramuscular (IM)	0–6 mo	Atropine or glycopyrrolate
	6–12 mo	Atropine or glycopyrrolate + pentobarbital
	Over 12 mo	Atropine or glycopyrrolate + pentobarbital + morphine or meperidine
Oral (PO)	0–12 mo	None
	Over 12 mo	Atropine or glycopyrrolate + diazepam + meperidine

Dosage

Drug	Route	Dosage
Atropine	IM, PO	0.02 mg/kg; minimum 0.15 mg, maximum 0.5 mg
Glycopyrrolate	IM, PO	0.01 mg/kg to maximum 0.35 mg
Pentobarbital	IM	3.0–4.0 mg/kg; maximum 120 kg
Morphine	IM	0.05–0.10 mg/kg; maximum 10 mg
Meperidine	IM, PO	1.0–2.0 mg/kg; maximum 100 mg
Diazepam	PO	0.2 mg/kg

During anesthesia, monitoring of heart tones with a precordial stethoscope, a continuous electrocardiogram (lead 2), continuous measurement of rectal temperature with a thermistor probe, and assessment of arterial pressure by the Riva-Rocci or ultrasonic Doppler method are mandatory for all age groups. For children in poor physical condition or those undergoing extensive surgery, inserting a plastic cannula into an artery for continuous direct measurement of arterial pressure as well as for blood sampling is usually indicated.

National anesthesia machine standards call for a device to measure continuously the inspired oxygen concentration and for safety devices that preclude the delivery of a hypoxic gas mixture to the patient. The pulse oximeter accurately and precisely measures arterial oxygen saturation (SaO_2), even when mean systemic arterial pressures are as low as 30 mm Hg; skin pigmentation does not affect its reading. The unheated sensor can be attached to an infant's finger, hand, or foot for many hours without replacement and remains accurate without harming the infant's skin. Continuously measuring end-tidal expired carbon dioxide concentration by infrared or mass spectrometry and pulse oximetry can noninvasively provide important information about the child's gas exchange. Mass spectrometry may also semicontinuously assess inspired and end-tidal carbon dioxide, oxygen, nitrous oxide, and volatile anesthetics such as halothane, enhancing both the efficacy and safety of anesthesia.

Shock from hypovolemia may occur suddenly, and cardiac arrest ensue (Sec. 5.41). Being aware of the infant's approximate blood volume (80–90 mL/kg in the newborn, 75 mL/kg in the older infant) and immediately replacing losses exceeding 10–15% of that volume can prevent hypovolemic shock. Blood for rapid infusion should be warmed to 37° C immediately before use because rapid infusion of cold blood may produce cardiac arrest. When the anticipated losses exceed one third of the patient's estimated blood volume, CPD (citrate-phosphate-dextrose) blood less than 10 days old should be used because older blood becomes extremely acidotic (pH 6.5–6.7) and depleted of clotting factors. Serial arterial pH, pCO_2, and electrolyte determinations will detect the acidosis, hypocalcemia, and hyperkalemia that may be associated with rapid, massive blood replacement. Selecting the appropriate blood products and balanced electrolyte solutions often permits restoration of intravascular volume without using whole blood.

Continuous monitoring of body temperature is essential during general anesthesia. In modern air-conditioned operating rooms inadvertent hypothermia (colonic temperature under 35° C, 95° F) develops frequently in small infants undergoing laparotomy or thoracotomy and is associated with ventilatory depression, peripheral vasoconstriction, and a moderate metabolic acidosis in the immediate postanesthetic period. Overhead radiant heaters and circulating warm water mattresses, as well as heated humidification of inspired gases, can minimize this thermal stress. **Malignant hyperpyrexia** (MH), the abrupt and unexplained rise in body temperature above 41° C (105.8° F) during or following (immediately or after several hours) inhalation anesthesia or administration of succinylcholine, occurs in children over 1 yr of age and in young adults. Typically, there is also tachypnea, tachycardia, and hypertension. The overall mortality rate approaches 75% unless detected at the outset and treated. Successful management demands immediate recognition of a rapid rise in temperature, cessation of anesthesia, and hyperventilation with oxygen. Treatment also includes packing the patient in ice, ice-water gastric lavage, rapid infusion of intravenous fluids at 5–10 times the maintenance rate until adequate urine output is established, intravenous administration of sodium bicarbonate (4–7 mEq/kg), and dantrolene (1 mg/kg to a total of 10 mg/kg). The patient at risk of MH by prior personal or family history requires consultation with an anesthesiologist

well in advance of the day of operation. Preparation for such patients involves purging of the anesthesia machine with oxygen for 12 hours, selecting anesthetic agents and adjuvant drugs least likely to trigger MH, and often providing prophylactic therapy with dantrolene.

5.49 POSTANESTHETIC RECOVERY

Recovery room facilities and nursing must be available to provide constant surveillance of airway patency, adequate ventilation, and circulatory stability. Infants less than 6 mo of age should remain in the recovery room for a period of at least 2 hr to ensure full recovery of respiratory control, neuromuscular function, and upper airway reflexes. Common sequelae of general anesthesia in infants and children include postanesthetic excitement, vomiting, and pain. Postanesthetic excitement occurs most frequently in patients who have undergone painful procedures involving the head and neck and the abdomen; intravenous narcotics in an appropriate dose are most effective in managing this complication. Vomiting occurs commonly following myringotomy, tonsillectomy, procedures on the eyes, and intra-abdominal operations. It can sometimes be relieved with intravenous diazepam or phenothiazines in small doses. For control of severe pain, such as that associated with extensive orthopedic procedures, morphine (0.05–0.10 mg/kg intramuscularly) should provide relief for at least 3 hr.

Patients with upper airway anomalies, operations in the pharynx or upper airway, or a history of upper airway obstruction during sleep require exceptionally more careful and longer observation. They may develop lethal airway obstruction when sedated and should be observed in an intensive care unit for 24 hr.

Following tracheal intubation, patients between 6 mo–6 yr of age may develop subglottic edema, especially if they have a history of croup or recent upper respiratory infection, which can often be relieved by inhaling aerosolized racemic epinephrine (0.2%) in addition to supportive measures, including receiving humidified oxygen and intravenous fluids. Intravenous corticosteroids appear to have no beneficial effect. Rarely, orotracheal intubation followed by nasotracheal intubation or tracheostomy may be required for 2–5 days to guarantee an adequate airway. Malignant hyperpyrexia may also occur in the immediate postanesthetic period; therefore, careful monitoring of temperature remains important.

JOHN J. DOWNES
RUSSELL C. RAPHAELY

Betts EK, Downes JJ: Anesthesia. In: Welch KJ, Randolph JG, Ravitch MM, et al (eds): Pediatric Surgery. 4th ed. Chicago, Year Book Medical Publishers, 1986, pp 50–67.
Gregory GA (ed): Pediatric Anesthesia. Vol 1, 2. New York, Churchill-Livingston, 1983.
Keenan RL, Boyan CP: Cardiac arrest due to anesthesia. A study of incidence and causes. JAMA 253:2373, 1985.
Salem MR, Bennet EJ, Schweiss JF, et al: Cardiac arrest related to anesthesia. Contributing factors in infants and children. JAMA 223:238, 1975.
Sessler DI: Malignant hyperthermia. J Pediatr 109:9, 1986.
Smith RM: Anesthesia for Infants and Children. 4th ed. St. Louis, CV Mosby, 1980.
Swedlow DB, Stern S: Continuous non-invasive oxygen saturation monitoring in children with a new pulse-oximeter. Crit Care Med 11:228, 1983.
Yelderman M, New W: Evaluation of pulse oximetry. Anesthesiology 59:349, 1983.

Infant Apnea

Kurth CD, Spitzer AR, Broeunle AM, et al: Postoperative apnea in former premature infants. Anesthesiology 63:A475, 1985.
Liu LMP, Cote CJ, Goudsouzian NG, et al: Life-threatening apnea in infants recovering from anesthesia. Anesthesiology 59:506, 1983.
Richards JM, Alexander JR, Shinebourne EA, et al: Sequential 22-hour profiles of breathing patterns and heart rate in 110 full-term infants during their first 6 months of life. Pediatrics 74:763, 1984.
Steward DJ: Preterm infants are more prone to complications following minor surgery than are term infants. Anesthesiology 56:304, 1982.

5.50 DRUG THERAPY*

Pediatric pharmacology is concerned with pharmacokinetics and pharmacodynamics in the developing individual. *Pediatric pharmacotherapeutics* combines basic and clinical pharmacology with knowledge of the impact of disease upon pharmacokinetic and dynamic factors to develop dosage recommendations and other information essential to the safe medicinal treatment of infants and children. Although extensive preclinical and clinical evaluations for safety and efficacy of drugs are required in the United States, the same drugs evaluated for adult use are frequently not evaluated for infant and child use. Therefore, the safe and effective use of drugs for infants and children continues to be a major problem.

In the past, children's recommended doses were frequently extrapolated from adult doses by using various age-related formulas. However, no consistent age-based relationship exists between a safe, effective dose for an adult and one for an infant or child. Rational pediatric dose recommendations are based on either controlled clinical studies or empirical information gleaned from extensive clinical experience with infants and children. In either case, average dosages should be calculated on the basis of the patient's weight or body surface area (Fig. 29–1). The physician must always remember that recommended "average" doses may need to be adjusted for a particular patient owing to that individual's unique drug disposition and pharmacodynamic response characteristics.

5.51 DRUG DISPOSITION AND METABOLISM

In humans, a drug's actions depend on a number of factors that must be understood before rational therapeutics can be practiced. The effects of most drugs are reversible and depend on their concentration at the site of action. A drug's concentration and temporal course of action are determined by the dose administered and by its *pharmacokinetic characteristics* (absorption, distribution, metabolism, and excretion). *Pharmacodynamic factors*, such as the drug's interaction with biologic receptors and other mechanisms of action, are also basic to the therapeutic or toxic effects produced. Pharmacokinetic and pharmacodynamic characteristics vary according to the patient's stages of maturation, which present variations that may have important therapeutic implications.

During the early months of life some drugs administered orally may be absorbed more completely than at any other time in life; the absorption of others may be impeded. This variation may be related to changes in gastric pH and emptying time which occur during development. The unpredictable eating habits and exercise patterns of children and adolescents may also modify absorption of orally administered drugs. At different ages, anatomic, physiologic, and behavioral factors can each lead to variations in absorption.

Several factors determine the distribution of drugs in the body. The size of the drug molecule and its charge at physiologic pH influence the ease with which it passes through body membranes. Because of their specialized nature and structure, membranes vary in their permeability to individual drug molecules. Blood flow to individual organs and tissues is also an important determinant of drug distribution. Other factors include the relative size of the various tissue compartments, the ratio of lean body mass to total body weight, and the affinity of the drug for proteins in various tissues.

Protein binding is especially important in influencing the distribution of drugs. Drugs having a high affinity for extravascular binding sites, such as digoxin, which binds to myocardial and skeletal muscle, selectively concentrate in tissues outside the vascular compartment. Conversely, many drugs are bound, in varying degrees, to plasma proteins. Acidic drugs, such as salicylate and phenobarbital, bind primarily to albumin. Basic drugs, such as theophylline and morphine, associate with several plasma proteins, including albumin, α_1-acid glycoprotein, and the lipoproteins. The affinity basic drugs have for plasma proteins is generally less than the affinity highly bound acidic drugs have for albumin. A drug molecule bound to a plasma protein is not free to move across membranes and distribute into extravascular spaces. The apparent volume of distribution, V_d, of such a drug will depend on the concentration of available protein binding sites in the vascular compartment and the binding affinity of the drug for those sites. The binding of many drugs to plasma proteins is decreased during infancy compared with later childhood or adult life. Decreased binding cannot be explained totally on the basis of decreased plasma protein concentrations and appears to be due, in part, to qualitative differences between plasma proteins of infants and adults. The presence of increased concentrations of endogenous ligands such as bilirubin and free fatty acids, which compete for albumin binding sites, may also reduce drug binding in newborn infants. Drug binding equal to that of adults generally occurs in normal infants by 3–6 mo of age.

Drugs that are water soluble at physiologic pH are primarily excreted unchanged in the urine, e.g., penicillin and aminoglycoside antibiotics. Excretion rates are directly proportional to the rates of glomerular filtration and tubular secretion. During the neonatal period, renal clearance is approximately 5% that of adults but approaches mature levels by 6–12 mo. Prepubescent children typically have glomerular filtration rates, corrected for body surface area, that are 1.2 to 1.5 times that of adults; these rates decrease to adult levels by early adulthood. The elimination of drugs that are excreted primarily by the kidney parallels these age-related changes in renal function.

Many drugs are highly lipid-soluble compounds which are filtered by the glomerulus but are reabsorbed so completely in the renal tubules that they would persist in the body in an active form for long periods of time if not modified chemically by enzymatic reactions. The two major categories of drug metabolizing reactions are nonsynthetic (oxidation, reduction, and hydrolysis) and synthetic (conjugation). The *nonsynthetic reactions* are catalyzed by mixed-function oxidases, which are fixed to the membranes of the endoplasmic reticulum. The resulting products may be less active, equally active, or more active pharmacologically than the parent compound. *Synthetic reactions* generally result in the conversion of drugs or their (nonsynthetic) metabolic products into highly polar compounds that can be excreted in either the bile or the urine. Drug metabolism occurs in various tissues, including blood, lung, kidney, gastrointestinal tract, and liver. However, the principal site of biotransformation is the liver.

Drug metabolism changes both quantitatively and qualitatively during physiologic growth and development. Furthermore, the quantitative changes may occur at different times from pathway to pathway. For example, while the hydroxylation and glucuronide conjugating processes are generally decreased at the time of birth, methylation, sulfation, and acetylation pathways are usually well developed in newborn infants. Variation in the rate of drug metabolic processes is

---

*Consult Table 29–1A and B for drugs and dosages.

usually assumed to imply that there is a deficit in metabolic capacity at some immature stages. However, during periods of growth and development the capacity to metabolize some drugs may be markedly increased. Thus, in prepubescent children phenytoin, phenobarbital, and theophylline may each be eliminated at rates that are 2- to 6-fold greater than those found in adults.

When quantitative changes take place they result in qualitative differences in the end metabolites produced. For example, infants up to about 6 mo of age methylate theophylline to caffeine, an active product, since the oxidative pathways are poorly developed. Later, as these pathways mature, at about 6 mo, the active metabolites are no longer produced in significant concentrations and are rapidly cleared from the body after each dose of theophylline. Thus, age as well as size must be considered in dose calculations.

Knowledge about the ontogeny of factors controlling pharmacodynamic responses is limited. Cholinergic receptors have been functionally identified in human fetal tissues as early as the 8th week of gestation. Sensitivity to acetylcholine stimulation does not change through the 2nd trimester, although the effector capacity, expressed as smooth muscle tension, increases 4-fold. Components of the adrenergic receptor system have been demonstrated in human fetuses as early as 12–22 wk of gestation and increase with gestational age. Function of the α-adrenergic receptors generally develops later than that of the β-adrenergic ones. The presence of functional receptors in the developing human, coupled with the results of animal experiments, suggest that receptors in the CNS may be particularly vulnerable to the effects of drugs during specific periods of immaturity in prenatal and postnatal life. Exposure to certain drugs during these susceptible periods of development could have long-lasting or even permanent behavioral effects on the individual; the term "behavioral teratology" has been used to describe such effects.

Time Course of Drug in the Body. Since the pharmacologic effects of most drugs are reversible, both the time of onset and intensity of effect of a drug are proportional to the concentration of drug at any point in time. Maintaining the drug concentration within a prescribed range is important to achieving and maintaining a desired therapeutic effect with minimal risk of toxicity. Drug concentration is a dynamic function of the rates of administration and elimination. The ability to predict drug concentrations with some degree of confidence is useful, especially when prescribing drugs for which optimal therapeutic concentrations are relatively close to potentially toxic concentrations, i.e., low *therapeutic index*. Pharmacokinetic relationships quantitatively describe the change in amount or concentration of drug in the body with time, predict the concentration at any time after a dose, and facilitate the calculation of an approximate dose to achieve the desired concentration. Serum or plasma concentration is usually used to establish both the drug's concentration and its observed pharmacologic effect, since the serum or plasma level generally reflects the quantity of administered drug in the body.

The elimination (metabolism and excretion) of most drugs can be described mathematically as a first-order or exponential process, e.g., a constant fraction of the drug in the body is removed/unit time. The absolute amount of drug eliminated/unit time is proportional to the amount of drug in the body at any given moment and, therefore, changes as the amount of drug in the body changes.

The simplest mathematical expression of the change in drug concentration with time is $C = C_0 e^{-Kt}$, where C is the drug concentration at time T, C_0 is the concentration at time 0 if the drug were instantaneously administered and distributed in the body, e is a constant with the value 2.71828, K is the fraction of drug eliminated/unit of time (elimination rate constant), and t is the time after the dose. Although this equation oversimplifies the time course of drug elimination, it works well for most drugs in clinical practice. The graphic representation of this equation is shown in Figure 5–12 where K is represented by the slope of the logarithm of the serum concentration; the concentration decreases by one half every half-life. Half-life and elimination rate constant are related according to the equation $t_{1/2} = \dfrac{0.693}{K}$, where 0.693 is the natural logarithm of 2.

The *apparent volume of distribution* (V_d) is important when relating drug concentration to dose. This volume has no anatomic or physiologic meaning but is a theoretical volume into which the drug would distribute if it existed in the same concentration throughout the body as it does in serum or plasma where it is being measured. The apparent volume of distribution may be expressed by the equation $V_d = \dfrac{D}{C} e^{-Kt}$ where D is the dose of drug (other terms are defined above). Another useful concept in describing drug disposition is *clearance* (Cl), which represents the theoretical volume from which the drug is totally removed/unit time; clearance is the product of the apparent volume of distribution and the elimination rate constant, i.e., $Cl = V_d \times K$.

When the clearance of the drug is known and the desired concentration is determined, a dosing schedule to provide that concentration can be calculated. The concentration at any time after beginning dosing is described by the equation $C = \dfrac{D}{Cl \times \tau} (1 - e^{-Kt})$, where D is each dose, τ is dosing interval, and t is the time since initiating dosing. This relationship is shown graphically in Figure 5–13. A steady-state concentration is achieved following repetitive dosing for at least five half-lives at which time the term e^{-Kt} approaches 0 and the equation simplifies to $C_{ss} = \dfrac{D}{Cl \times \tau}$ where C_{ss} represents the mean steady-state concentration for that dose.

The latter equation can be rearranged to $D = C_{ss} \times Cl \times \tau$ to determine the dose required to provide a desired steady-state concentration. Since doses are usually administered intermittently, the drug concentration rises and falls around the average concentration. The average steady-state concentration is determined by the size of the dose, whereas the degree of fluctuation is determined by the length of the dosing

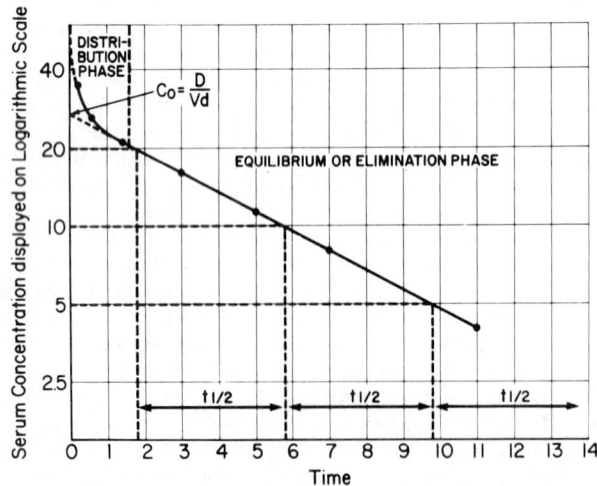

Figure 5–12. Time course of concentration of drug after administration of a single dose by the intravenous route. C_o and $T_{1/2}$ can be determined from such a graph and V_d and K can be calculated as noted in text.

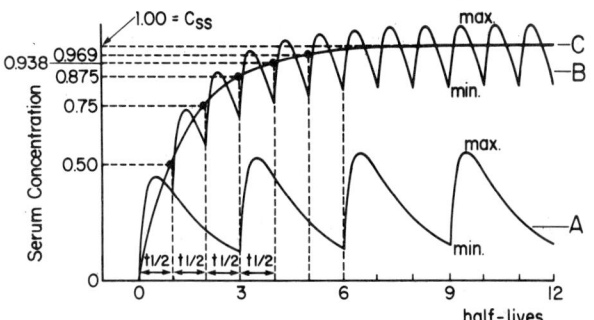

Figure 5–13. Repeated dosing at various constant dosing intervals. C represents the time course of serum concentration during constant intravenous infusion of a drug. After constant infusion for 5 half-lives the concentration reaches 96.9% of C_{ss}. In A, a fixed dose is administered (by the oral or intramuscular route) at a dosing interval of $3 \times T_{1/2}$. In B, the same dose and route are used but the dosing interval $= T_{1/2}$. Note that in a correct dosage regimen the same C_{ss} should be achieved by an appropriate dose irrespective of the route of administration, and the concentration maxima and minima should lie within the therapeutic range. The combination of an initial loading dose with subsequent doses offers the advantage of achieving an effective drug concentration rapidly and maintaining it safely, when administering a drug with a long $T_{1/2}$.

interval in relation to the half-life of the drug. In general, a drug should not be administered less frequently than once every half-life, to avoid excessive fluctuations in concentration.

The disposition of a few drugs cannot be accurately described with simple first-order kinetics. For example, phenytoin, salicylate, and alcohol exhibit saturation kinetics to which the concepts of half-life and clearance do not apply. Plasma concentrations of other drugs may sequentially decrease at several apparent rates: an early rapid decline followed by one or more slower rates of decline. Such patterns of concentration change must be described by multiexponential equations that are beyond the scope of this section.

5.52 INDIVIDUALIZATION OF DRUG DOSAGE

The response to an average recommended drug dose varies considerably among individuals even when the dose is corrected for body weight, surface area, or stage of maturation. This variation in response is due both to differences in rates of drug elimination and to pharmacodynamic response. Pathophysiologic states may also alter drug clearance or response. Such interindividual variability frequently requires adjusting the dosage regimens for specific patients, especially when prescribing drugs with a low therapeutic index. For some drugs, such as dopamine or furosemide, the dosage may be adjusted according to their immediate and readily quantitated effects. For other drugs, dosage adjustments may be guided by measuring the concentration of drug in plasma or serum. When a concentration-effect correlation can be defined, a concentration range within which a majority of patients will experience the desired effect and a concentration range within which a majority will suffer undesired effects can be determined.

Recent advances in analytical technology have made it possible to measure a variety of drugs rapidly in small blood samples. Monitoring plasma concentrations is particularly useful for evaluating inadequate therapeutic responses, suspected drug toxicities, and potential drug-drug interactions; for guiding dosage adjustments of drugs, either those with a low therapeutic index or those administered to patients with impaired elimination; and for managing a patient with known

or suspected drug overdose. Alternatively, measuring plasma concentrations of certain drugs is sometimes of little clinical use because (1) some drugs can be safely administered in relatively large doses to ensure adequate concentrations, i.e., they have a high therapeutic index; (2) some drugs produce an immediate and readily quantified pharmacologic effect; and (3) some drugs exist for which no readily defined relationship exists between plasma concentrations and pharmacologic effect.

When measuring drug concentrations, it is important to keep in mind the pharmacokinetic characteristics of the drug in question so that samples are obtained at appropriate times in relation to the dosing schedule and concentrations are properly interpreted to avoid serious therapeutic errors. The optimal range of plasma or serum concentration of drugs commonly used in pediatric pharmacotherapeutics is catalogued in Table 5–28. However, any therapeutic regimen

Table 5–28. Therapeutic Range (Serum Concentration) for Some Drugs Used in Pediatric Practice

Antiarrhythmic/cardiotonic			
Digoxin			
Newborns and infants (birth–1 year)	0.0008–	0.0025	µg/mL
Children and adolescents	0.0008–	0.0016	µg/mL
Lidocaine	1.5 –	6	µg/mL
Procainamide	4 –	8	µg/mL
Propranolol	0.02 –	0.2	µg/mL
Quinidine	1 –	5	µg/mL
Anticonvulsants			
Carbamazepine	4 –	12	µg/mL
Clonazepam	0.02 –	0.07	µg/mL
Ethosuximide	40 –	100	µg/mL
Phenobarbital	10 –	40	µg/mL
Phenytoin	10 –	20	µg/mL
Trimethadione (metabolized to dimethadione. This may attain levels of 500–1000 µg/mL on long-term use)	6 –	40	µg/mL
Valproic acid	50	–150	µg/mL
Antimicrobial agents			
Amikacin	15 –	25	µg/mL
Carbenicillin		around 100	µg/mL
Chloramphenicol	10 –	25	µg/mL
Gentamicin	4 –	10	µg/mL
Isoniazid	2 –	10	µg/mL
Kanamycin	15 –	25	µg/mL
Metilmicin	4 –	10	µg/mL
Tobramycin	4 –	10	µg/mL
Antipyretic/analgesic/anti-inflammatory			
Acetylsalicylic acid (measured as salicylate)			
Antipyretic (short-term treatment)	50	–150	µg/mL
Antiarthritic (long-term use)	100	–300	µg/mL
Acetaminophen (short-term use)	50	–100	µg/mL
Meperidine	0.150 –	0.600	µg/mL
Phenylbutazone	40 –	80	µg/mL
Propoxyphene	0.05 –	0.2	µg/mL
Psychoactive drugs			
Amobarbital		around 5	µg/mL
Chloral hydrate	5 –	10	µg/mL
Chlordiazepoxide	1 –	3	µg/mL
Chlorpromazine	0.04 –	0.3	µg/mL
Diazepam	0.15 –	0.06	µg/mL
Imipramine	0.05 –	0.16	µg/mL
Pentobarbital		around 1	µg/mL
For therapeutic coma	5 –	40	µg/mL
Miscellaneous			
Chlorothiazide	2 –	2.5	µg/mL
Theophylline	10 –	20	µg/mL

Table 5–29. Drug Interactions of Potential Importance in Pediatric Practice

Drugs interfering with gastrointestinal absorption of other drugs

Oral administration of:	*Interferes with absorption of:*
antacid	phenothiazines
	salicylate
	sulfonamides
antacid (aluminum-containing)	isoniazid
	digoxin
	tetracyclines
barbiturate	griseofulvin
kaolin-pectin	lincomycin
iron (ferrous)	tetracyclines
salicylate	fenoprofen
	indomethacin

Displacement of drug from protein binding site

Drug causing displacement	*Drug displaced*
phenylbutazone	phenytoin
phenytoin	thyroid hormone
salicylate	methotrexate
	naproxen
	phenytoin
sulfonamides	methotrexate
	phenytoin
quinidine	phenytoin
nalproate	digoxin*
	phenytoin

Drugs with additive effect

Drugs increasing the action	*Drugs in which action is increased (effect triggered)*
digitalis glycosides	beta-adrenoceptor–blocking agents (bradycardia)
diazoxide	beta-adrenoceptor–blocking agents (bradycardia)
diuretics (potassium-losing)	corticosteroids (potassium depletion)
	curariform drugs (neuromuscular blockade)
ethanol (acute intoxication)	barbiturates (CNS depression)
	chloral hydrate (sedation)
	diazepam (CNS depression)
	meprobamate (CNS depression)
	salicylate (gastrointestinal bleeding)
phenothiazine	antihypertensives (hypotension)
	morphine (hypotension)
propranolol	phenothiazines (hypotension)
	phenytoin (cardiac depressant)
	quinidine (negative inotropic action)
	reserpine (sympathetic blockade)
	skeletal muscle relaxants (neuromuscular blockade)
quinidine	phenothiazines (cardiac depressant)
	skeletal muscle relaxants (neuromuscular blockade)
reserpine	beta-adrenoceptor–blocking agents (bradycardia)
tricyclic antidepressants	chlordiazepoxide (sedation)
	sympathomimetic amines (hypertensive crisis)

Drug-drug interaction by enhancement of the metabolism of one drug by another (induction of the drug-metabolizing enzyme system)

Drug causing induction	*Drug of which metabolism is increased (pharmacologic effect diminished)*
barbiturates (especially phenobarbital)	corticosteroids
	chloramphenicol
	clonazepam
	digoxin
	doxycycline
	estrogens
	phenothiazines
	phenytoin
	tricyclic antidepressants
	testosterone
carbamazepine	phenytoin
	valproic acid
phenytoin	corticosteroids
	diazepam
	thyroxine
	metapyrone
	primidone
salicylate	fenoprofen

(Drugs causing induction of their own metabolism: chlordiazepoxide, chlorpromazine, hexobarbital, meprobamate, pentobarbital, phenobarbital, phenylbutazone, phenytoin [weak effect], probenecid)

Table 5-29. Drug Interactions of Potential Importance in Pediatric Practice *(Continued)*

Drug-drug interaction by inhibition of metabolism of one drug by another

Drug causing inhibition	*Drug of which metabolism is reduced (risk of toxicity increased)*
allopurinol	azathioprine
	cyclophosphamide
	mercaptopurine
barbiturates (in large dose)	phenytoin
chloramphenicol	phenytoin
phenothiazines (especially chlorpromazine)	phenytoin
cymetidine	carbamazepine
	diazepam
	phenobarbital
	phenytoin
	propranolol
	theophylline
diazepam	phenytoin
erythromycin	theophylline
isoniazid	phenytoin
para-aminosalicylic acid	isoniazid
phenytoin	primidone
propoxyphene	carbamazepine
sulfonamides	phenytoin
valproic acid	phenobarbital
	phenytoin

Facilitation of a common adverse effect through combined use

aminoglycoside + second aminoglycoside or ethacrynic acid or furosemide	nephrotoxicity and ototoxicity
aminoglycoside + cephalosporin	nephrotoxicity, acute renal failure
aminoglycoside + polymyxin	nephrotoxicity
amphotericin B + digitalis glycoside	cardiac arrhythmia (hypokalemia)
cephaloridine + ethacrynic acid	nephrotoxicity
cephaloridine + furosemide	nephrotoxicity
corticosteroid + indomethacin	gastrointestinal ulceration
digitalis glycoside + sympathomimetic amine	cardiac arrhythmia
diuretic (K-losing) + digitalis glycoside	digitalis toxicity
isoniazid + rifampin	hepatotoxicity
phenytoin + isoniazid	neurotoxicity
tetracycline + diuretic	nephrotoxicity
tricyclic antidepressant + phenothiazine	cardiotoxicity
valproic acid + other anticonvulsants	neurotoxicity

*Precise mechanism of interaction unknown

should be based on the patient's needs and individual responses to the specific drug in addition to measurements of concentrations.

Unique Problems of Drug Administration. Although it may be assumed that drugs given intravenously are usually administered rapidly and completely, this is not always true, especially in infants and small children. The rate of delivery and the time to infuse the total dose of an intravenously administered drug depend on the flow rate of the intravenous fluid, the dead space of the system into which the drug dose is injected, and the volume in which the drug is diluted. Because standard intravenous fluid delivery systems, including their tubing, are designed for adults, they contain a large volume/unit length, which introduces a relatively large dead space resulting in substantial infusion delays when operated at the slow flow rates used for infants and children. For example, a dose of gentamicin placed in the volume chamber (Buretrol or Metriset) of an intravenous system and administered with a flow rate of 25 mL/hr will not begin to infuse into the infant or small child until 1 hr after dosing, and it will take approximately 3 hr to infuse 90% of the dose. Such slow infusion rates may profoundly affect both the serum concentration and the therapeutic effect of the drug. These problems can be circumvented by infusing the drug into the distal intravenous line by a separate pump through a Y-site or stopcock and by using low volume extension tubing between the site of drug injection and the patient.

5.53 SPECIAL PROBLEMS OF DRUG TOXICITY

See also Sec. 10.53.

Problems Linked to Growth and Development. A drug's effect on normal development must be considered when planning therapeutic regimens for pediatric patients. The increased incidence of kernicterus among jaundiced infants who were given drugs that displaced bilirubin from its intravascular binding sites is a widely appreciated example of such pediatric drug toxicity (Sec. 8.44-8.45). Other adverse reactions specific to growing organisms that may make a drug approved for use in adults hazardous to infants and children include the damaging effects of tetracyclines upon permanent dentition when administered before completion of amelogenesis, and the possible adverse effect on statural growth owing to treatment with steroid hormones, amphetamine, or methylphenidate.

Drug-Drug Interactions. When two or more drugs are administered to the same patient, their absorption, distribution, metabolism, excretion, and effect of each may be modified by their combined interaction (Table 5-29). Not all drug interactions are dangerous, but most lead either to suboptimal efficacy or to increased toxicity of one or more of the drugs that have been combined. Therefore, the effect of each drug on the others of the regimen should be carefully considered.

Any drug can potentially produce an adverse reaction which

usually represents an extension of its expected pharmacologic effects. Some adverse effects are referred to as *idiosyncratic* since their occurrence cannot be predicted from knowing the drugs' usual effects. This type of adverse effect frequently takes the form of a complex of symptoms that may mimic naturally occurring syndromes (Table 5–30).

Pharmacogenetics. Inheritance may influence drug response, since genetic variation can probably be expected for all of the processes involved in drug disposition. The variety of specific examples of genetically determined variations in drug metabolism include hemolysis upon exposure to certain drugs in patients with glucose-6-phosphate dehydrogenase (G-6-PD) deficiency; prolonged paralysis after receiving succinylcholine in patients with abnormal pseudocholinesterase isozymes; differences in rate of acetylation of isoniazide, procainamide, and various sulfonamides; variations in oxidative drug metabolism, e.g., debrisoquine, sparteine, and antipyrine; genetically determined methyl conjugation; and

---

Table 5–30. Some Syndromes Produced as Side Effects of Drug Therapy*

Erythema multiforme and Stevens-Johnson syndrome†
  barbiturates
  codeine
  ethosuximide
  penicillins
  phenobarbital
  phenytoin
  salicylates
  sulfonamides
  tetracyclines
  thiazides

Erythema nodosum
  penicillins
  sulfonamides

Exfoliative dermatitis
  barbiturates
  penicillins
  phenytoin
  sulfonamides

Extrapyramidal symptomatology
  butyrophenones (haloperidol)
  diazoxide
  phenothiazines

Hemolytic anemia
associated with G6PD deficiency:
  acetylsalicylic acid (in large doses)
  chloramphenicol
  dimercaprol
  nalidixic acid
  nitrofurantoin
  para-aminosalicylic acid
  primaquine
  probenecid
  quinidine
  sulfonamides (including salicylazosulfapyridine)
  water-soluble vitamin K analogues

associated with positive Coombs test:
  cephalosporins
  chloramphenicol
  insulin
  isoniazid
  methicillin
  methyldopa
  para-aminosalicylic acid
  penicillins (in high doses)
  rifampin
  sulfonamides

Mental depression
  amphetamine withdrawal
  clonidine
  methyldopa
  phenothiazines
  prednisone (more commonly results in euphoria)
  propranolol
  reserpine
  tetrahydrocannabinol

Photosensitivity (phototoxic and photoallergic reactions can occur coincidentally or concomitantly)
photoallergic (sensitization during first exposure, allergic reaction on continued exposure or re-exposure):
  antihistamines
  phenothiazines
  sulfonamides
  sunscreens (para-aminobenzoic acid)
  tetracyclines
phototoxic (manifestations appearing 6 to 18 hr after exposure):
  antibacterial soaps (halogenated salicylanilides)
  coal tar and derivatives (perfumes, colognes, plants)
  griseofulvin
  nalidixic acid
  phenothiazines
  sulfonamides
  tetracyclines

Pseudomembranous colitis
  ampicillin
  chloramphenicol
  clindamycin
  lincomycin
  tetracyclines

Retrobulbar (optic) neuritis
  chloramphenicol
  clioquinol (iodochlorhydroxyquinoline)
  ethambutol
  isoniazid
  penicillamine
  phenothiazines

Serum sickness–like syndrome
  acetylsalicylic acid
  griseofulvin
  hydralazine
  penicillins
  sulfonamides
  thiouracil derivatives

Systemic lupus erythematosus
  hydralazine
  isoniazid
  penicillamine
  procainamide

Toxic epidermal necrolysis (Lyell syndrome, Ritter disease, scalded skin syndrome)
  acetylsalicylic acid
  allopurinol
  barbiturates
  methotrexate
  penicillins
  phenylbutazone
  phenytoin
  sulfonamides
  thiazides

---

*Hepatitis and nephritis syndromes, as well as fever and seizures, may be caused by a variety of agents and are not listed here. Consult a standard textbook of pharmacology for such relationships.
†Associated, but causality not established.

deficient glutathione synthesis leading to increased susceptibility to toxic products of oxidative metabolism. Studies of human twins have also demonstrated that both the plasma half-lives of many drugs and the rate constants for drug metabolite formation are much more similar in monozygotic than in dizygotic twin pairs. Whenever either an unexpected drug effect or toxicity is observed in a patient, the possibility that pharmacogenetic factors underlie such a reaction should be considered.

Drugs in Human Milk. Virtually all drugs administered to lactating women are secreted to some extent into their milk and may be ingested by the nursing infant. Although drug use should be minimal during lactation, a few drugs have been reported to adversely affect the nursing infant (Sec. 8.6 and Table 8–4).

5.54 PRESCRIBING PRACTICES

Factors such as taste, smell, color, consistency, and cost may affect the degree to which patients comply with their therapeutic drug regimen. Using generic names in prescribing drugs can sometimes reduce the cost for an individual patient, but the prescribing physician must be certain that the generic brands afford equal bioavailability, bioeffectiveness, and patient acceptability. Complete data are not available on many drugs used in pediatrics.

Drugs familiar to the practitioner should be prescribed for the desired therapeutic effect. Newer preparations which are congeners of established agents and which have no major therapeutic or monetary advantage should be avoided; many are more expensive and most have slightly different therapeutic actions or toxic potentials than the original drugs with which they were designed to compete. Newer agents should be substituted for established drugs only after extensive clinical experience has demonstrated their added benefits.

Prescriptions should direct the dispensing of enough drug to treat the patient but not enough to leave a significant amount after the prescribed course of therapy is over. Parents should be instructed to discard residual doses to protect against accidental poisoning or improper self-medication at a later date. Simplified regimens should be employed whenever possible, and single ingredient preparations should be prescribed whenever appropriate. Complex regimens that require frequent dosing with one or another of several agents should be avoided since they frequently lead to over- or under-administration of the drugs by the parents or older child.

Compliance. Little is known about the factors that determine the degree of compliance with a physician's instructions in an individual family. However, many studies have shown that patients frequently do not take medication consistently or in the manner intended and prescribed. Moreover, patients frequently take medications not recommended or prescribed by the physician. Compliance may be maximized in many instances by careful orientation of the family to the nature of the child's illness, to the action of the drugs prescribed, and to the importance of following the instructions precisely. If instructions are written down clearly and in detail for the family and if the regimen results in as little bother and interference as possible with the family living schedule, particularly the parental sleep habits, it probably will be followed with greater fidelity by more families.

SANFORD N. COHEN
RALPH E. KAUFFMAN
LEON STREBEL

Avery GS (ed): Drug Treatment. Principles and Practice of Clinical Pharmacology and Therapeutics. 2nd ed. New York, ADIS Press, 1980.
Boreus LD: Principles of Pediatric Pharmacology. New York, Churchill Livingstone, 1982.
Committee on Drugs, American Academy of Pediatrics: The transfer of drugs and other chemicals into breast milk. Pediatrics 72:375, 1983.
Melmon K, Morrelli HF (eds): Clinical Pharmacology. Basic Principles in Therapeutics. 2nd ed. New York, Macmillan, 1978.
Roberts RJ: Drug Therapy in Infants. Philadelphia, WB Saunders Co., 1984.
Shope JT: Medication compliance. Pediatr Clin North Am 28:5, 1981.
Weinshilboum RM: Human pharmacogenetics. Fed Proc 43:2295, 1984.
Yaffe SJ (ed): Pediatric Pharmacology: Therapeutic Principles in Practice. New York, Grune and Stratton, 1980.

5.55 PEDIATRIC IMAGING

All pediatric imaging techniques require an understanding of each child's medical problems and the special anatomic and physiologic characteristics of the maturational stage of the child. New imaging modalities must be evaluated in terms of their diagnostic yield compared with conventional radiologic techniques, of their hazards due to any sedation or anesthesia they require, of their need for physical restraint and/or the presence of pain or discomfort during the examination, of the length and degree of radiation exposure they require (Table 5–31), and of their cost effectiveness. The patient's benefits from the proposed procedure should exceed the expected untoward effects.

Conventional radiography generally yields static images, and pathophysiology is inferred rather than shown directly, although image-intensified fluoroscopy reveals structures in motion. Sometimes, particularly in the skeletal system, the radiologic examination is equivalent to a gross pathologic examination. Most well-established radiologic techniques will remain in general use for the foreseeable future, but, after eight decades of refinement, many new imaging modalities are now available that offer direct insights into pathophysiologic processes.

Exposure times of radiographic examinations should be short, to limit radiation and to avoid motion artifacts. The greatest reduction in radiation exposure results from carefully considering whether or not the examination is truly needed. However, equipment that uses automatic coning and permits manual reduction of the exposed area by the technologist is important for careful collimation of the beam and for gonadal shielding. Table 5–31 gives the range of various medical and nonmedical radiation exposures.

Young infants, unable to cooperate, may require immobilization or sedation, but children capable of understanding should receive appropriate explanations to facilitate their cooperation. As the scan times for computed tomography have decreased, sedation is less necessary, especially in examining the head; however, it is still frequently required up to age 4, and its use carries some risk.

The *relationship of age to radiologic diagnosis* of disease is important in pediatrics. Many abdominal diseases frequently seen in children are rare or nonexistent in the adult. Intraperitoneal masses tend to be cystic and originate from the bowel, mesentery, ovary, or omentum. Among retroperitoneal non-neoplastic masses, hydronephrosis (Sec. 17.40) and, in newborns, multicystic dysplastic kidney (Sec. 17.34) are common. The most frequent neoplasms in this area are Wilms tumor (Sec. 16.13) and neuroblastoma (Sec. 16.11); two thirds of patients with Wilms tumor are less than 3 yr old at diagnosis, and three fourths of neuroblastomas are found before 5 yr of age. Ovarian teratoma, a tumor that makes up

Table 5–31. **Range of Radiation Doses Received in Various Medical and Nonmedical Activities**

Type of Radiation	Rads, Rems (Very Approximate)	Time	Where Received
A. Medical radiation			
Chest film, newborn	0.004	Millisec	Skin entrance dose; exit dose much less
CT, contiguous slices, child	1	Sec	Skin of circumference of scanned volume
Lateral of lumbosacral spine, adult	1.1	Sec	Skin entrance dose; exit dose much less
Cardiac catheterization	10	Hr	Skin entrance dose; exit dose much less
Curative radiotherapy	7000	Wk	Tumor and adjacent structures
B. Nonmedical radiation			
Natural background at sea level	0.08	Yr	Whole body
Some professional jet pilots and flight crews, from cosmic rays	1	Yr	Whole body
Residents of certain areas of India with radioactive soil	3	Yr	Whole body
Radiation workers, permitted dose	5	Permitted per yr	Radiation badge
LD_{50}, nuclear warfare	450	Min	Whole body

only 10% of ovarian tumors in the adult, is the most common solid ovarian tumor in the child (Sec. 16.23). Simple (follicular) cysts are probably the most prevalent ovarian lesions of early life (Sec. 16.23). Pancreatic carcinoma, often seen in the adult, is very rare in childhood; post-traumatic and postinflammatory pseudocysts are much more frequent. Masses in the liver include abscesses, cysts, primary neoplasms, vascular lesions, and metastases. Biliary disease is probably more common in children and adolescents than previously thought. Biliary calculi are frequent in children after certain major surgical procedures, such as the repair of scoliosis. Ultrasonography has shown that the gallbladder may become markedly but transiently dilated in the presence of infection elsewhere.

Acute appendicitis (Sec. 12.62) is common in children; approximately 70% of children under 5 yr of age with acute appendicitis have a perforation when first seen. The resulting abscesses occur anywhere in the peritoneal cavity, particularly in the pelvis, and are difficult to delineate by conventional radiography; ultrasonography and computed tomography often help in difficult chronic cases, although they are rarely indicated in the acute stage of appendicitis.

The neonate suffers a variety of abnormalities of the central nervous system not encountered in later life. Ultrasonography delineates intracranial hemorrhage (Sec. 8.23) with great precision and can also be used to quantify ventricular dilation. However, brain tumors, a significant fraction of pediatric neoplasms (Sec. 21.22), are frequently infratentorial, and delineation of the posterior fossa remains a problem even for modern computed tomography; magnetic resonance imaging holds great promise here.

A variety of lesions may be present in the thorax of the infant or child. Leukemia (Sec. 16.4–16.7) may involve mediastinal lymph nodes and the thymus. Lymphoma, neuroblastoma, rhabdomyosarcoma of the thoracic wall or diaphragm, and malignant teratoma also occur. Cystic lesions such as bronchogenic cysts (enteric cysts) may cause tracheobronchial or esophageal obstruction. Anomalies of the great vessels (Sec. 14.18–14.24) may be defined by esophagography, ultrasonography, conventional or digital subtraction arteriography, or computed tomography. Magnetic resonance imaging permits visualization of the cardiac chambers and the great vessels without the use of contrast material.

SPECIFIC MODALITIES

Conventional Radiography and Fluoroscopy. At the Children's Hospital in Boston, 75% of the radiologic examinations are conventional multiple projections, tomography, fluoroscopy with dynamic or static recording of images, and procedures associated with the introduction of contrast material into a vessel or hollow viscus. Approximately one third of chest examinations are now done with bedside equipment because the children's illnesses preclude their being moved. Nuclear medicine, ultrasonography, computed tomography, arteriography, and interventional techniques comprise the remaining 15% of the total; however, these techniques consume 65% of the radiologists' time.

Conventional radiography is used to localize and characterize most skeletal injuries. Trauma to the central nervous system, the spine, and the solid thoracic and abdominal viscera often requires definition by ultrasonography, computed tomography, or nuclear medicine. Ultrasonography has substantially reduced the need to perform excretory urograms. Barium studies of the gastrointestinal tract remain important, although endoscopy is beginning to displace this modality. For example, esophagitis and early inflammatory bowel disease are best defined by endoscopy. However, plain roentgenographic films remain the best technique for diagnosing intestinal obstruction and many chest diseases, especially those involving upper and lower airways. The addition of fluoroscopy allows the function of the airway to be evaluated, as, for example, in obstruction by a foreign body. Barium esophagography is also frequently useful, bronchography only occasionally so.

Nuclear Medicine. Advances in equipment and radiopharmaceuticals have increased the usefulness of nuclear medicine in pediatrics over the last decade. Scintigraphy, the formation of static and dynamic images from gamma ray emissions caused by the breakdown of small quantities of radioactive agents administered to the patient, is frequently helpful in demonstrating the anatomy of a lesion and is particularly useful in adding functional information when the anatomy has already been shown by other methods. Hepatobiliary agents, for example, can show both hepatocyte function and biliary flow. Nonabsorbable radionuclides can now be used to evaluate gastrointestinal reflux. Gallium accumulated in abscesses, in other inflammatory lesions, and in certain tumors can be used for their identification; however, gallium's long half-life requires caution in its use.

Many new radionuclides have very short half-lives. Iridium-191m ($t_{1/2}$ = 4.95 sec), useful in radionuclide angiocardiography, is now available in a few centers using osmium generators. Serial images in many angulations can be obtained with a dramatic decrease in radiation exposure compared with radiotracers having longer half-lives. This iridium isotope is useful in quantifying right to left shunts and in measuring the ventricular ejection fraction. Other agents permit the accurate assessment of myocardial perfusion.

A major change has occurred in the mix of nuclear medicine examinations over the past decade. Because of the development of computed tomography and ultrasonography, radionuclide brain scans are now uncommon. However, as the scintigraphic delineation of osteomyelitis, other benign disorders, and primary and metastatic bone tumors has been refined, bone scans have become more numerous. Magnification scintigraphy has been recently used in intraoperatively localizing osteoid osteoma and in examining specimens for adequacy of removal. A small decrease in examinations of the liver and spleen reflects the increased application of ultrasonography and computed tomography for those organs. The total number of genitourinary examinations (renal scans, voiding cystography, and scrotal scintigraphy) is now about 35% of the nuclear medical workload. Radionuclide cystography for following patients with vesicoureteral reflux (Sec. 17.39) is being used much more frequently because of its high sensitivity and extremely low radiation exposure. Technetium-labeled dimercaptosuccinic acid (DMSA) demonstrates the renal cortex, permits the measurement of regional renal function, and distinguishes normal cortical tissue from cysts and tumors. Rapidly excreted technetium-labeled diethylenetriaminepenta-acetic acid (DTPA) is especially useful in hypertension and in obstructive and reflux nephropathy. This agent allows accurate quantification of the glomerular filtration rate without the need for collecting urine. Technetium-labeled compounds may soon replace iodinated orthoiodohippurate in determining effective renal plasma flow.

Ventilation-perfusion scans of the lung using xenon-133, intravenously and by inhalation, are helpful in evaluating patients with cystic fibrosis, airway obstruction, bronchopulmonary dysplasia, bronchiectasis, and pectus excavatum. Intravenous technetium-99m monoaggregates show regional lung perfusion well.

Radioisotope labeling of monoclonal antibodies has been used for detecting osteosarcoma and neuroblastoma and is being evaluated for use in tumor therapy.

Ultrasonography. This method of forming images by recording and visualizing the movements of high frequency sound waves as they are reflected off the interfaces of structures that impede sound waves differentially is an important diagnostic technique. Contrasts between the properties and efficacy of computed tomography and those of ultrasonography in the pediatric abdomen are given in Table 5–32. Ultrasonography is most commonly used to evaluate the neonatal brain, the liver and biliary system, and the kidney and to detect and evaluate intra-abdominal, pelvic, and retroperitoneal masses. It is also used to facilitate the placement of biopsy needles and nephrostomy tubes.

Because of high mortality and morbidity from intracranial hemorrhage (Sec. 8.23), ultrasonography is prognostically important. It may also be important in excluding intracranial hemorrhage in the differential diagnosis of obscure neurologic illness. Because the maneuverability of the transducer makes examination easier, real-time ultrasonography is the preferred technique at the bedside. The brain is readily displayed through the acoustic window provided by the anterior fontanel, where the lack of bone permits the use of higher frequency transducers, which provide better resolution.

Intraoperative ultrasonography through the intact or incised dura is used for the exact localization and tissue characterization of masses in the brain. Ultrasonography can guide the placement of shunt catheters.

Ultrasonography is also applicable to a wide range of abdominal problems, except for those of the gastrointestinal tract (although some mural lesions can be seen). If a duplication of the bowel (Sec. 12.34) is large enough (1.5–2 cm), it can be recognized by the liquid within it. Whether a duplication can be differentiated from a mesenteric or omental cyst is an unsettled issue, although duplications are usually smaller. The intrahepatic ducts (if dilated), the gallbladder, and the hepatic vessels can be visualized. Primary and metastatic hepatic tumors (Sec. 16.22) over 1 cm in diameter can usually be detected, and the liver parenchyma can be characterized to some extent. Ultrasonography can be used to guide liver biopsies and determine liver size. Examining the spleen is less satisfactory because of the closeness of the overlying ribs, but its size, the effects of trauma, and the presence of cysts can be shown. Dilatation of the main pancreatic duct, inflammatory and traumatic pancreatitis, and pseudocysts can be seen (Sec. 12.69).

Ultrasonographically evaluating the *urinary tract* is becom-

Table 5–32. Properties and Functions of Computed Tomography and Ultrasonography as Applied to Visualizing Children's Abdomens

Computed Tomography	Ultrasonography
Records and quantifies differences in x-ray absorption	Records differences in acoustical impedance
CT superior to ultrasonography	
Images conform to standard anatomic presentations	Less true; images less meaningful to the uninitiated
"Contrast enhancement" will distinguish between structures of similar x-ray density but different vascularity	No such ability
Few difficulties caused by gas, bone	Major image problems from gas and bone
Useful throughout abdomen; intestinal gas of infants is helpful	Difficulties in left upper quadrant because of ribs, in midabdomen because of gas
Image quality moderately dependent on operator's skill	More dependent
Data semipermanently available for re-analysis	At present, data ephemeral except for images on tape or film
CT inferior to ultrasonography	
Usually takes more time for examination	Usually takes less time
More expensive	Less expensive
Ionizing radiation; consequent small hazard	No proven hazard from ultrasound signal
Sedation often required to age 4	Seldom required
Substantial image problems caused by motion, respiration, metal	Minor problems
No bedside capability	Considerable bedside capability
Some difficulty identifying fluid as such	Less difficulty
Dependence on perivisceral fat for organ delineation; scanty in infants and young children	No dependence; children's leanness an advantage
Fewer pixels per body part in small patients; corresponding lack of resolution	Little loss of resolution because of small size
Little ability to assess diaphragmatic motion, vascular pulsation	Diaphragmatic motion and vascular pulsations readily seen
Useful throughout abdomen	Especially useful in liver, pelvis, kidneys

ing increasingly important. Recognizing a first urinary tract infection (Sec. 17.38) was formerly followed by both voiding cystourethrography and intravenous urography. Now, if the voiding study is negative, ultrasonography of the kidneys is done; intravenous urography is necessary only if cystourethrography or ultrasonography is positive. Ultrasonography shows renal anatomy well, even when function is diminished. It is very valuable in the diagnosis and sequential evaluation of hydronephrosis. Visualizing a dilated ureter allows vesicoureteral reflux and ureterovesical obstruction to be distinguished from ureteropelvic obstruction. When a retroperitoneal mass is suspected, a plain film of the abdomen plus ultrasonography is a reasonable screening protocol. Obstructions of, perirenal fluid collections around, and alterations in size and shape of transplanted kidneys can be shown.

In the pelvis, cystic and solid neoplasms and inflammatory disease are readily detected. Pregnancy and its complications are revealed without the hazard of ionizing radiation.

Because images can be obtained in many planes, evaluating intra-abdominal vessels is possible. Extension of Wilms tumor into the inferior vena cava and right atrium can be shown. Visualizing the aorta and its branches helps to determine the precise location and extent of masses. Enlarged lymph nodes can be seen, and the staging of certain malignancies is possible.

In the abdomen, ultrasonography's ability to discriminate between a solid structure and one partially or completely filled with liquid is a major advance. Whether liquid is transudate or exudate is not always determinable, although the presence of particulate material in a cystic mass suggests exudate or hemorrhage. The technique also helps to localize abscesses and stones in the biliary tract and kidney during surgery.

Ultrasonographically examining the bones and peripheral soft tissues is at an early stage of development. Fluid can be recognized in the hip joint, and at times the nature of the fluid is suggested. Early detection of congenital dislocation of the hip (Sec. 23.2) is possible when the large amount of cartilage in the region makes radiographic demonstration difficult; the subsequent follow-up examination of the region is easier than with roentgenography. Soft tissue masses in the extremities can be shown to be solid, liquid, or mixed.

Echocardiography has revolutionized cardiac diagnosis. The ability to assess septal defects, the relationships and size of the great vessels, intracardiac masses, and myocardial contractility makes this a highly useful diagnostic procedure. Its noninvasiveness is particularly well suited to follow-up examinations.

Computed Tomography (CT). This modality is a method of body section roentgenography that produces a cross-sectional image made by rotating a roentgen tube and a detector located opposite the tube around the patient's body. A computer then manipulates the x-ray absorption data to produce the image. CT has dramatically changed the diagnostic evaluation of the brain: pneumoencephalography and ventriculography, both painful and dangerous procedures, are now rarely performed, and arteriography is performed infrequently except when arteriovenous malformations and other highly vascular tumors are being considered. Even with CT, however, there are difficulties: thick, dense bones such as the petrous pyramids produce artifacts; many tumors have indistinct margins; and visualizing the structures in the posterior fossa is difficult. Computed tomography is central to diagnosing and managing hydrocephalus (Sec. 21.12). It is very useful in intraspinal disease, particularly after non-ionic contrast material has opacified the subarachnoid space. Evaluating the vertebral column by CT, i.e., complex fractures and malformations, is particularly effective. However, CT seldom finds spinal illness not already signaled by plain films or isotope scans.

Computed tomography of the neck and trunk is particularly useful in showing the extent and defining the character of masses such as neuroblastomas, Wilms tumors, lymphomas, and abscesses. In children, most computed tomographic examinations of the thorax are investigations of primary or metastatic malignancy; pulmonary metastases are particularly well shown by CT. Although granulomas and other confusing nodular shadows abound in an adult, a child or adolescent having a malignancy capable of metastasizing to the lungs who is shown to have a round pulmonary nodule 4 mm or larger in diameter probably has a metastasis.

Using intravenously injected contrast material leads to opacification not only of the major vessels but also of the capillaries and extracellular fluid, which is particularly helpful in evaluating the abdomen, where the material allows masses previously concealed within solid organs to be seen. Calcification is exquisitely visible by CT, frequently before it can be seen by ordinary radiography. Introducing contrast material into the gastrointestinal tract prior to most abdominal studies is necessary to distinguish loops of bowel from enlarged lymph nodes and other tumors (Table 5–32).

Masses in peripheral soft tissue are well evaluated by CT. Ultrasonography may suggest the character of the lesion, but intravenously enhanced CT will often show the vascularity of the lesion and the displacement of surrounding vessels more accurately. The relationship of a mass to specific muscle bundles and nerves can often be exquisitely demonstrated. The method is also helpful in determining the intramedullary extent of bone tumors, although it is often impossible to know where the tumor stops and edema or hemorrhage starts. Although CT may identify the extent of bone destruction and medullary involvement in osteomyelitis, adequate plain films are more important.

Computed tomography is also of great value in certain interventional techniques, such as draining abdominal and retroperitoneal abscesses.

Digital Subtraction Angiograms. These are formed by the computer subtraction of precontrast radiographic images from images obtained after intravascular injection of opaque contrast material. This type of angiography has a role in the investigation of pediatric vascular abnormalities, specifically of the aorta and its major branches. Abnormalities of the pulmonary vasculature and in pulmonary perfusion can also be shown. The method is a viable alternative to biplane cine angiography and requires less contrast material during cardiac catheterizations for congenital heart disease. However, motion artifacts are a problem, and sedation is often mandatory.

Magnetic Resonance Imaging. This modality yields cross-sectional, longitudinal, and oblique images formed from signals emitted by a patient placed in a strong magnetic field to which an electromagnetic impulse of the proper resonant frequency is applied. Magnetic resonance shows blood flow, hemorrhage, and myelinization of the brain better than CT; however, calcification is less well seen. Delineating masses in the chest is easier with magnetic resonance, because large vessels are readily displayed without intravenous contrast material. The method has been used to show the effects of chemotherapy and radiation therapy on tumors and to delineate osteomyelitis and a variety of bone marrow disorders in children. Echoplanar imaging has been reported as a promising dynamic imaging technique for the heart.

JOHN A. KIRKPATRICK, JR.
N. THORNE GRISCOM

Cohen MD, Klatte EC, Baehner R, et al: Magnetic resonance imaging of bone marrow disease in children. Radiology 151:715, 1984.
Dickinson DF, Wilson N, Partridge JB: Digital subtraction angiography in infants and children with congenital heart disease. Br Heart J 51:485, 1984.

Fletcher BD, Scoles PV, Nelson DA: Osteomyelitis in children: Detection by magnetic resonance. Radiology 150:57, 1984.

Ghelman B, Visorita VJ: Postoperative radionuclide evaluation of osteoid osteomas. Radiology 146:509, 1983.

Haller JO, Schneider M: Pediatric Ultrasound. Chicago, Year Book Medical Publishers, 1980.

Hurwitz RA, Traves S, Kuruc A: Right ventricular and left ventricular ejection fraction in pediatric patients with normal hearts: First pass radionuclide angiocardiography. Am Heart J 107:726, 1984.

Johnson MA, Pennock JM, Bydder GM, et al: Clinical NMR imaging of the brain in children: Normal and neurologic disease. Am J Roentgenol 141:1005, 1983.

Kaufman RA, Towbin R, Babcock DS, et al: Upper abdominal trauma in children: Imaging evaluation. Am J Roentgenol 142:449, 1984.

Kirkpatrick JA: Advantages and disadvantages of nuclear medicine, ultrasound and CT in pediatric radiology. *In:* Margulis AR, Burhenne HJ (eds): Alimentary Tract Radiology. 3rd ed. St Louis, CV Mosby, 1983.

Kirks DR: Practical Pediatric Imaging. Diagnostic Radiology of Infants and Children. Boston, Little, Brown and Co, 1984.

Kuhns LR: Computed tomography of the retroperitoneum in children. Radiol Clin North Am 19:495, 1981.

Novick G, Ghelman B, Schneider M: Sonography of the neonatal hip. Am J Roentgenol 141:639, 1983.

Rosen PR, Treves ST, Ingelfinger J: Hypertension in children: Increased efficacy of Tc 99m succimer in screening for renal disease. Am J Dis Child 139:173, 1985.

Stanley P, Atkinson JB, Reid BS, et al: Percutaneous drainage of abdominal fluid collections in children. Am J Roentgenol 142:813, 1984.

Straub WH (ed): Manual of Diagnostic Imaging. A Clinician's Guide to Clinical Problem Solving. Boston, Little, Brown and Co, 1984.

Sweet EM: The impact of new imaging systems on pediatric radiology. Clin Radiol 34:361, 1983.

Wagner ML, Singleton EB, Egan ME: Digital subtraction angiography in children. Am J Roentgenol 140:127, 1983.

6

PRENATAL DISTURBANCES

PRENATAL FACTORS IN DISEASES OF CHILDREN

GENETIC FACTORS

Genetic abnormalities are a common cause of disease, handicap, and death among infants and children. Genetic disease accounts for the primary diagnosis of 11–16% of patients admitted to the pediatric units of teaching hospitals. One percent of newborn infants have a hereditary malformation, and 0.5% have an inborn error of metabolism or an abnormality of the sex chromosomes that causes no physical abnormalities and that can be detected only by specific laboratory tests.

The types of biochemical abnormalities that have been identified as causes of genetic disease include: substitution of a single amino acid (e.g., sickle cell disease, Sec. 15.18) or synthesis of extra amino acid residues (e.g., hemoglobin Constant Spring) in a protein molecule; deficient activity of an enzyme located normally in the lysosomes, mitochondria, or extracellular space (e.g., phenylketonuria due to deficiency of dihydropteridine reductase, Sec. 7.2, and Ehler-Danlos syndrome, type VII due to deficiency of procollagen peptidase, Sec. 24.17); lack of production of a specific protein or protein sugar complex (e.g., macular corneal dystrophy due to failure to synthesize keratan sulfate proteoglycan); or defective biosynthesis (e.g., of the C_1 esterase inhibitor in hereditary angioneurotic edema).

Many genes have been localized to specific chromosomes. Recombinant DNA technology now makes gene mapping possible, so that gene deletions, rearrangements, and the substitution of a few single bases can be identified more readily from alterations in restriction enzyme patterns. New methods for staining human chromosomes and identifying subtle duplications and deficiencies of chromosomal material have also enlarged the understanding of human chromosomal abnormalities.

A more complete understanding of the basic defect in many of the genetic diseases has altered current clinical classifications. For example, different types of hemophilia are now identified by the antigen level and the clotting activity of factor VIII. Homocystinuria, once considered a single disease, has been shown to be the manifestation of several different metabolic abnormalities. Glucose-6-phosphate dehydrogenase deficiency has been found to result not from a single genetic abnormality but possibly from over 100 separate genetic errors, mostly due to substitutions of one amino acid in this enzyme molecule. The lethal type of osteogenesis imperfecta, once considered a single disorder, has been shown to be caused by several different alterations of the collagen gene, including internal deletions in the gene's structure, its failure to properly form the collagen triple helix, and failure to secrete the precursors of collagen from cells. The identification of genetic markers, called restriction length polymorphisms, that are close to mutant genes is making it possible to trace mutant genes in diseases such as Huntington disease, hemophilia B, and thalassemia, through successive generations.

Four categories of genetic defects have been identified in man: the single mutant gene, abnormalities of the chromosomes, multifactorial inheritance, and cytoplasmic inheritance. Other genetic abnormalities have been postulated but not proved, e.g., delayed mutation expressed in response to environmental factors, or from a deletion in a chromosome that accentuates the effect of an adjacent gene or permits the expression of the effect of a mutant recessive gene on the homologous chromosome.

In clinically appraising and managing the child with an inherited disorder, three phases are critical: (1) recognizing that the condition is inherited, (2) identifying the pattern of inheritance, and (3) clarifying the clinical nature of the disorder, which includes understanding the risk of the disease's occurrence in siblings or other members of the family. Recognition that a condition is hereditary may be difficult when the patient has no affected relatives. The physician should be familiar with the different types of genetic diseases and be able to identify their patterns of inheritance using appropriate references such as *Mendelian Inheritance in Man* by McKusick, which catalogues conditions caused by single mutant genes. No catalogue is available for disorders attributed to multifactorial inheritance; their recognition depends on the physician's knowledge of these disorders. Only for chromosomal abnormalities is there a laboratory test for providing visible evidence of the underlying genetic disorder (Sec. 6.8).

6.1 SINGLE MUTANT GENES

Each single mutant gene exhibits one of the four patterns of mendelian inheritance: autosomal recessive, autosomal dominant, X-linked recessive, and X-linked dominant. Table 6–1 lists some of the common diseases with each of these inheritance patterns. This method of grouping genetic diseases is often helpful in understanding the clinical presentation of a disorder. Concepts such as the basic structure of the DNA molecule and the transmission of genetic information, initially to messenger RNA and then to the formation of a specific polypeptide, help in explaining the basis for diseases such as the various disorders of hemoglobin structure in which the primary abnormalities include amino acid substitutions and deletions, elongated globin chains, and fused or

Table 6–1. **Incidence of Diseases Due to Single Mutant Genes***

Genetic Disease	Frequency of Heterozygote	Number of Affected Individuals per Million Births
Autosomal Recessive		
Adrenogenital syndrome		15
Albinism, tyrosinase negative		25
Albinism, tyrosinase positive		25
Alpha$_1$-antitrypsin deficiency, SZ Pi type		240 } whites in Sweden*
ZZ		600
Cystic fibrosis	4% (U.S. whites)	270 (whites)
Galactosemia		25
Hemoglobin		
S-S (sickle cell anemia)	8% (U.S. blacks)	1600 (U.S. blacks)
S-C	(3% of U.S. blacks have hemoglobin A-C)	1200 (U.S. blacks)
		600 (U.S. blacks)
S-β thalassemia	1% (U.S. blacks)	100 (U.S. blacks)
β thalassemia	Up to 16% of Italians	400 (U.S. citizens of Mediterranean origin)
Metachromatic leukodystrophy		25
Hurler syndrome α-iduronidase deficiency		25
Sanfilippo syndrome		20
Phenylketonuria		70 (whites)
Tay-Sachs disease	3% (U.S. Jews)	400 (U.S. Ashkenazi Jews)
Autosomal Dominant		
Achondroplasia		100
Acrocephalosyndactyly (Apert syndrome)		6
Aniridia		5–10
Dentinogenesis imperfecta		8000
Facioscapulohumeral muscular dystrophy		4
Huntington chorea		50
Hyperlipoproteinemia, type II (familial hypercholesterolemia)		10,000
Marfan syndrome		15
Neurofibromatosis		303
Polycystic kidneys (all types)		4000
Retinoblastoma		50
Thanatophoric dwarfism		15
Tuberous sclerosis		10
Waardenburg syndrome		250
X-Linked Recessive Diseases		
	Frequency of female carriers	
Bruton agammaglobulinemia		10–15
Ocular albinism		10–15
Amelogenesis imperfecta		10
Fabry disease		2–5
Color blindness (deutan)		6% of males
(protan)		2% of males
Diabetes insipidus, nephrogenic		0.1
Glucose-6-phosphate dehydrogenase deficiency (African type or A-minus variant)	24% of American black females	10-14% of black Americans
Chronic granulomatous disease		1–5
Duchenne muscular dystrophy		200–220
Factor VIII deficiency (hemophilia A)		100–120
Factor IX deficiency (hemophilia B; Christmas disease)		20–30
Hunter syndrome		20
Ichthyosis		200
Retinitis pigmentosa		1–5

Data from Benirschke K, Carpenter G, Epstein C et al: *In* Brent RL, and Harris MI (eds): Prevention of Embryonic, Fetal and Perinatal Disease. Washington, D.C., DHEW Pub. No. (NIH) 76–853, 1976, pp 219–261.
*Data from Sveger T: N Engl J Med *294*:1316, 1976.

"hybrid" globin chains. Other concepts explaining the mechanisms for the occurrence of genetic abnormalities that are apparent in the study of microorganisms, such as defective function of repressor genes and regulator genes, are not yet applicable to understanding human genetic diseases.

In discussing single mutant genes a number of special terms are used. The 23 chromosomes in the sperm combine with the 23 chromosomes in the egg to form a *zygote* having 23 *pairs* of chromosomes. The *gene locus* is the particular location of a specific gene in a specific chromosome. Recent studies show that the coding portions of a gene, such as the beta globin gene, are interrupted by *intervening sequences* of DNA of variable lengths. These intervening sequences are not represented in the mature messenger RNA that corresponds to the gene. Each gene has an analogue with a similar location in the homologous (other of a pair) chromosome; the identical pair of loci are called *homologous loci*. The genes at the homologous loci are called *alleles*. Allelic genes are analogous (i.e., affect the nature of the same characteristic) but are often not identical; extensive variation may be observed in many of the different types of serum proteins among people of the same as well as different races. In view of the genetic variation that exists at many gene loci, it is arbitrary to consider some genes as mutant; usually the distinction is that the mutant gene has a major, harmful effect. When a person has a mutant gene at a locus in one chromosome but not at the homologous locus of the other, the person is *heterozygous* for that mutant gene. If the mutant gene does not affect the heterozygous individual, it is called a *recessive gene*. If the mutant gene has an effect in the heterozygous state, it is a *dominant gene*. A person having the same mutant gene at both homologous loci is *homozygous* for that gene. Autosomal recessive genes manifest their clinical effect only in the *homozygote*. The distinctions between recessive and dominant genes become arbitrary when identifying the heterozygote by biochemical testing or when the heterozygote only mildly expresses the disorder.

Each mendelian pattern of inheritance has characteristics that may be useful in establishing a diagnosis or in planning family studies that may be important for a clear explanation to the parents of an affected child.

6.2 AUTOSOMAL RECESSIVE INHERITANCE

The pedigree illustrating this pattern of inheritance (Fig. 6–1) shows the following characteristics: the child of 2 heterozygous parents has a 25% chance of being homozygous (that is, 1 chance in 2 of inheriting the mutant gene from each parent: $1/2 \times 1/2 = 1/4$); males and females are affected with equal frequency; the affected individuals are almost always born in only 1 generation of a family; the children of the affected (homozygous) person are all heterozygotes; the children of a homozygote can be affected only if the spouse is a heterozygote, a rare event because of the low incidence of most adverse recessive genes in the general population.

If the frequency of an autosomal recessive disease is known, the frequency of the heterozygote or carrier state can be calculated from the Hardy-Weinberg formula: $p^2 + 2pq + q^2 = 1$, in which p is the frequency of one of a pair of alleles and q is the frequency of the other. For example, if the frequency of cystic fibrosis among white Americans is 1 in 2500 (p^2), then the frequency of the heterozygote (2 pq) can be calculated: if $p^2 = 1/2500$, then $p = 1/50$ and $q = 49/50$; $2pq = 2 \times 1/50 \times 49/50$ or approximately 1/25 (or 3.92%).

Every human probably has several rare, harmful, recessive genes. Since these mutant genes are frequently not identifiable by laboratory tests, the heterozygous adult usually learns about his or her harmful recessive genes after the birth of a homozygous (and therefore affected) child. Related parents are much more likely to be heterozygous for the same harmful recessive genes because they have a common ancestor. Consanguineous matings are rare in the United States and in many other countries. Therefore, few genetic studies have been carried out to establish the overall risk for healthy but related parents. Based on the information available, the risk for parents who are first cousins of having a child with a birth defect is about double the 4% risk faced by healthy, unrelated parents.

6.3 AUTOSOMAL DOMINANT INHERITANCE

The pedigree in Figure 6–2 shows that both males and females are affected, that transmission occurs from one parent to child, and that the responsible mutant gene can arise by spontaneous mutation. The risk is 50% that an offspring of the affected person will inherit the chromosome that contains the mutant gene.

6.4 X-LINKED RECESSIVE INHERITANCE

The pedigree in Figure 6–3 shows that only males are clinically affected; that affected males are related through carrier females; that all daughters of affected males are carriers of the mutant gene; and that affected males do not have affected sons but may have affected grandsons born to carrier females. The female carrier has a 50% chance of giving her chromosome that bears the mutant gene to each of her children. In other words, each daughter of a carrier has a 50% chance of being a carrier, and each son has a 50% chance of

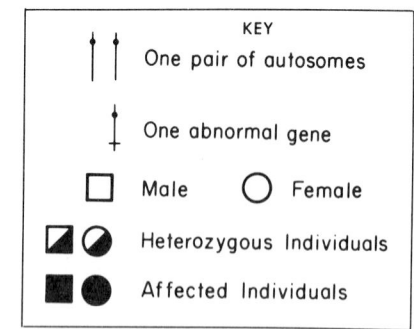

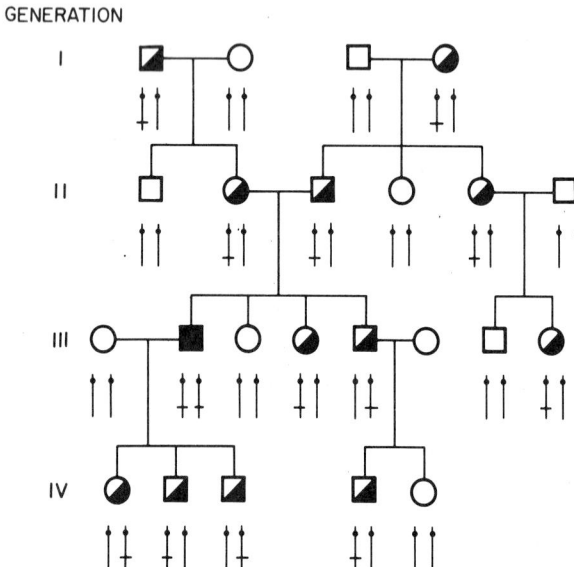

Figure 6–1. Autosomal recessive inheritance.

GENERATION

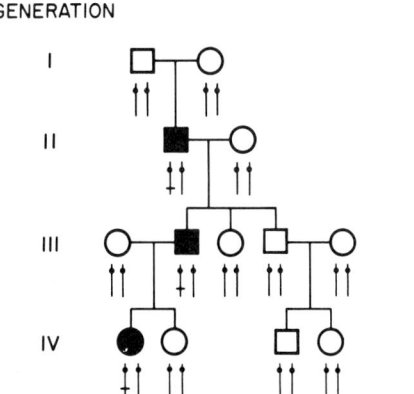

Figure 6–2. Autosomal dominant inheritance. (See Figure 6–1 for key.)

inheriting the mutant gene and having the disease that it causes. Therefore, in each pregnancy the female carrier has a 25% chance of having an affected son.

Initially, both X chromosomes of a female zygote are active. Random inactivation of portions of one X in each cell occurs early in fetal development. The inactivated X, which replicates later than the active X, is the sex chromatin mass or Barr body, which may be observed in the nucleus of a cell near the nuclear membrane. This random inactivation, also called *lyonization*, protects the carrier female from the effect of the X-linked recessive mutant gene because there is as much chance that the X chromosome which carries the mutant gene will be inactivated as that the other X chromosome will. Therefore, the carrier expresses the effect of the mutant gene in an average of 50% of her cells. For this reason the female carrier of classic hemophilia will have a reduced level of factor VIII activity but a level not nearly as low as that in her affected son or brother.

6.5 X-LINKED DOMINANT INHERITANCE

Very few X-linked dominant genes have been identified in humans. Two examples are vitamin D-resistant rickets and the Melnick-Needles syndrome of multiple malformations. The pedigree in Figure 6–4 shows the essential characteristics: both males and females are affected, but males are often more

severely affected; the disorder is transmitted from generation to generation; all daughters of an affected father will be affected, but none of his sons.

6.6 MULTIFACTORIAL INHERITANCE

The term multifactorial inheritance refers to the process in which a disease or abnormality is the result of the additive effect of one or more abnormal genes and environmental factors (Sec. 6.7). These disorders include some of the most common malformations as well as medical conditions such as allergic disorders, schizophrenia, and some types of hyperlipidemia (Table 6–2 and Sec. 7.39–7.49). The number of genes involved is unknown. Some investigators have postulated that the genes involved are "minor genes," which individually are not harmful but whose cumulative effect is harmful; others postulate that genes that exert a major effect are also involved. Few of the environmental factors have been identified in humans, but studies of conditions caused by multifactorial inheritance in animals emphasize their relevance. Some of the environmental factors identified in humans include seasonal variation in the occurrence of the disorder, increased frequency in families living in poor socioeconomic conditions, and associations with an altered uterine environment. (See Table 6–15.) Considerable data must be available on many affected persons and their families before the disease or malformation can be attributed to multifactorial inheritance. This term should not be used simply because the reason for familial occurrence is poorly understood.

Some of the features of multifactorial inheritance are similar to mendelian inheritance of single mutant genes, e.g., the incidence of specific conditions varies according to racial background; this racial predisposition persists after migration to other countries.

Most of the features of multifactorial inheritance, however, are quite different from those observed in mendelian inheritance of a single mutant gene:

1. There is a similar rate of recurrence (usually 2–10%; Table 6–2) among all first-degree relatives (parents, siblings, and offspring of the affected infant). For example, if a couple

GENERATION

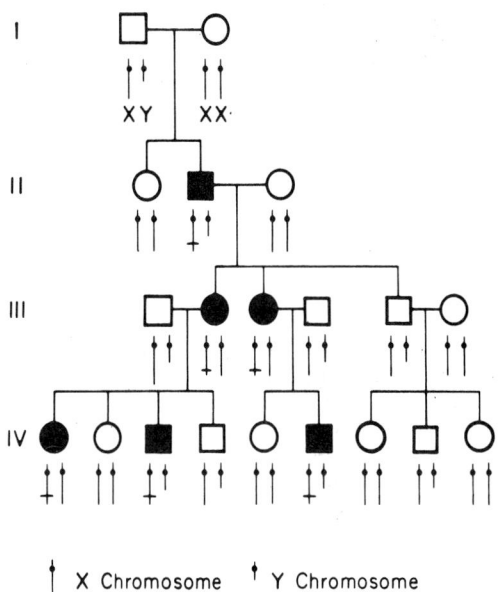

† X Chromosome † Y Chromosome

Figure 6–4. X-linked dominant inheritance. (See Figure 6–1 for key.)

GENERATION

† X Chromosome † Y Chromosome ⊙ Carrier Female

Figure 6–3. X-linked recessive inheritance. (See Figure 6–1 for key.)

Table 6–2. Genetic Disorders Attributed to Multifactorial Inheritance

Abnormality	Race	Prevalence in General Population (%)	Risk of Recurrence Among Family Members of an Affected Individual (%)		
			Siblings	Offspring	Identical Twin
Malformations					
Cardiac defects					
Ventricular septal defect		0.23	4.4	3.7	
Atrial septal defect		0.1 (1/1000)	3.3	3.5 (parents)	
Patent ductus arteriosus		0.05	1.4	2.8	
Tetralogy of Fallot		0.03	1.0	1.6	
Cleft lip and palate	Whites	0.13 (1/750)	3.9	3.5	31
	Blacks	0.04			
	Navajos	0.2			
	Japanese	0.16			
Cleft palate	Whites	0.05 (1/2000)	3.0	6.2	40
	Blacks	0.04			
	Navajos	0.03			
Club foot (talipes equinovarus)		0.01	2.9		33
Dislocation of hip, congenital		0.07 (1/1400)	4.3		35
Hirschsprung disease		0.02 (1/5000)	3.8*		
			12.5†		
Hypospadias	Whites	0.8 (1/120)	7.0	6.0	
	Blacks	0.2 (1/500)			
Legg-Perthes disease		0.07 (Canada)	3.7*		
			4.3†		
Meningomyelocele, anencephaly, encephalocele	Whites	0.3 (1/330) (London)	4.4	3.0	21
		0.14 (1/700) (Boston)	2		
	Jews	0.08			
	Blacks	0.07			
	Puerto Ricans	0.2			
Pyloric stenosis		0.2 (1/500) (London)	3.2*	25.4‡	22
			6.5†	4.2§	
Other Diseases					
Ankylosing spondylitis			7.0*		
			2.0†		
Atopic disease		2–3	5.8		24
Psoriasis		1–2	7.8		63
Schizophrenia		1–3	6–12	10	40

* = If brother affected.   ‡ = If mother affected.
† = If sister affected.   § = If father affected.

has had one child with cleft lip and palate, the risk that the next one will be affected is about 4%; if one parent has cleft lip and palate, the chance that the 1st child will have the same malformation is also about 4%.

2. Some disorders have a sex predilection. For example, pyloric stenosis is much more common in males, whereas congenital dislocation of hips is much more common in females.

3. If there is an altered sex ratio, the affected person of the sex less likely to be affected is much more apt to have affected children. For example, a woman who had pyloric stenosis as an infant has a 25% chance of having a child similarly affected; the risk for the children of the father who had pyloric stenosis is only 4%.

4. The likelihood that both of identical twins will be affected with the same malformation is less than 100% but much greater than the chance that both nonidentical twins will be affected. The frequency of concordance for identical twins ranges from 21 to 63% for the disorders listed in Table 6–2. This distribution contrasts with that of mendelian inheritance, in which identical twins always share a disorder due to a single mutant gene.

5. The risk of recurrence in subsequent pregnancies depends on the outcome in previous pregnancies. For example, the risk of recurrence for cleft lip and palate is 4% for a couple with 1 affected child, but 9% after they have had 2 affected children.

6. The risk of abnormality in offspring is directly related to the severity of the malformation. For example, the infant who has congenital intestinal aganglionosis of a long segment of bowel has a greater chance of having an affected sibling than the infant who has aganglionosis of only a small segment.

6.7 GENERAL CLINICAL PRINCIPLES IN GENETIC DISORDERS

The Negative Family History. A child with a genetic disease or malformation is usually the only known affected member of his or her family. This reflects the fact that the rates of recurrence are very low for common abnormalities of the chromosomes and for conditions attributed to multifactorial inheritance. For example, the recurrence risk for Down syndrome associated with trisomy-21 is 1%; for conditions attributed to multifactorial inheritance it varies from 2 to 10% (Table 6–2). The recurrence risk for disorders with a mendelian pattern of inheritance is much higher (e.g., 25% for autosomal recessive disorders), but in small families it is more likely that an autosomal recessive disorder will affect only 1 of 3 or 4 children rather than 2. In the case of autosomal dominant disorders, the child may be affected by a spontaneous genetic mutation rather than by inheriting the mutant gene from an affected parent. Generally speaking, a negative family history may be misleading.

Environmental Factors. Since the family history is usually negative for the disorder under consideration, the parents often blame themselves and look for environmental factors that might have been the cause. The physician should anticipate their feelings of guilt and carefully discuss the events, including medications taken, to which congenital disorders may be attributed inappropriately by parents.

Genetic Heterogeneity. A single clinical manifestation may have more than one cause. An elevation in serum phenylalanine may be associated with classic phenylketonuria (either the absence or deficiency of phenylalanine hydroxylase); absence or deficiency of the enzyme pteridin reductase; or deficient biopterin synthesis. Arachnodactyly may be an isolated characteristic of a tall, thin person, or it may be a feature of a number of genetic disorders, including Marfan syndrome and contractural arachnodactyly.

Pleiotropism. Some genetic disorders have many different features, all of which are the pleiotropic effect of a single mutant gene. For example, in classic galactosemia, cataracts, hepatomegaly, malabsorption, neonatal sepsis, and mental deficiency are all related to deficiency of the transferase enzyme, which is the primary effect of the underlying autosomal recessive mutant gene. In neurofibromatosis, café-au-lait spots, subcutaneous nodules, solid tumors, scoliosis, and mental deficiency are caused by a single autosomal dominant gene.

Variable Expression. Publications often present the extreme manifestations of a clinical disorder but rarely describe its milder forms. The clinician must appreciate that 2 or 3 café-au-lait spots may be either innocent birth marks or the earliest signs of neurofibromatosis in which additional features may become manifest at an older age. This diagnostic dilemma can be resolved only by a careful diagnostic evaluation and sometimes long-term follow-up. In the case of hereditary disorders without progressive changes, such as the Treacher Collins syndrome (mandibulofacial dysostosis), the affected child may have microtia, severe hearing loss, colobomas of the lower eyelids, and marked maxillary hypoplasia, while the affected parent may have only mild hearing loss, a downward slant of the palpebral fissures, and a decreased number of lashes on the lower eyelid.

Not Everything Familial Is Genetic. Environmental factors, such as infection and teratogens (see Table 6–15) may simulate genetic conditions; on occasion two or more children of healthy parents may be affected.

Establishing the Pattern of Inheritance Requires Extensive Data. Data from a small number of families cannot establish a pattern of inheritance. For example, when a presumed genetic disorder has occurred in a son and daughter of healthy parents, it is often concluded that each child is homozygous for an autosomal recessive mutant gene. However, a familial chromosomal abnormality and multifactorial inheritance could also cause the same pattern. Similarly, the pattern of occurrence in families with a disorder due to multifactorial inheritance may simulate mendelian inheritance; e.g., the parent and child with cleft lip and palate mimic autosomal dominant inheritance. With the rate of recurrence·among parents and siblings only 4% for Caucasians, almost all children with cleft lip and palate are the only affected members of their families. Data on hundreds of families were needed to establish multifactorial inheritance as the basis for the disorder and to exclude the possibility of mendelian inheritance.

LEWIS B. HOLMES

de Grouchy J: The human gene map: A review. Biomed Pharmacother 37:159, 1983.

Egger J, Wilson J: Mitochondrial inheritance in a mitochondrially mediated disease. N Engl J Med 309:142, 1983.

Fraser FC: The multifactorial/threshold concept: Uses and misuses. Teratology 14:267, 1976.

Gusella JF, Wexler NS, Conneally PM, et al: A polymorphic DNA marker genetically linked to Huntington's disease. Nature 306:234, 1983.

Hall JG, Powers EK, McIlvaine RT, et al: The frequency and financial burden of genetic disease in a pediatric hospital. Am J Med Genet 1:417, 1978.

Harris H, Hopkinson DA, Robson EB: The incidence of rare alleles determining electrophoretic variants: Data on 43 enzyme loci in man. Ann Hum Genet (London) 37:237, 1974.

Orkin SH, Kazazian HH, Antonarakis SE, et al: Linkage of beta-thalassemia mutations and beta-globin gene polymorphisms in human beta-globin gene cluster. Nature 296:627, 1982.

Scriver CR, Claw CL: Phenylketonuria: Epitome of human biochemical genetics. N Engl J Med 303:1336, 1394, 1980.

Woo SLC: Prenatal diagnosis and carrier detection of classic phenylketonuria by gene analysis. Pediatrics 74:412, 1984.

General

McKusick V: Mendelian Inheritance in Man: Catalogs of Autosomal Dominant, Autosomal Recessive and X-Linked Phenotypes. 5th ed. Baltimore, Johns Hopkins University Press, 1978.

Vogel F, Motulsky AG: Human Genetics: Problems and Approaches. New York, Springer-Verlag, 1979.

Watson JD, Tooze J, Kurtz DT: Recombinant DNA: A Short Course. New York, Scientific American Books, WH Freeman, 1983.

6.8 CHROMOSOMES AND THEIR ABNORMALITIES

Scientific and technologic advances permitted Hsu and Levan in 1952 to accurately observe human chromosomes and Tjio and Levan in 1956 to discover that the correct systemic chromosome number in humans is 46. In 1959 Lejeune observed that patients with Down syndrome have 47 chromosomes, including an extra chromosome 21 (trisomy 21). These seminal observations were rapidly followed by the discovery of other trisomies in congenital malformation syndromes, abnormalities in the number of sex chromosomes in Klinefelter and Turner syndromes, and the first detection of chromosomal mosaics and abnormalities of chromosome structure. Cytogenetic abnormalities are now recognized as important etiologic factors in human disease. During the ensuing 25 years, laboratory procedures were developed to identify precisely the individual chromosomes (and chromosomal segments), enabling the interpretation of complex chromosomal rearrangements as well as minor morphologic variations. These techniques have also led to more accurate clinical diagnosis as well as to more precise genetic counseling.

Because chromosome studies are complicated and expensive, candidates for these procedures must be carefully identified. The most important clinical indications are congenital malformations, especially if more than one system is involved, and mental retardation of unknown origin. Some of the more common features of children with chromosome abnormalities are odd facies, abnormal ears, heart and kidney malformations, abnormal hands and feet, simian creases, a single crease on the 5th finger, and low birthweight. It has been estimated that about 1 in 150 newborn infants has a chromosomal abnormality. Table 6–3 lists the incidence of various chromosomal abnormalities in liveborn infants.

In addition, the fact that 50–60% of the products of early spontaneous abortion have a chromosomal abnormality suggests that at least 10% of human conceptions have a karyotypic abnormality. At 16–18 wk of gestation, the incidence of chromosomal abnormalities as detected by amniocentesis is greater than in liveborn infants, suggesting the loss of additional cytogenetically unbalanced fetuses in mid- and late pregnancy. Approximately 90% of karyotypically abnormal conceptions do not survive pregnancy. Of the chromosomal abnormalities observed in liveborn infants, about half involve the autosomes and half the sex chromosomes. Chromosomal abnormalities are associated with approximately 50% of cases of primary amenorrhea, 10% of male sterility, and 20% of mental retardation, and are found in the vast majority of neoplastic cells. Their discoverable frequency should increase as more accurate methods for detection of minor structural alterations become available.

METHODOLOGY

Cell Culture. The small lymphocyte, which is readily stimulated to divide with the plant mitogen phytohemagglutinin (PHA), is commonly used for chromosome investigation. The dividing cells are arrested in metaphase and the chromosomes are dispersed and air dried.

Cultures of fibroblasts may be necessary for studies of mosaicism and biochemical defects. For diagnosing blood dyscrasias, bone marrow preparations are best, but chromosomes of peripheral blood myelocytes can be used. The methodology for culturing amniotic fluid cells is similar to that for fibroblasts. Cytogenetic analysis is complete in 2–3 wk.

A much more rapid method for fetal chromosome analysis, chorionic villus biopsy, consists of obtaining a small sample of chorionic villi by ultrasonically guided transcervical suction biopsy followed by directly observing chromosomes in the sample or in cells cultured from the sample. The procedure is performed at 8–11 weeks of gestation, and results are generally available before the end of the 1st trimester. The safety of the procedure has not been fully evaluated.

Chromosome staining methods have been largely supplanted by the development of techniques that can yield characteristic patterns of alternating light and dark (or bright and dull) bands for each chromosome. These bands appear to be associated with the composition of base pairs forming the DNA, as well as the distribution of the various histone and non-histone proteins along the length of the chromosome. Staining with quinacrine derivatives or similar compounds, followed by microscopic investigation using an ultraviolet

light source, produces fluorescent bands called *Q bands*, while corresponding *G bands* are produced by a modified Giemsa staining procedure. Another method, using Giemsa or acridine orange, produces staining intensities opposite to Q and G bands, which are called reverse or *R bands*. All qualified cytogenetic laboratories now use at least one of these banding methods to assure a reliable diagnosis. Other procedures available in more advanced laboratories include C-banding to stain constitutive heterochromatin found near the centromere of each chromosome; a *C-band* stain (G-11) specific for No. 9; NOR, using ammoniacal silver to stain the nucleolar organizing regions of satellited chromosomes; and SCE, a procedure that reveals exchanges between sister chromatids.

An important newer development consists of examining chromosomes during late prophase, at which time they are much less contracted than at metaphase when they are commonly examined. This procedure allows the analysis of 600–1400 bands as opposed to the usual 200–400, permitting the discovery of very small deletions and duplications.

Karyotyping. Chromosomal DNA replicates during the S stage of interphase, but the double-structured nature of the chromosomes becomes clearly visible only at the beginning of mitosis; each chromosome consists of two identical long thin strands called sister chromatids, which coil progressively tighter, giving the appearance of short, thick arms held together by the centromere. At metaphase, when they are at their shortest length, the chromosomes are photographed and arranged in pairs. This systematized arrangement from a single cell is referred to as a karyotype. Only "banded" karyotypes are acceptable for diagnoses, and most laboratories study 10–40 metaphase karyotypes per subject. If mosaicism is suspected, more cells, as well as cells of other tissues, should be analyzed. When finer details are required, prophase or prometaphase chromosomes are examined because they are longer and show more bands.

6.9 THE NORMAL KARYOTYPE

The diploid number of human chromosomes is 46, consisting of 23 pairs; 23 is the haploid number found in the gametes. At metaphase each chromosome, consisting of 2 chromatids, has a characteristic morphology determined by the position of the centromere, or primary constriction, which delineates the long and short arms (Fig. 6–5A). Examples of the three normal characteristic shapes are Nos. 1, 3, and 16 (*metacentric*), Nos. 4 and 5 (*submetacentric*), and Nos. 21 and 22 (*acrocentric*). The short arms of all acrocentric chromosomes except the Y have a secondary constriction and satellite. Following the accurate identification of each chromosome, accomplished on the basis of size, morphology, and banding pattern, a number system was agreed upon (Fig. 6–6).

A few morphologic variants have been observed in the normal karyotype with conventional stains. Best known are elongation of the paracentromeric region in the long arm of Nos. 1, 9, and 16, extended or deleted short arms or enlarged satellites of acrocentric chromosomes, and a secondary constriction on the short arm of No. 17 (Figs. 6–5B and 6–7). The Y chromosome may also vary in length and shape. Although the banding patterns are constant for each chromosome, normal variants have been revealed by fluorescent stains, e.g., variation in intensity of fluorescent bands near the centromeres of chromosomes 3 and 4 and satellites on the acrocentric chromosomes (Fig. 6–7). The variation in length of the Y chromosome is the result of extension or loss of the brilliant Q band, which appears to have no effect on the phenotype. Morphologic variants were first observed in abnormal subjects and thought to be associated with disease, but it soon became apparent that they were inherited in

Table 6–3. Incidence of Chromosomal Abnormalities among Liveborn Infants

Down syndrome (21-trisomy)	1/800
18-trisomy syndrome	1/8000
13-trisomy syndrome	1/20,000
Turner syndrome (females)	1/10,000
Klinefelter syndrome (males)	1/1000
Poly-X anomalies (females)	1/1000
XYY karyotype (males)	1/1000
Balanced structural rearrangement	1/520
Unbalanced structural rearrangement	1/1700
Fragile X (males)	1/2000
(females)	1/1000
Total	1/150

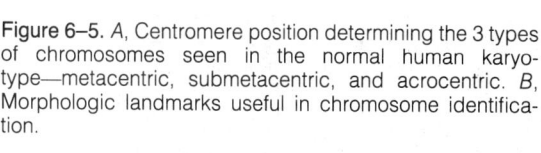

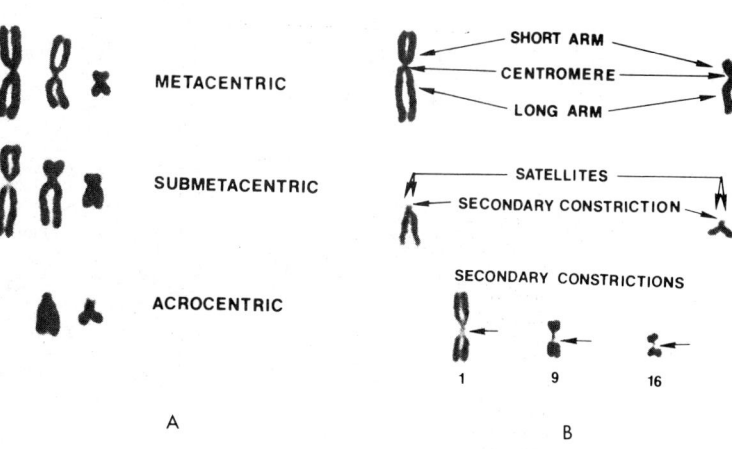

Figure 6–5. *A,* Centromere position determining the 3 types of chromosomes seen in the normal human karyotype—metacentric, submetacentric, and acrocentric. *B,* Morphologic landmarks useful in chromosome identification.

A

B

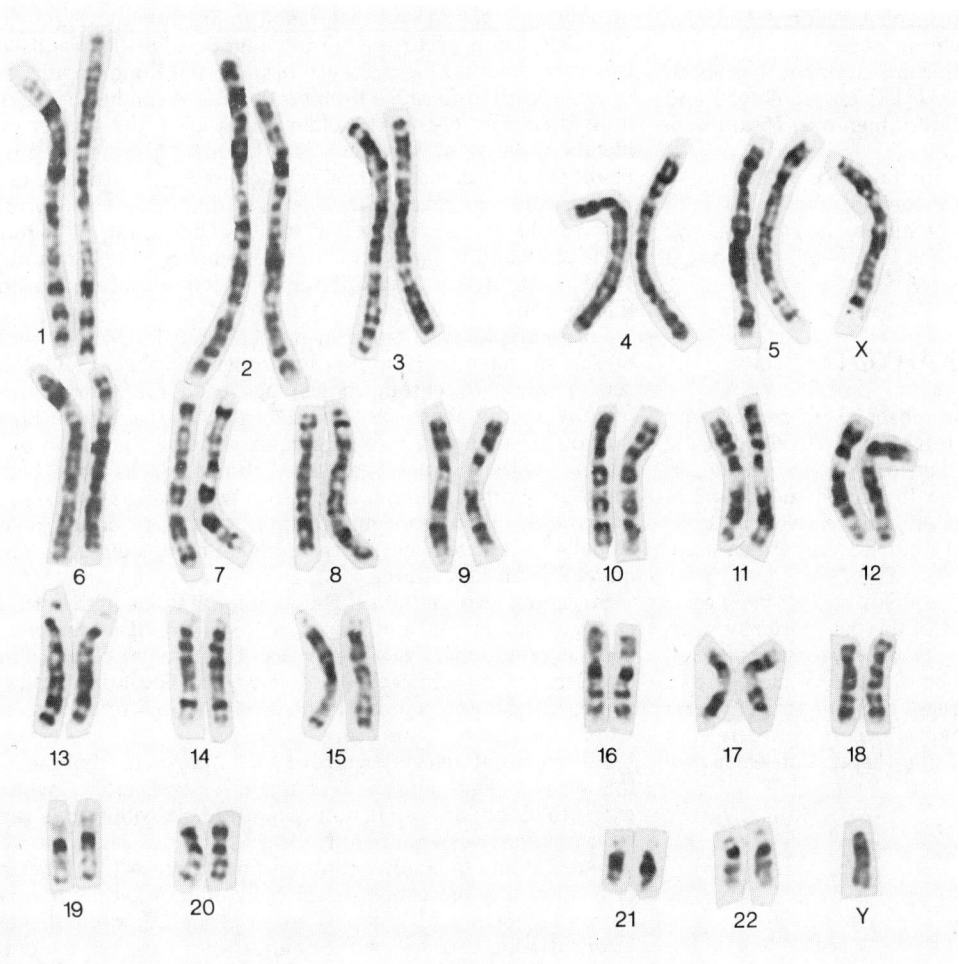

Figure 6–6. Karyotype of normal male with chromosomes in late prophase. The chromosomes are longer and a greater number of bands are seen than when chromosomes are photographed at metaphase.

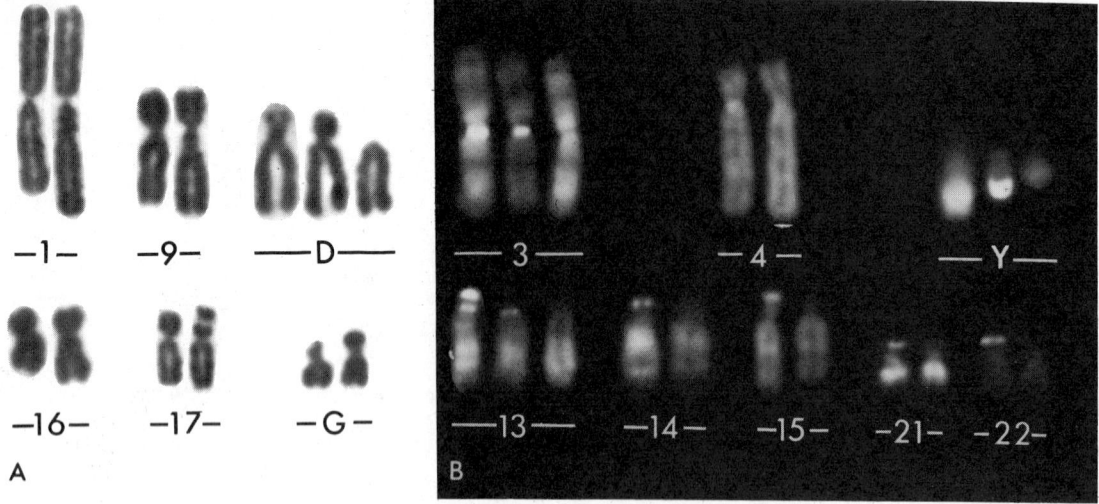

Figure 6–7. Some morphologic variants found in normal subjects. *A*, Chromosomes stained with aceto-orcein. The left-hand chromosome of each pair or triad is a usual or "nonmarker" chromosome. *B*, Chromosomes stained with quinacrine dihydrochloride showing differences in intensity of fluorescent bands among homologues.

mendelian fashion, and some occur in sufficiently high frequencies to be considered polymorphisms ("normal variants"). Therefore, they are useful genetic markers and also help to localize genes to specific chromosomes.

Cell-to-cell variation in chromosome number has been found in older people. A tendency exists for women 55 and older to lose an X chromosome and for men over 65 to lose a Y chromosome.

Another category of variation is the presence or absence of fragile sites. While most of these are not associated with specific syndromes, the presence of such a site near the end of the long arm of the X chromosome (Fig. 6–8) is associated with mental retardation.

6.10 ABNORMAL KARYOTYPES

Numerical Abnormalities. Chromosomal aberrations are divided into numerical and structural types. A cell with the exact multiple of the haploid number, e.g., 46, 69, 92, etc., is referred to as *euploid*. Euploid cells with more than the normal *diploid* number of 46 chromosomes are termed *polyploid*. Cells deviating from one of the euploid numbers are termed *aneuploid*.

The most common type of aneuploidy is *trisomy*, i.e., 3 homologous chromosomes instead of the pair normally present. Lack of a chromosome is called *monosomy* (for the affected pair). Aneuploid individuals may be trisomic for more than 1 pair of chromosomes or may even combine trisomy and monosomy. During meiosis, synapsis occurs between each chromosome and its homologue; after separation each proceeds to an opposite pole of the dividing cell. Failure of synapsis or failure to separate (*nondisjunction*) interferes with orderly segregation and may result in aneuploidy (Fig. 6–9). Nondisjunction occurring during mitotic division results in *mosaicism*, that is, the presence of more than one population of cells with differing chromosome numbers in the same individual (Fig. 6–10). The older the mother, the greater the likelihood of nondisjunction and trisomy. Monosomy may result from chromosome loss or *anaphase lag*, i.e., failure of a chromosome to reach either pole during anaphase, which also results in mosaicism (Fig. 6–10). The timing of mitotic nondisjunction in embryonic development may result in mosaicism with two or three different populations of cells present (Fig. 6–11).

Pure polyploidy is lethal in humans, but individuals with mosaicism have been known to survive. *Triploidy* (3 haploid sets, totaling 69 chromosomes) has been found most frequently among abortuses and stillbirths. It arises by fertilization of the ovum by two spermatozoa or by the union of a haploid with a diploid gamete. Tetraploid cells have been found in aborted material, in persons with malignant disease, and, rarely, in dysmorphic infants. *Tetraploidy* occurs occasionally in cultured cells, particularly amniotic fluid cells, and increases during culture.

Structural Aberrations. These abnormalities result from chromosome breaks and rearrangements. *Deletion syndromes*, such as cri-du-chat (5p−), may result from a simple deletion or from the inheritance of a deleted translocation chromosome. Interstitial deletions result from the loss of a segment within the chromosome arm (Fig. 6–12).

All structural defects require at least 2 chromosomal breaks followed by reunion of the broken ends. *Translocations*, which may be inherited or arise de novo, are most common. *Reciprocal translocations* result from the exchange of segments between 2 nonhomologous chromosomes (Fig. 6–12). Carriers of reciprocal translocations are usually phenotypically normal since they have a full complement of genes. Children of such "translocation carriers" will be abnormal if they receive only 1 of the 2 translocation chromosomes and thus become affected by duplication-deficiency syndromes (Fig. 6–13). Depending upon the amount of material duplicated or deficient, the aberration is referred to as *partial trisomy* or *partial monosomy*. A special type of translocation, the *centric fusion* or

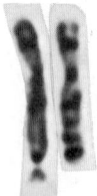

Figure 6–8. X chromosomes with the one on the left showing a fragile site near the lower end of the long arm (fra(X) (q28)).

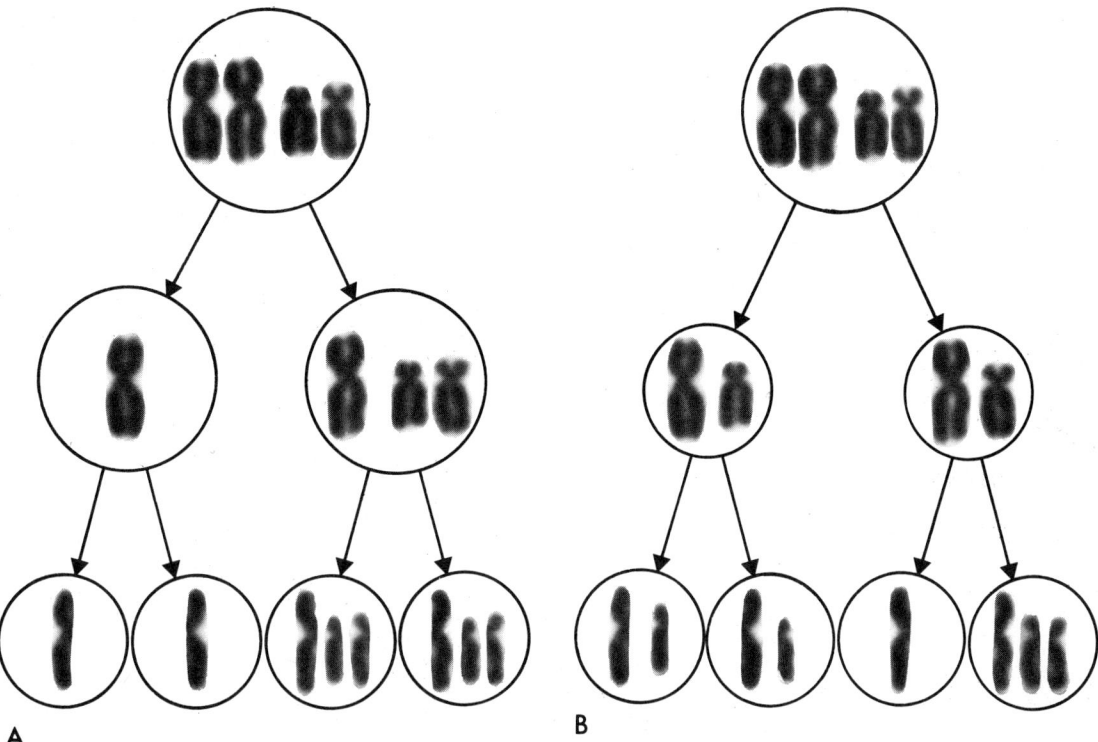

Figure 6–9. Nondisjunction during meiosis illustrated with 2 pairs of chromosomes. *A*, First division nondisjunction with failure of smaller homologues to separate gives rise to gametes with no small chromosome or with an extra one. *B*, Second division nondisjunction following division of centromere. Two newly formed chromosomes fail to separate in cell on the right.

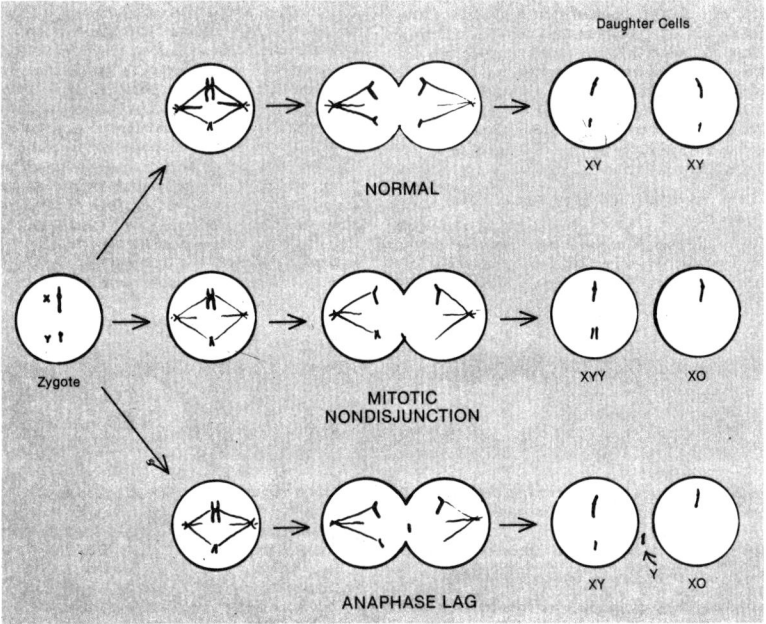

Figure 6–10. The formation of mosaicism. The X and Y chromosomes are used to illustrate two common errors leading to chromosomally abnormal cell populations. In normal mitosis (top) duplicated chromosomes separate and become incorporated into daughter cells. If one replicated chromosome fails to separate, mitotic nondisjunction occurs (middle). Occasionally, normal separation occurs, but one member fails to migrate. This is known as anaphase lag (bottom). (From Wisniewski LP, Hirschhorn K: Birth Defects 16 (6), 1980.)

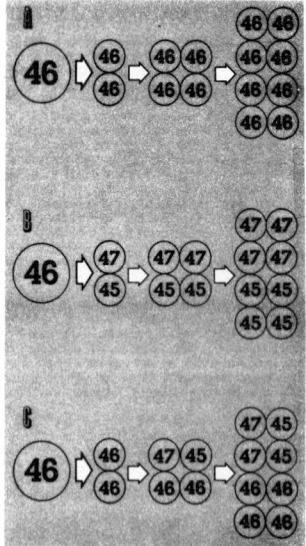

Figure 6–11. Relationship of the timing of mitotic nondisjunction to the proportion of abnormal cells in a mosaic embryo. *A*, Normal mitosis; all resulting cells contain 46 chromosomes. *B*, Error occurring during the first mitosis after conception; two types of cells subsequently compose the developing embryo (half containing 47 chromosomes, half containing 45). *C*, An error occurs after some growth has been achieved; three different cell populations result (cells with 45, 46, and 47 chromosomes). (From Wisniewski LP, Hirschhorn K: Birth defects 16 (6), 1980.)

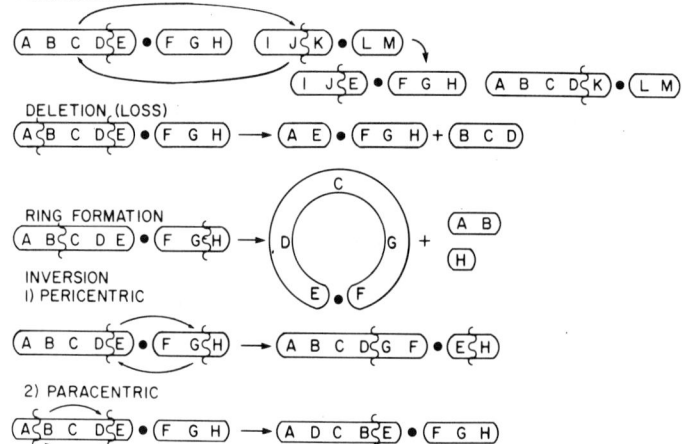

Figure 6–12. Mechanisms leading to structural chromosome abnormalities. These aberrations are dependent upon the occurrence of at least 2 breaks (symbolized by a wavy line).

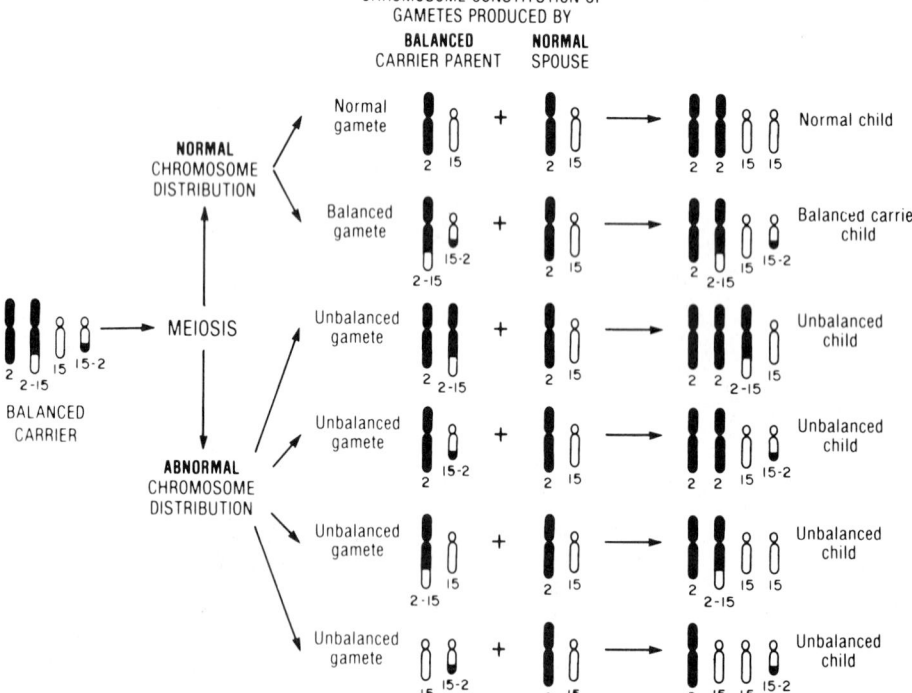

Figure 6–13. The inheritance of a 2/15 translocation. (From Wisniewski LP, Hirschhorn K: Birth Defects 16 (6), 1980.)

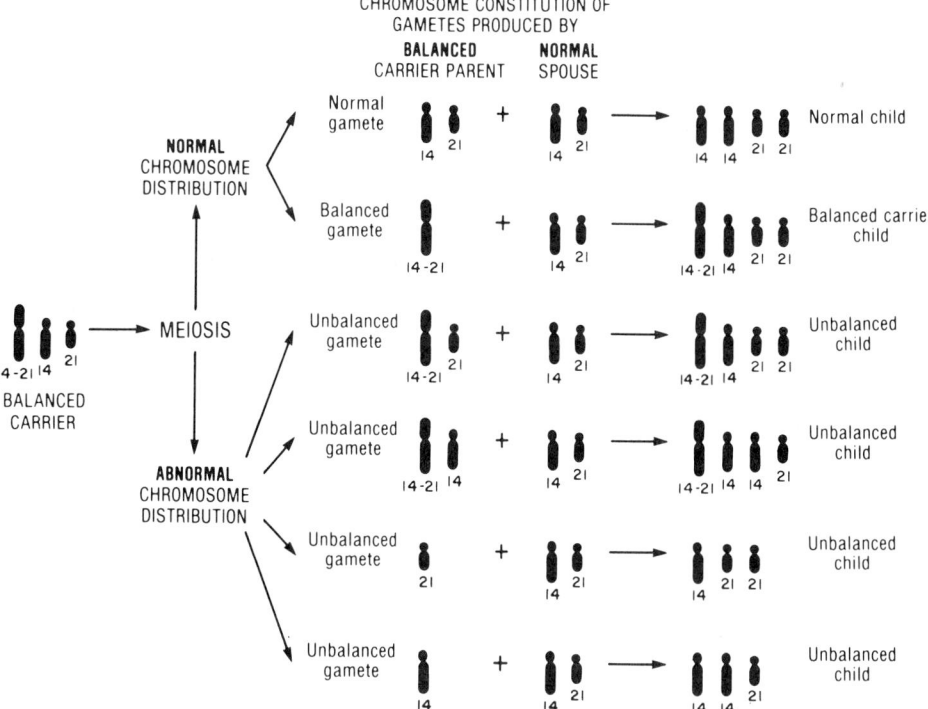

CHROMOSOME CONSTITUTION OF
GAMETES PRODUCED BY

Figure 6–14. The inheritance of a 14/21 centric fusion. Although this translocation can also result in abnormalities of chromosome 14 and monosomy 21, conceptions with these defects rarely, if ever, survive. (From Wisniewski LP, Hirschhorn K: Birth Defects 16 (6), 1980.)

Robertsonian translocation, involves acrocentric chromosomes in which the breaks occur adjacent to the centromeres of "recipient" and "donor" chromosomes. The centromere of the donor chromosome and the short arms of both chromosomes are usually lost. Centric fusion commonly involves No. 14 and No. 21 and therefore may result in Down syndrome (Fig. 6–14). Since the short arms of acrocentric chromosomes appear to be genetically inactive, the loss of material in such translocations has no apparent phenotypic effect on carriers.

Ring chromosomes are formed when both tips of a chromosome are broken and the ends of the centric fragment rejoin forming a chromosome with a deletion of both arms (Fig. 6–12). This unstable closed structure leads to difficulties in mitosis. *Inversions* (Fig. 6–12) of two types may result when the segment between 2 breaks in a single chromosome is inverted and the order of the genes reversed. Since an inversion may cause difficulty in synapsis, it may increase the risk of nondisjunction.

During meiosis, crossing over of genes between chromatids of homologous chromosomes is a normal phenomenon readily proved by the recombination or separation of genes originally linked on the same chromosome. Exchanges between chromatids may also occur during mitosis and may involve the chromatids of 2 homologous or nonhomologous chromosomes. Since at metaphase the sister chromatids have not yet separated, such exchanges result in *quadriradial* configurations that resemble crossroads. It is more difficult to prove the existence of *sister chromatid exchanges* (SCE) in mitotic cells because replicated chromatids carry identical genes and no unusual configurations are formed. This can be done with staining techniques. The various types of chromatid exchanges are found in breakage syndromes (Sec. 6.19) and in cells exposed to mutagenic agents.

NOMENCLATURE

The nomenclature for describing a karyotype has been standardized to avoid confusion. First, the total number of chromosomes, and second, the sex chromosome complement are recorded; then any aberration is described (Table 6–4). The short arm is referred to as *p* and the long arm as *q*. Any addition or loss of chromosomal material is denoted by a plus (+) or minus (−) sign placed before the chromosome number if a whole chromosome is involved and after a symbol if any increase or decrease in length is involved. Chromosomes involved in a translocation are written in brackets preceded by a *t*; e.g., t(14q21q) denotes the translocation most frequently found in Down syndrome. (Most children with Down syndrome, however, have three No. 21 chromosomes, the extra denoted as +21.)

Table 6–4. Some Representative Karyotype Notations

46,XY	Normal male karyotype
47,XX,+13	Female with 13-trisomy
47,XY,+21	Male with 21-trisomy (Down syndrome)
46,XY,−21,+t(21q21q)	Male with Down syndrome due to centric fusion-type translocation between 2 chromosomes 21, replacing 1 chromosome 21
45,XX,−14,−21, +t(14q21q)	Phenotypically normal female carrier of centric fusion-type translocation between chromosomes 14 and 21
46,XY,del(5p)	Male with cri du chat syndrome due to deletion of part of short arm of chromosome 5
46,XX,del(18q)	Female with deletion of all or a portion of the long arm of chromosome 18
46,XY,r(19)	Male with ring chromosome 19
45,X	Female with Turner syndrome due to monosomy X
47,XXY	Male with Klinefelter syndrome
46,X,i(Xq)	Female with Turner syndrome due to isochromosome for long arm of X chromosome
46,XY/47,XXY	Male with XY/XXY mosaic Klinefelter syndrome
46,XY,fra(X)(q28)	Male with fragile X syndrome

The regions within the chromosomes are now also delineated by their characteristic bands. Each chromosome arm is divided and subdivided into regions so that the breakpoints in chromosomal rearrangements can be identified and the aberration described with some accuracy. This nomenclature is complicated, and the clinician dealing with chromosomal disorders will often need to consult a cytogeneticist.

DERMATOGLYPHICS

Before the advent of human cytogenetics, the analysis of hand and footprints was used as one criterion for diagnosing Down syndrome. The subsequent development of techniques for chromosomal analysis has decreased their relative importance in the clinical assessment of patients suspected of having a chromosomal abnormality.

Dermatoglyphics refers to those configurations formed by the dermal ridges, not by the flexion creases. The most important landmarks are the patterns on the distal phalanges of the digits, the position of the triradius in the axis of the palm, and the pattern in the hallucal area of the soles. The size of a pattern is determined by counting the number of dermal ridges between the center or core of the pattern and the triradius that determines its periphery. Whorls usually have the highest ridge counts while an arch has a count of 0 since it has no triradius. Digital pattern size is important in certain syndromes.

There is a strong correlation between dermatoglyphics and chromosomes. Characteristic dermal patterns are established for trisomies 13, 18, and 21 and in 18 and G deletion syndromes. They are described under the respective syndromes.

CLINICAL ABNORMALITIES OF THE AUTOSOMES

ANEUPLOIDY

6.11 21-TRISOMY
(Down Syndrome; Mongolism)

The presence of an extra No. 21 chromosome results in the best recognized and most frequent human chromosomal syndrome (Fig. 6–15). The important clinical features are listed in Tables 6–5 and 6–6.

The incidence in the general population is 1 in 600–800 live births. Among all conceptuses, greater than twice this fre-

quency occurs, but more than half of the trisomy 21 fetuses are spontaneously aborted during early pregnancy. A high correlation exists between increasing maternal age and the nondisjunction resulting in the presence of an extra chromosome in the offspring. In New York State the frequency of 21-trisomic children rose from a low of 1 in 1925 births among mothers aged 20 yr to a high of more than 1% in women over 40 yr (Table 6–7). An incidence of more than 5% has been found among fetuses of mothers over 40 yr of age who have been screened by genetic amniocentesis.

Heteromorphisms on fluorescent staining have furnished

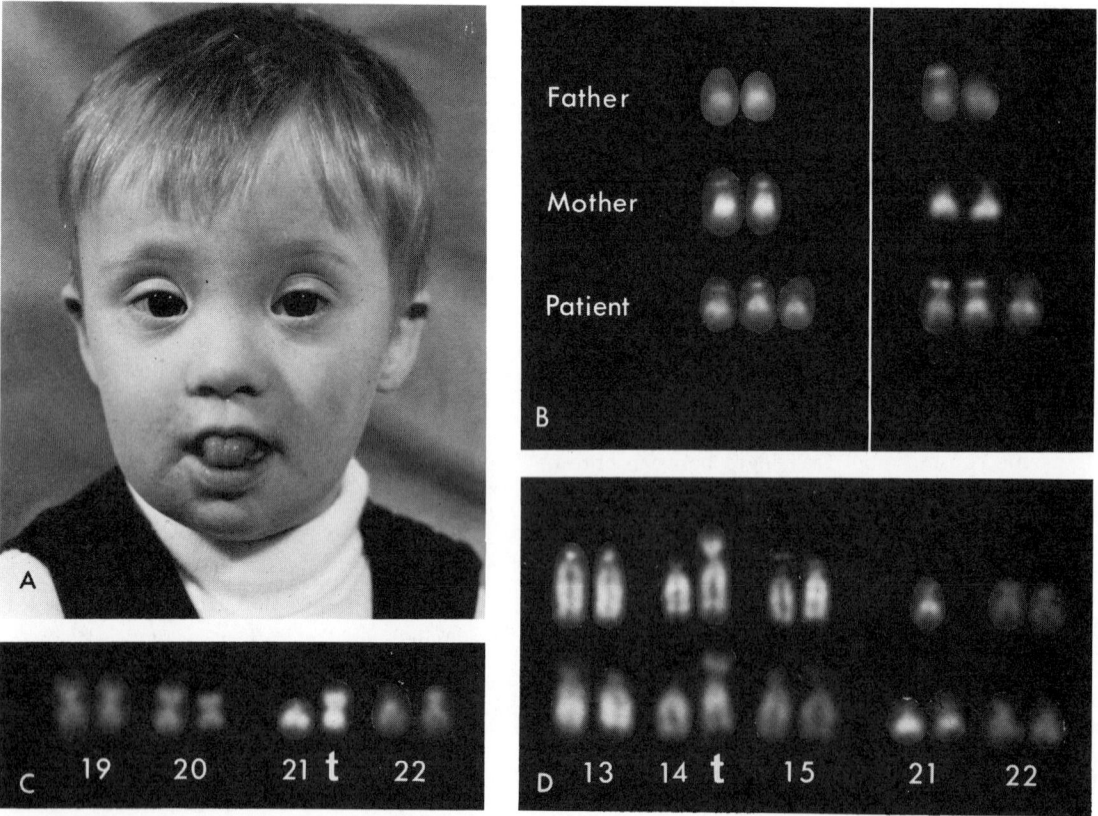

Figure 6–15. Partial karyotypes from patients with Down syndrome. *A,* Patient with trisomy 21. *B,* Chromosomes 21 from 2 patients and their parents. Left: 2 of a patient's chromosomes with brightly fluorescent satellites were transmitted by the mother. Right: 2 chromosomes with bright satellites resulted from paternal nondisjunction at second meiotic division. *C,* 21q21q translocation. *D,* 14q21q translocation in a mother (above) and her affected child (below).

Table 6-5. **Major Clinical Features of the Three Most Common Autosomal Trisomic Syndromes**

Characteristic Features	21-Trisomy	18-Trisomy	13-Trisomy
General	Mental retardation; hypotonia	Mental retardation; hypertonia; failure to thrive; preponderance of females; low birthweight	Mental retardation; failure to thrive; capillary hemangiomas; increased nuclear projections in neutrophils; persistent fetal hemoglobin; seizures; apneic episodes
Craniofacies	Flat occiput; oblique palpebral fissures; epicanthic folds; speckled irides (Brushfield spots); protruding tongue; prominent, malformed ears; flat nasal bridge	Prominent occiput; small features; micrognathia; low-set, malformed ears	Microcephaly; cleft lip ± palate; midline scalp defects; microphthalmia; colobomata; low-set malformed ears; apparent deafness
Thorax	Congenital heart disease, mainly septal defects, especially of the endocardial cushion	Congenital heart disease, mainly VSD* and PDA*; short sternum; diaphragmatic hernia	Congenital heart disease, mainly septal defects, PDA
Abdomen and pelvis	Decreased acetabular and iliac angles; small penis; cryptorchidism	Horseshoe kidney; small pelvis; cryptorchidism; limited hip abduction; inguinal or umbilical hernia	Polycystic kidneys; bicornuate uterus; cryptorchidism
Hands and feet	Simian crease; short, broad hands; hypoplasia of middle phalanx of 5th finger; gap between 1st and 2nd toes	Flexion deformity of fingers; short, dorsiflexed big toes; rockerbottom feet or equinovarus; phocomelia (rare)	Polydactyly; hyperconvex or hypoplastic fingernails; simian crease
Other features observed with significant frequency	High-arched palate; strabismus; broad, short neck; small teeth; furrowed tongue; intestinal atresia; imperforate anus; Hirschsprung disease	Cleft lip ± palate; ocular anomalies; simian crease; hypoplasia of fingernails; widely spaced nipples; webbed neck; single umbilical artery; tracheoesophageal fistula	Flexion deformity of fingers; single umbilical artery; shallow supraorbital ridges; micrognathia; retroflexible thumb; rockerbottom feet; omphalocele

*VSD = ventricular septal defect; PDA = patent ductus arteriosus.

cytologic proof for the parental origin of nondisjunction in a number of instances (Fig. 6–15B). Abnormal segregation is paternal in origin in approximately 10–20% of cases. There are two distribution curves for maternal age: the age-independent curve, which includes cases due to translocation and probably paternal nondisjunction, and the age-dependent curve.

The reason for the correlation between late maternal age and nondisjunction is unknown. It is thought to be due to some aspect of aging of the oocyte, which lives in suspended animation during meiotic division from late fetal life until that oocyte participates in ovulation. The incidences of both Down syndrome and maternal exposure to diagnostic roentgenograms of the abdomen correlate with maternal age. Virus-induced disturbance of chromosomal segregation has been suggested to account for the clustering of births of 21-trisomic infants following epidemics of infectious hepatitis. "Over-ripeness" of the ovum due to delayed fertilization because of decreased frequency of coitus with age has also been suggested. Significant increases in the frequency of thyroid autoantibodies also have been observed in patients and mothers. Finally, a genetic predisposition to nondisjunction could account for the repetition of 21-trisomy and other aneuploidy in some families.

The recurrence risk of trisomy to chromosomally normal parents is uncertain. Estimates range from increase in risk over the general population to a 50-fold increase in young mothers. Analysis of data using only chromosomally proven trisomy indicates that the risk of recurrence, regardless of maternal age, appears to be about the same as that for a mother who is over the age of 45 yr, i.e., 1/80. This increased risk may be due to undetected mosaicism in a parent or repeated exposure to the same environmental insult. In pregnancies subsequent to the birth of a 21-trisomic infant, the risk of recurrence can generally be estimated for counseling as 1% above the age related risk (Table 6–7), which is significant only for women under 37 yr.

Translocation Down syndrome. "Regular" trisomy comprises some 95% of cases of Down syndrome. Approximately 1% of cases are mosaic (this estimate is minimum since some mosaics probably remain undetected, particularly among phenotypically normal parents of trisomic offspring); the remainder are the result of translocation.

The majority of translocations giving rise to the Down syndrome consist of centric fusions between No. 21 and chromosomes 13, 14, or 15; approximately half of these are inherited. The vast majority are t(14q21q) (Fig. 6–15) and a few are t(15q21q). The rarity of t(13q21q) probably accounts

Table 6-6. **Important Dermatoglyphic Patterns and Flexion Creases Found in the Three Common Autosomal Trisomic Syndromes**

Areas	21-Trisomy	18-Trisomy	13-Trisomy
Digits	Ulnar loops on most fingers; radial loops on fingers 4 and 5	Arches on fingers and toes	—
Palms	Distal axial triradius or large *atd* angle	—	Distal axial triradius or large *atd* angle
Soles	Arch tibial or small loop distal in hallucal area	—	Arch fibular or arch fibular-S in hallucal area
Flexion creases	Simian crease; single crease on finger 5	Single crease on finger 5 or on all fingers	Simian crease

Table 6–7. **Estimated Rates of Down Syndrome (New York State Study)**

Maternal Age in Years*	Estimated Rate	Maternal Age in Years*	Estimated Rate
20	1/1925	35	1/365
21	1/1695	36	1/285
22	1/1540	37	1/225
23	1/1410	38	1/175
24	1/1300	39	1/140
25	1/1205	40	1/110
26	1/1125	41	1/85
27	1/1050	42	1/67
28	1/990	43	1/53
29	1/935	44	1/41
30	1/885	45	1/32
31	1/825	46	1/25
32	1/725	47	1/20
33	1/590	48	1/16
34	1/465	49	1/12

*Age at last birthday at delivery.
From Hook EB: Birth Defects *13*(3A):123,1977.

for the absence of 13-trisomy syndrome, which would be expected to occur among the offspring of phenotypically normal carriers of the 13q21q translocation. Carrier mothers produce three types of viable offspring: normal phenotype and karyotype, phenotypically normal translocation carrier, and the translocation trisomy-21 (Fig. 6–16). Theoretically, these three types of offspring should occur with equal frequency, but only 10% have been abnormal, probably because of an increased lethality to the unbalanced zygote or fetus. The expected frequency of one third affected has been observed, however, among fetuses studied early in gestation. Carrier fathers rarely have affected offspring, though they do produce both normals and carriers.

Only 5% of cases of translocation Down syndrome involving chromosomes 21 or 22 are inherited from a carrier parent.

The small metacentric translocation chromosome may represent centric fusion of chromosomes 21 and 22 or of two No. 21 chromosomes (Fig. 6–15C and D). All viable offspring from a t(21q21q) carrier would have Down syndrome. A t(21q22q) carrier, on the other hand, can produce carrier and normal as well as abnormal offspring.

Not all translocations producing Down syndrome are of the centric fusion type. Some have been reported with increased length of the long arm of one chromosome No. 21. Other patients with Down syndrome and apparently normal karyotypes may have a hidden translocation, i.e., part of No. 21 attached to a larger chromosome, which can be demonstrated by banding techniques. However, most children with Down syndrome and apparently normal karyotypes probably have mosaic patterns with low frequencies of trisomic cells.

The frequency of acute leukemia among individuals with Down syndrome is higher than in the general population; the majority are of the lymphoblastic type. The Philadelphia (Ph¹) chromosome found in patients with chronic myelogenous leukemia involves No. 22, in which the distal portion of the long arm has been reciprocally translocated to the long arm of chromosome 9.

A number of biochemical alterations have been reported in patients with Down syndrome, but most have not been consistent enough to provide useful genetic information. Several gene loci have been assigned to chromosome 21. Studies of two of these, the genes for the soluble form of the *superoxide dismutase* (SOD$_s$) and for the interferon receptor have revealed a dose relation proportional to the number of No. 21 chromosomes in a cell. The level of SOD$_s$ in cells from patients with trisomy 21 has been shown to be approximately 1.5 times normal.

6.12 18-TRISOMY SYNDROME

This is the second most common autosomal aberration, originally referred to as the E-trisomy syndrome until improved techniques permitted distinction between chromo-

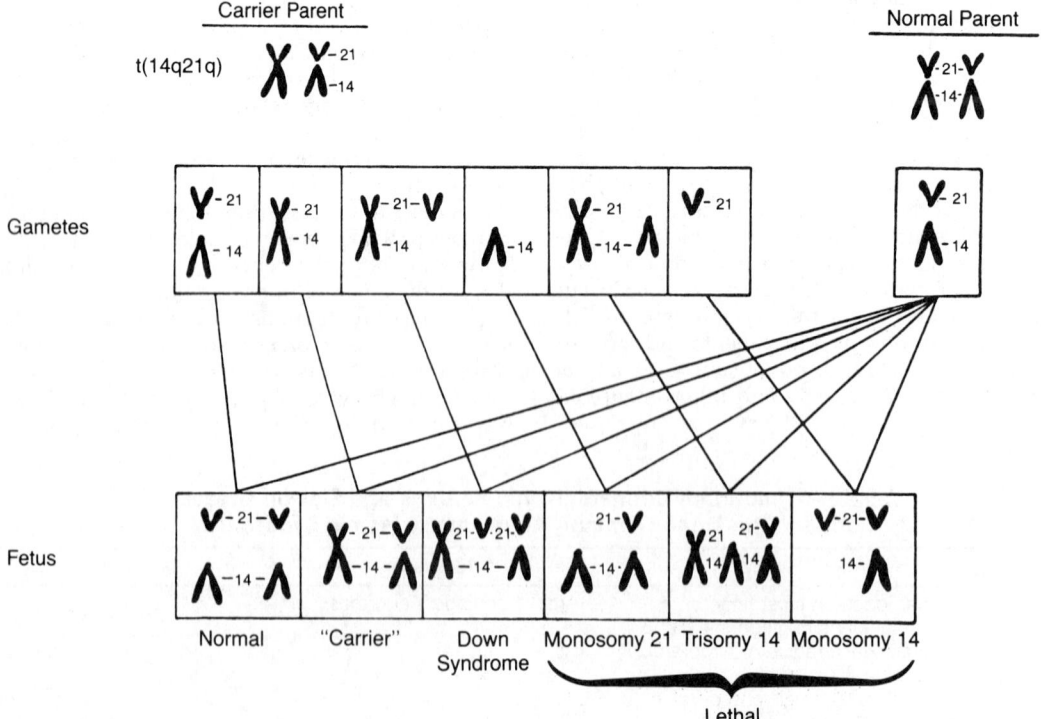

Figure 6–16. Possible outcomes of pregnancy in segregation products of a balanced carrier of a Robertsonian translocation.

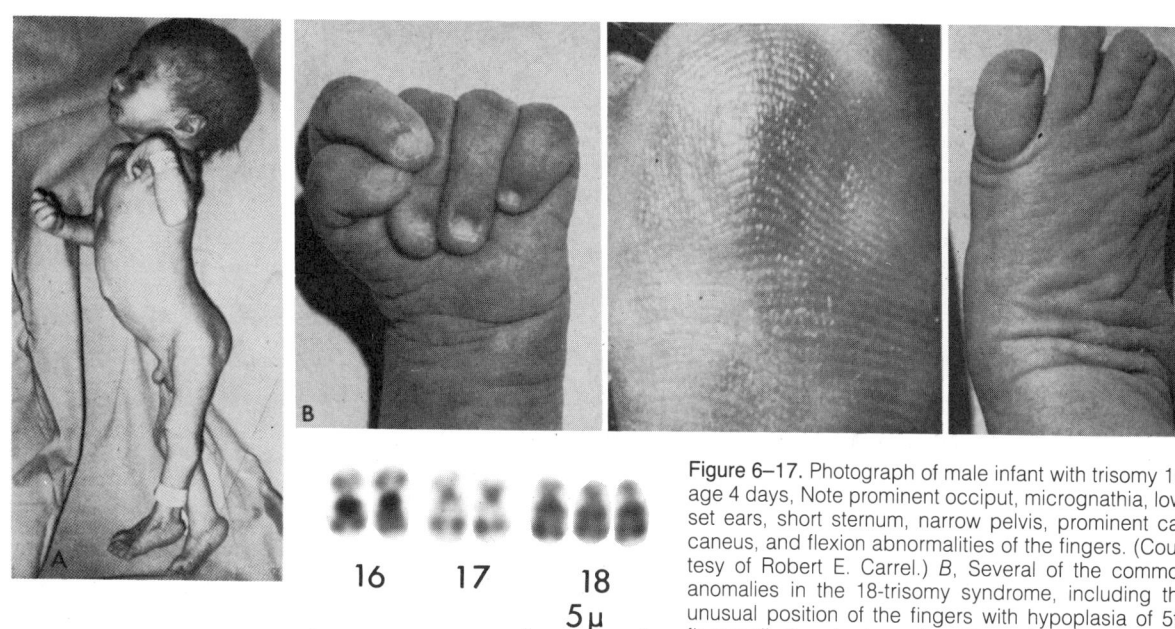

Figure 6–17. Photograph of male infant with trisomy 18, age 4 days, Note prominent occiput, micrognathia, low-set ears, short sternum, narrow pelvis, prominent calcaneus, and flexion abnormalities of the fingers. (Courtesy of Robert E. Carrel.) *B,* Several of the common anomalies in the 18-trisomy syndrome, including the unusual position of the fingers with hypoplasia of 5th fingernail; the simple arch pattern of the fingers; and the dorsiflexed hallux with hypoplasia of toenails. (From Smith DW: Am J Obstet Gynecol *90*:1055, 1964.) *C,* Partial karyotype of trisomy 18 prepared with modified Giemsa stain.

somes 17 and 18. Small, delicate facial features serve to distinguish children with 18-trisomy from other trisomics (Fig. 6–17). The principal clinical characteristics are listed in Tables 6–5 and 6–6.

Incidence is about 1 in 8000 births. Affected infants are usually born after term, but the birth weight is low. The sex ratio is 1 male to 4 females. Almost all have a cardiac malformation, a major factor in the characteristically early demise, most frequently within the first 3 mo of life. Exceptional long-lived patients have been reported, the oldest being 15 yr of age. As with 21-trisomy, advanced maternal age is etiologically important.

Translocations of Chromosome 18. These, though rare, have given rise to partial 18-trisomy syndromes, i.e., only part of one No. 18 chromosome is duplicated either by elongation of its long arm or by translocation to another chromosome. The diagnosis of partial trisomy has generally been based on the clinical picture, since in the absence of reciprocal translocation in one parent it has not been possible to confirm cytologically the origin of the extra chromosomal material. As with translocation Down syndrome, offspring of 6 different chromosomal types can result from segregation of the chromosomes of a carrier parent, but probably only 3 are viable: normal karyotype, balanced translocation carrier, and partial 18-trisomy, theoretically in equal proportions. Mosaics and double trisomics have also been reported.

6.13 13-TRISOMY SYNDROME

Chromosome No. 13 is found in triplicate in this syndrome. Trisomies for No. 14 and 15, which are similar in appearance, can be identified by differences in banding patterns (Fig. 6–18). The phenotypic features of the 13-trisomy syndrome are listed in Tables 6–5 and 6–6. The prognosis is grave as in the 18-trisomy syndrome. Most infants affected die in the 1st year of life, but at least one is known to be alive at 10 yr of age. The incidence is approximately 1 in 20,000 live births and it

increases with advancing maternal age. No sex predilection has been observed.

Translocations of Chromosomes No. 13, 14, and 15. Translocations involving chromosome 13 have been more frequently reported than have those of No. 18, probably because of the greater tendency of acrocentric chromosomes to break and rearrange and the ease of identification due to chromosome length. Most are formed by centric fusion, but some consist of two chromosomes attached in tandem to form a very long acrocentric chromosome. The pattern of inheritance is similar to that of other Robertsonian translocations discussed above.

There are many large pedigrees with phenotypically normal subjects who have 45 chromosomes, including a centric fusion of No. 13 or 14, but such a carrier has a risk of less than 1% of producing trisomic offspring; larger chromosomes with symmetric arm lengths tend to segregate in an orderly fashion, giving rise to karyotypically normal individuals or balanced carriers. However, spontaneous abortion and infertility are encountered with increased frequency and the abortuses are probably effective trisomics for No. 14.

6.14 22-TRISOMY SYNDROME

Patients with an additional small acrocentric chromosome but without the clinical signs of Down syndrome were originally interpreted as having 22-trisomy, XYY, or partial trisomy resulting from deletions of larger chromosomes. However, with the aid of marker chromosomes and fluorescent banding, it has been possible to identify 22-trisomy in some of these patients. They have a clinical syndrome characterized by mental and growth retardation; microcephaly; micrognathia; preauricular skin tags, appendages, and/or sinuses; low-set and/or malformed ears; cleft palate; congenital heart disease; finger-like or malopposed thumbs; and deformed lower limbs. 22-Trisomy is seen less frequently than 21-trisomy in spite of the similarity in size and shape of the chromosomes, probably because of greater loss of 22-trisomics during pregnancy.

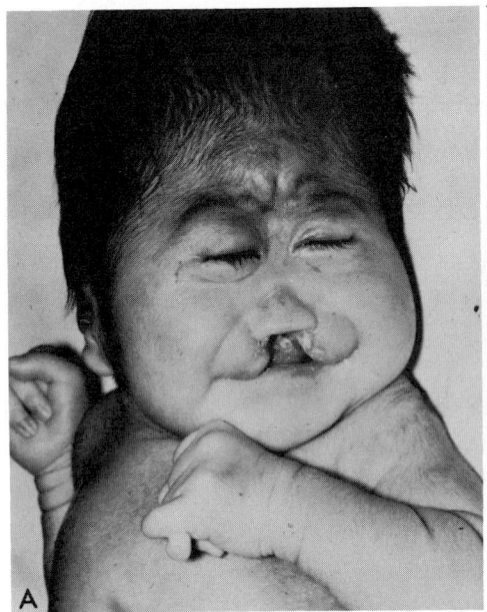 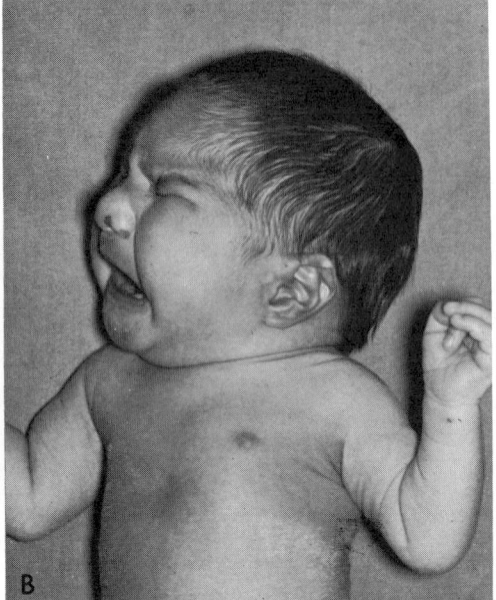

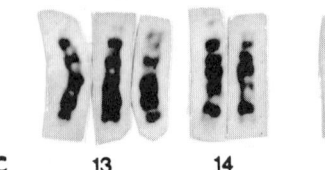

C   13   14   15

Figure 6–18. *A* and *B,* Female infants with 13-trisomy syndrome. Note midline cleft of the lip and palate, microcephaly, hypotelorism, microphthalmus, bulbous nose, polydactyly, and overlapping of fingers. Scalp defects (not shown) are also present. (Courtesy of Miriam G. Wilson.) *C,* Partial karyotype showing chromosomes No. 13, 14, and 15 stained with the trypsin-Giemsa method.

Table 6–8. **Major Clinical Features of the Trisomy-8 and Trisomy-9 Syndromes**

Feature	Trisomy-8	Trisomy-9
General	Mental retardation, short stature, decreased weight, vertebral anomalies	Mental retardation
Craniofacies	Dysmorphic skull, prominent forehead, dysplastic ears, strabismus, plump nose with broad base, low-set ears, everted lower lip, high palate, cleft soft palate, micrognathia	Microcephaly, abnormal cranial sutures, prominent forehead, deep-set eyes, protuberant ears, prominent nose, fishmouth, micrognathia
Thorax	Congenital heart disease	Congenital heart disease
Abdomen and pelvis	Urinary tract anomaly, narrow pelvis	Urinary tract anomaly
Limbs	Patellar dysplasia, limited joint mobility, deep flexion creases on palms and soles	Congenital hip/knee dislocation, clinodactyly, digital hypoplasia, nail hypoplasia, syndactyly, simian palmar creases, absent B and C palmar digital triradii

6.15 TRISOMY INVOLVING OTHER AUTOSOMES

Accurate identification of chromosomes has led to the description of new autosomal trisomy syndromes due to trisomy-8 and trisomy-9 (Table 6–8). Full (i.e., not in mosaic association with a chromosomally normal cell line) trisomies for other chromosomes have also been reported, but documentation is lacking. Trisomy for virtually every autosome has been documented in the products of early spontaneous abortion; most full trisomies are probably lethal. Partial trisomy (duplication or duplication-deficiency state) for almost all the autosomes produced by segregation of a translocation or inversion has been described, as has partial trisomy for an unattached segment of an autosome.

6.16 AUTOSOMAL MONOSOMY

Several cases of monosomy involving chromosome 21 or 22 have been reported, but few have been adequately documented as complete monosomy. Syndromes produced by deletion (partial monosomy) of part of the long arm of chromosome 21 or 22 have been well documented, as have deletions of parts of other chromosomes (Table 6–9).

STRUCTURAL ABERRATIONS

6.17 TRANSLOCATIONS

These are the most common structural aberrations. Exchange of segments between two nonhomologous chromosomes is known as a *reciprocal* or *balanced translocation*. Although early reports of translocations suggested the presence of *simple translocations*, i.e., a segment of one chromosome broken off and attached to the unbroken end of the recipient chromosome, no convincing evidence exists for the occurrence of simple translocations in humans.

In phenotypically normal individuals translocations are assumed to be *reciprocal* and *balanced* since loss or gain of chromatin material usually results in an abnormal phenotype. An exception is the balanced (Robertsonian, Sec. 6.10) translocation discussed above. Unbalanced karyotypes associated with *duplication-deficiency syndromes* are found among the offspring of carriers of balanced translocations (Fig. 6–13).

Except for translocation resulting in well-known clinical syndromes, it is difficult and often impossible, even with the aid of banding patterns, to identify with certainty the origin of excess chromosomal material in the absence of a reciprocal translocation in a parent. Another exception is the translocation of a large segment of the X chromosome that can be positively identified by the X chromatin or thymidine-labeling pattern. When a parent is a translocation carrier, the origin of the extra (trisomic) or missing (monosomic) chromosomal material can be accurately determined, and the delineation of new clinical syndromes becomes possible. Banding techniques can identify small duplications and deletions in karyotypes that were thought to be normal with conventional stains.

Syndromes have been described as the result of partial trisomy (duplication) for chromosomes 1q, 2p, 2q, 3p, 3q, 4p, 4q, 5p, 6q, 7q, 9p, 9q, 10q, 12p, 14q, 18q, and 22q. The best known and most frequently documented partial trisomy is the 9p-trisomy syndrome (Fig. 6–19). Translocation of the short arm of chromosome 9 to a variety of autosomes has been reported, and many kindreds have been described in which reciprocal translocations are carried by many members and transmitted through several generations. Characteristic features include mental retardation, microcephaly, hypertelorism, oblique palpebral fissures, enophthalmos, bulbous nose, downward slanting mouth, low-set protruding ears, and single palmar crease.

The most commonly observed reciprocal translocation occurs between the long arms of 11 and 22 (Fig. 6–20). A number of the offspring of balanced carriers of this translocation (t[11;22]) have 47 chromosomes, the extra one consisting of a part of both chromosomes 11 and 22. These infants show microcephaly, a wide face with a short flat nose, a prominent philtrum, microretrognathia, cleft palate, low set abnormal ears with preauricular pits and tags, a micropenis, heart defects, renal anomalies, anal anomalies, and dislocated hips. They therefore share abnormalities with children with trisomy 22 and those with partial trisomy of the long arm of No. 11. The phenotypic results of translocations depend on the parts of the chromosomes involved, so that new syndromes are constantly being described.

Although all chromosomes are subject to breaks that result in structural aberrations, the chromosomes most frequently involved in translocations appear to be the acrocentrics of chromosomes 13, 14, 15, 21, and 22, probably because of their close association as nucleolar organizers—i.e., the stalks of the satellites have the capacity to organize diffuse nucleolar material into one or more compact bodies during interphase. These translocations and their modes of transmission have been discussed in the respective sections under *Aneuploidy*.

6.18 DELETIONS

Chromosomal deletions are associated with several clinical syndromes. Some lead to a less severely affected phenotype than do trisomies. Clinical features of the more common deletions are listed in Table 6–9.

Table 6–9. **Important Clinical Features**

Feature	4p –	5p –	9q –	11p –
General	LBW,* severe MR,* delayed ossification	LBW, MR, catlike cry	MR	MR, growth retardation
Craniofacies	Microcephaly, hypertelorism, epicanthus, ptosis, colobomata, beaked nose, short broad philtrum, cleft palate, micrognathia, simple ears	Microcephaly, round face, hypertelorism, epicanthus, antimongoloid palpebral fissure, micrognathia, low-set malformed ears, preauricular tags	Trigonocephaly, upward slanting palpebral fissures, epicanthal folds, depressed nasal bridge, anteverted nares, long philtrum, low-set ears, high palate, micrognathia, short and webbed neck	Aniridia
Thorax		CHD* (occasional)	Widely spaced nipples, cardiac murmur	
Pelvis and abdomen	Inguinal hernia, sacral dimples, hypospadias, cryptorchidism	Inguinal hernia, diastasis recti, small iliac wings		Wilms tumor, gonadoblastoma, ambiguous genitalia in males
Hands and feet		Short metacarpals or metatarsals, partial syndactyly, pes planus, simian crease	Long fingers, square nails	

*CHD = Congenital heart disease; LBW = low birthweight; MR = mental retardation; TRC = total ridge count.

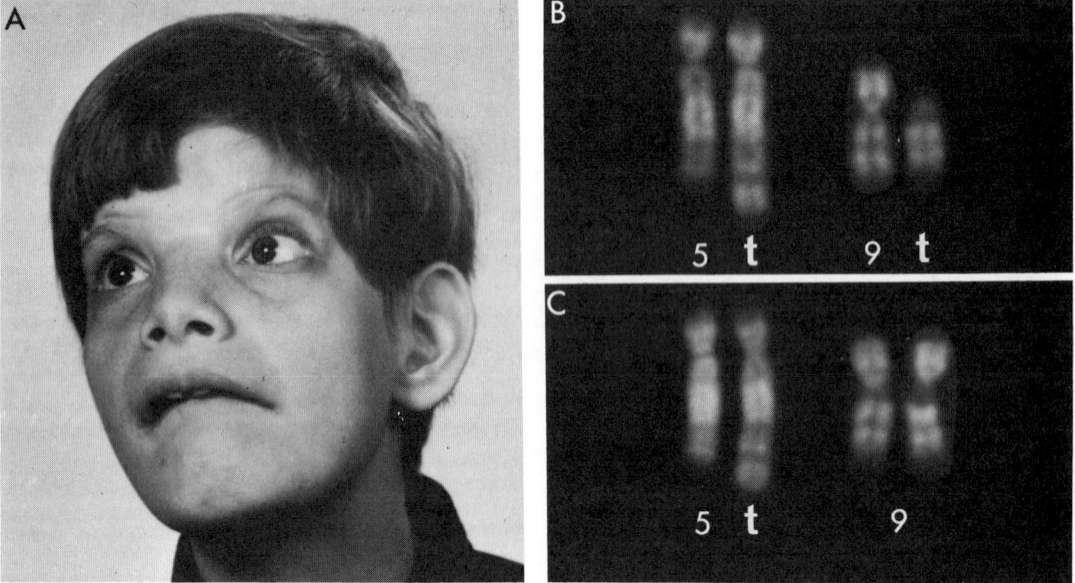

Figure 6–19. *A*, Patient with 9p-trisomy syndrome showing some of the characteristic features: hypertelorism, bulbous nose, downward slanting mouth, low-set protruding ears. *B*, Balanced t(5q/9p) translocation carried by mother. *C*, Unbalanced translocation resulting in 9p-trisomy syndrome in above patient. t = translocation chromosome.

of the Deletion Syndromes

13q −	18p −	18q −	21q −	22q −
LBW, severe MR, failure to thrive	LBW, variable MR, short stature, Turner syndrome–like stigmata	LBW, severe MR, seizures, hypotonia	MR, hypertonia, skeletal malformations, growth retardation	MR, hypotonia
Microcephaly; trigonocephaly; flat, wide nasal bridge; hypertelorism; ptosis, epicanthus, microphthalmia, colobomata; retinoblastoma; micrognathia	Hypertelorism, epicanthus, flat nasal bridge, micrognathia, low-set, large floppy ears	Microcephaly, ophthalmologic defects, carp-shaped mouth, apparently protruding mandible, atretic ear canals	Microcephaly, downward-slanting palpebral fissures, high palate, large and/or low-set ears, prominent nasal bridge, micrognathia	Microcephaly, high palate, large and/or low-set ears, epicanthal folds, ptosis of eyelids, bifid uvula
CHD		CHD (occasional), supernumerary ribs		
Hip dysplasia, cryptorchidism		Small penis, cryptorchidism, hypoplastic genitalia in females	Pyloric stenosis, inguinal hernia, hypospadias, cryptorchidism	
Hypoplastic or absent thumbs, clinodactyly of 5th fingers, syndactyly of toes	Stubby hands with high-set thumbs, partial webbing of toes, large digital patterns with high TRC*	Long, tapering fingers; abnormal implantation of toes; large digital patterns with high TRC	Nail anomalies	Syndactyly of toes, clinodactyly

Chromosomes 4 and 5 (4p − and 5p − Syndromes). The cri du chat syndrome (5p−) (Fig. 6–21A) is so named because the cry of affected infants resembles that of a kitten and is characterized by high-pitched, tense phonation. This distinguishing trait probably accounts for the apparently greater frequency of 5p − compared to other deletions. However, the typical cry tends to disappear in late infancy, and a similar cry has been noted on occasion in other retarded infants. Most cases arise sporadically, but reciprocal translocation is sometimes present in a parent. Ring chromosomes with loss of material from both ends may produce the same syndrome.

Patients with a deletion of chromosome 4 (Fig. 6–21B) are much more severely malformed and retarded and do not have the typical cry. The clinical signs are listed in Table 6–9.

Chromosome 9 (9p − Syndrome). A small number of infants have been described with deletion of the short arm of chromosome 9 (Table 6–9).

Chromosome 11 (11p − Syndrome). Deletion in the short arm of chromosome 11, always including band 11p13, results in aniridia and is frequently associated with Wilms tumor. Additional abnormalities include mental and growth retardation, ambiguous genitalia in the male patients, and gonadoblastoma in some of the patients. Most cases occur de novo but occasionally familial chromosomal rearrangements are responsible (Table 6–9).

Chromosome 13 (13q − Syndrome). A deletion of the long arm of chromosome 13, including band 13q14, is associated with retinoblastoma (Sec. 16.20). Other clinical findings depend on the amount of the chromosome deleted. These are listed in Table 6–9.

Chromosome 18 (18p − and 18q − Syndromes). Deletions of chromosome 18 take 3 forms: loss of the entire short arm, 18p−; loss of part of the long arm, 18q−; and deletions of both ends to form a ring, r(18). Patients with 18p − are phenotypically extremely variable. A few are severely affected, with arrhinencephaly, cyclopia, or cleft lip and palate, but most have only minor malformations and are only moderately retarded (Table 6–9 and Fig. 6–22). Turner syndrome is often suspected. On the other hand, children with 18q − are severely retarded and have more characteristic malformations (Fig. 6–23). Children with a ring chromosome 18 have phenotypic features of both short and long arm deletions since the ends of both arms of the chromosome are lost during ring formation.

A number of characteristics are common to the three types of deletion. Prognosis for survival seems to be good. IgA deficiency has been noted in some patients. Large dermal patterns are present on the digits, mainly whorls, giving a very high total ridge count similar to that seen in the Turner syndrome. This is in sharp contrast to 18-trisomy syndrome, in which the presence of arches results in a very low ridge count.

Chromosomes 19, 20, 21, 22. Deficiencies in these chromosomes have resulted mainly in formation of ring chromosomes. Loss of material from the long arm has occurred in some subjects, but deletions compatible with life may often be too small to identify unless a ring is formed. *Aberrations* in chromosomes 19 and 20 were first reported only in studies of aborted material and patients with blood dyscrasias, but a few patients with severe mental retardation have now been described; others with deletions in only some of their cells (mosaics) appear to be phenotypically normal.

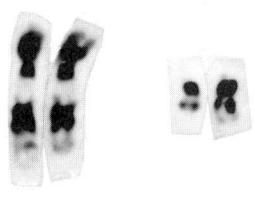

t11   t12

Figure 6–20. Translocation between the long arms of chromosomes 11 and 22 (t(11; 22) (q23; q11)).

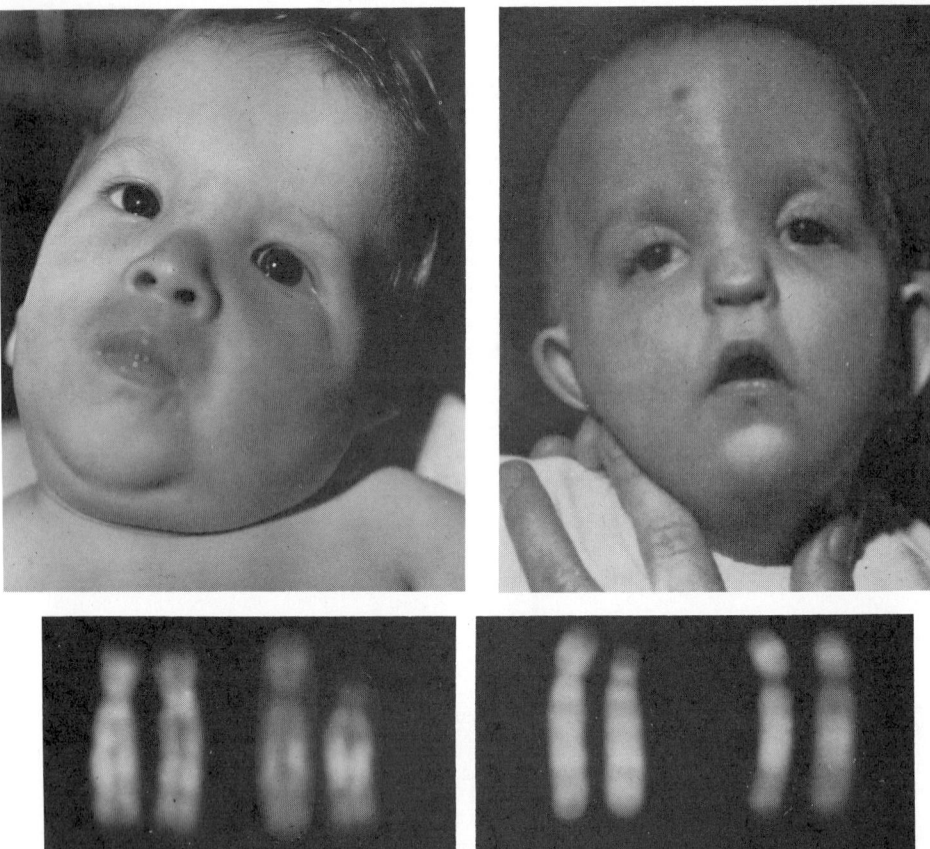

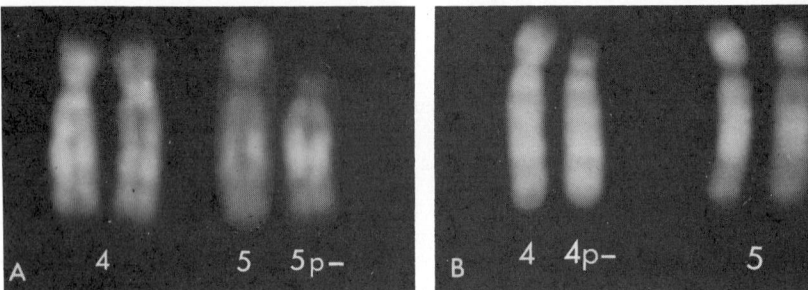

Figure 6–21. Patients with partial deletion of short arm chromosomes No. 4 and 5. *A*, An 8 mo old boy with cri du chat syndrome and deletion of part of the short arm of one chromosome No. 5 (5p−). *B*, 1 yr old boy with partial deletion of the short arm of one chromosome No. 4. (Courtesy of W. R. Breg.)

Figure 6–22. Patient with 18 short arm deletion, 18p−

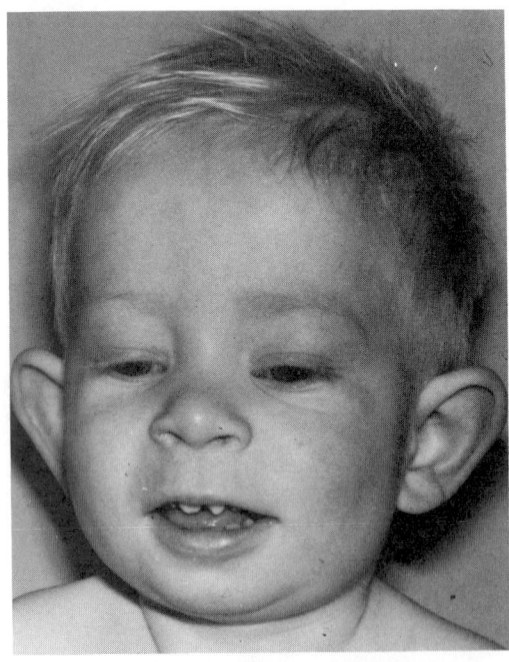

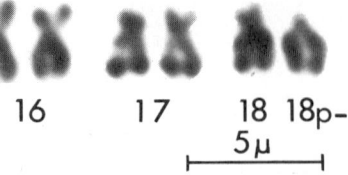

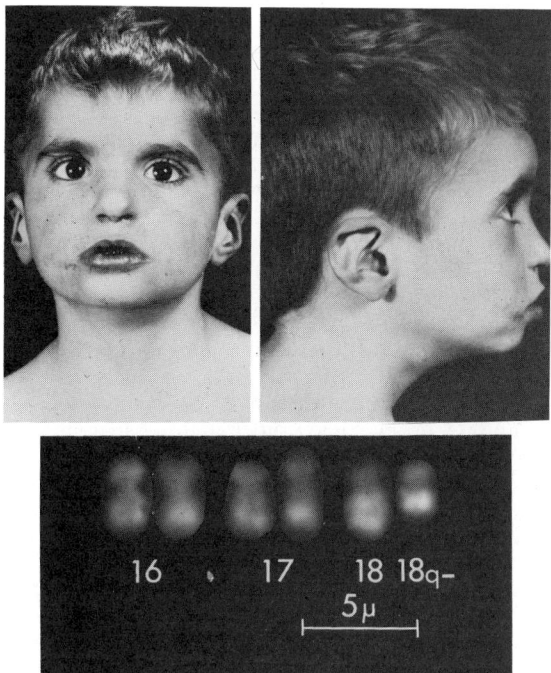

Figure 6–23. Patient with partial deletion of long arm of chromosome No. 18. (Courtesy of P. S. Gerald and W. Wertelecki.) Partial karyotype showing 18q−, stained with quinacrine dihydrochloride.

Because many more cases have been described with *deletions* of chromosomes 21 and 22, two syndromes have emerged, one attributed to 21q− and the other to 22q−. The phenotypic features of these syndromes, some of which are shared by both, are enumerated in Table 6–9. Since some of the clinical signs of chromosome 21 deletions are variations of those of the Down syndrome, this syndrome has also been referred to as "antimongolism."

6.19 BREAKAGE SYNDROMES

Chromosomal breakage, structural rearrangements, and aneuploidy have been reported as inconsistent findings during viral diseases such as measles, chickenpox, and infectious hepatitis. Specific rearrangements have been described in a number of neoplastic diseases, primarily leukemias and lymphomas. These include the following translocations with their associated conditions: acute myelogenous leukemia, t(8; 21); chronic myelogenous leukemia, t(9; 22) (Philadelphia chromosome); acute promyelocytic leukemia, t(15; 17); acute monocytic leukemia, t(11; 19); Burkitt lymphoma, t(8; 14), t(8; 22), and t(2; 8). In Burkitt lymphoma the break point in the long arm of chromosome 8, common to the three observed translocations, occurs at the site of the oncogene c-myc, while the break points in chromosomes 14, 22, and 2 occur at the sites of the genes for immunoglobulin (14: heavy chains; 22: lambda light chains; 2: kappa light chains). It is probable that these rearrangements put the oncogene under the regulation of the immunoglobulin genes, causing inappropriate activity of factors leading to abnormal growth of the cells. It is likely that other translocations will be shown to work in an analogous fashion.

There is a group of autosomal recessive diseases with high frequencies of chromosome breaks and rearrangements, together with an increased risk of leukemia and other malignancies: Bloom syndrome (congenital telangiectatic erythema with dwarfism, Sec. 24.14), constitutional aplastic pancytopenia (Fanconi anemia, Sec. 15.31), ataxia-telangiectasia (Louis-Bar syndrome, Sec. 10.19 and 21.20), and xeroderma pigmentosum (Sec. 24.14).

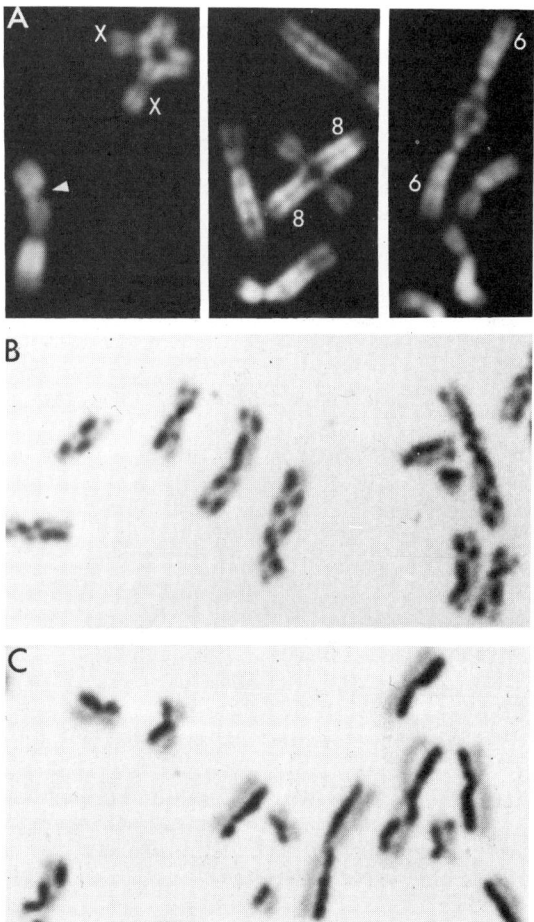

Figure 6–24. Partial spreads showing chromosome aberrations in cells from patient with Bloom syndrome, compared with a normal subject. *A*, Fluorescent-stained spreads with quadriradial figures formed by homologous chromosomes, typical of this syndrome. *B*, Harlequin effect resulting from high frequency of sister chromatid exchanges (SCE) in cells of patient with Bloom syndrome, treated with 5-bromo-deoxyuridine (BrdU). *C*, Low rate of sister chromatid exchanges in cells of normal subject.

In addition to breaks and gaps, the characteristic chromosomal aberration of Bloom syndrome is the quadriradial, formed by the exchange of chromatid segments, usually between 2 chromosomes of the No. 6–12 and No. 19–20 groups. In almost all cases the breaks occur at corresponding sites in homologous chromosomes (Fig. 6–24). The number of sister chromatid exchanges is much higher in cultured cells from affected children than in cells from homozygous normals or heterozygotes for the Bloom syndrome allele.

In the Fanconi pancytopenia syndrome endoreduplication and a variety of gaps, breaks, and rearrangements involving nonhomologues as well as homologues have been observed. The number of sister chromatid exchanges per cell is lower than that found in the cells of normal subjects. Chromosomal studies of the Louis-Bar syndrome have revealed an increase in gaps and breaks, an increase in rearrangements such as dicentrics and abnormal monocentrics, and the presence of distinct, stable cell subpopulations (clones) with translocations involving particularly chromosome 14.

Chromosomal gaps, breaks, and rearrangements have not been seen in xeroderma pigmentosum, but chromosomally abnormal clones have been observed in cultured skin fibroblasts from affected patients. An increased number of ultraviolet light-induced chromosome breaks and sister chromatid exchanges occur in cultured lymphocytes.

6.20 THE SEX CHROMOSOMES

The normal sex chromosome complement in the female is XX and in the male XY. The following sections deal with departures from that norm. In the Q-banded karyotype, the Y is ordinarily the most brightly fluorescent chromosome. The brightly fluorescent segment of the long arm may be greatly extended or completely deleted (Fig. 6–7B) without producing any discernible phenotypic effect. The only clinically relevant gene loci known to occupy the Y chromosome are those involving male sex determination; they are found in the pale-fluorescing region of the short arm.

6.21 SEX CHROMATIN

Tests for sex chromatin most often utilize cells scraped from the buccal mucosa, the *buccal smear*. Other tissues used include vaginal epithelial cells, hair root sheath cells, and cells from amniotic fluid. Because of limitations described below, X- and Y-chromatin determinations should not be relied upon for the definitive diagnosis of an abnormal sex chromosome constitution. However, such determinations may be useful, along with chromosomal analysis by banding techniques, in genetic studies and in identification of structural rearrangements of the sex chromosomes.

X-CHROMATIN

Because females have two X chromosomes, they have two alleles for each X-linked gene; the male, with a single X, is therefore hemizygous for each X-linked allele. The lack of quantitative differences between the two sexes in the products of X-linked genes suggests *dosage compensation*. Lyon provided evidence that one of the two X chromosomes in the cells of females becomes genetically inactive in early embryonic life. In each cell of a normal female the active X, whether paternally or maternally derived, is determined at random, but, once it is determined, all progeny of a particular cell will have the same active X. Thus each cell, whether in a male or a female, contains only one genetically active X chromosome (the *Lyon hypothesis*). The genetic consequence is that all females are mosaic for any heterozygous alleles located in the X chromosome. The cytologic manifestation of the inactive X is the *X-chromatin mass* or *"Barr body,"* found at the periphery of the resting or interphase nucleus (Fig. 6–25A). In a cell all X chromosomes in excess of one are inactive and form

X-chromatin masses. By counting the number of X-chromatin masses (in at least 100 cells), it is possible to obtain an index of the number of X chromosomes present in the cells of a subject, i.e., one more than the number of X-chromatin masses per cell. Because cell survival requires the presence of one entire active X chromosome, any X with a deletion always forms the X-chromatin mass.

Although it is generally stated that one X chromosome in a female cell is genetically inactive, it has been shown that the tip of the short arm of the otherwise inactive X remains genetically active. The loci in this region include those for the Xg blood group and for steroid sulfatase. It is believed that this region of the X has loci analogous to some on the short arm of the Y chromosome and that these regions on the X and the Y associate during meiosis, thereby allowing for exchange of genetic material. The area on the Y may include genes for masculinization which, if translocated to the X, could result in an XX male in the next generation (Sec. 6.26).

X-Chromatin in Turner Syndrome. Determining X-chromatin is a valuable diagnostic and screening technique only if its limitations are kept in mind. Some Turner syndrome patients who are X-chromatin-positive have two X chromosomes, one of which is structurally altered (Fig. 6–26). If X-chromatin determination were the sole cytologic basis for diagnosing Turner syndrome, then the presence of an X-chromatin mass would erroneously exclude the diagnosis. Almost 40% of patients having Turner syndrome are X-chromatin-positive.

Y-CHROMATIN

Q-banding has led to a second type of chromatin determination. In the interphase nucleus the Y chromosome remains tightly condensed and appears as a small, brilliantly fluorescent mass of chromatin (Fig. 6–25B). The number of Y-chromatin masses in a nucleus bears a 1:1 relation to the number of Y chromosomes present. However, the Y-chromatin test also has limitations. Some acrocentric chromosomes bear fluorescent satellites which are large and brilliant enough to resemble a Y-chromatin body in an interphase nucleus. Moreover, if all or most of the brilliantly fluorescent segment of the Y chromosome has been deleted, a Y-chromatin mass will not be detected.

ABNORMALITIES OF THE SEX CHROMOSOMES

These make up about half of all chromosomal abnormalities encountered in newborn infants (Table 6–3). Their consequences may be varied, but nearly all have some effect on gonadal function.

6.22 TURNER SYNDROME

See Sec 19.30 and 19.34 for clinical features.

Turner syndrome is defined as the spectrum of phenotypic features resulting from complete or partial monosomy of the *short arm* of the X chromosome. The most frequent abnormality, accounting for about 55% of cases, is complete monosomy-X, with a karyotype 45,X. Its frequency is approximately 1 in 10,000 live female births, but this figure represents only a small proportion of conceptuses with a 45,X karyotype, at least 95% of which are estimated to be spontaneously aborted. The 45,X karyotype is one of the most common chromosomal aberrations found among the products of spontaneous abor-

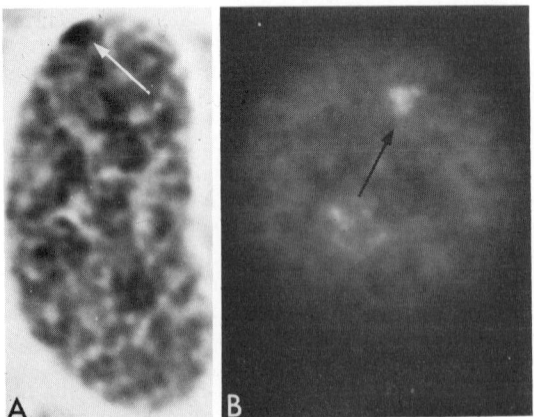

Figure 6–25. Sex chromatin bodies in interphase nuclei. *A*, X-chromatin mass (Barr body) seen at periphery of nucleus. *B*, Bright fluorescent Y-chromatin mass in nucleus of normal male.

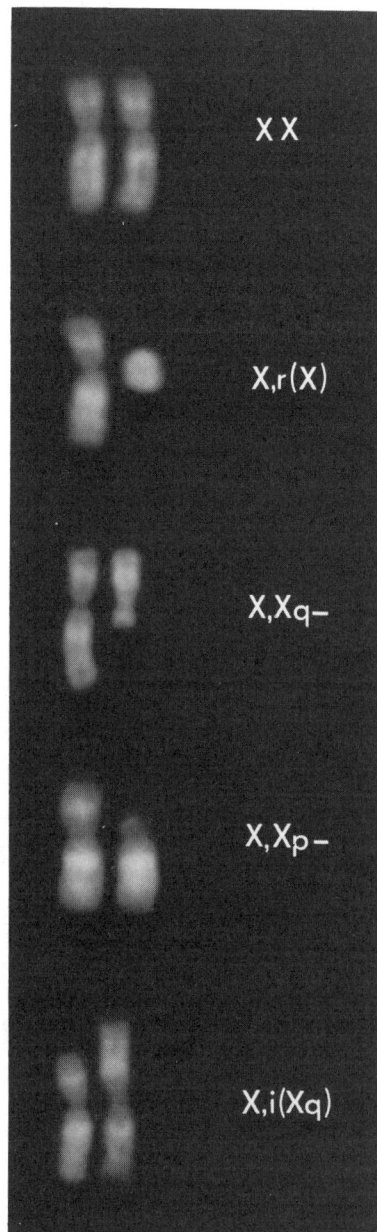

Figure 6–26. Structural aberrations of the X chromosome. Normal X chromosome on left of each pair. On right, from top to bottom: normal X, ring X, deletion of long arm, deletion of short arm, long arm isochromosome. All are X chromatin–positive.

Table 6–10. **Abnormalities of the Sex Chromosomes**

	Percent of Cases	Population Frequency
Turner syndrome		1/10,000 females
45,X	57	
Mosaics 45,X/46,XX;45,X/47,XXX, etc.	12	
Mosaics 45,X/46,XY	4	
46,X,i (Xq) including mosaics	17	
46,X,del (Xq) including mosaics	1	
Other [del (Xp), r(X), mosaics]	$\underline{9}$	
	100	
Klinefelter syndrome		1/1000 males
47,XXY	82	
48,XXXY	3	
49,XXXXY	<1	
Mosaics	8	
Other (XXYY, XXXYY)	$\underline{6}$	
	100	
Poly-X females		1/1000 females
47,XXX	98 +	
48,XXXX	Rare	
49,XXXXX	Rare	
Mosaics	$\underline{\text{Rare}}$	
	100	
Fragile X [fra(X)(q28)]		1/2000 males
		1/1000 females
Y-polysomy		1/1000 males
47,XYY	98 +	
Other (XXYY,XXXYY)	$\underline{\text{Rare}}$	
	100	

While mental retardation has not ordinarily been considered a feature of Turner syndrome, a recent review noted its presence in 18% of patients. In the absence of mental retardation, an abnormality in spatial perception has been reported in some cases. The characteristic dermatoglyphic feature is the large size of dermal patterns on the digits (high ridge count).

A mosaic karyotype is common in Turner syndrome; 45,X/46,XX is most frequent. In general, the presence of a

tion and is the only well documented chromosomal monosomy in humans. Turner syndrome may result from a number of abnormalities of the X chromosome other than 45,X (Table 6–10 and Fig. 6–26). The most frequently encountered structural aberration is the isochromosome of the long arm designated i(Xq). A metacentric X resembling the i(Xq) may be formed by a translocation following breaks in the paracentromeric regions of the short arms of two X chromosomes to form a dicentric. Simple deletion of the short arm of an X[del (Xp)] also produces Turner syndrome. However, patients with deletion of part or most of the long arm, while manifesting gonadal dysgenesis and its phenotypic results, do not have the other somatic features of Turner syndrome.

The characteristic features of Turner syndrome are listed in Table 6–11. Most important are short stature, gonadal dysgenesis with "streak" gonads, and primary amenorrhea.

Table 6–11. **Clinical Features of Turner Syndrome**

	Feature	Frequency (%)
General	Short stature	97
	Primary amenorrhea	96
	Sterility	>99
	Sexual infantilism	95
	Hypertension (primary)	27
	Mental deficiency	18
	Pigmented nevi	60
Craniofacies	Epicanthal folds	30
	High palate	45
	Defective vision	22
	Defective hearing	53
	Micrognathia	40
	Short neck	71
	Webbed neck	53
	Low nuchal hairline	73
Thorax	Pectus excavatum	38
	Shield chest	59
	Cardiac/vascular anomaly (e.g., coarctation of the aorta, aortic stenosis)	43
Abdomen	Urinary tract anomaly	43
Limbs	Peripheral lymphedema	41
	Cubitus valgus	58
	Short metacarpals or metatarsals	48
	Hypoplastic, hyperconvex nails	73

46,XX cell line in addition to the 45,X line mitigates the effects of X-monosomy. Secondary sex development, menses, and even fertility have been reported in patients with 45,X/46,XX mosaicism. Fertility has also been described in a few cases of nonmosaic 45,X Turner syndrome. One form of mosaicism, 45,X/46,XY (mixed gonadal dysgenesis, Sec. 19.30), predisposes the patient to gonadal neoplasia and is an indication for surgical removal of the gonads. A buccal smear for X-chromatin is misleading in 45,X/46,XY mosaicism since it does not reflect the presence of the XY cell line. Chromosomal analysis is needed in all patients suspected of Turner syndrome.

Unlike autosomal trisomy and 47,XXY Klinefelter syndrome, Turner syndrome is not associated with advanced maternal age, suggesting that the underlying mechanism can involve the loss of either a paternal or a maternal sex chromosome. In 75% of testable cases of 45,X Turner syndrome, the *paternal* X or Y is absent. The frequency of mosaic karyotypes implicates a postfertilization error in cell division as the cause of many cases. Once parents have had a child with Turner syndrome, their risk for producing a second affected infant is *not* increased.

6.23 KLINEFELTER SYNDROME

See Sec. 19.30 for clinical features.

Klinefelter syndrome is defined as the spectrum of phenotypic features resulting from a sex chromosome complement that includes two or more X chromosomes and one or more Y chromosomes (Table 6–12). The 47,XXY Klinefelter syndrome occurs in approximately 1 per 1000 liveborn males but very rarely among spontaneous abortuses. The syndrome with karyotypes other than 47,XXY is rare. The somatic features are few and nonspecific. It is not often detected in the prepubertal male unless found in an X-chromatin screening program of a population, such as the males in an institution for the mentally abnormal. One helpful diagnostic feature is the presence of small patterns on the digits with a low ridge count. Klinefelter syndrome is associated with advanced maternal age.

Klinefelter syndrome is not a serious pediatric problem because, aside from infertility, most affected males lead normal lives; they are not identified until they are examined more closely because of the infertility and are found to have small testes and azoospermia.

Somatic abnormalities are more common in the Klinefelter syndrome when it is caused by chromosomal abnormalities other than 47,XXY. A direct correlation is apparent between the increased likelihood and severity of mental retardation and increasing number of X chromosomes. A specific identifiable phenotype has been attributed to the 49,XXXXY karyotype (Table 6–13).

Table 6–12. Phenotypic Features of Klinefelter Syndrome with 47,XXY Karyotype

Feature	Frequency (%)
Histologic evidence of impaired spermiogenesis	100
Small testes	99
Azoospermia	93
Gynecomastia	55
Decreased facial hair	77
Decreased pubic hair	61
Decreased penile size	41
Decreased libido or potency	68
Decreased testosterone (plasma)	79
Increased gonadotropins (urine and plasma)	75
Mental retardation or abnormality	10

Table 6–13. Phenotypic Features of the 49,XXXXY Male

Feature	Frequency (%)
Skeletal abnormalities (radioulnar synostosis, coxa valga; rib anomalies; abnormal ossification centers in hands; fusion of vertebral arches; pseudoepiphyses in hands and feet; absent radial heads; short, bowed radius and ulna)	70
Genital anomalies	
Hypoplastic scrotum	70
Cryptorchidism	30
Small penis	85
Small testicles	80
Decreased or female distribution of pubic hair	40
Mental retardation	100
Facial features	
Upward slanting palpebral fissures	75
Epicanthal folds	80
Strabismus	57
Hypertelorism	87
Malformed ears	73
Broad nasal bridge	86
Depressed nasal bridge	68
Short neck	70
Increased frequency of digital arch patterns	

6.24 THE 47,XXX FEMALE

The 47,XXX karyotype occurs with the same frequency among females as does 47,XXY among males (1/1000). There is no characteristic phenotype, and affected females are usually identified by chance, as in X-chromatin screening programs, newborn surveys, or amniocentesis ordered for other reasons; or they may be identified when an unrelated chromosomal abnormality is discovered in a child or other relative of a proband in a family study. They usually have normal gonadal function and are fertile, but they may have offspring with an abnormal sex chromosome complement. 47,XXX females may also have an increased frequency of delayed motor and speech development, mild intellectual deficit, and disturbed interpersonal relationships. More than three X chromosomes have been found in females, the largest number being five X. As in males, mental retardation or psychiatric abnormality appears to increase in females with increasing numbers of X chromosomes.

6.25 THE XYY MALE

A stigma has become attached to the 47,XYY sex chromosome complement because of studies, carried out in a prison population, reporting an association with aggressive antisocial behavior. The other feature claimed to be characteristic of XYY males is tall stature. Another study, while finding an elevated crime rate, did not relate the criminal behavior to aggression. Difficult ethical problems are raised by such studies. Among children the XYY karyotype has occasionally been found in those referred for chromosomal analyses because of difficult personality problems in school. The frequency of XYY has been estimated from newborn surveys as 1 in 1000 live births. See also Sec. 19.30.

6.26 ATYPICAL SEX CHROMOSOME KARYOTYPES

46,XX in Phenotypic Males

A 46,XX karyotype has been reported in phenotypic males with characteristics resembling those of Klinefelter syndrome.

Their internal and external genitalia are male. Most affected males are discovered at or after puberty because of sterility or failure of development of secondary sex characteristics (Sec. 19.30).

The occurrence of an XX sex chromosome constitution in a phenotypic male is contrary to the concept that a Y chromosome is necessary for male sex determination and differentiation. Possible explanations for the phenomenon include (1) undetected 46,XX/46,XY chimerism or 46,XX/47,XXY mosaicism, (2) translocation of the male sex-determining segment of the Y to the X chromosome or to an autosome, and (3) a mutant gene or genes. Available evidence suggest that the second explanation is likely in most cases, although the first explanation cannot be completely ruled out. The translocation of the male-determining segment of the Y to the X could produce an apparently XX male by the inactivated X-chromatin mechanism. The occurrence in the same family of an XX male and an XX true hermaphrodite is consistent with the suggestion of a mutant gene that may produce sex reversal in the 46,XX person.

46,XY in a Phenotypic Female

See also Sec. 19.23, 19.34, and 19.40.

The XY sex chromosome constitution exerts an effect on the early embryo to cause the gonads and the internal and external genitalia to differentiate into the definitive genital apparatus of the male; otherwise the embryo will differentiate as a female. The influence of the XY chromosome constitution is not completely understood but is mediated through induction of testicular differentiation. Testicular Leydig cells then secrete testosterone, which is converted peripherally to dihydrotestosterone. Target cells must have the capacity to respond to testosterone and dihydrotestosterone. If any of these steps fails, then masculinization of the embryo will not occur and the infant may have a female genital phenotype. Female phenotype may be seen in a 46,XY infant as the result of (1) complete insensitivity of target tissue to androgen (testicular feminization), (2) testicular unresponsiveness to luteinizing hormone (LH) and human chorionic gonadotropin (hCG) (Leydig cell aplasia), (3) a severe defect in the biosynthesis of testosterone, and (4) the syndrome of XY pure gonadal dysgenesis (Swyer syndrome).

6.27 FRAGILE X SYNDROME

"Heritable fragile sites" form another category of clinically significant chromosome breaks. These sites, reported to exist on several chromosomes, manifest themselves as spontaneous breaks inherited in a mendelian fashion whose appearance may be enhanced by the use of special tissue culture media or specific pretreatments of the cells. The most important of such fragile sites occurs on the long arm of the X chromosome (band q27–28) (Fig. 6–8) and is associated with a syndrome of mental retardation, with or without macro-orchidism in males. The "fragile-X syndrome" may account for up to 30% of X-linked mental retardation in males and perhaps 10% of all mild mental retardation in females (heterozygotes). The assessment of the mentally retarded male is incomplete without testicular measurement and chromosome study for this X chromosome marker.

SPONTANEOUS ABORTIONS

Over 20%, and perhaps as many as 50%, of all conceptuses are spontaneously aborted, at least half because of chromosomal aberrations, the most common being aneuploidy. Loss of a sex chromosome has been found most frequently. Chromosomal banding techniques have resulted in the identification of trisomies for all chromosomes except No. 1. Trisomy 16 is the most common, followed by trisomies of the small and large acrocentrics with the notable exception of No. 13. Autosomal monosomies have not been found, probably due to their lethality prior to implantation. Another relatively common finding in abortuses is polyploidy, usually triploidy (69 chromosomes), a condition resulting either from fertilization of an ovum by two sperm (dispermy) or from retention of the second polar body. No evidence exists of an association of polyploidy or other types of aberrations with birth control pills. In about 5 to 10% of couples who have had two or more spontaneous abortions, one or the other parent carries a balanced translocation. Such couples deserve cytogenetic study, since they are also at risk for producing chromosomally abnormal offspring.

6.28 GENETIC COUNSELING IN CHROMOSOMAL DISORDERS

See Sec. 6.30.

With the many advances in cytogenetic procedures, counseling for chromosomal abnormalities is becoming more precise. The aberrant chromosome can usually be identified; small translocations, deletions, and inversions can often be distinguished. Fairly accurate risk figures can be given for inherited translocations. But the recurrence risks following aneuploidy and sporadic deletions and translocations are still based on empiric data.

Amniocentesis, with culture and karyotyping of cells obtained from amniotic fluid, has provided a practical tool to identify chromosomal defects in utero and, by selective abortion, to prevent the birth of chromosomally abnormal offspring. Because of the risks involved in this procedure (estimated as one fetal loss in 200 to 400 procedures), priority indications are situations in which a parent is known to be chromosomally abnormal, maternal age is over 35, or there has been a previous trisomic child. Physicians have a responsibility to ensure that mothers are aware of the availability of intrauterine diagnosis and of the increased risk of chromosomal aberrations related to maternal age.

Chorionic villus biopsy is in the process of being evaluated for its safety and accuracy (Sec. 6.30). If it proves to be more accurate and the risk of fetal loss proves to be higher than that from amniocentesis, it will primarily be used when there is a relatively high risk of an abnormal fetus.

Acknowledgments. Acknowledgment is made to Sophie Paciuc, Elizabeth Byrnes, and Paula R. Martens for the preparation of karyotypes. I am grateful to Drs. Maimon M. Cohen and Henry N. Nadler for permission to use portions of their chapter from the previous edition.

KURT HIRSCHHORN

Bergsma D (ed): Birth Defects Compendium. 2nd ed. New York, AR Liss, 1979.

Boué A, Boué J, Gropp A: Cytogenetics of pregnancy wastage. Adv Human Genet 14:1, 1985.

deGrouchy J, Turleau C: Clinical Atlas of Human Chromosomes. 2nd ed. New York, John Wiley & Sons, 1984.

Hamerton JL: Human Cytogenetics. Vols I and II. New York, Academic Press, 1971.

LeBeau MM, Rowley JD: Chromosomal abnormalities in leukemia and lymphoma. Adv Hum Genet 15:1, 1985.

Paris Conference (1971): Standardization in Human Cytogenetics. Birth Defects—Original Article Series. Vol 8. New York, The National Foundation—March of Dimes, 1971.

Paris Conference (1971) Suppl (1975): Standardization in Human Cytogenetics.

Birth Defects—Original Article Series. Vol II. New York, The National Foundation—March of Dimes, Suppl 1975.

Simpson JL: Disorders of Sexual Differentiation: Etiology and Clinical Delineation. New York, Academic Press, 1977.

Thompson MW: Thompson & Thompson Genetics in Medicine. 4th ed. Philadelphia, WB Saunders, 1986.

Turner G, Jacobs P: Marker (X)-linked mental retardation. Adv Human Genet 13:83, 1983.

Patient Education

Smith DW, Wilson AA: The Child with Down's Syndrome (Mongolism). Philadelphia, WB Saunders, 1973.

Wisniewski LP, Hirschhorn K: A Guide to Human Chromosome Defects. 2nd ed. Birth Defects: Original Article Series Vol 16(6), New York, March of Dimes Birth Defects Foundation, 1980.

6.29 CONGENITAL MALFORMATIONS

About 2% of newborn infants have a major malformation. The incidence is as high as 5% if one includes malformations detected later in childhood, such as abnormalities of the heart, kidneys, lungs, and spine. Malformations are more common among spontaneous abortuses; many of these are severe and may cause abortion. About 9% of perinatal deaths are due to malformations. Treatment of malformations is one of the common reasons children are hospitalized.

A simple and arbitrary terminology has evolved for describing malformations. A *major malformation* has serious medical, surgical, or cosmetic consequences. A *minor anomaly* and a *normal variation* have no serious consequences and are arbitrarily differentiated: a minor anomaly occurs in 4% or less of children of the same race, whereas a normal variation occurs more commonly in children of the same racial group. For example, the incidence of features such as simian crease, clinodactyly of the 5th finger, extra nipples, Brushfield spots, and sacral dimple varies with race (Table 6–14).

A *syndrome* refers to a recognized pattern of malformations considered to have a single and specific cause, such as the Holt-Oram syndrome, an autosomal dominant disorder with malformations of the heart and upper extremities. *Association* is used to indicate a pattern of malformations for which no specific etiology has been identified, such as the VATER association of *v*ertebral, *a*nal, *t*racheal, *e*sophageal, radial upper limb, and *r*enal anomalies. A *morphogenic complex* (which has also been called an *anomalad*) comprises a primary malformation and its derived structural changes (e.g., Pierre Robin syndrome of cleft palate, glossoptosis, and micrognathia) but does not specify a cause.

Etiology. In a prospective study of 30,681 newborn infants 810 major malformations (2.6%) occurred, 57% of which were attributed to genetic abnormalities. The infants had 0.2% of malformations attributed to chromosomal abnormalities, 0.1% to single mutant genes, 0.7% to multifactorial inheritance, and 0.5% to uncertain patterns of inheritance. The number of chromosomal abnormalities is less than the 0.6% incidence of all types of chromosomal abnormalities in newborn infants because many of the common disorders, such as 47,XXY, 47,XYY, and 47,XXX, have no detectable physical characteristics in the newborn infant. Teratogens and other environ-

mental factors were identified as causes of malformations in 0.4% of the infants or 16.0% of all malformations, an incidence lower than many clinicians expect. Teratogens include drugs and maternal conditions such as diabetes mellitus; other environmental factors include amniotic constrictive bands, vascular abnormalities, and oligohydramnios. Vascular abnormalities, including absence of arteries, an abnormal persistence of embryonic vessels, and occlusion of vessels, have been shown to be associated with some types of bowel atresia, hydranencephaly, absence of the pectoralis major muscle (Poland anomaly), and absence of long bones. Twinning is associated with a higher incidence of malformations than that in singletons; the acardiac infant syndrome occurs only in monozygous twins.

The causes of 27% of the 810 major malformations were not detected. Malformations of unknown cause include imperforate anus, megaloureter, Goldenhar syndrome, omphalocele, cloacal exstrophy, and diaphragmatic hernia through the foramen of Bochdalek.

Underlying Mechanisms. The understanding of malformations has been derived principally from the study of animals. Basic abnormalities identified include (1) abnormal cell shape; (2) abnormalities of the collagens or of the proteoglycans, major constituents of the extracellular matrix; (3) errors in circulation during fetal development; and (4) lack of appropriate death of cells during morphogenesis. An example of abnormal cell shape is the defect in the Bergmann glial cells which normally provide the latticework for migration of neuronal cells. When they are defective because of the autosomal recessive gene *weaver* in the mouse, hypoplasia of the cerebellum results. Several types of Ehlers-Danlos syndrome have been identified by clinical and genetic studies in humans; at least three have been shown to be due to different defects in collagen metabolism. For example, in type VI the collagen is deficient in hydroxylysine because of a deficiency of lysyl hydroxylase; in type VII there is an inability to convert procollagen to collagen; in type IV there is a lack of type III collagen.

The malformation *hemifacial microsomia* can be caused by a failure of the vascular supply to be transferred from the stapedial artery to the external carotid artery, a switchover that normally occurs during the 6th and 7th wk of gestation in humans. *Synostosis of bones* can be due to a lack of appropriate death of cells between the developing long bones in a limb. *Cleft palate* reflects a failure of the palate shelves to meet and fuse, a process in which death of cells in the epithelium must precede the fusion of the underlying palatal mesenchyme.

Clinical Evaluation. Any child with a major or with multiple minor malformations deserves diagnostic evaluation. This includes a history of defects in other family members and of any untoward events during the pregnancy as well as a thorough physical examination. In the examination, objective measurements should be used when a physical feature seems too long, short, narrow or wide. Many normal standards are included in Smith's *Recognizable Patterns of Human Malformation*. Chromosomal analysis by banding techniques should be obtained when there are multiple malformations, especially if

Table 6–14. Incidence of Minor Anomalies and Normal Variations in Newborn Infants

Physical Feature	White Infants (%) (N = 3989)	BLACK INFANTS (%) (N = 827)
Third sagittal fontanel	3.1	9.8
Epicanthal folds, bilateral	1.4	1.0
Brushfield spots, bilateral	7.2	0.2
Preauricular sinus, left or right	0.8	5.3
Extra nipple, left or right	0.5	4.6
Umbilical hernia	0.7	6.1
Sacral dimple	4.8	0.6
Clinodactyly of both 5th fingers	5.2	4.5
Simian crease, both hands	0.7	0.5
Syndactyly of toes 2 and 3, left or right	1.7	2.3

From Holmes LB: The Malformed Newborn—Practical Perspectives. Boston, Developmental Disabilities Council, 1976.

the infant is mentally retarded, is stillborn, or dies soon after birth (Sec. 6.8). For such studies on a deceased infant, cells obtained from biopsies of skin, gonad, thymus, or spleen grown in tissue culture are preferable to those obtained from a blood sample taken when the infant is moribund. The likelihood of finding a chromosomal abnormality in infants in the above categories is only 10–20%. Screening for metabolic diseases may be warranted in some malformed infants. Glutaric aciduria type II has been observed in some malformed infants, especially in association with polycystic kidneys.

The same clinical signs or malformations may be caused by a variety of genetic accidents. For example, the split-hand/split-foot syndrome, an unusual malformation in which there is a cleft in the middle of the hand, foot, or both, may be due to lack of development of the middle digits and metatarsals and metacarpals. The same deformity occurs in focal dermal hypoplasia, a multiple malformation syndrome, and in the autosomal dominant disorder in which the deformities are limited to the limbs.

Gorlin RJ, Pindborg JJ, Cohen MM Jr: Syndromes of the Head and Neck. 2nd ed. New York, McGraw-Hill, 1976.
Holmes LB: Inborn errors of morphogenesis. N Engl J Med 291:763, 1974.
Hootnick DR, Levinsohn EM, Randall PA, et al: Vascular dysgenesis associated with skeletal dysplasia of the lower limb. J Bone Joint Surg 62A:1123, 1980.
Machin GA: Chromosome abnormality and perinatal death. Lancet 1:549, 1974.
Mueller RF, Sybert VP, Johnson J: Evaluation of a protocol for post-mortem examination of stillbirths. N Engl J Med 309:586, 1983.
Poswillo D: The pathogenesis of the first and second branchial arch syndrome. Oral Surg 35:302, 1973.
Smith DW: Recognizable Patterns of Human Malformation. 3rd ed. Philadelphia, WB Saunders, 1982.
Sweetman L, Nyhan WL, Tranner DA, et al: Glutaric acidemia type II. J Pediatr 96:1020, 1980.
Tharapel AT, Summitt RL: A cytogenetic survey of 200 unclassifiable mentally retarded children with congenital anomalies and 200 normal controls. Hum Genet 37:329, 1977.
Van Allen MI, Hoyme HE, Jones KL: Vascular pathogenesis of limb defects. I. Radial artery anatomy in radial aplasia. J Pediatr 101:832, 1982.
Warkany J: Congenital Malformations. Chicago, Year Book Medical Publishers, 1971.

6.30 GENETIC COUNSELING

Genetic counseling is a communication process dealing with the human problems associated with the occurrence or risk of occurrence of a genetic disorder in a family. Many are unaware of their risks, while some request genetic information and counseling. The latter most commonly are couples whose first child has just been born with a birth defect or medical problem. Older couples also are frequently concerned about genetic risks and wish to learn about prenatal diagnosis. Others seek information prior to marriage or before having children because of medical problems of their relatives. The physician should recognize which birth defects and medical problems are hereditary and offer genetic information to all families, not just to those who request it. Genetic counseling becomes more complex when detection of carriers is possible or when the relevance of prenatal diagnosis must be explained.

PRINCIPLES OF GENETIC COUNSELING

The first step in genetic counseling is to make certain the diagnosis is correct. The physician must, for example, distinguish isolated cleft lip and palate (multifactorial inheritance) from cleft lip and palate with lip pits (autosomal dominant); distinguish Duchenne muscular dystrophy (X-linked recessive) from the Becker type of muscular dystrophy (X-linked recessive), the latter being much less severe; distinguish the perinatal type of infantile polycystic kidney disease (autosomal recessive) from unilateral multicystic kidney (nonhereditary).

With diagnosis established, the steps in the counseling process follow:

1. Have both parents present for the discussion (a teenager in the family should be offered the opportunity of a separate discussion).

2. Discuss the medical consequences of the defect; if relevant, the variability of associated features that might develop in future years should be explained.

3. Review the family history of each parent and identify any unrecognized genetic risks.

4. Review the interpretations the family has made or which have been offered by others to explain the condition under discussion.

5. Describe the genetic basis for the problem, using *visual aids* (pictures demonstrating phenotypic or other features of the problem, pictures of chromosomes, diagrams of patterns of inheritance) as much as possible.

6. Explain the genetic risks in terms the family can understand.

7. Outline the options available, such as having no children, having children and accepting the risks, adopting a child if possible, artificial insemination (this option is particularly pertinent in the case of all autosomal recessive disorders and serious paternal autosomal dominant disorders); note whether prenatal diagnosis is possible.

8. Provide the persons counseled with a summary of the issues discussed and, if possible, meet with them again to help them decide the option most appropriate for them.

9. Stay in contact with families previously counseled to provide new information that may become available, such as new methods for carrier detection in a parent or for prenatal diagnosis.

Often parents first become aware of their genetic risks after the birth of a child having a birth defect. Coping with this knowledge usually includes periods of denial, anger, and depression before it is assimilated and accepted. Each family's situation is different and their reaction to counseling unique. A frequent problem for families is conceptualizing the genetic abnormality, such as a single mutant gene, an abnormal chromosome, or, in the case of multifactorial inheritance, the interaction of several genes and environmental factors. In the case of chromosomal abnormalities, it may be advantageous to show the abnormal karyotype compared with a normal one. Another problem is the fact that most infants and children with a genetic disorder are the first affected member of the family. Parents may assume a problem cannot be hereditary if no other relatives are affected. It is helpful for the counselor to discuss in detail how healthy parents with no affected relatives can have a child with a hereditary disorder.

GENETIC COUNSELING WHEN DETECTION OF CARRIERS IS POSSIBLE

Genetic counseling is simplified, more specific, and probably more effective when the carrier state for the genetic abnormality in question can be identified by laboratory tests. Those at risk can be identified, and their relatives who were tested and found not to be carriers can be reassured. The concept of genetic risk is more concrete when an individual has a venipuncture and can be shown the test results in comparison with the normal. Carrier detection is possible for some biochemical disorders, for certain abnormalities of the chromosomes, and through DNA analysis techniques, such as gene mapping and the identification of a restriction length polymorphism that is closely linked to a mutant gene.

Biochemical Disorders. Persons heterozygous for some autosomal recessive inborn errors of metabolism and abnormalities of hemoglobin can be identified. These inborn errors include abnormalities such as hemoglobins S and C, thalassemia, Tay-Sachs disease, and α_1-antitrypsin deficiency. If the assay is appropriate for screening large numbers of individuals, testing high-risk populations may be conducted. This type of testing has been used to screen Jews of Eastern European origin for Tay-Sachs disease, persons of Mediterranean ancestry for thalassemia, and blacks for hemoglobins S and C. Screening for genetic diseases may have untoward psychologic effects by focusing on a racial or ethnic group. Another limitation of screening for heterozygotes is lack of easy access to prenatal diagnosis for couples who are both heterozygous. This is particularly true of the hemoglobin abnormalities for which placental venipuncture, a technique available in only a few medical centers, is required.

Females can be identified as heterozygous for several X-linked recessive metabolic disorders, such as glucose-6-phosphate dehydrogenase deficiency, Fabry disease (α-galactosidase deficiency), and hypoxanthine–guanine phosphoribosyl transferase deficiency. Detection of female carriers is less precise in the two most common X-linked recessive disorders, Duchenne muscular dystrophy and hemophilia A. Testing for the carrier of Duchenne muscular dystrophy has been indirect and has relied primarily on measuring the serum level of the muscle enzyme creatine phosphokinase (CPK). Only about 75% of known carriers can be identified by this method. Important factors in the testing are establishing a normal range for the laboratory being used, and testing women at risk at least 3–4 times, preferably in the resting state. The fact that the level of CPK in carriers is highest before age 30 and decreases thereafter presents another variable in the testing procedure. More accurate identification of carrier females and affected fetuses is being developed using DNA analysis; this is not useful in all families. Some investigators use other serum enzymes, such as lactate dehydrogenase (LDH), to detect carriers. In the affected male fetus the diagnosis cannot be made with adequate consistency to justify attempts at prenatal diagnosis. When proven female carriers are informed of their high risk of having affected sons, they often elect not to have more children.

The method for identifying women carrying the gene for hemophilia A has recently been improved by instituting the measuring of both the activity of factor VIII and the amount of factor VIII antigen that is present. This test effectively identifies about 80% of *known* carriers. In the 2nd trimester prenatal diagnosis by means of immunoradiometric assays for factor VIII on fetal plasma obtained by percutaneous ultrasound-guided blood sampling (PUBS) is available. However, this option cannot be used by families in which hemophiliac males have circulating cross-reactive material.

Chromosomal Translocations. When a child is abnormal because of an excess or deficiency of chromosomal material, the parents should be studied to identify whether or not either is the carrier of a balanced translocation. A carrier parent can then be counseled as to his or her risk of having children with an unbalanced translocation, and other blood relatives may be tested to see if they, too, are carriers. Related chromosomal abnormalities of the fetus of the carrier of a balanced translocation may be identified through culture of fetal cells obtained by amniocentesis.

GENETIC COUNSELING WHEN PRENATAL DIAGNOSIS IS POSSIBLE

Many couples seek genetic counseling to learn more about prenatal diagnosis. The most common indications for prenatal diagnosis are advanced maternal age (Table 6–7) and a previous child with either Down syndrome or anencephaly-meningomyelocele.

In general, prenatal diagnosis by amniocentesis is recommended for all women over the age of 35, as their risk of having a child with any type of chromosomal abnormality is at least 1%. There has been a steady decline over the last 25 yr in the percentage of infants with Down syndrome born to women over 35. Thus 80% of the infants with Down syndrome are now born to women under 35 yr of age, because this group is not routinely offered prenatal diagnosis as an option. Further, in about 1 of 5 instances, the extra No. 21 chromosome is derived from the father (Sec. 6.11).

Couples at risk for having children with metabolic diseases have a less common indication for prenatal diagnosis (Table 8–11). Metabolic testing on amniotic cells should be done by those laboratories experienced in conducting such assays on amniotic cells.

Prenatal diagnosis by *amniocentesis* is usually undertaken at 15–16 wk of gestation, when the uterus extends high enough out of the pelvis to facilitate the procedure. Ultrasonography is used to locate the placenta and to determine whether there is more than one fetus; the incidence of twin pregnancy is about 1 in 80. Using aseptic technique and local anesthesia, a 22-gauge spinal needle with trocar in place is inserted through the abdomen at the most favorable site, as indicated by the ultrasonogram, and advanced into the amniotic cavity. The trocar is removed and the first 2 mL of fluid is discarded to minimize the risk of contamination of the sample with cells from the mother's skin; then 10–30 mL of amniotic fluid is withdrawn into a second syringe, sealed in the syringe, and taken directly to the laboratory. The specimen is tested for the presence of fetal blood, and centrifuged to separate the fluid from the cells; the cells are then placed in tissue culture medium under sterile conditions in an incubator.

Fetal loss from amniocentesis is less than 0.5%. Three percent of women have transient cramps and leakage of amniotic fluid. In about 5% of instances the amniocentesis must be repeated, either because no amniotic fluid was obtained with the first amniocentesis or because there was insufficient growth of cells.

Results can be provided within 14–21 days of the amniocentesis. If the tests show that the fetus is abnormal and the parents elect to have the fetus aborted, most obstetricians prefer to terminate the pregnancy before 20 wk of gestation, although up to 24 wk is permissible by law in the United States.

Prenatal diagnosis based on chorionic villus sampling (CVS) at 9–11 wk of pregnancy is being evaluated. The tissue is obtained by inserting a sampling device through the cervix and up into the fetal placenta. The tissue obtained can be used for direct DNA analysis to identify hemoglobin abnormalities or for cell culture. The risk of fetal loss after CVS may be below 2%. Early amniocentesis at 12–14 wk of gestation is being developed as another alternative for prenatal diagnosis.

Tissues and Technical Procedures Used in Prenatal Diagnosis

The Cells in the Amniotic Fluid. The cells obtained by amniocentesis can be used for chromosomal analysis, biochemical assay, or DNA analysis. Two to 3 wk are needed for the cells to multiply and reach a number adequate for testing; it is more difficult to obtain good metaphase preparations from amniotic fluid cells than from peripheral lymphocytes. Chromosomal abnormalities such as polyploidy and mosaicism with both normal and abnormal cell lines are also more common in amniotic fluid cells obtained at 14–16 wk gestation than in cells of infants at birth.

The Amniotic Fluid. *Alpha-Fetoprotein (AFP).* The level of this constituent of amniotic fluid, which is synthesized by the fetal liver, gastrointestinal tract, and yolk sac, is increased whenever transudation across a thin membrane occurs, as in anencephaly, meningomyelocele, encephalocele, and omphalocele. The most common use of measuring AFP is to evaluate subsequent pregnancies of couples who have had a child with anencephaly, meningomyelocele, or encephalocele; omphalocele is not hereditary. AFP levels have also been used to identify the Meckel syndrome (an autosomal recessive disorder that includes encephalocele, polycystic kidneys, polydactyly, cleft lip and palate, and anomalies of the genitals and eyes) and congenital nephrosis (a rare autosomal recessive disorder).

The level of AFP is highest between 14 and 18 wk of gestation and falls steadily thereafter; it is important to obtain an estimate of gestational age by ultrasonography before amniocentesis. The concentration of AFP may be increased by the presence of fetal blood, fetal spontaneous abortion, fetal death, Rh sensitization, congenital nephrosis, and the presence of intestinal atresia. The measurement of acetylcholinesterase in amniotic fluid is helpful in confirming the presence of a neural tube defect and in eliminating false-positive elevations of AFP. The AFP level is often normal if a neural tube defect, such as meningocele or encephalocele, is covered by skin.

Routine prenatal screening of pregnant women by measuring the level of AFP in serum by radioimmunoassay is effective in identifying 80–90% of fetuses with anencephaly and meningomyelocele. This test is performed at 16–18 wk of pregnancy. An elevated value requires a second serum test. If the serum AFP is 2.5 times the median value on two occasions, the fetus is examined by ultrasonography and amniocentesis. In addition to neural tube defects, serum AFP screening will also identify the presence of other malformations such as omphalocele, growth retardation, and twinning. Current studies are evaluating whether low levels of serum AFP are reliable for detecting Down syndrome in fetuses.

Secretor Substance. Under certain conditions, either the presence or absence of the secretory substance in amniotic fluid can be used in some families to determine whether the fetus of an affected parent had myotonic dystrophy and whether the locus of the dominant gene is responsible for the secretor substance.

The amniotic fluid can also be analyzed for steroid hormones and has been used to diagnose congenital adrenal hyperplasia due to a deficiency of 21-hydroxylase.

Ultrasonography. Ultrasonography is used primarily to determine gestational age, to localize the placenta, to rule out multiple pregnancies, and to diagnose congenital malformations (Sec. 5.55 and 8.9–8.11).

Fetoscopy. Direct inspection of the fetus is possible, but the risk to the fetus is about 5%. It has been used for obtaining blood samples from placental vessels as well as for performing skin biopsies and liver biopsies. Fetoscopy has also been used to identify limb deformities. A difficulty with this technique is the small area that can be seen at one time. Improvements in ultrasonography and techniques of DNA analysis have decreased the need for blood sampling by fetoscopy.

Radiography. Roentgenograms of the fetus may be helpful when the fetus is at risk for a severe deficiency of the long bones, as in thrombocytopenia with radial aplasia, and to identify vertebral malformations, as in the Jarcho-Levin syndrome. However, this technique is being replaced by ultrasonography.

Genetic Counseling

Antley RM: Variables in the outcome of genetic counseling. Social Biology 23:108, 1976.
Leonard CO, Chase GA, Childs B: Genetic counseling: A consumer's view. N Engl J Med 287:433, 1972.
Lippman-Hand A, Fraser FC: Genetic counseling, provisions and reception of information. Am J Med Genet 3:113, 1979.
Zare N, Sorenson JR, Heeren T: Sex of provider as a variable in effective genetic counseling. Soc Sci Med 19:671, 1984.

Carrier Detection

Klein HG, Aledort LM, Bourma BN, et al: Detection of the carrier state of classic hemophilia. N Engl J Med 296:959, 1977.
Hutton EM, Thompson MW: Carrier detection and genetic counselling in Duchenne muscular dystrophy: A follow-up study. CMA Journal 115:749, 1976.
Munsat TL, Baloh R, Pearson CM, et al: Serum enzyme alteration in neuromuscular disorders. JAMA 226:1536, 1973.

Prenatal Diagnosis

Cuckle HS, Wald NJ, Lindenbaum RH: Maternal serum alpha-fetoprotein measurement: a screening test for Down syndrome. Lancet 1:926, 1984.
Haddow J, Macri JN: Prenatal screening for neural tube defects. JAMA 242:515, 1979.
Hill LM, Breckle R, Gehrking WC: The prenatal detection of congenital malformations by ultrasonography. Mayo Clin Proc 55:805, 1983.
Hobbins JC, Romero R, Gannum P, et al: Antenatal diagnosis of renal anomalies with ultrasound. Am J Obstet Gynecol 148:868, 1986.
Kidd VJ, Golbus MS, Wallace RB, et al: Prenatal diagnosis of α-1-antitrypsin deficiency by direct analysis of the mutation site in the gene. N Engl J Med 310:639, 1984.
Lowry RB, Jones DC, Renwick DHG, et al: Down syndrome in British Columbia, 1952–1973: Incidence and mean maternal age. Teratology 14:29, 1976.
Magenis RW, Overton KM, Chamberlain J, et al: Parental origin of the extra chromosome in Down's syndrome. Hum Genet 37:7, 1977.
Marion KP, Kassam G, Fernhoff PM, et al: Acceptance of amniocentesis by low-income patients in an urban hospital. Am J Obstet Gynecol 138:11, 1980.
Midtrimester amniocentesis for prenatal diagnosis: Safety and accuracy. JAMA 236:1471, 1976.
Old JM, Ward RHT, Petrou M, et al: First-trimester fetal diagnosis for hemoglobinopathies: three cases. Lancet 2:1413, 1982.
Schrott HG, Karp L, Omenn GS: Prenatal prediction in myotonic dystrophy; guidelines for genetic counseling. Clin Genet 4:38, 1973.

6.31 TERATOGENS

When an infant or child is malformed or mentally retarded, the parents often wrongly blame themselves and attribute the child's problems to events that occurred during pregnancy. Since infections occur and several drugs are often taken during many pregnancies, the pediatrician must evaluate the presumed viral infections and the drugs ingested to help parents understand their child's birth defect. The causes of about 40% of congenital malformations are unknown. While only a few agents teratogenic in humans are recognized at this time (Table 6–15), additional agents, e.g., valproic acid (used to treat convulsions) and isotretinoin (used to treat acne), continue to be identified.

Several generalizations can be made about teratogens. None is harmful to every exposed fetus; some drugs (e.g., phenytoins) and maternal conditions (e.g., diabetes mellitus) may cause only a 2- to 3-fold increase in the overall incidence of malformations. Since the increase caused by a teratogen may be relatively small, harmful effects may be difficult to demonstrate. In general, exposure during the 1st trimester of pregnancy is probably the most harmful. The exact age of the fetus when a particular drug is most harmful has been established only for thalidomide (days 34–50). Even less information is available on the effects of exposure during the 2nd and 3rd trimesters.

If a child has multiple structural malformations, such as polydactyly, cleft palate, meningomyelocele, or absence of a long bone, it is inappropriate to consider intrauterine infections as a possible cause. It is true that rubella infection in utero causes cardiac anomalies, but its other effects, such as

Table 6–15. **Teratogenic Agents in Humans**

Teratogen	Phenotypic Effect	Period of Greatest Sensitivity	Likelihood of Harmful Effect
Drugs Taken by Pregnant Mother			
Aminopterin or amethopterin (folic acid antagonist)	Hydrocephalus, craniosynostosis, shortened limbs, absent digits, mental deficiency	?	?
Diethylstilbestrol	Carcinoma and adenosis of vagina in exposed females; genitourinary anomalies in exposed males	First 2 months	>50% of females 25% of males
Iodides and propylthiouracil	Goiter, fetal hypothyroidism	?	?
Isotretinoin	Brain malformations, microtia, thymic hypoplasia, conotruncal heart defects	First trimester	>20-fold increase
Phenytoin	Heart defects, nail hypoplasia, growth retardation	First trimester	3-fold increase
Progestogens contaminated with testosterone	Masculinization of female fetus	Third trimester	?
Tetracyclines	Enamel dysplasia	Second and 3rd trimester	?
Thalidomide	Phocomelia, anomalies of ears, teeth, eyes, and intestine	Days 34–50 (menstrual age)	>90%
Valproic acid	Spina bifida, facial anomalies, developmental delay	First trimester	>20-fold increase
Warfarin (vitamin K antagonist)	Hypoplasia of nose, shortened digits, stippled epiphyses, mental deficiency in some	Weeks 6–8 (menstrual age)	?
Maternal Conditions			
Chronic, severe alcoholism	Growth retardation, mental deficiency, microcephaly, heart defects, flexion contractures	?	30–50%
Diabetes mellitus	Heart defects; all types of birth defects; sacral agenesis; anencephaly and spina bifida	?	3-fold increase
Lupus erythematosus	Congenital heart block	?	?
Phenylketonuria	Microcephaly, mental deficiency, heart defects	?	?
Smoking	Decrease in birthweight, abnormal placentation	?	?
Trace Metals			
Lead	Decrease in intelligence	?	?
Mercury	Microcephaly, spasticity, mental deficiency	?	?
Intrauterine Infections			
Cytomegalovirus	Microcephaly, mental deficiency	First trimester	?
Rubella	Heart defects, microcephaly, cataracts, deafness, mental deficiency	First trimester	15–40%
Toxoplasmosis	Macrocephaly or microcephaly, microphthalmia, mental deficiency	First trimester	?
Varicella	Skin scars, hypoplasia of limbs, microphthalmia, cataracts, mental deficiency	?	?
Uterine Factors			
Amniotic band deformity	Amputation or constriction bands on one or more extremities	?	?
Severe oligohydramnios	Lung hypoplasia, deformities caused by pressure from surrounding structures	Throughout	100%

microcephaly, cataracts, and deafness, are the results of infection of the tissues concerned, not structural malformations. Likewise, congenital toxoplasmosis may cause hydrocephalus, and intrauterine infection with cytomegalovirus may cause cerebral cysts. However, none of these intrauterine infections causes multiple major and minor *structural* malformations, as can be caused by chromosomal abnormalities, single mutant genes, and teratogenic drugs.

The mechanism of action is known or postulated for very few teratogens. Warfarin, an anticoagulant because it is a vitamin K antagonist, prevents carboxylation of gamma-carboxyglutamic acid (GLA). Inasmuch as this substance is a calcium-binding amino acid, normally part of the prothrombin molecule, deficiency of it interferes with normal clotting of blood. Gamma-carboxyglutamic acid is also present in human bones, and human fetuses exposed to warfarin in utero show abnormal cartilage, although the exact role of gamma-carboxyglutamic acid in chondrogenesis is unknown. Hypothyroidism

in the fetus may be caused by maternal ingestion of an excessive amount of iodides or of propylthiouracil; each interferes with the conversion of inorganic to organic iodides. Phenytoin may be teratogenic because of the accumulation of a metabolite due to deficiency of epoxide hydrolase.

Recognition of teratogens offers the opportunity for prevention of related birth defects. For example, if a pregnant woman is informed of the potentially harmful effects of alcohol on her unborn infant, she may be motivated to control this problem during pregnancy.

Physicians are often asked about the risks of exposure in utero to drugs that have not been proved to be teratogenic. These include caffeine, diazepam, LSD (lysergic acid), marijuana, heroin, blighted potatoes, aspirin, and phenothiazine derivatives, such as Bendectin. Current references should be consulted before drawing conclusions.

Genetic factors play a role in determining teratogenicity that may represent multifactorial inheritance in which the *inherited* factor is susceptibility to a teratogenic *environmental* factor. Variation in susceptibility to teratogens is apparent not only between different species of animals but also within species, e.g., different genetic strains of rats show different degrees of susceptibility to cortisone as a teratogenic agent that induces cleft palate in the rat fetus. The parents of a child with phenytoin-induced malformations have an increased risk of a subsequent child developing this drug-induced embryopathy in comparison to parents whose exposed children are not malformed. This increased risk may reflect a genetic difference in metabolizing phenytoin.

Other conditions are also teratogenic, such as amniotic constriction bands, oligohydramnios, and uterine constraint. Bands of amniotic tissue cause either amputation or constriction of one or more extremities in about 1 in every 5000 pregnancies. Oligohydramnios may result from bilateral renal agenesis, severe polycystic kidney disease, chronic leakage of amniotic fluid, and extrauterine pregnancy. Its consequences are lung hypoplasia, club foot deformity, a flattened face, and amnion nodosum.

Bellinger DC, Needleman HL: Lead and the relationship between maternal and child intelligence. J Pediatr 102:523, 1983.

Clarren SK, Smith DW: The fetal alcohol syndrome. N Engl J Med 298:1063, 1978.

DiLiberti JH, Farndon PA, Dennis NR: The fetal valproate syndrome. Am J Med Genet 19:473, 1984.

Dunn PM: Congenital postural deformities. Br Med Bull 32:71, 1976.

Fernhoff PM, Lammer EJ: Craniofacial features of isotretinoin embryopathy. J Pediatr 105:595, 1984.

Hall JG, Pauli RM, Wilson KM: Maternal and fetal sequelae of anticoagulation during pregnancy. Am J Med 68:122, 1980.

Heinonen OP, Slone D, Shapiro S: Birth Defects and Drugs in Pregnancy. Littleton, Mass., Publishing Science Groups, 1976.

Levy HL, Waisbren SE: Effects of untreated maternal phenyketonuria and hyperphenylalaninemia on the fetus. N Engl J Med 309:1269, 1983.

Litsey SE, Noonan JA, O'Connor WN, et al: Maternal connective tissue disease and congenital heart block. N Engl J Med 312:98, 1985.

Shepard TH: Catalog of Teratogenic Agents. 5th ed. Baltimore, The Johns Hopkins University Press, 1986.

Wilson JG, Brent RL: Are female sex hormones teratogenic? Am Obstet Gynecol 141:567, 1981.

6.32 RADIATION

Accidental exposure of pregnant women to radiation is a common cause for anxiety among women, their families, and their physicians, usually about whether the fetus will have birth defects or genetic abnormalities. It is unlikely that exposure to either diagnostic or therapeutic radiation will cause gene mutations; no increase in genetic abnormalities has been identified in the offspring exposed as unborn fetuses to the atomic bomb explosions in Japan in 1945.

Table 6–16. **Radiation Exposure of the Fetus**

	Millirads*
Roentgenogram of:	
Chest	1
Thoracic spine	11
Abdomen	221
Pelvis	210
Hips	124
Roentgenographic contrast studies	
Upper G.I. series	171
Barium enema	903
Cholangiogram	78
Intravenous pyelogram	588

*Due to variation in techniques these estimates may be exceeded. (From U.S. DHEW: Gonad Doses and Genetically Significant Dose from Diagnostic Radiology; U.S., 1964 and 1970. Washington, D.C., U.S. Government Printing Office, 1976.)

A more realistic concern is whether the exposed human fetus will show birth defects or a higher incidence of malignancy. The recommended occupational limit of maternal exposure to radiation from all sources is 500 millirads for the entire 40 wk of a pregnancy. Estimates of the gonadal exposure for the mother and the whole body exposure of the fetus from several common roentgenographic examinations are shown in Table 6–16. The limited data on human fetuses show that large doses of radiation (10,000–30,000 millirads) are harmful to the central nervous system.

Therapeutic abortion is often recommended when exposure exceeds 10,000 millirads. It is much more likely that a human fetus will be exposed to 1000–3000 millirads, an amount not shown to cause malformations. There is controversy as to whether this level of exposure is associated with an increased risk of developing cancer or leukemia. (See also Sec. 5.55 and Chapter 27.)

LEWIS B. HOLMES

Brent RL: Radiation teratogenesis. Teratology 21:281, 1980.

The Effects on Populations of Exposure to Low Levels of Ionizing Radiation (BEIR Report). Washington DC, National Academy of Sciences. National Research Council, November, 1972.

Griem ML, Meier P, Dobben GD: Analysis of the morbidity and mortality of children irradiated in fetal life. Radiology 88:347, 1967.

US Department of Health, Education, and Welfare: Gonad Doses and Genetically Significant Dose from Diagnostic Radiology: US., 1964 and 1970. Washington DC, US Government Printing Office, 1976.

Webster EW: On the question of cancer induction by small X-ray doses. Am J Roentgenol 137:647, 1981.

Yamazaki NJ: A review of the literature on the radiation dosage required to cause manifest central nervous system disturbances from in utero and postnatal exposure. Pediatrics 37:877, 1966.

6.33 DYSMORPHOLOGY—THE APPROACH TO STRUCTURAL DEFECTS OF PRENATAL ONSET

The field of dysmorphology has expanded dramatically as the number of recognizable patterns of malformation has more than tripled over the last 15 yr; new insights have been gained into the pathogenesis of various structural defects, the potential prenatal effect of various drugs, chemicals, and environmental agents has been better appreciated, and the number of defects in which prenatal detection is possible has increased. Because of their vast number, a listing of all known recognizable patterns of malformation will not be presented. Rather, this section will provide an approach to the child with the prenatal onset of structural defects. The approach is predicated upon the concept that the nature of the structural defects represents a clue to the time of onset, mechanism of injury, and possible etiology of the problem, all of which determine the necessary evaluation. This permits a systematic narrowing of the diagnostic possibilities so that other sections of this textbook or one of the basic compendiums on dysmorphology may be used to make a specific diagnosis.

Structural defects of prenatal onset can be separated into those which represent a *single primary defect* in development and those which represent a multiple malformation syndrome. In the majority of cases, the defect involves only a single structure, the child being otherwise completely normal. The seven most common single primary defects in development are congenital hip dislocation (Sec. 23.2), talipes equinovarus (Sec. 23.1), cleft lip with or without cleft palate (Sec. 12.5), cleft palate alone (Sec. 12.5), cardiac septal defects (Sec. 14.35), pyloric stenosis (Sec. 12.27), and defects in neural tube closure (Sec. 21.10). For most, the etiology is unknown, and counseling as to recurrence risk is difficult. However, most single primary defects are explained on the basis of multifactorial inheritance (Sec. 6.6), which carries a recurrence risk of between 2–5% for the next child of unaffected parents with one affected child.

The extent to which multifactorial inheritance contributes to the etiology of some of the less common single defects in development is unclear. The fact that single primary defects are etiologically heterogeneous implies that some have an environmental etiology and others result from dominantly or recessively inherited single altered genes. Craniosynostosis (Sec. 23.9) secondary to in utero constraint is an example of the former, whereas postaxial polydactyly (Sec. 23.8) illustrates the latter. Before multifactorial risk figures are used for counseling when a single primary defect is recognized, references should be consulted to determine whether other risk figures are available.

In contrast to the concept of the single primary defect in development, the designation *multiple malformation syndrome* is used when several observed structural defects all have the same known or presumed etiology. The defects usually include a number of anatomically unrelated errors in morphogenesis. Multiple malformation syndromes are caused by chromosomal abnormalities, by teratogens, and by single gene defects inherited in mendelian patterns. Risks of recurrence range from 0 in cases that represent fresh gene mutations or are caused by teratogens to 100% in the case of a child with the Down syndrome in which the mother is a balanced 21/21 translocation carrier (Sec. 6.11).

Single Primary Defects in Development. These defects are subcategorized according to the nature of the error in morphogenesis that has produced the observed structural defect: malformation, deformation, or disruption of developing structure. A *malformation* is a primary structural defect arising from a localized error in morphogenesis. A *deformation* is an alteration in shape and/or structure of a part which has differentiated normally. The term *disruption* is used for a structural defect resulting from destruction of a previously normally formed part. Of the deformations noted at birth, 90% will correct spontaneously; of those that do not, most can be corrected with early postural intervention. If correction of malformations or disruptions is at all possible, surgery is virtually always required.

Malformations. Most children with a localized malformation such as cardiac septal defect or pyloric stenosis are otherwise completely normal. Following surgical correction, prognosis is excellent. When neither dominant nor recessive inheritance is established, multifactorial recurrence risk factors (2–5%) apply to unaffected parents.

Deformations. The majority of deformations involve the musculoskeletal system and are probably caused by intrauterine molding. The pressure producing such molding may be intrinsic, due to neuromuscular imbalance within the fetus, or may be extrinsic, secondary to fetal crowding. In either case, the impaired ability of the fetus to kick results in decreased fetal movement, an important factor in development of the normal musculoskeletal system, particularly with respect to normal joint development. In addition, marked positional deformation of any body part can occur when the fetus is unable to change position and thus alter the direction along which potentially deforming forces are being directed. Intrinsically derived positional deformation of prenatal onset occurs in disorders involving muscle degeneration, such as the Steinert myotonic dystrophy syndrome, and disorders

involving motor neurons, such as Werdnig-Hoffmann disease (Sec. 22.2). Early defects in development of the central nervous system are more common causes of positional deformations and should be seriously considered whenever a structural defect is thought to be intrinsically derived.

Fetal crowding, the common cause of an extrinsically derived deformation of prenatal onset, is usually due to a decreased volume of amniotic fluid, a situation that occurs normally during the later weeks of gestation when the fetus is undergoing extremely rapid growth. However, it also occurs abnormally with diminished fetal urinary output and chronic leakage of amniotic fluid.

Other extrinsic factors associated with the development of deformations include breech presentation and the shape of the amniotic cavity. When a fetus is in the breech position, the legs may be trapped between the body and the uterine wall. In that position, the fetus is unable to kick optimally, resulting in a 10-fold increase in the incidence of deformations. The shape of the amniotic cavity, which has profound influence on the shape of the fetus that lies within it, is influenced by many factors, including uterine shape; volume of amniotic fluid; size and shape of the fetus; presence of more than one fetus; site of placental implantation; presence of uterine tumors; shape of the abdominal cavity, which is influenced by the pelvis, sacral promontory, and neighboring abdominal organs; and tightness of abdominal musculature.

Various forms of talipes and congenital hip dislocation are the most frequently observed congenital postural deformities. Most children with these deformations are otherwise completely normal, and their prognosis is excellent. Correction usually occurs spontaneously. However, recognizing that a structural defect represents a deformation does not always imply "normal" fetal crowding and should lead to careful consideration of other etiologic possibilities that might have far greater significance to the child. For example, since decreased fetal movement can be secondary to serious neurologic abnormalities, multiple joint contractures should alert the physician to the possibility of a malformation in central nervous system development. Although congenital hip dislocations and talipes have a 2–5% recurrence risk, the vast majority of deformations are the result of physiologic crowding and have a lower recurrence risk. Deformations that are due to pathologic crowding (e.g., uterine tumors or malformation) have a much higher recurrence risk unless the factors leading to crowding are altered prior to subsequent pregnancies. Deformations that are the result of an underlying malformation (e.g., renal agenesis) have a recurrence risk similar to that of the underlying malformation.

Disruption. These defects occur when there is destruction of a previously normally formed part. At least two basic mechanisms are known to produce disruption. One involves entanglement followed by the tearing apart and/or amputation of a normally developed structure, usually a digit, arm, or leg, by strands of amnion floating within amniotic fluid, i.e., amniotic bands (Sec. 24.5). The second involves the interruption of blood supply to a developing part leading to infarction, necrosis, and/or resorption of structures distal to the insult. If interruption of blood supply occurs early in gestation, the disruptive defect which is seen at term usually involves atresia or absence of a particular part. If the infarction occurs later, necrosis is more likely to be present. Examples of disruptive single primary defects for which infarctive mechanisms have been implicated include nonduodenal intestinal atresia, gastroschisis (Sec. 12.65), and porencephaly (Sec. 21.11). The extent to which disruption of a developing structure plays a role in dysmorphogenesis is unknown.

Genetic factors play a minor role in the pathogenesis of disruptions; most are sporadic events in otherwise normal families. The prognosis for a disruptive defect is determined entirely by the extent and location of the tissue loss. Thus a child with a limb amputation has an excellent prognosis for normal function, whereas a child with porencephaly does not.

Sequence. The pattern of multiple anomalies that occurs when a single primary defect in early morphogenesis produces multiple abnormalities through a cascading process of secondary and tertiary errors in morphogenesis is called a sequence. When evaluating a child with multiple anomalies, the physician must differentiate between multiple anomalies secondary to a single localized error in morphogenesis (a sequence) and a multiple malformation syndrome. In the former recurrence risk counseling for the multiple anomalies depends entirely upon the recurrence risk for the single localized malformation.

The words malformation, deformation, and disruption sequence are used to describe only the initiating error in morphogenesis of a sequence if it is known. For example, the Robin malformation sequence (Sec. 12.5) is a pattern of multiple anomalies, all of which are produced by a single prenatal onset defect in development, mandibular hypoplasia. Since the tongue is relatively small for the oral cavity, it drops back (glossoptosis), blocking closure of the posterior palatal shelves and causing a U-shaped cleft palate. Recognizing that all of the observed defects are due to a single localized error permits recurrence risk counseling based upon the single defect.

The patient depicted in Figure 6–27 has bathrocephaly, torticollis, facial asymmetry, a dislocated hip, and valgus anomalies of both feet resulting from compression of developing fetal parts. This pattern is the breech deformation sequence. Intrauterine crowding occurred because the large-sized infant was delivered from a breech position to a small, primigravida mother; recurrence risk is therefore negligible. Recognizing the deformational nature of the abnormalities is helpful with respect to prognosis. All of the problems should resolve spontaneously or with postural therapy.

In the amniotic band disruption sequence all of the cranio-

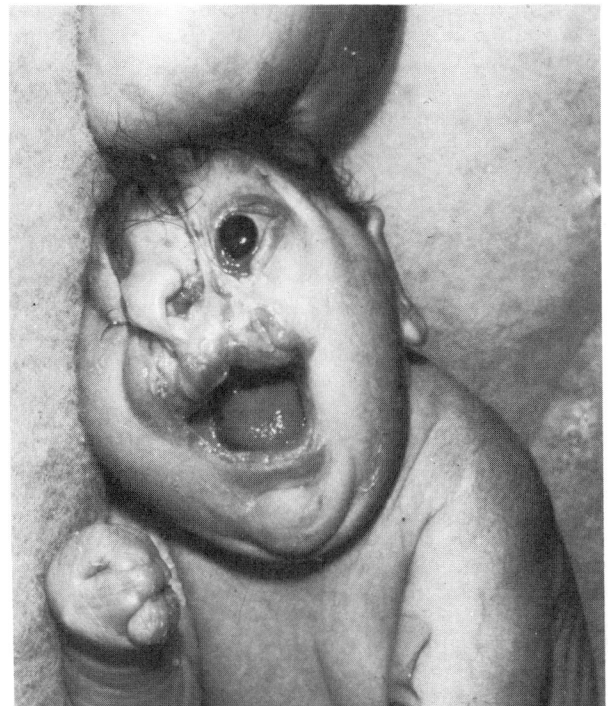

Figure 6–28. Amniotic band disruption sequence.

facial and limb defects are secondary to constrictions caused by entanglement in multiple fibrous strands of amnion extending from the placental insertion of the umbilical cord to the surface of the amnion-denuded chorion or floating freely within the chorionic sac (Fig. 6–28). These strands of amnion, which result from disruption of the normally formed membrane, can cause secondary defects through several mechanisms. Malformations occur if a strand of amnion interferes with the normal sequence of development; e.g., a strand of amnion may interrupt fusion of the facial processes so that a cleft lip results. Disruptions occur secondary to tearing apart of structures that have previously developed normally; e.g., an amniotic band might cleave areas in the developing craniofacies along lines not conforming to the normal planes of facial closure. Deformations due to fetal compression occur secondary to oligohydramnios and/or tethering of a fetal part. The former may result from rupture of both amnion and chorion, leading to chronic leakage of amniotic fluid. Tethering occurs when the fetus or one of its parts becomes immobilized by the constraining effect of an amniotic band so that it is unable to change positions and thus alter the direction along which potentially deforming forces are being directed. The recurrence risk is based upon the recurrence risk for amnion rupture; unaffected parents have not been reported to have given birth to more than one child affected with this disorder.

Multiple Malformation Syndromes. This category includes patients in whom one or more developmental anomalies of two or more systems have occurred, all of which are thought to be due to common etiology. Other than Down syndrome, with an incidence of 1:660, and XXY syndromes (1:500 males), none of these disorders occurs more frequently than 1 in 3000 live births.

Multiple malformation syndromes may be caused by chromosomal and genetic abnormalities and by teratogens. A number of these are associated with chromosome abnormalities (Sec. 6.8).

Disorders due to single mutant genes (dominant, or

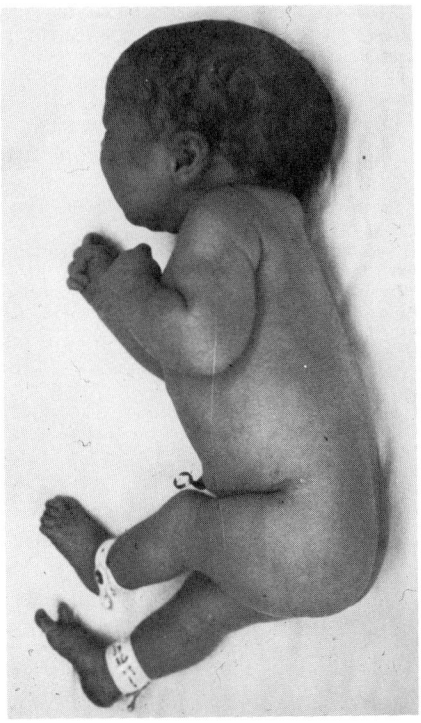

Figure 6–27. Breech deformation sequence.

X-linked in males) or to pairs of mutant genes (autosomal recessive) also cause a number of recognizable multiple malformation syndromes of prenatal onset. Their correct diagnosis depends on clinical recognitions, since in most cases there is no laboratory test to confirm the diagnosis. A family history of a similarly affected individual is extremely helpful. However, in many patients with multiple malformation syndromes of genetic etiology, the occurrence is sporadic and thus represents fresh gene mutations. In such situations, all family members are normal, and diagnosis depends entirely on evaluation of the patient's phenotype.

Disorders caused by teratogens include multiple malformation syndromes due to the effect of specific infections or of pharmacologic and/or chemical agents with which the embryo and/or fetus has come into contact during gestation. These conditions may be prevented prior to conception, particularly in the case of drugs and chemicals if the mother is aware that the agent in question can affect her baby. It is difficult, on the other hand, for a pregnant woman to avoid contact with all infectious agents.

A careful history of drug intake (Sec. 5.50–5.53) and chemical exposure (Sec. 28.16) should be obtained from the parents of all children with multiple malformation syndromes, especially when the etiology of the disorder is unknown. *A Catalog of Teratogenic Agents* by T. H. Shepard is an excellent reference for determining whether the agent the mother has been exposed to is a known teratogen.

Specific and easily distinguishable phenotypes do not exist for each of the infectious diseases which are commonly associated with altered fetal development, but intrauterine infection can frequently be suspected if there is an overall pattern of malformation (Sec. 8.68–8.73). Any patient should be suspected of having had an intrauterine infection if he or she is small for gestational age, developmentally delayed, or affected by microcephaly or hydrocephalus, ocular defects including microphthalmia, chorioretinitis, cataracts, and/or glaucoma, and hepatosplenomegaly and thrombocytopenia. Intrauterine infections have a wide spectrum of clinical manifestations from the severely affected newborn infant with multiple malformations to the child with no malformations who first manifests learning disabilities at school age.

There are also some well-recognized multiple malformation syndromes in which virtually all cases have been sporadic in otherwise normal families and the etiology is unknown. The *Cornelia de Lange syndrome*, the *Williams syndrome*, the *Prader-Willi syndrome*, and the *Rubinstein-Taybi syndrome* are the most common disorders in this category. Each occurs with a frequency greater than 1 per 10,000. Despite the lack of knowledge of etiology, experience with many children with each of these disorders has provided a vast amount of information that can be extremely helpful to parents in understanding their child's behavior and to educators in planning an appropriate curriculum. For example, a specific behavioral phenotype has been delineated for the de Lange syndrome; the parents' awareness that the child's aberrant behavior is "normal" for the de Lange syndrome rather than "their fault" can be extremely helpful in relieving their anxiety and guilt. For Williams syndrome, a characteristic psychologic profile that indicates delayed motor and perceptual development with relatively good verbal performance and sociability has been demonstrated. This knowledge of a child's particular strengths and weaknesses may allow educators to develop a curriculum that will give affected children a better chance to reach their potential.

Finally, there are certain nonrandom associations of malformations for which it has not been determined whether the pattern is a sequence or a syndrome. These are designated associations. One important clinical example is the VATER association. This acronym includes *v*ertebral defects, *a*nal atresia, *t*racheo*e*sophageal fistula with atresia, *r*adial upper limb hypoplasia, and *r*enal defects. Single umbilical artery and cardiac and genital anomalies also occur in this association. These defects are likely to occur together in almost any combination of two or more and usually represent a sporadic occurrence in an otherwise normal family.

The ultimate goal in evaluating a child with structural defects is making a specific overall diagnosis. When this is achieved, appropriate recurrence risk counseling for the parents, accurate prognostication about the child's future development, and an appropriate plan to help the child reach his or her potential usually are possible. When an overall diagnosis is lacking, the most that can be expected is a better understanding of the nature and onset of the problem, which often may be helpful to parents and to others dealing with the child.

KENNETH LYONS JONES

Bennett FC, Vanderveer B, Sells CJ: The Williams elfin facies syndrome: A psychological profile. Clin Res 25:170a, 1970.

Dunn PM: Congenital postural deformities. Br Med Bull 32:71, 1976.

Gorlin RJ, Cohen MM Jr, Pinburg JJ: Syndromes of the Head and Neck. 2nd ed. New York, McGraw-Hill, 1975.

Higginbottom MC, Jones KL, Hall BD, et al: The amniotic band disruption complex. Timing of amniotic rupture and variable spectra of consequent defects. J Pediatr 95:544, 1979.

Hobbins JC, Romero R, Grannum P, et al: Antenatal diagnosis of renal anomalies with ultrasound.

Johnson HG, Ekman P, Friesen W, et al: A behavioral phenotype in the deLange syndrome. Pediatr Res 10:843, 1976.

Kalter H, Warkany J: Congenital malformation, etiologic factors and their role in prevention. N Engl J Med 308:424, 1983.

Kazazian HH Jr: The nature of mutation. Hosp Pract, Feb, 1985, p 55.

McKusick VA: Mendelian Inheritance in Man. Catalog of Autosomal Dominant, Autosomal Recessive and X-linked Phenotypes. 5th ed. Baltimore, The Johns Hopkins University Press, 1978.

Shepard TH: A Catalog of Teratogenic Agents. 5th ed. Baltimore, The Johns Hopkins University Press, 1986.

Smith DW: Recognizable Patterns of Human Malformation. 3rd ed. Philadelphia, WB Saunders, 1982.

7

INBORN ERRORS OF METABOLISM

7.1 INTRODUCTION

Many disorders originate in mutational events that alter the genetic constitution of an individual, disrupting normal function. Hundreds of human hereditary biochemical disorders, termed "inborn errors of metabolism" by Garrod at the turn of the century, have been discovered, and they are continually being discovered.

Now modern biochemical genetics can describe how genetic information is translated into the synthesis of proteins having specific metabolic or structural properties (see Chapter 6). An inherited mutational event can result in the alteration of either primary protein structure or the amount of the specific protein being synthesized. In either case, the functional ability of the protein, whether it is an enzyme, receptor, transport vehicle, membrane pump, or structural element, may be relatively or seriously compromised.

If the process affected by an inborn error of metabolism is essential for well-being and if the degree of alteration is sufficient to affect the system, clinical consequences may result. Some genetic changes are clinically inconsequential and are responsible only for the many polymorphic differences that set individuals apart. Others produce changes that express themselves only under conditions that may not be encountered during the lifetime of an individual. Still others, however, produce a disease state, which may range from very mild to lethal. Most inborn errors of metabolism exhibiting clinical consequences manifest themselves (or can be detected) in the newborn period or shortly thereafter. It is also now possible to screen and detect many of these disorders in utero (Sec. 8.13).

This chapter covers primarily inborn errors of metabolism of amino acids, carbohydrates, lipids, purines and pyrimidines, heme pigments, mucopolysaccharides, and a few other enzymes and proteins of interest; the approach to diagnosis is emphasized. Discussions of the hemoglobinopathies and disorders of clotting mechanisms are presented in Chapter 15, defects of cellular transport in Sec. 12.59–12.60, defects of hormone synthesis in Chapter 19, and defects of immunoglobulin synthesis in Chapter 10.

Children with inborn errors of metabolism may present with one or more of a large variety of signs and symptoms (Table 7–1). These may include metabolic acidosis (Table 7–2), failure to thrive, developmental abnormalities, elevated blood or urine levels of a particular metabolite, e.g., an amino acid or ammonia, a peculiar odor (Table 7–3), or physical changes such as hepatomegaly. Diagnosis is facilitated by considering the neonatal period separately from children presenting later in life.

Neonatal Period. Inborn errors of metabolism causing *clinical manifestations* in the neonatal period are usually severe and are often lethal if proper therapy is not promptly initiated. Clinical findings are usually nonspecific and similar to those seen in infants with generalized infections. An inborn error of metabolism should be considered in the differential diagnosis of a severely ill neonatal infant, and special studies should be undertaken if the index of suspicion is high (Fig. 7–1).

Neonatal infants with metabolic disorders are usually normal at birth; however, signs and symptoms such as lethargy, poor feeding, convulsions, and vomiting may develop as early as a few hours after birth. A history of clinical deterioration in a previously normal neonate should suggest an inborn error of metabolism. This clinical course contrasts with most other genetic disorders or perinatal insults, which cause abnormalities from the time of birth. Occasionally, vomiting may be severe enough to suggest the diagnosis of pyloric stenosis, which is usually not present, although it has simultaneously occurred in such infants. Lethargy, poor feeding, convulsions, and coma may also be seen in infants with hypoglycemia (Sec. 8.57) or hypocalcemia (Sec. 5.34). Response to intravenous injection of glucose or calcium usually establishes these diagnoses. Since most inborn errors of metabolism are inherited as autosomal recessive traits, a history of consanguinity and/or death in the neonatal period in the immediate family should increase suspicion. Physical examination usually reveals nonspecific findings with most signs related to the central nervous system. Hepatomegaly, how-

Table 7–1. **Some Clinical Findings Often Associated with Inborn Errors of Metabolism**

Symptoms or Signs	Associated Diseases
Neurologic abnormalities	Almost all categories
Metabolic acidosis with ketosis	See Table 7–2
Pernicious vomiting	Isovaleric acidemia, urea cycle or amino acid defects, methylmalonic acidemia, propionic acidemia, PKU, valinemia, α-methylacetoacetic acidemia, adrenal insufficiency, carnitine deficiency, multiple acyl-CoA dehydrogenase deficiency
Liver disease	Tyrosinemia, glycogen storage, galactosemia, Wilson disease, hereditary fructose intolerance, α₁-antitrypsin deficiency, cystic fibrosis, hemochromatosis, lipidoses

Miscellaneous
  Clinical: dislocated lenses, renal stones, thrombosis, deafness, microcephaly, cataracts, hematuria, self-mutilation, abnormal urine odor (see Table 7–3) or color, coarse facies, persistent eczema, abnormal hair
  Laboratory: osteoporosis, rickets, hypoglycemia, unexplained jaundice, bony x-ray change, increased anion gap, ketoacidosis, abnormal liver function

Table 7–2. **Inborn Errors of Metabolism That May Have Metabolic Acidosis as a Major Component**

Disease	Major Metabolites (Acids)
AMINOACIDOPATHIES	
1. Maple syrup urine disease	α-Ketoisocaproic, α-keto-β-methylvaleric, α-ketoisovaleric, indoleacetic, ketones*
2. Isovaleric acidemia	Isovaleric, N-isovalerylglycine, β-hydroxyisovaleric, ketones*
3. 3-Methylcrotonylglycinuria	3-Methylcrotonylglycine, β-hydroxyisovaleric, 2-oxoglutaric, ketones*
4. 3-Hydroxy-3-methylglutaric aciduria	3-Hydroxyisovaleric, 3-methylglutaric, 3-methylglutaconic, 3-hydroxy-3-methylglutaric
5. α-Methylacetoacetic aciduria	α-Methyl-β-hydroxybutyric, α-methylacetoacetic, ketones*
6. Propionic acidemia	Propionic, propionylglycine, β-hydroxypropionate, methylcitric, ketones*
7. Methylmalonic acidemia	Methylmalonic, ketones*
8. Pyroglutamic acidemia	Pyroglutamic (5-oxoproline)
9. α-Ketoadipic aciduria	α-Ketoadipic, α-hydroxyadipic, α-aminoadipic,1,2-butenedicarboxylic
10. Glutaric acidemia	Glutaric, lactic, isobutyric, isovaleric, α-methylbutyric
11. Multiple carboxylase deficiency	α- and β-Hydroxybutyric, 3-hydroxyisovaleric, propionic, 3-methylcrotonylglycine, lactic ketones*
12. Hawkinsinuria	4-Hydroxycyclohexylacetic, hawkinsin
ORGANIC ACIDEMIAS	
13. Multiple acyl-CoA dehydrogenase deficiency (glutaric acidemia type II)	2-Ethylmalonic, adipic, glutaric, C8 and C10 dicarboxylic, ω-hydroxy acids, glutaric hexanoylglycine, ketones*
14. Ethylmalonic aciduria	2-Ethylmalonic, adipic
15. γ-Hydroxybutyric aciduria	γ-Hydroxybutyric
DEFECTS IN CARBOHYDRATE METABOLISM	
16. Diabetes mellitus	Lactic, ketones*
17. Fructose-1,6-diphosphatase deficiency	Lactic, pyruvic, ketones*
18. Succinyl-CoA transferase deficiency	Ketones*
19. Glycogen storage disease, type I	Lactic, pyruvic, ketones*
20. Pyruvate carboxylase deficiency	Lactic, pyruvic
21. Pyruvate dehydrogenase complex deficiency	Lactic, pyruvic

*Acetoacetic and β-hydroxybutyric.
Diagnosis of the diseases listed among the aminoacidopathies can be made through detection of the corresponding metabolite in urine by various techniques such as column or gas or high pressure liquid chromatography or by measuring enzyme activity in cultures of skin fibroblasts. Of the carbohydrate defects, only succinyl-CoA transferase deficiency can be detected in fibroblasts. Deficiency of fructose-1,6-diphosphatase can be demonstrated in white cells. Glycogen storage type I and pyruvate carboxylase defects must be detected in liver biopsies. In addition to the above, acidosis has been reported in a patient with acute tyrosinemia and in patients with oxalosis and renal tubular acidosis, in whom persistent acidosis is due primarily to a renal defect rather than being a direct effect of the metabolic error.

Table 7–3. Inborn Errors of Amino Acid Metabolism Associated with Abnormal Odor of Urine

Inborn Error of Metabolism	Urine Odor
Glutaric acidemia (type II)	Sweaty feet
Phenylketonuria	Mousy or musty
Maple syrup urine disease	Maple syrup
Isovaleric acidemia	Sweaty feet
β-Methylcrotonylglycinuria	Tomcat urine
Methionine malabsorption	Cabbage
Trimethylaminuria	Rotting fish
Tyrosinemia	Rancid, fishy, or cabbage
Oasthouse disease	Hoplike
Hawkinsinuria	Swimming pool

ever, is a common finding in a variety of inborn errors of metabolism. Occasionally, an unusual odor may offer an invaluable aid to the diagnosis (Table 7–3). A physician caring for a sick infant should smell the patient and his or her excretions; patients with maple syrup urine disease have the unmistakable odor of maple syrup in their urine and their bodies.

Diagnosis usually requires a variety of specific *laboratory studies.* Measuring serum concentrations of ammonia, bicarbonate, and pH is often very helpful to differentiate major causes of metabolic disorders (Fig. 7–1). Elevation of blood ammonia is usually due to defects in urea cycle enzymes. These infants with elevated blood ammonia commonly have normal serum pH and bicarbonate, and without measurement of blood ammonia they may remain undiagnosed and succumb to their disease.

Elevation of serum ammonia, however, has also been observed in some infants with certain organic acidemias. These infants are severely acidotic because of accumulation of organic acids in body fluids.

When blood ammonia, pH, and bicarbonate are normal, other aminoacidopathies such as hyperglycinemia and galactosemia should be considered; galactosemic infants may also manifest cataracts, hepatomegaly, ascites, and jaundice.

Most inborn errors of metabolism presenting in the neonatal period are lethal if specific *therapy* is not initiated immediately. Specific diagnosis, even in an infant in whom death seems inevitable, is of great importance for genetic counseling of the family. Therefore, every effort should be made to determine the diagnosis while the infant is alive; postmortem examination is usually not helpful.

Children after the Neonatal Period. Most inborn errors of metabolism that cause symptoms in the first few days of life exhibit milder variant forms having a more insidious onset. These forms may escape detection during the neonatal period, and the diagnosis may be delayed for months or even years. The early clinical manifestations in children with these forms are commonly nonspecific and may be attributed to perinatal insults.

Clinical manifestations such as mental retardation, motor deficit, and convulsions are the most constant findings in some of these children. There may be an episodic or intermittent pattern with episodes of acute clinical manifestations separated by periods of seemingly disease-free states. The episodes are usually triggered by a stress or a nonspecific insult such as an infection. The child may die during one of these acute attacks. An inborn error of metabolism should be considered in any child with one or more of the following

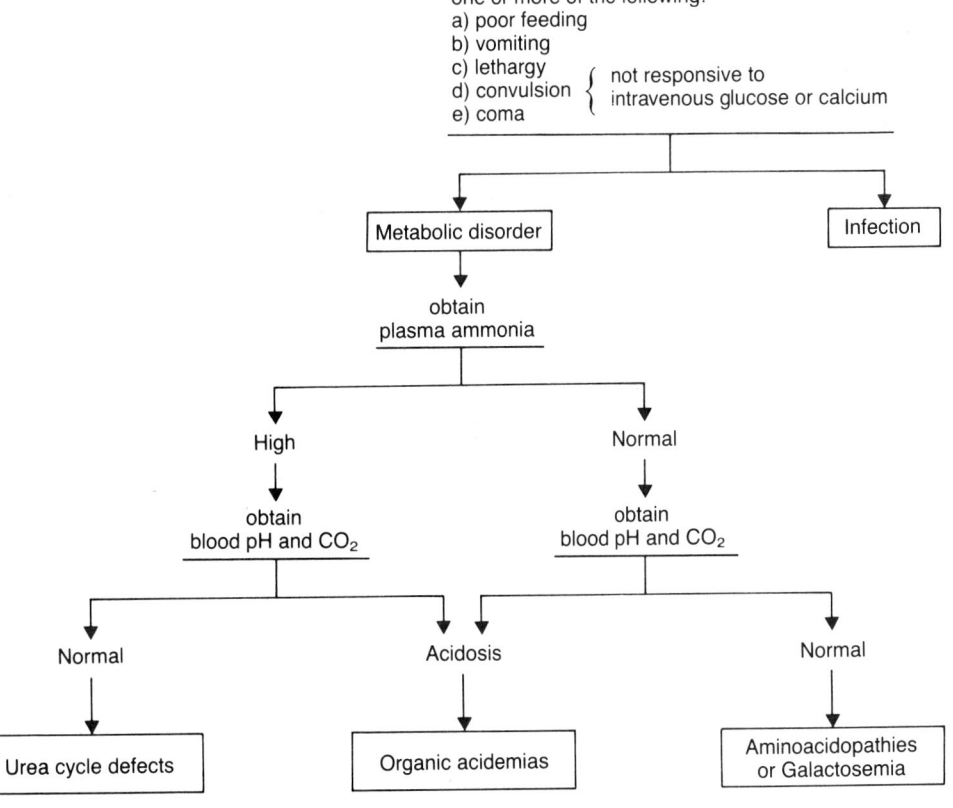

Figure 7–1. Clinical approach to a newborn infant with a suspected metabolic disorder. This schema is a guide to the elucidation of some of the metabolic disorders in newborn infants. Although some exceptions to this schema exist, it is appropriate for the large majority of cases.

manifestations: (1) unexplained mental retardation, developmental delay, motor deficits, or convulsion; (2) unusual odor, particularly during an acute illness; (3) intermittent episodes of unexplained vomiting, acidosis, mental deterioration, or coma; (4) hepatomegaly; or (5) renal stones.

Inborn errors of metabolism of a given pedigree run true to type. Thus, although symptomatology may vary among sib-lings, usually if one child in a family has the form of maple syrup urine disease manifested during the neonatal period, the next affected sibling will have the same defect, not the variant that occurs only intermittently later in childhood.

IRAJ REZVANI
VICTOR H. AUERBACH

DEFECTS IN METABOLISM OF AMINO ACIDS

7.2 PHENYLALANINE

Phenylalanine is an essential amino acid. Dietary phenylalanine not utilized for protein synthesis is normally degraded via the tyrosine pathway (Fig. 7–2). Deficiency of the enzyme phenylalanine hydroxylase, or of its cofactor tetrahydrobiopterin, causes accumulation of phenylalanine in body fluids. Several clinically and biochemically distinct forms of hyperalaninemia exist.

Classic Phenylketonuria (PKU). This form of the disorder is caused by the complete or near complete deficiency of phenylalanine hydroxylase. Excess phenylalanine is transaminated to phenylpyruvic acid or decarboxylated to phenylethylamine. These and subsequent metabolites, along with excess phenylalanine, disrupt normal metabolism and cause brain damage.

Clinical Manifestations. The affected infant is normal at birth. Mental retardation may develop gradually and may not be evident for a few months. It has been estimated that an untreated infant loses about 50 points in IQ by the end of the 1st year of life. Mental retardation is usually severe and most patients require institutional care. Vomiting, sometimes severe enough to be misdiagnosed as pyloric stenosis, may be an early symptom. Older untreated children become hyperactive with purposeless movements, rhythmic rocking, and athetosis.

On physical examination these infants are blonder than unaffected siblings; they have fair skin and blue eyes. Some may have a seborrheic or eczematoid skin rash, which is usually mild and disappears as the child grows older. These children have an unusual odor of phenylacetic acid, which has been described as musty, mousey, or wolf-like. There are no consistent findings on neurologic examination. However, most infants are hypertonic with hyperactive deep tendon reflexes. About one fourth of children have seizures, and more than 50% have EEG abnormalities. Microcephaly, prominent maxilla with widely spaced teeth, enamel hypoplasia, and growth retardation are other common findings in untreated children. The clinical manifestations of classic PKU are rarely seen in those countries in which neonatal screening programs for the detection of PKU are in effect.

Diagnosis. Infants with PKU are clinically normal at birth, and tests of their urine for phenylpyruvic acid may be negative in the first few days of life; accordingly, the diagnosis depends on measuring blood levels of phenylalanine. The bacterial inhibition assay method of Guthrie is widely used in the newborn period to screen for PKU. This test requires a few drops of capillary blood, which are placed on a filter paper and mailed to the laboratory for assay. Blood phenylalanine in affected infants may rise to levels necessary to render the Guthrie test positive as early as 4 hr after birth in the absence of any protein feeding. It is recommended, however, that the blood for screening be obtained after 72 hours of life and preferably after feeding proteins in order to reduce the possibility of false negative results. When this test indicates an elevated level of phenylalanine, the phenylalanine and tyrosine concentrations of the plasma should be measured. The criteria for diagnosis of classic PKU are: (1) a plasma phenylalanine level above 20 mg/dL; (2) a normal plasma tyrosine level; (3) increased urinary levels of metabolites of phenylalanine (phenylpyruvic and o-hydroxyphenylacetic acids); (4) an inability to tolerate an oral challenge of phenylalanine; and (5) a normal concentration of the cofactor tetrahydrobiopterin.

Treatment. The goal of therapy is to reduce phenylalanine and its metabolites in body fluids in order to prevent or minimize brain damage. This can be achieved by a diet low in phenylalanine; formulas low in this essential amino acid are now available commercially.* The administration of the low phenylalanine diet requires close nutritional supervision and frequent monitoring of the serum concentration of phenylalanine. The optimal serum level to be maintained probably lies between 2 and 9 mg/dL. Because phenylalanine is not synthesized in the body, "overtreatment," particularly in rapidly growing infants, may lead to phenylalanine deficiency, manifested by lethargy, anorexia, anemia, rashes, diarrhea, and even death; moreover, tyrosine becomes an essential amino acid in this disorder and its adequate intake must be assured. Dietary treatment should be started as soon after birth as the diagnosis is established.

The duration of diet therapy is controversial. Although rigid diet control may be relaxed after 6 yr of age, some form of restriction in dietary phenylalanine may be necessary indefinitely. The dietary management is almost inevitably complicated by emotional problems resulting from dietary restriction and the abnormal eating habits imposed upon child and family. The maintenance of adequate dietary control without psychologic problems is achieved with difficulty, and parents and children need continuous skillful and empathetic support and guidance.

Pregnancy in Mothers with PKU. Pregnant women with PKU who are not on a low phenylalanine diet have a higher risk of spontaneous abortion than the general population. Infants born to such mothers are often mentally retarded and may have microcephaly and/or a congenital heart anomaly. These complications seem to be related to high levels of blood phenylalanine. Prospective mothers who have PKU should be started on a low phenylalanine diet before conception, and every effort should be made to keep blood phenylalanine below 10 mg/dL throughout pregnancy.

Phenylketonuria due to Deficiency of Cofactor Tetrahydrobiopterin (BH₄). In about 2% of infants with hyperphenylalaninemia the defect resides in one of the enzymes necessary for production of BH_4. These infants deteriorate neurologically despite adequate control of serum phenylalanine because BH_4 is also the cofactor for tyrosine and tryptophan hydroxylases, which are essential for biosynthesis of the neurotransmitters dopamine and serotonin. BH_4 is synthesized from guanosine triphosphate, and at least three enzyme deficiencies leading

---

*Dietary management with this milk substitute is described in "Phenylketonuria"—Low Phenylalanine Dietary Management with Lofenalac, a pamphlet available from Mead Johnson Laboratories, Evansville, Indiana 47721.

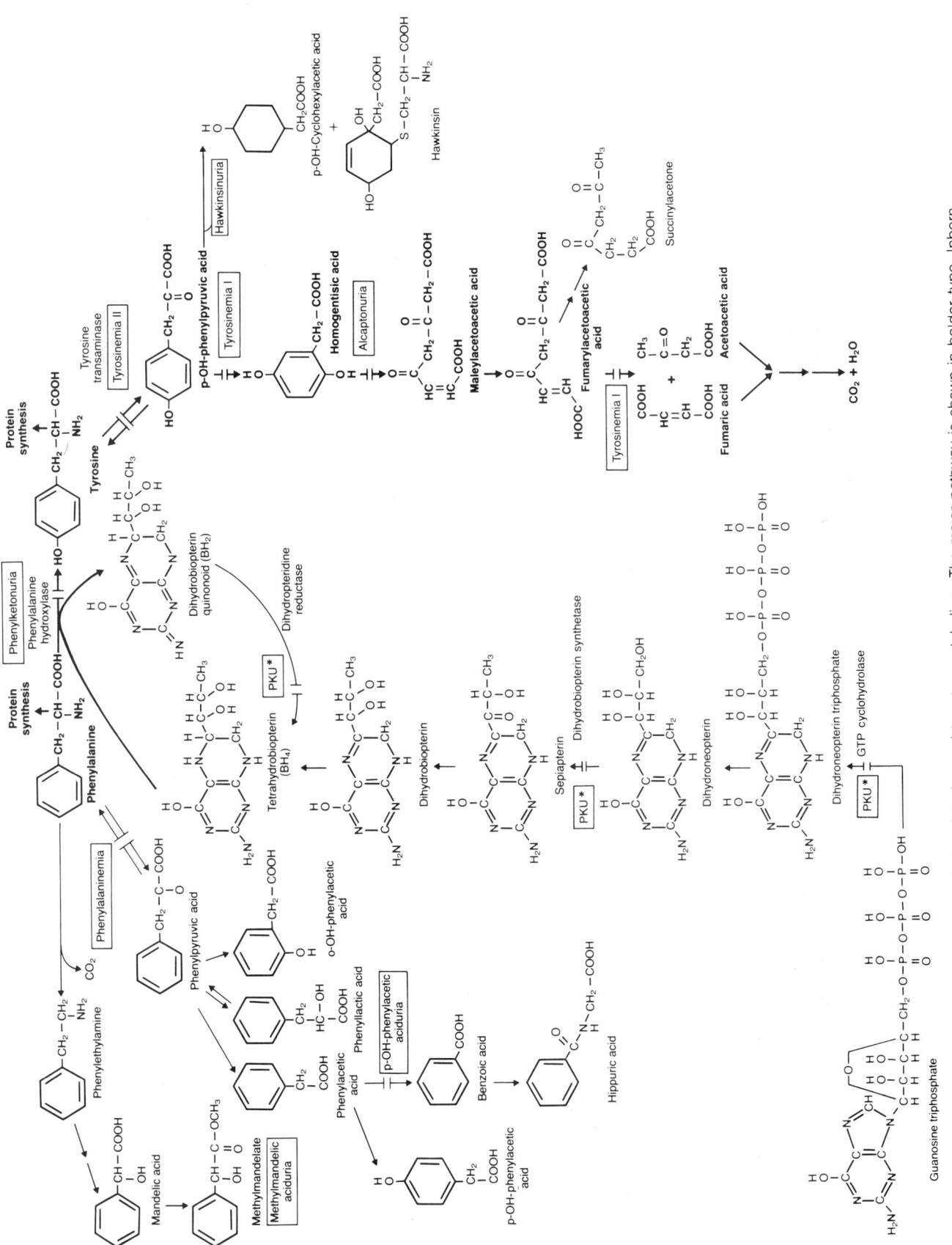

Figure 7-2. Pathways of phenylalanine and tyrosine metabolism. The major pathway is shown in bolder type. Inborn errors are depicted as bars crossing the reaction arrow(s). PKU⁺ refers to defects of BH₄ metabolism that affect the phenylalanine, tyrosine, and tryptophan hydroxylases. See Figures 7–3 and 7–5.

to deficiency of BH$_4$ have been described (Fig. 7–2). About half of the reported patients have had a deficiency of dihydrobiopterin synthetase and the other half have had a deficiency of dihydropteridine reductase. Only two patients with a deficiency of guanosine triphosphate cyclohydroxylase have been reported.

Clinical Manifestations. The majority of the infants are indistinguishable from those with classic PKU during the first few months of life. Neurologic manifestations develop despite adequate diet therapy.

Diagnosis. BH$_4$ deficiency and the responsible enzyme defect may be established by one of the following:

1. Measuring neopterin and biopterin in body fluids (urine, plasma, spinal fluid). In patients with biopterin synthetase deficiency there will be a marked elevation of neopterin and a concomitant decrease in biopterin (neopterin/biopterin ratio is high). In infants with reductase deficiency the ratio of neopterin/biopterin will be low.

2. BH$_4$ loading test: An oral dose of BH$_4$ (7–10 mg/kg) normalizes plasma phenylalanine in affected infants within 4–6 hr.

3. Enzyme assay: The activity of dihydropteridine reductase can be measured in many tissues such as liver, leukocytes, red cells, and cultured fibroblasts. Dihydrobiopterin synthetase can be measured in liver, kidney, and possibly red blood cells. GTP cyclohydrolase can be measured in liver and in phytohemagglutinin-stimulated lymphocytes.

Treatment. The long-term efficacy of various therapies is unknown and include:

1. Low phenylalanine diet. Although phenylalanine does not prevent neurological damage, such a diet in conjunction with the following therapies is recommended for at least the first 2 yr of life. High levels of phenylalanine inhibit synthesis of neurotransmitters.

2. Neurotransmitter precursors: Administering L-dopa and 5-hydroxytryptophan seems to be the most effective treatment and may prevent neurological damage if started early in life. *All patients with PKU and hyperphenylalaninemia should be tested for BH$_4$ deficiency.* Treatment started after 6 months of age, although resulting in some improvement, has not reversed existing neurological damage.

3. BH$_4$ replacement: Oral administration of the cofactor in small daily doses normalizes serum levels of phenylalanine. This compound, unless given at high doses (20–40 mg/kg/24 hr), does not readily cross the blood-brain barrier, and neurological damage may continue to progress.

Persistent Hyperphenylalaninemia. Occasionally identified are infants with hyperphenylalaninemia whose blood levels of phenylalanine are only slightly elevated; these concentrations are insufficient (less than 15–20 mg/dL) to result in the excretion of phenylpyruvic acid. Like infants with classic PKU, these patients presumably have a deficiency of the phenylalanine hydroxylase enzyme but with some residual enzyme activity; measured activity has ranged from 1 to 35% of normal, in contrast to the nondetectable enzyme activity found in classic PKU. These infants have been detected by screening tests in the neonatal period; they are asymptomatic and may develop normally without special dietary treatment. They should, however, be tested for the presence of the cofactor tetrahydrobiopterin, and if it is deficient they should be treated accordingly (see above).

For infants who have serum phenylalanine concentrations in the range of 10–20 mg/dL, with normal tyrosine values and no PKU, a simple reduction of dietary protein intake may be sufficient to control serum concentrations of phenylalanine; if this is not effective, specific restriction of dietary phenylalanine is indicated. All infants who are not treated with dietary restriction should be systematically monitored with repeated urine and blood tests and with developmental evaluations to establish the safety of continuing partial treatment or nontreatment. Periodic challenges with natural protein may be helpful in determining the need for continuing dietary restriction.

Transient Hyperphenylalaninemia. Moderately elevated levels of phenylalanine occur in transient tyrosinemia of the newborn infant (Sec. 7.3). When the infant's ability to oxidize tyrosine matures, the elevated levels of tyrosine and phenylalanine return to normal.

Absence of or delayed maturation of phenylalanine transaminase can also produce phenylalaninemia if the patient is being fed milk with a high protein content. Such infants cannot produce much phenylpyruvic acid even when their blood levels of phenylalanine approach 30 mg/dL; they have normal blood levels when fed milk products having the protein content of human milk.

Genetics and Prevalence. All defects causing persistent hyperphenylalaninemia and PKU are inherited as autosomal recessives. They have a collective prevalence of 1:10,000 to 1:20,000 live births, with classic PKU being the most common and GTP cyclohydrolase the rarest. Prenatal diagnosis and carrier detection is possible using specific genetic probes and chorionic villus biopsy.

Methylmandelic Aciduria. Ataxia, convulsions, and mental retardation have been associated with excretion of large amounts of methylmandelic acid. This compound results from the further oxidation of phenylethylamine, the decarboxylated product of phenylalanine. Symptoms are produced by high protein feeding and reduced by the restriction of protein to 0.5 gm/kg/24 hr.

Parahydroxyphenylacetic Aciduria. Patients with growth retardation who may also have cardiomegaly, hepatomegaly, hypotonia, and anemia are known to excrete excessive amounts of *p*-hydroxyphenylacetate. Excretion of the latter compound was influenced directly by the ingestion of phenylalanine but was independent of tyrosine intake. These patients excreted no appreciable amounts of hippurate. The latter was formed when benzoate was fed. A defect in the conversion of phenylacetic acid to benzoic acid and then to hippuric acid has been postulated (Fig. 7–2).

7.3 TYROSINE

Tyrosine, obtained from ingested protein and synthesized endogenously from phenylalanine, is used for protein synthesis and is a precursor of dopamine, norepinephrine, epinephrine, melanin, and thyroxine. Excess tyrosine is metabolized to carbon dioxide and water (Fig. 7–2). At least two distinct clinical entities are associated with a persistent increase in plasma concentrations of tyrosine, but only in tyrosinemia type II are signs and symptoms attributed to high levels of tyrosine in body fluids. In hereditary tyrosinemia type I the causal relationship with increased tyrosine levels remains unclear. There are also patients who present varied clinical findings and tyrosinemia but do not fit into any specific category, and a transient form of tyrosinemia is seen in newborn infants.

Tyrosinemia Type I (Tyrosinosis, Hereditary Tyrosinemia, Hepatorenal Tyrosinemia). In this condition a moderate elevation of serum tyrosine is associated with severe involvement of liver, kidney, and central nervous system. The pathogenesis of this disorder is controversial. Although deficiency of the enzymes *p*-hydroxyphenylpyruvic acid oxidase and fumarylacetoacetate hydrolase have been shown in these patients, it is unclear whether they are the causes of the condition or secondary to liver damage. Marked elevation of serum α-fetoprotein may occur in the cord blood before any elevation in serum tyrosine, indicating liver damage in utero before tyrosinemia and other clinical manifestations become evident.

Clinical Manifestations. There are two forms of the disease: the neonatal or acute form, which comprises most reported cases, and the chronic or late form. Intermediate forms also occur.

Infants having the *acute form* become symptomatic within the first 6 mo of life. Failure to thrive, developmental delay, irritability, vomiting, diarrhea, and fever are among the early manifestations. Hepatomegaly, jaundice, hypoglycemia, and bleeding tendencies, as manifested by melena, hematuria, and ecchymosis, are common findings. A cabbage-like odor of some infants is related to metabolites of methionine. Death from hepatic failure usually occurs before the 2nd yr of life.

In the *chronic form* clinical manifestations may not be present until after 1 yr of age. Failure to thrive, developmental delay, progressive cirrhosis, renal tubular dysfunction (Fanconi syndrome), and vitamin D–resistant rickets are characteristic. Death usually occurs by 10 yr of age from liver failure or hepatoma.

Tyrosinemia type I is an autosomal recessive trait. Most reported patients have a French-Canadian ancestry.

Laboratory Findings. These include normocytic anemia and marked elevations of serum bilirubin (both conjugated and unconjugated), serum transaminases (SGOT and SGPT), and α-fetoprotein. Plasma levels of tyrosine and other amino acids, especially methionine, are moderately increased. Generalized amino aciduria occurs. The presence of succinylacetoacetate and succinylacetone in serum and urine is diagnostic (Fig. 7–2). Liver histology is usually compatible with nonspecific cirrhosis. Hyperplasia of pancreatic islet cells is also a common finding.

Treatment. Diets low in tyrosine, phenylalanine, and methionine do not change the clinical course in most patients. However, because of their beneficial effect in some patients, a trial of diet therapy is indicated in all patients with this type of tyrosinemia. Liver transplant for patients who develop hepatoma appears promising.

Tyrosinemia Type II (Richner-Hanhart Syndrome, Oculocutaneous Tyrosinemia). This rare autosomal recessive disorder results in mental retardation, palmar and plantar punctate hyperkeratosis, and herpetiform corneal ulcers. Corneal lesions usually occur during the first few months of life and are presumed to be due to tyrosine deposition; skin lesions may develop later in life. Mental retardation is usually mild to moderate and may be associated with self-mutilation.

Significant hypertyrosinemia (20 to 50 mg/dL) and tyrosyluria are present. The condition is due to the deficiency of the cytosol fraction of hepatic tyrosine amino transferase (tyrosine transaminase). In contrast to tyrosinemia type I, liver and kidney functions, as well as serum concentrations of other amino acids, are normal.

Treatment with a diet low in tyrosine and phenylalanine has not only corrected the chemical abnormalities but has also resulted in dramatic healing of the skin and eye lesions. Mental retardation may be prevented by early dietary restriction of tyrosine.

Transient Tyrosinemia of the Newborn. In 0.5–10% of newborn infants, plasma tyrosine may rise to as high as 60 mg/dL during the first 2 wk of life. Most affected infants are premature and are receiving high protein diets. Lethargy, poor feeding, and decreased motor activity occurs in some of them, but most are asymptomatic, and come to medical attention because of a high blood phenylalanine level, rendering the Guthrie test for PKU positive. Tyrosinemia usually resolves spontaneously during the lst mo of life. The condition is presumably due to delayed maturation of p-hydroxyphenylpyruvic acid oxidase and is often corrected by administration of vitamin C. Since vitamin C is necessary for optimal func-

tioning of the oxidase, it is not surprising that tyrosinemia occurs in scurvy. Mild intellectual deficits have been reported in some of the fullterm infants with this disorder.

Other Types of Tyrosinemia. There are patients with tyrosinemia who cannot be placed in any unified category. For example, the first reported case of tyrosinemia was in a 49 yr old male with myasthenia gravis who excreted more than 1 g/day of p-hydroxyphenylpyruvic acid, as well as other oxidative products of tyrosine. Plasma tyrosine could not be measured at that time, and the site of enzyme deficiency remains speculative, although tyrosine loading in this patient and measurement of urinary metabolites helped establish that dihydroxphenylalanine was synthesized from tyrosine. A very similar patient has been reported subsequently in whom the activity of p-hydroxyphenylpyruvic acid oxidase was 5% of normal. This patient was mildly retarded and had a seizure disorder; plasma concentration of tyrosine was 11.6 mg/dL. At least four other reports note patients with tyrosinemia and mental retardation for whom the exact cause of elevated plasma tyrosine and its metabolites remains unclear.

Hawkinsinuria. This form of tyrosyluria (named after the first affected family described) is inherited as an autosomal dominant trait. All the affected individuals have been presumed to be heterozygous for the condition. Adults are without symptoms, but infants have severe metabolic acidosis, ketosis, failure to thrive, and a transient tyrosinemia. Infants respond well to a diet low in both phenylalanine and tyrosine and their clinical manifestations resolve spontaneously by about 1 yr of age. There is no mental retardation or liver disease.

Affected children and adults excrete p-hydroxyphenylpyruvic and p-hydroxyphenylacetic acids as well as two very unusual organic acids in their urine, 4-hydroxycyclohexylacetic acid (4-HCAA) and (2-L-cystein-S-yl-1-4, dihydroxycyclohex-5-en-1-yl)-acetic acid (hawkinsin) (Fig. 7–2). Both of these latter compounds arise from tyrosine and are presumed to be the unnatural products of a partial block of the enzyme p-hydroxyphenylpyruvic acid oxidase, whose normal product is homogentisic acid.

The activity of p-hydroxyphenylpyruvic acid oxidase is presumed to be absent or totally inactive in some of the forms of tyrosinemia described above; however, in hawkinsinuria it is postulated that all of the enzyme produced is capable of binding with p-hydroxyphenylpyruvic acid, but only the normal half can carry out the oxidative decarboxylation to the level of homogentisic acid. The abnormal half of the enzyme forms the usual substrate complex, resulting in an epoxide intermediate which is immediately released from the enzyme before the side chain can shift to form homogentisic acid. The epoxide is then either reduced to 4-HCAA or partially reduced and coupled with cysteine to form hawkinsin. The compounds would not be expected to be found in either heterozygotes or in homozygotes with an abnormal p-hydroxyphenylpyruvic acid oxidase. Hawkinsinuria is another example of the value of using one of nature's mistakes to investigate the intricacies of a biochemical pathway that might not be amenable to study in normal individuals.

Albinism. This metabolic defect, one of the oldest recognized in man, is described in the Bible. There are at least three major genetic forms: generalized albinism (also known as oculocutaneous albinism), which is inherited as an autosomal recessive; partial albinism, which is inherited as dominant; and albinism restricted to the eye, which is inherited as a sex-linked trait.

Oculocutaneous Albinism. Generalized albinism (Sec. 24.11) is a defect in the formation of the pigment melanin. There are at least 6 variants. In the most common form, tyrosinase is not active. In the 2nd type, tyrosinase is present in the melanosome; thus, tyrosine can be converted to dopa and then to dopa quinone, but the permease for the transport of tyrosine into the melanosome is presumably absent (Fig. 7–3). In both the tyrosinase negative and tyrosinase positive types of albinism neither melanin nor pheomelanin can be formed; single hair roots incubated in tyrosine can be used to differentiate these two variants, since in the former no melanin is synthesized in the hair bulb, whereas in the latter obvious darkening is noted. A third type, found among the Amish, is due to a defect in an unidentified enzymatic step between dopa quinone and melanin. Affected patients can produce pheomelanin, a yellowish pigment, from dopa quinone; they develop normal skin color, but their ocular signs persist through life.

Three additional rare forms have been described. In the *Chédiak-Higashi syndrome* (Sec. 10.32) the major features include incomplete oculocutaneous albinism, neutropenia, and susceptibility to pyogenic infections. The *Hermansky-Pudlak syndrome* is an autosomal recessive disorder characterized by oculocutaneous albinism and a hemorrhagic diathesis, in which there appears to be defective glutathione peroxidase activity. The *Cross syndrome* was first described in a consanguineous Amish family with four affected children, who presented with hypopigmentation, gingival fibromatosis, spasticity, athetoid movements, and microphthalmia.

Albinism occurs in all races, varying in incidence from 1 in 140 in the San Blas Indians of Panama to 1 in 100,000 in France. In the United States, the rate is approximately 1 in 20,000. It is transmitted as an autosomal recessive characteristic. Normal children have been born to parents both of whom had generalized albinism, but of different allelic forms.

In addition to extremely fair skin and fine silky hair, albinos have numerous ocular abnormalities. Traces of pigment may occur on the uveal borders, but it is absent from the iris, sclera, and fundus, and the iris appears gray or blue. Refractive errors, strabismus, nystagmus, and photophobia are common. Persistent loss of visual acuity and a red reflex are present in all tyrosinase-negative individuals. In tyrosinase-positive persons, the poor visual acuity may improve with age; the red reflex is found in white children and adults.

Other Forms. Partial albinism is characterized by localized areas of skin and hair devoid of pigment and is inherited as a dominant trait. In some instances a white forelock or a patch of depigmented hair elsewhere may be the sole manifestation.

In *albinism limited to the eye*, the depigmentation may be limited to the retina or may also involve the iris. Visual acuity is decreased, and nystagmus is present. Since this defect is sex-linked, this biochemical defect must be different from those occurring in generalized or oculocutaneous albinism. *Waardenburg syndrome* (Sec. 24.11) must be considered in the differential diagnosis of partial albinism.

Alcaptonuria. This disorder of tyrosine metabolism is characterized by accumulation in the body and excretion in the urine of homogentisic acid (Fig. 7–2) and its oxidation products. It is transmitted by an autosomal recessive gene. Defective activity of the enzyme homogentisic acid oxidase arrests the catabolism of tyrosine, and large amounts of homogentisic acid are excreted in the urine.

Urine from affected patients becomes black on standing because of oxidation and polymerization of homogentisic acid. The darkness of the stain increases with continued exposure to air; a dried diaper has a pitch-black stain. The abnormality is usually noted in infancy, but in some instances the dark urine has not been observed until the 2nd or 3rd decade of

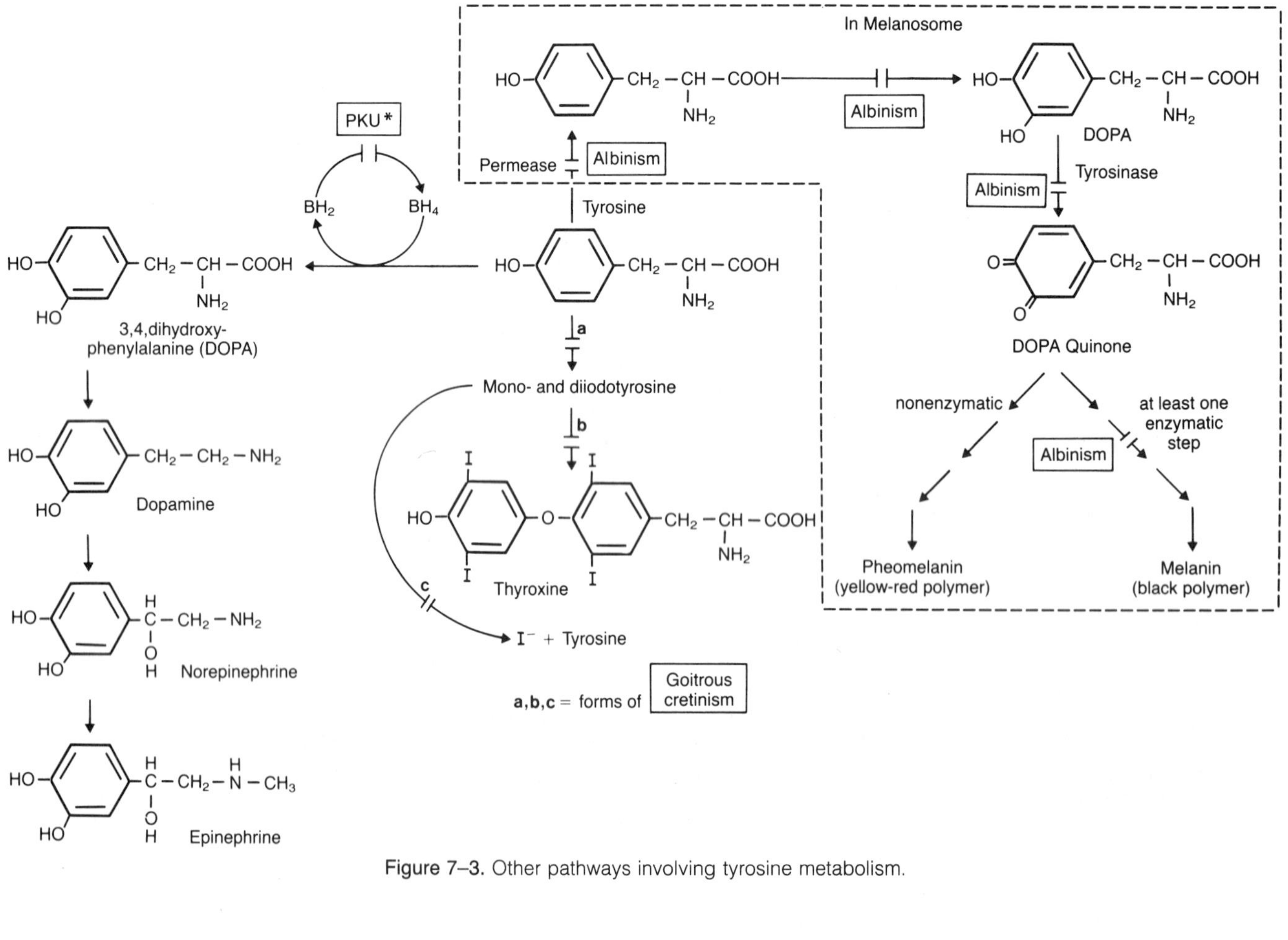

Figure 7–3. Other pathways involving tyrosine metabolism.

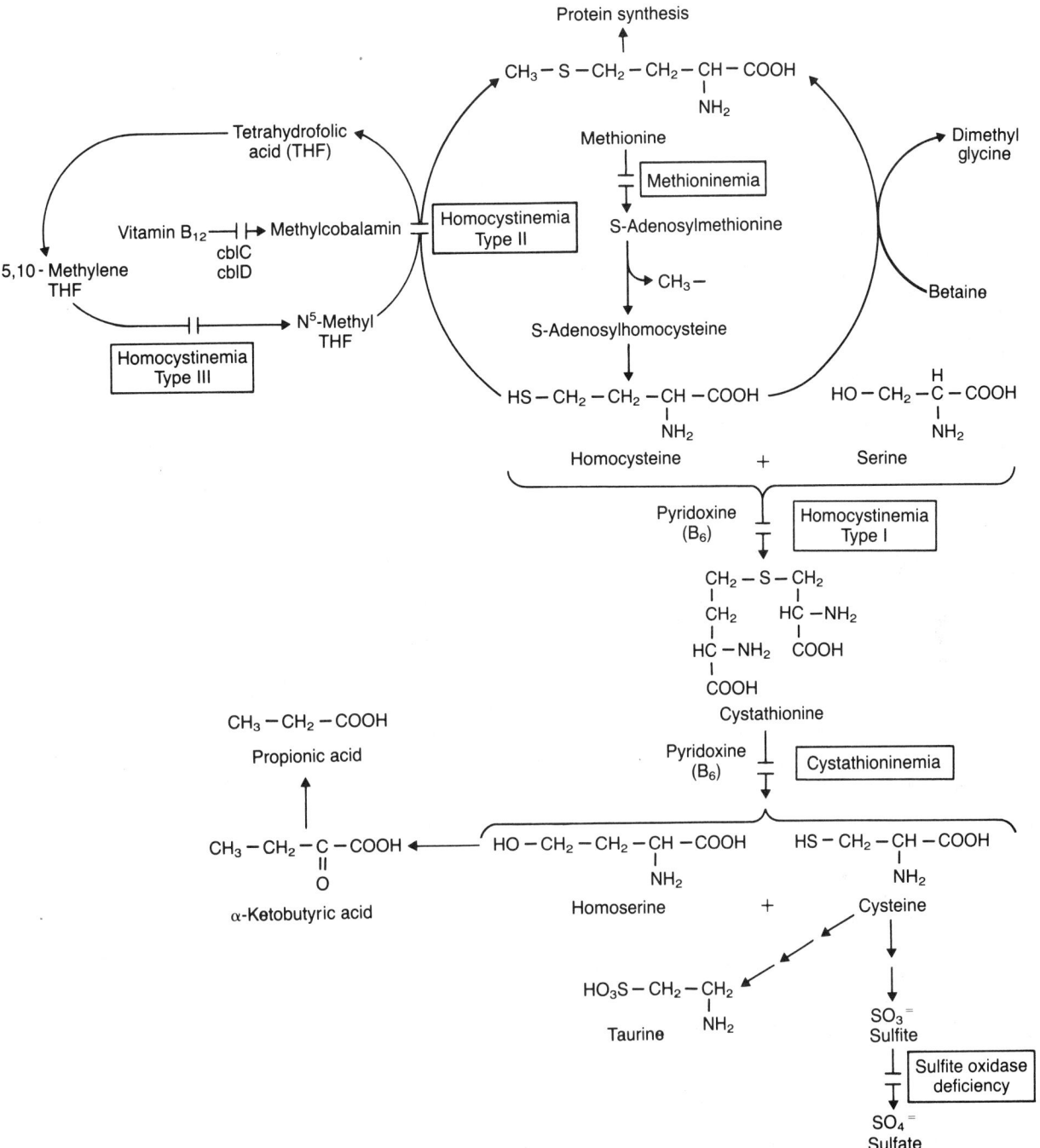

Figure 7–4. Pathways in the metabolism of the sulfur-containing amino acids.

life. The slow accumulation of the black polymer of homogentisic acid in cartilage and other mesenchymal tissues produces a black discoloration (*alcaptonuric ochronosis*) of the cheeks, nose, sclerae, and ears, which becomes evident by midadult life. Degeneration of pigmented cartilage leads to arthritis in about half of older patients with alcaptonuria. The connective tissue defects appear to be due to inhibition of the enzyme lysyl hydroxylase by homogentisic acid. The defect is otherwise asymptomatic.

The urine produces a positive reaction with Fehling or Benedict reagent. The dark urine of phenol poisoning and that associated with melanotic tumors do not have these reducing properties. Homogentisic acid does not react with glucose oxidase.

There is no effective treatment for this disorder.

Parkinsonism. Patients with parkinsonism and some with schizophrenia excrete *p*-tyramine or decarboxylated tyrosine.

The tyrosine hydroxylase of the brain requires the cofactor tetrahydrobiopterin for activity, and is distinct from the tyrosinase of melanocytes; both convert tyrosine to dopa. Tyramine may accumulate in the brain in excessive amounts if the reaction from tyrosine to dopa is blocked.

7.4 METHIONINE

The normal pathway for catabolism of methionine, an essential amino acid, produces S-adenosylmethionine, which serves as a methyl group donor for methylation of a variety of compounds in the body, and cysteine, which is formed through a series of reactions called transsulfuration (Fig. 7–4).

Homocystinemia (Homocystinuria). Most homocysteine, an intermediary compound of methionine degradation, is normally remethylated to methionine. This methionine sparing reaction is catalyzed by an enzyme that requires a metabolite of folic acid as a substrate and a metabolite of vitamin B_{12} as a cofactor (Fig. 7–4). Homocysteine ordinarily is not detectable in plasma or urine, but defects at 3 different enzymatic steps can produce homocystinemia and homocystinuria.

Homocystinemia type I, or *classic homocystinuria*, the most common inborn error of metabolism of methionine, is due to the deficiency of the enzyme cystathionine synthetase. The prevalence of this autosomal recessive condition is estimated at 1:200,000 live births. About 40% of these patients respond to high doses of vitamin B_6 and usually have milder clinical manifestations than those who do not respond to vitamin B_6 therapy.

Clinically, infants having homocystinemia type I are normal at birth. *Clinical manifestations* during infancy are nonspecific and may include failure to thrive and developmental delay. The diagnosis is usually made after 3 yr of age when subluxation of the ocular lens (ectopia lentis) occurs. Severe myopia, astigmatism, glaucoma, staphyloma, cataracts, retinal detachment, and optic atrophy are other ocular findings that may develop later in life. Progressive mental retardation is common. Normal intelligence, however, has been reported in some patients. Convulsions occur in about 3% of the patients. Patients with homocystinuria manifest skeletal abnormalities resembling those of the Marfan syndrome (Sec. 23.43): they are usually tall and thin with elongated limbs and arachnodactyly. Scoliosis, pectus excavatum or carinum, genu valgum, pes cavus, high arched palate, and crowding of the teeth are commonly seen. These children usually have fair complexions, blue eyes, and a peculiar malar flush. Generalized osteoporosis is the main roentgenographic finding. Thromboembolic episodes involving both large and small vessels, especially those of the brain, are common and may occur at any age.

Elevations of both methionine and homocysteine in body fluids are the *diagnostic laboratory findings*. Freshly voided urine should be tested for homocysteine, since this compound is unstable and may disappear as the urine is stored. Cysteine is low or absent in plasma.

Treatment with high doses of vitamin B_6 (200–1000 mg/24 hr) causes dramatic improvement in patients responsive to this therapy, but some patients may not respond because of folate depletion; therefore, a patient should not be considered unresponsive to vitamin B_6 until folic acid (1–5 mg/24 hr) has been added to the regimen. Restriction of methionine intake in conjunction with cysteine supplementation is recommended for all patients regardless of their response to vitamin B_6. Betaine (trimethylglycine), which also serves as a methyl group donor, lowers homocysteine levels in body fluids by remethylating homocysteine to methionine; this treatment has produced clinical improvement in patients unresponsive to vitamin B_6 therapy.

Patients with the other two types of homocystinemia have enzymatic defects that reside in the remethylation of homocysteine to methionine, have normal or low levels of methionine in body fluids, and have no ectopia lentis nor the skeletal abnormalities observed in type I homocystinemia.

Homocystinemia type II is due to the defect in the formation of methylcobalamin from vitamin B_{12}. Methylcobalamin is the cofactor for the enzyme 5-methyl-tetrahydrofolate methyltransferase, which catalyzes the remethylation of homocysteine to methionine. These patients also have methylmalonic acidemia (Sec. 7.7).

Homocystinemia type III is due to the deficiency of 5–10 methylene-tetrahydrofolate reductase, which is needed to produce 5-methyl tetrahydrofolate that provides the methyl group for the forming of methionine from homocysteine. At

least 14 patients with this deficiency have been reported. The severity of the enzyme defect and of the clinical manifestations varies considerably in different families. The complete absence of the enzyme activity results in neonatal apneic episodes and myoclonic seizures, which may lead rapidly to coma and death. Partial deficiency may result in a more chronic clinical picture manifested by mental retardation, convulsion, and spasticity. One 15 yr old developed schizophrenia and mental deterioration at age 11 yr. Treatment with folic acid, methionine, and vitamin B_6 has produced dramatic responses in some patients.

Hypermethioninemia. Abnormal elevations of plasma methionine occur in liver disease, tyrosinemia, and homocystinemia type I. Hypermethioninemia has also been found in premature and some fullterm infants on high protein diets, in whom it may represent delayed maturation of the enzyme methionine adenosyltransferase; lowering the protein intake usually resolves the abnormality. Hypermethioninemia due to the deficiency of hepatic methionine adenosyltransferase has also been reported. These children were diagnosed in the neonatal period during screening for homocystinuria and have remained asymptomatic for at least 6 yr.

Cystathioninemia. Cystathionine, an intermediate metabolite of methionine degradation that requires vitamin B_6 as a cofactor, is normally cleaved by cystathioninase to cysteine and homoserine (Fig. 7–4). Cystathioninase is not present in normal fetal and newborn liver, and thus cysteine becomes an essential amino acid during the newborn period, particularly in the premature infant.

Cystathioninuria occurs in patients with vitamin B_6 deficiency, liver disease (particularly when the liver damage is secondary to galactosemia), hepatoblastoma, neuroblastoma, ganglioblastoma, or defects in remethylation of homocysteine (homocystinuria types II and III).

Cystathioninase deficiency results in massive cystathioninuria and mild to moderate cystathioninemia; cystathionine is not normally detectable in blood. Deficiency of this enzyme is inherited as an autosomal recessive trait. Affected subjects with a wide variety of clinical manifestations have been reported. Lack of a consistent clinical picture and the presence of cystathioninuria in a number of normal persons suggests that cystathioninase deficiency perhaps is of no clinical significance. A majority of reported cases are responsive to oral administration of large doses of vitamin B_6 (100 mg or more/24 hr). Once cystathioninuria is discovered in a patient, vitamin B_6 treatment seems indicated, but its beneficial effect is not established.

7.5 CYSTINE

Cystinuria. (See also Sec. 17.47). This term refers to at least three closely related disorders that are inherited in an autosomal recessive manner. The homozygotes have excessive urinary loss of cystine, arginine, lysine, and ornithine. The urinary loss of cystine is associated with renal calculi.

Cystinosis. In this syndrome (Sec. 23.58) excessive storage of cystine crystals in the reticuloendothelial system and parenchymatous organs takes place. A specific transport system (presumably a genetically specific protein) which is normally responsible for the efflux of cystine from the lysosomes is absent or nonfunctional in persons with cystinosis. The disorder is transmitted as an autosomal recessive, and heterozygous carriers can be detected by the elevation of intracellular free cystine in peripheral leukocytes or in fibroblasts grown in tissue culture. When renal transplantation has been performed in patients with cystinosis, cystine accumulated even in the donor kidneys. However, the cystine was not deposited in the renal parenchymal cells (as is the case in the original kidneys) but was contained in macrophage which migrated from the host.

Sulfite Oxidase Deficiency. In the final step of cystine catabolism, inorganic sulfate is formed and excreted in the urine. A syndrome consisting of mental retardation, ataxia, seizures, and dislocated lenses is associated with the absence of inorganic sulfate in the urine. These children excrete large amounts of sulfite, thiosulfate, and S-sulfo-L-cysteine. The defect, inherited as an autosomal recessive, occurs in the molybdenum-containing enzyme sulfite oxidase (Fig. 7–4). At least three distinct variants exist, one of which involves the molybdenum cofactor.

Sulfite and metabisulfite are widely used by the food and beverage processing industry to preserve color, taste, and/or crispness. About 5% of asthmatic patients are very sensitive to sulfites contained in food and experience serious adverse reactions after ingesting small amounts of sulfite; some have died during acute attacks. Sensitive asthmatics have only 15% of the normal activity of sulfite oxidase in fibroblasts. The pathophysiology is unknown.

β-Mercaptolactate-Cysteine Disulfiduria. β-Mercaptolactate-cysteine disulfide, a derivative of cystine in which one of the two amino groups is replaced by a hydroxyl group, has been found in high concentration in the urine of a mentally retarded patient whose parents were siblings, in normal individuals, and in one mildly retarded individual having dislocated lenses. There were no other amino acid abnormalities.

Taurinuria. Taurine is normally excreted in the urine as an intermediate in the oxidation of cysteine. Individuals with camptodactyly due to a dominant gene have also been shown to excrete excess taurine (Fig. 7–4).

7.6 TRYPTOPHAN

Serotonin Deficiency. Serotonin, an important neurotransmitter, is formed by decarboxylation from 5-OH-tryptophan. The latter is formed from tryptophan by tryptophan hydroxylase, an enzyme which requires tetrahydrobiopterin as a cofactor. Defects in biopterin metabolism are discussed in Sec. 7.2; another consequence of any of these defects is an inability to synthesize serotonin. This explains, in part, why simply treating patients with PKU due to a biopterin defect with the usual low phenylalanine diet does not work.

Hartnup Disease. In this rare hereditary disorder there is a single defect in the transport of monoamino-monocarboxylic amino acids by intestinal mucosa and renal tubules.

Massive generalized aminoaciduria occurs. Plasma amino acid concentrations are not elevated; therefore the aminoaciduria must arise from faulty tubular reabsorption. The exception to this generalization is tryptophan, whose levels in plasma are abnormally low; impaired intestinal absorption results in its bacterial decomposition in the intestine to various indole and indoxyl derivatives, which are absorbed, detoxified, and excreted in the urine in abnormally large amounts.

Cutaneous photosensitivity is seen early in most affected children. Unprotected skin becomes rough and red after moderate exposure to the sun; with greater exposure, a rash identical to that of pellagra develops. Patients with Hartnup disease may also have cerebellar ataxia with involvement of the pyramidal tracts. During febrile illnesses, ataxia may develop without a rash. The clinical course is variable; severe cutaneous and nervous disturbances may alternate with periods of complete remission over many years. Mental deficiency, an incidental finding in the original kindred, has not been observed in other cases. The disease, transmitted by an autosomal recessive gene, must be considered in the differential diagnosis of pellagra.

The impaired intestinal absorption and urinary loss of tryptophan result in decreased synthesis of nicotinic acid. It is not surprising, therefore, that large doses of nicotinamide may cause sustained remission of the neurologic and cutaneous aspects of the disorder. Such remissions, however, may occur without therapy. The aminoaciduria and urinary excretion of indole compounds are not suppressed by such therapy, nor do they decrease during spontaneous remissions. High protein diets may compensate for the loss of amino acids.

Tryptophanemia. The catabolism of tryptophan (presumably in its conversion to formyl kynurenine) is involved in this disorder (Fig. 7–5). Patients may have mental retardation, dwarfism, cerebellar ataxia, and a pellagra-like rash similar to that seen in Hartnup disease. There is also tryptophanuria and moderate tryptophanemia without generalized aminoaciduria or indicanuria. No metabolites distal to the block are excreted even after a tryptophan load. Several instances of consanguinity suggest autosomal recessive inheritance.

Kynureninuria. An abnormality of tryptophan metabolism consistent with a partial block of kynurenine hydroxylase has been reported in a patient with scleroderma but with healthy relatives. Abnormal amounts of kynurenine and other tryptophan metabolites proximal to hydroxykynurenine (Fig. 7–5) were excreted in the urine both before and after administration of tryptophan. Pyridoxine did not affect the excretion pattern of tryptophan metabolites. Affected persons appear to be heterozygous for the condition.

Kynureninase Defects. *Hydroxykynureninuria*. Mild mental retardation, migraine-like headaches, and excretion of large amounts of kynurenine, 3-hydroxy-kynurenine, and xanthurenic acid have suggested a lack of kynureninase activity (Fig. 7–5). Signs and symptoms of nicotinic acid deficiency develop in the absence of added dietary nicotinic acid, since affected persons cannot synthesize it from tryptophan. Pyridoxine did not alter the excretion pattern of the tryptophan metabolites but did relieve the headaches.

Pyridoxine-Responsive Xanthurenic Aciduria. Children with pyridoxine deficiency may excrete several metabolites of tryptophan, mainly xanthurenic acid, since pyridoxal phosphate is the coenzyme for many enzymes involved in amino acid metabolism, including kynureninase. In pyridoxine-responsive xanthurenic aciduria, patients do not have anemia, convulsions, or pyridoxine deficiency. However, large doses of pyridoxine are required to normalize xanthurenic acid excretion, and liver biopsies have demonstrated that kynureninase does not bind with the coenzyme form of the vitamin.

Excessive excretion of hydroxykynurenine, kynurenine, and xanthurenic acid, corrected by pyridoxine, has been observed in five unrelated patients with chronic granulomatous disease.

Indicanuria. This occurs when tryptophan, poorly absorbed from the gastrointestinal tract, is converted there by bacterial action to indole. Indole is absorbed, oxidized, sulfated, and excreted as an indican (Fig. 7–5). Indicanuria is commonly observed whenever stasis in the bowels occurs, such as in constipation or in the "blind loop syndrome"; it also occurs in Hartnup disease in which tryptophan is poorly absorbed, and in phenylketonuria. The *blue diaper syndrome*, a familial disorder characterized by hypercalcemia, nephrocalcinosis, and indicanuria, derives its name from the fact that indican is oxidized to indican blue on exposure to air.

Hydrindicuria. The combination of mental retardation and persistent metabolic acidosis, presumably caused by hydroxyindole derivatives, has been associated with urinary indole pigments derived from tryptophan and phenylalanine metabolism. Laboratory manipulation of urine containing these abnormal indoles converts them to 5,6-dihydroxyindole (hydrindic acid); hence the name of the disorder (Fig. 7–5). Prolonged administration of antibiotics to halt indole forma-

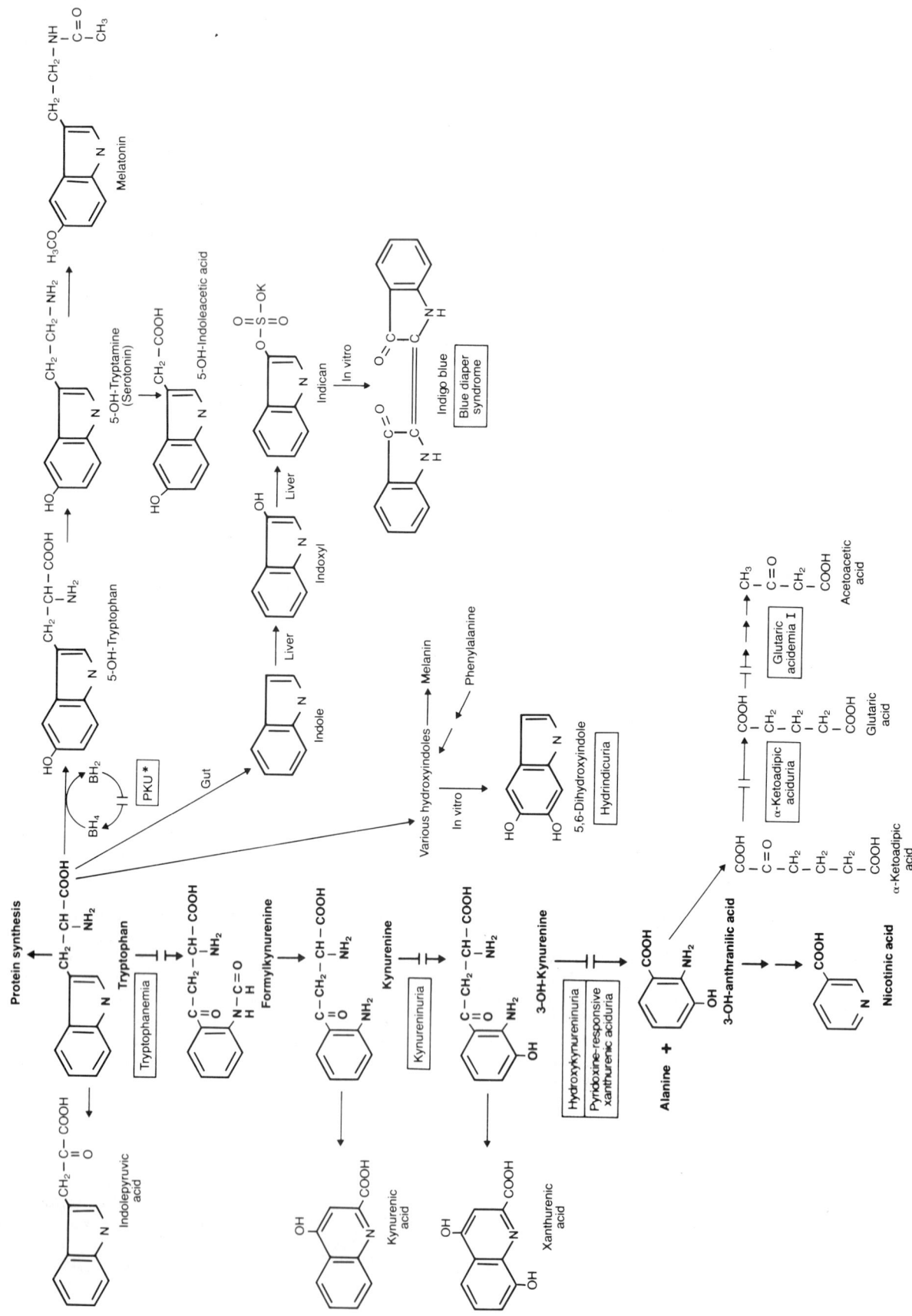

Figure 7–5. Pathways in the metabolism of tryptophan. The major pathway is shown in bolder type.

tion in the gut had no effect upon indole excretion, and loading tests showed an increase of urinary hydrindic acid after administration of phenylalanine and tryptophan.

Indolylacroylglycinuria. Indolylacroylglycine is formed by the conjugation of glycine with a molecule of tryptophan from which a molecule of ammonia has been removed to form a double bond. It is one of the many tryptophan metabolites excreted in Hartnup disease and has been found alone in a family with mental retardation. Administering neomycin usually temporarily eliminates the indolylacroylglycinuria; thus, it appears that bacterial metabolism produces the compound.

Glutaric Acidemia. See Sec. 7.16.

α-Ketoadipic Aciduria. See Sec. 7.16.

7.7 VALINE, LEUCINE, ISOLEUCINE, AND RELATED ORGANIC ACIDEMIAS

The early steps of the degradation of these three essential amino acids, the branched chain amino acids, are similar (Fig. 7–6). Although valine transaminase may be different from leucine-isoleucine transaminase, only one enzyme system is involved in the decarboxylation of their three keto acid derivatives. The intermediate metabolites are all organic acids, and deficiency of any of the degradative enzymes, except for the transaminases, causes acidosis; in such instances, the organic acids before the enzymatic block accumulate in body fluids and are excreted in the urine. These disorders cause severe metabolic acidosis, which usually occurs during the first few days of life. Although most of the clinical findings are non-specific, some manifestations may provide important clues to the nature of the enzyme deficiency. An approach to infants suspected of having an organic acidemia is presented in Figure 7–7. Definitive diagnosis is usually established by identifying and measuring specific organic acids and the enzyme assay.

Organic acidemias are not limited to defects in catabolic pathways of branched chain amino acids. Disorders causing accumulation of other organic acids include those derived from lysine (Sec. 7.16), those associated with lactic acid (Sec. 7.20), and dicarboxylic acidemia associated with defective fatty acid degradation (Sec. 7.54).

Leucine-Isoleucinemia. Failure to thrive, mental retardation, convulsions, retinal regeneration, and neural deafness have been associated with type II prolinemia and mild (twice normal) to marked (8 times normal) elevations of blood valine and, especially, isoleucine and leucine levels. Assays of leukocytes revealed no abnormalities of branched-chain ketoacid decarboxylase activities or of valine transaminase but a 50% reduction of isoleucine and leucine transaminase.

Valinemia. Mental deficiency and growth failure has been observed along with elevated levels of valine in plasma and urine. The urine neither contained ketoacids nor had the odor of maple syrup, and impaired transamination of valine was demonstrated in leukocytes.

The presence of valinemia and leucine-isoleucine as separate clinical entities suggests there may be more than one transaminase for these amino acids.

Maple Syrup Urine Disease (MSUD). Decarboxylation of leucine, isoleucine, and valine is accomplished by a complex enzyme system using thiamine pyrophosphate as a coenzyme. Deficiency of this enzyme system causes MSUD (Fig 7–6), named after the sweet odor of maple syrup found in body fluids, especially in urine. Several forms of this condition have been reported.

Classic MSUD. This form has the most severe *clinical manifestations.* Affected infants who are normal at birth develop poor feeding and vomiting during the 1st wk of life; lethargy and coma ensue within a few days. Physical examination reveals hypertonicity and muscular rigidity with severe opisthotonos. Periods of hypertonicity may alternate with bouts of flaccidity. Neurologic findings are often mistaken for generalized sepsis and meningitis. Convulsions occur in most infants, and hypoglycemia is common. However, in contrast to most hypoglycemic states, correcting the blood glucose does not improve the clinical condition. Routine laboratory studies are usually unremarkable except for severe metabolic acidosis. Death usually occurs in untreated patients within the first few weeks or months of life.

Diagnosis is often suspected because of the peculiar odor of maple syrup found in urine, sweat, and cerumen (Fig. 7–7). It is usually confirmed by amino acid analysis showing marked elevations in plasma levels of leucine, isoleucine, valine, and alloisoleucine (a stereoisomer of isoleucine not normally found in blood). Leucine levels are usually higher than those of the other three amino acids. Urine contains high levels of leucine, isoleucine, and valine and their respective ketoacids. These ketoacids may be detected qualitatively by adding a few drops of 2,4-dinitrophenylhydrazine reagent (0.1% in 0.1 N HCl) to the urine; a yellow precipitate of diphenylhydrazone is formed in a positive test.

Treatment of the acute state is aimed at quick removal of branched chain amino acids and their metabolites from the tissues and body fluids. Since renal clearance of these compounds is poor, hydration alone does not produce a rapid improvement. Peritoneal dialysis is the most effective mode of therapy and should be promptly instituted; significant decreases in plasma levels of leucine, isoleucine, and valine are usually seen within 24 hr of treatment. Attempts should also be made to stop the patient's catabolic state by providing sufficient calories intravenously or orally.

Treatment after recovery from the acute state requires a low branched-chain amino acid diet. Synthetic formulas devoid of leucine, isoleucine, and valine are now commercially available.* Since these amino acids cannot be synthesized endogenously, small amounts of them should be added to the diet; the amount should be titrated carefully by frequent plasma amino acid analysis. A clinical condition resembling acrodermatitis entropathica occurs in affected infants whose plasma isoleucine becomes very low; addition of isoleucine to the diet causes a rapid and complete recovery. Patients with MSUD should remain on the diet for the rest of their lives.

The long-term *prognosis* of the affected children remains guarded. Severe ketoacidosis, coma, and death may occur during any stressful situation such as infection or surgery. Mental and neurologic deficits are common sequelae.

Intermittent MSUD. In this form of MSUD seemingly normal children develop vomiting, odor of maple syrup, ataxia, lethargy, and coma during stress such as infection or surgery. During these attacks, laboratory findings are indistinguishable from those of the classic form and death may occur. Treatment of the intermittent variety is similar to that of the classic form. After recovery, although a normal diet is tolerated, one low in branched-chain amino acids is recommended. The activity of decarboxylase in patients having the intermittent form is much higher than in the classic form and may reach 8–16% of the normal activity.

Mild (Intermediate) MSUD. In this form affected children develop milder disease after the neonatal period. They are usually mildly to moderately retarded, have increased plasma levels of leucine, isoleucine, and valine, and excrete ketoacid derivatives of these amino acids in their urine. They usually have the odor of maple syrup. These children are commonly diagnosed during an intercurrent illness when signs and symptoms of classic MSUD occur. The decarboxylase activity is 2–8% of normal. Since patients with thiamine-responsive

---

*MSUD Formula, Mead Johnson Laboratories, Evansville, Indiana.

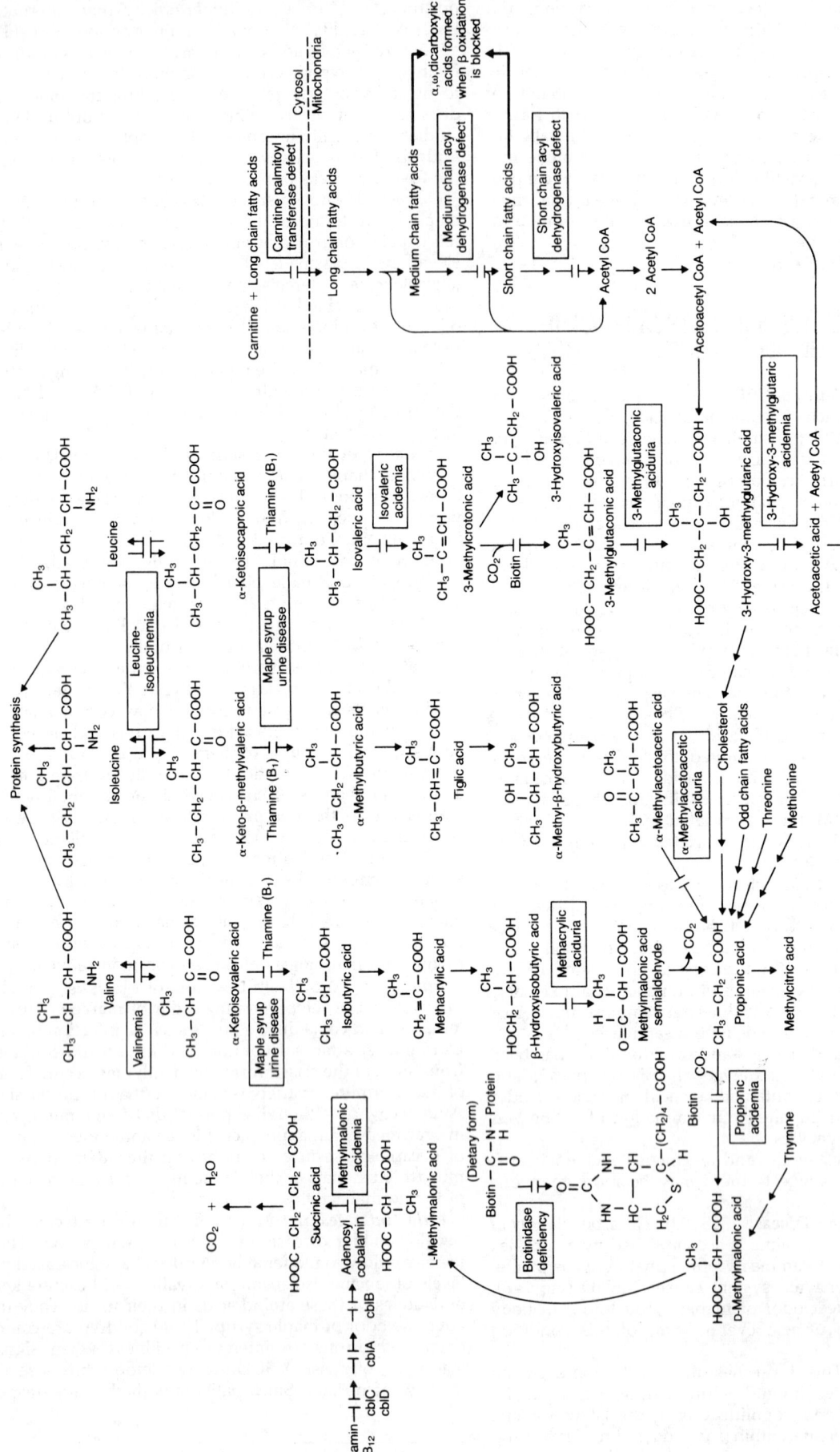

Figure 7–6. Pathways in the metabolism of the branched chain amino acids. Many of the intermediates (the organic acids) are metabolized via their coenzyme A (CoA) derivatives. For the sake of simplicity, this is not indicated in most of the cases.

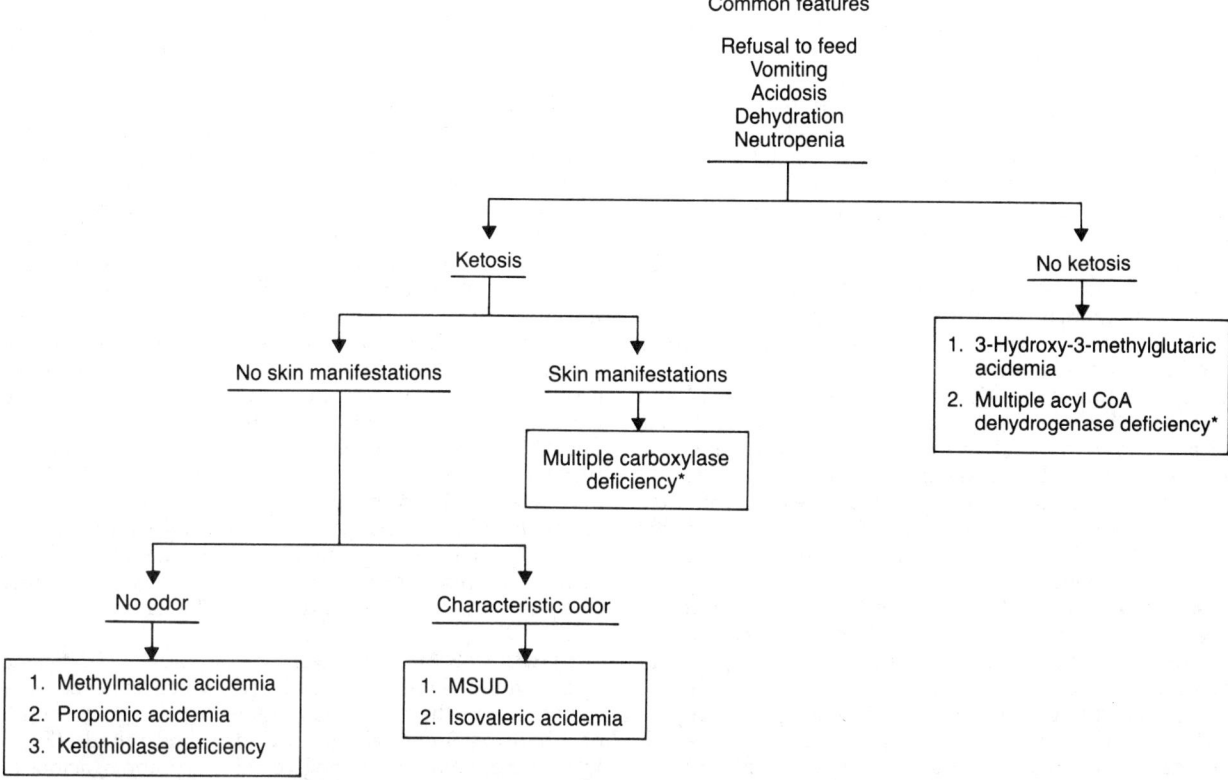

Figure 7–7. Clinical approach to infants with organic acidemia. Asterisks indicate disorders in which patients have a characteristic odor (see text).

MSUD usually have similar manifestations as in the mild form, a trial of thiamine therapy is recommended.

Thiamine-Responsive MSUD. Children with mild or intermittent forms of MSUD have been reported in whom treatment with high doses of thiamine results in dramatic clinical and biochemical improvement. Although some children have responded to 10 mg/24 hr thiamine, others require as high as 200 mg/24 hr for at least 3 weeks before a favorable response is observed.

Genetics and the Prevalence of MSUD. All forms of this disorder are inherited as an autosomal recessive trait. The severity of the enzyme deficiency may vary in different families. The mild and intermittent forms may be "double heterozygotes" with two different mutant alleles. Decarboxylase activity can be measured in leukocytes and fibroblasts, making it possible to diagnose heterozygotes and affected fetuses. The incidence in the United States is about 1:200,000; however, the gene is much more common among Mennonites.

Isovaleric Acidemia. This rare condition is due to the deficiency of isovaleryl CoA dehydrogenase, which catalyzes the conversion of isovaleric acid to 3-methylcrotonic acid in the leucine degradative pathway (Fig. 7–6).

Clinical manifestations include vomiting and severe acidosis in the first few days of life. Lethargy, convulsions, and coma ensue, and death may occur if proper therapy is not initiated. The vomiting may be severe enough to suggest pyloric stenosis. The characteristic odor of sweaty feet may be present (Fig. 7–7). A milder, less common form of the disease also exists in which the first clinical manifestation may not appear until the infant is a few months or a few years old.

Laboratory findings reveal severe ketoacidosis, neutropenia, thrombocytopenia, and, occasionally, pancytopenia. Hypocalcemia and moderate to severe hyperammonemia may be present in some patients. Increases in plasma ammonia may

suggest defects in the urea cycle. However, in the latter conditions the infant is not acidotic. Hyperglycinemia may be present in some patients.

Diagnosis is established by demonstrating marked elevations of isovaleric acid and isovaleryl glycine in body fluids, especially urine. Isovaleric acid is volatile and may disappear from the urine if the specimen is not handled properly; however, isovaleryl glycine is a stable compound, more reliable for diagnostic purposes. Measuring the enzyme in cultured skin fibroblasts confirms the diagnosis.

Treatment should aim at hydration, correction of metabolic acidosis (by infusing sodium bicarbonate), and removal of the excess isovaleric acid. Since isovaleryl glycine has a high urinary clearance, administering glycine (250 mg/kg/24 hr) is recommended to enhance formation of isovalerylglycine. Exchange transfusion and peritoneal dialysis may be needed if glycine fails to induce significant clinical and biochemical improvements. Patients should be kept on a low protein diet after recovery from the acute attack. Mental retardation is a common sequela, but normal development may be achieved with early and proper treatment.

Isovaleric acidemia is inherited as an autosomal recessive trait. The gene frequency in the general population is not known. Heterozygote detection and intrauterine diagnosis are not yet possible.

Multiple Carboxylase Deficiency (Defects in Utilization of Biotin). Biotin is a vitamin that acts as a cofactor for all carboxylases in the body: pyruvate carboxylase, propionyl CoA carboxylase, 3-methylcrotonyl CoA carboxylase, and acetyl CoA carboxylase. Two of these carboxylases are involved in metabolic pathways of leucine, isoleucine, and valine (Fig. 7–6). Dietary biotin is bound to protein (carboxylases), and free biotin is generated in the intestine by the action of biotinidase. Free biotin must form a covalent peptide bond with the apoprotein of the above carboxylases in order to render them active. This binding is catalyzed by holocarboxylase synthetase. Deficiencies in this enzyme or in biotinidase result in malfunction of all the carboxylases and in organic acidemia.

Holocarboxylase Synthetase Deficiency (Infantile Form of Multiple Carboxylase Deficiency). Infants with this rare autosomal recessive disorder become symptomatic in the 1st few weeks of life with vomiting, failure to thrive, acidosis, and ketosis. The urine may have a peculiar odor which is described as similar to tomcat urine. The finding that differentiates this disorder from other organic acidemias, especially propionic acidemia, is the skin manifestations, which include generalized erythematous rash with exfoliation and alopecia totalis (Fig. 7–7). Hypotonia and convulsions with abnormal EEG findings may also occur.

Laboratory findings include metabolic acidosis, ketosis, and the presence of organic acids such as lactic acid, propionic acid, 3-methylcrotonic acid and its glycine conjugate, and 3-hydroxyisovaleric acid in body fluids. Significant hyperammonemia has occurred in some patients. These infants may also have immunodeficiency manifested by a decrease in the number of T cells. Treatment with biotin (10 mg/24 hr) results in a dramatic response.

Biotinidase Deficiency (Multiple Carboxylase Deficiency—Juvenile Form). The absence of biotinidase causes biotin deficiency. Infants having this deficiency develop signs and symptoms similar to those seen in holocarboxylase synthetase deficiency, but, in contrast to the latter, symptoms appear later when the child is several months or several years old. The delay is presumably due to the presence of sufficient free biotin derived from the mother or the diet. Dermatitis, alopecia, ataxia, seizure, and immunodeficiency are common. Episodes of metabolic acidosis may also occur. The pattern of organic acids in body fluids resembles that of the holocarboxylase deficiency. These children respond dramatically to administration of free biotin (10 mg/24 hr). The prevalence of this condition is estimated at 1:40,000.

Multiple Carboxylase Deficiency due to Dietary Biotin Deficiency. Acquired deficiency of biotin may occur in infants receiving parenteral nutrition without added vitamins or in children with short gut or chronic diarrhea who are receiving formulas low in biotin. Excessive ingestion of raw eggs may also cause biotin deficiency since the protein avidin in egg white binds biotin and makes it unavailable for absorption. Infants with this deficiency develop dermatitis, alopecia, and moniliasis.

3-Methylcrotonyl Glycinemia. This glycine conjugate of a metabolite of leucine was found in the urine of a 4½ mo old girl who had symptoms similar to those of Werdnig-Hoffman disease but who died during the first year of life. Small amounts of this compound were excreted by her parents and two brothers. She also excreted 3-hydroxyisovaleric acid. Based on these findings, and the lack of response to low doses of biotin, it was concluded that a defect of the activity of 3-methylcrotonyl CoA carboxylase existed. However, this patient could also have had a defect of enzyme holocarboxylase synthetase.

3-Methylglutaconic Aciduria. Clinical manifestations have ranged from mild motor and speech retardation to severe neurological deficit with self-mutilation. Patients excrete large amounts of 3-methylglutaconic acid, an intermediate metabolite in the catabolism of leucine, in their urine. It is not clear whether the metabolic defect is the cause of the clinical manifestations.

Methacrylic Aciduria. Cysteine conjugates of methacrylic acid have been found in the urine of an infant who died with multiple skeletal, cardiac, and brain malformations. Methacrylic acid, a metabolite of valine, is nonenzymatically converted to β-hydroxyisobutyric acid. The defect in this disorder

is presumed to be at the level of β-hydroxyisobutyryl CoA deacylase, and it has been postulated that methacrylic acid, which binds with free sulfhydryl groups, is a teratogenic agent.

β-Ketothiolase Deficiency (α-Methylacetoacetic Aciduria). Normally in isoleucine degradation, α-methylacetoacetyl CoA is converted to acetyl CoA and propionyl CoA. Children excreting large amounts of α-methylacetoacetate, α-methyl-β-hydroxybutyrate, and the glycine conjugate of tiglic acid may be deficient in β-ketothiolase, which is responsible for this conversion. These children have intermittent acidosis, vomiting, lethargy, and coma, usually brought on by intercurrent infection; death has occurred during such an episode. Feeding additional isoleucine aggravates the conditions, whereas reduction of protein intake to 2 g/kg/24 hr ameliorates the clinical course. Amino acid and propionate levels are not elevated in blood or urine and there is no peculiar odor. A defect in isoleucine oxidation has been demonstrated in cultured skin fibroblasts.

A defect of β-ketothiolase activity has also been reported in an infant with ketotic glycinemia and hyperammonemia but no methylmalonic or propionic acidemia, though the clinical symptoms were those associated with the latter two findings (see below); a low protein diet (1.5 g/kg/24 hr) seemed beneficial.

3-Hydroxy-3-Methylglutaric Acidemia. The deficiency of hydroxymethylglutaryl CoA lyase, which catalyzes the terminal step in the catabolism of leucine, causes accumulation of 3-hydroxy-3-methylglutaric acid in body fluids (Fig. 7–6). Episodes of vomiting, hypoglycemia, hypotonia, acidosis, and dehydration may rapidly lead to lethargy, ataxia, and coma. Signs and symptoms often occur during an intercurrent infection. The onset of the disease may be in the first few weeks of life or may be as late as 2 yr of age. Hyperammonemia, hepatomegaly, and abnormal liver function tests may falsely suggest Reye syndrome. There is no ketosis (Fig. 7–7), since 3-hydroxy-3-methylglutaric acid is unable to be converted to acetoacetic acid and β-hydroxybutyric acid, and ketone bodies cannot be formed from any source since 3-hydroxy-3-methylglutaryl CoA is an obligatory intermediate in their formation (Fig. 7–6). Detection of high concentrations of 3-hydroxy-3-methylglutaric acid and more proximal intermediate metabolites of leucine catabolism confirms the diagnosis. Treatment of acute crises includes hydration and administration of sodium benzoate to reduce hyperammonemia. Exchange transfusion and peritoneal dialysis may be required if the clinical condition deteriorates. Restriction of protein and fat intake is recommended for long-term management of these patients.

Propionic Acidemia (Propionyl CoA Carboxylase Deficiency). Propionic acid is an intermediate metabolite of isoleucine, valine, threonine, methionine, odd chain fatty acids, and cholesterol catabolism. It is normally carboxylated to methylmalonic acid by the mitochondrial enzyme propionyl CoA carboxylase, which requires biotin as a cofactor (Fig. 7–6).

Clinical manifestations are nonspecific. The majority of the patients develop symptoms in the first few weeks of life. Poor feeding, vomiting, hypotonia, lethargy, dehydration, and clinical signs of acidosis progress rapidly to coma and death. Seizures occur in about 30% of affected infants. If an infant survives the first attack, similar episodes may occur during an intercurrent infection or following a high protein diet. Less frequently, the infant may come to medical attention later in life because of mental retardation without acute attacks of ketosis. The severity of clinical manifestations may also be variable within a family; in a kindred, a brother was diagnosed at 5 yr of age while his 13 yr old sister, with the same level of propionyl CoA carboxylase deficiency, was asymptomatic.

Laboratory findings reveal severe acidosis, ketosis, neutropenia, thrombocytopenia, and hypoglycemia. Moderate to severe hyperammonemia is commonly seen in these infants and may suggest genetic defects in the urea cycle enzymes. However, infants with defects in the urea cycle are usually not acidotic (Fig. 7–1). Hyperglycinemia is common in patients with propionic acidemia. Elevations in plasma and urinary levels of glycine have also been observed in patients with methylmalonic acidemia, isovaleric acidemia, and α-methylacetoacetic acidemia (ketothiolase deficiency). These disorders are collectively referred to as *ketotic hyperglycinemia*. Propionic acid and methylcitric acid (presumably made by the condensation of propionyl CoA with oxaloacetic acid) are markedly elevated in plasma and urine of infants with propionic acidemia. Measuring methylcitric acid is especially helpful in the diagnosis, since, unlike propionic acid which is volatile, methylcitric acid is a stable compound and does not disappear from the specimen during shipping and handling. Other intermediate metabolites of isoleucine catabolism, such as tiglic acid, tiglylglycine, and α-methyloacetoacetic acid, are found in urine.

The diagnosis of propionic acidemia should be differentiated from holocarboxylase synthetase deficiency (see above). Earlier reported patients with propionic acidemia responsive to biotin were later found to have holocarboxylase synthetase deficiency. The latter infants often have skin manifestations and excrete large amounts of lactic acid, 3-methylcrotonic acid, and 3-hydroxyisovaleric acid in addition to propionic acid. Holocarboxylase synthetase deficiency is biotin-responsive, and the affected infants usually can tolerate near normal protein loads with biotin therapy. Definitive diagnosis of propionic acidemia may be established by measuring the appropriate enzyme activity in leukocytes or cultured fibroblasts.

Treatment of acute attacks usually requires peritoneal dialysis or hemodialysis for removal of ammonia and other toxic compounds. Other measures to increase excretion of ammonia by the kidney (benzoate, etc.) should also be employed (Sec. 7.13). Dehydration and acidosis should be treated vigorously. Adequate calories with minimal amount of protein (0.25 to 0.5 g/kg/24 hr) should be provided intravenously or by intragastric tube to minimize the catabolic state. Although infants with true propionic acidemia are rarely responsive to biotin, this compound should be administered (10 mg/24 hr) to all infants during the initial attack and should be continued until a definitive diagnosis is established.

Long-term treatment is by a low protein diet (0.5 to 1.5 g/kg/24 hr). The infant's growth and biochemical parameters should be monitored closely. Stressful situations that may trigger acute attacks (such as infections) should be treated promptly and aggressively.

Long-term *prognosis* is guarded. Death may occur during an acute attack at any age. Normal psychomotor development is possible, but most children manifest some degree of permanent neurodevelopmental deficit.

The prevalence of propionic acidemia, an autosomal recessive trait, is unknown. Prenatal diagnosis has been accomplished by measuring enzyme activity in the cultured amniotic fluid cells.

Methylmalonic Acidemia. Methylmalonic acid, a structural isomer of succinic acid, is normally derived from propionic acid as part of the catabolic pathways of isoleucine, valine, threonine, methionine, and odd chain fatty acids. Two enzymes involved in the conversion of methylmalonic acid to succinic acid are methylmalonyl acid CoA racemase and methylmalonyl CoA mutase. The latter enzyme uses adenosylcobalamin, a metabolite of B_{12}, as a coenzyme (Fig. 7–6). Deficiency of the mutase or its coenzyme causes accumulation of methylmalonic acid and its precursors in body fluids. Deficiency of the racemase has not yet been conclusively identified.

After entering the cell, vitamin B_{12} or cobalamin undergoes enzymatic activation to form two coenzymes: adenosylcobalamin and methylcobalamin. The former is the coenzyme for methylmalonyl CoA mutase and the latter is the coenzyme for the remethylation of homocystine to methionine (Fig. 7–4). There are at least six genetically different defects that can cause methylmalonic acidemia. Two of the defects involve the mutase protein (apoenzyme) itself. These are designated *mut°*, meaning no enzyme activity and *mut⁻*, indicating partial absence of the mutase apoenzyme. The other four defects are in the pathway of cobalamin activation and have been called *cbl* A, *cbl* B, *cbl* C, and *cbl* D; the first two defects result in deficiency of adenosylcobalamin; whereas in *cbl* C and *cbl* D synthesis of both adenosylcobalamin and methylcobalamin is impaired. Patients with *mut°*, and *mut⁻*, *cbl* A, and *cbl* B variants have similar clinical and laboratory findings. Patients with *cbl* C and *cbl* D forms have a less severe clinical course than the other types and have homocystinuria in addition to methylmalonic acidemia. The most common variant is the *mut°* form.

Clinical manifestations of *mut°*, *mut⁻*, *cbl* A, and *cbl* B are similar to those of propionic acidemia. However, fulminating neonatal forms causing severe ketosis, acidosis, hyperammonemia, pancytopenia, coma, and death are more common in methylmalonic acidemia than in propionic acidemia. There is variation in the severity of the clinical manifestations, with asymptomatic patients having been identified by screening of newborn infants. These latter children were not responsive to vitamin B_{12}, tolerated a normal diet, and were mentally normal; two of them had deficiency of the mutase apoenzyme (*mut* variant).

Laboratory findings include ketosis, acidosis, anemia, neutropenia, thrombocytopenia, hyperglycinemia, and the presence of large quantities of methylmalonic acid in body fluids. Propionic acid and its metabolites 3-hydroxypropionic acid and methylcitric acid are also found in urine.

Patients with *methylmalonic acidemia and homocystinuria* (*cbl* C and *cbl* D variants) usually present with failure to thrive, mental retardation, seizure, and megaloblastic anemia during the first few months of life. In these infants, the concentration of methylmalonic acid in body fluids is lower than that found in the other forms. Homocystinuria is also less pronounced than in patients with cystathionine synthetase deficiency. Older patients with dementia, myelopathy, and speech disorders have also been reported.

Patients with dietary vitamin B_{12} deficiency or absence of intrinsic factor also produce detectable amounts of methylmalonic acid and homocysteine in addition to having megaloblastic anemia.

Treatment of patients with methylmalonic acidemia is similar to that of patients with propionic acidemia (see above), except that large daily doses (1 mg) of vitamin B_{12} are used instead of biotin. Although the majority of patients with the mutase apoenzyme deficiency do not respond to vitamin B_{12}, all patients should receive a trial of this vitamin therapy.

Long-term *prognosis* seems to depend on the type of enzymatic defect. Patients with the mutase apoenzyme deficiency (*mut°* and *mut⁻*) have a worse prognosis.

The condition is inherited as an autosomal recessive trait with a prevalence of about 1:60,000. Prenatal diagnosis has been accomplished by assay of the mutase enzyme in cultured amniotic cells.

7.8 GLYCINE

Glycine is a nonessential amino acid synthesized mainly from serine and threonine. The main catabolic pathway requires the complex glycine cleavage enzyme system to cleave the 1st carbon of glycine and convert it to carbon dioxide.

The 2nd carbon is transferred to tetrahydrofolate (THF) to form hydroxymethyltetrahydrofolate, which may either react with another mole of glycine to form serine (Fig. 7–8) or form methyltetrahydrofolate, which serves as a methyl group donor for many reactions in the body (Fig. 7–4).

Hyperglycinemia. Elevated levels of glycine in body fluids occur in patients having a number of inborn errors of metabolism, including propionic acidemia, methylmalonic acidemia, isovaleric acidemia, and ketothiolase deficiency. These disorders have been collectively referred to as *ketotic hyperglycinemia* because episodes of severe acidosis and ketosis occur. The pathogenesis of hyperglycinemia in these disorders is not fully understood, but inhibition of the glycine cleavage enzyme system by the various organic acids has been shown to occur in some of the affected patients. The term nonketotic hyperglycinemia is reserved for the clinical condition caused by the genetic deficiency of the glycine cleavage enzyme system (Fig. 7–8). In this condition hyperglycinemia is present without ketosis.

Nonketotic hyperglycinemia. The majority of patients with this disorder become ill during the first few days of life. The *clinical manifestations* of poor feeding, failure to suck, and lethargy may progress rapidly to a deep coma. Convulsions, especially myoclonic seizures, and hiccups are common. This disorder is usually fatal; current therapeutic measures may produce only transient improvement. Milder forms of the condition have also been reported; mental retardation, convulsions, and spasticity are frequent findings in these patients. Heterogeneity in clinical severity of the disease has also been observed within a given family.

Laboratory findings reveal moderate to severe hyperglycinemia and hyperglycinuria, and an increased glycine concentration in the spinal fluid. The high ratio of glycine concentration in the spinal fluid to that in blood has been used to differentiate nonketotic hyperglycinemia from other hyperglycinemic states. Plasma serine levels are usually low. Serum pH is usually normal. A variety of amino acid loading tests to establish precursor relationships have been uninformative, except that most affected children develop profound coma after a valine load. This test should therefore be avoided.

No effective *treatment* is known. Exchange transfusion, dietary restriction of glycine, and administration of sodium benzoate or folate have not altered the neurologic outcome. Drugs that counteract the effect of glycine on the neuronal cells, such as strychnine and diazepam, have been used; beneficial effects have been observed in some patients having the mild form of the condition.

Nonketotic hyperglycinemia appears to be inherited as an

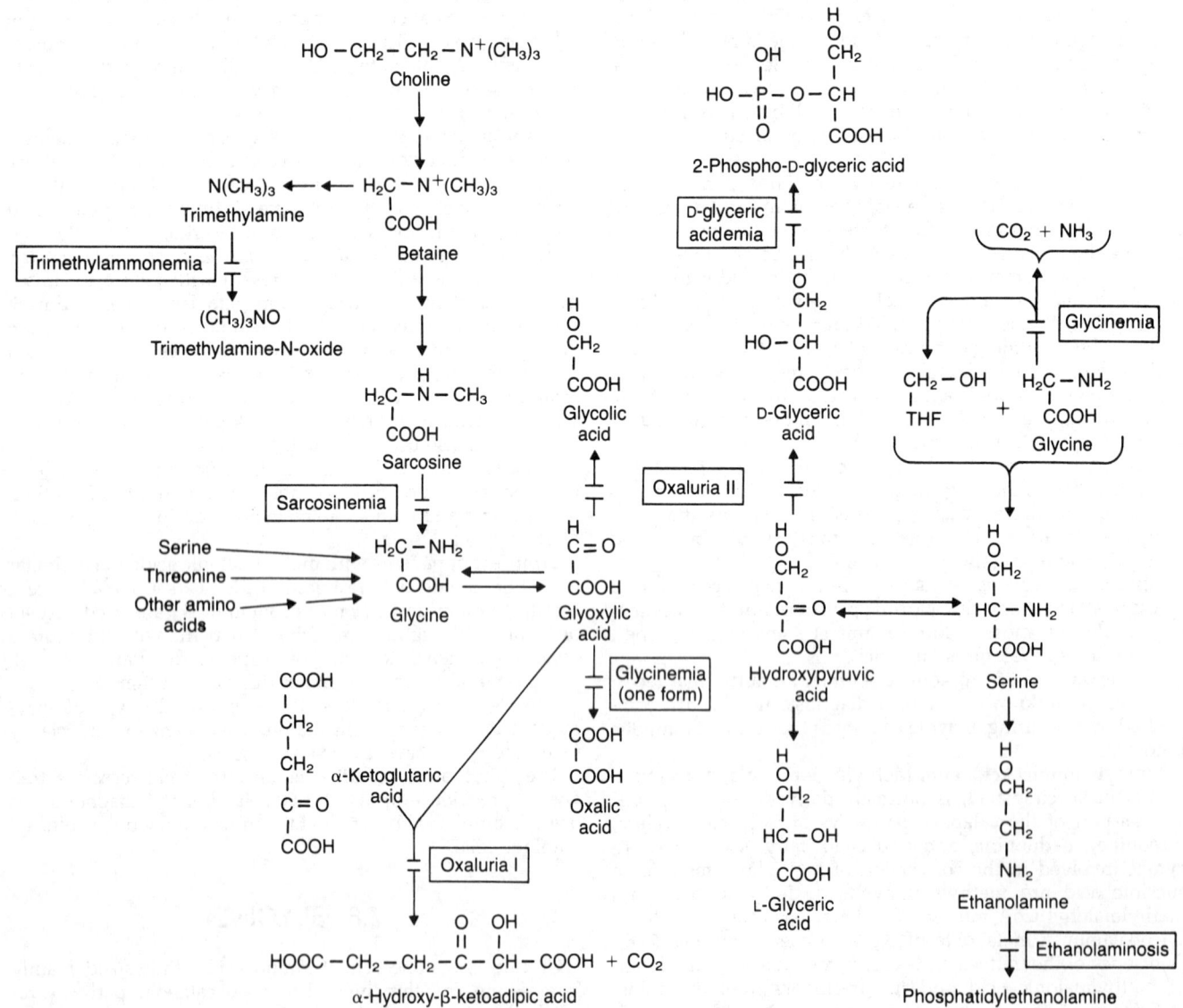

Figure 7–8. Pathways in the metabolism of glycine.

autosomal recessive trait and is more common in Finland than in any other part of the world. The enzyme system may be assayed in specimens obtained from liver or brain. Prenatal diagnosis has been accomplished by measuring glycine and serine levels in amniotic fluid.

Sarcosinemia. Increased concentrations of sarcosine (N-methylglycine) have been observed in both blood and urine, but no consistent clinical picture can be attributed to this metabolic defect. This is probably a recessively inherited inborn error involving sarcosine dehydrogenase, the enzyme that converts sarcosine to glycine (Fig. 7–8).

D-Glyceric Acidemia. Mental retardation has been associated with excretion of abnormal quantities of D-glyceric acid, normal amounts of oxalic acid, nonketotic glycinemia without acidosis. Normal plasma glycine with a persistent metabolic acidosis has also been observed in this disorder. There may be a block at D-glycerate kinase (Fig. 7–8) so that glycerate cannot be converted to 2-phospho-D-glycerate.

Trimethylaminuria. Trimethylamine is normally produced in the intestine from the breakdown of dietary choline and trimethylamine oxide by the bacteria. Eggs and liver are the main sources of choline, and fish is the major source of trimethylamine oxide. Trimethylamine thus produced is absorbed and is oxidized in the liver by trimethylamine oxidase to trimethylamine oxide, which is odorless, and is excreted in the urine. Deficiency of this enzyme results in massive excretion of trimethylamine in urine. Several asymptomatic patients with trimethylaminuria have been reported; there is a foul body odor which resembles that of a rotten fish. Restriction of fish, eggs, liver, and other sources of choline (such as nuts and grains) in the diet significantly reduces the odor.

Glycinuria and Glucoglycinuria. These are separate disorders of the renal tubules. Glycinuria is also observed in prolinemia and prolinuria, since a common transport system for proline, hydroxyproline, and glycine exists in addition to the specific renal transport system for glycine alone.

Hyperoxaluria and Oxalosis. Normally, oxalic acid is derived mostly from the oxidation of glycine via glyoxylic acid (Fig. 7–8) and, to a lesser degree, from the oxidation of ascorbic acid. Foods containing oxalic acid, such as spinach and rhubarb, are the main exogenous source of this compound. Oxalic acid cannot be further metabolized in man and is excreted in the urine.

Secondary hyperoxaluria may occur in a variety of acquired conditions such as pyridoxine deficiency and ingestion of ethylene glycol or high doses of vitamin C. *Primary hyperoxaluria* is a rare genetic disorder in which large amounts of oxalates accumulate in the body. Two enzyme deficiencies cause primary hyperoxaluria. The term *oxalosis* refers to deposition of calcium oxalate in parenchymal tissues.

Hyperoxaluria Type I. This is the most common form of primary hyperoxaluria. This rare condition, due to the deficiency of α-ketoglutarate glyoxylate carboligase, which converts glyoxylic acid to a α-hydroxy-β-ketoadipic acid, is inherited as an autosomal recessive trait (Fig. 7–8).

The majority of patients become symptomatic before 5 yr of age. The initial *clinical manifestations* are related to renal stones and nephrocalcinosis. Renal colic and asymptomatic hematuria lead to a gradual deterioration of renal function as manifested by growth retardation and uremia. Most patients die before 20 yr of age owing to renal failure. Acute arthritis is a rare manifestation and may be misdiagnosed as gout, since uric acid is usually elevated in patients with type I hyperoxaluria. Late forms of the disease presenting during adulthood have also been reported.

Treatment has been largely unsuccessful. In some patients, administering large doses of pyridoxine reduces urinary excretion of oxalate. Renal transplant in patients with renal failure has not improved the outcome in most cases because oxalosis has recurred in the transplanted kidney.

Hyperoxaluria Type II. This type is due to the deficiency of D-glyceric acid dehydrogenase, the same enzyme that converts glyoxylic acid to glycolic acid. In the absence of this enzyme, hydroxypyruvate (the keto acid of serine) is reduced to L-glyceric acid by lactic dehydrogenase. Clinically, these patients are indistinguishable from those with hyperoxaluria type I, except that renal failure has not been observed in the type II disorder; type II patients excrete large amounts of L-glyceric acid in urine in addition to oxalic acid. L-glyceric acid is not present in urine from normal subjects. The reason hyperoxaluria is present in these patients thought to be due to increased conversion from glyoxylic acid (Fig. 7–8).

7.9 SERINE

Ethanolaminosis. This disorder has occurred in patients with cardiomegaly, hypotonia, cerebral dysfunction, and clinical findings usually associated with glycogen storage disease, type II (Sec. 7.21). Patients have died before 2 yr of age. Many tissues contained material which stained with PAS and Best carmine. Glycogen content of the liver and heart was normal, as were all of the enzymes measured that are associated with the glycogenoses, the lipidoses, or the mucopolysaccharidoses. Ethanolamine was found in excessive amounts in liver and urine and was undetected in serum. There was a 70% reduction of activity of ethanolamine kinase (Fig. 7–8) in liver. Although it has been postulated that this disease represents a defect in the synthesis of phosphatidyl-ethanolamine, this disorder may represent a new type of polymer storage disease.

7.10 THREONINE

Threoninemia. Threonine is an essential amino acid that can be deaminated to α-ketobutyric acid or degraded to succinic acid via propionic acid. Periodic episodes of convulsions and developmental retardation have been associated with a marked elevation of threonine in urine and blood (up to 13 times normal in serum). The parents of an affected 8 mo old infant were related and had normal serum threonine levels. The site of the enzymatic defect is unknown.

7.11 PROLINE AND HYDROXYPROLINE

Proline and hydroxyproline are found in high concentration in collagen. Neither of these amino acids is normally found in urine in the free form except in early infancy. Excretion of "bound" hydroxyproline (dipeptides and tripeptides containing hydroxyproline) reflects collagen turnover and is increased in disorders of accelerated collagen turnover, such as rickets or hyperparathyroidism.

Prolinemia. Two types of prolinemia are known in which excessive amounts of proline are present in both blood and urine. Hydroxyproline and glycine are also excreted in abnormal amounts in urine because of inhibition of the common tubular reabsorption mechanism. In type I prolinemia the enzymatic defect involves proline oxidase (Fig. 7–9). In type II the defect is presumed to be in the enzyme of the next step, a dehydrogenase, since pyrrolidine carboxylic acid, as well as proline, accumulates abnormally. Type I has been associated with mild mental retardation, renal abnormalities, nerve deafness, and photogenic epilepsy. Type II was originally observed in a young child who had only mild mental retardation.

Many asymptomatic individuals with both types of prolinemia have now been described. Since prolinemia is apparently a coincidental finding in these patients, diet therapy may not be indicated.

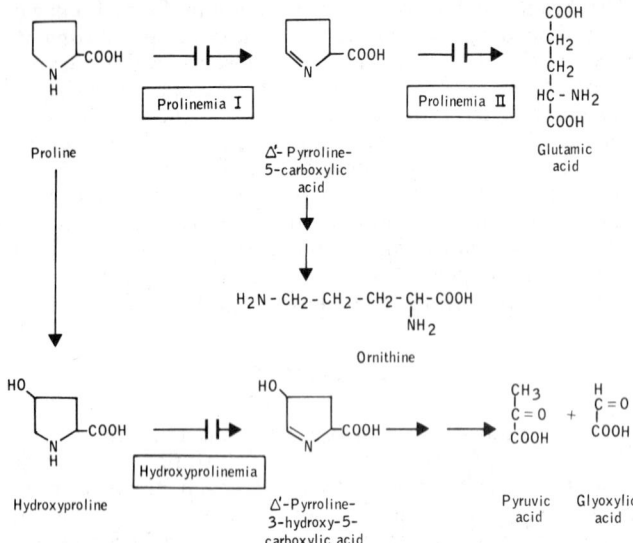

Figure 7–9. Pathways in the metabolism of the imino acids.

Hydroxyprolinemia. Mental retardation has been associated with excessive hydroxyproline in serum and urine. In hydroxyprolinemia, in contrast to prolinemia, excessive urinary excretion of proline and glycine, share the same transport mechanisms, does not occur. The defect is in hydroxyproline oxidase (Fig. 7–9), which is distinct from the corresponding enzyme that acts upon proline. The disorder is presumed to be inherited as an autosomal recessive. Normal adult siblings of an affected child have been reported to have hydroxyprolinemia.

Familial Iminoglycinuria. An asymptomatic defect in renal tubular reabsorption of proline is inherited as an autosomal recessive. Since proline, hydroxyproline, and glycine are all transported by a common mechanism, patients with familial iminoglycinuria also excrete the other two amino acids in abnormal amounts. The serum concentrations of these amino acids are normal. Many of the affected persons also have impaired intestinal transport of proline, and a few may be coincidentally mentally retarded. In a screening program persistent iminoglycinuria occurred in 15 of 200,000 infants, none of whom had any clinical abnormalities.

Prolidase Deficiency Syndrome. During collagen degradation, imidodipeptides are released and normally cleaved by blood prolidase. This autosomal recessive disorder results from a defect in this enzyme. A number of patients with excessive imidodipeptiduria have characteristic joint abnormalities, dermatitis with severe skin ulcers, skeletal and tendinous abnormalities, splenomegaly, frequent infections, and occasional retardation; an otherwise asymptomatic affected sibling of a known patient also has been reported.

7.12 GLUTAMIC ACID

A number of inborn errors are related to the metabolism of glutamic acid. Glutathione (γ-glutamylcysteinylglycine) is involved in a nonspecific amino acid transport system, particularly in the renal tubule and intestinal villus; the cyclical synthesis and degradation of glutathione play a role in the formation of dipeptides with glutamic acid of the amino acids to be transported.

Anemia Due to γ-Glutamylcysteine Synthetase Deficiency. Chronic hemolytic anemia, intermittent jaundice, mild neurologic symptoms, and progressive spinocerebellar degeneration, speech impairment, and myoclonic seizures, have oc-

curred with decreased γ-glutamylcysteine synthetase activity. The anemias noted in disorders of the γ-glutamyl cycle presumably result from lowered intracellular glutathione concentration, as a result of which red cell membranes become more susceptible to lipid peroxidation.

Anemia Due to Glutathione Synthetase Deficiency. Mild hemolytic anemia and intermittent jaundice but no neurologic findings have been associated with markedly decreased red cell glutathione synthetase acivity and glutathione levels.

Pyroglutamic Acidemia (Glutathione Synthetase Deficiency). Patients with this disorder excrete massive amounts (6–20 g/24 hr) of pyroglutamic acid (also known as 5-oxo-L-proline), an intermediate in the Meister γ-glutamyl cycle for the transport of amino acids (Fig. 7–10). In the neonatal period they may have hemolysis and severe metabolic acidosis. Progressive neurologic deterioration or apparently normal development may take place. Glutathione content and glutathione synthetase activity are quite low in red cells and fibroblasts. Overproduction, rather than underutilization, of pyroglutamic acid is the cause of the organic acidemia. This acidemia results from the release of feedback inhibition of the γ-glutamylcysteine synthetase by glutathione and the subsequent conversion of the overproduced γ-glutamylcysteine to pyroglutamic acid at a rate that exceeds the ability of 5-oxyprolinase to convert it back to glutamic acid. There is no explanation for the marked clinical contrast between pyroglutamic acidemia and the mild anemia of glutathione synthetase deficiency, though both lack activity of this enzyme. Patients with the latter condition may have only a red cell deficiency, whereas those with the former may have many tissues involved.

Pyroglutamic Acidemia (5-Oxyprolinase Deficiency). In contrast to the disorder described above, this form of pyroglutamic acidemia is due directly to the inability to degrade the compound, as is usually the case in other inborn errors of metabolism. Episodes of vomiting, diarrhea, and abdominal pain without metabolic acidosis may occur repeatedly from infancy to adolescence. Urinary pyroglutamic acid excretion up to 9 g/24 hr has been reported. 5-Oxyprolinase was markedly reduced in the patients' fibroblasts and leukocytes, whereas the level in their parents' fibroblasts was intermediate between those in patients and those in normal controls. Levels of other enzymes of the γ-glutamyl cycle were normal, as was the gluthathione content of erythrocytes.

Gluthathionemia. This disorder has been detected by routine screening of adults who excreted large amounts of gluthathione and had elevated serum gluthathione. γ-Glutamyl transpeptidase activity in cultured fibroblasts was very low (Fig. 7–10). Although this enzyme is necessary for nonspecific amino acid transport, renal excretion of amino acids is normal.

Vitamin B_6-Responsive Seizures. This diagnosis should be considered for children in whom seizures in early life are poorly controlled with conventional anticonvulsant therapy but in whom parenteral administration of vitamin B_6 results in dramatic improvement of both seizure activity and EEG abnormalities. Analysis of tissues from several of these patients revealed a decrease in glutamic acid decarboxylase activity that was reversed with addition of pyridoxal phosphate (vitamin B_6). Since this defect cannot be detected in fibroblasts, the diagnosis is usually made on the basis of a clinical response to vitamin B_6.

γ-Hydroxybutyric Acidemia. A defect of succinic semialdehyde dehydrogenase, inherited as an autosomal recessive disorder, leads to the increased production of γ-hydroxybutyric acid, a normal minor metabolite of γ-aminobutyric acid. Since both γ-amino- and γ-hydroxybutyric acid are thought to be neurotransmitters, it is interesting that the patients with this disorder so far described have presented with mild mental retardation, hypotonia, and ataxia of the trunk and limbs,

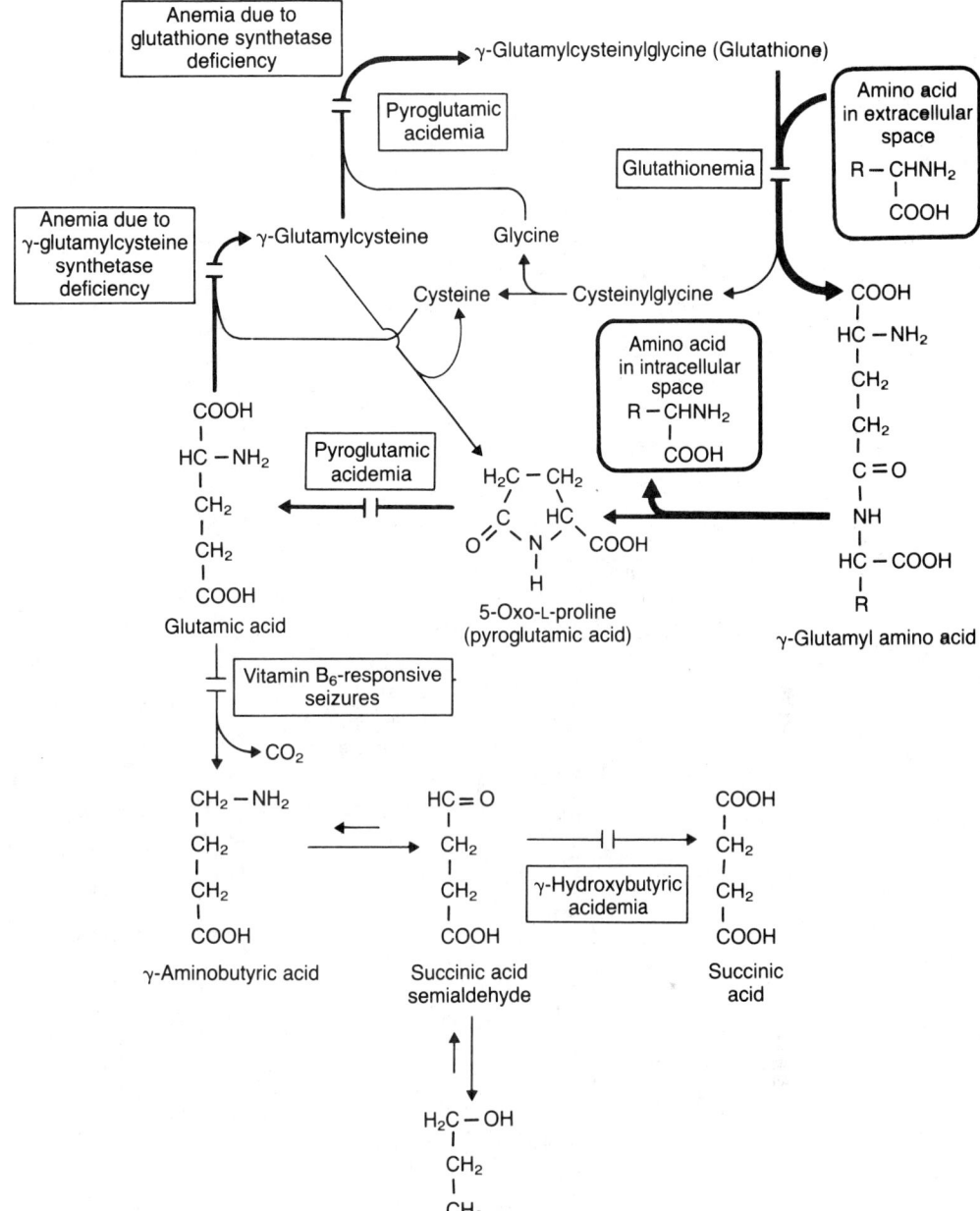

Figure 7–10. The γ-glutamyl cycle for nonspecific amino acid transport. Defects of glutathione synthesis and degradation are noted.

which is nonprogressive. With age there is an improvement in the clinical course; some of the patients have a dramatic improvement of cerebellar function. γ-Hydroxybutyric acid may be markedly elevated in plasma early on in the patient's course and fall toward normal with age. Large amounts may be found in the patient's urine and some may be present in cerebrospinal fluid.

Chinese Restaurant Syndrome. Monosodium glutamate (MSG), a widely used flavor enhancer, is one of the active components of soy sauce. It is responsible for the so-called Chinese restaurant syndrome. Certain individuals react to MSG by developing an acute syndrome that may last for 12 hr and consists of substernal pressure, headache, burning sensations, palpitations, and vomiting. Though there are no apparent sequelae in adults, animal experiments suggest possible central nervous system toxicity. This syndrome may be a benign, undefined inborn error of glutamate metabolism.

7.13 UREA CYCLE AND HYPERAMMONEMIA

Catabolism of amino acids results in the production of free ammonia, which is highly toxic to the central nervous system. Ammonia is detoxified to urea through a series of reactions known as the Krebs-Henseleit or urea cycle (Fig. 7–11). Five enzymes are required for the synthesis of urea: carbamyl-phosphate synthetase (CPS), ornithine transcarbamylase (OTC), argininosuccinate synthetase (AS), argininosuccinate lyase (AL), and arginase. A sixth enzyme, *N*-acetylglutamate synthetase, is also required for synthesis of *N*-acetylglutamate, which is an activator of the CPS enzyme. Individual deficiencies of these enzymes have been observed, and with an overall prevalence of 1:30,000 live births, they are the most common genetic causes of hyperammonemia in infants. In

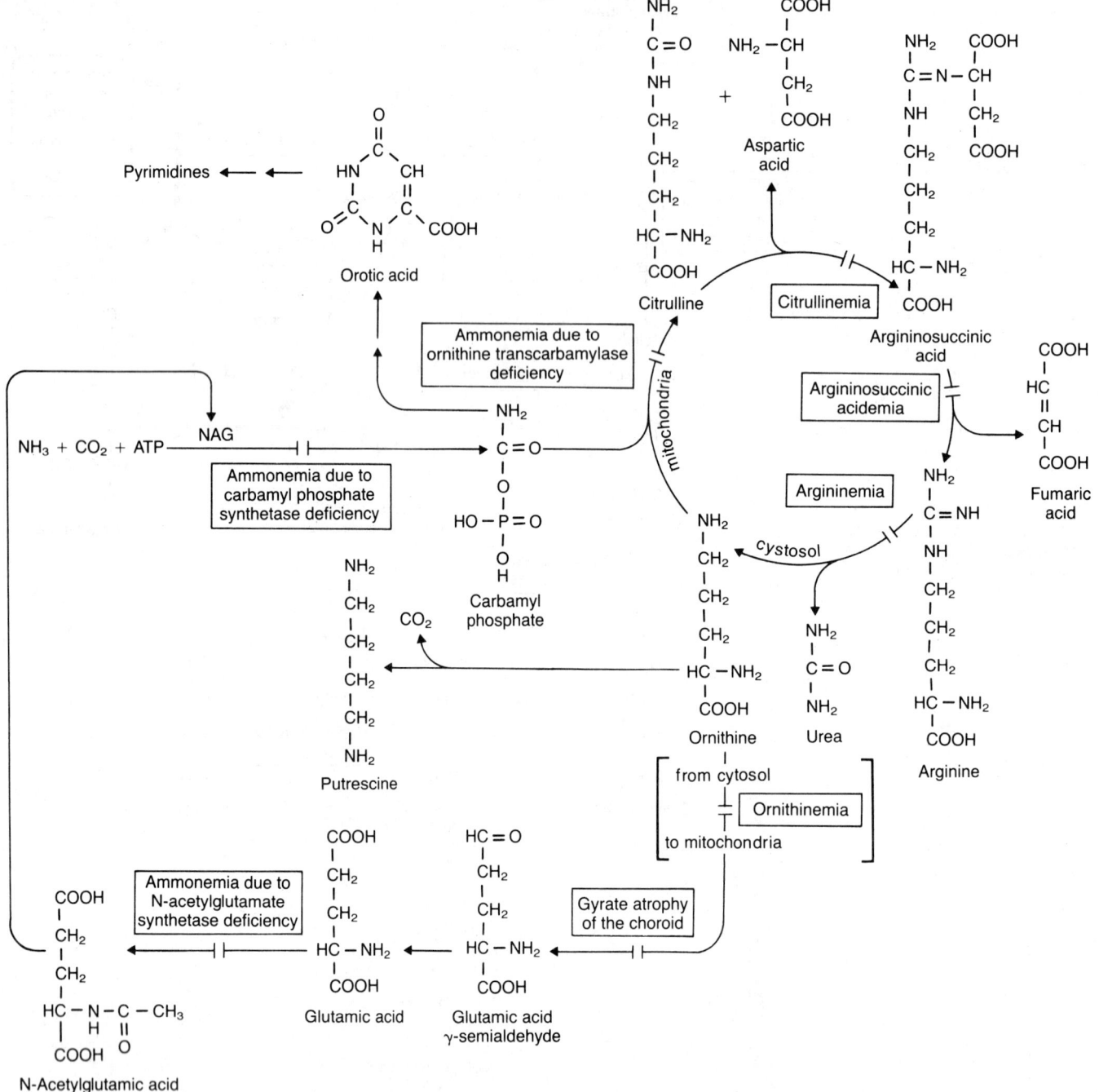

Figure 7–11. Pathways in the metabolism of ammonia and in the urea cycle.

addition to these genetic defects of the urea cycle enzymes, marked increases in plasma levels of ammonia have also been observed in other inborn errors of metabolism (Table 7–4). In this section only defects of the urea cycle enzymes and transient hyperammonemia of the newborn are discussed.

Clinical Manifestations of Hyperammonemia in Infants. Symptoms and signs are mostly related to the brain dysfunction and are similar, regardless of the cause of the hyperammonemia. In general, the affected infant is normal at birth but becomes symptomatic after a few days of protein feeding. Refusal to eat, vomiting, tachypnea, and lethargy quickly progress to a deep coma. Convulsions commonly occur. Physical examination may reveal hepatomegaly in addition to the neurologic signs of a deep coma.

Laboratory studies show no specific findings when hyperammonemia is due to the disorders of the urea cycle enzymes. In infants with organic acidemias, hyperammonemia is commonly associated with severe acidosis, neutropenia, and thrombocytopenia. Infants with hyperammonemia are often diagnosed as having a generalized infection and may succumb to the disease without a correct diagnosis. Autopsy is usually unremarkable. It is, therefore, imperative that plasma ammonia be measured in any ill infant whose clinical manifestations cannot be explained by an obvious infection.

Diagnosis. The main criterion for diagnosis is hyperammonemia. Plasma ammonia in the ill infant is usually above 400 μM (the upper limit of normal is 35–60 μg/dL). Blood urea nitrogen is usually low. An approach to the differential

Table 7-4. Inborn Errors of Metabolism Causing Hyperammonemia

Deficiencies of the urea cycle enzymes
  Carbamylphosphate synthetase (CPS)
  N-acetylglutamate synthetase
  Ornithine transcarbamylase (OTC)
  Argininosuccinate synthetase (AS)
  Argininosuccinate lyase (AL)
  Arginase

Organic acidemias
  Propionic acidemia (Sec. 7.7)
  Methylmalonic acidemia (Sec. 7.7)
  Isovaleric acidemia (Sec. 7.7)
  Ketothiolase deficiency (Sec. 7.7)
  Multiple carboxylase deficiency (Sec. 7.7)
  Fatty acid acyl CoA dehydrogenase deficiency (glutaric acidemia
    type II) Sec. 7.54)
  3-Hydroxy-3-methylglutaric acidemia (Sec. 7.7)

Lysinuric protein intolerance (Sec. 7.16)

Hyperornithinemia-hyperammonemia-homocitrullinemia syndrome
  (Sec. 7.13)

Periodic hyperlysinuria with hyperammonemia (?) (Sec. 7.16)

Transient hyperammonemia of the newborn (Sec. 7.13)

diagnosis of hyperammonemia is illustrated in Figure 7–12. Patients with deficiency of carbamylphosphate synthetase or of ornithine transcarbamylase have no specific abnormalities of plasma amino acids except for increased levels of glutamine, aspartic acid, and alanine secondary to hyperammonemia. A marked increase in urinary orotic acid in ornithine transcarbamylase deficiency differentiates this defect from that of the carbamylphosphate synthetase deficiency. Patients with deficiencies of argininosuccinic acid synthetase, argininosuccinic acid lyase, and arginase have marked increases in plasma levels of citrulline, argininosuccinic acid, and arginine respectively. Differentiation between carbamylphosphate synthetase and N-acetylglutamate synthetase deficiencies may require assay of the respective enzymes. Clinical response to oral administration of carbamylglutamate, however, suggests N-acetylglutamate synthetase deficiency.

Treatment of Acute Hyperammonemia. Acute hyperammonemia causing neurologic manifestations should be treated promptly and vigorously. The goal of therapy is to remove ammonia from the body and to provide adequate calories and essential amino acids to halt further breakdown of the endogenous proteins. Since ammonia has a very poor clearance from the kidney, its removal from the body must be expedited by dialysis and by formation of compounds with high renal clearance. Peritoneal dialysis is the most effective route for removal of ammonia; there is usually a dramatic decrease in plasma ammonia within a few hours of dialysis, and most infants normalize their plasma ammonia within 48 hr of initiation of dialysis. Hemodialysis is equally effective, but more experience in young infants is needed to show its safety and superiority over the peritoneal dialysis.

Administering sodium benzoate (250 mg/kg/24 hr) to form hippuric acid with endogenous glycine is probably the most effective way to detoxify and excrete ammonia. Hippuric acid is cleared from the kidney at 5 times the glomerular filtration rate. Phenylacetate (250 mg/kg/24 hr) is another compound

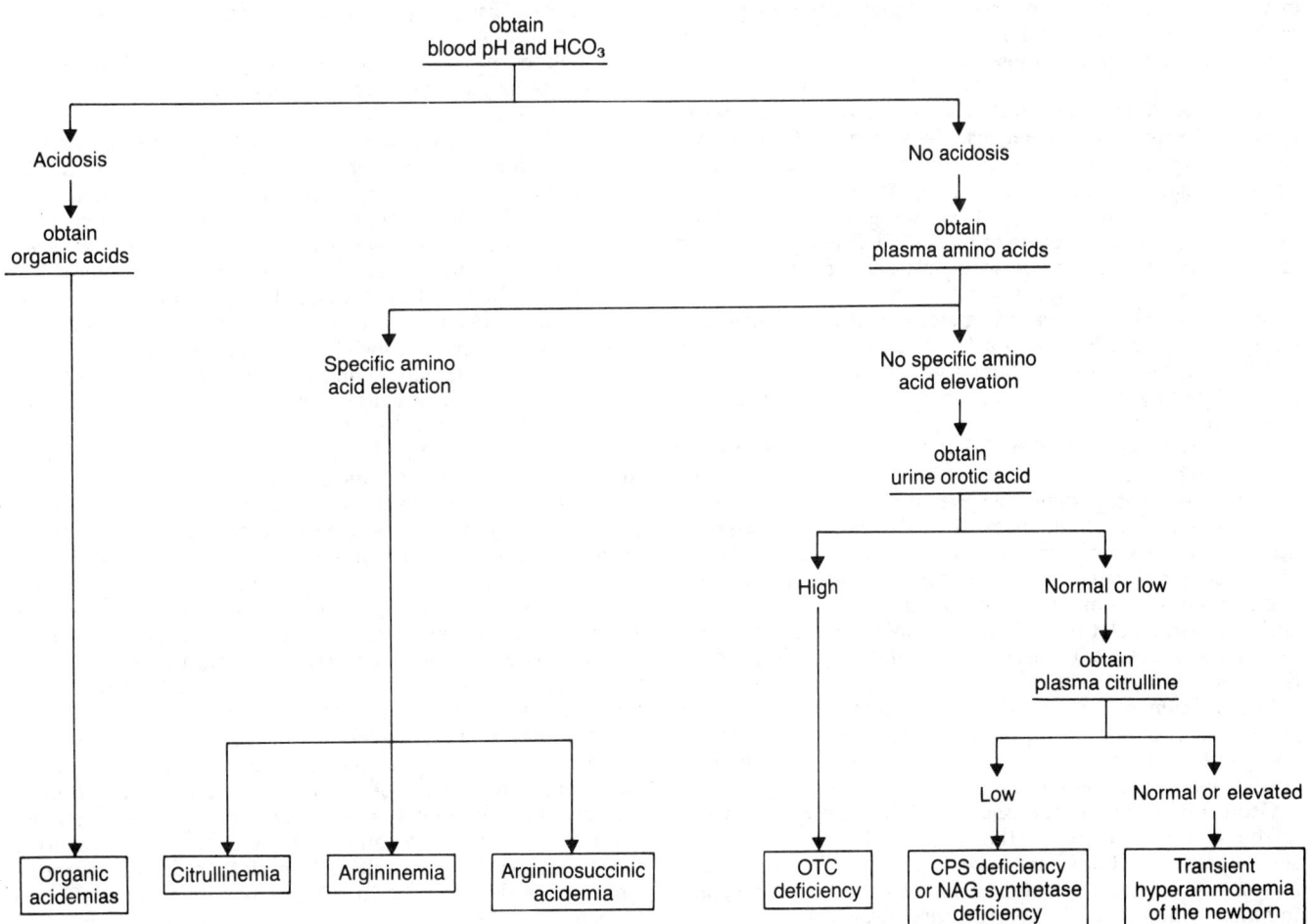

Figure 7–12. Clinical approach to a newborn infant with symptomatic hyperammonemia.

that conjugates with glutamine to form phenylacetylglutamine, which is also readily excreted by the kidneys.

Administering arginine (300–700 mg/kg/24 hr) also increases ammonia excretion by forming an intermediate metabolite of the urea cycle. In patients with citrullinemia or argininosuccinic aciduria, 1 mole of arginine can react with 1 or 2 moles of ammonia to form citrulline or argininosuccinic acid respectively. Renal clearance of these compounds, especially argininosuccinic acid, far exceeds that of ammonia. Patients with ornithine transcarbamylase deficiency may benefit from citrulline supplementation since 1 mole of citrulline can accept 1 mole of ammonia to form arginine. In patients with carbamylphosphate synthetase deficiency, neither arginine nor citrulline seem to facilitate nitrogen excretion. However, administering arginine is indicated because it becomes an essential amino acid in these patients.

Adequate calories should be provided intravenously or through a nasogastric tube. Small doses of protein (0.25–0.5 g/kg/24 hr), preferably composed of essential amino acids, are also needed to correct the catabolic state. To decrease the nitrogen load, keto analogues of essential amino acids have been used by some in place of the amino acid without beneficial effect. Adequate hydration must also be provided. To curtail possible production of ammonia by the intestinal bacteria, oral administration of neomycin and lactulose has also been advocated.

There may be considerable lag between the normalization of plasma ammonia and the improvement in neurological status of the patient. Several days may be needed before the infant becomes fully alert.

Long-Term Therapy. Once the infant is alert, therapy should be tailored to the underlying cause of hyperammonemia. In general, all patients require some degree of protein restriction (0.5–1.5 g/kg/24 hr) regardless of the enzymatic defect. Catabolic states triggering hyperammonemia should also be avoided.

Carbamyl Phosphate Synthetase (CPS) and N-Acetylglutamate Synthetase Deficiencies. Deficiencies of these two enzymes produce similar *clinical and biochemical manifestations*. Affected infants usually become symptomatic in the first few days of life with refusal to eat, vomiting, lethargy, convulsions, and coma. Late forms of the CPS deficiency, characterized by mental retardation with episodes of vomiting and lethargy, have also been reported.

Laboratory findings reveal hyperammonemia without an increase in any specific amino acids in plasma; marked elevations in plasma concentrations of glutamine and alanine are secondary to hyperammonemia. Urinary orotic acid is usually low or may be absent.

Treatment of patients with CPS deficiency is similar to that outlined above for hyperammonemia. Patients with N-acetylglutamate synthetase deficiency may benefit from oral administration of carbamylglutamate. It is, therefore, important to differentiate between these two enzyme deficiencies by assay of the enzyme activities in the biopsies obtained from the liver. In addition, an improvement in the patient's clinical and biochemical status following administration of carbamylglutamate favors a diagnosis of N-acetylglutamate synthetase deficiency.

CPS deficiency is inherited as an autosomal recessive trait; the enzyme is normally present in liver and intestine. N-acetylglutamate synthetase has been assayed only in liver specimens obtained at biopsy.

Ornithine Transcarbamylase (OTC) Deficiency. In this X-linked dominant disorder the hemizygote males are more severely affected than heterozygote females. The latter may have a mild disease or no clinical manifestations. It is probably the most common of all the urea cycle disorders.

Clinical manifestations in a male newborn infant are those of severe hyperammonemia; milder forms simulating Reye syndrome have also been observed, both of which indicate heterogeneity of the mutant gene. As with the carbamylphosphate synthetase deficiency, there is no increase in the plasma levels of any specific amino acid. Marked increase in urinary levels of orotic acid differentiates this condition from the CPS deficiency.

The *diagnosis* may be confirmed by assay of enzyme activity normally present only in liver. Perinatal diagnosis has been achieved by fetal liver biopsy. Treatment is similar to that of the CPS deficiency except that citrulline may be used in place of arginine.

Asymptomatic heterozygous female carriers may be identified by using an oral protein load, which increases plasma ammonia and urinary orotic acid levels. The asymptomatic female carriers have mild cerebral dysfunction compared with their unaffected siblings.

Argininosuccinic Acid Synthetase Deficiency (Citrullinemia). This disorder shows considerable clinical and biochemical heterogeneity. The spectrum of *clinical manifestations* range from lethal forms to asymptomatic ones. Mental retardation and neurologic deficit, however, are common findings even in the mild forms. Marked elevation in the plasma level of citrulline is diagnostic. Patients with argininosuccinic aciduria also show some increase in their plasma concentration of citrulline, as well as elevated levels of argininosuccinic acid. The *diagnosis* is confirmed by assay of the enzyme activity that is normally present in cultured fibroblasts. *Treatment* is similar to that of other urea cycle disorders.

Citrullinemia is inherited as an autosomal recessive trait. The severity of the mutant genes inherited from each parent is different in a given patient, indicating that most affected patients are "double or compound heterozygotes." Prenatal diagnosis is based on an assay of the enzyme activity in cultured amniotic cells.

Although *prognosis* is very poor for symptomatic neonates, patients with the mild disease usually do well on a protein restricted diet.

Argininosuccinate Lyase Deficiency (Argininosuccinic Aciduria). With a prevalence of 1:70,000 live births in the United States, this is the second most common of the urea cycle disorders after ornithine transcarbamylase deficiency. The severity of the *clinical and biochemical manifestations* varies considerably. In the neonatal form severe hyperammonemia develops in the first few days of life and mortality is usually high. In the subacute or late form the major finding is mental retardation, which is associated with episodic vomiting, failure to thrive, and hepatomegaly. Abnormalities of the hair (characterized by dry brittle hair) are of special diagnostic value. Microscopically, the hair appears similar to that seen in patients with trichorrhexis nodosa. Less severe hair abnormalities are also seen in patients with citrullinemia.

Laboratory findings reveal hyperammonemia, moderate elevation in liver enzymes, nonspecific increases in plasma levels of glutamine and alanine, moderate increase in plasma levels of citrulline (less than that seen in citrullinemia), and marked increase in plasma levels of argininosuccinic acid. In most amino acid analyzers, argininosuccinic acid appears within the isoleucine or methionine regions, which may cause confusion in the diagnosis. Argininosuccinic acid can also be found in large amounts in urine and spinal fluid. The levels in the spinal fluid are usually higher than those in plasma.

Treatment is similar to that for other urea cycle disorders. Argininosuccinate lyase deficiency, inherited as an autosomal recessive trait, is normally present in erythrocytes, liver, and cultured fibroblasts. Prenatal diagnosis is based on measuring the enzyme activity in cultured amniotic cells. Argininosuccinic acid is also elevated in the amniotic fluid of the affected fetuses.

Arginase Deficiency (Hyperargininemia). This second rarest of the urea cycle disorders (next to N-acetylglutamate synthetase deficiency) presents early with signs of vomiting, irritability, and developmental delay. Progressive spasticity with scissoring of the lower extremities, spastic diplegia, ataxia, choreoathetosis, and seizures are common findings in older children. Mental retardation is usually severe and progressive. Hyperammonemic episodes usually occur after 6 mo of age.

Laboratory findings reveal marked elevation of plasma arginine and urinary orotic acid. The diagnosis is confirmed by assaying arginase activity in erythrocytes. Arginase deficiency is inherited as an autosomal recessive trait, and intrauterine diagnosis can be made by assaying enzyme activity in fetal erythrocytes.

Transient Hyperammonemia of the Newborn. Although the plasma levels of ammonia in normal fullterm infants are within the normal limits of the older children, a majority of premature infants with low birthweights have a mild transient hyperammonemia (40–50 μM), which lasts for about 6–8 wk. These infants are asymptomatic, and follow-up studies up to 18 mo of age have not revealed any significant neurologic deficits.

Severe transient hyperammonemia has been observed in newborn infants. The majority of affected infants have been premature and have had mild respiratory distress syndrome. Hyperammonemic coma may develop within 2–3 days of life, and the infant may succumb to the disease if treatment is not started immediately. Laboratory studies reveal marked hyperammonemia (plasma ammonia as high as 4000 μM), with moderate increases in plasma levels of glutamine and alanine. Plasma concentrations of urea cycle intermediate amino acids are usually normal except for citrulline, which may be moderately elevated. The cause of the disorder is unknown. Urea cycle enzyme activities are normal. Treatment of hyperammonemia should be initiated promptly and continued vigorously. Recovery without sequelae is common, and hyperammonemia does not recur even with a normal protein diet.

Ornithine. Ornithine is one of the intermediate metabolites of the urea cycle that is not incorporated into natural proteins. Rather, it is generated in the cytosol from arginine and must be transported into the mitochondria, where it is used as a substrate for the enzyme ornithine transcarbamylase (OTC) to form citrulline. Excess ornithine is catabolized by two enzymes, ornithine 5-aminotransferase, which is a mitochondrial enzyme and converts ornithine to a proline precursor, and ornithine decarboxylase, which resides in the cytosol and converts ornithine to putrescine (Fig. 7–11). At least two genetic disorders result in hyperornithinemia: gyrate atrophy of the retina and hyperammonemia-hyperornithinemia-homocitrullinemia syndrome.

Gyrate Atrophy of the Retina and Choroid. This is an autosomal recessively inherited disorder due to the deficiency of the enzyme ornithine 5-aminotransferase. About half of the reported cases are from Finland. Clinical manifestations are limited to the eyes and include night blindness, myopia, loss of peripheral vision, and posterior subcapsular cataracts. These eye changes start between 5 and 10 yr of age and progress to complete blindness by the 4th decade of life. Atrophic lesions in the retina resemble cerebral gyri. These patients usually have normal intelligence. There is a 10 to 20 fold increase in plasma levels of ornithine. There is no occurrence of hyperammonemia and no increase in any other amino acids. Some patients respond to high doses of pyridoxine (500–1000 mg/24 hr) and low dietary arginine.

Hyperornithinemia-Hyperammonemia-Homocitrullinemia Syndrome (HHH Syndrome). In this rare autosomal recessive inherited disorder the defect is in the transport system of ornithine from the cytosol into the mitochondria, causing accumulation of ornithine in the cytosol and deficiency of ornithine inside the mitochondria. The former causes hyper-

ornithinemia and the latter results in disruption of urea cycle and hyperammonemia. Homocitrulline is formed from the reaction of mitochondrial carbamylphosphate with lysine, which occurs because of intramitochondrial deficiency of ornithine. Acute episodes of hyperammonemia in early infancy may result in coma. Failure to thrive, chronic vomiting, mental retardation, and seizures are common findings. No ocular lesions have been observed in these patients. Marked increases in plasma levels of ornithine and homocitrulline are usually diagnostic. Restriction of protein intake improves hyperammonemia. Ornithine supplementation may cause clinical improvement in some patients.

7.14 HISTIDINE

Histidinemia. In histidinemia the activity of the enzyme histidase, which normally converts histidine to urocanic acid, is deficient in liver and skin. As a result, histidine is transaminated to imidazolepyruvic acid, which appears in the urine along with excessive amounts of histidine (Fig. 7–13). Imidazolepyruvic acid, like phenylpyruvic acid, reacts with ferric chloride to produce a blue-green color. Many patients with histidinemia have been detected through screening tests for phenylketonuria, and some have been misdiagnosied as having PKU. Elevations in plasma levels of histidine are necessary for diagnosis, and a definitive diagnosis depends on measuring histidase activity of cornified epithelium or of liver.

Some affected persons have had impaired speech, a few were retarded in growth, and some were mentally retarded. The relation of these findings to histidinemia is unknown inasmuch as routine amino acid screening has uncovered a significant number of asymptomatic persons with histidinemia. The metabolic defect is transmitted as an autosomal recessive trait; in some families the heterozygous state can be identified by demonstrating decreased histidase activity in skin.

Evidence for genetic heterogeneity in histidinemia exists. In some affected children plasma levels of alanine as well as histidine were elevated for unknown reasons. In some families with histidinemia the level of histidase in skin is normal, and perhaps the defect in enzymatic activity is limited to the liver. Several children with Marfan syndrome also have histidinemia, but no relationship has been shown between these two genetic disorders.

Affected neonates do not excrete imidazole derivatives of histidine because there is a normal delay in the maturation of histidine transaminase.

Histidine and Folic Acid Metabolism. After histidine has been converted to urocanic acid, it is further metabolized to formiminoglutamic acid (FIGLU). The formimino group of this compound is normally transferred to folic acid, with the concomitant production of glutamic acid (Fig. 7–13). Measurement of the urinary excretion of FIGLU after loading with histidine has been used to detect folic acid deficiency states. Both FIGLU and urocanic acid are excreted by patients with megaloblastic anemia due to folic acid deficiency. Urocanic acid is also found in the urine of children with kwashiorkor.

Four distinct defects in folic acid metabolism have been delineated, in each of which the blood values of folic acid are normal or elevated. In the first, the enzyme formiminotransferase is deficient; the formiminoglutamic acid level is increased after administration of histidine. Mental retardation, microcephaly, and electroencephalographic abnormalities were frequent findings in some Japanese infants with elevated folate levels. Other patients with normal folate levels and no hematologic abnormalities or retardation excreted massive amounts of FIGLU. These children responded to folate by decreasing FIGLU excretion, and they may represent a harm-

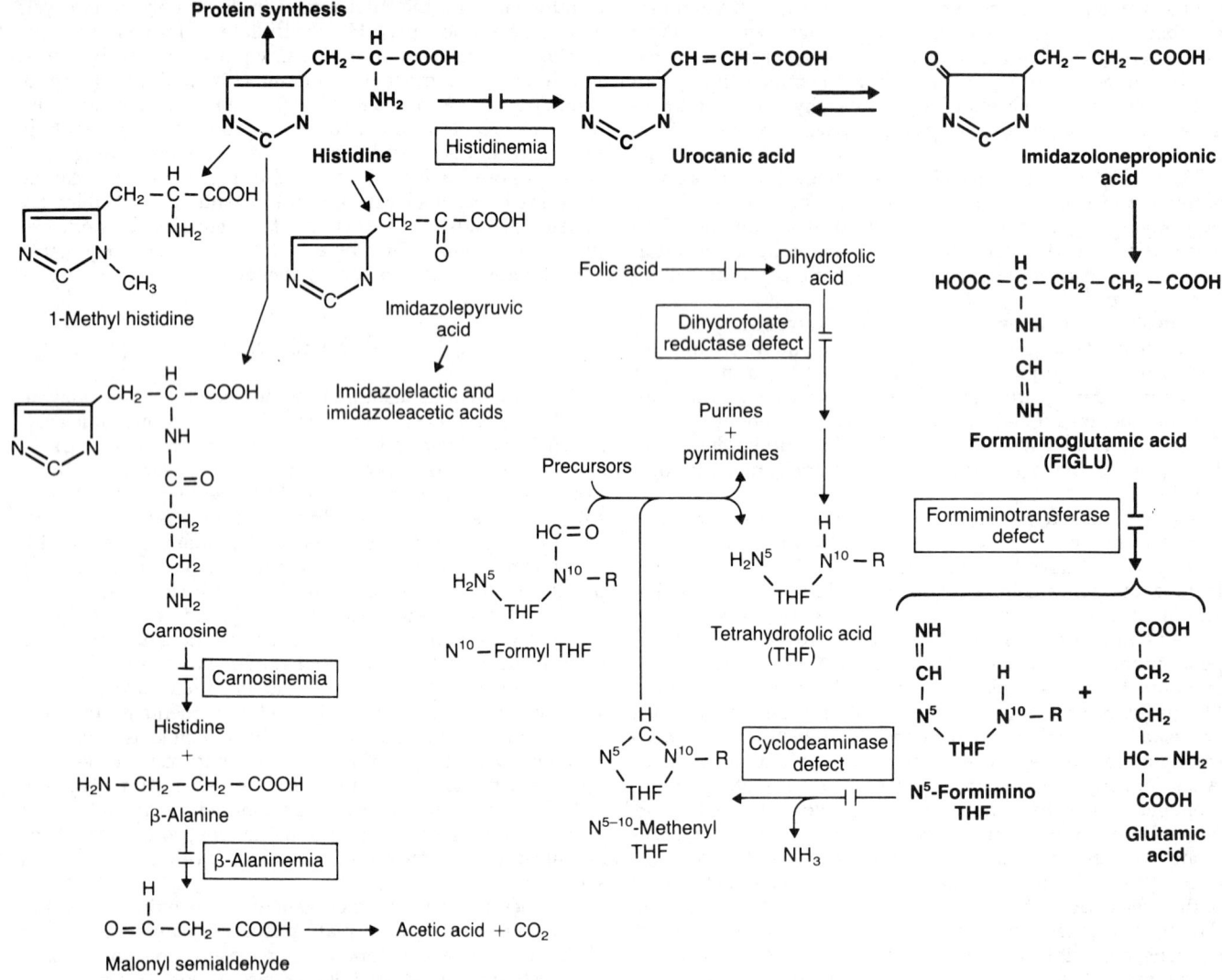

Figure 7–13. Pathways in the metabolism of histidine, beta amino acids, and folic acid. (THF is an abbreviation for tetrahydrofolic acid.) Major pathway is shown in bolder type.

less variant of formiminotransferase deficiency. The more severely affected Japanese patients may represent a double enzyme defect involving not only formiminotransferase but cyclodeaminase, the enzyme responsible for converting N^5-formimino-THF to N^5-N^{10}-methylene THF (Fig. 7–13). The second and third disorders are farther down the metabolic pathway and involve defects either in the enzyme that normally transfers the methyl group of N^5-methyltetrahydrofolate to homocysteine, forming methionine, or in the reductase which converts 5,10-methylene THF to N^5-methylene THF (Fig. 7–4 and Sec. 7.4). A fourth defect in folic acid metabolism results from decreased dihydrofolate reductase activity. Three children with megaloblastic anemia and normal serum folate levels responded hematologically to 5-formyl-tetrahydrofolic acid but not to folic acid; enzymatic analysis of liver tissue established that reductase activity was deficient.

Histidinuria. The urinary excretion of histidine normally increases in pregnant women. Histidinuria also occurs as an overflow phenomenon in patients with histidinemia. Isolated histidinuria without histidinemia, due to defective renal tubular reabsorption, has been found in 3 children whose parents and siblings were shown to be heterozygous for the defect.

Dipeptides of Histidine. Carnosine (β-alanylhistidine) and anserine (β-alanyl-1-methyl histidine) are peptides of histidine of unknown function found in muscle. These peptides, as well as 1-methyl histidine derived from anserine, occur in urine of normal persons, particularly after the ingestion of large amounts of turkey and chicken. Homocarnosine (γ-aminobutyryl-histidine) appears to be brain-specific since it is found only in the cerebrospinal fluid. In the disorders described below, the findings of the dipeptides of histidine in urine have been specific and independent of dietary intake.

Imidazole Aciduria. Excessive excretion of carnosine, anserine, and occasionally of homocarnosine (γ-aminobutyryl-histidine), as well as of histidine and 1-methyl histidine, has been associated with a form of cerebromacular degeneration resembling juvenile Tay-Sachs disease. Synthesis of the dipeptides appears increased. The genetic basis of the disorder is unclear; in the 3 families studied the cerebromacular degeneration was inherited on a recessive basis, whereas the histidine peptiduria appeared to be transmitted on a dominant one. Isolated increased excretion of 1-methyl histidine without 1-methyl histidinemia has been reported in 3 male siblings with precocious puberty who had no other clinical abnormality.

Serum Carnosinase Deficiency. Patients with serum carnosine deficiency usually have severe neurologic involvement with persistent carnosinuria but not carnosinemia. The defect is in the enzyme carnosinase, which normally hydrolyzes carnosine to histidine and β-alanine and can be assayed in plasma. The disorder appears to be recessively inherited.

Homocarnosinosis. Progressive spastic paraplegia, mental deterioration, retinal pigmentation, and cerebrospinal fluid homocarnosine concentrations that are 20 times normal characterize homocarnosinosis. The relationship of the biochemical abnormality to the mental deterioration remains obscure. Increased cerebrospinal fluid homocarnosine values have been found in parents of affected children and in some untreated phenylketonuria patients.

7.15 BETA-AMINO ACIDS

β-Alaninemia. Lethargy, somnolence, grand mal seizures, and death in infancy have been associated with persistent β-alaninemia at concentrations 2–4 times normal. Beta-alanine is derived from the hydrolysis of certain dipeptides and by the degradation of uracil. It is normally further metabolized by transamination to malonic acid, then to acetate and carbon dioxide. Evidence suggests a block in the transamination β-alanine. The increased urinary concentrations of β-aminoiso-butyric acid and taurine as well as of β-alanine suggest a common renal transport mechanism for the β-amino acids. The affected child also has increased concentration of γ-aminobutyric acid in cerebrospinal fluid, plasma, and urine. Neurologic symptoms have been attributed to the increase in β-alanine and the decrease in γ-aminobutyric acid within the brain. Abnormal urinary excretion of β-alanine and β-amino-isobutyrate has also been reported in a normal child with brittle hair, and what appears to be an isolated transport defect for β-alanine has been associated with physical and mental retardation.

β-Aminoisobutyric Aciduria. Excessive excretion of β-aminoisobutyric acid (BAIB) is a genetic variant in metabolism in a small percentage of the normal population. Affected persons are asymptomatic and excrete 100–300 mg of β-aminoisobutyric acid daily, in contrast to 10–40 mg in normal persons. The condition is transmitted by a recessive gene. In addition, β-aminoisobutyric aciduria occurs in a variety of illnesses in which there is tissue destruction and deoxyribonucleic acid is catabolized excessively. Normal persons fed large amounts of β-aminoisobutyric acid, a normal metabolite of both valine and thymine, can excrete it rapidly.

7.16 LYSINE

Lysine is an essential dibasic amino acid with a unique catabolic pathway, which starts with its condensation with α-ketaglutaric acid to form saccharopine rather than with its transamination. Saccharopine is then broken down to aceto-acetic acid through a series of reactions (Fig. 7–14). The first two enzymes involved in the catabolic pathway of lysine, α-ketoglutarate reductase and saccharopine dehydrogenase, are very likely part of a one-protein complex controlled by a single gene. In a minor pathway for the catabolism of lysine, transamination is the first step and pipecolic acid is formed (Fig. 7–14).

Hyperlysinemia. Marked elevations of plasma lysine may occur as a persistent or as a periodic disorder; the latter is also associated with hyperammonemia.

Persistent Hyperlysinemia. This rare, presumably autosomal recessive disorder, is due to the deficiency of the putative enzyme complex lysine ketoglutarate reductase/saccharopine dehydrogenase system. About 20 patients have been reported.

Clinical manifestations range from severe mental and physical retardation, joint laxity and convulsion to perfectly normal children (who were identified through routine screening).

Hyperlysinemia is not generally believed to be the cause of clinical manifestations in symptomatic patients.

Laboratory findings reveal hyperlysinemia, saccharopinemia, lysinuria, and saccharopinuria (saccharopine is not normally detected in blood or urine) in the majority of the patients. Affected persons with hyperlysinemia, but without saccharopinemia, have also been reported. In addition, homocitrulline and homoarginine are found in body fluids (Fig. 7–14). Combined deficiencies of the enzymes lysine ketoglutarate reductase and saccharopine dehydrogenase have been found in all patients having these measurements except one who had a complete deficiency of saccharopine dehydrogenase with mild decrease in lysine ketoglutarate reductase activity.

Hyperlysinemia/saccharopinemia is an example of a double deficiency of two sequential enzymes. Another example is the enzyme deficiency causing orotic aciduria (Sec. 7.51).

The need for treatment of patients with hyperlysinemia is controversial.

Periodic Hyperlysinemia with Hyperammonemia. Patients with this disorder have episodes of hyperammonemia and hyperlysinemia which may start in the newborn period. They are triggered by a diet high in lysine or in protein (2–3 g/kg/24 hr). A low protein diet normalizes plasma concentrations of lysine and ammonia. Patients may have increased levels of plasma arginine or citrulline during the attacks. Enzymes of the urea cycle were within normal limits in the original reports, but subsequently deficiency of enzyme argininosuccinic synthetase was reported. The basic defect in these patients is obscure but may be a deficiency of one of the urea cycle enzymes, because plasma lysine is elevated in some patients with deficiencies of the urea cycle enzymes.

α-Aminoadipic Acidemia. Normal children and children with multiple bony anomalies and learning disabilities who excrete large amounts of α-aminoadipic acid have been reported. No relationship could be established between the clinical abnormalities and the biochemical defect. Since lysine loads increased the α-aminoadipic acid excretion, the block is presumed to be an inability to convert α-aminoadipic to α-ketoadipic acid.

α-Ketoadipic Acidemia. Neonatal seizures, ichthyosis, mild metabolic acidosis, and subsequent marked retardation are associated with elevated α-ketoadipic acid levels in plasma and urine. A defect in the decarboxylation of α-ketoadipic to glutaric acid has been demonstrated. However, the same biochemical defects have been found in a clinically normal sibling of an affected patient, raising doubts as to any relationship between the metabolic defect and the mental retardation.

Glutaric Aciduria Type I. Glutaric acid is an intermediate in the degradation of lysine (Fig. 7–14), hydroxylysine, and tryptophan (Fig. 7–5). Glutaric aciduria type I, a rare autosomal recessive disorder caused by deficiency of glutaryl CoA dehydrogenase, should be differentiated from glutaric aciduria type II, a distinct clinical and biochemical disorder caused by multiple deficiencies of the acyl CoA dehydrogenases (Sec. 7.54).

Affected patients are normal at birth and may remain relatively asymptomatic in the first few months of life, but progressive mental and neurologic disturbances usually become evident after 3 mo of age. The hallmark of the disease is generalized spasticity with dystonia and choreoathetosis. Death may occur following a state resembling Reye syndrome.

Laboratory studies reveal mild metabolic acidosis and ketosis. High concentrations of glutaric acid are found in urine and in blood. Plasma amino acids are usually normal.

Treatment with a low protein diet (especially restricted in lysine and tryptophan) and with high doses of riboflavin (the coenzyme for glutaryl CoA dehydrogenase) causes a signifi-

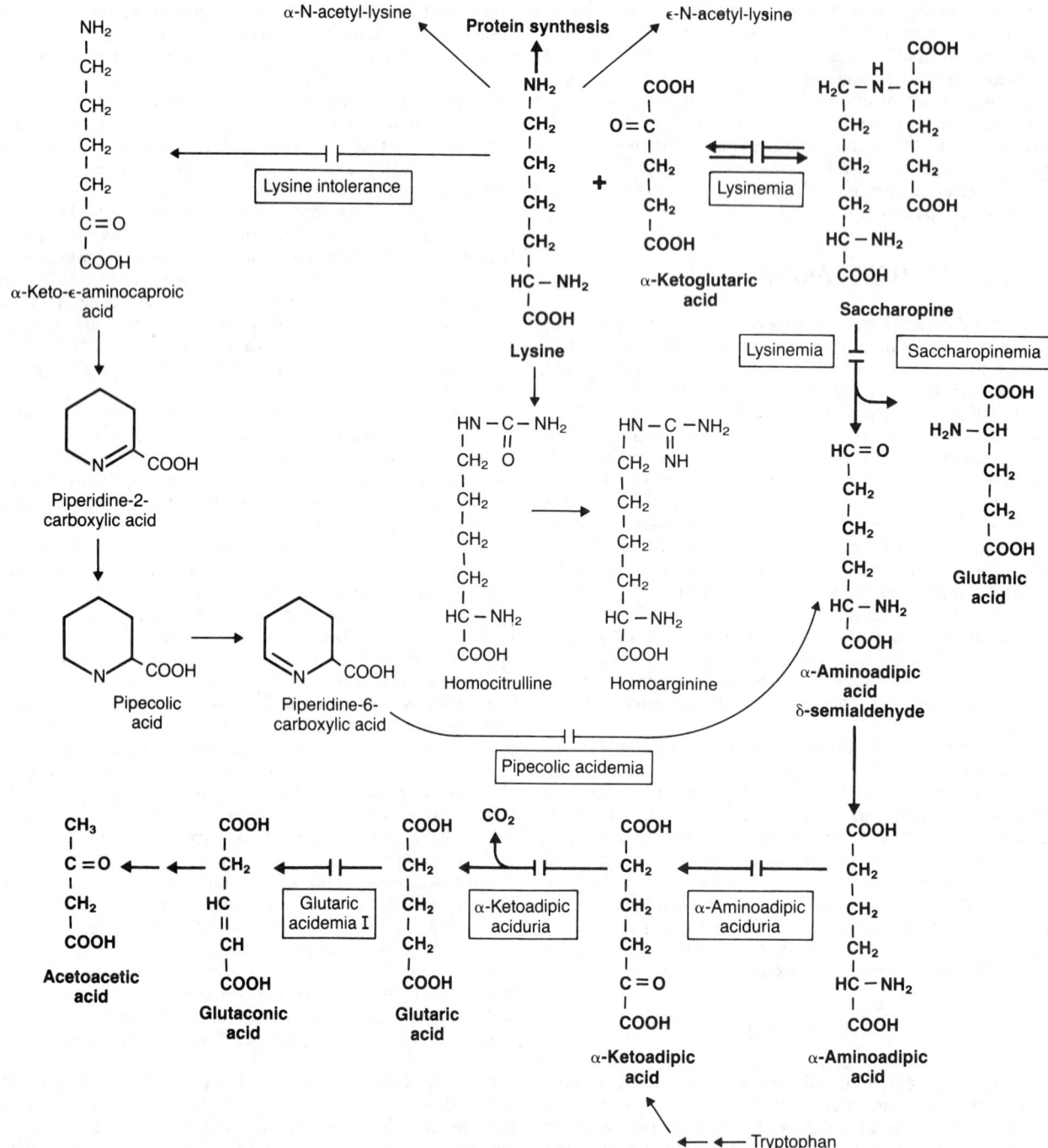

Figure 7–14. Pathways in the metabolism of lysine. Major pathways are shown in bolder type.

cant decrease in levels of glutaric acid in body fluids. Adding γ-aminobutyric acid (GABA) analogues to the therapeutic regimen has caused some clinical improvement in affected children.

Pipecolatemia (Pipecolic Acidemia). Pipecolic acid is one of the intermediate metabolites of the minor pathway of lysine catabolism (Fig. 7–14). Increased levels of pipecolic acid in body fluids have been noted in infants having signs and symptoms resembling those of the Zellweger syndrome (Sec. 7.54). Plasma levels of lysine, and other amino acids are normal. Cystic changes of the kidney and absence of hepatic peroxisomes, commonly seen in patients with Zellweger syndrome, are not present in patients with pipecolic acidemia. The defect in thought to be in the enzyme aminoadipic semialdehyde oxidase, which catalyzes the conversion of pipecolic acid to α-aminoadipic semialdehyde, but the pathogenesis remains unclear.

Lysinuria (Hyperdibasicaminoaciduria). The dibasic amino acids (lysine, arginine, ornithine, and cystine) share a common transport mechanism in the intestine and kidney. Several genetic variants have been described that can affect the renal reabsorption of one or more of these dibasic amino acids. In cystinuria (Sec. 7.5), all four amino acids are affected. Some patients who excrete lysine, arginine, and ornithine in excessive amounts have severe mental and physical retardation. Other mentally retarded individuals have been described with isolated defects of lysine transport or defects limited to lysine and arginine.

Lysinuric Protein Intolerance (Familial Protein Intolerance). This rare autosomal recessive disorder is due to a defect in transport of lysine, ornithine, and arginine in both kidney and intestine. Unlike patients with cystinuria, urinary excretion of cystine is not increased in these patients. Failure to thrive, refusal to feed, vomiting, and diarrhea are *clinical manifestations* in the first few months of life. Physical and mental retardation associated with episodes of hyperammonemic coma may develop later. Patients with this disorder have an aversion to protein and may have sparse, brittle hair, hepatomegaly, osteoporosis, and hyperlaxity of the joints.

Laboratory findings may reveal hyperammonemia, anemia, neutropenia, and thrombocytopenia. Plasma concentrations of lysine, arginine, and ornithine are usually low, but urinary excretion of these amino acids is increased tremendously. The mechanism of hyperammonemia may be related to the deficiency of arginine and ornithine; low levels of these amino acids slow down the urea cycle, and hyperammonemia ensues. *Treatment* with a low protein diet supplemented with arginine and citrulline has resulted in biochemical and clinical improvement.

Most reported cases are from Finland, where the prevalence has been estimated to be 1:60,000–1:80,000.

Hydroxylysinemia. Patients with a variety of symptoms (two had trisomy 21) have been reported with hydroxylysinemia. As hydroxylysine is usually not detectable in plasma, the small amount found in the plasma indicates that the defect is not one of renal absorption. The nature of the defect, presumably in the degradation of free hydroxylysine, is unknown.

Hydroxylysine-Deficient Collagen. Patients with the clinical appearance of Ehlers-Danlos syndrome (Sec. 24.17) have been shown to have collagen with an abnormally low hydroxylysine content. Some patients exhibited severe scoliosis, joint laxity, hyperextensible skin, and thin scars, while another had, in addition, clubbed feet, retinal detachments, peptic ulcer, and hiatal hernia. Measurements of the activity of the enzyme lysyl-protocollagen hydroxylase in cultured fibroblasts revealed approximately one eighth of the normal value.

IRAJ REZVANI
VICTOR H. AUERBACH

Ballard RA, Vinocur B, Reynolds JW, et al: Transient hyperammonemia of the preterm infant. N Engl J Med 299:920, 1978.

Batshaw ML, Brusilow SW: Asymptomatic hyperammonemia in low birth weight infants. Pediatr Res 12:221, 1978.

Batshaw ML, Brusilow S, Waber L, et al: Treatment of inborn errors of urea synthesis. N Engl J Med 306:1387, 1982.

Batshaw ML, Wachtel RC, Thomas GH, et al: Arginine-responsive asymptomatic hyperammonemia in the premature infant. J Pediatr 105:86, 1984.

Cederbaum SD: Disorders of lysine metabolism. *In:* Kelley VC (ed): Practice of Pediatrics. Vol 6. Philadelphia, Harper and Row, 1985.

Dhondt J-L: Tetrahydrobiopterin deficiencies: Preliminary analysis from an international survey. J Pediatr 104:501, 1984.

DiGeorge AM, Rezvani I, Garibaldi LR, et al: Prospective study of maple-syrup-urine disease for the first four days of life. N Engl J Med 307:1492, 1982.

Donn SM, Banagale RC: Neonatal hyperammonemia. Pediatr Rev 5:203, 1984.

Endo F, Kitano A, Uehara I, et al: Four-hydroxyphenylpyruvic acid oxidase deficiency with normal fumarylacetoacetase: A new variant form of hereditary tyrosinemia. Pediatr Res 17:92, 1983.

Gaull GE, Tallan HH, Lonsdale D, et al: Hypermethioninemia associated with methionine adenosyltransferase deficiency: Clinical, morphological and biochemical observations on four patients. J Pediatr 98:734, 1981.

Gibson KM, Jansen I, Sweetman L, et al: 4-Hydroxybutyric aciduria. A new inborn error of metabolism. III. Enzymology and inheritance. J Inher Metab Dis 7 (Suppl l):95, 1984.

Harpey JP, Rosenblatt DS, Cooper BA, et al: Homocystinuria caused by 5,10-methylenetetrahydrofolate reductase deficiency: A case in an infant responding to methionine, folinic acid, pyridoxine and vitamin B$_{12}$ therapy. J Pediatr 98:275, 1981.

Hayasaka K, Tada K, Kikuchi G, et al: Nonketotic hyperglycinemia: Two patients with primary defects of P-protein and T-protein, respectively, in the glycine cleavage system. Pediatr Res 17:967, 1983.

Hoganson G, Berlow S, Kaufman S, et al: Biopterin synthesis defects: Problems in diagnosis. Pediatrics 74:1004, 1984.

Holtzman NA, Kronmal RA, Van Doorninck W, et al: Effects of age at loss of dietary control on intellectual performance and behavior of children with phenylketonuria. N Engl J Med 314:593, 1986.

Hostetter MK, Levy HL, Winter HS: Evidence for liver disease preceding amino acid abnormalities in hereditary tyrosinemia. N Engl J Med 308:1265, 1983.

Kaufman S: Hyperphenylalaninemia caused by defects in biopterin metabolism. J Inher Metab Dis 8(Suppl 1):20, 1985.

Larsson A, Mattsson B, Wauters EA, et al: 5-Oxoprolinuria due to hereditary 5-oxoprolinase deficiency in two brothers—a new inborn error of the 8-glutamyl cycle. Acta Paediatr Scand 70:301, 1981.

Ledley FD, Levy HL, Shih VE, et al: Benign methylmalonic aciduria. N Engl J Med 311:1015, 1984.

Levy HL, Waisbren SE: Effects of untreated maternal phenylketonuria and hyperphenylalaninemia on the fetus. N Engl J Med 309:1269, 1983.

Levy HL: Phenylketonuria-1986. Pediatr Rev 7:269, 1986.

Matalon R, Naidu S, Hughes JR, et al: Nonketotic hyperglycinemia: Treatment with diazepam—a competitor for glycine receptors. Pediatrics 71:581, 1983.

Matsui SM, Mahoney MJ, Rosenberg LE: The natural history of the inherited methylmalonic acidemias. N Engl J Med 308:857, 1983.

McInnes RR, Arshinoff SA, Bell L, et al: Hyperornithinaemia and gyrate atrophy of the retina: Improvement of vision during treatment with a low-arginine diet. Lancet 1:513, 1981.

Meryash DL, Levy HL, Guthrie R, et al: Prospective study of early neonatal screening for phenylketonuria. N Engl J Med 304:294, 1981.

Msall M, Batshaw ML, Suss R, et al: Neurological outcome in children with inborn errors of urea synthesis. N Engl J Med 310:1500, 1984.

Mudd SH, Skovby F, Levy HL, et al: The natural history of homocystinuria due to cystathionine β-synthetase deficiency. Am J Hum Genet 37:1, 1985.

Ney D, Bay C, Schneider JA, et al: Dietary management of oculocutaneous tyrosinemia in an 11 year old child. J Dis Child 137:995, 1983.

Niederwieser A, Blau N, Wang M, et al: GTP cyclohydrolase I deficiency, a new enzyme defect causing hyperphenylalaninemia with neopterin, biopterin, dopamine, and serotonin deficiencies and muscular hypotonia. Eur J Paediatr 141:208, 1984.

Nyhan WL: Abnormalities in Amino Acid Metabolism in Clinical Medicine. Norwalk, CT, Appleton-Century-Crofts, 1984.

Reddi OS: Threoninemia—a new metabolic defect. J Pediatr 93:814, 1978.

Roth KS, Yang W, Forman JW, et al: Holocarboxylase synthetase deficiency. A biotin responsive organic acidemia. J Pediatr 96:845, 1980.

Shinnar S, Singer HS: Cobalamin C mutation (methylmalonic aciduria and homocystinuria) in adolescence. A treatable cause for dementia and myelopathy. N Engl J Med 311:451, 1984.

Starzl TE, Zitelli BJ, Shaw BW Jr, et al: Changing concepts: Liver replacement for hereditary tyrosinemia and hepatoma. J Pediatr 106:604, 1985.

Wilcken B, Hammond JW, Howard N, et al: Hawkinsuria, a dominantly inherited defect of tyrosine metabolism with severe effects in infancy. N Engl J Med 305:865, 1981.

Wilcken DE, Wilcken B, Dudman NP, et al: Homocystinuria—the effects of betaine in the treatment of patients not responsive to pyridoxine. N Engl J Med 309:448, 1983.

Woo SL: Prenatal diagnosis and carrier detection of classic phenylketonuria by gene analysis. Pediatrics 74:412, 1984.

Yokoi T, Honke K, Funabashi T, et al: Partial ornithine transcarbamylase deficiency simulating Reye syndrome. J Pediatr 99:929, 1981.

DEFECTS IN METABOLISM OF CARBOHYDRATES

7.17 INTESTINAL DEFECTS OF CARBOHYDRATE METABOLISM

Nutritional carbohydrates in man's diet include starch (the glucose polymers from plants) and glycogen (from animals), the disaccharides lactose and sucrose, and the monosaccharides glucose, galactose, and fructose (Sec. 3.4).

There are two forms of starch: amylose and amylopectin. Amylose consists of α-1,4 linked glucose units that form straight chains. In amylopectin, the straight chains are branched by an α-1,6 linkage in about every 30th α-1,4 linked glucose unit. Glycogen averages 1 α-1,6 branch point per 10 α-1,4 linked glucose units.

Amylases in saliva and pancreatic juice hydrolyze starch and glycogen to maltose, maltotriose, and α-dextrin (isomaltose). Maltose consists of 2 glucose units joined in α-1,4 linkage. Maltotriose consists of 3 such units. Alpha-dextrin consists of several glucose units linked by an α-1,6 bond and a few α-1,4 linkages. In lactose, carbon 1 of galactose is attached to carbon 4 of glucose. The reducing end of the glucose unit, carbon 1, remains free. Thus, lactose is a reducing sugar and gives a positive reaction with *Clinitest* but not with *Testape*. Strips of Testape, or of similar dipsticks such as Clinistix, contain glucose oxidase, which acts on free glucose only. Clinitest tablets contain cupric sulfate that is converted to cuprous oxide by reducing substances.

The reducing sugars include glucose, maltose, maltotriose, and α-dextrin, but not sucrose. In sucrose, the reducing end of glucose is linked to that of fructose. Thus, the reducing end of neither hexose is free to react, and sucrose is a nonreducing disaccharide.

The brush border of the intestinal villus cell exhibits the following **hydrolytic activities** (as demonstrated by hydrolysis of the substrates listed in parentheses): maltase (maltose, maltotriose), isomaltase (α-dextrin), lactase (lactose), and sucrase (sucrose). Glucose and galactose are actively transported across the intestinal epithelium.

Hydrolysis or transport can be impaired either on a genetically determined (primary) basis or as the (secondary) consequence of another disease, such as infectious gastroenteritis or cystic fibrosis. In either case the clinical syndrome of malabsorption may develop. We are concerned here only with primary malabsorption (see also Sec. 12.49). A deficiency of maltase has not been reported; deficency states of the other three hydrolases and of the mechanism for glucose-galactose transport are described in the following paragraphs.

Sucrase-Isomaltase Deficiency

Clinical manifestations of sucrase-isomaltase deficiency include chronic diarrhea and abdominal pain and discomfort that occur when the diet contains sucrose (table sugar) or starch, i.e., with most solid foods. If this diet is replaced by one containing lactose, the symptoms disappear. Milk is tolerated well, as is glucose; but the usual "clear liquid diet" of water containing table sugar, fruit juices or carbonated beverages, and applesauce may aggravate the diarrhea.

Orally administering a test dose (1–2 g/kg) of lactose, glucose, or galactose and of maltose produces a normal rise of blood sugar concentration that is not observed after ingestion of sucrose, which may be followed by explosive diarrhea. Stool pH is low because lactic acid is formed by the bacterial fermentation of the unabsorbed carbohydrates. Lactic acid maintains diarrhea, since it acts as an irritant and increases intraluminal intestinal osmolality.

Definite *diagnosis* depends on the demonstration of deficient activity of sucrase and isomaltase in a biopsy specimen of intestine. It is not known why both these enzymatic activities are defective together. Absence of steatorrhea and usually of villous atrophy serves to exclude celiac disease. Partial villous atrophy, if present, will revert to normal after *treatment* with a prolonged sucrose-free diet that is provided by milk, meat, fish, fowl, eggs, animal fat, glucose, vegetables, and cheese.

Lactose Intolerance

This syndrome is divided into at least three entities: familial lactose intolerance, congenital lactose intolerance, and late onset lactose intolerance.

Familial Lactose Intolerance. This rare, severe disorder is characterized by onset of vomiting after the initial feeding of milk or during the first few days of life. Intestinal lactase activity is normal. No enzymatic defect has been described.

Congenital Lactose Intolerance. Severe diarrhea, abdominal pain, and distention appear soon after birth when the diet begins to contain lactose. The symptoms disappear if milk is replaced by a "clear liquid diet." Steatorrhea may occur. Blood glucose concentrations increase normally after orally administering glucose or galactose but not after lactose, which may induce explosive diarrhea, flatulence, and intestinal discomfort. Lactic acid produces an acid stool pH and maintains the diarrhea.

Normal morphology is found in biopsies of the small intestine, which has a markedly deficient lactase activity. A lactose-free diet is effective treatment.

Late Onset Lactose Intolerance. Clinical and pathologic observations are similar to those in congenital lactose intolerance except that the disorder may appear gradually, beginning several years after birth. People of northern European ancestry do not seem to be affected, whereas up to 90% of members of some other races may be affected. For example, 1 of 10 white and 7 of 10 black American adults develop moderate symptoms of lactase deficiency when challenged with oral lactose, either as milk or in a lactose tolerance test (the dose is not more than 50 g of lactose, equivalent to 1 L of milk).

Children and adults may learn to adjust their diets so that the amount of dietary lactose is not greater than they can tolerate. Partial lactase deficiency may account for the relative mildness of symptoms in many persons.

Glucose-Galactose Malabsorption

Inheritance of glucose-galactose malabsorption is autosomal recessive. The affected newborn develops severe diarrhea, abdominal distention, and discomfort after the first feeding of glucose water or milk. Symptoms are not relieved by formulas containing sucrose or maltose. Symptoms disappear if a carbohydrate-free (CHO-free) formula is fed that has been fortified with fructose. A normal rise in blood glucose concentration occurs after orally administering fructose but not after lactose, glucose, or galactose.

The intestinal mucosa is morphologically normal, as is the activity of intestinal disaccharidases. The transport of glucose and galactose across the intestinal mucosa is thought to be defective.

Testing Procedures

Intestinal hydrolase deficiency is definitively diagnosed by measuring the specific enzymatic activity in a biopsy specimen. Techniques of peroral biopsy of intestinal mucosa and of hydrolase assay are readily available. In addition, simple bedside tests for sugar intolerance can be done on the liquid portion of a diarrheal stool. Immediately after collection, the liquid stool specimen is mixed with 2 volumes of water, and of this mixture, 15 drops are tested by Clinitest tablets for the presence of reducing sugars, and another drop is tested by Testape for the presence of glucose. A Clinitest reading of 0.5% or less is normal. Since sucrose is not a reducing sugar, it must be hydrolyzed prior to testing by boiling 1 part of liquid stool specimen in 2 parts of 0.1 N HCl for 2 min. After hydrolysis, the sucrose components, glucose and fructose, can be demonstrated by Clinitest.

In patients with sugar intolerance, the pH of the liquid stool specimen will likely be less than 6 and often less than 5.5 if there has been sufficient time for fermentation of the sugar by bacteria in the large bowel.

Peroral sugar tolerance tests are performed after several hours of fasting. The child drinks 50 g/m² of body surface of the suspected sugar in a 10% solution. Normally the blood sugar concentration is expected to increase by 30 mg/dL or more within the following 2 hr; and, perhaps more reliably, liquid stool specimens should not indicate the (increased) presence of the administered sugar. In disaccharidase deficiency the unresponsive blood sugar curves observed following administration of the disaccharide may be found normal after an equivalent mixture of the respective monosaccharide moieties is ingested.

7.18 DEFECTS IN INTERMEDIARY CARBOHYDRATE METABOLISM

The intracellular conversion of glucose, fructose, and galactose proceeds as shown schematically in Figures 7–15, 7–16, and 7–17. Defects of the enzymes that are identified by name in the three figures have been associated with the disorders listed in Tables 7–5, 7–6, and 7–7.

The demonstration of defective enzyme activity must serve as the basis of diagnosis and therapy in inborn errors of metabolism. However, an enzymatic defect affecting one tissue may not be demonstrable in another tissue for several reasons:

1. The defective enzyme may normally be absent as is glucose-6-phosphatase from muscle. Therefore, the deficiency of this enzyme in liver, kidney, and intestine of glycogen storage disease type I (GSD I) does not affect the skeletal muscle.

2. An enzymatic activity may reflect different enzyme proteins in different tissues. This is the case for glycogen synthetase, phosphorylase, or phosphorylase kinase. Thus, the deficiency of these enzymes in the livers of GSD 0, GSD VI, or GSD IX does not affect their activity in skeletal muscle.

3. There may not have been the opportunity to measure a defective activity in more than one tissue of the patient. Galactokinase deficiency of erythrocytes is likely to affect the liver. However, galactokinase has not been assayed in hepatic tissue of a patient with the defect of this enzyme in erythrocytes.

4. An enzyme may not be effective in vivo although the usual assay indicates in vitro activity. This is the case in GSD Ib (pseudo-GSD I) that has the clinical and biochemical manifestations of GSD Ia, except that in vitro activity of glucose-6-phosphatase in frozen liver specimens is normal.

5. The enzymatic deficiency demonstrable in vitro may be the result of an artifact. For example, the activity of liver phosphorylase is low or absent in autopsy tissue, even though it is normal in a postmortem biopsy specimen of the same patient.

7.19 DEFECTS WITHOUT LACTIC ACIDOSIS OR ABNORMAL GLYCOGEN STORAGE

Defects in Galactose Metabolism

See Table 7–5 and Figure 7–15.

Galactosemia: Deficiency of Galactokinase. This disorder is characterized by galactosemia, galactosuria, and cataracts without mental deficiency or aminoaciduria. Cataracts begin to form after birth when the diet contains galactose derived

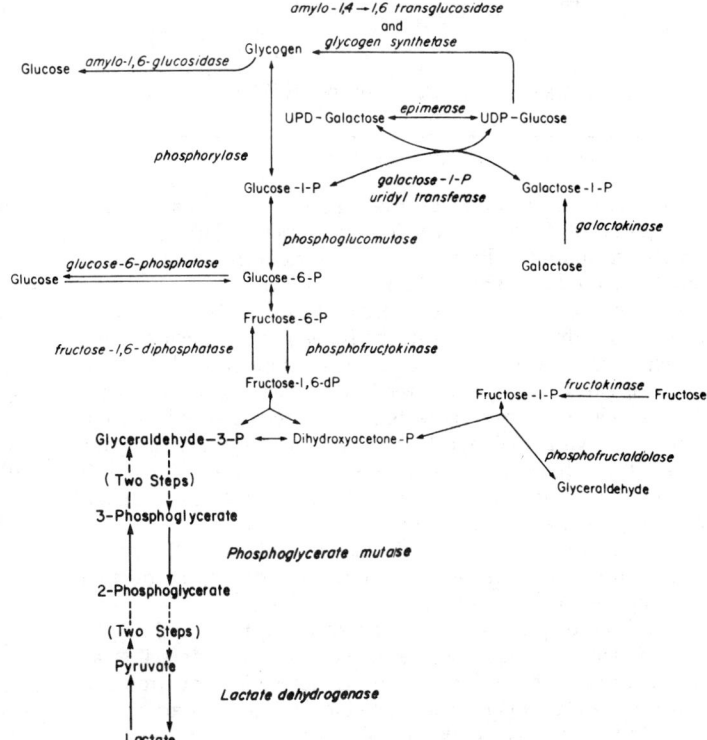

Figure 7–15. Pathway of cytoplasmic glycogen synthesis and degradation. Enzymes identified by name have been found deficient in diseases listed in Table 7–5.

Table 7–5. **Defects in Intermediary Carbohydrate Metabolism without Lactic Acidosis or Abnormal Glycogen Storage**

Enzyme Affected	Tissue Distribution of Defect	Symptoms and Signs	Comments
Galactokinase	Erythrocytes; presumably also liver (and other tissues) because administered galactose is not converted to glucose. Feasibility of prenatal diagnosis not established; generally not indicated	Cataracts growing since infancy may become recognized when vision fails in an otherwise normal schoolchild; no hepatomegaly, hepatotoxicity, aminoaciduria, or mental retardation; prognosis favorable	Galactokinase has not yet been assayed in liver of patients; increased concentrations of galactose and galactitol (but not of galactose-1-phosphate); galactose or galactitol may produce cataracts
Galactose-1-phosphate uridyl transferase	Liver, erythrocytes, intestine; prenatal diagnosis is feasible and indicated, with enzyme analysis of cultured cells of amniotic fluid	Onset at birth or later; vomiting, hypoglycemia, hepatomegaly, hepatic cirrhosis, splenomegaly, jaundice, cataracts, aminoaciduria, galactosuria, glucosuria, mental retardation; poor prognosis if untreated; galactose tolerance test unnecessary and dangerous	Increased intracellular concentration of galactose-1-phosphate and galactitol; galactose-1-phosphate responsible for hepatotoxicity and mental retardation, and galactitol for cataracts
Uridyl diphosphate galactose 4-epimerase	Erythrocytes, leukocytes, lymphocytes; liver, cultured fibroblasts, and stimulated lymphoblasts have normal enzyme activity	No signs of disease; no need for dietary exclusion of galactose, which is metabolized in the liver	Condition discovered during neonatal screening, since erythrocytic galactose-1-phosphate concentration elevated
Fructokinase	Liver, kidney, intestine	No symptoms; fructosuria usually an incidental finding; affected individuals healthy	Also known as benign or essential fructosuria; Testape (= glucose oxidase) negative, Clinitest positive; urine must *not* be basis for incorrect diagnosis of diabetes mellitus
1-Phosphofructaldolase	Liver, kidney, intestine; prenatal diagnosis not established	Hepatomegaly and hepatic cirrhosis; vomiting and hypoglycemia after fructose ingestion; aminoaciduria; prognosis fair to good with dietary elimination of fructose; fructose tolerance test not necessary for diagnosis, and may produce irreversible coma, especially in infants and young children	Also called hereditary fructose intolerance; leukocytes and erythrocytes not involved (they normally lack 1-phosphofructaldolase); heterogeneity suggested by fact that some patients may die in infancy whereas others do well on similar management
Phosphoglycerate mutase (M unit)	Muscle	Myoglobinuria, muscle pain, exercise intolerance	Only muscle isozyme is deficient (Type MM); brain isozyme (Type BB) is present
Lactate dehydrogenase (M unit)	Muscle, RBC, WBC	Myoglobinuria, easily fatigued after exercise	M isozyme subunit absent, H isozyme present

from the lactose in milk. By the time the diagnosis is made, elimination of dietary galactose may come too late to reverse cataract formation, although younger siblings of the patient may be helped and should be tested at birth.

Galactokinase catalyzes the initial phosphorylation of galactose. If its activity is deficient, the ingestion of galactose leads to increased concentration of galactose in blood and in urine, where it can be found as a reducing substance which is not glucose. Urine specimens tested for galactose should be collected following the ingestion of a galactose-containing formula. If an affected infant receives glucose water for a substantial period prior to the urine collection, galactose is absent from the urine and the diagnosis will be missed.

Postnatal institution of a galactose-free diet should prevent cataract formation. Since the children are otherwise normal, the prognosis can be good.

Definitive diagnosis is made by showing that erythrocytes are deficient in galactokinase activity, but the defect is assumed to involve the liver. Some galactose is converted into galactitol, which may be responsible for the cataract formation. Erythrocytic galactokinase activity in affected patients is below the limits of measurement; heterozygous parents and siblings have intermediate activity values. Inheritance is autosomal recessive. The incidence of the condition is about 1 in 40,000.

Galactosemia: Deficiency of Galactose-1-Phosphate Uridyl Transferase. "Classic" galactosemia is a serious disease with early onset of symptoms. The newborn infant normally receives up to 20% of caloric intake as lactose, which consists of glucose and galactose. Without the transferase the infant is unable to metabolize galactose-1-phosphate, whose accumulation injures the affected infant and perhaps the fetus in utero.

The diagnosis of uridyl transferase deficiency should be considered in newborn infants or older infants or children with any of the following *clinical manifestations*: jaundice, hepatomegaly, vomiting, hypoglycemia, convulsions, lethargy, irritability, feeding difficulties, poor weight gain, aminoaciduria, cataracts, hepatic cirrhosis, ascites, splenomegaly, or mental retardation. When the diagnosis is not made at birth, damage to the liver (cirrhosis) and brain (mental retardation) becomes increasingly severe and irreversible. Therefore galactosemia should be considered for the newborn or young infant who is not thriving or who presents any of the above findings.

Since galactose is injurious for persons with galactosemia, diagnostic tests dependent on administering galactose orally or intravenously cannot be used. Galactose administration results in high concentrations of intracellular galactose-1-phosphate, which can function as a competitive inhibitor of phosphoglucomutase. This inhibition transiently impairs the conversion of glycogen to glucose and produces hypoglycemia. Galactose-1-phosphate is responsible for hepatotoxicity and mental retardation, but galactitol causes cataracts. Deficiency of either galactokinase or uridyl transferase produces elevations of galactitol.

Light and electron microscopy of hepatic tissue reveals fatty infiltration, the formation of pseudoacini, and eventual macronodular cirrhosis. These changes are consistent with a metabolic disease, but do not indicate the precise enzymatic defect.

The preliminary *diagnosis* of galactosemia is made by demonstrating a reducing substance in several urine specimens collected while the patient is receiving human or cow's milk or another formula containing lactose. The reducing substance found in urine by Clinitest can be identified by chromatography or by an enzymatic test specific for galactose. Clinistix or Testape urine tests are negative since these test materials rely on the action of glucose oxidase, which is specific for glucose and nonreactive with galactose. The enzymatic defect is easily demonstrable in erythrocytes, which also exhibit increased concentrations of galactose-1-phosphate. Heterogeneity is manifested by partial enzymatic defects, which are now being found with increasing frequency. In the complete absence of uridyl transferase activity, very small amounts of galactose may still be metabolized by alternate pathways of no clinical significance in most patients.

The incidence of the disease is 1 in 50,000.

The term galactosemia, though adequate for the deficiencies of both galactokinase and uridyl transferase, generally designates the latter, for historical reasons.

An occasional infant with galactosemia may tolerate an unexpectedly large amount of food containing lactose, but this is rare. Usually galactose must be excluded from the diet early in life to avoid severe cirrhosis of the liver, mental retardation, cataracts, and recurrent hypoglycemia. With good dietary control the prognosis is generally good.

Deficiency of Uridyl Diphosphogalactose-4-Epimerase. There are two forms of this defect. Depending on the tissue distribution, the condition can be either completely asymptomatic or clinically identical to that of the classic form of galactosemia in which there is a deficiency of transferase activity.

In the benign form the defect is an incidental finding in an otherwise healthy individual without clinical manifestations. The liver is not enlarged, nor are there cataracts or abnormal neurologic findings. Growth and development are normal on an unrestricted normal diet. Patients may be discovered during a newborn screening to have increased concentration of erythrocyte galactose-1-phosphate; galactokinase and uridyl transferase activity is normal. Inheritance is autosomal recessive. The epimerase deficiency affects leukocytes, lymphocytes, and erythrocytes, but its normal activity in tissues other than blood cells may explain the normal tolerance for galactose and the absence of clinical symptoms. No treatment is required.

In patients with generalized epimerase deficiency, the epimerase activity is less than 10% of normal in fibroblasts, in addition to decreased activity in leukocytes and erythrocytes. Parents have about 50% of normal activity in their fibroblasts, consistent with an autosomal recessive mode of inheritance. The clinical manifestations and course are indistinguishable

from that of classical galactosemia including cataracts, hepatomegaly, jaundice, proteinuria, and the presence of a nonglucose reducing substance in the urine. Treatment is with a galactose free diet. Although this form of galactosemia is very rare, it must be considered in a symptomatic patient who has normal transferase activity.

Defects in Fructose Metabolism

See also Sec. 7.20.

Deficiency of Fructokinase (Benign Fructosuria). This condition is not associated with any clinical manifestations. It is an accidental finding usually made because the asymptomatic patient's urine contains a reducing substance. No treatment is necessary. Inheritance is autosomal recessive with an incidence of 1 in 120,000.

Fructokinase deficiency is present in liver, intestine, and kidney. Ingested fructose is not metabolized. Its level is increased in the blood, and it is excreted in urine, there being practically no renal threshold for fructose. Positive Clinitest tests and negative Clinistix tests reveal the urinary reducing substance not to be glucose. It can be identified as fructose by chromatography.

Deficiency of 1-Phosphofructaldolase (Hereditary Fructose Intolerance). This severe disease of infants appears with the ingestion of fructose-containing food. Either fructose or sucrose (table sugar), the disaccharide of glucose and fructose, may be added as a sweetener to baby foods or formulas. Symptoms may occur quite early in life, soon after birth if foods or formulas containing sucrose or fructose are then introduced into the diet. Early *clinical manifestations* may resemble those of galactosemia and include jaundice, hepatomegaly, vomiting, lethargy, irritability, and convulsions. A urinary reducing substance that is not glucose can be identified as fructose by chromatography.

The deficiency of 1-phosphofructaldolase is practically complete in the liver. Fructose-1-phosphate accumulates in hepatocytes and acts as a competitive inhibitor for phosphorylase in concentrations similar to those of intracellular glucose-1-phosphate. The resulting transient inhibition of the conversion of glycogen to glucose leads to severe hypoglycemia. Some affected children show severe reduction in the hepatic conversion of fructose-1,6-diphosphate in addition to that of fructose-1-phosphate. The concentration of fructose-1-phosphate may be reduced in body tissues by dietary elimination of fructose. However, fructose-1,6-diphosphate is an obligatory metabolite of glycolysis and gluconeogenesis and cannot be eliminated from the body by dietary means.

The severe reduction in the conversion of fructose-1,6-diphosphate in some children may result in *progressive liver disease* despite a fructose-free diet in patients who appear clinically well except for hepatomegaly and elevated levels of serum transaminases. Successive liver biopsies show increasing fatty infiltration and fibrosis, with focal cytoplasmic dissolution, and abnormal appearance of glycogen and mitochondria, and unusual plate-like and needle-like crystals in hepatocytes. The prognosis of fructose intolerance must be guarded in some patients, even with good dietary control. Without such control, the disease can result in death during infancy or early childhood. Some infants with hereditary fructose intolerance show fewer and relatively milder symptoms.

Fructose tolerance tests are contraindicated, since they may be followed by hypoglycemia, shock, and death.

Treatment requires completely eliminating fructose from the diet. This may be difficult since fructose is a widely used additive, found even in some aspirin preparations. Inheritance is autosomal recessive and the incidence (including a mild form in adults) is about 1 in 40,000.

Deficient Muscle Phosphoglycerate Mutase. This deficiency has occurred in an otherwise healthy adult exhibiting myoglobinuria and cramps after exercise. The patient was unable to increase blood lactic acid concentration after ischemic exercise, and a muscle biopsy showed normal glycogen concentration and enzyme activities except for low phosphoglycerate mutase activity due to the presence of small normal amounts of B (brain type) isozyme and absence of the M (muscle type) isozyme.

Deficient Muscle Type Lactate Dehydrogenase. The inability to synthesize the M unit of lactate dehydrogenase (LDH) is inherited as an autosomal recessive and resides on chromosome 11. Affected patients still possess the ability to make the H unit of the enzyme.

The main complaints are fatigue and myoglobinuria after strenuous exercise. There is slightly below normal activity of erythrocyte LDH with a disproportionately high ratio of creatine kinase to LDH activity. Ischemic work results in venous lactate below that of control subjects and venous pyruvate concentration is at least twice that of normal controls. Patients with deficient M type lactate dehydrogenase can convert muscle glycogen to pyruvate, which is then released into the bloodstream rather than converted to lactate.

7.20 DEFECTS IN INTERMEDIARY CARBOHYDRATE METABOLISM ASSOCIATED WITH LACTIC ACIDOSIS

The defects in carbohydrate metabolism associated with lactic acidosis are listed in Table 7–6; Figure 7–16 depicts the relevant metabolic pathways.

The normal lactic acid blood concentration is less than 18 mg/dL or 2 mM. Hyperlactic acidemia unrelated to an enzymatic defect occurs in hypoxemia. In this case the serum pyruvic acid concentration may remain normal (<1.0 mg/dL), whereas it is usually increased when hyperlactic acidemia results from an enzymatic defect. It is useful, therefore, to measure lactic and pyruvic acid in the same blood specimen and on multiple blood specimens obtained when the patient is symptomatic since dramatic and ultimately fatal hyperlactic acidemia can be intermittent. Thiamine (vitamin B_1) deficiency (as in alcoholism) also can be associated with life-threatening lactic acidosis that is correctable by thiamine administration. Thiamine participates in the pyruvate dehydrogenase reaction

(Fig. 7–16); this participation and lack of thiamine toxicity are the basis of thiamine treatment that is sometimes used for intractable lactic acidosis.

Deep sighing respirations of the Kussmaul variety should suggest acute metabolic acidosis from hyperlacticacidemia (Sec. 5.12). If not corrected, the acidosis can lead to coma, respiratory failure, cardiovascular collapse, renal insufficiency, and death (Sec. 5.41).

Hyperlacticacidemia occurs with those defects of carbohydrate metabolism that interfere with the conversion of pyruvate to glucose via the pathway of gluconeogenesis or to CO_2 and water via the mitochondrial enzymes of the citric acid cycle. The concentration of blood lactic acid should be determined in infants and children with unexplained acidosis, especially if the anion gap (Sec. 5.12) in blood is greater than 16 mM.

Deficiency of Glucose-6-Phosphatase. Glycogen storage disease type I (GSD I) is the only 1 of the 12 types of glycogenosis associated with significant lactic acidosis. In most patients the resultant recurrent metabolic acidosis is of minor clinical importance, but in some children it is a life-threatening condition. GSD I is discussed further in Sec. 7.21.

Deficiency of Fructose-1,6-Diphosphatase. These infants are symptom-free as long as their diet is limited to human milk. If they receive formulas or food containing fructose or sucrose, they develop intermittent attacks of hypoglycemia, shock, coma, convulsions, and a metabolic acidosis due to hyperlacticacidemia. In symptom-free intervals, physical examination may be normal except for hepatomegaly. If untreated, the disease can lead to psychomotor retardation or death. Inheritance is autosomal recessive.

Fructose-1,6-diphosphatase is 1 of the 4 key enzymes of gluconeogenesis. Its activity is markedly reduced or undetectable in hepatic biopsy specimens which show fatty infiltration and reduced glycogen concentration. Other enzymes of fructose metabolism, gluconeogenesis, or glycogen degradation are normal. The normal increase in blood glucose concentration after glucagon administration is found after 6 hr of fasting but not after 18 hr, which may indicate rapid exhaustion of stores of liver glycogen. Administering galactose produces a normal increase in concentration of blood glucose that is not observed after administering fructose, glycerol, or alanine. The latter substances may produce acute hypoglycemia and lactic acidosis; tolerance tests using them should be avoided. Fasting for more than 10 hr may cause hypoglycemia

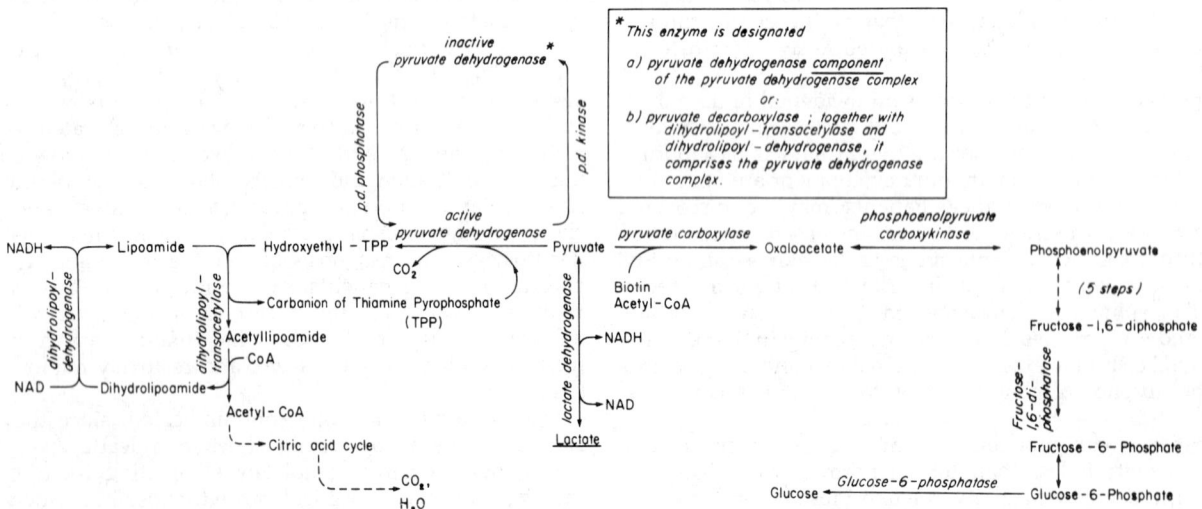

Figure 7–16. Enzymatic reactions of carbohydrate metabolism, deficiencies of which may give rise to lactic acidosis, pyruvate elevations, and/or hypoglycemia. Enzymes identified by name have been found deficient in diseases listed in Table 7–6.

Table 7–6. **Defects in Intermediary Carbohydrate Metabolism Associated with Lactic Acidosis**

Enzyme Affected	Tissue Distribution of Defect	Symptoms and Signs	Comments
Glucose-6-phosphatase	Liver, kidney, intestine	Lactic acidosis, hypoglycemia, tendency for hepatoma in later life (see Table 7–7)	Treatment (if necessary) by frequent small meals or by continuous night-time feeding, not by portacaval shunt and not by phenytoin or phenobarbital administration (see Table 7–7)
Fructose-1,6-diphosphatase	Liver	Infants with hypoglycemia, hyperventilation, convulsion, shock, elevated blood lactate, hepatomegaly; oral galactose converted to glucose; no conversion of fructose, alanine, or glycerol, which produce hyperlacticacidemia; may be fatal	Severe fatty infiltration of hepatocytes; hypoglycemia after oral fructose or glycerol (avoid such tolerance tests); hepatic glycogen concentration reduced to <1.4%; on diet free of fructose and sorbitol, mental and physical development will be normal
Pyruvate dehydrogenase component of the *pyruvate dehydrogenase complex*; or 1st enzyme (E_1) of the pyruvate dehydrogenase complex; or pyruvate decarboxylase	Liver, brain, white blood cells, cultured skin fibroblasts	Neurologic abnormalities from birth; increased blood concentration of pyruvate and lactate; death in infancy *or* Intermittent neurologic signs (ataxia, choreoathetosis); elevated blood lactate and pyruvate; normal psychomotor behavior and intelligence between attacks	In a patient with severe signs at birth who died at 6 mo, the enzymatic defect was complete; partial defect in an unrelated 9 yr old boy with intermittent symptoms, who was normal between attacks
Dihydrolipoyl-transacetylase; or 2nd enzyme (E_2) of the pyruvate dehydrogenase complex	Cultured skin fibroblasts (no other tissues analyzed)	Severe retardation; minimal blood pyruvate and lactate elevation; severe lactic acidosis on diet low in fat and high in carbohydrates	Data derived from cultures of skin fibroblasts in 1 patient suggest deficient activity of dihydrolipoyl transacetylase (not measured directly)
Dihydrolipoyl-dehydrogenase; or 3rd enzyme (E_3) of the pyruvate dehydrogenase complex	Liver, muscle, brain, kidney and "all tissues measured"; feasibility of prenatal diagnosis not established	In a male infant of consanguineous parents: at 2 mo of age, lethargy, hypertonia, optic atrophy, laryngeal stridor; twice normal blood pyruvate, lactate, and α-ketoglutarate concentration; not responsive to thiamine or dietary fat; death at 7 mo. In an unrelated 3 yr old girl of consanguineous marriage with severe neurologic disease, lactic acidosis, optic atrophy, and muscular hypotonia may have existed	Dihydrolipoyl-dehydrogenase can function in vitro as the 3rd component of the α-ketoglutarate dehydrogenase complex; simultaneously deficient activity of both dehydrogenase complexes may indicate that their 3rd components are similar, if not identical
Pyruvate carboxylase	Liver	In an 11 mo old boy, anorexia, vomiting, lethargy, retardation, elevation of blood lactate and pyruvate	Complete loss of activity of enzyme in liver; enzyme was not found in *normal* control leukocytes or in skin fibroblasts
		In an unrelated newborn girl, hypoglycemia, psychomotor retardation, increased blood concentration of pyruvate, lactate, and alanine; symptoms aggravated by high carbohydrate diet, ACTH, or anorexia, but controlled by a diet low in carbohydrate and protein, or by thiamine or by both	Total liver enzyme activity in this patient reduced by less than 50%; the result of complete loss of 1 of 2 "isoenzymes"
Pyruvate dehydrogenase phosphatase	Liver, muscle, not brain	In a newborn male, lactic acidosis, blood elevation of pyruvate, free fatty acid, alanine, ketone bodies; lethargy, irritability, generalized seizures, death at 6 mo	Incubation of liver of patient with ATP deactivates pyruvate dehydrogenase in normal manner; enzyme not reactivated under conditions effective in controls

Table continued on following page

Table 7–6. **Defects in Intermediary Carbohydrate Metabolism Associated with Lactic Acidosis** Continued

Enzyme Affected	Tissue Distribution of Defect	Symptoms and Signs	Comments
Congenital idiopathic lactic acidosis (no demonstrated enzyme defect)	Patients with this diagnosis usually have not had biochemical studies appropriate to all of the enzyme defects listed in this table	Convulsions, lethargy, hyperventilation, ataxia, vomiting, psychomotor retardation, muscular weakness, hypoglycemia, eye abnormalities, hepatomegaly; death in infancy or childhood, or intermittent attacks compatible with life	Diagnosis of "idiopathic lactic acidosis" requires demonstration that pyruvate dehydrogenase complex and gluconeogenic enzymes are normal; most patients so diagnosed have been incompletely studied
Leigh subacute necrotizing encephalopathy (SNE)	No enzyme defect consistently demonstrated as yet; total deficiency of liver pyruvate carboxylase in 1 patient (the 1st patient described in this table as having "pyruvate carboxylase deficiency")	Convulsions, lethargy, vomiting, psychomotor retardation, muscular weakness, blindness, etc.; fatal in infancy or longer lasting (some adults); symptoms do not distinguish SNE with certainty from several other entries in this table; an inhibitor in blood, CSF, and urine for thiamine pyrophosphate–adenosine triphosphate phosphoryl transferase (which catalyzes the reaction TPP + ATP ↔ TTP + ADP)	Comments on "congenital idiopathic lactic acidosis" apply; SNE and pyruvate carboxylase deficiency and "pyruvate dehydrogenase phosphatase deficiency showing cavitation and demyelination of basal ganglia" similar in autopsy findings in brain; the inhibitor is found in up to 10% of normal persons (significance uncertain)

and lactic acidosis. The clinical presentation may resemble "ketotic hypoglycemia" (Sec. 20.10). Untreated fructose-1,6-diphosphatase deficiency is a serious disease with a poor prognosis. Growth and development are normal if the diet is kept free of fructose, sucrose, and sorbitol and reasonably restricted in fat and protein.

Deficiency of Pyruvate Decarboxylase. This enzyme has also been designated the pyruvate dehydrogenase component or the 1st enzyme (E_1) of the pyruvate dehydrogenase complex. Its activity was undetected in a 1.3 kg newborn boy of 35 wk gestation who had tachypnea and neurologic signs and died at 6 mo of age despite attempts at dietary control. Plasma concentrations of pyruvate and lactate were high. In contrast, a 9 yr old boy had 20% of normal enzyme activity in cultured skin fibroblasts and white cells. He suffered intermittent episodes of cerebellar dysfunction and choreoathetoid movement, which began at 16 mo of age, occurred from 2 to 6 times a year, lasted a few hours to over 1 wk, and seemed to be triggered by febrile illnesses or other stresses. The episodes ranged in severity from generalized clumsiness to severe ataxia so incapacitating that locomotion was possible only by crawling. Serum concentrations of pyruvate, lactate, and alanine were moderately elevated during attacks, but normal between them, as was clinical appearance. Intelligence was normal. Dexamethasone relieved attacks but did not correct the blood chemical abnormalities.

Deficiency of Dihydrolipoyl Transacetylase. This enzyme is designated the 2nd enzyme (E_2) in the pyruvate dehydrogenase complex, and the only reported patient who might have had this defect was a 9 yr old boy with profound motor and mental retardation. Blood concentrations of pyruvate and lactate were normal when the patient was fasting, but rose to twice the level of controls by 2 hr after a normal meal. A diet high in carbohydrates but not fat (65% and 15%, respectively) precipitated severe lactic acidosis. Dietary thiamine had no effect. Two sisters of the patient had died with severe lactic acidosis; their brains were severely deficient in myelin, but there were no signs of active demyelination. The boy's cultured skin fibroblasts had reduced activity of the pyruvate dehydrogenase complex; activity of the pyruvate decarboxylase was normal. Since the α-ketoglutarate dehydrogenase complex was not defective and since there is evidence that

this complex includes an enzyme similar, if not identical, to E_3 of the pyruvate dehydrogenase complex, it can be inferred that E_2 may have been defective.

Deficiency of Dihydrolipoyl Dehydrogenase. The *clinical manifestations* of a deficiency of this 3rd enzyme (E_3) of the pyruvate dehydrogenase complex are severe and include lethargy, hypertonia, irritability, optic atrophy, hyperactive reflexes with muscular hypotonia, lower extremity spasticity, irregular respirations, and laryngeal stridor. Persistent lactic acidosis was not corrected by a diet high in thiamine or fat. Episodes of hypoglycemia may be relieved by alanine. There has been a history of consanguinity.

Laboratory findings include elevations of blood concentrations of pyruvate, lactase, and α-ketoglutarate. Liver function tests may be normal. Dihydrolipoyl dehydrogenase activity in tissues may be as low as 5% of normal. Activity of the pyruvate dehydrogenase complex (but not E_1) and the α-ketoglutarate dehydrogenase complex in liver, muscle, brain, kidney, and skin fibroblasts have also been decreased.

Pathology of the brain in one infant revealed cavitation and lack of myelination in basal ganglia, thalamus, and brain stem resembling Leigh syndrome.

Deficiency of Pyruvate Carboxylase. *Clinical manifestations* of this deficiency have varied from hypoglycemia in infancy to absence of clinical signs and symptoms during the first year of life. Usually psychomotor retardation becomes evident in the first year and may be severe and progressive, culminating in death. Clinical findings have included vomiting, irritability, lethargy, progressive motor and mental retardation, hypotonia, hyporeflexia, abnormal eye movements, optic atrophy, ataxia, and convulsions. There may be a history of psychomotor retardation and death of siblings whose clinical or pathologic findings suggested Leigh syndrome or who were undiagnosed.

Laboratory findings are characterized by elevated concentrations of blood lactate, pyruvate and alanine. Cerebrospinal fluid protein may be elevated. In one patient, although liver size was normal, glycogen in liver and muscle was increased; there was a normal increase of blood glucose concentration following glucagon administration.

Diagnosis is based upon demonstrating a pyruvate carboxylase deficiency in the liver; a partial defect has been reported in 1 of 2 liver pyruvate carboxylases. Activities of the 3 other gluconeogenic enzymes have been normal.

Treatment with thiamine has prevented episodes of acute metabolic acidosis and controlled the biochemical defect in some patients but has not affected the clinical outcome. Therapy with biotin and lipoic acid is ineffective.

Deficiency of Pyruvate Dehydrogenase Phosphatase. This deficiency has been found in a newborn boy who had a metabolic acidosis with high serum concentrations of lactate (up to 7 times normal), of pyruvate (2 times normal), and of free fatty acids (3 times normal). There was no hypoglycemia or hepatomegaly. The acidosis improved when the glucose intake was increased and that of fat decreased. Periods of clinical stability and moderate hyperlacticacidemia were interrupted every few days by episodes of severe lactic acidosis. Neurologic damage was evident, with lethargy, convulsions, hypotonia, and irritability. The patient died at 6 mo of age.

The pyruvate dehydrogenase component E_1 of the pyruvate dehydrogenase complex exists in an active and in an inactive form. E_1 is inactivated when it is phosphorylated by pyruvate dehydrogenase kinase in the presence of ATP. E_1 is stimulated by calcium. Pyruvate dehydrogenase phosphatase activity was reported deficient in liver and muscle but not brain of this child based on the observation that the addition of calcium to a homogenate of liver increased the activity of pyruvate decarboxylase in the patient by 4% and in a control by 50%. Deficiency of this activating phosphatase has been reported in another 7 mo old boy in whom brain autopsy findings were consistent with Leigh syndrome.

Carnitine Deficiency Syndrome. This can present with recurrent attacks of severe metabolic acidosis (hyperlactic acidosis and pyruvicacidemia), hypoglycemia, and hepatomegaly. Cardiomegaly may be present. Untreated, the patient may die during the crisis, but correction of acidosis and intravenous glucose may terminate the crisis, usually within 12–24 hr. Carnitine concentration is reduced in serum, muscle, and liver. Administration of L-carnitine (i.e., the carnitine isomer synthesized by the liver) seems to benefit some but not all of the patients, but administering DL-carnitine is without demonstrable benefit and may be harmful.

Carnitine deficiency exists on a genetic primary basis or it can be acquired secondary to some other condition. Either type can derive from various defects and result in various clinical manifestations. Genetic presentations have been asymptomatic and symptomatic with recurrent severe lactic acidosis and acute cardiac failure resulting in death. Carnitine deficiency, probably on an acquired basis, has presented in newborns with intrauterine growth retardation and in several patients with Fanconi syndrome. The latter occurred as part of type XI glycogenosis and the associated renal defect resulting in urinary loss of carnitine and severe hepatic fatty infiltration. This disappeared when the body carnitine was replenished by L-carnitine administration in an amount sufficient to compensate for the ongoing urinary loss.

Congenital Idiopathic Lactic Acidosis. This diagnosis should be considered when there is labored respiration in infancy associated with metabolic acidosis from hyperlactic acidemia. Liver and spleen may be enlarged. Convulsions, hypoglycemia, psychomotor retardation, and neurologic damage usually lead to death in infancy despite dietary administration of thiamine, biotin, steroids, lipoic acid, and other agents. Long-term survival in a few instances is possible.

There are increased serum concentrations of pyruvate, lactate, and alanine, as well as of other amino acids. Cerebral autopsy findings may show severe spongy degeneration and lack of myelination, or there may be only moderate or mild abnormalities.

A variety of deficiencies in enzymatic activities, including those reported above, may lead to lactic acidosis. In patients who have not been examined in a systematic way, excluding the defects described above, the diagnosis of congenital idiopathic lactic acidosis should probably not be used.

Leigh Subacute Necrotizing Encephalopathy (SNE). This condition is characterized by seizures, psychomotor retardation, optic atrophy, hypotonia, vomiting, abnormal movements, lethargy, and lactic acidosis. It is difficult to reliably distinguish this syndrome from many of the enzymatic deficiencies that are associated with lactic acidosis. Gliosis, cavitation, and capillary proliferation in brain stem, basal ganglia, and thalamus, critical criteria for a pathologic diagnosis, may be visible on CT scan. Similar lesions viewed as characteristic have been encountered in patients shown to have pyruvate carboxylase deficiency, or, in one case, defective pyruvate decarboxylase activity in skin fibroblasts. Another boy shown to have SNE by brain autopsy also had deficiency of pyruvate dehydrogenase phosphatase. The assessment of patients presenting symptoms and signs consistent with Leigh syndrome must include assays of enzymatic activities that result in lactic acidosis. These activities were normal in a 22 mo old boy who had the cerebral findings of Leigh syndrome associated with increased concentration of endorphin and norepinephrine in CSF and of enkephalins in cerebral cortex.

Thiamine is transiently effective in some patients with Leigh syndrome, but not in others. Its use was suggested by the report that extracts of blood, cerebrospinal fluid, and urine of patients with SNE inhibited thiamine pyrophosphate–adenosine triphosphate phosphoryl transferase. Thiamine in pharmacologic doses might have overridden this inhibitor, which is also reported to be found in the urine of as many as 10% of clinically normal persons. For further discussion see Sec. 21.18.

Attempts to correct hyperlactic acidemia with dichloroacetate, which inhibits the inactivating kinase for pyruvate dehydrogenase (E_1; Fig. 7–16), thereby maintaining dehydrogenase (E_1) activity, have been ineffective in a child with fatal lactic acidosis of unknown cause.

Acute, life-threatening hyperlactic acidemia can be corrected by the intravenous infusion of *tris-hydroxymethyl aminomethane* (THAM), which avoids the sodium overload of sodium bicarbonate administration. This treatment does not alter the poor prognosis for the majority of conditions that are associated with increased lactic and pyruvic acid.

7.21 THE GLYCOGEN STORAGE DISEASES (GSD)

These diseases are the result of metabolic errors leading to abnormal concentrations or structure of glycogen. The GSD or glycogenosis can be classified based on the identified enzymatic defects, or sometimes the distinctive clinical features (Table 7–7). The identification of a new type is useful only if the clinical or biochemical manifestations are sufficiently distinctive to permit their precise recognition in future patients. Fig. 7–17 depicts the relevant metabolic pathways. Table 7–8 indicates the concentrations of glycogen and the enzymatic activities found in liver and in skeletal muscle of normal individuals and of a patient representative of each type of glycogenosis.

Deficiency of Glycogen Synthetase (GSD 0). Early morning convulsions associated with hypoglycemia are typical symptoms. There is an associated hyperketonemia. Serum concentrations of lactate are normal when the patient is fasting, but are increased after administering glucose or after more than 12 hr of fasting. Hypoglycemia appears during such periods without food and is not responsive to glucagon. After administering glucose the blood glucose remains elevated for longer than usual. The diagnosis should be made expeditiously, since hypoglycemic episodes and mental retardation can be

Table 7–7. **Features of the Glycogen Storage Diseases, Types 0–XI (GSD 0–XI)**

Type, Enzyme Affected	Tissue Distribution of Excessive Glycogen and Enzyme Deficiency	Clinical Symptoms and Signs*	Comments Alternate Names
GSD 0 Glycogen synthetase	Liver but not muscle (other tissues not analyzed); glycogen depletion in liver; hepatic glycogen synthetase less than 2% of normal, but some hepatic glycogen (1%) demonstrable	Fasting hypoglycemia; prolonged hyperglycemia after a meal or glucose administration; mental retardation follows hypoglycemic convulsions—when these are avoided by frequent protein-rich meals, psychomotor development can be normal	*Aglycogenosis;* defect convincingly demonstrated in 2 unrelated families; early diagnosis and dietary treatment important for prevention of retardation; some children with "ketotic hypoglycemia" may have GSD 0
GSD Ia Glucose-6-phosphatase	Liver, kidney, intestine; frequent intranuclear glycogen seen in these organs not diagnostic; continuous nightime feeding by tube and pump may alleviate clinical symptoms; portacaval shunt risky and clinically disappointing; treatment with phenytoin or phenobarbital ineffective	Enlarged liver and kidneys; "doll face," stunted growth, normal mental development; tendency to hypoglycemia, lactic acidosis, hyperlipidemia, hyperuricacidemia, gout, bleeding; IV galactose or fructose not converted to glucose (caution: these tests may precipitate acidosis); abortive or no rise in blood glucose after SC epinephrine or IV glucagon; normal urinary catecholamines; prognosis fair to good	*Von Gierke disease, hepatorenal glycogenosis;* no involvement of skeletal or cardiac muscle, or of leukocytes or cultured skin fibroblasts (glucose-6-phosphatase not normally present in these tissues)
GSD Ib In vitro activity of glucose-6-phosphatase is normal	Activity of glucose-6-phosphatase is normal in frozen liver homogenate but is deficient in isotonic homogenate of fresh liver tissue that has never been frozen	Symptoms are as those of GSD Ia; in addition, frequent neutropenia	Transport defect for glucose-6-phosphate at microsomal membrane
GSD Ic In vitro activity of glucose-6-phosphatase can be demonstrated	Activity of glucose-6-phosphatase is normal in frozen liver homogenate but is deficient in isotonic homogenate of fresh liver tissue that has never been frozen	The patient, an 11 yr old girl, had hepatomegaly, brittle diabetes, frequent hypoglycemia	Transport defect for inorganic phosphate at microsomal membrane
GSD IIa, b Lysosomal acid α-glucosidase (deficient activity of acid α-1,4- and of α-1,6-glucosidase; the latter could be considered "lysosomal glycogen debrancher")	In the fatal, infantile, classic form (GSD IIa), glycogen concentration excessive in all organs examined; acid α-glucosidase deficiency was generalized in 1 patient; in others *normal* renal acid α-glucosidase; amniotic *fluid* (in contrast to cultured amniotic fluid cells) contains acid α-glucosidase activity even if the fetus has the disease	Clinically normal at birth, though minimal cardiomegaly, abnormal ECG, increased tissue glycogen, abnormal lysosomes in liver and skin, and acid α-glucosidase deficiency demonstrable at birth. Within a few months, marked hypotonia, severe cardiomegaly, moderate hepatomegaly; normal mental development; death usually in infancy (GSD IIa). Cases with involvement of muscle and liver but without cardiomegaly described in children and adults (GSD IIb). Normal blood glucose response to glucagon; normal urinary catecholamines	*Pompe disease, generalized glycogenosis, cardiac glycogenosis;* prenatal diagnosis *within* a few days after amniocentesis by the electron microscopic demonstration of abnormal lysosomes in *uncultured* amniotic fluid cells; for prenatal diagnosis by enzyme analysis, *cultured* amniotic fluid cells required, which also show the abnormal lysosomes GSD IIa: *infantile fatal form* GSD IIb: *late juvenile-adult form*
GSD III Amylo-1,6-glucosidase, "debrancher enzyme"	Liver, muscle, heart, etc., in various combinations; designated types IIIA through D; cultured amniotic fluid cells have diagnostic biochemical abnormality	Moderate to marked hepatomegaly; none to moderate hypotonia; none to moderate cardiomegaly, ECG rarely abnormal; no acidosis, hypoglycemia, or hyperlipemia; glucagon produces a normal rise in blood glucose after a meal but not after fasting; normal mental development; failure of liver or heart rare; normal urinary catecholamines; prognosis fair to good	*Limited dextrinosis, debrancher glycogenosis, Cori disease, Forbes disease;* prenatal diagnosis by enzyme assay of cultured amniotic fluid cells feasible but perhaps unnecessary, owing to the usual benign course

Table continued on opposite page

Table 7–7. Features of the Glycogen Storage Diseases, Type 0–XI (GSD 0–XI) *Continued*

Type, Enzyme Affected	Tissue Distribution of Excessive Glycogen and Enzyme Deficiency	Clinical Symptoms and Signs*	Comments Alternate Names
GSD IV Amylo-1,4→1,6-transglucosidase, "brancher enzyme"	Generalized (?); low to normal levels of abnormally structured glycogen (amylopectin-like molecules with fewer branch points than normal in animal glycogen)	Hepatosplenomegaly, ascites, cirrhosis, liver failure; normal mental development; death in early childhood	*Amylopectinosis, brancher glycogenosis, Andersen disease;* prenatal diagnosis of this incurable disease may be feasible and indicated by enzyme analysis of cultured amniotic fluid cells.
G5D V Muscle phosphorylase deficiency (congenital absence of skeletal muscle phosphorylase; phosphorylase-activating system intact)	Skeletal muscle; liver and myometrium normal	Temporary weakness and cramping of skeletal muscle after exercise; no rise in blood lactate during ischemic exercise; symptoms like those of type VII glycogenosis; normal mental development and urinary catecholamines; myoglobinuria in later life; fair to good prognosis	*McArdle syndrome;* liver and smooth muscle phosphorylase not affected; cardiac muscle phosphorylase not examined; prenatal diagnosis not feasible, does not seem indicated
GSD VI Liver phosphorylase deficiency (phosphorylase-activating system intact)	Liver; skeletal muscle normal; leukocytes unsatisfactory for diagnosis	Marked hepatomegaly, no splenomegaly; no hypoglycemia, acidosis, or hyperlipemia; no rise of blood glucose after SC epinephrine or IV glucagon; normal mental development; normal urinary catecholamines; good prognosis	Lack of glucagon-induced hyperglycemia distinguishes GSD VI from GSD IX; the latter shows a normal glucagon response; prenatal diagnosis not feasible, may not be indicated
GSD VII Phosphofructokinase	Skeletal muscle, erythrocytes (in initial report; other tissues not examined); not known whether cultured amniotic fluid cells are affected, but prenatal diagnosis not indicated	Temporary weakness and cramping of skeletal muscle after exercise; no rise in blood lactate during ischemic exercise; normal mental development; symptoms identical to those of type V glycogenosis; good prognosis	Reduction of phosphofructo-kinase activity severe in skeletal muscle, mild in erythrocytes, not established in other tissues; incapacity may be minimal
GSD VIII No enzymatic deficiency yet demonstrated; total liver phosphorylase normal but most is in inactive form (liver phosphorylase activity reduced because control lost over extent of phosphorylase activation)	Liver, brain; skeletal muscle normal; cerebral glycogen increased; electron microscopy shows some cerebral glycogen in the form of α-particles within axon cylinders and synapses	Hepatomegaly; truncal ataxia, nystagmus, "dancing eyes" may be present; neurologic deterioration progressing to hypertonia, spasticity, decerebration and death; urinary epinephrine and norepinephrine are increased during acute phase of disease, not in stationary end phase	Predominant clinical problem of the 3 patients with this presumptive diagnosis was progressive degenerative disease of brain
G5D IX a, b, c Liver phosphorylase kinase deficiency (total phosphorylase content normal but in inactive form, owing to the lack of phosphorylase kinase)	Liver; muscle tissue normal biochemically (in IXa and IXb) and microscopically; diagnosis not possible by using leukocytes, possible by using leukocytes; D-thyroxine induced liver phosphorylase kinase activity in 1 patient, but not in 2 others of a different family	Marked hepatomegaly, no splenomegaly; no hypoglycemia or acidosis; normal urinary catecholamines; normal rise in blood glucose after IV glucagon or SC epinephrine; prognosis good; treatment may not be necessary ("benign hepatomegaly" may disappear in early adulthood)	Liver phosphorylase can be activated in vitro by addition of exogenous kinase to the homogenate; not the human counterpart of muscle phosphorylase kinase deficiency in mice; normal glucagon response is a distinguishing feature vs GSD VI; GSD IXa, autosomal recessive; GSD IXb, X-linked recessive; prenatal diagnosis not demonstrated and is unnecessary *Table continued on following page*

Table 7–7. **Features of the Glycogen Storage Diseases, Type 0–XI (GSD 0–XI)** *Continued*

Type, Enzyme Affected	Tissue Distribution of Excessive Glycogen and Enzyme Deficiency	Clinical Symptoms and Signs*	Comments *Alternate Names*
GSD X Loss of activity of cyclic 3'5'-AMP–dependent kinase in muscle and presumably liver. (Total phosphorylase content of liver and skeletal muscle normal, but the enzyme completely deactivated in both organs; phosphorylase kinase activity 50% of normal, possibly owing to the loss of 3'5'-AMP–dependent kinase activity)	Liver and muscle (other organs not tested); identical biochemical findings were made in 2 muscle biopsy specimens taken 6 yr apart	Marked hepatomegaly; patient otherwise clinically healthy initially, but 6 yr after diagnosis mild recurrent muscle pain; no cardiomegaly or hypoglycemia; no rise in blood glucose after IV glucagon; the only individual known to have this condition not incapacitated at 12 yr of age	In vitro activation of the patient's phosphorylase occurs (1) under assay conditions not requiring 3'5'-AMP–dependent kinase, or (2) after the patient's muscle homogenate has been fortified with phosphorylase kinase–deficient mouse muscle that supplied 3'5'-AMP–dependent kinase; postulated defect restricted to the activity of the cyclic 3'5'-AMP–dependent kinase that phosphorylates phosphorylase kinase, other cyclic 3'5'-AMP–dependent phosphorylations being intact
GSD XI All enzymatic activities measured to date are normal (adenyl cyclase, 3'5'-AMP–dependent kinase, phosphorylase kinase, phosphorylase, debrancher, brancher, glucose-6-phosphatase)	Liver, or liver and kidney	Tendency for acidosis; markedly stunted growth; vitamin D–resistant rickets (that can be cured with high doses of vitamin D and oral supplementation of phosphate); hyperlipidemia, generalized aminoaciduria, galactosuria, glucosuria, phosphaturia; normal renal size; no rise in blood glucose after IV glucagon or SC epinephrine; urinary excretion of cyclic 3'5'-AMP increases markedly after administration of glucagon	Muscle usually not affected; GSD XI may include patients with glycogenoses with different enzymatic defects Patients exhibit noncystinotic Fanconi syndrome associated with secondary (acquired) carnitine deficiency

*IV, intravenous administration of; SC, subcutaneous administration of.

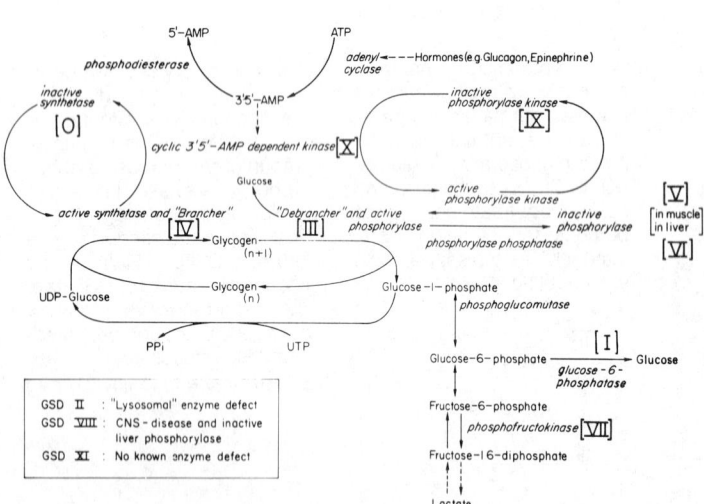

Figure 7–17. Pathway of phosphorylase activation and anaerobic glycolysis. Bracketed numbers refer to the type of glycogenosis in which the activity of the enzyme next to the number is defective. The various types are listed in Table 7–7.

Table 7–8. **Biochemical Analysis of Tissues in Glycogen Storage Diseases**

Cases	Glycogen Concentration % Wt. of Wet Tissue	Phosphorylase		Phosphorylase Kinase Active	Acid α-Glucosidase μmoles Glucose/ g/min	Amylo-1,6-Glucosidase*	Glucose-6-Phosphatase μmoles Phosphate/ g/min
		Total μmoles Phosphate/g/min	Active				
"Normal"							
Liver	2.5–6.0	44.3† ± 9.6	25.1 ± 6.5	100%	0.258 ± 0.093	3750 ± 490	4.7 ± 1.9
Muscle	0.1–1.5	78.0 ± 21.1	47.7 ± 13.2	100%	0.035 ± 0.011	7113 ± 553	
GSD Ia							
Liver	8.9	42	23	Normal	0.242	Normal	0
Muscle	0.6	59	38		0.041		
GSD Ib							
Liver	7.4	53	46	Normal	0.261	Normal	3.9; 0.9‡
Muscle	1.1	77	28		0.037		
GSD IIa							
Liver	8.8	47	26	Normal	0	Normal	3.2
Muscle	7.5	64	42		0		
GSD IIb							
Liver	11.5	45	29	Normal	0.026	Normal	5.4
Muscle	1.6	80	31		0.0		
GSD III							
Liver	9.3	40	19	Normal	0.210	45	2.9
Muscle	6.0	72	45		0.030	43	
GSD V							
Liver	4.5	48	26	Normal	0.260	Normal	3.8
Muscle	3.8	0	0	Normal or increased	0.028		
GSD VI							
Liver	7.6	2	1.8	Normal	0.176	Normal	3.4
Muscle	0.3	61	46		0.025		
GSD VIII							
Liver	12.0	43	6	Normal	0.312	Normal	5.1
Muscle	0.4	58	35		0.040		
GSD IXa							
Liver	9.9	46	2.3	<10%	0.155	Normal	3.7
Muscle	0.3	70	58	Normal	0.026		
GSD IXb							
Liver	10.5	44	0.8	<10%	0.318	Normal	2.6
Muscle	1.4	100	72	Normal	0.029		
GSD X							
Liver	10.5	39	0.1	Normal	0.292	Normal	6.8
Muscle	2.9	54	0	50% of normal§	0.044		
GSD XI							
Liver	10.8	53	37	Normal	0.243	Normal	5.1
Muscle	0.7	69	42	Normal	0.029	Normal	

*Glucose-^{14}C incorporated into -1,6-branch points expressed as cpm/mg glycogen/g tissue in 1 hr.

†Mean value ± 1 S.D.

‡In "frozen tissue" homogenate; in isotonic homogenate of "fresh tissue."

§Enzyme is demonstrable in GSD X only if I-strain mouse muscle and 3′5′-AMP have been added to homogenate of patient's muscle; in other types of GSD, the addition of mouse muscle is not needed.

avoided if the patient is given frequent meals rich in protein. The clinical picture is quite similar to that of ketotic hypoglycemia (Sec. 20.10), and patients with the latter diagnosis may benefit from an assay of hepatic glycogen synthetase. The persistent hyperglycemia and increase in serum lactate concentration after administration of glucose should reveal those with possible deficiencies of glycogen synthetase.

Glycogen synthetase activity is deficient in liver, but normal in muscle and in white and red blood cells. Glycogen concentration is low (less than 2%) but not absent in liver and normal in muscle. Differential involvement of tissues reflects the fact that different isozymes of glycogen synthetase exist for various tissues. The activation system for glycogen synthetase is normal.

A patient has been reported with deficiencies of glycogen synthetase, phosphorylase, and glucose-6-phosphatase in the liver. These additional deficiencies may be a postmortem artifact, or synthetase and phosphorylase may share certain peptide constituents, since 25% of normal phosphorylase activity was found in a liver biopsy.

Deficiency of Glucose-6-Phosphatase (GSD Ia). In GSD Ia, glucose-6-phosphatase activity is defective, and glycogen concentration is increased in liver, kidney, and intestine. *Clinical manifestations* are summarized in Table 7–7. Mild hypotonia is sometimes also reported in GSD Ia, but the disease does not have a primary effect on muscle, since muscle does not normally contain glucose-6-phosphatase. Marked hypoglycemia may be well tolerated; patients with blood glucose levels as low as 10 mg/dL may display normal behavior. Hyperlipidemia and hyperuricacidemia are marked. In adults the latter produces gout, which must be appropriately treated. There is a secondary impairment of platelet function, which may make bleeding a problem when biopsies are done. Young children with GSD Ia have impressive hepatomegaly, but liver involvement may be easily overlooked in the affected adult. In GSD Ia, the kidneys are moderately but consistently enlarged on roentgenographic examination, which helps to differentiate between GSD Ia and GSD III, in which renal size is normal.

Administering galactose or fructose does not produce an elevation of blood glucose concentration; tolerance tests with these sugars should not be done because they can lead to severe acidosis. Administration of fructose, but not of galactose, is followed by increased concentrations of serum insulin. Intravenous administration of glucagon is not followed by a normal rise in blood glucose, regardless of how recently the patient may have eaten. The glucagon tolerance test can, therefore, differentiate between GSD Ia and GSD III; in the latter the concentration of blood glucose will increase if glucagon is given 2 hr after a meal. Subcutaneous administration of epinephrine has no advantage over the glucagon tolerance test and may produce unpleasant side effects.

Acute lactic acidosis may be a recurrent and life-threatening problem. Portacaval shunt has been advocated for its prevention or control, but we have not encountered any patients who have benefited from the operation, which has been complicated by closure of the anastomosis and by development of cirrhosis or encephalopathy. Patients difficult to control can be managed successfully with continuous nighttime feedings by nasopharyngeal or gastrostomy tubes. Therapeutic success also has been reported with repeated daily drinking of a solution of uncooked cornstarch. With such dietary regimens, children grow satisfactorily, hepatomegaly recedes, and hypoglycemia and lactic acidosis become manageable. However, when the gastric tube feedings are discontinued, the pretreatment tolerance of hypoglycemia may have been lost. Disease-related post-treatment hypoglycemia may result in convulsions. Frequent meals have effects similar to those of gastric tube feedings and may suffice for clinical control. As patients grow older, their metabolic problems become less severe and more easily manageable. Neither phenobarbital nor phenytoin corrects the biochemical or clinical abnormalities in patients with glycogenoses.

In GSD Ia, hepatocytes contain many lipid droplets ranging in size from smaller than mitochondria to several times that of the nucleus, and the nuclei themselves frequently contain glycogen. Nuclear glycogenosis can also occur in GSD III, in diabetes mellitus, and in Wilson disease. Patients with GSD Ia have an increased incidence of hepatoma. Abdominal examination by ultrasound or CT scan every 6 to 12 months may be indicated. Prenatal diagnosis using amniotic fluid cells is not feasible since glucose-6-phosphatase is not normally present in cultured skin fibroblasts; nor can the enzyme be demonstrated in normal white cells.

GSD Ib (Pseudo-GSD I). Clinically GSD Ib is indistinguishable from GSD Ia, except that children with GSD Ib seem to have an increased incidence of neutropenia. Hepatic glycogen concentration is increased but glucose-6-phosphatase activity is normal in homogenates made of frozen liver tissue. The activity is decreased, however, in isotonic homogenates made from fresh liver tissue, suggesting a defect in the transport of glucose-6-phosphate across microsomal membranes of GSD Ib hepatocytes. Further evidence that this variant of GSD I is due to a microsomal membrane defect is the finding that when fresh liver homogenates from affected patients are treated with deoxycholate, the activity of glucose-6-phosphatase is normal; deoxycholate is known to break up microsomal membranes.

GSD Ic. Transport of glucose-6-phosphate into microsomes (which is defective in GSD Ib) normally occurs associated with transport of inorganic phosphates in the opposite direction. A deficiency in this phosphate transfer has recently been described in an 11 yr old girl with insulin-dependent diabetes (GSD Ic). Liver glycogen concentration was 9.4%, but since the patient had frequent hypoglycemic attacks, the increased glycogen concentration could have resulted from therapeutic glucose administration. The patient's clinical picture appeared similar to that of Mauriac syndrome in diabetic children.

Deficiency of Lysosomal Acid α-Glucosidase (GSD II). This disease, whose clinical manifestations are summarized in Table 7–7, occurs in at least two varieties, one affecting infants (GSD IIa), the other affecting older children and adults (GSD IIb). Both varieties have not occurred in members of the same family. Fibroblast studies have indicated that in a case of GSD IIa, the lysosomal acid α-glucosidase was structurally altered, whereas in a case of GSD IIb the amount of the enzyme was reduced. Abnormal lysosomes are the morphologic hallmark of GSD II. The gene for acid α-glucosidase is localized on chromosome 17.

GSD IIa. This is the classic form of generalized glycogenosis and is always fatal, usually within 2 yr after birth. Affected children appear clinically healthy at birth with normal muscle tone and liver size. Heart size and electrocardiogram are marginally abnormal. However, after a few weeks or months at home, the infant becomes completely flaccid. Sucking becomes weak, respirations shallow, and the cardiac silhouette huge. The liver is typically only moderately enlarged. The patients are alert and normally intelligent. The mouth is kept open and the tongue thrust forward, perhaps more because of air hunger than macroglossia; the resulting facial expression is characteristic. Aspiration pneumonia leads to chronic pulmonary infiltrates, and bronchial compression by the large heart leads to atelectasis. Death is due to failure of respiratory muscles. There is hardly any other condition in which such extreme cardiomegaly and muscular weakness occur in an infant who appears normal at birth. Blood glucose concentrations are normal, as are tolerance tests with glucagon and other carbohydrate test substances.

GSD II is the only lysosomal disease among the glycogenoses; the other types of GSD are associated with defects of enzymes located in the cytoplasm. The deficient acid α-glucosidase is a glycogen-degrading enzyme associated with the lysosomal fraction of tissue homogenates. Figure 7–18 indicates that fusion of a primary lysosome with an autophagic vacuole normally creates a secondary lysosome. If the primary lysosome is deficient in a lysosomal enzyme (such as α-glucosidase), then the secondary lysosome may become engorged with the material (such as glycogen) that should have been degraded by the defective enzyme. Besides deficiencies of enzymes other errors in lysosomal mechanisms may be present, such as membrane defects. In GSD IIa the deficiency of lysosomal acid α-glucosidase produces intracellular vesicles (so-called "abnormal lysosomes") engorged with glycogen (Fig. 7–19) in cells of liver, muscle, heart and most other tissues of the body. Deficient acid α-glucosidase activity is also associated with the formation of glycogen filled "abnormal lysosomes" in cells of placenta and skin of children with I-cell disease (Mucolipidosis type II, ML II; Sec. 7.38).

Increased glycogen concentrations are found in many tissues of affected children. The deficiency of the lysosomal enzyme for glycogen degradation can explain the membrane-bound accumulations of glycogen in lysosomes, but it does not explain the excessive accumulation of glycogen in the cytoplasm of heart and muscle cells. This cytoplasmic glycogen accumulates, despite the fact that it is probably in contact with the normal glycolytic enzymes of cytoplasm, none of which are known to be defective in GSD II.

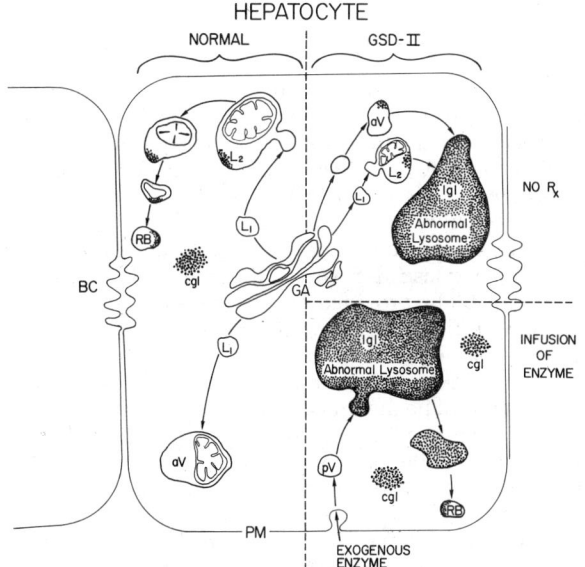

Figure 7–18. The lysosomal mechanism. During treatment of GSD IIa (right lower quarter), the exogenous enzyme is admitted to the cell in a pinocytotic vesicle (pV) and initiates the degradation of lysosomal glycogen (lgl) after the pinocytotic vesicle has fused with the abnormal lysosome. The cytoplasmic glycogen (cgl) is not degraded because it is shielded from the exogenous enzymes by the membrane of the pinocytotic vesicle that, presumably, derives from the plasma membrane (PM). Without treatment (right upper quarter), GSD IIa hepatocytes are characterized by the accumulation of membrane-surrounded glycogen (lgl) because the primary lysosome is deficient in lysosomal acid α-glucosidase.

aV, autophagic vacuoles that fuse with L_1, resulting in secondary lysosomes (L_2); BC, bile canaliculus; cgl, cytoplasmic glycogen; GA, Golgi apparatus; L_1, primary lysosomes containing acid hydrolases; L_2, secondary lysosomes; lgl, lysosomal glycogen; PM, plasma membrane; pV, pinocytotic vesicle; RB, residual bodies.

(From Hug G: Glycogen storage disease. Birth Defects 12:157, 1976.)

The excessive tissue glycogen as such may not be a cause of death; for example, the same 7-fold increase in muscle glycogen was found in a clinically healthy girl at birth and 2 yr later in tissue obtained post mortem. Glucagon and epinephrine can mobilize cytoplasmic liver glycogen to produce a rise in blood glucose concentrations, but cannot produce this effect if cytoplasmic liver glycogen is depleted. The lysosomal glucogen can be mobilized from hepatocytes by administering purified glycogen-degrading enzymes of fungal origin, resulting in the disappearance of abnormal lysosomes. However, the normalization of hepatic ultrastructure was not clinically beneficial for the patient. Bone marrow transplantation of a boy with GSD IIa resulted in engraftment of blood cell lines, but the patient died of GSD IIa 5 mo after the procedure.

The prenatal diagnosis of GSD IIa can be made by electron microscopic examination of cells obtained at amniocentesis (see below).

GSD IIb. These patients begin to have weakness of skeletal muscle later in life than those with GSD IIa. In some the disease is compatible with a normal life span, though it may demand a sedentary life style. In other patients, death from respiratory failure can occur during the 3rd or 4th decade. Cardiomegaly is absent and the electrocardiogram is normal. The diagnosis is based on electron microscopic examination of skin biopsy showing "abnormal lysosomes" packed with glycogen particles.

Some cases cannot be explained on the basis of defective

activity of lysosomal acid α-glucosidase. For example, a patient who died of unrelated hypertension at 24 yr of age had a deficiency of acid α-glucosidase consistent with GSD IIa. Glycogen concentration was increased in all tissues except heart, though cardiac α-glucosidase activity was deficient. Heart muscle appeared normal on light microscopy; electron microscopy revealed occasional abnormal lysosomes but no excess of glycogen in cytoplasm.

Deficiency of "Debrancher" Activity (GSD III). Clinical manifestations are summarized in Table 7–7. In GSD III, hepatomegaly can be as impressive as in GSD I. When generalized this disorder affects muscle and heart, but either organ may be clinically involved to a varying degree. Some patients resemble children with muscular dystrophy. Electrocardiographic abnormalities and moderate cardiomegaly are usually found; the size of the kidneys is normal. Patients with GSD III restricted to the liver usually do well. Hypoglycemia is rare and does not present a clinical problem. There may be recurrent pneumonia, but the long-term prognosis is usually good. The serum concentrations of uric acid, lactate, ketones, and lipids are normal. Blood glucose concentration increases if glucagon is given 2 hr after a meal in GSD III but not in GSD I, whereas blood glucose levels remain flat in both glycogenoses when glucagon is administered after overnight fasting. These clinical and laboratory findings distinguish GSD III from GSD I.

For "debranching" of the glycogen molecule, two enzymatic reactions need to occur in sequence after phosphorylase activity has reduced the outer chains of the glycogen molecule to within 4 glucose units of the 1,6 branch point. The first reaction is that of a transferase that transfers 3 glucose units of the branched outer chain into the straight outer chain. The

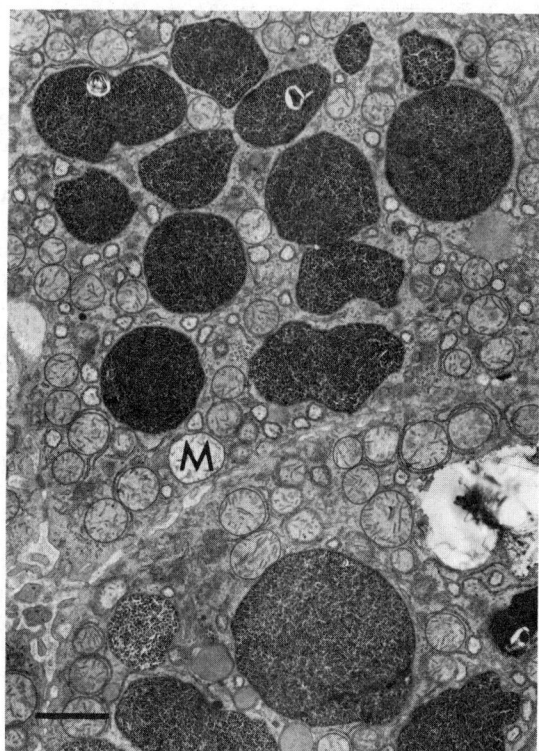

Figure 7–19. Liver autopsy specimen of GSD IIa. "Abnormal lysosomes" with lysosomal glycogen (tightly packed black particles) are ubiquitous, but cytoplasmic glycogen is missing. The absence of cytoplasmic glycogen indicates that this specimen was obtained after starvation and/or epinephrine treatment, or autopsy. M, mitochondria, (Bar: 2 μm).

glucose molecule at the branch point becomes exposed and accessible to the action of α-1,6-glucosidase, which removes it. Both the transferase and the α-1,6-glucosidase activities are deficient in the livers of patients with GSD III. In some the activity of transferase in muscle may be low, whereas that of α-1,6-glucosidase remains normal. The overall effect in either liver or muscle is a loss of "debrancher" activity. Both enzymatic activities may be retained in muscle, with the defect being limited to the liver.

Most frequently GSD III is a generalized disease, with glycogen concentrations increased and "debranching" activity deficient in every (examined) tissue. In generalized GSD III, the concentration of glycogen in muscle may reach the same levels as in GSD II, though patients with the former may be symptom-free and those with the latter are markedly hypotonic. In GSD III, starvation induces the degradation of glycogen to within 4 units of the branch point. Glycogen with such short outer chains is called a limit dextrin; hence *limit dextrinosis* is an alternative designation for GSD III. Light microscopic appearance of liver in GSD III is similar to that of GSD I except that GSD III exhibits formation of fibrous septa, more extensive nuclear glycogenosis, and a paucity of intracellular lipid droplets. Hepatic cirrhosis does not usually develop in GSD III; the fibrous septa usually remain stable.

Deficiency of "Brancher" Activity (GSD IV). This defect is clinically characterized by hepatomegaly and splenomegaly. Progressive portal fibrosis leads to hepatic cirrhosis, ascites, and death in childhood from liver failure. Treatment with corticosteroids may induce temporary remission. Affected children may be candidates for liver transplantation.

Hepatic symptoms are associated with reduced rather than increased concentrations of tissue glycogen. The glycogen resembles amylopectin, since it has fewer than the normal number of branch points. This may be the consequence of deficiency of branching enzyme, though one would expect a defect of this enzyme to result in the synthesis of amylose, the glucose polymer with no branch points. The cirrhosis may be the result of the amylopectin-like glycogen, since this glucose polymer is not normally even transiently present in the liver. The limit dextrin of GSD III may not have this effect because it is a transient form normally encountered during synthesis and degradation of glycogen.

Deficiency of Muscle Phosphorylase (GSD V) (McArdle Syndrome). This disorder exhibits a wide clinical spectrum, varying from almost no symptoms to recurrent myoglobinuria, attacks of rhabdomylosis, and unremitting muscle pain. The muscular pains and cramps after exercise that characterize GSD V are differentiated from muscle cramps related to more common causes by the ischemic exercise test.

The test requires inflation of a blood pressure cuff on the upper arm to above the arterial pressure. The patient is then asked to squeeze a rubber ball with the hand of the same arm about once every sec. The healthy person will easily squeeze 70–110 times, with some discomfort but without cramping of the muscle or residual symptoms after deflation of the blood pressure cuff. In the patient with GSD V, muscle cramps may limit the squeeze to 20–30 movements. When the cuff is released, the cramps persist, with the hand in a tetanic position (wrist bent, fingers extended) that cannot be corrected by the patient or by the examiner. After several min there is gradual release of the cramp, but pain may persist for 24–48 hr. In the healthy person, blood samples taken from the antecubital vein of the ischemic arm during the exercise will show a rise in serum lactate, which does not occur in GSD V because of the inability to produce lactate from glycogen. The diagnosis of GSD V also has been made using nuclear magnetic resonance (NMR) by measuring pH, ATP, and phosphocreatine concentration following both aerobic and ischemic exercise. A clinical picture consistent with McArdle syndrome, including recurrent rhabdomylosis, has also occurred in patients with carnitine palmityl transferase deficiency.

Skeletal muscle is without phosphorylase activity. The activity in liver and smooth muscle is normal. The system of phosphorylase activation is intact; patients may have 3 times the normal activity of muscle phosphorylase kinase. Glycogen concentration is increased in muscle, but usually not above 4%. Histologically, much of the excessive glycogen is deposited in the cytoplasm beneath the sarcolemma. In patients with phosphorylase deficiency, the energy for muscle contraction can still be provided by glucose entering the myocyte, which may suffice for energy requirements at rest when there are not symptoms. Peak demands for energy, however, which can ordinarily be met by supplemental breakdown of muscle glycogen, cannot be met in GSD V because of the phosphorylase defect resulting in pain and cramping during and after exercise, with little or no production of lactic acid. The ischemic exercise worsens the situation by interrupting the normal supply of oxygen and glucose.

Treatment with a high protein diet has been reported.

Deficiency of Liver Phosphorylase (GSD VI). In GSD VI, hepatomegaly may be massive. Otherwise, the affected children are without symptoms and lead normal lives, though there may be some elevation of serum lipids and transaminases (Table 7–7). Most patients do not have hypoglycemia. The blood glucose concentration does not increase after glucagon administration; this finding can be used to separate GSD VI from GSD IX, in which glucagon tolerance curves are normal. Separation from GSD I can be made on clinical evidence. The hepatomegaly may recede as the children grow older.

The low activity of the hepatic phosphorylase system is consistent with but not diagnostic of GSD VI, since low activity may result from a number of defects within the phosphorylase activation system. The diagnosis rests on demonstrating a deficiency in the liver phosphorylase enzyme itself. Leukocyte phosphorylase may also be affected but cannot be relied upon for diagnosis. By light microscopy, slight formation of fibrous septa is seen in portal areas of the liver. Whether this minimal change remains stationary or progresses to cirrhosis in adulthood is unknown. Phosphorylase activity, glycogen concentration, and histologic appearance are normal in muscle.

Deficiency of Phosphofructokinase (GSD VII). The symptoms of GSD VII resemble those of GSD V but the muscle pain and cramping after exercise may be somewhat less severe. The disease has been tolerated by a young man who plays tennis for pleasure.

Phosphofructokinase is deficient in skeletal muscle but not in the liver; it is only partially defective in erythrocytes. Since this key glycolytic enzyme affects the use of both glycogen and glucose in muscle, it is surprising that the deficiency may cause fewer symptoms than a deficiency in phosphorylase, which affects only the utilization of glycogen. The concentration of glycogen in muscle is moderately elevated, and its distribution is subsarcolemmal, like that observed in GSD V and GSD X.

Progressive Brain Disease and Deactivated Liver Phosphorylase without Demonstrated Enzyme Defect (GSD VIII). Hepatomegaly is apparent soon after birth. However, the *clinical features* unique for GSD VIII among the glycogenoses are related primarily to the central nervous system (Table 7–7). The infant develops nystagmus and rolling of the eyes, ataxia, and truncal tremor. The patient becomes hypotonic and then spastic; spasticity may become severe. Gradually the patient loses rapport with the environment, becomes unresponsive and bedridden, develops swallowing difficulties, and may die of aspiration pneumonia. Urinary excretion of epinephrine and norepinephrine may be increased. The glucagon tolerance test is normal.

Glycogen concentration is increased in liver and cerebral biopsies; it has been normal in muscle and in the other tissues examined. Electron microscopy of cerebral biopsies reveals increased amounts of glycogen, in the form of α particles that are about 10 times wider than the β particles usually found in brain. Liver phosphorylase activity is low. Cerebral enzymes have not been assayed. The low activity of the hepatic phosphorylase system does not reflect a deficiency of phosphorylase enzyme or of any other specific enzyme in the hepatic system of phosphorylase activation. This is indicated by the normal glucagon tolerance curve and also by the fact that in vivo the phosphorylase activity increases to normal within 2 min after the administration of glucagon or epinephrine to the patient. The low phosphorylase activity observed in a liver specimen obtained before glucagon administration can be increased to normal in vitro by the patient's own liver homogenate. Accordingly, the affected child appears to suffer from impaired control of phosphorylase activation.

Deficiency of Liver Phosphorylase Kinase (GSD IX). This defect occurs in three forms that differ in their pattern of inheritance and tissue distribution. GSD IXa follows an autosomal recessive pattern of inheritance, and GSD IXb is sex-linked recessive. Otherwise, these two forms are indistinguishable. Skeletal muscle is not affected and is normal biochemically (Table 7–7) and morphologically. In GSD IXc, with autosomal recessive inheritance, the phosphorylase kinase activity of liver and muscle is deficient. Hepatomegaly is massive in early life but recedes as the children grow older; it may disappear completely in teenagers or adults, though the liver can remain somewhat large. Transaminases are minimally elevated. GSD IX can be classified as a benign hepatomegaly except in patients who also have defective debrancher activity. Glucagon produces a normal rise in blood glucose concentration that serves to distinguish it from GSD VI, in which the glucagon tolerance curve remains flat. Affected children require no treatment, except perhaps in rare instances of combined deficiencies.

The concentration of liver glycogen is increased and phosphorylase activity is low, as is the case in GSD VI. In GSD IX, however, the low activity of phosphorylase results from a deficiency in phosphorylase kinase. Other enzymes of the activating system, including phosphorylase, are normal. Cultured skin fibroblasts and leukocytes have been reported to be affected but are undependable for diagnosis.

Deficiency of Cyclic 3′5′-AMP-Dependent Kinase (GSD X). The single patient with this condition had marked hepatomegaly at 6 yr of age, when the clinical picture was indistinguishable from GSD IX except that her blood sugar curve remained flat after intravenous administration of glucagon (Table 7–7). She had no skeletal muscular symptoms at this time, but 6 yr later she complained of muscular pain, cramping after exercise, and a minimal degree of persistent muscular weakness. The ischemic exercise test was normal and hepatomegaly persistent. The patient is doing well without specific therapy.

Liver glycogen concentration was high and hepatic phosphorylase activity was low. Concentration of glycogen in muscle was increased to 2–4%. Light and electron microscopy showed increased glycogen deposition in liver and skeletal muscle cells. Muscle phosphorylase was present only in the inactive form, whereas normally 60–80% of total phosphorylase is in the active form. GSD X reflects a deficiency in activity of cyclic 3′5′-AMP-dependent kinase. It is interesting that the complete inactivation of muscle phosphorylase in GSD X is clinically well tolerated, whereas the complete lack of muscle phosphorylase in GSD V is characterized by cramps and pains. This difference may be due to the ability of inactive

phosphorylase b to degrade glycogen in the presence of adenylic acid (5′-AMP), which is normally found in muscle tissue.

Hepatic Glycogenosis with Stunted Growth (GSD XI). This disorder is characterized by a greatly enlarged liver and markedly stunted growth (Table 7–7). Serum transaminase and lipid levels may be elevated. Affected children develop severe hypophosphatemic rickets early in life unless they receive oral phosphate supplementation and 50,000 units or more of vitamin D daily. Orally administering phosphate alone to the extent necessary for correction of the hypophosphatemia may heal the florid rickets, but adequate growth is not attained through this regimen. The marked rachitic bone changes are due to Fanconi syndrome characterized by urinary loss of phosphate, amino acids, glucose, and galactose that can occur in these children. Administering arginine raises the level of growth hormone in serum. After puberty the hepatomegaly may recede (although hepatic glycogen concentration remains increased) and the growth rate may increase (although the ultimate body height remains far below normal). However, after puberty the serum phosphate concentration remains normal without supplementation with phosphate or vitamin D.

Glycogen concentration is markedly increased in liver and kidney but normal in muscle. All measured hepatic glycolytic enzyme activities have been normal. Administering glucagon did not increase the blood glucose concentration, but did increase urinary excretion of cyclic AMP that is usually induced by glucagon administration. Glucose concentration decreased after the oral administration of 1.75 g/kg of galactose, an amount that normally is followed by a significant increase of blood glucose. Conversely, orally administering an equivalent amount of fructose was followed by the normal increase of blood glucose concentration. It seems reasonable to postulate that patients with GSD XI have a functional deficiency of hepatic phosphoglucomutase, despite the fact that the activity of this enzyme has been reported to be normal in vitro.

Prenatal Diagnosis of GSD

The glycogenoses generally follow an autosomal recessive pattern of inheritance, except for GSD IXb, in which inheritance is sex-linked recessive. They should be detectable in the fetus through assay of cultured amniotic fluid cells when these cells normally produce the particular enzyme under study. This criterion is not fulfilled for GSD I since glucose-6-phosphate is not found in normal cultured amniotic fluid cells. GSD I, GSD III, GSD VI, GSD IX, and GSD X may not be candidates for prenatal diagnosis because most of the affected children with these conditions lead near normal lives. In GSD IIa and GSD IV, on the other hand, antenatal diagnosis has been made through assay of cultured amniotic fluid cells (Sec 6.30). Acid α-glucosidase activity has been present in all amniotic fluid specimens tested, even in GSD IIa. Although several weeks may be needed to culture the amniotic fluid cells, prenatal diagnosis of GSD IIa is feasible within 3 days after amniocentesis through electron microscopic examination of uncultured amniotic fluid cells, which show abnormal intracellular lysosomes that are not present in heterozygous or normal fetuses.

Concurrent Deficiencies of Enzymes in Patients with GSD

The prognosis may be altered from that of an isolated deficiency when two or more enzyme activities are deficient in the same patient. For example, in patients with deficiencies of liver debrancher or phosphorylase there is usually a delicate fibrosis that does not progress. However, in a patient with both defects the fibrosis may progress to frank clinical cirrhosis. Alternatively, an occasional combination of defects may mitigate or ameliorate the problem, though this might not be readily appreciated. Alternatively, a defect may be compensated for by increased activity of a normal biochemical collateral pathway. For example, one would expect a deficiency of phosphohexoisomerase to result in arrested glycolysis and severe illness. That this does not happen suggests that the defective interconversion of glucose-6-phosphate and fructose-6-phosphate can be bypassed by way of the pentose phosphate shunt.

DEFICIENCY OF XYLULOSE DEHYDROGENASE
(Essential Benign Pentosuria)

This benign condition is characterized by a reducing substance in the urine of an otherwise healthy individual. Care should be taken not to mistake the reducing substance for glucose. The pentose in the urine reacts with *Clinitest* but not with glucose oxidase test papers such as *Testape* or *Clinistix* dipsticks.

L-Xylulose dehydrogenase converts L-xylulose (which can arise from D-glucuronate) to xylitol. Xylitol is converted to D-xylulose, which becomes D-xylulose-5-phosphate and enters the pentose phosphate shunt. Deficiency of this enzyme leads to increased concentration of L-xylulose in blood and urine. This rare defect is most common in Jews. No therapy is required.

Pentosuria can be observed in normal individuals if the dietary pentose intake is increased, as with the excessive ingestion of fruit containing pentose. Under these circumstances there may be urinary excretion of xylose and arabinose up to 200 mg/24 hr in normal individuals.

DEFICIENCY OF ACID α-MANNOSIDASE
(Mannosidosis)

The appearance of the patient with mannosidosis is similar to that in Hurler syndrome (Sec 7.24). The liver and spleen are enlarged in this lysosomal disease; the lymphocytes contain vacuoles. Skeletal roentgenograms reveal structural abnormalities (dysostosis multiplex). Infections are frequent, especially of the middle ear and lungs. There may be corneal or lenticular opacities and psychomotor retardation is usually present. No treatment is available.

Acid α-mannosidase activity is deficient in body fluids and tissues. Mannose-containing macromolecules are stored in the abnormal liver lysosomes, which resemble those of the Hurler syndrome. Mannosidosis exists in heterogeneous forms.

DEFICIENCY OF ACID α-FUCOSIDASE
(Fucosidosis)

See Sec. 7.27.

BLOOD GROUP SUBSTANCES

Blood group antigens are glycolipids or glycoproteins, depending upon whether they are cellular or soluble, respectively. In the synthesis of specific antigens, basic or fundamental macromolecules undergo modification through various transferases that are determined by genes designated H, A, B, Le, and so on. Gene H defines an enzyme that attaches fucose to the basic macromolecule in preparation for action by the other transferases. The attachment of this fucose molecule establishes the blood group O. Absence of the gene H results in a rare blood group (Bombay). The transferase dependent on gene A permits attachment of N-acetylgalactosamine. Macromolecules so modified become blood group A antigens. The transferase dependent on gene B attaches galactose, which defines group B antigens. To complete the synthesis of the respective antigen the attachment of several units of fucose (6-deoxy-L-galactose) is required. The exact sites and positions of these fucose units codetermine antigen specificity within the ABO and Lewis systems of blood group substances.

Incorporation of fucose is also decisive for whether an individual will secrete blood group substances into various body fluids, such as saliva. "Secretors" have the activity of a particular fucosyltransferase, whereas "nonsecretors" do not. The incidence of nonsecretors varies from 40% in black Americans to 25% in whites and to near zero in American Indians.

Patients with fucosidosis have the Lewis antigens in more than 5 times their usual concentration. The accumulation of this macromolecule may occur because the deficiency of α-fucosidase in tissues of such patients impairs the disposal of fucose units that reside in the Lewis antigen.

7.22 DIAGNOSTIC PROCEDURES IN DEFECTS OF METABOLISM OF CARBOHYDRATES

Clinical awareness is essential to the diagnosis of the child who may have an inborn error of carbohydrate metabolism. A limited number of tests may provide a preliminary assessment (Table 7–7). The ultimate diagnosis depends on biochemical analysis of tissues which provides the basis of treatment (Table 7–8).

The tissue to be examined should be obtained preferentially from the organ or organs showing clinical signs of abnormality. Liver biopsy using the Menghini needle does not carry undue risks for the patient so long as adequate precautions are taken. However, needle biopsy provides only about 20 mg of tissue, which may not be enough for definitive studies. The interest of the patient may, therefore, be better served by open biopsy, which has the added advantage of providing easy access to specimens of skeletal muscle of the abdominal wall.

Although analysis of white blood cells is valuable in selected instances, such as the determination of the carrier state of GSD IIa, our experience suggests that examination of blood cells is only complementary to analysis of tissues of solid organs. Fibroblast cultures of skin biopsy specimens are of limited reliability.

Detailed advice on how to procure and handle specimens shipped to special laboratories should be obtained from the collaborating laboratory *before* the biopsy is made.

7.23 THERAPY OF DEFECTS IN METABOLISM OF CARBOHYDRATES

For many of these conditions no treatment is effective; for others, none is necessary. The clinician's role may be limited to supportive care (Sec. 2.70 and 2.71) or to genetic counseling (Sec. 6.7 and 6.30).

In a few conditions dietary regimens may offer some help; for some they are lifesaving (galactosemia, fructose intolerance, etc.). Future therapies depend upon research to find ways of replacing specific enzymes, adding pharmacologic doses of cofactors (vitamins, etc.) to the diet, or compensating for the enzymatic defect with hormones or drugs.

Enzyme replacement has been carried out by transplanting normal kidneys into patients with Fabry disease (Sec. 7.28) and normal cultured fibroblasts into patients with Hunter or Hurler disease (Sec. 7.24). In Fabry disease, the transplanted normal kidney may provide a "filter" for circulating trihexoside with enough α-galactosidase to initiate its degradation. In Hurler disease transplanted normal cultured fibroblasts have been unsuccessful. Bone marrow transplantation has been therapeutically effective in children with some lysosomal disease, in particular in various types of mucopolysaccharidoses (7.24). It did not benefit a patient with GSD IIa nor did infusion of fungal α-glucosidase.

GEORGE HUG

Aynsley-Green A, Wiliamson DH, Gitzelmann R: Hepatic glycogen synthetase deficiency: Definition of the syndrome from metabolic and enzyme studies on a nine-year-old girl. Arch Dis Child 131:573, 1977.
Barranger JA, Brady RO (eds.): The Molecular Basis of Lysosomal Storage Disorders. New York, Academic Press, 1984.
Beratis NG, LaBadie GU, Hirschhorn K: Characterization of the molecular defect in infantile and adult acid α-glucosidase deficiency fibroblasts. J Clin Invest 62:1264, 1978.
Brandt NJ, Terenius L, Jacobsen BB, et al: Hyper-endorphin syndrome in a child with necrotizing encephalomyelopathy. N Engl J Med 303:914, 1980.
Brown WJ, Farquhar MG: The mannose-6-phosphate receptor for lysosomal enzymes is concentrated in cis Golgi cisternae. Cell 36:295, 1984.
Chen Y-T, Cornblath M, Sidbury JB: Cornstarch therapy in type I glycogen storage disease. N Engl J Med 310:171, 1984.
DeVivo DC, Haymond MW, Obert KA, et al: Defective activation of the pyruvate dehydrogenase complex in subacute necrotizing encephalomyelopathy (Leigh disease). Ann Neurol 6:483, 1979.
Durand P, Borrone C, Gatti R: On genetic variants in fucosidosis. J Pediatr 89:688, 1976.
Farrell DF, Clark AF, Scott CR, et al: Absence of pyruvate decarboxylase activity in man: A cause of congenital lactic acidosis. N Engl J Med 292:1082, 1975.
Garibaldi LR, Canini S, Suporti-Furga A, et al: Galactosemia caused by generalized uridine disphosphate galactose-4-epimerase deficiency. J Pediatr 103:927-930, 1983.
Gitzelmann R, Steinmann B, Mitchell B, et al: Uridine diphosphate galactose 4'-epimerase deficiency. IV. Report of eight cases in three families. Helv Paediatr Acta 31:441, 1976.
Greene HL, Slonim AE, O'Neill JA, et al: Continuous nocturnal intragastric feeding for management of type I glycogen storage disease. N Engl J Med 294:423, 1976.
Gröbe H, von Bassewitz DB, Dominick HC, et al: Subacute necrotizing encephalomyelopathy: Clinical, ultrastructural, biochemical and therapeutic studies in an infant. Acta Paediatr Scand 64:755, 1975.
Hug G, Chuck G, Walling L, et al: Liver phosphorylase deficiency in glycogenosis type VI: Documentation by biochemical analysis of hepatic biopsy specimens. J Lab Clin Med 84:26, 1974.
Hug G, Schubert WK, Chuck G: Phosphorylase kinase of the liver: Deficiency in a girl with increased hepatic glycogen. Science 153:1534, 1966.
Hug G, Schubert WK, Soukup S: Treatment related observations in solid tissues, fibroblast cultures and amniotic fluid cells of type II glycogenosis, Hurler disease and metachromatic leukodystrophy. Birth Defects 9(2):160, 1973.
Hug G, Soukup S, Ryan M, Chuck G: Rapid prenatal diagnosis of glycogen storage disease type II by electron microscopy of uncultured amniotic-fluid cells. N Engl J Med 310:1018, 1984.
Kornfeld M, LeBaron M: Glycogenosis Type VIII. J Neuropathol Exp Neurol 43:568, 1984.
Lerner A, Iancu TC, Bashan N, et al: A new variant of glycogen storage disease type IXc. Am J Dis Chil 136:407, 1982.
Mehler M, DMauro S: Late-onset acid maltase deficiency. Arch Neurol 33:692, 1976.
Reitman ML, Varki A, Kornfield S: Fibroblasts from patients with I-cell disease and pseudo-Hurler polydystrophy are deficient in UDP-N-acetylglucosamine: glycoprotein N-acetylglucosaminylphosphotransferase activity. J Clin Invest 67:1574, 1981.
Robinson BH, Taylor J, Sherwood WG: Deficiency of dihydrolipoyl dehydrogenase: A cause of congenital lactic acidosis. Pediatr Res 11:1198, 1977.
Saul R, Ghidoni JJ, Molyneux RJ, et al: Castanospermine inhibits α-glucosidase activities and alters glycogen distribution in animals. Proc Natl Acad Sci 82:93, 1985.
Slonim AE, Goans PJ: Myopathy in McArdle's syndrome: Improvement with a high-protein diet. N Engl J Med 312:355, 1985.

7.24 DISORDERS OF MUCOPOLYSACCHARIDE METABOLISM

The mucopolysaccharidoses are a group of inherited disorders caused by incomplete degradation and storage of acid mucopolysaccharides (glycosaminoglycans). The clinical manifestations result from the accumulation of mucopolysaccharides in various organs. Specific degradative lysosomal enzyme deficiencies have been identified for all the mucopolysaccharidoses.

The mucopolysaccharides are polyanionic polymers, most of which contain alternating carbohydrate residues of N-acetylhexosamine and uronic acid. Although the acid mucopolysaccharides are closely related as a group, individual compounds differ in their distribution in the body's tissues. Dermatan sulfate, heparan sulfate, and keratan sulfate are the major mucopolysaccharides involved in the pathogenesis of the mucopolysaccharidoses. The structural differences of the mucopolysaccharides explain the need for various lysosomal enzymes required for their degradation.

Since the mucopolysaccharides are major components of the intercellular substance of connective tissue, bony changes are characteristic of the mucopolysaccharidoses. The skeletal deformities seen in roentgenograms are referred to as **dysostosis multiplex.** The central nervous system also may be affected, leading to progressive mental retardation. In addition, the cardiovascular system, liver, spleen, tendons, joints, and skin may be involved. The degree of disability and overall prognosis in each of the mucopolysaccharidoses is determined by the extent of the physical and mental involvement.

The mucopolysaccharidoses follow an autosomal recessive mode of inheritance, with the exception of Hunter syndrome, which is inherited as an X-linked recessive trait. They are suspected on the basis of clinical and radiological manifestations, and the diagnosis is confirmed by finding increased urinary excretion of mucopolysaccharides and the deficiency of a specific enzyme. Table 7–9 lists the various mucopolysaccharidoses, the specific products excreted in urine, and the enzyme deficiencies.

Hurler Syndrome (MPS I-H). This syndrome is the most severe of the mucopolysaccharidoses. Its relentless progression usually results in death by the early teenage years.

Etiology and Pathology. The basic defect in Hurler disease is a deficiency of alpha-L-iduronidase, which leads to the accumulation of the dermatan and heparan sulfates in tissues and their urinary excretion. Almost every tissue in the body is affected, with widespread occurrence of vacuolated, or "gargoyle," cells, containing lysosomes engorged with mucopolysaccharide. In the brain, lipid storage also occurs with the mucopolysaccharide accumulation. There is unusual hyalinization of collagen and separation of the collagen bundles. These changes lead to joint deformities and stiffness, thickened meninges, hydrocephalus, peripheral nerve compression, and a tendency to develop hernias. As the disease progresses, narrowing of the coronary arteries, thickening of the cardiac valves and endocardium, and stiffening of the myocardium may lead to congestive heart failure. The constricted thorax contributes to the clinical deterioration of these patients.

Clinical Manifestations. Infants with Hurler syndrome appear normal at birth, and during the 1st year of life only slight developmental delays are noted. Physical examination, however, reveals hepatosplenomegaly, exaggerated kyphosis,

Table 7–9. **The Mucopolysaccharidoses**

Disease	Urinary Mucopolysaccharides	Enzyme Deficiency
Hurler syndrome	Dermatan sulfate Heparan sulfate	α-L-Iduronidase
Scheie syndrome	Dermatan sulfate	α-L-Iduronidase
Hurler-Scheie syndrome	Dermatan sulfate	α-L-Iduronidase
Hunter syndrome	Dermatan sulfate Heparan sulfate	Iduronosulfate sulfatase
Sanfilippo syndrome A	Heparan sulfate	Sulfamidase
Sanfilippo syndrome B	Heparan sulfate	α-N-Acetylglucosaminidase
Sanfilippo syndrome C	Heparan sulfate	Acetyl CoA: α-glucosaminide N-acetyltransferase
Sanfilippo syndrome D	Heparan sulfate	N-Acetylglucosamine-6-sulfate sulfatase (specific for heparan sulfate only)
Morquio syndrome A	Keratan sulfate Chondroitin-6-sulfate	N-Acetylgalactosamine-6-sulfate sulfatase and galactose-6-sulfatase
Morquio syndrome B	Keratan sulfate	β-Galactosidase
Maroteaux-Lamy syndrome	Dermatan sulfate	N-Acetylgalactosamine-4-sulfate sulfatase (arylsulfatase B)
β-Glucuronidase deficiency	Chondroitin 4/6 sulfate	β-Glucuronidase
Keratan and heparan sulfaturia	Keratan sulfate Heparan sulfate	N-Acetylglucosamine-6-sulfate sulfatase (specific for keratan sulfate and heparan sulfate)

persistent nasal discharge, and noisy breathing. The facial features become progressively coarser after the 1st year of life (Fig. 7–20). The head is large and dolichocephalic, with frontal bossing and prominent sagittal and metopic sutures. The bridge of the nose is depressed, and the nose is broad and flat. Clouding of the corneas becomes evident at about 1 yr of age. Umbilical and inguinal hernias are common. Children afflicted with this disease regress developmentally, and mental retardation becomes obvious. The downhill course continues rapidly after the 2nd or 3rd year of life. These children become immobile, their joints become progressively stiff and contracted, and they usually die by their early teens.

Roentgenographic Changes. Roentgenograms of patients with Hurler syndrome reveal dysostosis multiplex, which includes a large dolichocephalic skull and thickened calvarium. There may be hyperostosis of the cranium, and the sella turcica may be boot- or "J"-shaped. The medial third of the clavicle is thickened. The vertebral bodies are ovoid in the lower thorax and upper lumbar regions. They develop beak-like projections on their lower anterior margins, while their upper portions remain hypoplastic (Fig. 7–21). This results in the gibbus deformity commonly seen in these patients. The ribs are spatulated or oar-shaped, and the pelvis shows flaring of the iliac bones, with shallow acetabulae. Roentgenograms of the hips show progressive coxa valga deformity, sometimes resembling the findings of aseptic necrosis. Roentgenograms of the hands show tapering of the terminal phalanges and widening at the distal and tapering at the proximal ends of the metacarpals. The 5th metacarpal is the first to show these changes (Fig. 7–22). In the long bones, particularly of the upper extremities, irregular widenings associated with areas of cortical thinning and expansion of the medullary cavity are seen. Occasionally, there may be cortical thickening. The radius curves toward the ulna, and the articular surfaces of the radius and the ulna face one another, forming a "V" (Fig. 7–22). The humerus may be angulated and the glenoid fossa, like the acetabulum, may be shallow. Severe growth retardation is common in these children.

Diagnosis. The diagnosis of Hurler syndrome is suggested by the presence of the relevant clinical and roentgenographic findings. Urinary excretion of dermatan and heparan sulfates provides further support. Although there are helpful screening methods for quantifying the mucopolysaccharides in the urine, definitive diagnosis requires detection of alpha-L-iduronidase deficiency in white blood cells, serum, or cultured skin fibroblasts.

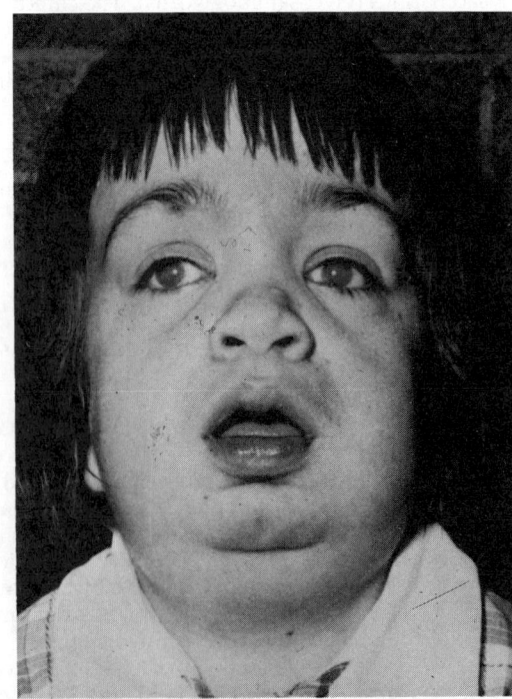

Figure 7–20. Typical appearance of a patient with Hurler syndrome.

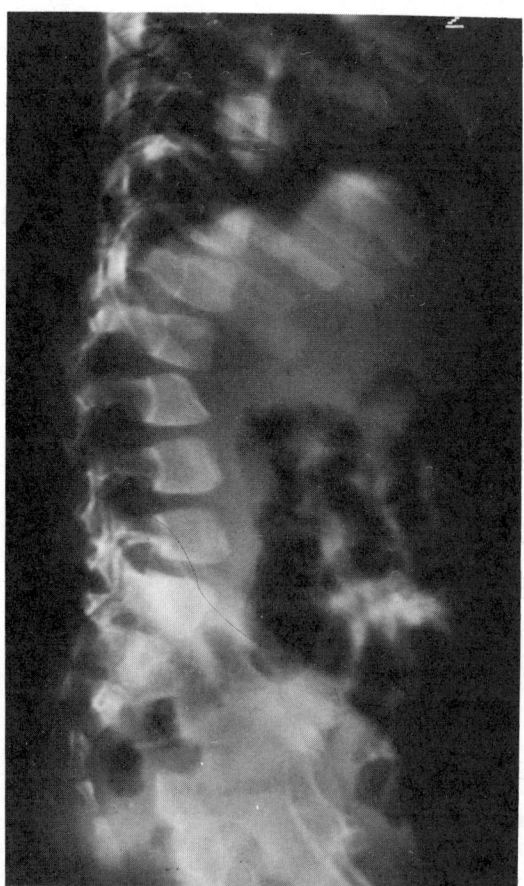

Figure 7–21. Lateral spine roentgenogram of patient with Hurler syndrome.

Scheie Syndrome (MPS IS). This syndrome is the mildest of the mucopolysaccharidoses. It is a distinct clinical and genetic entity; the enzyme deficiency, alpha-L-iduronidase, is the same as in Hurler syndrome but is specific for dermatan sulfate, which accumulates in tissues and is excreted in excessive amounts in urine.

Clinical Manifestations. Patients with this disease have normal intelligence, mild facial coarsening with striking prognathism, joint stiffness typified by claw hands, and carpal tunnel syndrome. Corneal clouding is a constant feature which leads to loss of visual acuity. Aortic regurgitation is common. The clinical features do not appear until after 5 yr of age, and the disease is compatible with close-to-normal life expectancy. The patient with Scheie syndrome reaches normal height.

Roentgenographic Changes. Findings on roentgenography include mild dysostosis multiplex, without the vertebral changes or the gibbus deformity seen in Hurler disease. There is coxa valga and slight radial and ulnar obliquity with "V" formation of their articular surfaces.

Diagnosis. Early clinical diagnosis is more difficult in Scheie than in Hurler syndrome because the somatic changes are mild and mental retardation is not present. The detection of urinary dermatan sulfate is helpful, but the diagnosis is confirmed by demonstrating a deficiency of alpha-L-iduronidase in white blood cells or in cultured skin fibroblasts.

Hurler-Scheie Syndrome (MPS IH/IS). Few reports exist of patients with this syndrome.

Etiology. The basic defect is alpha-L-iduronidase deficiency specific for dermatan sulfate, which is excreted in urine and stored in the liver, spleen, and other tissues. It has been suggested that the Hurler-Scheie syndrome is a genetic com-

pound of two recessive genes, analogous to hemoglobin SC disease, but recent work indicates it is best explained as an allelic mutation of the iduronidase gene.

Clinical Manifestations. Patients develop mild coarseness of facial features, corneal clouding, shortness of stature, joint contractures, hepatosplenomegaly, hernias, and cardiac valvular lesions, primarily mitral insufficiency (Fig. 7–23). Mental development is normal. The clinical features, which usually develop in the first 2 yr of life and in early childhood, are often mistaken for manifestations of a variety of skeletal defects causing growth retardation. The disease is compatible with long life.

Roentgenographic Features. Roentgenograms of patients with this syndrome reveal severe dysostosis multiplex with findings identical to those seen in Hurler syndrome, except that there is no gibbus.

Diagnosis. Diagnosis is based upon the findings of dermatan sulfate in the urine and alpha-L-iduronidase deficiency. The clinical pattern of onset of joint involvement and the severity of skeletal deformities distinguishes Hurler-Scheie from Scheie disease.

Hunter Syndrome (MPS II). This syndrome is the only X-linked disorder among the mucopolysaccharidoses. It is milder than Hurler syndrome with respect to the skeletal and mental defects, although the mucopolysaccharides, dermatan and heparan sulfate, stored in tissues and excreted in the urine are similar in the two diseases. The enzyme deficient in tissues is iduronosulfate sulfatase, but there is a considerable phenotypic heterogeneity; there is no biochemical or enzymatic difference between the severe form of the disease, designated *type A*, and the mild disease, *type B*.

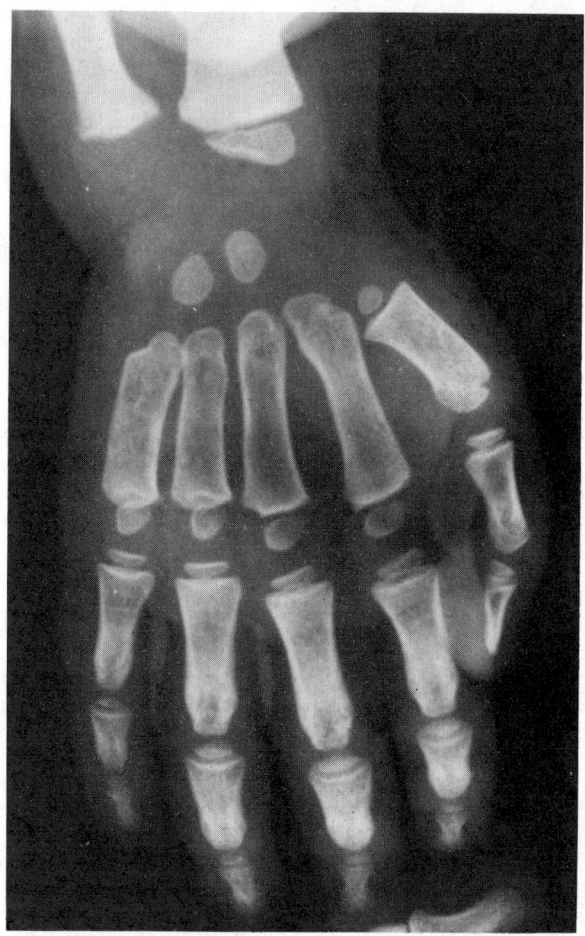

Figure 7–22. Roentgenogram of hand of patient with Hurler syndrome.

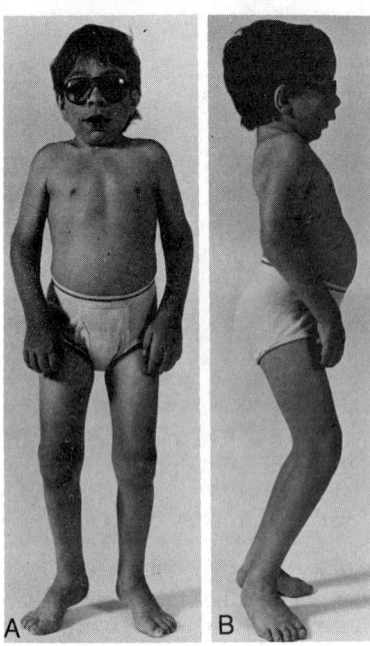

Figure 7–23. A patient with Hurler-Scheie syndrome with normal intelligence. Note the joint stiffness of all extremities.

Type A. This is the "classic" form of Hunter syndrome. Coarseness of facial features, short stature, joint stiffness, hepatosplenomegaly, and hernias are common clinical manifestations. Mental retardation is severe. Progression of the disease process is slower and the dysostosis multiplex is milder than in Hurler syndrome. Corneal clouding is usually absent, but hearing loss is very common. Skin changes also are frequent, including small raised papules over the skin of the shoulders, the scapulas, and the lower back. Cardiac involvement often occurs. Patients usually do not have gibbus deformity, although mild kyphosis may be present in some. Life expectancy for these patients is usually into the late teens or early twenties.

Type B. This syndrome is a far milder disease than *type A,* even though the enzyme deficiency and urinary mucopolysaccharides are the same. Retardation is usually lacking, or very minimal. The physical features are similar to, but milder than, those in type A, and patients have a longer life expectancy.

Diagnosis. The physical features, dysostosis multiplex, and dermatan and heparan sulfaturia suggest either Hurler or Hunter syndrome, but sex-linked inheritance is specific to the latter. Enzyme studies showing iduronosulfate sulfatase deficiency in serum, white blood cells, or cultured fibroblasts confirm the diagnosis of Hunter syndrome. Other sulfatases should be examined, since multiple sulfatase deficiency can be confused with Hunter syndrome.

Sanfilippo Syndrome (MPS III). This syndrome is a distinct entity, based on clinical findings and the excessive urinary excretion of exclusively heparan sulfate. The coarse facial appearance and skeletal involvement are milder than in the Hurler and Hunter syndromes. There are four enzymatic variants, distinct deficiencies all leading to the same phenotype and mucopolysacchariduria. Heparan sulfate is stored in tissues, and its accumulation is responsible for the neuronal damage and atrophy underlying the profound mental retardation associated with the disease.

Clinical Manifestations. The clinical features of the Sanfilippo syndrome in early life are not very striking. Affected children have delayed developmental milestones, and are usually very hyperactive. By the end of the first decade there

is rapid neurologic deterioration; their gait becomes unsteady, and they become bed ridden. Most of the children die in their middle teens. Mental retardation, some joint stiffening, hepatosplenomegaly, hernias, and dysostosis multiplex are common, but dwarfism and corneal clouding are rare.

Patients manifest dysostosis multiplex typical of the mucopolysaccharidoses. The large bones are not as severely involved; the obliquity of the radius and ulna and the tapering of the proximal ends of the metacarpals are very mild.

Diagnosis. Sanfilippo syndrome should be considered in the presence of heparan sulfaturia, hepatosplenomegaly, mental retardation, and dysostosis multiplex. Screening tests for urinary mucopolysaccharides usually give positive results, but not as consistently as in the Hurler or Hunter syndromes. The different enzymatic variants can be confirmed by specific enzyme assays provided by special laboratories.

Sanfilippo A Syndrome (MPS III A). Sulfamidase is deficient in this disease, which can be assayed using cultured skin fibroblasts or peripheral blood leukocytes.

Sanfilippo B Syndrome (MPS III B). This form is characterized by alpha-N-acetylhexosaminidase deficiency, which can be assayed on serum, white blood cells, or cultured skin fibroblasts.

Sanfilippo C Syndrome (MPS III C). This syndrome is caused by a deficiency of acetyl CoA:alpha-glucosaminide N-acetyltransferase. The assay requires cultured fibroblasts or white blood cells.

Sanfilippo D Syndrome (MPS III D). This deficiency of N-acetylglucosamine-6-sulfatase is specific for heparan sulfate. The enzyme is assayed using a substrate prepared from heparin.

Morquio Syndrome (MPS IV). This disorder is characterized by keratan sulfaturia and skeletal dysplasia. Keratan sulfate is stored in tissues together with chondroitin-6-sulfate. The keratan sulfaturia may decrease with age, but it is always above the normal range. There are two enzyme defects that lead to identical phenotypes in this syndrome.

Clinical Manifestations. The syndrome is associated with severe somatic manifestations and lack of mental involvement. At birth it may not be recognized. Joint laxity and shortness of stature first appear at about 1 yr of age. Skeletal abnormalities include flat vertebrae (platyspondyly universalis), short neck, genu valgum, flat feet, large and unstable knee joints, large elbow joints, and large wrists with ulnar deviation. The platyspondly leads to short trunk and short stature. The odontoid process is underdeveloped; early on, this may cause atlantoaxial subluxation or translocation, with spinal cord compression. Corneal clouding also may be apparent at an early age. There is mid-face hypoplasia with a depressed nasal bridge and protrusion of the mandible, which give these patients a permanent grin. Hepatosplenomegaly is not as pronounced as in the other mucopolysaccharidoses, but it is usually present. Cardiac manifestations are secondary to respiratory failure caused by kyphoscoliosis and restricted chest movements, although aortic regurgitation may complicate the Morquio syndrome. Teeth are severely affected and have very thin enamel. Hearing loss may result from recurrent otitis media. Variation in the clinical manifestations are common, and very mild cases may be encountered. Patients usually die in their 3rd or 4th decade of life from cor pulmonale caused by the severe abnormalities of the chest and spine.

Roentgenographic Changes. In the 1st year of life, roentgenograms may reveal only mild changes in patients with Morquio syndrome. The vertebral bodies show height loss and anterior tongue-like projections. At 2 yr the platyspondyly becomes evident. The hypoplasia of the odontoid process can be clearly seen in tomographic studies. The skull and sella turcica are mildly involved. The long bones are shortened, and the metaphyses appear irregular. There is progressive distortion of the epiphyseal metaphyseal plates. The pelvis shows wide acetabulae with progressive subluxation or dislocation of the femoral heads. The metacarpal bones are short and wide with conical tapering of their proximal ends. The distal ends of the radius and ulna face one another, similar to the obliquity seen in other mucopolysaccharidoses. These changes, especially the coxa valga and the changes in the wrists and lumbar spine, should differentiate Morquio syndrome from other skeletal dysplasias.

Diagnosis. The spondyloepiphyseal dysplasias may mimic Morquio syndrome both clinically and roentgenographically. Screening tests for acid mucopolysaccharides in the urine of these patients can be negative; therefore, quantitative rather than qualitative isolation methods are preferred. The urinary finding of keratan sulfaturia, morever, is also found in the Kniest syndrome. Therefore, enzyme determinations are essential for differentiating Morquio syndrome from other conditions. There are two enzyme deficiencies:

MORQUIO SYNDROME, TYPE A (MPS IV A). This syndrome is caused by a deficiency of N-acetylgalactosamine-6-sulfate sulfatase, an enzyme that also degrades galactose-6-sulfate.

MORQUIO SYNDROME, TYPE B (MPS IV B). In this syndrome β-galactosidase is deficient. An important clinical difference between the two syndromes is the lack of enamel hypoplasia in type B. In other respects, including roentgenograms of the spine, the two forms may be indistinguishable. Morquio syndrome type B should not be confused with GM1 gangliosidosis, which also is associated with β-galactosidase deficiency, but clinically resembles Hurler syndrome.

Keratan and Heparan Sulfaturia (MPS VIII). A single case of this unusual form of mucopolysacchariduria has been described. The patient was a male who was noted to have developmental delay at 18 mo of age. At 2½ yr he was severely retarded, bedridden, and blind. He had scaphocephaly and mild pectus excavatum but no organomegaly; corneal clouding was not noted. Roentgenographic studies showed dysostosis multiplex, without the platyspondyly seen in Morquio syndrome.

Urinary studies showed excessive excretion of both keratan and heparan sulfates. Enzymatic assays revealed normal activity for both of the known Morquio enzyme defects. N-acetylglucosamine-6-sulfate sulfatase specific for a substrate prepared from keratan sulfate was deficient. This enzyme defect is different from that of Sanfilippo D, in which N-acetylglucosamine-6-sulfate sulfatase deficiency is specific for heparan sulfate only.

Maroteaux-Lamy Syndrome (MPS VI). The Maroteaux-Lamy syndrome resembles Hurler disease clinically, but does not involve mental retardation. There are two clinical types: the severe form is designated *type A*, and the milder form, with less pronounced skeletal deformities, is designated *type B*.

Clinical Manifestations. Coarse facial features are typical of this syndrome. The head is enlarged, and the neck and trunk are short. The chest shows pectus carinatum deformity. Claw hands and other joint contractures are common. The abdomen protrudes owing to hepatosplenomegaly (Fig. 7–24). Umbilical hernias and corneal opacities are frequent. Mental ability is usually not impaired, although hydrocephalus and increased intracranial pressure are sometimes associated with Maroteaux-Lamy disease. Cardiac involvement includes mitral insufficiency and aortic regurgitation. The roentgenographic findings are those of dysostosis multiplex seen in Hurler syndrome.

Diagnosis. The elevated urinary mucopolysaccharide in Maroteaux-Lamy syndrome is almost exclusively dermatan sulfate, and N-acetylglucosamine-4-sulfate sulfatase (arylsulfatase B) is the deficient enzyme. Types A and B have the same mucopolysacchariduria and the same enzyme defi-

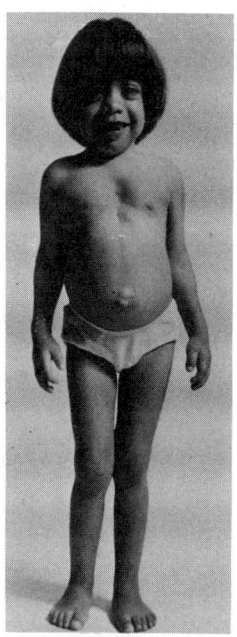

Figure 7–24. A patient with Maroteaux-Lamy syndrome with normal intelligence. The elbows, wrists, and fingers show typical joint stiffness. The abdomen is protuberant with umbilical hernia.

ciency. The findings of somatic changes resembling those of Hurler syndrome, normal mental development, and dermatan sulfaturia suggest either Maroteaux-Lamy or Hurler-Scheie syndrome. Deficiency of arylsulfatase B in white blood cells or cultured fibroblasts confirms the diagnosis of Maroteaux-Lamy syndrome.

Beta-Glucuronidase Deficiency (MPS VII). Patients with this disease have clinical and skeletal features of mucopolysaccharidoses with hepatosplenomegaly, umbilical hernia, thoracolumbar gibbus, and mental retardation. Variations in the phenotypic expression of this enzyme defect have been reported; some patients have a clinical course similar to that of Hurler disease, whereas others have had no mental retardation and a very mild course. The roentgenographic changes are those of dysostosis multiplex. The severity of the bony changes may vary, but at times are indistinguishable from those seen in Hurler disease.

The biochemical findings are characterized by the mucopolysacchariduria of chondroitin 4/6 sulfate. The definitive diagnosis is made by establishing β-glucuronidase deficiency in white blood cells or in cultured skin fibroblasts.

DIFFERENTIAL DIAGNOSIS OF THE MUCOPOLYSACCHARIDOSES

Diseases with dysostosis multiplex and physical features of the mucopolysaccharidoses are summarized in Table 7–10.

Multiple sulfatase deficiency (Sec. 7.31) may mimic the mucopolysaccharidoses in its clinical manifestations, roentgenographic findings, and the presence of mucopolysacchariduria. The mental and neurological deterioration is usually more rapid than in the Hurler or Hunter diseases and often resembles metachromatic leukodystropy. Severe ichthyosis, a constant feature, and hepatomegaly should raise the suspicion of multiple sulfatase deficiency in a patient suspected of having a mucopolysaccharidosis. Urinary screening for mucopolysaccharides and sulfatides is usually positive.

GM1 gangliosidosis (generalized gangliosidosis) (Sec. 7.25) shares clinical features of lipid and mucopolysaccharide storage diseases. Clinically, patients with the infantile severe form of generalized gangliosidosis are mentally retarded and

Table 7–10. Diseases to be Considered in the Differential Diagnosis of the Mucopolysaccharidoses

Syndrome	Biochemical Findings	Enzyme Deficiency	Genetics
GM$_1$ gangliosidosis	GM$_1$ stored in tissues. "Keratan sulfate–like" glycoprotein stored in tissue and excreted in urine	β-Galactosidase	Autosomal recessive
Mannosidosis	Mannose containing glycopeptides excreted in urine and stored in tissues	α-Mannosidase	Autosomal recessive
Fucosidosis	Fucose containing oligosaccharides and glycopeptides are stored in tissues and excreted in urine	α-Fucosidase	Autosomal recessive
Aspartylglucosaminuria	Aspartylglucosamine in urine and tissues	Aspartylglucosaminidase	Autosomal recessive
Mucolipidosis I	Sialic acid containing oligosaccharides are excreted in urine and stored in tissues	α-Sialidase	Autosomal recessive
Mucolipidosis II "I" cell disease	Very high levels of acid hydrolases, e.g., β-hexosaminidase in urine and serum. Very low levels of the same enzymes in cultured fibroblasts	UDP-N-Acetylglucosamine: N-acetylglucosamine-1-phosphotransferase	Autosomal recessive
Mucolipidosis III	Same as mucolipidosis II	Same as in mucolipidosis II	Autosomal recessive
Mucolipidosis IV	No consistent findings	Sialidase in some cases	Autosomal recessive
Multiple sulfatase deficiency	Heparan sulfate and sulfatides in urine and tissues	Arylsulfatases A, B, and C, sulfamidase, iduronosulfatase	Autosomal recessive
Kniest syndrome	Keratan sulfaturia	None known	Autosomal dominant
Spondyloepiphyseal dysplasias	No consistent biochemical findings	None known	Several forms: autosomal dominant, recessive, and X-linked

hypotonic and have hepatosplenomegaly. In over 50% there is a macular cherry-red spot.

Mannosidosis (Sec. 7.21) is characterized by psychomotor retardation, hearing loss, coarse features with Hurler-like facial appearance, hepatosplenomegaly, muscular hypotonia, and mild dysostosis multiplex. There is no mucopolysacchariduria but mannose-rich oligosaccharide is found in the urine.

Patients with *fucosidosis* (Sec. 7.27) show coarse facial features, hepatosplenomegaly, severe psychomotor retardation, and dysotosis multiplex. There is no mucopolysacchariduria, and fucose-containing oligosaccharide is stored in tissues and excreted in urine.

Aspartylglucosaminuria (AGU) has frequently been confused with the Hurler or Hunter syndromes. Children with this disease appear normal at birth, but progressively develop coarse facies with broad nose, depressed nasal bridge, thick lips, and antiverted nostrils. Other features include short neck, cranial asymmetry, scoliosis, hepatosplenomegaly, and urinary excretion of aspartylglucosamine.

The *mucolipidoses* must also be distinguished from the mucopolysaccharidoses. Patients with mucolipidosis I (Sec. 7.38) share many clinical and roentgenographic features with the Hurler syndrome, including the skeletal deformities. However a macular cherry-red spot is frequently a characteristic feature of this disorder. Neurologic deterioration is progressive, and is often associated with myoclonic seizures, muscle atrophy, choreoathetotic movements, and nystagmus. Urinary mucopolysaccharides are normal, and sialic acid–bound oligosaccharides are excreted in increased quantities.

Mucolipidosis II: "I" Cell Disease (Sec. 7.38) is often confused with Hurler or Hunter syndromes. The "I" cell disease is distinguished from the Hurler syndrome by the rapid psychomotor retardation and early death. Gingival hyperplasia is characteristic in early life. The thorax is small, and cardiac valvular disease is frequent. Corneal clouding is not a feature. Periosteal bone formation is observed in the long bones during the first 6 mo of life, and there is no mucopolysacchariduria.

Mucolipidosis III (Sec. 7.38), a milder form of mucolipidosis

II, is characterized by mild mental retardation and joint stiffness; the skeletal defects are not as pronounced as in I cell disease. The diagnosis depends on findings of coarse facial features, lack of mucopolysacchariduria, elevated hydrolases in serum and urine, and depressed levels of these enzymes in cultured fibroblasts.

Mucolipidosis IV (Sec. 7.38) is characterized by corneal clouding and mental retardation without mucopolysacchariduria.

The *spondyloepiphyseal dysplasias* (Sec. 23.15) are commonly confused with the mucopolysaccharidoses, particularly with the Morquio syndrome. These diseases lack mucopolysacchariduria.

The *Kniest syndrome* (Sec. 23.15) may be recognized at birth, and usually is confused with Morquio syndrome. The full expression of the syndrome becomes obvious after the 1st year of life and includes short trunk and limbs, large head with depressed nasal bridge, stiffness of fingers and other joints, short neck, bell-shaped chest, tibial bowing, cleft palate, retinal detachment, deafness, and hernias. Later in life exaggerated lordosis and kyphoscoliosis become apparent. Radiographic findings include generalized osteoporosis with poor modeling. The Kniest syndrome is characterized by keratan sulfaturia, which may also occur with the Morquio syndrome. The specific enzyme defects, e.g., N-acetylgalactosamine-6-sulfate sulfatase or β-galactosidase, which are characteristic of Morquio syndrome, are normal in the Kniest syndrome.

REUBEN MATALON

Dorfman A, Matalon R: The mucopolysaccharidoses (a review). Proc Natl Acad Sci USA 73:630, 1976.
Matalon R: Mucopolysaccharidoses. In: Gershwin ME, Robbins DL (eds): Musculoskeletal Diseases of Children, New York, Grune and Stratton, 1983.
McKusick VA: The mucopolysaccharidoses. In: Heritable Disorders of Connective Tissue. 4th ed. St. Louis, CV Mosby, 1972.
McKusick VA, Neufeld EF: The mucopolysaccharide storage diseases. In: Stanbury JB, Wyngaarden JB, Fredrickson DS, et al (eds): The Metabolic Basis of Inherited Disease. 5th ed. New York, McGraw-Hill, 1983.

DEFECTS IN METABOLISM OF LIPIDS

LIPIDOSES

The lipidoses or lipid storage diseases, a group of genetic diseases involving the accumulation of lipids in one or more of the body's organs, are usually due to a defect in their catabolism. Some of these disorders are associated with characteristic foamy histiocytes on examination of the bone marrow (Fig. 7–25) (Niemann-Pick disease, Gaucher disease, G_{M1} gangliosidoses type I, fucosidosis); others are not (Tay-Sachs disease, Krabbe disease, metachromatic leukodystophy). Patients in the latter group show other characteristic changes in cells where the lipids accumulate, such as in nervous tissue. The signs and symptoms for each syndrome vary with the defect and site of lipid accumulation. The amount of storage depends on the organ involved and on the amount of catabolism required for maintenance of normal chemical composition.

Although most patients with lipidoses have low activity of a required enzyme, others are missing a sphingolipid activator protein needed for lipid-enzyme interaction. These latter patients may clinically resemble those with a mutation in the enzyme, but the confirming diagnostic test is difficult to perform and limited to the expertise and facilities of a few laboratories. Clinical variants are reported with increased frequency and many do not fit the textbook descriptions of a given syndrome, though they are enzymatically closely related. In other cases a sign thought to be pathognomonic for a given disease has been found in patients with other syndromes. The diffuse angiokeratomatosis of Fabry disease, for example, has also been found in patients with fucosidosis and with glycoprotein sialidase deficiency.

When a symptom (or a group of symptoms) could indicate a genetic lipidosis, a confirming test should be requested from an experienced laboratory. In most of the diseases to be described, the definitive diagnosis can be made from blood (serum and leukocytes) or a biopsy of skin which can be cultured and subsequently assayed. Usually frozen serum or leukocytes can be shipped or heparinized blood can be sent at room temperature for preparation of leukocytes in a laboratory that has been readied for such procedures. Skin biopsies can also be sent by air mail for culturing, or a flask of cultured cells can be sent for subsequent subculturing and assaying.

When a diagnosis has been made in a child, other family members should be screened since studies on the parents, siblings, and other relatives can provide important genetic information. Carriers of most of the lipidoses can be reliably identified; these studies can assist in genetic counseling and in alleviation of fear and guilt. Prenatal diagnosis should be available to couples at risk. Diagnosis of most lipid storage diseases can be made at 9–10 wk gestation from chorionic villus samples; uncultured villi, sent frozen, and cultured trophoblasts can be used. The risks to mother and fetus from this procedure are still being evaluated. Amniocentesis at 14–16 wk, followed by culturing of the cells is recommended if ambiguous numbers are obtained from the chorionic villus sample. The accuracy of prenatal studies should be confirmed by study of the aborted fetus or delivered infant. It should be noted that among the few laboratories that do these tests, conditions of enzyme assay vary, and activity levels reported for controls, patients, and carriers have not been standardized.

The sphingolipids have as their basic structure the long-chain amino diol sphingosine (sphingenine), in which the C-2 and C-3 carbon atoms have the D-configuration (Fig. 7–26). The amino group of sphingosine usually has a long-chain fatty acid attached to it. This derivative is called ceramide. The C-1 hydroxyl group of ceramide can be substituted with a variety of different compounds to produce the different sphingolipids. For example, attachment of galactose in a beta-linkage to ceramide at C-1 creates galactosylceramide (commonly called galactocerebroside). Galactosylceramide with a sulfate group of C-3 of the galactose moiety is called sulfatide. Both these glycosphingolipids are found primarily in white matter.

Attachment of glucose in a beta-linkage to C-1 of ceramide produces glucosylceramide (glucocerebroside). Free glucosylceramide is found in small amounts in normal tissues but is stored to great amounts in tissues of patients with Gaucher disease. Glucosylceramide is a portion of most larger glycosphingolipids and gangliosides. All degradation of these glycosphingolipids takes place sequentially from the nonreducing end of the molecule toward the lipid portion. Deficiency in enzyme activity results in the storage of the compound (or compounds) behind the block. In addition to the primary storage product, other lipid compounds may be stored because of secondary factors.

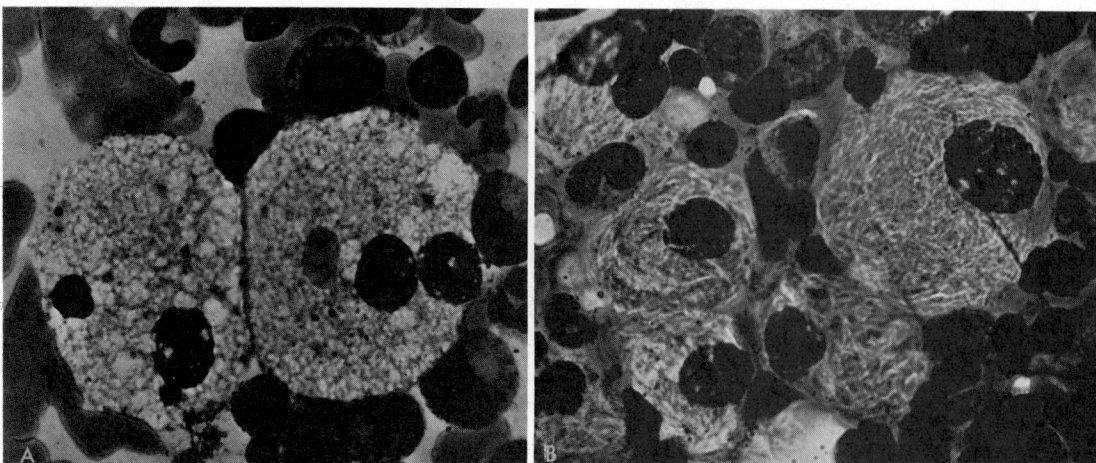

Figure 7–25. Smears from bone marrow aspirations (Giemsa stain) showing characteristic cells of Neimann-Pick disease (*A*) and Gaucher disease (*B*). Note the bubbly, vacuolated appearance of the Niemann-Pick foam cells, as contrasted with fibrillar texture of the Gaucher cell cytoplasm.

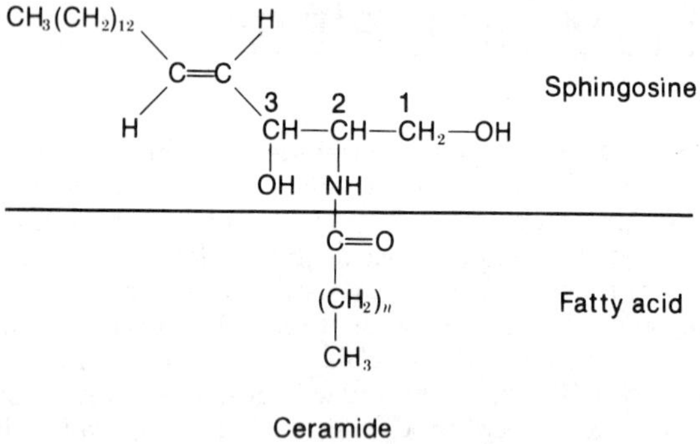

Figure 7–26. Basic structure of sphingolipids. All additions to ceramide are made through the hydroxyl group of carbon atom 1: Glycosphingolipids = Ceramide plus one or more sugars attached to C-1. Gangliosides = Glycosphingolipids plus one or more sialic acid residues. Sphingomyelin = Ceramide plus phosphorylcholine attached to C-1.

7.25 G_{M1} GANGLIOSIDOSES

These are a group of lysosomal disorders with variable clinical findings. G_{M1} ganglioside is a monosialoganglioside found in normal cerebral gray and white matter and in lesser quantities in the viscera. It is also formed during the normal catabolism of polysialogangliosides (Fig. 7–27).

G_{M1} **ganglionsidosis type 1 (generalized gangliosdosis)** is a severe cerebral degenerative disease with onset soon after birth. Edema and weakness and, in most cases, facial features not unlike those seen in Hurler syndrome and I-cell disease (mucolipidosis II) are observed. In many cases hepatosplenomegaly, joint stiffness, umbilical and inguinal hernias, (hyperacusis, and cherry red spot of the macula occur. Developmental retardation is severe. Roentgenographic changes of dysostosis multiplex are often found. Death usually occurs before 2 yr of age from respiratory infections.

Patients with G_{M1} **gangliosidosis type 2** usually have an onset of ataxia at 1–2 yr of age, with cessation of psychic and

motor development. Within the next 6 mo deterioration leads to an unresponsive state. There is little, if any, enlargement of the liver or other organs. Roentgenographic changes are minimal. Death usually occurs at 3–10 yr of age from bronchopneumomia.

Patients with significantly different phenotypes but the same enzymatic defect have been described. Two siblings, 19 and 25 yr, presented before 5 yr of age with clumsiness and mild roentgenographic bone changes but with normal intelligence. They developed dysarthria and mild CNS involvement as young adults. Other patients with β-galactosidase deficiency have severe bone involvement suggestive of Morquio syndrome (mucopolysaccaridosis type IV). These children have normal intelligence. Other patients with moderate to severe mental retardation have survived until the 3rd or 4th decade. Another group of patients with myoclonus, cherry-red spot in the macular region, and dementia has been recently demonstrated to have a deficiency of both β-galactosidase and glycoprotein sialidase activities. They may be missing a protein required for aggregating these enzymes into a stable, high molecular weight complex.

All patients with G_{M1} gangliosidosis have a profound *deficiency of acid β-galactosidase activity* in their leukocytes and cultured skin fibroblasts. In most suspected cases the use of a synthetic β-galactoside substrate to measure β-galactosidase activity can confirm the diagnosis. This enzyme is active with many β-galactoside–containing substrates in the body. The major compounds include the G_{M1} ganglioside, glycoproteins (and oligosaccharides derived from them), and keratan sulfate–like mucopolysaccharides. Depending on the particular mutation in the enzyme, failure to hydrolyze some or all of these potential substrates results in storage. Patients with G_{M1} gangliosidosis type 1 have little, if any, activity toward all potential substrates; hence severe involvement of brain, viscera, and bone occurs. Patients with connective tissue involvement paramount might be expected to have more residual β-galactosidase activity toward G_{M1} ganglioside and less toward keratan sulfate–like mucopolysaccharides. Type 1 patients store G_{M1} ganglioside in brain (10 times normal in gray matter)

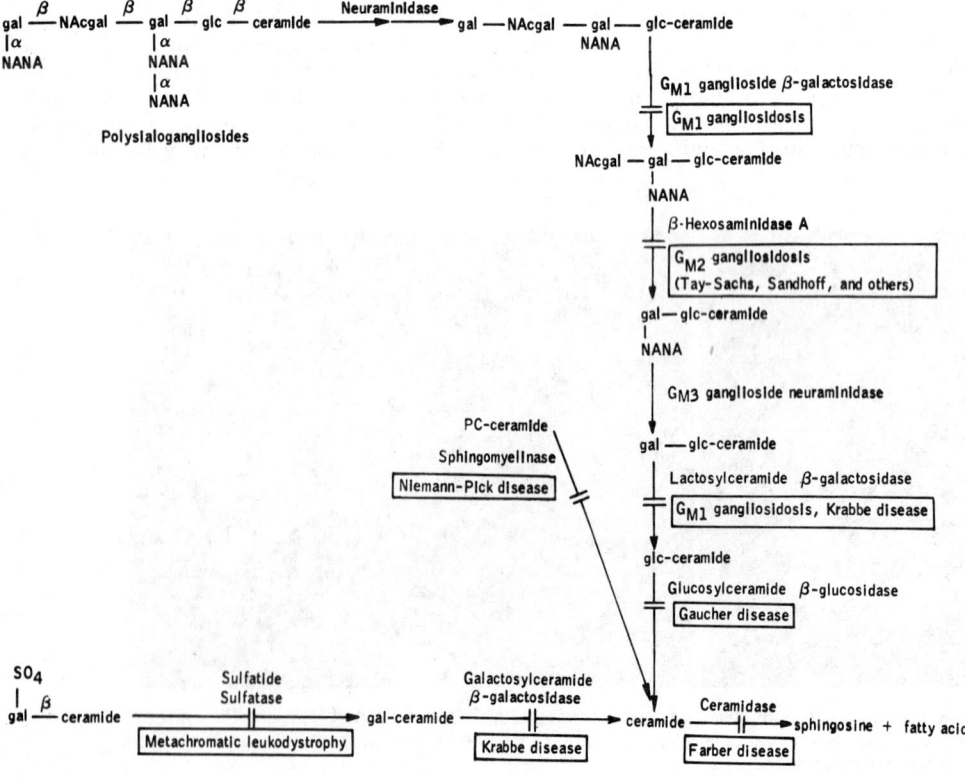

Figure 7–27. Pathways in the metabolism of sphingolipids found in nervous tissues. The name of the enzyme catalyzing each reaction is given with the name of the substrate acted upon. Inborn errors are depicted as bars crossing the reaction arrows, and the name of the associated defect or defects is given within the nearest box. The gangliosides are named according to the nomenclature of Svennerholm. Anomeric configurations are given only at the largest starting compound.

gal, galactose; glc, glucose; NAcgal, N-acetyl-galactosamine; NANA, N-acetyl-neuraminic acid; PC, phosphorylcholine.

and viscera (20–50 times normal in liver), and keratan sulfate–like mucopolysaccharides and oligosaccharides in the viscera. The less severe forms have less storage of β-galactoside-terminal complex carbohydrates.

In type 1 patients the neurons and the hepatic, glomerular, and renal tubular cells are vacuolated. Foamy histiocytes are found in all viscera. Storage in brain results in heavy damage to nerve cells, with demyelination and gliosis. Involved nerves show cytoplasmic membranous bodies, similar to those seen in Tay-Sachs disease. Secondary damage to white matter causes a decrease in the amount of cerebrosides and sulfatides found at autopsy. Similar, but milder, changes are found in juvenile forms of G_{M1} gangliosidosis. Few mildly affected patients have been examined in detail.

The *diagnosis* of all forms of G_{M1} gangliosidosis depends on demonstrating a deficiency of acid β-galactosidase activity. The type 1 form may be initially confused clinically with certain mucopolysaccharidoses or mucolipidoses. In most cases of G_{M1} gangliosidosis, mucopolysacchariduria does not occur and the enzymatic testing in leukocytes or fibroblasts confirms the diagnosis. Patients with Hurler and Hunter syndromes may have low acid β-galactosidase activities in their livers, due to secondary mucopolysaccharide storage. Tests on the parents will show about half normal β-galactosidase activity, indicating the autosomal recessive inheritance. Prenatal diagnosis using cultured amniotic fluid cells and chorionic villus samples has been successful in all clinical types of β-galactosidase deficiency. There is no treatment for these syndromes, though some orthopedic procedures may help older patients with bone problems. The prognosis of the older patients in unknown.

7.26 G_{M2} GANGLIOSIDOSES

See also Sec. 21.18.

This group of genetic diseases includes cases of cerebral degeneration in which the storage of G_{M2} ganglioside and related glycosphingolipids is due to deficiencies of specific hexosaminidases or sphingolipid activator protein required for their catabolism (Figs. 7–27 and 7–28).

Tay-Sachs disease or **G_{M2} gangliosidosis type 1,** also known as infantile amaurotic familial idiocy, involves *pathologic changes* mostly restricted to the central nervous system, though neurons throughout the body contain the characteristic membranous cytoplasmic bodies. With time, neurons are lost. There is proliferation of microglial cells, which are also swollen and filled with large granules. The spinal cord may have similar changes, with anterior horn cells more affected than those of the posterior and lateral horns. In the eye macular changes result in the cherry-red spot seen in most patients. The liver and other organs show membranous cytoplasmic bodies with electron microscopy, though there may be little actual storage. Foam cells are not usually found in the bone marrow. The failure of hexosaminidase A to degrade G_{M2} ganglioside results in the 100-fold increase of this ganglioside found in the brains of children with Tay-Sachs disease. G_{M2} ganglioside is a minor component of normal brain, but it is in the degradative pathway for the major brain gangliosides.

The classic *clinical manifestations* of the onset of this disease include psychomotor retardation and deterioration after 4–6 mo of normal development and a startle response to sound. Hypotonia, loss of interest in surroundings, poor head control, and apathy also occur early. A cherry-red spot in the macula may be found later. Seizures begin later, and in advanced stages of illness the child has little response to external stimuli. The head enlarges and in the final stage is obviously macrocephalic. No visceromegaly is found. Many cases are found in families of Eastern European Jewish heri-

tage, but the diagnosis should not be excluded from consideration in non-Jewish or nonwhite children.

The *diagnostic test* for Tay-Sachs disease is measurement of the hexosaminidase A isoenzyme component of serum, leukocytes, tears, hair roots, or cultured skin fibroblasts. Total hexosaminidase activity may be normal, but an almost total deficiency of activity of the "A" component usually makes up over 50% of the total hexosaminidase activity, which is diagnostic. Carriers have been identified among people with no familial history of Tay-Sachs disease and among couples at risk so that genetic counseling can be initiated. Over 500,000 healthy people have been screened. Ashkenazi Jews have a carrier frequency of about 1 in 25. It is recommended that all Jewish couples of Eastern European ancestry be advised that tests for the carrier state are available and the prevention of this fatal disease is possible. Prenatal diagnosis is possible using chorionic villi and amniotic fluid samples.

Little can be done for the affected child other than supportive care for recurrent infections in the late stages of the disease. Death usually occurs by 3–4 yr. Carriers have no symptoms.

Sandhoff disease, or **G_{M2} gangliosidosis type 2** (or 0 variant), is the result of total deficiency of hexosaminidase activity (both A and B isoenzymes of hexosaminidase are missing). This leads to the storage not only of G_{M2} ganglioside in the brain but also of other β-hexosaminide terminal glycolipids, glycoproteins, and oligosaccharides in brain and viscera. The clinical symptoms are similar to those seen in Tay-Sachs disease but with additional visceral involvement. The brain contains a 100- to 200-fold increase in G_{M2} ganglioside and a 50- to 100-fold increase in G_{A2}, the asialo-derivative of G_{M2}. The liver, kidneys, and spleen have greatly increased amounts of globoside, the major glycosphingolipid of red blood cells (Fig. 7–28). The lack of hexosaminidase A and B activity prevents the degradation of all these glycosphingolipids (Figs. 7–27 and 7–28). The diagnosis of Sandhoff disease can be made with serum, plasma, leukocytes, or cultured skin fibroblasts. Carriers can be identified using the same tissues, and prenatal diagnosis is possible. There is no increased incidence in Eastern European Jewish families.

Juvenile G_{M2} gangliosidosis or **type 3** has a later onset than either Tay-Sachs or Sandhoff disease. Ataxia and progressive psychomotor retardation begin at 2–6 yr of age. Loss of speech, progressive spasticity, athetoid posturing of hands and extremities, and minor motor seizures develop. Death occurs between 5 and 15 yr. Organomegaly, bony deformities, and foam cells are not found. Blindness occurs in the later stages of this disease. Neuronal lipidosis is prominent and G_{M2} ganglioside is stored because of a partial deficiency of hexosaminidase A. Diagnosis, identification of carriers, and prenatal diagnosis are available through measurement of hexosaminidase A activity.

Some patients suspected of having G_{M2} gangliosidosis have been found to have normal hexosaminidase activity when the usual diagnostic tests are done. However, defect in G_{M2} ganglioside metabolism can be demonstrated in cerebrospinal fluid, where G_{M2} ganglioside is greatly increased. Two types of patients have been delineated: one type (called A^MB variant) has a defect in hexosaminidase A diagnosed using a new sulfated fluorogenic substrate or the natural substrate; the other type (called AB variant) has a decreased concentration in the required sphingolipid activator protein in cultured skin fibroblasts and possibly in leukocytes. Prenatal diagnosis of these variant forms should be possible.

Adult patients with low hexosaminidase activity have been found. Some of these patients have a variant form of spinocerebellar degeneration (ataxia, muscle atrophy, pes cavus, foot drop, spasticity, dysarthria, and normal intelligence), while others have psychotic behavior. These unusual findings

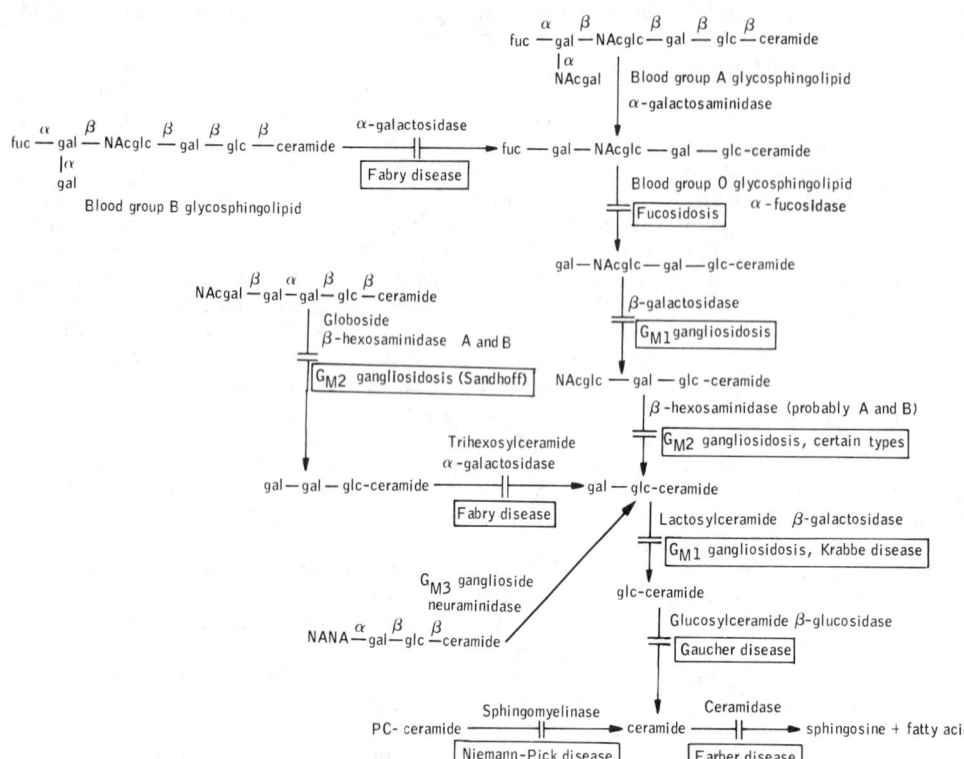

Figure 7–28. Pathways in the degradation of sphingolipids found in visceral organs and red or white blood cells. See also legend for Figure 7–27. Additional abbreviations: fuc, fucose; NAcglc, N-acetylglucosamine.

result from different mutations in the α and β subunits making up hexosaminidase A.

7.27 FUCOSIDOSIS

Fucosidosis has at least two clinical presentations, both having signs and symptoms found in other lysosomal storage diseases. All clinical types have a deficiency of lysosomal α-fucosidase activity resulting in the storage of fucose-containing glycosphingolipids (Fig. 7–28) in the visceral organs and of fucose-containing oligosaccharides and glycoproteins in the brain and viscera. Fucose is a component of glycoproteins and glycolipids with blood group activity (A, B, H, and Lewis) and of other glycoproteins, including immunoglobulins, ceruloplasmin, transferrin, and some hormones.

Pathologically hepatocytes are dense and osmophilic, containing multilayered lamellar structures in fingerprint patterns. The Kupffer cells are filled with granular and multilamellar structures. Electron microscopy of liver reveals vacuoles similar to those seen in Hurler syndrome. In the central nervous system every nerve cell is enlarged, with a round to oval eccentric nucleus. The cells appear empty or filled with granular, weakly basophilic, and PAS-positive material. There is neuronal loss, and the remaining neurons are vacuolated, as are the glial cells. Myelination is affected, and the pathologic picture resembles that of sudanophilic leukodystrophy. Macrophages are numerous in liver and white matter. Cultured skin fibroblasts show clear vacuoles that sometimes show lamellar inclusions.

Most *clinical manifestations* are related to the abnormal accumulation of glycosphingolipids and glycoproteins in liver, heart, and brain. There is evidence also of lysosomal storage in vascular endothelium, eccrine sweat gland epithelium, and fibrocytes. The more severely affected patients have severe psychomotor retardation, neurologic signs including convulsions, and bony deformities evident before the end of the 1st yr of life (fucosidosis type I). Myocarditis and cardiomegaly may occur. Short stature, macroglossia, coarse facial features,

frontal bossing, spastic ataxia, hepatomegaly, splenomegaly, increased levels of sodium chloride in sweat, and delayed development are also reported. Skeletal changes include lumbar kyphosis, contractures of hips, knees, ankles, and elbows, and deformities of ribs. Patients with fucosidosis type II may also have an onset in early childhood, but the course is slower. These patients initially have less severe psychomotor and neurologic signs, but severe mental retardation comes in the later stages. They also tend to have normal sweat electrolytes, less severe bone changes, and no hepatosplenomegaly. Skin lesions resembling the angiokeratoma corporis diffusum seen in Fabry disease usually appear at 5–7 yr of age.

The clinical picture of both types of fucosidosis may suggest a mucopolysaccharidosis or mucolipidosis. Urine does not contain mucopolysaccharides but rather fucose-containing oligosaccharides. Most patients have characteristic vacuolated lymphocytes. *Diagnosis* is confirmed by a total deficiency of α-fucosidase activity in white blood cells or cultured skin fibroblasts. Serum levels of this enzyme are low, but some normal people have very low α-fucosidase activity in serum. Carriers are detected by means of white blood cells and cultured skin fibroblasts. Inheritance is autosomal recessive. Prenatal diagnosis has been reported using cultured amniotic fluid cells. A high incidence has been noted in Italians and Spanish-Americans.

Treatment is only supportive. Dehydration and repeated respiratory infections of the more severely affected patients require attention. Patients with the more severe form usually die before 10 yr of age, whereas those with the less severe form may live into the 3rd decade.

7.28 FABRY DISEASE

This disease, formerly called *angiokeratoma corporis diffusum*, is an X-linked lipidosis. Affected males have the complete clinical syndrome, whereas heterozygous females may have one or more manifestations which can present serious health problems. Purple punctate angiokeratomas in the "bathing suit" area were once thought to be pathognomonic for Fabry disease, but identical skin lesions have now been found in patients with certain types of fucosidosis and sialidosis. Patients without skin lesions or corneal opacities have also been determined to have Fabry disease.

Fabry disease is caused by the deficiency of α-galactosidase activity, which is responsible for the degradation of α-galactosyl terminal glycolipids. The main storage product is trihexosylceramide, formed from the action of β-hexosaminidase on globoside, the major red blood cell glycosphingolipid (Fig. 7–28). Further degradation of trihexosylceramide requires a specific α-galactosidase (called α-galactosidase A) which is missing in this syndrome. Another storage product is digalactosylceramide, which is found mainly in kidney tissue. In those patients having blood group B an additional storage product may be found, but this has not been correlated with a more severe clinical picture. Storage of trihexosylceramide and digalactosylceramide takes place in visceral organs, especially in heart muscle and in renal tubules and glomeruli. Additional storage is evident in all vascular epithelia, the pituitary gland, autonomic neurons of the diencephalon and brain stem, the mesenteric and submucosal plexus of the gastrointestinal tract, and most skeletal muscles. Examination of the affected tissues reveals fine sudanophilic, PAS-positive granules and foamy storage cells. Bone marrow has shown granular material in histiocytes, with no evidence of anemia or other hematologic manifestations.

Storage of lipid material in the blood vessels leads to most of the clinical manifestations. Fabry disease is not a disease of early childhood, but many patients are discovered before 10 yr of age because of complaints of pain in extremities, lack of sweating, unexplained proteinuria, attacks of fever, and the presence of a few purple skin lesions. With progression, there are complaints related to easy fatigability (due to storage in skeletal muscle), poor vision (corneal opacities, tortuosity of retinal and conjunctival vessels, and cataracts), and high blood pressure (due to continued vascular storage). This storage eventually leads to cardiac or renal failure in the 3rd or 4th decade of life. Psychologic disturbances have been reported and are probably due to decreased blood flow and thrombus formation in brain.

Increased levels of trihexosylceramide can be found in biopsy samples, urinary sediments, and cultured skin fibroblasts, but *diagnosis* depends upon measuring decreased α-galactosidase activity in plasma, urine, white blood cells, tears, or cultured skin cells using the synthetic substrate 4-methylumbelliferyl-α-D-galactoside. Cultured amniotic cells permit prenatal diagnosis. Heterozygous females can be identified using serum, white blood cells, and cultured skin fibroblasts.

Though this disease can be quite benign until the 2nd or 3rd decade, it can also lead to early death due to cardiovascular complications. Pain in the extremities, reported by almost all patients, has been treated with diphenylhydantoin (200 mg/24 hr) or carbamazepine (200 mg/24 hr) with variable success. Treatment of renal failure by dialysis and renal transplantation has had limited success and attempts to supply the missing enzyme using whole plasma and purified α-galactosidase are experimental.

Inheritance is X-linked, and many carrier females have some symptoms. A family history of early male deaths with the above symptoms should suggest Fabry disease. There seems to be no ethnic group at increased risk.

7.29 GAUCHER DISEASE

Gaucher disease includes three clinically distinct genetic entities involving the storage of glucosylceramide (glucocerebroside) in the reticuloendothelial system, often splenomegaly, variable bone involvement, and the characteristic "Gaucher cell" in bone marrow aspirates and in visceral organs (Fig. 7–25 B). The types of Gaucher disease are called type 1, adult, chronic, or non-neuropathic; type 2, acute neuropathic or infantile; and type 3, subacute neuropathic or juvenile. Unfortunately, these names do not alway reflect the age of onset of symptons or the severity of the disease. Some "adult" patients have obvious bone problems and splenomegaly leading to splenectomy before the end of the 1st decade, whereas others are not diagnosed until the 8th decade.

Gaucher cells are characteristic of the disease, though similar cells are found in cases of myelogenous leukemia and there have been rare cases of confirmed Gaucher disease without this typical cell in bone marrow. These fusiform histiocytes are 15–85 μ in size and have one or more small dense nuclei eccentrically located. They have a blue staining cytoplasm with the appearance of wrinkled silk as opposed to the foamy cells fround in other lipidoses. Gaucher cells are derived from reticular or sinusoidal endothelial cells and are found in bone marrow, spleen, liver, lungs, lymph nodes and occasionally the brain of patients who die of infantile Gaucher disease. These cells stain positive with PAS and strongly for acid phosphatase.

All the clinical problems in these patients appear to be caused by the storage of glucosylceramide due to deficiency of a specific β-galactosidase activity required for its degradation. Glucosylceramide is a portion of larger glycosphingolipids which is generated during the degradation of gangliosides, of red and white blood cell glycolipids, and of endogenous membrane glycosphingolipids (Figs. 7–27 and 7–28). The reason for the great variation in clinical picture among patients is not clear as all patients are deficient in the same enzymatic activity. Within families, however, the clinical picture is relatively consistent; adult and infantile forms of Gaucher disease do not usually occur in the same family.

Splenomegaly is the initial *clinical manifestation* in most patients, with spleens weighing over 5000 g not unusual in adults. The liver is usually enlarged and liver failure may occur. Patients with infantile Gaucher disease have severe involvement of the central nervous system, with decreased brain size, neuronal degeneration, and active neuronophagia. There is loss of neurons in the spinal cord. Skeletal complications are common, especially in the adult type, with fractures of the femoral neck and vertebral bodies and sometimes aseptic necrosis of the femoral head.

The onset of **infantile Gaucher disease** usually occurs within the 1st few months of life with hepatosplenomegaly, slow development, strabismus, swallowing difficulties, laryngeal spasm, opisthotonos, and a picture of "pseudobulbar palsy." Recurrent aspiration and chronic bronchopneumonia usually lead to death at 6–18 mo. The **juvenile form of Gaucher diseases** is less well defined; most cases have been reported in certain areas of Sweden. Dementia, often accompanied by behavior changes, seizures, and extrapyramidal and cerebellar signs, becomes evident in late childhood. Most patients have the **chronic or adult type**, but the clinical picture can vary greatly. Usually hypersplenism in early childhood causes anemia and thrombocytopenia. Bone pain and joint swelling also occur. Pathologic fractures are a major problem in some patients, whereas others have few or no osseous difficulties. Roentgenograms help identify osseous complications. Some adult patients have a yellow or patchy brown pigmentation in the exposed areas of the body and pingueculae of the conjunctiva. Liver necrosis and severe pulmonary involvement may rarely be found, with possibly a higher incidence in the black population.

Preliminary *diagnosis* of Gaucher disease is based on the clinical picture and the identification of Gaucher cells in bone marrow. Serum acid phosphatase levels are greatly elevated. Most patients with Gaucher disease show an elevation of glucosylceramide content in visceral organs. All patients have less than 20% of normal activity of glucosylceramide β-galactosidase in leukocytes and cultured skin fibroblasts, whereas carriers have about 60% of normal activity. Prenatal diagnosis can be made for all types of Gaucher disease using chorionic villi and amniotic fluid cells. Type 1 (adult) Gaucher disease is most common in Ashkenazi Jewish people, but all ethnic groups are affected. Inheritance is autosomal recessive.

Treatment by total or partial splenectomy has been used to control the anemic and hemorrhagic symptoms of hypersplenism, and orthopedic supervision can help manage bone involvement. Episodes of bone pain can be helped by rest, analgesics, and possibly the brief use of steroids. Problems in the hip joint may be serious and require surgery. No treatment is available for the infantile or juvenile forms; only supportive treatment for infections and feeding problems can be given. Attempts to treat Gaucher disease by transplantation of spleen, kidney, and bone marrow have been made, with limited success. Enzyme replacement therapy has not provided long-term improvement. It is hoped that recent success in cloning the β-glucosidase gene will lead to effective therapy in the future.

7.30 NIEMANN-PICK DISEASE

This disorder is a group of genetic diseases in which sphingomyelin and, secondarily, cholesterol are stored in many organs. Basically, four subtypes are recognized: (1) classic Niemann-Pick disease (type A according to Crocker), showing storage in viscera and severe CNS degeneration in infancy (with foam cells in bone marrow [Fig. 7–25] and severe deficiency of sphingomyelinase activity); (2) type B, showing severe visceral involvement in infancy (with foam cells in bone marrow and severe deficiency of sphingomyelinase activity); (3) juvenile types, showing moderate visceral involvement and variable CNS degeneration in early childhood (with foamy and/or sea-blue histiocytes in bone marrow and partial sphingomyelinase deficiency in certain tissues); and (4) other patients with evidence of sphingomyelin storage who have normal sphingomyelinase activity and few, if any, neurologic abnormalities.

The disabilities of patients with *classic infantile Niemann-Pick disease* stem from extensive storage of sphingomyelin and cholesterol (and some glycosphingolipids, secondarily) in liver, spleen, and lungs, with less marked storage in brain. The brain, though, shows a marked increase in G_{M2} and G_{M3} gangliosides. Clinical onset typically comes after a period of normal development lasting several months, with a slowing of motor and mental progress and hepatomegaly, followed by general deterioration of neurologic functions and health. Examination of bone marrow, blood, and organs reveals foamy cells loaded with lipid. Deterioration continues to a vegetative state, and death usually occurs before 4 yr of age. Cherry-red spots in the macula are found in about 50% of the cases. Many of these patients are Jews of Eastern European ancestry.

Patients with the less frequently occurring *type B form*, who have visceral involvement only, show pronounced storage of sphingomyelin and cholesterol in visceral organs and foam cells in the marrow. Health problems related to this storage may be mild or severe. The lack of nervous system involvement in these patients is unexplained. Sphingomyelinase levels in visceral organs and cultivated skin fibroblasts are at the same low levels as in type A patients.

The *juvenile types* present a variety of symptoms. Early jaundice may be followed by relatively normal development until 5–7 yr of age when unsteadiness of gait, ataxia, problems in vertical gaze, learning difficulties, emotional lability, and dementia become evident. The course is progressive at a variable rate, death occurring in the 1st, 2nd, or 3rd decade. Hepatosplenomegaly is not always evident, though some patients have evidence of excess sphingomyelin in the liver. This group includes some patients with disease previously labeled type C or D Niemann-Pick disease and some with forms of sea-blue histiocyte syndrome. Sphingomyelinase levels are normal or partially deficient, with activities varying from tissue to tissue.

Some *adult patients* store sphingomyelin in visceral organs with no serious health problems or neurologic deterioration occurring. These patients do not have the severe sphingomyelinase deficiency reported for type B individuals. Their prognosis is unknown; some have lived past the 5th decade.

Pathologically large lipid-laden foam cells are found in all groups of patients with sphingomyelin lipidosis. These cells differ from "Gaucher cells" and resemble the nondescript foam cells of G_{M1} gangliosidosis and other lipidoses. Sea-blue and/or foamy histiocytes are found in increased numbers in a juvenile form of sphingomyelin lipidosis, as well as in other lipidoses and unrelated diseases. Hepatosplenomegaly is marked in most types, especially in the infantile forms. Lymph nodes, adrenal glands, and lungs frequently show evidence of storage. The brain is smaller than normal, with most regions atrophic. the neurons of the cortex and deep gray matter show marked distention of the cytoplasm and loss of Nissl bodies. Purkinje cells are reduced in the cerebellum, and myelin and axonal fibers are reduced in cerebellar white matter. The juvenile and later-onset forms of Niemann-Pick disease show many of the same findings but to a lesser degree. The brain may reveal no significant pathologic changes, but cirrhosis of the liver may be found.

The *diagnosis* of infantile Niemann-Pick disease should be suspected in any infant failing to thrive, with upper respiratory infections, hepatosplenomegaly, and impaired development. In both type A and type B enzymatic assays to confirm a deficiency of sphingomyelinase can be done with leukocytes or cultured skin fibroblasts. Because the level of this enzyme activity is low in normal leukocytes, cultured skin fibroblasts are preferred. Carriers can be identified in fibroblast cultures, and prenatal diagnosis can be done with cultured amniotic fluid cells. All forms of Niemann-Pick disease are inherited in an autosomal recessive manner.

The juvenile forms are less well understood with respect to the relationship between specific sphingomyelinase deficiencies and sphingomyelin storage. Some patients have a partial deficiency of sphingomyelinase in cultured skin fibroblasts (15–50% of normal versus 0–2% of normal for groups A and B). Cultured cells from some patients show decreased ability to catabolize exogenous sphingomyelin given in the medium. Recently a defect in the ability to esterify cholesterol has been demonstrated in the cultured cells from these patients. Further studies of this latter group of patients are needed to correlate symptoms and signs, storage, and enzyme levels before accurate diagnosis, carrier identification, and prenatal diagnosis are available.

No treatment for this group of diseases has been effective.

7.31 METACHROMATIC LEUKODYSTROPHY

See also Sec. 21.19.

Metachromatic leukodystrophy (MLD) has four clinical forms; three with variable age of onset and a deficiency of arylsulfatase A activity and one form with a juvenile presentation and a deficiency of a required sphingolipid activator protein (SAP-1). Arylsulfatase A and SAP-1 are required for the degradation of sulfatide (Fig. 7–27). Late infantile MLD usually has its clinical onset in the 2nd yr of life. The first signs are genu recurvatum and impairment of motor function. Patients with juvenile MLD present ataxia and intellectual deterioration at 5–20 yr of age. Patients with the adult type of MLD present ataxia, weakness, dementia, and psychosis after 20 yr of age. Deposits of sulfatide are found in the peripheral and central nervous systems, as well as in kidney and gallbladder (where some is naturally found).

White matter from the brains of patients with MLD undergo demyelination with the deposition of many metachromatic bodies, which stain strongly positive with PAS and alcian blue. Oligodendroglial cells are markedly reduced in number. Neuronal inclusions are also reported in nerve cells in the midbrain, pons, medulla, retina, and spinal cord. Demyelination occurs in the peripheral nervous system. Biopsies of sural nerve stained with acid cresyl violet show many brown metachromatic deposits containing granules which accumulate in the perinuclear cytoplasm of Schwann cells and in perivascular histiocytes. All involved areas show a loss of oligodendroglial elements.

The late infantile form of MLD is the most common. Initial *clinical manifestations* consist of disturbances of gait and slowed development. Examination reveals reduced or absent tendon reflexes, weakness, and hypotonia. Within months or years the child will have gradual onset of nystagmus, cerebellar and Babinski signs, dementia, tonic seizures, optic atrophy, and quadriparesis. Juvenile patients have many of the same symptoms seen in the late infantile form but with a slower progression. Adult patients may initially present psychiatric problems, including emotional lability, apathy, and change of character, followed by mental deficiency. Eventually, abnormal tendon reflexes, speech difficulties, muscular weakness, ataxia, tremor, and auditory and visual problems become evident. There is progressive dementia and optic atrophy.

Diagnosis is based on the clinical picture and the findings of decreased nerve conduction velocities, increased cerebrospinal fluid protein, metachromatic deposits in biopsied segments of sural nerve, and metachromatic granules in urinary sediment. No hepatosplenomegaly, bone involvement, or foam cells exist in the bone marrow. Confirmation is based on enzymatic studies on leukocytes and on cultured skin fibroblasts, which show deficient sulfatide sulfatase or arylsulfatase A activity (as measured with an artificial substrate). Enzymatic studies do not differentiate between the clinical types of MLD. However, they can be differentiated by measuring the ability of their cultured fibroblasts to metabolize carbon-14 sulfatide presented in the medium. SAP-1–deficient patients can be diagnosed by measuring the concentration of SAP-1 using monospecific antibodies in leukocytes and cultured skin fibroblasts. A low level of cross-reacting material is found. Enzymatic studies on family members confirm the autosomal recessive pattern of inheritance. Some carriers of MLD have arylsulfatase A levels near those found in affected children. Therefore, parents of affected children should be checked for their carrier status before prenatal testing is undertaken to avoid abortion of a nonaffected but low-activity carrier. This problem can be prevented by measuring the metabolism of carbon-14 sulfatide in cultured amniotic fluid cells or cultured trophoblasts. Low carriers look like controls, while true patients show little if any metabolism of the added sulfatide. Prenatal diagnosis can be done for the late infantile and juvenile forms of this syndrome.

There is no *treatment* for any form of MLD; only supportive care can be given. Attempts have been made to treat young patients having MLD with bone marrow transplantation. Although normal enzyme levels can be achieved in peripheral blood, no clear evidence indicates a change in the neurological deterioration. Patients with the late infantile form usually live 2–4 yr after the diagnosis; those with the juvenile form live 4–6 yr after diagnosis. Some with the adult form have lived to the 5th decade.

Multiple sulfatase deficiency is another autosomal recessive disease with deficiency of arylsulfatase A (along with arylsulfatases B and C). There is accumulation of sulfatides, glycosaminoglycan sulfates, steroid sulfates, and gangliosides in cerebral cortex. The neurologic picture is similar to late infantile MLD, but slight bony involvement may suggest a mucopolysaccharidosis. There is severe ichthyosis. Examination of urine for mucopolysaccharides is positive. There is a striking abnormality of granulation in the leukocytes, and enzymatic studies will confirm the diagnosis.

7.32 KRABBE DISEASE

See also Sec. 21.19.

Krabbe disease, or globoid cell leukocystrophy, is a progressive cerebral degenerative disease affecting primarily white matter. A high incidence occurs in persons of Scandinavian descent. Inheritance is autosomal recessive. The name globoid cell comes from the globular distended multinucleated bodies found in the basal ganglia, pontine nuclei, and cerebellar white matter.

Pathologically these globoid cells are found clustered around blood vessels; they have a lacy, pink cytoplasm (with hematoxylin-eosin stain) and prominent staining of intracellular material with PAS. The pathologic abnormalities are almost entirely restricted to white matter of nervous tissue. There may, however, be some damage to cortical gray matter but without the intense intraneuronal deposition usually observed in other cerebral lipidoses. Visceral organs are usually not involved because of the paucity of galactosylceramide lipids.

There is severe unexplained demyelination throughout the brain, though the myelin that remains has a normal glycolipid composition. Some investigators feel that an abnormal myelin is made initially, which is subject to easier degradation. The patients with later onset forms of Krabbe disease may have had normal myelin that functioned adequately until some event (possibly a viral infection) started the degradative process. As the myelin is degraded by way of lysosomal enzymes, the lack of galactosylceramide β-galactosidase (galactocerebrosidase) activity results in the preservation of galactosylceramide; this results in globoid cell formation (Fig. 7–27).

The *clinical onset* usually occurs before 6 mo of age, with irritability, hypertonicity, bouts of hypothermia, mental regression, and possibly optic atrophy and seizures. Within 9–12 mo there is increased hypertonicity, opisthotonos, hyperpyrexia, blindness, and seizures. In the final stage the patient is blind, deaf, spastic, and decerebrate, with death occurring usually before 2 yr of age. In forms of this disease with later onset, patients may reach late infantile developmental milestones before loss of vision and motor regression become evident. Other patients appear normal until 3–4 yr of age. Some have lived until 20 yr of age. An adult is rarely found to have the same enzymatic defect.

Most patients with Krabbe disease will have elevated spinal fluid in protein levels (values of 100–500 mg/dL are not unusual). As in MLD, there is a decrease in velocity of nerve conduction. All patients have a severe deficiency of galactosylceramide β-galactosidase activity in leukocytes or cultured skin fibroblasts. Carriers have approximately half normal galactocerebrosidase activity in leukocytes and cultured skin fibroblasts. A few normal adults have been found to have low levels of galactosylceramide β-galactosidase activity; they appear to be carriers of the Krabbe defect, showing less than 15% of normal activity by the in vitro test.

Patients with onset before 6 mo rarely live longer than 2 yr. Feeding, seizures, and aspiration pneumonia increasingly become problems. There is no treatment. Genetic counseling is appropriate. Prenatal diagnosis is possible using cultured amniotic cells and chorionic villus samples.

7.33 FARBER DISEASE

Farber disease (lipogranulomatosis) is an autosomal recessive disorder characterized by widely disseminated granulomas containing foam cells. There are numerous subcutaneous nodules and plaques, and symptoms include arthropathy, hoarseness, irritability, and poor growth and development. Deformed and painful joints are common and may simulate rheumatoid arthritis. Most patients die in the 2nd yr with respiratory infections and malnutrition; a few live into the 2nd decade with few, if any, neurologic problems. A neonatal presentation may include corneal clouding, hepatosplenomegaly, and joint contractures without subutaneous nodules.

The foam cells within the granulomas contain PAS-positive material (possibly gangliosides); lymph nodes, liver, kidneys, and lung contain 10- to 60-fold excesses of free ceramide. Ballooning of neurons in the central and autonomic nervous systems is also reported. Visceral organs are not usually enlarged, though electron microscopic examination of liver cells reveals osmophilic deposits surrounding electron-lucent material in a dense granular matrix. Kupffer cells and liver macrophages contain dense bodies with an osmophilic matrix. Most patients have increased spinal fluid protein and excrete excess ceramide in the urine.

This disease results from a deficiency of acid ceramidase activity. Ceramide is the lipid component of all sphingolipids and is formed during the degradation of many glycosphingolipids and sphingomyelin (Figs. 7–27 and 7–28). The deficiency of acid ceramidase has been demonstrated in kidney, cerebellum, and cultured skin fibroblasts. A partial deficiency in acid ceramidase activity is found in some heterozygotic persons. Prenatal diagnoses have been made using cultured amniotic fluid cells. No effective treatment is available; some improvement of joint function has been associated with the use of chlorambucil.

7.34 WOLMAN DISEASE AND CHOLESTERYL ESTER STORAGE DISEASE

Wolman disease, or primary familial xanthomatosis with involvement of the adrenals, is an autosomal recessive disease marked by severe failure to thrive, diarrhea, vomiting, and abdominal distention with hepatosplenomegaly and calcification of the adrenals. Storage of lipid in histiocytic foam cells produces the hepatosplenomegaly. Onset occurs in the 1st few weeks of life. Death usually occurs within 6 mo due to cachexia complicated by peripheral edema. Foam cells are found in bone marrow and other visceral organs, including intestinal villi. Hepatocytes stained with oil red O show vacuolation. There is evidence of storage of cholesterol and/or cholesteryl esters in liver cells, Kupffer cells, and histiocytes. Spleen and intestines also show evidence of storage. Neurons show changes like those in sudanophilic leukodystrophy. Storage in intestinal tissues can add to the nutritional problems; a large excess of cholesteryl esters and triglycerides may occur in these organs.

Examining bone marrow reveals a large number of lipoid cells. Roentgenograms of the abdomen show enlargement and calcification of the adrenals. Leukocytes and cultured skin fibroblasts studies indicate acid esterase (acid lipase) deficiency. Patients have no measurable activity with a variety of suitable substrates. Carriers of this disease can be identified by enzyme assays in leukocytes and cultured skin fibroblasts, and prenatal diagnosis has been accomplished using cultured amniotic fluid cells. There is no effective treatment.

Cholesteryl ester storage disease is a relatively mild genetic disorder characterized by liver enlargement, short stature, chronic gastrointestinal loss of blood of uncertain etiology, and chronic anemia. Hyperlipidemia is found in most patients. Foam cells and sea-blue histiocytes occur in the bone marrow, and lipids accumulate in the lamina propria of the intestine. Neurologic symptoms are minimal. Levels of cholesteryl esters are markedly elevated in liver, those of triglycerides only moderately elevated. A marked deficiency of cholesteryl ester hydrolase and triglyceride hydrolase has been found (as in Wolman disease). The hyperlipidemia predisposes the patient to atherosclerosis. Measuring acid lipase activity can confirm a diagnosis and presumably identify carriers of this autosomal recessive disease. A patient treated with phenobarbitone (30 mg b.i.d.) showed improvement in his malaise and jaundice.

7.35 ADRENOLEUKODYSTROPHY

Adrenoleudodystrophy (ALD) is an X-linked disorder associated with progressive demyelination of cerebral white matter and adrenal insufficency. The *clinical manifestations*, including change in behavior, loss of vision, gait disturbances, and dysarthria and dysphagia, are usually noted from 3–12 yr of age. Neonatal onset forms have been described in males and females. The disease progresses rapidly with death in 1–4 yr from onset. Symptoms of Addison disease, including melanoderma, hypotension, and a failure of ACTH to induce a rise in plasma cortisol, are noted after the initial diagnosis. Later onset forms are recognized in which adrenal insufficiency is associated with slowly progressive paresis and peripheral neuropathy. Patients with this slowly progressing form called *adrenomyeloneuropathy* (AMN) may survive to the 4th or 5th decade.

Diagnoses have been made in suspected males by examining biopsy samples from brain, adrenals, conjunctiva, and skin. Examining the fatty acid composition from the total lipid extract of cultured skin fibroblasts reveals higher levels of C_{26} fatty acids in patients and mothers of patients when compared to controls or to other metabolic diseases involving lipid metabolism; the ratio of C_{26} to C_{22} is reported. This method identifies the cultures from patients with both ALD and AMN, confirming the close association of these two syndromes. In both ALD and AMN characteristic inclusions consisting of electron-dense leaflets enclosing an electron-lucent space are found in the cerebral white matter, peripheral nerves, and adrenal cortex. There is an accumulation of C_{24}–C_{30} fatty acids in the involved tissues in both disorders. The C_{26}:C_{22} ratio in mothers of ALD patients was between that found in patients and controls. There is impaired oxidation of very long chain fatty acids in leukocytes, cultured skin fibroblasts, and amniocytes. This method should allow diagnosis of patients from only a skin biopsy and allow prenatal diagnosis in cultured amniotic fluid cells from at risk pregnancies.

Treatment with cortisone acetate (15 mg/24 hr) and phenytoin (150 mg/24 hr) has been beneficial in some cases of ALD. Dietary restriction of very long chain fatty acids is not likely to change the course of the disease.

7.36 REFSUM DISEASE

Most patients with Refsum disease (phytanic acid storage disease or heredopathia atactica polyneuritiformis) have the onset before 20 yr of age of failing vision (night blindness), anosmia, ichthyosis, weakness in extremities, and unsteady gait. The liver and kidneys are severely infiltrated with neutral fat. Plasma contains a large amount of phytanic acid (a 20-carbon branched-chain acid), which may constitute 5–30% of the total fatty acids. The larger size of phytanic acid, in contrast to the size of other fatty acids, may distort cell membranes and result in nerve degeneration. Refsum disease is inherited as an autosomal recessive trait.

Most patients are identified before 20 yr of age, although some have not presented until after age 50 yr. Almost all patients have retinitis pigmentosa, peripheral polyneuropathy, and cerebellar ataxia, and they may have dramatic exacerbations associated with ill-defined febrile illnesses, surgical procedures, or pregnancy. Lengthy periods of remission are not unusual. Diagnosis is indicated from clinical findings, increased spinal fluid protein (average 275 mg/dL), and elevated phytanic acid (up to 25 µg/mL) in the plasma. Phytanic acid is oxidized in cultured skin fibroblasts at 1–2% of the normal rate. Heterozygotes can be identified. There appears to be a high incidence among Norwegians.

Treatment is possible through dietary elimination of precursors of phytanic acid. These include dairy products, ruminant fats, and other foods containing chlorophyll (to exclude phytol). With reduction of the content of phytanic acid in plasma and tissue there is some amelioration of the neuropathy in some patients. Supportive physiotherapy and orthopedic devices may help patients cope with neuropathy; extraction of cataracts may be indicated. Death due to cardiac and respiratory complications usually occurs before the 5th decade.

7.37 NEURONAL CEROID-LIPOFUSCINOSES

See also Sec. 21.7 and 25.4.

The neuronal ceroid-lipofuscinoses encompass a group of genetic diseases including Batten disease, Spielmeyer-Vogt disease, Jansky-Bielschowsky syndrome, Kufs disease, and three types of amaurotic familial idiocy. All are inherited as autosomal recessive diseases. Persons affected by this group of diseases have neuronal storage of autofluorescent lipopigments of the ceroid-lipofuscin type, with relatively normal ganglioside patterns. The age of onset is 2–5 yr in late infantile type, 8–12 yr in the juvenile type, and over 20 yr in the adult type. In most of the younger patients (2–12 yr of age) clinical onset is marked by seizures, visual disturbances, intellectual retardation, and ataxia. Myoclonus and seizures can become refractory to all anticonvulsant medications. Blindness, with macular degeneration and retinitis pigmentosa, is common in the later stages of these syndromes. The course is variable, younger patients usually surviving 3–5 yr and juvenile patients 6–8 yr after initial signs. Adult patients present with ataxia and dementia or signs of involvement of basal ganglia and dementia.

In a patient suspected of having the disorder the diagnosis is usually based on finding abnormal neurons in a rectal or brain biopsy. There is a severe loss of neuronal perikarya, which contain granules that stain with Sudan black B and PAS and give positive reactions with all stains for ceroid or lipofuscin. The cytoplasm of many neurons contains variable numbers of irregularly shaped cytoplasmic inclusions called "curvilinear bodies." Other inclusions have the appearance of "fingerprint profiles." Studies of peripheral lymphocytes and skin or conjunctival biopsies in young patients will often reveal characteristic cytoplasmic inclusions, obviating the need for brain or rectal biopsy.

The clinical findings resemble those of other cerebral degenerative diseases, such as G_{M1} and G_{M2} gangliosidoses and the leukodystrophies, in which there are deficiencies of a specific lysosomal hydrolase. The exact protein defect in the ceroid-lipofuscinoses has not yet been determined. Carriers cannot yet be accurately identified. Prenatal diagnosis of neuronal ceroid lipofuscinosis has been made by identifying characteristic curvilinear bodies in uncultured amniocytes.

Seizure control should be attempted since uncontrolled seizures tend to hasten the course. No procedures have been successful in preventing death from aspiration pneumonia in the severely handicapped child.

7.38 MUCOLIPIDOSES

Patients with mucolipidoses exhibit clinical features of both lipidoses and mucopolysaccharidoses (Sec. 7.24). Despite their name, there is little evidence of true storage of lipids or mucopolysaccharides in the organs of affected patients. Technically, fucosidosis, G_{M1} gangliosidosis, and multiple sulfatase deficiency are mucolipidoses because there is evidence for storage both of lipids (as glycosphingolipids) and of glycosaminoglycans in various organs. All of the mucolipidoses are inherited as autosomal recessive traits.

Mucolipidosis (ML-I), lipomucopolysaccharidosis, or sialidosis type 2 (infantile onset) produces symptoms in the first year of life. There are Hurler-like features, with dysostosis multiplex, moderate mental retardation, visceromegaly, corneal clouding, cherry-red spot, seizures, vacuolated lymphocytes, and coarse fibroblast inclusions, but no mucopolysacchariduria. Sialic acid terminal oligosaccharides are excreted in large amounts in the urine. Kupffer cells and hepatocytes are vacuolated, and sural nerve biopsy reveals metachromatic myelin degeneration. These patients are deficient in glycoprotein sialidase activity. Ganglioside sialidase is normal. Carriers can be identified and prenatal diagnosis can be made using cultured amniotic cells.

ML-II or I-cell disease is manifest within the first few months of life. The clinical pattern somewhat resembles Hurler syndrome and G_{M1} gangliosidosis (type 1). Affected patients may have congenital dislocation of the hips, inguinal hernias, hypertrophy of the gums, restriction of motion in the shoulders, generalized hypotonia, thick and tight skin, and hepatomegaly. The coarse facial features become more conspicuous with age. Characteristic bone changes related to severe dysostosis multiplex occur, leading to a cloaking of the appearance of long tubular bones, to shortening of vertebral bodies, and to other significant changes in the pelvis, hands, ribs, and skull. Death from pneumonia or congestive heart failure usually occurs at 2–8 yr of age.

Urinary mucopolysaccharides are normal but sialyloligosaccharides are elevated. Fibroblast cultures reveal characteristic inclusions, which initially set this disease apart from the mucopolysaccharidoses. Enzyme studies show greatly increased lysosomal enzymes in serum, whereas values in leukocytes are near the normal range. Activities of almost all lysosomal enzymes are deficient in cultured skin fibroblasts, whereas the culture medium has an excess of these enzymes when compared with that of control fibroblast lines. The primary defect in ML-II and ML-III is a deficiency of a specific N-acetylglucosaminyl phosphotransferase which phosphorylates newly formed lysosomal enzymes. In the absence of these phosphate groups, which serve as part of a recognition marker, the newly synthesized enzymes do not get into the lysosomes but are excreted from the cell. This specific enzyme's activity can be measured in fibroblast cultures and this will provide a specific diagnostic test for patient and carrier identification and for prenatal diagnosis.

ML-III or pseudo-Hurler polydystrophy is a milder form of ML-II. After possibly delayed early psychomotor development, affected 3–4 yr old may present progressive joint stiffness, short stature, mild dysostosis multiplex, mild gingival hyperplasia, and normal urinary mucopolysaccharide levels. Corneal clouding or nystagmus may be present. The IQ may range from normal to as low as 50. The prognosis is unknown; some patients have attained the 3rd decade of life. Orthopedic treatment may be indicated in some cases. As in I-cell disease, serum lysosomal enzymes are elevated, and cultured skin fibroblasts reveal characteristic inclusions and decreased activities for many lysosomal enzymes. Measurement of UDP-N-acetylglucosamine-1-phosphotransferase activity using exogenous substrate shows more residual activity than in ML-II. Prenatal diagnosis is possible through examination of cultured amniotic fluid cells.

ML-IV is a recently described mucolipidosis. Most cases reported so far have occurred in children of Ashkenazi Jewish descent. Soon after birth affected children present bilateral corneal opacities and strabismus. After 6 mo hypotonia and psychomotor retardation become more evident. There is no skeletal dysplasia or excess excretion of mucopolysaccharides in the urine. There are grossly abnormal storage bodies in the cells of liver, brain, conjunctiva, and fibroblasts. The prognosis is uncertain. One patient has reached 24 yr of age. Treatment to correct the corneal opacities may improve the vision, but no other treatment is available.

Diagnosis is based on examining fibroblast cultures for the characteristic lamellated multivesicular membrane bodies. Patients have been found to have a partial deficiency of ganglioside sialidase activity. Although some obligate heterozygotes have less than normal activity, it is still not proven whether this is the primary defect. Prenatal diagnosis is made by examining cultured amniotic fluid cells for characteristic storage bodies.

Sialidoses is the name given to a group of disorders in which patients have a deficiency of sialidase (neuraminidase) activity when certain glycoprotein, oligosaccharide, or synthetic sialic acid-containing derivatives are used as substrates. Ganglioside sialidase activity is normal. The clinical manifestations of disease in these patients vary greatly, from those presenting in the 1st yr of life (mucolipidosis I, sialidosis type 2, infantile onset) to those having myoclonus, cherry-red spot, and vision loss but near normal intelligence (sialidosis type 1) presenting in the 1st or 2nd decade and surviving until the 4th decade. One group of patients having a clinical picture between these two types (sialidosis type 2, juvenile onset) has been mistaken for unusual forms of G_{M1} gangliosidosis because low β-galactosidase activity has also been found in certain tissues. All types excrete sialyloligosaccharides in urine and store sialic acid–containing derivatives in cultured cells.

The sialidoses can be enzymatically diagnosed in cultured fibroblasts and leukocytes, and prenatal diagnoses have been made. Carriers can be identified.

DAVID WENGER

Banerjee A, Burg J, Conzelmann E, et al: Enzyme-linked immunosorbent assay for the ganglioside G_{M2}-activator protein. Hoppe-Seyler's Z Physiol Chem 365:347, 1984.

Barranger JA, Murray GJ, Ginns EI: Genetic heterogeneity of Gaucher's disease. In: Barranger JA, Brady RO (eds): Molecular Basis of Lysosomal Storage Disorders. New York, Academic Press, 1984, p 311.

Crandall BF, Philippart M, Brown WJ, et al: Mucolipidosis IV. Am J Med Genet 12:301, 1982.

Crocker AC, Farber S: Niemann-Pick disease. A review of 18 patients. Medicine 37:1, 1958.

Fujibayashi S, Inui K, Wenger DA: Activator protein deficient metachromatic leukodystrophy: Diagnosis in leukocytes using immunologic methods. J Pediatr 104:739, 1984.

Inui K, Emmett M, Wenger DA: Immunological evidence for a deficiency of an activator protein for sulfatide sulfatase in a variant form of metachromatic leukodystrophy. Proc Natl Acad Sci USA 80:3074, 1983.

Johnson WG: The clinical spectrum of hexosaminidase deficiency diseases. Neurology 31:1453, 1981.

Lowden JA, O'Brien JS: Sialidosis: A review of human sialidase deficiency. Am J Hum Genet 31:1, 1979.

Moser HW, Moser AE, Trojak JE, et al: Identification of female carriers of adrenoleukodystrophy. J Pediatr 103:54, 1983.

O'Brien JS: The gangliosidoses. In: Stanbury JB, Wyngaarden JB, Fredrickson DS, et al (eds): The Metabolic Basis of Inherited Disease. New York, McGraw-Hill, 1983, p 945.

O'Reilly RJ, Brochstein J, Dinsmore R, et al: Marrow transplantation for congenital disorders. Semin Hematol 21:188, 1984.

Poenaru L, Kaplan L, Dumez J, et al: Evaluation of possible first trimester prenatal diagnosis in lysosomal diseases by trophoblast biopsy. Pediatr Res 18:1032, 1984

Reitman ML, Varki A, Kornfeld S: Fibroblasts from patients with I-cell disease and pseudo-Hurler polydystrophy are deficient in uridine 5'-diphosphate-N-acetylglucosamine: glycoprotein N-acetylglucosaminylphosphotransferase activity. J Clin Invest 67:1574, 1981.

Suzuki K, Suzuki Y: Galactosylceramide lipidosis: Globoid cell leukodystrophy (Krabbe's disease). In: Stanbury JB, Wyngaarden JB, Fredrickson DS, et al (eds): The Metabolic Basis of Inherited Disease. New York, McGraw-Hill, 1983, p 857.

DISORDERS OF LIPOPROTEIN METABOLISM AND TRANSPORT

The Framingham and other similar studies have demonstrated that the higher the plasma cholesterol level, the greater the risk of myocardial infarction secondary to the premature development of atherosclerosis. However, until recently there were no clinical trials that conclusively proved that efforts to reduce plasma cholesterol had any beneficial effect on the incidence of atherosclerotic heart disease. In 1984, the Lipid Research Clinics Coronary Primary Prevention Trial showed that for every 1% drop in plasma cholesterol obtained by cholestyramine therapy, there was a 2% reduction in the incidence of myocardial infarction. Therefore, children at risk for developing premature atherosclerosis in adulthood because they have inherited one or more genes for hypercholesterolemia should be identified early in life, in order to try to reduce the associated risk of early heart disease. Hypertriglyceridemia, also known to be associated with the early development of atherosclerosis, is generally considered to be a less significant risk factor than hypercholesterolemia. These sections present an overview of the metabolism and transport of cholesterol and triglycerides, an assessment of "normal" plasma levels of these lipids, a description of the primary (i.e., genetic) and secondary defects of lipoprotein metabolism that can result in abnormal lipid levels in children, and a discussion of the diagnosis and management of pediatric patients with these disorders.

Plasma Lipoprotein Metabolism and Transport. Cholesterol and triglycerides are transported in the circulation in macromolecular complexes termed *lipoproteins*; the protein components of the complexes are called apolipoproteins. Dietary lipoproteins (chylomicrons) are formed in, and secreted by, the small intestine; other lipoproteins (e.g., very low density lipoproteins) are synthesized in the liver; still others (high density lipoproteins) reach their mature form in the circulation after exchange of components with other circulating lipoproteins or with tissues.

Transport of Exogenous (Dietary) Lipids (Fig. 7–29). After ingestion of a fat-containing meal and hydrolysis by intestinal and pancreatic lipases, free fatty acids and cholesterol are re-esterified in the intestinal epithelium to form triglycerides and cholesteryl esters, respectively. These lipids are then packaged together with phospholipids, free cholesterol, and at least two apolipoproteins (apoA-I and apoB-48) to form *chylomicrons*, which are secreted into the intestinal lymph and pass through the thoracic duct into the peripheral circulation. In the circulation, chylomicrons acquire additional apolipoproteins, mainly apoE and several forms of apoC. Triglycerides, which constitute most of the chylomicron mass, are immediately hydrolyzed by lipoprotein lipase at the capillary endothelium. The free fatty acid products of this hydrolysis are transferred primarily to adipose tissue for storage as triglyc-

CHYLOMICRON PATHWAY

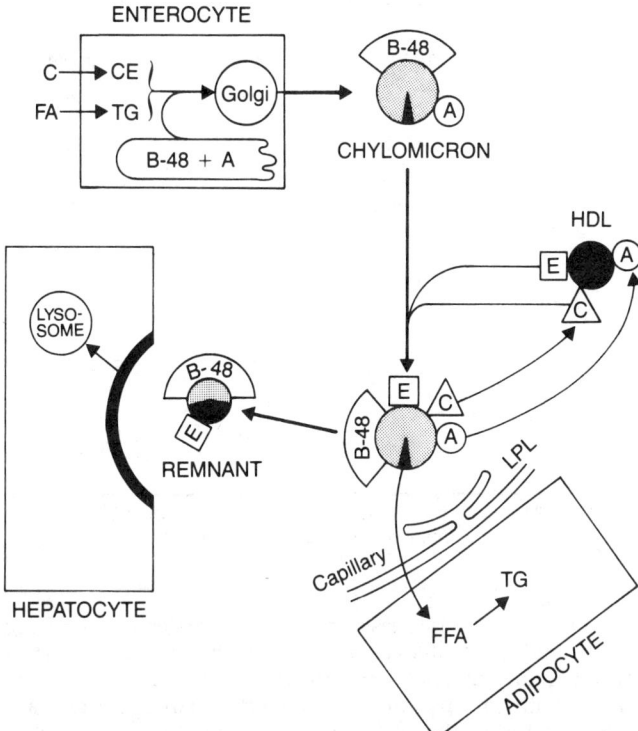

Figure 7–29. Pathway of chylomicron metabolism in human plasma. Fatty acids (FA) and cholesterol (C) are esterified in the intestinal mucosa to form triglycerides (TG) and cholesteryl esters (CE), respectively. They combine with apoA and apoB-48 to form chylomicrons, which are secreted into the circulation; TG (shaded area) and CE (black area). Chylomicrons undergo lipolysis in the capillary endothelium near adipose tissue and muscle tissue, losing TG via lipoprotein lipase (LPL), gaining apoE from HDL and losing apoA and apoC to HDL. The resulting chylomicron remnants are taken up by hepatic apoE receptors for degradation by lysosomes. (Adapted from Havel RJ: Med Clin North Am 66:319, 1982.)

erides or to muscle tissue for beta-oxidation. The lipoprotein particles, now smaller and more dense because they have lost most of their triglyceride content, are called *chylomicron remnants*. They have retained virtually all of their cholesteryl ester content and transferred some of their apolipoproteins (apoC and apoA-I) primarily to *high density lipoproteins* (HDL); and they have become enriched with respect to their apoB-48 and apoE content. These remnants are recognized, bound, and internalized in part via hepatic membrane receptors specific for the apoE on the particles. By this mechanism, dietary cholesterol is delivered to the liver, where it plays a role in the regulation of hepatic cholesterol metabolism. Under normal circumstances, chylomicrons and their remnants are very short-lived in the circulation; following a 12 hr fast, there are normally no lipoproteins of dietary origin remaining in the plasma.

Transport of Endogenous Lipids from the Liver (Fig. 7–30). The liver secretes a class of lipoproteins called *very low density lipoproteins* or VLDL, which contain free and esterified cholesterol, triglycerides, phospholipids and a characteristic set of apolipoproteins, notably apoB-100, apoC, and apoE. Like chylomicrons, VLDL exchange apolipoproteins with other circulating particles and deliver triglycerides to adipose tissue via lipoprotein lipase. In the process, they become smaller and more dense and are termed VLDL remnants or *intermediate density lipoproteins* (IDL). Some of these remnant particles are taken up via a hepatic cell membrane receptor, while

some proportion undergo conversion to *low density lipoproteins* (LDL); this latter process involves removal of the remaining triglycerides and all apolipoproteins except apoB-100 and results in a particle that is almost entirely made up of cholesteryl esters and apoB-100. A specific LDL receptor is present on most cell membranes that recognizes, binds, and internalizes LDL. By this mechanism, LDL particles can deliver cholesterol to extrahepatic tissues to serve their requirements for membrane synthesis; in addition, tissues involved in steroid hormone synthesis can meet their cholesterol needs by receptor-mediated uptake of LDL. LDL particles can circulate in the plasma for several days.

HDL and Reverse Cholesterol Transport. In contrast to chylomicrons and VLDL, which are secreted into the circulation as mature particles, HDL are secreted from the liver and small intestine as nascent discoidal particles composed primarily of phospholipids and proteins (apoE and apoA). The particles accept cholesterol from VLDL and LDL, as well as from tissues; this cholesterol is esterified via the lecithin:cholesterol acyltransferase (LCAT) reaction. Part of the cholesteryl ester is stored in the core of HDL, making it a

VLDL-LDL PATHWAYS

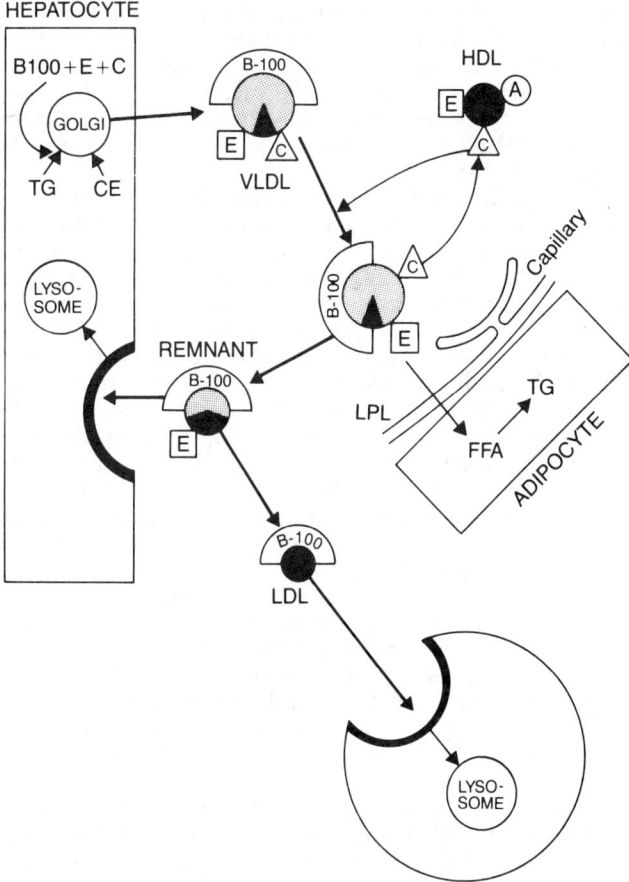

Figure 7–30. Pathways of VLDL and LDL metabolism in human plasma. Triglycerides (TG) and cholesteryl esters (CE) are combined with apoB-100, apoC, and apoE in the liver, and the secreted as VLDL: TG (shaded area) and CE (black area). VLDL undergo lipolysis in the capillary endothelium near adipose tissue and muscle tissue, losing TG via lipoprotein lipase (LPL). The resulting VLDL remnants are either converted to low density lipoproteins (LDL) for transport to peripheral cells via LDL receptor-mediated uptake, or are taken up by hepatic receptors. (Adapted from Havel RJ: Med Clin North Am 66:319, 1982.)

Table 7–11. **Plasma Cholesterol and Triglyceride Levels (mg/dL) in Childhood and Adolescence**

Age	Total Cholesterol		LDL Cholesterol		HDL Cholesterol		Total Triglyceride	
	Mean	5th–95th Percentile	Mean	5th–95th Percentile	Mean	5th–95th Percentile	Mean	5th–95th Percentile
Cord	68	42–103	29	17–50	35	13–60	34	14–84
6 mo	132	89–185	73	40–111	51	23–88	80	45–169
1 yr	145	99–193	81	49–121	51	22–81	73	42–158
<1–4 yr								
Male	155	114–203	—	—	—	—	56	29–99
Female	156	112–200	—	—	—	—	64	34–112
5–9 yr								
Male	155	125–189	93	63–129	56	38–74	52	28–85
Female	164	131–197	100	68–140	53	36–73	64	32–126
10–14 yr								
Male	160	124–202	97	64–132	55	37–74	63	33–111
Female	160	125–205	97	68–136	52	37–70	72	39–120
15–19 yr								
Male	153	118–191	94	62–130	46	30–63	78	38–143
Female	159	118–207	96	59–137	52	35–74	73	36–126

Data for cord blood, 6 mo, and 1 yr from Frerichs RR et al: Circulation 54:302, 1976. Data for <1–4 yr. Children from Tables 6, 7, 20, and 21, and all other data from Tables 24, 25, 32, 33, 36, and 37 in The Lipid Research Clinics Population Studies Data Book, Vol. 1, 1980.

spherical particle, while part of it is transferred back to VLDL and LDL. Sincle LDL and remnants of VLDL metabolism can be taken up by the liver, this provides a way for returning tissue-derived cholesterol to the liver (reverse cholesterol transport). HDL itself can also be metabolized by the liver and may provide another vehicle for the return of tissue-derived cholesterol to the liver. The liver can then excrete cholesterol in bile.

Plasma Lipid and Lipoprotein Levels. Table 7–11 presents normal plasma cholesterol and triglyceride levels. During the first few months of life, cholesterol levels increase largely because of changes in LDL. Over the next 15–20 years, there is little change in the total cholesterol level, which averages 150–165 mg/dL in both males and females. LDL cholesterol levels remain slightly under 100 mg/dL in both males and females during this period. HDL cholesterol levels are comparable in males and females early in life; they remain essentially constant in females but decline markedly in males during the second decade to a level that is maintained through adulthood. Plasma triglyceride levels, on the other hand, tend to rise transiently in both males and females in the first year, fall to a mean of 50–60 mg/dL in the ensuing few years, and then rise to a mean of approximately 75 mg/dL by age 20 years. In early adulthood, there is a marked rise in plasma cholesterol that is due almost exclusively to an increase in LDL cholesterol. The rate of increase over the next 30 years is greater in males than in females. When coupled with their lower HDL cholesterol levels and their higher triglyceride levels, this puts men at much greater risk than women for atherosclerotic heart disease, at least up to the age of 50–60 years.

Generally, a patient is classified as hyperlipidemic if his or her lipid level is above the 95th percentile, corrected for age and sex. Therefore, hypercholesterolemia could be defined as a fasting cholesterol level greater than 200 mg/dL for both males and females in the first 2 decades (Table 7–11). However, the National Institutes of Health Consensus Development Conference on Lowering Blood Cholesterol (1984) recommended designating anyone 2–19 yr old with a plasma cholesterol level greater than 170 mg/dL (the 75th percentile)

as being at "moderate risk" and those greater than 185 mg/dL (the 90th percentile) as being at "high risk" for premature cardiovascular disease. Early treatment of hypercholesterolemia in both groups was recommended, since lifestyle and dietary patterns that influence cholesterol levels are often developed in the childhood years.

Information about family history of premature myocardial infarction or sudden death (before the age of 50 in male relatives and 60 in female relatives), hyperlipidemia, and xanthomas should be obtained. If a child has a strong family history of early heart disease, total cholesterol, HDL cholesterol, and total triglycerides should be measured. The LDL cholesterol level can be estimated from the following equation:

$$\text{LDL cholesterol} = \text{total cholesterol} - [\text{HDL cholesterol} + (\text{total triglycerides} \div 5)],$$

assuming that the sample is obtained in the fasting state, and that the total triglyceride level is less than 400 mg/dL. Lipid measurements on other family members may be necessary to establish a specific diagnosis.

Some investigators believe that all children should be screened to determine whether they have hypercholesterolemia. However, since major dietary modifications before 2 yr of age are not recommended, we suggest that total plasma cholesterol be measured after the age of 2 yr, or at least by the preschool examination. If elevated, the plasma cholesterol level should be remeasured, HDL cholesterol and triglyceride levels obtained, and LDL cholesterol calculated.

Hypertriglyceridemia can be defined as a fasting triglyceride level greater than the 95th percentile, i.e., above 100 mg/dL in the 1st decade of life, and between 130 and 150 mg/dL in the 2nd decade, since triglyceride levels increase with age. Although elevated triglyceride levels per se do not represent an independent risk factor for premature cardiovascular disease, levels above the 95th percentile can be a marker for some patients with genetic forms of hyperlipoproteinemia. The pediatrician should always obtain a careful history for evidence of premature heart disease in the families of these children. If the elevated level is confirmed by repeated measurement, it warrants further investigation.

HYPERLIPOPROTEINEMIAS

Extensive epidemiological data and clinical findings in man and experimental studies in animals relate the premature development of atherosclerosis to persistent hyperlipoproteinemia. Elevation of LDL for any reason is a risk factor for early myocardial infarction, although the precise mechanisms by which this occurs are not entirely clear. It is known that macrophages and smooth muscle cells invade the arterial wall during the process of atherogenesis; these cells serve as scavengers, taking up many different kinds of lipoproteins through unregulated receptor-mediated processes, resulting in the formation of foam cells characteristic of the early atherosclerotic lesion.

One-third of patients who have suffered their first myocardial infarction before the age of 50 yr in men and 60 yr in women have hyperlipoproteinemia, and about one half of these are due to a dominantly inherited disorder of lipoprotein metabolism.

PRIMARY GENETIC DEFECTS

7.39 FAMILIAL HYPERCHOLESTEROLEMIA (FH)

Heterozygous FH. This dominantly inherited disease affecting lipoprotein metabolism (and hence plasma lipid levels) occurs with a frequency of at least 1 in 500 in the population and is the most common form of inherited hyperlipidemia recognized in childhood. The molecular defects responsible for this disorder are known, and there are at least eight separate allelic mutations in the gene for LDL receptors that impair the receptor-mediated uptake of LDL from the circulation (Fig. 7-30). Most patients with FH are heterozygous for one of these alleles and have approximately half normal and half defective receptors, resulting in marked elevation of the plasma LDL cholesterol level from birth, which persists throughout life.

Clinical manifestations of FH, the most important of which is premature coronary atherosclerosis, do not typically develop until the 3rd or 4th decade. The peak incidence of myocardial infarction in affected men is in the 4th–5th decades; by age 60, 85% have suffered a myocardial infarction. In women, the mean age of onset is about 10 yr later. Most adult patients present with a strong family history of premature coronary artery disease and tendon xanthomas (nodular swellings involving the Achilles and other tendons due to cholesteryl ester deposition in macrophages) as well as deposits in the soft tissue of the eyelid (xanthelasmas) and in the cornea (arcus corneae). These signs are rarely present in pediatric patients with heterozygous FH, except for tendon xanthomas which may be seen in 10–15% of them as an initial clinical manifestation in the 2nd decade. Achilles tendinitis in a teenager should suggest the diagnosis of FH.

Diagnosis of FH is supported by a strong family history of early myocardial infarctions, tendon xanthomas, and total plasma cholesterol levels greater than 300 mg/dL in affected adults. Affected children usually have total cholesterol levels above 250 mg/dL, with LDL cholesterol above 200 mg/dL.

Treatment by weight control has relatively little impact on the plasma cholesterol level in heterozygous FH. A diet (NIH Diet 2) low in cholesterol (250–300 mg/day) is indicated, and the patient should receive no more than 30% of total calories from fat (approximately 10% each of polyunsaturated, monounsaturated, and saturated). Although this may produce a significant reduction (by as much as 15%) in LDL cholesterol, diet alone will not return the LDL cholesterol level to normal. Consequently, cholestyramine or colestipol resin is recommended to further reduce LDL cholesterol. These nonabsorb-able drugs interrupt the enterohepatic cycle through the binding of bile acids in the intestine; they have the additional benefit of inducing LDL receptors in the liver. Most children tolerate this medication quite well; the side effects of constipation and abdominal discomfort usually can be managed effectively. Both drugs may interfere with the absorption of fat-soluble vitamins; supplements may be required, and assessment of plasma vitamin A levels and prothrombin time may be indicated. Cholestyramine is available in 9 g packets (equivalent to 4 g of active drug). The dose of drug varies with age and with the severity of hypercholesterolemia, ranging from as little as ½ packet (2 g active drug) b.i.d. before meals and increasing to the adult dose (3–4 packets b.i.d. or 24–32 g/day). Up to 3 packets b.i.d. (24 g/day) can be well tolerated by teenagers and may reduce LDL cholesterol by 50–100 mg/dL. Colestipol is available in 5 g packets, all of which is active drug; dosage is similar to that of cholestyramine. If the LDL cholesterol persists above the 95th percentile, nicotinic acid, which is used in adults, should be considered. In addition, plasmapheresis is quite effective when performed every 2–3 wk.

Homozygous FH. A rare patient (about 1 per million) with severe FH is either homozygous for one abnormal allele or is a compound heterozygote for two alleles that impair LDL receptor function. Homozygotes have plasma cholesterol levels of 600 mg/dL or higher from birth. They have unique planar cutaneous xanthomas over the knees, elbows, and buttocks, which are often evident at birth and always by 6 yr of age. Tendon xanthomas, xanthelasmas, and arcus corneae are virtually always present. Coronary atherosclerosis frequently has its onset before 10 yr of age; most patients die of complications of myocardial infarction before 30 yr.

Drugs and diet do not have a major impact. Consequently, regular plasmapheresis and aggressive therapies such as ileal bypass surgery and portacaval shunt have been attempted with some success. Liver transplantation has been successful in a few cases. Another promising therapy is LDL-apheresis, the specific removal of LDL by plasmapheresis through affinity columns.

7.40 POLYGENIC HYPERCHOLESTEROLEMIA

There are many families in which high LDL cholesterol levels appear to be inherited, but the moderate degree of hypercholesterolemia, the lack of physical stigmata (such as tendon xanthomas), and the less severe family history of coronary artery disease do not support the diagnosis of FH. In some, familial combined hyperlipidemia (Sec. 7.45) is the cause, while in others, there may be other genetic causes for their hypercholesterolemia. Possibly a combination of one or more genes interacting with one or more environmental factors (e.g., diet) explains some of these cases. Nevertheless, the hypercholesterolemia is an indication for obtaining a careful family history for evidence of coronary artery disease and determining whether HDL or LDL cholesterol is increased. If LDL cholesterol is elevated, the patient should be managed as described above for heterozygous FH. In addition to diet, weight control and regular exercise should be emphasized, and the patient should be warned about the added risk attributable to smoking. If LDL cholesterol remains elevated despite these measures, the use of cholestyramine or colestipol is recommended.

7.41 FAMILIAL HYPERALPHALIPOPROTEINEMIA

Unlike elevation of other lipoproteins, elevation of plasma HDL cholesterol has a protective effect against the development of atherosclerotic heart disease, presumably because of its role in reverse cholesterol transport. The inherited elevation of HDL cholesterol has been described by Glueck as a longevity syndrome in families that appear to be at a lower than normal risk for the development of premature atherosclerosis. Therefore, HDL cholesterol levels should be measured in children with moderate hypercholesterolemia. Those with hyperalphalipoproteinemia have HDL cholesterol levels at the upper end of the normal distribution, and their LDL cholesterol levels will often be within normal limits.

7.42 FAMILIAL (ENDOGENOUS) HYPERTRIGLYCERIDEMIA

This disorder occurs with a frequency of 2–3 per 1000 adults but is found in at least 5% of patients suffering a myocardial infarction before the age of 60. The increased risk of premature atherosclerosis with familial hypertriglyceridemia is, however, significantly less than that associated with familial hypercholesterolemia or familial combined hyperlipidemia. It can be diagnosed only by family studies, which commonly show elevation of the fasting plasma triglyceride level in the range of 200–500 mg/dL, not associated with hyperchylomicronemia, and occurring in a dominantly inherited fashion. There are families with endogenous hypertriglyceridemia in which some members have, in addition, hyperchylomicronemia (see Sec. 7.43). Only 10–20% of children in families with familial hypertriglyceridemia have elevated triglycerides before the age of 20, while 50% of adults (i.e., those who have inherited the gene) will be affected with hypertriglyceridemia. Obesity, insulin resistance, hyperinsulinemia, glucose intolerance, and hyperuricemia are often associated findings. Although the precise metabolic defect is unknown, there may be more than one cause, since some studies have demonstrated overproduction of VLDL and others have demonstrated reduced clearance of VLDL in patients with familial hypertriglyceridemia.

Children can usually be managed with weight reduction and use of a diet controlled in carbohydrate content (45% of calories), modified in fat, and moderately cholesterol-restricted (NIH Diet 4). The risk/benefit ratio does not ordinarily justify drug intervention.

7.43 ENDOGENOUS AND EXOGENOUS HYPERLIPIDEMIA (HYPERLIPOPROTEINEMIA TYPE 5)

Patients with this rare disorder (<1 in 5000) have marked elevations of both chylomicron and VLDL triglycerides. Clinical findings include eruptive xanthomas, lipemia retinalis, pancreatitis, and abnormal glucose tolerance associated with hyperinsulinism. The disorder is usually not expressed in childhood, but several families have been found in which the unidentified defect(s) is expressed early in life. The treatment is primarily weight control and dietary modification (NIH Diet 5). Carbohydrate restriction may also be required to reduce endogenous overproduction of VLDL triglycerides. Patients should avoid alcohol and restrict fat intake. Aggressive dietary measures should be tried before drug therapy is considered to reduce the VLDL triglyceride level.

7.44 EXOGENOUS HYPERTRIGLYCERIDEMIA (HYPERCHYLOMICRONEMIA)

Lipoprotein Lipase (LPL) Deficiency. This is an extremely rare (<1 in 100,000) autosomal recessive disorder. Although demonstrable shortly after birth, the massive elevation of plasma triglycerides (1000 mg/dL to over 4000 mg/dL) is clinically silent and is often not discovered until the patient's blood is sampled for another reason; the chylomicronemia is

striking. Clinical manifestations include eruptive xanthomas over the trunk, lipemia retinalis, mild hepatosplenomegaly, and recurrent bouts of pancreatitis. The hyperchylomicronemia results from a failure of hydrolysis of chylomicrons due to genetic deficiency of lipoprotein lipase on the endothelial surface of the capillaries. The diagnosis of LPL deficiency is made by measuring the enzyme activity in plasma after administration of heparin (post-heparin lipolytic activity).

ApoC-II Deficiency. The clinical and laboratory manifestations of genetic deficiency of apoC-II, a cofactor for LPL, are similar to those of LPL deficiency. The diagnosis is made by isoelectric focusing of VLDL proteins.

In both of these disorders, patients are not at risk for early development of atherosclerosis, but recurrent bouts of pancreatitis can be life-threatening. Therapy for these disorders is aimed at making the diet low enough in long-chain fatty acids (no more than 15 g regular food fat/day for children under 12 years) to keep the patient asymptomatic and free of recurrent bouts of pain. Using medium-chain triglyceride (MCT) oil in food preparation serves both to make the diet more palatable and to provide sufficient calories for growth. MCTs are absorbed directly into the portal vein and are transported to the liver without requiring chylomicron formation and transport through the systemic circulation. None of the presently available hypolipidemic drugs have any sustained effect.

7.45 FAMILIAL COMBINED HYPERLIPIDEMIA

This familial multiple lipoprotein type of hyperlipoproteinemia is probably the most frequent inherited disorder of lipoprotein metabolism (as high as 1 per 100) and is associated with a high risk of myocardial infarction. In this dominantly inherited disease, approximately one third of the hyperlipidemic family members have hypertriglyceridemia, one third have hypercholesterolemia, and one third have elevations of both cholesterol and triglycerides. The lipid elevations tend to be modest, often fluctuating around the 95th percentile. In addition, the lipoprotein abnormalities can change from time to time in the same affected individual. This disorder is not usually associated with tendon xanthomas, but obesity, hyperinsulinism, and glucose intolerance are frequently found in adults. Although 50% of adults with an affected parent will have hyperlipoproteinemia, affected children may not manifest significant hypercholesterolemia and/or hypertriglyceridemia until the 2nd or 3rd decade owing to gradual gene expression. The risk of premature heart disease is considerable, although lipid levels may be only moderately elevated; 25–50% of patients suffer a myocardial infarction prior to age 50. The reasons for the varied expression of hyperlipidemia are unclear, but the disease is known to be associated with overproduction of VLDL. Patients with this type of hyperlipidemia should be treated similarly to patients with heterozygous FH. Dietary intervention should be aimed at controlling the hypercholesterolemia, with or without controlled carbohydrate intake to reduce hypertriglyceridemia.

7.46 FAMILIAL DYSBETALIPOPROTEINEMIA (HYPERLIPOPROTEINEMIA TYPE 3)

This rare condition is characterized by abnormal plasma lipoproteins designated "beta VLDL" or "floating beta lipoproteins." The presence of planar xanthomas along the palmar creases of the hands (xanthoma striata palmaris) is virtually diagnostic. Other clinical features include tuberoeruptive xanthomas of the trunk, tuberous xanthomas over the elbows and knees, and tendinous xanthomas. Coronary artery disease as well as peripheral vascular disease are commonly found. The specific genetic abnormality is a mutation that alters the structure of apoE, decreasing the binding of apoE-containing lipoproteins to the liver receptor (Figs. 7–29 and 7–30) and thereby retarding the uptake of chylomicron and VLDL remnants. There are three common alleles at the apoE gene locus, resulting in six phenotypes of apoE which can be distinguished by isoelectric focusing of VLDL proteins. One of these phenotypes, designated apoE 2/2, occurs in about 1% of the population, but over 90% of patients with familial dysbetalipoproteinemia have this phenotype. Since familial dysbetalipoproteinemia is quite rare (less than 1 per 1000 adults), the majority of individuals with apoE 2/2 appear to tolerate this clearance disorder well. If they overproduce chylomicrons (e.g., because of dietary indiscretion) or VLDL (e.g., because of a gene for another familial hyperlipidemia), their clinical disease can be fully expressed.

The diagnosis can be made on the basis of clinical manifestations or by demonstrating abnormal lipoproteins by electrophoresis. The abnormal chemical composition of the particles also can be demonstrated. The cholesterol content of VLDL in these patients is high; the ratio of their VLDL cholesterol to total triglycerides is greater than 0.3. ApoE phenotyping is not generally available but can be performed in specialized laboratories.

Familial dysbetalipoproteinemia is one of the only inherited hyperlipidemias which is exquisitely sensitive to dietary intervention. Weight loss to a level appropriate for height can often cause the lipid levels to return to normal. The diet should be carbohydrate-controlled (35–40% of calories), modified in fat (40% of calories with an increased proportion of polyunsaturated to saturated fat), and reduced in cholesterol (NIH Diet 3). There is little experience with drug treatment of this disorder in children, but adults with familial dysbetalipoproteinemia whose lipid elevations fail to respond to dietary intervention have been treated with fibric acid derivatives.

SECONDARY HYPERLIPIDEMIAS

Much of the hypertriglyceridemia and, to a smaller extent, hypercholesterolemia seen in clinical practice is secondary to exogenous factors or underlying clinical disorders. Obesity, for example, is probably the major cause of mild elevations of plasma triglycerides, and the hypertriglyceridemia is frequently normalized following a return to desirable weight. Weight loss also reduces cholesterol levels in the overweight.

Other pediatric conditions associated with hypertriglyceridemia include diabetes mellitus, renal disease (nephrotic syndrome, uremia, maintenance dialysis, and renal transplantation), hypothyroidism, and occasionally other endocrine and metabolic disorders, such as type I glycogen storage disease. Secondary causes of hypercholesterolemia include hypothyroidism, nephrotic syndrome, and congenital biliary atresia.

Excessive alcohol intake is a well-known cause of hypertriglyceridemia in adults and should be considered in teenagers. Oral contraceptives generally increase triglyceride levels, with varying effects on LDL and HDL cholesterol levels. Other drugs that raise triglyceride levels are thiazide diuretics and some beta-adrenergic blocking agents.

Treatment of the underlying condition or removal of the offending drug is usually the first management approach to the patient with secondary hyperlipidemia. If the elevated lipid level persists, however, consideration must be given to the possibility that the patient has an underlying primary form of hyperlipoproteinemia, and therapy appropriate to the particular disease should be initiated.

7.47 HDL DEFICIENCY STATES (HYPOALPHALIPOPROTEINEMIA)

Low levels of HDL cholesterol are associated with an increased risk of atherosclerosis, and high levels appear to be protective. Most patients with extremely low levels of HDL cholesterol (less than 10 mg/dL plasma) have an inherited HDL deficiency state, such as *Tangier disease*.

Homozygotes for *Tangier disease* have HDL particles that are structurally abnormal and present in markedly reduced concentrations. Associated lipoprotein abnormalities include extremely low apoA-I and low apoA-II levels, low to normal LDL cholesterol levels, and high plasma triglyceride levels. The major clinical manifestations, some of which can be detected in childhood, result from deposition of cholesteryl esters in a number of tissues: enlarged yellowish tonsils, splenomegaly, peripheral neuropathy, hepatomegaly, lymphadenopathy, and diffuse corneal infiltration. Heterozygotes have approximately 50% of normal levels of HDL cholesterol, apoA-I, and apoA-II but none of the clinical manifestations noted above. Coronary artery disease, however, is common in both homozygotes and heterozygotes for *Tangier disease*, but only after the age of 40 yr. The precise molecular defect is unknown, but abnormalities in apoA-I synthesis and metabolism have been identified.

Other rare inherited HDL deficiency states have been described (apoA-I and apoC-III deficiency, HDL deficiency with planar xanthomas, fish-eye disease) that share some of the features of *Tangier disease*. There is no specific treatment for these disorders, but a diet restricted in fat is recommended.

In view of the numerous observations that HDL cholesterol levels tend to be low in patients with premature coronary artery disease, attempts have been made to identify other inherited causes of reduced HDL. Families have been described with low (50% of normal) HDL cholesterol levels apparently segregating in an autosomal dominant fashion, and associated with premature vascular disease. There have been few systematic clinical studies of familial hypoalphalipoproteinemia, and it is not known whether therapies that act on HDL levels in the general population (i.e., exercise, moderate alcohol intake) will influence HDL cholesterol levels in this group of patients.

7.48 ABETALIPOPROTEINEMIA AND HYPOBETALIPOPROTEINEMIA

Abetalipoproteinemia is a rare autosomal recessive disease characterized in childhood by fat malabsorption and diarrhea, retinitis pigmentosa, cerebellar ataxia, and acanthocytosis. All forms of apoB are absent from plasma; thus, homozygotes have no detectable chylomicrons, VLDL, or LDL, and their plasma cholesterol and triglyceride levels are extremely low (usually less than 30 mg/dL). Heterozygotes have no known clinical or biochemical abnormalities. The underlying defect in abetalipoproteinemia is unknown but likely involves an abnormal synthesis or secretion of apoB-containing lipoproteins. The clinical manifestations are directly referable to the failure of transport of lipids and lipid-soluble vitamins. Treatment is symptomatic. Large doses of vitamin E may retard the progress of neurologic and retinal degeneration; water-soluble vitamin A and vitamin K may alleviate symptoms of night blindness and coagulopathy, respectively. Restriction of dietary long-chain fat may lessen the diarrhea. MCT oil may help maintain caloric balance.

Hypobetalipoproteinemia is distinguished from abetalipoproteinemia because it is apparently inherited as an autosomal dominant trait. Homozygotes are clinically similar to patients with abetalipoproteinemia. Heterozygotes have low plasma cholesterol and low-to-normal triglyceride levels, but are otherwise usually asymptomatic.

7.49 LECITHIN:CHOLESTEROL ACYLTRANSFERASE (LCAT) DEFICIENCY

Deficiency of this plasma enzyme is associated with markedly reduced levels of cholesteryl esters in lipoproteins. This deficiency results in alterations of virtually all of the plasma lipoproteins: HDL and LDL cholesterol levels are low; triglycerides are generally high; and lipoproteins have abnormal electrophoretic mobility. Clinically, LCAT deficiency presents early in childhood. Corneal opacities, anemia, and proteinuria have been commonly demonstrated; sea-blue histiocytes in bone marrow and spleen have been reported. This rare disorder (probably less than 1 per million) can be diagnosed by measuring LCAT activity in plasma. There is no specific treatment, although transfusion therapy, renal transplantation, and corneal transplantation have been tried. Dietary management includes stringent fat restriction.

JEAN A. CORTNER
PAUL M. COATES

Assmann G: Lipid Metabolism and Atherosclerosis. Stuttgart, FK Schattauer Verlag, 1982.
Bilheimer DW, Goldstein JL, Grundy SM, et al: Liver transplantation to provide low-density-lipoprotein receptors and lower plasma cholesterol in a child with homozygous familial hypercholesterolemia. N Engl J Med 311:1658, 1984.
Brown MS, Goldstein JL, Fredrickson DS: Familial type 3 hyperlipoproteinemia. *In*: Stanbury JB, Wyngaarden JB, Fredrickson DS, et al (eds): The Metabolic Basis of Inherited Disease. 5th ed. New York, McGraw-Hill, 1983, p 655.
The Dietary Management of Hyperlipoproteinemia. A Handbook for Physicians and Dietitians. NIH Publication No. 78–110, 1978.
The Framingham Study: An Epidemiologic Investigation of Cardiovascular Disease. NIH Publication No. 76–1083, 1976.
Frerichs RR, Srinavasan SR, Webber LS, et al: Serum cholesterol and triglyceride levels in 3,446 children from a biracial community. The Bogalusa heart study. Circulation 54:302, 1976.
Glueck CJ, Gartside P, Fallat RW, et al: Longevity syndromes: Familial hypo-beta- and familial hyperalphalipoproteinemia. J Lab Clin Med 88:941, 1976.
Goldstein JL, Brown MS: The low density lipoprotein pathway and its relation to atherosclerosis. Ann Rev Biochem 46:897, 1977.
Goldstein JL, Brown MS: Familial hypercholesterolemia. *In*: Stanbury JB, Wyngaarden JB, Fredrickson DS, et al (eds): The Metabolic Basis of Inherited Disease. 5th ed. New York, McGraw-Hill, 1983, p. 672.
Goldstein JL, Schrott HG, Hazzard WR, et al: Hyperlipidemia in coronary heart disease: genetic analysis of lipid levels in 176 families and delineation of a new inherited disorder, familial combined hyperlipidemia. J Clin Invest 52:1544, 1973.
Grundy SM: Hypertriglyceridemia: Mechanisms, clinical significance, and treatment. Med Clin North Am 66:519, 1982.
Havel RJ: Approach to the patient with hyperlipidemia. Med Clin North Am 66:319, 1982.
Kane JP, Malloy MJ: Treatment of hypercholesterolemia. Med Clin North Am 66:537, 1982.
Lipid Research Clinics Population Studies Data Book. Vol. 1, The Prevalence Study. NIH Publication No. 80–1527, 1980.
Lipid Research Clinics Program: The Lipid Research Clinics Coronary Primary Prevention Trial Results. I and II. JAMA 251:351, 365, 1984.
Malloy MJ, Kane JP: Hypolipidemia. Med Clin North Am 66:469, 1982.
Nikkilä EA: Familial lipoprotein lipase deficiency and related disorders of chylomicron metabolism. *In*: Stanbury JB, Wyngaarden JB, Fredrickson DS, et al (eds): The Metabolic Basis of Inherited Disease. 5th ed. New York, McGraw-Hill, 1983, p. 622.
Schaefer EJ: Clinical, biochemical, and genetic features in familial disorders of high density lipoprotein deficiency. Arteriosclerosis 4:303, 1984.

DEFECTS IN METABOLISM OF PURINES AND PYRIMIDINES

Purines and pyrimidines are heterocyclic nitrogen-containing compounds. Combinations of purines and pyrimidines with ribose or deoxyribose and with phosphate create nucleotides. Combined with ribose and phosphate (hence, ribonucleotide), purines and pyrimidines form the elements of ribonucleic acid (RNA); combined with deoxyribose and phosphate (deoxyribonucleotides), they form deoxyribonucleic acid (DNA). The ability to synthesize the purine ring de novo is virtually universal among living organisms. The final product of purine metabolism in man is uric acid.

Other than uric acid, the purines recognized to have clinical importance are adenine and guanine. The important pyrimidines are thymine, cytosine, and uracil. The importance of nucleotides as components of DNA rests on the genetic function of this material. RNA is of central importance in the regulation of protein synthesis and as a component of such important energy-producing compounds and nucleotide cofactors as ATP, UDPG, NAD and NADP, and others.

7.50 DISORDERS OF PURINE METABOLISM

Gout. The hallmark of gout is the elevation of serum uric acid concentration. This disease primarily affects adults and rarely occurs in children except those with type I glycogen storage disease (GSD I), in whom hyperuricemia routinely occurs and gouty arthritis and tophi appear in adolescence (Sec. 7.21.) When hyperuricemia and gout occur in childhood, they are almost always secondary to another disorder.

Elevations of uric acid concentration in serum can result from several general metabolic disturbances. Certain patients have an abnormally active production de novo of uric acid;

others have reduction in the renal clearance of uric acid; and some represent combinations of these two major factors.

At least 95% of gouty arthritis is seen in postpubertal males. In a very small group of patients, the activity of the enzyme hypoxanthine guanine phosphoribosyl transferase (Fig. 7–31) is reduced to only a few per cent of normal (a total deficiency leads to the Lesch-Nyhan syndrome). In another group of patients overproduction of uric acid and hyperuricemia can be traced to an abnormally high activity of the enzyme phosphoribosylpyrophosphate synthetase or PRPP synthetase (Fig. 7–32). In both of these situations, the increased availability of PRPP leads to an increase in the endogenous production of uric acid. Both enzymes are genetically transmitted as X-linked recessives. The increased availability of PRPP is the mechanism that also leads to hyperuricemia in type I glycogen storage disease; some of the reduction in uric acid clearance in GSD I may also be due to the hyperlactic acidemia, which reduces the renal clearance of uric acid.

Whether or not a patient with elevated levels of uric acid in serum develops gouty arthritis largely depends on the severity and duration of hyperuricemia.

Lesch-Nyhan Syndrome. Boys with this syndrome are usually normal at birth. The first abnormality consistently noted is a delay in motor development in the first few months of life. Later, extrapyramidal choreoathetoid movements appear, and hyperreflexia, ankle clonus, and spasticity of the legs develop. The most striking clinical abnormality is the dramatic, compulsive self-destructive behavior usually observed. Older children begin to bite and chew their fingers, lips, and buccal mucosa, leading to mutilation. It is not the result of inability to feel pain but of a compulsive urge that appears so

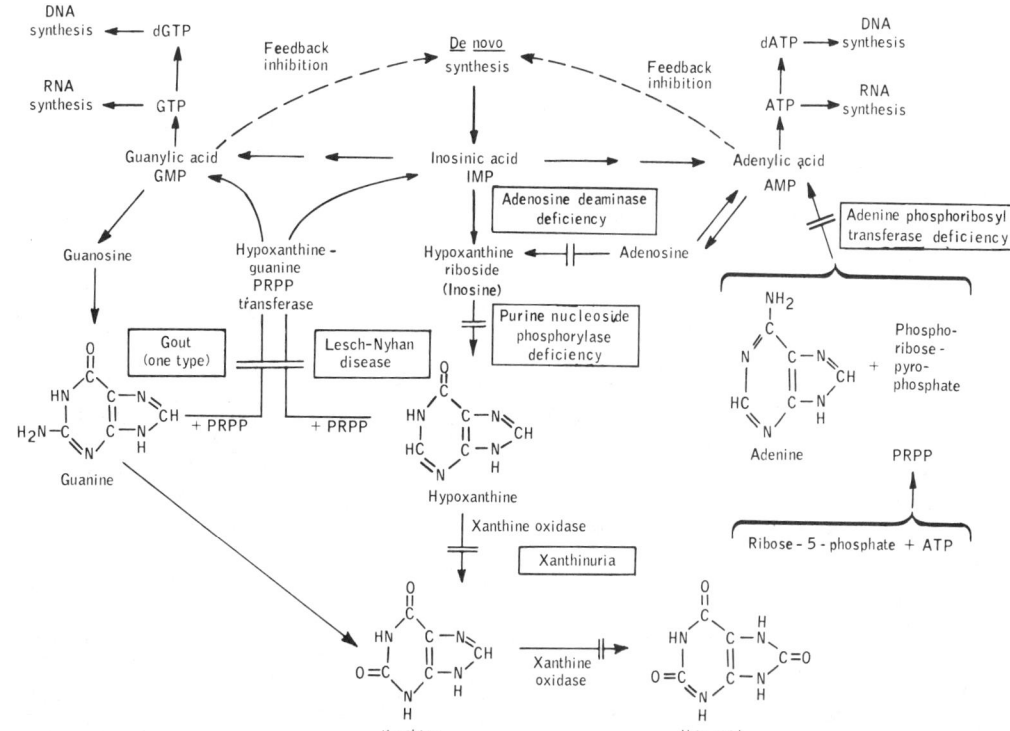

Figure 7–31. Pathways in purine metabolism and salvage.

irresistible that it is necessary to restrain the patients. Gouty tophi and gouty arthritis are also sometimes seen in older children with the Lesch-Nyhan syndrome. Tophi result from the accumulation of sodium urate crystals in subcutaneous and other tissues; they occur over the extensor surfaces of the elbows, knees, fingers and toes.

In the Lesch-Nyhan syndrome, serum uric acid concentrations are commonly in the range seen in the adult with gout (10–12 mg/dL); there are marked increases in the production of uric acid and in its urinary excretion. There is an almost total absence of hypoxanthine guanine phosphoribosyltransferase activity in many tissues, including erythrocytes and fibroblasts. This enzyme is important to the "purine salvage" pathway, through which hypoxanthine and xanthine can be converted to nucleotides, inosinic acid, and guanylic acid (Fig. 7–31). When this enzymatic pathway is not operative, PRPP synthetase activity increases and PRPP accumulates within

the cell, giving rise to accelerated purine production de novo and to excesses of uric acid. The salvage pathway may be important in the synthesis of nucleotides within the brain; when this pathway is inactive, the brain may be unable to synthesize required nucleotides.

This syndrome is transmitted as an X-linked condition. Fibroblasts cultured from biopsies of skin of mothers of patients with Lesch-Nyhan syndrome consist of 2 cell populations, 1 normal and 1 deficient in the crucial enzyme, lending support to the Lyon hypothesis (Sec. 6.4–6.5).

The introduction of cloned genes into patients with Lesch-Nyhan syndrome is currently being considered as an experimental, potentially curative treatment.

Other Abnormalities of Uric Acid Metabolism. Hyperuricemia is commonly encountered in situations of a marked increase in cell number and cell destruction, as in myeloproliferative disease. The excess of uric acid results from an

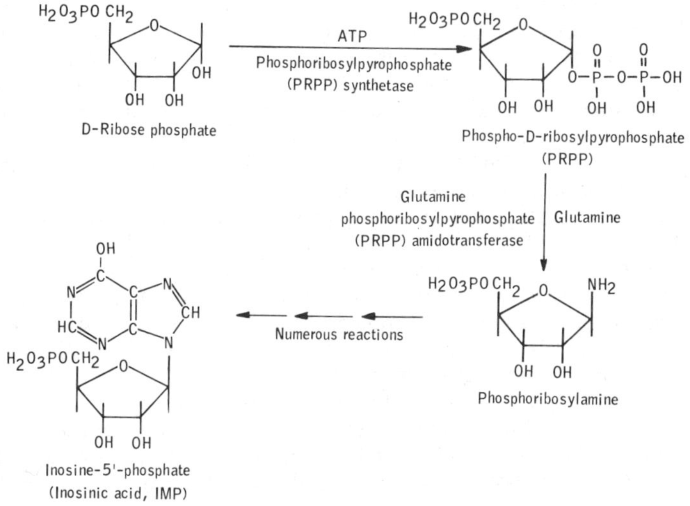

Figure 7–32. Early steps in the biosynthesis of the purine ring.

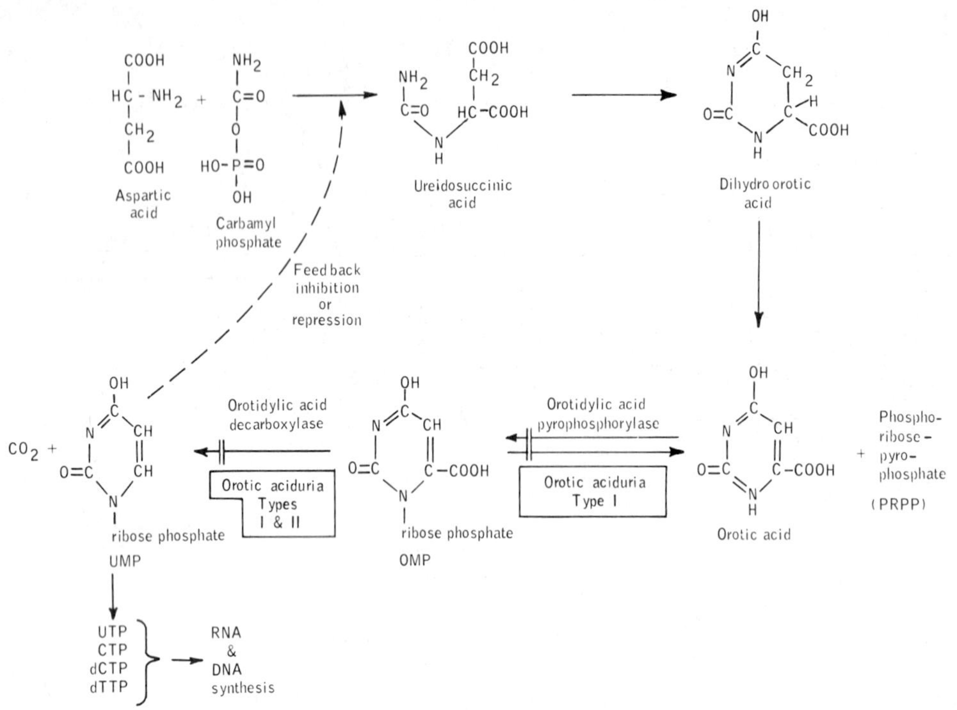

Figure 7-33. Pathways in pyrimidine biosynthesis.

increased intensity of degradation of nucleotides to purine end products (uric acid). In the treatment of acute leukemia or lymphoma masses, the sudden lysis of cells may provoke hyperuricemia and hyperuricosuria with clinical consequences (Sec. 16.3).

Hyperuricemia may occur in any condition in which renal clearance is reduced. When the serum concentrations of β-hydroxybutyrate and acetoacetate are increased, as in starvation and diabetic ketoacidosis, there are elevations of serum uric acid concentrations related to reduction in renal clearance. Commonly used drugs, such as salicylates, in low doses, may reduce renal clearance and produce hyperuricemia. Down syndrome patients regularly display modest hyperuricemia. All of these variables must be weighed in the interpretation of serum uric acid concentrations in children.

Hypouricemia due to an increase in renal clearance of uric acid occurs in proximal renal tubular diseases (e.g., Fanconi syndrome). In a clinically normal patient, hypouricemia has been caused by an isolated defect of renal tubular reabsorption of uric acid; the same defect is found in Dalmatian dogs. Hypouricemia is also a prominent feature of xanthinuria and nucleoside phosphorylase deficiency (see below).

Treatment of Hyperuricemia. Several approaches are used. The avoidance of foods high in purines (such as sweetbreads) is of modest benefit. Drugs that increase the renal clearance of uric acid are also recommended. Probenecid is effective in increasing uric acid clearance and may be used to treat hyperuricemia in patients with normal renal function. Allopurinol, an inhibitor of xanthine oxidase, is also widely used. In persons with no known enzymatic defect in purine biosynthesis, this drug reduces total purine production, increases the excretion of the oxypurines (xanthine and hypoxanthine), and reduces the excretion of uric acid. In Lesch-Nyhan syndrome, allopurinol treatment reduces uric acid concentrations (and ameliorates gouty arthritis and tophi); there is no effect on the severe neurologic problems.

For any patient with hyperuricosuria, whether as a result of increased synthesis de novo or of drug therapy, it is essential that high urine volumes be maintained and that urine pH be kept near neutrality (7.0). This can ordinarily be done effectively with a balanced mixture of salts, such as Polycitra, which is usually more effective than bicarbonate. The importance of adjusting the urine pH to 7.0 is illustrated by the fact that at pH 5.0 the solubility of uric acid is 15 mg/dL, whereas at pH 7.0 the solubility is 200 mg/dL.

The hyperuricemia associated with type I glycogen storage disease, like other significant hyperuricemias, should be treated; it does not respond to probenecid, but does respond appropriately to allopurinol.

Xanthinuria. Xanthine is the immediate precursor of uric acid. It is formed directly from certain purines, whereas hypoxanthine is an intermediary formed from others. The oxidations of hypoxanthine to xanthine and of xanthine to uric acid are mediated by xanthine oxidase, which is found in liver and intestinal mucosa (Fig. 7-31).

Xanthinuria is uncommon. Serum uric acid levels in affected persons are virtually undetectable (0.1-0.8 mg/dL). There are low levels of hypoxanthine and uric acid in both plasma and urine; the amount of uric acid in urine falls to 0 with a purine-free diet. Xanthine is even less soluble than uric acid in urine; accordingly, some patients with xanthinuria have had *urinary calculi* composed of pure xanthine. The stones are radiolucent, except that slight radiopacity was reported in one instance when the stone contained 5% calcium phosphate. Some patients with muscular pain after exertion were shown to have deposits of xanthine crystals in muscles. Jejunal biopsies of affected patients show no activity of xanthine oxidase toward xanthine and only about 5% of normal activity toward hypoxanthine. Xanthine stones have also been reported as a rare consequence of allopurinol administration. The enzymes xanthine oxidase and sulfite oxidase require molybdenum as a cofactor. A single patient has been recognized to have **molybdenum deficiency** and simultaneous deficiencies of xanthine oxidase and sulfite oxidase. All patients with xanthinuria should maintain a high fluid intake, dietary restriction of purines, and alkalinization of the urine. The solubility of xanthine in urine at pH 5.0 is 5 mg/dL, and at pH 7.0 it is 13 mg/dL.

Adenosine Deaminase Deficiency. In nearly half of patients with severe combined immunodeficiency (SCID), a deficiency of adenosine deaminase activity has been demonstrated (Sec. 10.22).

Nucleoside Phosphorylase Deficiency. Deficiencies of this enzyme are associated with marked deficiencies of cellular but normal humoral immunity (Sec. 10.22).

7.51 DISORDERS OF PYRIMIDINE METABOLISM

Orotic Aciduria. Orotic acid is an intermediate metabolite in the synthesis of pyrimidines. Orotic aciduria is a rare disorder of children, resulting from a block in the further metabolism of orotic acid. Affected children have megaloblastic anemia unresponsive to therapy with vitamin C, folic acid, or vitamin B_{12}; they excrete up to 1.5 g/24 hr of orotic acid and form orotic acid crystals in urine. Although these patients are retarded in their growth and development, the hematologic manifestations are the more dramatic clinical features, because vigorous synthesis of RNA and DNA is so necessary for normal hematopoiesis. Corticosteroid treatment may result in general improvement, but disappearance of abnormalities in the marrow or of the excretion of orotic acid occurs only when pyrimidine compounds found beyond the metabolic block are administered.

In most patients with orotic aciduria, orotidylic acid pyrophosphorylase and orotidylic acid decarboxylase are deficient (Fig. 7–33). A patient who lacked only the decarboxylase was clinically indistinguishable from patients with the more usual genotype. The absence of two sequential enzymes in most patients with orotic aciduria suggests that the enzymes share some common subunit. These enzyme deficiencies have been demonstrated in liver, leukocytes, erythrocytes, and fibroblasts grown in culture. Heterozygotes have approximately half the normal level of activities of both enzymes.

The administering of pyrimidine derivatives lowers the urinary excretion orotic acid. This effect indicates that enzymes in the pathway leading to orotic acid synthesis are under feedback inhibition control. The hematologic response is directly due to the provision for DNA and RNA synthesis of essential material that cannot be made de novo.

Orotic acid excretion is increased in the urine of children who have primary genetic defects in the urea cycle. These defects result from additional carbamyl phosphate (usually utilized in urea synthesis) that is shunted into de novo pyrimidine synthesis, leading to an apparent overproduction of orotic acid. Orotic aciduria is also seen in nucleoside phosphorylase deficiency.

R. RODNEY HOWELL

Willis R, Jolly DJ, Miller AD, et al: Partial phenotypic correction of human Lesch-Nyhan (hypoxanthine-guanine phosphoribosyltransferase–deficient) lymphoblasts with a transmissible retroviral vector. J Biol Chem 259:7842, 1984.
Zegers BJ, Stoop JW: Therapy in adenosine deaminase and purine nucleoside phosphorylase deficient patients. Clin Biochem 16:43, 1983.

OTHER DEFECTS OF ENZYMES AND PROTEINS

Some inborn errors of metabolism cannot be assigned naturally to systems, such as those involved in amino acid, carbohydrate, lipid, pigment, purine, or pyrimidine metabolism. These other defects involving the soluble proteins and formed elements of blood and certain proteins and enzymes of other organs or tissues will be discussed in the following sections.

The absence of any given protein in a specific individual or the presence of an abnormally migrating protein by electrophoretic and chromatographic techniques is prima-facie evidence for the existence of an inborn error of metabolism. Also, immunologic recognition systems depend upon the presence of a variety of cell surface macromolecules under genetic control, e.g., HLA antigens and the association of various markers with different diseases. Further, a large array of receptor proteins are found in and on cells that mediate hormonal action. Inborn errors of such protein moieties also occur.

7.52 DEFECTS IN PLASMA PROTEINS

Analbuminemia. Plasma albumin maintains the oncotic pressure of blood and serves as a vehicle for the transport of many normal blood constituents. A few persons have been observed in whom no circulating albumin cound be demonstrated. Some were asymptomatic; others exhibited only slight edema. The disorder may be genetic. Periodic administrations of albumin result in disappearance of edema, but usually no treatment is necessary. The lack of symptoms in analbuminemia may be the result of lifelong compensations in fluid dynamics that patients with such disorders as nephrosis or protein-losing enteropathy are unable to make.

Haptoglobin Deficiency. Haptoglobin is an α-2-globulin that binds free hemoglobin. There are numberous phenotypic variations (polymorphism) in the types of haptoglobins among normal persons, which are under genetic control. With severe hemolytic anemia, haptoglobin levels may be greatly decreased or absent. Healthy persons have been found who have no demonstrable circulating haptoglobin without apparent ill effect.

Abetalipoproteinemia. See Sec. 7.48.

Analphalipoproteinemia (Tangier Disease). See Sec. 7.47.

Absence of Transferrin. Transferrin, or siderophilin (a β-2 globulin), is a plasma protein that has a prominent role in the transport of iron. The only recorded instance of a congenital absence of transferrin at birth involved a physically retarded girl with hepatomegaly, splenomegaly, and anemia sufficiently severe to require multiple transfusions. The anemia did not respond to any treatment. Iron was absorbed from the intestinal tract and transported to the tissues. Erythrocytes were hypochromic, and the marrow contained many immature erythroblasts. Liver biopsy revealed cirrhosis and siderosis. Antibodies to transferrin developed after multiple transfusions. Sudden death at 7 yr of age was attributed to hemosiderosis. Both parents had lower than normal amounts of transferrin, suggesting autosomal recessive transmission.

C1 Esterase Inhibitor. See Sec. 10.26 and 10.28.

Complement Deficiencies. See Sec. 10.25–10.29.

α-Antitrypsin Protein Deficiency. See Sec. 12.79 and 13.87.

Transcobalamin II Deficiency. Two different serum proteins bind vitamin B_{12}. One of these, transcobalamin I (an α-globulin), has been reported deficient in two siblings without clinical or hematologic sequelae. Deficiency of the other protein, transcobalamin II (a β-globulin), was associated with severe megaloblastic anemia and neurologic manifestations in several infants. No abnormalities were found in reactions involving the coenzyme forms of vitamin B_{12}, homocysteine methyltransferase, and methylmalonyl CoA mutase (Sec. 7.7). Treatment consists of parenterally administering large doses of vitamin B_{12}.

7.53 DEFECTS IN PLASMA ENZYMES

Pseudocholinesterase. Pseudocholinesterase is found in plasma, liver, and neural tissue; its physiologic function is poorly understood.

Numerous presumably allelic forms of the altered enzyme are known, in some, enzyme activity is reduced or absent. Homozygotes for each form and mixed heterozygotes are known. About 1 in 25 persons is heterozygous for one or another of these defects.

The 1 person in 3000 who is homozygous for one of these genes is ordinarily asymptomatic. However, the enzyme participates in the destruction of a commonly used muscle relaxant, succinylcholine. Normally this drug is rapidly destroyed by pseudocholinesterase and therefore has a transient effect. Persons homoyzgous for mutant pseudocholinesterase degrade the drug very slowly or not at all and apnea results, lasting for hours. Artificial respiration with endotracheal intubation is required. The period of apnea can be shortened by transfusion with normal plasma.

Another genetic alteration of pseudocholinesterase has been described which leads to increased enzyme activity and hence to resistance to the pharmacologic effects of succinylcholine.

Lecithin-Cholesterol Acyltransferase Deficiency. See Sec. 7.49.

Carnosinase Deficiency. See Sec. 7.14.

γ-Glutamyl Transpeptidase Deficiency. A moderately retarded adult with increased levels of glutathione in blood and urine has been shown to have a deficiency of serum γ-glutamyl transpeptidase, which catalyzes the first step in the degradation of glutathione. There was no other abnormality in amino acid excretion. This serum enzyme produced in the liver appears to be under different genetic control from that synthesized in the renal tubule and intestine.

Hypophosphatasia. Several isoenzymes in plasma have alkaline phosphatase activity. The one presumably derived from bone is markedly low in homozygous individuals who excrete large amounts of phosphoethanolamine and have a defect of ossification leading to severe bone disease (Sec. 23.53).

Elevated Alkaline Phosphatase. Elevated serum alkaline phosphatase levels (2–10 times normal) usually indicate either liver or bone disease. However, increases (2–4 times normal) also occur in otherwise normal families owing to a genetic alteration.

7.54 DEFECTS OF PROTEINS IN OTHER TISSUES

Alcoholism. (Also see Sec. 9.4.) The physiologic response to ethanol varies from individual to individual and shows marked racial differences. A high percentage of Orientals who exhibit facial flush after the ingestion of alcohol and are very sensitive to its effects lack the low K_m variant of the enzyme aldehyde dehydrogenase. The levels of this cytoplasmic form of hepatic aldehyde dehydrogenase with the lower K_m for ethanol are much lower in alcoholics than in control individuals. It is not know whether this finding is cause or effect.

Many severely malnourished alcoholics develop Wernicke-Korsakoff syndrome as a result of low thiamine intake. Transketolase, one of a number of enzymes which requires thiamine pyrophosphate as a coenzyme, has a higher K_m for the cofactor in these patients than in normal controls. The other thiamine-requiring enzymes are unaffected. This may represent a genetic predisposition for thiamine dependency not manifest under good nutritional conditions.

Menkes Kinky Hair Syndrome. This sex-linked disorder is characterized by abnormal hair, growth retardation, progressive neurologic degeneration, and death in the first few years of life. Defective absorption of copper and decreased levels of ceruloplasmin and copper in plasma occur. If copper is administered intravenously to these patients, the synthesis of ceruloplasmin develops rapidly. Analysis of mitochondria from brain and muscle has revealed a diminished content of the copper-containing enzyme cytochrome oxidase (cytochrome a + a_3), which may be secondary to the defect in copper absorption. Fibroblasts cultured from patients with this disease consistently have elevated copper concentrations compared with normal fibroblasts.

Molybdenum Cofactor Deficiency. Sulfite oxidase deficiency (Sec. 7.5) and xanthinuria (Sec. 7.50) have been associated with ocular abnormalities (dislocated lenses, Brushfield spots, and nystagmus), neurologic findings (tonic-clonic seizures), and mental retardation. The defect is an inability to form the molybdenum-pterin–containing cofactor whose presence is required for the activity of both enzymes. Treatment consists of restricting sulfur-containing amino acids and administering allopurinol.

Myoglobin. Myoglobin, a heme protein found in muscle, is responsible for the intracellular transport of oxygen. Two variants of myoglobin have been identified, and the changes in amino acid sequence producing myoglobinopathies are analogous to the changes responsible for the hemoglobinopathies. Patients have been heterozygous for the normal and for the aberrant molecules. Neuromuscular diseases have not been found in these families.

Spectrophotometric analyses of myoglobin from a number of patients with various neuromuscular diseases have revealed consistent changes in those with the sex-linked form of pseudohypertrophic muscular dystrophy (Duchenne) and the persistence of fetal myoglobin in a patient with facioscapulohumeral dystrophy. Fetal myoblobin has also been found in a patient with recurrent myoglobinuria. The myoglobin isolated from patients with progressive spinal muscular atrophy and the limb-girdle type of muscular atrophy is normal spectrometrically. Myoglobinuria may also occur in a number of disorders of muscle metabolism such as deficient phosphorylase activity (Sec. 7.21), deficient phosphofructokinase activity (Sec. 7.19), deficient phosphoglycerate mutase activity (Sec. 7.19), deficient lactate dehydrogenase activity (Sec. 7.19), and absent carnitine palmityl transferase activity (see below).

X-Linked Ichthyosis. See Sec. 24.16 for discussion of steroid sulfatase deficiency.

Xeroderma Pigmentosum. See Sec. 24.14.

Dynein Arm Deficiency. The absence of this specific ATPase is discussed in Sec. 13.63.

Macular Corneal Dystrophy. This autosomal recessive condition results in progressive opacity of the cornea due to deposition of an abnormal keratan sulfate in the stromal layers. This keratan sulfate proteoglycan contains an excess of oligosaccharides and appears to be a precursor for normal corneal keratan sulfate proteoglycan. Thus, it is presumed that this disorder is due to an inborn error in which the enzyme that would normally "process" the keratan sulfate proteoglycan is absent or inactive. The presence of a precursor proteoglycan which has not been processed is thought to give rise to the opacity.

Receptor Proteins. Most, if not all, communications between cells, within the same organ, or across organ systems are mediated by specific proteins found on the surface of the cell receiving the message. An increasing number of inborn errors involving receptor proteins have been described. The receptor for low density lipoprotein (LDL) is an example (Sec. 7.39). Another example is the absence of functional receptor for the hormone vitamin D_3 which leads to vitamin D–dependent rickets type II (Sec. 23.46). One form of diabetes mellitus is due to a defect in the specific receptor for insulin (Sec. 20.1).

Pancreatic Enzyme Deficiencies. A number of patients have been described in whom malabsorption appears to result from a specific enzymopathy involving a pancreatic enzyme or proenzyme (Sec. 12.68). They have none of the pulmonary or electrolyte abnormalities of cystic fibrosis (Sec. 13.97).

A syndrome with inability to produce trypsin, lipase, and amylase in conjunction with hematologic evidence of bone marrow dysfunction has also been described (Sec. 12.68).

Lipase Deficiency. Congenital inability to form sufficient active pancreatic lipase leads to malabsorption of lipids and fatty (and sometimes malodorous) stools. Treatment with pancreatin is effective.

Trypsinogen Deficiency. Severe malnutrition, growth failure, and hypoproteinemic edema resembling kwashiorkor are associated with lack of the ability to synthesize pancreatic trypsinogen. As a result, chymotrypsin and carboxypeptidase activities are also low since these enzymes need to be formed from the corresponding proenzymes by trypsin activity. Treatment with a protein hydrolysate diet and exogenous pancreatic enzymes is recommended.

Amylase Deficiency. Less defined deficiencies of pancreatic amylase activity have been described in at least two children with malabsorption who did not have cystic fibrosis. One of the children also had reduced trypsin activity.

Intestinal Enterokinase Deficiency. Enterokinase, an enzyme secreted by the small intestine, initiates the reactions for the conversion of the pancreatic proenzymes to their active forms. Both the clinical findings in and recommended treatment for deficient enterokinase activity in children are identical to those described above for trypsinogen deficiency. Many if not all of the cases originally described as trypsinogen deficiency may be instances of enterokinase deficiency, with the lack of trypsin activity secondary to inability to form trypsin from trypsinogen.

Collagen Metabolism. Collagen refers to a group of fibrous proteins that hold the body together and constitute about one fourth of its total protein. Collagens are the major structural proteins of skin, tendons, cartilage, and bone. Collagen contains large amounts of glycine, hydroxylysine, and hydroxyproline. Although the primary structure of the various collagens is under genetic control, the formation of collagen from procollagen and post-translation hydroxylation of lysine and proline, as well as the addition of various carbohydrate side chains, is controlled by a number of specific enzymes. A growing number of disorders involve collagen metabolism at one stage or another; among these are the numerous variants of both osteogenesis imperfecta (Sec. 23.36) and Ehlers-Danlos syndrome (Sec. 24.17), and Marfan syndrome (Sec. 23.43).

Primary genetic defects in the coding for a particular collagen molecule (usually resulting from a deletion of a large segment of the molecule) are responsible for types I, II, and III *osteogenesis imperfecta* and for types IV and VII *Ehlers-Danlos syndrome*. A deficiency of the enzyme procollagen peptidase is the cause of type VII Ehlers-Danlos syndrome, while a deficiency of lysine hydroxylase has been shown to cause type VI. Excessive additions of mannose to collagen have been implicated in type III osteogenesis imperfecta. *Marfan syndrome* is known to be due to an abnormal crosslinking of collagen fibers, but the enzymatic deficiency is unknown. In type IX Ehlers-Danlos syndrome and in Menkes syndrome lysine oxidase activity is deficient, secondarily due to defective copper metabolism.

As alteration of the gene for type II collagen (insertion of a large segment of DNA) has also been demonstrated in a patient with achondroplasia, presumably leading to an abnormal collagen molecule and suggesting the autosomal dominant mode of inheritance.

Defects of Fatty Acid Degradation. The most commonly encountered organic acidemia is due to the production of

lactic acid (Sec. 7.20). Abnormal production of a number of other organic acids, such as methylmalonic, oxalic, β-hydroxy, β-methylglutaric, or α-methylacetoacetic, are each due to different defects in the degradation of a number of amino acids, (Sec. 7.6–7.8). Another group of patients excrete α, ω-dicarboxylic acids and ω-hydroxycarboxylic acids with between 6 and 10 carbon atoms each, as well as large amounts of glutaric acid (C-5). This group has been called *glutaric acidemia type II* to distinguish the defects from the glutaric acidemia resulting from defects in the further metabolism of lysine and tryptophan (Sec. 7.6 and 7.16). The defect in this group of patients is a deficiency of short and medium chain fatty acid acyl CoA dehydrogenase, an enzyme responsible for the first step in the normal β-oxidation of the fatty acids which lead to a shortening of the fatty acid by two carbon atoms. With deficient dehydrogenase activity an unusual ω-oxidation occurs, first forming an ω-hydroxy fatty acid then a dicarboxylic acid (Fig. 7–6).

Patients with **glutaric acidemia type II** are usually normal and present with episodic attacks of severe hypoglycemia (blood glucose <10 mg/dL). No ketosis is present, and response to administered glucose is rapid. Many of the patients have had siblings who have died in early childhood or infancy with similar attacks. After the elimination of other known causes of hypoglycemia it is usually found that large amounts of the unusual organic acids are excreted in the urine. Some of the patients have become hypoglycemic within 24 hr after the administration of a ketotic diet, although fasting for the same length of time was without clinical effect. The enzyme deficiency can be measured in cultured skin fibroblasts.

Two other patients have been described with a presumed but unproven defect in short chain fatty acid acyl CoA dehydrogenases. They had ketosis and hyperammonemia in addition to hypoglycemia and excreted not only the C-6 dicarboxylic acid but ethylmalonic acid as well. One patient was intolerant of oral medium chain triglycerides, and treatment consisted of a low fat diet.

Carnitine Metabolism. Carnitine, γ-trimethylamino-β-hydroxybutyric acid, is produced in the liver. It is required for the transport of long chain fatty acids across the inner mitochondrial membrane to the site for their subsequent catabolism to CO_2 or ketone bodies. Before a long chain fatty acid can be transported it must be attached to the carnitine by an enzyme, fatty acyl CoA carnitine transferase. A number of patients have been described who, due to dietary reasons or to some other underlying disease, are deficient in carnitine. Patients who have an organic acidemia due to a defect of fatty acid oxidation or of amino acid metabolism also become carnitine deficient as they excrete large amounts of the organic acid in question as the carnitine ester. Dietary carnitine deficiency can mimic nonketotic hypoglycemia and should be ruled out before this diagnosis is made. A smaller group of patients have an inborn error of metabolism.

Carnitine Palmityl Transferase Deficiency. This enzyme was markedly reduced in two brothers who, although otherwise normal, had repeated episodes of myoglobinuria; in one an acute episode of myoglobinuria resulted in renal failure.

Renal Tubular Defect for Carnitine Reabsorption. Children have presented with cardiomegaly as the principal sign of a renal tubular defect resulting in wastage of carnitine into the urine. They are markedly deficient in circulating carnitine. Dietary treatment with large amounts of carnitine (174 mg/kg/day) rapidly reversed the cardiomegaly and returned the children to good health, but without treatment death may occur.

Myopathic and Systemic Carnitine Deficiency. Other patients with a genetic disorder but without a demonstrated enzymatic defect fall into two categories. The first group exhibit symptoms involving only muscle, especially muscle weakness. Carnitine levels are normal in serum but low in muscle, and muscle enzymes are released into the blood. Such patients accumulate fat within the muscle fibers as a direct result of their inability to transport fatty acids into, and oxidize them in, the muscle mitochondria despite the presence of acyl CoA carnitine transferase and the enzymes of fatty acid oxidation. The second group of patients exhibit systemic deficiency of carnitine and may have central nervous system involvement. The disorder is severe, and about half the patients studied have died during an acute episode.

Two additional patients with what was thought to be recurrent Reye syndrome had systemic carnitine deficiency. A 3 yr old boy, whose brother had died in coma at the same age, had storage of neutral fat in muscle, liver, and nerve tissue. After 6 mo of treatment with carnitine his tissues no longer had lipid accumulation and his clinical condition was markedly improved. The second patient was an 11 mo old girl with muscle weakness, hypoglycemia, vomiting, and lethargy. Muscle biopsy revealed fatty infiltration and during an acute attack showed fatty degeneration, but another obtained when the patient was clinically well was normal. Therapy with oral carnitine for 18 mo did not raise muscle carnitine or improve muscle strength. A provocative 18 hr fast resulted in vomiting and lethargy. It is thought that a variety of defects in either the synthesis of carnitine or its transport into muscle cells may be responsible for these forms of the disorder.

Myoadenylate Deaminase Deficiency. Patients with muscle cramps, easy fatigability, and muscle pain upon exercise who lack adenylate deaminase in striated muscle have been described. Symptoms may first occur at any time from infancy to adulthood. The enzyme normally converts AMP to IMP (inosine-monophosphate) with the liberation of ammonia. The IMP formed is then normally recycled back to AMP. In the absence of AMP deaminase activity this cycle is broken and nucleotides are lost from the muscle cell, leading to impaired activity. Patients have no blood ammonia production upon ischemic forearm exercise, which distinguishes these patients from those with either McArdle disease (Sec. 7.21) or deficient muscle phosphoglycerate mutase or muscle lactic acid dehydrogenase (Sec. 7.19) who cannot produce lactic acid upon ischemic forearm exercise.

Uncoupling of Phosphorylation and Oxidation (Luft Disease). Adults with easy fatigability since childhood, who have high oxygen consumption and basal metabolic rates with completely normal thyroid function, have been demonstrated to have uncoupling or loose coupling of phosphorylate and oxidation in muscle mitochondria. This leads to heat production, but little ability to do work, similar to what occurs in hibernating mammals who have large deposits of brown fat containing many mitochondria. Newborn humans also have some brown fat, which is thought to function the same way and produce so-called "nonshivering" heat; the amount of brown fat in the human decreases with age. The genetic defect is presumed to be at the level of the as yet inadequately understood mitochondrial enzyme that captures the energy of the proton gradient during its synthesis of ATP. In one patient there was an increase in mitochondrial ATPase activity which was barely increased further by the uncoupling agent, 2,4-dinitrophenol; loss of calcium from the mitochondria was also demonstrated despite normal uptake from the cytosol.

Mitochondrial Myopathies. (See also Sec. 22.6.) Many patients with muscle weakness and lactic acidosis brought on by mild exercise do not have any of the disorders described either in Sec. 7.20 or immediately above. In many of these patients the muscle fibers appear "ragged red" on trichrome staining and abnormal muscle mitochondria are seen with electron microscopy. A variety of loci along the electron transport chain of the mitochondria have been implicated in different patients with pure mitochondrial myopathies as well as in patients with a variety of accompanying neurological disorders. These include the NADH–coenzyme Q reductase system, cytochrome b, cytochrome c oxidase, and mitochondrial ATPase, as well as some undefined steps in patients in whom all of the above have been shown to be normal. The range of clinical manifestations, even within a given biochemical variant, is wide. Some patients go for many years without any signs or symptoms, others become sick at an early age, and still others have been described with a form that is rapidly fatal in the neonatal period. The patients with mitochondrial myopathies may have partial or complete deficiencies limited to muscle or deficiencies with wide tissue distribution.

Succinyl-CoA, 3-Keto-Acid CoA-Transferase Deficiency. Acetoacetate and β-hydroxybutyrate cannot be further metabolized unless the acetoacetate is activated by the addition of a molecule of coenzyme A, which is donated by succinyl CoA via a specific transferase. Deficiency of this transferase is associated with severe ketoacidosis and death in infancy or early childhood. Consanguinity of some parents suggests the probability of autosomal recessive inheritance.

Acatalasia. Catalase is found in most tissues, including the erythrocytes. Persons with a decrease of catalase activity in all tissues, to less than 1% of normal, can be detected through the demonstration that blood placed in contact with hydrogen peroxide turns brown and does not produce the oxygen bubbles usually seen. The disorder is heterogeneous; some instances appear to be mutations of the controller gene. In all instances the mode of inheritance is autosomal recessive; the heterozygote can be detected by quantitative catalase assays. Of the two main types, the Japanese variants have oral gangrene (**Takahara disease**), whereas the Swiss variants are asymptomatic. A genetic strain of mice with acatalasia is known; catalase encapsulated in semipermeable membranes has been used successfully in their treatment.

Storage of Glutamyl Ribose-5-Phosphate. A mentally and physically retarded boy who died of renal failure at 8 yr of age had glutamyl ribose-5-phosphate stored in brain and kidney lysosomes. This compound is normally part of the linkage between histones and poly (ADP-ribose) and is thought to accumulate because of an X-linked deficiency of the enzyme ADP-ribose protein hydrolase.

Aspartylglycosaminuria. The compound 2-acetamido-1 (β-L-aspartamido)-1,2-dideoxyglucose (AADG) is a substituted hexose that forms one of the linkage points between the carbohydrate moiety and the amino acid groups of many glycoproteins. Large quantities of urinary AADG (as well as other compounds containing AADG) have been found in some patients with mental retardation, petit mal seizures, or manic-depressive psychosis. Other patients have had vacuolated lymphocytes, facial and osseous features similar to those of the mucopolysaccharidoses, hepatomegaly, and lenticular opacities. The defect is in the lack of the enzyme, normally demonstrable in seminal fluid, that hydrolyzes AADG to glucosamine and aspartic acid. The lysosomal enzyme is deficient in liver, brain, and spleen.

Acid Phosphatase Deficiencies. Two groups of patients have been reported with either decreased or absent activity of lysosomal acid phosphatase. Patients with partial activity of this phospholipid degrading enzyme have a clinical picture characterized by intermittent vomiting, hypotonia, lethargy, opisthotonos, terminal bleeding, and death within the 1st year of life. Patients with total deficiency exhibit the same symptoms and died in infancy. The enzyme involved is distinct from the normal acid phosphatase found in semen or elaborated by prostatic carcinoma.

True Cholinesterase. True cholinesterase, an enzyme essential for neural and muscular function, is also found in erythrocytes, where its function is unknown. There are no clinical manifestations associated with decreased erythrocyte cholinesterase activities. Deficiency of true cholinesterase at the neuromuscular end-plate may account for the defect in myotonia congenita (Sec. 22.6).

Syndromes with Impaired Leukocyte Function. See Sec. 10.36–10.40.

Zellweger syndrome. This autosomal recessive degenerative disease affects brain, kidney, and liver. The major findings are severe hypotonia and a peculiar facies with death usually occurring in the 1st year of life. The biochemical defect is the absence of peroxisomes and, consequently, of the enzymes that these originally contain. Affected patients have a decreased ability to synthesize various phospholipids such as phosphatidylethanolamase plasmalogen. One enzyme in particular, dihydroxyacetone phosphate acyltransferase, is found only in peroxisome and is very low in fibroblasts and leukocytes of patients with this disorder. This enzyme is necessary for the synthesis of ether lipids.

VICTOR H. AUERBACH

Blass JP, Gibson GE: Abnormality of a thiamine-requiring enzyme in patients with Wernicke-Korsakoff syndrome. N Engl J Med 297:1367, 1977.

Clark JB, Hayes DJ, Morgan-Hughes JA, et al: Mitochondrial myopathies: Disorders of the respiratory chain and oxidative phosphorylation. J Inher Metab Dis 7 (Suppl 1):62, 1984.

DiMauro S, Bonilla E, Lee CP, et al: Luft's disease. Further biochemical and ultrastructural studies of skeletal muscle in the second case. J Neurol Sci 27:217, 1976.

Engle AG, Rebouche CJ: Carnitine metabolism and inborn errors. J Inher Metab Dis 7(Suppl 1):38, 1984.

Gregersen N: Fatty acyl-CoA dehydrogenase deficiency: Enzyme measurement and studies on alteration stability. J Inher Metab Dis 7(Suppl 1):28, 1984.

Heymans HSA, Schutgens RBH, Tan R, et al: Severe plasmalogen deficiency in tissues of infants without peroxisomes (Zellweger syndrome). Nature 306:69, 1983.

Mantagos S, Genel M, Tanaka K: Ethylmalonic-adipic aciduria. In vivo and in vitro studies indicating deficiency of activities of multiple acyl-CoA dehydrogenases. J Clin Invest 64:1580, 1979.

Pike JW, Dokoh S, Haussler MR, et al: Vitamin D_3-resistant fibroblasts have immunoassayable 1,25-dihydroxyvitamin D_3 receptors. Science 224:879, 1984.

Prockop DJ, Kivirikko KI: Heritable diseases of collagen. N Engl J Med 311:376, 1984.

Rhead WJ, Amendt BA, Fritchman KS, et al: Dicarboxylic aciduria: Deficient [1-14C] octanoate oxidation and medium-chain acyl-CoA dehydrogenase in fibroblasts. Science 221:73, 1983.

Strom CM: Achondroplasia due to DNA insertion into the type II collagen gene. Pediatr Res 18:226A, 1984.

Thoene J, Wolf B: Biotinidase deficiency in juvenile multiple carboxylase deficiency. Lancet 2:398, 1983.

Waber LJ, Valle D, Neill C, et al: Carnitine deficiency presenting as familial cardiomyopathy: A treatable defect in carnitine transport. J Pediatr 101:700, 1982.

Williams JC, Butler IT, Rosenberg HS, et al: Progressive neurologic deterioration and renal failure due to storage of glutamyl-ribose-5-phosphate. N Engl J Med 311:152, 1984.

DEFECTS IN HEME PIGMENT METABOLISM

This section describes defects of iron and heme pigments. The defects involving melanin and bilirubin are discussed elsewhere (Sec. 7.3, 8.44, and 12.51).

7.55 THE PORPHYRIAS

This group of syndromes is characterized biochemically by errors in pyrrole metabolism and clinically by photodermatitis and visceral and neuropsychiatric complaints. Incidence is estimated 1.30,000 in the general population. Table 7–12 classifies them according to the organ system in which the error in metabolism is localized: *erythropoietic* and *hepatic* forms are recognized. Most of the porphyrias have a dominant mode of inheritance. Family studies and close surveillance through adolescence to identify cases in the latent stage are essential, since most deaths occur during the late adolescent and early adult years and are attributable to delays in diagnosis that may lead to inappropriate and harmful therapy. Porphyrins should be determined in both urine and stool in all members; in cases of photosensitivity, measurements of erythrocyte protoporphyrin are also necessary. With early diagnosis, proper fluid and dietary therapy, and avoidance of contraindicated drugs, the prognosis for survival and symptomatic relief during acute visceral attacks is good. Enzyme diagnosis using blood, leukocytes, or skin is possible in most of the heritable forms of porphyria.

Relation of Abnormal Heme Biosynthesis to Disease States. Heme is the prosthetic group of hemoglobin, myoglobin, catalase, peroxidase, and the cytochromes (including P450). Synthesis of heme is regulated by negative feedback control. It is formed via the metabolic pathway shown in Figure 7–34, which is common to all mammalian cells, each cell synthesizing its own heme for the formation of its own particular hemoproteins. The initial step, formation of δ-aminolevulinic acid (ALA),* is mediated by ALA synthase (Fig. 7–34). This mitochondrial enzyme is inductible, and its availability is rate-limiting for the entire process.

*See Table 7–13 for key to abbreviations used in this section.

Table 7–12. The Porphyrias

Hepatic Porphyrias
Acute intermittent porphyria (AIP, Swedish genetic porphyria)
Porphyria variegata (PV, South African genetic porphyria)
Hereditary coproporphyria (HCP)
The cutaneous porphyrias (PCT, porphyria cutanea tarda)
Hereditary types
Acquired (but possible genetic predisposition associated with alcoholism, etc.)
Toxic (hexachlorobenzene-induced)

Erythropoietic Porphyrias
Protoporphyria (P)
Congenital erythropoietic porphyria (CEP)

Four basic porphyrin isomers are known and are designated as types I, II, III, and IV. Mammalian hemoproteins only contain type III porphyrin isomers. Protoporphyrin (PROTO) 9 is a type III isomer. Infinitesimal quantities of type I isomers are formed as byproducts of heme synthesis.

The basic genetic defects in the dominantly inherited forms of *hepatic porphyria* associated with neurovisceral manifestations are partial deficiencies (approximately 50%) of porphobilinogen deaminase in *acute intermittent porphyria* (AIP), coproporphyrinogen oxidase in *hereditary coproporphyria* (HCP), and *protoporphyrinogen oxidase* in *porphyria variegata* (PV). These deficiencies are found in all latent cases, but alone they are not associated with neurovisceral attacks. Table 7–13 shows characteristic pyrrole excretion patterns during exacerbation and remission of symptoms in the various porphyrias. About 90% of AIP heterozygotes are symptom-free and may never show increased excretion of ALA and PBG in urine. Nevertheless, they are thought to be at risk for clinical attacks if exposed to certain drugs and other factors known to exacerbate hepatic porphyrias. Table 7–14 contains a partial list of porphyria-inducing substances. Clinical expression is uniformly associated with increased activity of hepatic ALA

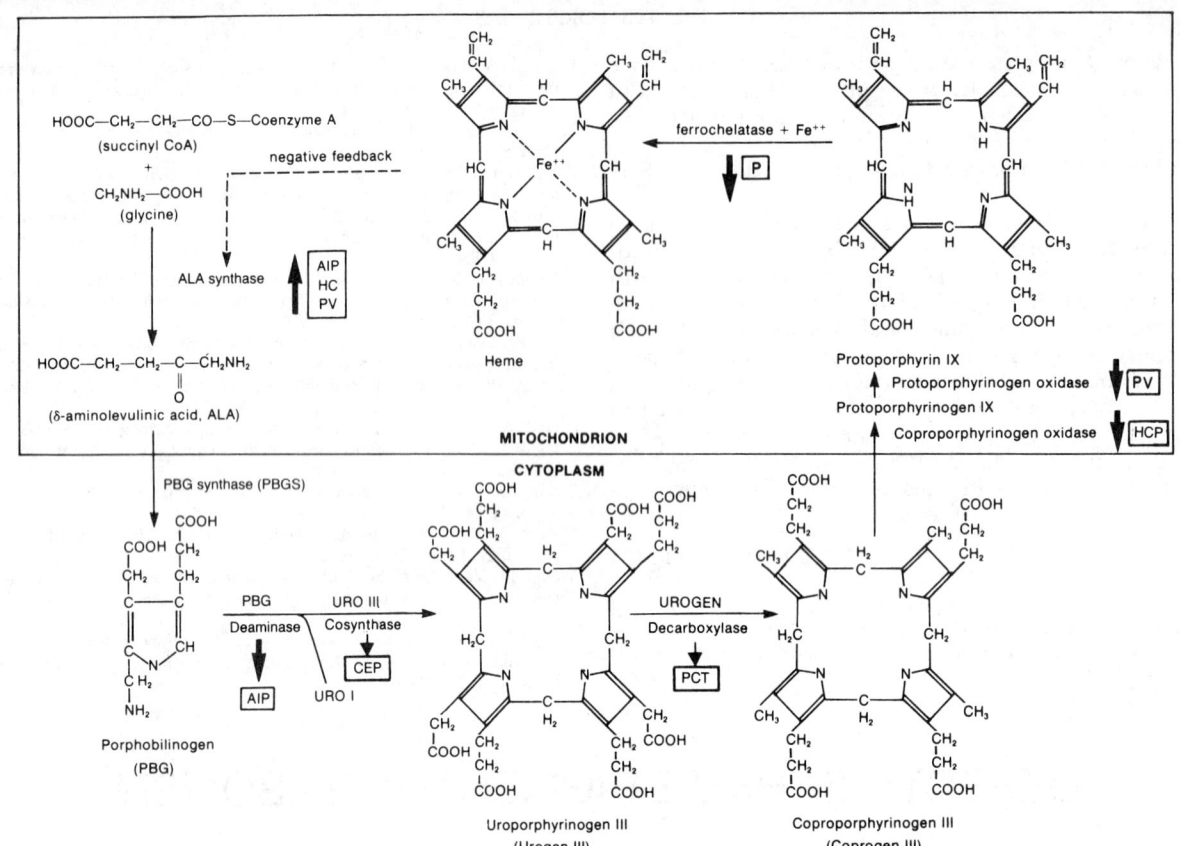

Figure 7–34. Intracellular organization of biosynthesis of heme. The initial and final steps in heme synthesis occur within the mitochondria. ALA is released in the cytoplasm. The metabolites formed in the cytoplasm are those found in the plasma and urine. ALA synthase is the rate-limiting enzyme. Only the fully reduced porphyrin intermediates UROGEN III and coproporphyrinogen (COPROGEN) III are utilized for heme formation. These colorless, unstable substances do not exhibit fluorescence. Oxidation stabilizes porphyrin molecules and renders them fluorescent. Those portions of UROGEN and COPROGEN not utilized for heme synthesis are oxidized to UROs I and III and COPROs I and III, and it is in this form that these porphyrins are usually detected in the tissues and excreta. PBG and ALA are also colorless and do not fluoresce; they are measured by chemical methods. Lead (Pb) inhibits PBGS and ferrochelatase (see Chapter 28).

Table 7–13. Clinical Syndromes and Pyrrole* Excretion Patterns in Heritable Forms of Porphyria

		Hepatic Porphyrias				Erythropoietic Porphyrias	
		Acute Intermittent Porphyria	Porphyria Variegata	"Porphyria Cutanea Tarda"	Hereditary Coproporphyria	Protoporphyria†	Congenital Erythropoietic Porphyria
Transmission		——————— Autosomal dominant ———————					Recessive
Onset of clinical manifestations		—— Puberty or later ——		—— Early childhood ——			Infancy
Acute visceral and neurologic attacks‡		Present	Present	Present	Present	Absent	Absent
Cutaneous lesions		Absent	Present	Present	?Absent	Present	Present
Pyrrole excretion§ during acute visceral and neurologic attacks	*Urine*						
	ALA, PBG¶	+ + + +	+ + + +	±	+ to + +		
	URO, COPRO	± to + + +	± to + + +	±	+ to + +		
	Feces						
	COPRO,	0	+ + + +	+ + + +	+ + + +		
	PROTO	0	+ + + +	+ + +	±		
Pyrrole excretion§ during remission of visceral and neurologic symptoms	*Urine*						
	ALA, PBG	±	0	±	0	0	0
	URO, COPRO	±	0	0	±	0	+ + + +
	Feces						
	COPRO,	0	+ + + +	+ + + +	+ + + +	±	+ + +
	PROTO	0	+ + + +	+ + + +	0	+ + +	±

*ALA is strictly a heme precursor and not a pyrrole. PBG is a monopyrrole. URO, COPRO and PROTO are tetrapyrroles.
†Erythrocyte PROTO grossly increased in protoporphyria.
‡In each group rare cases have been observed before puberty.
§Increased URO in feces found in some cases of each group.

¶ALA — δ-aminolevulinic acid.
PBG — porphobilinogen.
UROGEN — uroporphyrinogen.
URO — uroporphyrin.
COPROGEN — coproporphyrinogen.
COPRO — coproporphyrin.
PROTO — protoporphyrin.

Table 7–14. Partial List of Agents Used to Induce Chemical Hepatic Porphyria in Animals

Chemicals
Allylisopropylacetamide
Hexachlorobenzene
3,5-dicarbethoxy-1,4-dihydrocollidine

Drugs

Glutethamide	Griseofulvin
Barbiturates	Chloroquine
Sulfonamides	Diphenylhydantoin
Valproic acid	Tolbutamide

Endogenous Sex Steroids
Potent porphyrin-inducing activity

C-19 Steroids	C-21 Steroids
Etiocholanolone	Pregnanediol
Etiocholandiol	Pregnanolone
Etiocholandione	11-Ketopregnanolone
Etiocholanone-17	17-OH Pregnanolone

Weak porphyrin-inducing activity

Testosterone	Estrone
Progesterone	Estriol
Estradiol	

*For a more complete list of unsafe, potentially unsafe, probably safe, and safe drugs for patients with AIP, HCP and PV see the following reference:
Kappas A, Sassa S, Anderson KE: The porphyrias. In: Stanbury JB, Wyngaarden JB, Fredrickson DS, et al (eds): The Metabolic Basis of Inherited Disease. 5th ed. New York, McGraw-Hill, 1983, p 1344.

synthase, which can be induced in AIP, HCT, and PV by steroid hormones, certain of their metabolites, drugs (particularly those requiring hepatic P450 for their metabolism), and inadequate nutritional intake of carbohydrates and protein. With regard to endogenous steroid metabolism, the majority of patients with clinically manifest AIP have shown a 50% reduction in hepatic 5-α steroid reductase, which favors compensatory formation of 5-β steroid metabolites. Many 5-β steroid metabolites are more potent inducers of ALA synthase than their corresponding 5-α epimers. The same subtle alteration in hepatic steroid metabolism has also been demonstrated in HCP and PV. Glucuronide conjugates of porphyrin-inducing drugs and steroid metabolites do not induce ALA synthase, emphasizing the importance of maintaining good liver function. The hypertension and tachycardia seen in neurovisceral attacks are associated with increased levels of catecholamines. The roles of sex steroid metabolites as potent inducers of hepatic porphyria may explain why the onset of neurovisceral symptoms is so regularly delayed until after puberty. Reduced activity of hepatic tryptophan pyrrolase, a heme dependent enzyme, may play an important role in neurovisceral attacks.

There are two *erythropoietic porphyrias*. The basic genetic defect in *congenital erythropoietic porphyria* (CEP) is a partial deficiency of uroporphyrinogen III cosynthase, which results in excessive formation of URO I (Fig. 7–34). Atypical cases of CEP are now recognized. URO I accumulates within the nuclei of defective erythroblasts, diffuses into the circulation, is deposited in various tissues, including teeth and bone, and is excreted in the urine as a mixture of URO I and coproporphyrin (COPRO) I, with URO I predominant.

Protoporphyria is characterized by excessive amounts of free PROTO 9 in marrow reticulocytes and circulating erythrocytes, in which it has a short half-life and readily diffuses into plasma, skin, and liver. In iron deficiency and lead poisoning, which do not involve photosensitivity, the metalloporphyrin zinc protoporphyrin is found in erythrocytes rather than

"free" PROTO 9. Activity of ferrochelatase is diminished in erythroid cells in the bone marrow and possibly in liver in *protoporphyria*. This results in substantial accumulation of PROTO 9 in circulating erythrocytes and liver. Excess PROTO 9 is excreted in feces but not in urine. There is a reciprocal relationship between caloric intake and PROTO excretion, similar to the "glucose effect" found in the hepatic porphyrias (see below).

The urinary excretion of PBG and ALA does not normally exceed 3 mg/day. The qualitative Hoesch test for PBG (see below) is positive only with a pathologic excess of PBG. Porphyrins normally appear in the excreta in very small amounts: fecal COPRO and PROTO should not exceed 100 μg/g of dry feces/day; COPRO appears in urine at a rate of 2.2 μg/kg (1 μg/lb) of body weight/day. Infections and accelerated erythropoiesis cause a 2- to 3-fold increase in urinary COPRO; hepatitis (infectious and toxic), a 10- to 40-fold increase in urinary COPRO; and lead intoxication, a 10- to 40-fold increase in both ALA and COPRO in urine. Porphyria may cause up to 1000-fold increases in pyrrole excretion. In acquired porphyria COPRO always exceeds URO in urine, but in the heritable forms the quantity of URO in urine usually exceeds COPRO if both are present. Increased fecal porphyrins virtually always indicate a heritable form of porphyria.

Relation of Metabolic Errors to Clinical Manifestations. *Photosensitizing Effects of Porphyrins.* Some but not all the skin lesions of both erythropoietic and certain hepatic porphyrias are due to the photosensitizing effect of URO. Erythema, edema, and vesiculation of the exposed skin result when persons with increased uroporphyrinemia are irradiated with a combination of near ultraviolet (400 nm) and infrared (2600 nm) monochromatic lights. Protoporphyria is apparently unique among photosensitive dermatitides in that very brief exposure to sunlight can quickly cause intense pain and sensation of heat in the exposed skin. Repeated exposures to near ultraviolet light lead to urticarial and chronic eczematoid lesions. All the heme precursors (Fig. 7–34) have been injected into both healthy and porphyric human subjects without demonstrable adverse effect other than photosensitization.

Toxic and Experimental Hepatic Porphyria. Some drugs and chemicals used experimentally to produce hepatic porphyria (Table 7–14) affect P450, an inductable hemoprotein with short biologic half-life and rapid turnover rate. Phenobarbital, for example, increases the requirement for P450; on the other hand, allylisopropylacetamide increases its destruction. Such findings suggest that patients with heritable hepatic forms of porphyria (AIP, HCP, PV) may not be able to adjust the metabolism of P450 to the effects of the drugs, insecticides, other chemicals, and nutritional and hormonal factors.

Diagnosis and Management of the Porphyrias. *Clinical Manifestations.* Though the porphyrias are generally genetically determined and the basic metabolic errors are present from birth, clinical symptoms are rare before puberty in the hepatic forms. Three groups of clinical manifestations are recognized: cutaneous, visceral, and neuropsychiatric. Their onset is insidious, but once they occur, the complaints tend to run an undulating course throughout the remainder of the patient's life. The principal clinical syndromes and patterns of pyrrole excretion encountered in the porphyrias are summarized in Table 7–13.

Acute exacerbations of *dermal lesions* occur with exposure to sunlight. Visceral and neurologic complaints, which almost invariably occur together, may be precipitated by infection, menstruation, pregnancy, alcohol, barbiturates, and other agents (Table 7–14). The skin lesions are bothersome and may be disfiguring, but the acute visceral and neurologic problems threaten life. The relative frequency of various abnormal clinical findings encountered during an acute attack are shown in Figures 7–35 and 7–36; none are pathognomonic. Early diagnosis depends upon recognizing the sequence in which the clinical manifestations appear, intensify, and abate, and upon demonstrating excess pyrroles in the excreta. Colicky abdominal pain and varied neuropsychiatric symptoms are the usual presenting complaints. Enzymatic assays must substantiate the diagnosis.

Colicky abdominal pain, the initial symptom of an acute attack in most patients, is most frequently in the epigastrium or right iliac fossa but may be located anywhere in the abdomen or pelvis. There is considerable variation in its intensity; the pain tends to worsen in an undulating manner over a period of days. Severe colic may persist for hours, often causing the patient to writhe about or assume bizarre positions in bed. Vomiting and constipation develop shortly in all but the mildest attacks. Examination of the abdomen and pelvis reveals minimal signs, which seem insignificant compared with the patient's pain. Diffuse abdominal tenderness is usually present, but does not localize; rigidity and muscle spasm are rare. Leukocytosis and fever are often present. The acute visceral pain of porphyria has been confused with virtually every acute surgical condition of the abdomen, various painful gynecologic disorders, and "hysteria." In the absence of other features and objective findings characteristic of these other conditions, the presence of tachycardia and hypertension makes porphyria a likely diagnosis.

Pain, weakness, and paresthesia in back and limb muscles uncommonly occur as presenting complaints in the absence of abdominal pain. *Personality changes* are observed in most patients suffering from visceral attacks, but they are rarely the predominating features. Patients are variously described as depressed, nervous, hysterical, lachrymose, or "peculiar." These traits wax and wane with the severity of the pain. In severe colic, mental confusion, hallucinations, and disorientation are often present.

After the patient with acute intermittent porphyria or porphyria variegata has had an exacerbation characterized by abdominal pain, vomiting, constipation, tachycardia, and, in more severe cases, hypertension, the end of the attack may often be heralded by the return of blood pressure, pulse and weight to normal.

The urine is usually colorless at first, although PBG is always present in high concentration and is diagnostic. If the

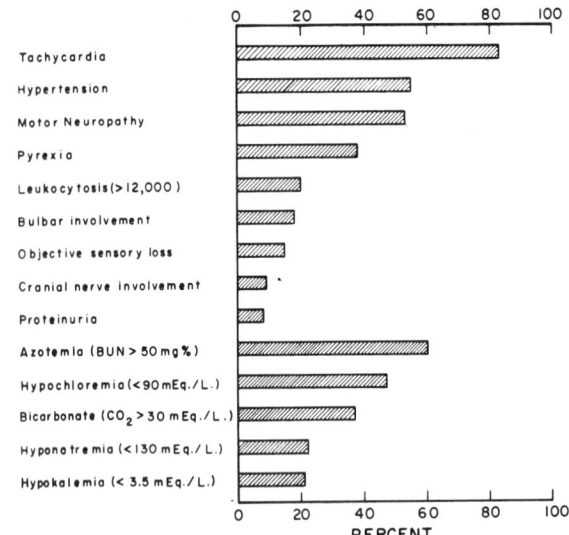

Figure 7–36. The acute attack of porphyria—relative frequency of signs and pertinent laboratory findings. (Adapted from Eales L: S Afr J Lab Clin Med 9:151, 1963.)

attack progresses, and especially if barbiturates are given, the urine usually becomes red, increasing motor restlessness is noted, and neurologic manifestations, rarely present initially, soon appear. These neurologic manifestations take the form of unpredictable, spotty weakness or paralysis, with diminished or absent tendon reflexes, and pain and tenderness in the involved muscle groups. These neurologic signs are attributable to patchy demyelination of peripheral nerves. Muscle paralysis is an ominous sign. Ill-advised abdominal or pelvic surgery may be quickly followed by catastrophic paralysis and coma. Weakness and paralysis may persist for months after the other features of an acute attack have subsided. Death, when it occurs, usually results from quadriparesis or respiratory failure.

A profound disturbance in water and electrolyte homeostasis occurs with severe attacks of porphyria. The serum is hypotonic, with reduced concentrations of sodium and chloride (Fig. 7–36). The urine is hypertonic, in part because of excessive loss of sodium, which is attributed to inappropriate secretion of antidiuretic hormone. The severity of neurologic injury may be related to the degree of hyonatremia. Hypocalcemia and hypomagnesemia may occur with or without tetany.

Burgundy red urine in the porphyric patient, due to the presence of URO, is a constant finding in congenital erythropoietic porphyria and a frequent finding in patients with cutaneous manifestations of hepatic porphyria.

A variety of *dermal lesions* occur in porphyria. Exposure to sunlight produces vesicles, bullae, and edema on the exposed skin. These photosensitive lesions are prone to secondary infection and heal slowly, with chronic scars which become hyperpigmented. In some patients such lesions may also follow minor mechanical trauma and exposure to indoor sources of ultraviolet light. Macules, papules, eczematous plaques, and urticaria are also seen.

Nearly all patients with cutaneous forms of porphyria eventually have hypertrichosis and a violaceous hue to their skin. These changes develop insidiously over the years and are most prominent on the exposed parts of the body.

Differential Diagnosis. Porphyria must be included in the differential diagnosis of essential hypertension, hyperthyroidism, painful gynecologic disorders, "hysteria," psychosis, all surgical conditions of the abdomen, lead poisoning, and

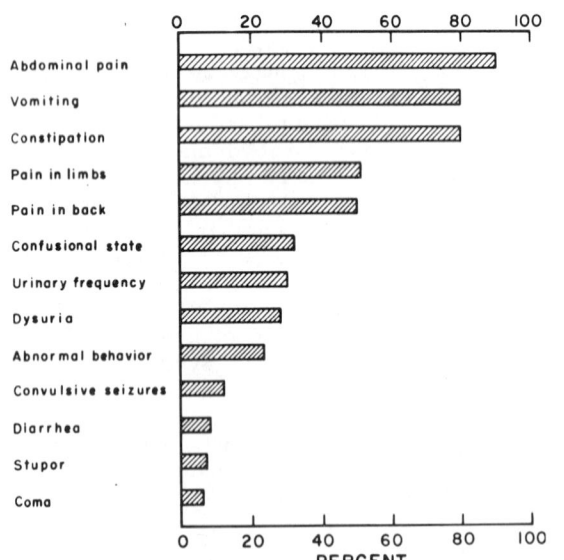

Figure 7–35. The acute attack of porphyria—relative frequency of symptoms. (Adapted from Eales L: S Afr J Lab Clin Med 9:151, 1963.)

hereditary tyrosinemia. Whenever a diagnosis of such surgical conditions as ulcer, gallbladder disease, or appendicitis cannot be made with confidence, a Hoesch test for PBG should be done prior to surgical exploration. Cutaneous porphyria should be included in the differential diagnosis of photosensitive dermatitides.

Laboratory Diagnosis. Accurate diagnosis requires examination of both urine and feces, and, in the case of erythropoietic protoporphyria, of blood (Table 7–13). The excreta of patients and their relatives must be examined to establish the type of pedigree and to identify latent cases. When possible, enzymatic diagnosis should be carried out in all family members. In the hepatic porphyrias, pyrrole excretion patterns may vary according to the presence or absence of visceral symptoms. Porphyrin excretion may be increased 1000-fold or more over the normal values. The red color imparted to urine by URO must be distinguished from that due to urates, bile, anthrocyanin (from beets), melanin, eosin, hemoglobin, or myoglobin.

The Hoesch test for PBG is simple, specific, and virtually always positive in acute visceral attacks. The test can be performed at the bedside as follows:

To 1 mL of Hoesch reagent (2 g of *p*-dimethylaminobenzaldehyde in 100 ml of 6 N hydrochloric acid) add 1–2 drops of *freshly voided* urine. An instantaneous cherry-red color at the top of the solution, which spreads throughout the solution on brief agitation, is specific for abnormally high amounts of porphobilinogen (PBG). False-positive results due to urobilinogen do not occur. Hoesch reagent is stable for 9 mo.

Newer simplified methods for measuring porphyrins in blood (primarily PROTO) should facilitate the clinical diagnosis of protoporphyria and possibly of other porphyrias associated with photosensitive dermatitis.

Treatment. Disturbances in water and electrolyte homeostasis are not usually seen in mild attacks, but they should be anticipated and the patient treated expectantly. When profound disturbances are present, restricting water and carefully replacing the sodium deficit may result in dramatic clinical improvement. Blood gases should be routinely monitored. Poor ventilation in depressed patients and respiratory paralysis may occur and require cardiopulmonary assistance. The infusion of hemin* to repress ALA synthase is associated with a dramatic clinical improvement and may be lifesaving in severe acute attacks. This drug is limited in availability and is usually reserved for severe acute cases in which glucose administration is not associated with very prompt improvement.

Because many chemical agents are capable of inducing porphyria, drug therapy must be approached with extreme caution. Pain and restlessness can be controlled with morphine and chloral hydrate. Cortisone and chlorpromazine may be beneficial in some cases, without obvious effect in others, and deleterious in a few. Adequate caloric and nitrogen intakes should be restored as rapidly as possible.

Successful long-term management requires careful control of infections and absolute avoidance of alcohol and of the drugs listed in Table 7–14. A calorically adequate diet high in carbohydrate content, adequate in protein, and low in fat is beneficial. Many patients fear precipitating colicky episodes and indulge in food fads. In some women, attacks are clearly related to the menstrual cycle; some have been treated with ovulatory suppressants, androgens, and even oophorectomy, with apparent beneficial results. Oral contraceptives in the

lowest effective dosage have been beneficial in some but not all cases of acute intermittent porphyria; they are contraindicated in pedigrees with dermal symptoms. A new approach using the long-acting agonist of luteinizing hormone–releasing hormone may prevent cyclical attacks of AIP associated with the menstrual cycle. Persons with latent or manifest hepatic porphyria should wear "Medic Alert" bracelets.

The cutaneous lesions are usually satisfactorily managed by avoiding excessive exposure to sunlight. When this is inadequate, *red veterinary petrolatum* applied to the skin may be beneficial. This ointment protects the skin from radiation in the near ultraviolet zone; the usual commercial sunscreens do not.

Infants of mothers with hepatic porphyria may have increased pyrrole excretion during the neonatal period; this *passive porphyria* is not associated with any symptoms. The infant's excretion of pyrroles soon returns to normal.

Acquired Hepatic Porphyria

The acquired forms of hepatic porphyria are clinically indistinguishable from the hereditary cutaneous syndromes (Table 7–13). Visceral manifestations are minimal or absent, and dermal features are usually less severe in the acquired disease, often being limited to hyperpigmentation and hypertrichosis. Acquired porphyria may occur as a rare complication of chronic alcoholism, cirrhosis, tumors involving the liver, and such systemic diseases as Hodgkin disease, disseminated lupus, and leukemia. Red urine due to the presence of URO is usually the clue leading to diagnosis.

Variants of Genetic Porphyria

Congenital erythropoietic porphyria is one of the rarest inborn errors of metabolism. Vastly increased amounts of URO I are found in bone marrow, circulating erythrocytes, plasma, urine, and feces. Lesser amounts of COPRO I are also found in the excreta. The excretion of other pyrroles is normal. The accumulation of URO I in the tissues (including the teeth) and the associated hemolytic anemia account for all the clinical manifestations of this disease. The photodermatitis of this disease is devastating, often causing severe permanent disfigurement. Splenomegaly results from the hemolytic anemia; splenectomy is beneficial in some cases. The excretion of urine that is burgundy red as passed, or becomes so upon exposure to light, begins at birth or shortly thereafter and continues for life.

Protoporphyria begins during childhood and continues through adult life. Symptoms that occur are pain, sensation of heat, and, following exposure to sunlight, two types of skin lesions, (1) an urticarial response that resolves without chronic dermal changes and (2) erythema and edema followed by an eczematous eruption on the exposed parts. This eczematous eruption is chronic rather than recurrent and leaves considerable scarring. These patients also have dull, opaque fingernails without lunulae. Increased amounts of PROTO 9 are always found in erythrocytes, and usually in feces.

Though the major symptoms are due to photosensitivity, a more important prognostic factor may be slowly progressive liver disease, culminating in cirrhosis and hepatic failure. Iron deficiency and other conditions stimulating erythropoiesis should be prevented, good nutrition maintained, hepatic function monitored, and hepatotoxic chemicals avoided. Rigorous avoidance of sunlight is indicated. Tolerance to sunlight is improved in most patients by long-term treatment with β-carotene, pure preparations of which are without side effects other than a usually mild carotenemia. β-Carotene is less effective in other forms of porphyria (CEP, PCT).

---

*Hemin for injection (Panhematin) is licensed and available on request from Abbott Laboratories, but it should be used only by physicians who are experienced in treating porphyria and practicing in hospitals where the necessary diagnostic and monitoring techniques are available.

Among the hepatic porphyrias the visceral, neurologic, and dermal manifestations and the pattern of pyrrole excretion are usually constant within a given pedigree. However, one pedigree varies considerably from another. The features of four typical variants are shown in Table 7–13. Of these, *acute intermittent porphyria* and *porphyria variegata* are the most common. In kindreds with acute intermittent ("Swedish") porphyria, visceral and neurologic attacks are most frequent and severe in females of childbearing age. In such kindreds, acute attacks often occur without obvious precipitating factors. The occurrence of visceral attacks before puberty is rare. The disorder has an autosomal dominant mode of transmission.

In kindreds with porphyria variegata, "South African porphyria," symptoms are most common between puberty and the 5th decade of life. Skin lesions are relatively more common in males, and acute visceral attacks are more frequent in females. Barbiturates often precipitate severe acute visceral attacks. There is an autosomal dominant mode of transmission; 50% of adult members of an affected family have a constant increase in excretion of porphyrins in the feces whether or not symptoms occur.

Hereditary coproporphyria is transmitted as an autosomal dominant. Clinically, it resembles acute intermittent porphyria, except that symptoms may begin during childhood. They may be chronic "nervousness" and other psychiatric complaints, with or without recurrent abdominal pain. The unique biochemical feature of this disease is increased fecal excretion of COPRO III. Urinary COPRO III may or may not be increased. In the majority of cases severe visceral attacks are provoked by barbiturates and possibly by other anticonvulsant and tranquilizing drugs; during such attacks urinary excretion of ALA, PBG, and COPRO III is increased as a consequence of reduced activity of coproporphyrinogen oxidase. Photosensitivity has been described in only 1 of 30 cases.

Patients with *porphyria cutanea tarda* (PCT) can be divided into three groups: (1) sporadic patients, (2) patients with evidence of autosomal dominant inheritance, and (3) patients with disease due to exposure to halogenated aromatic hydrocarbons. In familial cases the defect is partial deficiency of uroporphyrinogen decarboxylase in liver, erythrocytes and possibly in other tissues. The disease may be clinically manifest during childhood. When feasible, phlebotomy to reduce excess iron in the liver is the standard treatment for PCT and induces remissions in many patients. Alcohol must be avoided. Offending environment agents must be identified and removed in chemically induced cases of PCT.

Two unrelated male teenagers with symptoms characteristic of AIP and virtually complete absence of erythrocyte PBG synthase activity have recently been described. Family studies showed partial deficiency of this enzyme, suggesting an autosomal recessive mode of inheritance. Unlike in lead poisoning, PBG synthase activity in AIP could not be restored in vitro with sulfhydryl reagents.

7.56 HEREDITARY METHEMOGLOBINEMIAS

The iron of both oxygenated and deoxygenated hemoglobin is normally in the ferrous state, which is essential for its oxygen-transporting function. Oxidation of hemoglobin iron to the ferric state yields methemoglobin, which is nonfunctional and imparts a chocolate hue to the blood; in sufficient concentration it causes cyanosis. The blood of healthy persons contains methemoglobin, but the intraerythrocytic methemoglobin-reducing system maintains its concentration at less than 2% of the total hemoglobin. "Normal" methemoglobin has a characteristic spectral absorption band at 632 nm, which is abolished by treating the blood sample with cyanide. This test is specific for assaying methemoglobin produced by exposure to certain chemicals such as aniline dyes but yields erroneous results when hemoglobin M type pigments are present. Hemoglobin electrophoresis after oxidation with potassium ferricyanide is needed to identify the M hemoglobins. Among familial methemoglobinemias both recessive and dominant patterns of inheritance are recognized; each form involves a distinct metabolic error.

Hereditary Methemoglobinemia with Deficiency of NADH Cytochrome b5 Reductase. Reduction of methemoglobin in normal erythrocytes can be effected by four systems: ascorbic acid, reduced glutathione, tetrahydropterin, and NADH cytochrome b5 reductase. The system involving NADH cytochrome b5 reductase is by far the most active.

In hereditary methemoglobinemia with a recessive pattern of inheritance, there is complete absence of the system involving NADH cytochrome b5 reductase. The methemoglobin formed has the spectral and chemical properties of "normal" methemoglobin. Methylene blue is therapeutically effective because it is reduced to leucomethylene blue by both glutathione and NADPH diaphorase; leucomethylene blue, in turn, can reduce "normal" methemoglobin to hemoglobin.

Clinically, the disorder is characterized by cyanosis, the intensity of which varies with season and diet. The time at onset of the cyanosis also varies; in some patients it appears at birth, in others as late as adolescence. Despite the fact that up to 50% of the total circulating hemoglobin may be in the form of nonfunctional methemoglobin, there is little or no cardiorespiratory distress except on exertion. About 10% of these patients show an almost total absence of this enzyme. When the brain is involved, there is neurologic dysfunction, mental retardation, and early death.

Daily oral *treatment* with ascorbic acid (200–500 mg in divided doses) gradually reduces the quantity of methemoglobin to about 10% of the total pigment and alleviates the cyanosis as long as therapy is continued. Chronic high dosage of ascorbic acid has been associated with hyperoxaluria and renal stone formation. Methylene blue given intravenously (1–2 mg/kg) promptly eliminates both methemoglobin and cyanosis, and this effect can be maintained by the daily oral administration of methylene blue (3–5 mg/kg).

Hereditary Methemoglobinemia Associated with Abnormal Methemoglobins (Hemoglobin M Diseases). The dominantly transmitted forms of methemoglobinemia are collectively known as the hemoglobin M diseases. After all the hemoglobin pigment in a blood sample is oxidized to methemoglobin by treatment with potassium ferricyanide, the abnormal methemoglin M type pigments can be separated from normal methemoglobin by means of starch gel electrophoresis. The several hemoglobin M pigments have substitutions of abnormal amino acid residues in the globin chains. Dissimilar substitutions have been found in different pedigrees. This situation is analogous to that of other hemoglobinopathies (hemoglobin S, hemoglobin C, and others). The abnormal amino acid residue in each of the hemoglobin M pigments probably lies in a portion of the globin chain in close proximity to the prosthetic heme group where it can alter the properties of the heme moiety. Thus, cyanosis is probably due to the unusual stability of the methemoglobin form of the M hemoglobins. This hypothesis would also explain the variable response of patients to ascorbic acid and methylene blue as well as the abnormal spectral properties and differing response to cyanide treatment of various hemoglobin M pigments. Among the several hemoglobin M pedigrees examined, five different hemoglobin M pigments have been identified: HbM$_B$ (abnormal α chain), HbM$_S$ (abnormal β chain), HbM$_{M-1}$ (abnormal β chain), HbM$_{M-2}$, and HbM$_1$ (abnormal α chain). The entity previously described as "congenital sulfhemoglobinemia" may fall within the hemoglobin M disease group.

Clinically, methemoglobinemia of the hemoglobin M type should be suspected when family studies suggest an autosomal dominant pattern of inheritance and when the blood of the cyanotic patient does not show the absorption band at 632 nm, which is characteristic of normal methemoglobin. The patient's methemoglobin may or may not react with cyanide to yield a normal cyanomethemoglobin absorption curve. This finding varies with the pedigree. In these diseases the quantity of methemoglobin does not exceed 25% of the total hemoglobin; the cyanosis, although persistent from early infancy, is not associated with any disability. There may be a compensatory polycythemia. Affected members of some pedigrees do not respond to ascorbic acid or methylene blue (hemoglobin M_B and hemoglobin M_{M-1}). Fortunately, alleviation of cyanosis is not essential in the hemoglobin M diseases.

7.57 HEMOCHROMATOSIS

The term hemochromatosis refers to impairment of the structure and function of organs (primarily liver, pancreas, heart, gonads, skin, and joints) due to excessive storage of iron, mainly as hemosiderin in the parenchymal cells. *Idiopathic hemochromatosis* has an autosomal recessive mode of inheritance, with full clinical disease limited largely to adult males. The nature of the metabolic defect is unknown. Untreated cases eventually exhibit the classic triad of hepatic cirrhosis, slate or bronze pigmentation of the skin, and diabetes mellitus. Demonstration of massive iron overload distributed in parenchymal rather than in reticuloendothelial cells through elevated serum iron, saturated iron-binding capacity, highly elevated serum ferritin, and needle biopsy of the liver establishes the diagnosis. All siblings of index cases should have HLA typing and the above blood studies to identify heterozygotes and homozygotes in the latent stage, since early detection improves prognosis. Alcohol and excessive iron intake should be avoided. Excess iron stores are removed preferably by repeated phlebotomy.

A number of chronic anemias requiring repeated transfusions are associated with *secondary hemochromatosis*. In such cases chelation therapy with deferoxamine in conjunction with other measures to minimize iron intake are beneficial.

J. JULIAN CHISOLM, JR.

Anderson KE, Spitz IM, Sassa S, et al: Prevention of cyclical attacks of acute intermittent porphyria with a long-acting agonist of luteinizing hormone–releasing hormone. N Engl J Med 311:643, 1984.

Becker DM, Kramer S: The neurological manifestations of porphyria: A review. Medicine 56:411, 1977.

Bloomer JR, Phillips MJ, Davidson DL, et al: Hepatic disease in erythropoietic protoporphyria. Am J Med 58:869, 1975.

Bothwell TH, Charlton RW, Motulsky AG: Idiopathic hemochromatosis. In: Stanbury JB, Wyngaarden JB, Fredrickson DS, et al (eds): The Metabolic Basis of Inherited Disease. 5th ed. New York, McGraw-Hill, 1983.

Brenner DA, Bloomer JR: The enzymatic defect in variegate porphyria: Studies with human cultured skin fibroblasts. N Engl J Med 302:765, 1980.

Dean G, Barnes HD: The inheritance of porphyria. Br Med J 2:89, 1955.

Doss M, von Tiepermann R, Schneider J, et al: New type of hepatic porphyria with porphobilinogen synthase defect and intermittent acute clinical manifestation. Klin Wochenschr 57:1123, 1979.

Hellman ES, Tschudy DP, Bartter FC: Abnormal electrolyte and water metabolism in acute intermittent porphyria. Am J Med 32:734, 1962.

Kappas A, Sassa S, Anderson KE: The porphyrias. In: Stanbury JB, Wyngaarden JB, Fredrickson DS, et al (eds): The Metabolic Basis of Inherited Disease. 5th ed. New York, McGraw-Hill, 1983.

Lamon J, With TK, Redeker AG: The Hoesch test: Bedside screening for urinary porphobilinogen in patients with suspected porphyria. Clin Chem 20:1438, 1974.

Lamon JM, Frykholm BC, Hess RA, et al: Hematin therapy for acute porphyria. Medicine 58:252, 1979.

Mathews-Roth MM, Pathak MA, Fitzpatrick TB, et al: Beta carotene therapy for erythropoietic protoporphyria and other photosensitivity diseases. Arch Dermatol 113:1229, 1977.

Runge W, Watson CJ: Experimental production of skin lesions in human cutaneous porphyria. Proc Soc Exp Biol Med 109:809, 1962.

Sassa S, Solish G, Levere RD, et al: Studies in porphyria, IV. Expression of the gene defect of acute intermittent porphyria in cultured human skin fibroblasts and amniotic cells: Prenatal diagnosis of the porphyric trait. J Exp Med 142:722, 1975.

Schwartz JM, Reiss AL, Jaffe ER: Hereditary methemoglobinemia with deficiency of NADH cytochrome b5 reductase. In: Stanbury JB, Wyngaarden JB, Fredrickson DS, et al (eds): The Metabolic Basis of Inherited Disease. 5th ed. New York, McGraw-Hill, 1983.

Stein JA, Tschudy DP: Acute intermittent porphyria: A clinical and biochemical study of 46 patients. Medicine 49:1, 1970.

Welland FH, Hellman ES, Collins A, et al: Factors affecting the excretion of porphyrin precursors by patients with acute intermittent porphyria. I. The effect of diet. II. The effect of ethinyl estradiol. Metabolism 13:232, 251, 1964.

Winslow RM, Anderson WF: The hemoglobinopathies. In: Stanbury JB, Wyngaarden JB, Fredrickson DS, et al (eds): The Metabolic Basis of Inherited Disease. 5th ed. New York, McGraw-Hill, 1983.

EPILOGUE

The number of inborn errors of metabolism being recognized is constantly increasing, partly because of the clinical and biochemical identification of new syndromes. In addition, many disorders, such as phenylalaninemia and the glycogenoses, once thought to result from single enzymatic defects but presenting a broad spectrum of clinical manifestations, can be subdivided biochemically into several distinct clinical entities, each with a different enzymatic error.

The detection of many inborn errors of metabolism early in life makes it possible to initiate fetal or neonatal treatment or to interrupt pregnancy. In some instances large-scale screening detection programs are being carried out. For many conditions, particularly those associated with mental retardation (e.g., phenylketonuria), the earlier the detection takes place and effective diet therapy is instituted, the better is the prognosis. Other inborn errors are amenable to treatment with massive amounts of particular vitamins to overcome an enzymatic error when the mutant enzyme no longer effectively binds the cofactor derived from the vitamin, e.g., pyridoxine in one form of cystathioninemia. Replacing missing enzymes, a logical approach, has had limited success. In cystic fibrosis the extracellular enzyme required for proper digestion can be administered conveniently, though the underlying defect is not ameliorated. A number of partially successful trials have been reported wherein a purified enzyme was injected directly into an individual who lacked it.

There is now reason to anticipate that with increasing knowledge of genetic mechanisms it will be possible in the future to alter the genetic constitution of an individual and to ameliorate some of the clinical manifestation of some inborn errors of metabolism.

VICTOR H. AUERBACH
Associate Editor for Chapter 7

General

Bergsma D (ed): Birth Defects; Atlas and Compendium. Baltimore, Williams and Wilkins, 1973.

Bondy PK, Rosenberg LE: Metabolic Control and Disease. 8th ed. Philadelphia, WB Saunders, 1980.

Callahan JW, Lowden JA (eds): Lysosomes and Lysosomal Storage Diseases. New York, Raven Press, 1981.

Hers HG, vanHoof F (eds): Lysosomes and Storage Diseases. New York, Academic Press, 1973.

McKusick VA: Mendelian Inheritance in Man. 6th ed. Baltimore, Johns Hopkins Univ Press, 1983.

Stanbury JB, Wyngaarden JB, Fredrickson DS, et al (eds): The Metabolic Basis of Inherited Disease. 5th ed. New York, McGraw-Hill 1983.

Stryer L: Biochemistry. 2nd ed. San Francisco, WA Freeman, 1981.

8

THE FETUS AND THE NEONATAL INFANT

Although the "neonatal period" defines the first 4 wk of life after birth, both fetal and neonatal life form a continuum during which human growth and development are affected by genetic and by intrauterine and extrauterine environmental factors. For example, maternal toxemia may decrease the rate of fetal growth and cause an increased incidence of neonatal hypoglycemia. Social, economic, and cultural influences also affect this continuum. Low economic status is frequently associated with prematurity, which is correlated to high rates of morbidity and mortality, not only in the neonatal period, but throughout infancy. In the United States, the significantly higher nonwhite neonatal and infant mortality rate over that of white infants (Fig. 8–1) reflects such socioeconomic factors. Although social influences, such as physicians' reluctance to live in poverty areas, affect the availability of medical care to those most needing it, the failure of many mothers in these areas to use available prenatal and preventive medical care effectively also contributes to fetal and infant morbidity and mortality. Their failure results, in part, from inadequate public health education, from their lack of money to pay for the care, and from limited access to health facilities and providers. Social factors leading to illegitimate births and cultural practices, such as the use of drugs, also increase the incidence of fetal and neonatal disease.

Neonatal mortality has progressively decreased (Fig. 8–1); it is highest during the first 24 hr of life, then accounting for about 40% of deaths under 1 yr of age. Further reduction of mortality and related morbidity depends primarily on preventing the birth of low birthweight infants, prenatal diagnosis, and early treatment of diseases that result from factors

Table 8–1. **Principal Causes of Neonatal Mortality**

Cause	Percentage of Deaths
Congenital anomalies	15
Immaturity (unqualified)	13
Asphyxia of newborn (unspecified)	12
Respiratory distress syndrome or hyaline membrane disease	21
Respiratory infection	2
Nonrespiratory infection	4
Complications of pregnancy and labor	19
Other	14

From Seigel DG, Stanley F. *In:* Quilligan EJ, Kretchmer N (eds): Fetal and Maternal Medicine. New York, John Wiley and Sons, 1980.

acting during gestation and at delivery (Table 8–1). *Perinatal mortality* designates fetal and neonatal deaths influenced by prenatal conditions and circumstances surrounding delivery. It is often defined as deaths of fetuses and infants from the 20th wk of gestational life through the 28th day after birth.

Perinatal and infant mortality rates vary by country; they are lowest in the Scandinavian countries, Japan, and the Netherlands, and highest in the developing countries. Even though socioeconomic, cultural, and, perhaps, geographic factors may be the most important influences that determine perinatal mortality, autopsy findings on liveborn infants indicate that perinatal mortality may be further reduced by prophylactic health measures. The number of low birthweight infants primarily determines neonatal and infant mortality rates and significantly contributes to childhood morbidity. In the United States the low birthweight rate has not followed the declining mortality rates; the number of both the low birthweight (2500 g or less) and the very low birthweight (1500 g or less) are higher in this country than in a dozen other developed countries. This fact suggests a major need for prevention programs.

Successful and timely provision of high quality care to perinatal patients requires not only excellence in the performance of health professionals but also a system that facilitates coordinated teams linking the prenatal care of expectant mothers in their communities with special programs for high risk pregnancies and infants. Regional perinatal programs should provide continuing education and consultation in both the community and the referral center and transportation for pregnant women and newborn infants to appropriate hospitals; they should also include a regional center with facilities, equipment, and personnel for obstetric and neonatal intensive care.

Fetal and neonatal deaths contribute about equally to perinatal mortality. The obstetrician has a central role in reducing perinatal mortality and morbidity. Recently, intrapartum fetal deaths have declined more than antepartum fetal deaths, which may reflect an increase in use of fetal monitoring

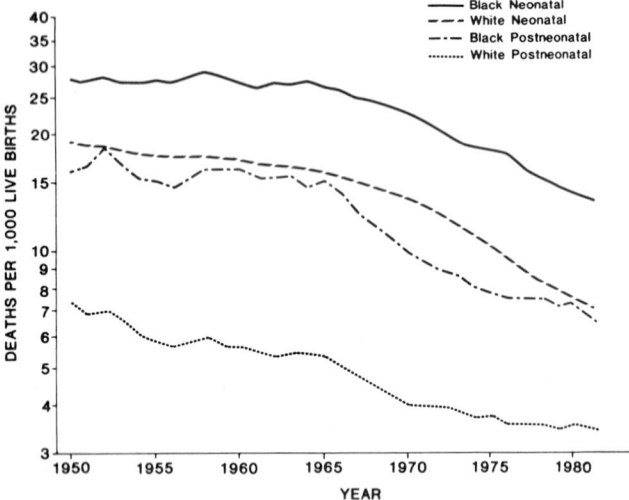

Figure 8–1. Trend in neonatal and postneonatal mortality, United States, black and white, 1950 to 1981. Data modified from presentation of J. Kleinman at International Symposium on Perinatal and Infant Mortality, Bethesda, MD, August 1984. (Source: National Center for Health Statistics, computed by Division of Vital Statistics.)

during labor and a more liberal use of cesarean section for fetal distress and other obstetric complications. It also emphasizes the need for the ability to predict the maturity and functional reserve of the fetus prior to labor. In order to identify as early as possible those fetuses and infants at greatest risk, the obstetrician and pediatrician must effectively interact to anticipate perinatal problems and to take prompt preventive and therapeutic measures.

Along with the need to lower perinatal mortality rates is the need to reduce the incidence of handicaps among high risk infants. Since both mortality and permanent neurologic sequelae are largely caused by the same or similar disturbances, research and public health measures directed at reducing perinatal mortality should also reduce the conditions contributing to the incidence of handicaps. For example, reducing the high incidence of mental retardation among infants whose births required vigorous and prolonged resuscitation mandates the early diagnosis of fetal asphyxia, appropriate obstetric management, and optimal resuscitation. How-

ever, some injury may be unavoidable; retinal damage may occur among those who had prolonged exposure to high concentrations of oxygen in the immediate postnatal period during which attempts were made to reduce the risk of hypoxic brain damage.

Committee to Study the Prevention of Low Birthweight: The Prevention of Low Birthweight. Division of Health Promotion and Disease Prevention. Institute of Medicine, National Academy of Sciences. Washington, DC, National Academy Press, 1985.

Koops B, Morgan L, Battaglia F: Neonatal mortality risk in relation to birthweight and gestational age: Update. J Pediatr 101:969, 1982.

Lee KS, Paneth N, Gartner L, et al: Neonatal mortality: An analysis of recent improvement in the United States. Am J Pub Health 70:15, 1980.

Shapiro S, McCormick M, Starfield B, et al: Relevance of correlates of infant deaths for significant morbidity at 1 year of age. Am J Obstet Gynecol 136:363, 1980.

Sinclair J, Tudehope D: Birth weight, gestational age and neonatal risk. In: Fanaroff A, Martin R (eds): Behrman's Neonatal-Perinatal Medicine. St Louis, CV Mosby, 1983.

Wigglesworth JS: Monitoring perinatal mortality. Lancet 2:684, 1980.

8.1 THE NEWBORN INFANT

See also Chapter 2.

The neonatal period is a highly vulnerable time for the infant, who is completing many of the physiologic adjustments required for extrauterine existence. The high neonatal morbidity and mortality rates attest to the fragility of life during this period; in the United States, of all deaths occurring in the first year, two thirds are of newborn infants. Deaths during the first year mark an annual rate unequaled until the 7th decade.

The infant's intrauterine to extrauterine transition requires many biochemical and physiologic changes. No longer dependent on maternal circulation via the placenta, the newborn's pulmonary function is activated for the self-sufficient exchange of oxygen and carbon dioxide. Also becoming activated are the neonatal gastrointestinal function for adsorbing food, the renal function for excreting wastes and maintaining chemical homeostasis, the liver function for neutralizing and excreting toxic substances, and the function of the immunologic system for protecting against infection. Unsupported by the maternal placental system, the neonatal cardiovascular and endocrine systems also adapt for self-sufficient functioning. Many of the newborn's special problems are related to poor adaptation following birth due to asphyxia, premature birth, life-threatening congenital anomalies, or adverse effects of delivery.

8.2 THE HISTORY IN NEONATAL PEDIATRICS

The medical history of the neonatal infant should aim toward (1) identifying early those diseases in which disability may be prevented by prompt treatment, (2) anticipating conditions that may be of later importance, and (3) uncovering possible causative factors that may help to explain any pathologic condition regardless of its immediate or future significance. A detailed family history should be elicited and recorded for every newborn infant; the events of labor, delivery, anesthesia, and the immediate postpartum period are especially important.

8.3 PHYSICAL EXAMINATION OF THE NEWBORN INFANT

Many physical and behavioral characteristics of the normal newborn infant are described in Sec. 2.3–2.5, which should be reviewed before reading this section.

The initial examination of the newborn infant should be performed as soon as possible after delivery to detect abnormalities and to establish a baseline for subsequent examinations. For high risk deliveries this examination should take place in the delivery room and focus on congenital anomalies and pathophysiologic problems that may interfere with a normal cardiopulmonary and metabolic adaptation to extrauterine life. Following a stable delivery room course, a second, more detailed examination should be performed within 24 hr of birth. In healthy infants the mother should be present during this examination; even minor, seemingly insignificant anatomic variations should be explained, since she may become disturbed at her or other relatives' later discovery of them or she may think the physician is not giving them adequate consideration. However, explaining any problem has the potential for unduly alarming otherwise unworried parents unless it is carefully and skillfully done. No infant should be discharged from the hospital without a final examination, since certain abnormalities, particularly heart murmurs, often appear or disappear in the immediate neonatal period, or there may be evidence of having just acquired disease. Pulse, respiratory rate, weight, length, head circumference, and dimensions of any visible or palpable structural abnormality should be recorded.

Examining the newborn requires patience, gentleness, and procedural flexibility. Thus, if the infant is quiet and relaxed at the beginning of the examination, palpation of the abdomen or auscultation of the heart should be performed first before other, more disturbing manipulations.

General Appearance. Physical activity may be absent during the relaxation of normal sleep or decreased by the effects of illness or drugs; the infant may be either lying with extremities motionless, to conserve energy for the effort of difficult breathing, or vigorously crying with accompanying activity of arms and legs. Both active and passive muscle tone and any unusual posture should be recorded. Coarse, tremulous movements with ankle or jaw myoclonus are more common and less significant in newborn infants than at any other age. Such movements tend to occur when the infant is active, whereas convulsive twitching usually occurs in a quiet state. Edema may produce a superficial appearance of good nutrition. Pitting after applied pressure may or may not be present, but the skin of the fingers and toes will lack the normal fine wrinkles when puffed with fluid. Edema of the eyelids commonly results from irritation from administering silver nitrate. Generalized edema may occur with prematurity, hypoproteinemia secondary to severe erythroblastosis fetalis (hydrops fetalis), congenital nephrosis, Hurler syndrome, or unknown cause. Localized edema suggests a congenital malformation of the lymphatic system; when confined to one or more extremities of a female infant, it may be the presenting sign of Turner syndrome (Sec. 19.35).

Skin. Vasomotor instablity and peripheral circulatory sluggishness are revealed by deep redness or purple lividity in the crying infant, whose color may darken profoundly with closure of the glottis preceding a vigorous cry, and by harmless cyanosis (acrocyanosis) of the hands and feet, especially when these are cool. Mottling, another example of general circulatory instability, may be associated with serious illness or related to a transient fluctuation in skin temperature. An extraordinary division of the body from forehead to pubis into red and pale halves is **harlequin color change,** a transient and harmless condition. Significant *cyanosis* may be masked by the pallor of circulatory failure; alternatively, the relatively high hemoglobin content of the first few days and the thin skin may combine to produce an appearance of cyanosis at a

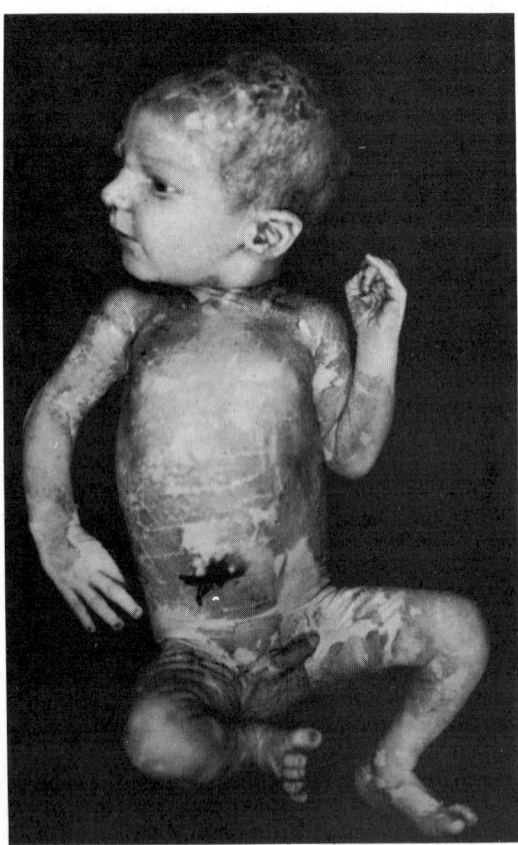

Figure 8–2. Placental dysfunction syndrome, stage III. Note long, thin infant with loose, peeling, parchment-like skin, alert expression, staining of skin and nails. (From Clifford: Advances in Pediatrics. Vol 9. Chicago, Year Book Medical Publishers, Inc.)

Table 8–2. Disorders Associated With a Large Anterior Fontanel

Achondroplasia	Osteogenesis imperfecta
Apert's syndrome	Prematurity
Athyrotic hypothyroidism	Pyknodysostosis
Cleidocranial dysostosis	Rubella syndrome
Hallerman-Streiff syndrome	Russell-Silver syndrome
Hydrocephaly	Trisomies 13, 18, 21
Hypophosphatasia	Vitamin D deficiency rickets
Intrauterine growth retardation	

higher paO$_2$ than in older children. Localized cyanosis is differentiated from ecchymosis by the momentary pallor following pressure. The same maneuver also helps in demonstrating *icterus*, possibly significant but unnoticed if the skin is suffused with blood. *Pallor* may represent asphyxia, anemia, shock, or edema. Early recognition of anemia may lead to a diagnosis of erythroblastosis fetalis, of liver rupture, subdural hemorrhage, or fetal-maternal or twin-twin transfusion. Without being anemic, postmature infants tend to have paler skin than do term or premature infants.

The vernix and common transitory capillary hemangiomas of the eyelids and neck are described in Chapter 24. Slate blue, well demarcated areas of pigmentation are seen over the buttocks, back, and sometimes other parts of the body in over 50% of black infants and occasionally in white ones. These have no known anthropologic significance despite their name, **mongolian spots;** they tend to disappear within the first year. The vernix, skin, and especially the cord may be stained a brownish yellow if the amniotic fluid has been colored by passage of meconium during or before birth, usually because of intrauterine anoxia. The skin of the premature infant is thin and delicate and tends to be deep red; in extremely premature infants, the skin appears almost gelatinous. Fine, soft, immature hair—lanugo hair—frequently covers the scalp and brow and may also cover the face in the premature infant. Lanugo hair has usually been lost or replaced by vellus hair in the term infant. Tufts of hair over the lumbosacral spines suggest an underlying abnormality such as an occult spina bifida, sinus tract, or tumor. The nails are rudimentary in the very premature, but they may protrude beyond the fingertips in infants born past term. Post-term infants may have a peeling, parchment-like skin (Fig. 8–2), a severe degree of which suggests ichthyosis congenita (Sec. 24.16).

Many neonates develop small, white, occasionally vesiculopustular papules on an erythematous base 1–3 days after birth. This benign rash, *erythema toxicum,* persists for as long as 1 wk and is usually distributed on the face, trunk, and extremities (Sec. 24.3). *Pustular melanosis,* a benign lesion seen predominantly in black neonates, is present at birth as a vesiculopustular eruption around the chin, neck, back, extremities, and palms or soles; it lasts 2–3 days. Both lesions need to be distinguished from more dangerous vesicular eruptions such as herpes simplex (Sec. 8.71) and staphylococcal disease of the skin (Sec. 8.67).

The **skull** may be molded, particularly if the infant is the firstborn and if the head has been engaged for a considerable time. The parietal bones tend to override the occipital and the frontal bones. The head of an infant born by cesarean section or from a breech presentation is characterized by its roundness. The suture lines and the size and tension of the anterior and posterior fontanels should be determined digitally. Great variation in the size of the fontanels exists at birth; if small, the anterior fontanel usually tends to enlarge during the first few months of life. Persistence of excessively large anterior and posterior fontanels has been associated with several disorders (Table 8–2). Soft areas **(craniotabes)** are occasionally found in the parietal bones at the vertex near the sagittal suture; they are more common in premature infants and in infants exposed to uterine compression. Although usually insignificant, if they persist, their possible pathologic cause should be investigated. Soft areas in the occipital region suggest the irregular calcification and wormian bone formation associated with osteogenesis imperfecta, cleidocranial dysostosis, lacunar skull, cretinism, and, occasionally, Down syndrome. Transillumination of the abnormal skull in a dark room or examination by ultrasound or CT scan will rule out hydranencephaly or porencephaly (Sec. 21.11).

The general appearance of the **face** should be noted with regard to dysmorphic features, such as epicanthal folds, widely spaced eyes, microphthalmia, long philtrum, and low-set ears, often associated with congenital syndromes. The face may be asymmetric from a 7th nerve palsy, from hypoplasia of the depressor muscle at the angle of the mouth, or from an abnormal fetal posture (Sec. 12.1); when the jaw has been held against a shoulder or an extremity during the intrauterine period, the mandible may deviate strikingly from the midline. The skull of the premature infant may suggest hydrocephalus because of the relatively larger brain growth compared to that of other organs.

The **eyes** often open spontaneously if the infant is held up and tipped gently forward and backward. This maneuver, a result of labyrinthine and neck reflexes, is more successful for inspecting the eyes than forcing the lids apart. Conjunctival and retinal hemorrhages are not by themselves seriously significant. The pupillary reflexes are present after 28 wk gestation. The iris should be inspected for colobomata and heterochromia. A cornea greater than 1 cm in diameter in a term infant suggests congenital glaucoma and requires prompt ophthalmologic consultation. The presence of bilateral red reflexes suggests the absence of cataracts or of intraocular pathology (Sec. 25.11–25.13).

Deformities of the pinnae of the **ears** are occasionally seen. Unilateral or bilateral preauricular skin tags occur frequently; if pedunculated, they can be ligated tightly at the base, and dry gangrene and slough will result. The tympanic membrane, easily seen otoscopically through the short, straight external auditory canal, normally appears dull gray. The **nose** may be slightly obstructed by mucus accumulated in the narrow nostrils.

The normal **mouth** rarely shows precocious dentition, with *supernumerary teeth* in the lower incisor position or aberrantly placed; these teeth are shed before the deciduous ones erupt. Alternatively, neonatal teeth occur in Ellis–van Creveld, Hallermann-Strieff, or other syndromes. Premature eruption of deciduous teeth is even more unusual. The **soft** and **hard palate** should be inspected for a hidden cleft and the contour noted if the arch is excessively high or the uvula bifid. On the hard palate on either side of the raphe may be temporary accumulations of epithelial cells called **Epstein pearls.** Retention cysts of similar appearance may also be seen on the gums. Both disappear spontaneously, usually within a few weeks of birth. Clusters of small white or yellow follicles or ulcers on an erythematous base may be found on the anterior tonsillar pillars, most frequently on the 2nd–3rd day of life. Of unknown cause, they clear without treatment in 2–4 days. There is no active salivation. The **tongue** appears relatively large; the **frenulum** may be short, but rarely, if ever, is this a reason for cutting it. Occasionally, the sublingual mucous membrane forms a prominent fold. The **cheeks** have a fullness on both the buccal and the external aspects due to the accumulation of fat making up the **sucking pads.** These pads, as well as the labial tubercle on the upper lip, disappear when suckling ceases. A marble-size buccal mass is usually fat necrosis.

The **throat** of the newborn infant is hard to see because of the arch of the palate; however, it should be clearly viewed because it is easily possible to miss posterior palatal or uvular clefts. The tonsils are small.

The **neck** appears relatively short. Abnormalities are not common; they include goiter, cystic hygroma, branchial cleft rests, and lesions of the sternocleidomastoid muscle which are presumably traumatic (Sec. 22.6). Redundant skin or webbing in a female infant suggests Turner syndrome (Sec. 19.35). Both clavicles should be palpated for fractures.

Much can be learned about the **lungs** by observation of breathing. Variations in rate and rhythm are characteristic, fluctuating according to physical activity, state of wakefulness, or presence of crying. Because fluctuations are rapid, the respiratory rate should be counted for a full minute with the infant in the resting state, preferably asleep. Under these circumstances the usual rates for normal term infants are 30–40/min; for premature infants they are higher and fluctuate more widely. Rates consistently over 60/min during periods of regular breathing usually indicate cardiac or pulmonary disease. The premature infant may breathe with a Cheyne-Stokes rhythm, known as periodic respiration, or with complete irregularity. Periodic respiration is rare in the first 24 hr of life. Irregular gasping, sometimes accompanied by spasmodic movements of the mouth and chin, strongly indicates serious impairment of respiratory centers.

The breathing of newborn infants is almost entirely diaphragmatic, so that during inspiration the soft front of the thorax usually draws inward while the abdomen protrudes. If the baby is quiet, relaxed, and of good color, this "paradoxical movement" does not necessarily signify insufficient ventilation. On the other hand, labored respiration is important evidence of respiratory distress syndrome, pneumonia, anomalies, or mechanical disturbance of the lungs. A weak groaning, whining cry, or **grunting** often accompanies expiration in severely disturbed respiration.

Normally, the breath sounds are bronchovesicular. Suspected pulmonary pathology due to diminished breath sounds, rales, or percussion dullness should always be followed up with a chest roentgenogram.

The size of the **heart** is difficult to estimate owing to normal variations in the size and shape of the chest. The location of the heart should be determined to detect dextrocardia. There may be transitory murmurs. Congenital heart disease may not initially produce the murmur that will be present later; only a 1:12 chance exists that a murmur heard at birth represents congenital heart disease. Evaluating the heart by roentgenography, echocardiography, and electrocardiography is essential when the possibility of significant lesions exists. The pulse may vary normally from 90/min in relaxed sleep to 180/min during activity. The still higher rate of paroxysmal tachycardia may be counted better on an electrocardiogram than by ear. Premature infants, whose resting heart rate is usually 140–150/min, may have a sudden onset of **sinus bradycardia. Pulses** should be palpated in the upper and lower extremity on both admission and discharge from the nursery.

Blood pressure measurements may be a valuable diagnostic aid (Sec. 14.1). The *auscultatory method* is often satisfactory, provided the stethoscope head is small enough. The *Doppler method*, using a transducer in the cuff, transmits and receives ultrasound waves. By detecting movements of the arterial wall, it more accurately measures systolic and diastolic pressures. Other methods include the *palpatory method*, in which the systolic blood pressure is understood to be the point at which the pulse distal to the cuff becomes palpable during deflation, and the *flush method*, in which first compressing the extremity renders the area below the cuff relatively bloodless, and then, while deflating the cuff, the mean pressure is recorded at the point flushing appears in the arm or hand below the cuff. Each is disadvantageous in that the pulse pressure is not obtained and that the reading lies between the systolic and diastolic pressures obtained by the auscultatory method. Continuous or intermittent direct measurement of blood pressure using an umbilical artery catheter may be indicated in special circumstances for infants under close observation in an intensive care unit (Fig. 8–3).

In the **abdomen** the liver is usually palpable, sometimes as much as 2 cm below the rib margin. Less commonly, the spleen tip may be felt. The approximate size and location of each kidney can usually be determined on deep palpation. Unusual masses should be investigated immediately by ultrasonography. Hydronephrosis, renal dysplasia, renal embryoma, ovarian cysts, and intestinal duplications are the most common masses encountered. Abdominal distention at or shortly after birth suggests either obstruction or perforation of the gastrointestinal tract, often due to meconium ileus; later distention suggests lower bowel obstruction, sepsis, or peritonitis. A scaphoid abdomen in the newborn suggests diaphragmatic hernia. At no other period of life does the amount of air in the gastrointestinal tract vary so greatly, nor is it usually so great under normal circumstances. The abdominal wall is normally weak (especially in premature infants), and **diastasis recti** and umbilical hernias are common, particularly among black infants.

The **genitalia** and **mammary glands** normally respond to transplacentally obtained maternal hormones to produce enlargement and secretion of the breasts in both sexes and prominence of the female genitalia, often with considerable nonpurulent discharge. These transitory manifestations require observation but no interference. Imperforate hymen may result in **hydrometrocolpos** and a lower abdominal mass. The normal scrotum is relatively large; its size may be increased by the trauma of breech delivery or by a **transitory hydrocele,** which is distinguished from a hernia by palpation and transillumination. The testes should be in the scrotum or palpable in the canals. The male black infant usually has dark pigmentation of the scrotum before the rest of the skin assumes its permanent color.

The prepuce of the newborn infant is normally so tight and adherent that no information can be obtained as to later need for circumcision. Severe hypospadias or epispadias should always lead one to suspect the presence of abnormal sex chromosomes (Sec. 19.30) or that the infant is actually a masculinized female with enlarged clitoris, since this may be

the first evidence of the adrenogenital syndrome (Sec. 19.23). Erection of the penis is common and has no significance. Urine is usually passed during or immediately after birth; a period without voiding may normally follow. However, about 95% of preterm and term infants void within 24 hr.

Some passage of **meconium** usually occurs within the first 12 hr after birth; 99% of term infants and 95% of premature infants will pass meconium within 48 hr of birth. **Imperforate anus** is not always visible and may require evidence obtained by the gentle insertion of the little finger or a rectal tube. Roentgenographic study is required. The dimple or irregularity of skinfold often normally present in the sacrococcygeal midline may be mistaken for an actual or potential pilonidal sinus.

In examining the **extremities** the effects of fetal posture (Sec. 23.1) should be noted so that their cause and usual transitory nature can be explained to the mother. This is particularly important after breech presentations. The suspicion of a fracture or nerve injury associated with delivery is more commonly aroused by observing the extremities in spontaneous or stimulated activity than by any other means. The ·hands and feet should be examined for polydactyly, syndactyly, and abnormal dermatoglyphic patterns such as a simian crease.

The hips of all infants should be examined to rule out a congenital dislocation (Sec. 23.2).

Neurologic Examination. See Sec. 2.3 and 21.3.

ORDINARY CARE OF THE NEWBORN INFANT

The basic requirements of the newborn infant are: immediate assistance at birth when needed, primarily to *establish respiration;* and subsequent assistance in obtaining *adequate nutrition,* in maintaining a *normal body temperature,* and in *avoiding contact with infection.* The environment meeting these requirements should also provide constant care by a nursing and medical staff alert to any signs of specific illness and should keep to a minimum the time the mother and infant are separated. The care of full term and premature infants differs only in the degree of emphasis on each of these requirements.

8.4 ROUTINE DELIVERY ROOM CARE

The low risk infant should be placed head downward immediately after delivery in order to clear the mouth, pharynx, and nose of fluid, mucus, blood, and amniotic debris by gravity; gentle suction with a bulb syringe or soft rubber catheter may also be helpful in removing this material. Wiping the palate and pharynx with gauze may lead to abrasions and the development of thrush, pterygoid ulcers (Bednar aphthae), or, rarely, tooth bud infection with maxillary osteomyelitis and retrobulbar abscess formation. If infants appear to be in satisfactory condition, they may be given to their mothers for immediate bonding and nursing. If there is any concern about respiratory distress, they should be placed under a warmer, with their head dependent. As a guide to prognosis and to the need for particularly close observation or care in the delivery room and nursery, the Apgar method of scoring is of practical value at 1 and 5 min (Table 8–3). *The score taken at 1 min is an index of asphyxia and of the need for assisted ventilation;* the 5 min score is a more accurate index of likelihood of death (Fig. 8–4) or neurologic residual. Infants with prolapsed cord or delayed delivery and evidence of intrauterine asphyxia should receive prompt resuscitation and close observation subsequently (Sec. 8.29) The stomachs of infants delivered by cesarean section may contain more fluid

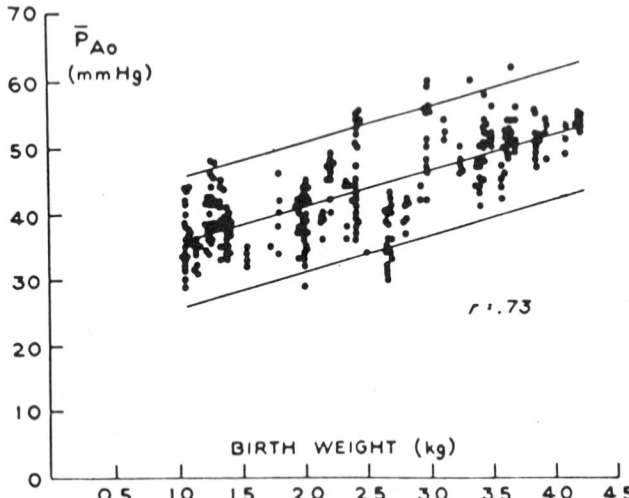

Figure 8–3. Linear regression and 95% confidence limits of mean aortic blood pressure in infants between 2 and 12 hr of age. (From Kitterman J, Philbs R, Todey W: Pediatrics 44:959, 1969.)

Table 8–3. **Evaluation of the Newborn Infant**

Sign	0	1	2
Heart rate	Absent	Below 100	Over 100
Respiratory effort	Absent	Slow, irregular	Good, crying
Muscle tone	Limp	Some flexion of extremities	Active motion
Response to catheter in nostril (tested after oropharynx is clear)	No response	Grimace	Cough or sneeze
Color	Blue, pale	Body pink, extremities blue	Completely pink

Sixty sec after the complete birth of the infant (disregarding the cord and placenta) the 5 objective signs above are evaluated, and each is given a score of 0, 1, or 2. A total score of 10 indicates an infant in the best possible condition.
Modified from Apgar V: Current Res Anesth Analg 32:260, 1953.

than those of infants delivered vaginally. Their stomachs should be emptied by gastric tube to prevent aspiration of gastric contents.

Maintenance of Body Heat. Relative to body weight, the body surface of the newborn infant is approximately 3 times that of the adult, and in low birthweight infants the insulating layer of subcutaneous fat is thinner. The estimated rate of heat loss in the newborn is approximately 4 times that of an adult. Under the usual delivery room conditions (20–25° C), an infant's skin temperature falls approximately 0.3° C/min, and the deep body temperature approximately 0.1° C/min during the period immediately after delivery, resulting usually in a cumulative loss of 2–3° C in deep body temperature (corresponding to a heat loss of approximately 200 kcal/kg). The heat loss occurs by *convection* of heat energy to the cooler surrounding air, by *conduction* of heat to colder materials on which the infant is resting, by heat *radiation* from the infant to other nearby solid objects, and by *evaporation* from moist skin and lungs (a function of alveolar ventilation).

Term infants exposed to cold after birth may develop metabolic acidosis, hypoxemia and hypoglycemia, and increased renal excretion of water and solutes owing to their efforts to compensate for heat loss. They augment heat production by increasing the metabolic rate and oxygen consumption and, indirectly, by releasing more norepinephrine, which results in nonshivering thermogenesis through oxidation of fat, particularly of brown fat. In addition, muscular activity may increase. Hypoglycemic or hypoxic infants cannot increase their oxygen consumption when exposed to a cold environment and their central temperature decreases. After labor and vaginal delivery, many newborn infants have a mild to moderate metabolic acidosis for which they may

compensate by hyperventilating, which is more difficult for depressed infants and infants exposed to cold stress in the delivery room. Therefore, it is desirable to ensure the infant is dried and either wrapped in blankets or placed under a warmer while having skin to skin contact with the mother. Since carrying out resuscitative measures on a covered infant or one enclosed in an incubator is difficult, a radiant heat source should be used to immediately receive the baby.

Antiseptic Skin and Cord Care. To reduce the incidence of skin and periumbilical infections, the entire skin and cord should be cleansed in the delivery room or upon admission to the nursery with sterile cotton soaked in warm water and/or a mild soap solution. The infant may be rinsed with water at body temperature if care is taken to avoid chilling. The baby is then dried and wrapped in sterile blankets and taken to the nursery. To lessen the chance of carrying pathogenic organisms into the nursery, the outer blanket can be discarded at the nursery door. Total body exposure (i.e., while bathing) to detergent solutions containing 3% hexachlorophene over prolonged periods may be neurotoxic, particularly in infants of less than 35 wk gestation or 1200 g weight or those with abraded skin, and is not recommended. At 2–4 hr of life, a single bath with a 3% hexachlorophene solution followed immediately by a thorough rinse, significantly reduces the rate of *Staphylococcus aureus* colonization. When a high staphylococcal risk exists in a nursery or when a baby has a minor skin infection, such baths may be used with discretion. Nursery personnel should continue to use hexachlorophene-containing detergents or similar effective agents for routine handwashing. Rigidly enforcing hand-to-elbow washing for 2 min in the initial wash and 15–30 sec in the second wash is recommended for staff and visitors enter-

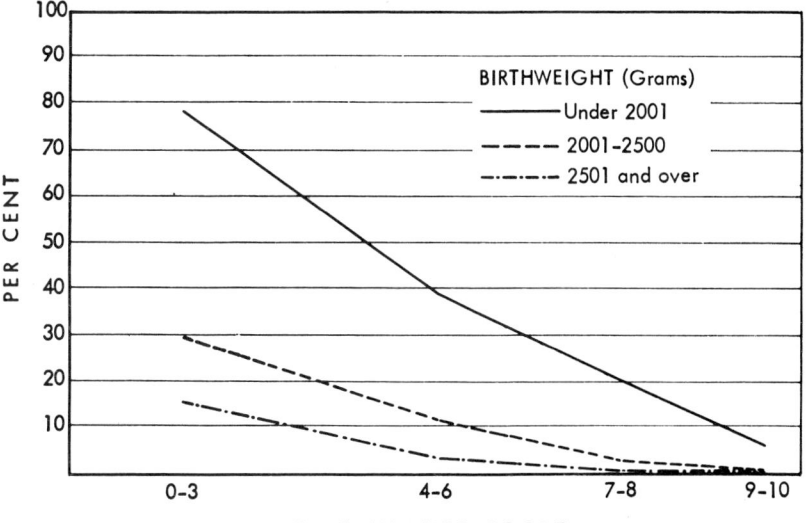

Figure 8–4. Mortality (percentage) during first 28 days of life of infants with various Apgar scores recorded at 5 min, arranged according to birth weight. (From Drage JS, Berendes J: Pediatr Clin North Am 13:635, 1966.)

ing the nursery. Shorter but equally thorough washes between handling infants also should be required. Initial and daily painting of the umbilical cord stump with a bactericidal dye also may be used until hospital discharge in an attempt to reduce bacterial colonization.

Other Measures. The **eyes** of all infants must be protected against gonorrheal infection by instilling 1% *silver nitrate* drops, the best-proved therapy; erythromycin drops are an alternative which is also effective against chlamydial conjunctivitis. This may be delayed during the initial short alert period following birth to promote bonding, but once applied, drops should not be rinsed out. Also see Sec. 8.64.

Though hemorrhage in the newborn may be due to factors other than *vitamin K deficiency,* an intramuscular injection of 1.0 mg of water-soluble vitamin K$_1$ is recommended for all infants immediately after birth to prevent any coagulation defect related to vitamin K deficiency. Larger amounts may predispose to the development of hyperbilirubinemia and kernicterus and should be avoided. Administering vitamin K to the mother during labor is not recommended.

8.5 NURSERY CARE

Non–high risk infants may be taken after the delivery room examination to the ''regular'' newborn nursery or placed in the mother's room if the hospital has a rooming-in arrangement.

The bassinet, preferably of clear plastic to allow for easy visibility and care, should be cleaned frequently. All professional care should be given in the bassinet, including the physical examination, clothing changes, temperature-taking, skin cleansing, and other procedures that, if performed elsewhere, would establish a common contact point and possibly provide a channel for cross infection. The clothing and bedding should be minimal, only those needed for the infant's comfort; the nursery temperature should be kept at approximately 24° C (75° F). The infant's temperature should be taken once by rectum and thereafter in the axilla; although the interval between temperature taking depends on many circumstances, it need not be shorter than 4 hr during the first 2–3 days and 8 hr thereafter. Axillary temperatures of 36.0–37.0° C (96.5–98.5° F) are within normal limits. Weighing at birth and daily thereafter is sufficient.

Vernix is spontaneously shed within 2–3 days, much of it adhering to the clothing, which should be completely changed daily. The diaper should be checked before and after feeding and when the baby cries; it should be changed when wet or soiled. Meconium or feces should be cleansed from the buttocks with sterile cotton moistened with sterile water. The foreskin of the male infant should not be retracted.

8.6 PARENT-INFANT BONDING

See also Sec. 2.3.

Normal infant development depends partly on a series of affectionate responses exchanged between a mother and her newborn infant binding them psychologically and physiologically. This bonding is facilitated and reinforced by the emotional support of a loving husband and family. The attachment process may be important in enabling some mothers to provide loving care during the neonatal period and subsequently during childhood. It is initiated before birth with the planning and confirmation of the pregnancy and with the growing acceptance of the fetus as an individual. After delivery and during the ensuing weeks, visual and physical contact between mother and baby triggers a variety of mutually rewarding and pleasurable interactions such as the mother's touching the infant's extremities and face with her fingertips

Table 8–4. Drugs and Breast Feeding

Probably Safe	Drugs to Avoid
Acetaminophen	Anthroquinones (laxatives)
Aldomet	Antineoplastic agents†
Ampicillin	Atropine
Antihistamines*	Birth control pills
Aspirin	Bromocriptine†
Chlorpromazine*	Bromides
Codeine*	Calciferol
Digoxin	Cascara
Dilantin	Clemastine†
Furosemide	Cimetidine†
Haloperidol*	Chloramphenicol†
Hydralazine	Danthron
Indomethacin	Diethylstilbestrol†
Methadone*	Dihydrotachysterol
Phenobarbital*	Ergots†
Prednisone	Estrogens
Propranolol	Ethanol
Propylthiouracil	Gold salts†
Theophylline	Immunosuppressants†
Warfarin	Iodides†
	Meprobamate†
	Methimazole†
	Metronidazole
	Narcotics
	Phenindione†
	Primidone
	Radiopharmaceuticals†
	Reserpine
	Tetraycline†
	Thiouracil†

*Watch for sedation.
†Absolute contraindication for breast feeding.

and encompassing and gently massaging the infant's trunk with her hands. Touching the infant's cheek elicits responsive turning toward the mother's face or toward the breast with nuzzling and licking of the nipple, a powerful stimulus for prolactin secretion. The infant's initial quiet alert state provides the opportunity for eye to eye contact, particularly important to the loving and possessive feelings of many mothers for their babies. The infant's crying elicits the maternal response of touching the infant and speaking in a soft, soothing, higher-toned voice. Initial contact between mother and infant should take place in the delivery room, and opportunities for extended intimate contact should be provided within the first hours after birth. Delayed or abnormal maternal-infant bonding, occuring because of prematurity, infant or maternal illness, birth defects, or family stress, may harm infant development and maternal caretaking ability. Hospital routines should be designed to encourage parent-infant contact.

Nurseries and Breast Feeding. See Sec. 3.10 and 3.11 for full discussion of breast and formula feeding, respectively. Many hospital practices contribute to breast feeding difficulty by enforcing 4-hr feeding schedules, limiting nursing time, using only one breast at a feeding, washing nipples with substances other than water, delaying the first feeding, and using heavy intrapartum sedation.

Hospital practices that encourage successful breast feeding include immediate postpartum mother-infant contact with suckling, rooming-in, demand feeding, inclusion of fathers in prenatal breast feeding education, and support from experienced women. Nursing at least 5 min at each breast is reasonable and allows the baby to obtain most of the available breast contents and to provide effective stimulation for increasing milk supply. Nursing episodes should then be extended according to the comfort and desire of mother and infant. A confident and relaxed mother, supported by an encouraging home and hospital environment, is likely to nurse well.

Drugs and Breast Feeding. Maternal medications may affect the production and safety of breast milk (Table 8–4). Most commonly used medications, such as antihypertensive agents, are safe, but each should be investigated if used during breast feeding. Sedatives may result in the infant's sedation. When fresh breast milk is fed by tube or bottle, bacteriologic evaluation of stored milk should be performed within 24 hr.

Gussler JD, Briesemeister LH: The insufficient milk syndrome: A biocultural explanation. Medical Anthropology 4(2), 1980.
Klaus MH, Kennell JH: Care of the mother, father and infant. *In:* Behrman's Neonatal-Perinatal Medicine. St Louis, CV Mosby, 1983.
Lawrence RA (ed): Counseling the Mother on Breast-Feeding. Report of the Eleventh Ross Roundtable on Critical Approaches to Common Pediatric Problems. Columbus, Ohio, Ross Laboratories, 1980.

8.7 HIGH RISK PREGNANCIES

Pregnancies in which factors exist that increase the likelihood of abortion, fetal death, premature delivery, intrauterine growth retardation, fetal or neonatal disease, congenital malformations, mental retardation, or other handicaps are termed high risk pregnancies (Table 8–5; also see Sec. 8.14). Some factors, such as ingestion of a teratogenic drug in the first trimester, are causally related to the risk; others, such as hydramnios, are associations that alert the physician to the existence of the risk or risks. Based on their history, 10–25% of pregnant patients can be identified as "high risk"; over half of all perinatal mortality and morbidity is associated with these pregnancies. Though assessing antepartum risk is important to reducing perinatal mortality and morbidity, some women become high risk only during labor and delivery; therefore, careful monitoring is critical throughout the intrapartum course.

Identifying high risk pregnancies is important not only because it is the first step toward prevention, but also because therapeutic steps may often be taken to reduce the risks to the fetus or neonate if the physician knows of the potential for difficulty. Good prenatal care reduces the incidence of low birthweight infants.

Genetic Factors. The occurrence of chromosomal abnormalities, congenital anomalies, inborn errors of metabolism, mental retardation, or any familial disease in blood relatives increases the risk of the same condition in the infant. Because many parents recognize only obvious clinical manifestations of genetically determined diseases, specific inquiry should be made about any disease affecting one or more blood relative(s).

Maternal Factors. The lowest neonatal mortality rate occurs in infants of mothers 20–30 yr of age. Both teenage pregnancies and those among women over 35 yr of age, particularly primiparous women, carry an increased risk for intrauterine growth retardation, fetal distress, and intrauterine death.

Maternal illness (Table 8–6); multiple pregnancies, particularly those involving monochorionic twinning; and certain drugs (Sec. 8.12) increase the risk for the fetus.

Polyhydramnios and *oligohydramnios* indicate high risk pregnancies. Although there is a rapid turnover rate, during normal pregnancy the amniotic fluid volume gradually increases at a rate of less than 10 mL/day until about the 34th wk of pregnancy, after which it slowly diminishes. The volumes vary widely in normal pregnancy; term volume may be 500–2000 mL. A volume estimated at greater than 2000 mL in the 3rd trimester constitutes polyhydramnios, and a volume estimated at less than 500 mL indicates oligohydramnios.

Acute polyhydramnios is rare, usually associated with premature labor and delivery before 28 wk. Chronic polyhydramnios is commonly diagnosed in the 3rd trimester by the discrepancy between uterine size and gestational age; occasionally it goes undiagnosed until the patient has a dysfunctional labor or an abnormally large amount of amniotic fluid is noted during delivery. Ultrasonography may establish the

Table 8–5. Factors Associated with High Risk Pregnancy

Demographic factors
- Lower socioeconomic status
- Marital status: unwed mothers
- Maternal age
  - Gravida less than 16 yr of age
  - Primigravida 35 yr of age or older
  - Gravida 40 yr of age or older
- Maternal weight: nonpregnant weight less than 45 kg (100 lb) or more than 90 kg (200 lb)
- Stature: height less than 157 cm (62 in)
- Malnutrition
- Poor physical fitness

Past pregnancy history
- Grand multiparity: 6 previous pregnancies terminating beyond 20 wk gestation
- Antepartum bleeding after 12 wk of gestation
- Premature rupture of membranes, premature onset of labor, premature delivery
- Previous cesarean section or mid- or high-forceps delivery
- Prolonged labor
- Previous infant with cerebral palsy, mental retardation, birth trauma, central nervous system disorder or congenital anomaly
- Reproductive failure: infertility, repetitive miscarriages, fetal loss, stillbirth, or neonatal death
- Delivery of preterm (less than 37 wk) or post-term (more than 42 wk infant)

Past or present medical history
- Hypertension or renal disease or both
- Diabetes mellitus (overt or gestational)
- Cardiovascular disease (rheumatic, congenital, or peripheral vascular)
- Pulmonary disease producing hypoxemia and hypercapnia
- Thyroid, parathyroid, and endocrine disorders
- Idiopathic thrombocytopenic purpura
- Neoplastic disease
- Hereditary disorders
- Collagen diseases
- Epilepsy

Additional obstetric and medical conditions
- Toxemia
- Asymptomatic bacteriuria
- Anemia or hemoglobinopathy
- Rh sensitization
- Habitual smoking
- Drug addiction
- Chronic exposure to any pharmacologic or chemical agent
- Multiple pregnancy
- Rubella or other viral infection
- Intercurrent surgery and anesthesia
- Placental abnormalities and uterine bleeding
- Abnormal fetal lie or presentation, fetal anomalies, oligohydramnios, polyhydramnios
- Abnormalities of fetal or uterine growth or both
- Maternal trauma during pregnancy
- Maternal emotional crisis during pregnancy

Table 8–6. Maternal Noninfectious Disease Affecting the Fetus

Maternal Disorder	Fetal or Neonatal Effects
Cholestasis	Preterm delivery
Cyanotic congenital heart disease	Intrauterine growth retardation
Diabetes mellitus	Large for gestational age infant, hypoglycemia, hypocalcemia, immaturity
Endemic goiter	Neonatal hypothyroidism
Graves disease	Transient neonatal thyrotoxicosis
Hyperparathyroidism	Hypocalcemia
Hypertension	Intrauterine growth retardation, stillbirth
Hypoparathyroidism	Hypercalcemia
Idiopathic thrombocytopenia	Thrombocytopenia, bleeding
Immune neutropenia	Fetal neutropenia
Malignant melanoma	Placental metastasis
Myasthenia gravis	Transient neonatal myasthenia
Myotonic dystrophy	Neonatal myotonic dystrophy
Obesity	Large for gestational age infant, hypoglycemia
Preeclampsia-eclampsia (toxemia)	Intrauterine growth retardation, stillbirth, asphyxia
Phenylketonuria	Microcephaly, mental retardation
Renal disease	Intrauterine growth retardation, abortion
Rhesus immunization	Fetal anemia, hydrops
Rickets	Hypocalcemia, rickets
Sickle cell anemia	Intrauterine growth retardation
Systemic lupus erythematosus	Congenital heart block, transient rash, anemia, leukopenia, thrombocytopenia, pericardial effusion

diagnosis before labor. Polyhydramnios is associated with maternal diabetes (especially if severe), congenital malformations (Table 8–7), erythroblastosis fetalis, and multiple gestations (especially monochorionic twins); even without known maternal or fetal disease the association correlates with an increased perinatal mortality. Anencephaly and hydrocephaly are frequently associated congenital anomalies. The incidence of atresias of the upper intestinal tract, which presumably interfere with the reabsorption into the circulation of swallowed amniotic fluid, is also increased. When polyhydramnios occurs with erythroblastosis fetalis, hydrops fetalis is usually present.

Aplasia or hypoplasia of the fetal kidneys is often associated with oligohydramnios, presumably because fetal urine has not been formed. Oligohydramnios, whatever its cause, be-

Table 8–7. Fetal Malformations Frequently Associated With Polyhydramnios or Oligohydramnios

Polyhydramnios	Oligohydramnios
Anencephaly (in approximately 20% of cases)	Renal agenesis
Meningocele and encephalocele	Ureteral dysplasia
Esophageal or duodenal atresia	Urethral atresia
Klippel-Feil syndrome	Pulmonary hypoplasia
Cleft palate and harelip	Amnion nodosum
Achondroplasia	
Diaphragmatic defects	
Lung anomalies	
Multiple anomalies (not central nervous system)	
Hydrocephaly	
Trisomy 18 or 21	
Nonobstructive hydronephrosis	

fore the last few weeks of pregnancy may result in mechanically induced abnormalities of the fetal limbs. It is also associated with pulmonary hypoplasia, which can result in respiratory insufficiency and neonatal death.

Obstetric factors are understandably important because fetuses weighing more than 2500 g make up a very high proportion of the total fetal deaths, and neonatal mortality is greatest during the first 24 hr after delivery. A pregnancy should be considered high risk when the uterus is inappropriately large or small. A uterus large for the estimated stage of gestation suggests multiple fetuses, hydramnios, or an excessively large infant; an inappropriately small one suggests retardation of intrauterine growth. Rupture of membranes earlier than 24 hr before delivery carries a risk of fetal infection. Prolonged and difficult labors increase the risks of mechanical and hypoxic damage. The risk of neonatal death in uncomplicated labors lasting 24 hr or less is approximately 0.3%; it increases 6-fold in labors lasting over 24 hr and 20-fold (to 6%) in those over 30 hr. A tumultuous short labor, with a precipitate delivery, increases the risk of birth asphyxia and intracranial hemorrhage. Placental separation at any time prior to delivery and abnormal implantation or compression of the cord increase the possibility of brain damage from fetal anoxia; brown or muddy amniotic fluid suggests that meconium has been passed during an episode of fetal anoxia.

Although the safety of any type of delivery depends upon the skill of the obstetrician, additional hazards accompany particular methods and also result from the circumstances that dictated them. Neonatal deaths following deliveries by mid and high forceps, breech extraction, and version are likely to be related to traumatic intracranial injury; those following vaginal delivery and cesarean section are more apt to be due to anoxia.

Infants born by cesarean section present problems possibly relating to the unfavorable obstetric circumstance that necessitated the operation or to prolonged maternal anesthesia. In normal term pregnancies, when there is no indication of fetal distress, delivery through the abdomen carries a greater risk than delivery through the birth canal. However, controversy exists regarding the safest type of delivery for the nondistressed viable immature fetus, especially in a breech presentation; cesarean section may involve less risk than the "stress" of labor and the potentially anoxic effects of uterine contractions during vaginal delivery. A small percentage of mature infants delivered by cesarean section have some degree of respiratory difficulty for 1–2 days. Although transient tachypnea is the most frequently associated problem, hyaline membrane disease may develop, particularly in infants born to diabetic mothers or following asphyxia.

Anesthesia and analgesia affect the fetus as well as the mother; mild maternal hypoxemia or hypotension may result in severe fetal hypoxia and shock. Skilled use of medication avoids severe fetal narcosis while securing the benefits of gentle and unhurried delivery. Even skilled administration often results in a mildly depressed infant whose crying and breathing may be delayed 1–2 min and who may be somewhat inactive for several hr. When anesthesia and analgesia are carelessly used or when their milder effects are added to already unfavorable fetal circumstances such as prematurity, anoxia, or trauma, the result may be catastrophic.

Barden T: Premature Labor. *In* Fanaroff A, Martin R (eds): Behrman's Neonatal-Perinatal Medicine. St Louis, CV Mosby, 1983.

Bargs V, Benacerraf B, Frigoletto F: Second trimester oligohydramnios. A predictor of poor fetal outcome. Ob Gyn 64:608, 1984.

Berkowitz R: High Risk Pregnancy—1980. Clin Perinatol 7:Entire issue, 1980.

Bottoms S, Rosen M, Sokol R: The increase in the cesarean section rate. N Engl J Med 302:559, 1980.

Campbell S, Kurjak A: Comparison between urinary estrogen assay and serial ultrasonic cephalometry in assessment of fetal growth retardation. Br Med J 4:336, 1972.

Cyr RM, Usher RH, McLean FH: Changing patterns of birth asphyxia and trauma over 20 years. Am J Obstet Gynecol 148:490, 1984.

Duchon M, Gyves M, Merkatz I: Diabetes in pregnancy. In Fanaroff A, Martin R (eds): Behrman's Neonatal-Perinatal Medicine. St Louis, CV Mosby, 1983.

Mann LI, Tejani NA, Weiss RR: Antenatal diagnosis and management of the small-for-gestational age fetus. Am J Obstet Gynecol 129:995, 1974.

Niswander K, Elbourne D, Redman C, et al: Adverse outcome of pregnancy and the quality of obstetrical care. Lancet 2:827, 1984.

Queenan J: Polyhydramnios and oligohydramnios. In Fanaroff A, Martin R (eds): Behrman's Neonatal-Perinatal Medicine. St Louis, CV Mosby, 1983.

Zuspan F: Preeclampsia-eclampsia. In Fanaroff A, Martin R (eds): Behrman's Neonatal-Perinatal Medicine. St Louis, CV Mosby, 1983.

8.8 THE FETUS

Fetal life begins with the completion of organogenesis at about the 12th wk of gestation. Genetic and environmental influences may affect the embryo and fetus at any time during development; the fetal genome itself plays a role in development and fetal survival. Gene mutations and environmental factors may influence selection and expression of genes.

The father's health may affect the motility of the spermatozoon and its ability to penetrate the ovum. The mother's health and state of nutrition may affect ovulation, the viability of the ovum and the zygote, and the availability of an adequate site for implantation; women who suffer from malnutrition or debilitating illness have diminished fertility and often diminished frequency of menstruation. Exposure of the embryo or fetus to drugs, chemicals, infectious disease, or other noxious influences may result in structural malformations or aberrant fetal growth. The general health and nutrition of the mother, and possibly her emotional health during pregnancy, also affect the fetus; the infants of malnourished mothers may weigh less and be slightly shorter at birth than those of mothers with adequate nutrition. Illness of the mother may result in miscarriage, fetal death, fetal growth retardation or premature delivery.

The major emphases in fetal medicine are (1) assessing fetal growth and maturity; (2) evaluating fetal well-being or distress; (3) assessing the effects of maternal disease on the fetus; (4) evaluating the fetal effects of drugs administered to the mother; and (5) identifying and treating fetal disease or anomalies. Increasing knowledge of fetal physiology has paved the way for effective fetal therapy, intervention during fetal distress, and improved adaptation of the newborn infant, particularly of the premature one, to extrauterine life. Some aspects of human fetal growth and development are summarized in Sec. 2.2.

8.9 FETAL GROWTH AND MATURITY

Fetal growth is usually assessed by ultrasonography as early as the 12th wk, but the assessment is more likely to be required between 18–20 wk. Serial determinations of the biparietal diameter are most helpful; head to abdomen circumference ratios may also be useful. Femur length and total intrauterine volume measurements are occasionally indicated. An estimate of gestational age by dating of the last menstrual period should also be obtained. Two patterns of fetal growth retardation have been identified: continuous fetal growth 2 standard deviations below the mean for gestational age and a normal fetal growth curve that abruptly slows or flattens later in gestation (Fig. 8–5).

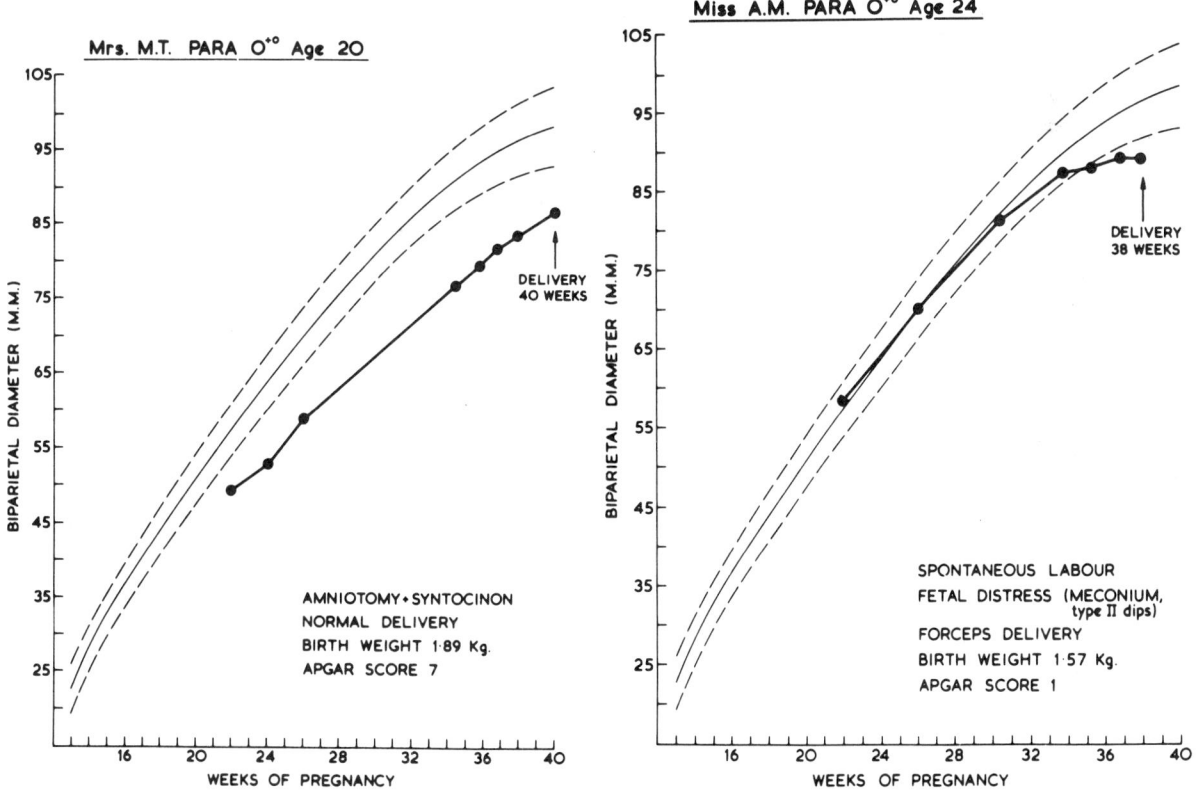

Figure 8–5. *A*, Example of "low profile" growth retardation pattern. Uneventful pregnancy and labor. Baby cried at 1 min and did not develop hypoglycemia. Birth weight was below the 5th percentile weight for gestational age. *B*, Example of "late flattening" growth retardation pattern. Typical history of preeclampsia, intrapartum fetal distress, low Apgar score, and postnatal hypoglycemia. Birth weight was below the 5th percentile weight for gestational age. (From Campbell S: Clin Obstet Gynecol 1:41, 1974.)

Fetal maturity is usually estimated by determining the amniotic fluid surfactant content (Sec. 8.13 and 8.32). Determining the extent of calcification by ultrasound (placental maturity index), detecting the first audible fetal heart tones (16–18 wk), and observing initial fetal movements (18–20 wk) may also aid in evaluating the maturity of the fetus.

8.10 FETAL DISTRESS

Fetal distress is usually associated with abnormal heart rate or rhythm, acidosis, and hypoxia secondary to maternal hypotension, or a cord accident. The causes of antepartum fetal distress include maternal diseases that reduce oxygen transport to the fetus due to maternal hypoxemia (e.g., anemia, cyanotic heart disease), uteroplacental insufficiency (e.g., hypertension, pre-eclampsia, abruptio placenta), or fetal disease (e.g., erythroblastosis, nonimmune hydrops).

Prior to labor, direct measurement of fetal pH or pO₂ is not possible, so indirect tests to evaluate fetal well-being are used. The *Non-Stress Test* (NST) monitors the presence and number of fetal movements, the degree of heart rate acceleration accompanying these movements, and the beat-to-beat variability of the heart rate. The presence of fetal movement, heart rate acceleration, and beat to beat variability are reassuring. The *oxytocin challenge test* (OCT) consists of the intravenous maternal infusion of oxytocin to produce three uterine contractions over 10 min; if this results in three late decelerations (see below), the fetus is judged to be at risk. The biophysical profile is also used to evaluate risk (Table 8–8).

Fetal distress during labor may be detected by monitoring fetal heart rate, uterine pressure, and fetal scalp blood pH (Fig. 8–6).

Continuous fetal heart rate monitoring detects abnormal cardiac patterns by instruments that compute the beat-to-beat fetal heart rate from a fetal electrocardiogram signal. Signals are derived from an electrode attached to the fetal presenting part or the mother's abdomen; from an ultrasonic transducer placed on the maternal abdominal wall to detect continuous ultrasonic waves reflected from the contractions of the heart; or from a phonotransducer placed on the mother's abdomen. Uterine contractions are simultaneously recorded from an amniotic fluid catheter and pressure transducer or from a tocotransducer applied to the maternal abdominal wall overlying the uterus.

Fetal heart rate patterns show various characteristics, some of which suggest fetal distress. Baseline fetal heart rate is the average rate between uterine contractions, which gradually decreases from about 155 beats/min in early pregnancy to about 135 beats/min at term; the normal range at term is 120–160 beats/min. **Tachycardia** (over 160 beats/min) is associated with early fetal hypoxia, maternal fever, maternal hyperthyroidism, maternal β-sympathomimetic or atropine therapy, fetal anemia, and some fetal arrhythmias. The latter do not generally occur with congenital heart disease and tend to resolve spontaneously at birth. **Fetal bradycardia** (less than 120 beats/min) occurs with fetal hypoxia, the placental transfer of local anesthetic agents and beta adrenergic blocking agents, and, occasionally, heart block associated with congenital heart disease.

Normally, the baseline fetal heart rate is variable, with long-term changes of 3–5 cycles/min as well as short-term beat-to-beat variation. This variability may be decreased or lost with fetal hypoxemia or the placental transfer of drugs such as atropine, diazepam, promethazine, magnesium sulfate, and most sedative and narcotic agents. Prematurity and fetal tachycardia may also diminish beat-to-beat variability.

Periodic accelerations or decelerations of fetal heart rate in response to uterine contractions may also be monitored (Fig. 8–6). **Early deceleration** (type I dips), associated with head compression, is a repetitive pattern of slowing, synchronous with and proportional to, the amplitude of the uterine contraction. **Variable deceleration** (associated with cord compression) is characterized by variable shape, onset and occurrence with consecutive contractions, and the return to baseline at or after the conclusion of the contraction. **Late deceleration** (type II dips), associated with fetal hypoxemia, occurs repetitively after a uterine contraction is well established, is proportional to its amplitude, and persists into the interval following contractions. The late deceleration pattern is usually associated with maternal hypotension or excessive uterine activity, but may be a response to any maternal, placental, umbilical cord, or fetal factor that limits effective oxygenation of the fetus. Early signs of fetal distress include mild late deceleration, loss of baseline variability, and increasing baseline rate.

Fetal scalp blood sampling during labor through a slightly dilated cervix may aid in confirming fetal distress suspected on the basis of variations in fetal heart rate or the presence of meconium in the amniotic fluid. The proper use of this technique may result in the earlier delivery of depressed infants having a better chance of successful resuscitation, increased survival, and less morbidity. Alternatively, when continuous fetal heart rate monitoring or general clinical evaluation suggests that a fetus is at risk, a normal fetal scalp blood sample may help to avert obstetric intervention.

Women reasonably comfortable and pain-relieved during

Table 8–8. **Technique of Biophysical Profile Scoring**

Biophysical Variable	Normal (score = 2)	Abnormal (score = 0)
Fetal breathing movements	At least 1 episode of at least 30 sec duration in 30 min of observation.	Absent or no episode of ≥30 sec in 30 min.
Gross body movement	At least 3 discrete body/limb movements in 30 min (episodes of active continuous movement considered as a single movement).	Two or fewer episodes of body/limb movements in 30 min.
Fetal tone	At least 1 episode of active extension with return to flexion of fetal limb(s) or trunk. Opening and closing of hand considered normal tone.	Either slow extension with return to partial flexion or movement of limb in full extension or absent fetal movement.
Reactive fetal heart rate	At least 2 episodes of acceleration of ≥15 bpm and at least 15 sec duration associated with fetal movement in 30 min.	Less than 2 accelerations or acceleration <15 bpm in 30 min.
Qualitative amniotic fluid volume	At least 1 pocket of amniotic fluid that measures at least 1 cm in 2 perpendicular planes.	Either no amniotic fluid pockets or a pocket <1 cm in 2 perpendicular planes.

From Manning F, Morrison I, Lange I, et al.: Clin Perinatol 9:285, 1982.

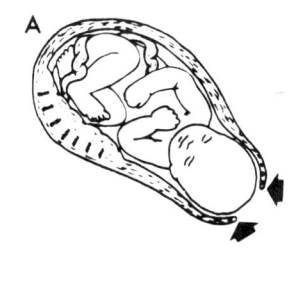

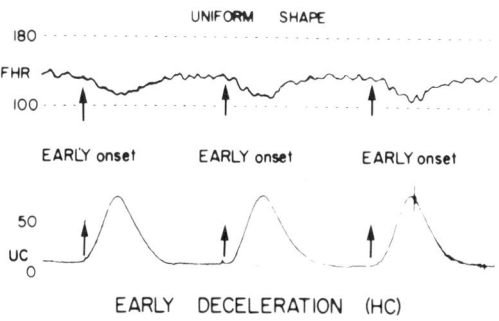

HEAD COMPRESSION

EARLY DECELERATION (HC)

Figure 8–6. Patterns of periodic fetal heart rate decelerations. Tracing in *A* shows early deceleration which occurs during the peak of uterine contractions and is due to pressure on the fetal head; *B*, late deceleration due to uteroplacental insufficiency; *C*, variable deceleration due to umbilical cord compression. Arrows denote time relation between onset of FHR changes and uterine contractions. (From Hon EH: An Atlas of Fetal Heart Rate Patterns. New Haven, CT, Harty Press, Inc., 1968.)

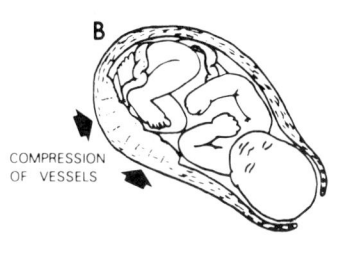

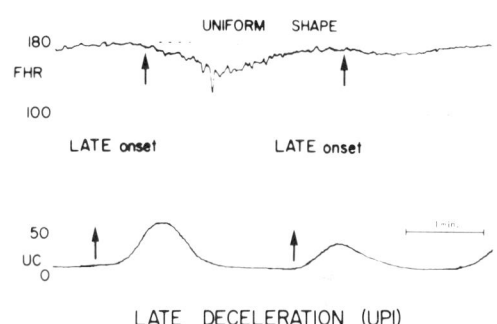

UTEROPLACENTAL INSUFFICIENCY

LATE DECELERATION (UPI)

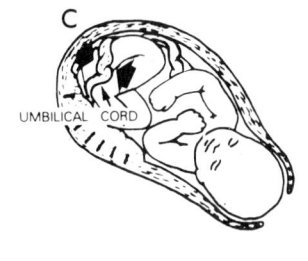

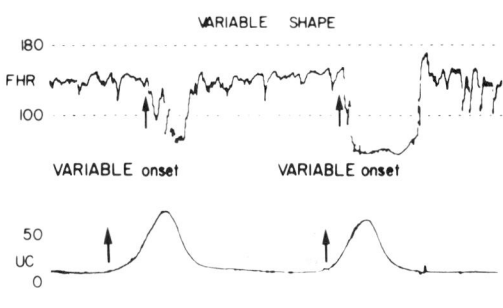

UMBILICAL CORD COMPRESSION

VARIABLE DECELERATION (CC)

labor and delivery usually exhibit an early mild respiratory alkalosis due to hyperventilation and, just before delivery, a mild metabolic acidosis due to a lactic acid accumulation that occurs toward the end of labor. However, pain or stress may produce severe hyperventilation, which markedly reduces maternal and subsequent fetal pCO_2; such a reduction may mask fetal acidosis. Fetal scalp blood pH and pCO_2 levels fall between values measured in the umbilical vein and artery, in most instances giving a reasonable estimate of systemic fetal acid-base values. Fetal scalp blood pH in normal labor decreases from about 7.33 early in labor to approximately 7.25 at the time of vaginal delivery; the base deficit is about 4–6 mEq/L. Changes in the buffer base may be particularly helpful in assessing fetal status, since they correspond to fetal lactic acid accumulation and do not occur as rapidly as changes in fetal pCO_2, which may be influenced by maternal ventilation as well as by placental diffusion.

Fetal hypoxia and circulatory insufficiency result in a mixed placental respiratory and metabolic acidosis that often, but not invariably, can be detected by the determination of pH, base deficit, and carbon dioxide tension in blood obtained from the fetal scalp. A pH less than 7.25 strongly suggests

fetal distress, and a pH of less than 7.20 is an indication for early delivery. A high correlation between fetal acidosis and fetal hypoxia exists, as indicated by the birth of depressed infants with low Apgar scores.

Normal scalp blood pH values are associated with normal continuous fetal heart rate patterns and accurately indicate the absence of recent moderate to severe hypoxia. In contrast, low scalp blood pH values frequently correlate with severe variable deceleration or late deceleration alone and with loss of beat-to-beat variability or baseline tachycardia associated with these deceleration patterns. However, a wide range of pH is found with these patterns. Accordingly, heart rate–uterine contraction monitoring should be used as a screening technique, and acid-base analysis of fetal scalp blood and maternal blood should be obtained to properly evaluate many types of fetal heart rate abnormalities.

Complications of fetal scalp sampling and internal monitoring devices are relatively uncommon, but include bleeding (usually due to an underlying coagulation defect), puncture of the fontanel, and scalp abscesses with or without adjacent osteomyelitis. Abscesses may be due to *Staphylococcus aureus* or gram-negative rods; more often they are sterile.

8.11 MATERNAL DISEASE AND THE FETUS

Infectious Diseases. Almost any maternal infection with severe systemic manifestations may result in miscarriage, stillbirth, or premature labor. Whether these results are due to infection of the fetus or are secondary to stress is not always clear. Maternal hyperthermia during infections may be associated with an increased incidence of congenital anomalies. Regardless of the severity of the maternal infection, certain agents frequently infect the fetus with serious sequelae. Such fetuses are frequently small for gestational age. Some infections, such as rubella, may also produce congenital malformations if they occur during the period of organogenesis. Maternal infections that cause disease in the fetus or newborn infant include *Borrelia burgdorferi* (Lyme disease), *Chagas disease*, *chickenpox* or *herpes zoster*, *Coxsackie B viruses*, *cytomegalovirus, hepatitis, herpes simplex, listeriosis, malaria* (miscarriage, premature delivery), *mumps* (fetal death and possibly endocardial fibroelastosis), *parvovirus, poliomyelitis* (abortion, congenital paralysis) *rubella, rubeola* (miscarriage, prematurity, fetal measles, possibly congenital malformations), *smallpox* (fetal smallpox), *streptococcus syphilis, toxoplasmosis, tuberculosis* (congenital tuberculosis), *vaccinia or vaccination* (fetal vaccinia), *vibrio fetus* (miscarriage, prematurity, meningitis), and *Western equine encephalitis* (encephalitis).

Noninfectious Diseases (Table 8–6). *Maternal diabetes* may result in organomegaly, hypertrophy and hyperplasia of the beta cells of the fetal pancreas, and metabolic derangements in the neonate (Sec. 8.56). A high incidence of intrauterine death exists after the 36th wk of gestation in unmonitored mothers. *Toxemia* of pregnancy, chronic hypertension, and renal disease result in small fetal size for gestational age, prematurity, and intrauterine death, all probably due to diminished uteroplacental perfusion. Uncontrolled maternal *hypothyroidism* or *hyperthyroidism* is responsible for relative infertility, a tendency to abort, premature labor, and fetal death. Maternal *immunologic diseases,* such as idiopathic thrombocytopenic purpura, systemic lupus, myasthenia gravis, and Graves disease, all of which are mediated by IgG autoantibodies which cross the placenta, frequently result in a transient illness in the newborn. Untreated maternal *phenylketonuria* results in miscarriage, congenital malformations, and injury to the brain of the nonphenylketonuric fetus.

8.12 MATERNAL MEDICATION AND THE FETUS

The effects of drugs taken by the mother vary considerably, especially in relation to the time in pregnancy when they are taken. Miscarriage or congenital malformations result from maternal ingestion of teratogenic drugs during the period of organogenesis. Some drugs may be synergistic in producing their teratogenic effects. Maternal medications taken later, particularly during the last few weeks of gestation or during labor, tend to affect the function of specific organs or enzyme systems, adversely affecting the neonate rather than the fetus (Tables 8–9 and 8–10). Individual genetic make up may deter-

Table 8–9. **Maternal Medications That May Adversely Affect the Fetus**

Drug	Effect on Fetus	Dependability of Evidence
Accutane (isotretinoin)	Facial-ear anomalies, heart disease	Suggestive
Adrenal corticosteroids	Cleft palate	Doubtful
Alcohol	Congenital anomalies, IUGR*	Conclusive
Aminopterin	Abortion, malformations	Conclusive
Amphetamines	Congenital heart disease, IUGR	Suggestive
Azathioprine	Abortion	Suggestive
Busulfan (Myleran)	Stunted growth, corneal opacities, cleft palate, hypoplasia of ovaries, thyroid, and parathyroids	Doubtful
Caffeine	Spontaneous abortion, stillbirth, anomalies, or premature birth	Doubtful
Chloroquine	Deafness	Suggestive
Cigarette smoking	Low birthweight for gestational age	Suggestive
Cyclophosphamide	Multiple malformations	Suggestive
Dicumarol	Fetal bleeding and death, hypoplastic nasal structures	Conclusive
Lithium	Cyanotic heart disease	Suggestive
Meclizine (Bonine)	Congenital malformations	Doubtful
Mepivacaine	Bradycardia, death	Conclusive
6-Mercaptopurine	Abortion	Suggestive
Methimazole	Goiter	Conclusive
Methyltestosterone	Masculinization of female fetus	Conclusive
17-Alpha-ethinyl-19-nortestosterone (Norlutin)	Masculinization of female fetus	Conclusive
Penicillamine	Cutis laxa syndrome	Suggestive
Phenytoin (Dilantin)	Congenital anomalies, IUGR, tumor	Conclusive
Progesterone	Masculinization of female fetus	Suggestive
Propranolol	Hypoglycemia, bradycardia, respiratory depression	Suggestive
Propylthiouracil	Goiter	Conclusive
Quinine	Abortion, thrombocytopenia, deafness	Suggestive
Radioactive iodine (^{131}I)	Destruction of fetal thyroid	Conclusive
17-Alpha-ethinyl testosterone (Progestoral)	Masculinization of female fetus	Conclusive
Stilbestrol (diethylstilbestrol [DES])	Vaginal adenocarcinoma in adolescence	Conclusive
Streptomycin	Deafness	Suggestive
Tetracycline	Retarded skeletal growth	Suggestive
	Pigmentation of teeth, hypoplasia of enamel	Conclusive
	Cataract, limb malformations	Doubtful
Thalidomide	Phocomelia, other malformations	Conclusive
Trimethadione and paramethadione	Abortion, multiple malformations, mental retardation	Conclusive
Tolbutamide	Congenital malformations	Doubtful
Valproate	Spina bifida	Suggestive
Vitamin D	Supravalvular aortic stenosis, hypercalcemia	Doubtful

*IUGR = intrauterine growth retardation.

Table 8–10. **Maternal Medications That May Adversely Affect the Newborn Infant**

Anesthetic agents (volatile)—central nervous system depression
Adrenal corticosteroids—adrenocortical failure (rare)
Ammonium chloride—acidosis (clinically inapparent)
Aspirin—neonatal bleeding, prolonged gestation
Bromides—rash, CNS depression
Captopril—cardiovascular instability
Caudal anesthesia with mepivacaine (accidental introduction of anesthetic into scalp of baby)—bradypnea, apnea, bradycardia, convulsions
CNS depressants (narcotics, barbiturates, tranquilizers) during labor—central nervous system depression
Cephalothin—positive direct Coombs test reaction
Coumarin derivatives—high perinatal mortality, anomalies
Dilantin—bleeding diathesis (vitamin K deficiency)
Hexamethonium bromide—paralytic ileus
Indomethacin—persistent fetal circulation
Intravenous fluids during labor, e.g., salt-free solutions—electrolyte disturbances, hyponatremia, hypoglycemia
Iodides—neonatal goiter
Isoxsuprine—ileus, hypocalcemia, hypoglycemia, hypotension
Magnesium sulfate—respiratory depression, meconium plug, hypotonia
Morphine and its derivatives (addiction)—withdrawal symptoms (poor feeding, vomiting, diarrhea, restlessness, yawning and stretching, dyspnea and cyanosis, fever and sweating, pallor, tremors, convulsions)
Naphthalene—hemolytic anemia (in glucose-6-phosphate dehydrogenase [G-6-PD]–deficient infants)
Nitrofurantoin—hemolytic anemia (in G-6-PD–deficient infants)
Oxytocin—hyperbilirubinemia
Phenobarbital—bleeding diathesis (vitamin K deficiency)
Primaquine—hemolytic anemia (in G-6-PD–deficient infants)
Propranolol—hypoglycemia, bradycardia, apnea
Reserpine—drowsiness, nasal congestion, poor temperature stability
Sulfonamides (long-acting)—interfere with protein binding of bilirubin; kernicterus at low levels of serum bilirubin
Sulfonylurea—refractory hypoglycemia
Thiazides—neonatal thrombocytopenia (rare)
Vitamin K (excessive amounts)—hyperbilirubinemia

mine susceptibility to some drugs. In addition, the effects of drugs may be evident immediately in the delivery room or may be delayed, such as with the development of genital lesions in female offspring of women exposed to diethylstilbestrol during pregnancy or childhood tumors following fetal alcohol or phenytoin exposure. Consumption of drugs in pregnancy is frequent; surveys indicate that 90% of pregnant patients have taken at least 1 drug. The average mother has taken 4 drugs other than vitamins or iron during pregnancy; 4% have taken 10 or more drugs.

In view of the limits of the current knowledge of fetal effects from maternal medication, no drugs should be prescribed during pregnancy without weighing the maternal need against the risk of fetal damage.

8.13 IDENTIFICATION OF FETAL DISEASE (INTRAUTERINE DIAGNOSIS)

See Sec 8.10 for discussion of fetal distress.

Diagnostic procedures may be used for identifying disease in the fetus when interruption of the pregnancy is considered and when direct treatment of the fetus is possible. In a broader context, the family history, reproductive history of the mother, and course of the pregnancy may lead to the nonspecific diagnoses of "high risk pregnancy" and "high risk infant" (Sec. 8.7 and 8.15).

Amniocentesis, the transabdominal withdrawal of amniotic fluid during pregnancy for diagnostic purposes (Table 8–11), is frequently done to determine the timing of the delivery of fetuses with erythroblastosis fetalis or the need for a fetal transfusion. It is also done for genetic indications, usually between the 16th and 18th gestational weeks. The amniotic fluid may be directly analyzed for amino acids, enzymes, hormones, and abnormal metabolic products; uncultivated amniotic fluid cells may be subjected to sex chromatin analysis and Y chromosome fluorescence to detect male fetuses at risk for sex-linked disorders, such as hemophilia and progressive muscular dystrophy; and amniotic fluid cells may be cultivated to permit detailed cytologic analysis for the prenatal detection of chromosomal abnormalities and DNA-gene or enzymatic analysis for the detection of inborn metabolic errors. Analysis of amniotic fluid may also help in identifying neural tube defects (elevation of α-fetoprotein), adrenogenital syndrome (elevation of 17-ketosteroids and pregnanetriol), and thyroid dysfunction. In addition, direct viewing of the fetus by transabdominal amnioscopy has been used to diagnose fetal anomalies and to facilitate sampling of fetal blood for detecting hemoglobinopathies, hemophilia, and thrombocytopenia.

The best available chemical indices of fetal maturity are provided by determinations of amniotic fluid creatinine and lecithin, which reflect the maturity of fetal kidney and lung, respectively. Lecithin (L) is produced in the lung by type II alveolar cells and eventually reaches the amniotic fluid via the effluent from the trachea. Until the middle of the 3rd trimester, its concentration nearly equals that of sphingomyelin (S); thereafter, S remains constant in amniotic fluid while L increases. By 35 wk, on the average, the L/S ratio is about 2:1 and indicates lung maturity.

Earlier lung maturation may occur when there is severe premature separation of the placenta, premature rupture of the fetal membranes, narcotic addiction, or maternal hypertensive and renal vascular disease. A delay in pulmonary maturation may be associated with hydrops fetalis or maternal diabetes without vascular disease. The likelihood of hyaline membrane disease is greatly reduced with L/S ratios of 2 or more to 1, although hypoxia, acidosis, and hypothermia may increase the risk despite this "mature" L/S ratio. However, 20–25% of infants with L/S ratios less than 2:1 will not have hyaline membrane disease. Maternal and fetal blood have an L/S ratio of about 1:4; thus, contamination will not alter the significance of a ratio of 2:1 or more. Meconium contamination, storage, and centrifugation all may reduce the reliability of the L/S ratio. An alternative bubble stability or shake test is also used as an index of a "mature" level of pulmonary surfactant; after diluting amniotic fluid with isotonic saline and then shaking with 95% ethanol, varying degrees of bubble formation develop. The greater the dilution (1:2, 1:3, 1:4) that results in a complete ring of bubbles, the lower the risk of hyaline membrane disease.

A determination of saturated phosphatidyl-choline (L) or phosphatidyl-glycerol (PG) concentrations in amniotic fluid may be more specific and sensitive predictors of hyaline membrane disease, especially in high risk pregnancies such as occur with diabetes.

Table 8–11. **Applications of Amniocentesis During Pregnancy**

Biochemical and cytogenetic studies in early pregnancy
Diagnosis and prognosis of erythroblastosis fetalis
Diagnosis and treatment of polyhydramnios
Direct fetal visualization and blood sampling
Intravascular fetal transfusion of platelets or blood
Studies of amniotic fluid circulation
Determinations of fetal maturity
Induction of labor
Instillation of pharmacologic agents for treatment of the fetus

Although amniocentesis can be carried out with little discomfort to the mother, there is, even in experienced hands, a small risk of direct damage to the fetus, of placental puncture and bleeding with secondary damage to the fetus, of stimulating uterine contraction and premature labor, of amnionitis, and of maternal sensitization to fetal blood. The earlier in gestation amniotic puncture is done, the greater the risk to the fetus. The risks can be reduced by using ultrasound B scan for placental localization. The procedure should be limited to those cases in which the potential benefits of the findings will outweigh the risk.

Ultrasonography, using a pulsed sound of high resolution and short wavelength inaudible to humans, is used to obtain serial, accurately measurable images of the fetus. Two-dimensional B-scan sonographic display techniques are used to determine the dimensions of the fetal head (cephalometry), thorax, and abdomen to estimate maturity and diagnose intrauterine growth retardation or death (Sec. 8.9); to localize the placenta prior to amniocentesis so that it can be avoided; to identify a placenta previa or a hydatidiform mole; to diagnose fetal position and number; to diagnose fetal hydrops; and to detect congenital abnormalities. The low energy levels employed in pulsed or continuous ultrasound have no detectable effect on tissue culture, on chromosomes, or on the infants. Although more than 95% of fetuses whose biparietal diameters measure 9.5 cm or more by ultrasonography are of at least 37 wk gestational age, this does not assume mature lungs. Combining biparietal diameter and abdominal circumference estimates enhances the ability to detect intrauterine growth retardation before delivery. Sonography also has been used successfully to diagnose anencephaly, hydrocephaly, meningocele, polycystic kidneys, omphalocele, gastroschisis, diaphragmatic hernia, dextrocardia, congenital heart disease, hydrops, gastrointestinal obstruction, and large fetal neoplasms.

Roentgenographic examination is a diagnostic procedure now rarely chosen to estimate fetal maturity or to establish a fetal diagnosis. The distal femoral epiphysis may appear as early as 32 wk and is nearly always present by 40 wk, while the proximal tibial epiphysis may appear as early as 36 wk and is present in 50–75% of fetuses at 40 wk. Ultrasonography is more accurate before 36 wk of gestation and avoids the remote risks of genetic or developmental injury from diagnostic radiation. Roentgenograms may be indicated to detect bony or calcific abnormalities such as achondroplasia, infantile cortical hyperostosis, osteogenesis imperfecta, or meconium peritonitis. Lipid-soluble contrast medium injected into the amniotic fluid (amniography) can be used to outline the fetal soft tissues and diagnose congenital anomalies.

The *concentration of estriol* in the urine of pregnant women reaches levels 100–1000 times greater than that of nonpregnant women as a result of the production of androgen precursors (mainly dihydroepiandrosterone sulfate) in the fetal adrenal, their hydroxylation in the fetal liver and conversion to estriol in the placenta, and the conjugation of estriol in the maternal liver. The 24 hr urine estriol excretion increases throughout pregnancy with a surge during the last 4–8 wk. Abnormally low serial urinary estriol determinations and depressed plasma unconjugated estriol levels are associated with fetal death; maternal diabetes, hypertension, renal disease, or toxemia; prolonged pregnancy; intrauterine growth retardation; anencephaly; fetal adrenal insufficiency; and maternal drug therapy (corticosteroids, ampicillin, Mandelamine, dihydroxyanthraquinone derivatives). Placental sulfatase deficiency, a rare disorder affecting male infants, results in low estriols but no other abnormality. Estriol determinations should only be used to complement nonstress testing or the biophysical profile.

8.14 TREATMENT AND PREVENTION OF FETAL DISEASE

Managing fetal diseases continues to depend on coordinated advances in accuracy of diagnosis; in understanding of fetal nutrition, pharmacology, immunology, and pathophysiology; in the availability of antimicrobial and especially antiviral drugs; and in therapeutic procedures. Progress in providing specific treatments for accurately diagnosed diseases has been slow (Table 8–12).

Fetal syphilis is most always present in untreated maternal disease and can be specifically and safely treated (Sec. 11.49). Fetal mortality and prematurity associated with maternal bacterial urinary tract infections can be reduced with appropriate antibiotic treatment of the mother. Immunization has effectively reduced fetal mortality and morbidity from rubella (Sec. 4.1 and 11.62).

The incidence of sensitization of Rh negative women by Rh positive fetuses has been reduced by the prophylactic administration of Rh(D) immune globulin to mothers early in pregnancy and after each delivery or abortion, thus reducing the frequency of hemolytic disease in their subsequent offspring. Fetal erythroblastosis (Sec. 8.47) may now be accurately diagnosed by amniotic fluid analysis and treated with intrauterine intraperitoneal or intravenous transfusions of packed Rh negative blood cells to maintain the fetus until mature enough to have a reasonable chance of survival.

Fetal asphyxia or distress may now be diagnosed with moderate success (Sec. 8.10). Treatment, however, remains limited to supplying the mother with high concentrations of oxygen, positioning the uterus to avoid vascular compression, and operative delivery before severe fetal injury occurs.

Pharmacologic approaches to fetal immaturity (e.g., administration of steroids to the mother to accelerate fetal lung maturation and to decrease the incidence of hyaline membrane disease [Sec. 8.32] in prematurely delivered infants) are promising. Inhibiting labor with β-sympathomimetic tocolytic agents is successful in some patients with premature labor.

Table 8–12. Fetal Therapy

Disorder	Treatment
Maternal PKU	Phenylalanine restriction
Fetal galactosemia	Galactose-free diet
Mixed carboxylase deficiency	Biotin
Methyl malonic acidemia	B$_{12}$
Neural tube defects	Folate, multivitamins (?)
Hypothyroidism	Thyroid hormone
Adrenal genital syndrome	Corticosteroids
ITP (Idiopathic thrombocytopenic purpura)	Corticosteroids? Fetal platelets transfusion
Paroxysmal tachycardia	Digoxin, verapamil, procainamide, quinidine, propranolol
Withdrawal syndrome	Methadone
Pulmonary immaturity	Corticosteroids
Fetal distress	Tocolysis, oxygen, maternal position
Premature labor	Tocolysis
Toxoplasmosis	Spiramycin
Syphilis	Penicillin
Tuberculosis	Antituberculosis drugs
Group B streptococcus	Ampicillin
Maternal diabetes	Tight insulin control
Erythroblastosis fetalis	Intrauterine transfusion
Hydrocephalus	Ventricular catheter placement (?)
Hydronephrosis	Nephrostomy
Urethral obstruction	Suprapubic catheter

Treating definitively diagnosed fetal genetic disease or congenital anomalies consists of parental counseling and/or abortion; rarely, high dose vitamin therapy for a responsive inborn error of metabolism (e.g., biotin-dependent disorders) or fetal surgery to relieve obstructive genitourinary tract anomalies may be indicated. The nature of the defect and its consequences as well as ethical concerns of parents, society, and the physician must be considered.

Frantz T, Lindback T, Skjaeraasen J, et al: Phospholipids in amniotic fluid. II. Lecithin fatty acid patterns related to gestation, maternal disease and fetal outcome. Acta Obstet Gynecol Scand 54:33, 1975.
Freeman RK: The use of the oxytocin challenge test for antepartum clinical evaluation of uteroplacental respiratory function. Am J Obstet Gynecol 121:481, 1975.
Fuchs F: Prevention of premature birth. Clin Perinatol 7:3, 1980.
Gabert HA, Bryson MJ, Stenchever MA: The effect of cesarean section on respiratory distress in the presence of a mature lecithin-sphingomyelin ratio. Am J Obstet Gynecol 115:366, 1973.
Garite T, Freeman R: Antepartum stress test monitoring. Clin Obstet Gynecol 6:295, 1979.
Gluck L, Kuolvich MU, Borer RC Jr, et al: Interpretation and significance of the lecithin-sphingomyelin ratio in amniotic fluid. Am J Obstet Gynecol 120:142, 1974.
Golbus M, Harrison M, Filly R: Prenatal diagnosis and treatment of fetal hydronephrosis. Semin Perinatol 7:81, 1983.
Golbus M, Loughman W, Epstein C, et al: Prenatal genetic diagnosis in 3000 amniocenteses. N Engl J Med 300:157, 1979.
Goodlin R (ed): Fetal monitoring. Semin Perinatol 5, 1981.
Hobbins J, Mahoney M: Fetoscopy in continuing pregnancies. Am J Obstet Gynecol 129:440, 1977.
Hobbins J, Grannum P, Berkowitz R, et al: Ultrasound in the diagnosis of congenital anomalies. Am J Obstet Gynecol 134:331, 1979.
Hon EH, Zannini D, Quilligan EJ: The neonatal value of fetal monitoring. Am J Obstet Gynecol 122:508, 1975.
Johnson M, Pretorius D, Clewell W, et al: Fetal hydrocephalus: Diagnosis and management. Semin Perinatol 7:83, 1983.
Liley AW: Liquor amnii analysis in management of pregnancy complicated by rhesus sensitization. Am J Obstet Gynecol 82:1359, 1961.
Low JA, Panchow SR, Worthington D, et al: The incidence of fetal asphyxia in six hundred high-risk monitored pregnancies. Am J Obstet Gynecol 121:456, 1975.
Manning F, Morrison I, Lange I, et al: Antepartum determination of fetal health. Composite biophysical profile scoring. Clin Perinatol 9:285, 1982.
Olson EB, Jr, Harline JV, Schneider JM, et al: The use of amniotic bubble stability, L/S ratio, and creatinine concentration in the assessment of fetal maturity. Am J Obstet Gynecol 122:755, 1975.
Pitkin RM: Estimation of fetal maturity. In: Fanaroff A, Martin R (eds): Behrman's Neonatal-Perinatal Medicine. St Louis, CV Mosby, 1983.
Pleet H, Graham J, Smith D: Central nervous system and facial defects associated with maternal hyperthermia at 4–14 wk gestation. Pediatrics 67:785, 1981.
Porreco R, Young P, Cousins L, et al: Reproductive outcome following amniocentesis for genetic indications. Am J Obstet Gynecol 143:653, 1982.
Report of the International Fetal Surgery Registry: Catheter shunts for fetal hydronephrosis and hydrocephalus. N Engl J Med 315:336, 1986.
Tejani N, Maran LI, Bhakthavathsalan A, et al: Correlation of fetal heart rate–uterine contraction patterns with fetal scalp blood pH. Obstet Gynecol 46:392, 1975.
Zuspan F, Quilligan E, Lams J, et al: NICHD Consensus Development Task Force Report: Predictors of intrapartum fetal distress—the role of electronic fetal monitoring. J Pediatr 95:1026, 1979.

8.15 THE HIGH RISK INFANT

Infants particularly at risk during the neonatal period should be identified as early as possible in order to decrease neonatal morbidity and mortality (see also Sec. 8.7). The term *high risk* infant designates infants who should be under close observation by experienced physicians and nurses. Usually needed for only a few days, such observations may range from a few hours to several weeks. Some institutions find it advantageous to provide a special or transitional care nursery for high risk infants, often within the labor and delivery suite. This facility should be equipped and staffed similarly to a neonatal intensive care area, where well but high risk term infants can be observed and cared for immediately after birth without being separated from their mothers.

Infants in the high risk category are listed in Table 8–13.

Examination of a fresh *placenta, cord,* and *membranes* may alert the physician to a newborn infant at high risk. Fetal blood loss may be indicated by placental pallor, **retroplacental hematoma,** and tears of a velamentous cord or of chorionic blood vessels supplying succenturiate lobes. **Placental edema** and subsequent deficiency of immunoglobulin G in the newborn may be associated with feto-fetal transfusion syndrome, hydrops fetalis, congenital nephrosis, or hepatic disease. **Amnion nodosum** (granules on the amnion) and **oligohydramnios** are associated with pulmonary hypoplasia and renal agenesis, and small whitish **nodules** on the cord suggest a candida infection. **Short cords** occur with chromosome abnormalities and omphalocele. **Chorioangiomas** are associated with prematurity, abruptio, polyhydramnios, and intrauterine growth retardation. **Meconium staining** suggests asphyxia and the risk, of pneumonia, and opacity of the fetal placental surface suggests infection. **Single umbilical arteries** are associated with an increased incidence of congenital abnormalities.

Many high risk infants are born prematurely, have low weight for gestational age, have significant perinatal asphyxia, or are born with life-threatening congenital anomalies without exhibiting previously identified risk factors. Generally speak-

Table 8–13. High Risk Infants

1. Birth before 37 wk or after 42 wk gestation
2. Birthweight <2500 or >4000 gm
3. Deviations in expected size for stage of development (see Fig. 8–7 and Sec. 8.17)
4. History of fetal or neonatal sibling deaths or serious illness
5. Poor condition at delivery (Apgar 0–4 at 1 min) or resuscitation required at delivery or subsequently
6. History of maternal infection or other illness during pregnancy (Table 8–6), premature rupture of membranes, severe social problems (e.g., teenage pregnancy, drug addiction), absent or late prenatal care, abnormal gestational weight gain, prolonged infertility, four or more previous pregnancies, 35 yr or more maternal age (especially if primiparous), or ingestion of drugs listed in Tables 8–9 and 8–10
7. Multiple pregnancy or gestation commencing within 6 mo of a previous pregnancy
8. Delivery by cesarean section or any unusual obstetrical complication, including hydramnios, abruptio placentae, placenta previa, or abnormal presentation
9. Significant malformation or suspicion of malformation
10. Anemia or blood group incompatibility
11. Severe maternal emotional problems, such as hyperemesis gravidarum
12. Serious accidents or general anesthesia during pregnancy

ing, for any given duration of gestation, the lower the birth weight, the higher the neonatal mortality, and, for any given weight, the shorter the gestational duration, the higher the neonatal mortality (Fig. 8–7). The highest risk of neonatal mortality occurs among infants who weigh less than 1000 g at birth and whose gestation was less than 30 wk. The lowest risk of neonatal mortality occurs among infants with birthweights of 3000–4000 g whose gestational age was 38–42 wk. As birthweight increases from 500 to 3000 g, a logarithmic decrease in neonatal mortality occurs; for every wk increase in gestational age from the 25th to 37th wk, the neonatal

GRAMS

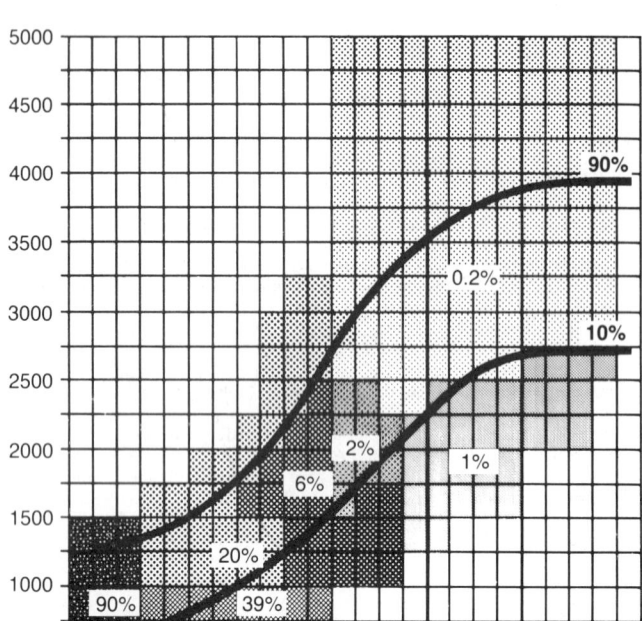

24 26 28 30 32 34 36 38 40 42 44 46

Pre-Term | Term | Post-Term

WEEKS OF GESTATION

Figure 8–7. Neonatal mortality risk based on actual data from 14, 413 live births at the University of Colorado Health Sciences Center from 1974 to 1980. (From Koops B, Morgan L, Battaglia F: J Pediatr 101:969, 1982.)

mortality rate decreases approximately one half. Nevertheless, approximately 40% of all *perinatal deaths* occur after 37 wk of gestation in infants weighing 2500 g or more; many of these deaths occur in the period immediately before birth and are more readily preventable than those of smaller and more immature infants. In addition, neonatal mortality rates rise sharply for infants weighing over 4000 g at birth and for those whose gestational period is 42 wk or longer. Since neonatal mortality largely depends on birth weight and gestational age, Fig. 8–7 helps to quickly identify high risk infants. However, this analysis is based on total live births and, therefore, describes the mortality risk only *at birth*. Because most neonatal mortality occurs within the first hours and days after birth, the outlook improves dramatically with increasing postnatal survival.

Battaglia FC, Frazier TM, Hellegers AE: Birth weight, gestational age and pregnancy outcome with special reference to the high birth weight, low gestational age infant. Pediatrics 37:417, 1966.
Behrman RE, Babson GS, Lessel R: Fetal and neonatal mortality in white middle class infants. Am J Dis Child 121:486, 1971.
Behrman RE: Prevention of low birthweight: A pediatric perspective. J Pediatr 107:842, 1985.
Bjerkedahl T, Bakketeig L, Lehmann EH: Percentiles of birth weights of single live births at different gestational periods. Acta Pediatr Scand 62:449, 1973.
Hobel C: Better perinatal health: U.S.A. Lancet 1:31, 1980.
Tanner JM, Lejarraga H, Turner G: Within-family standards for birth weight. Lancet 2:193, 1972.
Whitby C, DeCates C, Robertson N: Infants weighing 1.8–2.5 kg: Should they be cared for in neonatal units or postnatal wards? Lancet 1:322, 1982.

8.16 MULTIPLE PREGNANCIES

Incidence. The reported incidence of twins is highest among blacks and East Indians, followed by North European whites, and is lowest among the Mongolian races. Specific rates include: Belgium, 1:56, American blacks, 1:70; Italy, 1:86; American whites, 1:88; Greece, 1:130; Japan, 1:150; China,

1:300. Differences in the incidence of twins mainly involve fraternal (polyovular) twins. Triplets are estimated to occur in 1 of 86^2 pregnancies and quadruplets in 1 of 86^3 pregnancies in the United States. The incidence of females increases with the number of fetal products of a multiple pregnancy.

Etiology. The occurrence of monovular twins appears to be independent of genetic influences. Polyovular pregnancies are more frequent beyond the second pregnancy, in older women, and in families with a history of polyovular twins. They may result from simultaneous maturation of multiple ovarian follicles, but follicles containing two ova have been described as a genetic trait leading to twin pregnancies. Twin-prone women have higher levels of gonadotropins. Polyovular pregnancies occur in many women treated for infertility with human pituitary or gonadotropins.

Conjoined twins (Siamese twins) probably result from relatively late monovular separation, as does the presence of two separate embryos in one amniotic sac. The latter condition has a high fatality rate due to obstruction of the circulation secondary to intertwining of the umbilical cords. The prognosis for conjoined twins depends on the possibility of surgical separation.

Superfecundation, the fertilization of an ovum by an insemination that takes place after one ovum has already been fertilized, and *superfetation,* the fertilization and subsequent development of an ovum when a fetus is already present in the uterus, have been proposed as a reason for differences in size and appearance of certain twins at birth.

Monozygotic versus Dizygotic Twins. Identifying twins as monozygotic or dizygotic (monovular or polyovular) is important because studying monozygotic twins is useful in determining the relative influence of heredity and environment on human development and disease. Twins not of the same sex are dizygotic. In twins of the same sex, zygosity should be determined and recorded at birth through careful examination of the placenta or later through comparison of physical characteristics, detailed blood typing, or tissue typing.

Examination of the Placenta. If the placentas are separate, they are always dichorionic, but the twins are not necessarily dizygotic since initiation of monovular twinning at the first cell division or during the morula state may result in two amnions, two chorions, and even two placentas. One third of monozygotic twins are dichorionic and diamniotic.

An apparently single placenta may be present with either monovular or polyovular twins. Yet inspecting the polyovular placenta usually reveals a separate chorion for each fetus that crosses the placenta between the attachments of the cords and two amnions. Separate or fused dichorionic placentas may be disproportionate in size. The fetus attached to the smaller placenta or portion of placenta is usually smaller than its twin or is malformed. Monochorionic twins may be presumed to be monovular. They are usually diamnionic, and, almost invariably, the placenta is a single mass.

Placental vascular anastomoses occur with high frequency only in monochorionic twins. In monochorionic placentas, the fetal vasculature is usually joined, sometimes in a very complex manner. The vascular anastomoses in monochorionic placentas may be artery-to-artery, vein-to-vein, or artery-to-vein. They are usually well enough balanced so that neither twin suffers. Artery-to-artery communications cross over placental veins, and when anastomoses are present, blood can readily be stroked from one fetal vascular bed to the other. Vein-to-vein communications are similarly recognized and less common. A combination of artery-to-artery and vein-to-vein anastomoses is associated with *acardiac fetus.* In rare cases one umbilical cord may arise from the other after leaving the placenta. In such instances the twin attached to the secondary cord is usually malformed or dies in utero. Table 8–14 lists the more frequent changes associated with a large uncompensated arteriovenous shunt from the placenta of one twin to that of the other; twins of widely discrepant size are usually monochorionic.

In the **fetal transfusion syndrome,** an artery from one twin delivers blood that is drained through the vein of the other. The latter becomes plethoric and large while the former is anemic and small sized. Maternal hydramnios in a twin pregnancy suggests the fetal transfusion syndrome. Anticipating this possibility by preparing to transfuse the donor twin or to bleed the recipient twin may be life-saving. Death of the donor twin in utero may result in generalized fibrin thrombi in the smaller arterioles of the recipient twin, possibly as the result of transfusion of thromboplastin-rich blood from the macerating donor fetus. The surviving twin may develop disseminated intravascular coagulation.

Postnatal Identification. *Physical criteria* for determining monovular twins are (1) both must be the same sex; (2) their features, including ears and teeth, must be obviously alike (but they need not resemble one another more than the lateral halves of one individual); (3) their hair must be identical in color, texture, natural curl, and distribution; (4) their eyes must be of the same color and shade; (5) their skin must be of the same texture and color (nevi may be differently apportioned and distributed); (6) their hands and feet must be of the same conformation and of similar size; and (7) their anthropometric values must show close agreement.

Detailed blood and tissue typing can prove that twins are monozygotic.

Prognosis. Most twins are born prematurely, and maternal complications of pregnancy are more common than with single pregnancies. Although there is a significant increase in perinatal mortality among monochorionic twins, there is no significant difference between the neonatal mortality rates of twin and single births in comparable weight groups. Yet, since most twins are premature by weight, their overall mortality is higher than that of single births. The perinatal mortality of twins is about four times that of singletons. The incidence of malformations incompatible with life is greater in multiple than in single pregnancies. There is also an increased incidence of ruptured vasa previa and velamentous insertion of the umbilical cord, with an associated higher risk of bleeding during labor. Monoamniotic twins have an increased likelihood of entangling their cords, which may lead to asphyxia. If one of the fetuses is macerated, the live twin is usually delivered first. Theoretically, the second twin is more subject to anoxia than is the first because the placenta may separate after the birth of the first twin and before the birth of the second. In addition, the delivery of the second twin may be difficult, since it may be in an abnormal presentation, uterine tone may be decreased, or the cervix may begin to close following the first twin's birth. A growth retarded twin is at high risk for hypoglycemia. Notable differences in size at birth of monovular twins usually disappear by the time the infants are 6 mo of age.

Treatment. Prenatal diagnosis enables the obstetrician and the pediatrician to anticipate the birth of infants who are at high risk because of twinning. Close observation is indicated during labor and in the immediate neonatal period so that prompt treatment of asphyxia or fetal transfusion syndrome can be initiated. The decision to perform an immediate blood transfusion in a severely anemic "donor twin" or to perform a partial exchange transfusion of a "recipient twin" must be based on clinical judgment.

Benirschke K, Chung KK: Multiple pregnancy. N Engl J Med 288:1276, 1329, 1973.
McCarthy BJ, Sachs BP, Layde PM, et al: The epidemiology of neonatal death in twins. Am J Obstet Gynecol 141:252, 1981.
Rausen AR, Seki M, Strauss L: Twin transfusion syndrome. A review of 19 cases studied at our instituion. J Pediatr 66:613, 1973.
Soma H, Yoshida K, Tada M, et al: Fetal abnormalities associated with twin placentation. Teratology 12:211, 1975.

8.17 PREMATURITY AND INTRAUTERINE GROWTH RETARDATION

Definitions. Liveborn* infants delivered before 37 wk from the first day of the last menstrual period are termed *premature* by the World Health Organization. "Premature" is also often

*Live birth is defined by the World Health Assembly (1950) as "the complete expulsion or extraction from its mother of a product of conception . . . which, after such separation, breathes or shows any other evidence of life such as beating of the heart, pulsation of the umbilical cord, or definite movement of the voluntary muscles, whether or not the umbilical cord has been cut or the placenta is attached." This definition is approved by the American Public Health Association.

Table 8–14. Characteristic Changes in Monochorionic Twins With Uncompensated Placental Arteriovenous Shunts

Twin on	
Arterial Side—Donor	Venous Side—Recipient
Oligohydramnios	Polyhydramnios
Small premature	Large premature
Malnourished	Well nourished
Pale	Plethoric
Anemic	Polycythemic
Hypovolemia	Hypervolemic
Hypoglycemia	Cardiac failure
Microcardia	Cardiac hypertrophy
Glomeruli small or normal	Glomeruli large
Arterioles thin-walled	Arterioles thick-walled

used to denote immaturity. More recently, infants of extremely low birthweight, i.e., less than 750 g, have been referred to as immature neonates. Historically, prematurity was defined by a birthweight of 2500 g or less, but today infants who weigh 2500 g or less at birth, "low birthweight infants" (LBW), are considered to be premature with a shortened gestational period, to be intrauterine growth retarded for their gestational age, or both. Prematurity and *intrauterine growth retardation* (IUGR) are associated with increased neonatal morbidity and mortality. Ideally, the definitions of low birthweight should be set for individual populations as genetically and environmentally homogeneous as possible to obtain. Fig. 8–7 presents variations in neonatal mortality based on birthweight with respect to gestational age.

Incidence. During 1981, 6.8% of live births in the United States weighed 2500 g or less; the rate for whites was 5.7%, and the rate for blacks was 12.5%. Only about one third of LBW infants have a gestational age of 37 wk or more. At LBW rates above 10%, the majority of LBW infants have IUGR and are commonly referred to as being *small for gestational age* (SGA); at LBW rates of 5–7%, the majority are *appropriate for gestational age* (AGA). Except for term LBW infants, SGA infants generally have lower neonatal and postneonatal mortality than AGA infants.

The Very Low Birthweight (VLBW) Infant. This designation refers to infants weighing 1500 g or less; they constituted about 1.2% of all births in the United States in 1981.

The modest decline in the LBW rate in the past decade has been primarily due to a reduction in the number of term moderately low birthweight (MLBW) infants (1501–2500 g). However, VLBW infants still account for about half of the neonatal deaths, and their survival rate is directly related to birthweight, with about 2% survivors at 501–600 g and 85–95% survivors at 1251–1500 g. Perinatal care and improved survival rate of these VLBW infants has assumed great importance because their survival rate has a significant impact on overall premature mortality rates and on the large commitment of resources required to achieve lower mortality in the VLBW infant. Their decrease in mortality has probably not been associated with increased severe morbidity. However, compared with larger infants, VLBW infants have a higher incidence of rehospitalization during the first year of life for causes such as inguinal hernias, infections, treatment of chronic sequelae of prematurity, and psychosocial disorders.

Factors Related to Premature Birth and Low Birthweight. It is difficult to separate completely factors associated with prematurity from those associated with IUGR. (See also Sec. 8.7, 8.11, and 8.12.) A strong positive correlation exists between both premature birth and IUGR and low socioeconomic status. In families of low socioeconomic status there are relatively high incidences of maternal undernutrition, anemia, and illness; inadequate prenatal care; drug addiction; obstetric complications; and maternal histories of reproductive inefficiency (relative infertility, abortions, stillbirths, premature or

Table 8–15. Factors Often Associated with Premature Birth

Maternal	Placental
Erythroblastosis fetalis	Abruptio placentae
Incompetent cervix	Amnionitis
Preeclampsia	Placenta previa
Severe maternal illness	Polyhydramnios
Urinary tract infection	Premature rupture of membranes
Fetal	**Iatrogenic**
Congenital malformations	Unknown
Multiple pregnancy	

Table 8–16. Factors Often Associated With Intrauterine Growth Retardation

Fetal
Chromosomal disorders (e.g., autosomal trisomies)
Chronic fetal infections (e.g., cytomegalic inclusion disease, congenital rubella, syphilis)
Radiation injury
Multiple gestation
Pancreatic aplasia

Placental
Decreased placental weight or cellularity or both
Decrease in surface area
Villous placentitis (bacterial, viral, parasitic)
Infarction
Tumor (chorioangioma, hydatidiform mole)
Placental separation
Twin transfusion syndrome (parabiotic syndrome)

Maternal
Toxemia
Hypertensive or renal disease or both
Hypoxemia (high altitude, cyanotic cardiac or pulmonary disease)
Malnutrition or chronic illness
Sickle cell anemia
Drugs (narcotics, alcohol, cigarettes, antimetabolites)

low weight infants). Other associated factors such as illegitimacy, teenage pregnancies, close spacing of pregnancies, and mothers who have borne more than four previous children are also encountered more frequently. Systematic differences in fetal growth have also been described in association with maternal size, birth order, sibling weight, social class, maternal smoking habit, and other factors. The degree to which the variance in birthweights among various populations is due to environmental (extrafetal) rather than to genetic differences in growth potential is difficult to determine.

The *premature birth* of infants whose low birthweight is appropriate for their preterm gestational age is generally associated with medical conditions in which there is inability of the uterus to retain the fetus, interference with the course of the pregnancy, premature separation of the placenta, or a stimulus to effective uterine contractions prior to term (Table 8–15). *Intrauterine growth retardation* is associated with medical conditions that interfere with the circulation and efficiency of the placenta, with the development or growth of the fetus, or with the general health and nutrition of the mother (Table 8–16). Many factors are common to both prematurely born and low birthweight infants with IUGR.

Assessment of Gestational Age at Birth. Compared with the premature infant of appropriate weight, the infant with retarded intrauterine growth has a reduced birthweight and appears to have a *disproportionately larger head relative to body size*; infants in both groups lack subcutaneous fat. In some infants (e.g., those with nonbacterial infections or chromosomal anomalies), birthweight and brain growth are severely affected; this is referred to as symmetrical growth retardation. In general, neurologic maturity (e.g., nerve conduction velocity) correlates with gestational age despite reduced fetal weight.

Physical signs may be useful in estimating gestational age at birth. Commonly used, the Dubowitz scoring system is accurate to ±2 wk (Fig. 8–8, 8–9, and 8–10). An infant should be presumed to be at high risk of mortality or morbidity if a discrepancy exists between estimation of gestational age by physical examination, the mother's estimated date of last menstrual period, and fetal ultrasonic evaluation.

Spectrum of Disease in Low Birthweight Infants. Immaturity tends to increase the severity but reduce the distinctiveness of the clinical manifestations of most neonatal dis-

EXTERNAL SIGN	SCORE				
	0	1	2	3	4
Edema	Obvious edema of hands and feet; pitting over tibia	No obvious edema of hands and feet; pitting over tibia	No edema		
Skin texture	Very thin, gelatinous	Thin and smooth	Smooth; medium thickness; rash or superficial peeling	Slight thickening; superficial cracking and peeling, especially on hands and feet	Thick and parchmentlike; superficial or deep cracking
Skin color (infant not crying)	Dark red	Uniformly pink	Pale pink; variable over body	Pale; only pink over ears, lips, palms, or soles	
Skin opacity (trunk)	Numerous veins and venules clearly seen, especially over abdomen	Veins and tributaries seen	A few large vessels clearly seen over abdomen	A few large vessels seen indistinctly over abdomen	No blood vessels seen
Lanugo (over back)	No lanugo	Abundant, long and thick over whole back	Hair thinning, especially over lower back	Small amount of lanugo and bald areas	At least half of back devoid of lanugo
Plantar creases	No skin creases	Faint red marks over anterior half of sole	Definite red marks over more than anterior half, indentations over less than anterior third	Indentations over more than anterior third	Definite deep indentations over more than anterior third
Nipple formation	Nipple barely visible; no areola	Nipple well defined; areola smooth and flat; diameter <0.75 cm	Areola stippled, edge not raised; diameter <0.75 cm	Areola stippled, edge raised; diameter >0.75 cm	
Breast size	No breast tissue palpable	Breast tissue on one or both sides <0.5 cm diameter	Breast tissue both sides; one or both 0.5 to 1.0 cm	Breast tissue both sides; one or both >1 cm	
Ear form	Pinna flat and shapeless, little or no incurving of edge	Incurving of part of edge of pinna	Partial incurving whole of upper pinna	Well-defined incurving whole of upper pinna	
Ear firmness	Pinna soft, easily folded, no recoil	Pinna soft, easily folded, slow recoil	Cartilage to edge of pinna, but soft in places, ready recoil	Pinna firm, cartilage to edge; instant recoil	
Genitalia Male	Neither testis in scrotum	At least one testis high in scrotum	At least one testis down in scrotum		
Female (with hips half abducted)	Labia majora widely separated; labia minora protruding	Labia majora almost cover labia minora	Labia majora completely cover labia minora		

Figure 8–8. External characteristics of the Dubowitz examination. Physical criteria are recorded and a final score is obtained following addition of each category's score. (From Dubowitz L, Dubowitz V: Gestational Age of the Newborn. Reading, MA, Addison-Wesley Pub Co Inc, 1977.)

their birthweight; this may be related to chronic intrauterine stress accelerating pulmonary maturity. Problems encountered in SGA or IUGR infants include perinatal asphyxia, hypoglycemia, hypothermia, pulmonary hemorrhage, meconium aspiration, necrotizing enterocolitis, polycythemia, and illnesses related to congenital anomalies, syndromes, or infections. The prognosis for these infants depends on the etiology of their growth retardation and on the acute management of these potentially lethal neonatal problems. Head circumference less than the 10th percentile at birth and abnormal neurologic examination in the newborn period are associated with poor growth, later microcephaly, and neurologic deficit.

Hemorrhage (Sec. 8.22, 8.23, 8.49, and 15.50), whether associated with trauma, asphyxia, infection, or defect of clotting mechanism, is frequent and often severe in low birthweight infants. Subcutaneous ecchymoses and subepen-

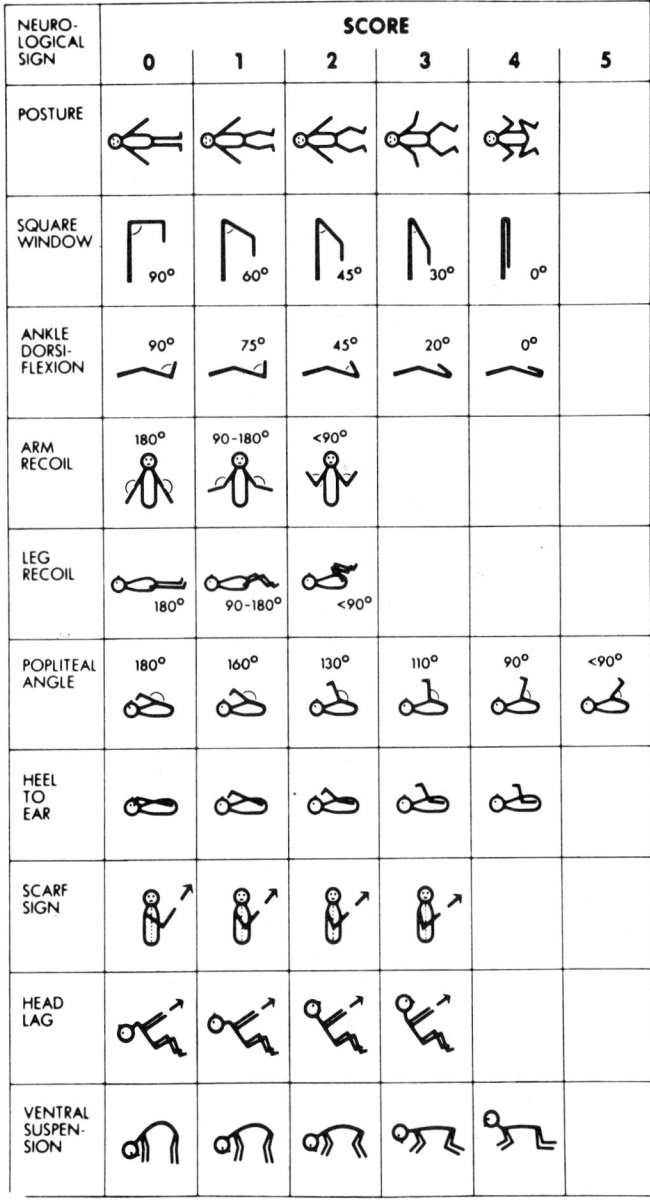

Figure 8–9. Neurologic characteristics of the Dubowitz examination. Neurologic criteria are recorded and added to a final score as performed for the physical assessment. (From Dubowitz L, Dubowitz V: Gestational Age of the Newborn. Reading, MA, Addison-Wesley Pub Co Inc, 1977.)

eases. The principal causes of death among infants are hyaline membrane disease, intraventricular hemorrhage, septicemia, asphyxia, birth injuries (principally cerebral), and malformations; prematurity itself should not be considered a cause of death in an infant born alive. The major causes of death at term are asphyxia, infection, anomalies, and aspiration pneumonia.

Although there is substantial overlap, the incidence of certain neonatal risks varies with birthweight, gestational age, and birthweight for gestational age. Problems of major clinical significance associated with *premature birth* include respiratory distress (hyaline membrane disease, pulmonary hemorrhage, aspiration syndrome, congenital pneumonia, pneumothorax, bronchopulmonary dysplasia), recurrent apnea, hypoglycemia, hypocalcemia, hyperbilirubinemia, anemia, edema, cerebral anoxia, circulatory instability, hypothermia, bacterial sepsis, and disseminated intravascular coagulopathy. In addition, preterm infants frequently have weak and/or uncoordinated ability to feed, prolonged failure to gain weight, and late metabolic acidosis.

Infants *with IUGR (SGA)* are a very heterogeneous population, even when those with congenital anomalies or congenital infections are not included. They tend to have neonatal problems related more to their gestational age than to their birthweight. In addition, preterm SGA infants have a lower incidence of hyaline membrane disease than expected for

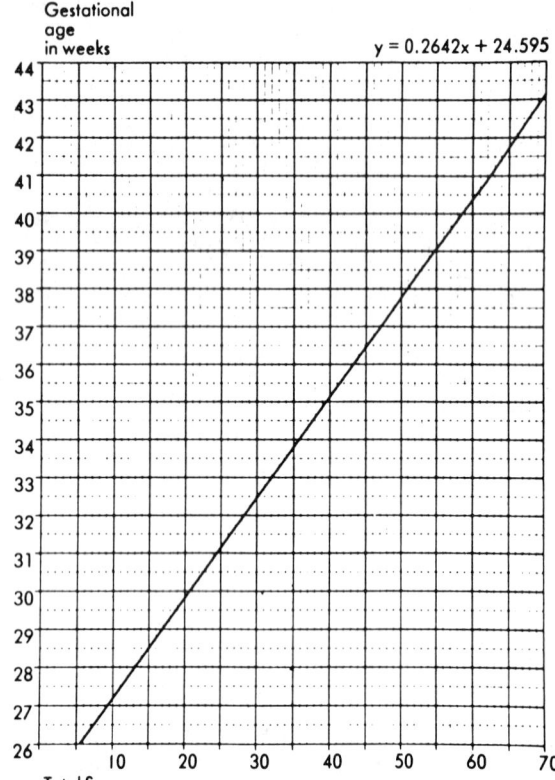

Figure 8–10. Both the external physical criteria score and that for the neurologic criteria are added together and gestational age (± 2 wk) may be read off this graph. (From Dubowitz L, Dubowitz V: Gestational Age of the Newborn. Reading, MA, Addison-Wesley Pub Co Inc, 1977.)

$y = 0.2642x + 24.595$

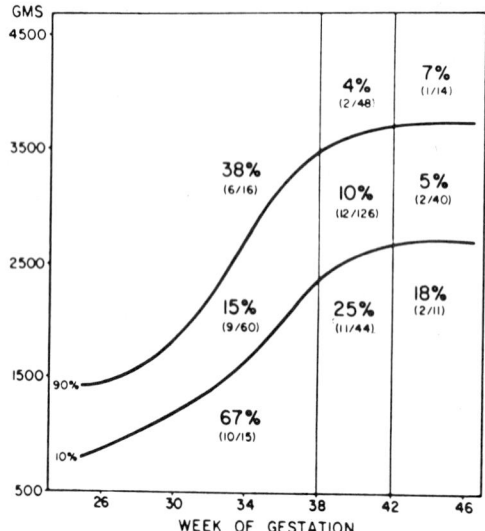

Figure 8–11. Incidence of hypoglycemia by birth weight, gestational age, and intrauterine growth. (From Lubchenco LO [ed]: The High Risk Infant. Philadelphia, WB Saunders, 1976.)

dymal and intraventricular hemorrhage are frequent. Increased capillary fragility, vulnerable arterial and venous capillary networks in friable periventricular germinal tissue, hypernatremia, and increased vascular pressures may be contributing causes. Sudden shock and collapse during the first few days of life are often due to massive **intraventricular hemorrhage** (Sec. 8.22 and 8.23), which occurs predominantly in very small premature infants. It is uncommon in infants who weigh more than 2000 g at birth or are of more than 34 wk gestational age. Less severe degrees of hemorrhage may be associated with lethargy, seizures, apnea, and an acute decline of the hematocrit. Small intraventricular or subependymal hemorrhage may go undetected. Pulmonary hemorrhage has a similar pattern of increased incidence and high mortality in preterm infants, especially those who are SGA.

Hyaline membrane disease (respiratory distress syndrome) occurs most frequently, and mortality is highest, in infants of shortest gestation, and the incidence and mortality fall progressively with increasing gestational age. It is rare in large infants born at or near term, except in those delivered by cesarean section or born to diabetic mothers (Sec. 8.32).

Congenital malformations (Sec. 6.29) occur with a greater frequency in infants of low birthweight than in all live births. There is a higher malformation rate both in preterm babies and in fullterm SGA infants; those with the slowest intrauterine growth rates have the highest incidence of malformations. Breech presentation is common. The incidence of ventricular septal defect is much higher in infants of birthweight less than 2500 g and gestational age less than 34 wk than among larger or older infants. Infants with chromosome anomalies (e.g., trisomy 21, trisomy 18) and those with congenital rubella infection have a high incidence of congenital heart disease and tend to be SGA. Infants with meconium ileus, intestinal

obstruction, gastroschisis, and omphalocele are often born prematurely, especially if hydramnios is present.

Patent ductus arteriosus in LBW infants is discussed in Sec. 14.46.

Hypoglycemia may occur in 15% of premature and up to 67% of infants with IUGR (Fig. 8–11). Early feeding and intravenous glucose have reduced its incidence to less than 5% (see Sec. 8.56, 8.57, and 20.6.)

Hyperglycemia is a common problem in extremely premature infants receiving excessive intravenous glucose infusions (over 10 mg/kg min).

Recurrent apnea (Sec. 8.31), the cessation of breathing for more than 20 sec or long enough to produce cyanosis or bradycardia, has a very high incidence in infants under 1500 g or under 32 wk gestational age (Table 8–17).

Necrotizing enterocolitis (Sec. 8.43) occurs most commonly in infants of low birth weight. The highest incidence is among babies weighing less than 1500 g, but it may also occur in term, normal weight infants.

Retrolental fibroplasia (*retinopathy of prematurity*) occurs in premature infants treated with oxygen at concentrations above ambient air levels (Sec. 25.13). The increased arterial oxygen tensions that result may lead to severe damage to the immature retina. The eyes of premature infants exposed to oxygen should be examined after recovery from the illness requiring oxygen therapy, before discharge, and at 3 mo after discharge; retinal surgery has been proposed for severe detachment. The practice of administering oxygen only in the amounts and for

Table 8–17. **Etiologies of Apnea**

Gastrointestinal: gastroesophageal reflux

Infections: sepsis, meningitis, necrotizing enterocolitis

Metabolic: ↓ glucose, ↓ calcium, ↓ pO₂, ↑ environmental temperature, ↑ ammonia, ↕ sodium

Vascular: hypotension, hypertension, anemia, dehydration

CNS: drugs, hemorrhage, seizures, reflex, sleep state, immaturity

Respiratory: airway obstruction, alveolar collapse, chest wall instability, laryngeal reflex, intrapulmonary pathology

Idiopathic

the duration of time absolutely necessary for relieving respiratory distress, apnea, hypoxemia, or cyanosis, along with the frequent monitoring of arterial oxygen tensions, has significantly reduced the incidence of this disease and the partial or complete blindness that may result from it. The exact level or duration of elevated arterial pO_2 that results in injury is unknown, but arterial oxygen tensions should be kept between 50 and 80 mm Hg. Immaturity is an important contributing factor and may rarely be the only identifiable cause. Hypercarbia is another risk factor. Ambient light may also be a factor. The risk of hypoxic brain injury from too little oxygen must be balanced against the risk of retrolental fibroplasia from too much oxygen. The prophylactic administration of vitamin E may ameliorate the severity of injury in some infants (Sec. 15.13); however, its use has also been associated with an increased incidence of sepsis, necrotizing enterocolitis, and other serious systemic toxic effects.

Kernicterus (Sec. 8.44, 8.45) associated with hyperbilirubinemia occurs in 2–20% of autopsies of premature infants. High incidences are probably the result of inappropriate treatment, such as the administration of large amounts of vitamin K analogues to mothers in labor or to newborn infants and the use of sulfisoxazole as chemoprophylaxis. Very low birthweight infants are at increased risk, particularly if they have meningitis; in these immature infants bilirubin levels as low as 10 mg/dL may be dangerous.

Immaturity of anatomic structure or physiologic and biochemical functions is an index of the relative inability of the preterm infant to survive. Deficiencies in these functions affect the infant's ability to withstand demands that do not exist in the protective intrauterine environment, such as control of body heat, pulmonary function, nutrition, disposal of metabolic waste, immunologic function, and detoxification and excretion of toxic substances. The immature infant's respiratory function is limited by the underventilation of perfused alveoli and insufficient surface-active lipid surfactant to prevent collapse of alveoli. Underdeveloped airways and pulmonary tissue and persistence of fluid in the lung result in increased resistance to air flow. The ability to minimize heat loss in response to cold stress is proportional to body size. Decreased stores of hepatic and myocardial glycogen compromise the immature infant's ability to withstand a moderate degree of asphyxia. Renal blood flow, glomerular filtration, and tubular functions are decreased. The cardiopulmonary circulation is transitional between that of a fetus and that of an adult; increased shunting through the ductus arteriosus and foramen ovale may occur in response to stress, hypoxia, or polycythemia and result in circulatory insufficiency or underperfusion of vital organs.

Nursery Care. At birth the same measures for clearing the airway, initiating breathing, caring for the cord and eyes, and administering vitamin K are required for immature infants as for those of normal weight and maturity (Sec. 8.4). Special care is required to maintain a patent airway and avoid potential aspiration of gastric contents. Additional considerations are (1) need for incubator care and heart rate and respiration monitoring, (2) need for increased oxygen, and (3) need for special attention to the details of feeding. Safeguards against infection can never be relaxed. Everyone involved must be aware that routine procedures that disturb these infants may result in hypoxia. Finally, the need for the parents to regularly and actively participate in the infant's care in the nursery, the need for instructing the mother in the at-home care of the infant, and the question of prognosis for later growth and development require special consideration. There can be significant untoward effects on the development of a normal mother-infant relationship as a consequence of separation during the neonatal period; these effects may contribute to subsequent behavioral and physical abnormalities, e.g., fail-

ure to thrive and deprivation syndromes, child neglect, and abuse (Sec. 5.38).

Incubator Care. Modern incubators conserve body heat through provision of a warm atmospheric environment and standard conditions of humidity. They also may provide a regulated oxygen supply and reduced atmospheric contamination if they are scrupulously cleaned. The survival of LBW and sick infants is greater when they are cared for at or near their *neutral thermal environment.* This is a set of thermal conditions, including air and radiating surface temperatures, relative humidity, and air flow, at which heat production (measured as oxygen consumption) is minimal and the infant's core temperature is within the normal range. It is a function of the size and postnatal age of infants; larger, older infants require lower environmental temperatures than smaller, younger infants. The optimal incubator temperature for minimal heat loss and oxygen consumption for the unclothed infant is that which will maintain the infant's core temperature at 36.5–37.0° C. This depends on an infant's size and maturity; the smaller and more immature the infant, the higher the environmental temperature required. A plexiglass heat shield or head caps and body clothing may be required when incubator care alone is insufficient to keep a small premature infant warm.

Maintaining a relative humidity of 40–60% aids in stabilizing body temperature by reducing heat loss at lower environmental temperatures; by preventing drying and irritation of the lining of respiratory passages, especially during the administration of oxygen and following or during endotracheal or nasotracheal intubation; and by thinning viscid secretions and reducing insensible water loss from the lungs.

Administering oxygen to reduce the risk of injury from hypoxia and circulatory insufficiency must be balanced against the risks of hyperoxia to the eyes (retinopathy of prematurity) and oxygen injury to the lungs. When possible, oxygen should be administered by a head hood, CPAP apparatus, or endotracheal tube to maintain stable and safe inspired oxygen concentration. Although the presence of cyanosis, tachypnea, and apnea are definite clinical indications whose treatment should include only the amount of oxygen needed to eliminate these signs, the potential harm from hypoxia or hyperoxia cannot be minimized without monitoring the oxygen tension (pO_2) of arterial blood and, based on laboratory analysis, continuously readjusting the concentration of oxygen administered. The development of the transcutaneous oxygen electrode for routine clinical management of these infants has significantly improved the effectiveness of oxygen monitoring. Capillary blood gases are inadequate for estimating arterial oxygen levels.

If an incubator is not available, the general conditions of temperature and humidity control outlined above can be attained by the intelligent use of radiant warmers, blankets, heating lamps, heating pads, and warm water bottles, and by control of the temperature and humidity of the room. It may be necessary to administer oxygen temporarily by face mask or through an intubation tube.

The infant should be removed from the incubator only when the gradual change to the atmosphere of the nursery does not result in a significant change of the infant's temperature, color, or activity.

Feeding. The method of feeding each LBW infant should be individualized. It is important to avoid fatigue and the aspiration of food by regurgitation or by the feeding process. No feeding method will avoid these problems unless the person feeding the infant has been well trained in the method. Oral feedings (nipple) should not be initiated or should be discontinued in infants with respiratory distress, hypoxia, circulatory insufficiency, excessive secretions, gagging, sepsis, central nervous system depression, immaturity, or signs of serious illness. These infants will require parenteral or gavage feedings to supply calories, fluid, and electrolytes.

Large premature infants can often be fed by bottle or at the breast. Since the effort of sucking is usually the limiting factor, breast feeding is less likely to succeed until the infant matures. Bottle feeding of expressed breast milk may be a temporary alternative. In *bottle feeding*, effort may be reduced by use of special small, soft nipples with large holes. The process of oral alimentation requires, in addition to a strong suck, the coordination of swallowing, epiglottal and uvular closure of the larynx and nasal passages, and normal esophageal motility, a synchronized process that is usually absent prior to 34 wk gestation.

Smaller or less vigorous infants should be fed by *gavage*: a soft plastic tube of No. 5 French external and approximately 0.05 cm internal diameters with a rounded atraumatic tip and two holes on alternate sides is preferable. The tube is passed through the nose until approximately 2.5 cm (1 in) of the lower end is in the stomach. The free end of the tube is then placed under water. If bubbles appear with each expiration, the catheter is in the trachea and must be reinserted into the proper position. The free end of the tube has an adapter into which the tip of a syringe is fitted, and the measured amount of feeding is allowed to flow in slowly by gravity. Such tubes may be left in place for 3–7 days before replacement by a similar tube through the alternate nostril. Occasionally an infant has enough local irritation from an indwelling tube that he or she may gag or that troublesome secretions may gather around it in the nasopharynx. In such instances a catheter may be passed through the mouth by a skilled person and removed at the end of each feeding. Change to bottle or breast feeding may be instituted gradually as soon as the infant displays general vigor adequate for oral feeding without fatigue.

Continuous nasogastric and nasojejunal feedings have also been used successfully in LBW infants unable to ingest adequate calories by bottle or gavage owing to poor suck, uncoordinated swallowing, and delayed gastric emptying. Intestinal perforation has occurred during nasojejunal feedings.

Gastrostomy feeding is contraindicated in premature infants because of an associated increase in mortality, except as an adjunct to the surgical management of specific gastrointestinal conditions. Partial or total *intravenous alimentation* for premature infants should not be routinely used as a substitute for oral or gavage feedings, but rather only for situations when the latter are contraindicated by the infant's condition.

INITIATION OF FEEDING. The main principle in the feeding of premature infants is to proceed cautiously and gradually. Careful early feeding of glucose or formula tends to reduce the risk of hypoglycemia, dehydration, and hyperbilirubinemia without the added risk of aspiration, provided the presence of respiratory distress or other disorders does not present an indication for withholding oral feedings and administering electrolytes, fluids, and calories intravenously.

If the infant is vigorous, making sucking movements, and in no distress, oral feeding may be attempted, although most infants under 1500 g require initial tube feeding because they are unable to coordinate sucking and swallowing. A suggested schedule is to begin with 1–2 mL of a sterile solution of 5% glucose in water for infants under 1000 g; 2–4 mL for infants between 1000 and 1500 g; and 5–10 mL for infants over 1500 g. If the beginning amount is 1 mL, feedings may be given hourly for the first 8 hr, increasing the amount by 1 mL at every other feeding. Feedings may then be given every 2 hr, with an increment of 2 mL at every other feeding until 12 mL is reached. Once glucose in water feedings have been tolerated, formula feeding may be substituted within 12 hr. Standard commercial formulas with caloric density of 20 kcal/oz are satisfactory for most premature infants. Amounts of formula

may then be gradually increased so that the intake is approximately 150 mL/kg/24 hr. If the infant still seems hungry or fails to gain weight, the amounts should be further increased. The expected weight increments for infants of various birth weights can be projected from Fig. 8–12. Certain infants with small gastric capacities fail to gain on tolerated amounts of formula containing 20 kcal/oz. In such instances more frequent feedings may be given to increase the total daily intake or the caloric content may be increased incrementally to as high as 30 kcal/oz. To avoid dehydration care must be taken when using these hypercaloric high solute formulas.

Infants of 1000–1500 g may be given glucose in water feedings (formula after the first 2–3 feedings) every 2–3 hr, with 2–4 mL increments at every other feeding depending on how successfully the infant tolerates the changes. With infants over 1500 g the interval may be 3–4 hr with 4–8 mL increments.

Regurgitation, vomiting, abdominal distention, or residuals from prior feedings in the early stages of the feeding schedule should arouse suspicion of sepsis or intestinal obstruction; later, these are indications to drop back in the schedule and increase subsequent feedings slowly and to evaluate for more serious problems. Weight gain may not be achieved for 10–12 days, and a daily intake of 130–150 mL/kg or higher may be necessary for some infants. Alternatively, in vigorous infants whose feeding schedule is advanced rapidly in calories or volume, weight gain may appear within a few days.

When tube feeding is used, the contents of the stomach should be aspirated before each feeding. If only air or small amounts of mucus are obtained, the feeding is given as planned. If greater than 10% of the previous feeding is obtained, it is advisable to reduce the amount of the feeding and to proceed more gradually with subsequent increases.

The digestive enzyme systems of infants greater than 28 wk gestation are mature enough to permit adequate digestion and absorption of protein and carbohydrate. Fat is less well absorbed due primarily to inadequate amounts of bile salt; unsaturated fats and the fat of human milk are absorbed better than those of cow's milk. Weight gain of infants weighing under 2000 g at birth should be adequate when human milk or "humanized" milk (40% casein and 60% whey) with a protein intake of 2.25–2.75 g/kg/24 hr is fed. These two alternatives should provide all amino acids essential for premature infants, including tyrosine, cystine, and histidine. Higher protein intakes may be well tolerated and generally safe, especially for older, rapidly growing infants. However,

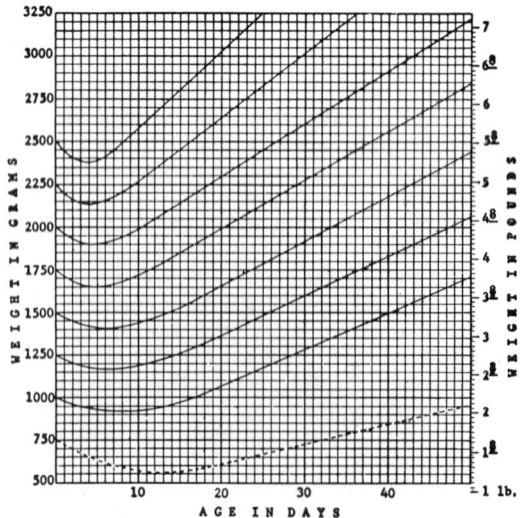

Figure 8–12. Grid for recording weights of premature infants. The average weight increments are indicated on the basis of weight at birth. (From Dancis J, et al: J Pediatr, Vol 33.)

protein intakes as high as 4.5 g/kg/24 hr may be hazardous: although linear growth may be promoted, high protein formulas may cause abnormal plasma aminograms; elevations in blood urea nitrogen, ammonia, and sodium concentrations; metabolic acidosis (cow's milk formulas); and untoward effects on neurologic development. Further, the high protein and mineral contents of balanced cow's milk formulas of high caloric content constitute a large solute load for the kidney, a fact important in maintaining water balance, especially in the infant with diarrhea or fever.

Breast milk may not always be optimal for infants under 1000 g, since these infants require more calcium, phosphorus, and protein than is present in pooled, banked breast milk. Premature breast milk obtained from the infant's mother may be more appropriate; specialized premature formulas may also be used.

Although formula in amounts necessary for adequate growth probably contain sufficient amounts of all vitamins, the volume of milk sufficient to satisfy requirements may not be ingested for several weeks. Therefore, LBW infants should be given supplemental vitamins. Since requirements for these infants have not been precisely established, the recommended daily allowances for term infants should be given (Chapter 3). Further, these infants may have a special need for certain vitamins. Intermediary metabolism of phenylalanine and tyrosine depends, in part, upon vitamin C. Decreased fat absorption with increased fecal fat loss may be associated with decreased absorption of *vitamin D*, other fat soluble vitamins, and calcium in premature infants. VLBW infants are particularly prone to develop rickets, but their total intake of vitamin D should not exceed 1500 IU/24 hr. *Folic acid* is essential for the formation of DNA and production of new cells; serum and erythrocyte levels decrease in preterm infants over the first few weeks of life and remain low for 2–3 months. Therefore, supplementation is recommended, though it does not result in improved growth or increased hemoglobin concentration. Deficiency of vitamin E is associated with increased hemolysis and, if severe, with anemia in premature infants. Vitamin E functions as an antioxidant to prevent peroxidation of polyunsaturated fatty acids in red blood cell membranes; its need may increase because of the increased membrane content of these fatty acids. Vitamin K deficiency is discussed in Sec. 3.33.

In the LBW infant, physiologic anemia due to postnatal suppression of erythropoiesis is exacerbated by smaller fetal iron stores and greater expansion of blood volume resulting from a more rapid growth compared with the term weight infant's; therefore, the anemia develops earlier and reaches a lower ultimate level. Fetal or neonatal blood loss accentuates this problem. Iron stores, even in the VLBW neonate, are usually adequate until the infant's birthweight has doubled. In addition, iron supplementation during the period when these infants are at risk for vitamin E deficiency (less than 34 wk post-conception age) may enhance hemolysis and reduce vitamin E absorption. Therefore, vitamin E supplementation may be discontinued once the birthweight doubles, at which time iron supplementation (2 mg/kg/24 hr) should be started.

The properly fed premature infant may have from 1–6 daily stools of semisolid consistency; a sudden increase in their number, the appearance of occult or gross blood, or a change to a watery consistency is more reason for concern than any arbitrarily stated frequency.

The premature infant should not vomit or regurgitate. He or she should be satisfied and relaxed after a feeding but may normally show the activity of hunger shortly before the next one.

Fluid Requirements. These vary according to gestational age, environmental conditions, and disease states. Assuming minimal water losses in stool of infants not receiving oral fluids, their water needs are equal to insensible water loss, renal solute excretion, and any unusual ongoing losses. Insensible water loss is indirectly related to gestational age; the very immature preterm infant (<1000 g) may require as much as 2–3 mL/kg/hr, partly because of thin skin, lack of subcutaneous tissue, and a large exposed surface area. Insensible water loss is increased under radiant warmers, during phototherapy, and in the febrile infant. It is diminished when the infant is clothed, is covered by a plexiglass inner heat shield, breathes humidified air, or approaches term. Larger premature infants (2000–2500 g) nursed in an incubator may have an insensible water loss of approximately 0.6–0.7 mL/kg/hr.

Fluids also need to be administered to permit excretion of the urinary solute load, e.g., urea, electrolytes, phosphate. The amount varies with dietary intake and the anabolic or catabolic state of nutrition. High solute load formulas, high protein intake, and catabolism increase the end products that require urinary excretion and thus increase the requirement for water. Renal solute loads may vary between 7.5–30 mOsm/kg. Newborn infants, especially those of very low birthweight, also are less able to concentrate urine, thus their fluid intake required to excrete solutes increases.

Water intake in term infants is usually begun at 60–70 mL/kg on day 1 and increased to 100–120 mL/kg by day 2–3. Smaller, more premature infants may need to be started with 70–100 mL/kg on day 1 and advanced to 150 mL/kg or more by day 3–4. Fluid volumes should be titrated individually, although it is unusual to exceed 150 mL/kg/24 hr. Daily weights, urine output and specific gravity, and serum urea nitrogen with electrolytes should be monitored carefully to detect abnormal states of hydration, since clinical observations and physical examinations are poor indicators of the state of hydration of premature infants. Conditions that increase fluid losses, such as glycosuria, the polyuric phase of acute tubular necrosis, and diarrhea, may place additional strain on kidneys that have not yet developed their maximum capacity to conserve water and electrolytes, the results of which may be severe dehydration. Alternatively, fluid overload may lead to edema, congestive heart failure, and a patent ductus arteriosus.

Total Parenteral Nutrition. When oral feeding is impossible for prolonged periods of time, total intravenous alimentation may provide sufficient fluid, calories, electrolytes, and vitamins to sustain growth of LBW infants. This technique has been lifesaving for infants who have had intractable diarrheal syndromes or extensive resection of bowel. Infusions may be administered through an indwelling central vein catheter or through a peripheral vein.

The goal of parenteral alimentation is to deliver enough nonprotein calories to allow the infant to use most of the protein for growth. The infusate should contain synthetic amino acids of 2.5 g/dL and hypertonic glucose in the range of 10–25 g/dL in addition to appropriate quantities of electrolytes, trace minerals, and vitamins. The initial daily infusion should deliver 10–15 g/kg/24 hr of glucose and increase gradually to 25–30 g/kg/24 hr when glucose alone is used to meet the full requirements of 100–120 nonprotein kcal/kg/24 hr. If a peripheral vein is used, it is advisable to keep the glucose concentration below 12.5 g/dL. Intravenous fat emulsions such as Intralipid (11 kcal/g) may be used to provide calories without an appreciable osmotic load, thereby decreasing the need for infusion of the higher concentrations of glucose by central or peripheral vein and usually preventing the development of essential fatty acid deficiency. Electrolytes, trace minerals, and vitamin additives are included in amounts approximating established intravenous maintenance requirements. The content of each day's infusate should be determined after carefully assessing the infant's clinical and biochemical status. Slow and continuous infusion is advisable.

A well trained pharmacist using a laminar flow hood should mix all solutions.

After a caloric intake of greater than 100 kcal/kg/24 hr is established by total parenteral intravenous nutrition, LBW infants can be expected to gain about 15 g/kg/24 hr, with positive nitrogen balances of 150–200 mg/kg/24 hr, if there are not multiple operative procedures, episodes of sepsis, or other severe stress. This goal usually can be achieved and the catabolic tendency during the first week of life reversed with subsequent weight gains by peripheral vein infusions of 2.5 g/kg/24 hr of an amino acid mixture, 10 g/dL of glucose, and 2–3 g/kg/24 hr of Intralipid.

The complications of intravenous alimentation are related to both the catheter and the metabolism of the infusate. Sepsis is the most important known problem of central vein infusions and can be minimized only by meticulous catheter care and aseptic preparation of the infusate. *Staphylococcus aureus*, *Staphylococcus epidermidis*, and *Candida albicans* are the common infecting organisms. Treatment for staphylococcal infection includes appropriate antibiotics. If infection persists, the line must be removed. Thrombosis, extravasation of fluid, and accidental dislodgment of catheters have also occurred. Sepsis is rarely attributable to peripheral vein infusions, but phlebitis, cutaneous sloughs, and superficial infection occasionally occur. The **metabolic complications** include hyperglycemia from the high glucose concentration of the infusate, which may lead to an osmotic diuresis; dehydration; azotemia; hypoglycemia from a sudden accidental cessation of the infusate; hyperlipidemia and possibly hypoxemia from intravenous lipid infusions; and hyperammonemia, which may be due to high levels of ammonia in fibrin hydrolysates or the lack of arginine in casein hydrolysates. Cholestatic jaundice has also been noted. Hyperchloremic acidosis occurs in infants receiving synthetic amino acids, unless there is an appropriate balance between cationic and anionic amino acids and salts. Abnormal elevations of blood amino acid levels are an additional potential hazard. If intravenous fat emulsions are not used, essential fatty acid deficiency may also occur. When the infusion is given through a peripheral vein, the osmolality of the solution may limit the length of time an infusion site can be used while, at the same time, it may require greater volumes of fluid than can be tolerated. Continuous chemical and physiologic monitoring of infants receiving intravenous alimentation is indicated because of the frequency and seriousness of complications.

Intravenous Supplementation of Tolerated Oral Feedings. Glucose, amino acid mixtures, and lipid emulsions alone or in combination may be infused into peripheral veins when sufficient calories cannot be provided to LBW infants by oral feeding alone. Some infants weighing less than 1500 g may regain their birthweight sooner and have fewer apneic episodes with a supplemental infusion containing sources of nitrogen. Increases in weight, length, and head circumference approaching those expected in utero have been achieved with mixtures of protein hydrolysate, glucose, and Intralipid. Although the complications of both techniques may occur, the combination of nutrient delivery methods allows smaller volumes of enteral feedings, thus decreasing the risk of aspiration.

Prevention of Infection. Premature infants have an increased susceptibility to infection, which requires having personnel rigorously wash hand-to-elbow before and after handling the infant, taking measures to reduce contamination of food and objects coming in contact with the infant, preventing air contamination, avoiding overcrowding, and limiting direct and indirect contacts with nursery personnel and other infants. No one with an infection should be permitted into the nursery. However, the risks of infection must be balanced against the disadvantages of limiting the infant's contacts with the family, which may be detrimental to the infant's ultimate development; early and frequent participation by parents in the nursery care of their infant does not significantly increase the risk when preventive precautions are maintained. Prophylactic administration of gamma globulin to premature infants has not proved to be beneficial, despite their lower levels of immunoglobulin.

Preventing infection from being transmitted from infant to infant is difficult because often neither term nor premature newborn infants manifest clear clinical evidence of an infection early in its course. If a unit admits infants born outside that hospital, it should be presumed that they are infected until 72 hr of observation in a special nursery or an incubator with an individual air supply proves otherwise. When epidemics occur within a nursery, cohort nursing and isolation rooms should be employed in addition to routine antiseptic care.

The most important factor in the successful care of premature infants is the skill, experience, and number of the nursing staff. It is the responsibility of the physician to insist on an optimal amount of expert nursing.

Immaturity of Drug Metabolism. Renal clearances for almost all substances excreted in the urine are diminished in newborn infants, but more so in premature ones. Intervals between doses may, therefore, need to be extended when administering drugs excreted chiefly by the kidney. Serum creatinine levels may help determine the appropriate dosage. For instance, highly satisfactory levels of penicillin, gentamicin, and kanamycin are maintained on doses given at 12 hr intervals. Drugs detoxified in the liver or requiring chemical conjugation before renal excretion should also be given with caution and in doses smaller than usual. When possible, blood levels should be obtained for potentially toxic drugs, especially if renal or hepatic dysfunction is present. Decision as to the choice and dose of antibacterial agents and route of administration should be made on an individual rather than on a routine basis, owing to the dangers of (1) development of infections with organisms resistant to antibacterial agents, (2) destruction or inhibition of intestinal bacteria which manufacture significant amounts of essential vitamins (e.g., vitamin K and thiamine), and (3) possibility of harmful interference in important metabolic processes.

Many drugs apparently safe for adults on the basis of toxicity studies may be harmful to newborn infants, especially premature ones. Oxygen and a number of drugs have proved toxic to premature infants in amounts not harmful to term infants (Table 8–18). Thus, administering any drug, particularly in large doses, without pharmacologic testing in premature infants, should be carefully undertaken after weighing risk against benefit.

Prognosis. There is now a 95% or greater chance of survival for infants born weighing between 1501 and 2500 g, but those weighing less still have a significantly higher mortality (see Fig. 8–7). Intensive care has extended the period during which a VLBW infant is likely to die from complications of perinatal disease, such as bronchopulmonary dysplasia, necrotizing enterocolitis, or secondary infection. The mortality rate of LBW infants who survive to be discharged from the hospital is higher than that of term infants during the first 2 yr of life. Because many of these deaths are attributable to infection they are at least theoretically preventable. There is also an increased incidence of failure to thrive, the sudden infant death syndrome, child abuse, and inadequate maternal-infant bonding among premature infants. Abnormalities in cardiorespiratory regulation due to immaturity or to complications of underlying perinatal disease and significant health risks associated with poverty also contribute to the high mortality and morbidity of these infants. Congenital anatomic anomalies are present in approximately 3–7% of LBW infants.

In the absence of congenital abnormalities, central nervous

Table 8–18. Adverse Reactions to Drugs Administered to Premature Infants

Drug	Reaction
Sulfisoxazole	Kernicterus
Chloramphenicol	Gray baby—shock
Vitamin K analogues	Jaundice
Novobiocin	Jaundice
Hexaclorophene	Encephalopathy
Benzyl alcohol	Acidosis, collapse, intraventricular bleeding
Intravenous vitamin E	Ascites—shock
Phenolic detergents	Jaundice
NaHCO$_3$	Intraventricular hemorrhage
Amphotericin	Anuric renal failure
Reserpine	Nasal stuffiness
Indomethacin	Oliguria, hyponatremia
Tetracycline	Enamel hypoplasia
Tolazoline	Hypotension
Calcium salts	Subcutaneous necrosis
Aminoglycosides	Deafness
Enteric gentamicin	Resistant bacteria
Prostaglandins	Seizures, diarrhea
Phenobarbital	Altered state, drowsiness
Morphine	Hypotension
Diuretics	Hypochloremia, hypokalemia

system injury, VLBW or marked IUGR, physical growth of LBW infants tends to approximate that of term weight infants during the second year; this occurs earlier in premature infants of larger birth size. VLBW infants may not catch up, especially if they have severe chronic illness, insufficient nutritional intake, or an inadequate caretaking environment. Premature birth in itself may prejudice later development. In general, the greater the immaturity and the lower the birthweight, the greater the likelihood of intellectual and neurologic deficit (Fig. 8–13). Small head circumference at birth may be similarly related to poor neurobehavioral prognosis. The incidence of neurologic and developmental handicap in VLBW infants ranges from 10–20%, including cerebral palsy (3–6%), moderate to severe hearing and visual defects (1–4%), and learning difficulties (20%). Mean global I.Q. is 90–97, and 76% have normal school performance. Many surviving LBW infants have hypotonia prior to 8 mo corrected age, which improves by the time they are 8 mo–1 yr. This transient hypotonia is not a poor prognostic sign.

Mothers of low socioeconomic status are more apt to have LBW babies who tend to develop less well than do those in better postneonatal environments. Major neurologic defects were found to be uncommon in a prospective study of full-term small-for-dates (IUGR) infants, although compared with appropriate-for-gestation term infants, they had an increased incidence of minimal cerebral dysfunction (hyperactivity, short attention span, learning difficulties), electroencephalographic abnormalities, and speech defects.

Behavior and personality problems may be more common in children born prematurely than in those born at term. The extent to which isolated care in early infancy, a defect in development of the normal maternal-infant relationship, and understandable parental anxiety and overprotectiveness may foster an abnormal emotional environment for the growing infant is unknown. However, avoiding unnecessarily prolonged hospitalization and encouraging parental visiting and participation in the nursery care of the infant might reasonably be expected to decrease such a possible untoward effect.

Discharge From Hospital. Before discharge, a premature infant should be taking all nutrition by nipple, either bottle or breast. Growth should be at steady increments of approximately 10–30 g/day. Temperature should be stabilized in an open crib. There should have been no recent apnea or brady-

cardia, and oxygen and parenteral drug administration should have been discontinued. Infants previously treated with oxygen should have an eye examination to determine the presence, stage, or absence of retrolental fibroplasia, while all LBW infants should have a hearing test, and those who had indwelling umbilical arterial catheters should have their blood pressure measured to check for renal vascular hypertension. A hemoglobin level or hematocrit should be determined to evaluate possible anemia. If all major medical problems have resolved and the home setting is adequate, premature infants may then be discharged when their weight approaches 1900–2100 g; close follow-up and easy access to health care providers are essential for early discharge protocols. Alternatively, if the medical or social environment is not ideal, high risk neonates transported to neonatal intensive care units whose major illness has resolved may be returned to their hospital of birth for an additional period of hospitalization.

Home Care. While the infant is in the hospital the mother should be instructed in caring for the baby after discharge. This program should include at least one visit to her home by someone capable of evaluating domestic arrangements and of advising about any needed improvements.

8.18 POST-TERM INFANTS

Post-term infants are those born after 42 wk of gestation, calculated from the mother's last menstrual period, irrespective of weight at birth. This designation is often used synonymously with the term "postmature" for infants whose gestation exceeds the normal 280 days by 7 days or more. Approximately 25% of all pregnancies end on or after the 287th day of gestation, 12% on or after the 294th day, and 5% on or after the 301st day. The cause of post-term birth or postmaturity is unknown. Large size of the infant correlates poorly with late delivery, but it does correlate with large size

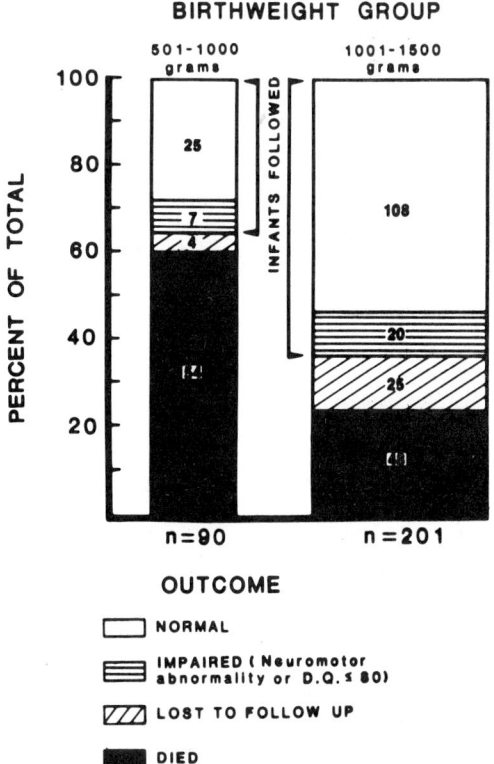

Figure 8–13. Prognosis of very low birth weight infants followed to a mean of 2 yr conceptual age at Rainbow Babies and Childrens Hospital, Cleveland, Ohio. (N Engl J Med 301:1162, 1979.)

of either parent, multigravidity, or a prediabetic or diabetic state in the mother.

Clinical Manifestations. Post-term infants may be clinically indistinguishable from term infants, but some have received the designation postmature because of appearance and behavior suggesting those of an infant 1–3 wk of age. These post-term, postmature infants are often of increased birthweight and are characterized by the absence of lanugo, decreased or absent vernix caseosa, long nails, abundant scalp hair, white parchment-like or desquamating skin, and increased alertness. If *placental insufficiency* occurs, the amniotic fluid and fetus may be meconium stained, and abnormal fetal heart rates may be observed; the infant may have growth retardation. Although this syndrome is frequently confused with postmaturity, *only about 20% of infants with placental insufficiency syndrome are post-term.* The majority affected are term and preterm infants, particularly those small for gestational age who are the infants of toxemic mothers, older primigravidas, and women with chronic hypertension. The placentas are often small or poorly attached. This syndrome has been postulated to result from degenerative changes in the placenta which progressively reduce oxygen and nourishment to the fetus.

Those infants born post-term in association with presumed placental insufficiency may have a variety of physical signs: desquamation, long nails, abundant hair, pale skin, alert faces, and loose skin, especially around the thighs and buttocks, giving them the appearance of having recently lost weight; meconium-stained nails, skin, vernix, umbilical cord, and placental membranes. (see Fig. 8–2).

Prognosis. When delivery is delayed 3 wk or more beyond term, there is a significant increase in mortality, which in some series has approximated three times that of a control group of infants born at term. Mortality has been lowered markedly through improved obstetric management. Primiparity and maternal age over 35 yr appear to increase the mortality rates.

Treatment. Careful obstetrical monitoring, including nonstress testing, biophysical profile, or oxytocin challenge tests, usually provides a rational basis for choosing a course of nonintervention, induction of labor, or cesarean section. Cesarean section may be indicated in older primigravidas who go more than 1–2 wk beyond term, particularly if there is evidence of fetal distress. Meconium aspiration pneumonia or hypoxic encephalopathy are treated symptomatically.

8.19 LARGE FOR GESTATIONAL AGE

See also Sec. 8.56.

Neonatal mortality rates decrease with increasing birthweight until approximately 4000 g, after which mortality increases. These oversized infants are usually born at term, but preterm infants with weights high for gestational age also have a significantly higher mortality than infants of the same size born at term; maternal diabetes and obesity are predisposing factors. Infants who are very large, regardless of their gestational age, have a higher incidence of birth injuries, such as cervical and brachial plexus injuries, phrenic nerve damage with paralysis of the diaphragm, fractured clavicles, cephalhematomas, subdural hematomas, and ecchymoses of the head and face. The incidence of congenital anomalies, particularly congenital heart disease, is also higher than in term infants of normal weight. Intellectual and developmental retardation is statistically more common in high birthweight term and preterm infants than in babies of appropriate weight for gestational age.

INFANT TRANSPORT

With the advent of regionalized care of high risk neonates, increasing numbers of sick infants are being transported to neonatal intensive care units in hospitals at which they were not born. Ideally, high risk mothers should be transported to and delivered at centers where these specialized units are located. Neonatal transport should include consultation about the infant's problem and care before transport, ease of access to the transport team, and transport and stabilization by the team before moving the infant. Securing an airway, providing oxygen, assisting with infant ventilation, antimicrobial therapy, and providing a warmed environment plus placing intravenous or arterial lines or chest tubes should all be initiated if indicated prior to transport. Infant and maternal records, laboratory reports, and a tube of clotted maternal blood should also be provided. Before departing, the mother should be briefly reassured and allowed to see the stabilized infant, if practical; the father should follow the transport vehicle to the unit. The transport officer or nurse should also call ahead to inform the receiving unit about the nature of the patient's illness.

The transport vehicle should be equipped with appropriate medicines, fluids, oxygen tanks, catheters, chest tubes, endotracheal tubes, laryngoscopes, and an infant warming device. It should be well illuminated and have ample room for emergency procedures and monitoring equipment. With efficient transport and appropriately educated nursing and medical staff at the referring hospitals, the mortality of "outborn" neonates should be no higher than that of those born within the tertiary care center.

American Academy of Pediatrics: Hospital Care of Newborn Infants. Evanston IL, The Academy, 1983.

Anderson T, Muttart C, Bieber M, et al: A controlled trial of glucose versus glucose and amino acids in premature infants. J Pediatr 94:947, 1979.

Bell E, Warburton D, Stonestreet B, et al: Effect of fluid administration on the development of symptomatic patent ductus arteriosus and congestive heart failure in premature infants. N Engl J Med 302:598, 1980.

Bryan MH, Wei P, Hamilton JR, et al: Supplemental intravenous alimentation in low birth weight infants. J Pediatr 82:940, 1973.

Chen JS, Wong PWK: Intestinal complications of nasojejunal feeding in low birth weight infants. J Pediatr 85:109, 1974.

Chernick V, Raber MB: Electrical hazards in the newborn nursery. J Pediatr 77:143, 1970.

Cross KW, Hey EN, Kennard DL, et al: Lack of temperature control in infants with abnormalities of the CNS. Arch Dis Child 46:437, 1971.

Driscoll J: Care of the newborn. *In:* Fanaroff A, Martin R (eds): Behrman's Neonatal-Perinatal Medicine. St Louis, CV Mosby, 1983.

Driscoll J: Physical examination. *In:* Fanaroff A, Martin R (eds): Behrman's Neonatal-Perinatal Medicine. St Louis, CV Mosby, 1983.

Du JN, Oliver TK Jr: The baby in the delivery room; a suitable microenvironment. JAMA 207:636, 1967.

Duc G: Assessment of hypoxia in the newborn; suggestions for a practical approach. Pediatrics 48:469, 1971.

Fanaroff AA, Wald M, Gruber HS, et al: Insensible water loss in low birth weight infants. Pediatrics 50:236, 1972.

Gaudy GM, Adamsons K, Cunningham N, et al: Thermal environment and acid base homeostasis in human infants during the first hours of life. J Clin Invest 43:751, 1964.

Gaull GE, Rassin DK, Raiha NCR, et al: Milk protein quantity and quality in low-birth-weight infants. III. Effects on sulfur amino acids in plasma and urine. J Pediatr 90:348, 1977.

Gordon HH, Levine SJ, McNamara H: Feeding of premature infants; a comparison of human and cow's milk. Am J Dis Child 73:442, 1947.

Heird W, Anderson T: Methods of nutrient delivery for the low birth weight infant. *In:* Fanaroff A, Martin R (eds); Behrman's Neonatal-Perinatal Medicine. St Louis, CV Mosby, 1983.

Heird W, Okamoto E, Anderson T: Nutritional requirements of the low birth weight infant. *In:* Fanaroff A, Martin R (eds): Behrman's Neonatal-Perinatal Medicine. St Louis, CV Mosby, 1983.

Hittner HM, Hirsch NJ, Rudolph AJ: Assessment of gestational age by examination of the anterior vascular capsule of the lens. J Pediatr 91:455, 1977.

Hittner HM, Rudolph AJ, Kretzer FL: Suppression of severe retinopathy of prematurity with vitamin E supplementation. Ophthalmology 91:1512, 1984.

Johnson L, Bowen FW, Abbasi S, et al: Relationship of prolonged pharmacologic serum levels of vitamin E to incidence of sepsis and necrotizing enterocolitis in infants with birth weight 1500 grams or less. Pediatrics 75:619, 1985.

Kinsey VE, Arnold HJ, Kalina RE, et al: PaO$_2$ levels and retrolental fibroplasia: A report of the cooperative study. Pediatrics 60:655, 1977.

Kliegman R, King K: Intrauterine growth retardation: Determinants of aberrant fetal growth. *In:* Fanaroff AA, Martin RJ (eds): Behrman's Neonatal Perinatal Medicine. St Louis, CV Mosby, 1983.

Lubchenco LO, Hausman C, Boyd E: Intrauterine growth in length and head circumference as estimated from live births at gestational ages from 26 to 42 weeks. Pediatrics 37:403, 1966.

Niswander KR, Gordon M: Collaborative Perinatal Study; The Women and Their Pregnancies. Philadelphia, WB Saunders, 1972.

Perlstein H, Edwards NK, Sutherland JM: Apnea in premature infants and incubator air temperature changes. N Engl J Med 282:461, 1970.

Philips JB, Dickman HM, Resnick MB, et al: Characteristics, mortality and outcome of higher-birth weight infants who require intensive care. Am J Obstet Gynecol 149:875, 1984.

The Prevention of Low Birthweight. Report of the Committee to Study the Prevention of Low Birthweight. Division of Health Promotion and Disease Prevention. Institute of Medicine. Washington, DC, National Academy of Sciences, National Academy Press, 1985.

Roy R, Sinclair J: Hydration of the low birth weight infant. Clin Perinatol 2:393, 1975.

Sargal S, Rosenbaum P, Sjoskopj B, et al: Outcome in infants 501 to 1000 gm birth weight delivered to residents of the McMasters Health Region. J Pediatr 105:989, 1984.

Sauer P, Visser M: The neutral temperature of very low birth weight infants. Pediatrics 74:788, 1984.

Shapiro S, McCormick MC, Starfield BH, et al: Relevance of correlates of infant deaths for significant morbidity at 1 year of age. Am J Obstet Gynecol 136:363, 1980.

Shapiro S, McCormick MC, Starfield BH, et al: Changes in morbidity associated with decreases in neonatal mortality. Pediatrics 72:408, 1983.

Speidel B: Adverse effects of routine procedures in preterm infants. Lancet 1:864, 1978.

Tiffany FM, Dabiri CM, Hallock N, et al: Developmental effects of prolonged pregnancy and postmaturity syndrome. J Pediatr 90:836, 1977.

Van den Berg BJ, Yerushalmy J: The relationship of the rate of intrauterine growth of infants of low birth weight to mortality, morbidity and congenital anomalies. J Pediatr 69:531, 1966.

DISEASES OF THE NEWBORN INFANT: PREMATURE AND FULL-TERM

The child's physician should appreciate the wide variety of disorders that may originate in utero, during birth, or in the immediate postnatal period, and the need to distinguish them according to their time of onset, etiology, and place of origin. The disorders may represent genetic mutations, chromosomal aberrations, or acquired diseases and injuries.

8.20 CLINICAL MANIFESTATIONS OF DISEASE DURING THE NEONATAL PERIOD

Recognizing disease in the newborn infant depends on knowledge about the disorder and evaluation of a limited number of relatively nonspecific clinical signs and symptoms.

Central cyanosis usually indicates respiratory insufficiency, which may be due to pulmonary conditions or may be secondary to central nervous system depression from drugs, intracranial hemorrhage, or anoxia. If it is due to the former, respirations tend to be rapid and may be accompanied by retraction of the thoracic cage. If it is due to the latter, respirations tend to be irregular and weak and often slow. Cyanosis persisting for several days, unaccompanied by obvious signs of respiratory difficulty, suggests cyanotic congenital heart disease or methemoglobinemia. Cyanosis from congenital heart disease may, however, be difficult to distinguish clinically from cyanosis caused by respiratory disease. Episodes of cyanosis also may be the presenting sign of hypoglycemia, bacteremia, meningitis, shock, or persistent fetal circulation. Peripheral acrocyanosis is common and usually does not warrant concern.

Pallor, in addition to anemia or acute hemorrhage, should suggest hypoxia, hypoglycemia, sepsis, shock, or adrenal failure.

Convulsions (Sec. 21.7) usually point to a disorder of the central nervous system and suggest asphyxia, intracranial hemorrhage, cerebral anomaly, subdural effusion, meningitis, hypocalcemia, hypoglycemia, and rarely, pyridoxine dependency, hyponatremia, hypernatremia, inborn errors of metabolism, drug withdrawal, or familial seizures. They may also be the first sign of bacteremia or other severe infection and may occur as a nonspecific sign in any severe illness, particularly if there is circulatory insufficiency. Seizures beginning in the delivery room or shortly thereafter may be due to unintentionally injecting maternal local anesthetic into the fetus. Convulsions may also result from administering large amounts of hypotonic fluids to the mother shortly before and during delivery, with subsequent hyponatremia and water intoxication occurring in the infant.

Convulsions (seizures) should be distinguished from jitter-iness which may be present in normal newborns, in infants of diabetic mothers, in those who experienced birth asphyxia or drug withdrawal, and in polycythemic neonates. Jitteriness resembling simple tremors may be stopped by holding the infant's extremity; it often depends on sensory stimuli, and is not associated with abnormal eye movements. Seizures in premature infants are often subtle and associated with abnormal eye or facial movements; the motor component is often that of tonic extension of the limbs, neck, and trunk. Term infants may have clonic or myoclonic movements but may also manifest more subtle seizure activity. *Apnea* may be the first manifestation of seizure activity, particularly in a premature infant.

Lethargy may be a manifestation of infection, asphyxia, hypoglycemia, sedation from maternal analgesia or anesthesia, cerebral defect, and, indeed, of almost any severe disease including inborn errors of metabolism. Lethargy appearing after the second day should, in particular, suggest infection.

Irritability may be a sign of discomfort accompanying intraabdominal conditions, meningeal irritation, infections, congenital glaucoma, or any condition producing pain. As in later infancy, the eardrums should always be examined as a possible source of pain.

Hyperactivity, especially of the premature infant, may be a sign of hypoxia, pneumothorax, emphysema, hypoglycemia, hypocalcemia, central nervous system damage, drug withdrawal, thyrotoxicosis, or discomfort due to a cold environment.

Failure to feed well is seen in most sick newborn infants and should always occasion a careful search for infection and other abnormal conditions.

Fever may be the result of too high an environmental temperature due to weather, overheated nurseries or incubators, or too many clothes or bedclothes. It is also seen in "dehydration fever" of newborn infants. If these causes of fever can be eliminated, then serious infection (pneumonia, bacteremia, viremia, meningitis) must be considered, although such infections often occur without provoking a febrile response in newborn infants. An unexplained *fall in body temperature* may accompany infection or other serious disturbances of the circulation or central nervous system. A sudden servo-controlled increase in incubator temperature to maintain body temperature is often associated with sepsis.

Periods of *apnea,* particularly in the premature infant, may be associated with a variety of disturbances (see Table 8–17). When apneas reoccur within intervals no longer than 20 sec or are associated with cyanosis or bradycardia, they warrant an immediate diagnostic evaluation.

Jaundice during the first 24 hr of life should be considered to be due to erythroblastosis fetalis until proved otherwise.

Septicemia (especially in the low birthweight infant), cytomegalic inclusion disease, the congenital rubella syndrome, and toxoplasmosis should also be considered, especially if there is an increase in plasma direct-reacting bilirubin.

Jaundice after the first 24 hr may be "physiologic," or may be due to septicemia, hemolytic anemia, galactosemia, hepatitis, congenital atresia of the bile ducts, inspissated bile syndrome following erythroblastosis fetalis, syphilis, herpes simplex, or congenital infections. (See Sec. 8.44–8.45)

Vomiting during the first day of life suggests obstruction in the upper digestive tract or increased intracranial pressure. Roentgenographic studies are indicated when obstruction is suspected. Vomiting also may be a nonspecific symptom of an illness such as septicemia. It is a common manifestation of overfeeding or inexperienced feeding technique, pyloric stenosis, milk allergy, duodenal ulcer, stress ulcer, or adrenal insufficiency. Infants placed in body casts for orthopedic treatment often vomit transiently. Vomitus containing dark blood is usually a sign of life-threatening illness; the benign possibility of swallowed maternal blood should also be considered. Bile-stained vomitus strongly suggests obstruction below the ampulla of Vater.

Diarrhea may be a symptom of overfeeding, acute gastroenteritis, malabsorption, or a nonspecific symptom of infection. It may be seen in conditions accompanied by compromised circulation of part of the intestinal or genital tract, such as mesenteric thrombosis, necrotizing enterocolitis, strangulated hernia, intussusception, and torsion of the ovary or testis.

Abdominal distention, usually a sign of intestinal obstruction or an intra-abdominal mass, may also be seen in infants with enteritis, ileus accompanying sepsis, respiratory distress, or hypokalemia.

Failure to move an extremity or part of it suggests fracture, dislocation, or nerve injury. It is also seen in osteomyelitis and other infections that cause pain on movement of the affected part.

CONGENITAL ANOMALIES

Congenital anomalies are a major cause of stillbirths and neonatal deaths, but are perhaps even more important as causes of physical defects and metabolic disorders. (Anomalies are discussed in general in Chapter 6 and specifically in the chapters on the various systems of the body. For congenital mental defects, see Chapter 2; for congenital metabolic and chemical disorders, see Chapter 7; and for immunologic deficiency disorders, see Chapter 10.) Early recognition of anomalies is important for planning care; for some, such as tracheoesophageal fistula, diaphragmatic hernia, choanal atresia, and intestinal obstruction, immediate medical and surgical therapy is essential for survival. Parents are likely to be assailed by anxiety and guilt upon learning of the existence of a congenital anomaly and will require sensitive counseling.

8.21 BIRTH INJURY

The term *birth injury* is used to denote avoidable and unavoidable mechanical and anoxic trauma incurred by the infant during labor and delivery. These injuries may result from inappropriate or deficient medical skill or attention, or they may occur, despite skilled and competent obstetric care, independently of any acts or omissions of the parents. In order to avoid later misunderstandings, recriminations, or parental guilt, it is important to counsel parents who have a child with a residuum from birth trauma or anoxia about this broad use of the term "birth injury." The definition does not include injury from amniocentesis, intrauterine transfusion,

scalp vein sampling, or resuscitation procedures, all of which are discussed elsewhere.

The incidence of birth injuries has been estimated at 2–7/1000 live births. Predisposing factors include macrosomia, prematurity, cephalopelvic disproportion, dystocia, prolonged labor, and breech presentation. Although the incidence has decreased in recent years, in part owing to refinement in obstetric techniques and judgment, birth injuries are still an important problem, since frequently even transient injuries readily apparent to the parents result in anxiety and questioning that require supportive and informative counseling. Some injuries may be latent initially, but later result in severe illness or sequelae.

8.22 CRANIAL INJURIES

Caput succedaneum is a diffuse, sometimes ecchymotic, edematous swelling of the soft tissues of the scalp involving the portion presenting during vertex delivery. It may extend across the midline and across suture lines. The edema disappears within the first few days of life. Analogous swelling, discoloration, and distortion of the face are seen in face presentations. No specific treatment is needed, but if there are extensive ecchymoses, early phototherapy for hyperbilirubinemia may be indicated. *Molding* of the head and overriding of the parietal bones are frequently associated with caput succedaneum and become more evident after the caput has receded, but disappear during the first weeks of life. Rarely, a hemorrhagic caput may result in shock and require blood transfusion.

Erythema, abrasions, ecchymoses and *subcutaneous fat necrosis* of facial or scalp soft tissues may be seen after forceps deliveries. Their location depends on the area of application of the forceps. Ecchymoses may be seen after manipulative deliveries and occasionally in premature infants for no discernible reason.

Subconjunctival hemorrhages are frequent, and *petechiae* of the skin of the head and neck are common. All are probably secondary to a sudden increase in intrathoracic pressure during passage of the chest through the birth canal. Parents should be assured that they are temporary and the result of *normal* hazards of delivery.

Cephalohematoma (Fig. 8–14) is a subperiosteal hemorrhage, hence always limited to the surface of 1 cranial bone. There is no discoloration of the overlying scalp, and swelling is usually not visible until several hours after birth, since subperiosteal bleeding is a slow process. An underlying skull fracture, usually linear and not depressed, is occasionally associated with cephalohematoma. Cranial meningocele may

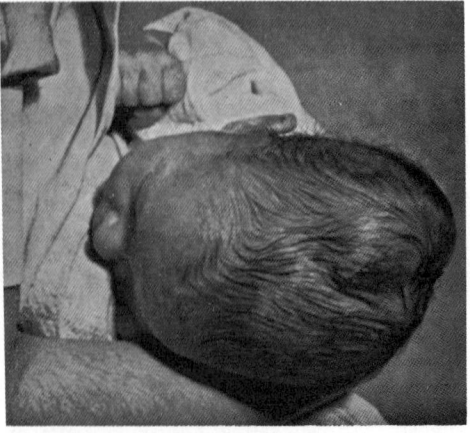

Figure 8–14. Cephalohematoma of the right parietal bone.

be differentiated from cephalohematoma by pulsation, increased pressure on crying, and the roentgenographic evidence of bony defect. Most cephalohematomas are resorbed within 2 wk–3 mo, depending on their size. They may begin to calcify by the end of the second week. A sensation of central depression suggesting underlying fracture or bony defect is usually encountered on palpation of the organized rim of a cephalohematoma. A few remain for years as bony protuberances and are detectable roentgenographically as widening of the diploic space; cyst-like defects may persist for months or years. Despite these residuals, cephalohematomas require no treatment, although phototherapy may be necessary to ameliorate hyperbilirubinemia. Incision and drainage are contraindicated because of the risk of introducing infection in a benign condition. A massive cephalohematoma may rarely result in blood loss severe enough to require transfusion. It may also be associated with a skull fracture and intracranial hemorrhage.

Fractures of the skull may occur as a result of pressure from forceps or from the maternal symphysis pubis, sacral promontory, or ischial spines. Linear fractures, the most common, cause no symptoms and require no treatment. Depressed fractures are usually indentations of the calvarium similar to a dent in a ping-pong ball; usually they are a complication of forceps delivery. The infant may be asymptomatic unless there is associated intracranial injury; it is advisable to elevate such depressions to prevent cortical injury from sustained pressure. Fracture of the occipital bone with separation of the basal and squamous portions almost invariably causes fatal hemorrhage owing to disruption of the underlying sinuses. It may result during breech deliveries from traction on the hyperextended spine of the infant with the head fixed in the maternal pelvis.

8.23 INTRACRANIAL (INTRAVENTRICULAR) HEMORRHAGE

Intracranial hemorrhage may result from trauma or asphyxia and, rarely, from a primary hemorrhagic disturbance or congenital vascular anomaly. Traumatic hemorrhage is especially likely when the fetal head is large in proportion to the size of the mother's pelvic outlet; when for other reasons the labor is prolonged; when there are breech or precipitate deliveries; or when there is injudicious mechanical interference with delivery. The proper use of forceps may decrease the incidence of intracranial bleeding in prolonged hard labors. Intracranial hemorrhages often involve the ventricles **(intraventricular hemorrhage)** of premature infants delivered spontaneously without apparent trauma.

In premature infants, subependymal and intraventricular hemorrhages are common. Subarachnoid and intracerebral bleeding are less common. The highly vascularized periventricular subependymal germinal matrix is a particularly vulnerable region in the fetus and premature infant during the first week of life. Hypoxic-ischemic injury or neonatal circulatory disturbances such as hypervolemia and hypertension, pneumothorax, or shock may result in thrombosis and/or bleeding, and intraventricular hemorrhage. Excessive use of sodium bicarbonate and elevated carbon dioxide tension have also been associated with intraventricular hemorrhage in premature infants. Massive subdural hemorrhages, often associated with tears in the tentorium cerebelli or less frequently in the falx cerebri, are rare but encountered more often in fullterm than in premature infants.

Primary hemorrhagic disturbances and vascular malformations usually give rise to subarachnoid or intracerebral hemorrhage. Intracranial bleeding may be associated with disseminated intravascular coagulopathy or idiopathic thrombocytopenia.

Clinical Manifestations. Intraventricular and subependymal hemorrhages may be present at birth in premature infants and occasionally are immediately symptomatic, but clinical manifestations usually appear later within the first 3 days of life. The most common symptoms are diminished or absent Moro reflex, poor muscle tone, lethargy, apnea, and somnolence. In premature infants with intraventricular hemorrhage there is often a precipitous deterioration on the second or third day of life. Periods of apnea, pallor, or cyanosis, failure to suck well, abnormal eye signs, a high-pitched, shrill cry, muscular twitchings, convulsions, decreased muscle tone, paralyses, metabolic acidosis, and a decreased hematocrit or its failure to increase after transfusion may be the first indications. The fontanel *may* be tense and bulging. Retinal hemorrhage, ocular palsies, inequality in size of and failure of the pupils to react to light, nystagmus, or hyperpyrexia may be observed. Severe neurologic depression progresses to coma after more severe intraventricular hemorrhages, with extension to the cerebral cortex and ventricular dilation. In a small percentage there may be no clinical manifestations.

Diagnosis. This is based chiefly on the history, the clinical manifestations, and the course. Since nonlocalizing signs of intracranial hemorrhage are identical with those caused by cerebral edema or anoxia, before carrying out any diagnostic procedure, the physician should weigh the chance of helping the patient against the risk of the procedure. In the absence of an obstetric history of intrapartum hemorrhage, of other signs of bleeding, of extensive bruising in the infant, or of iatrogenic removal of large quantities of blood, a significant fall in hematocrit should suggest the diagnosis of intracranial hemorrhage or that of subcapsular hemorrhage of the liver. Cerebral ultrasonography is the method of choice in diagnosing intracranial hemorrhage in the neonatal infant; computed tomography may be similarly useful. Four levels of increasing severity of hemorrhage have been defined by ultrasound for LBW infants: grade I is bleeding confined to the subependymal matrix; grade II indicates intraventricular bleeding; grade III includes grade II plus intraventricular dilation; and grade IV includes grade III plus intracerebral bleeding. Prognosis is poorest with grade III and grade IV hemorrhage, especially in the presence of coma. CT scan is indicated for term infants, since ultrasound may not reveal intraparenchymal hemorrhage. Lumbar puncture is indicated in the presence of signs of increased intracranial pressure or deteriorating clinical condition to identify gross subarachnoid hemorrhage or to rule out the possibility of bacterial meningitis; the cerebrospinal fluid usually has elevated protein levels with many red blood cells. Not infrequently there is hypoglycorrhachia and a mild lymphocytosis. Apnea, bradycardia, or circulatory insufficiency may occur as a consequence of the physical manipulation of performing a lumbar puncture in a premature infant. *Subdural hemorrhage* is more common in larger term infants and is often chronic; it usually presents at 1–2 mo with anemia, seizures, and a bulging fontanel. Subdural taps may be lifesaving.

Since a small amount of bleeding into the cerebrospinal fluid often occurs in the course of normal and even cesarean deliveries, small numbers of red blood cells or slight xanthochromia in subarachnoid fluid does not necessarily indicate significant intracranial hemorrhage. Conversely, the subarachnoid fluid may be absolutely clear with severe subdural or intracerebral hemorrhage occurring when there is no communication with the subarachnoid space.

Prognosis. Intrapartum death may occur in the more severe cases; postnatally, fatalities usually occur within the first week resulting from central nervous system depression and respiratory failure. If an infant survives, recovery may be complete, or there may be permanent residuals, mainly cerebral palsy and posthemorrhagic hydrocephalus. Prior to the availability of cerebral ultrasonography or the CT scan, the diagnosis in the surviving or asymptomatic patient was rarely certain.

Because the majority of parents both realize and fear the possibility of cerebral residuals following intracranial hemorrhage or cerebral anoxia, it is usually wisest to give them an opportunity to air their anxiety in a frank discussion of the problem, during which their questions should be invited rather than suppressed or evaded. As optimistic an attitude as possible, consistent with the physician's opinion of the prognosis of the individual case, should be maintained.

Prevention. Prophylactic measures include continuing improvements in obstetric and pediatric management; many instances of traumatic intracranial hemorrhage are avoidable. Wide swings of blood pressure and pCO_2 should be avoided. In addition, judicious use of sodium bicarbonate is indicated.

Treatment. The infant should be handled as infrequently and as gently as possible and maintained in an incubator that allows good temperature control, continuous observation, and easy administration of oxygen for cyanosis. Phenobarbital or other anticonvulsant drugs in appropriate doses may be used to control convulsive movement. A small dose of vitamin K_1 oxide (Sec. 8.49) and a transfusion of fresh frozen plasma are indicated in the presence of hemorrhagic disease of the newborn. The management of disseminated intravascular coagulopathy is discussed in Sec. 15.50. Disagreement persists about the advisability of serial spinal punctures for relieving intracranial pressure and for removing blood to reduce its irritant effect on the cerebral cortex or to prevent possible interference with the normal resorptive mechanisms for cerebrospinal fluid. Neurosurgical procedures are not indicated unless hydrocephalus is uncontrolled by other measures, such as repeated lumbar punctures.

Cerebral edema may result in any or all of the clinical signs produced by intracranial hemorrhage. Trauma and asphyxia are the most common causes. It is usually not possible to establish this diagnosis during life except by inference from the history. Anterior fontanel pressure may be monitored externally to detect changes in intracranial pressure, but the technique is not generally available or well established. Treatment includes avoidance or correction of dilutional hyponatremia. The indications for and benefits of reducing increased intracranial pressure from edema by removal of cerebrospinal fluid, by the parenteral administration of dexamethasone (10 mg/m^2 initially, then 5 mg/m^2 every 6 hr), by hyperventilation, or by intravenous infusions of mannitol in neonatal infants have not been established. They may be indicated if an infant's condition is deteriorating with rapidly progressing neurologic signs.

8.24 SPINE AND SPINAL CORD

Strong traction exerted when the spine is hyperextended or when the direction of pull is lateral, or forceful longitudinal traction on the trunk while the head is still firmly engaged in the pelvis, especially when combined with flexion and torsion of the vertical axis, may produce fracture and separation of the vertebrae. Such injuries, rarely diagnosed clinically, are most likely to occur when difficulty is encountered in delivering the shoulders in cephalic presentations and the head in breech presentations. The injury occurs most commonly at the level of the 7th cervical and 1st thoracic vertebrae. Transection of the cord may occur, but hemorrhage and edema may produce neurologic signs indistinguishable from those of transection, except that they are not permanent. There is complete paralysis of voluntary motion below the level of injury, although the persistence of a withdrawal reflex mediated through spinal centers distal to the area of injury is frequently misinterpreted as representing voluntary motion. If the injury is severe, the infant who, from birth may be in poor condition due to respiratory depression, shock, or hypothermia, may deteriorate rapidly to death within several hours before neurologic signs are obvious. Alternatively, the course may be protracted with symptoms and signs appearing at birth or later in the first week; immobility, flaccidity, and associated brachial plexus injuries may not be recognized for several days. Constipation may also be present. Some infants survive for prolonged periods, their initial flaccidity, immobility, and areflexia being replaced after several weeks or months by rigid flexion of extremities, increased muscle tone, and spasms.

The differential diagnosis includes amyotonia congenita and myelodysplasia associated with spina bifida occulta. The survivors' treatment is supportive, and they often remain permanently injured. When there is compression from a fracture or dislocation, the prognosis is related to the time elapsing before the compression is removed.

8.25 PERIPHERAL NERVE INJURIES

Brachial Palsy. Injury to the brachial plexus may cause paralysis of the upper arm with or without paralysis of the forearm or hand or, more commonly, paralysis of the entire arm. These injuries occur when lateral traction is exerted on the head and neck during delivery of the shoulder in a vertex presentation, when the arms are extended over the head in a breech presentation, or when there is excessive traction on the shoulders.

In **Erb-Duchenne paralysis** the injury is limited to the 5th and 6th cervical nerves. The infant loses the power to abduct the arm from the shoulder, to rotate the arm externally, and to supinate the forearm. The characteristic position consists of adduction and internal rotation of the arm with pronation of the forearm. The power of extension of the forearm is retained, but the biceps reflex is absent; the Moro reflex is absent on the affected side (Fig. 8–15). There may be some sensory impairment on the outer aspect of the arm. The power in the forearm and the hand grasp are preserved unless

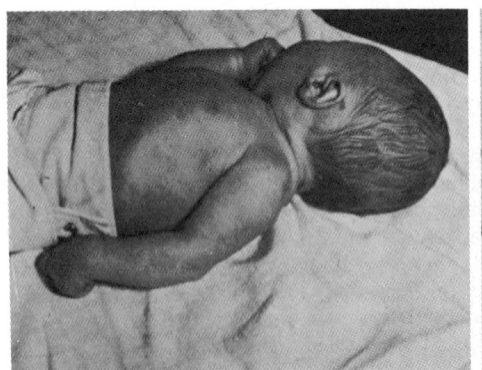
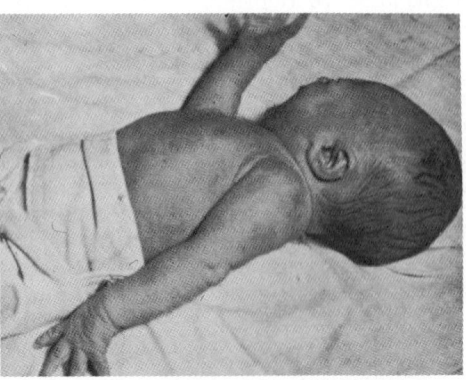

Figure 8–15. Brachial palsy of the left arm (asymmetric Moro reflex.)

the lower part of the plexus is also injured; the presence of the hand grasp is a favorable prognostic sign. When the injury includes the phrenic nerve, alteration of the diaphragmatic excursion may be observed fluoroscopically.

Klumpke paralysis is a rarer form of brachial palsy; injury to the 7th and 8th cervical nerves and the 1st thoracic nerve produces a paralyzed hand and ipsilateral ptosis and miosis if the sympathetic fibers of the 1st thoracic root are also injured.

The mild cases may not be detected immediately after birth. Differentiation must be made from cerebral injury; from fracture, dislocation, or epiphyseal separation of the humerus; and from fracture of the clavicle.

The *prognosis* depends on whether the nerve was merely injured or was lacerated. If the paralysis was due to edema and hemorrhage about the nerve fibers, there should be a return of function within a few months; if due to laceration, permanent damage may result. The involvement of the deltoid is usually the most serious problem and may result in a shoulder drop secondary to muscular atrophy. In general, paralysis of the upper arm has a better prognosis than paralysis of the lower arm.

Treatment consists of partial immobilization and appropriate positioning to prevent development of contractures. In upper arm paralysis, the arm should be abducted 90 degrees, with external rotation at the shoulder and with full supination of the forearm and slight extension at the wrist with the palm turned toward the face. This may be done with a brace or splint during the first 1–2 wk. Immobilization should be intermittent through the day while the infant is asleep and between feedings. In lower arm or hand paralysis, the wrist should be splinted in a neutral position and padding placed in the fist. When the entire arm is paralyzed, the same treatment principles should be followed. Gentle massage and range of motion exercises may be started by 7–10 days of age. Infants should be followed closely with active and passive corrective exercises. If the paralysis persists without improvement for 3–6 mo, neuroplasty and tendon transfers offer hope for partial recovery but are usually not advisable before 3–4 yr of age when muscle development can be adequately assessed.

Phrenic Nerve Paralysis. Phrenic nerve injury with diaphragmatic paralysis must be considered when cyanosis and irregular and labored respirations develop. Such injuries, usually unilateral, are associated with ipsilateral upper brachial palsy. Because breathing is thoracic in type, the abdomen does not bulge with inspiration. Breath sounds are diminished on the affected side. The thrust of the diaphragm, which often may be felt just under the costal margin on the normal side, is absent on the affected side. The *diagnosis* is established by fluoroscopic examination, which reveals the elevation of the diaphragm on the paralyzed side and seesaw movements of the two sides of the diaphragm during respiration.

There is no specific *treatment*; the infant should be placed on the involved side and given oxygen if necessary. Initially, intravenous feedings may be needed; later, progressive gavage or oral feedings may be started depending on the infant's condition. Pulmonary infections are a serious complication. Recovery usually occurs spontaneously by 1–3 mo; rarely, surgical plication of the diaphragm may be indicated.

Facial Nerve Palsy. Usually, facial palsy is a peripheral paralysis that results from pressure over the facial nerve in utero from efforts during labor or from forceps during delivery. Rarely nonobstetric, it may result from nuclear agenesis of the facial nerve. Peripheral paralysis is flaccid and, when complete, involves the entire side of the face, including the forehead. When the infant cries, there is movement on only the nonparalyzed side of the face, and the mouth is drawn to that side. On the affected side the forehead is smooth, the eye cannot be closed, the nasolabial fold is absent, and the

corner of the mouth droops. The forehead will wrinkle on the affected side with central paralysis, since only the lower two thirds of the face is involved. Usually there are also other manifestations of intracranial injury, most commonly a 6th nerve palsy. The *prognosis* depends upon whether the nerve was injured by pressure or whether the nerve fibers were torn. Improvement occurs within a few weeks in the former instance. Care of the exposed eye is essential. Neuroplasty may be indicated when the paralysis is persistent. Facial palsy may be confused with the absence of the depressor muscles of the mouth, which is a benign problem.

Other peripheral nerves are seldom injured at birth, except when they are involved in fractures or hemorrhages.

8.26 VISCERA

The **liver** is the only internal organ other than the brain injured with any frequency during birth. The damage usually occurs from pressure on the liver during delivery of the head in breech presentations. Large infant size, intrauterine asphyxia, coagulation disorders, extreme prematurity, and hepatomegaly are contributing factors. Incorrect cardiac massage is a less frequent cause. The liver is ruptured with formation of a subcapsular hematoma. The infant usually appears normal for the first 1–3 days. Nonspecific signs related to loss of blood into the hematoma may appear early and include poor feeding, listlessness, pallor, jaundice, tachypnea, and tachycardia. A mass may be palpable in the right upper quadrant. The hematoma may be large enough to cause anemia. Shock and death may occur if the hematoma breaks through the capsule into the peritoneal cavity, reducing pressure and allowing fresh hemorrhage. Early suspicion and diagnosis and prompt supportive therapy can decrease the mortality of this disorder. Surgical repair of a laceration may be required.

Rupture of the spleen may occur alone or in association with rupture of the liver. The causes, complications, treatment, and prevention are similar.

Although **adrenal hemorrhage** occurs with some frequency, especially after breech delivery, its cause is undetermined: it may be due to trauma, anoxia, or severe stress, as in overwhelming infections. Calcified central hematomas of the adrenal have been identified roentgenographically or at autopsy in older infants and children, suggesting that not all adrenal hemorrhages are immediately fatal. In severe cases the diagnosis is usually made at post mortem examination. The symptoms are profound shock and cyanosis. There may be a mass in the flank with overlying skin discoloration; jaundice may also develop. If adrenal hemorrhage is suspected, abdominal ultrasonography may be helpful and treatment for acute adrenal failure may be indicated (Sec. 19.22).

INJURY OF THE STERNOCLEIDOMASTOID

See Torticollis, Sec. 23.6.

8.27 FRACTURES

Clavicle. This bone is fractured during labor and delivery more frequently than any other bone; it is particularly vulnerable when there is difficulty in delivery of the shoulder in vertex presentations and of the extended arms in breech deliveries. The infant characteristically does not move the arm freely on the affected side; crepitus and bony irregularity may be palpated and occasionally discoloration is visible over the fracture site. The Moro reflex is absent on the affected side, and there is spasm of the sternocleidomastoid muscle with obliteration of the supraclavicular depression at the site of the fracture. In greenstick fractures there may be no limitation of movement and the Moro reflex may be present. Fracture of the humerus or brachial palsy may also be responsible for limitation of movement of an arm and absence of a Moro reflex on the affected side. The *prognosis* is excellent. *Treatment,* if any, consists in immobilization of the arm and shoulder on the affected side. A remarkable degree of callus develops at the site within a week and may be the first evidence of the fracture.

Extremities. In fractures of the long bones spontaneous movement of the extremity is usually absent. The Moro reflex is also absent from the involved extremity. There may be associated nerve involvement. Satisfactory results for a fractured humerus are obtained with 2–4 wk of immobilization by strapping the arm to the chest, by applying a triangular splint and a Velpeau bandage, or by application of a cast. For fracture of the femur, good results are obtained with traction-suspension of both lower extremities, even if the fracture is unilateral; the legs, immobilized in a spica cast, are attached to an overhead frame. Splints are effective for treatment of fractures of the forearm or leg. Healing is usually accompanied by excess callus formation. The *prognosis* is excellent for fractures of the extremities. Fractures in preterm infants are related to osteopenia (Sec. 8.54).

Dislocations and **epiphyseal separations** rarely result from birth trauma. The upper femoral epiphysis may be separated by forcible manipulation of the infant's leg as, for example, in breech extraction or after version. There is swelling, slight shortening, limitation of active motion, painful passive motion, and external rotation of the leg. The diagnosis is established roentgenographically. The prognosis is good for the milder injuries, but coxa vara frequently results from extensive displacement.

Nose. The most prevalent injury of the nose is a dislocation of the cartilaginous portion of the septum from the vomerine groove and the columella. The infant may have difficulty in nursing and some impairment in nasal respiration. On physical examination, the nares appear asymmetrical and the nose flattened. An oral airway rarely is needed, and surgical consultation should be obtained for definitive treatment.

8.28 HYPOXIA-ISCHEMIA

Anoxia is a term used to indicate the consequences of a complete lack of oxygen owing to a number of primary causes. *Hypoxia* refers to an arterial concentration of oxygen that is less than normal, and *ischemia* refers to blood flow to cells or organs that is insufficient to maintain their normal function. *Hypoxic-ischemic encephalopathy* is the primary cause of permanent damage to central nervous system cells, which may result in death or which may be manifest later as cerebral palsy or mental deficiency. Its prevention and treatment are those of the basic conditions that cause it; death and disability may sometimes be prevented through symptomatic treatment with oxygen or artificial respiration and the correction of associated metabolic acidosis with sodium bicarbonate.

Etiology. Fetal hypoxia may result from (1) inadequate oxygenation of maternal blood as a result of hypoventilation during anesthesia, cardiac failure, or carbon monoxide poisoning; (2) low maternal blood pressure as a result of the hypotension that may complicate spinal anesthesia or that may result from compression of the vena cava and aorta by the gravid uterus; (3) inadequate relaxation of the uterus to permit placental filling as a result of uterine tetany caused by excessive administration of oxytocin; (4) premature separation of the placenta; (5) impedance to the circulation of blood through the umbilical cord as a result of compression or knotting of the cord; and (6) placental inadequacy from numerous causes, including toxemia and postmaturity.

After birth, hypoxia may result from (1) anemia severe enough to lower the oxygen content of the blood to a critical level due to severe hemorrhage or hemolytic disease; (2) shock severe enough to interfere with the transport of oxygen to vital cells from adrenal hemorrhage, intraventricular hemorrhage, overwhelming infection, or massive blood loss; (3) a deficit in arterial oxygen saturation from failure to breathe adequately postnatally, due to a cerebral defect, narcosis, or injury; and (4) failure of oxygenation of an adequate amount of blood from severe forms of cyanotic congenital heart disease or deficient pulmonary ventilation.

Pathology. The pathologic changes of hypoxia-ischemia are principally those caused by congestion and increased capillary permeability. Congestion and petechiae are found in all organs but are especially noticeable in the pleura, pericardium, thymus, adrenals, brain, and meninges. Cerebral edema is common. Gross subarachnoid, intraventricular, or adrenal hemorrhage may be present without demonstrable tearing of blood vessels. Histologic study of the brain and liver, particularly the right lobe, may reveal cellular regenerative changes similar to those produced experimentally by anoxia. Fetal hypoxia is characterized pathologically by the additional finding of large amounts of amniotic debris in the respiratory passages. Pathophysiologically, within minutes of the onset of total fetal hypoxia there is bradycardia, hypotension, decreased cardiac output, and severe metabolic as well as respiratory acidosis. The initial circulatory response of the fetus is with increased shunting through the ductus venosus, ductus arteriosus, and foramen ovale with transient maintenance of perfusion of the brain, heart, and adrenals in preference to the lungs (due to pulmonary vasoconstriction), liver, kidneys, and intestine.

Clinical Manifestations. The signs of hypoxia in the *fetus* are usually noted a few minutes to a few days before delivery. The fetal heart rate slows, and the beat to beat variability declines. Continuous heart rate recording may reveal a variable or late (type II dips) deceleration pattern (Fig. 8–6), and scalp blood analysis may show a pH less than 7.20. The acidosis is made up of varying degrees of metabolic and/or respiratory components. Particularly in the infant near term, these signs should lead to the administration of high concentrations of oxygen to the mother and immediate delivery to avoid fetal death or central nervous system damage.

At *delivery* the presence of yellow, meconium-stained amniotic fluid and vernix caseosa is evidence that there has been fetal distress, probably hypoxic. At birth these infants are frequently depressed and fail to breathe spontaneously. During the ensuing hours they may remain hypotonic or change from hypotonia to extreme hypertonia, or their tone may appear normal. Pallor, cyanosis, apnea, slow heart rate, and unresponsiveness to stimulation also are signs of hypoxic-ischemic encephalopathy. Cerebral edema may develop during the next 24 hr and result in profound brain stem depression. During this time seizure activity may occur which may be severe and therefore refractory to the usual doses of anticonvulsants. Although most often a result of the hypoxic-ischemic encephalopathy, seizures in asphyxiated newborns may also be due to hypocalcemia and hypoglycemia.

In addition to central nervous system dysfunction, congestive heart failure and cardiogenic shock, persistent fetal circulation, respiratory distress syndrome, gastrointestinal perforation, hematuria, and acute tubular necrosis are also associated with perinatal asphyxia.

After delivery hypoxia is due to respiratory failure and circulatory insufficiency (Sec. 8.32 and 8.29).

Prognosis. Most of the deaths and cerebral damage that result from hypoxic-ischemic encephalopathy are probably due to late fetal or postnatal periods of hypoxia. Early detection of fetal distress signs by continuous monitoring of fetal heart rate and by serial determinations of acid-base balance in fetal scalp blood samples during labor may significantly decrease this morbidity and mortality by providing improved criteria for obstetric intervention in labor (Sec. 8.10). Although the incidence of asphyxia is higher in the more premature infants, the increased risk of death from it is greater in more mature infants, e.g., increased over 100–fold for those greater than 36 wk gestation. Survival is directly related to gestational age, central nervous system depression, or coma; and postasphyxial seizures are associated with a poor prognosis.

8.29 PEDIATRIC EMERGENCIES IN THE DELIVERY ROOM

The most common and important emergency related to the newborn infant in the delivery room is the failure to initiate and maintain respirations. Less frequent, but of major importance, are shock, severe anemia (Sec. 8.21–8.23 and 15.34), plethora (Sec. 8.48), convulsions (Sec. 21.7), and management of life-threatening congenital malformations (Sec. 6.29).

Respiratory Distress and Failure. Disorders of respiration in the newborn infant can be categorized as either *central nervous system failure*, representing depression or failure of the respiratory center, or *peripheral respiratory difficulty*, indicating interference with the alveolar exchange of oxygen and carbon dioxide (Table 8–19). Cyanosis occurs in both groups. The respiratory problems encountered in the delivery room are most frequently those of airway obstruction and of depression of the central nervous system with the absence of adequate respiratory effort.

Respiratory distress in the presence of good respiratory effort should lead to an immediate consideration of peripheral causes; *it is an indication for a roentgenographic examination of the chest,* if this is at all possible.

If respiratory movements are made with the mouth closed but the infant fails to move air in and out of the lungs, bilateral **choanal atresia** (Sec. 13.24) or other obstruction of the upper respiratory tract should be suspected. The mouth should be opened, and the mouth and posterior pharynx cleared of secretions by gentle suction. An oropharyngeal airway should be inserted and the source of the obstruction sought immediately. If effective respiratory flow is not produced by opening the infant's mouth and clearing the airway, laryngoscopy is indicated. With obstructive malformations of the epiglottis, larynx, or trachea, an endotracheal tube should be inserted; prolonged endotracheal intubation or tracheostomy may be required. Respiratory failure from depression or

injury of the central nervous system may require continuous artificial ventilation with a face mask and bag or through an endotracheal tube.

Hypoplasia of the mandible (Pierre Robin syndrome) (Sec. 12.5) with posterior displacement of the tongue may result in symptoms similar to those of choanal atresia, which may be temporarily relieved by pulling the tongue forward. A scaphoid abdomen suggests a **diaphragmatic hernia** or **eventration,** as does asymmetry of contour or movement of the chest or shift of the apical impulse of the heart; these latter manifestations are also compatible with tension pneumothorax.

Causes of peripheral respiratory difficulty are discussed in Sec. 8.30–8.40.

Failure to Initiate or Sustain Respiration. This usually originates in the central nervous system due to asphyxia; immaturity in itself is seldom a causative factor except in VLBW infants (< 1000 g). Intrapulmonary problems, such as the pulmonary hypoplasia associated with Potter syndrome and severe organized intrauterine pneumonia, may at times result in poorly sustained ventilation. The lungs in these infants are very noncompliant, and efforts to begin respirations may be inadequate to start sufficient ventilation.

Narcosis results from heavy doses of morphine, Demerol, barbiturates, reserpine, or tranquilizers administered to the mother shortly before delivery or from maternal anesthesia, given during the second stage of labor. The infant is cyanotic at birth and slow to cry or breathe; when respiration is established, it is extremely slow.

Narcosis should be avoided by using appropriate analgesic and anesthetic practices. Treatment includes initial physical stimulation and securing a patent airway. If effective ventilation is not initiated, artificial breathing with a mask and bag must be instituted. At the same time, if depression is due to morphine or its derivatives, Narcan (naloxone hydrochloride), 0.01 mg/kg, should be given by intravenous, subcutaneous, or intramuscular routes. Ventilation is essential prior to and during the administration of this antidote. If depression is due to other anesthetics or analgesics, artificial respiration should be continued until the infant is able to sustain ventilation. Central nervous system stimulant drugs should not be used as they are ineffective and may be harmful.

Prenatal or **perinatal hypoxia,** whatever the cause, if sufficiently severe, will produce brain stem depression and secondary apnea, which is unresponsive to sensory stimulation. Death due to apnea may be prevented by resuscitation, provided the basic cause of the hypoxia can be eliminated

Table 8–19. **Respiratory Distress and Failure in Newborn Infants**

Type	Manifestations	Clinical Entity
Central nervous system failure	Apnea Slow, irregular, gasping respiratory efforts	Narcosis Prenatal or perinatal hypoxia Intracranial hemorrhage or trauma CNS anomalies
Peripheral respiratory difficulty	Rapid respiratory rate Increasing respiratory rate Chest lag Intercostal retraction Subcostal retraction Xiphoid retraction Chin tug Expiratory grunt Frothing at lips	Primary atelectasis Hyaline membrane disease Aspiration of amniotic fluid containing formed elements Pneumonia Airway obstruction Diaphragmatic hernia Lung cysts Lobar emphysema Pneumothorax Aspiration of food or mucus Congestive heart failure

within a reasonable time while artificial respiration, if necessary, is being carried out. External cardiac massage, correction of acidosis, and circulatory support with drugs may be important adjuncts to ventilation. Hypothermia as a means of temporarily reducing metabolic needs for oxygen during the period of hypoxia is contraindicated.

Intracranial hemorrhage and **trauma** are discussed in Sec. 8.22 and 8.23. **Central nervous system anomalies** are rarely responsible for respiratory failure.

Resuscitation. Failure to breathe spontaneously within 1 min of birth is an indication for resuscitation. If the central mechanism can be revived, the infant will be more effective in ventilating the lungs safely than will any available artificial technique.

After the upper and central airway has been cleared as adequately as possible by removing accumulated liquid contents, resuscitation should start with simple, gentle physical stimulation such as slapping the soles of the feet with a finger. If this is unsuccessful, the upper respiratory passage should be suctioned again and a flow of oxygen directed at the infant's face. If the infant has an Apgar score of 4 or less, or if the pulse rate is less than 80 beats/min, artificial respiration or pulmonary inflation is indicated. Administration of 100% oxygen at 16–20 cm of H_2O pressure for 1–2 sec, added to stimulus of chemoreceptors, initiates a gasp in about 85% of patients. If the Apgar score is 2 or less or if a gentle flow of oxygen at pressures up to 25 cm of H_2O administered either steadily or in puffs through a face mask does not produce first an improved color and tone and then subsequent, spontaneous respiratory movements, direct laryngoscopy and endotracheal intubation are indicated which should include suctioning of the lower respiratory passages and an attempt to inflate the lungs by applying short bursts of oxygen at higher pressures. Pressures of greater than 25 cm of H_2O may rupture the lung but may be required if lower pressures are ineffective in a noncompliant lung.

Maintaining the circulation through closed chest cardiac massage at a rate of 100 or more/min is an important adjunct to artificial respiration in infants in circulatory collapse with bradycardia (< 100 beats/min) or unpalpable or weak femoral pulses. This must be synchronized with ventilation with 100% oxygen at a rate of 30–40 inflations/min. Laryngoscopy, intubation, and cardiac massage should be carried out skillfully by trained, technically adept personnel, one of whom should be in every delivery room.

Mouth-to-mouth breathing has been successful in resuscitating some infants but may be harmful owing to the possible occurrence of alveolar rupture from uncontrolled pressures or to introduction of infection.

After the airway has been cleared and adequate ventilation provided, severely asphyxiated and acidotic infants often require the slow (1 mL/min) administration of sodium bicarbonate (1–2 mEq/kg) through an umbilical catheter to correct the associated metabolic acidosis; a solution containing 0.5 mEq of sodium bicarbonate/mL is used. It may also be necessary to administer epinephrine (0.1 mL/kg of a 1:10,000 solution) via intravascular or endotracheal tube injection to combat hypotension, bradycardia, or poor cardiac output. The umbilical vein should be used if a catheter cannot be inserted into the artery, as this procedure is easier during emergency conditions. Intracardiac injection of epinephrine is a last resort. Respiratory stimulants are contraindicated.

Shock. Circulatory insufficiency may present at birth as a result of internal hemorrhage; fetal bleeding during gestation, labor, or delivery (e.g., feto-fetal or feto-maternal transfusion syndrome); bleeding from the fetal circulation secondary to a placental tear during amniocentesis; excessive bleeding from a severed or torn umbilical cord; or severe hemolytic anemia. Clinical manifestations include signs of respiratory distress; cyanosis; pallor; flaccidity; cold, mottled skin; tachycardia or

bradycardia; hepatosplenomegaly; and, rarely, convulsions. **Edema** and hepatosplenomegaly also may suggest hydrops fetalis or congestive heart failure without shock. Shock from overwhelming infection may also be present after birth.

Supportive treatment with type O, Rh negative blood, plasma, or electrolyte solutions is indicated for hypovolemia. Oxygen should be administered and metabolic acidosis corrected with sodium bicarbonate. β-Sympathomimetic agents such as dopamine or dobutamine may be needed to support cardiac output and blood pressure. The diagnosis and treatment of erythroblastosis fetalis is discussed in Sec. 8.47. If infection is present, appropriate antibiotics must be started as soon as possible.

After supportive measures have stabilized the infant's condition, a specific diagnosis should be established and appropriate continuing treatment instituted.

Apgar V, James LS: Further observations on the newborn scoring system. Am J Dis Child 104:419, 1962.
Behrman RE, James LS, Klaus MH, et al: Treatment of the asphyxiated newborn infant. J Pediatr 79:981, 1969.
Bergman I, Bauer, RE, Barmada MA, et al: Intracerebral hemorrhage in the full term neonatal infant. Pediatrics 75:488, 1985.
Chevalier RL, Campbell, F, Brenbridge AG: Prognostic factors in neonatal acute renal failure. Pediatrics 74:265, 1984.
Daniel SS, James LS: Abnormal renal function in the newborn infant. J Pediatr 88:856, 1976.
Dray JS, Kennedy C, Berendes H, et al: The Apgar score as an index of infant morbidity. A report from the collaborative study of cerebral palsy. Dev Med Child Neurol 8:141, 1966.
Ergander U, Eriksson M, Zetteretrom R: Severe neonatal asphyxia. Acta Paediatr. Scand. 72:321, 1983.
Finer NN, Robertson CM, Peters RN, et al: Factors affecting outcome in hypoxic ischemic encephalopathy in term infants. Am J Dis Child 137:21, 1983.
French CE, Waldstern G: Subcapsular hemorrhage of the liver in the newborn. Pediatrics 69:204, 1982.
Gregory G: Resuscitation of the newborn. Anesthesiology 43:225, 1975.
Hayden CK, Shattuck KE, Richardson CJ, et al: Subependymal germinal matrix hemorrhage in full-term neonates. Pediatrics 75:714, 1985.
Holden KR, Mellits ED, Freeman JM: Neonatal seizures. I. Correlation of prenatal and perinatal events with outcome. Pediatrics 70:165, 1982.
Kreusser KL, Tarby TJ, Kovmar E, et al: Serial lumbar punctures for at least temporary amelioration of neonatal posthemorrhagic hydrocephalus. Pediatrics 75:719, 1985.
Lees MH: Cyanosis of the newborn infant. J Pediatr 77:484, 1970.
MacDonald H, Mulligan J, Allen A, et al: Neonatal asphyxia. I. Relationship of obstetric and neonatal complications to neonatal mortality in 38,405 consecutive deliveries. J Pediatr 96:898, 1980.
Mangurten HH: Birth injuries. In Fanaroff A and Martin R (eds): Behrman's Neonatal-Perinatal Medicine. St Louis, CV Mosby, 1983.
McDonald MM, Koops, BL, Johnson ML, et al: Timing and antecedents of intracranial hemorrhage in the newborn. Pediatrics 74:32, 1984.
Mellits ED, Holden KR, Freeman JM: Neonatal seizures. II. A multivariate analysis of factors associated with outcome. Pediatrics 70:177, 1982.
Ment LR, Scott DT, Ehrenkranz RA, et al: Neonates of ≤1,250 grams birth weight: Prospective neurodevelopmental evaluation during the first year post-term, Pediatrics 70:292, 1982.
Mulligan J, Painter M, O'Donoghue P, et al: Neonatal asphyxia. II. Neonatal mortality and long term sequelae. J Pediatr 96:903, 1980.
Oliver TK Jr, Demis JA, Bates GD: Serial blood-gas tensions and acid-base balance during the first hour of life in human infants. Acta Pediatr 50:346, 1961.
Papile L, Munsick-Bruno G, Schaefer A: Relationship of cerebral intraventricular hemorrhage and early childhood neurologic handicaps. J Pediatrics 103:273, 1983.
Schrager GO: Elevation of depressed skull fracture with a breast pump. J Pediatr 77:300, 1970.
Silverman SH, Liebow SG: Dislocation of the triangular cartilage of the nasal septum. J Pediatr 87:456, 1975.
Syzmonowicz W, Yu VYH: Timing and evolution of periventricular hemorrhage in infants weighing 1250g or less at birth. Arch Dis Child 59:1, 1984.
Syzmonowicz W, Yu VYH, and Wilson FE: Antecedents of periventricular hemorrhage in infants weighing 1250 g or less at birth. Arch Dis Child 59:13, 1984.
Tzipora D, Skidmore MB, Fong KW, et al: Incidence, severity, and timing of subependymal and intraventricular hemorrhages in preterm infants born in a perinatal unit as detected by serial real-time ultrasound. Pediatrics 71:541, 1983.
Volpe J: Neonatal seizures. Clin Perinatol 4:43, 1977.
Volpe J, Pasternak JF: Parasagittal cerebral injury in neonatal hypoxic-ischemic encephalopathy: Clinical and neuroradiologic features. J Pediatr 92:472, 1977.
Zelson C, Lee SJ, Pearl M: The incidence of skull fractures underlying cephal-hematomas in newborn infants. J Pediatr 85:371, 1974.

DISTURBANCES OF ORGAN SYSTEMS

RESPIRATORY TRACT

Disturbances of respiration in the immediate postnatal period may have originated in utero, in the delivery room, or in the nursery. A wide variety of pathologic lesions may be responsible for one or more of the signs of respiratory distress or failure (Table 8–19); cyanosis is common and, if respiratory embarrassment is severe, pallor may also be present. It is occasionally very difficult to distinguish cardiovascular from respiratory disturbances on the basis of clinical signs alone. Signs of respiratory distress in the newborn infant may suggest hyaline membrane disease (idiopathic respiratory distress syndrome), aspiration syndrome, pneumonia, sepsis, congenital heart disease, congestive heart failure, choanal atresia, hypoglycemia, hypoplasia of the mandible with posterior displacement of the tongue, macroglossia, malformation of the epiglottis, malformation or injury of the larynx, cysts or neoplasms of the larynx or chest, pneumothorax, lobar emphysema, pulmonary agenesis or hypoplasia, congenital pulmonary lymphangiectasis, Wilson-Mikity syndrome, tracheoesophageal fistula, avulsion of the phrenic nerve, hernia or eventration of the diaphragm, intracranial lesions, neuromuscular disorders, and metabolic disturbances. *Any sign of postnatal respiratory distress is an indication for a roentgenogram of the chest.*

8.30 TRANSITION TO PULMONARY RESPIRATION

The establishment of adequate lung function at birth is related to gestational age or maturity. Fluid filling the fetal lung must be removed, functional residual capacity (FRC) established and maintained, and a ventilation-perfusion relationship developed that will provide optimal exchange of oxygen and carbon dioxide between alveoli and blood (Sec. 13.3, 13.6, 13.8).

The First Breath. During vaginal delivery intermittent compression of the thorax facilitates removal of lung fluid. Surfactant in the fluid enhances aeration of the gas-free lung by reducing surface tension, thereby lowering the pressure required to open alveoli. Nevertheless, the pressures required to inflate the airless lung are higher than those needed at any other period of life; they range from 10–70 cm of H_2O for 0.5–1.0 sec intervals compared with about 4 cm for normal breathing in term infants and adults. Most infants require the lower range of opening pressures. Higher pressures necessary to initiate respiration are required to overcome the opposing forces of surface tension (particularly in small airways) and the viscosity of liquid remaining in the airways, as well as to introduce about 50 mL of air into the lungs, 20–30 mL of which remains after the first breath to establish the FRC. Most of the liquid in the lung is removed by the pulmonary circulation, which increases many fold at birth as all of the right cardiac output perfuses the pulmonary vascular bed. The remainder of the fluid is removed by the pulmonary lymphatics, expelled by the infant, swallowed, or aspirated from the oropharynx; this removal may be impaired following cesarean section or neonatal sedation.

The stimuli responsible for the first breath are multiple and their relative importance uncertain. They include a fall in pO_2 and pH and a rise in pCO_2 owing to the interruption of the placental circulation, a redistribution of cardiac output after the umbilical cord is clamped, a decrease in body temperature, and a variety of tactile stimuli.

Compared to the term infant, the LBW infant having a very compliant chest wall may be at a disadvantage in accomplishing the first breath. The FRC is least in the most immature infants, reflecting the presence of atelectasis. Abnormalities in the ventilation-perfusion ratio are greater and persist for longer periods of time, as does gas trapping. There may be a low paO_2 (40–50 mm Hg) and elevated $paCO_2$, reflecting atelectasis, intrapulmonary shunting, and hypoventilation. The smallest immature infants have the most profound disturbances, which may resemble respiratory distress syndrome.

Breathing Patterns in Newborns. During sleep in the first months of life, normal full-term infants may have infrequent episodes when regular breathing is interrupted with short pauses. This **periodic breathing** pattern, shifting from a regular rhythmicity to intermittent apnea, is more common in the premature infant, who may have apneic pauses of 5–10 sec followed by a burst of rapid respirations at a rate of 50–60/min for 10–15 sec. There is rarely an associated change in color or heart rate, and it often stops without apparent reason. Periodic breathing persists intermittently usually until premature infants are about 36 wk of gestational age. An increase in inspired oxygen concentration or external physical stimulation will often convert periodic to regular breathing. There is no prognostic significance to periodic breathing, a normal characteristic of neonatal respiration.

8.31 APNEA

Periodic breathing must be distinguished from prolonged apneic pauses, since the latter are associated with serious illnesses. Apnea may be due to airway obstruction, diminished ventilatory drive, or both. (See also Sec. 13.5 and 13.9.) Apnea of short duration may occur in normal term infants; its incidence and duration is greatest in the first week of life and during active sleep. Apnea may also occur in premature infants in the absence of identifiable disease or as a complication of spontaneous or iatrogenic neck flexion; in preterm infants serious apnea is often defined as cessation of respiration for greater than 10–20 sec with or without bradycardia or cyanosis. Periodic breathing may precede a series of apneic spells; both patterns often occur in the same infant. Bradycardia, cyanosis, or both are almost invariably associated with significant apnea, and there is frequently marked hypoxemia with a lesser degree of carbon dioxide retention; these pauses occur most often from the second to sixth days of life but may occur earlier or later. The sudden onset of apnea in a previously well child beyond the second week of life is a critical event and warrants immediate investigation.

Physical stimulation of the infant is often adequate to get the infant breathing again. In severe cases, assisted ventilation with a bag and mask may be necessary to terminate an episode. Oxygen should be administered to treat hypoxia, and airway obstruction should be relieved. Apnea of prematurity which is not secondary to any identifiable cause should be treated with theophylline. Loading doses of 5 mg/kg followed by 1–2 mg/kg every 8–12 hr by oral or intravenous routes should be used with close monitoring of vital signs, the clinical course, and drug levels. Continuous positive airway pressure (CPAP) is an alternate to theophylline. When apnea is due to other diseases, specific therapy for the disorder is indicated, in addition to relieving airway obstruction and providing adequate oxygenation.

Aranda J, Turmen T: Methylxanthines in apnea of prematurity. Clin Perinatol 6:87, 1979.

Hoppenbrouwers T, Hodgman JE, Harper RM, et al: Polygraphic studies of normal infants during the first six months of life: III. Incidence of apnea and periodic breathing. Pediatrics 60:418, 1977.

Kattwinkel J: Neonatal apnea: Pathogenesis and therapy. J Pediatr 90:342, 1977.

8.32 HYALINE MEMBRANE DISEASE
(Idiopathic Respiratory Distress Syndrome)

Incidence. This condition is a major cause of death in the newborn period. An estimated 50% of all neonatal deaths result from hyaline membrane disease or its complications; it accounts for 10,000–40,000 deaths each year.

The clinical incidence is difficult to determine due to differing diagnostic criteria. Hyaline membrane disease occurs primarily in premature infants; incidence is inversely proportional to the gestational age and birthweight. It occurs in about 60% of infants less than 28 wk of gestational age, in 15–20% of those between 32–36 wk, in about 5% beyond 37 wk, and rarely at term. An increased frequency is associated with infants of diabetic mothers, delivery before 37 wk gestation, multiple pregnancy, cesarean section delivery, precipitous delivery, asphyxia, and a history of prior affected infants.

Etiology and Pathophysiology. The failure to develop a functional residual capacity (FRC) and the tendency of affected lungs to become atelectatic correlate with high surface tensions and the absence of surfactant. The major constituents of surfactant are dipalmityl-phosphatidylcholine (lecithin), phosphatidylglycerol, two apoproteins, and cholesterol. With progressive gestational age increasing amounts of phospholipids are synthesized and stored in type II alveolar cells. These active agents are released into the alveoli, reducing the surface tension and helping to maintain alveolar stability by preventing the collapse of small air spaces at end-expiration. However, the amounts produced or released may be insufficient to meet postnatal demands because of immaturity. Surfactant is present in high concentrations in fetal lung homogenates by 20 wk of gestation but does not reach the surface of the lung until later. It appears in the amniotic fluid between 28–38 wk. Mature levels of pulmonary surfactant are usually present after 35 wk.

Surfactant synthesis depends in part, on normal pH, temperature, and perfusion. Asphyxia, hypoxemia, and pulmonary ischemia, particularly in association with hypovolemia, hypotension, and cold stress, may suppress surfactant synthesis. The epithelial lining of the lung may also be injured by high oxygen concentrations, poor drainage of the upper airway, and the effects of respirator management, resulting in further reduction in surfactant.

Alveolar atelectasis, hyaline membrane formation, and interstitial edema make the lungs less compliant, requiring greater pressure to expand the small alveoli and airways. In these immature infants, the lower chest wall is pulled in as the diaphragm descends and the intrathoracic pressure becomes negative, thus limiting the amount of intrathoracic pressure that can be produced; the result is a tendency to atelectasis. The highly compliant chest wall of the preterm infant offers less resistance than that of the mature infant against the natural tendency of the lungs to collapse. Thus, at end-expiration, the volume of the thorax and lungs tends to approach the residual volume, leading to atelectasis.

Deficient synthesis or release of surfactant, together with small respiratory units and compliant chest wall, produces atelectasis, resulting in perfused but not ventilated alveoli, which causes hypoxia. Decreased lung compliance, small tidal volumes, increased physiologic dead space, increased work of breathing, and, eventually, insufficient alveolar ventilation results in hypercarbia. The combination of hypercarbia, hypoxia, and acidosis produces pulmonary arterial vasoconstriction with increased right to left shunting through the foramen ovale and ductus arteriosus and within the lung itself. Pulmonary blood flow is reduced, with ischemic injury to the cells producing surfactant and to the vascular bed, resulting in an effusion of proteinaceous material into the alveolar spaces (Fig. 8–16).

Pathology. The lungs appear deep purplish red and are liver-like in consistency. Microscopically, there is extensive atelectasis with engorgement of the interalveolar capillaries and lymphatics. A number of the alveolar ducts, alveoli, and respiratory bronchioles are lined with acidophilic, homogeneous, or granular membranes. Amniotic debris, intra-alveolar hemorrhage, pneumonia, and interstitial emphysema are additional but inconstant findings; interstitial emphysema may be marked when an infant has been ventilated with a method that employs increased end-expiratory pressure. The characteristic hyaline membranes are rarely seen in infants dying earlier than 6–8 hr after birth.

Clinical Manifestations. Signs of hyaline membrane disease usually appear within minutes of birth, although they may not be recognized for several hours until rapid, shallow respirations have increased to 60 or more/min. The late onset of tachypnea should suggest other conditions. Some patients require resuscitation at birth because of intrapartum asphyxia or initial severe respiratory distress. Characteristically tachypnea, prominent (often audible) grunting, intercostal and subcostal retractions, nasal flaring, and duskiness are seen (Table 8–19). There is increasing cyanosis, often relatively

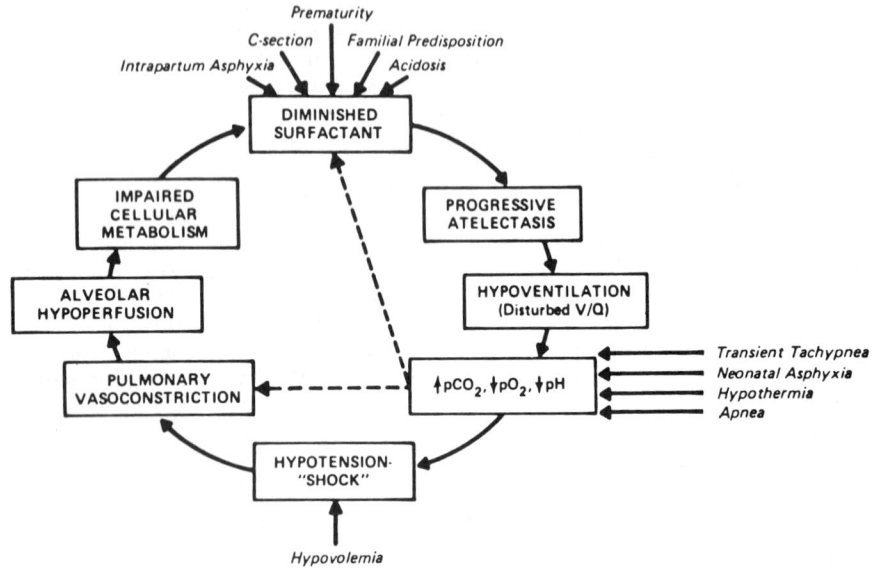

Figure 8–16. Contributing factors in the pathogenesis of hyaline membrane disease. Potential "vicious circle" perpetuating hypoxia and pulmonary insufficiency. (From Farrell P, Zachman R, *In:* Quilligan EJ, Kretchmer N (eds): Fetal and Maternal Medicine. New York, John Wiley and Sons, 1980.)

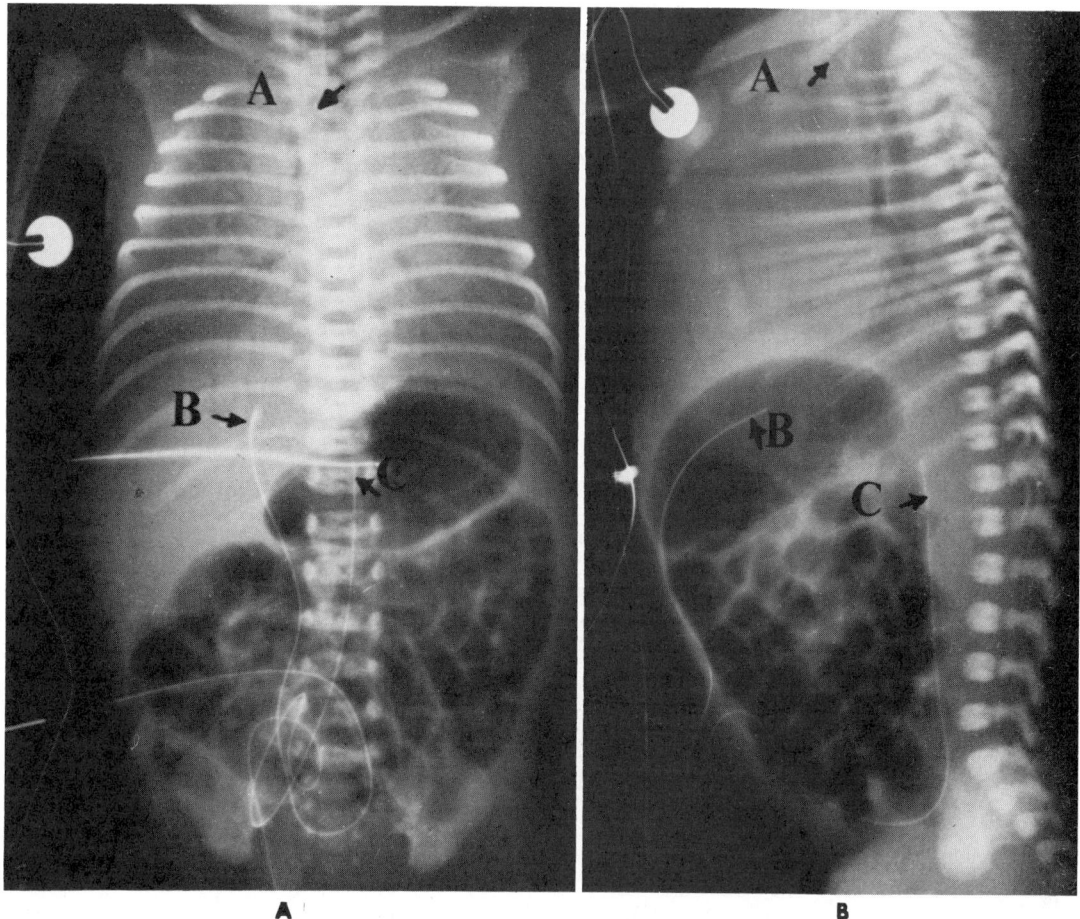

Figure 8–17. Infant with hyaline membrane disease. Note granular lungs, air bronchogram, and air filled esophagus. Anteroposterior (A) and lateral (B) roentgenograms are needed to distinguish umbilical artery from vein catheter and to determine appropriate level of insertion. The lateral view clearly identifies that the catheter has been inserted into an umbilical vein and is lying in the portal system of the liver. A, endotracheal tube; B, umbilical venous catheter at the junction of the umbilical vein, ductus venosus and portal vein; C, umbilical artery catheter passed up the aorta to T-12. (Courtesy Walter E. Berdon, Babies Hospital.)

unresponsive to oxygen administration. Breath sounds may be normal or diminished with a harsh tubular quality, and, on deep inspiration, fine rales may be heard, especially over the lung bases posteriorly. The natural course is characterized by progressive worsening of signs of air hunger and dyspnea. If inadequately treated, blood pressure and body temperature may fall; fatigue, cyanosis, and pallor increase and grunting decreases or disappears as the condition worsens. Apnea and irregular respirations occur as infants tire and are ominous signs requiring immediate intervention. There may also be edema, ileus, and oliguria. Signs of asphyxia secondary to apnea or partial respiratory failure occur when there is rapid progression of the disease. The condition may progress to death in severely affected infants, but in milder cases, the symptoms and signs may reach a peak within 3 days, after which gradual improvement sets in. Death is rare after 3 days, except among infants whose fatal course has been forestalled by treatment.

The course may be dramatically altered by supportive therapy directed at maintaining adequate oxygenation, circulation, acid-base balance, and nutrition. Even in severe cases, clinical recovery may be complete within 10 days–2 wk. Alternatively, the natural course may be attenuated with persistence of mild to severe signs and superimposed complications associated with the treatment, such as pneumothorax, patent ductus arteriosus, or bronchopulmonary dysplasia.

Diagnosis. The clinical course, roentgenogram of the chest, and blood gas and acid-base values help to establish the clinical diagnosis. Roentgenographically, the lungs may have a characteristic, but not pathognomonic, appearance which includes a fine reticular granularity of the parenchyma and air bronchograms which are often more prominent early in the left lower lobe because of the superimposition of the cardiac shadow (Fig. 8–17). Occasionally, the initial roentgenogram is normal, only to develop the typical pattern at 6–12 hr. There may be considerable variation among films, depending on the phase of respiration and the use of CPAP, often resulting in poor correlation between the roentgenograms and clinical course. The laboratory findings are characterized initially by hypoxemia and later by progressive hypoxemia, hypercarbia, and variable metabolic acidosis.

In the *differential diagnosis*, group B streptococcal sepsis may be indistinguishable from hyaline membrane disease. In pneumonia presenting at birth, the chest roentgenogram may be identical to that for hyaline membrane disease; gram-positive cocci in the gastric or tracheal aspirates and buffy coat smear, a positive test of urine for streptococcal antigen, and the presence of marked neutropenia may suggest this diagnosis. Cyanotic heart disease, persistent fetal circulation, aspiration syndromes, and congenital anomalies must also be considered. Transient tachypnea may be distinguished by its short and mild clinical course.

Prevention. Most important are the prevention of prematurity, including avoidance of unnecessary or poorly timed cesarean section, appropriate management of the high-risk pregnancy and labor, and the prediction and possible in utero treatment of pulmonary immaturity (Sec. 8.13). In timing cesarean section or inducing labor, estimation of the fetal head circumference by ultrasound and determination of the lecithin concentration in the amniotic fluid by the lecithin to sphingomyelin (L/S) ratio or shake test decrease the likelihood of delivering a premature infant. Intrauterine antenatal and intrapartum monitoring may similarly decrease the risk of fetal asphyxia, which is associated with an increased incidence and severity of hyaline membrane disease.

The administration of a synthetic corticosteroid to women who do not have toxemia, diabetes, or renal disease 48–72 hr before delivery of fetuses at 32 wk or less gestation significantly reduces the incidence and mortality from hyaline membrane disease. It may thus be appropriate to administer 1–2 doses of betamethasone intramuscularly to pregnant women whose lecithin in amniotic fluid indicates fetal lung immaturity and who are likely to deliver in 48–72 hr or whose labor can be delayed 48 hr or more.

Treatment. The basic defect requiring treatment is inadequate pulmonary exchange of oxygen and carbon dioxide; metabolic acidosis and circulatory insufficiency are secondary manifestations. Early supportive care of the low birthweight infant, especially in the treatment of acidosis, hypoxia, hypotension, and hypothermia, appears to lessen the severity of hyaline membrane disease. Therapy requires careful and frequent monitoring of heart and respiratory rates, arterial pO_2, PCO_2, pH, bicarbonate, electrolytes, blood glucose, hematocrit, blood pressure, and temperature. Umbilical artery catheterization is frequently necessary. Since most cases of hyaline membrane disease are self-limiting, the goal of treatment is to minimize abnormal physiologic variations and superimposed iatrogenic problems. The management of these infants is best carried out in a specially staffed and equipped hospital unit, the neonatal intensive care nursery.

The general principles for supportive care of any LBW infant should be adhered to, including gentle handling and minimal disturbance consistent with management. To avoid chilling and to minimize oxygen consumption, infants should be placed in an Isolette and core temperature maintained between 36.5 and 37° C (Sec. 8.17). Calories and fluids should be provided intravenously. For the first 24 hr, 10% glucose and water should be infused through a peripheral vein at a rate of 65–75 mL/kg/24 hr. Subsequently, electrolytes should be added and fluid volumes increased gradually to 120–150 mL/kg/24 hr (Sec. 5.22).

Warm humidified oxygen should be provided at a concentration sufficient initially to keep arterial levels between 60–80 mm Hg with stable vital signs to maintain normal tissue oxygenation while minimizing the risk of oxygen toxicity.

When the arterial oxygen tension cannot be maintained above 50 mm Hg at inspired oxygen concentrations of 70% applying *continuous positive airway pressure* (CPAP) at a pressure of 6–10 cm of H_2O by nasal prongs or head box or *continuous negative chest pressure* (CNCP) is indicated, which usually produces a sharp rise in arterial oxygen tension. Although the course may be protracted, the amount of pressure required usually decreases abruptly at about 72 hr of age and the infant can be weaned from CPAP shortly thereafter. If an infant on CPAP cannot maintain an arterial oxygen tension above 50 mm Hg while breathing 100% oxygen, assisted ventilation is required.

Infants with severe hyaline membrane disease or those who develop complications resulting in persistent apnea may require assisted ventilation. Reasonable indications for its use are (1) arterial blood pH <7.20; (2) arterial blood pCO_2 ≥60 mm Hg; (3) arterial blood pO_2 ≤50 mm Hg at oxygen concentrations of 70–100%; or (4) persistent apnea.

The simplest method of assisted ventilation is the intermittent use of a **mask and bag resuscitator,** usually as an adjunct to nasal CPAP, for 5 min out of every 20 min or another time

regimen adapted to the needs of the individual infant. A patient-cycled constant positive-pressure with variable volume or a constant volume with variable pressure **respirator** with a nasotracheal tube in place is widely used, but its use has been accompanied by serious upper airway complications, especially when nursery personnel are inexperienced. Negative-pressure respirators are advantageous in that they require neither mask nor endotracheal tube and may be associated with a lower incidence of chronic lung disease. However, their construction makes them difficult to use on very low birthweight infants. In general, the extent to which the morbidity and mortality of severe hyaline membrane disease can be reduced with mechanical ventilation and the frequency with which complications secondary to the use of respirators can be minimized are directly related to a high level of skill and experience continuously practiced and maintained by an intensive care team that regularly cares for critically ill newborn infants. High frequency jet and oscillator ventilation are experimental treatments that theoretically may reduce airway pressure and improve oxygenation.

Although controlled studies have not shown a decrease in mortality as a result of **correcting the acidosis** associated with hyaline membrane disease, the severity of the disease seems to be lessened, and the risks of pulmonary vasoconstriction, ventilation-perfusion abnormalities, untoward shunting through the foramen ovale or ductus arteriosus, hypotension, and arrhythmias are probably diminished. These risks are increased when acidosis is coupled with hypoxia.

Respiratory acidosis may require short-term or prolonged assisted ventilation. In severe respiratory acidosis and hypoxia, treatment with sodium bicarbonate may exacerbate hypercarbia. With hypoventilation and hypercarbia a complicating intracranial hemorrhage may also occur.

Metabolic acidosis in hyaline membrane disease may be a result of perinatal asphyxia and hypotension and is often encountered when an infant has required resuscitation (Sec. 8.29). The dosage of bicarbonate may be estimated as follows:

$$HCO_3^- \text{ needed (mEq)} = HCO_3^- \text{ deficit or}$$
$$\text{base excess (mEq/L)} \times HCO_3^- \text{ space (L)}$$

The values recommended for the HCO_3^- space range from 20–60% of the body weight, with 30% being the most frequently used. When 60% is used, it is advisable to give only one half of the calculated dose initially. The dose may be given over a 10–15 min period through a peripheral vein with the acid-base determination repeated within 30 min, or it may be administered over several hours. More often, 1–2 mEq/kg of sodium bicarbonate is initially administered. In an emergency, an umbilical catheter may be used. Alkali therapy may result in skin sloughs from infiltration, increased serum osmolarity, hypernatremia, and liver injury when concentrated solutions are administered rapidly through an umbilical vein. The risk of complications is diminished when the circulation is adequately supported. More than 8 mEq/kg/24 hr of sodium bicarbonate should rarely be given unless serum sodium levels are normal and urine output adequate. In the presence of hypernatremia with edema, oliguria, or congestive heart failure, infusion of 0.3 M tris-hydroxymethyl aminomethane (THAM) at a rate of 1 mL/min, to provide 1.0 mL/kg for each pH unit below 7.4, may be preferred to bicarbonate.

Monitoring of *aortic blood pressure* through an umbilical arterial catheter or by Doppler technique may be useful in managing the shock-like state that may occur during the first hour or so after premature birth of an infant who has been asphyxiated or who has developed respiratory distress (see Fig. 8–3). Radiopaque catheters should always be used, and their position checked roentgenographically after insertion (see Fig. 8–17). The tip of an umbilical artery catheter should lie just above the bifurcation of the aorta (L3–L5) or above the celiac axis (T6–T10). Placement and supervision should be done by skilled and experienced personnel. Catheters should be removed as soon as there is no indication for their continued use, i.e., when paO_2 is stable and the FiO_2 is less than 40%.

Periodic monitoring of arterial oxygen and carbon dioxide tension and of pH is an important part of the management; if assisted ventilation is being used, it is essential. Blood should be obtained from the umbilical or radial artery. Temporal artery lines are contraindicated because of cerebral emboli. Tissue pO_2 and pCO_2 may also be estimated continuously from transcutaneous electrodes. Capillary blood samples are of limited value for determining pO_2 but may be useful for evaluating pCO_2 and pH.

Owing to the difficulty of distinguishing some group B streptococcal or other infections from hyaline membrane disease, routinely administering antibacterial agents is advocated by some but rejected by those more fearful of increasing the numbers of resistant organisms. If used, penicillin or ampicillin with kanamycin or gentamicin is suggested, depending on the recent pattern of bacterial sensitivities in the hospital where the infant is being treated (Sec. 8.59 and 8.60).

Tracheal administration of a saline suspension of artificial surfactant within the first day has been reported to rapidly reduce the inspired oxygen requirement and roentgenographic abnormalities; this therapy requires further evaluation before it can be recommended.

Complications of Hyaline Membrane Disease and Intensive Care. The most serious complications of **tracheal intubation** are asphyxia from obstruction of the tube, cardiac arrest during intubation or suctioning, and the subsequent development of subglottic stenosis. Other complications include bleeding from trauma during intubation, difficult extubation requiring tracheostomy, ulceration of the nares due to pressure from the tube, permanent narrowing of the nostril from tissue damage and scarring from irritation or infection around the tube, erosion of the palate, avulsion of a vocal cord, laryngeal ulcer, papilloma of a vocal cord, and persistent hoarseness, stridor, or edema of the larynx.

Measures to reduce the incidence of these complications include skillfully observing the infant; using polyvinyl endotracheal tubes that do not contain tin, which is toxic to cells; using a tube of the smallest practicable size to reduce local ischemia and pressure necrosis; avoiding frequent changes of the tube; avoiding motion of the tube in situ; avoiding too frequent or vigorous suctioning; and avoiding infection through meticulous cleanliness and frequent sterilization of all apparatus attached to or passed through the tube. The personnel inserting and caring for the endotracheal tube should be experienced and skilled.

The risks of **umbilical arterial catheterization** include vascular embolization, thrombosis, spasm, and perforation, ischemic and/or chemical necrosis of abdominal viscera; infection; accidental hemorrhage; and impaired circulation to a leg with subsequent gangrene. Although at necropsy the reported incidence of thrombotic complications varies from 1 to 23%, aortography has demonstrated that clots form in or about the tips of 95% of catheters placed in an umbilical artery. Aortic ultrasound can also be used to investigate the presence of thrombosis. The risk of a serious clinical complication from umbilical catheterization is probably between 2 and 5%.

Transient blanching of the leg may occur during catheterization of the umbilical artery. It is usually due to reflex arterial spasm, the incidence of which is lessened by using the smallest available catheters, particularly in very small infants. The catheter should be removed immediately; catheterization of the other artery may then be attempted. Persistent spasm after removal of the catheter may be relieved by warming the opposite leg. Blood sampling from a radial artery may simi-

larly result in spasm or thrombosis, and the same treatment is indicated. Intermittent severe spasm or unrelieved spasm may respond to the cautious local infusion of tolazoline (Priscoline), 1–2 mg injected intra-arterially over 5 min. Accidentally lodging the catheter in a smaller artery, either blocking it completely or causing unrecognized local vascular spasm, may result in gangrene of the organ or area supplied by the vessel. To prevent this complication, the catheter should be removed promptly if blood cannot be obtained through it.

Serious hemorrhage on removal of the catheter is rare. Thrombi may form in the artery or in the catheter; their incidence is lowered by use of a smooth-tipped catheter with a hole only at its end, by rinsing the catheter with a small amount of saline solution containing 1 unit of heparin/mL or by continuously infusing a solution containing 1 unit/mL of heparin. The risks of thrombus formation with potential vascular occlusion can also be reduced by removing the catheter when there are early signs of thrombosis, such as narrowing of pulse pressure and disappearance of the dicrotic notch. Some prefer to use the umbilical artery for blood sampling only, leaving the catheter filled with heparinized saline between samplings. Renovascular hypertension may occur days to weeks following umbilical arterial catheterization in a small number of neonates.

Umbilical vein catheterization is associated with many of the same risks as artery catheterization. In addition, there is an association with subsequent liver cirrhosis from portal vein thrombosis. Other long-term risks of catheterization of the umbilical artery or umbilical vein are as yet unknown.

The toxicity to the retina from elevated concentrations of oxygen administered for prolonged periods has been amply demonstrated. (Sec. 8.17).

Oxygen is toxic to the lung, particularly if administered by means of a positive pressure respirator, resulting in **bronchopulmonary dysplasia** (see also Sec. 8.38). Instead of showing improvement on the 3rd–4th day, consistent with the natural course in survivors, some infants who have been on prolonged intermittent positive pressure breathing using increased concentrations of oxygen roentgenographically show a worsening of their pulmonary condition (Fig. 8–18A). Respiratory distress persists and is characterized by hypoxia, hypercarbia, oxygen dependency, and the development of right heart failure. The chest roentgenogram is described as gradually changing from a picture of almost complete opacification with air bronchogram and interstitial emphysema to one of small, round, lucent areas alternating with areas of irregular density resembling a sponge (Fig. 8–18B). In the histologic picture at this stage (10–20 days after beginning oxygen therapy) there is less evidence of hyaline membrane formation, progressive alveolar coalescence with atelectasis of surrounding alveoli, interstitial edema, coarse focal thickening of the basement membrane, and widespread bronchial and bronchiolar mucosal metaplasia and hyperplasia. This corresponds with a severe maldistribution of ventilation. Most surviving neonates with persistent roentgenographic changes recover by 6–12 mo with about normal pulmonary function, but some require prolonged hospitalization with oxygen, diuretics, digitalization, bronchodilators, and chest physiotherapy and may have respiratory symptoms persisting through infancy. Right heart failure and viral necrotizing bronchiolitis are major causes of death. Pathology reveals cardiac enlargement and pulmonary changes consisting of focal areas of emphysematous alveoli with hypertrophy of the peribronchial smooth muscle of the tributary bronchioles, some perimucosal fibrosis and widespread metaplasia of the bronchiolar mucosa, thickening of basement membranes, and separation of the capillaries from the alveolar epithelial cells.

Extrapulmonary extravasation of air is another frequent

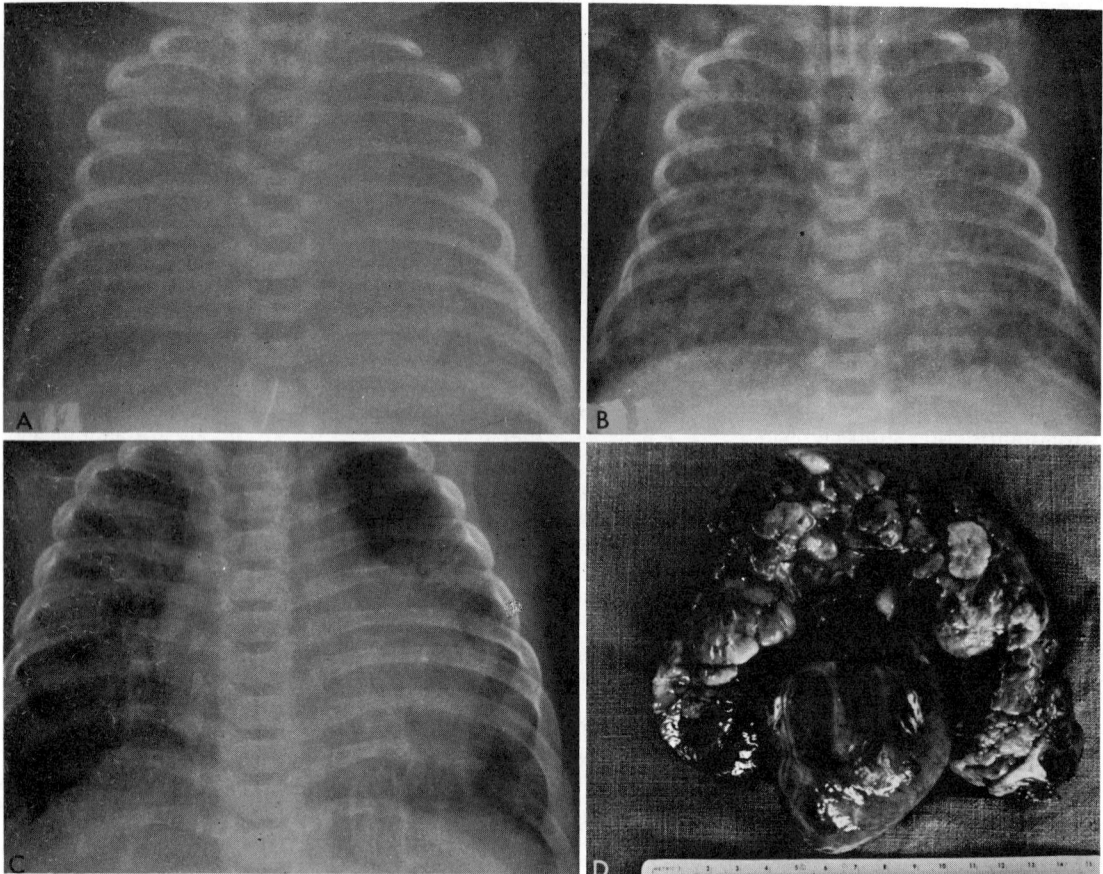

Figure 8–18. Pulmonary changes in infants who were treated in the immediate postnatal period for the clinical syndrome of hyaline membrane disease with prolonged, intermittent positive pressure breathing with air containing 80 to 100% oxygen. *A*, A 5 day old infant with nearly complete opacification of lungs. *B*, A 13 day old infant with "bubbly lungs" simulating the roentgenographic appearance of the Wilson-Mikity syndrome. *C*, A 7 mo old infant with irregular, dense strands in both lungs and cardiomegaly. *D*, Large right ventricle and cobbly, irregularly aerated lung of an infant who died at 11 mo of age; this infant also had a patent ductus arteriosus. (From Northway WH Jr, Rosan RC, Porter DY: N Engl J Med 276:357, 1967.)

complication of the management of hyaline membrane disease (Sec. 8.37).

There may be clinically significant shunting through a **patent ductus arteriosus** in some neonates with hyaline membrane disease, the delayed closure being due to associated hypoxia, acidosis, increased pulmonary pressure secondary to vasoconstriction, systemic hypotension, immaturity of these infants, and local release of prostaglandins which dilate the ductus. The manifestations may include (1) persistent apnea for unexplained reasons in an infant recovering from hyaline membrane disease; (2) an active heaving precordium, bounding peripheral pulses, and a systolic or to-and-fro murmur; (3) carbon dioxide retention; (4) increasing oxygen dependency; (5) roentgenographic evidence of cardiomegaly and increased pulmonary vascular markings; (6) enlarged left atrium demonstrated by echocardiography; and (7) hepatomegaly. Most infants respond to general supportive measures including diuretics and fluid restriction. In selected patients in whom spontaneous closure does not occur but in whom there is progressive deterioration despite supportive and cardiotonic treatment, indomethacin, 1–3 doses of 0.2 mg/kg at 12–24 hr intervals for 48 hr, may induce pharmacologic closure by inhibiting prostaglandin synthesis. Indications for surgical closure are discussed in Sec. 14.46.

Anemia secondary to frequent withdrawal of blood samples may also occur as a complication of intensive care. The cumulative amount of blood withdrawn should be carefully recorded. Some of its replacement by transfusion may be indicated if more than 10–15% of estimated total blood volume

is removed or if there is a significant decrease in the hematocrit. Oxygen-dependent infants should have their hematocrit maintained above 40%.

Prognosis. Early provision of intensive observation and care to high risk newborn infants can significantly reduce morbidity and mortality due to hyaline membrane disease and other acute neonatal illnesses. However, good results depend on experienced and skilled personnel, specially designed and organized regional hospital units, equipment, and the lack of complications, such as severe fetal or birth asphyxia, intracranial hemorrhage, or irremediable congenital malformation.

Overall mortality for low birthweight infants referred to intensive care centers is steadily declining; about 50% of those under 1000 g survive and the mortality progressively decreases at higher weights with over 95% of sick infants weighing more than 2500 g surviving. Although 85–90% of all infants surviving hyaline membrane disease after requiring ventilatory support with respirators are normal, the outlook is much better for those above 1500 g; about 80% of those under 1500 g have no neurologic or mental sequelae. The long-term prognosis for normal pulmonary function in most infants surviving hyaline membrane disease is excellent.

Avery ME: The argument for prenatal administration of dexamethasone to prevent respiratory distress syndrome. J Pediatr 104:240, 1984.
Avery M, Fletcher B, Williams R: The Lung and Its Disorders in the Newborn Infant. 4th ed. Philadelphia, WB Saunders, 1981.
Barr PA, Sumners J, Wirtshafter D, et al: Percutaneous peripheral arterial cannulation in the neonate. Pediatrics (Suppl) p 1058, 1977.

Behrman RE: The use of acid-base measurements in clinical evaluation and treatment of the sick neonate. J Pediatr 74:632, 1969.

Carlos W, Chatburn R, Martin R, et al: Decrease in airway pressure during high frequency jet ventilation in infants with respiratory distress syndrome. J Pediatr 104:101, 1984.

Cherniack NS: Sleep apnea and its causes. J Clin Invest 73:1501, 1984.

Coates AL, Desmond K, Willis D, et al: Oxygen therapy and long-term pulmonary outcome of respiratory distress syndrome in newborns. Am J Dis Child 136:892, 1982.

Corbet AJ, Adams JM, Kenny JD, et al: Controlled trial of bicarbonate therapy in high-risk premature newborn infants. J Pediatr 91:771, 1977.

Edwards DK, Wayne DM, Northway WH Jr: Twelve years' experience with bronchopulmonary dysplasia. Pediatrics 59:839, 1977.

Fitzhardinge PM, Pope J, Arstikaitis M, et al: Mechanical ventilation of infants of less than 1500 grams' birth weight: health, growth, neurologic sequelae. J Pediatr 88:531, 1976.

Gerhardt T, Bancalari E: Apnea of prematurity: 1. Lung function and regulation of breathing. Pediatrics 74:58, 1984.

Gerhardt T, Bancalari E: Apnea of prematurity: II. Respiratory reflexes. Pediatrics 74:63, 1984.

Gitlin JD, Parad R, Taeusch WH: Exogenous surfactant therapy in hyaline membrane disease. Semin Perinatol 8:272, 1984.

Gluck L, Kulovich M: Lecithin-sphingomyelin ratios in amniotic fluid in normal and abnormal pregnancy. Am J Obstet Gynecol 115:539, 1973.

Green TP, Thompson TR, Johnson DE, et al: Diuresis and pulmonary function in premature infants with respiratory distress syndrome. J Pediatr 103:618, 1983.

Gregory G, Kitterman J, Phibbs R, et al: Treatment of the idiopathic respiratory distress syndrome with continuous positive airway pressure. N Engl J Med 284:1333, 1971.

Guilleminault C, Coons S: Apnea and bradycardia during feeding in infants weighing >2000 gm. J Pediatr 104:932, 1984.

Heldt GP, Mellroy MB, Hansen TN, et al: Exercise performance of survivors of hyaline membrane disease. J Pediatr 96:995, 1980.

Henderson-Smith DJ, Pettigrew AG, Campbell DJ: Clinical apnea and brainstem neural function in preterm infants. N Engl J Med 308:353, 1983.

Ingram D, Pendergrass E, Bromberger P, et al: Group B streptococcal disease. Am J Dis Child 134:754, 1980.

Jacob J, Edwards D, Gluck L: Early onset sepsis and pneumonia observed as respiratory distress syndrome. Am J Dis Child 134:766, 1980.

Krauss A: Assisted ventilation: A critical review. Clin Perinatol 7:61, 1980.

Merrett TA, Farrell PM: Diminished pulmonary lecithin synthesis in acidosis: Experimental findings as related to the respiratory distress syndrome. Pediatrics 57:32, 1976.

Miller, MJ, Carlo WA, Martin RJ: Continuous positive airway pressure selectively reduces obstructive apnea in preterm infants. J Pediatr 106:91, 1985.

Northway WH, Rosan RC, Porter DB: Pulmonary disease following respiratory therapy. N Engl J Med 276:357, 1967.

Robert MF, Neff RK, Hubbell JP, et al: Association between maternal diabetes and the respiratory distress syndrome in the newborn. N Engl J Med 294:357, 1976.

Shelly S, Kovacevic M, Paciga J, et al: Sequential changes of surfactant phosphatidylcholine in hyaline membrane disease of the newborn. N Engl J Med 300:112, 1979.

Southall DP, Richards JM, Rhoden KJ: Prolonged apnea and cardiac arrhythmias in infants discharged from neonatal intensive care units: Failure to predict an increased risk for SIDS. Pediatrics 70:844, 1982.

Stahlman M: Newborn intensive care: success or failure. J Pediatr 105:162, 1984.

Stahlman M, Hedvail G, Lindstrom D, et al: Role of hyaline membrane disease in production of later childhood lung abnormalities. Pediatrics 69:572, 1982.

Stewart AL, Reynolds EOR: Improved prognosis for infants of low birth weight. Pediatrics 54:724, 1974.

Stocker JT, Madewell JE: Persistent interstitial pulmonary emphysema: Another complication of the respiratory distress syndrome. Pediatrics 59:847, 1977.

Thibeault DW, Emmanoulides GC, Nelson RJ, et al: Patent ductus arteriosus complicating the respiratory distress syndrome in preterm infants. J Pediatr 86:120, 1975.

Thibeault D, Hall I, Sheehan M, et al: Postasphyxial lung disease in newborn infants with severe perinatal acidosis. Am J Obstet Gynecol 150:393, 1984.

8.33 TRANSIENT TACHYPNEA OF THE NEWBORN

Transient tachypnea, occasionally termed **respiratory distress syndrome type II,** usually follows uneventful normal preterm or term vaginal delivery or cesarean delivery. It may be characterized only by the early onset of tachypnea, sometimes with retractions, or expiratory grunting and, occasionally, cyanosis that is relieved by minimal oxygen. Patients usually recover rapidly within 3 days, although they may rarely appear severely ill and have a more protracted course. The lungs are usually clear without rales or rhonchi, and the chest roentgenogram shows prominent pulmonary vascular markings, fluid lines in the fissures, overaeration, flat diaphragms, and, occasionally, pleural fluid. Hypoxemia, hypercapnia, and acidosis are uncommon. Distinguishing the disease from hyaline membrane disease may be very difficult; the distinctive features of transient tachypnea are its sudden recovery, and the absence of a roentgenographic reticulogranular pattern on air bronchography. The syndrome is believed to be secondary to slow absorption of fetal lung fluid. Discontinuing oral feeding may be necessary to avoid the risk of aspiration and to treat with oxygen, but usually no other treatment is required.

Avery ME, Gatewood OB, Brumley G: Transient tachypnea of newborn. Possible delayed reabsorption of fluid at birth. Am J Dis Child 111:380, 1966.

Gross TL, Sokol RJ, Kwong MS, et al: Transient tachypnea of the newborn: The relationship to preterm delivery and significant neonatal morbidity. Am J Obstet Gynecol 146:236, 1983.

Sundell H, Garrott J, Blankenship WJ, et al: Studies on infants with type II respiratory distress syndrome. J Pediatr 78:754, 1971.

8.34 ASPIRATION OF FOREIGN MATERIAL
(Fetal Aspiration Syndrome; Aspiration Pneumonia)

During prolonged labors and difficult deliveries, infants often initiate vigorous respiratory movements in utero because of interference with the supply of oxygen via the placenta. Under such circumstances the infant may aspirate amniotic fluid containing vernix caseosa, epithelial cells, meconium, or material from the birth canal, which may block the smallest airways and interfere with alveolar exchange of oxygen and carbon dioxide. Pathogenic bacteria frequently accompany the aspirated material, and pneumonia may ensue; but even in the noninfected cases respiratory distress accompanied by roentgenographic evidences of aspiration is seen (Fig. 8–19).

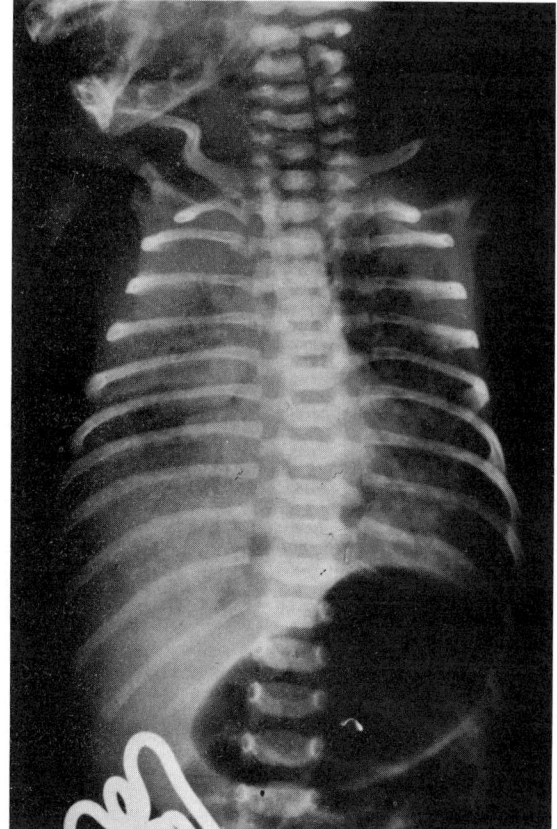

Figure 8–19. Fetal aspiration syndrome (aspiration pneumonia). Note the coarsely granular pattern with irregular aeration typical of fetal distress from aspiration of materials such as vernix caseosa, epithelial cells, and meconium contained in amniotic fluid.

Pulmonary aspiration of foreign material may also occur in the newborn infant due to tracheoesophageal fistula, esophageal and duodenal obstructions, gastroesophageal reflux, improper feeding practices, the administration of medicines, and improper handling and placement of infants in their cribs.

The contents of the stomach should be aspirated through a soft rubber catheter just before operation or other procedures requiring anesthesia or significantly disturbing an infant. Once aspiration has occurred, treatment consists of general and respiratory support and treatment of pneumonia (Sec. 8.60).

Goodwin SR, Graves SA, Haberkern CM: Aspiration in intubated premature infants. Pediatrics 75:85, 1985.

8.35 MECONIUM ASPIRATION

Meconium-stained amniotic fluid is seen in 5–15% of births, but this syndrome usually occurs in term or post-term infants. Usually, but not invariably, there has been fetal distress and hypoxia with passage of meconium into the amniotic fluid. These infants are frequently meconium-stained and depressed and require resuscitation at birth. Either in utero or more often with the first breath, thick meconium is aspirated into the lungs. The resulting small airway obstruction may produce respiratory distress within the first hours with tachypnea, retraction, grunting, and cyanosis in severely affected infants. Partial obstruction of some airways may lead to pneumothorax, pneumomediastinum, or both. Prompt treatment may delay the onset of respiratory distress, which may consist only of tachypnea without retractions. Overdistention of the chest may be prominent. The condition usually improves within 48 hr, but when its course requires assisted ventilation, it may be severe and its potential for mortality high. Tachypnea may persist for many days or even several weeks. The typical chest roentgenogram is characterized by patchy infiltrates, coarse streaking of both lung fields, increased anteroposterior diameter, and flattening of the diaphragm. Arterial pO_2 may be low, and if hypoxia has occurred, metabolic acidosis is usually present. The mortality of meconium-stained infants is considerably higher than that of nonstained infants, and meconium aspiration accounts for a significant proportion of neonatal deaths. Residual lung problems are rare, but the ultimate prognosis depends on the extent of central nervous system injury from asphyxia and the presence of associated problems such as persistence of the fetal circulation.

Treatment of meconium aspiration should begin in the delivery room with the atraumatic removal of oropharyngeal and tracheal meconium. Endotracheal tube insertion and suction are indicated when there is meconium staining. Supportive care for respiratory distress should be provided as indicated. The oxygenation benefit of positive end-expiratory pressure (or CPAP) must be weighed against its increasing the risk of air leaks. Ventilation at high rates to produce a metabolic alkalosis may be beneficial. Hydrocortisone therapy is not of benefit.

Gregory GA, Gooding CA, Phibbs RH, et al: Meconium aspiration infants; a prospective study. J Pediatr 85:848, 1974.
Marshall R, Tyrala E, McAlister W, et al: Meconium aspiration syndrome: Neonatal and follow-up study. Am J Obstet Gynecol 131:672, 1978.
Murphy JD, Vawter GF, Reid LM: Pulmonary vascular disease in fetal meconium aspiration. J Pediatr 104:758, 1984.

8.36 PERSISTENT FETAL CIRCULATION
(Primary Pulmonary Hypertension)

This syndrome occurs in term or post-term infants following meconium aspiration, asphyxia, sepsis, polycythemia, or in-dependent of any apparent cause. Profound hypoxia with a large right to left shunt, tachypnea, and cyanosis often suggest congenital heart disease (Sec. 14.12). The chest roentgenogram shows clear lung fields and a normal heart size. Echocardiogram shows elevated right ventricular time intervals suggesting increased pulmonary vascular resistance. Reversible pulmonary arterial hypertension may respond to conventional respirator settings, but hyperventilation to attain a $pCO_2 = 20$ mm Hg and pH = 7.5–7.6 may be needed to elevate the PaO_2. Pavulon may be needed to produce adequate ventilation; fluids and pressors may be needed to maintain systemic blood pressure. Intravenous tolazoline (1 mg/kg) may result in pulmonary artery dilation and improved oxygenation; it may also produce systemic hypotension. The prognosis for survivors is good.

Fox W, Duara S: Persistent pulmonary hypertension in the neonate: Diagnosis and management. J Pediatr 103:505, 1983.
Gersony W: Neonatal pulmonary hypertension: Pathophysiology, classification and etiology. Clin Perinatol 11:517, 1984.
Levin DL, Weinberg AG, Perkin RM: Pulmonary microthrombi syndrome in infants with unresponsive persistent pulmonary hypertension. J Pediatr 102:299, 1983.

8.37 EXTRAPULMONARY EXTRAVASATION OF AIR
(Pneumothorax, Pneumomediastinum, and Pulmonary Interstitial Emphysema)

Asymptomatic pneumothorax, usually unilateral, is estimated to occur in 1–2% of all newborn infants; symptomatic pneumothorax and pneumomediastinum are less common. Pneumothorax is more common in males than in females and in term and post-term infants than in premature ones. The incidence is increased among infants with lung disease, such as meconium aspiration and hyaline membrane disease; in those who have had vigorous resuscitation or are receiving assisted ventilation, especially if high inspiratory pressure or a continuous elevation of end-expiratory pressure is used; and in infants with urinary tract anomalies.

Etiology and Pathophysiology. The most common cause of pneumothorax is overinflation resulting in alveolar rupture. It may be "spontaneous" or idiopathic or secondary to underlying pulmonary disease, such as lobar emphysema or rupture of a congenital or pneumonic cyst; to trauma; or to a "ball-valve" type of bronchial or bronchiolar obstruction resulting from aspiration. Air from a ruptured alveolus escapes into the interstitial spaces of the lung where it may cause *interstitial emphysema* and/or dissect along the peribronchial and perivascular connective tissue sheaths to the root of the lung. If the volume of escaped air is great enough, it may follow the vascular sheaths to cause mediastinal emphysema or a rupture with subsequent pneumomediastinum, pneumothorax, and subcutaneous emphysema. There may also be right to left shunting with persistent circulation through a collapsed area of lung. Rarely, increased mediastinal pressure may compress pulmonary veins at the hilum, interfering with venous return to the heart and cardiac output. On occasion, air may embolize into the circulation, producing cutaneous blanching, air in intravascular catheters, an air-filled heart on chest roentgenograms, and death.

Tension pneumothorax occurs if an accumulation of air within the pleural space is sufficient to elevate intrapleural pressure above atmospheric pressure. A unilateral tension pneumothorax results in impaired ventilation not only in the collapsed lung but also in the normal lung by a mediastinal shift to the other side. Compression of the vena cava and torsion of the great vessels may interfere with venous return.

Clinical Manifestations. The physical findings of *asymptomatic pneumothorax* are hyper-resonance and diminished breath sounds over the involved side of the chest with or without tachypnea.

Symptomatic pneumothorax is characterized by respiratory distress, which varies from only an increased respiratory rate to severe dyspnea, tachypnea, and cyanosis. Irritability and restlessness or apnea may be the earliest signs. The onset may be sudden or gradual; an infant may rapidly become critically ill. The chest may appear asymmetric with increased anteroposterior diameter and bulging of the intercostal spaces on the affected side, and there may be hyper-resonance and diminished or absent breath sounds. The heart is displaced toward the unaffected side, and the diaphragm is displaced downward, as is the liver with right-sided pneumothorax. Since both sides are affected in approximately 10% of patients, symmetry of findings does not rule out pneumothorax. In tension pneumothorax there may be signs of shock, and the apex of the heart is pushed away from the affected side. Rupture tends to occur early in meconium aspiration and later in hyaline membrane disease when the infant is beginning to make more vigorous efforts with improving lung compliance, or it may be a complication of assisted ventilation.

Pneumomediastinum occurs in at least 25% of patients with pneumothorax and is usually asymptomatic. The degree of respiratory distress depends on the amount of trapped air. If it is great, there is bulging of the midthoracic area, the neck veins are distended, and the blood pressure is low. The last two findings are the result of blockage of the circulation by compression of the systemic and pulmonary veins. Although few clinical signs may exist, subcutaneous emphysema in the newborn infant is almost pathognomonic of pneumomediastinum.

Pulmonary interstitial emphysema (PIE) may precede the development of a pneumothorax or may occur independently, resulting in increasing respiratory distress due to decreased compliance, hypercarbia, and hypoxia. Progressive enlargement of blebs or air may result in cystic dilatations and respiratory deterioration resembling pneumothorax. In severe cases PIE precedes the development of bronchopulmonary dysplasia (BPD). Avoidance of high inspiratory or mean ventilatory pressures may prevent the development of PIE. Treatment may include bronchoscopy if there is evidence of mucus plugging, selective intubation of the involved bronchus, oxygen, and general respiratory care, and high-frequency jet ventilation.

Diagnosis. Pneumothorax and pneumomediastinum should be suspected in any newborn infant who shows signs of respiratory distress or who displays restlessness or irritability, or has a sudden change in condition. The diagnosis is established roentgenographically with the edge of the collapsed lung standing out in relief against the pneumothorax (see Fig. 13.19), and in pneumomediastinum with hyperlucency around the heart border and between the sternum and the heart border (Fig. 8–20). Transillumination of the thorax is often helpful in the emergency diagnosis of pneumothorax; the affected side transmits excessive light.

Pneumopericardium may be asymptomatic requiring only general supportive treatment but usually presents as sudden shock with tachycardia, muffled heart sounds, and poor pulses suggesting tamponade, which requires prompt evacuation of entrapped air. **Pneumoperitoneum** from air dissecting through the diaphragmatic apertures may also be confused with perforation of an abdominal organ.

Treatment. Without a continued air leak, asymptomatic and mildly symptomatic small pneumothoraces require only close observation. Frequent small feedings may prevent gastric dilatation and minimize crying, which can further compromise ventilation and worsen the pneumothorax. Breathing 100% oxygen accelerates the resorption of free pleural air into the blood by reducing the nitrogen tension in blood, with a resultant nitrogen pressure gradient from the trapped air into the blood, but the benefit must be weighed against the risks of oxygen toxicity. With severe respiratory or circulatory embarrassment, emergency needle aspiration is indicated. If there is adequate time, a chest tube should be inserted and attached to underwaterseal drainage. Severe localized interstitial emphysema may respond to selective bronchial intubation. Judicious use of Pavulon in infants fighting the ventilator may reduce the incidence of pneumothorax.

Chernick V, Avery ME: Spontaneous alveolar rupture at birth: Pediatrics 32:816, 1963.
Hall RT, Rhodes PG: Pneumothorax and pneumomediastinum in infants with idiopathic respiratory distress syndrome receiving CPAP. Pediatrics 55:493, 1975.
Primhak RA: Factors associated with pulmonary air leak in premature infants receiving mechanical ventilation. J Pediatr 102:764, 1983.

8.38 INTERSTITIAL PULMONARY FIBROSIS
(Wilson-Mikity Syndrome; Bronchopulmonary Dysplasia; Pulmonary Insufficiency of the Premature)

See also Sec. 8.32 for discussion of bronchopulmonary dysplasia.

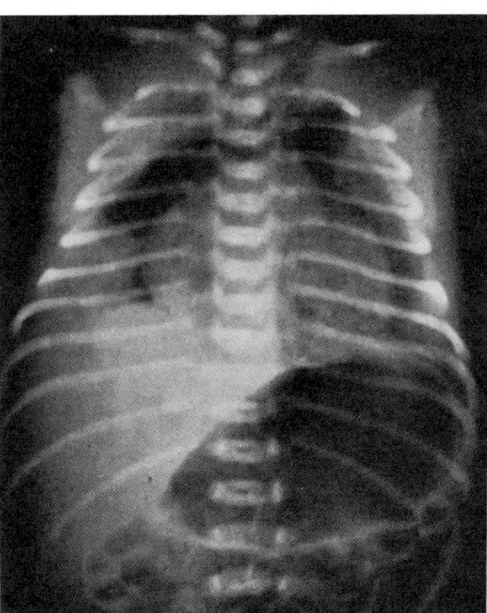
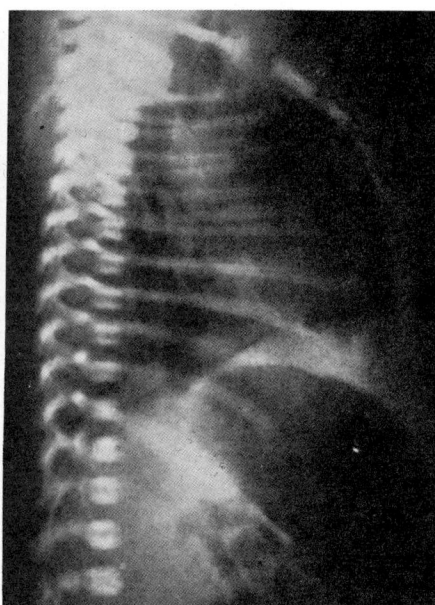

Figure 8–20. Pneumomediastinum in a newborn infant. Anteroposterior view demonstrates compression of lungs and the lateral view shows bulging of the sternum, each resulting from distention of the mediastinum by trapped air.

Wilson and Mikity described a pulmonary syndrome of premature infants, usually of less than 32 wk gestation and birthweights below 1500 g, characterized by insidious onset of dyspnea, tachypnea, retractions, and cyanosis during the first month of life. Rare cases that have been reported in full-term infants are those usually having a history of meconium aspiration or oxygen administration. Viral infections also have been implicated.

Several variations on the clinical presentation have been described with similar roentgenographic findings. Some infants have respiratory distress at birth that is occasionally severe, resembles hyaline membrane disease, and requires oxygen; these may be cases of bronchopulmonary dysplasia. Others have a more gradual development of dyspnea and cyanosis. Others have no early respiratory symptoms or history of exposure to oxygen, and the onset of symptoms is at several weeks of life.

Cough, wheezing, and rales may develop, but fever occurs only with concomitant infection. There may be collapse of a lobe or lung; other complications are right-sided heart failure, osteoporosis, and rib fractures. The symptoms usually increase over 2–6 wk with increasing oxygen dependency persisting for several months, followed by gradual resolution or progressive respiratory and cardiac failure. Infants who recover from the severe form may have an increased number of lower respiratory tract infections in the first year of life. The most characteristic features of this syndrome are roentgenographic. Early, they include bilateral coarse reticular streaky infiltrates and, often, overexpansion of the lungs with small areas of emphysema that develop into multicystic lesions. Subsequently, the cysts enlarge and coalesce to give a hyperlucent, bubbly appearance (Fig. 8–18C). The roentgenograms tend to clear gradually over months to several years. The roentgenographic changes in Wilson-Mikity syndrome may be indistinguishable from those of bronchopulmonary dysplasia.

The syndrome must be differentiated from pneumonia due to cytomegalovirus, *Pneumocystis carinii*, or chlamydia pneumonia, and from cystic fibrosis. *Chronic pulmonary insufficiency of prematurity* is initially different from bronchopulmonary dysplasia. Usually a VLBW infant without respiratory distress syndrome develops severe apnea on day 2–5. Atelectasis and a reduced functional residual capacity follows requiring treatment with CPAP or mechanical ventilation. With prolonged ventilation, a picture of bronchopulmonary dysplasia intervenes.

Treatment consists of supportive measures: oxygen for cyanosis, bronchodilators, diuretics for cardiac failure, acid-base correction, and assisted ventilation when indicated. Prophylaxis with vitamin E or A does not decrease the incidence or severity of bronchopulmonary dysplasia. Steroids may have a temporary beneficial effect in BPD, but hypertension and infection are serious side effects.

Abman SH, Wolfe RR, Accurso FJ, et al: Pulmonary vascular response to oxygen in infants with severe bronchopulmonary dysplasia. Pediatrics 75:80, 1985.

Burr BH, Guyer B, Todres ID, et al: Home care for children on respirators. N Engl J Med 309:1319, 1983.

Kao LC, Warburton D, Cheng MH, et al: Effect of oral diuretics on pulmonary mechanics in infants with chronic bronchopulmonary dysplasia: Results of a double-blind crossover sequential *trial*. Pediatrics 74:37, 1984.

Saldanha RL, Cepeda EE, Poland RL: The effect of vitamin E prophylaxis on the incidence and severity of bronchopulmonary dysplasia. Pediatrics 101:89, 1982.

Toce SS, Farrell PM, Leavitt LA, et al: Clinical and roentgenographic scoring systems for assessing bronchopulmonary dysplasia. Am J Dis Child 138:581, 1984.

Wilson MG, Mikity VG: A new form of respiratory distress in premature infants. Am J Dis Child 99:489, 1960.

LOBAR EMPHYSEMA

See Sec. 13.86.

8.39 LUNG CYSTS

Most lung cysts observed during the neonatal period are acquired as the result of rupture of alveoli by overinflation or infection, often staphylococcal. Congenital cysts are rare; they may be solitary or multiple, air- or fluid-filled, and are believed to result as a developmental anomaly of the bronchial buds (Sec. 13.49). Infants with congenital or acquired cysts may be asymptomatic or present with tachypnea and dyspnea at birth or any time thereafter or with recurrent or persistent pneumonia. Air-filled cysts on the surface of the lung, whatever their origin, sometimes rupture and cause pneumothorax. This is particularly true of multicystic disease. Since most cystic areas discovered only on roentgenographic examination will disappear spontaneously, treatment, which is surgical removal, should be reserved for those causing severe respiratory distress.

8.40 PULMONARY HEMORRHAGE

Massive pulmonary hemorrhage is present in 15% of neonates who come to autopsy in the first 2 wk of life. The reported incidence at autopsy varies from 1 to 4 per 1000 live births. About three fourths of the patients weigh less than 2500 g at birth.

Most infants in whom pulmonary hemorrhage is demonstrated at autopsy have had symptoms of respiratory distress indistinguishable from those of hyaline membrane disease. The onset may occur at birth or be delayed several days. One fourth to one half of affected infants cough up or regurgitate material containing old or fresh blood from the nose, mouth, or endotracheal tube. Roentgenographic findings are varied and nonspecific, ranging from minor streaking or patchy infiltrates to massive consolidation.

The cause of massive pulmonary hemorrhage is usually not identified; the incidence is increased in association with acute pulmonary infection, severe asphyxia, hyaline membrane disease, assisted ventilation, congenital heart disease, erythroblastosis fetalis, hemorrhagic disease of the newborn, kernicterus, inborn errors of ammonia metabolism, and cold injury. Although in the majority of instances bleeding into other organs is observed at autopsy, bleeding other than through the nostrils and mouth is relatively rare during life and should suggest the possibility of an additional bleeding diathesis such as disseminated intravascular coagulation (Sec. 15.50). Bleeding is predominantly alveolar in about two thirds of cases and interstitial in the rest. In some infants the pulmonary hemorrhage represents hemorrhagic pulmonary edema due to severe left-sided heart failure from hypoxia.

The little information available that describes the prognosis of infants who bleed through the mouth or nostrils suggests that it is extremely poor. Death occurs in the first 48 hr of life in two thirds of the infants who come to autopsy. Treatment includes blood replacement, positive end-expiratory pressure, and epinephrine aerosols.

Cole VA, Norman ICS, Reynolds EOR, et al: Pathogenesis of hemorrhagic pulmonary edema and massive pulmonary hemorrhage in the newborn. Pediatrics 51:175, 1973.

Trompeter R, Yu VYH, Aynsley-Green A, et al: Massive pulmonary haemorrhage in the newborn. Arch Dis Child 51:123, 1975.

CONGENITAL PULMONARY LYMPHANGIECTASIA

See Sec. 13.51.

CHYLOTHORAX

See Sec. 13.103.

8.41 DIGESTIVE SYSTEM

Vomiting. Infants may vomit mucus, often blood-streaked, in the first few hours after birth. This vomiting rarely persists after the first few feedings; it may be due to irritation of the gastric mucosa by material swallowed during delivery. If the vomiting is protracted, gastric lavage with physiologic saline solution may relieve it.

Vomiting is a relatively frequent symptom during the neonatal period. In the majority of instances it is simply regurgitation from overfeeding or from failure to permit the infant to eructate swallowed air. (See Sec. 12.21 for discussion of gastric emptying and gastroesophageal reflux.) When vomiting occurs shortly after birth and is persistent, the possibilities of intestinal obstruction and increased intracranial pressure must be considered. A history of maternal hydramnios suggests upper intestinal atresia.

Obstructive lesions of the digestive tract occur most frequently in the esophagus and intestines (Chapter 12). Vomiting from esophageal obstruction occurs with the first feeding. The diagnosis of **esophageal atresia** can be suspected if there is unusual drooling from the mouth and if resistance is encountered in the attempt to pass a catheter into the stomach. Diagnosis should be made before the infant chokes on oral feedings and risks aspiration pneumonia. Infantile **achalasia** (cardiospasm), a rare cause of vomiting in the newborn infant, is demonstrable roentgenographically by obstruction at the cardiac end of the esophagus, without organic stenosis. Regurgitation of feedings owing to continuous relaxation of the esophageal-gastric sphincter, **chalasia,** is a cause of vomiting, which can be controlled by keeping the infant in a semi-upright position.

Vomiting from *obstruction of the small intestine* usually begins on the first day of life and is frequent, persistent, usually nonprojectile, copious, and, unless the obstruction is above the ampulla of Vater, bile-stained; it is associated with abdominal distention, visible deep peristaltic waves, and reduced or absent bowel movements. **Malrotation** with obstruction from midgut volvulus is an acute emergency that must be considered. Upright roentgenographic films of the abdomen will show the distribution of air in the intestine and often aid in locating the site of the obstruction; malrotation may be identified by contrast studies. Normally, air can be demonstrated roentgenographically in the jejunum by 15–60 min, in the ileum by 2–3 hr, and in the colon by 3 hr after birth. Persistent vomiting may occur with congenital *hernia of the diaphragm* (Sec. 12.65). The vomiting of **pyloric stenosis** may begin any time after birth but does not assume its characteristic pattern before the 2nd–3rd wk. Vomiting may occur with many other disturbances that do not obstruct the digestive tract, such as celiac disease, milk allergy, adrenal hyperplasia of the salt-losing variety, septicemia, meningitis, and urinary tract infections.

Thrush (Oral Candidosis). Thrush of the mouth occurs in healthy infants; later, it is rare except in debilitated infants and children and in those receiving antibiotic or immunosuppressive therapy.

Transmission of the infection from maternal vaginal moniliasis to the infant's oral mucosa is the primary means of infection in healthy newborns. Secondary cases develop in the hospital nursery, presumably owing to contact with infected infants and contaminated supplies or caretakers.

Oral thrush in an otherwise healthy infant is usually a self-limited infection, but treatment is advised, especially in the presence of candidal diaper rash. (Sec. 12.9.)

Diarrhea. See Sec. 5.24, 8.63, 11.8, 11.25, 12.13, and 12.40.

Constipation. More than 90% of newborn infants pass meconium within the first 24 hr, and most of the remainder do so within 36 hr; the possibility of intestinal obstruction should be considered in any infant who does not. Intestinal atresia or stenosis, congenital aganglionic megacolon, milk bolus obstruction, meconium ileus, or meconium plugs may present as constipation. Constipation not present from birth, but appearing during the first month of life, suggests congenital aganglionic megacolon, cretinism, or anal stenosis. It must be kept in mind that infrequent bowel movements do not necessarily mean constipation. A breast-fed infant usually has frequent bowel movements, whereas a formula-fed infant may have 1–2 movements a day or every other day.

Meconium Plugs. Lower colonic or anorectal plugs (Fig. 8–21) having a water content lower than normal may cause intestinal obstruction. Rarely a firm mass of meconium may form elsewhere in the intestine and cause intrauterine intestinal obstruction and meconium peritonitis unrelated to cystic fibrosis. Anorectal plugs may also cause intestinal ulceration and perforation. The plug may be evacuated by irrigation with isotonic sodium chloride solution. Enemas with the iodinated contrast medium, *Gastrografin,* will usually cause passage of the plug, presumably because the high osmolarity (1900 mOsm/L) of the medium draws fluid rapidly into the intestinal lumen and loosens inspissated material. Since this rapid loss of fluid into the bowel may result in acute dehydration and shock, it is advisable to dilute the contrast material with an equal amount of water, to correct any existing dehydration, and to provide intravenous fluids during and for several hours after the procedure. *After removal of a meconium plug the infant should be observed closely for the possible presence of congenital aganglionic megacolon.*

8.42 MECONIUM ILEUS IN CYSTIC FIBROSIS

In the newborn infant impaction of meconium causes intestinal obstructions often associated with cystic fibrosis. The absence of pancreatic enzymes limits normal digestive activities in the intestine, and meconium is left in a viscid, mucilaginous state. It clings to the intestinal wall and is moved with difficulty. The inspissated and impacted meconium fills the intestinal canal but is most concentrated in the lower ileum.

Clinically, the pattern is that of congenital intestinal obstruction with or without intestinal perforation. Abdominal distention is prominent, and persistent vomiting soon occurs. Infrequently one or more inspissated meconium stools may be passed shortly after birth.

The differential diagnosis involves other causes of intestinal obstruction; an exact diagnosis cannot be made except at laparotomy. A presumptive diagnosis can be made on the basis of a history of cystic fibrosis in a sibling, by palpation of doughy or cordlike masses of intestines through the abdominal wall, and by the roentgenographic appearance. Roentgenographically, in contrast to the generally evenly distended intestinal loops above an atresia, the loops may vary in width and not be as evenly filled with gas. At points

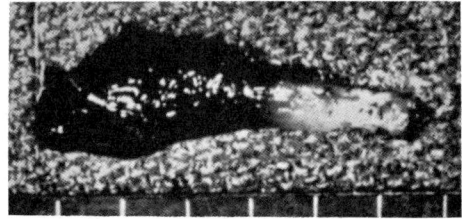

Figure 8–21. Anorectal plug, from child who had not passed meconium for 2 days after birth, is indistinguishable from normal plug. Pale end was adjacent to anus. (From Emery JL: Arch Dis Child, Vol 32.)

of heaviest meconium concentration the infiltrated gas may create a bubbly granular appearance (Fig. 8–22 and 8–23). A negative sweat test in the neonatal period may not rule out cystic fibrosis.

The case fatality rate is high, but a number of infants have survived the neonatal period; their subsequent prognosis depends on the basic disturbance, cystic fibrosis (Sec. 13.97).

Treatment is high Gastrografin enemas as described under Meconium Plugs in the previous section. If they are unsuccessful or if there is reason to suspect a perforation of the bowel wall, laparotomy is performed and the ileum opened at the point of greatest diameter of the impaction. The inspissated meconium is removed by gentle and patient irrigation with warm isotonic sodium chloride solution introduced through a fine catheter which may be passed between the impaction and the bowel wall.

Meconium Peritonitis. Perforation of the intestine may occur in utero or shortly after birth. Either the tear may be sealed by natural processes relatively quickly with only a small amount of meconium escaping, or the meconial contents may largely be emptied into the peritoneal cavity. Such perforations occur most often as a complication of meconium ileus in infants with cystic fibrosis, but occasionally the perforation is due to a meconium plug or intestinal obstruction of another cause.

When the intestinal perforation is spontaneously sealed and only a small amount of meconium has escaped, the event may never be detected, except when some of the meconial particles become calcified and are later fortuitously discovered on roentgenograms of the abdomen. Alternatively, the clinical picture may be dominated by the signs of intestinal obstruction or peritonitis. Characteristically there is abdominal distention, vomiting, and absence of stools. The treatment is primarily elimination of the intestinal obstruction and drainage of the peritoneal cavity.

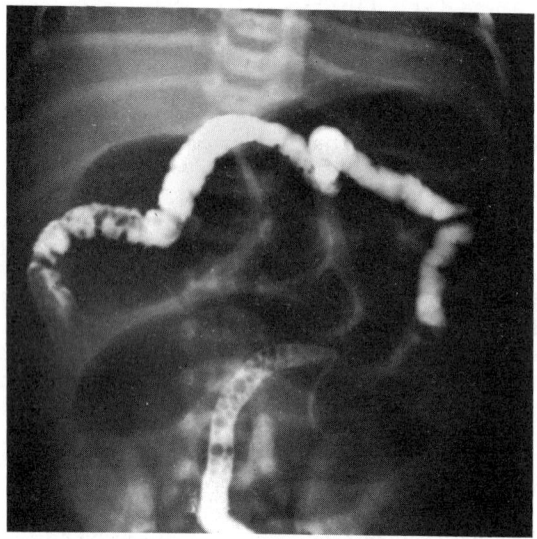

Figure 8–23. Meconium ileus. The colon, outlined by contrast material, is small because meconium has not reached it.

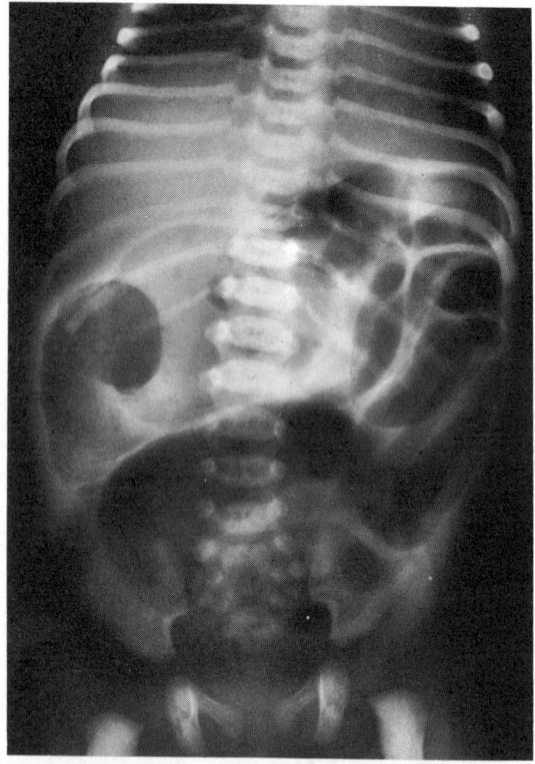

Figure 8–22. Meconium ileus. Impacted meconium with small amounts of air interspersed throughout it in loops of intestine on the right side of abdomen; intestinal loops above this impaction are greatly distended.

8.43 NEONATAL NECROTIZING ENTEROCOLITIS (NEC)

This serious disease of the newborn is of unknown etiology and characterized by varying degrees of mucosal or transmural necrosis of the intestine. No particular race or sex is unduly susceptible to the disease. Incidence ranges from 1 to 5% of admissions to neonatal intensive care units. Since the very small, ill newborn infant is particularly susceptible to NEC, a rising incidence in recent years may reflect improved survival of this high risk group of patients. The disease does occur occasionally in term infants.

Pathology and Pathogenesis. Many factors may contribute to the development of a necrotic segment of intestine, the gas accumulation in the submucosa of the bowel wall, and progression of the necrosis leading to perforation, sepsis, and death. The distal ileum and proximal colon are involved most frequently. Some form of perinatal stress, especially asphyxia or hypothermia, is thought to predispose the infant to intestinal ischemia. A variety of other factors such as polycythemia, hypertonic milk or medicines, or too rapid feeding protocols may contribute to mucosal injury and subsequent infection leading to bowel necrosis. NEC may occur in premature infants without stress, particularly during epidemics. The clustering of cases suggests a primary role for an infectious agent; *Clostridium difficile, C. perfringens, Escherichia coli,* and rotavirus have commonly been recovered from cultures.

Clinical Manifestations. Onset usually occurs in the first 2 wk but can be as late as 2 mo of age. Meconium is passed normally, and the first signs are abdominal distention with gastric retention. Obvious bloody stools are seen in 25% of patients. The onset is often insidious, and sepsis may occur before an intestinal lesion is suspected. There is a wide spectrum of illness from mild with only guaiac positive stools to severe with peritonitis, bowel perforation, shock, and death. Progression may be rapid, but it is unusual to progress from mild to severe after 72 hr.

Diagnosis. A very high index of suspicion in managing infants at risk is essential. Plain abdominal roentgenograms may demonstrate pneumatosis intestinalis, a finding that is diagnostic of NEC in the newborn infant; 50–75% of patients have pneumatosis when treatment is started. Portal vein gas is a sign of severe disease, and pneumoperitoneum indicates a perforation.

The differential diagnosis of NEC includes specific infections (systemic or intestinal), obstruction, and volvulus. Cultures and roentgenograms may be diagnostic. Barium enemas are contraindicated in these patients because of the risk of bowel perforation.

Treatment. Intensive therapy is advisable for suspected as well as diagnosed cases. Cessation of feeding, nasogastric decompression, and intravenous fluids with careful attention to acid-base and electrolyte balance are very important. Once cultures are taken of blood, stool, and cerebrospinal fluid, systemic antibiotics (Sec. 11.4) should be started. When present, umbilical catheters should be removed, and ventilation should be assisted if distention is contributing to hypoxia and hypercapnia. If hypotension develops, resuscitation with blood, plasma, or crystalloid is essential.

The patient's course should be monitored by frequent cross-table lateral abdominal roentgenograms in search of perforation and by hematocrit, platelet, electrolyte, and acid-base determinations. Gown and glove isolation and grouping infants at similar increased risk into cohorts separate from other infants should be instituted to contain an epidemic.

A surgeon should be consulted early in the course of treatment. Evidence of perforation is usually an indication for resection of necrotic bowel. Peritoneal drainage may be helpful for the patient in extremis with peritonitis who is unable to withstand bowel resection.

Prognosis. Medical management fails in about 20% of patients in whom there is pneumatosis intestinalis at diagnosis; of these, at least 25% die. Strictures develop at the site of the necrotizing lesion in about 10% of patients. No long-term problems with intestinal obstruction have been noted as a sequela of NEC unless a massive resection is necessary.

Kliegman R, Fanaroff A: Necrotizing enterocolitis. N Engl J Med 310:1093, 1984.
Kosloske A: Pathogenesis and prevention of necrotizing enterocolitis: A hypothesis based on personal observation and a review of the literature. Pediatrics 74:1086, 1984.

8.44 JAUNDICE AND HYPERBILIRUBINEMIA IN THE NEWBORN

Jaundice is observed during the first week of life in approximately 60% of term infants and 80% of preterm infants. The color usually results from the accumulation in the skin of unconjugated, nonpolar, lipid-soluble bilirubin pigment (indirect-reacting) formed from hemoglobin by the action of heme oxygenase, biliverdin reductase, and nonenzymatic reducing agents in the reticuloendothelial cells; it may also be due, in part, to the deposition of the pigment after it has been converted in the liver cell microsome by the enzyme uridine diphosphoglucuronic acid (UDPGA) glucuronyl transferase to the polar, water-soluble ester glucuronide of bilirubin (direct-reacting). The unconjugated form is neurotoxic for infants at certain concentrations and under various conditions.

Jaundice should be considered a sign of risk for the infant; the degree of danger it may represent depends on factors that affect the production, metabolism, excretion, and distribution of bilirubin after birth.

Etiology. The newborn infant's metabolism of bilirubin is in transition from the fetal stage, during which the placenta is the principal route of elimination of the lipid-soluble bilirubin, to the adult stage, during which the water-soluble conjugated form is excreted from the hepatic cell into the biliary system and then into the gastrointestinal tract. Jaundice may be caused or increased by any factor that (1) increases the load of bilirubin to be metabolized by the liver (hemolytic anemias, shortened red cell life owing to immaturity or to transfused cells, increased enterohepatic circulation, infection); (2) may damage or reduce the activity of the enzyme (hypoxia, infection, possibly hypothermia and thyroid defi-

ciency); (3) may compete for or block the enzyme (drugs and other substances requiring glucuronic acid conjugation for excretion); or (4) leads to an absence of or decreased amounts of the enzyme or to reduction of bilirubin uptake by the liver cell (genetic defect, prematurity). The risk of toxic effects from elevated levels of bilirubin in the serum is increased by factors that reduce the retention of bilirubin in the circulation (hypoproteinemia, displacement of bilirubin from its binding sites on albumin by competitive binding of drugs such as sulfisoxazole, acidosis, hyperosmolality, increased free fatty acid concentration secondary to hypoglycemia, starvation, or hypothermia), or by factors that increase the permeability of the blood-brain barrier or nerve cell membranes to bilirubin or the susceptibility of brain cells to its toxicity such as asphyxia, prematurity, and infection. Early feeding decreases and dehydration increases the serum levels of bilirubin. Meconium has 1 mg bilirubin/dL and may contribute to jaundice by the enterohepatic circulation. Drugs such as oxytocin and chemicals employed in the nursery such as phenolic detergents may also produce hyperbilirubinemia.

Clinical Manifestations. Jaundice may be present at birth or may appear at any time during the neonatal period, depending on the condition responsible for it. *Its intensity bears no clinically dependable relation to the degree of hyperbilirubinemia,* particularly in infants receiving phototherapy (Sec. 8.45). Therefore, bilirubin determinations should be done on all jaundiced infants. Jaundice resulting from deposition of indirect bilirubin in the skin tends to appear bright yellow or orange; jaundice of the obstructive type (direct bilirubin), a greenish or muddy yellow. This difference is usually apparent only in severe jaundice. The infant may be lethargic and feed poorly. Signs of kernicterus rarely appear on the first day of jaundice.

Differential Diagnosis. Jaundice present at birth or appearing within the first 24 hr of life may be due to erythroblastosis fetalis, concealed hemorrhage, sepsis, cytomegalic inclusion disease, rubella, or congenital toxoplasmosis. Jaundice in infants who have received intrauterine transfusions may be characterized by an unusually high proportion of direct-reacting bilirubin. Jaundice which first appears on the 2nd or 3rd day is usually "physiologic," but may represent a more severe form called *hyperbilirubinemia of the newborn.* Familial nonhemolytic icterus (Crigler-Najjar syndrome) also is seen initially on the second or third day. *Jaundice appearing after the 3rd day and within the first wk should suggest septicemia as a likely cause;* it may be due to other infections, notably syphilis, toxoplasmosis, and cytomegalic inclusion disease. Jaundice secondary to extensive ecchymosis or hematoma may occur during the first day or later, especially in premature infants. Polycythemia may lead to early jaundice.

Jaundice initially noted after the first week of life suggests breast milk jaundice, septicemia, congenital atresia of the bile ducts, hepatitis, rubella, herpetic hepatitis, galactosemia, congenital hemolytic anemia (spherocytosis), or possibly the crises of other hemolytic anemias (such as pyruvate kinase and other glycolytic enzyme deficiencies, thalassemia, sickle cell disease, hereditary nonspherocytic anemia), or hemolytic anemia due to drugs (as in congenital deficiencies of the enzymes glucose-6–phosphate dehydrogenase, glutathione synthetase, reductase, or peroxidase).

Persistent jaundice during the first month of life suggests the so-called inspissated bile syndrome (which may follow hemolytic disease of the newborn), hyperalimentation-associated cholestasis, hepatitis, cytomegalic inclusion disease, syphilis, toxoplasmosis, familial nonhemolytic icterus, congenital atresia of the bile ducts, or galactosemia. Rarely, physiologic jaundice may be prolonged for several weeks, as in infants with hypothyroidism or pyloric stenosis.

Regardless of the gestational age or time of appearance of

jaundice, significant hyperbilirubinemia requires a complete diagnostic evaluation, which should include the determination of the direct and indirect bilirubin fractions, hemoglobin, reticulocyte count, blood type, Coombs test, and an examination of the peripheral blood smear (Table 8–20). Indirect reacting bilirubinemia, reticulocytosis, and a smear demonstrating evidence of red cell destruction suggest hemolysis; in the absence of blood group incompatibility, nonimmunologically induced hemolysis should be considered. If there is direct-reacting hyperbilirubinemia, hepatitis, cholestasis, inborn errors of metabolism, cystic fibrosis, and sepsis are diagnostic possibilities. If the reticulocyte count, Coombs test, and direct bilirubin are normal, physiologic or pathologic indirect hyperbilirubinemia may be present.

Physiologic Jaundice (Icterus Neonatorum). Under normal circumstances, the level of indirect-reacting bilirubin in umbilical cord serum is 1–3 mg/dL and rises at a rate of less than 5 mg/dL/24 hr; thus, jaundice becomes visible on the 2nd–3rd day, usually peaking between the 2nd and 4th days at 5–6 mg/dL and decreasing to below 2 mg/dL between the 5th and 7th days of life. Jaundice associated with these changes is designated "physiologic" and is believed to be the result of breakdown of fetal red cells combined with transient limitation in the conjugation and excretion of bilirubin by the liver.

Among premature infants the rise in serum bilirubin tends to be the same or a little slower than in term infants but of longer duration, which generally results in higher levels, the peak being reached between the 4th–7th days (Fig. 8–24); the pattern depends upon the time required for the preterm infant to achieve mature mechanisms for the metabolism and excretion of bilirubin. Usually, peak levels of 8–12 mg/dL are not reached until the 5th–7th day, and jaundice is infrequently observed after the 10th day.

The diagnosis of physiologic jaundice in term or preterm infants can be established only by excluding known causes of jaundice on the basis of history and clinical and laboratory findings (Table 8–20). In general, a search to determine the cause of jaundice should be made if (1) it appears in the first 24 hr of life; (2) serum bilirubin is rising at a rate greater than 5 mg/dL/24 hr; (3) serum bilirubin is greater than 12 mg/dL in full-term or 14 mg/dL in preterm infants; (4) jaundice persists after the first week of life; or (5) direct-reacting bilirubin is greater than 1 mg/dL at any time.

Genetic and *ethnic factors* may affect the severity of physiologic jaundice resulting in pathologic hyperbilirubinemia.

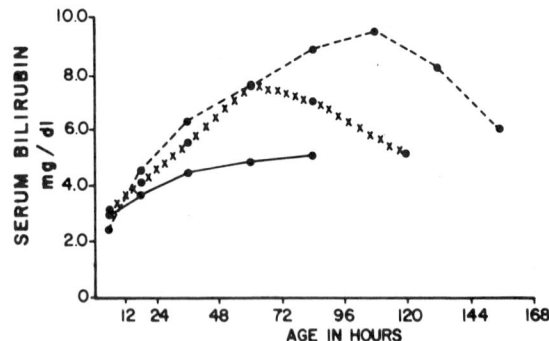

Figure 8–24. Mean serum bilirubin in relation to age in 3 groups of infants. ----: preterm, birthweight < 2500 g (AGA); xxxx: term, birthweight < 2500 g (SGA); ———: term, birthweight ≥ 2500 gm (AGA). AGA = appropriate for gestational age; SGA = small for gestational age. (From Behrman RE (ed): Neonatology. St. Louis, CV Mosby, 1973.)

Mean peak serum unconjugated bilirubin concentrations in Chinese, Japanese, Korean, and American Indian full-term newborns are approximately double those of other populations. The incidence of kernicterus is increased in Oriental and in Greek infants from Lesbos and Rhodes independent of hemolysis from the increased incidence of G-6-PD deficiency.

Pathologic Hyperbilirubinemia. Jaundice and its underlying hyperbilirubinemia are considered pathologic if their time of appearance, duration, or pattern of serially determined serum bilirubin concentrations varies significantly from that of physiologic jaundice; or if the course is compatible with physiologic jaundice but other reasons exist to suspect that the infant is at special risk from the neurotoxicity of unconjugated bilirubin. It may not be possible to determine precisely the etiology for an abnormal elevation of unconjugated bilirubin, especially in premature infants; hence, the term **hyperbilirubinemia of the newborn** is used for those infants whose primary problem is probably a deficiency or inactivity of bilirubin glucuronyl transferase rather than an excessive load of bilirubin for excretion.

The *significance* of hyperbilirubinemia lies in the high incidence of kernicterus associated with serum bilirubin levels over 18–20 mg/dL in term infants. The correlation between serum bilirubin levels and kernicterus or milder forms of brain

Table 8–20. **Diagnostic Features of the Various Types of Neonatal Jaundice**

Diagnosis	Nature of Van den Bergh Reaction	Jaundice Appears	Jaundice Disappears	Peak Bilirubin Conc. mg/dL	Peak Bilirubin Conc. Age in Days	Bilirubin Rate of Accumulation mg/dL/day	Remarks
1. "Physiologic jaundice":							1. Usually relates to degree of maturity
Full-term	Indirect	2–3 days	4–5 days	10–12	2–3	<5	
Premature	Indirect	3–4 days	7–9 days	15	6–8	<5	
2. Hyperbilirubinemia due to metabolic factors, etc.:							2. Metabolic factors: hypoxia, respiratory distress, lack of carbohydrate
Full-term	Indirect	2–3 days	Variable	>12	1st wk	<5	Hormonal influences: cretinism,
Premature	Indirect	3–4 days	Variable	>15	1st wk	<5	hormones Genetic factors: Crigler-Najjar syndrome, transient familial hyperbilirubinemia Drugs: vitamin K, novobiocin
3. Hemolytic states and hematoma	Indirect	May appear in 1st 24 hr	Variable	Unlimited	Variable	Usually >5	3. Erythroblastosis: Rh, ABO. Congenital hemolytic states: spherocytic, nonspherocytic. Infantile pyknocytosis Drugs: vitamin K. Enclosed hemorrhage—hematoma
4. Mixed hemolytic and hepatotoxic factors	Indirect and direct	May appear in 1st 24 hr	Variable	Unlimited	Variable	Usually >5	4. Infection: bacterial sepsis, pyelonephritis, hepatitis, toxoplasmosis, cytomegalic inclusion disease, rubella Drugs: vitamin K
5. Hepatocellular damage	Indirect and direct	Usually 2–3 days	Variable	Unlimited	Variable	Variable can be >5	5. Biliary atresia; galactosemia; hepatitis and infection as in (4)

From Brown AK: Pediatr Clin North Am 9(No. 3):589, 1962.

injury in infants with erythroblastosis fetalis probably holds for all newborn infants who develop bilirubin concentrations beyond the physiologic range for their weight and gestational age, independent of the etiology of the jaundice. Low birthweight infants develop kernicterus at lower levels (10–12 mg/dL) in association with asphyxia, respiratory distress syndrome, hypoglycemia, acidosis, sepsis, and meningitis. Sulfisoxazole also increases susceptibility to kernicterus at relatively low levels (12–15 mg/dL) of serum bilirubin.

Fewer than 3% of term infants without blood group incompatibility develop bilirubin levels greater than 15 mg/dL. Sixteen percent of white and 8% of black infants of low birthweight (presumably preterm) achieve these levels. Unconjugated hyperbilirubinemia has also been associated with the administration of vitamin K_3 or novobiocin, trisomy 21, polycythemia, and maternal diabetes.

Jaundice Associated with Breast Feeding. An estimated 1 of 200 breast-fed term infants develops significant elevations in unconjugated bilirubin between the 4th and 7th days of life, reaching maximum concentrations as high as 10–27 mg/dL during the 3rd wk. If breast feeding is continued, the hyperbilirubinemia gradually decreases and then may persist for 3–10 wk at lower levels. If nursing is discontinued, the serum bilirubin level falls rapidly, usually reaching normal levels within a few days. Cessation of breast feeding for 2–4 days results in a rapid decline in serum bilirubin, after which nursing can be resumed without a return of the hyperbilirubinemia to its previously high levels. These infants have no other sign of illness, and kernicterus has not been reported. The milk of some of these mothers contains 5-β-pregnane-3α,20-β-diol or nonesterified long-chain fatty acids, which competitively inhibit glucuronyl transferase conjugating activity. In others, the milk contains a glucuronidase which may be responsible for jaundice. This syndrome must be distinguished from an accentuated unconjugated hyperbilirubinemia in the first week of life in breast fed infants.

Transient Familial Neonatal Hyperbilirubinemia. Severe unconjugated hyperbilirubinemia leading to kernicterus may occur rarely in the first 2 days of life because of a glucuronyl transferase-inhibiting factor present in the serum of mother and infant.

Neonatal Hepatitis. See Sec. 12.73 and 12.74.
Congenital Atresia of the Bile Ducts. See Sec. 12.74.
Inspissated Bile Syndrome. See Late Complications in Sec. 8.47.

8.45 KERNICTERUS

Kernicterus is a neurologic syndrome resulting from the deposition of unconjugated bilirubin in brain cells. The risk in infants with erythroblastosis fetalis is directly related to serum bilirubin levels, and it is probably similar for infants with hyperbilirubinemia of whatever cause.

The precise blood level above which indirect-reacting bilirubin or free bilirubin will be toxic for an individual infant is unpredictable, but kernicterus is rare in term infants with serum levels under 18–20 mg/dL. The duration of exposure necessary to produce toxic effects is also unknown. There is some evidence that motor disturbances in later childhood are more common among newborn infants whose total serum bilirubin rises above 15 mg/dL. *The less mature the infant, the greater the susceptibility to kernicterus.* Factors that potentiate the movement of bilirubin into brain cells and its adverse effects on them are discussed in Sec. 8.44. In exceptional circumstances kernicterus in premature infants with serum bilirubin concentrations as low as 8–12 mg/dL has been associated with an apparently cumulative effect of a number of these factors.

Clinical Manifestations. Signs and symptoms of kernicterus

usually appear 2–5 days after birth in term infants and as late as the 7th day in premature ones, but hyperbilirubinemia may lead to the syndrome at any time during the neonatal period. The early signs may be subtle and indistinguishable from those of sepsis, asphyxia, hypoglycemia, intracranial hemorrhage, and other acute systemic illnesses in the neonatal infant. Lethargy, poor feeding, and loss of the Moro reflex are common initial signs. Subsequently, the infant may appear gravely ill and prostrated with diminished tendon reflexes and respiratory distress. Opisthotonos, with bulging fontanel, twitching of face or limbs, and a shrill high-pitched cry may follow. In advanced cases convulsions and spasm occur, with the infant stiffly extending his or her arms in inward rotation with fists clenched. Rigidity is rare at this late stage.

Many infants who progress to these severe neurologic signs die; the survivors are usually seriously damaged, but may appear to recover and for 2–3 mo manifest few abnormalities. Later in the first year of life opisthotonos, muscular rigidity, irregular movements, and convulsions tend to recur. In the second year opisthotonos and seizures abate but irregular, involuntary movements, muscular rigidity, or, in some infants, hypotonia increase steadily. By 3 yr of age the complete neurologic syndrome is often apparent, consisting of bilateral choreoathetosis with involuntary muscle spasm, extrapyramidal signs, seizures, mental deficiency, dysarthric speech, high-frequency hearing loss, squints, and defective upward movement of the eyes. Pyramidal signs, hypotonia, and ataxia occur in a few infants. In mildly affected infants the syndrome may be characterized only by mild to moderate neuromuscular incoordination, partial deafness, or "minimal brain dysfunction," occurring singly or in combination; these problems may be inapparent until the child enters school.

Pathology. The surface of the brain is usually pale yellow. On cutting, certain regions are characteristically stained yellow by unconjugated bilirubin, particularly the corpus subthalamicum, hippocampus and adjacent olfactory areas, striate bodies, thalamus, globus pallidus, putamen, inferior clivus, cerebellar nuclei, and cranial nerve nuclei. Nonpigmented areas may also be damaged. Loss of neurons, reactive gliosis, and atrophy of involved fiber systems are found in late disease. The pattern of injury has been related to the development of oxidative enzyme systems in various regions of the brain and overlaps with that found in hypoxic brain damage. Evidence favors the hypothesis that bilirubin interferes with oxygen utilization by cerebral tissue, possibly by injuring the cell membrane; antecedent hypoxic injury increases the susceptibility of brain cells to injury. Gross bilirubin staining without hyperbilirubinemia or the specific microscopic changes of kernicterus may not be the same entity.

Incidence and Prognosis. Using pathologic criteria one third of infants with untreated hemolytic disease and bilirubin levels in excess of 20 mg/dL will develop kernicterus. The incidence at autopsy of hyperbilirubinemic premature infants is 2–16% and is related to the risk-factors discussed in Sec. 8.44. Reliable estimates of the frequency of the clinical syndrome are not available because of the wide spectrum of manifestations. Overt neurologic signs have a grave prognosis; 75% or more of such infants die, and 80% of affected survivors have bilateral choreoathetosis with involuntary muscle spasm. Mental retardation, deafness, and spastic quadriplegia are common. Infants at risk should have screening hearing tests.

Treatment of Hyperbilirubinemia. Irrespective of etiology, the goal of therapy is to prevent the concentration of indirect-reacting bilirubin in the blood from reaching levels at which neurotoxicity may occur; it is recommended that exchange transfusion and/or phototherapy be used to keep the maximum total serum bilirubin below the levels indicated in Table

8–21. The risk of injury to the central nervous system from bilirubin must be balanced against the risk inherent in the treatment for each infant. The criteria for initiating phototherapy are not generally agreed on. Since phototherapy may require 12–24 hr to have a measurable effect, it must be started at bilirubin levels below those indicated in Table 8–21. When identified, the underlying cause of the icterus should be treated, e.g., antibiotics for septicemia. Physiologic factors that increase the risk of neurologic damage should also be treated, e.g., correction of acidosis.

Exchange Transfusion. This widely accepted treatment should be repeated as frequently as necessary to keep indirect bilirubin levels in the serum under 20 mg/dL in full-term infants. (See Exchange Transfusion in Sec. 8.47.) A variety of factors may alter this criterion in either direction in an individual patient. Appearance of clinical signs suggesting kernicterus is an indication for exchange transfusion at any level of serum bilirubin. A healthy full-term infant may tolerate a concentration slightly higher than 20 mg/dL with no apparent ill effect, whereas a sick premature infant may develop kernicterus at a significantly lower level. A level approaching that considered critical for the individual infant may be an indication for exchange transfusion during the first day or two of life when a further rise is anticipated but not on the 4th day in term infants or on the 7th day in premature infants, when an imminent fall may be anticipated as the conjugating mechanism becomes more effective.

Phototherapy. Clinical jaundice and indirect hyperbilirubinemia are reduced on exposure to a high intensity of light in the visible spectrum. Bilirubin absorbs light maximally in the blue range (from 420 to 470 nm). Bilirubin in the skin absorbs light energy, which by photoisomerization converts the toxic unconjugated bilirubin into unconjugated isomers that are excreted in the bile (4Z,15E-bilirubin) and urine (lumirubin), and by autosensitization involving singlet oxygen may result in oxidation reactions producing breakdown products that are excreted by the liver and kidney without need for conjugation.

The use of phototherapy with fluorescent light bulbs has decreased the need for exchange transfusion in low birthweight infants without hemolytic disease and in infants with hemolysis as well as for repeated exchange transfusion of infants with hemolytic disease. However, when there are indications for exchange transfusion, phototherapy should not be used as a substitute.

Phototherapy is indicated only after establishing the presence of pathologic hyperbilirubinemia. The basic cause(s) of the jaundice should be treated concomitantly. The effectiveness of phototherapy in lowering serum bilirubin levels varies inversely with the rate and degree of hemolysis, if present, and varies directly with the often unpredictable degree of activity of glucuronyl transferase.

Normal infants receiving phototherapy for 1–3 days have peak serum bilirubin concentrations about one half those of untreated infants. In premature infants without significant hemolysis serum bilirubin usually declines 1–3 mg/dL after 8–12 hr of exposure, and peak levels attained may be decreased by 3–6 mg/dL. The therapeutic effect depends on the light energy emitted in the effective range of wavelengths, the distance between the lights and the infant, and the amount of skin exposed, as well as on the rate of hemolysis and in vivo metabolism and excretion of bilirubin. It is not known whether phototherapy prevents kernicterus or milder forms of brain injury associated with bilirubin toxicity. Available commercial phototherapy units vary considerably in the spectral output and intensity of radiation emitted; therefore, the dose can be accurately measured only at the skin surface. Dark skin does not reduce the efficacy of phototherapy.

Phototherapy is applied continuously and the infant is turned frequently for maximal skin exposure. It should be discontinued as soon as the indirect bilirubin concentration has been reduced to levels considered safe in view of the infant's age and condition. Serum bilirubin levels and hematocrits should be monitored every 4–8 hr in infants with hemolytic disease or those with bilirubin levels near the range considered toxic for the individual infant. Others, particularly older infants, may be monitored at 12–24 hr intervals. Monitoring should continue for at least 24 hr after cessation of phototherapy, since unexpected rises of serum bilirubin sometimes occur and require further treatment. Skin color cannot be relied on for evaluating the effectiveness of phototherapy; the skin of babies exposed to light may appear almost without jaundice in the presence of marked hyperbilirubinemia. The infant's eyes should be closed and adequately covered to prevent exposure to light (excessive pressure from an eye bandage may injure the closed eyes, or the corneas may be excoriated if the infant can open his or her eyes under the bandage). Body temperature should be monitored, and the infant should be shielded from bulb breakage. If feasible, irradiance should be measured directly, and details of the exposure should be recorded (type and age of bulbs, duration of exposure, distance from light source to infant, and so forth). *In the infant with hemolytic disease, care must be taken not to overlook developing anemia, which may require transfusion.*

Complications of phototherapy include loose stools, rashes, overheating and dehydration, chilling from exposure of the infant, and "bronze baby syndrome." Phototherapy is contraindicated in the presence of porphyria. Eye injury or nasal occlusion from the bandages is uncommon.

The term **bronze baby syndrome** refers to a dark, grayish brown discoloration of the skin sometimes noted in infants undergoing phototherapy. Almost all infants observed with this syndrome have had a mixed type of hyperbilirubinemia with significant elevation of direct-reacting bilirubin and often with other evidence of obstructive liver disease. The discoloration may last for many months.

Wide clinical experience suggests that long-term adverse biologic effects of phototherapy are absent, minimal, or unrecognized. However, those employing phototherapy should remain alert to these possibilities and avoid its unnecessary use since untoward effects on DNA have been demonstrated in vitro.

Phenobarbital. Phenobarbital enhances the conjugation and excretion of bilirubin. Its administration will limit the development of physiologic jaundice in the newborn infant when

---

Table 8–21. **Recommended Maximal Permissible Total Serum Bilirubin Concentrations (mg/dL)***

Birthweight Category (g)†	Uncomplicated Course	Complicated Course‡
Less than 1250	13	10
1250–1499	15	13
1500–1999	17	15
2000–2499	18	17
2500 and up	20	18

*Direct-reacting bilirubin concentrations are not subtracted unless they amount to more than 50% of the total serum bilirubin concentration. This table is applicable during the first 28 days of life.

†Equivalent gestational age categories may be used in lieu of birth weight for small for gestational age (SGA) infants.

‡Complications include perinatal asphyxia and acidosis, postnatal hypoxia and acidosis, significant and persistent hypothermia, hypoalbuminemia, meningitis and other significant infections, hemolysis, hypoglycemia, and signs of clinical or CNS deterioration.

From Gartner LM. *In:* Behrman RE (ed): Neonatal-Perinatal Medicine. St. Louis, CV Mosby, 1977.

administered to mothers in a dose of 90 mg/24 hr prior to delivery or to infants at birth in a dose of 10 mg/kg/24 hr. However, since its effect on bilirubin metabolism is usually not manifest until after several days of administration, since it is less effective than phototherapy in lowering serum bilirubin concentrations, and since it may have an untoward sedative effect and does not add to the response to phototherapy, phenobarbital is not recommended for treating jaundice in the neonatal infant.

Andres JM, Mathis RK, Walker WA: Liver disease in infants; Part I: Developmental hepatology and mechanisms of liver dysfunction. J Pediatr 90:686, 1977.

Broderson R: Bilirubin transport in the newborn infant, reviewed with relationship to kernicterus. J Pediatr 96:349, 1980.

Cashore W, Stern L: The management of hyperbilirubinemia. Clin Perinatol 11:339, 1984.

Drew JH, Kitchen WH: The effect of maternally administered drugs on bilirubin concentration in the newborn infant. J Pediatr 89:657, 1976.

Ennever JF, Knox I, Denne SC, et al: Phototherapy for neonatal jaundice: In vitro clearance of bilirubin photoproducts. Pediatr Res 19:205, 1985.

Gartner L, Lee K: Unconjugated hyperbilirubinemia. In Fanaroff A, Martin R (eds): Behrman's Neonatal-Perinatal Medicine, St Louis, CV Mosby, 1983.

Gollan JL, Knapp AB: Bilirubin metabolism and congenital jaundice. Hosp Prac 20:83, 1985.

Kivlahan C, James EJP: The natural history of neonatal jaundice. Pediatrics 74:364, 1984.

Mathis RK, Andres JM, Walker WA: Liver disease in infants; Part II: Hepatic disease states. J Pediatr 90:864, 1977.

National Institute of Child Health and Human Development: Randomized, controlled trial of phototherapy for neonatal hyperbilirubinemia. Pediatrics (Suppl)75:385, 1985.

Nilsen ST, Finne PH, Bergsjo P, et al: Males with neonatal hyperbilirubinemia examined at 18 years of age. Acta Paediatr Scand 73:176, 1984.

Nwaesei CG, Aerde JV, Boyden M, et al: Changes in auditory brainstem responses in hyperbilirubinemic infants before and after exchange transfusion. Pediatrics 74:800, 1984.

Ritter DA, Kenny JD, Norton HJ, et al: A prospective study of free bilirubin and other risk factors in the development of kernicterus in premature infants. Pediatrics 69:260, 1982.

Scheidt PC, Mellito ED, Hardy JB, et al: Toxicity to bilirubin in neonates: Infant development during the first year in relation to maximum neonatal serum bilirubin concentration. J Pediatr 92:292, 1977.

Turkel S, Guttenberg M, Moynes D, et al: Lack of identifiable risk factors for kernicterus. Pediatrics 66:502, 1980.

Turkel S, Miller CA, Guttenberg M, et al: A clinical pathologic reappraisal of kernicterus. Pediatrics 69:267, 1982.

THE BLOOD

8.46 ANEMIA IN THE NEWBORN INFANT

The normal cord hemoglobin is 14–20 g/dL (HCT 43–63%) at term birth and 1–2 g/dL less in 28–30 wk premature infants. Determinations of less than the normal range for birthweight and postnatal age are defined as anemia (Tables 29–2 and 14–3).

Anemia at birth is manifest by pallor, congestive heart failure, or shock (Fig. 8–25). It is usually caused by hemolytic disease of the newborn but may also be the result of tearing or cutting of the umbilical cord during delivery, abnormal cord insertions, communicating placental vessels, placenta previa or abruptio, or hemorrhage from the fetal side of the placenta. The last may be caused by accidental incision of the placenta in the course of cesarean section or by so-called transplacental hemorrhage. Anemia at birth may also occur in one of twins with conjoined placental circulation, in which case the anemic twin "bleeds into" the other twin. Rarely, scalp blood sampling for fetal distress may result in anemia.

Transplacental hemorrhage, with bleeding from the fetal into the maternal circulation, is probably more common than is generally recognized and, unless severe, is usually not sufficient to cause clinically apparent anemia at birth. The cause of transplacental hemorrhage is not clear, but its occurrence has been proved by demonstrating significant amounts of fetal hemoglobin and red cells in the maternal blood on the day of delivery.

Acute blood loss usually results in severe distress at birth, initially with normal hemoglobin level, no hepatosplenomegaly, and the early onset of shock. In contrast, chronic blood loss in utero produces marked pallor, less distress, low hemoglobin level with microcytic indices, and, if severe, congestive heart failure.

Anemia appearing in the first few days after birth is also most frequently the result of hemolytic disease of the newborn. Other causes are hemorrhagic disease of the newborn, bleeding from an improperly tied or clamped umbilical cord, large

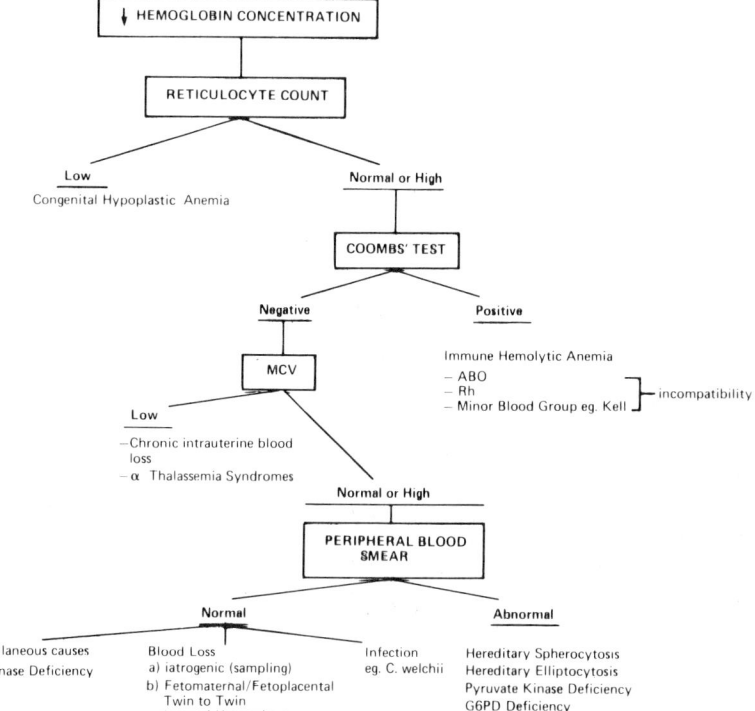

Figure 8–25. Diagnostic approach to anemia in the newborn infant. (From Blanchette V, Zipursky A: Clin Perinatol 11:489, 1984.)

cephalohematoma, intracranial hemorrhage, or subcapsular bleeding from rupture of the liver, spleen, adrenals, or kidneys. Rapid decreases in hemoglobin or hematocrit values during the first few days of life may be the initial clue to these conditions.

Later in the neonatal period delayed anemia from hemolytic disease of the newborn, with or without exchange transfusion or phototherapy, may be seen. Vitamin K (as Synkayvite) in large doses may cause anemia in premature infants, which is characterized by inclusion bodies (Heinz bodies) in the erythrocytes. Congenital hemolytic anemia (spherocytosis) occasionally appears during the first month of life, and hereditary nonspherocytic hemolytic anemia has been described during the neonatal period secondary to deficiency of such enzymes as G-6-PD and pyruvate kinase. Bleeding from hemangiomas of the upper gastrointestinal tract or from ulcers caused by aberrant gastric mucosa in a Meckel diverticulum or duplication is a rare source of anemia in the newborn. Repeated blood sampling of infants requiring frequent monitoring of blood gases and chemistries may also produce anemia. Deficiency of minerals such as copper may cause anemia in infants on total parenteral nutrition.

A further "physiologic" decrease in hemoglobin content is noticed at 8–12 wk in term infants (hemoglobin 11 g/dL) and at about 6 wk in premature infants (7–10 g/dL). Treatment of any significant anemia (less than 8 g of hemoglobin/dL) present at or shortly after birth consists not only in eliminating its cause, if it is still present, but also in transfusing small amounts of packed red blood cells (10–15 mL/kg; 2 mL/kg raises hemoglobin about 1 g/dL).

8.47 HEMOLYTIC DISEASE OF THE NEWBORN
(Erythroblastosis Fetalis)

Erythroblastosis fetalis results from the transplacental passage of maternal antibody active against red cell antigens of the infant, leading to an increased rate of red cell destruction. It continues to be an important cause of anemia and jaundice in newborn infants despite the development of a method of prevention of maternal isoimmunization by Rh antigens. Although more than 60 different red cell antigens capable of eliciting an antibody response in a suitable recipient have been identified, significant disease is associated primarily with the D antigen of the Rh group and with incompatibility of ABO factors. Rarely, hemolytic disease may be caused by C or E antigens or by other red cell antigens, such as C^w, C^x, D^u, K(Kell), M, Duffy, S, and Kidd. Anti-Lewis antibodies do not cause disease.

Hemolytic Disease of the Newborn Due to Rh Incompatibility

The Rh antigenic determinants are genetically transmitted from each parent and determine the Rh type and direct the production of a number of blood group factors (C, c, D, d, E, and e). Each factor can elicit a specific antibody response under suitable conditions; 90% are due to D, the remaining to C or E.

Pathogenesis. Isoimmune hemolytic disease from D antigen is approximately three times more frequent in whites than in blacks. When Rh positive blood is infused into an Rh negative woman through error or when small quantities (usually more than 1 mL) of Rh positive fetal blood containing D antigen inherited from an Rh positive father enter the maternal circulation during pregnancy, with spontaneous or induced abortion, or at delivery, antibody formation against D may be induced in the unsensitized Rh negative recipient mother. Once immunization has occurred, considerably smaller doses

of antigen can stimulate an increase in antibody titer. Initially, a rise of antibody in the 19S gamma globulin fraction occurs, which later is replaced by 7S (IgG) antibody; the latter readily crosses the placenta, causing hemolytic manifestations.

Hemolytic disease rarely occurs during a first pregnancy, since transfusions of Rh positive fetal blood into an Rh negative mother tend to occur near the time of delivery, too late for the mother to become sensitized to transmit antibody to the infant before delivery. The fact that 55% of Rh positive fathers are heterozygous (D/d) and may have Rh negative offspring and that only 50% of pregnancies have fetal to maternal transfusions reduces the chance of sensitization as does small family size, in which the opportunities for its occurrence are fewer. Finally, the capacity of Rh negative women to form antibodies is variable, some producing low titers even after adequate antigenic challenge. Thus, the overall incidence of isoimmunization of Rh negative mothers at risk is low, with antibody to D detected in less than 10% of those studied, even after five or more pregnancies; only about 5% ever have babies having hemolytic disease.

When mother and fetus are also incompatible with respect to groups A or B, the mother is protected to a degree against sensitization by the rapid removal of Rh positive cells from her circulation by her anti-A or anti-B, which are IgM antibodies and which do not cross the placenta. Once the mother is sensitized, the infant is likely to have hemolytic disease. There is a tendency for the severity of the illness to worsen with successive pregnancies. The possibility that the first affected infant after sensitization may represent the end of the mother's child-bearing potential for Rh positive infants argues urgently for the prevention of sensitization when this is possible. Such prevention consists of injection into the mother of anti-D gamma globulin (RhoGam) immediately following the delivery of each Rh positive infant (see below).

Clinical Manifestations. A wide spectrum of hemolytic disease occurs in affected infants born to sensitized mothers, depending on the nature of the individual immune response. The severity of the disease may range from only laboratory evidence of mild hemolysis (15% of cases) to severe anemia with compensatory hyperplasia of erythropoietic tissue, leading to massive enlargement of the liver and spleen. When the compensatory capacity of the hematopoietic system is exceeded, profound anemia results in pallor, signs of cardiac decompensation (hepatosplenomegaly, respiratory distress), massive anasarca, and circulatory collapse. This clinical picture, termed **hydrops fetalis,** frequently results in death in utero or shortly after birth; it may also occur from other etiologies (Table 8–22). Failure to initiate spontaneous effective ventilation owing to pulmonary edema or bilateral pleural effusions results in birth asphyxia; following successful resus-

---

Table 8–22. Etiologies of Hydrops Fetalis

Hematologic: Rh incompatibility, rarer blood group incompatibility, α-thalassemia, twin-twin transfusion, feto-maternal hemorrhage
Infections: syphilis, cytomegalovirus, toxoplasmosis, Chagas disease, leptospirosis
Cardiovascular: paroxysmal atrial tachycardia, congestive heart failure, arteriovenous malformation, umbilical vein thrombosis
Tumors: congenital neuroblastoma, placental chorioangioma
Pulmonary: pulmonary lymphangiectasia, cystic adenomatoid malformation, hypoplasia
Hepatorenal: hepatitis, nephrosis, renal vein thrombosis, urethral atresia
Metabolic: maternal diabetes mellitus, Gaucher disease, achondroplasia
Idiopathic
Multiple severe congenital anomalies

citation, severe respiratory distress may ensue. Petechiae, purpura, and thrombocytopenia may also be present in severe cases reflecting decreased platelet production or the presence of concurrent disseminated intravascular coagulation.

Jaundice is usually absent at birth because of placental clearance of lipid-soluble unconjugated bilirubin, but in severe cases bilirubin pigments stain the amniotic fluid, cord, and vernix caseosa yellow. Icterus is generally evident within the first day of life since the infant's bilirubin-conjugating and excretory systems are unable to cope with the load resulting from massive hemolysis. Indirect-reacting bilirubin therefore accumulates postnatally and may rapidly reach extremely high levels which represent a significant risk of bilirubin encephalopathy. There may be a greater risk of developing kernicterus from hemolytic disease than from comparable nonhemolytic hyperbilirubinemia, although the risk in an individual patient may only be a function of the severity of illness (anoxia, acidosis, and so on). Hypoglycemia occurs frequently in infants with severe isoimmune hemolytic disease and may be related to hyperinsulinism and hypertrophy of the pancreatic islet cells in these infants.

The availability of techniques for improved intrauterine diagnosis of the severity of disease in an affected fetus has led to the development of obstetric criteria for induced premature delivery. This development has decreased the incidence of fetal death from the disease and increased the frequency of premature infants with clinical erythroblastosis, who also have the added risk of neurologic damage from the combination of immaturity and hyperbilirubinemia.

Infants born after intrauterine transfusion for prenatally diagnosed erythroblastosis are generally severely affected, since the indications for the transfusion are evidence of already severe disease in utero. Such infants usually have very high (but extremely variable) cord levels of bilirubin, which reflects the severity of hemolysis and its effects on hepatic function. Anemia from continuing hemolysis may be masked by the prior intrauterine transfusion, and the clinical manifestations of erythroblastosis may be superimposed upon various degrees of immaturity due to spontaneous or induced premature delivery.

Laboratory Data. Prior to treatment, the direct Coombs test is usually positive. Anemia is usual. The cord blood hemoglobin varies, usually proportionally to the severity of the disease; with hydrops fetalis it may be as low as 3–4 g/dL. Alternatively, despite hemolysis, it may be within the normal range owing to compensatory bone marrow activity. The blood smear usually shows polychromasia and a marked increase in nucleated red blood cells. The reticulocyte count is increased. The white blood cell count is usually normal but may be elevated, and there may be thrombocytopenia in severe cases. The cord bilirubin is usually between 3–5 mg/dL; only rarely is there a substantial elevation of direct-reacting (conjugated) bilirubin. The indirect-reacting bilirubin rises rapidly to high levels in the first 6 hr of life.

After intrauterine transfusions the cord blood may show a normal hemoglobin concentration, negative direct Coombs test, predominantly type O Rh negative adult red cells, and a relatively normal smear. Marked elevation of both indirect- and direct-reacting bilirubin levels has been reported in these infants.

Diagnosis. The definitive diagnosis of erythroblastosis fetalis requires demonstration of blood group incompatibility and of corresponding antibody bound to the infant's red cells.

Antenatal Diagnosis. In Rh negative women a history of previous transfusions, abortion, or pregnancy should suggest the possibility of sensitization. Expectant parents' blood types should be tested for potential incompatibility and the maternal titer of IgG antibodies to D should be assayed at 12–16, 28–32, and 36 wk. The presence of measurable antibody titer at the beginning of pregnancy, a rapid rise in titer, or a titer of 1:64 or greater suggests significant hemolytic disease, although the exact titer correlates poorly with the severity of disease. If a mother is found to have antibody against D at a titer of 1:16 or greater at any time during a subsequent pregnancy, the severity of fetal disease should be monitored by amniocentesis. Higher titers suggest a more severely affected fetus and the need for earlier amniocentesis. If there is a history of a previously affected infant and/or a stillbirth, an Rh positive infant is usually equally or more severely affected than the previous infant, and the severity of disease in the fetus should be followed by serial amniocenteses. Ultrasonography is indicated to determine if there is hydrops fetalis.

Amniocentesis. Spectrophotometric analysis of bilirubin pigments in amniotic fluid obtained by direct transabdominal uterine aspiration after placental localization by ultrasound has proved to be a generally safe and reliable way of predicting the severity and progress of fetal hemolysis. In the affected fetus there is a positive deviation from the normal straight line curve of optical density of the amniotic fluid, measured at wavelengths from 350–700 nm and plotted on semilogarithmic paper. The peak of density deviation from the normal occurs at 450 nm (ΔOD450) and is used as an index of the risk of intrauterine death and severity of anemia when plotted against gestational age and compared with the outcome of a population of affected infants. The risk is categorized by "zones"; the infants at highest risk are in zone 3.

Postnatal Diagnosis. Immediately after the birth of any infant to an Rh negative woman, blood from the umbilical cord or from the infant should be examined for ABO blood group, Rh type, hematocrit and hemoglobin, and reaction of the direct Coombs test. If the Coombs test is positive, baseline serum bilirubin should be measured, and a commercially available red cell panel should be used to identify red cell antibodies that are present in the mother's serum, both of which are done not only to establish the diagnosis but also to ensure the selection of the most compatible blood for exchange transfusion, should it be necessary. The direct Coombs test is usually strongly positive in clinically affected infants and may remain so for a few days up to several months.

Treatment. The main goals of therapy are (1) to prevent intrauterine or extrauterine death from severe anemia and its complications and (2) to avoid neurotoxicity from hyperbilirubinemia.

Treatment of the Unborn Infant. The survival of moderately and severely affected fetuses has been markedly improved by inducing labor between 33–34 wk when repeated amniocenteses show flat or rising ΔOD450's in high zone 2 or zone 3. When the chance is small that a severely affected fetus will survive to a gestational age compatible with early delivery and neonatal survival, an intrauterine intraperitoneal or intraumbilical venous transfusion of erythrocytes compatible with the mother's blood may be indicated. A judgment must be made whether, at a particular gestational age, the risk of death from erythroblastosis or from premature delivery is greater than the risk of death during or immediately following the procedure. Additional indications for intrauterine transfusion include several optical density readings in zone 3, especially if the trend is increasing and there is a family history of stillbirths, hydrops fetalis, or severely affected infants. Some use hydrops fetalis as an indication for intrauterine transfusion.

Treatment of the Liveborn Infant. The birth should be attended by the physician who will care for the affected infant afterward. Fresh, low titer, group O, Rh negative blood, cross-matched against the maternal serum, should be immediately available. If clinical signs of severe hemolytic anemia (pallor, hepatosplenomegaly, edema, petechiae, or ascites) are evident at birth, immediate supportive therapy, temperature stabilization, and monitoring before proceeding with exchange transfusion may save some severely affected infants, though hydropic babies rarely survive. Such therapy should include correction of acidosis with 1–2 mEq/kg of sodium bicarbonate; a small transfusion of compatible packed red cells to correct anemia; volume expansion for hypotension, especially in those with hydrops; and provision of assisted ventilation for respiratory failure.

Exchange Transfusion. When the infant's clinical condition at birth does not require an immediate full or partial exchange transfusion, the decision to perform one should be based on a judgment that there is a high risk of rapidly developing a dangerous degree of anemia or of hyperbilirubinemia. The predictive criteria for this judgment include a cord blood hemoglobin of 10 mg/dL or less, verified by an equally low capillary blood hemoglobin (which tends to be higher than that of cord or venous blood), or a cord bilirubin of 5 mg/dL or greater. Some physicians consider previous kernicterus or severe erythroblastosis in a sibling, reticulocyte counts greater than 15%, and prematurity to be further factors supporting a decision for early exchange transfusion.

The hemoglobin, hematocrit, and serum bilirubin levels should be measured at 4–6 hr intervals at first, with extension to longer intervals if and as the rate of change diminishes. The decision to perform an exchange transfusion is based on the likelihood that the trend of bilirubin levels plotted against hours of age indicates that the serum bilirubin will reach the level indicated in Table 8–21, above which there is an increased risk of kernicterus. Ordinary transfusions of compatible Rh negative red cells may be necessary to correct anemia at any stage of the disease up to 6–8 wk of age when the infant's own blood-forming mechanism may be expected to take over. Weekly determinations of hemoglobin or hematocrit should be done until a spontaneous rise has been demonstrated.

Careful monitoring of the serum bilirubin level is essential until a falling trend has been demonstrated in the absence of phototherapy (Sec. 8.45). Even then, an occasional infant, particularly if premature, may experience an unpredicted significant rise in serum bilirubin as late as the 7th day of life. Attempts to predict the attainment of dangerously high levels of serum bilirubin, based on observed levels exceeding 6 mg/dL in the first 6 hr or 10 mg/dL in the second 6 hr of life or on rates of rise exceeding 0.5–1.0 mg/dL/hr, can be unreliable. Indices of free bilirubin and bilirubin binding have not yet been shown to be routinely reliable aids in evaluating the risk associated with hyperbilirubinemia.

Blood for exchange transfusion should be as fresh as possible. Heparin or citrate-phosphate-dextrose (CPD) may be used as anticoagulants. If the blood is obtained before delivery, it should be taken from a type O, Rh negative donor with a low titer of anti-A and anti-B and should be compatible with the mother's serum by indirect Coombs test. After delivery, blood should be obtained from an Rh negative donor whose cells are compatible with both the infant's and the mother's serum; when possible, type O donor cells are usually employed, but cells of the infant's ABO blood type may be used when the mother has the same type. A complete crossmatch, including indirect Coombs test, should be performed prior to the second and subsequent transfusions. Blood should be gradually warmed to and maintained at a temperature between 35 and 37° C throughout the exchange transfusion. It should be kept well mixed by gentle squeezing or agitation of the bag to avoid sedimentation; otherwise, the use of supernatant serum with a low red cell count at the end of the exchange will leave the infant anemic. Whole blood should be used rather than packed red cells. The infant's stomach should be emptied prior to transfusion to prevent aspiration,

body temperature should be maintained, and vital signs monitored. A competent assistant should be present to help monitor, tally the volume of blood exchanged, and perform emergency procedures.

The umbilical vein is cannulated, using strict aseptic technique, with a polyvinyl catheter to a distance no greater than 7 cm in a full-term infant. When free flow of blood is obtained, the catheter is usually in a large hepatic vein or the inferior vena cava. Exchange should be carried out over a 45–60 min period, alternating aspirations of 20 mL of infant blood and infusions of 20 mL of donor blood. Smaller aliquots (5–10 mL) may be indicated for sick and premature infants. The goal should be an exchange of approximately 2 blood volumes of the infant (2×85 mL/kg). If heparinized blood is used, 0.45 mL (4.5 mg) of a 1% solution of protamine sulfate may be injected intravenously at the conclusion of the transfusion for each dL of blood exchanged.

Administering albumin before an exchange transfusion is not recommended because of conflicting results concerning the increased efficiency of bilirubin removal that may result, the risk of redistribution of bilirubin from areas of innocuous deposition into the nervous system, the potential bilirubin-displacing effect of stabilizers added to injectable preparations of human serum albumin, the risk of resulting hypervolemia, and the increased difficulty in interpreting subsequent bilirubin levels that results from albumin-binding of bilirubin in the vascular space.

The venous pressure should be measured intermittently during an exchange transfusion if the catheter is in the vena cava; elevated umbilical venous pressure (higher than 10 cm H_2O) may occur among infants with severe hemolytic disease and hydrops fetalis or those born after intrauterine transfusions. This may represent congestive heart failure. The pressure is usually falsely elevated as the result of faulty catheter placement, pulmonary disease, or high intra-abdominal pressure from ascites. Direct or indirect measurement of blood pressure is important for detecting hypovolemic hypotension or in diagnosing hypertension which may occasionally occur with exchange transfusion.

Infants with acidosis and hypoxia from respiratory distress, sepsis, or shock may be further compromised by the significant acute acid load contained in citrated (CPD) blood which usually has a pH between 6–7. The subsequent metabolism of citrate may result in a later metabolic alkalosis if CPD blood is used. Fresh heparinized blood avoids this problem. However, blood exposed to radiant heat during transfusion may become acidotic and hemolysed, resulting in a decreased hematocrit and an increased potassium concentration. During the exchange, the blood pH and paO_2 should be serially monitored, since infants often become acidotic and hypoxic during exchange transfusions. Symptomatic hypoglycemia may occur before or during exchange transfusion in moderately to severely affected infants; it may also occur 1–3 hr after exchange.

After exchange transfusion the bilirubin level must be determined at frequent intervals (every 4–8 hr), as bilirubin may rebound 40–50% within hours. Repeated exchange transfusions should be carried out to keep the indirect fraction from exceeding the levels indicated in Table 8–21. Symptoms suggestive of kernicterus are mandatory indications for exchange transfusion at any time.

The risk of death from exchange transfusion performed by experienced physicians is less than 1%. However, with the decreasing use of this procedure because the use of phototherapy is prevalent and because sensitization is being prevented, the general level of competence is decreasing. Thus, it may be best to concentrate this mode of treatment in neonatal referral centers.

Late Complications. The infant with hemolytic disease

and/or who has had an exchange or an intrauterine transfusion must be observed carefully for the development of anemia and cholestasis. Treatment with supplemental iron and/or blood transfusion may be indicated. A mild graft-versus-host syndrome may be manifested as diarrhea, rash, hepatitis, and eosinophilia.

Inspissated bile syndrome refers to the rare occurrence of persistent icterus in association with significant elevations of direct as well as indirect bilirubin in infants with hemolytic disease. The cause is unclear but the jaundice clears spontaneously within a few weeks or months.

Portal vein thrombosis may occur among children who have been subjected to exchange transfusion as newborn infants. It is probably associated with prolonged, traumatic, or septic umbilical vein catheterization.

Prevention of Rh Sensitization. The risk of initial sensitization of Rh negative mothers has been reduced from between 10–20% to less than 1% by intramuscular injection of 300 μg of human anti-D globulin (1 mL of RhoGAM) within 72 hr of delivery or abortion. This quantity is sufficient to eliminate approximately 10 mL of potentially antigenic fetal cells from the maternal circulation. Large fetal-to-maternal transfer of blood may require proportionately more RhoGAM, which, when administered at 28–32 wk and again at birth (40 wk), may be more effective. The use of this technique, combined with improved methods of detecting maternal sensitization and quantitating the extent of the fetal to maternal transfusion, plus the use of fewer obstetric procedures that increase the risk of such fetal to maternal bleeding (versions, manual separation of the placenta, and so on) should further reduce the incidence of erythroblastosis fetalis.

Hemolytic Disease of the Newborn Due to A and B Incompatibility

Major blood group incompatibility between mother and fetus usually results in milder disease than does Rh incompatibility. Maternal antibody may be formed against B cells if the mother is type A or against A cells if the mother is type B. However, usually the mother is Type O and the infant is A or B. Although ABO incompatibility occurs in 20–25% of pregnancies, hemolytic disease develops in only 10% of such offspring and usually the infants are of type A_1, which is more antigenic than A_2. Low antigenicity of the ABO factors in the fetus and newborn infant may account for the low incidence of severe ABO hemolytic disease relative to the incidence of incompatibility between the blood groups of mother and child. Although antibodies against A and B factors occur without prior immunization ("natural" antibodies), these are ordinarily present in the 19S (IgM) fraction of gamma globulin, which does not cross the placenta. However, univalent, incomplete (albumin active) antibodies to A antigen may be present in the 7S (IgG) fraction, which does cross the placenta, so that A–O isoimmune hemolytic disease may be seen in firstborn infants. Mothers who have become immunized against A or B factors from a previous incompatible pregnancy also exhibit antibody in the 7S gamma globulin fraction. These "immune" antibodies are the primary mediators in ABO isoimmune disease.

Clinical Manifestations. Most cases are mild, with jaundice as the only clinical manifestation. The infant is not generally affected at birth; pallor is not present and hydrops fetalis is extremely rare. Liver and spleen are not greatly enlarged, if at all. Jaundice usually appears during the first 24 hr. Rarely, it may become severe with symptoms and signs of kernicterus rapidly developing.

Diagnosis. A presumptive diagnosis is based on the presence of ABO incompatibility, a weakly to moderately positive direct Coombs test, and spherocytes in the blood smear,

which may at times suggest the presence of hereditary spherocytosis. Hyperbilirubinemia is often the only other laboratory abnormality. The hemoglobin level is usually normal but may be as low as 10–12 g/dL. Reticulocytes may be increased to 10–15%, with extensive polychromasia and increased numbers of nucleated red cells. In 10–20% of affected infants the unconjugated serum bilirubin level may reach 20 mg/dL or more unless phototherapy is employed.

Treatment. Phototherapy may be effective in lowering serum bilirubin levels (Sec. 8.45). Otherwise, treatment is directed at correcting dangerous degrees of anemia or hyperbilirubinemia by exchange transfusions with blood of the same group as that of the mother (Rh type should match the infant's). The indications for this procedure are similar to those previously described for hemolytic disease due to Rh incompatibility.

Other Forms of Hemolytic Disease

Blood group incompatibilities other than Rh or ABO (c, E, Kell [K], and so on) account for less than 5% of hemolytic disease of the newborn. The direct Coombs test is invariably positive, and exchange transfusion may be indicated for hyperbilirubinemia and anemia. Congenital infections, such as cytomegalic inclusion disease, toxoplasmosis, rubella, and syphilis, may present with hemolytic anemia, jaundice, hepatosplenomegaly, and thrombocytopenia, but the direct Coombs test is negative, and there are usually other distinguishing clinical findings. Homozygous α-thalassemia may present with severe hemolytic anemia and a clinical picture resembling hydrops fetalis; it can be distinguished by a negative direct Coombs test and characteristic clinical and laboratory findings (Sec. 15.23–15.26). Anemia and jaundice may occur in infancy from hereditary spherocytosis (Sec. 15.13) and, if untreated, can result in kernicterus. Hemolytic anemia producing jaundice in the first week of life may also be secondary to congenital deficiencies in red cell enzymes, such as pyruvate kinase or glucose-6-phosphate dehydrogenase (G-6-PD).

8.48 PLETHORA IN THE NEWBORN INFANT
(Polycythemia)

See also Sec. 15.30.

Plethora or apparent cyanosis associated with abnormally high hemoglobin and hematocrit values has been reported with and without clinical findings suggestive of placental insufficiency syndrome. Polycythemia is defined as a central hematocrit value of 65% or more. Anorexia, lethargy, cyanosis, and convulsions may appear on the 2nd and 3rd days of life. Hyperbilirubinemia, necrotizing enterocolitis, respiratory distress, and persistent fetal circulation are associated problems. The pathophysiology of the condition is not clear but may, in part, be related to the increased viscosity of the blood. Plethora may also be due to a "placental transfusion" in the recipient twin of monozygotic twins with parabiotic placental circulations. It also may occur in large "cushingoid" infants of diabetic mothers, Down syndrome, adrenogenital syndrome, neonatal Graves syndrome, and Beckwith syndrome.

The *treatment* of symptomatic plethora of the newborn is phlebotomy and replacement with saline or albumin. A partial exchange transfusion to reduce the hematocrit to 50% is a technically simpler and therapeutically more effective approach. The volume exchanged is calculated from the formula:

$$\text{Volume of exchange (mL)} = \text{Blood volume} \times \frac{\text{Observed} - \text{desired HCT}}{\text{Observed HCT}}$$

8.49 HEMORRHAGE IN THE NEWBORN INFANT

Hemorrhagic Disease of the Newborn. A moderate decrease of factors II, VII, IX, and X normally occurs in all newborn infants by 48–72 hr after birth, with a gradual return to birth levels by 7–10 days of age. This transient deficiency of vitamin K–dependent factors probably is due to lack of free vitamin K in the mother, immaturity of the infant's liver, and absence of bacterial intestinal flora normally responsible for synthesis of vitamin K. Rarely among term infants and more frequently among premature infants there is an accentuation and prolongation of this deficiency between the 2nd and 5th days of life, resulting in spontaneous and prolonged bleeding. Breast milk is a poor source of vitamin K, and hemorrhagic complications have appeared more commonly in breast-fed than cow's milk–fed infants. This form of hemorrhagic disease of the newborn, which is responsive to vitamin K therapy, must be distinguished from disseminated intravascular coagulopathy and from rarer congenital deficiencies of one or more of the other vitamin K–dependent factors or of factor V which are unresponsive to vitamin K (Sec. 15.45).

Hemorrhagic disease of the newborn resulting from severe transient deficiencies of vitamin K–dependent factors is characterized by bleeding that tends to be gastrointestinal, nasal, subgaleal, intracranial, or a result of circumcision. The prothrombin time, blood coagulation time, and partial thromboplastin time are prolonged, and the levels of prothrombin (II) and factors VII, IX, and X are significantly decreased. Bleeding time, fibrinogen, factors V and VIII, platelets, capillary fragility, and clot retraction are normal for maturity. Administering 1 mg of natural oil-soluble vitamin K intramuscularly at the time of birth prevents the fall in vitamin K–dependent factors in full-term infants but is not uniformly effective in the prophylaxis of hemorrhagic disease of the newborn in premature infants. The disease may be effectively treated with an intravenous infusion of 1–5 mg of vitamin K_1, with improvement of coagulation defects and cessation of bleeding within a few hr. However, serious bleeding, particularly in premature infants or those with liver disease, may require a transfusion of fresh frozen plasma or whole blood. The mortality rate is low among treated patients.

A particularly severe form of deficiency of vitamin K–dependent coagulation factors has been reported in infants born to mothers receiving anticonvulsive medications during pregnancy (phenobarbital and phenytoin). There may be severe bleeding with onset within the first 24 hr of life, usually corrected by vitamin K_1, although in some the response is poor or delayed. A prothrombin time (PT) should be obtained on cord blood and the infants given 1–2 mg of vitamin K intravenously. If the PT is greatly prolonged and fails to improve, then 10 mL/kg of fresh frozen plasma should be given.

Concentrated forms of vitamin K–dependent coagulation factors should be avoided in this group of infants because they may carry considerable risk of transmitting serum hepatitis.

Other forms of bleeding may be clinically indistinguishable from hemorrhagic disease of the newborn responsive to vitamin K but are neither prevented nor successfully treated with it. A clinical pattern identical to that of hemorrhagic disease of the newborn may also result from any of the **congenital defects in blood coagulation** (Sec. 15.43–15.46). Hematomas, melena, and postcircumcision and umbilical cord bleeding may be present; only 5–35% of factor VIII and IX deficiencies become clinically apparent in the newborn period. Treatment of the rare congenital deficiencies of prothrombin and factors V, VII, and X requires fresh whole blood or specific factor replacement.

Disseminated intravascular coagulopathy in newborn infants results in consumption of coagulation factors and bleeding. The infants are often premature; the clinical course is frequently characterized by hypoxia, acidosis, shock, hemangiomas, or infection. Treatment is directed at correcting the primary clinical problem, such as infection, and at interrupting consumption and replacing clotting factors. The prognosis is poor regardless of therapy (Sec. 15.50).

Infants with central nervous system or other bleeding constituting an *immediate threat to life* should receive a small transfusion of fresh, compatible whole blood or plasma, as well as vitamin K, as soon as possible after blood has been drawn for coagulation studies, which should include determining the number of platelets.

The so-called **swallowed blood syndrome,** in which blood or bloody stools are passed, usually on the 2nd or 3rd day of life, may be confused with hemorrhage from the gastrointestinal tract. The blood may be swallowed during delivery or from a fissure in the mother's nipple. Differentiation from gastrointestinal hemorrhage is based on the fact that the infant's blood contains mostly fetal hemoglobin, which is alkali-resistant, whereas swallowed blood from a maternal source contains adult hemoglobin, which is promptly changed to alkaline hematin upon the addition of alkali. Apt devised the following test for this differentiation:

(1) Rinse a bloodstained diaper or some grossly bloody stool with a suitable amount of water to obtain a distinctly pink supernatant hemoglobin solution. (2) Centrifuge the mixture. Decant the supernatant solution. (3) To 5 parts of the supernatant fluid add 1 part of 0.25 normal (1%) sodium hydroxide. Within 1–2 min a color reaction takes place: a yellow-brown color indicates that the blood is maternal in origin; a persistent pink, that it is from the infant. A control test with known adult or infant blood, or both, is advisable.

Widespread **subcutaneous ecchymoses** in premature infants at or immediately after birth are apparently a result of fragile superficial blood vessels rather than of a coagulation defect. Administering vitamin K_1 to the mother during labor has no effect on their incidence. Occasionally, an infant is born with petechiae or a generalized bluish suffusion limited to the face, head, and neck, which are probably the result of venous obstruction caused by sudden increases in intrathoracic pressure during delivery. It may take 2–3 wk for such suffusions to disappear.

Neonatal Thrombocytopenic Purpura. See Sec. 15.48.

Barnard D: Inherited bleeding disorders in the newborn infant. Clin Perinatol 11:309, 1984.

Blanchette V, Zipursky A: Assessment of anemia in newborn infants. Clin Perinatol 11:489, 1984.

Chaou W, Chou M, Eitzman DV: Intracranial hemorrhage and vitamin K deficiency in early infancy. J Pediatr 105:880, 1984.

Desjardins L, Blaychman M, Chintu C, et al: The spectrum of ABO hemolytic disease of the newborn infant. J Pediatr 95:447, 1979.

Grannum P, Copel J, Plaxe S, et al: In utero exchange transfusion by direct intravascular injection in severe erythroblastosis fetalis. N Engl J Med 314:1431, 1986.

Gross S, Stuart M: Hemostasis in the premature infant. Clin Perinatol 4:259, 1977.

Holzgreve W, Curry C, Golbus M, et al: Investigation of nonimmune hydrops fetalis. Am J Obstet Gynecol 150:805, 1984.

Lane PA, Hathaway WE: Vitamin K in infancy. J Pediatr 106:351, 1985.

Liley AW: Liquor amnii analysis in management of pregnancy complicated by rhesus sensitization. Am J Obstet Gynecol 82:1359, 1961.

Motohara K, Matsukura M, Matsuda I, et al: Severe vitamin K deficiency in breast-fed infants. J Pediatr 105:943, 1984.

Mountain KR, Hirsch J, Gallus AS: Neonatal coagulation defect due to anticonvulsant drug treatment in pregnancy. Lancet 1:265, 1970.

Peddle L: The antepartum management of the Rh sensitive woman. Clin Perinatol 11:251, 1984.

Phibbs RH, Johnson P, Kitterman JA, et al: Cardio-respiratory status of erythroblastotic newborn infants; III. Intravascular pressures during the first hours of life. Pediatrics 58:484, 1976.

8.50 GENITOURINARY SYSTEM

See also Chapter 17.

One or both kidneys are often easily palpable in the newborn infant. When both are palpable and similar, there is usually no particular diagnostic problem, but when only one kidney can be felt, the impression that it is larger than normal or is displaced by an intrinsic or extrinsic mass frequently arises. Fetal lobulation may contribute to this impression. Usually the problem resolves itself as the kidney becomes progressively less easily palpable during the early months of life. Since palpable enlargement or displacement of the kidney in the newborn may be due to hydronephrosis, neuroblastoma or an embryoma, or a cystic malformation, ultrasound examination is indicated. During the neonatal period moderate elevation of the blood urea nitrogen does not necessarily signify renal disease, and elevations may occur in association with polycystic disease and hydronephrosis without necessarily implying a poor prognosis. The urine may also contain casts and cellular elements simply as a manifestation of dehydration.

Thrombosis of the Renal Vein. See Sec. 8.56.

8.51 THE CRANIUM

See Anencephaly, Microcephaly, Craniosynostosis, and Hydrocephalus in Chapter 21.

8.52 THE SKIN

Skin disorders of the newborn are covered in Chapter 24.

Mastitis Neonatorum. Engorgement of the breasts is physiologic in newborn infants. Infection may be initiated by undue manipulation of the breasts and is manifest by redness, local heat, swelling, and pain. Fever and other general symptoms may also be present. The prognosis is favorable unless septicemia develops. *Staphylococcus aureus* and *Escherichia coli* are causative agents. Prophylaxis consists in avoiding the manipulation of or other trauma to the engorged breasts. Treatment includes systemic antibiotic therapy and hot compresses applied locally. If an abscess develops, it should be incised and drained.

Scar formation after infection may distort the nipple and impair the secretory power of the mammary gland in a female later in life.

THE EYE

See Chapter 25.

8.53 THE UMBILICUS

Umbilical Cord. The cord contains the two umbilical arteries, the vein, the rudimentary allantois, the remnant of the omphalomesenteric duct, and a gelatinous substance called Wharton jelly. The sheath of the umbilical cord is derived from the amnion. Its arteries have a strong contractile capacity; that of the vein is less so, since it retains a fairly large lumen after birth. When the cord sloughs, portions of these structures remain in the base. The blood vessels are functionally closed but are patent anatomically for 10–20 days. The arteries become the lateral umbilical ligaments; the vein, the ligamentum teres; and the ductus venosus, the ligamentum venosum. During this interval the umbilical vessels are potential portals of entry for infection. The umbilical cord usually sloughs

within 2 wk. *Delayed separation of the cord,* greater than 1 mo, has been associated with neutrophil chemotactic defects and overwhelming bacterial infection.

A **single umbilical artery** is present in about 5–10/1000 births; the frequency is about 35–70/1000 twin births. Approximately one third of infants with a single umbilical artery have congenital abnormalities, usually more than one, and many such infants are stillborn or die shortly after birth. Trisomy 18 is one of the more frequent abnormalities. Since many abnormalities are not apparent on gross physical examination, it is important that at every delivery the cut cord and the maternal and fetal surfaces of the placenta be inspected. The number of arteries present should be recorded as an aid to the early suspicion and identification of abnormalities in such infants.

Patency of the omphalomesenteric duct may be responsible for an intestinal fistula, prolapse of the bowel, polyp, or a Meckel diverticulum (Sec. 12.34).

A *persistent urachus* (urachal cyst) is due to failure of closure of the allantoic duct. Patency should be suspected if there is a clear, light yellow, urine-like discharge from the umbilicus.

Congenital Omphalocele. An omphalocele is a herniation or protrusion of abdominal contents into the base of the umbilical cord. In contrast to the more common umbilical hernia, the sac is covered with peritoneum without overlying skin. The size of the sac that lies outside the abdominal cavity depends on its contents. There is herniation of intestines into the cord in about 1 of 5000 births, and of liver and intestines in 1 of 10,000 births. The abdominal cavity is proportionately small, because the impetus to grow and develop is deficient. Immediate surgical repair, before infection has taken place and before the tissues have been damaged by drying or by rupture of the sac, is essential for survival. Silastic, Mersilene, or similar synthetic material may be used to cover the viscera if the sac has ruptured or if excessive mobilization of the skin would be necessary to cover the mass and its intact sac. Omphalocele, macrosomia, and hypoglycemia suggest Beckwith syndrome (Sec. 8.57).

Tumors. Tumors of the umbilicus are rare; they include angioma, enteroteratoma, dermoid cyst, myxosarcoma, and cysts of urachal or omphalomesenteric duct remnants.

Hemorrhage. Hemorrhage from the umbilical cord may be due to trauma, to inadequate ligation of the cord, or to failure of normal thrombus formation. It may also indicate hemorrhagic disease of the newborn, septicemia, or local infection. The infant should be observed frequently during the first few days of life so that, if hemorrhage does occur, it will be detected promptly.

Granuloma. The umbilical cord usually dries and separates within 6–8 days after birth. The raw surface becomes covered by a thin layer of skin, scar tissue forms, and the wound is usually healed within 12–15 days. The presence of saprophytic organisms delays separation of the cord and increases the possibility of invasion by pathogenic organisms. Mild infection may result in a moist granulating area at the base of the cord with a slight mucoid or mucopurulent discharge. Good results are usually obtained by cleansing with alcohol several times daily.

The persistence of exuberant granulation tissue at the base of the umbilicus is common. The tissue is soft, vascular and granular, and dull red or pink, and it may have a seropurulent secretion. The *treatment* is cauterization with silver nitrate; it should be repeated at intervals of several days until the base is dry.

Umbilical granuloma must be differentiated from **umbilical polyp,** a rare anomaly resulting from persistence of all or part of the omphalomesenteric duct or of the urachus. The tissue of the polyp is firm and resistant, bright red, and has a mucoid secretion. If there is a communication with the ileum or bladder, small amounts of fecal material or urine may be discharged intermittently. Histologically the polyp consists of intestinal or urinary tract mucosa. Treatment is surgical excision of the *entire* omphalomesenteric or urachal remnant.

Infections. Inflammation in the umbilical region, which may be caused by any of the pyogenic bacteria, is especially serious because of the danger of hematogenous spread or extension to the liver or peritoneum. Venous phlebitis may develop later, resulting in portal hypertension and cirrhosis. The general manifestations may be minimal even when septicemia or hepatitis has resulted. Daily baths or daily application of triple dye to the umbilical stump and surrounding skin may reduce the incidence of umbilical infection. *Treatment* includes prompt antibacterial therapy and, if there is abscess formation, surgical incision and drainage.

Umbilical Hernia. Often associated with diastasis recti, umbilical hernia is due to an imperfect closure or weakness of the umbilical ring. Common especially in low birthweight and black infants, it appears as a soft swelling covered by skin that protrudes during crying, coughing, or straining and can be reduced easily through the fibrous ring at the umbilicus. The hernia consists of omentum or portions of the small intestine. The size of the defect varies from less than 1 cm in diameter to as much as 5 cm, but large ones are rare.

Treatment. Few medical problems have given rise to more contradictory opinions and practices than has the management of umbilical hernia in infancy. Most umbilical hernias that appear before the age of 6 mo will disappear spontaneously by 1 yr of age. Even large hernias (5–6 cm in all dimensions) have been known to disappear spontaneously by 5–6 yr of age. Strangulation is extremely rare. There is considerable agreement that "strapping" is ineffective. Surgery is not advised unless the hernia persists to the age of 3–5 yr, causes symptoms, becomes strangulated, or becomes progressively larger after the age of 1–2 yr.

8.54 METABOLIC DISTURBANCES

HYPERTHERMIA IN THE NEWBORN
(Transitory Fever of the Newborn; Dehydration Fever)

Elevations of temperature (38–39° C or 100–103° F) are occasionally noted on the 2nd–3rd day of life in infants whose clinical course has been otherwise satisfactory. This disturbance is especially likely to occur in breast-fed infants whose intake of fluid has been particularly low or in infants exposed to high environmental temperatures, either in an incubator or in a bassinet near a radiator or in the sun.

The infant may be restless, and there may be a precipitous drop in weight. However, there may not be a consistent relation between the fever and the extent of weight loss or inadequacy of fluid intake. The urinary output and frequency of voiding diminish. The skin may lose some of its elasticity, and the fontanel may be depressed. The infant appears unhappy and takes fluids avidly. The apparent vigor of the infant contrasts with the usual appearance of "being sick" in the presence of infection. Rarely there may be marked tachypnea and tachycardia as the infant attempts to increase heat loss by way of the respiratory tract to compensate for a sudden increase in environmental temperature. The rise in temperature may be associated with an increase in serum protein and sodium and hematocrit. The possibility of local or systemic infection should be evaluated. Administering oral or parenteral fluids or lowering the environmental temperature leads to prompt reduction of the fever and alleviation of symptoms.

A *more severe form of neonatal hyperthermia* occurs among both newborn and older infants when they are warmly dressed for outdoor low temperatures that do not exist in their immediate indoor environment. The diminished sweating capacity of the newborn infant is a contributing factor. Warmly dressed infants left near stoves or radiators, traveling in well heated automobiles, or left with bright sunlight shining directly on them through the windows of a closed room or automobile are likely victims. Overclothing in hot weather, especially when the infant is left in the sun, is a less common cause. Body temperature is often as high as 41–44° C (106–111° F). The skin is hot and dry, and initially the infant usually appears flushed and apathetic. This stage may be followed by stupor, grayish pallor, coma, and convulsions. Hypernatremia may contribute to the convulsions. The mortality and morbidity rates (brain damage) are high. Hyperthermia has been associated with sudden infant death. The condition is prevented by dressing the infant in clothing suitable for the temperature of the *immediate* environment. In the newborn infant exposure of the body to usual room temperature or immersion in tepid water usually suffices to bring the temperature back to normal levels. Older infants may require cooling for a longer time by repeated immersions or by use of a water-cooled mattress or other apparatus for induction of hypothermia. Attention to possible fluid and electrolyte disturbance is essential.

NEONATAL COLD INJURY

Neonatal cold injury usually occurs among infants in inadequately heated homes during damp cold spells when the outside temperature is in the freezing range. The presenting features are apathy, refusal of food, oliguria, and coldness to touch. The body temperature is usually between 29.5–35° C (85–95° F), and immobility, edema, and redness of the extremities, especially of the hands, feet, and face, are observed. Bradycardia and apnea may also occur. The facial erythema frequently gives a false impression of health, delaying recognition that the infant is ill. Local hardening over areas of edema may lead to confusion with scleredema. Rhinitis is common, as are serious metabolic disturbances, particularly hypoglycemia and acidosis. Hemorrhagic manifestations are frequent; massive pulmonary hemorrhage is a common finding at autopsy. Treatment consists of warming with scrupulous attention to recognizing and correcting metabolic imbalances, particularly hypoglycemia. Prevention consists in providing adequate environmental heat. The mortality rate is about 25%; about 10% of the survivors have evidence of brain damage.

EDEMA

Generalized edema occurs in association with hydrops fetalis and in the offspring of diabetic mothers. In the premature infant edema is often a consequence of a decreased ability to excrete water or sodium, although some have considerable edema without identifiable reason. Infants with hyaline membrane disease may become edematous without congestive heart failure. Edema of the face and scalp may result from pressure from the umbilical cord around the neck, and transient localized swellings of the hands or feet may similarly be due to intrauterine pressures. Edema may be present with heart failure due to congenital cardiac lesions; a lag in renal excretion of electrolytes and water may result in edema when there has been a sudden, large increase in intake of electrolytes, particularly with feeding of concentrated cow's milk formulas. High protein formulas also may cause edema owing to the excessive solute load, particularly in premature infants. It is difficult to show a relation between low serum protein or low hemoglobin and the occurrence of edema in older premature infants. Edema also occurs in association with anemia and vitamin E deficiency in premature infants. Rarely, *idiopathic hypoproteinemia* with edema lasting weeks or months is observed in term infants. The cause is unclear, and the disturbance is benign. Persistent edema of one or more extremities may represent congenital lymphedema (Milroy disease) or, in females, *Turner syndrome*. Generalized edema with hypoproteinemia may be seen in the neonatal period with congenital nephrosis and rarely with Hurler syndrome or after feeding hypoallergenic formulas to infants with cystic fibrosis of the pancreas. *Sclerema* is described in Sec. 24.17.

HYPOCALCEMIA (TETANY)

See Sec. 5.33.

Osteopenia of Prematurity. Very small premature infants with chronic illnesses often develop a rickets-like syndrome with pathologic fractures and demineralized bones. There may be associated cholestasis and vitamin D or calcium malabsorption; urine calcium loss due to diuretics; and poor calcium, phosphorus, or vitamin D intake, or aluminum toxicity. The treatment of fractures requires immobilization and administration of calcium, phosphorus, and vitamin D. Appropriate formulas for prematures should provide a more optimal intake of calcium, phosphorus, and vitamin D and promote bone mineralization. See also Sec. 3.29, 3.30, 5.33, 19.17, and 23.46.

HYPOMAGNESEMIA

Rarely, hypomagnesemia of unknown etiology may occur in the newborn infant, usually in association with hypocalcemia. It may also be associated with insufficient stores of skeletal magnesium secondary to deficient placental transfer, decreased intestinal absorption, neonatal hypoparathyroidism, hyperphosphatemia, renal loss, a defect in magnesium and calcium homeostasis, or an iatrogenic deficiency due to loss during exchange transfusion or insufficient replacement during total intravenous alimentation. It has also been observed in uremic infants. Infants of diabetic mothers may have serum magnesium levels that are lower than normal. The clinical manifestations of hypomagnesemia are indistinguishable from those of hypocalcemia and tetany and may, in fact, be secondary to the accompanying hypocalcemia.

Hypomagnesemia occurs when serum magnesium levels fall below 1.5 mg/dL, although clinical signs usually do not develop until serum magnesium levels fall below 1.2 mg/dL. During exchange transfusion with citrated blood, which is low in magnesium ion because of binding by citrate, the serum magnesium drops about 0.5 mEq/L; approximately 10 days are required for a return to normal. In noniatrogenic hypomagnesemia the serum magnesium may be less than 0.5 mEq/L. The serum calcium in either instance is usually at levels seen in hypocalcemic tetany, but the serum phosphorus value is normal or high. Since the hypocalcemia accompanying hypomagnesemia is inadequately corrected by administering calcium, hypomagnesemia should also be suspected in any patient with tetany not responding to calcium therapy.

Immediate *treatment* consists of the intramuscular injection of magnesium sulfate. For newborn infants 0.25 mL/kg of a 50% solution daily usually suffices. The accompanying hypocalcemia usually corrects itself as the hypomagnesemia is relieved. The same daily dose can be given for oral maintenance therapy. Four to five times higher doses may be required in malabsorptive states. In most cases the metabolic defect is transient, and treatment can be discontinued after 1–2 wk. A few patients appear to have a permanent form of the disease that requires continuous oral supplementation

with magnesium to prevent recurrence of hypomagnesemia.* No residual damage to the central nervous system is evident after prompt treatment.

HYPERMAGNESEMIA

Hypermagnesemia may occur in newborn infants of mothers treated with magnesium sulfate for eclampsia. At high serum levels the central nervous system is depressed and totally paralyzed so that artificial respiration is required. Toxicity may also result from magnesium sulfate enemas. Lower levels may result in hypoventilation, hypotension, lethargy, flaccidity, and hyporeflexia. The upper limit of normal magnesium is 2.8 mg/dL, but serious symptoms occur at levels above 5 mg/dL. Hypermagnesemia may be associated with failure to pass meconium (meconium plug syndrome). Exchange transfusion has been used as a means of rapid removal of magnesium ion from the blood. Calcium salts and diuresis have also been used. Recovery appears to be complete.

OTHER METABOLIC DISEASES

A number of inborn errors of metabolism may be manifest during the neonatal period; these include phenylketonuria, galactosemia, the urea cycle defects, methylmalonic acidemia, and maple syrup urine disease (see Chapter 7). Pyridoxine deficiency and dependency are considered in Sec. 3.26.

NARCOTIC ADDICTION AND WITHDRAWALS

Physiologic addiction to narcotics exists in most infants born to actively addicted mothers, since opiates cross the placenta. It may be manifest even before birth by increased activity of the fetus when the mother feels the need for the drug or develops withdrawal symptoms. Heroin and methadone are the drugs most frequently involved, but withdrawal syndromes also occur with alcohol, phenobarbital, pentazocine, codeine, propoxyphene, cocaine, and diazepam.

Pregnancy in an addict or alcoholic is, by definition, a high risk. Prenatal care is usually inadequate, and there is a higher incidence of venereal disease, toxemia, premature rupture of the membranes, breech presentations, prolapsed cords and limbs, preterm and small for gestational age infants, and prenatal morbidity and mortality.

Heroin addiction results in 50% incidence of low birthweight infants, half of whom are small for gestational age. Infections, maternal undernutrition, and a direct fetal growth inhibiting effect have been causally implicated. The rate of stillbirths is increased, but not the incidence of congenital anomalies. *Clinical manifestations* of withdrawal occur in 50–75% of infants, usually beginning within the first 48 hr, depending on the daily maternal dose (<6 mg/24 hr is associated with no or mild symptoms); duration of addiction (>1 yr has a greater than 70% incidence of withdrawal); and time of last maternal dose (there is a higher incidence if within 24 hr of birth). Symptoms rarely appear as late as 4–6 wk of age. The incidence of hyaline membrane disease and hyperbilirubinemia may be decreased in low birthweight infants of heroin addicts; hyperventilation leading to respiratory alkalosis or accelerated production of surfactant may explain the former, and enzyme induction of glucuronyl transferase, the latter.

---

*Four mL/kg/24 hr of the following solution:
Magnesium chloride (MgCl$_2$ × 6 H$_2$O) 4.0 g (39.6 mEq)
Magnesium citrate (MgHC$_6$H$_5$O$_7$ × 5 H$_2$O) 6.0 g (39.6 mEq)
Water to 100 mL
Solution provides approximately 0.8 mEq of magnesium/mL.

Tremors and hyperirritability are the most prominent symptoms. The tremors may be fine or jittery and indistinguishable from those of hypoglycemia but are more often coarse, "flapping," and bilateral; the limbs are often rigid, hyperreflexic, and resistant to flexion and extension. Irritability and hyperactivity are generally marked and may lead to skin abrasions. Other signs include tachypnea, diarrhea, vomiting, high-pitched cry, fist sucking, poor feeding, and fever. Sneezing, yawning, myoclonic jerks, convulsions, abnormal sleep cycles, nasal stuffiness, apnea, flushing alternating rapidly with pallor, and lacrimation are less common. The *diagnosis* is generally established by the history and clinical presentation. Examining the urine for opiates may reveal only low levels during withdrawal, but quinine, which is often mixed with heroin, may be present in higher concentrations. Hypoglycemia and hypocalcemia should be excluded.

Methadone addiction has produced an increasing number of infants with withdrawal symptoms, the incidence varying from 20–90%. In general, mothers taking methadone have better prenatal care than those taking heroin; however, there is a high incidence of multiple drug abuse, including alcohol, barbiturates, and tranquilizers, and they are often heavy smokers. There is no increased incidence of congenital anomalies. The average birthweight of infants of mothers taking methadone is higher than that of infants of heroin-addicted mothers; the *clinical manifestations* are similar except that the former group has a higher incidence of seizures (10–20%) and of late onset (2–6 wk of age) of symptoms and signs.

Alcohol withdrawal is uncommon. The infants of women who have been drinking immediately before delivery may have alcohol on their breath for several hours, since it rapidly crosses the placenta, and blood levels in the infant are similar to those in the mother. Infants who develop withdrawal symptoms often become agitated and hyperactive with marked tremors lasting for 72 hr, followed by about 48 hr of lethargy before return to normal activity. Seizures may develop.

Phenobarbital withdrawal usually occurs in full-term, appropriate for gestational age infants of addicted mothers. Symptoms begin at a median age of 7 days (range 2–14 days). There may be a brief acute stage consisting of irritability, constant crying, sleeplessness, hiccups, and mouthing movements, followed by a subacute stage that may last 2–4 mo consisting of voracious appetite, frequent regurgitation and gagging, episodic irritability, hyperacusis, sweating, and a disturbed sleep pattern.

Cocaine withdrawal is unusual; pregnancy may be complicated by premature labor, abruptio placentae, and fetal asphyxia. Infants have abnormal neurobehavioral manifestations.

Treatment of heroin and methadone withdrawals has been successful using various combinations of narcotics, sedatives, and hypnotics. Therapy is indicated for seizures, for diarrhea, or for such irritability that normal sleep and feeding patterns are disturbed and weight gain is poor. Methadone withdrawal may require larger amounts of medication for longer periods than heroin withdrawal to control clinical manifestations. Phenobarbital, 8–10 mg/kg/24 hr in 4 divided doses, can effectively reduce irritability and prevent seizures. It is as effective as chlorpromazine, 2.2 mg/kg/24 hr, divided into 3–4 doses. It is usually not necessary to administer either drug for more than 5 days, but on occasion it may be necessary to treat for as long as 6 wk. Patients with severe autonomic symptoms may require gradually diminishing doses of methadone or paregoric for 2–10 wk. Paregoric at a beginning dose of 3–5 drops given every 3–6 hr, increased to 5–10 drops every 4 hr if necessary, depending on the size and response of the infant, will abolish most withdrawal symptoms, especially diarrhea. The dose and duration of therapy may be adjusted according to the clinical response. Parenteral administration of fluids may be necessary to prevent aspiration or dehydration until the symptoms are brought under control. Narcotic and phenobarbital withdrawal requires swaddling, frequent feedings, and protection from noxious external stimuli.

Current mortality is not over 5%, and with early recognition and treatment may be negligible. *Prognosis* for normal development is affected by the adverse circumstances of high risk pregnancy and delivery and by the environment to which the infant is returned after recovery.

Fetal Alcohol Syndrome. High levels of alcohol ingestion during pregnancy can be damaging to embryonic and fetal development. A specific pattern of malformation identified as the *fetal alcohol syndrome* has been documented, and major and minor components of the syndrome are expressed in 1–2 infants/1000 live births. Both moderate and high levels of alcohol intake during early pregnancy may result in alterations in growth and morphogenesis of the fetus; the greater the intake, the more severe the signs. Infants born to heavy drinkers have twice the risk of abnormality compared with those born to moderate drinkers; 32% of infants born to heavy drinkers demonstrated congenital anomalies, compared with 9% in the abstinent and 14% in the moderate group.

The characteristics of the fetal alcohol syndrome include (1) prenatal onset and persistence of growth deficiency for length, weight, and head circumference; (2) facial abnormalities, including short palpebral fissures, epicanthal folds, maxillary hypoplasia, micrognathia, and thin upper lip; (3) cardiac defects, primarily septal defects; (4) minor joint and limb abnormalities, including some restriction of movement and altered palmar crease patterns; and (5) delayed development and mental deficiency varying from borderline to severe. The severity of dysmorphogenesis may range from severely affected infants with full manifestations of the fetal alcohol syndrome to those mildly affected with only a few manifestations.

The detrimental effects may be due to the alcohol itself or to one of its breakdown products. Some evidence suggests that alcohol may impair placental transfer of essential amino acids and zinc, both necessary for protein synthesis, which accounts for the intrauterine growth retardation.

The *management* of these infants may be difficult, since no specific therapy exists. The infants may remain hypotonic and tremulous despite sedation, and the prognosis is poor. Counseling with regard to recurrence is important. *Prevention* is achieved by eliminating alcohol intake after conception.

LATE METABOLIC ACIDOSIS

Between 5 and 40% of preterm low birthweight infants develop a metabolic acidosis during the 2nd or 3rd wk of life. Usually there is no history of asphyxia, respiratory distress, or other problems, and the infants are vigorous. However, they often have received cow's milk formulas of high protein and casein content shortly after birth and have had a delayed start of postnatal weight gain. Blood base excess values range from -10 to -16 mEq/L, and pCO_2 values are usually less than 40 mm Hg. The condition probably represents an abnormally high rate of endogenous acid formation. Treatment includes administering $NaHCO_3$ and changing to a formula of lower protein content with a whey:casein ratio of 60:40.

Chasnoff I, Burns W, Schnolls S, et al: Cocaine use in pregnancy. N Engl J Med 313:666, 1985.

Clarren SK, Alvord EC Jr, Sumi SM, et al: Brain malformation related to prenatal exposure to ethanol. J Pediatr 92:64, 1978.

Kildeberg P: Late metabolic acidosis of premature infants. *In* Winters RW (ed): The Body Fluids in Pediatrics. Boston, Little, Brown and Co, 1973.

Madden J, Payne T, Miller S: Maternal cocaine abuse and effects on the newborn. Pediatrics 77:209, 1986.

Nervez CT, Shott RJ, Bergstrom WH, et al: Prophylaxis against hypocalcemia in low birth weight infants receiving bicarbonate infusion. J Pediatr 87:439, 1975.

Neuman L, Cohen S: The neonatal narcotic withdrawal syndrome. Clin Perinatol 2:99, 1975.

Ovellette EM, Rosett HL, Rosman P, et al: Adverse effects on offspring of maternal alcohol abuse during pregnancy. N Engl J Med 297:528, 1977.

Scriver CR, Feingold M, Mamanes P, et al: Screening for congenital metabolic disorders in the newborn infant: Congenital deficiency of thyroid hormone and hyperphenylalaninemia. Pediatrics 3(Suppl):389, 1977.

Streissguth AP, Herman CS, Smith DW: Intelligence, behavior and dysmorphogenesis in the fetal alcohol syndrome: A report of 20 patients. J Pediatr 92:363, 1978.

Tsang R, Steichen J, Brown D: Perinatal calcium homeostasis: Neonatal hypocalcemia and bone demineralization. Clin Perinatol 4:385, 1977.

8.55 THE ENDOCRINE SYSTEM

The endocrinopathies are discussed in Chapter 19. The purpose of this section is to call attention to those endocrine disturbances that may be identified at birth or during the first month of life.

Pituitary dwarfism is usually inapparent at birth, although panhypopituitary male infants may present with neonatal hypoglycemia and micropenis. Conversely, constitutional dwarfs usually demonstrate length and weight consistent with prematurity when born after a normal gestational period; otherwise their physical appearance is normal.

Thyroid deficiency may be apparent at birth in genetically determined **cretinism** or in infants of mothers treated with thiouracil or its derivatives during pregnancy. Constipation, prolonged jaundice, lethargy, or poor peripheral circulation as shown by persistently mottled skin or cold extremities should suggest cretinism. The early diagnosis and treatment of congenital deficiency of thyroid hormone may be greatly facilitated by screening all newborn infants for this deficiency.

Temporary *hyperthyroidism* may occur at birth in the infants of mothers with hyperthyroidism or of those who have been receiving thyroid medication.

Transient *hypoparathyroidism* may be manifest as tetany of the newborn.

The *adrenal gland* is subject to numerous disturbances, which may become apparent and require lifesaving treatment during the neonatal period. Acute adrenal *hemorrhage* and failure may be seen after breech or other traumatic deliveries or in association with overwhelming infection. *Adrenocortical hyperplasia* is suggested by vomiting, diarrhea, dehydration, convulsions, shock, or phallic or clitoral enlargement. Since the condition is genetically determined, newborn siblings of patients with the salt-losing variety of adrenocortical hyperplasia should be observed closely for manifestations of adrenal insufficiency. *Congenitally hypoplastic adrenal glands* may also give rise to adrenal insufficiency during the first few weeks of life. Female infants with webbing of the neck, lymphangiectatic edema, hypoplasia of the nipples, cutis laxa, low hairline at the nape of the neck, low-set ears, high-arched palate, deformities of the nails, cubitus valgus, and other anomalies should be suspected of having *gonadal dysgenesis*.

Transient *diabetes mellitus* (Sec. 20.5) is rare and seen only in the newborn. It usually presents as dehydration, loss of weight, or acidosis in small for gestational age infants.

8.56 INFANTS OF DIABETIC MOTHERS

The control of diabetes mellitus with insulin has led to the survival of increasing numbers of diabetic women who bear children. Their infants and the infants of women who later develop diabetes share certain distinctive morphologic characteristics, including large size, macrosomia, and high morbidity risks. Diabetic mothers have a high incidence of poly-

hydramnios and their fetal mortality rate, which is high at all gestational ages, especially so after 32 wk, is 10 times that of nondiabetic mothers. Fetal wastage throughout pregnancy is associated with poorly controlled maternal diabetes, especially ketoacidosis and congenital anomalies. Diabetic mothers produce an excess of high birthweight infants at all gestational ages and, if complicated with vascular disease, of low birthweight infants at 37–40 wk gestations. The neonatal mortality rate is over five times that of infants of nondiabetic mothers and is higher at all gestational ages and in every birthweight for gestational age category; the relative risk is highest in infants of normal and high birthweight.

Pathophysiology. No single physiologic or biochemical event explains the diverse clinical manifestations. The probable pathogenic sequence is that maternal hyperglycemia causes fetal hyperglycemia, and the fetal pancreatic response leads to fetal hyperinsulinemia; fetal hyperinsulinemia and hyperglycemia then cause increased hepatic glucose uptake and glycogen synthesis, accelerated lipogenesis, and augmented protein synthesis. Related pathologic findings are the hypertrophy and hyperplasia of the pancreatic islets with a disproportionate increase in the number of β cells; increased weights of the placenta and infant organs except for the brain; myocardial hypertrophy; increased amounts of cytoplasm in liver cells; and extramedullary hematopoiesis. Hyperinsulinism produces fetal acidosis, which may result in an increased rate of stillbirth. The separation of the placenta suddenly interrupts glucose infusion into the neonate without a proportional effect on the hyperinsulinism, resulting in hypoglycemia and attenuated lipolysis during the first hours after birth.

Hyperinsulinemia has been documented in infants of gestational diabetic mothers and in those of insulin-dependent diabetic mothers without insulin antibodies. The former group also have significantly higher fasting plasma insulin levels than normal newborns despite similar glucose levels; they respond to glucose with a prompt elevation of plasma insulin and assimilate a glucose load more rapidly. Following arginine administration, they also have an enhanced insulin response and increased disappearance rates of glucose, compared with normal infants. In contrast, fasting glucose utilization rates are diminished. The lower free fatty acid levels in infants of insulin-dependent diabetic mothers probably also reflect their hyperinsulinemia. With good prenatal diabetic control, the incidence of macrosomia has decreased.

Although hyperinsulinism is probably the main cause of hypoglycemia, the diminished epinephrine and glucagon responses that occur may be contributing factors. Cortisol and human growth hormone levels are normal.

Clinical Manifestations. The infants of diabetic and gestational diabetic mothers often bear a surprising resemblance to each other (Fig. 8–26). They tend to be large and plump owing to increased body fat and enlarged viscera, with puffy, plethoric facies resembling those of patients who have been receiving a corticosteroid. These infants may, however, also be of normal or low birthweight, particularly if delivered before term or if there is associated maternal vascular disease.

The infants tend to be "jumpy," tremulous, and hyperexcitable during the first 3 days of life, although hypotonia, lethargy, and poor sucking also may occur. They may have any of the diverse manifestations of hypoglycemia. Early appearance of these signs is more likely to be related to hypoglycemia and later appearance related to hypocalcemia; these abnormalities also may occur together. Perinatal asphyxia or hyperbilirubinemia may produce similar signs. Rarely, hypomagnesemia may be associated with the hypocalcemia.

About 75% of infants of diabetic mothers and 25% of infants of mothers with gestational diabetes develop hypoglycemia

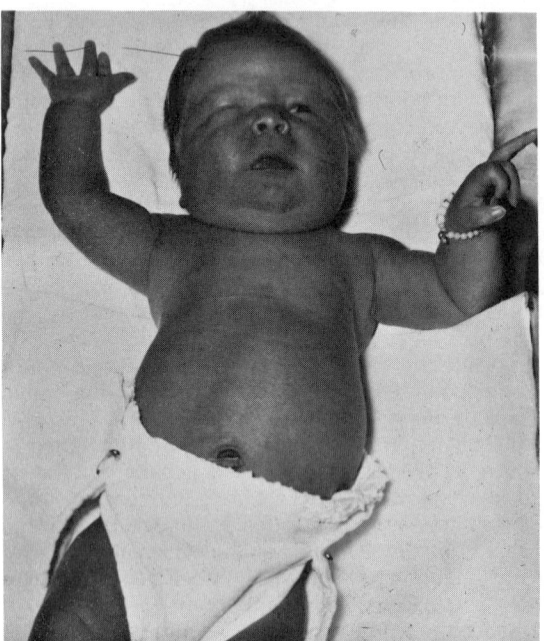

Figure 8–26. Large, plump, plethoric infant of a gestational diabetic mother. Baby was born at 38 wk of gestation but weighed 9 lb 11 oz (4408 gm). Mild respiratory distress was the only symptom other than appearance.

(<35 mg/dL glucose), but only a small percentage of these infants become symptomatic. The probability of an infant developing hypoglycemia increases and the glucose levels are likely to be lower at higher cord or maternal fasting blood glucose levels. Usually, the nadir in the infant's blood glucose concentration is reached between 1 and 3 hr; spontaneous recovery may begin by 4–6 hr.

Many infants of diabetic mothers develop tachypnea during the first 5 days of life, which may be a transient manifestation of hypoglycemia, hypothermia, polycythemia, cardiac failure, transient tachypnea, or cerebral edema from birth trauma or asphyxia. A greater incidence of hyaline membrane disease appears in infants of diabetic mothers than in infants of normal mothers born at comparable gestational age; the greater incidence is possibly related to an antagonistic effect between cortisol and insulin on surfactant synthesis.

Cardiomegaly is common (30%), and heart failure occurs in 5–10% of infants of diabetic mothers. Asymmetrical septal hypertrophy may occur and become manifest as idiopathic hypertrophic subaortic stenosis.

Neurologic development and ossification centers tend to be immature and correlate with the brain size (which is not increased) and gestational age rather than with total body weight. There is also an increased incidence of hyperbilirubinemia, polycythemia, and renal vein thrombosis; the latter should be suspected in the presence of a flank mass, hematuria, and thrombocytopenia.

The incidence of congenital anomalies is increased 3-fold in infants of diabetic mothers; cardiac and lumbosacral agenesis are most common. These infants may also develop abdominal distention due to a transient delay in the development of the left side of the colon, the *small left colon syndrome.*

Prognosis. The subsequent incidence of diabetes mellitus in infants of diabetic mothers is increased over that of the general population. Physical development is normal, but oversized infants may be predisposed to obesity in childhood that may extend into adult life. Disagreement persists about whether or not a slightly increased risk of impaired intellectual

development exists unrelated to hypoglycemia; symptomatic hypoglycemia probably increases the risk.

Treatment. Management of these infants should be initiated before birth by frequent prenatal evaluation of all pregnant women with overt or gestational diabetes, by evaluation of fetal maturity, and by planning delivery of these infants in hospitals where expert obstetric and pediatric care is continuously available. Regardless of size, all infants of diabetic mothers should initially receive intensive observation and care. Asymptomatic infants should have a blood sugar determination within 1 hr of birth and then every hr for the next 6–8 hr; if clinically well and normoglycemic, oral or gavage feedings initially with sterile water or 5% glucose water, followed by milk formula, should be started at 2–3 hr of age and continued at 3 hr intervals. If any question arises about an infant's ability to tolerate oral feeding, the feeding should be discontinued and glucose given by peripheral intravenous infusion at a rate of 4–8 mg/kg/min. Blood glucose values under 35 mg/dL should be treated, even in asymptomatic infants, with intravenous infusions of glucose sufficient to keep the blood levels well above this level. Bolus injections of hypertonic glucose should be avoided, as they may cause further hyperinsulinemia and potentially produce rebound hypoglycemia. Managing hypoglycemia in sick or symptomatic infants is discussed in the following section. For treatment of *hypocalcemia* and *hypomagnesemia,* see Sec. 8.54; for *hyaline membrane disease* treatment, see Sec. 8.32; for treatment of *polycythemia,* see Sec. 8.48.

8.57 HYPOGLYCEMIA

Also see Sec. 20.6–20.15.

Hypoglycemia is present when an infant's blood glucose concentration is significantly lower than the mean for a population of infants of similar age and weight. In term infants, lowered glucose concentration is defined as plasma concentrations of less than 35 mg/dL in the first 72 hr and 45 mg/dL subsequently; in low birthweight infants, it is less than 25 mg/dL (Fig. 8–11). Whole blood glucose values are 5 mg/dL lower. Glucose is the major source of energy throughout fetal life, although ketones, amino acids, and lactate constitute additional sources of nutrients during gestation. The rate of fetal glucose uptake is related to the maternal blood glucose level; the fetal blood level is approximately two thirds that of the mother. After they are abruptly removed from the constant placental infusion of glucose, full-term infants usually stabilize their blood levels between 50 and 60 mg/dL during the first 72 hr of life, and low birthweight infants at lower levels.

Four pathophysiologic groups of neonatal infants are at high risk of developing hypoglycemia: (1) Infants of mothers with diabetes mellitus or gestational diabetes, infants with severe erythroblastosis fetalis, insulinomas, β cell nesidioblastosis, functional β cell hyperplasia, Beckwith syndrome (see below) and panhypopituitarism seem to suffer from hyperinsulinism. (2) Infants with intrauterine growth retardation or those who are preterm may have experienced intrauterine malnutrition resulting in reduced hepatic glycogen stores and total body fat; the smaller of discordant twins (especially if discordant by 25% or more in weight with a weight of less than 2.0 kg), polycythemic infants, infants of toxemic mothers, and infants with placental abnormalities are particularly vulnerable. (Other factors in the development of hypoglycemia in this group include abnormal insulin responsiveness, impaired gluconeogenesis, diminished free fatty acids, increased brain/liver weight ratio, low cortisol production rates, and possibly increased insulin levels and decreased output of epinephrine in response to hypoglycemia.) (3) Very immature or severely ill infants may develop hypoglycemia due to increased metabolic needs disproportionate to substrate stores and calories supplied; low birthweight infants with respiratory distress syndrome, perinatal asphyxia, polycythemia, hypothermia, and systemic infections, as well as infants in heart failure with cyanotic congenital heart disease, are at increased risk. The interruption of intravenous infusions, particularly those with high glucose concentrations, may also result in the precipitous onset of hypoglycemia. (4) Rare infants with genetic or primary metabolic defects, such as galactosemia, glycogen storage disease, fructose intolerance, propionic acidemia, methylmalonic acidemia, tyrosinemia, maple syrup urine disease, and leucine sensitivity, are also susceptible.

The overall frequency of hypoglycemia is 2–3/1000 live births but appears to be significantly higher among intrauterine growth retarded infants, especially those with a complicated prenatal history or severe illness. The incidence among infants of diabetic mothers may be as high as 75%. It is lower in infants of gestationally diabetic mothers.

Clinical Manifestations. In contrast to the frequency of chemical hypoglycemia, the incidence of symptomatic hypoglycemia is highest in small for gestational age infants (see Fig. 8–11). These infants usually fall into category 2 or 3 of the above pathophysiologic groupings, and some are referred to as having *transient symptomatic idiopathic neonatal hypoglycemia*. Because many of the symptoms also occur together with other conditions such as infections—especially sepsis and meningitis; central nervous system anomalies, hemorrhage, or edema; hypocalcemia and hypomagnesemia; asphyxia; drug withdrawal; apnea of prematurity; congenital heart disease; or polycythemia—and because some may be seen in normoglycemic well infants, the exact incidence of symptomatic hypoglycemia has been difficult to establish. It probably varies between 1 and 3 per 1000 live births with about 5–15% of growth retarded infants being affected.

The onset of symptoms varies from a few hours to a week after birth. In approximate order of frequency there are jitteriness or tremors, apathy, episodes of cyanosis, convulsions, intermittent apneic spells or tachypnea, weak or high-pitched cry, limpness or lethargy, difficulty in feeding, and eye-rolling. Episodes of sweating, sudden pallor, hypothermia, and cardiac arrest and failure also occur. There is frequently a clustering of episodic symptoms. Because these clinical manifestations may result from a variety of causes, it is critical to determine whether they disappear with the administration of sufficient glucose to raise the blood sugar to normal levels; if they do not, other diagnoses must be considered.

Treatment. When seizures are not present, an intravenous bolus of 200 mg/kg (2 mL/kg) of 10% glucose is effective in elevating the blood glucose concentration. In the presence of convulsions 4 mL/kg of 10% glucose as a bolus injection is indicated.

Following initial therapy a glucose infusion should be given at 8 mg/kg/min. If hypoglycemia recurs, the infusion rate should be increased until 15–20% glucose is employed. If intravenous infusions of 20% glucose are inadequate to eliminate symptoms and maintain constant normal blood glucose concentrations, hydrocortisone (2.5 mg/kg/6 hr) or prednisone (1 mg/kg/24 hr) should also be administered. Blood glucose should be measured every 2 hr after initiating therapy until several determinations are above 40 mg/dL. Subsequently levels should be obtained every 4–6 hr and the treatment gradually reduced and finally discontinued when the blood glucose has been in the normal range and the baby asymptomatic for 24–48 hr. Treatment is usually necessary for a few days to a week, rarely for several weeks. Diazoxide, epinephrine, and fructose are not of established benefit. Epinephrine and fructose may produce lactic acidosis. If neonatal hyperinsulinism is present, as in nesidioblastosis, and unresponsive

to steroids and glucose given for a sufficient time, diazoxide and Sus-Phrine may be employed.

Surgery is the definitive treatment for *nesidioblastosis* and *islet cell adenomas*; glucagon plus somatostatin has been a helpful adjunct in some cases.

Infants who are at increased risk of developing hypoglycemia should have their blood glucose measured within 1 hr of birth and subsequently every 1–2 hr for the first 6–8 hr, then every 4–6 hr until 24 hr of life. Normoglycemic high risk infants should receive oral or gavage feedings with formula started at 1–3 hr of age and continued at 2–3 hr intervals for 24–48 hr. An intravenous infusion of glucose at 4 mg/kg/min should be provided if oral feedings are poorly tolerated or if *asymptomatic transient neonatal hypoglycemia* develops.

Prognosis. Prognosis for life is good. Hypoglycemia recurs in 10–15% of infants after adequate treatment. Some have been reported as late as the age of 8 mo. Recurrences are more common if intravenous fluids extravasate or are too rapidly discontinued before oral feedings are well tolerated. Children who later develop ketotic hypoglycemia have an increased incidence of neonatal hypoglycemia. Prognosis for normal intellectual function must be guarded, since prolonged and severe hypoglycemia may be associated with neurologic sequelae and death. Symptomatic infants with hypoglycemia, particularly low birthweight infants and large-sized infants of overtly diabetic mothers, have a worse prognosis for subsequent normal intellectual development than do asymptomatic infants.

Hypoglycemia with Macroglossia
(Beckwith Syndrome)

Beckwith described a syndrome of intractable neonatal hypoglycemia occurring in infants with macroglossia, large size, visceromegaly, mild microcephaly, omphalocele, facial nevus flammeus, a characteristic earlobe crease, and renal medullary dysplasia. The visceromegaly involves chiefly the liver and the kidneys in which there is a noncystic hyperplasia. Some infants are also polycythemic. Hyperinsulinemia has been demonstrated. Treatment is that of hypoglycemia; in this syndrome hypoglycemia may be severe and persist for several months. The prognosis is poor.

Severe hypoglycemia has also been demonstrated in extremely high birthweight infants who do not have the anomalies present in Beckwith syndrome. These *infant giants* weigh from 3.8 to 5.3 kg, and, in some, pancreatic hyperplasia has been described.

ROBERT M. KLIEGMAN
RICHARD E. BEHRMAN

Adam P: Infant of a diabetic mother: Energy imbalance between adipose tissue and liver. Semin Perinatol 2:329, 1978.

Cornblath M, Schwartz R: Carbohydrate Metabolism in the Neonate. 2nd ed. Philadelphia, WB Saunders, 1976.

Cowett R, Schwartz R: The infant of the diabetic mother. Pediatr Clin North Am 29:1213, 1982.

Haworth JC, Dilling LA: Relationship between maternal glucose tolerance and neonatal blood glucose. J Pediatr 89:810, 1976.

Kalhan S, Savin S, Adam P: Attenuated glucose production rate in newborn infants of insulin dependent diabetic mothers. N Engl J Med 296:375, 1977.

Kolvisto M, Blanco-Sequiros M, Krause N: Neonatal symptomatic and asymptomatic hypoglycemia; a follow up study of 151 children. Dev Med Child Neurol 14:603, 1972.

Lilien L, Pildes R, Srinivasan G, et al: Treatment of neonatal hypoglycemia with minibolus and intravenous glucose infusion. J Pediatr 97:295, 1980.

Pildes RS, Cornblath N, Warren I, et al: A prospective controlled study of neonatal hypoglycemia. Pediatrics 54:5, 1974.

Sosenko I, Kitzmiller J, Loo S, et al: The infant of the diabetic mother. Correlation of increased cord C-peptide levels with macrosomia and hypoglycemia. N Engl J Med 308:859, 1979.

8.58 INFECTIONS OF THE NEWBORN

GENERAL CONSIDERATIONS

Infections are a frequent and important cause of morbidity and mortality in the neonatal period (Chapter 1 and Sec. 4.4.). As many as 2% of fetuses are infected in utero, and up to 10% of infants are infected during delivery or the first month of life. Inflammatory lesions are found in about 25% of newborn infant autopsies; these lesions are second only to hyaline membrane disease in frequency.

Several general factors contribute to the frequency and severity of neonatal infections and emphasize the importance of early and accurate diagnosis and appropriate therapy. First, a variety of organisms, including bacteria, viruses, fungi, protozoa, chlamydia, and mycoplasma, are etiologic agents. Second, with the increasing complexity of neonatal intensive care, gestationally younger and lower birthweight newborns are surviving and remaining in the high risk for infection environment for a longer duration. Third, the presenting clinical manifestations in the neonate with infection may be subtle and may mimic the features of other common diseases during this period. As a result, the diagnosis of infection is often missed or delayed until the process has become widespread. Fourth, many routine laboratory tests available to aid in the diagnosis of infection are imprecise or do not provide the rapid results needed. Fifth, the newborn infant's host resistance mechanisms, particularly those of the sick premature infant, may be immature and easily overcome by invading microorganisms. Infections, therefore, may become fulminant and cause death within a few hours or days, despite appropriate and intensive antimicrobial therapy. Sixth, many bacterial infections are caused by organisms relatively resistant to antibiotics, particularly the gram-negative enteric bacilli. These infections are difficult to treat, and the dose of antibiotics that can safely be used is limited by toxic side effects. Finally, with the exception of herpes simplex virus, antiviral chemotherapy is not available for the viruses commonly infecting the neonate.

Frequency and Specific Predisposing Factors. Table 8–23 lists the frequency of the most common infections in the newborn infant and, when the fetus is infected in utero, the frequency of infection in the mother during pregnancy. A variety of maternal and neonatal factors are associated with increased frequency or severity of infections. Mothers susceptible to certain pathogens (e.g., rubella or cytomegalovirus) may acquire an acute primary infection and transmit the microorganism transplacentally to the fetus. On the other hand, mothers who are immune (e.g., to measles or a particular strain of group B streptococcus) have antibody in their serum that can pass transplacentally and provide passive protection for the neonate against infection after birth. During epidemic periods, the incidence of maternal and congenital disease may be several-fold higher. The use of vaccines against maternal infections, such as rubella, has reduced the frequency of congenital infections. Much higher rates of vaginal colonization with group B streptococcus and genital infection with herpes simplex virus occur in women with multiple sexual partners; the rates of infection in neonates born to such women are correspondingly higher.

An important variable in the increased risk of neonatal sepsis in infants born of mothers with prolonged rupture of membranes is the development of ascending infection of the amniotic fluid, which then leads to congenital aspiration pneumonia (Sec. 8.34, 8.35, and 13.69) in the fetus and subsequent neonatal sepsis. However, amniotic and fetal infection can occur with rupture of membranes for less than 24 hr, and membranes may be ruptured for more than 24 hr without infection developing. Maternal urinary tract infections are also associated with an increased incidence of disease in the neonate. The maternal genital tract may be colonized with a wide variety of organisms that do not necessarily cause disease in the mother, but may result in a heavy inoculum for the neonate at the time of birth and cause significant illness during the newborn period. These organisms include group B streptococcus, *Escherichia coli* (particularly the K1 capsular antigen-containing organisms), gonococcus, *Listeria*, chlamydia, *Candida*, herpes simplex virus, and cytomegalovirus. Difficult or traumatic delivery is associated with an increased frequency of neonatal infections.

The most important neonatal factor predisposing to infection is prematurity or low birthweight; there is a 3- to 10-fold higher incidence of sepsis, meningitis, or urinary tract infection in these infants than in full-term normal birthweight infants. Males have an approximately 2-fold higher incidence of sepsis, meningitis, and urinary tract infections than females, suggesting the possibility of a sex-linked factor in host susceptibility. Resuscitation at birth, particularly if it involves endotracheal intubation, insertion of an umbilical vessel catheter, or both, is associated with increased risk of bacterial infection. The presence of underlying diseases, such as hyaline membrane disease, or congenital defects, such as meningomyelocele, predisposes to infection by acting as a portal of entry for organisms or by compromising host resistance. The majority of infants cared for in a neonatal intensive care unit are exposed to a variety of diagnostic and therapeutic procedures that may also compromise host defenses and provide a portal of entry for organisms. In addition, these infants may be exposed to antibiotic-resistant organisms carried on the hands of personnel or on contaminated equipment.

Epidemiology and Pathogenesis. Infections in the newborn infant may be acquired in utero (congenital), at the time of birth (natal), or after birth and during the neonatal period (postnatal). The transplacental route is the most common means by which microorganisms reach the fetus in utero. Some viruses, *Toxoplasma gondii*, *Treponema pallidum*, and occasionally bacteria are transmitted by this route. Infection acquired in utero may result in resorption of the embryo, abortion, stillbirth, congenital malformation, intrauterine growth retardation, premature birth, acute disease in the

Table 8–23. Approximate Frequency of Infections in the Mother During Pregnancy and in the Newborn Infant

Infectious Agent	Approximate Frequency	
	Mother per 1000 Pregnancies	Neonate per 1000 Live Births
Bacterial infections		
Sepsis	—	1–5
Meningitis	—	0.2–0.5
Urinary tract infection	—	1–10
Viruses		
Cytomegalovirus		
During pregnancy	10–70	6–34
Perinatal	30–130	20–70
Rubella		
Epidemic	20–40	3–7
Nonepidemic	0.1–2.0	0.1–0.7
Postvaccine	0.03–0.7	0.03–0.2
Hepatitis B	1–160	0–61
Herpes simplex	1–10	0.03–0.3
Protozoa		
Toxoplasma gondii	1–10	1–6

immediate neonatal period, or an asymptomatic but persistent infection that can cause neurologic sequelae later in life (Table 8–24). Most infections acquired by the newborn infant during birth are the result of aspiration of infected amniotic fluid or vaginal secretions, which can result in colonization of the upper respiratory tract or true infection of the lower respiratory tract. The most common organisms causing infection at this time are group B streptococcus, E. coli, Neisseria gonorrhoeae, and herpes simplex virus, which often result in acute, fulminant, systemic infections; Candida albicans and chlamydia, which usually cause less severe infection limited to the mucous membranes; and cytomegalovirus, which tends to result in asymptomatic infections. Symptoms of infections acquired during birth are usually apparent within a few days after birth, except those that have long incubation periods (e.g., chlamydia and cytomegalovirus). Those acquired after birth are the result of environmental exposure in either the hospital or the community. The respiratory or the gastrointestinal tract is the primary route of infection in the latter, while the umbilicus, a surgical wound, a trachea with an endotracheal tube in place, or the site of an intravascular catheter may be the portal of entry in a hospitalized neonate.

Clinical Manifestations. Infection in the newborn infant may simulate other common diseases, may be subtle or nonspecific, and may involve a number of organ systems (Table 8–25). In addition, infections with different microorganisms may have overlapping patterns so that it is usually not possible to make a definitive diagnosis of a specific etiologic agent from clinical features alone. Finally, in the majority of congenital infections no symptoms are evident at birth.

Diagnosis. The maternal history may provide important clues to the diagnosis of infection in the newborn infant. Congenital hepatitis B virus infection is much more common in mothers with acute hepatitis than in asymptomatic chronic carriers. However, virtually all of the primary infections due to cytomegalovirus and toxoplasma and half of those due to rubella are asymptomatic in the pregnant woman. A history of painful genital ulcers or of genital herpes in a sexual partner should suggest neonatal herpes, and the occurrence of prolonged rupture of the fetal membranes, maternal peripartum infection, or complications during labor or delivery should suggest the possibility of early onset bacterial sepsis.

Definitive diagnoses of a specific infection usually require recovery of an etiologic agent from body fluids or tissues, particularly from sites of infection. In the infant with sus-

Table 8–24. Viral, Parasitic, and Spirochetal Agents Associated With Fetal and Infant Morbidity and Mortality

Pathogen	Fetus	Neonatal Disease	Congenital Defects	Late Sequelae
Rubella virus	Abortion	Low birthweight, hepatosplenomegaly, petechiae, osteitis	Heart defects, microcephaly, cataracts, microphthalmia	Deafness, mental retardation, thyroid disorders, diabetes, degenerative brain tissue, autism
Cytomegalovirus	—	Anemia, thrombocytopenia, hepatosplenomegaly, jaundice, encephalitis	Microcephaly, microphthalmia, retinopathy	Deafness, psychomotor retardation, cerebral calcification
Varicella-zoster virus	—	Low birthweight, chorioretinitis, congenital chickenpox or disseminated neonatal varicella, possibly zoster	Limb hypoplasia, cortical atrophy, cicatricial skin lesions	Fatal outcome due to secondary infection
Picornaviruses				
Coxsackie virus	Abortion	Mild febrile disease, exanthems, aseptic meningitis, disseminated disease, multiple organ involvement (CNS, liver, heart), gastroenteritis	Possible congenital heart disease, myocarditis	Neurologic deficits
Echovirus	—			
Poliovirus	Abortion	Congenital poliomyelitis		Paralysis
Herpes simplex virus	Abortion	Disseminated disease, multiple organ involvement (lung, liver, CNS), vesicular skin lesions, retinopathy	Possible microcephaly, retinopathy, intracranial calcifications	Neurologic deficits
Western equine virus	—	Congenital encephalitis	—	Neurologic deficits
Measles virus	Abortion	Congenital measles	—	—
Vaccinia virus	Abortion	Congenital vaccinia	—	—
Variola virus	Abortion	Congenital variola	—	—
Hepatitis B virus	—	Asymptomatic HB$_s$Ag positive infection, low birthweight, rarely acute hepatitis	—	Chronic hepatitis, persistent HB$_s$Ag positive
Mumps virus	Abortion	Possible association with endocardial fibroelastosis		—
Influenza virus	Possible abortion	—		
Toxoplasma gondii	Abortion	Low birthweight, hepatosplenomegaly, jaundice, anemia	Hydrocephalus, microcephaly	Chorioretinitis, mental retardation
Treponema pallidum	—	Skin lesions, rhinitis, hepatosplenomegaly, jaundice, osteitis	—	Interstitial keratitis, frontal bossing, saber shins, tooth changes
Malaria	—	Hepatosplenomegaly, jaundice, anemia, poor feeding, vomiting	—	

Table 8–25. Clinical Manifestations of Infection in the Newborn Infant

General
  Fever, hypothermia
  "Not doing well"
  Poor feeding
  Lethargy
  Scleredema

Cardiovascular System
  Pallor, cyanosis, mottling, cold, clammy skin
  Hypotension

Gastrointestinal System
  Abdominal distention
  Anorexia, vomiting
  Diarrhea
  Hepatomegaly

Central Nervous System
  Irritability
  Tremors, seizures
  Hyporeflexia
  Abnormal Moro reflex
  Irregular respirations
  Full fontanel

Respiratory System
  Apnea, dyspnea
  Tachypnea, retraction
  Flaring, grunting
  Cyanosis

Hematologic System
  Jaundice
  Splenomegaly
  Pallor
  Petechiae, purpura
  Bleeding

pected bacterial sepsis, samples of spinal fluid, blood, and urine should be obtained for culture and other laboratory tests. Gram-stained smears of spinal fluid, urine, or material from sites of infection may provide an immediate tentative diagnosis of bacterial infection and can assist in the choice of initial antibiotic therapy. Within hours the antigens of group B streptococcus or K1 strains of *E. coli* can be identified in the spinal fluid or urine by counterimmunoelectrophoresis (CIE) or latex agglutination. Since the prognosis and the duration of antibiotic therapy are quite different in the infant having sepsis alone as compared with the infant having sepsis complicated by meningitis, and since neonates with urinary tract infection can present a picture resembling sepsis in the absence of bacteremia, the infant with suspected sepsis should have a complete evaluation.

The usual samples obtained for virus isolation are urine for cytomegalovirus; throat swab for rubella, herpes simplex, and enteroviruses; vesicle fluid for herpes simplex and varicella-zoster viruses; spinal fluid for herpes simplex, rubella, and enteroviruses; and stool for enteroviruses. Viral cytopathic effect in tissue culture may be evident within a few days with some viruses (herpes simplex, enteroviruses) but not for a week or more with others (cytomegalovirus, rubella, varicella-zoster virus). Hepatitis B virus antigen is demonstrable in serum by a variety of techniques (Sec. 8.70). Serologic tests are usually used in addition to virus isolation to diagnose viral infection in newborn infants, e.g., the TORCH (Toxoplasmosis, Other, Rubella, Cytomegalovirus, Herpes simplex) screen. Serologic testing is the primary means used for diagnosis of rubella (Sec. 11.62) and *Toxoplasma gondii* (Sec. 11.107). Since the antibodies measured in the TORCH screen are predominantly IgG, they are passed from mother to fetus and are found at approximately the same level in maternal sera and in cord blood or samples from the newborn infant. Serum levels obtained from the infant at the age of 4–5 mo will show a significant drop if the antibody was passively transferred from the mother but remain the same as in the neonatal period or even rise if active infection is present in the neonate. Although quantitative elevation of IgM in cord blood or early neonatal sera (IgM is not passed transplacentally under normal circumstances) has been used as a screening test to identify neonates with an intrauterine infection, there is a high rate of both false-positive and false-negative results. Furthermore, the test does not identify a specific etiologic agent. However, presence of IgM against specific antigens

(cytomegalovirus, rubella, toxoplasma, herpes simplex, syphilis) can be used to make an etiologic diagnosis with a single serum specimen obtained during the neonatal period.

Routine laboratory tests may assist in diagnosing infection in the newborn infant. In neonatal sepsis, increases in the absolute band neutrophil count and the immature/mature neutrophil ratio and thrombocytopenia often occur within the first 24 hr after onset of symptoms. White blood cells may also contain vacuoles and toxic granulation. Thrombocytopenia also occurs in congenital cytomegalovirus, rubella, toxoplasma, and spirochetal infections. Erythrocyte sedimentation rate and C-reactive protein are elevated in most neonates with systemic bacterial infection. However, delays in the development of an abnormal test and the time required to perform the laboratory test have reduced their usefulness. Although inflammatory cells are present in sections of umbilical cord and increased numbers of neutrophils are seen in smears of gastric aspirates obtained within hours of birth in many infants with early onset sepsis, a high incidence of false-positive results occurs. Roentgenographic examination is the primary method of diagnosing suspected pneumonia, septic arthritis, or osteomyelitis.

Because of the rapidity with which bacterial infections can become fulminant and life-threatening in this age group and the lack of a definitive diagnostic test short of bacteriologic cultures, a high index of suspicion should be maintained when the history or clinical circumstances indicate an increased risk of bacterial infection. If sepsis, pneumonia, or meningitis is suspected, treatment should be initiated after appropriate cultures have been obtained and diagnostic laboratory studies performed. The decision to continue antibiotics for a full course of therapy will depend on the results of cultures and on other laboratory tests and on the course of the illness.

Nosocomial Nursery Infections. Epidemics of infectious illness due to a variety of bacterial and viral agents have occurred in nurseries and neonatal intensive care units. Although the most common nosocomial infections are surface infections (ECG lead abscesses, omphalitis, conjunctivitis, pyoderma), there is also a significant incidence of serious infections such as pneumonia, bacteremia, surgical wound infection, urinary tract infection, and meningitis. *Staphylococcus aureus* has been a major cause of hospital-acquired infections and has resulted in outbreaks of pustules and cellulitis, pneumonia, septicemia, and the staphylococcal scalded skin syndrome (Sec. 8.67). Group A beta hemolytic streptococcus has caused a low grade granulating omphalitis, cellulitis, pneumonia, septicemia, and meningitis, while enteropathogenic *Escherichia coli* have caused outbreaks of diarrheal disease. A number of gram-negative enteric bacteria including *E. coli*, *Klebsiella pneumoniae*, *Pseudomonas aeruginosa*, *Proteus mirabilis*, *Serratia marcescens*, and *Flavobacterium meningosepticum* have resulted in epidemics of pneumonia, sepsis, and meningitis. Clusters of cases of fulminant viral infection consisting of hepatitis, encephalitis or aseptic meningitis, and myocarditis have been observed with Coxsackie and ECHO viruses. Adenovirus has caused cases of upper respiratory infection and gastrointestinal disease, whereas respiratory syncytial virus, parainfluenza virus, and influenza viruses have resulted in predominantly lower respiratory tract disease (pneumonia and bronchiolitis).

The occurrence of a similar clinical illness due to the same organism in several infants from the same nursery unit over a short period of time should suggest the possibility of an epidemic. In full-term infants whose nursery stay is usually only 2–3 days, the illness may not manifest itself for several days or weeks after discharge, making it difficult to recognize a nursery-acquired infection or a clustering of similar cases suggesting a nursery-associated outbreak. It may also be possible to demonstrate that one organism has caused the illness.

When a nursery epidemic outbreak occurs the following steps should be taken: (1) Cultures should be obtained from infants and, depending on the pathogen, from nursery personnel to identify additional cases, those incubating the disease, or asymptomatic carriers. Even during an outbreak of staphylococcal disease in a nursery, most infant carriers are asymptomatic. (2) All symptomatic and asymptomatic infants colonized with the epidemic strain should be isolated, and a cohort system should be maintained until all infants are discharged from the unit. (3) Systemic antibiotic therapy is required for infants with significant disease, while topical antibiotics may be used for asymptomatic carriers of *S. aureus*; oral antibiotic therapy is necessary for infants colonized with enteropathogenic *E. coli*, and triple dye should be applied to the umbilicus for a group A streptococcus outbreak. In some instances antibiotic treatment of nursery personnel may be required. (4) The extent of the epidemic should be defined. If the outbreak is confined to only a few infants in a single room in the nursery, limited infection control measures may be adequate. However, more extensive steps may be required if a number of areas or numerous infants or personnel are involved. If the outbreak is extensive and serious disease results, closure of the nursery to new admissions may be required until the outbreak is brought under control. (5) Culturing the environment for reservoirs of pathogens may be necessary in selected instances. Faucet aerators, sink traps and drains, eyewash solutions, resuscitation equipment, and humidification apparatus have been the source of outbreaks due to *P. aeruginosa, Serratia marcescens*, and *Flavobacterium meningosepticum*.

Davies PA, Gothefors LA: Bacterial Infections in the Fetus and Newborn Infant. Philadelphia, WB Saunders, 1984.
Hanshaw JB, Dudgeon JA, Marshall WC: Viral Diseases of the Fetus and Newborn. Philadelphia, WB Saunders, 1985.
Harris H, Wirtschafter D, Cassady G: Endotracheal intubation and its relationship to bacterial colonization and systemic infection of newborn infants. Pediatrics 58:816, 1976.
Hemming VG, Overall JC Jr, Britt MR: Nosocomial infections in a newborn intensive care unit: Results of forty-one months of surveillance. N Engl J Med 294:1310, 1976.
Hill RR, Hunt CE, Matsen JM: Nosocomial colonization with Klebsiella type 26 in a neonatal intensive care unit associated with outbreak of sepsis, meningitis and necrotizing enterocolitis. J Pediatr 85:415, 1976.
McCracken GH Jr: Perinatal bacterial diseases. In: Feigin RD, Cherry JD (eds): Textbook of Pediatric Infectious Diseases. Philadelphia, WB Saunders, 1981, p 747.
Overall JC Jr: Viral infections of the fetus and neonate. In: Feigin RD, Cherry JD (eds): Textbook of Pediatric Infectious Diseases. Philadelphia, WB Saunders, 1981, p 684.
Plotkin S, Starr S: Perinatal infections. Perinatol Clin North Am 8:entire issue, 1981.
Remington JS, Klein JO: Infectious Diseases of the Fetus and Newborn Infant. Philadelphia, WB Saunders, 1983.

8.59 SEPSIS AND MENINGITIS

Neonatal sepsis is a clinical syndrome characterized by symptomatic systemic illness and bacteremia. Asymptomatic bacteremia may also occur in the neonate. Meningitis is present when the spinal fluid contains increased cells and protein, a low sugar, and bacteria or bacterial antigens. Sepsis and meningitis are considered together, because their etiology, epidemiology, and pathogenesis have many common features and the clinical manifestations are similar. Suspected sepsis and/or meningitis is one of the most frequent diagnoses considered by the physician caring for sick newborn infants.

Etiology and Epidemiology. The most common organisms causing disease are *Escherichia coli* and group B streptococcus (which together usually account for 50–75% of cases), *Staphylococcus aureus*, enterococcus, *Klebsiella-Enterobacter* sp., *Pseu-*

domonas aeruginosa, Proteus sp., *Listeria monocytogenes*, and anaerobic organisms. Recently, coagulase-negative staphylococci and candida species have emerged as important pathogens, particularly in low birthweight infants who have required intravascular catheters. Early-onset disease presents as a fulminant process involving multiple organs in the 1st wk of life, while late-onset disease is often manifested as meningitis after the 1st wk. In the former there are usually associated maternal factors, and the organisms are acquired from infected amniotic fluid or on passage through the birth canal, while in the latter the infant may acquire infection in the community or from a number of sources in the hospital. *E. coli* and group B streptococcus may be responsible for either early or late onset of infection, whereas staphylococci, *Klebsiella-Enterobacter* sp., *P. aeruginosa, Candida*, sp., and *Serratia* sp. more commonly cause late-onset disease. Organisms that are the major cause of septicemia and meningitis in the older infant and child—*Hemophilus influenzae* type b, *Streptococcus pneumoniae*, and *Neisseria meningitidis*—are infrequent etiologic agents of disease in the neonatal period (Sec. 11.12, 11.13, and 11.19–11.21).

Clinical Manifestations. The usual manifestations of sepsis are temperature instability, jaundice, respiratory distress, hepatomegaly, abdominal distention, anorexia, vomiting, and lethargy. Similar findings may occur with meningitis, along with convulsions and irritability. Bulging fontanel and stiff neck are absent in 75% or more of the neonates with meningitis. The initial signs of sepsis or meningitis may be subtle. Often the mother or nurse states that the infant "doesn't look well" or "feeds poorly." A high index of suspicion is important, particularly in a neonate with a history of one or more of the risk factors referred to in Sec. 8.58.

Diagnosis. The diagnosis of sepsis or meningitis depends upon the isolation of the etiologic agent from the blood, cerebrospinal fluid (CSF), urine, or other body fluids. Blood for culture should be obtained from a peripheral vein, since blood collected from indwelling vascular catheters gives a high incidence of false-positive results. Osteomyelitis and septic arthritis of the hip have been associated with femoral vein puncture, which is rarely indicated. Two blood cultures often aid in interpreting possible bacterial contaminants; but because antibiotic therapy should be instituted promptly, a single sample will suffice for the diagnosis so that therapy may proceed at once. As little as 0.5–1.0 mL may be adequate when smaller volumes of blood culture media are used. Culture of the urine is important, since the kidney can be seeded with organisms during bacteremia, resulting in positive urine cultures. The neonate with an isolated urinary tract infection can also present a clinical picture resembling sepsis.

Infants with meningitis usually have CSF cell counts greater than $100/mm^3$ with a neutrophil predominance, although the cell count may be considerably less. The protein concentration in the CSF of normal neonates may be as high as 150 mg/dL, particularly in the premature, but in patients with meningitis, levels of several hundred to a few thousand are usually observed. Since hypoglycemia can occur in neonates, it is important to obtain a simultaneous blood sugar in order to interpret hypoglycorrhachia. In meningitis the CSF glucose is usually lower than 40 mg/dL and less than 50% of a simultaneous blood level. A Gram-stained smear of CSF may facilitate an immediate diagnosis and a prediction as to the likely etiologic agent.

Cultures of other body sites should be performed whenever the clinical situation indicates that they may provide useful information: needle aspirate of cellulitis or an abscess; swab of purulent discharge from the eye, umbilicus, or surgical wound. Cultures of the external ear canal, axilla, gastric aspirate, or throat are usually not helpful, since it is difficult to differentiate colonization from true infection.

Treatment. Once the diagnosis of sepsis or meningitis is suspected and once appropriate cultures have been obtained, antibiotic therapy should be instituted immediately. Initial treatment should consist of ampicillin and gentamicin or another aminoglycoside by the intravenous or intramuscular route. Doses of the commonly used antibiotics are provided in Table 8–26. The choice of an aminoglycoside is influenced by (1) where the infection was acquired and (2) what the antibiotic susceptibility pattern of gram-negative enteric organisms is in a particular nursery or newborn intensive care unit. Gram-negative infections acquired from the mother or in the community are more likely to be susceptible to kanamycin, whereas gentamicin (or even tobramycin or amikacin) may be required for infections acquired in the newborn intensive care unit. When the history or the presence of necrotic skin lesions suggests the possibility of *Pseudomonas* infection, initial therapy should be ticarcillin and gentamicin. When staphylococcal sepsis is suspected, treatment should be initiated with methicillin or nafcillin and gentamicin.

Once the pathogen has been identified and the antibiotic sensitivities determined, the most appropriate drug(s) should be selected. With most of the gram-negative enteric bacteria and with enterococcus both a penicillin (ampicillin or carbenicillin) and an aminoglycoside (gentamicin, kanamycin, or one of the newer aminoglycosides) should be used since synergism has been demonstrated with this combination of antibiotics in a substantial proportion of the strains. Ampicillin alone is adequate for *Listeria*, whereas penicillin will suffice for group B streptococcus and most anaerobes. The combination of nafcillin and gentamicin is synergistic against staphylococcal infections.

Third generation cephalosporins, such as cefotaxime or moxalactam, are valuable additions for treating neonatal sepsis and meningitis because (1) the minimal inhibitory combinations for gram-negative enteric bacilli are much lower than for the aminoglycosides; (2) there is excellent penetration into

CSF in the presence of inflamed meninges; and (3) much higher doses than of the aminoglycosides can be given, since toxicity is quite limited. The end result is much higher bactericidal titers in serum and CSF than is achievable with ampicillin/aminoglycoside combinations. However, these cephalosporins have only modest activity against *S. aureus*; moxalactam is relatively ineffective against group B streptococci; *Listeria* and enterococci are resistant to both drugs. Because moxalactam has caused problems with coagulation and bleeding in adults, most authorities currently recommend use of cefotaxime as the third generation cephalosporin for neonates.

Sepsis therapy should be continued for a total of 10–14 days or for at least 5–7 days after clinical response, when there is no evidence of deep tissue involvement or abscess formation. Blood culture 24–48 hr after initiation of therapy should be negative. If the culture is positive, change in therapy may be indicated or the possibility of an occult abscess should be considered. Treatment of meningitis should be continued for at least 3 wk; longer treatment may be necessary if the clinical response is poor or if the spinal fluid cell count, protein, and sugar do not demonstrate a satisfactory response. Response to therapy in meningitis should be followed by serial lumbar punctures until cultures are negative. It is not unusual for spinal fluid cultures to continue positive for 3–4 days with gram-negative enteric bacteria, whereas group B streptococcus and *Listeria* are usually negative in 1–2 days. Mortality and neurologic sequelae rates are no better with intrathecal or intraventricular gentamicin plus parenteral ampicillin and gentamicin than with parenteral therapy alone in treating gram-negative enteric neonatal meningitis. Randomized trials with parenteral moxalactam versus ampicillin plus amikacin and open trials with cefotaxime in gram-negative enteric neonatal meningitis have indicated that these third generation cephalosporins are at least as effective as ampicillin/aminoglycoside combinations. Since the cephalosporins

Table 8–26. **Dosages of Antibiotics Commonly Used in Newborns**

| Antibiotics | Routes of Administration | Dosages (mg/kg/24 hr) and Intervals of Administration | | | |
| | | Body Weight <2000 g | | Body Weight >2000 g | |
		Age 0–7 days	>7 days	Age 0–7 days	>7 days
Amikacin	IM, IV	15 div q12h	30 div q8h	20 div q12h	30 div q8h
Ampicillin,	IV, IM				
Meningitis		100 div q12h	150 div q8h	150 div q8h	200 div q6h
Other diseases		50 div q12h	75 div q8h	75 div q8h	100 div q6h
Cefazolin	IV, IM	40 div q12h	40 div q12h	40 div q12h	60 div q8h
Cefotaxime	IV, IM	100 div q12h	150 div q8h	100 div q12h	150 div q8h
Cephalothin	IV	40 div q12h	60 div q8h	60 div q8h	80 div q6h
Chloramphenicol*	IV, PO	25 once daily	25 once daily	25 once daily	50 div q12h
Erythromycin	PO	20 div q12h	30 div q8h	20 div q12h	30–40 div q8h
Gentamicin	IM, IV	5 div q12h	7.5 div q8h	5 div q12h	7.5 div q8h
Kanamycin	IM, IV	15 div q12h	30 div q8h	20 div q12h	30 div q8h
Methicillin	IV, IM				
Meningitis		100 div q12h	150 div q8h	150 div q8h	200 div q6h
Other diseases		50 div q12h	75 div q8h	75 div q8h	100 div q6h
Mezlocillin	IV, IM	150 div q12h	225 div q8h	150 div q12h	225 div q8h
Nafcillin	IV	50 div q12h	75 div q8h	50 div q8h	75 div q6h
Penicillin G,	IV				
Meningitis		100,000 U div q12h	150,000 U div q8h	150,000 U div q8h	200,000 U div q6h
Other diseases		50,000 U div q12h	75,000 U div q8h	50,000 U div q8h	100,000 U div q6h
Penicillin G,	IM				
benzathine		50,000 U (one dose)	50,000 U (one dose)	50,000 U (one dose)	50,000 U (one dose)
procaine		50,000 U once daily	50,000 U once daily	50,000 U once daily	50,000 U once daily
Ticarcillin	IV, IM	150 div q12h	225 div q8h	225 div q8h	300 div q6h
Tobramycin	IM, IV	4 div q12h	6 div q8h	4 div q12h	6 div q8h
Vancomycin	IV	30 div q12h	45 div q8h	30 div q12h	45 div q8h

*Serum levels are highly variable. Chloramphenicol should be given to newborns only if serum levels can be monitored.
Adapted from McCracken GH Jr, Nelson JD: Antimicrobial Therapy for Newborns. New York, Grune and Stratton, 1983.

have higher bactericidal titers and lower toxicity, many authorities recommend cefotaxime as the treatment of choice for gram-negative enteric meningitis.

Supportive treatment, including management of fluid and electrolyte balance, ventilatory assistance, fresh whole blood transfusion, white cell transfusions, exchange transfusions, treatment for DIC, support of blood pressure with inotropic agents such as dopamine, dobutamine, or steroids, and other measures, is an important adjunct to antibiotic therapy. Appropriate management of complications, such as surgical drainage of a deep abscess, fluid restriction for inappropriate antidiuretic hormone secretion, and anticonvulsant therapy for seizures, should be instituted when they occur.

Prognosis. Current mortality rates in neonatal sepsis range from 10 to 40% and in meningitis from 15 to 50%. Rates vary depending on the time and manner of disease onset, the etiologic agent, the degree of prematurity, the presence and severity of associated disease, and the particular nursery or newborn intensive care unit. Significant neurologic sequelae, including hydrocephalus, mental retardation, blindness, hearing loss, motor disability, and abnormal speech patterns, occur in 30–50% of the survivors of neonatal meningitis. Milder sequelae, such as perceptual difficulties, learning disability, and behavioral problems may also occur.

Prevention. Increased and improved prenatal care, the establishment of a program to deliver high risk mothers at medical centers with newborn intensive care facilities, and the development of modern transport equipment may ameliorate maternal and neonatal factors predisposing to neonatal infection. Controlled studies have not established the efficacy of prophylactic use of antibiotics when there has been premature rupture of membranes, maternal peripartum infection, respiratory distress syndrome, exchange transfusion, surgical procedures in the neonate, or insertion of an umbilical catheter. Regular cleaning and decontamination of nursery equipment, emphasis on sound handwashing principles, regular surveillance for infection in nurseries and newborn intensive care units, and rapid identification and control of common source outbreaks are important in reducing the risk of infection. Vaccines against group B streptococcus and the K1 antigen-containing strains of *E. coli* are being developed for use in the mother to provide passive protection for the neonate.

Baley JE, Kliegman RM, Fanaroff AA: Disseminated fungal infections in very low-birth-weight infants: Clinical manifestations and epidemiology. Pediatrics 73:144, 1984.

Bell WE, McGuinness GA: Suppurative central nervous system infections in the neonate. Semin Perinatol 6:1, 1982.

Christensen R, Rothstein G, Anstall M: Granulocyte transfusions in neonates with bacterial infection, neutropenia and depletion of mature marrow neutrophiles. Pediatrics 70:1, 1982.

Dudley MN, Barriere SL: Cefotaxime: Microbiology, pharmacology and clinical use. Clin Pharmacol 1:114, 1982.

Freedman RM, Ingram DL, Gross I, et al: A half century of neonatal sepsis at Yale. Am J Dis Child 135:140, 1981.

Feigin RD: Neonatal meningitis: Problems and prospects. Hosp Pract 18:175, 1983.

Hill HR: Host defenses in the neonate: Prospects for enhancement. Semin Perinatol 9:2, 1985.

Kafetzis DA, Brater DC, Kapiki AN, et al: Treatment of severe neonatal infections with cefotaxime. Efficacy and pharmacokinetics. J Pediatr 100:483, 1982.

Kovatch AL, Wald ER: Evaluation of the febrile neonate. Semin Perinatol 9:12, 1985.

McCracken GH Jr, Mize SG: A controlled study of intrathecal antibiotic therapy in gram-negative enteric meningitis of infancy. J Pediatr 89:66, 1976.

McCracken GH Jr, Threlkeld N, Mize S, et al: Moxalactam therapy for neonatal meningitis due to gram-negative enteric bacilli. JAMA 252:1427, 1984.

Munson DP, Thompson TR, Johnson DE, et al: Coagulase-negative staphylococcal septicemia: Experience in a newborn intensive care unit. J Pediatr 101:602, 1982.

Sarff LD, Platt LH, McCracken GH Jr: Cerebrospinal fluid evaluation in neonates: Comparison of high risk infants with and without meningitis. J Pediatr 88:473, 1976.

Siegel JD: Neonatal sepsis. Semin Perinatol 9:20, 1985.

Siegel JD, McCracken GH Jr: Sepsis neonatorum. N Engl J Med 304:642, 1981.

Starr SE: Antimicrobial therapy of bacterial sepsis in the newborn infant. J Pediatr 106:1043, 1985.

8.60 PNEUMONIA

Pneumonia (Sec. 13.66–13.68), an important cause of morbidity and mortality in the newborn infant, is the most common inflammatory lesion found at autopsy in the neonatal period. Although pathologic evidence of pulmonary inflammatory disease is evident in 15–20% of stillborns and 20–30% of neonatal deaths, not all of the inflammatory disease is due to infection, and its role as a cause of death is often unclear. Pneumonia due to infection may be acquired *transplacentally* as one component of a generalized intrauterine infection caused by cytomegalovirus, rubella virus, *Toxoplasma*, *Listeria*, and *T. pallidum* (Sec. 8.68–8.69, 11.34, 11.49, and 11.107); *natally* by aspiration of infected amniotic fluid or birth canal secretions with onset of illness during the first few days of life (Sec. 8.34), most commonly associated with group B streptococcus (Sec. 8.66), gram-negative enteric bacilli (Sec. 8.58), chlamydia (Sec. 11.56), and herpes simplex virus (Sec. 8.71); and *postnatally* with symptoms usually not evident until after several days of life, caused by *Staphylococcus aureus* (Sec. 8.67, 13.66), *Pseudomonas aeruginosa* (Sec. 11.30), *Klebsiella*, and *Serratia* sp. (Sec. 13.66), and respiratory viruses (Sec. 11.67).

Pneumonia acquired transplacentally or perinatally is often termed *congenital pneumonia*, and is frequently associated with prolonged rupture of the membranes, chorioamnionitis, prolonged labor, premature labor, or fetal distress.

A diffuse, bilateral, interstitial pneumonitis in infants 6–12 wk of age, due to *Chlamydia trachomatis*, *Pneumocystis carinii*, cytomegaloviris, or perhaps *Ureaplasma urealyticum*, has recently been described. Onset is slowly progressive, and infants are afebrile but may have profound respiratory distress including hypoxia and apnea. The clinical manifestations of infection with these microorganisms are similar; laboratory diagnosis is required to determine the specific etiologic agent.

Low birthweight infants on ventilators often develop new infiltrates on the chest roentgenogram that are associated with deterioration in the respiratory status and that sometimes are accompanied by temperature instability and elevation of the white count. Determining whether this condition is true infectious pneumonia or segmental atelectasis is difficult, but the infants are usually treated with antibiotics for a presumed bacterial infection.

Pathology. Pneumonia in early infancy is usually bronchopneumonia in type, occasionally interstitial or lobar.

Clinical Manifestations. Infants with natal or postnatal pneumonia may initially exhibit nonspecific signs of illness such as poor feeding, lethargy, irritability, poor color, a rise or sudden fall in body temperature, abdominal distention, sudden loss or gain in weight, and the general impression that they are doing less well than before. Signs of respiratory distress, including tachypnea, flaring of the alae nasi, grunting, tachycardia, apnea, accentuation of periodic breathing, and retraction of the suprasternal, intercostal, and subcostal spaces, may rapidly ensue or be somewhat delayed.

Dullness to percussion is difficult to elicit but, when present, suggests extensive consolidation or effusion. Auscultation may reveal fine, crackling rales in any portion of the lung or decreased breath sounds, but often these may not be present, even with extensive pneumonia. It is important to auscultate the chest with the baby crying as well as quiet, since rales frequently are heard only at the end of the deep inspirations that come with crying in the newborn. Areas of hyperresonance may indicate compensatory emphysema. Roentgenograms of the chest are often helpful and are essential to distinguish pneumonia from other causes of respiratory distress.

An acute, often fulminant, form of group B streptococcal pneumonia associated with septicemia may present within the 1st day of life, or later, with respiratory distress, sometimes with shock, or with the sudden deterioration of an infant receiving assisted ventilation. The roentgenogram may be typical for bronchopneumonia or show a diffuse atelectasis resembling hyaline membrane disease.

Tracheal aspirate and blood cultures are helpful in making an etiologic diagnosis.

In the afebrile interstitial pneumonitis syndrome of neonatal infants, tracheal aspirates or nasopharyngeal swabs should be obtained for chlamydial culture or immunofluorescent stain of a smear, serum should be obtained for detection of pneumocystis antigen, and tracheal secretions should be obtained for culture of ureaplasma and cytomegalovirus.

Treatment. Since the etiologic agents of bacterial pneumonia are the same as for sepsis and meningitis, similar antibiotic regimens are used. Chlamydial pneumonia is treated with erythromycin or trimethoprim/sulfamethoxazole; pneumocystis pneumonia is treated with trimethoprim/sulfamethoxazole, and pneumonia involving *Ureaplasma* infection with erythromycin.

Ablow RC, Driscoll SG, Effmann EL, et al: A comparison of early onset group B streptococcal neonatal infection and the respiratory distress syndrome of the newborn. N Engl J Med 294:65, 1976.
Beem MD, Saxon E, Tipple MA: Treatment of chlamydial pneumonia of infancy. Pediatrics 63:198, 1979.
Dworsky ME, Stagno S: Newer agents causing pneumonitis in early infancy. Pediatr Infect Dis 1:188, 1982.
Sherman MP, Chance KH, Goetzman BW: Gram's stains of tracheal secretions predict neonatal bacteremia. Am J Dis Child 138:848, 1984.

8.61 OSTEOMYELITIS AND SEPTIC ARTHRITIS

See also Sec 11.14 and 11.15.

Because of the unique nature of the blood supply to the skeletal system in the neonate and young infant, these two infections often occur together. During the first several months of life capillaries penetrate the epiphyseal plate and provide a direct communication between the metaphysis of the bone and the joint space. In addition, the capsules of the hip and shoulder joints attach distal to the metaphysis of the femur and humerus, respectively. Therefore, infections beginning in the metaphysis, the site of initial involvement in osteomyelitis, can readily spread to involve the joint space and vice versa. Although osteomyelitis and septic arthritis usually occur as a result of hematogenous seeding during the course of a bacteremia, extension from a subcutaneous infection (osteomyelitis of the calcaneus associated with multiple heel punctures for blood samples) or by direct inoculation during a procedure (septic arthritis of the hip associated with a femoral puncture) have been reported.

Etiology. *Staphylococcus aureus* is the causative agent in 85% of infants with osteomyelitis. Other causative organisms include group A and B streptococcus and pneumococcus; gram-negative bacteria are rarely encountered. In septic arthritis *S. aureus* is a frequent causative organism, and gram-negative enteric bacteria, *Candida*, and *Neisseria gonorrhoeae* are not uncommon etiologic agents.

Clinical Manifestations. There may be little or no sign of systemic illness. Diminished spontaneous movement, pain on passive motion of the affected limb, or localized swelling may be noted. In the more severe form systemic manifestations of sepsis predominate, and multiple skeletal sites are often involved. The long bones and the major joints of the extremities are the most commonly involved areas.

Diagnosis. Roentgenographic examination demonstrates soft tissue swelling followed by necrosis of bone, with rarefaction and periosteal elevation in the metaphyseal area. The radionuclide bone scan may be positive early in the course of osteomyelitis when roentgenograms show no or minimal change, but false negative results occur in 40–50% of cases. Widening of the joint space may be observed in septic arthritis, and subluxation of the hip or shoulder joint is occasionally seen. Direct aspiration of the joint space or the subperiosteal area is indicated in all cases and may provide an immediate diagnosis. Orthopedic consultation should be obtained. Gram stain and culture of any aspirated material should be performed and blood cultures obtained. The peripheral white count is often not helpful, but the sedimentation rate may be elevated in infants with osteomyelitis.

Treatment. The choice of initial antibiotic agents should be guided by the Gram stain. If gram-positive cocci are seen, treatment should be initiated with methicillin or nafcillin plus gentamicin; if gram-negative organisms are present, therapy should consist of ampicillin and gentamicin. Once the results of culture and antibiotic sensitivity are known, treatment should be continued with the appropriate drug(s). The antibiotics should be given by the intravenous or intramuscular route in the doses indicated in Table 8–26 for at least 3–4 wk after defervescence. Because of insufficient data about reliability and clinical efficacy of oral antibiotics in neonates, this route of administration should not be used. Direct instillation of antibiotic into the joint space or bone is not indicated as adequate levels are achieved with parenteral therapy. In general the infected bone or joint space should be drained by either aspiration or surgical incision. The hip and shoulder joints, in particular, require drainage since purulent material under pressure within the joint capsule can occlude the vascular supply and result in necrosis of the bone. The affected extremity should be immobilized until inflammation has subsided and roentgenographic evidence of healing is present.

Prognosis. Although death is infrequent, long-term morbidity may be significant. Chronic osteomyelitis, skeletal and joint deformities, or disturbed bone growth may occur in 25–50% of cases, particularly if the hip or knee is involved.

Edwards MS, Baker CJ, Wagner ML, et al: An etiologic shift in infantile osteomyelitis: The emergence of the group B streptococcus. J Pediatr 93:578, 1978.
Fox L, Sprunt K: Neonatal osteomyelitis. Pediatrics 62:535, 1978.
Marcy SM: Bacterial infections of the bones and joints. In: Remington JS, Klein JO (eds): Infectious Diseases of the Fetus and Newborn Infant. Philadelphia, WB Saunders, 1983.
Nelson JD: Follow up: The bacterial etiology and antibiotic management of septic arthritis in infants and children. Pediatrics 50:437, 1972.
Ogden JA: Pediatric osteomyelitis and septic arthritis: The pathology of neonatal disease. Yale J Biol Med 52:423, 1979.
Weissberg ED, Smith AL, Smith DH: Clinical features of neonatal osteomyelitis. Pediatrics 53:505, 1974.

8.62 URINARY TRACT INFECTION

See also Sec. 17.38.

Urinary tract infection occurs in 0.1–1% of newborn infants. The incidence is much higher in low birthweight infants and is about three times more common in males than females. Over 75% of the infections are due to *Escherichia coli*; the remainder are caused by other gram-negative enteric bacilli (*Klebsiella*, Enterobacter, and *Proteus* sp.) and gram-positive cocci (enterococci, *Staphylococcus aureus*, and *S. epidermidis*). The major route of neonatal infection is hematogenous invasion. The incidence of anatomic obstructive lesions is around 5%.

Clinical Manifestations. The signs are varied and nonspecific. Infants may present a picture resembling sepsis, or there may be an insidious onset consisting of low grade fever, irritability, and failure to gain weight. Some infants may be completely asymptomatic, while others may have localized signs such as balanitis, urethritis, a weak urinary stream, or a large flank mass.

Diagnosis. The diagnosis is confirmed by a positive urine culture. Since collecting a satisfactory clean catch urine specimen is often difficult, obtaining an uncontaminated urine by suprapubic aspiration is advised. In infants who appear septic, blood and CSF cultures should also be obtained. Although pyuria is not a reliable indicator of infection in the neonate, the presence of white cells in the urine on a routine urinalysis should be evaluated for possible infection.

Treatment and Prognosis. If the infant with a urinary tract infection has signs of sepsis, the antibiotic regimens outlined in Sec. 8.59 should be used. The urine culture should be negative in 36–48 hr in a successfully treated patient. If cultures continue positive, an obstructive lesion or an abscess should be suspected. Therapy is continued for 10–14 days in the uncomplicated case. Recurrent infections may occur in 20–25% of patients, usually within the first few months after the initial episode, and should be treated with a full course of antibiotics. Therefore, follow-up urine cultures should be obtained.

Every infant with a documented urinary tract infection should have ultrasonic and/or roentgenologic evaluation of the urinary tract (Sec. 5.55), but unless the infant fails to respond to antibiotic therapy, this should be deferred until recovery from the acute stages of the illness and attainment of a few weeks of age. Vesicoureteral reflux can occur during the acute disease and clear with resolution of the infection, and excretion of the dye used in the intravenous pyelogram may be inadequate to provide proper visualization during the first 1–2 wk of life. Infants with obstructive lesions should be referred for urologic evaluation for potential corrective surgery.

Abbott GD: Neonatal bacteriuria: A prospective study in 1,460 infants. Br Med J 1:267, 1972.
Bensman A, Baudon J, Jablonski J, et al: Uropathies diagnosed in the neonatal period: Symptomatology and course. Acta Paediatr Scand 69:499, 1980.
Bergstrom T, Larson H, Lincoln K, et al: Studies of urinary tract infections in infancy and childhood: Eighty consecutive patients with neonatal infection. J Pediatr 80:858, 1972.
Edelmann CM Jr: The prevalence of bacteriuria in full term and premature newborn infants. J Pediatr 82:125, 1973.
Ginsburg CM, McCracken GH: Urinary tract infections in young infants. Pediatrics 69:409, 1982.
Littlewood JM: Sixty-six infants with urinary tract infection in the first month of life. Arch Dis Child 47:218, 1972.
Nelson JD, Peters PC: Suprapubic aspiration of urine in premature and term infants. Pediatrics 36:132, 1965.

8.63 DIARRHEA

Although a pathogen is identified in only a small percentage of neonates with diarrhea, the possibility of nursery epidemics of infectious diarrhea involving many infants with a potentially life-threatening illness is a serious risk (Sec. 11.8). The neonate is usually infected at the time of birth by organisms present in maternal stool or after birth by spread of organisms from other infected infants on the hands of personnel. Outbreaks of diarrheal disease in nurseries have occurred due to *Escherichia coli*, salmonella, echovirus, rotavirus, and adenovirus.

Onset of the illness may be either slow and insidious or abrupt. Often, a period of listlessness and poor feeding is followed by vomiting and then diarrhea. Stools are initially yellow and loose, then become watery, green, and mucoid as they increase in frequency. The most serious aspect of disease is fluid loss with resultant dehydration and electrolyte disturbances; small premature infants may lose sufficient fluid into

the bowel lumen to cause hypovolemic shock prior to the development of clinically significant diarrhea. Management of diarrhea occurring in a nursery includes maintenance of fluid and electrolyte balance, antibiotics when appropriate, and the prevention of spread of the disease to other infants (Sec. 8.58) by an emphasis on good handwashing techniques, discharge of culture-positive infants from the hospital as soon as their condition allows, and follow-up stool cultures on patients who have received a course of therapy.

Anders BJ, Lauer BA, Paisley JW: Campylobacter gastroenteritis in neonates. Am J Dis Child 135:900, 1981.
Barton LL, Pickering LK: Shigellosis in the first week of life. Pediatrics 52:437, 1973.
Blacklow NR, Cukor G: Viral gastroenteritis. N Engl J Med 304:397, 1981.
Boyer KM, Peterson NJ, Farzaneh I, et al: An outbreak of gastroenteritis due to E. coli 0124 in a neonatal nursery. J Pediatr 86:919, 1975.
Kapikian AZ, Kim KW, Wyatt RG, et al: Human reovirus-like agent as the major pathogen associated with winter gastroenteritis in hospitalized infants and children. N Engl J Med 294:965, 1976.
Kaslow RA, Taylor A Jr, Dweck HS, et al: Enteropathogenic Escherichia coli infection in a newborn nursery. Am J Dis Child 128:797, 1974.
Marcy SM, Guerrant RL: Microorganisms responsible for neonatal diarrhea. In: Remington JS, Klein JO (eds): Infections of the Fetus and Newborn Infant. Philadelphia, WB Saunders, 1983, p 917.
Steinhoff MC: Rotavirus: The first five years. J Pediatr 96:611, 1980.

8.64 CONJUNCTIVITIS

See also Sec. 25.9.

Conjunctivitis is frequently encountered in the newborn infant, secondary to inflammation caused by silver nitrate and to infection with *Neisseria gonorrhoeae*, *Chlamydia trachomatis*, and *Staphylococcus aureus*. Less common causes include infection with group A or B streptococcus, *Pseudomonas aeruginosa*, other bacteria, or herpesvirus hominis type 2. *N. gonorrhoeae*, *C. trachomatis*, group B streptococcus, and herpesvirus hominis are acquired on passage through a colonized or infected birth canal; other bacteria are usually acquired after birth. Prematurity and prolonged rupture of membranes are associated with an increased incidence of conjunctivitis due to the organisms acquired at birth.

Clinical Manifestations. The onset of inflammation caused by silver nitrate drops is usually within 6–12 hr after birth, with clearing by 24–48 hr. The usual incubation period for conjunctivitis due to *N. gonorrhoeae* is 2–5 days and for that due to *C. trachomatis*, 5–14 days. The time of onset of disease with other bacteria is highly variable.

Gonococcal conjunctivitis begins with mild inflammation and a serosanguineous discharge. Within 24 hr the discharge becomes thick and purulent, and tense edema of the eyelids with marked chemosis occurs. If proper treatment is delayed, the infection may spread to involve deeper layers of the conjunctivae and the cornea. Complications include corneal ulceration and perforation, iridocyclitis, anterior synechiae, and rarely panophthalmitis. Conjunctivitis caused by *C. trachomatis* (inclusion blennorrhea) may vary from mild inflammation to severe swelling of the eyelids with copious purulent discharge. The process involves mainly the tarsal conjunctivae; the corneas are rarely affected. Conjunctivitis due to *S. aureus*, *P. aeruginosa*, or other organisms is similar to that produced by *C. trachomatis*.

Diagnosis. Conjunctivitis appearing after 48 hr should be evaluated for a possibly infectious cause. Gram stain of the purulent discharge should be performed and the material cultured. If a viral etiology is suspected, a swab should be submitted in tissue culture media for virus isolation. In chlamydial conjunctivitis the diagnosis is made by examining Giemsa-stained epithelial cells scraped from the tarsal conjunctivae for the characteristic intracytoplasmic inclusions, by isolating the organisms from a conjunctival swab using special tissue culture techniques, or by immunofluorescent staining of conjunctival scrapings for chlamydial inclusions.

Treatment. Treatment of the infant in whom gonococcal ophthalmia is suspected and the Gram stain shows characteristic organisms should be initiated immediately with aqueous penicillin G, given intravenously or intramuscularly in a dosage of 100,000–150,000 units/kg/24 hr in 2–3 divided doses for 5–7 days. In addition, the eye should be irrigated with saline every 10–30 min at first and gradually increasing to 2 hr intervals, until the purulent discharge has cleared. Some advocate the use of penicillin G or chloramphenicol as eye drops immediately after each saline irrigation. Inclusion blennorrhea is treated with oral erythromycin for 2 wk. Staphylococcal and *Pseudomonas* neonatal conjunctivitis are treated with systemic antibiotics plus local saline irrigation, with or without topical use of antibiotics.

Prognosis and Prevention. Prior to the institution of silver nitrate prophylaxis at birth, gonococcal ophthalmia was a common cause of blindness or permanent eye damage. If properly applied, this form of prophylaxis is highly effective. Drops of 1% silver nitrate are instilled directly into the open eyes at birth using wax or plastic single dose containers. Saline irrigation is unnecessary but, if performed, should not be done until after the silver nitrate solution has been in contact with the eye for at least 15 sec.

Antigonococcal prophylaxis with silver nitrate has little effect on chlamydial ophthalmia. With prompt recognition and appropriate therapy, only a small percentage of such patients have demonstrable corneal scarring, rarely associated with any visual disturbance. Because of the increasing recognition of chlamydial infections, possible alternatives to silver nitrate prophylaxis of ophthalmia neonatorum include 1% tetracycline or 0.5% erythromycin ointment, which are active against *C. trachomatis* as well as *N. gonorrhoeae*, or a single intramuscular injection of aqueous penicillin (50,000 units in term or 20,000 units in preterm infants).

American Academy of Pediatrics: Prophylaxis and treatment of neonatal gonococcal infections. Pediatrics 65:1047, 1980.

8.65 OTITIS MEDIA

See also Sec. 13.40.

Acute otitis media in the newborn period presents a special diagnostic problem, because the signs and symptoms of disease are subtle and nonspecific and the tympanic membrane is difficult to examine. In examining the eardrum, it is important to determine its mobility since the tympanic membrane may appear dull and thickened in the normal infant. Nonspecific signs and symptoms include irritability and/or lethargy, decreased appetite or failure to thrive, mild respiratory symptoms, and low grade fever. Infants may be asymptomatic.

Otitis media occurs more frequently in preterm than in term infants. In contrast to older children, the etiologic agents isolated during the first 6 wk of life from about one third of infants with otitis media include *E. coli, K. pneumoniae, P. aeruginosa*, group B streptococci, and *S. aureus. S. pneumoniae* and *H. influenzae*, the most common pathogens in older children, are found in approximately one third of the cases. In the remainder, nonpathogens are isolated or no organism is found.

The initial therapy of a neonate definitively diagnosed as having otitis media but in whom sepsis is also considered should be that of neonatal sepsis. In an asymptomatic infant ampicillin or amoxicillin may be started, but the infant should be carefully reevaluated in 2–3 days to determine that the middle ear disease has responded. The therapeutic regimen should optimally be based on tympanocentesis in order to

identify the specific etiologic agent, and there should be careful follow-up to prevent the development of chronic middle ear disease.

Bland R: Otitis media in the first six weeks of life, diagnosis, bacteriology, and management. Pediatrics 49:187, 1972.
De Sa D: Infection and amniotic aspiration of middle ear in stillbirths and neonatal deaths. Arch Dis Child 48:872, 1973.
Klein, JO: Bacterial infections of the respiratory tract. In: Remington JS, Klein JO (eds): Infectious Diseases of the Fetus and Newborn Infant, Philadelphia, WB Saunders, 1983, p 736.
Shurin PA, Howe VM, Pelton SI, et al: Bacterial etiology of otitis media during first six weeks of life. J Pediatr 92;893, 1978.

8.66 GROUP B STREPTOCOCCUS

In some medical centers this organism is the leading cause of sepsis and meningitis in neonates; in others, group B streptococcal infections are rarely seen. The reasons for these differences in frequency are unknown (also see Sec. 11.16).

Epidemiology. Infants are commonly infected on passage through a birth canal colonized with group B streptococcus. Although maternal cervical and/or vaginal colonization rates vary from 5–30%, depending on the geography and the nature of the population sampled, group B streptococcus rarely results in clinically significant diseases in the mother. Colonization of the throat or umbilicus in newborn infants occurs at a rate of 30–50%, but only approximately 1 in 50–100 colonized infants gets systemic disease. The organism can also be transmitted to neonates after birth on the hands of personnel; nosocomial nursery outbreaks have been reported.

Clinical Manifestations. Two patterns of illness in the neonate have emerged: early-onset disease with fulminant pneumonia and sepsis and late-onset disease that is insidious and manifests primarily as meningitis. However, these patterns may vary considerably and may merge: infants have been seen early with meningitis and late with sepsis. The *early-onset disease* is associated with a high incidence of maternal obstetric complications, such as prolonged rupture of membranes, difficult traumatic delivery, or maternal peripartum fever. Characteristically, the infant's birthweight is low and respiratory distress begins within hours of birth and rapidly worsens. The clinical and roentgenographic features closely resemble those of hyaline membrane disease; infants with group B streptococcal infection often have prolonged rupture of membranes (>12 hr), gram-positive cocci in the tracheal aspirate, and low white blood cell counts, especially in the first 12 hr. In many cases, a rapid downhill course brings death in 12–24 hr despite intensive support therapy and high intravenous doses of appropriate antibiotics. Mortality rates range from 40 to 60%, and the organisms usually can be cultured from multiple body fluids and orifices.

The *late-onset* disease usually presents more slowly with the features characteristic of meningitis: fever, lethargy, vomiting, and a bulging fontanel. Other forms of late-onset disease may occur, such as septic arthritis, osteomyelitis, and cellulitis. Asymptomatic bacteremia has also been reported. Mortality rates in group B streptococcal meningitis range from 15 to 20%, with neurologic sequelae in 30 to 50% of survivors.

Diagnosis. Group B streptococcus infection is established by isolation of the organism from blood, CSF, or urine. A rapid diagnosis can be made using counterimmunoelectrophoresis or latex agglutination on these fluids. Although a number of infants with early-onset disease may have leukopenia, thrombocytopenia, or both, peripheral blood counts are not usually helpful. The most important aspect of diagnosis is maintaining a high index of suspicion. When the diagnosis is strongly considered, antibiotic therapy should begin promptly after appropriate cultures have been obtained.

Treatment. Although virtually all strains of group B streptococcus are sensitive to penicillin or ampicillin, many authorities recommend a penicillin/aminoglycoside combination for the initial treatment of serious infections. Ampicillin and gentamicin have been demonstrated to be synergistic against group B streptococcus in vitro and in experimental animal infections, and isolates from patients with a poor clinical response to ampicillin alone have been found to be penicillin tolerant organisms. Combination therapy should be continued for the first several days until there is a good bacteriologic and clinical response. Penicillin or ampicillin alone could then be used for a total treatment course of 10–14 days for uncomplicated bacteremia, 2–3 wk for meningitis and septic arthritis, and 3–4 wk for osteomyelitis.

Because of the high mortality rates particularly in the early-onset disease, chemo- or immunoprophylaxis of the colonized mother or infants at risk has been considered but not generally accepted because of lack of efficacy, expense, and risks. Treatment of babies with intramuscular penicillin at the time of birth has also not been established. Absence of protective antibody against the group B streptococcus in both the infected infant and the maternal sera has been noted. Efforts are underway to develop a vaccine to immunize mothers and provide passive protection for the neonate. In addition, use of hyperimmune gamma globulin for intravenous administration is being evaluated.

Anthony BF, Okada DM: The emergence of group B streptococci in infections of the newborn infant. Ann Rev Med 28:355, 1977.

Baker C: Summary of the workshop on perinatal infections due to group B streptococcus. J Infect Dis 136:137, 1977.

Baker C, Edwards MS: Group B streptococcal infections. In: Remington JS, Klein JO (eds): Infectious Diseases of the Fetus and Newborn Infant. Philadelphia, WB Saunders, 1983, p 820.

Hodes HL: Penicillin prophylaxis and neonatal streptococcal disease. Hosp Pract 15:115, 1980.

Howard JB, McCracken GH Jr: The spectrum of group B streptococcal infections in infancy. Am J Dis Child 128:815, 1974.

Pyati SP, Pildes RS, Jacobs NM, et al: Early penicillin in infants <2000 grams with early onset GBS: Is it effective? Pediatr Res 16:1019, 1982.

Siegel JD, McCracken GH, Threlkeld N, et al: Single dose penicillin prophylaxis against neonatal group B streptococcal infections. N Engl J Med 303:769, 1981.

Yow MD, Mason EO, Leeds LJ, et al: Ampicillin prevents intrapartum transmission of group B streptococcus. JAMA 241:1245, 1979.

8.67 STAPHYLOCOCCUS

See also Sec. 11.17 and 13.66.

During the first 5 days of life, 40–90% of infants are colonized by staphylococcal organisms. Periodic epidemics of neonatal staphylococcal infection are related in part to differences in the capacity of different strains to colonize and cause disease.

Despite the high colonization rates with *S. aureus* in neonates, the incidence of disease in the absence of epidemics is probably no more than 1–3/1000 live births. The most common source of infection for the newborn infant is medical personnel. Although those with clinically evident staphylococcal infections are more likely to disseminate the organism, asymptomatic carriers are extremely common and may be infectious on occasion. Medical personnel can carry staphylococci on their skin, in their anterior nares, axillae, or perineal areas.

Clinical Manifestations. *S. aureus* is associated with a wide spectrum of clinical disease. Skin lesions (especially pustules and cellulitis), the most frequent manifestation, are found mainly in the diaper area, axillae, groin, neck, and umbilicus and, in males, the site of circumcision. Staphylococcal scalded skin syndrome or Ritter's disease is a generalized manifestation of a local staphylococcal infection. The initial focus of infection may be in the umbilicus, site of circumcision, conjunctiva, or oropharynx. A scarlatiniform rash may precede the development of superficial bullae, which readily rupture. Large areas of epidermis desquamate, leaving a raw, weeping, red, "scalded"-appearing surface (see Fig. 24–40). Light rub-

bing of the skin results in wrinkling and separation of the outer layers of the epidermis (Nikolsky sign). The disease is usually caused by coagulase-positive, phage group II (3A, 3C, 55, 71) *S. aureus* which produces an exfoliative toxin. Intact, fluid-filled bullae are usually sterile and lack inflammatory cells. After rupture, staphylococci may often be isolated from the raw, denuded surface of the skin. The lesions heal without scarring over 7–10 days.

Other clinical manifestations of staphylococcal disease in the neonate include septicemia without focal disease, pneumonia (Sec. 8.60, 11.17, and 13.66), osteomyelitis, septic arthritis, breast abscess, conjunctivitis, and otitis media.

A number of host defense mechanisms in the sick neonate may be compromised, and organisms of relatively low virulence, such as *S. epidermidis* (Sec. 11.18), may cause disease, particularly in the presence of a foreign body like a shunt for hydrocephalus, an umbilical catheter, or a central venous catheter. If a neonate has clinical evidence of infection and *S. epidermidis* is a consistent or the only isolate from appropriate cultures, it should be considered the pathogen.

Prevention and Treatment. There is little evidence that caps, masks, and gowns contribute significantly to control of infection in a nursery unit except when isolating an infant with known infection. However, vigorous enforcement of handwashing techniques, short-term use of hexachlorophene washes, and the application of antibiotic agents or triple dye to the umbilical cord decrease colonization rates.

Although milder forms of skin lesions may be treated with local cleansing, antibiotic therapy should be given to any infant who does not respond readily to local treatment or who develops signs of extensive disease or systemic illness. Penicillinase-resistant semisynthetic penicillins should be used except when staphylococci are resistant to these drugs. Under these circumstances systemic vancomycin therapy should be instituted.

Dunkle L, Naqvi S, McCollum R, et al: Eradication of epidemic methicillin-gentamicin resistant *Staphylococcus aureus* in an intensive care nursery. Am J Med 70:455, 1981.

Johnson JD, Malachowski NC, Vosti KL, et al: A sequential study of various modes of skin and umbilical care and the incidence of staphylococcal colonization and infection in the neonate. Pediatrics 58:354, 1976.

Kaslow RA, Dixon RE, Martin SM, et al: Staphylococcal disease related to hospital nursery bathing practices—a nationwide epidemiologic investigation. Pediatrics 51:418, 1973.

Melish ME, Glasgow LA: The staphylococcal scalded-skin syndrome. Development of an experimental model. N Engl J Med 282:1114, 1970.

Mortimer AE Jr, Lipsitz PJ, Wolinsky E, et al: Transmission of staphylococci between newborns. Importance of the hands of personnel. Am J Dis Child 104:289, 1962.

Shinefield HR: Staphylococcal infections. In: Remington JS, Klein JO (eds): Infectious Diseases of the Fetus and Newborn Infant. Philadelphia, WB Saunders, 1983, p 882.

Shuman RM, Leech RW, Alvord EC Jr: Neurotoxicity of hexachlorophene in the human. I. A clinical-pathological study of 248 children. Pediatrics 54:90, 1974.

LISTERIA

See Sec. 11.34.

8.68 CYTOMEGALOVIRUS (CMV)

See also Sec. 11.68.

This ubiquitous agent usually results in subclinical infections in the healthy adult or child but may cause serious disease in the immunologically immature or compromised host. The fetus or newborn may acquire CMV infection congenitally by transplacental transmission, perinatally by aspiration of infected genital secretions, and postnatally from breast milk or blood transfused from seropositive donors. Transmission among infants in an intensive care setting is quite rare. Congenital infection may occur in fetuses of mothers with either a primary or a recurrent (reactivated latent) infection. However, only 15% of infants born to mothers with primary CMV infection during pregnancy have clinical evidence of CMV disease during the neonatal period; none of those born to mothers with recurrent CMV have CMV-related symptoms. Perinatal and breast milk–acquired CMV infections rarely cause disease in the neonate, but blood transfusion–transmitted infections have caused disease in 80–90% of infants and death in 20–25%.

Clinical Manifestations. Congenital CMV infection or cytomegalic inclusion disease may be a systemic illness characterized by intrauterine growth retardation, hepatosplenomegaly, jaundice, petechial rash, chorioretinitis, cerebral calcifications, and microcephaly (Fig. 8–27). However, this severe form of the disease represents less than 10% of congenitally infected neonates. The majority of infections are asymptomatic in the neonatal period. Hepatomegaly is usually associated with hyperbilirubinemia and with moderate elevations of the serum transaminase and alkaline phosphatase activities; direct involvement of the liver is indicated by isolation of virus and the presence of multinucleated giant cells and characteristic intranuclear inclusions. Extramedullary hematopoiesis may cause organomegaly in the absence of hepatitis. Although the duration of hepatosplenomegaly may vary from several months to several years, CMV does not cause persistent active hepatitis. A generalized, usually pinpoint, petechial rash is found in approximately 50% of severely involved infants. The virus appears to affect the bone marrow directly, causing a thrombocytopenia that may clear in 48–72 hr or persist for weeks to months. Significant bleeding, however, rarely occurs.

Infection of the central nervous system results in the most severe sequelae. Microcephaly is found with increasing frequency in severely involved infants and, when associated with cerebral calcification, carries a high probability of psychomotor retardation. The cerebral calcifications are typically periventricular in distribution, in contrast to the more diffuse patterns observed in congenital *Toxoplasma* infection; these patterns, however, are not diagnostic. Microcephaly may not become apparent for several months. The eye is less commonly involved in congenital cytomegalovirus infection than in rubella or toxoplasmosis. Chorioretinitis occurs in approximately 25% of the severely involved infants; strabismus and optic atrophy may occur. Microphthalmia and corneal opacities are rare. CMV can also directly infect the stucture of the inner ear, resulting in deafness. Ear involvement may be unilateral or bilateral and can be progressive. The majority of infants with congenital CMV infection are asymptomatic during the neonatal period. However, these inapparent infections result in hearing loss and impaired intellectual functioning in at least one third of involved infants.

CMV infection associated with blood transfusion is characterized by a septic appearance, hepatosplenomegaly, gray pallor, pneumonitis, a deteriorating respiratory status, and atypical lymphocytosis. The disease occurs in sick premature infants who are long-term residents of an intensive care unit, usually at 1–2 mo of age. Blood transfusions from seropositive donors have been associated with this syndrome. Whenever possible only CMV seronegative donors should be used for blood transfusions in neonates.

Diagnosis. The virus can be cultured from urine. TORCH screen antibody assays, that measure predominantly IgG, require two serum specimens for accurate diagnosis: one in the neonatal period and one at 4–6 mo of age. A falling CMV antibody titer indicates transplacental passage of antibody from mother to fetus, whereas a stable or rising titer supports congenital, perinatal, or postnatal infection. Demonstration of CMV-specific IgM antibody in neonatal serum can be diagnostic.

Treatment and Prevention. Antiviral drugs transiently suppress viruria but have no lasting effect on CMV neurologic disease. Useful infection control measures include (1) isolation of infants known to be infected with CMV, (2) good handwashing and personal hygiene habits in personnel caring for infected infants, and (3) use of blood from only CMV-seronegative donors for neonatal transfusion. Work is in progress toward a live, attenuated CMV vaccine.

Hanshaw JB, Dudgeon JA, Marshall WC: Viral Diseases of the Fetus and Newborn. Philadelphia, WB Saunders, 1985.
Kumar ML, Nankervis GA, Gold E: Inapparent congenital cytomegalovirus infection; a followup study. N Engl J Med 288:1370, 1973.
Stagno S, Reynolds DW, Amos CS, et al: Auditory and visual defects resulting from symptomatic and subclinical congenital cytomegalovirus and Toxoplasma infections. Pediatrics 59:669, 1977.
Stagno S, Reynolds DW, Huang E, et al: Congenital cytomegalovirus infection: Occurrence in an immune population. N Engl J Med 296:1254, 1977.
Yeager AS, Grumet FC, Hafleigh EB, et al: Prevention of transfusion-acquired cytomegalovirus infections in newborn infants. J Pediatr 98:281, 1981.

8.69 RUBELLA

See also Sec. 11.62.

The rubella syndrome represents a prototype for congenital viral infections. During maternal infection rubella virus can cross the placenta, infect the fetus, and result in death of the conceptus or birth of an infant with congenital rubella. The chronically infected infant who acquired the infection in utero may be a source for maintaining the virus during periods when few cases are recognized in the community. Immunization with the live attenuated rubella vaccine has resulted in a decreased incidence of congenital rubella.

Pathogenesis and Pathology. Maternal viremia may lead to seedings of the placenta. The placenta, in turn, may serve as a source of virus for the fetus. The gestational age of the conceptus at the time of infection is a critical factor in determining the outcome. Prior to the 8th wk of gestation, 50–80%

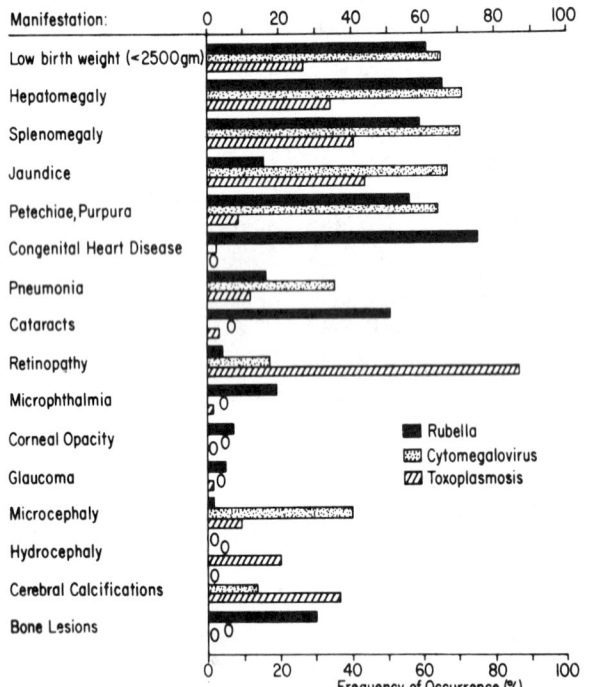

Figure 8–27. Manifestations of symptomatic congenital rubella, cytomegalovirus, and toxoplasma infections. (From Overall JC Jr, *In*: Feigin RD, Cherry JD (eds): Textbook of Pediatric Infectious Diseases. Philadelphia, WB Saunders, 1981.)

of fetuses exposed to maternal rubella become infected; by the 2nd trimester no more than 10–20% of infants become infected, and during the 3rd trimester infection of the fetus is relatively uncommon.

Early in pregnancy the clinical manifestations of fetal infection are more severe, and multiple organ involvement is more frequent. Regardless of the degree of involvement, however, fetal infection is usually chronic and infants with congenital rubella may carry the virus in the nasopharynx, urine, cerebrospinal fluid, stool, eye, bone marrow, and peripheral leukocytes for extended periods of time.

Necrosis of vascular endothelium is common and may lead to vascular obstruction with secondary damage to organs. Direct lysis of cells by rubella virus may occur in involved organs, particularly myocardial and skeletal muscle cells, and epithelial cells of the lens and inner ear. There is only a minimal infiltration of inflammatory cells, a characteristic which may be noted in a number of other viral infections of the fetus. Hepatocellular disease with necrosis, giant cell formation, bile stasis, and fibrosis occurs, as well as hepatic biliary obstruction.

Clinical Manifestations. Congenital rubella may range from a subclinical to severe disease involving multiple target organs and numerous anomalies. Infants of mothers with known or suspected rubella should be followed carefully throughout childhood since asymptomatic infants with chronic subclinical infection may subsequently develop defects or have specific organ involvement. The frequency of clinical manifestations identified in symptomatic infants during the neonatal period is illustrated in Fig. 8–27. The incidence of thrombocytopenic purpura is relatively high as one group of patients was selected on the basis of the presence of purpura; the frequency of purpura in most series ranged from 15–50%. Thrombocytopenia usually resolves spontaneously during the 1st mo of life, but it is often found in severely affected infants with multiple organ involvement and congenital anomalies. Of 58 patients with purpura in one series, 35% died during the 1st yr of life, in contrast to an overall mortality rate of only 13% during the first 18 mo of life for the total series of 271 children with the rubella syndrome. Death is rarely due to hemorrhage, although the thrombocytopenia may be profound.

Signs of congenital heart disease are observed frequently in the neonatal period. There also may be a viral interstitial pneumonia characterized by cough, tachypnea, and respiratory distress. The primary presenting syndrome may be respiratory; in one series, six of seven patients with this syndrome died during the 1st yr of life as a result of their pulmonary disease. Low birthweight for gestational age is common and is believed to result from intrauterine growth retardation. Direct involvement of the liver by rubella virus may result in neonatal hepatitis, evidenced by hepatomegaly, a predominantly direct-reacting hyperbilirubinemia, and elevations of alkaline phosphatase and serum transaminase activities.

Cataracts, the most characteristic ocular lesion, may not be recognized until after the neonatal period. The retina also may be involved and lesions may be widespread, mottled, or blotchy, with black pigmentary deposits that are variable in size and location—the "salt and pepper" retinitis. Retinal function is usually not adversely affected. Bone lesions are another typical finding but also may exist in isolation; they consist of small linear areas of radiolucency and increased bone density in a longitudinal axis of the metaphyseal area in the long bones of the upper and lower extremities. The abnormality usually resolves by 2–3 mo of age. The lesions may be differentiated from those observed in congenital syphilis by the absence of periosteal reaction.

Central nervous system involvement is frequent in symptomatic infants. Lethargy, irritability, disturbances of tone, and bulging fontanel are common. Seizures may occur but often are not observed until after the neonatal period. Elevation of protein in the cerebrospinal fluid is common, but elevation of cell counts is less frequent; rubella virus may often be isolated from the cerebrospinal fluid. The extent of impairment in infants at 18 mo of age is not predictable on the basis of clinical symptomatology or virus isolation in the 1st few weeks of life. Severe involvement is more frequent, however, in infants with seizures and with high levels of protein in the cerebrospinal fluid during the neonatal period.

The majority of infected infants may be asymptomatic in the newborn period. However, as many as 70% will subsequently develop evidence of congenital rubella. The most significant delayed manifestations include hearing loss (87% of 426 referred infants in whom hearing was tested), congenital heart disease (46%), mental retardation (39%), and cataract or glaucoma (34%). Children thought to have normal hearing when tested early in life have subsequently been found to have hearing loss when they reached school age. The hearing loss may be profound and a major contributor to speech impairment and learning disabilities. The lesions of the heart may not become significant until after the neonatal period; those occurring most commonly, in order of frequency, are patent ductus arteriosus, pulmonary artery stenosis, valvular pulmonic stenosis, aortic arch anomalies, and ventricular septal defect. Children may have more than one cardiac defect. Mental retardation, when present, is frequently severe. Cerebral dysfunction and psychiatric disorders, including reactive behavior disorder and infantile autism, also have been recorded. Other late sequelae are increased frequency of diabetes, thyroid dysfunction, and development of progressive rubella encephalitis.

Diagnosis. Although a history of an illness compatible with rubella in the mother during pregnancy may suggest the diagnosis, from one half to two thirds of the cases of maternal rubella are clinically inapparent. When congenital rubella is suspected, the diagnosis should be confirmed by virologic or serologic methods (Sec. 11.5 and 11.62). Virus may be isolated from throat, urine, or CSF. If the eye is involved, a conjunctival swab may be a source for virus isolation. The congenitally infected infant usually maintains high levels of IgG antibody against rubella throughout the first years of life. A small number of infected infants, however, may have a gradually declining antibody titer to the rubella virus during the first several years of life, apparently having lost their own capacity to respond to the rubella virus antigen. Demonstration of IgM antibody specific for rubella may also establish the diagnosis.

Treatment. There is no specific chemotherapy for rubella virus. For discussion of immunization, see Sec. 4.1 and 11.62.

Alford CA Jr, Griffiths PD: Rubella. In: Remington JS, Klein JO (eds): Infectious Diseases of the Fetus and Newborn Infant. Philadelphia, WB Saunders, 1983.
Chess S, Fernandez P, Korn S: Behavioral consequences of congenital rubella. J Pediatr 93:699, 1978.
Cooper LZ: Congenital rubella in the United States. In: Krugman S, Gershon AA (eds): Infections of the Fetus and the Newborn Infant. New York, AR Liss Inc, 1975.
Desmond MM, Fisher ES, Vorderman AL, et al: The longitudinal course of congenital rubella encephalitis in nonretarded children. J Pediatr 93:584, 1978.
Hanshaw JB, Dudgeon JA, Marshall WC: Viral Diseases of the Fetus and Newborn. Philadelphia, WB Saunders, 1985.
Horstmann DM: Rubella. Clin Obstet Gynecol 25:585, 1982.
Orenstein WA, Bart KJ, Hinman AR, et al: The opportunity and obligation to eliminate rubella from the United States. JAMA 251:1988, 1984.
Peckham CS, Martin JAM, Marshall WC, et al: Congenital rubella deafness: A preventable disease. Lancet 1:258, 1979.

8.70 HEPATITIS

The etiologic agent responsible for neonatal hepatitis frequently cannot be identified (Sec. 12.74 and 12.80). Hepatitis A appears to be transmitted across the placenta relatively rarely. Although non-A–non-B hepatitis may be transmitted from an infected mother to her offspring, infants exposed in utero are either uninfected or have only mild transient abnormalities of liver chemistries. Hepatitis B, on the other hand, is a common infection to which infants may be exposed during the perinatal period and presents a management problem (see Sec. 11.76). Other etiologic agents are cytomegalovirus, rubella, enteroviruses, syphilis, and toxoplasmosis.

An infant may be exposed through a number of different circumstances: (1) the mother may be asymptomatic but a chronic carrier of HB_sAg, (2) the mother may have active hepatitis B virus infection during pregnancy, or (3) the mother may have chronic active hepatitis. The rate of transplacental transmission appears to vary directly with the presence of the e antigen, Hb_eAg. Antibody also may develop against HB_eAg, and the presence of anti-HB_e in the serum of the mother is associated with a lower rate of transmission of the infection to her offspring. The infant born to the mother who has acute hepatitis faces a different risk. When maternal hepatitis occurs during the 1st or 2nd trimester, only a small percentage of infants become infected, whereas 25–76% become infected with the virus when maternal hepatitis occurs during the 3rd trimester or near delivery time. Although hepatitis B virus may cross the placenta causing infants to be born with antigenemia, most infants who acquire hepatitis B virus from mothers with acute hepatitis do not have Hb_sAg in their cord blood but rather develop antigenemia by 6–12 wk of age, suggesting that transmission occurs at delivery or shortly thereafter. Postpartum transmission of hepatitis B virus may infrequently occur by other routes since HB_sAg has been found in saliva, breast milk, urine, and stool.

Clinical Manifestations. Maternal hepatitis B has not been associated with congenital malformations, miscarriages or stillbirths, or intrauterine growth retardation. However, it has been correlated with prematurity, particularly during the last trimester of pregnancy. Infants exposed to maternal hepatitis B (1) become HB_sAg-positive and remain asymptomatic but develop persistent antigenemia with evidence of chronic liver involvement; (2) become Hb_sAg-positive, remain asymptomatic, or develop mild hepatitis and then recover with clearance of their antigenemia; (3) become HB_sAg-positive and develop severe fulminant hepatitis with liver necrosis and death; or (4) never acquire hepatitis B virus infection. Differences in the time of exposure, the route of inoculation, and the size of the viral inoculum may explain this wide variation in the time of antigenemia in the infected neonate.

The most common sequence of events in infants who acquire hepatitis B virus is to remain asymptomatic and become a chronic carrier, i.e., HB_sAg-positive. These children have persistently elevated transaminase levels but usually show no clinical evidence of liver disease. Biopsy specimens, however, indicate persistent hepatitis and evidence of ongoing liver disease. Long-term follow-up of these children is not available.

A small number of infants born either to mothers with acute hepatitis or to carrier mothers may become HB_sAg-positive at any time during the 1st yr of life. These infants may have mild or no clinical signs of hepatitis, clear their antigenemia, and recover. Although most neonatal infections with hepatitis B virus are benign during infancy, a small number of infants have severe fulminant disease with massive liver necrosis and die; such cases may follow transfusions during the neonatal period or occur in infants of chronic carrier mothers. Several families have also been reported in which more than one infant born to the same carrier mother developed fulminant fatal neonatal hepatitis B.

Prevention and Treatment. See Sec. 11.76.

Centers for Disease Control: Postexposure prophylaxis of hepatitis B. MMWR 33:285, 1984.

Crumpacker CS: Hepatitis. In: Remington JS, Klein JO (eds): Infectious Diseases of the Fetus and Newborn Infant. 2nd ed. Philadelphia, WB Saunders, 1983.
Okada K, Kamiyama I, Inomata M, et al: e Antigen and anti-e in the serum of asymptomatic carrier mothers as indicators of positive and negative transmission of hepatitis B virus to their infants. N Engl J Med 294:746, 1976.
Stevens CE: Viral hepatitis in pregnancy: The obstetrician's role. Clin Obstet Gynecol 25:577, 1982.
Stevens CE, Toy PT, Tong MJ: Perinatal hepatitis B virus transmission in the United States: Prevention by passive-active immunization. JAMA 253:1740, 1985.
Tong MJ, Thursby M, Rakela J, et al: Studies on the maternal-infant transmission of the viruses which cause acute hepatitis. Gastroenterology 80:999, 1981.
Vyas GN, Blum HE: Hepatitis B virus infection: Current concepts of chronicity and immunity. West J Med 140:754, 1984.

8.71 HERPES SIMPLEX VIRUS (HSV)

HSV (Sec. 11.65) may cause severe disease in the neonate with high mortality and devastating sequelae. Three quarters of the cases are due to HSV type 2 and are acquired during passage through an infected birth canal. However, since 70% of these maternal genital infections are asymptomatic or are not recognized clinically, the option of performing a cesarean section to prevent neonatal infection may not be considered. The remaining 25% of neonatal herpes is caused by HSV type 1, largely acquired from maternal genital or oral lesions, paternal or other family member oral herpes, or nosocomial transmission from other infected babies. Transmission of HSV to a neonate from the cold sore of hospital personnel has not been demonstrated. Rarely HSV may cross the placenta, infect the fetus, and result in congenital malformations.

About 50% of infants delivered vaginally to mothers with primary genital herpes at the time of delivery will develop neonatal herpes, whereas 4% or less born to mothers with recurrent lesions will have neonatal HSV disease. The risk in neonates born to mothers with asymptomatic shedding is unknown.

Clinical Manifestations. Neonatal herpes simplex infections may produce a spectrum of manifestations ranging from a local infection in the skin, eye, or mouth to encephalitis or a generalized disease involving multiple target organs. Virus is rarely found in the absence of signs or symptoms. One half of the infants have the disseminated form, which involves the liver and adrenal glands and may produce a clinical picture resembling bacterial sepsis. In approximately 60% of infants the virus affects the central nervous system; death may occur before neurologic symptoms are apparent. Onset occurs usually within the 1st wk of life but may be seen at birth or as late as 3 wk of age. The initial signs are usually nonspecific and include fever, lethargy, poor feeding, irritability, and vomiting; convulsions, jaundice, apneic spells, cyanosis, respiratory distress, and hepatosplenomegaly are frequently observed. Clinical evidence of central nervous system involvement includes irritability, bulging fontanel, focal or generalized seizures, flaccid or spastic paralysis, opisthotonos, decerebrate rigidity, or coma. Involvement of the central nervous system in the absence of lesions in the skin, mouth, or eye is unusual but has been seen with subsequent development of the other manifestations. Infants with disseminated infection in multiple organs or those with central nervous system involvement alone tend to have a poor prognosis with high mortality or major sequelae. Often the disease progresses rapidly to death following a deteriorating neurologic status.

The skin and mucous membranes are the most common sites of involvement with this virus; 80% of patients present with skin vesicles, conjunctivitis, or ulcerative lesions of the mouth. Importantly, 75% of infants that present with infection limited to these areas will progress to more serious disease (CNS involvement or disseminated infection). Because of this progression of localized disease, infants with neonatal herpes should receive systemic antiviral chemotherapy, regardless of the extent of the infection at the time of diagnosis.

Diagnosis. The best method of diagnosis is isolation of infectious virus in tissue culture. Vesicles are the most productive site for sampling; but the virus has been recovered from mouth or conjunctival swabs, CSF, buffy coat, and biopsies of tissues. Sensitive tissue culture lines demonstrate characteristic viral cytopathic effect within 1 day in 50% of the specimens and within 2 days in 80%. Development of antigen detection systems may shorten the time for diagnosis.

Treatment and Prevention. A cesarean section is indicated for mothers with a known genital infection at the time of delivery. This is more likely to decrease the risk when performed before, or less than 4 hr after, rupture of the membranes. Mothers with a history of recurrent herpes who have been followed with serial viral cultures during the latter stages of pregnancy can be safely delivered vaginally, if the last culture prior to delivery is negative and there are no lesions or prodrome of an episode at the time of delivery. An infant born to a mother with genital herpes should be isolated and cultures of the infant obtained to determine whether infection has occurred.

Adenine arabinoside (vidarabine, ara-A), 15–30 mg/kg/24 hr delivered as a single 12 hr infusion, has reduced the mortality of neonatal herpes from 62 to 35%, and has increased normal survivors from 19 to 43%. Comparison trials between ara-A and acyclovir are in progress.

Corey L, Adams HG, Brown ZA: Genital herpes simplex virus infections: Clinical manifestations, course, and complications. Ann Intern Med 98:958, 1983.

Corey L, Holmes KK: Genital herpes simplex virus infections: Current concepts in diagnosis, therapy, and prevention. Ann Intern Med 98:973, 1983.

Grossman JH, Wallen WC, Sever JL: Management of genital herpes simplex virus infection during pregnancy. Obstet Gynecol 58:1, 1981.

Nahmias AJ, Keyserling HL, Kerrick GM: Herpes simplex. In: Remington JS, Klein JO (eds): Infectious Diseases of the Fetus and Newborn Infant. 2nd ed. Philadelphia, WB Saunders, 1983.

Overall JC Jr: Genital and perinatal herpes simplex virus infections. In: De la Maza (ed): International Symposium on Medical Virology. Philadelphia, Franklin Institute Press, 1985.

Sullivan-Bolyai J, Hull HF, Wilson C, et al: Neonatal herpes simplex virus infection in King County, Washington. JAMA 250:3059, 1983.

Whitley RJ, Nahmias AJ, Visintine AM, et al: The natural history of herpes simplex virus infection of mother and newborn. Pediatrics 66:489, 1980.

Whitley RJ, Yeager A, Kartus P, et al: Neonatal herpes simplex virus infection: Follow-up evaluation of vidarabine therapy. Pediatrics 72:778, 1983.

8.72 ENTEROVIRUSES

The enteroviruses (Sec. 11.77) are responsible for a wide spectrum of clinical manifestations in both mothers and neonates. Congenital infection by the transplacental route is infrequent. More commonly, infants are infected during the birth process or in the neonatal period. After delivery, infection is acquired in the same fashion as with older children and adults. When enterovirus disease occurs in a nursery setting, infected infants should be isolated and infection control techniques carefully followed.

There is no convincing evidence that Coxsackie virus and echovirus infections result in fetal loss. Congenital anomalies have not been reported with poliovirus or echovirus, but maternal Coxsackie virus infections may be associated with urogenital, digestive, and cardiovascular anomalies. See Sec. 11.77 for discussion of illnesses in newborn infants.

Cherry JD: Enteroviruses. In: Remington JS, Klein JO (eds): Infectious Diseases of the Fetus and Newborn Infant. 2nd ed. Philadelphia, WB Saunders, 1983.

Dagan R, Jenista JA, Menegus MA: Clinical, epidemiological, and laboratory aspects of enterovirus infection in young infants. In: De la Maza LM: International Symposium on Medical Virology. Philadelphia, Franklin Institute Press, 1985.

8.73 VARICELLA-ZOSTER

The newborn may be exposed to varicella-zoster virus in utero or in the immediate postpartum period by the occurrence of either varicella or zoster in the mother or through contact with other neonates or medical personnel (Sec. 11.66). Although fetal wastage has not been statistically associated with maternal varicella, individual cases of abortion or stillbirth have been reported with lesions in the placenta and multiple fetal organs. A small number of infants delivered to women with a history of varicella during the first 15 wk of gestation have had a similar constellation of malformations at birth (low birthweight, hypoplastic limbs or digits, cicatricial skin lesions, cortical atrophy, growth retardation, delayed motor development, ocular abnormalities, enhanced susceptibility to infections).

Clinical Manifestations. Varicella can be acquired congenitally when maternal chickenpox occurs within 21 days prior to delivery. Disease in the infant is seen in approximately 25% of the maternal infections. When the onset in the neonate is at 0–4 days of life, usually reflecting the occurrence of varicella in the mother more than 5 days prior to delivery, the disease may follow a severe course, with a mortality of 25–30%. When clinical signs of varicella occur at 5–10 days of age, the course usually is benign and fatalities rare. This amelioration may relate to the time of exposure of the fetus and the transfer of maternal antibody. Chickenpox may also be acquired by neonatal exposure, but spread within the nursery is rare and the disease is generally mild. The majority of infants exposed by nonmaternal sources probably have acquired maternal antibody and thus are protected against this virus. A diagnosis can usually be made by the characteristic distribution of vesicular lesions which closely resembles that in older children and a history of maternal or postnatal exposure. The differential diagnosis includes disseminated herpes simplex, impetigo, contact dermatitis, and the hand-foot-mouth syndrome.

On rare occasions zoster has been reported in infants, although varicella-zoster has not been isolated from any of these cases. The recovery of herpes simplex virus from at least one neonate with zoster indicated that the diagnosis should be made with caution and that cultures for virus isolation should be obtained.

Zoster immune globulin and pooled immune serum globulin can attenuate or prevent varicella when administered early during the incubation period. Infants born to mothers who have had varicella near the time of delivery should receive zoster immune globulin or, if that is not available, 0.6–1.2 mL/kg of normal immune serum globulin as soon as possible. With onset of maternal or neonatal varicella, the mother and infant should be isolated to prevent spread to susceptible individuals. Antiviral chemotherapy with adenine arabinoside (vidarabine, ara-A) or acyclovir may be considered in neonates with severe varicella.

JAMES C. OVERALL, Jr.

Brunell PA: Fetal and neonatal varicella-zoster infections. Semin Perinatol 7:47, 1983.

Hanshaw JB, Dudgeon JA, Marshall WC: Viral Diseases of the Fetus and Newborn. Philadelphia, WB Saunders, 1985.

Siegel M, Fuerst HT, Peress NS: Comparative fetal mortality in maternal virus diseases. A prospective study on rubella, measles, mumps, chickenpox and hepatitis. N Engl J Med 274:768, 1966.

Young NA, Gershon AA: Chickenpox, measles, and mumps. In: Remington JS, Klein JO (eds): Infectious Diseases of the Fetus and Newborn Infant. 2nd ed. Philadelphia, WB Saunders, 1983.

9

SPECIAL HEALTH PROBLEMS DURING ADOLESCENCE

See also Sec. 2.9 and 2.30.

Overview. Although adolescents (those 11–20 yr of age) constituted 17% of the United States population during 1980–1981, they were responsible for only 11% of physician office visits. The majority of these visits were for acute rather than chronic conditions, in contrast with all other age groups, for whom chronic illness or nonillness health care predominated.

Younger adolescents had higher rates of office visits than older ones, and females in the 15–20 yr age group had higher rates than comparably aged males, primarily because of gynecologic or obstetric care. Younger adolescents differed from older ones also in reasons for their medical visits. For the younger ones, the leading reason was respiratory illness (21%), followed by routine examinations (17%) and injuries or poisonings (16%). For older adolescents, the leading reasons, after routine examinations (24%), included diseases of the skin and subcutaneous tissue (14%), followed by diseases of the respiratory system, injury, and poisoning (13% each).

Thirty-five percent of adolescents' office visits were made to general practitioners and family physicians; 29% of 11–14 yr olds and only 8% of 15–20 yr olds made office visits to pediatricians. The low rate of use of private physicians may reflect the general good health of adolescents or their different patterns of use of physicians. Whatever the cause, the result is that physicians, particularly pediatricians, have less opportunity to evaluate and counsel teenagers than their true health status warrants.

Data from the National Health Examination Survey of 1966–1970 showed that 20% of presumably healthy 12–17 yr olds had previously undiagnosed health problems. These were primarily related to the rapid growth and maturation that characterizes puberty and included such problems as scoliosis (Sec. 23.5), slipped capital femoral epiphysis (Sec. 23.2), Osgood-Schlatter disease (Sec. 23.3), goiter (Sec. 19.13), and acne (Sec. 24.31). In addition, a number of health problems regarded as "adult" in the past are actually present during adolescence, albeit in preclinical form, e.g., hypertension, hypercholesterolemia, and carcinoma-in-situ of the cervix, may be detected during adolescence.

Violence, including accidents, homicides, or suicides, accounts for 70% of all adolescent deaths. Neoplasms (7%) and infectious diseases or diseases of a congenital nature (7%) account for an additional, small proportion of deaths. Among the neoplasms, testicular tumors and tumors of bone or lymphatics are those most prevalent. The birth rate has leveled off for all other age groups but continues to rise for young adolescents, who also lead the nation in reported cases of sexually transmitted disease, such as gonorrhea and chlamydia. Certain of the non–sexually transmitted infectious diseases, including rubella, rubeola, infectious mononucleosis, and toxic shock syndrome, now have their peak incidence among adolescents. Health-destructive behavior, such as cigarette and marijuana smoking and abuse of alcohol and other drugs (often in combination with driving), continue to be serious problems for adolescents. Eating disorders, such as anorexia nervosa and bulimia, are increasing in prevalence and are reported to affect 1% of 16–18 yr old females in the United States.

9.1 ACCIDENTS

See also Sec. 5.37, 5.43, 5.44, and 28.3–28.11.

Automobile and motorcycle accidents are the leading causes of adolescent morbidity and mortality. Sixteen to 19 yr olds comprise 8% of the population but account for 17% of vehicular fatalities. Sixty-three percent of automotive deaths among adolescents involve passengers in cars driven by adolescents. Alcohol is a factor underlying most of these fatalities, along with failure to use seat belts in cars or helmets while riding motorcycles. Most accidents involve male rather than female adolescents and occur between 4 hr before and 4 hr after midnight. Lowering of the drinking age to 18 yr has been associated with a 5% increase in fatal automotive accidents. Sports injuries and drownings are also important causes of morbidity and mortality. Pediatricians have the opportunity to prevent adolescent accidents by offering anticipatory guidance to young people and by influencing legislation aimed at raising the drinking age and enforcing seat belt and helmet use.

PSYCHOSOCIAL PROBLEMS

9.2 DEPRESSION

See also Sec. 2.43.

Adolescence is a time of heightened emotionality, hypothetical thinking, and further development of empathetic feelings, especially towards peers. As a result, mood swings from the depths of depression to the heights of elation are common. It is often difficult to decide which sad-looking adolescent is at risk for true depression or even suicide. The hallmark of the youngster at risk is the persistence of the depressed mood, the absence of corresponding periods of elation, an inability to function, and the expression of hopelessness and helplessness. Puig-Antich suggests that the depressed mood should be considered persistent if it lasts for at least 3 consecutive hours for 3 or more periods each week.

Assessing the adolescent's functional status should focus on school performance and on peer and family interactions. Symptoms of depression may include declining school grades, an increase in school absenteeism or truancy, use of alcohol or drugs, accident-proneness, and pervasive boredom. On the other hand, persistent euphoria, if coupled with "acting-out" behavior, such as promiscuity, may be indicative of "masked depression." Eating and sleeping disturbances are not as pervasive in adolescents as in adults but may be quite severe. Insomnia, and especially difficulty in initially falling asleep, sometimes to the extent of sleeping all day and remaining awake at night without ever feeling rested, is a common sign of depression in adolescents. A family history of depressive illness should increase concern, particularly if family history includes a suicide.

When evaluating the adolescent suspected of depression, it is useful to inquire about future plans. The youngster who has none or who responds that he or she "won't be here much longer" is obviously at risk for suicide. Less dramatic, but often effective, is a question about the desire to change anything in one's life. An answer in the affirmative warrants a follow-up question as to what steps, if any, have been taken to make such changes. When severe depression is revealed or suspected, the physician should ask if the patient has ever felt so sad that death was considered a preferable alternative to living. If answered in the affirmative, questions about the existence of a plan for self-destruction should be asked. The patient who has a suicide plan must be immediately evaluated by a psychiatrist. The patient having no suicide plan will not be harmed by such questioning and is often relieved to have an opportunity to discuss his or her concerns with an obviously caring physician. The physician should not be misled by the adolescent who suddenly appears cheerful after a period of depression. Rather than a sign of improvement, such a change may accompany the youngster's resolution of ambivalence and the decision to resolve sadness by suicide.

Mattsson describes five forms of adolescent depression in order of increasing pathology:

1. *Normal depressive mood swings.*

2. *Acute depressive reactions.* These occur normally following death of or separation from a loved one and are the equivalent of a healthy grief response. Although feelings of mournfulness may preoccupy the adolescent for weeks or months, there is a gradual move toward resolution and restoration of normal functioning. If such an adolescent denies suicidal thoughts and if evidence of increased risk-taking behavior is lacking, the primary care physician may manage the situation by close observation.

3. *Neurotic depressive disorders.* These may follow lack of resolution of a grief reaction and are characterized by feelings of hopelessness and helplessness and self-incrimination and guilt in relationship to the lost individual, by difficulty in concentration and withdrawal from school and social contacts, and by interference with normal sleeping, eating, and activity. A desire to join the deceased may be elicited upon careful questioning. This form of depression must be managed by a psychiatrist.

4. *Masked Depression.* In this variant of the neurotic depressive disorder, the youngster deals with his or her feelings of despair by denial and somatization. "Acting-out" behavior, such as running away from home, school truancy, multiple accidents, and substance abuse may be manifestations of this form of depression, as may the appearance of headaches, abdominal pain, or other physical complaints. Psychiatric management is indicated.

5. *Psychotic depressive disorders.* Impaired reality testing, thought distortion, and delusions of guilt may be present in addition to characteristics already described. Referral for psychiatric treatment is mandatory.

9.3 SUICIDE

See also Sec. 2.44.

Suicide is the third leading cause of death among 15–19 yr olds in the United States, and has been increasing in incidence over the past two decades. Female adolescents lead male adolescents in the incidence of suicide attempts, but males outnumber females in completed suicides. Native Americans and Asian Americans have a higher suicide rate than the general population. The chronically ill adolescent is also at increased risk for suicide as a result of feelings of impotence, diminished competence, or of alienation of loved ones.

The method of suicide most commonly used by teenagers is ingestion of medication. The medication may be the patient's own or often that of a parent with whom there has been conflict. The drug most commonly used in suicide attempts is a tricyclic antidepressant, suggesting the advisability of prescribing a "bubble-pack" or similar unit-dose form of packaging when there is any concern that it or any other medication may be used in a suicide attempt. Hanging, shooting, wrist-slashing, or other more violent methods are used more often by males and by those most intent on completing the act. However, it is often difficult to assess the seriousness of the intent by the actual potency of the method. An adolescent who ingests a pharmacologically benign medication (such as an antibiotic) may be as serious about committing suicide as is the one who consumes a substance that is obviously toxic. Medical lethality correlates poorly with seriousness or intent, but there is a good correlation between the latter and the patient's expectation of lethality, which is often inaccurate.

Other factors to be considered in assessing seriousness of a suicide attempt are the extent of premeditation and the likelihood of rescue. The adolescent who impulsively grabs a bottle from the medicine cabinet after announcing that he or she plans to commit suicide is generally less serious about actually doing so than is the one who has carefully planned the event, particularly if rescue was unlikely. Leaving a suicide note suggests premeditation and should be considered a sign of serious intent. An attempt by a teenager with a family history of suicide is particularly serious. Any attempt or gesture should be regarded as serious, however, regardless of apparent intent, since most completed suicides occur among persons who have made earlier attempts or gestures.

Whenever an adolescent makes a suicide attempt, it should be considered a desperate effort at conflict resolution. Merely attending to its pharmacologic or surgical sequelae, as is usually the case in hospital emergency rooms, does little to assist in constructive resolution of the conflict; fewer than one third of families of adolescents who attempt suicide actually follow up with recommendation for referral made after a brief emergency room evaluation. On the other hand, provision of short-term hospitalization effectively accomplishes this goal by providing a secure setting for the patient, by impressing parents with the need to attend to the underlying problems, and, most importantly, by facilitating psychosocial assessment upon which to base a recommendation for appropriate therapy or referral. Consultation with a skilled psychiatrist is mandatory in the assessment of every teenager who makes a suicide attempt.

9.4 SUBSTANCE ABUSE

Background and Etiology. The use of mind-altering substances for medicinal, social, and religious purposes has characterized the human race throughout recorded history. Nor is such use by teenagers a new phenomenon. The increased complexity of modern society, as well as increased availability of a wide variety of drugs, has contributed to increased use by adolescents and awareness of physical and psychosocial sequelae by health professionals. In our society, drug use serves a variety of purposes for the adolescent. For the individual aspiring to attain adult status, the use may be symbolic of maturity and of facilitating the negotiation of independence from parental domination. Peer group acceptance, stress-reduction, escapism, and rebellion against the establishment are other functions possibly served by drug use. In addition, the developing teenager, seeking to explore the limits of his or her new cognitive abilities and emotionality may attempt to do so through hallucinogenic agents.

With so many diverse functions of adolescent adaptive development served by drug use, its popularity is not surprising; and intervention strategies for preventing or stopping drug use by this age group must consider alternatives that meet these developmental needs. Drug use in the form of alcohol, marijuana, or both, is experienced at some time by more than 90% of teenagers; accordingly, it is not useful to think of teenagers as either drug users or not. Rather, the clinician should approach each youngster individually to assess the role of drug use in his or her life and to assess the effects of specific drugs on physical and functional parameters. Because it is apparently much easier to resist pressures to use drugs than to stop once begun, efforts should be focused on prevention.

Continued use of a drug after the first experience with it usually suggests serious underlying problems. For example, drug use is more prevalent among depressed teenagers and among those prone to problem behavior. No single factor distinguishes "problem" adolescent drug users from those whose drug involvement does not portend major problems, but weighing an aggregate of multiple variables may be helpful (Table 9–1). The type of drug used (e.g., marijuana versus heroin), the circumstances of use (e.g., alone or in a group setting), the frequency and timing of use (e.g., daily before school versus rarely on a weekend), the premorbid personality (depressed versus happy), and the general functional status of the teenager should be considered in evaluating any adolescent found to be using a drug of abuse. In addition, the use of any psychoactive substance in conjunction with the operation of a motor vehicle is sufficient reason for immediate intervention to prevent harm to the using teenager and others.

Epidemiology. Use of illicit drugs declined from a peak of 39% in 1979 to 32% in 1983; much of the decline during this period is due to a decrease in current use of marijuana from 37% to 27% and in annual prevalence from 51% to 42%. Active daily use of marijuana is now at its lowest level (5.5%). There has also been a marked decline in the use of amphetamines, methaqualone, and LSD and the continuation of a gradual long-term decline in the use of barbiturates, tranquilizers, and PCP. Heroin use has leveled off at less than 1%, and inhalant use at 4%. However, the use of cocaine has doubled between 1975 and 1979; rates in western and northeast sectors of the United States are double those in the southern and north central regions.

Nonprescription stimulants and diet pills have a lifetime prevalence of 15–20% and 31%, respectively. Of particular concern is a 45% lifetime prevalence for use of diet pills among adolescent females (see Sec. 9.6).

Alcohol is clearly the most widely abused substance; 93% of high school seniors report having used it at some time,

69% within the previous month, and 5.5% report everyday use. The rate of binge drinking (five or more drinks in a row) during the prior 2 wk is about 41%. Male-female differences in usage rates have narrowed.

Smoking tobacco on a daily basis has decreased from 29% in 1977 to 20% by 1981. Slightly more adolescent females than males smoke regularly (13.6% versus 13.1%, respectively), the reverse of earlier patterns. Future educational plans correlate significantly with smoking patterns; 8% of college-bound seniors smoke half a pack or more daily compared with 21% of those who do not plan to go to college. Use of "smokeless" tobacco by male adolescents is a recent and growing phenomenon.

In summary, approximately two thirds of teenagers in the United States try some illicit drug before they finish high school; 40% have used some illicit drug other than marijuana. About 1 in 5 high school seniors smokes cigarettes daily, and about 1 in 20 drinks alcohol on a daily basis.

Longitudinal studies indicate that the time of greatest risk for initiation of cigarette smoking and for using alcohol and marijuana is before the age of 20; the greatest risk for using illicit drugs other than cocaine is before the age of 21 yr. Marijuana use begins to decline at age 22.5, but use of cigarettes continues to climb at least through the age of 25.

Among 10th–12th graders, 25% of males and 16% of females qualified as "problem drinkers" in 1972. "Problem drinking" was defined as (1) having within the previous year been drunk six or more times; or (2) within the same period having on two or more occasions experienced negative consequences of drinking in three or more life-areas among the following: difficulty with teachers, friends, or parents; criticism from dates; and trouble with police or driving a car while under the influence of alcohol. Among the males who were problem drinkers during adolescence, half were no longer in this category by young adulthood; for the females, only 25% of the original problem drinker group remained so classified during young adulthood. Among those who were not problem drinkers during adolescence, 40% of males and 20% of females became problem drinkers as young adults. Although problem drinking during adolescence was correlated with other concurrent problem behaviors, such as smoking marijuana and engaging in sexual intercourse, it was not significantly correlated with negative consequences in later life. These longitudinal studies by Jessor suggest the need for caution in predicting postadolescent development and attainment on the basis of earlier behavior and the need for avoiding the premature labeling of adolescents as problem drinkers, since this might adversely influence their development.

Longitudinal studies have also indicated that marijuana use is predictive of later use of hard drugs, primarily in those who begin its use at a young age. A New York study found that alcohol use was experienced by 20% before the age of 10 yr and by 50% by 14 yr of age; that marijuana use began to

Table 9–1. **Assessing the Seriousness of Adolescent Drug Abuse**

	0	+1	+2
Age	>15	<15	
Sex	Male	Female	
Family history of drug abuse		Yes	
Setting of drug use	In group		Alone
Affect before drug use	Happy		Sad
School performance	Good/improving	Always poor	Recently poor
Use before driving	None		Yes
History of accidents	None		Yes
Time of week	Weekend	Weekdays	
Time of day		After school	Before school
Type of drug	Marijuana, beer, wine	Hallucinogens, amphetamines	Whiskey, opiates, cocaine, barbiturates

Total score: 0–3 less worrisome; 3–8 serious; 8–18 very serious.

climb at approximately 13 yr; and that cigarette use began to rise at about 11 yr. The pattern for onset of use of psychedelics parallels that of marijuana, whereas that for cocaine shifts to an older age group (8% by age 18 and 30% by age 24). Of potential importance to preventive efforts is the finding that although males outnumber females in the magnitude of illicit drug use, psychoactive substances are prescribed more often for females, beginning in early adolescence and continuing through adulthood.

Pathophysiology. Physical growth and development during puberty may be adversely affected by using drugs or alcohol. For example, one third of adolescent females who use heroin have secondary amenorrhea, even in the absence of weight loss. The higher incidence of menstrual abnormalities results from greater vulnerability of the hypothalamic-pituitary-ovarian axis in the maturing individual. Endogenous opiates block release of gonadotropin-releasing hormone; a similar effect may occur from exogenous opiates. Amphetamines interfere with stage 4 sleep and may impair the intimate relationship between sleep and augmentation of secretion of gonadotropins during early adolescence. Deriving calories largely from alcohol during the peak of the pubertal growth spurt deprives the body of the protein necessary for normal growth of muscles.

The metabolism of certain drugs may be affected by coincident abuse of illicit drugs or alcohol (Table 9–2). Induction of hepatic smooth endoplasmic reticulum by barbiturates or alcohol may accelerate the metabolism and enhance the excretion of substances requiring glucuronidation. Therefore, estrogen-containing oral contraceptives taken by a young woman who abuses barbiturates or alcohol may leave her vulnerable to pregnancy. Conversely, use of estrogen will increase the risk of intoxication from alcohol as a result of decreased ethanol metabolism. The potentiating interaction of alcohol and barbiturates must also be considered when prescribing anticonvulsant medications. A more immediate and dramatic interaction occurs when metronidazole is ingested by an alcohol-abusing adolescent because of the antagonistic effect of alcohol on acetaldehyde.

Psychosocial Sequelae. Youth may engage in robbery, burglary, drug-dealing, or prostitution for the purpose of acquiring the money necessary to buy drugs or alcohol. Regular use of any drug will eventually diminish ability to function adequately in school, to hold a job, or to operate a motor vehicle. An "amotivational" syndrome has been described in chronic marijuana users who lose interest in age-appropriate activities.

Prevention. It is important to anticipate that the normally developing adolescent will experiment with some agent at some point and to attempt to delay that event as long as possible, limit the amount used, and prevent any use while the adolescent is operating a motor vehicle. Educational efforts based on scare techniques have not been successful, whereas those that present unemotional, factual information about medical complications of drug use have had some beneficial impact. Strategies that teach young adolescents to resist peer pressure to smoke, by the use of trained peer counselors using role-playing techniques, have significantly reduced smoking in the few studies of middle-class youngsters thus far evaluated.

Opiates. Opiate abuse by adolescents has decreased considerably over the past decade, but the magnitude and variety of its medical sequelae warrant continued attention by the pediatrician. Heroin and methadone are most subject to abuse by adolescents. Heroin produces euphoria and analgesia. It is hydrolyzed to morphine, which undergoes hepatic conjugation with glucuronic acid before excretion, usually within 24 hr of administration. It can be detected by thin layer chromatography up to 48 hr following administration.

The route of administration influences the timing of onset of action. When the drug is inhaled ("snorting"), it requires almost 30 min until the desired effect is achieved. By the subcutaneous route ("skin-popping"), the effect is achieved within minutes; and when injected intravenously ("mainlining"), it has an almost instantaneous effect. A larger dose can also be administered by the intravenous route. Tolerance is developed first to the euphoric effect, but it is rare for an individual to develop a tolerance to the inhibitory effect on smooth muscle, typically manifested by constipation or miosis.

Clinical Manifestations. The pharmacologic effects of heroin or its adulterants, combined with the conditions and route of administration, are responsible for the manifestations in major organ systems.

The *cerebral effects* include the sought-after euphoria, diminution in pain, and a sleep-like EEG pattern. Coma, depressed respiration, miosis, and tachycardia are also characteristically found. Seizures and increased intracranial pressure may complicate overdoses. An effect on the hypothalamus is suggested by the lowering of body temperature. In addition, the lack of sterile technique in injection may lead to multiple cerebral microabscesses, usually caused by *Staphylococcus aureus*.

Transverse myelitis of the thoracic segments may occur in patients resuming heroin use after a period of abstinence, suggesting a possible hypersensitivity reaction. Rarely, Guillain-Barré syndrome and toxic amblyopia, the latter presumably due to the quinine additive, are found in heroin addicts. Brachial and lumbosacral plexitis and poly- and mononeuropathies, the latter manifested by ankle or wrist drop, are the more common peripheral neurologic findings.

Acute *rhabdomyolysis* with myoglobinuria may follow intravenous injection of heroin and is manifested by generalized muscle tenderness, edema, and marked weakness of extremities. **Necrotizing fasciitis** is a rare complication after inadvertent subfascial injections of heroin. Another rare complication is **contractures** of the fingers resulting from infection and scarring medial to the proximal interphalangeal joint following injection into the small veins of the hand, such injections being necessitated by sclerosis of the larger veins or to avoid detection by authorities.

Table 9–2. **Interactions Between Alcohol and Prescription Drugs**

Additive (Reduce Dose)	Cross-Tolerant (Need Higher Dose)	Antagonistic (Antabuse-Like Effect)
Salicylates	Chloroform	Metronidazole
Acetaminophen	Fluorinated anesthetics	Isoniazid
Antihypertensives	Ether	Chloramphenicol
Anticoagulants (acute intoxication)	Anticoagulants (chronic intoxication)	Griseofulvin
Antihistamines		Cefamandole
Barbiturates		
Benzodiazepines	Phenytoin	Moxalactam
Phenothiazines		
Propoxyphene		

Vasodilation is a major cardiovascular manifestation related to the method of administration of the drug. Lack of antisepsis with parenteral administration is responsible for **endocarditis**, with a high incidence of infection with coagulase-positive *Staphylococcus aureus*, involvement of the tricuspid valve, and high mortality. Rare complications of parenteral heroin administration include arteriovenous fistula, arterial and venous thrombosis, embolism, necrotizing arteritis, and mycotic aneurysm.

Respiratory depression is caused by heroin's effect on the central nervous system and is characterized by alveolar underventilation with a fall of arterial oxygen tension and saturation. In addition, particles of cotton fibers or nonsoluble adulterants inadvertently injected with the heroin cause **granulomatosis** and **pulmonary fibrosis**, which may lead to pulmonary hypertension and a decrease in lung volume and diffusing capacity. **Pulmonary edema** is common with the overdose syndrome and may follow intranasal as well as parenteral administration. It is always found in those who die of heroin overdose, but it may also be an incidental roentgenologic finding in an otherwise asymptomatic adolescent heroin abuser. Pulmonary infections have not been prominent in this age group.

The most common *dermatologic lesions* are the so-called tracks, the hypertrophic linear scars that follow the course of large veins. Smaller, discrete peripheral scars resembling healed insect bites may be easily overlooked. The adolescent who injects heroin subcutaneously may have fat necrosis, lipodystrophy, and atrophy over portions of extremities. Attempts at concealment of these stigmata may include amateur tattoos in unusual sites. Abscesses secondary to unsterile techniques of drug administration are commonly found.

The mechanism for the reported *loss of libido* in heroin users is unknown. The female heroin user may resort to prostitution to support the habit, adding to other hazards the risks of sexually transmitted disease and of pregnancy.

Urinary retention and *constipation* may occur. The practice of swallowing the cotton used as a filter for heroin solutions or of concealment of heroin in a swallowed condom or balloon may cause intestinal obstruction or sudden, often fatal, overdose if the container breaks.

The *abstinence or withdrawal syndrome* starts after the addicted individual has been without heroin for 8 hr or more and lasts for 24–36 hr. The earliest sign is yawning, followed by lacrimation, mydriasis, insomnia, "gooseflesh," cramping of the voluntary musculature, hyperactive bowel sounds and diarrhea, tachycardia, and systolic hypertension. Grand mal seizures are rare in adolescent addicts.

A short course of diazepam is effective and safe for heroin **detoxification**. An oral dose of 10 mg every 6 hr for 3 days is recommended for those with mild withdrawal symptoms (i.e., no evidence of gastrointestinal hypermotility or change in vital signs), administered within 24 hr of the last dose of heroin or prophylactically for those known to be addicted. For moderate withdrawal symptoms (i.e., evidence of gastrointestinal effect or change in vital signs), treatment is begun with the intramuscular administration of 2 doses of 10 mg of diazepam given 4 hr apart followed by the oral regimen. For severe withdrawal, 10 mg of diazepam is administered intramuscularly every 4 hr for a 24 hr period, followed by oral administration. Insomnia is not eliminated by this regimen, but hypnotics should be avoided because of their lack of efficacy and potential for abuse.

An alternative to diazepam for detoxification is methadone. This synthetic opiate is effective by the oral route and is pharmacologically similar to heroin except for its lack of euphoric effect. An initial oral dose of 10 mg is administered and repeated every 6 hr (not to exceed 40 mg daily) if withdrawal symptoms reappear or do not abate. On the 2nd day, the same dose is administered; thereafter, the daily dose is reduced by 20%. Treatment should not extend beyond 21 days, since only licensed methadone maintenance programs are authorized to provide prolonged administration. Neither the safety nor the dosage of methadone has been established for children or adolescents.

The *overdose syndrome* is an acute reaction following administration of an opiate. It is the leading cause of death among drug users. The rapidity of onset, the finding of eosinophilia after recovery, and the fact that it occurs only in those who have used the drug previously suggest a hypersensitivity mechanism. The clinical signs include stupor or coma, miotic pupils (unless severe anoxia has occurred), respiratory depression, cyanosis, and pulmonary edema. The differential diagnoses include central nervous system trauma, diabetic coma, hepatic (and other) encephalopathy, and Reye syndrome, as well as overdose of alcohol, barbiturates, PCP, or methadone. Diagnosis is facilitated by the intravenous administration of the opiate antagonist naloxone, 0.01 mg/kg (a vial of 0.4 mg usually suffices for an adolescent), which causes dilatation of pupils constricted by the opiate; diagnosis is confirmed by finding morphine in the serum. Treatment consists of maintaining adequate oxygenation and continued administration of naloxone every 5 min as necessary to improve and maintain adequate ventilation. Naloxone may have to be continued for 24 hr if methadone, rather than shorter-acting heroin, has been taken.

Laboratory Findings. Hepatic enzyme activities are frequently elevated in heroin users, the majority of whom have serologic evidence of hepatitis B viral infection. Elements of chronic aggressive hepatitis on biopsy and persistence of enzyme abnormalities suggest a poor prognosis. Elevations in immunoglobin (IgM) levels are consistently noted in parenteral heroin users, and IgA level elevations are also reported in those who inhale the drug. Abnormal serologic reactions are also common, including false-positive VDRL and latex fixation test results. Lymphocyte response to stimulation by mitogens may also be depressed; this may relate to an association with acquired immune deficiency syndrome (Sec. 10.23).

Hallucinogens. A number of naturally occurring and synthetic substances have been used by adolescents for their hallucinogenic properties. Some that enjoyed popularity in the 1970's such as LSD, have been shunned by the current generation who prefer others that are equally dangerous; phencyclidine, certain mushrooms, and jimsonweed may cause serious toxicity and even death.

Phencyclidine (PCP, sternyl, angel dust, "hog," "peace pill," "sheets"). The popularity and toxicity of this arylcyclohexylamine are related in part to its ease of synthesis in home laboratories. Bacterial contamination may cause cramps, diarrhea, and hematemesis. PCP is thought to potentiate adrenergic effects by inhibiting neuronal re-uptake of catecholamines. It is available as a tablet, liquid, or powder that may be used alone or sprinkled on cigarettes ("joints"). The powders and tablets generally contain 2–6 mg of PCP, whereas joints average 1 mg for every 150 mg of tobacco leaves, or approximately 30–50 mg per joint.

Clinical manifestations are dose related. Euphoria, nystagmus, ataxia, and emotional lability occur within 2–3 min after smoking doses of 1–5 mg and last for hours. Hallucination may involve bizarre distortions of body image that often precipitate panic reactions. With doses of 5–15 mg a toxic psychosis may occur, with disorientation, hypersalivation, and abusive language lasting for more than 1 hr. After oral ingestion of 15 mg or more, the patient usually becomes comatose within 30–60 min, with alternating periods of wakefulness and with dystonic posturing, muscular rigidity, or myoclonic jerks. Hypotension, generalized seizures, and cardiac arrhythmias commonly occur with plasma concentrations from 40–200 µg/dL. Death has been reported during psychotic delirium, resulting from hypertension, hypotension, hypothermia, seizures, or trauma. The coma of PCP may be distinguished from that of the opiates by the absence of respiratory depression; the presence of muscle rigidity, hyperreflexia, and nystagmus; and lack of response to naloxone. PCP psychosis may be difficult to distinguish from schizophrenia. In the absence of history of use, analysis of urine must be depended on.

Treatment of the PCP-intoxicated patient includes placement in a darkened, quiet room on a floor pad, safe from injury. Diazepam, in a dose of 10–20 mg orally or 10 mg intramuscularly every 4 hr may be helpful if the patient is agitated and not comatose. Ammonium chloride, 500 mg every 6 hr, may be administered orally or by nasogastric tube to maintain urinary pH at 5.5–6, which enhances urinary clearance of PCP. Supportive therapy of the comatose patient is indicated with particular attention to hydration, which may be compromised by PCP-induced diuresis.

Mushrooms. These contain ibotenic acid, muscimol, and similar toxins causing both cholinergic and anticholinergic effects in addition to the desired euphoria and hallucinations. The adverse effects are usually self-limited and do not require therapy. Those mushrooms containing psilocybin and related antiserotonergic indoles cause LSD-like reactions and may require treatment with diazepam for resulting agitation. Because most hallucination-seeking adolescents are not expert mycologists, mushrooms with other toxic and even fatal effects may be accidentally ingested (Sec. 28.2). Treatment by inducing vomiting and by administering activated charcoal is advisable when there is any possibility of such ingestion.

Jimsonweed (*Datura stramonium*). This is also known as devil's weed," "locoweed," "stinkweed," and thornapple and grows wild throughout the United States. The seeds, which appear in the autumn, contain alkaloids including hyoscyamine, as well as atropine and scopolamine. One hundred seeds, the upper limit of contents of a single pod, contain the equivalent of 6 mg of atropine. Ingestion of the seeds or other plant parts produces dose-related CNS and other anticholinergic effects ranging from restlessness, disorientation, and the desired hallucinations at the lower dose range, to lethargy and coma and rarely, convulsions. The presence of dry mouth, dry hot skin, fever, mydriasis, cycloplegia, urinary retention, and sinus tachycardia, in conjunction with delirium and visual or auditory hallucinations, should alert the physician to the possibility of jimsonweed intoxication. In addition to supportive care, physostigmine salicylate, an anticholinesterase, is indicated for treatment of hypertension, convulsions, severe hallucinations, and supraventricular tachyarrhythmias. This agent is administered slowly by the intravenous route over a 2–5 min period in an initial dose of 1–2 mg. This dose can be repeated in 20 min. Should cholinergic symptoms result from physostigmine administration, atropine sulfate may be given in a dose of 0.5 mg for each mg of physostigmine.

Volatile Substances. The practice of inhaling a variety of euphoriants has enjoyed popularity among adolescents for centuries. The first well-described documentation relates to an "epidemic" of ether sniffing by Irish teenagers in the 19th century. More recently, the easy availability and low cost of substances such as airplane glue, freons, paint thinners, and gasoline have provided a wide range of potential hallucinogens and a broad spectrum of complications relating to chemical toxicity, to the method of administration (e.g., in plastic bags, with resultant suffocation), and to the often dangerous setting in which the inhalation occurs (e.g., inner-city rooftops).

Airplane glue continues to be a problem among young adolescents. Toluene, its main ingredient, is rapidly excreted

in the urine as hippuric acid, with the residual detectable in the serum by gas chromatography. The glue is inhaled via the nose or mouth and causes relaxation and rather pleasant hallucinations for up to 2 hr. Tolerance and physical dependence may occur, but this has not been documented. Toxicity of the chemical is acute and chronic. Death in the acute phase may result from cerebral edema, pulmonary edema, or myocardial toxicity. Chronic use may cause pulmonary hypertension, restrictive lung defects or reduced diffusion capacity, peripheral neuropathy, acute rhabdomyolysis, hematuria, tubular acidosis, and possibly cerebral and cerebellar atrophy.

Gasoline sniffing is popular among rural adolescents and Native American youth and may cause ataxia, nausea, and loss of consciousness. Euphoria followed by violent excitement and coma may result from prolonged or rapid inhalation. The long-term effects of chronic exposure include irreversible encephalopathy, bone marrow aplasia (from contained benzene), and lead encephalopathy when the gasoline contains tetraethyl lead.

Inhalation of *aerosol products*, such as hair sprays, deodorants, frying-pan lubricants, and cocktail glass chillants has also become popular. The method of dispensation involves fluorocarbon propellants (freons), which have been implicated in cardiac sensitization to epinephrine, resulting in arrhythmias and death following inhalation.

A variety of *volatile nitrites* such as amyl nitrite, butyl nitrite, and related compounds marketed as room deodorizers are used as euphoriants, enhancers of musical appreciation, and aphrodisiacs among older adolescents and young adults. They may result in headaches, syncope, and lightheadedness; in profound hypotension and cutaneous flushing followed by vasoconstriction and tachycardia; in transiently inverted T waves and depressed S-T segments on ECG; and in methemoglobinemia, increased bronchial irritation, and increased intraocular pressure. The potential for producing carcinogenic nitrosamines has not been fully evaluated.

Marijuana and Alcohol. These popular substances of abuse among adolescents share a number of psychopharmacologic qualities. Both decrease short-term memory, reaction time, and fine coordination and produce mental clouding; 300 mg of cannabis is equivalent to about 70 g of alcohol.

Marijuana (THC, "pot," "weed," "hash," "grass"). This is synthesized from the resin of the *Cannabis sativa* plant, which flourishes in temperate and hot, dry climates. The tetrahydrocannabinol (THC) fraction of the resin is responsible for its hallucinogenic properties and has been synthesized (delta-9-THC). THC is rapidly absorbed by the nasal or oral routes, producing a peak of subjective effect at 10 min and 1 hr, respectively. Marijuana is generally consumed as a "reefer" or "joint," made by rolling the crushed plant material in paper. Although there is great variation in content, each marijuana cigarette contains approximately 1 g of marijuana, or 20 mg of delta-9-THC.

Clinical manifestations, in addition to the desired elation and euphoria, include impairment of short-term memory, poor performance of tasks requiring undivided attention (such as those involved in driving), loss of critical judgment, and distortion of time perception. Visual hallucinations and perceived body distortions rarely occur, but there may be "flashbacks" or recall of frightening hallucinations experienced under marijuana's influence, which usually occur during stress or with fever. Body temperature may be lowered. Tachycardia is apparent within 20 min of smoking marijuana and is followed by transient systolic and diastolic hypertension (½ hr later), which disappears by 3 hr. Tachypnea is observed only in the experienced user. In placebo-controlled studies of experienced users, smoking marijuana caused decreases in forced expired volume, maximal mid-expiratory flow rate, airway conductance, and diffusing capacity. Reduction in bronchospasm may also occur. Both delta-9-THC and marijuana (smoking a single "joint") cause a significant fall in intraocular pressure, lasting up to 5 hr in both healthy persons and patients with glaucoma.

Dose-related suppression of plasma testosterone levels and spermatogenesis that results from smoking marijuana for a minimum of 4 days/wk for 6 mo prompts concern over the potential deleterious reproductive effects of smoking marijuana before completing pubertal growth and development. Smoking marijuana for 1 wk also decreases glucose tolerance. The antiemetic effect of oral THC or smoked marijuana, which is often followed by appetite stimulation, is the basis of the drug's use in patients receiving cancer chemotherapy. Although the possibility of teratogenicity and carcinogenesis has been raised because of findings in animals, there is no evidence for such effects in humans, nor is there proof of physiologic dependency.

Alcohol. Adolescent drinking has increased over the past decade and poses a threat to the normal functioning of the teenager as well as to the lives of those potentially jeopardized by drunken drivers. The usual progression is from beer to wine to hard liquor, although regional differences may alter this pattern. Four ounces of hard liquor (86 proof) consumed on an empty stomach produces a plasma ethanol level of approximately 65 mg/dL in an adult male of average weight and 80 mg/dL in a premenstrual female of adult weight. The legal definition of intoxication in most statutes is a blood ethanol level of 100 mg/dL (0.10%).

PATHOPHYSIOLOGY. Alcohol (ethyl alcohol, or ethanol) is rapidly absorbed from the stomach, transported to the liver, and metabolized by two pathways. The primary pathway involves removal of two hydrogen atoms to form acetaldehyde, a reaction catalyzed by alcohol dehydrogenase through reduction of a cofactor NAD. The removed hydrogen atoms supply energy (7.1 kcal/g of alcohol) and contribute to the excess synthesis of triglycerides, a phenomenon that is responsible for producing a fatty liver, even in those who are well-nourished. Engorgement of hepatocytes with fat causes necrosis, triggering an inflammatory process (alcoholic hepatitis), which is followed by fibrosis, the hallmark of cirrhosis. Early hepatic involvement may result in elevations in gamma-glutamyl transpeptidase and serum glutamic-pyruvic transaminase; cirrhosis has been reported in Native American adolescents. The second metabolic pathway, which is utilized at high serum alcohol levels, involves the microsomal system of the liver, in which the cofactor is reduced NADPH. The net effect of activating this pathway is to decrease metabolism of drugs that share this system, resulting in their accumulation, enhanced effect, and possible toxicity; e.g., drinking alcohol and ingesting tranquilizers results in potentiation of each (Table 9–2).

CLINICAL MANIFESTATIONS. Alcohol acts primarily as a central nervous system depressant producing euphoria, grogginess, talkativeness, and impaired short-term memory. It also increases the pain threshold and the time needed to brake a car under simulated driving conditions. Alcohol's ability to produce vasodilation and hypothermia is also centrally mediated. At very high serum levels, respiratory depression occurs. Alcohol's inhibitory effect on pituitary release of antidiuretic hormone is responsible for its diuretic effect.

The most common gastrointestinal complication of alcohol use is acute erosive gastritis, which is manifested by epigastric pain, anorexia, vomiting, and guaiac-positive stools. Less commonly, vomiting and midabdominal pain may be caused by acute alcoholic pancreatitis; diagnosis is confirmed by the finding of elevated serum amylase and lipase activities.

Physiologic dependence on alcohol may develop in the adolescent who uses it on a daily basis over a period of weeks. In such individuals, alcohol deprivation may precipitate a **withdrawal syndrome** whose manifestations are generally mild, occurring within 8 hr of the last dose of alcohol and lasting no longer than 48 hr in the untreated patient. Anxiety, tremor, insomnia, and irritability are common symptoms. Only rarely do severe reactions occur in older adolescents who have been drinking steadily for 1 yr or more; these consist of auditory or visual hallucinations, hyperthermia, delirium, and seizures occurring 48 hr or more after the last drink. Treatment of the alcohol withdrawal or abstinence syndrome involves employment of drugs that are cross-tolerant with alcohol but that have a longer duration of action, such as benzodiazepine derivatives, of which chlordiazepoxide (Librium) is the most popular. The usual initial regimen consists of an oral dose of 25 mg every 6 hr. If a satisfactory effect is not achieved, the dose is repeated at 2 hr intervals. Once symptomatic relief is obtained, the dose is tapered by 25 mg daily.

The **alcohol overdose syndrome** should be suspected in any teenager who appears disoriented, lethargic, or comatose. While the distinctive aroma of alcohol may assist in diagnosis, confirmation by blood analysis is recommended. At levels above 200 mg/dL the adolescent is at risk of death, and levels above 500 mg/dL (LD_{50}) are usually associated with a fatal outcome. Because there is a high correlation between serum and breath analyses, the latter method may be reliably used. The usual mechanism of death is respiratory depression; artificial ventilatory support must be provided until the liver can eliminate sufficient amounts of alcohol from the body. In a patient without alcoholism, it generally takes 20 hr to reduce the blood level of alcohol from 400 mg/dL to zero. Dialysis should be considered when the blood level is higher than 400 mg/dL. When the level of depression appears excessive for the reported blood level, head trauma or ingestion of other drugs should be considered as possible confounding factors.

Cocaine has become less expensive and is now widely used by adolescents. The alkaloid extracted from the leaves of the South American *Erythroxylon coca* is supplied as the hydrochloride salt in crystalline form. It is rapidly absorbed from the nasal mucosa, detoxified by the liver, and excreted in the urine as benzoyl ecgonine. Its half-life is slightly more than 1 hr, yet social custom often dictates its repeated administration every 15 min. The perceived effect of "snorting" cocaine may be influenced by some of the many diluents now being added to or actually substituted for the drug (heroin, amphetamines, PCP, or fillers such as mannitol or quinine).

Recently the smoking in pipes or cigarettes of the cocaine alkaloid ("free basing") sometimes mixed with tobacco, marijuana, or parsley, or as a paste or solid ("crack"), has become a popular method of use. The effects appear to be exaggerations of those achieved by other routes. Accidental burns are potential complications of this practice.

Cocaine causes euphoria, increased motor activity, decreased fatigability, and occasionally, paranoid ideation. The sympathomimetic properties of cocaine are responsible for tachycardia, hypertension, and hyperthermia. The chronic user may develop tolerance to these physiologic effects, and psychologic dependence may occur. Rapid addiction to "crack" has been reported. Moreover, "crack" may cause cardiac arrhythmias, coronary insufficiency, and sudden death. Autopsies have shown myocardial contraction bands.

Cigarette Smoking. There are immediate and long-term potential sequelae for the more than 13% of adolescents who smoke cigarettes and for the increasing numbers of adolescent females who smoke. The severity of atherosclerosis is correlated with the duration of smoking, placing those who begin smoking during adolescence at higher risk than those whose cigarette smoking begins during adulthood. In eight states in 1984, for the first time, the incidence of lung cancer in women exceeded that of breast cancer, reflecting the increasing prevalence of smoking among women. The adverse health effects of smoking may also be evident even during adolescence itself and include: an increased prevalence of chronic cough, phlegm production, and wheezing; in pregnancy, an average decrease in fetal weight of 200 g, which, in addition to the correlation of low birthweight and teenage pregnancy, leads to increases in perinatal morbidity and mortality; an increased risk of myocardial infarction due to smoking in combination with ingestion of estrogen-containing oral contraceptives; and an influence on the metabolism of endogenously produced hormones and drugs such as phenacetin, theophylline, and imipramine. In addition, laboratory tests may be affected by smoking: white blood cell count, hemoglobin, hemocrit, mean corpuscular volume (MCV), and platelet aggregation are increased; and serum creatinine, albumin, globulin (in females), and uric acid (in males) are decreased.

9.5 SLEEP DISORDERS

The maturational changes in sleep patterns during adolescence have only recently begun to be described. There is an increase in daytime sleepiness and a decrease in sleep latency between sex maturation stages (SMRs) 3 and 4, and a secretory spurt of gonadotropins and growth hormone with each completed sleep cycle during early puberty, a pattern not found at any other time of life. This normal pattern of sleep augmentation of gonadotropin secretion is disturbed in anorexia nervosa (Sec. 9.6) and possibly in other situations associated with significant weight loss. The clinical association of sleep disorders with depression has long been appreciated, but its physiologic bases are only beginning to be understood; shortened REM latency appears to be common in such patients.

Narcolepsy often first becomes symptomatic during adolescence. The syndrome includes (1) attacks of REM sleep during wakefulness, with excessive daytime sleepiness; (2) hypnagogic hallucinations, and frightening and recurring visual hallucinations; (3) cataplexy, the sudden inhibition of tone of a muscle group with the effects dependent on the muscle group involved; and (4) sleep paralysis, a paralysis of voluntary musculature while falling asleep.

The *sleep apnea-hypersomnia syndrome* also may first become symptomatic during adolescence and consists of increased daytime sleepiness following multiple episodes of brief nighttime waking after each of the obstructive apneic spells.

Insomnia affects 10–20% of adolescents. The etiology may be depression or the delayed sleep phase syndrome in which the difficulty lies in falling asleep, rather than awakening once sleep has begun. According to Anders, "Adolescents may be particularly susceptible to this syndrome, because the changing social demands, which result in later bedtimes, interact with the changing neuroendocrine secretion patterns of puberty, which affect sleep state relationships."

9.6 ANOREXIA NERVOSA AND BULIMIA

The incidence of anorexia nervosa and bulimia has increased in the past two decades; 1 in every 100 16–18 yr old females has such an eating disorder. There is a bimodal distribution with one peak at 14.5 yr and the other at 18 yr. The increased incidence has occurred in all Western countries, with sporadic reports from other nations; affected females outnumber males by 5–10 to 1. Although initially reported only in middle and upper class white patients, anorexia nervosa now also occurs in smaller numbers among those from the lower classes and among nonwhite ethnic groups. Bulimia is undoubtedly more common; a recent survey reported that 13% of all university students responding to a questionnaire had major symptoms of bulimia. An increased incidence of eating disorders among primary relatives of those with anorexia nervosa and bulimia suggests a familial basis.

Definitions and Diagnoses. The criteria for the diagnosis of *anorexia nervosa* include (1) intense fear of becoming obese, which does not diminish as weight loss progresses; (2) disturbance of body image, e.g., claiming to "feel fat" even when emaciated; (3) weight loss of at least 25% of original body weight or, for patients under 18 years of age, if weight loss from original body weight plus weight gain projected from growth charts reaches 25%; (4) refusal to maintain body weight over a minimal normal weight for age and height; and (5) absence of known physical illness that would account for weight loss.

Anorexia nervosa is further characterized by amenorrhea, excessive physical activity in the face of apparent inanition, denial of hunger, and preoccupation with food preparation, frequently accompanied by bizarre eating behaviors and often by studiousness and academic success. Most patients are described as having been "model children" prior to the onset of the illness. Patients are subdivided into the restrictor and bulimia subgroups; restrictors severely limit their intake of carbohydrate and fat-containing foods, whereas bulimics tend to eat in binges and then purge themselves of food by self-induced vomiting or use of cathartics or both. The binge-purge pattern may also occur in youngsters who have normal weight or are slightly obese.

Bulimia, or binge eating, may alternate with anorexia nervosa or exist as a separate syndrome. The criteria for the diagnosis of *bulimia* include (1) recurrent episodes of binge eating (rapid consumption of a large amount of food in a discrete period of time, usually less than 2 hr); (2) at least three of the following: (a) consumption of high caloric, easily digested food during a binge, (b) inconspicuous eating during a binge, (c) termination of such eating episodes by abdominal pain, sleep, social interruption, or self-induced vomiting, (d) repeated attempts to lose weight by severely restrictive diets, self-induced vomiting, or use of amphetamines, cathartics or diuretics, and (e) frequent weight fluctuations of greater than 10 lb, owing to alternating binges and fasts; (3) depressed mood and self-deprecating thoughts following eating binges; and (4) absence of anorexia nervosa or evidence of any physical disorder.

Etiology and Psychodynamics. Eating disorders commonly begin as dieting behavior not unlike that seen in many other adolescent women, but those women having anorexia nervosa gradually progress to profound weight loss with emaciation. The premorbid psychiatric characteristics of those patients who develop this disorder include excessive dependency, developmental immaturity, isolation, obsessive-compulsive traits, and constriction of affect. Their families are described as having difficulty with problem solving and as being intrusive and overprotective. The onset of anorexia nervosa and bulimia at the time of puberty has prompted psychoanalysts to regard them as defenses against emerging sexuality, problems in identity development, or disorders of mood accompanied by manic or depressive symptomatology. Bulimic patients may have greater sensitivity to interpersonal relationships and more labile affect than those with anorexia nervosa. Different subgroups of these disorders may be dynamically and prognostically different. The biogenic amine neurotransmitter abnormalities found in some patients with anorexia nervosa may provide new insights into its etiology and pathogenesis.

Complications. Anorexia nervosa and bulimia are associated with disturbances in almost every organ system, although it is uncertain which disorders are primary and which are the result of severe malnutrition. The death rate in anorexia nervosa is approximately 10%, and is usually caused by severe electrolyte disturbance, cardiac arrhythmia, or congestive heart failure in the recovery phase.

Bradycardia and postural hypotension are not uncommon, with pulse rates as low as 20/min; both improve with nutritional therapy. A variety of ECG abnormalities are common, including low voltage, T-wave inversion and flattening, ST-segment depression, and supraventricular and ventricular dysrhythmias; some are preceded by a prolonged Q-T interval. Death from congestive heart failure occurs late and may result from unduly rapid rehydration and refeeding. If daily weight gain is limited to 0.1–0.4 kg this complication is rare.

Sleep disturbances occur in some anorexics and include a short REM latency time, similar to that often found in depressed patients. Problems of thermal regulation, particularly *hypothermia* are very common (15% of our patients had temperatures below 95° F [35° C]). Hypothermia also occurs in some bulimics of normal weight. Disorders of the hypothalamic-pituitary-ovarian axis are manifested as *amenorrhea* associated with immature patterns of secretion of luteinizing hormone. These findings may represent a primary hypothalamic defect, rather than being secondary to weight loss (which also causes amenorrhea), since amenorrhea antedates weight loss in one third to one half of patients with anorexia nervosa and since a similar proportion fail to resume menses when normal weight is restored. Evidence for hypothalamic-pituitary-adrenal axis dysfunction includes increased secretion of cortisol, loss of diurnal variation in its secretion, and failure of dexamethasone to suppress cortisol secretion. Abnormal dexamethasone suppression test results often persist after weight rehabilitation. Growth hormone secretion is abnormally high in these patients. Thyroid stimulating hormone (TSH) levels are normal, T_4 and T_3 are low, and reverse T_3 is elevated, presumably in adaptation to a lowered basal metabolic rate due to malnutrition and carbohydrate deprivation. *Peripheral edema*, in the absence of congestive heart failure or hypoproteinemia, may occur, due to inappropriate secretion of antidiuretic hormone (ADH).

Elevations of blood urea nitrogen (BUN) may reflect dehydration and decreased glomerular filtration rate (GFR), but normal levels may be found under these same conditions because of low protein intake. Findings of mild proteinuria, hematuria and pyuria, with negative urine cultures, generally resolve with proper rehydration.

Bone marrow hypoplasia is common in patients having anorexia nervosa with leukopenia, anemia, and (rarely) thrombocytopenia. Low erythrocyte sedimentation rates are also common, perhaps reflecting low fibrinogen production secondary to malnutrition.

Constipation is a very common complication in anorexia nervosa, and *esophagitis* is common in bulimia with vomiting. Perforation has been reported from nasogastric tube insertion in patients who refuse to eat. Elevations in amylase levels may be associated with bilateral parotid swelling or with frank pancreatitis in those who vomit.

Electrolyte imbalance results from vomiting, from "waterloading" (a practice of drinking large amounts of water in order to achieve an agreed-upon weight gain), and/or from abuse of diuretics or laxatives. Potassium depletion, associated with a hypochloremic alkalosis, is very common. Abnormalities of calcium, magnesium, and phosphorus metabolism may result from laxative abuse, secondary either to malabsorption or to use of preparations containing phosphate.

Patients having anorexia nervosa are remarkably resistant to infection, considering their degree of inanition; studies of their immunologic status have been normal. The fact that protein intake is relatively good in these otherwise malnourished persons may contribute to this finding.

The skin in anorexia nervosa is dry, and lanugo hair is often seen. Hair loss often occurs in the refeeding phase.

Treatment and Prognosis. Systematic, controlled studies of therapy for these disorders are not available. Most of the current regimens combine psychotherapy (individual and family), behavior modification techniques, and nutritional rehabilitation. Pharmacologic therapy (primarily with antidepressant medications) may be added to these treatment regimens. Many patients, especially those with moderate or severe weight loss, require hospitalization in the initial phase of management.

The short-term success rate is generally about 70%. The frequent occurrence of medical complications and the possibility of death (about 6%) during the acute or rehabilitation phase, mandates that a physician knowledgeable about physiology participate in the management team. The long-term prognosis is variable, depending primarily on the magnitude and treatability of the underlying personality problems. Eating problems or psychiatric impairment, or both, may persist in about 50% of the patients.

PROBLEMS RELATED TO ADOLESCENT SEXUALITY

9.7 PREGNANCY

For women aged 15–19 the pregnancy rate in the United States fell from a peak of 97.3 births/1000 in 1957 to 52/1000 in 1980. However, this reduction in birth rate was accomplished largely through increased use of abortion, rather than through prevention of pregnancy; and the current rate remains among the highest for developed countries. Additional cause for continuing concern stems from the fact that the rate of out-of-wedlock births in this age group increased by 190.1% from 1960–1977. Among those whose pregnancies went to term, from 1971–1976, there was an increase of 7% of teenaged mothers who chose to keep their babies rather than place them for adoption. In addition, from 1973–1978, there was a 5% increase in pregnancies among those under the age of 15 yr, who are at increased risk for obstetrical and perinatal complications such as toxemia, postpartum hemorrhage, postpartum infection, and low birthweight and stillborn infants. (See also Sec. 2.30.)

Adolescent mothers are less likely to marry or achieve a high school education and are more likely to be unemployed and to have a larger number of children than those women who postpone childbearing until after the age of 20 yr. Children born to teenaged mothers have an increased risk of experiencing an accident within the home and of being hospitalized for that or another condition before the age of 5 yr.

As most pregnancies in adolescents are unintended, there is a need to assist young people in prevention of pregnancy. Fewer than half of teenagers use any form of contraception at the time of first intercourse and the birth control methods they do use are rarely effective ones. The lag between becoming sexually active and seeking effective contraception usually exceeds 1 yr, resulting in nearly 40% of sexually active teenagers becoming pregnant within 2 yr of initiating intercourse.

The physician rarely has an opportunity for primary prevention of pregnancy, since discussions of abstinence usually fall on deaf ears; on the other hand, stimulating a young girl who has a boyfriend to think about whether she feels ready for intercourse may be useful if done in a nonjudgmental manner. For the already sexually active adolescent, information about, access to, and motivation to use contraception are necessary for successful pregnancy prevention. Motivation is difficult to achieve, since many girls who have been sexually active without getting pregnant assume that they are sterile and are unlikely to use any contraceptive method until they are made to feel vulnerable to an unwanted pregnancy. Alternatively, those who have gotten pregnant in the past and thus proved their fertility may shun contraception, promising abstinence or expressing fear that their fertility has been impaired from abortion, infection, or some less well-founded concern. Therefore, it is important to inquire about the reason any sexually active female thinks she has not gotten pregnant.

Once it is established that the teenager is not pregnant, that intercourse is likely to continue, and that the patient accepts the fact that she is at risk for pregnancy, efforts should be directed toward providing the most effective and safest contraceptive method. In order to enhance the likelihood of compliance once the method is prescribed, the physician must learn about the frequency and circumstances of intercourse; past experience and compliance with both contraceptive and noncontraceptive chronic medications; the partner's attitudes about various methods; and parents' knowledge and attitudes about contraception. In the United States currently physicians may provide contraception to minors without parental knowledge, but in choosing a method it is useful to know whether the parents are aware of their daughter's sexual activity.

9.8 CONTRACEPTION

All methods of birth control should be available to the adolescent, but the risk(s) of each method must be weighed against the significant risk of pregnancy. For contraception to be successful every effort should be made to individualize the method to the needs of each patient. The risks, benefits, and indications for each of the available methods follow.

Barrier Methods

Condom. There are no major side effects associated with condom use. However, its effectiveness in preventing pregnancy is low, with 15 pregnancies/100 woman-years of use by adult women in the United States. Comparative figures are not available for adolescents, but in this age group acceptance of this method is limited by the male partner's perceived decrease in sensitivity. A 1979 study found that only 23% of 15–19 yr old females reported that their partner ever used a condom. Condoms used in this country are thicker than those marketed in other countries, where they enjoy widespread use. The main advantages of condoms are their low price, availability without prescription, little need for advance planning, and effectiveness in preventing transmission of sexually acquired diseases (Sec. 9.9).

Diaphragm. The diaphragm prevents sperm from gaining access to the cervix, while placing spermicidal jelly in a position to be effective. Aside from rare instances of contact vaginitis caused by the latex or by the powder used to preserve the diaphragm, there are no adverse side effects associated with its use. Possible teratogenicity from absorption of spermicides has not been supported by recent studies. However, the diaphragm is effective in only 85% of women who use it properly over a 1 yr period of time. In a study of adolescents who were highly motivated to avoid pregnancy, however, diaphragm use was associated with only 2 pregnancies/100 woman-years. Adolescents may object to the messiness of the jelly or to the fact that diaphragm insertion may interrupt the spontaneity of sex, or they may express discomfort about touching their genitalia. At Stanford University this method is used by 21% of sexually active women students, compared with only 3.5% of 15–19 yr old inner-city youth.

A diaphragm must be individually fitted by a trained physician or nurse practitioner. Once fitted, the same diaphragm may be used for 3 yr unless extreme weight gain or loss or pregnancy occurs. After the proper diaphragm is selected, the teenager should be given instructions and ample opportunity to learn to insert and remove it before leaving the office.

Cervical Cap. This method is currently under evaluation.

After proper fitting, this rubber cap remains affixed to the cervix by suction for 1–3 intermenstrual days. Like the diaphragm, it must be used in conjunction with spermicidal jelly.

Spermicides

A variety of agents containing the spermicide nonoxynol-9 are available as foams, jellies, creams, or effervescent vaginal suppositories. Each must be placed in the vaginal cavity shortly before intercourse and reinserted prior to each ejaculation in order to be effective. Contact vaginitis is a rare side effect. Possible teratogenicity from absorption of this agent has not been supported by recent investigation. Effectiveness is about the same as with barrier methods (only about 85%), but nonoxynol-9 has the added advantage of being gonococcocidal and spirocheticidal.

Combination Methods

The conjoint use of condom by the male and spermicidal foam by the female adolescent is extremely effective; the failure rate is only 2%, without any of the potential side effects and complications associated with use of other forms of contraception having comparable efficacy. This combination also prevents sexually transmitted diseases. The contraceptive sponge, which incorporates the theoretical advantage of barrier and spermicides, has recently been marketed over the counter, but its efficacy is only about 85% and toxic shock syndrome (Sec. 11.18) has been reported in users.

Hormonal Methods

Hormonal contraceptive methods currently employ either an estrogenic substance in combination with a progestin, or a progestin alone. The estrogen-progestin combination prevents the surge of luteinizing hormone, inhibiting ovulation; progestin alone may prevent ovulation but is not as reliable. It does, however, affect fallopian tube transport and the composition of cervical mucus in such a way as to make fertilization and/or implantation less likely.

Combination Oral Contraceptives. The "pill" contains 80, 50, or 35 μg of estrogenic substance, typically either mestranol or ethinyl estradiol. Thrombophlebitis, hepatic adenomas, myocardial infarction, and carbohydrate intolerance are some of their more serious potential complications. These are, however, exceedingly rare in adolescents. The risk of cardiovascular complications is limited almost exclusively to women over the age of 35 and is highest in those who smoke cigarettes.

Some long-range beneficial effects of estrogen use include decreased risks of benign breast disease, of ovarian cystic disease, and of anemia. Adolescents taking estrogen-containing oral contraceptives also have higher levels of high density lipoproteins than controls. Inhibition of ovulation and/or the suppressant effect of estrogens on prostaglandin production by the endometrium make oral contraceptives effective in preventing dysmenorrhea (Sec. 9.10).

The potential inhibiting effect of estrogens on epiphyseal growth is not a problem, either because the amount in oral contraceptives is small or because they are taken at a time when most growth has been completed. However, postpill amenorrhea, persisting for up to 18 mo after discontinuation of use, occurs with greater frequency in adolescents than in adults. The increased risk may not be due to age alone but may reflect oligomenorrhea or low body weight (less than 47 kg), or both, prior to initiation of use of the pill. Acne may be worsened by some and improved by other oral contraceptive preparations. *Contraindications* to using estrogen-containing oral contraceptives include hepatocellular disease; migraine headaches; diabetes mellitus; and any condition in which hypercoagulability may be a problem (e.g., replaced cardiac valve, thrombophlebitis, sickle cell anemia, and so on), owing to the increased levels of factor VIII and decreased production of antithrombin III.

Despite these potential problems, the pill is the most reliable contraceptive method available, with a pregnancy rate in the range of 0.8/100 woman-years. Some side effects can, without sacrificing their efficacy, be minimized by use of low estrogen content preparations. With the use of 35 μg preparation, however, there may be a higher incidence of breakthrough bleeding, which may lead to noncompliance.

All-Progestin Contraceptives. These are available for the adolescent in whom use of estrogen is potentially deleterious (e.g., those with liver disease, replaced cardiac valves, or hypercoagulable states). They are less reliable in inhibiting ovulation and are associated with a pregnancy rate of 2.4/100 woman-years. Acceptance by adolescents is limited by the necessity to take the pill daily and the higher incidence of amenorrhea, or by increased bleeding.

An injectable progestin, medroxyprogesterone (Depo-Provera), is highly effective in birth control. It needs to be administered only once every 3 mo, its anovulatory action is completely reversible, and the cessation of menses is coterminous with its use. This agent is particularly appropriate for adolescents who have difficulty with compliance or for mentally retarded teenagers. It is not, however, available as a contraceptive in the United States, because of concern over a reported association with increased risk of benign breast tumors in experimental animals. Worldwide, it is the leading birth control method.

Recently, a new delivery system for the long-acting progestational agent, levonorgestral or "Norplant," has been extensively tested. The active ingredient is contained in a small silastic tube, which is implanted subcutaneously and is easily removable. The contraceptive potency remains for 5 yr. This agent is not available commercially in the United States, and its use in teenagers has not been explored.

Postcoital Contraception. Unprotected midcycle intercourse carries a pregnancy risk of 2–30%. The risk may be reduced or eliminated by intervention within 72 hr after unprotected intercourse by either hormonal or mechanical methods. The "morning after" pill, DES (diethylstilbestrol), although effective, should be avoided because of its potential teratogenic effect (Sec. 18.4). If begun within 72 hr of unprotected intercourse, ethinyl estradiol, 2.5 mg twice daily for five days, appears equally effective, but its potential effect on a fetus is unknown and it may produce nausea and vomiting. Ovral, which combines norgestrel and ethinyl estradiol, is another promising postcoital combination oral contraceptive, administered in a dose of 2 pills initially and two additional 2 pills 12 hr later.

Intrauterine Devices (IUD). IUD's are small, flexible, plastic objects introduced into the uterine cavity through the cervix. They differ in size, shape, and the presence or absence of pharmacologically active substances (such as copper or progesterone). Their mechanism of action is uncertain, although it is known that they render the endometrium unsuitable for implantation by inducing a local polymorphonuclear leukocyte response, that they induce production of prostaglandins E_2 and F_{2a}, and that they stimulate uterine contractility. IUD's are effective in preventing pregnancy in 97–99% of women. Those women who become pregnant with an IUD in place, however, are at greater risk for having an ectopic pregnancy, especially if the IUD is a progesterone-containing one; have increased menstrual bleeding and dysmenorrhea (although the progesterone-containing ones reportedly decrease dysmenorrhea); and are at increased risk of infection, including the risks of septic abortion and death. The highest risk is associated with use of the Dalkon Shield, which has been removed from the market. Infection risk varies among the other types of IUD's, but is highest with the progesterone-containing ones. The small amount of copper that leaches out of the copper-containing IUD's may be bactericidal. Young patients and those with multiple sexual partners are also at increased risk of infection. The increased risk of infection should limit prescription of an IUD to those teenagers who require passive contraception as a last resort.

9.9 SEXUALLY TRANSMITTED DISEASES

Adolescents have the highest rate of sexually transmitted disease of any age group. This results from sexual experimentation characteristic of their psychosocial development, as well as from certain aspects of their physical development. During puberty, increasing levels of estrogen cause the vaginal epithelium to thicken and cornify, and the cellular glycogen content to rise causing vaginal pH to fall. These changes increase the resistance of the vaginal epithelium to penetration by certain organisms (including gonococcus) and its susceptibility to others (such as *Candida albicans* and *Trichomonas*). As a result of these physiologic changes, gonococcal infection becomes primarily cervical, and susceptibility is greatest during menses, when the pH is 6.8 to 7.0. At this time in the cycle infection is most likely to ascend to the endometrium, fallopian tubes, and peritoneum. The emergence of β-lactamase–producing, penicillin-resistant strains of gonococcus and the presence of asymptomatic disease in males has hampered attempts to control transmission.

The failure to use any contraceptive method or the use of oral contraceptives are behaviors conducive to the transmission of venereal organisms. Adolescents are typically reluctant to consider the possibility that a potential sexual partner may have a venereal disease or to discuss the problem with physicians. In caring for sexually active adolescents it is necessary to test for sexually transmitted disease, which is often asymptomatic, to look for others if one is found, to consider the problem of noncompliance when deciding upon a treatment regimen (which usually means favoring parenteral administration of medication), to find and treat the sexual partner, and to make every effort to preserve fertility, which may require trials of intensive parenteral therapy for salpingitis or tubo-ovarian abscess. Although diagnosis and therapy are often necessarily carried out within the context of a confidential relationship between physician and patient, the need to report certain sexually transmitted diseases to health department authorities should be clarified at the outset. Most health departments will not violate confidentiality if assured that treatment and case finding have already been accomplished, and that the patient can be expected to follow through in a responsible, mature manner.

Gonorrhea. (See also Sec. 11.22.) Gonorrhea is the most commonly reported sexually transmitted disease among adolescents. Its incidence has risen more rapidly in 15–19 yr olds than in any other age group, reaching 1500 cases/100,000 in 1979. Infection occurs via the urethral, cervical, anal, pharyngeal, or conjunctival route. An initial inflammatory response is followed either by resolution with a fibrous response, by extension along mucosal planes to adjacent organs (endometrium, fallopian tubes, peritoneum, and liver capsule in the female or urethra, prostate, and epididymis in the male), or by hematogenous dissemination to cause arthritis, dermatitis, or rarely, meningitis or endocarditis.

Penicillin is the drug of choice for the treatment of gonorrhea. However, additional antibiotic coverage is often indicated because of the high frequency of coexisting chlamydial and anaerobic infections along with gonococcal infection, the difficulty in diagnosing the former agents, and the increasing incidence of resistant organisms. For prophylaxis (e.g., administered to a rape victim or partner of a known case), 4.8 million units of aqueous procaine penicillin G should be given intramuscularly, with 1 g of probenecid orally. The same dosage regimen may suffice for local infection (cervicitis, urethritis, prostatitis, or epididymitis) but tetracycline (500 mg orally four times daily for 7 days) or doxycycline (100 mg orally twice daily for 7 days) should be added. Teenagers who refuse injection may be treated with a single oral dose of 3.5 g ampicillin, combined with 1 g probenecid, and doxycycline (100 mg orally twice daily for 7 days). This approach is slightly less effective than penicillin therapy and will not adequately treat incubating syphilis should this be present. The oral medication should be taken in the presence of the nurse or physician to ensure compliance. The patient's sexual partner should be treated also.

Acute pelvic inflammatory disease (PID), which includes endometritis, salpingitis, parametritis, or peritonitis, may similarly involve multiple agents. The hospitalized patient should receive doxycycline (100 mg) plus cefoxitin (2.0 g) intravenously twice daily for at least 4 days and at least 48 hr after improvement is noted, followed by oral doxycycline (100 mg twice daily) to complete a 10–14 day treatment schedule. Ambulatory treatment should consist of cefoxitin (2.0 g intramuscularly) or amoxicillin (3.0 g orally) or ampicillin (3.5 g orally) or aqueous procaine penicillin G (4.8 million units intramuscularly at two sites), each accompanied by probenecid (1.0 g orally) and followed by doxycycline (100 mg orally, twice daily) for 10–14 days.

Adolescents with gonococcal ophthalmia should be hospitalized and treated with aqueous penicillin G (10 million units intravenously for 5 days). Irrigation of the eyes with saline or buffered ophthalmic solutions may be used to eliminate discharge. Patients should be carefully monitored for ocular complications.

Disseminated gonococcal infection should be treated with aqueous crystalline penicillin G (10 million units intravenously each day) for at least 3 days followed by amoxicillin or ampicillin (500 mg orally 4 times daily) to complete at least 7 days of therapy; or amoxicillin (3.0 g) or ampicillin (3.5 g) each with probenecid (1 g orally) followed by amoxicillin or ampicillin (500 mg orally 4 times daily) for at least 7 days; or cefoxitin (1 g intravenously 4 times daily) for at least 7 days; or cefotaxime (500 mg intravenously 4 times daily) for at least 7 days.

Persistence of infection after any of the above courses of therapy suggests the presence of penicillinase-producing or chromosomally mediated resistant strains of *Neisseria gonorrhoeae*, which require treatment with spectinomycin (2.0 g intravenously) or ceftriaxone (250 mg intramuscularly) both followed by tetracycline or doxycycline in doses as indicated above. For patients in whom tetracyclines are contraindicated or not tolerated, a single dose regimen may be followed by erythromycin base or stearate 500 mg orally 4 times daily for 7 days or erythromycin ethylsuccinate 800 mg 4 times daily for 7 days.

In the case of penicillin sensitivity, local infection may be treated with spectinomycin (2 g intramuscularly); and pelvic infection with doxycycline (200 mg intravenously, followed by 100 mg orally twice daily for 10 days). Penicillin sensitivity in the pregnant adolescent with gonorrhea poses a serious therapeutic dilemma, since neither spectinomycin nor tetracyclines are approved for use during pregnancy. Although there is rare potential for cross reactivity, ceftriaxone (250 mg intramuscularly) and erythromycin base (500 mg) or erythromycin ethylsuccinate (800 mg) orally 4 times daily for 7 days may be used under such circumstances.

Syphilis. (See also Sec. 11.49.) This infection is rare in adolescents, but the serious consequences of lack of treatment and the ease of serologic diagnosis suggest the advisability of screening for syphilis in high risk adolescents, e.g., those who are pregnant, sexually promiscuous, homosexual, delinquent, or have evidence of another sexually transmitted disease. The Venereal Disease Research Laboratory test (VDRL) is the most sensitive and least specific of the serologic tests for syphilis. False positives may occur in teenagers who are intravenous abusers of drugs, as well as in those who have liver disease of any etiology, collagen-vascular disease, or infectious mononucleosis. A positive test should be confirmed by a more specific test such as the Treponema Pallidum Immobilizing (TPI) test.

Following a rape, prevention of syphilis can be accomplished with the same regimen as for prevention of gonorrhea. In the infected adolescent the most common manifestations of syphilis include condyloma latum or lesions on the palms and soles, or both.

Chlamydia. (See also Sec. 11.56.) Known cases of sexually transmitted infection with *Chlamydia* have increased dramatically in adolescents over the past decade, most likely owing to increased availability of diagnostic testing rather than to a true increase in incidence. The majority of cases of urethritis formerly considered to be nongonococcal are now known to be chlamydial in origin, as are approximately one half of cases of salpingitis. Moreover, all of the complications of gonococcal infection, such as perihepatitis, conjunctivitis, sterility, and so on, occur as potential sequelae of chlamydial infection. For this reason laparoscopy with tubal puncture and culture has become the optimal approach to etiologic diagnosis in salpingitis. If this is not feasible, therapy should cover both gonococcal or chlamydial etiologies. Treatment with doxycycline, 200 mg intravenously initially, followed by 100 mg orally twice daily for 10 days should suffice for chlamydia. *Lymphogranuloma venereum* (LGV), caused by an agent related to *Chlamydia trachomatis* (Sec. 11.59), should be considered in the differential diagnoses of lesions of the genitalia, inguinal lymphadenopathy, and rectal bleeding, purulent proctitis, or rectal structure. The sexual history is, therefore, a mandatory part of the evaluation of adolescents thought to have inflammatory bowel disease.

Chancroid. The need for a biopsy to diagnose chancroid may contribute to its apparent rarity. It appears in adolescents often enough to be readily recognized. The initial lesion is a vesicopustule that rapidly breaks down to form a painful, purulent, sharply delineated ulcer without induration. This latter feature and its painful nature distinguishes it from the syphilitic chancre with which it shares a similar genital distribution. Autoinoculation may result in multiple lesions, and unilateral painful lymphadenopathy is not uncommon. Chancroid is treated with tetracycline, 1 g orally daily for 10 days, and with oral sulfisoxazole, 4 g daily for 10 days. Problems of compliance and the need to treat sexual partners should be addressed.

Genital Herpes. (See also Sec. 11.65.) The possibility of preventing herpes infection through use of a condom should be stressed in counseling sexually active adolescents or those found to have the disease. Appearance of the characteristic herpetic lesion may be preceded by exquisite sensitivity and sharp pain radiating from the perineum, along the course of affected nerve routes. Topical acyclovir may palliate and shorten the symptomatic and shedding phases in primary infections. Its use in recurrent cases is less satisfactory but may be tried in the absence of alternative therapy. Systemic therapy is being evaluated and may prove superior. Routine, yearly Papanicolaou (Pap) smears are necessary following infection, because this is a premalignant agent. Cervical cultures may be positive for herpesvirus in asymptomatic sexually active adolescents, suggesting that Pap smears should also be obtained routinely from such adolescents.

Condyloma acuminatum. This is caused by a DNA-containing papovavirus that propagates in the epidermis of the genitalia or in the perianal region, giving rise to cauliflower-like, grey papules, which often become confluent, macerated, or secondarily infected. When genital mucous membranes are involved, however, the appearance is that of smooth, fleshy protuberances which may be confused with sarcoma botryoides. The lesions are typically multiple and spread by local extension as well as by autoinoculation, the latter producing "kissing" lesions on opposing surfaces, such as the buttocks or labia. Local therapy with podophyllin, 20% benzoin, is recommended. To avoid sclerosis, instructions to the patient should stress the importance of washing thoroughly with soap and water 6 hr after application, or sooner if there is a burning sensation.

Trichomonas. This infection is probably sexually transmitted; it rarely occurs in those who do not engage in sexual intercourse. The symptomatic female patient will have a frothy vaginal discharge. Although males may harbor the organism, they have few clinical manifestations. Hematospermia has been reported in an adult. Diagnosis is based on identification of trichomonads on microscopic examination of a mixture of the discharge with saline. The treatment of both sexual partners with metronidazole (a single dose of 1.5 g orally) is advised, unless pregnancy is suspected. The adolescent should be cautioned about the adverse effect (abdominal pain and vomiting) of alcohol ingestion within 24 hr of metronidazole administration.

Hemophilus (Gardnerella) vaginalis. This is associated with the production of an often foul-smelling vaginal discharge that gives off a fishy odor when KOH is added to a wet preparation, and with the appearance of "clue cells" (epithelial cells ringed with the rod shaped organism on the periphery). The organism is frequently found in vaginal smears from asymptomatic women, but when other etiologic explanations are not found, treatment with metronidazole, 1.5 g orally (see above for precautions), may bring relief.

9.10 MENSTRUAL PROBLEMS OF ADOLESCENTS

Amenorrhea

Primary amenorrhea indicates that menarche has never occurred, whereas *secondary* amenorrhea refers to cessation of menses for more than 3 mo after regular menstrual cycles have been established. In order to diagnose primary amenorrhea it must be ascertained that the patient has passed the age at which menarche normally occurs. This requirement is not as simple as it may first seem. Menarche occurs at an average age of 12.3 yr, but the range of normal is quite broad, extending from approximately 10–16 yr. A better approximation can be made if the sexual maturity rating (SMR) is used as the reference standard rather than chronologic age (Sec. 2.9 and 2.30); 10% of girls have menarche while at SMR 2, 20% at SMR 3, 60% at SMR 4, and 10% at SMR 5. Accordingly, the determination of whether or not an individual girl may be properly considered to have primary amenorrhea should first be based on assessing her stage of pubertal development; if she has not entered puberty by the expected time, or if pubertal development is completed without the onset of menses, she should be evaluated more thoroughly even if her chronologic age is within the normal range. Similarly, the close concordance between the ages of menarche of daughters, mothers, and siblings suggests that the diagnosis of primary amenorrhea be entertained when there is more than 1 year's discrepancy between the patient's age and the age when menarche occurred in either mother or sister, even if the patient's age falls within the normal range for menarche.

The onset and continuation of normal menstrual cycling is dependent on the functional and anatomic integrity of (1) the hypothalamus, together with higher centers, including possibly the pineal; (2) the anterior pituitary; (3) the ovary; and (4) the uterus. Accordingly, evaluation of the adolescent with amenorrhea should include consideration of abnormalities at any of these levels. The only difference in approach between primary and secondary amenorrhea is that in the former, congenital abnormalities such as gonadal dysgenesis, the triple-X syndrome, isochromosomal abnormalities, testicular feminization syndrome, and, rarely, true hermaphroditism must be considered. The finding of elevated levels of follicle-stimulating hormone (FSH) and luteinizing hormone (LH) suggests primary gonadal failure, and chromosome analysis will often elucidate its cause. Once such a diagnosis is made, management includes use of estrogen and progesterone to produce development of secondary sex characteristics and cyclic bleeding if a uterus is present. The purpose is to help the patient to feel like her peers, as well as to prevent later osteoporosis. (See also Sec. 6.22.)

Primary amenorrhea may be caused by chronic illnesses, particularly those associated with malnutrition or tissue hypoxygenation (such as diabetes mellitus, inflammatory bowel disease, cystic fibrosis, or cyanotic congenital heart disease). In most cases the illness will have been previously diagnosed, but occasionally amenorrhea is the first manifestation. Accordingly, a general physical examination, complete blood count, and erythrocyte sedimentation rate should be included in the evaluation of any patient with amenorrhea. Amenorrhea may be the first sign of a central nervous system tumor, most commonly craniopharyngioma (Sec. 21.22 and 19.1).

Abnormalities of the thyroid gland, typically hyperthyroidism, may be first suspected when delayed sexual maturation and amenorrhea occur, even in the absence of other signs and symptoms. Determination of TSH, T_4 and T_3 levels should assist in establishing this diagnosis. Anorexia nervosa may be confused with hyperthyroidism, because weight loss, hyperactivity, and personality changes are seen in both. In anorexia nervosa, amenorrhea may be either primary or secondary (Sec. 9.6).

When primary amenorrhea is accompanied by advanced pubertal development (i.e., SMR 5), either polycystic ovary syndrome or a structural anomaly of the müllerian duct system should be suspected. Imperforate hymen is the most common anomaly and is associated with recurrent (monthly) abdominal pain, and, after some time has passed, by a midline lower abdominal mass, the blood-filled vagina (hematocolpos). Diagnosis is made when inspection of the introitus reveals a bulging hymen with bluish discoloration. If the obstruction is at the level of the cervix, the blood-filled uterus (hematometrium) will be felt on bimanual examination. Agenesis of the cervix or uterus is rare but occurs in patients with sacral agenesis. Serum levels of gonadotropins are normal; diagnosis is made on ultrasonography.

When amenorrhea occurs with signs of virilization (clitoridomegaly, hirsutism, or excessive acne), adrenal or ovarian pathology is suspected. The adrenal causes are discussed in Sec. 19.21 and 19.23 and consist of cortical tumors and, very rarely, of late-onset congenital adrenal hyperplasia. Measurement of the 24 hr excretion of urinary 17-ketosteroids and serum testosterone levels will assist in diagnosis. Ovarian causes of virilization include a Sertoli-Leydig cell or lipoid cell tumor, both of which are rare and the *polycystic ovary syndrome (PCO)*, which is not. In fact, although the classic presentation of PCO in the adult is amenorrhea in association with virilization, the young adolescent with PCO may have amenorrhea or oligomenorrhea with no signs of masculinization. Levels of 17-ketosteroid secretion may be normal or elevated. Patients with PCO have normal serum levels of FSH and marked elevations of LH levels (usually 2–3 times higher). In adolescents with PCO, laparoscopic biopsy may reveal normal ovarian tissue or the histologic findings typical of the adult picture, consisting of cysts and thickened tunica albuginea. Management differs between adult and adolescent patients. The former typically requires assistance with hirsutism or infertility (managed by wedge-biopsy), whereas the adolescent with PCO may, by administration of combination oral contraceptives, be spared the masculinizing effects of this condition, as well as the risk of endometrial carcinoma from continued exposure to estrogens unopposed by progesterone.

In the adolescent with **secondary amenorrhea** the first diagnosis to be considered is pregnancy. This possibility may also, albeit rarely, cause primary amenorrhea, if fertilization of the first ovum occurred before menses. A history of sexual intercourse, nausea, and breast tenderness, and findings on physical examination of increased pigmentation of nipples and linea alba, cyanosis and softening of the cervix, and enlarged uterus form the classic picture. Measurement of serum β-subunit human chorionic gonadotropin (HCG) level is the most sensitive and specific test for pregnancy.

Ingestion of drugs, both licit and illicit, may cause amenorrhea, and in the case of phenothiazines, even a false positive pregnancy test in urine. Some drugs, including phenothiazines and certain antihypertensives, may cause galactorrhea, further mimicking pregnancy.

Psychogenic factors have been implicated in amenorrhea. It is often difficult to separate psychologic from nutritional factors, since weight loss is a confounding variable in many situations, such as depression, anorexia nervosa, or the stress of leaving home or being incarcerated. Under conditions of extreme stress, such as the threat of annihilation that dominated life in concentration camps, the incidence of amenorrhea was highest in adolescents.

Evaluation of the adolescent with amenorrhea should include a thorough history and physical examination, a complete blood count, erythrocyte sedimentation rate, and pregnancy test, and if these are negative, serum levels of gonadotropins (LH and FSH), prolactin, TSH, T_4 and T_3, lateral roentgenographic examination of the skull or CT scan, and, under certain circumstances, chromosome studies and determination of urinary levels of 17-ketosteroids. Ultrasonography can often be useful in assessing the presence and size of uterus and ovaries and of tumors and cysts. In approximately half of reported cases, ovarian biopsy at the time of exploratory laparoscopy has assisted in making a diagnosis.

Determination of the cause of amenorrhea may permit corrective intervention. When the condition is not amenable to remediation, consideration should be given to establishing regular pseudomenses to help the adolescent feel like her peers. If a vaginal smear is positive for estrogen effect, regular cycling can be accomplished using medroxyprogesterone in a dose of 10 mg orally for 5 days, every 6–12 wk. In a patient with gonadal dysgenesis, conjugated estrogens must first be given in an oral dose of 0.625 mg for 3 wk, followed by medroxyprogesterone (10 mg orally on days 17–21 of the cycle).

Menometrorrhagia

Excessive menstrual bleeding is one of the few gynecologic emergencies of adolescence. Bleeding may be so severe as to cause hypovolemia and anemia in a frightened young patient. Accordingly, diagnosis and therapy must be accomplished expeditiously, while providing supportive reassurance.

Excessive menstrual bleeding is most often secondary to the anovulatory cycles that normally occur in the 1st yr postmenarche. Without ovulation, the effect of estrogens on the endometrium is unopposed by that of progesterone,

resulting in continued endometrial proliferation with eventual massive shedding. This common condition has been termed **dysfunctional uterine bleeding.** The prolonged estrogen effect also serves to inhibit the LH surge responsible for ovulation, thus perpetuating the problem. Imbalance between FSH and LH, with the former higher than the latter, is often found, along with evidence of anovulation on measurement of basal body temperature.

Treatment of dysfunctional uterine bleeding is indicated only when blood loss is significant. The goal is to correct the imbalance between estrogen and progesterone, while providing hemostasis. One approach to treatment is the immediate oral administration of 25 mg of Enovid. Some patients may become nauseated with Enovid, but the rapidity of effect (within 2 hr) has much to recommend it. Thereafter, the dose is reduced by 5 mg daily until a daily dose of 5 mg is reached. This is maintained for 21 days from the day treatment began. If bleeding recurs at any point, the previous day's dose is resumed, and tapering of the dose stopped until there is no further bleeding. A normal menstrual period should begin approximately 2 days after the last pill is taken. On the 5th day of this bleeding, a 2 mo course of conventional oral contraceptive therapy should be begun. This could be continued if there were need for contraception, with due consideration of the increased risk of postpill amenorrhea in adolescents who have had anovulatory cycles prior to initiation of treatment with these compounds. Emans and Goldstein have suggested an alternative to the use of high doses of Enovid. They propose oral administration of Ortho-Novum (2 mg) or Enovid-E (2.5 mg) every 4 hr until the bleeding slows or stops, after which it is administered twice daily until the calendar pack is finished.

In the rare patient whose bleeding is not controllable by one of the above methods, an endometrial curettage may be indicated. This procedure is common in adult women with menometrorrhagia, but the rarity of endometrial carcinoma and the usual efficacy of hormonal therapy in adolescents renders this procedure unnecessarily invasive under most circumstances.

Far less often, excessive vaginal bleeding may result from other pathologic conditions, such as bleeding diatheses, endocrinopathies, complications of medications, trauma, infection, or pregnancy.

Among the congenital coagulopathies, **von Willebrand disease** should be considered in the adolescent whose first menstrual period is excessive. The finding of a prolonged bleeding time suggests this diagnosis, which is characterized by a defect of platelet adhesiveness and by lower than normal levels of factor VIII (Sec. 15.43–15.46). The fact that estrogen raises factor VIII levels makes therapy with this hormone appropriate in the management of patients with this condition and underscores the necessity for performing diagnostic studies on blood obtained prior to institution of this therapy. Management is the same as for dysfunctional uterine bleeding (see above), with the exception that administration of oral contraceptives may be required for the entire menstrual life of the patient.

An acquired bleeding diathesis as a result of ingestion of therapeutic doses of aspirin is relatively common, and results from disruption of platelet adhesiveness, secondary to the effect of the acetyl moiety on release of adenosine diphosphate. A history of use of aspirin within 14 days of menses suggests this possibility and warrants a trial of aspirin avoidance.

Thrombocytopenia secondary to toxins, marrow infiltration, hypersplenism, or idiopathic thrombocytopenic purpura may accompany or be complicated by menometrorrhagia. Management is the same as that for dysfunctional uterine bleeding (see above), but platelet transfusions may be needed also.

Exogenous hormones, such as oral contraceptives used improperly, may cause excessive vaginal bleeding, so that careful and sensitive history taking is an important part of evaluation of a patient with this symptom.

Hypothyroidism may cause excessive vaginal bleeding, which is in some cases the presenting symptom. The characteristically low level of T_4 may be altered by estrogen therapy used to stop the bleeding, but free T_4 levels should remain low and TSH elevated. Rarely, hyperthyroidism, adrenal dysfunction, diabetes mellitus, or estrogen-secreting ovarian tumors may result in increased vaginal bleeding. The bleeding caused by adenocarcinoma of the vagina is typically scant (Sec. 18.4).

In contrast with the conditions described thus far, menometrorrhagia resulting from trauma, infection, or pregnancy is typically accompanied by pain. Lacerations of the genital tract may result from first or forceful intercourse or athletics, such as waterskiing. The circumstances of the injury may be embarrassing or frightening for the patient, requiring supportive and sensitive history taking. Surgical intervention by a gynecologist is usually needed if bleeding is secondary to trauma or to pregnancy.

Since approximately 15% of adolescent pregnancies terminate in spontaneous abortion, this possibility should be considered in every instance of painful excessive vaginal bleeding. In addition to history and physical examination, a β-subunit HCG pregnancy test should be obtained, as this remains positive up to 15 days following an abortion. Other tests typically revert to negative within 5–8 days. Involvement of a gynecologist is necessary once the diagnosis of spontaneous abortion is confirmed. Rarely, ectopic pregnancy may present with abnormal vaginal bleeding.

Dysmenorrhea

Painful menstrual cramps are experienced by nearly two thirds of postmenarchal teenagers in the United States. More than 10% of this group miss a day or more of school, making dysmenorrhea the leading cause of short-term school absenteeism in female adolescents. Dysmenorrhea may be primary or secondary, the former being the more common. *Dysmenorrhea* is *secondary* when there is an underlying structural abnormality of the cervix or uterus, a foreign body such as an IUD, endometriosis, or endometritis. In endometriosis implants of endometrial tissue are found ectopically within the peritoneal cavity. With the increased availability of laparoscopy, endometriosis is being diagnosed with increasing frequency among adolescents. Characteristically, severe pain occurs at the time of menses. The location of pain depends on the site of the implants. Some patients respond favorably to treatment with oral contraceptives, whereas the more severe cases are treated with Danazol, an antigonadotropin. A pelvic examination must be done in adolescents with dysmenorrhea; and if no basis for secondary amenorrhea is found, a diagnosis of primary dysmenorrhea may be entertained.

Primary dysmenorrhea occurs in the absence of any underlying anatomic abnormality. For this reason, it was long erroneously considered to be emotional in origin. Those suffering from primary dysmenorrhea have been found to have higher levels of prostaglandins $F_{2\alpha}$ and E_2 than pain-free controls. These substances, produced by the endometrium, stimulate the myometrium to contract, producing pain. Symptomatic relief occurs when prostaglandin synthetase inhibitors are administered. If given prior to a menstrual period, or shortly after it begins, these agents can stop prostaglandin production before it produces pain. Administration of a rapidly absorbed prostaglandin synthetase inhibitor, such as naproxen sodium, is effective for this purpose. Two tablets of 275 mg each are taken with the onset of menses, and one tablet is taken every 6–8 hr thereafter for the first 24 hr. It is rare that medication is needed beyond the first day. For the teenager with dysmenorrhea who requires contraception, oral contraceptive therapy may be indicated. It is not certain whether the beneficial effect of the contraceptives derives from their ability to inhibit ovulation and hence eliminate progesterone production from the corpus luteum or from their ability to limit endometrial proliferation and hence the production of prostaglandins.

Premenstrual Syndrome

A complex of physical signs and behavioral symptoms that occur during the second half of the menstrual cycle and that resolve with onset of menses has been called the premenstrual or "PMS" syndrome. Included are: breast fullness and tenderness; bloating; fatigue; headache; increased appetite, especially for sweets and salty foods; irritability and mood swings; depression; inability to concentrate; tearfulness; and tendencies to violence. It is estimated that one third of women in the reproductive age group have PMS, but the absence of objective findings makes this difficult to corroborate. It does not appear to be as common among adolescents as among adults, nor does it seem related to dysmenorrhea, which is much more common in the lower age group. The popular use of vitamin B_6 and progesterone supplementation has not been based on evidence of effectiveness, nor has a theoretical basis for their use been substantiated. Short-term use in adults of a gonadotropin-releasing hormone agonist has been supported by carefully controlled studies, but long-term effects and complications have not yet been evaluated, making its use in adolescents premature.

Toxic Shock Syndrome

See Sec. 11.18.

9.11 THE BREAST

As an earlier and obvious sign of puberty (Sec. 2.9 and 2.30), breast development is often the focus of attention and often a cause of anxiety, particularly when there is *asymmetry*. In most instances, a padded bra will suffice until catch-up growth occurs in the smaller breast. Rarely, asymmetry is so marked as to create self-consciousness and interfere with self-image. Under those circumstances, consideration may be given to corrective surgery. Both augmentation and reduction mammoplasty are possible, each with advantages and disadvantages. The former necessitates implantation of a foreign substance, whereas the latter may cause considerable blood loss and the possibility of later cutaneous hyposensitivity. In no case should surgery be considered prior to completion of breast growth, which coincides with achievement of SMR 5.

The most common breast disorder in adolescents is the presence of a *mass* within breast tissue. Hein found that 80% of adolescent girls discovered the mass on their own, with or without prior instruction on self-examination (Sec. 16.24). The majority of masses in adolescents are benign cysts or fibroadenomas. One biopsy series found 71% to be fibroadenomas, 11% abscesses, and 2% cystosarcoma phylloides, a low-grade malignancy.

Cysts vary in size over the course of a menstrual cycle, so that a patient should be reexamined 2 wk after the initial examination. Persistence of the mass, or its enlargement over 3 menstrual cycles is an indication for surgical consultation. Aspiration, usually attempted under local anesthesia, often results in curative drainage if the mass proves to be a cyst. If no fluid is forthcoming, an excisional biopsy is indicated. This should be done through a circumareolar incision to prevent what might otherwise be perceived as a disfiguring scar. Since carcinoma of the breast is rare in adolescence and the possible long-term sequelae of mammography serious, this procedure is not advised for this age group.

Gynecomastia (Sec. 19.33) occurs in approximately one third of normal males during early puberty and often causes concern, which may or may not be voiced. This symptom is often associated with serious misconceptions relating to masculinity or to marijuana use, which calls for factual information and reassurance that it is usually transient. Rarely is it of such magnitude or persistence as to warrant surgery.

Nipple discharge in adolescents is usually due to local stimulation, use of medications, including oral contraceptives, or pregnancy, and rarely results from pituitary or breast neoplasm or infection. Examination of the discharge assists in diagnosis, since benign conditions are associated with a milky or grumous (sticky and thick) discharge, infection with a purulent one, and intraductal papilloma or cancer with a serous, serosanguineous or bloody discharge. Elevation of the serum prolactin level may be found in the amenorrhea-galactorrhea syndromes associated with use of certain antihypertensive medications, oral contraceptives, or tranquilizers, or with pituitary neoplasms. The last possibility is evaluated with computed tomography or magnetic resonance imaging. The possibility of breast neoplasm is an indication for cytologic examination of the discharge and for surgical consultation. Infection in the non–breast feeding adolescent is rare, and in our own experience has been secondary to a human bite or diabetes mellitus. Culture of the discharge is indicated, followed by appropriate antibiotic therapy (usually directed against *Staphylococcus aureus*); surgical drainage is rarely necessary.

9.12 SKIN PROBLEMS

The skin responds as a secondary sex characteristic during puberty, reflecting increased levels of androgens by increased size and secretions of sebaceous follicles and apocrine glands. The most common manifestation of these phenomena is the production of acne. The pathogenesis, clinical picture, and management of acne is discussed in Sec. 24.31. As adolescents become preoccupied with their appearance, acne assumes greater importance to the patient than might be warranted by its medical significance. For that reason, it is appropriate to offer treatment that may enhance self-image, even to the youngster whose acne appears mild. Special considerations in the treatment of acne in this age group include the need, before instituting therapy with either tetracycline or cis-retinoic acid, to be sure that the female patient is not pregnant; that she is alerted to the possibility that chronic tetracycline therapy may cause vaginal infection with *Candida*; and that acne may be worsened or improved by oral contraceptives, depending on the type.

The skin of the adolescent is influenced not only by the hormonal concomitants of puberty but also by psychosocial factors. For example, sexual experimentation may result in a sexually transmitted disease with dermatologic manifestations (Sec. 9.9); stress may be manifested by trichotillomania; contact sports (most notably wrestling) may be associated with *Herpes simplex* infection; and drug abuse may cause skin lesions (Sec. 9.4). These examples should remind the clinician of the need for careful psychosocial assessment when evaluating a skin problem.

9.13 ORTHOPEDIC PROBLEMS

Puberty is associated with rapid growth of long bones, open epiphyses, and increased traction at sites of insertion of muscles, all of which contribute to the increased incidence and unique types of orthopedic problems of this age group. Sports participation is an added risk factor (Sec. 5.37 and 23.12–23.13), particularly when teams are configured on the basis of chronologic rather than developmental age. Conditions such as slipped capital femoral epiphysis (Sec. 23.2), Osgood-Schlatter disease (Sec. 23.3), idiopathic scoliosis (Sec. 23.5), and costochondritis of the sternoclavicular junction (Tietze syndrome, Sec. 10.86) are most common in adolescents. Osteogenic sarcoma is also common in this age group. Infection of bone and joints, although generally less common in adolescents than in younger children, but may occur as a complication of disseminated *gonococcemia* (Sec. 11.22) or as osteomyelitis in patients with sickle cell anemia (Sec. 15.18). Viral infections, such as rubella and infectious mononucleosis, are more apt to cause arthralgia in adolescents than in younger children.

9.14 DELIVERY OF HEALTH CARE TO ADOLESCENTS

In providing health care to adolescents, the physician must combine familiar elements of the "well-child" visit with others, drawn from the practice of adult medicine, which acknowledge the patient's maturation. Accordingly, prevention of physical and psychologic dysfunction is addressed through examination, education, and anticipatory guidance, as well as by immunization.

Functional status is assessed through taking an age-appropriate history and performing physical examination and laboratory testing using instruments, techniques, and standards devised for the appropriate age group. Dysfunction is addressed through age-appropriate interventions. Throughout, a balance is struck between the adolescent's need for autonomy, privacy, and confidentiality and the parents' concern and desire to be informed. Judgment is necessary also in weighing the adolescent's need to have a specific acute problem addressed against the physician's wish to utilize an episodic or rare medical contact with the teenager for the purposes of education, prevention, and screening, which are often time-consuming processes.

Legal Issues. In the United States the right of a minor to consent to treatment without parental knowledge is governed by state laws. In all states currently, the right of minors to seek and consent to treatment is granted when there is suspicion of a sexually transmitted disease. As such diseases are often asymptomatic, this provision in the various public health codes is generally interpreted as enabling the physician to perform a pelvic examination on any sexually active adolescent solely upon her consent. In many states, adolescents may consent to receive care for drug abuse or mental health problems. The minor's right to obtain contraceptives has not been reviewed by the Supreme Court, but the minor's right to privacy has been upheld (except in a recent Supreme Court decision allowing for searches in schools). Accordingly, most states permit the provision of contraceptives to teenagers upon their own consent. Recent attempts at restricting programs funded under Title X to provision of contraception only after informing parents have not been legislated, but the publicity received by the proposal has left many teenagers with the mistaken notion that their parents will be informed if they seek birth control from any physician. The right of an adolescent to obtain an abortion without parental consent or over parental objection is unsettled.

With the exception of Delaware, which has an age limit of 17 yr, all other states require that an individual be 18 yr of age or more in order to consent to blood donation. Organ donation by a consenting minor generally requires parental consent as well as a court order, to ensure that there is no alternative adult donor, that the transplant is necessary to save the life of the recipient, and that the adolescent donor will not suffer physically or psychologically as a result of the procedure.

In addition, minors are exempt from the requirement of parental consent for medical treatment under the following circumstances: (1) in the case of *emancipated minors*, those who live away from home, are no longer subject to parental control, are economically self-supporting, are married, or are members of the military; (2) in *emergencies* a minor may be treated without consent of parents if, in the physician's judgment, the delay resulting from attempts to contact them would jeopardize the life or health of the minor; and (3) on invoking the *Mature Minor Rule*. An emerging trend in law is the recognition that many minors are sufficiently mature to understand the nature of their illness and the potential risks and benefits of proposed therapy, and that they should, therefore, receive or reject such treatment upon their own consent. In these cases, the physician should document that the adolescent has acted in a responsible manner.

The growing number of cases involving charges of sexual misconduct against male physicians suggests that a chaperone should be present whenever an adolescent female patient is examined. The need for a chaperone for the interaction of a female physician with a male adolescent patient has not yet become an issue.

Screening. These tests should be done only if they are cost-effective. This determination for the adolescent patient involves knowledge of the prevalence of the target condition, as well as the cost, which must include possible psychologic and physical sequelae. Screening for trivial conditions or for those for which there is no immediate intervention should be avoided, lest their discovery deepen the early adolescent's natural tendency to feel flawed or imperfect. During late adolescence, however, it may be appropriate to perform screening tests for genetic disease carrier states in preparation for marriage. Reference standards for this age group should be available before a screening test is performed on an adolescent, in order to avoid the erroneous conclusion of pathology when none exists. Gender and stage of puberty should determine the timing and choice of screening maneuvers (Tables 9–3 and 9–4).

Laboratory Tests. During early adolescence, a screening urinalysis and urine culture are indicated for the female. The presence of polymorphonuclear leukocytes in the urinary sediment suggests the possibility of cervicitis, vaginitis, urethritis, or an asymptomatic infection of the urinary tract, the last a common finding in adolescent girls.

The frequency of iron-deficiency anemia following menarche mandates a yearly hematocrit in female adolescents. The reference standard for this test will change with progression of puberty, as estrogen suppresses erythropoietin.

Androgens cause the hematocrit to rise during male pu-

Table 9–3. Package of Care—The Well Adolescent Visit I—Early Adolescence (Tanner 1 and 2)

	Females	Males
Screening Physical	Hematocrit Urine culture screen Rubella titer (once) Tuberculin	— — —
Psychosocial	Self-image Depression Peer interaction (including sexuality) School performance Substance abuse	Self-image Depression Peer interaction (including sexuality) School performance Substance abuse
Health Promotion	Self-examination of breasts Nutrition counseling	Self-examination of scrotum Nutrition counseling
Prevention	Smoking Cycle safety Automotive passenger safety Immunization update (see Table 4–5)	Smoking Cycle safety Automotive passenger safety Immunization update (see Table 4–5)
Anticipatory Guidance	Developing independence Dealing with peer pressure Confidentiality Variations in growth and development Dating Preparation for menarche	Developing independence Dealing with peer pressure Confidentiality Variations in growth and development Dating —
Physical Examination Special attention to:	Blood pressure Height, weight Skinfold thickness — Stage of sexual development Scoliosis Goiter Acne — Tibial tubercle Gait	Blood pressure Height, weight Skinfold thickness Grip strength Stage of sexual development — — Acne Gynecomastia Tibial tubercle Gait
Symptomatic Treatment (anything revealed by the above +)	Acne Dysmenorrhea	Acne —

From Litt IF: Adolescent health care. *In* Green M, Haggerty RJ (ed): Ambulatory Pediatrics III. Philadelphia, WB Saunders, 1984.

Table 9–4. **Package of Care—The Well Adolescent Visit II—Mid–Late Adolescence (Tanner 3–5)***

	Females	Males
Screening		
Physical	Vision testing Hearing testing Genetically transmitted diseases	Vision testing Hearing testing Genetically transmitted diseases
If sexually active	Pap smear VDRL Gonorrhea culture	— VDRL Gonorrhea culture
Prevention	Automotive safety Venereal disease prevention Prevention of pregnancy	Automotive safety Venereal disease prevention Prevention of pregnancy
Anticipatory Guidance	Planning for marriage Vocational/educational planning Cults Becoming a health-care consumer	Planning for marriage Vocation/educational planning Cults Becoming a health-care consumer
Physical Examination	Breast masses — Vaginal discharge Pregnancy	Gynecomastia Testicular tumor Urethral discharge —
Treatment	Corrective surgery (after growth complete)	Corrective surgery (after growth complete)

*Incremental with items listed for Early Adolescence.
From Litt IF: Adolescent health care. *In* Green M, Haggerty RJ (ed): Ambulatory Pediatrics III. Philadelphia, WB Saunders, 1984.

berty, so that the SMR 1 male has a hematocrit averaging 39%, whereas the one who has completed puberty (SMR 5) will have an average value of 43%.

A *rubella titer* is indicated for all female adolescents, followed by immunization of those found not to have evidence of protective antibody, regardless of immunization history (Sec. 4.1). Alternatively, immunization of all female adolescents might be rationalized on the basis of its cost-efficiency, efficacy, and the low rate of complications in nonimmunocompromised patients. Accidental immunization of pregnant women with this vaccine has not been associated with production of fetal anomalies, but it is still prudent to withhold immunization until one is satisfied that the patient is not pregnant (Sec. 9.7). Tuberculin (or PPD) testing yearly is important in adolescents, as puberty has been shown to exacerbate tuberculosis in those not previously treated.

Sexually active adolescents should undergo screening for sexually transmitted diseases (STD's), regardless of symptoms. Papanicolaou smears are indicated in sexually active females, regardless of age, as various studies have detected a rate of early neoplastic changes between 5–35/1000 adolescents who have engaged in sexual intercourse. Obtaining two successive cervical scrapes increases the yield of positive smears by 26.3% over that obtained for a single cervical specimen.

When screening tests for carrier states for genetic defects are performed, age-appropriate counseling should be immediately available to ensure an opportunity to have questions answered and unspoken fears allayed.

The use of *spirometry for adolescents who smoke*, may over time serve as a deterrent if deterioration of respiratory status can be demonstrated.

Audiometry. Highly amplified music of the kind enjoyed by many adolescents is known to elevate audiometric threshold. Therefore, an audiogram should be performed yearly during adolescence, even if earlier tests have been normal.

Vision Testing. The pubertal growth spurt may extend to the optic globe, resulting in elongation and myopia in genetically predisposed individuals. Vision testing should be performed, therefore, in order to detect this problem before it affects school performance.

Blood Pressure Determination. Criteria for the diagnosis of hypertension are based on age-specific norms that reflect increases associated with pubertal maturation (Sec. 14.88). When a patient's reading is more than 2 standard deviations

higher than the mean for age, he or she is suspected of having hypertension, whatever the absolute reading. It is important that the proper technique be used (Sec. 14.1).

Most adolescents found to have elevations in blood pressure will be shown ultimately to have labile hypertension, a condition in which the search for etiology will be futile. Since about half of those with onset of labile hypertension in adolescence will have sustained hypertension as adults, they need close follow-up. Proscription of salty foods and of adding salt to diet may be useful in influencing the natural history of the condition, but compliance with such a suggestion during adolescence is unlikely. Antihypertensive medication is not indicated for labile hypertension.

If blood pressure readings below 2 standard deviations for age are found, conditions such as anorexia nervosa or Addison's disease should be considered.

Scoliosis. Approximately 5% of male and 10–14% of female adolescents have mild curvature of the spine, 2–4 times the rate in younger children. Scoliosis typically becomes manifest at or near the peak of the height/velocity curve (Sec. 2.9), at approximately 12 yr in females and 14 yr in males. Curves measuring in excess of 10 degrees should be followed by an orthopedist until growth is completed (Sec. 23.5).

Breast Examination. Examination of the female adolescent's breasts is performed in order to detect masses (Sec. 9.11), to stage progress of sexual maturation (Sec. 2.9–2.10 and 2.30), and to provide reassurance about development to the patient as well as to teach the technique of self-examination with the hope that this practice will continue into the later years of higher risk.

Scrotum Examination. The age of peak incidence of germ cell tumors of the testes is late adolescence and early adulthood. For that reason, palpation of the testes may have an immediate yield and should serve as a model for instruction of self-examination. As varicoceles often appear during puberty, such an examination provides an opportunity to explain and reassure the patient about this entity (Sec. 16.23).

Psychosocial. Some questions offer a relatively effective and economical way to open discussion with the adolescent regarding psychosocial issues. Such questions may deal with: *peer relationships* (e.g., "Do you have a best friend with whom you can share even the most personal secret?"); with *self-image* (e.g., "Is there anything you would like to change about yourself?" or "What do you consider to be your best features?"); with *depression* (e.g., "What do you see yourself doing five years from now?" or "Are you ever so sad that you think of dying?"); with *school* (e.g., "How are your grades this year compared with last?" and "How many days have you been absent from school this year compared with last?"); with *personal decisions* (e.g., "Are you feeling pressured to engage in any behavior you do not feel you are ready for?" or "Is there anything you would like to change in your relationship with your boyfriend, your father, and so on?"); or with an *eating disorder* (e.g., "Do you ever feel that food controls you rather than vice versa?"). If the responses to any of these questions suggest that problems exist, standardized tests are available for more thorough probing, or interviewing in greater depth may elucidate the problem (see Table 9–1).

Interviewing the Adolescent. (See also Sec. 2.30.) It is often difficult to establish open communication with the adolescent patient, unless a prior relationship existed with the physician. Even under that circumstance, the previously comfortable relationship may change with the advent of adolescence, as parents often find it does when their child becomes an adolescent. The teenager may now wish more privacy than that usually available in the pediatrician's office, and the pediatrician may appear judgmental to a teenager having some conflict with his or her own parents. Adolescents often imagine that through the process of physical examination the physician can detect evidence of behaviors such as smoking, drinking, masturbation, and so on.

The physician who takes time to listen, avoids judgmental statements and use of street jargon, and gives evidence of respect for the adolescent's emerging maturity will have an easier time communicating with him or her. The use of open-ended rather than closed-ended questions will further facilitate history taking (e.g., Q: "Do you get along with your father?" [leading] A: "Yes;" *versus* Q: "What would you like to change in your relationship with your father?" [open-ended] A: "I would like to stop him from always putting me down, especially in front of my friends.") Giving adolescents "the floor" so that they might express concerns and the reasons for seeking medical attention is effective as well.

After the teenager's agenda is addressed, the physician may wish to define the boundaries of the physician-patient relationship. In such a relationship, the former agrees to provide confidentiality, except if in so doing the well-being of the patient or of another person may be jeopardized, and the adolescent, in turn, agrees to act maturely and responsibly *vis à vis* medical care.

Health Enhancement. The health status of adolescents may be enhanced by the application of principles of prevention and anticipatory guidance. Prevention of infectious disease is a traditional pediatric role and for the adolescent includes immunization as well as counseling. For example, boosters of DT should be given at the age of approximately 15 yr, or 10 yr after the last booster; immunization against rubella should be given to females without evidence of protective serum titers, and mumps vaccine should be given to males who have not previously been immunized and who have not had the clinical disease. The prevention of sexually transmitted diseases (Sec. 9.9) and of pregnancy (Sec. 9.8) are important issues to be addressed in sexually active adolescents of both sexes. All of these needs challenge the clinician to develop skills in the assessment of the adolescent's health status and health needs at all levels, from molecular to social, from which health problems can be identified or anticipated.

IRIS F. LITT

Psychosocial Problems

Depression/Suicide

Beck AT, Beck R, Kovacs M: Classification of suicidal behaviors: 1. Quantifying intent and medical lethality. Am J Psychol 132:285, 1975.

Mattsson A: Adolescent depression and suicide. *In*: Friedman SB, Hoekelman RA (eds): Behavioral Pediatrics. New York, McGraw-Hill, 1980.

McAnarney ER: Suicidal behavior of children and youth. Pediatr Clin North Am 22:595, 1975.

Puig-Antich J, Rabinovich H: Major child and adolescent psychiatric disorders. *In*: Levine MD, Carey WB, Crocker AC, Gross RT (eds): Developmental-Behavioral Pediatrics. Philadelphia, WB Saunders, 1983, pp 865–890.

Substance Abuse

Jessor R, Chase JA, Donovan JE: Psychosocial correlates of marijuana use and problem drinking in a national sample of adolescents. Am J Public Health 70:604, 1980.

Jessor R, Jessor SL: Adolescence to young adulthood: A twelve-year prospective study of problem behavior and psychosocial development. *In*: Mednick S and Horway M (eds): Longitudinal Research in the United States. New York, Praeger, 1984.

Johnston LD, O'Malley PM, Bachman JG: Highlights from Drugs and American High School Students, 1975–1983. USDHHS, PHS, Alcohol, Drug Abuse and Mental Health Administration, 1984.

Kandel DB, Logan JA: Patterns of drug use from adolescence to young adulthood: 1. Periods of risk for initiation, continued use, and discontinuation. Am J Public Health 74:660, 1984.

Kolodny RC, Masters WH, Kolodner RM, et al: Depression of plasma testosterone after chronic intensive marijuana use. N Engl J Med 290:872, 1974.

Lieber CS: The metabolism of alcohol. Sci Am 234:25, 1976.

Litt IF, Cohen MI: The drug-using adolescent as a pediatric patient. J Pediatr 77:195, 1970.

Disorders of Sleep

Anders TF, Keener MA: Sleep-wake state development and disorders of sleep in infants, children, and adolescents. *In*: Levine MD, Carey WB, Crocker AC, Gross RT (eds): Developmental-Behavioral Pediatrics. Philadelphia, WB Saunders, 1983.

Anorexia Nervosa

Bruch H: The Golden Cage: The Enigma of Anorexia Nervosa. Cambridge, Harvard University Press, 1978.

Steiner H: Anorexia nervosa. Pediatr Rev 4:123, 1982.

Problems Related to Adolescent Sexuality

Breast

Hein K, Dell R, Cohen MI: Self-detection of a breast mass in adolescent females. J Adol Health Care 3:15, 1982.

Pregnancy and Contraception

Alan Guttmacher Institute: Teenage Pregnancy: The Problem That Hasn't Gone Away. New York, Alan Guttmacher Institute, 1981.

Hatcher RA, Stewart GK, Stewart F, et al: Contraceptive Technology, 1983–1984. 13th ed. New York, Irvington Publishers, 1983.

Sorensen RC: Adolescent Sexuality in Contemporary America. New York, World, 1973.

Menstrual Problems

Emans SJH, Goldstein DP: Pediatric and Adolescent Gynecology. Boston, Little, Brown, 1977.

Litt IF: Menstrual problems during adolescence. Pediatr Rev 4:203, 1983.

Litt IF: Toxic shock syndrome—An adolescent disease. J Adolesc Health Care 4:270, 1983.

Delivery of Health Care to Adolescents

Holder AR: Legal Issues in Pediatrics and Adolescent Medicine. New York, John Wiley & Sons, 1977.

Litt IF: Adolescent health care. *In*: Green M, Haggerty RJ (eds): Ambulatory Pediatrics III. Philadelphia, WB Saunders, 1984.

10

IMMUNITY, ALLERGY, AND RELATED DISEASES

10.1 THE IMMUNOLOGIC SYSTEM

The immunologic system is the segment of host defenses that includes macrophages, leukocytes, lymphocytes, and the complement system. Together with physical barriers, such as an intact integument and motile cilia, its primary function is to protect against invasion by infectious agents. The major costs of this protection are allergy, autoimmunity, and rejection of organ transplants.

PHYSIOLOGY

Source of Cells. The hematopoietic and lymphoid systems develop from multipotential precursors. In early intrauterine life the fetal liver serves as the repository for lymphoid precursor cells. The bone marrow is populated later, and in extrauterine life serves as the major source of the precursor cells.

Differentiation. Lymphoid stem cells differentiate into two major lines: the T cells and the B cells, which have different functions in their protective roles (Table 10–1). T cells are so named because of their intimate association with the thymus gland, which is their site of differentiation, and B cells because of their relationship to the bursa of Fabricius in chickens and the bone marrow in humans. There is evidence that the fetal

Table 10–1. **Functions of T and B Cells**

Role of T Cells
- T helper function
- T suppressor function
- T killer function
  - Containment of acidfast bacteria
  - Containment of certain viral infections after establishment (rubeola, varicella, herpes, cytomegalovirus, Epstein-Barr virus, "slow" viruses)
  - Containment of fungal infections (especially *Candida*)
  - Containment of protozoan infections
  - Rejection of allografts (and possibly tumors)
  - Graft versus host disease (GVHD)
  - Contact dermatitis

Role of B Cells
- Synthesize and secrete major classes of immunoglobulin, which:
  - Protect against staphylococcus, streptococcus, hemophilus, pneumococcus reinfection (or infection in immunized persons)
- Neutralize viruses to prevent initial infection
- Act as barriers along gastrointestinal and respiratory passages
- Initiate killing of microorganisms by macrophages and null cells
- Cause the secretion of vasoactive amines from mast cells and basophils
- Actively lyse cells of autologous origin or engage in antigen-antibody complex disease
- Interfere with T killer cell activity by directly or indirectly blocking the reaction

Adapted from Horowitz SD, Hong R: The Pathogenesis and Treatment of Immunodeficiency. Basel, S. Karger, AG, 1977.

liver assumes the bursal function in humans. The individual cell lines mature and acquire capabilities of subspecialization within the two major sites. It is thought that most of the steps involved in the *early differentiation* of B cells are independent of antigenic stimulation and reflect an intrinsic capability of the cells to acquire a certain degree of maturation, at which time the cells are ready to react with antigen. Appropriate interaction with antigens leads to a number of steps that are collectively referred to as *terminal differentiation* and that lead to the immune state.

Terminal differentiation is probably highly dependent upon divalent cations and cyclic nucleotides. Antigen binding to surface receptors of the lymphocytes probably affects intracellular ratios of cyclic guanosine monophosphate (cCMP) to cyclic adenosine monophosphate (cAMP). Depending upon the degree of perturbation of its surface (e.g., by antigen), a lymphocyte may be triggered to further proliferate or, in some cases, to be placed in a resting or nonreactive state (e.g., to yield memory or tolerance). Receipt of antigen on the surface of lymphocytes can also effect the influx of calcium ions. This induces the series of events that constitute terminal differentiation, which probably takes place in peripheral lymphoid organs such as the lymph node, spleen, and organized lymphoid tissues of the gastrointestinal tract.

Cellular interactions and proliferative and differentiative events are enhanced and perhaps wholly dependent upon factors released by lymphocytes and macrophages. In some cases, these factors (interleukins, growth or differentiation factors, and some of the interferons) are being produced by recombinant DNA techniques. Certain deficiency states may be ascribed to lack of one or more of these factors. Clinical use of these agents to augment immunity has begun.

Hormones produced by the thymus gland are important in the terminal differentiation of T cells and probably in promoting normal maturation and proliferation of thymus cells. In some cases the effects of thymectomy can be reversed by the injection of these hormonal substances. Both thymosin fraction V, a crude extract obtained from calf thymus, and synthetic polypeptides have been used. A synthetic substance termed facteur thymique serique (FTS) by French workers has raised IgA and IgE levels to normal in patients with ataxia-telangiectasia. A fraction termed alpha 7 is reported to give encouraging results in patients with lung cancer. As more purified fractions become available and their precise roles become better defined, widespread use of thymic hormones may result in clinical benefits.

Traffic. Since the events of the immune process, from differentiation to the receipt of antigen and elaboration of immune products, take place in different areas of the body, the lymphocytes must be quite motile. They circulate freely through the major lymphoid channels, the thoracic duct, and the vascular tree, but their movement into and from the lymphoid organs is highly controlled. For example, cells that leave the thymic parenchyma apparently do not re-enter this

Table 10–2. **Levels of Immunoglobulins**

	IgG (mg/dL)	IgM (mg/dL)	IgA (mg/dL)	IgE (IU/mL)
Serum				
Newborn	1031 ± 200*	11 ± 5	2 ± 3	0–7.5
6 mo	427 ± 186	43 ± 17	28 ± 18	—
12 mo	661 ± 219	54 ± 23	37 ± 18	—
24 mo	762 ± 209	58 ± 23	50 ± 24	137 ± 147
8 yr	923 ± 256	65 ± 25	124 ± 45	251 ± 167
16 yr	946 ± 124	59 ± 20	148 ± 63	330 ± 212
Adult	1158 ± 305	99 ± 27	200 ± 61	200†
Secretions				
Colostrum	10	61	1234	—
Stimulated parotid saliva	0.036	0.043	3.9	—
Unstimulated whole saliva	4.86	0.55	30.4	—
Jejunal fluid	34	70	—	—
Seminal fluid	510	90	116	—
Cerebrospinal fluid				
Normal	3 ± 1	0	0.4 ± 0.5	—
Purulent infection	9	4	4	—
Viral infection	4	0.5	1	—

*Mean ± 1 standard deviation.
†Values up to 800 IU/mL are normal.
Adapted from Clin Immunobiol 3:13, 1976.

site of primary differentiation. The traffic pattern appears to be controlled by chemical groupings on the surface of the lymphocytes. Removal of surface carbohydrate or protein moieties alters the traffic pattern.

Ontogeny. The newborn is immunologically quite competent. Fetal studies have shown various types of T cell function beginning as early as 7.5 wk of intrauterine life. By 8–9 wk lymphoid infiltration into the thymus begins; at 12 wk the thymus resembles the mature organ. Even premature infants can reject skin grafts.

Circulating B cells have been detected as early as 13 wk after conception; secretory capability is probably present for all major classes of immunoglobulins by the 20th wk. Extensive synthesis and secretion of antibody do not occur, owing to the relatively sheltered antigenic environment of the fetus. IgM antibodies are first to develop; increased levels of IgM can, therefore, be taken as evidence of intrauterine infection. Serum IgM usually rises to adult levels by 1 yr of age, IgG by about 4 yr, and IgA in adolescence (Table 10–2).

Cellular Events. The production of immune cell lines following exposure to antigens requires cellular interaction involving both T and B cells and macrophages. Physical contact between at least 2 of these cell types is probably necessary. Receptor molecules on the surfaces of the T and B cells are able to recognize antigens. The B cell receptor is classic antibody, but the nature of that on the T cell is uncertain. Macrophages can adsorb antibody molecules onto their surfaces. Simply put, antigen can be thought of as a ligand which binds 2 or more cells together. Following interaction initiated by this event, the cells are rendered immune and can then exert their protective action upon re-exposure to the antigen. The details of developing immunity are much more complex and appear to involve the activation of other groups, such as histocompatibility antigens and complement receptor molecules, which are also present on cell surfaces.

Transplantation (histocompatibility) antigens play important roles in the development of normal immune responses. It appears that their biologic role is to define the initial cellular interactions that control the ultimate immune response. Soluble antigens do not immediately stimulate the T cells; they must first be ingested and processed by macrophages and other antigen-processing cells. The antigens are subsequently re-expressed on the cell surface, but in close association with

(or perhaps even physically modified as a part of) one of the transplantation antigens. The T cell becomes sensitized to this transplantation foreign antigen complex and will give an immune reaction only when it sees both together again in the future. It is not sensitized to either alone. In this way, transplantation antigens serve as important modulators of the immune response, promoting certain cellular reactions and forbidding others. An immunodeficiency disease is associated with absence of surface transplantation antigens (bare lymphocyte syndrome).

It is thus clear that the cell lines involved in the immune response carry molecules on their surfaces which control their behavior. The ability to detect some of these has provided a system of markers, which serve to differentiate T from B cells. The functional significance of some of the surface moieties is known; the importance of others, unknown. Through the use of specific antibodies produced by hybridomas, extensive typing of mononuclear cells is now available. These reagents make possible rapid quantitation of lymphocyte subsets. Characterization of lymphoid tumors in terms of these subsets is now being carried out, since it is thought that surface markers of tumor cells represent normal differentiation antigens and that lymphomas or leukemias can be considered malignant expansions of lymphocytes arrested at certain stages of normal development. This classification is useful in determining prognosis and provides guides for therapy (Table 10–3).

The events triggered within T cells by surface reactions are not fully understood. The events involved in the synthesis and secretion of immunoglobulins by B cells are schematically pictured in Figure 10–1. Basically, receipt of the appropriate signals on the surface of a B cell creates an internal signal that sets into motion the machinery which synthesizes immunoglobulin. After the assembly of the full immunoglobulin molecule, including the chains necessary for polymerization and carbohydrate groups that may be necessary to control traffic, the molecule is secreted into the lymph and thence enters the blood stream so it may bathe the areas of need and combine with the appropriate antigen.

Amplification. This term describes the augmentation, by various collaborative processes, of the protective effect of antigen-binding by B and T lymphocytes. Amplification is necessary for complete elimination of infectious agents. Com-

Table 10–3. **Mononuclear Cell Markers**

Cell Lineage	Marker*	Comment
B cell		
Stem cell		
Pre-B cell	Cytoplasmic IgM	
Mature B cell	Surface IgM, D, A, E, G	Denotes synthetic capacity
	B1, BA-1, B4	Early and mature B cells; leukemias
	BA-2	Mostly leukemic cells; few peripheral cells
	Epstein-Barr virus	Receptor for infectivity
	Fc receptors (for various Ig's)	Involved in regulation of Ig levels
	Complement receptors	
	DR	Also on activated T cells and macrophages
	CD10 (CALLA, J5, BA-3)	Most non T, non B leukemias now shown to be of B cell origin
T cell		
Thymocyte	CD1 (T6)	Specific for cortical thymocytes; not normally in blood
Mature	CD2 (T11)	Cells bear sheep erythrocyte receptor; most T cell malignancies
	CD3 (T3)	All mature T cells; most T cell chronic leukemias
	CD4 (T4, Leu 3a)	Inducer T cell subset; most chronic T cell leukemias
	CD8 (T8, Leu 2a)	Cytotoxic/suppressor T cell subset; few T cell leukemias
	Fc receptors†	Involved in regulation of Ig levels
	Leu 11	Natural killer cells (probably a T cell subset); also on neutrophils
Macrophage‡		
	CD9 (BA-2)	Present on most non T, non B leukemias
	CD11	Also on granulocytes; some acute myelogenous leukemias
	CDw14 (MY4)*	Exclusive for monocytes; some acute myelogenous leukemias
	Mac 120 (Leu M2)	Most monocytes; important in antigen presentation
	Leu M1	Nearly all granulocytes as well; stains Reed-Sternberg cells

*MY, B, BA, Leu: designations of commercially available hybridoma antiserum.

†Cells showing receptors for Fc of IgM (T mu cells) and IgG (T gamma cells), formerly thought to be helper and suppressor cells, respectively. Recent studies do not confirm these earlier impressions.

‡Macrophages commonly adsorb Igs on their surface so the presence of certain markers does not necessarily reflect macrophage synthesis of that product.

mon modes of amplification include processes that lyse infectious agents or produce a granulomatous response. Amplification of the protective function of B cells is accomplished chiefly by activation of the complement system, that of the T cells chiefly by lymphokines, though both B and T cells secrete lymphokines. It is doubtful that complement amplifies the protective function of T cells to any significant degree.

Lymphokines may have direct toxic effects (Table 10–4) or act indirectly as in the case of migration inhibitory factor (MIF), one of the best studied of the lymphokines. MIF attracts

macrophages to an area where T cells have combined with an antigen; the macrophages then destroy the infectious agent through the release of lysosomal enzymes. They also release products that may lead to the formation of granulomas and may store or carry antibody. Primary quantitative or qualitative deficiencies in macrophages, though poorly defined at present, may conceivably impair host defenses.

The biologic effects of one of the lymphokines, interleukin 1 (IL-1), have been extensively studied. IL-1 is also known as endogenous pyrogen, leukocytic endogenous mediator, lymphocyte activating factor, and mononuclear cell factor. It is unclear whether it is a single factor or a series of related factors. It is produced primarily from phagocytic cells and is responsible for many laboratory and clinical features of acute phase reactions, such as the fever and myalgias associated with many aggressive immunologic disorders.

The effect of IL-1 upon the immune response is largely due to its stimulation of T cells to secrete interleukin 2 (also known as T cell growth factor), which supports growth of effector T cell populations. In this way, massive mobilization of T cells is brought about.

T Cell Subpopulations. The versatility of the immune system depends on the actions of subpopulations of the T and B cells. The major T cell subgroups currently defined are helper, suppressor, and killer cells. *Helper cells* are necessary in the initial responses to antigen, especially to generate IgG and IgA; some IgM antibodies are formed in the absence of T helper cells. The immune response, because of its potential for harm as well as good, must be modulated to prevent hyperimmune reactions. It is thought that T *suppressor cells* serve a homeostatic role in keeping the immune response within a tolerable level. T *killer cells* are the effector cells of the thymus-dependent system. They combine with antigen to initiate the cytotoxic mechanisms that kill invading organisms.

T cells and their products are primarily concerned with acidfast bacteria, certain viral infections (e.g., rubeola, varicella, herpes, cytomegalovirus), and fungi. T cells are also the major immune factor involved in rejection of organ transplants and are responsible for the graft-versus-host reaction (Sec. 10–21). The major immunopathologic mechanism in contact dermatitis is thought to be mediated by the T cell.

B Cell Subpopulations. Subspecialization of B cells has not been as well defined as for T cells, but surface marker analysis (Table 10–3) suggests that subpopulations also exist for B cells. The B cell products (immunoglobulins) are divided into 5 major classes (isotypes), each of which is produced by a different cell line. Immunoglobulins are active against staphylococci, streptococci, *H. influenzae,* and pneumococci and are important in the initial prevention of such viral infections as rubeola, varicella, and hepatitis. They can do little, however, to control an established viral disease.

Table 10–4. **Lymphokines**

B cell growth and differentiation factors
Chemotactic factor (for eosinophils, monocytes, neutrophils)
Clonal inhibitory factor
Gamma interferon
Interleukin 1 (IL-1)
Interleukin 2 (IL-2, T cell growth factor)
Lymph node permeability factor
Macrophage activation factor
Macrophage aggregation factor
Migration inhibition factors (for leukocytes and macrophages)
Mitogenic factor
Skin-reactive factor
Suppressor factors
T cell-replacing factor
Transfer factor

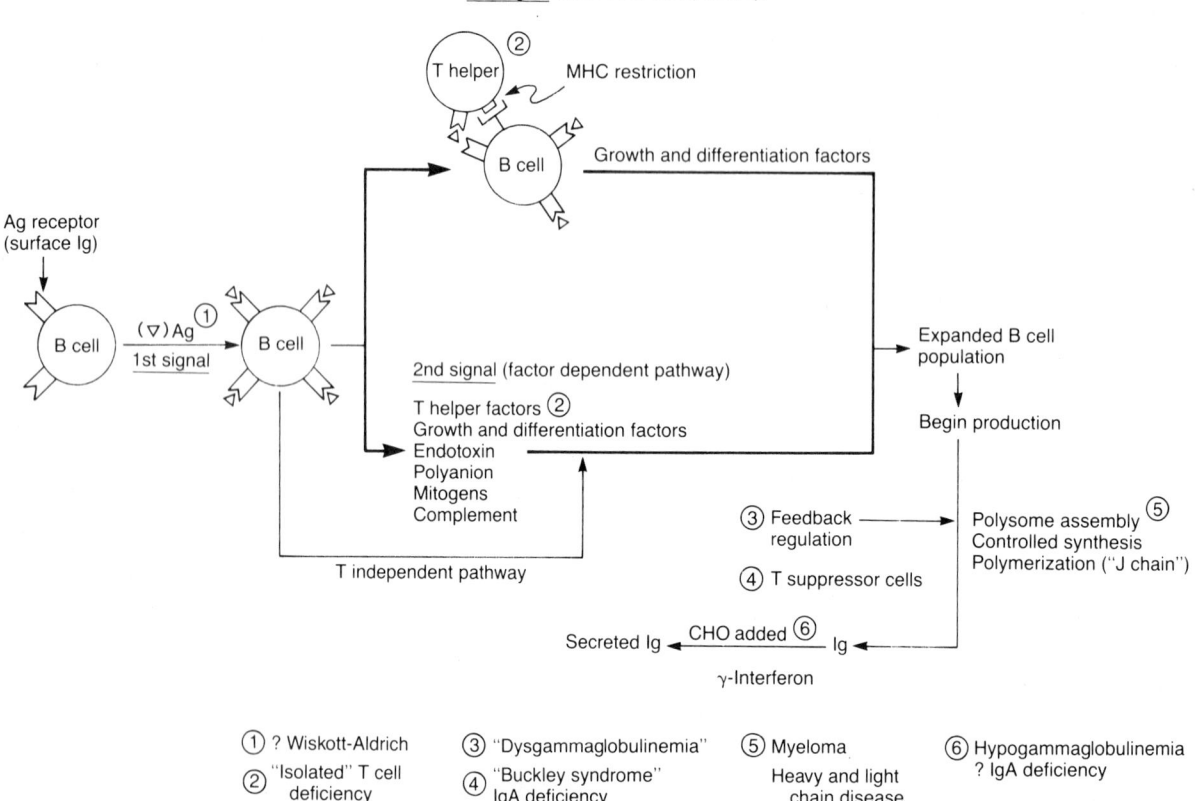

Figure 10–1. Mechanism of activation of synthesis and secretion of immunoglobulins. The numbers indicate points where a fault could result in clinical disease. Proposed disease correlates are shown at the bottom of the figure (see text).

Typical immediate hypersensitivity reactions such as hay fever and asthma are mediated by B cells, as are antigen-antibody complex disease and such disorders as autoimmune hemolytic anemia.

The 5 major classes of immunoglobulins (Igs) are IgM, IgG, IgA, IgD, and IgE. Their chemical characteristics and biologic functions are summarized in Table 10–5.

IgM can be considered the first line of defense. It is the Ig first formed in response to antigen, is found most commonly in the vascular space, and has high efficiency in the functions that enhance immunity, such as complement fixation, agglutination, and opsonic activity. IgG has a long half-life and can cross the placenta, features supporting passive immunization and recall immunity. IgA protects mainly secretory surfaces (gastrointestinal tract and eyes) where exposures to antigens are nonvascular and conditions such as acid secretion, presence of proteolytic enzyme, and intestinal motility may impair antibody activity. IgE effects the release of pharmacologically active agents from mast cells that cause asthma, hay fever, and anaphylaxis. The role of IgD is not fully known. It is primarily a lymphocyte receptor; the amounts detected in the serum probably represent effete receptors shed from young lymphocytes. The unique structural characteristics of IgD may promote cross-linking of receptors on cell surfaces, with potent modulation of cellular responses.

Secretory IgA and IgE play a major role in the immune status of inhabitants of underdeveloped countries, where antibiotic therapy, nutrition, and general hygiene are less than optimal. Since breast feeding is a major means of providing long-lasting protection in these countries, weaning is followed by increased death rates from infection. In addition to secretory IgA, breast milk delivers macrophages and perhaps T cells to the infant. IgE is a major factor in the elimination of parasites. Macrophages armed with IgE antiparasite immune complexes are especially effective in eliminating parasitic infestation. These two defenses have become

Table 10–5. **Properties of Immunoglobulins**

| | | IgA | | | | |
	IgG	Serum	Secretory	IgM	IgD	IgE
Molecular weight	140,000	160,000	370,000	900,000	160,000	197,000
Complement fixation	+	−	?	+	−	−
Placental passage	+	−	−	−	−	−
Secreted by mucous surfaces	±*	±*	+	±†	?	±
Fixes to homologous skin and mast cells	−	−	−	−	−	+
"Blocking antibody"	+	?	+	?	?	?
Polymer formation	−	+	+	+	−	−

*In inflammatory conditions. + = positive; ± = weak or intermittent; − = negative.
†Frequently in selective IgA deficiency.
From Hong R: Immunobiol 1:29, 1972.

less critical in developed countries, where persons with no detectable secretory IgA or IgE can sometimes enjoy normal health.

The immunoglobulins are structurally modified for these subspecialized activities. All show the same chemical structure of two heavy and two light polypeptide chains. The combining site on the antibody, where antigen combines with the antibody molecule, is formed by both chains and found in a portion of the molecule known as the *Fab fragment*. Two identical Fab fragments are found in each monomeric molecule of immunoglobulin. A 3rd fragment (Fc) is composed of two portions of heavy chain and contains the structures that determine the biologic characteristics of the immunoglobulin (complement fixation, placental passage, and so on) and the unique determinants that differentiate one Ig from another. For example, the Fab fragments of IgG and IgA are virtually identical, but the Fc portions are quite dissimilar.

IgM and secretory IgA are polymers. The polymerization is probably initiated intracellularly by a short polypeptide chain known as the *J chain*. The IgA found in secretions (gastrointestinal, genitourinary, biliary, tears, saliva) has, in addition, a fragment known as *secretory component* (SC). IgA exists in a monomeric form in serum and in dimeric form in secretions.

Each isotype includes subgroups. Four are known for IgG (IgG$_1$, IgG$_2$, IgG$_3$, IgG$_4$) and two for IgA (IgA$_1$, IgA$_2$). Other isotypic subgroups are less well defined. Different subgroups respond preferentially to various antigens (e.g., IgG$_2$ to polysaccharides, IgG$_1$ and IgG$_3$ to Rh antigens). IgG$_4$ cannot fix complement. Most secretory IgA is of the IgA$_2$ subgroup. The subgroups provide fine tuning of the immune response. In some patients, absence of one or more subgroups leads to clinical states somewhat different from classic panhypogammaglobulinemia.

Macrophages. Macrophages, once regarded as scavenger cells without much specificity of function, have been found to play an important role in the acquisition of immunity and tolerance and serve a key role in the effector mechanisms of T cells. Disorders of macrophages and phagocytes are considered in Sec. 10.30 to 10.40.

ASSESSMENT OF T AND B CELLS

10.2 T CELLS

A preliminary assessment of T cell function can be made from the peripheral blood lymphocyte count, lateral roentgenogram of the chest, and skin tests for delayed hypersensitivity. More definitive studies require laboratories where T cell surface markers are identified, lymphocytes are stimulated in vitro, and morphologic studies of the thymus and other lymphoid tissues can be performed. It is noteworthy that ordinary viral infections can markedly influence tests of T cell function. Repeated tests are necessary to confirm significant deficiencies of the T cell system.

Normally blood contains more than 1500 lymphocytes/mm³; each is less than 10 μ in diameter. In some T cell deficiencies, the number of lymphocytes may be normal or even elevated, and the lymphocytes are large (>10 μ in diameter) and have a loose chromatin network in the nucleus and a much greater amount of pale bluestaining cytoplasm. Monocytosis, eosinophilia, and neutropenia are commonly associated with T cell deficiency. In a patient who has not been stressed, the roentgenographic absence of a thymus suggests thymic deficiency, but this is often difficult to assess.

Positive delayed skin reactions (e.g., to tuberculin or *Candida*) help to establish the presence of normal T cell function if they are not the result of nonspecific irritation at the test site. Negative skin tests are inconclusive evidence for deficient T cell function, particularly in younger children with limited antigenic experience.

More specialized tests attempt to measure the capabilities of T cell subpopulations and can differentiate between deficiencies at various levels of T cell development or between different phases of the immune response, e.g., at the stage of recognition of antigen (affector defect) or at the stage of killer cell function (effector function). Patients may lack only some of the T cell capabilities. Performance and interpretation of T cell evaluation requires skill, patience, and experience. A list of T cell tests and their interpretation is given in Table 10-6. No single test serves as an appropriate general screening test of the integrity of T cells.

The number of T cells in blood can be counted through use of monoclonal antibodies. Sera specific for the major subsets of human mononuclear cells have been developed (see Table 10-3), and quantitative measurement of the various types is possible. These measurements generally provide the clinician with the same sort of information derived from quantitative measurements of immunoglobulin. Total absence of any particular subset indicates a marked deficiency; in most cases, however, there is simply a lower than normal number, the full significance of which requires further analysis.

A measurement of overrated significance is the ratio of helper to suppressor cells (T4/T8 ratio). In the acquired immunodeficiency syndrome (AIDS), a major feature of advancing disease is a loss of nearly all T4 cells. Inversion of this ratio (normally >1.0) is characteristic of patients with AIDS as they move into the terminal phases of disease. A reversed T4/T8 ratio is not, however, a priori diagnostic of AIDS, nor is it an absolute sign of serious T cell deficiency. A reversal of ratio may be due to increases of T8 cells, to problems in handling of the specimen, or to mild intercurrent infections. In infants with AIDS, the T4/T8 ratio is not always depressed.

Further assessment of T cell funtion is accomplished by observation of in vitro responses. The three major types of responses displayed by T cells are proliferation, cytotoxicity, and immunoregulatory. The latter two can be correlated with in vivo events, but the first bears little, if any, relation to the functions of the T cell in vivo. Substances used for study of proliferation include mitogens (usually plant substances which stimulate T cells to divide), allogeneic cells (cells from unrelated persons), and antigens. Proliferative responses to mitogens merely prove that a responsive population is present, but since the biologic function of that population is not

Table 10–6. Tests of T Cells

Test	Significance
Mitogen stimulation	Undefined T cells proliferate (concanavalin A preferentially stimulates T suppressor cells)
Allogeneic stimulation	T cells can recognize transplantation antigens Of value in predicting acceptance of bone marrow transplant and severity of GVHD
Antigen stimulation	Best correlate of in vivo T cell ability to provide protection from infection
Cell-mediated lympholysis	In vitro correlate of ability to control viral infections and transplant rejection capability
Co-culture with B cells & pokeweed mitogen	Helper and suppressor functions of Ig synthesis and secretion
Lymphokine assays	Effector amplification
Thymopoietin, thymosin, FTS (facteur thymique serique)	Hormonal activity

well delineated, this information provides little more than the monoclonal surface marker. Patients with profound immunodeficiency who will die of overwhelming infection may show good proliferative responses to phytohemagglutinin or to allogeneic cells. Of the proliferative responses, those to specific antigens are the best predictors of the ability to resist infection. Cytotoxic assays show the ability of the lymphocytes to kill a defined target, usually after a period of stimulation by the target in vitro (i.e., a sensitization phase). Since this process simulates fairly closely what occurs in vivo, these assays are useful in defining T cell capability. Finally, T cells can be added to mixtures of other cells engaging in an in vitro immune response. The ability of added cells to support the test is taken as an indicator of helper activity, and their ability to decrease the response as a measure of suppressor activity.

The stimulation of lymphocytes by certain substances such as concanavalin A generates a large number of T cells capable of inhibiting other T cell responses. For example, supernatants of such stimulated cultures (or the stimulated cells themselves) will inhibit a mixed leukocyte culture reaction or the synthesis of immunoglobulin by B cells. Concanavalin A-stimulated cells serve as a suppressor T cell assay.

Isolated T cells can be added to purified B cell preparations, after which T-dependent proliferative processes or the synthesis of immunoglobulin is used as a T helper cell assay.

The ability of T lymphocytes to secrete lymphokines can also be assessed, but the tests are difficult to perform and require reagents that are not widely available. Interpretation of the results of T cell tests and the assessment of T cell function are primarily functions of research laboratories.

Morphology. The normal *thymus* consists of lobules with a rich zone of thymocytes at the outer border and a less intensely staining zone containing many epithelial elements in the center. These two areas are easily separated from each other at a corticomedullary cleavage plane. Within the medulla are whorl-like bodies known as *Hassall corpuscles*. Absence of one or more of these features is found in various abnormalities of the T cell system. In the *profound defects*, there are virtually no normal areas; the gland consists only of reticular cells in a loose structure with broad fibrous bands. Hassall corpuscles and lymphoid elements (thymocytes) are conspicuously absent. The gland is very small, about 2–3% of normal size; often it does not descend into the mediastinum but remains high in the neck. In *less severe deficiency*, the thymus may appear to be involuted with a few remnants of normal structure. Some thymic abnormalities involve only mass (hypoplasia or aplasia), sometimes with a small gland of perfectly normal architecture.

In *lymph nodes*, the zone of lymphocytes situated just below the layer of follicles and germinal centers at the periphery is populated by T cells. This area is poorly developed and cell-depleted in isolated deficiency of the T cell system. In addition, although B cell follicles may sometimes be seen, formation of germinal centers does not occur. In the *spleen*, a collar of T lymphocytes surrounds the arterioles; absence of lymphocytes in this area is consistent with thymic deficiency.

10.3 B CELLS

B cells as well as T cells can be enumerated in blood. The most commonly employed markers are the IgM molecules present on the surface of B lymphocytes. Approximately 10% of mononuclear cells in the blood carry these markers and also IgD. Other immunoglobulin classes are represented rarely, if at all. Other markers of B cells are listed in Table 10–3; their physiologic significance is as yet unknown.

The most commonly employed test of B cell function is quantitative measurement of serum immunoglobulin levels. A common error in using the single radial diffusion method is overinterpretation of slightly low values. Normal values for immunoglobulins vary greatly (several fold) and increase over a period of several years from low values in infancy until adult levels are attained. Normal values also vary from laboratory to laboratory; it has been suggested that immunoglobulin levels be expressed in international units after comparing one's local values to an international reference standard.* The laboratory diagnosis of immunodeficiency states requires stringent standards for the diagnosis of deficiency and correlation with the clinical picture.

Most states of true B cell immunodeficiency in children show IgG values under 200 mg/dL, and IgA and IgM are undetectable. An unusual form of B cell deficiency is associated with higher than normal levels of IgM (dysgammaglobulinemia). These high values are in part artifactual due to the more rapid diffusion of some of the IgM that is present as a low molecular weight monomer (rather than as the normal heavier polymer); rapid diffusion causes a large precipitin ring to develop, suggesting a higher than actual level of IgM.

Extremely high or at least normal values of one or more of the immunoglobulins are seen also in unusual forms of combined T and B cell deficiency. In these cases, the immunoglobulins classically show restricted electrophoretic mobility resembling that of myeloma proteins. Affected patients are usually immunologically inert; no specific antibodies can be detected either before or after antigenic stimulation. In cases of IgG subgroup deficiency, the total IgG levels are within normal limits, but individual subgroups are absent.

The pattern of various immunoglobulin levels in serum is diagnostically uninformative, but some hints of the underlying or associated process can occasionally be found. Markedly elevated levels of IgA are often seen with thymic deficiency. Low levels of IgG and IgA in association with near-normal IgM values, as opposed to the immunoglobulin levels typical of hypogammaglobulinemia (e.g., IgG = 150 mg/dL, IgA = 0 mg/dL, IgM = 5 mg/dL), should suggest intestinal loss of protein. In such cases the levels of albumin and transferrin will also show marked diminution. Similar changes are also seen in the hypoproteinemic states of nephrosis and in cases of lymphangiectasia.

In selective deficiency of IgA, tests utilizing radial immunodiffusion present a special problem. Because of increased permeability of the gastrointestinal tract secondary to the deficiency of IgA, more dietary antigens are absorbed. As a result, higher levels of antibodies are formed to foodstuffs, especially to milk proteins. Precipitating antibodies to bovine proteins cross-react with many antisera (e.g., goat) used as anti-immunoglobulin reagents. As a result, in the diffusion analysis a band interpreted as goat antihuman IgA precipitating with serum IgA is actually human antibovine IgG precipitating goat IgG in cross-reaction. The interpretation would be that the patient has detectable levels of IgA when, in fact, he or she has none. The error can be avoided by the use of rabbit antisera to human IgA for quantitation or by testing the patient's serum in immunoelectrophoretic analysis in which no arc will be seen in the IgA region.

Ambiguous values of immunoglobulins require evaluation of immunoglobulin function for full interpretation. This is accomplished by measuring antibody response to specific antigens. One can use antigens to which the patient was exposed naturally (blood group substances, common bacteria) or as a result of immunization procedures (tetanus, diphtheria), or antigens purposefully injected to measure the response. Of the latter, bacteriophage φχ 174† is probably most

---

*The standard is available from NCI Immunoglobulin Reference Center, 6715 Electronic Dr., Springfield, VA 22151. The conversion units are as follows (μg/IU): IgG, 80.4; IgA, 14.2; IgM, 8.47.

†Assessment is available by arrangement with R. J. Wedgwood, M. D., Department of Pediatrics, University of Washington School of Medicine, Seattle, WA 98195.

informative; in cases of suspected B cell deficiency, the diagnosis can be made even at birth because normally even newborns will eliminate the phage by immune clearance. The transferred IgG levels of the mother offer no problem in interpretation, as they might if only quanitative levels were measured. Furthermore, there are different patterns of response which serve to define more precisely the nature of the B cell defect. *It is to be emphasized that live viruses other than φχ 174 should never be given to a patient suspected of immunodeficiency until the immune system is known to be normal, as severe disease or death may ensue.*

B lymphocytes stimulated with pokeweed mitogen and cultured in the presence of normal T cells will synthesize and secrete immunoglobulin. B cells that bear immunoglobulin on the surface (SIg cell) are in the early presecretory stage; the surface molecules are lost after the cell responds to the antigen and undergoes terminal differentiation enabling it to secrete the specific antibody. A study of the lymphocyte surface markers and the response to pokeweed mitogen can define the level at which the defect occurs in many cases. For example, SIg cells are usually absent in X-linked agammaglobulinemia but present in normal numbers in late onset common variable immunodeficiency. In the latter, pokeweed mitogen will not induce further differentiation. X-linked agammaglobulinemia can be thought of as an early defect due to lack of B cells; common variable immunodeficiency can be thought of as a failure of B cells to undergo terminal differentiation.

In some patients with common variable immunodeficiency, excessive T suppressor cell activity is found. Their T cells, incubated with normals, will completely prevent induction by pokeweed mitogen of synthesis and secretion of IgG, IgA, and IgM. In other patients deficiency of T helper cells is found. Thus, complete evaluation of B cells requires assessment of modulating influences as well as of the capability of the patient's lymphocytes to synthesize immunoglobulins.

Morphology. The thymus can be assumed to be normal in classic "pure" B cell deficiency disorders, of which congenital hypogammaglobulinemias of the X-linked or autosomal recessive types are prime examples. The thymus is abnormal in cases associated with paraprotein-like immunoglobulins. The lymph nodes show deficient or absent follicle formation, and germinal centers are absent in cases of deficient production of immunoglobulins. In selective deficiency of IgA there may be a compensatory increase of IgM-producing cells in the lamina propria of the intestine.

DISEASES DUE TO IMMUNOLOGIC DEFICIENCY

10.4 PRIMARY IMMUNODEFICIENCY

It is convenient to think of diseases as primarily involving the T cell or B cell systems, or both. In each case the clinical presentation and treatment are different. Generally, disorders of the T cell system are associated with a much graver prognosis than are those of the B cell system. Combined immunodeficiency involving both T and B cells carries the worst prognosis; if of the severe variety, death in the first 2 yr of life is the rule. Some patients with pure B cell disorders remain clinically well without any therapy.

Clinical differentiation between primary T or B cell deficiency cannot be made with certainty, but certain clinical features suggestive of involvement of particular systems are listed in Table 10–7.

Unusual response to usually benign infectious agents, or infection with unusual organisms, is a feature of immunodeficiency; this may occur in isolated T or B cell diseases or in combined disorders. The major organisms involved in immunodeficient patients are *Pneumocystis carinii*, cytomegalovirus, rubeola, and varicella; each often results in fatal pneumonia. Pneumonitis caused by any of these agents should suggest immunodeficiency.

There is an increased incidence of malignancy among patients with immunodeficiency. Explanations for this include increased susceptibility to infection by an oncogenic virus, the cancer as another expression of the basic genetic fault, and a failure of immune surveillance. The last explanation is based on the theory that T cells eliminate newly formed populations of malignant cells as they arise, considering them foreign transplants. An alternative hypothesis attributes the high incidence of lymphoid malignancy to failure of feedback control of antigen-induced lymphoproliferation. Since immunodeficient patients do not make antibody or other normal immune products following receipt of antigen, the stimulated aberrant lymphoid elements continue to respond by proliferation, with repeated cell divisions increasing the likelihood of random malignant mutation.

Epstein-Barr virus (EBV) is particularly associated with oncogenesis in immunodeficient states. EBV can transform human B lymphocytes into cell lines capable of long-term survival in tissue culture; premalignant clones may be perpetuated in vivo as well. In the immunodeficient host, these clones are not eliminated because of T killer cell deficiency. Genetic and other environmental factors may also play a role. In patients at risk, the appearance of markedly enlarged nodes and persistent daily fever spikes is an ominous sign. Abnormal lymphocytes can be found in the bone marrow or peripheral smear. Central nervous system symptoms of a mass lesion are common. Infiltrates of transformed B lymphocytes are often found in enlarged lymph nodes or spleen or in intestinal lymphoid nodules. These may consist of immunoblasts or small cleaved follicular center cells and may histologically resemble malignant cells. They can usually be shown to be polyclonal and may resolve spontaneously or following immunotherapy. The proliferation may be so massive that death can result from mass effects, or evolution into a monoclonal malignant tumor may occur.

10.5 PRIMARY B CELL DISEASES

Clinically, the hypogammaglobulinemic syndromes can be divided into panhypogammaglobulinemia, selective deficiencies of immunoglobulins, and deficiencies of immunoglobulin subgroups.

10.6 PANHYPOGAMMAGLOBULINEMIA
(Congenital Agammaglobulinemia; Bruton Disease)

Panhypogammaglobulinemia involving all 3 major classes of immunoglobulins is usually congenital in origin. X-linked (Bruton disease), autosomal recessive, sporadic, and "late-onset" forms are seen, but such differentiation is of little help in defining etiology, management, or prognosis. Since some patients with congenital deficiency remain amazingly asymptomatic until later in life, the term late-onset does not imply an acquired or secondary disorder. Most late-onset diseases are in the category termed common variable immunodeficiency (Sec. 10.7).

Clinical Manifestations. Panhypogammaglobulinemia presents a history of repeated infections caused by pneumococ-

Table 10–7. **Clinical Symptoms of Immunodeficiency**

Suggestive of T cell defect
    Systemic illness following vaccination with any live virus or BCG; unusual life-threatening complication following infection with ordinarily
        benign viruses (e.g., giant cell pneumonia with rubeola; varicella pneumonia)
    Chronic oral candidosis after 6 mo of age
    Chronic mucocutaneous candidosis
    Features (fine, thin hair, short-limbed dwarfism with characteristic roentgenographic features of cartilage-hair hypoplasia [CHH])
    Intrauterine graft-versus-host disease — most characteristic feature is scaling erythroderma and total alopecia (absence of eyebrows
        quite striking)
    Graft-versus-host disease after blood transfusion
    Hypocalcemia in newborn (DiGeorge syndrome, especially with characteristic facies, ears, and cardiac lesion)
    Small (less than 10μ diameter) lymphocyte count persistently less than 1500/mm^3; must rule out gastrointestinal loss or loss from
        lymphatics

Suggestive of B cell defect
    Recurrent proven bacterial pneumonia, sepsis, or meningitis
    Nodular lymphoid hyperplasia

Suggestive of B and T cell defect (combined immunodeficiency disease [CID])
    Features of all above except chronic mucocutaneous candidosis and nodular lymphoid hyperplasia
    Features of Wiskott-Aldrich syndrome (draining ears, thrombocytopenia, and eczema)
    Features of ataxia-telangiectasia

Suggestive of immunodeficiency without clearly implicating T or B cell defect
    Pneumocystis carinii pneumonia
    Intractable eczema
    Ulcerative colitis in infants less than 1 yr of age
    Intractable diarrhea
    Unexplained hematologic deficiency (RBC, WBC, platelet)
    Severe generalized seborrheic dermatitis (Leiner disease) suggests C5 deficiency; seborrhea common in combined immunodeficiency
        disease
    Recurrent pyogenic infections seen in C3 deficiency

Suggestive of biochemical defect
    Features of combined immunodeficiency with characteristic bony lesions (adenosine deaminase deficiency)
    Features of Diamond-Blackfan aplastic anemia (nucleoside phosphorylase deficiency)

Suggestive of abnormality of polymorphonuclear leukocytes
    Primarily skin infections (if associated with asthma, eczema, and coarse facies, think of Buckley syndrome*)
    Chronic osteomyelitis with *Klebsiella* or *Serratia* species, draining lymph nodes (chronic granulomatous disease)

Suggestive that deficiency is secondary
    Concomitant or preceding viral infection
    Lymphoid malignancy (chronic lymphatic leukemia, Hodgkin disease, myeloma)

*Buckley RH, et al: Pediatrics 49:59, 1972.
Modified from Hong R, *In*: Rose NR, Friedman H (eds): Manual of Clinical Immunology. Washington, D.C., American Society for Microbiology, 1976.

cus, staphylococcus, and *H. influenzae*. Conjunctivitis secondary to *H. influenzae* is especially annoying. In older patients, chronic sinusitis is common, sometimes as the only complaint. Chronic pulmonary disease, with eventual bronchiectasis, pulmonary fibrosis, and cor pulmonale, characterizes adult disease. Fatal encephalitis and chronic viremia following echovirus, type 30, and other viral infections have been reported.

Autoimmune disorders are common. An increased frequency of malignancy also occurs (Sec. 10.4).

Skin disorders are unusually frequent in patients with immunodeficiency; intractable eczema and dermatomyositis have been reported. Eczema, recurrent skin abscesses, a history of allergy, and coarse facies occur with extremely elevated serum IgE values and leukocyte dysfunction.

Diagnosis. In panhypogammaglobulinemia levels of IgG seldom exceed 200 mg/dL in childhood; IgA and IgM are barely, if at all, detectable. During the first 3 mo of life, the high levels of maternally derived IgG can make the diagnosis difficult, but normal levels of IgA and IgM will virtually rule out significant hypogammaglobulinemia. Inguinal lymph nodes are easily detected in normal infants, even at birth; the palpation of normal lymph nodes, along with visible tonsillar tissue, speaks strongly against the diagnosis of hypogammaglobulinemia. A rare syndrome of enlarged lymph nodes and histiocytosis-like skin lesions (Omenn disease) is discussed in Section 10.17. Criteria defining significant infections should

be stringent. Upper respiratory infections are a common feature of the first few years of life, and as many as 9–10/yr may occur normally. Unless there is also a verified history of repeated bacterial pneumonias or other severe infections, frequent upper respiratory infections are not an indication to investigate the patient exhaustively for immunodeficiency.

Treatment. This consists of the intramuscular injection of immune serum globulin (ISG) prepared by alcohol precipitation (Cohn Fraction II). A dose calculated to produce a serum level of 300 mg/dL is given (a loading dose of 1.4 mL/kg, followed by 0.7 mL/kg every 4 wk). For a larger person the large size of an individual dose may require shortening the interval to weekly and reducing the size of each dose proportionately. Local pain at the site of the injection can be partially controlled by mixing a small amount of local anesthetic with the immune serum globulin in the syringe.

Preparations consisting primarily of IgG are now available for intravenous administration. With these it is now possible to attain near normal levels of IgG and to maintain therapeutic levels in adults in a simple, well tolerated manner. Earlier use of plasma to maintain high levels in adults and older children has been abandoned because of concerns with contamination by hepatitis viruses or by AIDS-related viruses.

Chronic infection of the central nervous system is occasionally seen in B cell deficiencies. In an affected patient daily intravenous administration of IgG resulted in dramatic control of symptoms; relapse followed cessation of therapy. Chronic thrombocytopenia and hemolytic anemia sometimes occur as complications of hypogammaglobulinemia. Intravenous administration of gamma globulin has controlled these conditions in both immunodeficient and immunocompetent states.

Anaphylaxis may complicate either intramuscular or intravenous gamma globulin therapy, especially the latter. Close monitoring of the patient during infusion is necessary. The cause of these reactions is the existence of small aggregates of immunoglobulin that resist the chemical modification procedures. A rare cause is the paradoxical production of anti-IgA antibodies in some hypogammaglobulinemic patients. ISG is highly enriched for IgG, but all preparations of gamma globulin have significant amounts of IgA and IgM (5-10%).

Chronic pulmonary disease is an ever-present danger in panhypogammaglobulinemia. Pulmonary function should be tested at least annually in all patients over 10 yr old, unless symptoms or roentgenograms suggest that earlier assessment should be performed. Unremitting pulmonary disease is probably a sign of failure of intramuscular therapy with gamma globulin and an indication for intravenous or plasma therapy. This approach is entirely empiric. Daily prophylaxis with 10 mg/kg of trimethoprim and 50 mg/kg of sulfamethoxazole in 2 divided doses may also be helpful in selected cases.

10.7 COMMON VARIABLE IMMUNODEFICIENCY

This catch-all term encompasses most immunodeficiency states with a prominent B cell component and a minimal or no T cell defect. It excludes X-linked agammaglobulinemia (Bruton disease). Usually, the onset of symptoms is later than that of Bruton disease, and both sexes are involved. Otherwise, the clinical picture is indistinguishable from that of congenital agammaglobulinemia. The later onset was originally thought to indicate an acquired causation, but examples of familial incidence and the finding of autoimmune diseases in a high percentage of first-degree relatives implicate a genetic mechanism.

The major difference in laboratory studies between these patients and those with Bruton disease is the finding of circulating B cells. This group of diseases does not, therefore, represent a failure of differentiation from stem cells. Inadequate T helper function, excess suppressor T cell function, and autoantibodies to T or B cells have been found. Attempts to correct some of these faults, in particular the excess suppression, have not been very successful. As the patients grow older, increasingly significant T cell abnormalities develop.

About 25% of patients with common variable immunodeficiency have significant malabsorption, most commonly involving vitamin B_{12}. *Giardia lamblia* infestation is especially common. Lactose intolerance, disaccharidase deficiency, villous abnormalities, and nodular lymphoid hyperplasia may be seen. Infiltration of spleen, lung, and skin with noncaseating granulomas is common. Their cause is unknown, but corticosteroid therapy will usually cause marked reduction in their size and number.

SELECTIVE DEFICIENCIES

Selective deficiencies of IgA or IgM have been well studied; that of IgE, whether or not associated with ataxia-telangiectasia, remains of unknown clinical significance. Only one case of selective total deficiency of IgG has been described, but deficiencies of subgroups are well known.

10.8 Selective Deficiency of IgA

IgA is the major immunoglobulin protecting the respiratory, gastrointestinal, and other secretory areas. As a result of its deficiency, recurrent respiratory infections and chronic diarrheal syndromes may occur. A striking association with autoimmune disorders, especially systemic lupus erythematosus and rheumatoid arthritis, is seen. The autoimmunity is believed to result from uncontrolled access of antigenic substances to the lymphoid system via the gastrointestinal tract, with undue stimulation causing generation of antigen-antibody complexes. Another reason for the association may be the profound dependency of the IgA system on intact thymic function, a deficiency in production of IgA implying a thymic abnormality. One such defect, lack or deficiency of T suppressor cells, could predispose to autoimmunity.

Some patients with selective deficiency of IgA show spontaneous recovery. Two patients with deficiency of serum IgA have gradually acquired normal levels after 3-5 yr without any specific therapy. Since all IgA-deficient patients studied to date possess normal numbers of nonsecreting lymphocytes bearing IgA molecules and since, in one study, these cells could be stimulated in vitro to become secreting cells, the potential for spontaneous recovery may exist in all patients. Selective deficiency of IgA may also be produced by external factors, e.g., by administration of phenytoin.

Patients with selective *total* deficiency of IgA have normal capacity for synthesizing IgG antibody, and their B cells can respond vigorously to most antigens. If such patients receive IgA from any source, formation of anti-IgA antibody is quite likely since their immune systems treat IgA as a foreign protein. ISG is a common source, resulting from the frequent and, in our opinion, injudicious practice of empirically administering immune serum globulin as a prophylactic measure to children with frequent respiratory infections, which are usual in patients with total absence of IgA. ISG contains amounts of IgA that are adequate to sensitize the child with total deficiency of IgA but not to protect against agents that cause respiratory infections. If blood or blood products containing significant amounts of IgA are then administered to such IgA-sensitized patients, fatal anaphylaxis may result; ISG should not, therefore, be administered without justification to children with frequent upper respiratory infections. Furthermore, patients known to have total IgA deficiency should not receive blood or blood products without first determining that they have no anti-IgA antibodies in their sera.

Selective IgA deficiency may be inherited in either autosomal recessive or autosomal dominant manner. Often siblings of patients with panhypogammaglobulinemia show selective IgA deficiency. Selective IgA deficiency has an unexplained association with a chromosome 18 abnormality. The structural genes for immunoglobulins do not seem to be present on chromosome 18.

Although serum IgA and secretory IgA appear to be under separate control, virtually all patients with serum IgA deficiency also have secretory IgA deficiency. Occasionally, a patient with deficiency of serum IgA will show IgA-staining plasma cells in the intestine. In these cases, full evaluation of the capability to produce secretory IgA in the gastrointestinal or respiratory tracts has not been carried out. It is not known, therefore, whether the number of IgA-producing cells was normal throughout the secretory system or whether their rate of synthesis of secretory IgA was adequate for protection. IgA function in the secretions is most critical, but as a practical matter in most situations measurement of serum IgA predicts the status of secretory IgA. Patients with deficiency of secretory IgA in the face of normal levels of serum IgA have been found to have a deficiency of secretory component (Sec. 10.9).

If symptoms warrant, determination of secretory IgA status must be made regardless of the level of IgA in the serum.

It has been reported that the severity or likelihood of respiratory disease in IgA deficiency is best correlated with an associated IgG subgroup defect. IgG2 or IgG4 deficiency may also increase the risk for lymphoproliferative disease. In one large series, nearly one half of patients with IgA deficiency had concomitant IgE deficiency.

IgA deficiency is probably not often an isolated defect, but may be associated with a number of other defects of the T and B cell systems. Assessment of affected patients must include sufficient general evaluation of IgG subgroups and of the T cell system to determine the extent of involvement.

10.9 Selective Deficiency of Secretory Component (SC)

Secretory component is a protein produced by epithelial cells in many parts of the body. It is found on all molecules of IgA secreted into the lumen of the intestine; it may play an important role in the transport of IgA, and perhaps of IgM, from the site of synthesis in the plasma cells of the lamina propria. Absence or deficiency of secretory component has been reported in 5 of 8 children with sudden infant death syndrome (SIDS). Two children with deficiency of secretory component have had chronic diarrhea; these patients also had a deficiency of secretory IgA but normal levels of serum IgA.

10.10 Selective Deficiency of IgM

This primary deficiency state has a frequency of approximately 1:1000 in the general population. Affected patients tend to succumb to rapid hematogenous spread of bacterial infections; atopy and splenomegaly have also been noted. Whipple disease, regional enteritis, and lymphoid nodular hyperplasia have also been observed with increased frequency.

Patients should be treated aggressively with antibiotics at the first sign of infection. It has been recommended that their blood relatives also be treated at the first sign of infection if their serum IgM status is unknown.

10.11 IgG Subgroup Deficiency

Generally speaking, in IgG subgroup deficiency the total levels of IgG are normal but the heterogeneity of its electrophoretic mobility may appear to be restricted. When tests of specific antibody formation are made, antibody formation to some antigens but not to others appears. Clinically, the patients show the same increased susceptibility to infection characteristic of panhypogammaglobulinemia, and some, but not all, will respond to gamma globulin therapy.

10.12 PRIMARY T CELL DISEASES

When T cell function is compromised but B cells function normally, infections are primarily fungal or viral. Chronic interstitial pneumonia, nasal discharge, and neutropenia are other features associated with T cell deficiency. The major types of T cell defects in which the immunoglobulins are measurable (and usually functional) are the DiGeorge syndrome, Nezelof syndrome, cartilage-hair hypoplasia, some cases of adenosine deaminase deficiency, and nucleoside phosphorylase deficiency.

10.13 DiGEORGE SYNDROME

The thymus arises from the 3rd and 4th pharyngeal pouches in common with the parathyroid. An embryologic defect in these structures causes a combined deficiency of the thymus and parathyroids in association with congenital defects of the aortic arch and heart. Hypoplastic mandible, defective ears, and a short philtrum also occur. A characteristic feature is the marked variability of expression of the syndrome, with clinical symptoms ranging from minimal thymic deficiency with spontaneous acquisition of normal T cell function to involvement so severe that B cell deficiency is also present. Post mortem examination of thymuses from patients with DiGeorge syndrome reveals variable degrees of hypoplasia, but usually the architecture is preserved. To meet the definition of DiGeorge syndrome, the disorder must include both parathyroid deficiency (with lack of parathormone) and T cell dysfunction. Other features may or may not be present.

Hypocalcemia in the neonatal period is frequently the initial presentation. Should this occur, careful examination for associated facial and cardiac features should be made. Chest roentgenograms may be informative since sufficient stress to cause disappearance of the normal thymic shadow has usually not occurred. If hypocalcemia is mild, the diagnosis may first be made in the cardiac clinic. Zellweger syndrome may be confused with DiGeorge syndrome; lack of peroxisomes characterizes the former.

Thymic transplantation has been successful in treatment of DiGeorge syndrome, but it must be remembered that cure may be spontaneous. Thymus implanted in a cell-impermeable Millipore chamber may also result in normalization of T cell tests, suggesting that humoral ("hormonal") factors play an important role in reconstitution.

10.14 NEZELOF SYNDROME

The absence of parathyroid or cardiac involvement differentiates Nezelof syndrome from DiGeorge syndrome. The presence or absence of specific antibodies was not determined in Nezelof's original studies. Newer concepts of the role of the thymus in expression of the B cell system make this an important distinction. We prefer to classify patients with immunoglobulins of known specificity in the face of T cell deficiency as having Nezelof syndrome and believe them to be quite different from those whose immunoglobulins are measurable but are of nondefined specificity. The latter group of patients frequently do not produce all three major classes, and electrophoretic abnormalities are common. We believe that this group should be considered a variant of combined B and T cell deficiency.

10.15 CARTILAGE-HAIR HYPOPLASIA

Patients with cartilage-hair hypoplasia (CHH) have a unique form of bone dysplasia, short-limbed dwarfism, sparse hair lacking a central pigmented core, and neutropenia. The patients were first found in an Amish population, but cases occur in other ethnic groups. Only a small percentage of short-limbed dwarfs show the immune defect; furthermore, even though testing implies a virtual absence of T cell function, susceptibility to infection is limited and the major agents involved are vaccinia or varicella virus. Chronic candidosis, for example, is not a feature of this T cell deficiency.

Little information is available on the response of cartilage-hair hypoplasia to therapy. Bone marrow transplantation has been performed in one case, with apparent benefit.

COMBINED T AND B CELL DISEASE

In these disorders, both T and B cell functions are profoundly depressed. Originally, it was thought that combined T and B cell disease was best explained by a lesion of stem cells at the point in their development immediately preceding differentiation into T and B cells. B cell differentiation is highly thymus dependent, however, and at least some combined B and T cell disorders are probably caused by a primary thymic deficiency.

10.16 COMBINED IMMUNODEFICIENCY DISEASE (CID)

The term severe combined immunodeficiency originally described a syndrome that began in infancy and usually resulted in death by 2 yr of age. Milder forms have now been observed, and early death is not inevitable. When the disorder involves both T and B cell systems, the disease is more severe than with either separate defect; the infectious processes that occur are of the varieties that characterize either deficiency state.

If combined immunodeficiency disease (CID) is defined as a disorder in which both T and B cell functions are diminished, *absence* of products of either system is not an absolute requirement for diagnosis. For example, patients with E-rosette cells but no other normal T cell functions and those with some or all classes of immunoglobulins but no detectable antibody activity ("cellular immunodeficiency with immunoglobulin") may also be included in the category of combined immunodeficiency disease. Certainly, the susceptibility to infection and disease seems to be as great in these children as in those with no detectable lymphocytes or immunoglobulins.

In addition to the symptoms already discussed for isolated deficiencies, a number of features are characteristic of CID. Wasting, whether or not associated with chronic diarrhea, is common. If diarrhea is present, it is recalcitrant to therapy and total parenteral alimentation may be required. Unusual skin eruptions, total alopecia, excessive seborrhea, cutaneous laxity manifested by redundant skin folds, large umbilical hernias, and hyperelastic joints are also seen. One form of CID is associated with short-limbed dwarfism, caused by metaphyseal or spondyloepiphyseal dysplasia.

Hematologic abnormalities include thrombocytosis, neutropenia, anemia, monocytosis, and eosinophilia. Monocytosis and eosinophilia may occur in response to overwhelming infections such as pneumocystic pneumonia.

CID can be successfully treated with transplantation of bone marrow, with apparently complete and long-lasting reconstitution of both B and T cell systems. The successful transplants have come from siblings who are matched at the major histocompatibility locus most important in determining the severity of graft-versus-host reaction, the HLA-D locus. Only about 25% of siblings can be expected to match. Recently, two methods have been developed for transplanting marrow from haploidentical donors (usually parent to child). The mature T cells in the marrow inoculum can be removed by treatment of the marrow either with soybean lectin (usually with a sheep red blood cell-rosetting step) or with monoclonal antibody(ies) directed against mature T cells. Marrow so treated will produce little or, at worst, controllable graft-versus-host disease. Failure of engraftment is more common with these techniques, suggesting that the histocompatibility differences are sufficient to incite a primitive rejection reaction by a host with virtually absent immunity. In such cases, immunosuppression of the host is necessary, even though testing of his or her T cell function indicates profound impairment. The need for T cell ablation prior to transplantation greatly complicates haploidentical bone marrow transplantation, but several successes have followed this procedure.

No significant benefit has resulted from treatment with transfer factor or thymic hormone. Transplants of fetal liver, fetal liver combined with fetal thymus, fetal thymus alone, or cultured thymic epithelium (CTE) have shown promise in some cases; it may be that for different varieties of CID different approaches are necessary.

Pneumocystis infection is responsive to either pentamidine isethionate or trimethoprim-sulfamethoxazole; prophylaxis with the latter is advisable in a patient with CID until curative transplantation of bone marrow is established. Treatment of cytomegalovirus, rubeola, and varicella infections is unsatisfactory. Zoster immune globulin is indicated to prevent infection upon exposure of a susceptible immunodeficient patient to varicella. In varicella pneumonia or overwhelming varicella, therapy with acyclovir is effective.

10.17 COMBINED IMMUNODEFICIENCY DISEASE AND LETTERER-SIWE SYNDROME
(Omenn Disease)

A chronic skin eruption, hepatosplenomegaly, eosinophilia, and histiocytic infiltration of the lymph nodes occur in one variety of CID. The marked histiocytosis has led to reports of immunodeficiency and Letterer-Siwe syndrome occurring together. However, the skin eruptions of Letterer-Siwe syndrome, with its extreme seborrhea and characteristic histiocytic infiltration, are actually quite different from any form of CID. Furthermore, in Letterer-Siwe syndrome there is no immunodeficiency unless cytotoxic drugs have been given. CID of the Omenn type is one of the few forms of severe immunodeficiency in which there is marked deficiency of both T and B cell systems but easily palpable lymph nodes. Usually, many of the tests of lymphocyte function are normal; thus, the diagnosis may require thymic biopsy for confirmation. A deficiency of the ectoenzyme 5'-nucleotidase may be characteristic of Omenn disease. *Pneumocystis* pneumonia is a common presenting symptom. The rash is often actually a manifestation of a chronic graft-versus-host disease.

10.18 WISKOTT-ALDRICH SYNDROME

This is an X-linked recessive disorder characterized by thrombocytopenia, draining ears, and eczema. Serum IgA and IgE levels are markedly elevated, IgM is diminished, lymphopenia is common, and malignant reticuloendotheliosis is a common terminal event. A characteristic laboratory finding is small (approximately half-size) platelets. A defect in glycosylation of surface proteins may play a significant role in pathogenesis.

The reason for susceptibility to infection in Wiskott-Aldrich syndrome is unknown. Although the most striking immunologic abnormality consistently found is an inability to form antibodies to carbohydrate antigens, poor responses to other antigens are found as the disease progresses. Detailed study may show mild dysfunction of T cells but less than in the usual forms of T cell deficiency. The defects increase with time so that originally normal findings give way to abnormal responses; immunoglobulin levels change to a characteristic hyper-IgA, hypo-IgM pattern; and abnormalities of lymphoid tissues occur.

Bone marrow transplants have been successful in patients with Wiskott-Aldrich syndrome. Because the immunity is not nearly so profound as in CID, early attempts at transplantation with minimal or modest immunosuppression were unsuccessful. Administration of busulfan or total body-irradiation is required at the very least, and more may be required, especially if a haploidentical donor is used.

Splenectomy may control the thrombocytopenia in situations in which bone marrow transplantation cannot be done; for maximal benefit it must be done early in the course of the disease.

10.19 ATAXIA-TELANGIECTASIA

Ataxia-telangiectasia (AT) is characterized by ataxia, ocular and cutaneous telangiectasia, chronic sinopulmonary disease, endocrine abnormalities, and variable B and T cell deficiency. Deficiency of IgA and IgE, singly or together, constitutes the most common B cell abnormality. The disease may be due to a common embryologic fault resulting in failure of mesoderomoentodermal interactions, leading to telangiectasia, neurologic disease, and lymphoid abnormalities. The finding of elevated alpha-fetoprotein and carcinoembryonic antigen in virtually all patients with ataxia-telangiectasia is consistent with an abnormal process of embryogenesis. Since only fetal-type cells synthesize these proteins, continued postnatal production suggests an arrest at a fetal stage. In some as yet undefined way, similar arrests involving the many and varied organ systems in ataxia-telangiectasia could lead to the manifestations observed. Some workers have found evidence for autoimmune reactivity against various organ systems, including brain and thymocytes, implying autoaggression as a factor in the pathogenesis.

Patients with AT have a defect in DNA repair mechanisms, which probably accounts for the high incidence of chromosomal breaks observed in AT karyotypes. The defect in repair is confined to x-ray-induced damage; UV radiation damage is repaired appropriately. This defect precludes x-ray or radiomimetic therapy in the treatment of malignancy in AT. It is possible that error-prone repair may be related to the clinical symptoms. It has been suggested that the defective DNA repair is indicative of the basic defect in differentiation.

The disease is inherited as an autosomal trait, probably recessive. Cerebellar ataxia is usually the first neurologic sign; intellectual development is normal at first, but seems to arrest at about the 10 yr level. A mask-like facies with excessive drooling gives a remarkable similarity of appearance to affected patients. The telangiectases are most obvious in the sclerae, although involvement of the ear, lateral aspect of the nose, and antecubital and popliteal fossae is common.

Deficiency of both IgA and IgE may be seen in 50–70% of cases; isolated IgE deficiency may occur in another 20–40%. Selective IgA deficiency is also found in high frequency. Variable degrees of T cell deficiency progressively worsen with time, and death from malignant lymphoma is a common terminal event.

10.20 CHRONIC MUCOCUTANEOUS CANDIDOSIS

This chronic, indolent candidosis involves mucous membranes and spreads peripherally onto the skin. Satellite patches may occur on the trunk and extremities; onychomycosis may be present. Some patients have associated endocrine deficiencies, with hypoadrenalism, hypoparathyroidism, and hypothyroidism among the most common. Initially, these patients show increased susceptibility to infection with *Candida* only, with normal ability to resist other infectious agents. Gradually, however, their general immunity wanes, and infection occurs from other opportunistic organisms.

The immunologic background for chronic mucocutaneous candidosis is varied. The usual tests may show defects of T cell immunity, deficiency of migration inhibitory factor (MIF), selective IgA deficiency, or biotin deficiency. In some patients no abnormalities have been found.

Intravenous administration of amphotericin is effective, but symptoms frequently recur upon cessation of therapy. In recalcitrant cases, clotrimazole, transfer factor, leukocyte infusions, and thymosin have all been used with variable degrees of success. An especially effective anti-candidal agent is ketoconazole. It is important to remember that endocrinopathy, e.g., acute adrenal insufficiency, may occur at any time.

10.21 GRAFT-VERSUS-HOST DISEASE (GVHD)

This complication of T cell deficiency states occurs when a patient receives immunocompetent (T killer) cells with ordinary blood transfusions or bone marrow transplants. More rarely, it may occur in utero following transfusion for erythroblastosis fetalis or as a result of passage of maternal cells across the placenta into the fetal circulation. In the intrauterine situation, whether the affected fetus must be T cell deficient or not is not known. The rarity of GVHD in the normal population and its frequent occurrence among immunodeficient patients suggest that intrauterine graft-versus-host disease probably does not occur in normal fetuses.

Graft-versus-host disease may be acute or chronic. The *acute* variety is usually seen in recipients of blood or bone marrow from donors who differ at the HLA-D locus; the event most often occurs when a blood transfusion is unwittingly given to a T cell deficient patient. It may rarely occur after transplants of fetal tissue. Occasionally GVHD is associated with blood product infusions in leukemic patients. It remains a rare event, however, and probably occurs only when a number of chance events happen simultaneously. *Chronic* GVHD is seen with intrauterine transfusions, after transplantation from HLA-D matched bone marrow donors (especially in leukemia), and after transplants of fetal liver or fetal thymus.

Acute GVHD begins 7–14 days after grafting and is generally heralded by a skin eruption. This can be maculopapular or, in more explosive cases, can resemble *"scalded skin syndrome."* Periportal necrosis of the liver, coagulation necrosis of the epidermis, and lesions of the crypts of the gastrointestinal tract are the characteristic histologic findings. When the source of killer T cells is from an HLA-D incompatible donor, death can result. When the donor is HLA-D compatible, the syndrome can vary from a fleeting skin rash and transient elevation of liver enzymes to a severe but usually nonfatal disease. GVHD has an unusual capacity to activate latent virus infections. If the patient harbors cytomegalovirus, CMV infection may overwhelm the patient before immunologic reconstitution occurs. *Pneumocystis* pneumonia often becomes manifest early in the post-transplant period, probably for the same reason.

The chronic disease is characterized by a scaling erythroderma, alopecia, and failure to thrive.

Control of GVHD has improved in recent years. High-dose corticosteroid therapy, monoclonal anti-T cell antibody, and antithymocyte or antilymphocyte globulin have been used in various combinations. In some cases, total control of symptoms has been attained.

10.22 SECONDARY IMMUNODEFICIENCY DISEASES

In these disorders the primary cause is clearly outside the lymphoid system. The immune elements are involved either as part of a generalized process or as a result of some aspect of the primary disease which directly attacks or consumes the lymphoid products.

Adenosine Deaminase (ADA) and Nucleoside Phosphorylase (NP) Deficiency. These are the first biochemical defects having immunodeficiency as an associated feature. Adenosine deaminase–deficient patients have usually combined immunodeficiency disease, but isolated defects of the thymus system are known. Nucleoside phosphorylase deficiency usually presents first as an isolated T cell defect, but NP deficiency eventually results in B cell deficiency as well. These biochemical defects cause immunodeficiency because products accumulated as a result of an inability to catabolize purines have a toxic effect on lymphocytes. ADA catalyzes the conversion of adenosine to inosine; in its absence, levels of lymphocyte ATP, cyclic AMP, and their deoxyanalogues increase. NP catalyzes the reversible conversion of inosine to hypoxanthine, guanosine to guanine, and xanthosine to xanthine. A breakdown in normal catabolic processes results in the accumulation of inosine and guanosine. Whether these or other metabolites are the actual toxic factors is unknown as yet, but the notion of slow toxic attrition of the lymphoid system appears to be valid. Characteristically, a period of normal lymphoid function is followed by a gradual waning of immunity.

The diagnosis is established by measurement of enzyme levels in erythrocytes. It can also be suspected when the clinical history suggests an "acquired" defect of late onset and, in NP deficiency, from finding low serum uric acid levels. Characteristic splaying of the ends of the ribs and "squaring off" of the scapulae are seen in ADA deficiency. In NP deficiency, the metabolic defect may result in megaloblastic anemia, pure red cell aplasia, or spastic tetraparesis.

Repeated blood transfusions have been effective in managing some patients with ADA deficiency. In NP deficiency this form of treatment in a single reported case was without benefit. Another patient with NP deficiency responded to thymosin injections, but development of allergy to the hormone required cessation of the medication.

Transplantation of cultured thymus fragments offers additional help in management. Bone marrow transplantation is curative.

Loss of Immunologic Materials. Loss of protein, hence of immunoglobulins, may occur from the genitourinary and gastrointestinal tracts and from the lymphatic system. In *nephrotic syndromes* the glomerular sieve allows the escape of IgG and IgA but retains the larger molecules of IgM, which remain at near-normal levels. Manufacture of antibody is unimpaired, and susceptibility to infection is not increased (the susceptibility of nephrotic children to pneumococcal peritonitis appears to be related, in part, to ascites and to lack of previous experience with the specific type of pneumococcus responsible for the infection in addition to factors discussed in Sec. 17.27). The situation with *protein-losing enteropathy* is analogous. Both are characterized by hypogammaglobulinemia associated with edema or hypoalbuminemia. Loss of immunologic materials from the *lymphatic system*, whether due to congenital malformations of the lymphatic vessels or to surgical accidents, includes loss of lymphocytes as well as of circulating immunoglobulins. The lymphocyte count may drop to one third of normal, and all three major classes of immunoglobulins may fall to one half of normal levels. Tests of T cell function show abnormal lymphocyte responses in vitro and retention of allogeneic skin grafts for up to 2 yr. Resistance to infections is surprisingly unimpaired, except in chylothorax; lymphangiectasia involving the thoracic cavity is associated with more infectious problems than that of other areas of the body.

Nutritional Deficiency. In *protein-calorie malnutrition*, disseminated herpes infections and gram-negative sepsis are common. Death from measles may occur. Lymphopenia is marked, in vitro lymphocyte responses are defective, and tonsils and thymus are small. Usually B cell function is only slightly diminished; IgE may be markedly elevated.

Immune cellular functions are dependent upon divalent cations. For example, internal movement of calcium ions causes proliferation of lymphocytes, and immunodeficiency has been described in association with copper, zinc, iron, and calcium abnormalities. Acrodermatitis enteropathica is due to zinc malabsorption; chronic candidosis may be associated with biotin deficiency.

Chemical or Physical Immunosuppression. The widespread use of immunosuppressive drugs in autoimmune disorders and transplantation has led to a number of immunologic deficiency states; cytotoxic agents employed in cancer chemotherapy have also produced such states. Pre-existing immunity usually persists at pretreatment levels unless the dosage of medication is extremely high.

The addition of irradiation to chemotherapy adds significantly to the mortality of leukemic patients from infections. Deficiencies of both T and B cell systems are found. Immunologic recovery may require as much as 1 yr after such therapy has stopped.

When antilymphocyte serum or globulin is employed, marked depression of T cell functions is seen, with an associated increased incidence of fungal, protozoal, and viral infections.

Viral Infections. Intrauterine infections may cause altered development of lymphoid cells and organs, such as the thymus, in which primary differentiation takes place. B cell deficiency may occur following infection with Epstein-Barr virus. The disease (Duncan disease) appears to be X-linked, and the initial bout of Epstein-Barr virus infection is unusually severe and fulminant. The association of viral infection with the acquired immunodeficiency syndrome (AIDS) is discussed in Sec. 10.23.

RICHARD HONG

Ammann AJ, Hong R: Disorders of the T cell system. *In:* Stiehm ER, Fulginiti VA (eds): Immunologic Disorders in Infants and Children. 2nd ed. Philadelphia, WB Saunders, 1980, p. 286.

Hadden JW, Stewart WE (eds). The Lymphokines. Clifton, NJ, Humana Press, 1981.

Horowitz SD, Hong R: The Pathogenesis and Treatment of Immunodeficiency. Basel, S Karger, 1977.

Moretta L (ed): Lymphocytes. I. Sem Hematol 21:223, 1984.

Moretta L, Fauci AS (eds): Lymphocytes. II. Sem Hematol 22:1, 1985.

Ochs HD, Wedgwood RJ: Disorders of the B cell system. *In:* Stiehm ER, Fulginiti VA (eds): Immunologic Disorders in Infants and Children. 2nd ed. Philadelphia, WB Saunders, 1980, p. 239.

Oxelius VA: Chronic infections in a family with hereditary deficiency of IgG2 and IgG4. Clin Exp Immunol 17:19, 1974.

Purtillo DT: Epstein-Barr virus-induced oncogenesis in immune deficient individuals. Lancet 1:300, 1980.

Reinherz EL, Geha R, Rappeport JM, et al: Reconstitution after transplantation with T-lymphocyte-depleted HLA haplotype-mismatched bone marrow for severe combined immunodeficiency. Proc Natl Acad Sci USA 79:6047, 1982.

Reisner Y, Kapoor N, Kirkpatrick D, et al: Transplantation of severe combined immunodeficiency with HLA-A, B, D, Dr incompatible parental marrow cells fractionated by soybean agglutinin and sheep red blood cells. Blood 61:341, 1983.

Rosen FS, Cooper MD, Wedgwood RJP: The primary immunodeficiencies (First of two parts). N Engl J Med 311:235, 1984.

Rosen FS, Cooper MD, Wedgwood RJP. The primary immunodeficiencies (Second of two parts). N Engl J Med 311:300, 1984.

Shannon KM, Ammann AJ: Acquired immune deficiency syndrome in childhood. J Pediatr 106:332, 1985.

10.23 ACQUIRED IMMUNODEFICIENCY SYNDROME (AIDS)

Introduction. The acquired immunodeficiency syndrome (AIDS) has become important in the differential diagnosis of immunodeficiency disease in infants and children. Epidemiologic studies suggest that AIDS may be acquired by infants from mothers who are carriers of the infectious agent and that it may be transmitted by means of transfusions of blood or of blood products such as antihemophilic globulin. Sexual activity is the most common means of transmission among adults, but is relatively rare among sexually active adolescents. There is as yet no cure for AIDS, but early recognition and treatment may mitigate morbidity and perhaps postpone death.

Etiology. AIDS was first recognized in 1980 as a distinct syndrome of acquired immunodeficiency in young homosexual males, with Kaposi sarcoma and opportunistic infection as striking features. There had been a sudden increase in the incidence of these abnormalities in previously healthy males and in widely separated geographic areas (New York and San Francisco). Epidemiologic studies indicated a relationship between life style and risk of AIDS. Major risk factors include male homosexuality with multiple sex partners, especially the passive partner in rectal intercourse, and intravenous drug abuse. Persons of Haitian origin may also be at increased risk. The pattern of transmission, which is similar to that of infectious hepatitis, and the association of AIDS with blood transfusions provide evidence for an infectious etiology. Several patients with hemophilia A were reported who developed opportunistic infection or Kaposi sarcoma and additional studies indicated that the majority of patients with hemophilia A who had received factor VIII concentrate therapy had immunologic abnormalities similar to those found in AIDS. Other evidence for an infectious cause of AIDS was its transmission to some infants born to mothers with risk factors for AIDS, such as intravenous drug abuse or Haitian ancestry.

Viruses associated with AIDS infection have included Epstein-Barr virus, hepatitis B virus, adenovirus, and cytomegalovirus. Some of these viruses have also been associated with minor degrees of immunodeficiency in patients who do not have AIDS, but it is unlikely that they produce severe immunodeficiency in more than a few patients. In 1984, three groups of investigators, in Paris, in Bethesda, and in San Francisco, isolated retrovirus from patients with AIDS. The viruses were termed human T-cell lymphotropic virus-III (HTLV-III), lymphadenopathy-associated virus (LAV), or AIDS-associated retrovirus (ARV); they are probably identical or at least belong to the same species of retrovirus. The virus is now called human immunodeficiency virus (HIV). Recent epidemiologic data, supported by antibody testing and virus isolation techniques, indicate that a retrovirus is the most likely cause of AIDS. On the other hand, infection by a single viral agent does not explain all of the features of AIDS, such as the diverse immunologic abnormalities, the severity of infection in certain populations, or the association of Kaposi sarcoma only in certain risk groups.

Pathophysiology. The normal immune system has four major components: T-cells, B-cells, complement, and phagocytic activity. AIDS produces a generalized disturbance of regulatory pathways, with aberrations of all four major components.

A reversal of the ratio of helper to suppressor T cells (normally > 1.0) is characteristic of AIDS. An altered helper/suppressor T cell ratio does not necessarily indicate T cell immunodeficiency, since it is also observed following acute viral infections in normal individuals, but the persistence of this abnormality in patients with AIDS suggests a more permanent regulatory defect. As the disease progresses, functional abnormalities of T cells appear; they include abnormal responses of lymphocytes to antigens, mitogens, and allogeneic cells. T cells may also fail to produce normal amounts of such lymphokines as interleukin 2 and interferon.

Abnormal T cell regulation may result in abnormalities in the B cell system. Typically, patients with AIDS have elevated levels of IgG, IgM, and IgA. This "polyclonal hypergammaglobulinemia" is frequently associated with an inability to form specific antibody following immunization with antigens to which the patient has been recently exposed.

Patients with AIDS have increased amounts of circulating immune complexes, which are probably the consequence of chronic infection with one or more microbial agents. Abnormal monocyte chemotaxis, antigen processing, and cytotoxicity are found in some patients.

Opportunistic infection is the major cause of death in AIDS. The second most common cause of death is malignancy, especially Kaposi sarcoma. Children and adults with AIDS have similar types of opportunistic infections, with the exception of venereal diseases. In children with AIDS, Kaposi sarcoma is less malignant than in adults. At autopsy, the histologic appearance of the thymus and lymphoid tissue is consistent with chronic infection and is not typical of primary immunodeficiency disease. Unique histologic abnormalities in children with AIDS include extensive lymphoid infiltration of the lung (diffuse lymphoid interstitial pneumonitis), which may be related to Epstein-Barr virus.

The time from exposure to the putative infectious agent to the development of AIDS may be as short as 3 months or as long as 5 years. The reasons for the wide range in the incubation period are unknown; they may relate to the presence or absence of other infections or to pre-existing immunodeficiency, e.g. prematurity, viral immunosuppression.

Clinical Manifestations and Diagnosis. The majority of infants and children with AIDS are born to mothers who have risk factors such as Haitian ancestry or intravenous drug abuse. An important feature of this form of AIDS is that the mothers, who may be clinically well, have evidence of immunologic dysregulation, such as depressed helper/suppressor T cell ratios and abnormalities of T cell function. Both mothers and infants have antibodies to AIDS-associated retrovirus. Several infants born to the same mother have developed AIDS, and AIDS has occurred in some infants born by cesarean section.

Affected infants may be small for gestational age and may fail to thrive. Microcephaly may be present. Symptoms usually occur within the first 3 to 6 months of life, but may be delayed for as long as 5 years. Hepatosplenomegaly, lymphadenopathy, failure to thrive, and chronic interstitial pneumonia (especially *pneumocystis carinii* infection) are frequent manifestations. Recurrent otitis media, chronic sinopulmonary infection, *Candida* infection of the mucous membranes, and chronic diarrhea also occur. A feature of AIDS in children that is infrequently found in adults is chronic parotid swelling. Kaposi sarcoma is uncommon in children with AIDS.

The diagnosis of transfusion-associated AIDS may be difficult, owing to the prolonged incubation period (up to 5 years) following exposure. Once such AIDS is recognized, an investigation of both the recipient(s) and donor(s) should be instituted, since donor blood is frequently distributed to several recipients. Studies of transfusion-associated AIDS indicate that platelet transfusions may be more closely associated with the development of AIDS than with the administration of other blood products. Not all persons who receive blood transfusions from a donor with AIDS will develop AIDS.

More than 80% of patients with hemophilia who receive factor VIII concentrate therapy develop antibodies to AIDS-associated retrovirus. Such patients have immunologic abnormalities that are similar to those found in patients with AIDS or in those who have AIDS-associated risk factors. Initial reports of patients with hemophilia who developed AIDS highlighted the occurrence of *Pneumocystis carinii* pneumonia and Kaposi sarcoma. A subgroup of such patients develop chronic lymphadenopathy, with recurrent fevers, night sweats, weight loss, chronic diarrhea, and hepatosplenomegaly. Biopsy of lymph nodes provides no specific cause for the chronic lymphadenopathy. Patients with hemophilia who receive factor VIII concentrate therapy also may have evidence of other viral infections, such as Epstein-Barr virus, hepatitis B, or cytomegalovirus.

Exposure to a risk factor must lead to suspicion of the diagnosis of AIDS. These risk factors include intravenous drug abuse, Haitian ancestry, homosexuality, exposure to infectious material from a person with AIDS or with an AIDS risk factor (e.g., blood transfusion), or having a mother with risk factors. It has been suggested that infants or children be considered to have AIDS if they have: (1) a risk factor associated with AIDS, (2) polyclonal hypergammaglobuline-mia, (3) T cell immunodeficiency, and (4) evidence of infection with AIDS-associated retrovirus. The distinctive immunologic profile of T cell immunodeficiency associated with polyclonal hypergammaglobulinemia and antibody to AIDS-associated retrovirus is not found in other primary or secondary immunodeficiency disorders.

The laboratory studies most useful in the diagnosis of AIDS include quantitative measurement of immunoglobulin levels to detect the elevated levels of IgG, IgM, and/or IgA; examination of peripheral blood mononuclear response to mitogen or antigens to detect T cell immunodeficiency; and quantitation of helper and suppressor T cells to determine if a reduced helper/suppressor cell ratio is present (see also Sec. 10.2). Most patients with AIDS fail to make specific antibody following immunization. Additional immunologic abnormalities include the presence of circulating immune complexes, decreased lymphocyte cytotoxicity, decreased production of interleukin 2 and interferon, and decreased natural killer cell activity.

Prevention. In most risk groups it is difficult to prevent AIDS. A mother with risk factors associated with AIDS may have one or more infected offspring, and once she is infected she may become a chronic carrier. Many of the blood donors who have risk factors associated with AIDS are relatively asymptomatic and may consider themselves to be "normal."

Reducing exposure to the infectious agent is essential. Most blood banks have instituted screening programs to exclude as blood donors persons with AIDS-associated risk factors. Antibody testing for AIDS-associated retrovirus (HTLV-III, LAV, ARV) has been instituted in most blood banks. Screening is effective in detecting antibody, but it does not detect donors who may be antigen (virus) positive and antibody negative. Methods are being investigated to inactivate retrovirus in factor VIII concentrate in an attempt to reduce the risk to patients with hemophilia. It is hoped that recombinant DNA factor VIII therapy will become available for treatment of hemophilia. The physician should advise patients with risk factors associated with AIDS that these contribute to the development of a potentially fatal disease for which there is no treatment. Appropriate changes in life style should then be undertaken. Recent evidence suggests that AIDS may be transmitted by heterosexual intercourse, but there is as yet no evidence that AIDS is transmitted by means of saliva or other secretions or excretions.

Treatment. AIDS is an irreversible disease. Supportive measures are required for the treatment of opportunistic infection (Sec. 11.11) and for the prevention of additional infections (Table 10–8), which may further compromise the patient. Measures necessary for isolation and identification of the cause of infection may include open lung biopsy; this is the best means of establishing a diagnosis of *Pneumocystis carinii* pneumonia (Sec. 13.68), a primary cause of interstitial pneumonia in patients with AIDS. *Pneumocystis carinii* infection should be treated with pentamidine and trimethoprim/sulfamethoxazole. Combination therapy is felt by many investigators to be more effective than the use of a single agent. Patients with AIDS should be treated prophylactically with trimethoprim/sulfamethoxazole from the time of diagnosis. A high percentage of patients with AIDS develop a maculopapular rash, cytopenia, and fever when receiving trimethoprim/sulfamethoxazole. These reactions may be so severe as to prevent the use of this agent either in therapy or prophylaxis. Interstitial pneumonia may also be caused by cytomegalovirus or Epstein-Barr virus. Life-threatening chronic diarrhea with *Cryptosporidium* may also occur (Sec. 11.103).

Chronic candidosis may be resistant to standard antifungal agents and require treatment with ketoconazole; this agent must be used cautiously, since it may produce hepatitis.

Table 10–8. Principal Agents of Infection of Patients with Acquired Immunodeficiency Syndrome (AIDS)

Viruses
AIDS-related retrovirus (HIV, HTLV-III, LAV, ARV)
Herpesvirus (types 1 and 2)
Cytomegalovirus
Varicella
Adenovirus
Epstein-Barr
Hepatitis B

Fungi
Candida albicans
Cryptococcus neoformans

Protozoa
Pneumocystis carinii
Toxoplasma gondii
Isospora sp (including *I. cryptosporidium*)
Giardia lamblia
Entamoeba histolytica

Other Microorganisms
Mycobacteria
Mycobacterium tuberculosis
M. avium intracellulare
M. kansasii
Legionella sp

Spirochetes
Treponema sp (including *T. pallidum*)

Bacteria
Campylobacter sp
Neisseria sp (including *N. gonorrhoeae*)
Shigella sp
Salmonella sp
Streptococcus pneumoniae
Staphylococcus aureus
Various gram negative organisms

Amphotericin B is needed for severe systemic fungal infections. Children with AIDS have an increased incidence of severe bacterial infections due to *Streptococcus pneumoniae*, various gram-negative organisms, *Staphylococcus aureus*, and other agents. Intravenous administration of gamma globulin, 100–200 mg/kg monthly, may help prevent both bacterial and viral infections. Supportive measures should address such results of chronic infection as anemia, thrombocytopenia, weight loss, and malnutrition. As in patients with primary immunodeficiency disease, all blood products administered to patients with AIDS should be irradiated to prevent graft versus host reaction and should have a negative test for antibodies to cytomegalovirus. Routine childhood immunizations should be avoided in patients with AIDS.

Attempts to correct the immunologic abnormalities of patients with AIDS through bone marrow transplantation or the use of thymic factors and interleukin 2 have been unsuccessful. Several experimental antiviral agents are under investigation. Most of these, such as azidothymidine, are inhibitors of reverse transcriptase.

Prognosis. Long-term follow-up of patients with AIDS indicates that the mortality approaches 80–90% at the end of three years; the rate in infants is similar to that in adults. Prolonged survival may occur in patients with limited manifestations, such as chronic lymphadenopathy.

Counseling. Susceptibility to AIDS has not been associated with any specific genetic factor such as histocompatibility antigens. The occurrence of the disease in more than one child in a family suggests vertical transmission of an infectious agent rather than horizontal transmission or a genetic factor. Infants born to mothers with risk factors for AIDS should be evaluated periodically for at least 5 yr to determine if they have antibody to AIDS-associated retrovirus or if they have developed immunologic abnormalities; in either case, appropriate prophylactic measures should be instituted.

ARTHUR J. AMMANN

Ammann AJ: Is there an acquired immune deficiency syndrome in infants and children? Pediatrics 72(3):430, 1983.
Ammann AJ, Schiffman G, Abrams D, et al: B cell immunodeficiency in acquired immunodeficiency syndrome. JAMA 251:1447, 1984.

Curran JW, Lawrence DN, Jaffe H, et al: Acquired immunodeficiency syndrome (AIDS) associated with transfusions. N Engl J Med 310:492, 1984.
Gallo RC, Salahuddin SZ, Shearer GM, et al: Frequent detection and isolation of cytopathic retroviruses (HTLV-III) from patients with AIDS and at risk for AIDS. Science 224:500, 1984.
Oleske JM, Minnefor AB, Cooper R, et al: Immune deficiency syndrome in children. JAMA 249(17):2345, 1983.
Rubinstein AM, Sicklick A, Gupta L, et al: Acquired immunodeficiency with reversed T4/T8 ratios in infants born to promiscuous and drug addicted mothers. JAMA 249:2350, 1983.
Scott GB, Buck BE, Letterman JG, et al: Acquired immunodeficiency syndrome in infants. N Engl J Med 310:76, 1984.

COMPLEMENT AND ASSOCIATED DISEASES

10.24 COMPLEMENT

It was noted in the late 19th century that certain bacteria could be killed in vitro by fresh serum from animals immunized against the organism. Serum heated to 56° C for 30 min or allowed to age for several days at room temperature, however, lost its bactericidal capacity although its antibodies were retained. Addition to the heated serum of small amounts of fresh serum from unimmunized animals (itself incapable of effecting killing) restored bactericidal ability. Thus, bacteriolysis was shown to require both specific antibody and a nonspecific, heat-labile principle, now termed *complement*. Within a few years it was known that complement consisted of more than one factor; by the 1960's nine components were known, one of which had three subcomponents. By the early 1970's a second major pathway of activation of complement, the *alternative* or *properdin pathway*, had been described. The latter system contains three unique factors. In addition, five regulators that control activity of either or both pathways have been identified in serum, and two such regulatory proteins have been found on the surface of cells. The original system of 11 factors is now referred to as the classical pathway of complement. The term *complement system* generally refers to both pathways, which interact and depend upon each other for their full activity. All of the 19 serum components and regulators are proteins. Together they make up about 10% of the globulin fraction of serum.

Increasing knowledge of the components of complement and their biochemistry has led to our understanding that the system acts as the principal mediator of the inflammatory response and plays an essential role in host defense against infection.

Nomenclature. The terminology applied to complement is cryptic but logical and consists of only a few rules: The components have been assigned numbers in the order of their discovery and are preceded by the letter C. Unfortunately, the first four components do not interact in the sequence in which they were discovered, but rather in the order C1423. The remaining components react in the appropriate numerical order, C56789. C1 has 3 subcomponents, C1q, C1r, and C1s. Fragments of components resulting from cleavage by other components acting as enzymes are assigned small letters (a, b, c, d, or e); with the exception of C2 fragments, the smaller piece that is released into surrounding fluids is assigned the letter "a," and the major part of the molecule, bound to other components or to some part of the immune complex, is assigned "b," e.g., C3a and C3b. When a component is activated (becomes an active enzyme), a bar is placed above the number, e.g., $C\bar{1}$.

Components of the alternative pathway have been assigned letters: B, D, and P (properdin). Factor B has an active form denoted $\overline{Bb}$. C3 (in particular, its major fragment, C3b) is a component of both the classical and alternative pathways.

General Concepts. Complement is a *system* of interacting proteins. The biologic functions of the system depend upon the interaction of individual components, which occurs in sequential fashion. This has been referred to as a "cascade," in analogy to the clotting system of blood; activation of each component (except the 1st) depends upon activation of the prior component or components in the sequence.

Interaction occurs along two pathways: the classical pathway, in the order antigen-antibody-C142356789; and the alternative pathway, in the order activator-(antibody)-properdin system-C356789. Antibody accelerates the rate of activation of the alternative pathway, but some activation can occur on appropriate surfaces in the absence of antibody. The classical and the alternative pathways interact with each other through the ability of both to activate C3.

The interaction of the early-acting components of complement (C1423) results in the generation of a series of active enzymes, $C\bar{1}$, $C\overline{42}$, and $C\overline{423}$. Thus, "activation" refers to transformation of the component into part of an active enzyme. In contrast, the interaction among C5b, C6, C7, C8, and C9 is nonenzymatic. In the case of C1, activation is a result of its interaction with antibody. Activation of C4, C2, C3, and C5, as well as factor B of the alternative pathway, is secondary to cleavage by a preceding component or components. Thus, activation of early components generates enzymes that fix to the antigen-antibody complex and catalyze a reaction on the next component, whereas later acting components (C6-C9) adsorb to the complex or the underlying cell by an interaction that depends on a change in their configuration.

These basic principles can be illustrated by a more detailed analysis of the activation sequence.

Sequence of Activation. The sequence in which the components of the classical pathway interact, the interdigitation between classical and alternative pathways, the chemical and some functional by-products of these reactions, and the regulators of the system are summarized in Figure 10–2.

The sequence begins with fixation of C1, by way of C1q, to the Fc (Sec. 10.1), nonantigen-binding part of the antibody molecule after antigen-antibody interaction. The C1 tricomplex changes configuration, and the C1s subcomponent becomes an active enzyme, "$C\bar{1}$ esterase."

C-reactive protein (CRP), which reacts with "C carbohydrate" from microorganisms and is elevated in certain inflammatory states, can substitute for antibody in the fixation of C1q and initiate reaction of the entire sequence. Thus, C-reactive protein functions like antibody though it can combine with only a few specific "antigens" and its size and structure are quite different. This reaction has the potential of initiating inflammation in the absence of antibody. Other agents that can activate C1 directly, without a requirement for antibody, include certain RNA viruses, uric acid crystals, the lipid A component of bacterial endotoxin, and the membranes of certain intracellular organelles.

In the next two steps of the classical pathway, polypeptide fragments are split from C4 and C2 during their activation

THE COMPLEMENT SYSTEM

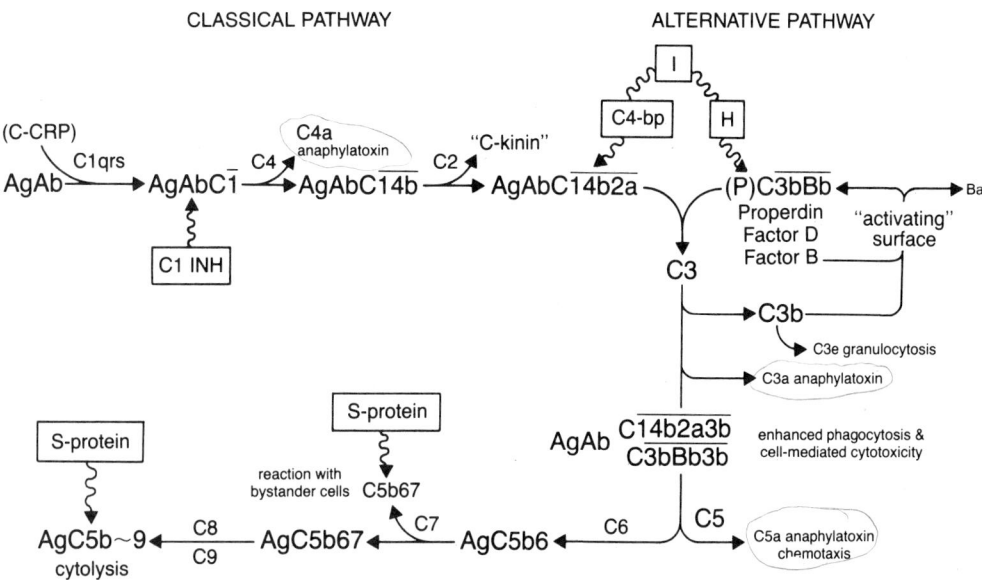

Figure 10–2. Sequence of activation of the components of the classical pathway of complement and interaction with the alternative pathway. Ag = antigen (bacterium, virus, tumor cell, or erythrocyte); Ab = antibody (IgG or IgM classes only); C-CRP = C carbohydrate–C-reactive protein; C1 INH = C1 inhibitor; I = factor I, C3b inactivator; C4-bp = C4-binding protein; H = factor H, β1H. Regulator proteins are each enclosed in a box.

and fixation by the enzymatic action of C1. One of these appears to be a kinin-like peptide that can induce vascular permeability and edema through direct action on postcapillary venules. The peptide C4a has *anaphylatoxin* activity; it reacts with mast cells to release the chemical mediators of immediate hypersensitivity, including histamine. Fixation of C4b to the complex permits it to adhere to a variety of mammalian cells, including neutrophils, monocytes, and erythrocytes, a phenomenon termed *immune adherence.*

Cleavage of C3 and generation of C3b is the next step in the sequence and the most crucial in terms of biologic activity. Cleavage of C3 can be achieved through C142, the "C3 convertase" of the classical pathway, or through the C3 convertase of the alternative pathway, C3bBb (see below). Once fixed to the complex, C3b permits adherence of the antigen-antibody complex to cells with receptors for C3b (complement receptor 1, CR1), including B lymphocytes, erythrocytes, and phagocytic cells (neutrophils, monocytes, and macrophages), leading, in the last case, to phagocytosis. Without C3 bound to them, phagocytosis of most microorganisms in vitro, especially by neutrophils, is very inefficient. The severe pyogenic infections that occur commonly in C3-deficient patients indicate that without C3, phagocytosis is also inefficient in vivo. The biologic activity of C3b is controlled by cleavage by factor I (C3b inactivator) to C3bi, which is further degraded by factor I and serum or tissue enzymes to C3c, which is released, and C3d, which stays bound. C3bi promotes phagocytosis on binding to the C3bi receptor (CR3) on phagocytes. A receptor for C3d (CR2) exists on B lymphocytes and K cells. Further cleavage of C3c creates C3e, which induces release of granulocytes from bone marrow.

The peptide C3a, generated when C3 is acted upon by either pathway, has anaphylatoxin activity. The action of C423 or of the alternative pathway "C5 convertase" on C5 releases C5a, a powerful anaphylatoxin that can react with neutrophils, macrophages, mast cells, smooth muscle cells, and certain T cells to induce release of a variety of mediators of inflammation. This same peptide serves as a potent chemical attractant for phagocytic cells.

The "membrane-attack" sequence leading to cytolysis begins with the attachment of C5b to C423, the C5-activating

enzyme (or to the alternative pathway enzyme). C6 is bound to C5b without being cleaved, stabilizing the activated C5b fragment. The C5b6 complex then dissociates from C423 and reacts with C7. C5b67 complexes must attach to the cell membrane promptly or lose their activity and remain in the fluid phase. Next, C8 binds, and the C5b678 complex then promotes the addition of multiple C9 molecules. The C9 polymer of 12–18 molecules forms a transmembrane channel, and lysis ensues.

Control mechanisms act at several points to prevent the system's consuming itself in activity that is unnecessary or deleterious to the host. An α-2 globulin, C1 inhibitor (C1 INH), inhibits C1s enzymatic activity and, thus, the cleavage of C4 and C2. Activated C2 has a half-life of about 8 min at 37° C, and this relative instability limits the effective life of C42 and C423. The alternative pathway enzyme that activates C3, C3bBb, also has a short half-life, though it can be prolonged by the binding of properdin (P) to the enzyme complex. Serum contains the protein "anaphylatoxin inactivator," an enzyme that cleaves the carboxyterminal arginine from both C3a and C5a, thereby markedly reducing their anaphylatoxic activity and the chemotactic activity of C5a. Factor I inactivates C4b and C3b, thus serving as an important means of controlling both pathways. Factor H(β1H) accelerates inactivation of C3b by I. An analogous factor, C4 binding protein (C4-bp), accelerates cleavage of C4b by factor I. Two protein constituents of cell membranes, CR1 and decay accelerating factor (DAF), promote the disruption of C3 and C5 convertases assembled on those membranes. Serum lipoproteins or circulating C8 can inhibit attachment of the C5b67 complex to cell membranes. Attachment to the cell can be inhibited by the binding to C5b67 of S-protein, so called because it interacts with the membrane binding site (S) of the C5b67 complex. S-protein also inhibits the polymerization of C9, which limits the formation of the transmembrane channel and, thereby, lysis.

Alternative Pathway. The alternative pathway can be activated by C3b generated through classical pathway activity, through leukocyte proteases released by degranulation, or perhaps through activation of thrombin or plasmin during blood coagulation. It can also be activated by a form of C3 created by low grade, spontaneous reaction of native C3 with a molecule of water, which occurs constantly in plasma. Once formed, C3b or this hydrolyzed C3 can bind to any nearby cell or to factor B. Factor B attached to C3b in the plasma or on the surface of a particle can be cleaved to Bb by D, which exists as an active proteolytic enzyme. The complex C3bBb becomes an efficient C3 convertase, which generates more C3b through an "amplification loop" (Fig 10–2). P can bind to C3bBb, increasing stability of the enzyme and protecting it from inactivation by factors I and H, which serve to modulate the loop. Cleavage of B releases Ba, which has weak chemotactic activity.

Certain materials promote alternative pathway activation if C3b is fixed to their surface, e.g., teichoic acid from bacterial cell wall, endotoxic lipopolysaccharide, or immunoglobulin aggregates, especially of the IgA class. This activation depends on the ability of the C3bBb enzyme complex to escape the efficient control otherwise exercised by factors I and H. The surface of rabbit red blood cells also protects C3bBb from inactivation. This phenomenon serves as the basis for an assay of serum alternative pathway activity. Endotoxin may alter normally "nonactivating" cell surfaces in vivo so that C3bBb is relatively protected from inactivation, which may partially explain the activation of the alternative pathway in patients with gram-negative bacteremia. Sialic acid on the surface of microorganisms or cells prevents formation of an effective alternative pathway C3 convertase by promoting activity of I and H.

Although C3bBb can activate C3 efficiently on only a limited variety of surfaces, significant activation of C3 can occur through this pathway, and the resultant biologic activities are qualitatively the same as those achieved through activation by C142, as illustrated in Figure 10–2.

Participation in Host Defense. Specific activities of the complement system in host defense against infection are summarized in Table 10–9. Neutralization of virus by antibody can be enhanced with C1 and C4. When antibody concentrations are low, the additional fixation of C3b to the viral antigen-antibody complex through the classical or alternative pathway improves neutralization; C5 and C6 add little to the effect. Complement may, therefore, be particularly important in the early phases of a viral infection when antibody is limited. Antibody and complement can also eliminate infectivity of at least some viruses, with the production of typical complement "holes" in the virus, as seen by electron microscopy. Animal RNA tumor viruses interact directly with human C1q in the absence of antibody with resulting activation of the classical pathway and lysis of the virus. This may be a natural resistance mechanism that limits the infectivity of these viruses in man.

Table 10–9. **Activities of Complement**

Components or Fragments	Functional Activity
C14, C1423	Neutralization of viruses
C4a, C3a, C5a	"Anaphylatoxin" (mediator release, capillary dilation)
C3a	Suppression of antibody response
C3b	Opsonization; enhancement of cell-mediated cytotoxicity; solubilization of immune complexes
C3 cleavage product (C3e)	Induction of granulocytosis
C5a	Chemotaxis of neutrophils, monocytes, eosinophils; enhancement of antibody response
C1 ~ 5 (? additional components)	Endotoxin inactivation
C1 ~ 9	Lysis of viruses, virus-infected cells, tumor cells, mycoplasma, protozoa, spirochetes, and bacteria

C4a, C3a, and C5a can bind to mast cells and leukocytes and thereby trigger release of histamine and other mediators, leading to vasodilatation and to the swelling and redness of inflammation. C5a is the major chemical stimulus for the influx into inflammatory sites of neutrophils, monocytes, and eosinophils, all of which can efficiently phagocytize microorganisms coated (opsonized) with C3b. Inactivation of cell-bound C3b by cleavage to C3d removes its opsonizing activity. Fixation of C3b to a target cell can enhance its lysis by a "killer" cell in an antibody-dependent, cell-mediated cytotoxicity system.

Insoluble immune complexes can be solubilized in vitro by incubation in complement, apparently by disruption of the orderly antigen-antibody lattice by C3b. This finding is probably related to the immune complex disease found in patients who lack C1, C4, C2, or C3.

The complement system may be involved in certain aspects of B and T lymphocyte-mediated specific immunity. Binding of C3b- and C3d-coated particles to B lymphocytes can be shown in vitro. C3a appears to suppress antibody formation, whereas C5a appears to enhance this response. C3e, a cleavage product generated during the inactivation of C3, induces an increase in circulating granulocytes.

Neutralization of endotoxin in vitro and protection from its lethal effects in experimental animals require later-acting components of complement, at least through C6. Finally, activation of the entire complement sequence can result in lysis of virus-infected cells, tumor cells, and most types of microorganisms. Bactericidal activity of complement has not appeared to be important to host defense except for the occurrence of infections with *Neisseria* in patients lacking later-acting components of complement (Sec. 10.25).

Fearon DT: Complement. J Allergy Clin Immunol 71:520, 1983.
Hugli TE: Complement and cellular triggering reactions. Fed Proc 43:2540, 1984.
Müller-Eberhard HJ, Miescher PA: Complement. Berlin, Springer-Verlag, 1985.
Pangburn MK: Activation of complement via the alternative pathway. Fed Proc 42:139, 1983.
Smith TF, Johnston RB Jr: The complement system: Implications for pediatrics. In: Moss AJ (ed): Pediatrics Update. New York, Elsevier, 1981, p. 305.

DISEASES OF THE COMPLEMENT SYSTEM

10.25 PRIMARY DEFICIENCIES OF COMPLEMENT COMPONENTS

Congenital deficiencies of all 11 component proteins of the classical pathway and of factor D of the alternative pathway have been described (Table 10–10).

Complete **deficiency of C1q** has been detected in children with a syndrome of septicemia or meningitis, skin infections, and a florid maculopapular rash. Biopsies of the rash have shown deposition of immune complexes in the basal epidermis or walls of small blood vessels. **C1q dysfunction** has been found in persons with complete deficiency of C1q activity but only partially decreased amounts of an antigenically altered C1q molecule in their sera. Some family members have had a systemic lupus erythematosus-like syndrome; others were healthy.

Patients with C1q, C1r, C1s, C3, C4, and C2 **deficiencies** have had a high incidence of vasculitis syndromes (Table 10–10), especially systemic lupus erythematosus or a lupus-like syndrome in which antinuclear antibody may be undetectable. A few patients with **C3, C5, C6, C7, or C8 deficiency** have had such a disorder, but recurrent infections are much more likely to be the major problem in this group. The reason for the concurrence of deficiencies of components of complement and these "autoimmune" diseases is not known; but if these diseases originate as infections, the association may be a

Table 10–10. **Genetic Deficiencies of Complement Components**

Deficient Component	Associated Clinical Findings	
	*Collagen-Vascular Disease**	*Infections*
C1q	SLE, dermal vasculitis, MPGN, DLE	Recurrent bacterial, fungal—dermatitis, meningitis
C1q dysfunction	SLE	
C1r	CGN, SLE, dermal vasculitis	Pneumonia,† meningitis†
C1s	SLE	
C4	SLE, H-S purpura,† Sjögren syndrome†	Bacteremia,† meningitis†
C2	SLE, DLE, CGN, MPGN, H-S purpura, dermal vasculitis, dermatomyositis†, ITP†	Recurrent septicemia, especially pneumococcal; meningitis; pneumonia
C3	MPGN, SLE, dermal vasculitis	Severe, generalized bacterial
C5	SLE†	Disseminated gonococcal or meningococcal; pyoderma†; meningitis†
C6	SLE,† DLE,† MPGN,† Sjögren syndrome†	Disseminated gonococcal or meningococcal
C7	SLE,† scleroderma,† ankylosing spondylitis,† RA†	Disseminated gonococcal and/or meningococcal
C8	SLE†	Disseminated gonococcal or meningococcal
C9		Meningococcal meningitis†
Factor D		Recurrent sinusitis, bronchitis; bronchiectasis

*CGN = chronic glomerulonephritis; DLE = discoid lupus erythematosus; H-S = Henoch-Schönlein; ITP = idiopathic thrombocytopenic purpura; MPGN = membranoproliferative glomerulonephritis; RA = rheumatoid arthritis; SLE = systemic lupus erythematosus.
†Finding reported uncommonly in patients with this deficiency.

result of absence of one or more of the host defense properties described in Table 10–9. Complement facilitates elimination of immune complexes; inefficiency of this process is an alternative explanation.

Several patients with **C2 deficiency** have had repeated life-threatening septicemic illnesses, most commonly due to pneumococci. Most have not had problems with increased susceptibility to infection, presumably because of the protective function of the alternative pathway. A depression of factor B levels to about 50% of normal can occur in conjunction with C2 deficiency, however, and persons with deficiency of both proteins might be at particular risk.

Since C3 can be activated by C142 or by the alternative pathway, a defect in the function of either pathway can be compensated, at least to some extent. Without C3, however, the chemotactic fragment from C5 is not generated, and opsonization of bacteria is inefficient. Some organisms must be well opsonized in order to be cleared, and **congenital absence of C3** has been associated with recurrent, severe pyogenic infections due to pneumococci and meningococci. Some C3-deficient patients have had sluggish neutrophilic responses to infection, in agreement with reports that C3e, a cleavage factor of C3, elicits an increase in blood neutrophils.

The first patient found to have homozygous **C5 deficiency** was a girl who developed classic systemic lupus erythematosus in late childhood and had a lifelong history of recurrent pyogenic infections, especially of the skin, perhaps because of the absence of the critical chemotactic factor split from C5. Generation of chemotaxis by her serum in vitro was markedly depressed. Other patients have had recurrent disseminated gonococcal infection or multiple episodes of meningococcal meningitis. Some infants with Leiner disease (generalized seborrheic dermatitis, severe diarrhea, and recurrent infections due to enteric bacteria and staphylococci) have had **dysfunction of C5,** with decreased opsonization of yeast by their serum. Serum from these infants had normal hemolytic complement activity, but purified C5 from 1 patient behaved abnormally in special studies of this component. The defect appears to be familial.

About half of the approximately 90 individuals reported to have congenital **C6, C7,** or **C8** deficiencies have had meningococcal meningitis or extragenital gonococcal infection. About 10% have had a collagen-vasular disease. It is not clear why patients with deficiency of one of the late-acting components suffer a particular predisposition to neisserial infections; it may be that serum bacteriolysis is uniquely important in defense against this organism, but some persons with such a deficiency have had no significant illness.

Identical twin sisters had **isolated deficiency of factor D** of the alternative pathway. Both had recurrent sinusitis and bronchitis; one also had bronchiectasis. Hemolytic complement activity in their serum was normal, but alternative pathway activity was markedly deficient.

C1q dysfunction and deficiencies of C1r, C4, C2, C3, C5, C6, C7, C8, C9, factor I, and factor H appear to be transmitted as an "autosomal codominant" trait; i.e., each parent transmits a gene that codes for synthesis of half the serum level of the component. The mode of transmission of C1q and C1s deficiency has not been clear. Properdin deficiency appears to be transmitted as an X-linked trait.

10.26 PRIMARY DEFICIENCIES OF COMPLEMENT CONTROL PROTEINS

Congenital deficiencies of five proteins (four serum and one cell-associated) that control activity of the complement system have been described (Table 10–11).

Factor I deficiency was originally reported as a deficiency of C3 due to its hypercatabolism. The first patient described had suffered a series of severe pyogenic infections similar to those seen with agammaglobulinemia or congenital deficiency of C3. Further studies indicated that the primary deficiency was that of factor I, an essential regulator of the alternative pathway. This deficiency permits prolonged existence of C3b in the C3 convertase of the alternative pathway, $\overline{C3bBb}$, resulting in constant activation of the alternative pathway and cleavage of more C3 to C3b, in circular fashion. Intravenous infusion of plasma or purified factor I induced a prompt rise in serum C3 concentration in the patient and a return to

Table 10–11. **Genetic Deficiencies of Complement Control Proteins**

Deficient Component*	Associated Clinical Findings†
C1 INH	Angioedema, SLE
Factor I	Severe pyogenic infections
Factor H	Hemolytic-uremic syndrome
Properdin	Meningococcal meningitis
C3b receptor (CR1)‡	SLE

*INH = inhibitor.
†SLE = systemic lupus erythematosus.
‡CR1 = complement receptor 1.

normal of in vitro C3-dependent functions such as opsonization.

One of the first reported patients with **factor H deficiency** had hemolytic-uremic syndrome; the other was healthy. Persons with **properdin deficiency** have had a predisposition to meningococcal meningitis. All reported patients have been male, and their families have had a striking history of male deaths due to meningitis. The predisposition to infection in these patients indicates a requirement for the alternative pathway in host defense against bacterial infection. This predisposition does not exist in the presence of antibody since the classical pathway is normal in their serum. Neither the patients nor members of their families have had collagen-vascular disease.

The receptor for C3b (complement receptor 1, CR1) on cell surface membranes assists in the disruption of C4b- or C3b-bearing immune complexes that the cell encounters in the plasma or on the surface of adjacent cells. Patients with systemic lupus erythematosus (SLE) and their asymptomatic family members have a partial **deficiency of CR1,** which appears to be inherited as an autosomal codominant trait. This deficiency could increase the risk of developing immune complex disease and, thereby, contribute to the pathogenesis of SLE.

Hereditary angioedema occurs in persons born without the ability to synthesize normally functioning C1 inhibitor. In 85% of affected families the affected members have markedly reduced concentrations of inhibitor (5–30% of normal); in the other 15% normal or elevated concentrations of an immunologically cross-reacting but nonfunctional protein occur. Both forms of the disease are transmitted as autosomal dominant traits.

In the absence of this α_2-globulin, activation of C1 leads to uncontrolled $\overline{C1s}$ activity, with breakdown of C4 and C2 and release of a vasoactive peptide (kinin) from one or both of these substrates. Episodic, localized, nonpitting edema results from the vasodilatory effects of the kinin on the postcapillary venule. The mechanism by which C1 is activated in these patients is not known.

Swelling of the affected part accumulates rapidly, without urticaria, itching, discoloration, or redness, and often without severe pain. Swelling of the intestinal wall, however, can lead to intense abdominal cramping, sometimes with vomiting or diarrhea; concurrent subcutaneous edema is often absent, and patients have undergone abdominal surgery or psychiatric examination before the true diagnosis was made. Laryngeal edema can be fatal. Attacks last 2–3 days, then gradually abate. They may occur at sites of trauma, after vigorous exercise, with menses, or with emotional stress. Attacks can begin in the first 2 yr of life but are usually not severe until late childhood or adolescence. The condition can be acquired in association with lymphoid cancer. Systemic lupus erythematosus has been reported in patients with the congenital disease (Sec. 10.27 and 10.28).

10.27 SECONDARY DEFICIENCIES OF COMPLEMENT

Partial deficiency of C1q has occurred in patients with *severe combined immunodeficiency disease* or *hypogammaglobulinemia*, apparently secondary to the deficiency of IgG, which normally binds reversibly to C1q and prevents its rapid catabolism.

Serum from patients with *chronic membranoproliferative glomerulonephritis* contains a protein termed *nephritic factor* (NeF) that promotes activation of the alternative pathway. Nephritic factor is an IgG antibody to the C3-cleaving enzyme of the alternative pathway, $\overline{C3bBb}$, that protects the enzyme from inactivation. The result is increased consumption of C3. Serum C3 concentrations vary widely from patient to patient, how-

ever. Pyogenic infections, including meningitis, may occur if the serum C3 level drops below about 10% of normal. This disorder has been found in children and adults with *partial lipodystrophy*. It is not known whether the lipodystrophy is a cause or a result of the NeF-C3 abnormality. An IgG nephritic factor that binds to and protects $\overline{C42}$, the classical pathway C3 convertase, has been described in *acute postinfectious nephritis* and in *systemic lupus erythematosus*. The consumption of C3 that characterizes poststreptococcal nephritis and lupus could be due to this factor, to activation of complement by immune complexes, or to both.

Newborn infants are known to have mild to moderate deficiencies of most components of the classical pathway of complement and of factor B and properdin. Opsonization and generation of chemotactic activity in serum from full-term newborns can be markedly deficient through either the classical or the alternative pathway. Complement activity is even lower in preterm infants than in full-term babies. Patients with *malnutrition* or *anorexia nervosa* may also have significant depletion of components and functional activity of complement. Although synthesis of components is depressed in these conditions, serum from some patients with malnutrition also appears to contain immune complexes that could accelerate depletion. Severe chronic *cirrhosis of the liver* may also result in decreased synthesis of C3.

Patients with *sickle cell disease* have normal activity of the classical pathway, but some have defective function of the alternative pathway in opsonization of pneumococci, in bacteriolysis and opsonization of salmonellae, and in lysis of rabbit erythrocytes. Similar defects have been described in about 10% of individuals who have undergone *splenectomy* and in some patients with β-*thalassemia major*. The underlying mechanism for the defects in alternative pathway function in these disorders has not been fully defined. Children with *nephrotic syndrome* may have subnormal serum opsonizing activity in association with decreased serum levels of factor B.

Immune complexes, including those initiated by microorganisms or their by-products, may induce consumption of components of complement. Activation occurs primarily through fixation of C1 to antibody and, thereby, initiation of the classical pathway. In *systemic lupus erythematosus*, immune complexes activate the classical pathway, and C3 is deposited at sites of tissue damage, including kidneys and skin; depressed synthesis of C3 is also seen. Formation of immune complexes and consumption of complement have been demonstrated in *lepromatous leprosy, subacute bacterial endocarditis, infected ventriculojugular shunts, malaria, infectious mononucleosis, dengue hemorrhagic fever,* and *acute hepatitis B*. Nephritis or arthritis may develop as a result of deposition of immune complexes and activation of complement in these infections. The syndrome of *recurrent urticaria, angioedema, eosinophilia, and hypocomplementemia* secondary to activation of the classical pathway may be due to circulating immune complexes. Circulating immune complexes and decreased C3 have been reported in some patients with *dermatitis herpetiformis, celiac disease, primary biliary cirrhosis,* and *Reye syndrome*.

In patients with *bacteremic shock*, bacterial products appear to initiate direct activation of the alternative pathway. *Intravenous injection of iodinated roentgenographic contrast medium* can induce a rapid and significant activation of the alternative pathway, which may explain at least some of the reactions that occur in 5–8% of patients undergoing this procedure.

Burns can induce massive activation of the complement system, especially the alternative pathway, within a few hours after injury. Generation of C3a and C5a occurs, which stimulates neutrophils and induces their sequestration in the lung. These events may play an important part in the development of shock lung after burn injury. *Post-perfusion syndrome* may have a similar pathogenesis, since cardiopulmonary bypass can activate serum complement, with release of C3a and C5a. In patients with *erythropoietic protoporphyria* or *porphyria cutanea tarda* exposure of the skin to light of certain wavelengths activates complement, generating chemotactic activity. Phototoxicity is associated histologically with lysis of capillary endothelial cells, mast cell degranulation, and the appearance of neutrophils in the dermis.

Paroxysmal nocturnal hemoglobinuria results from an acquired deficiency of decay-accelerating factor in a subpopulation of erythrocytes and leukocytes. In the absence of this membrane protein, C3b that is deposited on the cells from serum in continuous low-grade fashion is not efficiently broken down by factor I. This permits the alternative pathway C3 convertase, $C\overline{3bBb}$, to develop effectively on the cell surface; the membrane attack complex (C5~9) forms and lysis ensues.

10.28 DIAGNOSIS OF DISORDERS OF THE COMPLEMENT SYSTEM

Testing for total hemolytic complement activity (CH_{50}) is a useful screening procedure for most of the diseases of the complement system. A normal result in this assay depends on the ability of all 11 classical pathway component proteins to interact and lyse antibody-coated erythrocytes. The dilution of serum that lyses 50% of the cells determines the end point. In congenital deficiencies of C1 through C8, the CH_{50} value will be about 0; in C9 deficiency, the value will be approximately half normal. Values in the acquired deficiencies will, of course, vary with the severity of the underlying disorder. This assay will not detect deficiencies of the alternative pathway components B, D, or properdin. Deficiency of factors I or H (Sec. 10.25) will permit consumption of C3, with partial reduction in the CH_{50} value.

In *hereditary angioedema*, depression of C4 and C2 during an attack significantly reduces the CH_{50}. Serum concentrations of C4 and C3 can be determined by radial immunodiffusion. In hereditary angioedema, C4 is characteristically low and C3 normal. Concentrations of C1 inhibitor can be determined with antibody, but a normal result can be anticipated in about 15% of cases (Sec. 10.26). Since C1 acts as an esterase, the specific diagnosis can be made by showing increased capacity of patients' sera to hydrolyze synthetic esters.

Decreased serum concentrations of both C4 and C3 suggest activation of the classical pathway by immune complexes. In contrast, decreased C3 and normal C4 levels suggest activation of the alternative pathway. This difference is particularly useful in distinguishing nephritis secondary to complex deposition from that due to NeF (nephritic factor). In the latter condition and in deficiency of factor I, factor B is consumed, and its serum concentration is low as measured by radial immunodiffusion. Alternative pathway activity can be measured with a relatively simple and reproducible hemolytic assay that depends on the capacity of rabbit erythrocytes to serve as both an "activating" (permissive) surface and a target of alternative pathway activity.

A defect of complement function should be suspected in any patient with collagen-vascular disease or chronic nephritis, or with recurrent pyogenic infections, neisserial infections, or septicemia. Complement disorders are frequently detected by means of the relatively simple hemolytic complement assay; this procedure should always be available as a screening test.

10.29 MANAGEMENT OF DISORDERS OF THE COMPLEMENT SYSTEM

Regular infusions of plasma have been an effective deterrent to infections in children with *C5 dysfunction*. Since these patients make C5 (though it is nonfunctional), they should not generate antibody that would nullify the effect of the infused C5 and perhaps induce anaphylaxis or a serum sickness reaction. The same argument might be invoked for the use of plasma infusions to treat the variant of the *hereditary angioedema* in which patients have nonfunctional C1 inhibitor, but substrate for C1 (C4 and C2, the source of vasoactive kinin) would be infused along with normal C1 inhibitor and might precipitate or accentuate an attack. Adults with this disease respond to danazol, a synthetic androgen with weak virilizing and mild anabolic potential. The drug, given orally, increases the level of C1 inhibitor 3- to 4-fold and prevents attacks. It has not been recommended for use in children.

Only supportive management is available for other primary diseases of the complement system. Purified components are not available, and if they were, the risk of inducing antibody to them would probably preclude their long-term use. It should be emphasized, however, that identification of a specific defect in the complement system may have an important impact on a patient's health. Concern for the associated complications (Table 10–10) should encourage vigorous diagnostic efforts and earlier institution of therapy, including the obtaining of cultures and institution of antibiotic treatment with the onset of unexplained fever. Immunization of the patient and family members with bacterial capsular polysaccharides should also be considered. As defects are carefully characterized, the likelihood of specific therapy may improve.

RICHARD B. JOHNSTON, JR.

Congenital Deficiencies

Altenburger KM, Johnston RB Jr: The complement system and its disorders in man. In: Chandra RK (ed): Primary and Secondary Immunodeficiency Disorders. Edinburgh, Churchill Livingstone, 1983, p. 113.

Donaldson VH, Rosen FS: Hereditary angioneurotic edema: A clinical survey. Pediatrics 37:1017, 1966.

Ellison RT III, Kohler PF, Curd JG, et al: Prevalence of congenital or acquired complement deficiency in patients with sporadic meningococcal disease. N Engl J Med 308:913, 1983.

Hosea SW, Santaella ML, Brown EJ, et al: Long-term therapy of hereditary angioedema with danazol. Ann Intern Med 93:809, 1980.

Hyatt AC, Altenburger KM, Johnston RB Jr, et al: Increased susceptibility to severe pyogenic infections in patients with an inherited deficiency of the second component of complement. J Pediatr 98:417, 1981.

Ross SC, Densen P: Complement deficiency states and infection: Epidemiology, pathogenesis and consequences of neisserial and other infections in an immune deficiency. Medicine 63:243, 1984.

Sjöholm AG, Braconier J-H, Söderström C: Properdin deficiency in a family with fulminant meningococcal infections. Clin Exp Immunol 50:291, 1982.

Thompson RA, Haeney M, Reid KBM, et al: A genetic defect of the C1q subcomponent of complement associated with childhood (immune complex) nephritis. N Engl J Med 303:22, 1980.

Wilson JG, Wong WW, Schur PH, et al: Mode of inheritance of decreased C3b receptors on erythrocytes of patients with systemic lupus erythematosus. N Engl J Med 307:981, 1982.

Secondary Deficiencies

Anderson DC, York TL, Rose G, et al: Assessment of serum factor B, serum opsonins, granulocyte chemotaxis, and infection in nephrotic syndrome of children. J Infect Dis 140:1, 1979.

Corry JM, Polhill RB Jr, Edmonds SR, et al: Activity of the alternative complement pathway after splenectomy: Comparison to activity in sickle cell disease and hypogammaglobulinemia. J Pediatr 95:964, 1979.

Edwards KM, Alford R, Gewurz H, et al: Recurrent bacterial infections associated with C3 nephritic factor and hypocomplementemia. N Engl J Med 308:1138, 1983.

Gelfand JA, Donelan M, Hawiger A, et al: Alternative complement pathway activation increases mortality in a model of burn injury in mice. J Clin Invest 70:1170, 1982.

Halbwachs L, Leveillé M, Lesavre PH, et al: Nephritic factor of the classical pathway of complement: Immunoglobulin G autoantibody directed against the classical pathway C3 convertase enzyme. J Clin Invest 65:1249, 1980.

Johnston RB Jr, Altenburger KM, Atkinson AW Jr, et al: Complement in the newborn infant. Pediatrics 64:781, 1979.

Lim HW, Poh-Fitzpatrick MB, Gigli I: Activation of the complement system in patients with porphyrias after irradiation in vivo. J Clin Invest 74:1961, 1984.

Nicholson-Weller A, March JP, Rosenfeld SI, et al: Affected erythrocytes of patients with paroxysmal nocturnal hemoglobinuria are deficient in the complement regulatory protein, decay accelerating factor. Proc Natl Acad Sci USA 80:566, 1983.

Notarangelo LD, Chirico G, Chiara A, et al: Activity of classical and alternative pathways of complement in preterm and small for gestational age infants. Pediatr Res 18:281, 1984.

THE PHAGOCYTIC SYSTEM AND ASSOCIATED DISEASES

10.30 PHYSIOLOGY OF THE PHAGOCYTIC SYSTEM

The phagocyte system consists of sessile mononuclear cells (macrophages) and circulating polymorphonuclear and mononuclear leukocytes. Adequate numbers of properly functioning phagocytes are critically important for host defense against microbial disease.

Source and Storage of Phagocytes. Phagocytic leukocytes develop from pluripotent stem cells in the bone marrow. Leukocytes and erythrocytes are produced at nearly equal rates, but the shorter life of leukocytes (hours instead of months) results in the usual 2000:1 erythrocyte:leukocyte ratio in the circulation. Polymorphonuclear neutrophils enter the circulation as highly differentiated mature phagocytes; monocytes, as immature cells. Both cell types circulate in the blood for a short time (4–10 hr) and migrate into tissues.

On leaving the circulation, mononuclear phagocytic cells develop into macrophages with unique morphologic and metabolic characteristics, depending on where they reside. Macrophages are present in the spleen, liver, lungs, lymph nodes, intestine, skin, kidneys, and central nervous system. Circulating mononuclear phagocytes also migrate into areas of inflammation, usually after infiltration by neutrophils, and are essential for "walling off" an infectious process and forming granulomas. Macrophages are the primary phagocytic cells in breast milk.

A large reserve of mature neutrophils is normally stored in the bone marrow and marginated in the circulation. Inflammation stimulates mobilization of these reserves and causes rapid multiplication of precursor cells and accelerated differentiation; enormous numbers of neutrophils are produced during acute infections. Circulating factors released from peripheral leukocytes regulate production and release of phagocytic cells by the bone marrow.

Chemotaxis. Neutrophils and monocytes respond to inflammatory stimuli by adherence to capillary walls and by diapedesis into tissues. Once in tissues, phagocytic cells respond to inflammatory mediators and/or microbial factors by increased activity (chemokinesis) and movement toward the highest concentration of chemoattractant (chemotaxis). Chemotaxis involves perturbation of sequential segments of cell membrane with shifts in calcium concentration and change in surface charge; cytoplasmic contractile proteins, actin and myosin, polymerize into microfilaments, and locomotion ensues. Once phagocytic cells reach a site of bacterial invasion, the invaders must be recognized as "non-self" and the complex process of phagocytosis begins.

Phagocytosis. Factors that prepare bacteria for phagocytosis are opsonins (primarily specific antibacterial antibodies and complement components) that neutralize antiphagocytic factors on bacterial surfaces and function as ligands, binding bacteria to phagocytes. Phagocytic cells have membrane receptors for the Fc portion of antibodies and for activated fragments of complement, primarily C3b and C3bi. When recognition and attachment occur, contractile proteins are activated, and microbes or other particles are surrounded by pseudopods. When the phagocytic cell membrane completely surrounds the particle, a phagocytic vacuole is formed which migrates toward the nucleus; granular contents are contributed to the phagocytic vacuoles, and oxidative metabolism is stimulated.

Oxygen is consumed during phagocytosis and is univalently reduced to superoxide or divalently reduced to hydrogen peroxide. There is a shift of glucose metabolism to the hexose monophosphate pathway, and halides are oxidized. The rapid killing of most bacterial and fungal species requires the interaction of reactive oxygen molecules, myeloperoxidase (a constituent of cytoplasmic granules), and halides within phagocytic vacuoles. Critical factors required for this microbicidal activity are oxygen, reduced pyridine nucleotides, oxidase activity with electron transport via flavoproteins, cytochrome b, and quinone. An intact oxidative response can be identified either by nitroblue tetrazolium reduction or by chemiluminescence. Figure 10–3 represents the metabolic changes in human polymorphonuclear neutrophils during phagocytosis.

DISEASES ASSOCIATED WITH DISORDERS OF THE PHAGOCYTES

10.31 CHRONIC GRANULOMATOUS DISEASE OF CHILDHOOD

Chronic granulomatous disease (CGD) is a syndrome of recurrent bacterial or fungal infections associated with defective microbicidal capacity of phagocytic cells and abnormal oxidative metabolic responses during phagocytosis. The morphology of the neutrophils and monocytes and specific humoral and cell-mediated immunity are normal in patients with CGD.

Etiology. CGD occurs in both boys and girls; abut 20% of reported patients are girls. There is evidence for X-linked inheritance in most boys with the disease: intermediate defects of neutrophil function are found in mothers and female relatives, among whom two populations of neutrophils can

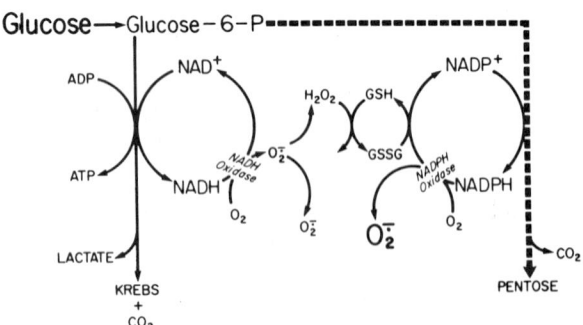

Microbicidal Metabolism of Phagocytes

Figure 10–3. Oxidative metabolic response during phagocytosis. Augmentation of hexose monophosphate shunt activity during phagocytosis is depicted by the heavy dashed line. Oxidase activity simulated during phagocytosis results in oxygen uptake, and electrons from NADH and NADPH result in production of superoxide (O_2^-) and hydrogen peroxide (H_2O_2). These reactive oxygen radicals are associated with the microbicidal activity of phagocytic cells.

ADP = adenosine diphosphate, ATP = adenosine triphosphate, GSH = reduced glutathione, GSSG = oxidized glutathione, KREBS = Krebs cycle, NAD = oxidized nicotinamide adenine dinucleotide, NADH = reduced nicotinamide adenine dinucleotide, NADP = oxidized nicotinamide adenine dinucleotide phosphate, NADPH = reduced nicotinamide adenine dinucleotide phosphate.

be distinguished on incubation with nitroblue tetrazolium (NBT). Carrier females rarely suffer severe infections, but several mothers of patients with CGD have had dermal infiltrates of lymphocytes similar to those seen in discoid lupus erythematosus.

The pattern of genetic transmission in most female patients with CGD appears to be autosomal recessive. When chemiluminescence is used as a measure of oxidative metabolism during phagocytosis, X-linked transmission in female as well as male patients with CGD is suggested. Markedly depressed neutrophil chemiluminescence (less than 2% of control) may be found in female patients, and their mothers and female relatives may have an intermediate chemiluminescence response during phagocytosis. Fathers and unaffected male siblings are always normal.

The Lyon hypothesis could explain X-linked transmission in females with CGD. Two distinct populations of neutrophils have been identified using the histochemical NBT dye reduction assay or autoradiographic technique for detection of bacterial iodination during phagocytosis in mothers of both male and female patients with CGD. Disproportionate inactivation of the normal X chromosome may result in a large population of defective phagocytic cells and clinical manifestations of CGD in females.

Certain patients with CGD lack Kell antigens on their erythrocytes (MacLeod phenotype), a condition making it exceedingly difficult to obtain compatible blood for transfusion; boys lack Kell antigen on their leukocytes, a deficiency suggesting that Kell antigens may be closely associated with membrane factors activating oxidative metabolism in phagocytic cells. Male patients with CGD also lack neutrophil cytochrome b, which is necessary for electron transport and reduction of oxygen to superoxide. Female patients with CGD who are not carriers have neutrophil cytochrome b, suggesting separate abnormalities of leukocyte oxidative metabolism among patients with phenotypic CGD.

Pathogenesis. Recognition and phagocytosis of bacteria occur normally in phagocytic cells of patients with CGD, but the ingested microbes are not killed. Bacterial multiplication is inhibited, but intracellular bacteria survive and infections persist. Phagocytosis does not result in increased oxygen uptake, hexose monophosphate shunt activity, chemiluminescence, or generation of reactive oxygen radicals in neutrophils, monocytes, or macrophages. When oxygen radicals are provided by ingested microbes that produce hydrogen peroxide (e.g., streptococci or pneumococci) or by particle-associated oxidases, CGD neutrophils kill bacteria at normal rates.

Defects in oxidative metabolism and production of reactive oxygen radicals during phagocytosis are the essential defects in CGD. Stimulation of nicotinamide adenine dinucleotide (NADH) and nicotinamide adenine dinucleotide phosphate (NADPH) oxidase activities normally occurs when the plasma membrane of phagocytes is perturbed by particle attachment and electrons are provided for the reduction of oxygen to reactive electronically excited states (superoxide and hydrogen peroxide). NADH and NADPH oxidases are present in phagocytic cells with CGD, but increased activity is not stimulated during phagocytosis. The "trigger" of oxidase activity is absent or electron transport is abnormal in these cells.

Clinical Manifestations. Children with CGD usually have increased numbers of serious infections during the 1st year of life. The areas of body infected are those constantly challenged with bacteria. Eczematoid lesions are frequently present around the nose and mouth, with development of purulent adenitis that requires surgical drainage. Hepatosplenomegaly is a nearly universal finding, and staphylococcal abscesses of the liver occur with discouraging frequency. Osteomyelitis is common and may affect the small bones of the hands and feet as well as long bones. Gram-negative

species such as *Serratia marcescens* are frequently found in bone lesions as well as in soft tissue abscesses; accordingly, aggressive attempts to obtain material for culture are necessary to determine appropriate antibiotic treatment.

The infecting organisms include a variety of gram-positive and gram-negative bacteria. The predominant gram-positive organism is *Staphylococcus aureus*; *Serratia marcescens*, *Klebsiella*, and *Pseudomonas cepacia* are frequently identified gram-negative organisms. Catalase-negative species (e.g., *S. pneumoniae*, *H. influenzae*, and streptococci) rarely cause serious infections in patients with CGD since these organisms produce hydrogen peroxide and are killed by the defective phagocytic cells.

Pneumonitis occurs commonly in patients with CGD. Lung infiltrates persist for several weeks in spite of appropriate antibiotic therapy, and residual changes are visible on chest roentgenogram for many mo. Typical etiologic agents include *S. aureus* and gram-negative bacilli, but *Aspergillus fumigatus* has become an extremely serious problem in recent years.

Granulomatous lesions or obstructive complications may involve any organ. Obstruction of the gastric antrum is common and must be considered if there is persistent vomiting in a patient with CGD. Biopsy material from the vicinity of abscesses or inflammatory lesions usually contains collections of macrophages with cytoplasmic lipoid material.

Treatment. See Sec. 10.40.

10.32 CHÉDIAK-HIGASHI SYNDROME

The Chédiak-Higashi syndrome (CHS) is an autosomal recessive disease characterized by recurrent infections, partial oculocutaneous albinism, photophobia, nystagmus, and neutrophils with giant cytoplasmic granules. The onset of symptoms usually occurs in early childhood, and death from infection or malignancy often results before the patient reaches 10 yr of age. The clinical course may be rapidly progressive in infancy, or it may be quiescent with recurrent minor infections until an "accelerated" phase later in childhood. Neurologic abnormalities include long tract and cerebellar involvement, peripheral neuropathies, and mental retardation.

Abnormal granules are found in the cytoplasm of all blood and bone marrow leukocytes (polymorphonuclear neutrophils, eosinophils, basophils, and monocytes). The granules contain both azurophilic and specific granular material such as lysosomal enzymes, peroxidase, and acid phosphates. Abnormal granules and inclusions are also found in lymphocytes, erythrocytes, cultured skin fibroblasts, and platelets. As the disease progresses, anemia, thrombocytopenia, and absolute leukopenia frequently develop. At autopsy, widespread histiocytic infiltrations of almost all tissues of the body may be found. Histiocytes as well as neurons and renal tubular epithelium contain cytoplasmic inclusions. Neutrophils of patients with CHS have defective chemotaxis, degranulation, and intracellular killing. The impaired chemotactic responsiveness has been demonstrated in vivo with Rebuck inflammatory skin window techniques and in vitro with the Boyden chamber assay.

The rate of phagocytic particle uptake and the ingestion capacity of leukocytes from patients with CHS are increased in relation to normal cells, and hexose monophosphate shunt activity (as measured by oxidation of [1-^{14}C]-glucose) is twice normal in both the resting and the phagocytizing state. Degranulation, however, is abnormal, since the giant lysosomes do not rupture into phagocytic vacuoles. Fifteen minutes after bacterial ingestion little peroxidase is found on the phagosomes. Unlike neutrophils from patients with CGD, cells from patients with CHS are significantly abnormal in intracellular killing of catalase-negative organisms (e.g., streptococci). Killing of *Escherichia coli* and *Candida albicans* by neutrophils from patients with CHS is abnormal during the first 20 min of incubation but returns to normal with longer incubation. The belief that degranulation and chemotaxis are dependent on intact microtubular function suggests that abnormal microtubular function may lead to defective function of the neutrophils. Microtubular function is regulated by the cyclic nucleotide guanosine 3':5'-cyclic phosphate (cyclic GMP), and cholinergic agents elevate intracellular cyclic GMP and enhance microtubule assembly in normal human neutrophils. These same agents improve the function of leukocytes from patients with CHS. Intraleukocytic concentrations of adenosine 3':5'-cyclic phosphate (cyclic AMP) may be markedly elevated in patients with CHS; an infant treated with ascorbic acid (200 mg/24 hr) had levels of cyclic AMP in the normal range, but such therapy has not improved the prognosis.

10.33 MYELOPEROXIDASE DEFICIENCY

The diagnosis of hereditary myeloperoxidase deficiency is based on the complete absence of peroxidase-positive granules on smears of neutrophils and monocytes stained histochemically for peroxidase. Eosinophil peroxidase is present in normal amounts. The metabolic response of myeloperoxidase-deficient neutrophils during phagocytosis is different from that of neutrophils in CGD; there are normal or increased consumption of oxygen, oxidation of [1-^{14}C]-glucose, production of superoxide anions, and reduction of NBT, all of which are depressed in neutrophils from patients with CGD. The chemiluminescence response and killing of intracellular bacteria are initially depressed in myeloperoxidase-deficient neutrophils during phagocytosis. Delayed bacterial killing does not appear to be a handicap to the defense of the host against bacterial infection, however, since patients with myeloperoxidase deficiency are not abnormally susceptible to bacterial infections. On the other hand, neutrophils from patients with congenital absence of myeloperoxidase cannot kill intracellular *C. albicans*; several patients with myeloperoxidase deficiency have had serious and prolonged *Candida* infections.

10.34 GLUCOSE-6-PHOSPHATE DEHYDROGENASE (G-6PD) DEFICIENCY

This deficiency is a relatively common, genetically determined error of metabolism that primarily affects erythrocyte function (Sec. 15.17). Fortunately, profound deficiency (less than 5% of normal values) is quite rare, and only deficiency of this magnitude is associated with defective neutrophil function, phenotypically similar to that of CGD (with recurrent infections and granulomatous lesions due to *S. aureus* or gram-negative bacteria). G-6PD activity is necessary for an increased hexose monophosphate shunt response during phagocytosis, which, in turn, is required for maintenance of adequate cellular levels of reduced pyridine nucleotide NADPH (the source of electrons for conversion of oxygen to superoxide) and for continued function of the glutathione system. Accordingly, lack of substrate rather than lack of enzyme activity is the basis for defective respiratory metabolic response during phagocytosis in G-6PD deficient phagocytes.

10.35 DEFECTIVE GLUTATHIONE SYSTEM

The glutathione system plays an essential role in detoxifying the reactive oxygen metabolites that are formed in abundance during phagocytosis. Neutrophils from affected members of a family with neutrophil glutathione reductase deficiency had a normal initial burst of oxidative metabolism during phagocytosis, but after a few minutes there was an abrupt halt in metabolism and cell death. Further evidence for a protective role of glutathione was the observation that a patient with glutathione synthetase deficiency had neutropenia during infections; leukocytes accumulate large amounts of hydrogen peroxide, which damage the cells, and neutropenia is the result. Glutathione peroxidase deficiency has been described in patients with CGD, but most patients with CGD have normal glutathione peroxidase activity.

10.36 TRANSIENT DISORDERS OF LEUKOCYTE BACTERICIDAL FUNCTION

These have been identified in patients with several clinical conditions (Table 10–12) such as overwhelming infection after severe burns or trauma. In these conditions there is a correlation between morphologic abnormalities of blood neutrophils and defective bactericidal function. Neutrophils that are vacuolated or contain toxic granules and Döhle bodies have defective bactericidal capacity. There is return to normal phagocytic function when patients recover clinically.

10.37 DEFECTIVE PHAGOCYTIC CELL CHEMOTAXIS

Abnormal locomotion of phagocytic cells has been identified in many patients with recurrent serious infections. Dysfunction may result from cellular defects, from inhibitors of chemotaxis in circulation, or from deficiency of chemotactic factors (Table 10–13). Abnormal locomotion of neutrophils may be the basis of neutropenia in certain patients. Patients with the so-called *lazy leukocyte syndrome* have normal neutrophils in the bone marrow, but these display abnormal random migration and chemotaxis. The defect appears to be in the capacity for locomotion from bone marrow into the circulation. Clinical manifestations include stomatitis and infections of the skin and upper respiratory tract.

NEWBORN INFANTS

Neutrophils from newborn infants have a depressed response to chemotactic stimuli and are less deformable than neutrophils from older children. These defects combined with a small bone marrow reserve of neutrophils may be related to increased susceptibility to severe infections.

HYPERIMMUNOGLOBULIN E RECURRENT INFECTION (JOB) SYNDROME

A clinical syndrome characterized by unusual susceptibility to serious staphylococcal disease, chronic skin lesions similar to eczema, and "cold" abscesses was reported in 1966 as "Job syndrome." Later, two boys with chronic dermatitis and recurrent severe lung, skin, and joint abscesses due primarily to staphylococci were found to have extremely elevated levels of IgE, suggesting a possible association between dermatitis, extremely elevated levels of IgE, and susceptibility to severe staphylococcal infection. Many, but not all, patients with very high levels of immunoglobulin E and recurrent infection have depressed chemotaxis of neutrophils and monocytes. Typically, these patients have recurrent severe staphylococcal

Table 10–12. **Disorders of Bactericidal Function of Leukocytes**

Chronic granulomatous disease	Bilobed nucleus and absent specific granules in neutrophils
Chédiak-Higashi syndrome	
Absent glucose-6-phosphate dehydrogenase	Myelogenous leukemia
	Trisomy 21 (Down syndrome)
Myeloperoxidase deficiency	Severe burn injury
Protein-calorie malnutrition	Overwhelming infection
Leukocyte alkaline phosphatase deficiency	Viral infection
	Cryoglobulinemia

Table 10–13. Disorders of Chemotaxis

Cellular Defects

Chédiak-Higashi syndrome	Kartagener syndrome
Panhypogammaglobulinemia	Anchor disease
Neutropenia	Shwachman syndrome
Hyperimmunoglobulin E	Microtubule abnormality
Hyperimmunoglobulin A	Ichthyosis
Chronic renal failure	Trisomy 21 (Down syndrome)
Acrodermatitis enteropathica	Measles
Mannosidosis	Severe eczema with
Leukemia	infections

Circulating Inhibitors

Wiskott-Aldrich syndrome	Periodontitis
Rheumatoid arthritis	Bone marrow transplant
Hodgkin disease	Cirrhosis
IgA myeloma	Felty syndrome
Chronic mucocutaneous	
candidosis	

Deficient Production of Chemotactic Factor

Absent C5	Abnormal activation of C3
Hageman factor abnormality	Immunoglobulin deficiency
Systemic lupus erythematosus	

infections, cellulitis, subcutaneous abscesses, and deep muscle abscesses.

Patients with hyperimmunoglobulin E syndrome frequently have red hair, but the clinical association of recurrent severe staphylococcal infections, defective phagocytic cell chemotaxis, and hyperimmunoglobulin E occurs in males and females, adults and children, and persons of all hair colors. There appears to be little primary association between defective chemotaxis and eczema or atopic dermatitis, but this abnormality of phagocyte function is found in eczematous patients who have hyperimmunoglobulin E and recurrent severe infections. Neutrophil and monocyte chemotaxis is highly variable in patients with hyperimmunoglobulin E syndrome; neutrophil chemotactic responsiveness may be low, slightly depressed, or normal. Material from lesions in patients with Job syndrome does contain neutrophils, but delay in accumulation of phagocytic cells may be related to pathogenesis of lesions. Monocytes spontaneously produce inhibitors of neutrophil chemotaxis. Patients generally develop severe bacterial infections during the first months of life, and pulmonary lesions are especially serious since pneumatoceles develop. Surgical removal of affected lung tissue has been a frequent necessity. A genetic basis for this disease is suggested since recurrent infections and extremely elevated levels of IgE have been identified in several family members.

Patients with Job syndrome have antibodies to *Staphylococcus aureus* of the IgE class in their serum; indeed, IgE antibodies to bacterial antigens were first demonstrated in these patients. Microbial species other than *Staphylococcus aureus* may produce serious infections. Occurrence of cryptococcal meningitis and *Pneumocystis carinii* pneumonia in patients with extremely elevated levels of IgE suggests an underlying defect in cell-mediated immunity.

OTHER DISORDERS OF LEUKOCYTE LOCOMOTION

Patients with *immotile cilia (Kartagener) syndrome* (Sec. 13.63) are highly susceptible to recurrent sinusitis and lower respiratory infections, and often demonstrate abnormal neutrophil chemotaxis. Abnormal respiratory tract ciliary function and chemotaxis may also be found in patients without Kartagener syndrome, but abnormal cilia suggest that neutrophil locomotion and ciliary activity have a common physiologic basis. Abnormal neutrophil chemotaxis and phagocytosis have been described in infants with *delayed separation of the umbilical cord* and recurrent serious bacterial infections and defective neutrophil adherence (Anchor disease or *glycoprotein 180 deficiency*)

(Table 10–13). These infants lack a neutrophil surface membrane glycoprotein (mol. wt. ~ 180). Monoclonal antibody techniques have enabled investigators to identify this glycoprotein as a receptor for complement opsonins. This glycoprotein is also involved in adherence of neutrophils, since affected cells do not adhere to glass or plastic in vitro. Abnormal adherence may be related to profound granulocytosis in patients.

Patients with *Shwachman syndrome* (Sec. 12.68) have pancreatic insufficiency and metaphyseal chondroplasia, are susceptible to recurrent infections, and have depressed neutrophil chemotaxis. Parents also have abnormal chemotaxis; accordingly, neutrophil dysfunction, like other features of Shwachman syndrome, may be inherited as a recessive characteristic.

TRANSIENT DISORDERS OF NEUTROPHIL LOCOMOTION

Transient disorders of neutrophil chemotactic responsiveness have been reported in several clinical conditions (Table 10–13). For example, depressed neutrophil locomotion was found in children with measles, but it returned to normal with resolution of the rash and clinical improvement. Chemotaxis may be abnormal in bone marrow transplant recipients during graft-versus-host reactions, and transient chemotactic disorders are present in patients with overwhelming bacterial infections. Children with severe protein-calorie malnutrition have depressed neutrophil chemotaxis and increased susceptibility to bacterial, fungal, and viral infections. Since these children have decreased antibody production, decreased cell-mediated immunity, low levels of complement components, and defective intraleukocyte killing of bacteria and fungi, they have increased susceptibility to infections.

10.38 INHIBITORS OF CHEMOTAXIS

The clinical features are similar in patients with cellular defects of neutrophilic chemotaxis and in patients with circulating inhibitors of chemotaxis: recurrent severe infections of the skin and lower respiratory tract. Polymeric IgA may be a chemotactic inhibitor, since a circulating inhibitor of chemotaxis has been identified in several patients with increased levels of IgA. This immunoglobulin is cytophilic for neutrophils. Other plasma factors inhibiting chemotaxis have been identified in diverse clinical conditions (Table 10–13). For example, patients with Wiskott-Aldrich syndrome have high circulating levels of lymphocyte-derived chemotactic factors that inhibit chemotactic responsiveness of neutrophils and monocytes. Physiologic inhibitors of chemotaxis are present in normal plasma, and the levels of these normally occurring plasma proteins may be elevated in certain conditions, such as Hodgkin disease. Increased levels of circulating chemotactic factor inhibitors may also contribute to the lack of delayed-type hypersensitivity in certain conditions such as cirrhosis or sarcoidosis. Monocytes may be prevented from migrating to the site of skin test antigen as a result of circulating inhibitors, thereby preventing a delayed-type hypersensitivity response in spite of normal recognition of antigen.

10.39 DEFICIENCY OF CHEMOTACTIC FACTORS

The absence of potential chemotactic factors can result in abnormal chemotaxis. Since most of the well-characterized chemotactic factors are components of the complement system, it is not surprising that patients with deficient or abnormal function of complement have chemotactic abnormalities. These include absence of C3 and C5 and hypercatabolism of C3. There are frequent serious infections of multiple organ systems with encapsulated gram-positive and gram-negative bacteria in patients with abnormalities of complement. Depressed immunoglobulin levels as well as deficient complement results in abnormal chemotaxis, since the generation of biologically active factors from complement requires the participation of immunoglobulin.

Chemotactically active C3 and C5 fragments of complement are produced via the alternative complement pathway as well as via the classical pathway. Accordingly, patients with deficient early components of complement (C1, C4, C2) do not have unusually severe or recurrent microbial infections. Patients with C5 deficiency, however, have serious chronic infections that respond poorly to antimicrobial therapy. Plasma from patients with C5 deficiency has normal opsonic function (since C3 is the primary source of complement-related opsonic activity) but nearly absent chemotactic activity (Sec. 10.24).

10.40 TREATMENT OF DISEASES ASSOCIATED WITH DISORDERS OF THE PHAGOCYTES

The identification of defective intracellular bacterial killing in phagocytic cells from patients with CGD has resulted in improved therapy of patients with disorders of the phagocytic system. Patients are highly susceptible to recurrent serious lesions of soft tissues and bones caused by staphylococci, gram-negative aerobes, and fungi. The diversity of microbial agents that cause severe disease in these patients makes prevention difficult, and every effort must be made to identify infectious microorganisms. Early, aggressive, and prolonged antimicrobial therapy is necessary for treatment. Surgical intervention is often required for abscesses developing in patients with phagocyte dysfunction. The presence of "saprophytic" or "poorly virulent" organisms in lesions is as serious as that of highly pathogenic species in these patients.

Patients with defective chemotaxis associated with underlying systemic illnesses often demonstrate improved resistance to infection when the underlying disorder is corrected. For example, when eczematoid skin lesions are improved, there is less danger of deep abscesses. Recovery of phagocytic cell function often coincides with clinical recovery in patients with severe eczema, trauma, or overwhelming infection.

Chronic anemia is common in CGD, but blood transfusions may be hazardous because these patients possess a very rare red cell genotype of the Kell system called K_0. Transfusion almost inevitably leads to isoimmunization.

Transfusion of leukocytes from normal donors may be used as adjunct therapy when life-threatening infections do not respond to antibiotic therapy in patients with CGD and other disorders of the phagocytic cells. The successful replacement of myelocytic precursor cells with bone marrow from HLA- and mixed lymphocyte-identical normal donors has the theoretical capacity to cure patients with disorders of phagocytic cells. Patients with CGD and with glycoprotein 180 deficiency have received bone marrow transplants.

PAUL G. QUIE

Chemotaxis

Donabedian H, Gallin JI: Two inhibitors of neutrophil chemotaxis are produced by hyperimmunoglobulin E—Recurrent infection syndrome mononuclear cells exposed to heat killed Staphylococci. Infect Immun 40:1030, 1983.
Gallin JI, Quie PG (eds): Leukocyte Chemotaxis: Methods, Physiology, and Clinical Implications. New York, Raven Press, 1978.
Gallin JI, Wright DG, Malech HL, et al: Disorders of chemotaxis. Ann Intern Med 92:520, 1980.
Schopfer K, Boerlocher K, Price P, et al: Staphylococcal IgE antibodies, hyperimmunoglobulin E and staphylococcus infection. N Engl J Med 300:835, 1979.
Snyderman R, Pike MC: Disorders of leukocyte chemotaxis. Pediatr Clin North Am 24:377, 1977.

Phagocytic Cell Function

Babior BM: Oxygen-dependent microbial killing by phagocytes. N Engl J Med 298:659, 1978.
Cohn ZA, Morse SI: Functional and metabolic properties of polymorphonuclear leukocytes. I. Observations on the requirements and consequences of particle ingestion. J Exp Med 111:667, 1960.
Elsback P, Weiss J: A re-evaluation of the roles of the O_2-dependent and O_2-independent microbicidal systems of phagocytes. Rev Inf Dis 5:843, 1983.
Klebanoff SJ, Clark RA (eds): The Neutrophil: Function and Clinical Disorders. Amsterdam, Elsevier/North Holland, 1978.
Root RK, Cohen MS: The microbicidal mechanisms of human neutrophils and eosinophils. Rev Inf Dis 3:565, 1981.

Chronic Granulomatous Disease

Johnston RB Jr: Recurrent bacterial infections in children. N Engl J Med 310:1237, 1984.
Mills El, Rholl KS, Quie PG: X-linked inheritance in females with chronic granulomatous disease. J Clin Invest 66:332, 1980.
Quie PG, White JG, Holmes B, et al: In vitro bactericidal capacity of human polymorphonuclear leukocytes: Diminished activity in chronic granulomatous disease of childhood. J Clin Invest 46:668, 1967.
Quie PG, Davis AT: Disorders of the polymorphonuclear phagocytic system. In: Stiehm ER, Fulginiti V (eds): Immunologic Disorders in Infants and Children. 2nd ed. Philadelphia, WB Saunders, 1980, p 349.
Segal AW, Cross AR, Garcia RC, et al: Absence of cytochrome b-245 in chronic granulomatous disease. A multicenter European evaluation of its incidence and relevance. N Engl J Med 308:245, 1983.

Chédiak-Higashi Syndrome

Blume RS, Wolff SM: The Chédiak-Higashi syndrome. Studies in four patients and a review of the literature. Medicine 51:247, 1972.
Boxer LA, Watanabe AM, Rister M, et al: Correction of leukocyte function in Chédiak-Higashi syndrome by ascorbate. N Engl J Med 295:1041, 1976.

Other Disorders

Anderson DC, Schmalstieg FC, Arnout MA, et al: Abnormalities of polymorphonuclear leukocyte function associated with a hereditable deficiency of a high molecular weight surface glycoprotein (GP 138). J Clin Invest 74:536, 1984.
Eliasson R, Mossberg B, Camner P, et al: The immobile cilia syndrome: A congenital ciliary abnormality as an etiologic factor in chronic airway infections and male sterility. N Engl J Med 297:1, 1977.

ALLERGIC DISORDERS

Allergic disorders are adverse physiologic reactions resulting from the interaction of antigen with humoral antibody and/or lymphoid cells. This definition precludes the use of the term allergy for disorders in which immunologic mechanisms have not been demonstrated. For example, adverse reactions following food or drug ingestion in some individuals may resemble typical allergic reactions, without any evidence of an immunologic basis. In some instances a biochemical basis for the reaction can be identified, as in diarrhea following milk ingestion in individuals with disaccharidase deficiency. When there is no reason to suspect that allergy is responsible for signs or symptoms, the use of immunologic methods in diagnosis or treatment is irrational.

The terms antigen and allergen are often used interchangeably, but not all antigens are good allergens or vice versa. For example, tetanus and diphtheria toxoids are highly antigenic but are only rarely responsible for adverse reactions. On the other hand, ragweed pollen protein, one of the most potent allergens, is not a particularly potent antigen by immunologic criteria. Most naturally occurring allergens share several common characteristics. They are protein in part, are acidic with isoelectric points between 2–5.5, and have molecular weights of 10,000–70,000 daltons. Molecules smaller than 10,000 daltons would be unable to bridge adjacent IgE antibody molecules on the surface of mast cells, a requirement for release of the mediators of the allergic reaction. Molecules larger than 70,000 daltons would encounter difficulties in traversing mucosal surfaces and reaching IgE-forming plasma cells.

The use of the term atopy or atopic in designating an allergic reaction implies a hereditary factor expressed as susceptibility to hay fever, asthma, and eczematoid dermatitis in the families of affected individuals. The atopic patient has a predisposition to selectively synthesize IgE antibodies to common environmental antigens. IgE production is under genetic control, and there appears to be an association between HLA histocompatibility types and IgE-mediated hypersensitivity responses. In experimental models, the IgE antibody response is regulated by antigen-specific helper and suppressor T cells which secrete IgE-binding factors that potentiate or suppress the reaction. Atopic individuals may differ from nonatopic individuals in their ability to regulate IgE antibody production or to dispose of allergens coming in contact with mucosal surfaces. They may also have defective control of mediator release or generation, or have impaired mediator inactivation processes.

The formation of IgE antibodies is revealed in atopic persons by "wheal and flare" reactions upon skin testing with allergenic extracts. However, the capacity to form IgE antibody is not limited to atopic individuals, since IgE is found in the serum and on mast cells of virtually all normal individuals. Under intense allergen exposure, as in certain occupations, or in response to particular allergens, such as ascaris, nonatopic individuals may form large quantities of allergen-specific IgE antibodies. Atopic persons, however, form IgE antibodies on exposure to such common environmental substances as pollens and house dust, and this distinguishes them from the nonatopic. Among patients with asthma, hay fever, or eczema we can identify "highly atopic" subjects and others with lesser atopic tendencies.

10.41 IMMUNOLOGIC BASIS OF ATOPIC DISEASE

The lymphoid system has a primary role in immunity to infections and in the elimination of malignant cells. Paradoxically, the same system is responsible for a broad spectrum of diseases and much chronic illness, ranging from relatively mild conditions like ragweed hay fever to such serious disorders as disseminated lupus erythematosus. Attempts to modulate the deleterious effects resulting from antigen-antibody or antigen-lymphocyte interaction by immunosuppression of the lymphoid system may result in serious infections or in the development of malignancy.

Allergic reactions in man may be completely reversible or produce permanent pathologic change. The extent of tissue damage depends upon both the character of the antigen and the target organs involved, but perhaps most important may be the nature and degree of involvement of various components of the immune system, which include antibodies, lymphoid and other hematopoietic cells (especially mast cells and eosinophils), the complement system, and a variety of physiologically active molecules generated or released as a result of interactions of antigen with antibodies or with lymphoid cells.

It is useful to characterize immunologic reactions in terms of the reactants involved in order to appreciate the mechanism by which injury occurs (Gell and Coombs classification). Immunologically mediated tissue injury may occur as a result of the interaction of humoral antibody with antigen or of the interaction of antigen with lymphocytes (cell-mediated or delayed-type hypersensitivity). Humoral antibody-antigen reactions are recognized in three forms, two of which occur on the surface of cells and the third in the extracellular fluids.

Of the two reactions occurring on the surface of the cells, the first type mediated by IgE (immediate type or anaphylactic hypersensitivity) is of greatest interest to the allergist. In this circumstance, circulating basophils and tissue mast cells, the latter strategically located around blood vessels, become "sensitized" through the binding of IgE antibodies to their surface receptors. This is the initial event in the production of immune tissue injury following allergen interaction with cell-bound IgE antibody molecules; the ultimate outcome of the reaction depends on a broad spectrum of secondary events involving various types of lymphoid cells, inflammatory cells, mediator-producing cells, and the soluble products derived not only from all of these cells but from other tissues (platelets, endothelial cells) at the site of the reaction. For example, in particularly intense allergen-induced reactions in the skin (and probably also in the lung), the initial wheal and flare does not entirely disappear but is replaced by an inflammatory lesion that reaches its maximal size at 6–12 hr and disappears in 24–72 hr. This late cutaneous response depends upon recruitment of inflammatory cells (polymorphonuclear leukocytes, eosinophils, and mononuclear cells) by chemotactic factors released in the early response.

The terms reaginic IgE, IgE reagins, and homocytotropic antibodies refer to molecules with activities against specific allergens, such as ragweed pollen, whereas "nonspecific" IgE molecules are found in the serum and tissues of all normal individuals. The "normal" role of IgE antibody appears to be to defend the host against tissue-invasive parasites. In man the ability to induce antigen-specific release of mediators from mast cells and basophils is principally confined to antibodies of the IgE class.

IgE antibodies, like IgA antibodies, are synthesized by plasma cells located predominantly under mucosal surfaces and particularly in the respiratory and gastrointestinal tracts. IgE-forming plasma cells arise following antigen-stimulated differentiation of B cells or their precursors.

Chemical modifications of antigens used in immunotherapy of allergic diseases have been shown to suppress IgE responses (Sec. 10.46). While the control of IgE antibody production is better known for animals than for man, there is good reason to believe that similar mechanisms occur in the human. The association of IgE responses with HLA-linked Ir genes has been shown for several allergens (ragweed antigen Ra3 and HLA-A2, ragweed antigen Ra5 and HLA-B7, rye grass antigen I and HLA-B8). Once formed, IgE antibody becomes reversibly bound or "fixed" to surface receptors of mast cells and basophils. The binding of IgE to its receptor involves the C4 and C3 domains of the Fc portion of the immunoglobulin molecule. In nonatopic individuals, only 20–50% of the receptors are occupied by IgE molecules. Atopic individuals with high serum IgE concentrations have a larger percentage, up to almost 100%, of their basophil and mast cell receptors occupied by IgE. Once binding of IgE occurs, the basophils and mast cells may be considered "sensitized"; and upon subsequent contact with antigen specific for the bound IgE, a cascade of biochemical reactions occurs (activation of methyltransferases, phospholipid methylation, Ca^{++} influx, and activation of the phospholipid diacylglycerol cycle). This results in fusion of the mast cell granules with the mast cell plasma membrane, resulting in release of pharmacologically active substances (such as histamine), known as chemical mediators. The released mediators act on tissue receptors to cause symptoms in the patient. The reaction is largely reversible; the mast cells and basophils participating in the reaction are not lysed, and the effects of mediators are only temporary. Though aggregated IgE can fix late components of the complement system through an alternative pathway, participation of the complement system in IgE-mediated hypersensitivity disorders has not been shown.

The usual tests for inhalant or food sensitivity make use of the reaction that occurs on the surface of mast cells between antigen and IgE antibody. Small amounts of extracts of pollens, molds, danders, and foods are introduced into the patient's skin by scratch, puncture, or intradermal techniques. If IgE antibody specific for the test antigen is bound to the subject's mast cells, the interaction of injected antigen with cell-bound IgE will release histamine, a potent vasoactive agent that causes increased capillary permeability and dilation and axon reflex stimulation, leading to the familiar wheal and flare reaction. The prototypic *anaphylactic* or *IgE-mediated* disease is ragweed hay fever.

In the *second type of interaction* between antigen and antibody at cell surfaces, IgG or IgM immunoglobulins react with antigenic determinants* that either are integral parts of the cell membrane or have become adsorbed to or incorporated into the membrane. In contrast to the IgE or anaphylactic type of reaction, this second kind of reaction activates the complement system in most instances, and the involved cell is destroyed. An example of this type of immunologic injury occurs when incompatible red blood cells are transfused. The recipient's isohemagglutinins (antibodies directed against determinants on the surface of the red cells) react with the incompatible cells, the complement system is activated, and sequential action of complement proteins leads to lysis of the cell. Analogous immune injury may involve platelets or leukocytes. In the case of drug-induced immune hemolytic anemias, various other mechanisms are also involved ("innocent bystander," drug adsorption).

The *third immunopathologic mechanism* of tissue injury involving humoral antibody and antigen occurs in the extracellular spaces. At certain ratios of antigen to antibody, antigen-antibody complexes are formed which are "toxic" to tissues in which they are deposited. For example, complexes may lodge in the filtering organs of the body (such as the kidney or lung) or infiltrate the walls of small blood vessels, activating the complement cascade. There is release of biologically active substances, including factors that are chemotactic for polymorphonuclear (PMN) leukocytes, which are attracted to the site. With phagocytosis of the complexes, the polymorphonuclear leukocytes are lysed, and basic proteins and proteolytic enzymes are released that damage tissue. Immune complex disease is responsible for up to 90% of immunologic glomerulonephritis in humans.

Toxic complex injury involves cooperation between different antibodies in the production of tissue injury. The deposition of immune complexes containing IgG_1, IgG_2, IgG_3, and IgM in small blood vessels in the kidney in experimental serum sickness in animals depends on an increase in the permeability of these vessels. This is brought about by histamine liberated in the course of a simultaneous interaction of IgE antibody and antigen, which leads to "leakiness" of the capillaries and prepares them to receive the toxic complexes. Such deposition can be largely prevented by pretreatment with antihistamine drugs in the animal model.

In *cell-mediated* or *delayed-type hypersensitivity* pathologic changes follow interaction of antigen with T lymphocytes of

at least two of the five presently identified functional subclasses (helper cells, suppressor cells, amplifier cells, cytotoxic cells, and lymphokine-producing cells). The basis for the tissue injury in classic cell-mediated immune reactions is not completely understood, but it is clear that macrophages and cytotoxic cells play major roles. Both basophils and eosinophils are involved in the evolution of delayed-type hypersensitivity reactions, and they and the inflammatory cells that they attract may also contribute to tissue injury. Contact allergy (poison ivy, chemical-induced contact dermatitis) is the prototype of allergic disease mediated by delayed-type hypersensitivity. Drug reactions with involvement of liver, lung, and kidney may be further examples of T cell–mediated disease. Cell-mediated immunity is involved in certain infiltrative hypersensitivity lung diseases in which granuloma formation is a pathologic feature.

10.42 CHEMICAL MEDIATORS OF ALLERGIC REACTIONS AND MECHANISMS OF RELEASE

Mast cells play the central role in immediate hypersensitivity responses. Considerable heterogeneity probably exists among populations of mast cells and basophils in the human; differences among these metachromatically staining cells can be measured by morphologic, immunologic, biochemical, and functional criteria. Mast cells and basophils are involved not only in IgE-mediated reactions but also in other chronic inflammatory disorders, e.g., inflammatory bowel disease, rheumatoid arthritis, parasitic infections.

The critical triggering event in mast cell degranulation and release of chemical mediators of allergic injury is the cross-linking of receptor-bound IgE antibodies (which may be viewed as an extension of the receptor) by multivalent specific antigen. Although antigen is usually the principal factor in causing the approximation of IgE receptors, this can be accomplished in the absence of antigen or even of IgE antibody, e.g., by purified antibody to the IgE receptor itself. Other stimuli can also cause mast cell activation without involvement of antigen and cell-bound IgE. These include products of activation of the complement system (C3a, C5a), kinins, neutrophil-derived lysosomal basic proteins, and a lymphokine. Whatever the nature of the mast cell surface signal that acts as the degranulation stimulus, a series of biochemical reactions takes place that results in granule discharge. Activation of a serine esterase, utilization of intracellular energy stores, calcium influx or remobilization of intracellular calcium, changes in the mast cell cytoskeleton such as polymerization of microtubules, and activation of actinomycin fibrils have all been observed during mediator release. Changes in membrane phospholipid metabolism also occur, including methylation and activation of phospholipases and generation of phospholipid byproducts, which participate in the fusion of the mast cell granules with the cell membrane, leading to extrusion of the granules. Once discharged from the mast cell, the granules, which are relatively water insoluble, remain intact for hours. The preformed mediators, such as histamine, eosinophil chemotactic factor (ECF-A), and other chemotactic factors, are rapidly eluted from the granule matrix and act immediately on local tissues—smooth muscles and endothelial cells in blood vessels. Another set of mediators which are preformed but granule associated (e.g., heparin, arylsulfatase B, enzymes such as trypsin and chymotrypsin, and inflammatory factors) are thought to be responsible for the late phase reaction; these mediators express their activity either while part of the intact granule or only after the granule begins to dissolve. A further set of mediators that are newly generated from a variety of tissues have major roles in allergic disorders (Table 10–14). These include products of arachidonic

---

*An antigenic determinant or epitope is a restricted portion of an antigen molecule that determines the specificity of an antigen-antibody reaction. Antigenic determinants may consist of only 4 or 5 amino acid residues. In complex antigens found in nature, such as pollens, there may be several hundred determinants on the surface of an antigen molecule, each capable of initiating immune responses and reacting with specific antibody.

Table 10–14. **Mast Cell Products**

Mediator	Structural Characteristics	Functions/Activities
I. Predominant Smooth Muscle Contracting and Vasoactive Activities		
Histamine (preformed)	5–β–Imidazolylethylamine MW 111	H_1 receptors: Increase in venular permeability Contraction of smooth muscle Increase in cyclic GMP levels Generation of prostaglandins Increase in nasal mucus production Positive chemokinetic effect on neutrophils and eosinophils* Positive chemotactic effect on neutrophils and eosinophils Bronchial irritant receptor stimulation Pruritus
		H_2 receptors: Increase in vascular permeability Increase in gastric acid secretion Positive chemokinetic effect on neutrophils and eosinophils Negative chemotactic effect on neutrophils and eosinophils Inhibition of T-cell responses Inhibition of basophil (not mast cell) mediator response Augmentation of gastric acid secretion Stimulation of airway mucus secretion Increase in cyclic AMP Increase in chronotropic and inotropic effects on heart
Arachidonic acid (newly formed)	Leukotrienes (LTC$_4$, LTD$_4$, LTE$_4$)—SRS-A (lipoxygenase-dependent derivatives of arachidonic acid) MW 400–600	Smooth muscle contraction and bronchostriction, particularly of peripheral airways Airway mucus secretion Vasoconstriction of large arteries (LTC$_4$) Increase in microvascular permeability
Platelet activating factor (PAF) (newly formed)	AGEPC (acetyl-glyceryl-ether-phosphorylcholine) MW 551 (hexadecyl) MW 523 (octadecyl)	Aggregation of platelets and secretion of amines Neutrophil aggregation and enzyme release Production of prostaglandins and thromboxanes by platelets Increase in vascular permeability Mimics physiologic and intravascular sequelae of IgE-mediated human systemic anaphylaxis
PGI$_{2\alpha}$ (prostacyclin) (newly formed)		Relaxation of smooth muscle Vasodilation
PGD$_2$ (newly formed)		Contraction of smooth muscle Bronchoconstriction Vasodilatation (skin) Chemokinesis of granulocytes Chronotropic effect on heart Increase in vascular permeability Sneezing Rhinorrhea
PGF$_{2\alpha}$ (newly formed)	Products of oxidative metabolism of arachidonic acid via cyclo-oxygenase pathway	Bronchoconstriction Chronotropic effect on heart
PGE$_2$ (newly formed)		Relaxation of smooth muscle Bronchodilatation Vasodilatation

Table continued on following page

Table 10–14. **Mast Cell Products** *Continued*

Mediator	Structural Characteristics	Functions/Activities
T$_x$A$_2$ (thromboxane A$_2$) (newly formed)		Bronchoconstriction Vasoconstriction Platelet aggregation
II. Predominant Chemotactic Activities		
ECF-A-tetrapeptides (preformed)	Val/Ala-Gly-Ser-Glu MW 400–500	Chemotactic attraction and deactivation of eosinophils Increase in eosinophil complement receptors
ECF-oligopeptides (preformed)	Peptides MW 1500–3000	Chemotactic attraction and deactivation of eosinophils and mononuclear leukocytes
HMW-NCF (preformed)	Neutral protein MW 600,000	Chemotactic attraction and deactivation of neutrophils
Hydroxy-eicosa-tetraenoic acids (HETE's)	Lipid-derived factors (newly generated via lipoxygenase pathway of arachidonic acid metabolism)	Chemotaxis and chemokinesis of eosinophils and neutrophils
Hydroxy-hepta-decatrienoic acid (HHT)	MW 300–400	Chemotaxis and chemokinesis of eosinophils and neutrophils
LTB$_4$	MW 400	Chemotaxis of neutrophils and eosinophils Release of lysosomal enzymes Adherence Aggregation Superoxide generation Inhibition of proliferation and synthetic activity of T cells
III. Enzymes†		
Chymase (preformed)	Protein MW 25,000	Proteolysis of chymotrypsin substrates
Arylsulfatases (preformed)	Protein A MW 100,000 B MW 60,000	Inactivation of leukotrienes (LTC, LTD, and LTE)
N-Acetyl-β-D-glucosaminidase (preformed)	Protein MW 150,000	Cleavage of glycosaminoglycans
Tryptase (preformed)	Protein MW 140,000	Proteolysis Generation of C$_{3a}$ Degradation of kininogen
β-Glucuronidase (preformed)	Protein MW 300,000	Cleavage of glucuronide residues
β-D-Galactosidase (preformed)	Protein MW 400,000	Cleavage of galactoside Cleavage of Hageman factor Cleavage of kinin from kininogen
IV. Structural Components		
Heparin (preformed)	Acidic proteoglycan MW 60,000 (human)	Anticoagulation (antithrombin III binding activity) Anticomplementary activity (at several sites) Augments inactivation of histamine

*Chemotactic migration requires a concentration gradient from the stimulus side. Movement in the absence of a gradient of the stimulus is termed "positive chemokinesis."

†Not all of these enzymes have been identified in the human; however, known analogues exist.

acid metabolism, vasoactive and smooth muscle contractile leukotrienes (LTC_4, LTD_4, LTE_4), the polymorphonuclear leukocyte-stimulating and T lymphocyte suppressing leukotriene LTB_4, the prostaglandins, prostaglandin-generating factor of anaphylaxis (PGF-A), and the thromboxanes.

The relationship of changes in cyclic nucleotides (cAMP and cGMP) to the process of mast cell activation-secretion is basic to the mechanism of drug action in IgE-mediated disorders. Mast cell mediator release may be dependent on a fall in intracellular cAMP, a rise in cGMP, or both. There may be separate pools of cAMP that may be increased by pharmacologic agents acting independently, but only one agent impedes the activation-secretion process.

Factors Not Mast-Cell–Derived That Participate in Immediate-Type Hypersensitivity Diseases

Eosinophil-derived molecules of potent biologic activity may contribute to tissue injury in IgE-mediated and other diseases. *Eosinophil major basic protein* (MBP) causes dose-dependent epithelial damage in guinea pig trachea and in human bronchial epithelium. MBP also stimulates histamine release from human basophils and causes a wheal and flare reaction when injected into human skin. In a variety of in vitro systems (bacteria, parasites, tumor cells), *eosinophil peroxidase* (EPO) causes injury. Both eosinophil-derived neurotoxin (EDN) and eosinophil cationic protein (ECP) have been shown to damage myelinated cells in animals.

Kinins are another system of proteins activated in inflammatory processes that have amplifier and effector properties. Their activities include chemotaxis, increased vascular permeability, and smooth muscle contraction. Bradykinin, a nonapeptide, is the most important product of the kinin system. The kinin, complement, and clotting systems are interrelated. Activation of Hageman factor (Factor XII) is the initial step in kinin generation and amplification, with positive feedback loops resembling those in the complement pathway. Hageman factor is activated by tissue injury by a number of agents, including IgG aggregates and immune complexes. Hageman factor and complexes of high molecular weight kininogen and prekallikrein and high molecular weight kininogen and factor XI are bound. Hageman factor appears to autoactivate to form activated Hageman factor (HF_a), which converts prekallikrein to kallikrein. Kallikrein digests high molecular weight kininogen to liberate the vasoactive peptide bradykinin. Bradykinin has potent contractile effects on smooth muscle, causes increased vascular permeability, and dilates peripheral arterioles. It also stimulates pain receptors. At least two other plasma kinins have biologic activities similar to those of bradykinin. The role of bradykinin in allergic disease is uncertain. Several patients with cold urticaria have had increased concentrations of bradykinin in plasma.

Platelet activating factor (PAF), a phospholipid, is synthesized by a variety of hematopoietic, lymphoid, and endothelial cells after appropriate in vitro stimulation. PAF has a variety of potent biologic actions and may have a role in anaphylaxis and cold urticaria.

Serotonin (5-hydroxytryptamine) is a vasoactive amine that, in experimental animals, induces contraction of smooth muscle and increases vascular permeability. Ninety percent of the body's stores of serotonin are found in the gastrointestinal tract, with the remainder divided between central nervous system and platelets. Serotonin is lacking from human mast cells. Serotonin has been reported to induce bronchoconstriction in asthmatics but not in normal persons, but it has no significant role in immediate hypersensitivity in humans. Its distinctive association is with diarrhea in the *carcinoid syndrome*.

While not mediators in the same sense as products released from mast cells or basophils, certain components of the complement system have activities that may contribute to allergic reactions. (1) Aggregated IgE can initiate complement system activity in vitro through the alternative pathway; this probably does not occur in vivo because of the large quantities of IgE required. (2) Certain "split" or "cleavage" products of the complement cascade, C3a and C5a, can induce mediator (histamine) release from basophils and from mast cells in the skin, producing wheal and flare reactions. C3a and C5a have been termed *anaphylatoxins* because they release histamine and resemble components of serum capable of causing guinea pig anaphylaxis. C5a and to a much lesser extent C3a are chemotactic for various leukocytes. Neutrophils attracted to the site of complement activation by C5a may degranulate, releasing basic lysosomal proteins that trigger mediator liberation from mast cells. The result in the skin is urticaria mimicking an antigen-IgE reaction. Small N-formylated peptides, derived from bacterial products, also possess potent granulocyte chemotactic activity and may operate in a manner similar to that of C5a to cause urticaria. (3) A kinin-like peptide derived from C2 as a result of reduced functional activity of the inhibitor of C1-esterase (C1s) is thought to mediate the angioedema observed in hereditary angioedema (HAE).

From the above considerations it is evident that the signs and symptoms of typical, immediate-type allergic reactions, such as anaphylaxis, though most often involving the IgE mechanism, may result from non-IgE immunologic mechanisms or from nonimmunologic mechanisms.

Gleich GJ, Loegering BS, Adolphson CR: Eosinophils and bronchial inflammation. Chest 87 (suppl.):105, 1985.
Goetzl EJ, Paxan DG, Goldman DW: Immunopathogenic roles of leukotrienes in human diseases. J Clin Immunol 4:79, 1984.
Grandel KE, Farr RS, Wanderer AA, et al: Association of platelet-activating factor with primary cold urticaria. N Engl J Med 313:405, 1985.
Ishizaka K: Regulation of IgE synthesis. Annu Rev Immunol 2:159, 1984.
Ishizaka T, Ishizaka K: Activation of mast cells for mediator release through IgE receptors. Prog Allergy 34:188, 1984.
Katz HR, Stevens RL, Austen KF: Heterogeneity of mammalian mast cells differentiated in vivo and in vitro. J Allergy Clin Immunol 76:250, 1985.
Wasserman SI: Mediators of immediate hypersensitivity. J Allergy Clin Immunol 72:101, 1983.

10.43 GENERAL AND SPECIFIC METHODS OF DIAGNOSIS

Allergic History. Careful inquiry is the most important method of diagnosis in allergic diseases. After the general medical history has been obtained, information of particular interest to the allergist is sought, such as whether the patient's symptoms are perennial or seasonal. Seasonal symptoms suggest an etiologic role for seasonal allergens, such as pollens, whereas perennial symptoms suggest exposure either to multiple seasonal allergens or to factors to which the child is exposed throughout the year, such as dust and animal danders. Questions concerning the home environment should focus on the heating system, composition of furniture and rugs, the furnishings in the child's bedroom (pillows, mattress, rugs, drapes, etc.), and the presence of pets. Are symptoms continuous or intermittent? Are they subject to diurnal variation? Has a change of location had any effect? These questions help to identify particular etiologic agents. In assessing the role of foods, it is important to distinguish between what the parents have actually observed following ingestion of a food and what they may have been told by a physician, possibly on the basis of skin tests to foods, which are subject to misinterpretation (Sec. 10.56). One must be particularly critical in interpreting cause and effect relationships when foods are concerned, since it is easy for parents to arrive at erroneous conclusions based on inconsistent relationships between ingestion of a particular food and the appearance of symptoms. The value of properly conducted double-blind food challenges cannot be overemphasized. Significant improvement in symptoms following the use of antiallergic drugs such as antihistamines, sympathomimetics, theophylline, or corticosteroids supports the notion that an allergic reaction is the basis of symptoms; on the other hand, symptoms having a nonimmunologic basis may also respond to such therapy.

In Vitro Tests. A white blood cell count and a differential count are useful in establishing whether *eosinophilia* is present. A total eosinophil count gives a more accurate determination. Eosinophils are subject to a diurnal rhythm, their numbers being highest in the early morning. Because eosinophilia may be intermittent, two to three normal results should be obtained before it is judged that eosinophilia is not present. Eosinophilia in excess of 5% on smear or of 250 cells/mm³ is considered elevated. Eosinophilia of respiratory tract secretions in a patient with rhinorrhea or cough is a useful diagnostic sign. A smear of nasal secretions or bronchial mucus is easily prepared and stained on a microscopic slide, preferably with an eosin-methylene blue stain (Hansel stain). A finding of more than 5–10% eosinophils supports the diagnosis of allergic rhinitis. Eosinophils in bronchial mucus strongly suggest asthma. Blood eosinophilia in allergic conditions does not generally exceed 15–20%, but may occasionally be as high as 35% in allergic children in the absence of other disorders known to cause eosinophilia. Other than atopic disorders, eosinophilia is associated most commonly with metazoan parasitoses, drug reactions, and a number of infiltrative pulmonary disorders. Corticosteroids cause eosinopenia for up to 6 hr following a dose; the timing of collection of a blood specimen should be appropriately adjusted.

A number of in vitro immunologic tests are of value in allergy diagnosis, such as measurement of the total and specific IgE content of serum and determining the sensitivity of the patient's leukocytes for antigen-induced histamine release. Quantification of total IgE can be accomplished by the paper radioimmunosorbent test (PRIST). Table 10–15 shows the serum concentrations of IgE in normal subjects of different ages. Mean concentrations of IgE in atopic persons are higher than normal, though a significant number of allergic individuals have normal or low IgE concentrations. In

Table 10–16. Disorders Associated With Increased Serum Concentrations of IgE

Allergic (extrinsic) asthma (40–60% of patients)
Bronchopulmonary aspergillosis
Pulmonary hemosiderosis
Hyperimmunoglobulin E syndrome (increased IgE, dermatitis, susceptibility to infection)
Wiskott-Aldrich syndrome
Some T cell immunodeficiency states
Hodgkin disease
IgE myeloma
Atopic dermatitis associated with allergic rhinitis and/or asthma
Bullous pemphigoid
Chronic acral dermatitis
Parasitic infestations (Ascaris, Toxocara, Necator, Echinococcus, and Capillaria)

suspected but atypical forms of atopic dermatitis, however, the finding of grossly elevated IgE levels, which are very common in active atopic dermatitis, will support the diagnosis. The finding of increased total IgE levels during infancy provides useful information regarding the likelihood of subsequent development of atopic diseases. Table 10–16 shows disorders associated with increased concentrations of serum IgE.

Determination of IgE levels against specific antigens is available for ragweed, grass, house dust, other inhalants, and various foods through the radioallergosorbent test (RAST). The principles of the RAST are shown in Figure 10–4. A comparison of RAST and skin testing in the diagnosis of IgE-mediated disorders is seen in Table 10–17.

There is good correlation among RAST results, other in vitro tests that measure specific antibody (such as the leukocyte histamine release test), mucous membrane provocation tests, and the likelihood of symptoms upon exposure to the allergen under study. There is, however, considerable interlaboratory and even intralaboratory variability in RAST results, even on the same specimen. Selection of a reliable laboratory is essential. Unfortunately, inappropriate use of RAST may be made by physicians unqualified and unskilled in comprehensive evaluation of allergic diseases. But to a physician who is competent to administer the tests and interpret the results, allergy skin testing is the method of choice to detect specific IgE antibody sensitization.

Table 10–15. Levels of Serum IgE Immunoglobulin of Normal Subjects at Different Ages*

Age	Range (IU/mL)	Geometric Mean (± 2 SD) (IU/mL)
0 days	<0.1–1.5	0.22 (0.04–1.28)
6 wk	<0.1–2.8	0.69 (0.08–6.12)
3 mo	0.3–3.1	0.82 (0.18–3.76)
6 mo	0.9–28.0	2.68 (0.44–16.26)
9 mo	0.7–8.1	2.36 (0.76–7.31)
1 yr	1.1–10.2	3.49 (0.80–15.22)
2 yr	1.1–49.0	3.03 (0.31–29.48)
3 yr	0.5–7.7	1.80 (0.19–16.86)
4 yr	2.4–34.8	8.58 (1.07–68.86)
7 yr	1.6–60.0	12.89 (1.03–161.32)
10 yr	0.3–215	23.66 (0.98–570.61)
14 yr	1.9–159	20.07 (2.06–195.18)
18–83 yr	1–178	21.20 (Modal values 10–20 IU/mL)†

*Ages 0–14 years adapted from Kjellman, N-IM, Johansson SGO, Roth A: Clin Allergy 6:51, 1976; ages 18–83 years adapted from Nye L, Merrett TG, Landon J, White RJ: Clin Allergy 1:13, 1975. The method used was a double antibody assay.

†Modal values — the most common values observed.

Radio Allergo Sorbent Testing

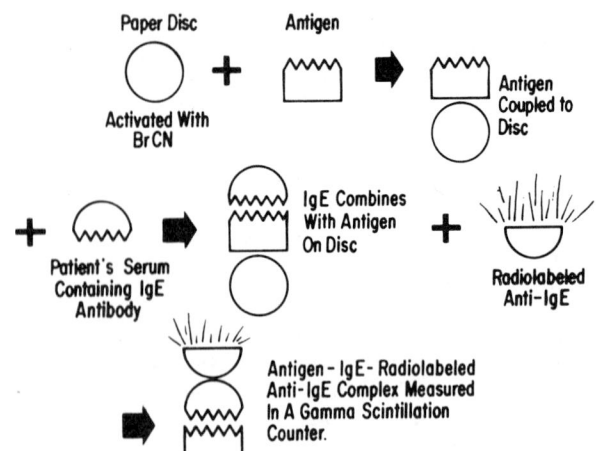

Figure 10–4. The principle of the radioallergosorbent test (RAST). The final step measures the amount of radiolabeled anti-IgE bound, which varies with the amount of IgE in the patient's serum that is specific for the test antigen.

Table 10–17. RAST versus Skin Testing in Diagnosis of IgE-Mediated Allergy

Radioallergosorbent Test (RAST)	Skin Test
Advantages	
Safe; convenient; semi-quantitative	Immediate results
Not influenced by drugs	Broad selection of
Useful in testing infants and patients	allergens
with widespread dermatitis or	Relatively inexpensive
dermographism	High degree of sensitivity
Allergens on disk stable	
Good correlation with clinical	
symptoms, skin testing by end-point	
dilution, bronchial challenge, and in	
vitro leukocyte-histamine release	
Disadvantages	
Limited selection of allergens	Allergens labile in dilute
Considerable interlaboratory variability	solution
Overinterpretation of low RAST scores	Influenced by drugs
Encourages "remote" or "mail order"	Risk of systemic reaction
practice of allergy	Liable to misinterpretation,
Expensive	particularly
	overinterpretation

Modified from Yunginger JW, Gleich GJ: Pediatr Clin North Am 22:3, 1975.

In the *leukocyte histamine release test*, the patient's leukocytes are tested for their sensitivity to antigen-induced histamine release. For example, when leukocytes (actually, basophils) from persons with ragweed hay fever are exposed to various concentrations of ragweed antigen E (the major allergen of ragweed pollen), they will, under appropriate in vitro conditions, release histamine into the suspending medium. The leukocytes of individuals with high degrees of cell sensitivity release histamine on exposure to very small amounts of specific antigen, whereas leukocytes with lesser degrees of cell sensitivity require higher concentrations of antigen for release of comparable amounts of histamine. There is reasonably good correlation between sensitivity of leukocytes to histamine release on exposure to ragweed antigen, the amount of ragweed-specific IgE antibody measured by RAST, the titer of passive transfer (P-K) activity, mucous membrane provocation testing with ragweed extract, and clinical sensitivity to ragweed on environmental exposure.

In Vivo Tests. Determination of allergic reactivity through direct *skin testing* of the patient is an important tool in the diagnosis of IgE-mediated sensitivity. A small quantity of allergenic extract is introduced into the skin by scratch, prick/puncture, or intracutaneous technique. If the patient's mast cells have IgE antibodies specific for the allergen on their surfaces, an allergen-IgE interaction will trigger biochemical events that culminate in release of histamine and other mediators from the mast cell. The histamine acts upon histamine receptors in small vessels, causing increased permeability and dilatation and axon reflex stimulation, which are observed clinically as the wheal and flare reaction. A biphasic late-phase reaction has also been described; this reaction begins with an influx of neutrophils over a 2–8 hr period and is followed by a mononuclear infiltrate at 24–48 hr. The late-phase reaction is due to slow elution of inflammatory factors from mast cell granules; these attract neutrophils and mononuclear cells to the site. The latter cells release the products that are responsible for late-phase tissue injury. The immediate wheal and flare reaction in skin indicates that specific IgE antibody is present also on the mast cells in the tissue of the clinically affected organ. *It does not indicate that the patient will necessarily have clinical symptoms on exposure to the allergen.* Significant numbers of atopic persons have no symptoms following natural exposure to allergens that give positive wheal and flare reactions on skin testing. As a general rule, the larger the size of the wheal and flare reaction, the more likely is the test antigen to be clinically relevant. But one must be cautious not to overinterpret skin test results.

Positive skin tests obtained by the puncture technique correlate better than intracutaneous tests with measurements of specific IgE antibody and with appearance of clinical symptoms upon exposure to the allergen being tested. With the intracutaneous technique, only those positive tests obtained with high dilutions (weak concentrations) of extract have as high correlations. If only concentrated solutions of allergenic extract (e.g., 1 to 100 or 1 to 10 weight/volume) elicit positive intracutaneous tests, the results will more often than not be of little clinical significance. Overinterpretation of such reactions has led to overuse of allergenic extracts in immunotherapy in the United States.

Various drugs, extracts that contain irritant materials or substances that are too concentrated, and improper technique can induce histamine release from tissue mast cells on a nonimmunologic or "toxic" basis. The resulting wheal and flare reaction cannot be differentiated from that which occurs as a result of IgE-allergen interaction, and IgE sensitivity may be mistakenly inferred. Other drugs may inhibit full expression of clinically relevant positive skin tests. Among these are certain adrenergic drugs such as epinephrine and ephedrine and the antihistamines, particularly such potent ones as hydroxyzine. These drugs should be withheld prior to skin testing (ephedrine for at least 12 hr and antihistamines for at least 24 hr). To make sure that the skin is capable of reacting to endogenously released histamine, a positive histamine control (histamine phosphate, 1%) should always be used. Corticosteroids to the equivalence of 60 mg of prednisone/24 hr have no appreciable inhibitory effects on IgE-mediated wheal and flare reactions and need not be withheld prior to skin testing.

The *passive transfer test* (Prausnitz-Küstner [P-K] test), in which serum from an allergic individual is injected intracutaneously into a nonallergic recipient and the injection sites subsequently skin tested, is now used only in research.

Because the appearance of symptoms on natural exposure may not correlate well with results of skin testing, *provocation testing* by direct exposure of the mucous membrane of the affected organ to the suspected allergen (usually in the form of an extract of the material) has received considerable attention, particularly in Scandinavian countries. Mucous membrane provocation testing has been used mostly in asthma, to a lesser extent in allergic rhinitis. As commonly performed, the test requires that increasing concentrations of extracts of various allergens be inhaled by the patient after nebulization with a suitable device. A positive response will be manifested by an increase in airway obstruction as monitored with an instrument that measures expiratory flow rate. The patient's degree of sensitivity should be determined by skin tests prior to provocation testing to permit appropriate initial concentrations of allergic extract to be used. With reasonable precautions the method is safe, and the results of provocation testing correlate well with clinical data. It is time consuming, however, and not suitable for general use in office or clinic. Bronchial challenge testing may be most useful in patients who have many positive skin tests, and it will guide selection of those allergens that may be most clinically significant for inclusion in an immunotherapy extract mixture. Selection in this way permits a greater concentration of the more clinically significant allergens in the mixture than would be possible if all the allergens possibly implicated by ordinary skin testing were to be included. Recent studies have shown excellent correlations between the results of provocative bronchial challenge testing, RAST, and quantitative intradermal skin tests (end-point dilution method); accordingly, bronchial challenge is principally reserved for research purposes. On the other hand, bronchial provocative testing with methacholine and histamine is valuable when the degree of airway reactivity in asthma must be determined and when the diagnosis of asthma is uncertain.

The utility of *provocation testing with foods* and other substances (allergens and even chemicals) using subcutaneous injection and/or sublingual administration is controversial. Symptoms referable to various organ systems are said by some to be provoked by positive tests and then "neutralized" by the injection of *weaker* concentrations of extract of the same foods that provoked the reactions, a response difficult to understand on immunologic or other grounds. In patients who have IgE-mediated sensitivity to a food, symptoms can often be provoked when the food is ingested or injected; "neutralization" of such a reaction has not been convincingly shown.

Provocation and neutralization techniques are currently unproven methods of allergy diagnosis and treatments; their validity has yet to be established by well designed studies.

Bierman CW, Pearlman DS (eds): Allergic Diseases of Infancy, Childhood and Adolescence. Philadelphia, WB Saunders, 1980.
Ellis EF (ed): Symposium on Pediatric Allergy. Pediatr Clin North Am. Philadelphia, WB Saunders, 1975.
Ellis EF (ed): Symposium on Pediatric Allergy. Pediatr Clin North Am. Philadelphia, WB Saunders, 1983.
Middleton E Jr, Reed CE, Ellis EF (eds): Allergy: Principles and Practice. St. Louis, CV Mosby, 1983.
Patterson R (ed): Allergic Diseases: Diagnosis and Management. Philadelphia, JB Lippincott, 1980.
Sly RM: Textbook of Pediatric Allergy. New Hyde Park, NY, Medical Examination Publishing Co, 1985.

10.44 PRINCIPLES OF TREATMENT OF ALLERGIC DISORDERS

Successful management of allergic disorders is based upon four principles: avoidance of allergens or irritants, pharmacologic therapy, immunotherapy (hypo-sensitization or desensitization), and prophylaxis.

When clinically relevant allergens are identified by history and judicious use of allergy skin tests, their elimination or *avoidance* will be all that is needed in many cases of IgE-mediated disease. For example, if history and skin testing indicate reactivity to such household inhalants as house dust or molds, or dog or cat dander is contributing to the patient's symptoms, these allergens should be eliminated. The recommendation that a family pet be removed from a home is frequently difficult to implement, since in some families pets seem to be as much a part of the family's social fabric as children. When the allergic disorder is a serious one, such as asthma, and when the child has a positive skin test to the dander of the pet, parents can generally be persuaded to remove the animal. When skin tests to danders are negative, the problem may be more difficult; most allergists feel that elimination of potentially sensitizing pets from the household of the allergic child is desirable on prophylactic grounds.

Instructions for preparation of an "allergen-free" indoor environment, emphasizing the bedroom, are found in standard allergy texts and are distributed by manufacturers of allergenic extracts. It is mandatory that exposure to certain environmental irritants known to trigger symptoms in allergic children, particularly tobacco smoke, be avoided. In significant numbers of patients, much can be accomplished by proper application of environmental control measures and appropriate use of pharmacologic agents without resort to immunotherapy.

Pharmacologic therapy is a major element in management of allergic diseases (Sec. 10.45). The drugs used have specific roles in the interruption of pathways leading to tissue damage as a consequence of antigen-antibody interaction. Certain drugs, for example, modulate the antigen-induced release of mediators (histamine, leukotrienes); others affect tension of smooth muscle; and others prevent the migration to the site of an allergic reaction of inflammatory cells having the potential for producing tissue injury. In some patients with rhinitis and asthma in whom there is no evidence that immunologic factors are involved, avoidance of allergens or attempts to increase the tolerance to allergens by immunotherapy are fruitless. Drug therapy, on the other hand, will be effective whether or not an allergic mechanism is involved. Patients with nonimmunologic or nonallergic asthma may respond as well to drug treatment as those in whom allergy plays a major role.

Immunotherapy is used for allergic disorders mediated by IgE antibody-antigen interactions that involve allergens that can either not be or only partially be avoided (Sec. 10.46).

If a predisposition to form IgE antibodies to substances of "high" allergic potential is an important characteristic of the atopic state, then *prophylaxis* through the prevention of exposure of infants and children at risk has a rational basis. It is appropriate, therefore, to recommend breast feeding infants born into families with strong histories of hay fever, asthma, or atopic dermatitis and to delay for at least 6 mo the introduction of solid foods into the diet of such infants, with special attention to foods of high allergic potential, such as eggs, wheat, fish, and peanut butter. The nursing mother should avoid highly allergenic foods in her diet, since there is evidence that the breast-fed infant can become sensitized to antigens (foods) in breast milk. It is not definitively established whether postponing cow's milk feeding in an atopic infant can prevent the development of cow milk allergy, of allergic diseases in general, or of atopic dermatitis in particular, though there is some evidence of such effects. There are no prospective studies that convincingly indicate that avoidance of environmental exposure of atopic infants and children to inhalant allergens (e.g., dog and cat dander) will lessen the likelihood of their sensitization, though such a result seems intuitively reasonable.

10.45 PHARMACOLOGIC THERAPY

Much relief can be provided children suffering from allergic diseases through the appropriate use of drugs, of which the most useful are of five distinctive types: adrenergics, theophylline, antihistamines, cromolyn sodium, and corticosteroids.

Adrenergics. These agents exert their activity by combining with specialized receptor areas on cell surfaces. Adrenergic receptors are subject to regulation in terms of numbers and properties by a variety of hormonal and other influences. The two general types of adrenergic receptors are termed α and β. With several exceptions, drugs that affect α receptors cause physiologic responses that are excitatory, whereas drugs that influence β receptors produce inhibitory responses. In a given tissue the response to a drug depends both upon the relative numbers of α and β receptors and upon the intrinsic properties of the drug (i.e., whether it stimulates predominantly α receptors, β receptors, or both). The identification of adrenergic receptors has been made possible largely through the development of drugs that specifically block various classes of these receptors. The adrenergic blocking agents have, in turn, become important in therapy of diseases in which it is advisable to block the physiologic responses resulting from stimulation of given receptors.

Variations in sensitivity of β receptors in different organs to β agonists (stimulants) and differences in response to β blocking drugs of diverse chemical structure have led to separation of β receptors into two subclasses, β_1 and β_2; β_1

receptors have approximately equal affinity for epinephrine and norepinephrine, whereas β_2 receptors have an approximately 10-fold higher affinity for epinephrine than for norepinephrine. Agents with greater β_2-selective activity can provide effective bronchodilation in asthma without the significant increase in heart rate that may occur with isoproterenol or epinephrine, since the latter drugs stimulate both bronchial β_2 receptors and cardiac β_1 receptors, producing cardioacceleration. β_2 selectivity is a relative phenomenon, however, and some patients will develop typical β_1 responses (e.g., cardioacceleration) after administration of a putative β_2-selective agent. The recent identification of β_2 receptors in the heart may explain this effect. Selective β_2 drugs have essentially no α-adrenergic activity and thus no pressor effect; accordingly, the patient does not develop the pallor that may occur with epinephrine administration. Recently, α-adrenergic receptors have been subclassified into α_1 and α_2 subtypes; these have wide distribution and mediate different effects. Stimulation of α_1 receptors contracts vascular and airway smooth muscle.

Although experiments in vitro with human tissues have shown that adrenergic drugs can inhibit allergen-induced mediator release from mast cells and basophils, their use in allergic disorders depends principally upon their effects on smooth muscle in blood vessels and in the bronchial airways. For example, stimulation of α-adrenergic receptors reduces edema of nasal mucous membranes through vasoconstriction and decreases the permeability of venules and capillaries, whereas β-adrenergic stimulation causes smooth muscle relaxation, which relieves at least one component of obstruction of the airway in asthma.

Adrenergic drugs include catecholamines (epinephrine, isoetharine, isoproterenol, and bitolterol [colterol]) and noncatecholamines (ephedrine, albuterol, metaproterenol, terbutaline and fenoterol). The former group are rapidly inactivated by enzymes found in the gastrointestinal tract and liver; accordingly, the use of epinephrine and isoproterenol is limited largely to injection, inhalation, and topical application to mucous membranes. Ephedrine, the oldest of the noncatecholamine sympathomimetics, has relatively weak β-stimulant activity and a significant incidence of adverse side effects, principally involving the central nervous system. Newer noncatecholamine adrenergic agents (metaproterenol, terbutaline, and albuterol), which may also be given orally, have somewhat longer duration of action (up to 6 hr) than ephedrine (4 hr), and have relatively selective activity on the β_2 receptors in the airways, with less of the cardiovascular effects of isoproterenol and epinephrine. Since several-fold lower doses of adrenergic drugs are effective when the agents are given by the aerosol rather than the oral route, aerosol administration is preferred wherever possible, in order to minimize adverse drug effects.

Recently, autoantibodies against β_2 adrenergic receptors have been identified in patients with allergic rhinitis and asthma, and the presence of these autoantibodies has been associated with β-adrenergic hyporesponsiveness. β_2 receptor autoantibodies are not solely responsible for the etiology of these disease states, but they may account for some of the abnormalities in autonomic function that have been encountered.

Adverse side effects of adrenergic drugs may include: skeletal muscle tremor, cardiac stimulation, worsening of hypoxemia, increased airway obstruction, central nervous system stimulation, gastrointestinal disturbances, and tolerance (subsensitivity, refractoriness).

Methylxanthines (Theophylline). Theophylline is the only methylxanthine used in the treatment of asthma; it is a major therapeutic agent for treatment both of acute and of chronic asthma. Its mode of action is uncertain. It is no longer held

that it is inhibition of cyclic AMP phosphodiesterase, since the concentrations necessary to demonstrate this effect are toxic in vivo. Moreover, other potent phosphodiesterase inhibitors (e.g., papaverine) are ineffective in asthma. Other possible modes of action include adenosine antagonism, an effect on calcium flux across cell membranes, prostaglandin antagonism, and enhancement of binding of cAMP to a cAMP-binding protein.

In order to use theophylline effectively and safely, the physician needs to be aware of the following:

Both the therapeutic and toxic effects of theophylline are related logarithmically to the serum concentration. *Measurement of serum theophylline concentration* is an important element in effective and safe use of the drug. Methods for theophylline analysis are specific, sensitive, rapid, and require only a small serum sample; they should be available in all hospitals. A 15-minute, non-instrumental method for determination of theophylline level in finger prick blood (AccuLevel) gives excellent results.

Pharmacokinetics. Both the rapidly absorbed and most (but not all) sustained-release (S-R) formulations of theophylline are, for all practical purposes, completely bioavailable. Rapidly absorbed preparations may be given with food without significant effect on rate or extent of absorption, but absorption characteristics of S-R products may be altered when they are administered with a meal and either accelerated or delayed, depending upon the product. Accordingly, unless the physician wishes to take advantage of the fact that food delays absorption of a specific S-R product (e.g., Theolair), these products are best given 30 minutes before meals. The ultra-slow release formulations may be incompletely bioavailable when given to patients with rapid gastrointestinal transit times (particularly in children). The absorption from a S-R product can vary from time to time, even in the same patient, leading to confused interpretation of serum concentration data. Occasionally, a "trough" theophylline level will be higher than that in a specimen drawn at a time thought to represent a "peak" level.

The marketed S-R products differ in theophylline-release characteristics, and care must be exercised in switching from one product to another. Substitution of a generic for a proprietary preparation without the physician's or patient's knowledge is a potential source of problems.

Despite these limitations, S-R formulations of theophylline represent an advance in dealing with the fluctuations in serum concentrations seen with rapidly absorbed products, particularly in young patients who metabolize the drug rapidly. Even with the S-R products, patients who metabolize theophylline rapidly may have unacceptable fluctuations in serum theophylline level if the drug is given at 12 hr rather than 8 hr intervals. Theophylline absorption is slower during nighttime hours; accordingly, administration every 12 hr may produce higher early morning levels than those later in the day.

Following its absorption, about 60% of theophylline is bound to protein (somewhat less in prematures). Free theophylline is distributed rapidly into body fluids, equilibration between serum and tissues being complete within 1 hr following intravenous injection. Salivary concentrations are about 60% of those in serum. Estimates of serum theophylline concentration derived from analysis of *appropriately collected* saliva samples are accurate enough for most clinical purposes. Theophylline distributes freely into umbilical cord blood, breast milk (not clinically significant for the infant) and cerebrospinal fluid.

Theophylline is metabolized by biotransformation in the liver via a cytochrome P_{448}-dependent microsomal mixed-function oxidase. Metabolism occurs via both first order (linear) and non-linear capacity-dependent processes. Some patients show disproportionate dose-dependent changes in theophylline serum concentration, particularly at the higher doses, owing to the non-linear elimination. About 10–15% of theophylline is excreted unchanged in urine (50% in prematures). There is substantial intersubject variation in the rate of theophylline body clearance. Intrasubject variations in clearance also occur. As with other drugs eliminated by hepatic metabolism, many environmental and disease factors alter the rate of elimination (Table 10–18). Most of the factors listed tend to decrease clearance, with increased theophylline concentration and risk of adverse effect. The clinical relevance of the factors vary: cigarette smoking, intercurrent disease, some drugs (macrolide antibiotics, cimetidine) have a significant effect, whereas others are probably of little clinical relevance (phenobarbital, protein/carbohydrate dietary content, ingestion of charcoal-broiled meats).

Pharmacodynamics. The logarithmic relationship between the theophylline bronchodilator effect and serum concentration in the 5–20 mcg/mL range is now well documented. The serum concentration that provides optimal bronchodilator effect probably varies from patient to patient. The physician should use the patient's response rather than the theophylline blood level as a guide. Some patients receive good bronchodilator effect with serum concentrations of less than 10 mcg/mL; in such cases, there is no need to increase the theophylline dose.

Toxicity. Theophylline toxicity is re-emerging as a major clinical problem, as theophylline is being more widely used and used in regimens requiring higher doses. Signs and symptoms of theophylline intoxication vary from mild nausea to severe seizures and death. Gastrointestinal symptoms are the earliest to appear and generally precede the more serious central nervous system manifestations of toxicity. Uncommonly, seizures may appear as the first sign of theophylline intoxication. Disturbances in cardiac rate, most often tachycardia and rhythm disturbances (various conduction abnormalities), are commonly observed with serious toxicity. Signs and symptoms of theophylline intoxication are, by and large, serum concentration-dependent, but concentrations associated with symptoms of serious toxicity vary widely. In adults with seizures the mean serum concentration has been reported to be approximately 50 mcg/mL with a range of 20–70 mcg/mL. Several infants with theophylline-induced seizures have been reported to have very high serum theophylline

concentrations (180 mcg/mL in one case) with no apparent permanent sequelae. Healthy adolescents who ingest theophylline in suicide attempts appear to tolerate very high theophylline serum concentrations (over 100 mcg/mL) with no permanent sequelae if treated appropriately. On the other hand, children who survive serious theophylline intoxication may be left with severe brain damage that resembles the sequelae of anoxic encephalopathy.

Treatment of theophylline intoxication should begin with measures designed to induce emesis (e.g., administration of ipecac, if the patient is not already vomiting) and/or gavage, followed by a slurry of 30 g of activated charcoal to absorb the theophylline remaining in the gastrointestinal tract. When S-R theophylline has been ingested, repeated administration of charcoal at 2–3 hr intervals is advisable. The addition of a non-absorbed saline cathartic has also been recommended, to decrease intestinal transit time when S-R products have been ingested. Peritoneal dialysis has been used to remove theophylline from intoxicated patients, but hemoperfusion using a specially prepared charcoal column is the method of choice. The indications for charcoal hemoperfusion are not completely defined; they will depend both upon the serum concentration and upon clinical considerations.

Antihistamines. These are drugs of diverse chemical structure that compete with histamine for receptors in various tissues. Two histamine receptors are now recognized, H_1 and H_2. Until recently, only H_1-receptor blockers were used in treatment of allergic disorders. It now appears that a combination of H_1 and H_2 antagonists may be beneficial in some patients with chronic urticaria and in treatment of anaphylactoid reactions such as those due to intravenous injections of contrast media for urography. Cimetidine, an H_2 antagonist, inhibits delayed-type hypersensitivity skin responses, suggesting that H_2-receptor blocking agents may modulate cell-mediated immune injury. The H_1-type antihistamines, as a group, are nitrogenous bases with aliphatic side chains that resemble histamine. The side chains are attached to cyclic or heterocyclic rings of various configurations. The antihistamines may be classified as follows:

Type I—ethylenediamines (tripelennamine [Pyribenzamine]), (methapyrilene [Histadyl, Copyronil]).

Type II—ethanolamines (diphenhydramine [Benadryl]), (carbinoxamine [Clistin, Rondec]).

Type III—alkylamines (chlorpheniramine [Chlor-Trimeton, Teldrin, Novahistine, Demazin]), (brompheniramine [Dimetane, BromFed]), (triprolidine [Actidil, Actifed]).

Type IV—piperazines (cyclizine [Marazine]), (meclizine [Bonine]).

Type V—piperidines (cyproheptadine [Periactin], azatadine [Trinalin]).

Type VI—phenothiazines (promethazine [Phenergan]).

Hydroxyzine (Atarax, Vistaril), which has potent antihistaminic activity, does not belong to any of the six types listed. Two new antihistaminic agents (terfenadine and astemizole) are effective in suppressing the signs and symptoms of allergic rhinitis, do not cross the blood-brain barrier, and have less sedative effects than other antihistamines. *The antihistamines may be found alone or in combination* in the above commercial preparations.

In general, the H_1 antagonists are rapidly absorbed after oral administration, with onset of action within 30 min, peak plasma concentration within 1 hr, and complete absorption within 4 hr. Antihistamines are eliminated by biotransformation in the liver; little nonmetabolized drug is found in urine. Some antihistamines (diphenhydramine and chlorcyclizine) stimulate liver microsomal drug-metabolizing enzymes in animals and may accelerate their own metabolism and that of other drugs. There have been relatively few pharmacokinetic studies of the antihistamines; most of the prescribing patterns

Table 10–18. Factors Influencing Theophylline Clearance

Factors	Decreased	Increased
Age	Prematures Neonates ? Age >50 years	Age 1–16 years
Weight	Obesity (in relation to total body weight)	
Diet	Dietary methylxanthines High carbohydrate	Low carbohydrate High protein Charcoal-broiled meats
Habits		Cigarette smoking (tobacco or marijuana)
Drugs	Troleandomycin Erythromycin Cimetidine Influenza vaccine	Phenytoin Phenobarbital Isoproterenol (intravenous) Terbutaline Rifampin
Disease	Cirrhosis Congestive heart failure Chronic obstructive pulmonary disease Acute pulmonary edema Acute viral illnesses	

are empirically based upon clinical experience. Diphenhydramine (Benadryl) has a relatively short serum half-life of 3–4 hr. Yet the drug is effective in suppression of wheal and flare response to allergy skin testing for over 24 hr. Thus, with this antihistamine there appears to be little correlation between serum concentration and therapeutic effect in the tissue. A study of chlorpheniramine in children showed a mean serum half-life of 13.7 hr (range 6–34 hr). Significant suppression of clinical symptoms of allergic rhinitis was observed for as long as 30 hr after injection of a single dose, at which time chlorpheniramine was not detectable in the serum. Data indicate that chlorpheniramine, brompheniramine, and hydroxyzine may not need to be given 3 or 4 times a day, but that twice or even once a day may suffice. In addition to histamine antagonism, the antihistamines have pharmacologic effects on exocrine secretions, the central nervous system, and the cardiovascular system.

Since antihistamines act as competitive antagonists, they are more effective in preventing than in reversing the action of histamine. To be effective, they must be administered in such dosage and at such intervals as will keep tissue histamine receptor sites saturated. Histamine is released explosively at the site of an IgE-mediated reaction; accordingly, antihistamines are less potent in antagonizing the effects of endogenous than of exogenous histamine. Their relative inefficacy in asthma is related both to this and to the fact that mediators of bronchoconstriction other than histamine are involved in allergic reactions in the lung. Many antihistamines possess anticholinergic activity, which is valuable in allergic rhinitis for controlling rhinorrhea. Anticholinergic activity may account for the occasional asthmatic patient who seems to have a favorable response to antihistamines. A well designed study has shown that in children with asthma, in the usual doses given for hay fever, antihistamines usually had neither favorable nor deleterious effects on the course of asthma.

There is little reason to choose one antihistamine over another. The ethanolamines (e.g., diphenhydramine) and the phenothiazines seem to have greater sedative effects than the alkylamines (e.g., chlorpheniramine); accordingly, if excessive sedation is noted, substitution of a drug from another group or of one of the newer non-sedating agents may be tried. The physician should learn to use one or two of these drugs effectively rather than occasionally use each of a large number of different drugs.

In general, antihistamines are extraordinarily safe and are sold without prescription. They have adverse effects, however, particularly in high dosages. Sedation is the most common side effect, to which some tolerance develops. Combinations of antihistamines with other central nervous depressants (e.g., alcohol) should be avoided. In high doses or in certain sensitive patients, the anticholinergic properties of antihistamines cause undesirable adverse reactions. These include excitation, nervousness, tachycardia, palpitations, dryness of the mouth, urinary retention, and constipation. Seizures are common in antihistamine poisoning. Skin eruptions, blood dyscrasias, fever, and neuropathy are rarely observed.

Cromolyn Sodium (Sodium Cromoglycate). Cromolyn sodium is the disodium salt of 1,3,-bis (2-carboxychromon-5-yloxy)-2-hydroxypropane. It is a chemical analogue of the drug khellin, which has smooth muscle-relaxing properties. It is soluble in water, but insoluble in lipids; only 1% is absorbed from the gastrointestinal tract. The drug is administered as a powder (Intal) with a special turboinhaler, the Spinhaler, or as a 1% (20 mg/2 mL) solution. It is used principally in asthma but has some value in allergic rhinitis and conjunctivitis and in vernal conjunctivitis. It has been used with varying results in aphthous ulcers, food allergy, systemic mastocytosis, ulcerative colitis, and chronic proctitis.

The drug has no bronchodilator properties; it is not, therefore, used in treatment of acute attacks but is given prophylactically, in a 20 mg dose 2–4 times/day. Cromolyn has no antimediator or anti-inflammatory properties. It prevents both antibody-mediated and non-antibody-mediated mast cell degranulation and mediator release. This effect may be due to the ability of cromolyn to block antigen-stimulated calcium transport across the mast cell membrane. Cromolyn inhibition of histamine release may also occur by regulation of phosphorylation of a mast cell protein. The drug also has weak phosphodiesterase inhibitor activity. Cromolyn appears to reduce airway hyperreactivity by a mechanism that is not yet understood. It inhibits bronchoconstriction produced by non-immunologic stimuli such as frigid air, exercise, and sulfur dioxide. These stimuli do not cause release of mast cell-derived mediators; accordingly, cromolyn may directly affect neural control of the airway.

Cromolyn is of greatest value in allergic or extrinsic asthma, but patients with nonallergic or intrinsic asthma who use it may also improve. Patients with mild degrees of asthma respond more favorably than those with severe disease. About 70% of asthmatic patients receive some benefit from inhalation of the drug. The incidence of toxic reactions to cromolyn is extremely low; dry throat and transient bronchoconstriction have been the most frequently reported side effects. The latter is most likely due to inhalation of the dry powder into irritable airways and is not an intrinsic effect of the drug itself. Rare reports have associated urticaria, angioedema, and pulmonary eosinophilia with the use of cromolyn. There are no known contraindications to its use except that in some patients, during an acute attack of asthma, the powder may act as an airway irritant.

Corticosteroids. Corticosteroids are the most potent drugs available for treatment of allergic disorders. Following administration of a well absorbed tablet of prednisone, peak plasma concentration is attained at 1–2 hr. The systemic availability of the drug is over 80% of the oral dose. Regardless of the route of administration, there is interconversion of prednisone and prednisolone (the active form), with prednisolone concentrations 4–10 times those of prednisone. There appears to be little effect of liver disease or renal insufficiency on the conversion of prednisone to prednisolone or on prednisolone disposition. The volume of distribution, metabolic clearance, and renal clearance of prednisone increase with increasing dose, owing to the partially saturable binding of prednisolone to transcortin in plasma, which provides more unbound drug at higher plasma concentrations of this steroid.

Some effects of prednisolone are evident within 2 hr after oral or intravenous administration (fall in peripheral eosinophils and lymphocytes); others may be delayed 6–8 hr or longer (e.g., hyperglycemia and improvement in pulmonary function in asthmatics). The delayed responses reflect the indirect mechanism of action of glucocorticoids. Steps leading to activity include (1) simple diffusion through the cell membrane, (2) binding to cytosol glucocorticoid receptors (found in most mammalian cells), (3) translocation of the steroid-receptor complex to the nucleus, (4) binding of the complex to chromatin which affects nuclear gene expression, and (5) subsequent synthesis of messenger RNA and proteins with enzyme activity. It is the newly synthesized enzymes that mediate the effects of glucocorticoids. The biologic half-life of the steroid is determined by the turnover time of the newly synthesized enzymes, not by steroid plasma concentrations. Plasma half-lives of commonly used steroids vary from 1.5–5 hr, while biologic half-lives vary from 8–54 hr.

Pharmacokinetic studies of prednisolone have shown no differences in distribution, protein binding, plasma clearance, or disposition of unbound drug between males and females or adults and children. Steroid-dependent asthmatics do not differ from normal individuals in prednisolone binding, distribution, or clearance. Clinically significant drug interactions occur with phenobarbital and phenytoin, both of which increase steroid clearance.

The anti-inflammatory actions of glucocorticoids result from: (1) alteration in leukocyte number and activity (redistribution, suppression of migration to sites of inflammation, decreased response to mitogens, decreased cytotoxicity, and suppression of delayed hypersensitivity responses in the skin); (2) suppression of mediator release (decreased histamine synthesis and release, decreased synthesis of prostaglandins and other products of arachidonic acid metabolism); (3) enhanced response to agents which increase cAMP (PGE_2 and histamine via the H_2 receptor); and (4) enhanced response to catecholamines (increased synthesis of β-adrenergic receptors, increased availability of epinephrine due to decreased extraneuronal uptake of catecholamines). Humoral antibody synthesis is little affected by glucocorticoids in the dosage usually given for treatment of allergic disorders. Chronic corticosteroid administration may lower total immunoglobulin concentrations.

The short-term use of corticosteroids in self-limited allergic conditions such as contact dermatitis due to poison ivy, or severe rhinoconjunctivitis due to IgE-mediated allergy to pollens or for occasional episodes of severe asthma is not associated with significant adverse effects. Long-term use, on the other hand, particularly if daily administration is required, may have substantial and undesirable side effects. In children the most common is suppression of linear growth. Posterior subcapsular cataracts develop occasionally in children on long-term steroid therapy.

Before any decision is made to initiate long-term corticosteroid therapy, all other modalities of management should be tried. Despite such measures, a small proportion of allergic children, most having asthma, will have severe and continuing symptoms which interfere with normal school attendance, play activities, sports participation, and the like. The judicious use of glucocorticoids, particularly in alternate-day regimens, can produce substantial improvement in such children with little adverse effect.

A few considerations in the systemic use of corticosteroids bear emphasis. (1) When given in equivalent anti-inflammatory doses, available drugs do not differ qualitatively in anti-inflammatory effects. Adverse effects are related to dose, dosing interval, and duration of treatment. Prednisone or prednisolone is the preferred drug for oral administration, and methylprednisolone or hydrocortisone for intravenous use. Other steroids with longer duration of biologic activity have greater propensities for certain adverse effects, are not suitable for alternate-day therapy, and are more expensive. (2) When corticosteroid therapy is initiated, a sufficient amount should be given in 3–4 divided doses to bring the disease under control. As soon as this is accomplished, an attempt should be made to adjust the dose and the dosing interval to suppress activity of the disease without adverse effects. Whenever possible, alternate-day regimens using prednisone or prednisolone should be tried. In the alternate-day regimen, the drug is given as a single dose every 48 hr between 6:00–8:00 A.M. If daily steroid medication is required, a single dose is given, again between 6:00–8:00 A.M.; this regimen mimics endogenous cortisol secretion and causes less suppression of the hypothalamic-pituitary-adrenal axis and other adverse side effects than the same daily dose of drug given in divided doses. When exacerbations of asthma occur during low dose maintenance therapy, high dose suppressive therapy in divided dosage will be indicated for a few days, with prompt return to low dose alternate-day treatment as soon as the acute process is brought under control.

A new generation of surface-active corticosteroids is available for aerosol administration to corticosteroid-dependent asthmatics. Their high surface activity enables them to be given in minute doses having little systemic effect in the usual regimens. The relative merits of low-dose alternate-day steroids and aerosol corticosteroids are still under study.

Altounyan REC: Review of clinical activity and mode of action of sodium cromoglycate. Clin Allergy 10(Suppl):481, 1980.
Berman BA: Cromolyn: past, present and future. Pediatr Clin North Am. 30:915, 1983.
Bernstein IL: Cromolyn sodium in the treatment of asthma: changing concepts. J Allergy Clin Immunol 68:247, 1981.
Editorial: Histamine H_1 and H_2 antihistamines, and immediate hypersensitivity reactions. J Allergy Clin Immunol 63:371, 1979.
Fauci AS, Dale DC, Balow JE: Glucocorticosteroid therapy: Mechanism of action and clinical considerations. Ann Intern Med 84:304, 1976.
Harper TB, Strunk RC: Techniques of administration of metered-dose aerosolized drugs in children. Am J Dis Childr 135:218, 1981.
Hendeles L, Weinberger M, Johnson G: Monitoring serum theophylline levels. Clin Pharmacokinet 3:294, 1978.
Hendeles L, Weinberger M: Theophylline, a "state of the art" review. Pharmacotherapy 3:2, 1983.
Jack D, Harris DM, Middleton E Jr: Adrenergic agents. In: Middleton E Jr, Reed CE, Ellis EF (eds): Allergy: Principles and Practice. St. Louis, CV Mosby, 1978, p 404.
Morris HG: Mechanisms of action and therapeutic role of corticosteroids in asthma. J Allergy Clin Immunol 75:1, 1985.
Ogilvie RI: Clinical pharmacokinetics of theophylline. Clin Pharmacokinet 3:267, 1978.
Rebuck AS, Gent M, Chapman KR: Anticholinergic and sympathomimetic combination therapy of asthma. J Allergy Clin Immunol 71:317, 1983.

10.46 IMMUNOTHERAPY

Historical Aspects. Immunotherapy (hyposensitization) was introduced in 1912 as a treatment for hay fever induced by grass pollen upon the mistaken notion that the symptoms observed in patients were from a toxin in the pollen and that favorable results obtained with pollen extract injections were due to antitoxin. The original technique has been modified remarkably little.

Immunologic Changes. In the early weeks following the institution of regular injections of ragweed pollen extract, IgE antibody against ragweed pollen antigen increases; as treatment is continued, however, the titer of anti-ragweed IgE antibody decreases. In untreated patients with ragweed hay fever, a rise and a fall of anti-ragweed IgE occur during the year; the rise occurs with the seasonal exposure to ragweed. Injection therapy appears to blunt this anamnestic rise. With continuing treatment, ragweed antibodies of the IgG class ("blocking" or "antigen-binding") appear in the serum; the ultimate titer achieved is related to the quantity of ragweed extract injected but does not necessarily correlate with clinical changes, if any occur.

A further change with therapy involves histamine release from leukocytes (basophils) on challenge in vitro with ragweed antigen E. Leukocytes from treated individuals require exposure to increased amounts of antigen E in order to release the same amount of histamine as prior to therapy. Leukocyte preparations from some treated patients behave as if they have been completely desensitized and do not at any concentration release histamine upon challenge by ragweed antigen E. The basis for this change in cell sensitivity is unknown; it does not appear to be related to titers of either ragweed IgE or IgG. There is thought to be some intrinsic change in receptors for IgE or in the biochemical pathways leading to histamine release. Changes in ratios of helper to suppressor T cells in control of B cells have been reported in experimental animals undergoing immunotherapy, and to a lesser extent in humans. In experimental animals, immunotherapy inhibits the late phase of the IgE reaction in skin and lung. In animals it is possible both specifically to suppress IgE antibody production and to induce tolerance to certain chemically modified or conjugated antigens.

Studies of Efficacy. Critical review of studies of treatment of ragweed hay fever with ragweed extract injections leads to the conclusion that *some* patients receive *some* degree of benefit. Data supporting the efficacy of grass and tree pollen and house dust mite immunotherapy in rhinitis induced by these allergens are less substantial, but the results appear similar to those with ragweed. Substantial proof of efficacy of immunotherapy in asthma, despite its widespread use, is lacking, although there is some evidence that it may be beneficial in asthma induced by house dust or grass pollen. The possibility of prevention of the late phase of the IgE reaction in the lung by immunotherapy provides further rationale for its use. Before immunotherapy can be adequately assessed as a treatment for allergen-precipitated asthma or recommended for widespread use, additional carefully controlled, well designed studies must be done. Immunotherapy with bee venom in patients with anaphylactic sensitivity to bee venom antigen has been shown to protect against anaphylaxis upon subsequent sting in a convincing double-blind study.

The cost of immunotherapy, its inconvenience, the possibility of making the disease worse, and other factors must be considered. There is no acceptable evidence for efficacy of injection therapy with allergens other than those noted above. Specifically, the injection of danders (cat, dog, horse), molds, bacterial vaccines, or food extracts has not been shown to influence favorably the course of rhinitis or asthma.

Indications, Materials, and Procedure. Immunotherapy is indicated in patients suffering from allergic rhinitis, IgE-mediated asthma, or allergy to stinging insects. Atopic dermatitis and food allergy are not improved by immunotherapy. A patient is a candidate for a trial of immunotherapy when good correlation exists between symptoms and exposure to an inhalant allergen that cannot be adequately avoided, when the patient has evidence of IgE-mediated allergy by either in vivo (skin testing) or in vitro (RAST) criteria, and when disabling symptoms are not easily controlled with medication. There should also be a reasonable likelihood of good compliance with the regimen, since treatment involves injections of allergenic extracts at regular intervals for several years.

Aqueous extracts are used most commonly. Alum-precipitated pollen extracts and alum-precipitated pyridine-extracted extracts (Allpyral) do not appear to offer any substantial advantages over aqueous extract therapy. Furthermore, the immunogenicity of certain Allpyral extracts (ragweed in particular) has been questioned by several groups of investigators. Allergenic extracts are considered drugs by the FDA, but standards of potency exist for only a few. Extracts have been sold in the United States for diagnosis and therapy that were totally lacking in allergenic activity when tested by the RAST inhibition methods. Some of the antigens in allergenic extracts (e.g., ragweed antigen E) are quite labile. Methods of extraction, antigen concentration, and storage temperature are all critical factors in the activity and shelf life of an allergenic extract. Pollen extracts are being modified in attempts to reduce their allergenicity without reducing their immunogenicity. Allergens polymerized with gluteraldehyde retain their immunogenicity but are less allergenic. Thus, the initial dose of extract may be substantially increased, the maintenance dose can be reached in about 2 mo compared with 5–6 mo with conventional therapy, and there is a greatly reduced incidence of local and systemic reactions. Such modified extracts are not yet available in the United States.

In practice, immunotherapy with aqueous extracts involves the repeated injection of increasing amounts of extract until the patient reaches an "optimal" maintenance dose. The dose considered optimal is often arbitrary; clinical trials involving ragweed have reported better results with "high dose" than with "low dose" treatment. High dose therapy is possible only when a limited number of allergens are included in the extract. No more than 4–5 allergens should be included in a single injection. Children tolerate the same doses as adults.

The injections are given 1–3 times/wk until the patient reaches the maintenance dose, usually after 5–6 mo. In the "rush" method of immunotherapy used in Scandinavia, the initial injection period is compressed into a few days with apparently satisfactory results. The interval between injections is then extended to 2, 3, and then 4 wk. If more than 4 wk elapse between injections, the subsequent dose is reduced to avoid the possibility of a systemic reaction. There is little reason to continue weekly injections for prolonged periods of time. During the course of the initial injections, the patient is observed carefully for evidence of excessive local reactions. Large local reactions are thought to predict systemic reactions, but this is uncertain. If an extensive local reaction or a systemic reaction occurs, the subsequent dose is reduced and then cautiously increased according to the patient's tolerance. Failure to see a local reaction at any time indicates either that the patient is not allergic to the constituents of the extract or that the extract is inactive.

Perennial treatment, in which injections are given throughout the year, is preferred to preseasonal treatment, in which the treatment regimen is renewed each year, beginning several months prior to the pollen season. During the pollen season the maintenance dose of extract is unchanged except for the patient who develops systemic reactions, presumably due to combined exposure to seasonal and injected allergen. For such patients, the dose may need to be reduced.

The optimal duration of treatment is not known and probably differs from patient to patient. Many allergists believe that if the patient is significantly improved after 3 yr of therapy, it is reasonable to discontinue the injections and observe for recurrence of symptoms. Some children have received "allergy shots" for many years with no evidence that they have been beneficial. Immunotherapy should not be continued if there is no substantial improvement in the condition for which the patient is being treated. Since skin test reactivity changes little during the early years of immunotherapy, it is unnecessary to retest the child yearly.

Precautions and Adverse Reactions. Allergenic extracts should *always* be administered in a physician's office where treatment of a systemic reaction or of anaphylactic shock is readily available. The patient should always remain under observation for at least 20 min after each injection since life-threatening reactions are most likely to occur within this time. Occasionally children will have delayed symptoms; for example, an exacerbation of asthma may occur in the evening of the day on which an injection of extract was given. Rarely, because of distance from a physician's office, it may be necessary to administer allergenic extracts in another setting. Under such circumstances, however, the non-physician who administers an injection must be prepared to treat a systemic reaction. Except for the possibility of constitutional reactions, no short- or long-term adverse effects of administration of allergenic extracts to children are known.

Editorial: A re-evaluation of immunotherapy for asthma. Am Rev Resp Dis 129:657, 1984.
Hendrix SG: A multi-institutional trial of polymerized whole ragweed for immunotherapy of ragweed allergy. J Allergy Clin Immunol 66:486, 1980.
Norman PS: An overview of immunotherapy: Implications for the future. J Allergy Clin Immunol 65:87, 1980.
Patterson RO: Clinical efficacy of allergen immunotherapy. J Allergy Clin Immunol 64:155, 1979.
Sadan N, Rhyne MB, Mellits ED, et al: Immunotherapy of pollenosis in children: Investigation of the immunologic basis of clinical improvement. N Engl J Med 280:623, 1969.
Warner JO, Soothil JF, Price JF, Hey EN: Controlled trial of hyposensitization to dermatophagoides pteronyssines in children with asthma. Lancet 2:912, 1978.

RESPIRATORY ALLERGY

The respiratory tract is the organ system most frequently affected by allergic disorders during childhood.

10.47 ALLERGIC RHINITIS

Seasonal allergic rhinitis, seasonal pollinosis, and hay fever all describe a symptom complex seen in children who have become sensitized to windborne pollens of trees, grasses, and weeds. Estimates indicate that 5–9% of children in unselected samples meet diagnostic criteria. Prevalence increases with age; ragweed hay fever is rarely observed before 4–5 yr of age.

In *perennial allergic rhinitis* the patient has symptoms year round. The causative agents, when they can be identified, are generally found to be allergens to which the patient is exposed more or less continually, though exposure may vary during the year. Indoor inhalant allergens are implicated most often, such as house dust, feathers, and danders of household pets; in certain climates, particularly where the humidity is high, mold spores are frequent offenders. In an occasional patient foods appear to cause symptoms of allergic rhinitis. Some patients are said to be able to ingest certain foods with impunity except during a pollen season, when ingestion causes an aggravation of nasal symptoms.

Diagnosis. The symptoms of allergic rhinitis include sneezing, which is frequently paroxysmal; rhinorrhea, which is often watery and profuse; nasal obstruction; and itching of the nose, palate, pharynx, and ears. Itching, redness, and tearing of the eyes may also occur, causing severe discomfort.

The typical case of allergic rhinitis presents bilateral nasal obstruction resulting from edema of the mucous membranes. Frequently, redundant mucosa is piled up on the floor of the nose. The mucous membranes are bluish in hue and rather pale, and a clear mucoid nasal discharge is seen. The child often has mannerisms involving the nose, which stem from itching or from attempts to increase the airway. The child wrinkles the nose (rabbit nose), and may rub it in characteristic ways (allergic salute). Rubbing in an upward direction may lead to a horizontal crease on the dorsum of the nose near the tip. Dark circles under the eyes may be seen in some patients; these have been attributed to venous stasis resulting from interference with blood flow through edematous nasal mucous membranes. Mouth breathing is common. The diagnosis of allergic rhinitis is substantiated by the finding of a predominance of eosinophils in a smear made of the nasal secretions. A nasal smear is best prepared by having the child blow the nose into wax paper; the mucus sample is then transferred to a glass slide and stained selectively for eosinophils.

Differential Diagnosis. *Eosinophilic non-allergic rhinitis* has recently been described. It occurs principally in adults. Symptoms are perennial, like those of allergic rhinitis; the mucous membranes are pale, and polyps and/or sinus disease are frequently associated. Eosinophils are found in the nasal smear, and allergy skin tests are generally negative. *Primary nasal mastocytosis*, with onset most often in adulthood, presents with perennial nasal blockage and rhinorrhea. Mast cells are found in the nasal smear, and allergy skin tests are negative. *Neutrophilic (infectious) rhinitis* occurs during the early years of childhood when allergic rhinitis is uncommon; there are complaints of chronic rhinorrhea and nasal blockage, principally during the cold weather months. Nasal secretions are commonly mucopurulent, and the nasal smear shows neutrophils, bacteria, and debris. A posterior pharyngeal discharge is often present. X-ray studies of the maxillary sinuses frequently show evidence of sinusitis. The condition appears to result from recurrent viral respiratory illnesses complicated by bacterial infections, but the possibility of underlying disease such as humoral antibody deficiency, immotile cilia syndrome, or cystic fibrosis should be considered. *Vasomotor rhinitis* designates a poorly understood disorder, presumably due to an imbalance of autonomic nervous system control of mucosal vasculature and mucous glands, in which symptoms suggest allergic rhinitis but an allergic etiology cannot be identified. Nasal obstruction is the predominant symptom, with minimal itching, sneezing, and rhinorrhea. The obstruction appears to be aggravated by environmental changes, such as in temperature or humidity, and by exposure to such irritants as tobacco smoke and other non-immunologic inhalants. The patients characteristically do not have eosinophils in their nasal secretions.

Other causes of nasal obstruction include *unilateral choanal atresia* in infants who characteristically have a unilateral nasal discharge, *deviated septum, hypertrophy of the adenoids, encephalocele* and *nasal polyposis*. Nasal polyposis occurs in as many as 20% of children with cystic fibrosis. Fewer than 0.5% of patients in a typical allergy practice will have nasal polyps on a simple allergic basis. Nasal polyposis occurs in *ciliary dyskinesia syndrome* (immotile cilia syndrome, Sec. 13.63) and in *immunologic deficiencies*. The syndrome of nasal polyps, asthma, and aspirin intolerance is known as *triad asthma*. A foul-smelling, unilateral purulent, or blood-tinged purulent nasal discharge in a child suggests a *foreign body*. A persistent blood discharge always suggests *malignancy;* nasal obstruction with epistaxis in a male in late childhood or early adolescence suggests *benign nasopharyngeal fibroma*, also known as *angiofibroma*. Nasal obstruction occurs in *hypothyroidism*. Adolescents may suffer from *rhinitis of pregnancy*. A profuse, clear nasal discharge should suggest *cerebrospinal fluid rhinorrhea*, which can be confirmed by measuring the level of glucose in the fluid. Excessive use of vasoconstrictor nose drops or sprays can lead to *rhinitis medicamentosa*, in which nasal obstruction can be severe. Reserpine can produce marked nasal congestion.

Swelling of the mucous membranes of the sinuses frequently occurs with allergic rhinitis in childhood and may be seen in roentgenograms of the involved sinuses, occasionally with fluid levels. The sinuses appear abnormal so often on roentgenography, not only in children with allergic rhinitis but also in those with viral upper respiratory infections and in entirely asymptomatic children, that such examination must be carefully interpreted. Sinus infection may complicate allergic rhinitis; the symptoms generally are fullness, discomfort, and persistent mucopurulent nasal and pharyngeal discharge.

Treatment. Treatment of either seasonal or perennial allergic rhinitis includes avoidance of exposure to suspected allergens, immunotherapy for those who cannot avoid them or can only partially avoid them, and drug therapy.

Avoidance. It is difficult or impractical to avoid exposure to seasonal pollens, but a great deal can be done to eliminate exposurea to such indoor inhalant factors as house dust, danders, and molds. Control of house dust, with special attention to the child's bedroom, often ameliorates symptoms in the dust-allergic child. Elimination of exposure to danders and feathers is mandatory for a child with perennial allergic rhinitis when these factors appear to contribute to the symptoms. For the child sensitive to indoor molds, avoidance of damp basements and the application of measures designed to discourage mold growth in the house frequently lead to good results. These measures include dehumidifiers, air conditioners with efficient filters, and air cleaning devices, either the electronic precipitator type or one containing an HEPA filter. A 1:750 solution of Zephiran chloride is an effective agent in controlling mold growth. In areas that can be closed off, such as damp cellars, volatilization of paraformaldehyde

(25–50 g, depending upon the size of the area to be treated) from several open jars is also frequently effective in inhibiting growth of mold. For infants with persistent rhinorrhea and nasal obstruction, an elimination diet has been recommended, with particular avoidance of cow's milk. Such diets are only rarely effective, but a brief period of dietary manipulation is innocuous and should be given a trial.

Immunotherapy is discussed in Sec 10.46.

Drug Therapy. Relief can usually be obtained in allergic rhinitis by the appropriate use of drugs. *Antihistamines* are useful, especially in the treatment of the seasonal variety of allergic rhinitis (Sec. 10.45). To achieve the desired effects, it is frequently necessary to increase the dosage beyond that routinely recommended. Nasal itching, sneezing, and rhinorrhea are usually well controlled by antihistamine therapy, whereas nasal obstruction is relieved to a lesser degree. Since antihistaminic agents generally have long half-lives, they need not be given more than twice a day. The major adverse side effect of antihistamine therapy is somnolence, which usually lessens with continued use. Sometimes it requires a change to another class of antihistamine. Non-sedating antihistamines (astemizole, terfenadine) should be tried in patients who experience undue sedation from conventional agents.

If nasal obstruction is particularly troublesome, *sympathomimetics* such as pseudoephedrine or phenylpropanolamine may be tried alone or in combination with an antihistamine. Nose drops or sprays containing sympathomimetic drugs should be avoided except for short-term use; continued use may lead to progressively severe nasal obstruction due to rebound vasodilatation. Treatment of this latter complication requires complete cessation of use of medicated nose drops and the substitution of nose drops of physiologic saline solution.

Cromolyn nasal solution (4%) is useful both in seasonal and in perennial allergic rhinitis. In children with hay fever, use of the nasal spray is best begun prior to the pollen season. The dose varies from 1–2 sprays in each nostril, given 3–6 times per day. As with the powder, cromolyn nasal solution is used prophylactically (Sec. 10.45).

By far the most effective treatment of allergic rhinitis is topical use of *corticosteroids.* Beclomethasone (Vancenase or Beconase) or flunisolide (Nasalide) should be used in children whose nasal symptoms are resistant to antihistamine-decongestant therapy. A dose of 2 inhalations in each nostril 3–4 times a day is given initially. After 3–4 days, as symptoms improve, the dose and frequency of use are reduced until a minimal effective dosage, on the order of 1–2 inhalations once or twice a day, is reached and continued as maintenance therapy. Occasionally, temporary use of corticosteroid eye drops is necessary in a child with hay fever and particularly severe eye symptoms.

For children who suffer from persistent neutrophilic (infectious) rhinitis with or without sinusitis, a 2-week course of a broad spectrum antibiotic (such as amoxicillin) frequently gives good results. Nasal irrigation with a warm saline solution using a bulb syringe or with an adaptation of the Water Pik device (1 tsp. of salt to a full reservoir of warm water) is helpful symptomatically in patients with the non-allergic form of chronic rhinitis.

Broder I, Higgins MW, Matthews KP, et al: Epidemiology of asthma in allergic rhinitis in a total community, Tecumseh, Michigan. IV, Natural history. J. Allergy Clin Immunol 54:100, 1974.

Meltzer EO, Zeiger RS, Schatz M, Jalowayski AA: Chronic rhinitis in infants and children: Etiologic, diagnostic and therapeutic considerations. Pediatr Clin North Am 30:847, 1983.

Mullarkey MF, Hill JS, Webb DR: Allergic and non-allergic rhinitis: Their characterization with attention to the meaning of nasal eosinophilia. J Allergy Clin Immunol 65:122, 1980.

Mygind N: Nasal Allergy. Oxford, Blackwell Scientific Publications, 1978.

10.48 ASTHMA

Asthma is a leading cause of chronic illness in childhood, responsible for a significant proportion of school days lost because of chronic illness. It is estimated that 5–10% of children will at some time during childhood have signs and symptoms compatible with asthma. Prior to puberty about twice as many boys as girls are affected; thereafter, the sex incidence is equal. Asthma can lead to severe psychosocial disturbances in the family. With proper treatment, however, much relief can be provided. There is no universally accepted definition of asthma; it may be regarded as a diffuse, obstructive lung disease with (1) hyperreactivity of the airways to a variety of stimuli and (2) a high degree of reversibility of the obstructive process, which may occur either spontaneously or as a result of treatment.

Both large (>2 mm) and small (<2 mm) airways may be involved to varying degrees. Irritability or hyperreactivity of the airways, while not limited to asthmatics, appears to be an intrinsic part of the disease and is present to some degree in all subjects. This hyperresponsiveness manifests itself as bronchoconstriction following exercise; on natural exposures to strong odors or irritant fumes such as sulfur dioxide (SO_2), tobacco smoke, or cold air; and upon intentional exposures in the laboratory to inhalations of parasympathomimetic agents such as methacholine (Mecholyl) or histamine. This heightened airway irritability is a sensitive objective indicator of asthma, and is present to some degree when patients are asymptomatic, free of physical findings, and have normal findings on spirometry. Airway hyperreactivity relates to the overall severity of the disease. It may vary from patient to patient but generally is stable over time in the same patient except for temporary fluctuations; increased reactivity occurs during viral respiratory infections, following exposure to air pollutants and to allergens or to occupational chemicals in sensitized individuals, and following administration of β-receptor antagonists. An acute decrease in airway irritability is observed following administration of β-receptor agonists, theophylline, and anticholinergics, and after chronic administration of cromolyn or corticosteroids, systemic or inhaled.

Data regarding the inheritance of asthma are most compatible with polygenic or multifactorial determinants. Lability of bronchoconstriction with exercise has been found concordant in identical twins but not in dizygotic twins. Bronchial lability in response to exercise testing also has been demonstrated in healthy relatives of asthmatic children. Whether airway hyperreactivity is genetically determined or acquired as a result of airway insults has not been established.

Epidemiology. Asthma may have its onset at any age; about 80–90% of asthmatic children have their first symptoms before 4–5 yr of age. The course and severity of asthma are difficult to predict. The majority of affected children have only occasional attacks of slight to moderate severity, managed with relative ease. A minority will develop severe, intractable asthma, usually perennial rather than seasonal, which is incapacitating and significantly interferes with school attendance, play activity, and day-to-day functioning. The relationship of age of onset to prognosis is uncertain; studies of Williams and McNichol in Australia found that most severely affected children have onset of wheezing during the 1st yr of life and a family history of asthma and other allergic diseases (particularly atopic dermatitis). These children may have growth retardation unrelated to corticosteroid administration, chest deformity secondary to chronic hyperinflation, and persistent abnormalities on pulmonary function testing.

The prognosis for young asthmatic children is generally good. Ultimate remission will be dependent in significant part upon growth in the cross-sectional diameter of the airways. Longitudinal studies indicate that about half of all asthmatic children will be virtually free of symptoms by the time they reach adulthood. Whether the hyperirritability of their airways ever disappears is unknown; abnormal responsiveness to methacholine inhalation in former asthmatics has been found up to 20 yr after symptoms have abated.

Pathophysiology. The three elements that contribute to airway obstruction in asthma are spasm of smooth muscle; edema and inflammation of the mucous membranes lining the airways; and intraluminal exudation of mucus, inflammatory cells, and cellular debris. The obstruction produces increased airway resistance that lowers forced expiratory volumes and flow rates, premature closure of the airways, hyperinflation of the lungs, increased work of breathing, and changes in the elastic properties and frequency-dependent behavior of the lung. Although the airway obstruction is diffuse, it typically is non-uniform from one part of the lung to another. The perfusion of inadequately ventilated portions of the lung leads to abnormalities in blood gases, particularly decreased pO_2. Early in the course of an acute asthmatic attack, arterial pCO_2 is commonly decreased because of hyperventilation. As the obstructive process worsens, net alveolar hypoventilation supervenes, pCO_2 rises, and when buffer mechanisms are exhausted, blood pH falls. Pulmonary hypertension, right ventricular strain, and impaired left ventricular filling may be observed.

Etiology. Asthma is a complex disorder involving biochemical, autonomic, immunologic, infectious, endocrine, and psychologic factors in varying degrees in different individuals. The control of the diameter of the airways may be considered a balance of neural and humoral forces (Fig. 10–5). Neural bronchoconstrictor activity is mediated through the cholinergic portion of the autonomic nervous system. Vagal sensory endings in airway epithelium—termed cough or irritant receptors, depending upon their location—initiate the afferent limb of a reflex arc, which at the efferent end stimulates bronchial smooth muscle contraction. On the neural bronchodilator side a non-adrenergic inhibitory system (purinergic) is found like that in the ganglion cells of the myenteric plexus. Humoral factors favoring bronchodilation include the endogenous catecholamines which act on β-adrenergic receptors to produce relaxation in bronchial smooth muscle. When humoral substances such as histamine and leukotrienes are released through immunologically mediated reactions, they produce bronchoconstriction, either by direct action on smooth muscle or by stimulation of the vagal sensory receptors described above.

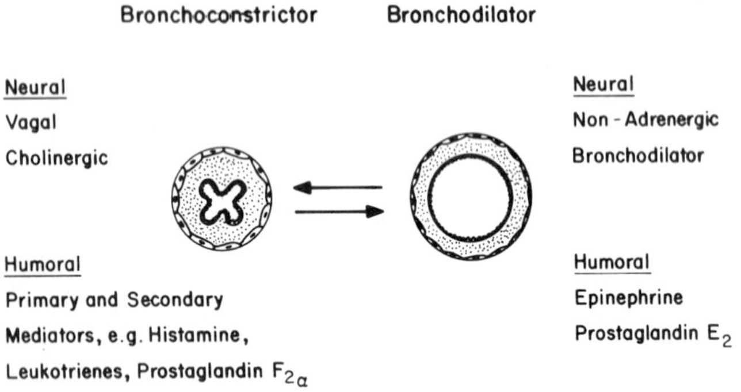

Figure 10–5. The figure shows only the factors that influence smooth muscle tone and control of airway diameter. While acute bronchoconstriction ("bronchospasm") in response to environmental stimuli is principally due to smooth muscle contraction, mucosal edema and inflammation play a major role in the airway obstruction of chronic asthma. In particular the so-called late-phase asthmatic response is due to airway inflammation secondary not only to the action of vasoactive and smooth muscle contractile mediators but also to tissue injury resulting from infiltration of cellular elements, e.g., neutrophils, eosinophils, and others.

One theory (Szentivanyi) considers asthma to be due essentially to abnormal β-adrenergic receptor-adenylate cyclase function, with decreased adrenergic responsiveness. Reports of decreased numbers of β-adrenergic receptors on leukocytes of asthmatics may provide a structural basis for hyporesponsiveness to β-agonists. Alternatively, increased cholinergic activity in the airway has been proposed as a fundamental defect in asthma, perhaps due to some intrinsic or acquired abnormality in irritant receptors, which seem in asthmatics to have lower than normal thresholds for response to stimulation. Neither theory reconciles all the data. In individual patients a number of factors generally contribute in varying degrees to the activity of the asthmatic process.

Immunologic Factors. In some patients with so-called *extrinsic or allergic asthma,* attacks follow exposure to environmental factors such as dust, pollens, danders, and foods. Often but not always, such patients have increased concentrations both of total IgE and of specific IgE against the allergen implicated. In other patients with clinically similar asthma, no evidence of IgE involvement can be found; skin tests are negative and IgE concentrations low. This form of asthma, which is seen most often in the first 2 yr of life and in older adults ("late onset" asthma), has been called *intrinsic or non-immunologic,* but no differences in general immunologic reactivity have been found between the intrinsic and extrinsic groups. In view of the scant evidence that the fundamental abnormality in asthma is immunologic, the interests of many patients, particularly children, have not been well served by narrow or excessive emphasis on the role of allergy in their disease, with overutilization of immunotherapy.

Viral agents are the most important infectious provocateurs of asthma. Early in life respiratory syncytial virus (RSV) and parainfluenza virus (PV) are most often involved; in older children rhinoviruses have also been implicated. Influenza virus infection assumes importance with increasing age. Viral agents may act to initiate asthma through stimulation of afferent vagal receptors of the cholinergic system in the airways. An IgE response to RSV has been reported to occur in infants and children with RSV-associated wheezing but not in those whose RSV respiratory disease is without associated wheezing.

Endocrine Factors. Asthma may worsen in relation to menses, particularly premenstrually, or may have its onset in women around the menopause. It improves in some children at puberty. Little else is known of the role of endocrine factors in the etiology or pathogenesis of asthma. Thyrotoxicosis increases the severity of asthma; the mechanism is unknown.

Psychologic Factors. Asthma is influenced to a considerable extent by emotional factors, and emotional incidents are important precipitants of symptoms in many children and adults, but "deviant" emotional or behavioral characteristics are not significantly more common among asthmatic children than among children with other chronic disabling illnesses. On the other hand, the effects of severe chronic illness such as asthma on children's views of themselves, their parents' views of them, or their lives in general can be devastating. Emotional or behavioral distubances are related more closely to poor control of asthma than to the severity of the attack itself; accordingly, skillful medical intervention can have important impact.

Clinical Manifestations. The onset of an attack of asthma may be acute or insidious. Acute episodes are most often brought on by exposure to irritants such as cold air and noxious fumes (tobacco smoke, wet paint) or exposure to allergens or simple chemicals, e.g., aspirin or sulfites. When airway obstruction develops rapidly in a few minutes, it is most likely due to smooth muscle spasm in large airways. Attacks precipitated by viral respiratory infections are slower in onset, with gradual increases in frequency and severity of cough and wheezing over a few days. The signs and symptoms of asthma include cough, which sounds tight and is nonproductive early in the course of an attack; wheezing, tachypnea, and dyspnea with prolonged expiration and use of accessory muscles of respiration; cyanosis; hyperinflation of the chest; tachycardia and pulsus paradoxus, which may be present to varying degrees depending upon the stage and severity of the attack.

When the patient is in extreme expiratory distress, the cardinal sign of asthma, wheezing, may be strikingly absent; in such patients, only after bronchodilator treatment gives partial relief of the airway obstruction can enough movement of air occur to evoke wheezing. Shortness of breath may be so severe that the child has difficulty walking or even talking. The patient may assume a hunched-over, tripod-like sitting position which makes it easier to breathe. Expiration is typically more difficult because of premature expiratory closure of the airway, but many children complain of inspiratory difficulty as well. Abdominal pain is common, particularly in younger children, and is due presumably to the strenuous use of abdominal muscles and the diaphragm. The liver and spleen may be palpable because of hyperinflation of the lungs. Vomiting is not uncommon and may be followed by temporary relief of symptoms.

During a severe attack respiratory effort may be great, and the child may sweat profusely; a low grade fever may develop simply from the enormous work of breathing; fatigue may become severe. Between attacks the child may be entirely free of symptoms and have no evidence of pulmonary disease on physical examination. A barrel chest deformity is a sign of the chronic, unremitting airway obstruction of severe asthma. Clubbing of the fingers is rarely observed in uncomplicated asthma, even in severe cases. Clubbing suggests other causes of chronic respiratory illness, particularly cystic fibrosis.

Diagnosis. Recurrent episodes of coughing and wheezing, particularly accentuated by exercise, are so characteristic of asthma that the diagnosis is easily made in the majority of cases. There are, however, a significant number of young children with asthma who have a persistent chronic nonproductive cough, particularly at night after going to bed, who cough and become short of breath on exercise, but in whom wheezing has not been documented. A diagnosis of "allergic cough," "allergic bronchitis," "wheezy bronchitis," or "chronic bronchitis" is often erroneously made. Pulmonary function testing, sometimes in conjunction with exercise challenge if the child is old enough to cooperate (usually around 6 yr of age), is useful in arriving at the correct diagnosis. Furthermore, when treated by measures that are specific for asthma, affected children show remarkable improvement, strongly suggesting that the cough is a sign of asthma. Williams and McNichol in their long-term study of asthmatic children were unable to separate those diagnosed as having "wheezy bronchitis" from those considered to have asthma. Both groups had similar family histories of atopic disease and increased incidences of hay fever, eosinophilia, and positive allergy skin tests when compared with controls.

Laboratory Evaluation. Eosinophilia of the blood and sputum occurs with asthma. Blood eosinophilia above 250–400 cells/mm³ is usual. Asthmatic sputum is grossly tenacious, rubbery, and whitish. With an eosin-methylene blue stain, numerous eosinophils and the granules from disrupted cells may be seen. Few diseases in children other than asthma are likely to present eosinophilia in sputum. Sputum cultures are generally not useful in asthmatic children, since bacterial superinfection is rare and cultures are frequently contaminated with oropharyngeal organisms. Serum protein and immunoglobulin concentrations are generally normal in asthma except that IgE levels may be increased.

Allergy skin testing is useful in identifying potentially important environmental allergens (Sec. 10.43).

Inhalation bronchial challenge testing is occasionally done to explore the clinical significance of allergens implicated by skin testing, but since there is excellent correlation between RAST results and bronchial challenge testing, the latter procedure is only rarely indicated. Where the diagnosis of asthma is uncertain, testing for heightened sensitivity to inhalation of Mecholyl and histamine may be helpful in children old enough to cooperate in pulmonary function testing.

The response of the asthmatic to *exercise testing* is quite characteristic (Sec. 13.19).

Every child suspected of having asthma should have *roentgenograms of the chest* with posteroanterior and lateral exposures. Lung markings are commonly increased in asthma. Hyperinflation occurs during acute attacks and may become chronic when airway obstruction is persistent. Atelectasis is very common during acute exacerbations and is particularly likely to involve the right middle lobe, where it may persist for months.

Pulmonary function testing (Sec. 13.19) is valuable in the evaluation of children in whom asthma is suspected. In those known to have asthma, such tests are useful in assessing the degree of airway obstruction and the disturbance in gas exchange, in measuring response of the airways to inhaled allergens and chemicals (bronchial provocation testing), in assessing the response to therapeutic agents, and in evaluating the long-term course of the disease. Assessments of pulmonary function in asthma are most valuable when made before and after administration of an aerosol bronchodilator; with this procedure the degree of reversibility of the airway obstruction at the time of the testing can be determined (Sec. 13.8 and 13.19).

In mild cases of asthma in remission, no abnormalities may be detected. In others a variety of abnormalities may be found. Total lung capacity (TLC), functional residual capacity (FRC), and residual volume (RV) are increased. Vital capacity (VC) is usually decreased. Dynamic tests of air flow, forced vital capacity (FVC), forced expiratory volume in 1 sec (FEV$_1$), and maximum expiratory flow between 25–75% of the vital capacity (FEF$_{25-75}$) may also show reduced values which tend to normalize following administration of aerosolized bronchodilators. With the availability of small, relatively inexpensive instruments that measure peak expiratory flow rate (Mini-Wright Peak Flow Meter, Healthscan), it is feasible to monitor expiratory flow rate at home 2–3 times a day, year round. This gives the physician an objective measurement of the degree of airway obstruction between office visits. Fall in peak expiratory flow predicts the onset of an exacerbation and encourages early intervention with additional drug therapy.

Determination of arterial blood gases and pH is important in evaluation of the patient with asthma, during an exacerbation requiring hospitalization. During remission pO$_2$, pCO$_2$, and pH may been normal. In symptomatic periods, low pO$_2$ is regularly found and may persist days to weeks after an acute episode is over. pCO$_2$ is generally low during the early stages of an asthmatic attack. As the obstruction worsens, pCO$_2$ rises; this is an ominous sign. Blood pH remains normal (or sometimes slightly alkalotic owing to hyperventilation) until the buffering capacity of the blood is exhausted, and then acidosis develops.

Differential Diagnosis. Most children who have recurrent episodes of coughing and wheezing will be shown to have asthma. Other causes of airway obstruction include congenital malformations (of the respiratory, cardiovascular, or gastrointestinal systems), foreign bodies in the airway or esophagus, infectious bronchiolitis, cystic fibrosis of the pancreas, immunologic deficiency disease, hypersensitivity pneumonitis, allergic bronchopulmonary aspergillosis, and a variety of rarer conditions that compromise the airway, including endobronchial tuberculosis, fungal diseases, and bronchial adenoma. Very rarely in the United States, tropical eosinophilia and other parasitic infections may involve the lung and mimic asthma.

Asthma in Early Life. Wheezing in the infant merits special mention because it is common and presents substantial diagnostic and therapeutic problems. A significant number of children subsequently shown to have asthma have had symptoms of obstructive airway disease early in life (39% under 1 yr of age and 57% under 2 yr of age in one series).

A number of anatomic and physiologic peculiarities of early life predispose to obstructive airway disease: (1) a decreased amount of smooth muscle in the peripheral airways compared to adults may result in less support; (2) mucous gland hyperplasia in the major bronchi compared to adults favors increased intraluminal mucus production; (3) disproportionately narrow peripheral airways up to 5 yr of age result in decreased conductance relative to adults and render the infant and young child vulnerable to disease affecting the small airways; (4) decreased static elastic recoil of the young lung prediposes to early airway closure during tidal breathing and results in mismatching of ventilation and perfusion and hypoxemia; (5) highly compliant rib cage and mechanically disadvantageous angle of insertion of diaphragm to rib cage (horizontal vs oblique in the adult) increase diaphragmatic work of breathing; (6) decreased number of fatigue-resistant skeletal muscle fibers in the diaphragm leave the diaphragm poorly equipped to maintain high work output; (7) deficient collateral ventilation with the pores of Kohn and the Lambert canals deficient in number and size. The infant and young child are therefore predisposed to the development of atelectasis distal to obstructed airways. The combination of the above factors with the normal susceptibility of infants and children to viral respiratory infections renders this age group particularly vulnerable to lower respiratory tract obstructive disease.

The clinical, roentgenographic, and blood gas findings in asthma and bronchiolitis are quite similar. It is helpful to remember that the incidence of bronchiolitis due to respiratory syncytial virus peaks during the first 6 mo of life, principally during the cold weather months, and that second and third attacks are uncommon. Some clinicians have proposed using the response to epinephrine to help decide whether an episode is asthma or bronchiolitis, with a favorable response favoring asthma. The validity of this test has not been established; the degree of response may be related more to the severity of the obstructive process than to its underlying nature. Trials of epinephrine or other bronchodilators are worthwhile, however, as will be discussed below.

The onset of symptoms is rather typical; many parents come to recognize and dread the sequence of events that leads to severe respiratory distress. In typical cases, previously well infants or young children will develop what seems to be a cold with rhinorrhea, rapidly followed by irritability, a tight cough, tachypnea, and wheezing. The symptoms may progress with frightening rapidity and often require hospitalization.

During infancy, respiratory tract infections with viruses or chlamydia may cause symptoms of airway obstruction that can be confused with asthma. Bacterial infections of the lower airway are rare, and the concept that allergic reactions to bacteria cause asthma is unproved. A child with recurrent episodes of coughing and wheezing associated with bacterial infections should be investigated for cystic fibrosis or immunologic deficiency. Chronic aspiration due to swallowing dysfunction (usually in developmentally delayed children) or to gastroesophageal reflux also may cause recurrent cough and wheezing in early life. In these infants symptoms of respiratory distress often occur with or shortly after feeding and a chest roentgenogram is commonly abnormal. Rarer causes of obstructive airway disease in early life include obliterative bronchiolitis (usually a sequela of a severe viral insult, most often adenovirus), and bronchopulmonary dysplasia.

The role of food allergy as a major cause of obstructive airway symptoms during early life is controversial. Positive skin tests for IgE-mediated sensitivity to foods are unusual in infancy, and elimination diets and provocative food tests rarely give consistent results. The temporary elimination of milk, wheat, eggs, and chocolate from the diet of the asthmatic patient is recommended by some practitioners.

For an infant who has had several episodes of obstructive airway disease, a history of asthma, hay fever, or atopic dermatitis in mother, father, or siblings is an important predictor of subsequent obstructive airway problems. Eczema is also frequently associated with the subsequent appearance of asthma. Eosinophilia greater than 400 cells/mm³ (and especially greater than 700 cells/mm³) and high serum IgE concentrations predict continuing respiratory tract problems.

Treatment. The principles of avoidance of allergens outlined under treatment of allergic rhinitis also serve the child with asthma. The hyperreactivity of the asthmatic airway as an additional factor is dealt with by minimizing exposure to nonspecific irritants such as tobacco smoke and to strong odors such as wet paint and disinfectants, and by avoiding ice cold drinks and rapid changes in temperature and humidity. Maintenance of humidified air is important in dry, cold climates in the winter. If the clinical history suggests IgE-mediated sensitivity to inhalant factors that cannot be avoided or can be only partially avoided, immunotherapy should be considered; its indications and evidence for its efficacy in asthma are discussed in Sec. 10.46.

Pharmacologic therapy is the mainstay of treatment of asthma. Oxygen administered by mask or nasal prongs at 2–3 L/min is indicated in most children during an acute attack of asthma. Not only is the pO_2 almost always reduced during an acute episode, but drugs used in therapy (isoproterenol or intravenous aminophylline) may cause a further fall in pO_2 secondary to worsening of ventilation-perfusion mismatching, which occurs because these agents cause pulmonary vasodilatation and/or increased cardiac output. Injection of epinephrine has been the treatment of choice for acute asthma for many years, but bronchodilator aerosols are preferred.

When epinephrine is used, a dose of 0.01 mL/kg of the 1:1000 (1.0 mg/mL) concentration of the aqueous preparation may be given. It may be necessary to repeat the same dose once in 20 min to obtain optimal relief. In infants and small children a dose of 0.05 mL is often effective. The unpleasant side effects of epinephrine (pallor, tremor, and headache) can frequently be minimized if doses of no more than 0.2–0.3 mL are given at any age. Terbutaline, a more selective β_2 agonist (Sec. 10.45), is available in an injectable form and is an alternative to epinephrine. The usual dose of 0.0035–0.005 mL/kg of the 1:1000 (1.0 mg/mL) concentration does not cause peripheral vasoconstriction, may produce less cardioacceleration than epinephrine (debatable), and has a longer duration of activity, up to 4 hr.

In children old enough to use them effectively, inhalation of bronchodilator aerosols is rapidly effective in relieving the signs and symptoms of asthma. Aerosols have the advantage that substantially less drug is given than would be required by the subcutaneous route; the unpleasant side effects of injected drugs such as epinephrine are avoided. Isoetharine 1% (Bronkosol) in a dose of 0.5 mL in 2 mL of saline is aerosolized from a plastic nebulizer with a source of compressed air (or preferably oxygen). Metaproterenol (Alupent) 5% solution may be used as an alternative to isoetharine in a dose of 0.25 ml, diluted as above.

If the response to epinephrine and/or bronchodilator aerosol (both may be tried) is not satisfactory, aminophylline may be given intravenously in a dose of 5 mg/kg over 5–15 min at a rate no greater than 25 mg/min. This dose (which will increase the serum theophylline concentration by no more than 10 μg/mL at the peak) is safe in the patient who has had no theophylline in the past few hours. Studies have shown that theophylline serum concentrations obtained at the time of arrival in the emergency room are almost always low enough to permit the administration of the dose recommended above. If, however, there is reason to believe that the patient may already have a significant serum theophylline concentration, the intravenous dose may be reduced by half to avoid the possibility of theophylline toxicity.

Most acute exacerbations of asthma respond to the treatment regimen described above. Unless the patient either is corticosteroid dependent or has had corticosteroids in the recent past, administration of steroids as part of the emergency room treatment program is unnecessary. In borderline cases, however, where the decision is made to send the child home rather than to hospitalize, the prescription of prednisone in decreasing doses over 5–7 days may hasten resolution of the exacerbation and causes no harm. The patient should be discharged from the emergency room with sufficient oral medication to continue therapy at home and appropriate arrangements made for follow-up. Good ambulatory management will almost always reduce the need for emergency room visits for acute attacks.

Status Asthmaticus

If a patient continues to have significant respiratory distress despite administration of sympathomimetic drugs and theophylline, the diagnosis of status asthmaticus should be considered. Status asthmaticus is a clinical diagnosis defined by increasingly severe asthma not responsive to drugs that are usually effective. A patient in whom the diagnosis is made should be admitted to a hospital, preferably to an intensive care unit, where the condition can be carefully monitored. A respiratory score should be determined initially (Table 10–19) and monitored at regular intervals. An indwelling arterial line may be indicated. Baseline complete blood count and serum electrolytes should be measured. Since hypoxemia and acid-base disturbances predispose to cardiac arrhythmias and potentially cardiotoxic drugs (theophylline, adrenergics) will be used, cardiac monitoring is almost always indicated. Analysis of arterial blood for pO_2, pCO_2, and pH is indicated. For these determinations well arterialized capillary blood is adequate

but less desirable than arterial blood, particularly if the patient has received epinephrine, which constricts the peripheral vascular bed.

Patients in status asthmaticus are invariably hypoxemic. Oxygen in carefully controlled concentrations is therefore always indicated to maintain tissue oxygenation. In the face of hypercapnia, particular care should be taken to administer oxygen continuously and not intermittently. It may be administered very effectively by nasal prongs or mask at a flow rate of 2–3 L/min. A concentration of oxygen sufficient to maintain a PaO_2 of 70–90 torr is optimal. A mist tent should not be used; the water does not reach the lower airway to any significant extent, and mists have an irritant effect on the airways of many asthmatics, leading to coughing and worsening of the wheezing. Furthermore, it is not possible to adequately observe a patient who is enveloped in a dense fog.

Dehydration may be present, owing to inadequate fluid intake, greatly increased insensible water loss due to tachypnea, and the diuretic effect of theophylline. Care should be taken not to overhydrate the patient, since increased secretion of antidiuretic hormone occurs during status asthmaticus, promoting fluid retention, and since the large negative peak-inspiratory pleural pressures that occur in children favor accumulation of fluid in the interstitial spaces around the small airways. No more than 1–1.5× maintenance levels of fluid should be given. Sodium bicarbonate, 1–3 mEq/kg, should be administered every 4–6 hr or more often if signs of metabolic acidosis appear.

Bronchodilator therapy initiated in the emergency room should be continued. Aminophylline, 4–5 mg/kg, should be given intravenously over 20 min every 6 hr. Alternatively, a 6 mg/kg loading dose followed by constant infusion in a dose of 0.75–1.25 mg/kg/hr may be administered. If the patient has received aminophylline intravenously in the emergency room, the loading dose should be omitted. It is essential to adjust the aminophylline dose by monitoring serum theophylline concentrations, since there are many physiologic derangements that occur during the course of status asthmaticus that may affect the disposition of theophylline. If the every-6-hr regimen is used, a serum sample should be obtained 1 hr after the intravenous injection and just before the next dose. During constant infusion, theophylline concentration should be monitored at least at 1, 12, and 24 hr as a basis for dose adjustments. A steady state serum concentration of approximately 12–15 μg/mL should be sought. Adrenergic drugs are best administered by aerosol as previously described. Bronchodilator treatments may be repeated every 2–3 hr or more often if necessary. Since the response to bronchodilators in status asthmaticus is by definition inadequate and short lived, we have repeated aerosol treatments as often as every 10–15 min in the very distressed patient who, by blood gas and other criteria, is not yet a candidate for intubation and assisted ventilation. In such a patient isoproterenol is often administered intravenously with gratifying results. Cardiac monitoring in this circumstance is essential. The drug is administered with a constant infusion pump in a dose of 0.1 μg/kg/min for 10–15 min; if the patient does not improve clinically, the dose is increased by 0.1 μg/kg/min for another 10–15 min. The dose may be increased by a similar increment until clinical or blood gas improvement occurs or the heart rate exceeds 200 beats/min. Blood gases should be measured before each incremental increase. This form of therapy has been used most effectively when the PaO_2 is less than 40 torr and the patient is resistant to all other drugs and very distressed.

Corticosteroids, such as methylprednisolone (Solu-Medrol) or hydrocortisone (Solu-Cortef), should be administered in large doses (2 mg/kg of prednisone, or its equivalent, every 4–6 hr). Because it has less effect on mineral metabolism when given in high doses and has lower cost for equivalent anti-

Table 10–19. Respiratory Scoring System

	0	1	2
PaO_2 (torr)	70–100	≤70 in room air	≤70 in 40% O_2
Cyanosis	None	In room air	In 40% O_2
$PaCO_2$ (torr)	<40	40–65	>65
Pulsus paradoxus (torr)	<10	10–40	>40
Use of accessory muscles of respiration	None	Moderate	Marked
Air exchange	Good	Fair	Poor
Mental status	Normal	Depressed or agitated	Coma

Interpretation of respiratory scoring system:
0–4   No immediate danger
5–6   Impending respiratory failure
7 or greater   Respiratory failure

At the 5–6 range, all those caring for patients in respiratory failure should be notified that there is a patient who may require assisted ventilation. (Modified from Wood DW, et al: J Allergy Clin Immunol 4:261, 1968.)

inflammatory dose, methylprednisolone is preferred to hydrocortisone.

Treatment is guided by serial measurement of blood gases and pH every few hours, or more often if indicated. If gas and pH analysis both indicate that respiratory failure is impending, an anesthesiologist should be alerted and facilities and equipment for nasotracheal intubation and respiratory support with a volume-cycled respirator should be available.

Sedation of patients with status asthmaticus is hazardous unless careful monitoring of blood gases is done. If sedation is necessary, chloral hydrate is the safest drug to use. The best sedative for the patient is the presence of a competent, compassionate physician and nurse at the bedside. Chest roentgenograms should be obtained in all cases and repeated as indicated to detect complications such as mediastinal emphysema or pneumothorax. Routine administration of antibiotics has not been shown to alter the course of status asthmaticus in children or the incidence of infectious complications.

Day-to-Day Management of the Asthmatic Child

On the basis of history, physical examination, laboratory data, pulmonary function testing, and need for medication, patients may be classified as having mild, moderate, or severe asthma. The day-to-day management of these different degrees of illness will vary.

Mild Asthma. Children with mild asthma have attacks of varying frequency, up to once a week, which are not severe and which respond to bronchodilator treatment within 24–48 hr. Generally, medication is not required between attacks when the child is essentially free of symptoms of airway obstruction. Children with mild asthma have good school attendance, good exercise tolerance, and little or no interruption of sleep by asthma. They have no hyperinflation of the chest; their chest roentgenograms are essentially normal. Pulmonary function testing may show mild, reversible airway obstruction, with none to minimal degrees of increased lung volume.

Moderate Asthma. Children with moderate asthma have symptoms more frequently than those with mild disease and often have cough and mild wheezing between exacerbations. School attendance may be impaired, exercise tolerance will be diminished because of coughing and wheezing, and the child may lose sleep at night, particularly during exacerbations. Such children will generally require continuous rather than intermittent bronchodilator therapy to achieve satisfactory control of symptoms. Continuous corticosteroid therapy is not required. Hyperinflation may be evident clinically and roentgenographically. Signs of airway obstruction on physiologic testing are more marked than in the mild group; lung volumes may be increased.

Severe Asthma. Children with severe asthma have virtually daily wheezing and more frequent and more severe exacerbations; they require recurrent hospitalization, which is rarely required for mild or moderate asthma. Severely affected children may miss significant amounts of school, have their sleep interrupted often by asthma, and have poor exercise tolerance. They have chest deformities due to chronic hyperinflation which is evident on roentgenograms. Bronchodilator medication will be required continuously, and regimens may include the regular systemic or aerosol administration of corticosteroids. Physiologic testing will show more severe airway obstruction than in mild or moderate asthma, less reversibility in response to aerosol bronchodilators, and more severe disturbances of lung volumes.

Children with mild asthma should receive bronchodilator medication only when symptomatic, and most exacerbations may be satisfactorily treated with adrenergic agents, preferably by aerosol (isoetharine, albuterol, metaproterenol, terbutaline, fenoterol, or bitolterol), or by injection (aqueous epinephrine). Patients too young to use an inhaled bronchodilator may be given an adrenergic agent in a liquid formulation for oral use. Theophylline may be added to an oral regimen when indicated. Drug therapy usually can be discontinued after a few days. Exercise-induced asthma is most effectively prevented by inhalation of an adrenergic drug immediately before exercise.

For children with moderate asthma who require round-the-clock therapy, two inhalations of an adrenergic aerosol every 4–6 hr often suffices. Alternatively, theophylline may be used. Dose and dosing regimen should be individualized and, if required, monitored by measurement of plasma theophylline concentrations. Some experienced allergists reserve monitoring for those patients who fail to have a favorable bronchodilator response or who have symptoms of toxicity (gastrointestinal or central nervous system) with average dosages. When sustained-release (S-R) formulations of theophylline are used, the peak plasma concentration (assuming a constant fraction of drug is absorbed, which may not be the case) occurs 3–4 hr after the dose, at which time a blood sample for monitoring should be obtained. Blood sampling should be delayed until after a day or so of therapy with S-R drugs to assure that a steady state has been achieved. Some children can be successfully treated on an every 12 hr schedule, but others metabolize theophylline particularly rapidly and will experience marked fluctuations in serum concentration. These peaks and troughs of concentration will be minimized by dividing the 24-hour dose into equal 8-hour doses.

Younger children (aged 1–9 yr) generally eliminate theophylline more rapidly than older children and adolescents and hence require a higher daily dose on a mg/kg basis. Nonetheless, it is safest to begin with a dose of 14–16 mg/kg/24 hr in all children. If this dose is well tolerated, one may increase by 25% increments at 3–4 day intervals to a maximum of 24 mg/kg/24 hr at 1–9 yr of age, to 20 mg/kg/24 hr from 9–12 yr, and 18 mg/kg/24 hr from 12–16 yr. If adequate control of symptoms is not achieved at the maximum doses or adverse effects become evident, adjustment in the dosing regimen must be guided by determination of serum theophylline concentration.

Rapidly absorbed liquids and uncoated tablets, while suitable for children with mild asthma who require a few days of therapy for an exacerbation, have no place in the therapeutic regimen of children who require round-the-clock theophylline therapy because wide fluctuations in serum theophylline concentrations are observed when rapidly absorbed products are used. Which of the sustained-release products to use will depend upon the dosage form (tablet vs capsule) and the amount of drug needed (Table 10–20). Capsule formulations that can be opened are virtually tasteless, should not be

Table 10–20. Selected Sustained-Release (SR) Theophylline Preparations

Dosage Form	Brand Name	Manufacturer	Anhydrous Theophylline Content
Tablets*	Theo-Dur	Key	100, 200, 300 mg
Tablets	Theolair-SR	Riker	200, 250, 300 mg 500 mg
Tablets	Uniphyl	Purdue-Frederick	200, 400 mg
Tablets	Theo-24	Searle	100, 200, 300 mg
Capsules†	Slo-Phyllin Gyrocaps	Rorer	60, 125, 250 mg
Capsules	Slo-Bid Gyrocaps	Rorer	50, 100, 200 mg 300 mg
Capsules	Theo-Dur Sprinkle	Key	50, 75, 125 mg 200 mg
Capsules	Somophyllin-CRT	Fisons	100, 200, 250 mg 300 mg

*All tablets are scored, to permit adjustment of dosage.

†Capsules may be opened and the contents mixed with *moist* food; they are particularly useful in young children.

chewed, and may be mixed with *moist* food, and are particularly suitable for young children. Crushing a sustained-release tablet destroys its constant release properties. Exacerbations of asthma in patients receiving round-the-clock theophylline medication should be treated with adrenergic drugs, as described above for children with mild asthma. If satisfactory control of asthma is not achieved with theophylline or an adrenergic aerosol alone, they should be used in combination.

Cromolyn powder inhaled 4 times a day from a Spinhaler is useful in some children with mild to moderate asthma. A solution of cromolyn is now available for home nebulization regimens for young children subject to recurrent attacks of asthma induced by viral infection during winter. Cromolyn and Bronkosol solutions may be mixed together in the nebulizer for ease of administration.

In certain children with mild or moderate degrees of asthma, significant flareups occur from time to time which may require the use of corticosteroids for a few days. Early use of steroids in the child who is known to become severely ill may reduce the need for hospitalization. Early intervention with bronchodilator drugs (with or without steroids, depending upon the clinical setting) is important in the management of all asthmatic children, regardless of the severity of their conditions. Steroids should be given in adequate doses (1–2 mg/kg/24 hr of prednisone in 2–3 doses) and should be discontinued as quickly as possible, for example, within 5–7 days; a long "weaning" period following an acute attack of asthma is unnecessary. In patients who only rarely require steroid administration, return of normal hypothalamic-pituitary-adrenal function is hastened by the *prompt* discontinuation of the drug when the acute episode is over.

In a minority of children who have severe asthma despite the management outlined above, unacceptable degrees of coughing and wheezing persist, which severely limit the child's play activities and school attendance. In such children the judicious administration of corticosteroids on an alternate-day basis or as an inhaled aerosol frequently results in significant amelioration of symptoms and allows the child to lead a normal life without suffering the adverse effects of corticosteroids. If alternate-day therapy is indicated because of either chronic disability or the severity or frequency of attacks of status asthmaticus, the patient is given 5–7 days of intensive daily therapy and then switched to an alternate-day regimen with a short-acting steroid (prednisone, prednisolone, or methylprednisolone). A 12 yr old child might be given 60 mg, 40 mg, 30 mg, 20 mg, and 10 mg of prednisone/24 hr over a 5 day period for an exacerbation of asthma, to be followed by alternate-day therapy at a dose of 20 mg/24 hr given as a single dose at 7–8 A.M. every 48 hr. If the patient responds well to this regimen, the prednisone may be reduced by 5 mg per dose at 10–14 day intervals until the lowest dose compatible with acceptable control of symptoms is reached, usually 5–10 mg on alternate days. Concurrent therapy with adrenergic drugs, theophylline, and/or cromolyn should be continued since this reduces the dose of steroid required. Low-dose alternate-day therapy is associated with minimal adverse effects and, thus, may be justified in a disease that can be life-threatening and capable of causing chronic invalidism. Use of steroid therapy should *not*, however, substitute for or delay comprehensive management of the disease.

Inhalational corticosteroids, such as beclomethasone dipropionate (Vanceril, Beclovent) and triamcinolone (Azmacort), may provide an alternative to the use of every-other-day oral corticosteroid medication. Beclomethasone, which is effective in microgram (µg) doses is rapidly inactivated in the liver into metabolites devoid of glucocorticoid activity. Accordingly, systemic effects in children given less than 420 µg/24 hr (usual dose is 2 inhalations or 84 µg 4 times a day) are minimal. Oropharyngeal candidosis rarely occurs. Its frequency is diminished by rinsing the mouth after inhaling the aerosol.

Effective use of inhaled steroid requires a degree of compliance by the patient not often found in children under 6–7 yr of age. Studies of adults who have received beclomethasone for up to 7 years have shown no evidence of epithelial atrophy or thinning of underlying connective tissue, but long-term adverse effects of the drug on the pharynx and airways are unknown.

Emotional tensions surrounding asthma are best handled by unhurried discussion of the child's difficulty with the parents, by avoidance of overdramatization of the child's illness, and by careful examinations with the parents of those areas in which parent and child seem to be in conflict. The use of tranquilizers or sedatives as a substitute for more direct attempts to solve emotional problems should be avoided. As the asthma is brought under control, the emotional climate is often improved.

Asthma education programs, for example, ACT (*Asthma Care Training*) and Superstuff, are being used in comprehensive asthma management. Their goal is to increase knowledge of asthma and its treatment on the part of both the child and parent, to improve communication within the family and with the physician and nurse, to improve compliance with the treatment plan, and to decrease the need for use of emergency room or hospital.

Blair H: Natural history of childhood asthma. Arch Dis Child 52:613, 1977.

Boushey HA, Holtzman MJ, Shelan JR, et al: State of the art. Bronchial hyperreactivity. Am Rev Respir Dis 121:389, 1980.

Editorial: Airways reactivity and asthma: significance and treatment. J Allergy Clin Immunol 74:21, 1984.

Editorial: Bronchial asthma—what are those inflammatory cells doing there anyway? J Allergy Clin Immunol 75:239, 1985.

Ellis EF: Asthma in childhood. J Allergy Clin Immunol 72:526, 1983.

Ellis EF, Middleton E Jr: Asthma in childhood. *In*: Lichtenstein LM, Fauci AS (eds): Current Therapy in Allergy and Immunology, 1983–84. St. Louis, CV Mosby Co, 1983.

Friedman R, Ackerman M, Wald E, et al: Asthma and bacterial sinusitis in children. J Allergy Clin Immunol 74:185, 1984.

Furukawa CT, Shapiro GG, Bierman CW, Pierson W: A double-blind study comparing the effectiveness of cromolyn sodium, a sustained-release theophylline in childhood asthma. Pediatrics 74:453, 1984.

Gurwitz D, Mindorff C, Levison H: Increased incidence of bronchial reactivity in children with a history of bronchiolitis. J Pediatr 98:551, 1981.

Hopp RJ, Bewtra AK, Nair NM, Townley RG: Specificity and sensitivity of methacholine inhalation challenge in normal and asthmatic children. J Allergy Clin Immunol 74:154, 1984.

Isles AF, Newth CJL: Pharmacokinetics of a sustained-release theophylline preparation in infants and pre-school children with asthma. J Allergy Clin Immunol 75:377, 1985.

Lewis CE, Rachelefsky G, Lewis MA, et al: A randomized trial of A.C.T. (Asthma Care Training) for kids. Pediatrics 74:478, 1984.

Marion RJ, Creer TL, Reynolds RVC: Direct and indirect costs associated with the management of childhood asthma. Ann Allergy 54:31, 1985.

McIntosh K, Ellis EF, Hoffman LS, et al: The association of viral and bacterial respiratory infections with exacerbations of wheezing in young asthmatic children. J Pediatr 82:578, 1973.

Norrish M, Tooley M, Godfrey S: Clinical, physiological and psychological study of asthmatic children attending a hospital clinic. Arch Dis Child 52:913, 1977.

Oseid S, Edwards AM (eds): The Asthmatic Child in Play and Sport. London, Pitman, 1983.

Weinberger M, Hendeles L, Ahrens R: Clinical pharmacology of drugs used for asthma. Pediatr Clin North Am 28:47, 1981.

Weiss ST, Tager IB, Speizer FE, Rosner B: Persistent wheeze. Its relation to respiratory illness, cigarette smoking and level of pulmonary function in a population sample of children. Am Rev Resp Dis 122:697, 1980.

10.49 ATOPIC DERMATITIS
(Infantile or Atopic Eczema)

Atopic dermatitis is an inflammatory skin disorder characterized by erythema, edema, intense pruritus, exudation, crusting, and scaling. In the acute stages intraepidermal vesiculation (spongiosis) is present. There appears to be a genetically determined predilection. Infants with atopic dermatitis tend subsequently to develop allergic rhinitis and asthma.

About 80% of patients with atopic dermatitis have serum IgE concentrations increased 5–10-fold over normal. There is conflicting evidence as to whether the level of IgE is related to either the severity or the extent of the dermatitis. The concentration of IgE does, however, fluctuate with the stage of the disease, serial studies finding that the level returns to normal when the disease has been quiescent for several years. The high levels of IgE have not been satisfactorily explained. It is by no means established that atopic dermatitis is primarily an IgE-mediated allergic disorder; in fact, it is often difficult to demonstrate a role for allergens, whether foods or inhalants, in the pathogenesis of eczema. Moreover, the relationship of atopic dermatitis to allergy or immunology is made more uncertain by reports that IgE does not seem to be increased in affected patients who have neither family history nor clinical evidence of rhinitis or asthma.

The typical dermal manifestation of the interaction of IgE antibody with antigen is the hive (wheal and flare) rather than the erythematous papule of atopic dermatitis; and, while patients with atopic dermatitis frequently possess IgE antibody specific for inhalants or food allergens, it is not generally possible to induce skin lesions of atopic dermatitis by intradermal injection of the suspected allergen. Typical lesions of atopic dermatitis may occur in individuals with X-linked agammaglobulinemia, who are virtually without IgE.

Increased concentrations of IgE in atopic dermatitis may be related to a deficiency of IgE "suppressor" T cell function. Impairment of cell-mediated immunity in some patients with atopic dermatitis is indicated by (1) absence of the reactions of delayed hypersensitivity upon intradermal skin testing with certain antigens; (2) inability to be sensitized with potent contact sensitizers (e.g., dinitrochlorobenzene [DNCB]); (3) diminished proliferative response of lymphocytes to mitogens such as phytohemagglutinin (PHA); and (4) decreased numbers of T lymphocytes in peripheral blood as measured by sheep red cell rosette formation.

The hyperreactive skin of atopic dermatitis differs from normal skin in its response to a variety of physical and pharmacologic stimuli. For example, a light mechanical stroke results within 1 min in a white line with a surrounding blanched area. This phenomenon ("white dermographism") is not seen in normal skin. Involved skin has abnormal rates of cooling and warming in response to temperature changes, particularly in flexural areas. Paradoxical responses occur to injections of various pharmacologic agents, such as histamine, acetylcholine ("delayed blanch phenomenon"), and nicotinic acid ester. Adrenergic responses are decreased in lymphocytes and granulocytes in atopic dermatitis, suggesting that autonomic imbalance may be a basis for the abnormalities in the skin. The abnormal reactivity of the skin has a counterpart in the airway hyperreactivity of asthma; in both disorders such hyperreactivity seems to be an intrinsic part of the disease, independent of immunologic factors.

Clinical Manifestations. Atopic dermatitis typically occurs in three stages with fairly distinctive features. The disease most often *begins in infancy,* usually during the first 2–3 mo of life. The onset is sometimes delayed until the 2nd or 3rd yr. The earliest lesions are erythematous weepy patches on the cheeks, with subsequent extension to the remainder of the face, neck, wrists, hands, and extensor aspects of the extremities. Involvement of flexural areas characteristically appears later but may occur as popliteal and antecubital dermatitis in early life.

Pruritus is marked; the affected infant makes incessant efforts to scratch by rubbing the face on bedclothes and against the sides of the crib. This trauma to the skin rapidly leads to weeping and crusting; secondary infection is common and may be extensive.

The onset of dermatitis frequently coincides with the introduction of certain foods into the infant's diet, particularly cow's milk, wheat, or eggs. In many infants, however, a prime role of reaginic sensitivity in pathogenesis of the eruption is hard to prove. On the other hand, a recent well designed study of a group of infants and children with atopic dermatitis and high IgE serum concentrations (median age 11 yr), found that 54% developed cutaneous symptoms after food challenges. There is unequivocal evidence of reaginic sensitivity in certain infants who have urticaria, colic, and a diffuse erythematous flush following ingestion of the offending food. The erythematous flush appears to be accompanied by intense itching, which results in scratching and then in the appearance of the skin lesions characteristic of eczema. The major role of scratching in the production of skin lesions has been demonstrated when one extremity has been encased in surgical dressings and the other left uncovered; the lesions of atopic dermatitis occur only in the uncovered extremity.

Atopic dermatitis shows a tendency to *remission at 3–5 yr of age.* In most cases the disease will become quiescent by the age of 5 yr; in some, a mild to moderate eczema may persist in the antecubital and popliteal fossae, on the wrists, behind the ears, and on the face and neck. During childhood, antecubital and popliteal involvement becomes common; extensor surfaces of the extremities may still be actively affected. With increasing age there is a tendency toward *drying and thickening of the skin* in the involved areas, particularly in the antecubital and popliteal fossae, and on the neck, forehead, eyelids, wrists, and the dorsa of the hands and feet. The face takes on a whitish hue (as increased capillary permeability and dilatation result in edema and blanching of surrounding tissues), sometimes called the "mask of atopic dermatitis." Hyperpigmentation of the skin, scaling, and lichenification (a particular kind of papular thickening of the skin, with accentuation of the normal surface lines) become prominent. There is a marked tendency toward lasting remission in the 4th and 5th decades of life.

Diagnosis. When pruritus is intense and the lesions characteristic, the diagnosis of atopic dermatitis may be easy. A family history of asthma, hay fever, or atopic dermatitis, the finding of elevated serum IgE concentrations and of reaginic antibodies to a variety of foods and inhalants, the presence of eosinophilia, and the demonstration of white dermographism support the diagnosis. Some patients have accentuated lines or grooves below the margin of the lower eyelids (atopic pleat, Dennie line, or Morgan fold) and an increased number of creases of the skin of the palm. The skin has a tendency to lichenify in response to chronic irritation or rubbing, a phenomenon that is not seen in normal persons. Generalized dryness of the skin, even in uninvolved areas, and sparsity of the hair of the lateral portion of the eyebrows, thought to be secondary to chronic rubbing, are also characteristic.

Differential Diagnosis. The eczematoid skin reaction characterized by erythema, edema, exudation, crusting, and scaling is not specific for atopic dermatitis. In infants and children the differential diagnosis includes seborrheic dermatitis, scabies, primary irritant dermatitis, allergic contact dermatitis, infectious eczematoid dermatitis, ichthyosis, phenylketonuria, acrodermatitis enteropathica, histiocytosis X, and two primary immunologic deficiency disorders: the Wiskott-Aldrich syndrome and X-linked agammaglobulinemia.

Seborrheic dermatitis typically begins on the scalp, often as "cradle cap," and involves the ear and contiguous skin, the sides of the nose, and eyebrows and eyelids with greasy, brownish scales. These are usually distinguished easily from the erythematous, weeping, crusted lesions of infantile atopic dermatitis, but sometimes during the first few months of life it is difficult to distinguish clearly between seborrhea and atopic dermatitis, particularly when the face is primarily involved. Seborrhea in infancy has a shorter course than that of atopic eczema and responds much more rapidly to treatment. The difficulty in differentiating the 2 conditions is reflected in the use of the term seborrheic eczema by some dermatologists. In infancy, *scabies* may be confused with atopic dermatitis. The location of the lesions helps differentiate the two. Atopic dermatitis most often begins on the cheeks and does not involve the palms and soles, whereas scabies commonly starts with large papules on the upper back and with vesicles on the palms and soles. The mite of scabies or its ova can be seen in scrapings from the vesicles.

Primary irritant dermatitis is a nonallergic reaction due to various irritants and most common in infancy in the diaper area. The location and rapid response of lesions to therapy indicate the correct diagnosis.

The lesions of *allergic contact dermatitis* (poison ivy is the prototype) are usually limited to sites of exposure to the offending allergen and do not typically involve the flexural areas. Occasionally, contact dermatitis is superimposed upon atopic dermatitis when sensitization occurs to chemicals used in treating the latter, such as neomycin, the parabens (used as preservatives in many ointments), or iodochlorohydroxyquin (Vioform).

Infectious eczematoid dermatitis is most often seen as a result of discharge of purulent material from a draining ear or other site of infection. The typical location of the lesions and rapid response to therapy support the diagnosis.

In *ichthyosis vulgaris*, dryness of the skin may lead to confusion with atopic dermatitis, but the scales in ichthyosis are usually larger than those in atopic dermatitis, and the pruritus of ichthyosis, if any, is generally mild. The two disorders may be associated. Infants and children with *untreated phenylketonuria* develop an eczematous dermatitis often confused with atopic eczema. The rash of phenylketonuria is responsive to a diet low in phenylalanine.

Histiocytosis X (Letterer-Siwe disease) and *acrodermatitis enteropathica* are serious systemic diseases occurring early in life. Failure to thrive is prominent. Hemorrhagic manifestations are common in the eczematous eruption of histiocytosis X. In acrodermatitis the skin around the oral, nasal, genitourinary, and rectal orifices is typically involved.

Patients with Wiskott-Aldrich syndrome and X-linked agammaglobulinemia may have an eczema that is indistinguishable from atopic dermatitis.

Complications. During early infancy and childhood, secondary infection of the lesions of atopic dermatitis with bacterial or viral agents is common. Staphylococci and β-hemolytic streptococci are the bacterial agents most often recovered from infected lesions. Herpes simplex (Kaposi varicelliform eruption) is also of particular concern. Infants and children with eczema should not be exposed to adults with herpes simplex infection ("cold sores"). Generalized vaccinia (eczema vaccinatum) should no longer be a problem. Keratoconus is occasionally seen in children with atopic dermatitis, perhaps owing to chronic rubbing of the eyelids. Cataracts occur in 5–10% of adults with severe atopic dermatitis but are rarely seen during childhood.

Treatment. Effective treatment of atopic dermatitis requires control of the environmental precipitants of the itch-scratch-itch cycle that perpetuates the disease, beginning with avoidance of ingestant, injectant, contactant, and atmospheric factors that are known or can be shown to trigger itching or scratching. Extremes of temperature and humidity should be avoided. A warm climate of moderate humidity appears to be optimal for the majority of patients. Sweating leads to itching and to aggravation of the disease. Exposure to sunlight and salt water is of benefit to many patients.

Garments should be made of a smooth-textured cotton; wool should be avoided. Infants should not be allowed to crawl on wool carpeting.

For the dry skin of atopic dermatitis, use of soaps and detergents that defat the skin should be avoided as much as possible. Bathing should be kept to a minimum. The purpose of bath oil or other creams applied to the skin is to seal water into the skin; used correctly, bath oil is added to the tub after the patient has soaked for 20 min. Used thus, bath oil seals the moisture in the hydrated skin instead of excluding it as would occur if the oil were added before the patient enters the bath. The same principle applies to application of creams and lotions; they should be applied to the damp skin following a bath. Should bathing appear to make the patient worse, a nondrying cleansing agent such as Cetaphil, a commercially available nonlipid lotion, can be used.

If it appears that a food or other ingestant makes itching worse, then that food must be excluded from the diet. Skin testing by the prick method is useful in *excluding* IgE-mediated food hypersensitivity. *Positive* skin tests must be assessed by properly controlled food challenges (Sec. 10.56). Arbitrary exclusion of numerous foods from the diets of infants with atopic dermatitis without clear evidence that they are involved in the disease is irrational and can lead to malnutrition. The possible contribution of inhalant factors must be evaluated with the same critical concern.

Local therapy is the mainstay of management of atopic dermatitis. During acute flare-ups of the disease, wet dressings (e.g., Burow solution, 1:20) have an antipruritic and anti-inflammatory effect. Topical corticosteroid lotions or creams may be applied between changes of wet dressings. The continuous application of wet dressings also has the advantage of immobilizing and protecting the affected parts and preventing scratching. Unless scratching can be controlled, it will be almost impossible to manage the disease successfully, particularly during infancy and early childhood. Fingernails must be kept cut as short as possible; restraints for the elbows to keep the hands from the face are sometimes necessary to control scratching at night. Itching is difficult to control with drugs. Drugs with both sedative and antihistaminic activity, such as diphenhydramine (Benadryl), hydroxyzine (Atarax, Vistaril), or promethazine (Phenergan), appear to be of greatest value. In some patients aspirin has a marked antipruritic effect.

When infection is present, antibiotics should be given systemically. Antibiotics in topical medicaments not only are of little therapeutic value but can lead to sensitization to the agents applied, particularly in the case of neomycin. The possibility of superimposed contact sensitization must be considered when there is a sudden exacerbation of atopic dermatitis to which a topical medicament has been applied. Parabens, mercurial compounds, and lanolin can all cause contact sensitization.

After the acute phase has subsided, topical application of corticosteroid creams and ointments is of great value in management of the disease. Their cost may be a serious problem. Cost can be reduced by purchasing relatively concentrated preparations in bulk, which the pharmacist can dilute to half strength with Aquaphor or Eucerin, rather than purchasing equivalent material in 15 or 30 g amounts. Small amounts of steroid rubbed in well at frequent intervals give better results than large amounts applied only infrequently. Percutaneous absorption of corticosteroid occurs but is not generally clinically significant. Long-term topical use of steroids leads to an increase in growth of hair in some patients and to atrophy of the skin. The more potent topical steroids should not be applied to the face.

Systemic administration of corticosteroids is generally not required in treatment of atopic dermatitis in infancy and childhood except in the most severely affected patients. Such treatment is effective in clearing the skin, but its withdrawal is often associated with reactivation of the dermatitis. Alternate-day therapy can be used successfully in the majority of such cases.

Topical treatment with corticosteroids has largely superseded the use of coal tar preparations. Tars stain clothes and skin, and compliance of the patient in their use is often poor. However, newer preparations, Estargel (Westwood) and Psorigel (Owen), are effective and more acceptable cosmetically. Tars are considerably less expensive for long-term topical use than corticosteroids. Coal tar is photosensitizing, and occasionally its use results in a sterile, pustular folliculitis.

Prognosis. With adequate control of factors known to trigger itching, appropriate local treatment, and understanding support for the parents of a child for whom no immediate cure is to be expected, reasonable control of atopic dermatitis can generally be achieved.

Atherton DJ: The role of food in atopic eczema. Clin Exp Dermatol 8:227, 1983.

Ferguson AC, Salinas FA: Elevated IgE immune complexes in children with atopic eczema. J Allergy Clin Immunol 74:678, 1984.

Rasmussen JE: Recent developments in the management of patients with atopic dermatitis. J Allergy Clin Immunol 74:771, 1984.

Sampson HA: Role of immediate food hypersensitivity in the pathogenesis of atopic dermatitis. J Allergy Clin Immunol 71:473, 1983.

Sampson HA, Albergo R: Comparison of results in skin tests, RAST and double-blind placebo-controlled food challenge in atopic dermatitis. J Allergy Clin Immunol 74:26, 1984.

Sampson HA, Jolie PL: Increased plasma histamine concentration after food challenges in children with atopic dermatitis. N Engl J Med 311:372, 1984.

10.50 URTICARIA
(Hives)

Clinical Manifestations. Urticaria, or hives, is a common skin disorder characterized by usually well circumscribed but sometimes coalescent, localized, or generalized erythematous raised skin lesions (wheals or welts) of various sizes. The lesions may be intensely pruritic or itch little, if at all. The individual hive usually resolves within 48 hr, but new ones may continue to appear singly or in crops. When urticaria persists for longer than 6–8 wk, the condition is arbitrarily deemed chronic. Urticaria has been attributed to edema of the upper corium due to dilatation and increased permeability of the capillaries.

In angioedema (angioneurotic edema) the deeper layers of skin or submucosa and subcutaneous or other tissues are involved; the upper respiratory tract and the gastrointestinal tract are common target organs. The distinction between urticaria and angioedema is frequently not clear; the lesions appear to differ only in the depth of tissue involvement.

Incidence. As many as 20% of persons experience hives at some time during life. Urticaria is somewhat more frequent in females than in males.

Pathogenesis. The principal noncytotoxic mechanism by which urticaria and angioedema are produced involves the interaction of antigen with mast cell- or basophil-bound IgE antibodies. The release of histamine from these cells causes vasodilatation and increased vascular permeability and stimulates an axon reflex, which produces a typical wheal and flare reaction. Leukotrienes may contribute to the edema of the IgE-mediated reaction. A second mediator pathway for urticaria involves the complement system. Two complement component split products, C3a and C5a, act as anaphylatoxins (Sec. 10.24) and trigger histamine release from mast cells and basophils by direct action on the cell surfaces, independent of antibodies. C3a and C5a can be generated through both the classical and the alternative complement pathways. A third mediator pathway involves the plasma kinin-forming system of the coagulation scheme. Bradykinin is at least as potent as histamine in increasing vascular permeability. Both non-IgE immunologic reactions and non-immunologic events can produce urticaria and angioedema when they activate the complement and kinin-forming systems.

Etiology. A clinical classification of urticaria is given in Table 10–21.

Table 10–21. Types of Urticaria

Due to ingestants (IgE mechanism in some cases)
  Foods, particularly fish, shellfish, nuts, and peanuts; food additives; Drugs
Due to contactants (IgE mechanism in some cases)
  Plant substances (e.g., stinging nettle)
  Drugs applied to the skin
  Animal saliva
Due to injectants (IgE mechanism in some cases)
  Drugs (particularly penicillin), transfused blood, therapeutic antisera, insect stings and bites, allergenic extracts
Due to inhalants (IgE mechanism)
  Pollens, danders, and ? molds
Due to infectious agents (mechanism unknown)
  Parasites
  Viruses (e.g., hepatitis, infectious mononucleosis)
  ? Bacteria
  ? Fungi
Due to physical factors (mechanism mostly unknown)
  Cold urticaria
  Pressure urticaria
  Solar urticaria
  Aquagenic urticaria
  Dermographism
  Vibratory angioedema
Episodic angioedema with eosinophilia (? a distinctive entity)
Cholinergic urticaria
Associated with systemic diseases (mechanism mostly unknown)
  Collagen-vascular
    Cutaneous vasculitis
    Serum sickness–like disease
  Malignancy
  Hyperthyroidism
  Urticaria pigmentosa (systemic mastocytosis)
Associated with genetic disorders (various mechanisms)
  Familial cold urticaria
  Hereditary angioedema
  Amyloidosis with deafness and urticaria
  C3b inactivator deficiency
Chronic urticaria and angioedema (mechanism unknown)
Psychogenic urticaria (existence as an entity uncertain)

Differential Diagnosis. With a few exceptions no laboratory tests establish or exclude the diagnosis of urticaria and angioedema. Allergy skin testing is generally not helpful. In the absence of any clue suggesting an ingestant etiology, elimination diets are not generally useful. The diagnosis is clinical and requires that the physician be aware of the various forms of urticaria. A carefully taken history will usually allow the type to be identified. Except when there are obvious associations with IgE-mediated reactions, naming the "cause" of urticaria may be difficult. When a causative factor is identified, it will most often be a food or drug; in chronic urticaria, identification is accomplished in no more than 5–10% of cases.

Some forms of urticaria need special mention. *Papular urticaria* is usually seen in small children, generally on the extremities and other exposed parts at the site of insect bites. *Cholinergic urticaria* appears as wheals 1–2 mm in diameter surrounded by large areas of erythema (flares) and frequently involves the skin in the neck area. It is brought on by exercise, by hot showers, and in some instances by anxiety. Affected individuals seem to have an increased sensitivity to cholinergic mediators, which can be demonstrated when an intradermal injection of 0.01 mg of methacholine (Mecholyl) in 0.1 mL of saline produces a localized hive surrounded by smaller, satellite lesions. Urticaria is probably due more often to *viral infection* than is commonly appreciated. It is particularly associated with hepatitis, especially during the prodromal stages, and with infectious mononucleosis. Viral infections can also produce *erythema multiforme*, often confused with urticaria, in which typical iris or target lesions are seen and mucosal involvement is common. In some patients typical hives appear to change spontaneously into lesions of erythema multiforme, which can be a sign of drug allergy (Sec. 5.53).

Urticaria pigmentosa typically occurs during the first few years of childhood and has a distinctive presentation. *Systemic mastocytosis* is a serious form of urticaria pigmentosa in which mast cells infiltrate skeleton, liver, spleen, and lymph nodes. In adults, and rarely in children, urticaria may be associated with *malignancy* or *collagen-vascular disorders.*

Cold urticaria is the most common form due to physical factors. Urticarial lesions, which may be either pruritic or described as painful or burning, appear upon exposure to cold and are confined to the exposed parts of the body. The lesions develop not only on exposure to cold weather but also with local application of cold. The cooling of skin associated with evaporation upon emerging from water can produce urticaria. Swimming in cold water is hazardous; death may occur in patients so exposed. There are two forms: a primary acquired form and a familial form. Cold urticaria may be seen in adults with such systemic diseases as cryofibrinogenemia, cryoglobulinemia, cold-agglutinin disease, and secondary syphilis. In some cases of primary acquired urticaria, the phenomenon has been passively transferred using purified IgE and IgM fractions of serum from affected patients. After appropriate cold challenge there are also increased concentrations of histamine, eosinophil, and neutrophil chemotactic factors; platelet activating factor in venous blood draining the challenge site is also present. Primary acquired cold urticaria appears and disappears spontaneously; in some cases, its onset occurs with a viral illness.

Hereditary angioedema (HAE), a potentially life-threatening form of angioedema (Sec. 10.26 and 10.28) is the most important familial form of angioedema.

A syndrome of *episodic angioedema*, urticaria and fever with associated eosinophilia, has recently been described in both adults and children. In contrast to other hypereosinophilic syndromes, this entity has a benign course.

Treatment. In most instances urticaria is a self-limited illness requiring little treatment other than that aimed at relieving the associated pruritus. Antihistamines are the drugs of first choice. Diphenhydramine (Benadryl), 1.25 mg/kg, or hydroxyzine, 0.5 mg/kg, may be given every 4–6 hr as required.

In particularly acute situations epinephrine 1:1000, 0.1–0.2 mL, gives rapid relief of itching. Hydroxyzine (0.5 mg/kg every 4–6 hr) is the drug of choice for cholinergic and chronic urticaria. The combined use of H_1- and H_2-type antihistamines has been reported to be beneficial in chronic urticaria. Cyproheptadine (Periactin) (2–4 mg every 8–12 hr) is especially useful as a prophylactic agent in cold urticaria. Cyproheptadine produces appetite stimulation and weight gain and perhaps other central nervous system–endocrine effects in some patients. Sun screens are the only effective treatment for solar urticaria. Corticosteroids have varying results in chronic urticaria; the doses required to control the urticaria are often so large that they cause serious side effects. Chronic urticaria does not often respond favorably to dietary manipulation, but a diet that includes only foods of low allergenic potential and that eliminates all food colors (tartrazine, FD&C yellow #5, in particular) and additives is worth a 1–2 wk trial. Unfortunately, chronic urticaria may persist for years. For treatment of hereditary angioedema, see Sec. 10.26 and 10.28.

Jorizzo JL, Smith ED: The physical urticarias: An update and review. Arch Dermatol 118:194, 1982.

Juhlin L: Recurrent urticaria: Clinical investigation of 330 patients. Br J Dermatol 104:369, 1981.

Kaplan AP: The pathogenic basis of urticaria and angioedema: Recent advances. Am J Med 70:755, 1981.

Matthews K: Management of urticaria and angioedema. J Allergy Clin Immunol 66:347, 1980.

Twarog FJ: Urticaria in childhood: Pathogenesis and management. Pediatr Clin North Am 30:887, 1983.

Wanderer AA, St. Pierre J-P, Ellis EF: Primary acquired cold urticaria: Double-blind study of treatment with cyproheptadine, chlorpheniramine, and placebo. Arch Dermatol 113:1375, 1977.

10.51 ANAPHYLAXIS

Definition. The term anaphylaxis describes sudden life-threatening reactions which are most often, but not necessarily, immunologic. Many anaphylactic reactions are the result of IgE-mediated sensitivity to foreign substances, most commonly drugs. Anaphylaxis is uncommon in children. It most commonly follows penicillin administration and Hymenoptera sting. The frequency may be higher in atopic persons. Fatal anaphylaxis follows about 1 in 7.5 million injections of penicillin and 1 in 8.6 million urograms.

Etiology. Virtually any foreign substance is capable of producing anaphylaxis under appropriate circumstances. Drugs, sera, allergenic extracts, venom of stinging insects, foods, injectable agents for roentgenographic contrast studies, and hormone preparations have all produced anaphylactic reactions. Recurrent idiopathic anaphylaxis and exercise-induced anaphylaxis are well documented clinical entities in adults, but are rare in children.

Pathogenesis. In the person who has developed IgE-mediated anaphylactic sensitivity to an antigen, subsequent administration of even minute amounts of the antigen may result in an explosive antigen-antibody reaction with massive release of chemical mediators such as histamine. The action of the mediators on various tissue receptors throughout the body produces the symptoms observed. Histamine plays a central role in the pathogenesis of human anaphylaxis, but other vasoactive substances (arachidonic acid metabolites, kinins, platelet-activating factor) may also have roles. Decreased levels of factor V and factor VIII have been reported, suggesting consumption of coagulation factors due to intravascular coagulation. Several patients studied during severe episodes of systemic anaphylaxis have had low levels of high molecular weight kininogen, C3, and C4. When an immunologic mechanism cannot be identified (anaphylactoid reactions), it is presumed that mediator release occurs as a direct effect of the causative agent on basophils and mast cells or perhaps by activation of the alternative complement pathway, with generation of anaphylatoxins (see above).

Clinical Manifestations. Anaphylactic reactions are characteristically explosive, particularly when the antigen is injected. Surviving patients describe a "feeling of impending doom." The more rapidly symptoms appear after administration of the foreign material, the more serious is the reaction. Often the first symptom noted is a tingling sensation around the mouth or face, followed by a feeling of warmth, difficulty in swallowing, and tightness in the throat or chest. The patient becomes flushed; urticaria and angioedema then appear, along with varying degrees of hoarseness, inspiratory stridor, dysphagia, nasal congestion, itching of the eyes, sneezing, and wheezing. Abdominal cramps, diarrhea, and contractions of the uterus and other organs of smooth muscle may also occur. The patient may lose consciousness and, on examination, be found hypotensive, with feeble heart sounds, bradycardia, and sometimes an arrhythmia. Cardiorespiratory arrest and death may ensue. In fatal cases death has most often resulted from acute upper airway obstruction, though profound circulatory collapse may occur without upper airway obstruction.

Treatment. Treatment of anaphylaxis depends on anticipation that the event may occur and being prepared for it. In particular, physicians who administer allergenic extracts must be ready to treat this life-threatening complication of immunotherapy. If, for example, a generalized reaction follows an injection of pollen extract into an upper extremity, aqueous epinephrine 1:1000, 0.2–0.3 mL, should immediately be administered subcutaneously into the other arm and a tourniquet placed above the site of injection of extract. An additional injection of epinephrine may be administered subcutaneously at the site of injection to retard absorption. An intravenous infusion must be started immediately to administer aminophylline should bronchoconstriction occur and to facilitate administration of drugs (epinephrine 1:10,000) and volume expanders for hypotension. Measurement of central venous pressure is a valuable guide to plasma volume expansion therapy. Oxygen sould be administered by mask, and if there is upper airway obstruction (stridor, hoarseness), the patient may need prompt intubation or a tracheostomy. Diphenhydramine (25–50 mg) should be given intravenously. Corticosteroids are not useful as emergency drugs, but may be useful in preventing the recurrences of symptoms during the 12–24 hr following the acute reaction. Serious anaphylactoid reactions to intravenous radio-contrast media are less common in children than in adults, but occasionally occur. A prophylactic regimen has been developed for patients known to be at risk by virtue of previous reactions. They should be pretreated with prednisone, 50 mg orally every 6 hr for 3 doses, ending 1 hr before the procedure. Diphenhydramine, 50 mg, is given 1 hr before the procedure. This regimen prevents adverse reactions of any degree in over 90% of high-risk patients.

The incidence of drug-induced anaphylaxis would drop substantially if drugs were given only when indicated and only by the oral route unless some compelling reason for injection exists. Not only is anaphylactic sensitivity more easily induced by injection of drugs than by oral administration, but in the sensitized patient anaphylaxis occurs more commonly following parenteral than oral administration. The incidence of anaphylaxis following Hymenoptera stings can be reduced significantly by the appropriate use of venom immunotherapy (Sec. 10.46 and 10.54).

Delage C, Irey NS: Anaphylactic deaths: A clinicopathologic study of 43 cases. J Forensic Sci 17:525, 1972.
Greenberger PA, Patterson R, Simon R, et al: Pretreatment of high-risk patients requiring radio-contrast media studies. J Allergy Clin Immunol 67:185, 1981.
Sheffer Al, Tong AKF, Murphy GF, et al: Exercise-induced anaphylaxis: A serious form of physical allergy. J Allergy Clin Immunol 75:479, 1985.
Smith PL, Kagey-Sobotka A, Bleechner ER, et al: Physiologic manifestations of human anaphylaxis. J Clin Invest 66:1072, 1980.

10.52 SERUM SICKNESS

The serum sickness syndrome is a characteristic systemic immunologic disorder that follows the administration of foreign antigenic material.

Etiology. The disorder was first described in 1905 by von Pirquet and Schick as a consequence of antitoxin therapy for such diseases as diphtheria and tetanus. The illness was shown to be due to an adverse reaction to the serum proteins of the animal in which the antitoxin was prepared. Therapeutic antisera of animal origin, especially equine, are still occasionally used, but today the major cause of the serum sickness syndrome is drug allergy, particularly that due to penicillin. Cases have also followed use of other therapeutic agents, including human gamma globulin, and even Hymenoptera stings. Preparations of immune globulin of human origin are available for treatment of diphtheria and tetanus (and prophylaxis of rabies) in humans, but antitoxins for treatment of crotalid envenomation and clostridial intoxication (botulism, gas gangrene) are still prepared in the horse.

Pathogenesis. Serum sickness is the classic example of "immune complex" disease in the experimental animal. After a single large dose of isotopically labeled antigen is injected into the rabbit, the symptoms of serum sickness occur coincidentally with the appearance of antibody formed against the injected antigen, at a time when the latter is still present in the circulation. Antigen-antibody complexes formed under conditions of moderate antigen excess lodge in small vessels and in filtering organs throughout the body (deposition being aided in the rabbit by the actions of IgE antibody, basophils, and platelet-activating factor and by the release of vasoactive amines that increase the permeability of blood vessels); these complexes activate the complement sequence. Complement components bound at the site of complex deposition promote accumulation of neutrophils through at least two general processes: adherence of neutrophils to the site of bound complement and chemotactic activity of the C567 complex and C3a and C5a fragments. Tissue injury results from the liberation of toxic molecules from the neutrophils. In this animal model, healing of the lesions occurs following elimination of the complexes from the circulation.

There are certain differences between the rabbit model and serum disease in humans; for example, glomerulonephritis is a major lesion in the rabbit but generally develops in humans only with severe serum sickness.

Serum sickness demonstrates how the differing biologic activities of the several species of antibodies formed against a complex antigen may be responsible for diverse parts of the clinical picture; the urticaria of serum sickness is thought to be due to IgE antibody molecules reacting with horse serum proteins, whereas the joint symptoms are thought to occur as a result of deposition of antigen-antibody complexes of the IgG and IgM classes. In both rabbits and humans it is suspected that histamine release from basophils and mast cells, mediated by IgE antibodies, facilitates the deposition of immune complexes through increases in vascular permeability.

Clinical Manifestations. Typically the symptoms of serum sickness begin 7–12 days following injection of the foreign material. Fever and malaise are almost always present, as are cutaneous eruptions. Urticaria, usually generalized, is a common finding. A characteristic serpiginous, erythematous, pruritic eruption on the hands and feet has been reported. Edema, particularly around the face and neck, fever, myalgia, lymphadenopathy, arthralgia, and/or arthritis involving multiple joints, and gastrointestinal complaints also occur. Intense pruritus accompanying the urticaria is the most distressing symptom in many patients. The site of injection of the foreign material generally becomes red and swollen, commonly 1–3 days before systemic symptoms appear. If there has been earlier exposure or previous allergic reaction to the same foreign antigen, symptoms may appear in accelerated fashion, within 1–3 days following injection, or as anaphylaxis. The disease generally runs a self-limited course, and the patient recovers in 7–10 days. Carditis and glomerulonephritis rarely occur; the most serious complications of serum sickness are Guillain-Barré syndrome and peripheral neuritis, especially involving the brachial plexus (C5–C6).

Laboratory Manifestations. The blood leukocyte and eosinophil counts are variable; marked thrombocytopenia is often found. Mild proteinuria and microscopic hematuria may be seen. Plasma cells have been found in blood. The erythrocyte sedimentation rate is often increased. A sheep cell agglutinin titer of the Forssman type is usually elevated. Serum complement levels (C3 and C4) are variably depressed and may fall to low concentrations around the tenth day. C3a anaphylatoxin may be increased. In serum sickness due to horse serum proteins, antibodies of the IgG, IgA, IgM, and IgE classes may be found directed against various horse serum proteins. Direct immunofluorescence studies of skin lesions often reveal immune deposits of IgM, IgA, IgE, or C3.

Treatment. Patients generally respond well to aspirin and antihistamines. When the symptoms are particularly severe, corticosteroids have been used with great efficacy. High doses are given and rapidly reduced as the patient improves.

Prevention. The use of horse serum or other animal serum in therapy should be limited to cases for which no alternative is available. When only equine antitoxin is available, skin tests should be employed prior to administration of serum, beginning with a puncture test using a 1:10 dilution. If the reaction is negative, one may then begin intradermal testing with 0.02 mL of a 1:10,000 dilution. If there is no reaction, a subsequent skin test should be performed with a 1:1000 dilution. If a negative result again is obtained, a final intradermal test with a 1:100 dilution of horse serum is done. A negative reaction to the strongest solution indicates that anaphylactic sensitivity to horse serum is very unlikely; skin tests do not predict the likelihood of development of serum sickness.

Occasionally, a patient will require horse serum therapy who has evidence of anaphylactic sensitivity to horse serum by virtue of either a previous reaction or a positive immediate wheal and flare skin test. In such a case the antitoxin can be successfully administered by a process of rapid desensitization. Some allergists prefer to medicate the patient with epinephrine and antihistamines prior to beginning the desensitization procedure. Others prefer not to mask possible evidence of a reaction at an early stage when it still might be of a minor degree and serve as a warning to proceed more slowly with the desensitization. The desensitization process is begun with 0.1 mL amounts of antitoxin, diluted to 1:100,000–1:10,000, depending upon an estimate of the degree of the patient's sensitivity, and injected intravenously at 20 min intervals. If the patient tolerates the previous injection without adverse reactions, the amount administered may be doubled every 20 min. Generally, the entire amount of antitoxin can be administered safely over a 4–6 hr period. The desensitization, unfortunately, is transient, and the patient will often regain his or her previous anaphylactic sensitivity within a few months. Administration of methylprednisolone in doses of 1–1.5 mg/kg/day has not prevented the development of serum sickness.

Editorial: Serum sickness and immune complexes. N Engl J Med 311:1435, 1984.
Lawley TJ, Bielory L, Gascon P, et al: A prospective clinical and immunologic analysis of patients with serum sickness. N Engl J Med 311:1407, 1984.
Mannik M: Physicochemical and functional relationships of immune complexes. J Invest Dermatol 74:333, 1980.

10.53 ADVERSE REACTIONS TO DRUGS

See also Sec. 5.53.

Definition. An adverse reaction to a drug may be defined as any unwanted consequence of administration of the agent during or following a course of therapy. Adverse reactions fall into two broad categories: those dependent upon pharmacologic mechanisms and those dependent upon immunologic mechanisms. The majority of adverse drug reactions are pharmacologic; the Boston collaborative drug surveillance program found only 6% to have an allergic basis. In a study of hospitalized children who suffered adverse drug reactions, no more than 15% were thought to be of an allergic nature.

Certain generalities apply to adverse drug reactions: (1) Virtually any organ system may be involved. (2) After the neonatal period, children are less often affected than adults. (3) The incidence of reactions increases almost exponentially with the number of drugs given simultaneously. (4) Certain diseases predispose to adverse drug reactions, particularly those in which multiple drug therapy is common (cardiovascular and infectious diseases and psychiatric illnesses). Diseases that affect organs responsible for absorption (gastrointestinal tract), metabolism (liver), or excretion of drugs (kidney) also increase the likelihood of adverse reactions. (5) The pharmacokinetic properties of a drug (for example, the extent of protein-binding) also affect the incidence of adverse reactions.

Classification. Adverse drug reactions can be classified in terms of their underlying mechanisms. *Toxicity* may result from a high concentration of drug in the body due to excessive intake—accidental or intentional—or to abnormalities in absorption, metabolism, or excretion of the drug. Various diseases, genetic factors, or drug interactions may permit accumulation of a drug. Some patients for unknown reasons have excessive pharmacologic responses *(intolerance)* to average drug doses. The signs and symptoms are generally intensifications of the expected pharmacologic effects of the agent.

Side effects are undesirable but essentially unavoidable effects of drugs and largely reflect the fact that a given drug rarely affects only one tissue. When theophylline is given as a bronchodilator agent in asthma, for example, central nervous system stimulation is considered a side effect, though this latter effect of theophylline warrants its use in neonatal apnea. *Secondary effects* of drugs are those not related to their primary pharmacologic actions. An example is disturbance of the bacterial flora of the intestine as a consequence of antibiotic therapy. In drug *idiosyncrasy* the signs and symptoms of the reaction are unrelated to the known pharmacologic properties of the agent, sometimes because of metabolic abnormalities. An example is the hemolytic anemia that follows ingestion of primaquine in patients with glucose-6-phosphate dehydrogenase (G-6-PD) deficiency (Sec. 15.17).

Drug interactions are discussed in Sec. 5.53 (Table 5–29).

Allergic drug reactions occur on the basis of recognized models of immune injury. These include (1) IgE-mediated reactions; (2) cytotoxic reactions resulting from hapten binding to cell membranes and subsequent reaction with anti-hapten antibodies; (3) immune complex reactions in which drug-antibody immune complexes with affinity for cell membranes activate the complement system, resulting in cell membrane damage; (4) reactions due to autoantibody formation; and (5) reactions due to cell-mediated mechanisms. Most drugs are simple chemicals with molecular weights under 1000 and are rarely immunogenic. Substances with low molecular weights may act as haptens and become immunogenic after covalent chemical bonding with tissue proteins to form drug-protein conjugates. Hapten-protein complex formation is necessary for the macrophage–T cell–B cell interaction that leads to formation of hapten-specific humoral antibodies and cellular immunity. In general, only drugs (or their degradative or metabolic products) with sufficient chemical reactivity to bind irreversibly with proteins are capable of inducing hypersensitivity reactions. The major impediment to both study and diagnosis of drug allergy is that the chemically reactive substance is often not the native drug itself but a metabolic or degradative product. Since little is known about the metabolic fate of many drugs in common use, it is often impossible to identify the chemically reactive intermediates necessary for investigative or diagnostic use.

The complexities of understanding allergic reactions to drugs are illustrated by considering the penicillin model. Benzyl penicillin (penicillin G) has produced a wide variety of allergic reactions, including systemic responses such as anaphylaxis, serum sickness, and vasculitis; hematologic disorders, including hemolytic anemia, thrombocytopenia, and granulocytopenia; a broad spectrum of dermatologic entities; pulmonary disease; and renal disease. Under physiologic conditions, both in vivo and in vitro, a number of highly protein-reactive compounds are formed from penicillin. These metabolic products become immunogenic following conjugation with tissue proteins as described above. The penicilloyl group, formed by the combination of benzyl penicillenic acid with amino groups of proteins, is the antigenic determinant formed in largest amounts. Ninety-five per cent of all benzyl penicillin that conjugates with tissue proteins in vivo forms benzylpenicilloyl haptenic groups (BPO), and thus benzyl penicillin has been designated the "major" haptenic determinant of penicillin hypersensitivity. A large percentage of persons who have been treated with penicillin possess antibodies to the benzylpenicilloyl determinant, but most will not develop symptoms of penicillin allergy. BPO-specific IgE antibodies can be detected through a benzylpenicilloyl-polylysine skin test reagent in which BPO haptenic groups are attached to a "backbone" of lysine. Benzylpenicilloyl polylysine is available as a skin test reagent and for coupling to cyanogen bromide-activated disks in the RAST.

Unfortunately, the most feared consequence of **penicillin allergy**, anaphylaxis, is not due to IgE sensitization to the major BPO haptenic group but to less well defined, so-called minor haptenic determinants. These include penicilloate, penilloate, and penicillenate and its oxidation products. Though only 5% or less of the benzyl penicillin that reacts with proteins forms minor haptenic determinants, these have major clinical significance; unfortunately, antigens with minor determinant specificity are not readily available for testing either in vivo or in vitro.

Allergy to benzyl penicillin is further complicated by the development of related semisynthetic penicillins and cephalosporins which share a degree of immunologic cross-reactivity. Among the penicillins, the specificity of the antibody formed by the patient (e.g., whether directed toward the 6-amino-penicillin acid core common to all penicillins or directed toward a unique determinant on a distinctive side chain) determines the degree of cross-allergenicity. Thus, some patients allergic to benzyl penicillin can tolerate the semisynthetic penicillins and vice versa. While substantially different structurally, penicillin and cephalosporins share the highly protein-reactive beta-lactam ring structure. Cases of anaphylaxis following administration of cephalosporins to patients with penicillin allergy are uncommon, but have occurred. Adverse reactions to ampicillin occur in upwards of 10% of patients who receive the drug and merit special consideration. The ampicillin rash is nonurticarial and appears in about 90% of patients with infectious mononucleosis, and also in patients with hyperuricemia. That the rash causes no other ill effects and typically disappears with continuing therapy casts doubt upon its immunologic nature; the pathogenesis of ampicillin rash remains an enigma.

Clinical Manifestations. Rashes are the most common manifestation of adverse drug reactions in children. Urticarial, exanthematous, and eczematoid eruptions predominate, but almost any morphology can be seen: exfoliative dermatitis (penicillin, sulfonamides, phenothiazines, anticonvulsants), bullous dermatoses (including epidermal necrolysis), erythema multiforme, Stevens-Johnson syndrome (sulfonamides, penicillin, barbiturates, anticonvulsants, phenytoin in particular), petechial eruptions, Lyell syndrome (penicillin, barbiturates, anticonvulsants, isoniazid), acneiform eruptions (iodides in postpubertal patients), lichenoid eruptions, photodermatitis (demethylchlortetracycline and phenothiazines), and fixed drug eruptions.

Renal or pulmonary disease following drug therapy rarely occurs during childhood. There have been occasional reports of interstitial nephritis associated with phenytoin that have in vitro evidence of a cellular immune reaction. In a child being treated with nitrofurantoin, fever, cough, and pulmonary infiltration strongly suggest an adverse drug reaction.

When a child who has received prolonged antimicrobial therapy has persistent fever without other cause, drug fever should be considered. Drug fever is often suspected but rarely proved and does not generally occur as the sole manifestation of an adverse drug reaction. Often there is a concomitant rash. The diagnosis is easily made when the drug is discontinued and defervescence occurs within 24–48 hr.

Immunologically mediated drug-induced reactions involving the liver are extremely rare in children, unlike in adults. The same is true for drug-induced disorders of granulocytes and platelets; the overwhelming majority of these are toxic.

Diagnosis. Diagnosis of an allergic drug reaction rests most often on a carefully taken history. Urticaria or angioedema following use of a drug is more relevant than nondescript rashes, for the former are the expression of IgE-mediated reactions. Even under the best of circumstances, however, a definitive diagnosis of an allergic drug reaction is frequently difficult to establish.

Only in the case of penicillin is there any indication that in vivo skin tests detect anaphylactic sensitivity. Skin testing with benzylpenicilloyl-polylysine (BPL; PrePen) (Wm. H. Rorer, Inc., Ft. Washington, PA) and penicillin G will identify the overwhelming majority of children who are at risk of anaphylactic reactions following penicillin administration. The BPL is tested in a concentration of 6.0×10^{-5} M (as supplied by the manufacturer), first by prick or puncture test and, if negative, then by intradermal test according to the manufacturer's instructions. Benzyl penicillin (penicillin G) supplied as potassium penicillin G for injection, USP 1,000,000 U/vial, is freshly diluted with saline to a concentration of 10,000 U/mL. Penicillin G is first tested by prick or puncture and then by intradermal technique up to a final concentration of 10,000 U/mL. If the skin tests (interpreted in the same way as skin tests with pollen or other allergenic extracts) are negative, anaphylaxis is highly unlikely, and, if there is a compelling reason to do so, treatment may be initiated with a small test dose, usually one tenth of the usual dose, given either intravenously or orally. It is, however, impossible to exclude anaphylactic sensitivity due to other haptenic determinants formed in vivo from penicillin for which no skin test reagents are available. Furthermore, penicillin skin tests are predictive only of anaphylaxis and not of serum sickness or other reactions associated with use of the drug.

Patch testing to determine delayed hypersensitivity to a drug is helpful; it should be carried out by someone familiar with the technique to avoid both false-positive and false-negative reactions due to improper procedure.

In vitro testing for drug allergy is principally carried out with the use of RAST for detection of BPO-specific IgE antibodies. RAST for the other haptenic determinants of penicillin allergy is not available. As is the case with other allergens, the properly performed skin test is preferred to RAST on the basis of speed, sensitivity, and cost. Search for serum antibodies to formed elements of the blood in patients with what appear to be drug-induced blood disorders is rarely productive. Assays of cellular immunity have been used in the investigation of drug allergy. Their validity in this context has not been established.

Treatment of Drug Reactions. Treatment of a drug reaction depends upon its mechanism and the clinical manifestations produced. Discontinuation of the drug is indicated in most cases. Under certain conditions, and especially in infants and small children who develop rashes while receiving antibiotics, the circumstances may support a decision to continue administration of the drug until the etiology of the rash becomes clear. If, for example, an infant or small child with a febrile illness develops an exanthematous and nonurticarial rash on first exposure to penicillin, ampicillin, or another antibiotic, the rash is much more likely that of a viral illness than a cutaneous manifestation of allergy to the drug. Rather than labeling the child allergic to the drug on tenuous grounds and compromising its future use, it may be reasonable to continue therapy for a further period while the course of the rash is observed. If the history suggests that an adverse reaction has a pharmacologic basis, the drug may be introduced again at a later date, at a lower dosage or a longer interval between doses, while the serum concentration of the drug is measured, if possible. Ampicillin presents a special problem. There is little to suggest an allergic basis to the rash. However, many physicians will discontinue the ampicillin. If there are special circumstances that dictate the need for the drug, therapy may be continued with the expectation that the rash will disappear and no other problems develop. On the other hand, *if an allergic etiology is likely, the drug should not be reintroduced into the patient,* and an alternative drug should be sought. An exception to this principle arises with penicillin in special circumstances. Desensitization to penicillin of anaphylactically sensitive individuals has been carried out successfully without harm in instances in which penicillin therapy was mandatory (in infectious endocarditis [SBE], for example). The procedure essentially is the same as that previously described for horse serum.

Treatment of systemic anaphylaxis is discussed in Sec. 10.51.

As noted, drug allergy in children is most commonly manifested in the skin. The eruptions are generally self-limited and disappear when the drugs are discontinued. Treatment is therefore symptomatic. Antihistamines are most useful for urticarial rashes. Diphenhydramine (Benadryl) and hydroxyzine (Atarax, Vistaril) possess antihistaminic and sedative properties, which may be useful. It may be necessary to give from 1.5–2 times the ordinarily recommended dose to achieve satisfactory control of symptoms. Epinephrine 1:1000 in doses of 0.1–0.3 mL provides short-term relief. For a more sustained effect, a suspension of epinephrine (Sus-Phrine) in doses of 0.1–0.2 mL may be given subcutaneously every 6 hr. Corticosteroids are reserved for severe cases not relieved by the foregoing measures. The dose and dosage interval are determined by the severity of the reaction.

Prevention. To minimize adverse drug reactions, physicians should use drugs only when indicated, be wary of new drugs, and know the relationships between drugs. Concurrent use of two or more drugs should be avoided unless genuinely indicated. Oral administration is less sensitizing than parenteral and preferred whenever possible. Topical application should be avoided when possible because of increased risk of sensitization by this route. Drug interactions should be anticipated, and patients should be warned against self-medication.

Allergy Grand Rounds: Anaphylactoid reactions to radiocontrast material. J Allergy Clin Immunol 75:401, 1985.
Kaplan AP: Drug-induced skin disease. J Allergy Clin Immunol 74:573, 1984.
Matthews KP: Clinical spectrum of allergic and pseudoallergic drug reactions. J Allergy Clin Immunol 74:558, 1984.
Position Statement: Adverse effects and complications of treatment with beta-adrenergic agents. J Allergy Clin Immunol 75:443, 1985.
Saxon A: Immediate hypersensitivity reactions to beta-lactam antibiotics. Rev Infect Dis 5:S368, 1983.
Sheffer AL, Pennoyer DS: Management of adverse drug reactions. J Allergy Clin Immunol 74:580, 1984.
Sogn DD: Penicillin allergy. J Allergy Clin Immunol 74:589, 1984.
Sullivan TJ: Allergic reactions to antimicrobial agents: A review of reactions to drugs not in the beta lactam antibiotic class. J Allergy Clin Immunol 74:594, 1984.

10.54 INSECT ALLERGY

Also see Sec. 10.46.

Allergic reactions to insects are commonly seen in three clinical forms: (1) respiratory allergy secondary to inhalation of particulate matter of insect origin, (2) local cutaneous reactions to insect bites, and (3) anaphylactic reactions to stinging insects.

Etiology. Sensitization to antigenic material found in the debris and disintegrated bodies of dead insects may produce conjunctivitis, rhinitis, or asthma. Inhalation of scales from the wings of insects such as the mayfly, caddis fly, and moths is a particularly common cause of respiratory symptoms in the Great Lakes area, where large numbers of these insects appear each summer. Local cutaneous reactions commonly follow bites by mosquitoes, flies, and various bugs. Anaphylactic reactions of both immediate and delayed type due to insect allergy are almost entirely caused by Hymenoptera, including the bee family, the wasp, hornet, and yellow jacket family (the vespids), and the ant family. About 0.4–0.8% of persons give histories of systemic reactions to stinging insects, which cause about 40 deaths/yr in the United States.

Pathogenesis. Inhalant allergy to insects is in many cases due to IgE-mediated sensitivity to antigenic materials found in the insects' bodies. The antigenic components responsible for respiratory symptoms have not been thoroughly studied, but the allergenic material appears to reside usually in the cuticle or integument of the insect's body.

In the case of biting insects, the local reaction is frequently a wheal and flare lesion; it appears to be due to vasoactive or irritant materials deposited in the skin while the insect is feeding. There is no evidence for IgE involvement in the local reaction. The mechanism of late or persisting cutaneous reactions is unknown.

Stinging insect venoms have had at least eight or nine components identified, including vasoactive materials such as histamine, acetylcholine, and kinins, a number of enzymes (phospholipase A, hyaluronidase), apamine, melittin, and formic acid. Phospholipase A is the major allergen of honeybee venom. Some antigens in Hymenoptera venom and whole-body extracts are common to the Hymenoptera order; others are family-specific. There is substantial cross-reactivity among vespid venoms. The majority of patients who experience systemic reactions following Hymenoptera stings have IgE-mediated sensitivity to antigenic material in the venom. There are, however, patients with convincing histories of sting anaphylaxis in whom both skin tests and RAST to venoms are negative. Children may have a systemic reaction with the first sting.

Clinical Manifestations. The clinical findings in inhalant allergy due to insects are quite similar to those seen with the usual inhalant allergens such as pollens. Rhinitis, conjunctivitis, and asthma have all been described.

The cutaneous reactions to biting insects are most often urticarial but may be papular, vesicular, and erythematous, particularly as the lesion progresses. Lesions that resemble typical delayed hypersensitivity reactions are also seen.

Clinical reactions to stinging insects range in severity from minimal pain and local erythema to life-threatening anaphylactic episodes. Local reactions vary from a papule or wheal at the site of the sting to edema of an entire extremity. The clinical manifestations of anaphylaxis due to sensitivity to stinging insects are identical to those observed in anaphylactic reactions from other causes. The patient may develop generalized urticaria, symptoms particularly of upper and to a lesser extent of lower airway obstruction, and circulatory collapse. Children who suffer anaphylactic reactions are much less likely than adults to experience such life-threatening features as laryngeal edema, bronchoconstriction, or profound hypotension, but death may occur within a few minutes if appropriate measures are not taken. Serum sickness, nephrotic syndrome, vasculitis, neuritis, or encephalopathy may be seen as late sequelae of the reaction to stinging insects.

Diagnosis. The diagnosis is usually easily made on the basis of history and, in the case of biting insects, by examination of skin lesions. Papular urticaria, which is common in children, is almost always the result of insect bites, particularly of fleas and bedbugs.

Whole-body extracts should not be used for the diagnosis or treatment of Hymenoptera sensitivity. Their potency varies with the amount of venom antigen they contain, which varies with the content of venom sac material in the whole body preparation. Venoms of all 5 Hymenoptera (honeybee, vespids [yellow jacket, yellow hornet, white-faced hornet], and polistes [wasp]) are available for skin testing and treatment. The skin tests should be done in accordance with the manufacturer's recommendations. There is a consensus that appropriately performed skin testing with potent materials is useful in identifying persons at risk of systemic anaphylaxis, but venom skin test–negative subjects have been reported to develop anaphylaxis when stung. Moreover, in some investigators' experience, as many as 40% of skin test–positive, nonimmunized subjects may *not* experience anaphylaxis upon sting challenge. In vitro testing with RAST has not substantially improved the ability to predict anaphylaxis, as compared to skin testing. With venom RAST both false-positive and false-negative results have a 20% incidence.

Treatment. Immunotherapy is occasionally undertaken when it can be established that inhalant allergy is due to a specific insect such as the mayfly or caddis fly. Beneficial results from such treatment have not been thoroughly documented, and avoidance of the insect appears to be the preferred management.

For cutaneous reactions due to biting insects, treatment with topical medicaments to relieve itching and local discomfort and occasionally the systemic use of an antihistamine are all that is generally required. Mosquito extract immunotherapy is not recommended.

In case of an anaphylactic reaction following a Hymenoptera sting, the acute treatment is essentially that of anaphylaxis. Epinephrine 1:1000 in a dose of 0.2–0.3 mL subcutaneously will be effective in combating both upper (glottis) and lower airway obstruction and symptoms of peripheral vascular collapse. Blood volume expanders must be given for persistent hypotension. An antihistamine (e.g., diphenhydramine, 25–50 mg) may be given, although its efficacy has not been established. Corticosteroids are of little use in treatment of the acute systemic reaction but may be useful for treatment of sequelae.

Kits are available commercially for emergency use in case of anaphylaxis following insect sting. Each contains a syringe filled with epinephrine and an antihistamine tablet; persons who have had previous severe or anaphylactic reactions should have such a kit in their possession at all times. Patients at risk of anaphylaxis from an insect sting should also wear an identification bracelet (Medic-Alert) indicating their allergy.

Persons at risk from insect sting should avoid using perfumes or cosmetics and wearing bright or pastel-colored clothing when outdoors. They should always wear gloves when gardening and long pants or slacks and shoes when walking in the grass or through fields.

Venom immunotherapy has an uncertain status, because the natural history of venom reactivity is not adequately understood. IgE-mediated reactivity as measured by skin test or RAST may decline spontaneously in untreated patients. During the 1st months of venom therapy, venom-specific IgE antibodies increase by as much as 3-fold but usually fall to pretreatment levels over 1–2 yr of therapy. Whether the patient's clinical sensitivity is increased during the early course of immunotherapy is unknown. In children, who very frequently lose their venom-specific IgE antibodies without treatment, it is possible that immunotherapy may perpetuate their anaphylactic sensitivity. Venom-specific IgG antibody, which correlates with protection against anaphylaxis in the

majority of patients (there are exceptions), peaks at 2–4 mo following initiation of immunotherapy and declines according to the half-life of the immunoglobulin; therefore monthly injections of aqueous extracts are indicated. IgE antibodies may remain detectable for many years in the serum of treated patients. How long treatment needs to be continued is unknown. There is a consensus that those who experience severe systemic reactions (airway involvement or hypotension) and have a positive skin test should receive immunotherapy. At Johns Hopkins, a better than 95% success rate has been reported in treated patients intentionally challenged with a sting. For patients who, following stings, have urticarial or erythematous reactions which are not considered to be serious, especially in children, immunotherapy is not mandatory. Such patients should adopt avoidance procedures and carry an anaphylaxis kit. Immunotherapy is not indicated in patients with a history of sting anaphylaxis and negative skin test and RAST; one would not know which venom to use. Children with large local reactions, even with positive skin tests or RAST, do not need to be treated with immunotherapy, but considerable judgment is needed in this group. The incidence of side effects during the course of treatment is significant (50% of treated adults experience large local reactions and about 7%, systemic reactions). The incidence of both local and systemic reactions is much lower in children. A major problem, particularly for indigent patients, is the high cost (related to the difficulty in obtaining vespid and polistes venom) of venom immunotherapy. An estimate of the cost of treatment for the first year of a patient with multiple venom sensitivities is $400–$600.

Graft DF, Schuberth KC: Hymenoptera allergy in children. Pediatr Clin North Am 30:873, 1983.
Hunt KJ, Valentine MD, Sobotka AK, et al: A controlled trial of immunotherapy in insect hypersensitivity. N Engl J Med 299:157, 1978.
Lichtenstein LM, Valentine MD, Sobotka AK: Insect allergy: The state of the art. J Allergy Clin Immunol 64:5, 1979.

10.55 OCULAR ALLERGIES

Allergic reactions involving the eye occur much less commonly in children than in adults. The eye may be involved as part of a generalized allergic reaction, in urticaria and angioedema, for example, or the eye alone may be affected. Allergic reactions in the eye are known to occur on the basis of IgE-mediated allergy, as conjunctivitis in a child with ragweed hay fever, for example, or on the basis of a cell-mediated (delayed hypersensitivity) immune reaction, as is seen in contact dermatitis of the eyelids.

Eyelids. Eyelids are particularly prone to swelling because of their loose areolar connective tissue. Swelling may result from contact dermatitis to a variety of environmental substances. The lids are particularly involved because of the frequency with which offending contact sensitizers are carried to the eyelids with the hands. Occasionally, contact dermatitis appears as a result of sensitization to medication applied to the eyes. Cosmetics and topical ophthalmic medications head the list of sensitizing agents. Sulfonamides, neomycin, scopolamine and atropine, pilocarpine, and topical anesthetics have all been reported to cause contact sensitization. The lids become inflamed and indurated, and a scaly eczematoid reaction is evident. The conjunctiva becomes red, and a follicular conjunctivitis may develop.

Blepharitis is an inflammatory eczematous reaction of the eyelid margins, which may be caused by infection, allergy, or both. A chronic staphylococcal infection has been implicated as the major cause of chronic eczema of the eyelid margins. The lid margins, particularly of the lower lids, are affected with an itchy, scaly, erythematous eruption and the presence of exudate at the base of the lashes. This gives the appearance of "granulated eyelids." The eyelids may be crusted together in the morning. The diagnosis is confirmed by slit lamp examination.

Allergic Conjunctivitis. This frequently accompanies allergic rhinitis in patients with hay fever, particularly when it is due to pollens. In affected children, both eyes itch, the conjunctivae are reddened and edematous, and there may be profuse tearing. Rubbing of the eyes aggravates the condition. There is no photophobia or other signs of corneal involvement. On occasion, edema of the conjunctiva will be so severe that the conjunctiva will prolapse over the lower lid in a gelatinous-appearing mass that causes great concern to parents. The eye secretions are frequently watery but, if persistent, may appear purulent. Even discharges that appear purulent, however, contain predominantly eosinophils; these permit differentiation from infectious conjunctivitis, in which the discharge has mainly polymorphonuclear leukocytes and bacteria.

Atopic keratoconjunctivitis occurs in patients with atopic dermatitis, who have extreme ocular itching, red eyes, swollen and thickened eyelids, and, when the cornea is involved, photophobia. Keratoconus, thought to be due to repeated eye rubbing, is a complication.

Vernal Conjunctivitis. Vernal conjunctivitis is more common in children, with a 3:1 male:female predominance, than in adults (80% of patients are under 14 yr old at onset). It appears most often during the spring and summer. The disease affects both eyes and occurs in palpebral and limbal forms. In the *palpebral* form, which is most common, the tarsal plate of the upper lid presents a characteristic "cobblestone" appearance as a result of hyperplasia and thickening of the conjunctiva. A thick, ropy, whitish discharge may be present over the hypertrophied, giant papillae giving the "cobblestone" appearance. In the *limbal* form, the junction of the cornea and sclera is involved, with thickening and opacity of the tissue in the area. Whitish Trantas dots, which represent accumulations of eosinophils, are pathognomonic of the disease. Progression of the limbal form may scar the cornea and lead to blindness in the most severe cases. Symptoms of vernal conjunctivitis include lacrimation, extreme itching, burning, and a particularly distressing photophobia. The seasonal occurrence, the finding of eosinophils, and the frequent coexistence with other atopic diseases such as asthma, hay fever, and eczema suggest that IgE-mediated sensitivity is responsible for the condition; but a detailed study of patients with the condition usually fails to identify any specific etiologic agent, and immunotherapy is of little if any value. The etiology of vernal conjunctivitis is unknown. The symptoms and signs of vernal conjunctivitis are mimicked in a syndrome induced by the wearing of hard or soft contact lenses.

Treatment. Contact dermatitis of the lids is best managed by identification of suspected sensitizers and their elimination. Topical corticosteroids are of value in managing the acute reaction.

Blepharitis is best treated by good lid hygiene, using cotton-tipped applicators and half-strength baby shampoo mixed with water to remove scales and exudate, followed by the use of antistaphylococcal ointments. If an excessive reaction to the treatment results, steroids are applied topically for a few days. Since the disease tends to recur, regular lid care is in order, often for a lifetime.

Allergic conjunctivitis in the patient with hay fever generally responds well to topical application of sympathomimetics (naphazoline or phenylephrine) in the form of eye drops, cromolyn sodium 4% solution, or, in more severe cases, to eye drops or ointments containing corticosteroids. As noted below, steroids should be used in the eyes with caution.

Immunotherapy for allergic conjunctivitis in the absence of allergic rhinitis gives poor results.

Atopic keratoconjunctivitis requires the use of topical steroids, particularly if the cornea is involved. Referral to an ophthalmologist is indicated.

Vernal conjunctivitis may be treated with sparing use of corticosteroid eye drops or ointments. Medrysone (HMS), a topically active, poorly absorbed corticosteroid, in a dose of 1–2 drops 4 times/day, is particularly indicated in allergic conjunctivitis when there is involvement of only the superficial layers of the eye. The drug is less likely to cause increased intraocular pressure than the more readily absorbed preparations such as dexamethasone or methylprednisolone. Whenever topical steroids are used in the eye for more than a few days, intraocular pressure should be monitored. Cromolyn sodium in 4% solution, 1–2 drops 4 times a day, may provide modest relief of the symptoms of vernal conjunctivitis.

Allansmith MR: The Eye and Immunology. St. Louis, CV Mosby Co, 1982.
Friedlaender MH: Clues in the diagnosis of ocular allergy. Immunol Allerg Pract 7:35, 1985.
Friedlaender MH, Akumoto M, Kelley J: Diagnosis of ocular allergy. Arch Ophthalmol 102:1198, 1984.

10.56 ADVERSE REACTIONS TO FOODS

The incidence of adverse reactions to foods is not known and unquestionably varies in different parts of the world. The average United States diet contains many food antigens, chemical food additives, antibiotics, and other substances; accordingly, a significant frequency of adverse reactions to foods should not be surprising. Food reactions caused by allergic mechanisms are estimated to occur in from 0.3–0.7% of persons, but the prevalence of food allergy is a subject of substantial disagreement. In the majority of cases in which individuals react adversely to the ingestion of various foods, these reactions cannot be shown to have an immunologic basis. In these cases the use of immunologic methods of diagnosis (skin testing or provocative testing [injection or sublingual administration of food antigen]) is inappropriate. Treatment based upon immunologic principles is similarly unwarranted.

Etiology. Possible mechanisms for adverse reactions to foods are summarized in Table 10–22. There is little doubt that intact macromolecules may pass through the epithelium of the gastrointestinal tract and gain access to the systemic circulation, particularly during the first few months of life. Secretory IgA limits the intestinal absorption of intact macromolecules. Persons with IgA deficiency have higher levels of antibodies to cow's milk proteins and of immune complexes containing milk than do normal controls. IgE-mediated reactions are characteristically rapid in onset and may present as angioedema of the lips, mouth, uvula, or glottis; as general-

Table 10–22. Mechanisms of Adverse Reactions to Foods

Immunologic
  IgE mediated
  ? Toxic complex (α-gliadin)
  ? Cell (lymphocyte) mediated injury
Biochemical
  Enzyme deficiency (e.g., disaccharidase)
  "Hot dog" headache — nitrite sensitivity
  Tyramine headache
  "Toxic" effect — α-gliadin
Unknown
  Reactions to food additives (F.D. & C. colors and flavorings)

ized urticaria; as asthma; or occasionally as shock. In such cases the patient usually recognizes that the symptoms have followed ingestion of a certain food. Persons with such IgE-mediated food allergy are at constant risk of exposure to the offending food hidden in a food mixture. For example, a nut-sensitive individual may have a serious reaction to ingestion of a cookie coated with almond extract.

Individuals with IgE-mediated food reactions consistently show positive skin tests to the suspected food. In fact, skin testing itself, particularly if done by the intracutaneous technique, can precipitate the clinical reaction in individuals with anaphylactic allergy to a food. Foods that have the highest potential to cause IgE-mediated sensitivity are fish, shellfish, peanuts (a legume), various nuts and seeds, eggs, cow's milk, soy, wheat, and corn.

More difficult to diagnose are reactions that begin a few to 24 hr after ingestion of the offending food. Such reactions have been attributed without much convincing evidence to allergy to a digestive product of the food such as a proteose or polypeptide. The roles of antigen-antibody complexes and cell-mediated immunity (delayed hypersensitivity) in the pathogenesis of these late-occurring reactions are unknown.

A variety of reactions have been reported to follow ingestion of *cow's milk* by infants and children. In some cases an IgE mechanism has been established. In others, however, even with antibodies to milk proteins (particularly α-lactalbumin, β-lactoglobulin, and casein) present in sufficient quantities to be demonstrable by gel diffusion methods, no immunologic mechanism has been established. During the first year of life, vomiting and watery, blood-streaked, mucoid diarrhea may follow cow's milk ingestion. An enteropathy with loss of both protein and blood has been found in other young infants fed large volumes of whole pasteurized milk (but not heat-processed formula). In older infants ingestion of cow's milk has been associated with occult fecal blood loss, recurrent roentgenographic pulmonary infiltrates, and multiple precipitating antibodies to cow's milk proteins (Sec. 13.81). Some cases of pulmonary hemosiderosis are said to be responsive to withdrawal of milk from the diet.

Adverse reactions to milk due to *disaccharidase* deficiencies are discussed in Sec. 12.59.

A number of *enteropathies* with varying combinations of malabsorption, steatorrhea, hypoalbuminemia, and fecal blood loss have been reported due to cow's milk or wheat intolerance. Despite close associations between symptoms or signs and the feeding of these foods, a precise mechanism of immunologic injury has not been identified. It is not known whether wheat-sensitive individuals who have adverse symptoms from the gluten fraction of wheat are reacting to α-gliadin as a toxin or as an antigen in an immune-complex type of injury.

During the first 3 yr of life, rashes and diarrhea following ingestion of fruits and juices are common. There is no evidence of an immunologic mechanism. Other non-immunologic adverse reactions to foods principally in adults include headaches after ingestion of wine and cheese (tyramine), cured meat or "hot dog" headache (sodium nitrite), or the Chinese restaurant syndrome (monosodium glutamate). Affected persons apparently have idiosyncratic, but not allergic, reactions to these simple chemicals. In other cases non-immunologic adverse reactions may be due to food additives, particularly the dyes used in foods and drugs. A report of the National Advisory Committee on Hyperkinesis and Food Additives concluded that there was no direct causal connection between artificial food colors and flavors and hyperactivity in children.

Diagnosis. An etiologic diagnosis in a child suspected of an adverse food reaction requires careful objective study. Elimination from the diet for a period of 7–10 days of a food causing difficulty should generally result in improvement in the patient's symptoms. Reintroduction of the food, initially in small quantities and then in increasing amounts, should result in the return of symptoms in a reasonable period of time, within 7 days at most. If symptoms are produced, the food is eliminated from the diet for several months. Reintroduction of the food (except in cases of anaphylactic sensitivity) should be attempted at regular intervals. An equally critical diagnostic approach should be undertaken in children felt possibly to have "allergic tension-fatigue."

The critical testing of foods by the elimination and provocation method is difficult if either patient or parent anticipates an unfavorable reaction because of the emotional bias incident to the ingestion of the suspected food. Food challenges are best done in a blind manner, the food being given in a disguised form, for example, in opaque capsules or mixed with another food. When the patient's symptoms are present on a more or less continuous basis, the results of elimination of a given food are readily appreciated. On the other hand, when symptoms such as headache are only intermittent, results of elimination and provocation testing are frequently equivocal.

Skin testing utilizing properly prepared food antigens will reveal the presence of any IgE antibody to the test antigen. A negative prick skin test (less than 3 mm diameter wheal) with properly prepared potent food extracts will, for all practical purposes, rule out IgE-mediated allergy to the test food. On the other hand, a positive skin test does not necessarily indicate that the particular food causes symptoms. Positive tests, particularly if they do not correlate with the history, should be confirmed by food challenge. In anaphylactic food allergy, skin tests almost invariably show a positive reaction to the offending food, but in this instance the history alone usually establishes the diagnosis and skin testing is superfluous. Occasionally, a positive skin test to a food not previously suspected of causing trouble will be clinically corroborated when the history is re-examined in light of the positive test. All too often, undue attention paid to clinically irrelevant skin reactions to food extracts has led to very restricted diets with no attempt made to confirm the clinical importance of suspected foods through elimination and provocative testing. Overdiagnosis of food allergy has sometimes produced malnutrition in infants and children as well as anxiety and depression in mothers who have found it impossible to adhere to severely restrictive diets.

RAST assay has been used to detect IgE antibodies to foods. The correlation between clinical history, puncture skin test, and RAST is excellent for codfish, egg white, nuts, peanuts, and peas. Positive RAST and skin tests to cereals correlate poorly with the results of cereal challenge. RAST for soybeans and white beans is unreliable, apparently because of nonspecific binding of IgE to the RAST disk. RAST does not appear to offer any substantial advantage over skin testing with potent food extracts.

In the provocative/neutralizing method of diagnosis of food allergy, dilutions of food extracts are injected intracutaneously in an attempt to reproduce the patient's symptoms, which are then said to be relieved by successive intracutaneous injections of other dilutions of the same extract. The techniques vary among users of the method. For example, some users both "provoke" and "neutralize" by *sublingual* administration of the antigen solutions. The validity of all of these methods has not been established, and their use in diagnosis and therapy is unwarranted and experimental at best.

Treatment. The treatment of an adverse food reaction is directed at the clinical manifestations, which may be anaphylaxis, urticaria, diarrhea, rhinitis, asthma, and so on. Offending foods should be removed from the diet. If elimination diets are prescribed, care must be taken to ensure that they are nutritionally adequate. For reasons that are unclear, some children shown to be highly reactive to foods will become "tolerant" as they grow older; this is particularly likely in infants and small children. Foods most likely to become tolerated with the passage of time are cow's milk, eggs, and soy. Hypersensitivity to peanuts, nuts, and fish persists for long periods. Cautious reintroduction of offending foods into the diet may be tried, particularly in the case of those common foods that are difficult to avoid in the average diet. A few studies report that cromolyn sodium, 60–200 mg, given orally 30 min before a food challenge, has blocked the appearance of symptoms in food-sensitive individuals. Cromolyn sodium may be tried, therefore, in those rare instances when an offending food cannot be avoided. The cost of such therapy is high because of the large amounts of drug required. Immunotherapy by injection or sublingual or oral administration of extracts of offending foods is not efficacious.

RELATIONSHIP BETWEEN THE PEDIATRICIAN AND ALLERGIST

Many of the common conditions discussed above can be effectively managed by pediatricians comfortable with the principles of allergy diagnosis and treatment. Consultation with an allergist is indicated if the pediatrician is not qualified to undertake measures such as skin or pulmonary function testing or if the case is difficult. The referral should be made for the evaluation of the role that IgE-mediated allergy may be playing in the disease and not just for "skin tests and shots" since, not uncommonly, no evidence of IgE-mediated allergy will be found and anticipated "shots" will not be indicated. The best results are obtained for the patient when pediatrician and allergist are in frequent communication and work together harmoniously.

ELLIOT F. ELLIS

Atkins FM, Metcalfe DD: The diagnosis and treatment of food allergy. Ann Rev Nutr 4:233, 1984.
Atkins FM, Steinberg SS, Metcalf DD: Evaluation of immediate adverse reactions to foods in adult patients. I. Correlation of demographic, laboratory and prick skin test data with responses to controlled oral food challenge. J Allergy Clin Immunol 75:348, 1985.
Atkins FM, Steinberg SS, Metcalf DD: Evaluation of immediate adverse reactions to foods in adult patients. II. A detailed analysis of reaction patterns during oral food challenges. J Allergy Clin Immunol 75:356, 1985.
Bock SA: The natural history of food sensitivity. J Allergy Clin Immunol 69:173, 1982.
Bock SA, Buckley J, Holst A, et al: Proper use of skin tests with food extracts in diagnosis of hypersensitivity to food in children. Clin Allergy 7:375, 1977.
Hill DJ, Ford RPK, Skelton MJ, Hosking CS: A study of 100 infants and young children with cow's milk allergy. Clin Rev Allergy 2:125, 1984.
Savilahti E, Verkasalo M: Intestinal cow's milk allergy: pathogenesis and clinical presentation. Clin Rev Allergy 2:7, 1984.
Simon RA: Adverse reactions to drug additives. J Allergy Clin Immunol 74:623, 1984.

RHEUMATIC DISEASES OF CHILDHOOD
(Inflammatory Diseases of Connective Tissue, Collagen Diseases)

The disorders described in these sections are grouped together because of similarities in symptomatology and pathology; in general, they are associated with inflammatory changes in various connective tissues throughout the body. Included are:

I. Rheumatic Fever (Sec. 10.87)
II. Juvenile Rheumatoid Arthritis (JRA) (Sec. 10.58)
III. Ankylosing Spondylitis (Sec. 10.59)
IV. Spondyloarthropathies (Sec. 10.60)
V. Systemic lupus erythematosus (SLE) (Sec. 10.61) (for lupus nephritis see Sec. 17.7)
  A. Lupus phenomenon in the newborn (Sec. 10.62)
VI. The vasculitis syndromes (Sec. 10.63)
  A. Schönlein-Henoch vasculitis (Sec. 10.64 and for nephritis, see Sec. 17.12)
  B. Polyarteritis nodosa (Sec. 10.65)
    1. Infantile polyarteritis (Sec. 10.66)
    2. Kawasaki disease (Sec. 10.67)
    3. Wegener granulomatosis (Sec. 10.68)
  C. Takayasu arteritis (Sec. 10.69)
VII. Dermatomyositis (Sec. 10.70)
VIII. Scleroderma (Sec. 10.71)
  A. Morphea
  B. Progressive systemic sclerosis
IX. Rheumatic syndromes of uncertain classification
  A. Mixed connective tissue disease (Sec. 10.72)
  B. Fasciitis (Sec. 10.73)
X. Miscellaneous conditions associated with rheumatic symptoms or signs in children
  A. Benign rheumatoid nodules (Sec. 10.74)
  B. Erythema nodosum (Sec. 10.75)
  C. Lyme disease (Sec. 10.76)
  D. Sarcoidosis (Sec. 10.77)
  E. Stevens-Johnson syndrome (Sec. 10.78)
  F. Goodpasture syndrome (Sec. 10.79)
  G. Fibrositis-Fibromyalgia syndromes (Sec. 10.80)
  H. Relapsing nodular panniculitis (Sec. 10.81)
  I. Relapsing polychondritis (Sec. 10.82)
  J. Syndrome of neonatal fever, rash, and arthropathy (Sec. 10.83)
  K. Behçet syndrome (Sec. 10.84)
  L. Sjögren syndrome (Sec. 10.85)
XI. Non-rheumatic conditions mimicking rheumatic diseases (Sec. 10.86)

Certain diseases, discussed elsewhere, have features similar to these disorders, including: serum sickness (Sec. 10.52), glomerulonephritis (Sec. 17.5), the idiopathic nephrotic syndrome (Sec. 17.27), inflammatory bowel disease (Sec. 12.43), and thrombotic thrombocytopenic purpura (Sec. 15.48).

The causes and pathogenesis of rheumatic diseases of childhood are unknown, and precise diagnostic criteria are lacking. They usually appear as distinct entities, each generally presenting characteristic clinical manifestations. For example, rheumatoid arthritis is associated with chronic arthritis, dermatomyositis with inflammation of muscle and skin, scleroderma with induration of skin, and so on. Each of these diseases, however, can affect many organs, and overlapping symptoms and signs may at times make precise diagnosis difficult.

10.57 LABORATORY STUDIES IN THE RHEUMATIC DISEASES

Although laboratory studies are often helpful, few, if any, are diagnostic or specific for rheumatic diseases. These studies include tests for acute phase phenomena, rheumatoid factors, antinuclear antibodies, serum complement and its components, immune complexes, serum proteins and immunoglobulins, and histocompatibility antigens. Other tests that are also useful at times in evaluating patients include blood counts, urinalyses, joint fluid analyses, studies of renal and liver function, and various imaging techniques. Biopsies are frequently performed in rheumatic diseases; although tissue histology may provide confirmatory evidence of tissue involvement or aid in classification of disease, it is rarely diagnostic of any specific disease.

THE ACUTE PHASE PHENOMENA

The acute phase reactants are plasma constituents that appear or increase during the inflammatory state. They include the sedimentation rate, C-reactive protein, serum mucoproteins, various alpha globulins, gamma globulins, some complement components, and certain proteins such as transferrin. Because patients with rheumatic diseases have an active inflammatory process, acute phase phenomena or reactants are usually present during periods of active disease. Such tests are not invariably positive during inflammation, however, and their absence does not exclude the possibility of an active disease process. These tests are of little diagnostic usefulness since they may be positive in a wide variety of conditions associated with inflammation (such as malignancy, infection, tissue trauma, and tissue necrosis). At times, acute phase phenomena are helpful in following the course of disease in individual patients. The sedimentation rate is the most readily available test; rapid sedimentation rates result from increased plasma levels of serum fibrinogen, gamma globulins, or other proteins.

RHEUMATOID FACTORS

Rheumatoid factors are a group of antibodies that react with the Fc portion of IgG immunoglobulins. These antibodies are not specific for host immunoglobulin but may react with immunoglobulin from other individuals or from other species. Rheumatoid factors detected by standard agglutination techniques such as the latex agglutination test or the sheep cell agglutination test are IgM immunoglobulins; anti-immunoglobulin antibodies of the IgG, IgA, and IgE classes can also be identified by methods other than agglutination tests. The occurrence of rheumatoid factors in disease states such as chronic infections or in experimental situations such as hyperimmunization of animals suggests that protracted immune stimulation or chronic infection or inflammation may underlie their production.

Rheumatoid factors, particularly IgM factors detected by classic agglutination techniques, are strongly associated with classic adult rheumatoid arthritis; in such patients they are present in high titer and on serial tests throughout the course of disease. A small subgroup of patients with juvenile rheumatoid arthritis resembling classic adult rheumatoid arthritis also have rheumatoid factors. However, rheumatoid factors are neither specific for nor diagnostic of rheumatoid arthritis. They also occur in other rheumatic diseases (lupus erythematosus, scleroderma), chronic active hepatitis, chronic infections (such as bacterial endocarditis, parasitic infections), leukemia and lymphoid malignancies, and certain viral infections; in addition, they can be found following immunizations, open heart surgery, or organ transplantation as well as in normal aging human beings. Many children with transiently positive low titer rheumatoid factor tests have probably had antecedent viral illnesses. Rheumatoid factors do not in themselves cause disease, nor are they necessary for the occurrence of chronic synovitis; they may play a role in perpetuation of synovial inflammation in rheumatoid arthritis by forming immune complexes with immunoglobulins.

Antinuclear Antibodies (Antinuclear Factors). The antinuclear antibodies are a group of antibodies that react with various nuclear constituents, including deoxyribonucleoprotein (DNP), deoxyribonucleic acid (DNA), ribonucleoprotein (RNP), ribonucleic acid (RNA), SM antigen (a soluble nuclear protein antigen), and many others. Stimuli for production of these antibodies remain unknown. Antinuclear antibodies are not specific for organs, individuals, or species of cell origin. They are generally detected by immunofluorescent staining techniques using frozen tissue sections.

Antinuclear antibodies are neither entirely diagnostic of nor specific for any disease. They are found in almost all patients with systemic lupus erythematosus (SLE) but are also found in patients with rheumatoid arthritis and scleroderma. The syndrome called mixed connective tissue disease is defined by the presence of antibody to RNP. Nonrheumatic conditions associated with antinuclear antibodies include drug ingestion (e.g., anticonvulsants, procainamide, birth control pills), certain infections (notably EB virus infection), certain malignancies, and the normal aging process. High titers of antinuclear antibodies are most common in SLE and mixed connective tissue disease. Antibodies reactive with double-stranded DNA are usually found only in patients with active SLE.

The lupus erythematosus (LE) cell is the result of an antinuclear antibody reaction with DNP. When the reaction occurs in vitro with nuclei of peripheral blood cells, the nuclei are rendered susceptible to phagocytosis; the LE cell is a polymorphonuclear leukocyte that has ingested such a nucleus. This test to demonstrate LE cells is no longer in general use.

Complement. Complement consists of a group of serum proteins that mediate certain aspects of inflammation and cell injury (Sec. 10.24). Serum complement levels can be useful in indicating the activity of SLE and other diseases associated with formation of immune complexes; low serum complement levels reflect complement consumption by immune complexes and thus indicate active disease. Measuring total serum hemolytic complement activity is probably the most useful test. Measurement of individual complement components C3 or C4 determines only the amount of protein without regard to its biologic activity. Complement studies are not diagnostic of any disease except the rare hereditary deficiencies of complement components.

Immune Complex Determinations. Immune complexes of antigen and antibody are responsible for tissue damage in some rheumatic diseases (notably SLE) and also in a wide variety of other conditions (such as infectious diseases). However, these tests are of limited clinical usefulness in evaluating patients. The most commonly available methods are C1q binding and Raji cell assay. The ultimate role for such determinations remains to be defined.

Serum Proteins and Immunoglobulins. Elevated levels of gamma globulins and alpha$_2$ globulins are frequently found in patients with active inflammation; these tests are not specific. Most notable elevations are generally found in SLE. Elevations of one or more specific immunoglobulins may also be found in rheumatic disease patients; however, there are no diagnostic patterns. Serum albumin levels may be low in patients with chronic inflammation of various causes. Rarely, patients with immunodeficiency (especially IgA) or hypogammaglobulinemia appear with rheumatic disease states.

The Histocompatibility (HLA) System. Associations of histocompatibility antigens (HLA antigens) with certain diseases provide insights into genetically determined susceptibility to disease. Histocompatibility antigens are located on the surfaces of most human cells. Loci determining HLA antigens are located on the 6th chromosome; A, B, C, D, and DR types are now recognized. The HLA system is complex, with multiple alleles for each locus. The prevalences of various HLA alleles vary in different racial groups. HLA typing requires antisera of known specificity to type A, B, C, and DR loci and cells of known specificity to type D locus.

The biologic roles of HLA antigens, other than those determining tissue compatibility, are not fully known. The HLA system is closely linked to several genes important to the immune system, including loci determining synthesis of various components of complement and perhaps loci determining immune responsiveness. Since the HLA antigens are genetically determined traits that can be accurately identified, they can provide information both concerning disease associations (the occurrence of particular diseases in association with particular HLA antigens) and disease linkages (the passage of a trait along with HLA antigens from generation to generation within the same family, implying that the genes responsible for the trait are close to those of the HLA system on the 6th chromosome).

The strongest association of human disease with the HLA system is that of HLA B27 with ankylosing spondylitis; 95% of patients with ankylosing spondylitis have HLA B27, as compared with only 6% of a control white North American population. An individual carrying HLA B27 has 90 times greater relative risk of developing ankylosing spondylitis than one who does not carry HLA B27. An estimated 8–20% of adults with HLA B27 actually have ankylosing spondylitis or a related disease. Reiter syndrome, the spondylitis of inflammatory bowel disease and psoriasis, acute iridocyclitis, pauciarticular arthritis of teenage and adult patients, and the "reactive" arthritis following infections with salmonella, shigella, *Yersinia enterocolitica*, or *Campylobacter* are also associated with HLA B27. It is unknown whether susceptibility to these diseases is conferred by HLA B27 itself or by a linked genetic trait. The associations of these spondyloarthropathic diseases with HLA B27 hold true in various racial populations. No corresponding HLA D associations have been made for these diseases.

HLA B27 is associated with only one subgroup of childhood arthritis—that of older-onset pauciarticular patients (type II) who may well have early ankylosing spondylitis or other spondyloarthropathies. DRW8, DRW6, and DRW5 are associated with pauciarticular juvenile rheumatoid arthritis (type I) and chronic iridocyclitis, and DRW4 with rheumatoid factor-positive polyarthritis.

A different group of diseases is associated with HLA B8 and HLA DW3/DR3 in North American and European populations. These include chronic active hepatitis, celiac sprue, dermatitis herpetiformis with malabsorption, insulin-dependent diabetes mellitus, thyroiditis, Graves disease, Addison disease, myasthenia gravis, Sjögren syndrome, childhood dermatomyositis, and perhaps systemic lupus erythematosus. All of these diseases are characterized by chronic inflammation, often associated with formation of antibodies reactive with human tissues ("autoantibodies"). Risks for any of these diseases are relatively low for individuals carrying B8-DW3/DR3, and the D associations are stronger than the B associations. Histocompatibility studies have revealed heterogeneous subgroups in several of these diseases: for example, in diabetes mellitus (only insulin-dependent diabetes is associated with B8-DW3/DR3) and in dermatitis herpetiformis (only dermatitis herpetiformis with malabsorption is associated with B8-DW3/DR3). The specific HLA antigens associated with these diseases may vary among racial groups.

Other human diseases, notably multiple sclerosis and psoriasis, have yet other HLA B and D associations. Few diseases have been associated primarily with antigens in the A locus (one such disease is hemachromatosis). Adult-onset rheumatoid arthritis has an HLA-D association (DW4/DR4) but no known A, B, or C associations.

Human conditions *linked* to the HLA system or transmitted along with antigens of the histocompatibility system from generation to generation include deficiencies of the 2nd and 4th components of complement, congenital adrenal hyperplasia, and possibly, predisposition to ragweed hay fever.

HLA typing is not diagnostic of any disease but is useful in matching tissue donors to recipients. There is also a potential use in prenatal diagnosis of linked diseases such as deficiency of the 4th component of complement. Histocompatibility studies remain of great interest both in classifying diseases and in seeking genetic factors that predispose to disease. Explanations for the associations of histocompatibility antigens with specific diseases are unknown.

10.58 JUVENILE RHEUMATOID ARTHRITIS

Juvenile rheumatoid arthritis (JRA) is a disease or group of diseases characterized by chronic synovitis and associated with a number of extra-articular manifestations. Other names which we consider to be synonymous with this entity include Still disease, juvenile chronic polyarthritis, and chronic childhood arthritis. This disease differs from rheumatoid arthritis of adult onset in both articular and extra-articular manifestations.

JRA is an extremely variable disease that encompasses several broad clinical subgroups (Table 10–23). Rheumatoid factor–positive polyarticular disease most closely resembles adult-onset rheumatoid arthritis; rheumatoid factor–negative polyarthritis also occurs in adults. Pauciarticular disease type II resembles those diseases described in adults as "spondyloarthropathies" (including early ankylosing spondylitis, Reiter syndrome, and the arthritis of inflammatory bowel disease). Systemic-onset disease rarely occurs in adults, and pauciarticular disease type I with chronic iridocyclitis has not been described in adults. Recognition of these patterns is useful in diagnosis, follow-up, and appropriate care of children with chronic arthritis.

Etiology and Epidemiology. The etiology of rheumatoid arthritis and the mechanisms for perpetuation of chronic synovial inflammation in the disease are unknown. Two current hypotheses are that the disease results from infection with as yet unidentified microorganisms or that it represents hypersensitivity or "autoimmune" reaction to unknown stimuli. Various microorganisms have been isolated from rheumatoid synovium but none consistently. Organisms such as mycoplasma can cause chronic synovitis resembling rheumatoid arthritis in experimental animals. The possible roles of virus infections are under investigation. Evidence that immune mechanisms are involved in the pathogenesis is supplied by the association of rheumatoid factors (antibodies reactive with IgG) with adult-onset rheumatoid arthritis. Although these antibodies do not cause the disease, immune complexes of rheumatoid factor and immunoglobulin may perpetuate synovial inflammation and are responsible for the rheumatoid vasculitis seen in seropositive rheumatoid arthritis. The low levels of complement found in the synovial fluid of some rheumatoid patients and low serum complement levels in patients with rheumatoid vasculitis are consistent with such a mechanism. This mechanism fails, however, to explain all rheumatoid inflammation since chronic synovitis can occur in the absence of rheumatoid factors and with normal levels of complement in joint fluid. The occurrence of chronic arthritis in patients with IgA deficiency and hypogammaglobulinemia suggests that immunodeficiency may somehow predispose to rheumatoid arthritis; however, no blatant immunodeficiency has been identified in rheumatoid patients. Clinical onset may follow an acute systemic infection or physical trauma to a joint, but no direct relation to such events has been shown. Exacerbations may follow intercurrent illness or psychic stress.

Pauciarticular disease type II is frequently associated with a positive family history for ankylosing spondylitis, Reiter syndrome, acute iridocyclitis, or pauciarticular arthritis. Both

Table 10–23. **Subgroups of Juvenile Rheumatoid Arthritis**

	Polyarticular Rheumatoid Factor– Negative	Polyarticular Rheumatoid Factor– Positive	Pauciarticular Type I	Pauciarticular Type II	Systemic-Onset
Per cent of JRA patients	20-25	5-10	35-40	10-15	20
Sex	90% girls	80% girls	80% girls	90% boys	60% boys
Age at onset	Throughout childhood	Late childhood	Early childhood	Late childhood	Through childhood
Joints	Any Multiple	Any Multiple	Few Large joints: knee, ankle, elbow	Few Large joints: hip girdle	Any Multiple
Sacroiliitis	No	Rare	No	Common	No
Iridocyclitis	Rare	No	30% chronic iridocyclitis	10–20% acute iridocyclitis	No
Rheumatoid factor	Negative	100%	Negative	Negative	Negative
Antinuclear antibodies	25%	75%	90%	Negative	Negative
HLA studies	?	HLA DR4	HLA DR5, DRW6, DRW8	HLA B27	?
Ultimate morbidity	Severe arthritis, 10%–15%	Severe arthritis, >50%	Ocular damage, 10% Polyarthritis 20%	Subsequent spondylo- arthropathy, ?%	Severe arthritis, 25%

pauciarticular JRA type I and rheumatoid factor positive polyarthritis occasionally occur in one or more first degree relatives of affected children. Neither systemic-onset disease nor seronegative polyarthritis appears to be familial.

JRA is not rare; there are about a quarter million affected children in the United States. About 5% of all cases of rheumatoid arthritis begin in childhood, usually not before the 2nd birthday.

Pathology. Rheumatoid arthritis is characterized by chronic nonsuppurative inflammation of synovium. Microscopically, affected synovial tissues are edematous, hyperemic, and infiltrated with lymphocytes and plasma cells. Secretion of increased amounts of joint fluid results in effusions. Projections of thickened synovial membrane form villi which protrude into joint spaces; hyperplastic rheumatoid synovium may spread over and become adherent to articular cartilage (pannus formation). With continuing chronic synovitis and proliferation of synovium, articular cartilage and other joint structures may become eroded and progressively destroyed, though the mechanisms remain unknown. The duration of synovitis before joint damage becomes permanent varies; in general, lasting damage to articular cartilage occurs later in the course of JRA than in adult-onset disease, and many children with JRA never incur permanent joint damage despite prolonged synovitis. Joint destruction occurs more often in children with rheumatoid factor–positive disease or systemic-onset disease. Once joint destruction has commenced, erosions of subchondral bone, narrowing of the "joint space" (loss of articular cartilage), destruction or fusion of bones, and deformity, subluxation, or ankylosis of joints may result. Tenosynovitis and myositis may be present. Osteoporosis, periostitis, accelerated epiphyseal growth, and premature epiphyseal closure can occur adjacent to affected joints.

Rheumatoid nodules are less common in children than in adults, occur primarily in rheumatoid–factor positive children, and show fibrinoid material surrounded by chronic inflammatory cells. Pleura, pericardium, and peritoneum may show nonspecific fibrinous serositis; chronic constrictive pericarditis occurs rarely if ever. The rheumatoid rash appears histologically as a mild vasculitis, with a few inflammatory cells surrounding small vessels in subepithelial tissues.

Clinical Manifestations. *Polyarticular Onset Disease.* This is characterized by involvement of multiple joints, typically including the small joints of the hands (Figs. 10–6 and 10–7). Polyarticular disease unassociated with prominent systemic manifestations occurs in 35% of children with JRA. Two subgroups are included: *rheumatoid factor–negative polyarthritis* (20–25% of all JRA patients) and *rheumatoid factor–positive polyarthritis* (5–10% of all JRA patients). Rheumatoid factor–positive disease has an onset in late childhood, more severe

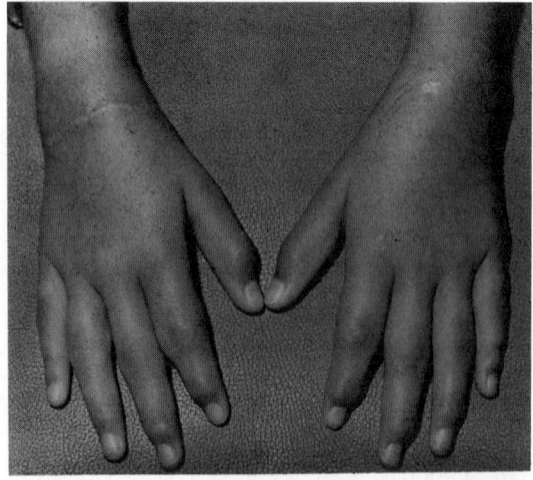

Figure 10–6. Hands and wrists of a girl with rheumatoid factor–negative polyarticular juvenile rheumatoid arthritis. Note symmetric involvement of the metacarpophalangeal joints, proximal interphalangeal joints, and distal interphalangeal joints. Both wrists are also affected.

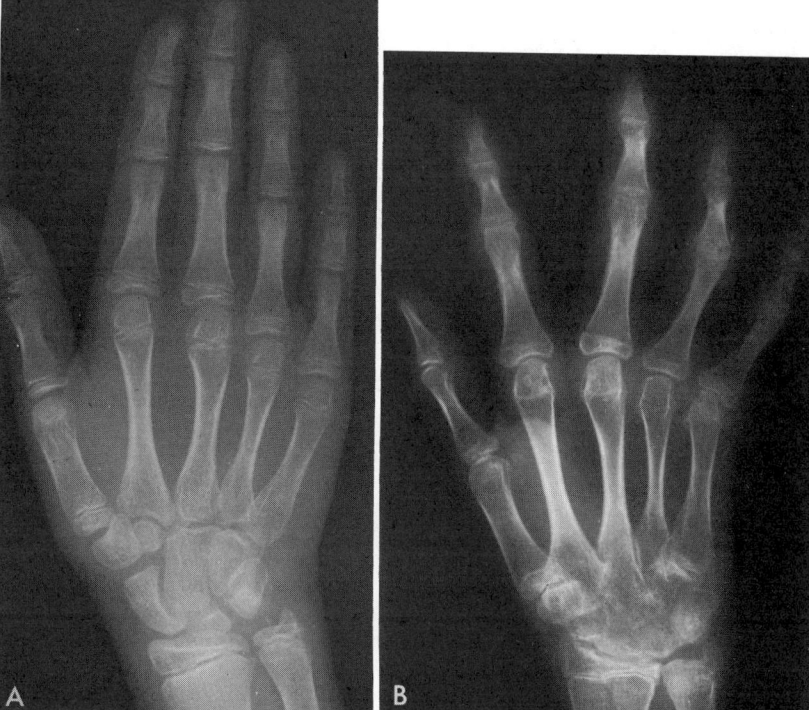

Figure 10–7. Progression of joint destruction in a girl with rheumatoid factor–positive juvenile rheumatoid arthritis despite doses of corticosteroids sufficient to suppress symptoms in the interval between *A* and *B*. *A*, Roentgenogram of hand at onset; *B*, roentgenogram 4 yr later, showing loss of articular cartilage and destructive changes in the distal and proximal interphalangeal and metacarpophalangeal joints and destruction and fusion of wrist bones.

arthritis, frequent rheumatoid nodules, and occasional rheumatoid vasculitis. Rheumatoid factor–negative disease may begin at any time during childhood, is frequently mild, and is rarely associated with rheumatoid nodules. More girls than boys are affected in both types of disease. Both the polyarticular pattern and the nature of the rheumatoid factor tests are generally established early in the course of disease.

Onset of arthritis may be insidious, with gradual development of joint stiffness, swelling, and loss of motion, or fulminant, with sudden appearance of symptomatic arthritis. Affected joints are swollen and warm but rarely red. Swelling results from periarticular edema, joint effusion, and synovial thickening. Some children have joint stiffness and discomfort before objective changes appear. Affected joints may be tender to touch and painful on motion; however, severe tenderness and pain are unusual, and many children do not complain of any pain in obviously inflamed joints. Limited joint motion is related early to muscle spasm, joint effusion, and synovial proliferation, and later to joint destruction and ankylosis or to contractures of soft tissues. Pronounced synovial proliferation may produce cystic swellings about affected joints; occasionally herniations of synovium and extravasation of synovial fluid occur into neighboring structures, particularly in the popliteal area (popliteal cyst). Morning stiffness and "gelling" following inactivity are characteristic of rheumatoid arthritis in children, as in adults. Young children, particularly those with polyarthritis, are often irritable and assume a typical posture of anxious guarding of their joints against movement (Fig. 10–8).

Arthritis, which may affect any synovial joint, often begins in large joints such as knees, ankles, wrists, and elbows. The involvement is often symmetrical. Inflammation of proximal interphalangeal joints produces spindling or fusiform changes of the fingers; metacarpophalangeal joint involvement is equally common, and distal interphalangeal joints may also be affected (Figs. 10–6 and 10–7). Arthritis of the cervical spine, characterized by neck stiffness and pain, occurs in about half the patients. Temporomandibular involvement with limited ability to open the mouth is common; the pain may be referred to as earache by young children. Hip involve-

ment occurs in at least half the children with polyarthritis, usually beginning later in the disease process. Destruction of the femoral heads may ensue; severe hip disease is a major cause of disability in late JRA (Fig. 10–9). Roentgenographic changes in the sacroiliac joints occur in some patients, usually in association with hip disease; the changes differ from those of ankylosing spondylitis and are not associated with involvement of the lumbodorsal spine. Rarely, cricoarytenoid arthritis causes hoarseness and laryngeal stridor. Involvement of sternoclavicular joints and costochondral junctions may cause chest pain.

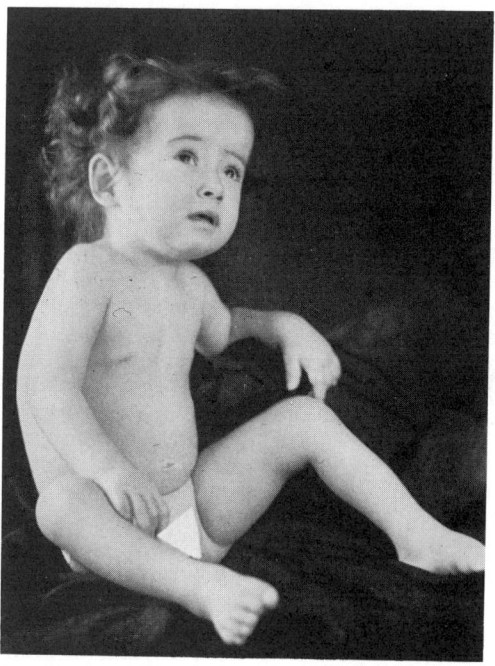

Figure 10–8. Characteristic posture of a child with juvenile rheumatoid arthritis, showing the anxious appearance and guarding of joints.

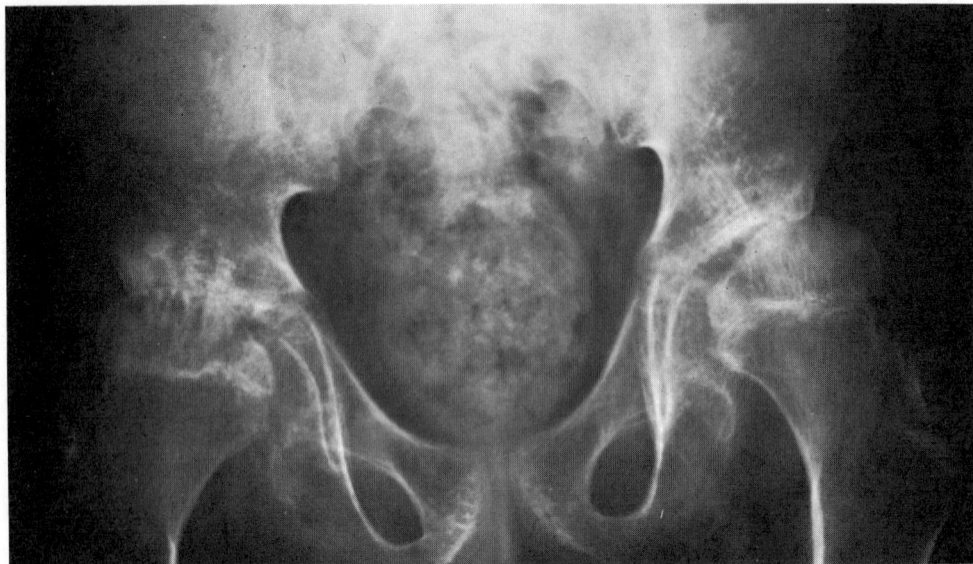

Figure 10–9. Severe hip disease in a 13 yr old boy with long-active, systemic-onset juvenile rheumatoid arthritis, showing destruction of femoral heads and acetabula, joint space narrowing, and subluxation of the left hip. The patient had received corticosteroids systemically for 9 yr.

Growth disturbances adjacent to inflamed joints may result in either overgrowth or undergrowth of the affected part. For example, increased leg length may follow chronic arthritis of the knee, and micrognathia after temporomandibular arthritis may be a late hallmark of JRA. Small, deformed feet may result from foot involvement in early childhood, and shortened fingers from early hand involvement.

Extra-articular manifestations are not so dramatic as in systemic rheumatoid arthritis. Most patients with active polyarticular disease have malaise, anorexia, irritability, and mild anemia. Low-grade fever, slight hepatosplenomegaly, and lymphadenopathy may be present. Pericarditis is infrequent and iridocyclitis rare. Rheumatoid nodules may occur over pressure points, usually in patients with positive agglutination tests for rheumatoid factor. Rheumatoid vasculitis occurs at times in rheumatoid factor–positive patients, as does Sjögren syndrome. Growth may be retarded during periods of active disease; growth spurts often occur with remission.

Pauciarticular Onset Disease. This illness is characterized by arthritis that remains limited to only a few joints for the first 6 months of the disease (Fig. 10–10). Large joints are primarily affected, and the distribution of arthritis is often asymmetrical or spotty. Two distinct subgroups are included: type I includes primarily girls who are young at onset and are at risk for chronic iridocyclitis; type II includes primarily boys who are older at onset and who are at risk for subsequent spondyloarthropathies.

Pauciarticular disease type I affects 35–40% of patients with JRA. Girls are predominantly affected, and the disease generally begins before the age of 4 yr. Tests for rheumatoid factors are negative, but 90% of patients have positive tests for antinuclear antibodies. HLA B27 is not associated. The most commonly affected joints are the knees, ankles, and elbows; occasionally, there is spotty involvement of other joints such as the temporomandibular joints, single toes or fingers, wrists, or neck. The hips and hip girdle are generally spared, and sacroiliitis is not associated. The clinical appearance and the synovial histology of affected joints are indistinguishable from those of polyarticular JRA. Eighty percent of children with type I pauciarticular onset disease continue to have limited joint involvement; however, 20% will later have additional joint involvement that may result in severe polyarthritis. There is currently no way of identifying either group early in the course of the disease. Although the arthritis may be chronic or recurrent, serious disability or joint destruction is uncommon. However, patients with pauciarticular disease type I are at high risk for eye complications; chronic iridocyclitis occurs in about 30% of such children at some time during the course of disease.

The *chronic iridocyclitis* of JRA is characteristically associated with early symptoms or signs, activity of arthritis, or elevated sedimentation rate. Occasionally, children note redness, pain, photophobia, or decreased visual acuity early in the course of iridocyclitis. One or both eyes may be affected. If initial involvement is unilateral, the other eye usually remains uninvolved. Iridocyclitis is sometimes the presenting manifestation of JRA but generally begins at or up to 10 yr after onset of joint complaints. Patients with iridocyclitis frequently have positive tests for antinuclear antibodies. The earliest signs of inflammation of the iris and ciliary body are increased numbers of cells and amounts of protein in the anterior chamber of the eye, changes detectable only by slit lamp examination. The ocular inflammation often remains active for years. Sequelae (Fig. 10–11) include posterior synechiae, complicated cataracts, secondary glaucoma, and phthisis bulbi (degeneration of the globe). Loss of vision may result; in severe cases permanent blindness occurs. Early detection and therapy before scarring occurs are important for preservation of vision. For this reason all children with pauciarticular disease should have slit lamp examinations 3–4 times yearly for the first 5 yr of disease regardless of the activity of the joint disease.

Other extra-articular manifestations are usually mild in pauciarticular JRA; low-grade fever, malaise, modest hepatosplenomegaly and lymphadenopathy, and mild anemia may be associated with active joint disease.

Pauciarticular disease type II affects 10–15% of patients with JRA. Boys are predominantly affected, and the onset is usually after the age of 8 yr. Family histories are often positive for pauciarticular arthritis, ankylosing spondylitis, Reiter disease, or acute iridocyclitis. Tests for both rheumatoid factors and antinuclear antibodies are negative; 75% of patients have HLA B27. Large joints are affected, particularly those of the lower extremities. Foot joints, temporomandibular joints, and upper extremity joints are involved at times. Heel pain or Achilles tendinitis is common, and there may be inflammation at the sites of tendon insertion into bone (enthetopathy). Hip girdle involvement is frequent early in the disease, and sacroiliitis can often be demonstrated on roentgenography. The peripheral arthritis is generally benign and often quite transient. Hip and foot pain may be severe at times, though, and may be incapacitating; such changes are often reversible with therapy.

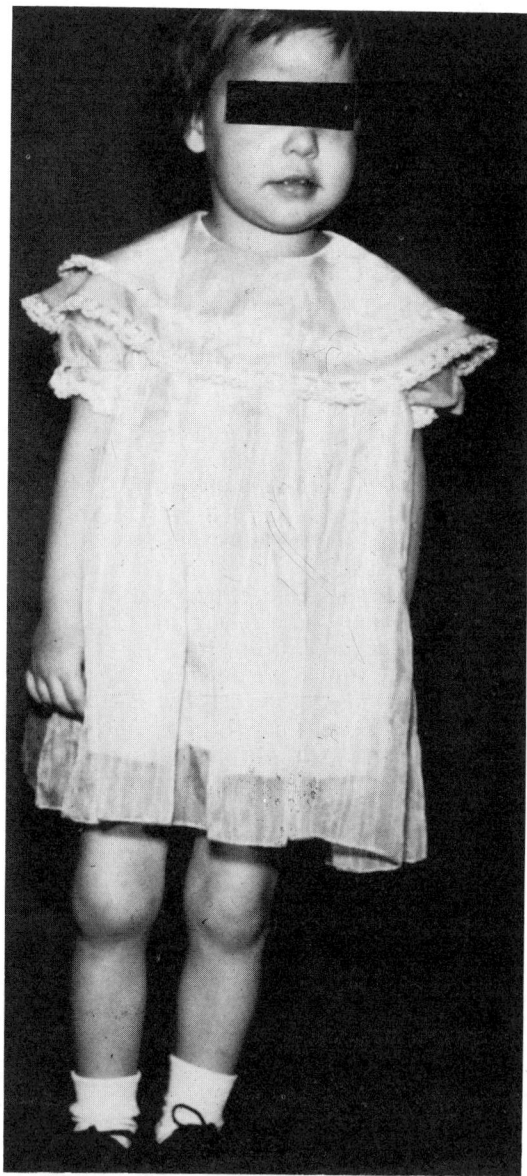

Figure 10–10. Characteristic appearance of a child with pauciarticular arthritis with onset in early childhood; note swelling of right knee.

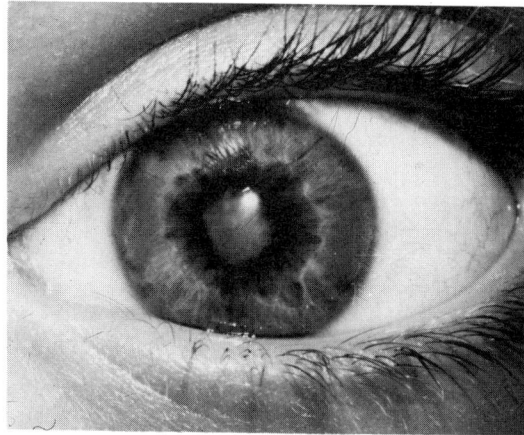

Figure 10–11. Chronic iridocyclitis of juvenile rheumatoid arthritis; extensive posterior synechiae have resulted in a small irregular pupil. There is a well developed cataract, and early band keratopathy can be seen at 3 and 9 o'clock position in the cornea.

As patients with pauciarticular disease type II are followed for years, some develop changes typical of ankylosing spondylitis with involvement of the lumbodorsal spine, changes consistent with Reiter syndrome (hematuria, urethritis, acute iridocyclitis, or mucocutaneous manifestations), or even inflammatory bowel disease. The ultimate morbidity for these children lies in the possible occurrence of any of these chronic spondyloarthropathies; the risks for such occurrences are not known. Children with pauciarticular disease type II need serial measurements of back flexion and chest expansion; 10–20% of them have self-limited attacks of *acute* iridocyclitis, which is associated with prominent early symptoms and signs of eye inflammation but few scarring residua.

Systemic-Onset JRA. Systemic JRA is characterized by prominent extra-articular manifestations (Table 10–24), particularly high fevers and rheumatoid rash. This type of disease occurs in 20% of patients with JRA. As many boys as girls are affected.

Systemic symptoms are generally the presenting manifestations of disease. The fever is intermittent, with daily or twice-daily elevations to 39.5° C (103° F) or higher and rapid

return to normal or subnormal levels (Fig. 10–12). Temperature elevations usually occur in the evening but sometimes in the morning as well. Shaking chills are frequently associated. Patients may seem alarmingly ill during the period of fever and surprisingly well during its remission. Rheumatoid rash (Figs. 10–13 and 10–14 [p. xxv]) is characterized by its appearance and by its evanescent, recurrent nature. It consists of small (several mm), pale, red-pink macules, often with central pallor; extensive lesions may coalesce. The rash is most frequently found on the trunk and proximal extremities but may occur anywhere on the body, including the palms and soles. It usually appears during febrile periods but may also be induced by skin trauma (isomorphic response), heat, and embarrassment. Hepatosplenomegaly and generalized lymphadenopathy occur in most children with active systemic disease. The degree of organomegaly may be marked. Mild hepatic dysfunction may be present, and lymph node histology may simulate lymphoma. About one third of affected children have pleuritis or pericarditis, often subclinical. Chest roentgenograms may show pleural thickening or small pleural effusions; pericardial effusion may be large and there may be electrocardiographic changes. The pericarditis of JRA is generally benign. Rarely, severe chest pain, dyspnea, or cardiac failure, with or without evidence of myocarditis, demands vigorous therapy. Occasionally, interstitial lung infiltrates occur with active systemic disease, but chronic rheumatoid lung disease rarely if ever occurs in children. A few children have episodes of severe abdominal pain during active disease.

Leukocytosis and even leukemoid reactions are common. Anemia is also common during active disease and is occasion-

Table 10–24. Manifestations of Systemic Juvenile Rheumatoid Arthritis

	%
High intermittent fever	100
Rheumatoid rash	95
Hepatosplenomegaly and/or lymphadenopathy	85
Pleuritis and/or pericarditis	60
Abdominal pain	20
Marked leukocytosis	85
Severe anemia	40
Rheumatoid factors	0
Antinuclear antibodies	0
Arthritis/arthralgia/myalgia during febrile periods	100
Chronic arthritis	90
Iridocyclitis	0

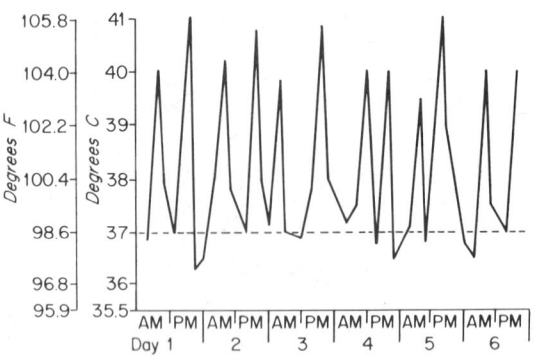

Figure 10–12. Characteristic fever of systemic juvenile rheumatoid arthritis; there are 1 or 2 daily temperature elevations to 39° C or greater, with rapid return of temperature to normal or subnormal levels.

ally profound. Disseminated intravascular coagulation and acute liver failure have been reported; whether these are manifestations of disease or of drug therapies (aspirin, gold) is not clear.

Most children with systemic JRA have joint manifestations at or within a few months of onset, but the arthritis may initially be overlooked because of the overwhelming systemic symptoms. Some patients initially have only severe myalgia, arthralgia, or transient arthritis. A few patients do not develop arthritis until months or years later. The pattern of joint involvement is ultimately polyarticular and resembles that described in polyarticular disease. The systemic manifestations generally run a self-limited course for several months but may recur. The real morbidity of systemic (polyarticular) JRA is arthritis that becomes chronic in some patients and persists after systemic symptoms have remitted. Systemic manifestations rarely recur after patients reach adulthood, even though chronic arthritis may persist.

Course and Prognosis. The major cause of morbidity in polyarticular and systemic JRA is chronic joint disease; in pauciarticular disease, the major morbidity is chronic iridocyclitis in type I patients and subsequent spondyloarthropathy in type II patients. The outcome is unpredictable in any individual patient. Even with severe systemic involvement, the disease is rarely life-threatening. There may be exacerbations and remissions, or symptoms may continue for years with mild arthritis causing little disability or, less commonly, with severe arthritis which progresses to joint destruction and permanent deformity. The disease does not always remit at puberty; some patients continue to have active arthritis into adulthood, and some have exacerbations after many years of apparently complete remission. Exacerbations may be associated with intercurrent illness; hepatitis and other forms of liver disease may be followed by transient remission of arthritis.

Patients with rheumatoid factor–positive polyarthritis and systemic-onset disease have the poorest prognosis for joint function. The overall prognosis is good, however. At least 75% of JRA patients eventually have long remissions without significant residual deformity or loss of function; a few are left with crippling joint deformities. Severe hip disease is particularly debilitating, as is loss of vision from iridocyclitis. Secondary amyloidosis (Sec. 26.2), generally heralded by proteinuria and diagnosed by demonstration of amyloid in tissues, may cause morbidity; in Europe amyloidosis affects about 5% of patients with JRA; in the United States this complication is very rare.

Laboratory Manifestations. There are no specific diagnostic tests. The sedimentation rate is usually, but not invariably, elevated during active disease. Anemia is common, usually

with low reticulocyte counts and negative Coombs test results; iron deficiency may also be present. The white blood cell count is often elevated; leukemoid reactions sometimes occur, particularly in systemic JRA, in which counts of 10,000–30,000/mm³ are the rule, and counts may sometimes be as high as 75,000/mm³. Thrombocytosis may occur, particularly in systemic-onset disease. Urinalyses are normal; during salicylate therapy a few erythrocytes and renal tubular cells may be seen. There may be an increase in the serum alpha-2 and gamma globulin fractions and a decrease in albumin. Any or all serum immunoglobulin levels may be elevated. *Antinuclear antibodies* are found in some children with rheumatoid-factor–negative (25%), rheumatoid-factor–positive (75%), or pauciarticular type I (90%) disease but are rarely if ever present in systemic or pauciarticular type II disease. The finding of antinuclear antibodies correlates with chronic iridocyclitis but not with severity of arthritis. LE cells can at times be demonstrated.

Rheumatoid factors are found in about 5% of children with JRA and correlate with older age at onset. Tests rarely convert from negative to positive despite long-active JRA. Positive tests are most commonly associated with polyarticular disease, late childhood onset, severe destructive arthritis, and rheumatoid nodules; rheumatoid vasculitis and Sjögren syndrome are also associated at times.

Histocompatibility studies are described above.

Synovial fluid in JRA is cloudy, may clot spontaneously, and usually contains increased amounts of protein. The cell count varies from 5000–80,000 cells/mm³; the cells are predominantly neutrophils. Levels of glucose may be low in the joint fluid; levels of complement may be normal or decreased.

Early *roentgenographic changes* consist of soft tissue swelling, osteoporosis, and periostitis about affected joints (Fig. 10–15). Regional epiphyseal closure may be accelerated and local bone growth increased or decreased. In long-active joint disease subchondral erosions and narrowing of cartilage spaces may occur, as may varying degrees of bony destruction and fusion. Late roentgenographic changes, e.g., in the wrist and hand (Fig. 10–7), are characteristic. Characteristic changes may occur in the neck, with narrowing and eventual fusion of neural arch joints (most frequently seen at C2 and C3, Fig. 10–16), erosions of the odontoid process, atlantoaxial sublux-

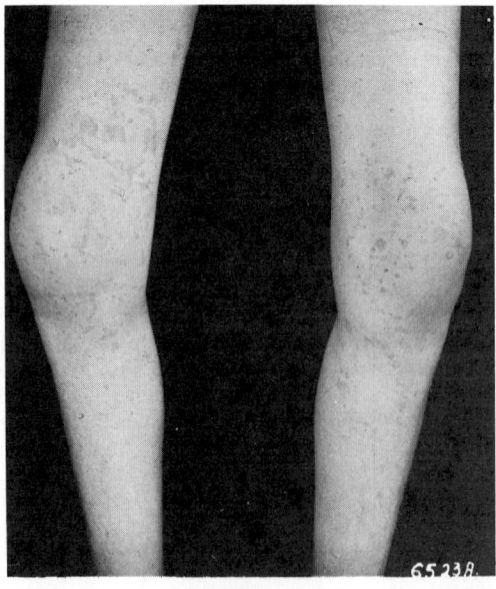

Figure 10–13. The rash of systemic-onset juvenile rheumatoid arthritis. (From Schaller JG, *In* Instructional Course Lectures, American Academy of Orthopedic Surgery, Vol XXIII. St. Louis, CV Mosby, 1974.)

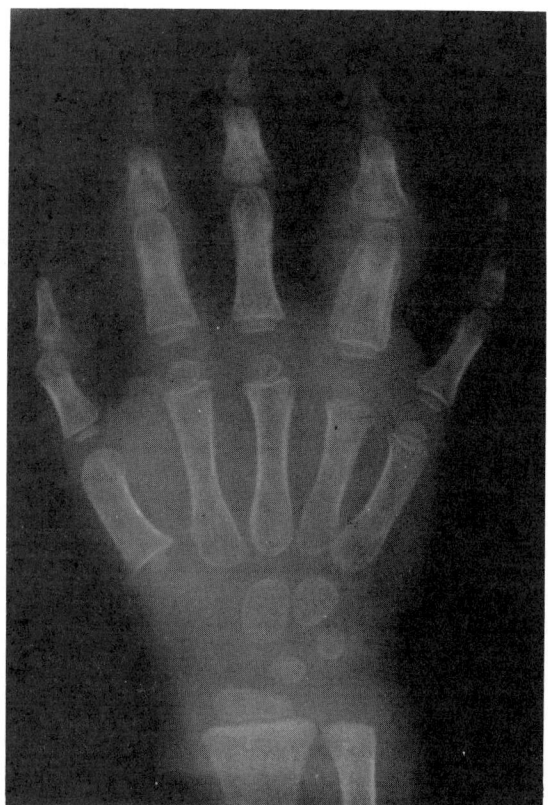

Figure 10–15. Early (6 mo duration) radiographic changes of JRA: soft tissue swelling and periosteal new bone formation appear adjacent to the 2nd and 4th proximal interphalangeal joints.

ation, and underdevelopment of vertebral bodies. Roentgenographic sacroiliitis resembling ankylosing spondylitis is often seen in pauciarticular disease type II.

Diagnosis and Differential Diagnosis. The diagnosis is clinical and depends on the persistence of arthritis or typical systemic manifestations for 3 or more consecutive months and on the exclusion of other diseases.

Early in the disease *pyogenic* or *tuberculous joint infection, osteomyelitis, sepsis,* or *arthritis associated with other acute infectious illnesses* may be considered. Culture of joint fluid, tuberculin testing and roentgenograms of affected joints are helpful. Arthritis of limited duration may occur in association with some viral infections and with rubella immunization. Gonococcal infection may result in arthritis. *Acute leukemia* and other malignancies occasionally present with pain and swelling of one or more joints and should be considered when onset is recent, particularly if severe anemia, thrombocytopenia, or abnormalities of peripheral white blood cells are present.

In *acute rheumatic fever* the transient, migratory nature of the arthritis and evidence of carditis help in differentiation. *Systemic lupus erythematosus* (SLE) and *mixed connective tissue disease* can cause arthritis indistinguishable from rheumatoid arthritis, but the joint changes are usually milder, and other clinical manifestations of lupus are usually present; however, antinuclear antibodies and occasionally LE cells occur in JRA as well as in SLE. *Ankylosing spondylitis* may present with arthritis of a few peripheral joints that is indistinguishable from JRA (particularly pauciarticular disease, type II) before characteristic involvement of the spine becomes manifest; the presence of early roentgenographic sacroiliac joint changes associated with pain in the low back and hip girdle is suggestive. *Reiter syndrome* (arthritis, urethritis, conjunctivitis) is

uncommon in children but should be considered in those with pauciarticular disease type II. The *vasculitis syndromes, dermatomyositis, ulcerative colitis, regional enteritis, psoriasis,* and *sarcoidosis* may be associated with arthritis similar to that of JRA but are generally distinguishable on clinical grounds. *Immunodeficiency diseases* may rarely be associated with chronic arthritis resembling JRA.

Various conditions such as *joint trauma, Legg-Perthes disease, Osgood-Schlatter disease,* and *slipped capital femoral epiphysis* may initially mimic JRA. *Acute toxic synovitis* of the hip is a self-limited condition of uncertain origin; JRA rarely begins in or affects solely the hip. *Pigmented villonodular synovitis,* an uncommon synovial overgrowth, usually affects only one joint.

Synovial biopsy may be useful, especially to exclude infection in monarticular disease; however, synovial histology does not distinguish among the various subgroups of JRA, various other rheumatic disorders, or even so-called postinfectious states.

Treatment. In planning therapy physicians must realize that although JRA may be of long duration and has no specific cure, the ultimate prognosis is good for most patients and life is rarely threatened. Management of affected children and their families tests the physician's sympathy, patience, empathy, and clinical skills. Unpredictable exacerbations are discouraging and make evaluating therapy difficult. There is an understandable tendency for parents to shop for medical help and to grasp for fad or quack cures. The chronic nature of the disease, on the other hand, may cause the discouraged family to give up supportive efforts, which may allow unnecessary crippling to occur.

The aims of immediate and long-term treatment are twofold: (1) to preserve joint function and to provide adequate care of extra-articular manifestations without iatrogenic harm; and (2) to support the family and child in achieving an optimal psychosocial adjustment. This requires the devoted attention of a primary physician and may require consultation with a variety of specialists.

A number of drugs can suppress the inflammatory process. Acetylsalicylic acid (aspirin) is the safest and most satisfactory; in doses sufficient to maintain blood levels of 20–30 mg/dL it usually alleviates both arthritis and systemic manifestations. Such blood levels can be reached by using doses of about 100 mg of aspirin/kg daily for children of 25 kg or less and total

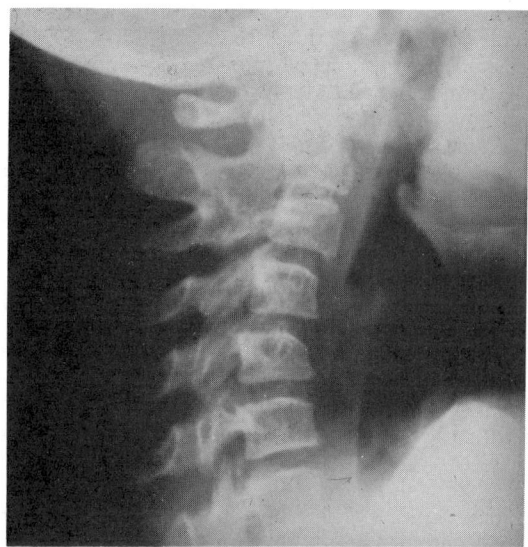

Figure 10–16. Cervical spine in long-active juvenile rheumatoid arthritis, showing fusion of neural arch between joints C2–C3, narrowing and erosions of the remaining neural arch joints, and resulting abnormal curvature.

daily doses of 2.4–3.6 g for older, heavier children. There is considerable individual variation in required doses, and patients must be watched carefully for toxicity. Full therapeutic response may require weeks to months. When dosage and response are determined and stabilized, the medication can be continued for years. Chronic therapeutic salicylate administration is relatively safe even in small children if physicians, patients, and parents are aware of the potential toxic effects. Intoxication from overdosage can be avoided if the dose is calculated with care and parents watch for the rapid or heavy breathing and drowsiness or other central nervous system changes that are often the earliest signs of salicylism in children. Tinnitus, a common complaint of adults with salicylism, is rarely noted by children. Salicylates should be given with food because of the possibility of gastric irritation. If patients complain of stomach ache, antacids can be added or buffered salicylate preparations or choline salicylate substituted for ordinary aspirin. Children with persistent gastrointestinal complaints should be investigated for peptic ulcer. Hemorrhagic phenomena and hypersensitivity reactions are rare with therapeutic doses of aspirin. Elevated activities of hepatic enzymes have been found in sera of patients with rheumatic diseases who were receiving large doses of salicylates; association of clinically significant liver disease is rare. Epidemiologic studies suggest that aspirin ingestion may be associated with Reye syndrome in children with either chickenpox or influenza; it may be wise to withdraw aspirin temporarily from children exposed to these infections.

A number of nonsteroidal anti-inflammatory agents are available for the therapy of arthritis in adults. These drugs are roughly as potent as aspirin in relieving pain and inflammation; some may provide particular relief for patients with spondyloarthropathies. These drugs include phenylbutazone, indomethacin, tolmetin, ibuprofen, naproxen, fenoprofen, and sulindac. Only tolmetin is currently labeled for use in children in the United States; it may provide a useful alternative to aspirin in some patients, and has few side effects.

There are few indications for systemic use of corticosteroids in JRA. They dramatically suppress symptoms, but do not induce permanent remission or prevent the occurrence of joint damage (Fig. 10–7). In addition, destruction of cartilage and aseptic necrosis of bone, particularly in the femoral heads, may be related to long-term steroid therapy (Fig. 10–9). Therapeutic doses of corticosteroids also cause adrenal suppression, may suppress growth, and may produce other potentially dangerous side effects. The dose required for suppression of symptoms is unpredictable and may actually increase with prolonged therapy.

Indications for corticosteroid use in JRA include severe systemic disease unresponsive to an adequate trial of salicylates and iridocyclitis uncontrolled by topical steroids. In the former, or in rare instances of cardiac decompensation from pericarditis or myocarditis, prednisone in initial doses of 1–2 mg/kg/24 hr is indicated. As soon as symptoms are suppressed, the dose should be decreased and the drug gradually discontinued under a cover of salicylates. With decreasing doses there is often transient rebound of symptoms, which should be waited out. Since the systemic manifestations of JRA generally run a self-limited course, prednisone can usually be successfully discontinued within weeks or months. In iridocyclitis unresponsive to topical steroid therapy, systemic administration is indicated in doses sufficient to suppress ocular inflammation, as monitored by slit lamp; single doses given daily or on alternate days may be sufficient. Therapy should be managed jointly with an ophthalmologist.

Corticosteroids should rarely be used for relief of joint manifestations alone since they neither cure arthritis nor prevent joint damage, and since their chronic side effects may be even less tolerable than the joint disease. Other reasonable therapeutic possibilities should always be exhausted first. If corticosteroids are used, every effort should be made to employ the lowest effective dose, to use alternate day or single daily dosage, and to minimize the period of treatment.

Gold salts have not been widely used in JRA but appear to be as effective as in adults, and no more toxic. They are useful if arthritis does not respond to an adequate trial of salicylates. Gold therapy requires weekly intramuscular injections, *each* preceded by careful evaluation for any signs of toxicity (rash, mucosal ulcers, leukopenia, thrombocytopenia, anemia, and proteinuria). Initially 2.5–5.0 mg of gold sodium thiomalate (Myochrysine) is given intramuscularly and repeated 1 wk later, followed by a maintenance dose of 1 mg/kg/wk intramuscularly; a maximum weekly dose of 25 mg is appropriate for children weighing 25–60 kg; 50 mg can be given to larger teenagers. Several months are required for therapeutic response, but if none has been noted after 20–24 weekly injections, the drug should be discontinued. If a response occurs, injections should be gradually spaced out to 3–4 wk intervals and continued indefinitely. *Continuous surveillance for side effects must be maintained throughout this therapy; their appearance is almost always an indication for discontinuing the drug.* Oral gold therapy has been tested in children but is not yet available for routine use.

Chloroquine and hydroxychloroquine may benefit some children with JRA but must be used with extreme care because of possible retinal toxicity; ophthalmologic examinations should be made every 3 mo. D-Penicillamine is a potentially toxic agent and still experimental. Although agents such as azathioprine, cyclophosphamide, and methotrexate have been advocated as therapeutic agents in rheumatoid arthritis, their use in children does not seem warranted until more is known of their long-term side effects. Chlorambucil and azathioprine may be effective in treating potentially fatal amyloidosis associated with JRA.

Physical and occupational therapy are important to improve motion and muscular strength about affected joints and to restore and maintain function of the patient as a whole. Patients and parents should be instructed in appropriate exercise programs to be carried out at home on a daily basis. Activities such as tricycle riding and swimming are beneficial and should be encouraged. Night splints for knees and wrists may aid in preventing and correcting deformity. Cylindrical casts or prolonged immobilization of joints should be avoided. Bed rest has little role in treatment. Children can usually set their own activity levels; in general, they should avoid only those activities that cause overtiring and joint pain. Orthopedic surgery is sometimes required to correct joint deformities. Synovectomy of selected joints is occasionally helpful but is not curative. Total replacement of destroyed joints, particularly hips and knees, is now possible when full growth has been attained. Injection of corticosteroids into selected joints may be helpful at times, but repeated injections should not be used. Micrognathia may require orthodontic management or oral surgery.

Iridocyclitis requires prompt diagnosis and therapy to preserve vision. The eyes should be examined at each medical visit. Ophthalmologic slit lamp examinations should be made at least once a year in children with systemic and polyarticular disease and 4 times yearly in children with pauciarticular disease. Parents should be cautioned to report at once any eye symptoms or decreased visual acuity. Therapy of iridocyclitis should be supervised by an ophthalmologist. Initially, it consists of topical use of steroids and dilating agents. Systemic use of steroids or subconjunctival injections should be used if prompt resolution of ocular inflammation is not achieved with topical agents. Frequent and long-term follow-up of eyes is essential. Ophthalmologic surgery may be required for chronic sequelae.

Children with JRA should be encouraged to lead as normal lives as possible. They and their parents need to know what to expect and to be treated optimistically. Affected children should not be led to believe that they are invalids but should be taught to be as self-sufficient as possible. With encouragement most can lead active lives, attend school, and participate in usual activities except strenuous sports. Long hospitalizations should be avoided. Children with residual handicaps need help in vocational planning.

10.59 ANKYLOSING SPONDYLITIS

Ankylosing spondylitis is characterized by stiffness and pain in the back, with involvement of sacroiliac joints and variable progression to joints and periarticular tissues of the lumbodorsal and cervical spine. About half of patients also have arthritis of peripheral joints. It is usually a disease of young and middle-aged adults but may begin in childhood, usually in males over 8 yr of age. There is striking association of ankylosing spondylitis with HLA antigen B27. The pathology of synovial tissue from affected joints is similar to that seen in rheumatoid arthritis.

Clinically, ankylosing spondylitis differs from rheumatoid arthritis in respect to: (1) characteristic involvement of sacroiliac joints and lumbodorsal spine, (2) predilection for males, (3) rarity of rheumatoid factor in affected adults, (4) extreme rarity of rheumatoid nodules, (5) high frequency of acute iridocyclitis, (6) occurrence of aortitis with resulting aortic insufficiency, and (7) significant familial incidence.

Clinical Manifestations. Peripheral arthritis may be the first manifestation and is often transient. Large joints, particularly those of the lower extremities, are affected most frequently. Heel pain is common, as is the occurrence of pain at various other sites at which tendons and ligaments attach to bone (enthetopathy). Shoulders, feet, and temporomandibular joints are also involved in a significant number of patients. Affected joints may be warm, swollen, and painful.

Characteristic involvement of sacroiliac joints and lumbodorsal spine may be present at the onset of disease or appear months to years later. Pain in the low back, hip girdles, and thighs is characteristic. The pain is often transient, more severe at night, and relieved by moving about. Stiffness in the low back with loss of normal spinal mobility follows (Fig. 10–17). Spinal involvement characteristically begins in the sacroiliac joints and ascends, involving the lumbar, the dorsal, and, finally, the cervical spine. In contrast, in JRA the neck is involved but the lumbodorsal spine spared. Decreased expansion of the chest, related to involvement of costovertebral joints, may occur early in disease. Low-grade fever, anemia, anorexia, fatigability, and growth retardation may occur. The family history is frequently positive for similar arthritis or for acute iridocyclitis.

Ankylosing spondylitis may arrest at any stage, or the entire spine may become involved over a number of years with loss of virtually all vertebral mobility. Prognosis for functional outcome is usually good if good posture is maintained. Deformity of peripheral joints is uncommon; some patients develop destructive hip disease. Acute iridocyclitis occurs in about 25% of patients at some time; aortitis has not been reported in children but occurs in a significant number of adults with ankylosing spondylitis.

Laboratory Manifestations. There are no specific laboratory tests. Although HLA B27 is present in 95% of patients, it is not diagnostic. Sedimentation rates may be elevated. Anemia similar to that of rheumatoid arthritis occurs. Rheumatoid factors are rarely found. Involvement of the sacroiliac joints is demonstrable roentgenographically (Fig. 10–18), usually within the first 3–4 yr; destruction is progressive, with even-

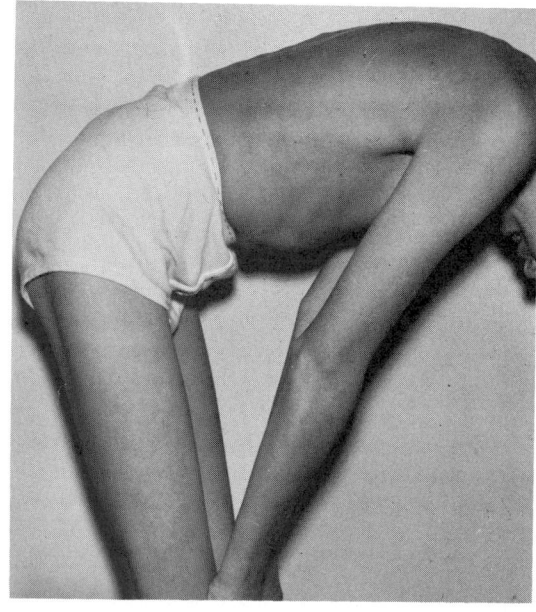

Figure 10–17. Loss of lumbodorsal spine mobility in a boy with ankylosing spondylitis: the lower spine remains straight when the patient bends forward.

tual obliteration of the joints. Characteristic roentgenographic changes in the lumbodorsal spine occur some years later.

Differential Diagnosis. Ankylosing spondylitis should be suspected in any child with persistent pain in hips, thighs, or low back, with or without peripheral arthritis. Roentgenographic changes in the sacroiliac joints are necessary for diagnosis, but several years may elapse before they appear. In differential diagnosis, *spinal cord tumors and other childhood malignancies, anatomic defects or infections of vertebrae or intervertebral discs, Scheuermann disease* and other orthopedic conditions of the spine must be considered in any child with persistent back pain. *Legg-Perthes disease* and *slipped capital femoral epiphysis* may cause persistent hip and thigh pain. *Ulcerative colitis, regional enteritis, psoriasis,* and *Reiter syndrome* may have associated spondylitis resembling ankylosing spondylitis.

Treatment. The aims of therapy are to relieve pain and to maintain good posture and function. For relief of pain, salicylates may suffice. Indomethacin and phenylbutazone may be helpful but must be used with caution in children and are

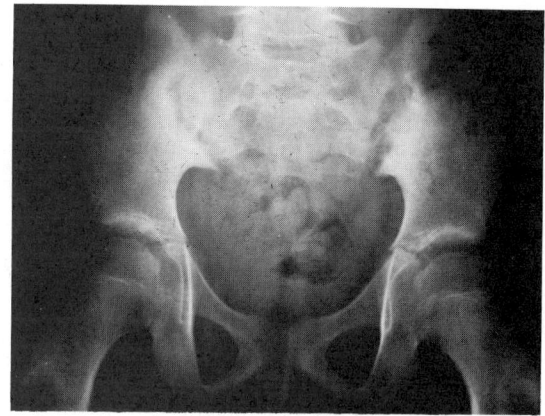

Figure 10–18. Well developed sacroiliitis in a boy with ankylosing spondylitis; both sacroiliac joints show extensive sclerosis, erosions of joint margins, and apparent widening of the joint space.

considered experimental agents. Other nonsteroidal agents may also prove useful; only tolmetin is now approved for use in children. Gold is not thought to be effective, and corticosteroid therapy is rarely, if ever, indicated. Radiation therapy is contraindicated. Maintenance of good posture is essential for preservation of good function; exercises designed to promote good posture and strengthen paraspinal muscles may be employed. A firm mattress or bed board should be used for sleeping, and thick pillows should be avoided.

10.60 OTHER SPONDYLOARTHROPATHIES IN CHILDREN

The spondyloarthropathies described in adults include those seronegative types of arthritis associated with sacroiliitis and spinal arthritis: ankylosing spondylitis, Reiter disease, psoriatic arthritis, the arthritis of inflammatory bowel disease, and the "reactive arthritis" of yersiniosis and other gastrointestinal infections. Although these types of arthritis are rarer in children than in adults, some of them, notably ankylosing spondylitis and Reiter disease, may sometimes be mislabeled as JRA during the childhood years. All of the spondyloarthropathies are associated with HLA B27, although not generally as strongly as is ankylosing spondylitis; all are associated neither with rheumatoid factors nor with antinuclear antibodies. The pathology of affected synovial tissues is not distinct from that of rheumatoid arthritis. Some of the spondyloarthropathies, notably Reiter disease and reactive arthritis, occur after identifiable environmental events such as infections with Shigella or Yersinia. Spondyloarthropathies may cluster in some families, with several family members having one or another of these types of arthritis; acute iridocyclitis may also be similarly associated. Except for psoriatic arthritis, the spondyloarthropathies affect boys and girls equally or have a male preponderance. Diagnoses of spondyloarthropathies rest on clinical grounds.

The pauciarticular disease type II subgroup of JRA probably represents early ankylosing spondylitis or one of the other spondyloarthropathies. Of the other JRA subgroups three are also seronegative (seronegative polyarthritis, systemic-onset JRA, and pauciarticular disease type I), but none is associated with sacroiliitis, HLA B27, or subsequent spondyloarthropathy.

Reiter Disease. In its full-blown form Reiter disease consists of sterile urethritis, arthritis, and ocular inflammation; other manifestations may include gastroenteritis and a variety of skin rashes. Males are predominantly affected. In young children Reiter disease has been reported following infections with Shigella, *Yersinia enterocolitica*, and Chlamydia; in older children, as in adults, Reiter disease has followed sexual exposure. Reiter disease is strongly associated with HLA B27, and the arthritis is generally pauciarticular, predominantly affecting large joints. Achilles tendinitis and heel pain are common. Some cases of pauciarticular disease type II may represent "partial" Reiter disease. The long-term prognosis of childhood-onset Reiter disease is unknown. The majority of children have recovered within a few months. However, some individuals can be expected to have subsequent ankylosing spondylitis, some will have recurrent or chronic arthritis, and some will have recurrent attacks of ocular or urethral inflammation. Diagnosis is clinical. Infectious urethritis and gonococcal disease must be excluded. Salicylates or one of the other nonsteroidal anti-inflammatory agents, as in pauciarticular JRA or ankylosing spondylitis, are used for treatment. Physical therapy also plays an important role in therapy. Patients need to be monitored for subsequent ankylosing spondylitis.

Arthritis of Inflammatory Bowel Disease. Both ulcerative colitis (Sec. 12.42) and regional enteritis (Sec. 12.43) can be associated with arthritis during childhood; about 10% of children with inflammatory bowel disease will at some time have joint manifestations. Affected children are generally older than 8 yr, and the arthritis generally affects a few large joints in a pauciarticular pattern. Periods of arthritis usually coincide with periods of active bowel disease or follow the appearance of identifiable bowel disease by months or years; in a few patients arthritis may be the 1st disease manifestation. The arthritis of inflammatory bowel disease in children follows two patterns, as it does in adulthood: most of the affected children have only peripheral arthritis, which waxes and wanes with activity of the bowel disease and causes neither joint destruction nor permanent joint deformity. However, a few children have early ankylosing spondylitis which may progress to disability regardless of control of the underlying bowel disease. For this reason it is important to follow children with inflammatory bowel disease for evidence of sacroiliitis or spinal arthritis. HLA B27 is associated with the ankylosing spondylitis but *not* with the peripheral arthritis of inflammatory bowel disease. Therapy for peripheral arthritis includes control of the underlying bowel disease, generally with corticosteroids, and the occasional additional use of salicylates or other nonsteroidal agents. If ankylosing spondylitis occurs, therapy should be given for that condition (Sec. 10.59).

Reactive Arthritis. Following gastrointestinal infection with *Yersinia enterocolitica*, Shigella, Salmonella, or Campylobacter, there may be a sterile arthritis, which generally affects a few joints in a pauciarticular fashion. Affected patients frequently have HLA B27. The relationship of such arthritis to Reiter disease and other spondyloarthropathies is unknown. The arthritis is generally transient and the ultimate outcome good. However, some affected patients may subsequently have chronic spondyloarthropathy. Any child with both gastroenteritis and arthritis should have appropriate stool cultures and serologic studies made.

Psoriatic Arthritis. Although psoriasis is a relatively common skin condition of children, psoriatic arthritis is uncommon during childhood. Girls are predominantly affected in a 2.5:1 ratio. Psoriatic arthritis in childhood is similar to that of adults. Arthritis begins in one or several joints, often in an asymmetric fashion. More than half of patients have involvement of distal interphalangeal joints; tendinitis is also common. In about half of patients, psoriasis precedes arthritis by months or years; in others the arthritis is the initial event, with psoriasis appearing later. Nail pitting is commonly associated. The prognosis of psoriatic arthritis in children appears to be good, though there are as yet few long-term studies. A few patients with psoriatic arthritis will develop the sacroiliitis and ankylosing spondylitis associated with HLA B27. Therapy of psoriatic arthritis is similar to that in adults; salicylates and other nonsteroidal anti-inflammatory agents are generally used. There is little experience with agents such as methotrexate in childhood psoriatic arthritis. As in JRA, physical and occupational therapy play important roles in maintaining good function.

10.61 SYSTEMIC LUPUS ERYTHEMATOSUS

Systemic lupus erythematosus (SLE) is a systemic disease characteristically affecting many organ systems. Its natural history is unpredictable; it is often progressive, terminating in death if untreated, but may remit spontaneously or smolder for many years. SLE in children is generally more acute and severe than in adults.

Etiology and Epidemiology. The cause is unknown. Many

observations support the hypothesis that SLE is a disease of altered immune regulation, perhaps genetically determined. Viruses may also play a role in pathogenesis. A variety of immune phenomena occur. Serum levels of immunoglobulins are increased. Antibodies are found that react with nuclear constituents (the antinuclear antibodies), and with ribonucleic acid, gamma globulin (rheumatoid factors), red blood cells (positive Coombs test), platelets, white blood cells, antigens used in serologic tests for syphilis (false-positive serology), and coagulation factors. There is also an association between inflammation and circulating immune complexes, particularly those of deoxyribonucleic acid (DNA) and antibodies reactive with DNA. Such immune complexes are deposited in tissues, fix complement, and initiate an inflammatory response that results in tissue injury. In SLE nephritis, for example, immunoglobulins and complement can be demonstrated in renal tissues by immunofluorescent techniques and DNA and anti-DNA antibodies eluted from affected glomeruli; active SLE with nephritis is associated with decreased levels of serum complement and with circulating antibodies reactive with DNA (Sec. 17.7).

The onset of exacerbations of disease may appear related to intercurrent infections; it is suspected that there is increased susceptibility to infections, perhaps on the basis of faulty immune mechanisms. Current evidence, including studies showing alterations in T and B lymphocyte function in patients with SLE, suggests that an immunodeficiency state may underlie the disease. It is sometimes familial and has affected identical twins; hypergammaglobulinemia, antinuclear antibodies, and other immune abnormalities have increased incidence in relatives of patients.

Lupus-like disease occurs following exposure to a number of drugs, notably hydralazine, sulfonamides, procainamide, and anticonvulsants. Drug-induced disease is generally mild and reversible when the inciting drug is withdrawn. Cutaneous manifestations and sometimes systemic manifestations may be exacerbated by sunlight.

The incidence is unknown, but the disease is not rare. SLE begins in childhood in 20% of cases, usually in children over 8 yr of age. Females are predominantly affected (8:1) in all age groups, except that in prepubertal patients, the sex incidence seems nearly equal. All races may be affected, with the prevalence perhaps higher in certain dark-skinned peoples including Blacks, Latin Americans, and some native American tribes.

Pathology. Changes occur at multiple sites and involve many organ systems. Characteristic masses of amorphous, purple-staining extracellular material are found in hematoxylin-stained affected tissues. These *hematoxylin bodies* probably represent degenerated cell nuclei similar to the inclusions of LE cells. Fibrinoid, an acellular, deeply eosinophilic material, is found in loose connective tissue or in walls of blood vessels of affected tissues. Fibrinoid is of uncertain composition, not specific for SLE, and is usually accompanied by a predominantly mononuclear inflammatory reaction. In the spleen perivascular fibrosis results in characteristic "onion ring" lesions around affected vessels. Granulomas are sometimes found in affected tissues. (See Sec. 17.7 for renal pathology.)

Clinical Manifestations. SLE may begin insidiously or acutely. Sometimes symptoms antedate the diagnosis of SLE by years. The most frequent early symptoms in children are fever, malaise, arthritis or arthralgia, and rash (Table 10–25). Fever occurs at some time in most affected children; it may be intermittent or sustained. Malaise, anorexia, weight loss, and debility are common.

Cutaneous manifestations occur in most affected children at some time. The "butterfly" rash (Fig. 10–19 [p. xxv]), an erythematous blush or scaly erythematous patches, involves the malar areas and usually extends over the bridge of the nose. The rash may be photosensitive, may spread to the face, scalp, neck, chest, and extremities, and may become bullous and secondarily infected. *Discoid lupus* (cutaneous manifestations only) is unusual in children. Other skin eruptions include distinctive erythematous macules and punctate lesions on the palms, soles, and fingertips; such lesions are secondary to vascular changes, and local infarction may occur. Raynaud phenomenon may be present. Vascular changes are seen at times in the nail beds. Macular and ulcerative lesions also occur on the palate and mucous membranes of the mouth and nose. Purpura, sometimes associated with thrombocytopenia, may appear on dependent or traumatized areas. Erythema nodosum and erythema multiforme are occasionally associated. Alopecia, from inflammation about hair follicles, may be patchy or generalized, and the hair coarse, dry, and brittle.

Arthralgia and joint stiffness are common and often occur without objective changes. Sometimes affected joints are warm and swollen, but persistent deforming arthritis is rare. Aseptic necrosis of bone, particularly in the femoral heads, occurs, presumably secondary to vasculitis. Tenosynovitis and myositis may also occur.

Polyserositis (pleurisy, pericarditis, and peritonitis) is characteristic. Hepatosplenomegaly and generalized lymphadenopathy are common. Cardiac involvement may be manifested by variable murmurs, friction rubs, cardiomegaly, electrocardiographic changes, or congestive heart failure, with myocarditis, pericarditis, or verrucous endocarditis (Libman-Sacks endocarditis) found at postmortem examination. Myocardial infarctions may cause death in relatively young patients, including children. Parenchymal lung infiltrates may occur; infection must be excluded, however, before pneumonia can be ascribed to SLE. Acute pneumonia, pulmonary hemorrhage, or chronic pulmonary fibrosis may occur. Involvement of the nervous system may cause personality changes, seizures, cerebrovascular accidents, and peripheral neuritis. Gastrointestinal manifestations include abdominal pain, vomiting, diarrhea, melena, and even bowel infarction secondary to vasculitis. Ocular changes may include episcleritis, iritis, or retinal vascular changes with hemorrhages or exudates (cytoid bodies). Most children have clinical renal involvement (Sec. 17.7).

Laboratory Manifestations. Antinuclear antibodies (ANA) should be demonstrable in all patients with active SLE and provide the best screening test for the disease; however, ANA also occur in many other conditions (Sec. 10.57). Claims for "ANA-negative lupus" remain to be verified. Antibodies to double-stranded DNA are relatively specific and are associated with active disease, particularly nephritis; DNA antibodies

Table 10–25. **Manifestations of Lupus in Children**

	% of Patients
Malaise, weight loss, growth retardation	96
Cutaneous abnormalities	96
Hematologic abnormalities	91
Fever	84
Nephritis	84
Musculoskeletal complaints	82
Pleural/pulmonary disease	67
Hepatosplenomegaly and/or lymphadenopathy	58
Neurologic disease	49
Cardiac abnormalities	38
Hypertension	33
Ocular abnormalities	31
Gastrointestinal symptoms	27
Raynaud's phenomenon	13

From Wallace C, Schaller JG, Emery H, et al: Arthritis Rheum 21:599, 1978.

thus provide a useful index of severity and activity. Serum hemolytic complement and some of its components (C3 is most frequently measured) are decreased in patients with severe active SLE, particularly in those with nephritis; measuring serum complement therefore provides another useful guide to the activity and severity of disease. Other antibodies may be demonstrated by biologic false-positive tests for syphilis or positive Coombs tests. Serum gamma globulin levels are usually elevated; alpha-2 globulin levels may be increased and albumin decreased. One or more of the individual immunoglobulins may be elevated. An increased prevalence of HLA B8 and DW3/DR3, and of DW2/DR2 has been reported in some series of lupus patients.

Anemia related to chronic inflammatory disease or hemolysis is common. Difficulties in typing and crossmatching blood may arise from the presence of erythrocyte antibodies. Thrombocytopenia and leukopenia occur frequently. Platelet antibodies may be demonstrable; idiopathic thrombocytopenic purpura (ITP) may be the first manifestation of SLE. The urine may contain red cells, white cells, protein, and casts. Renal insufficiency may produce elevated levels of blood urea nitrogen or creatinine and abnormal renal function studies.

Diagnosis and Differential Diagnosis. SLE may mimic any rheumatic disease and many other diseases as well. Diagnosis is clinical and is confirmed by laboratory tests; recent classification criteria have been proposed (Table 10–26). Antinuclear antibodies are always present even though they are not diagnostic; their absence makes the diagnosis unlikely. Antibodies to double-stranded DNA are virtually diagnostic but are present only in severe or widespread disease. LE cells are not always demonstrable. Hypergammaglobulinemia, positive Coombs test, false-positive test for syphilis, anemia, leukopenia, or thrombocytopenia, and signs of nephritis may also be diagnostically helpful. Serum levels of hemolytic complement and some of its components are lowered in some patients with active disease; absence of measurable hemolytic complement should suggest a possible complement deficiency. Renal biopsy may confirm the diagnosis, but histologic changes are not entirely specific. Thrombocytopenic purpura and hemolytic anemia may be presenting features; the differential diagnosis of these manifestations should include SLE.

Treatment. Therapy should be based on the extent and severity of disease in the individual patient. Patients must be thoroughly evaluated, particularly for renal involvement. The type and severity of the renal lesion should be determined by renal biopsy on patients with clinical evidence of nephritis. There is no specific therapy; drugs used to treat the disease suppress inflammation and perhaps suppress the formation of immune complexes and the activities of immunologically active effector cells (this latter mechanism is unproved). In general, patients should be treated to maintain clinical well-being and normal serum complement levels.

In patients with mild disease without nephritis, salicylates or other nonsteroidal agents should be used to provide symptomatic relief of arthritis and other discomforts. Careful follow-up for possible development of nephritis is important. Chloroquine and hydroxychloroquine are used in discoid and systemic lupus, but extreme care must be taken because of retinal toxicity. Topical use of corticosteroid preparations may suppress the facial rash. Systemic use of steroids in doses sufficient to suppress symptoms may be required. In patients with significant systemic involvement but without clinical nephritis and with normal serum complements and DNA antibodies therapy can also be symptomatic, with careful follow-up. Doses of corticosteroid sufficient to suppress symptoms should be given initially (1–2 mg/kg/24 hr may be required) and then tapered to the lowest suppressive dose. Antimalarial agents may be useful adjuncts in therapy. In patients with SLE and nephritis, therapy must be geared not only to maintain the clinical well-being of the patient but also to suppress the renal disease, as reflected by return of serum complement levels to normal and reduction of circulating antibodies to DNA. Large doses of corticosteroids for prolonged periods may be required; initial doses of prednisone of 1–2 mg/kg/24 hr are usual. All the undesirable side effects of steroid therapy may be expected if large doses are required for a significant period of time. Other schedules of steroid administration may be used, including intravenous pulses with large doses or alternate day dose schedules. Agents such as azathioprine, cyclophosphamide, or chlorambucil may be effective in suppressing severe SLE; however, such therapy must be used with extreme care. Little is known of the long-term effects of such drugs, particularly in children; side-effects include increased susceptibility to severe viral and other infections, gonadal suppression, and possible induction of malignancies. Such agents should never be used in mild SLE or in patients whose disease can be satisfactorily controlled with corticosteroids alone.

Seizures and other central nervous system manifestations should be treated with large doses of prednisone; they are generally associated with severe active disease. Central nervous system disease occurs episodically in SLE and may never recur if the patient is helped over the acute episode and the disease can be subsequently controlled.

Because of the possibility of drug-induced disease, inquiry should be made about possible offending agents; drugs known to be etiologically associated with SLE should not be used in patients with the disease.

Meticulous follow-up is of paramount importance in treating all patients with SLE and includes monitoring clinical, renal, and serologic status. Any signs of worsening disease should be promptly recognized and appropriately managed. Since there is no cure, the disease is potentially lifelong, and patients must be followed for years.

Table 10–26. 1982 Revised Criteria for Classification of Systemic Lupus Erythematosus

Malar rash
Discoid rash
Photosensitivity
Oral ulcers
Arthritis of 2 or more joints
Serositis
    Pleuritis or
    pericarditis
Renal disorder
    Persistent proteinuria or
    cellular casts
Neurologic disorder
    Seizures or
    psychosis
Hematologic disorder
    Hemolytic anemia or
    leukopenia or
    lymphopenia or
    thrombocytopenia
Immunologic disorder
    Positive LE cell preparation or
    anti-DNA antibody or
    anti-Sm antibody or
    false positive serologic test for syphilis
Antinuclear antibody

The proposed classification is based on 11 criteria. For the purpose of identifying patients in clinical studies, a person shall be said to have systemic lupus erythematosus if any 4 or more of the 11 criteria are present, serially or simultaneously, during any interval of observation.

(Tan EM, Cohen AS, Fries JF, et al: The 1982 revised criteria for the classification of systemic lupus erythematosus. Arthritis Rheum 25:1271, 1982.)

Prognosis. SLE has generally been considered a potentially or even uniformly fatal disease, particularly in children. Now, however, some children with milder disease are being recognized, and it is apparent that not all children have severe nephritis. Although spontaneous exacerbations and remissions occur, prolonged spontaneous remission is unusual in children. Therapy with antibiotics, corticosteroids, and anticancer drugs has prolonged survival and brightened the short-term prognosis for many patients with lupus. The 5 yr survival for children now approaches 90%. However, a significant number of patients still die later from the disease. Major causes of death in SLE patients today include nephritis, central nervous system complications, infections, pulmonary lupus, and myocardial infarctions. Whether the ultimate prognosis of severe lupus can be modified by vigorous therapy remains to be determined.

10.62 LUPUS PHENOMENA IN THE NEWBORN PERIOD

Infants of mothers with SLE may have transient manifestations of lupus in the newborn period, presumably mediated by transplacental factors. Transiently positive antinuclear antibody tests or LE cells are the most frequent abnormalities; there are generally no associated clinical manifestations, and the serologic abnormalities regress after several weeks. The most frequent clinical abnormality of infants born to mothers with SLE is a rash clinically and histologically typical of discoid lupus, which fades over a period of several months. Transient thrombocytopenia related to transplacental platelet antibodies, transient hemolytic anemia, and leukopenia also occur. SLE or other rheumatic disease can be identified in most mothers of infants with congenital heart block. The mechanism for this is unknown; the antinuclear antibody anti-Ro is associated (Sec. 14.72). Endocardial fibroelastosis has also been reported in infants of mothers with SLE. Few, if any, cases of true SLE in infants have been reported, but the late occurrence of SLE in young adults who had "transient" manifestations of lupus in the neonatal period has now been noted in several patients.

10.63 VASCULITIS SYNDROMES

In these syndromes of blood vessel inflammation the various patterns of disease depend on the size and location of affected vessels. When small nonmuscular vessels are involved, the disease takes the form of Schönlein-Henoch vasculitis (anaphylactoid purpura). With involvement of larger muscular arteries the disease is called polyarteritis nodosa; variants include infantile polyarteritis, Wegener granulomatosis, and probably Kawasaki disease. Some overlap of these syndromes occurs; vessels of various sizes may sometimes be involved in the same patients. In Takayasu arteritis the aorta and other great vessels are sites of inflammation.

Inflammation of blood vessels also occurs in other rheumatic disease in children, notably lupus erythematosus, dermatomyositis, and scleroderma; in hypertension; and in vessels exposed to local infection, trauma, or thromboemboli.

The causes of these disorders are unknown. Both Schönlein-Henoch vasculitis and polyarteritis may follow exposure to drugs or allergens. In serum sickness (sec. 10.52), vasculitis is caused by deposition of immune complexes. Polyarteritis nodosa has been associated with hepatitis B, vascular damage presumably being caused by immune complexes of the viral antigen and its antibody. In contrast to most other rheumatic diseases, Schönlein-Henoch vasculitis and polyarteritis nodosa predominantly affect males. In childhood Schönlein-Henoch vasculitis is the most commonly encountered type; polyarteritis and its variants are much rarer in children.

10.64 SCHÖNLEIN-HENOCH VASCULITIS
(Anaphylactoid Purpura)

This distinctive syndrome was described by Heberden before 1800; Schönlein in the 1830's described the typical rash and joint manifestations, and Henoch in the 1870's recognized the gastrointestinal and renal manifestations. Osler pointed out the similarity between this disease and the hypersensitivity reactions, erythema multiforme, and serum sickness. The skin lesion, which is usually purpuric, is the most obvious sign; the visceral lesions are less easily recognized but are far more serious. The primary manifestations are due to vasculitis of small blood vessels.

The cause is unknown. Allergy or drug sensitivity plays a role in some patients. The disease may follow an upper respiratory tract infection, sometimes streptococcal, but this sequence (or phenomenon) is of uncertain significance. The syndrome may occur at any age; it is more common in children than in adults, most cases occurring from 2–8 yr of age. Boys are affected twice as often as girls.

Pathology. In the skin small vessels of the corium are surrounded with an acute inflammatory reaction of polymorphonuclear and round cells; eosinophils and varying numbers of red blood cells may be present. Dermal IgA deposits have been demonstrated. Capillaries are most frequently involved, but small arterioles and venules may be affected. Scattered nuclear debris, edema, and swelling of collagen fibrils are found adjacent to affected vessels. Inflammation or hemorrhage at other sites may include synovium, the gastrointestinal tract, and the central nervous system. For the renal lesion, see Sec. 17.12.

Clinical Manifestations. Onset may be acute, with simultaneous appearance of several manifestations, or gradual, with sequential appearance of different manifestations over a period of weeks. Various combinations of symptoms and signs may occur. Malaise and low-grade fever are present in half the patients.

Skin lesions are present in all identified patients; it is not known whether visceral manifestations occur in the absence of rash. The lesions usually appear on the lower extremities but may involve buttocks, upper extremities, trunk, and face as well (Fig. 10–20 [p. xxv]). Dermatologic manifestations are extremely variable. The classic lesion begins as a small wheal or an erythematous maculopapule. Lesions initially blanch on pressure but later lose this feature and generally become petechial or purpuric. Purpuric areas evolve in the usual manner of ecchymoses, changing from red to purple, becoming rusty, and eventually fading. Skin lesions appear in crops, and at any time a variety may be present. In addition to these characteristic lesions, the various patterns of erythema multiforme and erythema nodosum may occur. Such rashes are rarely pruritic. Angioedema involving the scalp, eyelids, lips, dorsa of the hands and feet, back, and perineum is common and may be striking, especially in young children. Rarely an entire limb segment, such as the forearm, may be transiently swollen and tender.

Arthritis occurs in two thirds of affected children. Large joints, particularly knees and ankles, are most commonly involved. Affected joints may be swollen, tender, and painful on motion. Effusions may be present; joint fluid is serous, with leukocytosis, not hemorrhagic. Joint symptoms usually resolve after a few days without residual deformity or articular damage but may recur during the period of active disease.

Gastrointestinal symptoms appear in two thirds of affected children. The most common complaint is colicky abdominal pain, which may be severe and is often associated with vomiting. Stools show gross or occult blood in over half of patients, and hematemesis may occur. Failure to recognize this syndrome in children with sudden onset of acute abdominal pain may lead to unnecessary laparotomy. In such cases peritoneal exudate and enlarged mesenteric lymph nodes are usually found; segmental edema and hemorrhage into bowel wall may be present. Gastrointestinal roentgenograms may show decreased motility and segmental narrowing, presumably related to submucosal edema and hemorrhage. Rarely, intussusception, obstruction, or infarction and perforation of bowel may occur.

Renal involvement is potentially the most serious manifestation since it can result in chronic renal disease. It occurs in 25–50% of children during the acute phase, the frequency depending in part on the adequacy of examination. It is usually manifest during the first few weeks of illness but sometimes appears after other manifestations have become quiescent. Moderate azotemia and hypertension, and even oliguria and hypertensive encephalopathy, can occur. Most children with renal involvement recover, although some continue to have abnormal urinary sediment, with or without abnormal renal function; a few will have chronic renal disease within a few years of the acute phase.

A rare but potentially serious manifestation is central nervous system involvement, with seizures, pareses, and coma. Hepatosplenomegaly and lymphadenopathy may also occur during acute phases of the disease. Rarely, intramuscular hemorrhage, rheumatoid-like nodules, cardiac involvement, eye involvement, or testicular swelling and hemorrhage have been reported.

Prognosis is excellent in the absence of significant renal disease. The course is variable. Often the disease is mild, lasting a few days with only transient arthritis and a few pupuric spots. In more seriously affected children the average duration is 4–6 wk, but subsequent exacerbations and remissions may occur. Sometimes the illness may smolder for one or more years.

Laboratory Manifestations. Laboratory tests are not diagnostic. The sedimentation rate may be elevated. The white blood cell count is often increased, and eosinophilia may be present. Coagulation studies are normal. With renal involvement red cells, white cells, casts, and albumin are present in the urine. There may be gross or occult blood in the stools. Lupus erythematosus cells, rheumatoid factor, and antinuclear antibodies are not associated. Serum complement titers are normal or elevated. Serum levels of IgA may be elevated.

Diagnosis and Differential Diagnosis. The full-blown picture of Schönlein-Henoch vasculitis with rash, arthritis, and gastrointestinal and renal manifestations is characteristic. Diagnostic confusion may result when one symptom predominates or multiple system involvement is not recognized. The rash may suggest a *hemorrhagic diathesis* or *septicemia*; platelet counts, blood clotting tests, and cultures will exclude these possibilities. In addition, the patient with septicemia usually appears more acutely ill. When gastrointestinal manifestations predominate, the syndrome may suggest a number of *intra-abdominal emergencies*. The possibility of Schönlein-Henoch vasculitis should be considered in any child with acute abdominal pain and inquiry made for associated rash, nephritis, or arthritis. With prominent renal findings, *acute glomerulonephritis* may be suggested; other manifestations of Schönlein-Henoch vasculitis should allow differentiation. In children with chronic renal disease a history of acute Schönlein-Henoch vasculitis in the past should be sought. Differentiation from other rheumatic diseases is rarely difficult. In polyarteritis nodosa, peripheral neurologic changes and cardiac manifestations are more common, but clinical distinction from Schönlein-Henoch vasculitis may occasionally be difficult.

Treatment. There is no specific therapy. In the rare instance in which a specific allergen can be proved, the patient should be kept from contact with it. When the disease follows a bacterial infection, particularly streptococcal, the organism should be eliminated and, if the disease recurs, prophylaxis

considered. Symptomatic treatment only is indicated for arthritis, rash, edema, fever, and malaise. Salicylates will often alleviate these self-limited discomforts.

Intestinal hemorrhage, obstruction, intussusception, or perforation may be life-threatening in the acute phase; these complications may perhaps be prevented by the early use of corticosteroids. Therapy with prednisone in dosage of 1–2 mg/kg/24 hr is often associated with dramatic improvement. Corticosteroid therapy is also indicated for central nervous system manifestations. Acute renal failure should be managed in the same way as acute glomerulonephritis (Sec. 17.5). Therapy of severe nephritis with drugs such as corticosteroids, azathioprine, and cyclophosphamide remains experimental.

Prognosis. Rarely, death may occur during the acute phase from gastrointestinal complications (hemorrhage, intussusception, bowel infarction), acute renal failure, or central nervous system involvement. Chronic renal disease may cause later morbidity in a few patients. About 25% of children with initial renal involvement have persistence of abnormal urine sediment for years; the prognosis for these patients is unknown.

10.65 POLYARTERITIS NODOSA

Medium-sized and small arteries are the sites of inflammation in polyarteritis nodosa. The disease affects all age groups but is rare in childhood. Males are affected more frequently than females. The cause is unknown, but the disease has been reported to follow drug exposures. Hepatitis B antigen has been associated with a few cases as have streptococcal infections and serous otitis media.

Inflammation with polymorphonuclear leukocytes, eosinophils, and round cells may involve the entire vessel wall. Necrosis, thrombosis, or aneurysm formation may occur in affected vessels and result in infarction. Healed vessels become scarred or recanalized.

Clinical manifestations are diverse and depend on sites of vascular involvement. Signs of systemic illness such as fever, anorexia, lethargy, weakness, and weight loss are usually present. Arthralgia and arthritis are frequent; myalgia and myositis may be present. Various cutaneous manifestations are common and include erythematous rashes, nodular lesions, petechiae and purpuric spots, cutaneous ulcers, and edema. Rarely, gangrene of extremities occurs. Peripheral neuropathy, with pain, numbness, paresthesias, and muscle weakness, results from involvement of peripheral nerves adjacent to affected vessels. Abdominal pain, bleeding, ulcerations, and infarction can follow involvement of gastrointestinal vessels. Renal involvement may result in renal failure and death. Involvement of large renal vessels results in flank pain and gross hematuria, that of small vessels and glomeruli in microscopic hematuria, proteinuria, and cylindruria. Associated hypertension is usual. Inflammation of pulmonary vessels may cause cough, wheezing, pulmonary infiltrates, and pleuritis. Central nervous system manifestations include seizures, encephalitic symptoms, and stroke. Cranial nerve palsies and iridocyclitis may occur. Involvement of coronary vessels may produce tachycardia, congestive heart failure, and myocardial infarction; pericarditis may also be present. Orchitis and epididymitis are common.

There are no specific *laboratory tests*. The sedimentation rate may be elevated and acute phase reactants present. Anemia is common; eosinophilia is sometimes found. There may be gross or microscopic hematuria, and renal function studies may be deranged.

Polyarteritis nodosa is readily confused with many other diseases. Differentiation from other rheumatic diseases may be particularly difficult. The *diagnosis* is based primarily on clinical suspicion and on histologic changes in involved tissues on biopsy. Muscle biopsies may fail to identify vasculitis. Testicular biopsies are said to be helpful but are seldom done. Arteriography of liver or kidney may be helpful. The diagnosis in children is probably most frequently made at autopsy.

The prognosis is poor; death can occur from renal failure, heart failure, or severe gastrointestinal or central nervous system disease. Corticosteroids may suppress acute manifestations and lengthen survival. Anticancer drugs such as cyclophosphamide have occasionally achieved apparent success.

10.66 Infantile Polyarteritis

Polyarteritis in infants under 1 yr of age, though rare, presents a characteristic clinical pattern. Both sexes are affected. The cause is unknown, but, as in other forms of vasculitis, this disease has been reported in association with drug exposure (sulfonamides, penicillin). There is also a suggestive relation to immunization and to viral and bacterial illnesses.

The *pathology* is similar to polyarteritis in older patients, but fibrinoid necrosis of vessels is less prominent. On the basis of similar pathologic changes, a relationship between infantile polyarteritis and Kawasaki disease has been proposed.

Clinical manifestations usually begin with fever, rhinitis, conjunctivitis, and a macular erythematous rash, suggesting an acute viral infection, but the illness persists. Involvement of the coronary arteries has been the predominant manifestation in most patients, resulting in tachycardia, cardiomegaly, congestive heart failure, or pericarditis. The electrocardiogram may show right, left, or combined ventricular hypertrophy, as well as evidence of myocardial ischemia or infarction. At autopsy, aneurysms of coronary arteries are frequently found as well as myocardial infarcts and pericarditis. Aneurysms may perforate causing hemopericardium.

Other manifestations include renal involvement (abnormal urinary sediment), hypertension, decreased blood pressure in or ischemia of an extremity, central nervous system manifestations (nuchal rigidity, pareses, cranial nerve palsies, seizures), hepatosplenomegaly, lymphadenopathy, gastrointestinal symptoms, and cough. Involvement of vessels in skeletal muscle is uncommon, and muscle biopsy is of little diagnostic usefulness.

There are no specific *laboratory tests*. The white blood cell count is often elevated, with eosinophilia; sedimentation rates may be high. Diagnosis is usually made at autopsy, although awareness of this syndrome should permit presumptive clinical diagnosis. At autopsy widespread arteritis involving many organs has been found.

The prognosis is very poor, all reported cases having terminated in death within an average of 1 mo after onset. Death is usually sudden or related to progressive cardiac decompensation.

No satisfactory treatment has been found, but corticosteroid therapy appears worthy of trial.

10.67 Kawasaki Disease
(Mucocutaneous Lymph Node Syndrome)

This disorder of unknown etiology usually occurs in children under 5 yr of age. Although originally reported in Japanese children, worldwide distribution among many races is now recognized. It occurs sporadically or in epidemics, with an incidence of about 0.6/100,000 children (<5 yr)/yr in the United States. There is no evidence for person to person transmission.

Clinical Manifestations. Kawasaki disease is an acute inflammatory condition characterized by various combinations of several of the following features over a 1–3 wk period: prolonged high, often spiking, fevers; usually bilateral bulbar conjunctivitis; dry erythematous lips, strawberry tongue and injected oropharyngeal mucosa; nonpurulent primarily cervical lymphadenopathy; and skin lesions consisting of polymorphous macular erythematous rashes, erythema multiforme, and indurated edema and superficial desquamation of the skin of the hands and feet. In addition, many patients have serious cardiac involvement, with coronary arteritis, dilatation and aneurysm formation of affected vessels, myocarditis, arrhythmias, and coronary insufficiency. The regression or progression of these cardiac abnormalities is not predictable. A broad spectrum of other manifestations has also been observed such as arthritis (common), uveitis, irritability, cranial nerve palsies, encephalopathy, ataxia, hypertension, pulmonary infiltrates, gallbladder hydrops, ileus, hepatomegaly, and splenomegaly.

Laboratory Manifestations. Anemia, leukocytosis, and thrombocytosis often occur. Serum amylase activity and erythrocyte sedimentation rate may be elevated. There may be pyuria, proteinuria, and cerebrospinal fluid pleocytosis. Tests for rheumatoid factor and antinuclear antibody are negative. Serum complement may be normal or elevated.

Diagnosis. This rests on the clinical features, since there are no specific laboratory tests. Coronary artery vasculitis may be identified by echocardiography or arteriography, but electrocardiograms and chest roentgenograms may be normal even with advanced disease. Various infectious diseases, poststreptococcal disease, and Stevens-Johnson syndrome must be distinguished from Kawasaki disease.

Prognosis. Recovery is usually complete in those who do not develop coronary vasculitis, although second attacks do occur. Many patients have cardiac involvement but probably no more than 10% of those with aneurysms have fatal outcomes (1–2% of all patients), usually within 1–2 mo of onset.

Treatment. Salicylate is indicated during the febrile phase for symptomatic relief, but therapeutic serum concentrations of 20–30 mg/dL may be difficult to achieve, even with doses as high as 100 mg/kg/24 hr. This treatment does not prevent the development of coronary disease. Intravenous administration of gamma globulin may reduce the frequency of coronary artery abnormalities. Corticosteroids and anticoagulants are contraindicated.

10.68 Wegener Granulomatosis
(Lethal Midline Granuloma)

In this rare syndrome, destructive granulomatous lesions of the upper respiratory tract and lungs are associated with a systemic necrotizing vasculitis, most prominent in lungs and kidneys. The upper respiratory and pulmonary granulomas may predominate in some cases, antedating recognition of systemic vasculitis by years. Males are predominantly affected (2:1). The cause is unknown; as in other vasculitis syndromes, an association with drug sensitivity and allergy has been noted.

Respiratory symptoms are prominent *clinical manifestations*. Persistent nasal stuffiness and/or discharge may be an early symptom, with crusted or pustular lesions in the nares. Lesions are progressively destructive and may result in perforation of the nasal septum, obliteration of nasal sinuses, and ulcerations of the palate, pharynx, larynx, and trachea. Cough or hemoptysis may occur, and fever and prostration are common. Other frequently associated manifestations include arthritis, neuropathy, rash, splenomegaly, and severe progressive glomerulitis often terminating in renal failure. In cases with clinically inapparent systemic involvement, diffuse vasculitis may be found on post mortem examination.

There are no specific *laboratory manifestations*; eosinophilia may be present. Roentgenograms may reveal bone destruction in the nose and sinuses and pulmonary infiltrates suggestive of tuberculosis or neoplasm. Urinalyses usually show evidence of nephritis, and renal function studies may be abnormal.

Diagnosis is based on the clinical picture and confirmed by demonstration of granulomatous lesions of the respiratory tract and systemic vasculitis, particularly nephritis. Without therapy, the *prognosis* is poor. Patients with limited forms of the disease may have long survivals, but the destructive lesions of the upper respiratory tract may be disfiguring.

Treatment with corticosteroids may suppress systemic vasculitis and prevent progression of destructive lesions in the upper respiratory tract. Drugs such as azathioprine and cyclophosphamide may arrest the disease in some patients.

10.69 TAKAYASU ARTERITIS
("Pulseless Disease")

This uncommon condition, an inflammatory process involving the aorta and its major branches, occurs primarily in young women. Some cases have been reported in late childhood, a few in infants. Most reports are from Asia or Africa. The cause is unknown; associated congenital defects of great vessels have been recorded.

The underlying pathology is a segmental panarteritis of the aorta and its major branches. Smaller vessels are spared. Aneurysmal dilatation and rupture may occur. Involvement of the great vessels can cause weak or absent pulses in the upper extremities, hence, "pulseless disease." Blood pressure in the legs may exceed that in the arms, in contrast to coarctation of the aorta. Renal arterial involvement may cause renal ischemia, resulting in hypertension. Decreased brain blood flow can result in neurologic disturbances. Visual disturbances are common in older patients.

Associated rheumatic complaints have included arthritis, myalgia, pleuritis, pericarditis, fever, and rashes, sometimes antedating symptomatic aortitis by years. There are no specific laboratory data. Sedimentation rates and gamma globulin levels may be elevated; LE preparations may be positive. Angiography may demonstrate changes in affected vessels.

The condition should be considered in any child with obscure hypertension, particularly when fever and an elevated sedimentation rate are associated. The prognosis is variable. Some adults have survived; most children have died. No specific therapy is known. Corticosteroids have been used. Endarterectomy or nephrectomy may be warranted.

10.70 DERMATOMYOSITIS

This multisystem disease is characterized principally by nonsuppurative inflammation of striated muscle. Affected children usually have typical associated cutaneous lesions.

Etiology and Epidemiology. The cause of dermatomyositis is unknown. Cellular immune mechanisms may play a basic role in pathogenesis. Lymphocytes from patients with dermatomyositis release lymphotoxins and kill muscle cells in tissue culture. Immunoglobulin and complement deposition also occur in blood vessels of affected muscle. In adults but not in children there is a frequent association with malignancies (20% of patients). Preliminary studies suggest an association of childhood dermatomyositis with HLA B8/DR3.

Dermatomyositis is less common than rheumatoid arthritis, SLE, or Schönlein-Henoch vasculitis. It rarely begins before the 2nd year of life. Girls are affected more frequently than boys (3:2), and there is no familial or racial predilection.

Pathology. Lesions in skin, subcutaneous tissues, and muscles are irregularly distributed; care must be taken to choose an involved site for biopsy. The most prominent lesion in children is an occlusive vasculitis involving arterioles, venules,

and capillaries in connective tissues of skin, subcutaneous tissue, and muscle. In muscle there are patchy degeneration, atrophy, and regeneration of muscle fibers, interstitial edema, and proliferation of connective tissue. In affected skin there are thinning of the epidermis and edema and vasculitis in the dermis. Gastrointestinal tract vasculitis may produce mucosal ulcerations and tissue infarction. Mild renal glomerular changes have also been described.

Clinical Manifestations. Onset is usually insidious, with slowly developing muscle weakness, generally first apparent in proximal muscles of the extremities and trunk. The child may develop an awkward gait and slowly lose capacity for functions such as climbing stairs, riding a bicycle, and dressing. Affected muscles tend to be stiff and sore and sometimes brawny, indurated, and tender. Nonpitting edema and thickening of the skin and subcutaneous tissues may be present. Although myositis is generally most pronounced in proximal muscle, any muscles can be affected, with varying sites and degrees of atrophy. Severe involvement of palatorespiratory muscles may lead to respiratory difficulty, aspiration, and death. Arthralgia and arthritis sometimes occur.

The skin lesions are characteristic and often have a distinctive violaceous hue. The upper eyelids assume a pathognomonic violaceous discoloration (heliotrope eyelids) (Fig. 10–21 [p. xxv]). Periorbital and facial edema may be associated. A butterfly rash similar to that of SLE may be present. Lesions of palatal and nasal mucous membranes may be associated with the malar rash. The skin over extensor surfaces of joints, particularly the knuckles, knees, and elbows, becomes erythematous, atrophic, and scaly (Fig. 10–22 [p. xxv]). These areas later develop pigmentary changes resulting in hyperpigmentation or vitiligo. The capillaries of the nail bed may become tortuous or occluded. A dusky erythema may cover the upper trunk and proximal extremities. Other nonspecific skin changes may also occur. The skin over involved extremities may appear tight and glossy; in longstanding disease there may be cutaneous atrophy with binding of skin to underlying structures. Calcium may be deposited in affected subcutaneous tissues, muscles, and fascia; these deposits sometimes break down and are extruded in semisolid or solid form.

Low-grade fever is often present, and other evidence of systemic involvement such as lymphadenopathy, hepatosplenomegaly, and gastrointestinal manifestations may occur.

Laboratory Manifestations. Muscle inflammation is responsible for elevated serum levels of such enzymes as transaminases, creatine kinase, and aldolase. The electromyogram of affected muscles is abnormal. The sedimentation rate may be elevated or normal. Tests for rheumatoid factors and antinuclear antibodies are generally negative or of low titer. Urinalyses are usually normal. In patients with gastrointestinal involvement there may be gross or occult blood in the stool. Roentgenograms may reveal calcium deposits in soft tissues.

Diagnosis and Differential Diagnosis. In its typical form dermatomyositis should present little diagnostic difficulty. The combination of muscle weakness and characteristic rash, elevated serum levels of enzymes, and abnormal electromyogram is diagnostic; muscle biopsy is usually not necessary. In the differential diagnosis various neuromuscular disorders, such as poliomyelitis, Guillain-Barré syndrome, muscular dystrophy, and myasthenia gravis should be considered, as should illnesses having predominantly muscular lesions, such as trichinosis. Transient myositis has been reported in association with influenza and may occur with other viral infections as well. SLE, mixed connective tissue disease, juvenile rheumatoid arthritis, and scleroderma are distinguishable clinically and by laboratory tests. In the chronic phase, features of dermatomyositis and generalized scleroderma may overlap and thus make precise categorization difficult. When the onset is insidious, a period of observation may be needed to establish the diagnosis.

Treatment. During the acute phase, evaluation of palatorespiratory function may be lifesaving. If swallowing mechanisms are impaired, soft or liquid diets should be provided under close observation. The patient should be closely watched for possible deterioration in respiratory function. Constant nursing care is mandatory for any child with palatorespiratory involvement, and equipment for nasopharyngeal suction, endotracheal intubation, and tracheostomy should be available. A respirator may be required. The possibility of serious gastrointestinal manifestations during the acute phase of disease must also be considered.

Functional recovery depends on preserving adequate muscle strength and preventing crippling contractures. Corticosteroids effectively suppress the inflammatory process in most patients. Serial serum levels of transaminase, creatine kinase, or aldolase provide a helpful gauge of activity and therapeutic response. Prednisone in initial dosage of 1–2 mg/kg/24 hr (or 60 mg/M^2 of body surface area/24 hr) usually reduces enzyme levels toward normal values within 1–2 wk; clinical improvement with decreased pain and swelling in muscles and increasing muscle strength usually follows. When enzyme levels have declined to normal, the steroid dosage should be slowly decreased, with continued monitoring of the clinical course and serum enzyme levels. If the steroid dosage is reduced too rapidly, rebound in enzyme levels may occur; such rebounds are followed by deterioration in the clinical condition within a few weeks unless corticosteroid dosage is promptly increased. The lowest dose of steroids sufficient to suppress clinical symptoms and serum enzyme levels should be found and maintained for months. Steroid therapy can generally be discontinued in 1–2 yr. Steroid preparations such as triamcinolone and dexamethasone, which are associated with "steroid myopathy," should be avoided. Salicylates may occasionally be helpful as adjunctive drugs in relieving symptoms. For patients who do not respond to steroids, pulsed administration of steroids or drugs such as methotrexate or azathioprine may be used.

Physical therapy is essential to avoid contractures and to rebuild muscle strength. During the acute phase when muscle weakness is pronounced, passive exercises can be used to maintain range of motion. With clinical improvement active exercises to strengthen muscles should be added. Splints to maintain good limb position may be needed. Bed rest is not necessary, and immobilization without exercise should be avoided at all times. Skin hygiene, especially around the neck, skin creases, and axillae, is important.

Prognosis. In untreated patients mortality is about 40%. Most deaths are related to palatorespiratory involvement or such gastrointestinal complications as hemorrhage and perforation, and occur within 2 yr of onset. Otherwise, the disease slowly becomes inactive over several years and subsequent exacerbations are unusual. Infrequently, the disease may smolder for years. Most surviving patients are able to lead active lives, although they may have residual abnormalities. A few have severe contractures and crippling deformities. The course of dermatomyositis can be favorably modified by early, vigorous treatment with corticosteroids, and the prognosis in adequately treated children is good.

10.71 SCLERODERMA

Scleroderma ("hard skin"), a chronic inflammatory disturbance of connective tissue, classically involves skin but may also affect the gastrointestinal tract, heart, lung, kidney, and synovium. Cutaneous involvement may occur in focal patches (*morphea*), in a linear distribution (*linear scleroderma*), or in a generalized, symmetric distribution. The last is usually associated with systemic involvement (*progressive systemic sclerosis*) and is the usual adult form. Scleroderma in children usually has a patchy, focal distribution (morphea); systemic involvement is uncommon.

The disease is rare and of obscure origin. It affects girls more frequently than boys and may begin at any time during childhood. There is no familial predisposition.

Histology of affected cutaneous tissues shows increased thickness and density of dermal collagen with perivascular infiltrates of mononuclear cells.

Clinical Manifestations. *Morphea and Linear Scleroderma.* The first signs are patchy lesions of skin and subcutaneous tissues. These often have a linear pattern similar to the distribution of peripheral nerves and may occur primarily on one side of the body. During the early phases involved areas are slightly erythematous and edematous or have an atropic, shiny appearance. The child may complain of pain or a prickly sensation. As the disease progresses, the skin lesions become indurated with violaceous, sometimes elevated borders and pale, waxy-appearing centers. Lesions enlarge peripherally and may coalesce to involve an entire extremity or a large portion of the body. Extensive scarring and fibrosis of the involved area can occur with firm binding of cutaneous tissues to underlying structures ("hide-binding"). This may be severe enough to limit growth of the affected part and produce crippling contractures (Fig. 10–23). Chronically involved areas may be hyperpigmented or depigmented. Active disease may arrest over a period of months to years or may smolder for years. Prognosis for life is good in the absence of systemic involvement.

Progressive Systemic Sclerosis. Cutaneous involvement is symmetrical. It includes hands, feet and distal extremities and

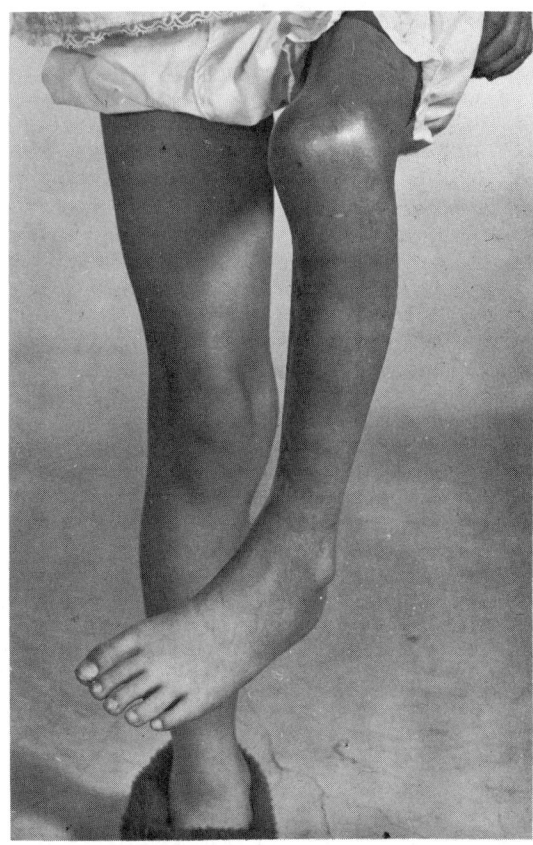

Figure 10–23. Extensive morphea involving the entire left leg, causing scarring, shortening, and flexion contractures. Note the shiny appearance and patches of hyperpigmentation and vitiligo of affected skin.

sometimes the trunk and face as well. Induration, pigmentary changes, and hide-binding of involved cutaneous tissues occur as with focal forms of the disease. Raynaud phenomenon and cutaneous ulcers may be associated. Synovitis, particularly about small hand joints, may mimic rheumatoid arthritis; tenosynovitis and nodules may occur about tendon sheaths. The disease may involve the gastrointestinal tract, heart, lungs, and kidneys. Systemic manifestations, particularly renal, cardiac, and pulmonary, may be fatal. Esophageal dysfunction may result in chronic aspiration pneumonia. Severe hypertension may occur.

Laboratory Manifestations. There are no specific laboratory tests. The sedimentation rate is frequently normal. Rheumatoid factors and antinuclear antibodies may be found in both focal and disseminated forms of the disease. Roentgenography may show dysfunction of esophageal and small bowel motility. Pulmonary function studies, electrocardiograms, and chest roentgenograms may disclose cardiopulmonary involvement. Urinalyses and renal function studies are abnormal in the presence of renal involvement.

Diagnosis. The clinical picture is characteristic in both morphea and progressive systemic sclerosis. The disease may bear some superficial resemblance to *dermatomyositis*, but absence of myositis and the characteristic rash of dermatomyositis should allow differentiation. *Subcutaneous fat necrosis* and *Weber-Christian nonsuppurative panniculitis* may be suggested in morphea, but the course and histology are distinctive. *Scleroderma adultorum*, a self-limited benign induration of subcutaneous tissues, occurs acutely, sometimes following streptococcal infection; subcutaneous tissues of the neck, upper trunk, and arms become indurated, but skin is spared.

Treatment. No specific therapy is known. Many therapeutic agents, including corticosteroids, salicylates, chelating agents, chloroquine, radiation, dimethyl sulfoxide, para-aminobenzoic acid, penicillamine, and anticancer drugs have been tried without clear-cut benefit. Systemic therapy with corticosteroids, penicillamine, or anticancer drugs may be tried for severe systemic disease. Topical corticosteroids have been used for morphea. Excision of local patches of morphea does not arrest the process. Vigorous physical therapy is important early in the course of morphea to prevent or minimize crippling contractures.

RHEUMATIC SYNDROMES OF UNCERTAIN CLASSIFICATION

10.72 MIXED CONNECTIVE TISSUE DISEASE

Mixed connective tissue disease is a syndrome combining features of SLE, rheumatoid arthritis, dermatomyositis, and scleroderma. It is characterized by high serum titers of antibody to ribonucleoprotein (so-called "ENA") and of speckled antinuclear antibody. *Clinical manifestations* include polyarthritis, sclerodermal skin changes, Raynaud phenomenon, fever, cardiac involvement (particularly pericarditis), rashes suggestive of either SLE or dermatomyositis, myositis, esophageal abnormalities, lymphadenopathy and organomegaly, pulmonary disease, and thrombocytopenia. Renal disease occurs in some patients, and neurologic abnormalities and parotitis have also been described. The *diagnosis* is made on recognizing the overlapping clinical symptoms and requires demonstrating serum antibodies to ribonucleoprotein and high titers of speckled antinuclear antibodies.

Initially this syndrome was thought to have a better *prognosis* than SLE and to be readily amenable to corticosteroid therapy. Although corticosteroid therapy does produce symptomatic improvement in many patients, and although life-threatening disease manifestations are perhaps not as common as in SLE, mixed connective tissue disease may be severe. The ultimate prognosis is unknown. The relationships of this syndrome to other rheumatic diseases are also unclear. Appropriate therapy consists of symptomatic treatment with corticosteroids, alertness to possible serious complications such as nephritis, physical therapy, and careful attention to function of the musculoskeletal system.

10.73 FASCIITIS
(Diffuse Fasciitis, Eosinophilic Fasciitis)

This unusual disorder is characterized by diffuse inflammation of fascial tissues. Long-term studies defining the extent and natural history of the disease are unavailable. It may be a variant of scleroderma. Although most patients have been adults, the disorder has occurred in children. Inflammation of fascial tissues occurs in the limbs and trunk; hands, feet, and face are generally spared. The onset may follow periods of heavy physical exertion. Affected tissues are swollen and tender; however, since the overlying skin is not affected, these areas appear puckered. Loss of musculoskeletal function and contractures may result. There has not been involvement of internal organs or Raynaud phenomenon. There are no diagnostic laboratory tests; tests for rheumatoid factors and antinuclear antibodies are generally negative. Some patients have striking eosinophilia (as high as 50%), and increased numbers of eosinophils may be found in affected tissues. Diagnosis is clinical and supported by biopsy evidence of fascial inflammation. Corticosteroids may be helpful, although long-term follow-up studies are not available.

MISCELLANEOUS CONDITIONS ASSOCIATED WITH RHEUMATIC SYMPTOMS OR SIGNS IN CHILDREN

10.74 BENIGN RHEUMATOID NODULES

Rheumatoid nodule-like lesions unassociated with rheumatic disease occasionally occur in children. Single or multiple lesions may be present over various sites, including the pretibial areas, dorsa of the feet, scalp, hands, and elbows; they may also appear over pressure points or after trauma, as do true rheumatoid nodules. Clinically, the nodules are subcutaneous or fixed to deeper tissues and resemble rheumatoid nodules. Histologically, these lesions show central areas of fibrinoid necrosis with surrounding histiocytes and mononuclear cells; they may resemble adult-type rheumatoid nodules or the intracutaneous lesions of granuloma annulare and may be associated with typical granuloma annulare.

The etiology of these nodules is unknown. Affected children are well and have no associated rheumatic complaints. Laboratory tests are normal; tests for rheumatoid factor and antinuclear antibodies are negative. The nodular lesions wax, wane, and may recur, but recurrences generally cease after months or years. This is a benign condition; affected children are not at increased risk for rheumatic disease, and no therapy other than reassurance is required.

The nodules associated with rheumatic disease (rheumatoid arthritis, acute rheumatic fever, scleroderma, SLE) rarely if ever occur as sole manifestations but rather appear with other signs of active rheumatic disease. Rheumatoid nodules in rheumatoid arthritis are generally accompanied by positive tests for rheumatoid factor.

10.75 ERYTHEMA NODOSUM

Erythema nodosum is characterized by the development of painful, indurated, shiny, red, hot, elevated, ovoid nodules 1–3 cm in diameter. They are most frequently distributed symmetrically over the shins (Fig. 10–24 [p. xxv]) but may also occur on the calves, thighs, buttocks, and upper extremities. Fever, malaise, and arthralgia may precede or accompany the rash, and hilar adenopathy may be present on chest roentgenograms. The skin lesions have a characteristic progression: over a period of several days they become protuberant and present a brilliant display of violaceous colors; after 1–2 wk, as induration decreases, a dull purple discoloration predominates and then fades in the manner of a large bruise, leaving a brown residuum. The lesions come in crops, usually over a period of 3–6 wk. The disease them becomes quiescent and rarely recurs. Erythema nodosum is uncommon in children under the age of 6 yr, becoming progressively more frequent up to the 3rd decade of life. Females are affected more frequently than males.

The lesions represent a reaction to a variety of stimuli. The eruption has been induced experimentally in patients with the disease by local injection of a single specific bacterial antigen. Epidemiologically, the disease was previously linked closely to tuberculosis, especially in Europe. In both the United States and Europe streptococcal infections are now more frequently implicated as stimuli. The eruption may also accompany sarcoidosis, histoplasmosis, coccidioidomycosis, and Yersinia infections, or the administration of some drugs, including birth control pills. It may also occur with such diseases as SLE, vasculitis, regional enteritis, and ulcerative colitis.

Search for a precipitating infection, drug, or underlying disease should be instituted. The sedimentation rate is usually elevated and other nonspecific evidences of inflammatory disease, such as acute phase reactants, are found. Suggestive etiologic evidence may include the demonstration of beta-hemolytic streptococci in throat cultures or a rising antistreptolysin O titer; conversion of a previously negative tuberculin, histoplasmin, or coccidioidin skin reaction; roentgenographic evidence of pulmonary tuberculosis or fungus disease; or evidence of an underlying disease such as SLE, inflammatory bowel disease, or sarcoidosis.

Salicylates are usually adequate for symptomatic relief of erythema nodosum. The skin lesions and the constitutional manifestations may respond to corticosteroids, but such therapy is usually not warranted in a self-limited disease and may be contraindicated because of the presence of underlying active infection.

JANE GREEN SCHALLER
RALPH J. WEDGWOOD

10.76 LYME DISEASE

Etiology. Lyme disease, a tick-borne illness, is characterized by a distinctive skin lesion (erythema chronicum migrans), carditis, meningitis, and arthritis and is caused by a spirochete *Borrelia burgdorferi*. These fastidious microorganisms have a world-wide distribution and are transmitted to man by ticks of the genus *Ixodes*. In the United States, three endemic areas are recognized: the coastal areas of the Northeast, Minnesota and Wisconsin in the Midwest, and parts of California, Oregon, Texas, and western Nevada in the West. These areas correspond to the distribution of the vectors, i.e., *I. dammini* in the Northeast and Midwest and *I. pacificus* in the West. Case reports from non-endemic regions in the United States suggest that the insect vector's range is expanding and/or that other hematophagous arthropods (Amblyomma americanum or "Lone Star tick") may be involved in transmission.

Epidemiology. Although a migrating annular lesion, erythema chronicum migrans (ECM), was described in a Swedish patient bitten by the ixodid tick *I. ricinus* in 1909, the initial description of ECM in the United States occurred in 1969. In 1975, investigators reported a number of individuals in Lyme, Connecticut with the entire clinical spectrum, including car-

ditis, arthritis, and meningitis, of what is now termed Lyme disease. The disease also occurs in Europe, where cases tend to be milder than those observed in the United States. A similar microorganism has been recovered from *I. ricinus* ticks, the vector of ECM in Europe, and from skin lesions, blood, joint fluid, and the CSF of infected patients.

Clinical Manifestations. The early cutaneous manifestation, erythema chronicum migrans, is an erythematous macule or papule. Approximately 30% of patients have a history of a tick bite at the site of the initial lesion, which usually within one week (3–32 days) develops into an expanding erythematous annular lesion with central clearing and often reaches a diameter of about 16 cm (3–68 cm). In some patients ECM is less characteristic, with an erythematous indurated center that may become vesicular or necrotic. These asymptomatic lesions may be located anywhere; however, the thigh, groin, and axilla are common sites. Several days after the initial lesion, many patients (50%) develop multiple secondary lesions. These are generally smaller, lack indurated centers, and are not associated with previous tick bites. Secondary lesions are uncommon in European patients. Additional dermatologic findings may develop and include a malar rash, conjunctivitis, and small evanescent red blotches and circles. Except for lethargy and fatigue, which may be constant and incapacitating, initial signs and symptoms are intermittent and include headache, fever, chills, and migrating musculoskeletal pains. Lymphadenopathy meningismus, encephalopathy, splenomegaly, hepatomegaly, and testicular swelling have also been described. During this early phase, non-specific laboratory abnormalities include a high sedimentation rate (50%), an elevated total serum IgM (33%), an increased serum glutamic oxaloacetic transaminase (19%), microscopic hematuria, and proteinuria. Regardless of treatment, these initial signs and symptoms resolve within 3–4 wk; however, dermatologic manifestations often recur.

The late manifestations of Lyme disease occur after a latent period of weeks to months, and may involve the central nervous system (10%), the cardiovascular system (8%), and/or the musculoskeletal system (80%). Symptoms are more severe and more protracted in patients with HLA DR-2. Neurologic abnormalities occur within 4 wk of the initial illness and typically resolve over 3 mo. A triad of symptoms occurs with some regularity—meningitis, cranial neuropathy (including Bell palsy), and peripheral radiculoneuropathy. However, these manifestations may occur alone. Less common neurologic manifestations include chorea, cerebellar ataxia, Guillain-Barré syndrome, pseudotumor cerebri, and demyelinating encephalopathy. Cerebrospinal fluid analysis reveals a mononuclear pleocytosis, a normal glucose level, and a modestly elevated protein level. Neurologic symptoms have long been recognized in patients with ECM by European clinicians, and have been referred to as tick-borne meningopolyneuritis, Bannwarth syndrome, and lymphocytic meningoradiculitis. When tested, these patients have high antibody titers to the responsible *Borrelia*. Cardiac abnormalities occur within 5 wk of the initial illness and include varying degrees of atrioventricular block (first degree, Wenkebach, or complete heart block), myopericarditis, left ventricular dysfunction, and/or cardiomegaly. Cardiac involvement is usually brief (3 days–6 wk) and rarely recurs. Joint manifestations occur within a week to 2 yr after the initial illness. Early symptoms include migratory arthralgias; arthritis begins months after the onset of the illness and typically involves the large joints, especially the knee. However, both large and small joints may be affected, and a minority of patients present with a symmetrical polyarthritis. Arthritis lasts for weeks to months and usually recurs for several years. Synovial fluid analysis finds white cell counts of 500–100,000 mm³, with a predominance of polymorphonuclear leukocytes, usually an elevated protein level, and slightly reduced C3, C4, and total hemolytic complement levels. In approximately 10% of patients, arthritis involving the large joints becomes chronic, with subsequent erosion of cartilage and bone. The risk of chronic arthritis appears related to the presence of B cell alloantigen DR-2. Transplacental transmission of *B. burgdorferi* has been documented and associated with congenital abnormalities, intrauterine death, premature birth, and developmental delay.

Diagnosis and Treatment. Diagnosis depends on recognition of signs and symptoms in a child living in an endemic area with or without a history of tick exposure. Confirmation of the clinical diagnosis requires serologic testing by indirect immunofluorescence or enzyme-linked immunosorbent assays. False positive serologic tests have been reported in patients with other treponemal infections or certain autoantibodies, and false negative tests may be found in the early stages of Lyme disease or following effective treatment with antimicrobial agents. Titers remain elevated for years. ECM and its associated symptoms resolve more rapidly in patients treated with penicillin or tetracycline than in patients receiving erythromycin. Moreover, studies suggest that early treatment with antimicrobial agents, particularly tetracycline, prevents the late complications of Lyme disease. Thus, in older children and adults, tetracycline (40 mg/kg/24 hr by mouth in 4 divided doses, not to exceed 1.0 gram daily) for at least 10 days and up to 20 days if symptoms persist or recur, is the treatment of choice. In younger children penicillin V (250 mg/24 hr in 4 divided doses) for the same duration is a satisfactory alternative regimen. In younger children with penicillin allergy erythromycin (40 mg/kg/24 hr in 4 divided doses) is recommended. High-dose intravenous penicillin therapy is effective for the established arthritis as well as the neurologic abnormalities of Lyme disease.

WILLIAM T. SPECK

10.77 SARCOIDOSIS

Arthritis resembling that of JRA may be a prominent feature of sarcoidosis, a chronic granulomatous disorder of uncertain etiology. One or multiple joints, generally large joints, may be affected. Although the arthritis may be chronic and indolent, joint destruction is rare. See discussion in Sec. 26.3.

10.78 STEVENS-JOHNSON SYNDROME
(Erythema Multiforme Exudativum)

This disorder is characterized by skin and mucous membrane lesions, fever, and systemic prostration.

The disease occurs in children and young adults and affects males more frequently than females. Onset often follows an upper respiratory tract infection. Evidence for an infectious agent, especially herpes virus or mycoplasma, has been inconclusive. Association of the syndrome with ingestion of drugs, including sulfonamides, anticonvulsants, penicillin, and barbiturates, has been observed. The LE phenomenon has been demonstrated in a few patients.

The hallmark of the syndrome is an erythematous papular skin lesion that enlarges by peripheral expansion and usually develops a central vesicle. This eruption may involve most cutaneous surfaces, including the palms and soles, but spares the scalp. Lesions may be scattered or confluent and may become bullous. New lesions appear for 1-2 wk after onset. Vesiculobullous lesions also occur on mucous membranes of the conjunctivae, nares, mouth, anorectal junction, vulvovaginal region, and urethral meatus. Lesions have been described in the larynx, trachea, bronchi, bladder, and gastrointestinal tract.

The rash is often preceded by fever and general malaise. Severe prostration may occur at the height of the syndrome. About one third of the affected patients have pulmonary

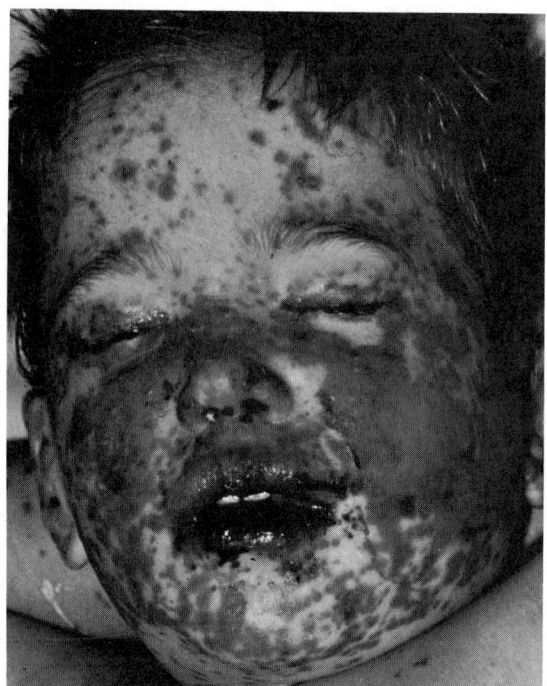

Figure 10–25. Cutaneous, oral, nasal, and conjunctival involvement in severe Stevens-Johnson syndrome.

involvement, with a harsh, hacking cough and patchy changes on the chest roentgenogram. Periarticular swelling has been described. Involvement of cardiovascular and renal systems does not usually occur. As the disease process reaches its peak, the patient presents a striking picture (Fig. 10–25). Stomatitis is particularly distressing; lesions erode, ulcerate, bleed, and crust. Meatal involvement may make urination painful. Conjunctivitis results in photophobia, and purulent conjunctival discharge may be profuse. Corneal ulcerations can occur, resulting in scarring and even blindness.

The mortality may be as high as 10% during the acute phase, particularly in patients with pulmonary involvement. Subsequently, the disease is self-limiting: skin lesions gradually subside without scarring in 1–4 wk; mucous membrane lesions may persist for months. In about 20% of patients the disease recurs, often in association with re-exposure to an offending drug.

During the acute phase symptomatic treatment is important. Fluid requirements are high. Cutaneous hygiene should be maintained to prevent secondary infection. Ophthalmologic consultation should be sought if serious conjunctivitis is present. Prednisone, 1–2 mg/kg/24 hr, is often used in children with serious disease. The efficacy of such therapy is not proved; it should be carefully supervised and is contraindicated whenever there is a possibility of herpetic infection of the eye. Appropriate antibiotic therapy is indicated if there is reasonable suspicion of infection with *Mycoplasma pneumoniae*.

10.79 GOODPASTURE SYNDROME

This combination of pulmonary alveolar hemorrhage and glomerulonephritis is a distinctive clinical entity, although there is some overlap with polyarteritis nodosa and with idiopathic pulmonary hemosiderosis. Young adult males are predominantly affected, but the disease also occurs in children. The cause is unknown. The disease often begins after an acute illness and has been associated with influenza. It has also followed exposure to certain drugs (e.g., penicillamine). Antibodies reactive with glomerular and alveolar basement membranes are involved in the pathogenesis.

The syndrome is characterized clinically by hemoptysis, anemia, and nephritis. Dyspnea, cough, malaise, and fever are often present, and rales and rhonchi may be heard on auscultation of the chest. Chest roentgenograms usually show bilateral flocculent infiltrates spreading from hilus to periphery of the lung fields. Hemosiderin-laden macrophages can be demonstrated in the sputum. Anemia, presumably related to pulmonary hemorrhage, is prominent. Urinalyses reveal varying degrees of proteinuria, hematuria, pyuria, and cylindruria. Azotemia is frequent; progressive renal failure often ensues. Histologically, focal glomerulitis or widespread glomerulonephritis occurs. Intra-alveolar hemorrhages, hemosiderin-laden macrophages, and thickening of alveolar septa are present in the lungs. Generalized vasculitis is not found; patients with concomitant vasculitis are usually considered to have polyarteritis nodosa.

The untreated disease is usually rapidly fatal. Therapy with plasmapheresis, corticosteroids, and anti-cancer drugs is effective in some patients. (Also see Sec. 17.11.)

10.80 FIBROSITIS-FIBROMYALGIA

Fibrositis-fibromyalgia is a poorly defined adult condition that has recently been described in children. Little is known of its physiology or pathology; a relationship to stress has been suggested in adults. There are no abnormal laboratory findings. The clinical manifestations are poorly defined musculoskeletal inflammation. Musculoskeletal pain can be reproduced by soft tissue pressure on a number of so-called trigger points. Fatigue, anxiety, insomnia, and headache frequently occur. This condition is neither progressive nor associated with chronic deformity. Therapy with reassurance, stress management, exercise, and perhaps non-steroidal anti-inflammatory agents may be helpful. The ultimate prognosis is unknown.

10.81 RELAPSING NODULAR NONSUPPURATIVE PANNICULITIS
(Weber-Christian Syndrome)

This rare disorder of unknown cause probably does not represent a single disease. Infection, drug reaction (especially to bromides and iodides), abnormal fat metabolism, and hypersensitivity have all been suggested as etiologic factors. It occurs in association with several rheumatic tissue diseases, with pancreatic disease, and with corticosteroid withdrawal. Adults are predominantly affected, although the syndrome has been reported in all age groups. Females are affected more frequently than males.

Histologically, there are foci of degeneration and inflammation in subcutaneous fat. Mesenteric, perivisceral, and periarticular adipose tissues may be affected; fatty metamorphosis of the liver and reticuloendothelial hyperplasia may occur. Laboratory findings are not specific. Leukopenia and elevated sedimentation rates may be present; rheumatoid factor, LE cells, and cryoglobulins have been observed.

Clinically, the disease is characterized by the appearance of crops of subcutaneous nodules on any part of the body; thighs, abdomen, breasts, and arms are most frequently involved. Nodules vary in size from mm to several cm and may be painful, with redness and warmth of the overlying skin. Nodules regress in days to weeks, usually leaving a pigmented depression. Fever is common, and a variety of rheumatic complaints may occur, including arthritis, arthralgia, and myalgia. Hepatosplenomegaly, abdominal pain, and episcleritis have been reported. Crops of nodules and systemic symptoms generally recur over long periods of time.

Diagnosis of Weber-Christian syndrome is based on the clinical picture and the histologic changes. Differential diagnosis includes erythema induratum, sarcoidosis, and postinjection subcutaneous fat necrosis. Fat necrosis with subcutaneous nodules, arthritis, and visceral involvement can occur as a manifestation of pancreatic disease, presumably from enzymatic action on fat cells.

No specific therapy is known. Symptomatic relief may occur after therapy with corticosteroids, chloroquine, or phenylbutazone. Patients with underlying pancreatic involvement are benefited by treatment of the pancreatic disease.

10.82 RELAPSING POLYCHONDRITIS

Relapsing polychondritis, one of the rarest of the rheumatic syndromes, has been described in few children. It consists of pain, swelling, destruction, and deformation of cartilaginous elements of the ears (both external and internal structures), nose, eyes, joints, laryngotracheobronchial systems, heart, and large blood vessels. Fever, malaise, and myalgia may be associated. Glomerulonephritis has been described. There are no characteristic laboratory tests. Diagnosis rests on the clinical picture and demonstration of cartilaginous inflammation on biopsy. This condition occasionally occurs in patients who have another established rheumatic disease such as vasculitis, rheumatoid arthritis, SLE or Sjögren syndrome. Death may result from cardiac or respiratory involvement. Therapy with corticosteroid and cytotoxic agents has been advocated, but their long-term benefits are unknown.

10.83 SYNDROME OF NEONATAL FEVER, RASH, AND ARTHROPATHY

This condition, characterized by high intermittent fevers, maculopapular rash, and systemic illness beginning in the 1st weeks of life, has been described in about 30 children in the last decade. Other features include meningoencephalitis (with pleocytosis and elevated protein in CSF), progressive mental retardation, chronic iridocyclitis, hepatosplenomegaly, and lymphadenopathy. The typical arthropathy is manifested by swelling, pain, and warmth in one or more joints; joint roentgenograms show periostitis and destruction of the ends of long bones. Patellas are usually enlarged. Affected children appear to have a characteristic facies with prominent foreheads.

Nothing is known of the etiology or pathogenesis of this syndrome. Although described in one set of siblings, it has not been familial in other reported instances. The condition superficially resembles systemic-onset JRA; however, the neonatal onset and the association of meningoencephalopathy, mental retardation, and chronic iridocyclitis as well as the nature of the arthropathy are distinctive. Treatment with non-steroidal agents and physical therapy may assist in musculoskeletal function, but does not slow progression of the disease. Progressive mental retardation and death in the 1st or 2nd decade of life have been noted, although the long-term prognosis is unknown.

10.84 BEHÇET SYNDROME

This disorder is characterized by recurrent oral and genital ulcers and eye inflammation. Arthritis, thrombophlebitis, neurologic abnormalities, skin lesions, fever, and colitis are associated clinical manifestations. It is rare in children, but may occur at any age and is worldwide in distribution.

The etiology is unknown. Pathologically, there is vasculitis of small and medium-sized arteries with cellular infiltration leading to fibrinoid necrosis and narrowing and obliteration of vessel lumens.

The clinical course is highly variable, with recurrent exacerbations and disease-free intervals of uncertain duration. The oral ulcers are usually the first manifestations, develop in almost all patients, persist for days to weeks, then heal without scarring. These painful necrotic ulcers (2–10 mm), surrounded by erythema, may occur singly or in crops over the oral-nasal cavity and upper airway. Genital ulcers occur in most patients and follow a parallel course. Ocular manifestations may involve any structure of the eye and are usually reversible, although they may progress to blindness. Arthritis is common, usually acute, recurrent, asymmetrical, and polyarticular involving large joints. Central nervous system abnormalities, such as meningoencephalitis, cranial nerve palsies, and psychosis, generally occur later in the course of the disease and have a poor prognosis. Skin manifestations are protean and occur in most patients. Laboratory findings are not diagnostic.

There is no effective treatment, although systemic prednisone (40–60 mg/24 hr), other immunosuppressive agents, and locally applied steroids may help some patients.

10.85 SJÖGREN SYNDROME

This chronic inflammatory, autoimmune disease, rare in children, is characterized by dry eyes (keratoconjunctivitis sicca, xerophthalmia), dry mouth (xerostomia), and associated connective tissue disorders. The salivary and lacrimal glands are progressively destroyed by infiltrating lymphocytes and plasma cells; a similar process may reduce secretions in the respiratory tract, vagina, and skin as well as the salivary and lacrimal glands.

Clinical manifestations include photophobia, burning and itching eyes, and blurred vision; painless unilateral or bilateral enlargement of parotid glands, decreased taste, dental caries, dysphagia, fissured tongue and angular cheilitis; decreased smell and epistaxis; and hoarseness, recurrent bronchitis, pneumonia, and chronic otitis. Rheumatoid arthritis and systemic lupus erythematosus are often associated collagen vascular diseases. A lymphoproliferative form may also occur. Diagnosis is based on clinical features supported by lip or glandular biopsy demonstrating lymphocytic infiltration; hypergammaglobulinemia, cryoglobulinemia, autoantibodies to nucleoprotein antigens (SS-B[La]), and immune complexes.

Treatment is symptomatic, with artificial tears, lozenges, and fluids to limit the damaging effects of decreased secretions. Corticosteroids are indicated only for severe functional disorders and life-threatening complications.

10.86 NON-RHEUMATIC CONDITIONS MIMICKING RHEUMATIC DISEASES OF CHILDHOOD

A large number of "non-rheumatic" conditions that can cause musculoskeletal complaints in children, with or without accompanying signs, must be considered in the differential diagnosis of childhood rheumatic diseases (Table 10–27).

Bacterial infections of bones and joints can cause pain and swelling about one or more joints, generally with accompanying fever and other systemic complaints (Sec. 11.14 and 11.15). Diagnosis may result from appropriate cultures, skin tests, and imaging techniques. *Viral* (Sec. 11.62) and *mycoplasmal* (Sec. 11.60) *infections* may be associated with transient arthritis which should not be confused with chronic rheumatic disease. *Discitis* (Sec. 23.5) or inflammation of the intravertebral discs and endplates of vertebral bodies may be confused with arthritis, although the pain in discitis is characteristically spinal; roentgenograms or bone scans may be diagnostic.

A number of childhood *malignancies* (Sec. 16.5 and 16.17–

16.18) can result in musculoskeletal involvement resembling arthritis, generally through a mechanism of infiltration of malignant cells about the joint capsules and periosteum or destruction of bone. Pain in affected joints is often severe and blood studies may reveal abnormal white blood cells (leukopenia or abnormal cellular forms), thrombocytopenia, anemia, or hyperuricemia. Bone roentgenograms may show metaphyseal rarefaction, periostitis, or lytic lesions. Suspicion of malignancy in a child with "arthritis" demands appropriate investigations, with oncologic consultation and biopsy of the bone marrow or other appropriate tissues.

Costochondral disease (*costochondritis*) is a relatively common disorder characterized by pain localized to the costosternal or costochondrial cartilaginous junctions. Although the pain may be of acute onset, sharp, darting, and of short duration, it usually evolves gradually as a dull aching pain lasting hours to days. It may be associated with a feeling of tightness due to muscle spasm and is generally not exacerbated by respiratory or other mild movements. There is often localized tenderness to palpation of one or more costal cartilages and a history of trauma or unaccustomed physical effort. The combination of pain, tenderness, swelling, and sometimes redness is referred to as *Tietze syndrome*. Discomfort usually persists

Table 10–27. Conditions Other Than Rheumatic Diseases Associated with Arthritis in Children

Infectious diseases
  Pyogenic arthritis
  Tuberculous arthritis
  Osteomyelitis with sympathetic joint effusion
  Virus-related arthritis
  Reactive arthritis
  Lyme Disease
  Other (e.g., mycoplasma arthritis)

Neoplastic diseases
  Leukemia
  Neuroblastoma
  Malignant histiocytosis
  Lymphoma, Hodgkin disease, reticulum cell sarcoma
  Rhabdomyosarcoma
  Osteogenic sarcoma
  Other primary bone tumors

"Orthopedic" conditions (noninflammatory conditions of bones and joints)
  Avascular necrosis syndromes (Legg-Calvé-Perthes disease, Kohler disease, Osgood-Schlatter disease, etc.)
  Toxic synovitis of the hip
  Slipped capital femoral epiphysis
  Trauma (child abuse fractures; joint, ligamentous, and muscle injuries, etc.)
  Chondromalacia patellae
  Congenital anomalies and genetically determined abnormalities of musculoskeletal system (e.g., muscular dystrophies, congenital subluxation of the hips, other congenital abnormalities of bones, joints, connective tissues, etc.)
  Tenosynovitis
  Discitis

Limb sympathetic dystrophy

Limb pains of childhood (growing pains)*

Hysteria, conversion reactions*

Miscellaneous conditions (sickle cell anemia, hemophilia, immunodeficiency-related arthritis, sarcoidosis, hypertrophic osteoarthropathy)

*These conditions may have associated symptoms suggesting arthritis; they do not produce or represent joint disease.

for only a few days or responds to mild analgesia and avoidance of strenuous activity. Severe episodes of Tietze syndrome may be relieved by corticosteroids or injection of procaine.

A number of *non-inflammatory conditions* can also mimic rheumatic diseases in children. Various orthopedic conditions such as bone fractures, soft tissue injuries, avascular necrosis syndromes, and slipped capital femoral epiphysis may mimic arthritis; roentgenograms or bone scans are generally diagnostic. In the *reflex sympathetic dystrophy syndrome* a limb or part of a limb is immobilized by severe pain; cutaneous hypersensitivity, osteoporosis, and signs of autonomic nervous dysfunction are characteristic. Successful therapy involves remobilization of the affected part. A number of congenital or genetically determined conditions can superficially resemble rheumatic diseases. For example, congenital myositis ossificans (fibrodysplasia ossificans congenita) is at times confused with dermatomyositis or scleroderma, and conditions such as *carpal-tarsal osteolysis* or *trichorhinophalangeal dysplasia* may suggest JRA. A positive family genetic history, the presence of associated dysmorphic features (for example, digital anomalies in congenital myositis ossificans or characteristic facial anomalies in trichorhinophalangeal dysplasia), or roentgenographic appearance of affected bones and joints (for example, lysis of the carpal and tarsal bones in carpal-tarsal osteolysis) may distinguish these entities (Sec 6.33).

Many other miscellaneous conditions may mimic childhood rheumatic diseases. Noteworthy are the hand-foot syndrome of sickle cell anemia and the arthropathy of hemophilia. In general, such conditions can be differentiated on the basis of historical or physical findings that do not appear to be entirely consistent with any of the rheumatic diseases.

JANE GREEN SCHALLER
RALPH J. WEDGWOOD

Patient Education

Arthritis in children. Arthritis Foundation, 3400 Peachtree Road NE, Atlanta, GA 30326. (Obtainable from the Arthritis Foundation or from its local chapter offices.)

Rodnan GP (ed): Primer on the Rheumatic Diseases. 8th ed, 1983. (Available in bound form from the Arthritis Foundation.)

General

Ansell BM (ed): Rheumatic Disorders in Childhood. Clin Rheum Dis 2(2), 1976.

Jacobs C: Pediatric Rheumatology for the Practitioner. New York, Springer Verlag, 1982.

Kelley WN, Harris ED, Ruddy S, et al (eds): Textbook of Rheumatology. 2nd ed. Philadelphia, WB Saunders, 1985.

McCarty DJ (ed): Arthritis and Allied Conditions: A Textbook of Rheumatology. 10th ed. Philadelphia, Lea & Febiger, 1984.

Juvenile Rheumatoid Arthritis

Ansell BM, Bywaters EGL: Diagnosis of "probable" Still's disease and its outcome. Ann Rheum Dis 21:253, 1967.

Bywaters EGL: Heberden Oration, 1966. Categorization in medicine: A survey of Still's disease. Ann Rheum Dis 26:185, 1967.

Laaksonen AL: A prognostic study of juvenile rheumatoid arthritis. Analysis of 544 cases. Acta Paediatr Scand (Suppl) 166:1, 1966.

Nepom BS, Nepom GT, Mickelson E, et al: Specific HLA-DR4 associated histocompatibility molecules characterize patients with seropositive juvenile rheumatoid arthritis. J Clin Invest 74:287, 1984.

Schaller JG: Juvenile rheumatoid arthritis. Pediatr Rev 2:163, 1980.

Schaller JG, Johnson GD, Holborow EJ, et al: The association of antinuclear antibodies with the chronic iridocyclitis of juvenile arthritis (Still's disease). Arthritis Rheum 17:409, 1974.

Schaller JG, Ochs HD, Thomas ED, et al: Histocompatibility antigens in childhood-onset arthritis. J Pediatr 88:926, 1976.

Schaller J, Wedgwood RJ: Is juvenile rheumatoid arthritis a single disease? A review. Pediatrics 50:940, 1972.

Silverman ED, Miller JJ, Bernstein B, et al: Consumption coagulopathy associated with systemic juvenile rheumatoid arthritis. J Pediatr 103:872, 1983.

Still GF: On a form of chronic joint disease in children. Med Chir 80:47, 1937. (Reprinted in Arch Dis Child 16:156, 1941.)

Ankylosing Spondylitis

Ebringer A, Shipley M (eds): Pathogenesis of HLA-B27 associated diseases. Br J Rheum 22 (Suppl 2), 1983.

Ladd JR, Cassidy JT, Martel W: Juvenile ankylosing spondylitis. Arthritis Rheum 14:579, 1971.

Schaller J, Bitnun S, Wedgwood RJ: Ankylosing spondylitis with childhood onset. J Pediatr 74:505, 1969.

Wilkinson M, Bywaters EGL: Clinical features and course of ankylosing spondylitis; as seen in a follow-up of 222 hospital referred cases. Ann Rheum Dis 17:209, 1958.

Spondyloarthropathies

Aho K, Ahvonen P, Lassus A, et al: HL-A 27 in reactive arthritis. A study of *Yersinia* arthritis and Reiter's disease. Arthritis Rheum 17:521, 1974.

Calin A, Marder A, Marks S, et al: Familial aggregation of Reiter's syndrome and AS. J Rheum 11:672, 1984.

Carroll WL, Balistreri WF, Brilli R, et al: Spectrum of Salmonella-associated arthritis. Pediatrics 68:717, 1981.

Jacobs JC, Berdon WE, Johnston AD: HLA B27–associated spondyloarthritis and enteropathy in childhood: Clinical, pathologic and radiographic observations in 58 patients. J Pediatr 100:521, 1982.

Keat A: Reiter's syndrome and reactive arthritis in perspective. N Engl J Med 309:1606, 1983.

Moll JM: Evolution of the psoriatic arthritis concept and its relationship to the spondyloarthritides. Clinical Rheum 1:157, 1982.

Russell AS: Reiter's syndrome in children following infection with *Yersinia enterocolitica* and *Shigella.* Arthritis Rheum (Suppl) 20:471, 1977.

Shore A, Ansell BM: Juvenile psoriatic arthritis—an analysis of 60 cases. J Pediatr 100:529, 1982.

Singsen BH, Bernstein BH, Koster-King KG, et al: Reiter's syndrome in childhood. Arthritis Rheum (Suppl) 20:402, 1977.

Systemic Lupus Erythematosus

Cook CD, Wedgwood RJ, Craig JM, et al: Systemic lupus erythematosus. Description of 37 cases in children and a discussion of endocrine therapy in 32 of the cases. Pediatrics 26:570, 1960.

Decker JL: The management of systemic lupus erythematosus. Arthritis Rheum 25: 891, 1982.

Estes D, Christian CL: The natural history of systemic lupus erythematosus by prospective analysis. Medicine 50:85, 1971.

Fish AJ, Blau EB, Westberg NG, et al: Systemic lupus erythematosus within the first two decades of life. Am J Med 62:99, 1977.

Jacobs JC: Systemic lupus erythematosus in childhood: Report of 35 cases, with discussion of seven apparently induced by anticonvulsant medication and of prognosis and treatment. Pediatrics 32:257, 1963.

Kukla LG, Reddy C, Silkalns G, et al: Systemic lupus erythematosus presenting as chorea. Arch Dis Child 53:345, 1978.

Lee HS, Mujais SK, Kasinath BS: Course of renal pathology in patients with systemic lupus erythematosus. Am J Med 77:612, 1984.

Lehman TJA, Hanson V, Singsen BH, et al: Serum complement abnormalities in ANA positive relatives of children with SLE. Arthritis Rheum 22:954, 1979.

Nepom BS, Schaller JG: Childhood systemic lupus erythematosus. Prog Clin Rheum 1:33, 1984.

Platt J, Burke B, Michael AF: Systemic lupus erythematosus in the first two decades of life. Am J Kid Dis 2:212, 1982.

Schur PH, Sandson J: Immunologic factors and clinical activity in systemic lupus erythematosus. N Engl J Med 278:533, 1968.

Singsen BH, Bernstein BH, King KK, et al: Correlations between changes in disease activity and the serum complement levels. J Pediatr 89:358, 1976.

Singsen BH, Fishman L, Hanson V: Antinuclear antibodies and lupus-like syndromes in children receiving anticonvulsants. Pediatrics 57:529, 1976.

Steinberg AD: Recent advances on the mechanisms and genetic aspects of systemic lupus erythematosus. Adv Nephrol 14:305, 1985.

Tan EM, Cohen AS, Fries JF, et al: The 1982 revised criteria for the classification of systemic lupus erythematosus. Arthritis Rheum 25:1271, 1982.

Wallace C, Schaller JG, Emery H, et al: Prospective study of childhood systemic lupus erythematosus. Arthritis Rheum 21:599, 1978.

Wallace C, Striker G, Schaller JG, et al: Renal history and subsequent course in childhood systemic lupus erythematosus. Arthritis Rheum 22:669, 1979.

Lupus Phenomena in the Newborn Period

Callen JP, Fowler JF, Kulick KB, et al: Neonatal lupus erythematosus occurring in one paternal twin. Arthritis Rheum 28:271, 1985.

Esscher E, Scott JS: Congenital heart block and maternal systemic lupus erythematosus. Br Med J 1:1235, 1979.

Jackson R, Gulliver M: Neonatal lupus erythematosus progressing into systemic lupus erythematosus: a 15 year follow-up. Br J Dermatol 101:81, 1979.

Lee LA, Bias WB, Arnett FC: Immunogenetics of the neonatal lupus syndrome. Ann Intern Med 99:592, 1983.

Lumpkin LR, Hall J, Hogan JD, et al: Neonatal lupus erythematosus: a report of 3 cases associated with anti-Ro/SS-A antibodies. Arch Dermatol 121:377, 1985.

Reed BR, Lee LA, Harmon C, et al: Autoantibodies to SSA/Ro in infants with congenital heart block. J Pediatr 103:889, 1983.

Schönlein-Henoch Vasculitis

Allen DM, Diamond LK, Howell DA: Anaphylactoid purpura in children (Schönlein-Henoch syndrome): Review with a follow-up of the renal complications. Am J Dis Child 99:833, 1960.

Austin HA, Balow JE: Henoch-Schönlein nephritis: Prognostic features and the challenge of therapy. Am J Kidney Dis 2:512, 1983.

Courahan R, Winterborn MH, White RHR, et al: Prognosis of Henoch-Schönlein nephritis in children. Brit Med J 2:11, 1977.

Levy M, Broyer M, Arsan A, et al: Anaphylactoid purpura nephritis in childhood: natural history and immunopathology. Adv Nephrol 6:183, 1976.

Meadow SR, Glasgow EF, White RHR, et al: Schönlein-Henoch nephritis. Q J Med 41:241, 1972.

Meadow SR, Scott DG: Berger disease: Henoch-Schönlein syndrome without the rash. J Pediatr 106:27, 1985.

Vernier RL, Worthen HG, Peterson RD, et al: Anaphylactoid purpura. Pathology of the skin and kidney and frequency of streptococcal infection. Pediatrics 27:181, 1961.

Polyarteritis Nodosa

Fager DB, Bigler JA, Simonds JP: Polyarteritis nodosa in infancy and childhood. J Pediatr 39:65, 1951.

Frohnert PP, Sheps SG: Long-term follow-up study of periarteritis nodosa. Am J Med 43:8, 1967.

Gocke DJ, Hsu K, Morgan C, et al: Vasculitis in association with Australia antigen. J Exp Med 134:330s, 1971.

Ronco P, Verroust P, Mignon F, et al: Immunopathological studies of PAN and Wegener's granulomatosis: A report of 43 patients with 51 renal biopsies. Q J Med 52:212, 1983.

Rose GA, Spencer H: Polyarteritis nodosa. Q J Med 26:43, 1957.

Infantile Polyarteritis Nodosa

Munro-Faure H: Necrotizing arteritis of the coronary vessels in infancy. Case report and review of the literature. Pediatrics 23:914, 1959.

Roberts FB, Fetterman GH: Polyarteritis nodosa in infancy. J Pediatr 63:519, 1963.

Kawasaki Disease

Burns JC, Glode MP, Clarke SH: Coagulopathy and platelet activation in Kawasaki syndrome: Identification of patients at increased risk for coronary artery aneurysms. J Pediatr 105:206, 1984.

Dean AG, Melish ME, Hicks R, et al: An epidemic of Kawasaki syndrome in Hawaii. J Pediatr 100:552, 1982.

Furusho K, Kamiya T, Nakano H, et al: High-dose intravenous gammaglobulin for Kawasaki disease. Lancet 2:1056, 1984.

Kawasaki T, Kosaki F, Okawa S, et al: A new infantile acute febrile mucocutaneous lymph node syndrome (MLNS) prevailing in Japan. Pediatrics 54:271, 1974.

Koren G, Rose V, Levi S, et al: Probable efficacy of high-dose salicylates in reducing coronary involvement in Kawasaki disease. JAMA 254:767, 1985.

Landing GH, Larson EJ: Are infantile periarteritis nodosa with coronary artery involvement and fatal mucocutaneous lymph node syndrome the same? Comparison of 20 patients from North America with patients from Hawaii and Japan. Pediatrics 59:651, 1977.

Leads from the MMWR: Multiple outbreaks of Kawasaki syndrome—United States. JAMA 253:957, 1985.

Meade RH, Brandt L: Manifestations of Kawasaki disease in New England. J Pediatr 100:558, 1982.

Newburger JW, Takahashi M, Burns JC, et al: The treatment of Kawasaki syndrome with intravenous gamma globulin. N Engl J Med 315:342, 1986.

Terai M, Ogata M, Sugimoto K: Coronary arterial thrombi in Kawasaki disease. J Pediatr 106:76, 1985.

Wegener Granulomatosis

Fauci AS, Haynes BF, Katz P, et al: Wegener's granulomatosis: prospective clinical and therapeutic experience with 85 patients for 21 years. Ann Intern Med 98:76, 1983.

Hall SL, Miller LC, Duggan EC: Wegener's granulomatosis in pediatric patients. J Pediatr 106:739, 1984.

Orlowski JP, Clough JD, Dyment PG: Wegener's granulomatosis in the pediatric age group. Pediatrics 61:83, 1978.

Takayasu Arteritis

Danaraj TJ, Wong HO, Thomas MA: Primary arteritis of the aorta causing renal artery stenosis and hypertension. Br Heart J 25:153, 1963.

Lee KS, Sohn KY, Hong CY, et al: Primary arteritis (pulseless disease) in Korean children. Acta Paediatr Scand 56:526, 1967.

Nakao K, Ideka M, Kimata SI, et al: Takayasu's arteritis. Clinical report of 84 cases and immunological studies of 7 cases. Circulation 35:1141, 1967.

Dermatomyositis

Banker BQ, Victor M: Dermatomyositis (systemic angiopathy of childhood). Medicine 45:261, 1966.

Bowyer SL, Blane CE, Sullivan DB, et al: Childhood dermatomyositis: Factors predicting functional outcome and development of dystrophic calcification. J Pediatr 103:882, 1983.

Crowe WE, Bove KE, Levinson JE: Clinical and pathogenetic implications of histopathology in childhood polydermatomyositis. Arthritis Rheum 25:126, 1982.

Pachman LM, Cooke W: Juvenile dermatomyositis: a clinical and immunologic study. J Pediatr 96:226, 1980.

Spencer-Green G, Crowe WE, Levinson JE: Nailfold capillary abnormalities and clinical outcome in childhood dermatomyositis. Arthritis Rheum 25:954, 1982.

Sullivan DB, Cassidy JT, Petty RE, et al: Prognosis in childhood dermatomyositis. J Pediatr 80:555, 1972.

Ziff M, Johnson RL: Polymyositis and cell-mediated immunity. N Engl J Med 288:465, 1973.

Scleroderma: Morphea and Progressive Systemic Sclerosis

Bradford WO, Cook CD, Vawter GF, et al: Scleroderma of childhood. J Pediatr 68:391, 1966.

Cassidy JT, Sullivan DB, Dabich L, et al: Scleroderma in children. Arthritis Rheum 20:351, 1977.

Chazen EM, Cook CD, Cohen J: Focal scleroderma. J Pediatr 60:385, 1962.

Chen Z-Y, Silver RM, Ainsworth SK, et al: Association between fluorescent antinuclear antibodies, capillary patterns and clinical features in scleroderma spectrum disorders. Am J Med 77:812, 1984.

Jaffe MO, Winkelmann RK: Generalized scleroderma in children. Arch Dermatol 83:402, 1961.

Steen VD, Medsgar TA, Rodnan GP: D-Penicillamine therapy in progressive systemic sclerosis (scleroderma). Ann Intern Med 97:652, 1982.

Suarez-Almazor ME, Catoggio LJ, Maldono-Cocco JA: Juvenile progressive systemic sclerosis: Clinical and serologic findings. Arthritis Rheum 28:699, 1985.

Mixed Connective Tissue Disease

Nimelstein HS, Brody S, McShane D, et al: Mixed connective tissue disease: a subsequent evaluation of the original 25 patients. Medicine 59:239, 1980.

Oetgen WJ, Boice JA, Lawless OJ: Mixed connective tissue disease in children and adolescents. Pediatrics 67:333, 1981.

Singsen BH, Bernstein BH, Komreich HK, et al: Mixed connective tissue disease in childhood. J Pediatr 90:893, 1977.

Singsen BH, Swanson VL, Bernstein BH, et al: A histologic evaluation of mixed connective tissue disease in childhood. Am J Med 68:710, 1980.

Fasciitis

Britt WJ, Duray PH, Dahl MV, et al: Diffuse fasciitis with eosinophilia: A steroid-responsive variant of scleroderma. J Pediatr 97:432, 1980.

Shulman L: Diffuse fasciitis with eosinophilia: A new syndrome. Arthritis Rheum 20:S205, 1977.

Benign Rheumatoid Nodules

Altman RS, Caffrey PR: Isolated subcutaneous rheumatic nodules. Pediatrics 34:869, 1964.

Burrington JD: "Pseudorheumatoid" nodules in children. Report of 10 cases. Pediatrics 45:473, 1970.

Mesara BW, Brody Gl, Oberman HA: "Pseudorheumatoid" subcutaneous nodules. Am J Clin Pathol 45:684, 1966.

Simons FER, Schaller JG: Benign rheumatoid nodules. Pediatrics 56:29, 1975.

Erythema Nodosum

A Group of Pediatricians: Aetiology of erythema nodosum in children. Lancet 2:14, 1961.

Blomgren SE: Erythema nodosum. Semin Arth Rheum 4:1, 1974.

Doxiadis SA. Erythema nodosum in children. Medicine 30:283, 1951.

Kirby JF, Kraft GH: Oral contraceptives and erythema nodosum. Obstet Gynecol 40:409, 1972.

Weinstein L: Erythema nodosum. Disease-A-Month. Chicago, Year Book Medical Publishers, June, 1969, p 1.

Lyme Disease

Schmid GP: The global distribution of Lyme disease. Rev Infect Dis 7:41, 1985.

Steere AC, Green J, Schoen RT, et al: Successful parenteral penicillin therapy of established Lyme arthritis. N Engl J Med 312:869, 1985.

Steere AC, Grodzick RL, Kornblatt AN, et al: The spirochetal etiology of Lyme disease. N Engl J Med 308:733, 1983.

Steere AC, Hutchinson GJ, Rahn DW, et al: Treatment of the early manifestations of Lyme disease. Ann Intern Med 99:22, 1983.

Steere AC, Malawista SE, Snydman DR, et al: Lyme arthritis: An epidemic of oligoarticular arthritis in children and adults in 3 Connecticut communities. Arthritis Rheum 20:7, 1977.

Stevens-Johnson Syndrome (Erythema Multiforme Exudativum)

Ashby DW, Lazar T: Erythema multiforme exudativum major. Lancet 1:1091, 1951.
Foy HM, Kenney GE, Koler J: *Mycoplasma pneumoniae* in Stevens-Johnson syndrome. Lancet 2:550, 1966.
Stevens AM, Johnson FC: A new eruptive fever associated with stomatitis and ophthalmia. Am J Dis Child 24:526, 1922.

Goodpasture Syndrome

Levin M, Rigden SPA, Pincott JR, et al: Goodpasture's syndrome: Treatment with plasmapheresis, immunosuppression and anticoagulation. Arch Dis Child 58:697, 1983.
McCombs RP: Diseases due to immunologic reactions in the lungs. N Engl J Med 286:1186, 1972.

Fibrositis-Fibromyalgia Syndromes

Yunus MD, Masi AT: Juvenile primary fibromyalgia syndrome: a clinical study of 33 patients and matched controls. Arthritis Rheum 28:738, 1985.

Relapsing Nodular Nonsuppurative Panniculitis

Case Records of the Massachusetts General Hospital: Case 17-1982. N Engl J Med 306:1035, 1982.
Sanford HN, Eubank DF, Stenn F: Chronic panniculitis with leukopenia (Weber-Christian syndrome). Am J Dis Child 83:156, 1952.
Winkelmann RK: Panniculitis in connective tissue disease. Arch Dermatol 119:336, 1983.

Relapsing Polychondritis

McAdam LP, O'Hanlan MA, Bluestone R, et al: Relapsing polychondritis: Prospective study of 23 patients and a review of the literature. Medicine 555:193, 1976.

Syndrome of Neonatal Fever, Rash and Arthropathy

Prieur AM, Griscelli C: Arthropathy with rash, chronic meningitis, eye lesions and mental retardation. J Pediatr 99:79, 1981.

Behçet Syndrome

Ammann AJ, Johnson A, Fyfe GA, et al: Behçet syndrome. J Pediatr 107:41, 1985.

10.87 RHEUMATIC FEVER

Rheumatic fever is a systemic disease involving more frequently the joints and the heart and less frequently the central nervous system, skin, and subcutaneous tissues. It has a tendency to recur; both initial and recurrent attacks are nonsuppurative complications of group A streptococcal upper respiratory infections. Although rheumatic fever is now less common in developed countries, the disease has not been completely eradicated and potentially is always serious because it may lead to permanent cardiac damage (rheumatic heart disease). In developing countries this disease remains a major health problem.

History. Rheumatic fever emerged as a separate entity in the 17th century under the name of "acute articular rheumatism." Although deformities of heart valves were noted frequently at autopsies, it was not until 1836 that the first clinical description of heart disease in patients with rheumatic fever was published by Bouilland. In 1931 the streptococcal etiology was proved by bacteriologic and epidemiologic studies; in 1939 Coburn and Moore showed that recurrences of rheumatic fever could be prevented by continual antistreptococcal prophylaxis; and a decade later Denny and Wannamaker demonstrated that adequate treatment of streptococcal pharyngitis with penicillin could prevent first rheumatic attacks.

Etiology and Epidemiology. Group A streptococcal infections of the upper respiratory tract are a prerequisite for the development of initial and recurrent attacks of rheumatic fever. Streptococcal skin infections lead to acute glomerulonephritis but rarely, if ever, to acute rheumatic fever; such infections are caused by group A serotypes that do not generally cause clinical pharyngitis. Also, the ASO response is often feeble following skin infections, presumably because skin lipids inhibit streptolysin O. However, it is not clear whether the site of infection is critical because of these differences or whether anatomic or other factors play a role.

Not all rheumatic fever patients have a history of a preceding upper respiratory infection, and not always are streptococci found on throat culture at the time of acute rheumatic fever, since the organisms often disappear from the pharynx during the 2–5 wk *latent* period between the upper respiratory infection and the onset of rheumatic fever. However, an elevated streptococcal antibody titer can be found in virtually all patients during the acute stage.

The rheumatic fever attack rate varies from 0.3% or less following sporadic streptococcal infections in the general population to approximately 3% documented during epidemics of untreated severe exudative pharyngitis. This suggests a relationship between the severity of the pharyngeal infection and the attack rate, although subclinical infections may also precede rheumatic fever.

Rheumatic fever occurs at all ages except infancy, but incidence peaks between 5–15 yr, a period when streptococcal infections are most frequent. In the United States rheumatic fever is seen in late winter and early spring, when streptococcal respiratory infections are most common. The disease occurs with about equal frequency in both sexes, and with no significant racial proclivity. However, a genetic factor may be involved since the illness runs in families and monozygotic twins have a higher concordance rate for rheumatic fever than dizygotic twins. Efforts to find a genetic marker that correlates with susceptibility, however, have thus far failed.

Environmental factors that promote the transmission of upper respiratory infections may account for the familial incidence of the disease. Rheumatic fever occurs in populations living in overcrowded conditions, a factor also promoting the spread of streptococcal infection. The incidence of rheumatic fever is higher among the poor. Improvement of socioeconomic conditions was associated with a decline in the incidence of rheumatic fever prior to the introduction of antibiotics. However, the acceleration of decline since 1945 is due specifically to earlier case detection, prevention of recurrences, and antibiotic treatment of upper respiratory infections. The annual incidence in the United States is now less than 1/100,000 childhood population.

Rheumatic fever occurs in all parts of the world, even in tropical countries where it was once thought to be rare. In contrast to economically advanced countries, many developing countries show rheumatic fever as the etiology in 30–40% of all heart disease and itself a major cause of morbidity and mortality. The recent increase of rheumatic fever in these countries is probably due to overcrowding that has come with industrialization and the migration from rural areas to urban slums, as well as the inadequacy of medical care.

Pathogenesis. Although the streptococcal etiology of rheumatic fever is established, how these organisms in the pharynx cause the varied, multisystemic manifestations of rheumatic fever is unknown. During the course of the disease streptococci cannot be found anywhere except in the upper respiratory tract. These organisms exude a large number of toxins and enzymes (extracellular products) which diffuse out from the site of infection, and some, such as streptolysin, are cardiotoxic in animals. However, none of these has been shown to have a direct toxic action in humans. Since many of the extracellular substances are antigenic and provoke an antibody response, one objection to the toxin theory is that any deleterious effect of these substances would be neutralized by circulating antibodies. However, in support of the theory it has been hypothesized that one of the extracellular products, streptolysin O, may exist as an antigen-antibody complex that subsequently dissociates, allowing streptolysin O to exert its toxic effect.

A more widely held theory regards rheumatic fever as an autoimmune disease. Several streptococcal antigens cross-react with human tissue antigens, and cross-reactive ("anti-heart") antibodies have been found in rheumatic fever patients. According to this hypothesis, streptococcal antigens, immunologically similar to human tissue antigens, may elicit antibodies capable of reacting not only with microbial products but also with the host's antigens. However, anti-heart antibodies have been found in individuals who do not develop rheumatic fever. Furthermore, immunologic cross-reactions between bacterial components and human tissues are a common biologic phenomenon, and whether they are the cause or the effect of tissue injury remains uncertain. Autoimmunity remains an attractive hypothesis but is by no means proven.

Pathology. During the acute stage of rheumatic fever, there is an exudative inflammatory reaction in the connective tissues of the heart, joints, and skin characterized by edema of the ground substance and by a cellular infiltration of lymphocytes and plasma cells. The inflammatory process may involve all segments of the heart. Within the myocardium there is cellular infiltrate in the interstitial tissues and damage to muscle cells. The valve leaflets are edematous and infiltrated mainly with lymphocytes. The mitral valve is far more frequently involved than any of the others. The serous surface of the pericardium is covered with a fibrinous exudate. On gross inspection the heart is dilated.

In joints there is swelling of the articular and periarticular structures with infiltration of the synovial membrane and serous effusion into the joint space. However, there is never erosion of joint surfaces or formation of pannus.

The changes seen during the acute stage are not diagnostic for rheumatic fever. This stage lasts for 2–3 wk and is followed by a proliferative phase that is essentially limited to the myocardium and endocardium. During this phase there is a perivascular aggregation of large, multinucleated cells arranged around an avascular core of fibrinoid material. This lesion is the myocardial *Aschoff body*, the pathognomonic lesion of rheumatic fever. Subsequently, fibrotic scarring occurs in the vicinity of Aschoff nodules. During the proliferative phase rheumatic vegetations made up of masses of eosinophilic material appear along the edge of the valves. These verrucous lesions, becoming progressively fibrotic, results in scarred, thickened valve cusps.

The histologic findings in the central nervous system are not characteristic of rheumatic fever, nor can they be correlated with the clinical findings. There is cellular degeneration and hyalinization of small blood vessels scattered throughout the cortex, cerebellum, and basal ganglia. No site is consistently involved.

Subcutaneous nodules contain a central area of fibrinoid necrotic material surrounded by fibroblasts and occasional lymphocytes. Their structure resembles the Aschoff body.

Clinical Manifestations. The clinical findings vary greatly and are determined by the site of involvement, the severity of the attack, and the stage at which the patient is first examined. The onset is usually acute when arthritis is the presenting manifestation and more gradual when carditis or chorea is the initial clinical feature.

Joint symptoms are the most common presenting complaint, occurring in about 75% of patients during the acute stage of rheumatic fever. The severity ranges from pain in a joint without objective findings, *arthralgia*, to frank *arthritis* with

swelling, redness, and heat. In rheumatic fever more than in any other joint disease, the pain is often disproportionate to the objective findings. Knees, ankles, elbows, and wrists are commonly affected, less often the hips, and rarely the small joints of hands and feet. Successive rather than concurrent involvement of joints results in the characteristic picture of *migratory* polyarthralgia or polyarthritis. If left untreated, each joint is inflamed for only a few days, and all joint symptoms usually disappear spontaneously in 3–4 wk, leaving no permanent deformities.

Carditis is the most serious manifestation of rheumatic fever because it can be fatal during the acute stage or cause permanent valvular damage. Carditis occurs in 40–50% in initial attacks. The highest incidence occurs in young children, but overall carditis is less frequent and less severe in the United States than it has been in the past.

The clinical picture is variable. Usually, rheumatic fever is heralded by fever and joint symptoms, and cardiac involvement is found on initial examination. At times, the cardiac findings are normal or equivocal at onset and become apparent after several days, or at most within 1–2 wk. Rarely is there a long delay in the appearance of carditis in acute onset rheumatic fever. Carditis may also present as an organic heart murmur in patients who initially appear with choreiform movements.

When carditis is the sole clinical manifestation, it can be difficult to determine when the attack began. Children have no symptoms referable to the heart unless pericarditis or heart failure is present. The history is vague. There is loss of appetite; the child appears pale and chronically ill and tires easily. The signs of cardiac involvement may be unequivocal, and often there is evidence of early heart failure. Carditis also can be entirely asymptomatic, so-called "silent carditis." This is a retrospective diagnosis when valvular heart disease, usually mitral stenosis, is discovered years later and other causes of acquired heart disease have been excluded.

Carditis should be suspected if there is tachycardia disproportionate to the degree of fever. However, the most distinctive sign of rheumatic carditis is a new significant murmur. An apical high-pitched, blowing, holosystolic murmur of at least grade II intensity indicative of mitral valvulitis is the most common heart bruit. It may be accompanied by a low-pitched mid-diastolic (Carey-Coombs) murmur. A decrescendo diastolic murmur along the left sternal border indicating aortic regurgitation is much less frequent. Enlargement of the heart, a pericardial friction rub or effusion, and congestive failure may be present at the onset or occur during the course of the acute attack.

The duration of rheumatic carditis varies from 6 wk to 6 mo. However, in patients with severe carditis the active rheumatic process may continue beyond 6 mo, so-called "chronic" rheumatic fever. Nowadays this occurs in a very small proportion of patients following an initial attack of rheumatic fever.

Chorea occurs in 10–15% of patients. It may be the only sign of rheumatic fever, or it may be associated with other manifestations such as carditis. Chorea is often heralded by emotional lability, deterioration in school performance, and poor coordination. Within 1–2 wk thereafter, involuntary, purposeless movements appear. These are random, nonrhythmic, rapid movements affecting any group of muscles but most often the face and upper extremities. The affected muscles are weak; at times the weakness is severe enough to resemble paralysis. The deep reflexes are variable, and there are no other neurologic findings.

Chorea is a self-limited condition with a variable course. Mild cases subside within a few weeks, but a 3 mo course is average; occasionally, choreiform movements continue for 6 mo to 1 yr.

Subcutaneous nodules are round, hard, freely movable painless swellings, usually overlying bone prominences. They occur in 1% of rheumatic patients, usually when severe carditis is present, and they often do not appear until several weeks after onset of the attack. *Erythema marginatum* is the characteristic skin rash of rheumatic fever. It occurs in fewer than 5% of patients. The lesions begin as slightly red, barely raised, nonpruritic macules that extend outward to form wavy lines or rings with sharp margins; they occur mainly over the trunk and inner surfaces of arms and legs. These lesions are evanescent and may come and go for several months.

Fever is usually present at the onset of an acute attack. It ranges from 38.3 to 40° C (101–104° F) without characteristic pattern. In children with an insidious onset the fever is low grade; it is completely absent in patients with pure chorea. *Abdominal pain* may precede other manifestations. The pain is not localized but can be severe enough to suggest a surgical condition. Spontaneous *epistaxis*, once frequent, is now rarely seen.

Laboratory Manifestations. Evidence of a recent streptococcal infection should be sought in every patient suspected of rheumatic fever. The throat culture may not be helpful for this purpose because by the time rheumatic fever develops, the culture is often negative. Tests for streptococcal antibodies are much more useful because they are specific for infections caused by these bacteria and antibodies usually reach their peak at about the time of onset of rheumatic fever. Approximately 80% have an elevated anti–streptolysin O (ASO) titer. Titers ranging from 200–300 units are common in healthy school-age children so that only levels of over 300 units are considered abnormal. Patients suspected of rheumatic fever who do not show an abnormal ASO titer should be tested for other streptococcal antibodies, e.g., anti–DNase B and anti–DPNase. If these tests are not available, there is a commercial multiple antibody test (Streptozyme); it is considered positive at dilutions over 1:200. The Streptozyme test should not be used in lieu of the ASO titer, which is the best standardized and most reproducible test available.

Because streptococcal antibody levels may begin to decline after 2 mo, titers in patients with insidious rheumatic carditis discovered several months after onset may have returned to normal levels. This is also true in patients with "pure" chorea since this manifestation may not appear until several months after streptococcal infection. There is no correlation between the height and duration of the antibody titer and the severity or persistence of rheumatic activity. Thus, once it has been established that the patient has an elevated titer, there is no reason to repeat antibody studies.

The tests generally used to measure the presence and degree of inflammatory process are the erythrocyte sedimentation rate (ESR) and C-reactive protein (CRP). Neither is specific for rheumatic fever, but they are useful for determining when the acute process has terminated. The CRP is somewhat more helpful because the sedimentation rate can be influenced by extraneous factors such as anemia. Mild to moderate anemia is common in active rheumatic fever; it is normocytic and normochromic.

Prolongation of the P-R interval occurs in about one third of the patients with acute rheumatic fever. While heart block can be a diagnostic aid, it is not of itself a sign of carditis and it has no prognostic significance. Other electrocardiographic changes include flattened or inverted T waves due to myocarditis as well as elevation of the S-T segment produced by pericarditis.

Roentgenograms of the chest are useful to detect cardiac enlargement and pericardial effusion. The echocardiogram is of limited value during the acute stage of the disease. Patients with rheumatic polyarthritis do not require roentgenograms of the joints.

Diagnosis. Since rheumatic fever may affect a number of organs and tissues, singly or in combination, no single clinical manifestation or laboratory test is characteristic enough to be diagnostic. The need to bring uniformity to the diagnosis led T. D. Jones to formulate diagnostic criteria based on combinations of clinical manifestations and laboratory findings (Table 10–28). Clinical signs that are most useful are designated *major manifestations* and include carditis, arthritis, chorea, subcutaneous nodules, and erythema marginatum. The term "major" relates to diagnostic importance and not to frequency, severity, or prognostic significance of the particular manifestation. Other signs and symptoms, while less characteristic, may still be helpful. These *minor manifestations* include fever, arthralgia, past history of rheumatic fever or rheumatic heart disease, prolongation of the P-R interval, and positive acute phase reactants. Two major or one major and two minor manifestations indicate a high probability of rheumatic fever.

Clinical criteria can neither encompass the full spectrum of a disease nor totally exclude overlapping conditions. Thus, not all bona fide rheumatic fever patients fit the criteria, especially if the attack is mild or patients are seen early in the course of the illness. There are also clinical conditions which fulfill the criteria but are not due to rheumatic fever. Nevertheless, the criteria are useful, especially for avoiding overdiagnosis. Many errors in diagnosis occur because the history, physical, or laboratory findings have been misinterpreted.

Differential Diagnosis. The frequent occurrence of combinations of rheumatic manifestations makes the diagnosis fairly straightforward in many cases. When the patient presents with a single clinical feature, the differential diagnosis varies according to the presenting manifestation.

Joint pains without objective findings, arthralgia, can be difficult to distinguish from *nonspecific limb pain*, a common complaint in children. Pains behind the knees and in calf muscles that awaken children at night (so-called growing pains) are not due to rheumatic fever. Abnormalities of the feet, patellar chondromalacia, osteochondroses, and other orthopedic conditions can simulate rheumatic arthralgia. Limb pains may also be an expression of a functional disorder. The sedimentation rate is a helpful screening test to distinguish many of these conditions from true rheumatic arthralgia.

Acute onset polyarticular *rheumatoid arthritis* can mimic rheumatic fever early in the course of the illness. Polyarthritis in children under 3 yr of age is almost always due to rheumatoid disease. It is less migratory, less responsive to salicylates, and often accompanied by a high intermittent fever, splenomegaly, lymphadenopathy, and an evanescent macular rash, none of which occur in rheumatic fever. Arthralgia and arthritis can occur during infections with *Yersinia enterocolitica, Salmonella, Shigella, rubella, viral hepatitis* and spirochetes (Lyme disease). *Hypersensitivity reactions, sickle cell*

Table 10–28. Jones Criteria (Revised) For Guidance in the Diagnosis of Rheumatic Fever

Major Manifestations	Minor Manifestations
Carditis	*Clinical*
Polyarthritis	Fever
Chorea	Arthralgia
Erythema marginatum	Previous rheumatic fever or
Subcutaneous nodules	rheumatic heart disease
	Laboratory
	Acute phase reaction
	ESR, leukocytosis
	C-reactive protein
	Prolonged P-R interval

Plus supporting evidence of preceding streptococcal infection: increased ASO or other streptococcal antibodies; positive throat culture for group A streptococcus; recent scarlet fever.

From Circulation 32:664, 1965.

disease, and *leukemia* can also cause periarticular pain and swelling and mimic rheumatic fever.

The most common diagnostic error related to the heart is misinterpretation of *innocent murmurs,* especially in children with ill-defined extremity pain and low grade fever. Innocent murmurs are common in children and are of two types: the ejection pulmonic systolic murmur and the musical parasternal systolic murmur. Since these murmurs are often loud, it is the quality, duration, and location rather than the intensity which distinguish them from the blowing pansystolic apical murmur of mitral regurgitation.

Viral myocarditis can usually be distinguished from rheumatic myocarditis since the latter is almost always accompanied by valvular disease and a significant murmur. An exception is the fulminant form of rheumatic myocarditis in very young children. Rheumatic pericarditis is also accompanied by other signs of carditis; when pericarditis is an isolated finding, a viral etiology should be suspected. Acute rheumatic carditis is rarely mistaken for congenital heart disease, although chronic rheumatic valvular disease can be confused with congenital abnormalities of the heart.

Abnormal movements due to other causes can be mistaken for Sydenham chorea when there is no other evidence of rheumatic fever. The repetitive stereotyped movements of *multiple tics* are fairly easy to distinguish from the random, jerky, choreiform movements. The *tic of Gilles de la Tourette* may resemble chorea at the onset, but its chronicity and other distinctive features soon distinguish it. *Huntington chorea* may start in childhood, but the movements tend to be choreoathetoid and there is a positive family history.

The significance of an elevated ASO has been a source of misdiagnosis. *An elevated ASO titer, no matter how abnormal, does not by itself confirm the diagnosis.* There must also be well documented clinical evidence of rheumatic fever. Questionable rheumatic manifestations plus an elevated ASO titer are insufficient for a diagnosis, but they may require careful observation of the patient.

Treatment. All patients with acute rheumatic fever should be placed at *bed rest,* if at all possible in a hospital. They should be examined daily to detect carditis, which almost always appears within 2 wk of onset. Thereafter, the duration and degree of bed rest should vary with the nature and severity of the attack. A guide for bed rest and ambulation is outlined in Table 10–29. In general, restrictions are continued until the rheumatic process has become quiescent. It is considered active when any of the following is present: joint symptoms, new organic murmurs, enlarging heart size, a sleeping pulse of greater than 100, or subcutaneous nodules. Heart failure in the absence of longstanding valvular disease is also a sign of activity. Persistence of an elevated ESR for more than 6 mo should not be considered a sign of rheumatic activity if no clinical signs are present.

Anti-inflammatory drugs are very effective for supressing the acute manifestations of rheumatic fever. However, in patients with arthralgia only or with mild arthritis, anti-inflammatory agents should be withheld and other analgesics used if needed. This is particularly wise when the diagnosis is uncertain since analgesics will not interfere with the development of migratory polyarthritis.

Patients with definite arthritis, or with carditis but no cardiomegaly, should be treated with salicylates: 100 mg/kg/24 hr in divided doses for the first 2 wk and 75 mg/kg/24 hr for the following 4–6 wk. Occasionally, 150 mg/kg/24 hr may be necessary to control arthritis.

Patients with carditis and cardiomegaly should be treated with prednisone, starting with a dose of 2 mg/kg/24 hr in divided doses. After about 2 wk, prednisone may be withdrawn, decreasing the daily dose at the rate of 5 mg every 2–3 days. When tapering is started, salicylates, 75 mg/kg/24 hr,

Table 10–29. Guide for Bed Rest and Ambulation in Patients with Acute Rheumatic Fever

Cardiac Status	Management
No carditis	Bed rest for 2 wk and gradual ambulation for 2 wk even if on salicylates
Carditis, no enlargement	Bed rest for 4 wk and gradual ambulation for 4 wk
Carditis, with enlargement	Bed rest for 6 wk and gradual ambulation for 6 wk
Carditis, with heart failure	Strict bed rest for as long as heart failure is present and gradual ambulation for 3 mo

should be added and continued for 1 mo after prednisone is stopped. Overlapping therapy reduces the incidence of post-therapeutic rebounds which may occur within 1–2 wk after anti-inflammatory drugs are discontinued. Laboratory rebounds and all but the most severe clinical rebounds are best left untreated.

The recommendations outlined above and in Table 10–30 limit the use of corticosteroids to patients with moderate to severe carditis because of the clinical impression that such patients respond more rapidly, tolerate steroids better than salicylates, and may be at less risk of death during the acute attack. However, most well controlled studies have failed to prove that treatment with steroids decreases the incidence of residual heart disease.

Mild heart failure can often be controlled by complete bed rest, oxygen, fluid restriction, and steroids. If severe failure is present, diuretics and digitalis are indicated. However, digitalis should be used with caution because some patients with acute myocarditis have an unusual sensitivity to digitalis.

Patients with chorea may benefit from barbiturates or chlorpromazine. More recently, haloperidol has been used, but no drug has proved uniformly effective. Steroids are not recommended unless there are also signs of an active rheumatic inflammatory process.

Prognosis. The sequelae of rheumatic fever are essentially limited to the heart and depend on the presence and severity of carditis. When there is no clinical evidence of carditis during the acute attack, complete recovery is the rule. The prognosis is also excellent if the findings are limited to prolongation of the P-R interval. When there is cardiac involvement, the incidence of residual heart disease is proportional to the severity of the carditis. Three quarters of the patients with congestive heart failure during the initial attack will have chronic valvular disease after 10 yr. On the other hand, when the cardiac findings are limited to a systolic murmur, only about 25% of the patients are left with residual heart disease. Thus, in patients with mild carditis, the number of patients who heal completely is remarkably high *if they remain free of recurrent attacks.*

Recurrences of rheumatic fever markedly influence the

Table 10–30. Recommended Anti-Inflammatory Agents For Acute Rheumatic Fever

Clinical Manifestations	Treatment
Arthralgia	Analgesics only
Arthritis only, and/or carditis without cardiomegaly	Salicylates 100 mg/kg/24 hr for 2 wk and 75 mg/kg/24 hr for 4–6 wk
Carditis with cardiomegaly or failure	Prednisone 2 mg/kg/24 hr for 2 wk and taper over 2 wk; salicylates 75 mg/kg/24 hr at 2 wk and continue for 6 wk

prognosis, and the availability of antistreptococcal prophylaxis is the main reason for improved outcome in recent years. Recurrences are more likely when the initial attack occurs early in life and when the attack includes carditis. They are more apt to occur in the years immediately after an attack, in patients with residual heart disease, and in those with previous recurrences.

Death during the acute attack has become exceedingly rare. The mortality from chronic rheumatic heart disease has also dropped markedly. The 10 yr mortality rate in a recent series was 4%, which contrasts with the 20–30% 10 yr mortality rate that prevailed prior to 1950.

Prevention. The attack rate after streptococcal infections in patients who have had rheumatic fever is much higher than in the general population. Therefore, once the diagnosis of rheumatic fever has been established, *continual antimicrobial prophylaxis* should be started to prevent streptococcal infections and recurrences of rheumatic fever. Intramuscular benzathine penicillin G, 1.2 million units every 4 wk, is the most effective prophylactic medication. It is the treatment of choice for *all* patients and especially for high risk patients, i.e., those with heart disease, those with a history of multiple attacks, or those unlikely to take oral medication regularly. There may be persistent pain for 1–2 days at the site of injection, but rarely does benzathine penicillin have to be discontinued for this reason. Allergic reactions in children are infrequent and generally mild.

Sulfadiazine is the drug of choice for the exceptional patient who cannot tolerate injections or who is allergic to penicillin. The dose is 0.5 g once daily in children less than 30 kg and 1.0 g in the others. Although reactions are rare, a blood count is advised after the first several weeks, and patients should be advised to report immediately the appearance of any rash.

Oral penicillin is also effective in a dose of 200,000 units twice daily. Patients on oral penicillin can be monitored for compliance by a simple urine test for penicillin. Oral penicillin, however, causes the emergence of resistant alpha streptococci in the mouth, whereas benzathine penicillin and sulfadiazine do not. Resistent alpha streptococci in the oral cavity are a potential hazard for patients with rheumatic heart disease since they are at risk for bacterial endocarditis.

Prophylaxis should be maintained at least throughout childhood and adolescence for a minimum of 5 years even in patients with no residual heart disease. Young adults with children in the home should also be urged to continue prophylaxis. The risk to individuals over 40 yr of age is very small, but lifetime prophylaxis is recommended if the patient has rheumatic valvular disease.

Initial attacks of rheumatic fever can be prevented by treatment of the preceding streptococcal pharyngitis. Ten days of antimicrobial treatment are required to achieve maximum cure rates. A single injection of benzathine penicillin is the most reliable treatment. A 10 day course of oral penicillin is effective, but it is less reliable because it depends on compliance. Patients who are allergic to penicillin should receive erythromycin for 10 days. Sulfonamides should not be prescribed since they fail to eradicate streptococci. The tetracyclines are also contraindicated because many strains of group A streptococci have become resistant to this antibiotic. None of the new antibiotics is more effective than penicillin, and most are much more expensive.

The prevention of first attacks of rheumatic fever is hampered by failure to recognize streptococcal pharyngitis, by the subclinical nature of many of these infections, and by the lack of easy access to medical care. Some of these difficulties have been overcome in recent years by the widespread use of throat cultures and greater availability of medical care through Medicaid and other programs. A study by Gordis in one city demonstrated a significant reduction in the incidence of first attacks of rheumatic fever after comprehensive care clinics were established in deprived areas and a concerted effort was made to identify and treat streptococcal infections. Because of the low risk of rheumatic fever at the present time, questions are being raised about the need to continue to pursue streptococcal infections as vigorously as in the past. However, evidence supports the view that a major reason for the recent dramatic decline is due to the widespread use of antibiotics for pharyngitis in children. An antistreptococcal vaccine is under development, but progress has been very slow.

MILTON MARKOWITZ

Community control of rheumatic heart disease in developing countries: A major public health problem. WHO Chronicle 34:336, 1980.

DiSciascio G, Taranta A: Rheumatic fever in children. A review. Am Heart J 99:635, 1980.

Gordis L: Effectiveness of comprehensive care programs in preventing rheumatic fever. N Engl J Med 289:331, 1973.

Inter-Society Commission for Heart Disease Resources: Prevention of rheumatic fever and rheumatic heart disease. Circulation 61:A–1, 1970.

Jones criteria (revised) for guidance in the diagnosis of rheumatic fever. Circulation 32:664, 1965.

Markowitz M, Gordis L: Rheumatic Fever. 2nd ed. Philadelphia, WB Saunders, 1972.

Stollerman GH: Rheumatic Fever and Streptococcal Infection. New York, Grune and Stratton, 1975.

United Kingdom and United States Joint Report: The natural history of rheumatic fever and rheumatic heart disease: Ten year report of a cooperative clinical trial of ACTH, cortisone and aspirin. Circulation 32:457, 1965.

Wannamaker LW: Medical progress: Differences between streptococcal infections of the throat and of the skin. N Engl J Med 282:23, 78, 1970.

11

INFECTIOUS DISEASES

GENERAL CONSIDERATIONS

11.1 FEVER OF UNKNOWN ORIGIN

Many physicians use the term fever of unknown origin (FUO) to describe the condition of any febrile child admitted to the hospital with neither an apparent site of infection nor a noninfectious diagnosis. In most of these children the development of additional clinical manifestations over a relatively short time period makes the infectious nature of the illness apparent. The term might better be reserved for children with (1) a history of fever of more than 1 wk duration, (2) fever also documented in the hospital, and (3) no apparent diagnosis after an investigation of 1 wk in the hospital.

The principal causes of FUO in children, using more restrictive criteria, are infections and collagen-vascular diseases. Neoplastic disorders should also be seriously considered, although most children with malignancies do not have fever alone. If the patient is receiving drugs, the possibility of drug fever should also be considered. This is not usually associated with other symptoms, and temperature remains elevated at a relatively constant level. Withdrawal of the drug is associated with resolution of the fever, generally within 72 hr (when drugs, such as iodides, are excreted over a prolonged period of time, fever may persist for up to 1 mo after drug withdrawal).

Most fevers of unknown or unrecognized origin result from common diseases that may be atypical in their presentations. In some cases the presentation of a fever of unknown origin is typical of the disease (juvenile rheumatoid arthritis), but a definitive diagnosis can be established only after prolonged observation because there are no associated findings on physical examination and all laboratory results are negative or normal.

In the United States the infectious diseases implicated most consistently in children with fever of unknown origin (by the above more rigorous definition) have been salmonellosis, tularemia, tuberculosis, rickettsial diseases, brucellosis, syphilis, leptospirosis, rat-bite fever, infectious mononucleosis, cytomegalic inclusion disease, and hepatitis.

Table 11–1 lists diseases that have presented as fever of unknown origin in children with sufficient frequency to merit serious consideration. Specific signs and symptoms of each of these diseases and methods of diagnosis are detailed elsewhere.

Juvenile rheumatoid arthritis and systemic lupus erythematosus are the collagen diseases associated most frequently with fever of unknown origin. Fever should be documented in the hospital by an individual who remains with the patient while the temperature is taken to rule out factitious fever. Prolonged and continuous observation of the patient is imperative. Repetitive evaluation including history, physical examination, and roentgenographic studies may be required.

Diagnostic Clues in the Child with Fever of Unknown Origin

History. A history of *exposure to wild or domestic animals* should be solicited. The incidence of zoonotic infections in the United States has been increasing, and they frequently are acquired from pets that are not overtly ill. For example, immunization of dogs against specific disorders such as leptospirosis may prevent canine disease but does not always prevent the animal from carrying and shedding leptospires which may be transmitted to household contacts. A history of ingestion of rabbit or squirrel meat may provide a clue to the diagnosis of oropharyngeal, glandular, or typhoidal tularemia.

A history of *pica* should be sought. Ingestion of dirt is a particularly important clue to infection with *Toxocara* (visceral larva migrans) or *Toxoplasma gondii* (toxoplasmosis).

A history of *travel* reaching back to the birth of the child should be sought. There may be re-emergence of malaria, histoplasmosis, and coccidioidomycosis years after visiting or living in an endemic area. It is important to ask about prophylactic immunizations and precautions taken by the individual against the ingestion of contaminated water or food during foreign travel (Sec. 4.5). Rocks, dirt, and artifacts from geographically distant regions which have been collected and brought into the home as souvenirs may serve as vectors of disease.

A *medication* history should be pursued rigorously. This should include over-the-counter preparations and topical agents, including eye drops (atropine-induced fever).

The *genetic background* of the patient also is important. Descendants of the Ulster Scots may have fever of unknown origin because they are afflicted with nephrogenic diabetes insipidus. Familial dysautonomia (Riley-Day syndrome, a disorder in which hyperthermia is recurrent) is more frequent among Jews than in other population groups.

Physical Examination. Sweating in a febrile child should be noted. The continuing absence of sweat in the presence of an elevated or changing body temperature suggests dehydration from vomiting, diarrhea, or central or nephrogenic diabetes insipidus. It also should suggest anhidrotic ectodermal dysplasia, familial dysautonomia, or exposure to atropine.

Red, weeping eyes may be a sign of collagen-vascular disease, particularly polyarteritis nodosa. Palpebral conjunctivitis in the febrile patient may be a clue to measles, coxsackieviral infection, tuberculosis, infectious mononucleosis, lymphogranuloma venereum, or cat-scratch or Newcastle disease virus infection. In contrast, bulbar conjunctivitis in a child with fever of unknown origin suggests leptospirosis.

Fever of unknown origin sometimes is due to hypothalamic dysfunction. A clue to this disorder is failure of pupillary constriction due to absence of the sphincter constrictor muscle of the eye. This muscle develops embryologically when hypothalamic structure and function also are undergoing differentiation.

Lack of tears or an absent corneal reflex may suggest fever from familial dysautonomia. A smooth tongue may reflect absence of fungiform papillae and also suggests this diagnosis.

Tenderness to tapping over the sinuses and teeth should be sought, and the sinuses should be transilluminated.

Oral candidosis may be a clue to various disorders of the immune system.

Table 11–1. Some Causes of Fever of Unknown Origin in Children

Bacterial diseases
  Abscesses: dental, liver, pelvic, perinephric, subdiaphragmatic
  Bacterial endocarditis
  Borrelliosis
  Brucellosis
  Leptospirosis
  Mastoiditis (chronic)
  Osteomyelitis
  Pyelonephritis
  Salmonellosis
  Sinusitis
  Tuberculosis
  Tularemia
Viral diseases
  Cytomegalic inclusion disease
  Hepatitis (chronic active)
  Infectious mononucleosis
Chlamydial diseases
  Lymphogranuloma venereum
  Psittacosis
Rickettsial diseases
  Q fever
  Rocky Mountain spotted fever
Fungal diseases
  Blastomycosis (nonpulmonary)
  Histoplasmosis (disseminated)
Parasitic diseases
  Babesiosis
  Malaria
  Toxoplasmosis
  Visceral larva migrans
Unclassified
  Sarcoidosis
Collagen vascular diseases
  Juvenile rheumatoid arthritis
  Polyarteritis nodosa
  Systemic lupus erythematosus
Malignancies
  Hodgkin disease
  Lymphoma
  Neuroblastoma
Miscellaneous disorders
  Anhidrotic ectodermal dysplasia
  Diabetes insipidus (non-nephrogenic and nephrogenic)
  Drug fever
  Factitious fever
  Familial dysautonomia
  Granulomatous colitis
  Infantile cortical hyperostosis
  Mucocutaneous lymph node syndrome (Kawasaki disease)
  Pancreatitis
  Periodic fever
  Serum sickness
  Thyrotoxicosis
  Ulcerative colitis

Fever blisters are common findings in patients with pneumococcal, streptococcal, malarial, and rickettsial infection. They also are common in children with meningococcal meningitis (which usually does not present as fever of unknown origin) but rarely are seen in children with meningococcemia. Fever blisters rarely are seen with salmonella or staphylococcal infections.

Repetitive chills and temperature spikes are common in children with septicemia (regardless of etiology), particularly when associated with renal disease, liver or biliary disease, endocarditis, malaria, brucellosis, rat-bite fever, or loculated collections of pus.

Hyperemia of the pharynx, with or without exudate, may suggest infectious mononucleosis, cytomegalic inclusion disease, toxoplasmosis, salmonellosis, tularemia, or leptospirosis.

The muscles and bones should be palpated carefully. Point tenderness over a bone may suggest occult osteomyelitis or bone marrow invasion from neoplastic disease. Tenderness over the trapezius muscle may be a clue to a subdiaphragmatic abscess. Generalized muscle tenderness suggests dermatomyositis, trichinosis, polyarteritis, or mycoplasma or arboviral infection.

Rectal examination may reveal pararectal adenopathy or tenderness and suggest a deep pelvic abscess, iliac adenitis, or pelvic osteomyelitis. A guaiac test should be obtained on any stool found on the examining finger; occult blood loss may suggest granulomatous colitis or ulcerative colitis as the cause of fever of unknown origin.

The general activity of the patient and the presence or absence of rashes must be noted.

Hyperactive deep tendon reflexes may suggest thyrotoxicosis as the cause of fever of unknown origin.

Laboratory Studies. These should make use of diagnostic tests most likely to provide a prompt definitive diagnosis; the general tendency to order a large number of tests in every child with fever of unknown origin according to a predetermined sequence may waste time and money. Alternatively, prolonged hospitalization for sequential tests may be more costly. The tempo of diagnostic evaluation should be adjusted to the tempo of the illness; haste may be imperative in a critically ill patient. But if the illness is more chronic, the evaluation can proceed more slowly and deliberately.

Routine *white blood cell counts* and *urinalyses* are generally of minimal diagnostic value in children who fulfill a rigorous definition of fever of unknown origin. An absolute neutrophil count below 5000 mm^3, however, is evidence against non-overwhelming bacterial infection other than typhoid. Conversely, patients with more than 10,000 polymorphonuclear leukocytes or more than 500 nonsegmented polymorphonuclear leukocytes/mm^3 have an 80% chance of having a severe bacterial infection.

An elevated *erythrocyte sedimentation rate* (>30 mm/hr, Westergren method) indicates inflammation and the need for further evaluation.

Blood cultures should be obtained aerobically and anaerobically. The isolation of leptospires, *Francisella*, or *Yersinia* may require selective media or specific conditions not routinely employed.

Tuberculin *skin testing* should be performed carefully with polysorbate 80 (Tween) stabilized purified protein derivative (PPD) which has been kept appropriately refrigerated.

Urine culture should be obtained routinely. Roentgenographic study of the urinary tract may be indicated.

Roentgenographic examination of the chest, sinuses, mastoids, or gastrointestinal tract may be suggested by specific historic or physical findings. Roentgenographic evaluation of the gastrointestinal tract for granulomatous colitis may be helpful in evaluating selected children with fever of unknown origin and no other localizing signs or symptoms.

Examination of the *bone marrow* may reveal leukemia; metastatic neoplasm; mycobacterial, fungal, or parasitic diseases; and histiocytosis or other storage diseases. If a bone marrow aspirate is performed, cultures for bacteria, *Mycobacterium*, and fungi should be obtained.

Serologic tests may aid in the diagnosis of infectious mononucleosis, cytomegaloviral disease, toxoplasmosis, salmonellosis, tularemia, brucellosis, leptospirosis, and, on some occasions, juvenile rheumatoid arthritis. For histoplasmosis, yeast and mycelial phase complement fixation tests may suggest the diagnosis. *Lymph node biopsies* and *exploratory laparotomies* seem helpful in children only when physical examination suggests they may be indicated.

Radioactive scans may be helpful in detecting osteomyelitis and abdominal abscesses. *Echocardiograms* may suggest the presence of vegetations on the leaflets of heart valves as in subacute bacterial endocarditis. Total body CT or MRI scanning permits the detection of neoplasms and collections of purulent material without the use of surgical exploration or radioisotopes.

Treatment. Fever and infection in children are not synonymous; antibiotics should not be used as antipyretics; empiric trials of medication should generally be avoided. An exception may be the use of antituberculous treatment in critically ill children with possible disseminated tuberculosis. Empiric trials of other antibiotics may be dangerous and can obscure the diagnosis of endocarditis, meningitis, parameningeal infection, or osteomyelitis. Hospitalization may be required for laboratory or roentgenographic studies which are unavailable or impractical in an ambulatory setting, for more careful observation, or for temporary relief of parental anxiety.

Prognosis. The child with fever of unknown origin has a better prognosis than that reported for adults, which suggest a mortality rate of 25–40%. In many cases no diagnosis can be established, but fever abates spontaneously. In as many as 25% of cases in which fever persists, the cause of fever will remain unclear even after thorough evaluation.

Feigin RD, Shearer WT: Fever of unknown origin in children. Curr Probl Pediatr 6:1, 1976.
Lorin MI: The Febrile Child: Clinical Management of Fever and Other Types of Pyrexia. New York, John Wiley & Sons, 1982.
Naiman JL, Bergman GE: Hematologic clues to systemic disease in childhood. Semin Hematol 12:287, 1975.

11.2 FEVER ASSOCIATED WITH DISEASES OF THE CENTRAL NERVOUS SYSTEM

Fever may be associated with a variety of diseases that affect the central nervous system (Table 11–2). In children,

Table 11–2. Diseases of the Central Nervous System with Which Fever May Be Associated

Acute bacterial meningitis
Viral meningitis: echovirus, coxsackievirus, poliovirus, mumps, herpes simplex, etc.
Mycoplasmosis
Leptospirosis
Syphilis
Tuberculosis
Sarcoidosis
Fungal meningitis: aspergillosis, North American blastomycosis, candidosis, cladosporiosis, coccidioidomycosis, cryptococcosis, histoplasmosis, paracoccidioidomycosis, phycomycosis (mucor), allescheriosis, alternariasis, cephalosporiosis, paecilomycosis, penicilliosis, rhinosporidiosis, sporotrichosis, torulopsosis, ustilagomycosis
Parasitic meningitis: cysticercosis, amebiasis, trichinosis, toxoplasmosis
Infectious encephalitis (usually viral, including herpes simplex, varicella, rubeola, rubella, infectious mononucleosis, arboviruses)
Acute hemorrhagic encephalitis
Subdural empyema
Ventricular empyema
Brain abscess
Intracranial or spinal epidural abscess
Thrombophlebitis (often associated with subdural empyema)
Encephalopathies: Reye syndrome, poisons (e.g., arsenic), metabolic disorders (thyrotoxicosis), uremia
Subdural hematoma
Intrathecal injections (chemical meningitis)
Serum sickness
Collagen-vascular diseases
Acute multiple sclerosis
Hemolytic-uremic syndrome

acute infection of the central nervous system is the most common cause of fever associated with signs and symptoms of central nervous system involvement.

Regardless of etiology, most patients with acute central nervous system infection present similar signs and symptoms, including fever, headache, nausea, vomiting, anorexia, restlessness, and irritability. Photophobia, back pain, nuchal rigidity, obtundation, stupor, coma, seizures, and focal neurologic signs also may be noted.

The neurologic expression of various parameningeal infections depends to some extent on the site of the lesion or lesions, which in turn is determined by the manner in which the intracranial or intraspinal infection was established. Ear infections may lead to epidural, subdural, or parenchymatous lesions of the adjacent temporal lobe or of the cerebellum. Infection of the frontal sinuses and, less often, of the maxillary sinuses may be followed by cerebral abscess, corticothrombophlebitis, or subdural empyema. Metastatic cerebral lesions may be solitary or multiple but usually occur in the distribution of the middle cerebral artery. Bacterial endocarditis leads most often to embolic occlusion of medium-sized vessels with subsequent infarction of the brain. This may result in secondary abscess formation or in the development of a mycotic aneurysm that may declare itself by a subarachnoid hemorrhage.

The diagnosis of acute bacterial meningitis and its differentiation from other central nervous system disorders associated with fever depend in large part upon careful examination of cerebrospinal fluid obtained by lumbar puncture. Cerebrospinal fluid findings characteristic of various central nervous system disorders associated with fever are shown in Table 11–3.

A variety of chemical or immunologic tests that may be performed upon cerebrospinal fluid, blood, or urine may aid in differentiating bacterial from viral infections of the central nervous system in patients whose bacterial and viral cerebrospinal fluid cultures are negative. (See Sections discussing specific etiologic agents.) Serum CRP measured by microquantitative techniques in patients with aseptic meningitis is generally less than 1.8 mg/dL, compared with the mean serum CRP of 17.5 mg/dL in patients with bacterial meningitis.

Unfortunately, in some cases a definitive diagnosis cannot be made on the basis of either clinical or cerebrospinal fluid findings, and a thorough search for foci of infection adjacent to or remote from the meninges must be performed. The extent of dysfunction of the nervous system must be defined by repeated neurologic examinations and appropriate laboratory studies. The presence of focal neurologic findings; a lymphocytic reaction within cerebrospinal fluid in which the glucose concentration is normal; associated infection of the ears, sinuses, or lung; or the presence of bronchiectasis or cyanotic heart disease should heighten suspicion of brain abscess, epidural or subdural infection, venous thrombophlebitis, or venous sinus thrombosis.

11.3 RASH

Rashes accompany many infectious diseases. They may be so characteristic of a particular disease that a specific diagnosis can be made without difficulty, but frequently the skin manifestations produced are common to many infections. Skin lesions may be the result of direct inoculation of the skin (e.g., anthrax or tularemia); hematogenous dissemination of microorganisms (e.g., septicemia due to meningococci or other bacteria); or contiguous spread from adjacent foci of infection (e.g., impetigo, herpetic lesions). The skin also may reflect the effect of toxins (e.g., scarlet fever), antigen-antibody reactions (e.g., rheumatic fever), or delayed hypersensitivity to the infecting agent (e.g., erythema nodosum).

Table 11–3. **Cerebrospinal Fluid Findings in Various Central Nervous System Disorders Associated with Fever**

Condition	Pressure (mm H$_2$O)	Leukocytes mm^3	Protein (mg/dL)	Glucose	Comments
Acute bacterial meningitis	Usually elevated	100–60,000 +; usually a few thousand; PMN predominate	Usually 100–500	Depressed compared with blood glucose; usually <40 mg/dL	Organism may be seen on Gram stain and recovered by culture
Partially treated bacterial meningitis	Normal or elevated	1–10,000; PMN usual but mononuclear cells may predominate if pretreated for extended period of time	100 +	Depressed or normal	Organisms may or may not be seen; in disease due to *H. influenzae*, organism may grow despite pretreatment; pretreatment may render sterile CSF of patients with pneumococcal and meningococcal disease
Tuberculous meningitis	Usually elevated; may be low due to block in advanced stages	10–500; PMN early but lymphocytes predominate through most of course	100–500; may be higher in presence of block	<50 mg/dL usual in most cases; decreases with time if treatment is not provided	Acid-fast organisms may be seen on smear; organism can be recovered in culture
Fungal meningitis	Usually elevated	25–500; mononuclear cells predominate except PMN early	25–500	<50 mg/dL, decreases with time if treatment is not provided	Budding yeast may be seen; organism may be recovered in culture; India ink preparation may be positive in cryptococcal disease
Syphilis (acute) and leptospirosis	Usually elevated	200–500, usually lymphocytes	50–200	Generally normal	Positive CSF serology; spirochetes not demonstrable by usual techniques of smear or culture; darkfield exam may be positive
Viral meningitis or meningo-encephalitis	Normal or slightly elevated	PMN early; rarely more than 1000 cells except in Eastern equine encephalomyelitis where counts of up to 20,000 have been recorded; mononuclear cells predominate during most of course	50–200	Generally normal; may be depressed to <40 mg/dL in various viral diseases, particularly mumps (15–20% of cases)	Enteroviruses may be recovered from CSF by appropriate viral cultures
Sarcoidosis	Normal or elevated slightly	0–100; mononuclear	40–100	Normal	No specific findings
Amebiasis	Elevated	500–20,000 +; PMN predominate	50–100	Normal or slightly depressed	Amebae may be seen rarely in CSF
Chemical (drugs, dermoids, cysts, myelography dye)	Usually elevated	100–1000 +; PMN predominate	50–100	20–40 mg/dL	Epithelial cells may be seen within CSF in some children with dermoids by use of polarized light
Subacute bacterial endocarditis with embolism	Normal or slightly elevated	0–100; mixed PMN and mononuclear cells	50–100	Normal	No organisms on smear or culture
Subdural empyema	Usually elevated	<100–5000; PMN predominate	100–500	Normal	No organisms on smear or culture of CSF unless meningitis also present; organism found on tap of subdural fluid

Table continued on following page

Table 11–3. Cerebrospinal Fluid Findings in Various Central Nervous System Disorders Associated with Fever
Continued

Condition	Pressure (mm H₂O)	Leukocytes mm³	Protein (mg/dL)	Glucose	Comments
Brain abscess	Usually elevated	10–200; fluid rarely acellular; lymphocytes predominate; if abscess ruptures into ventricle, PMN predominate and cell count may reach >100,000	75–500	Normal unless abscess ruptures into ventricular system	No organisms on smear or culture unless abscess ruptures into ventricular system
Cerebral epidural abscess	Normal to slightly elevated	0–500; lymphocytes predominate	50–200	Normal	No organisms on smear or culture
Spinal epidural abscess	Usually low, with spinal block	10–100; lymphocytes predominate	50–400	Normal	No organisms on smear or culture
Thrombophlebitis (sometimes with subdural empyema)	Normal or elevated	0–500; PMN and lymphocytes	50–200	Normal	No organisms on smear or culture
Acute hemorrhagic encephalitis	Usually elevated	0–1000; PMN predominate	100–500	Normal	No organisms on smear or culture
Collagen-vascular disease	Slightly elevated	0–500; PMN may predominate; lymphocytes may be present	100	Normal or slightly depressed	No organisms on smear or culture; LE preparation may be positive
Tumor, leukemia	Slightly elevated to very high	0–100+; mononuclear or blast cells	50–1000	May be depressed to 20–40 mg/dL	Cytology may be positive

PMN, polymorphonuclear leukocytes; CSF, cerebrospinal fluid; LE, lupus erythematosus cell.

Accurate diagnosis of patients with rashes presumed to be of infectious origin depends upon a careful history and an accurate, careful description of the skin lesions. Of specific interest are the nature and duration of any prodromal symptoms and an accurate description of the initial appearance and the evolution of the skin signs and symptoms. Pathognomonic signs (e.g., Koplik spots of measles) simplify diagnosis. In many cases the best the clinician can do is classify the disorder tentatively as viral, bacterial, or rickettsial or develop a list of a variety of infections that might be identified by appropriate cultural or serologic tests.

Rashes can be classified as macular eruptions, erythematous maculopapular eruptions, papulovesicular or bullous eruptions, petechial or hemorrhagic eruptions, ulcerative eruptions, and nodular eruptions. Many infections produce skin lesions that fall into more than one of these categories. Some infectious diseases and their agents are also associated with erythema multiforme eruptions or with erythema nodosum. In some patients, meningitis and pneumonia are associated with exanthems (Tables 11–4 and 11–5).

After an appropriate list of potential diagnoses has been assembled on the basis of the appearance of the skin lesions, further attempts to reduce the differential diagnosis can be made through use of pertinent historic data. In most cases the specific diagnosis can be made, sometimes only retrospectively, if appropriate cultures and serologic data are obtained. Antibiotic therapy for possible bacterial infections should be initiated promptly but only after cultures of blood

Table 11–4. Infectious Agents Associated with Exanthem and Meningitis

Agent	Illness
Herpes simplex virus 2	Recurrent genital herpes
Coxsackieviruses A2, A9, B1, B2, B4, B5	Enterovirus syndrome
Echoviruses 4, 6, 9, 11, 14, 17, 25, 33	Enterovirus syndrome
Colorado tick fever virus	Colorado tick fever
Reovirus 2	Respiratory infection
Neisseria meningitidis	Meningococcemia
Listeria monocytogenes	Listeriosis
Toxoplasma gondii	Toxoplasmosis

From Cherry JD, *In:* Feigin RD, Cherry JD (eds): Textbook of Pediatric Infectious Diseases. 2nd ed. Philadelphia, WB Saunders, 1987.

Table 11–5. Infectious Agents Associated with Exanthem and Pulmonary Involvement

Agent	Illness
Adenoviruses 7, 7a	Respiratory infection
Herpes simplex virus 1	Respiratory infection
Varicella-zoster virus	Chickenpox pneumonia
Epstein-Barr virus	Infectious mononucleosis
Coxsackievirus A9	Enterovirus syndrome
Echovirus 11	Enterovirus syndrome
Reovirus 3	Respiratory infection
Measles virus	Measles pneumonia and atypical measles
Chlamydia psittaci	Psittacosis
Mycoplasma pneumoniae	*M. pneumoniae* pneumonia
Neisseria meningitidis	Meningococcal pneumonia
Mycobacterium tuberculosis	Tuberculosis
Histoplasma capsulatum	Histoplasmosis
Cryptococcus neoformans	Cryptococcosis
Coccidioides immitis	Coccidioidomycosis

From Cherry JD, *In:* Feigin RD, Cherry JD (eds): Textbook of Pediatric Infectious Diseases. 2nd ed. Philadelphia, WB Saunders, 1987.

and skin lesions have been obtained. It is important to use media capable of supporting the growth of the organisms suspected of causing the infection. Skin biopsy may aid in the diagnosis of some of these disorders (e.g., rickettsial diseases or noninfectious papulovesicular eruptions). Vesicular or pustular skin lesions suspected to be due to viruses also should be cultured appropriately if the diagnosis cannot be established clinically. In some cases viruses may be recovered directly from the fluid of unruptured vesicles (e.g., varicella-zoster, herpes).

RALPH D. FEIGIN

Duncan WC: Cutaneous manifestations of infectious disease. In: Hoeprich PD (ed): Infectious Diseases. 2nd ed. Hagerstown, MD, Harper and Row, 1977.
Krugman S, Ward R, Katz SL: Infectious Diseases of Children. 6th ed. St. Louis, CV Mosby, 1977, p 472.

CLINICAL USE OF THE MICROBIOLOGY LABORATORY

The definitive diagnosis of an infectious disease requires analyses by a microbiology laboratory, which the clinician must supply with appropriate fresh specimens. Interaction between the physician and the laboratory should ensure that the specimens are tested for the suspected pathogens, that the results are correctly interpreted, and that appropriate antimicrobial agents are selected.

Laboratory diagnosis of an infection results from one of five methods, the selection of which often depends on the class of pathogenic agent suspected in the infection. The five methods are: (1) isolation of the agent; (2) detection of specific microbial antigens; (3) microscopic demonstration of the agent; (4) skin test for delayed type hypersensitivity; and (5) demonstration of specific antibody by serologic procedures.

11.4 LABORATORY DIAGNOSIS OF BACTERIAL INFECTIONS

Gram Stain. The examination of a Gram stain should be carried out on all fluids to be cultured. In addition to giving rapid results, the Gram stain may be useful in interpreting the subsequent cultural data.

Special Cultures. Most medically important bacteria can be cultivated on blood agar, chocolate agar, and eosin methylene blue or MacConkey agar. The frequency of recovery of anaerobic organisms has increased in recent years as media with low redox potentials have gained wide use. Thioglycollate broth, while an excellent general culture medium, will not foster growth of strict anaerobes. For collection of anaerobic cultures material should be transported to the laboratory in a capped syringe, or special swabs supplied in oxygen-free tubes should be used. In some cases clinical circumstances make it advisable to consult the microbiology laboratory in advance of sending a specimen.

Blood Culture. Culturing the blood is one of the most fruitful procedures in the diagnosis of bacterial disease. It should be done carefully *before* administration of antibiotics, using iodine-alcohol for skin disinfection. A number of different blood culture techniques are now available, most using 50–100 mL bottles containing broth nutritious for bacteria into which not more than 5–10 mL of blood are introduced. Sodium polyanethanol sulfonate is included in modern blood culture broth media to prevent coagulation and to inactivate leukocytes. Some blood culture bottles also contain an oxygen-free CO_2-enriched atmosphere that allows for the recovery of anaerobes. A more recent technique involves lysis of blood cells followed by inoculation of sediment obtained from centrifugation of the lysate. This method provides rapid detection, pathogen identification and antimicrobial susceptibility data, as well as quantitative blood culture results. Another recent technique depends on the detection of $[^{14}C]O_2$ released by bacteria from radioactively labeled substrates in the medium.

If an isolate is reported, blood cultures should be repeated to determine (1) whether treatment has been successful when the patient is already on antibiotics, and (2) whether the isolate is a contaminant when the organism reported is usually nonpathogenic. The question of whether an organism isolated from blood is a pathogen or a contaminant should be carefully considered, since nonpathogens may cause disease in hosts with compromised immune mechanisms.

Examination of Cerebrospinal Fluid. (See Table 11–3.) Fluid obtained by lumbar puncture or ventricular tap should be collected in sterile capped containers and transported quickly to the laboratory, where centrifugation is done to concentrate organisms. Gram stains of CSF sediment are helpful; the presence of organisms distinguishes bacterial from viral disease, but stains should not be relied on for the identification of a specific organism. Errors are possible, even by experienced technicians; it is better to use broad-spectrum initial therapy in life-threatening disease and to wait for the culture report before ordering specific treatment. Counterimmunoelectrophoresis and agglutination of antibody-coated latex beads are additional rapid, accurate methods for diagnosis. Specific antisera can be used to detect antigens of *H. influenzae* type b, *N. meningitidis*, *S. pneumoniae*, group B streptococci, and *E. coli* K1.

Urine Culture. Urine for culture and colony count can be obtained in midstream (clean catch), by catheterization, or by suprapubic puncture. The last method is the most reliable; urine so obtained should normally be sterile. Urine collected by catheter is likely to reflect infection if there are 10^4 organisms/mL or more. Clean-catch urine, if obtained after adequate cleansing, can be considered abnormal if more than 10^5 organisms/mL are present, and possibly abnormal if between 10^4 and 10^5 organisms/mL are counted. These limits apply only in uncomplicated urinary tract infection due to enteric gram-negative rods; different criteria may have to be used for gram-positive organisms, for yeasts, for patients in diuresis or with chronic pyelonephritis, or for patients on antibiotics. A Gram stain of unspun urine is helpful in predicting specimens with $>10^5$ cfu/mL. Clean-catch urine specimens from girls who have inadequately washed and specimens allowed to sit at room temperature for some time before being transported to the laboratory may result in unreliable cultures. If delay in transporting specimens is unavoidable, dip-slides coated with bacteriologic media, dipped promptly in the urine specimen as soon as it is passed, give reliable results for urine culture.

Culture of Feces. Rectal swabs or stool specimens are cultured either to identify common bacterial pathogens such as *Salmonella* and *Shigella* or to determine the predominant flora of the intestine in a patient with weakened host defenses whose endogenous flora may become pathogenic. Since feces contain mostly anaerobic bacteria, routine cultures identify only the predominant aerobic organisms among the billions of bacteria contained in each gram.

A number of organisms have recently been added to the

list of bacterial pathogens found in feces, including *Campylobacter spp.*, *Yersinia enterocolitica*, and *Clostridium difficile*.

Exudates and Transudates. Abscesses, pleural fluids, joint fluids, urethral exudates, and other miscellaneous exudates and transudates can be cultured directly on agar. In addition to cultures and stains, sugar and cell count determinations should be done on all transudates for the same reasons they are done on CSF.

Nasopharyngeal, Throat, and Skin Swabs. A dry rayon, Dacron, or calcium alginate swab is most efficient for collecting specimens from the skin and mucous membranes. Since drying rapidly destroys some pathogenic bacteria, swab specimens should be placed promptly in a transport medium. Now available are packaged swabs contained in a breakable ampule of transport medium that is crushed after the specimen is taken.

Interpretation of results of cultures from skin and mucous membranes is difficult because microbial flora are normally recovered from these areas. Some organisms are considered pathogenic wherever found, such as *Corynebacterium diphtheriae*, *Bordetella pertussis*, and *Neisseria gonorrhoeae*; others, such as *Streptococcus pyogenes*, *Neisseria meningitidis*, *Hemophilus influenzae*, or staphylococci, may be pathogenic or nonpathogenic, depending on circumstances. Still others, such as *Streptococcus viridans*, are rarely considered pathogenic. In respiratory tract disease there is little correlation between flora of the upper airway and that of the lower airway. Because sputum cultures are seldom reliable in children, tracheal aspirates and lung punctures are sometimes necessary for accurate diagnosis.

Fluorescent Techniques. Fluorescent antibody (FA) technique has increased the diagnostic scope of direct microscopy. Specific antisera are now available commercially for several common pathogens. In these sera the antibody molecules have been conjugated with a fluorescein dye. The specific dye-labeled serum is added to the smear containing the suspected organism, and the slide is microscopically examined for fluorescence under ultraviolet light. In the absence of specific fluorescein-labeled antisera, the indirect method is used: the smear is covered with the unlabeled specific antiserum, and time is allowed for antibodies to fix; the excess of unfixed antibody is washed off; and the slide is overlaid with a fluorescein-labeled antibody against gamma-globulin of the animal species in which the specific antiserum was made. The concentrated anti-gamma antibodies fluoresce at the sites of specific microorganism-antibody complexes. FA is used principally for identifying *Bordetella pertussis*, *Legionella pneumophila*, *Neisseria gonorrhoeae*, and group A streptococci. In the special case of *M. tuberculosis* no antibody is used; rather, the smears are stained with auramine-rhodamine, which is taken up by the organisms and fluoresces under UV light. This acid-fast fluorescent staining procedure is more sensitive but less specific than the Ziehl-Neelsen or Kinyoun acid-fast stain.

Serologic Tests. Bacteria are often serogrouped or serotyped through agglutination by specific antisera (sometimes attached to latex particles), but titration of serum antibodies is useful in only a few bacterial infections, some of which are caused by streptococci (Sec. 11.16), salmonella (Sec. 11.26), brucella (Sec. 11.31), legionnaires' bacillus (Sec. 11.42), and leptospira (Sec. 11.53). Slide tests such as Streptozyme (Wampole) rapidly and accurately detect antibodies to multiple exotoxins.

Antibiotic Sensitivity Tests. Most laboratories routinely test bacterial isolates for sensitivity to various antibiotics. The most prevalent technique of antibiotic testing is the agar disk diffusion method, in which a standardized inoculum of the organism is seeded onto a plate. Filter paper discs, each impregnated with an antibiotic, are placed on the agar surface, and after 18–24 hours of incubation, the zone of inhibition of bacterial growth around each disc is measured. Standard zone

diameters indicating sensitivity or resistance have been designated, according to previous tests correlating zone sizes and sensitivity by dilutions made in tubes of broth inoculated with bacteria. However, there are some pitfalls in the disc diffusion method. Small differences in zone diameter have large implications, and the control of inoculum size, the rate of diffusion of antibiotics, and the accurate measurement of zones are critical.

For more accurate measurement of antibiotic sensitivity, dilutions made in tubes or in wells on microtiter plates have come into wide use. Antibiotic dilutions in growth medium are prepared in steps through the range of attainable blood levels; then each tube or well is inoculated with a standardized suspension of the test organism. After 24 hr the tubes or wells are examined for turbidity; the lowest antibiotic concentration resulting in a clear tube or well indicates the bacteriostatic concentration of the particular antibiotic for the organism (minimal inhibitory concentration, or MIC). The tubes or wells are then subcultured to agar plates; the lowest concentration of antibiotic that yields a 99.9% decrease in organism viability is the bactericidal endpoint (minimal bactericidal concentration, or MBC).

Antibiotic sensitivities cannot be interpreted correctly except in the clinical pharmacologic context. Certain clinical situations, such as endocarditis or osteomyelitis, call for the use of bactericidal rather than bacteriostatic drugs. Although a staphylococcus might be sensitive to both semisynthetic penicillins and erythromycin, the former would be a better choice than the latter in a bloodstream infection. Toxicity of drugs must also be taken into account: the use of less toxic agents is preferable when possible. Finally, attainable blood and tissue levels are the true measure of clinical efficacy: polymyxin B gives good zones of inhibition in vitro, but the highest blood levels that can be tolerated are often insufficient to achieve sterilization; on the other hand, carbenicillin may appear ineffective in vitro, but the high blood levels that are possible with this drug and its synergism with certain other antibiotics, such as gentamicin, may make it useful even when in vitro results do not appear promising.

The bacteriostatic and bactericidal activity in the serum or other body fluids of a patient receiving antibiotics can be measured by inoculation of the organism originally isolated from the patient into dilutions of serum obtained at specified times after infection or infusion of antibiotics. The actual concentrations of certain antibiotics in the blood can be measured by immunologic assays or by microbiologic assays using susceptible stock strains of bacteria. These measurements are mandatory when patients with renal disease are treated with aminoglycosides or with vancomycin.

Office Bacteriology

Disposable materials have been developed so that rapid, inexpensive bacterial diagnosis can be made in the physician's office. Kits for detecting streptococci, gonococci, and urinary tract infection by culture are most widely used. The only additional purchase required is a small incubator. Unfortunately, quality control by testing of known positive cultures is seldom practiced, sometimes rendering office bacteriology inaccurate, unless both positive and negative results are periodically confirmed.

Every pediatrician should be able to do throat cultures for group A streptococci in the office to distinguish patients with pharyngitis who need antibiotic treatment from those who do not. A unit for this purpose with a built-in incubator is commercially available. An alternative is a separately purchased incubator and blood agar plates. A bacitracin disk (e.g., Taxo-A) should be placed on the plate after streaking; group A streptococci will usually be sensitive. Kits are now available for direct detection of Group A streptococcal antigens in pharyngeal swabs. Their place in diagnostic bacteriology is being evaluated.

In prepubertal vaginitis and in circumstances suggesting sexual abuse, cultures for gonococci should be obtained. Thayer-Martin medium, the basic medium that is available in convenient form, is selective by means of inhibitors to which some strains of gonococci may be sensitive. All putatively positive gonorrheal isolates should be confirmed at a standard bacteriology laboratory by cultures incubated aerobically in the presence of 5–10% CO_2.

Culture of urine is now simple and inexpensive with disposable units. In the usual outpatient circumstances in which clean-catch urine specimens may be delayed in reaching the laboratory, these units are more accurate than full-scale cultures. Some of the units are based on an agar-coated dipstick placed in the freshly voided urine. In all units the numbers of colonies can be quantitated by inspection and subcultures made for identification and for testing of antibiotic sensitivity. Several available dipstick methods diagnose urinary infection by detecting products of bacterial metabolism.

11.5 LABORATORY DIAGNOSIS OF VIRUSES

If viral disease is a diagnostic possibility when the patient is first seen, immediate steps should be taken to isolate the virus and obtain specimens for serologic evaluation.

Microscopic Observation. Electron microscopy and fluorescent-antibody techniques may provide rapid identification of viruses. Vesicle fluid examined by electron microscopy can distinguish smallpox (a poxvirus) from varicella (a herpesvirus). Smears of mucosal cells or urinary sediment stained by fluorescent antibody can identify the antigens of any virus for which there is a polyclonal or monoclonal animal antiserum, e.g., influenza and respiratory syncytial viruses. The antigens of hepatitis B and the rotavirus agents, which cause infantile gastroenteritis, can be conveniently detected by enzyme-linked immune serum assay (ELISA) or by radioimmunoassay (RIA) using specific antisera.

Cytologic examination aids in diagnosis when inclusion bodies or syncytia are found, for example, in the urine of patients infected with cytomegalovirus, or in the noses of patients with measles. Such demonstrations should be confirmed by actual isolation of the virus.

Isolation. Viruses require living cells for propagation; the cells used may be in live laboratory animals, embryonated hens' eggs, or human or animal cell tissue cultures. Since some viruses are difficult to isolate and many require a variety of culture systems for their isolation, the clinician should specify the type of virus or illness suspected.

Specimens should be delivered to the laboratory promptly. Throat and stool or rectal swab specimens should be submitted routinely. The best throat specimens are taken by vigorous throat swabbing, removing some superficial cells. For certain viruses, e.g., rubella, swabs should be taken from the nasal turbinates. The swab should be rinsed thoroughly in a transport medium containing antibiotics to inhibit bacterial growth, squeezed against the glass, and discarded. If the laboratory is reasonably close, specimens should be transported at 4° C.

Rectal swabs should not be heavily covered with feces since the antibiotics present in viral transport media may be insufficient to kill a large inoculum of bacteria. Rectal swabs should be collected even in respiratory and central nervous system syndromes, since many viruses replicate in the intestine as well as in target organs.

Cerebrospinal fluid is often positive during the acute stages of central nervous system inflammation. A small, extra amount of spinal fluid for viral diagnostic studies should be obtained at the initial lumbar puncture, and can be discarded if bacterial meningitis is diagnosed.

Urine culture for viruses is most useful for the isolation of cytomegalovirus, but urine is also a good source for isolation of mumps and adenoviruses. Urine should not be frozen but rather transported in ordinary ice.

Vesicular fluid can be cultured to distinguish among vaccinia, variola, varicella, herpes, and enteroviruses.

Blood is not routinely cultured for viruses, though viremia is part of cytomegalovirus, enterovirus, and other viral infections. The diagnosis of hepatitis B is made by demonstrating that the viral antigen is present in high titer in serum.

Serologic Tests. Serologic tests may be positive even when virus isolation fails. Correct diagnosis requires at least two blood specimens: the first should be obtained during the early acute phase of the disease ("acute serum"), the second ("convalescent"), 14–21 days later. If the second is taken earlier than 14 days, it is advisable to take a third blood specimen 4–6 wk after the onset, since the rise of antibodies may be delayed, especially in infants. If it is not possible to send blood to the laboratory promptly, serum may be removed for preservation by freezing. Whole blood should never be frozen. To establish the etiologic diagnosis, it is necessary to demonstrate a 4-fold rise in titer of antibody to an agent in the convalescent as opposed to the acute phase serum.

Although finding a substantial titer against a suspected agent in a single late acute or convalescent specimen of serum will not differentiate between a recent and a past infection, the following circumstances can define when single serum specimen studies strongly support a clinical diagnosis: (1) a high antibody level in comparison with that of the population in general; (2) particularly in neonates and in patients in the acute stage of hepatitis A, antibody in the IgM fraction; (3) antibody in the young infant not present in the mother; (4) antibody in both infant and mother that remains at the same level as the infant grows older; (5) in suspected mumps, the presence of antibody to the soluble ("S") fraction of the mumps virus in the acute serum (this antibody may be found as early as 2–3 days of the disease, when antibodies to the viral ("V") antigen may be absent or very low); and (6) in infectious mononucleosis, the presence of antibody to the early antigen found in cells infected by EB virus under specific conditions of preparation.

Methods of Detecting Antibody. Antibody can be detected by a variety of specific serologic methods; some are more appropriate than others for specific viruses. Complement-fixation (CF) antigens are available for a great range of viruses, and CF antibodies have the advantage of correlating with recent infection but may not persist. Neutralizing antibodies, on the other hand, remain for life; unless one has obtained serum early in the disease, a rise may be difficult to show. Furthermore, neutralization tests have the technical disadvantage of needing to be done in tissue cultures or in whole animals. Hemagglutination-inhibition (HI) antibodies correlate fairly well with neutralizing antibodies. Fortunately, many viruses such as the myxoviruses, rubella, and some enteroviruses can agglutinate erythrocytes. The presence of antibodies can be detected by the extent to which a particular serum specifically inhibits hemagglutination. Many of the viruses that agglutinate red cells will also cause red cells to be adsorbed onto the membranes of infected cell monolayers. Inhibition of adsorption is a particularly useful test for parainfluenza virus antibodies. Fluorescent antibodies (FA) can be detected by the indirect fluorescence technique (see above), which requires slides bearing cells infected with the specific virus against which antibodies are being sought. Indirect hemagglutination tests and latex agglutination are now in greater use in virology; these depend on the attachment of viral antigens to glutaraldehyde- or tannic acid–treated sheep erythrocytes or to latex beads. Radioimmunoassays and enzyme-linked immunoassays are also being used more widely.

11.6 LABORATORY DIAGNOSIS OF OTHER ORGANISMS

The diagnosis of *treponemal infection* relies on serologic procedures such as complement fixation, precipitin, and fluorescent antibody methods (Sec. 11.49–11.52). Darkfield examination of lesions of skin and mucous membranes may strongly suggest the diagnosis, but serologic confirmation is necessary. Leptospira can be cultivated directly in special media, but serologic tests are more generally available. Other spirochetes can be visualized directly.

Mycoplasma pneumoniae (Sec. 11.60) is an important cause of pneumonia and can be isolated on agar medium. Serologic tests on paired sera (by complement fixation, for example) are more often positive than cultures. If cold agglutinins are found in the blood, a presumptive diagnosis of mycoplasmal infection can be made, but both false negatives and false positives are common.

Chlamydiae are a cause of pneumonia and inclusion conjunctivitis in the infant (Sec. 11.57) and psittacosis, urethritis, and vaginitis in the sexually active patient (Sec. 11.56). The cytoplasmic inclusion bodies that characterize chlamydiae may be directly demonstrated by Giemsa stain or by FA staining. These organisms can also be isolated in tissue culture.

Ordinarily no attempt is made to culture *rickettsiae* (Sec. 11.85–11.92). Instead, diagnosis relies on nonspecific and specific serologic tests, all of which can be negative early in rickettsial infection.

Diagnosing *fungal disease* is often difficult (Sec. 11.93–11.98). Direct visualization of fungal elements in pus or exudates using various stains is particularly helpful in candidosis, cryptococcosis, and actinomycosis. Culture on Sabouraud dextrose agar is desirable for all fungi; *Candida* and other yeasts also grow well on ordinary bacterial media. Blood and bone marrow cultures are frequently positive in disseminated histoplasmosis.

Fungal serology, including precipitin, hemagglutinating, complement-fixing, and agglutinating antibody systems is widely used. Serologic tests are most valuable in candidosis, coccidioidomycosis, histoplasmosis, and blastomycosis. Cryptococcal antigen can be sought in serum or cerebrospinal fluid by latex slide agglutination.

Protozoan infection (Sec. 11.101–11.109) is identified mainly by direct visualization, for example, of amebae in feces, of *Pneumocystis carinii* in lung aspirates, or of sporozoans in blood. Serologic tests, however, are extremely valuable in the diagnosis of malaria, invasive amebiasis, and toxoplasmosis. Screening for toxoplasma antibodies is widely used to identify newborns with possible congenital infection.

Direct examination of stool or of other materials is the principal method of diagnosis of *helminthic infections* (Sec. 11.110–11.128). When tissue invasion occurs, as in trichinosis, echinococcosis, and toxocariasis, serologic procedures become crucial in efforts to identify the parasite before biopsy. These tests are done at the Centers for Disease Control in Atlanta, Georgia.

STANLEY A. PLOTKIN

Balows A, Hausler WJ: Diagnostic Procedures for Bacterial, Mycotic and Parasitic Infections. Washington DC, American Public Health Association Inc, 1981.

Belshe RB: Textbook of Human Virology. Littleton, MA, PSG Publishing Co, 1984.

Lennette EH, Balows A, Hausler WJ, et al: Manual of Clinical Microbiology. Washington, DC, American Society for Microbiology, 1980.

Lennette EH, Schmidt NJ: Diagnostic Procedures for Viral, Rickettsial and Chlamydial Infections. Washington, DC, American Public Health Association Inc, 1979.

11.7 ISOLATION MEASURES FOR INFECTIOUS DISEASES

The care of a patient with a communicable disease should include measures not only to prevent others from contracting it but also to protect the patient from secondary infection. Usually this involves individually prescribed isolation appropriate to the patient, the situation, and the disease (Table 11–6), rather than arbitrarily applied quarantine measures. *Patients on immunosuppressive drugs* should generally be isolated on "reverse precautions" (protecting the patient from contact with others) at the time of initiating the drug or when their *absolute neutrophil count* falls below 500 mm^3.

Isolation technique necessitates cooperation of physician, nurse, and family, and, in hospitals, of all personnel including those from laboratories, housekeeping, or maintenance who may come in contact with the patient or the patient's environment. An error in technique by any of these persons may defeat the efforts of the others.

The area occupied by the patient—whether a room in the home or an incubator, a room, or space in a ward in the hospital—constitutes a contaminated unit. The space between beds in open wards should be at least 2 m (6 ft). Anything which comes into contact with the unit area must also be considered contaminated. Isolation precautions for persons entering and leaving the unit area are based on "hand-and-gown technique"; all physicians and nurses should be familiar with an approved method. When the child is to be cared for by a nonprofessional attendant at home, adequate instruction should be provided.

Adequate hand washing before and after every contact with an infected patient or with anything in the contaminated area is essential in isolation technique. The clothing of attendants should be protected by clean or sterile gowns for each contact with the patient or contaminated objects. These must be donned, worn, removed, and disposed of in accordance with acceptable technique.

Infectious agents may also be transferred by air conduction. The control of airborne infection is difficult to achieve. Dust may be controlled through use of oils on floors; air sterilization with ultraviolet irradiation or an aerosol has limited effectiveness in reducing the spread of infection in institutions. Antibiotic treatment of bacterial infections is the most effective means for limiting their spread. Spread of *Legionella* through air-conditioning systems may be reduced by appropriate chlorination. Spread of *Pseudomonas* through humidifiers, incubators, and mechanical ventilators may be reduced by the addition of metallic copper to the water reservoirs and by frequent cleansing and changing of tubing.

The patient's unit must be properly equipped, and nothing should be taken into it that is not necessary or that cannot later be destroyed or decontaminated. Trays and dishes—or bottles for infants—should be sterilized after each use by boiling or autoclaving.

A bedpan should be provided for each patient. In the home a special bathroom reserved for the isolated area is a great convenience.

Bed linen and clothing, including diapers, should be adequately disinfected by washing in very hot water with an appropriate soap, detergent, or bactericidal chemical; in the home they should be boiled before being sent to the laundry.

Table 11–6. **Periods of Infectivity of Selected Infections**

Disease	Infective	Recommended Isolation
AIDS (acquired immune deficiency syndrome)	In current state of knowledge persons with AIDS, AIDS-related conditions (ARC), or seropositivity for HTLV-III antibody must be considered potentially infective to sexual and possibly other *intimate* contacts for life	Condoms during heterosexual or homosexual intercourse not proven effective but recommended; blood/body fluid precautions; avoid contact of mucous membranes or open wounds with blood or body fluids of affected persons; isolate affected persons who lack control of body secretions, who have open sores, or who bite others
Chickenpox (varicella)	1–2 days before rash until 5–6 days after onset, and all lesions are crusted; longer in patients with immune deficiency; may be longer in actively or passively immunized patients	Until all lesions are crusted; usually 5–6 days
Diphtheria	2–4 wk; 1–2 days after start of therapy	Until 2–3 consecutive cultures are negative
German measles (rubella)	Seven days before rash to 5 days after; up to 10–12 mo for congenital infection	None, except that women in the 1st trimester of pregnancy should not be exposed, nor should sexually active, nonimmune women in child-bearing years not using contraceptive measures
Hepatitis A (infectious hepatitis)	Variable; in feces up to 3 wk before and after jaundice; may be most communicable 1 wk before and 1 wk after onset of jaundice	Enteric precautions; emphasize personal hygiene; infected mothers may breast feed
Hepatitis B (serum hepatitis)	Variable; probably as long as HBsAg-positive	Blood/body fluid precautions as long as HBsAg-positive; emphasize personal hygiene
Hepatitis NANB (non-A–non-B)	Unknown Blood/body fluid precautions as long as clinically active; emphasize personal hygiene	
Measles (rubeola)	From 5th day of incubation through 4 days of rash	From onset of catarrhal stage through 3rd day of rash
Mumps	Up to 7 days before and 9 days after onset of parotitis or other manifestation	Until swelling subsides
Pertussis	From catarrhal stage through 4th wk	4 wk or until cough has ceased; protect infants from exposure
Poliomyelitis (enterovirus)	Shortly before and after onset; virus in throat for 1 wk after onset, in feces intermittently for 3–4 wk	Enteric precautions
Scarlet fever (scarlatina)	Variable; 1–2 days after start of therapy	One day after start of therapy
Smallpox (variola)	Onset of rash until all crusts are shed	Until all crusts are shed

The *hot* cycle of many home laundry machines is often adequate if the water is 70° C (158° F) or higher.

Secretions from the eyes, nose, mouth, and throat should be received on soft paper squares which are placed in a paper bag and burned.

All attendants should be in good health and free of infection of the respiratory and intestinal tracts.

Patients should be discharged from their units only after thorough bathing, including a shampoo, with soap and warm water. They should not return to the contaminated area.

Other materials, as well as the floor and furniture of the room, should be thoroughly washed with a disinfectant, and the room should be aired for at least 24 hr before being reoccupied.

Material in the unit area that cannot be burned is cleansed as follows: all clothing and linen as already described; mattresses and pillows aired for 6–8 hr, preferably on 2 successive days; all glass, rubber, china, enamelware, and any instruments (which permit it) boiled for 5–10 min, autoclaved, or wiped down with an antiseptic solution.

When a patient is taken to an operating or radiology room or is transferred to another unit, the accompanying attendant must wear a clean gown and the patient should be wrapped in a clean sheet. Equipment in the operating or radiology room that has been contaminated should be cleaned in the manner described for the unit.

R. JAMES MCKAY

DISORDERS CAUSED BY A VARIETY OF INFECTIOUS AGENTS

11.8 DIARRHEA

Diarrhea, one of the most frequent problems encountered by pediatricians (Sec. 4.4, 5.24, 8.63, 11.25, and 12.40), is defined as an increase in frequency, fluidity, and volume of feces; during the first 3 yr of life a child will experience an estimated 1–3 acute, severe episodes of diarrhea. Although most episodes of acute diarrhea subside within 72 hr with fluid administration and diet change, 1–4% of these episodes, worldwide, will be fatal.

Diarrhea may follow invasion of the intestinal mucosa (e.g., *Staphylococcus aureus*, enteroinvasive *E. coli*, *Shigella*, *Yersinia enterocolitica*, *Entamoeba histolytica*) or may be induced by exposure of the bowel to a microbial toxin (e.g., *Vibrio cholerae*, enterotoxigenic *E. coli, Shigella dysenteriae* type 1, *Clostridium perfringens, Salmonella, Staphylococcus aureus*). It also may be induced by adherence of bacteria to the mucosa of the gastrointestinal tract (*E. coli*) or infestation by *Giardia lamblia.*

Viruses are the major cause of wintertime diarrhea in infants. Rotavirus is the etiologic agent in over 50% of cases of acute diarrhea in children; other viruses causing diarrhea include parvovirus-like agents (Norwalk, Hawaii, and Montgomery), coxsackie-, echo-, and adenoviruses. More than two thirds of patients with rotavirus-associated diarrhea have a history of preceding or concurrent respiratory illness with rhinorrhea, cough, erythematous throat, or otitis media; most of these individuals are under 2 yr of age. Food does not appear to be a vector in transmission of this infection.

Common infections extrinsic to the gastrointestinal tract (pneumonia, otitis media) may also be accompanied by diarrhea. Diarrhea also occurs in association with a variety of anatomic defects, endocrinopathies, neoplasms, disorders accompanied by malabsorption, and inherited diseases (Table 11–7).

History and Physical Examination. A chief complaint of diarrhea should first be verified for accuracy (increase in number, volume, or fluidity of stools). The usual clinical manifestations of infectious diarrheas are presented in Table 11–8. A history of recent travel to Latin America may suggest diarrhea related to shigella, enterotoxigenic *E. coli* or amebiasis, and travel to the Rocky Mountains or Soviet Union may suggest giardiasis. A history of blood or mucus in the stool, abdominal pain, tenesmus, fever, abdominal mass, weight loss, or consumption of dairy products or contaminated meats or water should also be sought. The degree of dehydration and state of consciousness should be described specifically (Sec. 5.24). The presence or absence of arthralgia, arthritis, skin rashes, and bradycardia also may suggest var-

Table 11–7. Noninfectious Causes of Diarrhea

Feeding difficulty
Anatomic defects
    Malrotation
    Intestinal duplications
    Hirschsprung disease
    Fecal impaction
    Short bowel syndrome
Malabsorption
    Disaccharidase deficiencies
    Glucose-galactose monosaccharide malabsorption
    Cystic fibrosis
    Hereditary fructose intolerance
    Pancreatic insufficiency
    Abetalipoproteinemia
Endocrinopathies
    Thyrotoxicosis
    Addison disease
    Adrenogenital syndrome
    Hypoparathyroidism
Neoplasms
    Neuroblastomas
    Ganglioneuromas
    Pheochromocytomas
    Carcinoid
Miscellaneous
    Crohn disease (regional enteritis)
    Familial dysautonomia
    Immune deficiency diseases
    Protein-losing enteropathy
    Granulomatous colitis
    Ulcerative colitis
    Acrodermatitis enteropathica
    Niacin deficiency
    Methionine malabsorption syndrome
    Hartnup disease

Table 11–8. Usual Clinical Manifestations of Infectious Diarrheas

	Cholera	Enterotoxigenic E. coli*	Enteroinvasive E. coli*	"Enteropathogenic" E. coli	Shigella Diarrheic Form	Shigella Dysenteric Form	Salmonella	Rota (Reo-like) Virus
Site of action	Small bowel	Small bowel	Large bowel	? Small bowel	Small bowel	Large bowel	Small and Large bowel	Small bowel
Mechanism of action	Toxin	Toxin	Invasion	?	?	Invasion	?	?
Age	Any age	Any age	Any age	<1 yr	>2 yrs	Any age	Any age	<7 yrs
Diarrhea in household	+ +	?	?	0	+ +	+ +	+	+
Season	Epidemic	?	?	Fall	Fall	Fall	Any	Winter
Character of onset	Abrupt	Abrupt	Abrupt	Gradual	Abrupt	Gradual	Gradual	Abrupt
Vomiting	+ (Late)	+ +	0	+	+ +	+	+	+ +
Cramps	+ +	+ +	+ +	?	0	+ +	+	?
Tenesmus	0	0	?	?	0	+ +	+	?
Fever 39° C (102° F)	0	0	+ +	0	+ +	+	0	0
Convulsions	0	0	0	0	+ +	0	0	0
Anal sphincter tone	Normal	?	?	Normal	Lax	Lax	Normal	Normal
Stool: Volume	Large	Large	Small	Moderate	Large	Small	Moderate	Large
Consistency	Watery	Watery	Slimy	Slimy	Watery	Viscous	Slimy	Watery
Odor	Odorless	?	?	Musty	Odorless	Odorless	Foul	Odorless
Blood	0	0	+ +	+	0	+ +	0	0
Mucus shreds	+ +	+ +	+	0	+ +	0	0	0
Pus	0	0	+ +	+	0	+ +	+	0
Color	Colorless	Colorless	?	Green	Colorless	Bloody	Green/Brown	Colorless
Leukocytes	0	0	+ +	+	+	+ +	+ +	0
Bandemia†	?	?	?	+	+ +	+ +	0	0
Duration (untreated)	3–6 days	5–10 days	?	7–14 days	2–3 days	7–14 days	3–7 days	5–7 days

*Based on observations in adults.
†Refers to an increase in the percentage of bands on the peripheral blood smear.
?Insufficient data available.

0 Usually absent.
+ Sometimes present.
+ + Commonly present.

(Table prepared by John D. Nelson, M.D., and J. Patrick Hieber, M.D.)

11.9 ACUTE ASEPTIC MENINGITIS

ious etiologic diagnoses. The clinical findings coupled with a history of fluid intake, the frequency of urination, and an assessment of concurrent stool losses help to determine whether hospitalization is required.

Laboratory Diagnosis. The routine total and differential white blood cell count may be normal, increased, or decreased, but over 50% of the patients have 10–40% band forms in the differential counts.

The stool should be examined for volume, color, and consistency, and for the presence of mucus, blood, and leukocytes. Leukocytes may be noted by mixing a small amount of stool with 1–2 drops of methylene blue; generally, they are not seen when diarrhea is related to disease of the small bowel, but are observed in patients with salmonellosis, enteroinvasive *E. coli*, shigellosis, staphylococcal enterocolitis, *Entamoeba histolytica*, granulomatous colitis (regional enteritis), ulcerative colitis, and pseudomembranous enterocolitis. The stools of various patients should be cultured: patients with fecal leukocytes, hospitalized children, patients with persistent or chronic diarrhea, and individuals who have been exposed to others having diarrhea due to a bacterial pathogen. Examining the stool for ova and parasites should be individually carried out when the history, physical examination, course of the illness, or negative laboratory data suggest that a parasitic disease is possible. A diagnosis of *Giardia lamblia* can be made by examining the stool but may require examining a duodenal aspirate or a duodenal biopsy. Stool may be sent for immune fluorescent microscopy or enzyme-linked immunosorbent assay to confirm a diagnosis of infection by rotavirus.

Examination of stool pH, stool glucose content, and stool chloride concentration may be helpful. If the stool glucose content is low or stool pH is less than 5.5, various noninfectious causes of diarrhea should be considered. However, low stool pH may also be found in children with acquired lactase deficiency that has followed a persistent infectious diarrheal illness. Significant stool chloride losses occur in cholera; chloride losses of greater than 90 mEq/L of stool after fluid and electrolyte balance has been corrected strongly suggest congenital chloridorrhea.

Urine cultures may help in establishing a diagnosis of shigellosis, since this disorder may be complicated by bacteremia and urinary shedding of organisms, or in excluding urinary tract infection as a cause of nonspecific diarrhea. Blood cultures may be helpful in selected patients with salmonellosis or shigellosis.

RALPH D. FEIGIN
MARSHALL L. STOLLER

11.9 ACUTE ASEPTIC MENINGITIS

Acute aseptic meningitis, an inflammatory process of the meninges, is a relatively common illness caused by a large number of different factors. The cerebrospinal fluid is characterized by pleocytosis and the absence of microorganisms on Gram stain and on routine culture. In most instances the illnesses are self-limited; in some, however, the resulting diseases are severe and progressive and lead to disability and death.

Etiology. Etiologic agents and factors in aseptic meningitis are listed in Tables 11–9 and 11–10. Although in many instances the etiologic agent is not identified, clinical and research experience indicates that viruses are usually the responsible agents. Enteroviruses account for approximately 85% of all cases of aseptic meningitis; the most common specific types are coxsackievirus B5 and echoviruses 4, 6, 9, and 11. Other viruses are listed in Table 11–9. Arboviruses

Table 11–9. Etiologic Viruses in Acute Aseptic Meningitis Presented by Frequency of Occurrence in North America

Viruses	Frequency
Enteroviruses (coxsackieviruses, echoviruses, polioviruses, and others)	85%
Arboviruses* (Eastern equine encephalitis, Western equine encephalitis, Venezuelan equine encephalitis, St. Louis encephalitis, Powassan encephalitis, California encephalitis, Colorado tick fever)	5%
Mumps†	2%
Herpes simplex type 2	1%
Adenoviruses	<1%
Varicella-zoster	<1%
Epstein-Barr	<1%
Lymphocytic choriomeningitis	<1%
Encephalomyocarditis	<1%
Cytomegalovirus	<1%
Rhinoviruses	<1%
Measles	<1%
Rubella	<1%
Influenza viruses	<1%
Parainfluenza viruses	<1%
Rotaviruses	<1%
Live virus vaccines (measles, vaccinia, polio)	<1%

*In other areas of world many other arboviruses are important.
†In areas where mumps vaccine is not routinely used, this agent is a common cause of aseptic meningitis.

account for about 5% of cases, St. Louis and California encephalitides being the most common in the United States.

The most common cause of nonviral aseptic meningitis is partially and inappropriately treated bacterial disease (see below). *M. pneumoniae* is also a frequent cause of aseptic meningitis. Of the other etiologies listed in Table 11–10, the following are those most frequently seen: tuberculosis, leptospirosis, parameningeal bacterial infection, toxoplasmosis, Kawasaki disease, and malignancy.

Epidemiology. Since approximately 85% of cases of aseptic meningitis are due to enteroviral infections, the basic epidemiologic pattern reflects that of these agents. Hence, in temperate climates most cases occur in the summer and fall; infection with enteroviruses is spread directly from person to person, and the incubation period is usually 4–6 days. Epidemiologic considerations in aseptic meningitis due to agents other than enteroviruses may also depend upon season, geography, climatic conditions, animal exposures, and many other factors related to the specific pathogens.

Clinical Manifestations. The clinical course is usually characterized at least in part by the signs and symptoms of meningitis or meningoencephalitis (Sec. 11.13 and 11.77). The onset of illness is generally acute, although it may be insidious over a week or so or may be preceded by a nonspecific acute febrile illness of a few days' duration. The presenting manifestations in older children are headache and hyperesthesia, and in infants, irritability and resentment at being handled. Headache is most often frontal or generalized; adolescents frequently note retrobulbar pain. Fever, nausea, and vomiting are frequent, but convulsions are rare. Pain in the neck, back, and legs is common, as is photophobia. Preceding or accompanying exanthems may occur, especially with the echoviruses and coxsackieviruses. Examination often reveals nuchalspinal rigidity without significant localizing neurologic changes.

The manifestations may be limited to the meningeal and/or encephalitic pattern, as often occurs with the nonpolio enteroviruses (Sec. 11.77) and in some encephalitides caused by arboviruses (Sec 11.10); or, in other instances, the acute aseptic syndrome may be a phase, of varying importance, in a wide

Table 11–10. Clinical Conditions and Infectious Agents Other Than Viruses Associated with Aseptic Meningitis

Bacteria; meningitis
    M. tuberculosis
    Pyogenic—inadequately treated
    Leptospira sp. (leptospirosis)
    T. pallidum (syphilis)
    Borrelia sp. (relapsing fever and Lyme Disease)
    Nocardia sp. (nocardiosis)
Bacteria; parameningeal focus
    Sinusitis
    Mastoiditis
    Brain abscess
Rickettsia
    R. rickettsii (Rocky Mountain spotted fever)
Mycoplasma
    M. pneumoniae
    M. hominis
Chlamydia
    C. trachomatis
Fungi
    C. immitis (coccidioidomycosis)
    B. dermatitidis (blastomycosis)
    C. neoformans (cryptococcosis)
    H. capsulatum (histoplasmosis)
    C. albicans (candidosis)
Protozoa
    T. gondii (toxoplasmosis)
Other parasites
    Angiostrongylus cantonensis (eosinophilic meningitis)
    Trichinella spiralis (trichinosis)
Presumed infection
    Kawasaki disease
Malignancy
    Leukemia
    CNS tumor
Postvaccination
    Rabies
    Influenza
    Measles
Immune diseases
    Behçet syndrome
    Lupus erythematosus
Miscellaneous
    Heavy metal poisoning
    Intrathecal injections (contrast media, serum, antibiotics, etc.)
    Foreign bodies (shunt, reservoir)

variety of clinical disorders, such as in tuberculous meningitis, congenital syphilis, leptospirosis, leukemia, and so forth (Tables 11–9 and 11–10). The varied clinical manifestations of enteroviral aseptic meningitis are discussed in Sec. 11.77.

Laboratory Manifestations. The cerebrospinal fluid contains from a few to several thousand cells/mm³; early in the disease the cells are often polymorphonuclear; later they are chiefly mononuclear. No organisms are seen on direct smears (bacteria, mycobacteria, protozoans, nor yeasts), and there are normal to slightly elevated levels of protein. The glucose level is usually normal; decrease in glucose concentration can occur with medulloblastoma, leukemic infiltration, *M. pneumoniae* infection, inadequately treated bacterial meningitis, and tuberculosis and, rarely, with certain viral infections. The spinal fluid should be cultured for viruses, bacteria, fungi, and mycobacteria, and in some instances special examinations are indicated for protozoa, mycoplasma, and other pathogens. Careful examination of the spinal fluid is most important, especially to assure that stains used for smears do not introduce artifacts and that the tests used for glucose levels are accurate. A simultaneous blood glucose level should be taken at the time of spinal puncture. Specimens for viral culture should be obtained from the throat and feces. A serum specimen should be obtained early in the course of illness and then again 2–3 wk later for possible serologic studies. For special laboratory procedures used in the identification of viruses and other agents, refer to the sections on various diseases.

Differential Diagnosis. Careful analysis of the history and epidemiologic circumstances may point toward one of the specific causes listed in Tables 11–9 and 11–10. During the summer and autumn the presence of pleurodynia, herpangina, or unexplained febrile eruptions in the community suggests the possibility of coxsackieviral or echoviral infections; the coexistence of acute paralytic disorders in other patients suggests poliomyelitis; encephalitis in horses points to the possibility of an arbovirus infection; a history of swimming in waters contaminated by urine from infected animals may suggest leptospiral infection. Knowledge of clearcut exposure to or concurrent evidence of mumps or of one of the common exanthems may be helpful in the differential diagnosis.

The association of pneumonia or other respiratory illness preceding aseptic meningitis strongly suggests the possibility of *M. pneumoniae* as the etiologic agent.

Most difficult from the diagnostic, therapeutic, and prognostic points of view are instances of incipient or partially and/or inadequately treated bacterial (especially when due to *H. influenzae*) or mycobacterial meningitis. The clinical findings, the dosage of antibiotic previously used, and examination of spinal fluid by smear, latex agglutination, and other rapid antigen identification tests, culture, and glucose level may be helpful in bacterial meningitis. When tuberculous meningitis is suspected, a careful evaluation of contacts, an examination of an appropriately stained smear from the pellicle of the cerebrospinal fluid that was allowed to settle, and a positive tuberculin reaction may confirm that diagnosis as correct. Although combined bacterial and viral infection occur, examinations of CSF should be repeated when there is evidence of a double infection. The possibility that the observed meningeal reaction is of noninfectious origin should also be considered.

Treatment. Hospitalization is usually necessary because of the possibility of bacterial disease, which should be treated there, and because hydration frequently requires fluid therapy, which can best be furnished there. Treatment is symptomatic. Headache and hyperesthesia are treated with rest, analgesics, and a reduction in room light, noise, and visitors. Antipyretics are recommended for fever. If there is antecedent or concomitant respiratory illness, acetaminophen should be used rather than aspirin because the latter is associated with Reye syndrome. Codeine, morphine, and the phenothiazine derivatives, often used for pain and vomiting but rarely necessary in children, should be avoided since they may induce misleading signs and symptoms.

Several weeks after apparent recovery, careful neuromuscular assessment should be conducted to assure that muscular weakness is not a sequel. Bilateral audiometry is recommended, especially when mumps virus was involved.

Centers for Disease Control: Enterovirus Surveillance Report, 1970–79. Issued November 1981.

Cherry JD: Aseptic meningitis and viral meningitis. *In:* Feigin RD, Cherry JD (eds): Textbook of Pediatric Infectious Diseases. 2nd ed. Philadelphia, WB Saunders, 1987.

Cherry JD: Nonpolio enteroviruses: Coxsackieviruses, echoviruses, and enteroviruses. *In:* Feigin RD, Cherry JD (eds): Textbook of Pediatric Infectious Diseases. 2nd ed. Philadelphia, WB Saunders, 1987.

11.10 ENCEPHALITIS

Encephalitis is an inflammation of the brain, and the diagnosis can be established with absolute certainty only by the microscopic examination of brain tissue. In clinical practice the diagnosis is frequently made on the basis of neurologic manifestations and epidemiologic information without the aid of histologic material. When neurologic manifestations suggest encephalitis but inflammation of the brain has not occurred (such as in Reye syndrome), the condition is called an *encephalopathy*.

Usually when encephalitis occurs, it may be localized or other areas of the nervous system may also be involved, and diagnostic terms reflect this involvement: *acute cerebellar ataxia, meningoencephalitis, and meningoencephalomyeloradiculitis (Guillain-Barré syndrome)*.

Etiology. A classification of encephalitis by etiology and source is presented in Table 11–11. Many of the agents listed produce other illnesses and are discussed more fully elsewhere (see Index). Although only 370 of the 1441 cases of encephalitis reported to the Centers for Disease Control in 1978 had established causes, the seasonal pattern of disease in the United States indicates that the unidentified etiologic agents in the vast majority of cases are enteroviruses (Sec. 11.77) or arboviruses (Sec. 11.80–11.83). Of the 370 identified agents in 1978, 143 were arboviruses; 40, enteroviruses; 80, viruses of the common contagious diseases; and 77, herpesviruses. There was only one nonviral agent, a rickettsia.

Epidemiology. Since there are many different causes of encephalitis, no unified epidemiologic pattern exists. However, the vast majority of cases occur in the summer and fall, reflecting arboviral and enteroviral infections. Encephalitis due to arboviruses occurs in localized outbreaks and epidemics with boundaries determined by the range of particular mosquito vectors and the prevalence of natural reservoir animals. Although enteroviral encephalitis and aseptic meningitis usually occur in epidemics, sporadic cases also occur.

Sporadic cases of encephalitis occur in any season; epidemiologic considerations that must be reviewed in searching for the causative agent include geographic area; climatic conditions; animal, water, food, soil, and personal exposures; and host factors.

Arboviruses are zoonoses in which man, not being essential in the life cycle of arboviruses, is infected accidentally by an arthropod vector. Most commonly mosquitoes or other insects acquire arboviruses by biting infected birds, which often have prolonged viremia without illness. The insect vectors, though preferring birds, bite other vertebrates, including man and horses. Encephalitis in horses and mules ("blind staggers") may be the first indication of incipient trouble in an area; veterinarians are often the first to detect an impending epidemic. Although rural exposure is most common, urban and suburban outbreaks are also frequent.

Eastern equine encephalitis has a predilection for young infants; it is devastating, with high mortality and severe sequelae.

St. Louis virus encephalitis produces inapparent infection (demonstrated only by seroconversion) as well as disease and has a lower incidence of clinical disease in young children than in adolescents and adults.

Western equine encephalitis is frequently mild or clinically inapparent, demonstrated only by seroconversion. Mortality is much lower than with Eastern equine encephalitis, but sequelae may be severe.

California virus encephalitis outbreaks occur mostly in the midwestern United States. Severe illness is common, with important sequelae.

Powassan virus encephalitis is transmitted by the bite of infected wood ticks. More cases occur in Canada than in the United States, few of them in children.

Venezuelan equine encephalitis also occurs in the United States. Thus far the incidence has been low and the illness mild, though devastating outbreaks have occurred.

Enteroviruses (Sec. 11.77) are small RNA-containing viruses; 67 specific serotypes have been identified. The serotypes of poliovirus have become less important as agents of disease among well-vaccinated populations. Not all the coxsackievirus and echovirus serotypes have been definitely associated with neurologic disease. The severity of disease ranges from mild aseptic meningitis to severe encephalitis with death or significant sequelae. Epidemics, some devastating, have been observed among newborns in nurseries.

The *human herpesvirus group* consists of 4 DNA viruses of which man is the sole source: (1) herpes simplex types 1 and 2, (2) varicella-zoster virus, (3) cytomegalovirus, and (4) the Epstein-Barr virus (EBV). Any of these agents can cause encephalitis, as well as their more usual clinical syndromes. These viruses may become latent and induce late neurologic damage as a result of a variety of circumstances that compromise host resistance, especially conditions associated with depressed cellular immunocompetence (e.g., malignancy, immunodepressant drugs, organ transplants).

Herpes simplex types 1 and 2 are relatively frequent causes of sporadic acute encephalitis which may occur during primary contact with the virus or after an earlier primary infection, either subclinical or long forgotten. Herpesvirus encephalitis in newborn infants (Sec. 8.71) is part of a generalized viremia; the infection may be due to either type 1 ("oral") or type 2 ("genital") herpesvirus. In older patients herpes simplex virus may produce diffuse encephalitis or simulate brain abscess or fatal bulbospinal poliomyelitis, even when the patient's serologic status indicates a nonprimary infection. Characteristically, fluid obtained by nontraumatic spinal tap may contain erythrocytes. Progressive focal neurologic signs and evidence of localization by imaging techniques or electroencephalography are frequent and are indications for prompt brain biopsy and early therapy with adenine arabinoside or acyclovir (Sec. 11.65).

Varicella-zoster virus (VZV) may cause acute encephalitis in close temporal relationship to chickenpox. VZV is also capable of secluding itself in spinal and cranial nerve roots and ganglia as a latent or suppressed infection, to express itself later as herpes zoster.

Cytomegalovirus (CMV) may produce intrauterine infection with involvement of the central nervous system (Sec. 8.68 and 11.68). Severe cases may be recognized at birth, but more often subtle evidence of brain damage is not apparent for months or several years after birth. CMV may remain latent in various tissues and in leukocytes. Therefore, blood transfusions may be responsible for transmission of disease. Under situations compromising host immunity, recrudescence may occur.

Epstein-Barr virus (EBV) encephalitis may occur during infectious mononucleosis (11.69) but it also occurs without hematologic changes. There is no evidence that it may become latent in the nervous system.

Pathogenesis. The sequence of events varies with the agent of disease and with the host. In general, the viruses of encephalitis get into the lymphatic system, whether from ingestion of an enterovirus or from a mosquito or other insect bite. There multiplication begins, and seeding of the bloodstream leads to infection of several organs. At this stage (the extraneural phase) a systemic, febrile illness is present, but if further viral multiplication takes place in the seeded organs, a secondary propagation of large amounts of virus may occur. Invasion of the central nervous system is followed by clinical evidence of neurologic disease.

It is likely that neurologic damage is caused (1) by a direct invasion and destruction of neural tissues by actively multiplying viruses, or (2) by a reaction of the patient's nervous tissue to antigens of the virus. Neuronal destruction is probably due directly to viral invasion, while the host's vigorous tissue response probably results in demyelinization and vascular and perivascular destruction. Vascular damage leads to impaired circulation and to signs and symptoms. The deter-

Table 11–11. **Classification of Encephalitis by Etiology and Source**

I. Infections—viral
  A. Spread man to man only
    1. Mumps: frequent in an unimmunized population; often mild
    2. Measles: may have serious sequelae
    3. Enterovirus group: frequent all ages; more serious in newborns
    4. Rubella: uncommon; sequelae rare except in congenital rubella
    5. Herpesvirus group
       a. Herpes simplex (types 1 and 2): relatively common; sequelae frequent; devastating in newborns
       b. Varicella-zoster virus: uncommon; serious sequelae not rare
       c. Cytomegaloviruses—congenital or acquired: may have delayed sequelae in congenital CMV
       d. EB virus (infectious mononucleosis): not common
    6. Pox group
       a. Vaccinia and variola: uncommon, but serious CNS damage occurs
    7. Parvovirus (erythema infectiosum): not common
    8. Influenza A and B
  B. Arthropod-borne agents
    Arboviruses: spread to man by mosquitoes or ticks: seasonal epidemics depend upon ecology of the insect vector; the following occur in the U.S.A.:

Eastern equine	California
Western equine	Powassan
Venezuelan equine	Dengue
St. Louis	Colorado tick fever

  C. Spread by warm-blooded mammals
    1. Rabies: saliva of many domestic and wild mammalian species
    2. Herpesvirus simiae ("B" virus): monkeys' saliva
    3. Lymphocytic choriomeningitis: rodents' excreta

II. Infections—nonviral
  A. Rickettsial: in Rocky Mountain spotted fever and typhus; encephalitic component from cerebral vasculitis
  B. *Mycoplasma pneumoniae:* interval of some days between respiratory and CNS symptoms
  C. Bacterial: tuberculous and other bacterial meningitis; often has encephalitic component
  D. Spirochetal: syphilis, congenital or acquired; leptospirosis; Lyme disease
  E. Cat-scratch disease
  F. Fungal: immunologically compromised patients at special risk; cryptococcosis; histoplasmosis; aspergillosis; mucormycosis; candidosis; coccidioidomycosis
  G. Protozoal: *Plasmodium sp.; Trypanosoma sp.; Naegleria sp.; Acanthamoeba; Toxoplasma gondii*
  H. Metazoal: *trichinosis; echinococcosis; cysticercosis; schistosomiasis*

III. Parainfectious—postinfectious, allergic
    Patients in whom an infectious agent or one of its components plays a contributory role in etiology, but the intact infectious agent is not isolated in vitro from the nervous system. It is postulated that in this group the influence of cell-mediated antigen-antibody complexes plus complement is especially important in producing the observed tissue damage
  A. Associated with specific diseases (These agents may also cause direct CNS damage—see I and II above)

Measles	Rickettsial infections
Rubella	Pertussis
Mumps	Influenza A & B
Varicella-zoster	Hepatitis
Mycoplasma pneumoniae	

  B. Associated with vaccines

Rabies	Pertussis
Measles	Yellow fever
Influenza	Typhoid
Vaccinia	

IV. Human slow-virus diseases
    Accumulating evidence that viruses frequently acquired earlier in life, not necessarily with detectable acute illness, participate in later chronic neurologic disease (similar events also known to occur in animals) (see Chapter 21)
  A. Subacute sclerosing panencephalitis (SSPE); measles; rubella?
  B. Jakob-Creutzfeldt disease (spongiform encephalopathy)
  C. Progressive multifocal leukoencephalopathy
  D. Kuru (Fore tribe in New Guinea only)

V. Unknown—complex group
    This group constitutes more than two thirds of the cases of encephalitis reported to the Centers for Disease Control, Atlanta, Georgia. The yearly epidemic curve of these undiagnosed cases suggests that the majority are probably due to enteroviruses and/or arboviruses.

There is also a miscellaneous group that are based on clinical criteria: Reye syndrome is one current example. Others include the extinct von Economo encephalitis (epidemic from 1918 to 1928); myoclonic encephalopathy of infancy; retinomeningoencephalitis with papilledema and retinal hemorrhage; recurrent encephalomyelitis (? allergic or autoimmune); pseudotumor cerebri; and epidemic neuromyasthenia—Iceland disease.

An encephalitic clinical pattern may follow ingestion or absorption of a number of known and unknown toxic substances. These include ingestion of lead and mercury and percutaneous absorption of hexachlorophene as a skin disinfectant and gamma benzene hexachloride as a scabicide.

mination of how much of the damage to the central nervous system is inflicted directly by virus and how much represents immunologically mediated injury has therapeutic implications; agents to limit viral multiplication would be indicated for the former and agents to suppress the host's cellular immune response for the latter.

The etiology and pathogenesis of cases of inflammatory encephalitis in which there is no evidence of the direct or indirect involvement of any infectious agent are poorly understood.

Pathology. It is difficult to determine the etiology of encephalitis at autopsy, although morphologic identification of falciparum malaria, trypanosomiasis, and fungal encephalitis is possible. In viral encephalitides, the histopathologist may recognize rabies (Negri bodies) or an agent of the herpesvirus group (intranuclear inclusion bodies), but special viral studies are usually needed. Viral isolation and identification require that tissues be collected *without fixation in preservatives*.

Tissue sections of the brain generally are characterized by meningeal congestion and mononuclear infiltration, perivascular cuffs of lymphocytes and plasma cells, some perivascular tissue necrosis with myelin breakdown, neuronal disruption in various stages including ultimately neuronophagia, and endothelial proliferation or necrosis. A marked degree of demyelination with preservation of neurons and their axons is considered predominantly to represent "postinfectious" or "allergic" encephalitis. The cerebral cortex, especially the temporal lobe, is often severely affected by herpes simplex virus; the arboviruses tend to affect the entire brain; rabies has a predilection for the basal structures. Involvement of the spinal cord, nerve roots, and peripheral nerves is quite variable.

Clinical Manifestations. There is a wide range of severity of clinical manifestations even with the same etiologic agent. Some children may appear to be mildly affected initially only to lapse into coma and sudden death. Others may have their illness ushered in by high fever, violent convulsions interspersed with bizarre movements, and hallucinations alternating with brief periods of clarity and then emerge with relatively few sequelae.

Most commonly the initial manifestations resemble an undifferentiated acute systemic illness with fever, headache, or, in infants, screaming spells, abdominal distress, nausea, and vomiting. An associated mild nasopharyngitis is not common. As the temperature rises, there may be mental dullness eventuating in stupor; bizarre movements; convulsions; and nuchal rigidity, often not as pronounced as in purely meningitic illness. Focal neurologic signs may be stationary, progress, or fluctuate. Loss of bowel and bladder control and unprovoked emotional bursts may occur.

Specific forms or complicating manifestations of encephalitis include Guillain-Barré syndrome, acute transverse myelitis, acute hemiplegia, and acute cerebellar ataxia.

Acute cerebellar ataxia is characterized by an abrupt onset of truncal ataxia resulting in varying degrees of gait disturbance. Children with this illness will have tremulousness of the head and trunk when in the upright position and of the extremities when attempting to move them against gravity. The full-blown clinical pattern usually develops over 3–4 days to 1 wk, and the illness may last from a week to several months.

Diagnosis and Differential Diagnosis. A carefully recorded history is essential. It should take into account possible exposures over the past 2–3 wk to illnesses not only in other persons but also in animals (especially horses) and to possible contacts with mosquitos and ticks within remote areas as well as in the local community. Inquiry should also be made about recent injections of biologicals and of the possibilities of exposure to heavy metals, pesticides, or noxious substances.

The cerebrospinal fluid should be carefully examined to exclude other disorders that may respond to specific therapy. Smears for bacteria, appropriate rapid antigen identification tests, and cultures of the cerebrospinal fluid are mandatory; the history and clinical findings may indicate the need for acid-fast stain and culture of the sediment for mycobacteria. Other circumstances may indicate the need for excluding fungal or protozoal infection; atypical cells may require cytopathologic study to exclude neural neoplasms that may have presented acutely.

In viral encephalitis the cerebrospinal fluid is generally clear; the leukocyte count may range from none to several thousand, often with a significant percentage of polymorphonuclear cells initially, moderate or no elevation of protein, and an initially normal concentration of glucose relative to the simultaneously determined blood glucose concentration. Expert advice should be sought early for any patient suspected of having an encephalitic illness; and spinal fluid, blood, feces, and throat swabs should be collected and sent to a laboratory offering viral diagnostic services. An additional serum specimen should be collected 10–21 days later. Though these studies may not provide an immediate diagnosis, they may give early warning of an impending epidemic. If there is evidence for a specific virus, the patient can generally be assured of subsequent lasting immunity to that virus. The therapy also may be indicated by the preliminary results.

A patient with concurrent or recent mumps, measles, etc. (see Table 11–11, I, A) is at increased risk for developing encephalitis, and neurologic involvement may at times precede the development of other manifestations of the disease. For example, when mumps parotitis occurs without clinical evidence of involvement of the central nervous system, cerebrospinal fluid pleocytosis often indicates that such involvement is present; mumps meningoencephalitis commonly occurs without parotitis. In measles, some 40% of patients without clinical evidence of encephalitis have electroencephalograms suggestive of neurologic disturbance. The relation of acute non-neural diseases in early life to debilitating neural syndromes appearing in later life ("slow virus effects") is also important (see Table 11–11).

Occasionally patients who have traveled in Africa or Asia will present with bizarre systemic and central nervous system signs and symptoms from encephalitis due to viruses, trypanosomiasis, or falciparum malaria.

Immunologically compromised children (e.g., by lymphoma, cytotoxic drugs, acquired immunodeficiency syndrome, immunogenetic defects) are at increased risk, especially with respect to infections in which protective cell-mediated immunity is important (e.g., chickenpox, cytomegalovirus, fungal infections). Children with leukemia who have had prophylactic radiation to the central nervous system and intrathecal drugs may develop an acute meningoencephalitis *after* cessation of such prophylaxis and despite bone marrow remission.

Prevention. The widespread use of effective attenuated viral vaccines for measles, mumps, and rubella has almost eliminated central nervous system complications from these diseases in the United States. The control of encephalitis due to arboviruses has been less successful, as specific vaccines for the arbovirus diseases that occur in North America are not available. Control of insect vectors by suitable spraying methods and eradication of insect breeding sites is useful.

Treatment. With the exception of the use of adenine arabinoside or acyclovir for herpes simplex encephalitis (Sec. 11.65), treatment is nonspecific and empirical, aimed at maintaining life and supporting each organ system. The effectiveness of various recommended regimens has not been objectively evaluated.

Until a bacterial cause and, in particular, a brain abscess is substantially excluded, parenteral antibiotic therapy should be administered.

It is crucial to anticipate and be prepared for *convulsions, cerebral edema, hyperpyrexia, inadequate respiratory exchange, disturbed fluid and electrolyte balance, aspiration and asphyxia, abrupt cardiac and respiratory arrest of central origin,* and *cardiac decompensation. Disseminated intravascular coagulation* may be a complication.

All patients with severe encephalitis should be monitored in an intensive care unit (Sec. 5.39). In patients with evidence of increased intracranial pressure, placement of a pressure transducer in the epidural space is often indicated for monitoring intracranial pressure as a guide to therapy aimed at reducing cerebral edema. The risks of cardiac and respiratory failure or arrest are high. All fluids, electrolytes, and medications are initially given parenterally. In prolonged states of coma, parenteral alimentation is indicated. *Inappropriate secretion of antidiuretic hormone* is fairly common in acute central nervous system disorders, so that constant evaluation is required for its early detection. Normal blood levels of glucose, magnesium, and calcium must be maintained in order to minimize the threat of convulsions.

Phenobarbital, 5–8 mg/kg/24 hr, or phenytoin, 5–10 mg/kg/24 hr, may be given in an effort to prevent convulsions. The use of either of these drugs may make clinical assessment of progress difficult, but the importance of preventing convulsions is paramount (Sec. 21.7). If frequent or sustained convulsions appear, intravenous lorazepam (0.1–0.2 mg/kg) in a 3 min infusion may be necessary.*

A number of methods are proposed to minimize cerebral edema and to diminish the consequences of cerebral anoxia; these measures are difficult to evaluate and are generally reserved for patients with very severe illness whose condition appears desperate:

1. *Dexamethasone,* 0.4 mg/kg IV in an initial dose followed by 0.1 mg/kg/dose IV every 4 to 6 hrs is given. This large dose should be reduced gradually after a few days if recovery or improvement is evident. Dexamethasone probably should not be used in acute viral diseases because corticosteroids may potentiate the viral infection.

2. Other substances employed in an effort to reduce elevated intracranial pressure include: (a) *mannitol,* given intravenously, as a 20% solution in a dose of 1.5–2.0 g/kg over a 30–60 min period (this may be repeated every 8–12 hr†); and (b) *glycerol,* by nasogastric tube, using 0.5–1.0 mL/kg diluted with twice that volume of orange juice. This is nontoxic and may be repeated every 6 hr for an extended period of time.

Supportive and rehabilitative efforts are very important after the patient recovers. Motor incoordination, convulsive disorders, squint, total or partial deafness, and behavioral disturbances may appear only after an interval of time. Visual disturbances due to chorioretinopathy and perceptual amblyopia may also make a delayed appearance. Special facilities and, at times, institutional placement may become necessary.

Prognosis. Prognosis is guarded with respect to both immediate outcome and sequelae. Sequelae involving the central nervous system may be intellectual, motor, psychiatric, epileptic, visual, or auditory. Cardiovascular, pulmonary, hepatic, intraocular, and other systems may be permanently affected. The short-term and long-term prognoses depend to some extent on etiology and age. Young infants usually have severe disease and sequelae. In general, herpes simplex viruses carry a worse prognosis for survival and residual disability than do the enteroviruses. Fetal rubella encephalitis is

very ominous, as is acute generalized cytomegaloviral infection accompanied by encephalitis. The latter may be insidious, with evidence of disability deferred for some months.

JAMES D. CHERRY

Bryson YJ: Antiviral agents. *In:* Feigin RD, Cherry JD (eds): Textbook of Pediatric Infectious Diseases. 2nd ed. Philadelphia, WB Saunders, 1987.
Centers for Disease Control: Encephalitis Surveillance Annual Summary, 1978. Issued May 1981.
Cherry JD: Mycoplasma and ureaplasma. *In:* Feigin RD, Cherry JD (eds): Textbook of Pediatric Infectious Diseases. 2nd ed. Philadelphia, WB Saunders, 1987.
Cherry JD: Nonpolio enteroviruses: Coxsackieviruses, echoviruses and enteroviruses. *In:* Feigin RD, Cherry JD (eds): Textbook of Pediatric Infectious Diseases. 2nd ed. Philadelphia, WB Saunders, 1987.
Cherry JD: Viral meningoencephalitis and encephalitis. *In:* Feigin RD, Cherry JD (eds): Textbook of Pediatric Infectious Diseases. 2nd ed. Philadelphia, WB Saunders, 1987.
Monath TP, Tsai T: Arbovirus diseases of North America. *In:* Feigin RD, Cherry JD (eds): Textbook of Pediatric Infectious Diseases. 2nd ed. Philadelphia, WB Saunders, 1987.
Weiner LP, Fleming JO: Viral infections of the nervous system. J Neurosurg 61:207, 1984.

11.11 OPPORTUNISTIC INFECTIONS

The term opportunistic infection has come into increasingly wide use. Formerly it was mainly used to identify infections involving microbial agents that had little or no pathogenicity for the healthy individual but were able to adopt pathogenic roles in debilitated patients. Now it encompasses a broader range of organisms and sites of infection in patients suffering from malnutrition, low birthweight, and a variety of conditions associated with suppression of the immune system and with complications of modern medical care. Opportunistic infections are in large measure due to ordinarily nonpathogenic bacterial, viral, or fungal organisms commonly found in the environment or indigenous to the host. They usually result from an identifiable congenital, acquired, or environmentally induced increase in susceptibility of the host. Infections with common or rare pathogens may likewise be opportunistic in nature. Opportunistic infection should be anticipated as a possibility in every child with a derangement in host defense of any origin.

Decreased Protection by the Skin or Mucous Membranes. The skin and mucous membranes are important barriers to infection. The intact skin can destroy most bacteria with which it may be contaminated, and few microorganisms are able to penetrate it. Table 11–12 lists situations in which the barriers to infection provided by the skin and mucous membranes may be bypassed or compromised, as well as the organisms incriminated most frequently.

Shunts. Infection of the central nervous system occurs in 17–24% of children in whom cerebrospinal fluid is shunted to another site for absorption; the majority of these infections are acquired within the first 2 wks after surgery. With ventriculoperitoneal and ventriculoatrial shunts, staphylococci (65–75%) and gram-negative bacilli (6–19%) are the principal pathogens; gram-negative enteric organisms are responsible for over one third of ventriculoureteral shunt infections, while staphylococcal infections are rare at this site. There may be concomitant septicemia, wound infection, and peritonitis.

Underlying disease, lumbar puncture, ventricular taps, ventriculograms, and ventricular drainage unrelated to shunt surgery do not increase significantly the risk of development of infection. Shunts for renal dialysis and other purposes are also prone to infection.

Fever is an almost constant manifestation of shunt infection; erythema of the skin overlying the tubing used for diversion of cerebrospinal fluid is virtually diagnostic. Irritability and vague neurologic manifestations may be noted. Signs and

*Manufacturer's precaution: Efficacy and safety of parenteral lorazepam in children have not been established.

†Manufacturer's precaution: The use of mannitol in pediatric patients has not been studied comprehensively.

Table 11–12. **Opportunistic Infection in the Host Compromised by Changes in the Skin or Mucous Membrane Barriers to Infection or by Anatomic Defects**

Predisposing Causes: Defects in Anatomic Barriers	Opportunistic Organisms Isolated Most Frequently	Suggested Mechanisms
Cerebrospinal fluid shunts	*Staphylococcus epidermidis, Staphylococcus aureus, Bacillus* spp., diphtheroids	By-pass skin as barrier to infection; act as nidus for infection
Intravenous catheters	*Staphylococcus epidermidis, Bacteroides, Mimeae, Pseudomonas, Candida, Cryptococcus*	By-pass skin as barrier to infection; may serve as nidus for infection
Urinary catheters	*Pseudomonas* spp., *Serratia, Herellea, Staphylococcus epidermidis, Candida*	Serve as nidus for infection and new portal of entry for microorganisms
Inhalation therapy equipment	*Pseudomonas, Serratia*	Serve as new portal of entry; equipment and medication frequently contaminated with opportunistic organisms
Burns	*Pseudomonas, Serratia, Staphylococcus, Candida, Mucor*	Change ecology of skin flora and physicochemical properties of skin; neutrophil dysfunction, abnormal responses to antigenic stimulation, impairment of cellular immune (delayed hypersensitivity) responses
General surgery	*Staphylococcus epidermidis, Pseudomonas, Alcaligenes fecalis, Candida*	Prophylactic use of antibiotics alter normal flora
Cardiac surgery	*Staphylococcus epidermidis,* diphtheroids, *Mimeae, Pseudomonas, Candida, Aspergillus*	Prophylactic use of antibiotics may alter normal flora; foreign bodies inserted may serve as nidus of infection
Dermal sinus tracts	*Staphylococcus epidermidis,* diphtheroids	Skin by-passed as barrier to infection
Congenital and acquired cardiac defects	Viridans Streptococci, *Corynebacterium, Pseudomonas,* nonpathogenic *Neisseria*	Damaged tissue serves as nidus for infection

From Feigin RD, Shearer WT: J Pediatr 87:507, 1975.

symptoms of peritonitis may occur in patients who have had a ventriculoperitoneal shunt procedure. Children with infection of ventriculoatrial shunts generally have bacteremia, whereas blood cultures are less commonly positive and cerebrospinal fluid cultures may be negative in patients with infected ventriculoperitoneal shunts. When fever is observed in a child with a ventricular shunt, multiple blood cultures should be obtained. Direct aspiration of the shunt reservoir is a helpful diagnostic procedure and should be performed.

Hypocomplementemic glomerulonephritis is a well recognized complication of shunt infection. Most commonly, *Staphylococcus epidermidis* has been implicated as the organism associated with this syndrome.

Children with infected shunts should be treated with antibiotics specific for the offending organism. Prior to isolating and identifying the etiologic agent, treatment with penicillin and chloramphenicol should be given to cover for *S. epidermidis,* diphtheroids, and *Bacillus* species. In recent years many strains of *S. epidermidis* have become resistant to both penicillin and semisynthetic penicillin derivatives (methicillin, oxacillin, etc.) but have remained sensitive to cephalosporins. In institutions in which this resistance is a known problem, initial therapy should rather consist of a cephalosporin (cefazolin or cefamandole) and chloramphenicol. Alternatively, therapy with vancomycin and an aminoglycoside may be used. Usually, removal of the infected shunt is required. In fact, sterilizing the shunt with antibiotics alone may merely prolong morbidity and increase the duration of hospitalization. Defervescence occurs within 24–48 hr with immediate shunt removal but may last for a week or more if the shunt is not removed.

The temporal association of surgery with infection of shunts, particularly with staphylococci, has suggested the use of antibiotics prophylactically in the perioperative period, but controlled studies to evaluate their efficacy are not available.

Intravenous Catheters. Bacteremia or fungemia with organisms commonly found on the skin has been reported in 2–5% of patients with intravenous catheters. The infection and colonization rates for intravenous catheters are the same when the catheter remains in place for more than about 100 hr. A higher rate of septicemia is associated with prolonged intravenous catheterization used for total parenteral nutrition.

The hazard of extrinsic contamination can be decreased significantly by inspecting all bottles containing fluid for intravenous administration for cracks and turbidity immediately prior to use and by replacing daily all apparatus used for intravenous administration. Whenever possible, small needles rather than plastic catheters should be used. The intravenous site usually should be changed at least every 4 days.

Bacteremia related to intravenous therapy may occur in the absence of local signs of inflammation. More frequently, however, signs of inflammation or thrombosis are noted at the site of catheterization. When clinical signs suggest infection or when positive cultures are obtained, the suspect catheter should be withdrawn; bacteremia may resolve spontaneously without specific antibiotic therapy. The catheter tip should be cultured when withdrawn and blood cultures should be obtained. If clinical signs or positive cultures persist, appropriate antibiotics should be administered.

Urethral Catheters. Urethral catheterization, particularly with indwelling catheters, bypasses the mucosal barrier and frequently results in infection of the urinary tract (Sec. 17.38). *E. coli* are the bacteria most frequently involved. The elimination of "routine" indications for catheterization is an important preventive measure.

Inhalation Therapy Equipment. Opportunistic infection, particularly during the neonatal period, has been associated with the increasing use of respiratory life support systems. Reservoir nebulizers represent the greatest hazard. *Pseudomonas aeruginosa* and *Serratia marcescens* have been implicated most frequently. Risk of infection may be decreased by effective programs for surveillance and maintenance of respirators, nebulizers, and tubing used for inhalation therapy.

Burns. Opportunistic infections in children with burns (Sec. 5.28) may relate to interruption of the skin and mucous membrane barriers to infection, to long-term administration of antibiotics, and to prolonged intravenous or urinary catheterization. Septicemia with *Pseudomonas aeruginosa, Staphylococcus aureus,* and *S. epidermidis* is frequent. Burn injury has been associated with abnormal immune response to infection, such as neutrophil dysfunction, abnormal responses to specific antigens, and delayed rejection of homografts.

Surgery. Opportunistic infection should be considered whenever fever develops postoperatively. The organisms that may produce disease postoperatively are so varied that no single specific regimen appropriate for all patients can be given, although antibiotic coverage for staphylococci should be included. Cardiac surgery is especially associated with a significant risk of postoperative opportunistic infection, possibly related to extensive use of intravenous and intra-arterial catheters as well as of blood and blood products.

The risk of postoperative surgical infection has prompted many physicians to initiate antibiotic therapy prophylactically. The American Academy of Pediatrics has developed guidelines to reflect an emerging consensus on recommendations for prevention of surgical wound infections by antimicrobial prophylaxis in children.

Systemic prophylaxis is indicated when the benefits of preventing a wound infection outweigh the risks of drug reactions and emergence of resistant bacteria. Procedures in which the benefits justify the risks are those associated either with a significant risk of postoperative infection or those in which the consequences of infection may be catastrophic even if the risk of infection is low. The number of microorganisms within the wound upon completion of the procedure generally determines the probability of surgical wound infection. This has led to a classification of surgical procedures based on estimating bacterial contamination and risk of subsequent infection as follows:

1. Clean wounds are uninfected operative wounds in which no inflammation is noted and the respiratory, alimentary, and genitourinary tracts and the oropharynx are not entered. In addition, the procedure is elective and is one performed as

Table 11-13. Selected Prophylactic Treatment Regimens Useful When Indicated for Surgery or When Skin or Mucous Membrane Barriers Are Disrupted

Predisposing Cause	Prophylactic Regimen	Comments
Congenital or Acquired Cardiac Defects; dental and other procedures of the upper respiratory tract	1. Usual regimen: aqueous penicillin G 30,000 U/kg (840,000 U/m²) with procaine penicillin 20,000 U/kg (600,000 U/m²) IM 30–60 min prior to procedure, followed by penicillin V 250 or 500 mg (depending upon weight) PO q6h for 8 doses, *or* 1.0–2.0 g (depending upon weight) penicillin V PO 30–60 min prior to procedure and followed by 250–500 mg (depending upon weight) q6h PO for 8 doses 2. With penicillin allergy: erythromycin 20 mg/kg (560 mg/m²) PO 90–120 min prior to procedure and then 10 mg/kg (280 mg/m²) PO q6h for 8 doses 3. With cardiovascular prosthesis: parenteral penicillin as outlined in No. 1 above *plus* streptomycin 20 mg/kg (560 mg/m²) given simultaneously, followed by PO penicillin V 4. With cardiovascular prosthesis and penicillin allergy: vancomycin 20 mg/kg (560 mg/m²) IV 30–60 min prior to procedure, followed by erythromycin 10 mg/kg (280 mg/m² q6h PO for 8 doses	Intramuscular injections should be avoided in patients receiving anticoagulants
Gastrointestinal or genitourinary tract surgery or instrumentation	1. Aqueous penicillin G 30,000 U/kg (840,000 U/m²) IV or IM, or ampicillin 50 mg/kg (1.4 g/m²) IV or IM *plus* streptomycin 20 mg/kg (560 mg/m²) IM or gentamicin 2.0 mg/kg (60 mg/m²) IV or IM to be given 30–60 min prior to procedure. If streptomycin is used the dose should be repeated q12h for 2 doses or q8h for 2 doses. If gentamicin is used the dose should be repeated q8h for 2 doses. 2. With penicillin allergy: vancomycin 15 mg/kg (560 mg/m²) q6h IV *plus* streptomycin 20 mg/kg (560 mg/m²) IM with first dose to be given 30–60 min prior to procedure and repeated q12h for 2 doses	
Surgery for obstructive lesions of the urinary tract	Trimethoprim 2 mg/kg (56 mg/m²) and sulfamethoxazole 10 mg/kg (280 mg/m²) qD PO 3 days/wk *or* ampicillin 20 mg/kg (560 mg/m² qD PO *or* nitrofurantoin 2 mg/kg/24 hr (56 mg/m²/24 hr) PO	
Cleft palate surgery	Sulfisoxazole 50 mg/kg/24 hr (1.4 g/m²/24 hr) bid PO *or* ampicillin 20 mg/kg (560 mg/m²) qD PO *or* trimethoprim 2 mg/kg (56 mg/m²) and sulfamethoxazole 10 mg/kg (280 mg/m²) qD PO	
General surgery Head and neck	Ampicillin 20 mg/kg (560 mg/m²) q4h IV *or* cefazolin 12.5 mg/kg (350 mg/m²) q6h IV. First dose is given 30–60 min prior to procedure and treatment is continued for 2 days.	
Cardiovascular	Oxacillin 50 mg/kg (1.4 g/m²) q4–6h IV *or* cefazolin 12.5 mg/kg (350 mg/m²) q6h IV *or* vancomycin 20 mg/kg (560 mg/m²) q6h IV. First dose is given 30–60 min prior to procedure and treatment is continued for 2 days.	

Table continued on opposite page

primarily closed or drained with closed drainage. Operative incisional wounds following nonpenetrating trauma are included in this category. *In clean wounds prophylactic antimicrobial therapy is not recommended except in circumstances in which the consequences of infection are potentially life-threatening (e.g., implantation of a prosthetic foreign body such as a prosthetic heart valve; open heart surgery for repair of structural defects; surgery in patients who are immunocompromised as a result of an inherited disease or are receiving corticosteroids or chemotherapy for malignancy; and newborn infants).* Systemic antimicrobial agents have been recommended empirically for a clean procedure in patients with infection at another site.

2. Clean but potentially contaminated wounds are operative wounds in which the respiratory, alimentary, or genitourinary tract is entered under controlled conditions and does not have unusual contamination preoperatively. These include surgery involving the biliary tract, appendix, vagina, and oropharynx in which no evidence of infection or major break in technique is encountered. In clean but potentially contaminated procedures the risk of contamination is variable. *Recommendations for pediatric patients derived from data on adults suggest that prophylaxis may be provided for procedures in patients with obstructive jaundice and urinary tract surgery or instrumentation in the presence of bacteriuria or obstructive uropathy.*

3. Contaminated wounds include open, fresh, accidental wounds; major breaks in otherwise sterile operative technique; gross spillage from the gastrointestinal tract; and incisions in which acute nonpurulent inflammation is encountered. Dirty and infected wounds include old traumatic wounds with retained devitalized tissue and those in which clinical infection is apparent or in which the viscera have been perforated. *In contaminated and dirty or infected wound procedures, antimicrobial therapy is indicated.*

Prophylactic antimicrobial therapy for surgical procedures need not be initiated until within 2 hr of the surgical procedure (except for cesarean sections). Effective prophylaxis requires adequate concentrations of antibiotics in tissues during the surgical procedure. A single dose may suffice unless the procedure is very prolonged, requiring another dose intraoperatively to maintain adequate antimicrobial concentrations. Duration of antimicrobial prophylaxis may be as brief as 12 hours and should not extend beyond 24–48 hr.

The choice of antimicrobial agents is based on knowledge of the bacteria that most commonly cause infectious complications after a specified procedure, the susceptibility of the organisms likely to be encountered to the chosen drug, and the safety and efficacy of the drug. Effective prophylaxis correlates with a decrease in the total number of organisms within a wound rather than with their complete eradication. Thus, to be effective, the chosen agent should be active against the pathogens most likely to be present, not against every potential organism. Since therapeutic concentrations are required throughout the procedure, the intravenous route of administration generally is preferred. Suggested prophylactic antimicrobial regimens for various types of surgical procedures and for other disruptions in the skin and mucous membrane are listed in Table 11–13.

Dermal Sinus Tracts. Children with dermal sinus tracts that communicate with the subarachnoid space or neural tissue may develop meningitis due to *S. epidermidis* or other microflora of the skin.

Cardiac Defects. Both congenital cardiac defects and those

Table 11–13. Selected Prophylactic Treatment Regimens Useful When Indicated for Surgery or When Skin or Mucous Membrane Barriers Are Disrupted *Continued*

Predisposing Cause	Prophylactic Regimen	Comments
Gastroduodenal with pre-existing abnormal gastric motility	Cefazolin 12.5 mg/kg (350 mg/m²) q6h IV with first dose given 30–60 min prior to procedure and doses are continued for 2 days	Recommended only for patients with acute cholecystitis or ductal obstruction
Biliary tract obstructive disease	Cefazolin 12.5 mg/kg q6h IV or gentamicin 2.5 mg/kg q8h IV. First dose is given 30–60 min prior to procedure and doses are continued for 2 days.	
Colon	Oral: erythromycin 15–50 mg/kg (420–1400 mg/m²) and neomycin 25 mg/kg (700 mg/m²) PO given at 1 PM, 2 PM, and 11 PM the day prior to the procedure Parenteral: cefazolin 12.5 mg/kg (350 mg/m²) q6h IV *or* cefoxitin 40 mg/kg (1120 mg/m²) q4–6h IV *or* metronidazole 15–50 mg/kg/24 hr (420–1400 mg/m²/24 hr) q6h IV	Oral antibiotics are part of a preparative program lasting over several days; the parenteral medication is given in cases of emergency surgery or when the enteral route is prohibited. In cases of "dirty surgery," the antibiotics should be continued for a full therapeutic period
Appendix	Ampicillin 100–300 mg/kg/24 hr (2.8–8.4 g/m²/24 hr) q4h IM or IV, *or* cefazolin 25–50 mg/kg/24 hr (700–1400 mg/m²/24 hr) q6h IV, *or* metronidazole 15–50 mg/kg/24 hr (420–1400 mg/m²/24 hr) q6h IV	
Elective splenectomy	Pneumococcal vaccine prior to procedure	
Cerebrospinal fluid shunts	Methicillin, oxacillin, or nafcillin 100–200 mg/kg/24 hr q4–6h IV to be given for 2 days; first dose 30–60 min prior to procedure; *or* cefazolin 50 mg/kg/24 hr in 4 divided doses IV may be given for 2 days, first dose 30–60 min prior to procedure	
Burns	Penicillin 50,000 U/kg/24 hr (1.4 U/m²/24 hr) q4h IV or q6h PO; *plus* 0.5% silver nitrate solution or 10% mafenide acetate cream to area of burn with dressing changes	

See Table 11–12 for the organisms isolated most frequently and for suggested mechanisms by which infection may be initiated.

acquired through rheumatic fever or surgery, especially intracardiac shunts and prostheses, provide a nidus for opportunistic infection.

Inherited or Acquired Disorders Affecting Host Defense Systems (see also Chapter 10). These disorders, the organisms recovered most frequently, and the mechanisms that may be responsible for the infections are shown in Table 11–14.

Disorders of White Blood Cell Function or Number. Infection in patients with *chronic granulomatous disease* (Sec. 10.31) most often is due to catalase-positive organisms, such as *S. aureus,* many strains of *Pseudomonas, Proteus, Enterobacter, Salmonella,* paracolon bacillus, *Alcaligenes,* and some strains of *Herellea.*

Specific treatment should be dictated by the sensitivity patterns of the organisms producing the infection. When sepsis is suspected, parenteral treatment with a semisynthetic penicillinase-resistant penicillin and with gentamicin is recommended until results of culture are available. Drainage of abscesses is imperative. Continuous prophylactic antibiotic therapy with nafcillin or sulfonamide has been advocated by several groups.

Chédiak-Higashi syndrome has been associated with recurrent pyogenic infection related to defective bactericidal activity and abnormal chemotaxis (Sec. 10.32).

Opportunistic bacterial infection and septicemia have been seen repeatedly in children with all forms of *congenital* and *acquired neutropenia* and in those with a defect in polymorphonuclear leukocyte function. Treatment requires use of antibiotics (preferably bactericidal). Transfusions of white blood cells may be helpful temporarily in selected patients who are critically ill.

Congenital and Acquired Immunodeficiency Syndromes (Sec. 10.4 and 10.23). Disorders involving defective humoral or cellular immunity have been associated with recurrent infection, which are frequently due to opportunistic microorganisms. Treatment depends upon identifying the offending agent. An approach to preventing and treating opportunistic infections in B- and T-cell deficiency syndromes is presented in Table 11–15.

Acquired immunodeficiency syndrome (AIDS) is primarily discussed in Sec. 10.23 but is also presented here because of the importance of opportunistic infections in these patients. Of the almost 7000 patients with AIDS reported to the Centers for Disease Control by December, 1984, 72 were less than 13 yr of age; 50 of the 72 (69%) had *Pneumocystis carinii* pneumonia without Kaposi sarcoma, 4 (6%) had Kaposi sarcoma without *Pneumocystis* infection, and 2 had both. Sixteen (22%) had opportunistic infection with another organism.

Forty per cent of the children having AIDS came from families in which one or both parents had a history of drug abuse. Twelve children had received blood or blood products before the onset of their illness, and 4 had hemophilia. The median age at diagnosis of AIDS was 14 mo (range: 4–46 mo). Transfusion-associated AIDS in children was associated most commonly with transfusion given for medical problems associated with prematurity.

Pneumonia, meningitis, and encephalitis caused by Cytomegalovirus, *Toxoplasma gondii, Aspergillus, Candida, Cryptococcus, Nocardia, Strongyloides, Pneumocystis carinii, Cryptosporidium,* and atypical *Mycobacterium* are frequently reported. Esophagitis due to *Candida,* cytomegalovirus, or herpes simplex virus, progressive multifocal leukoencephalopathy, chronic enterocolitis due to cryptosporidiosis, or unusual extensive mucocutaneous herpes simplex of more than 5 wk duration also occurs. The diseases caused by the organisms that infect patients who have AIDS are described in greater detail in their respective sections of this text.

Cryptosporidiosis, caused by the intestinal protozoan parasite *Cryptosporidium,* is acquired by fecal-oral spread and is a special problem in patients with AIDS (Sec. 11.103). Patients

with normal immune function develop either asymptomatic or self-limited infection, whereas patients with abnormal immune function often develop chronic diarrhea that continues until death. The diarrhea is profuse and watery without blood. Other clinical manifestations of cryptosporidiasis include mild epigastric cramping pain, nausea, vomiting, anorexia, and low grade fever.

There is no effective treatment for cryptosporidiasis. Reversal of the underlying immunodeficiency ameliorates the infection. Hospital personnel caring for these AIDS patients should use isolation procedures similar to those recommended for patients with hepatitis B infections.

Malignancy, Immunosuppression, and Transplantation. Infection is a major problem and may be the terminal event for children with *cancer* (Chapter 16). Therapeutic maneuvers associated with a minimal risk of infection in the normal host (e.g., intravenous infusions, indwelling catheters, transfusions, use of respirators, broad-spectrum antibiotic therapy) become significant hazards to children with cancer.

The single most important factor that predisposes the child with cancer to infection is neutropenia (granulocyte count less than 1000/mm³). Granulocytopenia may be related to the primary disease or be the result of therapy. In some cases neutrophil function may be impaired in children with leukemia, both in relapse and remission, even though the number of circulating neutrophils is normal.

Although any agent may produce disease in children with malignancy, certain patterns emerge. Fever due to septicemia in patients with acute lymphocytic leukemia commonly involves gram-negative organisms, although in recent years the frequency of septicemia due to gram-positive organisms has increased. Protracted fever in patients with leukemia in relapse usually is the result of infection with fungal organisms. The majority of infections in patients with chronic lymphocytic leukemia and multiple myeloma are due to gram-positive organisms. When neutropenia develops in these patients, however, the incidence of gram-negative infection increases. Infections with intracellular organisms (*Listeria, Salmonella, Brucella,* mycobacteria, *Cryptococcus, Pneumocystis carinii*) are most prevalent in patients with Hodgkin disease. The lowest incidence of infection has been reported in children with solid tumors.

Infections also are responsible for significant morbidity and mortality in patients receiving *immunosuppressive therapy* for the management of malignancy, collagen vascular diseases, or transplantation. The microorganisms involved and the location of the infectious process depend, to some extent, upon the underlying disease process. In the immunosuppressed host, infection occurs more commonly with aerobic gram-negative than with aerobic or anaerobic gram-positive microorganisms.

Immunosuppressive therapy is an integral part of the process of *transplantation;* predictably, infections following transplantation are similar to those associated with immunosuppression. However, transplantation and the rejection process per se may also predispose the host to infection. Hill and associates noted that opportunistic microorganisms, including *Pseudomonas, Klebsiella, E. coli,* and staphylococci, were responsible for 75% of infections in a series of 123 patients who had received organ transplants (primarily renal). Infection with cytomegalovirus in recipients of transplanted organs is even more frequent; clinical or subclinical infection with this virus may be seen in 90% of patients at some time following transplantation.

An approach to the treatment and prevention of infection in the host compromised by malignancy, immunosuppression, or transplantation is shown in Table 11–16.

Cystic Fibrosis of the Pancreas. See Sec. 13.97.
Diabetes Mellitus. See Sec. 20.1.

Table 11–14. **Opportunistic Infection in Inherited and Acquired Disorders That Diminish Host Resistance**

Predisposing Causes: Inherited and Acquired Disorders of Inflammation or Immunity	Opportunistic Organisms Isolated Most Frequently	Suggested Mechanisms
Chronic granulomatous disease	*Staphylococcus*, gram-negative enteric organisms, *Serratia*, *Nocardia*	Impaired production of H_2O_2 with defective bactericidal function
Job syndrome	*Staphylococcus aureus*	Unknown
Myeloperoxidase deficiency	*Candida*	Failure to kill *Candida*
Glucose-6-phosphate dehydrogenase deficiency	*Staphylococcus*, *Serratia*	Deficient cellular NADH and NADPH; deficient HMPS activity; decreased H_2O_2 production; defect in bacterial killing
Chédiak-Higashi syndrome	Usual pyogens	Defective bactericidal activity, impaired chemotaxis, neutropenia
Congenital neutropenia	*Herellea*, *Serratia*, *Pseudomonas*, *Staphylococcus epidermidis*	Insufficient number of neutrophils
Complement deficiencies (C3, C3 inactivator)	Pathogens, i.e., *Streptococcus pneumoniae*, *Streptococcus pyogenes*, *Neisseria meningitidis*	Defective chemotaxis; impaired opsonization
Splenic insufficiency	*Streptococcus pneumoniae*, *Salmonella*	Defective opsonization; defective clearing of organisms
Sickle cell disease and other hemoglobinopathies	*Streptococcus pneumoniae*, *Salmonella*, *Edwardsiella*	Reticuloendothelial blockade; defective opsonization
Humoral immunodeficiency syndromes (predominantly B cell defects)	Bacterial pathogens, *Pseudomonas*	Reduced phagocytic efficiency; failure of lysis and agglutination of bacteria; inadequate neutralization of bacterial toxins
Cellular immunodeficiency syndromes (predominantly T cell defects)	*Mycobacterium*, *Listeria*, *Nocardia*, cytomegalovirus, varicella, *Cryptococcus*, *Candida*, *Pneumocystis*, *Strongyloides stercoralis*	Absence or impaired delayed hypersensitivity response; absent T cell cooperation for B cell synthesis of antibodies to T cell specific antigens
Severe combined immunodeficiency syndrome	Many bacteria, fungi, viruses, and *Pneumocystis*	Absence of T and B cell response
Acquired immunodeficiency syndrome	*Cytomegalovirus*, *Toxoplasma gondii*, *Candida*, *Pneumocystis carinii*, *Aspergillus*, *Nocardia*, *Strongyloides*, *Cryptococcus*, herpes simplex, *Cryptosporidium*	Retrovirus infection transmitted by blood that impairs T cell response of the host
Cancer	*Pseudomonas*, *Klebsiella*, *Escherichia coli*, *Listeria*, *Cryptococcus*, varicella-zoster, herpes simplex, *Pneumocystis*, *Mycobacterium*; incidence of infection with gram-negative organism increases in presence of neutropenia	Granulocytopenia; decreased neutrophil chemotaxis; decreased bacterial activity of neutrophils; lymphopenia, defective cell-mediated immunity; impaired antigenic response to challenge
Immunosuppression	*Pseudomonas*, *Klebsiella*, *Escherichia coli*, *Herellea*, *Serratia*, herpes simplex, varicella-zoster, cytomegalovirus, EB virus, papovavirus, hepatitis virus, *Candida*, *Aspergillus*, *Mucor*, *Cryptococcus*	Dependent upon agent utilized
Transplantation	*Staphylococcus*, *Pseudomonas*, *Klebsiella*, *Candida*, *Aspergillus*, *Nocardia*, *Pneumocystis*, cytomegalovirus, hepatitis virus, herpes simplex, varicella-zoster	Probably related to use of immunosuppressive agents
Malnutrition	Measles, herpes simplex, varicella-zoster, *Mycobacterium*	Impaired T cell function; reduction in complement activity; impaired migration of phagocytes; reduced bactericidal activity
Cystic fibrosis	*Staphylococcus*, *Pseudomonas*	Presence of ciliary dyskinesia factor; impaired phagocytosis of *Pseudomonas*
Polyendocrinopathy	*Candida*	Unknown
Nephrotic syndrome	*Streptococcus pneumoniae*, enteric bacteria	Unknown
Uremia	*Bacteroides*, *Serratia*, *Enterobacter*, *Staphylococcus*, *Candida*, *Mucor*, herpes simplex virus, varicella-zoster	Defects in early phases of inflammatory response; lymphopenia; impaired T cell function
Exudative enteropathy	*Streptococcus pneumoniae*, enteric bacteria, *Giardia lamblia*	Low levels of IgG; depressed T cell function in intestinal lymphangiectasia
Inflammatory bowel disease	*Candida*, *Mucor*, herpesvirus, varicella-zoster	Probably not related to basic disease but to use of corticosteroids
Collagen diseases	*Candida*, *Mucor*, *Aspergillus*, *Pneumocystis*, diphtheroids, *Listeria*, *Pseudomonas*, *Serratia*, *Staphylococcus*, *Nocardia*, cytomegalovirus, herpes simplex virus, varicella-zoster	Probably related to use of immunosuppressive agents; may relate to involvement of reticuloendothelial system

From Feigin RD, Shearer WT: J Pediatr 87:677, 1975.

Table 11–15. Infections in the Host Compromised by B- and T-Cell Immunodeficiency Syndromes

Immunodeficiency Syndrome	Approach to Treatment of Infections	Prevention of Infections
Humoral immunodeficiency syndromes (predominantly B-cell defects)	1. Gamma globulin 1.4 mL/kg 2. Vigorous attempt to obtain cultures prior to antimicrobial therapy 3. Incision and drainage if abscess present 4. Antibiotic selection based upon sensitivity reports	1. Maintenance gamma globulin (0.7 mL/kg/mo) administration 2. In chronic recurrent respiratory disease vigorous attention to postural drainage 3. In selected cases (recurrent or chronic pulmonary; middle ear) prophylactic administration of ampicillin or penicillin
Cellular immunodeficiency syndromes (predominantly T-cell defects)	1. Vigorous attempt to obtain cultures prior to antimicrobial therapy 2. Incision and drainage if abscess present 3. Attempt to use antimicrobial agent with the most narrow spectrum 4. Topical and nonabsorbable antimicrobial agents frequently useful	1. Prophylactic administration of trimethoprim-sulfamethoxazole for the prevention of *Pneumocystis carinii* pneumonia 2. Protective environments for some patients 3. Oral nonabsorbable antimicrobial agents to lower concentration of gut flora 4. No live virus vaccines or BCG 5. Careful tuberculosis screening
Combined immunodeficiency syndromes	1. Gamma globulin 1.4 mL/kg 2. Same as T-cell defects above	1. Gamma globulin maintenance 2. Same as T-cell defects above

Modified from Cherry JD, and Feigin RD, *In:* Stiehm ER, Fulginiti VA (eds): Immunologic Disorders in Infants and Children. Philadelphia, WB Saunders, 1980, p. 726.

Table 11–16. Infection in the Host Compromised by Malignancy, Immunosuppression, or Transplantation

Category	Approach to Treatment of Infections	Prevention of Infections
Malignancy	1. Appropriate Gram-stained smears and cultures (blood, urine, CSF, IV sites, wounds) even of minor lesions prior to the onset of therapy 2. When possible choose specific antibiotics for specific etiologic agents (employ bactericidal rather than bacteriostatic antibiotics) 3. When the etiology is not apparent initial therapy should be aimed at *Pseudomonas* and other gram-negative bacilli and *Staphylococcus aureus*; cefazolin and gentamicin (or another aminoglycoside antibiotic to which *Pseudomonas* is sensitive) is a good initial choice 4. Once therapy has been started allow ample time for effect; therapy should rarely be less than 7 days 5. Fresh frozen plasma, whole blood, and leukocyte transfusions are frequently helpful	1. Prophylactic administration of trimethoprim-sulfamethoxazole to prevent *Pneumocystis carinii* pneumonia 2. Avoidance of unnecessary hospitalization 3. Avoidance of antibiotics and catheters unless specifically indicated 4. Protective isolation in the hospital 5. Routine surveillance cultures (throat, stool, and axilla) at regular intervals 6. Use of zoster, vaccinia, and measles immune globulins if exposed 7. Pneumovax may be recommended for children with Hodgkin disease despite impaired antibody response 8. Penicillin prophylaxis should be given to splenectomized patients
Immunosuppression	Same as Malignancy, above	1. Avoidance of unnecessary hospitalization 2. Avoidance of antibiotics and catheters unless specifically indicated 3. Protective isolation in the hospital 4. Use of zoster, vaccinia, and measles immune globulins if exposed
Transplantation	Same as Malignancy, above	Same as Malignancy, above, plus: 1. Reduction of total bowel flora of microorganisms with nonabsorbable antibiotics 2. Removal from diet of items that contain microbial contamination 3. Possible use of special environmental units (laminar air flow rooms) for protective isolation

Modified from Cherry JD, Feigin RD, *In:* Stiehm ER, Fulginiti VA (eds): Immunologic Disorders in Infants and Children. Philadelphia, WB Saunders, 1980, p. 728.

Table 11–17. **Opportunistic Infection in Apparently Normal Children**

Organism	Frequent Types of Infection	Suggested Treatment
Actinomyces israelii	Cellulitis, pneumonia, osteomyelitis	Penicillin; alternate: tetracycline
Aeromonas hydrophila	Abscesses, cellulitis, diarrhea, peritonitis, pneumonia, septicemia, urinary tract infection	Chloramphenicol, gentamicin, kanamycin
Alcaligenes faecalis	Abscesses, cellulitis, otitis media, septicemia	Chloramphenicol, gentamicin, kanamycin
Bacteroides	Abscesses, peritonitis, septicemia	Chloramphenicol; alternate: clindamycin
Fusobacterium gonidia formans	Peritonsillitis, subdural empyema	Penicillin; alternates: tetracycline, erythromycin
Bacillus subtilis	Abscess, cellulitis, conjunctivitis, septicemia	Penicillin; alternate: chloramphenicol
Chromobacterium	Abscess	Carbenicillin; sensitivity varies and should be checked
Diphtheroids	Endocarditis, meningitis	Penicillin; alternate: erythromycin
Gaffkya tetragena	Meningitis	Penicillin
Hemophilus parainfluenzae	Endocarditis, meningitis, otitis media, septicemia	Ampicillin; alternate: chloramphenicol
HB group	Brain abscess, cellulitis, meningitis, otitis media, pneumonia	Chloramphenicol, tetracycline; alternate: ampicillin; sensitivity variable
Lactobacillus	Lung abscess	Check sensitivities
Mimae, Moraxella, Herellea	Cellulitis, conjunctivitis, endocarditis, meningitis, pneumonia, septicemia, septic arthritis, stomatitis	Gentamicin; alternate: kanamycin; oxidase-positive strains may be sensitive to penicillin
Nonpathogenic *Neisseria*	Meningitis, septicemia, otitis media	Penicillin, ampicillin
Nocardia	Osteomyelitis, pneumonia, septicemia	Sulfonamides or sulfonamides plus penicillin
Nonpathogenic *Pasteurella*	Brain abscess, meningitis	Penicillin, chloramphenicol
Pseudomonads	Abscesses, otitis media, pneumonia, septicemia	According to sensitivity studies
Serratia	Diarrhea, pneumonia, otitis media, osteomyelitis	Gentamicin; alternate: kanamycin or chloramphenicol according to sensitivity studies
Nonpathogenic *Spirillum*	Septicemia	Penicillin; alternate: tetracycline or chloramphenicol
Staphylococcus epidermidis	Meningitis, otitis media, osteomyelitis, septic arthritis, septicemia, urinary tract infection	Penicillin, or semisynthetic penicillin derivative if strain resistant to penicillin
Nonhemolytic streptococci	Abscess, cellulitis, endocarditis, gingivitis, pneumonia	Penicillin; alternate: erythromycin, ampicillin, or penicillin plus streptomycin
Vibrio	Abscess, pneumonia, septic arthritis	Chloramphenicol
Aspergillus	Abscess, endocarditis, pneumonia, osteomyelitis	Amphotericin B
Cryptococcaceae	Thrush, pneumonia, meningitis	Amphotericin B

From Feigin RD, Shearer WT: J Pediatr 87:852, 1975.

Protein-Losing or Exudative Enteropathy. This may accompany gastrointestinal infection, *Menetrier syndrome* (protein loss with giant hypertrophy of gastric mucosa), gluten-induced enteropathy, intestinal lymphangiectasia, kwashiorkor, Hirschsprung disease, gastrointestinal neoplasms, allergic gastroenteritis, regional enteritis, ulcerative colitis, jejunal malformations, gastrocolic fistula, angioneurotic edema, post-gastrectomy syndrome, congestive heart failure, constrictive pericarditis, and aminopterin administration. Infection with *Streptococcus pneumoniae*, enteric bacteria, and *Giardia lamblia* occurs with increased frequency in these patients. Increased susceptibility to infection may relate in part to the hypogammaglobulinemia that may result from intestinal protein loss. In patients with intestinal lymphangiectasia, lymphopenia and impaired homograft rejection also may occur.

Opportunistic Infection in the Apparently Normal Host. Infection by saprophytic microorganisms has been increasingly reported in normal, healthy children. The normal individual is at greatest risk of infection by organisms that constitute the indigenous flora of the host or by organisms commonly found in the environment during the neonatal period (Sec. 8.58).

Saprophytic microorganisms that have produced infection in normal children, the types of infection encountered most frequently, and the antibiotic therapy most likely to be effective (to be modified on the basis of specific sensitivity testing) are shown in Table 11–17.

Evaluation and Treatment. The principles are the same as those applied when infection is caused by organisms normally considered to be pathogenic. The physician should suspect and alert the laboratory to the possibility of opportunistic infection in certain clinical situations. In turn, the microbiologist must not regard the isolated saprophytic microorganism as a contaminant, particularly if it is recovered repeatedly from the same patient.

Once appropriate cultures and serologic tests designed to establish an etiologic diagnosis have been obtained, therapy should be initiated immediately. Prior to identification of a specific infectious agent, initial treatment should be guided by the disease process with which the patient is afflicted and the types of organisms most often responsible for infection in these individuals.

Prevention. Prevention is best accomplished by a program that permits the systematic identification of infection in hospitalized patients. Sources of infection and the microorganisms involved must be identified early to permit corrective measures. The principles of infection control should be taught to all individuals with responsibility for patient care. Unrestricted or routine use of antibiotics, particularly for prophylaxis, should be discouraged except in selected circumstances.

Centers for Disease Control: Morbidity and Mortality Weekly Report 33:661, 1984.

Cherry JD, Feigin RD: Infection in the compromised host. *In:* Stiehm ER, Fulginiti VA (eds): Immunologic Disorders of Infancy and Childhood. Philadelphia, WB Saunders, 1980, p 715.

Committee on Infectious Diseases, Committee on Drugs and Section on Surgery, American Academy of Pediatrics: Antimicrobial prophylaxis in pediatric surgical patients. Pediatrics 74:437, 1984.

DeClerck Y, DeClerck D, Rivard GE, et al: Septicemia in children with leukemia. Can Med J 118:1523, 1978.

Donaldson SS, Glatstein E, Vosti KL: Bacterial infections in pediatric Hodgkin's

disease: Relationship to radiotherapy, chemotherapy and splenectomy. Cancer 41:1949, 1978.
Fauci AS, Macher AM, Longo DL, et al: Acquired immunodeficiency syndrome: Epidemiologic, clinical, immunologic, and therapeutic considerations. Ann Intern Med 100:92, 1983.
Feigin RD, Shearer WT: Opportunistic infection in children. J Pediatr 87:507, 677, 852, 1975.
Hill RB Jr, Dahrling BE II, Starzl TE, et al: Death after transplantation; an analysis of sixty cases. Am J Med 42:327, 1967.

Navin TR, Juranek DD: Cryptosporidiosis: Clinical, epidemiologic, and parasitologic review. Rev Infect Dis 6:313, 1984.
Neiman PE, Reeves W, Ray G, et al: A prospective analysis of interstitial pneumonia and opportunistic viral infection among recipients of allogeneic bone marrow grafts. J Infect Dis 136:754, 1977.
Odio C, McCracken GH Jr, Nelson JD: CSF shunt infections in pediatrics. Am J Dis Child 138:1103, 1984.
Schoenbaum SC, Gardner P, Shillito J: Infections of cerebrospinal fluid shunts: Epidemiology, clinical manifestations and therapy. J Infect Dis 131:543, 1975.

BACTERIAL INFECTIONS

11.12 BACTEREMIA AND SEPTICEMIA

The terms bacteremia and septicemia refer to the presence of bacteria in the blood. In *bacteremia*, bacteria are recovered from blood cultures of a patient and may or may not be associated with disease. *Septicemia* is bacteremia associated with active disease, localized or systemic.

In some patients bacteremia or septicemia may be related to focal infection (e.g., pneumonia, osteomyelitis, endocarditis, meningitis), the presence of which can be suspected or confirmed rapidly by history, physical examination, and roentgenographic or other laboratory studies. In such cases, bacteremia or septicemia may be suspected with a high degree of likelihood; cultures should be obtained and administration of appropriate antibiotics started.

A clinical diagnosis of presumptive septicemia should be made when fever and the general appearance of the patient suggest serious illness. Shock and disseminated intravascular coagulation may be noted in patients with septicemia or in those with rickettsial, fungal, and viral diseases. Nevertheless, individuals with these clinical findings should always be managed as if septicemia were present; appropriate cultures should be obtained, and antibiotic therapy should be provided promptly by the intravenous route.

Septicemia without an apparent source of infection occurs most often in the newborn infant or the compromised pediatric host. The pathogenesis, diagnosis, and treatment of septicemia in these groups of infants and children are detailed in Sec. 8.59, 10.40, and 11.11.

Primary bacteremia, however, also occurs in normal infants and children. The precise frequency has not been determined by appropriate prospective studies, but available information suggests it occurs often. Bacteremia in the immunologically normal child without an obvious focus of infection frequently has been due to *N. meningitidis, S. pneumoniae, H. influenzae, S. pyogenes* (group A beta-hemolytic streptococci), *Escherichia coli,* and *Salmonella.* Bacteremia due to *E. coli* is particularly common in newborn infants and in children with pyelonephritis who have no symptoms or signs suggesting infection of the urinary tract. *Salmonella* bacteremia may occur in any child without any other signs and symptoms of salmonellosis but is most likely to occur in children with hemoglobinopathies. Rarely, *Francisella tularensis,* brucellae, and *Yersinia pestis* cause bacteremia in the absence of either symptoms or signs specifically suggestive of these infections.

Pneumococcal bacteremia occurs most frequently, usually in normal children 6–24 mo of age who do not appear to be seriously ill. Signs of an upper respiratory infection may be minimal or absent, and often no other sites of infection are identified. In most patients rectal temperature exceeds 38.9° C and the white blood cell count is more than 20,000/mm³. Blood culture should be obtained from children who fulfill these criteria. Many of these patients will improve without therapy, but the incidence of subsequent otitis media, pneumonia, and meningitis is greater in untreated children with this presentation than in children whose clinical illnesses do not fulfill these criteria. Therefore, children with pneumococ-

cal bacteremia who have not been treated and sent home should be recalled by the physician after receipt of the blood culture results. If they are now afebrile and well upon re-examination, they may be managed at home if the physician is confident that contact with the family can be maintained. Otherwise, another blood culture and treatment with oral penicillin in a dose of 50,000 units/kg/24 hr in 4 divided doses are appropriate. If the second blood culture is negative and the child remains well, treatment may be discontinued after 5 days; if it is positive, treatment should be continued for 10 days.

In a child with untreated pneumococcal bacteremia who reveals a focus of infection upon re-examination, a second blood culture should be obtained and the patient treated with penicillin provided in a dose, route, and duration appropriate to the disease process. If a child with pneumococcal bacteremia is re-examined and remains febrile but no focus of infection is yet apparent, the child should be hospitalized. In the hospital, blood cultures should be repeated and spinal fluid examined. The patient should be treated with aqueous penicillin intravenously and treatment modified subsequently according to the clinical course and results of culture of blood and spinal fluid.

Wright et al documented that most children with fever of 39.7° C or greater (103.5° F) who were over 3 mo. of age did not have bacteremia. A white blood cell count greater than 15,000/mm³ occurred more frequently in children with bacteremia than in those whose blood cultures were negative. The majority of children, however, with white blood cell counts greater than 15,000 cells/mm³ and with fever greater than 39.7° C had negative blood cultures; viruses were the causes of infection in a number of these children. These studies also suggest that a skilled clinician can differentiate as effectively as simple laboratory tests between children who may have bacteremia and those who do not. However, the economic and health costs of the failure to identify the few febrile children with bacteremia are greater than the costs of obtaining blood cultures on all of these children.

When a clinical diagnosis of septicemia is made for any patient beyond the neonatal period who exhibits no focus of infection, the patient should be hospitalized and blood cultures obtained. Examination of leukocyte-rich smears of peripheral blood stained with Gram or methylene blue stain is a rapid test of bacteremia, but the number of positive smears is relatively small compared with the total number of children with concomitantly positive blood cultures. Acridine orange–stained buffy coat smears identify a greater percentage of children with bacteremia or septicemia than does Gram stain of the buffy coat, and the technique requires less blood. A clean voided specimen of urine should be carefully examined and sent for culture. If physical findings are normal, a chest roentgenogram may disclose the focus of infection. If it and the urinalysis are normal, treatment may be initiated with ampicillin and a semisynthetic penicillinase-resistant penicillin (methicillin, oxacillin, nafcillin) intravenously, providing effective coverage for *S. aureus, S. pyogenes, S. pneumoniae,* most strains of *H. influenzae, N. meningitidis,* and *N. gonorrhoeae.*

Chloramphenicol may also be indicated for *H. influenzae*. See Sec. 11.13 for specific dosages, which should be similar to those used for meningitis.

In the compromised pediatric host or in the child with possible urinary tract infection and associated septicemia, a semisynthetic penicillinase-resistant penicillin and gentamicin should be used.

Kleiman MB, Reynolds JK, Schreiner RL, et al: Rapid diagnosis of neonatal bacteremia with acridine orange–stained buffy coat smears. J Pediatr 105:419, 1984.

McCarthy P, Jekel J, Dolan T: Temperature greater than or equal to 40° C in children less than 24 months of age: A prospective study. J Pediatr 59:663, 1976.

Teele D, Marshall R, Klein J: Unsuspected bacteremia in young children. Pediatr Clin N Amer 26:773, 1980.

Wright PF, Thompson J, McKee KT Jr: Patterns of illness in the highly febrile young child: Epidemiologic, clinical and laboratory correlates. Pediatrics 67:694, 1981.

11.13 ACUTE BACTERIAL MENINGITIS BEYOND THE NEONATAL PERIOD

Bacterial meningitis is presented as a clinical entity because its clinical manifestations commonly do not allow the clinician to distinguish among various etiologic agents, and its treatment, general supportive management and often initial antibiotic therapy are usually standard, irrespective of the specific infecting bacteria. The pattern of disease and its treatment during the neonatal period are generally distinctly different from those during later infancy and childhood and are, therefore, discussed separately, but the patterns may merge in early infancy (Sec. 8.59).

The incidence of bacterial meningitis is substantial and increasing (especially that due to *Haemophilus influenzae* type b and group B beta hemolytic streptococci). Mortality and morbidity are significant; reported deaths have decreased only about 50% over the past 50 years compared with 10- to 20-fold decreases in deaths from other infections of childhood.

Etiology. Among the factors that may predispose the host to bacterial infection or alter the response to an invading microorganism, young age is one of the most important. It is essential to remember, however, that most pathogens can produce disease in a patient of any age.

During the first 2 mo of life, the organisms that cause meningitis most frequently are those that reflect the maternal flora or the environment in which the infant has been placed, i.e., gram-negative enteric bacilli and the group B streptocci. An increasing number of cases caused by *Listeria monocytogenes* and *Haemophilus influenzae* type b in the neonatal period is being reported.

Most bacterial meningitis in children 2 mo–12 yr of age is due to *H. influenzae* type b, *Streptococcus pneumoniae*, or *Neisseria meningitidis*. Disease due to *H. influenzae* may occur at any age, but its frequency decreases beyond 5 yr of age. In children over 12, meningitis usually is due to *S. pneumoniae* or *N. meningitidis*. When host response has been compromised or anatomic defects are present, infections with other microorganisms, including *Pseudomonas*, staphylococci, salmonellae, or *Serratia*, become relatively more common than otherwise.

Epidemiology. Bacterial meningitis occurs more frequently in males than in females, especially in infancy. Conditions that lead to an increased incidence of respiratory infection appear to enhance that of bacterial meningitis.

***H. influenzae* Type b** (see also Sec. 11.20). Nonencapsulated strains of *H. influenzae* may be found in the throat or nasopharynx of up to 80% of children or adults; a smaller percentage carry *H. influenzae* type b. Carriage of type b occurs predominantly in children 1 mo–4 yr of age, when the

frequency of disease due to this organism is greatest, but data are insufficient to implicate prolonged carriage with subsequent development of septicemia and meningitis. The annual incidence of *H. influenzae* meningitis in the United States in children under 5 yr of age varies from 3 to 7 per 100,000; among Alaskan Eskimos or Navajo Indians, the annual incidence is as high as 40 and 170 per 100,000, respectively. The peak incidence is at 6–9 mo of age, and half of the cases occur in the first year. The highest attack rates are in November through January, but cases occur throughout the year, and there is a smaller increase in the spring. The risk of such disease occurring in a child exposed within the household or a day-care center to another with the disease is discussed in Sec. 11.20. Otitis media caused by *H. influenzae* type b, particularly if inadequately treated, appears to predispose to development of meningitis, and meningitis is regularly accompanied by bacteremia.

Streptococcus pneumoniae. The risk of developing septicemia and meningitis due to the pneumococcus depends, in part, upon the pneumococcal serotype. Meningitis most commonly is caused by serotypes 1, 3, 6, 7, 14, 18, 19, and 23. The risk is 5.5-fold greater in blacks than in whites, independent of income or population density. Fraser et al suggested that 1 in every 24 children with sickle cell disease may develop pneumococcal meningitis by 4 yr of age; this incidence is 36-fold greater than that in a black population without sickle cell disease and 314-fold greater than in white children.

Meningococcal Meningitis. See also Sec. 11.21.

Pathology. A meningeal exudate of varying thickness may be distributed widely with a tendency to accumulate around veins and venous sinuses, over the convexity of the brain, in the depths of the sulci, in the sylvian fissures, within the basal cisterns, and around the cerebellum. The spinal cord may be encased in pus. Ventriculitis (purulent material within the ventricles) is frequently observed. Subdural effusion and rarely empyema may occur.

Hydrocephalus is an uncommon complication of meningitis beyond the neonatal period. Most often it is of the communicating type and is the result of adhesive thickening of the arachnoid about the cisterns at the base of the brain. Less frequently, the aqueduct of Sylvius or the foramina of Magendie and Luschka are obstructed by fibrosis and reactive gliosis. Ventricular dilatation that ensues may be associated with necrosis of cerebral tissue due to the inflammatory process itself or to occlusion of cerebral veins or arteries.

Vascular and parenchymatous cerebral changes have been demonstrated at necropsy. These include polymorphonuclear infiltrates extending to the subintimal region of small arteries and veins, thrombosis of small cortical veins, occlusion of a major venous sinus, subarachnoid hemorrhages secondary to a necrotizing arteritis, and, rarely, necrosis of cerebral cortex in the absence of identifiable thrombosis of small vessels. Reactive microglia and astrocytes may be identified in the cerebral cortex.

Damage to the cerebral cortex reflecting the effects of vascular occlusion, hypoxia, bacterial invasion or toxic encephalopathy, or some combination of these factors, provides an adequate explanation for impaired consciousness, deficits in motor and sensory function, seizures, and later mental retardation that may be observed.

Pathogenesis. Bacterial meningitis most commonly is the result of hematogenous dissemination of microorganisms from a distant site of infection; bacteremia frequently precedes it or occurs concomitantly. Meningitis also may follow bacterial invasion from a contiguous focus of infection, e.g., paranasal sinuses or mastoids. Bacterial meningitis in children with otitis media generally follows bacteremia, though direct invasion may occur. Infection may spread to the meninges hematogenously in children with infective endocarditis, pneumonia, or thrombophlebitis.

Head trauma may precede bacterial meningitis; recurrent meningitis due to *S. pneumoniae* and *H. influenzae* has been noted following fractures through the paranasal sinuses. Direct invasion of the central nervous system also may occur from dermoid sinus tracts or meningomyeloceles where a direct communication between the skin and meninges is present; the infection is most commonly caused by skin organisms. Meningitis also may follow neurosurgical procedures, particularly those designed for diversion of cerebrospinal fluid, or may be a complication of osteomyelitis of the skull or vertebral column.

Infection of the central nervous system may be the result of special risks. The child with cystic fibrosis or with severe burns may develop meningitis due to *Staphylococcus aureus* or *Pseudomonas aeruginosa*. Children placed in a humidified atmosphere may develop septicemia and meningitis from organisms that proliferate in a moist atmosphere. Indwelling catheters used for parenteral alimentation, blood transfusion, or repeated venipunctures with contaminated equipment (as in narcotic addicts) predispose to infection by bacterial (and fungal) organisms, which generally are of low virulence for the normal host.

Congenital or acquired deficiencies in host response to infection may predispose to bacterial meningitis. Children with sickle cell anemia and other hemoglobinopathies experience meningitis due to *S. pneumoniae* and salmonellae more frequently than do normal children. Children with malignancies, particularly those involving the reticuloendothelial system, are prone to develop meningitis with organisms of low virulence. Central nervous system infection also has been noted with increased frequency in children with malnutrition, diabetes mellitus, and renal insufficiency.

Susceptibility to meningitis with *H. influenzae* type b is not due to a deficiency of bactericidal antibody to this organism. Children with *H. influenzae* meningitis have high titers of bactericidal antibody at the time of admission to hospital, and the titers do not increase during convalescence. However, the quantity of capsular polyribosephosphate (PRP) of *H. influenzae* type b to which the child has been exposed and the duration of exposure correlate directly with the frequency of complications or sequelae of *H. influenzae* meningitis. Antibody against polyribosephosphate appears to protect against *H. influenzae* infection. In general, such antibody is not found at the time of admission of children with *H. influenzae* meningitis, and its development correlates with protection from the disease. Few children under 1 yr of age develop this antibody.

The pathogenesis of subdural effusions in children with bacterial meningitis is discussed in Sec. 21.23.

Clinical Manifestations. Symptoms and signs of bacterial meningitis may be preceded by several days of upper respiratory or gastrointestinal symptoms. In some children, particularly young infants, signs of meningeal inflammation may be minimal; only irritability, restlessness, and poor feeding may be noted. Fever is usually but not invariably present.

Inflammation of the meninges generally is associated with nausea, vomiting, anorexia, nuchal rigidity, and occasionally photophobia. The older child may appear confused and may complain of back pain. Frequently, Kernig and Brudzinski signs are noted. Meningeal signs during the acute illness probably relate to inflammation of the pain-sensitive spinal nerves and roots. Increased intracranial pressure is common and may be reflected by complaints of headache in older children and by a bulging fontanel and diastasis of sutures in the infant. Papilledema is an uncommon finding in acute meningitis; when it is observed, occlusions of the venous sinuses, subdural empyema, or brain abscess should be suspected.

Often, there is inappropriate secretion of antidiuretic hormone. If the patient is given excessive amounts of water, a further increase in intracranial pressure occurs. Signs of excessive brain swelling also may develop, owing to a response to endotoxin.

Seizures occur in about 30% of children with bacterial meningitis. Seizures noted prior to or during the first several days of hospitalization are usually of no prognostic significance. When they are difficult to control or persist beyond the 4th hospital day, or develop for the first time late in the hospital course, permanent neurologic sequelae are more likely to occur.

Stupor, coma, and focal neurologic signs, when present at the time of hospital admission, are poor prognostic signs. The latter include transient or permanent paralysis of cranial nerves; deafness or disturbances in vestibular function, which are relatively common; and involvement of the optic nerve with blindness, which is rare. Paralysis of the 6th cranial nerve, usually transient, is noted frequently early in the course.

Collections of fluid in the subdural space (Sec. 21.23) have been demonstrated in up to 50% of infants during the acute illness. When appropriate corrections are made to normalize differences in age, the incidence of subdural effusion has been shown to be independent of the bacterial type causing the meningitis. The effusions appear to be more frequent in the very young, more readily detectable in infants, or both.

Subdural effusions may cause enlargement in head circumference or result in abnormal transillumination of the skull. Vomiting, seizures, focal neurologic signs, or persistent fever occur in children with bacterial meningitis without subdural effusions so frequently that one can rarely attribute their occurrence confidently to the subdural effusion per se.

Arthralgia and myalgia are noted in many children with bacterial meningitis. Transient arthritis may occur and is most common with meningococcal disease; arthritis may appear 7–10 days after the onset of illness. Joint effusions in these cases generally prove to be sterile; the arthritis presumably is the result of an antigen-antibody reaction.

Anemia due to hemolysis is more common with *H. influenzae* type b meningitis than with meningitis due to other bacteria. Petechial or purpuric lesions may be seen in 50% of children with meningococcal meningitis but also may accompany any infectious or noninfectious disease process in which vasculitis is noted.

Shock may be associated with any bacteremic illness. Profound hypotension has been noted in 9% of children with meningococcal and 5% of children with *H. influenzae* meningitis. Signs of disseminated intravascular coagulation may accompany hypotension in these patients.

Differential Diagnosis. Many of the signs and symptoms described above suggest meningeal or intracranial pathology, but none are pathognomonic of acute bacterial infection. Tuberculous meningitis, fungal meningitis, aseptic meningitis, brain abscess, intracranial or spinal epidural abscesses, bacterial endocarditis with embolism, subdural empyema with or without thrombophlebitis, and brain tumors may present with similar signs and symptoms. Differentiation of these disorders depends upon careful examination of cerebrospinal fluid obtained by lumbar puncture and additional immunologic, roentgenographic, and isotope studies delineated below.

Diagnosis. Lumbar puncture should almost *always* be performed when bacterial meningitis is suspected; cerebral edema may be a rare contraindication. Measurement of pressure is an important component of each cerebrospinal fluid examination. When the pressure is very high, only enough fluid should be removed to permit a careful examination. Compression of the jugular vein should be avoided unless compression of the spinal cord is suspected.

Cerebrospinal fluid should be examined immediately. The number of white blood cells should be determined in a counting chamber, and then, following centrifugation, a differential cell count should be performed on a Wright-stained smear of the sediment. Separate smears should then be made and Gram-stained for bacteria and Kenyoun-stained for mycobacteria.

If the lumbar puncture has been traumatic, a total cell count should be performed. The red blood cells then can be lysed with acetic acid and the count repeated. If the total number of white blood cells compared with the number of red cells is in excess of that in whole blood, one can assume the presence of cerebrospinal fluid pleocytosis.

Cerebrospinal fluid protein should be measured (it is usually elevated in bacterial meningitis). Cerebrospinal fluid glucose should be compared with the blood glucose concentration obtained concomitantly. In bacterial meningitis depression of CSF glucose and of the CSF:blood glucose ratio (normally about 2:3) is the rule.

Treatment of bacterial meningitis with antibiotics prior to initial lumbar puncture usually does not alter markedly the morphologic or chemical results obtained. Generally, in patients with H. influenzae meningitis, cerebrospinal fluid will not be sterilized by prior oral antibiotic therapy; this is not apt to be the case with pneumococcal or meningococcal disease.

Quellung and agglutination reactions can immediately identify various organisms if they are visible on smear and if appropriate type-specific antisera are available. Countercurrent immunoelectrophoresis (CIE) is useful for the rapid (within 1 hr) diagnosis of bacterial meningitis due to H. influenzae type b, S. pneumoniae, and N. meningitidis groups A, C, D, X, Y, Z, and W135. This technique can detect nonviable bacteria. It is imperative to use antisera with the greatest possible sensitivity and specificity in this technique. Cerebrospinal fluid, serum, and urine should be screened concomitantly; results are enhanced if urine is concentrated prior to screening. A negative CIE result does not exclude the diagnosis of bacterial meningitis. Latex agglutination also may be used for rapid etiologic diagnosis of H. influenzae meningitis. This technique, though somewhat more sensitive than CIE, yields false-positive results more frequently than CIE. An indirect enzyme-linked immunosorbent assay for the quantitation of type-specific antigen of Hemophilus influenzae type b also has been described and is more sensitive than CIE or latex agglutination; no false-positive reactions were noted. This test is more difficult to perform than CIE or latex agglutination and more time-consuming (4 hr). The limulus lysate assay may permit the identification of endotoxin from gram-negative organisms within cerebrospinal fluid. When meningitis is suspected, the cerebrospinal fluid should be cultured and a Gram-stained smear made even if it is crystal clear and acellular, since bacteria may be present before pleocytosis or chemical changes become apparent. The fluid should be cultured on a blood agar plate, on a chocolate agar plate, on Fildes or Leventhal medium, and in broth. In some cases a definitive diagnosis cannot be made from either the initial clinical or cerebrospinal fluid findings.

Blood cultures should be obtained in every patient and a thorough search made for foci of infection adjacent to or remote from the meninges. Cultures of the throat and nasopharynx have not been particularly helpful in identifying the pathogen.

When the number of bacteria in the blood is high, a Gram-stained or acridine orange–stained smear of the buffy coat may reveal microorganisms. If petechial lesions are present, a smear of the lesions following puncture with a small lancet may reveal microorganisms on Gram or acridine orange stain.

Roentgenograms of the chest, sinuses, skull, or spine should not be routine but may be helpful in disclosing a focus of infection in selected patients. Radioisotope scanning may also be helpful in selected patients; the pattern of distribution of radioactivity coincides with the accumulation of purulent material (Sec. 5.55).

Computed tomography (CT scan) detects ventricular dilatation, subdural effusion, decrease in brain mass, vascular lesions, and cerebral infarcts. Ventricular dilatation by CT scan may occur transiently in some children who do not develop hydrocephalus following recovery from their disease.

Prevention. *H. influenzae Meningitis.* See Sec. 4.1 and 11.20 for discussion of vaccine administration.

Prophylaxis is indicated for children under 4 yr of age who are family contacts of individuals with H. influenzae disease and for nursery school and day-care center contacts. The institution of prophylaxis in these latter settings may be deferred until two cases of invasive H. influenzae type b disease are noted within a period of 1 mo. Rifampin is the prophylactic agent of choice; the dosage is 20 mg/kg/24 hr once a day for 4 days (maximum dose, 600 mg/24 hr). Ampicillin should not be used because at the time that prophylaxis is instituted the sensitivity of the H. influenzae isolate may be unknown and the rate of eradication of nasopharyngeal carriage of H. influenzae, when these organisms are sensitive to ampicillin, is only 70%.

Meningococcal Infection. The use of chemoprophylaxis is reasonable in all household and day-care nursery contacts of a case of meningococcal infection. Schoolroom and hospital contacts usually are not given prophylaxis. Infections caused by sulfonamide-sensitive meningococci may be prevented by giving sulfadiazine orally in a dose of 0.5–1.0 g twice daily for 3–5 days. The prophylactic dose of rifampin is 600 mg twice daily in 4 doses in adults and 10 mg/kg/dose for 4 doses in children 1 mo–12 yr of age. A dose of 5 mg/kg every 12 hr for 4 doses can be used in children who are less than 1 mo of age.

Penicillin in dosage regimens practical for ambulatory patients has not proved to be effective prophylaxis for meningococcal disease.

Minocycline and rifampin are 80–90% effective in eradicating carriage of meningococci. However, frequent and significant vestibular reactions to even a single 100 mg dose of minocycline limit its prophylactic use. Rifampin-resistant strains may emerge in treated meningococcal carriers.

Four meningococcal polysaccharide vaccines are licensed in the United States: monovalent A, monovalent C, bivalent group A and C, and quadrivalent groups A, C, Y, and W135. An effective meningococcal serogroup B vaccine has not been prepared. A single dose of serogroup C vaccine is about 70% effective for a period of 6–9 mo in preventing meningococcal disease in children who are over 2 yr of age and is recommended in addition to rifampin prophylaxis for children 2 yr of age and above who are exposed within the household or day-care nursery to a confirmed case of serogroup C meningococcal disease. Meningococcal serogroup A vaccine is recommended, in addition to rifampin prophylaxis, for children 3 mo of age and above who are exposed within the household or day-care nursery to a confirmed case of serogroup A meningococcal disease.

Treatment. *Initial Therapy.* Immediate administration of an intravenous dose of 50–100 mg/kg of ampicillin and 25 mg/kg of chloramphenicol is usually indicated for clinically diagnosed bacterial meningitis after lumbar puncture but before laboratory evaluation of the cerebrospinal fluid. In some cases the cerebrospinal fluid may be visibly cloudy and therefore support a suspected diagnosis, since this cloudiness is rarely seen with viral meningitides other than that due to mumps. This is adequate initial treatment for meningococcus, pneumococcus, and most strains of H. influenzae and will prevent a significant number of deaths from the rapid progression of a potentially overwhelming infection.

Subsequent Therapy. The appearance of strains of *H. influenzae* type b resistant to ampicillin has required a change in the subsequent therapy given to children with bacterial meningitis. The identification of strains of *H. influenzae* resistant to chloramphenicol may require further changes in recommended therapy.

Generally, treatment should be initiated with ampicillin and chloramphenicol. Ampicillin is provided intravenously in a dose of 300 mg/kg/24 hr in 6 divided doses. Chloramphenicol is administered separately in a dose of 100 mg/kg/24 hr in 4 divided intravenous doses. If *N. meningitidis, S. pneumoniae,* or *H. influenzae* sensitive to ampicillin is identified, chloramphenicol is discontinued. If an ampicillin-resistant strain of *H. influenzae* is identified, ampicillin is discontinued.

Strains of *H. influenzae* type b that are resistant to ampicillin by a standardized disc susceptibility test should be reassessed by the tube-dilution method. Colorimetric assays permit the identification of β-lactamase production (suggesting resistance to ampicillin) within 15 min. Ampicillin resistance, however, may be mediated by a plasmid that does not affect β-lactamase activity. Thus, some β-lactamase–negative *H. influenzae* are resistant to ampicillin. For this reason, chloramphenicol *should not be discontinued* on the basis of a negative β-lactamase determination. A positive β-lactamase result indicates that ampicillin may be discontinued. Occasionally, both a β-lactamase–negative and a β-lactamase–positive organism can be isolated from the same site or from different sites of the same patient.

The appropriate antibiotic should be continued intravenously until the patient is afebrile for at least 3 days, and total duration of treatment should be at least 10 days for every patient. Although the use of oral chloramphenicol (75 mg/kg/24 hr) after several days of intravenous therapy has been suggested, we recommend using the drug intravenously for the entire course of therapy until data are available on the long-term sequelae of meningitis following use of oral chloramphenicol. If chloramphenicol is used orally after a period of intravenous administration, the patient should be hospitalized to ensure compliance, and serum concentrations should be monitored.

If clinical improvement is noted within 24 hr of treatment, a second examination of cerebrospinal fluid is not necessary. If clinical improvement is slower than anticipated or does not occur, a reexamination of cerebrospinal fluid may be indicated. A lumbar puncture need not be performed at the conclusion of treatment if the course is uneventful. If it is performed, the total number of cells usually is less than 50/mm³ (most are mononuclear). Cerebrospinal fluid protein concentration and the CSF:blood glucose ratio may not have returned to normal at the conclusion of treatment, but Gram stain should show no organisms, and cultures of cerebrospinal fluid should be sterile. Retreatment is mandatory if they are not, and may be necessary if more than 10% of the cells are polymorphonuclear leukocytes and if the CSF glucose or the CSF:blood glucose ratios are less than 30 mg/dL and 30%, respectively.

Strains of *H. influenzae* resistant to both ampicillin and chloramphenicol have been reported. To date, almost all isolates of *H. influenzae* (including ampicillin and chloramphenicol-resistant strains) have been sensitive to moxalactam at 0.25 μg/mL or less and to other third generation cephalosporins. Concentrations of moxalactam within CSF that are at least 4- to 8-fold greater than those required to kill all *H. influenzae* isolates can be achieved at doses of 200 mg/kg/24 hr.

A prospective randomized study comparing moxalactam with ampicillin and chloramphenicol has established that moxalactam (a loading dose of 100 mg/kg/24 hr followed by 200 mg/kg/24 hr in 4 divided doses intravenously) provides safe and effective therapy for *H. influenzae* type b meningitis and can be used in patients whose disease is caused by an isolate resistant to both ampicillin and chloramphenicol. Prophylactically administering vitamin K is recommended once a week, and bleeding times should be determined in patients who receive high doses of moxalactam for more than 3 days. Moxalactam *should not be used alone* as initial therapy for meningitis in children because of its relatively poor activity against *S. pneumoniae* and other gram-positive organisms.

Newer 2nd and 3rd generation cephalosporins (e.g., cefotaxime, ceftriaxone, cefuroxime) have been evaluated in relatively small numbers of children as therapy for *H. influenzae* resistant to ampicillin and chloramphenicol. When these drugs are given in doses of 150–200 mg/kg/24 hr in 4 divided doses intravenously, the outcome is similar to that of treatment with ampicillin or chloramphenicol. Cefotaxime, 200 mg/kg/24 hr in 4 divided doses intravenously, is recommended under these circumstances.

Despite appropriate antibiotic therapy and recovery of the patient, colonization of the nasopharynx by *H. influenzae* type b may persist. The American Academy of Pediatrics recommends that prior to or at the time of discharge, rifampin should be provided in a dose of 20 mg/kg/24 hr for 4 days (maximum dose, 600 mg/kg/24 hr) to prevent introduction or reintroduction of the organism into a household or day-care nursery.

When meningitis is due to *Streptococcus pyogenes* or *agalactiae,* ampicillin, as above, provides effective therapy. If meningitis is due to *Staphylococcus aureus* or *epidermidis* resistant to penicillin, use of oxacillin, methicillin, or nafcillin is indicated; 200 mg/kg/24 hr in 6 divided doses should be administered. The treatment of meningococcal meningitis is described in Sec. 11.21.

Supportive Care. This is vital and is directed toward the anticipation and prevention of complications. Pulse rate, blood pressure, and respiratory rate must be monitored frequently. A screening neurologic examination should be performed at the time of admission and daily thereafter.

Initially, to reduce the risk of aspiration, the patient should receive nothing by mouth, since vomiting may occur. In addition, delivery of all fluid intravenously during the early days of treatment ensures greater accuracy in measurements of intake and output. Every child with meningitis should be evaluated carefully for inappropriate secretion of antidiuretic hormone (ADH), seizure activity, and the development of subdural effusions (Sec. 21.23). Body weight, serum electrolytes, serum and urine osmolalities, and urine volume and specific gravity should be monitored.

If retention of fluid in excess of solute is suspected or documented, fluid administration should be restricted to 800–1000 mL/M²/24 hr. Fluid restriction is continued until it can be established that inappropriate ADH secretion is not a factor or has dissipated. The best indicators of retention of fluid in excess of solute are the body weight and serum sodium concentration. As serum sodium increases toward normal (140 mEq/L), fluid administration may be liberalized progressively to normal maintenance levels of 1500–1700 mL/M²/24 hr.

Head circumference should be measured, and the head should be transilluminated at the time of admission and daily thereafter. These simple techniques may detect possible development of subdural effusions, though an enlarging head may be due to other causes.

Treatment of subdural effusions should consist of subdural paracentesis only to curtail specific symptoms of increased intracranial pressure or to determine whether the effusions may be responsible for seizure activity or for the presence of focal neurologic signs. Usually, no subdural taps are required (Sec. 21.5 and 21.23).

When seizures are noted, a patent airway must be maintained and appropriate anticonvulsants administered. Sodium phenobarbital (7 mg/kg as an initial dose) may be administered parenterally. Seizure control may be sustained with phenytoin (5 mg/kg/24 hr) provided in 2 divided doses intravenously. Phenytoin generally does not depress the respiratory center to the same extent as phenobarbital; it may benefit the patient also by inhibiting secretion of ADH. Phenytoin should not be added to solutions containing glucose, in which this drug will precipitate. To terminate an episode of seizure activity, diazepam (Valium), 1 mg/yr of age to a maximum of 10 mg, may be given intravenously as a bolus.

Heparin therapy should be considered for patients with the syndrome of disseminated intravascular coagulation (Sec. 15.50).

Corticosteroids have been suggested as a therapeutic adjunct that may reduce cerebral edema and inflammation. In two controlled studies, however, steroids had no significant effect on the course or outcome of bacterial meningitis. An acute increase in intracranial pressure may necessitate the use of mannitol (Sec. 21.6).

Prognosis. Appropriate antibiotic therapy reduces the mortality rate for bacterial meningitis in children who are beyond the neonatal period to 1–6%, but as many as 50% of the survivors have some sequelae of their disease. Prognosis depends upon many factors: (1) age, (2) duration of illness prior to effective antibiotic therapy, (3) the specific microorganism causing disease, (4) number of organisms and/or quantity of capsular polysaccharide material present in the meninges and cerebrospinal fluid at the time of diagnosis, and (5) presence of disorders that may compromise host response to infection. For example, the case fatality rate of *H. influenzae* in the United States varies from 2 to 18%, depending on the facilities for rapid diagnosis, treatment, and supportive care. Generally, the younger the patient, the longer effective treatment is delayed, the greater the number of organisms and the larger the amount of capsular polysaccharide in the CSF at the initial lumbar puncture, the worse the prognosis.

Specific sequelae or complications include cranial nerve involvement, deafness, and blindness; hemi- or quadriparesis; muscular hypertonia; ataxia; permanent seizure disorders; and the development of obstructive hydrocephalus, mental retardation, hyperactivity, or language and learning disabilities. *Hearing impairment* can be detected in up to 29% of children following bacterial meningitis; 12% have a hearing impairment that may interfere with normal speech. Several prospective studies now have confirmed that *there is no correlation* between the loss of hearing and either the age of the patient at the onset of meningitis or the duration of illness prior to admission. Loss of hearing occurs early during the evolution of disease in many children and may not be prevented by early diagnosis and treatment. Tympanometry and hearing evaluation are recommended for all children following recovery. *Subdural effusions* (as noted above) are so frequent in young children that most can be considered a part of the general disease process rather than as a persistent or troublesome complication. *Brain abscess* following bacterial meningitis is rare; when it is found, the possibility that it preceded the development of meningitis must be entertained and a careful search for other sites of infection, e.g., endocarditis, should be initiated.

Approximately 40% of children have abnormalities detectable on neurologic examination at the time of discharge, but by 2 yr after discharge specific deficits are noted in only about 10%. In many patients even major neurologic defects such as hemi- or quadriparesis clear with time, suggesting the need to maintain cautious optimism in discussing long-term complications of meningitis with parents.

Bacteriologic relapse may follow treatment of meningitis, particularly that due to *H. influenzae* treated with ampicillin; relapse of *H. influenzae* meningitis after chloramphenicol treatment also has been reported. In almost all such cases failure occurred in patients who received a portion of treatment intramuscularly, a route now known to be unreliable.

Banch J, Fraser DW, Ajells G: Prevention of *Hemophilus influenzae* type b disease. JAMA 25:2381, 1984.

Deal WB, Sanders E: Efficacy of rifampin in treatment of meningococcal carriers. N. Engl J Med 281:641, 1969.

DeLemos RA, Haggerty RJ: Corticosteroids as an adjunct to treatment in bacterial meningitis. A controlled clinical trial. Pediatrics 44:30, 1969.

Dodge PR, Davis H, Feigin RD, et al: Prospective evaluation of hearing loss as a sequela of acute bacterial meningitis. N Engl J Med 311:869, 1984.

Feigin RD, Dodge PR: Bacterial meningitis: Newer concepts of pathophysiology and neurologic sequelae. Pediatr Clin North Am 23:541, 1976.

Feigin RD, Stechenberg BW, Chang MJ, et al: Prospective evaluation of treatment of *Hemophilus influenzae* meningitis. J Pediatr 88:542, 1976.

Gessert C, Granoff DM, Gilsdorf J: Comparison of rifampin and ampicillin in day care center contacts of *Haemophilus influenzae* type b disease. Pediatrics 66:1, 1980.

Kaplan SL, Catlin FI, Weaver T, et al: Onset of hearing loss in children with bacterial meningitis. Pediatrics 73:575, 1984.

Kaplan SL, Mason EO Jr, Mason SK, et al: Prospective cooperative trial of moxalactam versus ampicillin or chloramphenicol for treatment of *Haemophilus influenzae* type b meningitis. J Pediatr 104:447, 1984.

McCracken GH Jr, Ginsburg CM, Zweighaft TC, et al: Pharmacokinetics of rifampin in infants and children: Relevance to prophylaxis against *Haemophilus influenzae* type b disease. Pediatrics 66:17, 1980.

Munford RS, deVasconcelas ZJS, Phillips CJ, et al: Eradication of carriage of *Neisseria meningitidis* in families: A study in Brazil. J Infect Dis 129:644, 1974.

Murata R, and Vemura T: The diagnostic value of cerebrospinal fluid lactic acid levels in meningitis. Folia Psychiatr Neurol Jpn 35:175, 1981.

Peltola H, Kayhty H, Sivonen A, et al: *Haemophilus influenzae* type b capsular polysaccharide vaccine in children: A double-blind field study of 100,000 vaccines 3 months to 5 years of age in Finland. Pediatrics 60:730, 1977.

Peltola HO: C-Reactive protein for rapid monitoring of infections of the central nervous system. Lancet 1:980, 1982.

Pepple J, Moxon ER, Yolken RH: Indirect enzyme-linked immunosorbent assay for the quantitation of the type-specific antigen of *Haemophilus influenzae* b: A preliminary report. J Pediatr 97:233, 1980.

Sell SH: Long term sequelae of bacterial meningitis in children. J Pediatr Infect Dis 2:90, 1983.

Sell SHW, Merrill RE, Doyne EO, et al: Long-term sequelae of *Hemophilus influenzae* meningitis. Pediatrics 49:206, 1972.

Sell SHW, Webb WW, Pate JE, et al: Psychological sequelae to bacterial meningitis. Two controlled studies. Pediatrics 49:212, 1972.

Shackelford PG, Campbell J, Feigin RD: Countercurrent immunoelectrophoresis in the evaluation of childhood infections. J Pediatr 85:478, 1974.

Shapiro ED, Wald ER: Efficacy of rifampin in eliminating pharyngeal carriage of *Haemophilus influenzae* type b. Pediatrics 66:5, 1980.

Steele RW, and Bradsher RW: Comparison of ceftriaxone with standard therapy for bacterial meningitis. J Pediatr 103:138, 1983.

Ward JI, Fraser DW, Baraff LJ, et al: *Haemophilus influenzae* meningitis: A national study of secondary spread in household contacts. N Engl J Med 301:122, 1979.

OSTEOMYELITIS AND SEPTIC ARTHRITIS

See also Sec. 8.61.

Bacterial infections of bones (*osteomyelitis*) and of joints (*septic arthritis*) must be differentiated not only from each other but also from cellulitis; viral, rickettsial, fungal, and parasitic disease of bones and joints; collagen-vascular diseases; rheumatic fever; metabolic disorders; and malignancies.

Early diagnosis of osteomyelitis or septic arthritis in childhood depends upon a high index of suspicion; frequently the initial signs and symptoms may not even suggest an infectious etiology. As many as 30% of children with osteomyelitis are afebrile and have normal white blood cell counts when initially seen. Since chronic infection or other permanent debilitating sequelae may develop if diagnosis and treatment are delayed, appropriate antibiotics should be given prior to definitive diagnosis to children suspected of osteomyelitis or septic arthritis, as soon as cultures of the blood and of the joint and/or bone have been obtained.

Limping is a frequent presenting complaint, but the diagnosis of osteomyelitis or septic arthritis is often overlooked because of the absence of accompanying fever at the time of initial encounter. In one prospective study a diagnosis of osteomyelitis or septic arthritis was established in 25% of all children who presented to an emergency room with the chief complaint of unexplained limp. Unless some other reasonable explanation for limp can be established, a diagnosis of bone or joint infection must be seriously considered. Close observation, in the hospital if necessary, is essential until the diagnosis is clarified.

11.14 OSTEOMYELITIS

Acute osteomyelitis may occur at any age, but most often between 3 and 12 yr. It is twice as frequent in boys as in girls.

Etiology. Although coagulase-positive staphylococci are responsible for most infections, the proportion of infections caused by other organisms, particularly *H. influenzae* type b, the group B beta-hemolytic streptococcus, anaerobic microorganisms, and gram-negative enteric bacteria, may be increasing. *Mycobacterium tuberculosis* and coccobacilli of the HB group also cause osteomyelitis. Infectious lesions or other factors that predispose to the development of osteomyelitis include impetigo, furunculosis, infected lesions of varicella, infected burns, prolonged intravenous or central parenteral alimentation, drug addiction, and direct trauma to an area adjacent to the site of osteomyelitis. Patients with sickle cell disease and other hemoglobinopathies are particularly prone to osteomyelitis caused by salmonella or *Streptococcus pneumoniae*. Osteomyelitis secondary to dog or cat bites may be caused by *Pasteurella multocida*. *Pseudomonas* osteomyelitis most commonly follows puncture wounds of the foot.

Pathogenesis and Pathology. Osteomyelitis generally begins as a hematogenous abscess in the metaphysis. Subsequently, if untreated, this abscess ruptures subperiosteally, spreading along the shaft of the bone and possibly penetrating to the marrow cavity. The periosteum may separate and form a shell of new bone about the infected portion of the shaft. Pieces of dead bone are known as *sequestra*, and the new bone formed by the periosteum is known as an *involucrum*. In some cases the infectious process in the metaphysis ruptures into the joint cavity and a secondary suppurative arthritis develops.

Osteomyelitis is most commonly hematogenous in origin but may be secondary to direct invasion from a neighboring infected traumatic lesion or from an area of cellulitis. In infants osteomyelitis frequently is associated with septic arthritis (Sec. 8.61).

Clinical Manifestations. These vary with the age of the child affected and depend upon the differing nature of the vascular pattern of bone in infants up to 1 yr of age (Sec. 8.61), in children, and in adults. The course in older infants and young children may occasionally resemble that in the neonatal infant.

Hematogenous osteomyelitis in children beyond the neonatal period may occur as an abrupt illness with fever and systemic signs of toxicity or as a subacute illness in which local complaints at the site of involved bone dominate the clinical picture. Osteomyelitis localizes most often in the long bones. Osteomyelitis of the pelvis and small bones of the hands and feet, however, occurs with some frequency. There may be associated swelling, erythema, tenderness, and decreased movement of the involved part. When these findings are coupled with an elevated white blood cell count, elevated erythrocyte sedimentation rate, and roentgenographic evidence of bone disease, the diagnosis is established readily. In some patients, septic thrombophlebitis is associated with acute osteomyelitis. An increasing proportion of patients are presenting with less striking clinical findings, possibly reflecting suppression of disease by antibiotics administered for

another reason. Hematogenous osteomyelitis may involve the vertebrae. Clinically, vertebral osteomyelitis is notable because it has an insidious onset, vague symptomatology, and little or no associated fever or systemic toxicity. Patients may complain of back pain for several weeks with no other findings. Osteomyelitis of the cervical vertebrae may be manifested as torticollis. Vertebral osteomyelitis due to *Pseudomonas* has been reported among heroin addicts. Osteomyelitis of the pubis also has been described in patients who abuse drugs parenterally.

Diagnosis. Careful examination may reveal marked tenderness over the involved bone; the tender areas may be small and sharply defined. The total white blood cell count may be elevated but is normal so frequently that it is of no help in diagnosis. The erythrocyte sedimentation rate, although a nonspecific finding, frequently is elevated and is of help in monitoring the progress of the patient as well as in supporting the diagnosis.

Cultures of blood, of an aspirate of the soft tissue if there is cellulitis, and of the suspected site of bone involvement should be obtained prior to institution of antibiotic therapy. A tuberculin test should also be administered. A chest roentgenogram may be indicated for evidence of granulomatous disease, particularly with subacute or chronic osteomyelitis. Roentgenograms of the affected areas should be obtained but generally are normal during the acute phase (10–14 days). The radionuclide bone scan (Sec. 5.55), particularly with technetium-99m, is valuable in establishing a diagnosis of osteomyelitis in the face of negative roentgenographic studies and a normal white blood cell count. However, radionuclide imaging has several limitations; areas of increased uptake may be detected roentgenologically at an early stage of septicemia due to *S. aureus*, in which progression to osteomyelitis may not occur. Osteomyelitis has also been documented bacteriologically and histologically when bone scans were initially negative. Radionuclide imaging does not consistently permit the differentiation of cellulitis from osteomyelitis. Bone scanning with Tc-99m–polyphosphate performed following a fracture or bone surgery does not distinguish between bone repair and infection. Scanning with gallium-67 citrate may allow detection of osteomyelitis early and may be positive even when a Tc-99m–polyphosphate scan is negative since it accumulates in inflammatory exudates. Scans may remain positive for extended periods of time despite effective therapy; thus the extent of healing cannot be ascertained by scanning. Magnetic resonance imaging may reveal the existence of acute, subacute, or chronic osteomyelitis prior to changes in bone roentgenograms and at a time when computed tomographic and radionuclide studies are normal or equivocal.

Differential Diagnosis. Other disorders may mimic acute osteomyelitis: neoplastic diseases; histiocytosis; pancreatitis with lytic lesions of bone; scurvy; deep cellulitis; viral, rickettsial, fungal, and parasitic diseases of bones and joints; collagen-vascular diseases; rheumatic fever; metabolic disorders; and malignancies.

Treatment. Standard therapy consists of parenteral administration of antibiotics for 4–6 wk or longer. When administered systemically, the penicillins and cephalosporins penetrate infected bones adequately. The tissue concentrations of antibiotic obtained are independent of binding by serum protein and with appropriate dosage are several-fold greater than the minimal bactericidal concentrations for the commonly encountered pathogens. Management of suppurative bone infection may also include symptomatic therapy, immobilization in some cases, and adequate drainage of purulent material.

Treatment should be started as soon as the appropriate diagnostic studies are concluded. The initial choice of antibiotic may be based on the results of Gram stain of bone aspirate or biopsy and on other clinical considerations. Initial coverage should always be provided for penicillinase-producing staphylococci. In selected cases consideration may be given to treatment effective against the group B *Streptococcus* and *H. influenzae*. In patients with sickle cell disease, coverage for *Salmonella* and pneumococcus must be considered. Gram-negative enteric organisms may be present if there are soil-contaminated contiguous wounds. *Pseudomonas aeruginosa* should be considered in drug addicts, and *Candida, Aspergillus,* and *Rhizopus* in patients having compromised host defenses or receiving long-term parenteral hyperalimentation.

Recommended treatment for *Staphylococcus aureus* usually consists of methicillin, oxacillin, or nafcillin, in a dose of 200 mg/kg/24 hr in 6 divided doses *intravenously* for 4 wk; when such therapy has been provided, a treatment failure rate of 4% or less generally is found. In children who receive 3 wk of intravenous methicillin therapy, a 19% failure rate or progression to chronic osteomyelitis or to recurrent disease has been reported. After the 4-wk recommended period of treatment, decision to discontinue therapy should be based upon review of the course of the patient, roentgenographic evidence of healing, and a sedimentation rate that has returned to normal. Oral therapy may be provided after 4 wk of intravenous therapy for certain patients who are doing well but who have a persistently elevated erythrocyte sedimentation rate. In these patients dicloxacillin at a dose of 75 mg/kg/24 hr or oxacillin in a dose of 100–150 mg/kg/24 hr should provide adequate levels in bone.

Theoretically, it is possible to obtain serum levels of anti-staphylococcal antibiotics 10–20 times the minimal inhibitory concentration for the organism with high oral doses of certain antibiotics. This treatment has the advantage of shortening hospitalization significantly, but tolerance of the oral dose, compliance, and adequate follow-up, if the patient is discharged from the hospital, pose major problems. After an initial period of intravenous antibiotic therapy for 5–7 days, patients may be treated adequately by the oral route. Clindamycin in a dose of 30 mg/kg/24 hr, dicloxacillin 50–75 mg/kg/24 hr, cephalexin 100 mg/kg/24 hr, penicillin V 100 mg/kg/24 hr, and ampicillin 100 mg/kg/24 hr all have been demonstrated to provide adequate oral treatment of staphylococcal osteomyelitis.

Inadequate antibiotic therapy of osteomyelitis often leads to chronic disease and permanent orthopedic deformity. Therefore, if antibiotics are to be administered orally, the following conditions should exist: (1) patients should be hospitalized for the entire period of antibiotic therapy; (2) antibiotics should be provided parenterally for an initial period of 5–7 days; (3) satisfactory activity of the orally administered drug in vitro against the organism isolated from the individual patient must be demonstrated. Absorption of the oral drug should be assessed by measuring the patient's *serum bactericidal activity* against the pathogen. Dosage must be tailored to achieve a peak bactericidal titer of at least 1:8–1:16. The total duration of therapy must be based upon the clinical response of the patient, roentgenographic findings, and return of the sedimentation rate to 20 mm/hr or less. After antibiotics have been discontinued, patients may be discharged from the hospital but should be followed closely for the possibility of recurrence of disease.

Optimal treatment for subacute or chronic osteomyelitis has not been established. Adequate surgical excision of areas of necrotic bone is a critical component in the management of chronic osteomyelitis. Since antibiotics frequently must be provided for months or years, oral therapy at home may be the only practical mode of treatment. The addition of oral rifampin to other antibiotics has been of value in selected patients with chronic osteomyelitis due to *S. aureus*.

Prognosis. In appropriately managed patients, the prognosis of acute osteomyelitis has improved significantly. Progression to chronic disease is rare, as is mortality.

11.15 SEPTIC ARTHRITIS

Septic arthritis occurs most commonly during the 1st yr of life. It frequently follows infection of the skin or upper respiratory tract. Neonatal infection is discussed in Sec. 8.61.

Etiology. Staphylococci are frequent etiologic agents in all age groups. In the 2 mo to 4 yr old child, *Haemophilus influenzae* type b is now the most frequent etiologic agent, followed by staphylococci, streptococci, pneumococci, and meningococci. Primary meningococcal arthritis may occur in the absence of meningococcemia or meningitis. Beyond 2 yr of age, *S. aureus* predominates, though a great variety of other organisms may be involved. Sexually active adolescents may develop gonococcal arthritis or, occasionally, sterile inflammatory arthritis associated with gonococcal disease (Sec. 9.9).

Pathogenesis. Septic arthritis may result from hematogenous dissemination of bacteria, direct inoculation of organisms into the joint space, or contiguous spread of infection from surrounding soft tissues. In children under 2 yr of age, the metaphyseal plexus of veins traverses the epiphyseal plate; thus metaphyseal osteomyelitis is frequently complicated by concurrent septic arthritis in patients of this age.

Clinical Manifestations. The onset may be sudden, with systemic symptoms and fever. Local swelling may appear rapidly with pain and muscular rigidity. Erythema, tenderness, and warmth may also be noted, and generally there are fever, an increased leukocyte count, and an elevated erythrocyte sedimentation rate. The presenting complaint is frequently a limp; failure to include septic arthritis in the differential diagnosis because of the absence of fever at the initial examination is perhaps the most frequent diagnostic error.

Diagnosis. Rapid diagnosis of suppurative arthritis is best done by arthrocentesis if the presence of fluid is suspected or observed clinically or roentgenographically. It is important, if possible, to avoid traversing an overlying area of cellulitis in doing the joint tap since the underlying joint may be uninvolved and a deep cellulitis may be converted into septic arthritis.

The joint fluid should be examined grossly by Gram and Kenyoun stains and cultured aerobically and anaerobically. Protein and glucose determinations should be obtained. Blood cultures and a blood glucose concentration should be obtained concomitantly. Blood and/or joint cultures are positive in up to 85% of patients infected with *H. influenzae*. Joint fluid also may be sent to the laboratory for antinuclear antibody studies and for determination of hepatitis-associated antigen.

When septic arthritis is present, the joint fluid is usually purulent, the white blood cell count is markedly elevated (more than 50,000 cells/mm^3), the joint glucose concentration is depressed, and organisms are found in the Gram stain. Cultures of joint fluid that has the chemical and morphologic characteristics described may be negative in up to 30% of patients who have never received antibiotic therapy, since the fluid itself may exert a bacteriostatic effect. Blood cultures should always be obtained. In subacute or chronic septic arthritis, synovial biopsy may be helpful in distinguishing between an infectious and a noninfectious process.

Lactic acid concentration within joint fluid may be measured by a rapid enzyme technique and is a reliable method for establishing a diagnosis of septic arthritis in patients with negative synovial fluid cultures. In patients with septic arthritis, the mean (± 1 SD) synovial fluid lactic acid concentrations is elevated (11.6 ± 4.0 mmol/L) when compared with the concentrations in patients with noninfectious forms of arthritis (2.3–6.0 mmol/L).

If a diagnosis of septic arthritis cannot be established by joint aspiration but is still suspected, antibiotic therapy should be provided until repeated cultures of both joint fluid and blood prove to be negative. Concomitantly, diagnostic evaluation aimed at elucidating other possible causes of joint effusion should be initiated. Since septic arthritis may precede osteomyelitis, or osteomyelitis may be present but not demonstrable roentgenographically at the time that the diagnosis of septic arthritis is established, roentgenograms of the adjacent bone are usually indicated 10–14 days after therapy is initiated.

The hip joint presents special problems in diagnosis. In the neonate or young infant the clinical signs of hip involvement may be minimal. Warmth, erythema, and swelling may not be appreciated because of the considerable amount of soft tissue surrounding the joint. Pain on movement and refusal to move the limb may be the only signs.

Differential Diagnosis. Suppurative arthritis must be differentiated from deep cellulitis; viral, mycoplasmal, mycobacterial, and fungal arthritis; septic prepatellar bursitis (when the knee is the affected joint); acute rheumatic fever; rheumatoid arthritis or other collagen disease; toxic synovitis; Lyme arthritis; ulcerative colitis; granulomatous colitis; serum sickness; leukemia; Henoch-Schönlein (anaphylactoid) purpura; metabolic diseases affecting joints (e.g., ochronosis, Farber disease); and traumatic arthritis. As many as 10% of children who have joints involved have septic arthritis.

Treatment. When a diagnosis of septic arthritis has been established, the choice of antibiotics should be based upon the results of microscopic examination of a Gram-stained smear of the joint fluid and upon consideration of the agents likely to produce disease in a child of that particular age. Irrigation of the joint spaces with antibiotics is unnecessary except in cases of fungal arthritis. Surgical drainage should be performed immediately in an involved hip joint and seriously considered when the shoulder joint is involved. There are special characteristics of the hip joint which mandate drainage: (1) the joint capsule limits the amount of possible expansion, so that blood supply to the head of the femur may be compromised; (2) osteomyelitis in adjacent bone is a possibility because the articular cartilage covers only the articular surface of the head of the femur, making the periosteum of the neck subject to contact with the infected fluid.

The minimal duration of antibiotic therapy for septic arthritis is unknown. It is prudent to provide intravenous therapy for 14–21 days in most cases; septic arthritis of the hip should be treated for at least 4 wk.

Methicillin, oxacillin, or nafcillin, in a dose of 200 mg/kg/24 hr intravenously in 6 divided doses, is recommended for patients with suppurative arthritis due to *Staphylococcus aureus*. Disease due to *H. influenzae* should be treated with chloramphenicol in a dose of 100 mg/kg/24 hr in 4 divided intravenous doses and ampicillin in a dose of 200 mg/kg/24 hr in 6 divided doses. When and if the organism is shown to be sensitive to ampicillin, chloramphenicol may be discontinued; if the infection is resistant to ampicillin, only the chloramphenicol is continued.

Strains of *H. influenzae* resistant to both ampicillin and chloramphenicol have been reported. In such an instance, cefotaxime (150 mg/kg/24 hr) in 4 divided doses intravenously may be employed. When the infecting bacterium is one other than the two mentioned above, the antibiotic selected should be the one shown to be effective against it.

Therapy with oral antibiotics has been suggested for septic arthritis, and various antibiotics, including clindamycin, dicloxacillin, cephalexin, ampicillin, and penicillin have been tried. The precautions described under treatment of osteomyelitis should be followed if oral therapy is used.

If there is no evidence of clinical improvement within 48 hr, surgical drainage of the infected joint should be undertaken immediately. If an area of osteomyelitis adjacent to the infected joint is discovered by roentgenograms obtained 10–14 days after the initiation of antibiotic therapy, the antibiotic must be continued since the recommended duration of treatment for osteomyelitis (Sec. 11.14) to prevent possible chronic or recurrent disease is longer than that required for the treatment of septic arthritis.

Curtis GDW, Newman RJ, Slack MPE: Synovial fluid lactate and the diagnosis of septic arthritis. J Infect 6:239, 1983.
Fletcher BD, Scoles PV, Nelson AD: Osteomyelitis in children: Detection by magnetic resonance. Radiology 150:57, 1984.
Jackson MA, Nelson JD: Etiology and medical management of acute suppurative bone and joint infections in pediatric patients. J Pediatr Orthop 2:313, 1982.
Lisbona R, Rosenthall L: Observations on the sequential use of 99mTc-phosphate complex and 67Ga imaging in osteomyelitis, cellulitis, and septic arthritis. Radiology 123:123, 1977.
Nade S: Acute haematogenous osteomyelitis in infancy and childhood. J Bone Joint Surg 65:109, 1983.
Nordan CW, Fierer J, Bryant RF, et al: Chronic staphylococcal osteomyelitis: Treatment with regimens containing rifampin. Rev Infect Dis 5:5495, 1983.
Tetzlaff TR, McCracken GH Jr, Nelson JD: Oral antibiotic therapy for skeletal infections in children. II. Therapy of osteomyelitis and suppurative arthritis. J Pediatr 92:485, 1978.
Waldvogel FA, Vasey H: Osteomyelitis: The past decade. N Engl J Med 303:360, 1980.

11.16 STREPTOCOCCAL INFECTIONS

Streptococci are among the most common causes of bacterial infection in infancy and childhood. Group A streptococci, the most common *bacterial* cause of acute pharyngitis, also produce a large variety of other infections and nonsuppurative sequelae such as rheumatic fever (Sec. 10.87) and glomerulonephritis (Sec. 17.5). Infection during the first 3 mo of life with group B β-hemolytic streptococci has increased markedly during the past 5–10 yr.

Etiology. Streptococci are gram-positive spherical cocci, classified on the basis of their ability to hemolyze red blood cells: those with hemolysins producing complete hemolysis (*beta-hemolytic*), those producing partial hemolysis (*alpha-hemolytic*), and those producing no hemolysis (*gamma-hemolytic*).

Lancefield further separated the streptococci on the basis of differences in carbohydrate components (C-carbohydrate) within the cell wall; streptococcal groups A through H and K through T have thus been identified. The cell wall is composed of three distinct layers. The outer portion contains several antigenic proteins; the most important is M protein. Group A β-hemolytic streptococci can be divided into more than 55 immunologically distinct types that are based on differences in the M protein. M antigen is antiphagocytic and relates directly to virulence of the streptococcus.

Two other cell-wall proteins have been identified: T and R. More than 26 types have been recognized on the basis of T agglutination. Two immunogenically distinct R proteins also have been identified. The T and R antigens are unrelated to virulence.

Streptococci elaborate toxins, enzymes, and hemolysins. More than 20 extracellular antigens released by group A hemolytic streptococci growing in human tissues have been identified. The extracellular products of greatest clinical significance are erythrogenic toxins (A, B, and C), streptolysin O, streptolysin S, diphosphopyridine nucleotidase, streptokinases (A and B), deoxyribonucleases (A, B, C, and D), hyaluronidase, proteinase, amylase, and esterase. Erythrogenic toxins are responsible for the rash of scarlet fever. Generally, the elaboration of erythrogenic toxin depends upon bacteriophage infection (lysogeny) of the streptococcus. Streptolysin S is largely cell bound; recent evidence suggests that it exerts a leukotoxic action. Exposure to streptolysin O is followed by the development of antibodies that aid in the diagnosis of streptococcal infection. Elaboration of streptolysins S and O produces the clear zone of hemolysis permitting classification of the organisms as β-hemolytic strains. Streptokinases are immunogenic and induce antistreptokinase antibodies; their detection also may aid in the diagnosis of streptococcal disease. Hyaluronidase may play a role in permitting the spread of streptococci in human tissues.

Separation by type of hemolysis and Lancefield typing as methods of classifying streptococci are not mutually exclusive. Table 11–18 shows classifications by both methods and outlines the relationship of streptococci to human colonization and disease.

Group A Streptococci

Sequelae of group A β-hemolytic streptococcal disease (rheumatic fever, glomerulonephritis) are discussed in Sec. 10.87 and 17.5.

Epidemiology. Group A streptococci are normal inhabitants of the nasopharynx; prevalence rates vary from 15–20% throughout the year. The incidence of disease depends upon the age of the child, the season of the year, climate and geographic location, and the degree of contact with infected individuals.

Generally, incidence is lowest in the infant, who may be protected by transplacental acquisition of type-specific antibodies. Subsequently, the incidence increases and peaks from 10–18 yr of age. Streptococcal infection of the skin is most common in children under 6 yr; streptococcal pharyngitis is most common between 6 and 12 yr. The incidence of streptococcal pharyngitis is higher in temperate climates, and incidence and severity appear to increase in cold weather. Streptococcal skin disease is more prevalent in tropical climates and in warmer weather in temperate climates.

Group A β-hemolytic streptococci are spread from person to person or occasionally from animals to people. Infection may be spread by droplets; nasal and pharyngeal carriers are effective disseminators. Infection also may be spread by contact with skin lesions or transmitted by food, milk, and water.

Acquisition of streptococci generally is associated with crowding in the home, school, military installation, or other institution. Immunity, which is type-specific, may be induced either by carriage of the organism or by overt infection. The risk of streptococcal disease diminishes during adult life as immunity develops to the more prevalent serotypes.

Pathology. Streptococcal infection is associated with an acute inflammatory response. Local lesions are characterized by edema, hyperemia, and infiltration by polymorphonuclear

Table 11–18. Relationship of Streptococci Identified by Lancefield Grouping and Hemolytic Reactions to Sites of Human Colonization and to Disease

Lancefield Group	Species	Usual Reaction on Sheep Blood Agar	Usual Human Habitat	Most Common Human Disease
A	S. pyogenes	β	Pharynx, skin, rectum	Pharyngitis, erysipelas, impetigo, septicemia, wound infections, rheumatic fever, acute glomerulonephritis, necrotizing fasciitis, cellulitis, otitis media, meningitis, pneumonia, conjunctivitis, acute endocarditis
B	S. agalactiae	β	Pharynx, vagina	Puerperal sepsis, endocarditis, neonatal sepsis, meningitis, otitis media, osteomyelitis, pneumonia
C	S. equi equisimilis dysgalactiae zooepidemicus	β	Pharynx, vagina, skin	Wound infections, puerperal sepsis, cellulitis, endocarditis
D	S. faecalis* faecium* bovis* equinus	γ	Colon contents	Endocarditis, urinary tract infections, biliary tract infections, intestinal infection, peritonitis
E	S. infrequens	?	?	?
F	S. minutus anginosus	β	Mouth, pharynx	Sinusitis, meningitis, brain abscess, pneumonia
G	S. cariis	β	Pharynx, vagina, skin	Puerperal infection, skin or wound infection, endocarditis
H	S. sanguis†	α	Mouth	Endocarditis, brain abscess
K	S. salivarius†	α	Mouth	Endocarditis, sinusitis, meningitis, brain abscess
L	—	β or α	Mouth	Endocarditis, abscess, parotitis, neonatal sepsis
M	—	β or α	Mouth, pharynx, vagina	Endocarditis, septicemia
N	S. lactis cremoris	α or γ	Pharynx	?Meningitis, ?septicemia
O	—	α or β	Pharynx, conjunctiva, vagina	Pneumonia, endocarditis, septicemia
Nontypable	S. viridans	α	Pharynx	Endocarditis
Nontypable	S. mutans	α	Pharynx	Endocarditis

*"Enterococcus."
†These organisms are frequently isolated from the bloodstream as α-hemolytic streptococci. Along with many nongroupable α streptococci, they are often called S. viridans, a term that incorrectly implies a specific species. Nevertheless, as a group, they cause the majority of episodes of endocarditis and are usually, but not invariably, exquisitely sensitive to penicillin.
(Reproduced from Keusch GT, Weinstein L: Streptococcal Disease, Upjohn Company Publ.)

leukocytes. Pathologic changes in scarlet fever are related to the organisms and to toxin elaboration, which is responsible for the rash.

Pathogenesis. Streptococci proliferate rapidly following inhalation. Leukocytes are attracted to the mucosal surface, but the hyaluronic acid capsule and the M protein of streptococci exert antiphagocytic activity; if the organism is phagocytized, it may be killed promptly. Sometimes engulfment does not result in death because the polysaccharide-glycopeptide cell wall complex is resistant to enzymatic degradation. In addition, the organisms may elaborate leukotoxic DPNase and streptolysin S. Nonphagocytized streptococci may elaborate streptolysin O. The enzyme also has a leukotoxic effect. Lysis of leukocytes, erythrocytes, and host cells produces an inflammatory focus. Streptokinase may activate plasminogen in the inflammatory exudate. In turn, activated plasminogen may act on fibrin to provide nutrients for further bacterial growth. Production of hyaluronidase may aid in the spread of infection. If erythrogenic toxin is elaborated in an individual who does not possess immunity to the toxin, scarlet fever will result.

Clinical Manifestations. The most common infections caused by group A β-hemolytic streptococci involve the respiratory tract, skin, soft tissues, and blood.

Respiratory Tract Infection. See Sec. 13.26–13.29.

Scarlet Fever. This disease is the result of infection by streptococci that elaborate an erythrogenic toxin against which the host has no antibodies. The incubation period ranges from 1 to 7 days with an average of 3 days. The onset is acute, characterized by fever, vomiting, headache, pharyngitis, and chills. Abdominal pain may be present; when this is associated with vomiting prior to the appearance of the rash, an abdominal surgical condition may be suggested. Within 12–48 hr the typical rash appears.

Generally, temperature increases abruptly and may peak at 39.6–40° C (103–104° F) on the 2nd day and gradually returns to normal within 5–7 days in the untreated patient; it is usually normal within 12–24 hr after initiation of penicillin therapy. The tonsils are hyperemic and edematous and may be covered with exudate. The pharynx is inflamed and covered by a membrane in severe cases. The tongue may be edematous and reddened. During the early days of illness the dorsum of the tongue has a white coat through which the red and edematous papillae project (*white strawberry tongue*). After several days the white coat desquamates; the red tongue studded with prominent papillae persists (*red strawberry tongue*). The palate and uvula may be edematous, reddened, and covered with petechiae.

The exanthem is red, punctate, or finely papular. In some individuals it may be palpated more readily than it is seen, having the texture of gooseflesh or coarse sandpaper. The rash appears initially in the axillae, groin, and neck but within 24 hr becomes generalized. Punctate lesions generally are not present on the face. The forehead and cheeks appear flushed, and the area around the mouth is pale (*circumoral pallor*). The rash is most intense in the axillae and groin and at pressure sites. Areas of hyperpigmentation that do not blanch with pressure may appear in the deep creases, particularly in the antecubital fossae (*Pastia lines*). In severe disease, small vesicular lesions (*miliary sudamina*) may appear over the abdomen, hands, and feet.

Desquamation begins on the face in fine flakes toward the end of the 1st wk and proceeds over the trunk and finally to the hands and feet. The duration and extent of desquamation vary with the intensity of the rash; it may continue for as long as 6 wk.

Scarlet fever may follow infection of wounds (surgical scarlet fever), burns, or streptococcal skin infection. Clinical manifestations are similar to those described above, but the

tonsils and pharynx generally are not involved. A similar picture may be observed with certain strains of staphylococci that produce an erythrogenic toxin.

Scarlet fever must be distinguished from other exanthematous diseases, including measles (characterized by its prodrome of conjunctivitis, photophobia, dry cough, and Koplik spots), rubella (disease is mild, postauricular lymphadenopathy usually is present, and throat culture is negative), and other viral exanthems. With infectious mononucleosis there are generally pharyngitis, rash, lymphadenopathy, and splenomegaly as well as atypical lymphocytes. The exanthems produced by several enteroviruses can be confused with scarlet fever, but differentiation can be established by the course of the disease, the associated symptoms, and the results of culture. Roseola is characterized by the cessation of fever with the onset of rash and the transient nature of the exanthem. Severe sunburn can be confused with scarlet fever.

Pneumonia. See Sec. 8.66 and 13.66.

Skin Infections. The most common form of skin infection due to group A β-hemolytic streptococci is superficial pyoderma (**impetigo**) (Sec. 24.11).

Deeper soft tissue infections may occur secondary to impetigo. Streptococcal cellulitis is a painful, erythematous, indurated infection of the skin and subcutaneous tissues. Lymphangitis and regional lymphadenitis are common. Streptococcal soft tissue abscesses are rare but have occurred following immunization with contaminated needles. Fever and other systemic manifestations of disease may be noted.

Erysipelas. This is a cellulitis and acute lymphangitis of the skin which spreads marginally. The skin is erythematous and indurated; the margins of the lesions have a raised firm border. The skin lesion usually is associated with fever, vomiting, and irritability. These symptoms subside when progression of the rash ceases. In some cases streptococci break through the lymphatic barrier, and cellulitis, subcutaneous abscesses, bacteremia, and metastatic foci of infection are observed. Bacteremia and death have been associated with streptococcal cellulitis in the newborn infant; progression may be so rapid that there is no response to treatment with penicillin.

Bacteremia. See Sec. 11.12. Streptococcal bacteremia may follow localized streptococcal disease of the skin or respiratory tract and has been noted in children without an obvious focus of infection. Rarely, disseminated intravascular coagulation and peripheral gangrene occur. Hematogenous dissemination may result in *meningitis, osteomyelitis, arthritis,* or *pyelonephritis.* Rarely, *acute* or *subacute bacterial endocarditis* has been due to group A β-hemolytic streptococci.

Vaginitis. The β-hemolytic streptococcus is a common cause of vaginitis in prepubertal girls. There is usually a serous discharge and marked erythema and irritation of the vulvar area, accompanied by discomfort in walking and in urination. *Proctitis* is rare but may be seen in either sex.

Diagnosis. The diagnosis of streptococcal infection is suggested by characteristic clinical findings but established with certainty only by isolation of the organism.

Throat culture is the most useful laboratory aid in patients with acute tonsillitis or pharyngitis. A positive throat culture may indicate streptococcal pharyngitis, but hemolytic streptococci are common inhabitants of the nasopharynx in well children. Moreover, some children with a viral upper respiratory infection have positive throat cultures for β-hemolytic streptococci. Thus, isolation of a group A streptococcus from the pharynx of a child with pharyngeal infection does not necessarily indicate that the disease is caused by this organism. When streptococci are isolated from children with moderate or severe exudative pharyngitis who have petechiae on the palate and cervical adenitis, the diagnosis is more secure.

The immunologic response of the host following exposure

to streptococcal antigen can be assessed by measuring anti-streptolysin O (ASO) titers. An increase in ASO titer to greater than 166 Todd units occurs in more than 80% of untreated children with streptococcal pharyngitis within the first 3 wk following infection. This response may be modified or abolished by early and effective antibiotic therapy. ASO titers may be very high in patients with rheumatic fever; in contrast, they are weakly positive or not elevated at all in patients with streptococcal pyoderma; responses in patients with glomerulonephritis are variable. Group A β-hemolytic streptococci also may be recovered from the pharynx of asymptomatic individuals who develop an antibody response to this organism, indicating that subclinical infection has occurred.

Individuals with impetigo may react strongly to stimulation by other streptococcal extracellular products. Anti–DNase (deoxyribonuclease) B provides the best serologic test for streptococcal pyoderma. Most patients with streptococcal pharyngitis also develop elevated titers to this enzyme. Patients with pyoderma and pharyngitis also may develop antibody responses to hyaluronidase, but antihyaluronidase (AH) titers are elevated with less regularity than are ASO titers.

A response to DPNase (NADase, nicotinamide adenine dinucleotidase) may indicate present or past infection. This enzyme is made in particularly large quantities by serotypes 4, 12, and 49.

A 2 min inexpensive **Streptozyme*** slide test is designed to detect antibodies involved in all of the tests mentioned above. This test detects more patients with increased antibody titers than any other single test presently available. Nonspecific (false-positive) reactions have been limited in number, and the test is capable of detecting antibody responses early in the course of disease. However, the strength of the Streptozyme reagent varies from lot to lot, and it may not be specific for antibodies to extracellular products of group A streptococci, since a response to this test was observed in individuals with only non–group A strains isolated from their upper respiratory tracts. In patients with group A streptococci, the antibody response was comparable to but no greater than the ASO or anti–DNase B tests.

The white blood cell count may or may not be elevated. Leukocytosis may be noted in many bacterial and viral diseases; hence, this finding is nonspecific. Similarly, elevations in erythrocyte sedimentation rate and C-reactive protein do not help to establish a specific diagnosis.

Differential Diagnosis. Acute pharyngitis indistinguishable clinically from that caused by group A β-hemolytic streptococci may be caused by many viruses, including EB virus (infectious mononucleosis) and cytomegalovirus. A viral etiology may be suggested by failure to isolate streptococci and may be identified specifically by viral culture and serologic studies. Infectious mononucleosis may be suggested by clinical manifestations, the presence of atypical lymphocytes in the peripheral blood, and a rise in heterophile and EB viral antibody titers. Acute pharyngitis similar to that caused by β-hemolytic streptococci may be noted in patients with diphtheria, tularemia, and toxoplasmosis, and, rarely, in individuals with tonsillar tuberculosis, salmonellosis, and brucellosis. These diseases can be differentiated by appropriate cultures and serologic tests. An ulcerative pharyngitis may be noted in children with agranulocytosis, regardless of etiology.

Streptococcal pyoderma must be differentiated from staphylococcal skin disease. Often these bacterial species coexist. The lesions produced are clinically indistinguishable; distinction is made only by culture.

Streptococcal septicemia, meningitis, septic arthritis, and pneumonia present signs and symptoms similar to those produced by other bacterial organisms. The offending pathogen can be established only by culture.

Complications. Complications generally reflect extension of streptococcal infection from the nasopharynx. This may result in sinusitis, otitis media, mastoiditis, cervical adenitis, retropharyngeal or parapharyngeal abscess, or bronchopneumonia. Hematogenous dissemination of streptococci may cause meningitis, osteomyelitis, or septic arthritis. Nonsuppurative late complications include rheumatic fever and glomerulonephritis.

Prevention. Administration of penicillin will prevent most cases of streptococcal disease if the drug is provided prior to the onset of symptoms. Indications for prophylaxis are not clear. Generally, we have obtained throat cultures from children who are close family contacts of patients with streptococcal disease. If these cultures are positive, oral penicillin G or V, (400,000 units/dose) is provided 4 times each day for 10 days. Alternatively, 600,000 units of benzathine penicillin in combination with 600,000 units of aqueous procaine penicillin may be given as a single intramuscular injection. A similar approach may be used for institutional epidemics. Children exposed to an individual case at school may be observed carefully.

Management of carriers of group A β-hemolytic streptococci is controversial. It has been suggested that treatment of the carrier precludes the development of type-specific immunity, thereby leaving the individual susceptible to reinfection later in life. It is probably unnecessary to retreat asymptomatic convalescent patients with persistently positive throat cultures for group A streptococci, since they are generally carriers who do not have persistent or recurrent streptococcal infections.

No streptococcal vaccines are available for clinical use.

Treatment. Penicillin is the drug of choice for the treatment of streptococcal infections. All strains of group A β-hemolytic streptococci isolated to date have been sensitive to concentrations of penicillin achievable in vivo. Optimal treatment eradicates streptococci, prevents septic complications, and diminishes the likelihood of rheumatic fever and possibly of glomerulonephritis.

The goal of therapy is to maintain for at least 10 days blood and tissue levels of penicillin sufficient to kill streptococci. Children with streptococcal pharyngitis and simple pyoderma are customarily treated with 1.2–1.6 million units of penicillin daily in 4 divided doses; 800,000 units taken orally for 10 days is probably sufficient. Penicillin G or penicillin V may be employed; the latter is preferable because satisfactory blood levels are achieved even when the stomach is not empty. Amoxicillin given orally in a dose of 125 mg 3 times each day regardless of the weight of the child may be as effective as penicillin but is associated with a greater frequency of adverse reactions and with higher cost.

Erythromycin (40 mg/kg/24 hr), lincomycin (40 mg/kg/24 hr), clindamycin (30 mg/kg/24 hr), or cefadroxil monohydrate (15 mg/kg/24 hr) may be used for treating streptococcal pharyngitis in patients allergic to penicillin. Generally, relapse rates are greater with regimens other than penicillin. Tetracyclines and sulfonamides should not be used for treatment, although sulfonamides may be used for prophylaxis of rheumatic fever.

A single dose of 1,200,000 units of benzathine penicillin intramuscularly provides adequate therapy for streptococcal pharyngitis, circumventing the problem of patient compliance in use of an oral antibiotic. In addition, relapse rates are lower. Some have suggested that the clinical manifestations of streptococcal pharyngitis are of shorter duration if a combination of 600,000 units of procaine penicillin and 600,000 units of benzathine penicillin is given.

Patients with scarlet fever, streptococcal bacteremia, pneumonia, meningitis, deep soft tissue infections, erysipelas, or complications of streptococcal pharyngitis should be treated

---

*Wampole Laboratories.

parenterally with penicillin, preferably intravenously. The dose and duration of therapy must be tailored to the nature of the disease process, with daily doses as high as 400,000 units/kg/24 hr required in the most severe infections.

Prognosis. The prognosis for adequately treated streptococcal infections is excellent; most suppurative complications are prevented or readily treated. When therapy is provided promptly, nonsuppurative complications are prevented and complete recovery is the rule. In rare instances, particularly in the newborn infant or in children whose response to infection is compromised, fulminant pneumonia, septicemia, and death may occur despite usually adequate therapy.

Infections Due to Other Streptococci

In many centers the group B *Streptococcus* has become the leading cause of neonatal septicemia and meningitis (Sec. 8.59 and 8.66). Disease due to group B hemolytic streptococci has also become increasingly prevalent in infants 1–8 mo. of age, in whom the organism has been associated with septicemia, meningitis, pneumonia, acalculous cholecystitis, cellulitis, otitis media, osteomyelitis, and septic arthritis. Parenteral treatment with aqueous penicillin G is effective; the dose and duration depend upon the nature of the disease process. When systemic group B streptococcal disease is present, ampicillin plus an aminoglycoside (e.g., gentamicin) may be synergistic and enhance the efficacy of therapy in patients with this infection.

Human infection with streptococci of groups C to H and K to O, as well as with nontypable strains, has been reported in normal infants and children. The classification of these organisms and the infections with which they have been associated are shown in Table 11–18. Penicillin G provides effective therapy for non–group A streptococci, except for those belonging to group D (enterococci) and selected α-hemolytic strains; these organisms generally are susceptible to ampicillin. When endocarditis is caused by enterococci, therapy with ampicillin plus an aminoglycoside is recommended.

Infection with Lancefield group G streptococci has been recognized as an increasingly serious and frequent cause of human disease; endovascular infection, endocarditis, and septic arthritis are observed most frequently. Despite exquisite in vitro sensitivity to penicillin, in vivo responses have been disappointing. Therapy with ampicillin and an aminoglycoside is more efficacious than therapy with penicillin alone.

Non–group D α-hemolytic streptococci have been identified as an increasingly important cause of septicemia and meningitis in the newborn, although death due to these organisms is infrequent.

Bacterial endocarditis in children is commonly due to infection with *Streptococcus viridans*. A variant of this organism that requires vitamin B₆ or thiol compounds for optimal growth has also caused endocarditis in adults and children. It is important to know that supplemented media are needed for their isolation and sensitivity testing; spuriously low MIC's may be reported when nonsupplemented media are used. Some of these organisms are relatively tolerant to penicillin; therapy with penicillin and an aminoglycoside is recommended until results of sensitivity studies are available. In several instances these organisms have been resistant even to this combination of drugs but have been sensitive to clindamycin.

Broughton RH, Krafka R, Baker CJ: Non–group D alpha-hemolytic streptococci: New neonatal pathogens. J Pediatr 99:450, 1981.

Burech DL, Koranyl KI, Haynes RE: Serious group A streptococcal diseases in childhood. J Pediatr 88:972, 1976.

Feder HM Jr, Olsen N, McLaughlin JC, et al: Bacterial endocarditis caused by vitamin B₆–dependent viridans group streptococcus. Pediatrics 66:309, 1980.

Kaplan EL, Gastanaduy AJ, Huwe BB: The role of the carrier in treatment failures after antibiotic therapy for group A streptococci in the upper respiratory tract. J Lab Clin Med 98:326, 1981.

Kaplan EL, Howe BB: The sensitivity and specificity of an agglutination test for antibodies to streptococcal extracellular antigens: A quantitative analysis and comparison of the Streptozyme test with anti–streptolysin O and anti–deoxyribonuclease B tests. J Pediatr 96:367, 1980.

Lam K, Bayer AS: Serious infections due to group B streptococci. Am J Med 75:561, 1983.

Todd JK: Throat cultures in the office laboratory. Pediatr Infect Dis 4:265, 1982.

Wannamaker LW: Differences between streptococcal infections of the throat and of the skin. N Engl J Med 282:23, 78, 1970.

Wannamaker LW, Denny FW, Perry WD, et al: The effect of penicillin prophylaxis on streptococcal disease rates and the carrier state. N Engl J Med 249:1, 1953.

11.17 STAPHYLOCOCCAL INFECTIONS

For staphylococcal infections of the newborn, see Sec. 8.67.

Staphylococci are a common cause of pyogenic infections in infants and children. These organisms grow in clusters, aerobically or as facultative anaerobes. Strains are classified as *S. aureus* if they are coagulase-positive and as *S. epidermidis* if they are coagulase-negative, irrespective of their pigment production on solid media. Generally, strains of *S. aureus* produce a yellow pigment and those of *S. epidermidis*, a white pigment. Strains of *S. aureus* generally are mannitol-deoxyribonuclease– and acid phosphatase–positive and produce β hemolysis on blood agar. Strains of *S. epidermidis* generally are mannitol- and acid phosphatase–negative; production of β hemolysis on blood agar is variable.

Infections Due to *Staphylococcus aureus*

Staphylococcus aureus is the most common cause of pyogenic infection of the skin; it also may cause furuncles, carbuncles, osteomyelitis, septic arthritis, wound infection, abscesses, pneumonia, empyema, endocarditis, pericarditis, meningitis, and food poisoning.

Etiology. Disease may be the result of tissue invasion or reflect a reaction to a variety of toxins and enzymes elaborated by these organisms. Strains of *S. aureus* can be identified and classified by means of bacteriophage group typing. Group I (phage numbers 29, 52, 52A, 79, and 80); Group II (phage numbers 3A, 3C, 55, and 71); Group III (phage numbers 6, 7, 42E, 47, 53, 54, 75, 77, 83A, 84, and 85); Group IV (phage number 42D); and miscellaneous (phage numbers 81 and 187). If more precise identification is desired, a large panel of individual phages is required.

Many strains of *S. aureus* release *exotoxins*. Four immunologically distinct hemolysins have been identified. Alpha toxin may cause tissue necrosis, injure human leukocytes, and produce aggregation of platelets and spasm of smooth muscle. A beta hemolysin causes hemolysis of red blood cells incubated at 39° C and then exposed to cold, and a delta hemolysin is toxic to leukocytes. Little is known about gamma hemolysin other than that it also appears to act on cell membranes.

Leukocidin, produced by most strains of *S. aureus*, combines with the phospholipid of the cell membrane, producing increased permeability of the membrane, leakage of protein, and eventual death of the cell.

Exfoliative toxin, associated with phage group II staphylococci, is the cause of "scalded skin syndrome" (Ritter disease), bullous impetigo, and staphylococcal scarlatiniform eruption (Sec. 24.25).

Staphylococcal enterotoxins (types A, B, C, D, E, F) are elaborated by most strains of *S. aureus*. Ingestion of preformed enterotoxin A or B is associated with vomiting and diarrhea and in some cases with the development of profound hypotension (Sec. 28.1). Staphylococcal enterotoxins B, C, and F have been associated with toxic shock syndrome (Sec. 11.18).

A variety of *enzymes* may be released by staphylococci. Production of coagulase (causing plasma to coagulate) differentiates *S. aureus* from *S. epidermidis*. Other enzymes elaborated by staphylococci include staphylokinase (activator of plasma plasminogen), penicillinase or β-lactamase (inactivator of penicillin at the molecular level), hyaluronidase (spreading factor), lipase, and DNase.

Most strains of *S. aureus* possess an *agglutinogen* (protein A). This material can react with the Fc fragments of IgG molecules and causes hypersensitivity reactions in rabbits and guinea pigs. It also generates complement-derived chemotactic factors and has antiphagocytic properties. Several capsular antigens serve to block the agglutinating and opsonizing action of anticapsular antibodies.

Epidemiology. Most newborn infants are colonized within the first week of life (Sec. 8.67), and 20–30% of normal individuals carry *S. aureus* in the anterior nares at all times.

The organisms may be transmitted from the nose to the skin, where colonization seems to be more transient. Repeated recovery of *S. aureus* from the skin suggests repeated transfer rather than persistent skin colonization. Persistent umbilical and perianal carriage has been described.

Transmission of *S. aureus* generally occurs by direct contact or by spread of heavy particles over a distance of 6 ft or less. Spread by fomites is rare. Acquisition of staphylococci is dependent upon the efficiency of the disseminator and the susceptibility of the host. Heavily colonized individuals and perianal carriers are particularly effective disseminators. Newborn infants are extremely susceptible to staphylococci; the nasopharynx, skin, and umbilical stump are the most common sites of colonization. Handwashing between contacts with patients decreases the spread of staphylococci from patient to patient. Older children and adults are more resistant than the newborn infant to colonization.

Infection may follow colonization. Antibiotic therapy with a drug to which *S. aureus* is resistant favors both colonization and the development of infection. Other factors that increase the likelihood of infection include wounds, skin disease, ventriculoatrial shunts, intravenous or intrathecal catheterization, corticosteroid treatment, starvation, acidosis, and azotemia. Viral infections of the respiratory tract also may predispose to secondary bacterial infection with staphylococci.

Pathology. Suppuration is the hallmark of staphylococcal disease. Local multiplication of staphylococci within tissues produces necrosis and formation of abscesses. Elaboration of hyaluronidase may promote spread of the infection. Granulocytes appear in large numbers at the site of infection. Thrombosis of blood vessels and formation of fibrin clots may be noted. The developed local lesion is characterized by a necrotic center surrounded by a fibroblastic wall. Viable bacteria and leukocytes are within the abscess cavity. Rupture of the abscess results in bacteremia and disseminated disease.

Pathogenesis. The development of staphylococcal disease is related to resistance of the host to infection and to virulence of the organism. The intact skin and mucous membranes serve as barriers to invasion by staphylococci. A cellular factor that appears to be a mucopeptide, which can be extracted only from virulent strains of *S. aureus*, inhibits chemotaxis and accumulation of fluid at the site of infection. The ability of virulent staphylococci to establish disease may be related directly to their capacity to inhibit chemotaxis.

Protein A, present in most strains of *S. aureus* but not in *S. epidermidis*, reacts specifically with IgG1, IgG2, and IgG4. It is located on the outermost coat of the bacterium and can absorb serum immunoglobulin, preventing antibacterial antibodies from acting as opsonins and thus inhibiting phagocytosis. Leukocidin, causing degranulation of leukocytes, and staphylococcal hemolysin toxic to erythrocytes and leukocytes also contribute to the virulence of *S. aureus*.

Proliferation of staphylococci in the gastrointestinal tract is also controlled by the prevalence of other bacterial species. If this balance is upset during antibiotic therapy, resistant staphylococci may proliferate and invade the bowel wall. Elaboration of enterotoxin by staphylococci within the gastrointestinal tract or ingestion of preformed enterotoxins may produce disease in the absence of tissue invasion (Sec. 28.1).

The infant may acquire type-specific humoral immunity to staphylococci transplacentally. Older children and adults develop antibodies to staphylococci as a result of intermittent minor infections of the skin and soft tissues; the antistaphylococcal titer of serum generally increases after overt staphylococcal disease. The presence of antibody, however, does not always protect the individual from staphylococcal disease.

Formation of antibody and delayed hypersensitivity reactions can be induced by protein components of the cell wall, and by ribotol teichoic acid components of the organism. The specific protection afforded by antibodies to any of these components remains unclear.

Individuals with congenital or acquired defects in the complement system (required for chemotaxis), defective phagocytosis, and defective humoral immunity (antibodies required for opsonization) as well as those with an impaired intracellular bactericidal capacity are at increased risk of infection with staphylococci. Patients with chronic granulomatous disease, in which phagocytosis proceeds normally but killing of ingested bacteria is severely impaired, are particularly susceptible to staphylococcal disease. Impaired mobilization of polymorphonuclear leukocytes has been documented in children with diabetes mellitus and in healthy individuals following ingestion of alcohol.

Clinical Manifestations. These vary with the location of the lesions, which, though most commonly located on the skin, may involve any organ, the subcutaneous tissues, and the musculoskeletal system. The severity, in general, is related to septicemia (when present), to the site involved (e.g., usually less severe with a skin lesion than with pneumonia or meningitis), and to the elaboration of toxins (e.g., food poisoning). Although the nasopharynx and skin of a large number of persons in all segments of society are more or less constantly colonized with *S. aureus*, disease due to this organism is relatively uncommon. Lesions, especially those of the skin, are considerably more prevalent among persons living in low socioeconomic circumstances and particularly among those in tropical climates.

Individual staphylococcal disorders are covered elsewhere in appropriate sections of this book and cross-referenced in the following discussion.

Newborn. Nosocomial infections are discussed in Sec. 8.58, staphylococcal diseases in general in Sec. 8.67, sepsis and meningitis in Sec. 8.59, pneumonia in Sec. 8.60 and 13.66, otitis media in Sec. 8.65, conjunctivitis in Sec. 8.64 and 25.9, and osteomyelitis and septic arthritis in Sec. 8.61.

Skin. Pyogenic skin infections may be primary or secondary to wounds or may be a superinfection of other noninfectious skin disease, or of impetigo contagiosa, primarily of streptococcal origin.

Impetigo contagiosa, ecthyma, bullous impetigo, folliculitis, furuncles, carbuncles, staphylococcal scalded skin syndrome (Ritter disease), and a syndrome resembling the rash of scarlet fever are described in Sec. 24.25. An identical clinical picture may be seen in patients with wounds, especially burns (Sec. 5.44), secondarily infected with staphylococci. Nosocomial skin lesions, including pustules and cellulitis, are discussed in Sec. 8.58.

Respiratory Tract. Infections of the upper respiratory tract due to *S. aureus* are rare considering the frequency with which this area is colonized. Otitis media (Sec. 13.40) and sinusitis (Sec. 13.34) due to *S. aureus* may occur. Staphylococcal sinusitis is relatively common in children with cystic fibrosis or defects in white blood cell function. Suppurative parotitis is a rare infection, but *S. aureus* is a common cause. Staphylococcal tonsillopharyngitis (Sec. 13.33) is rare except in children whose response to infection has been compromised. Tracheitis that clinically resembles viral croup may be caused by *S. aureus*. Patients typically have high fever, leukocytosis and evidence of severe upper airway obstruction. Direct laryngoscopy or bronchoscopy shows a normal epiglottis with subglottic narrowing and thick purulent secretions within the trachea. Also see Sec. 13.53 for discussion of laryngotracheobronchitis.

Pneumonia (Sec. 8.60, 8.67, and 13.66) due to *S. aureus* may be primary or secondary to a viral infection. In children under 1 yr of age the onset may be heralded by expiratory wheeze briefly simulating bronchiolitis. More common are high fever, abdominal pain, tachypnea, dyspnea, and localized or diffuse bronchopneumonia or lobar disease. Staphylococci cause a necrotizing pneumonitis; hence empyema (Sec. 13.98), pneumatoceles, pyopneumothorax, and bronchopleural fistulas develop frequently. Occasionally, staphylococcal pneumonia produces a diffuse interstitial disease characterized by extreme dyspnea, tachypnea, and cyanosis. Cough may be nonproductive. Oxygen therapy may not significantly improve the oxygen saturation of the blood. Also see discussion of pneumonia in cystic fibrosis (Sec. 13.97).

Sepsis. See Sec. 11.12. Staphylococcal bacteremia and sepsis may be associated with any localized infection. The onset may be acute and marked by nausea, vomiting, myalgia, fever, and chills. Organisms may localize subsequently at any site but especially in the lung, heart, joints, bones, kidneys, and brain.

In some instances, especially when treatment of a local infection has been inadequate, disseminated staphylococcal disease occurs, characterized by fever, bone or joint pain, and urticarial, petechial, maculopapular, or pustular rashes. Less frequently, hematuria, jaundice, seizures, nuchal rigidity, and cardiac murmurs are noted. Leukopenia or leukocytosis, proteinuria, and red and white blood cells in the urinary sediment may be noted.

Muscle. Localized staphylococcal abscesses in muscle associated with elevation of muscle enzymes but without septicemia have been called tropical pyomyositis. Although this disorder has been reported most frequently from tropical areas, it also has occurred in the United States in otherwise healthy children. Multiple abscesses occur in 30–40% of cases. Prodromal symptoms may include coryza, pharyngitis, diarrhea, or prior trauma at the site of the abscess. Surgical drainage and appropriate antibiotic therapy are essential.

Adamski has documented generalized staphylococcal myositis with rhabdomyolysis but without suppuration in association with staphylococcal septicemia and elevation of serum levels of muscle enzymes. The infection responded to antibiotic therapy, but muscular wasting, weakness, and stiffness occurred.

Bones and Joints. *S. aureus* is the most common cause of osteomyelitis and septic arthritis in children (Sec. 8.61 and 11.15). Generally, disease is acquired hematogenously rather than by direct extension of infection from an adjacent skin or soft tissue lesion.

Central Nervous System. Meningitis (Sec. 8.59 and 11.13) due to *S. aureus* may follow bacteremia or occasionally result from direct extension of infection in patients with otitis media or osteomyelitis of the skull or vertebrae. Trauma or infection of meningomyeloceles also may predispose to *S. aureus* meningitis (Sec. 21.10). Staphylococcal infection following neurosurgical procedures most commonly is due to *S. epidermidis*. *S. aureus* can be recovered from about 25% of brain abscesses. *S. aureus* is also a common cause of spinal epidural abscess (Sec. 21.28). A staphylococcal etiology should be suspected more strongly in abscesses occurring in patients with known or possible staphylococcal bacteremia from whatever primary lesion.

Heart. Acute bacterial endocarditis (Sec. 14.74) may follow staphylococcal bacteremia and occur in the absence of valvular heart disease. Perforation of heart valves, myocardial abscesses, acute hemopericardium, purulent pericarditis (Sec. 14.82), and sudden death may ensue.

Kidney. *S. aureus* is a common cause of renal and perinephric abscess (Sec. 17.38). Urinary tract infection due to *S. aureus* is unusual.

Toxic Shock Syndrome. See Sec. 11.18.

Intestinal Tract. Staphylococcal enterocolitis follows overgrowth of normal bowel flora by staphylococci. This most commonly follows use of broad-spectrum oral antibiotic therapy. Diarrhea is associated with blood and mucus.

Food poisoning (Sec. 28.1) may be caused by ingestion of enterotoxins preformed by staphylococci contaminating foods. Two to 7 hr after ingestion of the toxin, sudden, severe vomiting begins. Watery diarrhea may develop, but fever is absent or low grade. Symptoms rarely persist longer than 12–24 hr. Rarely, shock and death may occur.

Diagnosis. The diagnosis of staphylococcal infection depends upon isolation of the organisms from skin lesions, abscess cavities, blood, cerebrospinal fluid, or other sites of infection. The organisms can be grown readily in liquid and on solid media. Following isolation, identification is made on the basis of Gram stain and coagulase and mannitol reactivity. Patterns of sensitivity to antibiotics can be assessed and the organism phage-typed if necessary for epidemiologic reasons.

Diagnosis of staphylococcal food poisoning generally is made on the basis of epidemiologic and clinical findings. Food suspected of contamination should be examined by Gram stain, cultured, and tested for enterotoxin. This last test can be done by the Centers for Disease Control. Teichoic acid antibodies in patients with *S. aureus* bacteremia can be measured by double diffusion in agar or by enzyme-linked immunosorbent assay. This test may be valuable in diagnosing patients with staphylococcal endocarditis or septicemia. Staphylococcal peptidoglycan is immunogenic in humans, and testing for IgG antibodies to it may be useful in the diagnosis of bacteremic staphylococcal infections.

Differential Diagnosis. Skin lesions due to *S. aureus* and those due to group A β-hemolytic streptococci may be indistinguishable. Staphylococcal pneumonia can be suspected on the basis of chest roentgenograms that may reveal pneumatoceles, pyopneumothorax, or lung abscess. These changes suggesting a necrotizing pneumonitis are not pathognomonic for staphylococcal infection and may be seen in patients with pneumonia due to other bacteria, including *Klebsiella* and many anaerobes. Fluctuant skin and soft tissue lesions also can be caused by many organisms, including *Mycobacterium*, *F. tularensis*, and various fungi and may be seen in patients with cat-scratch disease (Sec. 11.84).

Prevention. Staphylococcal infection is transmitted primarily by direct contact. *Strict attention to handwashing techniques* is the most effective measure for preventing the spread of staphylococci from one individual to another (Sec. 11.7). Use of a detergent containing an iodophor or of hexachlorophene is recommended. In hospitals or other institutional settings, all persons with acute staphylococcal infections should be excluded until they have been treated adequately. There should be constant surveillance for nosocomial staphylococcal infections within hospitals.

Food poisoning may be prevented by excluding individuals with staphylococcal infections of the skin from the preparation and handling of food. Prepared foods should be eaten immediately or refrigerated appropriately to prevent multiplication of staphylococci with which the food may have been contaminated.

Treatment. Antibiotic therapy alone is rarely effective in individuals with undrained abscesses or with infected foreign bodies. Loculated collections of purulent material should be relieved by incision and drainage. Foreign bodies should be removed, if possible. Therapy always should be initiated with a penicillinase-resistant antibiotic; in some areas, more than 90% of all staphylococci isolated, regardless of source, are resistant to penicillin.

For serious infections parenteral treatment is indicated; methicillin, oxacillin, and nafcillin are equally effective. Generally, a dose of 200 mg/kg/24 hr should be employed intravenously in 6 divided doses. Daily doses as high as 400 mg/kg/24 hr have been used without toxicity in selected patients.

The antibiotic employed as well as the dose, route, and duration of treatment is dependent upon the site of infection, the response of the patient to treatment, and the sensitivity of the organisms recovered from blood or from local sites of infection. In patients with staphylococcal pneumonia, intravenous treatment is recommended until the patient has been afebrile for 72 hr and other signs of infection have disappeared (Sec. 13.66). Oral therapy is continued for a total of 3 wk, longer in selected cases. The treatment of staphylococcal osteomyelitis (Sec. 11.14), meningitis (Sec. 11.13), and endocarditis (Sec. 14.74) are discussed in their respective sections. In all of these infections, oral treatment should be provided when parenteral therapy has been discontinued; dicloxacillin is penicillinase resistant, absorbed well orally, and quite effective. This drug is administered in a dose of 50–75 mg/kg/24 hr in 4 divided oral doses. Duration of oral therapy depends also upon the response of the patient as determined by the clinical, roentgenographic, and laboratory findings and by culture results. In selected patients with osteomyelitis, oral therapy may be required for 12 wk or longer, depending on the time it takes the erythrocyte sedimentation rate to return to normal.

Skin and soft tissue infection and minor upper respiratory infection may be managed by oral therapy alone or by an initial brief course of antibiotics provided parenterally, followed by oral medication. Dicloxacillin (25–50 mg/kg/24 hr), oxacillin (100 mg/kg/24 hr), or nafcillin (100 mg/kg/24 hr), each in 4 divided oral doses, provides excellent blood and tissue concentrations of these antibiotics. In very mild, localized skin infection, repeated cleansing with a mild antiseptic and use of topical antibiotics (bacitracin) may be effective. Penicillin should not be applied topically.

Penicillin G can be used to treat infections due to S. aureus if the organism proves sensitive to this antibiotic in vitro.

Individuals sensitive to penicillin and its derivatives must be treated with other antibiotics or desensitized to the penicillin derivative to be employed. About 5% of penicillin-sensitive children are also sensitive to cephalosporins. Clindamycin and lincomycin have proved effective for the treatment of skin, soft tissue, bone, and joint infections due to S. aureus. Clindamycin may be provided in 3–4 divided doses parenterally or orally (total daily dose 30–40 mg/kg/24 hr). Clindamycin and lincomycin should *not* be used to treat endocarditis, brain abscess, or meningitis due to S. aureus. Erythromycin, chloramphenicol, kanamycin, and gentamicin can be used but are inferior to the penicillins. Vancomycin can be used to treat penicillin-sensitive individuals with endocarditis, but serum levels of this antibiotic should be monitored when it is used. Peak serum concentrations should be 25–40 μg/mL. It can be administered in a dose of 10–15 mg/kg/dose given every 6 hr intravenously. Vancomycin also should be used to treat bacteremic staphylococcal infections when the organism is resistant to semisynthetic penicillin derivatives.

Staphylococcal infection of the central nervous system can be treated by vancomycin, chloramphenicol, or a combination of chloramphenicol and erythromycin, each by the intravenous route.

Prognosis. Untreated staphylococcal septicemia is associated with a mortality rate of 80% or greater. Mortality rates have been reduced to 20% by appropriate antibiotic treatment. Staphylococcal pneumonia can be fatal at any age but is more likely to be associated with high morbidity and mortality in young infants or in patients whose therapy has been delayed.

A total white blood cell count below 5000/mm³ or a polymorphonuclear leukocyte response of less than 50% is a grave prognostic sign. Prognosis also may be influenced by numerous host factors, including nutrition, immunologic competence, and the presence or absence of other debilitating diseases.

Adamski GB, Garin EH, Ballinger WE, et al: Generalized nonsuppurative myositis with staphylococcal septicemia. J Pediatr 96:694, 1980.

Boris M, Shinefield HR, Ribble JC: Bacterial interference: Its effect on nursery-acquired infection with *Staphylococcus aureus*. IV. Louisiana epidemic. Am J Dis Child 105:674, 1963.

Fine RN, Onslow JM, Erwin ML, et al: Bacterial interference in the treatment of recurrent staphylococcal infections in a family. J Pediatr 70:548, 1967.

Hieber JP, Nelson JD, McCracken GH Jr: Acute disseminated staphylococcal disease in childhood. Am J Dis Child 131:181, 1977.

Larinkari UM, Valtonen MV, Sarvas M, et al: Teichoic acid antibiotic test. Arch Intern Med 137:1522, 1977.

Liston SL, Gehrz RC, Siegel LG, et al: Bacterial tracheitis. Am J Dis Child 137:764, 1983.

Schoenbaum SC, Gardner P, Shillito J: Infections of cerebrospinal fluid shunts: Epidemiology, clinical manifestations, therapy. J Infect Dis 131:543, 1975.

Infections Due to *Staphylococcus epidermidis*

S. epidermidis is a normal inhabitant of the skin, throat, mouth, conjunctiva, vagina, and urethra. Rarely, it has been identified as a cause of meningitis, septicemia, osteomyelitis, or septic arthritis in normal, previously healthy children. More commonly, *S. epidermidis* has been identified as a cause of urinary tract infection; in one study this organism was responsible for 40% of such infections in children 11–16 yr of age.

Otitis media may be attributed to this organism if (1) the organism is grown on solid media from an aspirate obtained by needle tympanocentesis, (2) a swab of the external auditory canal obtained concomitantly fails to grow this organism, and (3) smears of exudate from the middle ear reveal this organism within polymorphonuclear leukocytes.

S. epidermidis is a common cause of infection in patients with shunts inserted for diversion of cerebrospinal fluid or with other foreign bodies that have been implanted. It is also a cause of subacute bacterial endocarditis after cardiac surgery.

Most infections with *S. epidermidis* are indolent and difficult to treat. Therapy must be guided by testing for sensitivity to various antibiotics; many isolates are resistant to penicillin. Selected isolates may be resistant to semisynthetic penicillins but unlike *S. aureus* may remain sensitive to cephalosporins. Vancomycin alone or combined with rifampin has proved to be effective therapy for septicemic *S. epidermidis* infection and for *S. epidermidis* meningitis associated with cerebrospinal fluid shunts. Sensitivity of *S. epidermidis* to various antibiotics should be assessed using tube dilution sensitivity tests.

RALPH D. FEIGIN

Hermansonn G, Bollgren I, Bergstrom T, et al: Coagulase-negative staphylococci as a cause of symptomatic urinary infections in children. J Pediatr 84:807, 1974.

Lowy FD, Hammer SM: *Staphylococcus epidermidis* infections. Ann Intern Med 99:834, 1983.

11.18 TOXIC SHOCK SYNDROME (TSS)

This syndrome is an acute, multisystemic disease characterized by high fever, hypotension, vomiting, abdominal pain, diarrhea, myalgias, nonfocal neurologic abnormalities, and an erythematous rash.

Etiology and Epidemiology. TSS was originally described in 1978 in seven children; from five of them a toxin-producing strain of *Staphylococcus aureus* phage group I was isolated. As new cases were reported, it soon became apparent that most of them (90%) were occurring in menstruating women who were using tampons in the presence of vaginal colonization and/or infection with toxin-producing strains of *S. aureus*. TSS, however, also continues to occur in children as well as in nonmenstruating women and in men. Although the disease has a worldwide distribution, relatively few cases have been reported outside the United States. There is a high recurrence rate (30%), with secondary cases being milder and occurring within 3 mo of the original episode; the overall mortality rate is 3%.

A majority of *S. aureus* strains isolated from confirmed cases are phage type 29/52, are noninvasive, do not adhere to vaginal epithelium, and produce a number of extracellular toxins. Two such toxins, staphylococcal enterotoxin F (SEF) and staphylococcal pyrogenic exotoxin C (PEC), reported to be responsible for the observed clinical manifestations of TSS, have subsequently been determined to be identical and are referred to as toxic shock syndrome toxin (TSS-1). However, TSS-negative strains have been isolated from patients with TSS, suggesting that other as yet unrecognized toxins play a role in TSS and that TSS-1 production is not essential to the pathogenesis of this illness.

Clinical Manifestations. The diagnosis of TSS is based on clinical manifestations (Table 11–19). The onset is abrupt with high fever, vomiting, and diarrhea and is often accompanied by sore throat, headache, and myalgias. A diffuse erythematous macular rash appears within 24 hr and may be associated with hyperemia of pharyngeal, conjunctival, and vaginal mucous membranes. Symptoms often include alterations in the level of consciousness, oliguria, and hypotension, which in severe cases may progress to shock and disseminated intravascular coagulation. Recovery occurs within 7–10 days and is associated with desquamation, particularly of palms and soles; hair and nail loss have also been observed.

There is no specific laboratory test; appropriate selective tests reveal involvement of multiple organ systems including the hepatic, renal, muscular, gastrointestinal, cardiopulmonary, and central nervous system. Vaginal cultures, prior to administration of antibiotics, usually yield *Staphylococcus aureus*.

Differential Diagnosis. Kawasaki disease (mucocutaneous lymph node syndrome) closely resembles TSS clinically. Both are associated with fever unresponsive to antibiotics, hyperemia of mucous membranes, and an erythematous rash with subsequent desquamation. Many of the clinical features of TSS, however, are absent or rare in Kawasaki disease, including diffuse myalgia, vomiting, abdominal pain, diarrhea, azotemia, hypotension, adult respiratory distress syndrome (Sec. 5.41), and shock. Kawasaki disease typically occurs in children under 5 yr of age; one might speculate that some cases of "adult Kawasaki disease" may be TSS. Scarlet fever, Rocky Mountain spotted fever, scarlet fever, leptospirosis, toxic epidermal necrolysis, and measles must also be considered in the differential diagnosis.

Prevention and Treatment. The low risk of acquiring TSS (6.2 cases/100,000 menstruating women) can be reduced by not using tampons or by using them intermittently during each menstrual period.

Management of adolescents suspected of having TSS includes the careful removal of any retained tampons at the time of initial cervical and vaginal cultures. Fluid replacement should be aggressive to prevent or treat cardiovascular collapse.

Parenteral administration of a beta-lactamase resistant antistaphylococcal antibiotic (e.g., nafcillin, oxacillin, methicillin) is recommended after appropriate cultures have been obtained. Antibiotic treatment is discontinued if cultures are negative for *Staphylococcus aureus*; however, positive cultures for this organism require prolonged treatment (parenteral followed by oral) until the organism has been eradicated from the vagina. Alternative antibiotics for patients allergic to penicillin include clindamycin, erythromycin, rifampin, and trimethoprim-sulfamethoxazole.

WILLIAM T. SPECK

Table 11–19. Clinical and Laboratory Characteristics of Toxic Shock Syndrome

Fever (temperature ≥ 38.9° C)

Rash (diffuse macular erythroderma)

Desquamation, 1–2 weeks after onset of illness, particularly of palms and soles

Hypotension (systolic blood pressure ≤ 90 mmHg in adults or < 5th percentile for age in children aged < 16 years, or orthostatic syncope)

Involvement of three or more of the following organ systems:
Gastrointestinal (vomiting or diarrhea at onset of illness)
Muscular (severe myalgia or creatine kinase level ≥ twice upper limits of normal for laboratory)
Mucous membrane (vaginal, oropharyngeal, or conjunctival hyperemia)
Renal (blood urea nitrogen level or serum creatinine level ≥ twice upper limits of normal for laboratory or ≥ 5 leukocytes per high-powered field, in the absence of urinary tract infection)
Hepatic (total bilirubin, serum glutamic oxaloacetic transaminase (AST) or serum glutamic pyruvic transaminase (ALT) activity ≥ twice upper limits of normal for laboratory)
Hematologic (platelet count ≤ 100 × 10⁹/L)
Central nervous system (disorientation or alterations in consciousness without focal neurologic signs when fever and hypotension are absent)

Negative results on the following tests:
Throat and cerebrospinal fluid cultures
Serologic tests for Rocky Mountain spotted fever, leptospirosis, and measles

Schlievert PM, Shands KN, Dan BB, et al: Identification and characterization of an exotoxin from *Staphylococcus aureus* associated with toxic-shock syndrome. J Infect Dis 143:509, 1981.
Shands KN, Schlech WF, Hargrett NJ et al: Toxic shock syndrome: Case control studies at the Centers for Disease Control. Ann Intern Med 96:895, 1982.
Shands KN, Schmid GP, Dan BB: Toxic shock syndrome in menstruating women: Association with tampon use and *Staphylococcus aureus* and clinical features in 52 cases. N Engl J Med 303:1436, 1980.
Todd J, Fishaut M, Kapral F, et al: Toxic-shock syndrome associated with phage-group I staphylococci. Lancet 2:1116, 1978.

11.19 PNEUMOCOCCAL INFECTIONS

The pneumococcus (*Streptococcus pneumoniae*), a normal inhabitant of the upper respiratory tract, can be an invasive pathogen.

Etiology. *Streptococcus pneumoniae* is a gram-positive, lancet-shaped, encapsulated diplococcus. In body fluids and tissues the organisms may be found as individual cocci or as chains. More than 80 serotypes are identified by their type-specific capsular polysaccharide. Antisera to some pneumococcal capsular polysaccharides cross-react with other pneumococcal types or with other bacterial species. Only smooth, encapsulated strains are pathogenic for humans. Virulence is related, in part, to the size of the capsule, but pneumococcal types with capsules of identical size may vary widely in virulence. Fully encapsulated strains (e.g., type 3) are extraordinarily virulent. Capsular material impedes phagocytosis; the mechanism is unclear.

C substance is a cell-wall antigen which is related to species rather than to specific pneumococcal serotypes. R antigen is a species-specific protein on or near the cell surface. A *type*-specific protein (M antigen) also has been detected, but it does not confer any significant antiphagocytic properties. Antibodies to the C, R, or M antigens produce only negligible immunity. In contrast, antibodies to the capsular polysaccharide are protective. The pneumococcus produces a hemolytic toxin called pneumolysin and a toxic neuraminidase. During autolysis pneumococci release a purpura-producing factor that causes dermal and internal hemorrhages when injected into rabbits. The role of these substances, if any, in the pathogenesis of human disease is unknown.

On solid media, the pneumococcus forms unpigmented, umbilicated colonies surrounded by a zone of incomplete (α) hemolysis. Pneumococcal capsules can be seen and the organisms typed by exposing them to homologous type-specific antisera that combine with their respective capsular polysaccharides, thus rendering the capsules refractile (quellung reaction).

Epidemiology. Many healthy individuals carry *S. pneumoniae* in their upper respiratory tracts. Serotypes 6, 19, and 23 constitute almost 50% of all isolates in children. These, plus types 3, 9, 11, 14, 15, and 18, account for 80% of all pneumococcal isolates. Frequently, the same serotype is carried continuously for extended periods (45 days–6 mo). Carriage of a particular serotype does not induce local or systemic immunity sufficient to prevent later reacquisition of the same serotype. Multiple serotypes may coexist in the same nasopharynx. Pneumococcal isolation rates peak during the first 2 yr of life and decline gradually thereafter; carriage rates are highest from December to April and lowest from July to September.

Streptococcus pneumoniae is the most frequent bacterial cause of bacteremia, pneumonia, and otitis media and the third most common cause of meningitis in infants and children. The peak incidence of meningitis occurs among infants 3 to 5 months of age, that of otitis media from 6 to 12 mo, and that of hospitalization for pneumonia from 13 to 18 mo of age. Males are more commonly affected than females, and blacks more than whites; the unusual susceptibility of black children is not entirely explained by the prevalence of sickle cell disease in that population.

Pneumococcal disease generally occurs sporadically. Its frequency and severity are increased in patients with sickle cell disease, asplenia, splenosis, deficiencies in humoral (B cell) immunity, and complement deficiencies.

Pathogenesis and Pathology. Pneumococci must invade to produce disease. Nonspecific host defense mechanisms, including the presence of other bacteria in the nasopharynx, generally limit the multiplication of pneumococci. Aspiration of secretions containing pneumococci is hindered by the epiglottic reflex and by the cilia of the respiratory epithelium, which continuously move infected mucus upward toward the pharynx. Whether disease develops when pneumococci reach the alveoli depends upon the outcome of the interaction of the bacteria with the alveolar macrophages.

Pneumococcal disease frequently follows a viral respiratory tract infection which may produce mucosal damage, diminish the epithelial ciliary activity, and depress the function of alveolar macrophages. Phagocytosis may be impeded by respiratory secretions. In the tissues pneumococci multiply and

spread via the lymphatics or bloodstream (bacteremia) or by direct extension from a local site of infection.

The severity of disease is related to the virulence and number of organisms causing bacteremia, and to the integrity of specific host defenses. Generally, a poor prognosis is associated with very large numbers of pneumococci in blood or with significant concentrations of capsular polysaccharide in the circulation; despite effective antibiotic therapy, patients with heavy antigenemia may have severe and protracted illness.

Deficiency of the terminal components of complement (C3–C9) has been associated classically with recurrent pyogenic infection which includes those caused by *S. pneumoniae*. C2 deficiency also appears to be associated with *S. pneumoniae* infection. The propensity for pneumococcal disease in asplenic persons is presumed to relate to deficient opsonization of the pneumococcus as well as to absence of the filtering function of the spleen on circulating bacteria. Pneumococcal disease is also more prevalent in patients with sickle cell disease and other hemoglobinopathies. Such patients become unable to activate C3 via the alternative pathway or to fix this opsonin to the pneumococcal cell wall. In summary, defective clearance of blood-borne bacteria in the nonimmune host, a decrease in antibody formation, and abnormal activation of the alternative pathway are additive factors that place the asplenic host at risk for overwhelming post-splenectomy infections. The efficacy of phagocytosis also is diminished in patients with B and T cell immunodeficiency syndrome because of a lack of opsonic anticapsular antibody and a failure to produce lysis and agglutination of bacteria. These observations suggest (1) that opsonization of the pneumococcus depends upon both the classical and the properdin (or alternative) complement pathways and (2) that recovery from pneumococcal disease depends upon the development of anticapsular antibodies which act as opsonins, thereby enhancing phagocytosis and ultimately killing the pneumococcus.

Low levels of factor B of the properdin pathway (and defective opsonization) occur in normal individuals during acute pneumococcal disease, suggesting that pneumococcal infection may develop in some individuals because of a transient pre-existing depression of factor B; alternatively, acute pneumococcal infection may be accompanied by consumption of this component of complement. In the normal host, regardless of the pathway of their activation, C3–C9 produce anaphylatoxic, chemotactic, and opsonic activities in serum, and each plays an important role in protection against pneumococcal infection.

In the lung and other body tissues the spread of infection is enhanced by the antiphagocytic properties of capsular-specific soluble substance; an edema-promoting factor also plays a role. In the lung, once infection is established, the alveoli are filled with acellular serous fluid. Soon thereafter polymorphonuclear leukocytes accumulate in the infected alveoli (consolidation), and phagocytosis of pneumococci may be noted. Macrophages subsequently replace the leukocytes in the exudate, and the lesion resolves. This sequence of events evolves over a period of 7–10 days but may be modified by appropriate antibiotic therapy or by administration of type-specific serum. The pathologic sequence in pneumococcal pneumonia is detailed in Sec. 13.66.

Clinical Manifestations. These are related to the site of infection; see pneumonia (Sec. 13.66), otitis media (Sec. 13.40), sinusitis and pharyngitis (Sec. 13.28), (Sec. 13.34), abscesses of the upper airway (Sec. 13.31–13.33), laryngotracheobronchitis (Sec. 13.53), peritonitis (Sec. 12.89), and bacteremia (Sec. 11.12). Local spread of infection may occur, causing empyema (Sec. 13.98), pericarditis (Sec. 14.82), mastoiditis (Sec. 13.40), epidural abscess (Sec. 21.23), or, rarely, meningitis. Bacteremia may be followed by meningitis (Sec. 11.13), septic arthritis (Sec. 11.15), osteomyelitis (Sec. 11.14), endocarditis (Sec. 14.74), and brain abscess (Sec. 21.23). Pneumococcal epiglottitis has been described in the immunocompromised host. Pneumococcal bacteremia in young children with unexplained fever but no localizing signs or symptoms is considered in Sec. 11.12. Subcutaneous abscesses rarely have been reported to follow occult pneumococcal bacteremia.

The incidence of pneumococcal bacteremia, meningitis, endocarditis, and endophthalmitis is increasing in infants under 1 mo of age.

Renal glomerular-capillary and cortical arteriolar thromboses have been associated with pneumococcal bacteremia. Localized gingival lesions, gangrenous areas of skin on the face or extremities, and disseminated intravascular coagulation have also been reported as manifestations of pneumococcal disease.

Diagnosis. This may be established by recovery of pneumococci from the site of infection or the blood. However, pneumococci found in the nose or throat of patients with otitis media, pneumonia, septicemia, or meningitis may not be related causally to their disease.

Blood cultures should be obtained in all children with pneumonia, meningitis, arthritis, osteomyelitis, peritonitis, pericarditis, or gangrenous skin lesions. It is also advisable to obtain blood cultures in children 6–24 mo of age with high fever and leukocytosis who have no localized signs of infection. Pneumococcuria, in most instances, represents seeding of the urine from a remote site of pneumococcal infection.

Pneumococci can be identified in body fluids as gram-positive, lancet-shaped diplococci. A direct quellung test utilizing pneumococcal omniserum (containing high titers of antibody to 82 pneumococcal types) may help to establish a definitive diagnosis rapidly. Early in the course of pneumococcal meningitis, many bacteria may be noted in a relatively acellular cerebrospinal fluid. Countercurrent immunoelectrophoresis of serum, cerebrospinal fluid, and urine, utilizing pneumococcal omniserum, may be helpful in establishing the diagnosis of pneumococcal meningitis or bacteremia. Pneumococcal antigen also may be detected in blood or urine of patients with localized pneumococcal disease (i.e., pneumonia, otitis media). Type-specific antisera enhance the sensitivity of this technique significantly; the diagnostic value of this technique is not affected significantly by previous antibiotic therapy. Countercurrent immunoelectrophoresis of sputum can be helpful in distinguishing between persons with pneumococcal pneumonia and those in whom colonization with the pneumococcus has occurred. This test generally is positive in the former and negative in the latter. Latex particle agglutination tests may also be helpful in rapidly establishing a diagnosis; they are more sensitive than countercurrent immunoelectrophoresis in detecting pneumococcal capsular polysaccharide antigen.

Leukocytosis generally is pronounced, with total white blood cell counts of 30,000/mm³ a common occurrence. The sedimentation rate may be elevated.

Prevention. See Sec. 4.1. Polyvalent pneumococcal vaccines have been tested. They have proved to be highly immunogenic and associated with a low level of untoward reactions. However, responsiveness to pneumococcal polysaccharide has been unpredictable in young children. An octavalent pneumococcal vaccine utilized in high risk children older than 2 yr of age has proved to be immunogenic and apparently protective against some fatal bacteremic pneumococcal infections. Pneumovax presently is recommended for children older than 2 yr of age with (1) asplenia regardless of etiology, (2) nephrotic syndrome, (3) sickle cell disease, and (4) related hemoglobinopathies. Immunization will not prevent pneumococcal disease related to serotypes not found in the vaccine; it will not invariably prevent morbidity and mortality from pneumococcal bacteremia even when the bacteremia is related to a pneumococcal strain that is serotypically identical to one of the vaccine strains.

Administration of gamma globulin to children with hypogammaglobulinemia (IgG less than 200 mg/dL) will diminish the frequency of pneumococcal bacteremia and meningitis but not of pneumococcal respiratory infections. Penicillin G or V, 25,000–50,000 units/kg/24 hr in 4 divided oral doses, may be given to patients who are asplenic or functionally asplenic or whose spleens have been removed. Controlled studies to document that this form of prophylaxis diminishes significantly the incidence of pneumococcal bacteremia in these patients are unavailable.

Treatment. Penicillin is the antibiotic of choice for pneumococcal disease. The dose and duration of treatment must be varied with the site of infection. The sections listed under Clinical Manifestations of the different types of infections should be consulted for specific treatments.

Pneumococci with a decreased susceptibility to penicillin (MICs of 0.2–0.4 μg/mL) have been isolated. Their existence makes it necessary to use high-dose penicillin therapy for patients with meningitis. Ideally, pneumococci isolated from the cerebrospinal fluid of patients with meningitis should be tested by tube dilution as a guide to appropriate therapy. When a pneumococcus is resistant to penicillin but sensitive to chloramphenicol, the latter drug is the treatment of choice. Strains of pneumococci resistant to many antibiotics and to sulfonamides have also been reported. Since no reliable predictions of future distribution or prevalence of these strains are possible, routine sensitivity tests should be performed on all pneumococcal isolates from blood and cerebrospinal fluid. In those areas where such strains are encountered, intravenous treatment with vancomycin (60 mg/kg/24 hr in 4 divided doses) may be required.

Erythromycin, cephalosporins, clindamycin, and chloramphenicol provide effective alternatives for patients allergic to penicillin. Clindamycin and cephalosporins should not be used in patients with pneumococcal meningitis or endocarditis. Sulfadiazine and sulfisoxazole also are effective in pneumococcal pneumonia. Tetracycline should not be used since many strains of pneumococci resistant to it have been reported.

Prognosis. This depends upon the integrity of host defenses, the virulence of the infecting organism, the age of the host, the site of infection, and the adequacy of treatment. See sections listed under Clinical Manifestations for specific diseases.

RALPH D. FEIGIN

Broome CV: Efficacy of pneumococcal polysaccharide vaccines. Rev. Infect Dis 3(Suppl):582, 1981.
Cowan MJ, Ammann AJ, Ward DW, et al: Pneumococcal polysaccharide immunization in infants and children. Pediatrics 62:721, 1978.
Istre GR, Humphreys JT, Albrecht KD, et al: Chloramphenicol and penicillin resistance in pneumonia isolated from blood and cerebrospinal fluid: A prevalence study in metropolitan Denver. J Clin Microbiol 17:472, 1983.
Jacobs NM, Lerdkachornsuk S, Metzger WI: Pneumococcal bacteremia in infants and children: A ten year experience at the Cook County Hospital with special reference to the pneumococcal serotypes isolated. Pediatrics 69:296, 1979.
Klein JO: The epidemiology of pneumococcal disease in infants and children. Rev Infect Dis 3:246, 1981.
Loda FA, Collier AM, Clezen WP, et al: Occurrence of *Diplococcus pneumoniae* in the upper respiratory tract of children. J Pediatr 87:1087, 1975.
Myers MG, Wright PF, Smith AL, et al: Complications of occult pneumococcal bacteremia in children. J Pediatr 84:656, 1974.
Paredes A, Taber LH, Yow MD, et al: Prolonged pneumococcal meningitis due to an organism with increased resistance to penicillin. Pediatrics 58:378, 1976.
Reed WP, Davidson MS, Williams RC Jr: Complement system in pneumococcal infections. Infect Immun 13:1120, 1972.
Sampson HA, Walchner AM, Baker PJ: Recurrent pyogenic infection in individuals with absence of the second component of complement. J Clin Immunol 2:39, 1982.

Topley JM, Cupidare L, Vaida S, et al: Pneumococcal and other infections in children with sickle cell–hemoglobin C (SC) disease. J Pediatr 101:176, 1982.

Weintrub PS, Schiffman G, Addiego JE Jr: Long term follow-up and booster immunization with polyvalent pneumococcal polysaccharide in patients with sickle cell anemia. J Pediatr 105:261, 1984.

Wright PF, Vaughn WK, Andrews C: Clinical studies of pneumococcal vaccines in infants: II. Efficacy and effect on nasopharyngeal carriage. Rev Infect Dis 3(Suppl):108, 1981.

11.20 HAEMOPHILUS INFLUENZAE

Epidemiology and Pathogenesis. *Haemophilus influenzae* is a fastidious, gram-negative, pleomorphic coccobacillus which requires factors X (hematin, heat stable) and V (phosphopyridine nucleotide, heat labile) for growth. Encapsulated strains are classified by the polysaccharides of the soluble capsular substance and designated as types a through f. Almost all serious, invasive infections in children are due to type b. Nonencapsulated strains (nontypable) are etiologic agents principally in upper respiratory tract infections, such as otitis media and sinusitis, but may also cause systemic infection in the neonate or in the immunocompromised child. *Haemophilus* is further classified biochemically into six biotypes; biotype 1 is the most common one isolated from blood and cerebrospinal fluid. *H. influenzae* type b can be further classified, using outer membrane proteins, into six major molecular weight categories that are useful for epidemiologic investigations. For example, utilizing this classification, it has been suggested that most children having recurrent invasive *H. influenzae* type b disease are reinfected with the same organism responsible for the first infection.

H. influenzae is usually endemic, but may be responsible for outbreaks of disease, particularly in day care centers or chronic care facilities. For about 30 days after onset of *H. influenzae* meningitis, the risk in household contacts is 585 times greater than the age-adjusted risk in the general population. The greatest risk of a secondary case is 6% in contacts under 1 yr of age; the risk in children under 4 yr of age is 2.1%. Thus, the risk of secondary cases of *H. influenzae* infection in household contacts under the age of 6 yr is very similar to the risk of secondary meningococcal disease in household contacts. The risk of secondary *H. influenzae* type b infection in day care centers appears to be less than that for household contacts. *H. influenzae* type b meningitis occurs more commonly in black and American Indian children than in white children; Hispanics have rates of infection 1.6 times that of whites. The highest incidence of systemic disease occurs among Alaskan Eskimos: 491 cases/100,000 children below 5 yr of age. Children with asplenia (congenital, surgical, and functional, as in sickle cell anemia) are also at great risk in acquiring serious *H. influenzae* infections.

Antibodies directed against the capsular polysaccharide play an important role in host defense. Anti-polyribophosphate (PRP) antibody is related in part to the opsonic activity of serum for *H. influenzae* type b; other antibodies directed against non-PRP antigens, such as outer membrane proteins, also play a role in opsonization. Both the classical and alternative complement pathways are important in the opsonization of *H. influenzae* type b. In addition, the macrophages of the reticuloendothelial system are critical components for intravascular clearance of *H. influenzae* type b. Less is known about immunity to nontypable strains of *H. influenzae*.

Children 18 mo or less of age demonstrate a poor or absent immunologic response to PRP antibody following either natural infection or immunization; *H. influenzae* type b capsular polysaccharide vaccine is not protective for children under 18 mo of age. Young children do not respond well to polysaccharide vaccines partly because purified polysaccharides are T-cell independent antigens. Anti-PRP response to both nat-ural infection and immunization appears to be partly under genetic control. When immunized with type b polyribosephosphate vaccine, children with allotype Km(1) fail to respond with antibody production to the extent noted in children without this allotype. The converse is true for meningococcus C polysaccharide vaccine. The frequency of the erythrocyte genotype MNSs is increased in children with *H. influenzae* type b epiglottitis compared with that in children with meningitis.

INFECTIONS DUE TO *HAEMOPHILUS INFLUENZAE* TYPE B

H. influenzae type b accounts for approximately 95% of serious infections due to *H. influenzae*. Other typable and nontypable strains infrequently account for serious systemic diseases but are commonly isolated from children with otitis media. The rapid diagnosis of *H. influenzae* type b can be accomplished by several laboratory techniques to detect capsular polysaccharide including countercurrent immunoelectrophoresis (CIE), latex particle agglutination, staphylococcal protein A coagglutination (Co-A), and enzyme-linked immunosorbent assays (ELISA).

Meningitis. See Sec. 11.13. *H. influenzae* type b is the leading cause of bacterial meningitis in the United States in children between ages 1 mo and 4 yr. Clinically, meningitis due to *H. influenzae* cannot be distinguished from that due to *Neisseria meningitidis* or *Streptococcus pneumoniae* and may be complicated by other infections due to this organism including pneumonia, arthritis, osteomyelitis, pericarditis, and endophthalmitis.

Acute Epiglottitis. See Sec. 13.53. This dramatic, potentially lethal condition usually occurs in children 2–7 yr old.

Pneumonia. See Sec. 13.66. The true incidence of *H. influenzae* pneumonia in children is unknown, but it appears to be more common in children 4 yr of age or less. The signs and symptoms of pneumonia due to *H. influenzae* cannot be distinguished from those due to other microorganisms, and associated infections such as otitis media, meningitis, and epiglottitis are common.

Septic Arthritis. See Sec. 11.15. *H. influenzae* type b is the most common organism responsible for septic arthritis in children 2 yr of age or less. Large joints, such as knee, hip, ankle, and elbow, are affected most commonly, and associated infections such as meningitis commonly occur. The signs and symptoms of septic arthritis due to *H. influenzae* type b are indistinguishable from those due to other organisms.

Cellulitis. *H. influenzae* type b is responsible for 5–14% of the cases of cellulitis in young children; over 85% of children with this type of cellulitis are 2 yr of age or younger. Frequently, these children have an upper respiratory infection which is followed by the acute onset of cellulitis. There is usually no prior history of trauma to the area of cellulitis. The head and the neck, particularly the cheek and the periorbital region, are the most common sites of infection. The lesion has generally indistinct margins and is tender and indurated. A violaceous or bluish purple color is common but not diagnostic. In buccal cellulitis an ipsilateral otitis media may be the focus of infection. Other infections such as meningitis and septic arthritis may complicate cellulitis. Blood cultures are positive, and *H. influenzae* type b may often be recovered directly from an aspirate with or without prior injection of 0.1 mL of a nonbacteriostatic sterile solution into the cellulitis. Cellulitis should be treated with intravenous ampicillin (150–200 mg/kg/24 hr in 4–6 divided doses) and chloramphenicol (50–75 mg/kg/24 hr in 4 divided doses) or cefuroxime (150 mg/kg/24 hr in 3 divided doses) until the patient is afebrile and the cellulitis has resolved; antibiotics should be continued until approximately 1 wk after all signs and symptoms have resolved. Depending on the sensitivities of the organism, ampicillin or chloramphenicol may be discontinued or a cephalosporin substituted (Sec. 11.13).

Osteomyelitis. See Sec. 11.14. *H. influenzae* type b is a relatively uncommon cause of osteomyelitis in children.

Pericarditis. See also Sec. 14.82. *H. influenzae* type b is the etiologic agent of bacterial pericarditis in up to 15% of children with this infection. The children are most commonly 2–4 yr of age and often have had an antecedent upper respiratory infection. Fever, respiratory distress, and tachycardia are constant findings. Associated infections also are very common. The etiologic diagnosis may be established by blood culture or by culture, Gram stain, or countercurrent immunoelectrophoresis of pericardial fluid. Ampicillin and/or chloramphenicol should be provided intravenously at dosages and for a duration similar to that of meningitis (Sec. 11.13). A pericardiectomy may be important to drain the purulent material effectively and prevent pericardial tamponade and constrictive pericarditis.

Bacteremia without an Associated Focus. See Sec. 11.1 and 11.12. Bacteremia due to *H. influenzae* type b may occur without any apparent focus of infection other than signs of an upper respiratory infection or pharyngitis. Although affected children may appear only mildly ill at the initial visit, they are at substantial risk of developing a serious infection such as pneumonia or bacterial meningitis.

Neonatal Disease. See Sec. 8.59–8.61. In the neonate nontypable *H. influenzae* is more common than type b. Septicemia, pneumonia and respiratory distress syndrome with shock, conjunctivitis, meningitis, mastoiditis, septic arthritis, and a congenital vesicular eruption have been reported.

Miscellaneous Infections. Urinary tract infection, epididymo-orchitis, cervical adenitis, acute glossitis, uvulitis, infected thyroglossal duct cysts, endocarditis, primary peritonitis, and periappendiceal abscess have been associated with *H. influenzae.*

Otitis Media. See Sec. 13.40.

Treatment. Ampicillin is the antibiotic of choice. Resistance to ampicillin is related primarily to production of a plasmid-mediated β-lactamase enzyme. The prevalence of ampicillin-resistant strains varies throughout the country and must be monitored in each region. Invasive infections presumably due to *H. influenzae* should be treated initially with chloramphenicol in addition to ampicillin. Invasive illnesses include meningitis (Sec. 11.13), pneumonia (Sec. 13.66), cellulitis (Sec. 11.20), epiglottitis (Sec. 13.53), septic arthritis (Sec. 11.15), and pericarditis (Sec. 11.13 and 11.20) but not otitis media (Sec. 13.40); the dosage regimen for each entity is discussed in their respective sections. Once an isolate is proved sensitive to ampicillin, chloramphenicol can be discontinued. β-Lactamase activity can be rapidly determined by a pH indicator system. If β-lactamase production is present, the isolate is considered resistant to ampicillin. If the β-lactamase test is negative, chloramphenicol should not be discontinued until disc or tube sensitivity tests prove that the isolate is sensitive to ampicillin, since a small percentage of β-lactamase negative strains may be resistant to ampicillin because of other mechanisms. In some patients a β-lactamase negative isolate can be recovered from one site and a β-lactamase positive isolate from another site; specific sensitivities of each isolate must be determined prior to discontinuing chloramphenicol. Strains of *H. influenzae* have also been reported to be resistant to chloramphenicol because of the production of a plasmid mediated acetyl-transferase. Cefotaxime, cefuroxime, ceftriaxone, moxalactam, and other third-generation cephalosporins hold significant promise for the treatment of such resistant *H. influenzae* infections because they are effective both in vitro against ampicillin- and chloramphenicol-resistant strains of *H. influenzae* and against infections due to ampicillin-resistant *H. influenzae* type b.

Prevention. A single dose of a vaccine consisting of purified capsular polysaccharide of *H. influenzae* type b should be administered to all children at 2 yr of age and to unimmunized children 2–5 yr of age, after which time the risk of infection decreases substantially because of acquired natural immunity. The vaccine may be given simultaneously with DPT, though at a different site. Serious vaccine reactions have not occurred. The vaccine should also be considered for 18–24 mo old children who are at increased risk of developing *H. influenzae* infections, such as those attending day care centers, those with anatomic or functional asplenia, native Americans, and children with malignancy who are immunosuppressed. Although the efficacy in 18–24 mo old children is not established, their high incidence of meningitis justifies the recommendation. These children should be given a second dose at 2 yr of age. Vaccines modified by conjugation with diphtheria toxoid and by using outer membrane proteins of *H. influenzae* to improve immunogenicity in young children are being evaluated.

Since the risk for secondary infection due to *H. influenzae* type b is equivalent to that of *N. meningitidis*, antibiotic prophylaxis has been suggested as one method of preventing secondary cases. Rifampin is recommended for all family contacts of individuals with *H. influenzae* disease; children (not the index case) less than 4 yr old should be given rifampin orally in a 20 mg/kg dose once daily (not to exceed 600 mg per day) for 4 consecutive days. Parents of children having invasive *H. influenzae* type b disease should be told there is an increased risk of secondary infection due to this organism in other young children in the same household, should be alerted to any signs or symptoms that might be related to such an infection, and should be instructed to seek prompt medical attention when such signs do appear. Parents of children exposed to a single case of systemic *H. influenzae* type b disease in a day care center or nursery school should be similarly warned.

INFECTIONS DUE TO *HAEMOPHILUS APHROPHILUS*

This tiny, gram-negative, nonmotile, pleomorphic coccobacillus may be confused with *H. influenzae* on stained smears. It must also be distinguished from other microaerophilic or fastidious gram-negative bacilli. *Haemophilus aphrophilus* has been isolated from gingival scrapings, interdental material, and tonsils. It has also been associated with pet contact, particularly dogs, and has been isolated from dog bite wounds.

A serious underlying illness is generally present in the patients with *H. aphrophilus* infection. The symptoms are those of the illness caused by the localization of the organism. Endocarditis occurs most frequently; less commonly, brain abscess, sinusitis, miscellaneous abscesses and infected wounds, pneumonia and/or empyema, septicemia, otitis media, septic arthritis, osteomyelitis, or meningitis may occur. Children with cyanotic congenital heart disease are at increased risk for brain abscess.

Standard disc susceptibility tests are not reliable for determining the in vitro antibiotic sensitivity of *H. aphrophilus*. Therefore, broth dilution tests are indicated for determining treatment of serious infections. In general, most strains are susceptible to chloramphenicol, tetracycline, and streptomycin. Susceptibility to penicillin, ampicillin, erythromycin, and cephalosporins is variable.

SHELDON L. KAPLAN
RALPH D. FEIGIN

Band JD, Fraser DW, Ajella G, et al: Prevention of *Haemophilus influenzae* type b disease. JAMA 251:2381, 1984.

Bieger RC, Brewer NS, Washington JA: *Haemophilus aphrophilus:* A microbiologic and clinical review and report of 42 cases. Medicine 57:345, 1978.

Echeverria P, Smith EWP, Ingram D, et al: *Haemophilus influenzae* b pericarditis in children. Pediatrics 56:808, 1975.

Faden HS: Treatment of *Haemophilus influenzae* type b epiglottitis. Pediatrics 63:402, 1979.

Ginsburg CM, Howard JB, Nelson JD: Report of 65 cases of *Haemophilus influenzae* b pneumonia. Pediatrics 64:283, 1979.

Granoff DM, Boise EG, Squires JE, et al: Histocompatibility leukocyte antigen and erythrocyte MNSs specificities in patients with meningitis or epiglottitis due to *Haemophilus influenzae* type b. J Infect Dis 149:373, 1984.

Granoff DM, Daum RS: Spread of *Haemophilus influenzae* type b: Recent epidemiologic and therapeutic considerations. J Pediatr 97:854, 1980.

Kaplan SL, Mason EO, Kvernland SJ, et al: Moxalactam treatment of serious infections primarily due to *Haemophilus influenzae* type b in children. Pediatrics 72:187, 1983.

Kenny JF, Isburg CD, Michaels RH: Meningitis due to *Haemophilus influenzae* type b resistant to both ampicillin and chloramphenicol. Pediatrics 66:14, 1980.

Lilian LD, Yeh TF, Novak GM, et al: Early onset *Haemophilus influenzae* sepsis in newborn infants: Clinical, roentgenographic and pathologic features. Pediatrics 62:299, 1978.

Marshall R, Teele DW, Klein JD: Unsuspected bacteremia due to *Haemophilus influenzae:* Outcome in children not initially admitted to hospital. J Pediatr 95:690, 1979.

Mason EO, Kaplan SL, Lamberth LB, et al: Serotype and ampicillin susceptibility of *Haemophilus influenzae* causing systemic infections in children: 3 years of experience. J Clin Microbiol 15:543, 1982.

Peltola H, Kayhty H, Sivornen A, et al: *Haemophilus influenzae* type b capsular polysaccharide vaccine in children: A double-blind field study of 100,000 vaccines 3 months to 5 years of age in Finland. Pediatrics 60:730, 1977.

Recommendations of the Immunization Practice Advisory Committee: Polysaccharide vaccine for prevention of *Haemophilus influenzae* type b disease. Morbid Mortal Weekly Rept 34:201, 1985.

Sell SH, Wright PF: *Haemophilus influenzae:* Epidemiology, Immunology, and Prevention of Disease. New York Elsevier Biomedical, 1982.

Ward JI, Fraser DW, Baraff LJ, et al: *Haemophilus influenzae* meningitis. A national study of secondary spread of household contacts. N Engl J Med 301:122, 1979.

INFECTIONS DUE TO NEISSERIAE

Neisseriae are gram-negative, nonsporulating, spherical or oval cocci. In smears prepared from clinical specimens or from cultures, they are commonly arranged in pairs (diplococci) and appear biscuit- or pear-shaped. Neisseriae are aerobic and can be recovered on blood agar. They are extremely sensitive to various physical and chemical agents and to drying; recovery is enhanced by use of appropriate media.

Neisseriae normally are found in the nasal and oral cavities, pharynx, vagina, and lower intestinal tract. Human disease most commonly is due to infection with *N. meningitidis* and *N. gonorrhoeae.* Neisseriae of low virulence, including *N. subflava, N. flavescens, N. sicca, N. mucosa, N. lactamica,* and *N. flava,* have been reported as causative agents of septicemia, meningitis, ophthalmitis, and endocarditis in normal children. In several instances petechial hemorrhages have been noted. In at least one case disseminated intravascular coagulation was associated with septicemia and meningitis due to *Branhamella catarrhalis,* a related organism (formerly *N. catarrhalis*).

Meningitis due to *B. catarrhalis* occurs more frequently in children than in adults; meningitis caused by chromogenic neisseriae (*N. subflava, N. perflava, N. flavescens,* and *N. flava*) has no predilection for children. The signs and symptoms of sepsis and meningitis caused by these low virulence organisms are similar to those of recognized pathogens. Penicillin or ampicillin provides effective treatment for them.

11.21 MENINGOCOCCAL INFECTIONS

Etiology. *Neisseria meningitidis* (meningococcus, *N. intracellularis*) may be recovered from the nasopharynx of healthy individuals. Disease occurs when organisms invade the bloodstream (meningococcemia) and then disseminate to other locations. The bacteria are commonly observed within polymorphonuclear leukocytes obtained from diseased areas. Various serogroups of *N. meningitidis* have been identified (types A, B, C, D, X, Y, Z, 29E, W135) and differentiated on the basis of specific capsular polysaccharides. The cell walls of meningococci contain lipopolysaccharide, which appears to be responsible for the endotoxin-like effect noted with meningococcemia.

Epidemiology. Carriage rates of *N. meningitidis* vary from 2–5% in healthy children to as high as 90% in groups of military personnel during epidemics. Children under 3 mo of age rarely develop meningococcal disease.

Meningococcal meningitis generally is a disease of children who acquire *N. meningitidis* from an adult carrier, usually in the same family. The disease has increasingly occurred following exposure within day care centers to children and adults who are carriers or who have infections. The estimated likelihood of meningococcal disease in family contacts, usually occurring simultaneously with the first case, is 1%. This rate is 1000-fold greater than the risk in the community. The risk of meningitis in day care center contacts of children with meningococcal disease is 1/1000. Age-specific attack rates per 100,000 population are greatest for infants under 1 yr; 80% of cases of meningococcal disease occur in children under 10 yr. In the United States, serogroup B has been most commonly associated with human disease (45% of isolates). Thirty-two per cent of isolates were group C; 18%, group Y; 2%, group A; and 3%, other serogroups. The incidence of serogroup C disease has increased, with epidemics occurring within closed populations where serogroup B disease has been endemic.

Pathogenesis. Initially, meningococci colonize the nasopharynx. Hematogenous dissemination occurs when the organism penetrates the mucosa and is transported by leukocytes to the bloodstream and, in turn, to other organs, including ears, eyes, lungs, joints, meninges, heart, and adrenal glands. Circulating serum antibodies and specific secretory IgA seem to be important in protecting the human host. Group-specific antimeningococcal antibody accumulates following prolonged carriage of meningococci. Nasopharyngeal carriage of nontypable meningococci, of those belonging to serogroups X, Y, and Z, or to lactose-fermenting meningococci evokes the production of bactericidal antibodies against groups A, B, and C. Bactericidal antibodies that cross-react with meningococci may also be induced by contact with unrelated gram-positive and gram-negative organisms. Presumably, meningococcemia is prevented in many individuals by these antibodies. The fetus may receive antibodies transplacentally; these persist up to the 3rd mo of life, after which they are generally undetectable until approximately 8 mo of age. Subsequently there is a gradual rise in the prevalence of antibodies; in one study 97% of children over 5 yr of age had antibody levels of 0.479 mg/mL or more. Group-specific hemagglutinating antibody has been detected in nasal washings of patients following recovery from meningococcal disease. Development of group-specific antimeningococcal secretory IgA antibody is associated with enhancement of the pharyngeal defense mechanism.

Pathology. Disease due to *N. meningitidis* is associated with an acute inflammatory response. Endotoxemia may be associated with diffuse vasculitis and disseminated intravascular coagulation. Small blood vessels may be filled with leukocyte-rich fibrin clots. Hemorrhage and necrosis may be noted in any organ system; bleeding into the adrenals may occur in patients with septicemia and shock (*Waterhouse-Friderichsen syndrome*).

Meningococcal infections occur more frequently in persons deficient in the terminal components (C5 through C9) of the complement system and in those with an existing complement-depleting disease. Fulminant meningococcal disease has also been reported in a family with an inherited deficiency of the alternative complement pathway component properdin.

The presence of the B27 histocompatibility leukocyte antigen complex is associated statistically with a predisposition for meningococcal disease. Recurrent meningococcal infection has been associated with a deficiency of IgG_2 subclass.

Clinical Manifestations. There are several patterns of presentation of meningococcemia. *Upper respiratory infection with bacteremia* is frequently observed during epidemics of meningococcal infection. This self-limited coldlike illness may resolve in a few days without further systemic or localizing signs. Maculopapular skin eruptions may occur in some of the affected children. Such meningococcal upper respiratory tract infections may also occur without bacteremia.

Alternatively, *acute meningococcemia* may also occur as an influenza-like illness with fever, malaise, myalgia, and arthralgia. Headache and gastrointestinal symptoms may also be noted. Within hours to days of the onset of clinical manifestations morbilliform, petechial, or purpuric lesions may develop. Hypotension, disseminated intravascular coagulation, oliguria and renal failure, and coma may occur. This septicemia may be *fulminant* with extensive rapidly progressive purpura and unrelenting shock, often with adrenal hemorrhage, and extensive hematogenous dissemination. On occasion, such patients seem unresponsive to any treatment. Acute meningococcemia is more often *nonfulminant*, of varying systemic severity, and responsive to appropriate antibiotics and supportive therapy. There may be dissemination to many different sites during acute meningococcemia. When meningitis follows hematogenous dissemination, lethargy, vomiting, photophobia, seizures, and other signs of meningeal irritation also may occur (Sec. 11.13). *Acute endocarditis, myocarditis,* and *pericarditis* also tend to be associated with acute meningococcemia. *Primary meningococcal pneumonia* also has been reported. *Endophthalmitis* is extremely rare, with symptoms of photophobia and ocular pain developing 1–3 days after the onset of septicemia or meningitis. Ciliary injection, exudate in the anterior chamber, and a swollen, muddy iris may be noted. Rarely, *vulvovaginitis,* urethritis, and pelvic inflammatory disease are due to *N. meningitidis.* Clinical manifestations include a white vaginal discharge, itching, and excoriation of the vulva. Meningococcal infections frequently reactivate latent infection with herpes simplex virus usually manifest as "cold sores."

Chronic meningococcemia is rare in children. When it occurs, it is characterized by anorexia, weight loss, chills, fever, arthralgia or arthritis, and maculopapular lesions. Purulent arthritis, while more common with chronic meningococcemia, may complicate any meningococcal infection accompanied by bacteremia. Acute nonsuppurative polyarthritis has been observed in some patients with meningococcal bacteremia. It occurs more frequently after 5 days or more of illness and may become apparent even in patients treated with appropriate antibiotics for *N. meningitidis. Erythema nodosum* may be observed. *Subacute meningococcal endocarditis* usually is associated with chronic meningococcemia.

Diagnosis. The diagnosis of meningococcal disease is established by culture of blood, cerebrospinal fluid, skin lesions, or other sites of infection. The nasopharynx also should be cultured, but isolation of meningococci from this site provides only presumptive evidence of infection. Petechial or papular lesions can be lanced and smeared to look for gram-negative diplococci. When meningitis is present, the morphologic and clinical characteristics of cerebrospinal fluid are those of an acute bacterial meningitis (Sec. 11.13). Cerebrospinal fluid culture may be negative if the lumbar puncture has been performed early in the course of disease or if the patient has received previous antibiotic treatment.

Blood, cerebrospinal fluid, and urine can also be evaluated by countercurrent immunoelectrophoresis. This technique can detect capsular antigen whether or not the organism is viable. Commercially available antisera for *N. meningitidis*, types A, C, and D, are effective. Commercial antisera for group B meningococci are unreliable. Antisera are also available for groups X, Y, and Z meningococci. Cerebrospinal fluid can be evaluated by the limulus lysate assay; a positive assay indicates the presence of endotoxin and suggests infection by a gram-negative organism. It does not, however, identify the etiologic agent.

Ancillary data may reveal thrombocytopenia, proteinuria, and hematuria. In patients with disseminated intravascular coagulation, decreased serum concentrations of prothrombin, factors V and VIII, and fibrinogen may be observed.

Differential Diagnosis. See Sec. 11.2 and 11.13 for discussion of related infectious and noninfectious diagnoses. The petechial or purpuric rash of meningococcemia (Fig. 11–1 [p. xxvi]) is similar to that noted in any patient with a disease characterized by generalized vasculitis. These include septicemia due to many gram-negative organisms; overwhelming septicemia with gram-positive organisms; bacterial endocarditis; Rocky Mountain spotted fever; infection with echoviruses, particularly types 6, 9, and 16; and coxsackieviruses, predominantly types A-2, A-4, A-9, and A-16. The morbilliform rash occasionally observed may be confused with any macular or maculopapular viral exanthem.

Complications. Meningococcal meningitis may be complicated by deafness, ataxia, seizures, blindness, paresis of cranial nerves 3, 4, 6, and 7, hemi- or quadriparesis, spinal cord infarction, obstructive hydrocephalus, and, rarely, brain abscess. Endophthalmitis, which can develop during the course of meningococcemia, is found more commonly in patients with meningococcal meningitis. Panophthalmitis and suppurative iridochoroiditis also may be observed.

Meningococcemia may be complicated by adrenal hemorrhage, encephalitis, arthritis, myocarditis, pericarditis, pneumonia, lung abscess, peritonitis, growth disturbance (extremely rare), and disseminated intravascular coagulation. Patients with hypotension and purpura may also have a "relatively" decreased adrenal response to ACTH.

Prevention. See Sec. 11.13.

Treatment. Aqueous penicillin G (penicillin V has only 10–25% the efficacy of penicillin G against meningococci and gonococci), 400,000 units/kg/24 hr, should be given intravenously in 6 divided doses. When the etiology is in doubt, ampicillin may be used (300 mg/kg/24 hr in 6 divided doses intravenously). Chloramphenicol sodium succinate, 100 mg/kg/24 hr intravenously in 4 divided doses, provides effective treatment for patients allergic to penicillin. Cefuroxime (200 mg/kg/24 hr), cefotaxime (200 mg/kg/24 hr), and ceftriaxone (100–150 mg/kg/24 hr) are all effective therapy for meningococcal disease and may be useful in patients who are allergic to penicillin. Cefotaxime and cefuroxime are given in 4 divided doses intravenously. Ceftriaxone is provided in 2 divided doses intravenously. Therapy for meningococcemia should be continued for at least 7 days *and* until the patient has been afebrile for 72 hr. If pericarditis, pneumonia, or other complications develop, more prolonged treatment may be necessary. Meningitis should be treated for at least 10 days *and* until the patient has been afebrile for at least 5 days.

Patients with acute meningococcal infections should be monitored carefully. Hourly or half-hourly blood pressure determinations are indicated during the 1st hours of treatment until the infection appears to be under control. White blood cell counts of 7000/mm³ or less or total blood eosinophil counts of over 25 cells/mm³ suggest overwhelming infection and impending shock, especially if purpuric lesions are present or beginning to appear. In this situation, immediate intravenous administration of hydrocortisone, 10 mg/kg, followed by 10 mg/kg/24 hr given in 4–6 divided doses for 24–48 hr may be beneficial but remains controversial.

If shock or disseminated intravascular coagulation develops, appropriate support of blood pressure with osmotically active fluids may be required (Sec. 5.41). Fresh whole blood, heparinization, or both may be helpful in hypotensive patients with disseminated intravascular coagulation (Sec. 15.50). For additional information concerning supportive care, see Sec. 11.13.

Prognosis. Mortality from acute meningococcemia may be as high as 15–20%. Mortality of patients with meningococcal meningitis is less than 3% in most major medical centers. Thus, survival of the untreated patient for the period of time required to develop meningitis is a good prognostic sign. Poor prognostic signs include the development of hypotension, coma, rapidly progressive purpura, disseminated intravascular coagulation, leukopenia, thrombocytopenia, high serum antigen concentrations, and a low sedimentation rate. Survival for 48 hr following initiation of therapy is a good prognostic sign. Later sloughing of skin over purpuric areas may occur but usually heals uneventfully.

Abildgaard CF, Corrigan JJ, Seeler RA, et al: Meningococcemia associated with intravascular coagulation. Pediatrics 40:78, 1967.
Altmann G, Egoz N, Bogokovsky B: Observations on asymptomatic infections with *Neisseria meningitidis*. Am J Epidemiol 98:446, 1973.
Center for Disease Control, The Meningococcal Disease Surveillance Group: Analysis of endemic meningococcal disease by serogroup and evaluation of chemoprophylaxis. J Infect Dis 134:201, 1976.
Ellison RT III, Kohler PF, Curd JG: Prevalence of congenital or acquired complement deficiency in patients with sporadic meningococcal disease. N Engl J Med 308:913, 1983.
Jensen AD, Naidoff MA: Bilateral meningococcal endophthalmitis. Arch Ophthal 90:396, 1973.
Lewis LS: Prognostic factors in acute meningococcemia. Arch Dis Child 54:44, 1979.
Munford RS, de Vasconcelas ZJS, Phillips CJ, et al: Eradication of carriage of *Neisseria meningitidis* in families; a study in Brazil. J Infect Dis 129:644, 1974.
Schaad UB: Arthritis in disease due to *Neisseria meningitidis*. Rev Infect Dis 2:880, 1980.
Wajchenberg B, Leme CE, Tambascin M: The adrenal response to exogenous adrenocorticotrophin in patients with infection due to *Neisseria meningitidis*. J Infect Dis 138:387, 1978.

11.22 GONOCOCCAL INFECTIONS

Gonorrhea, an acute infection caused by *Neisseria gonorrhoeae*, afflicts children of all ages. The dramatic increase in the number of reported cases, more than 400/100,000 population, coupled with an increasing proportion of isolates resistant to penicillin, makes this a disease of increasing importance. See also Sec. 9.9.

Etiology. *N. gonorrhoeae* are aerobic gram-negative diplococci, difficult to cultivate in vitro because of fastidious growth requirements. They grow best on chocolate agar to which vancomycin, colistimethate sodium, and nystatin (Thayer-Martin medium) have been added. This medium inhibits growth of organisms other than gonococci or meningococci. Gonococci grow best in an atmosphere of 2–10% carbon dioxide at pH 7.2–7.6 and at a temperature of 35–37° C. In clinical specimens the organism may be found within polymorphonuclear leukocytes.

N. gonorrhoeae can be subdivided on the basis of colony variation into 4 types. Pili can be visualized by electron microscopy on colony types 1 and 2 only, the types that produce human disease. Autotyping has permitted discrimination of approximately 20 types. Sixteen serotypes have been identified by antigenic specificity of the protein antigen in the outer membrane of the gonococcus.

Epidemiology. Gonorrhea is the most commonly reported infectious disease in the United States, at least 2 million cases each yr, one quarter in persons 10–19 yr of age.

In the newborn period gonorrhea generally is acquired during delivery or by contact with fomites. Young children may acquire disease through contact with infected parents or other caretakers. Most cases in adolescents follow venereal contact.

Pathology. An inflammatory response is initiated beneath the epithelium at the point of entry of the gonococcus. This response, apparently caused by endotoxin, is characterized by a yellow-white discharge containing polymorphonuclear leukocytes, serum, and desquamated epithelium. The discharge may block the ducts of paraurethral or vaginal glands and thus cause cysts or abscesses. In the untreated patient the inflammatory exudate is replaced by fibroblasts, and fibrous tissue may lead to stricture of the urethra.

Gonococci that invade the lymphatics and blood vessels may lead to inguinal lymphadenopathy; to perineal, perianal, ischiorectal, and periprostatic abscesses; and to disseminated gonococcal disease.

Pathogenesis. Gonococci can invade columnar epithelium, and even immature stratified squamous epithelium. Fully mature stratified squamous epithelium is resistant to invasion. On a mucosal surface (urogenital, conjunctival, pharyngeal, or rectal), gonococci adhere by means of hairlike protein structures (pili) that extend from the cell wall. The pili may protect the gonococcus from the action of antibody and complement and also may be responsible for antiphagocytic properties. Multiple capsular types may help to explain why multiple attacks of gonorrhea may occur. Local factors, such as the thickness of the vaginal wall and the pH of vaginal mucus, may influence the development of disease. The vaginal epithelium of prepubertal females is thin, and the pH of the vaginal mucin is alkaline, predisposing to vaginitis. The peroxidase-mediated bactericidal capacity of cervical secretions also is pH dependent and is least active during menses. Thus, extension of gonococcal disease from the cervix, as well as dissemination, is more likely to occur during menses. Disseminated infection more frequently follows pharyngeal or anorectal inoculation.

Antigonococcal secretory IgA antibody, sensitized lymphocytes, and serum antibodies have been detected in some but not all infected persons, principally in those with repeated infections and in asymptomatic female carriers. Apparently, these immune responses do not provide solid immunity to gonococcal disease; reinfection is common.

N. gonorrhoeae isolates from patients with disseminated gonococcal disease differ from other gonococcal isolates. They have unique nutritional requirements and are susceptible to lower concentrations of antibiotic agents. Moreover, sera from patients with uncomplicated gonorrhea are bactericidal for more strains of *N. gonorrhoeae* than sera from patients with disseminated gonococcal disease.

Clinical Manifestations. The clinical manifestations of gonococcal infection depend upon (1) the site of infection, (2) differences between strains of *N. gonorrhoeae*, and (3) the host response.

Asymptomatic Gonorrhea. The incidence of this form of gonorrhea in children has not been ascertained. In one study of females 12–19 yr of age admitted to a school for delinquents, the incidence of gonorrhea was 12%; most were asymptomatic. As many as 80% of adult women and 40% of adult men with gonorrhea apparently are asymptomatic. Asymptomatic rectal carriage of *N. gonorrhoeae* has been documented in 40–60% of females with genital infection and in 33–90% of such males (generally homosexuals). Asymptomatic pharyngeal infection has also been documented. Gonococci have been isolated from the oropharynx of young (2–9 yr of age) children who have been abused sexually by male contacts; oropharyngeal symptoms are usually absent. Individuals with asymptomatic gonorrhea are an important reservoir of infection and may develop disseminated disease.

Uncomplicated Gonorrhea. Genital gonorrhea has an incubation period of 2–5 days. Primary infection develops in the urethra of the male, the vulva and vagina of the prepubertal female, and the cervix of the postpubertal female. Neonatal ophthalmitis occurs in each sex.

Urethritis is characterized by a purulent discharge and by burning on urination. Gram-negative intracellular diplococci are demonstrable in the discharge.

The prepubertal female develops a vaginal discharge, and the vulva may be swollen, erythematous, and excoriated. Dysuria may be noted.

Symptomatic gonococcal cervicitis is characterized by purulent discharge, dysuria, and dyspareunia. The cervix may be inflamed and tender. Pain is not enhanced by moving the cervix, and the adnexae are not tender to palpation.

Gonococcal ophthalmitis may be unilateral or bilateral. The eyes are red and swollen and there is a purulent discharge. If the disease is not treated, corneal ulceration, opacification, and rupture may follow. See also Sec. 8.64 and 25.9.

Disseminated Gonococcal Disease. Hematogenous dissemination follows asymptomatic more commonly than symptomatic gonorrhea. The most common manifestations are arthritis, tenosynovitis, dermatitis, carditis, and meningitis.

Two forms of gonococcal arthritis have been described. The first is associated with fever, chills, skin lesions, and involvement of multiple large and small joints. Blood cultures frequently are positive, and, less commonly, *N. gonorrhoeae* may be recovered from the joint effusion. The second is associated with minimal systemic symptoms and signs, and monoarticular arthritis is more common; blood cultures tend to be negative, but the organism is commonly recovered from the joint effusion.

Dermatologic lesions may be macular, maculopapular, vesicular, pustular, or purpuric. The mucous membranes and scalp are generally spared. Lesions may be noted on the palms and soles. Rarely are gonococci recovered from the lesions.

Endocarditis is rare but often fatal. Arthritis or arthralgia may be initial symptoms. Both left- and right-sided endocarditis have been noted; aortic valve involvement is most frequent.

Meningitis with *N. gonorrhoeae* has been documented. Signs and symptoms are similar to those of any acute bacterial meningitis. (Sec. 11.13) Central nervous system infection with *N. gonorrhoeae* has been associated with the placement of ventriculoamniotic shunts. If this procedure is used, the mother must be monitored closely for cervical pathogens.

Diagnosis and Differential Diagnosis. A definite diagnosis of gonococcal disease depends upon isolation of *N. gonorrhoeae*. In the male with urethritis, a presumptive diagnosis can be made by identification of gram-negative intracellular diplococci in the urethral discharge. A similar finding in females is not sufficient since *Mima polymorpha* and *Moraxella* (normal vaginal flora) have a similar appearance. In some culture-positive cases, the Gram stain may be negative. Fluorescent staining is inaccurate; the antibody utilized cross-reacts with other species of *Neisseria* and other organisms. A rapid slide coagglutination test is now available (Phadebact gonococcus test) for identification of gonococci from culture media. The sensitivity is high (96–98%) for identification of gonococci in anogenital lesions of females and in urethral lesions of males.

Cultures should be obtained with noncotton swabs and should be placed immediately in a transport medium (Transgrow) or plated directly on Thayer-Martin medium. Colonies of *N. gonorrhoeae* are oxidase-positive. Further differentiation from oxidase-positive *Mima polymorpha* and *Neisseria lactamicus* (both found in normal vaginal and oral secretions) can be made by fluorescent antibody and sugar fermentation techniques; gonococci ferment only glucose.

Gonococcal urethritis and vulvovaginitis must be distinguished from other infections that produce a purulent discharge, including β-hemolytic streptococci, *Mycoplasma*, *Trichomonas vaginalis*, and *Candida*. Rarely, infection with herpesvirus type 2 may produce symptoms similar to those of gonorrhea. *Gonococcal arthritis* must be distinguished from other forms of septic arthritis as well as from rheumatic fever, rheumatoid arthritis, and arthritis secondary to rubella or rubella immunization.

Complications. Complications of gonorrhea result from the spread of gonococci from a local site of invasion. The time interval between primary infection and development of a complication varies from days to years. Endometritis may occur, especially during menses. It may be followed by salpingitis, pyosalpinx, hydrosalpinx, tubo-ovarian abscess, and eventual sterility. When gonococci gain access to the peritoneum, they may accumulate over the capsule of the liver to cause perihepatitis. The resultant right upper quadrant pain in association with signs of salpingitis is known as Fitz-Hugh–Curtis syndrome.

The most frequent complications of gonococcal urethritis in the male are prostatitis, epididymitis, and urethral strictures.

Gonococcal infection of joints may be associated with destruction of cartilage and ankylosis.

Gonococcal ophthalmitis may be associated with corneal ulceration, opacification, and blindness. Enucleation may be necessary.

All patients with gonorrhea should have a serologic test for syphilis at the time of diagnosis and 3 mo later (Sec. 11.49).

Prevention. Gonorrhea can be prevented by educational efforts and by initiation of bactericidal measures immediately following exposure. Prevention by immunization is not possible at present.

The use of a condom during intercourse helps to prevent acquisition of gonorrhea by the male; it also may prevent transmission of disease to his female partner. Vaginal foam, jelly, and cream contraceptives may also be effective in destroying gonococci.

Gonococcal ophthalmitis in the newborn infant can be prevented by instillation into the conjunctival sac of a 1% solution of silver nitrate shortly after birth (Sec. 8.64).

Treatment. Penicillin is the drug of choice for initial therapy of gonorrhea, although an increasing proportion of isolates of *N. gonorrhoeae* are relatively insensitive to penicillin (minimal inhibitory concentrations to penicillin are 0.5 μg/mL or higher), and some are resistant to tetracycline and penicillin. Cases of gonorrhea due to β-lactamase–producing gonococci (completely resistant to penicillin and ampicillin) have been reported within the United States.

Uncomplicated urethritis or vulvovaginitis can be treated with a single dose of aqueous procaine penicillin G, 100,000 units/kg intramuscularly, and probenecid, 25 mg/kg orally. Alternatively, amoxicillin, 50 mg/kg orally, with probenecid, 25 mg/kg (maximum 1.0 g), can be provided. For adults or children who weigh more than 45 kg (100 lb) the United States Public Health Service currently recommends injection of a single dose of 4.8 million units of aqueous procaine penicillin accompanied by 1.0 g of probenecid orally. Alternatively, ampicillin 3.5 g or amoxicillin 3.0 g (orally) with 1.0 g of probenecid (orally) can be used.

Tetracycline can be provided for allergic individuals over 8 yr of age in a dose of 40 mg/kg/24 hr orally in 4 divided doses for 5 days (total dosage 10 g), but single dose treatment with penicillin, ampicillin, or amoxicillin is recommended for patients who are not allergic to penicillin and are unlikely to complete the multiple-dose tetracycline regimen. Uncomplicated gonococcal disease in the penicillin-allergic child who is under 8 yr of age can be treated with erythromycin, 40 mg/kg/24 hr in 4 divided oral doses, for 7 days. Patients who are allergic to penicillin and who have gonococcal cervicitis, urethritis, epididymitis, or prostatitis may be treated with spectinomycin in a single dose of 2 g for men and 4 g for women administered once intramuscularly.

Patients with disseminated gonococcal disease should be hospitalized and treated with aqueous penicillin G intravenously, 100,000–200,000 units/kg/24 hr in 6 divided doses for 7–10 days. Allergic patients with disseminated gonococcal disease who are over 8 yr of age can be treated with tetracycline. An initial dose, 25 mg/kg, should be administered orally, followed by 40–60 mg/kg/24 hr in 4 divided doses for 7 days. When intravenous therapy is necessary, 15–20 mg/kg/24 hr of tetracycline should be given in 4 divided doses for 7 days. For children under 8 yr of age, disseminated disease can be treated with cephalothin, 60–80 mg/kg/day in 4 divided doses, intravenously for 7 days. Cephalothin should not be used in children with a previous history of anaphylaxis, urticaria, or exfoliative dermatitis associated with penicillin therapy.

Some studies suggest that trimethoprim-sulfamethoxazole may be effective for the treatment of gonococcal disease. Uncomplicated urethral gonococcal disease including infection caused by penicillin-resistant strains has responded to moxalactam in a single dose of 100 mg/kg (up to 1 g) intramuscularly. A single oral dose of cefaclor (3 g) has also provided effective therapy for the treatment in women of uncomplicated gonococcal infection caused by penicillinase-producing strains of *N. gonorrhoeae*. Single oral cefaclor doses of 40 mg/kg similarly may be effective in female children.

Infants born to mothers with known gonococcal infection should have immediate orogastric, rectal, and blood cultures. Aqueous penicillin G should be administered if cultures or Gram-stained smears reveal gonococci. Dosage and duration of therapy are determined by the clinical disease that develops. Patients with neonatal gonococcal ophthalmitis must be hospitalized (also see Sec. 8.64). Aqueous penicillin G, 50,000–75,000 units/kg/24 hr in 3 divided doses, is provided intravenously for 7–10 days. Saline irrigations of the eyes and instillation of penicillin, erythromycin, tetracycline, or chloramphenicol eyedrops may be utilized concomitantly.

Conjunctivitis caused by β-lactamase–producing *N. gonorrhoeae* has been treated effectively with cefotaxime, 100 mg/kg/24 hrs in 3 divided intravenous doses for 7 days.

Prognosis. Prompt diagnosis and adequate therapy virtually assure complete recovery from uncomplicated gonococcal disease. Complications and permanent sequelae may be associated with delayed treatment.

Center for Disease Control: Gonorrhea: Recommended treatment schedules, 1979: Morbidity and Mortality Weekly Reports, Vol. 28 (Jan. 19), 1979.

Dorqiswamy B, Hammerschlag MR, Pringle GF, et al: Ophthalmia neonatorum caused by β-lactamase producing *Neisseria gonorrhoeae*. JAMA 250:790, 1983.

Groothius JR, Bischoof ML, Jauregui LE: Pharyngeal gonorrhea in young children. Pediatr Infect Dis 2:99, 1983.

Litt IF, Edberg SC, Finberg L: Gonorrhea in children and adolescents: A current review. J Pediatr 85:595, 1974.

Thompson TR, Swanson RE, Weisner PF: Gonococcal ophthalmia neonatorum. Relationship of time of infection to relevant control measures. JAMA 228:186, 1974.

Tompkins DS, Nehaul BBG, Smith CAF, et al: Evaluation of the Phadebact Gonococcus Test in the identification of *Neisseria gonorrhoeae* in a routine diagnostic laboratory. J Clin Pathol 34:1106, 1981.

11.23 DIPHTHERIA

Diphtheria is an acute infectious disease caused by *Corynebacterium diphtheriae*. Generalized and localized clinical manifestations follow elaboration of toxin, an extracellular protein metabolite, by toxigenic strains of *C. diphtheriae*. Records suggest the recognition of diphtheria as early as the 4th century B.C.

Etiology. *C. diphtheriae* is an irregularly staining gram-positive, nonmotile, nonsporulating, pleomorphic bacillus. The club shape of the bacillus is not a true morphologic feature but a result of attempts to grow it under nutritionally inadequate circumstances (Loeffler medium). The bacillus is recovered most readily on media containing selective inhibitors that retard the growth of other microorganisms (tellurite).

Colonies of *C. diphtheriae* appear grayish white on Loeffler medium. On tellurite media, three colony types can be distinguished: mitis colonies are smooth, black, and convex; gravis colonies are gray and semirough; intermedius colonies are small and smooth and have a black center. These three types also display differences in fermentation and hemolytic reactions.

Both smooth and rough strains may be nontoxigenic or toxigenic; no differences have been detected in the exotoxins elaborated by the three strains of *C. diphtheriae*. Infection of *C. diphtheriae* by a bacteriophage carrying the gene for toxin production is required to render most strains toxigenic, but multiplication of phage is not a prerequisite for toxin production. The synthesis of toxin depends upon both genetic and nutritional factors. Toxin-producing cells apparently are those in which spontaneous induction of prophage to the phage occurs. Both toxigenic and nontoxigenic strains of *C. diphtheriae* can cause disease, but only strains that produce toxin are responsible for myocarditis and neuritis.

Epidemiology. Diphtheria occurs worldwide, but its incidence declined sharply following extensive use of diphtheria toxoid after World War II. From 1970 through 1976, an average of 248 cases of diphtheria were reported annually in the United States; since 1976, the average has been 56 cases. Mortality, however, has remained relatively constant at about 10% of cases.

The incidence of diphtheria peaks during the autumn and winter months. Eighty per cent of cases occur in unimmunized individuals under 15 yr of age, and the incidence is highest among the poor who reside in crowded conditions with limited access to health care.

Diphtheria is acquired by contact with either a carrier or a person with the disease. The bacteria may be transmitted by droplets spread by coughing, sneezing, or talking. Some reports suggest that diphtheritic infections of the skin predispose to respiratory colonization. Fomites and dust may also serve as vehicles of transmission.

Pathogenesis and Pathology. Diphtheria is predominantly initiated by entry of *C. diphtheriae* into the nose or mouth, and the bacilli remain localized on the mucosal surfaces of the upper respiratory tract. Occasionally, the skin or the ocular or genital mucous membranes serve as the site of localization. Following a 2–4 day period of incubation, strains infected with bacteriophage may elaborate toxin. This is initially adsorbed to the cell membrane and then penetrates it to interfere with protein synthesis within the bacterial cell. The toxin produces an enzymatic cleavage of nicotinamide adenine dinucleotide (NAD) with subsequent formation of an inactive transferase—adenosine diphosphoribose. Protein synthesis ceases because this enzyme is required for the transfer of amino acids from RNA to the elongating polypeptide.

Tissue necrosis is severe in the vicinity of colonization. The local inflammatory response coupled with the necrotic tissue produces a patchy exudate which initially can be removed. As toxin production increases, the area of infection widens and deepens, and a fibrinous exudate develops. A tough adherent membrane is formed that varies from gray to black, depending on the amount of blood it contains. In addition to fibrin, the membrane contains inflammatory, red blood, and superficial epithelial cells. Since the latter are an integral part of the membrane, attempts to remove it are followed by bleeding. The membrane sloughs spontaneously during the recovery period.

Edema of the soft tissues beneath the membrane may be extensive. Occasionally, secondary other bacterial infection (usually streptococcal) develops. The membrane and edematous tissue may encroach upon the airway and cause respiratory embarrassment or suffocation, if they extend to the larynx or tracheobronchial area.

Toxin produced at the site of infection is distributed via the bloodstream throughout the body. The toxin can damage any organ or tissue, but lesions of the heart, nervous system, and kidneys are particularly prominent. Although diphtheria antitoxin can neutralize circulating toxin or that adsorbed to cells, it is ineffective when cell penetration has occurred. There is a variable latent period before clinical manifestations appear. Myocarditis generally is observed 10–14 days after the onset of illness. Nervous system manifestations, particularly peripheral neuritis, usually do not appear for 3–7 wk.

The most prominent pathologic findings are toxic necrosis and hyaline degeneration of various organs and tissues. In the heart one may observe edema, congestion, and mononuclear cell infiltration of muscle fibers and the conducting system. A toxic neuritis with fatty degeneration of myelin sheaths may be noted. Liver necrosis may occur, possibly associated with hypoglycemia. Adrenal hemorrhage and acute tubular necrosis of the kidney are also noted in some cases.

Clinical Manifestations. The signs and symptoms of diphtheria will depend upon the site of infection and the immunization status of the host and upon whether or not toxin escapes into the systemic circulation.

The incubation period ranges from 1–6 days. Diphtheria is classified clinically by the location of the diphtheritic membrane (nasal, tonsillar, pharyngeal, laryngeal or laryngotracheal, conjunctival, skin, and genital). More than one anatomic site may be involved.

Nasal diphtheria initially resembles a common cold and is characterized by mild rhinorrhea and a paucity of systemic symptoms. Gradually, the nasal discharge becomes serosanguineous and then mucopurulent and excoriates the nares and upper lip. A foul odor may be noticed, and careful inspection will reveal a white membrane on the nasal septum (Fig. 11–2 [p. xxvii]). Slow absorption of toxin and the lack of systemic symptoms frequently delay diagnosis. This form of the disease occurs most often in infants.

Tonsillar and/or pharyngeal diphtheria begins insidiously. Anorexia, malaise, low-grade fever, and pharyngitis are noted initially. Within 1–2 days a membrane appears that may vary in extent according to the immune status of the host; in partially immune individuals a membrane may not develop. The membrane initially is thin and gray, resembling a spider web that gradually extends from the tonsil to the contiguous soft or hard palate; this characteristic distinguishes diphtheria from other forms of membranous tonsillitis. The adherent membrane may spread to cover the tonsils and pharyngeal wall (Fig. 11–3 [p. xxvii]) or progress into the larynx and trachea. Attempts to remove it are followed by bleeding.

Cervical lymphadenitis is variable, and when associated with edema of the soft tissues of the neck it may be so severe as to give the appearance of a "bull neck." The edema may obliterate the borders of the sternocleidomastoid muscle, the mandible, and the clavicle. The edema is brawny, pitting, warm, and tender. It occurs most commonly in children over 6 yr of age.

The course of pharyngeal diphtheria depends upon the extent of the membrane and the amount of toxin produced. In severe cases respiratory and circulatory collapse may occur. The pulse rate is increased disproportionately to the body temperature, which generally remains normal or slightly elevated. Palatal paralysis may occur. If it is unilateral, the palate deviates away from the paralyzed side; if bilateral, paralysis may eliminate the nasal quality of the voice and cause nasal regurgitation and cause difficulty in swallowing. Stupor, coma, and death may follow within 7–10 days. In less severe cases, recovery may be slow or may be complicated by myocarditis or neuritis. In mild cases the membrane sloughs in 7–10 days, and recovery is uneventful.

Laryngeal diphtheria generally represents a downward extension of the membrane from the pharynx. Occasionally, only laryngeal involvement is present. The clinical findings of noisy breathing, progressive stridor, and hoarseness are indistinguishable from those in other types of infectious croup. Suprasternal, subcostal, and supraclavicular retractions reflect severe laryngeal obstruction, which may be fatal unless alleviated. Occasionally acute and fatal obstruction may occur when a partially detached piece of membrane occludes the airway. In severe cases the membrane may extend downward and cover the entire tracheobronchial tree.

Cutaneous, vulvovaginal, conjunctival, and aural diphtheria also occur. *Cutaneous diphtheria* usually appears as an ulcer with a sharply defined border and a membranous base. It is more common in warmer climates and may serve as an important source of person-to-person transmission of diphtheria. *Conjunctival lesions* usually are limited to the palpebral conjunctiva, which appears red, edematous, and membranous; corneal erosion may occur. *Aural diphtheria* is characterized by otitis externa with a persistent purulent and frequently foul-smelling discharge.

Diagnosis. *Diagnosis should be made as promptly as possible on the basis of clinical findings. Any delay in therapy poses a serious risk to the patient.* Definitive diagnosis depends upon isolation of C. diphtheriae. Microscopic examination of material from diphtheritic lesions is unreliable; the fluorescent antibody technique may be used but is reliable only with experienced personnel.

Material from beneath the membrane or a portion of the membrane itself should be obtained for culture. C. diphtheriae is relatively resistant to drying; use of nonnutritive, moisture-reducing transport medium helps to prevent the overgrowth of other microorganisms. The laboratory should be notified about the suspicion of diphtheria so that appropriate Loeffler, tellurite, and blood agar media are inoculated. Diphtheria bacilli that are recovered should be tested for toxigenicity by inoculating two guinea pigs intracutaneously with a broth suspension of the microorganism. One of the animals is given diphtheria antitoxin prior to the intracutaneous challenge. An inflammatory lesion will appear at the site of inoculation in 24 hr and will become necrotic in 72 hr in the control animal. No skin reaction should occur in the animal given antitoxin.

Other laboratory studies are of little diagnostic value. The white blood cell count may be normal or elevated. Rarely, anemia may develop as a result of rapid hemolysis. In diphtheritic neuritis there may be a slight elevation of protein and, rarely, mild pleocytosis in the cerebrospinal fluid. Hypoglycemia, glycosuria, or both may reflect hepatic toxicity. An elevation in blood urea nitrogen may develop in patients with acute tubular necrosis. Electrocardiography may reveal arrhythmias or S-T segment and T-wave changes indicative of myocarditis.

Schick Test. This skin test is useful in determining the susceptibility of contacts and in the diagnosis of immunodeficiency.

Method: 0.1 mL (1/50 of a minimum lethal dose for a guinea pig) of a standard solution of diphtheria toxin is injected intracutaneously. In the absence of circulating antitoxin, a local inflammatory response characterized by erythema, swelling, and tenderness occurs and peaks at about 5 days after injection. If sufficient antitoxin is present, no reaction should occur. Many individuals become hypersensitive to the toxin itself or to other antigens in the toxin preparation. Therefore, a control injection of toxoid (0.005 Lf [limit flocculation unit]) is administered intradermally in the opposite arm. The individual who is immune but sensitive to the toxin preparation will react to both toxin and toxoid. These skin reactions generally are maximal at 48–72 hr and then fade into a positive Schick test, which persists for many days. If the individual has no antitoxin in his or her serum but is allergic to the toxoid, a reaction will be noted on both arms, but the reaction at the site of toxin injection will peak on day 5 and persist, whereas the reaction to toxoid will subside by 5–7 days. A positive Schick test consists of more than 10 mm of induration and indicates susceptibility to diphtheria.

Differential Diagnosis. Mild forms of nasal diphtheria in the partially immunized host may resemble the common cold. When a more serosanguineous or purulent nasal discharge is present, nasal diphtheria must be distinguished from foreign body in the nose, sinusitis, adenoiditis, or the "snuffles" of congenital syphilis. Careful examination of the nose with a nasal speculum, sinus roentgenograms, and serologic tests for syphilis should be helpful.

Tonsillar and/or pharyngeal diphtheria must be differentiated in particular from streptococcal pharyngitis and from infectious mononucleosis. The former is generally associated with more severe pain on swallowing, higher temperature, and a relatively nonadherent membrane limited to the tonsils. Pharyngeal diphtheria and streptococcal pharyngitis may coexist. Infectious mononucleosis is usually accompanied by lymphadenopathy and splenomegaly, atypical lymphocytes, and heterophile antibodies.

Nonbacterial membranous tonsillitis is usually characterized by a low white blood cell count, normal throat flora, and a course unaffected by antibiotics; primary herpetic tonsillitis, by gingivitis, stomatitis, and discrete lesions of the tongue and palate; and thrush, by lesions on the buccal mucosa and tongue and by absence of constitutional symptoms. Tonsillar and pharyngeal diphtheria also must be differentiated from blood dyscrasias, such as agranulocytosis and leukemia; from post-tonsillectomy faucial membranes, in which the membranes are stationary and do not spread; and from oropharyngeal involvement by *Toxoplasma*, cytomegalovirus, *Francisella tularensis*, and salmonellae. Vincent angina may be indistinguishable.

Laryngeal diphtheria must be differentiated from croup of other causes (Sec. 13.53), aspirated foreign bodies, peripharyngeal and retropharyngeal abscesses, and laryngeal papillomas, hemangiomas, or lymphangiomas. Direct laryngeal visualization in hospital under controlled conditions should be diagnostic provided that the child's condition does not demand an emergency tracheotomy.

Complications. Penicillin has significantly reduced the frequency of secondary bacterial complications. Nevertheless, respiratory obstruction and death may occur suddenly in young children with laryngeal or tracheal diphtheria. Edema of the neck may also compromise the airway. Myocarditis

(Sec. 14.77) may follow both severe and mild cases of diphtheria and is most common in patients with extensive local lesions and when there has been a delay in the administration of antitoxin. It generally occurs in the 2nd wk of the disease but may appear as early as the 1st or as late as the 6th wk. It is potentially the gravest of the complications and demands the most careful supervision and therapy. Complete bed rest is essential.

Neurologic complications generally appear after a variable latent period, are predominantly bilateral, and are usually motor rather than sensory. They usually resolve completely. Paralysis of the soft palate is most common, generally appearing in the 3rd wk. Ocular paralysis is most common during the 5th wk but may appear as early as the 1st wk. It may cause blurring of vision, difficulty with accommodation, and internal strabismus. Neuritis of the phrenic nerve may cause paralysis of the diaphragm, usually between the 5th and 7th wk. Paralysis of the limbs with loss of deep tendon reflexes and an elevation of cerebrospinal fluid protein may be noted; this complication is clinically indistinguishable from Guillain-Barré syndrome.

Rarely, 2–3 wk after onset of diphtheria the vasomotor centers may be affected and hypotension and cardiac failure ensue. Gastritis, hepatitis, and nephritis are frequent complications.

Prevention. *Immunization.* See Sec. 4.1.

Contacts. The immediate prevention of diphtheria depends upon isolation of the patient and upon management of contacts. The patient is infectious until diphtheria bacilli can no longer be cultured from the site of infection; three consecutive negative cultures are required before the patient is released from isolation.

Intimate contacts are likely to contract the disease if they are not immune. Culture samples from the nose and throat should be obtained. Previously immunized carriers should be given a booster injection of diphtheria toxoid *and* should be treated with aqueous procaine penicillin, 600,000 units daily for 4 days, benzathine penicillin, 600,000 units intramuscularly as a single dose, or erythromycin, 40 mg/kg/24 hr for 7–10 days. Nonimmunized asymptomatic carriers should have samples taken for culture, receive diphtheria toxoid and penicillin or erythromycin, and be examined daily by a physician. If daily surveillance is not possible, 10,000 units of diphtheria antitoxin may be administered intramuscularly. The risk of allergic reactions to horse serum limits the prophylactic use of antitoxin. When it is used, appropriate skin testing for sensitivity at a site separate from that of the toxoid injection should be carried out. The efficacy of chemoprophylaxis in preventing disease has not been established.

If a contact is experiencing symptoms, treatment for diphtheria is indicated. Prophylactic therapy should be carried out in nonimmunized contacts prior to receipt of the culture results.

Treatment. Treatment of diphtheria is predicated upon neutralization of free toxin and eradication of *C. diphtheriae* by the use of antibiotics. The only specific treatment is antitoxin of equine origin.

Antitoxin must be administered as early as possible by the intravenous route and in a dose sufficient to neutralize all free toxin. A single dose is used to avoid the risk of sensitization from repeated doses of horse serum. *Tests for sensitivity to horse serum must be performed* prior to administration of antitoxin. For this purpose, 0.1 mL of a 1:1000 dilution of antitoxin in isotonic saline can be given intracutaneously or placed in the conjunctival sac. A positive reaction (>10 mm of erythema at site of injection within 20 min or the development of conjunctivitis and tearing) necessitates desensitization. If a patient manifests sensitivity to horse serum, it should be given in slowly increasing doses at 20 min intervals. Several procedures have been recommended. One commonly employed regimen is:

0.05 mL of a 1:20 dilution subcutaneously
0.10 mL of a 1:20 dilution subcutaneously
0.10 mL of a 1:10 dilution subcutaneously
0.10 mL undiluted subcutaneously
0.30 mL undiluted intramuscularly
0.50 mL undiluted intramuscularly
0.10 mL undiluted intravenously

If no reaction has occurred, the remaining material is given by slow intravenous infusion. Reactions should be treated with aqueous epinephrine (1:1000) intravenously. Antitoxin dosage is empiric. Mild nasal or pharyngeal diphtheria can be treated with 40,000 units; 80,000 units for moderately severe pharyngeal diphtheria. Severe pharyngeal or laryngeal diphtheria should be treated with 120,000 units. The latter dose should also be given to patients with mixed clinical symptoms as well as to those with brawny edema or disease of longer duration than 48 hr.

Antibiotics are not a substitute for treatment with antitoxin but are needed to stop the production of diphtheria toxin. Penicillin and erythromycin are effective against most strains of *C. diphtheriae*. Penicillin may be given as aqueous procaine penicillin G, 600,000 units intramuscularly once daily for 7 days. Patients sensitive to penicillin should be given erythromycin in a daily dosage of 40 mg/kg/24 hr in 4 divided doses for 7–10 days. The end point of therapy is three consecutive negative cultures. Each of these antibiotics is also effective in eradicating group A β-hemolytic streptococci, which may complicate up to 30% of cases of diphtheria. Amoxicillin, rifampin, and clindamycin provided in appropriate dosage also may be effective. The carrier state has been treated effectively with benzathine penicillin G or oral erythromycin.

Supportive Treatment. Because of the frequency of myocarditis, bed rest is extremely important and should be required for 2–3 wk. Serial electrocardiograms should be obtained 2–3 times each wk for 4–6 wk to detect myocarditis as early as possible.

Hydration should be maintained and a high calorie liquid or soft diet provided. Secretions should be suctioned. The gag reflex and the quality of the voice should be checked regularly.

Laryngeal diphtheria may require relief of obstruction with a tracheostomy. This procedure should be carried out before the child has become exhausted.

Absolute bed rest must be enforced if myocarditis is detected. Sudden death has been precipitated by excessive activity. The patient with myocarditis may be digitalized if congestive heart failure develops. Digitalization for arrhythmias due to diphtheria may be contraindicated. In severe cases prednisone, 1–1.5 mg/kg/24 hr for 2 wk, has been shown to lessen the incidence of myocarditis.

Palatal and pharyngeal paralysis may be complicated by aspiration. Gavage via a polyethylene tube is indicated in these patients.

Immunization is necessary following recovery of the patient. At least half of the patients who recover from diphtheria do not develop adequate immunity and remain subject to reinfection.

Prognosis. Prior to the use of antitoxin and the availability of antibiotics, the mortality from diphtheria was 30–50%. Death was most common in children under 4 yr of age and often was the result of suffocation by the diphtheritic membrane. At present, the mortality is less than 5%, is most frequently associated with myocarditis, and is not associated with age.

The prognosis in all instances remains guarded until the child has recovered. Laryngeal obstruction may develop suddenly and unexpectedly. Myocarditis may be associated with congestive heart failure that responds poorly to digitalization. Occasionally, diphtheritic myocarditis is followed by permanent damage to the heart. Phrenic nerve paralysis may occur late and produce respiratory paralysis.

Generally, the prognosis in diphtheria depends upon the virulence of the organism, the location and extent of the diphtheritic membrane, the immunization status of the host, the rapidity with which medical care was sought and an accurate diagnosis suggested, the timeliness of treatment, and the adequacy of general nursing care.

Diphtheria caused by the *gravis* strain usually carries a poor prognosis. The more extensive the diphtheritic membrane, the more severe the disease. Laryngeal diphtheria is more likely to be fatal in infants or in patients whose respiratory status is not monitored closely. The development of amegakaryocytic thrombocytopenia or of myocarditis with atrioventricular dissociation heralds a poorer prognosis. If specific treatment is provided on the 1st day of disease, mortality may be reduced to less than 1%; delay in treatment until the 4th day may be associated with a 20-fold increase in mortality.

Nasopharyngeal persistence of *C. diphtheriae* may be noted in 5–10% of convalescing patients. Recovery is followed by immunity that is demonstrable for at least 1 yr after illness in 50% of patients. Second attacks are rare. Nevertheless, immunization should be carried out following recovery.

Belsey MA, Sinclair M, Roder MR, et al: *Corynebacterium diphtheriae* skin infections in Alabama and Louisiana. N Engl J Med 280:139, 1969.
Burch GE, Sun SC, Sohal RS, et al: Diphtheritic myocarditis. Am J Cardiol 21:261, 1968.
McCloskey RV, Eller JJ, Green M, et al: The 1970 epidemic of diphtheria in San Antonio. Ann Intern Med 75:495, 1971.
Miller LW, Older JJ, Drake J, et al: Diphtheria immunization. Effect upon carriers and the control of outbreaks. Am J Dis Child 123:197, 1972.
Morbidity and Mortality Weekly Report, Aug. 21, 1981, p 392.
Pappenheimer AM Jr: Diphtheria toxin. *In:* Ajl SJ, Kadis S, Montie TC (eds): Microbial Toxins, Vol 2B. New York, Academic Press, 1973.
Report of the Committee on Infectious Disease. 19th ed. Evanston Ill., American Academy of Pediatrics, 1982, p 71.
Tasman A, Minkenhof JE, Vink HH, et al: Importance of intravenous injection of diphtheria antiserum. Lancet 1:1299, 1958.
Zamiri I: Diphtheria today: Some experiences in Iran. Lancet 1:1222, 1970.

11.24 PERTUSSIS
(Whooping Cough)

Pertussis, meaning intensive cough, is an acute respiratory infection that can affect any susceptible host but is most common and serious in young children. The first description of an epidemic appeared in 1578; the etiologic agent was isolated in 1906 by Bordet and Gengou.

Etiology. Pertussis is usually caused by *Bordetella pertussis* (*Hemophilus pertussis*). A similar illness has been associated with infection by *B. parapertussis* and *B. bronchiseptica*. A sometimes indistinguishable clinical syndrome has also been associated with adenovirus infection (types 1, 2, 3, and 5). *B. pertussis*, and to a lesser extent *B. parapertussis*, are the etiologic agents that can be implicated in most unimmunized children with pertussis.

B. pertussis is a small, nonmotile, gram-negative rod with fastidious requirements for growth. It is recovered best on glycerin–potato–blood agar media (Bordet-Gengou) to which penicillin has been added to inhibit growth of other organisms. Freshly recovered organisms generally are an antigenic type designated phase I. Passage in culture may induce variant forms (phase II, III, or IV). *Phase I strains are required for transmission of disease and production of an effective vaccine. B. parapertussis* and *B. bronchiseptica*, morphologically similar to

B. pertussis, have similar requirements for growth but can be differentiated by specific agglutination reactions.

Epidemiology. Pertussis, one of the most contagious diseases, can produce attack rates of 97–100% in susceptible populations. Risk of disease is highest in children under 5 yr. In 1981, 6.5 per cent of cases in the United States were in individuals ≥15 yr of age. Mortality is greatest in young infants (during 1960–1967, 72% of reported deaths in the United States occurred in infants under 1 yr).

There is little seasonal variation. Females are affected more frequently than males. *B. pertussis* is rarely isolated from asymptomatic individuals; transmission of disease generally requires contact with a patient.

The incidence of pertussis remains high in developing countries. In the United States the incidence has decreased dramatically since the use of pertussis vaccine. Immunization reduces the incidence and mortality of pertussis, but immunity is neither complete nor permanent. Pertussis has recently been reported with increasing frequency in adolescents and medical personnel immunized appropriately during the first 6 yr of life. The possibility of nosocomial infection from hospital staff to patients has been suggested. Similarly, parents, older siblings, and other adults with waning immunity may become mildly infected and serve as the source of serious infection of unimmunized infants.

Pathology. The organisms multiply only in association with ciliated epithelium and produce various active substances or virulence factors (including toxins). There is congestion and infiltration of the mucosa with lymphocytes and polymorphonuclear leukocytes, and inflammatory debris accumulates in the lumen of the bronchi. Peribronchial lymphoid hyperplasia occurs early, followed by a necrotizing process that affects the midzonal and basilar layers of the bronchial epithelium. Bronchopneumonia develops with necrosis and desquamation of the superficial epithelium of small bronchi. Bronchiolar obstruction and atelectasis result from accumulation of mucus secretions. Bronchiectasis may develop and persist.

Pathologic changes have been described in brain and liver. Microscopic or gross cerebral hemorrhages may be noted, and cortical atrophy has been observed, possibly as the result of anoxia. Fatty infiltration of the liver may be noted with pertussis encephalopathy.

Pathogenesis. Inhalation of phase I organisms is followed by the development of agglutinins and of hemagglutination-inhibiting, bactericidal, complement-fixing, and immunofluorescent antibodies, but resistance to infection does not correlate with their presence. The existence of protective antigen in the cell wall of *B. pertussis* suggests that antibody directed against this antigen may offer protection from disease. An immunologically active material which correlates directly with immunity has not been identified in human sera.

The pili or surface appendages of *B. pertussis* and possibly an associated hemagglutinin apparently are responsible for its attachment to epithelial cells. In cell cultures, protective antibody to *B. pertussis* inhibits attachment. Secretions of persons immune to pertussis contain IgG and IgA with antipertussis activity. Such secretory IgA can inhibit bacterial adherence specifically, and prolonged resistance to infection may be mediated by serum IgG. Protection against pertussis that develops after infection depends upon secretory IgA antibodies that inhibit bacterial adherence to cilia or promote mucociliary discharge of bacteria. Protection is also conferred by serum antitoxin antibodies that inhibit fixation of toxins to receptor cells or that neutralize the toxins. These observations suggest that local and systemic humoral immunity plays an important role in human protection against pertussis.

A lymphocytosis-promoting factor presumably plays a role in human infection by mobilizing lymphocytes from lymphatic organs; both T and B lymphocyte populations are affected in a similar manner. However, this factor is not present in *B. parapertussis* infection, although lymphocytosis is prominent in children.

Clinical Manifestations. The incubation period of pertussis has a mean of 7 and a range of 6–20 days. Symptomatic illness is generally divided into three stages: catarrhal, paroxysmal, and convalescent. Illness generally lasts 6–8 wk. The clinical manifestations depend to some extent on the specific etiology of the syndrome as well as on the age and immunization status of the host. Illness due to *B. parapertussis* or *B. bronchiseptica* is less severe and of shorter duration than that described below.

Catarrhal Stage (1–2 wk). Symptoms of an upper respiratory infection predominate. Rhinorrhea, conjunctival injection, lacrimation, mild cough, and low grade fever are noted; a diagnosis of pertussis usually is not considered during this stage. Infants tend to have a profuse, viscid nasal discharge which may cause upper respiratory obstruction.

Paroxysmal Stage (2–4 wk or longer). Episodes of coughing increase in severity and number. Characteristically, repetitive series of 5–10 forceful coughs during a single expiration are followed by a sudden massive inspiratory effort which produces the *whoop* as air is inhaled forcefully against a narrowed glottis. Facial redness or cyanosis, bulging eyes, protrusion of the tongue, lacrimation, salivation, and distention of neck veins are prominent during the attack. Episodes of paroxysmal coughing may recur sequentially until the mucous plug obstructing the airway is dislodged. *Vomiting* in association with the paroxysms is characteristic enough that the child who vomits following coughing should be suspected of having pertussis, even in the absence of a whoop. The episodes are exhausting; it is not unusual for the patient to appear apathetic and to lose weight. Attacks may be triggered by yawning, sneezing, eating, drinking, and physical exertion or even by suggestion. Between attacks the patient may appear to be minimally ill and is usually comfortable. Some patients, especially infants, have no whoop.

Convalescent Stage (1–2 wk). Paroxysmal episodes of coughing and vomiting gradually decrease in frequency and severity. Cough may persist for several months. Infrequently, recurrent paroxysmal cough recurs for months or years with subsequent upper respiratory infections.

Physical examination is generally uninformative. In the paroxysmal stage petechial or conjunctival hemorrhages may be noted over the head and neck. In some patients diffuse rhonchi and rales are noted.

Diagnosis and Differential Diagnosis. Pertussis can be recognized readily during the paroxysmal stage of disease, if the diagnosis is considered. A history of contact with a known case is helpful.

The white blood cell count may be helpful. Leukocytosis (counts of 20,000–50,000 cells/mm³ of blood) with an absolute lymphocytosis is characteristic at the end of the catarrhal and during the paroxysmal stage of disease. The white cell count may not be as helpful in infants since they respond with lymphocytosis to many infections. Chest roentgenograms may show perihilar infiltrates, atelectasis, or emphysema.

Specific diagnosis depends upon recovery of the organism, best accomplished during the early phases of illness by culture of nasopharyngeal swabs obtained at the bedside (see Etiology). Cough plates are not recommended. Fluorescent antibody staining of pharyngeal specimens may provide a rapid specific diagnosis.

A serologic diagnosis of pertussis may be established by

measuring serum IgM, IgA, and IgG antibodies against *B. pertussis* using an enzyme-linked immunosorbent assay; it may be positive even when cultures are negative for *B. pertussis*. Conversely, some culture-positive patients, particularly infants less than 3 mo of age, may not develop measurable antibodies. An enzyme-linked immunosorbent assay has also been developed for detection of IgA antibody to *B. pertussis* in nasopharyngeal secretions; these antibodies appear during the 2nd or 3rd week of illness and persist for at least 3 mo. (This antibody is not induced by immunization.)

Spasmodic attacks of coughing may be observed in infants with bronchiolitis, bacterial pneumonia, cystic fibrosis, tuberculosis, and any lymphadenopathy causing extrinsic compression of trachea and bronchi. A foreign body may produce paroxysms of coughing but can often be distinguished by sudden onset of symptoms and by roentgenographic and endoscopic findings.

Infections with *B. parapertussis*, *B. bronchiseptica*, and adenoviruses may produce clinical syndromes indistinguishable from those of *B. pertussis*. Differentiation is based on isolating these agents and, for adenovirus, by demonstrating a rise in serum antibody.

Complications. The most frequent complication is pneumonia, which is responsible for more than 90% of deaths under 3 yr of age. Pneumonia may be related to *B. pertussis* itself, but more commonly it is caused by secondary bacterial invaders. Atelectasis may be secondary to mucous plugs. The force of the paroxysm may rupture alveoli and produce interstitial or subcutaneous emphysema. Bronchiectasis may develop.

Otitis media is common and is frequently due to *Streptococcus pneumoniae*. Pertussis also has been associated with activation of latent tuberculosis. Convulsions and coma may be a reflection of cerebral hypoxia related to asphyxia. Rarely, intraventricular and subarachnoid hemorrhage may be observed. Tetanic seizures may be associated with alkalosis related to persistent vomiting. Other complications include ulcer of the frenulum of the tongue, epistaxis, melena, subconjunctival hemorrhages, spinal epidural hematoma, rupture of the diaphragm, umbilical hernia, inguinal hernia, rectal prolapse, dehydration, and nutritional disturbances.

Prevention. See Sec. 4.1. Immunity to pertussis is not acquired transplacentally. Although detectable concentrations of agglutinins to pertussis are found in the serum of one third of newborn infants, there is no evidence that these antibodies prevent disease. Active immunity induced by vaccine has an efficacy of 70–90%.

The risk of serious neurologic complications following pertussis immunization in the United States has been estimated at about 1 in 180,000. Prematurity is not believed to increase the risk of seizures following pertussis immunization.

Contacts. Erythromycin is effective in preventing pertussis in newborn infants exposed to pertussis in a newborn nursery.

Close contacts less than 7 yr of age who have been immunized previously against pertussis should receive a booster dose of DTP unless a booster dose has been given within the preceding 6 mo. They also should be given erythromycin, 50 mg/kg/24 hr in 4 divided oral doses for 10 days. Children who are more than 7 yr of age and who have been immunized also should receive prophylactic erythromycin.

Persons in contact with a patient with pertussis who have not been immunized previously should receive erythromycin for 10 days after the contact has been broken. If the contact cannot be broken, erythromycin should be given until cough in the index patient has stopped or until the index patient has received erythromycin for 7 days. Although erythromycin eliminates carriage of pertussis, its effectiveness in preventing the development of disease is not established.

Treatment. Antibiotic therapy does not shorten the duration of the paroxysmal stage of the disease. Erythromycin (50 mg/kg/24 hr) or ampicillin (100 mg/kg/24 hr) may eliminate pertussis organisms from the nasopharynx within 3–4 days, thereby shortening the period of communicability. Erythromycin may abort or eliminate pertussis when given to patients in the catarrhal stage of the disease. Pertussis immune globulin has been used in children under 2 yr of age (1.25 mL daily for 3–5 doses); controlled studies have not documented its efficacy and it is not recommended.

Supportive care includes avoidance of factors that provoke attacks of coughing and maintenance of hydration and nutrition. Oxygen should be administered for respiratory distress, acute or chronic. Gentle suction to remove profuse, viscid secretions may be required, particularly in infants with pneumonia and significant respiratory distress.

Prognosis. Mortality rates have fallen to fewer than 10/1000 cases in the United States; they may reach 40% in infants under 5 mo. Most deaths are due to pneumonia or other pulmonary complications. The risk of chronic disease, including bronchiectasis, is unknown.

RALPH D. FEIGIN

Altemeier WA III, Ayoub EM: Erythromycin prophylaxis for pertussis. Pediatrics 59:623, 1977.
Baraff LJ, Cody CL, Cherry D: DTP-associated reactions: An analysis by injection site, manufacturer, prior reactions, and dose. Pediatrics 73:31, 1984.
Cherry JD: The epidemiology of pertussis and pertussis immunization in the United Kingdom and the United States: A comparative study. Curr Probl Pediatr 14:1, 1984.
Committee on Infectious Diseases, American Academy of Pediatrics: Pertussis vaccine. Pediatrics 74:303, 1984.
Kaplan JP, Schoenbaum SC, Weinstein MC, et al: Pertussis vaccine—an analysis of benefits, risks, and costs. N Engl J Med 301:906, 1979.
Nelson KE, Gavitt F, Batt MD, et al: The role of adenoviruses in the pertussis syndrome. J Pediatr 86:335, 1975.

11.25 INFECTIONS DUE TO DIARRHEOGENIC *ESCHERICHIA COLI*

Certain strains of *Escherichia coli* may cause acute diarrheal disease (see also Sec. 5.24 and 11.8). These organisms are classified as (1) enteropathogenic, (2) enterotoxigenic, (3) enteroinvasive, and (4) adherent. Historically enteropathogenic strains of *E. coli* (EPEC) have been associated with infantile diarrhea. Enterotoxigenic strains (ETEC) elaborate a toxin that may induce diarrhea. Enteroinvasive *E. coli* are capable of invading and destroying intestinal epithelial cells, thereby causing a dysentery-like illness similar to shigellosis. Enteroadherent *E. coli* heavily colonize the upper intestinal tract and may cause tissue damage and prolonged diarrhea.

E. coli are gram-negative, aerobic (facultatively anaerobic) rods that are generally motile. *E. coli* can be serotyped into many independent antigen groups; immune sera are directed to the O or somatic antigens (more than 150 groups) that are heat-stable, to the K-antigens (93 groups) that also are somatic antigens but heat-labile, and to the H (flagellar) antigens (52 groups) that are also heat-labile.

Epidemiology. During the 1940's and 1950's certain serotypes of *E. coli*, EPEC, were associated with outbreaks of diarrhea in hospital nurseries. Although these strains caused diarrhea when fed to volunteers, later studies revealed that EPEC serotypes could be isolated from individuals without diarrhea, and outbreaks of diarrhea did not necessarily occur in nurseries when EPEC serotypes were isolated.

Enterotoxigenic *E. coli* (ETEC), are the major cause of diarrhea in tourists (Sec. 4.5) and cause up to 4% of diarrheal disease in children in the United States. Higher percentages have been noted in Mexico City, Brazil, and the Philippines. Since a large inoculum of ETEC is required to cause disease, water or food sources of ETEC must be highly contaminated.

Enteroinvasive *E. coli* are not important causes of diarrhea in children in the United States, nor is person-to-person spread an important mode of transmission; outbreaks related to contaminated food have been reported.

Pathogenesis. The mechanism by which EPEC cause diarrhea is not completely understood. Some strains, which in large doses induce diarrhea in human volunteers, do not produce enterotoxins and are not invasive; others elaborate enterotoxin similar to *Shigella dysenteria* type 1 cytotoxin.

E. coli (ETEC) may produce heat-stable, heat-labile, or both types of enterotoxin. Genetic control for the production of either type of enterotoxin resides on transferable plasmids. Heat-labile enterotoxin, a high molecular weight antigenic protein, is closely related to the enterotoxin produced by cholera. It binds to G_{M1} ganglioside of epithelial cells as its receptor and activates cellular adenyl cyclase. The result is increased intracellular concentrations of cyclic AMP, which promote the net secretion of water and chloride. Heat-stable enterotoxin, a low molecular weight, poorly antigenic protein, activates guanylate cyclase, which also increases the secretory activity of the gastrointestinal tract. The genetic information that codes for antibiotic resistance may be carried on the same plasmid as that responsible for coding enterotoxin production. Thus, the widespread use of antibiotics may promote the distribution of both antibiotic-resistant and enterotoxigenic *E. coli*. Adhesion pili or fimbriae (colonization factors) contribute to the pathogenesis of diarrhea by some strains of ETEC by enabling the organism to attach to specific receptors on the enterocyte, thus promoting colonization of the small intestine.

Enteroinvasive *E. coli* are capable of invading and multiplying within the gastrointestinal epithelial cells much like *Shigella*. Local inflammation with hyperemia, edema, ulceration, and intraluminal exudate may result. The diarrheal stools may contain blood and mucus, and fecal leukocytes can be identified. Invasive *E. coli* usually are limited to serotypes O28, O32, O36, O112, O115, O143, O144, O147, O152, O164, and O214.

A 4th pathogenic mechanism for *E. coli* diarrhea involves adherence of bacteria to gastrointestinal epithelium with brush border damage and reduction in brush border enzymes but without invasion. Enteroadherent *E. coli* are usually EPEC serotypes.

Clinical Manifestations. In general, patients infected with EPEC have watery diarrhea with low grade fever and no other systemic symptoms. Stools may contain mucus but usually not blood. A patient may have 10–20 stools/day, and the gastroenteritis usually resolves spontaneously in 3–7 days. In young infants vomiting, dehydration, and electrolyte disturbances with acidosis may result.

The clinical picture of "traveler's diarrhea" due to ETEC is fairly typical (Sec. 4.5 and Table 4–6). Within 1–2 wk of arrival, the traveler may have the abrupt onset of acute watery diarrhea that may be explosive in nature with as many as 10–20 diarrheal stools/day. The diarrhea is frequently associated with severe abdominal pain or cramps, nausea, and vomiting; malaise and fever are variable. Disease due to the labile toxin may be less severe, with little or no complaint of abdominal pain or nausea and only low grade fever.

Patients with enteroinvasive *E. coli* diarrhea develop symptoms after an incubation period of approximately 18–24 hr. There is an abrupt onset of fever with severe diarrhea, urgency, and tenesmus. Bloody stools containing mucus may be present. Nausea, abdominal pain, myalgias, chills, and headache also may occur. *E. coli* that adhere to intestinal brush borders may be found more commonly in patients with protracted and chronic diarrhea. These children may demonstrate poor growth and do not tolerate enteral feeding.

Diagnosis. Enteropathogenic *E. coli* gastroenteritis may be suspected in outbreaks of diarrhea, particularly those occurring in nurseries. When the same serotype is isolated from the stools of many infected infants, a presumptive diagnosis may be made. In addition to the stool, nasopharynx, throat, and upper intestinal contents also may be colonized with the same serotype. Routine serotyping of *E. coli* for EPEC spectrum probably is not warranted except during outbreaks of diarrhea in nurseries or other enclosed populations. Detection of enterotoxigenic and enteroinvasive strains of *E. coli* requires special laboratory procedures that, at present, are usually performed only in certain research laboratories. The adherent form of *E. coli* diarrhea can only be diagnosed by intestinal biopsy.

Prevention. During institutional outbreaks of EPEC diarrhea, enteric precautions must be maintained. In nurseries a cohort system of admission should be instituted.

Although prophylactic therapy for traveler's diarrhea may be effective, the routine use of prophylactic antibiotics is not recommended because of the rapid emergence of resistant organisms as well as the possible adverse effects of the drugs (Sec. 4.5).

Treatment. In infants and children correction of fluid and electrolyte disturbances is the major element in therapy. (See Sec. 4.4, 5.24, and 11.8.)

Over-the-counter antidiarrheal preparations such as kaolin and pectins do not influence the frequency or the water content of stools in children with acute diarrhea. Diphenoxylate-atropine (Lomotil) also has no role in the treatment of diarrhea due to *E. coli*.

Neomycin, 100 mg/kg/24 hr, given in 3 divided doses orally for 3–5 days, is effective in the treatment of diarrhea due to EPEC, particularly among infants. Stool cultures become negative within 24 hr of therapy in approximately 75% of the children. A clinical response is generally noted when EPEC are eliminated from the stool. Relapse rates of 20% have been reported after therapy has been discontinued.

Antibiotic therapy of diarrhea due to ETEC has not been evaluated adequately in children. For travelers' diarrhea (about 60% was due to ETEC) trimethoprim-sulfamethoxazole or trimethoprim alone is effective therapy in adults when administered early; there are significantly fewer unformed stools and less abdominal pain and nausea compared with the patients given placebo. A similar approach in children seems reasonable.

Treatment of diarrhea due to enteroinvasive *E. coli* also has not been critically evaluated. In general, patients do not require hospitalization and are asymptomatic within 1 wk of onset of illness without antibiotic therapy. However, like *Shigella*, diarrhea due to enteroinvasive *E. coli* may respond to ampicillin when therapy is indicated.

Oral neomycin at a dose of 100 mg/kg/24 hr for 5–7 days and parenteral hyperalimentation both appear to be important in treating diarrhea due to enteroadherent *E. coli*.

SHELDON L. KAPLAN
RALPH D. FEIGIN

DuPont HL, Formal SB, Hornick RB, et al: Pathogenesis of *Escherichia coli* diarrhea. N Engl J Med 285:1, 1971.

DuPont HL, Reves RR, Galindo E, et al: Treatment of travelers' diarrhea with trimethoprim/sulfamethoxazole and with trimethoprim alone. N Engl J Med 307:841, 1982.

Echeverria P, Murphy JR: Enterotoxigenic *Escherichia coli* carrying plasmids coding for antibiotic resistance and enterotoxin production. J Infect Dis 142:273, 1980.

Klipstein FA, Rowe B, Engert RF, et al: Enterotoxigenicity of enteropathogenic serotypes of *Escherichia coli* isolated from infants with epidemic diarrhea. Infect Immunol 21:171, 1978.

Levine MM, Kaper JB, Black RE et al: New knowledge on pathogenesis of bacterial enteric infections as applied to vaccine development. Microbiol Rev 47:510, 1983.

Levine MM, Nalin DR, Hornick RB, et al: *Escherichia coli* strains that cause diarrhea but do not produce heat-labile or heat-stable enterotoxin and are noninvasive. Lancet 1:1119, 1978.

Moseley SL, Echeverria P, Seriwantana J, et al: Identification of enterotoxigenic *Escherichia coli* by colony hybridization using three enterotoxin gene probes. J Infect Dis 145:863, 1982.

Pickering LK: Antimicrobial therapy of gastrointestinal infections. Pediatr Clin North Am 30:373, 1983.

Rothbaum R, McAdams AJ, Giannella R, et al: A clinicopathologic study of enterocyte adherent *Escherichia coli*: A cause of protracted diarrhea in infants. Gastroenterology 83:441, 1982.

Ryder RW, Wachsmuth IK, Buxton AE, et al: Infantile diarrhea produced by heat stable enterotoxigenic *Escherichia coli*. N Engl J Med 295:849, 1976.

Sack RB: Enterotoxigenic *Escherichia coli*: Identification and characterization. J Infect Dis 142, 279, 1980.

Ulshen MH, Rollo JL: Pathogenesis of *Escherichia coli* gastroenteritis in man: Another mechanism. N Engl J Med 302:99, 1980.

11.26 INFECTIONS DUE TO SALMONELLAE

Salmonella organisms are important pathogens of humans and animals. Generally, human infections are caused by the ingestion of contaminated water or food. Currently, gastroenteritis due to *Salmonella* is one of the common infectious diseases in the United States, as it is worldwide. Although systemic infection with *Salmonella typhosa* (typhoid fever) is infrequent in the United States, it remains endemic and epidemic in many parts of the world.

Etiology. Salmonellae are motile, gram-negative, nonencapsulated, nonsporulating bacilli. The principal antigens are the flagellae (H) antigens, the cell wall (O) antigens, and the envelope (Vi) heat-labile antigens that block the O antigen-antibody agglutination. An elaborate typing scheme utilizing O and H antigens (Kaufman-White) has permitted the differentiation of over 2200 *Salmonella* serotypes. A system of nomenclature has been suggested in which all salmonellae are classified into three groups (*S. enteritidis, S. typhi,* and *S. choleraesuis*). The first group contains all salmonellae except the latter two. Each species, then, is classified as a bioserotype such as *S. enteritidis* bio *typhimurium.*

Salmonellae are resistant to many physical agents, but they can be killed by heating to 130° F (54.4° C) for 1 hr or 140° F (60° C) for 15 min. They remain viable at ambient or reduced temperatures for days and may survive for weeks in sewage, dried foodstuffs, pharmaceutical agents, and fecal material.

The properties of salmonellae responsible for their pathogenicity remain incompletely defined. The O antigen (an endotoxin) enhances resistance of the organism to phagocytosis; strains deficient in it are avirulent. The effects of endotoxin in the host may be responsible for certain manifestations of the systemic disease, but no evidence supports a role in gastroenteritis. Some serotypes have distinct host preferences and produce characteristic patterns of disease. *Salmonella typhosa* infects only man. Salmonellae of groups A and C are generally isolated from human sources, whereas *S. abortus equi* infects only horses. Despite this apparent propensity of strains to seek a particular host, 7 of the 10 types of *Salmonella* most commonly recovered from animal sources in the United States are among the 10 types most commonly isolated from humans.

NONTYPHOIDAL SALMONELLOSIS

Epidemiology. Opportunity to acquire an infection with one of the serotypes of *Salmonella* appears to be increasing; more than 30,000 culture-proven cases of salmonellosis are reported in the United States annually. The actual number of cases must be much greater. Of the reported cases, more than two thirds are in persons under 20 yr of age, with the higher attack rates in this age group predominantly among infants, young children, and males.

Meat and poultry products are the most common sources of salmonellae infection. Modern methods of feeding, holding, and transporting farm animals lead to contamination. On some farms the use of antibiotic-containing feed, especially for poultry, can lead to increased numbers of salmonellae and a high incidence of *Salmonella*-carrying chickens and turkeys. Large poultry processing plants must be particularly careful that a few infected birds do not contaminate conveyor belts, water baths, and other equipment, as this may cause unsuspected contamination of large numbers of chickens and turkeys.

Salmonella can infect many species of animals, but those of particular hazard to human health are meat-producing animals, poultry, and reptiles (particularly pet turtles). Most animal infections are asymptomatic. The prevalence of salmonellosis in chickens creates a high risk for contamination of eggs. Salmonellae can contaminate the shell surface, penetrate the egg, or be transmitted from an ovarian infection directly to the egg yolk. Pooling large numbers of eggs prior to freezing, drying, or use in the preparation of food materials increases the risk of human infection. All eggs utilized in processed foods should be pasteurized; up to 50% of poultry, 5% of beef, 16% of pork, and 40% of frozen egg products purchased in retail stores contain salmonellae. *Salmonella* introduced into kitchens on these contaminated foods may be transferred to other materials including utensils, table surfaces, and personnel. *Salmonella* can resist boiling within an egg for even 2–3 min. Contamination of equipment in processing plants has been responsible for outbreaks associated with baker's yeast, dried milk, dried coconut, cotton seed protein, and various dyes. Carmine red dye derived from female scale insects and larvae, sometimes used in hospitals for determination of intestinal transit time, has caused hospital outbreaks of salmonellosis. This dye is also used as an artificial coloring in drugs, foods, and cosmetics.

Humans are important carriers of *Salmonella* species and can cause localized epidemics of food poisoning by contaminating food at large gatherings such as picnics. Outbreaks in hospitals and nursing homes that are traced to a carrier are of considerable concern because of the increased morbidity and mortality observed in infants, young children, and the compromised host. Cross-contamination also can occur within institutions by means of contaminated fingers, clothes of the staff, or aerosols. Intrafamilial transmission of salmonellosis is a frequent occurrence. Improper refrigeration has led to multiplication of *S. kottbus* within donated breast milk. Contaminated marijuana has also been reported.

During the acute stages of infection, 10^6–10^9 salmonellae/g are excreted in stool; 70–90% of infected individuals will have a positive stool culture 2 wk following infection, about 50% at 4 wk, and 10–25% at 10 wk. The duration of *Salmonella* excretion is similar whether the infection has been asymptomatic or symptomatic but appears to be longer in infants than it is for older children. Excretion is prolonged by antibiotic therapy regardless of the agent used.

Pathogenesis and Pathology. There is limited information concerning the number of salmonellae required to cause disease in man. Infants and children may be infected by smaller numbers of organisms than adults, but the specific dose presumably varies widely depending upon the host and type or even subtype of *Salmonella* with which the host is infected.

Diarrhea initiated by *Salmonella* may be produced by several mechanisms. Many patients present with a nonspecific watery diarrhea clinically identical to that caused by enterotoxigenic *E. coli*; several toxins have been identified, but whether they are responsible for the excess intestinal fluid production in humans remains to be proved. It also has been suggested that *Salmonella* can initiate diarrhea by indirect stimulation of the energy system within epithelial cells, which allows these cells to secrete water and electrolytes. Prostaglandins released from the inflammatory exudate evoked by *Salmonella* may stimulate the adenylate cyclase–cyclic AMP system that would enable the epithelial cells to secrete fluid and electrolytes actively.

For *Salmonella* species to cause diarrhea, they must gain access to the mucosal lining of the small and large intestine. A stomach pH of 2 will kill swallowed salmonellae; there is no killing effect at pH 5. There are also nonspecific defense mechanisms within the intestinal tract that may adversely affect survival of salmonellae, e.g., rapid transit, lysozymes, and enzymes, but their role in preventing human disease is unknown.

Salmonellae can penetrate the superficial layers of the mucosal lining without destroying epithelial cells. A phagosome is created around the salmonellae in the epithelial cell, but no damage to the bacteria occurs as they travel through or between cells into the lamina propria. Serotypes that usually cause diarrhea evoke a polymorphonuclear leukocyte response in the lamina propria area. The infection extends no farther, and the patient develops only diarrhea. There may be low grade fever associated with diarrhea. The frequency of bacteremia is not known, but it is usually transient, and no metastatic phase of infection occurs in healthy individuals.

Systemic invasion by *Salmonella* is much more common in individuals at the extremes of age as well as in those with diseases that impair reticuloendothelial or cellular immune function. Children with sickle cell disease are prone to develop *Salmonella* septicemia and osteomyelitis. The numerous infarcted areas of the gastrointestinal tract, bones, and reticuloendothelial system may initially permit organisms greater access to the circulation from the intestine and then furnish an optimal environment for localization. The decreased phagocytic and opsonizing capacity of patients with SS hemoglobin disease also contributes to the enhanced infection rate. Individuals with chronic granulomatous disease of childhood or other white blood cell disorders have an increased propensity for infection. Possible defects in phagocytosis are also responsible for the chronic *Salmonella* bacteremia and bacilluria associated with chronic schistosomiasis (Sec. 11.122).

Clinical Manifestations. Gastroenteritis due to *Salmonella* has its peak incidence in the late summer and early fall, correlating with the number of foodborne outbreaks. Epidemics and sporadic cases involving small family units occur throughout the year.

The incubation period ranges from 8 to 48 hr. Onset often occurs the morning following an evening meal at which contaminated food was ingested. It is usually abrupt and is characterized by nausea, vomiting, and crampy abdominal pain followed by elimination of loose, watery stools, which occasionally contain mucus and blood. Vomiting is usually not severe and, when it does occur, is not protracted. Fever of 101–102° F is seen in as many as 70% of patients; however, chills are less frequent. Symptoms subside within 2–5 days in healthy individuals; in patients who are debilitated by the extremes of age, malignancy, or other illnesses or who are recipients of antibiotic therapy or corticosteroids, the illness may persist. Fatalities are rare (about 1%). Some patients remain afebrile and have only mild intestinal symptoms. Others develop severe disease with higher fever, headache, drowsiness, confusion, meningismus, and seizures. Moderate abdominal distention and severe, and even localized, pain with rebound tenderness may be manifest.

Septicemia, accompanied by chills and high fever, is more common in the first 3 mo of life than later. Symptoms of enteric fever are those described subsequently for typhoid fever but generally are shorter in duration and associated

with a lower mortality rate. Salmonellae can localize in any organ or tissue and cause a variety of disorders including pneumonia, empyema, abscesses, osteomyelitis, septic arthritis, pyelonephritis, and meningitis. *Salmonella choleraesuis* is associated with a greater incidence of septicemia and a higher mortality rate than is the case with other *Salmonella* organisms. It is also associated with chronic osteomyelitis resulting from asymptomatic bacteremia.

Complications. Complications of nontyphoidal salmonellosis are unusual and generally are limited to the extraintestinal lesions, such as those mentioned in the above paragraph. Children may develop *Salmonella*-reactive arthritis about 2 wk after the initial diarrheal episode. The arthritis tends to be polyarticular, with knees and ankles affected most frequently. Swelling and tenderness are more prominent features than joint erythema. The arthritis is frequently migratory with rapid recurrence and regression of symptoms. Exacerbations may be accompanied by fever and malaise. Sedimentation rates may be high, but white blood cell counts are minimally elevated. When joint effusions are tapped, they are sterile. Roentgenograms of the involved joints reveal only soft tissue swelling. There is a highly significant association between the presence of histocompatibility antigen HLA B27 and the postsalmonella reactive arthritis syndrome. Reiter disease (conjunctivitis, urethritis, and polyarthritis) also may be a complication (Sec. 10.60).

Diagnosis. A positive culture is necessary for diagnosis. Culture of the stool is positive more frequently than are specimens collected via rectal swabs. Bacteriologic results are enhanced by the incubation of the specimen in an enriched medium (e.g., tetrathionate broth) prior to plating on selective medium. Promising results have also been obtained with a rapid direct fluorescent antibody technique with specimens incubated in enrichment broth prior to examination. Although three consecutive negative stool cultures suggest that infection has ceased, excretion may be intermittent. Salmonellae can also be recovered from blood, urine, cerebrospinal fluid, or other tissues that are infected.

The stool of many individuals with *Salmonella* gastroenteritis contains polymorphonuclear leukocytes; these can be demonstrated by staining a freshly passed specimen with methylene blue. Mucus and red blood cells may also be present.

Serologic tests are helpful in the diagnosis of typhoid fever and other forms of *Salmonella* infection. A 4-fold or greater rise in serum titer is diagnostic, although as many as one third of patients may show insignificant increases in titer or no rise in titer at all. A titer change can be noted as early as 1 wk after the onset of disease. Some patients will have significant increases of O or H antibodies but not of both. A single titer of 1:320 or greater for O antibody, particularly in a child, should alert the physician to consider salmonellosis as the cause of infection. Patients with acute and chronic liver disease may have high O and H agglutinin titers, but these represent cross-reacting antibodies and may not signify salmonellosis.

Differential Diagnosis. *Salmonella* gastroenteritis must be distinguished from other viral and bacterial causes of diarrhea, including those caused by rotavirus, *E. coli*, *Shigella*, *Yersinia enterocolitica*, and *Campylobacter fetus*. Rarely, the clinical course and roentgenographic findings suggest ulcerative colitis, which should be excluded.

Treatment. Correction of dehydration and electrolyte disturbances (Sec. 5.19–5.24) as well as the symptomatic management of the patient are the most important aspects of the therapy of *Salmonella* gastroenteritis. Antibiotics do not eliminate susceptible salmonellae from the gastrointestinal tract and rarely, if ever, alter the clinical course. Antibiotics are indicated in gastroenteritis only for individuals at high risk for dissemination of disease to other organs or tissues (infants under 3 mo of age, children with immunologic deficiency, or those who are suffering a severe and protracted course).

Children with septicemia, enteric fever, or metastatic sites of infection should be treated with systemically administered ampicillin (200–300 mg/kg/24 hr), amoxicillin (100 mg/kg/24 hr), or chloramphenicol (50–100 mg/kg/24 hr for older children or 25 mg/kg/24 hr for newborn infants). The 24 hr dose of each of these drugs should be given in 4 divided doses at 6 hourly intervals. In vitro susceptibility of the organism should dictate the antibiotic to be used in each case. Resistance to chloramphenicol is unusual among salmonellae isolated in the United States but is relatively common among those recovered in other areas of the world. Twenty per cent of salmonellae isolated from humans in this country are resistant to ampicillin.

Some antibiotics have excellent bactericidal activity in vitro but not in vivo. Thus, the aminoglycosides, polymyxins, and tetracyclines should not be used for systemic *Salmonella* infections despite their in vitro activity. The cephalosporins can be effective in vitro and variously less effective in vivo; third generation drugs may be indicated when the infecting salmonella is resistant to ampicillin and chloramphenicol.

Prognosis. The prognosis for patients with *Salmonella* gastroenteritis is excellent except in very young infants or debilitated children with underlying disease. The prognosis for individuals with *Salmonella* meningitis or endocarditis is poor unless effective therapy is provided early.

11.27 TYPHOID FEVER
(Enteric Fever)

Epidemiology. From 300 to 500 new cases of typhoid fever are reported each year in the United States; the incidence has been declining steadily since 1900. The majority of reported cases are in persons under 20 yr of age. Several thousand chronic carriers of *Salmonella typhosa* are recorded in health departments throughout the country.

The typhoid bacillus infects only humans, and infected patients excrete *S. typhosa* in respiratory secretions, urine, and feces for variable periods of time. Chronic carriers are responsible for most of the disease in the United States. Characteristically, the implicated carrier is an adult who may have had an enteric illness and who has had contact, often as a preparer of food, with the index case. Long survival of *S. typhosa* in food facilitates transmission. Contaminated water generally involves inadequate plumbing or sanitation and is responsible for individual cases in the United States and for endemic disease in developing countries. Oysters and other shellfish cultivated in waters polluted by sewage are also a source of widespread infection.

Pathogenesis. Infection with *S. typhosa* always results in clinical disease. However, the reasons for differences in the pathogenicity of various strains of the bacilli as well as in the resistance of individual hosts to typhoid fever are largely unknown.

Virulent *S. typhosa* inhibit postphagocytic oxidative metabolism of neutrophils, resisting destruction by white cells. The bacilli then rapidly invade the bloodstream from sites of minimal inflammation; the upper small bowel is the predominant site of invasion. Monocytes, unable to destroy the bacilli early in the disease process, carry these organisms from the bloodstream into the mesenteric lymph nodes and other portions of the reticuloendothelial system where multiplication occurs within cells, producing inflammation in the lymph nodes, liver, and spleen.

The bacteria then re-enter the bloodstream from these sites. This secondary septicemia is usually prolonged, and many organs are seeded. The gallbladder is particularly susceptible and is infected from the liver via the biliary system or from the blood. Local multiplication of microorganisms in the wall of the gallbladder produces large numbers of salmonellae, which are discharged into the large intestine.

The lipopolysaccharide outside portion of the cell wall of salmonellae may act systemically as a pyrogenic endotoxin responsible for some of the signs and symptoms of infection and may act locally to induce the histologic changes in the intestine, liver, skin, and other tissues. However, circulating endotoxin is not usually demonstrable, probably because local concentrations of endotoxin indirectly stimulate the release of procoagulants from leukocytes, causing vascular damage and the release of clotting factor proteases.

Cell-mediated immunity is important in protecting the human host against typhoid fever. Decreased numbers of T lymphocytes occur in patients who are critically ill with typhoid fever. Carriers show impaired cellular reactivity to *S. typhosa* antigens in the leukocyte migration inhibition test, but they do not have a generalized depression of cell-mediated immunity; the carrier state may be a consequence of a specific defect in cell-mediated immune response to *S. typhosa*. In carriers of *S. typhosa,* a large number of virulent bacilli pass into the intestine daily without entering the epithelium of the host and are excreted in the stool.

Pathology. Morphologic changes of *S. typhosa* infection are less striking in younger children than in older children and adults. The mesenteric lymph nodes, liver, and spleen are hyperemic and generally reveal areas of focal necrosis. Hyperplasia of reticuloendothelial tissue with proliferation of mononuclear cells is the predominant finding. Hepatic cells may reveal cloudy swelling. The mucosa and lymphatic tissue of the intestinal tract are severely inflamed and necrotic. Ulceration that heals without scarring is common. Hemorrhages may occur. The inflammatory lesion may occasionally penetrate the muscularis and serosa of the intestine and produce perforation. A mononuclear response may be seen in the bone marrow associated with areas of focal necrosis. Inflammation of the gallbladder is focal, inconstant, and modest in proportion to the extent of local bacterial multiplication. Bronchitis is common. Inflammation also may be observed in the form of localized abscesses, pneumonia, septic arthritis, osteomyelitis, pyelonephritis, endophthalmitis, and meningitis. Bacteria may be observed in all organ systems.

Clinical Manifestations. The clinical pattern of typhoid fever *in infants* ranges from a mild gastroenteritis to a severe septicemia. Vomiting, abdominal distention, and diarrhea are common. The temperature may be variable but can be as high as 40.5° C (106° F). Seizures may occur. Hepatomegaly, jaundice, anorexia, and weight loss can be marked.

In older children the incubation period ranges from 5 to 40 days with an average of 10 to 20 days. It is followed by an irregular course characterized by fever, malaise, lethargy, myalgia, headache, and abdominal pain and tenderness. Diarrhea occurs in only half of the infected children at this stage of the disease; constipation occurs less frequently. Epistaxis may occur, and cough is common. Within a week the fever rises and becomes unremitting. Fatigue, anorexia, weight loss, cough, abdominal pain, and diarrhea increase in severity. The patient may become severely obtunded. Mental depression, delirium, and stupor all have been observed. The child now appears acutely ill, disoriented, and lethargic. At this stage of disease the spleen generally is enlarged, and abdominal tenderness is present. Abdominal distention may be appreciated, and rhonchi and scattered rales may be heard upon auscultation of the chest. A macular (rose spots) or maculopapular rash observable in as many as 80% of patients, occurs in the skin of the lower chest and abdomen, appearing in successive crops of lesions that are 1–6 mm in diameter and last 2–3 days. The paradoxical relationship of a high temperature and low pulse rate is observed less commonly in children than in adults. If no complications occur, the symptoms and physical findings resolve within 2–4 wk, but malaise and lethargy may persist for an additional 1–2 mo.

Complications. Intestinal perforation has been observed in 0.5–3% and severe hemorrhage in 1–10% of children with typhoid fever. Most complications occur during the second stage of disease and are generally preceded by a fall in temperature and blood pressure and an increase in pulse rate. Perforation rarely occurs without preceding hemorrhage, and the site is usually in the lower ileum. Perforation is accompanied by a marked increase in abdominal pain, tenderness, vomiting, and signs of peritonitis. Toxic encephalopathy and cerebral thrombosis are other complications. Acute cerebellar ataxia, aphasia, perceptive deafness, and transverse myelitis have been observed. Permanent sequelae appear to be rare. Peripheral and optic neuritis as well as chorea have been reported. Acute cholecystitis has been observed, often presenting as a toxic dilatation of the gallbladder. Thrombosis and phlebitis occur rarely. Pneumonia is common during the second stage of illness but often is caused by a superinfection related to organisms other than *Salmonella*. Pyelonephritis, endocarditis, and meningitis as well as osteomyelitis and septic arthritis occur rarely in the normal host. Septic arthritis and osteomyelitis occur more frequently in individuals with hemoglobinopathies.

Laboratory Data. A normochromic normocytic anemia may be associated with intestinal blood loss or toxic suppression of bone marrow. Blood leukocyte counts generally are low in relation to the fever and toxicity but seldom are less than 3000 cells/mm³. With pyogenic abscesses leukocytosis may reach 20,000–25,000/mm.³ Thrombocytopenia may be striking and persist for up to a week. Melena and proteinuria are common.

Diagnosis. *Microscopic examination of the stool* generally reveals a large number of leukocytes, most of which are mononuclear.

Bacteriologic cultures are diagnostic, but the identification of *S. typhosa* requires 3–5 days in most laboratories. Specimens grown on selective media and examined with fluorescein-labeled antibody to the Vi antigen may provide specific and rapid identification. Blood cultures are usually positive early in the disease, whereas urine and stool cultures become positive following the secondary septicemia. Cultures are positive in as many as 40% of children during the initial stage of typhoid fever. Cultures of the bone marrow and involved lymph nodes or other reticuloendothelial tissues often remain positive after the blood has been sterilized. Aspirates of the rose spots may be culture positive. Stool and urine of chronic carriers should be cultured, as bone marrow and blood cultures are not likely to be positive. Enteric carriers generally excrete 10⁶–10⁹ *S. typhosa* per gram of stool. In suspected cases with negative stool cultures, a culture of aspirated duodenal fluid to evaluate possible biliary infection may be helpful.

O and H antigens of *S. typhosa* are not unique to that serotype or even to salmonellae. Treatment with chloramphenicol may depress an antibody response; conversely, high titers of H agglutinins may result from prior typhoid immunization. Moreover, nonspecific agglutinins often are observed in the serum of individuals with underlying disease accompanied by macroglobulinemia. With these reservations, a 4-fold rise in agglutinin titer of a nonimmunized individual usually is diagnostic when performed in the same laboratory.

An increase in O agglutinins in an individual immunized more than 6 mo earlier also is suggestive of infection.

In the nonimmunized child who has lived in a nonendemic area, O agglutinin titers of greater than 1:160 are suggestive evidence of infection during the 1st wk of symptoms. Titers of Vi agglutinins of 1:5 or greater generally identify a chronic carrier in nonendemic populations.

Countercurrent immunoelectrophoresis has been used to detect serum *S. typhosa* antigen. An enzyme-linked immunosorbent assay (ELISA) has also been developed for detecting *S. typhosa* Vi antigen in urine; its high sensitivity and specificity suggest that it may be helpful in rapidly establishing a diagnosis.

Differential Diagnosis. During the initial stage of typhoid fever the clinical diagnosis may be bronchitis, bronchopneumonia, gastroenteritis, or influenza. Subsequently other infections caused by intracellular microorganisms, including tuberculosis, systemic fungal infections, brucellosis, tularemia, and rickettsial diseases as well as shigellosis and, where applicable epidemiologically, malaria, may need to be considered. Septicemia, leukemia, lymphoma, and Hodgkin disease also may be suggested. Concern about acute surgical disease of the abdomen may lead to unnecessary operative intervention.

Prognosis. The prognosis in typhoid fever depends upon the patient's age and previous state of health and the type of complications that may occur. Individuals who are not treated with antibiotics may die (10% of infants and a smaller percentage of older children succumb). Therapy with chloramphenicol has reduced the mortality rate to less than 1% in most areas. The presence of an underlying debilitating disease, perforation of the gastrointestinal tract, or severe hemorrhage increases the chances of death. Meningitis or endocarditis may be associated with high morbidity and mortality.

Relapse occurs in up to 10% of those who are not treated with antibiotics. Clinical manifestations of relapse generally become apparent about 2 wk after cessation of antibiotic therapy and resemble the acute illness. The relapse, however, is generally milder and more abbreviated. Multiple relapses in the same individual may occur.

Individuals who excrete *S. typhosa* 3 mo or more after infection are usually excreters at 1 yr and often for life. The risk of becoming a *chronic carrier* is low in children but increases with age. Up to 5% of acutely infected adults become chronic carriers; generally they have chronic gallbladder infections and excrete the organisms in their stool. Chronic urinary carriage also may occur but is rare except in individuals with schistosomiasis.

Treatment. The maintenance of appropriate fluid and electrolyte balance is essential. If shock or severe hemorrhage accompanies intestinal perforation, intravascular volume expansion is required.

Chloramphenicol is the antibiotic preferred by most infectious disease experts for the therapy of typhoid fever. It can usually be provided orally, but intravenous administration is indicated when the patient is acutely ill. It should not be administered by the intramuscular route. Doses of 50–100 mg/kg/24 hr are given to children and 25 mg/kg/24 hr to infants under 2 wk of age, divided into 4 doses and given at 6 hr intervals. Most children become afebrile within 7 days, but treatment of uncomplicated cases should be continued for at least 10–14 days or for 5–7 days following defervescence. In children who have underlying significant malnutrition and a high rate of complications, results have been improved by extending therapy for a period of 21 days. Complications including intestinal hemorrhage and perforation have been observed during therapy. Treatment with chloramphenicol may increase the chance of relapse and does not prevent development of the chronic carrier state.

Ampicillin therapy results in a slower clinical response and more treatment failures than does treatment with chloramphenicol. Patients who have a favorable response to ampicillin, however, are less likely to experience relapses or become chronic carriers. The dose of ampicillin is 100–200 mg/kg/24 hr divided at 6 hr intervals. Systemic administration is preferred.

Amoxicillin (100 mg/kg/24 hr given in equal divided doses at 6 hr intervals) provides results that are superior to those for ampicillin and equivalent to those obtained with chloramphenicol.

A combination of trimethoprim and sulfamethoxazole is also effective against typhoid fever (185 mg/m²/day TMP plus 925 mg/m²/day SMZ orally in 3 equally divided doses). However, patients respond less predictably than with chloramphenicol or ampicillin.

Illness due to chloramphenicol-resistant strains has been reported from Mexico, Southeast Asia, Mexico, and the Middle East. Most chloramphenicol-resistant strains are susceptible to ampicillin, amoxicillin, and trimethoprim-sulfamethoxazole, and therapy of such infections with these drugs is successful. Ampicillin-resistant strains have been noted, but these strains are sensitive to chloramphenicol or to trimethoprim-sulfamethoxazole.

Corticosteroid therapy has been suggested for individuals with severe toxemia or prolonged symptoms. It does not increase the incidence of complications if antibiotic therapy is adequate.

Platelet transfusions have been suggested to treat thrombocytopenia sufficiently severe to cause intestinal hemorrhage in patients for whom surgery is contemplated.

Up to 80% of carriers with chronic gallbladder infection can be cured by cholecystectomy even without antibiotic therapy. High dose ampicillin therapy provided for 4–6 wk has cured many carriers including some with cholecystitis.

Prevention. Typhoid fever stimulates host resistance by inducing a temporary nonspecific increase in phagocytic activity within the reticuloendothelial system as well as a more lasting enhancement of specific bactericidal activity in the form of type-specific antibodies. Antibodies slow extracellular bacterial multiplication and promote opsonization, but susceptibility to initial or subsequent attacks of typhoid fever does not correlate with the titers of antibodies to O, H, or Vi antigens. Reinfection occurs in 20–25% of adults exposed naturally or experimentally.

Parenteral vaccine is not indicated for routine use in children. Although available vaccines will prevent disease in most individuals exposed to small numbers of typhoid bacilli such as could occur with water-borne disease, exposure to a larger inoculum can overcome whatever immunity is induced by the vaccine. The indications for use of typhoid vaccine in the United States are as follows: (1) intimate exposure to a known household carrier; (2) an outbreak of typhoid fever in the community or an institution; and (3) travel to an endemic area, in an attempt to prevent disease acquired via contaminated water. However, children attending summer camps or traveling to endemic areas should not receive the vaccine. For children residing in endemic areas, the vaccine may provide some protection against water-borne disease, but a booster dose is not indicated, since field tests failed to show any increased protection when more than 1 dose was given. Immunity lasts at least 10 yr.

A dose of 0.5 mL administered subcutaneously is recommended for both primary and booster immunizations of individuals 10 yr or more of age; 0.25 mL is recommended for younger children. Local reactions, including fever, are common, and prophylactic administration of antipyretics in young children may be indicated. An intradermal dose of 0.1 mL may have immunogenicity and produce fewer side reactions than the larger subcutaneous dose; it may be used as a booster injection. Unacceptable reactions occur with the intradermal administration of acetone-extracted vaccine.

An oral vaccine containing the Ty 21 attenuated mutant strains of *S. typhosa* tested in Egypt had a protection rate of 95%, suggesting the importance of local immune responses. If further field trials are effective, this vaccine may gain widespread acceptance in areas where typhoid fever is endemic; it is not now licensed in the United States.

Control of *Salmonella* Infections. Attention to personal hygiene, hand washing, and sanitary practices is essential for personnel involved in the preparation of food and in patient care in order to minimize person-to-person and person-to-food transmission. Urine and feces of hospitalized patients should be handled with special precautions until three consecutive stool cultures are negative.

Every effort should be made to eradicate *Salmonella typhosa* from carriers. When these efforts are unsuccessful, the individuals must be kept under careful surveillance by local health departments and prevented from working in food and water processing plants, in kitchens, and in occupations related to patient care. Such individuals should be made aware of their potential contagiousness and the importance of hand washing and personal hygiene. Antibiotic therapy of exposed individuals is contraindicated; prophylactic ingestion of nonspecific antimicrobial agents (oxyquinolines) does not prevent infection.

Attention to the preparation of foodstuffs, the use of proper temperature for cooking, and the avoidance of holding potentially infected foods at warm temperatures are important control measures. The requirement that pets be certified as *Salmonella* free before sale would eliminate, to some extent, an unnecessary problem.

Typhoid fever can be controlled in endemic areas only by improved sanitation and housing and by the availability of pure water. Large scale immunization programs may reduce but will not eliminate this disease.

RALPH D. FEIGIN

Barrett TJ, Snyder JD, Blake PA, et al: Enzyme-linked immunosorbent assay for detection of *Salmonella typhi* Vi antigen in urine from typhoid patients. J Clin Microbiol 15:235, 1982.
Carrol WL, Balistreri WF, Brilli R, et al: Spectrum of *Salmonella*-associated arthritis. Pediatrics 68:717, 1981.
France GL, Mormer DJ, Steele RW: Breast-feeding and salmonella infection. Am J Dis Child 134:147, 1980.
Gianella RA: Importance of the intestinal inflammatory reaction on salmonella mediated intestinal secretion. Infect Immun 23:140, 1979.
Gianella RA, Formal SB, Dammin GJ, et al: Pathogenesis of salmonellosis. J Clin Invest 52:441, 1973.
Nelson JD: Antibiotic therapy for *Salmonella* syndromes. Am J Dis Child 135:1093, 1981.
Overturf G, Marton KI, Mathies AW: Antibiotic resistance in typhoid fever. N Engl J Med 289:463, 1973.
Ryder RW, Crosby-Ritchie A, McDonough B, et al: Human milk contaminated with *Salmonella kottbus*. JAMA 238:1533, 1977.
Weissbluth M, Shulman ST, Holson B: *Salmonella cholera-suis*: A distinctive bacterial pathogen. J Pediatr 98:423, 1981.
Wilson R, Feldman RA, Davis J, et al: Salmonellosis in infants: The importance of intrafamilial transmission. Pediatrics 69:436, 1982.

11.28 SHIGELLOSIS
(Bacillary Dysentery)

Shigellosis, an acute inflammatory disease of the gastrointestinal tract, is produced by *Shigella* bacteria. This illness may be characterized by fever, crampy abdominal pain, and loose or diarrheal stools that may contain mucus, pus, and blood.

Etiology. *Shigella* species are nonmotile, short, gram-negative rods biochemically characterized by very slow or absent fermentation of lactose. *Shigella* must be distinguished by other biochemical properties from those *E. coli* that do not ferment lactose or form gas. The genus *Shigella* is subdivided into four major groups (A, B, C, and D) by means of biochemical reactions and antigenic composition. Group A contains 10 serologic types, of which *Shigella dysenteriae* is the most important; this group is rarely encountered in the United States. *Shigella* Group B contains 6 serologic groups, of which *S. flexneri* is commonly isolated in the United States; Group C includes *S. boydii*, which is not common in the United States. *S. sonnei* is the single serotype in Group D; it accounts for over half of the *Shigella* isolates reported annually to the Centers for Disease Control.

Epidemiology. Shigellae are found worldwide. The highest incidence of shigellosis occurs in children 1–4 yr of age; it is more common during the late summer, but its seasonality is not as marked as that of *Salmonella*.

Man is the major reservoir for *Shigella*; there are no natural animal hosts, but flies may be vectors. The organism is transmitted principally by direct fecal-oral route; there have, however, been outbreaks of water-borne or food-borne disease. Spread of infection via inanimate objects, such as toys, also may occur. Persons in close contact in unsanitary conditions are at high risk for outbreaks of shigellosis. Institutionalized children are at particular risk, as are those in day care centers, who may transmit the disease to family members; a secondary attack rate of 25% has been recorded.

Pathogenesis. The ingestion of as few as 200 *Shigella* bacilli may result in infection, and *Shigella* can survive the acidity of gastric secretions for as long as 4 hr. *Shigella* must penetrate epithelial cells in order to induce infection. Once inside the epithelial cell, the organisms multiply in the submucosa and lamina propria. Local inflammation, edema, hyperemia, and epithelial cell dysfunction occur. Microabscesses form behind obstructed crypts, and superficial ulcers may lead to bleeding. A fibrinous exudate containing polymorphonuclear leukocytes covers the mucosal lining of the colon. Because of the superficial nature of the *Shigella* infection, intestinal perforation does not occur and bacteremia is unusual. These gastrointestinal changes resolve spontaneously within 4–7 days.

S. dysenteriae produces an enterotoxin that interrupts cytoplasmic protein synthesis, but its role in the pathogenesis of disease is unknown. Toxigenic strains that are noninvasive do not result in disease. In contrast, invasive nontoxigenic strains result in shigellosis. Virulent strains of *S. flexneri* and *S. sonnei* require the presence of a plasmid which codes for an I antigen related to the O-polysaccharide side chains on the *Shigella* lipopolysaccharide.

Clinical Manifestations. During the incubation period, usually 36–72 hr following ingestion, shigellae reach the colon. Then the patient may complain of crampy abdominal pain, the temperature may be greater than 40.0° C, and the patient may appear toxic. After 48 hr, diarrhea usually sets in; the child may have up to 20 stools/day containing blood and mucus. Later, bloody diarrhea may occur without fever or abdominal cramps. The child may have some lower abdominal tenderness to palpation without evidence of localization.

Shigellosis may mimic central nervous system infections such as meningitis and encephalitis, particularly when high fever is present with associated seizures. Seizures occur in 12–45% of children with *Shigella* gastroenteritis, and they are more likely to occur in children whose temperatures exceed 40.0° C. They are more common in children under 7 yr of age, particularly in those under 3 yr and in those children with a family history of a seizure disorder. Other symptoms may include headache, delirium, nuchal rigidity, fainting, and lethargy.

Fluid and electrolyte losses may result in dehydration, acidosis, and electrolyte disturbances. There may be complaints of urgency and tenesmus, and, particularly in patients with malnutrition, rectal prolapse and intussusception may occur.

Shigella may infrequently be responsible for infections in areas other than the gastrointestinal tract. Purulent conjunctivitis and vaginitis with blood-tinged purulent discharge may result from surface inoculation with contaminated fingers or objects. Bacteremia is rare, so that localized infections outside the intestinal tract are quite unusual. Systemic infections, such as pneumonia, meningitis, osteomyelitis, and arthritis, are most apt to be seen in infants and young children in populations where malnutrition is severe and common. In such instances, severe dehydration contributing to renal failure, at times to the hemolytic-uremic syndrome, may also be expected. Nonsuppurative arthritis may also occur, and Reiter syndrome has been associated with *S. dysenteriae* in HLA B27 positive children (Sec. 10.60). Mortality from *Shigella* septicemia is about 50%, and afebrile, dehydrated, and malnourished children who have had protracted diarrhea are at increased risk of bacteremia.

Diagnosis. *Shigella* should be considered a possible etiologic agent in any patient presenting with diarrhea, particularly those with accompanying fever. Stool stained with methylene blue should reveal leukocytes and red blood cells. The presence of leukocytes does not establish an etiologic diagnosis, nor does their absence exclude *Shigella* as the etiologic agent. There may be leukocytosis with abundant immature forms.

The diagnosis is established by isolating the organism from fresh stool or rectal cultures. Selected media such as xylose-lysine deoxycholate (XLD) and SS agar should be inoculated promptly with a fresh stool sample. If these media are not available, the stool should be placed in a buffered glycerol-saline solution for preservation prior to transport to a laboratory. Blood culture should be obtained from children who are severely ill with shigellosis. Shigellosis must be distinguished from other causes of dysentery such as enterotoxigenic *E. coli*, amebic dysentery, *Campylobacter fetus*, *Salmonella*, and rotavirus gastroenteritis, as well as from intussusception and acute appendicitis.

Treatment. Antibiotic treatment decreases the duration of excretion of *Shigella* as well as the duration of diarrhea. The choice of antibiotic depends upon the current sensitivities of this organism in the community. Resistance transfer factors are responsible for mediating multiple resistance to ampicillin, cephalosporins, chloramphenicol, aminoglycosides, sulfonamides, and tetracyclines. Susceptibility patterns may also vary between serotypes of *Shigella*. When *Shigella* strains are sensitive to ampicillin, it is effective at doses of 50–100 mg/kg/24 hr in 4 divided doses. Parenteral administration of ampicillin may be required initially. Amoxicillin, although better absorbed than ampicillin, is less effective. When ampicillin-resistant strains are suspected or proved, trimethoprim-sulfamethoxazole is the drug of choice (trimethoprim at 10 mg/kg/day and sulfamethoxazole at 50 mg/kg/day in 2 divided doses for 5–7 days).

Antibiotic therapy usually eliminates *Shigella* from the gastrointestinal tract. A long-term carrier state may rarely develop. In such instances lactulose, a synthetic derivative of lactose, will transiently decrease the excretion of *Shigella*. The metabolism of lactulose by normal gut flora results in an increased production of short chain fatty acids and a decrease in stool pH, both of which inhibit the growth of *Shigella*. Lactulose is ineffective for acute shigellosis, and drugs that decrease peristalsis are contraindicated. Fluid and electrolyte therapy is dependent upon the patient's state of hydration (Sec. 5.20–5.23).

Prognosis and Prevention. In most healthy children shigellosis is a self-limited illness which usually resolves spontaneously. Organisms occasionally can be cultured up to 3 mo following an acute episode. Increased morbidity and mortality may be seen in enclosed populations, such as those of mental institutions, or in countries where malnutrition is common.

Proper hygiene and environmental standards are the most important factors in preventing disease due to *Shigella*. Rigid handwashing is mandatory for individuals caring for children with shigellosis. In the hospital enteric precautions must be initiated promptly. No efficacious and reliable vaccine is available. Patients with shigellosis should be reported to public health officials.

SHELDON L. KAPLAN
RALPH D. FEIGIN

Barrett-Connor E, Connor JD: Extraintestinal manifestations of shigellosis. Am J Gastroenterol 53:234, 1970.
Blaser MJ, Pollard RA, Feldman RA: *Shigella* infections in the United States, 1974–1980. J Infect Dis 147:771, 1983.
Duncan B, Fulginiti VA, Sieber OF, et al: *Shigella* sepsis. Am J Dis Child 135:151, 1982.
Kowlessan M, Forbes GR: The febrile convulsion in shigellosis. N Engl J Med 258:520, 1950.
Murphy TV, Nelson JD: *Shigella* vaginitis: Report of 38 patients and review of the literature. Pediatrics 63:511, 1979.
Nelson JD, Kusmiesz H, Jackson LH: Comparison of trimethoprim-sulfamethoxazole and ampicillin therapy for shigellosis in ambulatory patients. J Pediatr 89:491, 1976.
Pickering LK, Evans DG, DuPont HL, et al: Diarrhea caused by *Shigella*, rotavirus, and *Giardia* in day-care centers: Prospective study. J Pediatr 99:51, 1981.

11.29 CHOLERA

Cholera, an acute intestinal disease, is caused by an enterotoxin elaborated by *Vibrio cholerae*, serotype 01. Its clinical course ranges from asymptomatic infection to the most severe form, *cholera gravis*, in which sudden, profuse, watery diarrhea results in hypovolemic shock, metabolic acidosis, and, if untreated, death.

Etiology. *V. cholerae* is a short, slightly curved, motile, gram-negative rod with a single polar flagellum. About 70 serotypes are known, and although many of them cause acute diarrhea, only the 01 serotype causes cholera. *V. cholerae* grows readily on a variety of media. *V. cholerae* 01 (and many other *V. cholerae* serotypes) produce opaque, yellow colonies on TCBS agar and can be recognized only by reactions with specific antisera. The two biotypes of *V. cholerae* 01 are classical and El Tor; each is separable into two serotypes, Ogawa and Inaba. Reversion of serotypes may occur during an epidemic.

Epidemiology. Cholera has been endemic in the Ganges delta throughout history, with annual epidemics in West Bengal and Bangladesh. From 1817 to 1926 the disease spread worldwide in six pandemics. A seventh pandemic, caused by the El Tor biotype, began in 1961 in Indonesia, and by 1977 had spread to most of Southeast and South Asia, the Middle East, Africa, Southern Europe, and the Western Pacific regions. By the end of 1985, 93 countries had been involved.

In the United States only a few laboratory-acquired cases were identified from 1911 to 1973, when a single indigenous case was reported in Texas. Since 1977, 44 infections have been identified, most of which occurred in Gulf states. All cases were traced to the consumption of seafood from the Gulf of Mexico. No other indigenous cases have been reported in other countries in the Western Hemisphere during the present pandemic.

Endemic and epidemic cholera often have a seasonal pattern. Contaminated water and food, especially shellfish, play a major role in transmission. African epidemics have often been observed following feasts and funeral gatherings at which rites were performed that facilitate transmission. Nosocomial outbreaks occur where overcrowding and poor sanitary conditions prevail. Secondary cases are rare in medical personnel who have had close contact with patients.

Persons with asymptomatic or mild infection play an important role in disseminating cholera. The ratio of asymptomatic or mild infections to severe disease is generally 5–7:1 in classical cholera and as high as 50–100:1 in El Tor cholera. A prolonged carrier state, with the gallbladder as the reservoir, has been documented in adults convalescing from El Tor cholera but has not been observed in children. Family contacts of hospitalized patients are frequently infected.

In endemic areas cholera is predominantly a disease of children; in rural Bangladesh attack rates are 5–10 times greater for children 2–9 yr than for adults. In infants, breast feeding provides protection and cholera is rare. Increasingly high titers of vibriocidal antibody occur with advancing age, suggesting that the lower attack rate for adults is due to immunity induced by recurrent exposure to *V. cholerae* 01 and that subclinical or asymptomatic reinfection probably occurs frequently. In contrast, when cholera spreads to a previously uninfected area, attack rates are usually equal for all age groups exposed.

Both human and nonhuman reservoirs of *V. cholerae* 01 may exist in endemic areas. The organism may be transmitted as a subclinical infection during interepidemic periods by persons who are asymptomatic or have mild disease; also, the El Tor biotype may survive for a prolonged time in an aquatic environment. Animals have no role in the human disease cycle.

Pathology and Pathophysiology. The site of infection is the small intestine, primarily the jejunum. After ingestion, the vibrios multiply in the lumen and adhere to the surface of epithelial cells underneath the mucous layer; here they elaborate an enterotoxic protein. The binding subunit of this enterotoxin attaches to a receptor (GM_1 ganglioside) on the surface membrane of epithelial cells. The active subunit then enters the cells and activates adenylate cyclase to produce increased amounts of cyclic adenosine monophosphate (cAMP). This leads to a decrease in active absorption of sodium and chloride in villus cells and an increase in active secretion of chloride by crypt cells, resulting in a net loss of water and electrolyte into the bowel. At least one other "toxic" factor involved in the pathogenesis of cholera may exist; this is suggested by studies in volunteers indicating that genetically engineered strains of *V. cholerae* 01 that lack the gene for toxin production can cause diarrhea.

Biopsy of the small intestine of a patient with cholera reveals an intact epithelium with minimal cellular response; emptying of goblet cells indicates an increase in mucus secretion. Slight edema of the lamina propria and moderate dilation of capillaries and lymphatics in tips of villi are also seen.

The diarrheal fluid lost is isotonic with plasma and has relatively high concentrations of bicarbonate and potassium. Stools from children with cholera contain more potassium and less sodium, chloride, and bicarbonate than stools from adults (Table 11–20). This fluid loss usually results in an isotonic deficit of sodium and water, potassium depletion, and acidosis due to deficit of base. Bicarbonate loss continues even when systemic acidosis develops. Although there is some impairment of activity of jejunal disaccharidases, including lactase, glucose absorption is usually preserved.

Clinical Manifestations. Typically, after an incubation period of 6 hr–2 days, a sudden onset of painless and profuse watery diarrhea occurs. In the most severe cases stools are passed frequently and effortlessly and have a rice-water appearance (i.e., clear fluid with only flecks of mucus visible), and a slight fishlike odor. In less severe cases the stool is more yellow in appearance. Periumbilical abdominal cramps occur in about 50% of cases; tenesmus is absent. Vomiting is common in severe cases, usually occurring after the onset of diarrhea. In about 25% of children, the rectal temperature is slightly elevated (38–39° C) on admission or in the first 24 hr of hospitalization.

Massive diarrhea can result in profound dehydration and circulatory collapse. In these severe cases, cholera gravis, the blood pressure falls and is often unobtainable, the radial pulse becomes imperceptible, respirations are rapid and deep, and urine flow ceases. The eyes and fontanel are deeply sunken; the skin is cold and clammy, with poor turgor; and the skin of the fingers becomes shriveled. Cyanosis and painful muscle cramps occur in the extremities, especially in the calves. The patient is restless and extremely thirsty. Lethargy, thick speech, and a somnolent state are common. Stool losses may continue for up to 7 days. Subsequent manifestations depend on the adequacy of replacement therapy. An early sign of recovery is usually the reappearance of bile pigment in the stool, after which the cessation of diarrhea is usually rapid.

Mild cases of cholera, considerably more common than those of cholera gravis as described above, usually present as simple diarrhea with little or no dehydration and are more common in children than in adults.

Diagnosis. Definitive diagnosis depends on isolating *V. cholerae* 01 from stool. Microscopic examination of stool usually reveals fewer than 5 polymorphonuclear cells/high power field. Retrospective diagnosis is possible by determining vibriocidal, agglutinating, and toxin-neutralizing antibodies whose peak titers usually occur 7–14 days after onset of illness. Vibriocidal and agglutinating antibody titers return to baseline levels 8–12 wk after onset; antitoxin titers remain elevated for up to 12–18 mo. A 4-fold or greater rise during acute disease or a fall in titer during convalescence is usually considered diagnostic. A 4-fold rise in vibriocidal antibody

also occurs after infection with other organisms, such as *Yersinia* and *Brucella*, making it imperative to interpret titers in light of clinical and epidemiologic findings. Illness with *V. cholerae* 01 is more likely to occur in persons with lower vibriocidal titers, although some with high titers will have severe disease. In endemic areas asymptomatic infection may also result in 4-fold rises in vibriocidal titer.

A diagnosis of cholera should be considered in a child with severely dehydrating diarrhea, especially when the patient has been in a cholera-infected area within 5 days of onset of illness. Severe cholera may be indistinguishable clinically from severe diarrhea produced by enterotoxigenic *Escherichia coli* or non-01 *V. cholerae*. Milder disease may be similar to that caused by other bacterial pathogens (e.g., *Salmonella*), or certain viruses (e.g., rotavirus).

Complications. These are more frequent and severe in children than in adults. Inadequate fluid replacement may lead to acute renal failure from tubular necrosis. Inadequate potassium replacement can result in cardiac arrhythmias, hypokalemic nephropathy, and paralytic ileus. Rarely, pulmonary edema has occurred in children treated with excessive and rapid fluid replacement without correction of severe acidosis. Transient tetany during correction of acidosis occurs infrequently. Prolonged drowsiness, coma, or convulsions may occur before or during treatment in as many as 10% of small children; these can be caused by marked hypoglycemia, but the reason is more often unknown. Hypoglycemia is preventable by including dextrose in replacement solutions. An increase in fetal deaths during the 3rd trimester of pregnancy has been observed principally in severely dehydrated patients who delay seeking hospital care.

Prevention. Avoidance of contaminated food and water is the best preventive measure. Commercially available cholera vaccine containing heat- or phenol-inactivated suspensions of classical Inaba and Ogawa strains of *V. cholerae* 01 is of low efficacy and provides only limited protection of short duration. High-potency vaccines have demonstrated 50–80% protection for up to 6 mo in endemic areas; no data are available on the efficacy of vaccine in newly infected areas, but it is likely that it is less in these areas where naturally acquired immunity is not present. Vaccine does not reduce the rate of inapparent infections and thus does not prevent transmission of cholera within families or in communities. Vaccination is not required for entry into the United States from a cholera-infected area (Sec. 4.5). A number of oral vaccines are being developed in an effort to enhance local immunity in the intestinal tract.

Chemoprophylaxis with tetracycline (for at least 2 days) in 2 daily doses of 500 mg for adults, 125 mg for children aged 4–13 yr, and 50 mg for children under 3 yr, reduces infection rates in household contacts. For ease of administration doxycycline in a single dose (300 mg in adults, 6 mg/kg in children below 15 yr) is the preferred tetracycline compound. Mass chemoprophylaxis in a large community is not advisable.

Table 11–20. Electrolyte Content of Cholera Stool and of Solutions Recommended for Intravenous and Oral Treatment of Children

| | Approximate Electrolyte Concentration (mm/L) | | | | | |
	Na	K	Cl	HCO₃	$C_6H_5O_7^{-3}$	Glucose
Cholera stool, adult	140	13	104	44	—	—
Cholera stool, child	101	27	92	32	—	—
Ringer's lactate solution*	130	4	109	28	—	—
Diarrhea treatment solution†	117	13	82	48	—	55
Oral glucose-electrolyte solution*‡	90	20	80	—	10	111

*Solutions recommended by World Health Organization.
†Prepared in g/L: NaCl, 4; Na acetate, 6.5 (or Na lactate, 5.4); KCl, 1; glucose, 10.
‡Prepared in g/L: NaCl, 3.5; $C_6H_5Na_3O_7$•2H₂O, 2.9; KCl, 1.5; glucose, 20. (2.5 g of NaHCO₃ may be used in place of $C_6H_5Na_3O_7$•2H₂O; this solution is referred to as ORS [Oral Rehydration Salts]).

Treatment. Successful management primarily requires prompt evaluation of dehydration (Sec. 5.21) and replacement of gastrointestinal losses of fluid and electrolytes (Sec. 5.19). Antibiotic therapy is adjunctive. Hospitalized patients do not require strict isolation but are more readily managed in a single unit. Enteric precautions should be carefully followed. When possible, patients should be weighed on admission, and subsequent stool output measured. A "cholera cot" made of canvas or burlap on a wooden frame with a plastic or rubber sheet extending through a 4–6 inch opening where the patient places the buttocks facilitates stool disposal and accurate measurement of stool volume. Urine output should be measured for at least 24 hr.

When a cholera patient is first seen, the extent of dehydration should be quickly determined (Sec. 5.21). Measurements of plasma specific gravity and serum electrolytes, especially bicarbonate, are helpful in planning fluid replacement. By the time dehydration is clinically apparent, a child has lost a significant amount of body fluid and electrolytes; the danger in treatment usually lies in underestimation of losses.

Patients with severe dehydration and hypovolemic shock should be given replacement fluids intravenously as promptly as possible (Sec. 5.38 and 5.41). Infants should receive about 70 mL/kg during the first 3 hr; if signs of dehydration persist, they should receive 20 mL/kg over the next 3 hr; older children and adults can usually be given the total amount of 100 mL/kg in 3–4 hr. The exact rate and amounts of fluids for replacement and maintenance should be adjusted in relation to continuous monitoring of the patient's state of hydration and stool losses. If no peripheral vein is available, the external jugular or femoral veins should be used rather than losing time by infusing fluid subcutaneously or intraperitoneally or by performing a cutdown. To avoid overhydration the neck veins should be monitored for distention, the lungs for rales of pulmonary edema, and the eyelids for edema. Table 11–20 indicates appropriate replacement fluids (see also Table 5–14). If Ringer lactate is used, potassium chloride should be added (10 mEq/L) or given orally if renal function is adequate. Isotonic saline can be used to correct hypovolemia if base, potassium, and glucose supplementations are given (Sec. 5.18–5.24).

Patients presenting with moderate to mild dehydration (e.g., with thirst alone or with diminished skin turgor and neck vein distention but without shock) may be given initial replacement fluid orally (Tables 5–15 and 11–20 and Sec. 5.17 and 5.24). The solution may be made using drinking water, but should be prepared daily to minimize bacterial contamination. Patients with moderate dehydration should be given 100 mL/kg of *oral rehydration salts (ORS) solution* over 4 hr; 50 mL/kg over the same time is given for mild dehydration. When a patient is tired, a nasogastric tube can be used to give fluid. Vomiting is not a contraindication to oral fluids; when it occurs, smaller amounts should be offered more frequently. In fewer than 1% of patients there is malabsorption of glucose from the oral fluid, with resultant worsening of diarrhea; in this situation the intravenous route must be used.

After replacement fluid has been given, *maintenance therapy* should be started to match insensible water loss (500–1000 mL/m² of body surface/24 hr in hot climates) and continuing diarrheal losses (Sec. 5.16). During the first few hours of treatment stool output is often minimal, but once shock is corrected, the diarrheal output generally increases to as much as 200–350 mL/kg/24 hr. In older children, hourly losses may be over 800 mL. Except for patients with very high rates of stooling and those with glucose malabsorption, continuing losses can usually be replaced with the oral glucose-electrolyte solution; they should receive 10–20 mL/kg/hr until diarrhea is distinctly decreased. If signs of dehydration reappear and losses cannot be adequately replaced orally, intravenous therapy should be instituted.

For patients with mild diarrhea the oral solution can be given at home at a rate of 100/mL/kg/24 hr until diarrhea stops. Breast-fed infants should be encouraged to breast feed ad libitum during maintenance therapy; other infants can be offered water or milk formula diluted with an equal volume of water, if desired.

Since cholera is endemic in many areas where malnutrition is common and there is evidence that most nutrients are absorbed during illness, an average diet for age should be started during maintenance therapy as soon as the patient can eat. This will help prevent further deterioration of nutritional status. Foods that are energy-rich and contain potassium should be given. For infants 4–6 mo of age or older who have not previously been given semisolid foods, this is a good time to start feeding such foods.

As soon as the patient is alert (within 2–6 hr), oral tetracycline should be given (50 mg/kg/24 hr every 6 hr for 2–3 days), although this may cause discoloration of teeth in children less than 8 yr old. Tetracycline shortens the duration and volume of diarrhea by 50–70% and the duration of carriage of vibrio organisms. Tetracycline-resistant strains of *V. cholerae* 01 are uncommon. Single dose doxycycline (6 mg/kg), furazolidone (5 mg/kg/24 hr given every 6 hr for 3 days), and erythromycin (30 mg/kg/24 hr given every 8 hr for 3 days) are as effective as tetracycline in decreasing duration and volume of diarrhea but are not as effective in shortening the period of excretion of vibrios. Both chloramphenicol (50 mg/kg/24 hr given every 6 hr for 2–3 days) and trimethoprim-sulfamethoxazole (as 8 mg/kg/24 hr of trimethoprim and 40 mg/kg/24 hr of sulfamethoxazole in 2 divided doses for 3 days) are beneficial but the latter is less so than tetracycline; most sulfonamides are ineffective. Parenteral antibiotic therapy is unnecessary. Antidiarrheal medications such as opiates, paregoric, other antimotility drugs, and steroids should not be used. Blood and plasma are not required.

Prognosis. The outcome of cholera in infants and children should be as favorable as it is in adults, in whom the overall mortality is less than 1%. The high mortality rates (20–70%) reported in earlier studies have been dramatically reduced by the improvements in fluid therapy.

MICHAEL H. MERSON

Carpenter CCJ Jr, Hirschhorn N: Pediatric cholera: Current concepts of therapy. J Pediatr 80:874, 1972.
Cholera and other vibrio associated diarrhoeas. WHO Scientific Working Group Report. Bull WHO 58:373, 1980.
Feachem R: Environmental aspects of cholera epidemiology. Parts I–III. Trop Dis Bull 78:676 and 866, 1981; 79:2, 1982.
Glass RI, Svennerholm AM, Stoll BJ, et al: Protection against cholera in breast-fed children by antibodies in breast milk. N Engl J Med 309:323, 1983.
Holmgren J: Actions of cholera toxin and the prevention and treatment of cholera. Nature 292:413, 1981.
Mahalanabis D, Watten RH, Wallace CK: Clinical aspects and management of pediatric cholera. In: Barua D, Burrows W (eds): Cholera. Philadelphia, WB Saunders, 1974.
Manual for the Treatment of Acute Diarrhoea. Geneva, World Health Organization, 1984.
Morris JG Jr, Black R: Cholera and other vibrioses in the United States. N Engl J Med 312:343, 1985.

11.30 INFECTIONS DUE TO *PSEUDOMONAS*

Pseudomonas lives abundantly in soil and water and is widespread throughout nature. It is also a common contaminant of moist environments within building structures, including hospitals. It is, however, a rare cause of disease in healthy infants and children beyond the newborn period. *Pseudomonas* can be responsible for serious disease among healthy, term newborn infants, often in an epidemic pattern; in such instances the mortality rate is apt to be high. Most infections, however, are among low birthweight infants who are otherwise at risk and in older infants and children with impaired host defenses, such as those with cystic fibrosis, immunodeficiency disorders, malignancies and other debilitating conditions, extensive burns, or malnutrition (especially in impoverished populations) and in those receiving immunosuppressive therapy (Sec. 11.11).

Etiology. There are a large number of identified *Pseudomonas* species, but only a few are pathogenic for man; of these, *P. aeruginosa* is by far the most common. Others, occasionally recognized as human pathogens, include: *P. cepacia, P. maltophilia, P. fluorescens, P. putrefaciens,* and *P. mallei,* the cause of glanders in horses (see below).

The pseudomonads are gram-negative bacilli and are strict aerobes. Since they can utilize any source of carbon, they multiply in most moist environments that contain minimal amounts of organic compounds. Strains from clinical specimens may produce beta-hemolysis on blood agar; more than 90% of strains produce a bluish-green phenazine pigment (blue pus) as well as fluorescein, which is yellow-green and fluoresces. These pigments diffuse into and color the medium surrounding the colonies. Strains of *Pseudomonas* can be differentiated from one another for epidemiologic purposes by serologic, phage, and pyocin typing.

Epidemiology. *Pseudomonads* frequently enter the hospital environment on the clothes, skin, or shoes of patients or hospital personnel. Colonization of any moist or liquid substance may ensue; for example, they may be found growing in distilled water, hospital kitchens and laundries, some antiseptic solutions, and equipment used for respiratory therapy. In some healthy persons, *Pseudomonas* is included in their usual intestinal flora.

Pathogenesis. The requirement of oxygen for growth may account for the lack of invasiveness of *Pseudomonas* after it has colonized or even infected the skin. It produces endotoxin that is extremely weak compared with that of other gram-negative bacilli, but it may initiate diarrhea. *Pseudomonas* also elaborates a number of extracellular products including lecithinase, collagenase, lipase, and hemolysins which may be responsible for localized necrosis of skin. One of the hemolytic factors is a heat-resistant glycolipid that may dissolve and destroy lecithin (surfactant), and that may in turn contribute to producing atelectasis in pulmonary infections caused by *Pseudomonas.* The pathogenicity of *P. aeruginosa* also depends upon its ability to resist phagocytosis, which seems to depend principally upon the production of toxins. The host responds to infection by producing antibodies to *Pseudomonas* exotoxin (exotoxin A) and lipopolysaccharide.

Clinical Manifestations. Although most clinical patterns relate to opportunistic infections (Sec. 11.11), *P. aeruginosa* introduced into a minor wound of a healthy child may be followed by cellulitis and a localized abscess that exudes green or blue pus. The characteristic skin lesions of *Pseudomonas,* whether due to direct inoculation or secondary to septicemia, begin as pink macules and progress to hemorrhagic nodules and eventually to areas of necrosis with eschar formation, surrounded by an intense red areola (*ecthyma gangrenosum*).

Multiplication of bacteria occurs locally, and occasionally septicemia, endocarditis, meningitis, corneal infections, orbital cellulitis, mastoiditis, folliculitis, pneumonia, or urinary tract infections may ensue in normal children. Rarely, *Pseudomonas* may be associated with gastroenteritis.

Otitis externa caused by *P. aeruginosa* may occur in swimmers who swim repetitively in pools contaminated by this organism.

Outbreaks of dermatitis and urinary tract infections caused by *P. aeruginosa* have been reported in healthy children following use of community swimming pools, recreational whirlpools, or family-owned hot tubs. Skin lesions develop several hours to 2 days following contact with these water sources. Skin lesions may be erythematous, macular, papular, or pustular. Illness may vary from a few scattered lesions to extensive truncal involvement. In some children, malaise, fever, vomiting, sore throat, conjunctivitis, rhinitis, and swollen breasts may be associated with dermal lesions.

Pseudomonads other than *P. aeruginosa* rarely cause disease in healthy children, but pneumonia and abscesses due to *P. cepacia,* otitis media due to *P. putrefaciens,* abscesses due to *P. fluorescens,* otitis media due to *P. stutzeri,* and cellulitis and septicemia due to *P. maltophilia* have been reported. Septicemia and endocarditis due to *P. maltophilia* have also been associated with intravenous abuse of drugs.

Shunts, Catheters, and Equipment. *Pseudomonas* septicemia may occur with indwelling intravenous or urinary catheters; pneumonia and septicemia occur in children receiving inhalation therapy. Peritonitis and septicemia have been associated with contaminated equipment used for peritoneal dialysis. Abscesses or meningitis may be related to dermal sinus tracts or dermoids that extend to or communicate with the meninges or neural tissue, or that extend to meningomyeloceles. *Pseudomonas* may produce acute or subacute endocarditis in children with congenital heart lesions or following cardiac surgery.

Burns and Wound Infection. The surfaces of wounds or burns are frequently populated by *Pseudomonas* and other gram-negative organisms; this does not necessarily imply infection but is a necessary prerequisite to invasive disease. Septicemia with *P. aeruginosa* is a major problem in the burned patient (Sec. 5.28 and 11.11.). It may be related to multiplication of organisms in devitalized tissues or associated with prolonged use of intravenous or urinary catheters. Administration of antibiotics may diminish the susceptible microbiologic flora but permit selected strains of *Pseudomonas* to flourish.

Cystic Fibrosis (Sec. 13.97). *P. aeruginosa,* especially the mucoid variety that produces an excessive amount of slime, can be recovered from the sputum of most children with cystic fibrosis. This does not necessarily imply infection and destructive pneumonitis related to this organism but rather the possibility of a relationship between the *Pseudomonas* and the patient with cystic fibrosis that permits permanent habituation. Usually, the tracheobronchial tree is chronically colonized, and the organism is rarely eradicated spontaneously or by antibiotic therapy. Mist tents and continuous broad-spectrum antibiotic therapy may also facilitate this relationship. *Pseudomonas* is chronically present and limited almost entirely to the lung; septicemia is rare.

Malignancy. Children with leukemia or other debilitating malignancies, particularly those who are receiving immunosuppressive therapy and who are neutropenic, are extremely susceptible to septicemia from invasion of the bloodstream by *Pseudomonas* with which the patient is already colonized (see Sec. 11.11). Anorexia, malaise, nausea, vomiting, diarrhea, and fever may be noted. A generalized vasculitis develops, and hemorrhagic necrotic lesions may be found in all organs, including skin, where they appear as purple nodules or ecchymotic areas which become gangrenous. Hemorrhagic or gangrenous perirectal cellulitis or abscesses may occur and be associated with ileus and profound hypotension.

Diagnosis and Differential Diagnosis. Diagnosis of *Pseudomonas* infection depends upon recovery of the organism from the blood, cerebrospinal fluid, urine, or needle aspirate of the lung or from purulent material obtained by aspiration of subcutaneous abscesses or areas of cellulitis.

Bluish, nodular skin lesions and ulcers with ecchymotic and gangrenous centers and bright areolae (ecthyma gangrenosum) have been considered to be virtually pathognomonic of *Pseudomonas* infection of the skin. Rarely, skin lesions clinically indistinguishable from those caused by *P. aeruginosa* may follow septicemia due to *Aeromonas hydrophila.*

Prevention. In part, this depends upon continuous surveillance of the hospital environment to identify and subsequently eradicate sources of the organism as quickly as possible. *Pseudomonas* may grow in distilled water, disinfectants, parenteral alimentation solutions, and medications. In newborn nurseries infection generally has been transmitted to the infants by the hands of personnel, from washbasin surfaces, from catheters and from solutions used to rinse suction catheters.

Strict attention to hand washing, particularly with an iodophor-containing liquid, before and between contacts with newborn infants may prevent or interdict epidemic disease. Growth of *Pseudomonas* on suction catheters can be prevented by rinsing catheters in a 3% solution of acetic acid. Meticulous care in the preparation of solutions for total parenteral alimentation and in the insertion and care of catheters as well as daily replacement of all apparatus used for intravenous administration greatly reduces the hazard of extrinsic contamination by *Pseudomonas* and other gram-negative organisms.

Prevention of follicular dermatitis caused by *Pseudomonas* contamination of whirlpools or hot tubs is possible by maintaining pool water at a pH of 7.2–7.8 and free chlorine concentration at 70.5 mg/L.

Burn patients may be actively immunized with a polyvalent *Pseudomonas* vaccine that reduces bacteremia and mortality. The administration of specific hyperimmune globulin also prevents septicemia. Infection also may be minimized by careful protective isolation, by the topical application of silver nitrate (0.5%) solution or 10% mafenide acetate cream, and by debridement of devitalized tissue.

Pseudomonas infection of dermal sinuses communicating with the cerebrospinal space can be prevented by early discovery and surgical repair. *Pseudomonas* infection of the urinary tract may be minimized or prevented by early identification and corrective surgery of obstructive lesions.

Treatment. Systemic infections with *Pseudomonas* should be treated promptly with an antibiotic to which the organism is sensitive in vitro. Response to treatment may be limited, and prolonged treatment may be necessary for systemic infection in the compromised host.

Septicemia usually should be treated with gentamicin in a dose of 5–7.5 mg/kg/24 hr in 3 divided doses. The higher dose may be used after the 1st wk of life. This drug may be given intramuscularly or intravenously (if it is infused slowly over a period of 1 hr). Carbenicillin (200–400 mg/kg/24 hr in 6 divided doses) or ticarcillin (200 mg/kg/24 hr in 6 divided doses intravenously) should be used concomitantly for a possible synergistic effect. Carbenicillin or ticarcillin alone is not recommended because strains of the organism rapidly become resistant to these agents. Tobramycin (3–5 mg/kg/24 hr) or amikacin (15–25 mg/kg/24 hr) in 3 divided doses intramuscularly or intravenously (over 1 hr) may be used to replace gentamicin in the therapeutic regimen. Polymyxin B and colistin (polymyxin E), previously widely used but now largely superseded by the preceding regimens, may still be useful in patients infected with strains of *Pseudomonas* resistant to other agents.

Many of the newer beta-lactam antibiotics possess variable degrees of activity against *P. aeruginosa*. In vitro, ceftazidime is the most active of these agents against *P. aeruginosa*, and it has also proved to be extremely effective in patients with cystic fibrosis (150–200 mg/kg/24 hr in 3 or 4 divided doses). Azlocillin and piperacillin also have proved to be effective therapy for selected strains of *P. aeruginosa* when combined with an aminoglycoside; they can be given in doses of 300 mg/kg/24 hr intravenously in 3 or 4 divided doses.

Meningitis should be treated with gentamicin and carbenicillin given intravenously as above. Concomitant intraventricular or intrathecal treatment with gentamicin (1–2 mg once daily, independent of body weight, until the cerebrospinal fluid is sterile) may be required.

Abscesses should be incised and drained. Failure to do so inhibits a favorable response to systemic antibiotic treatment.

Prognosis. This depends in large part upon the nature of the underlying disease; e.g., the leading cause of death in childhood leukemia is septicemia, and half of these cases are due to *Pseudomonas*. Likewise, *Pseudomonas* is recovered from the lungs of most children who die of cystic fibrosis and may be responsible for the deaths of many of them. The prognosis for normal development is poor in the few infants who survive *Pseudomonas* meningitis.

Disease Due to Other Pseudomonads

Glanders

Glanders is a severe infectious disease of horses due to *P. mallei* that is occasionally transmitted to man. It is relatively common in Asia, Africa, and the Middle East. The clinical manifestations include acute or chronic pneumonitis and hemorrhagic necrotic lesions of the skin, nasal mucous membranes, and lymph nodes.

Melioidosis

This rare disease of Southeast Asia is seen in the United States mainly in persons from endemic areas, including Vietnam. The causative agent is *P. pseudomallei*, an inhabitant of soil and water in the tropics. Infection follows inhalation of dust or direct contamination of abrasions or wounds. Melioidosis may present as a single primary skin lesion (vesicle, bulla, or urticaria). Pulmonary infection may be subacute and mimic tuberculosis. Occasionally, septicemia occurs and multiple abscesses are noted in various organs of the body. Myocarditis, pericarditis, endocarditis, intestinal abscess, cholecystitis, acute gastroenteritis, urinary tract infections, septic arthritis, paraspinal abscess, osteomyelitis, and generalized lymphadenopathy have all been observed. Melioidosis may also present as an encephalitic illness with fever and seizures; generally, antibiotic therapy results in recovery. The disease may remain latent and appear when host resistance is reduced, sometimes years after initial exposure.

Glanders and melioidosis are treated with tetracycline or chloramphenicol, supplemented with a sulfonamide, over a period of many months. Trimethoprim-sulfamethoxazole (6 mg/kg/24 hr of trimethoprim and 30 mg/kg/24 hr of sulfamethoxazole) in 2 divided doses may be utilized. Aminoglycosides and the penicillins are ineffective.

Feder HM Jr., Grant-Kels JM, and Tilton RG: *Pseudomonas* whirlpool dermatitis. Clin Pediatr 22:638, 1983.

Feigin RD, Shearer WT: Opportunistic infection in children. Parts I, II and III. J Pediatr 87:507, 677, 852, 1975.

Jones RJ, Roe EA, Gupta JL: Controlled trials of a polyvalent *Pseudomonas* vaccine in burns. Lancet 2:977, 1979.

Kercsmar CM, Stern RC, Reed MG, et al: Ceftazidime in cystic fibrosis: Pharmacokinetics and therapeutic response. J Antimicrob Chemother 12(Suppl A):289, 1983.

Liu PV: Biology of *Pseudomonas aeruginosa*. Hosp Pract Jan 1976, p 139.

Reed RK, Larter WE, Sieber OF Jr, et al: Peripheral nodular lesions in *Pseudomonas* sepsis: The importance of incision and drainage. J Pediatr 88:977, 1976.

Salmen T, Dwyer DM, Vorse H, et al: Whirlpool associated *Pseudomonas aeruginosa* urinary tract infections. JAMA 15:2025, 1983.

Schiotz PO, Nielsen H, Hoiby N, et al: Immune complexes in the sputum of patients with cystic fibrosis suffering from chronic *Pseudomonas aeruginosa* lung infection. Acta Path Microbol Sect C 86:37, 1978.

Sorensen RU, Stern RC, Polmar SH: Lymphocyte responsiveness to *Pseudomonas aeruginosa* in cystic fibrosis: Relationship to status of pulmonary disease in sibling pairs. J Pediatr 93:201, 1978.

11.31 BRUCELLOSIS
(Undulant Fever, Mediterranean Fever,
Goat's Milk Fever)

Brucellosis is an acute or chronic infectious disease of animals transmissible to man. Human infection is usually caused by one of the 4 main species of *Brucella* that may be transmitted from the cow, goat, hog, or dog. *Brucella* organisms also have been recovered from wild rats, field mice, wild guinea pigs, jack rabbits, ground squirrels, rams, camels, gazelles, water buffalo, chamois, deer, elk, bison, and fowl.

Etiology. Six *Brucella* species are known to be transmissible to man: *abortus* (cows), *melitensis* (goats), *suis* (hogs), *canis* (dogs), *ovis* (sheep and hares), and *neotomae* (desert wood rats). The organisms are small, gram-negative, nonmotile, non–spore-forming, nonencapsulated, and aerobic.

Epidemiology. Most cases of brucellosis in man result from direct contact with sick animals. Individuals working in food processing plants, dairy farmers, and others who have frequent contact with domestic animals are most commonly infected. Ingestion of unpasteurized milk, cream, butter, cheese, or ice cream from infected animals is usually the source of infection in man. The organism also may directly invade the eye, nasopharynx, and genital tract, but unbroken skin is resistant to invasion. Brucellae may remain viable up to 3 wk in a refrigerated carcass and can survive the curing of ham. The organisms are killed by pasteurization and cooking.

As a result of compulsory pasteurization of milk and control measures in cattle, the reported incidence declined to 0.1/100,000 persons in the 1970's. The disease is infrequent in children. In a seroepidemiologic investigation of *B. canis* antibodies, 67.8% of individuals tested were positive; 5.7% of newborn infants had antibodies by transplacental transfer. The high prevalence of *B. canis* antibodies in humans suggests that some unexplained febrile episodes in children who have intimate contact with dogs may be due to brucellosis. Human transmission of brucellosis has occurred only during the course of bone marrow transplantation. Congenital infections have not been reported.

Pathogenesis and Pathology. Brucellae are primarily intracellular parasites. The organisms are phagocytized by leukocytes and monocytes and are distributed throughout the reticuloendothelial system. Intracellular growth may take place in many cell types, including red blood cells.

Development of delayed or tuberculin-type hypersensitivity to brucella antigen is characteristic. It depends upon multiplication of living organisms; dead organisms, or fractions thereof, rarely produce sensitization.

The host responds to brucellosis by elaborating a variety of antibodies, including agglutinins, opsonins, bactericidins, precipitins, and complement-fixing antibodies. Multiplication of bacteria within the host appears to be essential for induction of immunity. Infection is followed by early development of specific serum IgM antibodies and then shortly by the appearance of IgG antibodies, which ultimately are preponderant.

Serum or plasma from normal individuals and from patients with acute brucellosis may, in the presence of complement, have nonspecific bactericidal activity against brucellae. In chronic infections, however, a specific inhibitor appears and prevents the lethal activity of the serum-complement system. The specific antibody that is produced acts as an opsonin and promotes phagocytosis by polymorphonuclear leukocytes and fixed phagocytes. Thus, brucellae are cleared rapidly from the blood of individuals with demonstrable antibodies. They are not killed, however; once sequestered within cells, they are protected from further bactericidal action of the blood. Smooth strains of *Brucella*, which are more virulent than rough strains, multiply within cells, including those obtained from immune individuals.

Smooth and intermediate strains of *Brucella* contain endotoxin, which does not appear to be important in the virulence of the organism but may be pathogenic after infection has been established.

All species of *Brucella* may produce granulomas in the liver, spleen, lymph nodes, and bone marrow. In addition, centrilobular necrosis and cirrhosis of the liver have been described. Granulomatous inflammation of the gallbladder, interstitial orchitis with scattered areas of fibroid atrophy, endocarditis with vegetations of the valves, granulomatous lesions of the myocardium, and involvement of the brain, kidney, and skin have also been noted.

Clinical Manifestations. The incubation period of brucellosis varies from a few days to several months. The onset may be sudden but most commonly is insidious. Subclinical illness in children in endemic areas is said to be relatively common. Prodromal symptoms include weakness, fatigue, anorexia, headache, myalgia, and constipation. As the disease progresses, evening elevations in temperature become increasingly prominent, with temperatures as high as 41–42.5° C (106–108° F). There may be chills, diaphoresis, epistaxis, abdominal pain, cough, and extensive weight loss.

Physical findings generally are limited to hepatomegaly, splenomegaly, and cervical and axillary lymphadenopathy. Pulmonary lesions may be demonstrable clinically and roentgenographically.

Chronic brucellosis may be difficult to detect. There may be fever, fatigue, myalgia, arthralgia, sweating, and nervousness, as well as anorexia and depressive or psychotic episodes. A maculopapular or, rarely, morbilliform rash may be observed. The bacteria may localize and be responsible for such disorders as uveitis, endocarditis, hepatitis, cholecystitis, epididymitis, prostatitis, osteomyelitis, encephalitis, and myelitis.

The white blood cell count may be normal, elevated, or reduced. Relative lymphocytosis is common, as is anemia.

Diagnosis. The most useful method for diagnosis is the brucella agglutination test; titers will be greater than 1:160 in most acute cases. Generally, the titer correlates with the activity of the infection, but brucella antigen in skin tests or food may produce an anamnestic response. Prozones of inhibition by blocking antibodies may obscure serum agglutination, but this can be avoided by use of the Coombs antiglobulin method. Cross-reactions occur with agglutinins against *F. tularensis*; thus tests against both should be performed. Later in the course of disease, the complement-fixation titer rises and usually is considered to be diagnostic if it is 1:16 or higher. An enzyme-linked immunosorbent assay that detects IgM, IgG, and total IgM plus IgG plus IgA antibodies against *Brucella* is being evaluated.

Skin tests, when negative, exclude infection, but they should not be performed if serologic studies are available, because the skin test antigen may stimulate production of antibody and thereby confuse subsequent serologic results.

Isolation of *Brucella* by culture provides a definitive diagnosis. Blood cultures are most productive in acute disease; cultures of infected tissues or abscesses also may be valuable. Cultures should be incubated under 10% carbon dioxide and should be incubated for at least 4 wk before they are discarded as negative.

Differential Diagnosis. Acute brucellosis can mimic many diseases, including tularemia, typhoid fever, rickettsial diseases, influenza, tuberculosis, histoplasmosis, coccidioidomycosis, and infectious mononucleosis. Chronic brucellosis may resemble malignant histiocytosis, lymphoma, or other neoplastic diseases. Appropriate historic, roentgenographic, and serologic and culture data help to differentiate these disorders. Biopsy of appropriate tissues may be required.

Complications. Complications are the result of localization of brucellae. Osteomyelitis, particularly suppurative spondylitis, is the most frequent complication. Acute suppurative arthritis also may be seen, but destructive joint disease is rare. Acute or subacute meningitis or encephalitis may occur early or late. Adhesive arachnoiditis has been observed.

Myocarditis and endocarditis are serious complications. A Herxheimer reaction may develop at the initiation of therapy.

Prevention. This depends upon avoidance of exposure to brucellae. Infection of domestic animals with which man has close contact can be prevented by immunization. In addition to immunization of animals and pasteurization of milk, periodic agglutination tests of milk and blood should be used to identify infected animals. Positive reactors should be slaughtered. Ingestion of unpasteurized milk and of products derived from unpasteurized milk or cream must be avoided.

Treatment. Brucellosis can be treated with tetracycline in a dose of 30–40 mg/kg/24 hr in 4 divided oral doses for 3–4 wk. If relapse occurs (and it may in as many as 50% of cases), the dose may be increased and streptomycin added in amounts of 15–30 mg/kg/24 hr in 2 equally divided doses administered every 12 hr for 14 days; the initial dose may be halved during the 2nd wk. Trimethoprim-sulfamethoxazole has been used with good results. Rifampin, 20 mg/kg/24 hr for 21 days, also has been shown to be effective, but it is preferable not to use it alone. Rifampin plus trimethoprim-sulfamethoxizole or moxalactam (150 mg/kg/24 hr) appears to be reasonable. Other third generation cephalosporins have been reported to be effective against *Brucella* in vitro, but clinical experience with the use of these drugs for this disease is scant.

Localized abscesses should be drained. Corticosteroids may reduce the risk of a Herxheimer reaction at the onset of therapy.

Patients with brucellosis should be encouraged to rest, and adequate dietary intake should be encouraged.

Prognosis. The mortality of untreated brucellosis is about 3%; recovery may require 6 mo. Prognosis following specific antibiotic therapy is excellent, and a prolonged course usually is due to a delay in diagnosis.

Boycott JA: Diagnosing brucellosis. Lancet 1:255, 1969.
Bradstreet CMP, Tannahil AJ, Pollock TM, et al: Intradermal test and serological tests in suspected brucella infection in man. Lancet 2:653, 1970.
Busch LA, Parker RL: Brucellosis in the United States. J Infect Dis 125:289, 1972.
Hall WH, Khan MY: Brucellosis. *In:* Hoeprich PD (ed): Infectious Disease. Ed 2. Hagerstown, Md., Harper & Row, 1977.
Street L Jr, Grant WW, Alva JD: Brucellosis in childhood. Pediatrics 55:416, 1975.
Young EJ: Human brucellosis. Rev Infect Dis 5:820, 1983.

11.32 YERSINIAL INFECTIONS

Three organisms of the *Yersinia* spp. are responsible for human disease: *Yersinia pestis* (formerly *Pasteurella pestis*), *Yersinia enterocolitica*, and *Yersinia pseudotuberculosis*. Disease caused by *Y. pestis* (plague) has played a prominent role in world history.

Plague

Although reports of plague are infrequent, a reservoir of plague infection exists in the rodent community throughout the western United States, extending into Canada and Mexico. This endemic area of infection is equivalent to any of the older plague foci of Europe and Asia and is a constant reminder that the threat of plague must be continually reviewed.

Etiology. *Yersinia pestis* is a nonmotile, nonsporulating, pleomorphic, gram-negative bacillus. The characteristic "safety pin" or bipolar appearance is demonstrated best in smears of infected secretions or tissue stained by the Giemsa method.

Epidemiology. Plague in domestic and wild animals occurs in two forms: enzootic and epizootic. *Enzootic plague* implies a stable rodent-flea cycle of infection which is found in a relatively resistant host population. Enzootic foci are inconspicuous and serve effectively as reservoirs of infection, as in the United States at the present time. *Epizootic plague* occurs when the disease is introduced into a highly susceptible mammalian population, causing a high mortality rate among infected animals.

Plague is transmitted to man by the bite of fleas which have sucked blood from infected animals, by the skinning and evisceration of infected animals, or by inhalation of infected droplets from a patient with pneumonic plague. Infrequent portals of entry include the pharynx and the conjunctiva. Transmission from animals to man usually causes bubonic plague and is referred to as *zootic plague*. Person-to-person transmission is called *demic plague*.

In the United States reported cases of plague have been increasing since 1966; two thirds have occurred in individuals under 25 yr of age. Infection is more common in males than in females (2:1).

Pathology and Pathogenesis. Plague bacilli ingested by the flea proliferate and eventually block the lumen of the proventriculus. These are regurgitated into dermal lymphatics of the human host by the flea and are then transmitted to regional lymph nodes, which become tender and enlarged (*buboes*). In *severe bubonic plague* the lymph nodes fail to filter out all multiplying bacilli which gain entrance to the efferent lymphatics and disseminate to the vascular system. Once entry into the blood stream has occurred, any organ of the body may be involved. Septicemia, meningitis, disseminated intravascular coagulation, and pneumonia (secondary) may develop.

Primary pulmonic plague may result from human-to-human transmission or from a laboratory accident. Droplets containing large numbers of virulent bacilli may be inhaled, causing severe pneumonia, septicemia, and, frequently, death within 24 hr.

When plague bacilli are introduced into man, they are susceptible to phagocytosis; those which survive are resistant to phagocytosis. The virulence of pneumonic plague may relate, in part, to the inhalation of such organisms.

The response of human tissues to *Y. pestis* generally is pyogenic; necrotic foci may develop within lymph nodes, spleen, and liver. Hemorrhagic lesions may also be found in many organs and tissues, particularly if disseminated intravascular coagulation develops.

Clinical Manifestations. The incubation period of bubonic plague is 2–6 days, and that of pneumonic plague is 1–72 hr.

The onset of *bubonic plague* may be acute or subacute. In the **subacute forms**, the initial findings are a tender lymphadenitis and associated lymphadenopathy. Patients are febrile but not particularly toxic in appearance. If treatment is delayed, septicemia may occur, associated with prostration, shock, and hemorrhagic pneumonitis.

Acute bubonic plague presents with high fever, tachycardia, and myalgia. The disease progresses to delirium, shock, and death within 3–5 days.

The course of *primary pneumonic plague* is even more virulent. Pulmonary signs and symptoms may be lacking until within 24 hr of death. Symptoms of plague include nausea, vomiting, abdominal pain, bloody diarrhea, and petechial and purpuric rashes.

During epidemics a *mild form* of the disease may occur in which lymphadenopathy and vesicular or pustular skin lesions develop, serious symptoms are absent, and recovery can occur without therapy.

Diagnosis. The diagnosis of nonepidemic plague depends upon a high index of suspicion. Sputum, blood, purulent exudates, and aspirates of lymph nodes should be examined by smears stained with Giemsa or Wayson stain and by culture. Serologic tests may be helpful in selected patients; passive hemagglutination antibody titers to Fraction I antigen of *Yersinia pestis* may be detectable by day 5 of illness; titers peak at 14 days.

Differential Diagnosis. Plague (mild form) may be confused with other disorders causing localized lymphadenitis and lymphadenopathy, including infection due to *S. aureus*, *S. pyogenes*, and *F. tularensis*. Septicemic plague may be indistinguishable clinically from any other form of overwhelming bacterial septicemia or from rickettsial diseases.

Prevention. A heat-killed vaccine prepared from *Y. pestis* may produce immunity. Routine vaccination is not recommended, even for individuals living in plague enzootic areas of the United States. Immunization may be useful for those whose occupation regularly brings them into contact with infected rodents or with the organism itself in the laboratory.

In the primary immunization of adults and children over 11 yr of age, an initial dose of 1.0 mL is followed in 4 wk by a second dose of 0.2 mL, and a third dose of 0.2 mL at 6 mo, and then by 3 booster doses at 6 mo intervals. Additional doses may be given at yearly intervals. For children under 11 yr of age, the doses are reduced in volume: children less than 1 yr receive one fifth of the adult dose and individuals 5–10 yr of age three fifths of the adult dose following the same immunization time schedule. If vaccinated individuals are exposed to plague, they should receive chemoprophylaxis, since the vaccine may not be completely protective, even in the presence of high antibody titers.

Primary prevention consists in environmental sanitation directed toward reducing rodent populations and their fleas. In endemic areas, the public must be educated to avoid burrows, to refrain from handling sick or dead rodents, to deflea household pets, and to eliminate trash near living areas. Patients with plague should be isolated until treated. Purulent exudates should be handled with rubber gloves. Face masks and goggles should be worn by medical personnel. *Y. pestis* may be found in feces; accordingly, stools of patients should be routinely disinfected before disposal.

Treatment. Streptomycin is bactericidal and can be used in a dose of 30 mg/kg/24 hr in 2–3 equally divided doses given intramuscularly for 5–10 days. Herxheimer reactions are not uncommon when streptomycin is given; thus this drug is usually reserved for pneumonic or septicemic forms of the disease. Tetracycline may be added after 2–3 days of streptomycin therapy in a dose of 30 mg/kg/24 hr in 4 divided oral doses and continued for 10 days. Chloramphenicol, 50 mg/kg/24 hr in 4 divided doses, can be substituted for tetracycline.

Bubonic plague can be treated with tetracycline (40 mg/kg/24 hr in 4 divided oral doses) for 10 days, or chloramphenicol (50 mg/kg/24 hr in 4 divided oral doses). In areas where streptomycin-resistant *Y. pestis* is found, chloramphenicol should be given to critically ill patients. Plague meningitis should be treated with chloramphenicol 100 mg/kg/24 hr in 4 divided doses intravenously for at least 10 days.

Contacts of patients with pulmonic plague should be quarantined and may be given tetracycline (20 mg/kg/24 hr) in 4 divided oral doses prophylactically for 10 days.

Prognosis. The mortality of untreated bubonic plague is 60–90%. Pneumonic plague is virtually 100% fatal if untreated.

When bubonic plague is treated early, the mortality rate is less than 10%. Prognosis in primary pneumonic plague is poor if specific treatment is not provided within 18 hr of onset of symptoms.

Yersinia enterocolitica and *Yersinia pseudotuberculosis*

Disease from these organisms is being recognized with increasing frequency.

Yersinia may be confused with coliform organisms. *Yersinia enterocolitica* and *Y. pseudotuberculosis* are oxidase-negative gram-negative rods which are motile at 22° C but not at 37° C. It is this last characteristic that aids in differentiating them from *Y. pestis* and Enterobacteriaceae. *Yersinia enterocolitica* and *Y. pseudotuberculosis* can be distinguished from each other by biochemical tests, by agglutination with specific antisera, and by the susceptibility of *Y. pseudotuberculosis* to specific bacteriophages. Serotypes 3, 8, and 9 of *Y. enterocolitica* and 1 of *Y. pseudotuberculosis* are the most frequent causes of disease in humans.

Yersinia enterocolitica has been recovered from many wild and domestic animals, raw milk, oysters, and water supplies. Infection from dogs and human-to-human spread have been documented. Infants and children are most commonly infected.

Y. enterocolitica has been associated with diarrhea, acute mesenteric adenitis, pharyngitis, abscesses, arthritis, osteomyelitis, hepatitis, carditis, meningitis, ophthalmitis, hemolytic anemia, Reiter syndrome, septicemia, glomerulonephritis, and rashes, including erythema nodosum. Septicemia has been reported after accidental overdose of oral iron in previously healthy children. Enhanced growth of *Y. enterocolitica* in the intestine after exposure of the organism to excess iron combined with damage to the intestinal mucosa by iron may have played a pathogenic role in this situation. Septicemia is associated with a case-fatality rate of nearly 50%, despite antibiotic treatment. With gastrointestinal disease, abdominal pain may be severe and simulate appendicitis. Ulceration of the small bowel has been described. Diarrhea is common and persistent, lasting 1–2 wk. The stool may be watery, mucoid, or bilious but generally is guaiac-negative. The stool of patients with diarrhea due to *Y. enterocolitica* may contain polymorphonuclear leukocytes. When it is severe there may be hypoalbuminemia and hypokalemia, suggesting extensive disruption of the small bowel mucosa. The duration of illness generally is 2–3 wk without treatment, but occasionally diarrhea may persist for several months.

Diagnosis may be established by identification of the organism in the stool. Passive hemagglutination tests may also confirm the diagnosis. Antibodies are detectable 8–10 days after the onset of illness and may persist for several months. Infants are less likely to have a serologic response than are older children.

Most strains of *Y. enterocolitica* are sensitive to streptomycin, tetracycline, chloramphenicol, and sulfonamides.

Yersinia pseudotuberculosis has been associated with mesenteric adenitis and terminal ileitis. Abdominal pain may be severe and suggest acute appendicitis. Septicemia is unusual but may occur. Postdiarrheal hemolytic-uremic syndrome has been reported, as have cases simulating Kawasaki disease. *Y. pseudotuberculosis* is generally sensitive to ampicillin, kanamycin, tetracycline, and chloramphenicol.

Kohl S: *Yersinia enterocolitica* infections in children. Pediatr Clin North Am 26:433, 1979.
Mann JM, Schaudler L, Cushing A: Pediatric plague. Pediatrics 69:762, 1982.

Marks MI, Pai CH, Lafleur L: *Yersinia enterocolitica* gastroenteritis: A prospective study of clinical, bacteriologic and epidemiologic features. J Pediatr 96:26, 1980.

Melby K, Slørdahl S, Gutteberg TJ, et al: Septicaemia due to *Yersinia enterocolitica* after oral overdoses of iron. Br Med J 285:467, 1982.

Poland JD: Plague. *In:* Hoeprich PD (ed): Infectious Diseases. 2nd ed. Hagerstown Md., Harper & Row, 1977.

11.33 TULAREMIA

Tularemia, an infectious disease caused by *Francisella tularensis (Pasteurella tularensis)*, varies in its clinical patterns in relation to the virulence of the bacterium and the route of infection. Infrequently the disease may run a subclinical course. Most often, however, it assumes one of five clinical forms: ulceroglandular (80%), glandular (refers to lymph nodes) (10%), oculoglandular (1%), oropharyngeal (relatively common in children), and typhoidal (6%).

Etiology. The organism is a short, non–spore-forming, nonmotile, unencapsulated, gram-negative bacillus which may be markedly pleomorphic in culture. Special containment facilities are recommended in handling cultures to avoid acquisition of disease.

Strains of *F. tularensis* are antigenically homogeneous, but virulence is variable. One strain (Jellison type A), found only in North America, is highly virulent for humans. A second strain (Jellison type B), found in North America, Europe, and Asia, is avirulent for rabbits and causes only mild disease in man.

Epidemiology. Tularemia is not an uncommon disease in the United States. No age group is immune. Most reported cases are from the West–South Central States, but a large outbreak occurred in Vermont in 1968.

F. tularensis has been recovered from over 100 types of mammals and arthropods. Type A bacteria generally are acquired from cottontail rabbits or ticks. Type B strains are more commonly acquired from rats, mice, squirrels, muskrats, beavers, moles, birds, and ticks. Tularemia may also be acquired from horseflies, deerflies, fleas, and lice.

Tularemia has been considered to be a disease of hunters, trappers, cooks, muskrat farmers, and others with occupational exposure to the organism. It may occur in children who have ingested food (rabbit or squirrel meat) or water contaminated with *F. tularensis* or who have been bitten by infected ticks, flies, or other vectors. In one outbreak in Baltimore, Maryland, tularemia pneumonia resulted from an aerosol established by children who beat a rabbit carcass with a stick.

Pathology and Pathogenesis. The host may be infected by inoculation through broken or intact skin or mucous membranes, ingestion (including penetration of the pharyngeal mucosa by ingested organisms), inhalation, or the bite of infected arthropod vectors. Within 48–72 hr after the organisms enter the skin, an erythematous maculopapular lesion may be noted, followed shortly by ulceration and regional lymphadenopathy. The organisms multiply and produce granulomas within lymph nodes. Subsequently, bacteremia may occur. Although any organ of the body may be involved, infection of the reticuloendothelial system is most prominent and common.

Pneumonia may follow inhalation of *F. tularensis*. An inflammatory reaction develops about the site of bacterial deposition, and necrosis of alveolar walls follows. The organisms that reach the lung are ingested by alveolar macrophages and enter first the hilar lymphatics and then the blood. A typhoidal form of tularemia results when the mastication of contaminated food releases *F. tularensis*, which is then inhaled.

F. tularensis is an intracellular parasite capable of surviving for extended periods of time within monocytes and other body cells. Although the immune response is usually persistent, chronic or relapsing disease may occur. Cell-mediated immunity may be of greater import than are circulating antibodies in determining complete recovery.

Clinical Manifestations. The incubation period varies from a few hours to a week. The onset is acute and characterized by myalgia, arthralgia, chills, fever of 40–41° C (104–106° F), nausea, vomiting, and diaphoresis. Headache is prominent and may be associated with photophobia. A generalized maculopapular rash is not unusual. Hematologic data are not discriminating; even the sedimentation rate can be normal. There may be transient proteinuria.

In the *ulceroglandular* form the primary maculopapular lesion is noted within 72 hr and ulcerates within 4–5 days. The ulceration is painful and requires about a month to heal. Regional lymphadenopathy occurs, usually without discernible intervening lymphangitis. The lymph nodes are tender and become fluctuant in about 25% of untreated cases. Generalized lymphadenopathy, splenomegaly, or both may develop.

Oropharyngeal tularemia is characterized by purulent tonsillitis and pharyngitis and occasionally by ulcerative stomatitis.

Glandular tularemia is similar to the ulceroglandular form, but no local lesion is apparent.

Oculoglandular disease is similar to the ulceroglandular form except that the primary lesion is a severe conjunctivitis accompanied by regional lymphadenitis.

The *typhoidal* form resembles typhoid fever. Fever is protracted, and cutaneous or mucous membrane lesions may not be apparent. A dry cough, severe retrosternal chest pain, and hemoptysis are common. Clinical evidence of bronchitis, pneumonitis, and/or pleuritis may be found in 20% of cases, and roentgenographic evidence of pulmonary involvement and nodular enlargement in the mediastinum is seen in the majority of instances. Splenomegaly is common, as is hepatic enlargement.

Meningitis, encephalitis, pericarditis, endocarditis, neuralgias, thrombophlebitis, and osteomyelitis have all been observed.

Diagnosis. The history and clinical manifestations may suggest the disease, particularly a history of ingestion of rabbit or squirrel meat, contact with rabbits, or bites by ticks, flies, or other vectors.

A preparation of phenolized organisms may be used for *skin testing*. Positive reactions may be observed by the 4th–7th day of infection. Skin test material may be obtained from the Rocky Mountain Laboratory of the National Institute of Allergy and Infectious Disease.

Culture of organisms is possible but requires appropriate media and is hazardous to inexperienced laboratory personnel. The organism may be isolated from blood, gastric washings, and drainage from wounds by culture or by inoculating guinea pigs intraperitoneally with these body fluids. Infected animals are even more hazardous to laboratory personnel than are cultures.

The *serum agglutination test* is reliable, although it usually is not positive until after the 1st wk of illness, and fatal cases have been reported in the absence of agglutinins. Agglutinins are first detectable between the 10th and 14th days. A titer of 1:80 or greater may be considered positive, but serially rising titers are of greater significance. Titers as high as 1:640 may be expected within another week and may be in excess of 1:1280 within the 2nd month. Low titers due to cross-reactions with brucella, heterophile, OX-19, and cholera vaccine have been reported.

A whole-blood lymphocyte stimulation test is now available. Initial evidence suggests that about 20% of infected persons will have a reaction within the 1st week and up to 97% within the 2nd week.

Differential Diagnosis. *Ulceroglandular tularemia* may resemble cat-scratch disease, infectious mononucleosis, sporotrichosis, plague, anthrax, melioidosis, glanders, rat-bite fever, or lymphadenitis due to *Streptococcus pyogenes* or *Staphylococcus aureus*. *Oropharyngeal tularemia* must be differentiated from the same diseases but also from acquired cytomegaloviral disease, acquired toxoplasmosis, and infection due to adenoviruses and herpes simplex.

Tularemic pneumonitis must be differentiated from other bacterial and nonbacterial pneumonias, particularly those due to mycoplasma, chlamydia, mycobacteria, fungi, and rickettsia. These distinctions can be made on the basis of isolation of the organisms.

Typhoidal tularemia must be differentiated from typhoid fever, brucellosis, and other severe septicemic illnesses.

Prevention. Avoidance of exposure to mammals and arthropod vectors that may be infected is most important. Rabbits that appear to be ill should be destroyed without direct handling. Rubber gloves should be worn to handle the flesh of wild animals. In areas infested with ticks, tight wristbands and boots are recommended. A careful search for ticks should be made as frequently as practical when one is within a wooded area and promptly upon departure. Ticks should be removed by an instrument or the gloved hand and should not be squeezed. The area of attachment should be cleansed with 70% ethanol.

An intradermal vaccine containing a live attenuated strain of *F. tularensis* is available. It is safe, and immunity persists for 3–5 yr. It has not been evaluated for use in children.

Treatment. Streptomycin, 30–40 mg/kg/24 hr in 2 divided doses intramuscularly for at least 7 days, is the treatment of choice. Tetracycline and chloramphenicol are also effective, but relapses are common with each of them. Retreatment with tetracycline has been effective.

Prognosis. Untreated ulceroglandular tularemia has a fatality rate of about 5%. Untreated patients who survive experience symptoms for 2–4 wk and a subsequent period of disability of 8–12 wk. Mortality in untreated patients may reach 30% if pneumonia develops. Recovery usually provides lifelong immunity. Second attacks may occur but are mild. Prognosis following infection with Jellison type B strains may be considerably better than that reported above. If treatment is provided promptly, recovery generally is rapid and fatality exceedingly rare.

Bloom ME, Shearer WT, Barton LL: Oculoglandular tularemia in an inner city child. Pediatrics 57:564, 1973.
Halsted CC, Kulasinghe HP: Tularemia pneumonia in urban children. Pediatrics 61:660, 1978.
Hughes WT: Tularemia in children. J Pediatr 62:495, 1963.
Miller RP, Bates JH: Pleuropulmonary tularemia. A review of 29 patients. Am Rev Resp Dis 99:31, 1969.
Syrjala H, Herva E, Ilonen J, et al: A whole blood lymphocyte stimulation test in human tularemia. J Infect Dis. In press.
Tyson HK: Tularemia: An unappreciated cause of exudative pharyngitis. Pediatrics 58:864, 1976.
Young LS, Bicknell DS, Archer BG, et al: Tularemia epidemic: Vermont, 1968. Forty-seven cases linked to contact with muskrats. N Engl J Med 280:1253, 1969.

11.34 LISTERIOSIS

During the last 50 yr, listeriosis has emerged as a septicemic or meningitic illness which most frequently affects the newborn infant and the compromised pediatric host. Human infections with *Listeria monocytogenes*, unlike those in animals, generally are characterized by a polymorphonuclear response in blood, cerebrospinal fluid, and other body tissues.

Etiology. *L. monocytogenes* is a small, gram-positive, non–spore-forming rod displaying tumbling motility at room temperature but not at 37° C. Generally, it produces beta-hemolysis on blood agar, but alpha-hemolysis has been observed.

Listeria can be divided into four serologic types on the basis of somatic (O) and flagellar (H) antigens. Groups I, III, and IV can be differentiated on the basis of the O antigens and group II on the basis of a distinctive H antigen. Major groups can be subdivided further. Most human disease is due to organisms belonging to groups I and IV.

On routine culture media *Listeria* frequently is mistaken for a diphtheroid and discarded as a nonpathogen. On Gram stains of clinical specimens, coccoid forms may be mistaken for streptococci. In poorly stained smears the cells may appear gram-negative and resemble *Haemophilus influenzae*.

Epidemiology. *Listeria* has been reported as a cause of disease in 42 domestic and feral mammalian and 22 avian species. It has been isolated from soil, where survival for more than 295 days has been recorded, and from streams, sewage, silage, dust, and slaughterhouse waste. It also has been recovered from the intestinal tract, vagina, cervix, nose, ears, and, rarely, blood or urine of apparently healthy humans. The role of healthy carriers in the perpetuation and transmission of *Listeria* remains ill defined.

In the newborn infant the organism may be acquired transplacentally or by aspiration or ingestion at the time of delivery. Older children may acquire it by inhalation or ingestion or, less commonly, by direct contact or venereal transmission. Transmission to humans by ingestion of unpasteurized milk has been strongly suggested. In some cases carriers may develop overt disease when their immune responses are altered by underlying disease (e.g., leukemia, lymphomas, Hodgkin disease) or by administration of immunosuppressive agents. Listeriosis has been reported in recipients of renal transplants, and outbreaks in hospital transplantation units have been presumed to occur by the respiratory route. Sporadic infection in immunosuppressed transplant recipients also may result from invasion of the blood stream by *Listeria* from sites of colonization in the gastrointestinal tract.

Pathology. *L. monocytogenes* produces disease in many organs, including liver, lung, adrenals, kidneys, and brain. The abscesses do not differ from those found in other pyogenic infections, but there may be granulomatous reactions and microabscess formation. Necrotizing changes may be noted in the kidneys and the lung, particularly in the bronchioles and alveolar walls.

Listeria produces a pyogenic meningitis and also may cause suppurative ependymitis, encephalitis, choroiditis, and gliosis.

Pathogenesis. *Listeria* is a facultative intracellular parasite. Cellular mechanisms are involved in the immune response to infection by these organisms. Any inherited or acquired disorder in which T cell function is impaired may predispose the host to infection by *Listeria*.

Listeriosis may develop at birth or be noted subsequently in the newborn infant or older child. Early-onset disease may be acquired transplacentally from a mother with subclinical or clinical infection. Infection acquired early in pregnancy may lead to abortion and, more commonly, if acquired later, to stillbirth or premature delivery.

Early-onset septicemic neonatal disease has been associated with maternal fever or other signs of maternal infection and frequently with recovery of serotypes Ia and Ib from mother and/or infant. The development of *late-onset* neonatal disease is not usually associated with maternal illness or carriage of the organism; epidemic neonatal disease has been described, presumably reflecting patient-to-patient transmission. Late-onset disease is primarily associated with recovery of serotype IVb and is predominantly a meningitis.

At any age all organs of the body may be involved after bloodstream invasion.

Clinical Manifestations. *Listeria* may cause septicemia and/or meningitis in infants and children. In the newborn infant, a spectrum of disease is apparent, and the clinical presentation depends upon the time and route of infection.

Early Onset. The liveborn infant with an infection acquired late in pregnancy may present acutely ill and expire within a few hours of birth. More often disease becomes apparent within the 1st wk of life. Whitish granulomas may be found on the mucous membranes and disseminated papules on the skin. Anorexia, lethargy, vomiting, jaundice, respiratory distress, pulmonary infiltrates, cyanosis, petechial rashes, evidence of myocarditis, and hepatomegaly have been noted. These infants frequently are premature, and the mortality rate is high. Septicemia and shock are common, and there may be associated meningitis (Sec 8.59).

Late Onset. The infant may appear well at birth and in the 1st wk but septicemia or meningitis may develop later during the neonatal period. Signs and symptoms are similar to those noted in any form of pyogenic meningitis (Sec. 8.59 and 11.13). Meningitis often occurs alone and the course may be indolent. However, there may be associated septicemia with a more fulminant presentation.

In older children meningitis or meningoencephalitis may be noted. Generally, no characteristics distinguish meningitis due to *Listeria* from that due to other causes. In some cases, however, the onset is subacute and characterized by headache, low grade fever, and malaise of several days' duration prior to the time that symptoms and signs referable to the central nervous system are first noted.

Meningitis may occur in association with conjunctivitis, otitis media, sinusitis, pneumonia, endocarditis, and pericarditis. An oculoglandular syndrome due to *Listeria*, characterized by keratoconjunctivitis, corneal ulceration, and regional lymphadenitis, also has been described. Listeriosis also may present as pneumonia, an influenza-like septicemic illness of pregnant women, endocarditis, localized abscesses, papular or pustular cutaneous lesions, conjunctivitis, and urethritis.

An infectious mononucleosis–like syndrome was the first disorder of humans with which *L. monocytogenes* was associated. The Paul-Bunnell heterophile antibody test is negative. The organism may be a secondary invader in the sense that the disease may be due to EB virus, but *L. monocytogenes* in some manner interferes with heterophil antibody production.

Diagnosis. The possibility of animal contact should be ascertained. *Listeria* infection should be suspected in the newborn who has signs and symptoms of septicemia, pneumonia, or meningitis and in children who have malignancies and are receiving immunosuppressive therapy. Appropriate materials for culture vary with the clinical diagnosis. If neonatal listeriosis is sought, cultures of the blood, cerebrospinal fluid, meconium, urine, and exudate expressed from an incised skin papule should be cultured. Cultures should also be obtained from the vagina and cervix of the mother and, if possible, from the placenta and lochia. Cerebrospinal fluid findings in cases of *Listeria* meningitis show a preponderance of polymorphonuclear leukocytes, elevated protein concentration, and depressed glucose.

The microbiology laboratory should be alerted when the possibility of listeriosis is considered so that confusion with diphtheroids can be minimized. Most strains of *Listeria* can be primarily isolated on conventional media within 1–2 days. Although a rise in agglutinins may occur 2–4 wk after the onset of infection, most investigators feel that serodiagnosis is unreliable because agglutinins to *Listeria* may be found in up to 90% of animals and man.

Differential Diagnosis. Listeriosis must be differentiated from bacterial septicemia and meningitis of other causes. In the rare cases in which atypical lymphocytes are noted, toxoplasmosis and infection due to EB virus, cytomegalovirus, and hepatitis viruses must be excluded.

Treatment. The sensitivity of strains of *L. monocytogenes* varies considerably. Most strains are sensitive by tube dilution in vitro to concentrations of erythromycin, tetracycline, pen-

icillin G, and ampicillin that can be achieved in vivo; many also are sensitive to chloramphenicol.

Usually, therapy should be initiated with ampicillin in a dose and route appropriate for the type of infection and the age of the patient. The sensitivity of each isolate should be tested and changes in therapy made if necessary. Tetracycline should not be used in pregnant women or in children under 8 yr of age because this drug may stain the teeth. Some strains of *L. monocytogenes* are resistant to ampicillin; in such instances a combination of ampicillin and gentamicin has proved effective.

Prognosis. If listeriosis is acquired transplacentally, the fetus is almost always aborted. The death rate of infants infected at or near term is greater than 50%. The mortality of listerial pneumonia noted within 12 hr of birth approaches 100%. Mortality varies from 20 to 50% if disease develops between 5 and 30 days of birth. Early treatment of septicemia and/or meningitis in immunologically competent older infants and children may be responsible for recovery in about 95% of instances. Mental retardation, paralysis, and hydrocephalus have been noted in survivors of *Listeria* meningitis.

Albritton WL: Neonatal listeriosis: Distribution of serotypes in relation to age at onset of disease. J Pediatr 88:481, 1976.

Dykes A, Baraff LJ, Herzog P: Listeria brain abscess in an immunosuppressed child. J Pediatr 94:72, 1979.

Gordon RC, Barrett FF, Yow MD: Ampicillin treatment of listeriosis. J Pediatr 77:1067, 1970.

Halliday HL, Hirata T: Perinatal listeriosis—a review of twelve patients. Am J Obstet Gynecol 133:405, 1979.

Larsson S: Epidemiology of listeriosis in Sweden 1958–1974. Scand J Infect Dis 11:47, 1979.

Stamm AM, Dismukes WE, Simmons BP, et al: Listeriosis in renal transplant recipients: Report of an outbreak and review of 102 cases. Rev Infect Dis 4:665, 1982.

11.35 ANTHRAX

Anthrax, a well-known infection of animals, is transmissible to humans. The name is derived from the Greek word for *coal* and refers to the characteristic black eschar in cutaneous forms of the disease.

Etiology. *Bacillus anthracis* is a nonmotile, encapsulated, spore-forming, gram-positive bacillus whose spores are formed under aerobic conditions. They are relatively resistant, surviving for years in soil and various animal products.

Epidemiology. The incidence of anthrax has decreased progressively in the United States since 1910; 80% of cases are the result of contact with goat hair, wool, or other animal products imported from Asia, Africa, and the Middle East. Worldwide, 10,000–100,000 cases occur each year. Skin infections have followed contact with commercially available products, including imported wool and shaving brushes.

Pathogenesis and Pathology. *Cutaneous anthrax* results from subepidermal inoculation of spores that multiply and produce toxin, resulting in necrosis of tissue and formation of a black eschar.

Pulmonary anthrax results from inhalation of spores into the alveolar spaces. After phagocytosis the spores are transported to regional lymph nodes where replication and production of toxin may ensue. Septicemia and, occasionally, meningitis and death may follow. Mediastinal nodes may become enlarged and hemorrhagic and compress the bronchi. Depression of the central nervous system due to toxin may occur. Primary pneumonitis is rare. Respiratory failure and death may follow thrombosis of pulmonary capillaries.

When spores are ingested, *gastrointestinal anthrax* may develop. The spores multiply and elaborate toxin, producing a necrotic lesion of the terminal ileum or cecum. Hemorrhage may follow.

Clinical Manifestations. The incubation period of *cutaneous anthrax* is usually 2–5 days. A small macule develops and rapidly becomes vesicular. As the initial lesion enlarges, the center becomes hemorrhagic and necrotic. A black eschar forms and enlarges. The eschar may be surrounded by vesicles and by firm nonpitting edema. Systemic symptoms include low-grade fever, malaise, and, occasionally, regional lymphadenopathy. Sometimes, atypical skin lesions may be the only cutaneous manifestation of disease; these may be small pinpoint black macules that never become vesicular. More than 90% of all cases of anthrax are cutaneous in form. Lesions on the arms are more common than those on the fingers; anthrax on the legs rarely occurs.

The incubation period of *pulmonary anthrax* is 1–5 days. Malaise, myalgia, and low-grade fever are noted initially. A nonproductive cough, rhonchi, and, after 2–4 days, severe respiratory stress may develop. Pulse, respiratory rate, and temperature increase; dyspnea and cyanosis may be severe. Moist rales, pleural effusion, and subcutaneous edema of the chest and neck may be noted. Death within 24 hr usually follows development of severe respiratory distress.

Gastrointestinal anthrax results from ingestion of contaminated meat. After an incubation period of 2–5 days, anorexia, nausea, vomiting, and fever occur, and there may be hematemesis and bloody diarrhea. Shock and death may occur.

Meningitis may follow untreated cutaneous anthrax. The skin has been implicated as the primary site of infection in more than 50% of cases, even though the skin lesion is no longer apparent. Cerebrospinal fluid of most patients is hemorrhagic but may be purulent. Cultures of cerebrospinal fluid generally are positive for *B. anthracis*. Encephalomyelitis and cortical hemorrhages may occur.

Diagnosis. This should be considered when there are typical skin lesions. Recovery of *B. anthracis* from the lesion confirms the diagnosis. Pulmonary anthrax may be identified by recovery of the organism from pleural fluid or, rarely, from sputum. A history of ingestion of contaminated meat should suggest gastrointestinal anthrax.

Differential Diagnosis. Cutaneous anthrax must be differentiated from skin lesions due to *S. aureus, F. tularensis, Y. pestis, P. aeruginosa, A. hydrophila*, and vaccinia.

Prevention. A cell-free vaccine is available for those at high risk of occupational exposure.

Treatment. The drug of choice is penicillin. Mild disease can be treated with penicillin V in a dose of 50,000 units/kg/24 hr in 4 divided oral doses, for 7–10 days. Moderate or severe cutaneous disease can be treated with procaine penicillin, 30,000–40,000 units/kg/24 hr, administered intramuscularly in 3 divided doses, for 7 days. Tetracycline, 15 mg/kg/24 hr in 4 divided doses orally for 7 days, can be used for persons sensitive to penicillin. The cutaneous lesion should be cleansed and covered; excision is not recommended and may lead to intensification of symptoms.

Pulmonary and meningeal anthrax are treated with aqueous penicillin G intravenously in a dose of 400,000 units/kg/24 hr in 6 divided doses for at least 10 days. Specific antitoxin has been used; a decrease in mortality from 28% to 6% in patients without meningeal or pulmonary anthrax has been attributed to it.

Prognosis. Despite antibiotic treatment the mortality rate in anthrax meningitis approaches 100%; that of pulmonary anthrax exceeds 90%. The mortality rate is 10–20% in untreated cutaneous anthrax but is less than 1% with penicillin treatment. The mortality rate of gastrointestinal anthrax is 25–50%.

Edwards MS: Anthrax. *In*: Feigin RD, Cherry JD: Textbook of Pediatric Infectious Diseases. Philadelphia, WB Saunders, 1981, pp 819–822.

Manios S, Kavaliotis I: Anthrax in children: A long forgotten potentially fatal infection. Scand J Infect Dis 11:203, 1979.

Plotkin SA, Brachman PS, Utell M, et al: An epidemic of inhalation anthrax, the first in the twentieth century. Am J Med 29:992, 1960.

11.36 TETANUS

Tetanus, an acute toxemic illness, is caused by a soluble exotoxin of *Clostridium tetani*. The toxin is ordinarily produced by the vegetative forms of the organism at a site of injury and is subsequently transported to and fixed within the central nervous system.

Etiology. *C. tetani*, an obligate anaerobe, is a gram-positive, nonencapsulated, slender, motile rod-shaped bacterium that forms terminal spores resembling drumsticks. The spores are resistant to many injurious agents, including boiling, but can be destroyed by autoclaving. They survive in soil for years if not exposed to sunlight, and may be found in house dust, salt and fresh water, and feces of many animal species. Spores and vegetative organisms may be found in the intestinal contents of humans. The vegetative forms of *C. tetani* are susceptible to heat and many disinfectants.

Tetanus bacilli are not invasive. Two toxins are produced, tetanospasmin and tetanolysin. The tetanospasmins produced by several antigenically different bacilli are immunologically identical. They are neurotoxins and are responsible for the clinical manifestations. Except for botulinum toxin, this diffusible protein is the most potent poison known; as little as 130 μg may be lethal for an adult.

Epidemiology. Tetanus occurs throughout the world; in developing countries it is an important cause of neonatal death. Morbidity and mortality rates in the United States have been decreasing since 1950, but case fatality rates have remained unchanged at 50–65% for the past 3 decades. Most reported cases occur between May and October; the highest incidence is in the southern states. Factors contributing to this distribution may include climate, prevalence of spores of *C. tetani* in the soil, and immunization practices. Attack rates for the United States are approximately 1 case/million/yr.

In the United States the incidence of tetanus has been higher in newborn infants than in older children; in 1975, however, the number of reported cases was greatest in children 1–5 yr of age. Males are affected more frequently than females in a ratio of 3:2. Mortality rates for females also have been lower than those for males of the corresponding age group. Newborn males and females are affected with equal frequency, and there is no seasonal variation in the distribution of cases. Most newborn infants with tetanus have been delivered outside a hospital to unimmunized mothers under unsterile conditions.

Pathogenesis. *C. tetani* is usually introduced into an area of injury as spores. Disease develops only after spores are converted to vegetative organisms, which produce tetanospasmin only under conditions of reduced ambient oxygen. Contamination of the umbilical cord is the common source of infection in the newborn infant. In older children it is usually by means of a traumatic injury. The risk is greatest from a deep puncture wound or an injury associated with tissue necrosis, conditions that favor toxin elaboration. Tetanus, however, has followed minor injuries, and occasionally no portal of entry is found. Under these circumstances it is presumed that spores previously introduced persisted in normal tissue for months or years and germinated when conditions were favorable. Alternatively, the site of infection may have been the gastrointestinal tract or the tonsillar crypts. Tetanus has followed use of contaminated sera, vaccines, or suture material.

Tetanospasmin may reach the central nervous system (1) by absorption at myoneural junctions followed by migration through perineural spaces of nerve trunks or (2) by transfer of lymphocytes to blood and then to the central nervous system.

Tetanospasmin acts on the spinal cord, the brain, the sympathetic nervous system, and the motor end plates in skeletal muscles. The toxin interferes with neuromuscular transmission by inhibiting release of acetylcholine from nerve terminals in muscle. Its effects on the spinal cord lead to dysfunction of polysynaptic reflexes. Within the central nervous system tetanospasmin is bound to gangliosides and suppresses inhibitory influences on the motor neurons and interneurons without directly enhancing excitatory synaptic action. The antidromic inhibition of evoked cortical activity is reduced, as it is in strychnine poisoning; this accounts for the associated hypertonicity, spasms, and seizures. The toxin also produces a fluctuating overactivity of the sympathetic nervous system, leading to tachycardia, labile hypertension, cardiac arrhythmias, peripheral vasoconstriction, profuse sweating, hypercarbia, and increased urinary excretion of catecholamines.

Toxin bound to tissue is neither dissociated nor neutralized by tetanus antitoxin. Antitoxin may prevent binding in the central nervous system if binding has occurred *only* in the periphery. It has no effect upon the germination of spores of *C. tetani* or multiplication of its vegetative organisms in tissues.

Pathology. *C. tetani* remain localized at the site of injury and elicit minimal tissue reaction. Local changes that may occur are secondary events. Pneumonia due to other microorganisms may be related to difficulty in clearing secretions. Degeneration of striated muscles occurs. The principal changes include loss of stripes, lysis and disappearance of myofibrils, and bleeding and rupture of muscle bundles. The changes in the intercostal muscles and diaphragm may contribute to ventilatory failure and also explain the myasthenia observed during convalescence. Vertebral fractures occur as a result of tetanic contractions.

Clinical Manifestations. The incubation period is usually 3–14 days after injury but may be as short as 1 day or as long as several months. There are three clinical forms: localized, generalized, and cephalic.

Localized tetanus produces pain and continuous rigidity and spasm of muscles in proximity to the injury; these symptoms may persist for weeks and disappear without sequelae. Occasionally, this pattern precedes development of the generalized disorder. Localized as well as a mild form of generalized tetanus occurs occasionally with chronic otitis media; *C. tetani* may be recovered from the middle ear fluid. The fatality rate of localized tetanus is about 1%.

Generalized tetanus is the most common form of the disease. The onset may be insidious, but trismus is the presenting symptom in over 50% of cases. Spasm of the masseter muscle may be associated with stiffness of the neck muscles and difficulty in swallowing. Restlessness, irritability, and headache are early manifestations. Spasm of the facial muscles produces a fixed sardonic grin (**risus sardonicus**). Shortly, tonic contractions of the somatic musculature become widespread. The lumbar and abdominal muscles may become rigid, and persistent spasm of the back muscles may result in opisthotonos. Tetanic seizures develop, characterized by sudden bursts of tonic contractions of various muscle groups, producing flexion and adduction of the arms, clenching of the fists, and extension of the lower extremities. Initially the spasms last for seconds to several minutes and are separated by periods of relaxation; with time, they become powerful and exhausting. Spasms may be precipitated by visual, auditory, or tactile stimulus. The patient is completely conscious during the clinical course and experiences intense pain. Apprehension is prominent. Spasm of the laryngeal and respiratory muscles may produce respiratory obstruction, and

cyanosis and asphyxia may ensue. Dysuria or urinary retention may be secondary to spasm of the bladder sphincter. Alternatively, there may be involuntary defecation and urination. Forcefulness of the contractions may produce compression fractures of the spine and hemorrhage into muscle. Peripheral neuropathy may result in weakness and sensory loss; such involvement is usually asymmetric; the nerves most commonly involved are the ulnar, median, and lateral popliteal. Electrophysiologic studies may initially reveal no conduction. Recovery occurs over weeks to months.

Fever is generally mild, but it may be as high as 40° C because of the energy generated by the tetanic seizures. Hyperhidrosis, tachycardia, hypertension, and cardiac arrhythmias may be manifest.

Signs and symptoms increase over 3–7 days, plateau during the 2nd wk, and abate gradually. Recovery is complete in 2–6 wk.

Cephalic tetanus is unusual. The incubation period is 1–2 days following otitis media or injuries to the head and face, including foreign bodies placed in the nose by the patient. Dysfunction of cranial nerves III, IV, VII, IX, X, and XI is the most prominent feature of the disease. Cranial nerve VII is affected most frequently. The cephalic pattern may be followed by generalized tetanus.

Tetanus neonatorum usually begins within 3–10 days after birth and is generalized in type. Progressive difficulty in sucking is associated with excessive crying. Difficulty in swallowing is soon apparent; the body becomes stiff, and spasms develop. Opisthotonos may be extreme or absent.

Diagnosis and Differential Diagnosis. The diagnosis of tetanus is made on clinical grounds. Most cases occur in individuals who are not immunized or in infants of unimmunized mothers. A history of trauma within the preceding 14 days is usual. This history, in conjunction with trismus, generalized muscular stiffness or rigidity, spasms, and a clear sensorium, is strongly suggestive of tetanus.

Routine laboratory studies are of little value. The white blood cell count is not remarkable. The cerebrospinal fluid is not abnormal, except that the pressure may be elevated by the muscular contractions. The electroencephalogram is normal, and electromyography is not distinctive. Wound cultures are positive for *C. tetani* in about one third of instances. Gram stains of material from the wound may or may not show *C. tetani*. Identification of the organism by Gram stain and anaerobic cultures is presumptive evidence of tetanus, but the absence of characteristic clinical manifestations does not mean that the patient has, or will develop, tetanus.

Tetanus must be differentiated from other local and systemic diseases. Trismus may be associated with alveolar, parapharyngeal, and retropharyngeal abscesses. These conditions can be differentiated by careful history, physical examination, and appropriate roentgenographic studies.

Poliomyelitis may be accompanied by stiffness and spasm early in the course of the illness; however, trismus is absent, flaccid paralysis develops, and the cerebrospinal fluid is usually abnormal (Sec. 11.77). Other forms of acute or postinfectious encephalitides rarely are associated with trismus, generally have abnormal cerebrospinal fluid findings, and display a clouded sensorium. Bacterial meningitis is also unaccompanied by trismus; examination of cerebrospinal fluid can establish or strongly suggest this diagnosis.

Both *rabies* and tetanus may follow animal bites, and trismus has been noted with the former. Rabid spasms tend to be intermittent and clonic rather than tonic, and pleocytosis may be noted. *C. tetani* is not a common inhabitant of the mouth of the dog. Tetanus toxoid may be given following dogbite to prevent tetanus.

A history of ingestion of poisons containing *strychnine* is most helpful in distinguishing this intoxication. Trismus is rare and, when it occurs, develops after the onset of generalized tonic activity. Usually, there is complete relaxation between convulsions. Trismus has also been noted in phenothiazine poisoning.

Tetany may be characterized by carpopedal spasm and laryngospasm, but trismus is rare. The diagnosis is confirmed by a low serum calcium concentration.

Complications. Complications of tetanus can be minimized by strict attention to supportive care and by appropriate therapy. Interference with pulmonary ventilation by respiratory muscle spasm and laryngospasm or by the accumulation of secretions may lead to aspiration pneumonia, atelectasis, mediastinal emphysema, or pneumothorax. The latter two conditions may be related to tracheostomy. Lacerations of the tongue or buccal mucosa, intramuscular hematomas, and vertebral fractures may result from severe tetanic seizures. If the course is prolonged, malnutrition and dehydration may develop unless strict attention is paid to fluid balance and caloric intake.

Prevention. Routine active immunization of children is discussed in Sec. 4.1. Immunization of previously nonimmune pregnant mothers will provide the newborn infant with protection immediately following delivery; preferably, tetanus immunization should be carried out prior to pregnancy.

Children who have not been immunized by 6 yr should receive a series of 3 doses of adult-type Td intramuscularly. The 2nd dose should be given 4–6 wk after the 1st, and the 3rd 6–12 mo after the 2nd. Thereafter, a Td booster should be given every 10 yr.

Preventive measures following injury must be dictated by the immunization status of the patient and by the characteristics of the injury. Immediate and thorough surgical treatment of wounds is mandatory. The wound should be cleansed, necrotic tissue and foreign bodies removed, and, if necessary, more extensive debridement performed. If active immunization has not been provided or if its status is unknown, *human tetanus immune globulin* (TIG) should be given intramuscularly in a dose of 250–500 units. If TIG is not available, *tetanus antitoxin* (TAT) of bovine or equine origin can be given in a dose of 3000–5000 units intramuscularly. Careful testing for sensitivity to TAT prior to its administration is mandatory; serum sickness may follow its use.

Tetanus toxoid should be given to initiate active immunity. It may be given at the same time as TIG or TAT, if it is administered in another site and in a separate syringe. If the child has had at least 4 DTP immunizations and 5 or more yr have elapsed since the 4th injection, a tetanus toxoid booster is indicated. If the wound has been neglected for more than 24 hr, TIG or TAT should also be provided. Fluid toxoid is preferred in this instance since it produces a more rapid secondary immune response than precipitated or adsorbed tetanus toxoids. If tetanus immunization is incomplete at the time of the wound, the remainder of the series of injections should be given.

Treatment and Supportive Care of Tetanus. The principal objectives of therapy are to remove the source of tetanospasmin, to neutralize circulating toxin, and to provide supportive care until tetanospasmin, which is fixed to neural tissue, can be metabolized. Supportive care must be intensive and performed meticulously.

Tetanus immune globulin of human origin, 3000–6000 units, should be given intramuscularly as soon as possible; it should not be given intravenously. Administration of TIG is not followed by allergy or anaphylaxis; higher and more persistent titers of antitoxin are produced than with antitoxin from nonhuman sources. Protective levels are obtained rapidly and decline slowly (half-life, 24 days). Repeated doses are not required. TIG has no effect on toxin fixed to neural tissue and does not penetrate the blood–cerebrospinal fluid barrier; it does neutralize toxin.

If TIG is not available and skin testing shows no hypersensitivity to TAT, it can be given in a single dose of 50,000–100,000 units: half the dose is given intramuscularly and half intravenously, with careful observation of the precautions detailed in the package insert. If sensitivity to TAT is demonstrated, desensitization should be carried out as described in the package insert.

Wounds should be cleansed and debrided if necessary. Foreign bodies must be removed and the wound left open. Surgical efforts should be delayed until the patient is sedated and antitoxin has been administered.

Antibiotic therapy may eradicate vegetative *C. tetani* organisms, which grow in areas of devitalized tissue where blood supply is poor or absent. For this reason large doses of penicillin G are favored in an effort to promote diffusion into the devitalized area. Penicillin G (200,000 units/kg/24 hr) may be used intravenously in 6 divided doses for 10 days. In patients who are sensitive to penicillin, tetracycline (30–40 mg/kg/24 hr, but not more than 2 g) in 4 divided oral doses for 10 days is effective.

Meticulous nursing care is imperative. The patient should be placed in a quiet environment and every effort made to control or eliminate auditory and visual stimuli. A respirator, oxygen, suction, and equipment for tracheotomy should be available. Although tracheotomy need not be considered a routine procedure, it should be performed prior to the development of severe involvement of respiratory muscles or laryngospasm.

Muscle relaxants should be given to all patients. Diazepam is effective in controlling hypertonicity and spasms. It may be used in a dose of 0.1–0.2 mg/kg every 3–6 hr intravenously or intramuscularly as needed. Dosages as high as 10–15 mg/kg/24 hr and plasma concentrations of 185–840 ng/mL have been required to control seizures in some children. Therapy for 2–6 wk may be required; the dose may be tapered as tetanic activity decreases. Chlorpromazine and mephenesin also have been utilized but seem to be less effective.

Neuromuscular blocking agents such as D-tubocurarine and pancuronium bromide (0.05 mg/kg/dose given every 2–3 hr intravenously as needed) have been used either to control seizures while sparing respiration or to produce complete respiratory paralysis which is then managed by artificial ventilation. The latter technique has produced the best survival rates but can be utilized only in centers where continuous intensive care and highly trained respiratory care teams are available (Sec. 5.38–5.39).

Patients receiving sedation and muscle relaxants must be monitored continually and suctioned frequently. Adequate ventilation must be ensured. Respiratory depression should be avoided and treated promptly if it occurs.

The patient should be weighed daily, and intake and output of fluids should be monitored carefully. An adequate intake of fluid, electrolytes, and calories should be maintained. The oral route may be used in some patients; generally, however, intravenous infusion and/or nasogastric intubation are required. In selected patients gastrostomy may be necessary. Meticulous care of the mouth, skin, bladder, and bowel is important.

The newborn infant has special problems relating to ventilation, hydration, and sedation. If possible, therapy should be aggressive and utilize endotracheal intubation, neuromuscular blocking agents, and assisted ventilation. Where facilities are not available, sedatives and muscle relaxants may be given orally. Syrup of chlorpromazine (3 mg every 6 hr), elixir of phenobarbital (10–20 mg every 6 hr), or elixir of mephenesin (130–160 mg every 6 hr) may be used.

Diazepam may be given intravenously in a dose of 0.3 mg/kg and repeated as needed to control severe spasms. Doses as high as 20 to 40 mg/kg/24 hr intravenously and plasma concentrations of 1950–5000 ng/mL have been required to control seizures in some infants.

The addition of pyridoxine (100 mg/24 hr) to conventional therapy decreases morbidity and mortality of *tetanus neonatorum*. This effect may occur because pyridoxine increases production of gamma-aminobutyric acid (GABA) at the nerve endings, which increases inhibitory responses and reduces spasms. Excision of the umbilicus is no longer recommended.

Prognosis. Case fatality rates of tetanus approximate 44–55%; rates for neonatal tetanus are 60% or greater.

Prognosis is affected by a number of factors. The highest mortality is found at the extremes of life; the lowest occurs in patients 10–19 yr of age (less than 20%). Extensive muscle involvement, high fever, and a short interval between injury and appearance of clinical manifestations correlate with high mortality rates. Patients who have localized disease or whose disease begins after a long incubation period as well as those who remain afebrile have a better chance of recovery. Fatalities in severe cases usually occur during the 1st wk of disease. Prognosis depends largely upon the quality of supportive care.

Cerebral palsy, paralysis, mental deficit, and behavioral disturbances have been noted in a few survivors of neonatal tetanus. Apnea and anoxia resulting from prolonged episodes of spasms appear to be a possible cause of brain damage.

Recovery from tetanus does not confer immunity; *active immunization of the patient following recovery is imperative.*

Adams JM, Kenny JD, Rudolph AJ: Modern management of tetanus neonatorum. Pediatrics 64:472, 1979.
Blake PA, Feldman RA, Buchanan TM, et al: Serologic therapy of tetanus in the United States. 1965–1971. JAMA 235:42, 1976.
Corbett JL, Kerr JH, Prys-Roberts C, et al: Cardiovascular disturbances in severe tetanus due to overactivity of the sympathetic nervous system. Anesthesia 24:198, 1969.
Gadoth N, Dagan R, Sandbank O: Permanent tetraplegia as a consequence of tetanus neonatorum. J Neurol Sci 51:273, 1981.
Godol JC: Trial of pyridoxine therapy for tetanus neonatorum. J Infect Dis 145:547, 1983.
Peebles TC, Levine L, Eldred MC, et al: Tetanus-toxoid emergency boosters; a reappraisal. N Engl J Med 280:575, 1969.
Shahani M, Dastur FD, Dastoor DH, et al: Neuropathy in tetanus. J Neurol Sci 43:173, 1979.
Stanfield JP, Gall D, Bracken PM: Single-dose antenatal tetanus immunization. Lancet 1:215, 1973.
Tekur U, Gupta A, Tayal G, et al: Blood concentrations of diazepam and its metabolites in children and neonates with tetanus. J Pediatr 102:145, 1983.
Weinstein L: Tetanus. N Engl J Med 289:1293, 1973.

OTHER CLOSTRIDIAL INFECTIONS

Clostridia other than *C. tetani* have been associated with a variety of disorders, including gas gangrene, food poisoning, necrotizing enteritis, and botulism. Some of these disorders are the result of elaboration of toxin by vegetative organisms.

11.37 GAS GANGRENE

Gas gangrene, an invasive anaerobic infection of soft tissues, including muscle, is characterized by extensive tissue necrosis, variable degrees of gas production, and profound toxemia.

Etiology. Six species of *Clostridium* are capable of producing gas gangrene: *C. perfringens* (formerly *C. welchii*), *C. novyi*, *C. septicum*, *C. histolyticum*, *C. bifermentans*, and *C. fallax*. These organisms are gram-positive rods that rarely produce spores; all are obligate anaerobes. In the vegetative form, during which they produce a variety of toxins, they can be destroyed by many chemical and physical agents. The most significant toxins are lecithinase (α-toxin), collagenase, hyaluronidase, leukocidin, deoxyribonuclease, protease, and lipase.

Epidemiology. Gas gangrene is uncommon in the United States. The incidence in postoperative wounds and civilian trauma is estimated at less than 0.1%. Spores of clostridia associated with gas gangrene may enter tissues from the soil or may gain entry from the gastrointestinal or female genital tracts, their sites of carriage in normal individuals.

Pathogenesis and Pathology. Development of gas gangrene depends on (1) contamination of a traumatized area with clostridia and (2) the presence of devitalized tissue with decreased oxidation-reduction potential. Trauma, ischemia, infection due to other bacteria, or the presence of a foreign body may induce an anaerobic environment. The toxins elaborated by multiplying clostridia are responsible for the gas gangrene syndrome. Lecithinases, particularly those elaborated by *C. perfringens*, destroy cell membranes and alter capillary permeability. A toxin produced by *C. histolyticum* can also digest tissues rapidly. Necrosis, thrombosis of regional blood vessels, and bacterial multiplication proceed, and gas (hydrogen and carbon dioxide) is liberated and may be palpated in the tissues. Edema and swelling intensify, and septicemia, shock, and death finally ensue.

Clinical Manifestations. The syndrome of *simple clostridial contamination* results from multiplication of clostridia in a wound, with little pain and no systemic reaction. Typical lesions appear deep and ragged; a foul-smelling, brownish-black, seropurulent exudate usually also appears. Healing proceeds slowly. Generally, anaerobic streptococci are recovered in addition to clostridia.

Anaerobic cellulitis may appear *de novo* or may complicate simple contamination; the incubation period is 3–4 days. Anaerobic cellulitis (gas abscess, localized gas gangrene, brown form of gas gangrene) is a clostridial infection of necrotic tissue already devitalized by ischemia or trauma. Healthy muscle remains uninvolved. Constitutional reactions are minimal. The wound appears dirty, has a foul odor, may be locally crepitant, and has a brownish, seropurulent discharge. Pain is minimal, and discoloration and edema of areas of skin surrounding the lesion are rare.

Anaerobic myonecrosis is the most serious form of gas gangrene. The incubation period may be as short as hours or as long as 1–2 mo; generally, it is less than 3 days. The onset is acute, beginning with pain, localized edema, and swelling in the region of the wound. The patient appears extremely ill, becomes pale, sweaty, and hypotensive, and may be agitated or delirious. Jaundice may be a late manifestation. The profuse serosanguineous discharge from the wound has a sweet odor. It contains numerous organisms but no polymorphonuclear leukocytes. Muscle at the site of infection may be edematous and pale; as the infection progresses, its color changes to brick red, contractility is lost, and bleeding from its surface ceases. Gas is minimal or absent. Invasion of the blood stream is an unusual complication of myonecrosis, but it may follow anaerobic endometritis (as in septic abortion or after prolonged rupture of membranes) or necrotizing infection of the gastrointestinal tract. Clostridial septicemia is not always clinically apparent, but it can lead to massive hemolysis, acute tubular necrosis, and death.

Infection by toxigenic clostridia also may involve the eye, brain, pleural cavity, lung, or liver. Gas gangrene may follow penetrating wounds of a variety of tissues that have been contaminated by soil.

Diagnosis and Differential Diagnosis. The diagnosis of clostridial infection must be made early and be based on clinical findings, especially the appearance of the site of infection. The specific clinical syndrome should be defined, since it dictates the choice of therapy. Large gram-positive rods may be found in smears of the discharge. *C. perfringens* does not sporulate in tissues, but other clostridia may do so. Toxigenic clostridia may be recovered by anaerobic cultures; their isolation does not necessarily indicate that they are causing the disease. Roentgenograms may help to document the presence and location of gas in tissues, as may crepitation in involved superficial tissues.

Two disorders must be differentiated from gas gangrene: *Postoperative synergistic gangrene* usually begins the 2nd wk after surgery or injury. An enlarging ulcer with a gray purulent center is surrounded by cellulitis. The lesion evolves slowly. Fever and anemia develop, and death may ensue. This disorder is due to the synergistic multiplication of *Staphylococcus aureus* and microaerophilic *Streptococcus* spp.

Necrotizing fasciitis, the second possible diagnosis, is an infection of subcutaneous tissues following surgery or trauma. This disease also is associated with *Streptococcus* spp. or with *Staphylococcus aureus*. Fever and hypovolemia occur, and death may follow within several days. In contrast to clostridial myositis, necrotizing fasciitis is characterized by hypesthesia or anesthesia of skin over the involved fascia, and the skin can be elevated readily from the necrotic fascia. No gas is found.

Prevention. The cornerstone of prevention is recognition of wounds prone to develop gas gangrene. Early, careful, and adequate debridement is imperative. All foreign bodies should be removed. Primary wound closure is best avoided. Penicillin G may be administered parenterally, but there is no evidence that its use will prevent gas gangrene in the absence of adequate surgery. There is no effective active immunization against gas gangrene.

Treatment. Surgical excision of infected tissue is indicated, as is penicillin G (250,000 units/kg/24 hr) in 6 divided doses intravenously to eradicate organisms not removed surgically. Chloramphenicol, erythromycin, and cephalosporins may be effective alternatives for patients allergic to penicillin.

Hyperbaric oxygen therapy may be helpful if suitable facilities are available. The value of polyvalent antitoxin in therapy of gas gangrene is unproved.

Altemeier WA, Fullen WD: Prevention and treatment of gas gangrene. JAMA 217:806, 1971.
Darke SG, King AM, Slack WK: Gas gangrene and related infection: Classification, clinical features, and aetiology, management and mortality: A report of 88 cases. Br J Surg 64:104, 1977.
Weinstein L, Barza MA: Gas gangrene. N Engl J Med 289:1129, 1973.

11.38 FOOD POISONING, NECROTIZING ENTERITIS, AND ANTIBIOTIC-ASSOCIATED PSEUDOMEMBRANOUS COLITIS DUE TO CLOSTRIDIA

Etiology. *C. perfringens* type A is a common cause of food poisoning (Sec. 28.1). Necrotizing enteritis is extremely rare; it is associated with ingestion of *C. perfringens* type F. Pigbel, an epidemic disease during periods of pig-feasting in New Guinea, has been related to ingestion of *C. perfringens* type C. Antibiotic-associated pseudomembranous colitis is related to elaboration of a toxin by *C. difficile*.

Epidemiology. Disease is acquired by ingestion of strains of *C. perfringens* capable of forming spores. These bacteria can be found in feces of normal individuals or animals and in raw meat. When food contaminated with *C. perfringens* is first cooled to temperatures that permit spores to survive and then is left to stand, vegetative organisms may grow, producing toxins. The symptoms produced after ingestion appear to be the result of both tissue invasion and toxin production.

Antibiotic-associated pseudomembranous colitis is the result of administration of an antibiotic that alters the flora of the gastrointestinal tract, permitting an overgrowth of *C. difficile* with elaboration of toxin that has cytopathic effects on the mucosa. This condition has been associated most commonly with clindamycin therapy, but it may also follow administration of other antibiotics (penicillin, ampicillin, cephalosporins, amoxicillin, tetracycline). *C. difficile* has been associated with outbreaks of diarrhea in day-care centers. Some of the affected children had received prior antimicrobial therapy for upper respiratory infections.

C. difficile has also been associated with both acute self-limited and chronic diarrheal illness in children who have never received antibiotic therapy.

Clinical Manifestations and Diagnosis. Within 12–24 hr following ingestion of food contaminated with *C. perfringens* type A, abdominal pain and diarrhea develop. Nausea and vomiting are rare. Fever is absent or low grade, and other constitutional symptoms are minimal. Duration of illness generally is 24–48 hr (Sec. 28.1).

Necrotizing enteritis, an illness caused by *C. perfringens* type F, has an acute onset characterized by severe abdominal pain, vomiting, diarrhea, and shock. Necrosis of gastrointestinal mucosa, associated with submucosal gas cysts, hemorrhage, and thrombosis of submucosal vessels, may occur and explain the severity of the disorder. Fatalities are common.

C. perfringens may be isolated by anaerobic cultures of contaminated food. They may also be recovered from the stools of infected patients. Tests to document toxin elaboration are available, and antibodies against *C. perfringens* enterotoxin can be measured in the serum following recovery.

Antibiotic-associated pseudomembranous colitis is characterized by abdominal pain, diarrhea with mucus and blood, and occasional intestinal perforation. Symptoms usually abate when the antibiotic that has played a causative role in the illness is discontinued. Pseudomembranous colitis has also been recorded in infants who had never received antibiotic therapy, but had *C. difficile* and its toxin in their stools. *C. difficile* has also been associated with epidemic necrotizing enterocolitis in neonatal intensive care units.

The diagnosis of antibiotic-associated pseudomembranous colitis can be made by recovery of *C. difficile* from the stools and documentation in vitro that the organism recovered produces a cytopathic toxin. An enzyme-linked immunosorbent assay for detecting antibodies to toxins A and B of *C. difficile* has also been developed. Available evidence suggests that patients develop serologic responses to one or both toxins.

Prevention. Disease can be prevented by cooking food thoroughly. If it is necessary for food to stand prior to ingestion, it should be stored at temperatures below 5° C or above 50° C.

Treatment. Gastroenteritis due to *C. perfringens* type A is usually self-limited. Adequate hydration should be maintained. Necrotizing enteritis and antibiotic-associated pseudomembranous colitis must be treated in hospital with appropriate fluids and electrolytes and by surgery designed to remove gangrenous portions of the bowel. The offending antibiotic must be discontinued when pseudomembranous colitis follows antibiotic administration. Antibiotics designed to prevent septicemia by organisms normally found in the gastrointestinal tract may be administered. Vancomycin, 2000 mg/1.73 m²/24 hr in 4 divided doses, has been well tolerated and effective in eliminating *C. difficile* and its toxin from the stools of affected children.

Bartlett JG, Chang TW, Gurwith M, et al: Antibiotic-associated pseudomembranous colitis due to toxin-producing clostridia. N Engl J Med 298:531, 1978.
Han VKM, Sayed H, Chance GW, et al: An outbreak of *Clostridium difficile* necrotizing enterocolitis: A case for oral vancomycin therapy. Pediatrics 71:935, 1983.
Johnson WD, Hook EW: Gastroenterocolitis syndromes. *In*: Hoeprich PD (ed): Infectious Disease. 2nd ed. Hagerstown, Md., Harper & Row, 1977.
Kim K, Dupont HL, Pickering LK: Outbreaks of diarrhea associated with

Clostridium difficile and its toxin in day-care centers: Evidence of person to person spread. J Pediatr 102:376, 1983.

Thompson CM, Gilligan PH, Fisher MC, et al: *Clostridium difficile* cytotoxin in a pediatric population. Am J Dis Child 137:271, 1983.

Viscidi B, Laughon BE, Yolken R: Serum antibody responses to toxins A and B of *Clostridium difficile*. J Infect Dis 148:93, 1983.

11.39 BOTULISM

Three forms of botulism have been described: (1) food-borne botulism (an intoxication resulting from improperly preserved food that contains preformed botulinum toxin; also see Sec. 28.1) (2) wound botulism (the result of wound infection by toxin-producing *C. botulinum* organisms); and (3) infant botulism (caused by germination of spores of *C. botulinum* in the gastrointestinal tract with toxin production in vivo).

Etiology. *C. botulinum* is a motile, anaerobic, gram-positive bacterium which produces heat-resistant spores. If the spores survive food-processing, they may germinate and elaborate toxins. Seven antigenically distinct toxins have been identified (A, B, C, D, E, F, and G). Types A, B, E, F, and G have been associated with human disease.

Epidemiology. *Infant botulism* usually occurs in children under 12 mo of age, has a peak onset from 2 to 6 mo, and is caused by types A and B strains. Sources for spores include soil, house dust, vacuum cleaner dust, honey, and possibly corn syrup. Although the distribution of cases has been widespread in the United States, the majority of patients have been reported from California, Pennsylvania, Hawaii, and Utah, clusters correlating roughly with areas where spore concentration of *C. botulinum* in the soil is high. Breast-fed white term infants were reported in one study to be at higher risk than bottle-fed ones.

Food-borne botulism is a worldwide problem that also continues to result in fatalities in the United States, with about 10 outbreaks/yr. Improperly home-preserved foods are the most frequent cause of intoxication in the United States. In North America botulism is most frequently associated with type A toxin; in Scandinavian countries, Japan, and Canada it is caused by type E toxin, and in Europe, by type B.

Wound botulism may follow contamination by *C. botulinum* with subsequent in vivo toxin production.

Pathogenesis. *Infant botulism* is caused by ingestion of spores of *C. botulinum* which colonize and germinate in the infant's intestinal tract, and elaborate toxins that are subsequently absorbed. Although spores are ubiquitous in soil and consumed regularly with foodstuffs, this sequence does not generally occur in older children or adults. *Food-borne botulism* results from intestinal absorption of preformed toxins ingested with improperly prepared foods. The toxins in *wound botulism* are produced at the sites of injury.

Toxins are probably transported by lymphocytes or blood to the motor nerve terminals and have varying affinities for binding to nervous tissue; type A is greater in binding affinity than type E, which is greater than type B. Type B toxin has been demonstrated in serum 3 wk after ingestion of contaminated food.

The toxin inhibits release of acetylcholine at the prejunction region of terminal nerve fibers. A suppressive effect on motor neurons in the spinal cord has also been demonstrated. In general, the effect of toxin on the brain is negligible, but terminals of cranial nerves are affected early, and patients may aspirate or develop asphyxia and cardiac arrhythmias.

Clinical Manifestations. The course of *infant botulism* may vary from mild constipation and poor feeding to severe neurologic deterioration and sudden death. Typically, a healthy-appearing afebrile infant becomes constipated, feeds poorly due to poor sucking and swallowing, develops weakness in crying and smiling, becomes hypotonic, and loses head control. Symmetrical, descending paralysis progresses over hours to days to sequentially involve muscles innervated by cranial nerves, the trunk, and the limbs. Ileus, bladder atony, ptosis, mydriasis, and decreased tearing and salivation may occur. Infants often require ventilatory support for respiratory failure. In contrast, the course in some patients may resemble that of the sudden infant death syndrome (Sec. 26.1).

Food-borne botulism usually has an incubation period of 12–36 hr, but this can range from several hours to a week. Nausea, vomiting, diplopia, dysphagia, dysarthria, and dry mouth are common manifestations. Weakness, postural hypotension, absent or diminished deep tendon reflexes, urinary retention, and constipation may develop. The patient remains alert at the outset but, with time, may become somnolent.

Physical examination generally reveals an afebrile patient with normal pulse rate. Ptosis, nystagmus, and paresis of extraocular muscles may occur. Pupils may be dilated and react sluggishly to light. Mucous membranes of the mouth, tongue, and pharynx are dry, and lacrimation may cease. Respiratory efforts may be impaired and progress rapidly to respiratory failure. Sensory examination is normal.

The course of *wound botulism* may be similar to that resulting from ingestion of toxins or may be milder and more prolonged and may vary depending on the nature of the contaminated wound.

Diagnosis and Differential Diagnosis. The diagnosis of infantile botulism is established by identification of *C. botulinum* organisms and/or toxin in the feces, since they are not part of the normal bowel flora of infants. The diagnosis of food-borne botulism is confirmed by demonstrating botulinal toxin in food the patient has ingested or in the patient's serum or stool. Wound botulism is diagnosed by demonstrating the organisms in the wound and/or the toxin in the blood. Inoculation of mice with serum from the affected patient identifies toxin by neutralization with specific known antitoxins. Serum antibodies to *C. botulinum* toxins A, B, and E have been detected using an enzyme immunoassay system.

Infant botulism's unique clinical presentation usually differentiates it from septicemia, myasthenia gravis, poliomyelitis, spinal cord injury, and metabolic disorders in infancy that may have some similar manifestations. The electromyogram may be similar to that observed with food-borne botulism.

Food-borne botulism must be differentiated from myasthenia gravis, poliomyelitis, Guillain-Barré syndrome, other forms of chemical or food poisoning, trichinosis, diphtheria, and various forms of electrolyte or mineral imbalance. A characteristic electromyographic pattern known as brief, small, abundant motor-unit action potentials (BSAP) frequently has been found. Its absence, however, does not exclude the diagnosis.

Myasthenia gravis is differentiated by the fatigability of muscle noted in this disease and by response to edrophonium chloride (Tensilon) or neostigmine. Guillain-Barré syndrome is associated with myalgia, paresthesias, occasional sensory deficits, and an elevated concentration of cerebrospinal fluid protein. Cranial nerve involvement is usually absent in other forms of food poisoning, and diarrhea is more prominent. Other infectious diseases, including poliomyelitis and encephalitis, are generally accompanied by fever, and cranial nerve involvement is less prominent than that noted in patients with botulism.

Prevention. Boiling for 10 min will destroy the toxin. A pressure cooker (115.5° C or 240° F) is required to kill spores of *C. botulinum*; pressure requirements vary with the food being processed.

Treatment. *Infant Botulism.* Treatment consists of continuous monitoring of vital signs and general intensive care, including appropriate respiratory and nutritional support. Recovery usually occurs over several weeks. Antitoxin is not routinely given because of its hazards and because intensive care alone is usually sufficient. Antibiotics do not shorten the clinical course or decrease intestinal colonization; aminoglycosides may exacerbate or accelerate paralysis, including respiratory failure.

Food-Borne Botulism. All individuals known to have ingested toxin should be hospitalized. Vomiting should be induced and gastric lavage initiated. Magnesium sulfate or other cathartics may be placed in the stomach at the conclusion of lavage. A high enema should be given to facilitate elimination of unabsorbed toxin.

Cardiac and respiratory function must be monitored carefully. Tracheostomy should be performed before respiratory impairment becomes severe.

Antitoxin has been efficacious. Three preparations of equine origin can be obtained in the United States on a 24 hr basis from the Centers for Disease Control, Atlanta, Georgia. The polyvalent preparation is preferred until the toxin type has been identified. Skin sensitivity testing is mandatory prior to administration.

Penicillin G is recommended to kill *C. botulinum*, which may continue to produce toxin. Aqueous penicillin G should be given parenterally in a dose of 50,000 units/kg/24 hr in 4–6 divided doses. Penicillin G may also be given orally in a dose of 1,600,000 units/24 hr in 4 divided doses after lavage has been concluded.

Hypotension should be treated with appropriate intravenous fluids; fluid and electrolyte balance must be maintained.

Wound Botulism. Adequate debridement and drainage of the wound must be performed. Supportive intensive care and administration of antitoxin and antibiotics are similar to the treatment given for food-borne botulism, except that efforts to remove toxin from the gastrointestinal tract are not indicated.

Prognosis. *Infant Botulism.* Most infants recover without sequelae if adequate intensive care and supportive therapy are provided. However, it has been speculated that up to 10% of sudden unexpected deaths in infancy are caused by botulism. Recovery from the clinical manifestations of infant botulism is not necessarily preceded by decreased colonization of *C. botulinum* or by a decreased quantity of toxin in the gastrointestinal tract.

Food-Borne Botulism. Severity of illness is directly proportional to the quantity of toxin ingested. A short incubation period is associated with more severe disease. The earlier the specific treatment is given, the better the prognosis. Recovery can be complete with appropriate supportive care.

Arnon SS: Infant botulism. Ann Rev Med 31:541, 1980.

Long SS: Epidemiologic study of infant botulism in Pennsylvania: Report of the Infant Botulism Study Group. Pediatrics 75:928, 1985.

Long SS: Infant botulism—a toxicoinfection. Infect Dis Newsletter (in press).

Merson MH, Dowell VR Jr: Epidemiologic, clinical and laboratory aspects of wound botulism. N Engl J Med 289:1105, 1973.

Morris JG Jr, Synder JD, Wilson R, et al: Infant botulism in the United States: An epidemiologic study of cases occurring outside of California. Am J Public Health 73:1385, 1983.

Robin LG, Dezfulian M, Yolken RH: Serum antibody response to *Clostridium botulinum* toxin in infant botulism. J Clin Microbiol 16:770, 1982.

Sonnabend O, Sonnabend W, Heinzle R, et al: Isolation of *Clostridium botulinum* toxin G and identification of type G botulinum toxin in humans. Report of five unexpected deaths. J Infect Dis 143:22, 1981.

Wilke BW Jr, Midura TF, Arnon SS: Quantitative evidence of intestinal colonization by *Clostridium botulinum* in four cases of infant botulism. J Infect Dis 141:419, 1980.

11.40 ANAEROBIC INFECTIONS OTHER THAN CLOSTRIDIAL

Advances in techniques for recovering anaerobic bacteria and an awareness of the possible role they play in clinical disease have permitted an assessment of the prevalence and significance of anaerobic microorganisms as a cause of infection.

Etiology. Anaerobic bacteria are present in soil and constitute a part of the normal human flora; they are found on all mucous membranes. In the mouth, in the vagina, and on the skin, anaerobic bacteria outnumber aerobic bacteria by 10 to 1; in the colon, by 100 to 1.

Anaerobic bacteria are microorganisms to which oxygen is toxic, but strains vary considerably in their ability to tolerate oxygen. Some strains survive in the presence of oxygen but grow better when the oxygen in their environment is reduced (*facultative anaerobes*). *Obligate anaerobes* do not grow on the surface of blood agar plates incubated aerobically or even in an environment enriched with CO_2. Obligate anaerobes predominate in the normal human flora. Anaerobic microorganisms can be classified as shown in Table 11–21.

Epidemiology. Blood, intra-abdominal sources, and soft tissues are the principal sites from which anaerobes are recovered during infection in infancy and childhood. Except in blood cultures, several anaerobes or both anaerobes and aerobes are recovered concomitantly from sites of infection.

Symptomatic anaerobic infection occurs infrequently in a general pediatric population. In a large prospective study, only 0.3% of blood cultures during a 1 yr period contained anaerobic organisms that were involved in the pathogenesis of the patients' diseases. In contrast, pathogenic aerobic microorganisms were recovered from 9% of the cultures. Anaerobes accounted for 5.8% of all bacteremic episodes (8.7% in the newborn period and 4.8% in children over 1 yr of age). Among the newborn infants whose disease was associated with bacteremia, 10.1% of the pathogens were anaerobes unassociated with aerobic bacteria.

The major clinical settings in which anaerobic infection of children might be anticipated are (1) birth following prolonged rupture of the membranes, amnionitis, or obstetrical difficulty; (2) peritonitis or septicemia associated with intestinal obstruction and perforation or with appendicitis; (3) disorders that impair the response of the host to infection; (4) subcutaneous abscesses and infections of the female genital tract; (5) orofacial infections; and (6) aspiration pneumonia.

Pathogenesis. Normally, anaerobes are of low virulence for humans. Their multiplication and invasion are favored by any means that removes oxygen from their environment or that otherwise lowers their oxidation-reduction potential. In some cases removal of aerobes facilitates anaerobic invasion. More frequently, however, aerobes facilitate establishment of anaerobic infection by destroying previously well-oxygenated tissue.

Anaerobic *pleuropulmonic disease* may be initiated by aspiration (general anesthesia, esophageal dysfunction, tonsillectomy, tooth extraction); preceding extrapulmonic anaerobic infection (otitis media, pharyngitis, bacterial endocarditis, peritonitis); penetrating chest wounds or open heart surgery; and systemic disease that impairs host response to infection. Anaerobic *brain abscesses* may follow chronic otitis media,

Table 11–21. Classification of Representative Anaerobes

Non–Spore-Forming Gram-Negative Bacilli
Bacteroides: B. fragilis, B. oralis, B. melaninogenicus, B. corrodens
Fusobacterium: F. nucleatum, F. varium, F. necrophorum, F. mortiferum

Spore-Forming Gram-Positive Bacilli
Clostridia: C. perfringens (welchii), C. tetani, C. botulinum, C. novyi, C. septicum, C. ramosum

Non–Spore-Forming Gram-Positive Bacilli: *Actinomyces, Arachnia, Bifidobacterium, Eubacterium, Propionibacterium, Lactobacillus*

Gram-Positive Cocci: *Peptococcus, Peptostreptococcus,* microaerophilic cocci

Gram-Negative Cocci: *Veillonella, Acidaminococcus, Megasphaera*

mastoiditis, sinusitis, lung abscess, congenital heart disease with right to left shunt, bacterial endocarditis, infections of the face or scalp, head trauma, or intracranial surgery.

Anaerobic *bacteremia* and/or *peritonitis* may be preceded by perforation of the large or small bowel, by appendicitis, gastroenteritis, or cholecystitis.

Neonatal anaerobic infection most commonly follows prolonged rupture of the fetal membranes or is associated with necrotizing enterocolitis.

Pathology. Abscess formation and widespread tissue destruction are associated with anaerobic infection. The specific pathology varies with the site.

Clinical Manifestations. Infections produced by anaerobic microorganisms occur in any part of the body.

Anaerobic infections of the *upper respiratory tract* are not unusual. Periodontal infection (trench mouth) is favored by poor dental hygiene or by malocclusion. The gingival tissues are inflamed and edematous, and a foul-smelling discharge may be elicited by pressing along the gums. Periapical abscesses or anaerobic osteomyelitis of the mandible or maxilla may develop.

Anaerobic microorganisms also may be involved in chronic sinusitis, otitis media, mastoiditis, peritonsillar and retropharyngeal abscesses, parotitis, and cervical lymphadenitis. Since potentially pathogenic aerobic organisms are generally recovered concomitantly, it is difficult to establish the precise role of anaerobes in these diseases.

Fusobacteria appear to be important in the development of **Vincent angina,** a tonsillar infection characterized by ulcers covered by a brown or gray foul-smelling exudate. Extensive tissue destruction has resulted in perforation of the carotid artery.

Ludwig angina is an acute cellulitis of the sublingual and submandibular spaces that tends to spread rapidly without lymph node involvement or abscess formation. Respiratory obstruction may require tracheotomy.

Anaerobic infection of the *lower respiratory tract* generally takes the form of necrotizing pneumonia, putrid empyema, or lung abscess. A history of aspiration can usually be elicited. Ordinarily, pneumonia develops first, and abscess formation results from liquefaction of lung tissue.

Anaerobic infection of the *central nervous system* may occur as brain abscess, subdural empyema, or septic thrombophlebitis of cortical veins and venous sinuses. The intracranial lesion may originate by direct spread from a contiguous infection or by hematogenous spread from a remote one. See Sec. 21.23 for a discussion of signs or symptoms of brain abscess. Purulent meningitis is rarely caused by anaerobes; recovery of anaerobes from the cerebrospinal fluid suggests brain abscess or subdural empyema.

Since the concentrations of anaerobes are normally highest in the lower gastrointestinal tract, it is not surprising that peritoneal spillage of gastrointestinal contents is associated with a high incidence of anaerobic intra-abdominal infection. Generally aerobes and anaerobes are recovered from peritoneal contents concomitantly.

Anaerobic bacteremia is clinically indistinguishable from aerobic bacteremia. Fever, leukocytosis, jaundice, hemolytic anemia, and shock may occur. Anaerobic bacteremia is frequently associated with disease of the gastrointestinal (e.g., necrotizing enteritis) and genitourinary (e.g., calculi) systems.

Anaerobic microorganisms also may cause osteomyelitis, septic arthritis, urinary tract infections, liver and subphrenic abscesses, lymphadenitis, skin and soft tissue infections, orbital cellulitis, and peritonsillar abscess. They have been recovered by needle tympanocentesis from the middle ear of children with chronic otitis media or with serous otitis media.

Diagnosis. The diagnosis of anaerobic infection depends upon (1) awareness of infections with which anaerobes are associated, (2) appropriate selection and collection of specimens for culture, and (3) use of media and techniques that will facilitate their recovery. Clinical specimens which should be routinely cultured for anaerobes include blood; bile; pericardial, peritoneal, pleural, or cerebrospinal fluid; abscesses; deep aspirates of wounds; transtracheal aspirates; and surgical specimens obtained from normally sterile sites.

Clinical clues to the diagnosis of anaerobic infection include the presence of a foul-smelling exudate or discharge, evidence of necrotic tissue or gangrene, infection located in proximity to a mucosal surface, gas in tissue or discharges, infection following an animal or human bite, infection associated with tissue destruction (trauma or malignancy), or infection that persists or follows prolonged use of aminoglycosides. Additional clues may include endocarditis with negative routine blood cultures, septic thrombophlebitis, or bacteremia associated with unexplained jaundice.

The following sites or specimens should not be cultured anaerobically except in rare cases: nose, mouth, throat, sputum, tracheostomy sites, bronchoscopic washings, gastric washings, feces, ileostomy or colostomy material, urine, vaginal swabs, or fistulas. Anaerobic microorganisms are normally found in these specimens and it is generally impossible to implicate them in a causative relationship with any disease process.

Bacteriologic clues that suggest infection with anaerobes include no growth on routine cultures (sterile pus); failure to grow aerobically but presence confirmed by Gram stain of the original exudate; growth in thioglycolate broth or on media containing 100 μg/mL of kanamycin, neomycin, or paromomycin; production of gas and foul odor in culture; and development of characteristic colonies on agar plates incubated anaerobically.

Rapid diagnosis of *Bacteroides* infection has been made utilizing an indirect immunofluorescence assay with specific antisera against the capsular polysaccharide of *B. fragilis* and pooled antisera against a number of serotypes of *Bacteroides* spp. Rapid diagnosis has also been achieved using gas-liquid chromatography of purulent material.

Treatment. The type of infecting anaerobe can usually be predicted from knowing the site of infection, and most anaerobes have predictable sensitivities to antibiotic agents. Therefore, appropriate drugs can often be selected before results of culture and sensitivity tests are available. The daily doses used to treat anaerobic infections are similar to those used to treat aerobic ones (see Table 29–1B). Duration of therapy, however, varies with the nature of the disease process.

Penicillin G is effective against virtually all gram-positive and most gram-negative anaerobes (except *B. fragilis*), and it should therefore be used to treat orofacial and pulmonary infections, unless beta-lactamase producing anaerobes are present. A combination of penicillin and chloramphenicol should be used to treat anaerobic bacteremia and anaerobic infections at other sites.

Most anaerobes are also susceptible to clindamycin, cefoxitin, and carbenicillin as well as chloramphenicol. However, erythromycin is effective only against anaerobic cocci, and clindamycin does not penetrate the blood-brain barrier and thus should not be used in place of chloramphenicol to treat brain abscesses. Cefoxitin is active against 80% of *B. fragilis* but is relatively inactive against species of *Clostridium* other than *C. perfringens*.

Metronidazole (30 mg/kg/24 hr parenterally or 40–50 mg/kg/24 hr orally) is also effective in treating anaerobic infections, especially meningitis and brain abscesses.

Kanamycin and gentamicin are not effective against anaerobes. However, synergisms between gentamicin and each of the following drugs—penicillin, clindamycin, and metronidazole—have been demonstrated for *B. melaninogenicus.* In addition, a combination of chloramphenical or clindamycin with gentamicin or kanamycin may be appropriate for mixed aerobic and anaerobic infections, particularly those involving the gastrointestinal tract, peritoneal cavity, genitourinary system, or retroperitoneal space.

Prognosis. In the neonatal period anaerobic bacteremia has been reported to have mortality rates varying from 4 to 37.5%, reflecting, in part, differences in patient population and the anatomic sites chosen for obtaining blood cultures. Positive anaerobic blood cultures obtained from the umbilical cord most likely reflect transient neonatal bacteremia occurring at the time of delivery rather than active infection.

Mortality associated with anaerobic infection is increased in patients with extensive tissue necrosis with inadequate debridement and in those with necrotizing enterocolitis.

Bartlett JG: Recent developments in the management of anaerobic infections. Rev Infect Dis 5:235, 1983.
Brook I: Anaerobic infections in childhood. Rev Infect Dis 6(Suppl 1):5187, 1984.
Brook I: β-Lactamase-producing bacteria recovered after clinical failures with various penicillin therapy. Arch Otolaryngol 110:228, 1984.
Chow AW, Leake RD, Yamauchi T, et al: The significance of anaerobes in neonatal bacteremia: Analysis of 23 cases and review of the literature. Pediatrics 54:736, 1974.
Klastersky J, Coppens L, Mombelli G: Anaerobic infection in cancer patients: Comparative evaluation of clindamycin and cefoxitin. Antimicrob Agents Chemother 16:366, 1979.
Law BJ, Marks MI: Excellent outcome of Bacteroides meningitis in a newborn treated with metronidazole. Pediatrics 66:463, 1980.
Tabaqchali S: Rapid techniques for the identification of anaerobic bacteria and presumptive diagnosis. Scand J Infect Dis (Suppl) 35:23, 1982.

11.41 *CAMPYLOBACTER* INFECTIONS

Three species of *Campylobacter* are known to cause disease in humans: (1) *Campylobacter fetus* ss. *fetus* (previously *C. fetus* ss. *intestinalis* or *Vibrio fetus,* referred to as *Campylobacter fetus)*; (2) *Campylobacter jejuni* (previously *C. fetus* ss. *jejuni* or *Vibrio jejuni)*; and (3) *Campylobacter coli* (previously *C. fetus* ss. *jejuni,* *Vibrio coli,* or related vibrios). Prior to 1947, *Campylobacter* species were best known as a cause of abortion in domestic animals. With the development of special isolation techniques, *Campylobacter* has now been established as a frequent cause of gastroenteritis in children.

Etiology. *Campylobacter* organisms usually appear as spirally curved, thin, gram-negative rods; they appear less often as short and S-shaped or as longer, multispiraled, filamentous organisms. In older cultures coccal forms may also be seen. The organisms are motile with single flagella at one or both poles.

Strains that affect humans can be divided into two groups on the basis of serologic cross-reactions. This division is useful when the serum of the patient can be tested against his or her own isolate. The majority of patients have elevated antibody titers (greater than 1:40 by hemagglutination or bacterial agglutination); paired acute and convalescent sera may show 4-fold titer increases.

Epidemiology. The epidemiology of human infections is only partially understood. Among the possible means of spread of infection are venereal transmission as a cause of perinatal disease; contamination of water and foodstuffs, including milk formulas; and direct close contacts with infected persons or domestic animals.

Pathogenesis and Pathology. The pathogenesis of systemic *Campylobacter* infections is unclear. Fewer than one third of patients have had documented environmental or occupational exposure. Attempts to identify an enterotoxin or to document invasive properties of *C. fetus* have not been successful. Extensive hemorrhagic ulcerations of the bowel wall and edema extending from the jejunum through the proximal ileum have been noted at autopsy, however.

Clinical Manifestations. The most common manifestation of systemic infection is *bacteremia* without evidence of localized infection. The majority of bloodstream isolates are *C. fetus.* The illness generally begins with fever, headache, and malaise. The fever, relapsing or intermittent, is associated with night sweats and chills and with weight loss when the illness is prolonged. Lethargy and confusion are common, but specific neurologic signs are unusual in the absence of cerebrovascular disease or meningitis. Abdominal pain is relatively frequent, but is infrequently accompanied by diarrhea and less so by hepatomegaly and icterus. Cough may occur, but pulmonary parenchymal involvement is unusual. Physical examination is generally unimpressive except for the appearance of illness. There may be a moderate leukocytosis.

Transient asymptomatic bacteremia that clears without antibiotic therapy has been noted, as has rapidly fatal septicemia. Prolonged bacteremia of 8–13 wk duration has also been reported with spontaneous remissions and relapses.

Endocarditis caused by *Campylobacter* infection has been observed in adults, mainly in males with pre-existing heart disease. An association with dental extractions was also noted; fatalities have occurred when patients have not received adequate antibiotic therapy.

Campylobacter infection has been linked to *meningitis* in both adults and children. Within the pediatric age range, it is seen mainly in the neonatal period. Most patients beyond the neonatal period have survived with antibiotic therapy.

Perinatal disease is suggested by the recovery of *Campylobacter* from the placenta and fetus of women who have had a febrile illness during pregnancy; the presence of *Campylobacter* is associated with previous abortion and/or previous premature delivery. In addition to meningitis, symptomatic gastroenteritis and asymptomatic bloody diarrhea have been reported in newborn infants. The mother may be symptomatic or asymptomatic at the time of delivery.

In 1977 Skirrow reported recovery of *C. jejuni* from the stool of 7.1% of 803 patients with diarrhea and from none of 194 patients without diarrhea. The incubation period of *Campylobacter* enteritis is estimated to be 2–11 days. Spread of infections within families and day care centers has been noted. Dogs with diarrhea and live or dressed chickens have been implicated as possible sources of infection. The incidence is similar to and perhaps greater than that caused by *Salmonella,* *Shigella,* or *Yersinia enterocolitica.* Fever and bloody stools occur in about 90% of the patients. Blood characteristically appears in the stools 2–4 days after the onset of symptoms. Over 90% of older children complain of abdominal pain; vomiting occurs in 30% of patients. The diarrhea is generally watery, profuse, and foul-smelling. Abdominal pain is periumbilical, and cramping may antedate other symptoms or persist after the stools return to normal. The organism may persist in stools for up to 7 wk in untreated patients but cannot be recovered after 48 hr of therapy with erythromycin. The disease may simulate appendicitis or intussusception.

The complications of *C. jejuni* enteritis include septic and reactive arthritis and mesenteric adenitis.

Thrombophlebitis has been reported in association with *C. fetus* bacteremia. A nonspecific febrile illness with prominent findings of thrombophlebitis should suggest this possibility. *Campylobacter* has also been reported to produce pericarditis, peritonitis, salpingitis, septic arthritis, lung abscess, and chest wall abscess.

Diagnosis. The diagnosis of *Campylobacter* enteritis is established by culture.

Treatment. Although uncomplicated *Campylobacter* enteritis may require only supportive therapy, erythromycin (40 mg/kg/24 hr) diminishes possible spread of disease within the household, day care center, or nursery school. It shortens the duration of bacterial shedding but fails to diminish significantly the duration of diarrhea. *Campylobacter* enteritis may also be treated with oral tetracycline (50 mg/kg/24 hr), furazolidone (5 mg/kg/24 hr), and oral neomycin (50 mg/kg/24 hr). Treatment of diarrheal disease should be provided for at least 1 wk.

Gentamicin may be the antibiotic of choice for the treatment of *Campylobacter* septicemia and nonenteric *Campylobacter* disease when the antibiotic sensitivity pattern is not known. Chloramphenicol should be considered for use in patients with meningitis. Treatment of systemic infections for 4 wk is recommended.

Most isolates are sensitive in vitro to gentamicin, kanamycin, chloramphenicol, and tetracycline; variable resistance has been reported to colistin, carbenicillin, and cephalothin.

Prognosis. *Campylobacter* septicemia in the immunocompromised host and in the newborn is associated with a high mortality rate. The rarity of cases precludes a precise estimate of mortality, particularly when early effective antimicrobial therapy is provided.

Prognosis of *Campylobacter* enteritis is good.

Blaser MJ, Taylor DN, Feldman RA: Epidemiology of *Campylobacter jejuni* infections. Epidemiol Rev 5:157, 1983.

Karmali MA, Fleming PC: *Campylobacter* enteritis in children. J Pediatr 94:527, 1979.

Pai CH, Gillis F, Toumanen E, et al: Erythromycin in treatment of *Campylobacter* enteritis in children. Am J Dis Child 137:286, 1983.

Skerman VDB, McGowan V, Sneath PHA: Approved lists of bacterial names. Int J System Bact 30:225, 1980.

Skirrow MB: *Campylobacter* enteritis: A "new" disease. Br Med J 2:9, 1977.

Torphy DE, Bond WW: *Campylobacter fetus* infections in children. Pediatrics 64:898, 1979.

11.42 LEGIONELLOSIS
(Legionnaires' Disease and Pontiac Fever)

Legionnaires' disease is a term initially used to describe an outbreak of pneumonia during a convention of the American Legion in Philadelphia in 1976; 221 of those attending were affected; 34 died. In 1977, McDade isolated a gram-negative rod, *Legionella pneumophila*, from lung tissue of patients who had died, and demonstrated a specific antibody response in living patients. Subsequently, outbreaks have occurred in widely scattered areas of the United States and elsewhere with varying case fatality rates.

The term legionellosis has been proposed to encompass the two recognized clinical forms of infection with *Legionella pneumophila*. One, first recognized in the Philadelphia outbreak, is known as **legionnaires' disease.** It is characterized on the basis of its relatively long incubation period and the severity of its viral-like pneumonic clinical pattern. The other form, known as **Pontiac fever** because of an outbreak in a Health Department in Pontiac, Michigan in 1968 (etiologically identified a decade later), has a shorter incubation period and an acute clinical course resembling influenza without pneumonia. No deaths from this form are known.

Etiology. Legionellaceae are fastidious, gram-negative organisms that are catalase-positive and nonfermentative. Five species are recognized as causes of bronchopneumonia: *L. pneumophila* (six serotypes), *L. micdadei*, *L. bozemanii*, *L. dumoffi*, and *L. longbeachae*. They may be differentiated by direct fluorescence antibody staining, by biochemical reactions, and by fluorescence under ultraviolet light.

Legionnaires' disease is caused only by *L. pneumophila*. Cell suspensions of the organism induce gelation of *Limulus* amebocyte lysate and are pyrogenic to rabbits. *L. pneumophila* survives for several months in distilled water and over 1 yr

in tap water maintained at room temperature. On agar the organism grows most rapidly at 35° C.

Epidemiology. The incidence of pneumonia due to *L. pneumophila* is estimated at 7–20 cases/100,000/yr in the United States. The risk of nosocomial infection is increased 2- to 3-fold in patients with cancer or other disorders of immunosuppression. Therapy with corticosteroids is a significant risk factor; several outbreaks have been noted among renal homograft recipients. Among patients with sporadic, community-acquired infection, diabetes mellitus therapy using diuretic agents has been noted as an apparent predisposing factor.

Only airborne spread of *L. pneumophila* has been documented. The bacterium has been recovered from central air conditioning systems as well as from stream water and mud. Person-to-person spread of legionnaires' disease has not been proved. However, hospital staff members who had direct or indirect contact with persons with legionnaires' disease had a higher prevalence (9.3%) of elevated serum antibody titers than did staff members without known exposure (3.7%). These observations and the presence of of *L. pneumophila* in respiratory secretions imply that person-to-person spread may occur in some circumstances.

Numerous common-source outbreaks of legionnaires' disease have been recognized; 0.5–5.0% of those exposed have been affected. This incidence contrasts sharply with outbreaks of Pontiac fever, in which the attack rate has been 95–100%. Many of the outbreaks of legionnaires' disease have been associated with large service buildings, including hotels and hospitals.

Data on legionnaires' disease in children are limited. In prospective studies of pneumonia in children the frequency of *Legionella* infection as determined by serologic study has ranged from 2.6 to 17.3%. On the basis of these data it appeared that pneumonia due to *L. pneumophila* occurs more frequently in children over 4 yr of age than in younger ones. In a retrospective survey of sera from 126 children less than 10 yr of age, seroreactivity was detected as early as 1 yr of age. Approximately 25% had titers above a level considered to be presumptive evidence of previous infection. It was speculated that infection with *L. pneumophila* might also be a cause of mild respiratory disease in infants and children. Among patients with cystic fibrosis a high prevalence of antibodies to *L. pneumophila* (approximately 30%) has also been noted.

Pathogenesis. Legionnaires' disease presumably begins with inhalation of *L. pneumophila*, which induces pneumonia after an incubation period of 2–10 days. The pulmonary infiltrate consists primarily of macrophages and polymorphonuclear leukocytes in alveolar spaces, fibrin, and proliferating alveolar lining cells. Terminal bronchioles may be involved, but the bronchi and proximal bronchioles are generally spared. The cellular infiltrate commonly becomes necrotic, but the underlying pulmonary structure usually remains intact. The resolution may not be complete; a residual defect in diffusing capacity may be related to the deposition of fibrin.

Bacteremia has been observed but involvement of other organ systems either directly or indirectly through elaboration of toxin has not been noted.

The pathogenesis of Pontiac fever syndrome is not understood. This disorder usually occurs within 24–48 hr after *L. pneumophila* is inhaled. The disorder is not fatal, and no pathologic data are available. It is not known whether bacterial proliferation is required to produce the syndrome.

Mechanisms of immunity to *L. pneumophila* are not well defined. Hotel staff members in the Philadelphia outbreak who had a high prevalence of elevated antibody titers to *L. pneumophila* serogroup 1 were apparently protected against disease; this suggests that humoral immunity may be effective. The role of cellular immunity is unknown.

Clinical Manifestations. Legionnaires' disease is a multisystemic illness characterized by pneumonia, high fever, chills, cough, chest pain, myalgia, headache, confusion, and diarrhea; there is laboratory evidence of hepatic involvement and renal disease. Renal failure may necessitate dialysis in 3% of patients. Seizures, acute cerebellar ataxia, meningitis, and erythema nodosum have also been described. The white blood cell count is usually normal or slightly elevated with an increased proportion of segmented polymorphonuclear leukocytes. The erythrocyte sedimentation rate is elevated.

The pneumonia progresses over the 1st wk of illness with daily temperatures of 39–40° C; with treatment subsequent resolution is gradual. Chest roentgenograms obtained early reveal patchy infiltrates that become nodular areas of consolidation and that coalesce in severe cases. Pleural effusion is usually small except in patients with impaired immunity, and in such patients pneumonic cavitation may occur. In the absence of specific therapy, mortality is about 15–20%; death usually results from progressive pneumonia. Weakness and shortness of breath may persist for months in some patients, and roentgenographic clearing of the pneumonia is slow.

Pontiac fever is characterized by high fever, myalgia, headache, and extreme debilitation that may persist for 2–7 days. Cough, diarrhea, confusion, and chest pain have been observed but are not prominent features. All patients known to have had this form of the disease have recovered completely.

Diagnosis and Differential Diagnosis. *Legionella* pneumonia must be distinguished from common bacterial pneumonias and from infections caused by *Mycoplasma pneumoniae, Coxiella burnetii, Chlamydia psittaci,* influenza, and other respiratory viruses. The diagnosis is established by isolating *L. pneumophila* in cultures from blood, pleural fluid, respiratory secretions, or lung tissue; by demonstrating it in respiratory secretions, lung tissue, pleural fluid, or urine by direct immunofluorescence or enzyme-linked, immunosorbent assay; or by demonstrating at least a 4-fold rise in antibody titer in paired serum specimens assayed by indirect immunofluorescence or other methods at a titer of more than 1:128. Serologic conversion commonly occurs by the 21st day but may not occur until the 6th wk. Cross reactions may occur with plague, tularemia, *M. pneumoniae, Rickettsia rickettsii,* and *Leptospira interrogans.*

Treatment. Therapy of legionnaires' disease is specific and supportive. The infection responds to erythromycin and to tetracycline. In epidemics mortality has been distinctly reduced by therapy with erythromycin. It is administered in a dose of 40 mg/kg/24 hr in 4 divided doses intravenously for 14 days (for patients other than neonates). Oral treatment with the same dose may also be used. Relapse has been reported in several patients when treatment was stopped after 14 days; if relapse is noted, therapy should be resumed.

It is recommended that rifampin, 15 mg/kg/24 hr, be reserved for combined therapy with erythromycin when the patient is not responding to intravenous erythromycin therapy alone.

Specific therapy is apparently not required for Pontiac fever.

Supportive therapy including supplemental oxygen and at times assisted ventilation may be required. Renal failure requires management of fluid and electrolyte balance and occasionally dialysis on a temporary basis. Vasoactive drugs may be of assistance in managing shock.

Prevention and Control. No method for preventing epidemics or sporadic cases of legionnaires' disease is known, but in some instances outbreaks can be stopped. When an epidemic is traced to a cooling tower or an evaporative condenser, the implicated source should be removed. Respiratory isolation of patients with legionnaires' disease is recommended, although person-to-person spread has not been proved.

Cohen ML, Broome CV, Paris A, et al: Fatal nosocomial legionnaires' disease: Clinical and epidemiologic characteristics. Ann Intern Med 90:611, 1979.
Fraser DW: Legionellosis. *In:* Feigin RD, Cherry JD (eds): Textbook of Pediatric Infectious Disease. Philadelphia, WB Saunders, 1981, pp 872–879.
Glick TH, Gregg MD, Berman B, et al: Pontiac fever: An epidemic of unknown etiology in a health department. I. Clinical and epidemiologic aspects. Am J Epidemiol 107:149, 1978.
Katz SM, Hosclaw DS Jr: Serum antibodies to *Legionella pneumophila* in patients with cystic fibrosis. JAMA 248:2284, 1982.
Muldoon RL, Jaecker DL, Kiefer HK: Legionnaires' disease in children. Pediatrics 67:329, 1981.
Orenstein WA, Overturf GD, Leedom JM, et al: The frequency of *Legionella* infection prospectively determined in children hospitalized with pneumonia. J Pediatr 99:903, 1981.
Van Arsdall JA II, Wunderlich HF, Melo JC: The protean manifestations of legionnaires' disease. J Infect 7:51, 1983.

11.43 PITTSBURGH PNEUMONIA AGENT

Etiology. In 1979 Pasculle et al reported the isolation of unique gram-negative, weakly acid-fast bacilli from the lung tissue of two renal transplant recipients who had pneumonia. This agent, designated tentatively as Pittsburgh pneumonia agent (PPA), is distinct from *Legionella pneumophila* as determined by bacteriologic, ultrastructural, tinctorial, and serologic analyses, and is now designated as *Legionella (Tatlockia) micdadei.* Subsequently, pneumonia due to the PPA was documented in 8 immunosuppressed patients.

Pathology. Touch-imprint smears of biopsied lung may reveal numerous polymorphonuclear leukocytes and many faintly staining, gram-negative bacilli. Many of the organisms are intracellular and are weakly acid-fast. A fibrinopurulent intra-alveolar infiltrate may be noted. Alveolar septa are congested, but the basic lung architecture usually is preserved. Bronchopneumonia or pneumonia with lobar consolidation has been observed.

PPA may be a contaminant of hot and cold water supplies; nosocomial infections have been traced to water storage tanks.

Clinical Manifestations. The patients described to date have been adults in whom pneumonia developed during hospitalization or within several days after discharge. It is not unreasonable to suspect, however, that this agent may also cause pneumonia in children who are immunosuppressed.

Initial clinical manifestations are mild. If fever is not present at the onset, it usually develops. There may be pleuritic pain, cough, and production of sputum. Disease has progressed in all patients despite treatment with broad-spectrum antibiotics and in several instances with antituberculous therapy as well. The hospital course of surviving patients was one of gradual, slow clinical improvement and even slower resolution of roentgenographic findings, which included patchy pneumonic infiltrates and nodular and well circumscribed ones as well as pleural effusions.

Diagnosis. This depends upon an awareness that this new agent has been described and a high index of suspicion of the possibility of this disease in patients who are immunosuppressed. Lung biopsies that reveal gram-indifferent or gram-negative bacilli that are also weakly acid-fast can be cultured in embryonated eggs or guinea pigs. *Legionella micdadei* can be identified by direct fluorescent antibody examination of lung tissue. Serum antibody to the PPA can be detected by an indirect fluorescent antibody (IFA) technique.

Treatment. Erythromycin has been suggested as the drug of choice; rifampin and trimethoprim-sulfamethoxazole appear to be efficacious in vitro. Most investigators suggest erythromycin as the drug of choice.

Prognosis. The prognosis is poor, a fact that may be related to the nature of the underlying disease and the abnormal state of the host rather than to the virulence of the organism.

RALPH D. FEIGIN

Cordes LG, Myerowitz RL, Pasculle AW, et al: *Legionella micdadei* (Pittsburgh pneumonia agent): Direct fluorescent-antibody examination of infected human lung tissue and characterization of clinical isolates. J Clin Microbiol 13:720, 1981.

Muder RR, Yu VL, Zuravleth JJ: Pneumonia due to Pittsburgh pneumonia agent: New clinical perspective with a review of the literature. Medicine 62:120, 1983.

Myerowitz RL, Pasculle AW, Dowling JN, et al: Opportunistic lung infection due to "Pittsburgh pneumonia agent." N Engl J Med 301:953, 1979.

Pasculle AW, Myerowitz RL, Rinaldo CR Jr: New bacterial agent of pneumonia isolated from renal-transplant recipients. Lancet 2:58, 1979.

11.44 ACTINOMYCOSIS

Actinomycosis, a chronic granulomatous disease of man and animals characterized by abscess formation, multiple draining sinuses, and subcutaneous spread of infection, is caused by an anaerobic actinomycete of the genus *Actinomyces*. The infection may involve the cervicofacial region, the thorax, the abdomen, and the pelvis, and disseminated actinomycosis has been described.

Etiology. *Actinomyces* are slow-growing gram-positive filamentous bacilli that are infrequently isolated in the laboratory because of their strict anaerobic requirements. Human disease is principally due to *A. israelii*; other species, including *A. naeslundii*, *A. viscosus*, and *A. odontolyticus*, have been incriminated.

Epidemiology. Actinomycosis is distributed worldwide but is decreasing in incidence in the United States. It is uncommon in children and more common in males than females by a ratio of 4:1. *Actinomyces* are not found free in nature but are normal inhabitants of the nasopharynx and gastrointestinal tract. Infection occurs when these bacteria enter damaged tissue following infection, trauma, or surgical instrumentation, usually producing concurrent infection with other anaerobic bacteria.

Pathology. Actinomycosis is characterized by areas of suppuration surrounded by extensive fibrosis. Sinus tract formation is common and may extend to the skin surface or into internal organs. "Sulfur granules" are scattered throughout the suppurative areas and appear in tissue secretions as rounded basophilic masses representing clumps of microorganisms cemented together and surrounded by reactive cells. These hard, yellow-white granules (diameter of about 2 mm) are more common in infections with *A. israelii* but have been observed in infections caused by other actinomyces, fungi, nocardia, and staphylococci.

Clinical Manifestations. *Cervicofacial actinomycosis*, the most common form of infection in children, is caused by microorganisms that gain access to the subcutaneous tissue of the neck from an infected tooth or after surgery or other trauma to the teeth and oral mucous membranes. An enlarging area of painless swelling is noted along the margin of the mandible from where the fluctuance gradually extends into the neck. The overlying skin becomes tense and develops a red or purple hue, and the mass is characteristically "woody" or indurated. With time, draining cutaneous fistulas appear, and the mass may temporarily decrease in size. Involvement of lymph nodes, the thyroid gland, and underlying bone is uncommon. Pain is minimal, and the child has no evidence of systemic disease. Roentgenographic examination is typically normal; however, with longstanding disease periosteal reaction and bone destruction become apparent.

Thoracic actinomycosis is uncommon in children; it occurs following aspiration of infected oral secretions or, less commonly, after extension of esophageal disease into the mediastinum. The clinical pattern is one of chronic pulmonary infection with fever, night sweats, weight loss, chest pain, productive cough, and hemoptysis. Extension of the pulmonary disease, which most often involves the lower lobes, may lead to pleural involvement; however, massive empyema and the classic findings of a draining chest-wall sinus discharging granules are rarely seen. Involvement of the heart and other mediastinal structures is uncommon. Roentgenographic examination is not characteristic but may demonstrate an extensive pulmonary lesion (at times with cavitation) involving the chest wall that may be associated with destruction of ribs, sternum, and shoulder girdle.

Abdominal actinomycosis may follow surgical treatment of an acute appendicitis or a perforated abdominal viscus and present as abdominal pain with fever, weight loss, and a palpable mass in the ileocecal region. Intra-abdominal extension occurs and may involve the entire abdomen. Diagnosis is often delayed. A small percentage of cases of actinomycosis involve the female pelvic organs; these characteristically occur in women using an intrauterine contraceptive device.

Diagnosis. The diagnosis of actinomycosis is established by demonstrating sulfur granules in biopsy material and/or gram-positive filamentous bacilli with branching hyphae in an area of suppuration and by isolating the actinomyces anaerobically.

Treatment. Prolonged antibiotic therapy, surgical drainage of abscesses, and excision of infected tissue are indicated. Massive doses of penicillin (400,000 units/kg/24 hr) given intravenously for 6–8 wk followed by oral penicillin (phenoxymethyl penicillin 2–4 g/24 hr) for an additional 6–12 mo are used to treat deep-seated infections. In patients allergic to penicillin, therapeutic success has been obtained with chloramphenicol, rifampin, erythromycin, tetracyclines, and clindamycin, alone or in combination.

Drake DD, Holt RJ: Childhood actinomycosis—report of 3 recent cases. Arch Dis Child 51:979, 1976.

Lerner PI: Susceptibility of pathogenic actinomycetes to antimicrobial compounds. Antimicrob Agents Chemother 5:302, 1974.

11.45 NOCARDIOSIS

Nocardiosis is a subacute or chronic suppurative disease of man and animals which occurs following inoculation of the skin, gastrointestinal tract, or lungs with a soil-borne actinomycete of the genus *Nocardia*. Infection in man usually presents as 1 of 4 distinct clinical syndromes: pulmonary, cutaneous, disseminated, and central nervous system disease.

Etiology. *Nocardia* species are aerobic, gram-positive, weakly acid-fast bacilli with delicate branching hyphae that appear microscopically as fragmented coccobacillary elements. These microorganisms are nonfastidious and grow over a wide temperature range (25–37° C) on a number of antibiotic-free culture media. *N. asteroides* is the dominant human pathogen in the United States and Europe and is most often responsible for systemic nocardiosis. Other human pathogens include *N. brasiliensis* and *N. caviae*, which are typically associated with localized infection of the skin and adjacent soft tissue. *N. farcinica*, an animal pathogen, may also infect man.

Epidemiology. Nocardiosis is being diagnosed with increasing frequency in the United States; it is estimated that 500–1000 culture-proven cases occur annually. Nocardiosis occurs at any age but is more frequent in adults; there is no particular geographic distribution; males are affected twice as often as females; and it occurs almost exclusively as an opportunistic infection in immunosuppressed patients. The respiratory tract is the initial site of involvement in 70% of cases.

Pathology. Nocardiosis produces a suppurative lesion characterized by tissue necrosis and abscess formation which microscopically resemble those of the common pyogenic bacteria. Branching filaments of *Nocardia* are often scattered throughout the area of suppuration; granule formation is uncommon. There is little localization other than an occasional wall of loose granulation tissue, and local spread involving the formation of satellite abscesses is common. Hematogenous dissemination from a pulmonary focus occurs in approximately one third of patients. The heart, liver, and spleen are occasionally sites of secondary infection, but the central nervous system is the site most often affected; this infection presents as a poorly encapsulated multilocular brain abscess.

Clinical Manifestations. In the United States nocardiosis typically presents as a subacute or chronic pulmonary infection in an immunocompromised patient with debilitating underlying disease. Pulmonary involvement begins as a confluent bronchopneumonia which progresses to consolidation, cavitation, pleural effusion, and empyema formation. The clinical findings include fever, night sweats, a productive cough, anorexia, weight loss, dyspnea, and chest pain. Without treatment, the course is chronic and may simulate tuberculosis. Clinical manifestations may also include tracheitis, bronchitis, pericarditis, and mediastinitis with obstruction of the superior vena cava. Extension through the chest wall and subcutaneous abscess formation are extremely rare. Patients whose disease is complicated by hematogenous dissemination may present with multiple subcutaneous abscesses and diffuse organ involvement. Brain abscesses may dominate the clinical picture and by extension lead to purulent meningitis. The cutaneous lesion is characterized by localized swelling involving the subcutaneous tissue with multiple sinus tracts that lead to the surface as well as to the bone. The purulent drainage through the sinuses may contain granules (compact colonies of microorganisms surrounded by reactive cells); their size, shape, and color may suggest the specific nocardial strain.

Diagnosis. The clinical manifestations may point to a diagnosis of nocardiosis. Branching gram-positive filamentous bacilli in sputum, bronchoscopic washings, pleural fluid, or material obtained by lung aspiration suggest the diagnosis of nocardiosis or actinomycosis. *Nocardia* are distinguished by the absence (usually) of granule formation and their acid-fast staining characteristics. Diagnosis by culture is difficult, especially in the case of heavily contaminated specimens.

Treatment and Prognosis. Sulfonamides (150 mg/kg/24 hr) in combination with appropriate surgical drainage of abscesses is the treatment of choice for nocardiosis. Antimicrobial susceptibility testing is helpful in selecting alternative therapeutic regimens when sulfonamides cannot be administered because of allergy or intolerance. Alternative drugs (cefotaxime, cefuroxime, minocycline, erythromycin, ampicillin, tobramycin, and amikacin) may be used in combination with sulfonamides in patients with serious, life-threatening infections. However, the efficacy of combination treatment for nocardiosis is not established. Therapy should be continued for a minimum of 6 wk, but sulfonamide administration is often continued for many months after apparent cure because nocardiosis tends to relapse. With sulfonamide therapy, the mortality rate for all forms of the disease has fallen from 75 to 40%; only 35% of patients with disseminated disease survive.

Curry WA: Human nocardiosis—a clinical review with selected case reports. Arch Intern Med 140:818, 1980.

Law BJ, Marks MI: Pediatric nocardiosis. Pediatrics 70:560, 1982.

Lerner PI, Baum GL: Antimicrobial susceptibility of *Nocardia* species. Antimicrob Agents Chemother 4:85, 1973.

Simpson GL, Stinson EB, Egger MJ, et al: Nocardial infections in the immunocompromised host: A detailed study in a defined population. Rev Infect Dis 3:492, 1981.

11.46 TUBERCULOSIS

The incidence of tuberculosis has decreased progressively, and sometimes dramatically, as the general standard of living and health status of children have increased in the United States, Europe, Japan, and other developed countries over the past century. In the United States it was the 8th leading cause of death by 1920 for children 1–4 yr of age, and by 1960 it was not one of the top 10 causes of death for any age group of children. This is in stark contrast to the persistent high incidence today in developing countries.

The modern epidemic of tuberculosis, "the white plague," began in the United Kingdom during the Industrial Revolution of the 18th century and spread to the United States, where the incidence peaked in the middle of the 19th century. The North American epidemic began in the northeast where European immigrants settled in overcrowded urban environments, spread west and south following the movement of settlers, and was particularly severe among American Indians and Eskimos, populations having minimal acquired immunity because of lack of exposure. Tuberculosis epidemics among these previously unexposed populations caused a secondary peak incidence of the disease in the early part of this century, but the incidence throughout the rest of the population began to decline owing to improved health status, increased immunity, and reduced urban overcrowding. This decline preceded the development of diagnostic and therapeutic tools. In the United States the incidence of childhood tuberculosis has remained constant since 1976, although the incidence in adults over 60 yr has increased so that they play a major role in spreading this disease.

Etiology. Tuberculosis is caused by tubercle bacillus, a member of the Mycobacteriaceae family, order Actinomycetales. In humans, the most common tubercle bacilli are *Mycobacterium tuberculosis*, responsible for most infections, and *M. bovis. M. africanum* is a rare cause of tuberculosis in West and Central Africa. Other "anonymous" or "atypical" mycobacteria exist as human pathogens and are discussed in Sec. 11.47.

All mycobacteria are aerobic, nonmotile, nonsporulating, pleomorphic rods. They are difficult to stain because of the high lipid content of their cell walls, and once stained they resist decoloration with acid-alcohol, the reason they are commonly described as being acid-fast. The Ziehl-Neelsen technique stains the bacilli red with carbolfuchsin dye so that they can be identified under oil immersion ($100\times$) against a background stained with methylene blue. The fluorochrome technique stains the mycobacteria with auramine-rhodamine dyes, which fluoresce yellow-green under ultraviolet light, allowing detection of the bacilli under low power ($25\times$) magnification; this increases sensitivity for identifying small numbers of bacilli in clinical specimens. The major disadvantage of the fluorochrome stain is that both viable and nonviable microorganisms become stained, preventing the assessment of the specimen's infectivity.

M. tuberculosis microorganisms are slow-growing; the average recovery time is 21 days, and occasional strains require 4–6 wk. Growth is best obtained using selective media incubated aerobically at 37° C in a carbon dioxide–enriched atmosphere. Growth can usually be detected within 2 wk by using radiolabeled nutrients in selective liquid media (Bactec radiometric system), but a major disadvantage of this system is that early speciation cannot be performed.

M. tuberculosis is differentiated from other mycobacterial strains by morphology of the colony, absence of pigment, production of niacin, ability to reduce nitrates, presence of a heat-labile catalase, and sensitivity to isoniazid. (*M. tuberculosis* strains resistant to isoniazid fail to produce niacin.) "Atypical" mycobacteria grow more rapidly than *M. tubercu-*

losis, produce no niacin, fail to reduce nitrates, produce heat-stable catalase, and are highly resistant to isoniazid. Newer techniques for rapidly classifying mycobacteria are based upon the detection of specific antigens using either agglutination reactions or enzyme-linked immunosorbent assays.

Epidemiology. The principal route of infection with *M. tuberculosis* is by the inhalation of contaminated droplets. (*M. bovis* can be transmitted by consumption of milk from infected cattle, but in developed countries, pasteurization of milk and elimination of diseased animals has nearly eradicated this route.) Droplets of aerosolized pulmonary secretions, produced by coughing and sneezing, are small enough to remain suspended in air and, when inhaled, can reach the terminal bronchioles and alveoli. The infectivity of these droplets depends on the number of microorganisms present, which is greatest in secretions from individuals with culture-positive sputum or cavitary pulmonary disease. Accordingly, primary infection in children (conversion to a positive tuberculin skin test) most often occurs following prolonged, close contact with an untreated adult with cavitary disease. Although genitourinary secretions from infected individuals may contain microorganisms, transmission following urine aerosolization is uncommon. Similarly, transmission following contact with infectious discharges (for example, drainage from open sinuses), contaminated objects, or household pets (dogs can acquire the infection from humans) is uncommon.

Immunology. The immune response to tuberculosis involves a series of interactions between the tubercle bacilli, specific lymphocyte subpopulations, and tissue macrophages. The various classes of antibodies produced during infection play no role in inhibiting bacterial growth or creating subsequent immunity. A cellular immune response begins after viable microorganisms are inhaled; pulmonary macrophages ingest the bacilli but are ineffective in killing them, and the bacilli proliferate. Infection subsequently spreads to the regional lymph nodes, followed by lymphatic and hematogenous dissemination and the establishment of many infected extrapulmonary foci.

Although the pulmonary macrophages do not kill the ingested microorganisms, macrophages are capable of processing mycobacterial antigens and presenting them to circulating T lymphocytes, which are activated by the antigens. These T lymphocytes proliferate and circulate throughout the lymphatic system and produce a number of soluble mediators, lymphokines. Lymphokines attract circulating lymphocytes and monocytes to sites of lymphocyte-antigen interaction, activate macrophages, and thereby enhance the intracellular killing of ingested microorganisms and promote differentiation of pulmonary macrophages into epithelioid cells and fibroblasts. In the presence of numerous tubercle bacilli, activated lymphocytes may also produce cytotoxic substances which, along with hydrolytic enzymes released from living and dead pulmonary macrophages, cause incomplete or caseation necrosis. In the lungs, liquefaction of this caseous material may cause the formation of cavities and a massive increase in the number of tubercle bacilli. Normally these immunologic processes occur over a 6–10 wk period and contain the primary infection and eliminate metastatic foci.

A number of factors can interfere with developing natural immunity, predisposing an individual to life-threatening infection. *Genetic* factors seem to influence morbidity and mortality. Studies of twins suggest concordance for severe infection in identical twins, and recent data indicate that severe infection is more common among individuals exhibiting certain HLA histocompatibility antigens. Although certain ethnic groups (American Indians and Eskimos) are predisposed to serious infection, these populations are also affected by *demographic* and *socioeconomic* variables. *Age* also affects the severity of infection: children under 3 yr of age have a high mortality rate due to miliary tuberculosis and meningitis. This may be the result of an immature immunologic response, or may reflect the relatively higher inoculum of infectious organisms received by a young child. A variety of factors that interfere with T-cell function also predispose to serious illness: *malnutrition*, various *infections* including rubeola and pertussis, *pregnancy*, *reticuloendothelial disease*, and *cancer* of the lymphatic system. Initial tuberculous infection may be more severe or dormant infection may be reactivated in patients treated with *immunosuppressive drugs*, including corticosteroids.

Diagnostic Skin Tests. The tuberculin skin test, which is based on the detection of delayed hypersensitivity to the antigens of *M. tuberculosis*, is a reliable diagnostic technique. An infected patient responds positively within 6–10 wk of infection. The test consists of an intradermally administered antigen preparation; a positive response is indicated by the appearance of induration, which results from migration of activated lymphocytes and macrophages to the site of antigen deposition. Two antigen preparations are available, *old tuberculin* (OT) and *purified protein derivative* (PPD). OT is a crude product prepared by heat sterilization of filtrates of culture medium containing *M. tuberculosis*. It is utilized only for multiple-puncture skin tests.

The PPD is a protein precipitate derived from OT. Its dosage is expressed in terms of tuberculin units (TU) using a single lot (PPD-S) as the biologic standard against which all PPD preparations are compared. (One TU is 0.00002 mg PPD-S.) Three dosage strengths are available: a first strength PPD (1 TU per 0.1 mL), an intermediate strength PPD (5 TU per 0.1 mL), and a second strength PPD (250 TU per 0.1 mL). Several precautions are taken to preserve the potency of PPD preparations. The protein derivative is provided as a dried powder to be diluted with buffered saline prior to use. To prevent absorption of protein to the walls of glass and plastic containers, a small amount of detergent (Tween 80) is added to the PPD diluent. In addition, after the solution has been prepared, it must be kept refrigerated (4° C) and be kept in the dark to preserve its potency. PPD, the preferred skin test antigen, is available for use in multiple-puncture skin tests and in the intracutaneous Mantoux test.

Several multiple-puncture skin tests are available and have been successfully used for mass screening of pediatric patients. These sensitive techniques lack specificity, so that patients with positive or doubtful reactions must be retested with the Mantoux test (see below). The *Tine test*, the most widely used multiple-puncture skin test, uses a disposable plastic unit with four stainless steel blades (tines) predipped in OT and is usually applied to the volar surface of the forearm after cleansing the skin with alcohol or acetone. The test is interpreted after 48–72 hr. A positive reaction consists of vesiculation with one or more papules measuring at least 2 mm in diameter. The *Aplitest* is similar to the Tine test, except that the four steel prongs are coated with PPD preserved in phenol. The *Heaf test* uses a special device (Heaf gun) that makes six simultaneous skin punctures 1 mm deep through a layer of concentrated PPD. The test is read 3–7 days afterward, and the presence of four or more papules constitutes a positive reaction. False-positive reactions are common for all of the multiple-puncture skin tests; therefore, all positive or doubtful reactions must be confirmed with a Mantoux test.

The *Mantoux test* is more difficult to administer than the multiple-puncture skin test, but because it delivers a defined amount of antigen, it is more reliable. One-tenth milliliter of intermediate strength PPD (5 TU) is injected intracutaneously into the volar surface of the forearm. A single-dose plastic syringe with a short needle (26 or 27 gauge) is used, with the beveled side up. A weal 6–10 mm in diameter should appear during the injection, and the withdrawal of the needle is delayed for a brief time in order to minimize leakage of PPD at the puncture site. The site of antigen injection is examined for induration after 48–72 hr. A 10 mm induration reaction after 48 hr indicates infection with the tubercle bacillus (erythema without induration is not considered a positive response); 5–10 mm of induration is considered "doubtful." A reaction of less than 5 mm induration in a well child is "negative," although anergy must be ruled out by demonstrating that the patient is able to show a positive skin test to mumps (after MMR vaccination) or to *Candida* antigen.

The most common cause of a "doubtful" response to the Mantoux is infection with "atypical" mycobacteria. PPD contains antigens common to nontuberculous strains of mycobacteria. This cross-reactivity is seen more frequently when a dose of 250 TU is used in the test. Under certain circumstances, reactions of 5 to 10 mm of induration might be termed "suspicious," and an indication for therapeutic intervention. For example:

1. In some areas of the United States, such as Alaska, atypical mycobacterial infections are uncommon, and so cross-reactivity is an unlikely cause of the doubtful response.

2. A response of less than 10 mm induration in a young infant should be considered "suspicious" if the patient has signs and symptoms compatible with tuberculosis or a history of contact with an active case.

False-negative responses to the Mantoux test can arise from a number of causes. A significant fraction of patients (as many as 20%) with culture-proven tuberculosis have negative skin test reactions during the early phase of their illness, even when skin testing is performed with 250 TU. The test itself can be inadequate because of loss of potency of the PPD from improper storage or bacterial contamination, improper administration of the antigen, or inadequate concentration (1 TU) of antigen. Any factor that interferes with lymphocyte activation and the delayed hypersensitivity reaction can prevent a patient from showing a positive response, including extremes in age (infants less than 6 mo), overwhelming illness of any type (including tuberculosis), coincident viral infections (rubeola and influenza), immunization with an attenuated virus vaccine, treatment with immunosuppressive agents (including corticosteroids), malnutrition, neoplastic disease (especially Hodgkin and non-Hodgkin lymphoma), sarcoidosis, and chronic renal failure.

False-positive responses to the Mantoux test can occur because of repeated skin testing with PPD or OT or because of prior immunization with bacillus Calmette-Guérin (BCG). Immunization with BCG may result in a tuberculin reaction that is difficult to distinguish from that due to *M. tuberculosis* infections. However, the positive response in the Mantoux test due to BCG immunization is induration, which rarely exceeds 10 mm and is strongest within the first few years after immunization. Accordingly, any reaction that exceeds 10 mm and occurs more than 3 years following immunization should be considered an indication of tuberculous infection.

CLINICAL FORMS OF TUBERCULOSIS
Intrathoracic

Pathogenesis and Pathology. Primary infection with tubercle bacilli usually occurs following inhalation of viable microorganisms. In the nonimmune child it is characterized at the cellular level by phagocytosis and intracellular multiplication of tubercle bacilli, spread from the pulmonary alveolus to regional lymph nodes, lymphadenitis and subsequent lymphatic/hematogenous dissemination, and the establishment of metastatic infection throughout the lung, the reticuloendothelial system, and other organ systems. In the absence of cell-mediated immunity, tissue damage is minimal, and signs and symptoms are absent. In most children the development

of acquired immunity over 6–10 wk results in healing and calcification of pulmonary and extrapulmonary foci. The surviving bacilli remain dormant indefinitely, particularly in the apical or subapical regions of the lung. Any condition, either local or systemic, that modifies cellular immunity may permit multiplication of dormant microorganisms and reactivation of pulmonary and/or extrapulmonary foci. Reactivation, which is also called postprimary or "adult tuberculosis," is most often a localized infection occurring in the presence of cell-mediated immunity, resulting in extensive tissue damage and producing signs and symptoms.

Primary Pulmonary Tuberculosis

Clinical Manifestations. In *older infants and children* (age 3–15 years) primary pulmonary tuberculosis is typically an asymptomatic illness identified in a child with a positive tuberculin skin test and often a normal chest roentgenogram. Constitutional symptoms, when present, are mild and nonspecific and include low grade fever of several days' duration, reduced appetite, and weight loss. *Erythema nodosum* and *phlyctenular keratoconjunctivitis* are rarely noted.

Additional symptoms may occur secondary to the massive lymph node involvement that is characteristic of primary infection, e.g., compression, obstruction, and/or erosion of mediastinal structures by enlarged lymph nodes. Nonpulmonary symptoms following subcarinal nodal enlargement and esophageal compression may include dysphagia and recurrent aspiration. Compression of major blood vessels may also occur, resulting in edema of an extremity or in the superior vena caval syndrome. Nodal compression of the recurrent laryngeal nerve or the phrenic nerve may be associated with vocal cord or diaphragmatic paralysis. Pulmonary symptoms secondary to enlargement of the paratracheal/parabronchial nodes include recurrent cough, stridor, and wheezing. Prolonged compression of these latter structures may result in lobar emphysema or segmental atelectasis of one or more lobes. Complete bronchial erosion accompanied by a discharge of caseum into the adjacent or distal airways may occur, resulting in signs and symptoms of acute pneumonia. However, in most children primary pulmonary infection is a mild, asymptomatic illness that resolves over a brief period of time with or without effective chemotherapy.

In *older children and adolescents* primary pulmonary tuberculosis commonly presents as an enlarging upper lobe infiltrate and cavitation in the absence of calcification and lymphadenitis. However, in some patients it may be associated with the adenitis and middle or lower lobe involvement seen in younger infants and children.

In *young infants and children* up to 3 yr signs and symptoms may coincide with hematogenous/lymphatic dissemination that is due to miliary-meningeal disease.

Diagnosis. Primary pulmonary tuberculosis is most often diagnosed in an asymptomatic infant by means of a positive tuberculin test. Routine laboratory examinations are not helpful. Roentgenographic examination of the chest is often normal; however, unilateral, often massive, hilar adenopathy with or without a small parenchymal focus in the lower or middle lung fields may be observed, and calcification may occur during the healing process. A diagnosis requires bacteriologic confirmation. Acid-fast bacilli may be found in sputum; these cultures are usually positive. However, microbial confirmation may be difficult in young infants with primary infection since infants may not cough and sputum, when produced, is usually promptly swallowed. Pulmonary secretions may be obtained using fiberoptic bronchoscopy. Examining gastric contents may replace sputum examination in young infants and should be carried out early in the morning in a fasting child, preferably upon awakening. Gastric contents are gently aspirated through a nasogastric tube and placed into a sterile container. Following this initial aspiration, the stomach should be lavaged with 30 mL of water and again aspirated. This material should be added to the initial specimen. This procedure should be repeated on at least two occasions on separate days. The material should be immediately transported to the laboratory for staining and culture.

Progressive Primary Pulmonary Tuberculosis

Progressive primary infection occurs when the primary focus of infection, instead of resolving, enlarges to involve the entire middle and/or lower lobes. It is uncommon except in immunosuppressed patients. Intrathoracic adenopathy is common, and cavitation, when present, may be associated with endobronchial dissemination to other portions of the lung. Symptoms are prominent and include elevated temperature, malaise, anorexia, weight loss, and productive cough. Physical findings and roentgenography demonstrate hilar adenopathy, middle or lower lobe pneumonia, and cavity formation. Diagnosis depends on bacterial confirmation.

Reactivation (Reinfection) Tuberculosis

Reactivation tuberculosis (also known as chronic or adult pulmonary tuberculosis) is uncommon in children, particularly when primary infection has occurred at less than 3 yr of age. Infection is often confined to the apical or posterior segments of the upper lobes or to the superior segments of the lower lobes, both of which contain conditions that favor the growth of tubercle bacilli disseminated during the lymphatic/hematogenous phase of primary infection. The initial infiltrate expands and undergoes cavitation, often in association with endobronchial dissemination. Intrathoracic lymphadenopathy is uncommon. The most prominent symptom is low grade fever, which may be associated with "night sweats" when defervescence occurs during sleep. Additional symptoms include malaise, fatigue, and weight loss. With the development of caseation necrosis, liquefaction, and cavitation, a productive cough develops, often associated with mild hemoptysis. Physical findings are usually confined to the apices of the lungs and consist of fine or post-tussive rales. The earliest roentgenographic change consists of a well-circumscribed, homogeneous shadow most commonly seen in the apex of the lung. As the infiltrate enlarges, it may result in lobar consolidation. Following liquefaction necrosis, the classic thick-walled cavities that lack air-fluid levels become visible.

Pleural Effusion

Pleural effusion due to discharge of tubercle bacilli into the pleural space from a subpleural focus is an uncommon complication of primary pulmonary tuberculosis. Pleural effusion may also be secondary to hematogenous dissemination; these effusions are often bilateral and associated with pericarditis and peritonitis. Although the pleural effusion frequently may resolve spontaneously, recognizing its tuberculous etiology is important; such effusions may be followed within a few years by reactivation tuberculosis, and this can be prevented by administering antituberculosis drugs. Effusions due to tuberculosis must be differentiated from effusions secondary to congestive heart failure, malignant disease, metabolic disturbances, or collagen vascular disease and the parapneumonic effusions caused by other infectious agents. Tuberculous effusions are exudates that have a specific gravity of 1.012 to 1.022, an elevated protein content (greater than 4 g/dL), high concentrations of LDH and adenosine deaminase, and a low glucose level (less than 30 mg/dL). Cytologic examination reveals an absence of mesothelial cells and a predominance of lymphocytes, although neutrophils may predominate early in the course. Acid-fast stains of the pleural fluid are usually negative, but positive cultures of fluid and pleural tissue may be obtained in more than half the cases. Repeated thoracentesis and centrifugation of large quantities of fluid increase the yield of positive cultures. Pleural biopsies should be obtained in all cases, preferably at the time of initial thoracentesis, since a biopsy specimen is difficult to obtain in the absence of pleural fluid. Histologic examination of the pleural tissue reveals granulomas in a majority of cases. In patients with a positive tuberculin skin test, a pleural effusion should always be considered tuberculous until proven otherwise. Similarly, an unexplained effusion in the presence of a negative tuberculin skin test mandates repeating the test within 2–3 wk. The natural history of these effusions is gradual resorption. Repeated thoracenteses and tube drainage are contraindicated.

Extrathoracic

Tuberculosis of the Upper Respiratory Tract

Involvement of the upper respiratory tract (larynx, epiglottis, pharynx, and middle ear) is now rare, although prior to the availability of effective chemotherapy it was a common complication of advanced pulmonary disease. It is still observed in developing countries. Children with laryngeal tuberculosis almost always have cavitary pulmonary disease, and symptoms include a croupy cough, sore throat, hoarseness, and pain on swallowing. Tuberculous otitis is associated with profound hearing loss, diffuse otorrhea, absence of pain, and pre- and/or postauricular adenopathy. Facial nerve involvement and mastoiditis are common. Otoscopic examination reveals a thickened tympanic membrane with one or more perforations. The treatment of upper respiratory tuberculosis depends on the extent of the concurrent pulmonary disease. A two-drug regimen consisting of isoniazid and rifampin for 18–24 mo is usually indicated. Surgical intervention is indicated in the presence of facial nerve paralysis, a subperiosteal abscess, and/or mastoiditis.

Tuberculosis of Lymph Nodes

The involvement of superficial and deep lymph nodes is common in tuberculosis. In children, the hilar nodes are the principal site of lymphadenitis, and local spread may involve the paratracheal, supraclavicular, deep cervical, and abdominal nodes. Adenitis secondary to a primary focus in an extremity is less common and results in inguinal or axillary lymphadenopathy. Adenopathy may follow the hematogenous or lymphatic dissemination of tubercle bacilli during the nonimmune phase of primary infection and affect superficial and deep lymph nodes. Superficial lymphadenitis, the most common form of nonrespiratory tuberculosis, is found most often in the head and neck and usually affects multiple nodes. Bilateral involvement is common. In order of decreasing frequency, it may involve the anterior and posterior cervical (scrofula), supraclavicular, and submandibular nodes and occasionally the preauricular and submental nodes.

Clinical Manifestations. The course of tuberculous lymphadenitis is insidious, but in children highly sensitive to tuberculin the illness may be acute with elevated temperature and perinodal inflammation. History often includes exposure to active tuberculosis. The tuberculin skin test is positive in most patients (90%), and the chest roentgenogram usually demonstrates evidence of primary pulmonary tuberculous. Occasionally lymph nodes may become very large and compress adjacent structures. Thus, mediastinal hilar adenopathy may result in compression of the trachea, bronchi, major blood vessels, recurrent laryngeal nerve, or thoracic duct. Enlargement of superficial lymph nodes may lead to rupture into surrounding tissue and formation of a cutaneous sinus tract. On physical examination, the nodes are nontender, firm, and discrete. Less often the nodes are fluctuant and adhere to overlying skin. Sinus tract formation is uncommon.

Diagnosis and Differential Diagnosis. A definitive diagnosis requires histologic and bacteriologic confirmation, which is best accomplished by total excisional biopsy of the involved node(s); excision of a caseous node or nodes may also limit the need for long-term antimicrobial treatment. Partial biopsy or needle aspiration is less satisfactory and may result in sinus tract formation. Histologic examination reveals non-caseating granulomas, and acid-fast stains are usually positive. Tuberculous and atypical mycobacterial lymphadenitis cannot be differentiated histologically; therefore, all biopsy material must be cultured in appropriate media.

Tuberculous lymphadenitis can be confused with other conditions. Although *M. tuberculosis* is the predominant cause of mycobacterial cervical adenitis in adults, the atypical mycobacteria cause most cervical adenitis in children. The differential diagnosis also includes lymphadenitis due to viruses, bacteria, fungi, toxoplasma, and the agent(s) causing cat scratch disease. Noninfectious causes of lymphadenopathy, including malignancy, sarcoidosis, and drug reaction (to phenytoin), must also be considered.

Treatment. Tuberculous lymphadenitis responds to therapy with isoniazid and either rifampin or ethambutol, prescribed for a minimum of 18 mo. Recent studies suggest that a 9 mo regimen of isoniazid and rifampin supplemented initially with ethambutol for 8 wk is an adequate regimen for adults with tuberculosis of the lymph nodes. Transient enlargement of nodes and/or the appearance of new nodes occurs in a minority of children during the initial phases of therapy but does not indicate failure of treatment or relapse. Residual nodes may be palpable following cure.

Miliary Tuberculosis

Miliary tuberculosis results from hematogenous spread of *M. tuberculosis* from an established focus, producing lesions that progress to necrosis and caseation in multiple organs. The granulomas are similar in size to and often resemble in appearance the millet seed, hence the term "miliary." In the era before chemotherapy, this was primarily a pediatric disease resulting from massive hematogenous dissemination of tubercle bacilli at the time of primary pulmonary infection and, along with meningitis, was responsible for most fatal cases of tuberculosis in infants and children. In developing countries where tuberculosis in children is common, miliary tuberculosis remains a disease of young children (more than one third of cases occur in children less than 3 yr) and usually presents within a year of primary infection. However, in the United States it is now more common in adults (more than one third of all cases occurring in individuals over 65 yr) with chronic disease and/or those receiving immunosuppressive therapy. Miliary tuberculosis also occurs in the acquired immunodeficiency syndrome (AIDS).

Clinical Manifestations. The onset in children is often abrupt and is characterized by temperature elevation (102–104° F), weakness, malaise, anorexia, and weight loss. Physical findings, which include lymphadenopathy, hepatomegaly, and splenomegaly, are nonspecific. Within weeks, respiratory signs and symptoms dominate the clinical picture; tachypnea, dyspnea, and cough are common and associated with diffuse rales over both lungs. Meningitis may be present, resulting in headache, lethargy, and nuchal rigidity. Less common physical findings include cutaneous metastasis and bilateral choroidal tubercles.

A different clinical picture is observed when small numbers of tubercle bacilli are discharged intermittently into the blood stream over an extended period of time. This condition, occurring more commonly in adults than in children, is designated *chronic hematogenous tuberculosis* or *protracted hematogenous tuberculosis*. It is characterized by continuous or intermittent fever, weakness, and weight loss extending over a period of weeks to months. Hepatomegaly, splenomegaly, and diffuse lymphadenopathy are common.

Diagnosis. Laboratory tests help little in diagnosing miliary tuberculosis. The white blood cell count may be normal, elevated, or depressed. Anemia and an elevated sedimentation rate are common. Monocytosis, thrombocytopenia, and evidence of disseminated intravascular coagulation are uncommon. There may be hyponatremia and hypokalemia, and abnormalities in liver function are common. The tuberculin skin test is usually positive, but patients may be anergic due to underlying immunosuppression or overwhelming disease. Thus, a negative skin test does not exclude the diagnosis. The chest roentgenogram is the single most important diagnostic test, typically revealing bilateral miliary infiltrates. However, it may be normal during the early stages, and roentgenographic examinations should be repeated when the index of suspicion is high.

Definitive diagnosis requires microbiologic evidence of *M. tuberculosis*. Accordingly, cultures of the urine, gastric aspirates, and cerebrospinal fluid must be obtained. A transbronchial lung biopsy with fiberoptic bronchoscopy, the diagnostic procedure of choice, will often reveal caseating and noncaseating granulomas and the presence of acid-fast bacilli. Culture of this material is usually positive.

Treatment. Isoniazid and rifampin combined with either ethambutol or streptomycin is indicated. If the organism is proved to be sensitive to isoniazid, a two-drug regimen consisting of isoniazid and either rifampin or ethambutol is continued for 12–18 mo. In severely ill patients with evidence of extensive pulmonary disease and hypoxemia, simultaneous administration of corticosteroids is indicated. However, there is no proof that treatment with corticosteroids improves survival.

Tuberculous Meningitis

Epidemiology. The incidence of tuberculous meningitis depends on the prevalence of tuberculosis. In the United States and other developed countries, the incidence has declined, but in the developing countries it remains a significant public health problem. Since tuberculous meningitis most often occurs in recently infected individuals, it has traditionally been considered a disease of infants and children, with symptoms developing within 6 mo of the primary pulmonary infection. However, in developed countries where the adult population includes a large number of tuberculin-negative individuals, it is primarily a disease of adults. Prior to the availability of effective therapy, tuberculous meningitis was invariably fatal, with most deaths occurring within weeks of initial presentation. While antimicrobial agents have improved the survival rate, serious sequelae are common.

Pathophysiology and Pathology. Metastatic foci of mycobacteria result from the hematogenous dissemination that occurs during the nonimmune phase of primary infection and/or miliary disease. In the central nervous system (CNS) these foci (tubercles) may be solitary, or may be scattered over the cerebral hemispheres and/or the meninges of the spinal cord. Tuberculous meningitis occurs when rupture of one or more of the subependymal tubercles or of a parameningeal focus (tuberculoma, spondylitis, otitis, or osteitis) discharges the tubercle bacilli and tuberculous antigens into the subarachnoid space. In an immune individual this results in a severe inflammatory reaction throughout the CNS. With time, a thick gelatinous exudate develops about the basal meninges, resulting in damage to cerebral arteries and veins, compression of the cranial nerves, and obliteration of the basal cisterns and ventricular foramina.

Clinical Manifestations. The symptoms are insidious and

involve three clinical stages: stage 1, a prodromal phase with nonspecific symptomatology; stage 2, the appearance of neurologic signs and symptoms; and stage 3, an alteration in the level of consciousness proceeding from stupor to coma. In children the earliest symptoms (stage 1) include apathy, mood changes, declining school performance, loss of appetite, nausea, vomiting, and low grade fever. Within a few weeks, neurologic signs and symptoms appear (stage 2). Irritability is increased, with older children complaining of headache. Neck stiffness accompanied by Kernig's and Brudzinski's signs may be present. Cranial nerve palsies are common and include ocular palsies (pupillary abnormalities, diplopia), facial palsy, decreased visual acuity, and deafness. Aphasia, slurred speech, disorientation, hemiplegia, ataxia, involuntary movements, and convulsions are not uncommon. Intracranial pressure, increased during this stage, may be associated with enlarging head circumference, a tense anterior fontanel, and, in older infants and children, papilledema. As the disease progresses (stage 3) evidence of diffuse cerebral dysfunction increases. In the terminal phase, children will demonstrate stupor, coma, decerebrate or decorticate posturing, irregular respiration, and/or fixed and dilated pupils.

Diagnosis. The most important factor in rapidly diagnosing tuberculous meningitis is maintaining a high index of suspicion in children with cerebrospinal fluid pleocytosis. The history often includes exposure to an individual with active tuberculosis, and the tuberculin skin test is usually positive. A negative skin test does not exclude the diagnosis even in a child with a positive mumps or *Candida* skin test and a negative reaction to second-strength PPD. Many children have evidence of concurrent pulmonary disease (hilar adenopathy, lower lobe infiltrate). Roentgenograms of the skull are normal unless the meningitis is associated with "split sutures" due to increased pressure or a calcified tuberculoma. CT scans often reveal periventricular lucencies, edema, infarctions, and hydrocephalus. Tuberculomas have been reported before, concurrent with or following tuberculous meningitis. Routine laboratory tests rarely help in establishing the diagnosis. Anemia and an elevated sedimentation rate are common. Hyponatremia and hypochloremia may be present when meningitis is complicated by the syndrome of inappropriate secretion of antidiuretic hormone.

Lumbar puncture reveals clear, colorless fluid under increased pressure. The cell count is elevated, although rarely exceeding 500 cells/mm,[3] having a predominance of lymphocytes; early in the course there may be a predominance of polymorphonuclear leukocytes. The spinal fluid glucose is below 40 mg/dL or less than half the value of a simultaneous blood glucose determination. The protein concentration is normal or slightly elevated (100–300 mg/dL) during the initial stages, but with time may exceed 1000 mg/dL. A low spinal fluid chloride concentration reflects a low serum chloride level due to prolonged vomiting or inappropriate secretion of antidiuretic hormone. Microscopic examination demonstrates acid-fast bacilli in 30% of patients. Bacilli may be better detected by allowing the cerebrospinal fluid to stand at room temperature for 24 hr and then staining the surface pellicle. Tubercle bacilli can usually be cultured from the spinal fluid. Culturing the sediment obtained following centrifugation of large volumes of cerebrospinal fluid increases the recovery of microorganisms. Measurement of cerebrospinal fluid adenosine deaminase activity, the radioactive bromide partition test, detection of bacterial metabolites by chromatographic techniques, and identification of soluble antigens and/or antibody by enzyme-linked immunosorbent assay and latex particle agglutination have been described but are not available in most laboratories.

Treatment. Isoniazid and rifampin are recommended by most authorities. Streptomycin or ethambutol is often added to this two-drug regimen during the initial 2 mo of treatment, after which treatment with isoniazid and rifampin is continued for an additional 10 mo. A four-drug regimen should be considered in children at risk for infection with drug-resistant organisms. Intrathecal medication (streptomycin or rifampin) is not indicated. Corticosteroids, however, are recommended during the initial phase of treatment (2–4 wk) despite the absence of well-controlled studies documenting their efficacy.

Prognosis. This is related to the patient's condition at the time of treatment. In stage 1 disease, a 100 per cent cure rate and low incidence of sequelae can be anticipated. In stage 2 illness, optimal treatment results in a cure rate of about 85%; neurologic defects can be demonstrated in approximately half the survivors. In stage 3 disease, a 50% survival has been reported, but most survivors have permanent handicaps.

Tuberculoma of the Central Nervous System

Tuberculomas are single or multiple, may appear at any time during the course of tuberculosis, and often present as a slowly expanding mass lesion. Symptoms include headache, visual or gait disturbances, and evidence of increased intracranial pressure. Skull roentgenograms may demonstrate calcifications in the tuberculoma (6%), and during the early stages the CT scan reveals a hypodense mass with ring enhancement and associated edema. Affected children usually have a history of exposure to active tuberculosis. A positive skin test and evidence of concurrent pulmonary disease (hilar adenopathy, lower lobe infiltrate, or pleural effusion) is present in a majority of affected children. Diagnosis is often confirmed at surgery; however, surgical removal is contraindicated, since most tuberculomas will resolve with medical management consisting of a three-drug regimen administered over 12–18 mo. Corticosteroids are usually administered during the first few weeks of treatment to decrease cerebral edema.

Tuberculosis of the Skin

See Sec. 24.25.

Tuberculosis of the Heart and Pericardium

Tuberculous pericarditis, a rare complication of childhood tuberculosis (see also Sec. 14.82), occurs secondary to rupture of a mediastinal lymph node into the pericardial space or to hematogenous dissemination. The signs and symptoms result from decreased cardiac output. Patients often present with fever, chest pain, dyspnea, and orthopnea. Physical examination reveals tachycardia, cardiomegaly, distant heart sounds, a pericardial friction rub, and, occasionally, a paradoxical pulse. Hepatomegaly and edema are common. The echocardiogram and electrocardiogram are abnormal due to the pericardial effusion. Evidence of extracardiac tuberculosis is uncommon, but the tuberculin skin test is invariably positive. Periocardiocentesis reveals clear fluid with cytologic and chemical abnormalities similar to those described for tuberculous pleuritis. The acid-fast stain is usually negative and the culture is positive for *M. tuberculosis* in less than half of the patients. Histologic examination and culture of pericardial tissue, which can be obtained at the time of a therapeutic pericardiocentesis, confirm the diagnosis. Treatment consists of isoniazid and either rifampin or ethambutol. Most authorities recommend a short course of corticosteroids in the hope of preventing constrictive pericarditis and the need for pericardial surgery.

Abdominal Tuberculosis

Gastrointestinal tuberculosis is uncommon in developed countries because of the early treatment of pulmonary tuberculosis, pasteurization of milk, and near-eradication of bovine tuberculosis. Disease is usually secondary to swallowing infectious respiratory secretions; the extent of pulmonary involvement correlates with the incidence of gastrointestinal tuberculosis. However, it can occur in the absence of pulmonary disease, presumably owing to spread from mediastinal or peritoneal lymph nodes.

Gastrointestinal tuberculosis may produce granulomatous disease with caseation necrosis throughout the gastrointestinal tract and involvement of regional lymph nodes. Infection of the esophagus and stomach, usually secondary to spread from caseous mediastinal or peritoneal lymph nodes, may present with dysphagia, abdominal pain, or pyloric obstruction. Involvement of the small intestine is more common and may be associated with obstruction, perforation, hemorrhage, fistula formation, and malabsorption. Tuberculosis of the cecum may be associated with a painful right lower quadrant mass, hemorrhage, and obstruction or diarrhea. Tuberculosis of the colon may be diffuse or localized and may present with a clinical picture indistinguishable from granulomatous or ulcerative colitis, resulting in obstruction, perforation, or hemorrhage. Anal involvement is uncommon and presents with abscess formation and fistulization. Tuberculosis is the most common cause of granulomatous hepatitis, which may be asymptomatic. Diagnosis of gastrointestinal tuberculosis requires histologic and bacteriologic examination of biopsy material obtained by endoscopy, exploratory laparotomy, or percutaneous needle biopsy.

Tuberculous peritonitis may occur with gastrointestinal tuberculosis secondary to rupture of a caseous abdominal lymph node, or less frequently secondary to spread from an intestinal focus or from the female genital tract. Symptoms include fever, anorexia, and intermittent or chronic abdominal pain. Weight loss and abdominal distention are common, and evidence of extraperitoneal tuberculosis is usually absent. The skin test is usually positive. Examination of the peritoneal fluid is rarely diagnostic (an exudative response with a predominance of lymphocytes); acid-fast bacilli are usually absent and the culture is positive in only 25 per cent of cases. Diagnosis requires histologic and microbiologic examination of biopsy material obtained by peritoneoscopy or laparotomy.

Treatment of gastrointestinal tuberculosis requires nutritional support and administration of antituberculous antibiotics. Most authorities recommend isoniazid and either rifampin or ethambutol for 12–18 mo.

Bone and Joint Tuberculosis

See Sec. 23.3 and 23.5.

Urogenital Tuberculosis

Urogenital tuberculosis, a late manifestation of primary pulmonary disease, most commonly involves the kidneys and is rare in children. Tubercle bacilli reach the renal cortex during the nonimmune hematogenous phase of primary infection and remain dormant for many years. Reactivation may subsequently occur with multiplication of the tubercle bacilli and resultant caseation, cavitation, and extension into the renal pelvis. The discharge of viable microorganisms into the renal collecting system may cause infection of the ureters, the bladder, and the urethra. In males, secondary infection may involve the seminal vesicles, prostate, and epididymis.

Clinical Manifestations. Many patients have inactive extragenital disease. Constitutional symptoms are uncommon and usually confined to the genitourinary system. Dysuria, frequency, and urgency may be the presenting symptoms. Flank pain and renal colic are uncommon. The tuberculin skin test is invariably positive, and most patients have hematuria and pyuria; proteinuria is uncommon. Intravenous urography is often abnormal and, depending on the extent of renal involvement, demonstrates cortical calcification, calyceal blunting, reflux, and hydronephrosis. Diagnosis requires bacteriologic

confirmation, which can be obtained in most patients by culturing morning urine specimens.

Tuberculous *orchitis* and *epididymitis* are rare in childhood, but when present they must be differentiated from infections due to nonmycobacterial pathogens.

Tuberculosis of the *female genital system* is also uncommon in children, but may involve the fallopian tubes (90%), the endometrium (50%) and/or the ovaries (20%). Infection of the cervix and vagina is extremely rare. Symptoms include pelvic discomfort, irregular menstruation, and vaginal discharge. Diagnosis requires histologic and microbiologic examination of endometrial tissue.

Treatment. Urogenital tuberculosis requires 12–18 mo of therapy with isoniazid and either rifampin or ethambutol.

Tuberculosis of the Eye

The most common sites of ocular involvement are the choroid, retina, iris, sclera, and cornea. Ocular infection is usually secondary to hematogenous dissemination of *M. tuberculosis,* and because of its vascularity, the uvea (iris, ciliary body, and choroid) is the tissue most often involved. Choroidal tubercles are the most common form seen in children. They appear as solitary or multiple gray to gray-white tubercles at the posterior pole of the eye. Acute tuberculous panophthalmitis and tuberculoma of the ciliary body are very rare. Tuberculous keratoconjunctivitis presents as a severe, often bilateral conjunctival infection. Differentiation of tuberculous from viral or bacterial (nonmycobacterial) infection is facilitated by the presence of preauricular lymphadenopathy and small ulcerative lesions present on the palpebral conjunctiva. Tubercle bacilli can frequently be recovered from these palpebral ulcerations. Ocular infection resulting from exogenous inoculation or extension from contiguous sites is uncommon.

CHEMOTHERAPY OF TUBERCULOSIS

Because studies determining both the duration of therapy and the most effective agent(s) have been performed primarily in adults, optimal chemotherapeutic treatment for children is not definitively established, and this situation is unlikely to change, given the smaller number of cases in children. The application of adult treatment regimens to pediatric patients often results in overtreatment of children because of the larger number of tubercle bacilli characteristic of adult cavitary disease. Although combination chemotherapy has been shown to enhance efficacy and to prevent the emergence of resistant strains in adults, a finding that has been applied to children, evidence in adults for shortening the duration of combination therapy is not considered sufficiently strong to modify the recommended prolonged course of chemotherapy for children.

Many children with tuberculosis can be adequately managed as outpatients. Hospitalization is recommended (1) when a repeat culture or biopsy is needed to establish the diagnosis, (2) for the initial treatment of extensive or life-threatening disease, (3) for initial treatment in young infants and children, (4) when surgical intervention or corticosteroid therapy is warranted, (5) for the treatment of severe drug reaction, (6) for treatment of coexisting illness requiring hospitalization, or (7) for initial treatment when family or social circumstances prevent adequate treatment from being obtained in the home. In this situation, the child should be discharged only after arrangements have been made to administer the medication under supervised conditions.

Antituberculosis Drugs

Isoniazid (INH), the drug of choice for tuberculosis, is included in all treatment regimens, unless the strain is suspected to be resistant. INH is usually administered orally as a single daily dose (10–20 mg/kg/24 hr) not to exceed 300 mg. At this dosage, determining whether patients are slow or rapid inactivators of INH is not necessary. It is well absorbed from the gastrointestinal tract, is widely distributed in body fluids and tissues, including the cerebrospinal fluid, and is metabolized in the liver and excreted via the kidneys.

Side effects of INH therapy are uncommon. Peripheral neuritis secondary to pyridoxine deficiency has been reported in adults but is extremely rare in children, in whom simultaneous administration of pyridoxine is not indicated. Hepatotoxicity, manifested as an asymptomatic transient elevation in liver enzymes, is uncommon when INH is administered to children without pre-existing liver disease. Thus, liver function need not be monitored except in those patients who have pre-existing liver disease or who are simultaneously receiving other hepatotoxic drugs (alcohol, phenytoin, rifampin, etc.). Less common side effects include gastrointestinal irritability, hypersensitivity reactions, and neurologic complications such as psychosis, confusion, and convulsions. Drug interactions with INH are rare; however, inhibition of the metabolism of diphenylhydantoin (phenytoin) and warfarin has been reported with high levels of INH.

Rifampin (RIF), a broad-spectrum antibiotic which is highly active against *M. tuberculosis*, is available in the United States as an oral preparation and is usually administered during the fasting state as a single daily dose (15–20 mg/kg/24 hr). RIF is well absorbed from the gastrointestinal tract, penetrates well into most tissues, including the cerebrospinal fluid, and is metabolized in the liver and excreted in urine and bile. Side effects are common and include an orange discoloration of tears (with permanent staining of soft contact lenses), urine, and saliva; gastrointestinal symptoms; and hepatotoxicity manifested as asymptomatic elevations in serum transaminase, particularly during the first few weeks of therapy. When RIF is administered with INH there is an increased risk of hepatotoxicity, which can be minimized by lowering the dose of INH to 10 mg/kg/24 hr. Intermittent administration of RIF has been associated with thrombocytopenia and leukopenia, and an "influenza syndrome" consisting of fever, headache, and malaise, and a "respiratory syndrome" associated with dyspnea and wheezing. RIF interferes with the metabolism of a number of drugs, including anticoagulants, oral contraceptives, corticosteroids, and oral hypoglycemic agents. It is also teratogenic in laboratory animals and is contraindicated during the first trimester of pregnancy.

Ethambutol (ETM) is active only against mycobacteria. It is administered orally as a single daily dose (15–20 mg/kg/24 hr), is distributed to various body tissues, but reaches low levels in the cerebrospinal fluid. ETM is excreted via the kidney in an active, unchanged state and, accordingly, high concentrations are found in the urine. Reversible ocular complications manifested as blurred vision, constriction of visual field, and color blindness have been reported in adults and can be minimized by limiting the maximum daily dose at 20 mg/kg. Many investigators feel that ETM is the ideal companion drug for INH (replacing the less effective PAS and the more expensive RIF) during initial treatment of older children and adults and that it is an ideal substitute when combined with RIF as an initial treatment when INH resistance is suspected. However, its use in younger children is limited by the lack of adequate pharmacokinetic data and by the difficulties involved in performing visual tests.

Streptomycin (STM) is substantially less effective than INH or RIF, but more effective than ETM against *M. tuberculosis*. For life-threatening tuberculosis, STM is usually administered as a daily intramuscular dose (20 mg/kg/24 hr) during the first few months of a three-drug regimen (INH, RIF, and STM). It diffuses rapidly into body fluids and tissues including tuber-

culous abscesses and caseous tissue, but it does not enter the cerebrospinal fluid unless meningitis is present. STM is filtered by the glomerulus and, unlike many other aminoglycoside antibiotics, rarely causes nephrotoxicity. The major toxic effect of STM is that it may cause damage to the eighth cranial nerve, especially to the vestibular division, resulting in vertigo, ataxia, and, less commonly, hearing loss.

Pyrazinamide (PZA), when combined with INH, is bactericidal against *M. tuberculosis*. The drug is administered orally in 2–3 divided doses (30–40 mg/kg/24 hr), is distributed to various body tissues, including the cerebrospinal fluid, and is excreted in the urine and bile. PZA's major limitations are its tendency to stimulate early drug resistance (which can be minimized by simultaneously administering other agents) and to produce hepatotoxicity manifested as abnormal liver function tests and jaundice. PZA use in children has been limited because pediatric pharmacokinetic data are scarce.

Para-aminosalicylic acid (PAS), the principal companion drug to INH for many years, has now been replaced by ETM and RIF. As an antituberculosis agent PAS is not very effective; however, it does reduce the development of resistance to other drugs. It is administered orally as a single daily dose or in two divided doses (200–300 mg/kg/24 hr). PAS is well absorbed from the gastrointestinal tract, is distributed to various body fluids and tissues, but not to the cerebrospinal fluid, and is excreted in the urine by glomerular filtration and tubular secretion. Its major side effect is gastrointestinal irritation manifested as nausea, vomiting, abdominal cramps, and diarrhea.

Ethionamide (ETH), a moderately effective agent for *M. tuberculosis*, is used most often as a companion drug for the retreatment of patients who have failed standard chemotherapy. Administered orally (15 mg/kg/24 hr) as a single daily dose, ETH is widely distributed throughout the body, including the cerebrospinal fluid. Gastrointestinal side effects are common and include nausea, vomiting, and abdominal pain due to the drug's direct effect upon the central nervous system. Use in children has been limited.

Single Drug Therapy

INH chemoprophylaxis is indicated for all asymptomatic tuberculin-positive people under 35 who have a normal chest film or a roentgenogram demonstrating inactive pulmonary disease. Treatment for 12 mo is recommended to prevent subsequent reactivation and systemic disease. For children who are at risk of becoming infected with INH-resistant strains (Asians, Haitians, etc.), careful follow-up is required when INH chemoprophylaxis is administered. Therapy with INH alone is also advised for patients at special risk of acquiring tuberculosis, e.g., children having household contact with known infectious cases, even if their skin test is negative. The usual practice is first to administer INH for 3 mo and then to repeat the skin test. If skin test conversion has occurred, a complete 12 mo course of INH is administered, but if the child's skin test reactivity has not been demonstrated and the source of the infection is no longer contagious, the INH treatment can be safely discontinued. INH prophylaxis may not be effective in preventing INH-resistant strains of *M. tuberculosis* from being transmitted.

Double or Triple Therapy

A satisfactory treatment for most forms of tuberculosis is a two-drug regimen, the most widely accepted of which is INH and RIF. When RIF is unavailable or when its high cost precludes its use, INH and ETM is an alternative. The usual duration of therapy for the two-drug regimens in children is 12 mo. Three-drug regimens are indicated as initial therapy in pediatric patients with potentially fatal disease such as miliary, meningeal, locally progressive, and chronic cavitary tuberculosis. The regimen most often used includes INH, RIF, and STM, with administration of the latter drug limited to the 1st month of therapy. A second indication for triple therapy is suspected INH resistance; a satisfactory regimen includes RIF, STM, and ETM.

Adult patients who have cavitary disease and a sputum that contains tubercle bacilli are noninfectious after 2 wk of chemotherapy that includes RIF. Similar criteria can be applied to infants and children. However, a longer period of isolation is suggested when close contacts include infants and children, or if drug resistance is suspected; under these circumstances, the infectiousness of each child must be decided individually.

PREVENTION

The prevention of tuberculosis depends upon (1) preventing contact with those who are actively infected, (2) providing chemoprophylaxis (see above), and (3) administering BCG to high-risk populations. General improvement in socioeconomic conditions is important to lowering the prevalence of this disease. The indications for immunization against tuberculosis by intracutaneous inoculation with BCG (bacillus Calmette-Guérin) remain controversial. The immunizing microorganism, an attenuated strain of M. bovis, was developed in the early part of the century and was subsequently demonstrated to decrease the incidence of tuberculosis, particularly in infants living in areas of high prevalence, and the mortality among tuberculosis-susceptible infants who had been immunized. However, some studies have not demonstrated this protective effect, possibly because of varying vaccine potency, improper preparation, storage, or administration of BCG, poor nutritional status of many vaccine recipients, and interference with vaccine-induced immunity by concurrent infection with nontuberculous mycobacteria.

BCG vaccination is recommended as a public health measure in developing countries with a high prevalence of tuberculosis (where skin test conversions exceed 1 per cent annually). Pre-BCG tuberculin skin testing is usually recommended, but because it is often impractical, vaccine is usually administered without prior skin testing. (Reactions to BCG in tuberculin-positive children are rarely serious.) In countries with a low prevalence of tuberculosis, BCG vaccination is recommended for children with negative skin tests who are repeatedly exposed to untreated or inadequately treated adults, and for children in subpopulations with a high infection rate and limited access to health care.

The vaccine should be stored in the dark and administered immediately following reconstitution. The recommended dose is 0.05 mL for neonates and 0.1 mL for infants and older children; it should be administered intradermally with syringe and needle. The preferred location of inoculation is the outer side of the upper arm at the insertion of the deltoid muscle. Percutaneous inoculation with a multiple-puncture apparatus and a concentrated vaccine is available. Administering BCG by jet injection is less effective and may cause severe local reactions. Following successful immunization, a small papule forms at the inoculation site, gradually enlarges, crusts, and disappears in 8–12 wk. Whenever possible, a tuberculin skin test should be administered 2–3 mo following BCG and a second vaccination administered to children who have a negative skin test. Side effects of BCG are uncommon and include cutaneous ulceration, localized lymphadenopathy and, less commonly, subcutaneous abscess formation, osteomyelitis, a lupoid reaction, dissemination, and death. Severe local reactions can be controlled with antituberculous drugs; however, such treatment inhibits the multiplication of BCG microorganisms and thus interferes with subsequent immunity, and, therefore, should be discouraged.

A major disadvantage of BCG vaccination is the production of sensitivity to tuberculin. In developing countries with a high risk of childhood infection, most individuals become tuberculin-positive during infancy, and the premature production of tuberculin sensitivity is of little consequence. In developed countries with a low risk of infection, the tuberculin skin test is an important public health tool for identifying cases of tuberculosis. The value of the tuberculin skin test outweighs the potential benefits of widespread administration of BCG, and many authorities discourage the routine administration of BCG vaccine in countries such as the United States.

TUBERCULOSIS DURING PREGNANCY

The potential hazards of ionizing radiation and antituberculosis chemotherapy for the pregnant woman and her unborn child have led to heavy reliance on tuberculin skin testing, limited use of roentgenographic examination, and caution in using drugs.

Tuberculosis Screening. Since pregnancy does not inhibit cutaneous reactivity to tuberculin, all women except those with a history of a previous positive reaction should be skin tested at the first antenatal visit. A positive skin test warrants further investigation of the patient, family members, and close contacts to diagnose active disease. In asymptomatic women having a positive skin test and normal physical findings, roentgenographic examination of the chest is deferred until they have completed the 1st trimester. In obtaining roentgenograms during pregnancy, avoiding portable equipment, which excessively scatters radiation, and shielding the abdomen minimizes the risk to the developing infant. Patients having positive skin tests and symptoms compatible with active disease and/or an abnormal physical examination should have an immediate roentgenogram of the chest.

Chemoprophylaxis. Pregnancy is a contraindication for isoniazid prophylaxis because of this drug's hepatotoxicity and because of the possible adverse effects of isoniazid on the developing fetus. Thus asymptomatic pregnant women having positive skin tests but whose chest roentgenograms show no active disease should not begin isoniazid prophylaxis until after their pregnancy.

Chemotherapy. Symptomatic pregnant women and/or those pregnant women who have roentgenographic evidence suggesting active disease should be hospitalized. Sputum and gastric aspirates should be collected, stained for acid-fast microorganisms, and cultured for M. tuberculosis. Women with sputum positive for acid-fast bacilli should begin immediate treatment with isoniazid, ethambutol, and pyridoxine. Rifampin is contraindicated during the first trimester of pregnancy. If stained smears fail to reveal microorganisms but the clinical history and roentgenograms suggest active disease, treatment should begin after sputum and gastric aspirates have been cultured. If cultures fail to reveal mycobacteria after 8 wk of incubation, treatment should be discontinued; however, close follow-up and repeated evaluation should continue throughout pregnancy and the immediate postpartum period.

Infants Born to Mothers with Active Tuberculosis

Since approximately 50 per cent of infants born to mothers with active pulmonary tuberculosis develop disease within the first year of life, prophylaxis is recommended. There is controversy, however, whether such treatment should consist of BCG immunization or isoniazid administration. The advantages of BCG administration include probable effectiveness, lack of toxicity, and the need for only a single injection which

Table 11–22. Management of Infants of Mothers with Positive Tuberculin Skin Test

Mother	Management of Infant
Asymptomatic	No immediate prophylaxis necessary; tuberculin test every 3 mo for 1 yr If positive, rule out active tuberculosis If active disease, begin therapy If no active disease, begin isoniazid prophylaxis* If negative tuberculin, retest annually
Past history of treated active tuberculosis, presumably asymptomatic	Same as above
X-ray consistent with questionable or minimally active disease†	Rule out congenital tuberculosis If present, begin therapy If not present, BCG‡ vaccination or isoniazid prophylaxis
Advanced pulmonary or extrapulmonary tuberculosis, or disseminated infection	Rule out congenital tuberculosis If present, begin triple therapy If not present, isoniazid for 1 yr, or isoniazid for 3 mo followed by chest x-ray and tuberculin; if both negative, give BCG; if tuberculin reactive and chest negative, give isoniazid; if chest positive, begin total therapy for 1 yr

*Isoniazid prophylaxis: 15–20 mg/kg/24 hr given as a single dose.
†Mothers with active disease should be treated and separated from their infants until noncontagious.
‡BCG is recommended when noncompliance and/or loss to follow-up examination is considered likely in situations in which the infant will be exposed to endemic tuberculosis in the environment. Immunization requires that 0.05 mL of BCG be injected superficially over the deltoid or triceps muscle. The infant is separated from the mother or other potentially contagious individuals until tuberculin positive (6–8 wk); if persistently negative, a 2nd dose of BCG is given. BCG should not be given during isoniazid prophylaxis because isoniazid inhibits multiplication of BCG. (After Weinstein L, Murphy T: Clin Perinatol 1:395, 1974.)

eliminates noncompliance and the need for follow-up examination. The disadvantages of BCG include variability of response in immunized individuals, limited value of subsequent tuberculin testing, and a necessary period of post-immunization separation of mother and infant prior to skin test conversion and protection. Isoniazid chemoprophylaxis has proved efficacious and permits continued use of tuberculin skin testing to document subsequent infection. Its major disadvantages are noncompliance in prophylactic medication and the lack of information on the pharmacology of isoniazid when administered during the neonatal period. Combining BCG immunization and isoniazid administration until skin test conversion is not recommended. However, the recent development of an isoniazid-resistant vaccine strain of *M. bovis* makes such an approach an attractive possibility.

The management approach outlined in Table 11–22 should be individualized for the newborn infant, taking into consideration the home environment and subsequent availability of the treated infant for follow-up evaluation.

WILLIAM T. SPECK

Abernathy RS, Dutt AK, Stead WW, et al: Short course chemotherapy for tuberculosis in children. Pediatrics 72:801, 1983.
Alvarez S, McCabe WR: Extrapulmonary tuberculosis revisited: A review of experience at Boston City and other hospitals. Medicine 63:25, 1984.
Bartelink AKM, Lenders JW, VanHerwaarden CL, et al: Fatal hepatitis after treatment with isoniazid and rifampicin in a patient on anticonvulsant therapy. Tubercle 64:125, 1983.
Begt BE, Ortbals DW, SantaCruz DJ, et al: Cutaneous mycobacteriosis: Analysis of 34 cases with a new classification of the disease. Medicine 60:95, 1981.
Dickinson DS, Bailey WC, Hirschowitz BI, et al: Risk factors for isoniazid (INH)-induced liver dysfunction. J Clin Gastroenterol 3:271, 1981.
Dutt AK, Stead WW: Present chemotherapy for tuberculosis. J Infect Dis 146:698, 1982.
Editorial: Antituberculous drugs in pregnancy. Lancet 2:1285, 1980.
Editorial: Scrofula today. Lancet 1:335, 1983.
Enarson DA, Dorken E, Grzybowski S: Tuberculous pleurisy. Can Med Assoc J 126:493, 1982.
Fairshter RD, Randazzo GP, Garlin J, et al: Failure of isoniazid prophylaxis after exposure to isoniazid-resistant tuberculosis. Am Rev Respir Dis 112:37, 1975.
Fox AD, Lepow ML: Tuberculin skin testing in Vietnamese refugees with a history of BCG vaccination. Am J Dis Child 137:1093, 1983.
Gow JG: The management of genitourinary tuberculosis. J Antimicrob Chemother 7:590, 1981.
Grzybowski S: Epidemiology of tuberculosis and the role of BCG. Clin Chest Med 2:175, 1980.
Harder E, Al-Kawi MZ, Carney P: Intracranial tuberculoma: conservative management. Am J Med 74:570, 1983.
Hsu KH: Thirty years after isoniazid. Its impact on tuberculosis in children and adolescents. JAMA 251:1283, 1984.
Kendig EL: Current status report: evolution of short-course antimicrobial treatment of tuberculosis in children, 1951–1984. Pediatrics 75:684, 1985.
Lai KK, Stottmeier KD, Sherman IH, et al: Mycobacterial cervical lymphadenopathy: Relation of etiologic agents to age. JAMA 251:1286, 1984.
Larrieu AJ, Tyers FO, Williams EH, et al: Recent experience with tuberculous pericarditis. Ann Thor Surg 29:464, 1981.
Molavi A, LeFrock JL: Tuberculous meningitis. Med Clin North Am 69:315, 1985.
O'Brien R, Long M, Cross F, et al: Hepatotoxicity from isoniazid and rifampin among children treated for tuberculosis. Pediatrics 72:491, 1983.
Ortbals BW, Avioli L: Tuberculosis pericarditis. Arch Intern Med 139:231, 1979.
Powell KE, Meador MP, Farer LS: Recent trends in tuberculosis in children. JAMA 251:1289, 1984.
Shan SA, Neff T: Miliary tuberculosis. Am J Med 56:495, 1974.
Sherman S, Rohwedder JJ, Ravikrishnan KP, et al: Tuberculous enteritis and peritonitis. Arch Intern Med 140:506, 1980.
Snider DE, Layde PM, Johnson MW, et al: Treatment of tuberculosis during pregnancy. Am Rev Respir Dis 122:65, 1980.
Tang L, Swash M: Tuberculosis of the nervous system: A modern problem. J Roy Soc Med 78:429, 1985.
Wasz-Hockert O, Donner M, Miettinen P, et al: Late prognosis in tuberculous meningitis. Acta Pediatr Scand 51(Suppl 141):1, 1963.

11.47 NONTUBERCULOUS MYCOBACTERIAL INFECTION

Nontuberculous, nonleprous *Mycobacterium* species (variously referred to as tuberculoid bacilli and as unclassified, anonymous, or atypical mycobacteria) are members of the family of Mycobacteriacae, whose staining and morphologic characteristics are similar to those of *M. tuberculosis*. They differ from the tubercle bacilli in their rate of growth, nutritional requirements, ability to produce pigments, enzymatic activity, temperature sensitivity, and resistance to antituberculous agents. Although more than 100 species of atypical mycobacteria are recognized, only 5 (*M. kansasii*, *M. avium-intracellulare*, *M. marinum*, *M. scrofulaceum*, and *M. chelonei*) are commonly associated with human disease.

Etiology and Epidemiology. Atypical mycobacteria are distributed worldwide and are ubiquitous in the environment, existing as saprophytes in soil and water, as pathogens in swine, birds, and cattle, and as part of the normal pharyngeal flora in many humans. Infection, which occurs following inhalation or inoculation, is relatively common in warm, humid, rural environments; in the United States infections occur most commonly in the southern states. Pulmonary infection in adult white males with chronic obstructive pulmonary disease is the most common clinical manifestation of atypical mycobacteria. Skin and soft tissue infections in infants and children occur less frequently, and disseminated disease is rare except in individuals with compromised immune function.

Classification. The pathogenic and nonpathogenic atypical mycobacteria were traditionally divided into four groups: Slow-growing microbacteria were classified as photochromogens (I), which form pigment following exposure to light; as scotochromogens (II), which form pigment in the dark; and as nonchromogens (III), which fail to produce pigment. Rapid-growing atypical mycobacteria form group IV. Now, because of improved ability to identify the individual species, they are identified by species. Biochemically and immunologically closely related strains are referred to as "complexes," e.g., the *M. fortuitum-chelonei* complex or the *M. avium-intracellulare-scrofulaceum* (MAIS) complex.

Pathology and Immunity. The histologic appearances of the pathologic lesions produced by the tuberculous and nontuberculous mycobacteria are often indistinguishable. When there are differences, the histologic lesion of atypical mycobacteria may resemble "nonspecific" inflammation more than it resembles granuloma formation, and the lesion, instead of caseating, may liquefy rather quickly. Definitive diagnosis requires isolation of microorganisms from clinical specimens. The immune response to infection with atypical mycobacteria has not been extensively studied; however, it is presumed to be similar to the interactions observed between the tubercle bacilli, lymphocyte subpopulations, and tissue macrophages. Skin testing has provided useful epidemiologic information but is of limited clinical value because the skin test antigens, no longer commercially available, are poorly standardized and lack sensitivity and specificity.

Clinical Manifestations. Lymphadenitis of the submandibular or anterior cervical nodes is the most frequent manifestation of atypical mycobacterial infection in children. Preauricular, posterior cervical, axillary, and inguinal nodes may also become involved. The initial pharyngeal lesion is rarely distinguished, and the cutaneous one may have disappeared or appear so insignificant as not to be recognized. Although children may appear sick and have high temperatures, affected children of 1 to 5 yr of age usually lack constitutional symptoms and have no history of exposure to tuberculosis. Lymph node involvement is invariably unilateral and the chest roentgenogram is normal. In the absence of treatment, the involved node(s) suppurate, rupture, and form a cutaneous sinus tract(s); chronic drainage resembles the classic scrofula of tuberculosis. In the United States, the *M. avium-intracellulare* complex and *M. scrofulaceum* are usually the responsible pathogens; however, *M. kansasii* is also recovered in a number of instances.

The differential diagnosis includes lymphadenitis due to viruses, other bacteria including *M. tuberculosis*, toxoplasma, and the agent(s) causing cat scratch disease. Noninfectious causes of lymphadenopathy must also be considered; these include malignancies, sarcoidosis, and drug reactions (phenytoin). The tuberculin skin test is usually negative (less than 10 mm of induration to PPD-S), although intermediate reactions (5–10 mm) are not uncommon. Definitive diagnosis requires excision of an involved node (removal of all involved nodes is not necessary) and recovery of the responsible pathogen. Surgery without chemotherapy is curative in 95 per cent of cases.

Cutaneous disease due to atypical mycobacteria occurs less frequently in children than superficial lymphadenitis. Infection usually follows percutaneous inoculation with fresh or salt water contaminated by *M. marinum* (formerly *M. balnei*). Within several weeks of exposure, a solitary nodule develops at the site of minor abrasions on elbows, knees, or feet ("swimming pool granuloma") and on the hands and fingers of fish fanciers ("fish tank granuloma"). The lesions eventually enlarge and ulcerate until they resemble the warty lesions seen in cutaneous tuberculosis. The lesions of a minority of patients resemble sporotrichosis; satellite lesions near the site of entry extend along the skin following the superficial lymphatics.

Diagnosis depends on isolating the responsible microorganisms from an excised granuloma. The cutaneous lesions usually heal spontaneously following incision and drainage, without other therapy. Heat treatment has been advocated because this pathogen is sensitive to higher temperatures. Antibiotic therapy is indicated for intractable cases. All isolates are resistant to isoniazid, but they are susceptible to rifampin, ethambutol, trimethoprim-sulfamethoxazole, and doxycycline. Extensive disease may be treated with rifampin and ethambutol for 6 mo. Corticosteroids are contraindicated because they enhance local spread.

M. ulcerans also causes cutaneous infection in children living in tropical countries (Africa, Australia, and South America). Infection follows percutaneous inoculation and presents as a painless, erythematous nodule on an extremity, which undergoes central necrosis and ulceration (Buruli ulcers). The lesion, which has a characteristic undermined edge, gradually expands and may result in extensive soft tissue destruction with secondary bacterial infection. Diagnosis depends on isolation of the responsible pathogen, and treatment requires extensive surgical excision.

Skin and soft tissue infections due to *M. fortuitum-chelonei* complex are rare in children, and usually follow percutaneous inoculation due to puncture wounds and minor abrasions. Clinical disease usually arises after a 3–4 wk incubation period and presents as a localized cellulitis or a draining abscess. Superficial infections usually resolve following surgical incision and open drainage; however, deep-seated infections require initial therapy with parenteral amikacin and cefoxitin combined with oral probenecid, pending susceptibility.

In unusual circumstances, the atypical mycobacteria may cause **bone and joint infections** that are indistinguishable from those produced by *M. tuberculosis*. Such infections usually result from operative incisions or accidental puncture wounds.

Pulmonary infection with *M. kansasii* is uncommon in children and can be mistaken for tuberculosis. The onset is usually insidious and consists of low grade fever, cough, night sweats, and general malaise. Thin-walled cavities are characteristic, but radiographic findings may resemble those of tuberculosis. Pulmonary infection should be treated with isoniazid, rifampin, and ethambutol for 12 mo, supplemented during the first 2 mo with biweekly streptomycin.

Disseminated disease may occur in individuals who have severe immunologic defects or who are receiving immunosuppressive therapy. In children, the responsible pathogens are usually the *M. avium-intracellulare* complex. Continuous bacteremia has been described in children having acquired immunodeficiency syndrome. Chemotherapy for *M. avium-intracellulare* disease usually includes isoniazid, rifampin, clofazimine, ethambutol, and amikacin or streptomycin.

JAMES B. BESUNDER
WILLIAM T. SPECK

Collins CH, Grange JM, Noble WC et al: *Mycobacterium marinum* infection in man. J Hyg (Lond) 94:135, 1985.

Saitz EW: Cervical lymphadenitis caused by atypical mycobacterium. Pediatr Clin North Am 28:823, 1981.

Schaad VB, Votteler TP, McCracken GH Jr, et al: Management of atypical mycobacterial lymphadenitis in childhood; a review based on 380 cases. J Pediatr 95:356, 1979.

Wallace RJ Jr, Swenson JM, Silcox VA, et al: Spectrum of disease due to rapidly growing mycobacteria. Rev Infect Dis 5:657, 1983.

Wolinsky E: Nontuberculous mycobacteria and associated disease. Am Rev Respir Dis 119:107, 1979.

11.48 LEPROSY (HANSEN DISEASE)

Leprosy, a chronic disease, is produced by infection with *Mycobacterium leprae* and by the ensuing host response. The organs most prominently affected are the skin and the peripheral nervous system, but upper respiratory, testicular, and ocular involvement are also relatively common. Man was long believed to be the sole host of *M. leprae*, but naturally acquired infection has recently been documented in armadillos in southeastern United States, and experimental infection has been established in primates, nude mice, and armadillos. These animal models have been crucial to a fuller understanding of leprosy.

Leprosy had been endemic throughout the world until late in the 19th century, when a striking drop in its incidence became evident in Northern Europe and North America, so that currently it is often erroneously thought of as being limited to tropical areas. The reasons for this decline are unknown, but it is notable that the decline coincided with a decrease in the incidence of tuberculosis and preceded the availability of antimycobacterial agents.

Chronic skin lesions, madarosis, sensory neuropathy resulting in the loss of digits or limbs, and paresis secondary to motor nerve dysfunction are among the sequelae of leprosy. The highly visible nature of these debilities led to the historical stigmatization of the "leper." The psychologic and sociologic sequelae of this stigma can be as debilitating as the disease itself and may result in delays in seeking medical attention. To combat this prejudice, the term "leprosy patient" has replaced the word "leper," and "Hansen disease" has become the accepted designation.

Etiology. *M. leprae* is an acid-fast bacillus of the family Mycobacteriaceae. Originally identified by Hansen in 1873, *M. leprae* was the first bacterial pathogen to be linked with a specific human disease. Koch's postulates, however, have never been fulfilled, since the bacterium has not been cultivated in vitro.

The exceedingly slow multiplication of *M. leprae* observed in animal models may partially explain the long incubation period seen in human disease. An incubation period of 3–5 years is believed to be typical. The rare occurrence of leprosy in infants as young as 3 mo of age suggests that *in utero* transmission may occur or that very short incubation periods may be possible in certain situations. Postulates to explain the mode of transmission include contact with desquamated infected epidermis, ingestion of infected breast milk, and bites of mosquitoes or other vectors. At the present, however, transmission via infected nasal secretions appears to be the basis for most infections. Extensive involvement of the nasopharynx manifested as chronic rhinitis is common in lepromatous disease.

Epidemiology. The World Health Organization estimated that worldwide there were 11 million cases of leprosy in 1975. This figure, however, must be considered as an underestimate, because of inadequate case finding and reporting. The insidious onset of the disease and the social stigma assigned to it delay medical consultation, and the lack of an inexpensive, simple diagnostic test makes confirmation of the diagnosis difficult. Conversely, the prevalence of leprosy may be overestimated when household contacts develop superficial fungal or other lesions that are inappropriately diagnosed as leprosy.

Most of the world's leprosy patients reside in Africa, India, Southeast Asia, and Central and South America. Prevalence rates vary widely between and within countries; the highest rates for entire countries are 25 or more cases per 1000 population, but rates as high as 200 cases per 1000 population have been found in small, hyperendemic pockets. Human-to-human transmission accounts for an overwhelming majority of cases; a high percentage of them occur in family members or in close contacts of known patients. Approximately 230 cases are reported annually in the United States, of which 90 per cent are in immigrants. The remaining 10 per cent develop in contacts in localized foci along the Gulf coast and in Hawaii and the Micronesian territories.

Leprosy occurs at all ages, but infections in infants are extremely rare; incidence rates peak during childhood and early adulthood in endemic areas.

Pathogenesis and Pathology. Individual leprosy bacilli are encased within a neutral glycolipid envelope and do not produce toxins. Most of the tissue damage and destruction results from the host immune response. Damage is mediated through many pathways, some of which are release of humoral mediators of inflammation by activated lymphocytes and macrophages, nerve compression by enlarging granulomata, and deposition of immune complexes. Multiple mechanisms may operate simultaneously or sequentially.

The site of entry of *M. leprae* into the human host is unknown. Primary respiratory or gastrointestinal tract involvement has not been documented prior to the appearance of lesions involving the skin and peripheral nerves. Growth and multiplication of *M. leprae* are maximal at 34–35° C. Nothing is known of the host immune responses in the initial period after infection, but skin testing (Mitsuda reaction, see below) and serologic studies suggest that up to 80–90% of those infected develop protective immunity without ever manifesting clinical disease. Most of the remaining patients, after a highly variable incubation period, develop typical skin lesions of *indeterminate leprosy*.

Fully developed clinical leprosy is classified into five categories that can be aligned upon a spectrum representing the range of intensity and efficacy of the cellular limb of the host immune response (see below and Table 11–23).

The beginning of the spectrum is *polar tuberculoid leprosy*, in which there is a vigorous and specific cell-mediated immune response. In tissue biopsies there are tightly organized granulomas composed of epithelioid cells and lymphocytes, but bacilli are scant or absent. Macrophages, when present, do not contain intracellular organisms. Caseation is rare. Nerve involvement is usually limited to cutaneous sensory nerve endings and to, at most, a single peripheral nerve trunk.

At the end of the spectrum is *polar lepromatous leprosy*, in which there is total and specific anergy to *M. leprae* both by skin testing and by in vitro assays of cell-mediated immunity. Large amounts of circulating and tissue-based antibody to mycobacterial antigens are present, but they afford no protective immunity. Bacilli are found in enormous numbers in the skin, nasal mucosa, and peripheral nerves. There is continual bacillemia as well as bacillary invasion of all major organs except the central nervous system. Tissue granulomas are poorly formed and are composed chiefly of loose aggregates of foamy histiocytes. Macrophages teeming with undigested bacilli (globi) are common. There is extensive, symmetric involvement of peripheral nerves, although the cutaneous nerve endings are usually spared.

An *M. leprae*–specific suppressor T-cell population is found in the circulation of patients with lepromatous leprosy, and increased numbers of suppressor T cells are found in their skin granulomas. T cells from lepromatous patients also produce less interleukin 2 and less gamma interferon following stimulation with *M. leprae* antigens than do T cells from tuberculoid patients or normal controls. These findings may relate to the underlying cellular defect that permits development of clinical leprosy in the susceptible individual.

Borderline or *dimorphous leprosy* is subdivided into three subclasses that lie between the tuberculoid and lepromatous categories on the clinical pattern spectrum. The number of bacilli present in tissues and the antibody titers to *M. leprae*

Table 11–23. Clinical, Histologic, Bacteriologic, and Immunologic Data of the Five Divisions of the Leprosy Spectrum

	Polar Tuberculoid (TT)	Borderline Tuberculoid (BT)	Borderline (BB)	Borderline Lepromatous (BL)	Polar Lepromatous (LL)
Skin lesions					
Number	1 to 3	Very few to moderate	Moderate	Moderate to many	Very many
Symmetry	Very asymmetrical	Asymmetrical	Asymmetrical	Slightly asymmetrical	Symmetrical
Anesthesia	Complete	Nearly complete	Moderate	Slight to nil	Nil
Nerve enlargement					
Cutaneous sensory nerves	Common	May occur	0	0	0
Peripheral nerves*	0 or 1	Common; asymmetrical	Common; asymmetrical	Moderately asymmetrical	Symmetrical
Skin histology					
Granuloma cell	Epithelioid	Epithelioid	Epithelioid	Histiocyte	Foamy histiocyte
Lymphocytes	+ + +	+ + +	+	± or + +	±
Dermal nerves	Destroyed	Mostly destroyed	Some visible	Visible	Easily visible
Bacillary index	0	0, 1, or 2	1, 2, or 3	4 or 5	5 or 6
Lepromin test					
(Mitsuda)	+ + +	+ +	± or 0	0	0
Reactions					
Erythema nodosum	0	0	0	Common	Very common
Reversal	0	Common	Very common	Very common	(rare)†

*Nerves of predilection: ulnar, median, lateral popliteal, facial, great auricular, and posterior tibial.

†Reversal reactions are occasionally seen in treated LL patients who have developed from borderline (BT, BB, or BL) in the absence of treatment.

Adapted from Waters, MFR: Leprosy. *In:* Beeson PB, et al (eds): Cecil Textbook of Medicine. 15th ed. Philadelphia, WB Saunders, 1979. Used by permission.

are inversely proportional to the degree of cell-mediated immunity.

Clinical Manifestations. *Indeterminate Leprosy (I).* This is the earliest clinically detectable form of leprosy. Although it is observed in only 10–20% of infected individuals, it is a stage through which most patients with advanced leprosy have passed. Usually there is a single hypopigmented macule, 2–4 cm in diameter, with a poorly defined border but having no erythema or induration. Anesthesia is minimal or absent, particularly if the lesion is on the face. Biopsied tissue may contain granulomas but bacilli are rarely demonstrable. The histopathology is not distinctive; the diagnosis is usually made by exclusion, in contacts (especially children) of leprosy patients. In 50–75% of patients with indeterminate leprosy, the lesions heal spontaneously; in the remainder, they progress to one of the classic forms. Thus, only 5–10 of every 100 infected individuals are likely to develop progressive leprosy (Table 11–23).

Polar Tuberculoid (TT). There is usually a single, large (often over 10 cm in diameter) lesion with a well demarcated, elevated erythematous rim. The interior of the lesion is flat, atrophic, hypopigmented, and anesthetic. Rarely there may be as many as four lesions. The closest superficial nerve is often impressively thickened. The ulnar, posterior tibial, and great auricular nerves are most commonly affected and are often referred to as the "nerves of predilection." Periodic examination of all leprosy patients and their contacts should include palpation of these six nerves. Without therapy, the lesion(s) tends to enlarge slowly, but documented instances of spontaneous resolution exist. The coloration of the rim slowly fades with therapy, and the induration resolves, resulting in a flat lesion with central hypopigmentation and a ring of postinflammatory hyperpigmentation. Loss of hair follicles, sweat glands, cutaneous nerve receptors, and of sensation in the central portion of the lesion is irreversible. Marked improvement should be apparent within 1–2 mo after

initiating therapy, but complete resolution may take up to 8–12 mo. There is an entity of "pure neural" tuberculoid leprosy, which presents as a mononeuropathy with prominent nerve thickening but no cutaneous lesions. Histopathology is mandatory to establish this diagnosis. Nerve trunk size varies widely, and overdiagnosis of "enlarged" nerves is common among inexperienced observers. Nodular or fusiform nerve thickening has greater diagnostic value than a palpable nerve that is smooth and symmetric.

Borderline Leprosy. The clinical and histologic criteria for the three subdivisions of borderline leprosy are less well defined than are those of the two polar categories (Table 11–23). In contrast to the tuberculoid and lepromatous patterns, those in the borderline divisions are more unstable. For example, host or bacterial factors can result in "downgrading" the clinical condition toward the lepromatous pattern or "upgrading" it toward the tuberculoid pattern. Therapy is the most common cause of upgrading reactions; downgrading can be seen in any condition that compromises host immunity, for example pregnancy. Clinical characteristics of the three generally accepted borderline subclasses are as follows:

In *borderline tuberculoid (BT)* leprosy the lesions are greater in number but smaller in size than in tuberculoid leprosy. There may be small satellite lesions around older lesions, and the margins of the borderline tuberculoid lesions are less distinct and the center is less atrophic and anesthetic. There is usually thickening of two or more superficial nerves.

In the *borderline (BB)* pattern the lesions are more numerous and more heterogeneous in appearance. They may become confluent, and plaques may be present. The borders are poorly defined, and the erythematous rim fades into the surrounding skin. There may be anesthesia, but hypesthesia is more common. Mild to moderate nerve thickening is common, but severe muscle wasting and neuropathy is unusual.

In the *borderline lepromatous (BL)* pattern, there are a large number of asymmetrically distributed lesions that are heterogeneous in appearance. Macules, papules, plaques, and nodules may all coexist. Individual lesions are small unless confluent. Anesthesia is mild and superficial nerve trunks are spared. The initial response to therapy is often dramatic; nodules and plaques flatten within 2–3 mo. With continued therapy the lesions become macular and almost invisible.

Polar Lepromatous Leprosy (LL). The lesions are innumerable, often confluent, and symmetric. Initially there may be only vague macules or even uniform, diffuse skin infiltrations without discernible lesions. As the disease progresses, the lesions become increasingly papular and nodular, so that with the diffuse thickening and infiltration of the skin, the characteristic leonine facies accompanied by loss of the eyebrows and distortion of the earlobes becomes apparent. Anesthesia of the lesions either does not occur or is mild, but a symmetric peripheral sensory neuropathy may develop. Chronic rhinitis is common, secondary to involvement of the mucosa of the nasopharynx. Testicular infiltration leading to azoospermia, infertility, and gynecomastia is common in adults but not in children. Bacilli are demonstrable in most internal organs other than the central nervous system, but tissue damage or interference with function is infrequent. Glomerulonephritis, when it occurs, is felt to be secondary to immune complex deposition rather than to infection per se. The initial response to therapy may be encouraging but is often followed by a long (2–5 yr) period of very slow improvement. In true polar lepromatous leprosy, the specific anergy to the leprosy bacillus persists despite therapy, thus making the patient theoretically susceptible to relapse if even a single viable bacillus remains at the end of therapy.

Reactional States. Acute clinical exacerbations are common in leprosy and are believed to reflect abrupt changes in the host-parasite immunologic balance. Although these reactional states do occur in the absence of therapy, they are especially common during the initial years of treatment. Three major variants are recognized:

Erythema nodosum leprosum (ENL) occurs in the majority of patients with polar lepromatous leprosy and in 25–40% of borderline lepromatous cases. Tender dermal nodules, clinically resembling erythema nodosum, are the hallmark of this syndrome. High fever, migrating polyarthralgia, orchitis, and increased activity in pre-existing cutaneous lesions complete the clinical picture. Circulating and tissue-based immune complexes are frequently present and may explain the resemblance to other immune complex disorders, but the underlying mechanism appears to involve the activation of a helper T cell subset. There is a strong tendency to recurrence and there is a risk of amyloidosis and renal failure if treatment is inadequate.

Reversal reactions are observed throughout the borderline range. Acute tenderness and inflammation at the site of existing cutaneous and neural lesions and the development of new lesions are the major manifestations. Fever and systemic toxicity are uncommon, but the acute neuritis can lead to irreversible nerve injury if not treated immediately. Reversal reactions constitute perhaps the only "medical emergency" related to leprosy per se. Patients should be instructed to contact their physicians immediately if signs of a reaction appear. A sudden increase in effective cell-mediated immunity with rapid killing of bacilli within nerve sheaths is the initiating event.

Lucio's phenomenon, a severe, necrotizing, cutaneous vasculitis, is uncommon; it occurs predominantly in patients of Mexican origin who have diffuse lepromatous leprosy. Conventional therapy for vasculitis has had only modest success, and fatalities are common. Experimental therapies, including plasmapheresis and cyclophosphamide, have been successful in isolated cases. The pathogenesis is unknown, although immune complexes almost certainly contribute.

Diagnosis. The critical factor in the diagnosis of leprosy is its inclusion in the differential diagnosis of a skin disorder in anyone who has resided in an endemic leprosy region. Anesthetic skin lesions with or without thickened peripheral nerves are virtually pathognomonic of leprosy. The finding of acid-fast bacilli in skin smears confirms the diagnosis, but such smears are usually negative in patients with indeterminate, tuberculoid, and borderline tuberculoid disease.

Lepromin is a suspension of killed *M. leprae* obtained from infected human or armadillo tissue. Following intradermal inoculation, early (48 hr, Fernandez reaction) as well as late (3–4 wk, Mitsuda reaction) reactions may be seen. The Mitsuda reaction, a granulomatous response to the antigen, is more consistent. Patients with tuberculoid leprosy have strongly positive (greater than 5 mm) responses, whereas patients with lepromatous leprosy do not respond. The test is not useful in the diagnosis of leprosy, since the majority of the population in both endemic and nonendemic leprosy areas will be Mitsuda-positive. Lepromin is not available in the United States.

Many diseases endemic in developing countries can mimic the appearance of leprosy; these include secondary syphilis, cutaneous leishmaniasis, yaws, and cutaneous fungal infections. None of these entities involves paresthesia/anesthesia localized to the skin lesions or causes thickening of peripheral nerves. The presence of nerve thickening with skin lesions also differentiates leprosy from primary neurologic disease. Indeterminate leprosy may present with minimal anesthesia, no nerve thickening, and equivocal histopathology suggesting a superficial fungal infection, particularly tinea versicolor. The diagnosis of indeterminate leprosy should be considered one of exclusion and will rarely be made in anyone other than a close contact of a known patient.

Treatment. Only three antimycobacterial agents have proven to be consistently effective.

Since the early 1940's, *dapsone* (diaminodiphenyl sulfone) has remained the cornerstone because of its low cost, minimal toxicity, and wide availability. Unfortunately, secondary resistance tends to develop when it is used as the sole agent and may appear after 10–15 yr of therapy. More worrisome is the increasing incidence of primary resistance, which has been reported in up to 30 per cent of newly diagnosed patients in Malaysia and Ethiopia. Dermatitis, hepatitis, and methemoglobinemia are the most common side effects; granulocytopenia is rare but potentially fatal. Dose-related hemolytic anemia, which can be severe, is seen in patients with glucose-6-phosphate dehydrogenase (G-6-PD) deficiency, methemoglobin reductase deficiency, or hemoglobin M. Available studies during pregnancy have not shown an increased risk of fetal abnormalities.

Rifampin is the most rapidly mycobacterial drug for *M. leprae,* achieving excellent levels inside cells where most leprosy bacilli reside. Resistance has been reported infrequently. The widespread use of rifampin has been limited by cost more than by toxicity. Hepatitis is the most common side effect that necessitates discontinuance.

*Clofazimine,** a phenazine dye with both antimycobacterial and anti-inflammatory activity, is particularly useful in cases of dapsone resistance or when recurrent reactional states have developed. The pharmacokinetics are poorly understood but the half-life is several days. The drug is avidly taken up by epithelial cells, a feature which may be important for its activity but which also results in cutaneous hyperpigmentation, ichthyosis, xerosis, and enteritis. The intense reddish-

*Thalidomide and clofazimine are available as investigational agents through the National Hansen's Disease Center, Carville, Louisiana. The National Hansen's Disease Center and its Regional Centers are available for consultation and assistance in patient management. The use of this service is strongly encouraged.

brown discoloration of the skin is cosmetically a deterrent to use and often results in discontinuation or poor compliance.

Delineation of the optimal therapeutic regimens for leprosy has been hampered by deficient patient compliance, the long durations of therapy required, and inadequacies in the long-term follow-up for late relapses. The following recommendations reflect the standard of practice among leprologists in the United States; they differ slightly from those of WHO, which largely reflect the economic realities in developing countries. The type and duration of treatment is determined by the number of bacilli in the skin, as estimated by smear or biopsy.

Paucibacillary patients (bacillary index $\leq 2+$: all indeterminate and polar tuberculoid and most borderline tuberculoid categories) should receive dapsone (2 mg/kg/24 hr up to 100 mg/24 hr) and rifampin (20 mg/kg/24 hr up to 600 mg/24 hr) for 1 yr, followed by dapsone alone for 1 yr for indeterminate leprosy and for 2–3 yr for tuberculoid and borderline tuberculoid leprosy. All patients with lepromatous or borderline lepromatous disease and most patients with borderline disease have large numbers of bacilli present in the skin (multibacillary leprosy). Common practice in the United States is to initiate treatment with dapsone and rifampin (same dosages as above) for the first 18–24 mo followed by dapsone alone for 10 yr in borderline disease, but lepromatous and borderline lepromatous disease may require therapy for life. The WHO recommends the addition of clofazimine (optimal dosage has not been determined for children; adult dose ranges from 100 to 300 mg/24 hr) to the dapsone/rifampin regimen in multibacillary cases, particularly in areas with a high prevalence of primary dapsone resistance. Recommendations concerning the necessary duration of therapy are arbitrary and controversial since there are no adequate evaluations of these new multi-drug regimens.

Therapy of reactional states can become very complicated and will generally require expert consultation. Erythema nodosum leprosum usually responds to corticosteroid therapy (1 mg/kg/24 hr of prednisone), but often relapses when the drug is discontinued. Clinical remission of acute and suppression of chronic erythema nodosum can be achieved with thalidomide.* *Thalidomide is absolutely contraindicated in women of child-bearing age*; otherwise it is much safer than corticosteroids for chronic use. The major side effect is fatigue. Pediatric dosages have not been established. Clofazimine is also useful in managing chronic erythema nodosum. Reversal reactions are optimally treated with corticosteroids. Alternate-day regimens may be effective in patients with frequent relapses.

Serial skin smears or repeat biopsies are useful in assessing response to therapy. Bacilli in the skin are quantitated on a logarithmic scale (bacillary index). Four to 8 yr of effective therapy is commonly required in lepromatous patients before the bacillary index becomes zero, but the appearance of the bacilli will gradually change, becoming first beaded and then fragmented. Persistence of intact bacilli in the skin or nerves during therapy suggests poor patient compliance or drug resistance and usually correlates with clinical failure or recrudescence. Drug sensitivity testing of *M. leprae* is difficult and not widely available but may be necessary to confirm suspected drug resistance.

Currently a WHO-sponsored trial is under way to evaluate immunotherapy through vaccination as an adjunct to chemotherapy.

---

*Thalidomide and clofazimine are available as investigational agents through the National Hansen's Disease Center, Carville, Louisiana. The National Hansen's Disease Center and its Regional Centers are available for consultation and assistance in patient management. The use of this service is strongly encouraged.

Prognosis. The prognosis for arresting progression of tissue and nerve damage is good, but recovery of lost sensory and motor function is variable and generally incomplete; hyperpigmentation, hypopigmentation, and loss of skin organs persist. Intercurrent reactional states, poor compliance, and emergence of dapsone resistance can all lead to clinical exacerbations or relapses necessitating close follow-up of patients. Much of the chronic debility results from repeated trauma to anesthetic digits and limbs. Careful counseling of patients and consultation with physical and occupational therapy services is essential for an optimal outcome.

Prevention. Two approaches are advocated for interrupting leprosy transmission in endemic areas. The first is directed at the risk of infection among household contacts of leprosy patients, especially those with multibacillary disease. It is based on regular periodic examination of contacts and early treatment at the first evidence of leprosy. Prophylactic therapy is reserved for special circumstances so that the inappropriate treatment of the 90–95% of contacts not expected to develop leprosy can be avoided.

The second approach to leprosy control has been establishment of partial herd immunity through vaccination. Experience to date, however, has not been promising.

One historical practice that has fortunately been abandoned is the forcing of leprosy patients into leprosariums. Mouse footpad inoculation studies have demonstrate that viability of *M. leprae* in skin biopsies falls sharply within 3 wk of initiating therapy with dapsone and rifampin. This rapid drop in infectivity combined with the high probability that family members have had prolonged exposure to the patient prior to the diagnosis makes physical isolation of leprosy patients unnecessary.

RICHARD A. MILLER
THOMAS M. BUCHANAN

Binford CH, Meyers WM, Walsh GP: Leprosy. JAMA 247:2283, 1982.

Bloom BR, Godal T: Selective primary health care: Strategies for control of disease in the developing world. V. Leprosy. Rev Infect Dis 5:765, 1983.

Bullock WE: Immunobiology of leprosy. *In:* Nahmias AJ, O'Reilly RJ (eds): Immunology of Human Infection. Part I: Bacteria, Mycoplasmae, Chlamydiae, and Fungi. New York, Plenum Medical Book Company, 1981, p 369.

Centers for Disease Control: Increase in prevalence of leprosy caused by dapsone-resistant *Mycobacterium leprae.* Morbid Mortal Weekly Report 30:637, 1981.

Ridley DS, Jopling WH: Classification of leprosy according to immunity: A five-group system. Int J Lepr 34:255, 1966.

Van Voorhis WC, Kaplan G, Sarno EN, et al: The cutaneous infiltrates of leprosy: Cellular characteristics and the predominant T-cell phenotypes. N Engl J Med 26:1593, 1982.

Young DB, Buchanan TM: A serological test for leprosy with a glycolipid specific for *Mycobacterium leprae.* Science 221:1057, 1983.

TREPONEMATOSES

11.49 SYPHILIS

Etiology. Syphilis is a systemic, communicable infection caused by *Treponema pallidum*, a long, slender, tightly coiled, motile spirochete with finely tapered ends belonging to the family Spirochaetaceae and the genus *Treponema*. The pathogenic members of this genus include *T. pallidum* (syphilis), *T. pertenue* (yaws), and *T. carateum* (pinta). Because these microorganisms stain poorly, detection in clinical specimens requires darkfield microscopy and/or immunofluorescent staining techniques. *T. pallidum* cannot be cultured in vitro, and laboratory isolation requires animal inoculation.

History and Epidemiology. The first recognized European epidemic and the initial description of syphilis as a distinct clinical entity occurred in Naples in the late 1400's. This outbreak was coincident with the invasion of that city by the French king, Charles VIII. The dispersal of Charles' mercenaries throughout Western Europe was responsible for the rapid spread of this new disease, "the great pox" (as distinguished from smallpox), throughout Europe over the next 3 yr. It was suggested that the European origin of the "new plague" was Charles' Spanish mercenaries who acquired the illness from a Spanish population infected by contacts with Columbus' crew, who themselves had become infected in Haiti.

Although the signs, symptoms, and venereal transmission of syphilis were recognized by the 1700's, early writers failed to distinguish between syphilis and gonorrhea. Ricord, in 1838, reporting on more than 2500 human inoculations, convinced the scientific community of the separate nature of syphilis and gonorrhea. The early 1900's introduced the age of modern syphilis management beginning with the almost simultaneous isolation of *Treponema pallidum*, the development of a serologic test for syphilis, and the introduction of arsenic and fever therapy. In the late 1930's and during World War II, major government programs to combat syphilis were initiated. In the United States, these programs and the availability of penicillin in the 1940's were responsible for cases decreasing annually from 106,000 in 1947 to 6500 cases a decade later. The incidence has subsequently increased; a total of 27,204 cases were reported during 1980, of which 277 were congenital.

Congenital (fetal) syphilis results from transplacental transmission of spirochetes; infant contact with a maternal chancre may rarely lead to postnatal infection. The risk of transplacental transmission varies with the stage of maternal illness. Thus, untreated pregnant women with primary and secondary syphilis and spirochetemia are more likely to transmit infection to their unborn infants than women with latent infection. Infected infants, however, have been delivered of women with latent infection. Transmission may occur throughout pregnancy, but it is most likely in the 3rd trimester.

Acquired syphilis results from sexual contact, transfusion of fresh blood, or accidental inoculation by needle stick. The incidence within the United States has increased by more than 50% over the past decade, largely among the sexually active, urban population, and especially so among promiscuous homosexual and bisexual males. Approximately 50% of homosexual males with AIDS (Sec. 10.23) also have serologic evidence of syphilis.

Clinical Manifestations. Congenital syphilis has traditionally been divided into early and late manifestations. The former appear during the first 2 yr of life as a result of active infection, whereas the latter appear years after birth and result from hypersensitivity phenomena and/or residual scarring. *Early congenital syphilis* is analogous to the secondary stage of acquired syphilis, and, accordingly, clinical manifestations are varied and protean. There may be no manifestations during the first few weeks or months of life; or generalized symptoms such as fever, anemia, failure to gain weight, restlessness, and irritability may be present from birth or shortly thereafter. Furthermore, these generalized symptoms may or may not include the "classic" skin and/or mucous membrane lesions; or local mucocutaneous lesions may be present in an infant who appears well.

The mucocutaneous lesions of congenital syphilis are varied, and several may appear in the same patient. A vesicular or bullous eruption and an erythematous maculopapular rash are characteristic. Each is initially more common on the hands and feet and may become generalized, darken, and eventually desquamate. Wart-like moist lesions at the mucocutaneous junction of the mouth, anus, and external genitalia (analogous to the condylomata lata of acquired syphilis) may also be present. The cutaneous lesions are highly infectious, often recur over a period of weeks or months, and eventually disappear. Mucous membrane involvement may be extensive and involve the nasal mucous membranes, and in about 10% of cases appears as a profuse, purulent, and blood-tinged nasal discharge ("snuffles") containing viable *T. pallidum*. This lesion, which appears during the 2nd wk of life, is often associated with excoriation of the nasal structures and upper lip, and heals spontaneously.

Hepatosplenomegaly is common (30%). Histologically, liver involvement includes bile stasis, fibrosis, and extramedullary hematopoiesis. Hyperbilirubinemia and elevated liver enzymes are common. Lymphadenopathy (5%) tends to be diffuse and resolve spontaneously; shotty nodes may persist.

Bone involvement is common (25%). Roentgenographic abnormalities include multiple sites of osteochondritis at the wrists, elbows, ankles, and knees; periostitis of the long bones and rarely the skull; widened and serrated epiphyseal lines; and, on occasion, separation of the epiphysis. The osteochondritis is painful, may be asymmetric, and often results in irritability and refusal to move the involved extremity (pseudoparalysis of Parrot). Osteochondritis of the hand (syphilitic dactylitis) resembles the hand-foot syndrome of sickle cell disease.

Histologic abnormalities involving one or all of the cellular elements of the bone marrow are common in congenital syphilis (20%). Thrombocytopenia is often associated with platelet trapping in an enlarged spleen. A Coombs-negative, hemolytic anemia is characteristic and may suggest blood group incompatibility. Leukocytosis at times may be extreme and present as a leukemoid reaction; on rare occasions, only monocytes may be involved.

Renal dysfunction is secondary to glomerulonephritis and/or the nephrotic syndrome (5%). Clinical abnormalities appear within the 1st few months of life and may include hypertension, hematuria, proteinuria, hypoproteinemia, hypercholesterolemia, and hypocomplementemia. They appear to be related to glomerular deposition of circulating immune complexes.

Less common clinical manifestations of early congenital syphilis include gastroenteritis, peritonitis, pancreatitis, pneumonia, eye involvement (glaucoma and chorioretinitis), and testicular masses.

The manifestations of *late congenital syphilis* have decreased in frequency since the availability of penicillin. They result from either chronic inflammation or a hypersensitivity reaction. Thus, skeletal changes due to persistent or recurrent periostitis and associated thickening of bone include: frontal bossing, a bony prominence of the forehead ("olympian brow"); unilateral or bilateral thickening of the sternoclavicular portion of the clavicle (Higoumenakis sign); an anterior bowing of the mid-portion of the tibia (saber shins); and scaphoid scapula, a convexity along its medial border. Dental abnormalities are common and include: (1) Hutchinson teeth, which are the peg- or barrel-shaped upper central incisors that erupt during the 6th yr of life; (2) abnormal enamel, which results in a notch along the biting surface (Fig. 11–4); and (3) mulberry molars, abnormal 1st lower (6 yr) molars,

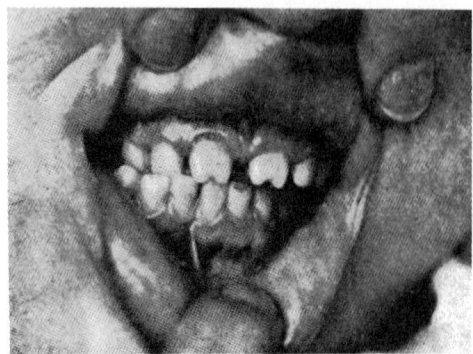

Figure 11–4. Hutchinson teeth in congenital syphilis.

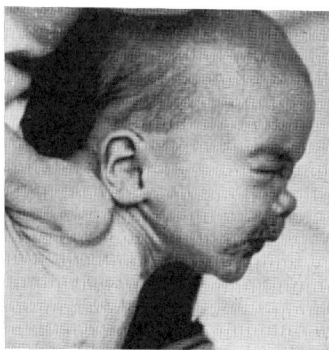

Figure 11-5. Saddle nose in early syphilis.

characterized by a small biting surface and an excessive number of cusps. Defects in enamel formation lead to repeated caries and eventual tooth destruction.

A saddle nose, a depression of the nasal root (Fig. 11-5), is a result of syphilitic rhinitis, which destroys the adjacent bone and cartilage. A perforated nasal septum is an associated abnormality. Rhagades are linear scars that extend in a spoke-like pattern from previous mucocutaneous lesions of the mouth, anus, and genitalia (Fig. 11-6). Juvenile paresis, an uncommon latent meningovascular infection, typically presents during adolescence with behavioral changes, focal seizures, and/or loss of intellectual function. Juvenile tabes with spinal cord involvement and cardiovascular involvement with aortitis are extremely rare.

Other clinical manifestations of late congenital syphilis may represent a delayed hypersensitivity phenomenon. These include unilateral or bilateral interstitial keratitis with symptoms such as intense photophobia and lacrimation, followed within weeks or months by corneal opacification and complete blindness. Less common ocular manifestations include choroiditis, retinitis, vascular occlusion, and optic atrophy. Eighth nerve deafness may be unilateral or bilateral, appears at any age, presents initially with vertigo and high tone hearing loss, and progresses to permanent deafness. Deafness, interstitial keratitis, and deformities of the teeth have been referred to as "Hutchinson triad." Clutton joint is a unilateral or bilateral synovitis involving the lower extremities (usually the knee) which presents as painless joint swelling with sterile synovial fluid; spontaneous remission usually occurs after a period of several weeks. Soft tissue gummas (identical with those of acquired disease) and paroxysmal cold hemoglobinuria are rare hypersensitivity phenomena.

Acquired syphilis is divided into various stages: incubating, primary, secondary, latent, and late syphilis.

Primary syphilis characteristically begins with a single painless papule at the site of inoculation 3-6 wk following contact.

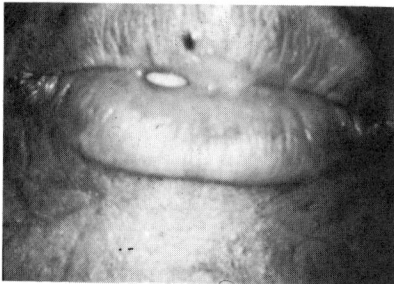

Figure 11-6. Rhagades as long-term residua of congenital syphilis.

The papule becomes indurated and eventually erodes leaving a shallow, clean based, painless ulceration with a firm raised border—the chancre. **Chancres** are most often on the external genitalia and may be multiple and may even go unrecognized. Sites of involvement include the cervix, mouth, rectum, and perineum. There are often associated bilateral, firm, painless, movable, nonsuppurative lymph nodes. In untreated patients the chancre spontaneously heals within 3-6 wk leaving a thin, atrophic scar.

Secondary syphilis begins 6-8 wk following the primary chancre. Clinical manifestations include a flu-like illness with low-grade fever, headache, malaise, anorexia, weight loss, sore throat, myalgias, arthralgias, and generalized lymphadenopathy. The initial cutaneous manifestation is an erythematous macular rash that begins on the trunk and upper portions of the extremities. This progresses to a generalized, nonpruritic, copper-colored, macular rash with a predilection for the palms and soles. The initial rash may also evolve into a maculopapular eruption, which may involve hair follicles and result in localized alopecia. Pustule formation (pustular syphilis) is uncommon. In warm, moist areas of the body (e.g., axilla, perineum, breast) papules may enlarge, coalesce, and erode to produce plaque-like lesions, **condylomata lata.** Similar lesions may develop on mucous membranes (mucous patches) and appear as oval, slightly raised erosions, covered with a grayish membrane and surrounded by a red areola. The cutaneous lesions of secondary syphilis are all highly infectious.

Noncutaneous manifestations result from multiple organ system involvement. These include meningitis (half of all patients with secondary syphilis have cerebrospinal fluid pleocytosis and elevated spinal fluid protein), hepatitis, glomerulonephritis (with or without nephrosis), bursitis, and/or periostitis. Laboratory abnormalities are common and reflect diffuse organ involvement.

In *latent syphilis* there is a positive antitreponemal antibody reaction (FTA-ABS or TPI). The patient appears to be without disease, although there is a history of prior untreated syphilis, exposure, and/or birth of a child with congenital infection. In the first year or so of the latent period, however, one may expect cutaneous relapses capable of infectivity in about 25% of patients, and in as many as 85% within the first 2 yrs. In the late phase there is no evidence of active disease, but the patient is seropositive, noninfectious, and resistant to reinfection. Approximately 60% of untreated patients with late latent syphilis remain asymptomatic; the remainder progress to late or tertiary syphilis.

Late syphilis is a slowly progressive inflammatory disease of adults that can affect any organ system. This stage of syphilis may be associated with gumma formation and the development of neurosyphilis and/or cardiovascular disease.

Diagnosis. Serologic tests for syphilis are either nonspecific nontreponemal (or "reagin") tests or specific antitreponemal tests. The former detect IgG and IgM antibody against a nonspecific lipoidal antigen of obscure origin, and the latter measure antibody specific for *T. pallidum*. In many laboratories the traditional nontreponemal Venereal Disease Research Laboratory (VDRL) slide test and Kolmer test have been replaced by the more sensitive nontreponemal rapid plasma reagin card test (RPRCT) or the automated reagin test (ART). These 2 tests, in addition to being rapid and inexpensive, offer the advantage of being capable of determining the level of disease activity; titers rise during active disease (including treatment failure or reinfection) and fall in adequately treated patients (Fig. 11-7). The rate of fall depends on both the time interval before initiation of therapy and the severity of illness. Serum usually becomes nonreactive within 1 yr of adequate therapy for primary syphilis and within 2 yr of adequate treatment for secondary disease. A small number of adequately treated patients, however, retain positive serology. A major disadvantage of the nontreponemal tests, particularly the VDRL, is that they are not specific for active infection and may be falsely positive, particularly in the presence of immunologic stimulation such as infection, immunization, collagen vascular disease, pregnancy, and drug addiction. Often these "biologic false-positive tests" for syphilis are low titered and their true nature is verified by demonstration of a negative specific antitreponemal test. Unfortunately, many conditions associated with false-positive nontreponemal tests also yield borderline positive antitreponemal tests (e.g., drug addiction, collagen vascular disease).

Despite their value as screening tests for primary and secondary syphilis, the nontreponemal tests may be used improperly in diagnosing congenital syphilis. For example, maternal antibody crosses the placenta, and accordingly a false-positive VDRL can occur in an uninfected infant delivered to a VDRL-positive mother. Passively acquired antibody is suggested when neonatal titers are significantly less (4-fold or less) than maternal titers and can be verified when antibody is no longer demonstrable by 3 mo of age. False-negative results may occur in infants who acquire infections late in pregnancy; such infants become seropositive in the postnatal period.

Two specific or anti-treponemal tests capable of detecting antibody to *T. pallidum* are available. The *T. pallidum immobilization test* (TPI), against which other antitreponemal tests are compared, measures the ability of test serum (antibody) plus complement to immobilize *T. pallidum*. Few laboratories maintain the viable spirochetes necessary for this test. The principal antitreponemal antibody test in clinical use is the *fluorescent treponemal antibody-absorption (FTA-ABS) test*, which is an indirect immunofluorescence test using fixed *T. pallidum* as the antigen to measure serum antitreponemal antibodies; it is sensitive and specific. Antibodies are detected early in infection and remain detectable in latent and late infections (Fig. 11–7). In general, treponemal tests are more sensitive than nontreponemal tests. False-positive reactions are uncommon but do occur in a few normal individuals during pregnancy and in patients with various diseases such as lymphoproliferative disorders, cirrhosis, collagen vascular disease, and drug addiction. The major disadvantages of this test are that its interpretation is subjective, its results cannot be quantitated, and, once positive, it remains so for life even with adequate therapy; it should not be used as a basis for monitoring the effectiveness of treatment. The FTA-ABS is subject to misinterpretation during the neonatal period because it also measures antitreponemal IgG antibody; seropositivity in an adequately treated mother results in a seropositive, uninfected

newborn. Follow-up titers will distinguish passively acquired antibody from disease-specific antibodies, the former becoming negative after the 6th mo of life. The *Treponema pallidum* hemagglutination assay (TPHA-TP) may prove superior to the FTA-ABS test, since it is inexpensive, is easy to perform, and does not require a fluorescent microscope; also, interpretation is not subjective. The test is less sensitive than the FTA-ABS test.

The significance of cerebrospinal fluid serology in both acquired and congenital syphilis remains controversial. Cerebrospinal fluid (CSF) antibodies, both "reagin" and treponemal, result from local production within the nervous system as well as by passive diffusion from serum. Thus, the CSF VDRL may be positive in congenital or in primary and secondary stages of acquired syphilis in the absence of central nervous system involvement. The recognition that maternal IgG antibodies may cross the placenta into the neonatal CSF by passive diffusion suggests that congenital neurosyphilis cannot be diagnosed solely on the basis of positive CSF serology; however, most authorities think that positive CSF serology in newborn infants warrants their treatment for neurosyphilis.

Darkfield microscopic examination or direct fluorescent antibody test of scrapings from primary lesions and moist, freshly scraped or swabbed congenital or secondary lesions can reveal *T. pallidum* and often permits a definitive diagnosis prior to the development of seropositivity. Antibiotics and antiseptics interfere with treponemal motility and accordingly interfere with the accuracy of darkfield examination. This technique is of limited value in detecting *T. pallidum* in oral lesions, since nonsyphilitic saprophytic spirochetes (*T. microdentium*) may contaminate the lesion and cannot be distinguished microscopically from *T. pallidum*. Placental examination by gross and microscopic techniques is useful in the diagnosis of congenital syphilis. The disproportionately large placentas are characterized histologically by focal proliferative villitis, endovascular and perivascular arteritis, and focal or diffuse immaturity of placental villi.

Treatment. *T. pallidum* is extremely sensitive to penicillin, and there is no evidence of increasing penicillin resistance. A serum concentration greater than 0.03 μg/mL of penicillin is needed to assure killing of spirochetes; microorganisms will regenerate if subinhibitory concentrations of penicillin (less than 0.0025 μg/mL) persist for more than 24 hr. Inhibitory levels of penicillin must be maintained for at least 7 days to assure complete cure; increasing the dose does not increase the efficacy of the treatment regimen. Table 11–24 presents appropriate therapeutic regimens for syphilis.

Incubating syphilis may be effectively treated with the currently recommended regimens for gonorrhea (Sec. 11.22). Because of the high risk of acquiring infection, "prophylactic treatment" should be given to anyone exposed to infectious syphilis within the preceding 3 mo regardless of serology. Follow-up serologic studies should be obtained in exposed seronegative individuals to establish the diagnosis and/or determine the adequacy of treatment.

Syphilis in Pregnancy. Routine serology for syphilis should be obtained during the 1st trimester and prior to delivery in high-risk populations. When clinical findings and/or serology suggest active infection or when the diagnosis of active syphilis cannot be excluded with certainty, treatment is indicated. Women who have been adequately treated in the past do not require additional therapy unless quantitative serology suggests evidence of reinfection (4-fold increase in titer). Congenital syphilis has been reported in infants of pregnant women whose syphilis has been treated, presumably adequately, with erythromycin or penicillin in late pregnancy. Hence, such infants should be considered untreated. The cephalosporins may be an effective alternative for women

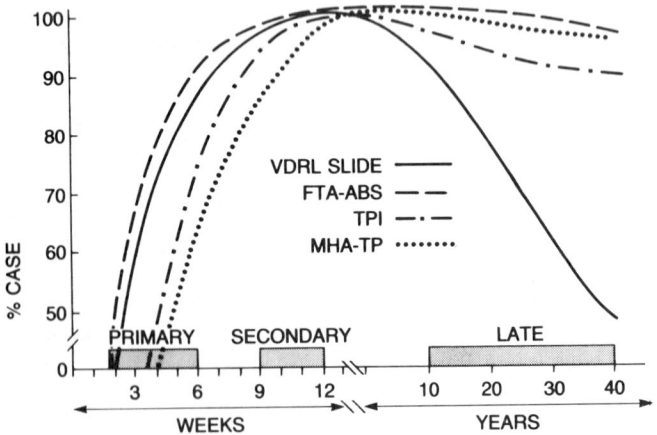

Figure 11–7. Serologic response in untreated syphilis.

Table 11–24. **Treatment of Syphilis**

Stage	Choice	Dosage	Alternatives
Early (primary, secondary or latent less than 1 yr)	Penicillin G benzathine *or* Penicillin G procaine	2.4 million U IM (30,000 U/kg) 600,000 U/day, IM for 8 days	Tetracycline HCl (500 mg oral qid × 15 days) Erythromycin (500 mg oral qid × 15 days)
Late (more than 1 yr duration)	Penicillin G procaine *or* Penicillin G benzathine	600,000 U/day, IM for 15 days 2.4 million U, IM weekly for 3 doses	Tetracycline HCl (500 mg oral qid × 30 days) Erythromycin (500 mg oral qid × 30 days)
Neurosyphilis	Penicillin G crystalline* *or* Penicillin G procaine†	12–24 million U/day, IV for 10 days 2,400,000 U/day, IM for 15 days	Tetracycline HCl (500 mg oral qid × 30 days) Erythromcyin (500 mg oral qid × 30 days)
Congenital CSF normal	Penicillin G benzathine *or* Penicillin G procaine	50,000 U/kg IM for 1 dose 50,000 U/kg/day for 10 days	
CSF abnormal	Penicillin G crystalline *or* Penicillin G procaine	50,000 U/kg/day, IM or IV for 14–21 days 50,000 U/kg/day, IM daily for 14–21 days	

*Followed by benzathine penicillin G, 2,400,000 U/week IM for 3 weeks.
†With probenecid, 500 mg PO qid for 10 days, followed by benzathine penicillin G, 2,400,000 U/week IM for 3 weeks.

allergic to penicillin; however, experience with these agents is limited. Chloramphenicol and tetracycline should not be administered during pregnancy.

Congenital Syphilis. Adequate maternal therapy eliminates the risk of congenital syphilis. Follow-up of all such infants, however, should continue until nontreponemal serologic tests are negative. The risk of giving penicillin to a newborn infant is minimal; therefore, whenever there is uncertainty concerning the adequacy of the mother's treatment, the infant should be treated.

An acute systemic febrile reaction, *Jarisch-Herxheimer reaction,* with exacerbation of lesions will occur in 15–20% of patients with acquired or congenital syphilis who are treated with penicillin. It is not an indication for discontinuation of penicillin therapy.

Prognosis. Untreated infection is associated with high perinatal mortality and morbidity. Thus, congenital syphilis results in intrauterine death in 25% of pregnancies and postnatal death in 25% of infected live-born infants. Although treatment during the later stages of pregnancy results in the birth of an uninfected infant, clinical findings of intrauterine infection may be present.

Curtis AC, Philpott DS: Prenatal syphilis. Med Clin North Am 48:707, 1964.
Fiumara PJ, Lessell S: Manifestations of late congenital syphilis: An analysis of 276 patients. Arch Derm 102:78, 1970.
Jaffe HW: The laboratory diagnosis of syphilis: New concepts. Ann Intern Med 83:846, 1975.
Oppenheimer EH, Hardy JB: Congenital syphilis in the newborn infant: Clinical and pathological observations in recent cases. Johns Hopkins Med J 129:63, 1971.

NONVENEREAL ENDEMIC CHILDHOOD SYPHILITIC DISEASES

Several variants of endemic syphilis are recognized by their geographic distribution. These include yaws, bejel, and pinta. Each is caused by a different strain of *Treponema,* and various factors modify their respective clinical patterns.

11.50 Yaws

Yaws is a chronic relapsing, nonvenereally transmitted disease caused by *Treponema pertenue,* a spirochete that cannot be differentiated microscopically or serologically from *T. pallidum.* It is primarily a disease of children living in rural areas of Africa, Southeast Asia, Australia, and South America. Transmission is by direct contact with an infectious lesion and is facilitated by overcrowding and poor personal hygiene. In 10% of untreated cases, there are late destructive changes in skin, bone, and cartilage.

Infection follows penetration of the causative organism through abraded skin. After an incubation period of several weeks an initial lesion (the "mother yaw") appears at the inoculation site as either a localized maculopapular rash, a small cluster of papules, or a large exudative papilloma. This lesion ulcerates before healing spontaneously, leaving behind a small hypopigmented scar. Following a period of weeks to months, a generalized papular eruption appears, often associated with generalized lymphadenopathy, anorexia, and malaise. Individual papules may enlarge and coalesce to form large papillomas and condylomas, disappear spontaneously, and/or ulcerate. Each ulcer is covered with a yellowish exudate containing treponemes. This polymorphic secondary eruption heals spontaneously without scarring; however, relapses are common and may extend over several years. The exacerbations are often associated with bone pain and underlying periostitis and/or osteomyelitis. Following the initial period of clinical activity the patient enters a long period of latency. This is followed by the appearance of tertiary lesions at puberty, which are often solitary and destructive. They present as painful papillomas on the hands and feet, gummatous skin ulcerations, and/or osteitis. Bony destruction and deformity are common, as are juxta-articular nodules, depigmentation, and painful hyperkeratosis (crab yaws) of the palms and soles.

Diagnosis depends on the clinical manifestations of the disease in an endemic area. Darkfield examination of cutaneous lesions and serologic tests for syphilis (VDRL, TPI, and

FTA-ABS) are confirmatory. Treatment consists of a single intramuscular injection of penicillin (1.2 million units of benzathine penicillin, IM), which cures the lesions of active yaws, renders them noninfectious, and prevents relapse.

Eradication of yaws from endemic foci may be accomplished by treating the entire population with penicillin. Patients allergic to penicillin may be treated with erythromycin or tetracycline.

11.51 Endemic Syphilis
(Bejel, Nonvenereal Childhood Syphilis)

Bejel affects children living in the Saharan regions of Africa and the Middle East. Infection with a strain of *T. pallidum* follows penetration of the spirochete through traumatized skin and/or mucous membranes. In experimental infections, a primary papule forms at the inoculation site after an incubation period of 3 wk; in human infection a primary lesion is almost never visualized. The initial clinical manifestations of the secondary stage of bejel are confined to the skin and mucous membranes and consist of highly infectious mucous patches on the oral mucosa and condyloma-like lesions on the moist areas of the body, especially the axilla and anus. These mucocutaneous lesions resolve spontaneously over a period of several months, but recurrences are common. The secondary stage is followed by a variable latency period before the onset of late or tertiary bejel. The late complications, identical to those of yaws, include gumma formation in skin, subcutaneous tissue, and bone, resulting in painful, destructive ulcerations, swelling, and deformity. Diagnosis is suspected on epidemiologic and clinical grounds and confirmed either by darkfield examination of skin and mucous membrane lesions, or by serologic testing (positive VDRL, TPI, and TBA-ABS). Differentiation from syphilis is extremely difficult in nonendemic areas. Bejel can be suspected by the absence of a primary chancre and lack of involvement of the central nervous and cardiovascular systems during the late stage. Treatment of early infection consists of a single dose of benzathine penicillin (1.2 million units, IM); late infection is treated with 3 injections, each of the same dose at intervals of 7 days. Patients allergic to penicillin may be treated with erythromycin or tetracycline.

11.52 Pinta

Pinta is a chronic, nonvenereally transmitted infection caused by *Treponema carateum*, a spirochete morphologically and serologically indistinguishable from other human treponemes. The disease is endemic in Mexico, Central America, northwestern South America, and parts of the West Indies. Infection follows direct inoculation of the treponeme through abraded skin. Following a variable incubation period of days, a primary lesion appears at the inoculation site as a small erythematous papule resembling localized psoriasis or eczema. The regional lymph nodes are often enlarged, and spirochetes can be visualized on darkfield examination of skin scrapings and/or of the involved lymph nodes. After a period of enlargement, the primary lesion disappears. Secondary lesions follow within 6–8 mo; they consist of small macules and papules on the face, scalp, and other exposed portions of the body. These pigmented lesions are scaly and nonpruritic and may coalesce to form large plaque-like elevations resembling psoriasis. In the late stage atrophic and depigmented lesions develop on the hands, wrists, ankles, feet, face, and scalp. Hyperkeratosis of palms and soles is uncommon. Diagnosis is confirmed by darkfield examination of early lesions and a serologic test for syphilis. Treatment consists of a single injection of long-acting penicillin (600,000 units of

benzathine penicillin). Tetracycline and erythromycin are satisfactory alternatives for patients allergic to penicillin.

Lyme Disease See Sec. 10.76.

11.53 LEPTOSPIROSIS

Etiology. Leptospirosis is a generalized infection of man and animals caused by spirochetes of the genus *Leptospira*. The pathogenic leptospires belong to a single species, *L. interrogans*, which contains more than 180 distinct serotypes arranged in 18 serogroups. The serogroups most often responsible for human infection in the United States include canicola, icterohaemorrhagiae, pomona, autumnalis, grippotyphosa, hebdomidis, and australis. A single serotype may produce a variety of distinct syndromes, and a single clinical manifestation, e.g., aseptic meningitis, may be caused by multiple serotypes.

Epidemiology. Leptospirosis is a zoonosis distributed worldwide. *Leptospira* infect many species of wild and domestic animals and have been isolated from birds, fish, and reptiles. The rat is the principal source of human infection; other important infective reservoirs include dogs, cats, livestock, and wild animals. Animal infection varies from inapparent to fatal; once infected, animals can excrete spirochetes in urine for extended periods of time. Survival of these organisms outside the human host is dependent upon the moisture content, temperature, and pH of the soil and/or water into which they are shed. The majority of human cases worldwide result from occupational exposure to rat-contaminated water or soil. In the United States, the major animal reservoir is the dog. Contact with spirochetes (principally *L. canicola*) frequently follows bathing and other outdoor recreational activities during summer months. *Leptospira* enter humans through moist and preferably abraded skin or exposed mucous membranes.

Pathophysiology. Following penetration of the skin, *Leptospira* enter the blood stream and are carried to all organs of the body. After an incubation period of 7–12 days, an initial "septicemic" phase begins in which *Leptospira* can be isolated from the blood, cerebrospinal fluid, and other tissues. Initial symptoms, which last approximately 2–7 days, are followed by a brief period of well-being and then a second or "immune" phase. With the appearance of circulating antibody during the immune phase, organisms are cleared from the blood and cerebrospinal fluid but may persist in the kidney, urine, and aqueous humor. Significant cell destruction has resulted in fatal renal failure.

Clinical Manifestations. Most cases of human leptospirosis are subclinical; inapparent infection is particularly common in high-risk occupational groups such as sewer workers and farmers and their families. Symptomatic infection may present as an acute febrile illness with nonspecific signs and symptoms (70%), as meningitis (20%), or as hepatorenal dysfunction (10%). The onset is typically sudden, and the illness tends to follow a biphasic course (Fig. 11–8).

Anicteric Leptospirosis. The onset of the initial or septicemic phase is abrupt, with fever, shaking chills, headache, malaise, nausea, vomiting, and severe and often debilitating muscular pain. Circulatory collapse is uncommon, but some patients have bradycardia and hypotension. Typically the child is lethargic, with mild to moderate dehydration. Additional physical findings include extreme muscle tenderness, most prominent in the lower extremities, the lumbosacral spine, and abdomen. Conjunctival suffusion with photophobia and orbital pain (in the absence of chemosis and purulent exu-

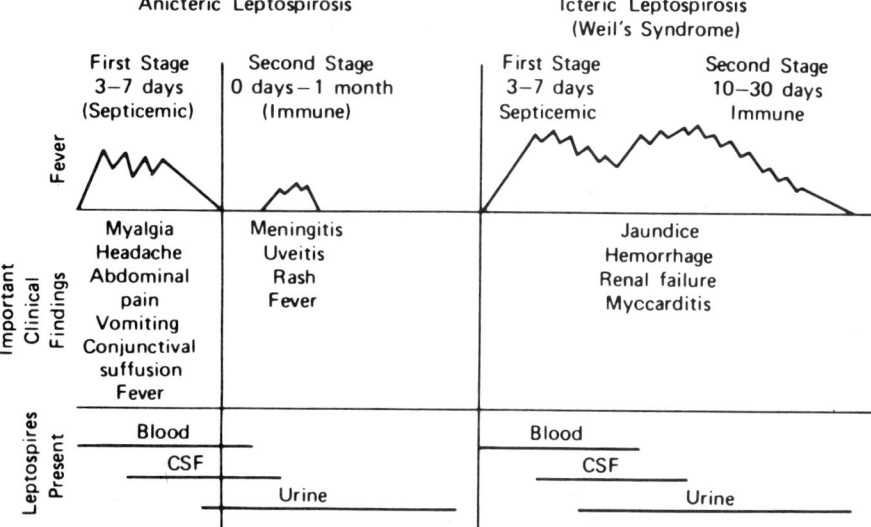

Figure 11–8. Stages of anicteric and icteric leptospirosis. Correlation between clinical findings and presence of leptospires in body fluids. (Reprinted with permission from Feigin RD, Anderson DC: CRC Crit Rev Clin Lab Sci 5:413, 1975. Copyright The Chemical Rubber Co., CRC Press, Inc.)

date), generalized lymphadenopathy, and hepatosplenomegaly may also be manifest. Cutaneous lesions are common (50%), usually consisting of a truncal erythematous or maculopapular rash, but they may be urticarial, petechial, purpuric, or desquamating. Less common manifestations include pharyngitis, pneumonitis, arthritis, carditis, cholecystitis, parotitis, orchitis, and otitis media. A mild febrile illness with a macular or maculopapular rash localized to the pretibial area (*pretibial* or *Fort Bragg fever*) has been associated with infection due to *L. autumnalis*.

The second or immune phase follows a brief asymptomatic interlude and is characterized by recurrence of fever. Aseptic meningitis is the hallmark of this phase. Despite abnormal cerebrospinal fluid profiles in 80% of infected children, only 50% have meningeal manifestations. Spinal fluid abnormalities include a modest elevation in pressure, a mononuclear pleocytosis rarely exceeding 500 cells/mm³ (polymorphonuclear leukocytes predominate initially), normal or slightly elevated protein, and normal glucose values. Encephalitis, cranial and peripheral neuropathies, papilledema, and paralysis are uncommon. Symptoms referable to the central nervous system resolve spontaneously within a week or so. Uveitis may occur during this phase; it can be unilateral or bilateral and is usually self-limited, rarely resulting in permanent visual impairment.

Icteric Leptospirosis (Weil Disease). This severe form of leptospirosis occurs in fewer than 10% of affected children. The initial manifestations are similar to those described for anicteric leptospirosis. The immune phase, however, is distinctive, being characterized by clinical and laboratory evidence of hepatic and renal dysfunction. In fulminating cases, hemorrhagic phenomena and cardiovascular collapse also occur. Hepatic abnormalities include right upper quadrant pain, hepatomegaly, direct and indirect hyperbilirubinemia, and elevated serum levels of liver enzymes. Renal manifestations are common, may dominate the clinical picture, and are the principal cause of death in fatal cases; all patients have abnormal urinalysis (hematuria, proteinuria, and casts), and azotemia is common, often associated with oliguria or anuria. Congestive heart failure is uncommon; however, abnormal electrocardiograms are present in 90% of affected children. Hemorrhagic manifestations are rare but when present may include epistaxis, hemoptysis, and gastrointestinal and adrenal hemorrhage. Thrombocytopenia and hypoprothrombinemia also occur.

Diagnosis. Leptospirosis should be considered in the differential diagnosis of any febrile illness when there is a history of direct contact with animals or with soil or water contaminated with animal urine, and especially when the onset is abrupt with chills and fever, myalgias, conjunctival suffusion, headache, and nausea and vomiting. Isolating the infecting organism from clinical specimens and/or a 4-fold rise in antibody titer in the presence of clinical symptoms compatible with leptospirosis establishes the diagnosis. A presumptive diagnosis is made in symptomatic children with stable titers of 1:100 or greater in two or more specimens, and in asymptomatic children exhibiting evidence of exposure and a seroconversion, i.e., a 4-fold rise in antibody titer in specimens obtained 2 or more wk apart.

Silver impregnation and fluorescent antibody techniques permit identification of *Leptospira* in infected tissue or body fluids. They may also be demonstrated by phase-contrast or darkfield microscopy; however, the skill required and the high frequency of artifacts limit their use. Unlike other pathogenic spirochetes, *Leptospira* are easily cultured on commercially available media. They can be recovered from the blood and/or cerebrospinal fluid during the first 10 days of illness and from urine after the 2nd wk. Because the number of *Leptospira* in clinical specimens is small and their growth rate is slow, multiple cultures should be obtained and incubated for 5–6 wk.

The diagnosis is most often established by serologic testing. A macroscopic slide-agglutination test utilizing killed antigen is the most useful screening test. A microscopic slide-agglutination test with a live or formalin-treated antigen may be used to determine antibody titer and tentatively identify the infecting serotype. Agglutinins usually appear by the 12th day of illness and reach a maximum titer by the 3rd wk. Low titers may persist for years. Approximately 10% of infected persons do not have detectable agglutinins, presumably because available antisera do not identify all *Leptospira* serotypes.

Treatment and Prevention. Despite the in vitro sensitivity of *Leptospira* to penicillin and tetracycline and the efficacy of these agents in experimental infection, their effectiveness in human leptospirosis remains controversial. It does appear that initiation of treatment before the 7th day will probably shorten the clinical course and decrease the severity of the infection. On this basis treatment with penicillin or tetracycline (in children over 12 yr) should be instituted as soon as the diagnosis is suspected. Parenteral penicillin G, 6–8 million units/m²/24 hr, in 6 divided doses for 7 days is recommended. In patients allergic to penicillin, tetracycline (10–20 mg/kg/day) should be administered orally or intravenously in 4 divided doses for 7 days.

Prevention of human leptospirosis is possible by rodent control and avoidance of contaminated water and soil. Immunization of livestock and family pets has been recommended as a means of eliminating animal reservoirs, but these programs have met with limited success. A formalin-killed polyvalent human vaccine has been utilized in "at risk" occupation groups in Europe and Asia; however, there have been no clinical trials to determine efficacy. Leptospirosis has been prevented in American servicemen stationed in the tropics by administering doxycycline, 200 mg once a week, as prophylaxis. This schedule may be similarly effective for the traveler entering a highly endemic area for a limited period.

Edwards GA, Domm BM: Human leptospirosis. Medicine 39:117, 1960.
Feigin RD, Anderson DC: Human leptospirosis. CRC Crit Rev Clin Lab Sci 5:413, 1975.
Heath CW Jr, Alexander AD, Galton MM: Leptospirosis in the United States. Analysis of 483 cases in man, 1949–1961. N Engl J Med 273:857, 1965.
Pace JL, Czonka GW: Endemic non-venereal syphilis (bejel) in Saudi Arabia. Br J Vener Dis 60:293, 1984.
Wong ML, Kaplan S, Dunide LM, et al: Leptospirosis: A childhood disease. J Pediatr 90:532, 1977.

11.54 RAT BITE FEVERS

Two distinctly different diseases are categorized under the term rat bite fever. These are spirillary and streptobacillary rat-bite fever. Both illnesses usually follow the bite or scratch of a rat; however, cases have been reported in the absence of a history of rodent exposure. Isolated case reports and several epidemics also have been described following the ingestion of raw milk contaminated by rats (*Haverhill fever*). The illnesses exist worldwide, with higher incidences reported in urban settings with poor sanitation and large rat populations. They are more common in children than adults and occur in approximately 10% of children bitten by wild rats.

SPIRILLARY RAT-BITE FEVER
(Sodoku)

This disease is caused by *Spirillum minor*, a short, tightly coiled, gram-negative spirochete that is present in the saliva

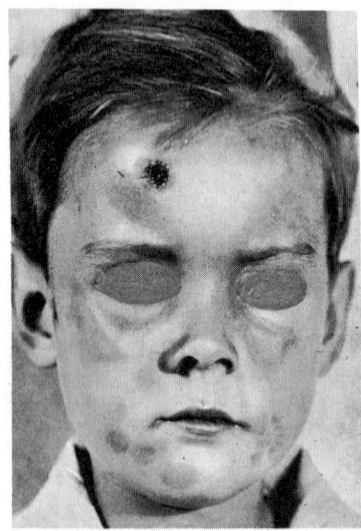

Figure 11–9. Sodoku: chancre-like indurated ulcer at bite site on forehead; secondary macular eruption of face.

of about 10% of healthy wild and laboratory rats. It cannot be grown consistently in commercially available media; laboratory isolation requires inoculation of mice and guinea pigs. However, it can be visualized by direct darkfield examination of infected lymph obtained from the inoculation site (preferably during the ulcerative phase) or from regional lymph nodes. Occasionally, the spirochete is visualized on peripheral blood smears.

Clinical Manifestations. The initial inoculation of spirochetes is followed by a long asymptomatic incubation period of 14–18 days. The wound appears to heal, but then becomes erythematous and indurated and eventually undergoes suppuration and eschar formation (Fig. 11–9). During this phase localized lymphangitis and lymphadenitis are observed in about 50% of affected children. At the onset there are fever, chills, severe myalgias, and a reddish-brown or purple macular rash (80%), typically beginning at the inoculation site and spreading to involve the entire body. In untreated children the fever persists for 3–4 days, at which time the constitutional symptoms subside, the rash disappears, and the inoculation site heals. This asymptomatic period persists for several days and is followed by a 2nd cycle of fever, rash, and constitutional symptoms. This relapsing pattern of illness may continue for months or years; however, the disease is eventually self-limiting. Fatalities are uncommon (1%) and have usually been associated with endocarditis.

Diagnosis. In patients with a history of a rat bite, the major differential diagnosis is etiologic: whether the infectious agent is *S. moniliformis* or *S. minor*. The long incubation period; the prompt initial healing of the primary wound followed by induration, ulceration, and eschar formation; and the absence of joint involvement suggest *S. minor* infection. The laboratory diagnosis depends on negative blood and joint fluid cultures for *S. moniliformis*, the presence of spirochetes on direct darkfield examination of tissue specimens, and recovery of spirochetes following animal inoculation.

Treatment. *S. minor* is extremely sensitive to penicillin; however, because this illness is often confused with rat bite fever due to *S. moniliformis*, which is more resistant to penicillin, and because dual infection has been described, large doses of procaine penicillin, i.e., 600,000 units of procaine penicillin G every 12 hr for 10 days, are recommended. In patients allergic to penicillin, tetracycline is a satisfactory alternative for children over 12 yr of age.

STREPTOBACILLARY RAT-BITE FEVER
(Haverhill Fever)

This form of rat-bite fever is caused by *Streptobacillus moniliformis*, an aerobic, nonmotile, pleomorphic, unencapsulated gram-negative bacillus, which can be isolated from the nasopharynx of about 50% of healthy wild and laboratory rats. The organism has also been isolated from mice, squirrels, dogs, cats, and weasels. *S. moniliformis* can be grown on commercially available artificial media. The morphologic characteristics of the pathogen, including the formation of L-forms devoid of cell wall, and the resistance to penicillin vary with the age of the inoculum and the components of the culture medium. Giemsa or Gram stain may reveal short rods, long chains, and/or long tangled filaments with fusiform swellings.

Clinical Manifestations. The incubation period is short, rarely exceeding 7 days. The onset is abrupt with fever and chills. Associated symptoms include severe myalgias, weakness, headache, and upper respiratory symptoms, most notably pharyngitis. A generalized rash and joint involvement appear within several days after the onset of fever. The rash may be maculopapular, petechial, and/or urticarial; most often it appears as a diffuse morbilliform rash involving the palms and soles. Joint involvement is common, consisting of a polyarticular, occasionally migratory arthritis and having a predilection for the small joints of the hands and feet. The initial inoculation site heals without suppuration, and lymphangitis and lymphadenitis are uncommon. In untreated patients the symptoms spontaneously resolve after several days, whereupon the illness assumes a relapsing course of paroxysms of fever, rash, and arthritis occurring at irregular intervals for several months; the illness is eventually self-limiting, and the mortality rarely exceeds 10%. Life-threatening complications include endocarditis and pneumonitis.

Diagnosis. In patients with a history of a rat bite or rodent contact, the major differential diagnosis involves the 2 forms of rat bite fever. In the streptobacillary form of infection the incubation period is short, the inoculation site heals without suppuration or eschar formation; lymphangitis and lymphadenitis are uncommon, and the responsible pathogen can be readily cultured from blood and joint fluid. Other bacterial infections to be considered in the differential diagnosis include disseminated gonococcal infection, chronic meningococcemia, and leptospirosis.

Treatment. Since the organism is relatively resistant to penicillin, initial therapy consists of 600,000 units of procaine penicillin G every 12 hr for 7–10 days. Streptomycin is effective in treating infections due to penicillin-resistant strains of *S. moniliformis* and should be considered as an alternative in children allergic to penicillin. Tetracycline has been used effectively in penicillin-allergic children over 12 yr of age.

11.55 RELAPSING FEVER
(Recurrent Fever, Louse-Borne Fever, Tick-Borne Fever)

Relapsing fever is an uncommon arthropod-borne infection characterized by recurrent episodes of fever. It is caused by spirochetes of the genus *Borrelia*, a fastidious microorganism with worldwide distribution that is transmitted to man by lice or ticks.

Etiology and Epidemiology. *Epidemic relapsing fever* is caused by *B. recurrentis* and is transmitted from man to man by the human body louse (*Pediculus humanus*). Following ingestion of an infective blood meal by the louse, the spirochetes penetrate its midgut, migrate to and multiply within the hemolymph, and remain viable throughout its life span (several weeks). Human infection occurs as a result of crushing lice during scratching, so that infected hemolymph is permitted to enter through the abraded skin. Louse-borne disease tends to occur in epidemics, often in association with typhus. It occurs more commonly during the winter, under circumstances which favor dissemination of body lice.

Endemic relapsing fever is caused by several species of *Borrelia* and is transmitted to man by ticks (genus *Ornithodorus*). Following ingestion of an infective blood meal, spirochetes invade all tissues of their arthropod hosts including salivary glands and reproductive tract. The latter permits transovarial passage of infected spirochetes, perpetuating arthropod infection in successive generations. Human infection occurs when saliva, coxal gland fluid, and/or excrement is released by the tick during feeding, thereby permitting spirochetes to penetrate skin and mucous membranes. *Ornithodorus* are distributed worldwide (including the western United States), prefer warm humid environments and high altitudes, and are found in rodent burrows, caves, and other nesting sites; rodents are the principal reservoirs. Infected ticks gain access to human dwellings on the rodent host. Human contact is often unnoticed, since these ticks are nocturnal feeders, have a painless bite, and detach immediately following a short blood meal.

Pathophysiology. The cyclic nature of relapsing fever is explained by the ability of *Borrelia* to continually undergo antigenic (phase) variation: multiple variants simultaneously evolve during the first relapse, with one type becoming predominant; and spirochetes isolated during the primary febrile episode differ antigenically from those recovered during a subsequent relapse. During febrile episodes, spirochetes enter the bloodstream, promote the development of specific IgM and IgG antibody, and undergo agglutination, immobilization, lysis, and phagocytosis. During remission, *Borrelia* disappear from the blood stream, and antigenic variants sequestered in the reticuloendothelial system and brain increase in number. The number of relapses in untreated patients depends upon the number of antigenic variants of the infecting strain.

Clinical Manifestations. Louse-borne disease has a longer incubation period, longer periods of pyrexia, fewer relapses, and longer remission periods than tick-borne disease. Each illness is associated with sudden onset of high fever, headache, photophobia, nausea, vomiting, myalgia, and arthralgia. Additional symptoms include abdominal pain, a productive cough, and mild respiratory distress. Bleeding manifestations are common and include epistaxis, hemoptysis, hematuria, and hematemesis. The child may be lethargic and often has a diffuse, erythematous, macular, and/or petechial rash over the trunk and shoulders. This rash is more common in louse-borne fever (25%), is of 1–2 days' duration, and occurs almost exclusively during the end of the primary febrile episode. There may also be lymphadenopathy, pneumonia, splenomegaly, and hepatomegaly with jaundice. Central nervous system manifestations may be the principal feature of late relapses in tick-borne disease; they include lethargy, stupor, meningismus, convulsions, peripheral neuritis, focal neurologic deficits, and cranial nerve paralysis. Myocarditis and hepatitis are not uncommon and may be responsible for death.

The initial symptomatic period characteristically ends with a crisis marked by abrupt diaphoresis, hypothermia, hypotension, bradycardia, profound muscle weakness, and prostration. In untreated patients subsequent relapses become shorter, symptoms are milder, and the afebrile remission period lengthens.

Diagnosis depends on demonstrating spirochetes in thin or thick blood smears stained with Giemsa or Wright stain. During afebrile remissions, spirochetes disappear from the blood.

Treatment and Prognosis. Oral or parenteral tetracycline, chloramphenicol, and erythromycin are the drugs of choice for louse-borne and tick-borne relapsing fever. In children under 12 yr of age chloramphenicol (50 mg/kg/24 hr) or erythromycin (50 mg/kg/24 hr) for a total of 10 days is recommended. For older children and young adults, tetracycline (500 mg every 6 hr) for 10 days has been effective. Single dose treatment with erythromycin or tetracycline (a single 500 mg oral dose) is efficacious in adults, but experience in children is limited.

Resolution of each febrile episode either by natural crisis or as a result of antimicrobial treatment is usually accompanied within 2 hr by the Jarisch-Herxheimer reaction, which is associated with clearing of the spirochetemia. Attempts to control this reaction by prior treatment with corticosteroids and/or antipyretics have met with limited success.

With adequate therapy the mortality rate for relapsing fever is below 5%. A majority of patients recover from their illness with or without treatment after the appearance of antiborrelial antibodies, which agglutinate, kill, or opsonize the spirochete.

No vaccine is available, and disease control requires avoidance or elimination of the arthropod vectors. In epidemics of louse-borne disease, dissemination can be prevented by good personal hygiene and delousing of persons, dwellings, and clothing with commercially available insecticides.

WILLIAM T. SPECK
PHILIP TOLTZIS

Butler T: Relapsing fever: New lessons about antibiotic action. Ann Intern Med 102:397, 1985.
Butler T, Jones PK, Wallace CK: *Borrelia recurrentis* infection. Single dose antibiotic regimens and management of Jarish-Herxheimer reaction. J Infect Dis 137:573, 1978.
Perine PL, Teklu B: Antibiotic treatment of louse borne relapsing fever in Ethiopia: A report of 377 cases. Am J Trop Med Hyg 32:1096, 1983.
Stoennerita DT, Larcen C: Antigenic variation in *Borrelia hermsii*. J Exp Med 156:1297, 1982.

11.56 CHLAMYDIAL INFECTIONS

History. Trachoma, an eye disease caused by *Chlamydia*, was first described in 1500 B.C. Neonatal conjunctivitis in association with maternal genitourinary chlamydial infection was reported in 1908. The chlamydiae responsible for psittacosis and lymphogranuloma venereum were isolated in 1930, but the closely related organism that causes trachoma was not successfully cultured until 1957. The spectrum of chlamydial disease was extended in 1977 by the description of a distinctive syndrome of pneumonia in young infants. Chlamydial genital infection is now found to be 2–3 times more common than gonorrhea.

Etiology. Chlamydiae are obligate intracellular parasites with discrete cell walls that are similar to those of gram-negative bacteria. They contain both RNA and DNA, are inhibited by some antibiotics, and do not stain red with Gram stain. Giemsa staining reveals typical cytoplasmic inclusion bodies lying close to the nucleus.

The genus *Chlamydia* is divided into two subgroups. Group A contains *Chlamydia trachomatis* and the agent of lymphogranuloma venereum, both of which infect mainly humans and usually produce local disease. Group B includes the agents of psittacosis/ornithosis and Reiter syndrome as well as those of feline pneumonitis, bovine encephalomyelitis, and sheep polyarthritis. Both groups have a common complement-fixing antigen, but microimmunofluorescence testing is species- and subclass-specific.

Epidemiology. Chlamydiae are distributed worldwide. Adult infection is spread venereally as urethritis or lymphogranuloma venereum, and from eye to hand to eye in trachoma. Infection of the newborn occurs during passage through the infected maternal birth canal.

Trachoma is associated with crowded and unsanitary living conditions. It continues to be a problem in American Indians living on reservations. Globally it is the leading cause of acquired blindness.

Chlamydiae are etiologic in about 40% of cases of nonspecific nongonococcal urethritis. *Chlamydia* also causes cervicitis, salpingitis, endometritis, and epididymitis and appears to be an important cause of tubal infertility. Infection rates of 20–30% have been observed in adolescents, some of whom were asymptomatic. A syndrome of acute salpingitis and perihepatitis (Fitz-Hugh–Curtis syndrome), formerly attributed to gonococcal infection, can be caused by *Chlamydia*.

Some cases of Reiter's disease (Sec. 10.60) are caused by *Chlamydia*. Rarely, *Chlamydia* can cause endocarditis, otitis media, choroiditis, or erythema nodosum.

About 12% of pregnant women are infected with chlamydiae; infection is more common in young women of low socioeconomic class. Infants born through an infected cervix have a 35% incidence of conjunctivitis; 20% develop pneumonia. Fifty per cent of exposed infants are culture positive

for *Chlamydia*, and 70% have seroconversion. The incidence of *Chlamydia* infection is estimated as 28/1000 live births. A fourth of all infants under 6 mo of age admitted to the hospital with lower respiratory disease and three fourths of all infants with afebrile pneumonia are infected with *Chlamydia*.

Chlamydia has been isolated from the lower respiratory tract of adults with severe bronchitis or diffuse interstitial pneumonia. Most of these patients were immunocompromised. In one study of young adults having pharyngitis, 20% had significant antibody responses to *Chlamydia*, 10% were positive for *Mycoplasma*, and only 9% for *Streptococcus*.

Psittacosis/ornithosis is transmitted by contact with infected birds such as parrots, parakeets, pigeons, turkeys, and ducks. Disease may be seen in children who purchase infected birds as pets. Person-to-person transmission has been documented in medical personnel caring for infected patients.

11.57 CHLAMYDIAL CONJUNCTIVITIS AND PNEUMONIA IN INFANTS

Clinical Manifestations. *Conjunctivitis* in the newborn usually begins in the 2nd wk of life but may occur as early as 3 days or as late as 5–6 wk. Infants typically are afebrile and alert, but develop purulent discharge from one or both eyes, swollen lids, and pseudomembranes. Routine bacterial cultures are negative. If untreated, the conjunctivitis most often subsides within 2–3 wk, but chronic mild infection is common. Response to appropriate topical antibiotics is prompt, but relapse is frequent.

A distinctive syndrome of *pneumonia* has been reported in infants infected with *Chlamydia*. These patients are usually seen at 3–16 wk of age but frequently have been sick for several weeks. The infant appears well and is afebrile but develops increasing tachypnea, with prominent cough. Physical examination reveals rales and at times wheezing. Conjunctivitis is present in about 50% of these infants.

Roentgenographically hyperinflation and diffuse interstitial or patchy infiltrates are evident. Moderate eosinophilia is common. pO_2 is decreased in arterial blood, but pCO_2 is normal. IgM and IgG are increased, sometimes to 2–4 times normal for age.

Deaths due to chlamydial pneumonia have not been reported. Organisms have been isolated from lung tissue obtained by biopsy: light microscopy shows necrotic bronchioles with alveolar and bronchiolar consolidation. Several infants with chlamydial pneumonia have also been infected with cytomegalovirus. Illness in these infants has not been clinically different from that with chlamydia alone.

Patients improve gradually without treatment, but symptoms and positive cultures for *Chlamydia* persist for weeks or months. Patients hospitalized with *Chlamydia* pneumonia or bronchiolitis show an increased incidence of chronic cough, wheezing, and abnormal lung function studies compared with controls.

Diagnosis and Differential Diagnosis. *Chlamydia* can be isolated in specially treated McCoy, hamster kidney, or HeLa cell lines. Testing for complement-fixing and microimmunofluorescent antibody is possible. Fluorescein-conjugated monoclonal antibody has been used in immunofluorescent tests on smears of urethral and cervical secretions for rapid diagnosis. Enzyme immunoassay (EIA) using chlamydial reticulate body antigen is available in a commercial kit to detect IgM against *Chlamydia*. It is less reliable with infant than with adult serum. Preliminary reports of an EIA using purified major outer membrane protein to detect antibody in infants are promising.

Intracytoplasmic inclusion bodies can sometimes be seen on Papanicolaou staining when *Chlamydia* cervicitis is present, but they are not pathognomonic. If conjunctivitis is present, the palpebral conjunctiva should be scraped with a blunt curette; loosened epithelial cells are fixed on glass slides and stained with Giemsa stain. Intracytoplasmic inclusions are easily seen. The diagnosis is usually made by a high index of suspicion in a patient with a compatible illness.

Chlamydia conjunctivitis must be differentiated from chemical conjunctivitis due to silver nitrate drops, which usually is seen while the infant is still in the nursery. Bacterial conjunctivitis caused by gonococcus or other bacterial can be identified by Gram stain and culture.

Pneumonia may be caused by a variety of bacteria or viruses. Bacterial pneumonia usually has an increased white blood cell count without eosinophilia. Blood cultures or lung taps are frequently positive for bacteria. Viral agents can be isolated with appropriate tissue culture techniques.

Treatment. *Conjunctivitis* responds to topical preparations of tetracycline or sulfonamides. Therapy should be continued for 2–3 wk. Relapses are common. A controlled study comparing the efficacy of oral therapy with erythromycin, 40 mg/kg/24 hr, with topical erythromycin showed no difference in response or recurrence. Nasopharyngeal carriage of *Chlamydia* was eliminated by oral therapy.

Chlamydial *pneumonia* responds to erythromycin in dosage of 40 mg/kg/24 hr or to sulfisoxazole (150 mg/kg/24 hr). Improvement is seen in 5–7 days and is associated with conversions of nasopharyngeal cultures to negative. Treatment should be continued for 3 wk.

Neonatal infection that stems from maternal cervical infection could be averted by preventing or treating the maternal disease. One gram of erythromycin daily for 14 days during the 3rd trimester is effective in eradicating the mother's infection. A similar treatment of her sexual partner is also necessary. For newborn infants, topical eye prophylaxis with erythromycin is another way to prevent conjunctivitis.

Genitourinary tract infections due to *Chlamydia* should be treated with tetracycline 0.5 g q.i.d. Urethritis should be treated for 5 days. Therapy should be continued for up to 3 weeks for more complicated infections.

11.58 PSITTACOSIS/ORNITHOSIS

This disease, caused by *Chlamydia psittaci*, is spread by psittacine and other birds. Infected particles are present in bird secretions and droppings. Infection can be present in apparently healthy birds. Those working in the poultry or pet bird industries or persons who have recently purchased a bird are especially at risk. Most cases occur in adults; mild cases are probably frequent but undiagnosed.

Onset of illness is usually abrupt, with chills, fever, severe headache, myalgia, weakness, and confusion. Pneumonia is frequent; anorexia, vomiting, photophobia, and splenomegaly are less frequent; hepatitis, pulmonary embolism, severe anemia, disseminated intravascular coagulation, erythema nodosum, and endocarditis occur rarely. The temperatures may reach 40.5° C (105° F).

Examination of the lungs may demonstrate rales; roentgenographically diffuse interstitial infiltrations are characteristic, and lobar consolidation is uncommon. The white blood cell count does not help in diagnosing the disease. Untreated, the patient may remain quite ill for 2–3 wk, gradually improving after that time. Mortality is less than 1%.

Pneumonia caused by other agents, such as *Mycoplasma*, influenza virus, or other viral agents, may present a similar clinical picture. A history of exposure to birds is suggestive. Isolation of *Chlamydia* from blood or sputum and/or a 4-fold rise in complement-fixing antibody is diagnostic. A presumptive diagnosis can be made on the basis of a single complement-fixing titer of at least 32. Relapses and reinfections occur, even in patients with high antibody titers.

Chlamydial infections are relatively infrequent in wild birds.

Crowding during shipment to the United States is mainly responsible for the widespread infection of imported birds. These birds are held in quarantine on arrival in the United States, and chlortetracycline is added to their feed for prophylactic treatment. This program, however, is not well administered, and animals have been shown to be infected when released from quarantine.

Tetracycline (30–40 mg/kg/24 hr) is the treatment of choice. Erythromycin (40 mg/kg/24 hr) can be used in children less than 8 yr but experience is limited. Treatment should be continued for 3 wk.

Control of fever and adequate oxygenation are important. Person-to-person spread has been documented on rare occasions. Hospitalized patients should be placed in respiratory isolation.

Beem MO, Saxon E: Respiratory tract colonization and a distinctive pneumonia syndrome in infants infected with *Chlamydia trachomatis*. N Engl J Med 296:306, 1977.

Beem MO, Saxon E, Tipple MA: Treatment of chlamydial pneumonia of infancy. Pediatrics 63:198, 1979.

Chacko MR and Lovchik JC: *Chlamydia trachomatis* infection in sexually active adolescents: Prevalence and risk factors. Pediatrics 73:836, 1984.

Chandler JW, et al: Ophthalmia neonatorum associated with maternal chlamydial infections. Tr Am Acad Ophthalmol Otolaryngol 83:302, 1977.

Harrison HR, Phil D, Taussig LM, et al: *Chlamydia trachomatis* and chronic respiratory disease in childhood. Pediatr Infect Dis 1:29, 1982.

Komaroff AL, Aronson MD, Pass TM, et al: Serologic evidence of chlamydial and mycoplasmal pharyngitis in adults. Science 222:927, 1983.

Myhre EB, Mardh PA: Unusual manifestations of *Chlamydia trachomatis* infections. Scand J Infect Dis Suppl 32:122, 1982.

Potter ME, Kaufmann AK, Plikaytis BD: Psittacosis in the United States, 1979. Morbid Mortal Weekly Rept 32:27SS, 1983.

Puolakkainen M, Saikku P, Leinonen M, et al: Chlamydial pneumonitis and its serodiagnosis in infants. J Infect Dis 149:598, 1984.

Tam MR, Stamm WE, Handsfield HH: Culture-independent diagnosis of *Chlamydia trachomatis* using monoclonal antibodies. N Engl J Med 310:1146, 1984.

Wolner-Hanssen P, Westrom L, Mardh PA: Perihepatitis and chlamydial salpingitis. Lancet 1:901, 1980.

11.59 LYMPHOGRANULOMA VENEREUM
(Lymphogranuloma Inguinale)

Lymphogranuloma venereum (LGV) is usually sexually transmitted, and the majority of children who have it have acquired it from an infected adult. The causative agent is related to *Chlamydia trachomatis* but differs in being more invasive.

Epidemiology. Lymphogranuloma venereum has been reported worldwide, but most frequently occurs in Southeast Asia and Central and South America. The reported incidence is much higher in males, reaching 20:1 in some series.

Pathology. Pathologic characteristics of the primary lesion are not specific and therefore do not help in establishing the diagnosis. Primary genital ulcers have an exudate of fibrin and contain cellular debris and polymorphonuclear leukocytes. The periphery of the ulcer contains large mononuclear and plasma cells as well. The lymph nodes that drain the infected area have characteristic stellate triangular abscesses, in the centers of which are polymorphonuclear leukocytes and macrophages. In older, healing lesions scars and sinus tracts may be expected.

Clinical Manifestations. If a primary genital lesion is considered the end point, the incubation period varies from 3 to 30 days. If such a lesion is undetected, the period from sexual contact to the development of adenopathy may be much longer.

The first manifestation is a small erosion, a papule or a pustule. In men it is usually on the coronal sulcus, frenulum, prepuce, glans, or shaft of the penis or on the scrotum. In women the most common sites are the posterior vaginal wall, cervix, or fourchette. Because the primary lesion is small and asymptomatic, it is frequently undetected. Rarely, extragenital primary lesions are noted; they too can usually be related to direct contact with infected genitals.

The secondary lesion, inguinal adenitis, develops 1–4 wk after the appearance of the primary lesion and is most often unilateral. Males often present with fever, toxicity, and inguinal adenopathy. The nodes are initially firm, tender, and movable. Later they become fixed to one another and to the overlying skin, which becomes erythematous and cyanotic, then scaly and edematous, preceding rupture of the nodes. Whether the rupture is spontaneous or surgical, a chronic sinus tract usually develops and drains for weeks or months. Rarely, the nodes resolve over a period of several months despite lack of treatment. Relapses of acute adenitis are common.

In women the anatomic site of the primary lesion determines the clinical location of the disease. Lesions of the upper third of the vagina and on the cervix drain to nodes between the external and internal iliac arteries; those of the middle third of the vagina, to nodes between the rectum and internal iliac arteries; those of the lower third of the vagina, to the pelvic and inguinal nodes.

Rectal drainage of blood, mucus, or pus secondary to rupture of perirectal nodes also occurs and may lead to fibrosis, scarring, and rectal stricture. The latter may result in periodic rectal bleeding and thin stools. Women may present initially with complications such as rectal stricture. Such symptoms are also especially common in homosexual males.

Untreated patients may develop elephantiasis of the genitalia and attendant soft tissue infections.

Like so many other sexually transmitted infections, lymphogranuloma venereum is a systemic disease and may be associated with fever, malaise, headache, anorexia, and other nonspecific symptoms. Rarely meningoencephalitis occurs, and *Chlamydia* are recovered from spinal fluid.

Hypergammaglobulinemia due to elevation of IgA and IgG is common. The white blood count and sedimentation rate are frequently elevated. Mild anemia, decreased albumin, elevated globulin, and elevated liver enzymes can also be seen. Autoimmune serum factors such as cryoglobulins, rheumatoid factor, antinuclear factor, positive Coombs test, and anticomplementary serum factors are present in most cases. Likewise, a false-positive serologic test for syphilis is common.

Diagnosis and Differential Diagnosis. Lymphogranuloma venereum must be considered in patients with the typical primary lesion; with enlarged, matted, and tender inguinal lymph nodes; and/or with proctitis, draining inguinal or perianal fistulas, and rectal strictures. It may mimic inguinal adenopathy of any cause, such as pyogenic infections, plague, tularemia, cat-scratch disease, chancroid, granuloma inguinale, syphilis, herpes genitalis, and rectal neoplasms. Other venereal diseases can, of course, coexist. Direct examination of the tissues may reveal the somewhat characteristic pathologic lesions as well as *Chlamydia* in the cytoplasm of the cells, which appear as blue inclusions with Giemsa stain. Aspirates from lymph nodes should be cultured.

Serologic tests, such as the complement-fixation reaction, are carried out with heat-stable group antigens. If a test is positive in a patient with a suspicious clinical history and findings, the diagnosis is strongly supported. The indirect immunofluorescence (IF) test is more sensitive but less available.

Prevention. Measures for preventing sexually transmitted diseases are applicable. There is no available vaccine.

Treatment. Tetracyclines are effective, as are sulfonamides and chloramphenicol, although resistance to the sulfonamides has been noted. Treated patients tend to have a shorter duration of the disease, less occurrence of sinus tracts, fewer relapses, and a decline in the complement-fixation titer. If there is a rise in titer after therapy, the patient should be retreated. The course of treatment should be 3–4 wk. Surgical excision or drainage is contraindicated because of the possible formation of sinus tracts. Response to therapy, although variable, is better in acute cases.

CAROL F. PHILLIPS

Banou L Jr: Rectal lesions of lymphogranuloma venereum in childhood. Am J Dis Child 83:860, 1952.
Becker LE: Lymphogranuloma venereum. Int J Dermatol 15:26, 1976.
Hieber JP: Infections due to *Chlamydia*. J Pediatr 91:864, 1977.
Jawetz E: Chemotherapy of chlamydial infections. Adv Pharmacol Chemother 7:235, 1969.
McLelland BA, Anderson PC: Lymphogranuloma venereum: outbreak in a university community. JAMA 235:56, 1976.
Thorsteinsson SB: Lymphogranuloma venereum: Review of clinical manifestations, epidemiology, diagnosis and treatment. Scand J Infect Dis Suppl 32:127, 1982.

11.60 MYCOPLASMAL INFECTIONS

Mycoplasma pneumoniae is the only mycoplasma species known to be pathogenic for humans. It is a major cause of respiratory infections in school-age children and young adults. The incidence of illness varies greatly with the age of the patient and the epidemicity of the organism. Clinically significant disease is unusual before the age of 4–5 yr; the peak incidence occurs from 10 to 15 yr. It has been estimated that *M. pneumoniae* causes 500,000 cases of pneumonia, 11,500,000 cases of tracheobronchitis, and 3,000,000 asymptomatic infections in the United States annually.

Etiology. *Mycoplasma pneumonia*, originally thought to be a virus and called the Eaton agent, was found to be a mycoplasma in the early 1960's. Mycoplasmas have no cell wall and are intermediate in size—larger than certain viruses, smaller than others. They can be grown on lifeless media and are, thus, the smallest free-living microorganisms known. Methods for isolation, propagation, and specific identification are highly technical and are performed routinely in only a few laboratories.

Epidemiology. *Mycoplasma pneumoniae* infections occur worldwide. In contrast to the acute, short-lived epidemics of some respiratory agents, those of *M. pneumoniae* are long-lasting and smoldering in character. They occur at irregular intervals with a tendency to begin in the fall.

The occurrence of mycoplasmal illness is dictated at least in part by the age and immune status of the patient. Overt illness is unusual before 4–5 yr of age; younger children appear to have frequent mild or subclinical infections, and reinfections appear to be common. In adults, previous infections, as demonstrated by the presence of circulating antibodies, prevent or ameliorate subsequent ones.

Mycoplasmal infections are not highly communicable, as evidenced by the slow rate at which susceptible family contacts may become infected; such periods may extend for weeks or months.

Pathology, Immunology, and Pathogenesis. Little information is available on the histopathologic features of *M. pneumoniae* disease, because it is rarely fatal. Peribronchiolar infiltrates of mononuclear and plasma cells and the intraluminal accumulation of polymorphonuclear leukocytes and sloughed epithelial cells are a part of a picture of interstitial pneumonia and acute bronchiolitis.

Electron microscopic studies of infected hamster lungs and exfoliated cells from human cases have demonstrated the attachment of *M. pneumoniae* by their specialized tip to ciliated epithelial cells. The organisms attach to cell surfaces and burrow down between cells, resulting in eventual sloughing of the cells, but intracellular organisms have not been found.

A variety of serologic responses occur following *M. pneu-*

moniae infection. Nonspecific cold hemagglutinins are usually the first antibodies detected and the first to disappear, but in some patients they are not present at any time. The presence of elevated titers of cold hemagglutinins and the height of the titer correlate with the severity of the illness. Specific immunologic reactions can be measured by a variety of techniques and persist for long periods of time.

Although the presence of circulating antibodies in humans can be correlated with protection against *M. pneumoniae* infections, studies in the hamster have shown that circulating antibody alone, in the absence of other forms of immunity, is incompletely protective. In hamsters most of the peribronchiolar mononuclear cells are laden with antibody. However, ablation of the T cell system with antithymocyte serum completely prevents the development of pneumonia. Thus, the disease produced by *M. pneumoniae* is very complex; the immunologic response of the host is responsible for the disease itself as well as for protection against it, depending on the qualitative and quantitative balance of humoral and cellular immunity.

Clinical Manifestations. Respiratory and nonrespiratory sites are involved in *M. pneumoniae* infections, but the lung is the primary site. The incubation period is thought to be 2–3 wk. The onset of illness is gradual and characterized by headache, malaise, and fever; cough is prominent, and sore throat is frequent. The severity of symptoms is usually greater than suggested by the physical signs that appear later in the disease. Rales, which are often fine and crackling and resemble those heard in asthma and bronchiolitis, are the most prominent sign; increased sputum production occurs frequently. *M. pneumoniae* can usually be isolated from the upper respiratory tract or sputum for several weeks to months after recovery.

Involvement of the respiratory tract other than the lungs also occurs, including undifferentiated upper respiratory tract infections, pharyngitis, croup, tracheobronchitis, and bronchiolitis. In addition, otitis media and bullous myringitis have been described.

Nonrespiratory sites of involvement include the skin, central nervous system, blood, heart, and joints. In contrast to the proved and constant relationship between *M. pneumoniae* and involvement of the respiratory tract, the association with nonrespiratory sites is unusual or tenuous. Skin lesions include maculopapular rashes, erythema nodosum, and the Stevens-Johnson syndrome. Meningoencephalitis and the Guillain-Barré syndrome have been reported. Hemolytic anemia is the most common hematologic disorder; thrombocytopenia and coagulation defects have also been described. Myocarditis, pericarditis, and a rheumatic fever–like syndrome are uncommon manifestations.

In general, *M. pneumoniae* illnesses are mild and hospitalization is infrequent. Fatal infections are rare. Complications are unusual, as is bacterial superinfection.

There is nothing diagnostic about the roentgenographic findings. Pneumonia is usually described as interstitial or bronchopneumonic; involvement is most common in the lower lobes. Significant amounts of pleural fluid are unusual, but patients with large effusions due to *M. pneumoniae* have been described. The white blood cell and differential counts are usually normal. Cultures of the throat or sputum on special medium may demonstrate *M. pneumoniae*. Cold hemagglutinins may be determined in acute-phase serum. Complement-fixing antibody tests, in which commercially available antigen is used, are satisfactory for usual diagnostic purposes. An antibody rise (or fall) in convalescent-phase serum obtained in 10 days–3 wk is diagnostic. Rapid diagnosis by fluorescent antibody or electron microscopic studies of exfoliated cells is still a research procedure.

Diagnosis. No specific clinical, epidemiologic, or laboratory observations permit a definite diagnosis of mycoplasmal infection early in the clinical course. Certain observations, however, are suggestive and can be helpful to the astute physician. For example, pneumonia in school-age children and young adults, especially if cough is a prominent finding, is always suggestive of *M. pneumoniae* disease. Cold hemagglutinins in a titer of 1:64 or greater support the diagnosis. The diagnosis can be confirmed by isolation of the organism and identification of specific antibodies. When *M. pneumoniae* can be confirmed in the community in a few patients, the probability of the existence of other mycoplasmal illnesses is greatly increased.

Prevention. At present no vaccine has been licensed for commercial use.

Treatment. *M. pneumoniae* is exceptionally sensitive to erythromycin and to the tetracyclines in vitro; because of the absence of a cell wall, the organism is resistant to the penicillins. Both erythromycin and the tetracyclines are effective in shortening the course of mycoplasmal illnesses. Erythromycin is the drug of choice in small children because of the toxic effects of the tetracyclines in this age group; it should be given in full therapeutic doses for several days after defervescence, usually a total of 7–10 days. For patients above the age of 8 yr tetracycline is an alternative choice. In spite of the efficacy of these drugs in ameliorating the clinical course, the organism is not eradicated.

Symptomatic treatment, including bed rest, analgesics and antipyretics, maintenance of fluid intake, and increased humidity, is indicated.

FLOYD W. DENNY

Clyde WA Jr: *Mycoplasma pneumoniae* respiratory disease symposium: Summation and significance. Yale J Biol Med 56:523, 1983.

Collier AM, Clyde WA Jr: Appearance of *Mycoplasma pneumoniae* in lungs of experimentally infected hamsters and sputum from patients with natural disease. Am Rev Resp Dis 110:765, 1974.

Denny FW, Clyde WA Jr, Glezen WP: *Mycoplasma pneumoniae* disease: Clinical spectrum, pathophysiology, epidemiology, and control. J Infect Dis 123:74, 1971.

Fernald GW, Clyde WA Jr: Immunologic responses to *Mycoplasma pneumoniae* infection. *In*: Bienenstock JB (ed): Immunology of the Lung. New York, McGraw-Hill, 1983, p 282.

Fernald GW, Collier AM, Clyde WA Jr: Respiratory infections due to *Mycoplasma pneumoniae* in infants and children. Pediatrics 55:327, 1975.

VIRAL INFECTIONS AND THOSE PRESUMED TO BE CAUSED BY VIRUSES

11.61 MEASLES
(Rubeola)

Measles, an acute communicable disease, is characterized by three stages: (1) an incubation stage of approximately 10–12 days with few, if any, signs or symptoms; (2) a prodromal stage with an enanthem (Koplik spots) on the buccal and pharyngeal mucosa, slight to moderate fever, mild conjunctivitis, coryza, and an increasingly severe cough; and (3) a final stage with a maculopapular rash erupting successively over the neck and face, body, arms, and legs and accompanied by high fever.

Etiology. Measles is an RNA virus of the family Paramyxoviridae, genus *Morbillivirus*. Only one antigenic type is known.

During the prodromal period and for a short time after the rash appears, it is found in nasopharyngeal secretions, blood, and urine. It can remain active for at least 34 hr at room temperature.

Measles virus may be isolated in cultures of human embryonic or rhesus monkey kidney tissue. Cytopathic changes, visible in 5–10 days, consist of multinucleated giant cells with intranuclear inclusions. Circulating antibody is detectable when the rash appears.

Infectivity. Maximal dissemination of virus is by droplet spray during the prodromal period (catarrhal stage). Transmission to susceptible contacts often occurs prior to diagnosis of the original case. An infected person becomes contagious by the 9th–10th day after exposure (beginning of prodromal phase), in some instances as early as the 7th day. Isolation precautions, especially in hospitals or other institutions, should be maintained from the 7th day after exposure until 5 days after the rash has appeared.

Epidemiology. Measles is endemic over most of the world. In the past, epidemics tended to occur irregularly, appearing in large cities at 2–4 yr intervals as new groups of susceptible children were exposed. Measles is very contagious; approximately 90% of susceptible family contacts acquire the disease. It is rarely subclinical. Prior to the use of measles vaccine, the age of peak incidence was 5–10 yr; most adults were immune. At present in the United States, measles occurs most often in teenagers and young adults who did not receive the live vaccine. Several large epidemics among college students have prompted many colleges to require proof of measles immunity from entering students. About 10% of Americans 15–25 yr of age and 5% of those 25–30 yr are estimated not to be immune to measles. Those over age 30 are virtually all immune. Since measles is still a common disease in many countries, infective persons entering this country may infect United States citizens, and Americans traveling abroad risk exposure there.

The many similarities among the biologic features of measles and smallpox suggest the possibility that measles may be eradicable. These features are: (1) a distinctive rash, (2) no animal reservoir, (3) no vector, (4) seasonal occurrence with disease free periods, (5) no transmissible latent virus, (6) one serotype, and (7) an effective vaccine. A prevalence of >90% immunization of infants has been shown to produce disease-free zones. In 1980, three fourths of all counties in the United States did not report a single case of measles.

Infants transplacentally acquire immunity from mothers who have had measles or measles immunization. This immunity is usually complete for the first 4–6 mo of life and disappears at a variable rate. Although maternal antibody levels are generally undetectable in the infant by usual testing performed after 9 mo of age, some protection persists which may interfere with immunization administered prior to 15 mo (Sec. 4.1). Infants of susceptible mothers have no such immunity and may contract the disease with the mother before or after delivery.

Pathology. The essential lesion of measles is found in the skin; in the mucous membranes of the nasopharynx, bronchi, and intestinal tract; and in the conjunctivae. Serous exudate and proliferation of mononuclear cells and a few polymorphonuclear cells occur around the capillaries. There is usually hyperplasia of lymphoid tissue, particularly in the appendix, where multinucleated giant cells up to 100 μ in diameter (Warthin-Finkeldey reticuloendothelial giant cells) may be found. In the skin, the reaction is particularly notable about the sebaceous glands and hair follicles. Koplik spots consist of serous exudate and proliferation of endothelial cells similar to those in the skin lesions. A general inflammatory reaction of the buccal and pharyngeal mucosa extends into the lymphoid tissue and the tracheobronchial mucous membrane. Interstitial pneumonitis due to measles virus takes the form of

Hecht giant cell pneumonia. Bronchopneumonia may be due to secondary bacterial infection.

In fatal cases of encephalomyelitis, perivascular demyelinization occurs in areas of the brain and spinal cord. In Dawson subacute sclerosing panencephalitis (SSPE), there may be degeneration of the cortex and white matter with intranuclear and intracytoplasmic inclusion bodies (Sec. 21.18).

Clinical Manifestations. The *incubation period* is approximately 10–12 days if the first prodromal symptoms are selected as the time of onset, or approximately 14 days if the appearance of the rash is selected; rarely it may be as short as 6–10 days. A slight rise in temperature may occur 9–10 days from the date of infection and then subside for 24 hr or so.

The *prodromal phase*, which follows, usually lasts 3–5 days and is characterized by low-grade to moderate fever, a hacking cough, coryza, and conjunctivitis. These nearly always precede Koplik spots, the pathognomonic sign of measles, by 2–3 days. An enanthem or red mottling is usually present on the hard and soft palates. **Koplik spots** are grayish white dots, usually as small as grains of sand, with slight, reddish areolae; occasionally they are hemorrhagic. They tend to occur opposite the lower molars but may spread irregularly over the rest of the buccal mucosa. Rarely they are found within the mid-portion of the lower lip, on the palate, and on the lacrimal caruncle. They appear and disappear rapidly, usually within 12–18 hr. As they fade, red, spotty discolorations of the mucosa may remain. The conjunctival inflammation and photophobia lead one to suspect measles before Koplik spots appear. In particular, a transverse line of conjunctival inflammation, sharply demarcated along the eyelid margin, may be of diagnostic assistance in the prodromal stage. As the entire conjunctiva becomes involved, the line disappears.

Occasionally, the prodromal phase may be severe, being ushered in by sudden high fever, at times with convulsions and even pneumonia. Usually the coryza, fever, and cough are increasingly severe up to the time the rash has covered the body.

The temperature rises abruptly *as the rash appears* and often reaches 40–40.5° C (104–105° F). In uncomplicated cases, when the rash appears on the legs and feet, within about 2 days, the symptoms subside rapidly; the subsidence includes a usually abrupt temperature drop. Patients up to this point may appear desperately ill, but within 24 hr after the temperature drop, they appear essentially well.

The rash usually starts as faint macules on the upper lateral parts of the neck, behind the ears, along the hairline, and on the posterior parts of the cheek. The individual lesions become increasingly maculopapular as the rash spreads rapidly over the entire face, neck, upper arms, and upper part of the chest within approximately the first 24 hr (Figs. 11–10 [p. xxvii] and 11–11). During the succeeding 24 hr it spreads over the back, abdomen, entire arms, and thighs. As it finally reaches the feet on the 2nd–3rd day, it begins to fade on the face. The fading of the rash proceeds downward in the same sequence in which it appeared. The severity of the disease is directly related to the extent and confluence of the rash. In mild measles the rash tends not to be confluent, and in very mild cases there are few, if any, lesions on the legs. In severe measles the rash is confluent, the skin being completely covered, including the palms and soles, and the face is swollen and disfigured.

The rash is often slightly hemorrhagic; in severe cases with a confluent rash, petechiae may be present in large numbers, and there may be extensive ecchymoses. Itching is generally slight. As the rash fades, branny desquamation and brownish discoloration occur and then disappear within 7–10 days.

The rash may vary markedly. Infrequently a slight urticarial, faint macular, or scarlatiniform rash may appear during the early prodromal stage and disappear in advance of the typical

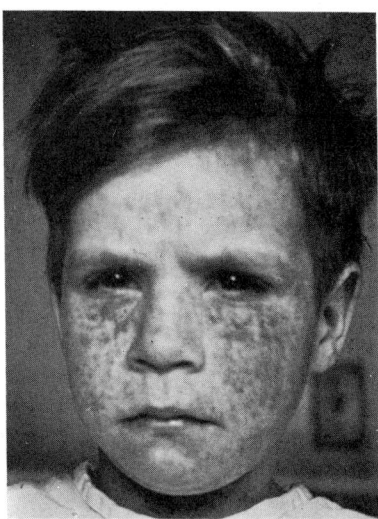
Figure 11–11. Purpuric rash of measles.

rash. Complete absence of rash is rare except in patients who have received human antibodies during the incubation period and possibly in infants under 8 mo of age who have appreciable levels of maternal antibody. In the hemorrhagic type of measles (black measles) bleeding may occur from the mouth, nose, or bowel. In mild cases the rash may be less macular and more nearly pinpoint, somewhat resembling that of scarlet fever or rubella.

Lymph nodes at the angle of the jaw and in the posterior cervical region are usually enlarged, and slight splenomegaly may be noted. Mesenteric lymphadenopathy may cause abdominal pain. Characteristic pathologic changes of measles in the mucosa of the appendix may cause obliteration of the lumen and symptoms of appendicitis. Changes of this type tend to subside with the disappearance of Koplik spots. Otitis media, bronchopneumonia, and gastrointestinal symptoms, such as diarrhea and vomiting, are more common in infants and small children (especially malnourished ones) than in older children.

The diagnosis of measles is frequently delayed in an adult because those providing health care for adults are not used to encountering the disease and rarely include it in the differential diagnosis. The clinical picture is similar to that seen in children. Liver involvement, with abdominal pain, mild to moderate elevation of SGOT, and occasionally jaundice, is common in adults. In developing countries, measles frequently occurs in infants less than 1 yr old; possibly because malnutrition is concomitant there, the disease is very severe and has a high mortality rate.

Diagnosis. This is usually made from the typical clinical picture; laboratory confirmation is rarely needed. During the prodromal stage multinucleated giant cells can be demonstrated in smears of the nasal mucosa. Virus can be isolated in tissue culture, and diagnostic rises in antibody titer can be detected between acute and convalescent sera. The white blood cell count tends to be low with a relative lymphocytosis. Lumbar puncture in patients with measles encephalitis usually shows an increase in protein and a small increase in lymphocytes. The glucose level is normal.

Differential Diagnosis. The rash of rubeola must be differentiated from exanthem subitum, rubella, infections due to echo-, coxsackie-, and adenoviruses, infectious mononucleosis, toxoplasmosis, meningococcemia, scarlet fever, rickettsial diseases, serum sickness, and drug rashes.

Koplik spots are pathognomonic for rubeola, and the diagnosis of unmodified measles should not be made in the absence of cough.

Roseola infantum (exanthem subitum) is distinguished from measles in that the rash of the former appears as the fever disappears. The rashes of rubella and of enteroviral infections tend to be less striking than that of measles, as do the degree of fever and severity of illness. Although cough is present in many rickettsial infections, the rash usually spares the face, which is characteristically involved in measles. The absence of cough and/or the history of injection of serum or administration of a drug usually serves to identify serum sickness or drug rashes. Meningococcemia may be accompanied by a rash somewhat similar to that of measles, but cough and conjunctivitis are usually absent. In acute meningococcemia the rash is characteristically petechial purpuric. The diffuse, finely papular rash of scarlet fever with a "gooseflesh" texture on an erythematous base is relatively easy to differentiate.

The milder rash and clinical picture of measles modified by gamma globulin or by partial immunity induced by measles vaccine, or in infants by maternal antibody, may be difficult to differentiate.

Complications. The chief complications of measles are otitis media, pneumonia, and encephalitis. Noma of the cheeks may occur in rare instances. Gangrene elsewhere appears to be secondary to purpura fulminans or disseminated intravascular coagulation following measles.

Pneumonia (Sec. 13.67) may be caused by the measles virus itself; the lesion is interstitial. Bronchopneumonia is more frequent, however; it is due to secondarily invading bacteria, particularly the pneumococcus, streptococcus, staphylococcus, and *Haemophilus influenzae.* Laryngitis, tracheitis, and bronchitis are common and may be due to the virus alone.

One of the potential dangers of measles is exacerbation of an existing *tuberculous process.* There may also be a temporary loss of hypersensitivity to tuberculin.

Myocarditis is an infrequent serious complication; transient electrocardiographic changes are said to be relatively common.

Neurologic complications are more common in measles than in any of the other exanthems. The incidence of *encephalomyelitis* is estimated to be 1–2/1000 reported cases of measles. There is no correlation between the severity of the measles and that of the neurologic involvement or between the severity of the initial encephalitic process and the prognosis. Rarely, encephalitis has been reported in association with measles modified by gamma globulin or by live attenuated measles virus vaccine. Infrequently encephalitic involvement is manifest in the pre-eruptive period, but more often the onset is 2–5 days after the appearance of the rash. The cause of measles encephalitis remains controversial. It is suggested that when encephalitis occurs early in the course of the disease, viral invasion plays a large role, although measles virus has rarely been isolated from brain tissue; encephalitis that occurs later is predominantly demyelinating and may reflect an immunologic reaction. In this demyelinating type the symptoms and course do not differ from those of other parainfectious encephalitides. Fatal encephalitis has occurred in children immunosuppressed for treatment of malignancies. Other central nervous system complications, such as Guillain-Barré syndrome, hemiplegia, cerebral thrombophlebitis, and retrobulbar neuritis, are rare.

Subacute sclerosing panencephalitis (Sec. 21.18) is due to measles virus.

A possible etiologic role of measles virus in multiple sclerosis has been suggested but not proved.

Prognosis. Case fatality rates in the United States have decreased in recent years to low levels for all age groups, largely because of improved socioeconomic conditions but also because of effective antibacterial therapy for the treatment of secondary infections.

When measles is introduced into a highly susceptible population, the results may be disastrous. Such an occurrence in the Faroe Islands in 1846 resulted in the deaths of about one fourth, nearly 2000, of the total population regardless of age.

At Ungava Bay, Canada, where 99% of 900 persons had measles, the mortality rate was 7%.

Prophylaxis. Quarantine is of little value because of the contagiousness during its prodromal stage, when measles may not be suspected.

Active Immunization. See also Sec. 4.1.

The response to live measles vaccine is unpredictable if immune globulin has been administered in the 3 mo preceding immunization. Anergy to tuberculin may develop and persist for 1 mo or longer after administration of live attenuated measles vaccine. A child with active tuberculous infection should be receiving antituberculosis treatment when live measles vaccine is administered. A tuberculin test prior to or concurrent with active immunization against measles is desirable.

Use of live measles vaccine is not recommended for pregnant women or for children with untreated tuberculosis. Live vaccine is contraindicated in children with leukemia and in those receiving immunosuppressive drugs because of the risk of persistent, progressive infection such as giant cell pneumonia. After exposure of these susceptible children to measles, measles immune globulin (human) should be given intramuscularly in a dose of 0.25 mL/kg as soon as possible. A larger dose may be advisable in children with acute leukemia, even those in remission. Measles vaccine can be given following exposure to the disease. Reactions are not increased, and measles may be prevented.

The use of inactivated (killed) virus vaccine is not recommended.

Passive Immunization. Passive immunization with pooled adult serum, pooled convalescent serum, placental globulin, or gamma globulin of pooled plasma is effective for prevention and attenuation of measles. Measles can be prevented by using immune serum globulin (gamma globulin) in a dose of 0.25 mL/kg given intramuscularly within 5 days after exposure but preferably as soon as possible. Complete protection is indicated for infants, for children with chronic illness, and for contacts in hospital wards and children's institutions. Attenuation may be accomplished by the use of gamma globulin in a dosage of 0.05 mL/kg. Gamma globulin is approximately 25 times as potent in antibody titer as pooled adult serum, and it avoids the risk of hepatitis. Attenuation is variable, and the modified clinical patterns may vary from those with few or no symptoms to those with little or no modification. Encephalitis may follow measles modified by gamma globulin.

After the 7th–8th day of incubation the amounts of antibody administered must be increased greatly for any degree of protection. If the injection is delayed until the 9th, 10th, or 11th day, slight fever may already have started and only slight modification of the disease may be expected.

Treatment. Sedatives, antipyretics for high fever, bed rest, and an adequate fluid intake may be indicated. Humidification of the room may be necessary for laryngitis or an excessively irritating cough, and it is best to keep the room comfortably warm rather than cool. The patient should be protected from being exposed to strong light during the period of photophobia. The complications of otitis media and pneumonia require appropriate antimicrobial therapy.

With complications such as encephalitis (Sec. 11.10), subacute sclerosing panencephalitis (Sec. 21.18), giant cell pneumonia, and disseminated intravascular coagulation (Sec. 15.50), each case must be assessed individually. Good supportive care is essential. Gamma globulin, hyperimmune gamma globulin, and steroids are of limited value. Currently available antiviral compounds are not effective.

Aicardi J: Acute measles encephalitis in children with immunosuppression. Pediatrics 59:232, 1977.
Brem J: Koplik spots for the record: An illustrated historical note. Clin Pediatr 11:161, 1972.
Cherry JD: The "new" epidemiology of measles and rubella. Hosp Pract 15:49, 1980.
Herman JJ, Radin R, Schneiderman R: Allergic reactions to measles (rubeola) vaccine in patients hypersensitive to egg protein. J Pediatr 102:196, 1983.
Jabbour JT, et al: Subacute sclerosing panencephalitis. JAMA 220:959, 1972.
Landrigan PJ, Witte JJ: Neurologic disorders following measles vaccination. JAMA 223:1459, 1973.
Laptook A, Wind E, Nussbaum M, et al: Pulmonary lesions in atypical measles. Pediatrics 62:42, 1978.
Modlin JF: Epidemiologic studies of measles, measles vaccine, SSPE. Pediatrics 59:505, 1977.
Panum PL: Observations Made During the Epidemic of Measles on the Faroe Islands in the Year 1846. Translated by AS Hatcher. New York, Delta Omega Society, American Public Health Association, 1940.
Payne FE, Baublis JV, Itabashi HH: Isolation of measles virus from cell cultures of brain from a patient with subacute sclerosing panencephalitis. N Engl J Med 281:11, 1969.
Ruuskanen O, Salmi TT, Halonen P: Measles vaccination after exposure to natural measles. J Pediatr 98:43, 1978.
Sabin AB, Arechiga AF, de Castro JF, et al: Successful immunization of infants with and without maternal antibody by aerosolized measles vaccine. JAMA 251:2363, 1984.
Starr S, Berkovich S: The effect of measles, gamma globulin modified measles and attenuated measles vaccine on the course of treated tuberculosis in children. Pediatrics 35:97, 1965.

11.62 RUBELLA
(German or Three-Day Measles)

Rubella is a common communicable disease of childhood characterized ordinarily by mild constitutional symptoms, a rash similar to that of mild rubeola or scarlet fever, and enlargement and tenderness of the postoccipital, retroauricular, and posterior cervical lymph nodes. In older children and adults the infection may occasionally be severe, with manifestations such as joint involvement and purpura.

Rubella in early pregnancy may cause severe congenital anomalies. The congenital rubella syndrome is an active contagious disease with multisystem involvement, a wide spectrum of clinical expression, and a long postnatal period of active infection with shedding of virus (Sec. 8.69).

Etiology. Rubella is caused by a pleomorphic, RNA-containing virus currently listed in the family Togaviridae, genus Rubivirus. The virus is usually isolated in tissue culture, and its presence is demonstrated by the ability of rubella-infected African green monkey kidney (AGMK) cells to resist challenge with enterovirus. During clinical illness the virus is present in nasopharyngeal secretions, blood, feces, and urine. Virus has been recovered from the nasopharynx 7 days before exanthem and 7–8 days after its disappearance. Patients with subclinical disease are also infectious.

Epidemiology. Humans are the only natural host of rubella virus, which is spread by oral droplet or transplacentally through congenital infection. Prior to institution of the rubella vaccine program, the peak incidence of the disease was in children 5–14 yr of age. Now most cases occur in teenagers and young adults. Large outbreaks have been reported among college students. Hospital epidemics among employees, with transmission to susceptible patients, have prompted some hospitals to require that employees having contact with patients be immune to rubella. Health care personnel in physicians' offices should also be screened for rubella antibody and, if necessary, immunized. Maternal antibody is protective for the first 6 mo of life. Boys and girls are equally affected. In closed populations, such as institutions and military barracks, almost 100% of susceptible individuals may become infected. In family settings the spread of the virus is less: 50–60% of susceptible family members acquire the disease. Many infections are subclinical, with a ratio of 2:1 inapparent to overt disease. Rubella usually occurs during the spring. It can be difficult to diagnose clinically since enteroviral and other rashes may produce a similar appearance. A single attack usually confers permanent immunity. Epidemics occurred every 6–9 yr before vaccine was available. Serologic studies prior to the use of rubella vaccine showed that about 80% of adult populations in the United States and other continents had antibody to rubella. In island populations, such as those of Trinidad and Hawaii, only 20% of adults screened had detectable antibody.

The epidemiology of the congenital rubella syndrome is discussed in Sec. 8.69. Infants with rubella are a source of infection for older children who are not immune and for nonimmune adults, including pregnant women and nursery personnel.

Clinical Manifestations. The incubation period is 14–21 days. The prodromal phase of mild catarrhal symptoms is shorter than that of measles and may be so mild as to go unnoticed. The most characteristic sign is retroauricular, posterior cervical, and postoccipital adenopathy. No other disease causes the tender enlargement of these nodes to the extent as does rubella. An enanthem may appear just before the onset of the skin rash. It consists of discrete rose spots on the soft palate that may coalesce into a red blush and extend over the fauces.

Lymphadenopathy is evident at least 24 hr before the *rash* appears and may remain for 1 wk or more. The exanthem is more variable than that of rubeola. It begins on the face (Fig. 11–12 [p. xxvii]) and spreads quickly. Its evolution is so rapid that the rash may be fading on the face by the time it appears on the trunk. Discrete maculopapules are present in large numbers; there are also large areas of flushing which spread rapidly over the entire body, usually within 24 hr. The rash may be confluent, particularly on the face. During the 2nd day the rash may assume a pinpoint appearance, especially over the trunk, resembling that of scarlet fever. Mild itching may occur. The eruption usually clears by the 3rd day. Desquamation is minimal. Rubella without a rash has been described.

The pharyngeal mucosa and the conjunctivae are slightly inflamed. In contrast to rubeola, there is no photophobia. Fever is slight or absent during the rash and persists for 1, 2, or occasionally 3 days. The temperature seldom exceeds 38.4° C (101° F). Anorexia, headache, and malaise are not common. The spleen is often slightly enlarged. The white blood cell count is normal or slightly reduced; thrombocytopenia is rare, with or without purpura. Especially in older girls and women, polyarthritis may occur with arthralgia, swelling, tenderness, and effusion but usually without any residuum. Any joint may be involved, but the small joints of the hands are affected most frequently. The duration is usually several days to 2 wk; rarely it persists for months. Paresthesia also has been reported. In one epidemic, orchidalgia was reported in about 8% of infected college-aged males.

The **congenital rubella syndrome** is discussed in Sec. 8.69. Subclinical intrauterine infection is common. The infant may appear normal at birth, but is infectious to nonimmune contacts. Some infants appear to do well for several months before developing severe illness characterized by interstitial pneumonia, rash, diarrhea, hypogammaglobulinemia, disorders of B and T cells, severe neurologic involvement, and death. Progressive panencephalitis has been reported in several adolescents with congenital rubella syndrome who had been functioning well prior to the onset of the panencephalitis.

Differential Diagnosis. Since similar symptoms and rashes can occur with many other viral infections (Sec. 11.3), rubella is a difficult disease to diagnose clinically except when the patient is seen during an epidemic. A history of having had rubella or rubella vaccine is unreliable; immunity should be determined by testing for antibodies. Particularly in its more severe forms, rubella may be confused with the mild types of scarlet fever and rubeola. *Roseola infantum* (exanthem subitum)

is distinguished from rubella by the severity of the fever and by the appearance of the rash at the end of the febrile episode rather than at the height of the signs and symptoms. *Drug rashes* may be extremely difficult to differentiate from rubella. The characteristic enlargement of the lymph nodes strongly supports rubella. In *infectious mononucleosis* a rash may occur which resembles that of rubella, and enlargement of the lymph nodes in each disease may lead to confusion. The hematologic findings in infectious mononucleosis should be sufficient to distinguish the 2 diseases. Enteroviral infections which are accompanied by a rash can be differentiated in *some* instances by respiratory and/or gastrointestinal manifestations and the absence of retroauricular adenopathy.

Diagnostic tests include isolation of virus from various tissues and serologic tests. Hemagglutination-inhibition (HI) antibody has been the usual method of determining immunity to rubella. Several newer tests including latex agglutination, enzyme immunoassay, passive hemagglutination, and fluorescent immunoassay appear to be equal or superior to the HI test in sensitivity. Rubella-specific IgM is present in the blood of affected newborn infants.

Complications and Prognosis. Complications are relatively uncommon in childhood. Neuritis and arthritis occur occasionally. Resistance to secondary bacterial infection is not altered significantly. Encephalitis similar to that seen with rubeola occurs in about 1/6000 cases. The prognosis of childhood rubella is good; that of congenital rubella varies with the severity of the infection (Sec. 8.69); only about 30% of infants with encephalitis appear to escape residual neuromotor deficits, including an autistic syndrome.

Prevention. In a susceptible person, **passive protection** from or attenuation of the disease may or may not be afforded by intramuscular injection of immune serum globulin (ISG) given in large dosage (0.25–0.50 mL/kg or 0.12–0.20 mL/lb) within the first 7–8 days after exposure. The effectiveness of immune globulin is not predictable. It apparently depends upon the antibody content of the product used and upon unknown factors. The value of ISG has been questioned also because in some instances rash was prevented and clinical manifestations were absent or minimal though viable virus was demonstrable in the blood. This form of prevention of rubella is not indicated, except in nonimmune pregnant women.

Since 1979 live-virus vaccine RA 27/3 (human embryonic lung fibroblasts of the WI-38 line) has been used exclusively for active immunization against rubella in the United States. RA 27/3 vaccine has many advantages over other rubella vaccines used in the past since it produces nasopharyngeal antibody and a wide variety of serum antibodies, provides better protection against reinfection, and more closely resembles the protection provided by natural infection. The vaccine virus is heat and light sensitive; therefore, the vaccine should be stored in the refrigerator at 4° C and used as soon as it is reconstituted. Vaccine is administered as a single subcutaneous injection. See Sec. 4.1 for routine immunization.

Antibody develops in about 98% of those vaccinated. While virus may persist, especially in the nasopharynx, and shedding occurs from 18–25 days after vaccination, communicability does not appear to be a problem.

The duration of persistence of rubella antibody following vaccination with RA 27/3 is uncertain but is probably lifelong. Preventive measures are of the greatest importance for the protection of the fetus. It is especially important that girls have immunity to rubella before the child-bearing age, either by contracting the natural disease or by active immunization. The immune status can be evaluated by appropriate serologic tests.

The rubella vaccine program in the United States calls for immunization of all boys and girls between the age of 15 mo and puberty and of nonpregnant postpubertal females who have been demonstrated to have a negative antibody test and can reasonably be relied upon not to become pregnant within 3 mo of immunization. Vaccination of infants under 15 mo is not recommended since persisting maternal antibody may interfere. This policy has successfully interrupted the usual epidemic cycle of rubella in the United States and decreased the reported incidence of congenital rubella syndrome. However, it has not resulted in a decrease in the percentage of women of childbearing age who are susceptible to rubella.

Some European countries have adopted a policy of immunizing only girls routinely at age 12 or older if they are found to be unprotected. This policy has not prevented epidemics of rubella but does appear to be increasing the level of immunity in women.

Pregnant women should not be given live rubella virus vaccine. No cases of serious malformations caused by rubella vaccine have been observed, although RA 27/3 vaccine virus was isolated from aborted material from 1 of 32 (3%) susceptible women who received the vaccine in early pregnancy. The risk of serious malformations when a susceptible women is immunized early in pregnancy with RA 27/3 vaccine is extremely small and should not ordinarily be a reason to interrupt the pregnancy. Other contraindications include immune deficiency states, severe febrile illness, hypersensitivity to vaccine components, and therapy with antimetabolites, corticosteroids, and steroid-like substances.

Clinical manifestations that may follow rubella immunization include fever, typical lymphadenopathy, rash, and arthritis and arthralgia. The last two occur more frequently in older girls and adult women and may last for weeks. Two unusual syndromes have been reported in association with rubella vaccine: one with paresthesia of the hand or arm that occurs at night lasts for up to 1 hr and may recur frequently during the night; the other is manifested by pain behind the knee and limitation of motion. Symptoms are worst in the morning, diminishing during the day. They may last for up to 5 wk. Both syndromes may recur.

Measles-mumps-rubella, measles-rubella, and mumps-rubella combined vaccines are also available and effective (Sec. 4.1).

Management of Pregnant Women Exposed to or Acquiring Rubella. Pregnant women, especially early in pregnancy but also during the entire gestational period, should avoid exposure to rubella regardless of history of the disease during childhood or of history of active immunization. Exposure of pregnant women to infants with congenital rubella syndrome should be especially guarded against because of prolonged shedding of virus. Risk of damage to the fetus decreases after the 14th wk of gestation.

Since approximately 80% of women in the child-bearing age are immune to rubella as a result of the natural infection or of immunization, women who may become pregnant should have their immune status to rubella determined.

If a pregnant woman whose immune status is unknown is exposed to rubella, an antibody test should be performed *immediately as an emergency measure.* If determined to be immune, she can be reassured that the pregnancy can be continued without added risk. If she is found to be susceptible and therapeutic abortion is unacceptable or unavailable to her, passive immunization with immune serum globulin (ISG), 20–30 mL intramuscularly, should be attempted immediately. Active immunization of pregnant women is not advised.

If exposure to rubella occurs in a susceptible pregnant woman to whom abortion is available and desirable because of significant potential hazard to the fetus, it is probably advisable to withhold ISG, and observe her carefully, and repeat the rubella antibody test. If rubella then develops at a stage of pregnancy at which she feels the risk is greater than she wants to assume or if serial antibody tests show that subclinical infection has occurred, abortion may be induced.

Reinfection. The incidence of reinfection on exposure of individuals serologically immune to wild virus is 3–10% among those demonstrating serologic immunity without a history of immunization, and 14–18% among those immunized with RA 27/3 vaccine. Infection has been demonstrated among the fetuses of reinfected pregnant women as well as among pregnant women who had received rubella vaccine. The relevance of reinfection of serologically immune pregnant women to the production of congenital malformations remains to be determined. Until these questions are answered, *all* pregnant women should make every effort to avoid exposure to rubella.

Treatment. Unless bacterial complications occur, treatment is symptomatic. Adamantanamine hydrochloride (amantadine) has been reported to be effective in vitro in inhibiting early stages of rubella infection in cultured cells. An attempt to treat a child having congenital rubella with this drug was unsuccessful. It is possible that the drug may be effective prophylactically or in the early incubation period of rubella, but no studies have been done. *Since amantadine is not recommended for pregnant women, its usefulness is very limited.*

Alford CA Jr, Neva FA, Weller TH: Virologic and serologic studies on human products of conception after maternal rubella. N Engl J Med 271:1275, 1964.

Chang TW: Rubella reinfection and intrauterine involvement (editorial). J Pediatr 84:617, 1974.

Clark M et al: Effect of rubella vaccination programme on serological status of young adults in United Kingdom. Lancet 1:1224, 1979.

Desmond MM, Wilson GS, Melnick JL, et al: Congenital rubella encephalitis: Course and early sequelae. J Pediatr 71:311, 1967.

Desmond MM, et al: The early growth and development of infants with congenital rubella. *In:* Woolman DH (ed): Advances in Teratology, Vol 4. New York, Academic Press, 1970, p 39.

Forrest JM, Menser MA, Burgess JA: High frequency of diabetes mellitus in young adults with congenital rubella. Lancet 2:332, 1971.

Greaves WL, Orenstein WA, et al: Clinical efficacy of rubella vaccine. Pediatr Infect Dis 2:284, 1983.

Gregg NM: Congenital cataract following German measles in the mother. Trans Ophthalmol Soc Aust 3:35, 1941.

Gregg NM, et al: The occurrence of congenital defects in children following maternal rubella during pregnancy. Med J Austr 2:122, 1945.

Horstmann DM, Liebhaber H, Le Bouvier GL, et al: Rubella. Reinfection of vaccinated and naturally immune persons exposed in an epidemic. N Engl J Med 283:771, 1970.

Lawless MR, Abramson JS, Harlan JE, et al: Rubella susceptibility in 6th graders: Effectiveness of current immunization practice. Pediatrics 65:1086, 1980.

Miller E, Cradock-Watson JE, Pollock TM: Consequences of confirmed maternal rubella at successive stages of pregnancy. Lancet 2:781, 1982.

O'Shea S, Best JB, Banatvala JE, et al: Development and persistence of class-specific antibodies in the serum and nasopharyngeal washings of rubella vaccines. J Infect Dis 151:89, 1985.

Plotkin SA, Klaus RM, Whitely JP, et al: Hypogammaglobulinemia in an infant with congenital rubella syndrome; failure of L-adamantanamine to stop virus excretion. J Pediatr 69:1085, 1966.

Rawls WE, Phillips CA, Melnick JL, et al: Persistent virus infection in congenital rubella. Arch Ophthalmol 77:430, 1967.

Rawls WE, Desmyter J, Melnick JL: Serologic diagnosis and fetal involvement in maternal rubella. JAMA 203:627, 1968.

Rudolph AJ, Yow MD, Phillips A, et al: Transplacental rubella infection in newly born infants. JAMA 191:843, 1965.

Tardieu M, Grospierre B, Durandy A, et al: Circulating immune complexes containing rubella antigens in late-onset rubella syndrome. J Pediatr 97:370, 1980.

Townsend JJ: Progressive rubella panencephalitis: Late onset after congenital rubella. N Engl J Med 292:990, 1975.

Weil ML: Chronic progressive panencephalitis due to rubella virus simulating subacute sclerosing panencephalitis. N Engl J Med 292:994, 1975.

Weiss DI, Cooper LZ, Green RH: Infantile glaucoma: A manifestation of congenital rubella. JAMA 195:105, 1966.

Wilkins J: Reinfection with rubella virus despite live vaccine-induced immunity. Am J Dis Child 118:275, 1969.

11.63 EXANTHEM SUBITUM
(Roseola Infantum)

Exanthem subitum is an acute, probably viral disease of infants and young children, usually occurring sporadically but occasionally in epidemics. It is unique in that the diagnostic rash and clinical improvement occur almost simultaneously. The disease is characterized by a period of high fever lasting 1–5 but usually 3–4 days, during which time there are insufficient clinical findings to explain the hyperpyrexia, and by an abrupt termination with a precipitous drop of the temperature to normal and the appearance of a generalized eruption, which fades quickly.

Etiology. Available evidence supports viral origin. Serum, heparinized blood, and throat washings obtained from patients on the 3rd day of fever and on the 1st day of the rash have been shown to be infective for susceptible infants and for monkeys. Typical disease resulted after an incubation period of 9–10 days in the infants. All attempts to isolate the etiologic agent have failed. No serologic tests are available, and nothing is known of the pathologic changes of the disease.

Epidemiology. The degree of contagiousness is not known. There is a tendency for the disease to occur in the spring and fall. It attacks both sexes equally. In the rare epidemics described, the incubation period was estimated to be 7–17 days, usually about 10 days. The epidemiologic pattern is not clear. The sporadic occurrence of exanthem subitum in early life and the rare occurrence of epidemics in older age groups suggest the possibility of an endemic spread in early infancy and childhood resulting in permanent immunity. Most of the cases occur from 6 to 18 mo of age. It is rare beyond 3 yr.

Clinical Manifestations. The onset is sudden with fever as high as 39.4–41.2° C (103–106° F); convulsions may occur at this time or later. Although the pharyngeal mucosa is slightly inflamed at times and there may be slight coryza, there are no typical signs. The outstanding feature is the absence of physical findings sufficient to explain the fever. Usually the child looks relatively well despite the degree of the fever. The diagnosis is suggested chiefly by excluding other infections, particularly those which at this age are the most common causes of high fever, such as otitis media, acute pyelonephritis, pneumonia, meningitis, and pneumococcal bacteremia.

During the first 24–36 hr of fever the white blood cell count may be as high as 16,000–20,000/mm³ with an increase in neutrophils. By the 2nd day leukopenia may become evident, with counts of 3000–5000 on the 3rd–4th day of fever. There may be an absolute neutropenia with a relative lymphocytosis, which may be as high as 90%. Occasionally, a large number of monocytes are present. The cerebrospinal fluid is normal.

The fever falls by crisis on the 3rd–4th day. As the temperature returns to normal, a macular or maculopapular eruption appears over the body, starting on the trunk, spreading to the arms and neck, and slightly involving the face and legs. The rash soon fades, rarely remaining as long as 24 hr. Desquamation is rare, and no pigmentation remains. In the rare epidemic outbreaks cases without a rash may be suspected, but a definite diagnosis cannot be made. Occasionally, the lymph nodes, especially in the cervical area, are enlarged, but not to the extent that they are in rubella.

Differential Diagnosis. Children with exanthem subitum present with the differential diagnosis of a fever of unknown origin (Sec. 11.1) until the rash appears and the fever drops precipitously. Rubella's other prodromal manifestations and the persistence of its fever after a rash appears usually distinguish it from exanthem subitum. *Rubeola* and *dengue* can be distinguished primarily by the time of appearance of their rash in relation to fever and other clinical findings. In rubeola, though there is usually a fever of variable degree for 3–4 days

just before the rash, the temperature becomes abruptly elevated to 39.4–40° C (103–104° F) at the time the rash appears and remains elevated for the next 2 days, when the rash fades rapidly. The lack of Koplik spots, severe coryza, conjunctivitis, and cough also helps to distinguish exanthem subitum from rubeola. *Pneumococcal bacteremia* may present with high fever and a well-appearing child. The white blood count is frequently elevated, and the blood culture is positive for pneumococcus. As a rule, distinguishing exanthem subitum from entero- and adenoviral diseases and drug reactions does not present a problem.

Prognosis. The prognosis is good except in the rare patient who has extreme hyperpyrexia or persistent seizures.

Prophylaxis and Treatment. No methods for shortening the course of the disease or for prophylaxis are known. In infants and young children who are prone to convulsions, administering a sedative at the time the sharp febrile onset of exanthem subitum appears may be effective as prophylaxis against such seizures. An antipyretic may be of help in partially reducing the fever and in allaying restlessness.

Berenberg S, Wright S, Janeway CA: Roseola infantum (exanthem subitum). N Engl J Med 241:253, 1949.
Burnstine RC, Paine RS: Residual encephalopathy following roseola infantum. Am J Dis Child 98:144, 1959.
Clemens HH: Exanthem subitum (roseola infantum): A report of eighty cases. J Pediatr 26:66, 1945.
Hellström B, Vahlquist B: Experimental inoculation of roseola infantum. Acta Paediatr 40:189, 1951.
Kempe CH, Shaw EB, Jackson JR, et al: Studies on the etiology of exanthem subitum (roseola infantum). J Pediatr 37:561, 1950.
Letchner A: Roseola infantum: A review of fifty cases. Lancet 2:1163, 1955.
McEnery JT: Postoccipital lymphadenopathy as a diagnostic sign in roseola infantum (exanthem subitum). Clin Pediatr 9:512, 1970.
Veeder BS, Hempelmann TC: A febrile exanthem occurring in childhood (exanthem subitum). JAMA 77:1787, 1921.
Zahorsky J: Roseola infantum. JAMA 61:1446, 1913.

11.64 ERYTHEMA INFECTIOSUM
(Fifth Disease)

Erythema infectiosum, a moderately contagious exanthematous disease affecting mainly children, is frequently called fifth disease because it was the fifth of five illnesses described exhibiting somewhat similar rashes. The other four diseases were rubella, measles, scarlet fever, and Filatov-Dukes disease, the last of which is now considered a mild atypical form of scarlet fever.

Etiology. A viral etiology is postulated. In 2 recent outbreaks in London, all 33 children and adolescents and 6 of 8 adults studied had IgM antibodies against human parvovirus.

Pathology. Edema and the presence of an infiltrate of lymphocytes comprise the changes occurring in the skin lesion.

Epidemiology. Infants and adults are affected infrequently. There is no sex predilection. The incubation period has been estimated from family studies to range from 7 to 28 days (average, 16 days). Community epidemics involving mainly school-age children have been described. Distribution is worldwide.

Clinical Manifestations. No prodromal symptoms usually appear. Fever is absent or low grade. The characteristic rash appears in three stages. The illness usually begins with the sudden appearance of livid erythema of the cheeks, giving the child a "slapped-cheek" appearance. An erythematous maculopapular rash then appears on the trunk and extremities; infrequently the body rash may precede the facial one. The rash fades with central clearing, giving a lacy or reticulated appearance (Fig. 11–13 [p. xxvii]); it is the most distinctive part of the disease. The rash lasts from 2–39 days (mean, 11 days), is frequently pruritic, and resolves without desquamation, but periodic recrudescences may occur with exercise, warm baths, rubbing of the skin, or emotional upset. Constitutional symptoms such as headache, pharyngitis, coryza, myalgia, arthralgia, and gastrointestinal disturbance are more frequent and more severe in adults.

Laboratory Data. No confirmatory laboratory tests exist.

Diagnosis. Erythema infectiosum must be differentiated from rubella, enteroviral diseases, systemic lupus erythematosus, atypical measles, and drug rashes.

Complications. Complications are rare. Arthritis, hemolytic anemia, pneumonitis, and encephalopathy have been reported.

Treatment. No treatment is indicated. Isolation is not required. Since the illness is mild and the duration of the rash may be prolonged, children with this disease should be allowed to attend school.

Anderson MJ, Jones SE, Fisher-Hoch SP, et al: Human parvovirus, the cause of erythema infectiosum (fifth disease)? Lancet 1:1378, 1983.

Balfour H: Fifth disease: Full fathom five. Am J Dis Child 130:239, 1976.

Hall CB, et al: Encephalopathy with erythema infectiosum. Am J Dis Child 131:65, 1977.

11.65 HERPES SIMPLEX

Herpesvirus hominis (HVH), a common parasite of man, has a variety of clinical manifestations involving the skin, mucous membranes, eye, central nervous system, and genital tract. It also causes generalized systemic disease. Two strains of the virus are identified: HVH-1 commonly infects skin and mucous membranes; HVH-2 primarily infects the genitalia.

Two types of infection are recognized:

1. *Primary* infection is the susceptible host's first experience with the virus, which in most instances is a subclinical infection; otherwise there are usually local superficial lesions (see below) accompanied by varying degrees of systemic reaction. In newborn infants and severely malnourished infants, a serious systemic infection, often without superficial lesions, may occur. Circulating antibodies develop in nonfatal cases.

2. *Recurrent* herpetic lesions represent reactivation of a latent infection in an immune host with circulating antibodies. Reactivation follows such nonspecific stimuli as changes in the external milieu (e.g., cold, ultraviolet light) or in the internal milieu (e.g., menstruation, fever, or emotional stress). The lesions tend to be localized and, generally, are not associated with systemic reactions.

Etiology. *Herpesvirus hominis* (HVH) is a DNA-containing virus. The virus readily infects a variety of animals, produces pocks on the chorioallantoic membrane of the embryonated hen's egg, and induces characteristic cytopathic changes in a variety of cells growing in monolayer tissue cultures. Two strains (HVH-1 and HVH-2) are recognized by biologic and antigenic characteristics.

Epidemiology. The virus develops an extremely compatible relationship with its host. In about 85% of instances the infection is subclinical; even when clinical manifestations are present, the host is only rarely seriously disabled. Under exceptional circumstances the primary infection may lead to institutional or family outbreaks of stomatitis. The incubation period is 2–12 days (average, 6 days). *The spread of infection appears to be determined by two factors: close bodily contact and trauma such as teething or a break in the skin.*

The higher incidence of HVH antibodies in lower socioeconomic groups correlates with crowded living conditions. The epidemiology differs for the two types of HVH. Detailed serologic studies have been done only in low income groups, in which most infants have transplacental antibody for about the first 6 mo of life. From 1 to 4 yr there is a sharp rise in antibodies to HVH-1 and then a much slower rate of acquisition up to 14 yr. At this time, there is a second sharp rise in antibodies, mostly to HVH-2. By adult life HVH antibodies are seen in by far the majority of persons in the lower socioeconomic groups: HVH-2 antibodies are found in up to 60% of the adults. The incidence of type 2 antibody in higher socioeconomic groups is about 10% and in nuns about 3%.

Once infected, the majority of people continue to carry the virus in a latent state and maintain an almost constant level of circulating antibodies. The initial level of antibodies reached after a primary infection may fall, and several subclinical reinfections may occur before a stable antibody level is established. Carriers may distribute the virus without having any manifest lesion. Herpes simplex virus can be isolated from the pharynx of about 5% of asymptomatic adults.

Pathology. The pathologic changes vary with the tissue infected. In general, a specific lesion is characterized by the presence of intranuclear inclusion bodies, homogeneous masses lying in the midst of a severely disorganized nucleus in which the basic chromatin has marginated to the nuclear membrane. Around the specific lesion there is always evidence of an acute inflammatory reaction. In the skin and mucous membranes the typical lesion is a unilocular vesicle. In the skin the vesicle is tense. Ballooned epithelial cells containing intranuclear inclusions can best be seen at the margins of the vesicle. The vesicular fluid contains infected epithelial cells, including multinucleated "virus" giant cells and leukocytes. In the corium there is no necrosis, but capillaries are dilated, and there is infiltration with mononuclear and polymorphonuclear cells. In the mucous membrane, because of maceration, there is early leakage of the vesicular fluid resulting in a collapsed vesicle, mainly filled with fibrin. The edematous roof cells form a gray membrane over the lesion.

In otherwise healthy persons, the lesions are confined to the skin and mucous membranes; viremia has rarely been described. Bloodstream spread of the virus with resultant widely disseminated disease is seen mainly in the newborn, in severely malnourished children, in persons with skin diseases such as eczema, and in those with defects in cell-mediated immunity. In these patients the virus spreads hematogenously from the portal of entry to susceptible organs. Virus increases within these organs, and secondary viremia occurs with evidence of extensive cell destruction. It is probable, however, that most cases of HVH-1 encephalitis other than in the newborn are caused by neurogenic transmission of the virus to the brain; HVH-2 infection is usually bloodborne. Healing begins with clearing of the viremia and decrease in the production of virus within the cells.

Clinical Manifestations. As indicated above, the herpes viruses characteristically produce a vesicular lesion. Only rarely is there a viremic distribution that results in widespread systemic disease or neurogenic transmission that leads to meningoencephalitis (see below and Sec. 11.10). Furthermore, although the occurrence of primary and recurrent lesions is an accepted characteristic of herpetic infection, their distinction clinically is often not possible without knowledge of the presence or absence of serum antibodies in the patient.

Lesions of the Skin and Mucous Membranes. On the skin the lesion consists of aggregates of thin-walled vesicles on an erythematous base. These rupture, scab, and heal within 7–10 days without leaving a scar except after repeated attacks or secondary bacterial infections; temporary depigmentation may occur in blacks. The local lesions may be preceded by mild irritation or burning at the local site or by severe neuralgic pain in the region. In children the vesicles often become secondarily infected, introducing *impetigo contagiosa* into the differential diagnosis. The lesions tend to recur at the same site, particularly at mucocutaneous junctions, but may occur anywhere.

Primary infection may, uncommonly, result in a generalized vesicular eruption in which the lesions are small and may continue to appear over a period of 2–3 wk. If the systemic manifestations are mild, the infection must be differentiated from varicella.

Traumatic lesions of the skin can be readily infected by the ubiquitous herpesvirus. Primary lesions can also occur on apparently unbroken skin, as, for example, on the chin of a drooling infant with herpetic stomatitis, in whom scattered isolated vesicles appear, in contrast to the grouped vesicles of recurrent attacks. When the skin of a limb is infected, vesicles appear in 2–3 days at the site of trauma. There is often centripetal spread along lymph channels causing enlargement of regional lymph nodes and scattered vesicles on the intervening undamaged skin. The final clinical picture may be mistaken for that of *herpes zoster,* especially if accompanied by neuralgic pain, unless the lesions are recognized as not being confined to a dermatome. The lesions heal slowly, often taking 3 wk; recurrences at the site of local trauma are common and may assume a bullous pattern. Wrestlers and medical personnel are prone to herpetic infections of superficial abrasions (herpes gladiatorum and herpetic whitlow). In the latter, infection of minor trauma about the nails leads to extremely painful, deep-seated spreading lesions with vesicles that resolve spontaneously in 2–3 wk. Similar lesions occur on the fingers of thumb suckers who are suffering from herpetic gingivostomatitis. Treatment is symptomatic only; the lesions should not be incised.

Acute Herpetic Gingivostomatitis (Acute Infectious Gingivostomatitis; Aphthous Stomatitis; Catarrhal Stomatitis; Ulcerative Stomatitis; Vincent Stomatitis). This primary infection, probably the most common cause of stomatitis in children 1–3 yr of age, can also occur in older children and adults. The symptoms may appear abruptly, with pain in the mouth, salivation, fetor oris, refusal to eat, and fever, often as high as 40–40.6° C (104–105° F). The onset may be insidious, fever and irritability preceding the oral lesions by 1–2 days. The initial lesion is a vesicle (Fig. 11–14), seldom seen because of its early rupture. The residual lesion is 2–10 mm in diameter and is covered with a yellow-gray membrane (Fig. 11–15). When this membrane sloughs, a true ulcer remains. Although the tongue and cheeks are most commonly involved, no part of the oral lining is exempt. Except in edentulous infants, acute gingivitis is characteristic of the disease and may precede the appearance of mucosal vesicles. Submaxillary lymphadenitis is common. The acute phase lasts 4–9 days and is self-limited. Pain tends to disappear 2–4 days before healing of the ulcers is complete. In some instances the tonsillar regions are involved early, and acute tonsillitis of bacterial origin or herpangina may be suspected. Failure of the lesion to respond to antibiotic therapy differentiates a bacterial infection, and

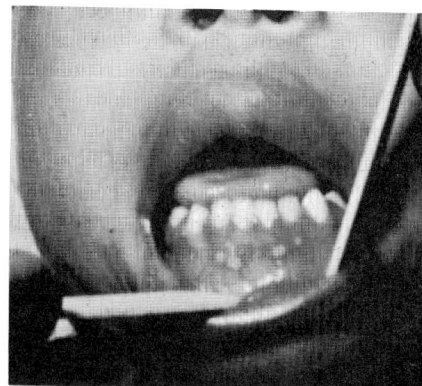

Figure 11–15. Herpetic stomatitis.

the spread of the vesiculation to the buccal mucosa rules out herpangina.

Recurrent Stomatitis. Localized lesions may occur on the palate in association with a febrile illness or on the mucosa adjacent to a lesion on the lip; recurrent aphthous ulcers, however, are not caused by herpesvirus. In some persons a generalized stomatitis recurs consistently 7–10 days after a recurrent herpetic lesion of the lip or elsewhere and is often accompanied by skin lesions of erythema multiforme.

Eczema Herpeticum (Kaposi Varicelliform Eruption; Juliusberg Pustulosis Vacciniformis Acuta). This, the most serious manifestation of "traumatic herpes," results from a widespread and usually primary infection of the eczematous skin with herpesvirus. The severity of this complication varies; the lesion may be so mild as to be overlooked, or it may be fatal. In a typical severe primary attack, vesicles develop abruptly in large numbers over the area of eczematous skin. They continue to appear in crops for as long as 7–9 days. Isolated at first, they later become grouped and may occur on adjoining areas of normal skin (Fig. 11–16). Wide denudation of the epidermis may occur. Scabs eventually form, and epitheliza-

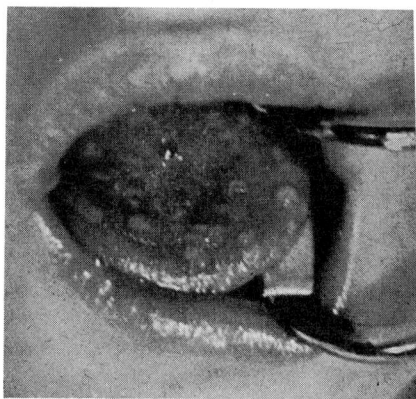

Figure 11–14. Lesions of herpetic stomatitis on the tongue.

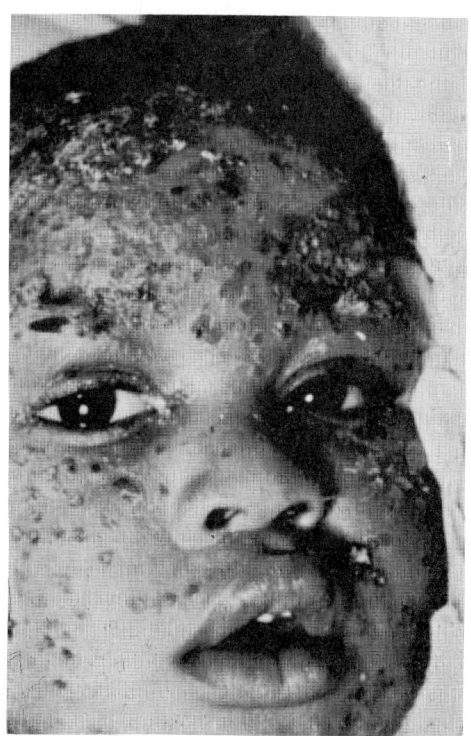

Figure 11–16. Eczema herpeticum.

tion occurs. The systemic reaction varies, but temperatures of 39.4–40.6° C (103–105° F) for 7–10 days are not uncommon. Recurrent attacks develop on chronic atopic skin lesions. Death may result from profound physiologic disturbances from loss of fluid, electrolytes, and protein through the skin, from dissemination of the virus to the brain and other organs, or from secondary bacterial invasion. A differentiation from *eczema vaccinatum* can usually be made by determining with reasonable certainty that the child has not been exposed to vaccinia and by the occurrence of crops of vesicles in herpes. The diagnosis can be accurately established by examination of vesicular fluid with the electron microscope. Herpes simplex virus cannot be differentiated from varicella-zoster by this method but can easily be distinguished from vaccinia and variola.

Ocular Lesions. Conjunctivitis and *keratoconjunctivitis* may occur as manifestations of either a primary or recurrent infection. The conjunctiva appears congested and swollen, but there is little, if any, purulent discharge. In primary infection the preauricular node is usually enlarged and tender. Cataracts, uveitis, and chorioretinitis have been described in newborn infants.

Corneal lesions may be superficial, in the form of a dendritic ulcer, or deep, as a disciform keratitis. The diagnosis is suggested by the presence of herpetic vesicles on the lids; it is established by the isolation of the virus. The highly contagious *epidemic keratoconjunctivitis* (shipyard conjunctivitis) due to any of several serotypes of adenovirus must be considered in the differential diagnosis.

Genital Herpes. Genital infections with herpesvirus occur most commonly in adolescents and young adults, are usually due to HVH-2, and are spread venereally. Five to 10% of cases are caused by HVH-1. When the patient has no antibody to either type of herpes (approximately 30% of cases), systemic symptoms such as fever, regional adenopathy, and dysuria are more likely to occur. In adult women, the vulva and vagina may be involved, but the cervix is the primary site of infection. Recurrence is common; when it involves only the cervix, it is frequently subclinical but this lesion can easily infect an infant during passage through the birth canal.

In males herpetic vesicles or ulcers are usually seen on the glans penis, prepuce, or shaft of the penis. The scrotum is less frequently involved.

Evidence suggests that HVH-2 may be a possible factor in the etiology of carcinoma of the cervix.

Systemic Infection. IN THE NEWBORN INFANT. See also Sec. 8.71. Most neonatal herpes is caused by HVH-2 acquired by passage through an infected birth canal or by ascension of virus into the uterine cavity after rupture of membranes.

Many of the infants with widespread systemic disease are born at low birthweight to young primiparas, many of whom have no readily available clinical evidence of genital herpes, although they are infected. Further, many of the infants do not have herpetic skin lesions, and some of them have other disorders, for example, hyaline membrane disease, bacterial pneumonia (with no apparent clinical response to antibiotics), and septicemia. It should be evident that detection of systemic herpetic infection in many infants will require a high degree of suspicion and resort to laboratory assistance (see below).

Manifestations that may be attributed to the herpetic infection per se usually appear within the first 2 weeks and include skin lesions at any site or those widely distributed, lethargy, poor feeding, persistent acidosis, hepatomegaly, pneumonitis, meningoencephalitis, and a bleeding diathesis. Untreated, the disease may progress to irreversible shock. Infants with meningoencephalitis are usually fullterm and develop clinical manifestations at 11–20 days.

About 70% of infants who present with only skin lesions progress to systemic involvement. When the disease remains

localized to the skin, eye, or mouth, mortality is low, but about 12% are neurologically impaired. Disseminated and central nervous system disease have a 40% mortality and a high incidence of significant neurologic residual, even when therapy has been provided. Delay in therapy is associated with a poor outcome.

IN SEVERELY MALNOURISHED INFANTS. The primary infection in infants who have severe protein malnutrition, as well as other *immunodeficiency disorders*, may be generalized and fatal. The clinical and pathologic findings are similar to those in the newborn infant (Sec. 8.71).

Meningoencephalitis. (See also Sec. 11.10.) Herpes encephalitis is seen in all age groups. HVH-2 is the usual cause in newborn infants, HVH-1 in older patients. The pathogenesis is unknown, but it can occur in patients who already possess antibody against herpes simplex. It is the most common type of nonepidemic encephalitis in the United States, has a high mortality rate, and in survivors frequently produces severe sequelae.

Laboratory Data. Microscopic examination of scrapings from lesions (Tzanck stain) reveals multinuclear giant cells and intranuclear inclusions. Immunofluorescent techniques applied to these specimens can be useful in diagnosing herpes infection and in differentiating the two types of herpes. Virus can be isolated from vesicles and from conjunctival swabs. Cerebrospinal fluid is positive for virus in about one third of infected neonates. Cerebrospinal fluid is rarely positive in older children with encephalitis; brain biopsy is required for a definitive diagnosis. Such cultures are usually positive in 1–4 days. Serologic tests are less helpful except for tests to determine herpes-specific IgM in the newborn infant.

Moderate polymorphonuclear leukocytosis occurs in acute herpetic gingivostomatitis, eczema herpeticum, and meningoencephalitis. In meningoencephalitis there are frequently red cells in the cerebrospinal fluid and an increase in lymphocytes, usually fewer than 100 but occasionally up to 1000/mm³; the protein level is elevated, and the sugar is within the normal range. Thrombocytopenia often occurs with systemic infection.

Diagnosis. The diagnosis is based on any two of the following: (1) a compatible clinical pattern; (2) isolation of the virus; (3) development of specific neutralizing antibodies; (4) demonstration of characteristic cells or histologic changes in scrapings or biopsy material.

Course and Prognosis. Primary localized infections with the herpesvirus are self-limited, usually lasting 1–2 wk. Mortality rates are high in newborn infants who also have systemic infection and in older infants who are severely malnourished. In patients with meningoencephalitis the prognosis for survival or for recovery without serious permanent residuals is guarded. Otherwise the prognosis is usually good. Arthritis has occurred. Attacks may frequently recur, but they seldom cause more than temporary inconvenience except in the eye, where they may eventually cause scarring of the cornea and blindness. Recurrent oral herpes lesions can be a significant problem in immunocompromised patients.

Treatment. Since neonatal herpes may be acquired during passage through an infected birth canal, cesarean sections are indicated in women with genital herpes who are close to term. If the membranes have been ruptured for longer than 4 hr, the risk of ascending infection increases, and cesarean section is less likely to protect the infant.

Topical therapy has been advocated for both labial and genital herpes. The psychologic effect of treatment is very strong; in one study of topical ether treatment of cold sores, 75% of treated and 77% of placebo controls reported reduction in the severity and duration of lesions. However, topical 5-iodo-2'-deoxyuridine (IDU), adenine arabinoside (vidarabine, ara-A), ether, and 2-deoxy-D glucose are not effective. Topical acyclovir (acycloguanosine; 9-[-2-hydroxyethoxymethyl] guanine) may decrease the period of viral shedding but has little effect on symptoms. Oral treatment with levamisole or lysine has not been shown to be effective.

Topical IDU or adenine arabinoside (vidarabine, ara-A) is usually effective in treating herpetic keratitis but does not reduce the recurrence rate. Topical corticosteroids may increase ocular involvement and should not be used.

Patients with primary genital infection who are treated with *oral acyclovir* (200 mg 5 times daily for 5 days) have significantly less pain, itching, and time to crusting; a shorter duration of viral shedding; and fewer new lesions compared with control patients. Those with recurrent genital infections who are treated similarly with oral acyclovir have a shorter duration of viral shedding and heal faster but do not have lessening of symptoms; therapy did not prevent recurrences.

Adenine arabinoside given intravenously in a dose of 15 mg/kg/24 hr for 10 days may be effective in herpes encephalitis and in local and disseminated neonatal disease. A controlled study of newborns in which 30 mg/kg/24 hr was used did not show any increase in efficacy. The drug is well tolerated; bone marrow depression occurs infrequently. The best results are obtained when treatment is started early. Patients under the age of 30 yr have a better prognosis than older patients. Recent studies showed no difference in the efficacy of acyclovir (10 mg/kg/dose given over 1 hr every 8 hr) and adenine arabinoside in treatment of herpes simplex virus infections in newborns. However, some herpes simplex viruses are resistant to acyclovir, and some infants and adults treated with acyclovir fail to develop neutralizing antibody against herpes virus. Some infants treated with acyclovir for cutaneous disease have developed encephalitis several weeks after therapy was stopped.

Some patients who responded to either adenine arabinoside or acyclovir have shown later neurologic deterioration; brain biopsy has shown postinfectious encephalopathy.

There are no reports of the use of antiviral compounds in patients with herpes stomatitis.

Many types of immunizing agents have been tried without success. Although inactivated herpes simplex vaccines may prevent recurrent infections, particularly those due to type 1, the possibility that herpesvirus may be oncogenic even when inactivated limits their usefulness.

Hyperimmune gamma globulin against type 1 or type 2 herpes simplex is not available. Treatment of infected newborns with high doses of gamma globulin has been recommended but has not proved helpful.

Symptomatic and supportive therapy is of great importance. In infants especially, eczema herpeticum and stomatitis may lead to severe dehydration, shock, and hypoproteinemia, requiring replacement of fluids, electrolytes, and proteins.

Oral lavage should be used for mouth care; Ceepryn 1:4000 or Zephiran 1:1000 may be useful. Local analgesics, such as viscous lidocaine or benzocaine lozenges, may allay pain and enable the older child to eat. Labial lesions may be made less painful by applying drying agents such as calamine lotion or glycerine with carbamine peroxide. Analgesics should be used systemically as required. Antibiotics are useful only in treating secondary bacterial infections.

Food and fluid intake will be facilitated by acquiescing to the child's whims. Ice-cold fluids or semisolids are often accepted when other food is refused. Recurrences are often due to emotional stress, which must be recognized and treated.

Arvin AM, Yeager AS, Bruhn FW, et al: Neonatal herpes simplex infection in the absence of mucocutaneous lesions. J Pediatr 100:715, 1982.

Overall JC, Whitley RJ, Yeager AS, et al: Prophylactic or anticipatory antiviral therapy for newborns exposed to herpes simplex infection. Pediatr Infect Dis 3:193, 1984.

Selby PJ, Jameson B, Watson JG, et al: Parenteral acyclovir therapy for herpes virus infections in man. Lancet 2:1267, 1979.

Straus SE, Takiff HE, Seidlin M, et al: Suppression of frequently recurring genital herpes. N Engl J Med 310:1545, 1984.

Whitley RJ, and NIAID Collaborative Antiviral Study Group: Interim summary of mortality in cases of herpes simplex encephalitis and neonatal herpes simplex virus infections: Vidarabine versus acyclovir. J Antimicrob Chemother 12(Suppl. B):105, 1983.

Whitley RJ, Yeager A, Kartus P, et al: Neonatal herpes simplex virus infection: Followup evaluation of vidarabine therapy. Pediatrics 72:778, 1983.

11.66 VARICELLA AND HERPES ZOSTER

Herpes zoster and chickenpox are different clinical manifestations of the same virus.

Etiology. The common viral agent is *Herpesvirus varicellae*, whose structure under the electron microscope is indistinguishable from that of *Herpesvirus hominis*. The virus can be grown in a variety of primary cultures of human and simian tissues. Serum antibodies in patients recovering from varicella react equally with the viral particles derived from varicella and herpes zoster vesicles.

The reasons for different clinical manifestations of the two diseases are not understood. Varicella may be the primary response of a susceptible host, whereas herpes zoster may be the response of partial immunity when a latent infection is activated by some exogenous factor, e.g., stress, trauma, malignancy, or radiation. One attack usually confers permanent immunity to generalized disease, but second episodes can occur, particularly in immunocompromised patients and in those who have received varicella vaccine. Second attacks are usually mild.

Pathology. The *skin lesions* of the two diseases are identical and cannot be distinguished histologically from those of herpes simplex. Although unusual in cases of average severity, necrosis with hemorrhage is sometimes found in the mucous membranes of the mouth, trachea, esophagus, and intestine.

In fatal cases of *varicella* intranuclear inclusions can be found in the endothelium of blood vessels. Intranuclear inclusions have been found in most organs of the body, including the salivary glands, the nervous system, and the myenteric plexus of the stomach and intestine. In the brain, perivenous demyelination is similar to that of other postinfectious encephalitides; necrosis of nerve cells and leptomeningitis have been described.

The characteristic lesions of *herpes zoster* are in the nervous system, particularly in the dorsal root ganglia. Early in the disease the cells of the dorsal ganglia of the affected dermatome contain intranuclear inclusions; later they become necrotic. As the disease progresses, evidence of inflammation and degeneration is found in the posterior roots and in the peripheral portions of the nerves. There may also be necrosis of nerve cells in the unilateral and segmental portions of the posterior horn (cf. poliomyelitis [Sec. 11.77], which involves the nerve cells of the anterior horn). Leptomeningitis occurs in the region of the involved nerves. Intranuclear inclusions have been found in the sympathetic ganglia, in the neurilemma cells of the nerve twigs in the corium, in the myenteric plexus, and in the walls of the bladder and other viscera.

VARICELLA
(Chickenpox)

Varicella is characterized by the appearance of successive crops of typical vesicles on the skin and mucous membranes, generally accompanied by a mild constitutional reaction.

Epidemiology. Ninety per cent of patients having this highly contagious disease are under 10 years of age; the peak incidence is 5–9 yr, but the disease may occur at any age, including the neonatal period. Secondary attack rates among susceptible household contacts is about 90%. About 96% of adults in the United States are immune. The complement-fixation test is the most widely available test to determine immunity, but it is not sensitive. Fluorescent antibody test against membrane antigen (FAMA), immunoadherence hemagglutination (IAHA), and enzyme-linked immunosorbent assay (ELISA) are more reliable but are not widely available. An intradermal skin test is being evaluated.

The disease is seen mainly from January to May. It is spread by direct contact, by droplet, or by airborne transmission. Infectious virus is present in the vesicles but, unlike the smallpox virus, is not contained in the crusts. Patients are infectious from about 24 hr before the appearance of the rash until all lesions are crusted (usually 7–8 days). Epidemics of chickenpox have been initiated by exposure to herpes zoster.

Clinical Manifestations. The incubation period varies from 11 to 21 days, and is most often 13 to 17 days. Prodromal symptoms usually precede the rash by 24 hr. There may be slight fever, malaise, or anorexia, accompanied at times by a scarlatiniform or morbilliform rash. It is characteristic of the specific rash to appear rapidly. Typically, it begins as crops of small, red papules which almost immediately develop into clear, often oval, "tear-drop" vesicles on an erythematous base; they are usually not umbilicated. The contents usually become cloudy within about 24 hr, when the vesicles are easily broken and become scabbed. Crops of widely scattered vesicles characteristically continue to appear for 3–4 days. Starting on the trunk, they spread to the face and scalp; distal parts of the extremities are involved minimally, if at all. The lesions concentrate in areas of skin pressure or irritation. Characteristically, at the height of the disease the eruption consists of papules, early and late vesicles, and crusts present at the same time (Fig. 11–17 [p. xxvii]). Rarely, in severe disease, the lesions appear as hard, pearly lumps (mostly at the same stage of development) and resemble those of smallpox. Pruritus is constant and annoying. Vesicles on the mucous membranes, particularly those of the mouth, rapidly become macerated and form a shallow ulcer. Less commonly, lesions are found on the genital mucous membranes and on the conjunctiva and the cornea, where they may endanger sight. Laryngeal involvement is rare. There may be generalized lymphadenopathy.

The severity of the disease varies from a few lesions and little evidence of systemic illness to many hundreds of lesions and extreme toxicity with temperatures that range from 39.4 to 40.6° C (103–105° F). Systemic manifestations occur only during the first 3–4 days, when the rash is erupting.

Infrequently, the rash becomes hemorrhagic in association with mild to severe thrombocytopenia, often with other complications, such as pneumonia, or in patients receiving immunosuppressive therapy. Purpura fulminans, which occurs about the end of the first week and is associated with gangrene, probably represents a Shwartzman-like reaction.

Varicella bullosa is an uncommon variant, seen mainly in children under 2 yr of age, in which many of the lesions appear as bullae instead of vesicles. The course of the disease is not changed.

Congenital varicella may be manifest at birth or appear within a few days when the mother has an active infection. When the mothers develop varicella within 5 days before or after delivery, about 17% of their infants develop disease; about 30% of these infants die. In contrast, infections acquired postnatally by young infants are usually mild.

Laboratory Data. There may be a mild leukocytosis. Giant cells can be demonstrated in scrapings from the floors of fresh vesicles. The virus can be isolated in human tissue cultures.

Diagnosis. Since the eradication of smallpox, the difficult distinction between mild smallpox and severe chickenpox has become moot. In contrast to smallpox (Sec. 11.67), chickenpox has a short, usually mild prodrome, and the superficial nonumbilicated skin lesions begin on the trunk, spreading peripherally, and may present all stages of development at once. The viruses are easily distinguished morphologically.

Complications. *Secondary bacterial infection* of skin lesions is the most common complication. *Thrombocytopenia* with hemorrhage into the skin and mucous membranes may occur; rare instances of internal hemorrhage from ulcerations or into an adrenal may be fatal.

Varicella *pneumonia* is uncommon in children, but 20–30% of adults have lung involvement. Recovery is usually prompt, but roentgenographic changes may persist for 6–12 wk in the more seriously ill. Fatalities have been reported. *Purpura fulminans* (Sec. 15.55) may occur following chickenpox. Lesions on the larynx may cause edema severe enough to produce respiratory distress. Myocarditis, pericarditis, endocarditis, hepatitis, glomerulonephritis, arthritis, and acute myositis of the limb muscles have been described. Keratitis and vesicular conjunctivitis are rare and usually benign. About 10% of cases of *Reye syndrome* occur following chickenpox. Infants whose mothers had varicella during the 1st trimester of pregnancy have been small for gestational age, have had congenital malformations, skin scarring, muscular atrophy, chorioretinitis or other ocular abnormalities, seizures, and mental retardation, and have been unusually susceptible to infection.

Postinfectious *encephalitis* is the most common central nervous system complication (Sec. 11.10). Cerebellar signs such as ataxia, nystagmus, and tremors are common. Encephalitis presenting mainly with cerebellar signs has a much better prognosis than when it presents with cerebral symptoms of convulsions and coma. Mortality varies from 5 to 25%. About 15% of survivors have such permanent sequelae as seizures, mental retardation, or behavior disturbances. Other central nervous system complications include Guillain-Barré syndrome, transverse myelitis, facial nerve palsy, optic neuritis with transient loss of vision, and a hypothalamic syndrome with obesity and recurrent fever. In contrast to herpes zoster, chickenpox virus has not been isolated from the central nervous system of patients having chickenpox who have subsequently died.

Children receiving corticosteroids or antimetabolites are at risk for severe, often fatal, chickenpox. Children with leukemia are at great risk, but deaths have occurred in children receiving steroids for acute rheumatic fever or nephrosis.

Prevention. A live attenuated varicella vaccine has been developed and tested in Japan. The vaccine is well tolerated, produces measurable levels of varicella antibody, is protective if given before or immediately after exposure to a contagious patient, and does not cause severe complications in children receiving corticosteroids. In one study, about 80% of leukemic children in remission developed antibody after 1 immunization; 90% responded to 2 doses. Some children developed mild to moderate rash; about 10% of these were infectious to others. Vaccine efficacy was 80% in children subsequently exposed to varicella. Those who developed clinical disease had mild illness. Because all herpesviruses produce latent disease and untoward effects may appear decades later, considerable thought needs to be given to the possible administration of this live vaccine, especially since varicella is generally a mild disease in childhood.

Passive immunity can be induced by administering zoster immune globulin (ZIG) or varicella-zoster immunoglobulin (VZIG). ZIG is a gamma globulin fraction of plasma with high titer of antibody obtained from patients recovering from herpes zoster infection; supply is very limited. VZIG is obtained from the plasma of normal donors having high levels of antibody against varicella-zoster. VZIG is as effective as ZIG and more available. VZIG is obtained through the American Red Cross. The dose is 125 units per 10 kg body weight. It is effective in preventing chickenpox when given within 72 hr of exposure. The recommended dose of ZIG is at least 5 mL intramuscularly, but doses as small as 2 mL have been effective in preventing infection in normal children.

Prophylaxis is indicated only in susceptible patients at high risk for developing severe varicella: those with immunodeficiency diseases, leukemia, or other malignancies or those on immunosuppressive drugs. Because these children are not protected by ZIG as completely as are normal children, larger quantities of high-titer ZIG or VZIG are required. VZIG should also be given to a newborn whose mother develops varicella within 5 days of delivery. Most adults are immune to chickenpox even if they have no history of having had the disease. Management of a presumably susceptible pregnant woman exposed to varicella is controversial. If possible, antibody testing should be done immediately. If test results are positive, the woman can be reassured. If they are negative or if antibody testing cannot be done, VZIG may be offered. It costs about $400 for an adult dose. Congenital malformations due to varicella are probably rare. Zoster has occurred in children exposed to varicella in utero.

Treatment. Symptomatic treatment should be directed to alleviating itching by using local and systemic antipruritic agents and sedation as required. The effects of scratching will be minimized if the patient wears mittens and keeps fingernails short. Daily changes of clothes and linen and antiseptic baths reduce the incidence of secondary bacterial infection. If secondary infection occurs, systemic antibiotic therapy is indicated. Because the use of aspirin in children with varicella increases the risk of developing Reye syndrome, other antipyretics should be used when symptomatic relief is necessary.

Treatment of varicella pneumonia is usually supportive. Antibiotics are indicated only if secondary bacterial infection occurs. Steroids and immune serum gamma globulin are not helpful.

Adenine arabinoside (vidarabine) has activity in vitro against viruses of the herpes group, and success has been reported when this drug, 15 mg/kg/24 hr, has been used to treat patients with severe varicella pneumonia. At this dose the drug does not have significant bone marrow toxicity or depress immune responses. Acyclovir (acycloguanosine, 9-[2-hydroxyethoxymethyl] guanine) is also effective; 500 mg/m²/dose given intravenously over a 1 hr period every 8 hr prevents the development of pneumonia or other visceral involvement in immunocompromised patients. The best results are obtained when therapy is begun before the 3rd day of illness.

In the hospital children with varicella should be isolated in rooms where air pressure is negative in relation to the hall. The room should have an air exhaust unit that prevents recirculation of air into the hospital, and the hall door should be kept closed.

Prognosis. The prognosis is usually good; fatalities are usually the result of complications.

HERPES ZOSTER
(Shingles)

Herpes zoster, an acute infection characterized by crops of vesicles and neuralgic pain, is usually confined to a dermatome.

Epidemiology. Herpes zoster is relatively uncommon under 10 yr of age, after which its incidence increases steadily with each succeeding decade. Second attacks occur in fewer than 1% of patients. The patient usually has a history of having had varicella. In some instances a mild case of varicella may have been misdiagnosed or there may have been exposure in utero or in the neonatal period that resulted in unrecognized disease. There is an increased incidence in patients with malignancies, in those receiving immunosuppressive drugs, and in children exposed to varicella in utero. The severity of herpes zoster increases with age. There is no sex, race, or seasonal predilection. The factors initiating an attack are not understood.

Clinical Manifestations. Herpes zoster has a pre-eruptive and a posteruptive phase. The illness usually starts with pain and tenderness along the involved dermatome, often accompanied by generalized malaise and fever. Within a few days groups of red papules appear, distributed along a dermatome or two adjacent ones. The individual lesions quickly vesiculate (Fig. 11–18), become pustular, dry up, and scab in the course of 5–10 days. The lesions tend to erupt first at a point nearest the central nervous system. Successive crops appear for 1–4 days, occasionally for 7 days, extending along the course of the nerve. The eruption clears in 7–14 days in most patients under 20 yr of age, but when vesicles continue to appear for 7 days or so, healing may be delayed up to 5 wk. The lesions, except in rare instances, are unilateral. Fever, pain, and tenderness usually continue throughout the period of progression. The regional lymph nodes are invariably enlarged. Although the dermatomes of the 2nd dorsal to the 2nd lumbar nerves are the most common sites for patients under the age of 20 yr, cephalic zoster and infection of the sacral nerves, producing lesions of the leg and genitalia, do occur in children. Transient paralysis of the affected part is a rare complication.

With infection of the 5th cranial nerve, any or several of its branches may be affected. With involvement of the ophthalmic branch, lesions may occur on the forehead with local loss of hair, on the nasal tip, and on the cornea (Fig. 11–19 [p. xxvi]); over the cheek and the homolateral palate with infection of the maxillary branch; and over the homolateral mandible and tongue when the mandibular branch is affected. Infection of the 7th nerve or the geniculate ganglion results in the *Ramsay Hunt syndrome*, paralysis of the facial nerve and vesicles in the external ear canal.

A generalized rash may accompany herpes zoster; this tends to occur in elderly patients or in children who have had a mild attack of varicella in early infancy. Occasionally the first vesicles of varicella in children may be distributed along a dermatome.

Laboratory Data. A mild cerebrospinal fluid lymphocytosis often occurs. Scrapings of the floors of vesicles in their initial stage contain virus giant cells.

Diagnosis. Diagnosing the disease may be difficult before the rash develops; the pain may resemble that of pleural, cardiac, or peritoneal origin, depending on the site of the lesion. When the rash appears, its distribution and characteristics together with the pain make the diagnosis relatively

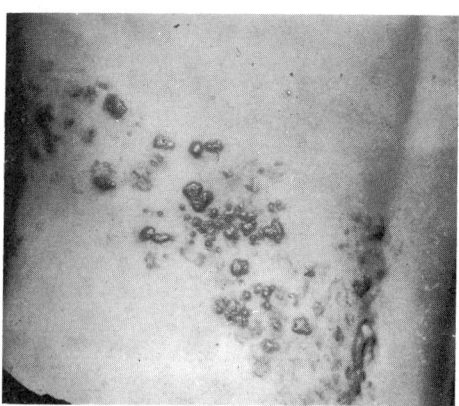

Figure 11–18. Herpes zoster. (Courtesy of Dr. Carrol S. Wright.)

simple. Occasionally, herpes simplex may simulate the distribution of herpes zoster.

Complications. Postherpetic pain does not occur in children, and ocular complications are rare. Keratitis and uveitis may follow 5th nerve involvement in adults. Secondary bacterial infection is possible in any of the lesions.

Prevention. Patients with zoster are infectious to those who have not had varicella. If hospitalization is required, they should be placed in isolation.

Treatment. Treatment is symptomatic. Soaks and calamine or other drying lotions may be helpful. Pain is seldom a problem in children. Aspirin is usually effective in controlling pain, but whether it alters the risk of Reye syndrome in patients with herpes zoster is unknown (see Varicella, above). Corticosteroids diminish the amount and duration of postherpetic neuralgia in adults without affecting the rate of healing of the skin lesions or increasing the number of complications.

Vidarabine (adenine arabinoside), 10 mg/kg/24 hr, given intravenously over a 12 hr period for 5 days, has been successfully used in treating immunocompromised patients with severe or disseminated zoster. Acyclovir, 500 mg/m^2/24 hr given in divided doses every 8 hr for 5 days, is also effective. Antiviral therapy speeds healing of the lesions, decreases pain, shortens time of viral shedding, and prevents the development of visceral lesions. Treatment or prophylaxis with zoster immune globulin is ineffective.

Course and Prognosis. In children the course is usually mild, and the ultimate prognosis is good. Immunocompromised patients can have delayed healing or dissemination of the virus to other skin areas or visceral organs.

Aronson MD, et al: Successful treatment of severe herpesvirus infections with vidarabine. JAMA 235:1339, 1976.
Balfour HH, McMonigal KA, Bean B: Acyclovir therapy of varicella-zoster virus infections in immunocompromised patients. J Antimicrob Chemother 12(Suppl B):169, 1983.
Bogger-Goren S, Baba K, Hurley P, et al: Antibody response to varicella-zoster virus after natural or vaccine induced infection. J Infect Dis 146:260, 1982.
Enders G: Varicella-zoster virus infection in pregnancy. Prog Med Virol 29:166, 1984.
Gershon AA, Steinberg SP, Gelb L, et al: Efficacy of live attenuated varicella vaccine in children with acute leukemia in remission. JAMA 252:355, 1984.
Gershon AA, Steinberg SP, Gelb L, et al: Clinical reinfection with varicella-zoster virus. J Infect Dis 149:137, 1984.
Griffith J, et al: The nervous system diseases associated with varicella. Acta Neurol Scand 46:279, 1970.
Leclair JM, Zaia JA, Levin MJ, et al: Airborne transmission of chickenpox in a hospital. N Engl J Med 302:450, 1980.
Preblud SR, Orenstein WA, Bart KJ: Varicella: Clinical manifestations, epidemiology and health impact in children. Pediatr Infect Dis 3:505, 1984.
Triebwasser J, et al: Varicella pneumonia in adults. Medicine 46:409, 1967.

11.67 SMALLPOX*
(Variola)

Smallpox, an acute communicable viral disease which, in past centuries, had been responsible for serious morbidity and high mortality rates worldwide, and in the past century was largely eliminated in industrialized countries by means of effective vaccination measures, no longer exists throughout the world. In 1958 the World Health Organization (WHO) began a campaign to eliminate smallpox from the world; at

---

*In view of the current assumption that smallpox has been eliminated as a disease of man on a worldwide basis, the editors have considered it reasonable to delete the clinical description of it from this edition of the textbook. Should the assumption not prove to be correct, and we share with all mankind the hope that it is correct, then appropriate coverage of smallpox will be replaced in subsequent editions. Meanwhile, we refer the reader to the 12th edition for clinical and other pertinent information on this disease.
—REB and VCV

that time there were about 250,000 cases of smallpox reported yearly. Massive organization, tireless efforts to investigate every suspected case and vaccinate susceptible contacts, and unprecedented cooperation between nations achieved this result by 1980.

The only remaining source of possible disease is laboratory accident, since seven carefully controlled laboratories in the world have stocks of variola virus. The WHO plans to stockpile large amounts of freeze-dried vaccine as insurance against any future outbreak of smallpox.

CAROL F. PHILLIPS

Kempe CH: The end of routine smallpox vaccination in the United States. Pediatrics 49:489, 1972.
Phillips CF: Smallpox; Vaccination against smallpox. In: Behrman RE, Vaughan VC III (eds): Nelson Textbook of Pediatrics. 12th ed. Philadelphia, WB Saunders, 1983, pp 759–763.

11.68 CYTOMEGALOVIRAL INFECTION

Cytomegalovirus infections, the most common congenital infections (Sec. 8.68), may be inapparent or, when acquired before, during, or after birth, may cause clinical manifestations of cytomegalovirus disease. When acquired after birth, they may also induce an illness resembling infectious mononucleosis, and they are frequently pathogenic among patients with impaired cellular immunity.

Etiology. Cytomegalovirus is a species-specific agent with the physicochemical and electron microscopic characteristics of herpesviruses.

Epidemiology. Cytomegaloviral infections are distributed worldwide, but the incidence of congenitally acquired infection is generally higher among populations having a lower standard of living. Twenty to 70% of women of childbearing age in the United States have serologic evidence of previous cytomegaloviral infection. Excretion of the virus in the urine can be demonstrated in 4–5% of pregnant women; cytomegalovirus is cervically shed in 10%, and 5–15% excrete it in their milk. The prevalence of congenital infection varies from 0.4 to 7.4%. In Japan, the majority of children become seropositive during infancy, as opposed to 10% in the United States.

Cytomegalovirus is not readily transmitted from one person to another, but when it is so transmitted, it usually follows intimate contact and is associated with inapparent infection. Epidemics have not been described. When infection is introduced into a household, however, it is likely that every susceptible family member will develop infection eventually, usually without having recognizable disease. The virus may be transmitted to the fetus following both primary and secondary or recurrent infection in the mother. Congenital infection is not uncommon among fetuses of women known to be seropositive prior to pregnancy, and it can occur in consecutive pregnancies. Neonatal disease in siblings is extremely rare, however. Acquired infection may result from contact with cytomegalovirus in cervical secretions during the 2nd stage of labor or from virus present in milk. Since virus is present in saliva, the upper respiratory tract, semen, leukocytes, milk, and feces as well as in urine, it is probable that contact with any of these infected sources can transmit the infection. Blood transfusion–associated cytomegaloviral mononucleosis has been described. Infection occurs more often in sexually promiscuous individuals. Most patients undergoing immunosuppressive therapy following renal homotransplantation develop active cytomegaloviral infection, which is more likely to be symptomatic if the recipient was seronegative prior to surgery. The virus may be present in the donor kidney even though the latter may show no histologic evidence of cytomegaloviral infection.

Pathology. The electron microscopic appearance of the cytomegalovirus particle is similar to that of varicella-zoster, Epstein-Barr, and herpes simplex virus particles. Light microscopy reveals large intranuclear inclusion bodies, especially in tissues having a high titer of virus. The large size of the inclusions in cells is sufficiently distinctive to permit a specific diagnosis, but tissue culture is a far more sensitive method for detecting cytomegalovirus.

Clinical Manifestations. *Congenital Infection.* Over 90% of infected newborns are asymptomatic, and observed illness varies in severity (Sec. 8.68).

Acquired Infection. As in congenital infection, cytomegaloviral infection acquired after birth is usually inapparent. There is evidence that some infants come in contact with maternal virus during the 2nd stage of labor and begin to excrete virus in the urine several wk later. Although infants acquiring infection under the cover of maternally acquired antibody usually do not have symptoms, the virus has been recovered in early infancy from patients with pneumonia, paroxysmal cough, petechial rash, hepatomegaly, and splenomegaly. The central nervous system is occasionally vulnerable to cytomegaloviral infection acquired after birth. Infantile spasms have not been implicated as a cytomegalovirus-induced abnormality. It is possible, however, that infectious polyneuritis has the same relationship to cytomegaloviral infection that it does to Epstein-Barr virus infection in patients with infectious mononucleosis. Chorioretinitis has been associated with acquired cytomegaloviral infection in immunosuppressed patients but otherwise is a rare manifestation of acquired disease.

In older children and adults, mononucleosis due to cytomegalovirus is the most common manifestation recognizable to the physician. Clinical presentation varies considerably, but malaise, myalgia, headache, anorexia, abdominal pain, hepatomegaly, and splenomegaly may be noted. Abnormal results of liver function tests are common. Pharyngeal edema, usually without exudate, is seen, but the anginal symptoms seen in infectious mononucleosis are either absent or are not striking. Fatigue can be extreme as well as extraordinarily persistent. Some patients require 12–15 hr of sleep/day. Fever and chills may last for 2 wk or longer, with daily spikes reaching 40° C (104° F) or higher. Atypical lymphocytosis is a consistent and early feature.

When blood products, particularly multiple units of fresh whole blood, are administered to seronegative recipients, post-transfusion cytomegaloviral mononucleosis may occur 3–4 wk later. Cytomegalovirus has been demonstrated in donor white blood cells. Administration of blood to preterm infants is frequently followed by gray pallor, respiratory distress, splenomegaly, atypical lymphocytosis, and cytomegaloviruria.

If ampicillin is administered, a maculopapular rash similar to that of patients with infectious mononucleosis has been observed. Abnormal serologic reactions, including cold agglutinins, antinuclear antibody, rheumatoid factor, and cryoimmunoglobulins, have been described in both infectious mononucleosis and cytomegaloviral mononucleosis.

Although there is little evidence that cytomegalovirus is an important cause of chronic hepatitis, the virus has been isolated from children and young adults with mildly abnormal liver function tests and from some with hepatomegaly, chronic hepatitis, granulomatous hepatitis, or cirrhosis of the liver. In some instances it is possible that patients with severe disease were more susceptible to the infection because of steroids administered to ameliorate chronic liver disease.

Diagnosis and Differential Diagnosis. *Congenital Infection.* The diagnosis of congenital infection may be made by isolating virus within 3 wk after birth, but since most infants do not

have symptoms in the newborn period, the test is not usually performed. If any infant followed for several months has a sustained complement-fixing, hemagglutination-inhibiting, or fluorescent antibody titer (IgG or IgM), strong evidence of congenital cytomegaloviral infection exists. Passively acquired antibody from the mother should be in a titer of less than 1:8 by 6 mo of age. An IgM level of 20 mg/dL or more in the cord serum suggests, but does not prove, that congenital infection is present. The presence of IgA antibody in the cord serum also suggests congenital infection.

Congenital cytomegaloviral infection must be distinguished from toxoplasmosis, rubella, herpes simplex, and bacterial sepsis.

TOXOPLASMOSIS. Cytomegaloviral disease in the neonate may resemble toxoplasmosis in striking detail, but the latter is more likely to be associated with microphthalmia, scattered cerebral cortical calcifications, hydrocephalus, and chorioretinitis. The demonstration of specific toxoplasmal antibody titers persisting beyond 6 mo of age or the presence of toxoplasmal IgM antibody in early infancy is tantamount to isolating the organism. Also see Sec. 11.107.

RUBELLA. In the neonatal period, congenital cytomegaloviral infection may be difficult to distinguish from congenital rubella. Both may be associated with a purpuric rash, jaundice, microcephaly, and deafness, but the presence of central cataracts is strong presumptive evidence for rubella. If all of these manifestations are associated with a congenital heart lesion, the probability of rubella is high. Specific laboratory tests for rubella virus or rubella IgM antibody or serial hemagglutination-inhibition antibody tests are required for a definitive diagnosis. The marked decrease in the incidence of rubella in recent years makes this diagnosis much less likely than that of cytomegaloviral infection. See also Sec. 8.69 and 11.62.

HERPES SIMPLEX NEONATORUM. Herpes simplex infection is usually transmitted to the infant during labor and has its onset 5–10 days after birth. The disease is often fulminant in character and may present as encephalitis, pneumonitis, or undiagnosed vesicular rash. The virus is readily isolated from vesicular lesions in a variety of tissue culture systems. Also see Sec. 8.71 and 11.65.

BACTERIAL SEPSIS. Infants with bacterial sepsis usually are more acutely ill than infants with cytomegalovirus disease and usually do not have a petechial rash. Although the diagnosis of sepsis rests on a positive blood culture, the decision to treat with antibiotic drugs must be made on the basis of the early clinical findings.

Acquired Infection. The diagnosis of cytomegaloviral infection in a patient with mononucleosis-like symptoms can be established by viral isolation as described above. Serologic determinations, such as the presence of specific immunofluorescent IgM antibody or a 4-fold rise or decline in complement-fixing antibody, must be interpreted with more caution than in the newborn period. In the fluorescent antibody tests for IgM, cross-reactions with Epstein-Barr virus occur. In addition, cytomegaloviral complement-fixing antibody may fluctuate widely in some normal subjects, making interpretation of this serologic test difficult. Patients with cytomegaloviral mononucleosis are heterophil antibody–negative.

INFECTIOUS MONONUCLEOSIS. Cytomegaloviral mononucleosis may be difficult to distinguish from heterophil antibody–negative infectious mononucleosis because both conditions occur in young adults with atypical lymphocytosis, sore throat, abnormal liver function tests, splenomegaly, and fever. The cytomegaloviral IgM fluorescent antibody test is positive in both cytomegaloviral and infectious mononucleosis, presumably because EB virus and cytomegalovirus share common antigens. A patient with cytomegaloviral mononucleosis generally sheds virus in the urine and upper respiratory tract.

Virus is also recoverable from peripheral leukocytes. EB virus antibody can be measured by several immunofluorescence techniques.

HEPATITIS A AND B. A jaundiced patient with cytomegaloviral mononucleosis may clinically resemble one with hepatitis A or B. A serum glutamic oxaloacetic transaminase level above 800 units is unusual for cytomegaloviral infections at any age, but it is common in icteric hepatitis A. Both conditions may be associated with mild atypical lymphocytosis. Jaundice in an adolescent or adult is more unusual with cytomegaloviral infections than with hepatitis virus infections; history of recent contact with a jaundiced person favors the diagnosis of hepatitis A. Hepatitis B surface antigen may be detected in the serum of most patients with hepatitis B. The latter virus may be transmitted in ways other than parenteral inoculation, including sexual and transplacental transmission.

Prevention. There is evidence that acquisition of cytomegaloviral infection may be prevented in specific situations, such as by using seronegative donors for kidney transplants or by avoiding the use of fresh blood, especially when multiple transfusions are required. The use of frozen and thawed red blood cells and the use of stored blood will also prevent CMV transmission. Usually, however, prevention is not possible; virtually everyone acquires this infection by the 5th decade of life. A vaccine is not available. A major concern is the capacity of some individuals to become reinfected even in the presence of humoral and cellular immunity. Congenital infection is rather common among infants of mothers seropositive prior to pregnancy. There is evidence that the long-term sequelae in infants born to mothers experiencing primary infections *during* pregnancy are more severe than those in infants born to mothers with evidence of infection *prior* to pregnancy.

Treatment. A number of antiviral agents have been used in the treatment of congenital and acquired cytomegaloviral infections, including deoxyuridine, cytosine arabinoside, adenine arabinoside, and acyclovir. Although virus excretion has been temporarily halted in some instances, no role in the treatment of these infections has been established. Furthermore, they are all potentially toxic, and their use for this purpose has not been approved by the U.S. Food and Drug Administration. Corticosteroids, interferon, interferon inducers, and transfer factor have either been inadequately studied or been shown not to affect the clinical course.

Prognosis. *Congenital.* If at birth an infant has recognizable symptoms of cytomegaloviral infection, the prognosis is fair for survival but guarded for normal psychomotor development. Approximately 90% of such infants will have some form of central nervous system sequelae such as low IQ, deafness, hypotonia, hypertonia, cerebral palsy, or microcephaly. Asymptomatic infants with viruria at birth may have diminished intelligence, hearing loss, and may perform poorly at school.

Acquired. The prognosis is excellent for most patients with cytomegaloviral mononucleosis. Rarely, however, individuals have had extraordinary fatigue, recurrent sore throats, and intermittent low-grade fever lasting as long as 2–3 yr. Patients with postperfusion and renal allograft–associated cytomegaloviral infections usually do well. A small number of patients develop severe pneumonitis, hemolytic anemia, or hepatitis, which may seriously impede recovery. A fatal outcome is not usually due to cytomegaloviral infection alone. Individuals with increased susceptibility to infections, such as those with Hodgkin disease and lymphomas, may have generalized cytomegaloviral infections terminally.

JAMES BARRY HANSHAW

Hanshaw JB, Dudgeon JA, Marshall WC: Viral Diseases of the Fetus and Newborn. Philadelphia, WB Saunders, 1985.
Hanshaw JB: Cytomegalovirus infection. *In*: Feigin RD, Cherry JD (eds): Textbook of Pediatric Infectious Diseases. Philadelphia, WB Saunders, 1985.
Ho M: Cytomegalovirus: Biology and Infection. New York, Plenum, 1982.
Stagno S, Pass RF, Dworsky ME, et al: Congenital cytomegalovirus infection: The relative importance of primary and recurrent maternal infection. N Engl J Med 306:945, 1982.
Weller TH: The cytomegaloviruses: Ubiquitous agents with protean clinical manifestations. N Engl J Med 285:203, 267, 1971.

11.69 INFECTIOUS MONONUCLEOSIS

Infectious mononucleosis is caused by Epstein-Barr virus (EBV), a member of the herpes group. Epithelial cells of the pharynx appear to be initial targets of the virus, but B lymphocytes soon become infected and are disseminated throughout the lymphatic system to most of the organs, where they proliferate until checked by activated T cells. In its full-blown form the illness is characterized by malaise, fever, sore throat, lymphadenopathy, hepatosplenomegaly, atypical lymphocytes in the peripheral blood, and a heterophil antibody response. The infection is often mild or even inapparent, but occasionally severe complications may be observed.

Etiology. EBV is indistinguishable morphologically from herpes simplex virus. It was originally observed by electron microscopy in cells cultured from specimens of Burkitt lymphoma, a neoplastic disease that occurs predominantly in central Africa. The original cultures were established by Epstein and Barr.

Until recently it was possible to transmit EBV only to lymphocytes or lymphoblast lines. There is now evidence that the virus infects in vivo and in vitro several types of epithelial cells. Although most of the atypical lymphocytes found in infectious mononucleosis are T lymphocytes, EBV infects only B lymphocytes. Infection of B lymphocytes in vitro with EBV enables them to grow indefinitely in culture (immortalization). Few, if any, of the immortalized cells synthesize virus but all harbor EBV genomes and express EBNA, the EBV-associated nuclear antigen. EBNA-positive B cell lines can be established also from the peripheral blood of seropositive donors indicating that immortalization of B lymphocytes may also occur in vivo.

Epidemiology. The epidemiology of infectious mononucleosis is related to the epidemiology of EBV. Infection with EBV occurs early in life in developing countries. In central Africa almost all children are infected by 3 yr of age, and in that environment typical infectious mononucleosis is practically unknown. In western countries the age at which EBV infection occurs is related to socioeconomic group. Adolescents are 60–80% seropositive, the more affluent being less likely to have been infected. Seropositivity increases with age until in the United States nearly all adults are positive. The seroconversion is particularly high during the high school and college years in upper middle class populations: at Yale University 15% of susceptibles developed antibodies to EBV each yr, and 65% of those infected had clinical infectious mononucleosis. Infectious mononucleosis occurs at all ages but only rarely under the age of 2 yr, when most EBV infections remain silent, or over the age of 40 yr, when most individuals are already immune. The overall incidence is approximately 50:100,000 persons/yr, but in young adults the incidence rises to about 1:1000/yr.

Transmission of EBV takes place by exchange of saliva from child to child, often in day care centers, or during kissing by young adults. The source of the virus may be parotid gland ductal cells and epithelial cells of the nasopharynx. Nonintimate contact does not lead to spread of EBV. EBV is excreted in the saliva in the cell-free state, particularly before and during the clinical disease, but also commonly for 6 mo after recovery and frequently longer. Healthy individuals with serologic evidence of past EBV infection excrete virus in 10–20% of cases, probably intermittently. Immunosuppressed patients who are seropositive often reactivate EBV, and about 60% shed the virus.

Clinical Manifestations. The incubation period of infectious mononucleosis in adolescents is 30–50 days. In children it may be shorter, but solid data are lacking. The onset is usually insidious and vague. The patient may complain of malaise, fatigue, headache, nausea, or abdominal pain. This prodromal period may last 1–2 wk. The complaints of sore throat and fever gradually increase until the patient seeks medical care. The sore throat is often accompanied by moderate to severe pharyngitis with marked tonsillar enlargement and even with exudates (Fig. 11–20 [p. xxvii]). The throat may resemble that of streptococcal pharyngitis, and the throat culture may be positive, but this phenomenon reflects the prevalence of inapparent streptococcal infection in normal populations. An enanthem consisting of petechiae at the junction of hard and soft palate is frequently seen. Fever is present in about 85% of patients and is usually in the moderate range, about 39° C (102° F).

The characteristic signs, aside from sore throat, are lymphadenopathy and hepatosplenomegaly. The posterior cervical nodes are most often enlarged, but other groups are also affected. Epitrochlear lymphadenopathy is particularly consistent with infectious mononucleosis. The liver is enlarged in only about a third of patients, but elevations of enzyme activities signifying anicteric hepatitis occur in 80%; frank jaundice, much less common, is seen in only about 5%. Splenomegaly is found in about half of patients, though extension to 2–3 cm below the costal margin, rather than massive enlargement, is the rule. On the other hand, splenic enlargement may be rapid enough to cause left upper quadrant discomfort and tenderness, which may be the presenting complaint.

Other clinical findings include edema of the eyelids and rashes. Rashes are usually maculopapular and have been reported in 3–15% of patients. Eighty per cent of patients with infectious mononucleosis will develop a rash if treated with ampicillin; the reason for this phenomenon is unknown.

The severe symptoms usually last 2–4 wk, followed by gradual recovery. Fatigue, malaise, and some disability are common complaints for several mo. Chronic infectious mononucleosis with persistently elevated EBV antibody titers has been described, but fatigue without evident explanation is more common. Second attacks of infectious mononucleosis caused by EBV have not been serologically documented. The prognosis for complete recovery is excellent if none of the severe complications described below ensue.

Symptomatic infection with EBV is more common in children than is generally believed. The disease may be clinically quite similar to that in older individuals, including development of heterophil antibodies. On the other hand, identification of current infections by viral serology (see below) has demonstrated that children may show less specific symptoms, such as tonsillitis, fever of unknown origin, or acute undifferentiated respiratory disease. The younger the child, the less typical the symptoms are likely to be, particularly hepatosplenomegaly and lymphadenopathy. Atypical lymphocytes are usually present. Under the age of 2 yr the great majority of primary EBV infections remain silent.

Some patients complain of intermittent fatigue, malaise, fever, and lymphadenopathy for a year or more after the onset of infectious mononucleosis. Their EBV-specific antibody profiles may show normal convalescent responses or may show slightly elevated titers of antibodies to viral capsid antigen (VCA) and to the R component of early antigen (EA) with low or undetectable levels of antibodies to Epstein-Barr nuclear antigen (EBNA) (see below). The variability of the symptoms and the difficulty in providing a firm laboratory diagnosis make a diagnosis of "chronic infectious mononucle-

osis" somewhat uncertain in these cases. However, a rare patient may develop a series of severe, life-threatening complications over the course of several years accompanied by excessively high antibody titers ($\geq$ 1:10,240) to VCA and to the D component of EA. Such cases of true chronic infectious mononucleosis have been treated with acyclovir.

Oncogenic Activity of EBV. EBV is almost certainly an initiator in the induction of Burkitt lymphoma (BL) in Africa and possibly also nasopharyngeal carcinoma (NPC) in Chinese populations. BL is found in restricted areas of tropical Africa, below certain elevations, that correspond with the distribution of malarial parasites. It is a type of lymphoma, often of the jaw, that has a median onset age of 5 yr. A large prospective study in Uganda found that children who later developed BL had high titers beforehand of antibodies to EBV VCA. BL occurs sporadically in many parts of the world, including the United States, but less than 20% of these cases are associated with EBV.

NPC, mainly a disease of adults, involves nasopharyngeal epithelium cells. It occurs at a very high rate only in Southeast Asia and among Eskimos. Occasionally, cases also occur in children 10–18 yr old. The presence of EBV genome in both BL and NPC tumor cells and the induction of lymphomas by EBV in New World monkeys strongly suggest that EBV causes certain cancers; but, in addition to the requisite infection, the occurrence of BL and NPC requires the existence of environmental cofactors.

Recently, polyclonal B cell lymphomas in immunologically compromised patients were shown to be EBV-associated; EBV DNA was demonstrated in the tumor and the tumor cells (expressed as EBNA). Such tumors were observed in genetic and acquired immunodeficiencies and in organ allograft recipients. Primary B-cell lymphomas in the CNS, an immunologically privileged site, may be EBV-associated.

Complications. The most feared complication of infectious mononucleosis is splenic rupture, which is said to occur most frequently during the 2nd wk of the disease. Rupture is commonly related to trauma, which often may be mild, sometimes involving mere medical palpation.

Swelling of the tonsils and pharynx may be so severe as to cause respiratory occlusion.

Neurologic involvement is more common than usually appreciated, and more serious. Convulsions, ataxia, and nuchal rigidity may be the first signs of disease. There may be meningitis with mononuclear cells in the cerebrospinal fluid, Bell palsy, transverse myelitis, encephalitis, or Guillain-Barré syndrome. The latter may produce complete paralysis and death, at times in the absence of other signs of infectious mononucleosis. Perceptual distortions of space and size, referred to as the "Alice in Wonderland" syndrome, may be a presenting symptom.

Myocarditis and interstitial pneumonia are common complications, both resolving in 3–4 wk. Hepatitis is so common that it is considered part of the disease.

A hemolytic anemia, often with a positive Coombs test and with cold agglutinins specific for red cell antigen *i*, may occur late in the illness. Thrombocytopenic purpura and even aplastic anemia may develop and confuse the diagnosis.

Rare complications include pancreatitis, parotitis, and orchitis. Reye syndrome may occur in the wake of the disease.

Severe, persistent, and sometimes fatal EBV infection has been identified in patients with familial, genetic disorders of the lymphoid system. These patients die either of disseminated lymphoproliferation involving multiple organs or of malignant lymphomas. One group of patients has been categorized as the X-linked lymphoproliferative syndrome, which occurs in males following EBV infection. In addition to disseminated lymphoproliferation, these patients may show unchecked fatal infectious mononucleosis, aplastic anemia, hypogammaglobulinemia, or malignant lymphoma. Other patients with a variety of cellular immune deficits, such as natural killer (NK) cell deficiency, also may suffer severe infections or EBV-induced malignancies. Rare cases of fatal disseminated infection have also been reported in previously immunocompetent hosts who develop lymphopenia during the disease.

Diagnosis. Confirmation of the diagnosis of infectious mononucleosis by laboratory means has now become precise.

Originally, the diagnosis could be made only on the basis of atypical lymphocytosis. Indeed, in more than 90% of cases there is leukocytosis of 10,000–20,000 cells/mm³, of which at least two thirds are lymphocytes; atypical forms usually account for 20–40% of the total number. The atypical cells are large with irregular shape and staining properties. They are mostly T cells, apparently responding to the presence of infected B cells. Mild thrombocytopenia (50,000–200,000/mm³) occurs in no fewer than 50% of patients, but only the rare case has values low enough to cause purpura.

The well-known serologic test for infectious mononucleosis has been the Paul-Bunnell-Davidsohn test for sheep red blood cell agglutination. This test is based on the fact that numerous abnormal antibodies, including those directed against antigens from animal tissues, are transiently found in persons with infectious mononucleosis. The antibody specific for infectious mononucleosis is in the IgM class. In order to distinguish the heterophil antibodies of infectious mononucleosis from others, serum is tested for sheep or, for greater sensitivity, horse red blood cell agglutination before and after absorption with ox red blood cells or guinea pig kidney cell suspension. In infectious mononucleosis the antibody titers to sheep or horse red blood cells remain after guinea pig kidney absorption but disappear after ox cell absorption. Titers greater than 1:28 or 1:40 (depending on the dilution system used) after absorption with guinea pig cells are considered positive. The sheep red blood cell agglutination test is likely to be positive only for several mo, but the horse red blood cell agglutination test may be positive for as long as 2 yr.

Other popular tests for heterophil antibodies use formalin-treated horse or sheep red blood cells for a rapid slide agglutination with commercially produced reagents. When the clinical situation is atypical, the slide test should be confirmed by the differential heterophil tube agglutination test or by the EBV-specific serologic tests.

Most children with typical infectious mononucleosis will have positive tests, but those under the age of 5 yr are more likely to be negative or to have lower titers than adults, and sensitive tests for heterophil antibodies are necessary for optimal results.

The specific serologic tests for EBV must be understood in the context of the structure of the virus particle. Replication of complete particles begins in the nucleus of infected cells, and virions then pass into the cytoplasm, where the viral nucleocapsid can be detected by immunofluorescence. If a patient's serum is applied to fixed-cell smears of lymphoblastoid cell lines infected with EBV, then, following exposure to fluorescein-conjugated antihuman IgG or antihuman IgM, antibodies of either class may be detected by fluorescent staining of the infected cells. IgG antibody to VCA is usually present in a titer greater than 1:160 at the time of acute disease. In addition, VCA-specific IgM antibodies are present in all cases when tested at the appropriate time, but may occasionally be missed since the IgM response is not long lasting. IgM antibody usually remains in evidence for 2–3 mo. Occasionally, EBV antibodies develop late; in such cases convalescent sera need to be tested.

Some lymphoblast lines do not produce viral capsid antigen or early antigens, but if these lines are superinfected with EBV, antigens are produced in the nucleus and cytoplasm by

abortive infection. These have been termed "early antigens" because during lytic infection they precede synthesis of viral particles. Antibodies to the "D," or diffuse-staining, component of the early antigens are found transiently in 80% of patients during the acute phase of infectious mononucleosis and reach high titers in patients with nasopharyngeal carcinoma. Antibodies to the "R," or cytoplasmic restricted, component emerge transiently in late convalescence from infectious mononucleosis and often attain high titers in patients with EBV-associated Burkitt's lymphoma, which in the terminal stage of the disease may be exceeded by antibodies to the D component. Antibodies to D or to R may be found also in immunoincompetent patients with activated persistent EBV infections.

Another serologic test useful for diagnosis is that for EBNA (EB nuclear antigen) antibodies. EB nuclear antigen is produced in every lymphoblast carrying EB viral genomes and is detected only by anticomplement immunofluorescence. Antibody will attach to the antigen and fix complement, which can then be detected by fluorescent antibody to complement. Antibody to EB nuclear antigen is the last to appear in infectious mononucleosis; thus, its absence when other antibodies are present implies recent infection, while its presence implies infection at least several weeks previously. Table 11–25 and Fig. 11–21 summarize the combinations of antibodies that would be expected in various situations.

EBV can be demonstrated in the nasopharyngeal secretions of patients by its capacity to transform cord blood lymphocytes in vitro. Aside from the fact that the test requires a long time, it is not clinically useful because 10–20% of healthy seropositives excrete EBV.

Differential Diagnosis. The patient with atypical lymphocytosis, lymphadenopathy, hepatosplenomegaly, and a positive heterophil test presents no problems in diagnosis. If a clinical picture suggestive of infectious mononucleosis is present but the heterophil tests are negative, four conditions should be considered: EBV infection without heterophil antibody response, cytomegaloviral infection, toxoplasmosis, and infectious hepatitis (hepatitis A). All four can be identified by serologic tests, including those for EBV, and virus isolation. Cytomegalovirus infection, a particularly common cause of an infectious mononucleosis–like illness in adults, is accompanied by negative heterophil tests.

Other conditions that occasionally cause confusion are mumps, adenoviral disease, rubella, and streptococcal sore throat because of facial edema, lymphadenopathy, rash, and positive throat culture, respectively. Although throat cultures for streptococci may be positive in infectious mononucleosis, they are no more often so than in any random population. Failure of a patient with "strep throat" to improve within 48 hr should evoke suspicion of infectious mononucleosis.

The most serious problem in diagnosis arises in the occasional case with low white blood cell counts, moderate thrombocytopenia, and even hemolytic anemia. In these cases bone marrow examination and hematologic consultation are war-

Table 11–25. **EBV Antibodies in Various Situations**

	Anti-VCA IgG	Anti-VCA IgM	Anti-EA(D)	Anti-EA(R)	Anti-EBNA
No previous infection	0	0	0	0	0
Acute infection	+	+	+/0	0	0
Recent infection	+	±/0	+/0	+/0	±/0
Past infection	+	0	0	0	+

0 = titer <10 or <2 for EBNA; + = ≥10 or ≥2 for EBNA; EA(D) = early antigen diffuse-staining; EA(R) = early antigen restricted staining; EBNA = Epstein-Barr nuclear antigen; VCA IgG = viral capsid antigen immunoglobulin G; VCA IgM = viral capsid antigen-specific immunoglobulin M.

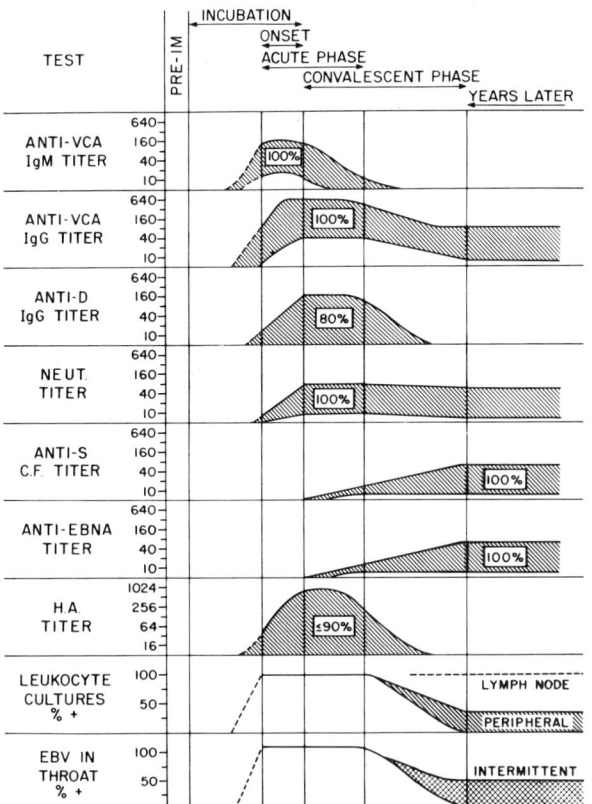

TEST					
ANTI-VCA IgM TITER	640 160 40 10				
ANTI-VCA IgG TITER	640 160 40 10				
ANTI-D IgG TITER	640 160 40 10				
NEUT. TITER	640 160 40 10				
ANTI-S C.F. TITER	640 160 40 10				
ANTI-EBNA TITER	640 160 40 10				
H.A. TITER	1024 256 64 16				
LEUKOCYTE CULTURES % +	100 50				
EBV IN THROAT % +	100 50				

Figure 11–21. Scheme of antibody responses, leukocyte cultures, and EBV assays in throat washings during the course of infectious mononucleosis. C.F. = complement fixing; D = diffuse-staining early antigen; EBNA = Epstein-Barr nuclear antigen; EBV = Epstein-Barr virus; H.A. = heterophile antibody; IM = infectious mononucleosis; NEUT. = neutralizing antibody; S = soluble complement-fixing antigen (probably identical with EBNA); VCA = viral capsid antigen.

ranted to rule out leukemia. Atypical lymphocytes may be found in cytomegaloviral infection, toxoplasmosis, infectious hepatitis, malaria, tuberculosis, typhoid, and mycoplasmal infection.

Treatment. There is no specific treatment for infectious mononucleosis. Short courses (under 14 days) of corticosteroids may be helpful in the event of pharyngotonsillar edema threatening to obstruct the airway, in hepatitis, or in severe abdominal pain due to splenomegaly or lymphadenopathy. Longer courses may be tried in hemolytic anemia, immune thrombocytopenia, or Guillain-Barré syndrome. There are no controlled data, however, showing efficacy of steroids in any of these conditions, and in view of the potential hazards of immunosuppression, steroids should not be used in the usual case of infectious mononucleosis.

The antiviral agent acyclovir is active in vitro against the replication of EBV, but has no effect on latency of the virus. Clinical trials have shown that excretion of EBV into the oropharynx ceases during acyclovir therapy but resumes as soon as the drug is stopped. In double-blind, placebo-controlled trials, more rapid subjective improvement, but no significant objective effects, were recorded in the patients treated with acyclovir. The drug has been reported to be beneficial in chronic infectious mononucleosis and EBV-associated polyclonal lymphoproliferation. Further exploration is indicated.

Withdrawal from athletic activity is indicated while splenomegaly is present, but bed rest is necessary only when the patient is toxic. As soon as there is definite improvement, the patient should be allowed to begin resuming normal activities.

Prognosis. If the rare occurrence of splenic rupture, severe central nervous system complications, or severe hemolytic anemia does not cause death in the acute period, the prognosis of immunocompetent patients is uniformly good for recovery. Recrudescence of illness during the first yr does occur, and fatigue is often present for months after the acute illness. On the whole, however, the patient should be strongly reassured of eventual complete recovery.

STANLEY A. PLOTKIN
WERNER HENLE

Biggar RJ, Henle G, Böcker J, et al: Primary Epstein-Barr virus infections in African infants. II. Clinical and serological observations during seroconversion. Int J Cancer 22:244, 1980.

Evans AS, Niederman JC, Cenabre LC, et al: A prospective evaluation of heterophile and Epstein-Barr virus–specific IgM antibody titers in clinical and subclinical infectious mononucleosis: Specificity and sensitivity of the tests and persistence of antibody. J Infect Dis 132:546, 1975.

Fleisher G, Lennette ET, Henle G, et al: Incidence of heterophil antibody responses in children with infectious mononucleosis. J Pediatr 94:723, 1979.

Henle W, Henle G, Horwitz CA: Epstein-Barr virus–specific diagnostic tests in infectious mononucleosis. Hum Pathol 5:551, 1974.

Horwitz CA, Henle W, Henle G, et al: Clinical and laboratory evaluation of infants with Epstein-Barr virus–induced infectious mononucleosis. Report of 32 patients aged 10 to 48 months. Blood 57:933, 1981.

Miller G: Epstein-Barr herpesvirus and infectious mononucleosis. Prog Med Virol 20:84, 1975.

Naegele RF, Champion J, Murphy S, et al: Nasopharyngeal carcinoma in American children: Epstein-Barr virus–specific antibody titers and prognosis. Int J Cancer 29:209, 1982.

Niederman JC, Evans AS, Subramanyan MS, et al: Prevalence, incidence and persistence of EB virus antibody in young adults. N Engl J Med 282:361, 1970.

11.70 MUMPS
(Epidemic Parotitis)

Mumps is an acute, generalized viral disease in which painful enlargement of the salivary glands, chiefly the parotids, is the usual presenting sign.

Etiology. The viral origin was established by Johnson and Goodpasture in 1934. The virus is a member of the paramyxovirus group, which also includes the parainfluenza, measles, and Newcastle disease viruses. Only one serotype is known. Primary cultures of human or monkey kidney cells are used for viral isolation. Cytopathic effect is occasionally observed, but hemadsorption is the most sensitive indicator of infection. Virus has been isolated from saliva, cerebrospinal fluid, blood, urine, brain, and other infected tissues.

Epidemiology. Mumps is endemic in most urban populations; the virus is spread from a human reservoir by direct contact, airborne droplets, fomites contaminated by saliva, and, possibly, by urine. It is distributed worldwide and affects both sexes equally; 85% of infections occur in children under the age of 15 yr. Epidemics occur at all seasons but are slightly more frequent in late winter and spring. Sources of infection may be difficult to trace because 30–40% of infections are subclinical. There has been a distinct decrease in the incidence since the introduction of mumps vaccine.

Virus has been isolated from saliva as long as 6 days before and up to 9 days after appearance of salivary gland swelling. Transmission does not seem to occur longer than 24 hr before appearance of the swelling or later than 3 days after it has subsided. Virus has been isolated from urine from the 1st–14th day after the onset of salivary gland swelling.

Lifelong immunity usually follows clinical or subclinical infection, although second infections have been documented. Transplacental antibodies seem effective in protecting infants during their first 6–8 mo. Infants born to mothers who have mumps in the week prior to delivery may have clinically apparent mumps at birth or develop illness in the neonatal period. Severity ranges from mild parotitis to severe pancreatitis. The serum neutralization test is the most reliable method for determining immunity but is cumbersome and expensive. A complement-fixing antibody test is available (see Diagnosis). The presence of V antibodies alone suggests previous mumps infection.

Pathogenesis. After entry and initial multiplication in the cells of the respiratory tract, the virus is blood-borne to many tissues, of which salivary and other glands seem to be the most susceptible.

Pathology. Little information is available concerning the lesions caused by mumps. In a parotid from which virus was isolated 70 hr after onset of the disease, the acini were well preserved, but there was periductal edema and lymphocytic infiltration extending slightly into the connective tissue. The main damage occurred in the ducts, ranging from slight epithelial swelling with a few polymorphonuclear cells in the lumen to complete desquamation of the epithelium and dilated lumens choked with debris. Cytoplasmic swelling was observed in some epithelial cells, but only rarely did one contain a large basophilic inclusion body. Other studies of parotid glands of patients with clinical mumps without viral isolation confirmed these general findings, although in some damage to the acini was observed. Changes in testes, when biopsies were taken within a day or two after onset of pain, have varied from the presence of mild interstitial edema and no disturbance of spermatogenesis, which occurs in the majority of instances, to focal destruction of epithelium, accompanied by extensive perivascular lymphocytic cuffing. The basic injury appeared to be vascular; irregular hemorrhages occurred in the more severe infections.

Clinical Manifestations. The incubation period ranges from 14–24 days, with a peak at 17–18 days. In children prodromal manifestations are rare, but may be manifest by fever, muscular pain (especially in the neck), headache, and malaise. The onset is usually characterized by pain and swelling in one or both parotid glands. The parotid swells characteristically: it first fills the space between the posterior border of the mandible and the mastoid and then extends in a series of crescents downward and forward, being limited above by the zygoma. Edema of the skin and soft tissues usually extends further and obscures the limit of the glandular swelling, so that the swelling is more readily appreciated by sight than by palpation. Swelling may proceed extremely rapidly, reaching a maximum within a few hours, although it usually peaks in 1–3 days. The swollen tissues push the ear lobe upward and outward, and the angle of the mandible is no longer visible. Swelling slowly subsides within 3–7 days but occasionally lasts longer. One parotid gland usually swells a day or two before the other, but swelling limited to one gland is common. The swollen area is tender and painful, pain being elicited especially by tasting sour liquids such as lemon juice or vinegar. Redness and swelling about the opening of the Stensen duct are common. Edema of the homolateral pharynx and soft palate accompanies the parotid swelling and displaces the tonsil medially; acute edema of the larynx has also been described. Edema over the manubrium and upper chest wall may occur, probably due to lymphatic obstruction. The parotid swelling is usually accompanied by moderate fever; normal temperatures are common (20%), but temperatures of 40° C (104° F) or more are rare.

Although the parotid glands alone are affected in the majority of patients, swelling of the submandibular glands occurs frequently and usually accompanies or closely follows that of the parotid glands. In 10–15% of patients only the submandibular gland(s) may be swollen. Little pain is associated with the submandibular infection, but the swelling subsides more slowly than that of the parotids. Redness and

swelling at the orifice of the Wharton duct frequently accompany swelling of the gland.

Least commonly the sublingual glands are infected, usually bilaterally; the swelling is evident in the submental region and in the floor of the mouth.

A maculopapular erythematous rash, most prominent on the trunk, occurs infrequently; rarely it is urticarial.

Complications. Viremia early in the infection probably accounts for the widespread complications.

Meningoencephalomyelitis. This is the most frequent complication in childhood. The true incidence is hard to estimate because subclinical infection of the central nervous system, as evidenced by cerebrospinal fluid pleocytosis, has been reported in over 65% of patients with parotitis. Clinical manifestations have been reported in over 10% of patients. The reported incidence of mumps meningoencephalitis is approximately 250/100,000 cases; 10% of these cases occurred in patients over 20 yr old. The mortality rate is about 2%. Males are affected 3–5 times as frequently as females. Mumps is one of the most common causes of aseptic meningitis (Sec. 11.9).

The pathogenesis of mumps meningoencephalitis has been described as (1) a primary infection of neurons and (2) a postinfectious encephalitis with demyelination. In the first type, parotitis frequently appears at the same time or following the onset of encephalitis. In the latter type, encephalitis follows parotitis by an average of 10 days. Parotitis may, in some cases, be absent. Aqueductal stenosis and hydrocephalus have been associated with mumps infection. Injecting mumps virus into suckling hamsters has produced similar lesions.

Mumps meningoencephalitis is clinically indistinguishable from meningoencephalitis of other origins (Sec 11.10 and 11.77). Moderate stiffness of the neck is seen, but the remainder of the neurologic examination is usually normal. The cerebrospinal fluid (CSF) usually contains fewer than 500 cells/mm^3, although occasionally the count may exceed 2000. The cells are almost exclusively lymphocytes, in contrast to enteroviral aseptic meningitis, in which polymorphonuclear leukocytes often predominate early in the disease. Mumps virus can be isolated from cerebrospinal fluid early in the illness.

Orchitis, Epididymitis. These lesions rarely occur in prepubescent boys but are common (14–35%) in adolescents and adults. The testis is most often infected with or without epididymitis; epididymitis may also occur alone. Rarely, there is a hydrocele. The orchitis usually follows parotitis within 8 days or so; it may also occur without evidence of salivary gland infection. In about 30% of patients both testes are affected. The onset is usually abrupt, with a rise in temperature, chills, headache, nausea, and lower abdominal pain; when the right testis is implicated, appendicitis may appear to be a diagnostic possibility. The affected testis becomes tender and swollen and the adjacent skin is edematous and red. The average duration is 4 days. Approximately 30–40% of affected testes atrophy. Impairment of fertility is estimated to be about 13%, but absolute infertility is probably rare.

Oophoritis. Pelvic pain and tenderness are noted in about 7% of postpubertal female patients. There is no evidence of impairment of fertility.

Pancreatitis. Severe involvement of the pancreas is rare, but mild or subclinical infection may be more common than is recognized. It may be unassociated with salivary gland manifestations and be misdiagnosed as gastroenteritis. Epigastric pain and tenderness, which are suggestive, may be accompanied by fever, chills, vomiting, and prostration. An elevated serum amylase value is characteristically present with mumps, with or without clinical manifestation of pancreatitis.

Nephritis. Viruria has been reported frequently. In 1 study of adults, abnormal renal function was observed at some time in every patient, and viruria was detected in 75%. The frequency of renal involvement in children is unknown. Fatal nephritis, occurring 10–14 days after parotitis, has been reported.

Thyroiditis. Although uncommon in children, a diffuse, tender swelling of the thyroid may occur about 1 wk after the onset of parotitis with subsequent development of antithyroid antibodies.

Myocarditis. Serious cardiac manifestations are extremely rare, but mild infection of the myocardium may be more common than is recognized. Electrocardiographic tracings revealed changes, mostly depression of the S-T segment, in 13% of adults in one series. Such involvement may explain the precordial pain, bradycardia, and fatigue sometimes noted among adolescents and adults with mumps.

Mastitis. This is uncommon in each sex.

Deafness. Unilateral, rarely bilateral, nerve deafness may occur; although the incidence is low (1:15,000), mumps is a leading cause of unilateral nerve deafness. The hearing loss may be transient or permanent.

Ocular Complications. These include *dacryoadenitis*, painful swelling, usually bilateral, of the lacrimal glands; *optic neuritis (papillitis)* with symptoms varying from loss of vision to mild blurring with recovery in 10–20 days; *uveokeratitis*, usually unilateral, with photophobia, tearing, rapid loss of vision, and recovery within 20 days; *scleritis; tenonitis*, with resultant exophthalmos; and *central vein thrombosis.*

Arthritis. Arthralgia associated with swelling and redness of the joints is an infrequent complication; complete recovery is the rule.

Thrombocytopenic purpura is infrequent.

Mumps Embryopathy. There is no firm evidence that maternal infection is damaging to the fetus; a possible relationship to endocardial fibroelastosis has not been established. Mumps in early pregnancy does increase the chance of abortion.

Diagnosis. The diagnosis of mumps parotitis is usually apparent from the symptoms and physical examination. When the clinical manifestations are limited to those of one of the less common lesions, the diagnosis is not so clear but may be suspected, especially during an epidemic. The routine laboratory tests are nonspecific; there is usually leukopenia with relative lymphocytosis, but complications often result in polymorphonuclear leukocytosis of moderate degree. An elevation of serum amylase is common; the rise tends to parallel the parotid swelling and then to return to normal within 2 wk or so. The etiologic diagnosis depends on isolation of the virus from the saliva, urine, spinal fluid, or blood or the demonstration of a significant rise in circulating CF antibodies during convalescence. Serum antibodies to the S antigen reach their peak early in about 75% of patients and are detectable at the time of the presenting symptoms. They gradually disappear within 6–12 mo; antibodies against the V or viral antigen usually reach a peak titer in about 1 mo, remain stationary for about 6 mo, and then slowly decline over the ensuing 2 yr to a low level, at which they persist. The presence of a high anti-S titer and a low anti-V titer during the acute stage of an otherwise undiagnosed meningoencephalitis, for example, would strongly suggest a mumps infection, which would be confirmed if a convalescent serum (taken 14–21 days later) revealed a 4-fold rise of anti-V antibodies accompanied by little change in the titer of anti-S antibodies.

Differential Diagnosis. This includes *parotitis* of other origin, as in the rare instances of coxsackievirus A and lymphocytic choriomeningitis infections, which can be distinguished only by specific laboratory tests; *suppurative parotitis*, in which pus can often be expressed from the duct; *recurrent parotitis*, a condition of unknown origin, but possibly allergic in nature, which has frequent recurrences and a characteristic sialogram; *salivary calculus*, obstructing either a parotid or, more commonly, a submandibular duct, in which the swelling is intermittent; *preauricular* or *anterior cervical lymphadenitis* from any cause; *lymphosarcoma* or other rare *tumors* of the parotid; *orchitis due to infections other than mumps*, e.g., the rare infections by coxsackievirus A or lymphocytic choriomeningitis viruses; and *parotitis due to cytomegalovirus* in immunocompromised children.

Treatment. Treatment of parotitis is entirely symptomatic. Bed rest should be guided by the patient's needs, but no statistical evidence indicates that it prevents complications. The diet should be adjusted to the patient's ability to chew. Orchitis should be treated with local support and bed rest. Mumps arthritis may respond to a 2 wk course of corticosteroids or a nonsteroidal anti-inflammatory agent. Salicylates do not appear to be effective.

Prophylaxis. *Passive.* Hyperimmune mumps gamma globulin is available but is not effective in preventing mumps or decreasing complications.

Active. The routine administration of live, attenuated mumps vaccine is discussed in Sec. 4.1. Vaccinated children usually do not develop fever or other detectable clinical reactions, do not excrete virus, and are not contagious to susceptible contacts. Rarely, parotitis can develop 7–10 days after vaccination. The vaccine induces antibody in about 96% of seronegative recipients and has a protective efficacy of about 97% against natural mumps infection. The protection appears to be long lasting. In one outbreak of mumps, several children who had been immunized with mumps vaccine in the past developed an illness characterized by fever, malaise, nausea, and a red papular rash involving the trunk and extremities but sparing palms and soles. The rash lasted about 24 hr. No virus was isolated from these children, but increases in the titer of mumps antibody were demonstrated.

CAROL F. PHILLIPS

Bistrian B, et al: Fatal mumps meningoencephalitis. JAMA 222:478, 1972.
Gordon SC, Lauter CB: Mumps arthritis: A review of the literature. Rev Infect Dis 6:338, 1984.
Quast U, Hennessen W, Widmark RM: Vaccine induced mumps-like disease. Develop Biol Standard 43:269, 1979.

11.71 INFLUENZA VIRAL INFECTIONS

Although usually given less attention than those of other respiratory viruses, influenza viral infections create a broad spectrum of illnesses causing significant morbidity and mortality in children.

Influenza Viruses. Influenza viruses are relatively large RNA *orthomyxoviruses*, which are grouped into three broad serologic types (A, B, and C), determined by the complement-fixing property of their ribonucleoprotein component (S antigen). The outer (glycoprotein) surface of influenza viruses contains spikelike projections which are responsible for antigenic characteristics that determine subtypes. On influenza A and B viruses the spikelike projections contain specific hemagglutinins and neuraminidase; neuraminidase antigen is not present on type C strains. Influenza A subtypes are identified by their hemagglutinin and neuraminidase antigens; antigens to 12 hemagglutinins (H1 to H12) and 9 neuraminidases (N1 to N9) are included in this system. Although antigenic variation occurs among influenza B viruses, formal subclassification utilizing neuraminidase antigens has not been done. Influenza A viruses are subject to two types of change: frequent minor antigenic changes are called antigenic "drift"; less frequent major changes are referred to as antigenic "shift." The most recent sustained shift in influenza A virus occurred in 1968 when A/Hong Kong/68 (H3N2) appeared. Subsequently, several drifts in the antigenic character of the virus have occurred (A/England/72, A/Port Chalmers/74, A/Victoria/75, A/Texas/77, A/Bangkok/79, and A/Philippines/82).

Shifts in influenza A viruses causing human disease may be cyclic; when a shift occurs, the previous viral subtype usually disappears from circulation. In the late fall of 1977 the expected shift of the influenza A subtype apparently occurred and in early 1978 epidemics of influenza due to an H1N1 serotype (A/USSR/77) occurred in many areas of the world. However, in contrast to predictions based upon past experiences, previous H3N2 influenza serotypes did not disappear but continued to cause epidemic disease. Since 1977 both H1N1 and H3N2 viral serotypes have remained in human circulation and have caused epidemic disease. Since 1977, several drifts in the antigenic character of the H1N1 virus have also occurred (A/Brazil/78, A/England/80, and A/Chile/83).

Antigenic drift, the result of point mutation, allows a growth advantage in the presence of antibody. Antigenic shift may arise by recombination between human and animal influenza viruses during chance simultaneous infections.

Influenza B strains undergo antigenic drift; antigenic shift has not been demonstrated.

Epidemiology. Severe pandemic influenza A resulting from antigenic shift occurs every 10–40 yr. Subsequently, epidemics of generally lesser intensity occur every 2–3 yr in association with antigenic drift. Major outbreaks of influenza B are more variable but tend to occur at 4–7 yr intervals. Antibody studies reveal that virtually all children have experience with influenza C virus by age 10 yr, but the epidemiologic patterns of this virus have not been determined. In a large urban area there is generally some influenza viral activity each year.

Influenza viruses have no geographic restrictions. Epidemics usually occur in cooler weather in temperate climates, and during the rainy season in the tropics. Small outbreaks of infections with an influenza A virus antigenically distinct (significant drift) from the one responsible for a terminating epidemic frequently herald the epidemic virus for the oncoming season.

Following the appearance of a new subtype of influenza A, the highest incidence of disease occurs in children 5–14 yr old, with an attack rate approaching 50%. In subsequent outbreaks with variants (drifts) of the same subtype, the attack rate in children of similar age drops to about 15%. In outbreaks of influenza B, the attack rate is generally higher in children than in adults.

Respiratory secretions of infected children contain large amounts of virus, and infection is transmitted directly from person to person by the airborne route or by fomites.

Pathology. Data about uncomplicated influenza in children are limited. The main site of cellular involvement is the mucous membrane of the respiratory tract, which shows extensive destruction of its ciliated epithelium. Influenza uncomplicated by secondary bacterial infection reveals marked desquamation of the tracheal epithelium as early as the 1st day after onset of symptoms. Cellular infiltration with lymphocytes, histiocytes, plasma cells, eosinophils, and polymorphonuclear leukocytes occurs, but to a lesser extent than might be expected on the basis of the extensive epithelial necrosis. Repair of the epithelium begins within 3–5 days. A pseudometaplastic response of undifferentiated epithelium up to 8 cell layers thick occurs, reaching its maximum within 9–15 days. After 15 days cilia reappear and mucus production resumes. With secondary bacterial involvement there is extensive inflammatory cell infiltration and destruction of the basal cell layer and the basement membrane, and consequently the regeneration of the ciliated epithelium is delayed.

In children dying of pneumonia the pulmonary findings have included peribronchiolar lymphocytic infiltration with mucus and cellular debris plugging the small bronchioles, necrosis of bronchiolar epithelium, and marked lymphocytic infiltration of the alveolar walls and interstitial lung tissue.

Although the main pathology in influenza lies in the respiratory tract, the heart, brain, or lymphoid tissues are occasionally involved in fatal cases. Toxic, focal, and diffuse forms of myocarditis have been noted. Cerebral edema is the most common central nervous system finding at autopsy. The lymph nodes of the tracheobronchial tree show extensive changes, including necrosis and disorganization of the germinal follicles.

Pathogenesis and Immunity. The incubation period is usually 2–3 days. The virus is commonly found in the respiratory tract, but in unusual instances viremia, viruria, and isolation of virus from extrapulmonary tissues have been noted. Immunity correlates better with secretory (IgA) nasal antibody than with circulating antibody, but high titers of serum antibody are usually protective.

Following natural infection with an influenza A virus, protection against reinfection with the particular viral subtype, even though antigenic drift may have occurred, lasts for several years. Subclinical reinfections, however, are common and tend to broaden the antibody response, allowing continued protection from disease.

When antigenic shift occurs within an influenza A virus, the previous influenza A antibody that a child may have is not protective. The duration of immunity to influenza B infections is less well known but appears quite variable. Although cell-mediated immune mechanisms can be demonstrated to be associated with influenza infections, their role in protection against and recovery from influenza viral infection is unknown. High levels of serum interferon are noted during influenza infections and may play a role in recovery.

Clinical Manifestations. The predominant manifestations are respiratory, although systemic complaints are usually an integral part of the picture. In general, characteristics of influenza A and B virus illnesses are similar, but they do demonstrate two distinct patterns based on age: manifestations in *older children* and those in *younger children.*

In *older children and adolescents* the manifestations are similar to those in adults (Table 11–26). The onset is abrupt with fever, flushed face, chills, headache, myalgia, and malaise. The temperature range is 39–41° C (102–106° F) and is usually inversely correlated with age; the severity of systemic symp-

Table 11–26. Relative Frequency of Symptoms and Signs during Classic Influenza in Older Children and Adolescents

	Occurrence*
Symptoms	
Chilly sensation	+ + + +
Cough	+ + +
Headache	+ + +
Sore throat	+ + +
Prostration	+ +
Nasal stuffiness	+ +
Diarrhea	+ +
Dizziness	+
Eye irritation or pain	+
Vomiting	+
Myalgia	+
Signs	
Fever	+ + + +
Pharyngitis	+ + +
Conjunctivitis (mild)	+ +
Rhinitis	+ +
Cervical adenitis	+
Pulmonary rales, wheezes or rhonchi	+

*+ + + + = 76% to 100%; + + + = 51% to 75%; + + = 26% to 50%; and + = 1% to 25%.

toms generally correlates directly with age. Dry cough and coryza are also early manifestations but may be overlooked because of the severity of the systemic manifestations. Sore throat occurs in over one half of cases and is usually associated with a nonexudative pharyngitis. Ocular symptoms include tearing, photophobia, and burning and pain on eye movement. During some outbreaks, diarrhea has occurred in about one third of the children and adolescents afflicted.

In uncomplicated influenza the fever usually persists for 2–3 days but may last up to 5 days. A biphasic temperature pattern may occur, however, even without secondary bacterial complications. By the 2nd–4th day, respiratory symptoms become more prominent, and the systemic complaints begin to subside. The cough is dry and hacking and usually persists for 4–10 days. Frequently, cough, in association with some degree of general malaise, persists for 1–2 wk after the illness has otherwise subsided. Illness due to influenza B virus tends to be associated with more prominent nasal and eye complaints and less prominent systemic ones than is the case with influenza A infections.

The leukocyte count and differential are usually normal, but leukopenia (<4500 cells/mm^3) occurs in about 25% of cases. Approximately 10% of older children and adolescents have clinical and roentgenographic evidence of pulmonary involvement.

In *younger children* the manifestations of influenza viral infections are frequently similar to manifestations resulting from other respiratory viruses (parainfluenza, respiratory syncytial, rhinovirus, and adenovirus) (Table 11–27). Laryngotracheitis, bronchitis, bronchiolitis, pneumonia, and the common cold all occur. Clinical descriptions of these illnesses are presented in Sec. 13.53–13.67. Laryngotracheitis resulting from influenza A infection is frequently severe and associated with a thick, tenacious tracheal exudate; a greater percentage of children with croup due to influenza A virus will require tracheostomy than children with similar illness resulting from other viral infections.

The onset of illness in the younger child is often a high fever, an appearance of moderate toxicity, and a clear nasal discharge. Febrile convulsions and vomiting are common. Mild diarrhea occurs in about 15% of cases, and otitis media

Table 11–27. **Relative Frequency of Clinical Manifestations of Influenza Viral Infections in Children Less than 5 Years of Age**

	Occurrence*
Major Clinical Category	
Upper respiratory illness	+ + + +
Laryngotracheitis	+
Bronchitis	+
Bronchiolitis	+
Pneumonia	+
Symptoms	
Cough	+ + + +
Anorexia	+ +
Coryza	+ +
Vomiting	+ +
Diarrhea	+
Sore throat	+
Signs	
Fever	+ + + +
Pharyngitis	+ + +
Cervical adenitis	+ +
Otitis media	+ +
Convulsions	+
Exanthem	+
Generalized adenitis	+

*+ + + + = 76% to 100%; + + + = 51% to 75%; + + = 26% to 50%; and + = 1% to 25%.

in almost one fourth. Fleeting erythematous, macular, or maculopapular discrete rashes occur frequently.

In the *neonate* with influenza viral infection, the sudden occurrence of fever, lethargy, poor feeding, and irritability suggests bacterial sepsis. Nasal discharge and other respiratory symptoms, however, appear early, so that the viral etiology can be suspected.

Acute myositis, particularly involving the gastrocnemius and soleus muscles, has been associated with influenza B viral infections in children. It occurs about 1 wk after onset of respiratory symptoms, usually after a brief period of clinical improvement. Acute parotitis has also occurred with influenza A infections.

Illness due to influenza C appears to be quite uncommon in children. It is characterized by fever, prolonged nasal discharge, sneezing, and cough and is generally less severe than are the influenza A and B infections.

Diagnosis and Differential Diagnosis. The etiologic diagnosis of a sporadic influenza viral respiratory infection is frequently difficult, although it may not be difficult during an epidemic. All age groups are clinically involved with febrile illnesses during influenza outbreaks, whereas with other agents, such as respiratory syncytial and parainfluenza viruses, illness in adults is only sporadic and not generally associated with fever.

The virologic confirmation of influenza viral infection is easy and relatively rapidly accomplished (72 hr) by standard virus isolation methods. Fluorescent antibody procedures and other rapid antigen identification techniques may provide a diagnosis within 24 hr. Retrospective diagnosis can be made by studying paired serum samples by complement fixation, hemagglutination inhibition, and other antibody techniques.

Complications. Complications frequently occur in influenza viral infections; many are variations of primary viral infection, e.g., myositis, parotitis, and severe croup. Secondary or superimposed bacterial infections are most important; otitis media, purulent sinusitis, and pneumonia are common. One must be constantly alert for their appearance and institute appropriate antibiotic therapy should any of them occur.

Complications relating directly to the primary viral infection include hemorrhagic pneumonia, encephalitis and other neurologic syndromes, myocarditis, sudden infant death syndrome, and myoglobinuria. Reye syndrome (acute encephalopathy and fatty degeneration of the liver) is most commonly associated with epidemic influenza B viral infection, but many cases have also occurred after influenza A (H1N1) infections. The pathogenesis of Reye syndrome is unknown, but administering salicylates to children and teenagers having influenza increases the risk of developing Reye syndrome (Sec. 12.82).

Prevention. Immunization with potent, antigenically up-to-date *inactivated influenza viral vaccines* is safe and effective. However, routine immunization of normal children or adults is not generally recommended. Vaccine should be given to those known to be at particularly high risk for complications, e.g., the elderly and children with: (1) cardiovascular disorders such as rheumatic, congenital, or hypertensive heart disease; (2) chronic bronchopulmonary disease such as tuberculosis, cystic fibrosis, asthma, and bronchiectasis; (3) chronic metabolic diseases such as diabetes mellitus; (4) chronic glomerulonephritis and nephrosis; and (5) chronic neurologic disorders, especially those associated with weak or paralyzed respiratory muscles.

Live vaccines have been successfully used in adults, and trials in children have shown some promise. Long-term studies assessing risks and benefits of more comprehensive immunization programs involving all segments of the population are needed.

Amantadine hydrochloride is effective prophylactically when administered prior to exposure to influenza A viruses. Minimal data are available supporting its pediatric efficacy and safety. The dose for children 1–9 yr of age is 4.4 to 8.8 mg/kg/24 hr with a maximum daily dose of 150 mg. For pediatric patients over 9 yr of age, the dose is 200 mg/24 hr.

Treatment. *Amantadine hydrochloride* is specifically active against influenza A viruses and has benefited adults when given early in the course of illness. The dose is the same as that for prophylaxis mentioned above.

Ribavirin is active against both influenza A and B viruses. When administered by aerosol it effectively shortens the course of influenza in college students. It is being evaluated and probably will be available for the treatment of severe influenza in the near future.

Since morbidity is frequently the result of cardiorespiratory problems, it is prudent to encourage bed rest in all but the mildest cases. Since pulmonary abnormalities may persist for a greater period of time than fever and other symptoms, it is also wise to insist upon restricted physical activity during convalescence.

Adequate fluid intake should be ensured; non–salicylate-containing antipyretics may be used for excessive fever. Parents should be advised not to administer aspirin to children suspected of having influenza (Sec 12.82). During convalescence the judicious use of codeine at bedtime will relieve cough. Although bacterial superinfections are common, prophylactic administration of antibiotics should be discouraged, but vigorous antibiotic therapy following appropriate culture is indicated at the first sign of bacterial infection.

Prognosis. The outcome is generally good, but the prognosis must be guarded in children with underlying problems that place them in the high-risk category. Anoxia associated with severe laryngotracheitis or pneumonia can result in brain damage. Neurologic complications are frequently but not invariably associated with a poor prognosis.

Belshe RB, Van Voris LP, Bartram J, et al: Live attenuated influenza A virus vaccines in children: Results of a field trial. J Infect Dis 150:834, 1984.

Centers for Disease Control: Reye syndrome—United States, 1984. Morbid Mortal Weekly Rep 34:13, 1985.

Centers for Disease Control: Influenza Report No 94, June 1984.

Centers for Disease Control: ACIP—Prevention and control of influenza. Morbid Mortal Weekly Rep 33:253, 1984.

Dagan R, Hall CB: Influenza A virus infection imitating bacterial sepsis in early infancy. Pediatr Infect Dis 3:218, 1984.

Davenport FM: Influenza viruses. In: Evans AS (ed): Viral Infections of Humans: Epidemiology and Control. 2nd ed. New York, Plenum Medical Book Co., 1982, p 373–396.

Delorme L, Middleton PJ: Influenza A virus associated with acute encephalopathy. Am J Dis Child 133:822, 1979.

Dykes AC, Cherry JD, Nolan CE: A clinical, epidemiologic, serologic and virologic study of influenza C virus infection. Arch Intern Med 140:1295, 1980.

Farrell MK, Partin JC, Bove KE: Epidemic influenza myopathy in Cincinnati in 1977. J Pediatr 96:545, 1980.

Glezen WP: Consideration of the risk of influenza in children and indications for prophylaxis. Rev Infect Dis 2:408, 1980.

Glezen WP: Serious morbidity and mortality associated with influenza epidemics. Epidemiol Rev 4:25, 1982.

Hall CB, Douglas RG, Gieman JM, et al: Viral shedding patterns of children with influenza B infection. J Infect Dis 140:610, 1979.

Katagiri S, Ohizumi A, Homma M: An outbreak of type C influenza in a children's home. J Infect Dis 148:51, 1983.

Lennon DR, Cherry JD, Morgenstein A, et al: Longitudinal study of influenza B symptomatology and interferon production in children and college students. Pediatr Infect Dis 2:212, 1983.

Mollooly JP, Barker WH: Impact of type A influenza on children: A retrospective study. Am J Publ Health 82:1008, 1982.

Wilson SZ, Gilbert BE, Quarles JM, et al: Treatment of influenza A (H1N1) virus infection with ribavirin aerosol. Antimicrob Agents Chemother 26:200, 1984.

Zahradnik JM, Cherry JD: Influenza viruses. In: Feigin RD, Cherry JD (eds): Textbook of Pediatric Infectious Diseases. 2nd ed. Philadelphia, WB Saunders, 1986.

11.72 PARAINFLUENZA VIRAL INFECTIONS

Parainfluenza viruses are common causes of respiratory illnesses in children and adults and are particularly associated with croup. They are relatively large RNA paramyxoviruses. Four serologic types cause disease in humans.

Epidemiology. By 3 yr of age almost all children will have been infected with parainfluenza type 3 virus, and the majority with types 1 and 2. Most infections with types 1, 2, and 3 are symptomatic, but the severity of illness varies markedly. Infection with type 4 virus is common, but most infections are asymptomatic. Symptomatic reinfections with types 1, 2, and 3 are common.

Infections with parainfluenza type 1 virus are frequently cyclic, with epidemics in the fall every 2nd year. There are also endemic patterns. Type 2 infections also tend to occur in fall epidemics. However, the pattern is more sporadic than with type 1, and type 2 virus may be absent from a community for several years.

Type 3 infection characteristically is endemic, with illness noted throughout the year.

There are no geographic limitations associated with parainfluenzal infections, which are most common in young children but also frequent in adults. Serious illness is more common in boys than in girls.

Infection is transmitted from person to person, by direct respiratory contact or by exposure to infected secretions.

Pathology. The hallmark of parainfluenza viral infection is replication of virus in the respiratory epithelium, usually without deeper invasion or systemic involvement. Limited pathologic data are available, only from cases representing the severe end of the spectrum of illness. In laryngotracheitis a marked inflammatory response of the glottic and tracheal surfaces occurs. In children dying of pneumonia, pathology has included peribronchiolar lymphocytic infiltration accompanied by plugging of small bronchioles by mucus and cellular debris, necrosis of bronchiolar epithelium, and marked lymphocytic infiltration of the alveolar walls and interstitial lung tissue.

Pathogenesis and Immunity. After experimental intranasal viral administration, the incubation period is 2–4 days. Although viremia may occur, symptomatology is mainly related to the direct involvement of the ciliated cells of the respiratory epithelium. Type 3 infections frequently occur in early life when transplacentally acquired specific serum antibody is present, and reinfection in older children and adults regularly occurs despite measurable serum antibody. Immunity correlates best with the presence of specific IgA nasal antibody, but high levels of serum antibody also reduce the risk of reinfection. The role of cell-mediated factors is unknown. However, the observation of a fatal giant cell pneumonia in children exhibiting cell-mediated defects suggests that T cell function may be important in clinical recovery. Although reinfection is common, illness is virtually always mild and upper respiratory.

Clinical Manifestations. The predominant manifestations are respiratory, although systemic manifestations are common. Eighty percent of these infections affect the upper respiratory tract. In children hospitalized for severe respiratory illness, parainfluenza viruses account for about 50% of the cases of laryngotracheitis and about 15% each of the cases of bronchitis, bronchiolitis, and pneumonia. Among the parainfluenza viruses, type 1 is the most frequent cause of laryngotracheitis, whereas type 3 accounts for the most cases of bronchitis, bronchiolitis, and pneumonia.

Clinical descriptions of laryngotracheitis, bronchitis, bronchiolitis, and pneumonia are presented in Sec. 13.53–13.67. The clinical manifestations of parainfluenza upper respiratory infections are listed in Fig. 11–22. Sore throat is a more common complaint in the older child. Fever is observed in only 20% of cases and its height is inversely related to age. Rashes that have been noted are discrete, erythematous, maculopapular lesions of short duration. Associated otitis media is probably most often the result of secondary bacterial infection.

The duration of viral illness is quite variable, with an average of about 5 days. The persistence of fever for more than 5 days suggests the onset of a superinfection, usually bacterial, such as otitis media or pneumonia.

Types 1 and 3 have been noted in association with acute parotitis and an illness indistinguishable from that due to mumps virus. A type 3 strain was isolated from the cerebrospinal fluid of an adolescent with Guillain-Barré syndrome. Reye syndrome has occurred in association with parainfluenza viral infections, and parainfluenza viruses have been recovered from victims of the sudden infant death syndrome.

Type 4 appears to be associated only with mild upper respiratory illness, which is usually afebrile.

Diagnosis and Differential Diagnosis. In an individual case, the clinical diagnosis of the etiology of respiratory illness is difficult. The differential diagnostic considerations in young children include influenza A virus in severe laryngotracheitis, respiratory syncytial virus in bronchiolitis, influenza A virus in bronchitis, and respiratory syncytial, influenza, and adenoviruses in pneumonia. In mild upper respiratory illnesses all the common respiratory viruses need to be considered (rhinoviruses, coronaviruses, adenoviruses, respiratory syncytial virus, influenza viruses, and selected enteroviruses); in the older patient *Mycoplasma pneumoniae* infection is a further possibility.

The most important clinical differential diagnostic consideration is that between laryngotracheitis and other acute upper airway obstructive diseases such as acute epiglottitis, angioneurotic edema, and foreign body.

The virologic confirmation of parainfluenza viral infections is relatively easy, provided proper attention is paid to the collection and transportation of the specimens for culture. Swabs containing respiratory secretions are best maintained in a small amount of transport media; they should be refrigerated and transported to the laboratory within 4 hr of collection without being exposed to sunlight. Parainfluenza viruses are isolated in monkey kidney tissue cultures; in the majority of instances results are available within 1 wk. The use of fluorescent antibody procedures on respiratory secretions may provide a diagnosis within 24 hr. Retrospective diagnosis can also be made by studying paired serum samples by complement fixation, hemagglutination inhibition, or neutralizing antibody techniques. However, serologic results may be difficult to interpret because of cross-reactions among paramyxoviruses.

Complications. Complications are relatively infrequent. Secondary bacterial infections are of most concern; otitis media and pneumonia are easily recognized and treated. Bacterial secondary infections in laryngotracheitis are usually manifest as tracheitis (Sec 13.54), bronchitis (Sec. 13.61), and pneumonia (Sec. 13.66). Progressive viral pneumonia has occurred in the immunocompromised host.

Prevention. No satisfactory vaccine is available.

Since the severity of illness with parainfluenza viruses is inversely related to age, it is prudent in some instances to discourage group care of infants and, when possible, to reduce unnecessary exposure of young children to respiratory infections of older children and adults.

Treatment. Careful attention to symptomatic care is important in managing severe laryngotracheitis, bronchiolitis, and pneumonia (Sec. 13.53–13.67). Since the exclusion of a bacterial etiology in parainfluenza viral pneumonia and severe bronchitis and bronchiolitis is often impossible, it may be reasonable to administer antibiotics. Therapy with cefuroxime is adequate because bacterial pneumonias would most likely be caused by *Haemophilus influenzae*, *Streptococcus pneumoniae*, and *Streptococcus pyogenes*. Secondary infection in laryngotracheitis may be caused by *Staphylococcus aureus* in addition to the above bacteria; this is also adequately treated with cefuroxime.

Ribavirin is active against parainfluenza viruses and is currently being investigated in children. It is administered by small-particle aerosol.

In parainfluenza viral upper respiratory illnesses, the prophylactic use of antihistamines, decongestants, and antibiotics should be discouraged, as they are expensive and of unproven effectiveness.

Prognosis. Parainfluenza viral infections are common, and the outcome with rare exceptions is good. Anoxia associated with severe laryngotracheitis or pneumonia can result in brain damage. Rarely death may result from cardiorespiratory arrest.

JAMES D. CHERRY

Denny FW, Murphy TF, Clyde WA Jr, et al: Croup: An 11-year study in a pediatric practice. Pediatrics 71:871, 1983.

Downham MAPS, Gardner PS, McQuillin J, et al: Role of respiratory viruses in childhood mortality. Br Med J 1:235, 1975.

Glezen WP, Frank AL, Taber LH, et al: Parainfluenza virus type 3: Seasonality and risk of infection and reinfection in young children. J Infect Dis 150:851, 1984.

Glezen WP, Loda FA, Denny FW: The parainfluenza viruses. *In:* Evans AS (ed): Viral Infections of Humans: Epidemiology and Control. 2nd ed. New York, Plenum Medical Book Co, 1982.

Hall CB: Parainfluenza viruses. *In:* Feigin RD, Cherry JD (eds): Textbook of Pediatric Infectious Diseases. 2nd ed. Philadelphia, WB Saunders, 1986.

Hall CB, Geiman JM, Breese BB, et al: Parainfluenza viral infections in children: Correlation of shedding with clinical manifestations. J Pediatr 91:194, 1977.

Powell HC, Rosenberg RN, McKellar B: Reye's syndrome: Isolation of parainfluenza virus. Arch Neurol 29:135, 1973.

Roman G, Phillips CA, Poser CM: Parainfluenza virus type 3 isolation from CSF of a patient with Guillain-Barré acute syndrome. JAMA 240:1613, 1978.

Zinserling A: Peculiarities of lesions in viral and mycoplasma infections of the respiratory tract. Virchow's Arch (Pathol Anat) 356:259, 1972.

Zollar LM, Mufson MA: Acute parotitis associated with parainfluenza 3 virus infection. Am J Dis Child 119:147, 1970.

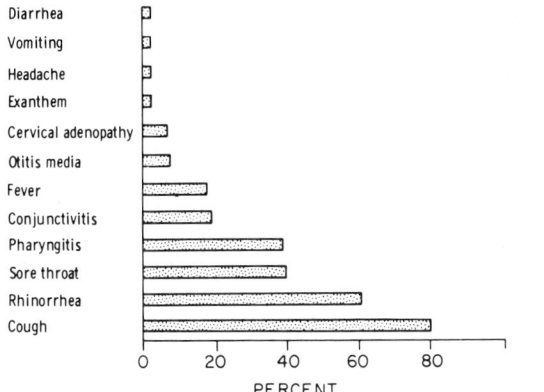

Figure 11–22. Signs and symptoms associated with parainfluenza viral upper respiratory infections.

11.73 INFECTIONS DUE TO RESPIRATORY SYNCYTIAL VIRUS

Respiratory syncytial virus (RSV) is the major cause of bronchiolitis (Sec. 13.64) and pneumonia in infants under 1 yr of age. It is the most important respiratory tract pathogen of early childhood.

Etiology. RSV is a medium-sized membrane-bound RNA virus that develops in the cytoplasm of infected cells and matures by budding from the plasma membrane. It belongs to the family *Paramyxoviridae*, along with parainfluenza and mumps viruses, but is classified in a separate genus, the pneumoviruses, because the diameter of its ribonucleoprotein helix is smaller. It contains no detectable hemagglutinin or neuraminidase, and it does not grow in embryonated eggs.

Although different strains of RSV show some antigenic heterogeneity, this variation is primarily seen in only one of the two surface glycoproteins, and the virus behaves in the human host like a single serotype.

RSV grows in a number of types of tissue culture, in which it produces characteristic syncytial cytopathology. Specimens for culture should be delivered rapidly and, if possible, on wet ice to the laboratory, since the virus is heat-labile and very susceptible to destruction by freezing and thawing. Tissue cultures also change spontaneously in their capacity to grow the virus with the characteristic cytopathology and therefore require frequent monitoring of cell lines for sensitivity.

Epidemiology. The occurrence of annual outbreaks and the high incidence of infection during the first months of life are unique among human viruses. RSV is distributed worldwide and appears in yearly epidemics. In temperate climates these epidemics occur each winter and last 4–5 mo. During the remainder of the year infections are sporadic and uncommon. Epidemics usually peak in January, February, or March, but peaks have been recognized as early as December and as late as June. At these times hospital admissions for bronchiolitis and pneumonia of infants under 1 yr of age increase and decrease in proportion to the number of RSV infections in the community. In the tropics, the epidemic pattern is less clear.

Placentally transmitted antibody may have some protective effect, particularly when present in high concentration. This may account for the fact that severe infections are uncommon in the first 4–6 wk of life. Nevertheless, serum antibody is apparently not fully protective, and the age at which an infant undergoes first infection depends significantly on the opportunities for exposure. It is estimated that in an urban setting about half the susceptible infants undergo primary infection in each epidemic. Thus, infection is almost universal by the 2nd birthday. Reinfection occurs at a rate of 10–20% per epidemic throughout childhood; the frequency is lower in adults. In situations of high exposure such as day care centers, attack rates are higher: nearly 100% for young infants and 60–80% for older infants.

Estimates of the severity of primary infections have emerged from studies of outbreaks in nurseries and institutions. Under these circumstances asymptomatic infection is rare. Most infants develop coryza and pharyngitis, usually with fever and occasionally with otitis. In 10–40% the lower respiratory tract is involved to a varying degree. Bronchitis, bronchopneumonia, and bronchiolitis all occur. Calculations based on hospital admissions in the United States and Britain yield a ratio of 1–3 infants hospitalized with bronchiolitis or pneumonia for every 100 primary infections with the virus.

Reinfection may occur as early as a few weeks after recovery but usually takes place during subsequent annual outbreaks. The severity of illness during reinfection is probably as much influenced by age as by prior experience with this virus, older children being generally less ill. Nevertheless, several instances of severe RSV bronchiolitis occurring twice in succession have been recorded.

Bronchiolitis is the most common clinical diagnosis in infants hospitalized with RSV infections, although the syndrome is often indistinguishable from RSV pneumonia in infants, and, indeed, the two frequently coexist. All RSV diseases of the lower respiratory tract (excluding croup) have their highest incidence in the 2nd mo of life and decrease in frequency thereafter. The syndrome of bronchiolitis becomes uncommon after the 1st birthday; acute infective wheezing attacks after that age are often termed "wheezy bronchitis," "asthmatoid bronchitis," or, simply, asthma attacks. Viral pneumonia, on the other hand, is a persistent problem throughout childhood, although RSV becomes less prominent as the etiologic agent after the first year. RSV is responsible for 45–75% of cases of bronchiolitis, 15–25% of childhood pneumonias, and 6–8% of cases of croup.

Bronchiolitis and pneumonia due to RSV are more common in boys than in girls by a ratio of about 1.5:1. Racial factors make little difference. Lower respiratory tract disease, however, occurs more often and earlier in life in low socioeconomic groups and under crowded living conditions.

The incubation period from exposure to first symptoms is about 4 days. The virus is excreted for variable periods, probably depending on severity of illness and immunologic status. Most infants with lower respiratory tract illness shed virus for 5–12 days after hospital admission. Excretion for 3 wk and longer has been documented. Spread of infection occurs when large infected droplets, either airborne or conveyed on hands, are inoculated in the nose or conjunctiva of a susceptible subject. RSV is probably introduced into most families by school children undergoing reinfection. Typically, in the space of a few days older siblings and one or both parents develop colds, while the infant becomes more severely ill with fever, otitis, or lower respiratory tract disease.

Hospital cross-infection during RSV epidemics is important. Not only do children infect one another, but also symptomatic infected adults have been implicated in the spread of the infection.

Pathology and Pathogenesis. Bronchiolitis is characterized by virus-induced necrosis of the bronchiolar epithelium, hypersecretion of mucus, and round cell infiltration and edema of the surrounding submucosa. These changes result in formation of mucous plugs obstructing bronchioles with consequent hyperinflation or collapse of the distal lung tissue. In interstitial pneumonia, infiltration is more generalized, and epithelial necrosis may extend to both the bronchi and the alveoli. In both diseases, but most commonly in bronchiolitis, infants are particularly apt to develop signs and symptoms of small airway obstruction because of the small size of the normal bronchioles.

Several facts suggest immunologic injury as a factor in the pathogenesis of bronchiolitis due to RSV: (1) infants dying of bronchiolitis have shown both immunoglobulin and virus in the injured bronchiolar tissues; (2) children who received a highly antigenic, inactivated, parenterally administered RSV vaccine developed, on subsequent exposure to wild RSV, more severe and more frequent bronchiolitis than did their age-matched controls; (3) bronchiolitis merges into asthma in older infants, and RSV is a frequently recognized cause of acute asthma attacks in children 1–5 yr old; and (4) IgE antibody directed toward RSV has been found in the secretions of convalescent infants with bronchiolitis. Nevertheless, despite continuing suspicion, a proven immunopathologic mechanism in bronchiolitis remains to be established.

It is not clear what role, in addition to the destructive effect of the virus and the attendant host response, is played by superimposed bacterial infection. In most infants with bronchiolitis, with or without interstitial pneumonia, clinical experience suggests that bacteria play an insignificant role. In severe cases or in infants with consolidative pneumonia, the possibility of pathogenic bacterial superinfection is somewhat greater.

Clinical Manifestations. The first signs of infection of the infant with respiratory syncytial virus are rhinorrhea and pharyngitis. Cough may appear simultaneously but more often after an interval of 1–3 days, at which time there may also be sneezing and a low-grade fever. Soon after the cough has developed, the child begins to wheeze audibly. If the disease is mild, the symptoms may not progress beyond this stage. Auscultation often reveals diffuse rhonchi, fine rales, and wheezes. Rhinorrhea usually persists throughout the illness, with intermittent fever. Roentgenograms of the chest are frequently normal.

If the illness progresses, cough and wheezing increase, and air hunger and evidence of hyperexpansion of the chest and of intercostal and subcostal retraction occur. The respiratory rate increases, and cyanosis occurs. Signs of severe, life-threatening illness are central cyanosis, tachypnea over 70/min, listlessness, and apneic spells. At this stage the chest may be greatly hyperexpanded and almost silent to auscultation because of poor air exchange.

Chest roentgenograms of infants hospitalized with RSV bronchiolitis are normal in about 10 per cent of cases; air trapping or hyperexpansion of the chest occurs in about 50%. Peribronchial thickening or interstitial pneumonia is seen in 50–80%. Segmental consolidation occurs in 10–25%. Pleural effusion is rarely, if ever, seen.

In some infants the course of the illness may be more like that of pneumonia. In these instances, the prodromal rhinorrhea and cough are followed by dyspnea, poor feeding, and listlessness, with a minimum of wheezing and hyperexpansion. Although the clinical diagnosis is pneumonia, wheezing is often present intermittently and the chest roentgenogram may show air trapping. In some infants the cough may be so severe and paroxysmal that the illness may mimic the pertussis syndrome.

Fever is an inconstant sign in RSV infection. Rash and conjunctivitis each occur in a few cases. In young infants, particularly those who were born prematurely, periodic breathing and apneic spells have been distressingly frequent signs, even with relatively mild bronchiolitis. Finally, it is likely that a small portion of deaths included in the category of sudden infant death syndrome (Sec. 26.1) are due to RSV infection.

Routine laboratory tests offer little helpful information in most cases of bronchiolitis or pneumonia due to respiratory syncytial virus. The white cell count is normal or elevated, and the differential count may be normal or shifted either to the right or left. Bacterial cultures usually grow normal flora. Hypoxemia is frequent and tends to be more marked than anticipated on the basis of the clinical findings. When it is severe, it is frequently accompanied by hypercapnia and acidosis.

Diagnosis. Bronchiolitis is a clinical diagnosis. The involvement of respiratory syncytial virus in any particular child's disease can be suspected with varying degrees of certainty from the season of the year and the presence of a typical outbreak at the time. Other features that may be helpful are the age of the child (aside from RSV, the only virus that attacks infants frequently during the first few mo of life is parainfluenza virus type 3) and the family epidemiology (colds in siblings and parents).

The diagnostic dilemma of greatest import is the question of possible bacterial or chlamydial involvement. When bronchiolitis is mild or when infiltrates are absent by roentgenogram, there is little likelihood of a bacterial component. In infants 1–4 mo of age, interstitial pneumonitis may be caused by *Chlamydia trachomatis* (Sec. 11.56). In this instance there may be a history of conjunctivitis, and the illness tends to be of subacute onset. Coughing is prominent; wheezing is not. There may also be eosinophilia. Fever is usually absent.

Consolidation without other signs or with pleural effusion is considered of bacterial origin until proved otherwise. Other signs pointing to bacterial pneumonia are depression of the white cell count in the presence of severe disease, ileus or other abdominal signs, high fever, and circulatory collapse. In such instances there is rarely any doubt about the need for antibiotics.

Definitive diagnosis of RSV infection is based on the detection of virus or viral antigens in respiratory secretions. The specimen should be put on ice, taken directly to the laboratory, and inoculated onto susceptible cell monolayers. Nasopharyngeal or throat swabs are probably of equal value. An aspirate of mucus from the child's posterior nasal cavity is preferable. A tracheal aspirate is unnecessary. Direct examination of nasal epithelial cells using fluorescent antibody techniques is of great value in the precise and rapid diagnosis of RSV infection.

Examination of acute and convalescent sera for a rise in antibody to RSV is often unrewarding, particularly in infants.

Prognosis. The mortality of hospitalized infants with RSV infection of the lower respiratory tract is about 2%. The prognosis is clearly worse in young, premature infants or those with underlying disease of the neuromuscular, pulmonary, cardiovascular, or immunologic systems.

Many children with asthma give a history of bronchiolitis in infancy. There is recurrent wheezing in 33–50% of children with typical RSV bronchiolitis in infancy. The likelihood of recurrence is increased in the presence of an allergic diathesis (eczema, hay fever, or a family history of asthma). In bronchiolitis over the age of 1 yr there is an increasing probability that, though it may be virus-induced, this is the first of multiple wheezing attacks that will later be called asthma.

Treatment. In uncomplicated cases of bronchiolitis, treatment is symptomatic. Humidified oxygen is usually indicated for hospitalized infants since most are hypoxic. Many infants are slightly to moderately dehydrated; therefore fluids should be carefully administered in somewhat greater than maintenance amounts. Often intravenous or tube feeding is helpful when sucking is difficult. Most infants seem to breathe better when propped up at an angle of 10–30 degrees.

Bronchodilators should not be routinely used. However, a trial of epinephrine should be made in wheezing children over 1 yr of age and bronchodilators administered if it is beneficial. Corticosteroids are not indicated except as a last resort in critical cases. Sedatives are rarely necessary.

In most instances antibiotics are not useful, and their indiscriminate use in presumed viral bronchiolitis and pneumonia should be discouraged. Interstitial pneumonia in infants 1–4 mo old may be chlamydial, and erythromycin (40 mg/kg/24 hr) may therefore be beneficial. When infants with interstitial pneumonia are older, or when consolidation is found, parenteral ampicillin (150–200 mg/kg/24 hr) may be used. In the critically ill child antibiotics are likewise indicated, though cultures or Gram stains may indicate the use of those other than ampicillin to cover staphylococci or ampicillin-resistant *H. influenzae.*

The antiviral drug ribavirin, delivered by small-particle aerosol and breathed, along with the required concentration of oxygen, for 20 out of 24 hours per day for 3–5 days, has a beneficial effect on the course of RSV pneumonia. It is probably indicated only in very sick infants or in high-risk infants, such as those with underlying cyanotic congenital heart disease or significant bronchopulmonary dysplasia, and should be administered early in the course of their infection (see Sec. 13.64).

Prevention. Within the hospital the most important preventive measures are aimed at blocking nosocomial spread. During RSV season high-risk infants should be separated from infants with respiratory symptoms. Separate gowns and gloves, and careful handwashing should be used for the care of all infants with suspected or established RSV infection.

Attempts to develop useful inactivated or attenuated vaccines have been unsuccessful. Indeed, the insufficiency of protection following natural RSV infection diminishes the likelihood that an attenuated vaccine will prevent subsequent disease. Breast milk, which contains antibody to RSV, may have some protective effect, but definitive proof is lacking to date.

KENNETH McINTOSH

Aherne W, Bird T, Court SDM, et al: Pathological changes in virus infections of the lower respiratory tract in children. J Clin Pathol 23:7, 1970.
Glezen WP, Paredes A, Allison JE, et al: Risk of respiratory syncytial virus infection for infants from low-income families in relationship to age, sex, ethnic group and maternal antibody level. J Pediatr 98:708, 1981.
Hall CB, Douglas RG Jr, Geiman JM, et al: Nosocomial respiratory syncytial virus infections. N Engl J Med 293:1343, 1975.
Hall CB, McBride JT, Walsh EE, et al: Aerosolized ribavirin treatment of infants with respiratory syncytial virus infection. N Engl J Med 308:1443, 1983.
Henderson FW, Collier AM, Clyde WA Jr, et al: Respiratory-syncytial-virus infections, reinfections and immunity: A prospective, longitudinal study in young children. N Engl J Med 300:530, 1979.
Kapikian AZ, Bell JA, Mastrota FM, et al: An outbreak of febrile illness and pneumonia associated with respiratory syncytial virus infection. Am J Hyg 74:234, 1961.
Kim HW, Arrobio JO, Brandt CD, et al: Epidemiology of respiratory syncytial virus infection in Washington, DC. I. Importance of the virus in different respiratory tract disease syndromes and temporal distribution of infection. Am J Epidemiol 98:216, 1973.
Loda FA, Clyde WA, Glezen WP, et al: Studies on the role of viruses, bacteria and M. pneumoniae as causes of lower respiratory tract infections in children. J Pediatr 72:161, 1968.
McIntosh K: Bronchiolitis and asthma: Possible common pathogenetic pathways. J Allergy Clin Immunol 57:595, 1976.
Parrott RH, Kim HW, Arrobio JA, et al: Epidemiology of respiratory syncytial virus infection in Washington DC. II. Infection and disease with respect to age, immunologic status, race and sex. Am J Epidemiol 98:289, 1973.
Simpson W, Hacking PM, Court SDM, et al: Radiological findings in respiratory syncytial virus infection in children. II. The correlation of radiological categories with clinical and virological findings. Pediatr Radiol 2:155, 1974.

11.74 ADENOVIRAL INFECTIONS

Adenoviruses cause 5–8% of acute respiratory disease in infants and children, including pneumonia. They also cause pharyngoconjunctival fever, follicular conjunctivitis, and epidemic keratoconjunctivitis. Only a third of the 37-plus serotypes have been associated with disease. Fatal infections are very rare. Recently, certain enteral adenoviruses have been recognized that may be responsible for about 4% of serious diarrhea in infants and children.

Etiology. Adenoviruses are DNA viruses of intermediate size, which are classified into subgenera A to G. Those in groups A to E are usually associated with respiratory tract infection and are identified in clinical specimens by inoculating human embryonic kidney, HEp-2, or HeLa cells and observing a typical cytopathic effect. ELISA and fluorescent antibody methods can detect adenovirus antigen prior to the cytopathic effect. Adenoviruses can also be cultured and characterized by electrophoresis and neutralization. Testing with the group complement-fixing antigen is a practical way to detect a seroresponse to adenovirus. The enteral adenoviruses (F, G) are primarily detected by electron microscopy; some will grow in 293 cell culture. The improved ability to grow these agents in cell culture should lead to the development of methods for rapid identification.

Adenovirus types 1, 2, 3, and 5 are highly prevalent in infants and children and are associated with rhinopharyngitis and exudative tonsillitis. Type 3 is typically associated with pharyngoconjunctival fever. Types 1, 3, 4, and 5 induce follicular conjunctivitis. Types 4 and 7, which cause 50–70% of acute respiratory disease in military recruits, are rarely found in children. A 7b genome type has been associated with severe, epidemic illness in infants in England and Sweden. Types 1, 2, 5, and 6 have been found as "latent" or "persistent" agents in surgically removed enlarged tonsils and adenoids. Whether their presence plays a part in the enlargement is speculative. Types 1 and 3 may be associated with pneumonia in young children and type 8 with epidemic keratoconjunctivitis. Adenoviruses have also been reported as causative or provocative agents in pertussis-like syndrome, hemorrhagic cystitis, mesenteric lymphadenitis, and intussusception. Adenoviruses in subgenera F and G have been associated with sporadic diarrhea in infants and children.

Epidemiology. Adenoviral infections are distributed worldwide. They occur year-round but are most prevalent in spring or early summer and again in midwinter in temperate climates. Over 60% of school-age children have antibodies against the more common types. Almost all adults have serum antibody against types 1–7. Infection with types 1 and 2 tends to occur early in childhood, with types 3 and 5, a bit later. Spread occurs by the respiratory and fecal-oral routes, and possibly by conjunctival inoculation.

Pathology. The oropharyngeal and perhaps nasopharyngeal mucous membranes are the tissues primarily affected early in acute infection. Pathologic changes in the respiratory epithelium include acidophilic nuclear inclusions, basophilic masses of cells, rosette formation, a mononuclear cell infiltrate, and focal necrosis of mucous glands.

Clinical Manifestations. The symptoms of most of the clinical syndromes associated with traditional adenoviral infection are localized to the pharynx, respiratory tract, and conjunctivae. The enteral adenoviruses are primarily associated with gastroenteritis.

Pharyngoconjunctival Fever. The features of this clinically distinct syndrome, occurring particularly in association with type 3 adenoviral infection, include fever, pharyngitis, conjunctivitis, cervical adenopathy, and rhinitis. A high fever is present in 90% of affected persons and lasts 4–5 days. About 75% of patients have enlargement and erythema of lymphoid tissue on the posterior pharynx and of the anterior pillars of the tonsillar fauces. Nonpurulent conjunctivitis occurs in 75% and is manifested by inflammation of both the bulbar and palpebral conjunctivae of one or both eyes. The cervical lymphadenopathy is predominantly posterior in distribution. In general, conjunctivitis tends to persist beyond the febrile period, and cervical lymphadenopathy is evident for several weeks after defervescence and subsidence of acute illness. Half of the patients have rhinitis with little rhinorrhea. Headache, malaise, and weakness are relatively common, and there is considerable lethargy after the acute stage.

Pharyngitis. Cases of rhinitis and pharyngitis with or without fever are not clinically distinctive, but pharyngitis is probably among the most common clinical manifestations of adenoviral infection. It is primarily associated with types 1, 2, 3, and 5, which are also found in a large proportion of children with exudative tonsillitis.

Conjunctivitis. Both epidemic keratoconjunctivitis, a problem primarily of adults, and acute follicular conjunctivitis may be caused by adenoviruses. Also, adenoviruses are frequently found in conjunctival scrapings or eye washings of patients with various eye diseases, including trachoma.

Pneumonia. Severe and at times fatal pneumonia in infants has been caused by adenoviruses. In most of these cases intranuclear inclusions have been present in the respiratory epithelial tissue. Seven to 9.5% of hospitalized cases of pneumonia in infants and children have been adenovirus-associated, primarily with the lower numbered serotypes.

Diarrhea. Systematic studies of acute diarrhea have rarely indicated traditionally cultivatable adenoviruses as etiologic agents. Enteral adenoviruses have also been reported in both sporadic and epidemic enteritis; respiratory manifestations are found in about half of the patients.

Intussusception, Mesenteric Lymphadenitis. The pathogenesis of intussusception is thought by many to include enlarged lymph nodes as an initiating factor. Adenoviruses have been recovered from mesenteric lymph nodes and also from a higher percentage of children with intussusception than from controls. Adenoviruses have also been visualized in the appendix of a child with intussusception and in the appendices of children with appendicitis. Whether these findings represent acute etiologic relationships or manifestations of a protracted intestinal latency is not clear.

Pertussis-like Syndrome. The common childhood adenoviruses have been found in cases simulating pertussis, both in the absence and the presence of *Bordetella pertussis* infection. Adenoviral infection is probably an uncommon cause of this syndrome. The finding of adenovirus in some cases may represent activation of a latent virus.

Hemorrhagic Cystitis. This is a syndrome with sudden onset of bacteriologically sterile hematuria, dysuria, frequency, and urgency (Sec. 17.38); the process subsides in 1–2 wk. Infection with adenovirus types 11 and 21 has been found in some of the affected children and young adults.

Diagnosis and Differential Diagnosis. Pharyngoconjunctival fever is clinically distinct, but most of the other syndromes of adenoviral infection are not distinctive enough to suggest the etiologic diagnosis.

Complications, Prevention, and Treatment. Some infants with adenoviral pneumonia have subsequently had bronchiectasis or lobar collapse. Immunization with unattenuated adenovirus types 4 and 7 in enteric capsules has been effective in military personnel. Such preparations are not available against the common childhood types of adenovirus. There is no specific treatment.

Brandt CD, Kim HW, Jeffries BC, et al: Infections in 18,000 infants and children in a controlled study of respiratory tract disease. II. Variation in adenovirus infections by year and season. Am J Epidemiol 95:218, 1971.

Fay HM, Grayston JT, Evans AS: Viral Infections of Humans. New York, Plenum Medical Books, 1976, pp 53–69.

Gary GW Jr, Herholzer JC, Black RE: Noncultivable adenoviruses associated with diarrhea in infants: A new subgroup of human adenoviruses. J Clin Microbiol 10:96, 1979.

Jackson GG, Muldoon RL: Viruses causing common respiratory infection in man. IV. Reoviruses and adenoviruses. J Infect Dis 128:811, 1973.

Nelson KE, Gavitt F, Batt MD, et al: The role of adenoviruses in the pertussis syndrome. J Pediatr 86:335, 1975.

Numazaki Y, Kumasaka T, Yano N, et al: Further study on acute hemorrhagic cystitis due to adenovirus type H. N Engl J Med 289:344, 1973.

Wadell G, Varsanyi TM, Lord A, et al: Epidemic outbreak of adenovirus 7 with special reference to the pathogenicity of adenovirus genome type 7b. Am J Epidemiol 112:619, 1980.

Wadell G, Hammarskjold M, Winberg G, et al: Genetic variability of adenoviruses. Ann NY Acad Sci 354:16, 1980.

Yolken RH, Lawrence F, Leister F, et al: Gastroenteritis associated with enteric type adenovirus in hospitalized infants. J Pediatr 101:21, 1982.

11.75 RHINOVIRAL INFECTIONS

Rhinoviruses, collectively the most common cause of the "common cold" in adults, represent a smaller proportion of infections in young children because of the frequency of other viral respiratory infections. Also rhinoviral infections in young children often do not produce respiratory illness. However, rhinoviruses spread readily, producing illness in nursery and other school groups, and these children provide a major link in their spread within families.

Etiology. There are 111 serologically distinct rhinoviruses, all members of the picornavirus family of small RNA viruses.

They are best identified by inoculating human embryonic kidney or human diploid cell cultures with nasal secretions from infected individuals and waiting to observe a cytopathic effect. Routine serologic testing for acquisition of antibody is not practical because of the multiplicity of types and infrequency of their cross-reactivity.

Several cross-sectional studies indicate that a low percentage of control children or children with diarrhea (1%) yield rhinoviruses at the time of sampling; similarly, only 2.2% of children with respiratory tract illness yield rhinoviruses. In longitudinal studies, however, 75% of pediatric rhinovirus infection is associated with illness, e.g., rhinitis and pharyngitis-bronchitis syndrome. Rarely have rhinoviruses been reported in connection with serious lower respiratory tract disease. They may precipitate asthma in children and chronic bronchitis in adults.

Epidemiology. Rhinoviruses are distributed worldwide with no predictable pattern of infection by serotype. Multiple types may be present in a community at one time.

In temperate climates the incidence of rhinoviral infection peaks in September and again in April or May, but some infections occur year-round. The peak incidence in the tropics occurs during the rainy season.

Rhinoviruses are recovered in highest concentration in nasal secretions, and experimental infection is most easily accomplished by nasal or conjunctival instillation. Infection via aerosol is less efficient. Virus persists for several hours in secretions on hands or other surfaces. Most transmission probably occurs by spread of nasal secretions to nose or eye by hand, occasionally by cough or sneeze.

Pathogenesis. The peak nasal inflammatory response occurs when virus growth is at its greatest, 2–4 days after experimental infection. Immune responses include specific nasal IgA and serum IgG antibody, which may contribute to modifying the illness and limiting viral shedding. Interferon and a nonspecific factor induced by infection with a heterotypic rhinovirus may be a part of the resistance mechanism. Usually the inflammatory response is limited to the nose, throat, and upper bronchial passages, but pneumonia has occurred.

Clinical Manifestations. The primary clinical response to rhinoviral infection, like that to most respiratory viral infections, is the "common cold" (see Sec. 13.27). There is an incubation period of 2–4 days; then sneezing, nasal obstruction and discharge, and sore throat ensue. Cough and hoarseness occur in 30–40% of cases. Headache and other systemic symptoms are not as common as in influenza. Fever is neither as frequent nor as high as in primary infections with respiratory syncytial virus, parainfluenza virus, or adenovirus. Symptoms are worse in the first 2–3 days of illness and last for a week in a majority of patients; they persist for over 14 days in 35 per cent of young children.

Complications. Complications of rhinoviral infection are like those of any infection causing edema and inflammation in the nasopharyngeal area. They include obstructive otitis media, sinusitis, local spread down the respiratory tract, and bacterial superinfection.

Diagnosis and Differential Diagnosis. Since other viral agents and β-hemolytic streptococci can produce the same manifestations, a clinical diagnosis can be only presumptive. Laboratory diagnosis is not practical under ordinary circumstances. If any question exists, bacterial cultures should be taken to exclude streptococcal infection.

Treatment and Prevention. There is no specific preventive or ameliorative treatment. Careful handwashing and avoidance of manual nose and eye manipulation is the best approach to reducing spread. For relief of acute symptoms, a mild analgesic and saline or decongestant nose drops may be used for a short time. Interferon has been reported in some studies to be of value in preventing rhinovirus infection, but other studies do not support this conclusion. Recent reports suggest that synthetic alpha-interferon administered by nose drops may have some effect against the rhinoviruses that produce the common cold in adults.

ROBERT H. PARROTT

Bloom HH, Forsyth BR, Johnson KM, et al: Relationship of rhinovirus infection to mild upper respiratory disease. JAMA 186:144, 1963.

Chanock RM, Parrott RH: Acute respiratory disease in infancy and childhood: Present understanding and prospects for prevention. Pediatrics 36:21, 1965.

Douglas RG Jr: The common cold—relief at last? N Engl J Med 314:115, 1986.

Gwaltney JM: In: Evans AS (ed): Viral Infections of Humans. New York, Plenum Medical Books, 1976, p 383.

Jackson GG, Muldoon RL: Viruses causing common respiratory infections in man. J Infect Dis 127:328, 1973.

Ketler A, Hall CE, Fox JP, et al: The Virus Watch Program: A continuing surveillance of viral infections in metropolitan New York families. VIII. Rhinovirus infections: Observations of virus excretion, intrafamilial spread and clinical response. Am J Epidemiol 90:244, 1969.

11.76 HEPATITIS

Hepatitis is a major health problem worldwide. In the United States there are estimated to be more than 70,000 cases yearly.

The viruses of hepatitis A, hepatitis B, and at least two other viruses causing hepatitis that is neither A nor B have been identified. Other as yet unidentified viruses may also cause hepatitis. In addition, cytomegalovirus (Sec. 11.68), Epstein-Barr virus (Sec. 11.69), rubella virus (Sec. 11.62), and enteroviruses (Sec. 11.77) may cause hepatitis. See also Sec. 12.80.

Etiology. *Hepatitis A (HA).* HA virus (HAV or enterovirus 72) can be demonstrated in human stool by a variety of immunologic techniques; both total and specific IgM antibody against HA virus (anti-HA) can also be measured by radio-immunoassay. Laboratory strains of HAV have been propagated in tissue culture.

Hepatitis B (HB, Hepadnavirus 1). This infection was first recognized by the detection of a viral antigen—the Australia antigen—in the blood of a hepatitis carrier. Electron microscopy initially revealed that the blood of carriers contained spherical and tubular particles, which were subsequently recognized to constitute the surface of the virion; hence, the structures originally designated Australia antigen are now referred to as hepatitis B surface antigen or HB_sAg; antibody directed against HB_s is designated anti-HB_s. A number of subtypes that have been useful in epidemiologic studies have been described for the HB_s antigen; they are referred to as a, y, w, d, r, and others.

Dane observed another larger virus-like particle in the serum of some patients with hepatitis B. This "Dane particle" is now known to represent the virion. The inner component or core of this virus is designated hepatitis B core antigen or HB_c. Antibody directed against HB_c is designated anti-HB_c.

The virus contains DNA, and DNA polymerase is found in the sera of some patients with hepatitis B, often in association with the HB_e antigen. HB_e antigen is an integral part of the core of HB virus and is associated with high infectivity. There appear to be three serotypes of HB_eAg. Antibody against HB_e is designated anti-HB_e (Table 11–28).

Hepatitis Viruses Other than HA or HB (Non-A–Non-B Virus). The delta (δ) agent ($HB_\delta Ag$) is an incomplete RNA virus that can multiply only in the presence of HBV. Infections may be concurrent, or δ agent can infect an individual persistently positive for HB_sAg. Transmission is usually by parenteral inoculation. Delta agent may result in fulminant hepatitis, and it also increases the likelihood of chronic liver disease in HB_sAg carriers. Epidemics have occurred among users of illicit parenteral drugs. Blood concentrates can also transmit the infection. Perinatal transmission is rare. Intrafamily and water-borne forms and parenterally transmitted varieties of non-A–non-B hepatitis also have been reported. Other, as yet unidentified, viral agents may play etiologic roles in this disorder.

Viruses That May Cause Hepatitis Incidentally. The liver is frequently involved in AIDS, in infectious mononucleosis, and in newborns infected with cytomegalovirus or herpesviruses. Cytomegalovirus in young adults may also cause a syndrome of hepatitis characterized by prolonged fever and development of atypical lymphocytes. Newborn infants with encephalomyocarditis due to coxsackievirus B usually have hepatic and pancreatic involvement. Coxsackieviruses have also been associated with a syndrome of hepatitis and myocarditis seen most commonly during adolescence. Fatal adenoviral pneumonia in infants has also been found to involve the liver. Hepatitis is common in congenital rubella and may occur in rare instances as a complication of varicella, mumps, measles, and other common infections. Newborn infants infected with echovirus 11 may also develop fatal hepatitis.

Epidemiology. That different agents cause hepatitis with characteristic incubation periods and different modes of transmission was recognized long before the agents were identified.

Hepatitis A (Infectious Hepatitis). This highly contagious disease is transmitted by person-to-person contact and occasionally by ingestion of contaminated food or water. In the United States, the number of reported cases occurring during each of the first three decades of life is approximately the same, but anicteric hepatitis is estimated to occur in over 80% of those infected who are under the age of 2 yr and in about half of those infected who are 3–4 yr old. The illness tends to be more severe in adults. Most infants are protected by maternal antibody during the early months of life.

The incubation period is approximately 4–6 wk from exposure until the appearance of jaundice. The highest titers of HAV in stool are found prior to onset of the rise in bilirubin.

Hepatitis A has no seasonal predilection. Seven year cycles of peak incidence have been described. Infection appears to occur at an earlier age under conditions of poor hygiene; the disease is endemic in underdeveloped areas. Common-source outbreaks from contaminated water or infected food or food handlers have been reported. Transmission by transfused blood, although rare, has also been documented. Infection has also been contracted from primates. Spread occurs readily between homosexuals and in day care centers. Personnel in

---

Table 11–28. **Components of Hepatitis B Virus (HBV)**

Antigens	Abbreviation	Antibodies Directed Against HBV Antigens
Hepatitis B surface antigen	HB_sAg	Anti-HB_s
— subtypes	HB_sAg/ayr; HB_sAg/adr; etc.	
Hepatitis B core antigen	HB_cAg	Anti-HB_c
Hepatitis B$_e$ antigen	HB_eAg	Anti-HB_e
Hepatitis B$_\delta$ antigen	$HB_\delta Ag$	Anti-HB_δ
Deoxyribonucleic acid polymerase	DNA polymerase	

day care centers and household contacts of attendees are at increased risk for HAV infection.

Hepatitis A during pregnancy or at the time of delivery does not appear to result in clinical disease in the newborn, in teratogenic effects, or in increased risk of abortion.

Hepatitis B (Serum Hepatitis). The term *serum hepatitis* refers to the most common method by which it is transmitted, but percutaneous or mucous membrane inoculation may also result in infection. Transmission has been documented between sexual partners and under the conditions of institutional living. A higher rate of infection is found among children with Down syndrome living in institutions than among those living at home with their families. Hepatitis B surface antigen (HB_sAg) can be demonstrated in saliva, feces, and other body secretions.

The incubation period of hepatitis B from exposure to the onset of jaundice is 2–5 mo. There is no seasonal prevalence.

The major mechanism of transmission is by inoculation with blood of carriers, which may contain large amounts of virus. Even a prick with a needle contaminated with a minute amount of blood from a carrier of hepatitis B virus can transmit infection; shared needles probably account for the high frequency of infection among drug users. Transfusion of infected blood carried a considerable risk of serum hepatitis prior to screening of blood donors and conversion from paid to volunteer donors. Patients who required frequent transfusions, e.g., those with hemophilia or thalassemia, had high rates of infection, as did those undergoing renal dialysis. There is an increased incidence of hepatitis B in families of patients on dialysis or receiving blood products frequently. Administering clotting factors prepared from pooled plasma may also transmit HBV and non-A–non-B viruses. Using heat-inactivated products may reduce the risk of infection with non-A–non-B viruses. Elimination of plasma from HB_s positive donors has reduced the risk of concentrates.

The transmission of hepatitis B from pregnant carriers of its surface antigen (HB_sAg) to their infants presents a special problem. The presence of HB_eAg in maternal carriers is highly correlated with transmission of hepatitis B infection to their offspring, but even HB_eAg negative mothers and mothers with anti-HB_e may have had affected infants. The older siblings of affected infants also have a high rate of HB_s and HB_eAg positivity. There is no increased risk of abortion or malformations following hepatitis during the 1st trimester of pregnancy.

HB_sAg has been inconsistently demonstrated in the breast milk of infected mothers. Breast feeding of unimmunized infants by infected mothers does not appear to confer a greater risk of hepatitis on their offspring than does artificial feeding, despite the possibility that cracked nipples may result in the ingestion of contaminated maternal blood by the nursing infant. Immunization of newborns decreases the risk even further.

During the neonatal period hepatitis B antigen is present in the blood of 2.5% of infants born to affected mothers, probably representing intrauterine infection. In most cases antigenemia appears later, suggesting that transmission occurred at the time of delivery; virus contained in amniotic fluid or in maternal feces or blood may be the source. Although most infants born to infected mothers become antigenemic from 2–5 mo of age, some infants of HB_sAg positive mothers are not affected until later in the 1st or even the 2nd yr of life.

Hepatitis B tends to be relatively milder in infants and children and probably is frequently unrecognized. Although newborn infants are rarely symptomatic, about 90% of those infected become chronic carriers. The risk of developing chronic liver disease or hepatocellular carcinoma later in life is increased in these infants. The carrier and HB_eAg positivity

rates appear to be highest in certain Asian Pacific island and Alaskan Eskimo groups in whom perinatal transmission is the most common means of perpetuating HBV. Individuals from these groups may be at increased risk of infecting their infants even after a number of generations have lived in the United States. Women born in Haiti or sub-Saharan Africa also are at increased risk of being HB_sAg positive and infecting their newborn infants.

Pathology. The acute response of the liver to virus injury hepatitis A or B virus is similar. Initially, balloon degeneration and necrosis of single or groups of parenchymal cells occur, starting in the center of the lobules. These are followed by infiltration of the parenchyma and portal areas with lymphocytes, macrophages, plasma cells, eosinophils, and neutrophils; in the later stages, lymphocytes predominate. Regeneration of parenchymal cells is evidenced by cells or clusters of cells containing mitotic figures. Later there are striking changes in the periportal areas, with widening due to infiltration of inflammatory cells, proliferation of bile ducts, and biliary stasis. In fulminating hepatitis there is total destruction of parenchyma with only the reticular framework of the liver remaining. The newborn infant responds to hepatic injury by forming giant cells.

By 3 mo after onset of clinical illness, liver morphology is generally normal. Persistence of significant histologic changes in patients with hepatitis B usually indicates the development of chronic liver disease.

The changes in *chronic persistent hepatitis* and *chronic active hepatitis* are discussed in Sec. 12.83. Cirrhotic changes are sometimes found.

Other organ systems are affected in hepatitis. Small intestinal tissue may show changes in villous structure. Renal, joint, and skin involvement may result from circulating immune complexes. A hypoplastic bone marrow may result in aplastic anemia.

Pathogenesis. Jaundice results from obstruction of biliary flow and damage to parenchymal cells. Elevations of both direct and indirect serum bilirubin are found. Intrahepatic obstruction to bile flow may result in acholic stools. Resumption of flow may deliver normal or increased amounts of bilirubin to the duodenum. Urobilinogen, a metabolite of bilirubin produced in the intestine, is normally reabsorbed. Damaged liver parenchymal cells may be unable to re-excrete this material, which subsequently appears in the urine. Elevated serum alkaline phosphatase, 5'-nucleotidase, or γ-glutamyl transpeptidase activities suggest biliary obstruction.

The release into blood of serum transaminases from damaged liver cells suggests the extent and duration of injury. Serum glutamic-pyruvic transaminase (SGPT) [alanine aminotransferase (ACT)] provides a more specific indicator of liver cell injury than does serum glutamic-oxaloacetic transaminase (SGOT) [aspartate aminotransferase (AST)]; injury to other cells such as erythrocytes, skeletal muscle cells, or myocardial cells may also cause rises in the SGOT. In severe liver injury, as in fulminating hepatitis, transaminases may fall to extremely low levels, indicating total destruction of parenchymal cells. Other enzymes, such as lactic dehydrogenase (LDH) may also be used to detect parenchymal cell injury.

Damage to liver cells may also be reflected in aberrations of their normal functions. Increased prothrombin time may result from their inability to synthesize proteins required for clotting. Obstruction to biliary flow reduces the flow of bile salts to the intestine, which normally facilitate fat absorption, including lipid-soluble vitamin K. Liver injury may also result in changes in carbohydrate, ammonia, and drug metabolism.

Clinical Manifestations. In adolescents and older children hepatitis tends to resemble the more severe disease seen in adults. Hepatitis A tends to be acute in onset, hepatitis B, insidious.

Hepatitis A typically presents at its onset with systemic complaints of fever, malaise, and digestive complaints of nausea, emesis, anorexia, intolerance of food and tobacco, and some abdominal discomfort. This prodrome may be mild or go unnoticed in children. Dull right upper quadrant pain or epigastric fullness may be exaggerated by exercise or jolting of any kind. Jaundice and dark urine usually appear after the onset of systemic symptoms, but they may be the presenting signs in children. Jaundice may be so subtle that it can be detected only by laboratory tests, or it may last overtly as long as 2–3 wk. Light or clay-colored stools may result from obstruction of biliary flow. Constipation from poor fluid intake is more common than diarrhea. Characteristic feelings of general discontent and depression are probably responsible for the cliché "a jaundiced view of life." Young infants may fail to gain weight. During convalescence, which may last several weeks, there is gradual return of appetite, exercise tolerance, and a feeling of well-being. Children tend to have less disability from hepatitis A than adults do, and their convalescence is usually shorter.

Hepatitis B may be heralded by arthralgia or skin eruptions, e.g., urticarial, purpuric, macular, or maculopapular rashes. Papular acrodermatitis, *Gianotti-Crosti syndrome,* may also occur. The course tends to be insidious and lasts somewhat longer than that of hepatitis A, although it may be characterized by many of the same manifestations. In some patients hematuria or proteinuria may appear during convalescence.

On physical examination, skin and mucous membranes are icteric, especially the sclera and the mucosa under the tongue. The liver is usually enlarged and tender to palpation. When the liver is not palpable below the costal margin, tenderness can be demonstrated by striking the rib cage over the liver gently with a closed fist. Splenomegaly and lymphadenopathy are common.

Asymptomatic hepatitis A and B are common, particularly in the very young. Of the infants born to mothers with hepatitis B who develop demonstrable antigenemia and elevated transaminases, few have clinical evidence of hepatitis.

Diagnosis. A history of jaundice in family contacts, friends, schoolmates, or day care center playmates or personnel, or travel to an endemic area may suggest the diagnosis. Accidental inoculation with blood of an infected person, drug abuse, and homosexual behavior should also arouse suspicion of hepatitis B. Children undergoing dialysis or who receive frequent transfusions of blood products, e.g., fibrinogen, factor VIII, or factor IX particularly, are also at high risk of hepatitis B infection.

The diagnosis may be substantiated by *laboratory data* indicating liver injury. Hyperbilirubinemia may occur without clinical jaundice. Direct and indirect serum bilirubin levels are elevated, the conjugated portion more so during the early stage of disease. Later, excretion of conjugated bilirubin resumes, and there is a relative increase of indirect bilirubin. Urobilinogen is increased in serum and, subsequently, in urine.

Rises in serum transaminases reflect injury to hepatic cells. In hepatitis A the transaminases usually reach a higher peak, often exceeding 1000 units, and decline more rapidly than they do in hepatitis B. Prolonged intermittent elevations are found in non-A–non-B hepatitis. With severe liver injury the prothrombin time is usually elevated. Biliary obstructive disease is manifested by elevated alkaline phosphatase, 5'-nucleotidase, or γ-glutamyl transpeptidase.

Mild leukopenia with a relative lymphocytosis and atypical lymphocytes may be observed during the first 2 wk of illness. IgM values may be elevated, particularly in hepatitis A. The sedimentation rate is usually elevated in hepatitis A and is often used as a method of following the course of the disease.

Acute and convalescent sera can be tested for the presence of anti-HAV. IgM anti-HAV is usually present at the onset of jaundice and is detectable for at least 6–8 wk. This test is also often useful in detecting subclinical cases among contacts. IgG anti-HAV appears a few weeks after onset and persists indefinitely. Hepatitis A virus can be demonstrated in stools for several days prior to and for up to 1 wk following the onset of jaundice.

A variety of antigen-antibody systems are available for confirming the diagnosis of hepatitis B (Table 11–29). HB$_s$Ag appears early in the disease and may disappear before the disappearance of jaundice. In carriers, however, HB$_s$Ag persists indefinitely. Anti-HB$_c$ is usually present soon after the onset of jaundice and then persists indefinitely. Anti-HB$_c$ or IgM anti-HB$_c$ may be the only marker present after HB$_s$Ag has disappeared or prior to the appearance of anti-HB$_s$, particularly in fulminant hepatitis. Anti-HB$_c$IgM has been less useful in young infants. DNA polymerase and HB$_e$Ag appear early, prior to the onset of icterus. Anti-HB$_e$ and then anti-HB$_s$ may appear during convalescence. During exacerbations, rises in anti-HB$_c$ are often observed. Serial samples tested simultaneously are often desirable for precise laboratory confirmation of hepatitis B.

HB$_e$Ag in a patient's serum denotes an increased risk of transmission of HBV infection. Donors or pregnant women who are HB$_s$Ag positive are more likely to transmit hepatitis B if they are also HB$_e$Ag positive.

Differential Diagnosis. Physiologic jaundice, hemolytic disease, and infection in neonates are usually easily distinguished from hepatitis (Sec. 8.44–8.47 and 8.59). After the immediate newborn period, infection remains an important cause of hyperbilirubinemia, but other causes are galactosemia, hypothyroidism, congenital defects in metabolism of bilirubin, biliary atresia, hepatitis associated with alpha$_1$-antitrypsin deficiency, and choledochal cysts. The introduction of pigmented vegetables into the infant's diet may result in carotenemia, which may be mistaken for jaundice.

In later infancy and childhood hemolytic-uremic syndrome may be mistaken initially for hepatitis (Sec. 17.13). Reye syndrome may suggest acute fulminating hepatitis. Jaundice may also occur with severe infection in older children, particularly in those with malignant disorders. Malaria, leptospirosis, or brucellosis may also cause hepatitis. In adolescents as well as in children with chronic hemolytic processes, gallstones may obstruct biliary drainage and cause jaundice. Cirrhosis, which may be associated with Wilson disease, cystic

Table 11–29. Tests for Infection with Hepatitis B Virus

Test	Preicteric	Icteric	Convalescent	Carriers
HB$_s$	+ + + +	+ +	+	+ +
Anti-HB$_s$		±	+ +	–
Anti-HB$_c$IgM		+ +	+ + +	
Anti-HB$_c$		±	+ + +	+
Anti-HB$_e$			+ +	+ or –
Bilirubin		+ + +		+ or –
Transaminase	+ + + +	+ + +	+ +	+ or –
DNA polymerase	+ + +	±		+ or –

fibrosis, Banti syndrome, and other causes, may sometimes present as hepatitis. The liver may be involved in collagen diseases, e.g., lupus erythematosus.

A variety of *medications* may produce jaundice; e.g., acetaminophen in excessive doses may cause liver damage, or other drugs may cause increased hemolysis, cholestasis, or hepatitis. Drugs well tolerated in normal children may cause problems in children with certain illnesses (Sec. 5.53).

Complications. Although most children recover uneventfully from hepatitis, a few suffer serious acute or chronic complications.

Acute Fulminating Hepatitis. See also Sec. 12.85. Some children develop a progressive course characterized by a rising serum bilirubin with peak levels exceeding 20 mg/dL, encephalopathy, bleeding, edema, and ascites. Drowsiness is followed by stupor and then by deep coma; clonus and hyperreflexia may be replaced later by loss of deep tendon, pupillary, and corneal reflexes. Transaminase levels may rise into the thousands and then return to normal or very low values. Blood ammonia is elevated and the electroencephalogram is usually abnormal. The full-blown disease may develop relentlessly over 1–2 wk or be more insidious. Liver biopsy reveals "bridging necrosis," areas of parenchymal necrosis that cross limiting plates, extending from the central vein of one lobule to another.

Acute fulminating hepatitis is more frequently associated with hepatitis B when there is coinfection or superinfection with δ agent than when there is infection with hepatitis B alone. The reported mortality is over 30%. Death from bacterial or fungal sepsis is not unusual. Treatment is aimed at sustaining the patient while providing the time for regeneration of hepatic cells.

Chronic Active Hepatitis (CAH). See also Sec. 12.83. Although the onset of jaundice may appear to be acute, careful questioning often reveals a more insidious course with a history of anorexia, nausea, emesis, and weight loss of several weeks' duration. The spleen as well as the liver is usually enlarged. Low-grade fever and joint complaints are frequent.

There is usually hypergammaglobulinemia, accompanied by the development of antinuclear, antiglomerular, antimitochondrial, and anti–smooth muscle antibodies and a positive Coombs test. HB_sAg is rarely found in children. Anemia and moderately elevated levels of both direct and indirect bilirubin are common. Transaminases are elevated and useful for following the response to therapy. Thrombocytopenia and prolongation of the prothrombin time are frequently found.

Aplastic Anemia. See also Sec. 15.32. Blood abnormalities characteristic of aplastic anemia may develop several weeks after the onset of hepatitis, at which time hepatic function and architecture may have returned to normal. The bone marrow shows various stages of aplasia; terminally, the marrow is replaced by fat. The prognosis of aplastic anemia associated with hepatitis has generally been poor.

Other. Nephrosis has developed in children with HBV infection. Renal biopsy has revealed membranous glomerulonephritis with deposition of complement and HB_eAg in glomerular capillaries. Studies in Asia and Africa reveal an association of HB_sAg in mothers with the development of hepatocellular carcinoma in their offspring during young adulthood.

Prevention. *Hepatitis A.* Hospitalized infected patients who are incontinent of stool or who are in diapers should be treated with *enteric precautions,* including isolation. Patients are contagious for about 1 wk following onset of jaundice. There is no need to isolate older children, but their stool and fecally contaminated materials should be treated with precautions, and handwashing should be strictly enforced.

Household contacts should receive 0.02 mL/kg of *immune globulin* (IG) as soon as the diagnosis made. This is effective in preventing clinical hepatitis, although many recipients have rises in transaminase, indicating that the infection is probably modified rather than prevented.

Immune globulin is not routinely recommended for sporadic nonhousehold exposure, e.g., protection of hospital personnel or schoolmates. It is possible to test for anti-HAV to establish immune status, and testing may be desirable when repeated exposure is anticipated.

Mass immunization of school children has been used when epidemics have been school centered. When a single case of hepatitis occurs in a day care center or in two families of children attending a day care center, IG should be administered to all children and personnel. It is also advisable to immunize family members of the children in diapers. Handwashing after changing diapers should be stressed at all times in day care centers.

HAV infection in pregnancy does not affect the newborn.

Prophylactic administration of immune serum globulin (0.06 mL/kg intramuscularly) is recommended for those traveling for extended periods in areas where hepatitis A is endemic. This larger dose will provide protection for a longer period, obviating the need to find a local health care provider who can administer IG.

A *vaccine* is not available.

Hepatitis B. CONTROL. A major advance in controlling the spread of hepatitis B is the use for transfusion of only donated blood shown by testing to be free of HBV. Isolation of hospitalized infected patients is not mandatory, but careful handling of blood, needles, and instruments contaminated with blood of infected patients is essential.

IMMUNIZATION. *Passive* immunization can be effectively provided by a dose of 0.06 mL/kg of hepatitis B immune globulin (HBIG). *Active* immunization can be provided by a vaccine prepared from HBV derived from blood (that is not associated with an increased risk of AIDS) or from a cloned DNA fragment coding for HB_sAg produced by yeast cells. When vaccination is indicated, a 3 dose regimen should be administered; the 2nd and 3rd doses should be given 1 mo and 6 mo after the 1st dose. For those under 10 yr of age half of the regular adult dose is recommended; a 40 μg dose should be used for patients on dialysis. Booster doses are required.

Children injected with or ingesting HB_sAg-contaminated blood should immediately be passively immunized with HBIG. This should be repeated in 1 mo. If reexposure is likely, active immunization should be started at the time of the first dose of HBIG; the second and third doses of vaccine are given at 2 and 6 months following the first dose. The second dose of HBIG is not needed.

If it is not known whether the blood is contaminated, a dose of HBIG should be given and the blood tested for HB_sAg; if negative, the subsequent treatment can be omitted. If the blood is positive, the risk of contracting hepatitis from the exposure is about 1 in 20; if the blood is from a high-risk patient (one with hepatitis or Down syndrome, someone of Asian or African descent, a patient on dialysis, etc) and the result of antigen testing is unknown, the risk is about 1 in 200.

Children or adolescents at high risk should receive HBV vaccine. This group includes those entering therapy programs that place them at increased risk, e.g., dialysis or frequent administration of blood products; those who have household or institutional contact with HB_sAg-positive individuals; and homosexuals.

Infants whose mothers are HB_sAg-positive or have had HBV infection during the 3rd trimester should receive 0.5 mL of HBIG when they receive eye prophylaxis or other routine newborn procedures. This can be best accomplished if mothers are tested prior to delivery in order to avoid delaying treatment while awaiting the test results and to allow those who are to attend the mother to protect themselves and others. The first of the 3 doses of hepatitis B vaccine should also be given at the same time at a site separate from that used for HBIG, using a different syringe. If medically indicated, the vaccine but not the HBIG may be delayed as long as 3 mo; if this is done, a 2nd dose of HBIG should be given at 3 mo. At 9 mo of age, vaccinees should be tested for HB$_s$Ag and for anti HB$_s$. Those who are antigenemic are vaccine failures and should be managed as carriers; those who are negative by both tests should receive another dose of the vaccine and the tests should be repeated one month later. Infants whose mothers are HB$_e$Ag-positive are at greatest risk of infection.

Pregnant women at increased risk, e.g., those of Asian or sub-Saharan origin, frequent recipients of blood products, intravenous drug users, and those with frequent exposure to individuals with liver disease or who have had liver disease, should be tested for the presence of HB$_s$Ag. If they test positive, their infants should be treated as above.

Although infants of HB$_s$Ag-positive mothers do not need to be isolated, the maternal blood that may be on their skin at delivery may contain HBV and should be removed by a gloved attendant by wiping.

Infants undergoing surgery or having a prolonged hospitalization should be tested for HB$_s$Ag. About 5% of blood specimens of infants who will develop HBV infections during the first 6 mo of life are likely to be positive at birth. Testing of cord serum is unreliable and not recommended.

Deinstitutionalized children having a tendency to bite others should be tested for HB$_s$Ag. If positive, measures may be needed to prevent infection of persons who might be bitten.

Health care providers likely to come into frequent contact with blood should be immunized.

Non-A–Non-B Hepatitis. The effectiveness of IG for prophylaxis of non-A–non-B hepatitis is unclear. Some evidence supports its use in doses similar to those used for HBIG in prophylaxis of HBV infection.

Treatment. Therapy for *uncomplicated hepatitis* is supportive (Sec. 12.80). Patients often find that a diet low in fat is more acceptable. Parents should be prepared to be tolerant of the child's anorexia. There is no evidence that rigid restriction of physical activity will speed recovery.

Occasionally, severe anorexia or emesis may necessitate intravenous therapy to prevent dehydration, but antiemetic preparations should be avoided since most are metabolized in the liver.

Corticosteroids are not indicated for uncomplicated hepatitis. See Sec. 13.83 for discussion of *chronic active hepatitis*.

The management of *acute fulminating hepatitis* is discussed in Sec. 12.85. The conventional strategy is to manage the patient's acute problems while awaiting the restoration of hepatic function. These problems include encephalopathy, bleeding, fluid retention and electrolyte disturbances, maintenance of adequate nutrition, and others.

The encephalopathy is managed, in part, by efforts to reduce blood ammonia levels, such as feeding with lactulose, administering neomycin to sterilize the bowel, and reducing protein intake. A variety of methods have been used to remove ammonia and toxic substances. Exchange transfusion occasionally produces dramatic results, but the effects are usually short-lived, and the effect on long-term survival is uncertain.

Electrolyte abnormalities may contribute to the encephalopathy. Low potassium levels are common; these may be aggravated by the use of diuretics. Metabolic alkalosis associated with hypokalemia may enhance ammonia diffusion into brain cells, thus potentiating the encephalopathy. It is essential that adequate intake of potassium be provided. Diuretics should

also be used with caution because of their tendency to cause hypovolemia.

Removal of ascites by paracentesis is indicated only when the fluid compromises pulmonary ventilation. Administration of serum albumin is sometimes required when low serum protein levels result in severe edema.

Bleeding may be serious enough to cause significant anemia, and bacterial breakdown of blood in the gastrointestinal tract may increase blood ammonia levels. The choice of packed cells or whole blood for transfusion will depend on the need to provide serum proteins. Vitamin K is generally ineffective in correcting a prolonged prothrombin time, even when given parenterally.

PHILIP A. BRUNELL

Alter HJ, Purcell RH, Holland PV, et al: Transmissible agent in non-A, non-B hepatitis. Lancet 1:459, 1978.

Alter HJ, Seeff LB, Kaplan PM, et al: Type B hepatitis: The infectivity of blood positive for e antigen and DNA polymerase after accidental needlestick exposure. N Engl J Med 295:909, 1976.

Athreya BH, Gorske AL, Myers AR: Aspirin-induced abnormalities of liver function. Am J Dis Child 126:638, 1973.

Beasley RP, Stevens CE, Shiao IS, et al: Evidence against breast-feeding as a mechanism for vertical transmission of hepatitis B. Lancet 2:740, 1975.

Blum AL, Stutz R, Haemmerli VP, et al: A fortuitously controlled study of steroid therapy in acute viral hepatitis. Am J Med 47:82, 1969.

Centers for Disease Control: Recommendations for protection against viral hepatitis. Morbid Mortal Weekly Rep 34:313, 1985.

Committee on Infectious Diseases, American Academy of Pediatrics: Prevention of hepatitis B virus infections. Pediatrics 75:362, 1985.

Derso A, Boxall EH, Tarlow MJ, et al: Transmission of HB$_s$Ag from mother to infant in four ethnic groups. Br Med J 1:949, 1978.

Dubois RS, Silverman A: Treatment of chronic active hepatitis in children. Postgrad Med J 50:386, 1974.

Gregory PB, Knauer CM, Kempson RL, et al: Steroid therapy in severe viral hepatitis: A double-blind, randomized trial of methylprednisolone versus placebo. N Engl J Med 294:681, 1976.

Hadler SC, et al: Hepatitis in day-care centers: A community-wide assessment. N Engl J Med 302:1222, 1980.

Levy RN, Sawitsky A, Florman AL, et al: Fatal aplastic anemia after hepatitis. N Engl J Med 273:1118, 1965.

Magnius LO, Lindholm A, Lundin P, et al: A new antigen-antibody system: Clinical significance in long-term carriers of hepatitis B surface antigen. JAMA 231:356, 1975.

Noble RL, Kane MA, Reeves SA, et al: Post transfusion hepatitis A in a neonatal intensive care unit. JAMA 252:2711, 1984.

Okada K, Kamiyama I, Inomata M: E antigen and anti-e in the serum of asymptomatic carrier mothers as indicators of positive and negative transmission of hepatitis B virus to their infants. N Engl J Med 294:746, 1976.

Provost PJ, Hilleman MR: Propagation of human hepatitis A virus in cell culture in vitro (40422). Proc Soc Exp Biol Med 160:213, 1979.

Repsher LH, Freebern RK: Effects of early and vigorous exercise on recovery from infectious hepatitis. N Engl J Med 281:1393, 1969.

Schenker S, Breen KJ, Hoyumpa AM: Hepatic encephalopathy: Current status. Gastroenterology 66:121, 1974.

Schumacher HR, Gall EP: Arthritis in acute hepatitis and chronic active hepatitis: Pathology of the synovial membrane with evidence for the presence of Australia antigen in synovial membranes. Am J Med 57:655, 1974.

Siegel M: Congenital malformations following chickenpox, measles, mumps, and rubella. JAMA 226:1521, 1973.

Siegel M, Fuerst HT: Low birth weight and maternal virus diseases: A prospective study of rubella, measles, mumps, chickenpox, and hepatitis. JAMA 197:680, 1966.

Steinberg SC, Alter JH, Leventhal BG: The risk of hepatitis transmission to family contacts of leukemia patients. J Pediatr 87:753, 1975.

Szmuness W, Stevens CE, Harley EJ, et al: Hepatitis B vaccine: Demonstration of efficacy in a controlled clinical trial in a high-risk population in the United States. N Engl J Med 303:833, 1980.

Takekoshi Y, Tanaka M, Miyakawa Y, et al: Free "small" and IgG-associated "large" hepatitis B e antigen in the serum and glomerular capillary walls of two patients with membranous glomerulonephritis. N Engl J Med 300:814, 1979.

US Public Health Service: Hepatitis B vaccine. Morbid Mortal Weekly Rep 30:423, 1981.

Villarejos VM, Visoná KA, Eduarte CA, et al: Evidence for viral hepatitis other than type A or type B among persons in Costa Rica. N Engl J Med 293:1350, 1975.

Weiss TD, Tsai CC, Baldassare AR, et al: Skin lesions in viral hepatitis: Histologic and immunofluorescent findings. Am J Med 64:269, 1978.

11.77 ENTEROVIRUSES

Enteroviruses—coxsackieviruses, echoviruses, and polioviruses—are responsible for significant and frequent human illnesses with protean clinical manifestations.

Etiology. Enteroviruses, a subgroup of picornaviruses, are small RNA viruses that retain activity for several days at room temperature and can be stored indefinitely at ordinary freezer temperatures ($-20°$ C). They are rapidly inactivated by heat ($>56°$ C), formaldehyde, chlorination, and ultraviolet light. There are several satisfactory systems for the primary recovery of enteroviruses from clinical specimens.

Epidemiology. Man is the only natural host of human enteroviruses. They are spread from person to person by fecal-oral and possibly oral-oral (respiratory) routes. Enteroviruses have been recovered from trapped flies, and probably this carriage contributes to the spread of human infections, particularly in lower socioeconomic populations having poor sanitary facilities.

Children are immunologically susceptible, and their unhygienic habits facilitate spread. Transmission occurs from child to child (via feces to skin to mouth) and then within family groups. Recovery of enteroviruses is inversely related to age, and prevalence of specific antibodies is directly related to age. The incidence of infections and the prevalence of antibodies do not differ between boys and girls, but significant disease is more common in boys.

In temperate climates viral infection peaks in August, September, and October, although some activity does occur during the winter months. No seasonal pattern is evident in the tropics. Infection and acquisition of postinfection immunity occur with greater frequency and at earlier ages among crowded, economically deprived populations.

Although there are 67 identified enteroviral types, most illness in the United States is due to about a dozen nonpolio enteroviral types. Recently, the most prevalent types have been echoviruses 4, 6, 9, 11, and 30, coxsackieviruses A9, A16, and B2 to B5, and enteroviruses 70 and 71. Studies of specimens from sewage and asymptomatic children during the present vaccine era reveal that the number of polioviral isolations (presumably vaccine strains) is greater than the number of nonpolio enterovirus isolations. This prevalence of vaccine viruses has not had an effect on the seasonal epidemiology of other enteroviruses.

Pathogenesis. Figure 11–23 shows a schematic diagram of the events of pathogenesis. Following initial acquisition of virus by the oral or respiratory route, implantation occurs in the pharynx and the lower alimentary tract. Within 1 day the infection extends to the regional lymph nodes. On about the 3rd day minor viremia occurs, involving many secondary sites. Multiplication of virus in these sites coincides with the onset of clinical symptoms. Illness can vary from minor to fatal infections. Major viremia occurs during the period of multiplication of virus in the secondary sites, usually lasting from the 3rd to the 7th day of infection. In many enteroviral infections central nervous system involvement occurs at the same time as other secondary organ involvement, but the occasional delay of central nervous system symptoms suggests that seeding occurred later in association with the major viremia or by another pathway such as autonomic nerve fibers. Cessation of viremia correlates with the appearance of serum antibody. The viral concentration in secondary sites begins to diminish on about the 7th day. However, infection continues in the lower intestinal tract for prolonged periods.

Pathology and Pathophysiology. The variation in the clinical signs of enteroviral infections reflects wide variations in pathology. Since pathologic material is generally available only from patients with fatal illnesses, accounting for only a small portion of all enteroviral infections, this discussion considers only the more severe manifestations.

Polioviruses. The *neuropathy* of poliomyelitis is due directly to virus multiplication and is usually pathognomonic. Not all affected neurons are killed. The injury may be reversible, and function may be restored within 3–4 wk after onset. There is little histologic evidence of meningeal reaction. Perivascular cuffing and some interstitial glial infiltration are present. Histologic sections generally reveal more widespread lesions of neuronal destruction than would be estimated from the clinical findings.

Neuronal lesions occur in the (1) spinal cord (anterior horn cells chiefly and to a lesser degree the intermediate and dorsal horn and dorsal root ganglia); (2) medulla (vestibular nuclei, cranial nerve nuclei, and the reticular formation, which contains the vital centers); (3) cerebellum (nuclei in the roof and vermis only); (4) midbrain (chiefly the gray matter, but also the substantia nigra and occasionally the red nucleus); (5) thalamus and hypothalamus; (6) pallidum; and (7) cerebral cortex (motor cortex). The following areas are spared: (1) the entire cerebral cortex *except* the motor area; (2) the cerebellum except the vermis and deep midline nuclei; and (3) the white matter of the spinal cord.

Extraneural pathology is usually a secondary phenomenon. Bronchopulmonary changes may occur, e.g., aspiration pneumonia, atelectasis, and purulent bronchitis, owing to impairment of cough and decreased thoracic movements. Respiratory failure results in respiratory acidosis and anoxic changes. The cardiovascular changes may result in hypertension, car-

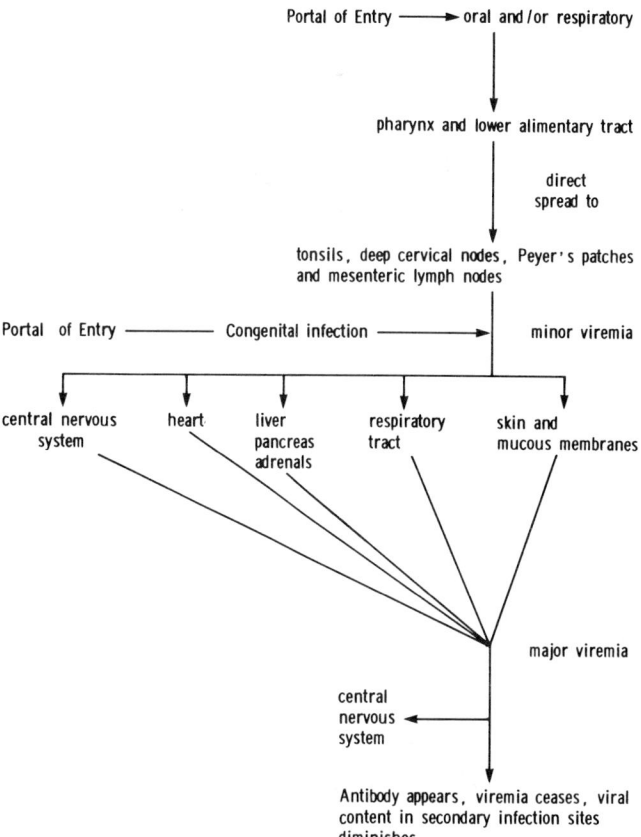

Figure 11–23. The pathogenesis of enteroviral infections. (Modified from Cherry JD, *In*: Remington JS, Klein JO (eds): Infectious Diseases of the Fetus and Newborn Infant. 2nd ed. Philadelphia, WB Saunders, 1983.)

diac failure, and pulmonary edema. Ulcerations in the alimentary tract may result in serious bleeding and occasional perforation. Prolonged immobilization leads to negative nitrogen and calcium balances, with urinary lithiasis, renal failure, hypertension with encephalopathy, and convulsions. Treatment itself may cause untoward complications, such as urinary tract infection (following catheterization), decubitus ulcers, and psychotic disturbances.

Coxsackieviruses A. Records of severe illnesses associated with coxsackieviruses A are rare, and no distinctive pathology has been described.

Coxsackieviruses B. The most common findings have been myocarditis and meningoencephalitis. Involvement of the adrenals, pancreas, liver, and lungs has also been noted. The *heart* is usually enlarged, with dilatation of the chambers or flabby musculature. The pericardium frequently contains some inflammatory cells; thickening, and edema, and focal infiltrations of inflammatory cells may be found in the endocardium. The myocardium is congested and contains infiltrations of a wide range of inflammatory cells. The involvement of the myocardium is often patchy and focal but occasionally diffuse. The muscle shows loss of striation as well as edema and eosinophilic degeneration. Frequently, muscle necrosis without extensive cellular infiltration is present. Lesions in *the brain and spinal cord* are focal rather than diffuse but frequently involve many different areas. The lesions consist of areas of eosinophilic degeneration of cortical cells, clusters of mononuclear and glial cells, and perivascular cuffing. The meninges are congested, edematous, and occasionally mildly infiltrated with inflammatory cells.

There are frequently areas of mild focal *pneumonitis* with peribronchiolar cellular infiltrations. The *liver* is often engorged and occasionally contains isolated foci of necrosis and mononuclear cellular infiltrations. In the *pancreas* occasional focal degeneration of the islet cells occurs. Mild to severe cortical necrosis and inflammatory cell infiltrates may be found in the *adrenals*.

Echoviruses. Hepatic necrosis has been observed in infections with echoviruses 6, 9, 11, 14, and 19. Other rare findings include adrenal and renal hemorrhage and interstitial pneumonitis.

Clinical Manifestations. *Poliovirus Infections.* When a susceptible person has been infected with poliovirus, one of the following responses may occur in this order of frequency: (1) asymptomatic infection occurs in 90–95% of those infected, (2) abortive poliomyelitis, (3) nonparalytic poliomyelitis, (4) paralytic poliomyelitis. A mild response may blend into a more severe form and result in a biphasic course ushered in by a minor febrile illness, then a symptom-free interlude of a few days succeeded by symptoms and signs referable to the nervous system.

ABORTIVE POLIOMYELITIS. A brief febrile illness occurs with one or more of the following symptoms: malaise, anorexia, nausea, vomiting, headache, sore throat, constipation, and unlocalized abdominal pain. Coryza, cough, pharyngeal exudate, diarrhea, and localized abdominal tenderness and rigidity are uncommon. The fever seldom exceeds 39.5° C (103° F), and the pharynx shows little despite the frequent complaint of sore throat.

NONPARALYTIC POLIOMYELITIS. The symptoms are those enumerated for abortive poliomyelitis, except that headache, nausea, and vomiting are more intense, and there is soreness and stiffness of the posterior muscles of the neck, trunk, and limbs. Fleeting paralysis of the bladder is not uncommon, and constipation is frequent. Approximately two thirds of the children have a short symptom-free interlude between the 1st phase (minor illness) and the 2nd phase (central nervous system or major illness). This 2-phase course is less common in adults, in whom the evolution of symptoms is more insidious. Nuchal and spinal rigidity should occur as a basis for the diagnosis of nonparalytic poliomyelitis during the 2nd phase.

Physical examination reveals *nuchal-spinal signs* and changes in superficial and deep reflexes. With cooperative patients the nuchal-spinal signs are first sought by active tests. The child is asked to sit up unassisted. If this causes undue effort, if the knees flex upward and the patient writhes a bit from side to side in sitting up and uses hands on the bed for the tripod supporting position, there is unmistakable spinal rigidity (Fig. 11–24). Still sitting, the patient is asked to flex chin to chest and is observed for nuchal rigidity. Alternatively, from the supine position, with knees held down gently, the patient is asked to sit up and kiss his or her knees (Fig. 11–25). If the knees draw up sharply or if the maneuver cannot be adequately completed, there is stiffness of the spine due to muscle spasm. If the diagnosis is still uncertain, attempts should be made to elicit Kernig and Brudzinski signs. Gentle forward flexion of the occiput and neck will elicit nuchal rigidity, which may precede spinal rigidity. *Head drop* may be demonstrated by placing the hands under the patient's shoulders and raising the trunk (Fig. 11–26). Normally the head follows the plane of the trunk, but in poliomyelitis it often falls backward limply. The head-drop sign is not due to true paresis of the neck flexors. In struggling infants it may be difficult to distinguish voluntary resistance from clinically important involuntary nuchal rigidity. One may place the infant's shoulders flush with the edge of the table, support the weight of the occiput in the hand, and then flex the head anteriorly (Fig. 11–27). Nuchal rigidity that persists during this maneuver may be interpreted as involuntary. When not closed, the anterior fontanel may be tense or bulging as in meningitis.

In the early stages the *reflexes* are normally active and remain so unless paralysis supervenes. Changes in reflexes, either increase or depression, may precede weakness by 12–24 hr; hence, it is important to detect them, especially in nonparalytic patients managed at home. The superficial reflexes, i.e., cremasteric and abdominal and the reflexes of the

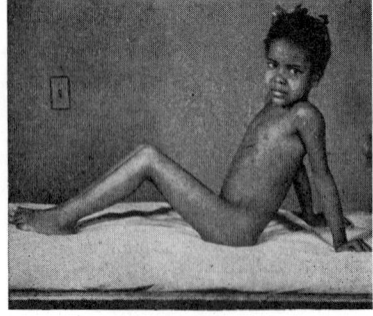

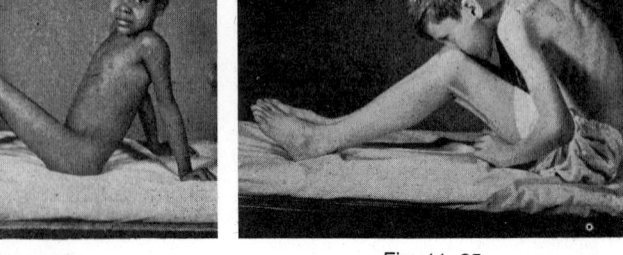

Fig. 11–24   Fig. 11–25

Figure 11–24. Tripod sign: characteristic position associated with stiffness of the spine. (From Steigman AJ: Pediatr Clin North Am, Vol 1, No 1A.)

Figure 11–25. Kiss-the-knee test: ability to complete the maneuver only by flexing the knee. Note tense appearance of the hamstrings. (From Steigman AJ: Pediatr Clin North Am, Vol 1, No 1A.)

Figure 11–26. Head-drop sign: the head fails to continue in the plane of the body when the shoulders are elevated. This child had nonparalytic poliomyelitis. Tripod and head-drop signs appear in nonparalytic and paralytic poliomyelitis. (From Steigman AJ: Pediatr Clin North Am, Vol 1, No 1A.)

Figure 11–27. Testing nuchal rigidity in uncooperative, struggling infant: Place the shoulders at the edge of the table, supporting the occiput manually. Flex anteriorly. Only true involuntary rigidity persists. (From Steigman AJ: Pediatr Clin North Am, Vol 1, No 1A.)

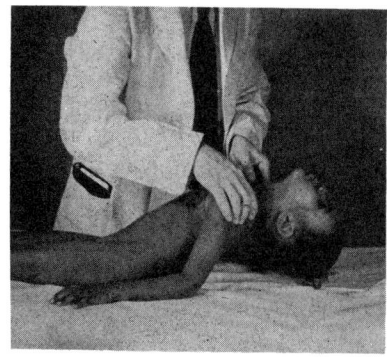
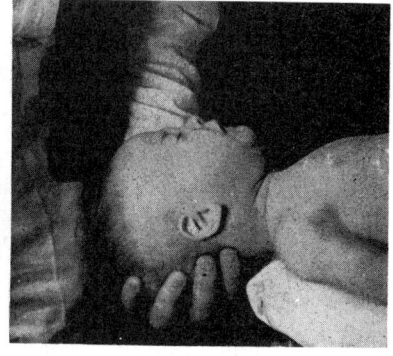

Fig. 11–26   Fig. 11–27

spinal and gluteal muscles, are usually the first to be diminished. The spinal and gluteal reflexes may disappear before the abdominal and cremasteric ones. Changes in the deep tendon reflexes generally occur 8–24 hr after depression of superficial reflexes and indicate impending paresis of the extremities. There is absence of tendon reflexes with paralysis. Sensory defects do not occur in poliomyelitis.

PARALYTIC POLIOMYELITIS. The manifestations are those enumerated for nonparalytic poliomyelitis plus weakness of one or more muscle groups, either skeletal or cranial. These symptoms may be followed by a symptom-free interlude of several days and then a recurrence culminating in paralysis. Bladder paralysis of 1–3 days' duration occurs in approximately 20% of patients, and bowel atony is common, occasionally to the point of paralytic ileus. In some patients muscular paralysis may be the initial presentation.

Flaccid paralysis is the most obvious clinical expression of the neuronal injury. The ensuing muscular atrophy is due to denervation plus the atrophy of disuse. The pain, spasticity, nuchal and spinal rigidity, and hypertonia early in the illness are probably due to lesions of the brain stem, spinal ganglia, and posterior columns. Respiratory and cardiac arrhythmias, blood pressure and vasomotor changes, and the like are reflections of damage to vital centers in the medulla.

On physical examination the distribution of paralysis is characteristically spotty. To detect mild muscular weakness, it is often necessary to apply gentle resistance in opposition to the muscle group being tested. In the *spinal form* there is weakness of some of the muscles of the neck, abdomen, trunk, diaphragm, thorax, or extremities. In the *bulbar form* there is weakness in the motor distribution of one or more cranial nerves with or without dysfunction of the vital centers of respiration and circulation. Components of both the preceding forms occur together in *bulbospinal poliomyelitis.* In the *encephalitic form* irritability, disorientation, drowsiness, and coarse tremors not explained by inadequate ventilation are noted; peripheral or cranial nerve paralysis coexists or ensues. Hypoxia and hypercapnia due to inadequate ventilation from respiratory insufficiency may produce disorientation without true encephalitis.

A number of components acting together may produce insufficiency of ventilation (Table 11–30), resulting in hypoxia and hypercapnia, which may produce profound effects on many other systems. Since respiratory insufficiency may develop rapidly, continued clinical evaluation is essential. Despite weakness of the respiratory muscles, the patient may respond with so much respiratory effort (associated with anxiety and fear) that overventilation may occur at the outset, resulting in respiratory alkalosis. Such effort is fatiguing and soon leads to respiratory failure.

Certain characteristic patterns of disease occur:

1. *Pure spinal poliomyelitis with respiratory insufficiency* involves tightness, weakness, or paralysis of respiratory muscles (chiefly the diaphragm and intercostals) without discernible clinical involvement of cranial nerves or vital centers. The cervical and thoracic spinal cord segments are chiefly affected.

2. *Pure bulbar poliomyelitis* involves paralysis of motor cranial nerve nuclei with or without involvement of the vital centers that control respiration, circulation, and body temperature. Involvement of the 9th, 10th, and 12th cranial nerves results in paralysis of the pharynx, tongue, and larynx with consequent airway obstruction.

3. *Bulbospinal poliomyelitis with respiratory insufficiency* affects the respiratory muscles with coexisting bulbar paralysis.

The clinical findings resulting from *involvement of the respiratory muscles* are (1) anxious expression; (2) inability to speak without frequent pauses, resulting in short, jerky, "breathless" sentences; (3) increased respiratory rate; (4) movement of the alae nasi and of the accessory muscles of respiration; (5) inability to cough or sniff with full depth; (6) paradoxical abdominal movements due to diaphragmatic immobility from spasm or weakness of one or both leaves; (7) relative immobility of the intercostal spaces, which may be segmental, unilateral, or bilateral. When the arms are weak, and especially when deltoid paralysis occurs, there may be impending respiratory paralysis since the phrenic nerve nuclei are in adjacent areas of the spinal cord. Observing the patient's capacity for thoracic breathing while the abdominal muscles are splinted manually will indicate minor degrees of paresis. Light manual splinting of the thoracic cage will help to assess the effectiveness of diaphragmatic movement.

The clinical findings of *bulbar poliomyelitis* with respiratory difficulty (other than paralysis of extraocular, facial, and

Table 11–30. Common Causes of Hypoxia and Hypercapnia in Poliomyelitis

1. Cranial nerves IX to XII involved, with
   a. Pharyngeal paralysis and pooling of secretions
   b. Laryngeal involvement—either spasm of laryngeal muscles or paralysis of vocal cords
   c. Lingual paralysis
   d. Tracheal accumulation of secretions due to inability to cough
   e. Aspiration of vomitus
2. Vital center involvement with
   a. Inefficient, irregular respiration
   b. Cardiovascular disturbance
   c. Hyperpyrexia causing increased oxygen consumption
3. Cervical and spinal cord involvement causing paresis of the primary and accessory muscles of respiration
4. Pulmonary complications, viz., pneumonia, atelectasis, edema
5. Contributory factors
   a. Panic
   b. Gastric dilatation
   c. Sedation
   d. Inadequate equipment, e.g., small-bore tracheostomy tubes, unsuitable respirator settings, and the like

masticatory muscles) include (1) nasal twang to the voice or cry due to palatal and pharyngeal weakness (hard-consonant words such as "cookie" or "candy" bring this out best); (2) inability to swallow smoothly, resulting in accumulation of saliva in the pharynx and indicating partial immobility (holding the larynx lightly and asking the patient to swallow will confirm immobility); (3) accumulated pharyngeal secretions, which may cause irregular respiration since each inspiration must be "planned" to avoid aspirating; the respirations may thus appear interrupted and abnormal even to the point of falsely simulating intercostal or diaphragmatic weakness; (4) the impossibility of effective coughing, with constant fatiguing efforts to clear the throat; (5) nasal regurgitation of saliva and fluids due to palatal paralysis, with inability to separate the oropharynx from the nasopharynx during swallowing; (6) deviation of the palate, uvula, or tongue; (7) involvement of vital brain stem centers, manifested by irregularity in rate, depth, and rhythm of respiration; by cardiovascular alterations which include blood pressure changes (especially increased), alternate flushing and mottling of the skin, and cardiac arrhythmias; and by rapid changes in body temperature; (8) paralysis of one or both vocal cords causing hoarseness, aphonia, and ultimately asphyxia unless recognized by laryngoscopy and managed by immediate tracheostomy; (9) the "rope sign," an acute angulation between the chin and larynx due to weakness of the hyoid muscles (the hyoid bone is pulled posteriorly, narrowing the hypopharyngeal inlet).

Nonpolio Enterovirus Infections (Table 11–31). Coxsackieviral and echoviral infections are exceedingly common, and their spectrum of disease is protean. Because many of the clinical-virologic associations are based upon a limited number of cases and because enteroviruses are frequently carried asymptomatically in the gastrointestinal tract for relatively long periods of time, some of the observed illnesses and coincidentally recovered viruses may not have a cause and effect relationship. However, repeated observations have confirmed many virus-illness associations, even though their occurrence has been sporadic.

ASYMPTOMATIC INFECTION. Coxsackieviruses and echoviruses can frequently be recovered from the stools of well children, but there are few data on the rate of asymptomatic infection with nonpolio enteroviruses. The isolation of enteroviruses from the stool cannot be equated with asymptomatic infection because illness, if it occurs, happens shortly after virus acquisition and is of short duration; a particular infection may have been associated with nonspecific illness 1–3 mo prior to collection of a stool specimen. In general, the more carefully clinical symptomatology is sought, the lower is the percentage of truly asymptomatic infections. Clinical expression is also inversely related to age and varies by viral type. Overall, probably fewer than 50% of all infections are asymptomatic.

NONSPECIFIC FEBRILE ILLNESS. This is the most common manifestation of coxsackieviral and echoviral infections. All viral types cause this clinical presentation, but the frequency varies considerably among the individual viruses. The onset of illness is usually abrupt and without prodrome. In young children the initial finding is fever and associated malaise. In older children headache and myalgia are usually also noted. The temperature ranges from 38.5 to 40° C (101–104° F) and has a mean duration of 3 days. In some instances the fever is biphasic; it occurs for 1 day, is absent for 2–3 days, and then recurs for an additional 2–4 days. In many young children the only manifestation of illness is fever, and its presence is discovered quite by chance by a parent. Malaise and anorexia are often related to the degree of temperature elevation, as is headache in older patients. The complaint of a sore or scratchy feeling in the throat is common, but an inflamed pharynx is

not seen. Nausea and vomiting occasionally occur at the onset of illness as does mild abdominal discomfort. A few mildly loose stools may be noted. Generalized myalgia is also noted. Findings on physical examination are generally benign. There may be minimal conjunctivitis, injection of the pharynx, and cervical lymphadenitis. The duration of illness varies from 24 hr to 6 days with an average of 3–4 days. The white blood cell count is normal.

RESPIRATORY MANIFESTATIONS (Table 11–31). Coxsackievirus A21 has produced epidemics of mild respiratory illness (*common cold*) in military populations, but epidemic disease has not been observed in children.

Pharyngitis, tonsillitis, tonsillopharyngitis, and *nasopharyngitis* are common clinical manifestations of coxsackieviral and echoviral infections; probably all enteroviruses on occasion cause mild pharyngitis. Pharyngitis is frequently associated with other clinical findings such as meningitis, pleurodynia, or exanthem. Although evidence of pharyngeal involvement may be present at the time of disease onset, the initial complaint is most often fever. Sore throat, coryza, and vomiting and/or diarrhea may also be noted. Examination of the tonsils and pharynx reveals varying degrees of erythema; in some, patches of exudate will be seen. The usual duration of uncomplicated pharyngitis is 3–6 days. The total white blood cell count may be normal or slightly elevated with a normal differential count.

Herpangina is usually characterized by the sudden onset of fever, although the initial temperature can be quite variable with a range from normal to 41° C (106° F). In general, the temperature tends to be higher in younger patients. Older children frequently complain of headache and backache. Vomiting occurs in about 25% of children under the age of 5 yr. In the majority of children the oropharyngeal lesions are present on the first examination at the time or shortly after fever is observed (Fig. 11–28 [p. xxvi]). The characteristic early lesions are small, 1–2 mm vesicles and ulcers. They start as papules, become vesicular, and then ulcerate in a short but variable time period. They are usually discrete with an average of 5 per patient; some patients have only 1 or 2 lesions; in others 14 or more may be noted. When seen early, the vesicular lesions enlarge over a 2–3 day period to 3–4 mm in size. Each vesicular and ulcerative lesion is surrounded by an erythematous ring which varies in size up to 10 mm in diameter. The major site of the lesions is the anterior tonsillar pillars. They also occur on the soft palate, uvula, tonsils, pharyngeal wall, and occasionally the posterior buccal surfaces. Aside from these lesions, the remainder of the throat appears either normal or minimally erythematous. Although occasionally noted in association with aseptic meningitis or other more severe enteroviral illness, most cases of herpangina are mild and without complication. The usual duration of signs and symptoms is 3–6 days.

Pleurodynia (Bornholm disease) is an epidemic disease, but sporadic cases do occur. Following an incubation period of about 4 days, there is sudden onset of fever and pain. The typical pain is located in the chest or upper abdomen, is muscular in origin, and is of variable intensity. Occasionally, the pain occurs in other areas of the body. It is often excruciatingly severe and sudden and associated with profuse sweating. The patient may appear pale and shock-like. The pain is spasmodic, with durations varying from a few minutes to several hours. Most commonly, the spasmodic periods last about 15–30 min. During spasms, the respirations are usually rapid, shallow, and grunting, suggesting pneumonia of pleural inflammation. Pleural friction rubs may be noted on auscultation, and they may appear and disappear with the coming and going of the pain episodes. Coughing, sneezing, or deep breathing makes the pain worse. In older children and adults the pain is described as stabbing or knife-like.

Table 11–31. Clinical Manifestations of Nonpolio Enteroviruses

Clinical Categories	Virus Types		
	Coxsackieviruses A	Coxsackieviruses B	Echoviruses and Enteroviruses
Nonspecific febrile illness	All types	All types	All types
Respiratory			
Common cold	Mainly 21, 24; rarely other types	Mainly 1–5; rarely 6	Mainly 2, 20; rarely other types
Pharyngitis (pharyngitis, tonsillitis, tonsillopharyngitis, and nasopharyngitis)	Probably all types; mainly 9	Probably all types; mainly 1–5	Probably all types; mainly 2, 4, 6, 9, 11, 16, 19, 25, 30
Herpangina	1–10, 16, 22	1–5	6, 9, 16, 17, 25
Lymphonodular pharyngitis	10		
Stomatitis and other lesions in the anterior mouth	5, 9, 10, 16	2, 5	9, 11, 20, 71
Parotitis	Coxsackievirus A not typed	3, 4	70
Croup	9	4, 5	4, 11, 21
Bronchitis		1, 4	8, 12–14
Bronchiolitis and asthmatic bronchitis	Many types	Many types	Many types
Pneumonia	9, 16	1–5	6, 7, 9, 11, 12, 19, 20, 30
Pleurodynia	1, 2, 4, 6, 9, 16	1, 2, 3, 5, 6	1–3, 6–9, 11, 12, 14, 16, 17, 18, 19, 23, 24
Gastrointestinal			
Nausea and vomiting	9, 16	2–5	2, 4, 6, 9, 11, 16, 19, 20, 22, 30
Diarrhea	2, 4, 6, 7, 9, 10, 14, 16	1–5	3, 4, 6, 7, 9, 11–14, 16–22, 25, 30, 71
Constipation	9	3–5	4, 6, 9, 11
Abdominal pain	9, 16	2–5	4, 6, 9, 11, 19, 30
Pseudoappendicitis			1, 8, 14
Peritonitis		1	
Mesenteric adenitis		5	7, 9, 11
Appendicitis		2, 5	
Intussusception		3	7, 9
Hepatitis	4, 9, 10, 20, 24	1–5	1, 3, 4, 6, 7, 9, 11, 14, 20, 21, 30
Reye syndrome	2	4	14, 22
Pancreatitis	9	3–5	
Diabetes mellitus		1, 2, 4, 5	
Acute hemorrhagic conjunctivitis	24		70
Pericarditis and myocarditis	1, 2, 4, 5, 7–10, 16	1–5	1, 4, 6–9, 11, 14, 17, 19, 22, 25, 30
Genitourinary			
Orchitis and epididymitis		1–5	6, 9, 11
Nephritis		4	6, 9
Hemolytic-uremic syndrome	4, 9	2–5	22
Pyuria, hematuria, or proteinuria		5	1, 6, 9
Myositis and arthritis	2, 9	4	9, 18, 24
Exanthem	2, 4, 5, 7, 9, 10, 16	1–5	1–7, 9, 11, 13, 14, 16–19, 22, 25, 30, 32, 33, 71
Neurologic manifestations			
Aseptic meningitis	1–14, 16–18, 21, 22, 24	1–6	1–9, 11–27, 29–33, 71
Encephalitis	2, 4–7, 9, 10, 16	1–5	1–9, 11–25, 27, 30, 33, 71
Paralysis (lower motor neuron involvement)	2, 4–7, 9–11, 14, 21	1–6	1–4, 6–9, 11, 12, 14, 16–19, 25, 27, 30, 31, 70, 71
Guillain-Barré syndrome and transverse myelitis	2, 4–6, 9, 16	1–4	6, 7, 19, 22, 70
Cerebellar ataxia	4, 7, 9	3, 4	6, 9, 16
Peripheral neuritis			9

When pain is localized to the abdomen, it is frequently crampy and suggests colic in the younger child. The child may double over and refuse to walk or move. Occasionally, the abdominal pain in association with a pale, sweaty, shock-like appearance suggests acute intestinal obstruction. Splinting and guarding of the abdomen also suggests appendicitis and peritonitis. Tenderness to some degree is present in areas of pain, but frank myositis with muscle swelling is not observed. Fever and pain usually last 1–2 days. Frequently, however, the illness is biphasic; after the initial febrile period the patient is asymptomatic for several days; then pain and fever recur. Rarely patients will have several recurrent episodes over a period of a few weeks. In these cases fever is less prominent during the recurrences.

In epidemics both children and adults are afflicted, with the majority of cases occurring in persons under 30 yr of age. Most children have other signs of enteroviral infection such as anorexia, nausea, vomiting, headache, and sore throat. Routine laboratory study is not very helpful. The white blood cell count is variable, but an increased percentage of polymorphonuclear neutrophils and band forms is frequent. The erythrocyte sedimentation rate is also inconsistent, with normal to extremely high values observed. The chest roentgenogram is most often normal.

Complications in pleurodynia are uncommon. Aseptic meningitis has been noted, and adult males have experienced orchitis. Myocarditis and pericarditis may also complicate pleurodynia.

The major etiologic agents in epidemic pleurodynia are coxsackieviruses B3 and B5; other associated viruses include coxsackieviruses B1 and B2 and echoviruses 1 and 6. Agents associated with sporadic occurrences are listed in Table 11–31.

A variety of nonpolio enteroviruses have been associated with sporadic instances of *parotitis, croup, bronchitis, bronchiolitis, asthmatic bronchitis,* and *pneumonia* as well as outbreaks of *lymphonodular pharyngitis, stomatitis,* and other lesions in the anterior mouth (Table 11–31). *Acute lymphonodular pharyngitis* is a unique enanthem associated with coxsackievirus A10 infection. The lesions have the typical distribution of herpangina; they are papular, discrete, 3 mm in diameter, and surrounded by a zone of erythema. They are whitish to yellowish and persist for 6–10 days.

GASTROINTESTINAL MANIFESTATIONS (Table 11–31). Gastrointestinal manifestations are common (7–30%) in enteroviral infections. *Vomiting* is a common manifestation of infections with many coxsackieviral and echoviral types, but it is rarely the major complaint of the patient or the parent. Except for the hand, foot, and mouth syndrome (coxsackievirus A16), in which vomiting is uncommon, this manifestation occurs in about 50% of all cases in epidemic enteroviral disease. Vomiting is most common in meningitis and least common in pleurodynia and uncomplicated exanthematous disease.

Diarrhea occurs commonly in coxsackieviral and echoviral infections as one of many manifestations of the systemic illness. It is rarely severe. In most instances loose stools occur for a 2–4 day period. The stools are rarely watery and never bloody and number at most 6–8/day.

Abdominal pain is also a common complaint in many enteroviral infections. About 10% of patients with coxsackievirus A16 (hand, foot, and mouth syndrome) complain of abdominal pain. Coxsackievirus and echovirus meningitis is associated with abdominal pain in about 25% of the cases. The severity of pain in enteroviral infections is quite variable and on occasion may suggest a surgical abdomen. The pain is most often periumbilical; it may be either constant or colicky. The associated fever is most often greater than 38.3° C (101° F).

Nonpolio enteroviruses have been associated with a variety of other gastrointestinal and abdominal complaints (Table 11–31). In most situations the findings are just one manifestation of a more typical enteroviral illness. The possible relationship with juvenile diabetes is based on observations of higher titers of serum antibody to coxsackievirus B4 within 3 mo of onset of disease than in controls, the recovery of coxsackievirus B4 from the pancreas of a previously healthy 10 yr old boy who died following diabetic coma, and serologic evidence of coxsackievirus B infections in patients at the time of onset of diabetes mellitus.

ACUTE HEMORRHAGIC CONJUNCTIVITIS. Conjunctivitis may be the dominant complaint. In the majority of epidemics, enterovirus 70 has been the etiologic agent. Acute hemorrhagic conjunctivitis has a sudden onset that is accompanied by severe eye pain and associated photophobia, blurred vision, lacrimation, erythema and congestion of the eye, and edematous and chemotic lids. There are subconjunctival hemorrhages of varying size and frequently a transient punctate epithelial keratitis, conjunctival follicles, and preauricular lymphadenopathy. Eye discharge is initially serous but becomes mucopurulent with secondary bacterial infection. Systemic symptoms (including fever) are rare. Occasionally, a picture suggestive of pharyngoconjunctival fever has occurred. A small number of patients have had a polyradiculomyeloneuropathy or paralytic poliomyelitis following enterovirus 70 acute hemorrhagic conjunctivitis. Persons 20–50 yr of age have the highest attack rates, and children are less often involved. Initially most epidemics occurred in coastal areas of tropical countries toward the end of hot rainy periods. More recently, outbreaks of disease have occurred in temperate climates, including many areas of the United States. Epidemics are explosive and are spread mainly by the eye-hand-fomite-eye route.

PERICARDITIS AND MYOCARDITIS. These manifestations have been noted in association with 27 different nonpolio enteroviruses (Table 11–31). The group B coxsackieviruses have been most frequently implicated, and B5 has been the most common causative agent. Of the echoviruses, type 6 has been most frequently associated with cardiac involvement. Hepatitis, pneumonia, nephritis, meningitis, and orchitis have also been occasional associated findings with coxsackievirus B. The mortality resulting from acute coxsackieviral and echoviral heart disease is significant. In nonfatal cases recovery is usually complete without residual disability; occasionally, constrictive pericarditis occurs as well as other sequelae.

GENITOURINARY MANIFESTATIONS (Table 11–31). Group B coxsackieviruses are second only to mumps as causative agents of *orchitis;* B5 is the most commonly associated virus, but B2 and B4 have also been implicated on many occasions. In almost all instances the orchitis is a secondary event, most commonly associated with pleurodynia. The illness is frequently biphasic; fever and pleurodynia or meningitis are followed by apparent recovery and then by orchitis about 2 wk after onset. Many patients also have *epididymitis.* In epidemics of disease due to group B coxsackieviruses, the occurrence of testicular involvement is quite variable. Generally orchitis is infrequent, but in one B2 outbreak 17% of the postpubertal males had orchitis and 7% also had epididymitis. Other genitourinary manifestations of nonpolio enteroviral infections include acute glomerulonephritis; mesangiolytic glomerulonephritis in an infant with immune deficiency; hemolytic-uremic syndrome; acute renal failure; pyuria, hematuria, or proteinuria; hemorrhagic cystitis; and vaginal ulcerative lesions.

MYOSITIS AND ARTHRITIS (Table 11–31). Myalgia is a common complaint accompanying many coxsackieviruses and echovirus illnesses. However, there is almost no direct evidence (demonstration of virus in muscle) or indirect evidence (muscle enzyme elevations) of muscle involvement in routine enteroviral illnesses. Coxsackievirus A2 has been associated with myositis, and coxsackievirus A9 and echovirus 18 have been associated with polymyositis. A dermatomyositis-like syndrome has been associated with immune deficiency and enteroviral infection. Arthritis has occurred rarely in enterovirus infection.

SKIN MANIFESTATIONS (Table 11–31). Nonpolio enteroviruses are a common cause of a large variety of skin manifestations. In the summer and fall they are the leading cause of exanthems. There is a marked variation in the rates at which exanthems occur among the various viral types and also among different age groups of the host. In general, the frequency is inversely related to the age of the infected patient, and several different agents can produce similar skin manifestations.

Coxsackievirus A16 is the major cause of the *hand, foot, and mouth syndrome*, which has a typically enteroviral pattern, with a short incubation period (4–6 days) and a summer and fall seasonal pattern. The clinical expression rate of the enanthem-exanthem complex is high, being close to 100% in young children, 38% in school children, and 11% in adults. The intraoral lesions are ulcerative and average about 4–8 mm in size. The tongue and buccal mucosa are most frequently involved. The hands are more commonly involved than the feet. Buttock lesions are also common, but these do not usually progress to vesiculation. The lesions on the hands and feet are usually vesicular and vary in size from 3 to 7 mm; they are generally more common on the dorsal surfaces but frequently occur on the palms and soles as well. They clear by absorption of the fluid in about 1 wk. Coxsackievirus A16 is frequently associated with subacute, chronic, and recurring skin lesions. Recently, enterovirus 71 has been the etiologic agent in several outbreaks of hand, foot, and mouth syndrome. Illness with this virus is frequently more severe than with coxsackievirus A16; aseptic meningitis, encephalitis, and paralytic disease are common.

Echovirus type 9 is the most prevalent nonpolio enterovirus, and *exanthem* is a common clinical manifestation. Nonspecific febrile illness and aseptic meningitis are the usual major manifestations of echovirus 9 infection. Exanthem occurs in about one third of the cases; 57% of children under 5 yr of age have rash, whereas only 6% of those over 10 yr of age have similar cutaneous findings. The rash is most frequently rubelliform, but in addition or as the sole manifestation, petechiae frequently occur. Rash and fever usually appear at about the same time, and frequently the illness closely mimics meningococcemia. The rash usually lasts 3–5 days.

NEUROLOGIC MANIFESTATIONS (Table 11–31). *Aseptic meningitis* due to enteroviruses occurs in epidemics and as isolated cases (Sec. 11.9). Epidemics have been most common with coxsackievirus B5 and echoviruses 4, 6, 9, and 11. In general, illness is more common in children than in adults. Virtually all patients have fever and pharyngitis; other respiratory manifestations are also common. Rash is common but varies with the specific viral agents; 30–50% of all patients with echovirus 9 meningitis will have exanthem. Except for the occurrence of rash, herpangina, pleurodynia, or myocarditis, there is little clinically that helps in identifying the etiology in a sporadic case of aseptic meningitis.

In addition to the clinical manifestations discussed in Sec. 11.9, there is commonly an erythematous, maculopapular, discrete rash. Frequently, particularly with echovirus 9 infection, the rash is petechial, thus suggesting meningococcemia. Pharyngitis is common. Generalized muscle stiffness or spasm is usually observed, although the degree varies considerably; Kernig and Brudzinski signs are positive in fewer than half the cases. Deep tendon reflexes are usually normal.

Cerebrospinal fluid examination reveals considerable variations among cases and in the same patient with repeated examination. Cerebrospinal fluid leukocyte counts vary from a few cells to a few thousand/mm³; the median is in the 100–150 cells/mm³ range. The percentage of neutrophils also varies

greatly. Initial examinations frequently reveal a predominance of neutrophils but rarely over 90% as seen in bacterial disease. Repeated cerebrospinal fluid examinations will demonstrate an increasing percentage of mononuclear cells. The cerebrospinal fluid protein is usually mildly elevated, and the glucose concentration is most often normal; rarely, hypoglycorrhachia occurs. Other routine laboratory studies are usually not diagnostically helpful.

The duration of illness is variable. In the majority of instances the temperature returns to normal within 4–6 days and disability due to neurologic involvement lasts 1–2 wk. Occasionally, a biphasic illness pattern occurs consisting of an initial period with fever, headache, nausea, vomiting, and muscle aches and pains of a few days' duration followed by general recovery; then the same symptoms return with more pronounced neurologic involvement.

About 2% of the reported cases of *encephalitis* (Sec. 11.10) in the United States are demonstrated to have an enteroviral etiology. This is probably an underestimate of the number of severe cases, which may total over 1000/yr. Echovirus type 9 is the most common cause of enteroviral encephalitis; other commonly associated enteroviral types are echoviruses 3, 4, 6, and 11 and coxsackieviruses B2, B4, and B5. In general the prognosis in encephalitis due to enteroviral infections is good, but fatalities have occurred in association with coxsackieviruses B3 and B6, echoviruses 2, 9, 17, and 25, and enterovirus 71.

Paralysis on the basis of anterior horn cell disease occasionally results from infection with nonpolio enteroviruses. Many coxsackieviruses and echoviruses have been associated with the *Guillain-Barré syndrome*. *Cerebellar ataxia* has been noted in association with coxsackieviruses A4, A7, A9, B3, and B4 and echoviruses 6, 9, and 16. *Peripheral neuritis* has been reported with echovirus 9 infection, and coxsackievirus A9 has been noted in association with a *focal encephalitis and acute hemiplegia*.

NEONATAL INFECTIONS. Nonpolio enteroviral infections in neonatal infants result in a wide variety of clinical manifestations ranging from asymptomatic infection to fatal encephalitis and myocarditis (Sec. 8.72).

Mild, nonspecific febrile illness may occur anytime during the 1st mo of life, most commonly in full-term infants following uneventful pregnancies and deliveries without complications. When the onset occurs after 7 days of age, a careful history frequently reveals a trivial illness in a family member. The onset of illness is characterized by mild irritability and fever. The temperature is usually in the 38–39° C (100.4–102.2° F) range, but occasionally it is higher. Poor feeding is frequently observed. One or two episodes of vomiting and/or diarrhea may occur in some babies. Bacterial disease must be strongly considered. The usual duration of illness is 2–4 days. Routine laboratory study is not helpful, but cerebrospinal fluid examination may reveal an increased protein concentration and leukocyte count indicative of aseptic meningitis.

The major diagnostic problem in neonatal enteroviral infections is the differentiation between bacterial and viral disease, both of which produce a *sepsis-like* illness characterized by fever, poor feeding, abdominal distention, irritability, rash, lethargy, and hypotonia. Other findings include diarrhea, vomiting, seizures, shock, hepatomegaly, jaundice, and apnea. The onset is marked by irritability, poor feeding, and fever followed within 24 hr by other manifestations. The duration of fever varies from 1 to 8 days but is usually 3–4 days. The total white blood cell count, number of neutrophils, and number of band form neutrophils are elevated in the majority of instances. The majority of mothers have evidence of a recent, febrile, virus-like illness. In addition, other factors often associated with bacterial sepsis, such as prolonged rupture of membranes, prematurity, and low Apgar scores, are unusual in enteroviral infections.

Most cases of *neonatal myocarditis* are due to coxsackievirus

B infections, and nursery outbreaks have occurred on several occasions. The illness is most commonly abrupt in onset, with listlessness, anorexia, and fever. A biphasic pattern is noted in about a third of the patients. Progression is rapid, and signs of circulatory failure appear in a 2 day period. If death does not occur, recovery is occasionally rapid but usually gradual over an extended period. Most patients have tachycardia, cardiomegaly, electrocardiographic changes, and transitory systolic murmurs; many show signs of respiratory distress and cyanosis. About one third of the infants will have signs suggesting neurologic involvement.

The initial clinical findings in *neonatal meningitis* or *meningoencephalitis* are similar to those in nonspecific febrile illness or sepsis-like illness. Most often the child is normal and then is noted to be febrile, anorectic, and lethargic. Jaundice is frequently noted in newborns, and vomiting occurs in neonates of all ages. Less common findings include apnea, tremulousness, and general increased tonicity. Seizures occasionally occur. Cerebrospinal fluid examination reveals considerable variation in protein, glucose, and cellular values. Findings are frequently similar to those observed in bacterial disease. Hypoglycorrhachia is noted in about 10% of newborns with enteroviral meningitis.

Hepatitis and rashes are occasionally associated with neonatal enteroviral infections.

Diagnosis. The clinical differentiation of enteroviral disease from treatable bacterial illnesses is frequently very difficult, although when all the circumstances of a particular illness are considered, enterovirus diseases often can be suspected on clinical grounds. The most important factors in clinical diagnosis are season of the year, geographic location, exposure, incubation period, and clinical symptoms. In temperate climates enteroviral prevalence is distinctly seasonal; therefore, disease is usually seen in the summer and fall and unlikely to be seen in the winter; in the tropics enteroviruses are prevalent throughout the year. A careful history of maternal illness is vitally important in neonatal disease. For example, a mother's nonspecific mild febrile illness that occurs in the summer and fall should suggest the possibility of severe neonatal illness. Certain findings (i.e., aseptic meningitis, paralysis, pleurodynia, herpangina, pericarditis, myocarditis) should alert the clinician to enteroviral illnesses. The short incubation period of enterovirus infections should be taken into consideration. Poliovirus infection should be considered in any unimmunized or incompletely immunized child with nonspecific febrile illness, aseptic meningitis, or paralytic disease.

Most viral diagnostic laboratories have facilities for recovering the majority of enteroviruses that cause illness. Tissue culture systems allow the isolation of polioviruses, group B coxsackieviruses, echoviruses, and coxsackieviruses A9 and A16. Enteroviral growth in tissue culture takes only a few days in many cases and less than a week in most; identification of type frequently takes much more time. A complete diagnostic isolation spectrum can be obtained using suckling mouse inoculation. Specimens for virus isolation should be obtained from the throat and rectum (feces) and any other clinically involved site. Virus isolation from all sites except the feces can usually be considered causally related to a specific illness. The demonstration of a neutralizing antibody titer rise to a virus recovered from the feces indicates recent infection and tends to indicate a causal role for the isolated virus. Serum should be collected and stored frozen as soon as possible after the onset of illness and then again 2–4 wk later.

Differential Diagnosis. The differential diagnosis of enteroviral infections depends upon the clinical manifestations. It is most important to distinguish bacterial diseases such as those commonly associated with pharyngitis, pneumonia, pericarditis, meningitis, and septicemia, although other viral illnesses must also be considered.

Paralytic Poliomyelitis. Conditions causing muscular weakness include the following:

1. *Infectious neuronitis* (Guillain-Barré syndrome) is the most common and difficult to distinguish from poliomyelitis. Generally, the fever, headache, and meningeal signs are less notable. Paralysis is characteristically symmetrical, and sensory changes and pyramidal tract signs are common but are absent in poliomyelitis. Characteristically, there are few cells but elevated globulin content in the cerebrospinal fluid.

2. *Peripheral neuritis*—postinjectional, toxic (lead, avitaminosis, and so forth), paralytic cranial herpes zoster, postdiphtheritic neuropathy—is excluded by history, sensory examination, and related findings.

3. Arthropod-borne viral *encephalitis*, *rabies*, and *tetanus* have been confused with bulbar poliomyelitis.

4. *Botulism* may closely simulate bulbar poliomyelitis; nuchal-spinal rigidity and pleocytosis are absent.

5. *Demyelinizing types of encephalomyelitis* are associated with or follow the exanthems and other infections or occur as an untoward sequel of antirabies vaccination.

6. *Tick-bite* paralysis is uncommon; meningeal signs are absent, and removal of the tick is followed by swift recovery.

7. *Neoplasms* originating in and around the spinal cord may rarely have a fairly abrupt onset.

8. *Familial periodic paralysis, myasthenia gravis,* and *acute porphyria* are uncommon causes of weakness.

9. *Hysteria* and *malingering* are rare in children.

Conditions causing pseudoparalysis do not present with nuchal-spinal rigidity or pleocytosis and include the following:

1. *Unrecognized trauma* from contusions, sprains, fractures, and epiphyseal separation is a common cause of diagnostic confusion.

2. *Nonspecific (toxic) synovitis* produces a limp, usually unilaterally; the hip and the knee are the most common sites. There may be low grade fever for several days.

3. *Acute osteomyelitis* has a more septic course; there is polymorphonuclear leukocytosis, with localized signs, positive blood culture, and, later, roentgenographic changes.

4. In *acute rheumatic fever* the clinical pattern is usually diagnostic.

5. *Scurvy* is revealed by history of inadequate intake of vitamin C and by roentgenographic changes in the bones.

6. *Congenital syphilitic osteomyelitis* of the acute painful type is found only in early infancy.

Other Enteroviral Illnesses. The differential diagnosis of other enteroviral syndromes (respiratory, pericarditis/myocarditis, exanthems, meningitis/encephalitis, and so forth) is presented in the respective sections of this book relating to the clinical category.

Complications. *Paralytic Poliomyelitis. Melena* severe enough to require transfusion may result from single or multiple superficial intestinal erosions; perforation is rare. *Acute gastric dilatation* may occur abruptly during the acute or convalescent stage, causing further embarrassment of respiration; immediate gastric aspiration and external application of ice bags are indicated. Mild *hypertension* of a few days' or weeks' duration is common in the acute stage, probably related to lesions of the vasoregulatory centers in the medulla and especially to underventilation. In the later stages, because of immobilization, hypertension may occur along with hypercalcemia, nephrocalcinosis, and vascular lesions. Dimness of vision, headache, and a light-headed feeling in association with hypertension should be regarded as premonitory of a frank *convulsion. Cardiac irregularities* are uncommon, but electrocardiographic abnormalities suggesting myocarditis are not rare. *Acute pulmonary edema* occurs occasionally, particularly in patients with arterial hypertension. *Pulmonary embolism* is uncommon despite the immobilization. Skeletal decalcification begins soon after immobilization and results in *hypercalciuria*, which in turn predisposes to *calculi*, especially when urinary stasis and infection are present. A high fluid intake is the only effective prophylactic measure. The patient should be mobilized as much and as early as possible.

Complications of enteroviral infections such as those associated with myocarditis or encephalitis are presented in other sections of this text.

Prevention. In the United States and other developed countries poliomyelitis has been virtually eliminated through the widespread use of either inactivated (IPV) or oral polio vaccines (OPV) (Sec. 4.1). However, in many areas of the world endemic and epidemic poliomyelitis is still a problem.

Attenuated viral vaccines for enteroviruses other than polioviruses are not available. However, passive protection with pooled human immune globulin (0.2 mL/kg intramuscularly) may be useful in preventing disease. This is worthwhile only in sudden and virulent nursery outbreaks. Pooled human immune globulin in most instances can be expected to contain antibodies against coxsackievirus types B1–B5, offering protection to those infants without transplacentally acquired specific antibody who have not yet become infected.

Treatment. *Poliomyelitis.* The broad principles of management are to allay fear, to minimize ensuing skeletal deformities, to anticipate and meet complications in addition to the neuromusculoskeletal ones, and to prepare the child and family for the prolonged treatment that may be required and for permanent disability when this seems likely. Patients with the nonparalytic and mildly paralytic forms may be treated at home. No antibiotics are effective against poliovirus, and human immune globulin is ineffective after the onset of illness.

For the **abortive form** simple analgesics, sedatives, an attractive diet, and bed rest until the child's temperature is normal for several days suffice. Avoidance of exertion for the ensuing 2 wk is desirable, and there should be a careful neuromusculoskeletal examination 2 mo later to detect any minor involvement.

Treatment for the **nonparalytic form** is similar to that for the abortive form, relief being indicated in particular for the discomfort of muscle tightness and spasm of the neck, trunk, and extremities. Analgesics are more effective when combined with the application of hot packs for 15–30 min every 2–4 hr. Hot tub baths are sometimes useful. A firm bed is desirable and can be improvised at home by placing table leaves or a sheet of plywood beneath the mattress. A footboard should be used to keep the feet at a right angle with the legs. Muscular discomfort and spasm may continue for some weeks, even in the nonparalytic form, necessitating hot packs and gentle physical therapy. Such patients should also be carefully examined 2 mo after apparent recovery to detect minor residuals that might cause postural problems in later years.

Most patients with the **paralytic form** require hospitalization. A calm atmosphere is desired. Suitable body alignment is necessary to avoid excessive skeletal deformity. A neutral position with the feet at a right angle, knees slightly flexed, and hips and spine straight is achieved by use of boards, sandbags, and, occasionally, light splint shells. Active and passive motions are indicated as soon as the pain has disappeared. Opiates and sedatives are permissible only if no impairment of ventilation is present or impending. Constipation is common, and fecal impaction should be prevented. When bladder paralysis occurs, a parasympathetic stimulant such as bethanechol (Urecholine), 5–10 mg orally or 2.5–5.0 mg subcutaneously, may induce voiding in 15–30 min; some patients do not respond, and others have nausea, vomiting, and palpitation. Bladder paresis rarely lasts more than a few days. If Urecholine fails, manual compression of the bladder and the psychologic effect of running water should be tried. If catheterization must be performed, strict asepsis is essential. An interesting diet and a relatively high fluid intake should be started at once unless there is vomiting. Additional salt should be provided if the environmental temperature is high or if the application of hot packs induces sweating. Anorexia is common initially. An indwelling polyethylene gastric tube may be necessary to ensure adequate dietary and fluid intake. The orthopedist and the physiatrist should see these patients as early in the illness as possible and assume responsibility before fixed deformities develop. The management of *pure bulbar poliomyelitis* consists of maintaining the airway and avoiding all risks of inhalation of saliva, food, or vomitus. Gravity drainage of accumulated secretions is favored by the head-low (foot of bed elevated 20–25 degrees) prone position with the face to one side. Aspirators with rigid or semirigid tips are preferred for direct oral and pharyngeal use, and soft flexible catheters may be used for nasopharyngeal aspiration. Fluid and electrolyte equilibrium is best maintained by intravenous infusion since tube or oral feeding in the first few days may incite vomiting. Later an indwelling polyethylene gastric tube may be used, and sips of sterile water may be given from a spoon with increments as indicated by ability to swallow. In addition to close observation for respiratory insufficiency, the blood pressure should be taken at least twice daily, since hypertension is not uncommon and occasionally leads to hypertensive encephalopathy. Patients with pure bulbar poliomyelitis may require tracheostomy because of vocal cord paralysis or constriction of the hypopharynx; the majority who recover have little residual impairment, although some patients exhibit mild dysphagia and occasional vocal fatigue with slurring of speech.

Impaired ventilation must be recognized early; mounting anxiety, restlessness, and fatigue are early indications for prompt intervention (Sec. 13.21). Tracheostomy is indicated for some patients with pure bulbar poliomyelitis, spinal respiratory muscle paralysis, and bulbospinal paralysis, since these patients are generally unable to cough, sometimes for many months. Mechanical respirators are often needed.

Nonpolio Enteroviruses. There is no specific therapy for any enterovirus infection. In severe, catastrophic, and generalized neonatal infection, it is probably advisable to administer immune globulin to the infant, but there is no evidence that this therapy is beneficial. Corticosteroids should not be given during acute severe enterovirus infections, such as neonatal myocarditis or encephalitis, although some authors believe this therapy has been beneficial to coxsackievirus myocarditis. These agents have deleterious effects in experimental coxsackievirus infections of mice. Since the possibility of bacterial sepsis cannot be ruled out in many instances of enteroviral infections, antibiotics should frequently be administered for the most likely potential bacterial pathogens. Therapy of myocarditis and meningoencephalitis is discussed in Sec. 14.76 and 11.10, respectively.

Prognosis. Mortality in large urban epidemics of poliomyelitis in the United States in the prevaccine era was 5–7%. Most deaths occur within the first 2 wk after onset. Mortality and the degree of disability are greater after the age of puberty. In general, the more extensive the paralysis in the first 10 days of illness, the more severe the ultimate disability. Unexpected improvement may appear soon after defervescence and again about 6 wk after onset, a time that corresponds to functional restoration of temporarily inactive neurons. The degree of functional recovery also depends upon the adequacy and promptness of therapy as related to proper body positioning, active motion, use of assistive devices, and, of great importance, the psychologic motivation to return to as full and normal a life as possible. A long-term follow-up study of adults with post-poliomyelitis neuromuscular symptoms has shown slowly progressive non–life-threatening muscle weakness, with a greater effect occurring in patients in whom poliomyelitis had caused severe disability and muscle weakness.

The prognosis in nonpolio enteroviral infections in the vast majority of instances is excellent. Morbidity and mortality are related almost entirely to cardiac and neurologic disease in older children and these same diseases accompanied by general disseminated infection in neonates.

JAMES D. CHERRY

General

Cherry JD: Enteroviruses. In: Remington JS, Klein JO (eds): Infectious Diseases of the Fetus and Newborn Infant. 2nd ed. Philadelphia, WB Saunders, 1983.

Cherry JD: Enteroviruses: Polioviruses (poliomyelitis), coxsackieviruses, echoviruses and enteroviruses. In: Feigin RD, Cherry JD (eds): Textbook of Pediatric Infectious Diseases. 2nd ed. Philadelphia, WB Saunders, 1987.

Melnick JL: Enteroviruses. In: Evans AS (ed): Viral infections of Humans; Epidemiology and Control. 2nd ed. New York, Plenum Medical Book Co, 1982, p 187.

Specific

Bodian D, Horstmann DM: Poliomyelitis. In: Horsfall FL, Tamm I (eds): Viral and Rickettsial Infections of Man. 4th ed. Philadelphia, JB Lippincott, 1965.

Centers for Disease Control: Enterovirus Surveillance Report, 1970–1979. Atlanta, issued November 1981.

Dagan R, Prather SL, Powell KR, et al: Neutralizing antibodies to non-polio enteroviruses in human immune serum globulin. Pediatr Infect Dis 2:454, 1983.

Dalakas MC, Elder G, Hallett M, et al: A long-term follow-up study of patients with post-poliomyelitis neuromuscular symptoms. N Engl J Med 314:959, 1986.

Jenista JA, Powell KR, Menegus MA: Epidemiology of neonatal enterovirus infection. J Pediatr 104:685, 1984.

Kaplan MH, Klein SW, McPhee J, et al: Group B coxsackievirus infections in infants younger than three months of age: A serious childhood illness. Rev Infect Dis 5:1019, 1983.

Moore M: Enteroviral disease in the United States, 1970–1979. J Infect Dis 146:103, 1982.

Wilfert CM, Thompson RJ Jr, Sunder TR, et al: Longitudinal assessment of children with enteroviral meningitis during the first three months of life. Pediatrics 67:811, 1981.

Yin-Murphy M: Acute hemorrhagic conjunctivitis. Prog Med Virol 29:23, 1984.

11.78 RABIES
(Hydrophobia)

Rabies is a viral infection of the central nervous system usually transmitted by contamination of a wound with saliva from a rabid animal and virtually 100% fatal once symptoms develop. It is a worldwide public health problem and a source of considerable terror for both exposed patients and their physicians.

Etiology. Rabies virus belongs to the rhabdovirus group. The viral particles resemble striated bullets. Inside the cylinder is the RNA-containing nucleocapsid. Antibodies to the nucleocapsid can be detected in infected animals, but only antibodies to the surface glycoproteins are neutralizing and protective. The surface carries a fringe of glycoprotein spikes that have hemagglutinating activity when present on the whole virion.

Epidemiology. Rabies is a widespread infection of warm-blooded animals. In North America rabies occurs principally in skunks, raccoons, foxes, and bats. In the United States cats are more likely than dogs to be rabid. However, for ecologic reasons, and because of foreign travel, the dog is the most common source of infection for human rabies cases.

In Central and South America dogs are the usual source of exposure. Vampire bats, which bite cattle, are an important part of the cycle of rabies in Latin America. Europe has had an epizootic of fox rabies, with many humans being bitten.

In Asia and Africa the principal problem is the rabid dog. Countries such as India, the Philippines, and Indonesia have large numbers of stray dogs, but social factors limit efforts at control of this important vector.

Recently the concept of rabies-free land areas has been promulgated. This permits health authorities in places like New York City to omit vaccination after most dog bites on the grounds that terrestrial rabies has been unknown there for years. Nevertheless, practically every state has rabies in rural wildlife; in 1982, 27 states reported canine rabies and 46 states reported rabid bats. The continent of Australia and many islands, including those of the United Kingdom and Hawaii, are totally free of rabies.

Knowledge about the local epidemiology of rabies is essential to the physician contemplating treatment of a human exposure. Unprovoked bites by bats or other wild animals will almost always require immunization; decisions regarding bites from domestic or pet animals should be made after discussion with public health veterinarians.

Pathogenesis and Pathology. The means by which rabies virus travels from the wound to the brain are only partially understood. Since the virus attaches to and penetrates cells rapidly in vitro, it is unlikely that it remains dormant in the wound for long periods of time. Moreover, although the virus has been shown to ascend axons from the periphery to the spinal cord, the speed of spread (3 mm/hr) is far too rapid to explain the long incubation period of the disease.

In animals the virus first multiplies in striated muscle. It may be hypothesized that antibody, interferon, and other host factors then act on the virus as it leaves striated muscle; if these factors are insufficiently protective, virus eventually attaches to the nerve. From then on, rabies may be inevitable. The possibility that the virus must overcome another barrier in passing from the first infected neuron to other neurons is indicated by electron microscopic studies of the brain, which demonstrate viral passage from cell to contiguous cell.

The basic lesion in the brain is neuronal destruction in the brain stem and medulla. The cerebral cortex is usually normal in the absence of prolonged anoxia before death. The hippocampus, thalamus, and basal ganglia often show neuronal destruction and glial infiltrates. The most severe pathology is evident in the pons and the floor of the 4th ventricle. The inspiratory muscle spasms that result in the striking symptom of hydrophobia may be due to destruction of brain stem neurons inhibitory to the neurons of the nucleus ambiguus, which control inspiration. Hydrophobia does not occur in other diseases since only rabies combines brain stem encephalitis with intact cortex and maintenance of consciousness.

The Negri body, long the pathologic hallmark of rabies, is a cytoplasmic inclusion found in neurons; it consists of clumped viral nucleocapsid. The absence of Negri bodies does not exclude rabies; fluorescent antibody stains of brain sections or smears may be positive in their absence.

Transmission. In animals as in humans rabies produces encephalitis as the principal symptom. After establishment of the encephalitis, however, the virus spreads down nerves from the brain. It multiplies in many organs but those important to transmission are the salivary glands. Not all rabid animals have virus in the saliva, and even when it is present, the quantity is variable. Skunks are particularly likely to have large amounts of virus in saliva. Although dogs may have virus in saliva for many days before symptoms occur, transmission to man from dogs who appeared normal for 10 days or more after a biting incident has not been reported. The variability of virus in saliva explains the fact that only about half of untreated bites by proven rabid animals will result in rabies.

Scratches by the claws of rabid animals are dangerous because animals lick their claws. Saliva applied to a mucosal surface such as the conjunctiva may be infectious.

Bat excreta contain enough rabies virus to pose danger of rabies to those who enter infested caves and inhale aerosols created by bats. Aerosols of rabies virus inadvertently produced in laboratories are dangerous to laboratory workers.

In general, if a biting animal does not die within 10 days, rabies is unlikely, although rarely a rabid terrestrial animal will recover from rabies. Bats, on the contrary, are often infected for long periods without showing symptoms.

Since the dog is the most important vector of rabies for people throughout the world, the following description by Blattner may be helpful:

In the dog symptoms may be considered under 2 general types, although it is not possible to separate them completely.

1. The "furious" type results from increased excitation of the central nervous system, with fever, hyperesthesia, and lack of appetite. The evidences of disease depend to a great extent upon the nature and training of the dog. The more aggressive dog will begin to snap and become excited and dangerous early in the course of the disease. The gentle dog in the early stages will more frequently seek seclusion and refuse food or will become excessively affectionate, after which it becomes agitated and restless. This is usually followed by irritability and snapping at strangers and a little later by snarling or snapping at imaginary objects and chasing and biting other animals. Finally, if free, it will run for miles, snapping at or biting all living things in its path until it falls paralyzed to the ground.

2. The "dumb" or paralytic type, despite its frequency (approximately 20%), is rarely recognized by the dog's owners, primarily because no agitation or excitement is seen. The course is far more rapid, paralysis occurring in any group of muscles, but particularly in the lower jaw and in the muscles of deglutition. In such cases the tongue hangs out of the mouth, continuously dripping saliva; sympathetic persons, suspecting a foreign body in the dog's throat, may expose their hands to the infective saliva in an effort to relieve the dog. Rapidly extending paralysis soon results in death; occasionally dogs die suddenly without signs of illness, and encephalitis with Negri bodies is found at autopsy.

Transmission of rabies by corneal transplant from patients with undiagnosed rabies encephalitis to healthy recipients has been recorded.

Clinical Manifestations. The incubation period of rabies is extremely variable. Exceptionally long incubation periods of 2 yr have been seen. On the other hand, an incubation period of only 9 days has followed severe exposure. Usually, the incubation period is 20–180 days with the peak at 30–60 days. The length is related to the site of the bite; shortest for bites on the head, longest for bites on the legs. It also tends to be shorter in children and in vaccinated individuals who nevertheless develop rabies.

There is usually a prodromal phase of rabies, lasting 2–10 days. Common nonspecific symptoms include fever, malaise, headache, anorexia, and vomiting. The patient may be troubled by ill-defined anxiety. A characteristic symptom at this stage is pain or paresthesia at the site of the wound.

The illness then enters an acute neurologic phase, of either the furious or paralytic variety, which lasts 2–10 days. In the former, hydrophobia is a pathognomonic sign. Attempts to swallow liquids, including saliva, result in spasms of the pharynx and larynx and aspiration into the trachea. Eventually a psychologic component exacerbates the spasms, and even the sight of water evokes terror. "Aerophobia" may be present and is considered by some also to be pathognomonic of rabies. Aerophobia is elicited by fanning a current of air across the face, which causes violent spasms of the pharyngeal and neck muscles.

The neurologic picture in the typical case may consist of bursts of hyperactivity, disorientation, and bizarre combative behavior, alternating with periods of lucidity. During the patient's lucid periods he or she may be aware of what is happening and able to articulate his or her fears. The facial expression of the patient is one of grim hopelessness.

Patients may also complain of pharyngeal pain, difficulty in swallowing, and hoarseness. Seizures are common, perhaps on the basis of hypoxia compounded by hyperventilation.

Some rabid patients develop meningismus or even opisthotonos. The cerebrospinal fluid may reflect meningeal irritation, with varying elevations of cells (predominantly lymphocytes) and protein, or may be normal. The peripheral white blood count often shows a polymorphonuclear leukocytosis.

In about 20% of patients, an ascending symmetric paralysis with flaccidity and decreased tendon reflexes dominates the entire acute phase. This course is particularly common after vampire bat bites. In the remainder of cases paralysis develops toward the end of the acute neurologic phase.

If the patient does not die of cardiorespiratory arrest during the acute stage, he or she slips into coma. With modern intensive care, life may be prolonged, but numerous complications occur during coma. Most significant is myocarditis, manifested by hypotension and arrhythmias. Rabies virus has been recovered from the heart, which shows inflammation at autopsy. Also prominent is pituitary dysfunction expressed as either diabetes insipidus or inappropriate secretion of antidiuretic hormone. As the patient continues in coma, the complications of intensive hospital care occur. Unless recovery begins within 2 wk the outcome will be fatal, although patients can be kept alive for months.

Diagnosis and Differential Diagnosis. When a patient has a history of having been bitten by an animal, paresthesias at the wound site, and hydrophobia, a clinical diagnosis of rabies is not difficult. Any disease in which there is encephalitis may occasionally cause confusion, such as those caused by arboviruses, enteroviruses, and *Herpes simplex*. However, if one finds signs of brain stem involvement in a patient whose sensorium is basically clear and who has no signs of a space-occupying lesion, other diagnoses can usually be set aside.

Paralytic rabies may be misdiagnosed as *Guillain-Barré syndrome, poliomyelitis,* or *postrabies vaccine encephalomyelitis.* Careful neurologic examination and analysis of the cerebrospinal fluid will often help rule out these diagnoses.

The spasms of *tetanus* may cause momentary diagnostic confusion, but trismus is not seen in rabies, and hydrophobia is not seen in tetanus. Botulism (wound or ingestion) will cause paralysis, but the absence of sensory changes should exclude rabies.

Perhaps the most confusing differential problem is *hysteria* in an individual who thinks he or she has rabies. Normal blood gases and the absence of variation in bizarre behavior will suggest pseudorabies.

Laboratory diagnosis is now possible before death. The virus may be demonstrated by fluorescent antibody stain of smears of corneal epithelial cells or sections of skin from the neck at the hairline. These tests are positive because virus migrates down the nerves from the brain; both the cornea and hair follicles are richly innervated. Autopsy examination of the brains of patients with fatal encephalitis should include fluorescent antibody tests for rabies.

Serologic diagnosis is also possible if the patient survives beyond the acute period. Neutralizing antibodies develop in both serum and cerebrospinal fluid and rapidly rise to extremely high levels, e.g., >100 International Units (IU). Vaccination, even with potent vaccine, is unlikely to raise titers above 20 IU.

Prognosis. Survival after infection is possible with intensive supportive care; however, almost all of these patients eventually die after prolonged courses.

Prevention of Rabies

Pre-exposure Prophylaxis. Vaccination of domestic dogs and elimination of strays have resulted in eradication of terrestrial rabies from many areas. If dog control were properly practiced, rabies could be suppressed in much of the world.

Those who are expected to be at risk, such as veterinarians, laboratory workers, and children going to rabies-enzootic areas, can be preimmunized. The new cell culture vaccine (see below) will produce virtually 100% response with 3 doses given at 0, 7, and 28 days. A titer of 0.3 IU has been accepted as protective, although some observations suggest the need for a higher titer.

Postexposure Prophylaxis. First, a decision must be made as to whether rabies prophylaxis is necessary. In many areas of the United States, rabies in mammals has been unknown for years. In those areas only bat bites call for treatment. Otherwise, the unprovoked bite of a wild animal should be considered rabid if the animal belongs to a species known to be a rabies host, such as a skunk, fox, raccoon, bat, or coyote. Rodents are very rarely carriers of rabies in the United States.

If a domestic animal such as a dog or cat is the offender, consideration must be given to the question of provocation, to the clinical appearance of the animal if apprehended, and to the rabies vaccination status of the animal. Difficulty in making decisions arises when the biting animal has run away after a seemingly unprovoked attack. Whether the animal was rabid or merely ill-tempered is often impossible to decide. When the animal is under observation, rabies treatment can be withheld until the animal acts abnormally, at which point it should be sacrificed and tested for rabies. However, a wild animal should be killed immediately and its brain examined for rabies antigen by the fluorescent-antibody technique.

Table 11–32 may help in making the often difficult decision whether to treat or not to treat.

If rabies prophylaxis is to be given after exposure, prevention depends on three complementary means of reducing the risk. Local treatment (see below) is designed to kill the virus by mechanical and virucidal action. Passive antibody (see below) then provides immediate blockage of attachment of virus to the nerve endings. However, passive antibody ultimately disappears and must be replaced by the active response provided by vaccine. The number of vaccine doses administered depends on its antigenic mass. The vaccine must not only produce a primary antibody response but also overcome the depressive effect of passive antibody on the immune response.

Local Treatment. The chief requirement of local treatment is that it be prompt and thorough. Simple mechanical removal by soap and water should be the first step, using copious amounts of solution. Catheters should be inserted for irrigation of puncture wounds. If the mechanical trauma of the local treatment is painful, procaine-type anesthetics may be used to infiltrate the area without adding risk.

The mechanical removal of virus may be followed by application of a virucidal solution such as 1% povidone-iodine or 70% alcohol. In an emergency, any alcoholic liquor of 86 proof or higher may be used. However, many authorities eschew antisepsis and depend on soap and water irrigation.

Passive Antibody. Passive immunization must be given to protect the patient until vaccination produces antibodies. Passive antibody is available in the form of equine antiserum (Sclavo) or human rabies immune globulin (Cutter and Merieux). The latter avoids serum sickness reactions to equine protein, which occur in about 5% of recipients of the animal product. The dose for human rabies immune globulin is 20 IU/kg. Up to half of the dose should be infiltrated subcutaneously at the site of bite or scratch; the remainder is injected intramuscularly into the arm or buttocks. The dose for equine antirabies serum is 40 IU/kg delivered in the same manner.

Passive immunization should be performed regardless of the interval between rabies exposure and treatment. However, if vaccine was previously started there is no need for passive immunization once 8 days have elapsed. Anaphylaxis is a possibility with the equine antiserum, and tests for hypersensitivity should be carried out in the usual manner (consult package insert). Steroids should be avoided in the treatment of reactions, since they cause activation of rabies virus in experimental situations.

Active Immunization. Early rabies vaccines were prepared in the central nervous system of animals. Their antigenicity was poor and multiple injections were required. As a result postvaccination encephalitis was a frequent problem. Animal nerve tissue vaccines are still in use in many places in the world.

Human diploid cell vaccine (HDCV) was developed to increase immunogenicity and safety. HDCV has had more than 10 yr of commercial use in Europe and more recently in the United States and has withstood the challenge of severe exposures to confirmed rabid animals in Iran, West Germany, and France. HDCV is now the only vaccine licensed in this country.

HDCV is more antigenic than previous vaccines; accordingly, the number of doses can be reduced from the traditional 14 or 21. The current recommendation in the United States is 5 doses at 0, 3, 7, 14, and 28 days. For pre-exposure vaccination of high-risk groups, inoculations are given at 0, 7, and 28 days. The schedule that has been used in Europe for postexposure vaccination consists of 6 doses (1 mL intramuscularly) at 0, 3, 7, 14, 30, and 90 days.

Reaction rates have been low, and neurologic reactions have been rare, probably because no nerve tissue is present in the cell culture used to grow the virus. Allergic reactions have occurred in less than 0.1% after primary vaccination, and systemic symptoms such as malaise and fever in only 5–15%, perhaps because the vaccine is made in human cell

Table 11–32. Postexposure Antirabies Treatment Guide

Animal	Evaluation of Animal at Time of Exposure*	Treatment of Exposed Human
Wild Skunk Fox Raccoon Coyote Bat	Regard as rabid	HRIG + V†
Domestic Dogs and Cats	Healthy Escaped (unknown) Rabid or suspect rabid	None‡ HRIG + V§ HRIG + V†

*An exposure is considered to be by bite, by scratch with claws, or by contamination with saliva of mucosal surfaces or skin that has been cut or abraded.

†Discontinue vaccine if fluorescent antibody tests of animal are negative.

‡Begin HRIG + V at first sign of rabies in biting dog or cat during holding period (10 days).

§In a rabies enzootic area, treat; in a rabies free area, no treatment may be indicated. V = Rabies vaccine; HRIG = Human rabies immune globulin.

These recommendations are only a guide. They should be used in conjunction with knowledge of the animal species involved, circumstances of the bite or other exposure, vaccination status of the animal, and presence of rabies in the region.

Modified from Public Health Service Advisory Committee Recommendations, Ann Intern Med 86:452, 1977.

culture. Nevertheless, administration of boosters results in an allergic reaction rate of 6%; accordingly, boosters are no longer routinely recommended, except following rabies exposure.

Treatment of Clinical Rabies. Large doses of interferon and antirabies serum have been advocated, but it is doubtful that these substances can affect rabies that has already spread to the brain.

                                                    STANLEY A. PLOTKIN

Anderson LJ, Sikes RK, Langkop CW, et al: Prophylactic immunization: Postexposure trial of a human diploid cell strain rabies vaccine. J Infect Dis 142:133, 1980.

Clark HF, Prabhakar ES: Rabies. In: Olsen RG, Krakowaka GS, Blakesle JR (eds): Comparative Pathobiology of Viral Diseases. Boca Raton, CRC Press, Vol II:165, 1985.

Houff SA, Burton RC, Wilson RW, et al: Human-to-human transmission of rabies virus by corneal transplant. N Engl J Med 300:603, 1979.

Iwasaki Y, Liu D-S, Yamamoto T, et al: The replication and spread of rabies virus in the human central nervous system. J Neuropathol Exp Neurol, in press.

Plotkin SA: Rabies vaccine prepared in human cell cultures: Progress and perspectives. Rev Infect Dis 2:433, 1980.

Plotkin SA, Clark HF: Committee on Immunization—prevention of rabies in man. J Infect Dis 123:227, 1971.

Public Health Service Advisory Committee on Immunization Practices: Rabies: Risk, management, prophylaxis, and immunization. Ann Intern Med 86:452, 1977.

Sureau P, Rollin P, Wiktor TJ: Epidemiologic analysis of antigenic variations of street rabies virus: Detection by monoclonal antibodies. Am J Epidemiol 117:605, 1983.

Turner GS: A review of the world epidemiology of rabies. Tr R Soc Trop Med Hyg 70:175, 1976.

Warrell DA: The clinical picture of rabies in man. Tr R Soc Trop Med Hyg 70:188, 1976.

Wiktor TJ, Koprowski H: Antigenic variants of rabies virus. J Exp Med 152:99, 1980.

World Health Organization: Guidelines for Dog Rabies Control. Geneva, March 1984.

11.79 SLOW REACTIONS OF THE HUMAN NERVOUS SYSTEM TO VIRUSES
(Slow Virus Infections)

Viruses are the causes of a group of central nervous system diseases that were previously regarded as degenerative or hereditary. These diseases are described as slow virus infections because the interaction between virus and host tissues that eventuates in disease takes place over a period of at least months and usually years. Once clinically manifest, these conditions progress rapidly and unremittingly, and are eventually fatal. Slow, therefore, refers to their long incubation period rather than to their course once clinical manifestations appear. Although viral replication occurs in various body organs, pathologic changes are seen only in the central nervous system.

The viruses involved have been categorized into *conventional viruses* and *unconventional viruses*. The conventional viruses that sometimes produce slow infections (measles [rubeola], rubella, and papovaviruses) possess the usual structural and biologic properties of viruses. The unconventional viruses are quite different from all other viruses in that they possess no nucleic acid cores, protein coats, or lipid envelopes and are, therefore, not recognizable as viruses by electron microscopy. They cannot be detected by cell culture techniques and induce no immunologic or inflammatory changes in the host. They are also unusually resistant to physicochemical inactivation. The evidence suggesting that these unconventional agents are viruses is that they pass through bacterial filters of small pore size and replicate in the reticuloendothelial system and later in the brains of experimental animals after parenteral inoculation. They probably constitute a new class of infectious

agents. The acronym prions (derived from proteinaceous infectious particles) has been proposed as a descriptive designation.

Slow Infections with Unconventional Viruses

The concept of slow virus infections of the nervous system of animals was proposed by Sigurdsson in 1954 as a result of his investigations of *scrapie*, a progressive degenerative and fatal neurologic disease of sheep and goats that, as the name suggests, causes the animals to rub and scratch. Infection with the scrapie agent, an unconventional virus, can be transmitted to small animals and serves as a model for slow virus infections associated with severe progressive neurologic disease in humans.

Spongiform Encephalopathies. The histopathology of scrapie and transmissible mink encephalopathy (another animal unconventional virus disease) closely resembles that seen in *kuru* and *Creutzfeldt-Jakob disease*, two degenerative neurologic diseases of humans caused by unconventional viruses. In these disorders intracytoplasmic vacuoles develop, resulting in neuronal degeneration and astrocytic gliosis. These changes are characterized as progressive spongiform encephalopathy.

Kuru. This heredofamilial degenerative disease of the central nervous system presents as a trembling ataxia (kuru means "trembling with fear") with progressive incapacity and death. It is confined to an area of the eastern highlands of Papua New Guinea, inhabited by the Fore tribe. By Fore custom the dead, including those dying of kuru, are eaten by female relatives. Participants in this practice of ritual cannibalism probably become infected by self-inoculation of infected brain tissue into dermal abrasions or mucosal surfaces. Because men do not participate, kuru occurs predominantly in women and in young children of both sexes who probably become inoculated with infected tissue by close association with their mothers during the ritual meal. With the decline in the practice of this custom, kuru has almost disappeared.

Several thousand cases have been documented in New Guinea, some occurring years later in persons who have migrated out of the endemic area. Kuru may appear in young children or after an incubation period of up to 18 yr. Brain tissue from subjects with kuru, when inoculated into chimpanzees, reproduces the disease after a latent period of 20 mo.

Creutzfeldt-Jakob Disease. This presenile dementia is predominantly a disease of older adults, although some affected patients in their 20's have been reported. It begins with vague psychic disturbances that progress within a few months to dementia accompanied by pyramidal and extrapyramidal tract signs, cerebellar dysfunction, and rigidity. Death soon occurs. Creutzfeldt-Jakob disease has a worldwide distribution. The prevalence rate in Europe and North and South America is estimated to be 1–2/million population.

The disease has been transmitted to animals by intracerebral and parenteral inoculation with brain tissue from affected humans. Direct human-to-human transmission was first observed when a cornea collected post mortem from a patient retrospectively diagnosed as having the disease was transplanted to a normal individual who developed the disease 18 mo later. Since then, cases have been connected with neurosurgical procedures, such as the insertion of electrodes sterilized with ethanol and formaldehyde into the brain, and with injections of growth hormone prepared from pooled human pituitary glands. The agent, as is true of kuru and of the viruses of scrapie and mink encephalopathy, withstands usual methods of chemical sterilization. Neurosurgeons, neuropathologists, and others, such as patients who have received human growth hormone of pituitary origin, may be at special risk of acquiring the disease. Preparation of growth hormone from pituitary glands has been discontinued. Tissues from patients with Creutzfeldt-Jakob disease should be handled with caution to prevent careless contamination of personnel and the environment. Equipment that has come in direct contact with tissues or blood from these patients should be autoclaved for 1 hr at a temperature ≥121° C before being discarded or prepared for reuse. When autoclaving is not practical, exposure of equipment to a solution of 1N sodium hydroxide for 1 hr is recommended. The natural route of transmission of this disease is unknown. Because it occurs in both a sporadic and familial form, it has been speculated that in some families there may be a genetic susceptibility to this slow virus infection.

Slow Infections with Conventional Viruses

These diseases are unusual late sequelae of commonly occurring infections with conventional viruses. The acute phase of these infections is not unusual. After a period of months or years, however, a neurologic illness appears that is usually progressive and fatal. These slow reactions to viruses are distinct from the early neurologic complications that sometimes occur during or shortly after the acute phase of viral infections (e.g., measles encephalitis).

Subacute Sclerosing Panencephalitis (SSPE). SSPE is a rare complication of infection with measles virus appearing 5–6 yr after the acute disease or after immunization with live measles vaccine virus. The illness begins with insidious changes in personality, behavior, and intellect. After weeks or months the steadily progressive course is characterized by dystonic and myoclonic movements, by convulsions, and terminally by decorticate rigidity. The estimated incidence of SSPE is 1 per 100,000 cases of natural measles and 1 per 1–2 million doses of attenuated measles vaccine. Therefore, the incidence of SSPE has declined as the use of measles vaccine has increased. Mean age of onset is 7–8 yr, but cases have been reported in children less than 2 and in adults over 20. The disease occurs 3–4 times more frequently in boys than in girls. Children who contract measles at an early age and who are intensely exposed, as in prolonged contact with an infected sibling, appear to be at increased risk.

The brain shows marked proliferation of astrocytes and microglial cells (hence the term sclerosing) along with demyelinization and intranuclear inclusion bodies. Perivascular cuffing and diffuse mononuclear infiltration of the gray and white matter are also observed. The isolation of a measles-like virus from the brain and the presence of high titers of measles virus antibody in the cerebrospinal fluid and serum are the basis for assuming that SSPE results from an unusual reaction between measles virus and the central nervous system. Cofactors appear to be involved, however, since the disease has a rural prevalence and occurs with increased frequency in developing countries. No cellular or humoral immune deficiencies have been identified in affected persons.

Progressive Rubella Panencephalitis (PRP). PRP is a chronic, progressive inflammatory disorder of the central nervous system that occurs as a late complication of either congenitally or postnatally acquired rubella. No cases have been associated with administration of rubella vaccines. The onset is usually in the 2nd decade, and the disease follows a protracted course over a period of several years. Patients exhibit slowly progressive cerebellar ataxia, spasticity, convulsions, and mental deterioration. PRP should not be confused with the encephalitis that frequently occurs as a component of the congenital rubella syndrome. The latter condition is either present at birth or develops during the 1st few months of life. Although this early form of encephalitis follows a variable course, the child's neurologic status usually stabilizes by or during the 2nd yr of life. PRP, in contrast, occurs many years later. The brain shows perivascular accumulations of lymphocytes and plasma cells, diffuse loss of neurons, and gliosis. Blood vessels of the central nervous system contain amorphous deposits similar to those seen in the blood vessels of children dying with congenital rubella. High titers of antibody against rubella virus are present in the serum and cerebrospinal fluid, and rubella virus has been isolated from the brain. No immunodeficiencies have been detected in patients with PRP. Rubella virus has an affinity for the central nervous system, and congenitally acquired infection can persist in certain tissues for months to years. The mechanisms by which this virus produces a progressive neurologic disease many years after initial exposure, however, are unknown. Immune complexes consisting of rubella virus antigen and anti-rubella antibodies have been detected in the blood and spinal fluid. Deposition of these complexes in blood vessels may be a pathogenetic factor in the cerebral vasculitis that occurs in this disease.

Progressive Multifocal Leukoencephalopathy (PML). The neuropathologic changes that occur in PML consist of noninflammatory foci of demyelinization and loss of oligodendroglia throughout the white matter. The oligodendroglia at the periphery of these foci contain intranuclear inclusion bodies that are filled with papovavirus-like particles, and strains of this group of viruses have been isolated from the brains of affected patients. Most patients with PML are adults who have pre-existing disorders associated with secondary immunodeficiency. The presenting neurologic signs depend upon the location of the foci of demyelinization. As these foci enlarge or coalesce, neurologic disability increases, and death usually occurs within 1 yr from onset of symptoms.

Although asymptomatic infections with papovaviruses are widespread, PML is a rare disease. Seroepidemiologic studies have shown that by adult life most persons have acquired this infection. Apparently when immune function is depressed by disease, an unusual reaction, manifest as PML, develops between brain tissue and papovaviruses in some infected persons. It is not known, however, whether PML results from activation of persistent central nervous system infection acquired earlier in life, or whether this disease represents the response of an immunodepressed host to first contact with these agents.

Slow Infections with Other Viruses. The slow virus infections that have been recognized are rare. Because of the potential for prevention, it is important to determine if slow infections with viruses play an etiologic role in other chronic diseases of higher prevalence such as multiple sclerosis, the dementias, and certain forms of cancer.

ALFRED D. HEGGIE

Aaby P, Bukh J, Lisse IM, et al: Risk factors in subacute sclerosing panencephalitis: age- and sex-dependent host reactions or intensive exposure? Rev Infect Dis 6:239, 1984.

Brockman JM, Kingsbury DT, McKinley MP, et al: Creutzfeldt-Jakob prion proteins in human brains. N Engl J Med 312:73, 1985.

Brown P, Gajdusek C, Gibbs CJ, et al: Potential epidemic of Creutzfeldt-Jakob disease from human growth hormone therapy. N Engl J Med 313:728, 1985.

Brown P, Gibbs CJ, Amyx HL, et al: Chemical disinfection of Creutzfeldt-Jakob disease virus. N Engl J Med 306:1279, 1982.

Brown P, Rohwer RG, Gajdusek DC: Sodium hydroxide decontamination of Creutzfeldt-Jakob disease virus. N Engl J Med 310:727, 1984.

Brown P, Salazar AM, Gibbs CJ, et al: Alzheimer's disease and transmissible virus dementia (Creutzfeldt-Jakob disease). Ann NY Acad Sci 396:131, 1982.

Chatigny MA, Prusiner SB: Biohazards of investigations of the transmissible spongiform encephalopathies. Rev Infect Dis 2:713, 1980.

Coyle PK, Wolinsky JS: Characterization of immune complexes in progressive rubella panencephalitis. Ann Neurol 9:557, 1981.

Gajdusek DC: Unconventional viruses and the origin and disappearance of kuru. Science 197:943, 1977.

Johnson RT: Viral Infections of the Nervous System. New York, Raven Press, 1982.

Merz PA, Rohwer RG, Kascak R, et al: Infection-specific particle from the unconventional slow virus diseases. Science 225:437, 1984.

Nathanson N: Slow viruses and chronic disease: The contribution of epidemiology. Pub Health Rep 95:436, 1980.

National Institute of Diabetes and Digestive and Kidney Diseases: Human growth hormone and Creutzfeldt-Jakob disease. NIH Publication No. 86–2793, 1986.

Prusiner SB: Prions: Novel infectious pathogens. Adv Virus Res 29:1, 1984.

Sanalang VE, Embil JA: Emergence of papovavirus in long term cultures of astrocytes from progressive multifocal leukoencephalopathy patients. J Neuropathol Exp Neurol 43:553, 1984.

ter Meulen V, Carter MJ: Measles virus: Persistency and disease. Prog Med Virol 30:44, 1984.

Wechsler SL, Meissner JC: Measles and SSPE viruses: Similarities and differences. Prog Med Virol 28:65, 1982.

Weil ML, Habashi JJ, Cremer NE, et al: Chronic progressive panencephalitis due to rubella virus simulating SSPE. N Engl J Med 292:994, 1975.

Zilber N, Rannon L, Alter M, et al: Measles, measles vaccination, and risk of subacute sclerosing panencephalitis (SSPE). Neurol 33:1558, 1983.

11.80 YELLOW FEVER

Yellow fever is an acute mosquito-borne infection characterized in its most severe form by fever, jaundice, proteinuria, and hemorrhage. Despite the availability of an effective vaccine for over 45 years, the disease remains a significant public health problem, particularly in West Africa, where large epidemics occur periodically, and in parts of tropical South America. The pediatrician practicing in North America needs to be able to provide appropriate advice regarding immunization of children travelling to endemic areas.

Etiology. Yellow fever is a member of the Flavivirus (Group B arbovirus) genus of the family Flaviviridae. Virus particles are of small size (35–45 nm in diameter) and contain an infectious single-stranded RNA genome. Human and non-human primate hosts acquire the infection by the bite of infected mosquitoes. After an incubation period of 3–6 days, virus appears in the bloodstream for 5–10 days and may serve as a source of infection for other mosquitoes. An incubation period of 1–2 weeks is required in the mosquito before it is capable of transmitting the virus.

Epidemiology. Figure 11–29 shows the present geographic distribution of endemic yellow fever. In the 19th and early 20th centuries, the disease occurred in the Caribbean, the United States, and parts of Europe; these areas, still infested with *Aedes aegypti* mosquitoes, are potentially receptive to the introduction and spread of the disease from the endemic zone. Yellow fever has never appeared in Asia. The incidence of officially reported cases in tropical America is approximately 200/yr, but the disease is significantly underreported. In West Africa, particularly large outbreaks have occurred periodically. In the Americas, adult males are the principal targets of yellow fever because they are exposed to infected mosquitoes while working in forested areas. In Africa, however, where epidemics occur in savannah village regions, children under 15 yrs have the highest incidence; there is an increasing immune barrier with age (due to naturally acquired and vaccine immunity). Transmission is highest during the rainy season (generally December–March in tropical America and July–November in West Africa). A significant factor that promotes the occurrence of yellow fever in some areas is the migration of nonimmune laborers and other populations into endemic regions.

In tropical forests, yellow fever virus is maintained in a transmission cycle involving monkeys and tree-hole breeding mosquitoes (*Haemagogus* spp. in the Americas, *Aedes africanus* in Africa). Persons entering the forest may be exposed, resulting in sporadic cases of jungle yellow fever. In Africa, the virus activity also occurs in moist savannah and savannah-forest transition areas, where other tree-hole breeding *Aedes* vectors present in high density transmit the virus between monkeys, between monkeys and humans, and between humans. Urban yellow fever, the result of human-to-human transmission by the domestic mosquito *Aedes aegypti*, occurs in villages and small towns in Africa, but has not been reported in the Americas since 1954.

Clinical Manifestations. Inapparent, abortive, or clinically mild infections are frequent, and some studies have suggested that children experience a milder disease than adults. Abortive infections, characterized by fever and headache, may go unrecognized except, at times, during epidemics.

In its full-blown form, yellow fever begins with sudden onset of fever, headache, myalgia, lumbosacral pain, anorexia, nausea, and vomiting. Physical findings during the early phase of illness, when virus is present in the blood, include prostration, conjunctival injection, flushing of face and neck, reddening of the tongue at the tip and edges, and a relative bradycardia. After 2–3 days, there may be a brief period of remission, followed in 6–24 hr by reappearance of fever, vomiting, epigastric pain, jaundice, dehydration, hemorrhage (particularly hematemesis), albuminuria, hypotension, signs of renal failure, delirium, convulsions, and coma. Between the 7th and 10th days death generally occurs. The fatality rate in severe cases approaches 50% but is only 10–20% in milder forms with jaundice. Some patients surviving the acute phase of illness may later succumb to renal failure or myocardial damage. Laboratory findings include leukopenia, prolongation of clotting, prothrombin, and partial thromboplastin times, thrombocytopenia, hyperbilirubinemia, elevation of serum transaminases, albuminuria, and azotemia. Hypoglycemia may be present in severe cases. EKG abnormalities (bradycardia, ST-T changes) have occurred.

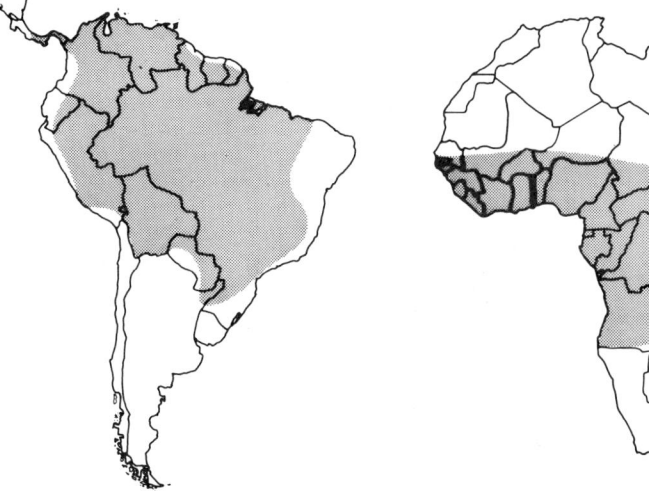

Figure 11–29. Endemic areas of yellow fever (shaded). Immunization of persons traveling to these regions is recommended, whether or not national health authorities require vaccination certificates.

Pathology and Pathophysiology. Histopathologic changes in the liver include: (1) coagulative necrosis of hepatocytes in the midzone of the liver lobule with sparing of cells around the portal areas and central veins; (2) eosinophilic degeneration of hepatocytes (Councilman bodies); (3) microvacuolar fatty change; and (4) minimal inflammation. The kidneys show acute tubular necrosis. Myocardial fiber degeneration and fatty infiltration are present. The brain may show edema and petechial hemorrhages. Direct viral injury to the liver, resulting in impaired biosynthesis and detoxification, is a central pathogenetic event. Hemorrhage results from decreased synthesis of vitamin K–dependent clotting factors and, in some cases, disseminated intravascular clotting. Renal dysfunction is attributed to hemodynamic factors (prerenal failure progressing to acute tubular necrosis). The roles of shock, systemic bacterial endotoxemia, and other conditions remain obscure.

Diagnosis and Treatment. Yellow fever should be suspected when fever, headache, vomiting and myalgia appear in residents of endemic areas or in unimmunized visitors who have recently traveled (within 2 wk prior to onset of symptoms) to those areas.

Mild yellow fever cannot be distinguished from a wide variety of other infections. Jaundice and hemorrhage may signal the presence of any one of several other diseases that must be differentiated; such possibilities include malaria, leptospirosis, viral hepatitis, Rift Valley fever, typhoid, rickettsial infections, and other viral hemorrhagic fevers. Specific diagnosis depends on tests for presence of virus or viral antigen in acute phase blood samples or on antibody determinations. Sera obtained during the first 10 days after onset of symptoms should be kept frozen, preferably in an ultra-low-temperature freezer ($-60°$ C) and shipped on dry ice for virus testing. Convalescent-phase samples for antibody tests are handled by conventional means. In handling acutely infected blood specimens, all clinical personnel must take care to avoid contaminating unimmunized personnel as well as laboratory equipment and operations.

Treatment is symptomatic and includes: (1) careful monitoring of vital functions, (2) reduction of fever by sponging or acetaminophen (avoid aspirin because of bleeding diathesis), (3) protection of the gastric mucosa (suction, antacids, cimetidine), (4) adequate nutritional intake and treatment of hypoglycemia (with intravenous 10–20% glucose), (5) avoidance of CNS depressant drugs, (6) correction of acid-base disturbances, and (7) treatment of hypotension and shock. If prerenal azotemia occurs, efforts should be made to increase renal perfusion by fluid challenge or (in presence of hypotension) by dopamine or dobutamine. If oliguric acute renal failure (acute tubular necrosis) is present, peritoneal dialysis may be indicated. If bacterial sepsis occurs as a complication, it should be treated with appropriate antibiotics. Bleeding diathesis, if severe, can best be managed by transfusion of fresh whole blood, fresh frozen plasma, or platelet concentrates. If DIC is documented, heparin may be indicated.

Prevention and Control. Yellow fever 17D is an extremely safe, live attenuated vaccine which should be administered as a single 0.5 mL subcutaneous injection at least 10 days before arrival in an endemic area (Fig. 11–29). All persons traveling to these areas should be considered for vaccination, but length of stay, exact locations to be visited, and likely environmental exposure may determine the specific risk and individual need for vaccination. If questions arise, information should be sought from the Centers for Disease Control, Atlanta, Georgia. For international travel certification, vaccination is valid for 10 years, although immunity lasts at least 40 years and is probably life-long. Vaccine should not be given to pregnant women or to persons with immunodeficiency syndromes. Vaccination of infants under 6 months of age should be avoided because the risk of encephalitis is greater for this age group. In persons with a history of egg allergy, vaccination should be avoided or a skin test should be performed to determine if there is a specific allergy to the material that would preclude vaccination.

THOMAS P. MONATH

Monath TP: Yellow fever. *In:* Warren KS, Mahmoud AF (eds): Tropical and Geographical Medicine. New York, McGraw-Hill, 1984, pp 636–651.
Monath TP, Craven RB, Adjukiewicz A, et al: Yellow fever in the Gambia, 1978–1979. Am J Trop Med Hyg 29:912, 1980.
Strode GK (ed): Yellow Fever. New York, McGraw-Hill, 1951.

11.81 DENGUE FEVER AND DENGUE-LIKE DISEASE

Dengue fever, a benign syndrome caused by several arthropod-borne viruses, is characterized by biphasic fever, myalgia or arthralgia, rash, leukopenia, and lymphadenopathy.

History. Epidemic dengue-like disease was described by David Bylon in Java in 1779 and a year later in Philadelphia by Benjamin Rush. Epidemics were common in temperate areas of the Americas, Europe, Australia, and Asia until early in the 20th century. Dengue fever and dengue-like disease are now endemic in tropical Asia, Northern Australia, tropical Africa, the Caribbean, and Central and parts of South America. Dengue fever occurs frequently among travelers.

Etiology. There are at least four distinct antigenic types of dengue virus. In addition, three other arthropod-borne (arbo) viruses cause similar or identical febrile diseases with rash (Table 11–33).

Epidemiology. Dengue viruses are transmitted by mosquitoes of the Stegomyia family. *Aedes aegypti*, a daytime biting mosquito, is the principal vector and all four virus types have been recovered from it. In most tropical areas *Aedes aegypti* is highly urbanized, breeding in water stored for drinking or bathing or in rain water collected in any container. Dengue viruses have also been recovered from *Aedes albopictus*, and outbreaks in the Pacific area have been attributed to *Aedes scutellaris*. These species breed in water trapped in vegetation. In Malaysia, dengue may be maintained in a cycle involving canopy-feeding jungle monkeys and *Aedes niveus*, which feeds on both monkeys and man.

Dengue outbreaks in urban areas infested with *Aedes aegypti* may be explosive; up to 70–80% of the population may be involved. Because *Aedes aegypti* has a limited range, spread of an epidemic occurs mainly through viremic human beings and follows main lines of transportation. Sentinel cases may infect household mosquitoes, with a large number of nearly simultaneous secondary infections giving the appearance of a contagious disease. Where dengue is endemic, children and susceptible foreigners may be the only persons to acquire overt disease, adults having become immune.

Dengue-like diseases may occur in epidemics. Epidemiologic features depend upon the vectors and their geographic distribution (Table 11–33). Chikungunya virus is widespread in the most populous areas of the world. In Asia, *Aedes aegypti* is the principal vector; in Africa other Stegomyia may be important vectors. In Southeast Asia, dengue and chikungunya outbreaks occur concurrently. Outbreaks of o'nyong-nyong and West Nile fever usually involve villages or small towns, in contrast to the urban outbreaks of dengue and chikungunya.

Pathology. Insufficient pathologic material has been obtained from virologically confirmed cases of dengue fever to permit a comprehensive description. Fatalities are rare with chikungunya and West Nile infections; those recorded have

Table 11–33. **Vectors and Geographic Distribution of Dengue-Like Diseases**

Togavirus Genus	Virus and Disease	Vector	Geographic Distribution
Alphavirus	Chikungunya	*Aedes aegypti* *Aedes africanus*	Africa, India, Southeast Asia
Alphavirus	O'nyong-nyong	*Anopheles funestus*	East Africa
Flavivirus	West Nile fever	*Culex molestus* *Culex univittatus*	Africa, Middle East, India

been ascribed to viral encephalitis, hemorrhage, or febrile convulsions (Sec. 11.82).

Clinical Manifestations. Manifestations vary with age and from patient to patient. In infants and young children the disease may be undifferentiated or characterized by a 1–5 day fever, pharyngeal inflammation, rhinitis, and mild cough. In outbreaks a majority of infected older children and adults have most of the findings described below.

After an incubation period of 1–7 days there is a sudden onset of fever, which rapidly rises to 39.4–41.1° C (103–106° F), usually accompanied by frontal or retro-orbital headache. Occasionally, back pain precedes the fever. A *transient*, macular, generalized rash that blanches under pressure may be seen during the first 24–48 hr of fever. The pulse rate may be slow relative to the degree of fever. Myalgia or arthralgia occurs soon after the onset and increases in severity. Involvement of the joints may be particularly severe in patients with chikungunya or o'nyong-nyong infection. From the 2nd–6th days of fever, nausea and vomiting are apt to occur, and generalized lymphadenopathy, cutaneous hyperesthesia or hyperalgesia, taste aberrations, and pronounced anorexia may develop.

One to 2 days after defervescence a generalized, morbilliform, maculopapular rash appears, which spares the palms and soles. It disappears in 1–5 days; desquamation may occur. Rarely there is edema of the palms and soles. About the time this second rash appears, the body temperature, which has previously fallen to normal, may become slightly elevated and establish the biphasic temperature curve.

Epistaxis, petechiae, and purpuric lesions are uncommon but may occur at any stage. Swallowed blood from epistaxis, vomited or passed by rectum, may be erroneously interpreted as gastrointestinal bleeding. Convulsions may occur during high fever, especially with chikungunya fever.

Infrequently, after the febrile stage, prolonged asthenia, mental depression, bradycardia, and ventricular extrasystoles may occur in children.

Laboratory Data. Pancytopenia may occur on the 3rd–4th days of illness; neutropenia may persist or reappear during the latter stage of the disease and may continue into convalescence. White blood cell counts as low as 2000/mm³ have been recorded. Platelets rarely fall below 100,000 cells/mm³. Venous clotting, bleeding and prothrombin times, and plasma fibrinogen values are within normal ranges. The tourniquet test infrequently is positive. Mild acidosis, hemoconcentration, increased transaminase values, and hypoproteinemia may occur during primary dengue virus infections, particularly in infants. Sinus bradycardia, ectopic ventricular foci, flattened T waves, and prolongation of the P-R interval may be observed electrocardiographically.

Diagnosis and Differential Diagnosis. *Clinical diagnosis* derives from a high index of suspicion and a knowledge of the geographic distribution and environmental cycles of causal viruses. Exposure to dengue may occur in hotels and during daytime shopping trips in epidemic or endemic areas. *Differential diagnosis* includes a number of viral respiratory and influenza-like diseases and the early stages of malaria, scrub typhus, hepatitis, and leptospirosis. Abortive forms of

these latter diseases modified by therapy or vaccine may never evolve beyond a dengue-like stage.

Four arboviral diseases have dengue-like courses but without rash: Colorado tick fever, sandfly fever, Rift Valley fever, and Ross River fever. Colorado tick fever occurs sporadically among campers and hunters in the Western United States; sandfly fever in the Mediterranean region, the Middle East, southern Russia, and parts of the Indian subcontinent; Rift Valley fever in North, East, Central, and South Africa; and Ross River fever is endemic in much of eastern Australia with epidemic extension to Fiji. In adults, Ross River fever often produces protracted and crippling arthralgia involving weight-bearing joints.

Because clinical findings vary and there are many possible causative agents, the term "dengue-like disease" should be used until a specific diagnosis is established. *Etiologic diagnosis* can be made by serologic study or by isolation of the virus from blood monocytes or serum. Blood for comparative antibody and viral studies should be obtained during the febrile period, preferably early, and during the convalescent phase, 14–21 days after onset. The acute phase serum or plasma may be frozen, optimally at −65° C or colder. Leukocytes should be refrigerated, not frozen. *Serologic diagnosis* depends on a 4-fold or greater increase in antibody titer in paired sera by hemagglutination-inhibition, complement-fixation, enzyme immunoassay, or neutralization test. It may not be possible to distinguish the infecting virus by serologic methods alone, particularly when there has been prior infection with another member of the same arbovirus group. Virus can be recovered from tissue culture or after intrathoracic inoculation of appropriate mosquitoes.

Prevention and Control. An attenuated vaccine for dengue type 1 and a killed vaccine for chikungunya are efficacious but not generally available. Prophylaxis consists of avoiding mosquito bite by use of insecticides, repellents, body-covering with clothing, screening of houses, and destruction of *Aedes aegypti* breeding sites. If water storage is mandatory, a tight-fitting lid or a thin layer of oil may prevent egg-laying or hatching. A larvicide, such as Abate [O,O'-(thiodi-p-phenylene) O,O,O'-tetramethyl phosphorothioate], available as a 1% sand-granule formation and effective at a concentration of 1 part/million, may be added safely to drinking water. Ultra-low-volume spray equipment effectively dispenses the adulticide malathion from truck or airplane for rapid intervention during an epidemic. Only personal antimosquito measures are effective against mosquitoes in the field, forest, or jungle.

Treatment. Treatment is supportive. Bed rest is advised during the febrile period. Antipyretics or cold sponging should be used to keep body temperature below 40° C (104° F). Analgesics or mild sedation may be required to control pain. Because of its effects on hemostasis, aspirin should not be used. Fluid and electrolyte replacement is required when there are deficits due to sweating, fasting, thirsting, vomiting, or diarrhea.

Prognosis. Primary infections with dengue fever and dengue-like diseases are usually self-limited and benign. Fluid and electrolyte losses, hyperpyrexia, and febrile convulsions are the most frequent complications in infants and young children. The prognosis may be adversely affected by passively acquired antibody or by prior infection with a closely related virus (Sec. 11.82).

Dengue in the Caribbean, 1977. Scientific Publication No. 375. Washington, D.C., Pan American Health Organization, 1979.

Halstead SB: Dengue: hematologic aspects. Semin Hematol 19:116, 1982.

Halstead SB: Selective primary health care: Strategies for control of disease in the developing world. XI. Dengue. Rev Infect Dis 6:251, 1984.

Schlesinger RW: Dengue Viruses. Virology Monograph 16. New York, Springer Verlag, 1977.

11.82 DENGUE HEMORRHAGIC FEVER/DENGUE SHOCK SYNDROME

(Philippine, Thai, or Singapore Hemorrhagic Fever; Hemorrhagic Dengue; Acute Infectious Thrombocytopenic Purpura)

Dengue hemorrhagic fever, a severe, often fatal, febrile disease caused by dengue viruses, is characterized by capillary permeability, abnormalities of hemostasis, and, in severe cases, a protein-losing shock syndrome. It is currently thought to have an immunopathologic basis.

Etiology. At least four distinct types of dengue virus (types 1–4) have been isolated from patients with hemorrhagic fever.

Epidemiology. Dengue hemorrhagic fever occurs where multiple types of dengue virus are simultaneously or sequentially transmitted. It is almost exclusively a disease of children. It is endemic in tropical Asia, where warm temperatures and the practice of water storage in homes result in large, permanent populations of *Aedes aegypti*. Under these conditions infections with dengue viruses of all types are common, and second infections with heterologous types are frequent. After 1 yr of age, 99% of patients with dengue shock syndrome have a secondary rise of antibody against dengue virus, indicating a previous infection with a closely related virus. Dengue hemorrhagic fever may occur during primary dengue infections, most frequently in infants whose mothers are immune to dengue.

In 1981 more than 10,000 children and adults were hospitalized in Cuba with dengue shock syndrome, and 158 died. The outbreak was caused by dengue 2, which had been preceded by an epidemic of dengue 1 in 1977. Severe cases occurred in individuals experiencing 2nd infections.

Nonimmune foreigners, adults or children, exposed to dengue virus during outbreaks of hemorrhagic fever have classic dengue fever or even milder disease. The differences in clinical manifestations of dengue infections between natives and foreigners in Southeast Asia are related more to immunologic status than to racial susceptibility. However, in the Cuban outbreak, dengue hemorrhagic fever/dengue shock syndrome attack rates were low in black children, possibly explaining the seeming absence of the syndrome in dengue-endemic areas of Africa.

Pathology. Usually no pathologic lesions are found to account for death. In rare instances, death may be due to gastrointestinal or intracranial hemorrhages. Minimal to moderate hemorrhages are seen in the upper gastrointestinal tract, and petechial hemorrhages are common in the interventricular septum of the heart, on the pericardium, and on the subserosal surfaces of major viscera. Focal hemorrhages are occasionally seen in the lungs, liver, adrenals, and subarachnoid space. The liver is usually enlarged, often with fatty changes. Yellow, watery, at times blood-tinged effusions are present in serous cavities in about three fourths of patients.

Microscopically, there is perivascular edema in the soft tissues and widespread diapedesis of red blood cells. There may be maturational arrest of megakaryocytes in bone marrow, and increased numbers of them are seen in capillaries

of the lungs, in renal glomeruli, and in sinusoids of the liver and spleen. Proliferation of lymphocytoid and plasmacytoid cells, lymphocytolysis, and lymphophagocytosis occur in the spleen and lymph nodes. In the spleen the germinal centers of the malpighian corpuscles are active and often necrotic. The thymus is depleted of lymphocytes. The liver shows varying degrees of fatty metamorphosis, focal midzonal necrosis, and hyperplasia of the Kupffer cells; there are non-nucleated cells with vacuolated acidophilic cytoplasm, resembling Councilman bodies, in the sinusoids. There is a mild proliferative glomerulonephritis. Biopsies of the rash reveal swelling and minimal necrosis of endothelial cells and subcutaneous deposits of fibrinogen. Dengue viral antigen has been found in extravascular mononuclear cells; on blood vessel walls; in Kupffer cells; in splenic, thymic, and lung macrophages; and in skin histiocytes.

Dengue virus is almost invariably absent in tissues at the time of death, with rare isolations reported from lymphatic tissues usually in infants under 1 yr who have experienced primary infections.

Pathogenesis. The pathogenesis is incompletely understood; epidemiologic studies suggest that it is usually associated with dengue type 2 infections. It is possible that prior exposure may promote cellular infection and enhance severity of the disease. Dengue 2 virus demonstrates enhanced growth in cultures of human mononuclear phagocytes prepared from dengue-immune donors or in cultures supplemented with non-neutralizing dengue antibody. Early in the acute stage of secondary dengue infections, there is rapid activation of the complement system. During shock, blood levels of C1q, C3, C4, C5–8, and C3 proactivator are depressed and C3 catabolic rates elevated. The blood clotting and fibrinolytic systems are activated and levels of factor XII (Hageman factor) depressed. Shock may be mediated by histamine released from mast cells by the peptides C3a and C5a. As yet, however, no specific mediator of vascular permeability in dengue hemorrhagic fever has been identified. A mild degree of disseminated intravascular coagulation, liver damage, and thrombocytopenia may produce hemorrhage synergistically. Capillary damage allows fluid, electrolytes, protein, and, in some instances, red blood cells to leak into extravascular spaces. This internal redistribution of fluid, together with deficits due to fasting, thirsting, and vomiting, results in hemoconcentration, hypovolemia, increased cardiac work, tissue hypoxia, metabolic acidosis, and hyponatremia.

Clinical Manifestations. The incubation period of dengue hemorrhagic fever is presumed to be that of dengue fever. The course is characteristic in the severely ill child. A relatively mild 1st phase with abrupt onset of fever, malaise, vomiting, headache, anorexia, and cough is followed after 2–5 days by rapid clinical deterioration and collapse. In this 2nd phase the patient usually has cold, clammy extremities, a warm trunk, flushed face, diaphoresis, restlessness, irritability, and mid-epigastric pain. Frequently, there are scattered petechiae on the forehead and extremities; spontaneous ecchymoses may appear, and easy bruisability and bleeding at sites of venipuncture are common. A macular or maculopapular rash may appear, and there may be circumoral and peripheral cyanosis. Respirations are rapid and often labored. The pulse is weak, rapid, and thready and the heart sounds faint. The liver may enlarge to 4–6 cm below the costal margin and is usually firm and somewhat tender. Fewer than 10% of patients have gross ecchymosis or gastrointestinal bleeding, usually following a period of uncorrected shock.

After a 24–36 hr period of crisis, convalescence is fairly rapid in the children who recover. The temperature may return to normal before or during the stage of shock. Bradycardia and ventricular extrasystoles are common during convalescence. Infrequently, there is residual brain damage due to prolonged shock or occasionally to intracranial hemorrhage.

In contrast to the fairly characteristic pattern in the severely ill child, secondary dengue infections are relatively mild in the majority of instances, ranging from an inapparent infection through an undifferentiated upper respiratory or dengue-like disease to an illness similar to that described above but without apparent shock.

Laboratory Data. The most common hematologic abnormalities during clinical shock are a 20% or greater increase in hematocrit over the recovery value, thrombocytopenia, mild leukocytosis (seldom exceeding 10,000/mm^3), prolonged bleeding time, and moderately decreased prothrombin level (seldom to less than 40% of control). Fibrinogen levels may be subnormal and fibrin split-products elevated.

Other abnormalities include moderate elevations of the serum transaminases, mild metabolic acidosis with hyponatremia, and, at times, hypochloremia, slight elevation of serum urea nitrogen, and hypoalbuminemia. Roentgenograms of the chest reveal pleural effusions in nearly all patients.

Diagnosis and Differential Diagnosis. In endemic areas hemorrhagic fever should be suspected in children having a febrile illness who exhibit a positive tourniquet test, hemoconcentration, thrombocytopenia, and hemorrhagic manifestations with or without shock. Appearance of pleural or peritoneal effusions and signs of shock are pathognomonic. Since many rickettsial diseases, meningococcemia, and other severe illnesses caused by a variety of agents may produce a similar clinical picture, the etiologic diagnosis should be made only when epidemiologic or serologic evidence suggests the possibility of dengue fever. Hemorrhagic manifestations have been described in other diseases of viral or presumed viral origin, including the clinically distinguishable hemorrhagic fevers described in Sec. 11.83.

In secondary dengue infections, there is a rapid and pronounced rise of both hemagglutination-inhibiting (HI) and complement-fixing (CF) antibodies to dengue antigen. There are usually high titers of HI antibody (1:640 or greater) and CF antibody (1:32 or greater) in both acute and convalescent serums. Antibodies of IgG class dominate in paired sera.

Prevention. Preventive measures are described in Sec. 11.81. The possibility exists that dengue vaccination may sensitize a recipient so that ensuing dengue infection may result in hemorrhagic fever. Vaccination with yellow fever 17D strain has no effect on the severity of dengue illness, although seroconversion rates to a dengue 2 vaccine were enhanced in yellow fever–immune persons.

Treatment. Management requires immediate evaluation of vital signs and degrees of hemoconcentration, dehydration, and electrolyte imbalance. Close monitoring is essential for at least 48 hr since shock may occur or recur precipitously early in the disease. Patients who are cyanotic or have labored breathing should be given oxygen. Rapid intravenous replacement of fluids and electrolytes can frequently sustain patients until spontaneous recovery occurs. When elevation of the hematocrit persists after replacement of fluids, plasma or plasma colloid preparations are indicated. Care must be taken to avoid overhydration, which may contribute to cardiac failure. Transfusions of fresh blood or of platelets suspended in plasma may be required to control bleeding; they should not be given during hemoconcentration but only after evaluation of hemoglobin or hematocrit values. Salicylates are contraindicated because of their effect on blood clotting.

Paraldehyde or chloral hydrate may be required for children who are markedly agitated. Use of pressor amines, α-adrenergic blocking agents, and aldosterone has not resulted in a significant reduction of mortality compared with that observed with simple supportive therapy. See Sec. 15.50 for treatment of disseminated intravascular coagulation. Steroids do not shorten the duration of disease or improve prognosis in children receiving careful supportive therapy.

Hypervolemia during the fluid reabsorptive phase may be life-threatening and is heralded by a fall in hematocrit with wide pulse pressure. Diuretics and digitalization may be necessary.

Prognosis. Death has occurred in 40–50% of patients with shock, but with adequate intensive care deaths should be less than 2%. Survival is directly related to early and intense management.

Bokisch VA, Top FH Jr, Russell PK, et al: The potential pathogenic role of complement in dengue hemorrhagic shock syndrome. N Engl J Med 289:996, 1973.

Cohen SN, Halstead SB: Shock associated with dengue infection. I. The clinical and physiological manifestations of dengue hemorrhagic fever in Thailand, 1964. J Pediatr 68:448, 1966.

Halstead SB: Dengue hemorrhagic fever, a public health problem and a field for research. Bull WHO 58:1, 1980.

Halstead SB: The pathogenesis of dengue. Molecular epidemiology in infectious disease. The Alexander D. Langmuir Lecture. Am J Epidemiol 114:632, 1981.

Halstead SB: Immune enhancement of viral infection. Prog Allergy 31:301, 1982.

Sangkawibha N, Rojanasuphat S, Ahandrik S, et al: Risk factors in dengue shock syndrome: A prospective epidemiologic study in Rayong, Thailand. I. The 1980 outbreak. Am J Epidemiol 1201:653, 1984.

Technical Guides for Diagnosis, Treatment, Surveillance, Prevention and Control of Dengue Haemorrhagic Fever. Geneva, World Health Organization, 1980.

11.83 OTHER VIRAL HEMORRHAGIC FEVERS

Viral hemorrhagic fevers are a loosely defined group of clinical syndromes in which hemorrhagic manifestations are either common or especially notable in severe illness. Both the etiologic agents and clinical features of the syndromes differ, but disseminated intravascular coagulation may be a common pathogenetic feature. A list of the more important viral hemorrhagic fevers is given in Table 11–34. Many other viral diseases may occasionally have similar hemorrhagic manifestations.

Etiology. Six of the viral hemorrhagic fevers are caused by arthropod-borne (arbo) viruses (Table 11–34). Four are togaviruses of the flavivirus group (KFD, OHF, DHF, and YF), and three are bunyaviruses (Congo, Hantaan, and RVF). Junin (AHF), Machupo (BHF), and Lassa (LF) are arenaviruses, a morphologic and ecologic viral group. Ebola (EHF) and Marburg viruses are enveloped, filamentous RNA viruses, which are sometimes branched, unlike any other known virus, and which are now termed filoviruses.

Epidemiology. With rare exceptions, the viruses causing viral hemorrhagic fevers are initially transmitted through a nonhuman agency. Since a specific ecosystem is required for viral survival, these are diseases of place. Although it is commonly thought that all viral hemorrhagic fevers are arthropod-borne, eight may be contracted from environmental contamination caused by animals or animal cells or from infected humans (RVF, AHF, BHF, CHF, LF, Marburg disease, EHF, and HFRS). Laboratory and hospital infections have occurred with many of these agents. Lassa fever and Argentine and Bolivian hemorrhagic fevers are reportedly milder in children than in adults. Dengue hemorrhagic fever (Sec. 11.82) and yellow fever (Sec. 11.80) are well-established pediatric problems. Features of the more common viral hemorrhagic fevers are summarized below.

Tick-Borne Hemorrhagic Fevers. CONGO-CRIMEAN HEMORRHAGIC FEVER (CHF). Sporadic human infection in Africa provided the original virus isolation. Natural foci are recognized in Bulgaria, western Crimea, and the Rostov-on-Don and Astrakhan regions; a somewhat similar disease occurs in Kazakstan and Uzbekistan. Index cases were followed by nosocomial transmission in Pakistan and Afghanistan in 1976, in the Arabian peninsula in 1983, and in South Africa in 1984. In the Soviet Union the vectors are *Hyaloma marginatum* and

Table 11–34. **Viral Hemorrhagic Fevers**

Mode of Transmission	Disease	Virus
Tick-borne	Congo-Crimean HF (CHF)* Kyasanur Forest disease (KFD) Omsk HF (OHF)	Congo Kyasanur Forest disease Omsk
Mosquito-borne†	Dengue HF (DHF) Rift Valley fever (RVF) Yellow fever (YF)	Dengue (4 types) Rift Valley fever Yellow fever
Infected animals or materials to humans	Argentine HF (AHF) Bolivian HF (BHF) Lassa fever (LF)* Marburg disease* Ebola HF (EHF)* Hemorrhagic fever with renal syndrome (HFRS)	Junin Machupo Lassa Marburg Ebola Hantaan

*Patients may be contagious; nosocomial infections are common.
†Chikungunya virus (Sec. 11.81) is associated at low frequency with petechiae, petechial hemorrhages, and epistaxis. More severe hemorrhagic manifestations have been reported in some studies.

H. anatolicum, which, along with hares and birds, may serve as viral reservoirs. Disease occurs from June to September, largely among farmers and dairy workers.

KYASANUR FOREST DISEASE (KFD). Human cases occur chiefly in adults in an area of Mysore State, India. The main vectors are two Ixodidae ticks, *Haemaphysalis turturis* and *H. spinigera.* Monkeys and forest rodents may be amplifying hosts. Laboratory infections are common.

OMSK HEMORRHAGIC FEVER (OHF). The disease occurs throughout the south central Soviet Union and in northern Rumania. Vectors may include *Dermacentor pictus* and *D. marginatus,* but direct transmission from moles and muskrats to humans seems well established. Human disease occurs in a spring-summer-autumn pattern, paralleling the activity of vectors. Omsk hemorrhagic fever occurs most frequently in persons with outdoor occupational exposure. Laboratory infections are common.

Mosquito-Borne Hemorrhagic Fevers. DENGUE HEMORRHAGIC FEVER AND YELLOW FEVER (DHF AND YF). See Sec. 11.82 and 11.80.

RIFT VALLEY FEVER (RVF). The virus causing Rift Valley fever is responsible for epizootics involving sheep, cattle, buffalo, certain antelopes, and rodents in North, Central, East, and South Africa. The virus is transmitted to domestic animals by *Culex theileri* and several *Aedes* species. Mosquitoes may serve as reservoirs by transovarial transmission. An epizootic in Egypt in 1977–78 was accompanied by thousands of human infections, principally among veterinarians, farmers, and farm laborers. Humans are most often infected during the slaughter or skinning of sick or dead animals. Laboratory infection is common.

Hemorrhagic Fever Transmitted Through Environmental Contamination. ARENAVIRAL DISEASE. The prototype arenavirus, lymphocytic choriomeningitis virus, establishes a persistent, tolerated infection in the young of the common house mouse, *Mus musculus,* which excretes virus continuously throughout life, contaminating food and fluids and creating a risk of airborne infection. There is evidence that Machupo and Junin viruses have similar host-parasite relationships with South American rodents as the Lassa virus has with African rodents.

ARGENTINE HEMORRHAGIC FEVER (AHF). Hundreds to thousands of cases occur annually from April through July in the maize-producing area northwest of Buenos Aires that reaches to the eastern margin of the Province of Cordoba. Junin virus has been isolated from the rodents *Mus musculus, Akodon*

arenicola, and *Calomys laucha laucha.* It infects migrant laborers who harvest the maize and who inhabit rodent-contaminated shelters.

BOLIVIAN HEMORRHAGIC FEVER (BHF). The recognized endemic area consists of the sparsely populated province of Beni in Amazonian Bolivia. Sporadic cases occur in farm families who raise maize, rice, yucca, and beans. In the town of San Joaquin a disturbance in the domestic rodent ecosystem may have led to an outbreak of household infection caused by *Calomys callosus,* ordinarily a field rodent. Mortality rates are high in young children.

LASSA FEVER (LF). Lassa virus has an unusual potential for human-to-human spread and has resulted in many small epidemics in Nigeria, Sierra Leone, and Liberia. Medical workers in Africa and the United States have also contracted the disease. Patients with acute Lassa fever have been transported by international aircraft, necessitating extensive surveillance among passengers and crews. The virus is probably maintained in nature in a species of African house rat, *Mastomys natalensis.* Rodent-to-rodent transmission and infection of humans probably operate via mechanisms established for other arenaviruses.

MARBURG DISEASE. Until recently, the world experience has been limited to 26 primary and 5 secondary cases in Germany and Yugoslavia in 1967 and to small outbreaks in Zimbabwe in 1975, in Kenya in 1980, and in South Africa in 1983. Transmission occurs by direct contact with tissues of the African green monkey, with infected blood, or with human semen. The reservoir and mode of transmission of the virus in nature are unknown.

EBOLA HEMORRHAGIC FEVER. Ebola virus was isolated in 1976 from a devastating epidemic involving small villages in northern Zaire and southern Sudan; smaller outbreaks have occurred subsequently. Outbreaks initially have been nosocomial. Attack rates have been highest in the 0–1 yr and 15–50 yr age groups. The virus resembles Marburg virus. The vertebrate reservoir and mode of transmission to man are unknown.

HEMORRHAGIC FEVER WITH RENAL SYNDROME (Epidemic Hemorrhagic Fever; Korean Hemorrhagic Fever). The endemic area includes Japan, Korea, far eastern Siberia, north and central China, European and Asian Russia, Scandinavia, Czechoslovakia, Rumania, and Bulgaria. Although the incidence and severity of hemorrhagic manifestations and the mortality are lower in Europe than in northeast Asia, the renal lesion is the same. Disease in Scandinavia, nephropathia epidemica, is caused by a different although antigenically related virus associated with *Clethrionomys glariolus*. Cases occur predominantly in the spring and summer. There appears to be no age factor in susceptibility, but because of occupational hazards, young adult men are most frequently attacked. Rodent plagues or evidences of rodent infestation have accompanied endemic and epidemic occurrences. Hantaan virus has been detected in lung tissue and excreta of *Apodemus agrarius coreae*. Antigenically related agents have been detected in laboratory rats, in urban rat populations around the world, and in the wild rodent *Microtus pennsylvanicus* in North America (Prospect Hill Virus). *Rodent-to-rodent and rodent-to-man transmission presumably occurs via the respiratory route.*

Clinical, Pathologic, and Laboratory Features. OMSK HEMORRHAGIC FEVER AND KYASANUR FOREST DISEASE. After an incubation period of 3–8 days, both diseases begin with sudden onset of fever and headache. In Omsk hemorrhagic fever there is moderate epistaxis, hematemesis, and a hemorrhagic enanthem but no profuse hemorrhage; bronchopneumonia is common. Kyasanur forest disease is characterized by severe myalgia, prostration, and bronchiolar involvement; it often presents without hemorrhage, but occasionally with severe gastrointestinal bleeding. Severe leukopenia and thrombocytopenia occur in both diseases. In many patients recurrent febrile illness may follow an afebrile period of 7–15 days. This second phase takes the form of a meningoencephalitis.

In Kyasanur forest disease, acute degeneration of renal tubules may correlate with the urinary changes noted. There may be focal liver damage. In both diseases vascular dilatation, increased vascular permeability, gastrointestinal hemorrhages, and subserosal and interstitial petechial hemorrhages occur.

CRIMEAN HEMORRHAGIC FEVER. The incubation period of 3–12 days is followed by a febrile period of 5–12 days and a prolonged convalescence. Illness begins suddenly with fever, severe headache, myalgia, abdominal pain, anorexia, nausea, and vomiting. After a day or more fever may subside until the patient develops an erythematous facial or truncal flush and injected conjunctivae. A second febrile period of 2–6 days then develops with a hemorrhagic enanthem on the soft palate and a fine petechial rash on the chest and abdomen. Less frequently, there are large areas of purpura and bleeding from gums, nose, intestine, lungs, or uterus. Hematuria and proteinuria are relatively rare. During the hemorrhagic stage there is usually tachycardia with weak heart sounds, and in some cases hypotension occurs. The liver is usually enlarged, but there is no icterus. In protracted cases central nervous system signs may include delirium, somnolence, and progressive clouding of consciousness. In convalescence there may be hearing and memory loss. Mortality ranges from 2–50%. Early in the disease leukopenia with relative lymphocytosis, progressively worsening thrombocytopenia, and gradually increasing anemia occur.

RIFT VALLEY FEVER (RVF). Most infections have been in adults, in whom disease is dengue-like. Onset is acute, with fever, headache, prostration, myalgia, anorexia, nausea, vomiting, conjunctivitis, and lymphadenopathy. The fever lasts 3–6 days and is often biphasic. Convalescence is often prolonged. In the 1977–78 outbreak, many patients died after showing signs including purpura, epistaxis, hematemesis, and melena. At autopsy there was extensive eosinophilic degeneration of the parenchymal cells of the liver.

ARGENTINE AND BOLIVIAN HEMORRHAGIC FEVER AND LASSA FEVER. The incubation period is commonly 7–14 days; the acute illness lasts for 2–4 wk. Clinical illnesses range from undifferentiated fever to the characteristic severe illness. Lassa fever is most often clinically severe in Caucasian subjects. Onset is usually gradual, with increasing fever, headache, diffuse myalgia, and anorexia. During the 1st wk there are frequently a sore throat, dysphagia, cough, oropharyngeal ulcers, nausea, vomiting, diarrhea, and pains in chest and abdomen. Pleuritic chest pain may persist into the 2nd–3rd wk of illness. In Argentine and Bolivian hemorrhagic fevers and less frequently in Lassa fever, a petechial enanthem appears on the soft palate 3–5 days after onset and at about the same time on the trunk. The tourniquet test may be positive.

In 35–50% of all patients these diseases may become severe, with persistent high fever, increasing toxicity, swelling of face or neck, microscopic hematuria, and frank hemorrhages from the stomach, intestines, nose, gums, and uterus. A syndrome of hypovolemic shock is accompanied by pleural effusion and renal failure. Respiratory distress due to outlet obstruction, pleural effusion, or congestive heart failure may occur. Ten to 20% of patients develop late neurologic involvement characterized by intention tremor of the tongue and associated speech abnormalities. In severe cases there may be intention tremors of the extremities, seizures, and delirium. The cerebrospinal fluid is normal. Prolonged convalescence is accompanied by alopecia and in Argentine and Bolivian hemorrhagic fevers by signs of autonomic nervous system lability, such as postural hypotension, spontaneous flushing or blanching of the skin, and intermittent diaphoresis.

Laboratory studies reveal marked leukopenia, mild to moderate thrombocytopenia, proteinuria, and, in Argentine hemorrhagic fever, moderate abnormalities in blood clotting, decreased fibrinogen, increased fibrinogen split-products, and elevated serum transaminases. Pathologically, there is focal, often extensive eosinophilic necrosis of liver parenchyma, focal interstitial pneumonitis, focal necrosis of the distal and collecting tubules, and partial replacement of splenic follicles by amorphous eosinophilic material. Usually bleeding occurs by diapedesis with little inflammatory reaction. Mortality is 10–40%.

MARBURG DISEASE AND EBOLA HEMORRHAGIC FEVER. After an incubation period of 4–7 days, illness begins abruptly with severe frontal headache, malaise, drowsiness, lumbar myalgia, vomiting, nausea, and diarrhea. Five to 7 days later a papular eruption begins on the trunk and upper arms; becomes generalized, often hemorrhagic, and maculopapular; and exfoliates during convalescence. The exanthem is accompanied by a dark red enanthem on the hard palate, conjunctivitis, and scrotal or labial edema. Gastrointestinal hemorrhage occurs as the severity of illness increases. Late in the illness, the patient may become tearfully depressed with marked hyperalgesia to tactile stimuli. In fatal cases, patients become hypotensive, restless, and confused and lapse into coma. Convalescent patients may develop alopecia and have paresthesias of the back and trunk. There is a marked leukopenia with necrosis of granulocytes. Disseminated intravascular coagulation and thrombocytopenia are universal and correlate with severity of disease; there are moderate abnormalities in clotting proteins and elevated serum transaminases and amylase. The mortality of Marburg disease is 25%; that of Ebola hemorrhagic fever, 50–90%.

HEMORRHAGIC FEVER WITH RENAL SYNDROME (HFRS). In most cases HFRS is characterized by fever, petechiae, mild hemorrhagic phenomena, and mild proteinuria, followed by relatively uneventful recovery. In 20% of recognized cases the disease may progress through 4 rather distinct phases. The *febrile phase* is ushered in with fever, malaise, and facial and truncal flushing, lasts 3–8 days, and ends with thrombocytopenia, petechiae, and proteinuria. The *hypotensive phase* of 1–3 days follows defervescence. Loss of fluid from the intravascular compartment may result in marked hemoconcentration. Proteinuria and ecchymoses increase. The *oliguric phase*, usually 3–5 days in duration, is characterized by a low output of protein-rich urine, increasing nitrogen retention, nausea, vomiting, and dehydration. Confusion, extreme restlessness, and hypertension are common. The *diuretic phase*, which may last for days or weeks, usually initiates clinical improvement. The kidneys show little concentrating ability, and rapid loss of fluid may result in severe dehydration and shock. Potassium and sodium depletion may be severe. Fatal cases manifest abundant protein-rich retroperitoneal edema and marked hemorrhagic necrosis of the renal medulla. Mortality is 5–10%.

Diagnosis. Diagnosis depends upon a high index of suspicion in endemic areas. In nonendemic areas histories of recent travel, recent laboratory exposure, or exposure to an earlier case should evoke suspicion of viral hemorrhagic fever.

In all viral hemorrhagic fevers the viral agent circulates in the blood at least transiently during the early febrile stage. The diagnostic specimens required for togaviruses and bunyaviruses are the same as those described in Sec. 11.81 for dengue fever. The principles for etiologic diagnosis of Argentine and Bolivian hemorrhagic fevers are similar; acute phase blood or throat washings from patients can be inoculated intracerebrally into guinea pigs, infant hamsters, or infant mice. Lassa virus may be isolated from the same specimens by inoculation into tissue cultures. In arenavirus infections, group-reactive complement-fixing antibodies and specific neutralizing antibodies appear in convalescent serum 3–4 wk after onset of illness. For Marburg disease and EHF, acute-phase throat washings, blood, and urine may be inoculated into tissue culture, guinea pigs, or monkeys. The virus is readily visualized by electron microscopy, its filamentous structure differentiating it from all other known agents. Specific complement-fixing and immunofluorescent antibodies appear during convalescence. The virus of HFRS is recovered from acute phase serum or urine by inoculating susceptible tissue cultures and identifying virus by use of fluorescent antibody, enzyme immunoassay, or neutralization tests.

Handling blood and other biologic specimens is hazardous and must be left to specially trained personnel. Blood and autopsy specimens should be placed in tightly sealed metal containers, wrapped in absorbent material inside a sealed plastic bag, and shipped on dry ice to laboratories with biocontainment level 4 facilities. Even routine hematologic and biochemical tests should be done with extreme caution.

Differential Diagnosis. Mild cases of hemorrhagic fever may be confused with almost any self-limited systemic bacterial or viral infection. More severe cases may suggest typhoid fever, epidemic, murine, or scrub typhus, leptospirosis, or a rickettsial spotted fever, for which, with the exception of leptospirosis, effective chemotherapeutic agents are available. Many of them may be acquired in geographic or ecologic locations similar to those that may provide exposure to a viral hemorrhagic fever.

Prevention. A form of inactivated mouse brain vaccine is said to be effective in preventing Omsk hemorrhagic fever. Inactivated Rift Valley fever vaccines are widely used to protect domestic animals and laboratory workers. Prevention of transmission by ticks includes careful examination of the skin after exposure with removal of any vectors found. Tight-fitting clothing that fully covers the extremities is helpful, as is the use of tick repellents. Disease transmitted from a rodent-infected environment can be prevented through methods of rodent control; elimination of refuse and breeding sites is particularly successful in urban or suburban areas. Congo-Crimean hemorrhagic fever, Lassa fever, Marburg disease, and Ebola hemorrhagic fever may be transmitted in hospital settings. Patients should be isolated until virus-free or for 3 wk following illness. Patients' urine, sputum, blood, clothing, and bedding should be disinfected. Disposable syringes and needles should be used. Prompt and strict enforcement of barrier nursing may be lifesaving. Case fatality among medical workers contracting these diseases is presently 50%.

Treatment. The principle involved in all these diseases, especially hemorrhagic fever with renal syndrome, is the reversal of dehydration, hemoconcentration, renal failure, and protein, electrolyte, or blood losses. The contribution of disseminated intravascular coagulation to the hemorrhagic manifestations is unknown, and the management of hemorrhage should be individualized. Transfusions of fresh blood and platelets are frequently given. Good results have been reported in a few cases following the administration of clotting factor concentrates. The efficacy of steroids, ε-aminocaproic acid, pressor amines, or α-adrenergic blocking agents has not been established. Sedatives should be selected with regard to the possibility of kidney or liver damage. The successful management of hemorrhagic fever with renal syndrome may require renal dialysis. Dramatic improvement in some cases of Lassa fever has been reported following administration of Lassa immune serum free of infectious virus.* Ribavirin is presently being evaluated for efficacy in Lassa fever.

SCOTT B. HALSTEAD

Casals J, Henderson BE, Hoogstraal H, et al: A review of Soviet viral hemorrhagic fevers, 1969. J Infect Dis 122:437, 1970.
International symposium on arenaviral infections of public health importance, 14–16 July 1975. Bull WHO 52:381, 1975.
Johnson KM, Halstead SB, Cohen SN: Hemorrhagic fevers of Southeast Asia and South America, a comparative appraisal. Prog Med Virol 9:106, 1967.
Lee HW, Lee MC, Cho LS: Management of Korean hemorrhagic fever. Med Prog Sept:15, 1980.
Monath TP: Lassa fever and Marburg virus disease. WHO Chron 28:212, 1974.
Pattyn SR: (ed): Ebola Virus Haemorrhagic Fever. Amsterdam, Elsevier/North Holland, 1978.
Simpson DIH: Viral haemorrhagic fevers of man. Bull WHO 56:819, 1978.

11.84 CAT SCRATCH DISEASE
(Cat Scratch Fever, Felinosis, Benign Lymphoreticulosis)

Cat scratch disease is a self-limited, regional lymphadenitis of children and young adults that is preceded by a primary skin lesion caused by the bite or scratch of a cat.

Pathology. The microscopic appearance of the involved lymph nodes, although not diagnostic, is sufficiently characteristic to suggest cat scratch disease. Three pathologic states have been described, progressing from reticulum cell hyperplasia to tubercle-like granuloma, which often contains Langerhans giant cells, and finally to microabscess formation; all stages may occur within a single node.

Etiology. The etiologic agent(s) of cat scratch disease has not been conclusively established. However, investigators have recently identified small, pleomorphic, gram-negative, silver staining, non–acid-fast bacilli in the lymphatic tissue of affected children. The distinct appearance of these microorganisms, their intracellular location, their abundance during the early stages of lymphadenitis, and their apparently specific immunofluorescent staining properties by fluorescein-tagged convalescent serum from patients with cat scratch disease implicate them as etiologic agents.

Epidemiology. Cat scratch disease has been reported from most parts of the world, occurring most often in temperate climates between September and February. Eighty per cent of diagnosed cases occur in patients under 20 yr of age; 95% have a history of a cat scratch or contact. The disease also has been reported following the scratch or bite of dogs and monkeys. This illness is limited to man; cats transmitting the

---

*Serum or immune serum globulin and information concerning dosage schedules may be obtained from the Centers for Disease Control, Atlanta, Georgia, or the World Health Organization, Geneva, Switzerland.

disease show no apparent illness and yield no infectious agent. Person-to-person transmission has not been reported.

Clinical Manifestations. A primary skin lesion develops at the scratch site in 50% of patients approximately 10 days (range 7–56 days) following inoculation. This painless, non-pruritic erythematous papule may pustulate before healing without scar formation. Regional lymphadenopathy occurs within 2 wk (range 7–61 days) of the primary lesion. The involved nodes, which are superficial and may reach 8–10 cm in diameter, are painful during the early stages of the disease. The axillary and epitrochlear nodes are the most often involved, followed by lymph nodes of the head and neck and the lower extremity. Lymphangitis has not been observed. Suppuration of involved nodes occurs in 30% of cases. Within 4–6 wk the nodes become less tender, and regress within 8 wk in the majority of cases. Constitutional symptoms, including malaise, anorexia, fatigue, and low-grade fever, appear during the period of regional lymphadenopathy in half of the affected individuals. Laboratory studies are often normal, although mild elevations in the erythrocyte sedimentation rate and in the absolute eosinophil count have been reported. Atypical presentations may include unilateral swelling of the preauricular lymph node (Parinaud syndrome) or the parotid gland, erythema nodosum, osteolytic lesions, thrombocytopenia purpura, and encephalitis.

Diagnosis. The diagnosis in a child with regional lymphadenopathy is based on fulfillment of 3 of the 4 following criteria: (1) a history of animal (usually a cat) contact, scratch, bite, and/or primary cutaneous lesion; (2) aspiration of sterile pus from an involved node; (3) characteristic histopathologic changes in an involved lymph node; and (4) a positive Hanger-Rose skin test. The skin test antigen is not commercially available but can be prepared from purulent material obtained from patients with cat scratch disease. The bloodless pus is diluted, 1 part in 4 parts isotonic saline; cultured for bacteria, mycobacteria, and fungi; and incubated for 72 hr at 60° C to inactivate hepatitis virus. The antigen may be refrigerated ($-20°$ C) for several mo without loss of potency. The skin test is performed by injecting 0.1 mL of the antigen intradermally. A positive test is defined as 5 mm or more of induration, or 10 mm or more of erythema at 48 hr. Positive skin tests have been observed in 90% of patients with cat scratch disease and in 5% of unaffected controls. Skin tests remain positive for years and rarely may produce an exacerbation of the disease consisting of worsening of systemic symptoms and transient enlargement of involved nodes.

Differential Diagnosis. Cat scratch disease must be differentiated from pyogenic, fungal, and tuberculous adenitis, atypical mycobacterial infection, brucellosis, plague, tularemia, lymphogranuloma venereum, rat bite fever, sarcoidosis, and lymphoma.

Treatment and Prognosis. This benign illness has an excellent prognosis. Aspiration may be indicated to resolve symptoms when the involved nodes become large, fluctuant, and extremely painful.

WILLIAM T. SPECK

Margileth AM: Cat scratch disease: Nonbacterial regional lymphadenitis. Pediatrics 42:803, 1968.
Wear DJ, Margileth AM, Hadfield TL, et al: Cat scratch disease: A bacterial infection. Science 221:1403, 1983.

11.85 RICKETTSIAE

Rickettsiae are small, fastidious, coccobacillary organisms with an ultrastructure closely resembling that of other gram-negative bacteria. They contain both RNA and DNA, divide by binary fission, and are inhibited by broad-spectrum antibiotics. Rickettsiae are unusual bacteria, however, in that they have an incomplete cell wall through which in the course of ontogeny they have lost essential enzymes; they therefore require an intracellular site for replication.

Rickettsiae are transmitted among mammal reservoirs by arthropod vectors. Humans are not an essential link in their natural cycle and become chance hosts when they are bitten by an infected vector or inhale the desiccated organism.

The rickettsial diseases of humans are separated into groups on the basis of clinical characteristics, insect vectors, etiologic agent, and epidemiology (Table 11–35). Rocky Mountain spotted fever is the rickettsial infection most frequently reported in the United States and accounts for nearly 90% of approximately 1000 cases/yr; small outbreaks of murine typhus, Q fever, rickettsialpox, and epidemic typhus make up the rest. In addition, occasional cases of boutonneuse or other spotted fevers are serologically confirmed in travelers who have been in Africa or to the Mediterranean. The presence of indigenous reservoirs and vectors, plus the continuous possibility of introduction of new strains of rickettsiae from other parts of the world, make the threat of new outbreaks in the United States a continuing concern. Tsutsugamushi fever (scrub typhus) occurs in areas of Japan and among the populations of India, Australia, Indonesia, and Malaya; it continues to be a hazard to those who enter endemic areas. Effective rickettsial vaccines are not available.

Pathogenesis. The fundamental lesion in rickettsial disease is a mononuclear vasculitis of small vessels with swollen endothelial cells and infiltration of the media, adventitia, and perivascular space. Any vessels may become involved, but those in skin, subcutaneous tissue, and brain are most commonly affected. In spotted fever, rickettsiae invade the media; in typhus, the endothelium is the site where organisms are found. Involved vessels have increased permeability resulting in local edema, diminished plasma volume, poor perfusion, and inadequate renal function. Thrombosis occurs in some vessels and the location and size of the resulting areas of infarction influence the type and severity of clinical manifestations. Various factors play a role in producing the vascular damage, including direct effect by invading rickettsiae, endotoxins or exotoxins, antibody- and cell-mediated immune mechanisms, and competition for essential nutrients by organism and host cell.

Q fever, which is not accompanied by a rash and does not require an insect vector, differs pathologically from the other rickettsial diseases. The principal, and usually the only, lesions occur in the lungs, where there is a patchy interstitial pneumonitis with copious exudate composed of fibrin and mononuclear cells. Alveolar walls, alveolar ducts, and terminal bronchioles are infiltrated by large, mononuclear cells.

Diagnosis. Human rickettsial infection is diagnosed early and most readily by the demonstration of specific rickettsial antigen in specimens of involved skin obtained by biopsy. Late diagnosis can be made by serologic tests employing either cross-reactive *Proteus* antigens or specific rickettsial reagents.

Immunofluorescent demonstration of rickettsiae in a typical petechial lesion stained with fluorescein isothiocyanate–labeled antibody reveals coccobacillary forms. This method has high specificity and reasonably good sensitivity; false negatives may occur if a vascular lesion is not included in the biopsy or if the patient has been treated with broad-spectrum antibiotics for 24 hr or longer. Antibiotic treatment should be started if the test is positive; if it is negative, the decision should be based on the overall clinical picture.

Serologic diagnosis (Weil-Felix reaction) is based on the observation that strains of *Proteus vulgaris* are antigenically similar to *Rickettsia prowazekii* and can be used for serum agglutination tests (Table 11–35). In epidemic typhus fever the agglutination to OX19 should reach a titer greater than 1:160 during the 2nd wk of illness; the OX2 and OXK titers should remain low. The agglutinin pattern observed with murine typhus is similar to that of epidemic typhus. Patients with Rocky Mountain spotted fever usually show a rise in antibody to OX19 of 1:160 or greater; some develop a high OX2 titer and little response to OX19; and others have persistently negative Weil-Felix tests. Proteus OXK agglutinin titers are high after tsutsugamushi disease. Convalescent serum from patients with Q fever or rickettsialpox does not agglutinate to significant titer the *Proteus* strains used in the Weil-Felix reaction. *Proteus* titers do not persist and are usually below a significant level within 3 mo after the illness.

Serologic procedures using rickettsial antigens in latex-agglutination, complement-fixation, or neutralization tests are more sensitive and specific than the Weil-Felix reaction and should be used to confirm the diagnosis of rickettsial infection. Unfortunately, the serologic confirmation is usually not possible until days 9–14 of the illness. A single titer of 1:160 or greater with *Proteus* antigen or a rickettsiae complement fixation titer of at least 1:16, or a 4-fold rise in titer by either test supports the diagnosis.

Rickettsiae may be cultured by inoculating susceptible experimental animals, tissue culture, or developing chick embryos, but culturing rickettsiae in the laboratory is extremely hazardous and has been the source of infection for many investigators. This is a task for a special laboratory with proper facilities.

Treatment. Tetracycline or chloramphenicol is usually curative if begun in adequate dosage on or before the 6th day of disease. The penicillins and other antibiotics are without effect, and the sulfonamides may make the patient worse by enhancing rickettsial replication. Final eradication of the microorganism depends upon the immune processes of the host.

The recommended dose of tetracycline is 40–50 mg/kg/24 hr given in 4 divided doses orally or intravenously. Chloramphenicol in a dose of 100 mg/kg/24 hr administered every 6 hr is the alternative form of treatment. The latter agent is preferable in patients with poor renal function. Antimicrobial therapy should continue until the patient has been afebrile 4–5 days, usually for a total course of 8–12 days.

Early diagnosis and proper antibiotic therapy are all that is necessary in the management of most rickettsial infections. Vigorous supportive therapy, parenteral fluids, transfusions, sedation, and oxygen are necessary for the severely ill. Glucocorticoids are not of proved benefit, but there are many who advocate their short-term, high-dosage use in patients with severe vasculitis.

Immunity. Prolonged immunity to specific rickettsial agents generally follows recovery from disease. A significant degree of cross-immunity to related organisms may result from infection with one member of the group; e.g., the individual who has had Rocky Mountain spotted fever is protected against other tick-borne spotted fevers. Immunity to epidemic and murine typhus is linked, but an attack of scrub typhus that confers good homologous immunity protects only transiently against heterologous strains of *Rickettsia orientalis*.

Chronic or recurrent infections with rickettsiae may occur. Brill disease is the well-known example; exacerbations of scrub typhus with repeated isolation of the same strain of *R. orientalis* have been observed. Cell-mediated immune mechanisms appear to play an important role in limiting the intracellular persistence of rickettsiae, but the mechanisms of immunity are still incompletely understood.

Prognosis. In general, mortality in children is less than in adults or the aged. Epidemics of typhus in the 19th century had an average mortality rate of 20%, ranging from less than 3% in the pediatric age group to 50% in those in their 5th decade of life. The pattern was similar in severe outbreaks of scrub typhus or Rocky Mountain spotted fever. Mortality rates are diminished by prompt diagnosis and administration of antibiotics; in the United States approximately 5–7% of patients less than 30 years of age die with Rocky Mountain spotted fever. Murine typhus, Q fever, and rickettsialpox are relatively mild diseases with low mortality rates, even when untreated. Mortality rates are higher in nonwhite populations; difficulty identifying the rash on pigmented skin and the availability of health care may contribute to this increased risk. Most deaths occur in the 2nd week of the illness, although with fulminant disease a fatal outcome may take place within 5 days.

Table 11–35. **Rickettsial Diseases of Man: Summary of Pertinent Information**

Group	Disease	Causative Agent	Arthropod Vector	Animal Host	Proteus Agglutination*	Geographic Distribution
Typhus	Epidemic typhus	*R. prowazekii*	Body louse Squirrel louse, flea	None Flying squirrel	OX19	Worldwide; United States
	Brill disease	*R. prowazekii*	None		OX19	Eastern cities of United States
	Murine typhus	*R. mooseri*	Rat flea, louse	Rat	OX19	Worldwide; southern states of United States
Spotted fever	Rocky Mountain spotted fever	*R. rickettsii*	Tick	Rodents, mammals	Variable OX2 or OX19	North and South America
	Rickettsial pox	*R. akari*	Mite	House mice	None	Eastern United States
Tsutsugamushi fever	Scrub typhus	*R. orientalis (tsutsugamushi)*	Mite	Rodents	OXK	Far East
Q fever	Q fever	*R. burnetii (Coxiella burnetii)*	Rarely ticks?	Ticks, cattle, sheep, goats	None	Worldwide; western United States

*Specific serologic procedures using rickettsial antigens in complement-fixation, agglutination, or neutralization tests are more reliable.

11.86 TYPHUS FEVER
(Epidemic Typhus; Louse-Borne Typhus)

Etiology and Transmission. Humans are the principal reservoir of *Rickettsia prowazekii*, the causative agent of epidemic typhus. The body or head louse becomes infected by feeding upon the blood of a person with rickettsemia. The ingested organisms multiply within the cells lining the alimentary tract of the insect and are eliminated in the feces. Contaminated feces may be introduced into a susceptible human host through abrasions or perforations in the skin, through the conjunctival sac, or through inhalation of dried, infected louse excreta present in the clothing, bedding, or furniture of a typhus patient. The infection usually occurs in winter and spring. In the United States there have been cases of epidemic typhus confirmed by serologic testing in which the flying squirrel *(Glaucomys volans)* is the apparent source of infection.

Clinical Manifestations. Typhus fever is usually a mild disease in children. The incubation period is less than 14 days. The clinical manifestations include fever, transient rash, and few constitutional symptoms, and are similar to those of Rocky Mountain spotted fever.

Brill disease is an unusual phenomenon in which a patient with a history of typhus suffers a recrudescence of the illness. Such an individual can infect lice and is a potential point of origin for a typhus epidemic.

Control. The immediate destruction of vectors with an insecticide is important in the control of an epidemic. Dust containing excreta from infected lice is capable of transmitting typhus, and care must be taken to prevent its inhalation.

11.87 MURINE TYPHUS
(Endemic Typhus)

Etiology and Transmission. Endemic typhus may be seen in most regions of the United States, but occurs particularly in Texas and the southeastern states. It usually occurs in the summer and fall.

Murine typhus is a disease of rats caused by *Rickettsia mooseri.* It is transmitted from rat to rat by the rat louse or flea. In both rat and insect vectors murine typhus is a mild disease with no apparent effect on life span. The eggs laid by infected fleas or lice do not transmit *R. mooseri* to the next generation. People acquire murine typhus when bitten by an infected rat flea, or by inhaling infected excreta of fleas.

Clinical Manifestations. Murine typhus is a mild, seldom fatal illness that can be distinguished from epidemic typhus only by special laboratory procedures (Sec. 11.85). The incubation period is about 8 days. Prodromal symptoms such as headache, arthralgia, and backache are followed by a gradually increasing temperature which may reach 41.1° C (106° F) in children and last 9–14 days. Any time from the 1st to the 8th day of fever, most often by the 5th day, the rash appears. The eruption begins on the trunk and spreads to the periphery, rarely involving the face, palms, or soles. Initially, the skin lesion is a dull red macule with ill-defined margins; it becomes slightly papular as it matures, persists for a short period, and rarely becomes purpuric. Twenty per cent or more of children may have no rash or such a transient one that it is not noted. Central nervous system symptoms are uncommon, as are peripheral vascular collapse and other complications.

Control. Control of murine typhus requires elimination of the rat reservoir, the insect vector, or both.

11.88 SCRUB TYPHUS
(Tsutsugamushi Fever; Mite Typhus)

Etiology and Transmission. *Rickettsia tsutsugamushi*, also known as *R. orientalis*, causes scrub typhus. The vectors that carry the agent are the larval forms of the chigger or trombiculid mites. *R. tsutsugamushi* has been isolated from many species of rodents; both mites and rodents serve as reservoirs. Scrub typhus has not been diagnosed in the United States.

Clinical Manifestations. The symptomatology of scrub typhus is similar to that of other rickettsial infections. The mite bite usually results in a local skin lesion which becomes either an eschar or a punched-out shallow ulcer. By the end of the 1st wk of illness a maculopapular rash develops on the chest and abdomen and gradually spreads to involve the entire body, but rarely the hands and face. Diffuse, tender adenopathy, greater in the region of the primary lesion, is common. The mortality rate when antibiotics are administered early is less than 5%.

Protective clothing and early treatment with broad-spectrum antibiotics are the most useful aids to prevention of death from scrub typhus.

11.89 ROCKY MOUNTAIN SPOTTED FEVER

Epidemiology. Spotted fever has been reported from all of the 48 contiguous states except Maine. More than half of the annual cases in the United States occur in the Southeast, including North and South Carolina, Virginia, and Tennessee. Fewer than 5% originate in the Rocky Mountain area. The highest incidence is in the 5–9 yr age group.

Etiology and Transmission. The causative agent of Rocky Mountain spotted fever, *Rickettsia rickettsii*, is maintained in nature by many hosts, including the ground squirrel, jackrabbit, chipmunk, wood rat, meadow mouse, and weasel; the animal hosts do not become ill. Transmission among animals and from animal to man occurs most commonly via the wood tick *Dermacentor andersoni* or the dog tick *Dermacentor variabilis*. Transovarial passage of *R. rickettsii* helps maintain the agent in tick populations.

A history of contact with ticks is helpful in reaching a diagnosis, but such information is obtained in only 50–60% of reported cases. An additional 25% may have been exposed to tick-infected woods or to dogs, but 15–20% cannot identify a source of infection. Most cases in the United States occur from April to September, when outdoor living and tick activity are maximum.

Clinical Manifestations. The incubation period in children varies from 1 to 8 days. The disease usually begins with such nonspecific symptoms as headache, fever, anorexia, and restlessness. The history may be helpful. Local reaction at the site of the bite is uncommon. Discrete, pale, rose-red macules or maculopapules appear 1–5 days after the onset of illness; in approximately 10% of cases there may be little or no rash. The rash characteristically begins peripherally on the ankles, wrists, or lower legs (Fig. 11–30) and then spreads, often rapidly, to involve the entire body, including the scalp, palms, and soles. Early, the rash fades with pressure, but after 1–2 days it becomes more purple, papular, and frequently pete-

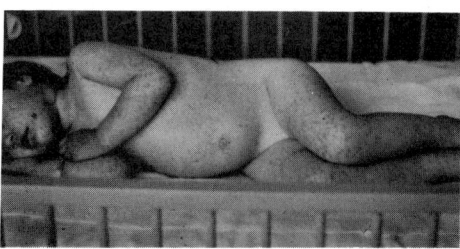

Figure 11–30. Patient with Rocky Mountain spotted fever. Note the greater concentration of skin lesions on the ankles, wrists, and lower legs. (Courtesy of William H. Wood, M.D., Cleveland.)

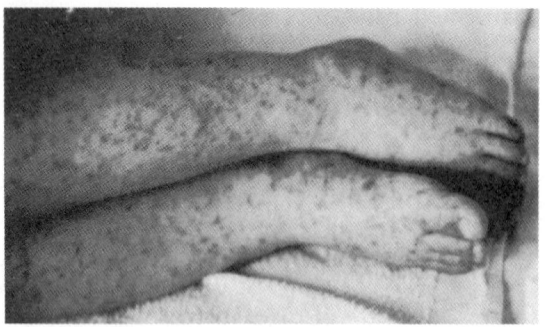

Figure 11–31. Ninth day of rash in Rocky Mountain spotted fever, showing hemorrhagic nature of rash and puffy edema of feet. (Courtesy of William H. Wood, M.D., Cleveland.)

chial (Fig. 11–31). Fever and headache persist; intense myalgia and malaise are frequent complaints. Splenomegaly is present in approximately 33% of patients and shock in 7–10%. Bizarre central nervous system symptoms, edema of the face, electrocardiographic evidence of myocarditis, renal involvement, peripheral collapse, and pneumonitis are the more severe manifestations. Thrombocytopenia is present in nearly half the patients and may be an important clue for early diagnosis. Patients with multiple coagulation disturbances (disseminated intravascular coagulation) constitute the group with highest risk of death. Fatality rates before the availability of antibiotics were 10–40%; with antibiotics the case fatality rate in children is 5–7%. Recovery in uncomplicated cases occurs in the 3rd wk, initiated by a fall in temperature and gradual subsidence of symptoms.

Laboratory Data. The clinical laboratory findings are not specific. See Sec. 11.85 for serologic tests.

Differential Diagnosis. Since the early manifestations are nonspecific, unless there is a high index of suspicion based on geographic location and season, the history of possible tick exposure may not be pursued and rickettsial disease not considered until the rash becomes apparent. In atypical cases when there is no rash or when other findings predominate, the correct diagnosis can be delayed. Jaundice, hepatomegaly, splenomegaly, abdominal pain, and vomiting with diarrhea are less common and very misleading manifestations of spotted fever. Infectious mononucleosis, rubella, atypical measles, enterovirus exanthems, meningococcemia, leptospirosis, mucocutaneous lymph node syndrome (Kawasaki disease), idiopathic thrombocytopenia, hepatitis, and Henoch-Schönlein purpura are frequently considered in the differential diagnosis of patients with Rocky Mountain spotted fever. The spread of rash from distal portions of the extremities to the trunk and face, with involvement of palms and soles, is often the clue that leads to the diagnosis. Negative blood cultures and normal spinal fluid are additional aids in reaching a correct diagnosis.

Control. The reservoirs and vectors of spotted fever are so numerous and widespread that removal of the source of infection is not feasible. Protection from tick bite is best accomplished by the use of proper wearing apparel plus tick repellents or, optimally, the avoidance during the tick season of areas known to be infested.

Ticks rarely transmit infection until they have fed for several hours; thus careful examination of children who have been playing in the woods and prompt removal of ticks may prevent disease. This is best accomplished with the use of gloves or forceps to protect the operator from being infected by the crushed insect. Application of a coating of petrolatum often provokes the tick to remove its mouth parts.

11.90 FIÈVRE BOUTONNEUSE

This relatively benign rickettsial spotted fever is limited almost exclusively to the countries surrounding the Mediterranean. Natives are infected early in life and develop long-lasting immunity; the visitor is vulnerable. *Rickettsia conorii*, the causal agent, is transmitted by the dog tick, *Rhipicephalus sanguineus*. As in rickettsialpox or scrub typhus, a local lesion known as tache noire, or primary eschar, develops, followed by a diffuse, maculopapular rash, which later becomes petechial. Severe systemic manifestations are uncommon. The diagnosis is usually made on the basis of the clinical symptoms in an exposed person with a primary skin lesion. Agglutinins to both OX19 and OX2 appear during the 2nd wk of the disease and may be used to confirm the diagnosis if the more specific complement-fixation test is not available. Antibiotic treatment is followed by rapid clinical improvement.

11.91 RICKETTSIALPOX

This febrile disease with varicelliform rash is caused by *Rickettsia akari* and transmitted by the mouse mite, *Allodermanyssus sanguineus*. The mite vector has been found in many cities of the United States. The illness is endemic in New York, and isolated cases have been reported from Boston, Philadelphia, and Cleveland.

Clinical Manifestations. Rickettsialpox is a mild illness characterized by an initial skin lesion followed by fever, chills, headache, and a papulovesicular rash. The initial lesion, presumed to be the site of the mite bite, has been observed in more than 90% of cases. It may be located anywhere on the body, beginning as a nontender, nonitching, firm, red papule, 0.5–2.0 cm in diameter. A deeply entrenched vesicle develops in the center of the papule and ruptures after several days, leaving a crusted, pigmented lesion or eschar which may persist 3 wk or longer. Adjacent lymph nodes become enlarged and tender, but do not suppurate.

The initial lesion is followed in 2–7 days by fever, headache, chills, and sweating. Temperature ranges from 39 to 40° C (102–105° F), but the patient remains oriented and does not appear severely ill. Within 24–72 hr after the onset of fever, scattered erythematous maculopapules appear over the body, showing no preference for trunk, head, or extremity. The lesions enlarge, become more papular, and develop vesicles on the summit of each papule. The secondary lesions (rash) resemble the initial lesion except that they are smaller in size and heal, without leaving scars, in 4–7 days. The duration of illness seldom exceeds 7–10 days. Complications, sequelae, and fatalities are rare.

Differential Diagnosis. The rash of rickettsialpox may be confused with that of chickenpox. In the latter the vesicles are superficial, thin, dewdrop lesions which appear in successive crops beginning on the chest. These differ from the deeply seated, randomly distributed firm vesicles of the rickettsial disease. The initial lesion and the presence of chills and fever before the rash may also help in differentiation. Other diseases to be considered include infectious mononucleosis, meningococcemia, Rocky Mountain spotted fever, and typhus.

Control. Preventive measures should include the eradication of rodent reservoirs as well as the mite vector.

11.92 Q FEVER

Q fever, a febrile disease without rash and often associated with an interstitial pneumonia, has been reported from all parts of the world.

Etiology and Transmission. Q fever occurs naturally in cattle, sheep, goats, and many wild animals. The causative agent, *Coxiella burnetii*, has been found in many species of ticks, in which it may pass from the adult through ova to progeny.

Experimentally, Q fever has been transmitted by insect bite and by inhalation. However, careful studies of outbreaks of the disease in human beings have failed to incriminate insect vectors, although this mode of transmission may be important among animals. Person-to-person spread is rare but can occur. In the endemic areas of California, human infections are related to contact with sheep or dairy cows. The main route of infection is inhalation of contaminated material from domestic animals which may be present in dust, hay, wool, or hides.

Milk may be another source of infection. *C. burnetii* has been isolated from raw milk sources and may survive pasteurization temperatures.

Clinical Manifestations. Q fever, as commonly recognized, is a disease of moderate severity with a duration in children of 2–3 wk. The onset is characteristically sudden, but in some instances symptoms may increase slowly in intensity. Malaise, fever, chilliness, and generalized weakness appear early, but the most prominent symptom is severe frontal headache, often associated with pain upon movement of the eyes. There is no rash. Cough may occur late in the 1st wk of illness, with blood-streaked sputum and chest pain. Pulmonary consolidation is usually patchy and in the peripheries of the lower lobes; hilar involvement is rare. Resolution is slow and may require 3–6 wk. Pleural effusion is infrequent. The mortality rate is less than 1%.

Differential diagnosis in the immunologically competent individual includes the long list of agents associated with the atypical pneumonia syndrome, such as mycoplasma, Epstein-Barr virus, psittacosis, and legionnaires' disease.

Control. Recognition of the disease in livestock should alert communities to the risk of infection. Milk from infected herds must be pasteurized at temperatures sufficient to destroy the rickettsiae. Special isolation measures are not necessary, since person-to-person spread of Q fever is rare.

ELI GOLD

Burgdorfer W, Anacker RL: Rickettsiae and Rickettsial Diseases. New York, Academic Press, 1981.

Fleisher G, Lennette ET, Honig P: Diagnosis of Rocky Mountain spotted fever by immunofluorescent identification of *Rickettsia rickettsii* in skin biopsy tissue. J Pediatr 95:63, 1979.

Heckemy KE: Laboratory diagnosis of Rocky Mountain spotted fever. N Engl J Med 300:859, 1979.

Wilfert CM, MacCormack JN, Kleeman K, et al: Epidemiology of Rocky Mountain spotted fever as determined by active surveillance. J Infect Dis 150:469, 1984.

Williams JC, Winkler HH: Molecular Biology of Rickettsiae. *In:* Lewe L, Schlessinger D (eds): Microbiology—1984. Washington, DC, American Society for Microbiology, 1984.

Woodward TE: Rocky Mountain spotted fever: Epidemiological and early clinical signs are keys to treatment and reduced mortality. J Infect Dis 150:465, 1984.

MYCOTIC INFECTIONS

11.93 BLASTOMYCOSIS

North American blastomycosis is an uncommon noncontagious granulomatous infection of the lungs, skin, bone, and genitourinary tract caused by the dimorphic saprophytic fungus *Blastomyces dermatitidis*.

Etiology. In infected tissue the yeast form of *B. dermatitidis* appears as spherical, multinucleated structures with thick, double refractile cell walls; each large daughter cell is attached to the parent by a broad-based neck.

Epidemiology. Blastomycosis occurs mainly in the southeastern United States and in the Mississippi, Ohio, and St. Lawrence River valleys. This endemic area includes the north central region of the United States and extends into Canada. Blastomycosis has also been reported in England, Africa, and India. Human infection occurs following inhalation of airborne spores from contaminated soil, which reach the lower respiratory tract and, after being converted to yeast forms during a long incubation period (30–45 days), establish a primary pulmonary infection. There is no age, sex, race, or occupational predilection.

Pulmonary Blastomycosis. This form most often occurs as an asymptomatic infection. The lack of an effective skin test antigen prevents a true estimate of its incidence. However, proof of subclinical infection has been obtained from studies of epidemic blastomycosis. Primary pulmonary blastomycosis may also present as a mild self-limited lower respiratory tract infection, a progressive or fulminant life-threatening pneumonia with or without extrapulmonary manifestations, or chronic pneumonia. In mild cases the child presents with low-grade fever, pleuritic chest pain, a nonproductive cough, and occasional hemoptysis. Roentgenographic examination reveals lobar consolidation and hilar adenopathy. In the progressive form of pneumonia, symptoms include high fever, night sweats, chills, anorexia, and dyspnea. Productive cough and hemoptysis are common. The physical examination reveals diffuse rales and signs of pulmonary consolidation. Roentgenographic examination demonstrates diffuse bilateral nodular basilar infiltrates. Cavitation and effusion are uncommon. Person-to-person transmission has not been documented.

Disseminated Blastomycosis. This form most often occurs in adults with chronic pulmonary infection. The skin is the most common site of extrapulmonary involvement and may be the presenting complaint in patients with asymptomatic or mild pulmonary disease. Solitary or multiple subcutaneous nodules of the face and trunk are characteristic of *cutaneous blastomycosis*. These appear initially as papules or pustules, which over a period of weeks or months progress to verrucous granulomas with erythematous, indurated, raised serpentine borders. The lesions advance centripetally with central scarring; regional lymphadenopathy does not occur. Other extrapulmonary sites of involvement include bone, joints, genitourinary tract (prostate, epididymis, and testes) and, on rare occasions, central nervous system, adrenals, thyroid gland, and liver.

Blastomycosis should be considered in the differential diagnosis in a patient from an endemic area presenting with a slowly responding or progressive pneumonia with or without involvement of the skin, bone, or genitourinary system. Skin tests lack specificity. A presumptive diagnosis requires serologic confirmation with enzyme immunoassay and/or complement fixation or identification of the yeast forms by histologic examination of biopsy material or by a wet mount preparation (with 10% potassium hydroxide) of exudate from sputum or abscesses. Definitive diagnosis requires isolation of the infecting organism.

Pulmonary blastomycosis may be a mild, self-limited illness requiring no specific treatment. However, progressive pulmonary disease with or without extrapulmonary dissemination is often fatal, and immediate therapeutic intervention is indicated. Cutaneous or chronic pulmonary disease is fatal in 20–30% of cases. Amphotericin B is the treatment of choice for progressive, disseminated, or chronic blastomycosis. In children a cumulative dose of 15–20 mg/kg up to a maximum of 2 g is effective in a majority of cases. Studies suggest that 2-hydroxystilbamidine is as effective as amphotericin B and should be considered as alternative therapy in patients who cannot tolerate amphotericin B. There is limited experience with the imidazole derivatives, however. Oral ketoconazole also appears promising, and recent studies suggest that it may replace amphotericin B as the initial treatment of blastomycosis that is not overwhelming.

Laskey WK, Sarosi GA: Blastomycosis in children. Pediatrics 65:111, 1980.
Macher A: Histoplasmosis and blastomycosis. Med Clin North Am 64:447, 1980.
Sarosi GA, Davies SF: Blastomycosis. Am Rev Resp Dis 120:911, 1979.

11.94 CRYPTOCOCCOSIS
(Torulosis, European Blastomycosis)

Cryptococcosis is an uncommon subacute or chronic fungal infection, often involving the central nervous system, caused by an encapsulated budding yeast, *Cryptococcus neoformans*. This fungus is surrounded by a polysaccharide capsule that contains antigenic determinants permitting identification of four serotypes, A, B, C, and D.

Epidemiology. *C. neoformans* is distributed worldwide, existing in nature as a soil saprophyte. The roosting sites of birds, particularly pigeons, provide the necessary conditions for luxuriant growth, and high rates of positive skin tests occur in individuals frequently exposed to pigeons. Cryptococcosis results from inhalation of spores, which germinate in the pulmonary tissue and may disseminate via the bloodstream to brain, meninges, bone marrow, and skin. It occurs sporadically, without any occupational predisposition, and is rarely associated with historical or roentgenographic evidence of respiratory involvement. There is an increased incidence of infection in patients receiving corticosteroids and in those with lymphoreticular malignancies (especially Hodgkin disease), sarcoidosis, the acquired immunodeficiency syndrome, and insulin-dependent diabetes. However, 50% of patients have no predisposing condition. The disease occurs in all age groups, affects males more often than females (3:1 ratio), and is more common in Caucasians.

Pathology. The characteristic lesion is a cyst-like cavity containing gelatinous material. Microscopic examination reveals clumps of cryptococci within the cyst and an inflammatory response consisting of macrophages, giant cells, and lymphocytes. In pulmonary cryptococcosis the common finding is a subpleural granuloma. In central nervous system disease multiple cystic lesions occur throughout the brain, particularly in the cortical gray matter and basal ganglia. Mass lesions are extremely rare.

Clinical Manifestations. *Pulmonary cryptococcosis* is uncommon in children, most often occurring in an immunosuppressed child as an influenza-like illness with low-grade fever, cough, pleuritic chest pain, and minimal sputum production. Physical examination may reveal diffuse rales. The chest roentgenogram demonstrates a varied pattern that may include a single pulmonary granuloma, apical cavities, pulmonary masses, interstitial pneumonitis, or pleural effusions. Routine laboratory studies are normal. Cultures of sputum and bronchial washings are occasionally positive, but invasive procedures may be needed to recover pathogens from tissues. *Cryptococcal meningitis* is the most common form of life-threatening cryptococcal infection and has a subacute or chronic presentation. Symptoms are intermittent and usually present for weeks to months; they include headache, 73%; mental changes, 45%; visual changes, 40%; nausea and vomiting, 33%; pain and stiffness of the neck and back, 33%; chills or fever, 30%; lethargy, weakness, and fatigue, 23%; ataxia, 20%; and aphasia or slurred speech, 13%. Physical examination may reveal nuchal rigidity, papilledema, hearing loss, motor weakness, cerebellar signs, and coma. Cerebrospinal fluid findings include an elevated opening pressure and protein concentration in 90% of cases, hypoglycorrhachia in 55%, and a mononuclear pleocytosis rarely exceeding 300 cells/mm^3.

The mortality rate is 50%. Treatment failure and early death are associated with underlying lymphoreticular malignancy; corticosteroid therapy; cerebrospinal fluid findings consisting of a high opening pressure, a low glucose level, fewer than 20 leukocytes/mm^3, and cryptococci seen in smear; cryptococci isolated from extraneural sites; and high titers of cryptococcal antigen in cerebrospinal fluid and serum. Forty per cent of survivors have residual neurologic deficits including visual loss, hearing defects, cranial nerve damage, motor impairment, personality change, and, on rare occasions, hydrocephalus.

Additional clinical manifestations include multiple papules, pustules, or small subcutaneous masses, most often located on the face or scalp, which eventually become necrotic and ulcerate; osteomyelitis and septic arthritis; lymphadenitis; endocarditis and pericarditis; renal abscesses; and prostatitis.

Diagnosis. Diagnosis depends on (1) histologic identification of cryptococci in biopsy specimens or body fluids, (2) recovery of *C. neoformans* following appropriate cultures, and/or (3) serologic demonstration of cryptococcal antigen. Histologically, appropriately stained organisms are yeast-like with narrow-based buds. The encapsulated yeast may be visualized in 50% of patients with meningitis after mixing sediment of the cerebrospinal fluid with an equal volume of India ink. Culture of *C. neoformans* produces creamy white mucoid colonies within 10 days of inoculation onto Sabouraud medium. Negative cultures of cerebrospinal fluid do not necessarily exclude the diagnosis of meningitis, as the often small numbers of organisms present necessitate repeated cultures of large volumes of centrifuged specimens. The latex agglutination technique detects cryptococcal polysaccharide capsular antigen in cerebrospinal fluid or serum in more than 90% of patients with cryptococcal meningitis.

Treatment. The mortality rate for cryptococcal meningitis is high (30%), relapse is frequent (20%), and a number of survivors (40%) are left with permanent neurologic sequelae. Most authorities recommend combined treatment with amphotericin B (0.3 mg/kg/24 hr) and oral 5-flucytosine (150 mg/kg/24 hr in 4 equally divided doses) as superior to treatment with amphotericin B alone (total dose of 30–40 mg/kg), which frequently results in irreversible nephropathy. Nevertheless, even with the lower dose of amphotericin, azotemia may occur with resulting accumulation of 5-flucytosine; accordingly, renal function and 5-flucytosine levels should be monitored. Toxic levels of 5-flucytosine result in leukopenia, thrombocytopenia, and diarrhea; the 5-flucytosine level should not exceed 100 µg/mL of serum. Weekly cultures of the cerebrospinal fluid should be obtained and treatment continued for a minimum of 6 wk or until cultures are negative for a period of 1 mo during therapy. Patients who fail to respond to this combined regimen or who relapse following appropriate therapy should receive intraventricular administration of amphotericin B. Alternative treatment regimens with oral, parenteral, or intraventricular miconazole or oral ketoconazole have been disappointing.

Bennett JE, Dismukes WE, et al: A comparison of amphotericin B alone and combined with flucytosine in the treatment of cryptococcal meningitis. N Engl J Med 301:126, 1979.

Diamond RD, Bennett JE: Prognostic factors in cryptococcal meningitis. Ann Intern Med 80:176, 1974.

Goodman JS, Kaufman L, Loenig MG: Diagnosis of cryptococcal meningitis. N Engl J Med 285:434, 1971.

Lewis JC, Rabinovich S: The wide spectrum of cryptococcal infections. Am J Med 53:315, 1972.

Salaki JS, Louria DB, Chmel H: Fungal and yeast infections of the central nervous system. A clinical review. Medicine 63:108, 1984.

11.95 MUCORMYCOSIS
(Phycomycosis, Zygomycosis)

The term mucormycosis refers to a group of invasive infections that spread across tissue planes and that are caused by dimorphic fungi of the class Zygomycetes and the order Mucorales. The principal human pathogens, *Rhizopus*, *Absidia*, and *Mucor*, are distributed worldwide, commonly grow on fruit and other food (e.g., bread mold), and are easily isolated from soil. The Mucorales grow on a variety of laboratory media as fluffy white, gray, or brownish molds following incubation at 37° C. In appropriately stained clinical specimens thick-walled, nonseptate, irregular right-angle branching hyphae are easily visualized.

Epidemiology. Exposure to spores of Mucorales is universal, but disease is uncommon. Infection is sporadic and almost exclusively limited to children who have underlying disease, e.g., diabetes mellitus (especially with acidosis), leukemia, or lymphoma; who have undergone organ transplantation and immunosuppression; or who have burns, renal failure, or malnutrition. An unusual epidemic of cutaneous mucormycosis was associated with use of Elastoplast bandages.

Clinical Manifestations. Mucormycosis follows inhalation or ingestion of spores germinate and invade the nasal, tracheal, and/or gastrointestinal mucosa. *Rhinocerebral mucormycosis*, the most common form of disease, typically occurs in children with poorly controlled diabetes. Infection begins in the nasal turbinates or hard palate and presents as a black eschar. Hyphae gradually extend, with involvement of the paranasal sinuses. Further extension through nerves, blood vessels, cartilage, and bone leads to involvement of the face, orbit, meninges, and brain. Initial symptoms of unilateral headache, nasal stuffiness, epistaxis, and facial numbness may progress to include periorbital cellulitis, with proptosis, loss of extraocular movements, and blindness. Intracranial extension may occur, resulting in occlusion of cerebral arteries and veins. Roentgenographic examination reveals diffuse clouding of the paranasal sinuses and extensive bony destruction; computed tomography delineates orbital involvement. Diagnosis depends on demonstrating hyphae in biopsy specimens; cultures are positive in only 15% of cases.

Pulmonary mucormycosis is an acute, life-threatening disease that occurs in immunosuppressed children with leukemia or lymphoma. Infection can occur in association with rhinocerebral mucormycosis or following inhalation of spores. In isolated pulmonary disease patients often present with a pulmonary infarction syndrome secondary to hyphal invasion and occlusion of pulmonary vessels: an acute onset of fever, pleuritic chest pain, and hemoptysis. Subsequent hematogenous dissemination with involvement of multiple organ systems is not uncommon. Roentgenographic examination may reveal a number of abnormalities including patchy infiltrates, lobar consolidation, cavity formation, and pleural effusion. Nodule formation, fungus balls, and mass lesions have also been reported. Diagnosis requires obtaining tissue for culture and histologic examination by transthoracic needle aspiration, transbronchial biopsy, and/or open lung biopsy.

Gastrointestinal mucormycosis is uncommon and in children is most often associated with malnutrition, kwashiorkor, or treatment with corticosteroids. Necrotic ulcers may involve the entire gastrointestinal tract, especially the stomach. Symptoms are acute and include bloody diarrhea, intestinal obstruction, and/or perforation.

Disseminated mucormycosis occurs in children with leukemia and lymphoma; is often associated with infections due to bacteria, viruses, and other pathogenic fungi; and is invariably fatal. Infection originates in the lung and disseminates to involve the brain and other organ systems. Neurologic manifestations are secondary to cerebrovascular invasion. Meningeal involvement is uncommon. Cultures of blood and cerebrospinal fluid are invariably negative, and diagnosis depends on the demonstration of fungus in the biopsy material.

Cutaneous mucormycosis occurs as a secondary infection following extensive burns and/or surgical procedures. It presents as an erythematous papule which ulcerates, leaving a black necrotic center. Diagnosis depends on biopsy, culture, and histologic examination of suspicious skin lesions.

Other reported infections with Mucoracea include endocarditis, bone marrow necrosis, and isolated renal infection.

Treatment. The treatment includes control of the underlying predisposing illness, reduction or elimination of immunosuppressive therapy, surgical resection of involved tissue, and intravenous administration of amphotericin B. The optimal dosage in children has not been established; however, in adults with extensive disease, treatment consists of 0.8–1.0 mg/kg/24 hr given over a 2–3 mo period. In superficial infection of the skin, debridement and topical therapy with amphotericin B have proved successful; however, with evidence of deep hyphal invasion, systemic therapy with amphotericin B is indicated.

Lehrer RI, Howard DH, Sypherd PS, et al: Mucormycosis. Ann Intern Med 93:93, 1980.

Meyer RD, Rosen P, Armstrong D: Phycomycosis complicating leukemia and lymphoma. Ann Intern Med 77:871, 1972.

Meyers BR, Wormser G, Hirschman SZ, et al: Rhinocerebral mucormycosis—premortem diagnosis and therapy. Arch Intern Med 139:557, 1979.

11.96 SPOROTRICHOSIS

Sporotrichosis is an uncommon chronic fungal infection caused by a dimorphic fungus, *Sporothrix schenckii*. It is distributed worldwide and exists in its saprophytic form in living, decaying, or dead vegetation. Disseminated infection is unusual but may follow inhalation or ingestion of spores. The cutaneous form is more common and results from intradermal inoculation of spores following contact with contaminated vegetation, e.g., sphagnum moss, barberry, rosebushes, and various species of grass. Consequently, it is often an occupational disease of farmers, horticulturalists, and others in continual contact with soil and vegetation. Epidemic sporotrichosis has been reported in adults and children following contact with straw and hay heavily contaminated with spores of *S. schenckii*. Human-to-human transmission has not been reported.

Pathology. Histologically, sporotrichosis is characterized by noncaseating granulomas and microabscess formation. Oval or cigar-shaped forms may be seen in stained biopsy material.

Clinical Manifestations. *Cutaneous sporotrichosis* is the most common form of disease in infants and children. *Lymphocutaneous sporotrichosis*, which accounts for more than 75% of reported cases, occurs after subcutaneous inoculation of spores. Following a variable and often prolonged incubation period (1–12 wk) an isolated, painless erythematous papule develops at the inoculation site, most often an extremity. The initial lesion enlarges and eventually ulcerates. Although infection may remain limited to the inoculation site, satellite lesions usually appear as multiple, painless, subcutaneous nodules extending along the lymphatic channels draining the initial lesion. These secondary nodules represent subcutaneous granulomas that attach to the overlying skin and ulcerate. Sporotrichosis does not heal spontaneously, and ulcerative lesions may persist for years unless appropriately treated. Systemic signs and symptoms are uncommon. Extracutaneous sporotrichosis is rare in children; pulmonary sporotrichosis, meningitis, osteomyelitis, septic arthritis, and disseminated disease have been reported in adults.

Diagnosis. Cutaneous sporotrichosis must be differentiated from the cutaneous forms of coccidioidomycosis, North American blastomycosis, histoplasmosis, tuberculosis, syphilis, anthrax, and tularemia. Histologic examination of biopsy material may demonstrate the organisms; however, a definitive diagnosis requires isolation of *S. schenckii* from infected tissue.

Treatment. Potassium iodide is the treatment of choice for cutaneous sporotrichosis. The solution is given orally (1 g/mL) beginning with 1–10 drops 3 times a day and increasing each dose by 1 drop/dose each day until a final dose of 10–40 drops 3 times a day is reached or until symptoms of iodism appear (skin eruptions, lacrimation, parotid swelling, nausea, vomiting). Treatment is continued for 1 mo after resolution of cutaneous lesions. Occasional patients have responded to oral ketoconazole; however, there are no comparative studies. Systemic administration of amphotericin B is required for extracutaneous infection.

Chandler JW, Kriel RL, Tosh FE: Childhood sporotrichosis. Am J Dis Child 115:368, 1968.
Dahl BA, Silberfarb PM, Sarosi GA, et al: Sporotrichosis in children. JAMA 215:1980, 1971.
Orr ER, Riley HD: Sporotrichosis in childhood: Report of ten cases. J Pediatr 78:951, 1971.

11.97 ASPERGILLOSIS

Aspergillosis refers to a group of diseases caused by a monomorphic fungus of the genus *Aspergillus* (*A. fumigatus*, *A. niger*, *A. flavus*, etc.), which is distributed worldwide in soil, water, and decaying vegetation. Although exposure to *Aspergillus* spores is frequent, disease is uncommon. Infection is most often acquired from inhalation of airborne spores which gain access to the paranasal sinuses or lower respiratory tract. Spores may also gain access to the body following ingestion, aspiration, or surgical instrumentation or following skin and wound contamination.

Aspergillus species are capable of producing invasive or local disease of pulmonary or nonpulmonary structures. Factors predisposing to invasive disease include (1) concomitant corticosteroid treatment, (2) cytotoxic chemotherapy, (3) recent or concurrent therapy with broad-spectrum antimicrobial agents, (4) leukopenia (<1000 cells/mm³), and (5) acute leukemia in relapse or acute rejection of a transplanted organ.

Hypersensitivity Syndromes

Atopic asthma may be precipitated by spores from *Aspergillus* species. Inhalation triggers an IgE-mediated response and bronchospasm. The clinical manifestations are nonspecific and include the acute onset of wheezing in the absence of pulmonary infiltrates or fever.

Allergic alveolitis occurs in nonatopic individuals after repeated exposure to organic dust. *Aspergillus* is one of many organic substances that results in this syndrome ("maltworkers lung"). The pathogenesis is unknown but it may represent an immune-complex disease of lung tissue. The clinical manifestations include fever, cough, and dyspnea, which occur within 4–6 hr following exposure to the offending antigen. Physical examination reveals rhonchi in the absence

of wheezing. Sputum and blood examinations do not show eosinophilia, and the chest roentgenogram reveals diffuse interstitial infiltrates. Persistent exposure gradually leads to irreversible pulmonary fibrosis.

Allergic bronchopulmonary aspergillosis often occurs in atopic children with a long history of asthma or other chronic pulmonary disease. The immune response to *Aspergillus* is mediated by IgG and IgE antibody directed against the fungus which colonizes the airways, producing a continued supply of antigen. Symptoms include recurrent episodes of wheezing, pulmonary infiltrates, and eosinophilia. Additional features include immediate skin reactivity and precipitating antibodies to *Aspergillus fumigatus*, elevated total serum IgE concentrations, and central bronchiectasis. Other less common manifestations are expectoration of brown mucous plugs, positive sputum cultures for *Aspergillus* species, and the demonstration of hyphal elements in bronchial secretions. Treatment with steroids, often for extended periods of time, is effective in eliminating signs and symptoms and preventing bronchiectasis. Administering systemic antifungal agents is not helpful.

Noninvasive (Saprophytic) Syndromes

Otomycosis is a benign condition characterized by pain, pruritus, and otorrhea in which *Aspergillus* species (e.g., *A. niger*) grow on the cerumen and cellular debris within the external auditory canal. The tympanic membrane is usually spared. Resolution follows curettage and topical antifungal therapy.

Sinusitis secondary to *Aspergillus* species most often involves the maxillary sinuses and presents with fever and pain over the involved sinus. Roentgenographic examination typically reveals a fungus ball lying free or attached to the mucosa of a chronically infected sinus. Curettage and drainage are the treatments of choice.

Aspergilloma follows colonization of poorly drained bronchi, cysts, or cavitary lesions within the pulmonary parenchyma by *Aspergillus* species that proliferate as a mass of hyphal elements (fungus ball). Aspergillomas occur primarily in the upper lobes of the lung and have been observed in pulmonary cavities of tuberculosis, histoplasmosis, and sarcoidosis. Mycelia may extend from the fungus ball into the wall of the cavity; however, extensive pulmonary invasion and hematogenous dissemination are uncommon. Affected children are often asymptomatic, although chronic cough and hemoptysis may occur. Diagnosis is established by roentgenographically demonstrating an air shadow outlining a pulmonary cavity which surrounds the fungus ball. Antifungal chemotherapy has little effect, and most clinicians follow asymptomatic patients, reserving surgical resection for those with recurrent or life-threatening hemoptysis.

Invasive Disease

Invasive pulmonary aspergillosis is an acute life-threatening infection occurring almost exclusively in immunosuppressed children. Predisposing factors include corticosteroid therapy, cytotoxic chemotherapy, recurrent or concurrent therapy with broad-spectrum antimicrobial agents, leukopenia (<1000 cells/mm³), and acute leukemia in relapse, or rejection of an organ transplant. Clinical manifestations mimic acute bacterial pneumonia. Temperature elevation, nonproductive cough, and dyspnea are common. Although radiographic examination may reveal lobar involvement or a miliary pattern, the more common finding is a peripheral patchy bronchopneumonia. Without treatment, these densities increase in size, extend toward the periphery, and undergo cavitation and/or abscess formation. Histologic examination reveals areas of pulmonary infarction secondary to thrombosis resulting from vascular invasion by *Aspergillus* spp. Thus, in some cases, the clinical presentation resembles pulmonary embolization and infarction. Pulmonary infection is often accompanied by dissemination (40%) to the brain, heart, liver, other viscera, and skin. The clinical course is usually fulminant, with an overall mortality of 80%.

The diagnosis is suggested by the clinical course of the illness, isolation of the fungus from pulmonary and/or nasopharyngeal secretions, negative culture for other pathogens, and failure to respond to antibacterial therapy. Cultures of the blood, CSF, bone marrow, and urine are rarely positive in disseminated disease. Attempts to diagnose *Aspergillus* infections serologically have been unrewarding, but recent techniques for identifying *Aspergillus* antigen by radioimmunoassay or CIE have been encouraging. Tissue should be obtained by transcutaneous needle aspiration, transbronchial biopsy, bronchial washings, and/or open lung biopsy for examination and culture.

Necrotizing pulmonary aspergillosis is a distinct clinical entity that may overlap with invasive pulmonary aspergillosis. Patients usually present with fever, a productive cough extending over a period of weeks to months, and signs of lower respiratory tract infection. Chest roentgenograms demonstrate infiltrative and cavitary disease typical of a chronic destructive lung process; cavity formation is often accompanied by the development of fungus balls. The diagnosis is suggested by the prolonged clinical course, the isolation of *Aspergillus* spp. from pulmonary secretions, negative cultures for other pathogens, and failure to respond to antibacterial and/or antimycobacterial therapy. The diagnosis is confirmed by pathologic evidence of tissue invasion and response to antimycotic therapy. Surgical therapy is reserved for patients unable to tolerate chemotherapy and/or those who have residual lung disease.

Successful management of invasive pulmonary aspergillosis depends on early diagnosis and treatment, remission of the underlying disease, and reversal, wherever possible, of drug-induced immunosuppression and bone marrow aplasia. Although the proper dose and duration of therapy in children is unknown, amphotericin B is recommended (0.3–0.5 mg/kg/24 hr for a minimum of 2 wk). The total dose is generally tailored to the extent of disease and the clinical progression or regression. Although synergism between amphotericin B and 5-flucytosine, tetracyclines, and rifampin has been demonstrated in vitro, there are limited data to support combination therapy. Miconazole and ketoconazole are nonfungicidal to *Aspergillus* spp. and, accordingly, have no role in treatment. The efficacy of granulocyte transfusions in neutropenic patients is not established.

Sinusitis due to *Aspergillus* spp. most often involves the maxillary sinuses. Two overlapping clinical entities exist. The more common presentation is low-grade fever, purulent rhinorrhea, facial fullness, and localized or referred pain. Roentgenographic examination reveals opacification with or without a fungus ball lying free or attached to the mucosa of chronically infected sinuses. Curettage and drainage are the treatments of choice. A more invasive sinusitis, often accompanied by lower respiratory tract involvement, occurs in immunosuppressed patients. Symptoms include fever, headache, localized pain, and purulent rhinorrhea, which may progress to swelling, proptosis, and paralysis of extraocular muscles. Roentgenographic examination reveals opacification and bony destruction. Surgical drainage and parenteral administration of amphotericin B is the treatment of choice.

Ocular infection typically occurs in immunocompromised patients, producing three categories of disease: (1) mycotic keratitis, in which fungi from an external source infect the cornea following trauma or superficial disease; (2) endogenous oculomycosis, which is intraocular infection secondary to

hematogenous dissemination; and (3) extension oculomycosis, which results from the extension of fungal disease into the orbit from adjacent tissue. Treatment includes surgical drainage and systemic antifungal therapy.

Endocarditis of normal, damaged, or prosthetic heart valves may produce large friable vegetations that obstruct the valve orifice and/or embolize to pulmonary or systemic arteries, resulting in metastatic foci of infection in the lungs, brain, kidney, and spleen. Treatment requires surgical removal of the infected valve and prolonged administration of amphotericin B.

WILLIAM T. SPECK
STEPHEN C. ARONOFF

Binder RE, Failing LJ, Pugath RD, et al: Chronic necrotizing pulmonary aspergillosis: A discrete clinical entity. Medicine 61:109, 1983.
Patterson R, Greenberger PA, Radin RC, et al: Allergic bronchopulmonary aspergillosis: Staging as an aid to management. Ann Intern Med 96:286, 1982.
Rinaldi M: Invasive aspergillosis. Rev Infect Dis 5:1061, 1983.
Weiner MH, Talbot GH, Gerson SL, et al: Antigen detection in the diagnosis of invasive aspergillosis. Ann Intern Med 99:777, 1983.

11.98 COCCIDIOIDOMYCOSIS
(San Joaquin Fever; Valley Fever; Desert Rheumatism; Coccidioidal Granuloma)

Etiology. Coccidioidomycosis is an infection caused by the fungus *Coccidioides immitis* found in the soil of the New World. The minute arthrospores of its mycelial saprophytic phase are inhaled or, rarely, enter through injured skin. In the infected host they round up into spherules (sporangia) which develop endospores. Liberation of the latter leads to formation of new spherules, which spread within a host but not to a new host. Viable C. *immitis* does occur in pulmonary cavities, often in the mycelial as well as spherule form, but no cases of person-to-person infection have been discovered. As they occur naturally, however, and on surface cultures, the arthroconidia of the saprophytic phase are highly infectious. Although isolation is unnecessary, precautions should be taken with dressings and casts over open lesions lest the mycelial arthroconidia develop as they do on surface cultures. Within the arid endemic areas of California's San Joaquin Valley, in scattered regions in northern and southern California, in central and southern Arizona, and even in southwestern Texas, many long-time residents have been infected, along with cattle, sheep, dogs, and wild rodents. Infection confers permanent immunity; where the population is stable, coccidioidomycosis is primarily a childhood infection.

Clinical Manifestations. Human infection takes three forms: (1) a benign, self-limited, primary infection (60% of infected persons show no clinical manifestations); (2) residual pulmonary lesions; and (3) a rare, disseminating, sometimes fatal disease. The disease tends to be milder in children; however, in those requiring medical attention, dissemination to bones and meninges is fairly common and approaches the incidence of these complications in adults. Maternal-fetal or -infant infection has been reported.

Primary Coccidioidomycosis. The incubation period varies from 1 to 4 wk, with an average of 10–16 days. Symptoms are influenzal in type; the onset may be insidious or abrupt with malaise, chills, and fever. Night sweats and anorexia are common. On occasion, there is a persistent dry cough and there may be a painful throat. There also may be headache, backache, and chest pain, which may vary from a mere sense of constriction to excruciating pleurisy.

A generalized, fine, macular erythema or urticarial eruption may appear within the 1st day or so. It may be evanescent and present only in the groin. Most frequently erythema nodosum with or without erythema multiforme occurs. These lesions develop at the time sensitivity to coccidioidin is maximal, 3–21 days after onset of symptoms. Skin lesions may occur, however, in persons otherwise asymptomatic. Other allergic manifestations, arthritis, and phlyctenular conjunctivitis may occur concomitantly.

Chest examination rarely discloses positive findings, even though roentgenography reveals extensive consolidation. Infrequently dullness, a friction rub, or fine rales may be detected. Pleural effusions occur at times and may be so massive as to embarrass respiration; they may develop without preceding respiratory symptoms.

Residual Pulmonary Coccidioidomycosis. Infrequently, a cavity may develop in an area of pulmonary consolidation during the primary infection and then regress. More often, however, after a variably prolonged period a persistent cavity may form. There are often no symptoms, and the diagnosis is made roentgenographically. Occasionally there is mild to moderate hemoptysis, which may recur and be alarming. Rarely, fatal hemorrhage has occurred. Dissemination of the fungus from cavities to other areas is rare. Pulmonary residual "granulomas" sometimes persist. They are not harmful but do pose problems of differentiation from tuberculosis or neoplasms. Infrequently, a chronic progressive fibrocavitary pulmonary disease is seen.

Disseminated or Progressive Coccidioidomycosis (Coccidioidal Granuloma). Certain persons lack ability to localize coccidioidal infection. Dissemination, which is rare and occurs mainly in males, especially in Filipinos, other Asians, and blacks, usually follows the initial illness within 6 mo, often without any interlude. This is analogous to progressive primary tuberculosis. Certain immunosuppressed states enhance dissemination or bring about relapse of apparently arrested coccidioidomycosis. Dissemination is enhanced if coccidioidal infection is acquired during the later stages of pregnancy. Skin lesions and cold abscesses, both subcutaneous and osseous, occur. Meningitis is the most serious of the disseminated lesions, being clinically similar to tuberculous meningitis. In whites it is not unusual for meningitis to be the only extrapulmonary lesion. Miliary dissemination and peritonitis may be distinguishable from tuberculosis only by demonstrating the causative agent, though coccidioidal peritonitis may present as a very mild disease. The mortality rate of untreated meningitis is practically 100%, but it is variable with other forms of disseminated coccidioidomycosis.

Diagnosis. Diagnosis of the disseminated infection may be established by biopsy or at autopsy. Sputum is generally so scanty in the primary infection that gastric lavage may be advisable, especially in children. If histologic examination demonstrates the characteristic double-contoured spherules with endospores and without budding, the diagnosis is certain. Demonstration of the fungus by culture and by animal inoculation is also diagnostic. Only especially qualified laboratories should undertake such hazardous procedures.

The sedimentation rate is rapid in both primary and disseminated infections and is helpful in evaluating clinical status. Eosinophilia is common and is proportionately higher with more severe infections. Serum alkaline phosphatase may be elevated in acute coccidioidomycosis even in the absence of obvious metapulmonary dissemination.

Skin Test. Tests with coccidioidin or the newer spherulin are specific except for occasional cross-reactions with histoplasmosis and blastomycosis. A positive reaction does not distinguish between a recent or old infection unless preceded within a reasonably short time by a negative test result. However, *a negative skin test does not rule out coccidioidal infection.* Coccidioidin is administered intradermally as 0.1 mL of a 1:1000, 1:100, or even 1:10 dilution. The reaction generally reaches its peak at 36 hr and should be read at 24 and 48 hr.

An area of induration more than 5 mm in diameter is positive. Patients with suspected coccidioidal erythema nodosum are likely to be hypersensitive and should receive the 1:1000 dilution. Patients with disseminated infections are much less sensitive; even a 1:10 dilution may not elicit a reaction. Dermal sensitivity to coccidioidin is less durable than to tuberculin. There is no danger of disseminating or activating a coccidioidal infection by a strong coccidioidin reaction, although there may be a systemic reaction as well as a local one. Coccidioidin does not evoke humoral antibodies in the human; therefore, the skin test may precede serologic tests and will provide information useful in their interpretation. However, negative skin tests should not preclude serologic tests.

Blood and Cerebrospinal Fluid Tests. Serum precipitins (IgM) and complement fixation (IgG) antibodies are detectable in early coccidioidomycosis and may persist with disseminated coccidioidomycosis. In general, the more severe the infection, the higher the complement fixation titer. Humoral antibodies are generally not demonstrable in asymptomatic acute infections. Rarely, serologic tests may be negative in active coccidioidomycosis, e.g., in the patient immunosuppressed for renal transplantation or by AIDS. The cerebrospinal fluid findings are similar to those of tuberculous meningitis (Sec. 11.46). Fixation of complement by cerebrospinal fluid occurs in 95% of patients with coccidioidal meningitis and is usually diagnostic. Occasionally, epidural coccidioidal lesions may also lead to complement fixation by the cerebrospinal fluid. Complement-fixing antibody may be detected in cisternal and lumbar fluid but be deceptively absent from the ventricular fluid. Antibodies detectable by complement fixation do not pass the blood-brain barrier but are found in cord blood at the same titer as in the mother's blood. Passively transferred antibody disappears from the infant within 6 mo.

Roentgenography. During the primary infection roentgenograms of the chest may not reveal pulmonary changes. Hilar adenopathy is frequent, and there may be single or multiple, sharply circumscribed or soft, feathery, small pulmonary densities or larger consolidated areas. Pulmonary cavities, when present, tend to be thin-walled. Pleural effusions are of variable extent. The osseous lesions, usually multiple and with a predilection for cancellous bone, often are widespread and are generally indistinguishable from those of tuberculosis.

Prevention. Avoidance of exposure to the spores is the only means for preventing infection. An available vaccine is of unproved value in humans.

Treatment. The treatment of *primary coccidioidal infection* consists of restriction of activity and symptomatic measures until the sedimentation rate returns to normal, precipitins vanish, the complement-fixing titer of serum decreases, and roentgenographic improvement is noted. Pulmonary cavities frequently close spontaneously. When a cavity persists or is located peripherally or there is recurrent bleeding or secondary infection, excision should be considered. Infrequently, bronchopleural fistulas or recurrent cavitation may occur as surgical complications; rarely, dissemination may result. When extensive thoracic surgery is required, therapy with amphotericin B may be desirable.

Amphotericin B, 0.5–1.0 mg/kg/24 hr given intravenously, is the mainstay of treatment of *disseminated coccidioidomycosis.* Once the full dose is achieved, it can be administered every other day or 2–3 times/wk in the face of reduced renal function due to its toxicity. Thrombophlebitis is common. Anemia due to the drug can be effectively treated with transfusions and terminates when treatment is stopped. Agranulocytosis is rare, and hepatic insufficiency develops occasionally, mainly in those with pre-existing liver damage. The drug should not be used in primary infections except when dissemination seems imminent. Although the response is occasionally dramatic in the disseminated form of the disease, generally treatment must be continued for months and, if possible, until improvement is reflected by a significant reduction (4-fold) in complement-fixing antibodies. An increase in sensitivity to coccidioidin is evidence of a favorable immunologic response. Immunologic reconstitution with leukocyte transfer factor (not yet fully evaluated) may be helpful in anergic patients.

Amphotericin B does not pass the blood-brain barrier in therapeutic amounts, but it may mask meningitis during intravenous treatment. Early treatment of coccidioidal meningitis is important, and intrathecal administration of the drug in doses of 0.5 mg 2–3 times/wk (gradually increased from a dose of 0.025 mg) is usually necessary. Arachnoiditis and transverse myelitis are hazards of intraspinal administration.

Cold abscesses should be drained, infected synovial membranes removed, and, if osseous lesions are accessible, excision considered. In these cases intravenous and local amphotericin B may be used, depending on extent of involvement.

Amphotericin B has been used to treat coccidioidomycosis during pregnancy without apparent adverse effect on the fetus.

Treatment of *coccidioidal meningitis* should begin with both intravenous and intrathecal or intraventricular administration of amphotericin B. Intrathecal administration into the cisterna magna is preferred. However, administering amphotericin in 10% glucose solution via the lumbar route with the patient's head tilted down at −30 degrees from the horizontal may reduce the incidence of serious arachnoiditis. Intravenous therapy may be discontinued when the physician feels confident that meningitis is the only extrapulmonary involvement, when the patient appears clinically well, and when laboratory findings support the clinical impression of improvement. Treatment should continue for at least 3 mo after the cerebrospinal fluid has normal cells, glucose, and protein and is negative on complement-fixation testing. Follow-up should include examination of the cerebrospinal fluid at intervals of 1–3 mo (and immediately if there is headache or any change in behavior or personality) for a period of at least 2 yr. Clinical surveillance should be continued for some years longer, as relapses have been noted as late as 3–5 yr after return of the CSF to normal.

Ketoconazole administered orally (in doses of approximately 3–15 mg/kg) is useful in treating disseminated nonmeningeal coccidioidomycosis that is not extensive nor progressing rapidly. It does not prevent dissemination from the primary pulmonary disease. Cutaneous and subcutaneous lesions are most responsive to this drug, synovial lesions next, and osseous lesions least responsive. Chronic pulmonary coccidioidal disease, cavitary or fibrocavitary, has not been consistently improved by ketoconazole or by amphotericin B. Oral ketoconazole has been used along with intrathecal amphotericin B or intraventricular miconazole for treating coccidioidal meningitis; although very high doses may penetrate the CSF, ketoconazole cannot be recommended in place of intrathecal amphotericin B or miconazole. Ketoconazole has been administered to children less than 2 yr of age, but the significance in children of the hepatic dysfunction and the inhibition of testosterone and adrenocorticoid synthesis noted in adults has not been adequately evaluated. Relapses have occurred in some patients after favorable clinical responses following therapy for more than a year.

The sole indication for the use of parenteral **miconazole** is intrathecal or intraventricular administration for suppression of coccidioidal meningitis.

DEMOSTHENES PAPPAGIANIS

General

Drutz DJ: Amphotericin B in the treatment of coccidioidomycosis. Drugs 26:337, 1983.
Einstein H (ed): Fourth International Symposium on Coccidioidomycosis. Washington, DC, National Foundation for Infectious Diseases, 1985.
Galgiani JN: Ketoconazole in the treatment of coccidioidomycosis. Drugs 26:355, 1983.
Harrison HR, Galgiani JN, Reynolds AF Jr, et al: Amphotericin B and imidazole therapy for coccidioidal meningitis in children. Pediatr Infect Dis 2:216, 1983.
Kafka JA, Catanzaro A: Disseminated coccidioidomycosis in children. J Pediatr 98:355, 1981.
Richardson HB, Anderson JA, McKay BM: Acute pulmonary coccidioidomycosis in children. J Pediatr 70:376, 1967.
Shafai T: Neonatal coccidioidomycosis in premature twins. Am J Dis Child 132:634, 1978.
Stevens DA (ed): Coccidioidomycosis: A Text. New York, Plenum Medical Book Co, 1980.
Stevens DA: Coccidioidomycosis and the indications for chemotherapy. Drugs 26:334, 1983.
Stevens DA: Miconazole in the treatment of coccidioidomycosis. Drugs 26:347, 1983.
Winn WA: The treatment of coccidioidal meningitis. The use of amphotericin B in a group of 25 patients. Calif Med 101:78, 1964.

Patient Education

Coccy (Coccidioidomycosis). The Facts. Published by the American Lung (Christmas Seal) Association and available through its local Chapter offices.

11.99 HISTOPLASMOSIS

Etiology. Histoplasmosis is a disease of man and animals caused by *Histoplasma capsulatum*. The mycelial or saprophytic form of this dimorphic fungus is distributed worldwide in soil. It grows on Sabouraud medium at room temperature (25° C) as white or tan fluffy colonies; small, budding, oval yeast forms are found in the infected tissue.

Epidemiology. Human histoplasmosis follows inhalation of airborne spores released by *H. capsulatum*. The saprophytic form grows best in soil heavily contaminated with avian and bat excreta. Birds, because of their high body temperature, are not infected but may carry the fungus on their feathers. However, bats may be infected and disseminate the fungus in their excreta. Chicken, starling, or blackbird roosts and hollow trees as well as bat-infested caves, lofts, attics, and bridges may be heavily contaminated and serve as a reservoir for human infection. Histoplasmosis occurs throughout the United States, is endemic in the Mississippi, Ohio, and Missouri River valleys, and is most common in Kentucky and Tennessee, where up to 90% of the population have a positive histoplasmin skin test reaction by the age of 20 yr. Other areas of high prevalence, often very local, occur in South America, Asia, and Europe. Focal outbreaks of epidemic histoplasmosis have been reported following cave exploration, excavation, demolition, or other dust-raising activities in heavily contaminated areas. A large outbreak occurred in Indianapolis in 1979, where an estimated 100,000 persons were infected, 15 of whom died from this disease. Histoplasmosis is not transmitted from person to person.

Pathogenesis and Pathology. Histoplasmosis usually occurs following inhalation of conidia, which reach the alveoli and transform into small budding yeast. During an initial period of multiplication, there is both a local spread to adjacent lymph nodes and transient dissemination from the pulmonary focus to organs throughout the body. In most patients these primary lesions enlarge and undergo caseous necrosis, fibrosis, and subsequent calcification. In the lung, calcification of a primary focus and adjacent lymph nodes may resemble the Gohn complex of primary pulmonary tuberculosis. Multifocal "buckshot" areas of calcification may also occur throughout the lungs, lymphatic tissue, and spleen. Two forms of progressive histoplasmosis occur in a small proportion of infected patients. *Disseminated histoplasmosis* occurs in infants and debilitated adults and in patients with defects in cell-mediated immunity. Yeast-laden macrophages infiltrate the entire reticuloendothelial system with extensive involvement of the bone marrow, liver, spleen, lungs, heart, adrenals, and brain. *Chronic pulmonary histoplasmosis* typically occurs in adult males and is associated with yeast invasion and multiplication in pre-existing emphysematous cavities, producing cavities, caseous necrosis, and fibrosis.

Clinical Manifestations. *Acute pulmonary histoplasmosis*, the most common form of disease, is classified as primary (initial infection) or secondary (reinfection) according to previous exposure history. The **primary** form is most often an asymptomatic disease in infants and young children, a positive histoplasmin skin test being the only manifestation of infection. The incubation period is 10–23 days, and the severity of symptoms, when present, corresponds to the concentration of inhaled conidia. Symptomatic primary acute pulmonary histoplasmosis presents as an influenza-like illness with abrupt onset of fever, malaise, myalgia, headache, and nonproductive cough. Physical examination is often normal; however, diffuse rales and mild hepatosplenomegaly have been described. Erythema multiforme and erythema nodosum occur in symptomatic and asymptomatic individuals, are more common in women, and are often accompanied by arthralgias and arthritis. Roentgenographic examination of the lungs during the acute illness is usually normal (75%), but a minority of patients may demonstrate small, patchy infiltrates with enlargement of hilar nodes. Abnormal chest roentgenograms may persist for several months, showing small nodular residues that eventually calcify. The illness is self-limited in most children; abnormal signs and symptoms, when present, rarely persist for more than 3 wk.

Secondary, or reinfection type, pulmonary histoplasmosis has the onset of symptoms within 3 days of exposure. They are similar but less severe and of shorter duration than in primary disease. The roentgenographic findings following reinfection consist of uniformly distributed miliary nodules indistinguishable from miliary tuberculosis, which resolve over several months without calcification.

Epidemic histoplasmosis has been reported in both endemic and nonendemic areas following massive exposure to dust heavily contaminated with spores of *H. capsulatum*. Clinical manifestations begin within 3–20 days following exposure and include an abrupt onset of high fever, chills, headache, malaise, and a nonproductive cough; pleuritic chest pain and dyspnea are common. Physical examination reveals diffuse rales often associated with minimal hepatosplenomegaly. Erythema nodosum and erythema multiforme appearing separately or together have been reported in young women during epidemics. Roentgenographic examination of the chest reveals pulmonary infiltrates, which may persist for several months. The prognosis is excellent, with spontaneous resolution of all signs and symptoms expected within weeks. Epidemic illness has, on rare occasions, led to disseminated disease in infants and children.

Chronic pulmonary histoplasmosis, a disease of middle-aged white male smokers with a history of chronic obstructive pulmonary disease, is uncommon in children. The onset is insidious and is characterized by cough, fever, and weight loss. Roentgenograms of the chest typically demonstrate upper lobe infiltrates, cavity formation, and calcified hilar nodes.

Disseminated histoplasmosis is an acute illness of infants, young children, and immunosuppressed patients which produces high morbidity and mortality; untreated, the outcome is uniformly fatal, having an average course of 4 wk. The illness begins as an acute pulmonary infection with fever, cough, and dyspnea and quickly progresses to involve multiple organ systems. Affected patients appear critically ill with persistent nausea, vomiting, abdominal pain, and diarrhea. Physical findings reveal generalized rales, diffuse lymphadenopathy, and impressive hepatosplenomegaly. Roentgenographic abnormalities often include a diffuse interstitial pneumonitis. Anemia, leukopenia, and thrombocytopenia are common and predispose to bleeding and/or secondary bacterial infection. Death is secondary to respiratory failure, uncontrolled gastrointestinal bleeding, disseminated intravascular coagulation, and/or bacterial sepsis. Subacute and chronic forms of disseminated disease have been reported in adults and may involve a single organ system.

Histoplasmoma and *mediastinal collagenosis* are rare in children, representing an exaggerated immune response. Histoplasmoma presents an enlarging, solitary pulmonary nodule with concentrated layers of fibrous tissue and calcium surrounding a healed primary focus; these nodules may reach 3–4 cm in diameter and must be differentiated from neoplasms. Mediastinal collagenosis is associated with fibrocalcification originating in a mediastinal node and extending through the mediastinum, resulting in entrapment and obstruction of mediastinal structures.

Diagnosis. Diagnosis of acute pulmonary histoplasmosis relies on conversion of the histoplasmin skin test, on seroconversion of the complement fixation assay, or on the immunodiffusion test. Sputum cultures are rarely positive, but in disseminated disease the organism can often be isolated from the blood, bone marrow, lymphatic tissue, or other biopsy material. In chronic cavitary disease, the fungus can often be recovered from sputum.

The skin test resembles the tuberculin test and is considered positive if an area of at least 5 mm of induration is observed at 48 hr. A positive reaction indicates previous sensitization to *H. capsulatum* but is not diagnostic of active disease. However, conversion from a negative to a positive reaction within a few weeks or a positive reaction in an infant suggests active infection. Skin testing has limited usefulness because of a large number of false negatives in patients with disseminated disease and late conversion following initial infection. Approximately 25% of patients with positive skin test will convert their serology from negative to positive after skin testing. Reactivity to histoplasmin antigen is relatively short lived, and conversion to a negative test occurs several years after primary infection.

Complement fixation titers are often helpful in diagnosing acute infection. An initial titer greater than 1:8 suggests active disease; only 25% of infected individuals will demonstrate a 4-fold increase between acute and convalescent titers. Cross-reaction with the serologic test for blastomycosis is common, and an initial titer of greater than 1:8 for *B. dermatitidis* in the absence of blastomycosis suggests acute infection with *H. capsulatum*. The immunodiffusion test with the M antigen has fewer false negatives than the standard complement fixation assay. Definitive diagnosis requires demonstration of the infecting organism by culture or histology.

Treatment. Amphotericin B is the treatment of choice for all life-threatening infections due to *H. capsulatum*. In acute pulmonary histoplasmosis in older children and adults, treatment is not indicated since the disease is often benign and self-limited. However, symptomatic pulmonary histoplasmosis in infants and young children (under 2 yr) may progress to disseminated disease; therefore a short course of amphotericin B (2 wk) is recommended. In disseminated histoplasmosis, treatment with amphotericin B is indicated. Although experience is limited in children, most authorities recommend a total dose of 30 mg/kg (see Sec. 11.98 for dosage regimen). Cultures often convert to negative within a few weeks; however, relapses are not uncommon, and repeated cultures to monitor the success or failure of chemotherapy are indicated.

In vitro studies demonstrate synergistic killing of *H. capsu-*

latum when amphotericin B is combined with rifampin, but clinical experience with this combination is limited.

Ketoconazole is a possible alternative but comparative studies in children are lacking, and the drug appears less effective than amphotericin B.

WILLIAM T. SPECK
STEPHEN C. ARONOFF

Goodwin RA, Des Prez RM: Histoplasmosis. Am Rev Resp Dis 117:929, 1978.
Goodwin RA, Shapiro JL, et al: Disseminated histoplasmosis: Clinical and pathologic correlations. Medicine 59:1, 1980.
Kauffman CA, Israel KS, et al: Histoplasmosis in immunosuppressed patients. Am J Med 64:923, 1978.
Macher A: Histoplasmosis and blastomycosis. Med Clin North Am 64:447, 1980.
Wheat J, French ML, Kohler RB, et al: The diagnostic laboratory tests for histoplasmosis. Ann Intern Med 97:680, 1982.

11.100 PARASITIC INFECTIONS

Infectious diseases due to protozoa and helminths are a major cause of morbidity and mortality in infants and children in many parts of the world. However, they have received relatively little attention compared with infections due to viral, bacterial, or fungal agents. Such neglect of parasitic diseases contrasts with their global significance; malaria alone claims more than a million lives of African children annually and is increasingly imported to Europe and North America. Parasites are endemic in many parts of the world; although they are more common in hot climates, no specific geographic area is spared. Recognition of these infections and their proper management are therefore essential. The major parasitic infections and their estimated prevalence, mortality, and morbidity are presented in Table 11–36.

The term "parasites" has been used historically and conventionally to refer only to those infectious organisms that belong to the animal kingdom, i.e., *protozoa, helminths,* and *arthropods.* Protozoa are unicellular organisms that multiply within their hosts and are therefore closely related to other infectious agents. In contrast, worms or helminths are multicellular and usually do not divide within the human host. These basic biologic differences between protozoa and helminths have important epidemiologic, clinical, and therapeutic implications.

The host-parasite relationship in protozoan and helminthic infections has several unique features. Infection and disease due to these agents must be clearly distinguished. When a parasite invades a host, it may die at once or survive without causing harm to the host (infection). Alternatively, it may survive and produce morbidity (disease) and possibly kill the host. Parasites have adapted through various evolutionary modifications to establish infections more commonly than disease and thus allow the development of a symbiotic relationship with their hosts. In addition, these organisms have evolved evasive mechanisms against host immune or protective responses. In respect to the host's well-being, parasites may cause disease by their physical presence or by competition with the host for specific nutrients. Disease may also result from the host's attempts to destroy the invaders, e.g., the host's immunopathologic reaction.

The sections on individual infections deal with the most important parasitic infections encountered in the pediatric age group. A deliberate attempt has been made to include only the most effective, reliable, and safe therapeutic agents.

Walsh JA, Warren KS: Selective primary health. An interim strategy for disease control in developing countries. N Engl J Med 301:967, 1979.
Warren KS, Mahmoud AAF: Tropical and Geographical Medicine. New York, McGraw-Hill, 1984.

PROTOZOA

INTESTINAL PROTOZOA

Protozoan infections of the intestine cause a wide variety of clinical syndromes, ranging from asymptomatic carrier states to severe disease associated with pathologic lesions in the gastrointestinal tract or other organs (Table 11–37). *Entamoeba histolytica* and *Giardia lamblia* cause important and clin-

ically well-defined pathologic lesions. Infections with less common organisms such as *Cryptosporidium, Balantidium coli,* and *Isospora hominis* are usually asymptomatic or associated with mild disease. Infections by the intestinal protozoa are usually acquired orally through fecal contamination of water or food, and they are more endemic in countries with unsanitary water conditions. *G. lamblia* and *Cryptosporidium,* how-

Table 11–36. **Estimated Worldwide Prevalence (In Thousands) of the Major Parasitic Infections in Relation to Associated Morbidity and Mortality**

Infection	Prevalence	Morbidity	Mortality
Protozoa			
Amebiasis	400,000	1500	30
Giardiasis	4000	1000–2000	0.1
Malaria	800,000	150,000	1200
Trypanosomiasis, African	1000	10	5
Trypanosomiasis, American	12,000	1200	60
Toxoplasmosis	800,000	10	0.1
Leishmaniasis	12,000	12,000	5
Helminths			
Ascariasis	1,000,000	1000	30
Hookworms	900,000	1500	50–60
Filariasis	300,000	500	20–50
Schistosomiasis	300,000	150,000	1200

Table 11–37. Important Intestinal Protozoan Infections of Children

Infection	Etiology	Transmission	Major Clinical Features	Diagnosis
Amebiasis	*Entamoeba histolytica*	Fecal-oral	Diarrhea-dysentery	Trophozoites or cysts in stools
			Liver abscess	Serology
Giardiasis	*Giardia lamblia*	Fecal-oral Person-to-person	Diarrhea Malabsorption	Cysts in stools Cysts or trophozoites in duodenal aspirate
Cryptosporidiosis	*Cryptosporidium*	Fecal-oral Person-to-person	Watery diarrhea	Oocysts in stools
Balantidiasis	*Balantidium coli*	Fecal-oral	Bloody diarrhea	Trophozoites or cysts in stools

ever, have recently been recognized as a major cause of epidemics of waterborne diarrhea in North America, and particularly in day care centers. *Cryptosporidium* infection is becoming a major cause of diarrhea in patients with acquired immunodeficiency syndrome (Sec. 11.11).

11.101 AMEBIASIS

Human infection with *Entamoeba histolytica* is prevalent worldwide; endemic foci are particularly common in areas with low socioeconomic and sanitary standards. *E. histolytica* parasitizes the lumen of the gastrointestinal tract and causes few or no disease sequelae in most infected subjects. In a small proportion of individuals the organisms invade the intestinal mucosa or may disseminate to other organs, especially the liver.

Etiology. Infection is established by ingestion of parasite cysts. These cysts measure 10–18 μm, contain 4 nuclei, and are resistant to environmental conditions such as low temperature and the concentrations of chlorine commonly used in water purification; the parasite can be killed by heating to 55° C. Upon ingestion, the cyst wall is digested, and the nuclei double in number to form 8 trophozoites. These are large, actively motile organisms that colonize the lumen of the large intestine and may invade its mucosal lining. Trophozoites have an average diameter of 20 μm; their cytoplasm consists of an outer clear zone and an inner densely granular endoplasm containing a spherical nucleus which has a small central karyosome and fine granular chromatin material. The endoplasm also contains vacuoles where, in cases of invasive amebiasis, erythrocytes may be seen. Two other species of nonpathogenic *Amoeba* may infect the human gastrointestinal tract: *E. coli* and *E. hartmanni*.

Epidemiology. The prevalence of amebic infections worldwide varies from 5 to 81%. Amebic dysentery due to invasion of the intestinal mucosa occurs in approximately 1–17% of infected subjects. Dissemination of the parasites to internal organs such as the liver occurs in an even smaller fraction of infected individuals and is less common in children than in adults.

Man is the natural host and reservoir of *E. histolytica*. The pattern of infection varies in different parts of the world. For example, infection acquired in India, Mexico, or Durban, South Africa, is more virulent than that from other locations. The definition of virulence, geographic strains, and pathogenicity of different amebae, however, is not clear.

Infection is transmitted via contaminated food and drinks. Food handlers carrying amebic cysts may therefore play a role in spreading the infection. Direct contact with infected feces also may be responsible for person-to-person transmission.

Pathogenesis and Pathology. Once *E. histolytica* trophozoites invade the intestinal mucosa, they produce tissue destruction (ulcers) with little local inflammatory response.

The organisms multiply and spread laterally underneath the intestinal epithelium to produce the characteristic flask-shaped ulcers. These lesions are commonly seen in the cecum, transverse, and sigmoid colon. Amebae may produce similar lytic lesions if they reach the liver (these are commonly called abscesses although they contain no granulocytes). *E. histolytica* occasionally disseminates to other extraintestinal sites such as the lungs and brain. The contrasts among the extent of tissue destruction by amebae, the absence of a local host inflammatory response, and the demonstration of systemic humoral (antibody) and cell-mediated reactions against the organisms remain a major scientific puzzle.

Clinical Manifestations. Most infected individuals are asymptomatic, and cysts are found in their feces. Tissue invasion occurs in 2–8% of infected individuals and may be related to the strain of parasites or the nutritional status and intestinal flora of the host. The most common clinical manifestations of amebiasis are due to local invasion of the intestinal epithelium and dissemination to the liver.

Intestinal amebiasis may occur within 2 wk of infection or be delayed for months. The onset is usually gradual with colicky abdominal pains and frequent bowel movements (6–8 movements/24 hr). Diarrhea is frequently associated with tenesmus. Stools are blood-stained and contain a fair amount of mucus with few leukocytes. Generalized constitutional symptoms and signs are characteristically absent. Acute amebic dysentery occurs in attacks lasting a few days to several weeks; recurrence is very common in untreated individuals. Occasionally, amebic dysentery is associated with sudden onset of fever, chills, and severe diarrhea, which may result in dehydration and electrolyte disturbances. In a few patients complications such as ameboma, extraintestinal extension, or local perforation and hemorrhage may occur. The characteristic flask-shaped ulcers with healthy intervening mucosa that occur in most cases may be detected by sigmoidoscopy in 25% of patients.

Hepatic amebiasis is a very serious manifestation of disseminated infection. Although diffuse liver enlargement has been associated with intestinal amebiasis, liver abscess occurs in fewer than 1% of infected individuals and may appear in patients with no clear history of intestinal disease. In children fever is the hallmark of amebic liver abscess. It is frequently associated with abdominal pain, distention, and an enlarged, tender liver. Changes at the base of the right lung, such as elevation of the diaphragm and parenchymal compression, may also occur. Laboratory examination shows a slight leukocytosis, moderate anemia, and no significant elevation of liver enzymes. Stool examination for amebae is negative in more than 50% of patients with documented amebic liver abscess. In most cases ultrasonography and isotope scans localize and delineate the size of the abscess cavity. Most patients have a single cavity in the right hepatic lobe. Amebic liver abscess may be associated with rupture into the peritoneum or thorax or through the skin when diagnosis and therapy are delayed.

Diagnosis. Diagnosis is based on detecting the organisms in stool samples or, rarely, in aspirates of a liver abscess. Several fresh stool samples should be examined by an experienced person. Whenever amebiasis is suspected, an additional stool sample may be preserved in polyvinyl alcohol for further identification and staining of the organisms. Material for microscopic examination may also be obtained by scraping the ulcerated areas of rectal mucosa. The indirect hemagglutination test may be helpful in invasive intestinal amebiasis and amebic liver abscess; diagnostic titers of ≥1:128 are reported in 98–100% of cases.

Treatment. All individuals with *E. histolytica* trophozoites or cysts in their stools, whether symptomatic or not, should be treated. Diloxanide furoate, a luminal amebicide, is the drug of choice for asymptomatic cyst passers. The recommended dose is 10 mg/kg/24 hr orally for 10 days. Toxicity is rare, but the drug should not be used in children under 2 yr of age.

Invasive amebiasis of the intestine, liver, or other organs requires the use of metronidazole, a tissue amebicidal drug; it is administered orally in a daily dose of 50 mg/kg for 10 days. Side effects of this drug include nausea, diarrhea, metallic taste in the mouth, and leukopenia; these are uncommon and disappear on completion of therapy. Metronidazole is also a luminal amebicide but less effective than diloxanide furoate for this purpose. Patients with invasive amebiasis should therefore receive an additional course of the latter drug following metronidazole therapy. If the case is severe or if metronidazole cannot be used, dehydroemetine is the recommended alternative therapeutic agent. It is administered by the subcutaneous or intramuscular route (never intravenously) in a dose of 1 mg/kg/24 hr for 10 days. Patients should be hospitalized when this drug is given because cardiac or renal complications may occur. If tachycardia, T wave depression, arrhythmias, or proteinuria develops, the drug should be stopped. A course of diloxanide furoate is also recommended following completion of dehydroemetine therapy. Amebic liver abscesses are treated with specific therapy as outlined above; however, aspiration of large lesions may be necessary if rupture is imminent or if the patient shows poor clinical response 4–6 days after administration of amebicidal drugs. Stool examination should be repeated 2 wk following completion of antiamebic therapy as a test of cure.

Control of amebiasis can be achieved by exercising proper sanitary measures. Regular examination of food handlers and thorough investigation of diarrhea episodes may identify the source of infection in some communities. There is no prophylactic drug for amebiasis.

11.102 GIARDIASIS

Infection with *Giardia lamblia* is a common worldwide cause of infectious diarrhea. The infection is more prevalent in children than in adults and is particularly significant in those with malnutrition or immunodeficiencies.

Etiology. *Giardia lamblia* infects man through ingestion of its cysts. The mature cyst, measuring approximately 8–10 μm, is thick walled and oval and contains 4 nuclei. They are passed in the stools of infected individuals and may remain viable in water for longer than 3 mo. Their viability is not affected by the normal concentrations of chlorine used to purify water for drinking. Upon reaching the upper small intestine, each *Giardia* cyst liberates 4 trophozoites. Trophozoites are piriform and measure 2–4 × 14 μ. The body of the trophozoite is divided longitudinally by 2 median rods and contains 2 oval nuclei anteriorly, a large sucking disc on the ventral surface, and a curved median body posteriorly. Each organism has 4 pairs of flagella.

Epidemiology. The prevalence in several parts of the world varies from 0.5–18%. Man was thought to be the only reservoir of *G. lamblia*, but it is now believed that the human parasite infects beavers and dogs as well. Person-to-person, waterborne, food-borne, and interspecies transmission may occur, possibly resulting in sporadic cases as well as in epidemics.

Although giardiasis has long been recognized as an important cause of chronic diarrhea in immunodeficient children, the relationship of the host immune system to susceptibility to infection and subsequent disease remains unclear.

Clinical Manifestations. Giardiasis is more frequently symptomatic in children than in adults. Symptoms occur in 40–80% of infected children; the most common presentation is diarrhea, weight loss, and failure to thrive. The onset of symptoms may be abrupt or gradual; the disease may be self-limited or capable of producing severe protracted diarrhea and malabsorption. Alterations in the digestive function of the brush border are common in those with protracted symptoms. Malabsorption of sugars (such as xylose and disaccharides), fats, and fat-soluble vitamins occurs in more than half of patients who have nonspecific morphologic abnormalities of the small intestinal mucosa similar to those seen in other malabsorptive disorders.

Diagnosis. *G. lamblia* trophozoites or cysts may be found in fecal samples obtained from infected children. As cyst excretion is irregular, examination of several fecal samples or duodenal contents may be needed. The Entero-test is an efficient, simple, and safe method for detecting *G. lamblia* in duodenal fluid of children.

Treatment. Furazolidone (8 mg/kg/24 hr for 10 days) is the drug of choice for children. Tinidazole has also been evaluated for treatment of infected children; a single oral dose of 50 mg/kg resulted in an 80% cure rate.

The recent increase of epidemics of giardiasis requires reexamination of sanitary practices. Water supply is the most important factor; its quality should be routinely monitored. The concentration of chlorine required for control, particularly in communities that are dependent on surface water but have no sand filtration, needs to be determined. Spread of infection in institutions can be prevented by identifying and properly treating asymptomatic carriers. No prophylactic medication prevents giardiasis.

11.103 CRYPTOSPORIDIASIS

Cryptosporidium, an intestinal protozoan initially described as a cause of significant diarrhea in calves and other farm animals, recently has been recognized as an important human pathogen causing watery diarrhea in immunocompetent individuals as well as in immunosuppressed patients, particularly those with AIDS (Sec. 10.23 and 11.11) or congenital immunodeficiencies. Infection is established by ingesting oocysts found in the feces of infected animals or humans. Excystation occurs in the gastrointestinal tract, and all subsequent development takes place at the surface of the intestinal epithelium. Recent stool surveys indicate that the prevalence of infection ranges from 4 to 7%. In day care center epidemics of diarrheal illness, up to 65% of children had cryptosporidium; additionally, 10–15% of stools examined from asymptomatic children in these centers were found to have this parasite.

The natural history of infection in immunocompetent patients suggests an incubation period of 2–7 days. Infection is characterized by the acute onset of watery diarrhea, nausea, and abdominal cramps. Infection is self-limited, lasting 10–14 days. In some, infection may be totally asymptomatic. In contrast, infection in immunosuppressed patients is associated with the development of profuse, watery diarrhea, resulting in weight loss and malnutrition; diarrhea may also become chronic with unrelenting severity.

Diagnosis is difficult. Special stool concentration and staining methods are required in the hands of experienced laboratory personnel. Parasites can also be identified on stained mucosal biopsy specimens, appearing as round eosinophilic bodies on the microvillus border.

Since the diarrheal illness due to cryptosporidiasis is self-limited in immunocompetent patients, no specific therapy is required. In some young infants supportive therapy with fluid and electrolytes may be necessary. Patients with immunodeficiencies have been treated with a wide variety of chemotherapeutic agents, but none showed consistent antiparasitic effect.

OTHER INTESTINAL PROTOZOA

Infection of children with *Balantidium coli* and other coccidia such as *Isospora* and *Sarcocystis* may be associated with vague gastrointestinal complaints such as abdominal pain, distention, and diarrhea. *B. coli* may, however, invade the intestinal mucosa, causing bloody diarrhea and ulcerations. Diagnosis of either infection is made by fecal examination. Therapy with metronidazole is recommended for symptomatic cases of balantidiasis.

ADEL A. F. MAHMOUD
BARBARA S. KAPLAN

Amebiasis

Adams EB, MacLeod IN: Invasive amebiasis. I. Amebic dysentery and its complications. Medicine 56:315, 1977.
Adams EB, MacLeod IN: Invasive amebiasis. II. Amebic liver abscess and its complications. Medicine 56:325, 1977.
Harrison RH, Crowe PC, Fulginiti VA: Amebic liver abscess in children: Clinical and epidemiologic features. Pediatrics 64:923, 1979.

Giardiasis

Craft JC: Giardia and giardiasis in childhood. Pediatr Infect Dis 1:196, 1982.
Craft JC, Murphy T, Nelson JD: Furazolidone and quinacrine. Comparative study of therapy for giardiasis in children. Am J Dis Child 135:164, 1981.
Kavousi S: Giardiasis in infancy and childhood: A prospective study of 160 cases with comparison to quinacrine (atabrine) and metronidazole (Flagyl). Am J Trop Med Hyg 28:19, 1979.
Rosenthal P, Liebman WM: Comparative study of stool examinations, duodenal aspiration and pediatric Entero-test for giardiasis in children. J Pediatr 96:278, 1980.

Cryptosporidiasis

Alpert G, Bell LM, Kirkpatrick CE, et al: Cryptosporidiosis in day care center. N Engl J Med 311:860, 1984.
Ma P, Soave R: Three step stool examination for cryptosporidiosis in 10 homosexual men with protracted watery diarrhea. J Infect Dis 147:824, 1983.
Navin TR, Juranek DD: Cryptosporidiosis: Clinical, epidemiologic, and parasitologic review. Rev Infect Dis 6:313, 1984.

SYSTEMIC PROTOZOAN INFECTIONS

11.104 MALARIA

Malaria results when erythrocytes are invaded by any of four species of protozoan parasites of the genus *Plasmodium*. It is characterized by high fever, which is often intermittent, and by anemia and splenic enlargement. Despite worldwide campaigns aimed at eradicating malaria through interruption of the life cycle of the parasite in the mosquito, the disease continues to be the principal health problem of warm climates. Frequently, malaria is imported to the temperate zone countries where, in the summer months, it may be spread by local mosquitoes.

For clinical and diagnostic purposes, malaria may be regarded as two disease entities: the more dangerous one, caused by *Plasmodium falciparum* and formerly termed "subtertian" or "malignant tertian malaria," can produce a variety of acute clinical manifestations and may, if untreated, be fatal within a few days of onset; the other, caused by *P. vivax* (benign tertian malaria), *P. ovale* (a rarity resembling *P. vivax*), or *P. malariae* (quartan malaria), is more typically paroxysmal and almost never fatal. Vivax and ovale infections may recur weeks after apparent cure of a primary attack, in contrast to the other two which, except in the case of drug-resistant falciparum strains, rarely recrudesce after standard treatment.

Etiology. Malaria is usually acquired from the bites of previously infected female anopheline mosquitoes. In other instances, malaria has developed following transplacental passage or after the transfusion of infected blood, both of which circumvent the pre-erythrocytic phase of the parasite's development in the liver. The usual evolution of the disease is as follows:

Pre-Erythrocytic Phase. The *sporozoites* injected into the blood stream by the biting mosquito reach the sinusoids of the liver and enter the cytoplasm of hepatic cells. Growth and nuclear division are rapid, and microscopic cysts (*schizonts*) containing *merozoites* are formed. Most of the cysts of all species rupture at the end of 6–15 days of development, liberating thousands of merozoites to penetrate red blood cells. However, a few *P. vivax* and *P. ovale* forms remain dormant in the liver for weeks or months, paving the way for relapses.

The incubation period (between the infecting mosquito bite and the presence of parasites in the blood) varies with the species; with *P. falciparum* it is 10–13 days; with *P. vivax* and *P. ovale*, 12–16 days; and with *P. malariae*, 27–37 days, depending on the size of the inoculum. Malaria transmitted by the transfusion of infected blood becomes apparent in a shorter time. Clinical manifestations of infection induced by any means may be suppressed for many months by subcurative treatment, particularly in the cases of vivax and quartan malaria.

Erythrocytic Phase. The merozoites that invade red blood cells appear first in stained smears as bluish rings or (*P. malariae*) bands of cytoplasm, with one or occasionally two red dots of nuclear chromatin. The growing parasites are named *trophozoites*, and appearing with them in the red cells are granules of yellow-brown pigment consisting of hematin derived from the hemoglobin consumed by the parasite to meet its protein requirements. The shape of the organism varies during growth until it becomes round and, with the scattered or clumped pigment, almost fills the red blood cell, which, in the case of *P. vivax*, is enlarged and stippled.

The nucleus of the parasite now divides asexually several times; its cytoplasm is arranged around the new nuclei, and the pigment aggregates into large clumps. This segmenter, or mature *schizont*, contains a varying number of merozoites, depending on the species. The erythrocytes containing these merozoites rupture, and naked merozoites, pigment, and erythrocytic debris are freed into the plasma. Those merozoites that escape inactivation by immunoglobulins or phagocytosis enter fresh red blood cells. Thus, an asexual cycle is begun each time a new crop of merozoites invades red cells. This cycle, the duration of which is of considerable clinical importance, lasts 48 hr in falciparum, vivax, and ovale malaria and 72 hr in quartan malaria. The malarial clinical paroxysm takes place only when enough cycles have occurred to produce the amount of parasitic material, pigment, and red cell debris required to induce febrile or other reactions.

Certain of the growing parasites fail to divide, the nucleus remaining intact during the period of maturation. They are differentiated into male or female forms called *gametocytes*, which are of no clinical importance but are capable of infecting mosquitoes feeding on the patient.

Mixed Infections and Broods. In mixed infections one species is usually responsible for the clinical pattern, with falciparum dominating vivax, and vivax dominating quartan; only when sufficient immunity is developed to the dominant strain does the other begin to produce clinical manifestations.

In an infection with a single species, distinct broods may develop. Since the merozoites in the liver are not released simultaneously and the erythrocytic schizonts do not all rupture at the same time, some groups of parasites begin their existence in red blood cells before or after the majority, often maturing in sufficient numbers to produce an independent clinical reaction. In vivax infections single broods will produce a febrile reaction every other day, whereas if two broods develop, there will be daily paroxysms; in falciparum malaria the classic picture of intermittent fever may likewise soon become disrupted.

Epidemiology. Only in regions where the people have gametocytes in their blood can anopheline mosquitoes become infected. Children may be especially important in this respect. Transmission of malaria occurs in most tropical and some temperate zones; although the United States, Canada, Europe, and Australia are at present free of indigenous malaria, focal outbreaks may occur through infection of local mosquitoes by travelers coming from endemic areas.

Congenital malaria, caused by transfer of the causative agent across the placental barrier, is rare. *Neonatal malaria,* on the other hand, is less uncommon and may result from mingling of infected maternal blood with that of the infant during the birth process.

Pathology and Pathophysiology. The extent of destruction of red blood cells depends upon the duration and severity of the infection. Hemolysis often leads to an increase in the serum bilirubin, and in falciparum malaria it may be sufficiently intense to result in hemoglobinuria **(blackwater fever).** In any malarial infection the degree of anemia is greater than that attributable solely to the destruction of cells by parasites. Autoantigenic changes produced in the red cell by the parasite probably contribute to hemolysis; these changes and increased osmotic fragility occur in all erythrocytes, whether infected or not. Hemolysis may also be induced by quinine or primaquine in persons with hereditary glucose-6-phosphate dehydrogenase deficiency.

The pigment extruded into the circulation upon red cell disintegration accumulates in the reticuloendothelial cells of the spleen, the follicles of which become hyperplastic and sometimes necrotic, in the Kupffer cells of the liver, and in the bone marrow, brain, and other organs. Deposition of sufficient pigment and of hemosiderin results in a slate-gray color of the organs.

The malignancy of falciparum malaria is peculiar to that species. The merozoites emerging from the liver are considerably more numerous than those of other species; there are as many in young children as in adults, so that children have a proportionately greater initial wave of infection. Young children are particularly prone to severe, often lethal, parasitemia.

Eight to 18 hr after the parasite has entered the red blood cells, these cells become increasingly sticky and tend to adhere to the endothelial lining of blood sinuses and vessels, especially when the circulation is slow. The sticky cell is thus fixed and unable to return to the general circulation, although the parasite within it matures in the normal manner. As more cells adhere, flow within the vessel is progressively impeded, and occlusion or even rupture may occur.

The site and extent of this interference with vascular function, coupled with a selective localization of parasitized cells in various organs or systems, are responsible for the variety of symptoms from falciparum infections. Thus, pneumonitis, encephalitis, or enteritis may be manifest when the bulk of the infection is in the lungs, brain, or intestinal tract, respectively. In the pregnant woman damage to the placenta may result in death of the fetus or in premature birth; infants born at full term to infected women have lower birth weights than those of infants born to uninfected mothers living under similar conditions.

The release of merozoites where the circulation is slowed facilitates the invasion of nearby red blood cells, so that falciparum parasitemia may be heavier than that of other species whose rupture of schizonts takes place in the active circulation. Whereas *P. falciparum* invades all erythrocytes irrespective of age, *P. vivax* attacks primarily reticulocytes,

and *P. malariae* invades mature red cells, features which tend to limit parasitemia of the latter two forms to less than 20,000 red cells/mm³. Falciparum infections in the nonimmune child may develop densities as high as 500,000 parasites/mm³.

Successful treatment stops the proliferation of parasites. Specific antibodies are associated with increased levels of immunoglobulin G in the serum of people repeatedly infected with a particular species. Antibody facilitates the phagocytosis of naked merozoites and of parasite-laden erythrocytes, which are ingested by reticuloendothelial cells, by large lymphocytes and neutrophils, and particularly by monocytes. These antibodies do not, however, interfere with development of the parasite in the liver. Passive immunity, occurring in infants born to mothers who have the disease, limits the severity of attacks of malaria for several weeks after birth. The beneficial effect of this transplacental humoral immunity may be enhanced by persistence of fetal hemoglobin and by a diet limited to milk (low in PABA, hence inimical to growth of parasites). Certain hemoglobinopathies are also protective and tend to be genetically selective in endemic malarious regions. *Plasmodium falciparum* may fail to mature in children with the sickle cell trait, and *P. vivax* in those with thalassemia and enzyme deficiencies; *P. falciparum* is unable to attain high densities in children deficient in glucose-6-phosphate dehydrogenase.

Clinical Manifestations. Children who acquire malaria fall into two groups: those having little or no immunity because of lack of previous contact with the disease, who become seriously ill unless treated; and those having a high degree of tolerance by about 10 yr of age due to repeated malarial infections in early childhood which they had survived, although there may be impaired growth and development. Tolerance to malaria also appears to be based on inherited factors that modify the severity of the disease; such tolerance is to be found mostly among Africans and persons of African descent. In the partially immune child heavy parasitemia may occur with few symptoms, or an intercurrent infection may initiate renewed activity of a quiescent malarial infection.

In a nonimmune child clinical signs usually appear 8–15 days after infection and may not be distinctive. Behavioral changes such as fretfulness, anorexia, unusual crying, drowsiness, or disturbances of sleep may be observed. Fever may be absent or increase gradually for 1–2 days, or the onset may be sudden with temperature up to 40.6° C (105° F) or higher, with or without prodromal chill. After varying periods of time, the temperature falls to normal or below, and sweating occurs.

The febrile paroxysm may be extremely short or may last for 2–12 hr; its characteristic pattern is usually obscured in children less than 5 yr of age. Complaints include headache, nausea, generalized aching, particularly of the back, and occasionally pain in the abdomen, when the spleen has swollen quickly and is tender. In vivax and quartan infections dominated by a single brood the fever is the characteristic manifestation, occurring at intervals of 48 hr in the former and 72 in the latter. If convulsions occur, they abate when the fever falls. Herpetic lesions of the mouth are not uncommon. The red blood cell count and hemoglobin level may decrease rapidly; leukopenia is variable, but monocytosis is common.

In falciparum infections the fever is less characteristic and may even be continuous; it may be overshadowed by severe manifestations related to the cerebral, pulmonary, intestinal, or urinary systems. Cerebral complications are evidenced by convulsions or coma, with few localizing neurologic signs and (unless bacterial or viral infections of the central nervous system are superimposed) a normal cerebrospinal fluid. In cases of algid malaria, coma is preceded in the child by shock. Persistent nausea and vomiting, an enlarged and tender liver, and progressive jaundice may evolve into hepatic failure; severe diarrhea may occur; or occasionally the signs of acute appendicitis may be imitated.

The spleen is more commonly enlarged in vivax than in falciparum infections; perisplenitis, infarction, and even rupture may occur, and after repeated attacks the spleen may become very large and hard. "Idiopathic splenomegaly" (so-called big-spleen disease of Africa) may constitute an abnormal immune response to *P. malariae* in malnourished children in developing countries. Enlargement of the spleen is accompanied by lymphocytic infiltration of liver sinusoids and an elevated fluorescent antibody titer for malaria, with or without scanty parasitemia.

Disturbances of renal function are shown by oliguria, and anuria may supervene. The *nephrotic syndrome* is associated with *P. malariae* in children inhabiting endemic malarious areas; the prognosis is poor. *Blackwater fever*, now rarely seen, is associated with *P. falciparum*: hemoglobinuria results from severe and sudden intravascular hemolysis, which may lead to anuria and to death from uremia.

Diagnosis. The diagnosis of malaria depends upon the identification of parasites in the blood. In falciparum malaria, only ring forms are likely to be seen initially, crescents (gametocytes) joining them after 10 days; up to 20% of the erythrocytes may be infected. All stages of the other species of parasites appear in the blood, but less than 1% of red cells will contain them.

In a blood smear the parasites within the red cells have red chromatin and bluish cytoplasm. In some leukocytes, particularly monocytes, remnants of phagocytized parasites and pigment may be seen. The parasites should first be looked for in thick blood films, since in light infections it may not be possible to find plasmodia in the thin film; the latter is best used for species differentiation. As parasites may not be seen at the height of the fever, examinations should be repeated preferably at intervals of 12 hr. The most suitable stain is Giemsa diluted 1:25 with distilled water preferably buffered to pH 7.0–7.2. Wright stain may be used, 0.75 g of the powder being repeatedly shaken for 2 days with 65 mL of pure methyl alcohol and 35 mL of pure glycerin.

The presence of species-specific antibodies associated with an elevated level of IgG, persisting for months or years after an acute attack, may be detected serologically, particularly by the indirect fluorescent antibody (IFA) test. A falsely positive Wassermann reaction will be found in many cases.

Prevention. Natural infection of humans does not occur where breeding of anopheline mosquitoes is prevented, where the adult mosquitoes are kept from contact with people by screens or bed nets, or where they are killed by natural enemies or insecticides before sporozoites have had time to mature. Children visiting endemic malarious areas should be screened from mosquitoes from dusk to dawn, but as this is rarely entirely effective, they should also be given one of the chemoprophylactic drugs *regularly* throughout their stay and for 6 wk thereafter. At least during this period, malaria should be suspected if febrile illness or chronic debility affects the child.

Chemoprophylactic drugs in common use are the following: the slightly bitter but extremely safe chlorguanide (proguanil), taken daily in amounts of 25 mg (to 2 yr), 50 mg (2–6 yr), or 100 mg (older than 6); the tasteless but more toxic pyrimethamine taken weekly in amounts of 6.25 mg (to 2 yr), 12.5 mg (2–6 yr), or 25 mg; and chloroquine or amodiaquine taken weekly in amounts of 37.5 mg of the base (to 1 yr), 75 mg (1–2 yr), 112.5 mg (2–6 yr), 150 mg (6–12 yr) or 300 mg. The bitterness of chloroquine diphosphate and sulfate may be disguised if the crushed tablet is mixed with a spoonful of jam or thick syrup. Commercially mixed syrups are available, but may not remain stable for long.

Unfortunately, resistance of *P. falciparum* to pyrimethamine and chlorguanide is widely distributed; therefore chloroquine

is generally preferred in prophylaxis. When resistance by *P. falciparum* to the latter compound also develops, as in northern South America, southeast Asia, the western Pacific, and eastern and central Africa, potentiating combinations of chlorguanide with dapsone (daily) or pyrimethamine with dapsone or with long-acting sulfonamides (weekly) may be indicated; however, their use for periods longer than 6 mo is discouraged because of possible side effects related to antifolate activity. Chloroquine should be taken concurrently each week to protect against *P. vivax*.

Treatment. Therapy falls into four categories: (1) specific chemotherapy for the attack, whether fresh infection, recrudescence, or relapse; (2) supportive treatment and management of complications; (3) specific chemotherapy to prevent late relapse of vivax or ovale infections; (4) specific chemotherapy to destroy or sterilize gametocytes, and thus to protect the community if mosquitoes are present.

1. Any of the drugs listed in Table 11–38 will effect a clinical cure of all types of malaria and provide a radical cure of falciparum and quartan malaria, unless drug-resistant parasites are present. Children who have inhabited malarious regions and through repeated and prolonged previous infections have acquired some immunity may be cured by one half of the quantities listed. Treatment must be repeated if vomiting occurs within 30 min of ingestion of drugs; persistent vomiting is an indication for parenteral therapy.

Although specific treatment should not usually be undertaken until the diagnosis has been established, many experienced physicians, when confronted with a critically ill or comatose child whose history is suggestive of malaria or exposure thereto, consider it advisable to administer quinine or chloroquine parenterally while awaiting the result of blood film examination.

Parenteral administration of chloroquine or quinine, although hazardous in children bordering on shock, is often essential for those who are vomiting persistently, who are in coma, or who cannot be induced to swallow the drugs even if the bitterness is concealed. Parenteral therapy with antimalarial drugs should be replaced by oral administration as soon as possible. Chloroquine may be given intravenously by slow drip in the quantity of 5 mg base/kg in 10 mL/kg of isotonic saline, infused over a 3–4 hr period, and should be repeated once, 6 hr later, if treatment still cannot be given by mouth. The volume of saline should be adjusted to the state of hydration of the patient, dehydrated children requiring 20 mL/kg, and overhydrated children 5 mL/kg. Administration of chloroquine intramuscularly is not recommended in small children, as it has occasionally precipitated convulsions and aggravated shock and resulted in death. It should not be given subcutaneously because of slow absorption by that route. Quinine dihydrochloride is administered intravenously in a dose of 10 mg/kg and may be repeated 12 hr later; it should be given well diluted (1 mg/mL) and slowly (during 1 hr). When quinine is not available in an emergency situation, quinidine may be used.

2. Supportive treatment includes that for hyperpyrexia. Particular attention should be paid to fluid and electrolyte needs (Sec. 5.32).

Metabolic requirements of the parasite rapidly deplete the reserves of glucose, vitamins, and coenzymes as well as of hemoglobin. Vitamin B_1 may be given, and when the acute phase is passed, ferrous sulfate should be prescribed for a considerable time. Transfusion of packed red cells may be beneficial to children who have had longstanding infections and consequently severe anemia (hemoglobin 5 gm/dL or less).

It is essential that children with severe falciparum infections receive fluids intravenously if dehydrated or in shock. Rapid expansion of the circulating blood volume with whole blood is more effective than with dextran, plasma, or glucose-saline

Table 11–38. **Treatment of Uncomplicated Malaria Attack**

Drug (USP)	Schedule	Dosage in mg Base (Chloroquine and Amodiaquine)* or mg Salt (Quinine)				
		Age Under 1 Yr	Age 1–3 Yr	Age 3–6 Yr	Age 6–12 Yr	Older Children
Chloroquine	Day 1—1st dose	75	100	200	300	450
or	6 hr later	75	75	150	150	300
Amodiaquine	6 hr later	37.5	75	75	100	150
	Day 2—1st dose	37.5	75	75	150	150
	6 hr later	—	—	—	—	150
	Day 3—1st dose	37.5	75	75	150	150
	6 hr later	—	—	—	—	150
Quinine	Daily†	167–250	250–333	333–583	583–1000	1000–2000

*Commercial tablets usually contain 250 mg of chloroquine diphosphate or sulfate, of which 150 mg is base; the quantity of base is stated on the label of the container, and should be prescribed as such.

†Given for 10 days in divided doses every 4 or 8 hr, as tolerated. Dosages indicated are multiples of the standard tablet containing 333 mg of quinine sulfate.

solution. Renal failure, which may require dialysis, is a rare development. When it is present, no more than one third of the conventional doses of antimalarial drugs should be given until the child is hydrated, out of shock, and urinating; quinine and primaquine are contraindicated in the presence of hemoglobinuria. The judicious use of chloroquine or amodiaquine is indicated for heavy parasitemia.

In the comatose stage of cerebral malaria, in addition to specific parenteral antimalarial treatment, dextran-75 may be useful for the prevention of intravascular sludging. Convulsions may be controlled with paraldehyde or barbiturates.

The nephrotic syndrome associated with quartan malaria is managed by the regimen described in Sec. 17.27, together with a course of chloroquine.

3. Late relapse of vivax or ovale malaria may occur up to 3 yr after the primary attack and may be prevented by treating the child with primaquine. Because primaquine given at the height of symptoms increases the tendency to vomit and may be immunosuppressive, it should not be given until the 3rd day of the concomitant clinical curative course of chloroquine, amodiaquine, or quinine. Primaquine is given for 14 days in a daily dose of 0.3 mg base/kg; for fear of possible side reactions some authorities prefer not to administer this drug to children aged less than 3 yr (or to pregnant women), but to treat the acute attack with chloroquine and then place the patients on a chemoprophylactic regimen for several months.

Children receiving primaquine should be watched for toxic manifestations such as methemoglobinemia, hemolytic anemia, hemoglobinuria in children with G-6-PD deficiency, neutropenia, and renal dysfunction. Hemolytic anemia may be particularly severe in G-6-PD deficient children of eastern Mediterranean or Asian descent, for whom two approaches to anti-relapse treatment are available: primaquine may be given once each wk for 8 wk in a dose of 0.9 mg base/kg; or primaquine may be omitted entirely and chemoprophylaxis given for several months following treatment of the acute attack with chloroquine. Quinacrine (mepacrine) should not be used simultaneously with primaquine. Other synthetic antimalarial drugs are relatively nontoxic in therapeutic doses.

4. Gametocytes, however, do not give rise to symptoms and disappear from the circulation soon after destruction of their asexual precursors by chloroquine, amodiaquine, or quinine. Gametocytes can be destroyed by a single dose of primaquine, 7.5 mg base for children aged 1–3 yr, 15 mg for those aged 4–6 yr, 30 mg for those aged 6 to 12 yr, and 45 mg for older children, or their further development in the mosquito inhibited by single doses of chlorguanide or pyrimethamine, provided the parasite is not resistant to these drugs.

Drug resistance is a growing concern. Many strains of *P. falciparum* are now resistant to chlorguanide and to pyrimethamine, but a greater problem is posed by the spread of resistance to chloroquine and amodiaquine in this species to northern South America, southeast Asia, the western Pacific, and eastern and central Africa. Some strains are also tolerant to quinine. These strains are being introduced into North America, Europe, and Australia, where focal summer outbreaks may infect children. Should the malarial attack not respond to chloroquine or amodiaquine, quinine should be used immediately. If this has only a temporary effect, the course should be repeated with the addition of sulfadiazine, 35 mg/kg every 6 hr for 5 days, and pyrimethamine, each day for 3 days, 6.25 mg (to 2 yr of age), 12.5 mg (2–6 yr), or 25 mg. An effective alternative is the full course of quinine, together with tetracycline hydrochloride, 10 mg/kg every 6 hr for 7 days. Tetracycline, which has a slow parasiticidal effect, should not be used unless accompanied by fast-acting quinine. In children less than 8 yr old, the potentially adverse dental effects of tetracycline should be considered.

Preparations combining sulfadoxine or sulfalene with pyrimethamine are generally effective as a single dose, the long-acting sulfonamide in the amount of 25 mg/kg and pyrimethamine 1.25 mg/kg. Rapidity of action is enhanced if quinine is also administered. A parenteral preparation is available, each mL containing 200 mg of sulfadoxine and 10 mg of pyrimethamine; children under 5 yr may be given 1 mL, those from 5–8 yr 2 mL, and older children 3 mL. Unfortunately *P. falciparum* in southeast Asia and South America is developing resistance to these combinations also. A new antimalarial, mefloquine, is coming into use on a restricted basis and is effective against these parasites with multiple drug resistance.

DAVID F. CLYDE

Bruce-Chwatt LJ (ed): Chemotherapy of Malaria. 2nd ed. Geneva, WHO, 1981.
Centers for Disease Control: General advice for travelers to malaria endemic areas. Centers for Disease Control, Atlanta, Georgia: Advisory Memorandum No. 88, 1986.
Hendrickse RG (ed): Paediatrics in the Tropics. Oxford, Oxford Medical Publications, 1981.
Jelliffe DB (ed): Child Health in the Tropics. 4th ed. London, E Arnold, 1974.
Quinn TC, Jacobs RF, Mertz GJ, et al: Congenital malaria: A report of four cases and a review. J Pediatr 101:229, 1982.

11.105 AMERICAN TRYPANOSOMIASIS
(Chagas' Disease)

This insect-transmitted infection is one of the major health problems of South America, largely because the primary infection, which occurs in children and young adults, frequently passes unnoticed and is essentially untreatable. In South America at least 24 million people are infected and 65 million exposed; infection occurs in every South American country and is particularly prevalent in Brazil, Argentina, Uruguay, Chile, and Venezuela. Infections also occur in Central America and in the Caribbean, and two cases have been reported in the United States, in Texans who had never left that state. No authenticated cases have been reported outside the Western Hemisphere.

The intermediate host infected with trypanosomes is a blood-sucking arthropod (reduviid) which is widespread in the endemic areas. In the United States, however, although infected bugs are found in all southwestern states and most southeastern states, these species are not important vectors of the disease for man since they have not become adapted to human dwellings, limiting opportunity for contact.

Etiology. American trypanosomiasis is a zoonosis caused by *Trypanosoma cruzi*, a protozoan parasite of the suborder Trypanosomatidae. It can be transmitted to man by blood-sucking insects of the genera *Triatoma, Rhodnius,* and *Panstrongylus.* Carlos Chagas was responsible for the initial description of the new disease and the discovery of its etiology, vectors, and reservoirs.

In the invertebrate host, *T. cruzi* grows extracellularly in two distinct forms. Epimastigotes multiply in the insect gut and within 1–2 weeks differentiate in the rectum of the insect into metacyclic trypomastigotes, the infectious forms for the mammalian host. These are released with the infected insect's feces when it defecates close to the site of its bite during or after feeding on the host's blood. They enter the host via the damaged skin or through contamination of mucous membranes. Once in the vertebrate host, the metacyclic trypomastigotes readily enter cells, where they replicate as amastigotes. Amastigotes then differentiate intracellularly into trypomastigotes, which are released into the vasculature, where they circulate as bloodstream-form trypomastigotes. These do not replicate until they enter another cell or are withdrawn by another insect vector.

Blood-form trypomastigotes appear in stained preparation as S-shaped flagellates 15–20 µm in length, with a flagellum emerging from the posterior end running along the parasite's body and emerging as free flagellum at the anterior end. A central nucleus and a large kinetoplast can be easily identified. Amastigotes of the vertebrate host appear as oval aflagellates of approximately 3–6 µm in diameter.

Epidemiology. *T. cruzi* infection originally occurred among wild mammals of the American continent and extended to humans when the reduviid insect vectors adapted to human dwellings, principally in rural and low socioeconomic areas. Reduviid bugs are variously known as wild bedbugs, cone-nose bugs, Mexican bedbugs, or assassin or kissing (based on the predilection to attack the face) bugs.

Adobe, mud, or cane housing with numerous cracks in the walls provides excellent shelter for reduviid bugs. Woodpiles near houses and the custom of keeping domestic animals near or within households provide easy access to human living quarters.

Animal reservoirs may play an important role in linking the wild domestic cycles of the parasite because of their habitat and their proximity to people. Dogs and cats are important domestic reservoirs of *T. cruzi;* in Panama and Costa Rica *Rattus rattus* is the main domestic reservoir. In the United States the most important wild reservoirs are opossums and raccoons, with infection rates of 17% and 2%, respectively.

The rarity of human infection in the United States may be due to low virulence of the organisms, the inefficiency of the insect vector, the better housing conditions of the human hosts, and the low adaptability of the North American species

to human dwellings. The prevalence of infection in reduviids has been estimated at 20–25% in the Southwest, but in southern Texas only 1.8% of unselected individuals had serologic evidence of infection.

Blood transfusions and congenital transmissions may also be responsible for *T. cruzi* infection. In Brazil, for instance, 15,000 new cases/year are attributed to transfusions, while 7,500 cases/year are the result of transmission by the congenital route. Accidental inoculation of laboratory workers has also occurred.

Pathogenesis and Pathology. The immune mechanisms involved in resistance to *T. cruzi* and control of the parasitism during the chronic phase of infection are not completely understood. The majority of infected individuals remain asymptomatic, although serologically positive; relatively few develop late complications. Despite the establishment of strong acquired immunity, there is no parasitologic cure, and procedures known to interfere with cell-mediated immune mechanisms increase the severity of infection by *T. cruzi.*

In the nonimmune host, macrophages provide a favorable environment for the growth and replication of the organisms; there they may be protected from certain aspects of the host's immune defense system, particularly in the acute phase. In contrast, in the immune host, macrophages become activated so that they are capable of destroying the interiorized organisms. Macrophages are activated by soluble products (lymphokines) of sensitized T lymphocytes which are stimulated by *T. cruzi* antigen.

IgG antibodies to *T. cruzi* are principally associated with the chronic phase of the infection, probably primarily in mediating immunophagocytosis and killing of the organisms by activated macrophages.

Depression of humoral and cell-mediated immune mechanisms during acute *T. cruzi* infection may be mediated by a subpopulation of thymus-derived lymphocytes. Accumulation of macrophages and lymphocytes is commonly seen during the phase of parasite multiplication and active inflammatory response in the heart and in the smooth muscles of the digestive tract, when muscle fibers and peripheral ganglia of the autonomic nervous system are damaged.

The histopathologic findings in acute Chagas' myocarditis consist of an infiltrate of mononuclear cells into the interstitial space, a degenerative process in myocardial fibers, and the appearance of the so-called pseudocysts. Changes in heart morphology depend upon the intensity of the inflammatory reaction.

In chronic Chagas' cardiomyopathy there are fibrotic foci, which may vary from a few small areas to larger fibrotic plates that thin the ventricular wall; degenerating myocardial fibers, usually in fibrotic areas; and infiltrates of mononuclear cells. When fibroblastic proliferation is extensive, the size of the heart increases and there is reduction of the thickness of the ventricular wall. These alterations are frequently associated with intramural thrombi, mainly at the apex of the left ventricle. Thinning of the ventricular wall by large fibrotic plates becomes the starting point for the formation of the aneurysms often found at the apex of the left ventricle or the posterior area of the mitral valve. Autoimmune reactions have been suggested as underlying these chronic lesions; e.g., antibodies against basement membrane structures could damage blood vessels and endocardium. Alternatively, the lesions could be explained by direct damage produced by the parasites and the resulting inflammation during the acute phase.

The histopathology of the hypertrophic, dilated esophagus and colon of patients with Chagas' disease shows the presence of a mononuclear cell infiltrate between smooth muscle cells and sometimes granuloma formation. A significant reduction of neurons in the myenteric plexus is also commonly seen and may produce the organomegalic syndromes.

Clinical Manifestations. Initially, the infection is often asymptomatic or the symptoms are very mild. This acute stage is followed by a long silent period, the asymptomatic chronic stage, which may last for decades. The disease may then progress to the chronic stage, presenting mainly with cardiac or intestinal manifestations. Approximately 10% of all serologically positive persons manifest chronic sequelae of the disease. There are differences in the clinical picture of disease as it occurs in different geographic localities, but the causes of these differences are unknown.

Acute American Trypanosomiasis. In most cases the clinical symptoms during the acute phase are either mild or absent, so that patients infrequently present a past history compatible with the acute disease. This rare presentation is mainly seen in children in endemic areas, particularly in the age range 0–2 years old, and coincides with local multiplication of the parasites at the site of entry and their subsequent hematogenous dissemination approximately 2–3 wk after infection. Initially, there may be local inflammation with heat, swelling, and redness of the area entered by the parasite. While 25% of individuals with symptomatic acute trypanosomiasis will have no local reactions, half will present with unilateral swelling of the eye (Romaña sign), and one fourth will develop a nodular skin lesion or a local tumor of the skin (chagoma). Enlargement of the local lymph nodes often accompanies these signs. With subsequent hematogenous dissemination of the organism, malaise, fever, muscular pain, and nontender enlargement of lymph nodes occur. A cutaneous morbilliform eruption, hepatosplenomegaly, and, less often, acute meningoencephalitis may be seen, particularly in infants. About 40% of these patients show electrocardiographic abnormalities such as tachycardia and arrhythmias. Mortality may approximate 10% and is related to heart failure or meningoencephalitis.

In transfusional transmission, the incubation period may be longer than in the vector-transmitted disease, sometimes reaching 4–5 mo. Congenital transmission has been usually associated with prematurity and high mortality at birth.

The majority of acute cases of Chagas' disease evolve over 2–3 mo into a subacute stage, and from this to an asymptomatic chronic stage.

Chronic American Trypanosomiasis. The chronic phase can be divided into an asymptomatic (indeterminate) form and a symptomatic form. The latter may involve cardiac and/or digestive manifestations, as well as other less frequent clinical syndromes. Over 40% of serologically positive cases are asymptomatic when assessed by routine examinations alone. However, when more sophisticated diagnostic methods are employed, or a long-term follow-up is undertaken, many of these patients are found to have clinical signs of disease. Patients within this group who have died suddenly have had foci of inflammation and fibrosis of the heart at postmortem examination. There are regional variations in the severity of the disease and in the distribution of the clinical forms. The young account for the greater number of patients in the asymptomatic group, and as age increases, the number of patients presenting with electrocardiographic abnormalities progressively increases.

Approximately 10–20% of patients with acute disease develop the chronic symptomatic form of Chagas' disease, and the prevalence of chronic cardiac and digestive manifestations is higher in patients who display the most severe acute manifestations. In endemic areas trypanosomiasis cardiomyopathy is the leading cause of cardiac disease and sudden death. In one large study, 82% of patients with chronic cardiomyopathy were 11–50 years of age. Males are more frequently affected than females.

Patients commonly present with symptoms and signs of congestive heart failure. The clinical course is one of gradually advancing myocarditis and cardiac failure with tachycardia, premature ventricular beats, enlargement of the heart, and various conduction defects. The most frequent electrocardiographic findings are partial or complete AV block and complete right bundle branch block. Signs of valvular damage and dysfunction are rare.

The incidence of organomegaly differs in the various endemic areas; it is particularly common in Brazil. Any hollow muscular viscus, but most commonly the esophagus and colon, may be involved. In 80% of 820 cases, dysphagia was the first symptom of megaesophagus. As dysphagia increases, nutritional impairment may occur. Dilation and enlargement of other hollow organs, such as the colon, ureters, or bronchi have been reported.

Diagnosis. Chagas' disease should be suspected in individuals who have lived in endemic areas and show suggestive symptoms and signs. A history of insect bites and their sequelae and the probable duration of infection are suggestive.

T. cruzi can be demonstrated in the peripheral blood of infected individuals, particularly during the acute stages of the infection. A drop of blood pressed by a cover slip and microscopically examined under high power may reveal the motile trypanosomes. Giemsa-stained blood or concentrated blood-pellet (Sec 11.106) smears should also be examined for the characteristic C-shaped organisms. The parasites may also be isolated by blood culture or demonstrated in the blood of mice injected with the patient's blood. Xenodiagnosis, or feeding the patient's blood to laboratory-reared reduviid bugs and examining their rectal contents 30–60 days later, is also an effective diagnostic method. The use of *T. cruzi* DNA hybridization assays is being evaluated.

Several serologic tests are available, e.g., precipitin, complement fixation, immunofluorescence, and more recently, an ELISA assay. These tests are largely used in patients with chronic disease when parasitologic techniques are less likely to demonstrate the organisms. About 80% of patients with chagasic heart disease and 90% of those with megaesophagus have positive complement-fixation tests. Cross-reactivity with other infections, however, may result in false positive reactions.

Treatment. There is no established and reliable therapeutic agent against *T. cruzi*. Nifurtimox (Lampit) is a promising compound effective in eradicating parasitemia in acute and possibly chronic American trypanosomiasis, but it is associated with severe side effects and must be given for periods of up to 60 days. Symptomatic treatment is needed in patients with chronic Chagas' disease; medical or surgical intervention may be necessary.

Control. This is based on educating people in endemic areas about the relation between bites from triatomine bugs and Chagas' disease. Residual insecticides such as dieldrin or lindane are highly effective in controlling the bug population when sprayed inside buildings, but these insecticides do not destroy the bug ova and should therefore be sprayed repeatedly at 2–4 week intervals. Razing adobe houses that harbor the insects and replacing them with adequately screened, more modern structures is indicated when feasible. Travelers should avoid sleeping in unscreened adobe houses in endemic areas. If this is unavoidable, bed nets should be used.

NADIA NOGUEIRA

Andrade ZA, Andrade SG, Olviera GB, et al: Histopathology of the conducting tissue of the host in Chagas' myocarditis. Am Heart J 95:316, 1978.
Coura JR: Evolutive pattern in Chagas' disease and the life span of *T. cruzi* in human infection. *In:* Pan American Health Org: New Approaches in American Trypanosomiasis Research. Scientific Publication No 318, 378, 1976.
Fife EH Jr: *Trypanosoma (Schizotrypanum) cruzi. In:* Krier JP (ed): Parasitic Protozoa. Vol. 1. New York, Academic Press, 1977, p 135.
Gonzalez A, Prediger E, Huecas M, et al: Minichromosomal repetitive DNA in

Trypanosoma cruzi: Its use in a high-sensitivity parasite detection assay. Proc Nat Acad Sci USA 8:3356, 1984.

Holt R, Mott KE, Silva JF, et al: Prevalence of parasitemia and seroreactivity to *Trypanosoma cruzi* in a rural population in Northeast Brazil. Am J Trop Med Hyg 28:461, 1979.

Spencer HC, Akain DS, Sulzer AJ, et al: Evaluation of the microenzyme-linked immunosorbent assay for antibodies to *Trypanosoma cruzi.* Am J Trop Med Hyg 29:179, 1980.

Texeira ARL: Chagas' disease: Trends in immunological research and prospects for immunoprophylaxis. Bull WHO 57:697, 1979.

11.106 AFRICAN TRYPANOSOMIASIS
(Sleeping Sickness)

The trypanosomiases of tropical Africa are a group of diseases of great social and economic importance. Human infections are caused by two subspecies of *Trypanosoma brucei,* *T. b. rhodesiense* and *T. b. gambiense,* which are morphologically indistinguishable but differ markedly in their epidemiology and the disease syndromes they cause. Infection with *T. rhodesiense* usually results in acute syndromes that run a rapid and, if untreated, fatal course, whereas *T. b. gambiense* infections usually run a more chronic course, resulting in the typical syndrome of sleeping sickness.

Information on the distribution, prevalence, and mortality rate of African trypanosomiasis is unreliable. Human trypanosomiasis in Africa occurs primarily in the region between latitudes 15° N and 15° S, which corresponds roughly to the area where the annual rainfall (500 mm or more) creates optimal climatic conditions for *Glossina* flies. *T. b. rhodesiense* infection is restricted to the eastern third of the endemic area in tropical Africa, stretching from Ethiopia to the northern boundaries of South Africa; *T. b. gambiense* occurs mainly in the western half of the continent's endemic region.

Etiology. Human infection is initiated by insect bite or by organisms penetrating intact mucous membranes or skin. The infective metacyclic forms of the trypanosomes are 15 μ long and possess no free flagella. One to 3 wk after a period of local multiplication in the skin, long and slender trypomastigote forms (12–42 μ) can be seen in the peripheral blood; intermediate and stumpy forms also occur. These are flagellated forms with a well developed undulating membrane. In the early stages of human infection, the organisms multiply rapidly in the blood and lymph nodes. They appear in waves in the peripheral blood, each wave being followed by a crisis when the organisms disappear owing to destruction of the trypomastigotes by host defense mechanisms. The reappearance of another population of organisms in the blood heralds the formation of a new antigenic variant, in response to which the host in turn forms a new "clone" of specific antibodies. *T. brucei* are capable of producing hundreds of antigenic variants. As the infection becomes chronic, fewer trypomastigotes are seen in the peripheral blood, but they can usually be recovered from lymph nodes. Invasion of the central nervous system occurs early in *T. b. rhodesiense* infections but late in the Gambian form.

The insect intermediate vectors are species of the tsetse flies of the genus *Glossina.* Both sexes of *Glossina* feed on human blood, but in nature only a small proportion of the insect population is infected. Inside the flies, the organisms localize in the posterior part of the midgut, where they transform in 3–4 days into a new trypomastigote form. These flagellates multiply enormously in the lumen of the insect's intestinal tract for about 10 days, then gradually migrate anteriorly where they attach to the walls of the salivary ducts and complete the final stages of development into the infective metacyclic forms. The life cycle within the tsetse fly takes 15–35 days; each fly infected with Rhodesian trypanosomes has been estimated to produce 40,000 infective organisms, of which only 300–450 are necessary to establish human infection.

Direct transmission to humans has also been reported. It is accomplished either mechanically through contact with the contaminated mouth parts of tsetse flies during feeding or congenitally to infants via the placenta of infected mothers.

Epidemiology. The insect intermediate vector plays a major role in determining the epidemiologic pattern of trypanosomiasis. Several *Glossina* species transmit the infection in different parts of tropical Africa. *Glossina* captured in endemic foci show a low rate of infection, usually under 5%. In the Rhodesian form, which usually runs an acute and often fatal course, chances of transmission to tsetse flies are greatly reduced. However, the ability of *T. b. rhodesiense* to multiply enormously in the blood stream of humans and to infect other species of mammals helps maintain its life cycle. *T. b. rhodesiense* infections found in wild mammals (bushbuck and hartebeest) are mainly transmitted by the so-called game tsetse flies.

T. b. gambiense infections usually run a chronic protracted course with very low levels of parasitemia. Because of low rates of infection in tsetse flies and the absence of animal reservoirs, the Gambian life cycle necessitates close and repeated contact between humans and insects to permit frequent biting. Important foci for transmission are therefore found where people habitually enter rivers to wash or to collect water.

Pathology. The initial entry site of the organisms soon develops into a hard, painful, red nodule, a "trypanosomal chancre." Histologically, it contains long, thin trypanosomes multiplying beneath the dermis and is surrounded by a lymphocytic cellular infiltrate. Dissemination into the blood and lymphatic systems follows, with subsequent localization in the central nervous system. The histopathologic lesions in the brain are those of meningoencephalitis, with increased cellularity of the pia-arachnoid due to lymphocyte infiltration and perivascular cuffing of the blood vessels by the same cell type. In chronic cases the appearance of morular cells (large, strawberry-like cells, supposedly derived from plasma cells) is the most characteristic finding.

Clinical Manifestations. The clinical presentations vary not only because of the two subspecies of organisms but also because of differences in host response in the indigenous population of endemic areas and in newcomers or visitors. Visitors usually suffer more from the acute symptoms and signs, but in untreated cases death is inevitable for natives and visitors alike. The clinical syndromes of African trypanosomiasis are best described as acute and chronic stages. Disease due to *T. b. rhodesiense* usually runs a more acute course, that due to *T. b. gambiense* a more protracted one.

Acute African Trypanosomiasis. The *site of the tsetse fly bite* may be the first presenting feature. A nodule or chancre develops in 2–3 days; within 1 wk it becomes a painful, hard, red nodule surrounded by an area of erythema and swelling. These nodules are commonly seen on the lower limbs but sometimes also on the head. They subside spontaneously in about 2 wk leaving no permanent scar. The *most common presenting features* of acute African trypanosomiasis occur at the time of invasion of the blood stream by the parasites, approximately 2–3 wk after the infection. Irregular episodes of fever, each lasting 1–7 days, are the usual early feature. Attacks may be separated by free intervals of days or even weeks. Headache, sweating, and generalized lymphadenopathy are frequently encountered along with the fever. Enlargement of lymph nodes is one of the most constant signs, particularly in the Gambian form. It most commonly affects the posterior cervical and supraclavicular groups. The lymphadenopathy is painless; the glands are moderately enlarged and are not matted together. Another common feature of trypanosomiasis in Caucasians is the presence of *blotchy, irregular, nonitching, erythematous macules* which may appear any time following the first febrile episode, usually within 6–8 wk. The majority of macules have a central normal skin area, giving the rash a circinate outline. This skin rash is seen mainly on the trunk and is evanescent, fading in one place only to appear at another site. Examination of the blood during this stage may show anemia, leukopenia with relative monocytosis, and elevated levels of IgM.

Neurologic symptoms and signs are generally nonspecific. They may precede invasion of the central nervous system by the organisms and present as irrational and inexplicable anxieties with frequent changes in mood. In untreated *T. b. rhodesiense* infections, invasion of the central nervous system occurs within 3–6 wk. It is associated with recurrent bouts of fever, weakness, and signs of acute toxemia. Tachycardia from myocarditis and neurologic symptoms such as irritability, insomnia, and personality or mood changes develop. Death occurs in 6–9 mo from secondary infection or cardiac failure.

Chronic African Trypanosomiasis. There is no precise time when cerebral symptoms begin in this disease. In the Gambian form they can be expected to appear within 2 yr after the onset of acute symptoms, although a general increase in drowsiness during the day and insomnia at night reflect the continuous nature of the pathologic processes. Progress is characterized by increasing anemia, leukopenia, and wasting of body musculature. Patients with chronic Gambian trypanosomiasis have an increased susceptibility to secondary infections.

Involvement of the central nervous system results in a chronic diffuse meningoencephalitis with no localizing symptoms, commonly known as *sleeping sickness.* Drowsiness and an uncontrollable urge to sleep are the major features of this stage of the disease and may become almost continuous in the terminal stages. Associated signs and symptoms also point to involvement of the basal ganglia. Tremor or rigidity with stiff and ataxic gait may occur. Psychotic changes occur in almost one third of untreated patients.

Diagnosis. Since the African trypanosomiases occur only in certain well defined areas of that continent, patients in other areas presenting with symptoms or signs of the disease should be questioned about their travel activities. Definitive diagnosis can be made during the early stages by examination of a fresh thick blood smear which will allow visualization of the motile active trypomastigote forms. Dried, Giemsa-stained smears should be examined for the detailed morphology of the organisms. If a thick blood smear is negative, a simple concentration method may help. Ten mL of heparinized blood are added to 30 mL of 0.87% ammonium chloride and the mixture centrifuged at 1000 g for 15 minutes. The sediment can then be examined fresh or by staining dried smears. Aspiration of an enlarged lymph node can also be used to obtain material for parasitologic examination. In every positive case a sample of CSF should also be examined for the organisms. In suspected cases when parasitologic diagnosis has failed, two rats should be inoculated intraperitoneally with 1 mL of blood; 2 wk later their blood should be examined for the parasites.

Treatment. The choice of chemotherapeutic agents depends on the stage of the infection and the causative organisms. The hematogenous forms of both Rhodesian and Gambian trypanosomiasis are susceptible to the action of suramin (Antrypol)* available as a 10% solution for intravenous administration. A test dose of 10 mg should first be administered intravenously to detect the rare idiosyncratic reactions of shock and collapse. The dose for subsequent injections is 20 mg/kg intravenously, repeated every 5–7 days for a total of 5 injections. Suramin is nephrotoxic; therefore urine should be

examined before each injection. The presence of marked proteinuria, blood, or casts is a contraindication for the completion of therapy with suramin. In these rare circumstances therapy should be continued by initiation of a course of melarsoprol,* or, in early cases without central nervous system invasion, pentamidine* may be used. Pentamidine, like suramin, is effective only against the hematogenous forms of the trypanosomes; moreover, its activity may be less certain in the Rhodesian form. It is administered intramuscularly as a 10% solution on alternate days for 5 doses. The dose for each injection is 3–4 mg/kg. Side effects of pentamidine are few; hypotension, faintness, and, occasionally, collapse may occur but can be reversed by administering epinephrine.

If invasion of the central nervous system has occurred, melarsoprol should be used. Melarsoprol contains 18.8% arsenic and is formed from the original arsenical melarsen oxide by the incorporation of dimercaprol (BAL). It is effective against all stages of both Gambian and Rhodesian trypanosomiasis but because of its arsenic content is restricted to use in patients with central nervous system involvement. It is administered intravenously as a 3.6% solution beginning with 0.4 mg/kg. The drug is given in 3 courses, each consisting of an injection on each of 3 successive days with a 1 wk interval between courses. According to the tolerance of the patient, the dose should be increased gradually to reach a maximum of 3.6 mg/kg for the 3rd course. Slight reactions such as fever and pains in the chest or abdomen may occur immediately or very soon after an injection of melarsoprol, but they are generally rare. The most important and serious of its toxic effects is encephalopathy and, less commonly, exfoliative dermatitis.

Control. The control of trypanosomiasis in endemic areas of Africa depends on recognition and effective therapy of human infections and on control of the vector. This is complicated by the fact that it involves cattle and humans and by the logistics of applying the available preventive measures.

Pentamidine has been used successfully as a prophylactic drug. A single injection of 3–4 mg/kg will give protection against Gambian trypanosomiasis for at least 6 mo. Its effect against the Rhodesian form, however, is not certain.

ADEL A. F. MAHMOUD

Foulkes JR: Human trypanosomiasis in Africa. Br Med J 283:1172, 1981.
Greenwood BM, Whittle HC: The pathogenesis of sleeping sickness. Trans Roy Soc Trop Med Hyg 74:716, 1980.
WHO: The African Trypanosomiases. Technical Report Series No. 635, 96 pp. Geneva, 1979.

11.107 TOXOPLASMOSIS

Infection with *Toxoplasma gondii*, an intracellular parasite, may result in toxoplasmosis. Two forms of toxoplasmosis exist; congenital infection is transmitted in utero, and acquired infection is most often asymptomatic.

Etiology. *T. gondii* is a coccidian protozoan. Its tachyzoites are oval or crescent-like, multiply only in living cells, measure $2–4 \times 4–7 \mu$, and are best stained with Giemsa or Wright stains. Tissue cysts, which may contain thousands of parasites, remain in tissues, especially the central nervous system and skeletal and heart muscle, for the life of the host. *Toxoplasma* can multiply in all tissues of mammals and birds, and its disease spectrum is expressed with remarkable similarity in different host species, perhaps because the parasite accommodates to an unparalleled variety of cells.

Only newly infected cats (and other Felidae) excrete *Toxoplasma* oocysts in their feces. The oocysts are infectious for all animals studied. *Toxoplasma* are acquired by susceptible cats,

---

presumably by eating infected meat. They multiply through schizogonic and gametogonic cycles in the distal ileal epithelium. Oocysts containing two sporocysts are excreted, and under proper conditions of temperature and moisture, each sporocyst matures into four sporozoites. For about 2 wk the cat excretes 10^5–10^7 oocysts per day, which, in a suitable environment, may retain their viability for a year or more. Oocysts sporulate 1–5 days after excretion and are then infectious. Oocysts are killed by drying, boiling, and exposure to some strong chemicals. Several isolations have been reported from soil and sand frequented by cats. This stage and tissue cysts are the sources of animal and human infections.

Epidemiology. *Toxoplasma* infection is ubiquitous in nature and is one of the most common latent infections of humans throughout the world. The incidence varies considerably among people and animals in different geographic areas. Significant antibody titers have been detected in 50–80% of residents of some localities but in fewer than 5% in others. The higher frequencies usually occur in warmer, more humid climates.

Infection is usually by the oral route via undercooked or raw meat that contains cysts or by ingestion of oocysts. Freezing meat to $-20°$ C or heating to 66° C renders the cysts noninfectious. Except for transmission by mother to fetus and, rarely, by organ transplant or transfusion, *Toxoplasma* are not communicated from person to person. The high incidence of subclinical infections in animals and humans makes it difficult to relate a human case to a specific animal.

Transmission to the fetus essentially occurs only when the infection is acquired by the mother during gestation. Congenital transmission from women infected prior to pregnancy is extremely rare. If only women without antibody at the beginning of pregnancy are considered, the risk of acquiring the infection during gestation in the United States is approximately 50 per 1000; the incidence of congenital infection is 1–2 per 1000 live births. Approximately 60% of mothers who go untreated will give birth to infected offspring.

The incidence of newly acquired infection in a population of pregnant women depends on the risk of becoming infected in that specific geographic area and the proportion of the population that has not been previously infected. Most mothers of children with congenital toxoplasmosis are unable to recall being ill during pregnancy. Approximately 10–20% will notice enlarged lymph nodes, most commonly in the cervical region.

Pathology. In the acute congenital and acquired forms of toxoplasmosis, histologic changes may be found in almost all tissues. In the congenital form, such changes are especially frequent in the central nervous system, the retina, and the choroid; retinochoroiditis occurs occasionally in acquired toxoplasmosis. During latent infection, *Toxoplasma* in tissues are seen as cysts with little or no associated tissue reaction. In acute infections, intracellular and, in areas of massive necrosis, extracellular tachyzoites may be noted. Gross or microscopic areas of necrosis may be present in many tissues, especially in heart, lungs, skeletal muscle, liver, and spleen. Areas of calcification occur in the brain in the congenital form but not in acquired cases. Characteristic lymph node changes occur. Examination of the placenta of infected newborns may reveal chronic inflammatory reactions, and cysts have been identified.

Clinical Manifestations. *Congenital Toxoplasmosis.* Clinical severity may vary, and not all fetuses in the same pregnancy are infected. Prospective studies by Desmonts and Couvreur provided data on the products of pregnancies in which susceptible women acquired the infection. The maternal infections characteristically were asymptomatic, and their offspring, contrary to previous impressions, often were not infected. In 176 such pregnancies, there were 55 infected, 110 uninfected (63%), and 11 possibly infected babies. Most infections were subclinical. Among the 6 stillbirths or neonatal deaths in this group, 2 were proved to be the result of congenital toxoplasmosis, and in the remaining 4 congenital toxoplasmosis was considered "possible." Among the 55 infected offspring, injury was severe in 9, mild in 11, and absent in 35.

The severely affected fetus may be stillborn, born prematurely, or born at term. Illness may be apparent at birth or may not become evident for some days. Manifestations include poor feeding, fever, maculopapular rash, petechiae (due to thrombocytopenia), lymphadenopathy, hepatomegaly, splenomegaly, icterus, hydrocephalus or microcephaly, microphthalmia, and convulsions. These may occur singly or in combination. Cerebral calcifications and chorioretinitis may be present at birth or appear later. The infection may terminate fatally in days or weeks or may become inactive, demonstrating residuals of varying degrees and combinations of hydrocephalus or microcephaly, chorioretinitis, ocular palsies, psychomotor retardation, and convulsive disorders. Only weeks or months after its apparent cessation may the full impact of the infection upon development become evident.

In a large series of cases of symptomatic congenital toxoplasmosis (Feldman), premature birth was common (31%), with a higher mortality rate (27%) than among infants born at term (12%). Chorioretinitis was noted in 99%, cerebral calcification in 63%, psychomotor retardation in 56%, and hydrocephalus or microcephalus in about 50% of these infants. Chorioretinitis was bilateral in 85%, but residual damage in some cases was as slight as a minute peripheral retinal scar or a single oculomotor palsy. Recurrent chorioretinitis, especially in early adolescence, which can be related to *Toxoplasma*, usually occurs in those with congenital infections.

The later in pregnancy the infection occurs, the higher the fetal infection rate but the less severe the manifestations. Though *Toxoplasma* may be responsible for premature birth, cerebral palsy, blindness, and mental retardation, it does not appear to be a prominent cause of any of them. Indeed, 86% of the pregnancies studied ended in either uninfected or asymptomatic offspring. However, of the 65–75% of infants whose infection is subclinical in the newborn period, the majority will develop untoward sequelae months or years later. In one study, 85% of such children developed sequelae (including chorioretinitis, mental retardation, or severe neurologic disability) over a mean follow-up period of 8 yr. The untoward sequelae were first recognized when the children were 1 mo to 9 yr of age.

Parasitemia probably occurs in all primary infections and is the presumed route by which the fetus acquires infection from its mother. Except for occasional instances of lymphadenopathy, clinical evidence of maternal infection is usually not discernible. Since the disease occurs in the offspring of only one pregnancy of a given mother, subsequent pregnancies may be undertaken without fear of its repetition.

Acquired Toxoplasmosis. Postnatally acquired toxoplasmosis is relatively common as an inapparent infection, usually without clinically expressed disease.

When clinical manifestations are apparent they may include almost any combination of malaise, fever, myalgia, maculopapular rash, localized or generalized lymphadenopathy, hepatomegaly, encephalitis, pneumonia, and myocarditis. Chorioretinitis (usually unilateral) occurs in fewer than 1% of cases. Symptoms may be evident from a few days to months, and most patients recover spontaneously.

Cases of generalized lymphadenopathy may resemble infectious mononucleosis, Hodgkin disease, or other lymphadenopathies. The most common manifestation is one or a few nodes in the cervical region. In the parapectoral area in women, the nodes are frequently considered tumors of the breast. Nodes may be tender but do not suppurate. Adenopathy may appear and disappear for as long as 1 yr. Because of the vagueness of this syndrome, the correct diagnosis is usually not considered, frequently resulting in an unnecessary node biopsy when appropriate serologic studies would have established the diagnosis.

Caution: Since the classical complement pathway is essential for the action of neutralizing antibody, sera naturally deficient in C2, C4, C5, C6, C7, or C8 cannot serve this function. Thus, individuals with any such complement deficiencies may be at greater risk of severe or fatal infections, whether congenital or acquired (See Sec. 10.25–10.29). They should be advised to eat only thoroughly cooked meat or that which has been well frozen and to avoid handling cat feces.

Laboratory Data. Congenital toxoplasmosis may be diagnosed in its active stage shortly after birth by demonstrating parasites in smears, or preferably cytocentrifuge preparations, from cerebrospinal and ventricular fluid sediments. These fluids may be xanthochromic and contain cells (sometimes eosinophils) and increased protein. Otherwise, identification depends upon isolation of the parasites in laboratory mice or in tissue culture. The inoculum should consist of unfrozen suspensions of fresh tissue or of sediment from body fluids. Organisms, especially cysts, may be found in sections of tissue.

The Sabin-Feldman dye test, which measures IgG antibody, is the most sensitive and reliable indicator of *Toxoplasma* antibody, requires live parasites, the classical complement pathway, and meticulous attention to detail. Dye test antibodies appear early in the course of infection and remain in high titer for months or years. Titers diminish gradually, but usually persist for life. In the sera of infants or young children with congenital infection and of their mothers, titers of 1:1000 to 1:16,000 are usual for at least some months. If the infant's antibodies have been acquired only by passive transfer, the titer will decrease by approximately one half per month. The same rate of decrease applies to both high titers and low titers. Thus, the common belief that all infants with a positive titer at 4–6 mo have congenital infection is incorrect. In some untreated, infected infants, antibody synthesis is delayed for 3–4 mo—their titers remain parallel to the expected titer of passively transferred maternal antibodies. In infants treated in the early weeks of life, antibody synthesis may be delayed by as long as 6–9 mo. In infected infants born to mothers who acquired their infection very near to the time of delivery, titers in the cord blood may be negative or very low during the first weeks of life.

The complement-fixation test may offer additional aid, but is available in only a few centers in the United States. It becomes positive more slowly so that early in the course there may be a strong positive dye but a negative complement-fixation reaction. The latter tends to decrease relatively quickly, so that within months or 1–2 yr after the initial illness there again may be a negative complement fixation and a positive dye reaction. An infant born with active disease and a positive dye test titer may have a negative complement-fixation reaction even though the mother has high titers by both procedures.

The recently introduced agglutination tests that employ either whole formalin-fixed tachyzoites or antigen-coated latex particles are sensitive and accurate for detection of IgG *Toxoplasma* antibodies. The indirect hemagglutination (IHA) test has some attractiveness because of its relative simplicity; titers rise later than they do in the dye or indirect fluorescent antibody (IFA) tests. For this reason, it should not be used to determine the presence of infection in the newborn or to screen pregnant women.

The IFA methods measure *Toxoplasma* antibodies of both the IgM and the IgG classes. Results of this test agree well with those of the dye test. The IgM-IFA test has been used for early identification of acquired infections; it is positive in only approximately 25% of infected newborns. More recently, a double sandwich IgM-ELISA method has been developed that detects approximately 75–85% of infected newborns. Screening cord bloods for elevated IgM levels may disclose cases of toxoplasmosis as well as other congenital infections, but about 75% of infants born with active toxoplasmosis will be negative by this test. If the diagnosis is strongly suspected, negative IgM test reactors should be restudied at 2–4 wk.

Differential Diagnosis. Any manifestation of congenital toxoplasmosis may occur in other diseases, especially that caused by cytomegalovirus (Sec. 8.68 and 11.68). Neither the cerebral calcification nor the chorioretinitis is pathognomonic. In the experience of one of us (H.F.), fewer than 50% of children under 5 yr of age with chorioretinitis satisfy the serologic criteria for congenital toxoplasmosis. Most of the other cases result from unknown causes. The clinical picture in the newborn infant also may be compatible with sepsis, syphilis, or hemolytic disease. In acquired cases, primary lymphadenopathic disease must be separated from toxoplasmosis.

Prevention. Since cats produce infective oocysts, there is great interest in them as a source of human infection, especially for the pregnant woman. Those women who have antibodies prior to pregnancy are safe from further difficulty. Those who do not have such antibodies, or who have not been tested, should be cautioned to eat only thoroughly cooked meat during pregnancy and to avoid handling cat litter, which should be disposed of daily to prevent sporulation of any freshly excreted oocysts. The cat litter box can be rendered noninfectious by disinfecting for 5 minutes with nearly boiling water. A cat known to have antibodies presents no problem. Cats kept indoors, maintained on prepared diets, and not fed fresh, uncooked meat also should present no problem. Pregnant women should avoid touching mucous membranes of mouth and eyes while handling raw meat or vegetables and should wash their hands thoroughly after handling them. They should wear gloves when working in the garden.

Treatment. A combination of pyrimethamine (Daraprim) and sulfadiazine or trisulfapyrimidines is superior to either drug alone and has been effective in interrupting acute disease; all infected newborns should be treated, whether or not they have clinical signs of the infection. Sulfadiazine should be administered in usual therapeutic dosage (see Table 29–1B) and pyrimethamine, 15 mg/m² or 1 mg/kg/24 hr. Because pyrimethamine has a half-life of 4–5 days, the drug may be administered every other day. In infants with severe disease it seems prudent to give the drug daily, at least for the first few weeks of therapy. The total daily dose of pyrimethamine should not exceed 25 mg, except that twice the calculated daily dose is usually prescribed for the initial 24–48 hr. Spiramycin, available through the Food and Drug Administration in the United States, is a macrolide antibiotic used widely in Europe to treat congenitally infected infants. Courses of 100 mg/kg/24 hr in three divided doses are usually given for 4–6 wk alternating with 21 day courses of the pyrimethamine-sulfonamide combination. Corticosteroids (prednisone 1.5 mg/kg/24 hr) may be added for patients with clinically active central nervous system infection or active macular involvement. Treatment should be continued arbitrarily for at least 6 mo.

Because both pyrimethamine and sulfonamides may produce severe leukopenia and/or thrombocytopenia, twice weekly leukocyte counts should be performed. The hematologic complications induced by pyrimethamine may be alleviated by the simultaneous administration of folinic acid (calcium leucovorin), which does not interfere with its antiparasitic activity. There is no evidence that the pyrimethamine-sulfonamide treatment affects encysted organisms. In newborn infants with active disease, the best that can be hoped for is that further damage will be prevented.

HARRY A. FELDMAN*
JACK S. REMINGTON

Couvreur J, Desmonts G, Tournier G, et al: Study of a homogeneous series of 210 cases of congenital toxoplasmosis in infants aged 0 to 11 months detected prospectively. Ann Pediatr 31:815, 1984.

Desmonts G, Couvreur J: Congenital toxoplasmosis: A prospective study of 378 pregnancies. N Engl J Med 290:110, 1974.

Dorfman RF, Remington JS: Value of lymph node biopsy in the diagnosis of acute acquired toxoplasmosis. N Engl J Med 289:878, 1973.

Frenkel JK, Weber RW, Lunde MN: Acute toxoplasmosis. Effective treatment with pyrimethamine, sulfadiazine, leucovorin, calcium, and yeast. JAMA 173:1471, 1960.

Naot Y, Desmonts G, Remington JS: IgM enzyme-linked immunosorbent assay test for the diagnosis of congenital Toxoplasma infection. J Pediatr 98:32, 1981.

Remington JS, Desmonts G: Toxoplasmosis. In: Remington JS, Klein JO (eds): Infectious Diseases of the Fetus and Newborn Infant. 2nd ed. Philadelphia, WB Saunders, 1983, pp 144–263.

Wilson CB, Remington JS: What can be done to prevent congenital toxoplasmosis? Am J Obstet Gynecol 138:357, 1980.

Wilson CB, Remington JS, Stagno S, et al: Development of adverse sequelae in children born with subclinical congenital Toxoplasma infection. Pediatrics 66:767, 1980.

11.108 LEISHMANIASIS

Infection with different species of *Leishmania* can cause cutaneous lesions, ulcerations of the oronasal mucosa, or visceral dissemination resulting in fatal complications. Leishmaniasis has a vast geographic distribution involving millions of people. Effective chemotherapeutic agents are available, and drug resistance is not uncommon.

Etiology. *Leishmania* are protozoal parasites existing in two morphologically distinct forms: flagellated promastigotes, which replicate extracellularly within the sandfly vector gut and also in axenic cultures; and amastigotes, which lack flagella and are obligate intracellular parasites of mononuclear phagocytes in the mammalian host. Female vector sandflies (certain *Phlebotomus*, *Lutzomyia*, and *Psychdopygus* species) become infected by ingesting *Leishmania*-infected macrophages while taking a blood meal. In the sandfly gut, amastigotes exit from the ingested host cells, transform into promastigotes, and replicate. Transmission occurs when promastigotes are subsequently injected into a susceptible host. They enter cells (probably tissue macrophages) in the host's skin, transform into amastigotes, replicate, and infect adjacent macrophages. Amastigote replication occurs locally. In cutaneous leishmaniasis local replication occurs, and in mucocutaneous and visceral disease dissemination (probably hematogenous) takes place.

Pathophysiology. *Leishmania* attach to mononuclear phagocyte surfaces by a complex process involving several ligands and probably requiring active participation of the parasite. Macrophage receptors for complement components, mannose, fibronectin, and (in the presence of antibody) the Fc portion of immunoglobulin G may play a role in the process. Once attached, the parasites enter by phagocytosis and become surrounded by a host plasma membrane–derived parasitophorous vacuole. Secondary lysosomes fuse with this vacuole (forming a phagolysosome) without apparent deleterious effects on the amastigotes. Different *Leishmania* species have different temperature optima for growth, which may explain why some species disseminate while others are restricted to the cooler parts of the body (skin).

Although amastigotes survive and replicate in quiescent mononuclear phagocytes, when these cells are "activated"

they can inhibit parasite replication and induce death. This host defense results primarily (if not exclusively) from direct contact between effector lymphocytes and infected macrophage and from lymphocyte secretion of macrophage-activating lymphokines such as gamma interferon; the intracellular demise of the parasite occurs without damage to the host cell. In some forms of leishmaniasis (e.g., visceral and diffuse cutaneous leishmaniasis), deficiency of host defense may be mediated by antibodies, immune complexes, or suppressor cells. Whether intrinsic features of the particular parasite species, the genetic composition of the host, or a complex specific interplay of parasite and host factors dictate disease outcome is unknown. Assessing this is complicated by the very large number of *Leishmania* species and by their changing taxonomy, especially at the subspecies level (complexes).

Clinical Manifestations. *Visceral Leishmaniasis.* This disease, also called kala-azar, is caused by species of *Leishmania* (*L. donovani* complex) that disseminate hematogenously, infecting macrophages in the liver, spleen, bone marrow, and lymph nodes. The infection is zoonotic in most areas. Dogs and other carnivores are the most common reservoirs. In India and East Africa man is thought to be the reservoir. The disease is found on all continents except Australia, and although epidemiologic features may differ widely, the important clinical features are generally similar in different geographic regions.

Typically, symptoms appear several weeks to 8 mo following the sandfly bite, although incubation periods of up to 10 yr have been reported. Lesions at the inoculation site are rarely observed when the patient first comes to medical attention. The course of the disease can be abrupt (as occurs frequently in young children) or insidious (especially in older children and adults). Fever is very common, and although it may have periodicity, the pattern is not diagnostically reliable. Vomiting, diarrhea, and a nonproductive cough accompany disease of abrupt onset. Infections with a more protracted course may be characterized by an initial 2–8 wk of fevers and nonspecific systemic complaints including weakness, anorexia, and vague abdominal problems. Thereafter, the fever may recede and the patient becomes weaker, and complains of symptoms related to an enlarged spleen, such as abdominal discomfort and early satiety. The most dramatic finding on physical examination is marked splenomegaly that may reach massive proportions. Hepatomegaly and less frequently lymphadenopathy are associated common features. With time, the hair thins and becomes brittle. The skin becomes dry and scaly and may acquire the gray, ashen appearance from which the name kala-azar ("black sickness") is derived. Petechiae, ecchymoses, and mild edema may appear; jaundice and ascites are rare.

The major complications leading to death, including hemorrhage and bacterial superinfection, result from a decrease in blood elements due to leishmanial infection of the bone marrow and hypersplenism. Anemia, leukopenia, and thrombocytopenia are common. Hypoalbuminemia, a marked polyclonal hypergammaglobulinemia (mostly IgG), circulating immune complexes and rheumatoid factor are associated laboratory findings. Immune complex glomerulonephritis with proteinuria and microscopic hematuria has been reported. Secondary amyloidosis and hepatic fibrosis leading to portal hypertension are unusual. Without treatment, death usually ensues within 2 yr as a result of infectious complications including pneumonia, dysentery, and septicemia, or of anemia or hemorrhage.

Post kala-azar dermal leishmaniasis (PKDL) develops in 3–20% of patients after treatment of the visceral infection. The lesions range from depigmented macules on the face and trunk to firm nodules appearing mostly on the nose and around the mouth. They may persist for months or years if untreated. A history of previous kala-azar and isolation of parasites from the lesions help establish this diagnosis.

Kala-azar should be suspected in endemic areas when patients present with enlarging spleens, pancytopenia (especially anemia), and hyperglobulinemia. It must be differentiated from malaria, miliary tuberculosis, salmonellosis, acute schistosomiasis, amebic liver abscess, and acute typhus. In the chronic stages it may mimic hepatosplenic schistosomiasis, brucellosis, tropical splenomegaly syndrome, chronic lymphocytic leukemia, lymphoma, malignant histiocytosis, and glycogen storage disease. PKDL may be confused with yaws, syphilis, and leprosy.

Cutaneous Leishmaniasis. This type of infection is traditionally divided into Old World (Mediterranean basin, Africa, India, China, Soviet Union, and Asia Minor) and New World (primarily Central and South America, excluding Chile and Uruguay). The former is caused by any of a number of species, including *Leishmania tropica* and *L. major;* the latter is caused by the *L. brasiliensis* and *L. mexicana* complexes. In most geographic areas, these parasites are maintained by transmission in nonhuman reservoirs, usually rodents, but human-to-human transmissions can also occur.

The characteristic skin lesion begins as an erythematous papule or macule that may ulcerate after several weeks. Unless superinfected with bacteria, the lesions are generally painless, nontender, and not pruritic. In some cases, lymphatic nodules may develop proximal to the lesion. Satellite lesions containing parasites may form adjacent to the primary one. In Old World cutaneous leishmaniasis, spontaneous healing usually occurs over a period of months. Certain specific clinical forms are recognized in distinct geographical areas. For example, the so-called chiclero's ulcer is found in the northern region of Central America and the Yucatan peninsula among workers who enter the rain forests to gather chicle gum. The lesion has a propensity to form on the pinna of the ear and may be destructive. Infection acquired in the forests of northern South America can lead to hyperkeratotic or papillomatous lesions that resemble secondary yaws ("pian bois" or forest yaws). Uta, a form acquired in the Peruvian Andes and Argentinian highlands, heals spontaneously.

Diffuse cutaneous leishmaniasis (DCL) is a rare form recognized primarily in Ethiopia, Venezuela, and the Dominican Republic. Multiple lesions form on the skin in association with anergy to leishmanial antigens. Defective host defense in these patients is also revealed by a paucity of lymphocytes and a large number of heavily infected macrophages in the lesions. Leishmania recidiva is another rare form found in areas of endemic *L. tropica* infection and manifested by lesions (usually facial) that resemble lupus vulgaris, which may persist for years. In contrast to DCL, the parasites may be difficult to identify in these lesions.

The differential diagnosis of cutaneous leishmaniasis includes tuberculosis and atypical mycobacteriosis of the skin, fungal infections, syphilis, yaws, leprosy, basal cell carcinoma, and sarcoid.

Mucocutaneous Leishmaniasis (Espundia). This is a complication of cutaneous leishmaniasis acquired in Central and South America. The rate of this complication varies in different geographic areas, from less than 1% to as high as 30% in southern Brazil. *L. brasiliensis brasiliensis* is most commonly responsible for this disease. The parasite spreads hematogenously, and the lesions in the oral and nasal mucosa may develop 1 mo to 24 yr (rare cases) after the initial cutaneous lesion. Coryza, nasal stuffiness, or epistaxis can be presenting complaints. Destructive lesions can involve the lips, tongue, soft palate, nasal septum and bridge, pharynx, larynx, and trachea. Destruction of the nasal septum can lead to perforation or to collapse that gives rise to the so-called tapir nose deformity. Erosion of the nose and lips can cause grotesque facial deformities. Involvement of the larynx, pharynx, or trachea can cause dysphagia and asphyxia. Aspiration pneumonia, wound infections, and bacterial meningitis are complications. Mucocutaneous leishmaniasis may resemble syphilis, yaws, histoplasmosis, paracoccidioidomycosis, sarcoidosis, basal cell carcinoma, and midline granuloma.

Diagnosis. When kala-azar is suspected, the diagnosis should be confirmed by biopsy or aspiration of an involved site. Using Giemsa-stained tissue and cultures, splenic aspirates are positive in 98% of cases, bone marrow aspirates in 54–86%, liver biopsy in 70%, and enlarged lymph nodes aspirates in up to 60%. By light microscopy, amastigotes appear in Giemsa-stained infected cells as round forms measuring about 2–5 μm in diameter with a characteristic large mitochondrion-associated mass of extrachromosomal DNA (the kinetoplast). Aspirated or homogenized biopsy material should be cultured for up to 4 wk on specialized media. Promastigotes can be observed as highly motile oblong bodies (20 μm long) in culture. Because of the risk of splenic rupture, especially in patients with a bleeding diathesis, splenic aspiration should be performed only by those experienced with this technique.

The Montenegro skin test (a test for cutaneous delayed type hypersensitivity response to a killed promastigote preparation called leishmanin) is negative in active kala-azar, only becoming positive after 6–8 wk of successful therapy. Leishmanin is not commercially available but can be obtained from the WHO Leishmaniasis Reference Center, Hadassah Hospital, Jerusalem, Israel. Serologic tests developed for the diagnosis of kala-azar include fluorescent antibody tests, indirect hemagglutination tests, direct agglutination tests, conventional ELISA, and dot ELISA tests. The indirect immunofluorescence antibody test and direct agglutination assay are available from the Centers for Disease Control (CDC), Atlanta, GA, United States. Serology should not be used to the exclusion of other diagnostic tests, since routine tests are not species-specific and may be falsely positive in patients infected with *Trypanosoma cruzi.*

Diagnosis of cutaneous leishmaniasis is best achieved by skin biopsy from the raised edge of a lesion; aspirates have also proved useful. Impression smears of biopsy material stained with Giemsa provide the most rapid diagnosis if amastigotes can be identified; identifying parasites on histologic sections may prove difficult. Some species identifiable on impression smears may fail to grow in culture. The Montenegro test generally becomes positive in 4–6 wk after infection and persists for years; in diffuse cutaneous leishmaniasis it is negative. In leishmaniasis recidiva the reaction is characteristically exuberant. Serology is unreliable in cutaneous leishmaniasis as titers are usually low. In mucocutaneous leishmaniasis organisms may be difficult to identify in tissue; the Montenegro test is generally positive. Antibody detected by immunofluorescence and direct agglutination assays are positive in 90% of such cases.

Treatment. The pentavalent antimonial (Sb^V) compounds sodium stibogluconate (Pentostam, 100 mg Sb/mL; available from CDC) and *N*-methylglucamine antimonate (Glucantime) are the preferred drugs for treating leishmaniasis. Both can be given intravenously or intramuscularly, and they appear to have similar efficacy and toxicities. Efficacy of treatment depends on the form of leishmaniasis being treated and on the geographic area where it was acquired. Resistance has been noted particularly in kala-azar acquired in East Africa, China, and the Mediterranean, and in diffuse cutaneous and mucocutaneous disease. All forms of visceral, mucocutaneous, and diffuse cutaneous leishmaniasis should be treated. Cutaneous disease acquired in the Old World usually is self-healing and requires treatment only if the lesion progresses, fails to heal in 3–5 mo, is disabling owing to its location, or is cosmetically embarrassing. The safest approach may be to treat all forms of cutaneous leishmaniasis acquired in Central and South America (except uta from Peru and Argentina), since most patients fail to heal spontaneously and some may be at risk for developing mucocutaneous disease. It is not established that treatment of the skin lesion prevents the subsequent development of mucocutaneous leishmaniasis. Therefore, patients should be followed even after successful treatment. PKDL and leishmaniasis recidiva are treated in the same way as primary infections.

Precise regimens are difficult to recommend since few careful comparisons have been reported. For most forms of leishmaniasis, 20 mg Sb^v/kg body weight (some suggest to a maximum of 850 mg/day) given once each day IM or IV for 20–30 days should be adequate. Shorter courses or lower doses might also be effective in some cases. For treatment failure or recurrence, repeated courses are recommended. Antimony is rapidly excreted by the kidney (80% in a few hours) with little accumulation in the tissue. Regimens using higher doses are being tested and appear to be well tolerated. Side effects of therapy occur relatively infrequently but include fever, rash, cough, and gastrointestinal irritation. Electrocardiographic changes such as T wave inversion and prolonged QT interval may herald the onset of arrhythmias. Renal insufficiency may develop and, thus, renal function should be followed; adjustment of dose or interval in patients with renal insufficiency may be advisable.

Resistant disease (such as mucocutaneous leishmaniasis) can be treated with amphotericin B or pentamidine. Amphotericin B is administered as for deep mycoses (Sec. 11.98). Patients with mucocutaneous leishmaniasis may require a total dose of 1–3 g; cutaneous disease can often be treated with less. Pentamidine administered intramuscularly, 2–4 mg/kg, 1–3 times/wk for 5–25 wk (depending on the nature of the illness) has been used as second line treatment. A variety of other agents (such as rifampin, trimethoprim-sulfamethoxazole, allopurinol, and ketoconazole) have been employed successfully in isolated cases or in a small series of patients. Their routine use cannot be recommended since carefully controlled trials have not been reported.

Splenectomy has been reported to be effective in advanced drug-resistent kala-azar. Its indications include drug resistance in the face of massive splenomegaly and symptomatic or disabling hypersplenism, especially in small children. Appropriate management of anemia, infection, and hemorrhage as well as good nutrition are essential for optimal care during this treatment. Cryosurgery, curettage, intralesional instillation of chemotherapeutic agents, and heat treatment have all had success in treatment of isolated cases of cutaneous disease, but they cannot be recommended as replacements for antimony treatment. Restorative plastic surgery and prostheses may be of great benefit to patients with mutilating mucocutaneous disease but should be performed only after an extended period of observation following treatment so that recurrence does not cause loss of the graft.

In evaluating responses to treatment, assessing both clinical and parasitologic parameters is important. Repeat aspirates or biopsies are useful in assessing a parasitologic "cure," but when the disease progresses despite apparent elimination of parasites, continued treatment may be necessary. Restoration of responsiveness to leishmanin and a fall in antileishmanial antibodies are useful indices of improvement in treatment of kala-azar.

Prevention. Prevention depends upon a detailed knowledge of the ecology of the reservoirs and vector of the various forms of leishmaniasis. Treating cases, decreasing human contact with the vector, destroying animal reservoirs, and vector control are important in reducing transmission. Insect repellents and fine mesh netting around beds can decrease exposure to sandflies. Travelers to endemic areas should be warned of the risk and instructed in methods for preventing acquisition of leishmaniasis. Spraying with residual insecticides has reduced the sandfly populations and controlled the disease in some areas; when insecticide spraying was instituted for malaria control in the Indian state of Bihar, the sandfly population was reduced to a level at which kala-azar was all but eliminated. Within a few years after such measures were ended, however, the disease returned in epidemic proportions. No chemoprophylactic agents are available. In the USSR, Iran, and Israel, a form of vaccination has been employed using live cultures of *L. tropica* or *L. major*, but complications preclude the widespread use of this measure. Since curing the infection appears to impart protection against reinfection with the homologous parasite species, developing an effective and safe vaccine should be possible. This holds the greatest promise for preventing leishmaniasis.

DAVID J. WYLER
HAROLD W. HOROWITZ

General

Greenblatt CL: The present and future of vaccination for cutaneous leishmaniasis. *In:* Mizrahi A (ed): New Developments with Human and Veterinary Vaccines. New York, Alan R. Liss, 1980, p 259.
Lainson R, Shaw JJ: Epidemiology and ecology of leishmaniasis in Latin-America. Nature (Lond) 273:595, 1978.
The Leishmaniases. Report of a WHO Expert Committee. WHO Tech Rep Ser 701:1, 1984.
Marinkelle CJ: The control of leishmaniasis. Bull WHO 58:807, 1980.
Pearson RD, Wheeler DA, Harrison LH, et al: The immunobiology of leishmaniasis. Rev Infect Dis 5:907, 1983.

Specific

Behforouz NC, Amirhakimi GH, Rezai HR, et al: Immunological findings on kala-azar in Iran. Trop Geogr Med 35:27, 1983.
Chulay JD, Bhatt SM, Muigai R, et al: A comparison of three dosage regimens of sodium stibogluconate in the treatment of visceral leishmaniasis in Kenya. J Infect Dis 148:148, 1983.
Jha TK: Evaluation of diamidine compound (pentamidine isethionate) in the treatment of resistant cases of kala azar in North Bihar, India. Trans R Soc Trop Med Hyg 77:167, 1983.
Kager PA, Rees PH, Manugu FM, et al: Clinical, hematological and parasitological response to treatment of visceral leishmaniasis in Kenya: A study of 64 patients. Trop Geogr Med 36:285, 1984.
Rees PH, Kager PA, Kyambi JM, et al: Splenectomy in kala azar. Trop Geogr Med 36:285, 1984.
Thakur CP: Epidemiological, clinical and therapeutic features of Bihar kala azar (including post kala azar dermal leishmaniasis). Trans R Soc Trop Med Hyg 78:391, 1984.

PNEUMOCYSTIS CARINII

See Sec. 13.68.

11.109 PRIMARY AMEBIC MENINGOENCEPHALITIS

Amebic meningoencephalitis is an acute, usually fatal infection of the central nervous system occurring primarily in children and young adults. In most cases there is a history of swimming in fresh water—ponds, lakes, or even heated pools, all of which may be heavily contaminated with algae or bacteria—which has put the patient in contact with the infectious agent.

Etiology and Epidemiology. Although free-living amebae occur ubiquitously in nature, the genera most often isolated from the central nervous system of infected humans are *Naegleria fowleri*, *Acanthamoeba*, and, on rare occasions, "unidentified" amebae. *Naegleria* are motile, freshwater amebae-flagellates, 10–20 μ in diameter, having a large nucleus, a prominent central karyosome, and large pseudopodia, which can be cultured on a number of laboratory media and on non-nutrient agar seeded with bacteria. Various species of *Acanthamoeba*, besides those found free-living in nature, also exist as part of the normal flora of the mouth and nasopharynx. Morphologically similar to *Naegleria*, they are 6–8 μ in diameter and have an abundant cytoplasm. *Acanthamoeba* are less motile than *Naegleria* and in clinical specimens can be confused with macrophages.

Human infection with *Naegleria* has been acquired through contact with tap water in Australia, thermally polluted water in Belgium, and swimming pools in Czechoslovakia. Most cases in the United States have occurred during summer months in children and young adults after swimming, diving, or water skiing in fresh water ponds and lakes. *Acanthamoeba* infection of the central nervous system is less common, but has a worldwide distribution. It is unassociated with previous aquatic activity, and occurs as an opportunistic infection in a debilitated and/or immunosuppressed patient.

Pathology. *Naegleria* gain access to the central nervous system through the nasal mucosa covering the cribriform plate and produce diffuse and extensive damage to the brain. Hemorrhagic necrosis of the olfactory nerves, the adjacent inferior frontal lobes, and the basilar surface of the cerebrum and cerebellum is common. Amebae mixed with neutrophils and macrophages can be found in the subarachnoid space, and in the superficial substance and small perivascular spaces of the brain. The inflammatory response in the meninges, as reflected in spinal fluid, includes the presence of a large number of polymorphonuclear leukocytes and an elevated protein level but a low glucose level. *Acanthamoeba* reach the central nervous system following hematogenous dissemination. The histopathologic findings consist of a granulomatous encephalitis with foci of hemorrhagic necrosis in the occipital, parietal, temporal, and (less often) frontal lobes. The upper portion of the spinal cord may be involved, and visceral lesions (lung, kidney, adrenals, etc.) are not uncommon. The inflammatory response of the meninges is minimal and reflected in the cerebrospinal fluid by lymphocytic pleocytosis, an elevated protein, and a normal or borderline low glucose.

Clinical Manifestations. *Naegleria* meningoencephalitis is an acute and rapidly progressive illness presenting with fever, headache, neck rigidity, vomiting, and lethargy within 5 days of exposure to fresh water. Symptoms rapidly progress over the first 24 hr with increasing lethargy, convulsions, and eventual coma. The clinical course is one of rapid deterioration and death. The typical course of acanthamoebic infection is that of a subacute or chronic meningoencephalitis with focal neurologic manifestations, e.g., hemiplegia, aphasia, visual disturbances.

Diagnosis. The cerebrospinal fluid in *Naegleria* infection is similar to that observed with purulent bacterial meningitis. The Gram stain and culture fail to reveal bacteria, but the motile amebae, often mistaken for lymphocytes, can be seen in a fresh wet-mount examination of uncentrifuged and nonrefrigerated cerebrospinal fluid. *Acanthamoeba* infection yields a cerebrospinal fluid consistent with aseptic meningitis; the amebae are not present in the cerebrospinal fluid but can be demonstrated by brain biopsy.

Treatment. Most cases of *Naegleria* meningoencephalitis have been fatal, and numerous amebicides have been tried unsuccessfully. Therefore, prevention by avoiding contact with contaminated water is essential. Three patients have been successfully treated with intravenous and intrathecal amphotericin B (two were simultaneously treated with oral rifampin and intravenous and intrathecal miconazole). *Acanthamoeba* are more sensitive than *Naegleria* to antimicrobial agents such as sulfanilamides, clotrimazole, and 5-fluorocytosine; amphotericin B is ineffective. Although these amebae are sensitive to a number of therapeutic agents, sufficient information is not available to identify the drug(s) most efficacious in human infection.

WILLIAM T. SPECK

Darby CP, Conradi SE, Holbrook TW, et al: Primary amebic meningoencephalitis. Am J Dis Child 133:1025, 1979.
Martinez AJ: Is *Acanthamoeba* encephalitis an opportunistic infection? Neurology 30:567, 1980.
Seidel JS, Harmatz P, Visvesvara GS, et al: Successful treatment of primary amebic meningoencephalitis. N Engl J Med 306:346, 1982.

HELMINTHS

NEMATODES
(Roundworms)

INTESTINAL NEMATODES

Infection with intestinal roundworms is the most common type of helminthiasis of humans. Although these infections are more prevalent in tropical and subtropical climates, individuals residing in temperate and cold regions are not spared. Children generally are more heavily infected than adults and are therefore more likely to suffer from the pathologic consequences of these infections. Intestinal nematodes may infect humans either directly by ingestion of mature eggs or indirectly via larval penetration of skin. With the exception of *Strongyloides stercoralis*, the adult stages of these nematodes live in the lumen of the intestinal tract and do not multiply in the human host. Although intestinal nematode infections are not usually associated with peripheral blood eosinophilia, increased eosinophil counts often develop during the phase of infection when parasite larvae migrate through host tissues. The more prevalent intestinal roundworm infections of children will be discussed according to their final location in the gut: small intestine (*Ascaris lumbricoides, Ancylostoma duodenale, Necator americanus,* and *Strongyloides stercoralis*), cecum (*Enterobius vermicularis*), and large intestine (*Trichuris trichiura*) (Table 11–39).

11.110 Ascariasis

Infection with *Ascaris lumbricoides* is the most prevalent human helminthiasis and produces an estimated 1 billion cases worldwide. Infection is most common in children of preschool or early school age. Ascariasis is ubiquitous; the greatest number of cases occur in countries having warmer climates. Nevertheless, there are approximately 4 million infected individuals, mainly children, in North America.

Etiology. The infective stage of *A. lumbricoides* is the mature larva-containing egg. It is broadly oval, has a thick shell with an outer mamillated covering, and measures approximately 40 × 60 μm (Fig. 11–32). Eggs are passed in the feces of infected individuals and mature in 5–10 days under favorable environmental conditions to become infective. After ingestion by the human host, larvae are released from the eggs and penetrate the intestinal wall before migrating to the lungs via the venous circulation. They then break through the pulmonary tissues into the alveolar spaces, ascend the bronchial tree and trachea, and are reswallowed. Upon their arrival in the small intestine, the larvae develop into mature adult worms (males measure 15–25 cm × 3 mm and females 25–35 cm × 4 mm). Each female has a life span of 1–2 yr and is capable of producing 200,000 eggs/day.

Epidemiology. Ascariasis, a soil-transmitted infection, depends on dissemination of eggs into environmental conditions

Table 11–39. **Important Intestinal Nematode Infections of Children**

Infection	Etiology	Mode of Transmission	Major Clinical Features	Diagnosis
Ascariasis	*Ascaris lumbricoides*	Eggs in soil	None, nutritional or obstructive lesions	Eggs in stools
Hookworms	*Ancylostoma duodenale, Necator americanus*	Larvae in soil	Anemia, hypoalbuminemia	Eggs in stools
Strongyloidiasis	*Strongyloides stercoralis*	Larvae in soil, autoinfection	Abdominal pain, diarrhea and malabsorption, dissemination	Larvae in stools or duodenal aspirate
Enterobiasis	*Enterobius vermicularis*	Fecal-oral, person-to-person, eggs in environment	Perianal itching	Eggs on perianal swabs
Trichuriasis	*Trichuris trichiura*	Eggs in soil	None	Eggs in stools

that are suitable for their maturation. Promiscuous defecation and use of human manure are the two most important unhygienic practices responsible for the endemicity of ascariasis. The mode of transmission to humans is hand to mouth; the fingers are contaminated by soil contact. Alternatively, food items (particularly those commonly consumed raw) become infected by human fertilizers or by flies. Endemicity of *A. lumbricoides* is aided by the extremely high egg output of worms and their resistance to unfavorable environmental conditions. Eggs have been shown to remain infective in soil for months and may survive cooler weather (5–10° C) for 2 yr. Transmission of ascariasis may occur seasonally or throughout the year.

Clinical Manifestations. Although disease sequelae occur in only a small proportion of infected individuals, they amount to a significant clinical problem because of the high incidence of ascariasis. Morbidity may be manifested during migration of the larvae through the lungs or be associated with the presence of adult worms in the small intestine. The pathogenesis of pulmonary ascariasis is not known, although a hypersensitivity phenomenon may be involved. Adult worms may cause disease by obstructing the gut or biliary tree and by affecting host nutrition. The nutritional status of children with ascariasis may be affected more by their socioeconomic and nutritional background than by the effects of the *Ascaris* infection.

Pulmonary ascariasis may occur following heavy exposure and is also common in individuals who live in areas with seasonal transmission of infection (seasonal pneumonitis). The most characteristic features are cough, blood-stained sputum, and eosinophilia. This Loeffler-like syndrome may be associated with transient pulmonary infiltrates. In children the differentiation of this syndrome from visceral larva migrans may be difficult, but abdominal symptoms or signs are very rare in pulmonary ascariasis.

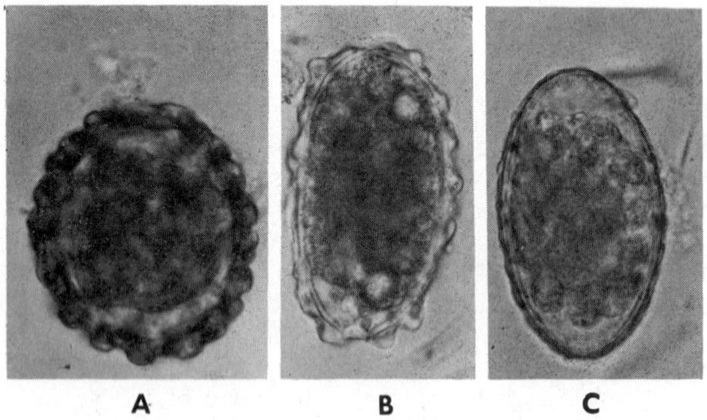

The presence of adult worms in the small intestine is associated with vague complaints such as abdominal pain and distention. Intestinal obstruction, although rare, may be due to a mass of worms in heavily infected children; the peak incidence occurs in children 1–6 yr old. The onset is usually sudden with severe colicky abdominal pain and vomiting which may be bile stained; these symptoms may progress rapidly and follow a course similar to acute intestinal obstruction of any other etiology. Migration of *Ascaris* worms into the biliary tract has also been reported, particularly occurring in China and the Philippines; the likelihood of this condition increases in heavily infected children. The onset is acute with colicky abdominal pain, nausea, vomiting, and fever. Jaundice is rarely seen.

Steatorrhea and diminished vitamin A absorption have occurred in some *Ascaris*-infected children. A study of Colombian children with moderate infections (30–50 worms) showed that administration of antihelminthic drugs was followed by decreased fat and nitrogen excretion and improved xylose absorption.

Diagnosis. Adult female worms deposit eggs which can be detected by direct fecal smear examination and quantified by the Kato thick smear method. Bisexual infections result in the excretion of mature fertile eggs, whereas infertile eggs are seen in individuals infected with female worms only (Fig. 11–32*B* and *C*). Diagnosis of pulmonary or obstructive ascariasis is based primarily on clinical data and a high index of suspicion.

Treatment. Several chemotherapeutic agents are effective against ascariasis; none, however, are useful during the pulmonary phase of the infection. Treatment, particularly of children with heavy infections, should be approached with caution. Piperazine salts (citrate, adipate, or phosphate) are administered orally in a daily dose of 50–75 mg/kg for 2 days. A single dose rather than 2 day regimens is effective in reducing worm loads in infected children. Since piperazine results in neuromuscular paralysis and a relatively rapid expulsion of the worms, it is the drug of choice for intestinal or biliary obstruction. Since sporadic hypersensitivity and neurotoxic reactions have been reported with piperazine derivatives, other drugs such as mebendazole (100 mg twice daily for 3 days) may be used for treating uncomplicated intestinal ascariasis. Rarely, surgical treatment may be needed in severe obstructive cases.

Control. Although ascariasis is the most prevalent worm infection worldwide, little attention has been given to its control, partly because of controversy concerning its clinical significance and also because of its unique epidemiologic

Figure 11–32. Fertilized (*A*) and unfertilized (*B, C*) eggs of *Ascaris lumbricoides*. (× 400.) The egg illustrated in *C* may be mistaken for that of a different nematode or of a trematode.

features. Attempts at reducing worm loads in humans by mass chemotherapy have shown some promise. Because of the high rate of reinfection, chemotherapy has to be repeated at 3–6 mo intervals. The feasibility and cost of such an undertaking will have to be evaluated before it can be widely accepted. Sanitary practices directed at treating human feces before it is used as fertilizer and providing hygienic sewage disposal facilities may be the most effective long-term preventive measures against ascariasis.

11.111 Hookworms

Three species of hookworms infect more than 900 million people: *Ancylostoma duodenale, Necator americanus,* and *Ancylostoma ceylonicum.* Infection is endemic in temperate, subtropical, and tropical areas of the world.

Etiology. Hookworm larvae are usually found in warm damp soil and infect the human host by penetrating the skin. Infection may also be acquired by drinking contaminated water. Larvae migrate to the venous circulation and are carried to the lungs, where they break into the alveolar spaces, migrate upward, and are then swallowed to reach their final habitat in the upper small intestine. Mature worms develop in 2–4 wk; they are grayish-white and slightly curved and measure 5–13 mm in length. The buccal cavity of *A. duodenale* has pointed, clawed teeth and that of *N. americanus* has two chitinous plates. These buccal structures help the mature worms attach to the jejunal mucosa and suck blood. In 6–9 wk worms reach sexual maturity and start to deposit eggs, which are excreted in the feces. Mature *A. duodenale* female worms produce about 30,000 eggs/day; daily egg production by *N. americanus* is 9000. The mean life span of adult hookworms is 1–3 yr, although they may occasionally survive up to 9 yr. Hookworm eggs are ovoidal and thin shelled and measure approximately 36×58 μm (Fig. 11–33). When freshly passed, these eggs contain 4 embryonic segments which mature into 1st stage larvae that hatch in 1–2 days under favorable environmental conditions. Larvae live in the soil for 1–2 wk, molt twice, and change into infective larvae capable of penetrating human skin.

Epidemiology. Humans are the primary host for the three species of hookworms. Endemicity of infection in any specific geographic location depends on suitability of environmental conditions for hatching of eggs and maturation of larvae, on fecal contamination of soil, and on human contact with contaminated soil. The optimal soil conditions are found in many parts of agrarian tropical countries and also in the southeastern part of the United States.

The morbidity of hookworm infections in endemic areas is sustained primarily by children. In one study half of the children were infected before age 5; 90% were infected by 9

yr of age. Intensity of infection increases up to age 6–7, then stabilizes for a few years. Newly infected children acquire a mean of 2 female worms; there is a net gain of 2.7 parasites/yr.

Pathology and Pathogenesis. Several factors may contribute to the morbidity of hookworm infection; these include worm burden, diet, race, and development of immunity in chronically infected individuals. Anemia, the major pathologic manifestation of infection, is affected primarily by the worm burden and the diet of the host.

Lesions due to hookworm may occur during the migratory phase of infection or may be related to the presence of adult worms in the small intestine. Ground itch or dermatitis results from larval invasion of skin and the subsequent inflammatory response. Mild pulmonary lesions similar to those described in ascariasis may occur during lung migration of larvae; it is questionable whether a Loeffler-like syndrome occurs. The presence of adult worms in the small intestine results in anemia and hypoalbuminemia. The severity of hookworm anemia is related to the intensity of infection and the host's iron balance. Blood loss varies with hookworm species; *A. duodenale* infection causes greater losses than *N. americanus.*

Clinical Manifestations. Infections are usually asymptomatic; significant clinical disease occurs in a small percentage of children in whom symptoms follow the chronologic order of worm migration in the host. Exposure of skin for the first time to infective larvae may lead to pruritus. Skin reactions vary from erythematous papules on primary exposure, which disappear within 1 wk, to vesiculation and generalized edema on subsequent infections, which may last 1–3 wk. Migration of the larvae through the lungs is associated with few, if any, specific symptoms or signs.

Symptoms of abdominal pain, loss of appetite, indigestion, postprandial fullness, and diarrhea have been attributed to the intestinal phase of hookworm infection. These clinical correlates are based primarily on observations of experimental infections in volunteers with heavy worm loads rather than on adequate studies of specific abdominal symptoms in natural hookworm infections. The significant disease sequelae of chronic hookworm infections include anemia, hypoalbuminemia, and edema. Hemoglobin concentrations under 5 g/dL have been associated with heart failure and sudden death. Hypoalbuminemia in excess of that anticipated from whole blood loss may also occur; the attendant decrease in plasma oncotic pressure may lead to edema.

Diagnosis. Direct examination of fecal smears for hookworm eggs provides a qualitative assessment of infection. The Kato thick smear offers a simple technique for quantitation of infection, but since hookworm eggs disappear within 1 hr of preparation, prompt examination of these smears is mandatory. Eggs of *A. duodenale* and *N. americanus* are morphologically indistinguishable; the only way to differentiate the species is to allow the eggs to hatch and examine the released larvae.

Treatment. Evaluation of intensity of infection and severity of anemia should precede therapy. In children with severe anemia (hemoglobin concentration under 5 g/dL) iron therapy should be given before antihelminthic drugs. Elemental iron is administered orally at a dosage of 2 mg/kg 3 times/day until anemia is corrected. In life-threatening anemia with signs of heart failure, diuretics followed by slow transfusion of packed red cells may be indicated. Mebendazole (100 mg orally twice a day for 2 days) or tetrachlorethylene (0.1 mL/kg and repeated at 4 and 8 day intervals) will eradicate or reduce the hookworm load.

Control. Eradication or control of hookworm infection depends on sanitation and mass chemotherapy. To allow cost-effective application of these two principles, the rate of worm acquisition, its life span, and the rate at which infection is lost have to be determined. Seasonal variations in transmission and the hookworm species must also be taken into

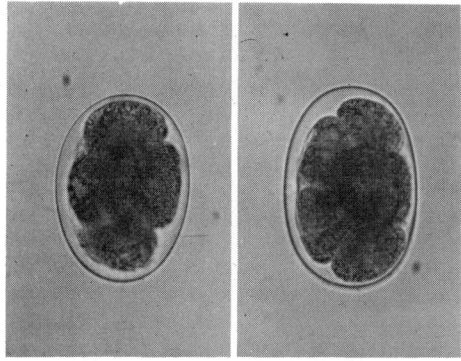

Figure 11–33. Eggs of hookworm *Necator americanus* in early cleavage as seen in freshly passed feces. (× 400.)

consideration. Eradication has been achieved in the southeast United States.

11.112 Strongyloidiasis

Infection with the nematode *Strongyloides stercoralis,* unlike that with other worms, may cause autoinfection with massive parasite invasion of the host and eventual death. This complication is more frequent in malnourished or immunosuppressed children. *S. stercoralis* infection is widely distributed throughout tropical and temperate regions, though it is less common than infection by other intestinal roundworms.

Etiology. Infected individuals pass larvae in their stools; these parasites may develop into free-living adults in the soil or change into infective filariform larvae. These latter forms penetrate human skin, pass via the blood stream to the lungs, and follow a pathway similar to hookworm and *Ascaris* larvae until they reach their final habitat in the upper small intestine. Mature female worms, which are larger than males (2.2 mm vs 0.7 mm in length), burrow into the intestinal mucosa and begin releasing eggs approximately 4 wk after infection. *S. stercoralis* eggs hatch rapidly, and small larvae (225 × 16 μm) are passed in feces. The larvae must undergo morphologic changes in soil to become infective, but these changes may also be accomplished as the parasites are being discharged from the body. Larvae are then capable of infecting the same individual by penetrating the intestinal wall or perianal skin. This unique feature of the *Strongyloides* life cycle allows the parasite to survive for many years inside the same host and occasionally to cause overwhelming infection.

Epidemiology. Man is the primary host of *S. stercoralis.* Transmission of infection and its endemicity depend on suitable soil and climatic conditions and poor sanitary habits. Close contact and poor personal hygiene may be important, since the prevalence of infection is much higher in institutions for the mentally retarded. Host factors such as nutrition and immune status may play a crucial role in the development of the hyperinfection syndrome.

Pathology and Pathogenesis. The initial penetration of skin by infective larvae usually produces no apparent pathologic lesions. Repeated skin invasion may, however, result in dermatitis; in cases in which autoinfection is established through the skin, a more extensive skin lesion, larva currens, may occur. A Loeffler-like syndrome with eosinophilia may be seen during migration of the larvae through the lungs. Eosinophilia may also occur when adult females burrow into the intestinal mucosa. Disseminated strongyloidiasis is a complex pathologic entity due to larval invasion of internal organs and complicating gram-negative bacteremia.

Clinical Manifestations. Signs and symptoms of strongyloidiasis occur in only a small percentage of infected individuals or in those with the hyperinfection syndrome. Pulmonary symptoms and skin lesions are usually mild and generally pass unnoticed. Pruritus with a papular erythematous rash may occur. Larva currens, a condition due to repeated skin invasion by larvae, is characterized by large erythematous urticarial lesions with rapidly moving edges. These are usually localized to an area within 30 cm of the anus and have a tendency to recur. The typical symptoms, which include abdominal pain, vomiting, and diarrhea, are caused by adult worms in the upper small intestine. These symptoms occur with uncertain frequency and may have an abrupt onset with periodic recurrences. Abdominal pain is often epigastric and may be burning, colicky, or dull in nature. Diarrhea with passage of mucus may alternate with periods of constipation. Chronic strongyloidiasis may result in a malabsorption-like syndrome with protein-losing enteropathy and weight loss. Blood eosinophilia is usually associated with and is often the only indication of the intestinal phase of infection.

Disseminated strongyloidiasis occurs in children with predisposing factors such as malnutrition or defects in cell-mediated immunity (lymphomas, Hodgkin disease, etc.). The onset is usually sudden, with generalized abdominal pain, distention, fever, and shock due to gram-negative septicemia. Massive invasion of internal organs by the parasite larvae causes extensive tissue destruction. Although leukocytosis may occur in these patients, eosinophilia is often absent.

Diagnosis. Intestinal strongyloidiasis is diagnosed by examining feces or duodenal fluid for the characteristic larvae. Several stool samples should be examined either by direct smear or by a concentration method such as formaldehyde-ether or that of Baermann. Alternatively, duodenal fluid obtained by the pediatric Entero test or aspiration may provide samples for definitive diagnosis. In children with hyperinfection syndrome, larvae may be found in sputum, gastric aspirates, or, rarely, in small intestinal biopsies. Strongyloidiasis should also be suspected in immunosuppressed patients who suddenly develop signs and symptoms consistent with disseminated infection. A recently described serologic test for *Strongyloides* antibodies may be more sensitive than parasitologic methods for diagnosing intestinal infection, but the utility of this assay in the hyperinfection syndrome has not been determined.

Treatment. The only available and effective therapeutic agent is thiabendazole. Treatment of infected children should aim at eradication of infection, and therefore subsequent stool examination is essential. Thiabendazole is administered orally in a dose of 25 mg/kg twice daily for 3 days. Courses of up to 2 wk may be needed in those with the hyperinfection syndrome.

Control. Sanitary practices designed to prevent soil and person-to-person transmission are the most effective control measures. Because the infection is uncommon, case detection and treatment are also advised. Individuals who will be subjected to immunosuppressive therapy should have a screening examination for *S. stercoralis* and, if infected, be treated with thiabendazole.

11.113 Enterobiasis
(Pinworm)

Enterobius vermicularis infection occurs worldwide and affects individuals of all ages and socioeconomic levels but is especially common in children. Living in congested districts, institutions, or families with pinworm infections predisposes to enterobiasis. The infection is essentially harmless and causes more social than medical problems in affected children and their families.

Etiology. Humans are infected by ingesting embryonated eggs which are usually carried on fingernails, clothing, bedding, or house dust. Eggs hatch in the stomach and larvae migrate to the cecal region where they mature into adult worms. *E. vermicularis* are small (1 cm) white worms; the gravid females migrate by night to the perianal region to deposit masses of eggs. Pinworm ova are asymmetric, are flattened on one side, and measure 30 × 60 μm (Fig. 11–34). After a 6 hr maturation period a single-coiled larva can be seen within each ovum. These larvae may remain viable for 20 days.

Epidemiology. Perianal irritation during oviposition by female worms induces scratching. Eggs carried under the fingernails are transmitted directly or disseminated in the environment to infect others. Man is the only natural host of *E. vermicularis.* The prevalence and intensity of infection are low in infants and young children and reach a peak in the 5–14 yr old age group; the prevalence decreases in adulthood because of either reduced exposure or acquisition of immunity.

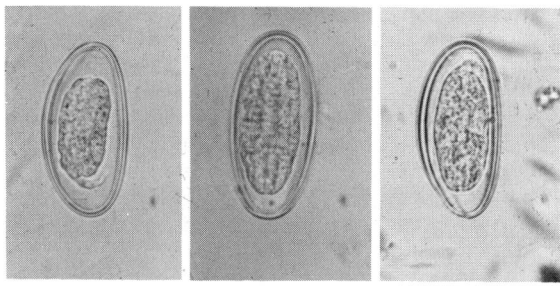

Figure 11–34. Eggs of *Enterobius vermicularis* in early developmental stages recovered from feces. (× 400.) One side of the shell is somewhat flat, but when viewed from above (center) it appears to be symmetrical and may be mistaken for a different species. When found in human feces, which is unusual, pinworm eggs contain a tadpole-stage embryo, whereas eggs recovered on a perianal swab contain a coiled larva that is more than twice the length of the egg.

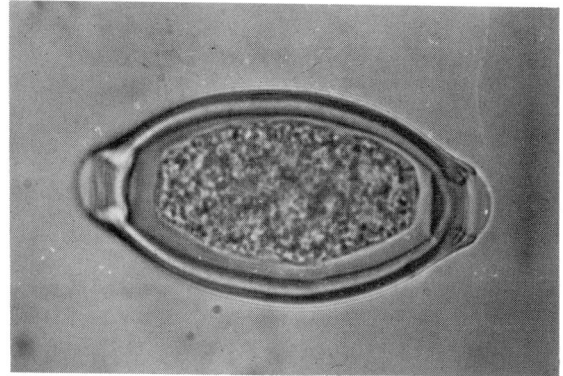

Figure 11–35. Egg of *Trichuris trichiura*, as seen in freshly passed feces. (× 1000.)

Clinical Manifestations. Many local and systemic signs and symptoms have been ascribed to *Enterobius* infection; however, a controlled study of infected children 2–12 yr old failed to document specific syndromes due to *E. vermicularis.* Symptomatic individuals most commonly complain of nocturnal anal pruritus and sleeplessness. The etiology and incidence of perianal and perineal irritation are unknown but may be related to the intensity of infection, to the psychiatric profile of the infected individual and his or her family, or to an allergic reaction to the parasite. Since tissue invasion does not occur in most cases of enterobiasis, eosinophilia is not observed. In a few cases, however, *E. vermicularis* has been recovered from ectopic sites such as the appendix, female genital tract, and peritoneal cavity.

Diagnosis. Definitive diagnosis is established by either finding the parasite eggs or recovering worms. Eggs can be easily detected on adhesive cellophane tape pressed against the perianal region early in the morning. Repeated examinations may be necessary, and in certain situations examination of all family members may be advised. If a worm is seen in the perianal region, it should be preserved in 75% ethyl alcohol until microscopic examination can be performed.

Treatment. Drug therapy should be given to all infected and symptomatic individuals; mebendazole (single oral dose of 100 mg for all ages) is recommended. Piperazine salts or pyrvinium pamoate may also be used. Repeated treatments every 3–4 months may be required in situations in which exposure is constant, e.g., children in institutions. While personal cleanliness is a useful general recommendation, there is no proof that it plays a significant role in control of enterobiasis.

11.114 Trichuriasis

Trichuris trichiura causes one of the most common worm infections of humans; approximately half a billion cases occur worldwide. Infection is more common in warm climates but does exist in North America.

Etiology. Infection is due to ingesting mature parasite eggs (Fig. 11–35), which are passed in the stools of infected individuals and mature in 2–4 wk if moisture and temperature conditions of the soil are optimal. Upon ingestion by man *Trichuris* eggs hatch, and larvae penetrate the small intestinal villi where they remain for 3–10 days before slowly moving down the bowel and maturing into adult worms. The final habitat of *T. trichiura* is the cecum and ascending colon. The body is divided into an anterior whip-like portion (hence the term whipworm) and a posterior bulky part and measures approximately 40 mm in length. The worms remain in the gut by anchoring the anterior portion of their body to the intestinal mucosa. Egg deposition by maturing females begins 1–3 mo after infection.

Epidemiology. Trichuriasis is most common in poor rural communities lacking sanitary facilities. Man is the primary host; the highest prevalence and intensity of infection are in children. Transmission of embryonated eggs occurs by contamination of hands, food, or drink. Eggs may also be carried by flies and other insects.

Clinical Manifestations. Most infected individuals are asymptomatic; however, vague abdominal complaints, colic, and abdominal distention have been associated with infection. Adult *Trichuris* suck approximately 0.005 mL of blood/worm/day. However, only heavy childhood infections produce mild anemia, bloody diarrhea, or, rarely, rectal prolapse. These cases are referred to as massive infantile trichuriasis and are often associated with shigellosis and protozoan infections of the gastrointestinal tract.

Diagnosis and Treatment. Examination of stool smears reveals the characteristic eggs of *T. trichiura.* An oral course of mebendazole (100 mg twice a day for 3 days) produces a cure rate of 70–90% and reduces egg output by 90–99%.

JAMES W. KAZURA
ADEL A. F. MAHMOUD

Ascariasis

Louw JH: Abdominal complications of *Ascaris lumbricoides* infestation in children. Br J Surg 53:510, 1966.
Pawlowski ZS, Arfaa F: Ascariasis. *In:* Warren KS, Mahmoud AAF (eds): Tropical and Geographical Medicine. New York, McGraw-Hill, 1984, p 347.
Spillman RK: Pulmonary ascariasis in tropical communities. Am J Trop Med Hyg 24:791, 1975.
Stephenson LS, Crompton DWT, Latham MC, et al: Relationship between *Ascaris* infection and growth of malnourished preschool children in Kenya. Am J Clin Nutr 33:1165, 1980.

Hookworms

Miller TA: Hookworm infection in man. Adv Parasitol 17:315, 1979.
Nawalinski T, Schad GA, Chowdhury AB: Population biology of hookworms in children in rural West Bengal. I. General parasitological observations. Am J Trop Med Hyg 27:1152, 1978.
Nawalinski T, Schad GA, Chowdhury AB: Population biology of hookworms in children in rural West Bengal. II. Acquisition and loss of hookworms. Am J Trop Med Hyg 27:1162, 1978.

Strongyloidiasis

Burke JA: Strongyloidiasis in childhood. Am J Dis Child 132:1130, 1978.
Grove DI, Blair AJ: Diagnosis of human strongyloidiasis by immunofluorescence using *S. ratti* and *S. stercoralis* larvae. Am J Trop Med Hyg 30:344, 1981.
Scowden EB, Schaffner W, Stone WJ: Overwhelming strongyloidiasis. Medicine 57:527, 1978.
Smith JD, Goette DK, Odom RB: Larva currens: Cutaneous strongyloidiasis. Arch Dermatol 112:1161, 1976.

Enterobiasis

Boyer A, Berdknikoff IK: Pinworm infestation in children; the problem and its management. Can Med Assoc J 86:60, 1962.

Weller TH, Sorensen CW: Enterobiasis: Its incidence and symptomatology in a group of 505 children. N Engl J Med 224:131, 1941.

Trichuriasis

Blumenthal DS: Intestinal nematodes in the United States. N Engl J Med 297:1437, 1977.

Jung RC, Beaver PC: Clinical observations on *Trichocephalus trichiurus* (whipworm) infestation in children. Pediatrics 8:548, 1951.

TISSUE NEMATODES

Tissue-dwelling nematodes infect over 800 million people worldwide. Although morbidity from these helminths primarily afflicts the populations of tropical and developing countries, inhabitants of regions with temperate climates may also be affected. These parasites have a complex life cycle which in most instances includes an intermediate invertebrate host. Childhood disease results mainly when children act either as an incidental host in whom the helminth does not undergo its normal development (*Toxocara sp., Dirofilaria sp.*) or as the definitive host (filariae, *Dracunculus medinensis).* Infections that are particularly common in childhood (visceral larval migrans) will be presented first and will be followed by a discussion of tissue nematodes that cause disease in individuals of all ages (cutaneous larva migrans, *Trichinella spiralis, D. medinensis*) or primarily in adults (human and animal filariae). The major characteristics of these infections are outlined in Table 11–40.

11.115 Visceral Larva Migrans
(Toxocariasis)

Visceral larva migrans is caused by infection with larvae of *Toxocara sp.* It occurs most frequently in children under the age of 10 yr and is characterized by fever, hepatomegaly, pulmonary disease, and eosinophilia.

Etiology. *Toxocara canis, T. cati,* and *Toxascaris leonina* are common parasites of dogs and cats that infect humans when the eggs of the helminth are ingested. Adult worms of *Toxocara sp.* reside in the gastrointestinal tract of dogs and cats and release large numbers of eggs which are passed in the feces. Ingestion of eggs by man is followed by larval penetration of the gastrointestinal tract and migration to liver, lung, and occasionally other sites (central nervous system, eye, kidney, and heart). *Toxocara* larvae do not develop beyond this stage in the human host.

Epidemiology. Visceral larva migrans is most common in children 1–4 yr of age, particularly those who engage in pica and have close contact with dogs and cats; ocular toxocariasis occurs most frequently in older children. Potential sources of infection are widely distributed in the canine and feline population (an estimated 20% of dogs in the United States excrete *Toxocara* eggs). These animals often defecate in areas where children play (24% of 800 soil samples taken from public parks in Great Britain were found to contain *Toxocara* eggs).

Pathology. *Toxocara* larvae usually elicit a granulomatous response characterized by large numbers of eosinophils, mononuclear cells, and tissue necrosis. These lesions are found in liver, lung, and other organs in which the helminth migrates. The inflammatory reaction is much less intense in the eye, where lesions consist mainly of mononuclear cells and a few eosinophils.

Clinical Manifestations. Major symptoms include fever (80%), cough with wheezing (60–80%), and seizures (20–30%). Respiratory distress may be severe enough to warrant hospitalization. Abdominal pain has been noted in occasional patients. Physical findings include hepatomegaly (65–87%), rales and/or rhonchi (40–50%), papular or urticarial skin lesions (20%), and lymph node enlargement (8%). These manifestations subside over a period of several months. Scattered patchy infiltrates are often seen on chest roentgenograms.

Patients with ocular toxocariasis most commonly present with decreased visual acuity (in 75% of cases) and occasionally with strabismus or periorbital edema. In one study unilateral blindness was noted in 6 of 17 patients. Most children do not have concurrent signs and symptoms of visceral disease. Funduscopic examination of the eye usually reveals solitary granulomatous lesions situated in the retina near the optic disc or macula. These may be mistaken for retinoblastomas and have led to inappropriate enucleation. Peripheral retinal lesions with vitreous bands and involvement of the iris have been documented in a few cases.

Diagnosis. The diagnosis is made on the basis of the clinical manifestations and serologic testing. The only reliable and specific test is an enzyme-linked immunosorbent assay (ELISA) which utilizes infective eggs of *T. canis* as antigen.

Table 11–40. **Tissue Nematode Infections of Children**

Infection	Etiology	Mode of Transmission	Major Clinical Syndromes	Diagnosis
Visceral larva migrans	*Toxocara canis, T. cati*	Eggs in soil	Wheezing and cough, hepatomegaly; many infections asymptomatic	Serology, clinical
Ocular toxocariasis	*Toxocara canis, T. cati*	Eggs in soil	Decreased visual acuity	Serology, clinical
Trichinosis	*Trichinella spiralis*	Larvae in undercooked meat	Myalgias, fever, diarrhea	Serology and larvae in muscle biopsy
Dracunculosis	*Dracunculus medinensis*	Larvae in freshwater crustaceans	Skin ulceration	Clinical, larvae in ulcer
Filariases	*Brugia malayi* and *Wuchereria bancrofti*	Mosquitoes and flies	Acute: lymphangitis; chronic: elephantiasis	Microfilariae in blood or tissues
	Onchocerca volvulus	Black fly	Dermatitis, blindness	Microfilariae in blood or tissues
	Loa loa	Tabanid	Calabar swelling	Microfilariae in blood or tissues
Tropical pulmonary eosinophilia	Microfilariae	Mosquito	Asthma, fever	Chest x-ray, eosinophilia, serology
Animal filariae	*Dirofilaria immitis, D. tenuis, Brugia beaveri*	Mosquito	Pulmonary coin lesions, subcutaneous nodules	Identification of parasite in tissue sections

This assay is positive (serum antibody titer ≥1:32) in 78% of cases of visceral larva migrans and in 45% of individuals with a clinical diagnosis of ocular toxocariasis. Eosinophilia (>500/mm³ blood) occurs in nearly all subjects with the visceral syndrome but is much less common with ocular disease. Nonspecific findings include elevations in serum gamma globulins and isohemagglutinins. Although larvae may be found upon examination of tissue sections, biopsy of liver or other organs is generally not indicated as clinical and laboratory data provide enough evidence to make the diagnosis.

Treatment. Therapy is not required in the majority of cases since the signs and symptoms are usually mild and subside over a period of weeks to months. When significant hypoxemia secondary to pulmonary disease occurs, however, the administration of anti-inflammatory drugs (prednisone, 5 mg/kg/24 hr until respiratory function improves) is beneficial. When disease is severe or when larvae lodge in critical locations, such as the eye, the use of drugs exhibiting possible larvicidal activity (diethylcarbamazine, 0.5 mg/kg/24 hr for 3 days, increased gradually to 3 mg/kg/24 hr for 21 days) has been advocated. There is disagreement about this approach, however, since dying larvae theoretically may incite an inflammatory response which produces more tissue damage than encapsulated, dormant parasites.

Control. Transmission of infection may be prevented by requiring children to wash their hands after playing with pets and instructing them to avoid areas where these animals defecate, particularly children with the habit of pica. Periodic deworming of dogs, especially puppies below the age of 6 mo, also decreases the likelihood of infection.

11.116 Cutaneous Larva Migrans
(Creeping Eruption)

Cutaneous larva migrans is caused by several larval nematodes not usually parasitic for man. *Ancylostoma braziliense* (a hookworm of dogs and cats) is the most common of these helminths, but other animal hookworms (*A. caninum, Uncinaria stenocephala,* and *Bunostomum phlebotosum*) and human parasites (*Necator americanus, Ancylostoma duodenale,* and *Strongyloides stercoralis*) may produce the disease. These organisms are widely distributed throughout tropical and subtropical areas of the world. In the United States infections are most prevalent in the South. Parasite eggs are deposited in the feces of animals and hatch to form infective larvae in warm moist areas, such as near vegetation on beaches or under porches. Man is infected when the skin comes in contact with these larvae.

Clinical Manifestations. After penetrating the skin, larvae localize at the epidermal-dermal junction and migrate in this plane, moving at a rate of 1–2 cm/day. The response to the parasite is characterized by raised, erythematous, serpiginous tracks which occasionally form bullae (Fig. 11–36 [p. xxvi]). These lesions may be single or multiple and are usually localized to an extremity, although any area of the body may be affected. As the organism migrates, new areas of involvement may appear every few days. Intense localized pruritus may be associated with the lesions.

Diagnosis and Treatment. Cutaneous larva migrans is diagnosed by clinical examination of the skin. Patients are often able to recall the exact time and location of exposure as the larvae produce intense itching at the site of penetration. If left untreated, the larvae die and the syndrome resolves within a few weeks to several months. Topical application of thiabendazole oral suspension or a 0.5 g tablet triturated with 5 g petroleum jelly may be used if symptoms warrant treatment.

11.117 Trichinosis

Human infection with *Trichinella spiralis* is fairly common worldwide. Infection is transmitted by ingestion of pork or other meat carrying the parasite. Sporadic epidemics have occurred in North America following ingestion of bear meat.

Etiology. Humans are infected by eating flesh contaminated with viable *Trichinella spiralis* larvae. This stage of the parasite excysts in the stomach and matures to form adult worms within the small intestine. Female *T. spiralis* release large numbers of newborn larvae which penetrate the gut wall and migrate to striated muscles or occasionally to other sites such as the central nervous system and heart. Larvae that enter muscle cells eventually become encysted and may remain viable for years. The life cycle in nature is maintained by hogs or other animals that ingest garbage containing carcasses of infected rodents.

Epidemiology. *T. spiralis* is found in all areas of the world except Australia and some islands in the South Pacific. Although infection was common in the United States in the past (4% of diaphragms examined post mortem in 1968 contained viable larvae), recent cases have been related to outbreaks from ingestion of undercooked homemade sausage, other pork products, or meat of bears, wild pigs, and walruses. Larvae are destroyed by cooking meat until there is no trace of pink fluid or flesh (this occurs at 55° C) or by storage in a freezer at −15° C for 3 wk. Smoked or salted meat may still contain viable parasites.

Pathology and Pathogenesis. Adult worms localize in the upper gastrointestinal tract and induce a mucosal inflammatory reaction characterized by a reduced villous:crypt ratio and the presence of eosinophils, neutrophils, and mononuclear cells. This response peaks within the 1st wk of infection, then gradually subsides as adult worms are expelled. In muscle cells migrating larvae elicit a reaction consisting of large numbers of eosinophils and mononuclear cells. These lesions may eventually calcify.

Clinical Manifestations. The signs and symptoms appear only in heavily infected individuals. Within the 1st wk adult worms in the upper gastrointestinal tract produce gastroenteritis and diarrhea associated with abdominal discomfort. Next, during larval invasion of muscle, periorbital or facial edema (80% of cases), and myalgias occur. Pain is associated with muscle activity; it is most common in the masseters, diaphragm, and intercostals. These signs and symptoms are first noted 10–14 days after infection and last for another 2–3 wk. Heart failure and arrhythmias may occur in patients with exceptionally heavy infections.

Diagnosis. Periorbital edema, myalgias, fever, and eosinophilia in an individual who gives a history of eating undercooked meat make the diagnosis of trichinosis likely. A history of similar illness in those sharing the food should be sought. Serologic studies such as the bentonite flocculation test (titer of 1:5 or greater) are confirmatory. Biopsy of muscle, usually the deltoid, may reveal larvae upon microscopic examination 3–4 wk after infection. Muscle enzymes such as creatine kinase and lactate dehydrogenase are elevated in 50% of patients.

Treatment. There is no clinically established therapy for the syndrome related to larval invasion of muscles. Thiabendazole (25 mg/kg/24 hr for 1 wk) is active primarily against adult worms and should therefore be given only to those individuals who were known to acquire the infection in the preceding 1–7 days. Corticosteroids may be used in critically ill patients, such as those with myocarditis or central nervous system damage, but evidence for their beneficial effect is equivocal.

11.118 Dracunculosis
(Guinea Worm Infection)

Dracunculosis occurs in all areas of the tropics and is especially common in India and West Africa. The parasite, *Dracunculus medinensis*, infects man when he swallows larva-containing microscopic crustaceans (copepods) living in communal water sites. Adult worms grow to a length of 1 meter or more and migrate through the subcutaneous tissues of the lower extremities (or occasionally other sites). An ulcer is produced where they penetrate the skin. The diagnosis is confirmed by identifying larvae contained in washings from the base of the lesion. Administering niridazole (12.5 mg/kg/24 hr for 10 days) or thiabendazole (50 mg/kg/24 hr for 3 days) diminishes the local inflammatory response and permits removal of the helminth. Infection may be prevented by avoiding ingestion of water that humans walk in or use for bathing. Boiling or chlorination kills the organism.

Filariases

Filariae are thread-like nematodes which may cause significant human morbidity. Disease due to infection with these organisms usually becomes evident years after exposure; it is thus uncommon for children to have clinically significant filariasis.

11.119 Malayan and Bancroftian Filariasis

Infection with *Brugia malayi*, *Brugia timori*, or *Wuchereria bancrofti* results in similar clinical syndromes characterized in the early stages by acute lymphangitis and lymphadenitis and later by lymphatic obstruction with hydrocele and elephantiasis. Over 200 million people in developing countries may be infected with these parasites.

Etiology. Filarial larvae are introduced into humans in secretions of biting mosquitoes. Over months to a year this stage of the helminth develops into adult worms which reside in the lymphatics. Sexually mature adult female worms release large numbers of microfilariae which circulate in the blood stream. The life cycle of the parasite is completed when mosquitoes ingest these organisms in a blood meal.

Epidemiology. Although as much as 80% of the population of endemic areas may be infected, fewer than 10–20% have clinically significant morbidity. Those who work in areas where there is repeated and chronic exposure to larvae-containing mosquitoes, such as in crowded urban areas with poor sanitation, are most at risk. *W. bancrofti* infection is distributed throughout tropical and subtropical Africa, Asia, and South America, while infection with *B. malayi* is restricted to the South Pacific and Southeast Asia. *B. timori* infection occurs in Indonesia.

Clinical Manifestations. The acute stage of infection is characterized by episodes of fever, lymphangitis of an extremity, headaches, and myalgias which last a few days to several weeks. This syndrome is most frequently observed in young people 10–20 yr old. Chronic manifestations of disease, such as hydrocele and elephantiasis, occur mostly in those over 30 and are a direct result of lymphatic fibrosis and obstruction to lymph flow. The presence of larvae (microfilariae) in the blood is not thought to have any pathologic consequences.

Diagnosis and Treatment. Demonstrating microfilariae in the blood is the only way to diagnose lymphatic-dwelling filariasis. Two mL of blood obtained at a time of day when the number of parasites in the circulation is expected to be highest (this varies with the geographic strain of filaria) should be filtered and examined for the organisms.

The use of antifilarial drugs must be individualized. Older patients with chronic lymphatic obstruction and those who remain in endemic areas will not benefit from specific therapy. Younger individuals with acute lymphangitis should be given a course of diethylcarbamazine (50 mg on day 1, 50 mg 2 and 3 times on days 2 and 3, respectively, then 10 mg/kg on days 4–21).

11.120 Onchocerciasis, Loiasis, and Tropical Pulmonary Eosinophilia

Infection with *Onchocerca volvulus* (onchocerciasis, river blindness) is a major cause of blindness in West Africa and Central America. The parasite is introduced into humans by blackflies of the genus *Simulium* which breed in rapidly running water; people who live or work near waterways are thus most likely to be infected. Most individuals are asymptomatic; those with chronic and heavy infections (usually men over 30 yr old) may suffer from pruritic dermatitis and eye disease (punctate keratitis, corneal pannus formation, chorioretinitis) due to the presence of microfilariae in subcutaneous and ocular tissues. Firm, nontender subcutaneous nodules containing adult parasites may also be palpable. *O. volvulus* infection is diagnosed by demonstration of parasites in skin snips removed from the buttocks or extremities or by visualization with a slit lamp of microfilariae in the cornea or anterior chamber of the eye. Children with symptomatic skin and/or eye disease should be treated with diethylcarbamazine as described for lymphatic filariasis (Sec. 11.119) and observed carefully for eye reactions (decreased visual acuity and iritis), increased pruritus with desquamation, and fever. If these reactions appear, corticosteroids should be administered. Because of the ocular side effects of diethylcarbamazine, asymptomatic lightly infected children who have left an endemic area should probably not receive this antihelminthic drug.

Loa loa infection occurs in the rain forest of West and Central Africa; the parasite is transmitted to human by tabanid flies. Adult worms migrate in the subcutaneous tissues and produce painful transient areas of localized edema known as calabar swellings, which tend to appear around the joints of the legs and arms. The parasite occasionally may be directly visualized in the conjunctiva, where it produces an intense inflammatory reaction. Microfilariae are present in highest concentrations in the peripheral circulation between 10 AM and 2 PM; identification in blood samples is diagnostic. Symptomatic individuals should be given gradually increasing doses of diethylcarbamazine as described for lymphatic filariasis (Sec. 11.119). Therapy should be discontinued and corticosteroids administered if fever, headache, or joint swelling occurs.

Tropical pulmonary eosinophilia (TPE) is a syndrome of filarial etiology in which microfilariae can be found in the lung and lymph nodes. It occurs only in subjects who have lived for at least several months in endemic areas of bancroftian or Malayan filariasis and is most common in Southeast Asia and the South Pacific. Although TPE has been observed in children, 20–30 yr old men are most likely to be affected. Patients present with paroxysmal nonproductive cough, occasional episodes of dyspnea, fever, weight loss, and fatigue. Rales and rhonchi are found on auscultation of the chest; roentgenographic examination may occasionally be normal but usually reveals increased bronchovascular markings, discrete opacities in the middle and basal regions of the lung, or diffuse miliary lesions. Recurrent untreated episodes may result in interstitial fibrosis and chronic respiratory insufficiency. In children hepatosplenomegaly and generalized lymphadenopathy are often seen. Eosinophilia (>2000/mm³ blood) with the appropriate history and symptoms suggests the diagnosis. Increased serum IgE levels (>1000 units/mL) and high titers of antimicrofilarial antibodies in the absence of blood-borne helminths should also be documented. Although microfilariae may be found in sections of lung or lymph node, biopsy is unwarranted in most patients. The clinical response to diethylcarbamazine (5 mg/kg/24 hr for 10 days) is the final criterion for diagnosis since in the majority of patients symptoms improve with this therapy. If they recur, a second course of the drug should be administered. Subjects presenting with chronic symptoms are less likely to show improvement than those who have been ill for a short time.

11.121 Infection with Animal Filariae

Humans may be infected with three types of animal filariae. *Dirofilaria immitis*, the heartworm, is found on all continents and is a common parasite of dogs in many parts of the United States. *D. tenuis*, *Brugia beaveri*, and other unclassified *Brugia sp.* have also been reported to infect man. These worms may be introduced into man by the bite of mosquitoes containing 3rd-stage larvae. The organisms, however, do not undergo normal development in the human host. *D. immitis* are trapped in the lung parenchyma after migrating for several months in the subcutaneous tissues. The pulmonary response consists of granulomas with eosinophils, neutrophils, and tissue necrosis. *D. tenuis* does not leave the subcutaneous tissues, while *B. beaveri* eventually localizes to superficial lymph nodes.

Most human infections with *D. immitis* are discovered incidentally when the chest roentgenogram reveals a solitary pulmonary nodule 1–3 cm in diameter. Definitive diagnosis and cure depend on surgical excision and identification of the nematode within the surrounding granulomatous response. *D. tenuis* and *B. beaveri* infections present as painful, rubbery 1–5 cm diameter nodules in the skin of the trunk, extremities, and orbit. Patients often report having been engaged in activities suggestive of exposure to infected mosquitoes, such as working in swampy areas. Diagnosis and management of these infections are similar to those of *D. immitis*.

JAMES W. KAZURA

Toxocariasis

Glickman LT: Toxocariasis. *In:* Warren KS, Mahmoud AAF (eds): Tropical and Geographical Medicine. New York, McGraw-Hill, 1984, p 431.
Greene BM, Taylor HR, Cupp EW, et al: Comparison of ivermectin and diethylcarbamazine in the treatment of onchocerciasis. N Engl J Med 313:133, 1985.
Huntley CC, Costas MC, Lyerly A: Visceral larva migrans syndrome: Clinical characteristics and immunologic studies in 51 patients. Pediatrics 36:623, 1965.
Schantz PM, Glickman LT: Toxocaral visceral larva migrans. N Engl J Med 298:436, 1978.
Zinkham WH: Visceral larva migrans. A review and reassessment indicating two forms of clinical expression: Visceral and ocular. Am J Dis Child 132:627, 1978.

Filariasis

Greene BM, Taylor HR, Cupp EW, et al: Comparison of ivermectin and diethylcarbamazine in the treatment of onchocerciasis. N Engl J Med 313:133, 1985.
Grove DI, Valeza FS, Cabrera BD: Bancroftian filariasis in a Philippine village: Clinical, parasitological, immunological and social aspects. Bull World Health Org 56:975, 1978.
Neva FA, Ottesen EA: Tropical (filarial) eosinophilia. N Engl J Med 298:1129, 1978.
Ottesen EA: Filariases and Tropical Eosinophilia. *In:* Warren KS, Mahmoud AAF (eds): Tropical and Geographical Medicine. New York, McGraw-Hill, 1984, p 390.
Taylor HR, Greene BM: Ocular changes with oral and topical diethylcarbamazine therapy of onchocerciasis. Br J Ophthal 65:494, 1981.

TREMATODES
(Flukes)

Parasitic trematodes form a group of important human infections that are endemic worldwide but are more prevalent in the less developed parts of the world. Trematodes are characterized by their complex life cycle; sexual reproduction of adult worms in the definitive host is followed by asexual multiplication by the larval stages in the intermediate host. This "alternation of generations" requires that flukes parasitize more than one host (often three) to complete their life cycle. The most important infections of humans are outlined in Table 11–41.

BLOOD FLUKES

11.122 Schistosomes

Five schistosome species infect man; these are *Schistosoma haematobium*, *S. mansoni*, *S. japonicum*, *S. intercalatum*, and *S. mekongi*. Schistosomiasis infects more than 200 million people, mainly children and young adults. With the necessity of developing irrigation projects, the infection is spreading as more suitable habitats for the snail intermediate host are created. *S. haematobium* is prevalent in Africa and the Middle East; *S. mansoni* in Africa, the Middle East, Caribbean, and South America; and *S. japonicum* in China, the Philippines, and Indonesia, with some sporadic foci in Japan and other parts of Southeast Asia. The other two less prevalent species are found in the Far East (*S. mekongi*) and West Africa (*S. intercalatum*).

Etiology. Humans are infected upon contact with water contaminated with cercariae, the infective forms of the para-

Table 11–41. Important Trematode Infections of Children

Infection	Etiology	Mode of Transmission	Major Clinical Syndromes	Diagnosis
Schistosomiasis	*Schistosoma haematobium*	Cercariae in fresh water	Hematuria, dysuria, and obstructive uropathy	Eggs in urine
	S. mansoni, *S. japonicum*	Cercariae in fresh water	Hepatosplenomegaly, portal hypertension	Eggs in feces
Clonorchiasis	*Clonorchis sinensis*	Metacercariae in fresh-water fish	Mainly asymptomatic	Eggs in feces
Opisthorchiasis	*Opisthorchis felineus* and *O. viverrini*	Metacercariae in fresh-water fish	Mainly asymptomatic	Eggs in feces
Fascioliasis	*Fasciola hepatica*	Metacercariae on aquatic vegetation	Early: fever, hepatomegaly, and eosinophilia Late: mainly asymptomatic	Eggs in feces
Fasciolopsiasis	*Fasciolopsis buski*	Metacercariae on aquatic plants	Mainly asymptomatic	Eggs in feces
Paragonimiasis	*Paragonimus westermani*	Metacercariae in freshwater crayfish or crabs	Hemoptysis, productive cough, and eosinophilia	Eggs in sputum or feces

site. These motile, forked-tail organisms emerge from infected snails and are capable of penetrating intact human skin within a few minutes. In the subcutaneous tissues cercariae change into another larval stage (schistosomula) and migrate to the lungs and finally the liver. Once they reach sexual maturation, adult worms migrate to specific anatomic sites characteristic of each schistosome species: *S. haematobium* adults are found in the vesical plexus, *S. mansoni* in the inferior mesenteric, and *S. japonicum* in the superior mesenteric veins. *S. intercalatum* and *S. mekongi* are found in the mesenteric vessels. Adult schistosome worms (1–2 cm in length) are different from most other flukes in that they exist as separate sexes; the female, however, accompanies the male in a groove formed by the lateral edges of its body. Upon fertilization, female worms begin oviposition in the small venous tributaries. The eggs of the three main schistosome species have characteristic morphologic features: *S. haematobium*, terminal spine; *S. mansoni*, lateral spine; and *S. japonicum*, smaller size with a short curved spine (Fig. 11–37). Eggs force themselves out of the blood vessels through surrounding tissues to reach the lumen of urinary tract or intestines, through which they are carried to the outside environment, where they hatch if deposited in fresh water. Motile miracidia emerge; they infect specific fresh water snail intermediate hosts and divide asexually. In 4–6 wk the infective cercariae are released in the water.

Epidemiology. Humans are the definitive host for the five clinically important species of schistosomes, although *S. japonicum* may infect some animals such as dogs and cattle. Transmission depends on disposal of excreta, the presence of specific intermediate snail hosts, and the patterns of water contact and social habits of the population. The distribution of infection in endemic areas shows that incidence increases with age to a maximum in the 10–20 yr age group, after which it declines. Furthermore, measuring intensity of infection (by egg count in urine or feces) demonstrates that heavy worm loads are usually found in the younger age groups. Schistosomiasis, therefore, is most prevalent and severe in children and young adults who are at maximal risk of suffering from its disease sequelae.

Pathology and Pathogenesis. The major pathologic lesions are associated with retention of eggs in the host tissues during the chronic stages of infection. Eggs may be trapped at sites of deposition (urinary bladder, ureters, intestine) or be carried by the blood stream to other organs, most commonly the liver and less often the lungs and central nervous system. The host response to these eggs involves local as well as systemic manifestations. Granulomas composed of lymphocytes, macrophages, and eosinophils surround the trapped eggs and add significantly to the size of tissue destruction. It has been shown that these granulomas are due to cell-mediated responses. Granuloma formation in the bladder wall and at the ureterovesical junction leads to the major disease manifestations of schistosomiasis hematobia: hematuria, dysuria, and obstructive uropathy. Intestinal as well as hepatic granulomas underlie the pathologic sequelae of the other schistosome infections: ulcerations and fibrosis of intestinal wall, hepatosplenomegaly, and portal hypertension due to presinusoidal obstruction of blood flow. Fibrosis usually follows the granulomatous process, adding to pathophysiologic changes. Granuloma formation undergoes modulation in chronically infected individuals with a decrease in size and diminution in pathologic sequelae, a phenomenon perhaps related to some of the systemic host responses (antibody, immune complexes, suppressor cells) which ultimately function as ameliorating factors. Protective immunity against schistosomiasis has been conclusively demonstrated in some animal species but not in man. The decrease in the prevalence and intensity of infection in the older age groups may be related to the development of immunity or to decreased water exposure.

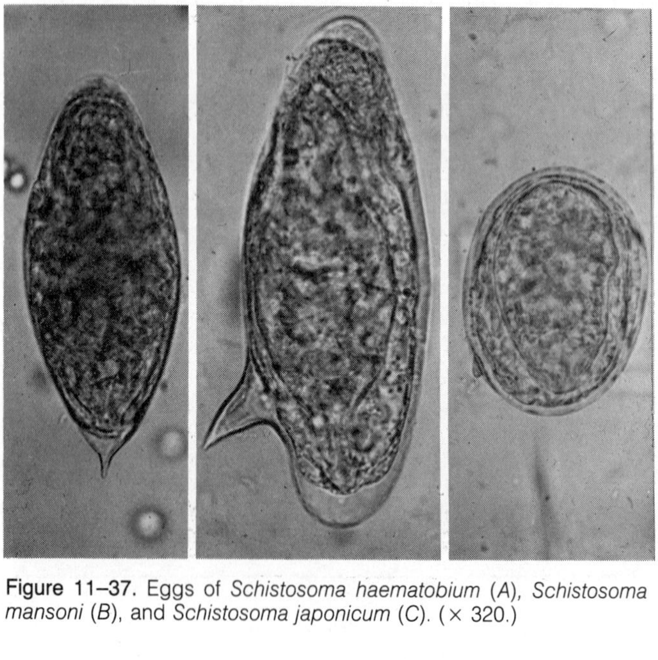

Clinical Manifestations. Most of the infected individuals suffer from no apparent ill health; symptomatology occurs mainly in those heavily infected. Cercarial penetration of human skin may result in a papular pruritic rash (swimmer's itch). It is more pronounced in previously exposed individuals and involves edema and massive cellular infiltrates in the dermis and epidermis. Katayama fever may occur, particularly in heavily infected individuals 4–8 wk after exposure; this is a serum sickness–like syndrome manifested by the acute onset of fever, chills, sweating, lymphadenopathy, hepatosplenomegaly, and eosinophilia. Its pathogenesis is unknown but may be due to immune complex formation.

Symptomatic children with chronic schistosomiasis haematobia usually complain of frequency, dysuria, and hematuria (often terminal). Urine examination shows erythrocytes, parasite eggs, and occasional leukocytes. In most endemic areas extensive pathologic lesions have been demonstrated in the urinary tract of more than half of infected children. The extent of disease is correlated to intensity of infection, but significant morbidity may occur even in lightly infected children. The terminal stages of schistosomiasis haematobia are associated with chronic renal failure, secondary infections, and cancer of the bladder in some endemic areas.

Children with chronic schistosomiasis mansoni, japonica, or mekongi may have intestinal symptoms; colicky abdominal pain and bloody diarrhea are the most common. The intestinal phase may, however, pass unnoticed, and the syndrome of hepatosplenomegaly, portal hypertension, ascites, and hematemesis may be the initial presentation. Liver disease is due to granuloma formation and subsequent fibrosis; there is no appreciable liver cell injury, and hepatic function may be preserved for a long time. Schistosome eggs may escape into the pulmonary vasculature causing hypertension and cor pulmonale. Furthermore, *S. japonicum* worms may migrate to the brain vasculature and produce seizures.

Diagnosis. Schistosome eggs are found in the excreta of infected individuals; quantitative procedures should be used to give an indication of intensity of infection. Urine should be collected around midday (time of maximal egg excretion) and 10 mL filtered through a nuclepore membrane for diagnosis of *S. haematobium* infection. Stool examination by the Kato thick smear procedure is the method of choice for diagnosis and quantification of other schistosome infections.

Figure 11–37. Eggs of *Schistosoma haematobium* (*A*), *Schistosoma mansoni* (*B*), and *Schistosoma japonicum* (*C*). (× 320.)

Treatment. Management of children with schistosomiasis should be based on intensity of infection and extent of disease. The drug of choice is praziquantel, which is effective against all schistosome species. It is administered orally as a single or divided dose of 40–60 mg/kg.

Control. Transmission in endemic areas may be decreased by reducing the parasite load in the population. The availability of oral, single dose, effective chemotherapeutic agents may help achieve this goal. Other measures, particularly improved sanitation and focal application of molluscicides, may be useful.

11.123 LIVER FLUKES
Clonorchiasis

Infection of bile passages with the Chinese or oriental fluke *Clonorchis sinensis* is endemic in China, other parts of Southeast Asia, and Japan. Humans acquire infection by ingestion of raw or inadequately cooked freshwater fish carrying the encysted metacercariae of the parasite under its scales or skin. These metacercariae excyst in the duodenum and pass through the ampulla of Vater to the common bile duct and bile capillaries, where they mature into hermaphroditic adult worms (3 × 15 mm). *C. sinensis* worms deposit small operculated eggs (14 × 30 μm), which are discharged via the bile duct to the intestine and feces (Fig. 11–38). The eggs mature and hatch, releasing motile miracidia. If these are ingested by specific snails, numerous cercariae develop, which may escape and encyst under the skin or scales of freshwater fish.

Most *C. sinensis*–infected individuals, particularly those with light infections, are asymptomatic. Localized obstruction of a bile duct and thickening of its walls may be the result of repeated local trauma and inflammation in heavily infected individuals. In these cases cholangitis and cholangiohepatitis may lead to liver enlargement and jaundice. In Hong Kong, cholangiocarcinoma in the Chinese population is associated with *C. sinensis* infection. Clonorchiasis may be diagnosed by examining feces or duodenal aspirates for the parasite eggs. Praziquantel is the drug of choice for treating clonorchiasis (25 mg/kg tid given for 1 day).

Opisthorchiasis

Infections with species of *Opisthorchis* are clinically similar to those with clonorchiasis. *O. felineus* and *O. viverrini* are common liver flukes of cats and dogs which may occasionally infect man through ingestion of metacercariae in freshwater fish. Infection with *O. felineus* is endemic in eastern Europe and Southeast Asia, and *O. viverrini* is found mainly in Thailand. Most individuals are asymptomatic; liver enlargement, relapsing cholangitis, and jaundice may be seen in heavily infected individuals. Diagnosis is based on recovering eggs from stools or duodenal aspirates. Praziquantel, in the same dosage as for clonorchiasis, is the drug of choice.

Fascioliasis

The sheep liver fluke *Fasciola hepatica* infects cattle, other ungulates, and occasionally man. Human infection has been reported from different parts of the world, particularly South America, Europe, Africa, China, and Australia. Although *F. hepatica* is enzootic in North America, human cases are extremely rare. Man is infected by ingestion of metacercariae attached to vegetations, especially wild watercress. In the duodenum the parasites excyst; penetrate the intestinal wall, liver capsule, and parenchyma; and wander for a few weeks before entering the bile ducts where they mature. Adult *F. hepatica* (1 × 2.5 cm) commence oviposition approximately 12 wk after infection; the eggs are large (75 × 140 μm) and

operculated, pass to the intestines with bile, and leave the body in the feces (Fig. 11–38). On reaching fresh water, the eggs mature and hatch into miracidia, which infect specific snail intermediate hosts to multiply into many cercariae. These then emerge from infected snails and encyst on aquatic grasses and plants.

Clinical manifestations usually occur either during the liver migratory phase of the parasites or after their arrival at their final habitat in bile canaliculi. The first phase is characterized by fever, right upper quadrant pain, and hepatosplenomegaly. Peripheral blood eosinophilia is usually marked. As the worms enter bile ducts, most of the acute symptoms subside. On rare occasions, patients may suffer from obstructive jaundice or biliary cirrhosis. *F. hepatica* infection is diagnosed by finding the characteristic eggs in fecal smears or duodenal aspirates. Praziquantel (25 mg/kg tid given for 1 day) is the recommended treatment.

11.124 INTESTINAL FLUKES

Several wild and domestic animal intestinal flukes, such as *Fasciolopsis buski* and *Heterophyes heterophyes*, may accidentally infect man. The clinical significance of most of these infections is doubtful and not fully understood. *Fasciolopsis buski* is endemic in the Far East. Humans are infected by ingesting metacercariae encysted on aquatic plants. They hatch and produce large flukes (1 × 5 cm) which inhabit the duodenum and jejunum. Mature worms produce operculated eggs that pass with feces; the organism completes its life cycle through specific snail intermediate hosts. Individuals with *F. buski* infection are usually asymptomatic; heavily infected subjects complain of diarrhea and abdominal pain and show signs of malabsorption. Diagnosis of fasciolopsis is made by fecal examination for eggs. As in other fluke infections, praziquantel is the drug of choice.

11.125 LUNG FLUKES
(Paragonimiasis)

Human infection by the lung fluke *Paragonimus westermani* occurs throughout the Far East, in localized areas of West Africa, and in several parts of Central and South America. The highest incidence of pulmonary paragonimiasis occurs in older children and adolescents 11 to 15 yr of age. Although *P. westermani* is found in many carnivora, human cases are relatively rare and seem to be associated with specific dietary habits such as eating raw freshwater crayfish or crabs. These crustaceans contain the infective metacercariae in their tissues;

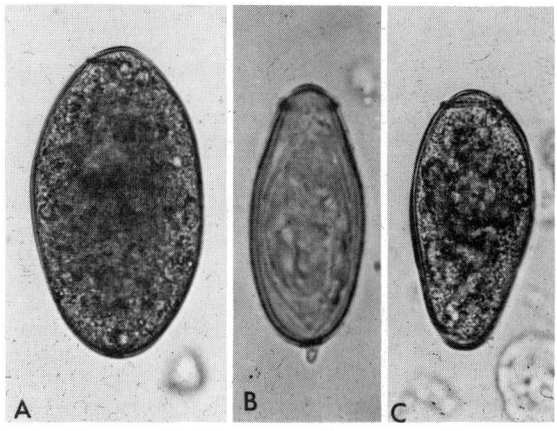

Figure 11–38. Eggs of liver flukes and a lung fluke. A, *Fasciola hepatica* (× 400). B, *Clonorchis sinensis* (× 1000). C, *Paragonimus westermani* (× 400).

they excyst in the duodenum, penetrate the intestinal wall, and migrate to their final habitat in the lungs. Adult worms (5 × 10 mm) encapsulate within the lung parenchyma and deposit brown operculated eggs (60 × 100 μm), which pass into the bronchioles and are coughed up (Fig. 11–38). Ova can be detected in the sputum of infected individuals or in their feces. If eggs reach fresh water, they hatch and undergo asexual multiplication in specific snails. The cercariae encyst in the muscles and viscera of crayfish and freshwater crabs.

Most individuals infected with *P. westermani* harbor low or moderate worm loads and are asymptomatic. In symptomatic infected children hemoptysis occurs in 98% of cases; other symptoms include cough and production of rust-colored sputum. There are no characteristic physical findings, but laboratory examination usually demonstrates marked eosinophilia. Chest roentgenogram often reveals small patchy infiltrates or radiolucencies in the mid-lung fields; however, the roentgenogram may be normal in one fifth of infected individuals. In rare circumstances lung abscess, pleural effusion, or bronchiectasis may be demonstrable. Extrapulmonary localization of *P. westermani* in the brain, peritoneum, intestines, or pleura may rarely occur. Cerebral paragonimiasis is seen primarily in heavily infected individuals living in highly endemic areas of the Far East; the clinical presentation resembles jacksonian epilepsy or cerebral tumors. Definitive diagnosis of paragonimiasis is made by finding eggs in fecal or sputum smears. The treatment of choice is praziquantel (25 mg/kg) given orally three times in 1 day.

Schistosomiasis

Domingo EO, Tiu E, Peters PA, et al: Morbidity in schistosomiasis japonica in relation to intensity of infection: Study of a community in Leyte, Philippines. Am J Trop Med Hyg 29:858, 1980.
Jordan P, Webbe G: Schistosomiasis: Epidemiology, Treatment and Control. London, Heinemann, 1982, p 361.
Mahmoud AAF, Siongok TKA, Ouma J, et al: Effect of targeted mass treatment on intensity of infection and morbidity in schistosomiasis mansoni: 3 year follow-up of a community in Machakos, Kenya. Lancet 1:849, 1983.
Siongok TKA, Mahmoud AAF, Ouma JH, et al: Morbidity in schistosomiasis mansoni in relation to intensity of infection: Study of a community in Machakos, Kenya. Am J Trop Med Hyg 25:273, 1976.
Warren KS, Mahmoud AAF, Muruka JF, et al: Schistosomiasis haematobia in Coast Province Kenya. Am J Trop Med Hyg 28:864, 1979.

Other Flukes

Bunnag D, Harinasuta T: Opisthorchiasis, clonorchiasis and paragonimiasis. In: Warren KS, Mahmoud AAF (eds): Tropical and Geographical Medicine. New York, McGraw-Hill, 1984, p 461.
Drugs for parasitic infections. Medical Letter 24:5, 1982.
Fischer GW, McGrew GL, Bass JW: Pulmonary paragonimiasis in childhood. JAMA 243:1360, 1980.

CESTODES
(Tapeworms)

Humans serve as the main definitive host of some of the cestodes, the segmented or tapeworms; other cestodes parasitize lower animals, human infection occurring only inci-

dentally. Most commonly adult worms parasitize the gastrointestinal tract, causing little or no clinical morbidity except when they interfere with host nutrition. Major clinical syndromes may occur, however, when man is infected with the larval stages of some cestodes which disseminate and can cause disease in any internal organ. The common cestode infections of children are outlined in Table 11–42.

11.126 TENIASIS AND DIPHYLLOBOTHRIASIS
(Giant Tapeworms)

There are three giant tapeworms that may cause human infection, and all three infections may be acquired by ingesting animal flesh that contains the larval stage of the parasites. *Taenia saginata* is found in all parts of the world and is particularly common in East Africa; in North America it is estimated to infect 23 persons/100,000 population. The exact prevalence of *T. solium* is not known but is reportedly less than that of *T. saginata*; the infection is most endemic in India, China, South Africa, Central Europe, and some parts of South America. Teniasis solium is not endemic in North America. *Diphyllobothrium latum* is endemic in regions with cold lakes such as Scandinavia, Northern Europe, Siberia, China, and North and South America. Parasitized fish may also be found in lakes at high altitudes in tropical areas, such as Central Africa.

Etiology. Man is infected by ingesting raw or undercooked flesh. Infective larvae of *T. saginata* are found in beef, those of *T. solium* in pork, and those of *D. latum* in freshwater fish. The cysticerci of taeniae or the plerocercoids of *D. latum* start their development upon reaching the human small intestine and mature in several months. Adult tapeworms consist of ribbon-like segments, approximately 1000 in *T. solium*, 2000 in *T. saginata*, and 4000 in *D. latum*. Mature worms vary in length from 4 to 10 meters. Mature segments may passively (*T. solium*) or actively (*T. saginata*) pass through the anus. Taenia eggs are rarely seen in stools. They are small (35 μm in diameter) and yellowish brown and contain hooklets in their center (Fig. 11–39). In contrast to *Taenia sp.*, *D. latum* segments usually deposit their eggs within the intestinal lumen, and they are easily seen in fecal smears of infected individuals. They are operculate and measure 45 × 75 μm (Fig. 11–40). When eggs of *Taenia sp.* are ingested by the appropriate host, they are digested and embryos emerge that penetrate the intestinal wall, disseminate throughout the tissues, and develop into mature infectious cysticerci. The cysticercus stage of *T. saginata* can be formed only in cattle. Ingestion of *T. solium* eggs by man may, however, occasionally lead to cysticercosis. Further development of *D. latum* eggs takes place in fish and crustacea; the infective forms finally lodge in the tissues of freshwater fish.

Epidemiology. Human infection by the giant tapeworms is most common in adults. Transmission is primarily related to nutritional habits, fecal disposal practices, and the methods used to feed domestic animals. Thorough cooking or freezing

Table 11–42. Important Cestode Infections of Children

Infection	Etiology	Mode of Transmission	Major Clinical Syndromes	Diagnosis
Teniasis	*Taenia saginata*	Cysticerca in beef	Passage of segments through anus	Microscopy of segments
	T. solium	Cysticerca in pork	Mainly asymptomatic	Microscopy of segments
Cysticercosis	*T. solium*	Ingestion of eggs	Space occupying lesion in brain, muscles, etc.	Clinical and serology
Diphyllobothriasis	*Diphyllobothrium latum*	Plerocercoid in freshwater fish	B$_{12}$ deficiency	Eggs in feces
Hymenolepiasis	*Hymenolepis nana*	Ingestion of eggs	Mainly asymptomatic	Eggs in stool
Echinococcosis	*Echinococcus granulosus*	Ingestion of eggs	Cysts in liver, lungs, brain, or bones	Clinical and serology

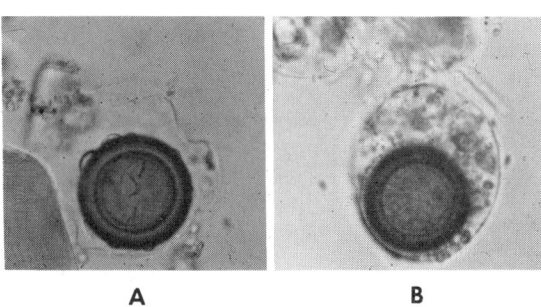

Figure 11–39. Eggs of *Taenia saginata* recovered from fresh feces. (× 400.) The cellular structure in which the egg develops while in the proglottid, more evident in *B* than in *A*, may be retained around the dark prismatic egg membrane which contains the larva. Usually evident in the larva are 3 pairs of hooklets (*A*), which occasionally may be seen in motion.

destroys the infective stages of these parasites. Adult worms may live for decades; human infection is usually due to only one worm and has no adverse effects. Infection with many worms or with the larval stage of *T. solium* may, however, produce serious clinical manifestations.

Clinical Manifestations. Infection with adult *T. saginata* or *T. solium* is almost always asymptomatic. These parasites do not compete to any significant degree for host nutrients. The most frequent sign in *T. saginata* infection is passage of motile segments through the anus. Although many abdominal symptoms have been associated with tapeworm infections, these correlations have not been based on properly controlled studies. Similar vague abdominal complaints have been associated with *D. latum* infection. The most important clinical sequela of this infection is vitamin B$_{12}$ deficiency. Adult worms absorb the vitamin at a fast rate and may cause megaloblastic anemia in infected individuals. In Finland it was estimated that 0.1% of an infected population developed anemia. Typical morphologic changes in the bone marrow and subacute spinal cord degeneration may be seen.

Human infection with the cysticercus stage of *T. solium* may be asymptomatic. However, heavy infection with localization of larvae in important anatomic areas, principally the brain, may lead to generalized or focal seizures and raised intracranial pressure. Eosinophilia is variable in patients with cysticercosis.

Diagnosis. Infection with *Taenia* worms is diagnosed by identification and morphologic characterization of adult segments. *D. latum* infection is usually identified by direct smear examination of feces. Cysticercosis may be diagnosed by a combination of clinical presentations, roentgenography and

CT scanning to detect cysts in brain or soft tissues, and serology. Hemagglutination titers are significantly elevated in 85% of individuals with cysticercosis.

Treatment. All three giant tapeworm infections are treated with a single oral dose of niclosamide (2 tablets [1 g] for children weighing 11–34 kg and 3 tablets [1.5 g] for those above 34 kg). Patients with megaloblastic anemia due to *D. latum* infection should be given vitamin B$_{12}$ and observed for neurologic complications. Symptomatic patients with cysticercosis are treated with praziquantel, 50 mg/kg/24 hr in 3 divided doses for 14 days.

11.127 HYMENOLEPIASIS
(Dwarf Tapeworms)

Infection with *Hymenolepis nana* is most common in children living in warm climates; the prevalence ranges from 0.3 to 2.9% in North America. Although most children harbor light infections that are not associated with symptoms or signs, young children are more likely to develop heavy worm loads, possibly secondary to autoinfection, and may present with abdominal pain or diarrhea.

Infection is acquired by ingesting eggs passed in feces of parasitized individuals. *H. nana* eggs are spherical or ovoid, measure 40 × 50 μm, and contain embryos with characteristic hooklets (Fig. 11–41). The ova hatch in the intestinal lumen and liberate embryos that mature into adult worms (1 × 40 mm); these usually reside in the ileum and begin oviposition in a few weeks. The eggs are carried to the outside via feces but may hatch inside the same host (autoinfection), increasing the intensity of infection. *H. diminuta*, a parasite of rodents, occasionally infects man. Adult worms are larger than *H. nana*, the life cycle is similar, and eggs are identical in shape but slightly greater in size.

The characteristic eggs of *H. nana* and *H. diminuta* may be found on fecal examination by direct smear or by concentration methods. Patients may be treated with niclosamide (same dose as for tapeworms). Praziquantel is also highly effective; in one study single doses of 25 mg/kg cured 94% of infected children.

11.128 ECHINOCOCCOSIS
(Hydatid Disease)

Human infection with the larval stage of the canine tapeworm *Echinococcus granulosus* occurs worldwide but is most prevalent in countries where sheep and cattle are raised. Endemic areas include Australia, South America, South Africa, the Soviet Union, and the Mediterranean region. Clinical disease occurs when hydatid cysts present as space-occupying

Figure 11–40. Eggs of *Diphyllobothrium latum* as seen in fresh feces. (× 400.) The operculum is usually evident.

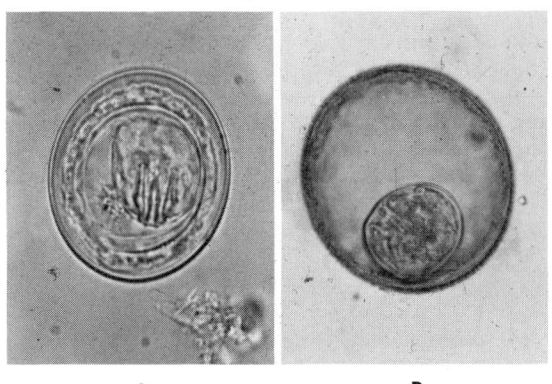

Figure 11–41. Eggs of *Hymenolepis nana* (A) (× 575) and *Hymenolepis diminuta* (B) (× 400).

lesions; these are most common in the liver, but other tissues, such as the lungs, brain, and bones, may also be affected.

Etiology. Domesticated dogs acquire the infection by eating parasitized viscera of sheep and cattle. Humans incidentally acquire infection with *E. granulosus* by ingesting parasite eggs that are discharged in the feces of infected dogs or wolves. Embryos escape from the eggs in the duodenum, penetrate its wall, and pass to the liver where they are usually trapped. If the embryos escape from the liver, they may seed the lungs or travel to other organs via the systemic circulation. Wherever the parasite embryos are trapped, they may be destroyed by the host response or develop into hydatid cysts. These cysts can grow in size up to 20 cm in diameter and are lined on the inside by a germinal layer, which forms multiple larval scolices and daughter cysts. *E. granulosus* infection in man cannot maintain the life cycle of the parasite as it is dependent on the death of the intermediate host and ingestion of larvae by dogs and wolves.

Epidemiology. *E. granulosus* transmission to humans is most common in regions of the world supporting major livestock industries. Infection is usually acquired by direct contact with dogs but may also occur by ingesting contaminated soil, vegetables, and water. The prevalence is highest in children; clinical manifestations, however, occur several years later. Another cycle of transmission to man occurs in North America, particularly in some areas of Alaska and Canada. The strain of *E. granulosus* endemic in these regions is found in the wolf, and larvae are found in large deer such as moose, reindeer, or caribou.

Clinical Manifestations. Most individuals with hydatid cysts are asymptomatic; clinical disease appears in a small proportion and is usually the result of the space-occupying nature of the cysts. When they occur in the liver, manifestations develop only when a cyst reaches large dimensions and presses on adjacent tissues and structures or is located in an area which obstructs blood flow, such as the porta hepatis. Since it takes several years for hydatid cysts to grow, clinical morbidity is usually detected in middle-aged or elderly patients. Symptoms occur earlier when the cysts are located in less well supported tissues like the brain and lung, where there is also an increased risk of rupture into adjacent structures. Dissemination of the daughter cysts may lead to serious infections in the peritoneal or pleural cavities. Approximately two thirds of hydatid cysts occur in the liver and one quarter in the lungs. In contrast to liver lesions, pulmonary hydatid cysts are commonly seen in children, who may present with hemoptysis, cough, or dyspnea. The cysts may rupture into the bronchial tree and spread by discharging their contents in respiratory secretions. Hydatid disease in the brain usually presents as space-occupying lesions; the most common presentation in bone is invasion with erosion and spontaneous fracture.

In some parts of North America, Europe, and Asia, another species of canine tapeworm, *E. multilocularis,* is found in foxes as well as domestic cats and dogs. Human infection with this parasite leads to the so-called malignant hydatid. Many small cysts occur in organs such as the liver; they multiply, spread quickly, and destroy adjacent normal tissues. The prognosis is grave, as measures to stop the spread of the infection are not available. Surgical intervention is hazardous.

Diagnosis and Treatment. Some cases of hydatid cyst may be discovered on routine roentgenographic examination of the chest or abdomen. Children in endemic areas with suggestive symptoms and signs should undergo roentgenographic and ultrasonic examination. The benign nature of the cyst may be confirmed by angiography. Serology may be helpful, particularly when antibodies to echinococcus antigen 5 are detected.

Once a presumptive diagnosis is made, the extent of disease must be assessed. Small or calcified liver cysts should be left alone; enlarging or symptomatic cysts should be removed surgically. In patients with pulmonary or bone cysts, surgical removal is also recommended. Care should be taken during the operative procedure not to disseminate the infection. It is therefore advisable to inject aqueous iodine or a concentrated salt solution into the cyst before its removal to kill the contained embryos. Recently, several reports have shown the efficacy of albendazole. If these observations are confirmed, administration of this drug may provide an alternative to surgical intervention in many patients, particularly those with liver cysts.

ADEL A. F. MAHMOUD

Pawlowski Z, Schultz MG: Taeniasis and cysticercosis. Adv Parasitol 19:269, 1972.
Saidi F: Surgery of Hydatid Disease. Philadelphia, WB Saunders, 1976.
Schantz PM: Echinococcosis (Hydatidosis). In: Warren KS, Mahmoud AAF (eds): Tropical and Geographical Medicine. New York, McGraw-Hill, 1984, p 487.
Schenone H: Praziquantel in the treatment of *Hymenolepis nana* infection in children. Am J Trop Med Hyg 29:329, 1980.
von Bonsdorff B: Diphyllobothriasis in Man. London, Academic Press, 1977, p 189.
Williams JF: Recent advances in the immunology of cestode infections. J Parasitol 65:337, 1979.

11.129 ARTHROPODS AND DISEASE

Arthropods (insects, spiders, ticks, etc.) produce disease in four ways: (1) certain arthropods elaborate venoms which they introduce into the human body; (2) some are blood-sucking ectoparasites; (3) others are tissue invaders; and (4) many arthropods are mechanical transmitters of pathogenic microorganisms, and others are obligate incubators and transmitters of disease-producing microorganisms.

VENENATING ARTHROPODS

This group includes centipedes, scorpions, spiders, ticks, mites, and several species of insects.

Centipedes. These arthropods have a pair of hollow jaws serving as fangs which introduce into the skin toxic substances elaborated in their heads. The venom is relatively weak, and, at most, even in an infant, will produce only an inflammatory reaction at the puncture site and mild lymphangitis. The affected areas may be treated with local compresses and an antiseptic.

Scorpions. Many species of scorpions, including the dangerous ones in the southwestern United States, Latin America, many areas in Africa, southern Europe, Israel, and India, have potent venom that is elaborated in the swollen caudal segment and introduced through the sharp, caudal sting into the skin of a person who accidentally steps on or otherwise makes contact with the animal.

The venom of some species produces only local tissue reaction (swelling at the puncture site is distinctive), while that of other species is primarily neurotoxic. The latter type contains several fractions, including hemolysins, endotheliolysins, and neurotoxins, and typically produces, in addition to an intense, aching pain and numbness radiating from the site of the injury and lymphadenitis, an ascending motor paralysis, convulsions resembling those observed in strychnine poisoning, a rapid weak pulse, excessive salivation, extreme thirst, and dysuria; at times there is evidence of acute pancreatitis. Deaths from scorpion stings occur, particularly in children under 4 yr of age.

Initially, the spread of venom from the site of the sting may be retarded by promptly applying a temporary tourniquet and (without incision) prolonged, but not excessive, cooling with ice packs. Standardized species-specific or group-specific antivenin is available for intramuscular administration.* Supportive treatment initially consists of infiltrating into the puncture wound a 2% solution of procaine containing 1:1000 epinephrine to relieve pain, then parenterally administering glucose and amino acid solutions. Shock should be treated with parenteral solutions (Sec. 5.41). Morphine and its derivatives are contraindicated because they synergistically increase the toxicity of scorpion venom as much as 7-fold. For irrational or convulsing patients, 6 mg/kg of sodium phenobarbital may be given as an initial parenteral dose in infants and children; subsequent doses of similar amounts are given at intervals of 20–30 min up to 4–5 administrations.

Applying creosote and oil as repellents or residual sprays of available organic insecticides to hiding places around homes and outbuildings reduces the number of scorpions and therefore the risk of stings.

Spiders. Nearly all spiders produce venoms to stun or kill their prey, but few species have fangs powerful enough or venom potent enough to endanger human beings as does the black widow spider of the United States, *Latrodectus mactans*. This black spider with variable red dorsal spots and an unmistakable red ventral spot attains a body length of 13 mm and a leg spread of 40 mm. Striking with a pair of anterior fangs, the spider may bite on chance contact or attack when her web is touched. An immediate, sharp pain occurs at the site, accompanied by a burning, swollen, inflamed area around the puncture wound. The venom enters the blood stream, producing in about 30 min dizziness, weakness, tremors, abdominal cramps, and, typically, a spastic contraction of the muscles, particularly those of the abdomen, simulating acute abdominal conditions and sickle cell crisis. Concomitant symptoms are rapid shallow respiration, tachycardia, and high arterial blood pressure. Acute nephritis may develop. Hemoglobinuria has been reported in small children. The double fang markings at the site of inoculation may provide a diagnostic clue, but diagnosis is usually made from the clinical history.

Treatment consists of intramuscular injection of standardized species- or group-specific antivenin.† Pain can be reduced by intramuscular or slow intravenous injection of a 10% solution of calcium gluconate, 0.05–0.1 mL/kg repeated as necessary, or by subcutaneous morphine sulfate, alone or with intramuscular phenobarbital. Prolonged hot baths are also effective. Barbiturates may be needed to allay muscle spasm and pain. Neostigmine bromide (USP) may also be used to reduce smooth muscle spasms. Acute symptoms usually abate after 24 hr, but there may be a long convalescence. Most deaths occur within 36 hr and are due to delay in supportive treatment or administering antivenin.

Species of the genus *Loxosceles*, which may have domestic habitats, produce necrotic arachnidism. *Loxosceles laeta* and *L. rufipes* in South America cause topical necrosis and, at times, systemic hemolysis. In the central and southern United States,

L. reclusa (brown recluse spiders) and related species (body 7–12 mm long, leg spread 30–40 mm; yellowish to reddish brown with 6 eyes and a dark, violin-shaped mark dorsally between the legs), inhabit dry cellars, closets, and outbuildings. They are not aggressive, but when crushed or entangled in clothing, both the male and the female bite, causing severe local pain, and the rapid development of an indurated wheal which transforms into a large violaceous sloughing ulcer that leaves a deep granulating base. Healing occurs very slowly over a period of weeks if the lesion is not excised. Systemic reactions vary but may include restlessness, fever, and sometimes a scarlatiniform rash; rarely, deaths have been reported. The venom contains a powerful necrotoxin. Parenteral administration of corticotropin will hasten healing of the wound.

Contact insecticides, such as lindane in kerosene sprayed on the spider's web, are lethal to *Latrodectus* and to *Loxosceles*.

Ticks and Mites. Ticks are macroscopic and mites microscopic arthropods with unsegmented flat or swollen bodies and 6 or 8 legs. Ticks are brown or gray, whereas mites may be colorless, reddish, or dark. Many species of ticks and several species of mites cause serious local irritation at the sites on the skin that they pierce to feed on blood or (chiggers) tissue fluid. The mites most irritating to children are chiggers ("red bugs") and rat or bird mites. Red bugs, encountered in grass, weeds, or undergrowth, produce intensely pruritic, gross, and hemorrhagic papular lesions which are frequently grouped in areas where clothing is snug. Rat and bird mites, leaving the nests of their hosts and invading human living areas, cause less prominent, widely dispersed lesions resembling mosquito bites. The local lesion at the site of attachment can be effectively treated by applying phenolated camphor solution in pure mineral oil or Quotane ointment containing dimethisoquin hydrochloride, or by coating chigger bites with collodion or nail polish. Dusting sulfur into socks and pants or rubbing dimethyl phthalate on the ankles and legs will usually prevent infestation with chiggers; repellents containing toluamide are also effective for ticks. Nonparasitic mites may be involved in house-dust allergy (*Dermatophagoides* spp. and others) and, infrequently, in contact dermatitis (grainitch, cheese, and produce mites).

Tick Paralysis. Certain ticks, including the Rocky Mountain wood tick and Eastern dog tick, after being attached for a number of days, introduce toxic saliva that may cause a flaccid ascending motor paralysis which usually begins in the legs. The entire body should be thoroughly searched for a tick that may be hidden in skin crevices or hair. Recovery is usually rapid and complete if the tick is removed promptly, but if it is allowed to remain, death may result from respiratory paralysis. Applying petrolatum or heat to induce the tick to detach will avoid the risk of leaving the imbedded mouth parts in the skin through forceful removal.

Insects. These include bees, wasps, ants, blister beetles, moth caterpillars, and many blood-sucking insects. The honeybee worker, unlike bumblebees and wasps, may leave the stinger imbedded in the skin; it should be scraped off carefully to avoid pressure on the attached poison sac. The venoms of bees, wasps, and ants are complex mixtures of peptides, proteins, and amines, including histamine and hyaluronidase. Hypersensitive people who go into shock require prompt administration of epinephrine and then a gradual desensitization (Sec. 10.54) to minimize subsequent reactions.

Blister beetles produce a painful blister when their juices are brought into contact with the skin. Ammonia will partly neutralize the blister fluid, and a corticosteroid ointment will ease the pain. Certain caterpillars elaborate venom in nettling hairs which, on contact with the skin or mucous membranes, produce an intense stinging sensation and a painful burn which heals slowly. Promptly washing with soap and water or alcohol is advisable, and a palliative such as calamine

*For sources of scorpion antivenins, contact the Information Officer, Centers for Disease Control, Atlanta, GA 30333 (tel. 404–329–3311) or the nearest Poison Control Center.

†Antivenin *Latrodectus mactans* (Merck Sharp and Dohme) is specific.

lotion, wet baking soda, or meat tenderizer may be applied. The pain is partially eased by a corticosteroid ointment, but systemic effects (e.g., from the puss caterpillar), which may be severe during the 1st day or longer, sometimes require sedation and bed rest.

Blood-Sucking Insects. Insects such as mosquitoes, gnats, deerflies, stable flies, fleas, lice, and assassin bugs introduce saliva into the skin while taking a blood meal. This foreign protein produces allergic manifestations in many persons. Antihistamines topically or orally may be palliative for insect bites and stings; specific desensitization may alleviate hypersensitivity. *Papular urticaria* in children may result from sensitivity to insect bites, particularly of fleas or bedbugs in the home, and requires appropriate control or protective measures. Repellents applied to exposed skin provide temporary protection out of doors; indoors, flying insects can be killed by household fly sprays or dichlorvos (DDVP)-impregnated plastic strips. For *pediculosis*, see Sec. 24.30.

TISSUE-INVADING ARTHROPODS

Important tissue-invading arthropods include the itch mite (*Sarcoptes scabiei*), which produces scabies; the chigoe (*Tunga penetrans*); and the maggots or larval stage of many species of filth flies and their relatives, which cause myiasis.

Scabies. See Sec. 24.30.

Chigoe Infestation. *Tunga penetrans*, a flea, is a common skin parasite of dogs, pigs, and barefooted persons in the American tropics and tropical Africa. The most common sites of human infestation are the spaces between the toes, into which the fleas burrow. The females swell to the size of a pea, producing painful, festering lesions. Gravid fleas should be removed with a sterile needle and the wound painted with tincture of iodine to kill the remaining fleas and eggs. Since infestation is usually acquired from direct contact between the bare foot and dust or dirt harboring fleas from dogs or pigs, well shod feet practically guarantee prevention.

Myiasis. This results from invasion of tissues and organs by the larvae (maggots or grubs) of various species of flies, which may be specific obligate parasites or semispecific or accidental facultative parasites. Myiasis may affect the skin, connective tissue, eye, nasopharynx, ear, intestines, or urethra; the clinical effects range from benign intestinal infestations or localized lesions to severe mutilation and even death from deep penetration into vital organs. Children are particularly vulnerable through either outdoor exposure or the ingestion of fly-contaminated food. The larvae are active, whitish, headless, segmented, and wormlike and are diagnostic when found imbedded in tissues or in freshly passed stools that have been protected from contamination by flies.

In specific myiasis the gravid fly deposits eggs or larvae on skin, hair, mucous membranes, or (tropical warble fly) carrier arthropods. The natural hosts are animals, and infestation of man is incidental. Individual larvae of the tropical warble fly (*Dermatobia hominis*) and fox, mink, and rodent parasites (*Wohlfahrtia* and *Cuterebra* species) produce furuncular lesions; horse bots (*Gasterophilus* species), a cutaneous creeping eruption; sheep bots (*Oestrus ovis*), conjunctival invasion; and cattle bots (*Hypoderma* species), deep migratory invasion; multiple larvae of the primary screwworm (*Cochliomyia hominivorax*) burrow deeply and destructively into the skin or head.

Semispecific and accidental myiasis may result from attraction of saprophagous flies to open lesions or soiled skin or from ingestion of food containing eggs or larvae of flies. Blowflies (species of *Calliphora*, *Lucilia*, *Phaenicia*, and *Cochliomyia macellaria*) and flesh flies (*Sarcophaga* species) are semispecific and most frequently involved, while other species,

including the house fly (*Musca domestica*), are rare accidental intestinal parasites.

Maggots burrowing into tissues or breeding in wounds should be removed as soon as possible. The lesions should be irrigated, treated with a bactericidal ointment, and covered with a sterile dressing. In intestinal myiasis, frequent saline purgation and enemas may be helpful. Young children, particularly those around stock farms, should be protected from flies by screening or mosquito netting, and any discharges from children's eyes, nares, or skin lesions should not be allowed to accumulate, since these attract myiasis-producing flies. Fly-control measures should be applied, especially around domestic animals and fur-breeding farms.

ARTHROPODS AS TRANSMITTING AGENTS OF DISEASE

Arthropods transmit disease-producing microorganisms to humans directly by mechanical means or indirectly as essential biologic hosts or incubators of pathogens.

Mechanical Transmitters. The most important mechanical transmitters are the filth flies, including the common housefly, the lesser houseflies, stable flies, greenbottles, bluebottles, blowflies, flesh flies, and fruit flies. During epidemics or times of gross pollution with human excreta of food and water, they are often responsible for transmitting typhoid and other salmonella infections, shigellosis, cholera, and amebiasis. Evidence is less conclusive that they play a conspicuous role in the spread of poliomyelitis and epidemic conjunctivitis. Cockroaches may also transmit enteric organisms to food.

Essential Transmitters. Arthropods that are biologic vectors of pathogens include (1) ticks (spotted fever, Q fever, Colorado tick fever, hemorrhagic fever, Lyme disease (Sec. 10.76), babesiosis, relapsing fever, and tularemia); (2) red mites (scrub typhus) and rat and mouse mites (murine typhus and rickettsial pox); (3) lice (epidemic typhus, trench fever, and relapsing fever); (4) fleas (plague, murine typhus, and several other infections); (5) mosquitoes (malaria, yellow fever, dengue, a number of viral encephalitides, filariasis, and tularemia); (6) sandflies (kala-azar, cutaneous and mucocutaneous leishmaniasis, Oroya fever, and pappataci fever); (7) *Glossina* (tsetse) flies (African trypanosomiasis); (8) black gnats (onchocerciasis); and (9) assassin bugs (Chagas' disease).

Children are particularly susceptible to these diseases. In some instances vaccine is protective, as in yellow fever, Rocky Mountain spotted fever, and typhus fever. In some, individual prophylaxis consists of avoiding endemic territory or using repellents or screens against the vectors. In certain diseases the only practical safeguard consists of dusting the exposed person's clothing with malathion or lindane, as in louse-borne typhus fever, or using these or other insecticides as residual sprays, as in areas of rodent plague. Another method of attack is the destruction of the reservoir host (rats in the case of plague and murine typhus). Vector arthropods constitute one of mankind's most serious challenges.

ALBERT MILLER

Baker EW, et al: A Manual of Parasitic Mites. New York, National Pest Control Association, 1956.
Blattner RJ: Necrotic arachnidism. J Pediatr 53:377, 1958.
DeBusk FL, O'Connor S: Tick toxicosis. Pediatrics 50:328, 1972.
Frazier CA: Diagnosis and treatment of insect bites. Clin Symp (Ciba) 20:75, 1968.
Frazier CA: Insect Allergy: Allergic and Toxic Reactions to Insects and Other Arthropods. St. Louis, WH Green, 1969.
Goldman L, Sawyer F, Levine A, et al: Investigative studies of skin irritation from caterpillars. J Invest Dermatol 34:67, 1960.

Haller JS, Fabara JA: Tick paralysis. Case report with emphasis on neurological toxicity. Am J Dis Child 124:915, 1972.

Harwood RF, James MT: Entomology in Human and Animal Health. 7th Ed. New York, Macmillan, 1979.

Horen WP: Insect and scorpion stings. JAMA 221:894, 1972.

James JA, Sellars WA, Austin OM, et al: Reactions following suspected spider bite. Am J Dis Child 102:395, 1961.

James MT: The Flies That Cause Myiasis in Man. Washington DC, US Department of Agriculture. Misc Publ No 631, 1947.

Maretic Z, Stanic M: The health problem of arachnidism. Bull WHO 11:1007, 1954.

O'Rourke FJ: The toxicity of black widow spider venom. In: Venoms. Washington DC, American Association for the Advancement of Science. Publ 44, 1956.

Reed HB Jr, Hackman RH, Fesmire FM: Variation in severity of loxoscelism. J Tenn Med Assoc 61:1097, 1968.

Ruebush TK, Juranek DD, Spielman A, et al: Epidemiology of human babesiosis on Nantucket Island. Am J Trop Med Hyg 30:937, 1981.

Schulze TL, Bowen GS, Bosler EM, et al: Amblyomma americanum: a potential vector of Lyme disease in New Jersey. Science 224:601, 1984.

Vorse H, Seccareccio P, Woodruff K, et al: Disseminated intravascular coagulopathy following fatal brown spider bite (necrotic arachnidism). J Pediatr 80:1035, 1972.

Wand M: Necrotic arachnidism: A new entity in the Northwest. Northwest Med 71:292, 1972.

12

THE DIGESTIVE SYSTEM

THE ORAL CAVITY

The condition of the oral cavity is important to the physical and psychologic health and sense of well-being of every child. Timely diagnosis and treatment require close cooperation between physicians and dentists. Many older children have regular dental examinations, but the oral problems of infants that require dental referral are recognized primarily through routine visits to physicians.

All children should receive a dental examination by 2 yr of age; an examination when a child's first teeth erupt is ideal. This provides an excellent opportunity to discuss dental disease when parental interest is high, to counsel about avoiding harmful practices, and to initiate measures to prevent dental caries (Sec. 12.6).

12.1 DEVELOPMENT OF THE TEETH

Initiation. The primary teeth form in dental crypts that arise from a band of epithelial cells incorporated into each developing jaw. By the 12th wk of fetal life each of these epithelial bands (the dental laminae) has five areas of rapid growth on each side of the maxilla and the mandible, seen as rounded, bud-like enlargements. Organization of adjacent mesenchyme takes place in each area of epithelial growth, and the two elements together are the beginning of a tooth.

The permanent teeth form in two groups. After the formation of the primary crypts another generation of tooth buds forms lingually from each side for the permanent incisors, cuspids, and premolars, which will erupt into sites previously occupied by primary teeth. This process takes place from about the 5th gestational mo for the central incisors to about 10 mo of age for the second bicuspids. Permanent molars, on the other hand, arise from extension of the dental laminae backward, beyond the site of the second primary molars. Bud-like enlargements form for the first, second, and third permanent molars at approximately 4 mo of gestation, 1 yr of age, and 4–5 yr of age, respectively.

Histodifferentiation-Morphodifferentiation. As the epithelial bud proliferates, the deeper surface invaginates, and a mass of mesenchyme becomes partially enclosed. Beginning with the crown, the epithelial cells assume the shape of the tooth they represent, and lay down the organic matrix for calcification of dentin. The vascular, nerve, and lymph structures (the dental pulp of the mature tooth) are confined in the mesenchyme of the hollow central portion of the tooth bud.

Calcification. The deposition of the inorganic mineral crystals of mature enamel and dentin takes place after the organic matrix has been laid down, from several sites of calcification that later coalesce. The characteristics of the inorganic portions of a tooth can be altered by (1) disturbances in formation of the matrix, (2) decreased availability of one or more of the minerals involved, or (3) the incorporation of foreign materials. Such disturbances may affect the color, texture, or thickness of the tooth surface.

Eruption. At the time of tooth bud formation, each tooth begins a continuous movement outward in relation to the

bone. The times of eruption of the human permanent teeth and the times of eruption and shedding of the primary teeth are listed in Table 2–10. The mandibular teeth usually erupt before the maxillary teeth, and those of girls generally earlier than those of boys.

12.2 ANOMALIES ASSOCIATED WITH TOOTH DEVELOPMENT

Both failures and excesses of tooth initiation are observed. *Anodontia*, or absence of teeth, occurs when no tooth buds form. Total anodontia often occurs with ectodermal dysplasia. Partial anodontia results from disturbance of a normal site of initiation (eg, the area of a palatal cleft), or from genetic failure (frequently familial) to code the formation of specific teeth. The third molars, maxillary lateral incisors, and mandibular second premolars are the teeth that most commonly fail to form. If the dental lamina produces more than the normal number of buds, *supernumerary teeth* occur, most often in the area of the maxillary central incisors. Since they tend to disrupt the position and eruption of the adjacent normal teeth, their identification as supernumerary teeth by roentgenographic examination is important. *Natal teeth* must be differentiated from supernumerary teeth (see below).

Disturbances during differentiation may result in gross alterations in dental morphology, such as *macrodontia* (large teeth) or *microdontia* (small teeth). The maxillary lateral incisors may assume a slender, tapering shape ("peg-shaped laterals").

Twinning, in which two teeth are joined together, is most often observed in the mandibular incisors of the primary dentition. It may result from gemination, fusion, or concrescence. Gemination is the result of division of one tooth germ to form a bifid or cloven crown on a single root with a common pulp canal; an extra tooth is then present in the dental arch. Fusion is the joining of incompletely developed teeth that, owing to pressure or trauma or crowding, continue to develop as one tooth. Fused teeth are sometimes joined through their entire length; in other instances a single wide crown is supported on two roots. Concrescence is the attachment of the roots of closely approximated adjacent teeth by an excessive deposit of cementum. This type of twinning, unlike the others, is found most often in the maxillary molar region.

Dens in dente (a "tooth in a tooth") is a roentgenographic finding in which the outline of a second dental structure is seen within a tooth of normal outward appearance. It results from an invagination in the lingual surface usually of a maxillary incisor, at the site of fusion between separate sites of calcification in the same tooth; an enamel-lined hollow space results.

Amelogenesis imperfecta, a dominant genetic trait, results in faulty production of the organic matrix. The teeth are covered by only a thin layer of abnormally formed enamel through which the yellow underlying dentin is seen, giving a darkened appearance to the dentition. Usually both primary and permanent teeth are affected. Susceptibility to caries is low, but the enamel is subject to destruction from abrasion. Complete coverage of the crown may be indicated for dentin protection and improved appearance.

Dentinogenesis imperfecta, or hereditary opalescent dentin, is an analogous condition in which the odontoblasts fail to differentiate normally and poorly calcified dentin results. The junction between the enamel and dentin is altered, the enamel has a tendency to flake away, and the exposed dentin is then susceptible to abrasion. The teeth are opaque and pearly, and the pulp chambers are obliterated by calcification. Both primary and permanent teeth are usually involved. Unless the crowns of these teeth are covered early and completely, the abrasion of chewing often reduces them to the level and contour of the supporting alveolar bone.

Localized disturbances of calcification that correlate with periods of illness or malnutrition are common and analogous to the growth disturbance lines often seen in roentgenograms of long bones. An example is the neonatal line commonly observed on the primary teeth and on the permanent central incisors and tips of cuspids at coronal levels consistent with the stage of calcification at birth. Two general disturbances of the surface of the enamel are also seen. Discoloration of the smooth surface, usually a more opaque white patch, is referred to as *hypocalcification.* A more severe disturbance, *hypoplasia,* may be manifest as pitting or as areas devoid of covering enamel. Hypoplasia is uncommon in the primary dentition because intrauterine stress is relatively infrequent compared with the frequent occurrence of illness during early infancy when the enamel of the outer third of the permanent incisors, cuspids, and first molars is forming. Dental restoration of such areas is desirable to eliminate the sensitivity of exposed dentin, to prevent caries, and to improve the appearance.

Mottled enamel is found in persons whose early life is spent in areas where the fluoride content of the drinking water is greater than 2.0 parts per million (ppm) and is probably due to ameloblastic dysfunction. It varies from small inconspicuous white patches to severe, brownish discoloration and hypoplasia; the latter changes are usually seen with fluoride concentrations of greater than 5 ppm.

Disturbances due to *mineral deficiency* are rare, but irregular dentin and enlarged pulp chambers have been observed with vitamin D resistant rickets, and hypoplasia has been observed with vitamin D deficient rickets.

Discolored teeth may result from incorporation of foreign substances into developing enamel. Neonatal *hyperbilirubinemia* may produce blue to black discoloration of the primary teeth, beginning at the neonatal line; the tips of the permanent first molars may also be affected. All *tetracyclines* are extensively incorporated into bones and teeth and, if administered during the period of formation of enamel, may result in brownish-yellow discoloration and hypoplasia of the enamel. Such teeth fluoresce under ultraviolet light. The period at risk extends from about the 4th mo of gestation to the 10th mo of life for primary teeth, and from about the 4th mo to the 16th yr of life for permanent teeth. Enamel is completely formed on all but the third molars by about 8 yr of age; accordingly, tetracyclines should not be prescribed for pregnant women or for children under 8 yr of age.

As the teeth penetrate the gums, inflammation and sensitivity sometimes occur *(teething).* The child may become irritable, and salivation may increase markedly. A blunt, firm object for the infant to bite usually provides some relief; incision of the gums is seldom indicated. There is no evidence that such systemic disturbances as low grade fever, facial rashes, or mild diarrhea can result from teething.

Delayed eruption of all teeth may indicate systemic or nutritional disturbances such as hypopituitarism, hypothyroidism, cleidocranial dysostosis, and rickets. Failure of eruption of single or small groups of teeth may stem from local causes such as malpositioning of teeth, supernumerary teeth, cysts, or retained primary teeth. Premature loss of primary predecessors is the most common cause of premature eruption of teeth. If the entire dentition is advanced for age and sex, an endocrine disorder should be considered.

Natal teeth are observed in approximately 1:2000 newborn infants; usually there are two in the position of the mandibular central incisors. Their attachment is generally limited to the gingival margin, with little root formation or bony support; such teeth should not be considered supernumerary until so identified roentgenographically. A natal tooth may be a prematurely erupted primary tooth, in which case early dental eruption may be expected.

Natal teeth may result in pain secondary to looseness and movement, and may produce maternal discomfort due to abrasion or biting of the nipple during nursing. There is danger of detachment with aspiration of the tooth. Since the tongue lies between the alveolar processes during birth, it may become lacerated, and occasionally the tip is amputated (Riga-Fede disease). Decisions regarding extraction of prematurely erupted primary teeth must be made on an individual basis; extraction requires careful dissection of the gingival attachment to prevent tearing of the tissue and excessive hemorrhage.

Exfoliation failure occurs when a primary tooth is not shed prior to the eruption of its permanent successor. The primary tooth should be extracted if the erupting permanent tooth becomes visible. This occurs most commonly in the mandibular incisor region.

12.3 DISORDERS OF THE TEETH ASSOCIATED WITH OTHER CONDITIONS

Osteogenesis imperfecta is usually accompanied by hereditary opalescent dentin, also termed "dentinogenesis imperfecta" (Sec. 12.2). Treatment usually involves covering the crowns.

In *cleidocranial dysostosis* orofacial variations include frontal bossing, mandibular prognathism, and a broadened base of the nose. Eruption of teeth is usually delayed. The primary teeth are abnormally retained, and the permanent teeth may remain unerupted. Supernumerary teeth are common, especially in the premolar area. Erupted teeth are free of hypoplasia, but variations in size and shape are common. The primary teeth and those permanent teeth which do erupt should be restored if they become carious. Patients with this disorder need extensive dental therapy in order to maintain efficient chewing.

In *ectodermal dysplasia* (Sec. 24.6) the teeth are totally or partially absent. Since alveolar bone does not develop in the absence of teeth, the alveolar processes are usually either totally or partially absent, and the resulting overclosure of the mandible causes the lips to protrude. Facial development is otherwise not disturbed. Teeth, when present, are small and conical in form. Aplasia of the buccal and labial mucous glands, leading to dryness and irritation of the oral mucosa, has also been observed. Persons with ectodermal dysplasia need either partial or full dentures. The vertical height between the jaws is thus restored, improving the position of the lips and facial contours. Masticatory function is restored, and eating habits are thereby improved.

Congenital syphilis affects differentiation of permanent teeth, resulting in screwdriver-shaped incisors, often with central notches in their incisive edges (Hutchinson incisors), and mulberry molars, with lobular occlusal surfaces and narrow, pinched crowns (Sec. 11.49).

12.4 MALOCCLUSION

The oral cavity can be viewed as a masticatory machine. The incisal edges of the anterior teeth are brought into opposition by mandibular closure for the purpose of biting off portions of large food items. The cusps of the opposing posterior teeth interdigitate and slide across each other to reduce foodstuffs to a soft, moist bolus. The cheeks and tongue force the food onto the areas of tooth contact.

The masseter and temporal muscles are the main forces of mandibular closure. Acting in conjunction with the internal pterygoid muscles, they produce high pressures of contact on opposing teeth. If a number of teeth meet simultaneously, the force is distributed over a large area of bone-to-tooth attachment. In malocclusion, when only a few teeth touch, the same force is exerted over a much smaller area. In adulthood, occlusal deformities are a leading cause of loss of teeth. Accordingly, preventive measures in childhood should be directed at establishing proper relationships between upper and lower dental arches for physiologic as well as cosmetic reasons.

Variations in growth patterns are classified into three main types of occlusion (Fig. 12–1). The occlusal relation is determined by observing the positions of the teeth when the jaws are closed and the heads of the mandibular condyles are in the most posterior position within the glenoid fossa. In class I (normal) the cusps of the posterior mandibular teeth interdigitate ahead of and inside the corresponding cusps of the opposing maxillary teeth. This relationship provides a normal facial profile. In class II the cusps of the posterior mandibular teeth are behind and inside the corresponding cusps of the maxillary teeth. This is the most common occlusal discrepancy; about 45% of the population exhibits some degree of this condition. An increased space between upper and lower anterior teeth encourages sucking and tongue-thrust habits. The appearance of a receding chin accompanies the retrognathia. In class III the cusps of the posterior mandibular teeth interdigitate a tooth or more ahead of their opposing maxillary counterparts. The anterior teeth are directly opposed, or the mandibular incisors protrude beyond the maxillary; a protruding chin accompanies prognathia.

Cross Bite. Normally the mandibular teeth are in a position just inside the maxillary teeth, so that the outside mandibular cusps or incisal edges meet the central portion of the opposing maxillary teeth. A reversal of this relation is referred to as a "cross bite."

Open and Closed Bites. If the posterior mandibular and maxillary teeth contact each other but the anterior ones are still apart, the situation is termed an "open bite." With the posterior teeth together, if the mandibular anterior teeth occlude inside the maxillary anterior teeth in an overclosed position, the situation is referred to as a "closed bite." Treatment consists of orthodontic correction; a few cases require orthognathic surgery. Optimal timing of treatment varies; earlier treatment generally allows some redirection of the growth pattern. Prognosis with early treatment is good except in severe cases.

Thumb Sucking. Various and conflicting theories have explained thumb sucking in children, and there are conflicting recommendations for its correction. Prolonged thumb sucking can cause flaring of the maxillary incisor teeth. More than half of children have had a thumb-sucking habit at some time. The prevalence of thumb sucking decreases steadily from the age of 2 yr to approximately 10% by the age of 5.

The likelihood of long-term effect on the developing dentition and face is controversial. Prognosis is good in children with procumbent incisors and acceptable occlusion of the molar and canine teeth; discontinuation of the habit will usually result in lessening of the incisor procumbency, with the possibility of an acceptable occlusion. Prognosis is mixed in children with procumbent incisors and a malrelationship of jaws or of posterior teeth; discontinuation of the habit will lessen the procumbency of the incisors but will not rectify an already deviant growth pattern. Prognosis worsens with continuation of the habit beyond the age of 6 yr. A variety of treatment protocols have been suggested. A common measure is the insertion of an appliance with modest extensions that serve as a reminder when the child attempts to insert the thumb. Greatest likelihood of success occurs in cases in which the child desires to stop.

12.5 DEVELOPMENTAL ABNORMALITIES WITH MULTIPLE DENTAL AND ORAL PROBLEMS

CLEFT LIP AND PALATE

Clefts of the lip and palate are distinct entities closely related embryologically, functionally, and genetically. Cleft of the lip appears to be due to hypoplasia of the mesenchymal layer, resulting in a failure of the medial nasal and maxillary processes to join. Cleft of the palate appears to represent failure of the palatal shelves to approximate or fuse.

Incidence and Epidemiology. The incidence of cleft lip with or without cleft palate is about 1:1000 births; the incidence of cleft palate alone is about 1:2500 births. The former is more common in males. Genetic factors are of more importance in cleft lip with or without cleft palate than in cleft palate alone.

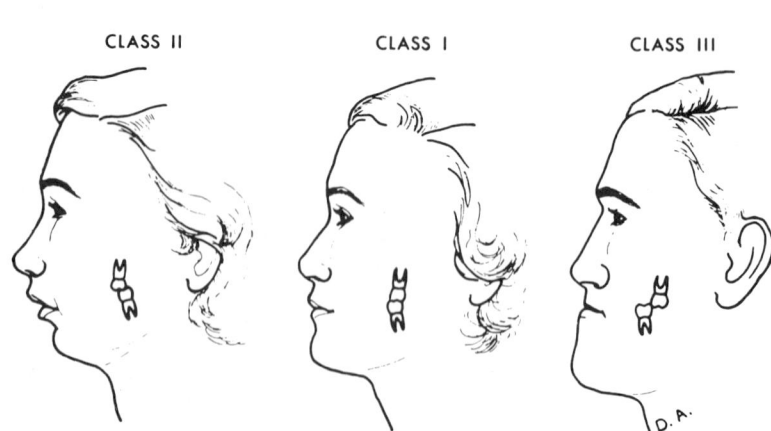

Figure 12–1. Angle classification of occlusion. The typical correspondence between the profile and molar relationship is shown. (From Moyers RE: Handbook of Orthodontics. 2nd ed. Chicago, Year Book Medical Publishers, 1963.)

The incidence of associated congenital malformations and of intellectual impairment are increased in children with cleft defects, especially in those with cleft palate alone. These findings are partially explained by an increased incidence of hearing impairment in children with cleft palate and by the frequency of cleft defects among children with chromosomal abnormalities. The risks of recurrence of cleft defects within families are discussed in Chapter 6.

Animal studies suggest that nongenetic influences may be responsible for clefts in a susceptible host at a critical period of organogenesis. Associated malformations are especially frequent in structures derived from the first branchial arch.

Clinical Manifestations. Cleft lip may vary from a small notch in the vermilion border to a complete separation extending into the floor of the nose. Clefts may be unilateral (more often on the left side) or bilateral and usually involve the alveolar ridge. Deformed, supernumerary, or absent teeth are associated. The nasal alar cartilage clefts of the lip are frequently associated with deficiency of the columella and elongation of the vomer, producing a protrusion of the anterior aspect of the cleft premaxillary process.

Isolated cleft palate occurs in the midline and may involve only the uvula or may extend into or through the soft and hard palates to the incisive foramen. When associated with cleft lip, the defect may involve the midline of the soft palate and extend into the hard palate on one or both sides, exposing one or both of the nasal cavities as a unilateral or bilateral cleft palate.

Treatment. The most immediate problem is feeding; a plastic obturator is fitted soon after birth to aid in control of fluids, provide a reference plane for suction, and provide stability for the lateral arch segments. Rapid growth of the dental arches requires the obturator to be refitted every few wk.

Surgical closure of a cleft lip is usually performed at 1–2 mo of age, when the infant has shown satisfactory weight gain and is free of any oral, respiratory, or systemic infection. Z-plasty is the most commonly used technique; a staggered suture line minimizes notching of the lip from retraction of scar tissue. A Logan clamp (a wire bow attached by adhesive to the cheeks) is applied immediately after the operation to take tension off the suture line. The initial repair may be revised at 4–5 yr of age. In many instances, corrective surgery on the nose is delayed until adolescence. Some surgeons will perform preliminary nasal surgery at the time of the lip repair. Cosmetic results depend on the extent of the original deformity, absence of infection, and skill of the surgeon.

Since clefts of the palate vary considerably in size, shape, and degree of deformity, the timing of surgical correction should be individualized. Criteria such as width of the cleft, adequacy of the existing palatal segments, the morphology of the surrounding areas (such as width of the oropharynx), and the neuromuscular function of the soft palate and pharyngeal walls affect the decision. The goals of surgery are the union of the cleft segments, intelligible and pleasant speech, reduction of nasal regurgitation, and avoidance of injury to the growing maxilla. In an otherwise healthy child, closure of the palate is usually done prior to 1 yr of age to enhance normal speech development. When surgical correction is delayed beyond the 3rd yr, a contoured speech bulb can be attached to the posterior of a maxillary denture so that contraction of the pharyngeal and velopharyngeal muscles can bring tissues into contact with the bulb to accomplish occlusion of the nasopharynx and help the child develop intelligible speech. Almost always the cleft crosses the alveolar ridge and interferes with the formation of teeth in the area. The missing elements of the dentition must be replaced by prosthetic devices; alterations of the positions of teeth may also be necessary.

Preoperative and Postoperative Management. Even the suspicion of infection is a contraindiction to operation. If the child is in good nutritional condition and in fluid and electrolyte balance, feeding may be permitted to within 6 hr of the operation (Sec. 5.31). During the immediate postoperative period special nursing care is essential. Gentle aspiration of the nasopharynx minimizes the chances of the common complications of atelectasis or pneumonia. The primary considerations in postoperative care are maintenance of a clean suture line and avoidance of strain on the sutures. For these reasons the infant is fed with a medicine dropper and the arms are restrained with elbow cuffs. A fluid or semifluid diet is maintained for 3 wk, and feeding is done with a dropper or spoon. The patient's hands as well as toys and other foreign bodies must be kept away from the palate.

Complications. Recurrent otitis media and hearing loss are frequent. Excessive dental decay is not unusual. Displacement of the maxillary arches and malpositions of the teeth usually require orthodontic correction.

Speech defects may be present or persist even after good anatomic closure of the palate. Such speech is characterized by emission of air from the nose and by a hypernasal quality when certain sounds are made. Both before and, at times, after palatal surgery, the speech defect is due to inadequacies in function of the palatal and pharyngeal muscles. The muscles of the soft palate and the lateral and posterior walls of the nasopharynx constitute a valve that separates the nasopharynx from the oropharynx during swallowing and in the production of certain sounds. If the valve does not function adequately, it is difficult to build up enough pressure in the mouth to make such explosive sounds as p, b, d, t, h, y, or the sibilants s, sh, and ch, and such words as "cats," "boats," and "sisters" are not intelligible. After operation or the insertion of a speech appliance, speech therapy may be necessary.

A complete program of habilitation for the child with a cleft lip or palate may require years of special treatment by a team consisting of pediatrician, plastic surgeon, otolaryngologist, pedodontist, prosthodontist, orthodontist, speech therapist, medical social worker, psychologist, child psychiatrist, and public health nurse. Ideally, the child's physician should be responsible for coordination of the use of specialists, and for parental counseling and guidance.

PALATOPHARYNGEAL INCOMPETENCE

The speech disturbance characteristic of the child with a cleft palate can also be produced by other osseous or neuromuscular abnormalities when there is an inability to form an effective seal between oropharynx and nasopharynx during swallowing or phonation. The abnormality may be in the structures of the palate or pharynx or in the muscles attached to these structures. In a child who has previously spoken normally, adenoidectomy may precipitate the speech defect when a submucous cleft palate has not been recognized. In such cases, the adenoid mass may have facilitated a seal when the elevated soft palate made contact with it, this becoming impossible after removal of the adenoids. If there is sufficient reserve neuromuscular function, compensation in palatopharyngeal movement may take place and the speech defect disappear, although often some symptoms of palatopharyngeal incompetence may persist. In other instances slow involution of the adenoids may allow for gradual compensation in palatal and pharyngeal muscular function. This may explain why a speech defect does not become apparent in some children who have a submucous cleft palate or similar anomaly predisposing to palatopharyngeal incompetence.

Clinical Manifestations. The symptoms of palatopharyngeal incompetence are similar to those of a cleft palate, although clinical signs vary. There may be hypernasal speech (especially noted in the articulation of pressure consonants such as p, b, d, t, h, v, f, and s); conspicuous constricting movement of the nares during speech; inability to whistle, gargle, blow out a candle, or inflate a balloon; loss of liquid through the nose when drinking with the head down; and otitis media and hearing loss. Oral inspection may reveal a cleft palate or a relatively short palate with a large oropharynx; absent, grossly asymmetric, or minimal muscular activity of the soft palate and pharynx during phonation or gagging; or a submucous cleft. The latter is suggested by a bifid uvula, by a translucent membrane in the midline of the soft palate (revealing lack of continuity of muscles), by palpable notching in the posterior border of the hard palate instead of a posterior nasal spinous process, or by forward or V-shaped displacement or grooving on the soft palate during phonation or gagging.

Palatopharyngeal incompetence may also be demonstrated roentgenographically. The head should be carefully positioned to obtain a true lateral view; one film is obtained with the patient at rest and another during continuous phonation of the vowel "u" as in "boom." The soft palate contacts the posterior pharyngeal wall in normal function, whereas in palatopharyngeal incompetence such contact is absent.

Treatment. In selected cases the palate may be repositioned or pharyngoplasty performed utilizing a flap of tissue from the posterior pharyngeal wall. Dental speech appliances have also been used successfully.

PIERRE ROBIN SYNDROME

This abnormality consists of micrognathia with glossoptosis (and pseudomacroglossia) and high arched or cleft palate. Posterior displacement of the attachment of the genioglossus muscle to the hypoplastic mandible prevents the normal anchorage of the tongue; in the supine child, under the influence of gravity, the tongue falls back, obstructing the pharynx. A postalveolar cleft of the hard and soft palates is a common but not constant feature, and in some instances the palate is high-arched.

The tongue is usually of normal size, but the floor of the mouth is foreshortened and the buccal cavity reduced in size. Obstruction of the air passages may occur, particularly on inspiration, and usually requires treatment to prevent suffocation. The infant should be maintained prone or partially prone so that the tongue falls forward to relieve respiratory obstruction. Temporary suturing of the ventral surface of the tongue to the lower lip is usually not necessary; nor is tracheostomy, since sufficient mandibular growth generally takes place within a few mo to relieve the glossoptosis. Use of splints and traction devices to pull the mandible forward has been unsuccessful. The feeding of infants with mandibular hypoplasia requires great care and patience but can usually be accomplished without resort to gavage. Often the growth of the mandible will achieve an essentially normal profile within 4–6 yr. Dental anomalies usually require individualized treatment.

MANDIBULOFACIAL DYSOSTOSIS
(Treacher Collins or Franceschetti Syndrome)

In this syndrome, the facial appearance is characterized by palpebral fissures sloping downward toward the outer canthi, colobomas of the lower eyelids, sunken cheekbones, blind fistulas opening between the angles of the mouth and the ears, deformed pinnas, atypical hair growth extending toward the cheeks, receding chin, and large mouth. Facial clefts, abnormalities of the ears, and deafness are common. The disorder is autosomal dominant, often with incomplete expression. The mandible is almost always hypoplastic; the undersurface is often pronouncedly concave, the ramus may be deficient, and the coronoid and condyloid processes are flat or even aplastic. The palatal vault may be either high or cleft. Infrequently, unilateral or bilateral macrostomia, or failure of embryonic fusion of the maxillary and mandibular processes, may occur. Dental malocclusions are frequent, owing to poor maxillary development and palatal deformity. The teeth may be widely separated, hypoplastic, or displaced or have an open bite. Orthodontic and routine dental treatments are indicated.

Unilateral hypoplasia of the mandible is sometimes part of a syndrome that includes partial paralysis of the facial nerve, macrostomia, blind fistulas between the angles of the mouth and the ears, and deformed ear lobes. Severe facial asymmetry and malocclusion develop because of the absence or hypoplasia of the mandibular condyle on the affected side. Congenital condylar deformity tends to increase with age. Early plastic surgery may be indicated to minimize the deformity.

Facial asymmetries resulting from excessive molding of the cranium or from displacement of the mandible during breech or face presentations are common and are usually self-correcting. Facial asymmetry due to injury of the growing cartilage or fracture of the condylar head during birth, infancy, or early childhood may be permanent. Traumatic injuries may occur during birth from obstetric forceps placed over the area or may result from blows on the chin during infancy and childhood.

Injuries, acute infections, or arthritis of the growing condylar cartilage may result in partial (fibrous) or complete (bony) ***ankylosis of the temporomandibular joint*** and failure of that side of the mandible to grow. The normal side, meanwhile, continues to grow and pushes the midline toward the affected side. The midline deviation is exaggerated during mouth opening. Roentgenograms of the affected side reveal an increased preangular notch or displaced condylar head. Bilateral injuries to the growing cartilage result in failure of the mandible and chin to grow downward and forward, causing the entire mandible to be retruded and smaller than normal.

12.6 DENTAL CARIES

Almost everyone in this country experiences dental caries to some degree, mostly during childhood and adolescence.

Etiology. The development of dental caries is dependent on critical inter-relationships between the tooth surface, dietary carbohydrates, and specific oral bacteria. The decay process is initiated by demineralization of the outer tooth surface, owing to formation of organic acids during bacterial fermentation of dietary carbohydrates. Incipient lesions first appear as opaque white spots; with progressive loss of tooth tissue, cavitation occurs.

An important experimental observation within the past two decades has been that dental caries has microbial specificity; that is, cariogenic potential resides in a group of oral streptococci collectively designated as *Streptococcus mutans*. Current knowledge indicates that these organisms initiate most dental caries of enamel surfaces. Once the enamel surface cavitates, other oral bacteria (in particular, the lactobacilli) invade the underlying dentin and cause further destruction of tooth structure through a mixed bacterial infection. An important approach toward prevention of dental caries would be to reduce or eliminate intraoral levels of *S. mutans*. Epidemiologic, chemotherapeutic, and immunologic approaches are currently under intense investigation.

A second important aspect of the etiology of dental caries relates to *frequency* of carbohydrate consumption. Frequency of ingestion is a more important determinant of development of dental caries than is the actual quantity of carbohydrate consumed. For example, cariogenic potential of a nursing bottle of apple juice that is sampled throughout the night or at nap times, or both, is quite different from that of the same volume of apple juice consumed at a single meal. Carbohydrates contained in food products retained orally for a long time may be more cariogenic than those in food products retained for short times (e.g., the sucrose in chewing gum is more cariogenic than the sucrose in cola beverages, as conventionally consumed).

Epidemiology. Dental caries is virtually ubiquitous. Recent investigations regarding its prevalence in the civilized world indicate that its severity has decreased markedly during the past two decades. This decrease is thought to be secondary to advances in prevention.

Clinical Manifestations. Dental caries usually begins in the pits and fissures of the occlusal (biting) surfaces of the molar teeth. Lesions of short duration cannot be diagnosed by inspection; they are usually detected by probing the affected pit or fissure. In contrast, pit and fissure caries of long duration can usually be detected by inspection, and usually present extensive cavitation of the occlusal surface. The second most frequent sites of caries are contact surfaces between the teeth. These areas are difficult to examine, even for the dentist, who usually depends on intraoral radiographs. Caries lesions are least frequently detected in the necks (cervical areas) of the teeth near the gingiva. Cervical decay is uncommon in children with mild to moderate caries but is usually present in instances of nursing bottle caries (Fig. 12–2).

Complications. Left untreated, dental caries will usually destroy most of the tooth and spread into contiguous tissues, causing pain and infection. Microbial invasion of the dental pulp (Fig. 12–3) precipitates an inflammatory response (pulpitis) that can elicit significant pain (toothache). Pulpitis can in turn progress to necrosis, with bacterial invasion of the alveolar bone (dental abscess; periapical abscess). This process may be quite painful and is associated with the complications of sepsis and facial cellulitis. Moreover, periapical infection of a primary tooth may disrupt normal development of the successor permanent tooth.

Treatment. Contemporary dental therapeutics can salvage the majority of severely carious teeth. When extraction is indicated, therapy must also address the problem that teeth surrounding the site of extraction will change their positions in the dental arch. This is of particular importance in the primary and mixed dentitions in order to prevent impaction or malposition of permanent successor teeth.

Clinical management of the pain and infection associated with untreated dental caries varies with the extent of involve-

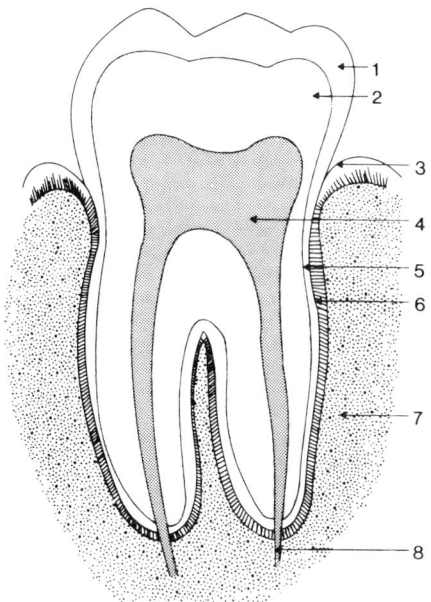

Figure 12–3. Basic dental anatomy: 1, enamel; 2, dentin; 3, gingival margin; 4, pulp; 5, cementum; 6, periodontal ligament; 7, alveolar bone; 8, neurovascular bundle.

ment and the medical status of the patient. In general, dental infection localized to the dentoalveolar unit can be managed by local measures (e.g., extraction, pulpectomy). Antibiotics are usually not indicated except in those patients with compromised host defenses, impaired wound healing, or risk for endocarditis. In contrast, antibiotics are routinely indicated for dental infections which have spread to structures outside the dentoalveolar unit. The oral route can usually be used for patients with unremarkable medical histories if the infection does not involve a vital area (e.g., buccal space). Should, however, the infection involve a vital area (e.g., submandibular space, which can lead to Ludwig angina; facial triangle, which can lead to cavernous sinus thrombosis; or periorbital space, which can lead to orbital involvement), parenteral routes are indicated. Parenteral routes are also indicated for patients with compromised host defenses, with impaired wound healing, or those at risk for endocarditis. Blood cultures should be obtained prior to initiating parenteral antibiotic therapy. Areas of fluctuance should be incised and drained. Exudate should be submitted for culture and Gram stain. Penicillin is the antibiotic of choice, except in patients with a history of allergy to this agent; erythromycin, clindamycin, and vancomycin are suitable alternatives for such patients. Finally, the offending tooth must be identified and local treatment instituted to ensure resolution of the infection.

Measures for control of pain are adjusted to the need of the patient. Combinations of acetaminophen with codeine given orally are usually adequate.

Prevention

Fluoride. The most effective preventive measure against dental caries is fluoridation of communal water supplies to approximately 1.00 ppm. Children born and reared in fluoridated communities have a 50 to 65% reduction in incidence of tooth decay. In fluoride-deficient areas similar caries prevention benefits are obtained from dietary fluoride supplements. The dosage schedule endorsed by the American Dental Association and the American Academy of Pediatrics is listed in Table 12–1; as indicated, dosage is based on the patient's age and the fluoride content of the water supply. The fluoride level of a water supply can usually be obtained by calling the local water board. Should the patient use a private water supply, it may be necessary for the physician or dentist to

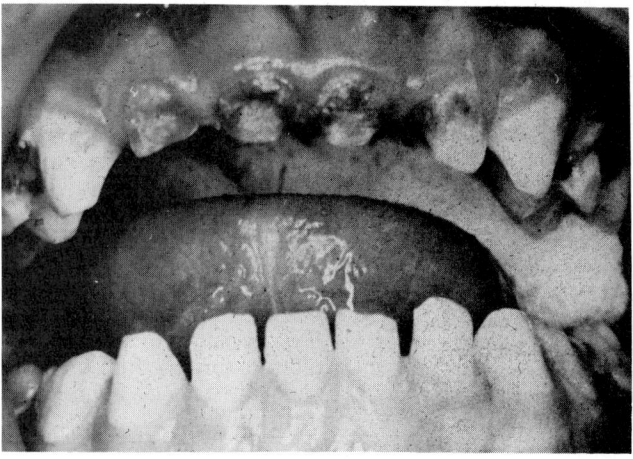

Figure 12–2. Nursing bottle caries.

Table 12–1. Recommended Daily Intake of Fluoride as Supplement to Normal Diet (mg F/day)

Age (yr)	Concentration of F (ppm) in water supply		
	0.0–0.3	0.3–0.7	>0.7
Birth to 2	0.25	0*	0*
2–3	0.50	0.25	0
3 and over	1.00	0.50	0

*0.25 mg for fully breast-fed infants.
Fluoride dosage regimen accepted by the American Academy of Pediatrics and the American Dental Association (1985).

facilitate a fluoride analysis. The patient's parents should be instructed to use a plastic container for the water specimen (a glass container may impair the accuracy of the fluoride assay). No fluoride prescription should be written for more than 120 mg of fluoride. This provides a daily supply of 1.0 mg fluoride for 4 mo. Even if a child ingested this entire supply, probably only mild gastric upset would ensue, which can be alleviated by an aluminum hydroxide preparation. Finally, the topical use of fluoride agents applied either professionally or by the patient are beneficial to children at high risk for caries (e.g., with xerostomia secondary to tumoricidal doses of head and neck radiation).

Oral Hygiene. Thorough daily brushing and flossing of the teeth helps to prevent dental caries and periodontal disease. Parents should receive professional instruction regarding oral hygiene techniques for children. Studies have shown that most children under 10 yr of age do not have the eye-hand coordination required for adequate oral hygiene; accordingly, parents should assume responsibility for brushing and flossing. The degree of parental involvement should be appropriate to the child's growing ability.

Diet. Decreasing the frequency of carbohydrate ingestion prevents dental caries. Parents and children should be encouraged to avoid between-meal snacks that contain carbohydrate. The use of gum, candy, and soft drinks containing sugar substitutes (mannitol, sorbitol, and aspartame [with precautions]) is an effective approach for the child with a "sweet tooth." In addition, infants should be weaned by 1 yr of age to avoid the problems of nursing bottle caries (see Fig. 12–2). Should this not be possible, bedtime and naptime nursing bottles should contain only water.

Sealants. Excellent oral hygiene and optimal fluoride therapy have minimal effect in preventing dental caries in the pits and fissures on the occlusal surfaces of the teeth. The use of sealants has been shown to be effective in the prevention of pit and fissure caries. Sealants are plastic coatings that are professionally applied to the occlusal surfaces of the posterior teeth.

Identification of High Risk Patients. Intact salivary gland function is the major host defense against dental caries. Without it, the patient is susceptible to rampant dental caries. Appropriate preventive therapy has been shown to minimize or eliminate development of dental caries in patients with Sjögren syndrome, Mikulicz disease, chronic graft-versus-host disease, and patients receiving long-term therapy with drugs that cause xerostomia.

12.7 PERIODONTAL DISEASES

The periodontium includes the gingiva, alveolar bone, and the periodontal ligament (see Fig. 12–3). Several distinct diseases of the periodontium occur during childhood and adolescence. These include gingivitis, acute necrotizing ulcerative gingivitis, herpetic gingivostomatitis, phenytoin-induced gingival overgrowth, juvenile periodontitis, and acute pericoronitis.

Gingivitis. Cessation of oral hygiene results in the accumulation of a dense bacterial mass (dental plaque) around the cervical areas of the teeth at the gingival margin (gum line). If not removed, this dental plaque will precipitate an inflammatory response of the gingiva, with reddening and swelling of the gingiva, spontaneous gingival hemorrhage, and fetor oris. These clinical signs may vary in severity. Such gingivitis may be localized or generalized; it is reversible when proper oral hygiene measures are instituted. Inability to resolve gingivitis by meticulous oral hygiene necessitates considering other problems in which gingivitis may be a presenting component (e.g., acute nonlymphocytic leukemia, diabetes mellitus, neutropenia, thrombocytopenia, scurvy, and hormonal changes associated with puberty and pregnancy).

Epidemiologic surveys indicate that over half of American school children will experience gingivitis. Gingivitis in healthy prepubertal children is much less likely to progress to periodontitis (resulting in loss of alveolar bone) than is gingivitis in adolescents and adults.

Acute Necrotizing Ulcerative Gingivitis (ANUG; Vincent infection; trench mouth). ANUG is a distinct periodontal disease prone to recurrence, the etiology of which is complex and not fully understood. The dramatic clinical response in its acute phase to penicillin indicates that bacteria are involved. The associated bacteriologic flora is composed of large numbers of oral spirochetes and fusobacteria; it is not clear, however, whether bacteria initiate the disease or are secondary invaders. ANUG develops primarily in young adults and adolescents. It rarely, if ever, develops in healthy children in developed countries. It occurs with surprising frequency, however, among children in southern India and certain African countries. Affected children usually have protein malnutrition. In these children, the lesion may not confine itself to the periodontium but may extend into adjacent tissues causing necrosis of facial structures (cancrum oris, or noma).

Clinical manifestations of ANUG include (1) necrosis and ulceration of erythematous gingiva, in particular the gingiva between the teeth; (2) an adherent grayish pseudomembrane over the affected gingiva; (3) fetor oris; (4) cervical lymphadenopathy; (5) malaise; and (6) fever. The disease is usually localized, the most common site being the periodontium associated with the mandibular incisor teeth. The condition may be mistaken for acute herpetic gingivostomatitis. ANUG is confined to the periodontium, however, and vesicle formation is not a feature. Dark field microscopy will demonstrate dense spirochete populations in smears of debris obtained from ANUG lesions.

Treatment of ANUG is divided into two phases. The acute phase is managed by antibiotic therapy (penicillin or erythromycin), local debridement, oxygenating agents (direct application of 10% carbamide peroxide in anhydrous glycerol four times a day), and analgesics. Dramatic resolution usually occurs within 48 hr. A second phase of treatment may be necessary if the acute phase of the disease has caused irreversible morphologic damage to the periodontium. Finally, current evidence indicates that this disease represents an endogenous rather than a communicable infection; accordingly, patients need not be managed as contagious.

Herpetic Gingivostomatitis (See Sec. 11.65). Phenytoin-Induced Gingival Overgrowth (PIGO, Dilantin Hyperplasia). The use of phenytoin in anticonvulsant therapy is associated with generalized enlargement of the gingiva. The etiology is complex, and not all factors are known. Current evidence indicates that phenytoin (diphenylhydantoin, DPH) and its metabolites are present in significant quantity in the gingiva of DPH-treated patients. DPH and its metabolites have a direct stimulatory action on gingival fibroblasts in vitro, resulting in accelerated synthesis of collagen. On the other hand, animal models and clinical studies indicate that PIGO does not complicate DPH therapy in most patients who maintain meticulous oral hygiene. This observation suggests that gingivitis plays a role in the pathogenesis of PIGO.

PIGO occurs in 10–30% of DPH-treated patients. Mild *manifestations* involve subtle gingival changes of no consequence to the patient. Severe manifestations may include (1) gross enlargement of the gingiva, sometimes to the point of covering the teeth; (2) edema and erythema of the gingiva; (3) secondary infection resulting in abscess formation; (4) migration of teeth; and (5) inhibition of exfoliation of primary teeth and subsequent impaction of permanent teeth. Severe PIGO may cause loss of optimal masticatory function and psychologic stress due to the cosmetic effects.

Treatment should be geared toward prevention. Ideally, the drug should be discontinued whenever possible. DPH-treated patients should receive regular dental follow-up. Meticulous oral hygiene prevents or minimizes PIGO in most instances. The severe form of PIGO is usually treated by gingivectomy; the lesion will recur, however, if excellent oral hygiene cannot be maintained.

Juvenile Periodontitis (JP). This rare disease is characterized by rapid alveolar bone loss and is associated with a flora composed of large numbers of *Capnocytophaga*, *Actinobacillus*, and *Bacteroides* species. Strains of *Actinobacillus* isolated from human lesions and inoculated into gnotobiotic rodents produced extensive alveolar bone loss in the experimental animals. In addition, the neutrophils of patients with JP have chemotactic and phagocytic defects; JP is associated with certain systemic diseases characterized by defects in neutrophil function (e.g., Down syndrome, diabetes mellitus, Chédiak-Higashi syndrome, and cyclic neutropenia). Collectively, these data suggest that JP occurs in patients who have impaired host defenses that facilitate colonization by highly periodontopathogenic flora.

JP is exceptionally rare in preschool children having only primary teeth. In older children it may be localized to the permanent incisors and 6-yr molars or may be generalized; the localized form may be associated with palmar and plantar hyperkeratosis (Papillon-Lefèvre syndrome). The gingiva is usually normal in appearance, but dental radiographs demonstrate alveolar bone loss. Affected teeth will demonstrate mobility, which varies with the severity of alveolar bone loss.

The rate of alveolar bone loss in JP is rapid. If left untreated, affected teeth will lose their attachment and exfoliate. Treatment approaches vary with the degree of involvement. Patients diagnosed at the onset of the disease are usually managed by local debridement, antibiotic therapy, and meticulous oral hygiene. Patients who have extensive alveolar bone loss at the time of initial diagnosis require extensive periodontal therapy that may include autologous osseous grafting. Prognosis depends on the degree of initial involvement and compliance with therapy.

Prevention of JP is not currently possible, but regular dental evaluations (one to two visits/yr) improve early detection and enhance the likelihood of favorable outcome. Patients with defects of neutrophil function should have such dental surveillance.

Acute Pericoronitis (AP). AP is an acute inflammation of the flap of gingiva that partially covers the crown of an incompletely erupted tooth. Mandibular third molars and less often second molars are common sites of AP. Accumulation of debris and bacteria between the gingival flap and tooth precipitates an inflammatory response. The flap of gingiva may become violently inflamed and edematous. Trismus and severe pain are common. Untreated cases may result in facial cellulitis and peritonsillar abscess, and fatalities have occurred in myelosuppressed patients.

Treatment of AP is in two phases. Treatment of the acute phase includes local debridement and irrigation, hot saline rinses, antibiotic therapy, and relief of the occlusion of the inflamed flap against the opposing jaw. When the acute phase has subsided, therapy is directed at preventing recurrences. This may include extraction of the tooth or resection of the gingival flap. Early recognition of the partial impaction of mandibular third molars and their subsequent extraction will prevent AP.

12.8 ORAL TRAUMA

Traumatic oral injuries may be conveniently categorized into three groups: (1) dental injuries; (2) soft tissue injuries (contusions, abrasions, lacerations, punctures, avulsions, burns); and (3) injuries to the body of the jaw bones (mandibular or maxillary fractures or both). This chapter will describe dental injuries. Basic texts of pediatric oral surgery offer complete reviews of the diagnosis and management of oral soft tissue injuries and facial fractures (see references).

DENTAL INJURIES

Approximately 10% of all young people between 18 mo–18 yr of age will sustain significant dental trauma. There appear to be three age periods of predilection: (1) preschool (1–3 yr), usually secondary to falls or child abuse; (2) school aged (7–10 yr), usually from bicycle and playground accidents; and (3) adolescents (16–18 yr), in whom dental trauma is generally secondary to fights, athletic injuries, and automobile accidents. Dental injuries are about twice as common among children with protrusion of teeth as among children with normal occlusion. Children with craniofacial abnormalities or neuromuscular deficits or both are also at increased risk for dental injury.

Dental trauma includes injuries to the hard dental tissues and pulp and injuries to the periodontal structure.

Injuries to Hard Dental Tissues and Pulp. Fractures of teeth are uncomplicated or complicated, in accordance with whether the fracture is confined to the hard dental tissues (uncomplicated) or extends through the pulp (complicated). Exposure of the pulp may result in its bacterial contamination, which can lead to infection and pulp necrosis. Pulp exposure complicates therapy and may lower the likelihood of a favorable outcome.

Traumatic blows to the mouth usually strike the maxillary incisor teeth, as they are the most anteriorly located. Fractures of the crowns and/or roots of these teeth are therefore common. Uncomplicated crown fractures are treated by covering exposed dentin and placing an esthetic restoration. Complicated crown fractures usually require endodontic (root canal) therapy. Crown-root fractures and root fractures usually require extensive dental therapy, which in the primary dentition may interfere with normal development of the permanent dentition; accordingly, these types of injury of the primary incisor teeth are usually managed by extraction of the fractured segments.

Oral injuries resulting in fractured teeth should be referred to a dentist as soon as possible. Furthermore, even when dentition appears intact following oral trauma, the patient should be evaluated soon by a dentist. The gathering of baseline data (radiographs; mobility patterns; responses to specific stimuli [percussion, electricity, hot, and cold]) enables the dentist to assess the likelihood of future complications. This may be especially important when the traumatic episode involves potential litigation.

Injuries to Periodontal Structures. These injuries usually present as mobile or displaced teeth or both. They account for approximately 20% of trauma to the permanent dentition and 70% of injuries to the primary dentition. Categories of trauma to the periodontium include (1) concussion, (2) subluxation, (3) intrusive luxation, (4) extrusive luxation, and (5) evulsion.

Concussion. Injuries that produce minor damage to the periodontal ligament are termed concussions. Teeth sustaining such injuries are without abnormal mobility or displacement but react markedly to percussion. This type of injury usually requires no therapy and resolves without complication. Primary incisors that sustain concussion may change color; this sign usually indicates pulpal degeneration and should be evaluated by a dentist as soon as possible.

Subluxation. This type of injury involves moderate damage to the periodontal ligament. Subluxated teeth exhibit mild to moderate horizontal mobility or vertical mobility or both. Hemorrhage is usually evident around the neck of the tooth at the gingival margin. There is no displacement of the tooth, so that a subluxated tooth retains its normal position in the dental arch. Many subluxated teeth need to be immobilized in order to ensure adequate repair of the periodontal ligament. Immobilization is facilitated by an acrylic splint. A few of these teeth will develop pulp necrosis; this type of injury should be referred to a dentist as soon as possible.

Intrusive Luxation. This type of injury is rare in the permanent dentition but is the most common injury to primary dentition. Intruded primary incisors may give the false appearance of being evulsed (Fig. 12–4). In order to rule out evulsion, an occlusal dental radiograph is indicated (Fig. 12–5). This type of injury should be referred to the dentist as soon as possible.

Extrusive Luxation. This type of injury is characterized by displacement of the tooth from its socket. The tooth is usually displaced to the lingual side, with fracture of the wall of the alveolar socket. These teeth need immediate treatment; the longer the delay, the more likely the tooth will consolidate in its ectopic position. Therapy is directed at reduction (repositioning the tooth) and fixation (acrylic splints). In addition, many such teeth become necrotic and require endodontic therapy. Extrusive luxation in the primary dentition is usually managed by extraction, since complications of reduction and fixation may result in problems with development of permanent teeth.

Evulsion. If evulsed permanent teeth are replanted within 30 min after injury, a greater than 90% success rate may be achieved; whereas if delay exceeds 2 hr, failure rate approaches 95%. The likelihood that normal reattachment will follow replantation is related to the viability of the periodontal ligament, and immediate therapy is directed at applying this principle. Parents confronted with this emergency situation can be instructed to:

1. *Find the tooth.*
2. *Rinse the tooth.* (Do *not* scrub the tooth. Do *not* touch the

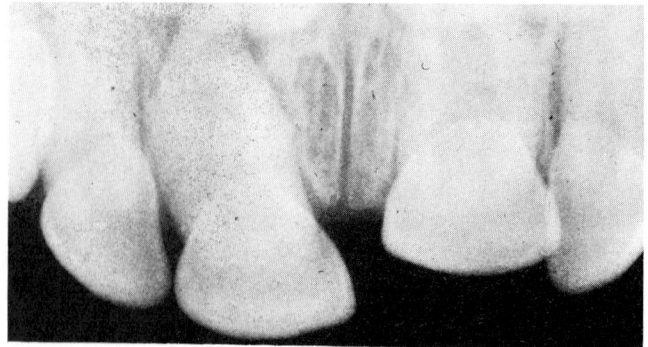

Figure 12–5. Occlusal radiograph documents intrusion of "missing tooth" presented in Figure 12–4.

root. After plugging the sink drain, hold the tooth by the crown and rinse it under running tap water.)

3. *Insert the tooth into the socket.* (Gently place it back into its normal position. Do not be concerned if the tooth extrudes slightly. If the parent or child is too apprehensive for replantation of the tooth, the tooth should be placed in cow's milk. Milk is the best transport medium to maintain periodontal ligament viability.)

4. *Go directly to the dentist.* (In transit, the child should hold the tooth in place with a finger. The parent should buckle a seatbelt around the child and drive safely. A quick stop may not only result in re-evulsion but also may introduce the complications of ingestion or aspiration.)

After the tooth is replanted, it must be immobilized (acrylic splint) to facilitate reattachment; endodontic therapy is usually required. The initial signs of complications associated with replantation may appear as early as 1 wk post-trauma or as late as several years later. Close dental follow-up is indicated for at least 1 yr.

Prevention. To minimize the likelihood of dental injuries:

1. Every child or adolescent who engages in contact sports should wear a mouth protector, which may be constructed by a dentist or purchased at any athletic goods store.

2. Helmets should be worn by children or adolescents with neuromuscular problems or seizures to protect the cranium during falls; they should also have face guards.

3. All children or adolescents with protruding incisors should be evaluated by a pediatric dentist or orthodontist.

Additional Considerations. Children with dental trauma have also sustained head trauma; accordingly, neurologic assessment is warranted. Tetanus prophylaxis should be considered with any injury that disrupts the integrity of the tissues lining the oral cavity. The possibility of child abuse should always be considered.

12.9 COMMON LESIONS OF THE ORAL SOFT TISSUES

Oropharyngeal Candidosis (OPC, Thrush, Moniliasis). Oropharyngeal infection with *Candida albicans* is not unusual in neonates who have contact with the organism in the birth canal. Transmission within the newborn nursery may reach epidemic proportions unless appropriate precautions are instituted. The lesions of OPC appear as white plaques covering all or part of the oropharyngeal mucosa. These plaques are removable from the underlying corium, which is characteristically inflamed and hemorrhagic. Discomfort associated with this infection may interfere with feeding. Diagnosis is confirmed by direct microscopic examination and culture of scrapings from lesions. OPC is usually self-limited in the healthy newborn infant, but treatment with nystatin

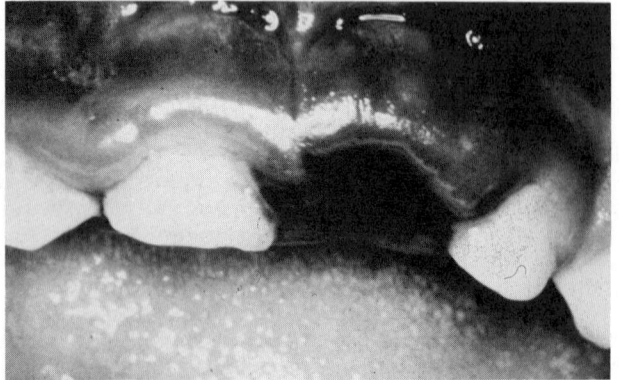

Figure 12–4. Intruded primary incisor that appears evulsed (knocked out).

(1,000,000 units four times a day, applied directly to the lesions) will hasten recovery and reduce the risk of spread to other infants.

OPC is also a major problem during myelosuppressive therapy. Recent data indicate that systemic candidosis (SC), a major cause of morbidity and mortality during myelosuppressive therapy, develops almost exclusively in patients who have had prior OPC. This observation implies that prevention of OPC should reduce the incidence of SC. A recent report describing the use of a multiagent regimen for OPC prophylaxis in children receiving bone marrow transplants indicated that the regimen was extremely effective in preventing OPC, SC, or candidal esophagitis. The multiagent regimen consisted of the following:

1. Debriding all mucous membrane surfaces within the oropharyngeal cavity with one povidone-iodine swabstick four times per day.

2. Swabbing all mucous membrane surfaces within the oropharyngeal cavity with one large cotton pledget saturated with 500,000 units of nystatin four times per day.

The povidone-iodine debridement preceded the nystatin application. Most of the patients were premedicated with intravenous narcotic analgesics in order to permit the procedure to be done thoroughly and quickly. No thyroid dysfunction was noted secondary to the iodine exposure. The multiagent regimen appears to be a safe and effective approach for OPC prophylaxis in myelosuppressed patients.

Finally, chronic OPC occurs in children who have certain endocrinopathies and nutritional deficiencies or who receive broad spectrum antibiotic therapy that alters the oral flora. In these situations, successful treatment depends also on correction of the underlying problem.

Aphthous Ulcers (Canker Sores). The aphthous ulcer is a distinct oral lesion, prone to recurrence. Its etiology is not known. Current data suggest that aphthous ulcers are a form of autoimmune disease. They may appear as either solitary or multiple ulcers. Common sites include the floor of the mouth, the ventral surface of the tongue, and the mucobuccal fold; they are found less frequently on the palate or buccal mucosa. The aphthous ulcer is generally less than 0.5 cm in diameter, with a depressed center and erythematous periphery. The lesion is usually covered by a yellowish-white fibrinous exudate. Many patients report prodromal symptoms such as burning, itching, or tenderness prior to the appearance of the ulcer. The lesions are painful and may make eating uncomfortable. Cold foods, particularly liquids, are usually better tolerated than hot. The use of oral analgesics relieves much of the discomfort associated with eating. Topical application of tetracycline to the lesion (three or four times/day) shortens healing to 2-4 days. This observation suggests that secondary infection may play a role in pathogenesis of the lesion. Lesions that persist for more than 14 days should be biopsied.

Epstein Pearls. Epstein pearls are small cystic lesions located along the midpalatine raphe in about 80% of neonates. These lesions arise from epithelium that was trapped during fusion of the palatal shelves. Treatment is not necessary; they disappear within a few weeks.

Bohn Nodules. Bohn nodules are small cystic lesions located along the buccal and lingual aspects of the mandibular and maxillary ridges of the neonate. These lesions arise from remnants of mucous gland tissue. Treatment is not necessary, as the nodules disappear within a few weeks.

Dental Lamina Cysts. Dental lamina cysts are small cystic lesions located along the crest of the mandibular and maxillary ridges of the neonate. These lesions arise from epithelial remnants of the dental lamina. Treatment is not necessary, they will disappear within a few weeks.

Mucocoele. The mucocoele usually appears as a raised bluish vesicle several millimeters in diameter. It occurs most commonly in the lower lip and rarely in the upper lip, palate, buccal mucosa, tongue, or floor of the mouth. It may persist for weeks or months prior to rupture, in which case it usually recurs. This lesion is caused by traumatic laceration of a minor salivary gland duct that permits accumulation of mucus in the soft tissues and subsequent proliferation of granulation tissue to sequestrate the mucus. Recurrences following surgical excision are largely the result of removing the mucocoele without extirpating the minor salivary gland that produced the extravasated mucus.

Fordyce Granules. Almost 80% of adults have multiple, yellowish-white granules in clusters or plaque-like areas on the oral mucosa, most commonly on the buccal mucosa or lips. Histologically, normal sebaceous glands are seen in the lamina propria and submucosa. The glands are present at birth, but they hypertrophy and first appear as discrete yellowish papules during the preadolescent period in approximately 50% of children. No treatment is necessary.

Herpangina. See Sec. 11.77.

Herpes Labialis (Cold Sore, Fever Blister). See Sec. 11.67.

Cheilitis. Dryness of the lips, followed by scaling and cracking and accompanied by a characteristic burning sensation, is common in children. It is usually caused by sensitivity to contact substances (from toys and foods) plus photosensitivity to the sun's rays. It is aggravated by the alternation of wetting with the tongue and drying by the wind, especially in cold weather. Cheilitis also often occurs in association with fever. Frequent application of a bland ointment facilitates healing and is also preventive.

Black Hairy Tongue (Lingua Nigra). This condition is characterized by an elongation of the filiform papillae into hair-like projections. It is generally concentrated in a triangular area in front of the V-shaped line of circumvallate papillae and is associated with accumulation of debris in that region. The patch may vary from brown to black. The condition is usually chronic, but will disappear with regular cleansing of the dorsal tongue.

Hairy tongue may also occur during prolonged antibiotic therapy, especially with oral troches. In addition, oral medications that contain bismuth may produce this benign condition.

Geographic Tongue (Migratory Glossitis). This benign and asymptomatic lesion is characterized by 1 or more smooth, bright red patches, often showing a yellowish, grayish, or whitish membranous margin upon the dorsum of an otherwise normally roughened tongue. The patches are areas in which the filiform papillae have become completely desquamated, leaving a smooth, slick surface. The patches may be single or multiple, discrete or confluent (map-like). They travel by extension of desquamation of the papillae at one edge and regeneration of normal papillae at the other. The condition may persist for weeks or months and then regress spontaneously, only to recur later.

Fissured Tongue (Scrotal Tongue). The fissured tongue is a malformation manifested clinically by numerous small furrows or grooves on the dorsal surface. The condition is painless except when food debris collects in the grooves and produces irritation. Regular debridement of the tongue's dorsal surface with a toothbrush helps to prevent this problem.

12.10 SALIVARY GLANDS

With the exception of mumps (Sec. 11.70), disease of the salivary glands is rare in children. Bilateral enlargement of the submaxillary glands may occur in cystic fibrosis, in malnutrition, and, transiently, during acute asthmatic attacks. Chronic vomiting and aspiration, as in achalasia, may be accompanied by enlargement of the parotids. Benign salivary gland hypertrophy has been associated with endocrinopathies; thyroid disease, diabetes, and disorders of the pituitary-adrenal axis are the most frequently encountered.

Newborn infants discharge saliva until swallowing and lip closure are effective. Later, when the irritation of teething is accompanied by increased oral activity, drooling may occur. In some children with neurologic impairment, drooling is never overcome. Increased secretion of saliva occurs as a reflex to anticipated feeding or pain, from irritative lesions in the mouth, in conjunction with nausea, after administration of mercurial compounds, and in encephalitis and chorea.

Recurrent Parotitis. Recurrent idiopathic swelling of the parotid gland may occur in otherwise healthy children. The swelling is usually unilateral, but both glands may be involved simultaneously or alternately; there may be up to 10 or more recurrences. There is little pain. The swelling is limited to the gland and usually lasts 2–3 wk. Subsidence is spontaneous and may be complete or partial. The incidence appears to be higher in the spring.

Suppurative Parotitis. This is usually due to *Staphylococcus aureus* and may be primary or a complication of parotitis due to another cause. It is usually unilateral and may be accompanied by fever. The gland becomes swollen, tender, and painful. Recurrent parotitis may be confused with suppurative parotitis. The latter responds to appropriate antibacterial therapy based on culture of pus obtained from the Stensen duct or by surgical drainage, which is infrequently required.

Ranula. Ranula is a cyst associated with a major salivary gland in the sublingual area. A ranula is a large, soft, mucus-containing swelling in the floor of the mouth. It occurs at any age, including infancy. The cyst should be excised and the severed duct exteriorized.

Xerostomia. Xerostomia (or dry mouth) may be associated with fever, dehydration, ingestion of drugs with anticholinergic activity, chronic graft-versus-host disease, Mikulicz disease, Sjögren syndrome, or tumoricidal doses of radiation when the salivary glands are within the field. Long-term xerostomia renders the patient highly susceptible to dental caries, which can be minimized or eliminated by appropriate preventive measures.

Salivary Glands Tumors. See Sec. 16.21.

12.11 DISEASES OF THE JAWS

Caffey Disease (Infantile Cortical Hyperostosis). See Sec. 23.42.

Osteomyelitis (Sec. 11.14 and 23.2). In the newborn infant, facial osteomyelitis tends to occur in the area of the premaxillary suture, but during childhood the mandible is the more common location. The infection is marked by swelling and redness of the oral mucosa or skin and is associated with pain, fever, and lymphadenopathy. Drainage should be established and the exudate cultured so that an appropriate antibiotic may be administered. Large sequestra may require surgical removal.

Reticuloendotheliosis (Histiocytosis X) (Sec. 26.5). Oral lesions may occur in any of the syndromes and may be an early manifestation. Lesions of the jaws may produce pain, swelling, loosening of teeth, and fetid breath. Healing is often delayed after dental extraction.

Neoplasms.

Benign Tumors. Ossifying fibroma is the most common benign tumor of the jaws. Growth is rapid prior to puberty, after which it may slow or cease. The lesion is painless; a unilateral soft tissue swelling is usually the first sign. Most patients do not require treatment, but if the lesion is extensive, curettage or further surgical correction may be required.

Cysts of the Jaw occur with multiple basal cell nevoid syndrome (Sec. 24.32).

Malignant Tumors. The malignant primary tumors of the jaws in children include Burkitt lymphoma, osteogenic sarcoma, lymphosarcoma, and, more rarely, fibrosarcoma (see Chapter 16).

ROBERT J. BERKOWITZ
DAVID C. JOHNSON

Baer PN: Periodontal Disease in Children and Adolescents. Philadelphia, JB Lippincott, 1974.
Enlow, DH: Handbook of Facial Growth. Philadelphia, WB Saunders, 1975.
Gorlin RJ, Pindborg JJ, Cohen MM Jr: Syndromes of the Head and Neck. 2nd ed. New York, McGraw-Hill, 1976.
Newbrun E: Cariology. Baltimore, Williams & Wilkins, 1978.
Sanders B: Pediatric Oral and Maxillofacial Surgery. St. Louis, CV Mosby, 1979.
Stewart RE, Barber TK, Troutman KC, et al: Pediatric Dentistry—Scientific Foundations and Clinical Practice. St. Louis, CV Mosby, 1982.

THE GASTROINTESTINAL TRACT

12.12 NORMAL DIGESTIVE TRACT PHENOMENA

Normal patterns of gastrointestinal development are mistaken easily for manifestations of significant disease. Processes involved in *ingestion of food* are well developed and coordinated at birth. The suckling infant encounters difficulties initially with solid foods, thrusting them forward with the tongue rather than back to the pharynx, but practice quickly corrects the problem. A relatively short lingual frenulum ("tongue-tie") is of no known functional significance. During suckling, infants swallow air; unlike older children they must be stimulated to burp during the course of feeding. Otherwise, gaseous gastric distention can interfere with intake. By 1 mo of age sweet and salty foods seem to be preferred.

Regurgitation of gastric content is very common in infants until 9–12 mo, when children normally become upright for much of the day. This incompletely understood phenomenon may accompany or follow several feedings each day; it usually resolves with time. If general health, growth, and development are unaffected and the complications of aspiration or esophagitis do not develop, there is no need for detailed investigation of such patients.

The *pattern of food intake* and *appetite* of children at different ages may seem bizarre to those who regularly consume three meals a day. Particularly distressing to parents, but normal, is the toddler's habit of gorging him- or herself after refusing to consume the daily requirements for a few days. Appetite fluctuates enormously. In periods of rapid growth during infancy and adolescence, appetite is usually voracious, whereas during the intervening years some children appear to eat almost nothing while they grow and gain weight normally.

The *number, color, and consistency of stools* vary greatly in the same infant and between infants of similar age regardless of diet or environment. After birth the first stools consist of meconium, a dark, viscous, gum-like material. When milk feedings begin, meconium is replaced by green-brown transition stools, often containing curds, and then in 4–5 days by yellow-brown milk stools. Stool frequency may vary from one to seven per day in babies who are otherwise perfectly well. Color of the stool is of little significance unless blood is present or bilirubin is absent. Some children are 2–3 yr of age before they have formed stools. Breast-fed infants tend to have infrequent yellow stools of loose consistency. Later, husks of vegetables like corn and peas and black "worm-like" threads from the surface of the peeled banana appear in stools after these foods have been eaten (see Sec. 3.13 and 8.41).

Abdominal findings in a normal young child may give rise to unnecessary concern. During the first 3–4 yr of life the abdominal musculature is relatively weak, the abdominal organs relatively large, and the lower spine lordotic so that the belly is protuberant but soft. Up to 2 yr a soft liver edge may be palpable up to 2 cm below the right costal margin. Although the spleen is not usually palpable, a soft tip may be felt in the course of an acute infection.

Blood loss from the digestive tract is never normal, but swallowed blood can easily be misinterpreted as enteric hemorrhage. Maternal blood may be ingested at the time of birth or later by the breast-fed baby when there is bleeding near the mother's nipple (Sec. 8.49). Children may also swallow their own blood from epistaxis or another source in the nasopharynx.

Jaundice occurs in about 20% of newborn term infants; the more prematurely born the baby, the higher the incidence. In most newborn infants jaundice results not from a specific disease but from a limited capacity of the immature liver during the early wk of life to conjugate the large quantities of hemoglobin breakdown products presented to it (Sec. 8.44).

12.13 MAJOR SYMPTOMS AND SIGNS OF DIGESTIVE TRACT DISORDERS

An understanding of the pathogenesis of major symptoms is useful in dealing with childhood gastroenterologic disorders because in many cases the cause is unknown and specific or curative treatment not available.

Disordered Ingestion. Abnormalities at several sites in the upper digestive tract can significantly compromise dietary intake.

Transfer Dysphagia. A complex sequence of neuromuscular events is involved in the transfer of foods to the upper esophagus. Suckling requires the lips to form a tight seal about the nipple while the tongue is displaced posteriorly. As the glottis closes to guard the airway, the soft palate raises to close the nasopharynx, the cricopharyngeal muscles relax, and food passes to the back of the pharynx. Solids similarly require a coordinated series of actions, and when they are consumed in large pieces, jaw movement and teeth become factors to consider. Salivary secretions, stimulated by the anticipation and act of ingestion, lubricate foods as they pass through the mouth. It is abnormalities of the muscles involved in the ingestion process (in their innervation, strength, or coordination) that usually cause transfer dysphagia in infants and children. In such cases, an oral-pharyngeal problem is almost always part of a more generalized neurologic or muscular problem. Occasionally, painful oral lesions, such as acute viral stomatitis or trauma, will interfere with ingestion. If the nasal air passage is seriously obstructed, the need for air will cause severe distress when suckling. Although severe structural, dental, and salivary abnormalities are relatively common potential handicaps, ingestion seems to proceed relatively well in the affected hungry child.

Dysphagia, Regurgitation. Swallowing is well coordinated at birth: primary peristaltic waves, initiated by swallowing, proceed down the length of the esophagus, while secondary waves which appear to empty the esophagus of residue are initiated by distention. Regurgitation can occur if swallowing is completely or partially obstructed by an intrinsic lesion in the esophagus or by an extrinsic lesion, in which case associated compression of the trachea may lead to stridor and cough. Primary motility disorders causing impaired peristaltic function and dysphagia are rare in children.

The lower esophageal sphincter (LES) helps to prevent reflux of gastric contents into the esophagus (Sec. 12.21). In general, if lower esophageal sphincter pressure is abnormally reduced, flow of gastric content in a retrograde direction will occur. In very young symptomatic patients there is a poor correlation between sphincter pressure and occurrence of gastroesophageal reflux. Hiatal hernia (Sec. 12.20) is probably not an important determinant of gastroesophageal reflux.

Continued exposure of the lower esophageal mucosa to gastric juice can cause esophagitis and, as a consequence, dysphagia and chronic blood loss. The chance of aspirating gastric juice is enhanced by underlying motility problems in the esophagus, particularly by dysfunction of the upper esophageal sphincter.

Anorexia. Hunger and satiety centers in man are probably located in the hypothalamus, and numerous pathways exist by which gastrointestinal diseases might depress appetite. Particularly important are afferents to the hypothalamus from the gut. For example, satiety is stimulated by distention of the stomach or upper small bowel, the signal being transmitted by sensory efferents which are especially dense in the upper gut. Chemoreceptors in the intestine, influenced by the presence and assimilation of nutrients, also affect afferent flow to the appetite centers. Impulses also reach the hypothalamus from higher centers possibly influenced by pain or the emotional disturbance of an intestinal disease. Other regulatory factors include hormones and plasma glucose, which in turn reflect intestinal function.

Vomiting. Vomiting occurs when violent descent of the diaphragm and constriction of the abdominal muscles force gastric content back up the esophagus. In humans, stimulation of a center in the medulla also can cause vomiting. Diseases in almost any system, particularly the brain, may cause vomiting.

Obstructions of the digestive tract in the stomach and beyond cause vomiting, probably mediated by visceral afferents reaching the vomiting center. If obstruction occurs below the second part of the duodenum, vomitus is often bile stained. Nonobstructive lesions of the digestive tract can also cause vomiting; most diseases of the upper bowel, pancreas, liver, or biliary tree are capable of provoking emesis. Furthermore, metabolic derangements such as those occurring in Reye syndrome may lead to severe, persistent emesis.

Diarrhea. Diarrhea can be defined as the excessive loss of fluid and electrolyte in stool (Sec. 5.24 and 11.8). The basis for all diarrhea is disturbed intestinal solute transport, since water movement across intestinal membranes is passive and determined by both active and passive fluxes of solutes, particularly sodium, chloride, and glucose. In most clinical situations epithelial abnormalities are the major known determinants of diarrhea; hypermotility is rarely a significant cause, and little is known about the roles of blood and lymphatic flow to the gut. Normally, all but a final small percentage of water absorption occurs in the small bowel; small bowel disease tends to cause voluminous diarrhea, whereas colonic diarrhea is less voluminous and characterized by alternating loose and formed or hard stools.

Disease may cause diarrhea by damaging the bowel wall or by elaborating secretagogues, which reach the epithelium via the circulation or from the bowel lumen. When the mucosa is damaged, not only may absorptive surface area be diminished but function of the remaining cells is often compromised. For example, in rotavirus enteritis, glucose transport is defective, disaccharidase and $Na^+ - K^+$ ATPase activities are reduced, and glucose-stimulated Na^+ transport is impaired in the small bowel epithelium after the virus invades the intestinal epithelium.

Other disorders can cause severe diarrhea without any effect on absorptive surface area or on the structure of the intestinal epithelium. Potent secretagogues produced in the gut lumen by *V. cholerae* and *E. coli* bind to the small intestinal brush border and stimulate adenylate cyclase activity, leading to accumulation of cyclic AMP in the epithelium. The result is a massive watery diarrhea characterized by brisk chloride secretion and impaired NaCl absorption, but preservation of the glucose-stimulated Na^+ absorption and $Na^+ - K^+$ ATPase activity that are defective in viral enteritis. Other secretagogues, such as the heat-stable toxin of *E. coli*, cause cyclic GMP accumulation with a similar result. Some intraluminal fatty acids and bile salts cause the colonic mucosa to secrete; the mechanism is unknown. This phenomenon may explain the diarrhea occurring with steatorrhea and with bile salt malabsorption secondary to resection of the distal ileum.

Constipation. Excessively infrequent and dry stools can arise from defects in filling or in emptying the rectum. Defective rectal filling occurs when colonic peristalsis is ineffective, e.g., in cases of hypothyroidism or opiate use, and when there is bowel obstruction caused either by a structural anomaly or by Hirschsprung disease. The resultant colonic stasis leads to excessive drying of stool and a failure to initiate reflexes from the rectum that normally trigger evacuation. Emptying the rectum by spontaneous evacuation depends on a defecation reflex initiated by pressure receptors in the rectal muscle. Stool retention therefore may also result from lesions involving these rectal muscles, the sacral spinal cord afferent and efferent fibers, or the muscles of the abdomen and pelvic floor. Disorders of anal sphincter relaxation also may contribute to fecal retention.

Constipation tends to be self-perpetuating, whatever its cause. Hard, large stools in the rectum become difficult and even painful to evacuate so that more retention occurs and a vicious cycle ensues. Distention of the rectum and colon lessens the sensitivity of the defecation reflex and the effectiveness of peristalsis. Eventually, watery content from the proximal colon may percolate around hard retained stool and pass per rectum unperceived by the child. This type of fecal soiling, involuntary *encopresis*, is frequently mistaken for diarrhea. Constipation does not per se have deleterious systemic organic effects. Urinary tract stasis may accompany severe longstanding cases and the problem itself may generate anxiety having a marked impact on the patient's emotional health.

Abdominal Pain. Individuals differ greatly in tolerance for and responses to intra-abdominal events, but any reported abdominal pain should always be assumed to be real. A specific cause is often difficult to determine, but the nature and location of a pain-provoking lesion can usually be determined from the clinical description. Two types of nerve fibers transmit painful stimuli in the abdomen: in skin and muscle, A fibers mediate sharp localized pain; and C fibers from viscera, peritoneum, and muscle transmit poorly localized, dull pain. These afferent fibers have cell bodies in the dorsal root ganglia, and some axons cross the mid-line and ascend to the medulla, mid-brain, and thalamus. Pain is perceived in the cortex of the postcentral gyrus, which can receive impulses arising from both sides of the body.

Visceral pain tends to be experienced in the dermatome from which the affected organ receives innervation. Painful stimuli originating in liver, pancreas, biliary tree, stomach, or upper bowel are felt in the epigastrium; pain from the distal small bowel, cecum, appendix, or proximal colon is felt at the umbilicus; and pain from distal large bowel, urinary tract, or pelvic organs is usually suprapubic. When pain is referred to

remote areas supplied by the same neurosegment as the diseased organ, the phenomenon usually means an increased intensity of the provoking stimulus. Parietal pain impulses travel in C fibers of nerves corresponding to dermatomes T6 to L1; such pain tends to be more localized and intense than visceral pain.

In the gut the usual stimulus provoking pain is tension or stretching. Inflammatory lesions may lower the pain threshold, but the mechanisms producing pain of inflammation are not clear. Tissue metabolites released near nerve endings probably account for the pain caused by ischemia. Perception of these painful stimuli can be modulated by input from both cerebral and peripheral sources. Psychologic factors are particularly important.

Gastrointestinal Hemorrhage. Bleeding may occur at any site in the digestive tract; the most common sites are the lower esophagus, stomach, duodenum, and colon. Usually, it is an erosion of the mucosa down to the vasculature that leads to hemorrhage, but vessel malformations or raised portal pressure also cause hemorrhage. Rarely, violent vomiting itself may cause mucosal tears and bleeding at the gastroesophageal junction (Mallory-Weiss syndrome). It is rare for clotting defects to cause gastrointestinal bleeding except in hemorrhagic diseases of the newborn.

When bleeding originates in the esophagus, stomach, or duodenum, it may cause **hematemesis.** When exposed to gastric or intestinal juices, blood quickly darkens to resemble coffee grounds; accordingly, the more massive and proximal the bleeding, the more likely it is to be red. Red blood in stools, **hematochezia,** signifies either a distal bleeding site or massive hemorrhage above the distal ileum. Moderate to mild bleeding from sites above the distal ileum tends to cause blackened stools of tarry consistency, **melena,** but major hemorrhages in the duodenum or above can cause melena.

Children can develop iron deficiency anemia from enteric blood loss even when occult blood is not found in stools on random testing. Bleeding into the gut rarely in itself causes gastrointestinal symptoms, although brisk duodenal or gastric bleeding may lead to nausea and vomiting. The breakdown products of intraluminal blood may tip the patient into hepatic coma if liver function is already compromised.

Abdominal Distention and Abdominal Masses. Enlargement of the abdomen can result from diminished tone of the wall musculature or from increased content—fluid, gas, or solid. Ascites, the accumulation of fluid in the peritoneal cavity, distends the abdomen both in the flanks and anteriorly when it is large in volume. This fluid shifts with movement of the patient and conducts a percussion wave.

Ascitic fluid is usually a transudate with a low protein concentration resulting from reduced plasma colloid osmotic pressure of hypoalbuminemia, from raised portal venous pressure, or from both. In cases of portal hypertension the fluid leak probably occurs from lymphatics on the liver surface and from visceral peritoneal capillaries, but ascites does not usually develop until the serum albumin level falls. For unknown reasons sodium excretion in the urine decreases greatly as the ascitic fluid accumulates so that additional dietary sodium goes directly to the peritoneal space, taking with it more water. When ascitic fluid contains a high protein concentration, it is usually an exudate caused by an inflammatory or neoplastic lesion.

When fluid distends the gut, either obstruction or imbalance between absorption and secretion should be suspected. Frequently, the factors causing fluid accumulation in the bowel lumen also cause gas to accumulate. The result may be audible gurgling noises. The source of gas is usually swallowed air, but the small amount normally produced by endogenous bacterial flora may increase considerably in malabsorptive states in which substrate reaches the lower intestine. Gas in the peritoneal cavity, which may cause a tympanitic percussion note even over solid organs like the liver, signals impending shock and/or sepsis since it indicates a perforated viscus.

An abdominal organ may enlarge diffusely or be affected by a discrete mass. In the digestive tract such discrete masses may occur in the lumen, in the wall, or in the mesentery. In the constipated child, mobile, nontender fecal masses are often found. The wall of the gut can be affected by anomalies, cysts, or inflammatory disease; gut wall neoplasms are extremely rare in children. The liver may enlarge diffusely in response to many disorders. Discrete liver masses may be islands of regenerating liver tissue in a cirrhotic liver; inflammatory and neoplastic masses also occur.

Jaundice (Sec. 8.44). Jaundice means yellow staining of tissues caused by accumulation of bilirubin. Excessive production of bilirubin results from excessive heme breakdown. If the load exceeds hepatocyte capacity to transport bilirubin, serum and tissue levels of unconjugated bilirubin rise. Bilirubin is taken up from plasma into the hepatocyte, bound to specific ligands, and unites with UDP glucuronide to form conjugated bilirubin diglucuronide. If the conjugation mechanism is defective or if cytoplasmic binding ligands are defective, unconjugated bilirubin accumulates in serum and tissues. This unconjugated bilirubin is relatively insoluble in serum and is largely bound to albumin; accordingly, it is not filtered by glomeruli and does not stain the urine. Normally, the excretion of relatively water-soluble conjugated bilirubin from the hepatocyte into canaliculi is rapid; it is this pigment that gives the yellow-green color to bile. After concentration by the gallbladder, bile normally reaches the intestinal lumen, where bilirubin remains conjugated until bacteria in the lower bowel deconjugate it. Urobilinogen is also produced in the terminal ileum, where it can be reabsorbed and excreted both in the urine and in bile. Defects in bilirubin excretion may occur in the hepatocyte itself or in the intrahepatic or extrahepatic collecting systems. The clinical manifestations of these excretory defects will include a rise in serum and tissue levels of conjugated bilirubin, the appearance of this soluble pigment in urine, and, depending on the degree of obstruction, a loss of pigmentation of stool and disappearance of urobilinogen from urine.

Berman NF, Holtzapple PG: Gastrointestinal hemorrhage. Pediatr Clin North Am 22:885, 1975.
Borison HL, Wong SC: Physiology and pharmacology of vomiting. Pharmacol Rev 5:193, 1953.
Cox KC, Ament ME: Upper gastrointestinal bleeding in children and adolescents. Pediatrics 63:408, 1979.
Dobbins WJ, Binder HJ: Pathophysiology of diarrhea: Alterations in fluid and electrolyte transport. Clin Gastroenterol 10:605, 1981.
Fitzgerald JF: Difficulties with defecation and elimination in children. Clin Gastroenterol 6:283, 1977.
Grand RJ, Watkins JB, Torti FM: Development of the human gastrointestinal tract. A review. Gastroenterology 70:790, 1976.
Gupta JM: Neonatal jaundice. Med J Aust 1:745, 1977.
Hall RJC: Normal and abnormal food intake. Gut 16:744, 1975.
Hamilton JR: Infectious diarrhea in children. Aust Pediatr J 15:25, 1979.
Pope CE II: The esophagus: Physiology. In: Sleisenger MH, Fordtran JS (eds): Gastrointestinal Disease. ed 2. Philadelphia, WB Saunders, 1978.

12.14 IMPORTANT CAUSES OF DIGESTIVE TRACT SYMPTOMS

In children gastrointestinal symptoms frequently can be attributed to non–digestive-tract disorders (Table 12–2). Particular note should be taken of cerebral and urinary tract diseases as causes of gastrointestinal symptoms since in young children the specific manifestations of these conditions may be subtle.

Important gastroenterologic causes of digestive tract symptoms are summarized in Table 12–3. This table deals with conditions likely to be encountered in North America and includes a few conditions in which digestive tract dysfunction is secondary to pathologic processes elsewhere.

J. RICHARD HAMILTON

Table 12–2. Important Non-Digestive-Tract Causes of Gastrointestinal Symptoms in Children

Anorexia
  Systemic disease (e.g., inflammatory, neoplastic)
  Iatrogenic—drug therapy, unpalatable therapeutic diets
  Depression
  Anorexia nervosa
Vomiting
  Increased intracranial pressure
  Infection (e.g., urinary tract)
Diarrhea
  "Parenteral" infection (e.g., respiratory, urinary)
  Uremia
Constipation
  Hypothyroidism
  Dehydration (e.g., diabetes insipidus, renal tubular lesions)
Abdominal pain
  Pyelonephritis, hydronephrosis, renal colic
  Pneumonia
  Pelvic inflammatory disease
  School phobia
Abdominal mass
  Ascites (e.g., nephrotic syndrome, neoplasm, heart failure)
  Discrete mass (e.g., Wilms tumor, hydronephrosis, neuroblastoma)
  Pregnancy
Jaundice
  Hemolytic disease

Table 12–3. **Important Gastroenterologic Disorders Causing Digestive Tract Symptoms**

Symptoms	In Infants	In Children
Dysphagia	Neuromuscular dysfunction (e.g., cerebral palsy) Esophageal atresia	Corrosive and foreign body damage Peptic esophagitis Achalasia
Regurgitation	Gastroesophageal reflux Feeding problem	Gastroesophageal reflux
Anorexia	Stomatitis Intestinal infection Celiac disease	Hepatitis Inflammatory bowel diseases Celiac disease

Vomiting	Congenital obstruction
	  Pyloric stenosis
	  Intestinal atresia
	Intussusception
	Intestinal infection
	Celiac disease
		Acute abdomen
		  Appendicitis
		  Pancreatitis
		Intestinal infection, food poisoning
		Intestinal obstruction—adhesions, volvulus
		Inflammatory bowel diseases
		Hepatitis
		Reye syndrome

Diarrhea	Intestinal infection Necrotizing enterocolitis Celiac disease Cystic fibrosis	Intestinal infection Inflammatory bowel diseases

Constipation	Bowel obstruction
	  Hirschsprung disease
	  Meconium ileus
		"Functional" constipation
		Meconium ileus equivalent

Abdominal pain	Infantile colic Intestinal infection Intussusception Volvulus	Appendicitis Intestinal infection Inflammatory bowel diseases Lactose intolerance Peptic ulcer Pancreatitis Cholecystitis
Hematemesis		Gastritis (aspirin ingestion) Esophagitis Esophageal varices Peptic ulcer Stress ulcer
Hematochezia or melena	Bacterial infection Necrotizing enterocolitis Anal fissure Meckel diverticulum Intussusception	Intestinal infection (bacterial, parasitic) Inflammatory bowel diseases Peptic ulcer Meckel diverticulum Colonic polyp Anal fissure
Abdominal mass Intestine	Distal bowel obstruction (Hirschsprung disease) Necrotizing enterocolitis Intestinal infection Celiac disease Cystic fibrosis Hernia (inguinal or umbilical)	Functional constipation Aerophagia Bowel obstruction Celiac disease Cystic fibrosis Intestinal infection
Peritoneum	Chylous ascites Peritonitis (bowel perforation)	Ascites Peritonitis
Hepatomegaly	Pancreatitis Cirrhosis Storage disease Neoplasm	Hepatitis Cirrhosis Passive congestion

Jaundice (hyperbilirubinemia)
  Unconjugated
  Mixed (conjugated, unconjugated)
	Breast feeding
	Perinatal infections
	Metabolic disorders
	  Galactosemia
	  Tyrosinemia
	  α_1-Antitrypsin deficiency
	Biliary atresia
		Gilbert disease
		Hepatitis (A, B, non-A–non-B)
		Chronic active hepatitis
		Drug reactions
		Metabolic disorders
		  Wilson disease
		  α_1-Antitrypsin deficiency
		Choledochal cyst

THE ESOPHAGUS

12.15 DEVELOPMENT AND FUNCTION OF THE ESOPHAGUS

The esophagus develops from primitive foregut, as two laryngotracheal grooves along its lateral wall fuse to separate the primitive esophagus from the anterior trachea. The function of the esophagus is to transport fluids and solids to the stomach and prevent their regurgitation.

Swallowing has been observed in utero at 20 wk gestation, and sucking and swallowing seem to be coordinated by 33–34 wk. The full-term newborn infant has short bursts of sucking following by swallows. Within a few days (or weeks if premature) the infant is able to swallow and breathe in a coordinated, rhythmic manner during prolonged bursts of sucking.

Swallowing is initiated by a sudden elevation of the posterior portion of the tongue, which thrusts the contents of the posterior pharynx into the esophagus. The laryngeal airway is protected by a simultaneous anterior superior displacement associated with closure of the laryngeal orifice, which is further protected by the epiglottis. The nasopharynx is closed off by the soft palate. Relaxation of the cricopharyngeal muscle facilitates entrance of food into the esophagus, and the bolus of food is propelled down the esophagus by peristaltic waves.

Three types of esophageal waves are described. A primary wave is initiated by a swallow and proceeds the length of the esophagus; secondary waves are usually initiated by local distention and serve to empty the esophagus of residual food or of gastric contents. Both of these waves empty the esophagus by propulsive efforts. In contrast, tertiary waves are nonpropulsive; they are abnormal if present in large numbers and can be associated with chest pains. The lower esophageal sphincter is a specialized segment of circular musculature in the distal 1–3 cm of the esophagus, where the intraluminal pressure is normally higher than that in the more proximal esophagus or in the stomach. This sphincter prevents gastroesophageal reflux but relaxes during deglutition to allow food to enter the stomach.

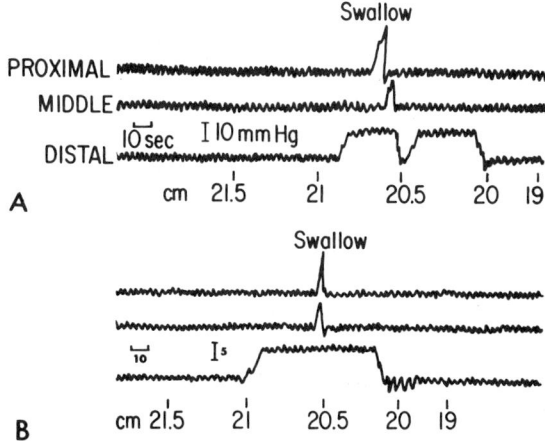

Figure 12–6. *A*, Pressures in the esophagus of a normal infant as recorded with a triple lumen catheter with recording tips 2.5 cm apart. When the distal recording tip was 21.5 cm from the gum line, it was within the lower esophageal sphincter. A swallow initiates a primary peristaltic wave. The pressure wave is detected first in the more proximal catheter and then the more distal one. A relaxation in the lower esophageal sphincter allows the food to enter the stomach. *B*, Abnormal manometric pattern in a patient demonstrating simultaneous pressure in the 2 proximal recording tips, characteristic of tertiary esophageal wave. There is no relaxation of the lower esophageal sphincter. Such a pattern is seen in patients with achalasia.

The *common symptoms* of esophageal disease are cough or choking with swallowing, regurgitation or vomiting, dysphagia, complete inability to swallow, pain on swallowing, and hematemesis. Each can be attributed to one or more defects in the complex coordination of the swallowing sequence. *Diagnostic evaluations* include conventional barium swallow roentgenographic studies, which may demonstrate masses impinging on the lumen or gastroesophageal reflux. Fluoroscopy can evaluate the dynamics of swallowing and reveal abnormalities that are present only transiently. Esophageal manometry permits quantitative measurements of pressures along the esophagus. The pressure in the lower esophageal sphincter is often decreased in patients with reflux, especially if esophagitis is present. In contrast, pressures are elevated, with poor relaxation, in achalasia (Fig. 12–6). Radionuclide scans can help to detect gastroesophageal reflux. In older children such scans can evaluate the efficiency of peristalsis in clearing liquid or a solid bolus from the esophagus. Measurement of intraluminal esophageal pH with a flexible 2 mm diameter pH probe in the distal esophagus is the most sensitive method to detect reflux of acid gastric contents. Esophagoscopy is especially useful in visualizing lesions on the mucosal surface and in detecting and removing foreign bodies. Flexible fiberoptic endoscopes permit direct examination and biopsy of the esophagus without general anesthesia.

12.16 DISORDERS OF THE ESOPHAGUS

12.17 ATRESIA AND TRACHEOESOPHAGEAL FISTULA

Esophageal atresia occurs in 1 in 3000–4500 live births; about one third of affected infants are born prematurely. In more than 75% of cases, a fistula between the trachea and distal esophagus accompanies the atresia (Fig. 12–7*A*). Less commonly, the esophageal atresia or tracheoesophageal fistula may occur alone (Fig. 12–7*B, C*) or in unusual combinations (Fig. 12–7*D, E*). These anomalies are thought to arise from defective differentiation of the primitive foregut into trachea and esophagus, defective growth of entodermal cells leading to atresia, and incomplete fusion of the lateral walls of the foregut to form tracheoesophageal fistula.

Clinical Manifestations. Atresia of the esophagus should be suspected (1) in cases of maternal polyhydramnios; (2) if a catheter used at birth for resuscitation cannot be inserted into the stomach; (3) if the infant has excessive oral secretions; or (4) if choking, cyanosis, or coughing occurs with an attempt at feeding. Suctioning of excess secretions from the mouth and pharynx frequently results in improvement, but symptoms quickly recur. Unfortunately, the diagnosis is often not made until after the baby has aspirated feedings. When a fistula connects the trachea and distal esophagus, air usually enters the abdomen, which often becomes tympanitic and may become so distended as to interfere with breathing. If a fistula connects the proximal esophagus to the trachea, the first attempt at feeding may lead to massive aspiration. Infants with atresia who have no fistula have scaphoid, airless abdomens. In the rare situation of fistula without atresia ("H type") (Fig. 12–7*C*) the usual sign is recurrent aspiration pneumonia, and diagnosis may be delayed for days or even months. Aspiration of pharyngeal secretions is almost universal among patients with esophageal atresia, but aspiration of gastric contents via a distal fistula causes a much more severe, life-threatening chemical pneumonitis.

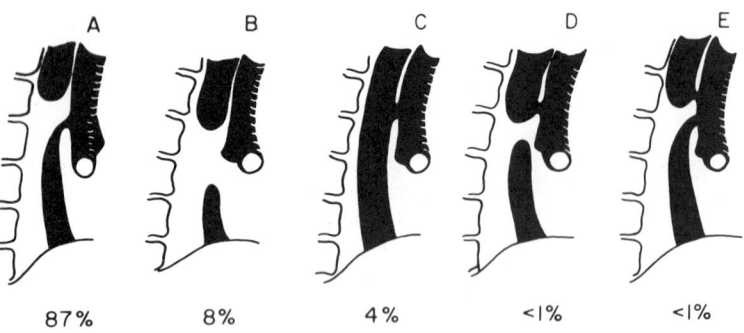

Figure 12–7. Diagrams of the 5 most commonly encountered forms of esophageal atresia and tracheoesophageal fistula, in order of frequency.

A	B	C	D	E
87%	8%	4%	<1%	<1%

At least 30% of infants with esophageal atresia have associated congenital anomalies, many of them potentially life-threatening. Cardiovascular anomalies are the most common. Other digestive tract defects (**duodenal stenosis,** imperforate anus, and so on) occur, along with urinary tract, skeletal, and central nervous system defects.

Diagnosis. Diagnosis of esophageal atresia is ideally made in the delivery room, since pulmonary aspiration is a major determinant of prognosis. Inability to pass a catheter into the stomach confirms the suspicion. Usually the catheter stops abruptly 10–11 cm from the upper gum line, and roentgenograms show a coiled catheter in the upper esophageal pouch (Fig. 12–8). Occasionally, plain roentgenograms of the chest show an esophagus dilated with air. The presence of air in the abdomen indicates a fistula between the trachea and the distal esophagus. Contrast medium used for roentgenography should be water soluble; less than 1 mL given under fluoroscopic control is sufficient to outline the blind upper pouch. The contrast medium should then be withdrawn to prevent overflow into the lungs and development of chemical pneu-

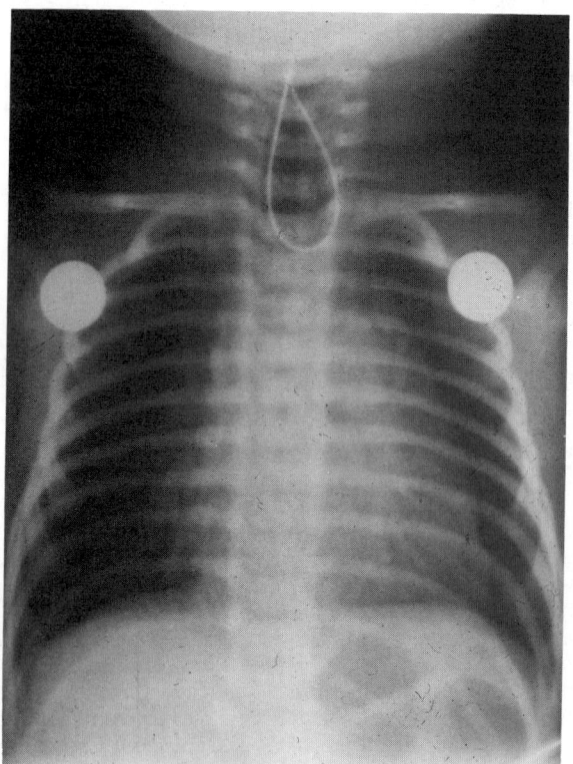

Figure 12–8. Roentgenogram of newborn infant with esophageal fistula. The coiled catheter outlines the upper blind pouch. The presence of air in the abdomen indicates a fistula to the distal esophagus.

monitis. "H type" fistulas (see Fig. 12–7C) can sometimes be demonstrated only with difficulty by cineradiography while the esophagus is filled with water-soluble contrast medium. The tracheal orifice of this type of fistula may be readily detectable at bronchoscopy.

Treatment. Esophageal atresia is a surgical emergency. Preoperatively, the patient should be kept prone to decrease any tendency of gastric contents to reach the lungs. The esophageal pouch should be kept empty by constant suction to prevent aspiration of secretions. Careful attention must be given to temperature control and respiratory function and to detection of any associated anomalies. Occasionally, the patient's condition requires that surgery be performed in stages, the first step usually being ligation of the fistula and insertion of a gastrostomy tube for feeding and the second being anastomosis of the two ends of the esophagus. Eight to 10 days after a primary anastomosis, oral feedings are usually tolerated. Esophagography at 10 days will help determine the adequacy of the anastomosis. Stenosis at the anastomotic site is common and may require dilatations. Persistent abnormal motility is always found in the distal esophagus; it predisposes to gastroesophageal reflux, aspiration, esophagitis, and stricture formation (see Sec. 12.21).

12.18 OTHER DISORDERS OF THE ESOPHAGUS

Laryngotracheoesophageal Cleft. Rarely, the larynx and upper trachea may fail to separate completely from the esophagus for a variable distance. Symptoms of the resultant laryngotracheoesophageal cleft are similar to those of tracheoesophageal fistula; aphonia should suggest the former. Roentgenographic diagnosis using contrast material is difficult; usually endoscopy is required.

External Compression. The most common masses impinging on the esophagus are enlarged lymph nodes in the subcarinal area, which may be due to tuberculosis, histoplasmosis, other forms of pulmonary suppuration, or lymphoma. Extrinsic pressure may also be caused by vascular anomalies in the mediastinum (Sec. 14.65).

Esophageal duplication cysts may cause esophageal compression. Their epithelium may come from any portion of the intestine, and they do not communicate with the esophagus unless there is ulceration from gastric mucosa in the cyst. Two thirds are on the right side of the esophagus. Rarely, duplication cysts may extend through the diaphragm and communicate with the intestine. Diagnosis is usually made by barium esophagography. *Neurenteric cysts* are esophageal duplication cysts that contain glial elements; vertebral anomalies usually accompany these cysts.

Congenital stenosis and webs are rare; their embryonic development is probably similar to that of atresia. Dysphagia usually first occurs when solids are introduced into the diet.

Table 12–4. Neuromuscular Disorders That May Cause Dysphagia

Cerebral palsy (more common)
Dermatomyositis
Infections—diphtheria, poliomyelitis, tetanus
Muscular dystrophy (more common)
Myasthenia gravis
Polyneuritis
Familial dysautonomia (Riley-Day) syndrome
Scleroderma
Specific cranial nerve defects (e.g., Moebius syndrome)
Werdnig-Hoffmann disease

The treatment is similar to that of the much more common strictures caused by peptic esophagitis, from which they must be distinguished (Sec. 12.22).

Dysphagia Due to Neuromuscular Disease. Many systemic, neurologic, and muscular disorders, may give rise to esophageal symptoms. These are listed in Table 12–4 and discussed elsewhere (see Index).

Cricopharyngeal Dysfunction. Spasm of the cricopharyngeal muscle or achalasia of the superior esophageal sphincter may cause intermittent dysphagia, and the increased pressure in the pharynx and upper esophagus may lead to development of a posterior pharyngeal diverticulum. Diagnosis of this idiopathic disorder is made by cineradiographic or manometric demonstration of a failure of the superior esophageal sphincter to relax during deglutition. Symptoms are relieved by myotomy of the cricopharyngeal muscle, analogous to the procedure used in hypertrophic pyloric stenosis (Sec. 12.27).

Cricopharyngeal incoordination of infancy is usually evident soon after birth. Sucking is normal, but affected infants tend to choke and aspirate with deglutition; they generally have small jaws that open poorly. Cineradiography shows repetitive to-and-fro movement of the contrast medium in the posterior pharynx. Careful feedings by spoon or gavage are required until the patient is about 6 mo of age, when symptoms abate. The cause of this disorder is unknown.

Bulbar palsy (supranuclear or lower motor neuron) may cause dysphagia. The child has poor sucking with liquids, and chews and swallows solid food with difficulty. With supranuclear bulbar palsy, the jaw jerk is exaggerated, and usually signs of generalized spastic cerebral palsy develop. Lower motor neuron disease with flaccid bulbar palsy and facial diplegia constitutes the Moebius syndrome.

Paralysis of the superior laryngeal nerve has been reported in neonates with dysphagia, diminished esophageal motility, a preference to lie with the head turned to one side, and, in some cases, unilateral facial weakness. The syndrome is thought to be caused when an unusual intrauterine position compresses the nerve between the thyroid cartilage and the hyoid bone. Spontaneous recovery occurs during the 1st yr.

Transient pharyngeal muscle dysfunction is often associated with palatal dysfunction, and may be due to delayed normal development or associated with cerebral palsy. Choking during feeding and dribbling of formula are the main symptoms. Paralysis of pharyngeal constrictors and a flaccid soft palate are noted in cineroentgenographic studies. Gavage feeding can prevent aspiration (the main complication) and may be required for only a few days or for many weeks. Affected infants often have generalized hypotonia, and other nervous system dysfunctions and developmental delays often become evident later.

12.19 ACHALASIA
(Megaesophagus)

Achalasia is a lack of relaxation of the lower esophageal sphincter with swallowing. A relative obstruction at the level of the sphincter is made worse by a lack of peristaltic waves in the esophagus (see Fig. 12–6B). The condition affects primarily adolescents and adults; children under the age of 4 yr comprise fewer than 5% of patients. The disease has been reported in siblings. Ganglion cells are frequently decreased in number and surrounded by inflammatory cells; a heightened response of esophageal muscles to metacholine has been interpreted as evidence of denervation hypersensitivity. Only in Chagas disease has the etiology been well established.

Clinical Manifestations and Diagnosis. Symptoms include difficulty in swallowing, regurgitation of food, cough from overflow of fluids into the trachea, and failure to gain weight. The diagnosis is usually made roentgenographically by demonstrating a persistently narrowed gastroesophageal junction and absence of propulsive peristaltic waves in the esophagus. If obstruction at the gastroesophageal junction persists, esophageal dilatation may become massive and air-fluid levels are often seen on an upright roentgenogram. Pulmonary infections, even bronchiectasis, may result from persistent aspiration of esophageal contents. In patients with advanced cases, retention of fluid and food in the esophagus may cause esophagitis. In rare instances, achalasia is associated with adrenal insufficiency.

Treatment. Transient relief of symptoms may occur after dilating the cardioesophageal junction with a mercury bougie. Permanent relief of symptoms usually follows surgical division of muscles at the cardioesophageal junction (Heller procedure). Alternatively, the sphincter may be forcefully dilated with a pneumatic bag placed in the cardioesophageal junction under fluoroscopy. Because the esophageal dysmotility cannot be reversed, any procedure that disrupts the sphincter and relieves the obstruction may allow gastroesophageal reflux, esophagitis, and occasionally stricture formation.

12.20 HIATAL HERNIA
(Partial Thoracic Stomach)

Herniation of part of the stomach into the thorax through the esophageal hiatus may be paraesophageal or sliding type (Fig. 12–9). In the paraesophageal hernia, the gastroesophageal junction is positioned normally, but a portion of the stomach herniates into the chest through a patent esophageal hiatus. Fullness after eating and upper abdominal pain are the usual symptoms; infarction of the herniated stomach is a rare complication. In the sliding variety, the gastroesophageal junction and a portion of the stomach lie within the chest.

Hiatal hernia is usually congenital in children and is frequently associated with gastroesophageal reflux. An association with other congenital malformations gives evidence of genetic factors. It is unknown whether the common hiatal

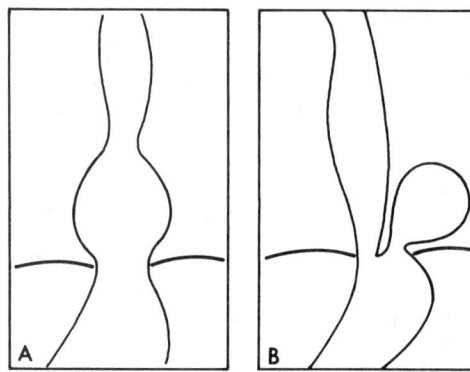

Figure 12–9. Types of esophageal hiatal hernia. *A*, Sliding hiatal hernia, the most common type; *B*, paraesophageal hiatal hernia.

hernias of adults represent lesions acquired in later life or ones present since infancy. Treatment is directed not at the hernia but at the gastroesophageal reflux.

12.21 GASTROESOPHAGEAL REFLUX
(Chalasia)

When the lower esophageal sphincter is not competent, excessive reflux of gastric contents may cause significant symptoms. The term *chalasia* describes free reflux across a dilated sphincter; in Europe the terms partial thoracic stomach or hiatal hernia are used.

Etiology. Many factors contribute to competency of the gastroesophageal sphincter and development of symptoms. In infants, unlike adults, hiatal hernia is frequently associated with gastroesphageal reflux. It has been shown that reflux may occur with increased intra-abdominal pressure, but more important mechanisms are a chronically lax sphincter or brief spontaneous decreases in sphincter tone. Reflux occurs frequently in normal persons after meals, and the swallowing of saliva to clear the esophagus of acid is an important mechanism for preventing esophagitis. The small reservoir capacity of the infant's esophagus predisposes to vomiting, a much less common problem in adolescents and adults.

Clinical Manifestations. The signs and symptoms relate directly to the exposure of the esophageal epithelium to refluxed gastric contents. In 85% of affected infants excessive vomiting occurs during the 1st wk of life; an additional 10% have symptoms by 6 wk. Symptoms abate without treatment in 60% by the age of 2 yr as the child assumes a more upright posture and eats solid foods, but the remainder continue to have symptoms until at least 4 yr of age.

About two thirds of patients will have delayed gastric emptying, and vomiting may be forceful because of pylorospasm. Aspiration pneumonia occurs in about one third of patients in infancy, and in those that persist until later childhood chronic cough, wheezing, and recurrent pneumonia are common. There may be rumination (see below). Growth and weight gain are adversely affected in about two thirds of patients. The major manifestation of esophagitis is hemorrhage; hematemesis occurs in some children, but rarely melena. Iron-deficiency anemia affects about 25% of patients, usually only with occult blood loss. Complaints of substernal pain are rare, but dysphagia may cause irritability and anorexia in advanced cases. In untreated patients, esophagitis leads to stricture formation in 5% of cases, and inanition and pneumonia lead to death in another 5%.

Diagnosis. In mild cases, a careful clinical assessment may be sufficient for diagnosis, which is confirmed by assessing the response to therapy. In severe or complex cases, the diagnosis can be confirmed by barium esophagography under fluoroscopic control. The finding of gastric folds above the diaphragm indicates the presence of a hiatal hernia (Fig. 12–10); in children these folds are more readily detected in a collapsed than in a full esophagus. Gastroesophageal reflux is an episodic event; accordingly, in many symptomatic patients significant reflux is not demonstrated initially by roentgenography. It is important to use enough barium to approximate the volume of a normal meal. Special maneuvering of the patient is not necessary. Normal children may have a small amount of reflux that is quickly cleared from the esophagus, but recurrent reflux is definitely abnormal. Strictures are easily demonstrated with barium esophagography. Severe esophagitis may be suspected when a ragged mucosal outline is seen on a roentgenogram, but esophagoscopy with biopsy is a superior diagnostic technique for this disorder. The severity and frequency of reflux can be documented by monitoring esophageal pH with a probe in the distal esophagus.

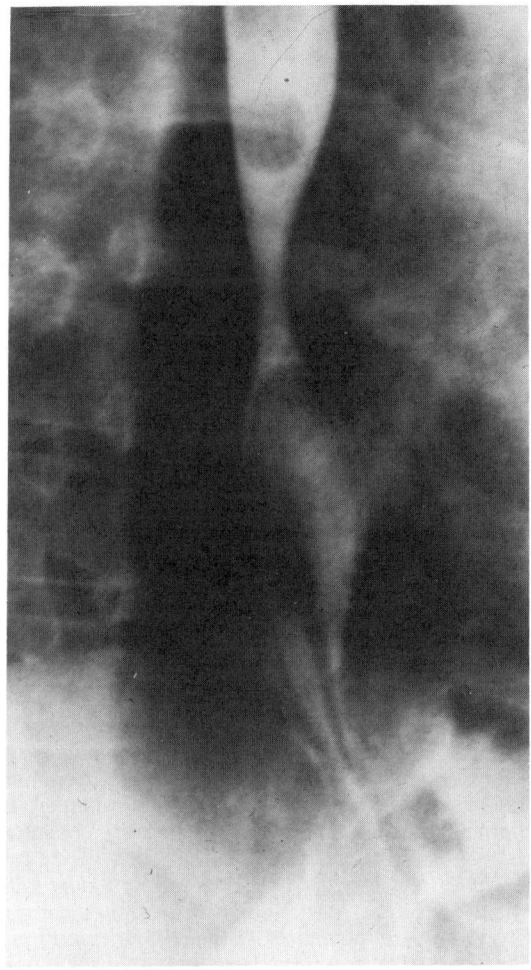

Figure 12–10. Barium esophagogram demonstrating tree gastroesophageal reflux. A stricture due to peptic esophagitis is present. Longitudinal gastric folds above the diaphragm indicate the presence of an associated hiatal hernia.

Treatment. The results of medical therapy are better in infants than in older children. In mild uncomplicated cases, keeping the child prone, thickening the feedings with cereal, and careful attention to burping are enough. In severe cases, the child should be maintained prone, with the head elevated 30° (Fig. 12–11). If esophagitis is present, frequent use of antacids, or cimetidine given four times a day (20–40 mg/kg/24 hr), can be helpful. Bethanechol in doses of 8.7 mg/m²/24 hr given before meals and at bedtime or metoclopramide (0.1 mg/kg/dose) before meals and at bedtime will accelerate gastric emptying and stimulate muscular activity in the esophagus. These drugs can lessen vomiting and encourage weight gain. The response to medical therapy may not be noticeable for as long as 2 wk; increased weight gain is often the first sign of improvement.

If symptoms do not respond to a 6 wk trial of intensive medical therapy, operative treatment is indicated; the medical trial may be shortened if recurrent aspiration and apnea are major problems. When stricture has occurred with reflux esophagitis, operation is indicated without a trial of positional therapy. Bouginage of strictures can provide temporary relief of dysphagia, but unless reflux can be prevented, the stricture will recur. Repeated bouginage is usually not needed if the reflux is controlled. The Nissen fundoplication or a variation of it is most often used in children; reflux is controlled in over 90% of cases. When the esophagus is severely shortened, an intrathoracic Nissen procedure is favored. Occasionally, stric-

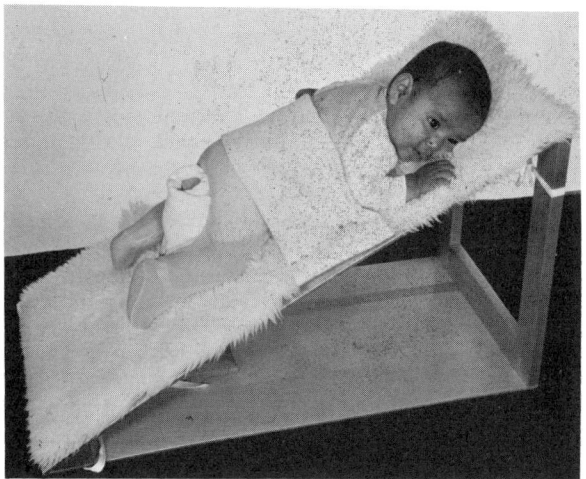

Figure 12–11. Child receiving positional treatment for gastroesophageal reflux. The child straddles a padded peg in the board and is thus kept in position.

ture formation is so extensive that colonic interpostion is required to replace a portion of the esophagus.

Rumination is an uncommon but serious form of chronic regurgitation that usually occurs during the latter half of the 1st yr, often with growth failure (see Sec. 5.36). The etiology is unknown. In some patients psychologic factors may be of prime importance. There are often abnormalities in the mother-child relationship, with an inability of the mother to develop a mature parental role. In some infants rumination is a repetitive self-stimulating behavior that develops when the infant has been deprived of soothing tactile, visual, or auditory stimulation. In some patients, gastroesophageal reflux or other abnormalities of esophageal function, or both, are major contributing factors; in others, abnormal esophageal function may only facilitate the development of rumination. Chewing movements and mouthing of the fingers often precede or accompany the regurgitation. Careful observation may disclose that the infant actively gags himself or herself with the tongue or fingers. A significant loss of nutrients may appear deceptively small; the infant often lies continuously in a small pool of regurgitated liquid. A barium swallow roentgenogram usually demonstrates easy reflux or a hiatal hernia and excludes other intestinal lesions such as esophageal stricture, achalasia, or duodenal ulcer.

In those cases in which a warm intensive relationship with the mother is lacking, efforts should focus on providing this for the infant. The establishment of regular eye contact is often associated with decreased regurgitation. Intensive medical therapy for gastroesophageal reflux should be instituted. If the patient does not improve, surgery for gastroesophageal reflux regularly stops rumination and initiates weight gain.

12.22 ESOPHAGITIS

Peptic esophagitis due to reflux of gastric acid, with pain, blood loss, and possibly stricture formation is the most common form of esophagitis.

Retroesophageal abscess usually represents extension of a retropharyngeal abscess downward; other causes are esophageal perforations, foreign bodies, spinal osteomyelitis, pleuritis, pericarditis, ulceration from an intubation or tracheostomy tube, diphtheria of the pharynx, or suppuration of mediastinal lymph nodes. The abscess forms behind and around the esophagus and often displaces it to one side, while at the same time it compresses the more firmly seated trachea.

The symptoms are dyspnea, a brassy cough, dysphagia, and, as the trachea is pushed forward, swelling of the neck. Pain and tenderness on palpation of the neck and cervical emphysema may be present. The increased retrotracheal space can be seen on lateral roentgenograms of the neck without the use of contrast medium; if the abscess is due to esophageal perforation, barium esophagography is contraindicated.

The abscess may rupture into the pleura, trachea, or lung. Death may result from pressure of the abscess upon the trachea with consequent asphyxia, or from an erosion into the great vessels of the neck with exsanguinating hemorrhage.

Prompt surgical drainage is indicated. If the abscess is high, the retroesophageal space may be opened in the neck along the anterior border of the sternocleidomastoid muscle. Drainage here is effective to the level of the fourth dorsal vertebra; for retroesophageal abscesses below this point posterior mediastinotomy is generally indicated. Antibiotic therapy is indicated, but such therapy may mask an advancing mediastinal infection; only serial lateral roentgenograms of the neck and chest will indicate the situation in the post-tracheal area.

Esophageal candidosis (moniliasis) usually occurs in patients receiving chemotherapy for hematologic or neoplastic diseases. Oral candidosis may be absent. Difficulty and pain on swallowing are prominent. Barium esophagography demonstrates a shaggy mucosal outline or numerous round filling defects, and esophagoscopy shows a friable mucosa with overlying whitish plaques. Treatment consists of ketoconazole 3–6 mg/kg/24 hr orally as a single daily dose, or nystatin 200,000 units orally every 2 hr. Amphotericin may be used in resistant cases. Administration of other antibiotics should be discontinued if possible. Prognosis is usually that of the underlying disease.

Diphtheria may involve the esophagus with extension of the membrane from the oropharynx (Sec. 11.23).

Tuberculosis rarely affects the esophagus; when it does, it usually extends directly from the larynx or contiguous lymph nodes.

Herpes simplex infection may cause acute esophagitis. Fever is common, and pain on swallowing is often so severe that no nutrients can be taken. Inspection usually shows typical vesicular lesions in the pharynx and endoscopy will demonstrate the same lesions in the esophagus. The illness often lasts only a few days. Viscous 2% lidocaine, 2–3 mL every 4 hr, offers symptomatic relief. With cases in severe immunocompromised patients, the use of adenine arabinoside may be considered.

Corrosive esophagitis most commonly follows ingestion of household cleaning products. Hydrochloric and sulfuric acid, bleaches, and strong bases in products used to clean ovens or unclog drains are the most common corrosives. A history of access to such substances in an infant or child with chemical burns of the hands, mouth, or other parts of the body strongly suggests the possibility of corrosive ingestion if that has not actually been observed. Following ingestion, the acute swelling and dysphagia clear in 2–4 wk. An asymptomatic period of weeks or even months may occur before the insidious formation of strictures leads to esophageal obstruction and the symptoms of dysphagia and vomiting.

Emergency management of probable ingestion involves oral administration of large quantities of fluid to flush away and neutralize the chemical. Gastric lavage is contraindicated (Sec. 28.3). Edema of the pharynx may require a tracheostomy. Esophagogastroscopy should be performed within 48 hr to assess the presence and/or severity of esophageal burns, since the absence of oral or pharyngeal lesions does not ensure absence of esophageal lesions. Rarely, the corrosive material may be transported to the stomach with few or no esophageal burns, while still causing severe gastritis, perforation, or late stricture formation.

Further therapy is unnecessary if no burns are detected by endoscopy. If esophageal burns are found, ampicillin and prednisone (2 mg/kg/24 hr in divided doses) are usually administered for 10 days. Prednisone may decrease subsequent stricture formation. Early detection and dilatation of developing strictures are an important part of continuing care. Occasionally, there is complete obliteration of the esophageal lumen, or stricture formation is so severe that dilatation is impossible. In such cases the involved portion of the esophagus is replaced at operation with a section of colon or a tube fashioned from the stomach.

The only truly effective management is prevention. Parents should keep corrosive compounds beyond the reach of children.

12.23 ESOPHAGEAL PERFORATION

This is usually caused by instrumentation for pre-existing disease. Spontaneous perforation may follow sudden increases in esophageal pressure, which occur with violent retching, in auto accidents, or even with compression in the birth canal. Ninety-five per cent of perforations occur on the left side of the distal esophagus in children, but occur more commonly on the right side in neonates. Common symptoms are vomiting followed by severe substernal pain, cyanosis, and shock. Esophagography shows extraluminal water-soluble contrast material.

Violent retching can tear the esophageal mucosa and submucosa, causing hematemesis (**Mallory-Weiss syndrome**). Esophagoscopy should differentiate this disorder from other more serious forms of upper gastrointestinal bleeding. In children, blood replacement is usually sufficient treatment for this self-limited disease.

12.24 ESOPHAGEAL VARICES

Esophageal varices may occur in children as a complication of portal hypertension. The principal signs are recurrent, profuse, bright red hematemesis, and tarry stools, with signs of intravascular volume depletion. Children with esophageal varices often have another source for acute gastrointestinal hemorrhage. Roentgenographic studies with barium may outline the varices, but esophagoscopy is more precise in diagnosis. Treatment of portal hypertension and acute gastrointestinal bleeding is discussed in Sec. 12.88.

12.25 FOREIGN BODIES IN THE ESOPHAGUS

Children swallow a variety of objects that can pass through the intestinal tract without complications. Objects that become lodged in the esophagus usually do so at one of three areas of physiologic narrowing: below the cricopharyngeal muscle; at the level of the aortic arch; or just above the diaphragm. Lodging of material at any other site should suggest coexistent esophageal disease.

Clinical Manifestations. The swallowing of a foreign body may provoke an attack of coughing and choking. Foreign bodies in the esophagus will usually cause pain, dysphagia (especially with solid foods), and occasionally dyspnea, owing to compression of the larynx. After an initial symptom-free period, edema and inflammation produce symptoms of esophageal obstruction. Pain, fever, and shock develop with perforation.

Diagnosis. Radiopaque foreign bodies are easily diagnosed. Coins and other flat objects will usually be seen on edge in a lateral film. Recognition of plastic and nonleaded glass objects is often difficult, but they can be detected with barium swallow roentgenography. The use of barium-soaked cotton to demonstrate the position of a foreign body is unnecessary and complicates therapy.

Treatment. The usual treatment is removal of the object under direct vision with esophagoscopy. Roentgenography should be repeated just prior to the procedure to make sure the foreign body has not passed into the stomach or been vomited. An alternative procedure is usually successful for blunt objects such as coins. A Foley catheter is inserted beyond the foreign body under fluoroscopic visualization. The balloon is inflated and catheter and foreign body are removed together while taking care that the object is not aspirated. Under no circumstance should attempts be made to force the foreign object into the stomach. The patient should be observed for 24 hr after removal of the foreign body for signs of obstruction or perforation.

JOHN J. HERBST

Esophageal Anomalies

Berdon WE, Baker DH: Vascular anomalies and the infant lungs: Rings, slings and other things. Semin Roentgenol 7:39, 1972.
Grossfeld JL, O'Neill JA, Clatworthy HW Jr: Enteric duplications in infancy and childhood: An 18 year review. Ann Surg 172:83, 1970.
Holder TM, Cloud DT, Lewis JE Jr, et al: Esophageal atresia and tracheoesophageal fistula. A survey of its members by the surgical section of the American Academy of Pediatrics. Pediatrics 34:542, 1964.

Hiatal Hernia and Gastroesophageal Reflux

Carre IJ: The natural history of the partial thoracic stomach (hiatus hernia) in children. Arch Dis Child 34:344, 1959.
Dodds WJ, Dent J, Hogan WJ, et al: Mechanisms of gastroesophageal reflux in patients with reflux esophagitis. N Engl J Med 307:1547, 1982.
Euler AR: Use of bethanechol for the treatment of gastroesophageal reflux. J Pediatr 96:321, 1980.
Jolley SG, Herbst JJ, Johnson DG, et al: Surgery in children with gastroesophageal reflux and respiratory symptoms. J Pediatr 96:194, 1980.

Rumination

Herbst JJ, Friedland GW, Zboralske FF: Hiatal hernia and "rumination" in infants and children. J Pediatr 78:261, 1971.
Richmond JB, Eddy E, Green M: Rumination: A psychosomatic syndrome of infancy. Pediatrics 22:49, 1958.
Sheagren TG, Mangurten HH, Brea F, et al: Rumination—a new complication of neonatal intensive care. Pediatrics 66:551, 1980.

Achalasia

Azizkhan RG, Tapper D, Eraklis A: Achalasia in childhood: A 20-year experience. J Pediatr Surg 15:452, 1980.
Berquist WE, Byrne WJ, Ament ME, et al: Achalasia: Diagnosis, management, and clinical course in 16 children. Pediatrics 71:798, 1983.

Swallowing and Dysphagia

Illingworth RS: Sucking and swallowing difficulties in infancy: Diagnostic problems of dysphagia. Arch Dis Child 44:655, 1969.
Utian HL, Thomas RG: Cricopharyngeal incoordination in infancy. Pediatrics 43:402, 1969.
Wolff PH: The serial organization of sucking in the young infant. Pediatrics 42:943, 1968.

Corrosive Esophagitis

Hollinger PH: Management of esophageal lesions caused by chemical burns. Ann Otolaryngol 77:819, 1968.
Viscomi GJ, Beekhuis GJ, Whitten CF: An evaluation of early esophagoscopy and corticosteroid therapy in the management of corrosive injury of the esophagus. J Pediatr 59:356, 1961.

Foreign Bodies

Brown LP: Blind esophageal coin removal using a Foley catheter. Arch Surg 96:931, 1968.
O'Neill JA Jr, Holcomb GW Jr, Neblett WW: Management of tracheobronchial and esophageal foreign bodies in childhood. J Pediatr Surg 18:475, 1983.

THE STOMACH AND INTESTINES

12.26 NORMAL DEVELOPMENT, STRUCTURE, AND FUNCTION OF THE STOMACH AND INTESTINES

Development. In gross and microscopic structure the gut matures relatively early in fetal life. In the 4 wk, 3 mm embryo, the primitive fore- and hindgut form a simple tube which rotates counterclockwise around the umbilical artery as the stomach and cecum become distinct. The tube then elongates quickly and protrudes into the umbilical cord. At 8 wk the caudal end becomes continuous with the rectum which has evolved from the cloaca, and at 10 wk the bowel rapidly re-enters the abdomen. Later, the colon achieves its mature conformation. Most structural anomalies are attributable to delay or aberration in this complex series of events.

The pyloric musculature of the stomach is seen by the 3rd mo of gestation, and parietal and chief cells appear by 14 wk. Intestinal-type cells found in the gastric mucosa gradually disappear during fetal life. Relatively mature villi are seen along the intestine by 12 wk, and by 20 wk the crypts are deep and the enterocytes columnar with some microvilli. Blood vessels and the nerve supply to the gut are fully developed by 12-13 wk. Intramural ganglia appear first at the fore end so that if their development is interrupted, the effect will be seen in the distal regions. Peristalsis has been recognized as early as 8 wk, but motility is usually not fully coordinated until near term. Lymphoid tissue has developed by 20 wk.

The gastrointestinal tract of the smallest premature baby appears relatively mature. Some functions develop relatively early in the fetal gut; others mature in postnatal life. For example, gastric acid secretion increases dramatically in the first 24 hr after birth; acid and pepsin secretion peak during the first 10 days and decrease from 10–30 days. Intrinsic factor secretion rises slowly during the first 2 wk of life, but at term circulating gastrin levels are inexplicably 2- to 3-fold higher than in adults.

Small intestinal function also matures during pre- and postnatal life. Epithelial glucose transport is detectable in the jejunum of the human embryo by 20 wk, but adult capacity may not be achieved for years. Disaccharidase activities are measurable in the human fetus at 12 wk; sucrase and maltase achieve maximal activities by the 24th and 32nd wk, respectively; but lactase activity rises later, reaching maximal fetal levels by 36 wk. In many children, particularly of black and oriental races, intestinal lactase activity begins to decline by 3 yr of age. Fetal intestine is involved in the daily turnover of a large amount of amniotic fluid, and there is significant activity of the Na pump in 10 wk old human fetal gut. Solute transport is probably adequate but marginal in premature infants and very young infants. Accordingly, relatively severe functional disturbances in response to small intestinal diseases can be anticipated, whereas older children can be expected to have significant reserve function.

Fat absorption is less efficient in term babies than in older children and even less efficient in premature infants than in those at term. An important determinant of these age-related changes is lower bile salt synthesis and transport rates in early life.

The human gut is capable of absorbing antigenically significant quantities of intact protein, particularly during the early weeks of life. The entry of potential protein antigens through the mucosal barrier in early life may play a role in later food- and microbe-induced symptoms.

Normal Structure. The serosal layer of the bowel wall is an extension of the peritoneum that extends distally as far as the rectum. There are two muscle layers, outer longitudinal fibers and inner circular ones; in the colon the longitudinal fibers form bands, or taeniae. The submucosa is a matrix for lymph and vascular plexuses, containing lymphoid cells and macrophages and, in the duodenum, Brunner glands. The mucosa of the small bowel is well designed to absorb nutrients since its absorptive surface has an area similar to that of a tennis court, owing to a multitude of constantly moving villi which extend into the lumen. In children these villi tend to be leaflike rather than finger-shaped projections; thus, the functional surface area of the small intestine probably increases with age. The colonic mucosal surface is flat, with numerous tubular crypts opening into the surface; in the rectum the surface is smooth. The lamina propria, a cellular layer just beneath the epithelium that contains cells capable of phagocytosis and immunoglobulin synthesis, provides a connective tissue core for the epithelium and its vascular supply. Lymphoid tissue is concentrated in Peyer patches, which become more numerous in the distal small bowel. There are four types of epithelial cells in the small intestine: the dominant cell type is the absorptive cell; goblet cells secrete mucus; endocrine cells secrete certain intestinal hormones; and in the crypts there are Paneth cells, whose function is unknown. The columnar absorptive cell is polarized with a microvillus "brush" border at the luminal surface to which a glycocalyx or "fuzz coat" is tightly adherent. Active cell division of the enterocytes occurs in the crypts, and as cells migrate up the villi, they differentiate. The jejunal epithelium is completely renewed in 5–6 days, providing a mechanism for rapid repair after injury; but in the very young infant the process may be slow. The epithelium over Peyer patches is not villous in contour. In some species, specialized "M" cells in the epithelium overlying Peyer patches play an antigen-sampling role, but neither the occurrence nor the function of such cells has been delineated in humans.

Normal Function. The stomach serves as a reservoir that delivers liquefied, blended, but minimally digested food to the intestine. It also secretes intrinsic factor, essential for the assimilation of vitamin B_{12} in the ileum. The small intestine must process not only ingested nutrients but also a large volume of water and shed epithelial cells. In adults the quantity of water entering the gut lumen is at least seven times the amount ingested.

Intraluminal digestion depends largely on the exocrine pancreas. Synthesis and secretion of bicarbonate and digestive enzymes are stimulated by secretin and cholecystokinin, which are released by the upper intestinal mucosa in response to various intraluminal stimuli, among them components of the diet. Digestion is an efficient, fast process, usually completed in the most proximal intestinal segment. Bile salts in the lumen facilitate digestion and are essential for the efficient delivery of products of lipid hydrolysis to the absorptive surface of the epithelium. Emulsification aids digestion, and long chain monoglycerides and fatty acids usually reach the epithelium in the form of mixed micelles with conjugated bile acids and phospholipid. Sterols such as vitamin D are particularly dependent on these micelles for their absorption; accordingly, diseases such as biliary atresia cause particular difficulties with vitamin D assimilation. Medium chain triglycerides available in certain specially designed therapeutic diets, on the other hand, do not require micelles, emulsification, or hydrolysis for their absorption.

Carbohydrate, protein, and fat are normally absorbed by the upper half of the small intestine; the distal segments represent a vast reserve of absorptive capacity. Most of the sodium, potassium, chloride, and water is absorbed in the small bowel. Bile salts and vitamin B_{12} are selectively absorbed in the distal ileum and iron in the duodenum and proximal jejunum.

Disaccharides are hydrolyzed by disaccharidases on the outer surface of the microvillus membranes, and resultant monosaccharides are actively transported across the cell, primarily to portal venous drainage. Dipeptides and probably larger peptides can be hydrolyzed at the brush border surface, but may also enter the cell intact before they contact peptidases. The small bowel has active transport pathways for specific groups of amino acids, similar to those seen in the renal tubule. Monoglycerides and fatty acids enter the epithelium intact; triglycerides are resynthesized, incorporated with phospholipid and lipoprotein into chylomicrons, and released into lymphatics. Medium chain triglycerides may be taken up intact and released into the portal stream. The entry of sodium with a protein carrier into the epithelial cell across the brush border is facilitated by glucose and certain amino acids, but the active Na pump associated with the $Na^+ - K^+ - ATPase$ system is in the basolateral cell membrane.

The colon extracts additional water and ions from the luminal contents in order to render the stools partially or completely solid. Stools can then be stored in the rectum until distention triggers a defecation reflex which, when assisted by voluntary relaxation of the external sphincter, permits evacuation.

J. RICHARD HAMILTON

Grand RJ, Watkins JB, Torti FM: Development of the human gastrointestinal tract; a review. Gastroenterology 79:790, 1976.
Gryboski JD: Gastrointestinal function in the infant and young child. Clin Gastroenterol 6:253, 1976.
Watkins JB: Mechanisms of fat absorption and the development of gastrointestinal function. Pediatr Clin North Am 22:721, 1975.

CONGENITAL AND PERINATAL ANOMALIES OF THE GASTROINTESTINAL TRACT AND INTESTINAL OBSTRUCTION

Many congenital and perinatal anomalies of the gastrointestinal tract may be responsible for partial or complete obstruction. The majority of the obstructions involve the rectum and anus or duodenum; the remainder are predominantly in the small intestine. The important anomalies are:

Pyloric stenosis
Duodenal atresia or stenosis (with or without annular pancreas)
Jejunal or ileal atresia or stenosis
Malrotation with or without volvulus neonatorum
Meconium ileus
Hirschsprung disease (aganglionic megacolon)
Imperforate anus
Duplications and diverticula

12.27 CONGENITAL (INFANTILE) HYPERTROPHIC PYLORIC STENOSIS

Pyloric stenosis affects approximately 1:150 male and 1:750 female infants; some believe it occurs more frequently in first-born male infants. Familial incidence is observed in about 15% of patients, but no specific pattern of inheritance has been established. Multifactorial inheritance is likely.

Etiology. The cause of pyloric stenosis is not known. Favoring a congenital origin are its high concordance in monovular twins, in contrast to binovular twins, and a slight association with hiatal hernia and esophageal atresia. There is probably, however, an undetermined, acquired factor involved in pathogenesis of the lesion. High levels of serum

gastrin have been found in affected infants, but it is not known whether this is a cause or a result of the condition.

Pathology and Pathophysiology. A diffuse hypertrophy and hyperplasia of the smooth muscle narrows the antrum of the stomach to a fine channel that easily becomes obstructed. The antral region is elongated, is thickened to as much as twice its normal size, and is of cartilaginous consistency. The muscular thickening is never confined to the isolated band of circular muscle fiber called the pyloric sphincter; it extends proximally well into the antrum, and ends distally quite abruptly where the duodenum begins. In response to outflow obstruction and vigorous peristalsis the stomach musculature becomes uniformly hypertrophied and dilates. Gastritis with bleeding may occur after prolonged stasis. As a result of vomiting the patient may become dehydrated and develop hypochloremic alkalosis.

Clinical Manifestations. Initially there is only regurgitation or occasional nonprojectile *vomiting*. The onset rarely occurs before 1 wk of age, usually in the 2nd-3rd wk; it is seldom delayed until the 2nd-3rd mo. The vomiting becomes projectile, usually within 1 wk after onset, and generally occurs during or shortly after feeding but at times up to several hours later. In some instances vomiting occurs after each feeding; in others it is intermittent. The infant is hungry and will take another feeding immediately. The vomitus consists only of gastric contents but may be blood-tinged; it is not bile-stained. The stools may become very small and infrequent, depending on the amount of food that reaches the intestinal tract.

Physical examination shows varying degrees of dehydration and lethargy depending on the metabolic state of the infant. Weight loss may occur. In advanced cases the baby may appear moribund and weight may decrease to a level below that at birth. Decreased elasticity of the skin and loss of subcutaneous tissue may occur. The eyes may be sunken and the fat pads of the cheeks lost so that the infant has a wrinkled, "old man" appearance.

Visible peristalsis, proceeding from the left upper quadrant toward the pylorus in the right upper quadrant of the abdomen, is most prominent immediately after feeding or just before vomiting (Fig. 12-12). The infant may appear uncomfortable, but distress is not prominent. Successful palpation of the abdomen requires patience since it depends on a totally relaxed anterior abdominal wall and an empty stomach. Continuous gentle gastric suction with a #10 nasogastric tube while simultaneously feeding the baby warm sugar solution will facilitate palpation of the "tumor." Palpation is best done from the infant's left side, and if the baby has pyloric stenosis, a mass can be felt in the epigastrium to the right of the midline, deep to the right rectus muscle, and under the edge of the liver. The tumor is hard, mobile, and nontender and feels like an acorn or olive; it is often best felt immediately after the baby has vomited. There is no need for barium

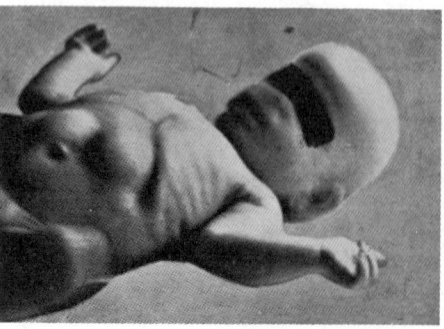

Figure 12–12. Gastric peristaltic waves of pyloric stenosis in an infant 3 wk of age. (Courtesy of Dr. Carl Wagner, Cincinnati.)

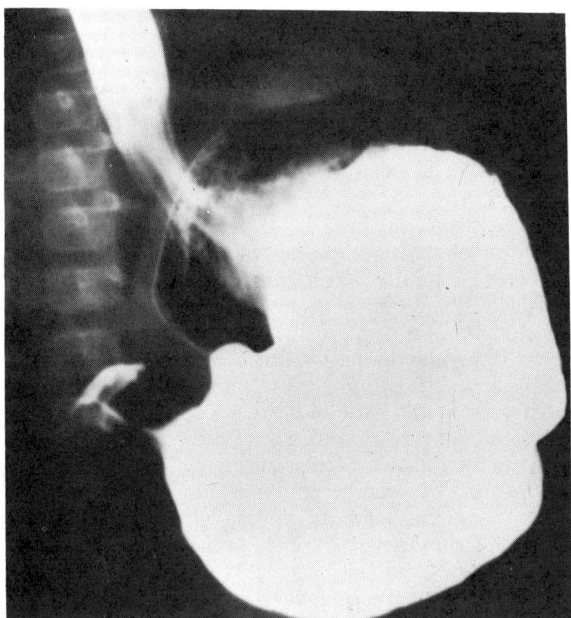

Figure 12–13. Barium in the stomach of an infant with projectile vomiting. The attenuated pyloric canal is typical of congenital hypertrophic pyloric stenosis.

studies once the tumor has been palpated. If the diagnosis of pyloric stenosis cannot be established after several examinations and is still suspected, an ultrasonic examination may be done. Measurements should be made of the diameter, thickness, and length of the pyloric muscle. The diagnosis is essentially a clinical one, confirmed by palpating the mass. No surgeon should undertake to operate for pyloric stenosis unless he or she has personally felt the tumor.

When a barium study is necessary, the appearance of hypertrophic pyloric stenosis is characteristic. There is a vigorously peristaltic stomach with delayed or no gastric emptying, a fine elongated pyloric canal seen as a single ("string sign") or sometimes a double line of barium, and an umbrella-shaped duodenal cap stretched out over the hypertrophied pylorus. Just proximal to the canal a curious diverticulum may be seen (Fig. 12–13).

Two to 9% of affected infants will have jaundice; the hyperbilirubinemia is thought to result from glucuronyl transferase deficiency or an increased enterohepatic circulation of bilirubin. It usually disappears within 72 hr after operative treatment.

Metabolic Alterations. Extensive and protracted vomiting in pyloric stenosis, as in other forms of high intestinal obstruction, may lead to critical deficits of potassium and sodium, which may be reflected by low values in the serum. Much more striking are the decrease in chloride concentration and increases in pH and in carbon dioxide content, which constitute the characteristic serum chemical changes of *hypochloremic alkalosis* (Sec. 5.25). Correction of these chemical changes requires replacement of sodium, chloride, and potassium. Intravenous administration of 5% glucose in isotonic sodium chloride solution, to which potassium chloride is added (to a concentration of 3–5 mEq/dL or 30–50 mEq/L), will gradually and satisfactorily replace the calculated deficits of potassium, chloride, and sodium. This will also avoid the danger of hyponatremia, which may ensue if hypotonic electrolyte solutions are used for replacement of fluid and electrolytes in dehydrated infants who have had protracted vomiting. The intravenous administration of ammonium chloride solution is contraindicated. The serum chloride level, which may vary from nearly normal to as low as 70 mEq/L, may be used as a rough index of potassium deficit; if the serum chloride is normal, the potassium deficit may be minimal and care should be taken not to overload the infant with this ion. Maintenance fluids should be given following correction of dehydration.

Differential Diagnosis. The usual case can be diagnosed by the characteristic clinical pattern and the identification of a pyloric mass. Infants who are exceptionally reactive to external stimuli, those fed by inexperienced or anxious caretakers, or those for whom an adequate maternal-infant bonding relationship has not been established may vomit frequently in the early weeks of life. Such infants may come to resemble infants with pyloric stenosis; the vomiting may be persistent and even projectile. Gastric waves are occasionally visible in small, emaciated infants who do not have pyloric stenosis. Chalasia of the esophagus and hiatal hernia usually result in vomiting in the 1st wk of life and can be differentiated from pyloric stenosis by palpation and roentgenographic studies. Adrenal insufficiency may simulate pyloric stenosis, but the absence of a palpable tumor and the metabolic acidosis and elevated serum potassium and urinary sodium concentrations of adrenal insufficiency aid in differentiation. Vomiting with diarrhea suggests gastroenteritis, but occasionally a patient with pyloric stenosis will have diarrhea. Infrequently, gastroesophageal reflux with or without a hiatal hernia may be confused with pyloric stenosis. Very rarely, a pyloric membrane or pyloric duplication may result in projectile vomiting, visible peristalsis, and, in the case of a duplication, a palpable mass.

Treatment. Surgical relief of the pyloric obstruction as soon as the diagnosis is established and the metabolic imbalances have been corrected is the treatment of choice. Well-hydrated infants without evidence of electrolyte imbalance may be operated on without delay; delays of 24–36 hr for replacement therapy without oral intake are indicated in severely dehydrated infants. At operation, after the stomach has been emptied by catheter, the seromuscular layer of the gastric antrum and pylorus is incised and the muscle split with a blunt instrument, allowing the mucosa to bulge between the split muscle (Fredet-Ramstedt pyloromyotomy). Four to six hours postoperatively, oral feedings are begun in small amounts and increased gradually. An acceptable regimen is to give 4 mL of 5% glucose in saline solution hourly for four feedings. If no vomiting develops, 8 mL is given hourly for the next four feedings; then a 4 hr schedule can be initiated with increasing volumes and formula gradually substituted for clear fluid until normal feedings are achieved, usually within 24–48 hr. We can generally begin normal feedings (formula or breast milk) on the day after the operation and discharge the patient that same day. If the infant is breast fed, it is advisable to place the infant at each breast for 1 min for the first postoperative feeding, thereafter increasing the time on each breast with each subsequent feeding. An alternative regimen is to maintain administration of intravenous fluids postoperatively, giving the infant nothing orally for 24 hr. Full feeding is then started. If vomiting occurs after feedings are begun, oral feedings are withheld for 4 hr, and the regimen is reinstituted from the beginning. Persistence of vomiting beyond the 5th postoperative day suggests an incomplete pyloromyotomy or possibly concomitant hiatal hernia or chalasia; occasional episodes of vomiting are not uncommon after operation, probably as the result of persisting gastritis. During an initial period of small feedings, intravenous administration of fluids is often required, depending on the fluid and electrolyte balance of the infant. Complete cessation of vomiting is the rule after operation, even though postoperative roentgenographic studies have shown that the pyloric canal may remain narrow for many mo in the asymptomatic infant. Hospitalization is not usually required beyond 48 hr postoperatively.

Nonsurgical Treatment. The slowness of improvement (2–8 mo), the higher mortality, and the current high cost and probable adverse effect on emotional development of prolonged hospitalization have led to a virtual abandonment of nonsurgical treatment for pyloric stenosis. If, for some reason, medical rather than surgical management is necessary, slow improvement will usually take place on a regimen of small, frequent feedings thickened with cereal, maintenance of a semi-upright position for 1 hr or so after feedings, sedation, administration of a cholinergic blocking agent, and parenteral administration of fluids as required. When there is epigastric distention before a feeding, emptying of the stomach by lavage may decrease the chance of vomiting.

Prognosis. When the diagnosis is made early in the course of the disease and the infant is properly prepared for operation, the operative mortality is less than 1%. Medical therapy has a higher mortality. Severe and prolonged undernutrition may have an untoward effect on subsequent development.

12.28 CONGENITAL INTESTINAL OBSTRUCTION

General Considerations. Intestinal obstruction occurs in approximately 1:1500 newborn infants. The cardinal signs are vomiting, abdominal distention, and failure to pass feces. Since a number of days may go by prior to full certainty that the infant has an obstructive lesion, early diagnosis depends on appreciation of the significance of vomiting and distention. *High intestinal obstruction* is characterized by vomiting, which tends to be persistent even when feedings have been stopped; distention may be absent. *Low obstruction* is characterized principally by distention, and vomiting may be only a later manifestation. When the obstruction is in the duodenum, symptoms may become manifest within a few hours; if it is in the large intestine, symptoms may be delayed for more than 24 hr.

From an anatomic standpoint congenital obstructive lesions of the intestines can be viewed as *intrinsic* (e.g., atresia, stenosis, meconium ileus, and aganglionic megacolon) or *extrinsic* (e.g., malrotation, constricting bands, intra-abdominal hernias, and duplications). An attempt should be made to locate the lesion preoperatively in order to guide the surgical approach.

When the obstruction is *complete*, there should be little difficulty in clinical recognition, but when it is *incomplete*, there may be considerable difficulty. Polyhydramnios is frequently an accompaniment of high intestinal obstruction, as it is of esophageal atresia. When polyhydramnios has been noted, the infant's stomach should be aspirated immediately after birth. Aspiration of 10–15 mL or more of gastric fluid, especially if it is bile-stained, is suggestive of a high intestinal obstruction.

Meconium stools may be passed initially if the obstruction is in the upper part of the small intestine.

Obstruction in the duodenum may cause epigastric distention and, at times, gastric waves similar to those of pyloric stenosis. The distention may not be persistent, however, since it may be relieved by vomiting. The vomiting may be projectile, and the vomitus will contain bile if the obstruction is below the ampulla of Vater, as it usually is.

Obstructions in the lower ileum, colon, or rectum cause more generalized distention, often with bulging of the flanks. When liver dullness is obliterated, there is a strong possibility that intestinal perforation has occurred. Onset of vomiting with lower bowel obstruction may be delayed a day. It may eventually become feculent.

When obstruction is *incomplete* (as, for example, with intestinal stenosis, constricting bands, duplications, and incomplete volvulus), signs (vomiting, abdominal distention, obsti-

pation) may appear shortly after birth or may be delayed an indeterminate time. They may approach in severity those of a completely obstructive lesion, or they may be sufficiently mild and infrequent as to be overlooked until either an acute episode or diagnostic studies disclose the lesion. Incomplete obstruction may present as urgent a need as complete obstruction for surgical intervention.

Valuable information on the location of congenital obstructive lesions in the intestine may often be obtained from flat and upright roentgenograms of the abdomen taken without use of contrast media. With completely obstructive lesions there will be distention of the bowel above the obstruction, and there may be a series of fluid levels with superimposed gas in the distended loops. Pneumoperitoneum may be seen, with free air in the subphrenic regions. Calcification within the peritoneal cavity will indicate meconium peritonitis. A characteristic "ground glass" appearance in the right lower quadrant with trapped bubbles of air within the obstructing meconium may be seen in patients with meconium ileus. A study of the colon with an enema containing radiopaque material may provide additional localizing information, especially in respect to the possibility of a misplaced cecum with malrotation of the intestine. Hirschsprung disease may be noted. Air is usually demonstrable roentgenographically in the stomach of the normal infant immediately after birth; within 1 hr air may reach the proximal portion of the small intestine and segments of the colon; air may become visible in the distal parts of the colon as early as the 3rd hr or as late as 18 hr.

Prognosis. If a complete obstruction is not relieved promptly, the clinical course progresses rapidly. Vomiting is persistent; dehydration, loss of weight, and prostration become severe, and the infant dies within a few days. When the obstruction is not complete, the infant may survive for weeks; minor obstructions may be compatible with life even without treatment. Recovery from both complete and incomplete obstructions can be expected in many instances with early diagnosis and appropriate management.

Treatment. Not every obstructive lesion is amenable to surgery, but infants can withstand massive resection of the small intestine when the lesion necessitates it. Preoperative preparation (including constant gastric aspiration) and postoperative care are of critical importance, especially in respect to correction of dehydration and electrolyte deficits and to the maintenance of fluid balance and nutrition by parenteral means (Sec. 5.31 and 8.17).

ATRESIA AND STENOSIS

Atresia (complete occlusion) and, less commonly, *stenosis* (partial occlusion) account for about one third of cases of intestinal obstruction. The obstructive lesion (excluding anorectal lesions) is more frequently in the ileum (50%) and duodenum (25%), less frequently in the jejunum, rarely in the colon, and almost never in the stomach. Infants with Down syndrome have an increased incidence of duodenal atresia and of imperforate anus. About 15% of intestinal atresias are multiple. The types of atresia are (1) a diaphragm-like occlusion of the lumen, (2) a blind end not in continuity with a distal segment, and (3) segments of bowel with cord-like connections.

12.29 CONGENITAL DUODENAL OBSTRUCTION

Etiology. Delayed vacuolization of the embryonic intestinal lumen is thought to account both for mucosal diaphragms within the duodenum and for duodenal atresia. Atresia may also be caused by vascular insufficiency.

Pathology. The atretic duodenum usually ends blindly just distal to the ampulla of Vater. Twenty to thirty per cent of affected infants have Down syndrome, and in 20% the common bile duct drains into the bowel beyond the site of atresia. Rarely, bile enters the bowel both proximal and distal to the site of the obstruction, especially when a duodenal diaphragm is present. After atresia, the second most common cause of congenital deodenal obstruction is incomplete rotation of the midgut, with the duodenum becoming obstructed by the misplaced peritoneal reflections of the preduodenal cecum. Volvulus neonatorum is a serious complication of malrotation and requires prompt relief. An annular pancreas, encircling the second portion of the duodenum, may compress and obstruct it partially or completely; this condition is almost always associated with an underlying duodenal stenosis. A **duodenal web,** mucosal diaphragm, or "windsock" may coexist with malrotation and should always be sought. Rarely, a preduodenal portal vein may compress and obstruct the anterior wall of the first part of the duodenum.

Clinical Manifestations. Vomiting of bile-stained material may occur shortly after birth or be delayed, especially with incomplete obstruction. Early, the epigastrium may be full with peristalsis observed, though there may be no abdominal distention. Down syndrome may be present, or a history of maternal hydramnios may be obtained. With prolonged vomiting a metabolic alkalosis with dehydration and electrolyte imbalance ensues. If the duodenum is atretic proximal to the ampulla of Vater, the vomitus will not contain bile. Any incomplete duodenal obstruction may result in the onset of symptoms beyond the neonatal period. Thus, a patient with duodenal stenosis may remain well for several mo, and

chronic duodenal ileus associated with malrotation may become evident even later.

Diagnosis. The diagnosis of duodenal obstruction may be made by studying the air pattern in supine and erect roentgenograms of the abdomen. Classically, a "double bubble" will be seen on the upright film as the air in the stomach and the distended duodenum rises to the top of each viscus and forms level lines at the fluid-air interfaces (Fig. 12–14), with contained gastric fluid and duodenal contents. With complete atresia no gas will be seen in the rest of the abdomen. A similar appearance may occur with malrotation, annular pancreas, and severe duodenal stenosis. If there is roentgenographic evidence of duodenal obstruction, a barium enema should be done as an emergency to determine whether a malrotation is present. If the cecum is undescended, it must be assumed that the duodenal obstruction is due to Ladd bands in association with malrotation and that volvulus neonatorum of the entire midgut may coexist.

Treatment. In duodenal atresia or stenosis the surgical procedures of choice are duodenoduodenostomy or duodenojejunostomy to bypass the obstruction. If obstruction is due to Ladd bands with malrotation, operation is necessary without delay. After division of the abnormal peritoneal folds or bands, the entire large intestine is placed within the left abdomen, with the small bowel on the right—the fetal position of nonrotation. Malrotation may also coexist with an intrinsic duodenal obstruction, such as a membrane or stenosis; this may be identified by passing a nasogastric balloon-tipped catheter into the jejunum below the site of obstruction, inflating the balloon, and slowly withdrawing the catheter. Annular pancreas is best treated by duodenoduodenostomy without dividing the pancreas, leaving as short a defunctioned loop as possible. Duodenal diaphragmatic obstruction is managed by duodenoplasty. The possibility exists that the common bile duct may open on the diaphragm itself.

12.30 ANOMALIES OF ROTATION
(Malrotation)

Incomplete rotation, or *malrotation of the intestine,* represents a failure of embryonic or fetal bowel to rotate to its normal position. The normal sequence is: (1) the cecum rotates around the superior mesenteric artery (which acts as an axis) counterclockwise from a position in the middle of the abdomen, below the stomach; (2) the colon, which lies on the left side of the abdomen, follows the cecum into the right upper quadrant and finally into the right lower quadrant; (3) when rotation is completed, the ascending and descending mesocolons fuse with the back of the abdomen, anchoring the mesentery from the ligament of Treitz obliquely downward to the cecal area. In some instances of complete rotation, fusion of the mesentery remains incomplete so that there is abnormal mobility of the midgut and colon.

Most often in malrotation the cecum fails to move into the right lower quadrant, and the bands fixing it to the posterior abdominal wall cross over and may obstruct the duodenum (Fig. 12–15). The narrow mesenteric stalk which suspends the small intestine in the area of the superior mesenteric vessels is liable to volvulus, resulting in intermittent or acute obstruction that may progress to strangulation. Obstruction occurs first at the duodenum, then at the lower end of the loop. *Volvulus* accounts for more than half of operations for intestinal obstruction in patients with the cecum in the right upper portion of the abdomen. This problem usually presents symptoms of acute or recurrent intestinal obstruction at birth or in the 1st yr of life. Occasionally, a child with malrotation presents the clinical picture of malabsorption, with relief following surgical repair. Nonrotation is associated with midgut volvulus, gastroschisis, omphaloceles, and hernias

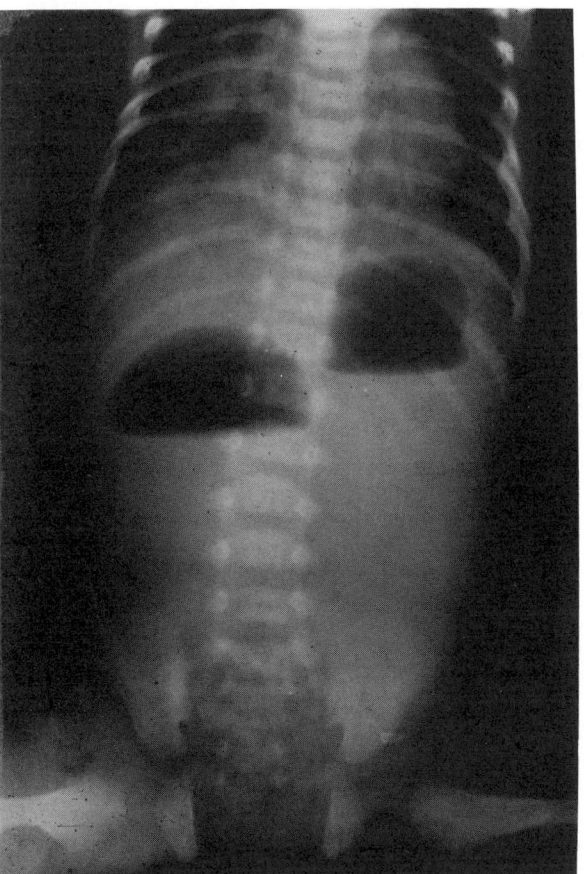

Figure 12–14. Abdominal roentgenogram of a newborn infant held upright. Note the "double bubble" gas shadow above and the absence of gas in the distal bowel in this case of congenital duodenal atresia.

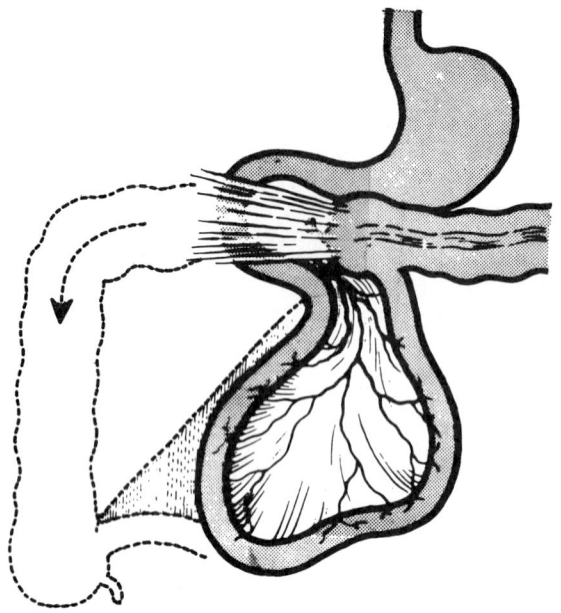

Figure 12–15. The mechanism of intestinal obstruction with incomplete rotation of the midgut (malrotation). The dotted lines show the course the cecum should have taken. Failure to rotate has left obstructing bands across the duodenum, and a narrow pedicle for the midgut loop, making it prone to volvulus. (From Nixon HH, O'Donnell B: The Essentials of Pediatric Surgery. Philadelphia, JB Lippincott, 1961.)

through the foramen of Bochdalek. Malrotation may be present with annular pancreas or with congenital atresia or stenosis of the duodenum.

Roentgenograms of the abdomen may show an abnormal colonic gas pattern, and barium enema confirms the abnormal position of the cecum. An upper gastrointestinal roentgenogram may show the ligament of Treitz to be shifted to the right. In acute obstruction, diagnosis occurs at laparotomy, and only an upright film of the abdomen is taken in order to disclose the gas and fluid shadows.

Management includes fluid therapy to combat shock and disturbance of body fluids and electrolytes, followed by laparotomy, at which the volvulus is unwound, transduodenal bands are divided, and the large intestine is straightened and placed in the left side of the abdomen with all the small bowel on the right.

12.31 JEJUNAL OR ILEAL OBSTRUCTION

These obstructions may result from atresia or stenosis, meconium ileus, Hirschsprung disease, intussusception, Meckel diverticulum, intestinal duplication, or strangulated hernia.

Pathology. The bowel in *ileal* or *jejunal atresia* ends blindly proximal and distal to an interruption in its continuity; there may even be a gap in the mesentery. With stenotic or "windsock" obstructions the bowel and mesentery are in continuity. The large size of the proximal obstructed loop of bowel contrasts greatly with that of the collapsed distal bowel. Rarely, atretic segments are multiple; this form has a familial incidence. Atresias, including reabsorption of gangrenous bowel, have been experimentally produced by intrauterine ligation of mesenteric vessels of fetal bowel.

Meconium ileus occurs in newborn infants with cystic fibrosis, but less than 10% of patients with the latter develop meconium ileus. The last 20–30 cm of ileum are collapsed and filled with pellets of pale-colored stool, above which a dilated loop of varying length appears obstructed by meconium with the consistency of thick syrup or glue. Peristalsis fails to propel this very viscid material forward, so that it becomes

impacted in the ileum. Volvulus, atresia, or perforation of the bowel may accompany meconium ileus. Perforation in utero produces meconium peritonitis. Intraperitoneal meconium can cause dense adhesions leading postnatally to adhesive intestinal obstruction and may rapidly become calcified.

In 3% of patients with *Hirschsprung disease* the aganglionic segment involves not only the entire colon but also terminal ileum. This condition causes a dilated small intestine with ganglionated but somewhat hypertrophied walls, a funnel-shaped transitional hypoganglionic zone, and a collapsed distal aganglionic bowel.

Clinical Manifestations. A history of hydramnios may be elicited with high jejunal atresias. In fibrocystic disease there may be a familial incidence. The obstructed patient may be born with abdominal distention from loops of meconium-filled bowel, or obstruction may develop shortly after birth and progress as the result of swallowed air. Distention often results from meconium peritonitis due to intrauterine perforation and leakage of meconium into the peritoneal cavity. The site of perforation usually seals in utero so that operative intervention after birth is seldom necessary, but if the perforation is still patent, increasing abdominal distention with free intraperitoneal air develops after birth, and an operation may be required. Vomiting may occur early, with bilirubin-stained vomitus. Infants with ileal or jejunal atresia may pass several surprisingly large meconium stools; with meconium ileus there is usually no stool. Pneumoperitoneum should be suspected if abdominal distention increases rapidly within the first 24 hr of life, if the liver is less dull to percussion, or if free fluid is evident within the abdomen.

Diagnosis. In meconium ileus plain films of the abdomen show a typical hazy or "ground glass" appearance in the right lower quadrant. Small bubbles of gas trapped in meconium are dispersed within this area. Furthermore, owing to their viscid contents, moderately dilated loops of bowel do not have the fluid levels usually seen roentgenographically on the erect projection. If there is meconium peritonitis, patchy calcification may be noted, usually in the flanks. Pneumoperitoneum is most readily seen as free air between liver and diaphragm on an upright roentgenogram of the abdomen; if there is a large amount of free air, the entire abdomen may look like a football from distention with air; the ligamentum teres is sometimes clearly visible in the midline.

It is impossible to distinguish consistently small bowel from large bowel by studying plain roentgenograms of the abdomen in newborn babies and infants. If plain roentgenograms are nonspecific, a barium or Gastrografin study of the colon may be needed to distinguish small from large intestine obstructions. A small colon, "microcolon," suggests disuse and the presence of obstruction proximal to the ileocecal valve. Gastrografin enemas should be used with caution in the diagnosis and treatment of meconium ileus because their hyperosmolality may result in dehydration and undue pressure may result in perforation.

Treatment. Patients with small bowel obstruction should be stable and in adequate fluid and electrolyte balance before operation or roentgenographic attempts at disimpaction unless volvulus is suspected. Infections should be treated with appropriate antibiotics. Prophylactic use of antibiotics is indicated.

Ileal or jejunal atresia requires resection of the dilated proximal portion of the bowel, followed by end-to-end anastomosis. If a simple mucosal diaphragm is present, jejuno- or ileoplasty with partial excision of the web is an acceptable alternative to resection. With meconium ileus, an attempt to reduce obstruction with a Gastrografin enema is usually indicated. The material should be allowed to flow around the pellets of stool in the terminal ileum and into the dilated proximal small bowel containing the obstructing meconium, where it will result in an outpouring of fluid from the bowel wall, dilution of the viscid meconium, and diarrhea. The enema may have to be repeated after 8–12 hr. Resection after reduction is not needed if there have been no ischemic complications.

About 50% of patients with meconium ileus do not adequately respond to Gastrografin enemas and will need laparotomy. A simple small ileotomy is done within a purse-string suture just large enough to allow the insertion of a #10 or #12 French catheter. The catheter is used to irrigate and remove the viscid contents of the bowel, using acetylcysteine as a mucolytic agent in concentrations of less than 5%. Once the contents have been aspirated, the purse-string suture is tied and a small drain placed near the ileostomy, making resections and anastomoses unnecessary.

At laparotomy for pneumoperitoneum colostomy or ileostomy may be needed at the site of perforation; if the perforation is of the stomach, duodenum, or upper jejunum, primary closure is preferred. Total parenteral nutrition may be required.

12.32 CONGENITAL MEGACOLON
(Hirschsprung Disease)

This is the most common cause of neonatal obstruction of the colon and accounts for about 33% of all neonatal obstructions. It is rare in premature infants. Occasionally there is a familial incidence. *Atresia* of the colon is extremely rare.

Etiology. There may be failure of migration of cells of the embryonic neural crest into the bowel wall or failure of craniocaudal extension of the myenteric and submucous plexuses within the wall.

Pathology. This disease results from absence of ganglion cells in the bowel wall, extending proximally from the anus for a variable distance. The aganglionic segment is limited to the rectosigmoid in 80% of patients; in 15% the colon is aganglionic from anus to hepatic flexure; and in 3% the entire colon lacks ganglion cells.

Incomplete parasympathetic innervation in the aganglionic segment of bowel results in abnormal peristalsis, constipation, and a functional intestinal obstruction. Proximal to the transition zone between normally and abnormally innervated bowel, muscular hypertrophy thickens the intestinal wall, and the intestine may become enormously dilated with retained feces and gas.

Clinical Manifestations. Early symptoms of megacolon range from complete acute neonatal obstruction to chronic constipation in the older child; sometimes there is diarrhea. There is often failure to thrive.

In newborn infants signs may be noted early, with failure to pass meconium, or may appear during the 1st wk and be those of partial or complete intestinal obstruction, with vomiting, abdominal distention, and failure to pass stools. Temporary relief of symptoms may occur after a rectal examination, which is characteristically followed by an explosive discharge of feces and gas. Bile-stained and even feculent vomiting may occur, and the infant may lose weight and become dehydrated. Diarrhea may be a prominent symptom in the neonatal period and be associated with symptoms of intestinal obstruction. Hypoproteinemia and edema may result from protein-losing enteropathy.

Episodes of constipation and diarrhea may alternate with periods of apparent normality. The diarrhea may develop into a fulminant **enterocolitis,** causing a profound dehydration and shock with fluid and electrolyte loss into the lumen of the obstructed bowel. This complication seems to be precipitated by gaseous and fecal colonic distention. *Clostridium difficile* has been implicated in the etiology. Unless energetically treated the condition tends to recur and may be fatal within 24 hr.

Hirschsprung disease in the older child causes chronic constipation and abdominal distention. The history often reveals increasing difficulty with the passage of stools, starting in the 1st few wk of life. A large fecal mass is palpable in the left lower abdomen, but on rectal examination the rectum is usually empty of feces. The stools, when passed, may consist of small pellets, be ribbon-like, or have a fluid consistency; the large stools and fecal soiling of patients with functional constipation are absent. In mild cases the nutrition may not be greatly disturbed; in severe cases there is likely to be loss of subcutaneous tissue and failure to grow. The wasted extremities and large, protruding abdomen of such patients create a typical appearance, which may be confused with that of the *malabsorption syndromes* (Sec. 12.49), especially when diarrhea is present. Hypochromic anemia may be present. Intermittent attacks of intestinal obstruction from retained feces may be associated with pain and fever.

Rarely (in ultrashort-segment Hirschsprung disease) the aganglionosis is confined to the internal anal sphincter and immediately adjacent anal canal and rectum. Affected patients may have encopresis, and unless a particularly low biopsy is done, ganglion cells may be found and the patient presumed to be normal.

Hirschsprung disease must be distinguished from the more common acquired megacolon (Fig. 12–16) of colonic inertia, chronic idiopathic constipation, obstipation, and so on (Table 12–5). Immature left colon syndrome (Sec. 8.56) may mimic Hirschsprung disease.

Diagnosis. A rectal biopsy by the punch or suction method that finds ganglion cells absent in the submucosa and intermuscular nerve plexuses with or without increased numbers of nerve fibers, is the only conclusive means of diagnosing megacolon. Because ganglion cells normally diminish in number in the more distal rectum and anal canal, biopsies should

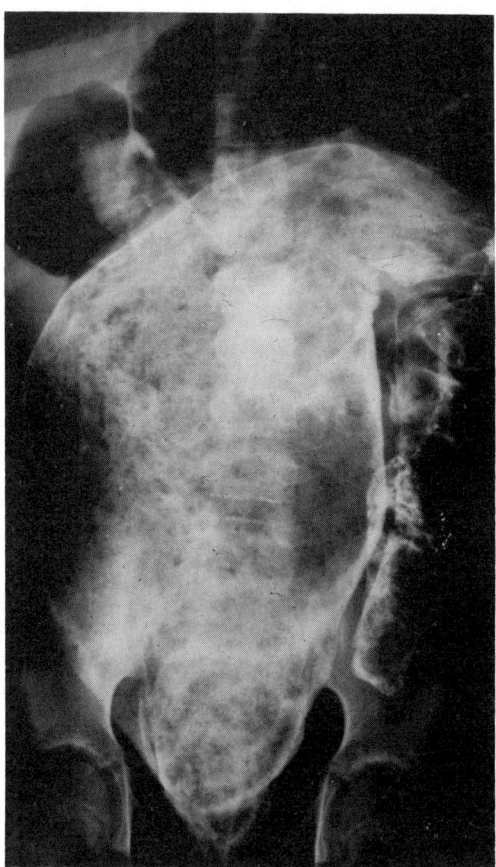

Figure 12–16. Barium enema in a 14 yr old boy with severe constipation. The enormous dilatation of rectum and distal colon is typical of acquired megacolon.

Table 12–5. Comparative Characteristics of Acquired Megacolon and Hirschsprung Disease

	Hirschsprung Disease	Acquired Megacolon
History		
From birth	Always	Never
Enterocolitis	Possible	None
Rectal bleeding	None	Possible
Coercive bowel training	Absent	Usually present
Encopresis (fecal soiling)	Never	Always
Size of stool	Normal, small	Huge
Examination		
Malnutrition	Possible	Absent
Abdominal distention + wide subcostal angle	Usual	Absent
Feces palpable abdominally	Usually	Often
Anal fissure	Never	Possible
Anal tone	Tight	Patulous
Feces in ampulla	Never	Packed with stool
Barium Enema		
Empty segment of rectum	Usually	Absent
Fecaloma in rectal ampulla	Absent	Always present
Delay in evacuation of barium	Usually	Absent
Biopsy		
Ganglion cells in plexuses	Absent	Present

Note: Ultrashort-segment Hirschsprung disease may have clinical features of acquired megacolon.

be taken no closer than 2 cm to the pectinate line. Nerve fibers in the bowel wall in Hirschsprung disease contain increased amounts of acetylcholinesterase; histochemical examination may facilitate interpretation of the biopsy.

Roentgenographic studies in the young infant with intestinal obstruction due to aganglionic megacolon show dilated loops of bowel throughout the abdomen on anteroposterior films taken in the erect position. In lateral erect films, rectal air, which is normally visible in the presacral area, is absent. The diagnostic findings on barium enema are (1) an abrupt change in caliber between the ganglionic and aganglionic sections of bowel (Fig. 12–17); (2) irregular "sawtooth" contractions of the aganglionic segment; (3) parallel transverse folds in the dilated proximal colon; (4) a thickened, nodular, edematous proximal colon associated with protein-losing enteropathy; and (5) failure to evacuate the barium. In infants a small amount of contrast material should be injected slowly through a small catheter, the tip of which is inserted barely beyond the anal sphincter while the patient, in an oblique position, is being observed under the fluoroscope; the characteristic abrupt transition in caliber may be missed if too much barium is used.

In the newborn infant with intestinal obstruction due to megacolon a barium enema will not always show the classic features as there may not have been time for the disparity in size to develop between the proximal colon and the distal aganglionic bowel. The roentgenographic appearances are even less typical when the entire colon lacks ganglion cells, though evacuation of the barium from the colon is usually delayed on a 24 hr roentgenogram.

Anorectal manometry, measured by distention of a balloon placed within the rectal ampulla, shows a fall of pressure in the internal anal sphincter in normal individuals but a striking rise in pressure in patients with megacolon. The accuracy of this diagnostic test is over 90% except in the neonate, in whom the test is less reliable.

In the older child the diagnosis will usually be made by the history of constipation since birth and the finding of an empty rectum. Confirmation is obtained on results of the barium enema (Fig. 12–17) and anal manometry. The roentgenographic appearance of megacolon may be misleading, however, either in terms of diagnosis or level of aganglionosis. In a suspected case, it is important not to cleanse the bowel prior to a barium enema so that the disparity in size between the ganglionic and aganglionic bowel is readily apparent.

Treatment. Once the diagnosis is unequivocally established in a neonate, operation is indicated. It is preferable to do a limited laparotomy with multiple biopsies, placing a colostomy in the most distal portion of normally ganglionated colon. Some surgeons perform a right transverse colostomy in the newborn without multiple biopsies, which is adequate for the usual case in which the aganglionic segment extends up to the rectosigmoid junction. If, however, the transition zone is at or proximal to the splenic flexure, then such a colostomy may need to be revised to bring the transverse colon down to the anus, thus avoiding excision of the intervening colon. Several excellent disposable infant stoma appliances are available to facilitate the management of the infant with a colostomy.

Attempts to postpone surgery by repeated colonic irrigations until the infant reaches a satisfactory size are not justified

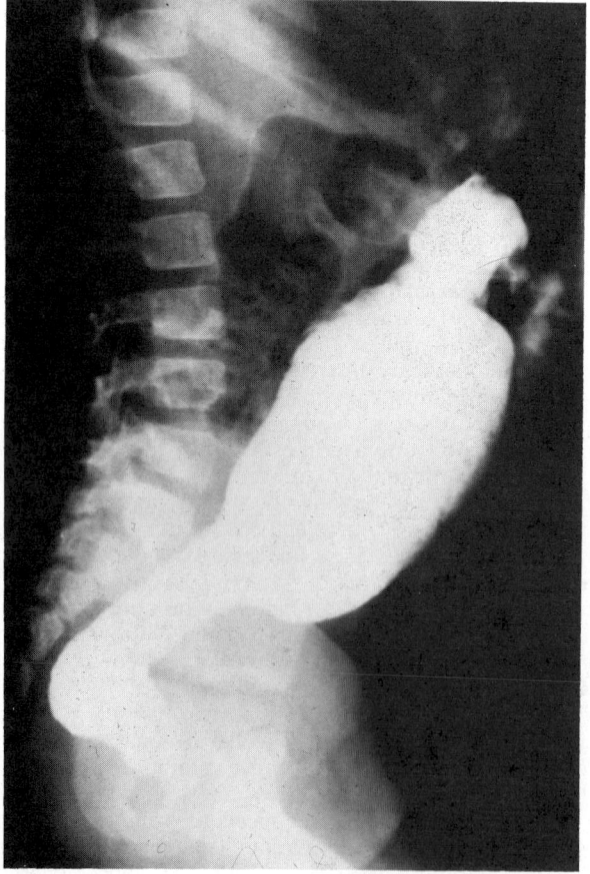

Figure 12–17. Lateral view of barium enema in a 3 yr old girl with Hirschsprung disease. The aganglionic distal segment is narrow with distended normal ganglionic bowel above it.

because of the risk of enterocolitis. With early colostomy the mortality from enterocolitis is 4%, in contrast to 33% if colostomy is done after the onset of enterocolitis.

When the infant is 6–12 mo of age a definitive pull-through operation is done using the Swenson, Duhamel, or modified Soave procedure. Surgical management consists of excising the aganglionic segment, and pulling the ganglionic intestine down through the anus anastomosing it to the anal canal within 2.5 cm of the pectinate line.

In most older children a preliminary colostomy is also advisable, with its closure after the later Swenson or Duhamel types of operation.

Ultrashort-Segmental Hirschsprung Disease. If the aganglionic segment is so short as to give rise to a clinical and roentgenographic picture almost indistinguishable from acquired megacolon, major surgery is unnecessary. Excision of a strip of internal anal sphincter (internal anal myectomy) is all that is usually required if nonoperative management is unsuccessful.

Total Colon Aganglionosis. When the entire colon is aganglionic, often together with a length of terminal ileum, ileal-anal anastomosis is the treatment of choice, preserving the aganglionic colon to facilitate water absorption, which helps the stools to become firm.

Prognosis. Results of treatment of Hirschsprung disease are generally satisfactory, with a great majority of patients achieving fecal continence. Because most cases are diagnosed and treated in the neonatal period, immediate postoperative continence is impossible to assess. Toilet training is usually delayed, and for several yr intermittent incontinence with diarrhea may occur, but with time most children become continent. Loperamide is useful in the management of diarrhea.

12.33 INTESTINAL PSEUDO-OBSTRUCTION

In this recently recognized condition, an apparent ileus causes intestinal obstruction. Cases occur sporadically and sometimes in families; the cause is unknown. The variability in clinical and pathologic patterns suggests that the syndrome may have several etiologies. In some cases, microscopy of the affected bowel has shown smooth muscle degeneration, in others neuropathic changes, and in still others, no abnormality.

In its severe form, the disorder begins in utero, causing fetal abdominal distention and maternal polyhydramnios. After birth, the distention, a silent abdomen, vomiting, and a failure to pass meconium are observed. When the disorder begins in infancy, there is often urinary stasis and retention. Symptoms can begin later in life, but this usually occurs before the age of 10 yr. By then, abdominal pain and malabsorption are usually noted.

The differential diagnosis in infants includes mechanical obstruction and Hirschsprung disease. In older children, collagen diseases, diabetic neuropathy, and celiac disease become considerations.

The course is usually chronic and remissions are extremely rare. No pharmacologic agent has been effective. Survival depends on total parenteral nutrition. In infants, surgical procedures to establish urinary drainage are often needed. No other surgical treatment is indicated unless a correctable lesion is identified. Most affected children die within 2 yr from complications related to the stasis in their gut and urinary tract or related to total parenteral nutrition.

12.34 DIVERTICULA AND DUPLICATIONS

These lesions consist of abnormal tissue, usually intestinal, in close relation to a part of the alimentary tract. In many there is ectopic gastric, pancreatic, duodenal, ileal, or colonic mucosa. These congenital anomalies may be due to abnormal formation of a part of an organ or duct or to failure of obliteration of one. If a diverticulum is anywhere but on the antimesenteric border, it is considered a dorsal enteric remnant.

With the exception of a Meckel diverticulum, congenital and acquired single and multiple diverticula of the intestinal tract are extremely rare in children. *Diverticulosis* (multiple outpouchings of the intestinal tract, usually in the colon) and *diverticulitis* (inflammation of diverticula) are essentially diseases of adult life.

Meckel Diverticulum

Two to three per cent of people have a Meckel diverticulum; the most common complication is bleeding. Other complications are rare.

In the embryo the intestine is linked to the yolk sac by the vitellointestinal duct. If this duct does not become completely atretic, it may persist in the form of a Meckel diverticulum. There may also be persistence of a fibrous cord from the Meckel diverticulum to the umbilicus, with cystic structures contained within the cord anywhere between the diverticulum and the peritoneal surface of the umbilicus. If the entire embryonic duct remains patent (persistent omphalomesenteric duct), there will be an enterocutaneous fistula; if the ileal end is closed, there is only mucoid secretion. A fibrous remnant of the vitelline artery may also persist as a band with the potential of causing intestinal obstruction.

Pathology. The Meckel diverticulum is usually 50–75 cm proximal to the ileocecal junction on the antimesenteric side of the intestine. The mucosal lining is the same as that of the adjacent ileum, but in at least 35% there is ectopic gastric or pancreatic tissue near the tip. This ectopic acid- or pepsin-secreting mucosa can cause an ulcer in the adjacent basal portion of the diverticulum or in the ileum to which it is attached. The erosion of the mucosa results in hemorrhage which may be massive. Much less frequently, diverticulitis occurs, usually without demonstrable cause, though rarely a foreign body may be found. Diverticulitis may lead to perforation and fecal peritonitis. Sometimes, the lesion is everted and may become the apex of an ileoileal intussusception. A *Littre hernia* is seen when the Meckel diverticulum is contained within an indirect inguinal hernia. The diverticulum itself may undergo volvulus, or a band attached to it may cause a volvulus of loops of small intestine, leading to gangrene.

Clinical Manifestations. Symptoms and signs from Meckel diverticulum can arise at any age but have peak incidence in the first 2 yr of life.

Painless rectal bleeding is the most common sign in children. There may be periodicity to the bleeding, as with peptic ulcer; usually it is acute, but rarely exsanguinating. Blood is often passed without stool; it is usually dark red, but if bleeding is brisk, it may be bright red. With mild recurrent bleeding iron deficiency anemia may develop that is refractory to iron therapy. Repeatedly positive tests for occult blood in stools of an anemic child suggest Meckel diverticulum.

Abdominal pain, when it occurs, may be acute and due to diverticulitis, with a clinical picture resembling that of acute appendicitis, or it may be vague and recurrent. Referral of the (ileal) pain to the umbilicus may suggest the true diagnosis. Perforation of an ulcer in the diverticulum may lead to peritoneal bleeding or inflammation. A Meckel diverticulum may become the leading point of an intussusception. The signs may also be those of incarcerated hernia, volvulus, appendicitis, or intestinal obstruction. A child (other than a newborn infant) who has intestinal obstruction without having had a previous operation, and who does not have an intussusception, most likely has a Meckel diverticulum or a fibrous remnant.

Diagnosis. In infancy the Meckel diverticulum with ectopic gastric tissue will often produce signs that require rapid and accurate preoperative evaluation. The diverticulum cannot be demonstrated by barium studies, but an accurate preoperative diagnosis is possible, owing to the fact that ^{99m}technetium is excreted by gastric mucosa; a negative ^{99m}Tc scan has a high correlation with absence of a Meckel diverticulum. A patent vitellointestinal duct and its communication with a loop of bowel will be shown by injection of radiopaque material into the fistula. Patients with Meckel diverticulitis may have an incorrect preoperative diagnosis of acute appendicitis, but correct diagnosis and treatment can be carried out at surgery.

Treatment. Excision of the diverticulum is the treatment of choice. If there is a peptic ulcer in the adjacent ileum, it will be necessary to excise the involved bowel together with the diverticulum.

Non-Meckelian Diverticula

These may occur in the duodenum, jejunum, ileum, or colon and are usually incidental roentgenographic or necropsy findings. Rarely, they may result in a clinical problem by causing mechanical pressure, becoming inflamed or ulcerated, or perforating.

Duplications

Dorsal Enteric Remnants

Duplication may result from a failure of normal regression of embryonic diverticula, persistence of transitory intestinal diverticula, median septum formation, errors of recanalization of epithelial plugs, or traction between adhering neural tube ectoderm or notochordal mesoderm and intestinal endoderm. The latter theory would account for the frequent occurrence of a band that extends from the duplicated intestine through the diaphragm and posterior mediastinum, gaining an attachment to the thoracic or cervical spine; this is often associated with vertebral anomalies, such as hemivertebrae or anterior spina bifida.

Pathology. Duplications are saccular or tubular structures, which have a smooth muscle wall and mucous membrane similar to some parts of the gastrointestinal tract. They are found on the mesenteric side of any segment of intestine and vary widely in size and length. Tubular structures vary in length from a few centimeters to duplication of virtually the entire small bowel. Their blood supply is the same as that of the adjacent bowel, precluding selective excision of the duplication. If saccular, the duplication is not lined by gastric mucosa; nor does it communicate with the lumen of normal bowel; thus peptic erosion of the intestine does not occur. The duplication may be so large that the intestine is stretched out over it and thereby obstructed. Less commonly, the duplication forms the apex of an intussusception or volvulus.

Tubular duplications have a gastric mucosal lining and are in communication with the adjacent bowel by one or more foramina. Acid secretion gains ready access to the unprotected normal small bowel and may cause a peptic ulcer, with bleeding or perforation.

Clinical Manifestations. Symptoms and signs usually arise during infancy and early childhood and include (1) obstruction of adjoining intestine by compression; (2) intestinal bleeding from peptic ulceration; (3) pain from secretory distention of a noncommunicating duplication; (4) gangrene of the bowel from obstruction of segmental vasculature; and (5) a movable mass palpated on routine examination of the abdomen. Duplications are most frequent in the ileum, ileocecal region, and esophagus but may occur in any part of the gastrointestinal tract. Duplications in the thorax (neurenteric cysts) are

usually of the esophagus or the stomach and only rarely communicate with either. They produce dysphagia and respiratory symptoms through esophageal and pulmonary compression and are demonstrable roentgenographically. Associated anomalies of vertebrae are common and often are at a higher level than the intrathoracic mass. Some intrathoracic duplications are lined by duodenal or jejunal mucosa.

Roentgenographic studies may show stenosis or compression of the intestinal lumen but more frequently are normal. An intrathoracic duplication is usually visible as a mediastinal mass in roentgenograms of the chest. Very rarely barium studies may fill a communicating duplication. As with Meckel diverticulum, and for the same reason, a ^{99m}Tc scan will demonstrate any ectopic gastric tissue.

Cystic Remnants of the Tail Gut

These lesions are found between the anus and the sacrum or coccyx and may be derivatives of that portion of the primitive archenteron extending caudal to the cloaca. Others consider these lesions to be duplications of the rectum or even teratoma. Symptoms are produced by the presence of a mass, which, if large, may obstruct the rectum. Such lesions must be distinguished from sacrococcygeal teratoma and anterior myelomeningocele.

Bilateral Duplications of Colon and Rectum

Several rare anomalies ("partial twinning") consist of doubling of the alimentary tract from where a Meckel diverticulum would be found down to the anus. There may also be doubling of the vagina or penis and bladder, and even the sacrum and lumbar vertebrae may be doubled.

12.35 ACQUIRED INTESTINAL OBSTRUCTION

Paralytic ileus is a major cause of acquired intestinal obstruction. It may complicate acute infections, electrolyte imbalance, or uremia. Pneumonia and gastroenteritis are probably the most frequent causes in infants, peritonitis (especially as a complication of perforated appendicitis) most frequent in older children. Ileus is likely to present as distention, with absence of bowel sounds and minimal pain.

Incarcerated inguinal hernias, complications related to Meckel diverticulum, and intussusception are the most frequent *mechanical causes* of intestinal obstruction in infants. Intestinal obstruction may also result from postoperative adhesions or those following recovery from acute peritonitis, and from chronic peritonitis, (e.g., tuberculous peritonitis). Other causes are duplications; foreign bodies in the intestine, including fecal concretions and inspissated meconium in the newborn infant; late obstruction by intraluminal contents in cystic fibrosis (pseudomeconium ileus); and masses of roundworms. Tumors of the bowel, including mesenteric cysts and polyps, may also be obstructive. Vomiting and abdominal distention may occur with either mechanical obstruction or ileus; severe colicky periumbilical pain and hyperactive, sometimes tinkling, bowel sounds are almost invariably found in the former.

In infants and children with intestinal obstruction, huge amounts of electrolyte-rich fluid are secreted into the lumen of the bowel. This may lead to severe fluid and electrolyte imbalances and to distention that compromises the circulation of a segment of intestine. With prolonged stasis this fluid becomes secondarily infected, often with putrefactive organisms, and the patient may have feculent vomiting (which should not be confused with true fecal vomiting, such as occurs with gastrocolic fistula or in coprophagy). A palpable distended single ("closed") loop and unexplained fever, leukocytosis, and anemia, together with abdominal tenderness, are ominous signs signifying strangulation. The development of gangrenous intestine may, however, be insidious.

12.36 INTUSSUSCEPTION

Intussusception occurs when a portion of the alimentary tract is telescoped into a segment just caudad to it. It is the most common cause of intestinal obstruction between 3 mo–6 yr of age; it is rare under 3 mo and decreases in frequency after 36 mo. A few intussusceptions reduce spontaneously or become autoamputated; if left untreated, most would lead to death.

Etiology and Epidemiology. The cause of most intussusceptions is unknown. The seasonal incidence has peaks in spring and autumn. Correlation with adenovirus infections has been noted, and the condition may complicate gastroenteritis. It is postulated that swollen Peyer patches in the ileum may stimulate intestinal peristalsis in an attempt to extrude the mass, thus causing an intussusception. At the peak age of incidence of this condition the infant's alimentary tract is also being introduced to a variety of new materials. In about 5% of patients recognizable causes for the intussusception are found, such as everted Meckel diverticulum, an intestinal polyp, duplication, or lymphosarcoma. Uncommonly, the condition will complicate Henoch-Schönlein purpura, with an intramural hematoma acting as the apex of the intussusception. Rarely, intussusception is postoperative, and then always ileoileal.

Pathology. Intussusceptions are most often ileocolic and ileoileocolic, less commonly cecocolic, and rarely exclusively ileal. Very rarely, the appendix forms the apex of an intussusception. The upper portion of bowel, the intussusceptum, invaginates into the lower, the intussuscipiens, dragging its mesentery along with it into the enveloping loop. Constriction of the mesentery obstructs venous return; engorgement of the intussusceptum follows, with edema, and bleeding from the mucosa leads to a bloody stool, sometimes containing mucus. The apex of the intussusception may extend into the transverse, descending, or sigmoid colon—even to the anus in neglected cases. After reduction of an idiopathic intussusception the portion of the bowel that had formed the apex of the intussusceptum is edematous and thickened, often with a dimple on the serosal surface that represents the origin of the lesion. Most intussusceptions do not strangulate the bowel within the first 24 hr but may eventuate in intestinal gangrene and shock.

Clinical Manifestations. In typical cases there is sudden onset, in a previously well child, of severe paroxysmal pain which recurs at frequent intervals and is accompanied by straining efforts and loud cries. Initially, the infant may be comfortable and play normally between the paroxysms of pain, but if the intussusception is not reduced, the infant becomes progressively weaker and lethargic. Eventually a shock-like state may develop, with an elevation of body temperature to as high as 41° C (106° F). The pulse becomes weak and thready, the respirations shallow and grunting, and the pain may be manifested only by moaning sounds. Vomiting occurs in most instances and is usually more frequent early. In the later phase the vomitus becomes bile-stained. Stools of normal appearance may be evacuated during the 1st few hr of symptoms. After this time fecal excretions are small or more often do not occur, and little or no flatus is passed. Blood generally is passed in the first 12 hr, but at times not for 1–2 days and infrequently not at all; 60% of infants will pass a stool containing red blood and mucus, the *currant jelly stool.* Some patients have only irritability and alternating or progressive lethargy.

Palpation of the abdomen usually reveals a slightly tender, sausage-shaped mass, sometimes ill defined, which may in-crease in size and firmness during a paroxysm of pain and is most often in the right upper abdomen, with its long axis cephalocaudal. If it is felt in the epigastrium, the long axis is transverse. About 30% of patients do not have a palpable mass. It is more readily located by bimanual rectal and abdominal palpation between paroxysms of pain. The presence of bloody mucus on the finger as it is withdrawn after rectal examination supports the diagnosis of intussusception. Abdominal distention and tenderness develop as intestinal obstruction becomes more acute. On rare occasions the advancing intestine prolapses through the anus. This prolapse can be distinguished from prolapse of the rectum by the separation between the protruding intestine and the rectal wall, which does not exist in prolapse of the rectum.

Ileoileal intussusception may have a less typical clinical picture, the symptoms and signs being chiefly those of small intestinal obstruction. *Recurrent intussusception* is uncommon. *Chronic intussusception*, in which the symptoms exist in milder form at recurrent intervals, is more likely to occur with or following acute enteritis and may arise in older children as well as in infants.

Diagnosis. The clinical history and physical findings are usually sufficiently typical for diagnosis. Plain abdominal roentgenograms may show a density in the area of the intussusception. A barium enema will show a filling defect or cupping in the head of barium where its advance is obstructed by the intussusceptum (Fig. 12–18). A central linear column of barium may be visible in the compressed lumen of the intussusceptum, and a thin rim of barium may be seen trapped around the invaginating intestine in the folds of mucosa within the intussuscipiens (coil-spring sign), especially after evacuation. Retrogression of the intussusceptum under the pressure of the enema and gaseous distention of the small intestine from obstruction are also useful roentgenographic signs. Ileoileal intussusception is usually not demonstrable by barium enema but is suspected because of gaseous distention of the intestine above the lesion.

Differential Diagnosis. It may be particularly difficult to diagnose intussusception in a child who already has *gastroenteritis*; a change in the pattern of illness, in the character of pain, or in the nature of vomiting, or the onset of rectal

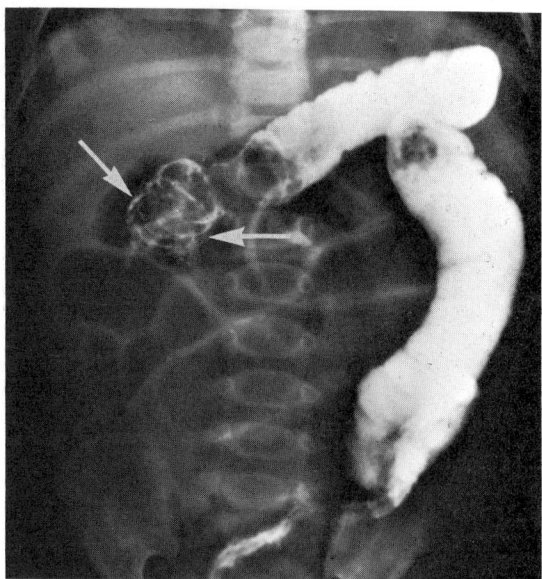

Figure 12–18. Intussusception in an infant. The obstruction is evident in the proximal transverse colon. Contrast material between the intussusceptum and the intussuscipiens is responsible for the coil-spring appearance.

bleeding should alert the physician. The bloody stools and abdominal cramps that accompany *enterocolitis* can usually be differentiated from intussusception because the pain is less severe and less regular, there is diarrhea, and the infant is recognizably ill between pains. Bleeding from *Meckel diverticulum* is usually painless. The intestinal hemorrhage of *anaphylactoid purpura* is usually, but not invariably, accompanied by joint symptoms or purpura elsewhere, and the colicky pain may be similar. Since intussusception may be a complication of this disorder, a barium enema may be required.

Treatment. Reduction of the intussusception is an emergency procedure to be carried out immediately after diagnosis and after rapid preparation for operation with fluids and blood for shock and water and electrolytes to replace losses. In over 75% of cases of short duration, when there are no signs of prostration, shock, or peritoneal irritation, it is possible to reduce the intussusception by hydrostatic pressure under fluoroscopic guidance and with the consultation and close proximity of a surgeon.

A nonlubricated Foley bag catheter is placed in the rectum and inflated. The buttocks are compressed tightly and taped together with adhesive plaster. A barium solution is then allowed to flow by gravity into the colon from a height of not more than 90 cm (3 ft) above the fluoroscopic table. *The abdomen is not touched during the procedure.* The column of barium and the filling defect with it advance slowly together in a proximal direction. Full reduction of the intussusception is manifest by free filling of the small intestine, disappearance of the mass, passage of flatus or feces, and improvement in the infant's condition. If doubt remains as to the completeness of reduction, an exploratory laparotomy is done immediately.

If there is clinical evidence of intestinal obstruction with abdominal distention, especially for 48 hr or longer, hydrostatic reduction of the intussusception should not be attempted because of the risk of perforating the intussuscipiens. In an ileoileal intussusception a barium enema is usually not diagnostic and reduction by the hydrostatic technique may not be possible. Such intussusceptions may develop insidiously as a complication of a laparotomy and require resection. A right-sided transverse paraumbilical or infraumbilical incision gives access to the ascending colon. If manual operative reduction is impossible or the bowel is not viable, resection of the intussusception will be necessary, with end-to-end anastomosis.

Prognosis. Untreated intussusception in infants is nearly always fatal; the chances of recovery are directly related to the duration of intussusception before reduction. The majority of infants will recover if the intussusception is reduced within the first 24 hr, but the mortality rate rises rapidly after this time, especially after the second day. Spontaneous reduction during preparation for operation is not uncommon.

At The Hospital for Sick Children, Toronto, the recurrence rate following barium enema reduction of intussusceptions is about 10%, following surgical reduction about 2–5%; none have recurred after surgical resection. It is unlikely that an intussusception caused by a lesion such as lymphosarcoma, polyp, or everted Meckel diverticulum will be successfully reduced by barium enema. With adequate surgical management, operative reduction carries a very low mortality rate in early cases.

Colonic Polyps

These lesions rarely cause obstruction and only when they constitute the lead point of a colocolic intussusception. Usually, they cause painless rectal bleeding. Consisting largely of granulation tissue and cystic spaces, they normally have relatively narrow pedicles; 80% of colonic polyps in children are single and within reach of a standard sigmoidoscope. There is no record of juvenile polyp becoming malignant. Most disappear spontaneously, presumably undergoing ne-

crosis from twisting of the pedicle. If within reach of the sigmoidoscope, a polyp is easily removed by intussuscepting it out of the anus and excising it. If beyond visualization by sigmoidoscopy, the mucosal lesions can be demonstrated by a double air/barium contrast study of the colon; if still present after prolonged observation by annual barium studies, lesions should be removed by use of a colonoscope. This approach is preferable to laparotomy and colotomy, but the latter may be necessary if the polyp has a broad sessile base.

HERNIAS

An *intra-abdominal* hernia occurs when loops of intestine are trapped by an anomalous fold of peritoneum created by malrotation or malfixation of the duodenum or colon to the posterior abdominal wall. Loops of intestine also may herniate through congenital defects of the mesentery, particularly near the terminal ileum. The symptoms and signs are those of intermittent or acute intestinal obstruction. Compression of the vasculature may produce gangrene of the intestine. Surgical reduction of the hernia and repair of the anomaly in order to prevent recurrence require knowledge of embryologic anatomy because of the danger of interference with intestinal blood supply. For extra-abdominal hernias, see Sec. 8.53, 12.65, and 12.89.

12.37 FOREIGN BODIES IN THE STOMACH AND INTESTINES

If ingestion of a foreign body is suspected, plain roentgenograms of the abdomen and chest are indicated; if an object is visible above the diaphragm, esophagoscopy or bronchoscopy may be needed to retrieve it (Sec. 12.25). An object that reaches the stomach will, in most instances, pass through the gastrointestinal tract without causing injury. Certain types of foreign bodies, however, are potentially dangerous. Needles, hairpins, or bobby pins pass easily through the esophagus on their long axis, but may be unable to round the turns of the duodenum, where they become fixed and eventually perforate the intestine. Such potentially dangerous foreign bodies can usually be removed gastroscopically. If safety pins are small, they will probably pass without difficulty, whether open or closed. If they are large, either closed or open, peroral removal is safe and is indicated.

If the foreign body has passed through the pylorus into the intestine, its progress should be observed by means of infrequent roentgenograms. There appears to be no need to have parents search the stools for the foreign body. If the object is benign (such as a coin), the second abdominal film need not be taken for a month, once it is known that there is nothing lodged in the esophagus. If serial roentgenograms show a foreign body to be moving progressively down the intestinal tract, perforation is not likely. If it remains stationary for several wk or is long or sharp, it should be removed either under fluoroscopy by a magnetized nasogastric tube or by laparotomy, owing to the dangers of ulceration and perforation of the bowel. If at any time such signs of perforation as tenderness, rigidity, pain, nausea, or vomiting develop, surgery is indicated immediately. The diet should be normal, with no change from that to which the child has been accustomed. Bizarre roughage, wool, or cotton diets are valueless and may be dangerous. Laxatives are contraindicated since the accelerated activity of the intestine may increase the danger of perforation.

Bezoars

Occasionally, infants and children, particularly if emotionally disturbed or mentally retarded, acquire the habit of swallowing hair from their heads or from dolls or brushes, or they may swallow fur, wool, or cotton from wearing apparel or blankets. This material is usually passed through the intestines, but when the habit is persistent, there may be an accumulation in the stomach with formation of a *hairball* or *trichobezoar*. The symptoms are indefinite, but indigestion and gastric distress may be present. The tumor mass is often palpable and may give a soft crackling sensation on palpation. A bald spot or sparse hair may be apparent. A roentgenogram after administration of barium may disclose a mass outlined by barium. A portion of the bezoar may be dislodged and subsequently become impacted in the intestine and cause obstruction. The diagnosis may be suspected from observation of the stool or of the child in the act of swallowing these materials. Surgical removal is indicated, and the child's mental and psychologic status should be evaluated.

Phytobezoars are accumulations of fibrous or mucilaginous materials as found in persimmons and various tar products. The accumulation is usually rapid compared with that of the hairball. Lactobezoars occur in the newborn.

12.38 MOTILITY DISORDERS

Chronic Duodenal Ileus, Superior Mesenteric Artery Syndrome, Cast Syndrome

This syndrome of intermittent or chronic functional obstruction of the duodenum is thought by some to result from compression of the third part of the duodenum between the superior mesenteric artery and the aorta (though the left renal vein curiously escapes this vise). Others consider it to result from loss of supporting fat to the second and third parts of the duodenum with normal or exaggerated lumbar lordosis effectively occluding the duodenum. Some cases occur as the result of incomplete rotation of the intestine.

Usually the patient is a tall, asthenic, visceroptotic adolescent female. A history of "bilious attacks" or other forms of episodic vomiting may be elicited. A barium study typically shows megaduodenum and rapid, churning, to-and-fro peristaltic movements. Dilatation of the duodenum usually ends just to the right of the midline. The stomach may also be dilated. If malrotation is suspected, a barium enema should be done to locate the cecum.

If patients can be nourished and the duodenum rested, most of them will be relieved of their obstruction. The simplest form of treatment consists of a prone knee-elbow position after meals, which allows the duodenum to fall away from the retroperitoneal structures which may be causing obstruction. Nasojejunal intubation and jejunal feeding for a period of several wk or total parenteral nutrition may allow periduodenal fat to accumulate, increasing the support of the duodenum and lessening the kinking at the duodenojejunal flexure. Metoclopramide has been reported helpful in management. If there is no relief despite compliant and prolonged conservative management, operation may become necessary. A Ladd procedure is the operation of choice; duodenojejunostomy is less satisfactory.

Pseudo-Obstruction

With increasing survival of *infants with gastroschisis*, more cases of intestinal pseudo-obstruction are being encountered. In these children innervation is normal, but the bowel seems unable to respond to the stimulation of distention with a normal wave of peristalsis. Treatment consists of complete rest of the bowel, using total parenteral nutrition. Gastrostomy may be necessary to prevent swallowed air from being ingested. Esophageal manometric studies may also demonstrate abnormal motility.

At least 15 cases of *congenital segmental dilatation* of the ileum, jejunum, or colon have been reported. A localized short segment of the small intestine is dilated and ineffective in propelling its contents into the adjacent normal distal bowel. The innervation of the bowel in the segment appears normal. The condition may cause acute neonatal intestinal obstruction or chronic obstruction, with great dilatation of the small bowel in an older child. Local resection of the dilated loop of bowel is effective treatment.

Intestinal pseudo-obstruction may also occur in the colon, with barium or Gastrografin studies demonstrating inertia of a segment of bowel. Treatment with parasympathomimetic drugs is not effective.

A colonic obstructive condition occurs in which the roentgenographic appearances are those of Hirschsprung disease but ganglion cells are present. If colostomy results in relief, excision of the roentgenographically abnormal segment may be indicated. Some newborn infants of diabetic mothers develop manifestations of bowel obstruction called *immature left colon syndrome;* a barium enema shows an appearance typical of megacolon, with the apparently aganglionic segment extending up to the splenic flexure or even beyond. Anal manometric studies and rectal biopsy are normal. The condition usually requires no specific treatment.

12.39 ANORECTAL MALFORMATIONS

Congenital anomalies of the anus and rectum are relatively common. Minor abnormalities occur in about 1:500 live births, major anomalies in 1:5000 live births. Anomalies associated with those of the rectum include malformations of the urinary tract, esophagus, and, less commonly, the duodenum. The most useful clinical classification separates "low" and "high" lesions in accordance with whether the rectum does or does not pass through the puborectalis muscle, which is a major portion of the levator ani muscle of defecation.

Embryology and Pathogenesis. The anus and rectum develop from the dorsal portion of the hindgut or cloacal cavity when lateral ingrowths of mesenchyme form the urorectal septum in the midline, separating the rectum and anal canal dorsally from the bladder and urethra ventrally. A small communication between the two systems, the cloacal duct, is closed by the 7th wk of gestation by a downgrowth of the urorectal septum. An ingrowth of mesoderm divides the cloacal membrane into the urogenital membrane ventrally and the anal membrane dorsally. During the 7th wk the urogenital portion of the original cloaca has acquired an external opening, but the anal membrane does not open until later. The anus develops by a fusion of the anal tubercles and an external invagination (the proctodeum), which deepens toward the rectum but is separated from it by the anal membrane. This membrane ruptures by the 8th wk of gestation.

Interference with the development of anorectal structures at varying stages gives rise to anomalies that range from anal stenosis and incomplete rupture of the anal membrane or anal agenesis (the "low" types) to complete failure of descent of the upper portion of the cloaca and failure of invagination of the proctodeum (the "high" types). Persistence of communication between the urinary and rectal portions of the cloaca results in fistulas, which are more common in the male. In the female, fistulas connect the rectum with the vagina more commonly than with the urinary system.

Since the muscle of the external anal sphincter is derived from exterior mesoderm, it is usually intact in infants with obstructive lesions of the anus and rectum.

Pathology. Supralevator "high" anomalies occur almost exclusively in males, and there is usually a rectourethral fistula between the rectum, which ends blindly, and the prostatic urethra. The bowel ends proximal to the puborectalis muscle, with absence of the internal anal sphincter; the puborectalis muscle is relatively ineffectual in sustaining rectal continence. Associated absence of all or part of the sacrum indicates likely faulty innervation of anal and urethral musculature, with likely development of continence. When these supralevator anomalies occur in girls, there is usually a fistulous communication between the rectum and the posterior vaginal fornix. **Rectal atresia** occurs when the proctodeum (anal canal) develops normally but fails to communicate with the rectum; the rectum may be separated by a substantial gap, or there may be only a mucosal diaphragm. There is no fistula. In rectocloacal anomalies the urethra opens anteriorly into a common cloacal (vaginal) channel and the rectum communicates posteriorly with the same channel. There is thus a single (cloacal) orifice on the perineum with neither rectum nor urethra visible. There is often a double vagina. **Cloacal exstrophy** is a complex mixture of exstrophy of the bladder, imperforate anus, maldevelopment or absence of the colon, and grossly malformed external genitalia. There may be an associated small omphalocele.

In translevator "low" anomalies the hindgut has transversed the levator ani muscle and the internal and external anal sphincters are well developed, with normal function. In males skin or membrane covers the anus, with an anteriorly placed fistulous opening onto the skin in the midline anterior to where the anus would be. This opening may be on the perineum, scrotum, or even the under surface of the penis. In females the anus is ectopic; it may be perineal, vestibular, or even (low) vaginal in location. An intermediate translevator anomaly with rectourethral fistula may also occur.

Associated anomalies are common. Significant urinary tract and vertebral abnormalities occur in about 50% of patients with high anorectal malformation and 25% of those with low types. Sacral anomalies may be important in prediction of later bowel or urinary functions.

Diagnosis. Evaluation of the newborn infant with an anorectal malformation should be directed first toward establishing whether a low or high lesion is present since initial treatment, definitive treatment, and prognosis differ for these two lesions.

Low lesions. Stenosis of the anorectal canal may occur at any point or extend its entire length. The constriction can be identified by digital and endoscopic examination. An *imperforate anal membrane* is readily identified as a thin translucent membrane which becomes progressively distended by the meconium just behind it.

More than 90% of the other low anomalies are associated with an external fistula to the perineum or vestibule. Fistulas may not be apparent at birth, but peristalsis will gradually force meconium through them. Repeated meticulous examinations during the first 24 hr of life will, in most cases, eventually detect a tiny speck of meconium at the opening of the fistula. Roentgenograms employing contrast media injected through a tiny catheter inserted into the fistula will confirm the diagnosis. In males, if meconium is seen at or anterior to the anus, a low anomaly is present. Folds of skin ("bucket-handles") may accompany high or low atresias. *Perineal pearls,* cystic accumulations of inspissated green or white mucus anywhere in the midline anterior to the anus and even extending onto the scrotum, always connote a covered anus. In females it is usually possible to insert a feeding tube into the ectopic anus to establish its presence and the direction of the anal canal and rectum. The presence of a dimple at the site of the anus does not indicate a low lesion.

High lesions. A poorly developed anal dimple, a rounded perineum, or vertebral anomalies suggest a high lesion. Passage of meconium or flatus in the urine is diagnostic of a rectourinary fistula and of a rectal pouch that ends above the puborectalis muscle. In most cases a lateral roentgenogram in the upside down position (Fig. 12–19) should be obtained when clinical distention becomes evident or after 18–24 hr of life. The infant should be held upside down for several min before the film is exposed, to allow the gas in the bowel to displace the meconium and proceed as far distally as possible. Stephens has suggested that the level of the levator ani muscle is represented by a line joining the symphysis pubis with the last segment of the sacrum; if the gas bubble is proximal to this line, the anomaly is a high one. Other methods of estimation involve the comparison of the level of the gas bubble with a comma-shaped ischium. A retrograde urethrocystogram will usually demonstrate the rectourethral fistula.

If none of the above measures clearly identifies the level of

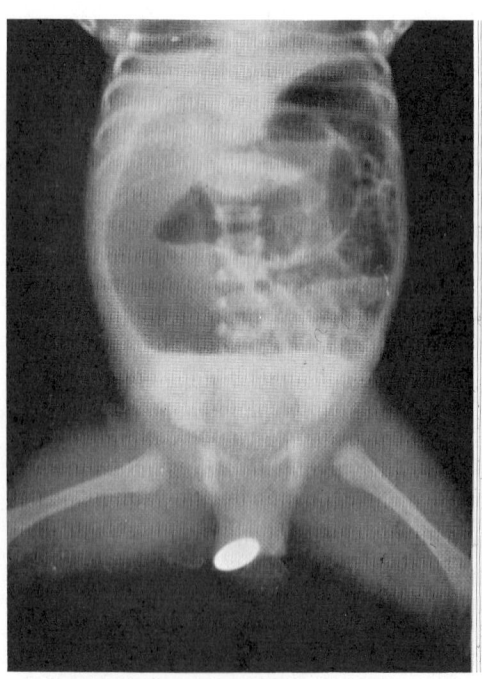
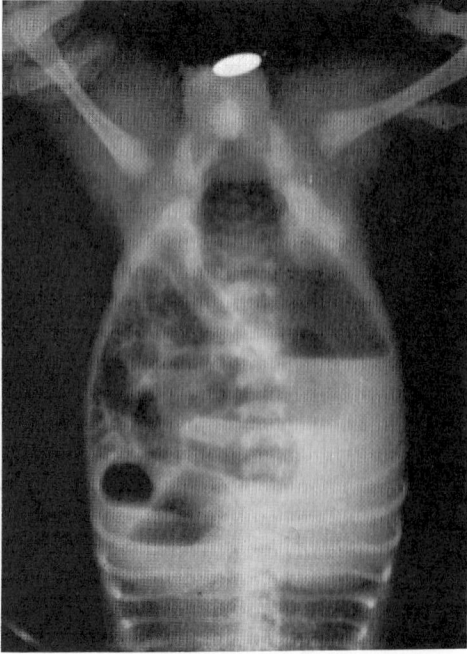

A   **B**

Figure 12–19. Wangensteen-Rice roentgenographic technique for demonstration of the position of the blind colonic pouch in the case of an imperforate or absent rectum. The infant is held head downward, causing the intestinal gas to rise to the blind end of the gut. *A,* Roentgenogram of child in upright position, showing transverse level of gas. The level of the obstruction is not demonstrated. *B,* The level of the obstruction is apparent when the roentgenogram is taken with the child in the inverted position. The site of the anus is marked by a lead disk.

the rectal pouch, it is safest to presume a high lesion. Blind exploration of the perineum in hopes of finding a low-lying rectal pouch should not be done.

Excretory urography or ultrasonography should be done in all cases and should precede definitive therapy in high lesions.

Treatment. Anal stenosis can generally be treated by digital or instrumental dilatations. All other forms of imperforate anus require surgical correction.

In the low types in females, since the bowel has the proper levator relationship, repair can be managed from below. These patients will be continent unless ill-advised operations are performed. There is no evidence that an anus placed 1 cm or so anterior to its normal position results in either urinary or genital infections or in major problems with parturition. Rarely, the anus will have to be transplanted dorsally when there is a low rectovaginal fistula. The "covered anus" in males and infrequently the vestibular ectopic anus in females will need the coverings of the anus incised in a dorsal direction and the mucosa sutured to the margins of the newly created anus. Postoperative regular dilatations for 1–2 mo may be necessary.

The high types are best treated by a preliminary transverse colostomy, with definitive repair in 6–12 mo. Careful positioning of the anus in relation to the external sphincter and of the bowel in the muscle complex is essential. Fistulas are also eliminated.

Surgical treatment of imperforate anus has recently been advanced by the development of the Pena procedure (posterior sagittal anorectoplasty). Using an electrical muscle-stimulating device, the entire pelvic musculature is reconstructed around a tapered neorectum after closure of the rectourethral fistula. The complex cloacal abnormalities encountered with high malformations in females also respond to this procedure.

The higher the blind pouch the more extensive the operation. Significant sacral anomalies are usually associated with deficient neurologic control of defecation, but with continuing care through the period of toilet training a satisfactory functional solution can usually be achieved. In a few instances there will be continuing problems due to stenosis, poor anal control, or poor guidance. In the postoperative period constipation rather than incontinence may be a problem. The lack of sensation of fecal material in the rectum leads to fecal impactions with paradoxic or overflow diarrheal stools and gives rise to the acquired type of megacolon. Early attention to ensure regular evacuations will prevent massive fecal impactions. As a rule, the child should be taught to defecate at a given time of day rather than await the urge. In some instances a daily enema may be needed.

Prognosis. All patients with low types of anorectal malformation should be continent. Patients with high anomalies on the other hand, may rarely be left with what is, in effect, a perineal colostomy. This form of incontinence, however, is more tolerable than abdominal colostomy in children and adolescents.

BARRY SHANDLING

Pyloric Stenosis

Bleicher MA, Shandling B, Zingg W, et al: Increased serum immunoreactive gastrin levels in idiopathic hypertrophic pyloric stenosis. Gut 19:794, 1978.
Blumhegen JD, Noble HGS: Muscle thickness in hypertrophic pyloric stenosis: sonographic determination. Am J Roentgenol 140:221, 1983.
Leahy A, Fitzgerald RJ: The influence of delayed feeding on postoperative vomiting in hypertrophic pyloric stenosis. Br J Surg 69:658, 1982.
Pollock WF, Norris WJ, Gordon HE: The management of hypertrophic pyloric stenosis at the Los Angeles Children's Hospital (a review of 1422 cases). Am J Surg 94:335, 1957.
Schärli AF, Sieber WK, Kiesewetter WB: Hypertrophic pyloric stenosis at the Children's Hospital of Pittsburgh from 1912 to 1967. J Pediatr Surg 4:108, 1969.
Touloukian RJ, Higgins E: The spectrum of serum electrolytes in hypertrophic pyloric stenosis. J Pediatr Surg 18:394, 1983.

Tunnell WP, Wilson DA: Pyloric stenosis: diagnosis by real-time sonography, the pyloric muscle length method. J Pediatr Surg 19:795, 1984.

Intestinal Atresias

Atwell JD, Klidian AM: Vertebral anomalies and duodenal atresia. J Pediatr Surg 17:237, 1982.
Daum R, Roth H, Schüler B, et al: The problem of congenital duodenal obstruction: a report of 123 cases. Z Kinderchir 35:125, 1982.
DeLorimier AA, Fondalsrud EW, Hays DM: Congenital atresia and stenosis of the jejunum and ileum. Surgery 65:819, 1969.
Fonkalsrud EW, DeLorimier AA, Hays DM: Congenital atresia and stenosis of the duodenum. A review compiled from members of the Surgical Section of the American Academy of Pediatrics. Pediatrics 43:79, 1979.
Louw JH: Resection and end-to-end anastomosis in the management of atresia and stenosis of the small bowel. Surgery 62:940, 1967.
Nixon HH, Tawes R: Etiology and treatment of small intestinal atresia: Analysis of a series of 127 jejunoileal atresias and comparison with 62 duodenal atresias. Surgery 69:41, 1971.

Malrotation

Dott NM: Anomalies of intestinal rotation: their embryology and surgical aspects, with report of 5 cases. Br J Surg 11:251, 1923.
Filston H, Kirks DR: Malrotation—the ubiquitous anomaly. J Pediatr Surg 16:614, 1981.
Ladd WE: Congenital obstruction of the duodenum in children. N Engl J Med 206:277, 1932.
Louw JH, Sender B, Shandling B: A rational approach to the surgical treatment of duodenal ileus. Afr J Lab Clin Med 3:249, 1957.
Stewart DR, Colodny AL, Daggett WC: Malrotation of the bowel in infants and children: a 15 year review. Surgery 79:716, 1976.

Meconium Ileus

Harberg FJ, Senekjian EK, Pokorny WJ: Treatment of uncomplicated meconium ileus via T-tube ileostomy. J Pediatr Surg 16:61, 1981.
Holsclas DS, Eckstein HB, Nixon HH: Meconium ileus: a 20-year review of 109 cases. Am J Dis Child 190:101, 1965.
Meeker IA, Kincannon WN; Acetyl cysteine used to liquify inspissated meconium causing intestinal obstruction of the newborn. Surgery 56:419, 1964.
Noblett HR: Treatment of uncomplicated meconium ileus by Gastrografin enema: a preliminary report. J Pediatr Surg 4:190, 1969.
Venugopal S, Shandling B: Meconium ileus: laparotomy without resection, anastomosis or enterostomy. J Pediatr Surg 14:715, 1979.
Wagget J, Bishop HC, Koop CE: Experience with Gastrografin enema in the treatment of meconium ileus. J Pediatr Surg 5:649, 1970.

Hirschsprung Disease

Bodian M, Stephens FD, Ward BIH: Hirschsprung's disease and idiopathic megacolon. Lancet 1:6, 1949.
Chow CW, Campbell PE: Short-segment Hirschsprung's disease as a cause of discrepancy between histological, histochemical and clinical features. J Pediatr Surg 18:167, 1983.
Duhamel B: Retrorectal and transanal pull-through procedure for the treatment of Hirschsprung's disease. Dis Colon Rectum 7:455, 1964.
Huntley CC, Schaffner L de S, Challa VR, et al: Histochemical diagnosis of Hirschsprung's disease. Pediatrics 69:755, 1982.
Ikeda K, Goto S: Diagnosis and treatment of Hirschsprung's disease in Japan. Ann Surg 199:400, 1984.
Loening-Baucke VA: Anorectal manometry: Experience with strain gauge pressure transducers for the diagnosis of Hirschsprung's disease. J Pediatr Surg 18:595, 1983.
Shandling B, Auldist AW: Punch biopsy of the rectum for the diagnosis of Hirschsprung's disease. J Pediatr Surg 3:386, 1968.
Soave F: Hirschsprung's disease: A new surgical technique. Arch Dis Child 39:116, 1964.
Swenson O, Neuhauser EBD, Pickett LK: New concepts of etiology, diagnosis and treatment of congenital megacolon (Hirschsprung's disease). Pediatrics 4:201, 1949.
Swenson O, Sherman JO, Fisher JH: Diagnosis of congenital megacolon: an analysis of 501 patients. J Pediatr Surg 8:587, 1973.

Pseudo-obstruction

Aneuras S, Christensen J: Recurrent or chronic intestinal pseudo-obstruction. Clin Gastroenterol 10:177, 1981.
Byrne WJ, Abel L, Euler AR, et al: Chronic idiopathic intestinal pseudo-obstruction syndrome in children: Clinical characteristics and prognosis. Pediatrics 90:585, 1977.

Meckel Diverticulum and Intussusception

Ein SH, Stephens CA: Intussusception: 354 cases in 10 years. J Pediatr Surg 6:1, 1971.
Hocking M, Young DG: Duplications of the alimentary tract. Br J Surg 68:92, 1981.

Mackey WC, Dineen P: A fifty year experience with Meckel's diverticulum. Surg Gynecol Obstet 156:56, 1983.

Mellish RWP, Koop CE: Clinical manifestations of duplication of the bowel. Pediatrics 27:397, 1961.

Ravitch MM: Intussusception. *In:* Pediatric Surgery, 3rd ed. Vol 2. Chicago, Year Book Medical Publishers, 1978, p 989.

Seagram CGF, Louch RE, Stephens CA, et al: Meckel's diverticulum: A 10 year review of 218 cases. Can J Surg 11:369, 1968.

Treves S, Grand RJ, Eraklis AJ: Pentagastrin stimulation of technetium-99m uptake by ectopic gastric mucosa in a Meckel's diverticulum. Radiology 128:711, 1978.

Polyps

Euler AE, Seibert JJ: The role of sigmoidoscopy, radiographs, and colonoscopy in the diagnostic evaluation of pediatric age patients with suspected juvenile polyps. J Pediatr Surg 16:500, 1981.

Jagelman DG: Familial polyposis coli. Surg Clin North Am 63:117, 1983.

Louw JH: Polypoid lesions of the large bowel in children. S Afr Med J 46:1347, 1972.

Mallam AS, Thomson SA: Polyps of the rectum and colon in children. Can J Surg 3:17, 1959.

Shermeta DW, Morgan WW, Eggleston J, et al: Juvenile retention polyps. J Pediatr Surg 4:211, 1969.

Motility Disorders

Bagwell CE, Filler RM, Cutz E, et al: Neonatal pseudoobstruction. J Pediatr Surg 19:732, 1984.

Fadda B, Maier WA, Meier-Ruge W, et al: Neuronal intestinal dysplasia—a critical 10-year analysis of clinical and bioptic results. Z Kinderchir 38:308, 1983.

Nguyen L, Shandling B: Segmental dilation of the colon: A rare cause of chronic constipation. J Pediatr Surg 19:539, 1984.

Puri P, Lake BD, Gorman F, et al: Megacystic-microcolon-intestinal hypoperistalsis syndrome: a visceral myopathy. J Pediatr Surg 18:64, 1983.

Shawis RN, Rangecroft L, Cook RCM, et al: Functional intestinal obstruction associated with malrotation and short small-bowel. J Pediatr Surg 19:172, 1984.

Tanner MS, Smith B, Lloyd JK: Functional intestinal obstruction due to deficiency of argyrophil neurones in the myenteric plexus. Arch Dis Child 51:837, 1976.

Young LW, Yunis EJ, Girdany BR, et al: Megacystis-microcolon-intestinal hypoperistalsis syndrome: Additional clinical, radiologic, surgical and histopathologic aspects. Am J Roentgenol 137:749, 1981.

Imperforate Anus

de Vries PA, Pena A: Posterior sagittal anorectoplasty. J Pediatr Surg 17:638, 1982.

Kiesewetter WB, Chang JHT: Imperforate anus: A five to thirty year follow-up perspective. Prog Pediatr Surg 10:111, 1977.

Kiesewetter WB, Nixon HH: Imperforate anus: Its surgical anatomy. J Pediatr Surg 2:60, 1967.

Lobe TE: Fecal continence following an anterior sagittal ano-enteroplasty in a patient with cloacal exstrophy. J Pediatr Surg 19:843, 1984.

Pena A, de Vries PA: Posterior sagittal anorectoplasty: important technical considerations and new applications. J Pediatr Surg 17:796, 1982.

Stephens FD: Congenital imperforate rectum, recto-urethral and recto-vaginal fistulae. Aust NZ J Surg 22:161, 1953.

12.40 INFECTIONS OF THE INTESTINE

See Sec. 11.8.

Diarrheal illness, most of it attributable to enteric infection, continues to kill millions of children each year. Where populations have access to good nutrition and sanitation, death rates are relatively low, but infectious diarrhea remains a major cause of illness in young children everywhere. The term "gastroenteritis" persists, but its use is usually inappropriate, because infections of the gastrointestinal tract generally affect the small or large intestine but not the stomach.

Etiology and Epidemiology. The major known causes of infectious enteritis in children are summarized in Table 12–6. In 20–30% of cases no specific pathogen is identified. In temperate climates human rotavirus (HRV) accounts for about 50% of all cases and for up to 80% of severe cases in infants during the winter; in the tropics a similar high incidence probably occurs in the rainy seasons. Parvo-like viruses have

Table 12–6. **Causes of Infectious Diarrhea in Children**

Viruses
   Human rotavirus (Sec. 11.8)
   Parvo-like viruses (Norwalk) (Sec. 11.8)
   Calci virus
   Astrovirus
   Adenovirus (enteric) (Sec. 11.74)
   Cytomegalovirus (Sec. 11.68)

Bacteria
   Shigella (Sec. 11.28)
   Campylobacter jejuni (Sec. 11.41)
   Salmonella (Sec. 11.26)
   Escherichia coli (Sec. 11.25)
      enterotoxigenic
      enteroinvasive
      enteroadherent
   Yersinia enterocolitica (Sec. 11.32)
   Vibrio cholerae (Sec. 11.29)
   Clostridium perfringens (Sec. 11.38)
   Aeromonas

Protozoa
   Giardia lamblia (Sec. 11.102)
   Entamoeba histolytica (Sec. 11.101)
   Cryptosporidium (Sec. 11.94)
   Dientamoeba fragilis

caused major community outbreaks of acute diarrhea (Norwalk, Hawaii, Montgomery County), and cytomegalovirus has been shown to infect the colon on occasion.

Bacterial pathogens probably cause 10–15% of cases of acute childhood diarrhea; this incidence rises in warm climates, particularly where sanitary conditions are poor. The most commonly identified bacterial pathogens in North American children are *Campylobacter jejuni* and various strains of the *Salmonella* and *Shigella* species. *Yersinia enterocolitica* is also relatively common, particularly in Eastern Canada and Europe. Some strains of *Escherichia coli*, a normal inhabitant of the distal bowel, are pathogenic, causing sporadic cases of acute enteritis, epidemic diarrhea (particularly in young infants), and traveler's diarrhea. Severe diarrhea in children has now been attributed also to enteroadherent strains of *E. coli*. The relative importance of *E. coli* strains as enteric pathogens in children is not yet defined.

Parasitic infections are discussed in Sec. 11.100. *Entamoeba histolytica* infections occur in all parts of the world, but they are usually found in subtropical climates. *Giardia lamblia* infestation is endemic in the tropics but is now common in children everywhere, especially in toddlers, particularly among those in day care centers. *Balantidium coli* infection is common in Latin America but rare in North America. *Cryptosporidium* may cause acute diarrhea, even in the immune-competent host. *Dientamoeba fragilis* appears to be capable of causing a mild transient diarrheal illness in children. Many worms can infest the gut, but they are generally not primary causes of enteritis and diarrhea.

Fungi, like bacteria, are normal inhabitants of the human gut. *Candida albicans* may cause local enteric disease and serve as a reservoir for disseminated infection in debilitated or immune-deficient patients.

Pathogenesis. Most of the diarrheogenic pathogens disturb intestinal function and cause diarrhea by invading the bowel wall or by elaborating an enterotoxin in the lumen. Adherence of an organism to the intestinal surface is an important determinant of its invasive potential. Of the enterotoxins, choleragen, produced by *V. cholerae*, has been the most intensively studied. It binds to the epithelial surface and activates the adenylate cyclase system, provoking intracellular accumulation of cyclic AMP, impaired absorption of sodium and chloride, and secretion of chloride; glucose-stimulated sodium absorption at the brush border remains intact (Sec. 11.29). Heat-labile *E. coli* enterotoxin acts similarly, but cyclic GMP mediates the secretory response to the heat-stable *E. coli* enterotoxin (Sec. 11.25).

Human rotavirus invades the upper intestinal epithelium, causing defective sodium and chloride absorption in the upper bowel; glucose-stimulated sodium transport and glucose absorption are impaired, but intracellular cyclic AMP levels are normal (Sec. 11.8). Some functional abnormalities that characterize viral enteritis appear to result from failure of normal cell differentiation during repair after the virus has been shed. Less is known about the pathogenesis of diarrhea caused by invasive bacteria; some seem to provoke an intestinal response similar to that caused by enterotoxins.

Sodium and chloride concentrations in stools of acute enterotoxigenic diarrhea approach those of plasma (100–130 mEq/L) and are much higher than those typical of invasive viral enteritis (30–50 mEq/L). Although glucose transport in acute viral enteritis is defective and disaccharidase activities reduced, large quantities of sugar are rarely found in stools during the acute disease since unabsorbed sugar is broken down by enteric bacteria.

Since the intestine possesses effective mechanisms to clear unwanted organisms in addition to the body's immunologic defenses, most enteric infections are brief, but infection may persist in the gut owing to a source of reinfection, to special properties of the organism involved, or to a defect in the host's defenses.

Clinical Manifestations. Diarrhea usually begins after 1–2 days of low grade fever and anorexia. In general, the younger infant or child has the more rapid onset and more severe symptoms. Vomiting is particularly common during the early stages of rotavirus enteritis; blood in stool is characteristic of invasive distal infections such as are caused by *Shigella* or *Campylobacter;* and crampy abdominal pain is a prominent feature of *Yersinia* and *Campylobacter* infections. Extraintestinal manifestations (erythema nodosum, arthritis, etc.) occur occasionally with *Yersinia* and *Campylobacter* enteritides. History rarely indicates a specific cause, such as a specific infectious contact, but historical data that reflect the impact of disease on fluid and electrolyte balance (e.g., the child's alertness, urinary output, and estimated fecal losses) are extremely useful.

Physical examination also should focus on findings indicative of fluid and electrolyte status. Acute weight loss, reduced skin turgor and fontanel tension, sunken eyes, and rapid pulse all point to severe fluid depletion. Abdominal distension may indicate pooling of intestinal secretions, which can be confirmed by a rectal examination that provokes a rush of fluid stool. Stool obtained in this way should be examined microscopically for the blood and pus of an invasive colonic infection, and biochemically for sugars suggestive of small bowel disease.

In children who are well at the onset, most enteritides heal within 1 wk. A small proportion of bacterial and protozoan infections persist for several weeks.

Diagnosis. It is appropriate to assume that all acute diarrheas in children, with or without vomiting, are caused by enteric infection. Disorders that may mimic enteritis early in their courses are pyloric stenosis, intracranial lesions and adrenal insufficiency if the infant is vomiting, "parenteral" diarrhea if there are loose stools of low volume, and intussusception if stools are bloody. If illness and diarrhea persist, chronic malabsorptive states (celiac disease, cystic fibrosis, etc.) and other chronic intestinal disorders (inflammatory bowel diseases, anomalies) should be considered.

Laboratory Data. The microbiologic diagnosis of each infection is discussed in Chapter 11. Electrolyte status assessment should be reserved for cases in which clinical evaluations suggest a problem; the most useful examinations are of urine and serum osmolality and serum concentration of Na, K, Cl, and HCO_3.

Treatment. The objectives should be to preserve fluid and electrolyte balance and to prevent deterioration of nutritional status while the disease runs its course. Experience with the World Health Organization oral rehydration solution (ORS) has clearly demonstrated the benefits of an orally administered, appropriately constituted, isotonic solution of glucose and electrolytes in young children with enteritis, even in those who are vomiting or dehydrated (see Sec. 5.22, 5.23, and 11.8).

J. RICHARD HAMILTON

Dobbins JW, Binder HJ: Pathophysiology of diarrhea. Alterations in fluid and electrolyte transport. Clin Gastroenterol 10:65, 1981.
Gall DG, Hamilton JR: Infectious diarrhea in infants and children. Clin Gastroenterol 6:431, 1977.
Hamilton JR: Treatment of acute diarrhea. Pediatr Clin North Am 32:419, 1985.
Tallett S, MacKenzie C, Middleton P, et al: Clinical, laboratory and epidemiological features of a viral gastroenteritis in infants and children. Pediatrics 60:217, 1977.

NONINFECTIVE INFLAMMATORY GASTROINTESTINAL DISEASE

12.41 ULCER DISEASE

Ulcer disease is much less common in children than in adults. In a New York county, a study found the annual incidence in children under 15 yr old to be 3.5/100,000, rising to 13.7/100,000 in boys by the age of 15, an incidence 3.8 times that of girls. In adults, the incidence rises to 3% after the age of 45 yr. It is convenient to discuss peptic ulcer disease and stress ulcers separately, although their treatment, methods of diagnosis, and biologic factors are similar.

Peptic Ulcers

Peptic ulcers occur mainly in the duodenum, less commonly in the stomach. In the 1st or 2nd yr of life, gastric and duodenal ulcers occur with similar frequency, but after 6 yr duodenal ulcers predominate.

Pathology and Pathophysiology. The etiology of peptic ulcer disease is uncertain, but a number of factors are important. A family history of ulcers can be found in 25–50% of patients with duodenal ulcers, and concordance for duodenal ulcer is 50% for monozygotic twins. Blood type O and high levels of pepsinogen I are associated with ulcer disease. Environmental factors such as climatic conditions, dietary habits, and emotional strain, also appear to be important.

The presence of gastric acidity is of major importance in the development of ulcer disease. Both adults and children with duodenal ulcer disease have increased acid secretion, but there is a large overlap with the normal range, and studies do not correlate acid secretion with ulcer size or duration of symptoms. In gastric ulcer disease acid output is often normal or low. Tissue resistance is an important variable in preventing ulcer formation; factors that lower resistance include anoxia, poor perfusion, and drugs. Salicylates, alcohol, and bile salts stimulate pepsinogen secretion, interfere with integrity of the mucosa, and favor ulcer formation. The rate of cell turnover and the type and the amount of mucus secretion are also thought to be important. In general, factors related to acid are most important in duodenal ulcers, whereas tissue resistance appears to be of greater importance in gastric ulcers.

Histologically, the ulcer may be very superficial, may erode deeply into the mucosa and submucosa, may penetrate a blood vessel and cause hemorrhage, or may cause perforation. It is usually surrounded by an infiltration of acute and chronic inflammatory cells. A very shallow ulcer is considered an abrasion. If inflammation and edema are extensive, acute or chronic gastric outlet obstruction may occur. Occasionally, a red, granular duodenal mucosa is seen on endoscopy; it is often diagnosed as duodenitis and treated as a developing ulcer. The relation of this lesion to symptoms or to eventual ulcer formation is unknown. Most duodenal ulcers occur in the posterior part of the bulb, and most gastric ulcers occur on the lesser curve or the antral area. Malignant gastric ulcers in children are exceedingly rare.

Clinical Manifestations. The manifestations of peptic ulcer disease are variable and often nonspecific, but include vomiting, gastrointestinal blood loss, pain, and a strong familial incidence. Of adults with dyspepsia symptoms thought to be compatible with ulcer disease, only about 15% will have ulcers on investigation. In children, the frequency of abdominal pain and the infrequent finding of ulcer disease suggest a similar situation.

Although the symptoms of ulcer disease are variable and easily confused with symptoms caused by other abdominal diseases or functional problems, certain presentations are particularly common at certain ages. In the 1st mo of life, the two main presentations are gastrointestinal hemorrhage and perforation. Most such ulcers will be stress ulcers (see below); and other disorders such as sepsis, heart disease, or respiratory distress will usually be present. It is likely that many ulcers with less dramatic symptoms go undiagnosed. Between the neonatal period and 2 yr of age, recurrent vomiting, slow growth, and gastrointestinal hemorrhage are the three major symptoms. In the preschool period, pain that is typically periumbilical and worse after eating is often elicited. Recurrent vomiting and intestinal hemorrhage are also common.

After 6 yr of age the clinical features of ulcer disease are similar to those in adults, and commonly include abdominal pain, acute or chronic gastrointestinal blood loss, a preponderance of males, and a strong family history of ulcer disease. The pain is often described as dull or aching in character, rather than sharp or burning as in adults. It may last from minutes to hours, and there are frequent exacerbations and remissions lasting from weeks to months. A history of typical ulcer pain with prompt relief following antacids is found in less than one third of affected patients. In patients with acute or chronic blood loss and penetration of the ulcer into the abdominal cavity or adjacent organs, symptoms of shock, anemia, peritonitis, or pancreatitis may occur.

Diagnosis. An upper gastrointestinal roentgenographic examination is the most useful regularly available test if symptoms are not acute. In approximately 25% of children with duodenal ulcers, the lesion will not be detected on the first examination, and even with double contrast examination, fewer than 40% of gastric lesions will be demonstrated. The duodenal bulb is often difficult to examine in infants because of its high posterior position. The ulcer crater should be demonstrated in multiple spot films, preferably in a distended bulb so as not to be confused with barium caught in normal mucosal folds. True deformity of the bulb is a good sign of past ulcer disease but does not ensure that current symptoms are due to ulcer disease or that an ulcer is present. Spasm of the bulb that relaxes and allows filling of the bulb is common in normal patients, and radiographic interpretations such as "duodenitis," "irritability of the bulb," and "pylorospasm" should not be interpreted as ulcer disease.

Gastroduodenoscopy is indicated when roentgenographic findings are questionable or absent in symptomatic patients, when symptoms persist despite radiographic evidence of healing, or with prolonged presence of an ulcer crater. In patients with acute upper gastrointestinal hemorrhage, if gastric lavage can clear the stomach of obscuring blood and clots, endoscopy is the diagnostic procedure of choice. Although direct visualization of the upper intestine has dramatically increased the precision of diagnosis of intestinal hemorrhage, there is no evidence that the increased accuracy has improved mortality.

Routine gastric acid analysis is not generally useful, as the values found in normal and abnormal patients overlap widely. In patients who have recurrent severe ulcers or multiple ulcers, serum gastrin levels should be measured to detect those who have Zollinger-Ellison syndrome.

In patients with active, severe upper intestinal bleeding, selective abdominal angiography may be indicated early in the diagnostic evaluation. Leakage of dye into the lumen from a bleeding ulcer can demonstrate the ulcer, and bleeding may be controlled by infusion of vasoconstrictors into vessels just proximal to the bleeding site or by therapeutic embolization of the bleeding vessels.

Treatment. The goal of therapy is to hasten healing of the ulcer, relieve pain, and prevent complications. Approximately 25% of children under the age of 6 yr will have recurrence of a primary ulcer, whereas 70% of older children will have recurrences as they enter adult life. Drugs such as aspirin or alcohol that predispose to ulcer formation and hemorrhage should be avoided. Tobacco smoking is associated with delayed healing. Recent studies in adults suggest that corticosteroids do not predispose to ulcers, but an increased incidence may be related to an underlying illness. The patient should eat a normal diet, avoiding only those foods that cause discomfort. Use of a bland diet or avoidance of cola drinks, coffee, or spiced foods has not been shown to decrease acid secretion or hasten healing.

Suppression of gastric acidity is the most important factor in treatment of ulcer disease, and antacids are the mainstay of medical management. Large doses hasten healing of duodenal ulcers in adults. The buffering ability of antacids varies greatly, and liquid forms are much more efficient than tablets, which must be thoroughly chewed for maximal efficiency. A quantity of antacid capable of buffering 100 mEq of stomach acidity/m^2 should be administered 1 and 3 hr after meals and at bedtime. This usually amounts to 15 mL/m^2 of the more concentrated liquid antacids. A bedtime snack should not be substituted, because food will stimulate acid secretion during the night. Intensive therapy with antacids should continue for 4–6 wk.

Most antacids are mixtures of magnesium hydroxide, magnesium trisilicate, and aluminum hydroxide. The magnesium compounds are effective but cause diarrhea. If diarrhea becomes a problem, intermittent use of antacids containing mainly aluminum hydroxide is warranted. Aluminum antacids bind with dietary phosphates and interfere with absorption. If large doses of aluminum hydroxide without phosphate are used over a prolonged period of time, it is possible to develop complications of phosphate depletion including anorexia, osteomalacia, and osteoporosis. Calcium antacids can cause increased acid secretion after their buffering effect has stopped. Sodium bicarbonate is a very effective acid buffer, but is not suitable for chronic use because of the large systemic alkaline and sodium load.

Cimetidine, a potent histamine H_2-receptor antagonist, blocks the secretion of gastric acid and is an alternative to frequent antacid administration. The usual recommended dose in children is 20–40 mg/kg/24 hr, administered four times a day with meals and at bedtime. Side effects are unusual but include gynecomastia and, on rare occasions, coma. Ranitidine in adult dosage of 150 mg twice a day is a newer H_2-receptor antagonist that appears to have fewer side effects and requires only twice a day dosage. Neither drug has been approved for use in children. These drugs have not been shown to be more effective in controlling gastric acidity than antacids, but are more convenient and do hasten the healing of ulcers. A single daily dose has been shown to be effective in preventing recurrence of ulcers.

Anticholinergic drugs can inhibit gastric acid secretion but are effective only when enough is given so that side effects of dry mouth or slightly blurred vision occur. It is often difficult to monitor these changes in children; these drugs are not, therefore, recommended as primary therapy.

Surgery is indicated in patients with perforation, intractable pain, chronic bleeding, or loss of over one third of the blood volume within 48 hr from a hemorrhage that could not be controlled through embolization of the bleeding vessel, as described above. Another indication for surgery is gastric outlet obstruction caused by edema and fibrosis around a chronic ulcer that is not improved after 72 hr of nasogastric drainage. Vagotomy and either pyloroplasty or antrectomy are the procedures most used in children.

Stress Ulcers

Stress erosions and ulcers are usually associated with physical trauma, burns, sepsis, hemorrhagic shock, or critical illness. These ulcers are usually acute; there is a lack of chronic inflammation and debris in the crater, and there are often multiple lesions. Stress ulcers occur with equal frequency in both sexes. They are more likely to occur in the duodenum and are often multiple.

Acute massive painless bleeding is frequently the first and only clinical manifestation of the ulcer. Partially because of the associated severe underlying disease, mortality is high, even if bleeding is controlled. Antacids or cimetidine can decrease the incidence of stress ulcers in adults who are at high risk. Accordingly, measures to control gastric acidity during periods of acute stress in children are recommended, especially in patients with massive burns or head injuries. Most of the ulcers that occur within the first 5 yr of life are stress ulcers.

The treatment for stress ulcers is similar to that for chronic peptic ulcer, especially with regard to antacid therapy. Often, bleeding will stop with iced-saline lavage. Blood replacement, avoidance of aspirin, and correction of coagulation defects in the acutely ill patient are critical elements of treatment. As noted previously, selective intra-arterial infusion of Pitressin or embolization therapy may control bleeding or at least allow stabilization of these very sick patients prior to surgery. Suture ligature of the bleeding sites combined with a vagotomy and pyloroplasty is usually the recommended surgical procedure.

Zollinger-Ellison Syndrome

This rare syndrome can cause multiple recurrent duodenal and jejunal ulcers and is occasionally associated with diarrhea. Gastric secretion is markedly increased in volume and acidity, and hypertrophy of gastric folds is often noted on radiography. Islet cell tumor or hypertrophy causes massive elevation in serum gastrin-like activity which stimulates secretion of acid; occasionally, other hormones that cause diarrhea may also be secreted. Chronic cimetidine therapy may control gastric acid secretion and reduce the need for complete gastrectomy. Symptoms can be controlled for long periods, even if these slow-growing tumors cannot be entirely removed.

JOHN J. HERBST

Ippoliti A, Walsh J: Newer concepts in the pathogenesis of peptic ulcer disease. Surg Clin North Am 56:1479, 1976.
Kumar D, Spitz L: Peptic ulceration in children. Surg Gynecol Obstet 159:163, 1984.
Lebenthal E: Peptic ulcer in children. Am J Gastroenterol 75:153, 1981.
Meyerovitz MF, Fellows KE: Angiography in gastrointestinal bleeding in children. Am J Roentgenol 143:837, 1984.

Peterson WL, Sturdevant RAL, Frankl HD, et al: Healing of duodenal ulcer with an antacid regimen. N Engl J Med 297:341, 1977.
Priebe JH, Skillman JJ, Bushnell LS, et al: Antacid versus cimetidine in preventing acute gastrointestinal bleeding. N Engl J Med 302:426, 1980.
Puri P, Boyd E, Blake N, et al: Duodenal ulcer in childhood: A continuing disease in adult life. J Pediatr Surg 13:525, 1978.
Robb JDA, Thomas PS, Orszulok J, et al: Duodenal ulcer in children. Arch Dis Child 47:688, 1972.
Sultz HA, Schlesinger EF, Feldman JG, et al: The epidemiology of peptic ulcer in childhood. Am J Publ Health 60:492, 1970.

12.42 IDIOPATHIC ULCERATIVE COLITIS

This chronic condition of unknown etiology affects the distal large bowel, extending proximally within the colon to a varying extent; in many patients the entire colon is affected. There is diffuse inflammation characterized by an infiltrate of neutrophils with crypt abscesses, but the lesion rarely extends beyond the mucosa into deeper layers. In its typical form, therefore, this lesion is distinct from that of Crohn disease (Sec. 12.43).

Epidemiology. Ulcerative colitis is relatively common in Jews and rare in black and oriental people. There is an unexplained concentration of cases in Western Europe and North America. The disease is relatively common among 1st degree relatives of patients, in patients with ankylosing spondylitis, and among persons with the histocompatibility antigen HLA-B27.

Clinical Manifestations. Symptoms begin before the age of 20 yr in about 15% of patients, occasionally in the newborn period, but usually not until the preadolescent years. The common symptoms are chronic diarrhea with fresh blood and copious mucus, fecal urgency, tenesmus, and lower abdominal cramps, particularly just before defecation. In most patients the onset is gradual; as diarrhea persists, anorexia develops with weight loss. At times, the onset is fulminant, with explosive bloody diarrhea, high fever and progression to peritonitis, and even perforation within days. If the symptoms are prolonged, particularly when nutrient intake has been poor, delayed growth and maturation occur, sometimes with secondary amenorrhea. The general impact of the disease is often reflected in the child's attendance and performance in school and at extracurricular activities.

Clinical signs of chronic ill health are usually evident at the time of diagnosis. The abdomen is tender, particularly along the left side, and bowel sounds are increased. There may be abdominal distention, and tenderness on rectal examination. In fresh stools blood is usually present with masses of leukocytes and mucus; anal fissures occur but perianal fistulas and abscesses are less common than with Crohn disease.

Extraintestinal manifestations are less common in children than in adults; but signs of arthritis are seen in about 10% of patients, usually involving large joints such as the knees, hips, or shoulders, which are tender, swollen, warm, and red. Spondylitis is more common with colitis than in noncolitic patients, but rare in children. Usually, arthritic activity parallels colitic activity, but joint signs may be severe in the presence of subtle intestinal symptoms. Erythema nodosum occurs in fewer than 5% of cases, usually when the colitis is active. Pyoderma gangrenosum, a necrotic lesion of the skin associated with ulcerative colitis, is very rare. Iritis, also rare, develops relatively late in the course of the disease. It is characterized by pain, conjunctival hyperemia in a perilimbal distribution, cells in the aqueous, deposits on the back of the cornea, and congestion of the iris. Coexisting hepatitis, also rare in children, usually causes a mixed hyperbilirubinemia with an enlarged firm liver. Unlike that of other extraintestinal features, the activity of hepatitis tends not to be related to the activity of the colonic disease. Finger clubbing occurs in fewer than 10% of patients and only with extensive disease. Peripheral edema (from excessive enteric protein loss), phlebitis, and hemolytic anemia are also associated with ulcerative colitis but are rare in childhood cases.

In the clinical assessment of these patients particular attention should be paid to psychologic status. Although emotional problems neither cause nor directly influence the course of the disease, they clearly exacerbate the child's symptoms. If the child and family are carefully evaluated initially, they can be better supported through a serious, chronic illness for which curative drug therapy is unavailable.

Differential Diagnosis. Infections are by far the most common causes of chronic intestinal inflammation (Table 12–7). The incidence of specific disorders varies with regions. A careful search for infectious contacts and microbiologic studies should be completed before a diagnosis of idiopathic ulcerative colitis is made. Infections that cause chronic colitis with pus and blood in stools include *Shigella, Salmonella, Yersinia enterocolitica, Campylobacter*, and *Entamoeba histolytica*. Ulcerative colitis is rare in infants, but necrotizing enterocolitis and intolerance of dietary protein (particularly cow milk) can cause colitis; furthermore, Hirschsprung disease may be complicated by colitis in infants. In older children Crohn disease is characterized by its segmental distribution, usually within small bowel, and involvement of all layers of the gut by a granulomatous inflammatory lesion. In anaphylactoid purpura or hemolytic-uremic syndrome, intestinal involvement may precede other manifestations, but evidence of a widespread vasculitis soon becomes apparent. Patients with pseudomembranous colitis have a typical sigmoidoscopic lesion, usually associated with use of an antibiotic.

Diagnosis. Clinical evaluation will usually suggest the diagnosis of an inflammatory bowel lesion, but further studies will be needed. Microbiologic studies should be guided by knowledge of possible contacts. If *Entamoeba histolytica* is suspected, both serologic and appropriate stool examinations are indicated. Longstanding infections with *Yersinia enterocolitica, Campylobacter jejuni*, and some *Salmonella* species may cause elevated serum antibody titers. *Clostridium difficile* enterotoxin assays should be carried out if antibiotic-associated colitis is suspected.

In idiopathic ulcerative colitis, colonoscopic examination demonstrates the typical diffuse inflammatory lesion of the rectum and distal colon. The mucosa is inflamed, granular, and extremely friable; ulcers are rarely seen in children. In the typical case, biopsy shows an inflammatory lesion characterized by polymorphonuclear infiltration and crypt abscesses. Even when a double contrast technique is used, a

Table 12–7. Chronic Inflammatory Disorders of the Intestine

Infections
  Salmonella
  Yersinia enterocolitica
  Campylobacter jejuni
  Tuberculosis
  Cytomegalovirus
  Entamoeba histolytica
  Trichuriasis
Others
  Particularly in infants
    Necrotizing enterocolitis
    Hirschsprung enterocolitis
    "Allergic" colitis
  All ages
    Idiopathic ulcerative colitis
    Crohn disease
    Anaphylactoid purpura
    Hemolytic-uremic syndrome
    Pseudomembranous (antibiotic-associated) enterocolitis
    Eosinophilic gastroenteritis
    Behçet syndrome

barium enema may be normal initially, but usually the examination shows a diffuse distal lesion; the process may extend proximally to involve the entire colon. Colonoscopy is more sensitive than roentgenographic techniques in detecting minor mucosal lesions and the proximal limits of disease. None of the roentgenographic, endoscopic, or biopsy abnormalities is specific for idiopathic ulcerative colitis.

Treatment. No curative medical therapy is available, but medications can reduce the activity of the inflammatory process and prevent recurrences.

Supportive measures are particularly important. In accordance with their ability to understand, the child and his or her parents must be given insight into the nature of the disease. In general, dietary restrictions have little place in treatment so long as a nutritious, balanced diet is provided. Some patients become seriously malnourished because of an inability to tolerate sufficient nutrient intake. Total parenteral nutrition is effective in restoring nutritional status, but does not usually affect the inflammatory process in the bowel. Encouragement should be given to the patient's living as full a life as possible. In general, mood-altering drugs and appetitic stimulants should not be used.

Controlled studies in adults show that chronic administration of *sulfasalazine* reduces the likelihood of exacerbation, even years after the onset of the disease. In a dose of 0.5 g/15 kg/24 hr (maximum 4 g) it rarely has side effects; anorexia or nausea can usually be reduced by using enteric-coated drug. Occasionally, neutropenia or a hypersensitivity reaction necessitates discontinuing the medication. Sulfasalazine interferes with folic acid absorption; long-term users should either have their folate status monitored or receive supplemental folate. A high incidence of reversible oligospermia and infertility has been associated with long term use of sulfasalazine; it should, nonetheless, be given on a regular, continuing basis to patients in whom the diagnosis of idiopathic ulcerative colitis is proved, unless contraindicated by its effects.

Recent clinical trials show a response to oral *5-aminosalicylic acid* (5-ASA) comparable to that to sulfasalazine. Limited experience with rectal use of 5-ASA in children suggests a possible role of these enemas in active distal ulcerative colitis.

Corticosteroids are most effective for treating active disease. For mild cases, particularly those with disease confined to the distal colon, soluble hydrocortisone or prednisolone may be used as an enema, 100 mg hydrocortisone or its equivalent for an adolescent, given slowly at bedtime for 6 wk, daily for the first 3 wk and then on alternate nights. If the patient deteriorates or does not improve within 10 days, oral administration should be added. Prednisone, 1–2 mg/kg/24 hr to a maximum daily dose of 60 mg/24 hr, is used for moderate to severe cases and those which fail to respond to enema therapy. Occasionally, with fulminant disease, the patient may be too ill to tolerate oral medication and will require an equivalent intravenous dose of hydrocortisone. Once begun, a 3–4 mo course of systemic medication should be given, in a full dose for 6 wk, then tapered by 5 mg/24 hr each wk. The changes in facial appearance and acne that occur in children receiving this medication vary in severity but are universally dreaded by young patients. Additional complications from long-term use are osteoporosis, cataracts, systemic hypertension, and growth retardation. Alternate-day administration of prednisone may avoid adrenal suppression, but it is often inadequate to control active disease.

Other medications are not of proven benefit. Sodium cromoglycate given by mouth in large doses has provided symptomatic relief to some patients. Azathioprine has been used in conjunction with prednisone in attempts to control activity with reduced steroid dosage.

The disease can be cured by *surgical resection* of the entire colon. Emergency colectomy may be indicated in cases of actual or impending perforation, massive hemorrhage, or the development of a carcinoma in the diseased bowel. The common indications for operative treatment of a child with ulcerative colitis are prolonged or debilitating symptoms, and particularly growth or maturational delay in the face of an extended trial of medical therapy. A difficult decision must be faced when the young patient is found to have active colitis 10 yr after onset of the disease. Because of the risk of carcinoma in the diseased colon most authorities advise colectomy for such patients, particularly if the disease is extensive. Otherwise, semiannual colonoscopy with multiple biopsies is necessary for early tumor recognition to be achieved.

For children the usual primary operative procedure is subtotal colectomy, leaving the rectal stump in situ. This limited resection has the advantages of being less traumatic, of allowing for improvement in general health (growth, etc.), and of preserving the option for a second-stage procedure. The patient's general condition usually improves after partial colectomy, but active disease invariably persists in the retained rectal stump. At a second operation the stump can be removed. Preliminary reports suggest success with a pull-through anastomosis that removes diseased mucosa but preserves bowel continuity. The incidence of fecal incontinence after this operation is reduced when the procedure includes creation of a reservoir in the distal segment. If continuity of the intestine is not restored after colectomy, a permanent conventional ileostomy may be maintained or a continent Koch pouch may be fashioned. This latter procedure allows the patient to drain an internal surgically created reservoir and eliminates the need for an ileostomy appliance, but requires fastidious care.

Prognosis. Most cases beginning in childhood are severe both in activity and in extent of involvement. Occasionally, a fulminant onset progresses to perforation of the colon before a diagnosis is made. The usual course is one of initial improvement on medication, followed by recurrent exacerbations. Occasionally, massive blood loss can be life threatening, but the most serious acute complication is toxic megacolon, a massive dilatation of the colon which signals impending perforation. Ulcerative colitis predisposes the patient to colonic cancer; the risk is only 3% in the 1st decade after onset but rises 20%/decade subsequently, unless the colon has been resected.

Ament M: Inflammatory disease of the colon: Ulcerative colitis and Crohn's colitis. J Pediatr 86:322, 1975.

Davidson M, Bloom AA, Kugler MM: Chronic ulcerative colitis of childhood: An evaluative review. J Pediatr 67:471, 1965.

Devroede GJ, Taylor WF, Saver WG, et al: Cancer risk and life expectancy in children with ulcerative colitis. N Engl J Med 285:17, 1971.

Edwards FC, Truelove SC: The course and prognosis of ulcerative colitis. III. Complications. Gut 5:1, 1964.

Ein SH, Lynch MJ, Stephens CA; Ulcerative colitis in children under one year: A twenty year review. J Pediatr Surg 6:264, 1975.

Gadacz TR, Kelly KA, Phillips SF: The continent ileal pouch: Absorptive and motor features. Gastroenterology 72:1287, 1977.

Hamilton JR, Bruce GA, Abdourhaman M, et al: Inflammatory bowel disease in children and adolescents. Adv Pediatr 26:311, 1980.

Martin LW, LeCoultre C, Schubert WK: Total colectomy and mucosal proctectomy with preservation of continence in ulcerative colitis. Ann Surg 186:477, 1977.

Toovey S, Hudson E, Hendry WF, et al: Sulphasalazine and male infertility: Reversibility and possible mechanism. Gut 22:445, 1981.

Werlen SL, Grend RJ: Severe colitis in children and adolescents: Diagnosis, course, and treatment. Gastroenterology 73:828, 1977.

12.43 CROHN DISEASE
(Regional Enteritis, Granulomatous Enterocolitis)

Crohn disease is a segmental transmural intestinal disease; it may involve one or more segments of gut from the mouth to the anus, but the distal ileum and colon are most commonly affected. The cause is unknown. The inflammatory process consists of noncaseating granulomas with regional lymphatic involvement. Fistulas may form between loops of bowel or from bowel to neighboring structures such as the skin or urinary tract. Early in the course biopsied tissue may not have granulomas, and findings may be identical to those of ulcerative colitis. Crohn disease and ulcerative colitis are the major causes of "nonspecific" *inflammatory bowel disease* (IBD), a term now reserved primarily for these 2 entities.

The incidence of Crohn disease has increased in Western Europe and North America in the past decade. Like ulcerative colitis, it is relatively common among Jews, 1st degree relatives of patients, and patients with ankylosing spondylitis and the histocompatibility antigen, HLA-B27.

Clinical Manifestations. Eighteen to 30% of cases of Crohn disease begin before the age of 20 yr, usually after 10 yr. The onset is usually subtle; many months may pass between the 1st symptoms and diagnosis. Crampy abdominal pain is the most common initial complaint, followed by diarrhea. Unlike patients with ulcerative colitis, about half of these patients have at onset nonintestinal problems such as fever, anorexia, growth failure, general malaise, and joint symptoms. Any teenager with chronic malaise and persisting growth problems, particularly with fever, should be suspected of having this condition. Chronic perianal lesions, even when there are no reasons to suspect primary bowel disease, are another early signal.

In time, most children with active Crohn disease develop abdominal pain and diarrhea. Pain from involvement of small intestine is often periumbilical or in the right lower quadrant rather than confined to the lower abdomen, as in ulcerative colitis. Stools are less explosive than in ulcerative colitis, and there is less tenesmus except when the distal segment is involved. Intestinal bleeding is rare but it can be massive.

Extraintestinal manifestations are similar to those of ulcerative colitis, but are more common with Crohn disease. Arthritis, usually affecting large joints, was reported in 18% of one pediatric series. Erythema nodosum, iritis, hepatitis, and phlebitis are rare; they tend to exacerbate and remit with the activity of the intestinal lesion. Finger clubbing occurs in about a third of patients with Crohn disease.

Differential Diagnosis. The usual causes of inflammatory bowel lesions are summarized in Table 12–7. The most important feature distinguishing Crohn disease from ulcerative colitis is that the distribution of the Crohn lesion is segmental, whereas, that of ulcerative colitis is diffuse and confined to the colon. Infections that are particularly likely to be confused with Crohn disease are those that involve the distal small bowel, e.g., *Yersinia enterocolitica*, which is common, and tuberculosis, which is rare in North America. *Yersinia* and anaphylactoid purpura may cause small intestinal abnormalities in barium studies similar to those found in Crohn disease. Intestinal manifestations of *Behçet syndrome* are identical to those of Crohn disease (see Sec. 10.84). Early in their courses, anaphylactoid purpura and hemolytic-uremic syndromes may closely mimic Crohn disease. All patients should be observed for skin lesions or renal lesions or both.

Diagnosis. A careful clinical evaluation will usually suggest a diagnosis of an inflammatory bowel lesion. An elevated erythrocyte sedimentation rate gives evidence of an active inflammatory process in more than 75% of patients at the time of diagnosis. Hemoglobin levels are mildly depressed and serum albumin levels reduced in about a third of cases.

If an inflammatory lesion is suspected and microbiologic studies exclude a specific infection, barium contrast roentgenograms of small and large bowel are needed to define the segments involved. Crohn disease is characterized by irregular mucosa or a cobblestone-like pattern, thickened bowel, and enteric fistulas, but it is the lesion's segmental distribution that is diagnostic. Detail may be better seen in the small bowel by injecting barium directly by tube into the duodenum, and, in the colon by using a double air-contrast technique.

Biopsies of rectal mucosa may show typical granulomas even if there is no gross evidence of distal segment involvement on sigmoidoscopy. Because involvement of the colon is often proximal, a rigid sigmoidoscope seldom reaches the diseased area. Colonoscopy, which allows visualization of the proximal colon from below, can be used to further define the limits of colonic Crohn lesions.

Treatment. Curative medical therapy is not available. A 30 yr recurrence rate of over 90% is reported after operative resection in Crohn disease.

Since medications are palliative at best, supportive measures are very important. The child and family must be helped to attain insight into the nature of this disease and its disabling symptoms. Therapy should be directed at enabling the patient to live as full a life as possible and creating an atmosphere in which the child does not consider himself or herself an invalid. For example, undue fatigue should be avoided but exercise encouraged. Usual household discipline should be exercised. Generally, a full nutritious diet should be encouraged; appetite stimulants and mood-altering drugs are unlikely to be helpful.

Placing the bowel "at rest" by use of total parenteral nutrition or by use of an elemental diet infused by nasogastric tube is usually effective in diminishing disease activity. These techniques are particularly effective for children with delayed growth and those with enteric fistulas. The enteral infusions are well tolerated unless there is very active disease, impending bowel obstruction, or severe psychologic disturbance. They can usually be given over 12 hr periods at night for 2 to 3 mo by patients at home.

Prednisone is indicated to treat acute exacerbations. For active small bowel disease 1–2 mg/kg/24 hr (maximum 60 mg) of prednisone should be given for 6 wk, after which gradual reduction of the dose should be attempted over a further 8–12 wk. If symptoms recur with decreased doses, the drug should be given at higher levels for a longer period. Alternate-day therapy is rarely effective in maintaining a remission. In some difficult cases the concomitant use of azathioprine, 2 mg/kg/24 hr, permits the reduction of steroid dose, but azathioprine should be used for no more than 1 yr, with careful monitoring of the white blood count. Sulfasalazine is not so beneficial in Crohn disease as in ulcerative colitis. Available data support its use (0.5 g/15 kg/24 hr up to 4 g/24 hr) for colonic Crohn disease, but the drug does not increase long-term remission rates or enhance the effect of corticosteroid. Metronidazole may be beneficial in some cases, particularly those with fistulas.

Because of high recurrence rates and in some cases extensive small bowel involvement, surgical resection for Crohn disease has less to offer than for ulcerative colitis. Massive hemorrhage, intestinal perforation, or persistent bowel obstruction will demand operative intervention as lifesaving; these emergencies are rare in children with Crohn disease. The question of operative resection usually arises around the issue of persisting debility, particularly when growth and maturation are delayed. Although recurrence appears to be inevitable, resection frequently permits an interval of good health, growth, and a return to full activity. The decision to operate will be based on the severity and duration of debility, the patient's age and potential for growth, and the response of the patient and family to the disease. Every effort should be made to arrange any elective resection for a time when nutritional status is satisfactory and the inflammatory process inactive.

Prognosis. The inflammatory activity of Crohn disease tends to remit and exacerbate through life without a consistent pattern. In most cases the region involved remains constant;

when extension occurs, it often appears to be a postoperative event. The natural course of this inflammatory process is to develop scar tissue resulting in bowel obstruction. Ileal disease leads almost inevitably to obstructive problems, but usually a decade or more after onset of the disease. The incidence of intestinal cancer is increased with longstanding Crohn disease but not nearly to the degree seen in ulcerative colitis.

Ament M: Inflammatory disease of the colon. Ulcerative colitis and Crohn's colitis. J Pediatr 86:322, 1975.
Gryboski JD, Spiro HM: Prognosis in children with Crohn's disease. Gastroenterology 74:807, 1978.
Hamilton JR, Bruce GA, Abdourhaman M, et al: Inflammatory bowel disease in children and adolescents. Adv Pediatr 26:311, 1980.
Kasahara Y, Tamaka S, Nishino N, et al: Intestinal involvement in Behçet's disease: Review of 136 surgical cases in the Japanese literature. Dis Col Rectum 24:103, 1981.
Kelts DG, Grand RJ, Shen G, et al: Nutritional basis of growth failure in children and adolescents with Crohn's disease. Gastroenterology 76:720, 1979.
Kirschner BS, Voinchet O, Rosenberg IH: Growth retardation in inflammatory bowel disease. Gastroenterology 75:504, 1978.
Morin CL, Roulet M, Roy CC, et al: Continuous elemental enteral alimentation in children with Crohn's disease and growth failure. Gastroenterology 79:1205, 1980.
Miller RC, Larson E: Regional enteritis in early infancy. Am J Dis Child 122:301, 1971.
Parkin JV, Wight DGD: Behçet's disease and the alimentary tract. Postgrad Med J 51:260, 1975.
Summers RW, Switz DM, Sessions JT, et al: National Cooperative Crohn's disease study: Results of drug treatment. Gastroenterology 77:847, 1979.

NEONATAL NECROTIZING ENTEROCOLITIS (NEC)
(See Sec. 8.43)

12.44 ANTIBIOTIC-ASSOCIATED (PSEUDOMEMBRANOUS) ENTEROCOLITIS

This potentially serious disorder associated with antibiotic administration presents a spectrum of illness ranging from mild diarrhea to pseudomembranous enterocolitis. The common etiologic factor is an enterotoxin-producing strain of *Clostridium difficile* in the lumen of the distal bowel.

Within 1 wk of starting oral antibiotic therapy the patient develops diarrhea. Many agents cause the problem, but clindamycin and ampicillin have been incriminated most often. The disease may run a fulminant course with increasing severity of diarrhea, bloody stools, and abdominal distention. In the severe form of the disease, sigmoidoscopy reveals a typical lesion: a patchy cream-white exudate, resembling a membrane, adherent to normal mucosa. Preceding abdominal surgery and underlying vascular disease increase the likelihood of a fulminant course. Enterotoxin-producing clostridia are found in the stools in these severe cases. The same organisms are found after antibiotic therapy in less severely ill children with diarrhea but no visible pseudomembrane formation.

Florid pseudomembranous enterocolitis requires emergency treatment. The possible offending antibiotics and oral food intake should be stopped, nasogastric suction begun, intravenous fluid and nutrients provided, and vancomycin or metronidazole given by mouth or nasogastric tube. Use of an appropriate antibiotic shortens the course in most cases and allows for return to usual oral intake within 1 wk. For affected children with mild diarrhea, stopping the causative antibiotic is usually sufficient. In the moderately severe case it is best to err on the aggressive side in therapy for this potentially fatal disease.

Bartlett JG: Antibiotic-associated colitis. Clin Gastroenterol 8:783, 1979.
Buts JP, Weber AM, Roy CC, et al: Pseudomembranous enterocolitis in childhood. Gastroenterology 73:823, 1977.

Fekety R, Kim K, Brown D, et al: Epidemiology of antibiotic associated colitis. Am J Med 70:906, 1981.
Keating JP, Frank AL, Barton LL, et al: Pseudomembranous colitis associated with ampicillin therapy. Am J Dis Child 128:369, 1974.
Tedesco FJ, Stanley RJ, Alpers DH: Diagnostic features of clindamycin-associated pseudomembranous colitis. N Engl J Med 290:84, 1974.

12.45 GASTROINTESTINAL SYMPTOMS IN ANAPHYLACTOID PURPURA

Two thirds of patients with anaphylactoid (Henoch-Schönlein) purpura have abdominal symptoms. Crampy abdominal pain may be very severe and precede any other manifestations of the disorder. The pain results from submucosal and subserosal hemorrhages, which may lead to small or large amounts of blood in the stools or to intussusception. In the acute disease barium contrast roentgenograms may show large filling defects in the bowel wall, suggestive of Crohn disease or a neoplasm. Diagnosis is made when the characteristic purpuric rash or renal manifestations develop.

Goldman LP, Lindenberg RL: Henoch-Schönlein purpura: gastrointestinal manifestations with endoscopic correlation. Am J Gastroenterol 75:357, 1981.
Silver DL: Henoch-Schönlein syndrome. Pediatr Clin North Am 19:1061, 1972.

12.46 GASTROINTESTINAL PROBLEMS IN HEMOLYTIC-UREMIC SYNDROME

This potentially fatal disorder may begin as an intestinal inflammatory disorder. Bloody diarrhea is frequently the first symptom. *Shigella*, *Campylobacter*, and enterotoxin-producing strains of *E. coli* have been isolated from stools of patients with hemolytic-uremic syndrome. Barium contrast roentgenograms show transient early filling defects, but the lesions may progress to stenosis. Diagnosis depends on the recognition of acute renal failure, hemolytic anemia, and thrombocytopenia, none of which may be apparent in the early stages.

Kaplan BS: The hemolytic-uremic syndrome. Pediatr Clin North Am 23:761, 1976.
Sawaf H, Sharp MJ, Youn KJ, et al: Ischemic colitis and stricture after hemolytic-uremic syndrome. Pediatrics 61:315, 1978.
Tochen ML, Campbell JR: Colitis in children with hemolytic-uremic syndrome. J Pediatr Surg 12:213, 1977.

12.47 DIETARY PROTEIN INTOLERANCE

Adverse reactions in the intestine can result from exposure to specific dietary proteins. In many cases these reactions appear to be allergic, but proof of an immunologic response is often lacking; in such cases the term *intolerance* seems appropriate. Because laboratory diagnostic criteria are not reliable, diagnosis is based on clinical responses to withdrawal and challenge with the potential dietary agent. Most cases are recognized in infants, and cow's milk is the usual incriminated food.

Cow's Milk Protein Intolerance

Because diagnostic criteria are uncertain, incidence is difficult to determine; in Sweden estimates range from 0.5–1.5%. This is largely a condition of infancy; a higher incidence is seen among infants fed cow's milk from birth than among those who are breast-fed initially. The incidence of allergic diseases (e.g., eczema, asthma) is increased in these patients and their family members.

Clinical Manifestations. Several gastrointestinal syndromes are attributed to cow's milk.

Acute Vomiting and Diarrhea. In young infants the usual onset is acute and characterized by vomiting and watery diarrhea which is often bloody, suggesting colitis. In its most fulminant form there is glottic swelling and anaphylactic shock, which, if untreated, can be fatal. The cellular exudate in stools often contains many eosinophils in addition to erythrocytes.

Chronic Diarrhea and Malabsorption. Diarrhea may be chronic, leading to general ill health, slow weight gain, and growth retardation. This chronic syndrome tends to occur in older infants and is associated with small bowel dysfunction (mild steatorrhea and malabsorption of d-xylose). Small intestine biopsies have shown patchy mucosal lesions of varying severity; there is shortening of villi, elongation of crypts, and an increase in intraepithelial lymphocytes and lamina propria cellularity, but single suction biopsy specimens may be normal. Most patients with this chronic syndrome have been reported from European centers.

Excessive Enteric Protein and Blood Loss. This syndrome has been reported mainly in older infants presenting with generalized edema, hypoproteinemia, and iron deficiency anemia. There may be diarrhea or no intestinal symptoms. In affected children excessive enteric loss of protein and blood ceases after withdrawal of milk. Often, the syndrome is associated with the change in feeding from milk formula to ordinary whole cow's milk.

Diagnosis. The diagnosis of milk protein intolerance is clinical. Acute symptoms should subside within 48 hr and chronic within 1 wk of complete withdrawal of milk. Caution and judgment must be exercised in rechallenging these patients with milk. In a young infant, particularly if an acute response is anticipated, the challenge should be carried out under observation, beginning with 1–5 mL of milk and increasing the dose progressively over a few days provided a response does not occur. For gastrointestinal responses to potential dietary antigens skin tests, circulating antibody titers, complement assays, and coproantibody titers are not of proven diagnostic value. In children with chronic symptoms some centers use mucosal biopsy to evaluate the response to challenge. It is important to rule out other conditions that may cause similar symptoms such as enteric infections, lactose intolerance, and other forms of nonspecific inflammatory bowel disease.

The syndromes described for cow's milk intolerance may occur also in response to **soy protein.** Some studies estimate that up to 50% of children intolerant to cow's milk are intolerant to soy. Since soy is not a commonly used food, most will not be exposed to soy unless they are first found intolerant to cow's milk. The approach to diagnosis is the same as for cow's milk.

Treatment. Prolonged breast feeding reduces the likelihood of later cow's milk intolerance. Treatment consists of removing the offending food from the diet. For the young infant the non–milk-containing dietary formulas consist of various soy feedings and hydrolyzed milk protein feedings. Many children with the enteric protein and blood loss syndrome will benefit by changing from fresh milk to processed (i.e., evaporated, powdered) milk. For rare cases of intolerance to many foods, oral administration of sodium cromoglycate has been reported to suppress intestinal symptoms and permit continued ingestion of the food.

Prognosis is variable. In many cases, food protein intolerances are transitory. About 50% of infants with the conditions described above have recovered within 1 yr and most of the remainder within 2 yr.

Ament ME, Rubin CE: Soy protein–another cause of the flat intestinal lesion. Gastroenterology 62:227, 1972.
Eastham EJ, Walker WA: Effect of cow's milk on the gastrointestinal tract: A persistent dilemma for the pediatrician. Pediatrics 60:477, 1977.
Fontaine SL, Navarro J: Small intestinal biopsy in cow's milk protein allergy in infancy. Arch Dis Child 50:357, 1975.
Goldman AS, Anderson DW, Sellers WA, et al: Milk allergy. Oral challenge

with milk and isolated milk protein in allergic children. Pediatrics 32:425, 1963.

Powell GK: Milk and soy-induced enterocolitis of infancy. J Pediatr 93:558, 1978.

Savilahti E, Kuitunen P, Visakorpi JK: Cow's milk allergy. *In:* Lebenthal E (ed): Textbook of Gastroenterology and Nutrition. New York, Raven Press, 1981.

Waldman TA, Wochner RD, Laster L, et al: Allergic gastroenteropathy: A cause of excessive gastrointestinal protein loss. N Engl J Med 276:761, 1967.

Walker-Smith JA, Harrison M, Kilby A, et al: Cow's milk sensitive enteropathy. Arch Dis Child 53:375, 1979.

12.48 EOSINOPHILIC GASTROENTERITIS

A rare form of inflammatory involvement of the intestine is characterized by infiltrates of eosinophils. Usually, the stomach and the upper small bowel are involved, but esophageal and distal intestinal lesions also occur.

The lesions normally cause abdominal pain, vomiting, diarrhea, and delayed growth and weight gain. Often, there are atopic symptoms, such as rhinitis and asthma and a peripheral eosinophilia, which suggest an allergic basis for the disorder. Excessive enteric protein loss may cause reduced serum albumin and immune globulin levels. Endoscopy may reveal an inflammatory lesion in the stomach, and duodenal biopsy shows eosinophilic congestion of the lamina propria and patchy villus shortening. Rarely, eosinophils infiltrate more deeply to cause bowel wall thickening and granuloma formation.

The disease usually runs a chronic debilitating course with sporadic severe exacerbations. A few patients are helped by elimination diets, but most require systemic administration of corticosteroids.

Cello JP: Eosinophilic gastroenteritis: A complex disease entity. Am J Med 67:1097, 1979.

Katz AJ, Golman H, Grand RJ: Gastric mucosal biopsy in eosinophilic (allergic) gastroenteritis. Gastroenterology 73:705, 1977.

Klein NC, Hargrove RL, Sleisenger MN, et al: Eosinophilic gastroenteritis. Medicine 49:299, 1970.

12.49 MALABSORPTIVE DISORDERS

The malabsorptive disorders include a number of gastrointestinal diseases with a wide range of clinical features that include defective assimilation of ingested nutrients. Those that cause maldigestion or malabsorption of many nutrients tend to share certain clinical manifestations: abdominal distention; pale, foul, bulky stools; wasting of muscles, particularly the proximal muscle groups; and retarded growth and weight gain (Fig. 12–20). *Celiac syndrome* or *malabsorption syndrome* has been used to describe these diseases. Over the years specific digestive tract disorders have been identified as causes of this *celiac syndrome*. One of these, a specific *gluten-induced enteropathy*, is called *celiac disease* or *celiac sprue*.

Major causes of generalized defects in absorption or digestion are summarized in Table 12–8, where those diseases that

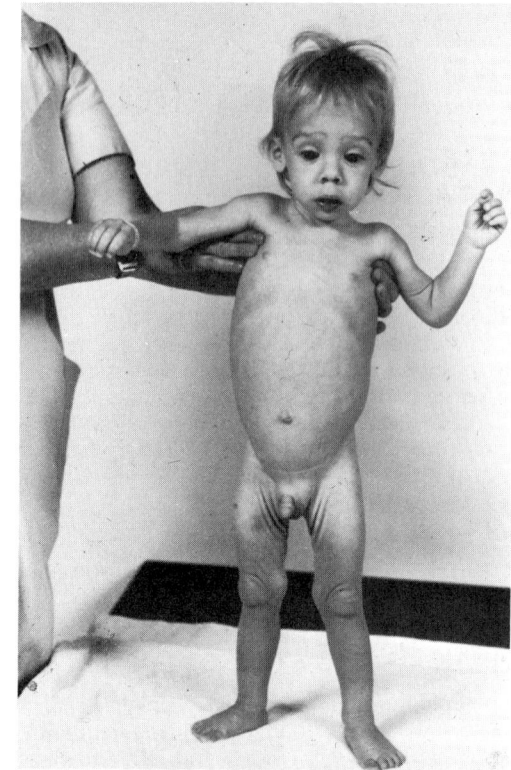

Figure 12–20. An 18 mo old boy with active celiac disease. Note the loose skin folds, marked proximal muscle wasting, and full abdomen. The child looks ill.

tend to occur relatively frequently in North America and Europe are separated from less common disorders.

Congenital disorders have been identified that involve only a single specific intestinal transport process. The clinical manifestations of these diseases often differ from those of the generalized malabsorptive state. Some cause intestinal symptoms, particularly diarrhea, but others may produce only nutritional deficiencies, without gastrointestinal symptoms. In Table 12–9 specific absorptive pathway defects are listed; only some of this latter group cause gastrointestinal symptoms, and all except the acquired disaccharidase deficiencies are rare.

EVALUATION OF PATIENTS SUSPECTED OF HAVING INTESTINAL MALABSORPTION

Many chronic nongastroenterologic diseases are capable of causing significant malnutrition and growth problems. For example, children with chronic renal disease or intracranial lesions may develop clinical manifestations very similar to

Table 12–8. **Generalized Malabsorptive States in Childhood**

	More Common	Less Common
Exocrine pancreas	Cystic fibrosis Chronic protein-calorie malnutrition	Shwachman-Diamond syndrome Chronic pancreatitis
Liver, biliary tree	Biliary atresia	Other cholestatic states
Intestine 　Anatomic defects	Massive resection Stagnant loop syndrome	Congenitally short gut
Chronic infection (± immune deficiency)	Giardiasis Coccidiosis	
Miscellaneous	Celiac disease Postenteritis malabsorption	Dietary protein intolerance (milk, soy) Tropical sprue Intestinal Whipple disease Idiopathic diffuse mucosal lesions

Table 12–9. Specific Defects of Digestive-Absorptive Function Occurring in Children

	Disease
Intestinal	
Fat	Abetalipoproteinemia
Protein	Enterokinase deficiency
	Amino acid transport defects (cystinuria, Hartnup disease, methionine malabsorption, blue diaper syndrome)
Carbohydrate	Disaccharidase deficiencies (congenital: sucrase-isomaltase, lactase; developmental: lactase; acquired: generalized glucose-galactose malabsorption)
Vitamin	Vitamin B_{12} malabsorption (juvenile pernicious anemia, transcobalamin II deficiency, Immerslund syndrome)
	Folic acid malabsorption
Ions, trace elements	Chloride-losing diarrhea
	Acrodermatitis enteropathica
	Menkes syndrome
	Vitamin D–dependent rickets
	Primary hypomagnesemia
Drug-induced	Salazosulfapyridine (folic acid malabsorption)
	Cholestyramine (Ca, fat malabsorption)
	Phenytoin (Dilantin) (Ca)
Pancreatic	Specific enzyme deficiencies
	Lipase
	Trypsinogen

those of children with malabsorptive states. Success in distinguishing those children with true malabsorptive diseases from patients with chronic nonspecific diarrhea or nongastrointestinal diseases causing small stature depends primarily upon clinical findings. Elements in the history and physical examination that help in assessment of many of these entities are presented in this section. More detailed descriptions of specific malabsorptive diseases are presented in subsequent sections.

Clinical Manifestations. Since many of the gastrointestinal diseases causing malabsorption are genetically determined, the family history often suggests the diagnosis. These congenital lesions usually cause symptoms early in infancy. Specific intestinal transport defects affect specific nutrients, and celiac disease is caused by a general response of the mucosa to dietary glutens. Besides the time of onset of symptoms and their relationship to dietary content and intake, aspects of the history that tend to be offered in great detail are of limited value. Descriptions of stools are highly subjective; quantity is of obvious interest, but color, odor, and consistency are of relatively little diagnostic significance. The relationship between diet and diarrhea must be logical to be meaningful; for example, if lactose is responsible for diarrhea, then one lactose-containing food should be as provocative as the next. Because diseases of many systems may produce clinical manifestations such as failure to thrive and abdominal distention suggestive of a malabsorptive state, a complete review of other systems is essential. Disorders of the central nervous system and urinary tract deserve particular attention.

The impact of symptoms on the child's general health is best assessed in terms of changes in body weight and length. Measurements should be related to earlier measurements and family patterns. Signs of malnutrition such as muscle wasting, edema, mouth sores, smooth tongue, and excessive bruising should be interpreted in the light of estimated nutrient intake. In cases of diarrhea, parents and physicians may limit the child's nutrient intake for prolonged periods, thereby inducing malnutrition which may be erroneously assumed to result from malabsorption.

A rectal examination is an important step in the initial examination of children suspected of having intestinal mal-

absorption. In addition to assessing the anus and rectum, this procedure provides immediate access to stool for gross, microscopic, and, in some cases, chemical analysis. Children with pancreatic insufficiency who are receiving a complete diet will have excessive triglyceride and undigested meat fibers in their stools; those with intestinal malabsorption will have crystalline aggregates of monoglyceride and fatty acid.

Laboratory Manifestations. *Absorptive Function.* Fat absorption can be quantitated by a *fecal fat balance* study comparing total losses to estimated dietary fat intake. If the patient is consuming appreciable quantities of fat (>20 g/day) and total collections are carried out for at least 4 days, excretion should not exceed 15% of intake in an infant or 10% in an older child. In hope of supplanting the unpleasant task of stool analysis, screening tests have been developed to assess absorption and to detect steatorrhea. The simplest is to measure fasting *serum carotene* concentration. In the presence of adequate dietary intake a result of <50 µg/dL suggests fat malabsorption and >100 µg/dL normal absorption; however, a significant number of false-positive and negative results occur with this screening test. In skilled hands, stool microscopy to assess directly the fat content of random stools compares favorably with other screening procedures for steatorrhea.

Carbohydrate absorption cannot be quantitated by simple balance procedures because sugars are broken down in the intestinal lumen by enteric bacteria. No more than a trace of sugar is found in normal stools except for those passed by breast-fed infants. An excess of sugar in fresh stool suggests sugar intolerance, but a lack of excess does not exclude the diagnosis. Random stool samples can be tested for reducing substance quickly and easily using commercially available tablets.* A result of >0.5% indicates abnormal absorption if the diet contains significant amounts of a reducing sugar. Most dietary sugars, except for sucrose, are reducing sugars; if sucrose is to be tested, it must first be hydrolyzed by heating the stool sample with HCl. Usually fresh stool of a patient with sugar intolerance will also have a pH of less than 6.0 because of the organic acids produced in the lumen by bacterial action on the unabsorbed sugar. The indirect method for measuring carbohydrate absorption is the *oral tolerance test.* An oral dose (0.5 g/kg body weight) of the sugar to be tested is given to the fasting patient and plasma concentration of glucose is measured at 15, 30, 60, and 120 min. A rise of at least 20 mg/dL glucose should occur normally after lactose and sucrose are given and at least 50 mg/dL when glucose is given. Many variables apart from digestion and absorption, however, can affect the results (e.g., rates of gastric emptying and glucose utilization). *Hydrogen concentrations in expired air* may be measured after an oral dose of sugar (2 g/kg body weight to 50 g maximum). If the sugar being tested is not absorbed in the upper small bowel, it reaches the distal intestine where enteric bacteria act on it to produce hydrogen gas, which is quickly absorbed and expired quantitatively. A rise in breath hydrogen exceeding 20 ppm during the first 2 hr is abnormal. Patients taking antibiotics and about 2% of the normal population do not have hydrogen-producing enteric flora.

Protein absorption cannot be accurately quantitated in routine clinical practice. Balance studies do not necessarily reflect assimilation because of endogenous sources of fecal protein, but *fecal nitrogen* can be measured as a rough guide. *Enteric protein loss* can be quantitated using an intravenous injection of $^{51}CrCl$ followed by measurement of the fecal excretion of the label in a 4 day collection of stool. A result exceeding 0.8% of the injected dose indicates excessive loss. *Fecal clearance of serum α_1-antitrypsin* also reflects enteric protein loss; as

---

*Clinitest, Ames Co.

measured on a 48 hr stool collection, clearance exceeding 15 mL/day is excessive.

Other nutrients that may be measured in blood include iron, the level of which will depend on transferrin concentration as well as on absorption; folic acid, the red cell concentration being a more accurate reflection of nutritional status than the serum concentration; serum calcium and magnesium; vitamin D and its metabolites; vitamin A; and vitamin B_{12}. In presence of apparent adequate intake, depressed concentrations of these will suggest inadequate absorption. It may take years to deplete stores of vitamin B_{12} after absorption is impaired.

Certain absorptive studies help to localize an intestinal lesion. Iron and *d-xylose*, a pentose minimally metabolized in man, are absorbed by the upper small bowel. A blood concentration of less than 25 mg/dL xylose 1 hr after a 14.5 g/m² body surface oral dose (up to 25 g) usually indicates a proximal intestinal mucosal lesion, but some false-negative and false-positive results are obtained using this technique. In the distal bowel, vitamin B_{12} is absorbed and bile salts are reabsorbed. *Vitamin B_{12} absorption* can be measured directly using the *Schilling test*, in which, after body stores of the vitamin are saturated, a tracer dose of radioactive B_{12} is given by mouth, with or without intrinsic factor, and urinary excretion measured over the next 24 hr. Defective absorption, shown by urinary excretion of less than 5% of the dose, occurs when an extensive length of distal ileum is resected or diseased, or when bacterial overgrowth occurs within the bowel lumen.

Diagnostic Procedures. MICROBIOLOGIC. The only common primary infection causing chronic malabsorption is giardiasis (Sec. 11.102). New techniques to fix and stain specimens have greatly improved the diagnostic value of examining stools for *Giardia* cysts. The trophozoite may be identified in fresh duodenal contents or the duodenal mucosa. When enteric clearing of bacteria is impaired, either from stasis of luminal contents or impaired immune function, colony counts from bacterial cultures of proximal intestinal juice may be very high.

HEMATOLOGIC. Blood smears may indicate iron deficiency. A megaloblastic smear suggests deficiency and therefore malabsorption of folic acid or of vitamin B_{12}. Acanthocyte transformation of erythrocytes occurs in abetalipoproteinemia. A blood smear may also suggest a lymphocyte defect or a neutropenia associated with Shwachman syndrome.

IMAGING PROCEDURES. These procedures are used primarily to identify local lesions in the abdomen. In children with malabsorptive disorders **plain roentgenograms** and **barium contrast** studies may suggest a site and cause of intestinal stasis. For example, the most common anomaly causing incomplete bowel obstruction is intestinal malrotation, a condition difficult to exclude without a barium enema to locate the cecum. In general, the small intestine should be examined with the use of large quantities of nonflocculating barium. Although flocculation of normal barium and dilated bowel with thickened mucosal folds have been attributed to diffuse malabsorptive lesions such as celiac disease, these abnormalities are nonspecific and of little diagnostic value. **Technetium (99Tc) scan** is an accurate technique with which to detect aberrant gastric mucosa such as might be present in a duplication or Meckel diverticulum, but these lesions rarely cause malabsorption. **Ultrasonography** can detect alterations in pancreatic mass, biliary tree abnormalities, and stones, even in infants with malabsorption. **Retrograde studies of the pancreatic and biliary tree** using contrast injection via endoscopy are reserved for rare cases requiring careful delineation of the biliary tree and pancreatic ducts.

SMALL BOWEL BIOPSY. Peroral suction biopsy of small intestinal mucosa is an important tool in the study of children with malabsorptive states. The demonstration of a typical diffuse mucosal lesion is prerequisite for the diagnosis of celiac disease, and a specific abnormality is seen in children with abetalipoproteinemia. Microscopic abnormalities may also be seen in the mucosa of patients with giardiasis, lymphangiectasia, gamma globulin deficiencies, viral enteritis, tropical sprue, and cow's milk or soy intolerance, and in some infants with idiopathic diffuse mucosal lesions.

Disaccharidase assays may be carried out on mucosa. If there is diffuse mucosal disease, these assays will be depressed, but specific congenital abnormalities may also be detected.

DISEASES CAUSING GENERALIZED MALDIGESTION OR MALABSORPTION

Cystic Fibrosis
(Fibrocystic Disease of the Pancreas, Mucoviscidosis)

See Sec. 13.97.

Shwachman-Diamond Syndrome
(Pancreatic Hypoplasia with Neutropenia)

See Sec. 12.68.

12.50 THE DIGESTIVE TRACT IN CHRONIC MALNUTRITION

Exocrine pancreatic function is much more susceptible to protein-calorie malnutrition than the intestine, and suppression of digestive enzyme secretion may occur relatively early in patients with primary malnutrition (Sec. 12.68). In developed countries where primary malnutrition is rare, chronic gastrointestinal disorders and their treatment are significant causes of malnutrition; undoubtedly, under these circumstances some degree of compromised pancreatic function develops. Children may be particularly at risk since their nutritional reserves are relatively meager. World-wide, exocrine pancreatic insufficiency is most often attributable to malnutrition, not to a primary pancreatic disease. Because 90% of functioning exocrine tissue must be lost before significant digestive problems develop in patients who are otherwise well, malnutrition is usually severe and prolonged before pancreatic insufficiency causes clinically apparent digestive defects.

The intestine is remarkably resistant to the effects of protein-calorie malnutrition. Patients with *kwashiorkor* may have a severely flattened small intestinal villus structure, but these abnormalities probably are attributable to coexisting infections and infestations. In *marasmus* villus structure is relatively preserved, though microvillus changes and intracellular electron microscopic abnormalities have been observed. Chronic malnutrition can lead to impaired immune function (Sec. 12.68); perhaps as a consequence, bacterial overgrowth of the upper intestine is seen in malnourished subjects.

When oral intake is completely withheld in experimental animals, intestinal mucosal mass and absorptive function diminish even when nutrient balance is maintained by the intravenous route. These changes can be reversed by small amounts of oral nutrient. Accordingly, there is a theoretical advantage in delivering nutrients via the gut rather than by vein. Also, because mucosal epithelial repair may be delayed in chronic malnutrition, convalescence from acute self-limited mucosal diseases such as viral enteritis may be prolonged in the malnourished state and shortened when nutrients are adequately provided.

Little is known about the effect of *specific nutritional deficiencies* on the pancreas or intestine; apart from potassium depletion causing ileus and severe dehydration causing constipation, available data suggest a relatively minor clinical effect of a wide range of specific deficiencies. Iron deficiency is associated with enhanced iron uptake at the mucosa and, in a few severe cases, occurrence of mucosal flattening. Deficiencies of vitamin B_{12} and folic acid may cause distortion of enterocyte morphology but no known serious functional abnormalities of gut. Some hypocalcemic states may be accompanied by steatorrhea and even by ion and water secretion, but this poorly understood relationship is not constant.

12.51 LIVER AND BILIARY DISORDERS

Steatorrhea occurs secondary to hepatobiliary disorders if bile flow to the duodenum is interrupted. When intraluminal bile salt concentrations fall below the critical micellar concentration, dietary fat cannot be efficiently assimilated, and because sterol absorption is especially dependent on bile formation, bone lesions secondary to vitamin D malabsorption are particularly likely to occur unless large supplements of the vitamin are given. Vitamin E malabsorption has been identified as an important factor in chronic neuropathies associated with severe chronic cholestasis. In general, steatorrhea is associated with severe obstructive jaundice such as occurs in biliary atresia, but on occasion other types of severe cholestasis cause steatorrhea.

12.52 INTESTINAL INFECTIONS CAUSING MALABSORPTION

Malabsorption is a rare consequence of primary intestinal infection. Only parasites with a propensity to chronic infestation cause malabsorption in the host who is not immunologically compromised. *Giardia lamblia* infestation is common in children, particularly toddlers, but a very small proportion of the infected patients develop malabsorption (Sec. 11.102). Children with immune deficiencies are particularly susceptible to *Giardia*, but even in these patients malabsorption affecting fat and sometimes disaccharides is mild. *Coccidiosis* due either to *Isospora belli* or to *I. hominis* in warm climates of the Southern Hemisphere can cause malabsorption and diarrhea (Sec. 11.98). *Intestinal hookworm*, although associated with malabsorption, is not thought to cause it.

12.53 IMMUNODEFICIENCY AND THE INTESTINE

See also Sec. 10.16 and 10.23.

The mechanisms for disturbed intestinal function in children with certain immunodeficiency states are not clear. Some patients are predisposed to infection with *Giardia lamblia*. Others with measurable abnormalities of intestinal function or structure do not have clearcut evidence of a specific enteric infection; yet it seems likely that defective resistance to enteric microflora lies behind their intestinal disorder. Diagnostic evaluation of these patients is complicated by the fact that some intestinal diseases may cause secondary immune deficiencies due to enteric losses of immunoglobulins and lymphocytes.

Congenital Sex-Linked Panhypogammaglobulinemia (Bruton). Mild intermittent diarrhea usually begins early and improves after 2 yr of age. Giardiasis is relatively common. Crypt abscesses may be seen in rectal biopsies of affected patients—yet they rarely experience colitic symptoms.

Hypogammaglobulinemia. Diarrhea is more common and more severe in children with acquired immunodeficiency disorders than in those with congenital sex-linked deficiency. By late childhood about 50% have diarrhea and many have steatorrhea. In some, a patchy shortening of jejunal villi is seen, but generalized disaccharidase deficiency may occur without marked structural abnormality. Nodular lymphoid hyperplasia is common, as seen on barium roentgenograms or mucosal biopsy, but asymptomatic.

IgA Deficiency. Isolated IgA deficiency, the most common primary immunodeficiency, only rarely causes intestinal symptoms. But giardiasis, ulcerative colitis, Crohn disease, and celiac disease all occur more frequently in affected persons than in the general population. These associations presumably reflect some compromise of the intestinal mucosal barrier.

Severe Combined Immunodeficiency (Swiss Type). Severe diarrhea and generalized malabsorption contribute substantially to the early high mortality in this disease. Disaccharidase deficiencies are common, and microscopic examination of the small bowel shows partial villous atrophy and PAS-positive macrophages in the lamina propria. Affected children may harbor organisms like rotavirus in their intestines for months.

Chronic Granulomatous Disease. Patients with this disease may have granulomas characterized by multinucleated giant cells and lipid histiocytes throughout the intestine, with diarrhea, malabsorption, and obstructive phenomena.

12.54 STAGNANT LOOP SYNDROME
(Blind Loop Syndrome)

These terms describe conditions associated with stasis of small intestinal contents, particularly in the upper regions. The cause of such stasis is usually incomplete bowel obstruction, which may be congenital (malrotation with duodenal bands, stenosis, or a diverticulum) or acquired (postoperative intestinal adhesions, longstanding Crohn disease). Stasis can also result when neuromuscular dysfunction impairs intestinal motility (intestinal pseudo-obstruction, hollow viscus myopathy). Whatever the cause, the sequence of pathophysiologic events is similar. Enteric bacteria, incompletely cleared by peristalsis, colonize the upper small bowel. These bacteria deconjugate bile salts, which leads to inefficient intraluminal processing of dietary fat and to steatorrhea; they bind vitamin B_{12}, interfering with its absorption; and they may damage the microvillus brush border membrane, diminishing disaccharidase activities.

In addition to symptoms of chronic incomplete bowel obstruction such as distention, pain, and vomiting, the patient may have pale, foul, bulky stools suggesting steatorrhea, a megaloblastic anemia from vitamin B_{12} deficiency, or diarrhea from disaccharidase deficiency. Clinical manifestations often do not suggest chronic intestinal obstruction, but laboratory investigations find the above functional abnormalities, as well as bacterial colonization of the upper intestine and deconjugated bile salts in the upper intestinal juice after a fatty meal. Barium contrast roentgenograms may reveal neither existence nor cause of obstruction.

Oral administration of an antimicrobial such as trimethoprim-sulfamethoxazole may be sufficient to control the problem temporarily. Definitive therapy may involve operative correction of incomplete bowel obstruction.

12.55 SHORT SMALL INTESTINE
(Short Gut Syndrome)

Congenital. Congenital shortness of the small bowel has been associated with intestinal malrotation and, in some cases, atresia. When the anomaly is severe, diarrhea and malabsorption begin at birth. Barium studies show a malrotated colon and a markedly shortened small bowel, but the villus structure is relatively mature. If the infant survives the early months, intestinal function improves in later years.

Massive Intestinal Resection. Acute illnesses sometimes necessitate removal of large portions of the small intestine. The newborn period is particularly hazardous in this regard. In young infants intestinal reserves permit loss of the colon or of short segments of small intestine, but problems in maintaining fluid and nutrient balance should be anticipated if more than 25% of the 200–300 cm of the newborn infant's small bowel is removed. Total parenteral nutrition now permits survival even when all but 20 cm is resected. Spontaneous improvement in absorptive and digestive function in the young infant can be expected over a 2 yr period after intestinal resection.

In general, loss of distal small bowel is more serious than loss of the proximal segment. The jejunum is relatively incapable of compensating for ileal loss since the ileum is the sole site for absorption of bile salts and vitamin B_{12}. Preservation of the ileocecal sphincter is advantageous to infants who have had extensive bowel resections; the sphincter impedes retrograde flow of colonic flora and prolongs contact of nutrients with the mucosa of the remaining small bowel.

After massive resection, gastric acidity and bacterial contamination of the intestinal lumen may compromise absorptive function. Hyperacidity is usually transient under these circumstances. If the terminal ileum is resected, excessive bile salt losses lead to malabsorption of dietary fats and fat-soluble vitamins. Bile salts reaching the colon may also provoke increased water and electrolyte secretion. If resection includes mid and distal jejunum as well as ileum, the patient may be unable to maintain positive fluid balance. Hyperoxaluria may occur after distal small bowel resections in which the colon is preserved, but resultant nephrolithiasis is rare during early childhood. Cell-mediated immunity is normal, but circulating immunoglobulin concentrations may be reduced after massive resection.

Often oral feeding cannot be tolerated for weeks after resection. In the interval the patient can be supported by intravenous nutrition. The diet to be offered depends on the patient's age and functional deficit. Initially, liquids or liquid formulas should be isotonic and given in frequent small amounts. Excessive water intake should be avoided, particularly at times when solids are being taken. When there is severe steatorrhea, long-chain fats should be restricted and medium-chain triglycerides substituted for them. Initially, dietary glucose may be better tolerated than disaccharides, but the concentration should not exceed 5 g/dL in order to maintain relative isotonicity of the feeding. Vitamin supplements are usually needed, and serum concentrations of calcium, magnesium, potassium, and phosphorus should be monitored and supplements given as required. If a large portion of the ileum is resected, monthly injections of 100 μg of vitamin B_{12} must be given for life, but it usually takes 2 yr or more for a deficiency to develop in the face of even a severe absorptive defect. Large doses of vitamin D may be necessary to prevent rickets. Prothrombin time should also be monitored as a basis for vitamin K supplementation. Antidiarrheal agents are rarely helpful in the management of massive bowel resection. Cholestyramine may reduce fecal water and sodium losses in infants with relatively short ileal resections by binding bile acids before they reach the colon, but if ileal resection is massive and steatorrhea severe, cholestyramine is likely to aggravate the problem. Theoretically, antacids should benefit infants with hyperacidity, but their value in this situation is unproved. Patients with bacterial contamination and stagnant loop syndrome will derive temporary benefits from oral antibiotics, but they may require additional surgery.

Successful management of young infants after massive resection requires a coordinated team approach. Along with the essential measures to maintain nutrient intake a concerted effort should be made to encourage mother-child bonding and to stimulate development. Studies suggest impressive preservation of intellectual function even in the most severely affected patients with early profound, prolonged malnutrition.

12.56 CELIAC DISEASE
(Celiac Sprue, Gluten-Induced Enteropathy, Nontropical Sprue)

An intolerance of the gluten of wheat and rye (celiac disease) is an important cause of the celiac syndrome in children. Its incidence ranges from 1:300 to 1:6000; accurate statistics are not available in North America, where in some regions the disease occurs as frequently as 1:2000 but in others much less frequently.

The intestinal damage is caused by a *permanent* intolerance to the gliadin fraction of gluten, a protein found in wheat and rye grains. There is uncertainty about the impact of barley and oats, but most patients tolerate moderate intakes of these grains. One theory of pathogenesis proposes that the mucosal lesion of celiac disease is due to an inborn mucosal enzyme defect which permits undigested toxic components of the gluten molecule to accumulate in the mucosa. A second theory attributes intestinal damage to immune reactions.

A predisposition to celiac disease is inherited, most likely as a mendelian dominant with incomplete penetrance. About 80% of celiac patients carry the HLA-B8 antigen compared with 22% of the normal population. Celiac disease and diabetes mellitus are more common among 1st degree relatives of patients than among controls.

Clinical Manifestations. The clinical features of celiac disease range from generalized severe intestinal malabsorption to normal or near normal health. Major manifestations are summarized in Table 12–10. The typical patient develops irritability, anorexia, and chronic diarrhea late in the 1st yr. The stools are pale and foul, the child underweight and perhaps short, with wasted muscles, particularly in the proximal groups. Additional physical signs may include mouth sores, a smooth tongue, excessive bruising, finger clubbing, and peripheral edema. However, the range of clinical findings among patients with celiac disease is extraordinarily wide so that "textbook" features should not be expected. At least 30% of patients are neither irritable nor anorexic; as many have problems with vomiting as with diarrhea, and some are constipated. The most constant features are decreased rates of weight gain and linear growth, which may persist without obvious gastrointestinal symptoms. Some patients who apparently have the same disease remain well throughout childhood only to develop typical symptoms as adults.

Laboratory Manifestations. Anemia is common; usually the patient is iron deficient, but blood folate levels may also be low. Vitamin B_{12} deficiency is seen only in severe, longstanding disease. Hypoalbuminemia and reduced circulating gamma globulin levels may result from poor intake, reduced absorption, and excessive loss.

Table 12–10. **Active Childhood Celiac Disease—42 Cases**

Symptoms	No. of Patients
Failure to thrive	36
Diarrhea	30
Instability	30
Vomiting	24
Anorexia	24
Foul stools	21
Abdominal pain	8
Excessive appetite	6
Rectal prolapse	3

Signs	No. of Patients
Height <25 percentile	30
Body weight <25 percentile	37
Wasted muscles	40
Abdominal distention	33
Edema	14
Finger clubbing	11

Most of the affected children eating significant amounts of fat have steatorrhea. A 4 day balance study usually finds fat excretion exceeding 10% of dietary intake. Stool microscopy usually reveals an excess of crystalline aggregates of fatty acid. There may also be reduced fasting serum carotene levels (<50 µg/dL), low serum 25-OH-vitamin D, calcium, and vitamin A levels, and prolonged prothrombin times. On the other hand, these latter measurements may be normal in patients with proven celiac disease.

Reflecting diffuse small bowel mucosal damage, the oral glucose tolerance test is usually flat, and the blood xylose concentration does not exceed 25 mg/dL after an oral load in children with active celiac disease, but false-negative and false-positive results are sufficiently common to make these tests unreliable. Gluten has been shown to injure celiac mucosa in organ culture, and this procedure may eventually be helpful diagnostically.

In barium contrast studies the small bowel is usually diffusely dilated, and the mucosal folds are coarse. Because these findings are nonspecific and inconsistent, roentgenograms are not indicated in the diagnostic evaluation of a suspected case unless a localized lesion is suspected. Bone films often show osteoporosis, but rickets is rare.

Pathology. The diffuse lesion of the upper small intestinal mucosa that characterizes celiac disease is seen in a peroral suction biopsy specimen. Short, flat villi, deepened crypts, and irregular vacuolated surface epithelium with lymphocytes in the epithelial layer are seen by light microscopy. Similar abnormalities occur in other conditions but none is likely to be confused with celiac disease. Invasive infections such as rotavirus enteritis, *Giardia lamblia*, or tropical sprue can cause villus flattening and elongated crypts but not the marked abnormalities of enterocytes. A flat mucosa occurs in kwashiorkor but may represent a response to infestation rather than to undernutrition. Tropical sprue, a poorly understood tropical enteropathy, can cause a lesion that is indistinguishable from that of celiac disease. Some cases of cow's milk protein or soy protein intolerance are associated with lesions similar to those of celiac disease in children. In immune deficiency and eosinophilic gastroenteritis, villi can be partially shortened. Infants with familial enteropathy have short villi, but the crypt dimensions are normal.

Diagnosis. This is based on finding the characteristic duodenal or jejunal mucosal lesion in a mucosal suction biopsy; on a clinical and laboratory response to a gluten-free diet; and on the reappearance of the lesion after gluten challenge. The final test may not be appropriate in some patients because of the risk from exacerbation of the disease. No gluten challenge should be made until at least 2 yr after therapy has been started, to allow for mucosal healing. It should be noted that once the mucosa has healed, moderate quantities (1–2 slices of bread/day) can be taken for months by many children with true celiac disease without symptoms occurring. It may take 2 yr for the mucosal lesion to reappear.

Children on a Gluten-Free Diet in Whom the Diagnosis of Celiac Disease Has Not Been Proved. If a child improves after a gluten-free diet is prescribed without a diagnosis proved by biopsy, the question arises whether improvement was spontaneous or a response to therapy. The child can be returned to a full gluten-containing diet and the response observed. If celiac disease seems a possible diagnosis, a peroral intestinal biopsy can be done when symptoms of malabsorption develop or when 2 yr have passed, at which time the diagnosis can be based on the development of a typical mucosal lesion. If the initial illness strongly suggests celiac disease, a gluten challenge can be deferred until the patient is at least 4 yr old when a challenge roughly equivalent to 1 slice of bread/day is usually tolerated without severe symptoms.

Treatment. All wheat and rye should be eliminated from an otherwise full diet. Most patients tolerate oats, at least in moderation. Although disaccharidase activities in the mucosa are diminished during active celiac disease, significant disaccharide intolerance is rare. A few patients who have definite lactase deficiency will benefit from a short period of disaccharide restriction. During the early months of therapy extra fat-soluble vitamins are advisable, and for those who are iron- or folate-deficient appropriate supplements should be given. Lifelong dietary treatment is a major undertaking and best carried out with the help of an experienced nutritionist and ample written instructions and recipes.

Prognosis. The clinical response to a gluten-free diet of a child with celiac disease is gratifying. Improvement of mood and appetite is followed by lessening of diarrhea. In most cases changes occur within 1 wk of starting therapy, but the response may occasionally be delayed. Older patients and very ill patients tend to respond slowly, but once in remission the celiac child should be treated as a well child. During preadolescence and adolescence, children with proven celiac disease seem to tolerate considerable quantities of dietary gluten without symptoms although the typical abnormalities reappear in their mucosa. No complications from long-term gluten-free diet treatment are recognized. In adult patients the incidence of intestinal malignancy is higher than in the normal population; the scant data available do not indicate that dietary therapy prevents the development of malignancy.

12.57 POST-ENTERITIS MALABSORPTION

Most children with chronic diarrhea and mild absorptive defects have none of the diseases listed in Tables 12–8 and 12–9. These patients, usually infants and toddlers, are rarely seriously ill but suffer from persistent small-intestinal symptoms after an initial acute illness which often resembles an enteric infection. The diagnosis of "toddler's diarrhea" is often attached.

Since the normal small intestine possesses mechanisms for rapid repair after acute damage, persistent malfunction suggests either continuing damage or failure of repair, owing to persisting infection or some other injury. Except for *Giardia lamblia*, however, most enteric pathogens are quickly shed after invading the mucosa unless the host has an immunodeficiency syndrome. Sugars, if inadequately assimilated, may accumulate in the lumen, where fermentation may produce organic acids that injure the mucosa. Proteins, particularly cow's milk protein, can cause immunologically mediated mucosal damage. Nutritional depletion may interfere with epithelial recovery after injury.

Clinical Manifestations. In children from 6 mo to 3 yr of age there is usually an acute onset of watery diarrhea with or without fever and vomiting followed by persistent loose stools. The patient's general health is good, but food intake and weight gain may be reduced, owing to imposed dietary restrictions. Diarrhea tends to worsen if the sugar intake is high; the stools contain excess sugar and organic acid, and the buttocks are excoriated. Usually there is diminished mucosal disaccharidase activity; if the damage is severe, glucose and ion transport are affected and there may be mild steatorrhea.

Treatment. Specific measures to accelerate healing of the bowel are not available. It is important that natural healing not be delayed by inappropriate measures. Excessive investigations may upset the child and accentuate parental anxiety. Inadequate nutrition will affect growth and may impair digestive tract repair and function (Sec. 12.49). Antidiarrheal medications may improve stool appearance in mild chronic cases, but they may also contribute to bowel stasis and persistent infection.

These patients and their parents need reassurance. Sugar intake, particularly in the form of fruit juices that are hyperosmolar, should be limited, diluted in half with water; when lactose intolerance occurs, milk intake should be limited or eliminated for a brief period. Adequate nutrition should be maintained using foods relatively low in sugar such as meats and cereals.

12.58 OTHER MALABSORPTIVE SYNDROMES

Tropical Sprue. The cause of this syndrome, which is confined to certain tropical regions, is unknown and perhaps multiple; it occurs in some Caribbean countries but not Jamaica and in Africa but not the southern half of the continent. It is characterized by generalized malabsorption associated with a diffuse lesion of the small intestinal mucosa.

Clinical Manifestations. Epidemics affect all ages but usually adults first. Fever and malaise precede the onset of watery diarrhea. Then, in a few days, the acute features subside and are followed by chronic malabsorption, intermittent diarrhea, and anorexia that lead eventually to severe malnutrition. Signs of malnutrition may include night blindness, glossitis, stomatitis, cheilosis, cutaneous and mucosal pigmentation, and edema. Muscle wasting is marked, and the abdomen often distended.

Laboratory studies usually demonstrate malabsorption of fat, sugars, and vitamin B_{12}. Biopsies of the small intestinal mucosa show varying degrees of villus shortening, increased crypt depth, round cell infiltration of the lamina propria, and irregularity and mild shortening of the surface epithelial cells. These pathologic changes are nonspecific and in their mild form are seen in healthy people in the same communities.

Treatment. Antidiarrheal agents, nutritional supplements (folic acid and vitamin B_{12}), and oral administration of broad spectrum antibiotics may result in rapid improvement of the intestinal lesion. This response to treatment suggests that enteric flora are involved in the pathogenesis of this syndrome.

Whipple Syndrome. This rare disease has been reported only once in a child. A rod-shaped bacillus may be the etiologic agent. The disease involves many organ systems; the small intestine is always affected, and malabsorption results. Common findings are arthralgia, fever, and polyserositis. Duodenal biopsy shows focal accumulation of PAS-positive macrophages, and bacilli may be seen in the lamina propria. Antibiotics produce dramatic improvement, but long-term therapy is necessary.

Intestinal Lymphangiectasia. This congenital generalized defect of the lymphatic system can involve the intestine extensively, causing steatorrhea, protein-losing enteropathy, edema, and lymphocytopenia. Usually, there is slight if any disturbance of bowel habit, and edema is the major clinical manifestation. Absorptive function, except long chain fat assimilation, is usually intact. Reduction of dietary long chain fats may reduce enteric protein loss; medium chain triglycerides can be substituted in the diet since they are transported by the portal stream.

Wolman Disease. This rare lethal lipidosis leads to lipid accumulation in many organs including the small intestine. In addition to vomiting and hepatosplenomegaly there may be steatorrhea as the result of lymphatic obstruction (Sec. 7.34).

Idiopathic Diffuse Small Intestinal Mucosal Lesions. Some infants have severe chronic malabsorptive states that do not fit into recognized disease patterns. Two idiopathic malabsorptive syndromes have been associated with lesions of the small intestine mucosa.

Infants with *familial enteropathy* are affected from birth by global malabsorption causing severe diarrhea and malnutrition. Unable to sustain adequate nutritional balance with oral feeding, they are dependent on total parenteral nutrition. Irrespective of nutrient intake, duodenal mucosal biopsy shows a profoundly flattened villus structure. Unlike celiac disease, the crypts are not elongated and epithelial mitotic activity is not increased. The condition appears to be due to a defect in intestinal epithelial renewal. In spite of aggressive supportive treatment including corticosteroids, most patients have died without improvement in intestinal function.

A second rare idiopathic syndrome of *persistent villus damage* causes serious chronic malabsorption in young infants, who develop severe generalized malabsorption after a few months of apparently good health. Initially, an acute illness is suspected, but the problem persists for months, even years. Dietary restrictions do not alter the course. The mucosal lesion is characterized by shortened villi, but, as in celiac disease, the crypts may be elongated and mitotic figures are plentiful. Corticosteroids may be beneficial.

Malabsorption Syndromes
General Reviews
Ament ME: Malabsorption syndromes in infancy and childhood. J Pediatr 81:685, 867, 1972.
Anderson CM: Malabsorption in children. Clin Gastroenterol 6:355, 1977.
Hamilton JR: Diarrhea and malabsorption in children. In: Sleisenger MH, Fordtran JS (eds): Gastrointestinal Disease. 2nd ed. Philadelphia, WB Saunders, 1978, p 336.
Wilson FA, Dietschy JM: Differential diagnostic approach to clinical problems of malabsorption. Gastroenterology 61:911, 1971.

Diagnostic Investigations
Barr RG, Perman JA, Schoeller DA, et al: Breath tests in pediatric gastrointestinal disorders: new diagnostic opportunities. Pediatrics 62:393, 1978.
de Silva M: Radiological investigation of small bowel disease in children. Med J Aust 1:819, 1971.
Drummey GD, Benson JA Jr, Jones CM: Microscopical examinations of the stool for steatorrhea. N Engl J Med 264:85, 1961.
Hill RE, Cutz E, Cherian G, et al: An evaluation of d-xylose absorption measurements in children suspected of having small intestinal disease. J Pediatr 99:245, 1981.
Hill RE, Hercz A, Corey MD, et al: Fecal clearance of alpha-1-antitrypsin. A reliable measure of protein loss in children. J Pediatr 99:416, 1981.
Katz AJ, Grand RJ: All that flattens is not sprue. Gastroenterology 76:375, 1979.
Kerry KR, Anderson CM: A ward test for sugar in the faeces. Lancet 1:981, 1964.
Magnus EM: Low serum and red cell folate activity in adult celiac disease. Am J Dig Dis 11:314, 1966.
McIntyre PA, Hahn R, Conley CL: Genetic factors in predisposition to pernicious anemia. Bull Johns Hopkins Hosp 104:309, 1959.
Shmerling DH, Farrer JCW, Prader A: Fecal fat and nitrogen in healthy children and in children with malabsorption or maldigestion. Pediatrics 46:690, 1970.
Townley RRW, Barnes GL: Intestinal biopsy in childhood. Arch Dis Child 48:480, 1973.

The Digestive Tract in Chronic Malnutrition
Barbesat GO, Hansen JDL: The exocrine pancreas and protein-calorie malnutrition. Pediatrics 42:77, 1968.
Brunser O: Effects of malnutrition on intestinal structure and function in children. Clin Gastroenterol 6:341, 1977.
Suskind RM: Gastrointestinal changes in the malnourished child. Pediatr Clin North Am 22:873, 1975.

Liver and Biliary Disorders
Atkinson M, Nordin BEC, Sherlock S: Malabsorption and bone disease in prolonged obstructive jaundice. Q J Med 25:299, 1956.
Hadorn B, Hess J, Troesch V, et al: Role of bile acids in the activation of trypsinogen by enterokinase: Disturbance of trypsinogen activation in patients with intrahepatic biliary atresia. Gastroenterology 66:548, 1974.
Kooh SW, Jones G, Reilly BJ, et al: Pathogenesis of rickets in chronic hepatobiliary disease in children. J Pediatr 94:870, 1979.

Short Small Intestine
Congenital
Hamilton JR, Reilly BJ, Morecki R: Short small intestine associated with malrotation. A newly described cause of intestinal malabsorption. Gastroenterology 56:124, 1969.

Acquired

Bohane TD, Haka-Ikse K, Biggar WD, et al: A clinical study of young infants after small intestinal resection. J Pediatr 94:552, 1979.

Valman HB: Long term effects and management of intestinal resection. In: Harris JT (ed): Essentials of Paediatric Gastroenterology. Churchill-Livingstone, London, 1977.

Wilmore DW: Factors correlating with a successful outcome following extensive intestinal resection in newborn infants. J Pediatr 80:88, 1972.

Young WF, Swain VAJ, Pringle EM: Long term prognosis after major resection of small bowel in early infancy. Arch Dis Child 44:465, 1969.

Stagnant Loop Syndrome

Bayes BJ, Hamilton JR: Blind loop syndrome in children. Acta Dis Child 44:76, 1969.

Gracey M: Intestinal microflora and bacterial overgrowth in early life. J Pediatr Gastroenterol Nutr 1:13, 1982.

Jonas A, Krishnan C, Forstner G: Release of disaccharidases from brush border membranes by extracts of bacteria obtained from intestinal blind loops of rats. Gastroenterology 75:791, 1978.

Soderlund S: Anomalies of midgut rotation and fixation. Clinical aspects based on sixty-two cases in childhood. Acta Pediatr 51:135, 1966.

Infections Causing Malabsorption

Ament ME: Diagnosis and treatment of giardiasis. J Pediatr 80:663, 1972.

Liebman WM, Thaler MM, Dehorimier A, et al: Intractable diarrhea of infancy due to intestinal coccidiosis. Gastroenterology 78:579, 1980.

Immune Deficiency States and the Intestine

Ament ME: Immunodeficiency syndromes and gastrointestinal disease. Pediatr Clin North Am 22:807, 1975.

Brown WR, Butterfield D, Savage D, et al: Clinical, microbiological and immunological studies in patients with immunoglobulin deficiencies and gastrointestinal disorders. Gut 13:441, 1972.

Katz AJ, Rosen F: Gastrointestinal complication of immunodeficiency syndromes. In: Immunology of the Gut. Ciba Foundation Symposium 46:243, 1977.

Walker WA, Hong R: Immunology of the gastrointestinal tract. J Pediatr 83:517, 711, 1973.

Celiac Disease

Anderson CM, Gracey M, Burke V: Celiac disease—some still controversial aspects. Arch Dis Child 47:292, 1972.

Cooper BT, Holmes GKT, Ferguson R, et al: Celiac disease and malignancy. Medicine 59:249, 1980.

Hamilton JR, McNeil LK: Childhood celiac disease: Response of treated patients to a small uniform daily dose of wheat gluten. J Pediatr 81:885, 1972.

Hamilton JR, Lynch MJ, Reilly BJ: Active celiac disease in childhood. Q J Med 38:135, 1969.

Young WF, Pringle EM: 110 children with celiac disease; 1950 to 1969. Arch Dis Child 46:421, 1971.

Post-enteritis Malabsorption

Gribbin M, Walker-Smith JA, Wood CBS: Delayed recovery following acute gastroenteritis. Acta Paediatr Belg 29:167, 1976.

Lifshitz F: Carbohydrate problems in paediatric gastroenterology. Clin Gastroenterol 6:415, 1977.

Manuel PD, Walker-Smith JA, Soeparto P: Cow's milk sensitive enteropathy in Indonesian infants. Lancet 2:1365, 1980.

Walker-Smith JA: Cow's milk intolerance as a cause of post-enteritis diarrhea. J Pediatr Gastroenterol and Nutr 1:163, 1982.

Tropical Sprue

Klipstein FA, Baker SJ: Regarding the definition of tropical sprue. Gastroenterology 58:717, 1970.

Santiago-Borrero PJ, Maldanado N, Horta E: Tropical sprue in children. J Pediatr 76:470, 1970.

Whipple Disease

Aust CH, Smith EB: Whipple's disease in a 3-month old infant. Am J Clin Pathol 37:66, 1962.

Intestinal Lymphangiectasia

Strober W, Wochner RD, Carbone PP, et al: Intestinal lymphangiectasia: A protein-losing enteropathy with hypogammaglobulinemia, lymphocytopenia and impaired homograft rejection. J Clin Invest 46:1643, 1967.

Vardy PA, Lebenthal E, Shwachman H: Intestinal lymphangiectasis: A reappraisal. Pediatrics 55:842, 1975.

Waldman TA, Wochner RD, Strober W: The role of the gastrointestinal tract in plasma protein metabolism. Am J Med 46:275, 1969.

Wolman Disease

Queloz JM, Capitanio MA, Kirkpatrick JA: Wolman's disease. Radiology 104:357, 1972.

Idiopathic Diffuse Small Intestinal Mucosal Lesions

Candy DCA, Larcher VF, Cameron DJS, et al: Lethal familial protracted diarrhea. Arch Dis Child 56:15, 1981.

Davidson GP, Cutz E, Hamilton JR, et al: Familial enteropathy. A syndrome of protracted diarrhea from birth, failure to thrive and hypoplastic villus atrophy. Gastroenterology 75:793, 1978.

DEFECTS OF SPECIFIC ENZYMES OR TRANSPORT PROCESSES INVOLVED IN DIGESTION OR ABSORPTION

12.59 ENZYME DEFICIENCIES

Enterokinase Deficiency

Congenital deficiency of this small-intestinal enzyme has been reported in a few children. The disease results in a complete absence of pancreatic proteolytic activity since enterokinase is an essential activator of pancreatic trypsinogens. Affected patients are ill from very early life with severe diarrhea and failure to thrive. Hypoproteinemia is common and may lead to edema. In duodenal juice tryptic activity is missing while lipase and amylase are normal; in vitro tryptic activity of the juice can be restored by the addition of enterokinase. Malabsorption of protein is the major defect, although mild steatorrhea has been reported. Pancreatic enzyme replacements restore normal digestive function.

Disaccharidase Deficiencies

The disaccharidases are located on the brush border membrane surface of the small bowel. Occasionally, congenital deficiencies occur, but abnormal disaccharidase activities have most often been the result of diffuse lesions of the intestinal epithelium, such as those of infection or celiac disease.

The response of the patient to significant disaccharidase deficiency (disaccharide intolerance) is similar whatever its cause or the enzymes involved. If disaccharide hydrolysis at the brush border is incomplete, the sugar accumulates in the distal intestinal lumen, where organic acids and hydrogen gas are produced. The excess intraluminal sugar and organic acids draw water into the lumen, leading to watery diarrhea with stools that are frothy, of low pH (<pH 6.0), that contain excess sugar, and tend to excoriate the buttocks. There may be bloating and borborygmi, but steatorrhea is rare. In some cases, particularly those beyond infancy, gas production causing crampy abdominal pain is the dominant problem, rather than diarrhea.

If the disaccharide involved is a reducing sugar (e.g., lactose), the standard Clinitest examination* will be 1+ or greater in most cases. Oral tolerance tests using the potential offending sugar have been employed for the clinical diagnosis of disaccharide intolerance, but these are unreliable. Disaccharidase activities can be assayed in mucosal biopsy specimens. Breath hydrogen excretion after an oral sugar load is a useful test for detecting disaccharide intolerance (Sec. 12.49).

Lactase Deficiency. *Congenital* absence of lactase has been reported in very few cases. The usual mechanism for primary lactose intolerance relates to the *developmental* pattern of lactase activity. Because lactase activity rises relatively late in fetal life and begins to fall after the age of 3 yr, intolerance to lactose can be anticipated in very premature infants and in older children and adults. Late decrease in lactase activity in childhood is common in blacks and Orientals, less common

---

*Ames Company.

in whites. Since lactase activity in the mucosa is at best marginal, this enzyme is particularly likely to be depleted *secondary to diffuse mucosal diseases* (Sec. 12.57).

Symptoms occur in response to ingestion of lactose, the sugar in milk. Watery diarrhea may result. A syndrome of recurrent, vague, crampy abdominal pain has also been attributed to lactose intolerance. School and preschool aged children develop episodic mid-abdominal pain. Usually, their general health is unaffected, and there is no obvious temporal relationship of pain to milk ingestion or to diarrhea. (See also Sec. 12.47.)

Treatment consists of removal of milk from the diet. In most cases the elimination need not be total; stopping milk ingestion as a beverage is important. A lactase preparation is available which for some children allows asymptomatic consumption of modest quantities of milk incubated with the added enzyme.

Sucrase-Isomaltase Deficiency. The only relatively common congenital deficiency of disaccharidase activities is a combined deficiency of sucrase and isomaltase. Symptoms usually begin when a sucrose-containing diet is started. There may also be some intolerance to starch, but since isomaltase acts only on the branch points of the starch molecule, isomaltase deficiency itself is relatively asymptomatic. The symptoms are bloating, watery diarrhea, and excoriation of buttocks. Recurrent abdominal pain has not been attributed to sucrose-isomaltose intolerance. Since sucrose is not a reducing sugar, its presence will not be detected in stool by Clinitest unless the specimen is first hydrolyzed with HCl. The morphology of the small-intestinal mucosa is normal, but enzyme assays show specific deficiencies of sucrase and isomaltase with normal levels of lactase and maltase. Breath testing usually demonstrates increased H_2 after sucrose ingestion. Affected patients improve quickly after dietary sucrose is reduced to minimal amounts.

12.60 DEFECTS OF ABSORPTION OR TRANSPORT

Glucose-Galactose Malabsorption. This rare congenital transport defect in brush border membrane glucose transport is inherited as an autosomal recessive trait. It also affects renal tubular epithelium to a mild degree. Acute viral enteritis and severe chronic diffuse mucosal damage also may impair the glucose-galactose carrier sufficiently to cause intolerance to these sugars. Usually, if mucosal damage is severe enough to impair glucose transport, other absorptive processes are affected.

The symptomatic response to sugar ingestion is similar whether the defect is congenital or secondary. Watery stools follow the ingestion of glucose, breast milk, or conventional formulas since most diet sugars are polysaccharides or disaccharides with glucose and/or galactose moieties. The patient may be bloated, and, if diarrhea persists, dehydration and acidosis can be severe. The stools are acidic and contain sugar. Glucose and galactose tolerance curves are flat. Patients with a congenital defect tolerate fructose normally; their small bowel function is normal in all other aspects, as are mucosal structure and disaccharidase activities.

Treatment consists of rigorous restriction of glucose and galactose and provision of a fructose-containing formula. Later in life limited amounts of glucose or sucrose may be tolerated.

Abetalipoproteinemia (Bassen-Kornzweig Syndrome). This relatively rare congenital disease, probably autosomal recessive, is characterized by fat malabsorption, acanthocytosis of erythrocytes, ataxic neuropathy, and retinitis pigmentosa. The underlying defect is not fully defined, but in the small bowel an absence of low density lipoproteins results in an inability to form normal chylomicrons and in defective release and transport of triglycerides from the enterocyte.

Affected patients are normal at birth but usually fail to thrive during the 1st yr. Stools are pale and bulky and the abdomen distended. Intellectual development is usually slightly retarded. After 10 yr of age development of ataxia, loss of deep tendon reflexes and the sense of position and vibration, and intention tremors reflects involvement of cerebellum, posterolateral columns, peripheral nerves, and basal ganglia. In adolescence an atypical retinitis pigmentosa develops. Mixed forms of the disorder (hypobetalipoproteinemia) occur.

Diagnosis rests on finding acanthocytes in the peripheral blood, very low serum levels of cholesterol (20–80 mg/dL), absent or minute levels of β-lipoprotein, and the typical marked lipid accumulation in villus enterocytes in the fasting duodenal mucosa. Usually, there is steatorrhea in younger patients, but other processes of assimilation are intact.

Specific therapy is not available. Large supplements of the fat-soluble vitamins A, D, E, and K, should be given. Massive doses of vitamin E (100 mg/kg/24 hr) may arrest the neurologic degeneration. Limiting long-chain fat intake may alleviate intestinal symptoms; medium-chain triglycerides can be used to supplement the fat intake.

Amino Acid Transport Defects. In several of the specific congenital disorders of amino acid transport (Chapter 7) defective intestinal amino acid transport occurs. Amino acid uptake into the intestinal mucosa is defective in *cystinuria*, but these patients have no gastrointestinal symptoms. In *Hartnup disease* malabsorption of tryptophan leads to ataxia, intellectual deterioration, and a pellagra-like skin rash. *Methionine malabsorption* is associated with episodes of diarrhea in fair-complexioned, retarded children whose urine has a sweet odor and contains excess α-hydroxybutyric acid. In the *blue diaper syndrome* tryptophan absorption is defective. *Lysine malabsorption* is reported in a case of hyperlysinuria.

Vitamin B₁₂ Malabsorption. Several rare congenital defects may affect assimilation of vitamin B_{12}. In *juvenile pernicious anemia* intrinsic factor production in the stomach is defective. Vitamin B_{12} malabsorption results, leading to megaloblastic anemia and growth failure. Gastric structure and function are otherwise normal.

Transcobalamin II deficiency is an inherited defect of a protein for intestinal transport of vitamin B_{12}. The result is severe megaloblastic anemia, diarrhea, and vomiting.

Imerslund has described patients in whom ileal absorption of vitamin B_{12} is defective. Ileal structure and function are otherwise normal. Megaloblastic anemia develops toward the end of the 1st yr. Proteinuria is commonly associated.

Treatment of these disorders is to administer vitamin B_{12} by injection: 1000 μg/wk for transcobalamin II deficiency, 100 μg/mo for the others.

Congenital Malabsorption of Folic Acid. A few patients have had folic acid deficiency in infancy as the result of a specific defect in folic acid assimilation. In addition to megaloblastic anemia, they have had cerebral degeneration.

Chloride-losing Diarrhea. This rare specific congenital defect of ileal chloride transport is associated with maternal polyhydramnios. The dominant symptom is severe watery diarrhea beginning at birth, the result of accumulation of chloride ion in the intestinal lumen. Watery diarrhea leads to dehydration and a severe electrolyte disturbance characterized by hypokalemia, hypochloridemia, and alkalosis, a most unusual pattern for a patient with chronic diarrhea. Other aspects of intestinal absorption are normal. Stools contain chloride in excess of the sum of sodium and potassium. There is no adequate treatment. Potassium supplements and some restriction of chloride intake are advisable.

Vitamin D Dependent Rickets. In this autosomal recessive disorder a specific defect in the metabolism of vitamin D causes malabsorption of calcium (Sec. 23.48). Intestinal function is otherwise normal.

Primary Hypomagnesemia. This specific intestinal transport defect in magnesium transport causes severe hypomagnesemia and, secondarily, hypocalcemic tetany in infancy. Other aspects of intestinal function are normal. The findings are reversed by large supplements of magnesium, which must be continued indefinitely.

Acrodermatitis Enteropathica. See also Sec. 24.12. This unusual constellation of clinical findings is due to zinc deficiency secondary to zinc malabsorption. Early in life the patient develops rashes around mucocutaneous junctions and on the extremities; alopecia, chronic diarrhea, and sometimes steatorrhea may occur. Untreated, the patient fails to thrive. Serum zinc concentration and alkaline phosphatase activity are low. Intestinal mucosal biopsies show Paneth cell inclusions that disappear after treatment. An oral supplement of zinc sulfate heptahydrate, 150 mg/24 hr, causes rapid healing of the skin lesions and improvement of diarrhea.

Menkes (kinky hair) Syndrome. This rare recessively inherited disorder is characterized by growth retardation, abnormal hair, cerebellar degeneration, and early death (Sec. 7.54). Its pathogenesis is unclear, but there is a widespread defect in cellular copper transport that affects the intestine as well as other tissues. Serum copper and ceruloplasmin levels are low, but cellular copper content is increased.

Drug-induced Absorptive Defects. Some drugs have a diffuse impact on the small intestinal epithelium. For example, methotrexate can cause arrest of enterocyte mitoses and result in a mucosal lesion; large doses of neomycin also affect mucosal structure. *Sulfasalazine* interferes with folic acid absorption. *Cholestyramine* binds bile salts and calcium in the intestinal lumen to cause hypocalcemia and steatorrhea. *Phenytoin* interferes with calcium absorption and can cause rickets.

J. RICHARD HAMILTON

Abetalipoproteinemia

Lee RS, Ahren E Jr: Fat transport in a β-lipoproteinemia. N Engl J Med 284:1261, 1969.
Muller DPR, Lloyd JK, Bird AC: Long-term management of abetalipoproteinemia. Arch Dis Child 52:209, 1977.
Scott BB, Miller JP, Losowsky MS: Hypobetalipoproteinemia: A variant of the Bassen-Kornsweig syndrome. Gut 20:163, 1979.

Enterokinase Deficiency

Hadorn B, Tarlow M, Lloyd JD, et al: Intestinal enterokinase deficiency. Lancet 1:812, 1969.

Amino Acid Transport Defects

Drummond KN, Michael AF, Ulstrom RA, et al: The blue diaper syndrome: Familial hypercalcemia with nephrocalcinosis and indicanuria. Am J Med 37:928, 1964.
Hooft G, Timmermand J, Snoeck J, et al: Methionine malabsorption syndrome. Ann Pediatr 205:73, 1965.
Milne MD: Hartnup disease. Biochemistry 111:3, 1969.
Morin CL, Thompson MW, Jackson SH, et al: Biochemical and genetic studies in cystinuria: Observations on double heterozygotes of genotype I/II. J Clin Invest 50:1961, 1971.
Whelan DT, Scriver CR: Hyperdibasicaminoaciduria: An inherited disorder of amino acid transport. Pediatr Res 2:525, 1968.

Disaccharidase Deficiencies

Ament ME, Perera DR, Esther L: Sucrase-isomaltase deficiency: A frequently misdiagnosed disease. J Pediatr 83:721, 1973.
Auricchio S, Rubino A, Murset G: Intestinal glycosidase activities in the human embryo, foetus and newborn. Pediatrics 35:344, 1965.
Barr RG, Levine MD, Watkins JB: Recurrent abdominal pain of childhood due to lactose intolerance. N Engl J Med 300:1449, 1979.
Gray GM: Carbohydrate digestion and absorption. Role of the small intestine. N Engl J Med 292:1225, 1975.
Harrison M, Walker-Smith JA: Reinvestigation of lactose intolerant children: Lack of correlation between continuing lactose intolerance and small intestinal morphology, disaccharidase activity and lactose tolerance tests. Gut 18:48, 1977.
Kretchmer N: Lactose and lactase. Sci Am 221:70, 1972.
Lifshitz F: Carbohydrate problems in paediatric gastroenterology. Clin Gastroenterol 6:415, 1977.

Glucose-Galactose Malabsorption

Fairclough PD, Clark ML, Dawson AM, et al: Absorption of glucose and maltose in congenital glucose-galactose malabsorption. Pediatr Res 12:1112, 1978.
Lindqvist B, Meeuwisse GW, Melin K: Glucose-galactose malabsorption. Lancet 2:666, 1962.
Schneider AJ, Kinter WB, Stirling CE: Glucose-galactose malabsorption. N Engl J Med 274:305, 1966.

Vitamin B₁₂ Malabsorption

Hall CA: Congenital disorders of Vitamin B₁₂ transport and their contribution to concepts. Gastroenterology 65:684, 1973.
Hitzig WH, Dohmann V, Pluss HJ, et al: Hereditary transcobalamin II deficiency: Clinical findings in a new family. J Pediatr 85:622, 1974.
Imerslund O: Idiopathic chronic megaloblastic anaemia in children. Acta Paediatr 49:Suppl 119, 1960.
MacKenzie IL, Donaldson RM, Trier JS, et al: Ileal mucosa in familial selective vitamin B₁₂ malabsorption. N Engl J Med 286:1021, 1972.

Folate Malabsorption

Lanzkowsky P: Congenital malabsorption of folate. Am J Med 48:580, 1970.

Chloride-Losing Diarrhea

Bieberdorf FA, Gorden P, Fordtran JS: Pathogenesis of congenital alkalosis with diarrhea. Implications for the physiology of normal ileal electrolyte absorption and secretion. J Clin Invest 51:1958, 1972.
Holmberg C, Perheentupa J, Launiala K, et al: Congenital chloride diarrhea. Arch Dis Child 52:255, 1977.

Vitamin D Dependent Rickets

Hamilton R, Harrison J, Fraser D, et al: The small intestine in vitamin D dependent rickets. Pediatrics 45:364, 1970.

Primary Hypomagnesemia

Paunier L, Radde IC, Kooh SW, et al: Primary hypomagnesemia with secondary hypocalcemia in an infant. Pediatrics 41:385, 1968.
Stromme JH, Nesbakken R, Normann T, et al: Familial hypomagnesemia. Acta Paediatr Scand 58:433, 1969.

Acrodermatitis Enteropathica

Bohane TD, Cutz E, Hamilton JR, et al: Acrodermatitis enteropathica, zinc and the Paneth cell. Gastroenterology 73:587, 1977.
Moynahan EJ: Acrodermatitis enteropathica: A lethal inherited human zinc-deficiency disorder. Lancet 2:399, 1974.

Menkes Syndrome

Danks DM, Stevens BJ, Campbell PE, et al: Menkes' kinky-hair syndrome. Lancet 1:110, 1972.

Drug-Induced Malabsorption

Franklin JL, Rosenberg HH: Impaired folic acid absorption in inflammatory bowel disease: Effects of salicylazosulfapyridine (Azulfidine). Gastroenterology 64:517, 1973.
Morijiri Y, et al: Factors causing rickets in institutionalized handicapped children on anti-convulsant therapy. Arch Dis Child 56:446, 1981.
Rogers AL, Vloedman DA, Bloom EC, et al: Neomycin-induced steatorrhea. JAMA 197:185, 1966.
Trier JS: Morphologic alterations induced by methotrexate in the mucosa of human proximal intestine. I. Serial observations by light microscopy. Gastroenterology 42:295, 1962.

12.61 IRRITABLE BOWEL SYNDROME
(Recurrent Abdominal Pain Syndrome)

The term *irritable bowel syndrome* embraces a wide spectrum of symptoms and signs that result from disordered and hyperreactive gastrointestinal function. A large number of illnesses of infants and children with intermittent or chronic diarrhea, vomiting, and abdominal pain fall into this category and need to be differentiated from the many specific organic lesions that may produce the same symptoms and signs.

Etiology. The cause of these reactive disturbances is unknown. One factor of importance is the high frequency of similar somatic symptoms in either parent or in other members of the family. The two most widely held views are (1) that the symptoms are stress-related or psychophysiologic (possibly including the sense of a learned maladaptive reinforcement of visceral response); and (2) that there is a disorder of autonomic function of the gastrointestinal tract, which has been shown to have increased transit time, heightened reactivity to cholinergic and other stimulating agents, hyperalgesia with distention of the bowel musculature, altered secretory patterns, and occasional but often inconsistent reactivity to certain foods. Data suggest that in patients who have a diarrhea-prone irritable bowel syndrome increased amounts of prostaglandin E_2 are secreted into the intestinal lumen. Histories of infantile colic are found in some affected children and are cited as examples of increased reactivity. Many of the affected children are observed to be sensitive, introspective, and insecure, but studies have not yet found any preponderant behavioral or psychosocial traits in these beyond some evidence of anxiety and depression. Various physical or emotional traumas, or both, are not uncommonly regarded as precipitating the onset or exacerbation of symptoms. The failure, however, of various studies with multiple testing methods to measure any specific psychopathology suggests that heightened gastrointestinal reactivity may be a central component of the syndrome. There is no sex difference until adolescence, when the incidence in females becomes higher than in males.

Clinical Manifestations. The predominant symptom in patients with the syndrome may be recurrent diarrhea, constipation, fecal incontinence, vomiting, or abdominal pain.

In the infant and toddler, "toddler's diarrhea" is common, with bouts of loose stools usually lasting a few days. The onset of symptoms may occur at any time between birth and the end of the 1st yr. The bowel movements are malodorous, runny, and severely irritating to the buttocks. Dehydration rarely occurs, and growth is usually normal unless dietary intake is restricted as a therapeutic measure. Some infants have intense thirst and drink large amounts of water. The diarrhea may be exacerbated by days of travel, holidays, and other periods of heightened stimulation. Findings on physical examination are usually normal, except for occasional abdominal distention and increased bowel sounds. The children appear healthy and are generally very active. Laboratory tests of intestinal function and general health are normal. If these children are hospitalized for study, the stools almost always become normal.

Treatment of toddler's diarrhea is limited. Most parents can be reassured that the diarrhea can be safely tolerated and is self-limited. In some instances, a decrease in fluid intake may be helpful. Other dietary manipulations are generally not helpful, and may result in nutritional deficits. In some instances, the fears of the family and the intensity of the diarrhea warrant some studies to assess the situation more thoroughly.

Recurrent abdominal pain of childhood as a form of the irritable bowel syndrome usually affects school aged children, with marked variability in time of occurrence, intensity, and duration. The pain can be very severe, in some instances mimicking an acute abdomen. Most patients hospitalized for observation of possible appendicitis that proves to be not present are later found to have the irritable bowel syndrome. The pain may be brought on by eating or have no relationship to eating, bowel movements, or any other particular experience. The pain generally occurs less frequently during sleep and has a common tendency to appear on arousal from sleep in the morning.

The pain is frequently described as periumbilical or epigastric, but the location can be quite variable. Failure to pass stools may last several days but is not usually more protracted. The stools are at times pellet-like and at other times unformed. There may be loud borborygmi and frequent passage of flatus.

In some children fecal incontinence or episodes of soiling undergarments may be the pervasive manifestation. Dysuria, urgency, and frequency also may occur, with no abnormality found in urine. Headaches, facial pallor, dizziness, and blurred vision are common and suggest a more generalized disturbance of autonomic function. On deep palpation of the abdomen there is often vague tenderness without muscle guarding, more frequently in the right and left lower quadrants and the epigastrium. This tenderness may be present even at times when the pain is absent. The sigmoid colon may be tender to palpation, and may reveal a row of scybala. On proctoscopy the mucosa is pale, with localized areas of hyperemia, prominent vascular markings, lymphoid hyperplasia, and a dilated rectal vault.

The *clinical course* may vary directly with such family crises as deaths, illnesses, and other events that threaten the child's sense of security. Since children with this syndrome do not readily communicate their feelings, the clinician may underestimate the intensity of the child's experience. Affected children commonly exhibit heightened sensitivity, low self-image, and an exaggerated concern for friends and family as indicators of feelings of insecurity; they often appear older than their years and relate particularly well to adults and younger children. School phobias, with poor academic performance and some degree of depression, are not uncommon.

Discussion with the child may help him or her to attain a new level of adaptation toward well-being. Hospitalization may at times be useful in showing that symptoms usually abate and in reducing the anxiety of both parents and child over the symptoms. Studies of the urinary and gastrointestinal systems may be necessary to reassure a worried family and child, even when negative results are expected. The pain should be accepted as real and not belittled or denied. Exploration of factors influencing the pain may be helpful. Strong, empathic relationships between physician and both child and family may be most helpful when environmental events and temperamental factors are prominent precipitating factors. Antispasmodics may benefit some children. A full nutritious diet with adequate fiber should be provided. Supplemental bulk agents may be of help in selected cases. Food does not, in general, play a major role, but any foods that repetitively seem to cause symptoms may be avoided.

The prognosis is variable; in some instances recurrent bouts of pain may continue into adulthood. Growth in self-understanding achieved over time and with supportive discussions may enable affected children to learn to tolerate the pain and to lead effective lives in spite of it.

GIULIO J. BARBERO

Apley J: The Child with Abdominal Pain. Ed 2, Oxford, Blackwell, 1975.
Barbero GJ: Recurrent abdominal pain in childhood. Pediatr Rev 4:29, 1982.
Davidson M, Wasserman R: The irritable colon of childhood (chronic non-specific diarrhea syndrome). J Pediatr 69:1027, 1966.
Galleo JR, Neustein S, Walker WA: Clinical aspects of recurrent abdominal pain in children. Adv Pediatr 27:31, 1980.
Raymer D, Weininger O, Hamilton JR: Psychological problems in children with abdominal pain. Lancet 1:439, 1984.

12.62 ACUTE APPENDICITIS

Acute appendicitis is the most common disease requiring abdominal surgery in childhood, and with trauma to viscera, intussusception, adhesive bowel obstruction, and lesions of the ovary, it is one of the few indications for emergency surgery in children over 2 yr of age. Diagnosis in children, however, can be difficult; more often in children than in adults appendicitis progresses to perforation because a physician has failed to recognize it. Preventable deaths of children from appendicitis still occur.

Epidemiology. The true incidence of acute appendicitis is unknown, but the annual rate of appendectomy is about 4 in every 1000 children under the age of 14 yr. A busy physician is likely to see two to three cases each yr, and an active pediatric emergency service may receive three to four each wk. Males predominate in most series. Appendicitis occurs in infancy and has been reported in the neonatal period, but it is unusual under the age of 2 yr and rare under 1 yr. Peak age incidence is in the teenage and young adult years. The frequency increases in autumn and spring.

Etiology. Acute appendicitis is almost always caused by some obstruction of the lumen. Hard concretions and appendiceal fecaliths are frequently found at the site of obstruction in inflamed appendices. The proximal portion of the appendix may be bound to the cecum by a congenital peritoneal fold (Jackson membrane), with a sharp kink and obstruction where the organ emerges from beneath the free border of this fold. The appendiceal mesentery can be so narrow that the distal portion of the appendix, with the mesentery, undergoes torsion, producing acute ischemic necrosis. Appendiceal obstruction has also been attributed to hyperplasia of the submucosal lymphoid tissue, presumably as a result of infection. Many resected appendices, both normal and diseased, contain pinworms, but parasites have not been proved to cause appendicitis. Fibrous stenosis resulting from earlier inflammation or a carcinoid tumor (argentaffinoma) may also predispose to appendicitis.

Nonobstructive appendicitis is rare; in some reported cases fecaliths have probably become dislodged. Both the clinical manifestations and the tissue changes are less severe in nonobstructive appendicitis, and resolution without perforation may occur.

Bacteriologic studies generally grow mixed intestinal organisms. Anaerobes are particularly important causes of intraperitoneal abscesses after perforation or surgery. Associated disease may delay the diagnosis of appendicitis and increase the risk of perforation, but it is doubtful that systemic infections predispose to or cause appendicitis.

Pathology. In the younger child the progression of the disease is generally so rapid that the first of three pathologic stages usually passes before medical attention is sought. First, when acute obstruction of the appendix occurs, the intraluminal pressure increases because the mucosal cells continue to elaborate mucus. Compression of mucosal vessels causes ischemia, necrosis, and ulceration. Second, bacterial invasion and infection of the appendiceal wall occur readily once the mucosa ulcerates. Inflammatory infiltrate appears within all layers, and fibrinous exudate is deposited on the serosa. Even before perforation is apparent, organisms can usually be cultured from the serosal surface of the appendix. Third, necrosis of the appendiceal wall results in perforation and fecal contamination of the peritoneum. Perforation usually occurs at the relatively ischemic tip or near the base where a fecalith has eroded through the wall.

In the older child the omentum and adjacent ileum usually adhere to the inflamed appendix prior to perforation and prevent widespread fecal spillage. The result is a localized abscess, usually in the right iliac fossa but occasionally low in the pelvis. Multiple foci of intraperitoneal sepsis and pleural empyema rarely complicate general peritonitis now because diagnoses are made early when treatment is more effective. Paralytic ileus or mechanical bowel obstruction may be associated, or the abscess may rupture, usually into an adjacent, adherent loop of intestine rather than into the general peritoneal space. Spontaneous recovery follows rupture of the abscess into the bowel lumen. In an infant or younger child appendicitis can progress quickly to perforation and general peritonitis since at this age the omentum is small and ineffective in localizing the infection.

Clinical Manifestations. Pain is invariably present. Initially, when the pathology is confined to the mucosa and muscular layers of the appendix, it is crampy and periumbilical. The colicky nature of the pain may reflect appendicular peristalsis directed at extruding the obstructing agent. When visceral and parietal peritoneal layers become involved in the inflammation, however, pain is localized to the area immediately overlying the appendix; it is commonly located in the right iliac fossa but may even be felt in the hypogastrium or within the pelvis if the appendix is pelvic, and in the loin if retrocolic. Movement such as jumping or driving over bumps in a car aggravates the pain. At this stage there is severe tenderness over the appendix, fever, tachycardia, and leukocytosis. While some older children may give the classic history described above, others locate the pain in the right iliac fossa throughout the illness. A young child will often hold a hand over the navel when asked to show where it hurts. In infancy, general irritability and a tendency to lie quietly with hips flexed may be the only indication of pain. The cramps of appendiceal obstruction are rarely severe. In fact, if an older child cries because of abdominal pain, he or she probably does not have appendicitis. The pain of peritoneal inflammation is made worse by any movement, such as a cough or a sudden turn. A patient who winces when jostled probably has peritoneal irritation.

Vomiting is almost always noted after the onset of the pain; it is not copious or frequent and is less common in older than in younger children. Anorexia is almost invariably present.

In children the duration of appendicitis before rupture is usually so short that there is insufficient time for constipation to develop. Diarrhea may suggest that cramps are due to gastroenteritis, but loose stools can also result from irritation of the colon by an adjacent, acutely inflamed appendix. Similarly, pelvic appendicitis can cause urinary frequency and urgency by irritating the bladder.

Sometimes a child with an acute retrocecal or retroiliac appendicitis will walk with an exaggerated lumbar lordosis and a slightly flexed hip due to spasm of the right psoas muscle.

Many children with acute appendicitis have previously had milder, self-limited attacks of a similar nature.

During history taking, it is helpful to observe the patient for pallor, flushing, physical activity, and abdominal movement. Pulse rate and rectal temperature should be obtained in advance. Jiggling the bed or gently shaking the child's thigh by a hand placed casually on the leg can suggest appendiceal inflammation if pain in the right lower abdomen results. Throughout the interview and examination it is important to proceed slowly, whenever possible distracting the child with appropriate conversation and never threatening with a sudden movement.

The physician should proceed directly to the specific abdominal examination leaving the remainder of the examination until later. First, the abdomen should be inspected for visible swelling and movements. If the child is old enough, compliance with a request to cough or to move the abdominal wall in and out will produce pain over any site of peritoneal inflammation. Palpation in younger children may be initiated by using a stethoscope as a light palpating instrument. The pressure on the abdomen with the instrument is gradually increased, and later the hand replaces the stethoscope. There should also be an attempt to elicit increased muscle tone, pressing gently in each quadrant, observing as well as feeling the resistance. Palpation must be gentle since voluntary splinting is the response to pain and involuntary tone cannot be assessed. The site of maximum tenderness is important; in the older child it is often well localized to the McBurney point, the junction between the lateral and middle thirds of the line joining the right anterior superior iliac spine and the umbilicus. In younger children localization to the right iliac fossa is usually all that can be detected. Pain produced in the appendiceal area by pressure elsewhere in the abdomen is a valuable sign in an anxious child. Rebound tenderness is a needlessly painful sign; eliciting it serves only to destroy the carefully built up relationship between the examiner and the child. It is also often falsely positive or negative. Bowel sounds may be depressed in appendicitis, silent with generalized peritonitis.

Atypical locations of the appendix cause difficulty in diagnosis. If it lies up the gutter, lateral to the cecum, the tenderness will be in the flank. A pelvic appendix may be reached only by rectum. Retroiliac appendicitis usually causes very poorly localized pain so that the diagnosis is unlikely to be made before perforation occurs. A posteriorly situated appendix lying on the psoas muscle will cause hip flexion, and pain may be produced by passive extension of the hip with the child lying on the left side (psoas sign). The most important physical sign is a constant, localized, significant degree of tenderness. The site of tenderness must not vary between examinations nor among examiners. An acutely inflamed but unruptured appendix should not give rise to tenderness of the entire hemiabdomen, nor should there be bilateral tenderness; an unduly extensive area of tenderness in the absence of perforation should call into question the diagnosis of appendicitis.

After the abdominal assessment the general examination is completed, leaving until last the essential rectal examination. For this, a mild hypnotic, such as one of the barbiturates, may occasionally facilitate the examination of a particularly upset child, but, if at all possible, hypnotics or sedatives should be avoided. Patience and gentle persistence are more effective aids in examination of an apprehensive child. In equivocal cases re-evaluation of the patient in 4–6 hr is helpful since the course of appendicitis is usually sufficiently rapid in children that 6 hr produces enough change to make the diagnosis. Even under ideal circumstances, up to 15% of operations for presumed acute appendicitis in children lead to the removal of noninflamed appendices.

Laboratory Data. A high white blood cell count suggests acute suppurative disease. Usually, there is neutrophilia with a shift to the left and absence of eosinophils. The teenager with early appendicitis is unlikely to have a count higher than 15,000/mm³, but the infant may show a leukocyte response of 20,000/mm³ or more even before perforation. Occasionally, the white count is depressed. Pyuria usually suggests urinary tract infection, particularly if there are bacteria in a fresh specimen, but an inflamed appendix lying across the ureter or irritating the bladder can also cause pyuria. Other hematologic or biochemical tests are not diagnostically useful but may be important in assessing a patient's general state.

Roentgenograms may detect intestinal obstruction, a calcified appendicolith, or pneumonia. Scoliosis concave to the right can be caused by an inflamed appendix, and a degree of paralytic ileus may be noted. In any case, the indications for surgery should be based, in almost all instances, on abdominal physical findings and not on roentgenograms.

Differential Diagnosis. The diffuse crampy pain and diarrhea of enteric infection usually distinguish it from appendicitis, but appendicitis may occur in a child who has had gastroenteritis for several days. The enteritis caused by *Yersinia enterocolitica*, an acute flare-up of *Crohn disease* or regional ileitis, and, infrequently, intussusception in an older child may produce right lower abdominal symptoms highly suggestive of appendicitis. Occasionally, Crohn disease may begin by mimicking appendicitis. Inflammation rarely complicates a *Meckel diverticulum*, but when it does, the clinical findings may be identical to those of appendicitis. Many children with viral or other infections have pain and tenderness in the appendiceal area and are assumed to have *mesenteric adenitis* (see below). However, ileocecal lymphadenopathy causing appendicitis-like symptoms is rare. An infected lesion on the ipsilateral lower limb or perineum may give rise to an external iliac adenitis with tenderness low down in the right iliac fossa. When generalized *viral infections* cause abdominal pain, it is usually midabdominal, worse upon eating, and associated with neutropenia. Early fever, headache, and chills favor a systemic infection, even if abdominal pain is noted later. *Pneumonia* involving the right lower lobe with diaphragmatic irritation may result in enough right-sided abdominal muscular rigidity and referred pain that appendicitis is suspected. Abdominal pain occasionally accompanies acute *streptococcal tonsillitis* or *pharyngitis* and can mimic appendicitis very closely, but these disorders may also occur with true appendicitis. *Acute rheumatic fever* can cause abdominal pain in its early stages. *Urinary tract infections* occasionally cause abdominal pain and tenderness; there should always be a careful urinary tract evaluation prior to appendectomy. *Diabetic ketoacidosis* frequently causes abdominal pain and vomiting, and in the undiagnosed diabetic can be confused with appendicitis. Urinalysis should lead to the correct diagnosis and must never be omitted prior to emergency surgery. *Bleeding from the right ovary*, a graafian follicle, or a persisting corpus luteum can also simulate appendicitis. *Primary peritonitis* is discussed in Sec. 12.89.

Abdominal pain is a common symptom of many hematologic disorders. It is associated with leukemia, especially in relapse. Appendicitis in patients with leukemia may be masked by immunosuppressant drugs. One should also suspect the diagnosis of appendicitis in a hemophiliac patient with abdominal pain. Sickle cell disease and anaphylactoid purpura (Henoch-Schönlein purpura) frequently cause severe abdominal pain (Sec. 10.64 and 15.47).

Treatment. Emergency appendectomy is the treatment for early acute appendicitis. Only under the most extreme circumstances should operation be delayed more than a few hr. Recovery is rapid and the child active in 3–4 days. Most surgeons recommend that the child with a localized appendiceal abscess receive adequate external drainage after appropriate preoperative correction of any fluid and electrolyte problems; at The Hospital for Sick Children, Toronto, however, only supportive care is provided until spontaneous drainage of the abscess occurs into an adjacent loop of a bowel, a process that rarely takes longer than 1 wk. Then 8–12 wk later appendectomy is carried out.

The child with generalized peritonitis due to appendiceal rupture requires intravenous hydration and correction of any electrolyte disturbance before surgery, because of substantial fluid loss into the abdominal space from an inflamed peritoneum. If there are no clinical signs of dehydration, lactated Ringer solution should be administered at a volume of 5% of the body weight. Half of the calculated need should be given in the first 1–2 hr, followed by the rest during and after the operation. If there are signs of dehydration, a volume equivalent to 7% of the body weight is administered; half of the deficit should be given preoperatively. For severe cases of dehydration 10–15% of the body weight is required as replacement. An adequate urinary output should be established before surgery.

It is essential that antibiotics be given before the operation when the appendix has ruptured to ensure adequate blood and tissue levels of the drugs used. Triple intravenous therapy using an aminoglycoside, ampicillin, and clindamycin or metronidazole or one of the newer cephalosporins is the treatment of choice. Appendectomy is necessary to limit continued fecal contamination of the peritoneum. Many surgeons use preoperative triple antibiotic therapy before any operation for appendicitis, discontinuing their use postoperatively if there was no perforation. After surgery a normal fluid and electrolyte balance should be maintained, and the stomach and bowel should be kept decompressed by effective nasogastric suction until intestinal activity returns.

Prognosis. The prognosis is excellent provided an appendectomy is performed before perforation has occurred, and good even after perforation. Among 550 children with generalized peritonitis from ruptured appendix managed at The Hospital for Sick Children, Toronto, three deaths (0.5%) occurred.

Complications. Since the institution of preoperative triple antibiotic therapy, postoperative infections have become far less common. The most common postoperative complication is infection of the wound. Pelvic, subphrenic, or other intra-abdominal suppuration is especially likely to develop after operation on a gangrenous, perforated appendix. Ultrasonography is a useful diagnostic aid at this stage. There is no urgent need for reoperation because of the development of intra-abdominal suppuration. Almost all pelvic abscesses will rupture into an adjacent loop of bowel and spontaneously resolve. It is virtually never necessary to drain these by the rectum. Subphrenic suppuration requires surgical drainage.

Prolonged paralytic ileus often follows generalized peritonitis; it may be aggravated by premature attempts at oral feedings.

Intestinal obstruction may occur as a postoperative complication. If this happens within 30 days of the appendectomy, nonoperative management is advisable. If obstruction occurs more than 30 days later and there is no evidence of ischemia of the bowel, nasogastric compression may be attempted for a short period (48 hr); if this is unsuccessful, a laparotomy will be necessary. A volvulus may be present, with gangrenous bowel caused by a single adhesion in the right lower quadrant. This complication may occur many yr after appendectomy. Pelvic peritonitis may rarely result in obstruction to the uterine tubes with consequent sterility.

The Appendix and Chronic Abdominal Pain. Obstruction of the vermiform appendix, whether by fibrous band, worms, or fecalith, used to be considered an important cause of recurrent or chronic abdominal pain, and many children were subjected to elective appendectomy for this reason. Some children may have been helped, but most continued to have pain and were belatedly diagnosed as having urinary tract pathology, gastrointestinal malfunction unrelated to the appendix, or psychophysiologic pain. Recurrent appendiceal obstruction is a rare cause of chronic or intermittent abdominal pain; an operation should be considered only after careful evaluation of these other possibilities. It is doubtful that chronic inflammation of the appendix ever occurs.

Acute Mesenteric Lymphadenitis. This ill-defined entity of uncertain nature or cause is frequently ascribed to associated acute infection of the upper respiratory tract and may initially simulate acute appendicitis. Both acute and chronic involvement of the mesenteric lymph nodes may be associated with infections of the appendix and the intestine.

BARRY SHANDLING
JAMES C. FALLIS

Apley J: The Child with Abdominal Pains. Ed 2. Oxford, Blackwell Scientific Publications, 1975.
Bartlett RH, Eraklis AJ, Wilkinson RH: Appendicitis in infancy. Surg Gynecol Obstet 130:99, 1970.
David IB, Buck JR, Filler RM: Rational use of antibiotics for perforated appendicitis in childhood. J Pediatr Surg 17:494, 1982.
Grosfeld JL, Weinberger M, Clatworthy HW: Acute appendicitis in the first two years of life. J Pediatr Surg 8:285, 1973.
Janik JS, Firor HV: Pediatric appendicitis. A 20-year study of 1640 children at Cook County Hospital. Arch Surg 114:717, 1979.
Johnson W, Borella L: Acute appendicitis in childhood leukemia. J Pediatr 67:595, 1965.
Leigh DA, Simmons K, Norman E: Bacterial flora of the appendix fossa in appendicitis and postoperative wound infection. J Clin Pathol 27:997, 1974.
McBurney C: Disease of the vermiform appendix. NY Med J 50:676, 1889.
Puri P, Rangecroft L, Servos G, et al: Perforated appendicitis in children: use of Metronidazole for the reduction of septic complications. Z Kinderchir 32:111, 1981.
Raffensperger JG, Seeler RA, Moncada R: The Acute Abdomen in infancy and Childhood. Chapters 10 and 12. Philadelphia, JB Lippincott, 1970.
Schwartz MZ, Tapper D, Solenberger RI: Management of perforated appendicitis in children: the controversy continues. Ann Surg 197:406, 1983.
Shandling B, Ein SH, Simpson JS, et al: Perforating appendicitis and antibiotics. J Pediatr Surg 9:79, 1974.
Stone HH, Sanders SL, Martin JD Jr: Perforated appendicitis in children. Surgery 69:673, 1971.
Wilkinson RH, Bartlett RH, Eraklis AJ: Diagnosis of appendicitis in infancy. Am J Dis Child 118:687, 1969.

12.63 SURGICAL CONDITIONS OF ANUS, RECTUM, AND COLON

In infants and children close inspection of the anal area is usually of greater value than a digital rectal examination. *Fissures* can be best identified by having the mother hold the infant's hips in acute flexion so that the examiner can separate the patient's buttocks, using both thumbs, gently stretching the anus and everting the lining to expose the fissure. On the other hand, in all cases of constipation, especially when an intrinsic or extrinsic rectal obstruction is possible, a digital examination is indicated, after assessing perianal sensation. Properly done, this should cause little or no discomfort to the patient. A well-lubricated finger is passed over the anus a few times to accustom the patient to the unusual sensation. Then the pulp of the index finger is pressed against the anus with increasing flexion of the interphalangeal joints and the finger slips easily into the anal canal.

ANAL FISSURE

A small slit or crack at the mucocutaneous line is a common acquired lesion in infancy and uncommon in the school aged child. Most anal fissures occur in the sagittal plane, usually dorsally in the midline. The cause is often not evident but may be secondary to constipation with passage of large hard stools, scratching induced by irritation from *Enterobius vermicularis* or eczema, or other perianal conditions.

Clinical Manifestations. Pain on defecation and, frequently, refusal to defecate are the principal manifestations. Bright red blood on the surface of the stool or on toilet paper and bleeding following defecation may be observed. The diagnosis is usually made by inspection of the anal area. The skin at the peripheral end of the fissure becomes swollen and forms a "tag." A history of prolapse of some tissue suggests a rectal polyp rather than a tag. Fissures also occur with Crohn disease. Sometimes, even after the fissure is healed the infant or child is afraid to defecate, anticipating anal pain; attempts are made to retain the stool.

Treatment. Most fissures will heal spontaneously if the local irritation is lessened or eliminated. Anal dilatation by the mother using a well-lubricated index finger twice daily for 1–2 wk will cure most anal fissures. A well-formed but not hard stool makes an excellent dilator of the anal canal and is attended by less psychic trauma than anal digital dilatation. The administration of laxatives to keep the stool fluid affords only temporary relief as eventually a more substantial stool must be passed with recurrence of the pain. If the patient is passing very hard stools, a mild stool softener may be useful, but the aim should not be to render the stools fluid. The addition of natural bran to the diet (1–3 tablespoons depending on the child's age) is of great value in softening the stool. Anesthetic ointment is traditionally prescribed, but it is often not helpful since it is most effective when applied 30 min before a bowel movement, which is impossible to predict. Washing the anal area with soap and water after every stool is important. Often the perianal skin is excoriated and inflamed, and sometimes multiple superficial anal fissures occur. In such cases an ointment or cream with a triamcinolone base is useful. Care should be taken to exclude the simultaneous presence of a fungal infection.

If there is no response to medical management or if the fissure has been present a long time, a minor operation may be indicated since excessively prolonged symptoms from a fissure may result in the development of acquired megacolon with fecal impaction and encopresis. The operation is done under general anesthesia and may consist of stretching the anus, excision of the fissure, or internal anal sphincterotomy, or of a combination of the three procedures. Minimal postoperative discomfort occurs; recurrence is unusual.

ANORECTAL ABSCESS

Perianal abscess may occur in young infants, often starting as a small perianal pustule from an infected diaper rash. The infection usually gains entrance to the ischiorectal fossa through the anal crypts and soon extends into the subcutaneous tissues and develops into a nodule, usually within 1.5 cm of the anus. The symptoms are pain and swelling. Defecation is painful, and the child is unable to sit comfortably. The temperature is usually not elevated unless the perirectal space is infected. A painful swelling overlies the ischiorectal fossa, with redness, heat, induration, and fluctuation. Treatment consists of immediate incision and drainage under anesthesia. In contrast to cervical lymphadenitis, it is not necessary to wait for fluctuation to develop before surgical drainage. Baths are helpful postoperatively. Antibiotics are not efficacious in the treatment of perianal abscess. After drainage, a persistent or intermittent discharge of purulent material from the site of drainage will indicate an anal fistula.

Ischiorectal suppuration in the older child or teenager and should suggest the possibility of Crohn disease or ulcerative colitis. The causative organism here, as with most perianal abscesses, is usually *E. coli*. The treatment is prompt surgical drainage.

ANAL FISTULA

Fistulas originating in the anus or rectum may be congenital or acquired and rarely may extend to and communicate with the urinary bladder, urethra, vagina, or perianal skin. Acquired fistulas are residuals of an abscess and usually open on the skin surface. There is frequently a history of one or more incisions into the abscess, of neglect, or of antibiotic treatment of the abscess.

Clinical Manifestations. An acquired fistula produces a recurrent painful swelling which subsides with a purulent discharge. An opening into the skin, into which a probe may be introduced, is found beside the anal orifice.

Treatment. No fistulas close spontaneously. Simple incision and unroofing of the fistulous tract is curative. Care must be taken not to injure the anal sphincter and cause incontinence.

HEMORRHOIDS

Hemorrhoids are very rare in infants and children. When they are encountered, an underlying cause may be present, such as a venacaval or mesenteric obstruction, cirrhosis, portal hypertension, or other reasons for venous obstruction. Occasionally, chronic constipation, fecal impaction, and straining at stool result in hemorrhoids. Operation is rarely indicated except for an acute external thrombus. The hemorrhoids generally subside when the primary condition is corrected.

PRURITUS ANI

Anal itching in childhood is generally secondary to enterobiasis, anal fissures, and other local inflammatory lesions, or to coarse or moist undergarments. Nocturnal itching may be the most frequent evidence of pinworm infestation. Treatment consists of eradication of the underlying cause and cleansing the anal area with a mild soap and drying it with a soft cloth or tissue. Powders or solutions such as witch hazel may be used. In small infants exposure to sunlight or dry heat is helpful when the anal area is inflamed.

PROLAPSE AND PROCIDENTIA OF THE RECTUM AND SIGMOID

Prolapse is abnormal descent of the mucous membrane of the rectum with or without protrusion through the anal orifice; *procidentia* is abnormal descent of all the coats of the rectum or sigmoid with or without protrusion through the anus. These conditions are most common from 3–5 yr of age. The anatomy of the infants' pelvis predisposes to rectal prolapse. Any sudden increase in intra-abdominal pressure, such as straining at bowel movements after prolonged sitting with the hips and knees flexed, may precipitate abnormal descent of the bowel wall. Malnutrition with absorption of ischiorectal fat is a contributory factor. Children with chronic malabsorption, particularly cystic fibrosis, are prone to develop prolapse. Protrusion at stool initially recedes spontaneously but later requires manual replacement. Bleeding and the passage of mucus may occur. The protruding mass varies from bright to dark red; it may be as much as 6 in long. In prolapse the striations or furrows radiate from the center of the anal aperture in contrast to the concentrically arranged rosette of procidentia. Both conditions must be differentiated from an intussusception with the apex presenting at the anus, and from juvenile rectal polyp presenting at the anus.

Treatment should be directed to dietary correction of constipation, to proper toilet training, and to the elimination of any underlying disturbance, such as parasitic infection, diarrhea, or polyps. Oral administration of stool softeners and having the child defecate with his or her feet off the floor may be helpful. Prolonged sessions on the toilet should be discouraged.

Reduction of protrusion is aided by pressure with warm compresses. An easy method of reduction is to cover the finger with a piece of toilet paper, introduce it into the lumen of the mass, and gently push it into the rectum. The finger is then immediately withdrawn. The toilet paper adheres to the mucous membrane, permitting release of the finger; the paper, when softened, is later expelled. Submucosal injection of sclerosants into the rectal ampulla is an effective means of preventing prolapse when repetitive attempts at medical therapy have failed. For intractable cases perineal operation may, on rare occasion, be indicated. In procidentia of the rectum and sigmoid, abdominal sigmoidopexy is required.

POSTANAL DIMPLE

A **postanal dimple** is seen relatively frequently in normal babies, located behind the anus, close to the upper limit of the natal cleft. It almost never requires treatment except when it is very deep and becomes the site of minor recurrent infections. If simple hygienic measures are inadequate, excision of the dimple may be necessary.

A dermal sinus is present when there is a communication between a postanal dimple and the sacrum or coccyx. Such a tract may be attached to the dural linings of the spinal canal. This lesion requires meticulous excision to prevent the development of postoperative meningitis.

A **pilonidal sinus** is an acquired condition that is not a sequel to or a complication of a postanal dimple. It consists of one or several pits dorsal to the anus and is usually seen in hairy youths. A pilondial sinus results from shed hairs piercing the skin in the natal cleft. This may follow undue friction of the buttocks, and during World War II it was called "jeep driver's disease." A similar condition is seen in the interdigital webs on the hands of barbers. The sinus tract may become obstructed, forming a *pilonidal cyst* or abscess. The physician is consulted when infection supervenes.

Pilonidal cysts and sinuses do not cause symptoms unless infected. Swelling, heat, redness, tenderness, and fluctuation over the sacrococcygeal region are characteristic of an infected sinus. Purulent material may be discharged from one or more openings. If infection occurs, drainage or total excision should be performed.

BARRY SHANDLING

Enberg RN, Cox RH, Burry VF: Perirectal abscess in children. Am J Dis Child 128:360, 1974.
Mentzer GG: Anorectal disease. Pediatr Clin North Am 3:113, 1956.
Stern RC, Izant RJ, Boat TF, et al: Treatment and prognosis of rectal prolapse in cystic fibrosis. Gastroenterology 82:707, 1982.

12.63 TUMORS OF THE DIGESTIVE TRACT IN CHILDREN

See also Sec. 16.21.

Juvenile Colonic Polyp. This is the most common tumor of the bowel in childhood. It is a hamartoma with no potential for malignancy. The lesion usually appears after the 1st yr and rarely persists beyond the age of 15. Approximately 80% are found in the distal large bowel, within reach of a sigmoidoscope; all but 10% are distal to the splenic flexure. Most are solitary. Rarely, multiple colonic juvenile polyps occur in families; these lesions are identical to those described above and are considered to be equally benign.

The typical *clinical manifestation* is painless rectal bleeding. Blood may be on the stool or mixed with it; the amount is usually modest. An iron deficiency anemia from occult blood loss may be the initial problem. There may be crampy pain if the lesion causes the bowel to intussuscept or if a polyp prolapses. Most polyps infarct spontaneously and are passed in stool.

The *differential diagnosis* includes other forms of polyposis (particularly the familial types), Meckel diverticulum, fissure in ano, and inflammatory problems including infection and other forms of colitis.

Diagnosis may be made by rectal examination. About one third of these polyps are within reach of the examining finger, but they are difficult to identify. Most are visible on sigmoidoscopy as smooth, pedunculated lesions containing gray-white cysts. An air-contrast barium enema may show lesions above the level of sigmoidoscopic examination. Fiberoptic colonoscopy, which permits visualization of the descending colon and often the transverse and proximal segments, is the preferred diagnostic procedure. A polyp observed at endoscopy should be biopsied to confirm its hamartomatous nature.

Treatment is conservative for this self-limited, nonmalignant problem except in rare cases in which hemorrhage is life-threatening. If the polyp can be reached with forceps, it can be removed per rectum using a speculum. More proximal polyps can be removed at colonoscopy by use of a snare. Laparotomy is recommended only for multiple proximal polyps that cannot be adequately assessed and treated by colonoscopy.

Familial Polyposis Syndromes. The rare familial syndromes associated with intestinal polyposis are important because they represent premalignant states which raise the fear of cancer in the patient or family.

Familial Adenomatous Polyposis Coli. This dominant premalignant condition with reduced penetrance is characterized by large numbers of of adenomatous lesions in the distal large bowel. The usual onset is late in the 1st decade of life or during the teens, but lesions may occur earlier. Initially, the polyps are asymptomatic and in many cases remain so. When symptomatic, they cause hematochezia, and occasionally crampy pain or diarrhea. Malignancy may develop during the teens.

The diagnosis should be suspected from the family history, but no technique yet permits prediction of the disorder in a young child of a proven case. Diagnosis is made by showing filling defects in a double contrast barium enema, or preferably by direct vision through a colonoscope. The polyps are usually numerous; biopsies show that they are adenomatous without the inflammatory and cystic findings of the juvenile polyp. For a child with a proven family history of polyposis coli, colonoscopy every 2 yr after 12 yr of age is recommended.

Treatment consists of a careful family survey, genetic counseling, and, for diagnosed cases, pancolectomy. Previously this approach has meant an ileostomy, but anastomotic procedures now permit restoration of bowel continuity with removal of all involved mucosa.

Peutz-Jeghers Syndrome. This rare dominantly inherited syndrome is characterized by mucosal pigmentation of the lips and gums, and hamartomas of the stomach and small bowel. The polyps are not premalignant. Deeply pigmented discrete freckles are seen at birth or appear during infancy on the lips and buccal mucosa, and even around the mouth. Evidence of intestinal lesions may come from bleeding, or from crampy pain associated with obstruction or intussusception.

Family studies and genetic counseling are important. Relatives may be found with either partial or complete manifestations of the syndrome. Intestinal lesions that are causing significant symptoms should be excised; involvement is usually too extensive to remove all the polyps.

Gardner Syndrome. This rare, dominantly inherited disorder is characterized by multiple intestinal polyps and tumors of the soft tissue and bone, particularly the mandible. The soft tissue lesions and osteomas may appear during childhood, but intestinal polyps usually do not become apparent until early adult life. These polyps may develop anywhere along the digestive tract and are premalignant. Accordingly, aggressive surgical treatment of the intestinal lesions is indicated.

Hemangioma of the Intestine. These rare benign lesions can cause massive, even fatal hemorrhage. The usual clinical manifestation is painless bleeding beginning in childhood. The blood loss can be subtle and chronic, or sudden and massive. Usually, there are no additional intestinal symptoms, but if intussusception occurs, there will be obstructive symptoms. About 50% of patients have cutaneous hemangiomas, and some have a family history of similar lesions. About half of these lesions are in the colon, where they may be seen by colonoscopy. During a period of bleeding selective mesenteric arteriography may be useful in locating a lesion.

Leiomyoma. This rare benign tumor occurs most commonly in stomach and jejunum. It remains asymptomatic for long periods, but if it extends into the lumen, it may cause intussusception.

Carcinoma. The fact that epithelial tumors of the digestive tract are extremely rare in children argues against an aggressive diagnostic approach to many gastrointestinal symptoms in this age group. Several conditions predispose to development of adenocarcinoma of the gut: familial polyposis, Gardner syndrome, idiopathic ulcerative colitis, and, to a lesser extent, Crohn disease and disorders associated with chromosomal breaks. In these disorders tumors are not usually seen until adult life.

The usual site of the lesion is the colon. Symptoms are general ill health, abdominal pain, an abdominal mass, and, less frequently, hemorrhage. The tumors are often relatively undifferentiated and highly malignant.

Lymphosarcoma of the Intestine. Of the malignancies of the digestive tract in children, most are lymphosarcomas (Sec. 16.21). The usual site is the lower small intestine. Manifestations are general ill health, abdominal pain, and anemia. Adults with longstanding celiac disease have a relatively high incidence of lymphosarcoma; a beneficial effect of dietary treatment on this relationship has not been proved.

Carcinoid Tumors. These tumors of the enterochromaffin cells of the intestine usually occur in the appendix in children and have very low grade malignancy. They cause symptoms similar to those of appendicitis and do not recur after resection, even when the tumor has extended to the muscularis and lymphatics.

Carcinoid tumors outside the appendix commonly metastasize, and the metastatic lesions give rise to the carcinoid syndrome, which is the result of pharmacologically active secretions produced by the tumor. These produce episodic intestinal hypermotility and diarrhea, vasomotor disturbances, and bronchoconstriction. The most important active agent is serotonin, and the diagnosis is usually made by finding high urinary levels of its metabolite 5-hydroxyindoleacetic acid. These functioning neoplasms are very rarely seen in children.

Abrahamson J, Shandling B: Intestinal hemangiomata in childhood and a syndrome for diagnosis: A collective review. J Pediatr Surg 8:487, 1973.
Bartholomew LG: Peutz-Jeghers syndrome. JAMA 183:901, 1963.
Berry CL, Keeling JW: Gastrointestinal lymphoma in childhood. J Clin Pathol 23:459, 1970.
Cohen SB, Pavlidos GP, Krush AJ, et al: Familial polyposis coli. Md State Med J 27:64, 1978.
Gardner EJ, Richards RC: Multiple cutaneous and subcutaneous lesions occurring simultaneously with hereditary polyposis and osteomatosis. Am J Hum Genet 5:130, 1953.
Holgerson LO, Miller RE, Zintel HA: Juvenile polyps of the colon. Surgery 69:288, 1971.
Mazier WP, Bowman HE, Ming Sun K, et al: Juvenile polyps of the colon and rectum. Dis Colon Rectum 17:523, 1974.
Mestel DL: Lymphosarcoma of small intestine in infancy and childhood. Am Surg 149:87, 1949.
Postlethwait RW: Gastrointestinal carcinoid tumors—a review. Postgrad Med 40:445, 1966.
Recalde M, Holyoke ED, Elias EG: Carcinoma of the colon, rectum and anal canal in young patients. Surg Gynecol Obstet 139:909, 1974.

Functioning Tumors Causing Diarrhea. Certain hormone-producing tumors may cause an increase in secretion leading to severe chronic diarrhea. The most common are those arising from the neural crest. *Neuroblastoma* or *ganglioneuroma* occurs most often in the adrenal gland but may develop anywhere along the sympathetic chain (Sec. 16.11). A diarrhea syndrome probably mediated by vasoactive intestinal peptide (VIP), a secretagogue produced by the tumor, is associated with about 10% of these lesions. Diarrhea is usually massive, causing fluid and electrolyte imbalance. Diagnosis is made by identifying the tumor and its secretory products, which include catecholamines and their metabolites. Pheochromocytomas do not cause diarrhea. Severe diarrhea is seldom associated with *Zollinger-Ellison syndrome* in children (Sec. 12.41); in this disorder the clinical manifestations are attributed to a gastrin-secreting pancreatic islet tumor. Rare non-gastrin-secreting pancreatic *islet tumors* may also cause diarrhea; the secretagogue may be a VIP.

Buchta RM, Kaplan JM: Zollinger-Ellison syndrome in a nine-year old child: A case report and review of this entity in childhood. Pediatrics 47:594, 1971.
Hamilton JR, Radde IC, Johnson G: Diarrhea associated with adrenal ganglioneuroma. New findings related to the pathogenesis of diarrhea. Am J Med 44:473, 1968.
Kaplan SJ, Holbrook CT, McDaniel HE, et al: Vasoactive intestinal peptide secreting tumors of childhood. Am J Dis Child 134:21, 1980.

Mitchell CH, Sinatra FR, Crast FW, et al: Intractable watery diarrhea, ganglioneuroblastoma and vasoactive intestinal peptide. J Pediatr 89:593, 1976.
Rambaud JC, Modigliani R, et al: Pancreatic cholera: Studies on tumor secretions and pathophysiology of diarrhea. Gastroenterology 69:110, 1975.

Nodular Lymphoid Hyperplasia. Lymphoid follicles in the lamina propria of the gut normally aggregate in Peyer patches. These areas appear as submucosal nodules which may be visible on barium contrast roentgenograms and mistaken for an abnormality. There are many more Peyer patches in the lower than the upper small bowel. In some patients lymphoid follicles become hyperplastic. The hyperplasia may occur in the colon or extend to the small bowel. Small bowel lesions are seen in cases of immunoglobulin deficiency, with and without *Giardia lamblia* infestation. Symptoms are mild. There may be rectal bleeding, diarrhea, and abdominal cramps beginning usually by 3 yr of age.

The major importance of this entity is the similarity of its manifestations to more serious disorders. Lymphoid hyperplasia resolves spontaneously and requires no specific treatment.

J. RICHARD HAMILTON

Hodgson JR, Hoffman HN, Huizenga KA: Roentgenologic features of lymphoid hyperplasia of the small intestine associated with dysgammaglobulinemia. Radiology 88:883, 1967.
Poley JR, Smith EL: Benign lymphatic hyperplasia of the rectum. South Med J 65:420, 1972.

12.65 HERNIAS

A hernia is a protrusion of the contents of a body compartment through the wall that normally encloses it. Hernias (or "ruptures") and hydroceles (Sec. 17.45) are the most common significant anomalies of children. The most common hernia of the groin in infancy and childhood is the indirect (congenital, infantile) inguinal hernia. Direct inguinal and femoral hernias are rare in children. Diaphragmatic and esophageal hiatal hernias are discussed in Sec. 12.80 and 12.88, omphaloceles and umbilical hernias in Sec. 8.53.

INDIRECT INGUINAL HERNIAS

Pathology and Pathogenesis. Late in fetal development the processus vaginalis, an outpouching of peritoneum originating at the internal inguinal ring, extends medially down each inguinal canal. Leaving the canal at the external ring, the processus enters the scrotum in the male, where it invests the developing testicle. Its lumen is normally obliterated before birth except for the portion enveloping the testicle. This part remains as a potential sac, the tunica vaginalis. In the female the processus extends from the external ring into the labium majus. If the proximal part of the processus vaginalis fail to close, a potential hernial sac is produced, into which an abdominal viscus may herniate or fluid collect. In the male the patent portion extends inferiorly a variable distance, sometimes into the scrotum; if it is continuous with the tunica vaginalis, a complete hernia is formed.

Inguinal hernias are particularly common in premature infants, presumably because curtailment of intrauterine development impaired the process of closure. When the testicle fails to descend (is cryptorchid), there is usually a large hernial sac, probably because something has arrested both testicular descent and closure of the peritoneal process. Children with multiple congenital anomalies, particularly those involving the lower abdomen, pelvis, or perineum, often have inguinal hernias as part of the complex.

Clinical Manifestations. Usually, a swelling is noted at the external ring, but it may extend for a variable distance downward into the scrotum or labium majus. The lump may be continually present or be apparent only with raised intra-abdominal pressure, such as when an infant cries or strains at stool. Sometimes a mass will appear suddenly in an infant and be associated with acute discomfort. In such circumstances, it may be difficult to distinguish acute hydrocele of the spermatic cord from incarcerated hernia. The former will have no gastrointestinal symptoms; in case of the latter, examination will reveal loops of bowel entering and leaving the internal inguinal ring. In the older child the mass typically appears at the end of an active day or with vigorous coughing. A hernia usually disappears when a baby relaxes with a bottle or when an older child lies down.

The diagnosis of inguinal hernia in infancy and childhood may be made from history alone, even if significant physical findings are absent when the child is seen by the doctor, so long as the typical swelling is described by a competent observer. Usually, however, it is preferable that the surgeon see and feel the lump for himself or herself to exclude the possibility of a retracted testis or another abnormality, and to decide whether the contents are intestinal or fluid alone.

Uncomplicated inguinal hernias in children rarely cause pain; pain in the groin is much more likely to represent hip disease than hernia. Occasionally, a baby will cry whenever the hernia is protruding, but usually the hernia protrudes because the child is crying. Sometimes there is fleeting inguinal discomfort or pain when the hernia or hydrocele first fills.

The older child with a hernia may have had a hydrocele in early infancy.

The observation of an inguinal or inguinoscrotal mass which is reduced either spontaneously or with manipulation is diagnostic. If the hernia is not present on initial inspection, inducing the baby to cry while the abdomen is firmly compressed is very likely to force it out. In the older child the hernia can usually be demonstrated by having the standing patient strain as the examiner manually compresses the abdomen. If these maneuvers fail to reveal a suspected hernia, the diagnosis may be supported by the finding of a thickened spermatic cord on the side in question. Introducing a finger into the external ring to detect a peritoneal impulse is of no value since the ring may be so large and the canal so short that an impulse is often readily palpable in the absence of herniation. Occasionally, a full bladder may occlude the internal inguinal ring and prevent elicitation of the physical findings of the hernia; emptying the bladder will enable the hernia to be demonstrated.

Treatment. The treatment of choice for inguinal hernia in infancy and childhood is herniorrhaphy. Some surgeons routinely explore the opposite inguinal region in cases of clinically unilateral inguinal hernias. There are no data, however, as to whether such a procedure may interfere with subsequent fertility. The author does not recommend routine bilateral exploration. For the older child surgical repair is carried out at the earliest convenient time. In a young infant an inguinal hernia should be repaired as soon as the patient's general condition is satisfactory, in order to remove the risk of incarceration. Except for premature or small-for-dates infants under the age of 6 mo, surgical repair may be done on an outpatient basis, provided appropriate facilities are available.

Supports and trusses designed to keep the abdominal contents from protruding into a hernial sac are not indicated.

Any inguinal hernia that cannot be reduced needs emergency surgical repair. Resection may be required if necrosis of bowel has occurred but is almost never necessary.

Although a bleeding tendency is generally a contraindication to surgery, the child with hemophilia should have his hernia repaired with appropriate coagulant therapy prior to and after operation (Sec. 15.43–15.46).

When associated with prematurity, a hernia should be repaired only after the infant gains strength and weight in the hospital. During this time the hernia should be carefully monitored and manually reduced as necessary. When the baby is big enough to go home, the hernia should be repaired in a facility accustomed to caring for small infants.

Complications. A hernia is incarcerated when its contents cannot be reduced and the contained bowel is obstructed. A hernia may seem irreducible on initial examination but prove to be reducible when manipulation is carried out by an experienced physician. Incarceration of an inguinal hernia is most likely to occur at the external inguinal ring and, with time, produces obstruction of the venous return from the herniated bowel and from the testis. This results in edema and progresses to venous infarction. The risk of incarceration is greatest in the youngest children. Cramps, bilious vomiting, and distention will occur with incarceration as the picture of intestinal obstruction develops. Irritability may be the only symptom of incarcerated hernia in an infant, and the diagnosis may be missed if the infant is not examined completely undressed.

Venous infarction of the testicle is a far more common complication of strangulation than intestinal ischemia, as the spermatic cord is readily compressed between the margin of the external ring and the hernial contents. A *Richter hernia* is a rare form of incarceration in which only a part of the bowel's circumference is pinched off within the hernia and intestinal obstruction does not develop.

Inguinal Hernias in Girls. About 10% of inguinal hernias in children occur in girls. In an infant girl the ovary is the organ most likely to herniate into the inguinal canal, where it is usually easily palpable as a movable almond-sized nodule. Although uncommon, infarction of the herniated ovary may occur because of torsion or compression of the pedicle. The inflamed abscess-like lesion which then develops in the groin is easily mistaken for inguinal lymphadenitis, but there are no lymph nodes in the anterior abdominal wall immediately above the inguinal ligament. In about 1% of operations on phenotypic girls for inguinal hernial repair, a testicle is discovered in the canal, abdomen, or labium majus. Closer examination reveals normal external genitalia, with the vagina a little shorter than usual. Rectal examination fails to reveal a uterus. Laparotomy in such instances reveals absence of female internal genital organs. The absence of chromatin bodies on buccal smear and appropriate chromosomal findings will indicate the diagnosis of testicular feminization (Sec. 19.29).

Prognosis. The prognosis following surgical repair of inguinal hernia in an infant or child is excellent. The complication rate is low and recurrences should be fewer than 1% following surgery.

BARRY SHANDLING

Hendren WH, Crawford JD: The child with ambiguous genitalia. Curr Probl Surg 1–64, Nov, 1972.

Holder TM, Ashcraft KW: Groin hernias and hydroceles. *In*: Pediatric Surgery, WB Saunders, 1980.

Janik JS, Shandling B: The vulnerability of the vas deferens (II): The case against routine bilateral inguinal exploration. J Pediatr Surg 17:585, 1982.

Kieseweter WB, Oh KS: Unilateral inguinal hernias in children: What about the opposite side? Arch Surg 115:1443, 1980.

McGregor DB, Halverson R, McVay CB: The unilateral pediatric inguinal hernia: Should the contralateral side be explored? J Pediatr Surg 15:313, 1980.

Mustard WT, Ravitch MM, Snyder WH, et al (eds): Pediatric Surgery. Ed 2. Chicago, Year Book Medical Publishers, 1969, Chapter 46.

Rescoria FJ, Grosfeld JL: Inguinal hernia repair in the perinatal period and early infancy: Clinical considerations. J Pediatr Surg 19:832, 1984.

Shandling B, Janik JS: The vulnerability of the vas (I). J Pediatr Surg 16:461, 1981.

THE EXOCRINE PANCREAS

12.66 DEVELOPMENT AND FUNCTION OF THE PANCREAS

Development. The pancreas appears at 5 wk of embryonic life as two outpouchings of the duodenum, ventral and dorsal. By 7 wk these pouches have rotated and fused to take up their established positions to the left of the duodenum, with the ventral derivative forming the posterior and lower portion of the pancreatic head drained by the duct of Wirsung and the dorsal derivative the body and the tail of the pancreas drained by the duct of Santorini. A variety of patterns arise from fusion of the two duct systems. The duct of Wirsung usually maintains its connection with the bile duct during rotation and opens into the papilla of Vater as the major excretory duct of the pancreas. The duct of Santorini usually fuses with and enters the major pancreatic duct, but in 10% of people it drains into the duodenum independently. The main pancreatic duct and the bile duct may also enter separately.

Exocrine and endocrine cells develop at the tips of the bifurcating duct systems, gradually filling the mesenchymal space between them. The exocrine cells form acinar glands, each drained by a small ductule connected through larger channels with the major duct system. Endocrine cells form nests in the interstices between acini. Zymogen granules containing pancreatic enzymes are present in exocrine cells at the 4th mo of gestation.

Function. Acinar cells secrete enzymes that degrade the macromolecular constituents of food to simpler compounds suitable for digestion and absorption by the intestine. α-Amylase splits the extended oligosaccharide chains of starch and other polysaccharides by cleaving α-1,4 glucosidic bonds and forming maltose, isomaltose, and small molecular weight dextrins with α-1,6 branch points. Proteolytic endopeptidases, trypsin, chymotrypsin, and elastase attack peptide bonds within proteins, producing smaller peptides that are ultimately degraded by aminopeptidases of the intestinal surface. The exopeptidases, carboxypeptidases A and B, cleave terminal amino acids from some of these peptides. Each of the proteolytic enzymes is secreted as an inactive proenzyme blocked in its function by a terminal peptide segment. Activation depends on the collision of the trypsin proenzyme, trypsinogen, with the intestinal brush border endopeptidase, enterokinase, which releases the blocking segment and permits trypsin to activate the proenzymes of the remaining proteases. In this way proteolytic activity is reserved for nutrients in the intestinal lumen and is absent within the pancreas and its ducts, where autodigestion of pancreatic tissue might occur. A phospholipase which might also digest pancreatic tissue is secreted similarly as an inactive precursor and activated by trypsin. Pancreatic lipase, which hydrolyzes long-chain triglycerides to monoglycerides and fatty acids, requires a cofactor, colipase, for its activity in the presence of physiologic concentrations of bile salts. The cofactor is secreted as a proenzyme and activated by trypsin; fat digestion, therefore, also depends to some extent on enterokinase.

The exocrine pancreas also secretes fluid and electrolytes. The daily volume is approximately 1500 mL in adults. Sodium and potassium concentrations are similar to those of plasma. Bicarbonate originates in the cells lining the smaller pancreatic ducts and rises to several times its concentration in plasma as pancreatic flow increases.

Secretion is under both hormonal and neurogenic control. Two hormones are elaborated by the epithelium of the upper intestine: cholecystokinin-pancreozymin, which primarily stimulates enzyme secretion; and secretin, which stimulates fluid and bicarbonate secretion. Cholecystokinin-pancreozymin also stimulates the release of enterokinase from the brush border of the intestinal epithelium into the lumen, enhancing the opportunity for contact of this activating enzyme with trypsinogen. Hormone secretion responds to food products and acid in the duodenum and is therefore closely regulated by requirements for the digestion of nutrients. Pancreatic secretion is also mediated by visceral efferent fibers of the vagus, which mimic cholecystokinin-pancreozymin in their effects.

The pancreatic response to cholecystokinin-pancreozymin is quite poor at birth or at 1 mo of age but is normal by the age of 2 yr. Pancreatic enzyme output is also less complete at birth than later. Amylase and lipase outputs are negligible as compared with adult values. In contrast, protease secretion is only moderately reduced. Studies indicate that a normal adult pattern of secretion is acquired by the age of 2 yr. Although it might be expected that infants would exhibit significant evidence of malabsorption, most appear to be capable of handling the starch and fat in their diet quite adequately.

Pancreatic function can be assessed by measuring the secretion of enzymes, fluid, and bicarbonate in response to administered hormones (exogenous response) or in response to food, fat, or amino acid in the intestine (endogenous response). For this purpose pancreatic juice must be obtained from a tube placed in the duodenum under fluoroscopic control. Exogenous and endogenous responses are not always equivalent, particularly when the intestinal mucosa is damaged and the cells are incapable of producing endogenous cholecystokinin-pancreozymin and secretin. A quantitative assessment of pancreatic secretory capacity can be achieved by perfusing the duodenum with fluid containing a nonabsorbable marker substance while stimulating secretory activity with an intravenous infusion of hormone. A second tube must be placed in the stomach to siphon off gastric contents to prevent their mixing with pancreatic secretions.

The digestive reserve of the pancreas is enormous. For example, approximately 98% of the organ's functional capacity must be lost before maldigestion of fat causes steatorrhea. Patients with such impairment have low plasma PABA levels and reduced urinary excretion of PABA in response to an oral test dose of N-benzoyl-L-tyrosyl-PABA, a compound that can be degraded only by chymotrypsin. They also have low serum trypsinogen levels. Their stools will usually, on microscopy, exhibit unhydrolyzed neutral fat droplets and excessive amounts of undegraded muscle fiber.

Enterokinase deficiency, a rare but important cause of infantile malnutrition and diarrhea, can be detected by examining duodenal juice for its ability to activate trypsinogen.

Gaskin KJ, Durie PR, Lee L, et al: Colipase and lipase secretion in childhood-onset pancreatic insufficiency. Gastroenterology 86:1, 1984.
Hadorn B: The exocrine pancreas. In: Anderson CM, Burke V (eds): Paediatric Gastroenterology. London, Blackwell Scientific Publications, 1975.
Go V, Hofmann A, Summerskill WH: Pancreozymin bioassay in man based on pancreatic enzyme secretion: Potency of specific amino acids and other digestive products. J Clin Invest 49:1558, 1970.
Lebenthal E, Lee PC: Development of functional response in human exocrine pancreas. Pediatrics 66:556, 1980.

12.67 ANOMALIES OF THE PANCREAS

Annular Pancreas. This rare anomaly occurs when a portion of the embryonic ventral pancreas remains behind as the rest of the organ rotates posteriorly during the 6th embryonic wk and the fusion of a complete pancreatic ring occurs around the duodenum.

The clinical manifestations depend on the degree of obstruction of the duodenum. Maternal polyhydramnios, complete or partial duodenal obstruction in the newborn period, symptoms of obstruction arising later in childhood and adult life, or no symptoms may be seen. Occasionally, obstruction of a bile duct causes episodes of biliary colic or pancreatitis. Roentgenograms show obstruction in the second part of the duodenum. Treatment is surgical bypass of the obstruction; the pancreas must not be dissected or divided.

Annular pancreas is often associated with other anomalies, including Down syndrome, intestinal atresia, malrotation, and imperforate anus. Manifestations of annular pancreas in adulthood frequently include peptic ulceration, pancreatitis, and jaundice.

Congenital cysts of the pancreas are usually multiple. They are asymptomatic and are frequently associated with polycystic involvement of other organs.

Ectopic pancreatic tissue (*pancreatic rests*) can occur in the stomach or small intestine. Usually asymptomatic, these lesions can cause hemorrhage, ulceration, and obstruction or even, in rare instances, can serve as a lead point for an intussusception.

PANCREATIC INSUFFICIENCY— CYSTIC FIBROSIS

See Sec. 13.97.

12.68 PANCREATIC INSUFFICIENCY NOT DUE TO CYSTIC FIBROSIS

Pancreatic Insufficiency with Neutropenia, Short Stature, and Bone Abnormalities (Shwachman Syndrome). This entity is 100 times less common than cystic fibrosis, but it is still the second most common pancreatic cause of malabsorption in children. The etiology is unknown. There is an associated defect in the chemotaxis of neutrophils. An autosomal recessive inheritance pattern best fits the instances in which more than one sibling in a family has been affected, but sporadic cases appear to be frequent.

Pancreatic acini are usually replaced by fat without fibrosis and with little damage to ducts or islets. Glandular loss must be variable, since some patients are able to digest and absorb fat quite effectively, particularly as they grow older. After stimulation with cholecystokinin and secretin, pancreatic enzyme output is invariably low, but in contrast to cystic fibrosis, water and bicarbonate secretion are well preserved. Neutropenia may be severe or mild, constant, episodic, or cyclic. Thrombocytopenia and hypoplastic anemia are common but rarely of concern. In the bone marrow maturation arrest in the granulocyte line and a reduction in committed granulocyte stem cells may occur but are not constant. In about 50% of patients bone roentgenograms reveal metaphyseal dyschondroplasia; the femoral head is often affected initially, but any metaphysis may be involved. Abnormally short ribs with flared anterior ends are a striking feature in some patients. In a few patients the thoracic cage is sufficiently narrow at birth to interfere with respiration. Linear growth rates are normal in the absence of severe malnutrition, but 80% of patients are shorter than the 3rd percentile for height. Bone age is appropriate for height. Mental activity is frequently subnormal, but few patients are severely retarded.

The diagnosis is usually made in infancy, when patients suffer most severely from recurrent infections and malabsorption. A normal sweat chloride level distinguishes these patients from those with cystic fibrosis. Other causes of malabsorption are usually excluded easily by the findings of pancreatic insufficiency and neutropenia. Occasionally, patients with severe malnutrition develop secondary pancreatic insufficiency and may have relatively low leukocyte counts. In such patients Shwachman syndrome can be excluded only by demonstrating a return of pancreatic function as malnutrition improves. Leukocyte mobility is impaired in both malnutrition and Shwachman syndrome.

There is no specific treatment. Pancreatic supplements are needed in infancy but may not be required later. Most patients survive infancy, and their subsequent course is often surprisingly mild.

Pancreatic agenesis has not been well documented pathologically. The term is used clinically to designate non-neutropenic pancreatic insufficiency in the newborn infant, associated with diabetes mellitus requiring insulin. Glucagon and pancreatic polypeptide are absent in plasma. Pancreatic agenesis is much less common than Shwachman syndrome.

Rare Syndromes Associated with Pancreatic Insufficiency. Pancreatic insufficiency occurs in patients with the Johanson-Blizzard syndrome (congenital aplasia of the alae nasi, deafness, dwarfism, absent permanent teeth, and malabsorption). Pancreatic dysfunction with extensive interstitial fibrosis occurs as part of a syndrome of sideroblastic anemia and vacuolization of marrow precursors.

Specific Pancreatic Enzyme Deficiencies. Rare cases are reported in which specific pancreatic enzymes appear to be congenitally deficient, but their documentation is incomplete. The children reported as having lipase deficiency may actually have had pancreatic hypoplasia (Shwachman syndrome). Reported cases of trypsinogen deficiency may be examples of enterokinase deficiency.

Secondary pancreatic insufficiency occurs in malnourished infants (as noted above) and in patients with severe enteropathies. In malnutrition the packaging of pancreatic enzymes may be compromised by the inability to support sustained protein synthesis, or secretory failure may result from decreased elaboration of stimulatory hormones. Enteropathies produce pancreatic insufficiency by destroying the cells which produce secretin and cholecystokinin-pancreozymin. In celiac disease, for example, patients are fully capable of producing a pancreatic response to exogenous hormone but unable to respond to the presence of acid or digestive products in the duodenum. An inadequate response to endogenous stimuli has been found in two males with idiopathic hypoparathyroidism, hypocalcemia, and steatorrhea.

Congenital Enterokinase Deficiency. See Sec. 12.48.

Anomalies

Montgomery RC, Poindexter MH, Hall GH, et al: Report of a case of annular pancreas of the newborn in two consecutive siblings. Pediatrics 48:148, 1971.
Ravitch MM: The pancreas in infants and children. Surg Clin North Am 55:377, 1975.

Pancreatic Insufficiency Not Due to Cystic Fibrosis

Aggett PJ, Cavanagh NPC, Matthew DJ, et al: Shwachman's syndrome. Arch Dis Child 55:331, 1980.
Heubi JE, Partin JC, Schubert WK: Hypocalcemia and steatorrhea—clues to etiology. Dig Dis Sci 28:124, 1983.
Hill RE, Durie PR, Gaskin KJ, et al: Steatorrhea and pancreatic insufficiency in Shwachman syndrome. Gastroenterology 83:22, 1982.
Howard CP, Go VL, Infante AJ, et al: Long-term survival in a case of functional pancreatic agenesis. J Pediatr 97:786, 1980.
Pearson HA, Lobel JS, Kocoshis SA, et al: A new syndrome of refractory sideroblastic anemia with vacuolization of marrow precursors and exocrine pancreatic dysfunction. J Pediatr 95:976, 1979.
Schussheim A, Choi SJ: Exocrine pancreatic insufficiency with congenital anomalies. J Pediatr 89:782, 1976.
Shwachman H, Diamond LK, Oski FA, et al: The syndrome of pancreatic insufficiency and bone marrow dysfunction. J Pediatr 65:645, 1964.

12.69 PANCREATITIS

Etiology. The pancreas is particularly susceptible to inflammation because its glands contain an arsenal of potentially destructive proenzymes which, when activated, rapidly digest pancreatic tissue. Activating enzymes are found in leukocytes, serum, and bacteria; any condition, therefore, that produces a local inflammatory response or causes retrograde infection of the pancreatic ducts may initiate a cascade of autodigestion. Table 12–11 lists causes of pancreatitis in children. Most cases occur after the age of 10 yr and are acute illnesses attributable to drugs, toxins, trauma, or viral illnesses. In about one case in five, no cause is apparent. The typical traumatic injury is a fall onto the handlebars of a bicycle, but any blunt trauma or abdominal operation will suffice. The incident may be trivial and the onset of pancreatitis somewhat delayed, so that the association with trauma can be easily missed without a careful history. Mumps is the most common cause of viral pancreatitis. Symptoms are usually associated with other signs of mumps and are rather mild. Although elevated amylase activity is found in approximately 50% of cases of Reye syndrome, often for a surprisingly prolonged period, pancreatitis is rarely a dominant feature.

Recurrent attacks of pancreatitis are relatively uncommon but create major diagnostic and therapeutic difficulties. Cholelithiasis and developmental anomalies of the biliary-pancreatic duct system are frequently found. Recurrent or chronic relapsing pancreatitis is a feature of hereditary pancreatitis, a rare autosomal dominant condition, reported chiefly in Caucasians from the United States. Both acute and recurrent pancreatitis may occur in patients with cystic fibrosis who have sufficient pancreatic tissue to support normal absorption.

Clinical Manifestations. The dominant symptom is abdominal pain, epigastric, steady, and possibly radiating to the back. Usually nausea and vomiting occur. The child lies on his or her side and is very still. The abdomen is full, tender, and quiet, and in some cases a mass is palpable. If the lesion is hemorrhagic, blue discoloration about the umbilicus may

Table 12–11. Etiology of Pancreatitis in Childhood

Idiopathic
Drugs and toxins
 Thiazides
 Furosemide
 Prednisone
 Alcohol
 Azathioprine
 Valproic acid
Trauma
Viral illnesses
 Mumps
 Hepatitis A and B
 Rubella
 Coxsackie B
 Influenza A
Reye syndrome
Disease and anomalies of the bile and pancreatic ducts
 Cholelithiasis
 Ascaris lumbricoides
 Choledochal cyst
 Duplication cysts
 Anomalous insertion of the common bile duct
 Nonfusion of dorsal and ventral pancreas
 Annular pancreas
Cystic fibrosis with normal fat absorption
Systemic illnesses
 Lupus erythematosus
 Periarteritis nodosa
 Hyperlipidemia, types I, IV, and V
 Hypercalcemia (hyperparathyroidism, etc.)
Hereditary pancreatitis

be seen. In severe cases pleural effusion and ascites may be found. Loss of large amounts of plasma into the pancreas and surrounding tissue may cause shock. High fever is an ominous sign associated with extensive pancreatic necrosis or abscess formation. In most instances symptoms improve gradually over 3–10 days. Prolonged abdominal discomfort or repeated attacks of pain over several wk may be associated with development of a pancreatic pseudocyst, which sometimes becomes palpable. Rarely, the finding of an unexplained abdominal mass is the initial sign of pancreatitis.

Laboratory Manifestations. The serum amylase activity is usually elevated within 12 hr of the onset but may return to normal within 24 hr. If ascitic or pleural fluid is obtained, it too will have high amylase activity. The ratio of the urinary clearance of amylase to that of creatinine is elevated, usually above 4.0, and is helpful in excluding nonpancreatic causes of hyperamylasemia such as mumps parotitis or macroamylasemia. There may be transient hyperglycemia and glycosuria. A low serum calcium level is a late and serious finding but rare in children. Plain roentgenograms of the abdomen may show dilated segments of small intestine in the vicinity of the pancreas (the sentinel loop), or generalized ileus. Calcification of the pancreas is rare in children except in hereditary pancreatitis. Roentgenograms of the stomach and duodenum may delineate large retroperitoneal pseudocysts which distort the duodenal loop or press forward against the stomach and into the lesser sac. Pancreatic ultrasonography is particularly helpful in detecting pseudocysts. It is also a sensitive technique for confirming the diagnosis of pancreatitis since the pancreatic density is low while the organ is inflamed and returns to normal with improvement. Endoscopic retrograde cholangiopancreatography (ERCP) may demonstrate obstructing stones, ductal narrowing or tortuosity, and unusual anatomic alignments. It is, therefore, an essential part of the investigation of patients with recurrent attacks of pancreatitis. Steatorrhea is an extremely rare consequence of chronic recurrent pancreatitis in children but may be seen after corrective surgery or in some cases of hereditary pancreatitis.

Treatment. The main goals of therapy are to put the pancreas at rest and to support the patient. The vigor with which these efforts are made should depend on the seriousness of the illness, but it is best to err on the safe side. Oral feedings should be stopped, constant nasogastric suction begun, and intravenous fluids and electrolytes given. In some patients total parenteral nutrition may be needed; in others blood or albumin is necessary to combat shock. Meperidine should be given for severe pain. The efficacy of anticholinergic agents and antibiotics is less certain, but they continue to be used in most centers. Oral feedings can be started very slowly once symptoms have subsided but should be discontinued if pain recurs. A pseudocyst can be treated conservatively with prolonged parenteral nutrition in its early acute stage in the hope that it will spontaneously resorb. Cysts which continue to enlarge or persist for 6 wk will usually require surgical drainage. When ductal abnormalities have been outlined by ERCP, patients often benefit from surgical techniques aimed at improving pancreatic drainage.

12.70 THE PANCREAS IN SYSTEMIC DISEASE

Acute and chronic changes in the pancreas are often associated with systemic diseases without producing clinical symptoms that lead to recognition of pancreatic involvement. Infiltration of the pancreas by leukemia, Hodgkin disease, and other lymphogranulomatous conditions is common. Severe congenital syphilis involving the pancreas causes widespread fibrosis. Fibrotic changes with extensive atrophy of acinar tissue result from chronic passive congestion of the pancreas in patients with longstanding cardiac decompensation. Miliary abscesses are associated with septicemia and tubercles with miliary tuberculosis. Neoplasms of the pancreas are rare in childhood.

GORDON FORSTNER

Pancreatitis

Craighead JE: The role of viruses in the pathogenesis of pancreatic disease and diabetes mellitus. Prog Med Virol 19:161, 1975.
Hendren WH, Greep JM, Patton AS: Pancreatitis in childhood: Experience with 15 cases. Arch Dis Child 40:132, 1965.
Jordan SC, Ament ME: Pancreatitis in children and adolescents. J Pediatr 91:211, 1977.
Kattwinkel J, Lapey L, di Sant'Agnese PA, et al: Hereditary pancreatitis: Three new kindreds and a critical review of the literature. Pediatrics 51:55, 1973.
Mallory A, Kern F: Drug-induced pancreatitis: A critical review. Gastroenterology 78:813, 1980.

Pseudocysts of the Pancreas

Bradley EL, Gonzalez AC, Clements JL: Acute pancreatic pseudocysts: Incidence and implications. Ann Surg 184:734, 1976.
Pena SDJ, Medovy H: Child abuse and traumatic pseudocyst of the pancreas. J Pediatr 83:1026, 1973.

LIVER AND BILIARY SYSTEM

12.71 DEVELOPMENT OF HEPATIC AND BILIARY STRUCTURE AND FUNCTION

Morphogenesis. The liver and biliary system originate from a cluster of cells that cap a ventral diverticulum in the primitive foregut. The hepatic anlage (pars hepatis) appears during the 4th wk of gestation as a duodenal diverticulum (Fig. 12–21). Within the ventral mesentery proliferation of cells forms anastomosing hepatic cords, with the network of primitive liver cells, sinusoids, and septal mesencyhme establishing the basic architectural pattern of liver lobule. The solid *cranial* portion of the hepatic diverticulum eventually forms hepatic glandular tissue and the intrahepatic bile ducts; the *caudal* portion (pars cystica) becomes the gallbladder, cystic duct, and common bile duct.

The hepatic lobules are identifiable at the 6th gestational wk. The liver reaches a peak relative size at the 9th wk, at

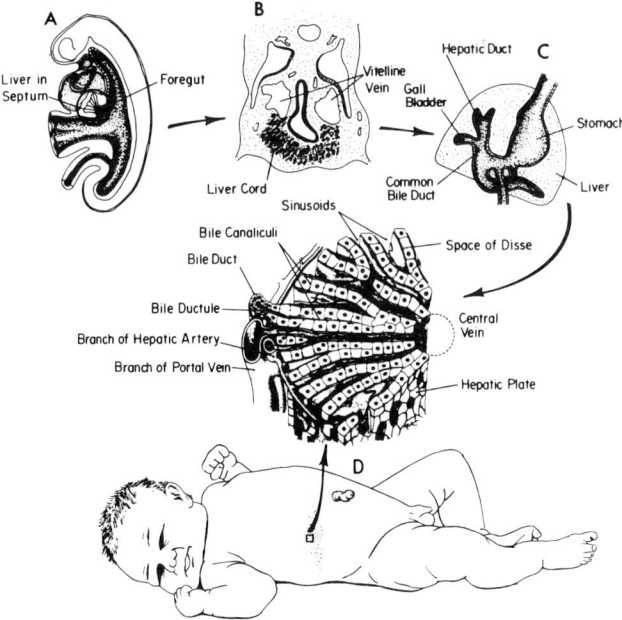

Figure 12–21. Hepatic embryogenesis. *A*, Ventral outgrowth of hepatic diverticulum from foregut endoderm in the 3.5 wk embryo. *B*, Between the two vitelline veins, the enlarging hepatic diverticulum buds off epithelial (liver) cords that become the liver parenchyma, around which the endothelium of capillaries (sinusoids) align (4 wk embryo). *C*, Hemisection of embryo at 7.5 wk demonstrating recanalization of the hepatic biliary tract. *D*, Three-dimensional representation of the hepatic lobule as present in the newborn. (Reproduced with permission from Andres JM, et al: J Pediatrics 90:686, 964, 1977.)

about 10% of the fetal weight. The bile canalicular structures, which include microvilli and junctional complexes are specialized loci of the liver cell membrane; these appear very early in gestation, and by 6–7 wk large canaliculi bounded by several hepatocytes are seen. The intrahepatic bile ducts are derived through branching of the hepatic duct; formation is complete by the 3rd mo. The cystic duct and the gallbladder are fully recanalized by the 7th–8th wk.

In the hepatic excretory (biliary) system, intercellular bile canaliculi empty into the smallest bile ductules, which unite to form interlobular bile ducts that follow the terminal branches of the portal vein. At the hilum of the liver the intrahepatic ducts leave the branches of the portal vein and merge to form the *extrahepatic* biliary system. The ducts of right and left lobes form the common hepatic duct. The common bile duct is formed from the merger of the common hepatic duct and cystic duct; it runs along the right edge of the lesser omentum, terminating as the intramural papilla of Vater. Union of the biliary tract with the pancreatic ducts forms the ampulla of Vater, which, with the sphincter of Oddi, regulates the flow of bile into the intestine, prevents entry of bile into the pancreatic duct, and inhibits reflux of intestinal contents into the ducts.

The transport and metabolic activities of the liver are facilitated by the structural arrangement of liver cell cords (Fig. 12–21*D*), which are formed by rows of hepatocytes, separated by sinusoids that converge toward the tributaries of the hepatic vein (the central vein) located in the center of the lobule. This establishes the pathways and patterns of flow for substances to and from the liver. Plasma proteins and other plasma components *secreted* by the liver arrive through the portal vein and the hepatic artery and pass through the sinusoids and past the hepatocytes to the systemic circulation at the central vein. Biliary components are transported via the series of enlarging channels from the bile canaliculi through the bile ductule to the common bile duct.

Bile secretion has been noted at the 12th gestational wk. The major components of bile vary with stage of development. Near term, cholesterol and phospholipid content is relatively low; and low concentrations of bile acids, the absence of bacterially derived (secondary) bile acids, and the presence of unusual bile acids reflect low rates of bile flow and immature bile acid synthesis.

Fetal hepatic blood flow is derived from the hepatic artery and from the portal and umbilical veins, which form the portal sinus. The portal venous inflow goes mainly to the right lobe of the liver; umbilical flow, primarily to the left. The ductus venosus shunts blood from the portal and umbilical veins to the hepatic vein, bypassing the sinusoidal network. The ductus venosus becomes obliterated when oral feedings are initiated. The oxygen saturation is lower in portal than in umbilical venous blood; accordingly, the right hepatic lobe has lower oxygenation and greater hematopoietic activity than the left. Sinusoidal endothelium is the site of large macrophages, which become the Kupffer (reticuloendothelial) cell network.

The liver constitutes 5% of body weight at birth, only 2% in the adult. Early in gestation (7th wk), hematopoietic cells outnumber functioning hepatocytes in the hepatic anlage. The hepatocytes are smaller (approximately 20 μm) than at maturity (30–35 μm) and contain less glycogen. Near term, the hepatocytes will dominate the organ, and cell size and glycogen content will increase. Hematopoiesis is virtually absent by the second postnatal month in full-term infants. As the density of hepatocytes increases with gestational age, the relative volume of the sinusoidal network decreases.

Ultrastructure. Our understanding of the anatomy of the hepatocyte (Fig. 12–22) has been made possible through electron microscopy and cell fractionation techniques. Various regions of the hepatocyte **plasma membrane** exhibit specialized functions. For example, bidirectional transport occurs at the sinusoidal surface, where materials reaching the liver via the portal system enter and compounds secreted by the liver leave the hepatocyte. Canalicular membranes of adjacent hepatocytes form bile canaliculi, which are bounded by tight junctions preventing transfer of secreted compounds back into the sinusoid. Abundant **mitochondria** are the sites of oxidation and metabolism of heterogenous classes of substrates, of fatty acid oxidation, of key processes in gluconeogenesis, and of storage and release of energy. The **nucleus** and **nucleolus** are surrounded by a pair of membranes, the outermost of which adjoins the **endoplasmic reticulum.** The latter is a continuous network of rough- and smooth-surfaced

tubules and cisternae, which are the site of various processes, including protein and triglyceride synthesis and drug metabolism. The endoplasmic reticulum is the major part of the **microsomal** fraction obtained by ultracentrifugation of liver homogenate. Low fetal activity of microsomal-bound enzymes accounts for a relative inefficiency of xenobiotic metabolism. The **Golgi apparatus** is active in protein packaging and possibly in bile secretion. Hepatocyte microbodies (**peroxisomes**) are single-membrane–limited cytoplasmic organelles that contain enzymes such as oxidases and catalase and that may play a role also in lipid and bile acid metabolism. The **cytoskeleton,** composed of actin filaments, is distributed throughout the cell and concentrated near the plasma membrane. Microfilaments and microtubules may play a role in receptor endocytosis, in bile secretion, and in maintaining the architecture and motility of the cell. **Lysosomes** contain numerous hydrolases and play a role in intracellular digestion.

In Reye syndrome, there are specific alterations in **mitochondria;** in Zellweger (cerebrohepatorenal) syndrome **peroxisomes** are absent; and in glycogenosis type II, a **lysosomal** hydrolase is absent.

Functional Development. Functions of the liver (hepatocytes) are summarized in Table 12–12. Several of these metabolic processes are immature in the healthy newborn infant, owing in part to the fetal patterns of activity of various enzymatic processes. Many hepatic functions are provided for the fetus by the maternal liver, which provides nutrients, serves as a route of elimination of metabolic end products, and is a site of biotransformations. Fetal liver metabolism is devoted primarily to the production of proteins for growth requirements. Toward term, primary functions become production and storage of essential nutrients, excretion of bile,

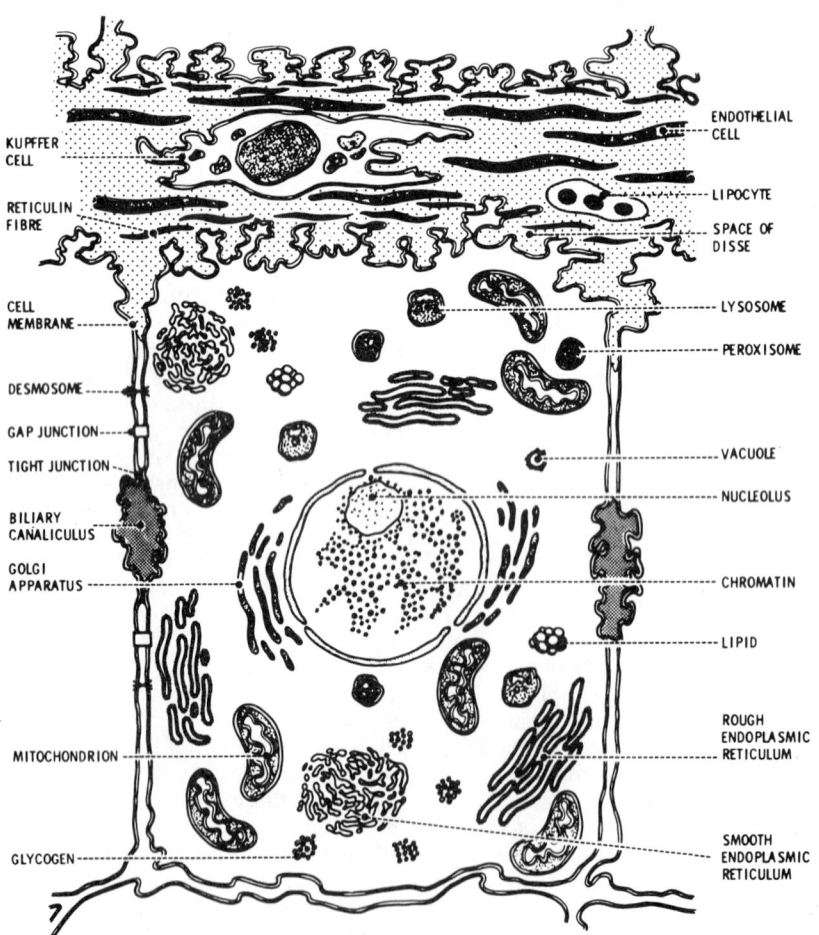

Figure 12–22. Hepatic ultrastructure, conceptualized. Electron microscopic appearance of a normal human liver cell. (Reproduced with permission from Sherlock S, *In* Diseases of the Liver and Biliary System, Chapter 1. Oxford, Blackwell Scientific, 1981.)

Table 12–12. **Functions of the Liver**

1. Nutrition—receives, processes, and stores nutrients absorbed from the digestive tract (amino acids, fatty acids, carbohydrates, cholesterol, and vitamins); releases metabolites on demand
2. Synthetic Function—produces plasma proteins (albumin, clotting factors, transport proteins); synthesizes binding proteins that modulate the circulating concentrations of calcium, magnesium, and drugs
3. Immunologic Function—involved in transport of immunoglobulins; antigens are cleared by Kupffer cells
4. Hematologic Function—synthesis and release of coagulation factors; clears activated coagulation factors
5. Detoxification—main site of metabolic conversion of endogenous and exogenous compounds
6. Excretory Function/Bile Acid Metabolism—synthesizes bile acids from cholesterol, secretes bile acids into the intestine, thereby regulating bile flow and allowing for efficient emulsification and absorption of dietary fat
7. Endocrine Function—serves as a major site of catabolism of thyroid and steroid hormones; insulin metabolism

and establishment of processes of elimination. Extrauterine adaptation involves de novo enzyme synthesis. Modulation of these processes depends on substrate and hormonal input via the placenta, and on dietary and hormonal input in the postnatal period.

METABOLIC FUNCTIONS OF THE LIVER

Carbohydrate Metabolism. The liver stores carbohydrate as glycogen, a polymer of glucose readily hydrolyzed to glucose. The newborn infant is entirely dependent on hepatic glycogen for glucose. Fetal glycogen synthesis begins at about the 9th wk of gestation, with glycogen stores most rapidly accumulated near term, when the liver will contain two to three times the amount of glycogen of adult liver. The majority of this stored glycogen is utilized in the immediate postnatal period. Reaccumulation will be initiated at about the 2nd wk of postnatal life, and glycogen stores will reach adult levels at approximately the 3rd wk in healthy full-term infants. The fluctuations in serum glucose concentration in preterm infants are due in part to the fact that efficient regulation of the synthesis, storage, and degradation of glycogen develops only near the end of full-term gestation. Dietary carbohydrates such as galactose are converted to glucose, but there is a substantial dependence on gluconeogenesis for glucose in early life, especially if glycogen stores are limited. Gluconeogenic activity is not present in the fetal liver.

Protein Metabolism. During the rapid fetal growth phase, specific decarboxylases that are rate-limiting in the biosynthesis of physiologically important polyamines have higher activities than in the mature liver. The rate of synthesis of albumin and secretory proteins in the developing liver parallels the quantitative changes in endoplasmic reticulum. Synthesis of albumin appears at approximately the 7th–8th wk in the human fetus and increases in inverse proportion to that of alpha-fetoprotein. By the 3rd–4th mo of gestation, the fetal liver is able to produce fibrinogen, transferrin, and low density lipoproteins. From this period on, fetal plasma will contain each of the major protein classes, at concentrations considerably below those achieved at maturity.

The **postnatal** patterns of development of various proteins are heterogeneous. Lipoproteins of each class rise abruptly in the 1st wk after birth, to reach levels which will vary little until puberty. Albumin concentrations are low in the neonate (approximately 2.5 g/dL), reaching adult levels (approximately 3.5 g/dL) after several months. Levels of ceruloplasmin and complement factors increase slowly to adult values during the first year. In contrast, transferrin levels at birth are similar to those of the adult, decline for 3–5 mo, and rise thereafter to

achieve their final concentrations. Low levels of activity of synthesis of specific proteins have implications for the nutrition of the infant: for example, a low level of cystathionase activity impairs the trans-sulfuration pathway by which dietary methionine is converted to cystine; accordingly, the latter must be supplied exogenously. Similar dietary requirements may exist for other sulfur-containing amino acids, such as taurine.

Lipid Metabolism. Fatty acid oxidation provides a major source of energy in early life and complements glycogenolysis and gluconeogenesis. The newborn infant is relatively intolerant of prolonged fasting, owing in part to a restricted capacity for hepatic ketogenesis. Rapid maturation of the ability of the liver to oxidize fatty acid occurs during the first few days of life. Milk provides the major source of calories in early life; this high fat, low carbohydrate diet calls on active gluconeogenesis to maintain blood sugar levels. When the glucose supply is limited, ketone body production from endogenous fatty acids may provide energy for hepatic gluconeogenesis and an alternative fuel for brain metabolism. Metabolic processes involving lipid and lipoprotein are predominantly hepatic; liver immaturity or disease affects lipid concentrations and lipoproteins.

Biotransformation. The newborn infant has a decreased capacity to metabolize and detoxify certain drugs, owing to underdevelopment of the microsomal component that is the site of the specific oxidative, reductive, hydrolytic, and conjugation reactions required for these biotransformations. The major components of the mono-oxygenase system, such as cytochrome P-450, NADPH, and cytochrome C–reductase, are present in low concentrations in fetal microsomal preparations. In the full-term infant, UDP-glucuronyl transferase and enzymes involved in the oxidation of polycyclic aromatic hydocarbons have very low activities. Age-related differences in pharmacokinetics vary. For example, the half-life of acetaminophen in a newborn is similar to that of an adult, whereas theophylline has a half-life of approximately 100 hr in the premature infant and 5–6 hr in the adult. Such physiologic variables taken together with factors such as binding to plasma proteins and renal clearance are important in determining drug dosage and in production of toxicity. Dramatic examples of the susceptibility of the newborn infant to drug toxicity are the responses to chloramphenicol (gray syndrome) or to benzoyl alcohol and its metabolic products, which involve ineffective glucuronide and glycine conjugation, respectively. The low concentrations of vitamin E, superoxide dismutase, and glutathione peroxidase in the fetal and early newborn liver lead to increased susceptibility to deleterious effects of oxygen toxicity through lipid peroxidation.

Conjugation reactions (which convert drugs or metabolites into forms that can be eliminated in bile) also are catalyzed by microsomal enzymes. For example, the newborn infant has decreased activity of UDP-glucuronyl transferase, which converts unconjugated bilirubin to the readily excreted glucuronide conjugate and which is the rate-limiting enzyme in the excretion of bilirubin. There is rapid postnatal development of transferase activity, even in prematurely born infants, irrespective of gestational age; this suggests that birth-related rather than age-related factors are of primary importance in the postnatal development of activity of this enzyme. The cord blood of normal full-term newborn infants contains no conjugated bilirubin. In infants with blood group incompatibility, however, both mono- and diglucuronide conjugates of bilirubin are found; this suggests that transferase activity can be prematurely induced by elevated concentrations of the substrate. Microsomal glucuronyl transferase activity can be stimulated also by the administration of phenobarbital or other inducers of cytochrome P-450.

Among other functional impairments in the newborn infant, transferase deficiency accounts for the transient rise in levels of unconjugated bilirubin after birth. In most newborn infants, the serum concentration of unconjugated bilirubin will reach a peak level between the 2nd–5th days of life, at approximately 6 mg/dL. Higher peak levels (10–12 mg/dL) may occur from the 5th–7th day of life in premature infants. Any superimposed factor, such as hemolysis, may cause a greater rise in serum bilirubin level. The diagnosis of "physiologic jaundice" requires exclusion of other precipitating or contributing factors (Sec. 8.44).

HEPATIC EXCRETORY FUNCTION

Hepatic excretory function and bile flow are closely related to bile acid excretion and recirculation. Inefficiency in the enterohepatic circulation of bile acids in the newborn infant may produce a phase of "physiologic cholestasis."

Bile acids are the major product of degradation of cholesterol. Their incorporation into mixed micelles with cholesterol and phospholipid creates an efficient vehicle for the solubilization and intestinal absorption of lipophilic compounds, such as dietary fats and fat soluble vitamins. The secretion of bile acids is the major determinant of bile flow in the mature animal. Accordingly, the maturity of bile acid metabolic processes affects overall hepatic excretory function, including biliary excretion of endogenous and exogenous compounds.

In humans, two of the bile acids (cholic and chenodeoxycholic acid—the primary bile acids) are synthesized in the liver. Prior to excretion, they are conjugated with glycine and taurine. In response to a meal, contraction of the gallbladder delivers bile acids to the intestine to assist in fat digestion and absorption. After mediating fat digestion, the bile acids themselves are reabsorbed from the terminal ileum through specific active transport processes. They return to the liver via portal blood, are taken up by liver cells, and are re-excreted in bile. In the adult, this enterohepatic circulation involves 90–95% of the circulating bile acid pool. Bile acids that escape ileal reabsorption reach the colon, where the bacterial flora, through dehydroxylation and deconjugation, produces the secondary bile acids, deoxycholate and lithocholate. In the adult the composition of bile reflects the excretion of not only the primary but also the secondary bile acids, which are reabsorbed from the distal intestinal tract.

In the neonate, there is inefficient ileal reabsorption and a low rate of hepatic clearance of bile acids from portal blood. The latter results in elevated serum concentrations of bile acids in healthy newborns, often to levels that would suggest liver disease in older individuals. The size of the bile acid pool in the neonate is about one half that of the adult, and the bile acid concentration in intestinal lumen is similarly decreased to levels in the proximal intestinal lumen that are frequently below the concentration required for micelle formation (2 mM/L); accordingly, absorption of dietary fats and fat soluble vitamins is inefficient. Transient phases of "physiologic cholestasis" and "physiologic steatorrhea" play a role in the nutrition of low birth weight infants but are of minor importance to healthy full-term newborns.

Beyond the neonatal period, disturbances in bile acid metabolism may be responsible for diverse effects on hepatobiliary and intestinal function (Table 12–13).

12.72 MANIFESTATIONS OF LIVER DISEASE

Pathologic Manifestations. Alterations in hepatic structure and function can be **acute** or **chronic,** with varying patterns of reaction of the liver to cell injury. The ultimate reaction is cell death, but the hepatocyte has a remarkable capacity for regeneration. Collagen is formed during the healing phase of

Table 12–13. Potential Sites for Disturbances in Bile Acid Metabolism

I. Defective bile acid **synthesis** may result from:
  A. Congenital impairment of hepatic synthesis
  B. Specific defects in bile acid synthesis as seen in:
    1. Cerebrotendinous xanthomatosis
    2. Intrahepatic cholestasis
      a. Qualitative abnormalities
      b. Quantitative abnormalities
  C. Acquired defects in bile acid synthesis (as observed in liver diseases such as hepatitis and cirrhosis)

II. Abnormalities of bile acid **delivery** to the bowel may be seen in:
  A. Celiac sprue (sluggish gallbladder contraction)
  B. Extrahepatic bile duct obstruction due to:
    1. Biliary atresia
    2. Stricture
    3. Stone
    4. Carcinoma

III. **Interruption** of the enterohepatic circulation of bile acids may occur with:
  A. An external bile fistula
  B. Ileojejunal exclusion for exogenous obesity or hypercholesterolemia
  C. Cystic fibrosis
  D. Contaminated small bowel syndrome (with bile acid precipitation, increased jejunal absorption and "short circuiting")
  E. Entrapment of bile acids in intestinal lumen by:
    1. Cholestyramine
    2. Trivalent cations (aluminum-containing antacids)
    3. Fiber

IV. Bile acid malabsorption
  A. Primary bile acid malabsorption (absent/inefficient ileal active transport)
    1. Intractable diarrhea (infancy)
    2. Irritable bowel (adults)
  B. Secondary bile acid malabsorption
    1. Ileal disease or resection
      a. Crohn disease
      b. Ileal resection
      c. Ileal bypass
      d. Radiation enteritis
      e. Postinfectious enteritis
    2. Exogenous bile acid administration (e.g., gallstone dissolution)
    3. Cystic fibrosis
  C. Tertiary bile acid malabsorption
    1. Postcholecystectomy
    2. Renal failure
    3. Drugs

V. Defective uptake or altered intracellular metabolism
  A. Parenchymal disease (acute hepatitis, cirrhosis)
    1. Regurgitation from cells
    2. Portosystemic shunting
  B. Cholestasis

cellular injury, with excessive growth of fibrous tissue becoming manifest as cirrhosis. The major pathologic responses of the hepatocyte, hepatic vasculature, and supporting tissue are as described subsequently.

Inflammation or **necrosis** of the hepatocytes can be due to viral infection, drugs, or toxins, immunologic disorders, or hypoxia. The evolving process will lead either to repair, to continuing injury with chronic changes, or in rare instances to massive hepatic damage or death.

Cholestasis is an alternative or concomitant response to injury. It is defined as the accumulation in serum of substances normally excreted in bile such as bilirubin, cholesterol, bile acids, and trace elements. A liver biopsy will demonstrate accumulation of bile and bile pigment in the parenchyma. In extrahepatic obstruction, bile pigment may be visible in the intralobular bile ducts or throughout the parenchyma as bile lakes or infarcts. Cholestasis may also be seen without evidence of bile duct obstruction, when hepatocyte injury or an alteration in hepatic physiology has led to a reduction in the rate of secretion of solute and water. Likely causes may include alterations in the ultrastructure or cytoskeleton of the hepatocyte, alterations in organelles responsible for bile secretion, alterations in enzymatic activity, or alterations in permeability of the bile canalicular apparatus. The end result is clinically indistinguishable from obstructive cholestasis.

Cirrhosis (defined by the presence of bands of fibrous tissue that link central and portal areas and form parenchymal nodules) is a potential end stage in any acute or chronic liver disease. Cirrhosis may be posthepatitic or postnecrotic, or may follow chronic biliary obstruction (biliary cirrhosis). Cirrhosis may be **macronodular** with nodules of varying sizes (up to 5 cm) separated by broad septae, or **micronodular**, with nodules of uniform size (less than 1 cm) separated by fine septae. There may also be mixed forms. The progressive scarring of cirrhosis leads to altered blood flow, with further impairment of liver cell function. In addition, the restriction of blood flow within the liver leads to portal hypertension.

Primary tumors of the liver are discussed in Sec. 16.22.

The liver may be **secondarily** involved in neoplastic (metastatic) and non-neoplastic (storage diseases and fat infiltration) and infectious processes. The liver may also be affected by chronic passive congestion of acute hypoxia, with hepatocellular damage.

Clinical Manifestations. *Hepatomegaly.* Enlargement of the liver can be due to several mechanisms (Table 12–14). Concepts of normal liver size have been based on age-related clinical indices, such as (1) the degree of extension of the liver edge below the costal margin, (2) the span of dullness to percussion, or (3) the length of the vertical axis of the liver, as estimated from imaging techniques. In children, the normal liver edge can be felt up to 2 cm below the right costal margin. In the newborn infant extension of the liver edge more than 3.5 cm below the costal margin in the right mid-clavicular line suggests hepatic enlargement. Measurement of *liver span* is carried out by percussing the upper margin of dullness and palpating the lower edge in the right mid-clavicular line; it may be more reliable than extension of liver edge alone, and the two measurements may correlate poorly.

The liver span increases linearly with body weight and age in both sexes. If percussion is used for both the upper and lower borders, the mean liver span is curvilinearly related to age. The span ranges from about 4.5–5.0 cm at 1 wk of age to approximately 7.0–8.0 cm in males and 6.0–6.5 cm in females by age 12 yr. The expected span of liver dullness in the midclavicular line in both sexes after 12 yr of age can be calculated as follows: in males, span (cm) = $0.032 \times$ weight (pounds) + $0.18 \times$ height (inches) − 7.86; in females, span (cm) = $0.027 \times$ weight (pounds) + $0.22 \times$ height (inches) − 10.75. These formulas are not accurate for newborns or younger children. In some persons, the lower edge of the right lobe of the liver extends downward (Riedel lobe) and may be palpable as a broad mass. Downward displacement of the liver by diaphragm or thoracic organs can create an erroneous impression of hepatomegaly.

Examination of the liver should include noting consistency, contour, tenderness, or the presence of any masses or bruits, as well as assessing splenic size.

Ultrasonography can often help in the evaluation of unexplained hepatomegaly; size and consistency can be assessed. Hyperechogenic, bright hepatic parenchyma can be seen with metabolic disease (glycogen storage disease) or fatty liver (owing to malnutrition or hyperalimentation, or following corticosteroid therapy).

Ultrasonography can also assess **gallbladder size.** Gallblad-

Table 12–14. Mechanisms of Hepatomegaly

1. Increase in the **number** or **size** of the cells in the liver
    a. Storage
        1. Fat in: Reye syndrome, malnutrition, obesity, metabolic liver disease, lipid infusion (total parenteral nutrition), cystic fibrosis, diabetes mellitus
        2. Specific lipid storage diseases: Gaucher, Niemann-Pick, Wolman syndromes
        3. Glycogen: glycogen storage diseases (multiple enzyme defects); total parenteral nutrition
        4. Miscellaneous: α_1-antitrypsin deficiency, Wilson disease, hypervitaminosis A, neonatal iron storage
    b. Inflammation
        1. Hepatocyte enlargement (hepatitis)
            viral—acute and chronic
            bacterial (sepsis, abscess, cholangitis)
            toxic
        2. Kupffer cell enlargement
        3. Inflammatory cells
    c. Infiltration
        1. Primary tumors
            hepatoblastoma
            hepatocellular carcinoma
            hemangioma
            focal nodular hyperplasia
        2. Secondary or metastatic tumors
            lymphoma
            leukemia
            histiocytosis
            neuroblastoma
            Wilms tumor
2. Increased size of **vascular** space
    a. Intrahepatic obstruction to hepatic vein outflow
        1. Veno-occlusive disease
        2. Hepatic vein thrombosis (Budd-Chiari syndrome)
        3. Hepatic vein web
    b. Suprahepatic
        1. Congestive heart failure
        2. Pericardial disease
            tamponade
            constrictive pericarditis
3. Increased size of **biliary** space
    Congenital hepatic fibrosis
    Caroli disease
    Extrahepatic obstruction
4. Idiopathic (? "benign")

der distension may be seen in sick infants who have sepsis. Gallbladder length normally varies from 1.5–5.5 cm (average 3.0) in infants to 4.0–8.0 cm in adolescents; width ranges from 0.5–2.5 cm (mean 0.8 in neonates) at all ages.

Jaundice. Yellow discoloration of the plasma, skin, and mucous membranes may be the earliest and only sign of hepatic dysfunction; it therefore requires urgent evaluation. Jaundice becomes clinically apparent in children and adults when the serum concentration of bilirubin reaches 2–3 mg/dL. In neonates, higher levels may be found without evident icterus. Icterus may be associated with dark urine or acholic (light-colored) stools during childhood.

Bilirubin occurs in plasma in four forms: (1) **unconjugated bilirubin** tightly bound to albumin; (2) **free or unbound bilirubin** (presumably the form responsible for kernicterus, since it can cross cell membranes); (3) **conjugated bilirubin** (the only fraction to appear in urine); and (4) **delta fraction** (bilirubin covalently bound to albumin), which appears in serum when hepatic excretion of conjugated bilirubin is impaired in patients with hepatobiliary disease. The delta fraction permits conjugated bilirubin to persist in the circulation and delays resolution of jaundice.

Measurement of serum bilirubin is usually via the van den Bergh (diazo) reaction. The terms "direct-reacting" and "indirect-reacting" bilirubin correspond roughly to **conjugated** and **unconjugated** bilirubin, respectively. Superior methods are available.

Jaundice in an infant or older child may reflect accumulation of either unconjugated or conjugated bilirubin. An increase in unconjugated bilirubin may indicate increased production, hemolysis, reduced hepatic removal, or altered metabolism of bilirubin (Table 12–15). Significant accumulations of conjugated bilirubin (greater than 20% of total) reflect decreased excretion by damaged hepatic parenchymal cells or disease of biliary tract, such as may be due to sepsis, endocrine or metabolic disease, inflammation of the liver, or obstruction. In most patients with diseases that tend to produce conjugated hyperbilirubinemia, a portion of the total bilirubin will be present in **unconjugated** form, with near parallel rises in both fractions.

Pruritus. Intense generalized itching may occur in patients with cholestasis, presumably owing to retained components of bile such as bile salts, as pruritus responds to bile acid-binding agents such as cholestyramine or to choleretic agents such as phenobarbital. Pruritus is unrelated to the degree of hyperbilirubinemia; deeply jaundiced patients may be asymptomatic.

Spider Angiomas. Vascular spiders, characterized by central pulsating arterioles from which small, wiry venules radiate, may be seen in patients with chronic liver disease.

Palmar Erythema. Blotchy erythema, most noticeable over the thenar and hypothenar eminences and on the tips of the fingers, may be due to vasodilatation and increased blood flow.

Xanthomata. The elevation of serum cholesterol associated with chronic cholestasis may cause the deposition of lipid in the dermis and subcutaneous tissue. Brown nodules may develop first over the extensor surfaces of the extremities; rarely, xanthelasma of eyelids develops.

Portal Hypertension. The portal vein drains the splanchnic area (abdominal portion of the gastrointestinal tract, pancreas, and spleen) into the hepatic sinusoids. Pressure is normally slightly higher (approximately 5–10 mm Hg) in the portal vein than in other venous systems in order to overcome the resistance of the sinusoidal system. Portal hypertension is defined as an increase in portal venous pressure to greater than 20 mm Hg; it may be due to (1) extrahepatic obstruction of the portal vein (presinusoidal), (2) intrahepatic disease (parenchymal), or (3) suprahepatic (outflow) obstruction. The most common cause of presinusoidal portal hypertension in children is portal vein thrombosis or cavernous transformation of the portal vein. Parenchymal disease such as hepatitis, infiltration, fatty liver, or cirrhosis can cause intrahepatic portal hypertension. Outflow obstruction may be associated with hepatic vein occlusion (such as veno-occlusive disease following bone marrow transplantation), venous thromboses, membranous obstruction of the inferior vena cava, or cardiac disease (such as heart failure or constrictive pericarditis). Portal hypertension produces an increase in collateral flow around the liver, with development of esophageal and other varices, which become potential sites of bleeding.

Ascites. Ascites may be associated with urinary tract anomalies, metabolic diseases (e.g., lysosomal storage disease), congenital or other heart disease, or hydrops fetalis. In patients with hepatic disease, sinusoidal blockade due to cirrhosis increases hydrostatic pressure and transudation of fluid; this may be abetted by hypoalbuminemia. The formation of ascites is poorly understood. Traditional theories have proposed that ascites occurs in cirrhotic patients when an imbalance of Starling forces in hepatic sinusoids and splenic capillaries leads to excessive formation of lymph; when the amount of lymph exceeds the capacity of the thoracic duct for drainage, lymph accumulates in the peritoneal space as ascites. A secondary contraction of circulating plasma volume is thought to account for the fact that while total plasma volume is increased, there is a reduced "effective" plasma volume owing to the ascites; renal tubular sodium retention is a secondary event. An alternative hypothesis postulates that inappropriate sodium retention by the kidneys is the primary event, with an expansion in plasma volume; this "overflow" of plasma volume becomes sequestered in the peritoneal space as ascites. These theories may not be mutually exclusive.

Encephalopathy. In acute or chronic liver disorders, metabolic abnormalities may produce an encephalopathy, with neuropsychiatric disturbances that may include neuromuscular dysfunction, altered mentation, altered consciousness, or coma. With chronic liver disease, hepatic encephalopathy

Table 12–15. Differential Diagnosis of Unconjugated Hyperbilirubinemia

I. Increased production of unconjugated bilirubin from heme
  A. Hemolytic disease (hereditary or acquired)
    1. Isoimmune hemolysis
      a. Rh-incompatibility
      b. ABO-incompatibility
      c. Other (Lewis, M,S, Kidd, Kell, Duffy)
    2. Congenital spherocytosis
    3. Hereditary elliptocytosis
    4. Erythrocyte enzyme defects:
      a. Glucose-6-phosphate dehydrogenase
      b. Pyruvate kinase
  B. Ineffective erythropoiesis
  C. Drugs
    1. Vitamin K
    2. Maternal oxytocin
    3. Phenol disinfectants
  D. Infection
  E. Enclosed hematoma
  F. Polycythemia
    1. Diabetic mother
    2. Fetal tranfusion (maternal, twin)
    3. Delayed cord clamping

II. Decreased **delivery** of unconjugated bilirubin (in plasma) to hepatocyte
    1. Right-sided congestive heart failure
    2. Portocaval shunt

III. Decreased bilirubin **uptake** across hepatocyte membrane
  A. Presumed enzyme deficiency (e.g., Gilbert)
  B. Competitive inhibition
    1. Breast-milk jaundice
    2. Lucey-Driscoll syndrome
    3. Drug inhibition
  C. Miscellaneous
    1. Hypothyroidism
    2. Hypoxia
    3. Acidosis

IV. Decreased **storage** of unconjugated bilirubin in cytosol (decreased Y and Z proteins)
    1. Competitive inhibition
    2. Fever

V. Decreased biotransformation (conjugation)
    1. Neonatal jaundice (physiologic)
    2. Inhibition (drugs)
    3. Hereditary (Crigler-Najjar)
      a. Type I (complete enzyme deficiency)
      b. Type II (partial deficiency)
    4. Hepatocellular dysfunction

VI. Enterohepatic recirculation
  A. Intestinal obstruction
    1. Ileal atresia
    2. Hirschsprung
    3. Cystic fibrosis
  B. Antibiotic administration
  C. Breast milk jaundice

may be recurrent and precipitated by intercurrent illness, drugs, bleeding, or electrolyte and acid-base disturbances.

Hepatic encephalopathy is characterized by profound neural inhibition, which may be due to an interaction between γ-aminobutyric acid (GABA, the primary inhibitory neurotransmitter) and GABA receptors on postsynaptic neurons. With hepatic failure, GABA produced by bacterial flora is not cleared from the blood but crosses the blood-brain barrier and produces inhibition. There may be a simultaneous decrease in excitatory neurotransmission. Other neuroactive or vasoactive compounds, such as glycine or amines, may be synergistic. Alternatively, roles are given to ammonia, to synergistic neurotoxins, or to "false neurotransmitters" with plasma amino acid imbalance.

Endocrine Abnormalities. Endocrine abnormalities are more common in adults with hepatic disease than in children. They reflect alterations in hepatic synthetic, storage, and metabolic functions, including those concerned with hormonal metabolism in the liver. For example, proteins such as those that bind hormones in plasma are synthesized, and steroid hormones are conjugated in the liver and excreted in the urine; failure of such functions may have clinical consequences. Endocrine abnormalities may also result from malnutrition or specific deficiencies.

Renal Dysfunction. There is a close relationship between liver and renal dysfunctions. Systemic disease or toxins may affect both organs simultaneously; parenchymal liver disease may produce secondary impairment of renal function, and vice versa. In hepatobiliary disorders, there may be renal alterations in sodium and water economy, impaired renal concentrating ability, and alterations in potassium metabolism. Ascites in patients with cirrhosis may be related to inappropriate retention of sodium by the kidney, with expansion of plasma volume, or to sodium retention mediated by diminished effective plasma volume.

Hepatorenal syndrome is defined as renal failure (azotemia and progressive oliguria) in a patient with cirrhosis (often with refractory ascites), in whom there is no other demonstrable cause of renal failure. This complication represents a complex sequence of compensation and decompensation in end-stage liver disease. The pathophysiology is poorly defined but seems to involve altered renal blood flow. Intense vasoconstriction of the renal cortical vessels is mediated by hemodynamic, humoral, or neurogenic mechanisms. The urinary sodium concentration is low and the sediment is normal. In management, a trial of volume expansion is warranted in order to exclude the possibility of prerenal azotemia secondary to volume depletion.

Miscellaneous Manifestations of Liver Dysfunction. Nonspecific signs of acute and chronic liver disease include (1) anorexia, often seen in the patient with anicteric hepatitis; (2) abdominal pain or distention; and (3) bleeding, which may be due to altered synthesis of coagulation factors (biliary obstruction with vitamin K deficiency or excessive hepatic damage) or to portal hypertension. There may be decreased synthesis of specific clotting factors, production of qualitatively abnormal proteins, or alterations in platelet number and function in the presence of hypersplenism. Altered drug metabolism may prolong the biologic half-life of commonly administered medications.

WILLIAM F. BALISTRERI

12.73 EVALUATION OF THE PATIENT WITH POSSIBLE LIVER DYSFUNCTION

Adequate evaluation of infant, child, or adolescent with suspected liver disease involves an appropriate and accurate history, a carefully performed physical examination, and skillful interpretation of signs and symptoms. Further evaluation will be aided by judicious selection of diagnostic tests (biopsy, imaging). Most "liver function tests" do not measure specific hepatic functions (Table 12–16). A rise in serum aminotransferase activity reflects liver cell injury; an increase in immunoglobulin level reflects an immunologic response to injury; or an elevation in serum bilirubin level may reflect any of several disturbances of bilirubin metabolism. The results of any single biochemical assay provide limited information, which must be placed in the context of the entire clinical and historic picture. In the future, more dynamic tests of hepatic function, such as clearance tests, may help define the severity of and monitor changes in liver dysfunction. Until then, the most cost-efficient approach is for the clinician to become familiar with the rationale, implications, and limitations of a selected group of tests, so that specific questions can be answered.

For a patient with suspected liver disease, evaluation addresses the following issues in sequence: (1) Is liver disease present? (2) If so, what is its nature? (3) What is its severity? (4) Is specific treatment available? (5) How can we monitor the response to treatment? and (6) What is the prognosis?

Biochemical Tests. Laboratory tests commonly used to confirm the suspicion of liver disease include measurements of serum bilirubin level and of aminotransferase and alkaline phosphatase activities often with determinations of prothrombin time and albumin level. These tests are complementary, and provide indices of synthetic and excretory functions and may suggest the nature of the disturbance (e.g., inflammation or cholestasis).

Acute liver cell injury (parenchymal disease) in viral hepatitis, drug or toxin-induced liver disease, shock, hypoxemia, or metabolic disease may best be reflected in marked increases in aminotransferase activities. Cholestasis (obstructive disease) involves regurgitation of bile components into serum; accordingly, the serum levels of total and conjugated bilirubin

Table 12–16. Analyses for Assessment of Hepatic Function

1. Substances produced or metabolized by the liver
   A. Substances **synthesized** by the liver
      1. albumin
      2. coagulation factors
      3. urea
   B. Substances **metabolized** by the liver
      1. drugs
      2. xenobiotics (caffeine)
      3. bilirubin
      4. lipids and lipoproteins
2. Substances **released** from damaged tissue
   A. Endogenous compounds (e.g., enzymes) released by damaged **hepatocyte**:
      1. aspartate aminotransferase (AST) (SGOT)
      2. alanine aminotransferase (ALT) (SGPT)
   B. Endogenous compounds **synthesized** at an increased rate and/or **released** by canalicular membrane and **bile duct** epithelium
      1. alkaline phosphatase
      2. γ-glutamyltransferase
      3. 5'-nucleotidase
3. Substances **cleared** by the liver
   A. Endogenous metabolites
      1. bile acids
      2. bilirubin
      3. ammonia
   B. Exogenous compounds
      1. indocyanine green
      2. aminopyrine
      3. galactose
4. Hepatic circulation

will be elevated. Elevations in serum alkaline phosphatase and gamma glutamyltransferase (GGT) activities are sensitive indicators of obstructive processes or of inflammation of the biliary tract.

The **severity** of the liver disease may be reflected in (1) *clinical signs* (occurrence of encephalopathy, apparent shrinkage of liver mass owing to massive necrosis, or onset of ascites) or in (2) *biochemical alterations* (hypoglycemia, electrolyte imbalance, continued hyperbilirubinemia, marked hypoalbuminemia, or prolonged prothrombin times unresponsive to parenteral administration of vitamin K).

Measurement of the conjugated and unconjugated fractions of serum bilirubin will help distinguish between elevations due to hemolysis and those due to hepatic dysfunction. A predominant elevation in the conjugated fraction provides a relatively sensitive index of hepatocellular disease or hepatic excretory dysfunction. Aminotransferase activities are highly sensitive to hepatocellular damage. Alanine aminotransferase (ALT, SGPT) is liver specific, whereas aspartate aminotransferase (AST, SGOT) is derived from other organs in addition to the liver. In most instances there are **parallel rises** in AST and ALT, but sometimes a differential rise or fall can provide useful information. The most marked rises of aminotransferase activities occur with acute hepatocellular injury, such as viral hepatitis, toxic injury, or Reye syndrome. Following blunt abdominal trauma, elevations in activity of these enzymes may provide an early clue to hepatic injury. In chronic liver disease or in intrahepatic and extrahepatic biliary obstruction, rises in aminotransferase activities may be less marked. In acute hepatitis the rise in ALT may be greater than that of AST; whereas in alcohol-induced liver injury, in fulminant echovirus infection, and in various metabolic diseases, predominant rises in AST have been reported.

Hepatic synthetic function is reflected in serum proteins and in prothrombin time. Examination of serum globulin concentration and of the relative amounts of the globulin fractions may be helpful. Gamma globulin levels are often high, and increased titers of smooth muscle antibody as well as antimitochondrial antibodies may be found in patients with chronic active hepatitis. A resurgence in alpha-fetoprotein levels may suggest hepatoma. Hypoalbuminemia due to depressed synthesis may complicate severe liver disease and serve as a prognostic factor. Cholesterol levels may be markedly elevated in patients with cholestasis, whether the cause be intra- or extrahepatic. On the other hand, with acute liver disease, such as hepatitis, serum cholesterol levels may be depressed. Deficiencies of factor V and of the vitamin K dependent factors (II, VII, IX, and X) may occur. When the prothrombin time is prolonged as a result of nutritional input or intestinal malabsorption of vitamin K, parenteral administration of vitamin K should correct it within 12 hr; unresponsiveness to vitamin K would suggest hepatic disease. Persistently low levels of factor VII are evidence of a poor prognosis in fulminant liver disease.

Serum levels of bile acids are sensitive indicators of hepatobiliary disease, especially in monitoring patients at high risk.

Interpretation of biochemical tests of hepatic structure and function must be made in the context of age-related changes. The activity of alkaline phosphatase varies considerably with age, reflecting predominantly the activity of the isoenzyme that originates in bone. Activity of the liver-specific isoenzyme or of 5′nucleotidase can be measured; the latter has a similar biliary origin and is not found in bone. An *isolated* increase in alkaline phosphatase may be benign if other liver function test results are normal. GGT exhibits high enzyme activity in early life that declines rapidly with age. Cholesterol concentrations increase throughout life.

Interpretation of serum ammonia values is uncertain, owing to variability in their physiologic determinants and to inherent difficulty in laboratory measurement. There is a transient elevation of the serum ammonia content in normal neonates; its causes are multifactorial, perhaps involving shunting of blood through the ductus venosus as well as metabolic immaturity.

Liver Biopsy. The morphologic features of specific hepatic diseases are sufficiently distinctive so that liver biopsy combined with clinical data can indicate an etiologic diagnosis in most cases. Tissue obtained by percutaneous liver biopsy can be used: (1) to provide a precise histologic diagnosis (in patients with neonatal cholestasis, chronic active hepatitis, Reye syndrome, intrahepatic biliary hypoplasia, congenital hepatic fibrosis, or portal hypertension); (2) for enzyme analysis to detect inborn errors of metabolism; and (3) for analysis of stored material (such as iron, copper, or specific metabolites). Serial assessments of hepatic status by liver biopsies can monitor responses to therapy or detect complications of treatment with potentially hepatotoxic agents such as aspirin, antimetabolites, or anticonvulsants.

In infants and children, needle biopsy of the liver is easily accomplished through percutaneous approach. The amount of tissue obtained, even in small infants, is usually sufficient for histologic interpretation, and for biochemical analyses (if the latter are deemed necessary). Percutaneous liver biopsy can be safely performed in infants as young as 1 wk of age. The usual percutaneous approach is transcostal and transdiaphragmic. The patient usually requires only sedation and *local* anesthesia. Contraindications include prolonged prothrombin time, thrombocytopenia, suspicion of a vascular, cystic, or infectious lesion in the path of the needle, and severe ascites. If administration of fresh frozen plasma or of platelet transfusions fails to correct a prolonged prothrombin time or thrombocytopenia, open surgical biopsy may be considered. The risk of development of a complication such as hemorrhage, hematoma, creation of an arteriovenous fistula, pneumothorax, or bile peritonitis is very small.

Hepatic Imaging Procedures. (See also Sec. 5.55.) Various techniques help define the size, shape, and architecture of the liver, including the intrahepatic and extrahepatic biliary trees. Such imaging may not provide precise histologic and biochemical diagnoses, but specific questions can be answered, such as whether hepatomegaly is related to accumulation of such material as fat or glycogen or is due to tumor or cyst. Such studies may direct further evaluation such as percutaneous biopsy and will make possible prompt referral of patients with biliary obstruction to the surgeon. Choice of imaging procedure should be part of a carefully formulated diagnostic approach, with avoidance of redundant demonstrations by several techniques.

A *plain roentgenographic study* may suggest hepatomegaly, but physical examination gives a more reliable assessment of liver size. The liver may appear less dense than normal with fatty infiltration, or more dense with deposition of heavy metals such as iron. A hepatic or biliary tract mass may displace an air-filled loop of bowel. Calcifications may be evident in the liver (parasitic and neoplastic disease), in the vasculature (with portal vein thrombosis), or in the gallbladder or biliary tree (gallstones). Collections of gas may be seen within the liver (abscess), biliary tract, or portal circulation (neonatal necrotizing enterocolitis).

Ultrasonography provides information about the size and composition of the liver. Increased echogenicity is observed with fatty infiltration, and mass lesions as small as 1–2 cm may be shown. Ultrasonography is more accurate than cholangiography in detecting stones in the gallbladder or biliary tree. Even in the neonate high frequency real-time ultrasonography can assess gallbladder size, detect dilatation of the biliary tract, or define a choledochal cyst. In infants with biliary atresia, the gallbladder is usually small or absent and the common duct not visualized. In patients with portal hypertension, ultrasonography can evaluate patency of the portal vein or demonstrate collateral circulation. Relatively small amounts of ascitic fluid can be detected.

Computed tomography (CT scan) provides information similar to that obtained by ultrasonography but is less suitable for use in patients under 2 yr of age because of the small size of structures, the paucity of intra-abdominal fat for contrast, and the need for heavy sedation or general anesthesia. The CT scan may be slightly more accurate in detection of focal lesions such as tumors, cysts, and abscesses and when coupled with injection of a contrast medium, may reveal a neoplastic mass density only slightly different from that of normal liver. When a hepatic tumor is suspected, CT is the best method to define anatomic extent, solid or cystic nature, and vascularity. CT can also reveal subtle differences in density of liver parenchyma, the average liver attenuation coefficient being reduced with fatty infiltration. Increases in density may occur with diffuse iron deposition or with glycogen storage. In differentiating obstructive from nonobstructive cholestasis, CT identifies the precise level of obstruction more frequently than ultrasonography. Either CT or ultrasonography may be used to guide fine needle biopsy or the aspiration of specific lesions.

Radionuclide scanning relies on selective uptake of a radiopharmaceutical agent. Commonly used agents include (1) technetium-99m-labeled sulfur colloid, which undergoes phagocytosis by Kupffer cells; (2) Tc-99m-iminodiacetic acid agents (PIPIDA, HIDA, etc.), which are taken up by hepatocytes and excreted into bile; and (3) gallium-67, which is concentrated in inflammatory and neoplastic cells. The anatomic resolution possible with hepatic scintiscans is generally less than that obtained with CT or ultrasonography.

The Tc-99m–sulfur colloid scan may detect focal lesions (such as tumors, cysts, or abscesses) greater than 2–3 cm in diameter. This scan may help evaluate patients with possible cirrhosis in whom hepatic uptake is patchy and in whom there is a shift of colloid uptake from liver to bone marrow.

The Tc-99m–substituted iminodiacetic acid dyes may differentiate intrahepatic cholestasis from extrahepatic obstruction in the neonate, as long as the serum bilirubin concentration is less than 5–6 mg/dL. Imaging results are best when scanning is preceded by a 5–7 day period of treatment with phenobarbital to stimulate bile flow. Following intravenous injection, the isotope is normally detected in the bowel within 1–2 hr. In the presence of cholestasis, excretion of the isotope is delayed; accordingly, serial scans should be made for up to 24 hr following injection. Early in the course of biliary atresia, hepatocyte function is usually good; uptake (clearance) occurs rapidly, but excretion into the intestine is absent. In contrast, uptake is poor in parenchymal liver disease, such as neonatal hepatitis, but excretion into the bile and intestine eventually ensues.

In older infants and children, HIDA or PIPIDA scintigraphy may also help to evaluate the gall bladder and bile ducts. In patients with acute cholecystitis, the gallbladder is not visualized, but the common duct is opacified.

Cholangiography, the direct visualization of the intrahepatic and extrahepatic biliary tree through use of opaque material, may be required in some patients to evaluate the cause, location, or extent of biliary obstruction. Percutaneous transhepatic cholangiography (PTC) with a fine needle is the technique of choice in infants and young children. The likelihood of opacifying the biliary tract is excellent in patients in whom CT or ultrasonography has shown dilated ducts.

Endoscopic retrograde cholangiopancreatography (ERCP) is an alternative method of examining the bile ducts in older children. The papilla of Vater is cannulated under direct vision through a fiberoptic endoscope, and contrast material is injected into the biliary and pancreatic ducts.

Selective angiography of the celiac, superior mesenteric, or hepatic artery may be employed to visualize the hepatic or portal circulation. Splenoportography has been largely replaced by this technique, in which both arterial and venous circulatory systems of the liver can be examined. Angiography is frequently required to define the blood supply of tumors prior to surgery and is useful in the study of patients with known or presumed portal hypertension. The patency of the portal system, the extent of collateral circulation, and the caliber of vessels under consideration for a shunting procedure can be evaluated.

FREDERICK J. SUCHY
WILLIAM F. BALISTRERI

DISEASES OF THE LIVER

12.74 NEONATAL CHOLESTASIS

Cholestasis, the prolonged elevation of serum levels of conjugated bilirubin, occurs in children most frequently in the 1st months of life. Neonatal cholestasis may be due to infectious, genetic, metabolic, or undefined abnormalities giving rise either to mechanical obstruction of bile flow or to functional impairment of hepatic excretory function and bile secretion (Table 12–17). An example of the former is stricture or obstruction of the common bile duct; biliary atresia is the prototypic functional obstructive abnormality. Functional impairment of bile secretion may result from damage to liver cells or to the biliary secretory apparatus. Neonates with cholestasis may be divided into those with extrahepatic and those with intrahepatic disease (Fig. 12–23). The clinical features of any form of cholestasis are similar. In an affected neonate, the diagnosis of some entities, such as galactosemia, sepsis, and hypothyroidism, is relatively simple. In most cases, however, the cause of cholestasis is more obscure. Differentiation among **extrahepatic biliary atresia,** idiopathic **neonatal hepatitis,** and **intrahepatic atresia** is often particularly difficult. The nosology is imprecise and diagnostic criteria uncertain.

Recent advances have improved our understanding of hepatic structure and function in early life, and several forms of neonatal cholestasis have been characterized within a new conceptual framework.

Mechanisms. Some of the histologic manifestations of hepatic injury in early life are not commonly seen in older

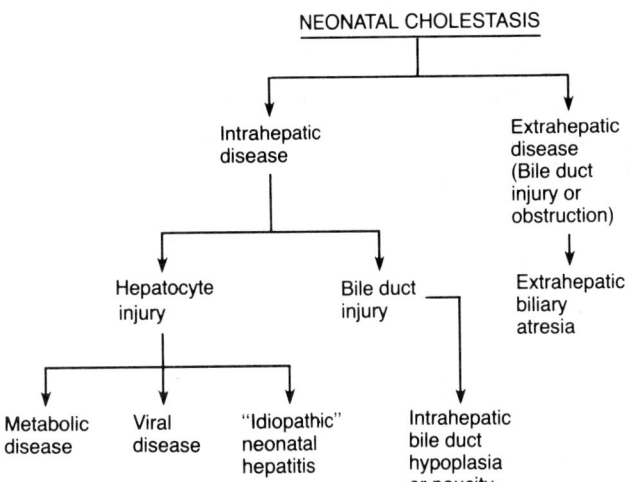

Figure 12–23. Neonatal cholestasis. Conceptual approach to the group of diseases presenting as cholestasis in the neonate. There are areas of overlap—patients with extrahepatic biliary atresia may have some degree of intrahepatic injury. Patients with "idiopathic" neonatal hepatitis may in the future be determined to have a primary metabolic or viral disease.

Table 12–17. Differential Diagnosis of Cholestasis in Early Life

I. Infectious
  A. Viral hepatitis
    1. Hepatitis B virus (? non-A, non-B virus)
    2. Cytomegalovirus
    3. Rubella virus
    4. Herpesvirus
    5. Varicella virus
    6. Coxsackievirus
    7. Echovirus
    8. Reovirus type 3
  B. Others
    a. Toxoplasmosis
    b. Syphilis
    c. Tuberculosis
    d. Listeriosis
II. Toxic
  A. Parenteral nutrition-related
  B. Sepsis (e.g., urinary tract) with endotoxemia
  C. Drug-related
III. Metabolic
  A. Disorders of **amino acid** metabolism
    1. Tyrosinemia
    2. Hypermethioninemia (?)
  B. Disorders of **lipid** metabolism
    1. Wolman disease
    2. Niemann-Pick disease
    3. Gaucher disease
  C. Disorders of **carbohydrate** metabolism
    1. Galactosemia
    2. Fructosemia
    3. Glycogenosis IV
  D. **Undefined/uncharacterized metabolic defect**
    1. α_1-Antitrypsin deficiency
    2. Cystic fibrosis
    3. Idiopathic hypopituitarism
    4. Hypothyroidism
    5. Zellweger (cerebrohepatorenal) syndrome
    6. Multiple acyl-CoA dehydrogenation deficiency (glutaric acid type II)
    7. Neonatal iron storage disease
    8. Indian childhood cirrhosis
    9. Trihydroxycoprostanoic acidemia
IV. Genetic/chromosomal
  A. Trisomy E
  B. Down syndrome
  C. Donahue syndrome (leprechaunism)
V. Intrahepatic diseases of unknown etiology
  A. Intrahepatic cholestasis—persistent
    1. "Idiopathic" neonatal hepatitis
    2. Alagille syndrome (arteriohepatic dysplasia)
    3. Intrahepatic biliary hypoplasia/paucity of intrahepatic bile ducts
    4. Byler disease
  B. Intrahepatic cholestasis—recurrent
    1. Familial benign recurrent cholestasis
    2. Associated with lymphedema (Aagenaes)
  C. Congenital hepatic fibrosis
  D. Caroli disease (cystic dilatation of intrahepatic ducts)
VI. Extrahepatic diseases
  A. Biliary atresia
  B. Biliary hypoplasia
  C. Bile duct stenosis
  D. Choledochal-pancreatico-ductal junction anomaly
  E. Spontaneous perforation of the bile duct
  F. Choledochal cyst
  G. Mass (neoplasia, stone)
  H. Bile/mucous plug ("inspissated bile")
VII. Miscellaneous
  A. Histiocytosis X
  B. Shock/hypoperfusion
  C. Associated with enteritis
  D. Associated with intestinal obstruction

individuals. For example, giant cell transformation of hepatocytes occurs frequently in infants with cholestasis and may be seen in any form of neonatal liver injury. It is more frequent and more severe, however, in intrahepatic forms of cholestasis (neonatal hepatitis or intrahepatic bile duct hypoplasia). The clinical and histologic findings thought to exist both in neonates with neonatal hepatitis and in those with extrahepatic biliary atresia have suggested that these diseases are manifestations of a single basic process, with an initiating insult causing inflammation of the liver cells or of the cells within the biliary tract. If bile duct epithelium is the predominant site of disease, cholangitis may result and lead to progressive sclerosis and narrowing of the biliary tree, the ultimate state being complete obliteration (**extrahepatic biliary atresia**). On the other hand, injury to liver cells may present the clinical and histologic picture of **neonatal hepatitis.** This concept does not account for all phenomena, but offers an explanation for well-documented instances of unexpected postnatal evolution of these disease processes; for example, infants initially regarded as having neonatal hepatitis, with a patent biliary system shown on cholangiography, have been later found to have extrahepatic biliary atresia.

The initial insult as well as the mechanisms that sustain the injury remain undefined, but there is a striking similarity between pathologic changes induced by infection with reovirus type 3 infection in weanling mice and the progressive postnatal fibrotic obliteration of the extrahepatic bile ducts in infants with biliary atresia and neonatal hepatitis. Serologic evidence of reovirus type 3 infection is found in a high percentage of infants with either extrahepatic biliary atresia or idiopathic neonatal hepatitis.

Functional abnormalities in the generation of bile flow may also play a role in neonatal cholestasis. Bile flow is directly dependent on effective hepatic bile acid excretion. During the phase of relatively inefficient liver cell transport and metabolism of bile acids in early life, minor degrees of hepatic injury may further decrease bile flow and lead to production of abnormal bile acids; or selective impairment of a single step in the series of events involved in hepatic excretion may produce the full expression of a cholestatic syndrome. A small number of cholestatic syndromes have a familial pattern; for example, Byler disease and benign recurrent cholestasis are presumably related to impaired membrane transport of bile acids. Defects in bile acid synthesis have been found in infants with intrahepatic cholestasis, such as Zellweger syndrome. A severe form of familial cholestasis has been associated with an aberration in the contractile proteins that comprise the cytoskeleton of the hepatocyte. Sepsis is known to cause cholestasis, presumably mediated by an endotoxin produced by *Escherichia coli.*

Evaluation. The clinical features of infants with neonatal cholestasis provide very few clues regarding etiology. Affected infants have icterus, dark urine, light or acholic stools, and hepatomegaly, all reflecting decreased bile flow owing either to liver cell injury or to bile duct obstruction. Hepatic synthetic dysfunctions may lead to hypoprothrombinemia and bleeding disorder; administration of vitamin K should be considered in initial management of cholestatic infants, in order to prevent hemorrhage.

The majority of infants with neonatal cholestasis will come to medical attention in the 1st mo of life. Prompt differentiation of conjugated from unconjugated hyperbilirubinemia is imperative, as the finding of cholestasis is more ominous. The initial step in identification of cholestasis is the finding that of the significantly elevated level of total bilirubin, more than 20% is direct-reacting bilirubin. The next step is the prompt recognition of any specific and/or treatable primary causes of cholestasis, such as *sepsis,* an *endocrinopathy* (hypothyroidism or panhypopituitarism), *nutritional hepatotoxicity* due to a specific metabolic illness (e.g., galactosemia), or other rare *metabolic diseases* (e.g., tyrosinemia). Recognition of such entities will allow institution of appropriate therapy and possibly prevent further injury.

Hepatobiliary disease may be the initial manifestation of homozygous α_1-antitrypsin deficiency or of cystic fibrosis. Neonatal liver disease may also be associated with infections due to agents of the TORCH complex. Hepatitis A and hepatitis B viruses rarely cause neonatal cholestasis. In up to 80% of infants with neonatal cholestasis, extensive evaluation will establish a diagnosis of either biliary atresia or neonatal hepatitis (Table 12–18).

Neonatal Hepatitis Syndrome (Intrahepatic Cholestasis). The term *neonatal hepatitis* implies intrahepatic cholestasis (Fig. 12–23), of which we can designate various forms:

1. **Idiopathic neonatal hepatitis** is a disease of unknown etiology having sporadic and familial varieties. It includes most of the cases of "neonatal hepatitis."

2. **Infectious hepatitis in a neonate** may be shown to be due to a specific virus, such as hepatitis B or cytomegalovirus. This accounts for a small percentage of cases of neonatal hepatitis syndrome.

3. Instances of **intrahepatic bile duct hypoplasia** or **bile duct paucity** form a heterogenous subset of cholestatic diseases that may appear as neonatal cholestasis.

Intrahepatic Bile Duct Hypoplasia or Paucity. Some syndromes characterized morphologically by intrahepatic cholestasis may be clinically manifest either as neonatal hepatitis (see above) or as cholestasis in an older child. As the patient matures, clinical and histologic features may suggest a specific syndrome. Many such cases are associated with bile duct hypoplasia or "paucity" (often erroneously called intrahepatic biliary atresia), which designates an absence or marked reduction in the number of interlobular bile ducts in the portal triads, with normal-sized branches of portal vein and hepatic arteriole. This unusual histologic feature represents either (1) congenital absence or partial failure to develop or (2) progressive atrophy or disappearance due to segmental destructive processes. Biopsy in early life will often reveal an inflammatory process involving the intralobular bile ducts. Subsequent biopsies then show subsidence of the inflammation with residual reduction in the number and diameter of bile ducts.

Recent observations suggest that it is possible to identify distinctive syndromes of isolated intrahepatic bile duct **paucity** and an **intact** extrahepatic biliary tree.

Alagille syndrome (arteriohepatic dysplasia) is the most common syndrome incorporating intrahepatic bile duct paucity. Serial assessment of hepatic histology often suggests progressive **destruction** of bile ducts. Clinical manifestations are expressed in varying degrees and may be nonspecific; they include unusual *facial characteristics* (broad forehead; deep-set, widely spaced eyes; long, straight nose; and underdeveloped

mandible). There may also be *ocular* abnormalities (posterior embryotoxon), *cardiovascular* abnormalities (usually peripheral pulmonic stenosis, sometimes tetralogy of Fallot), *vertebral arch* defects and failure of anterior vertebral arch fusion (butterfly vertebrae and increased interpeduncular distance), and tubulointerstitial *nephropathy*. Other findings such as growth retardation and defective spermatogenesis may reflect nutritional deficiency. Prognosis for prolonged survival is good, but the patients are likely to have pruritus, xanthomata, and neurologic complications of vitamin E deficiency.

Zellweger (cerebrohepatorenal) syndrome is a rare autosomal recessive genetic disorder marked by progressive degeneration of the liver and kidneys. The incidence is estimated to be 1:100,000 births; the disease is usually fatal within 6–12 mo. Affected infants have severe, generalized hypotonia and markedly impaired neurologic function with psychomotor retardation. There are an abnormal shape of the head and unusual facies, hepatomegaly, renal cortical cysts, stippled calcifications of the patellae and greater trochanter, and ocular abnormalities. Hepatic cells on ultrastructural examination show an absence of peroxisomes. Zellweger syndrome belongs to the category of "peroxisomal disorders." Biochemical abnormalities associated with absence of peroxisomal functions include (1) increased plasma levels of very long chain fatty acids, particularly hexacosanoic acid ($^C26:0$) and hexacosanoic acid ($^C26:1$); (2) elevated concentrations of trihydroxycoprostanic acid, an intermediate in bile acid synthesis; and (3) increased levels of pipecolic acid, an intermediate in lysine degradation. The biochemical alterations permit prenatal and early postnatal diagnosis and genetic counseling.

Bile duct hypoplasia with cholestasis, siderosis, and fatty degeneration is noted in *glutaric aciduria* type II (multiple acyl-CoA dehydrogenation deficiency); affected patients have features reminiscent of the cerebrohepatorenal syndrome and accumulate large quantities of carboxylic acid (and may, therefore, represent another "peroxisomal disease") (Sec. 7.54).

Byler disease is a rare familial form of fatal intrahepatic cholestasis and has apparently unique structural abnormalities in the bile canalicular membrane. Affected patients present failure to thrive, steatorrhea, pruritus, and rickets. Fatal cirrhosis gradually develops. In one form of idiopathic intrahepatic cholestasis (Aagenaes) recurrent cholestasis is associated with lymphedema of the lower extremities.

Extrahepatic Biliary Atresia

The term "biliary atresia" is imprecise, since the anatomy of abnormal extrahepatic bile ducts in affected patients varies markedly. There may be distal atresia with patent extrahepatic ducts up to the portal hepatis. This is a surgically **correctable** lesion, but it is uncommon. The most common form of extrahepatic biliary atresia (85% of cases) is obstruction of the ducts at or above the portal hepatis, which presents much more difficult problems in management.

Incidence. Biliary atresia has been detected in 1:10,000–15,000 live births, idiopathic neonatal hepatitis in 1:5,000–10,000. Intrahepatic bile duct atresia or hypoplasia appears much less commonly, in about 1:50,000–75,000 live births.

Differentiation of Idiopathic Neonatal Hepatitis from Biliary Atresia. It may be difficult to differentiate clearly infants with extrahepatic biliary atresia (who need surgical correction) from infants with neonatal hepatitis. No single biochemical test or imaging procedure is entirely satisfactory. Diagnostic schemata incorporate clinical, historical, biochemical, and radiologic features.

Patients with idiopathic neonatal hepatitis have a familial incidence of approximately 20%, whereas extrahepatic biliary atresia is unlikely to recur within the same family. Infants with biliary atresia have an increased incidence of other

---

Table 12–18. Initial Workup for Suspected Neonatal Cholestasis

1. History and physical examination: size and consistency of liver and spleen; presence of other anomalies (cardiac, renal, skin); stool color
2. Blood and urine analysis: fractionated serum bilirubin; serum bile acids; prothrombin time; alpha$_1$-antitrypsin phenotype; metabolic screen-urine/serum amino acids, urine reducing substances; thyroxine and thyroid-stimulating hormone; sweat chloride
3. Blood, urine, spinal fluid cultures
4. Serologic studies for evidence of infection (HBsAg, TORCH and VDRL)
5. Ultrasonography
6. Hepatobiliary scintigraphy
7. Liver biopsy

abnormalities, such as the polysplenia syndrome with abdominal heterotaxia, malrotation, levocardia, and intra-abdominal vascular anomalies. Neonatal hepatitis appears to be more common in premature, or small for gestational age infants. Persistently acholic stools suggest biliary obstruction, but patients with severe idiopathic neonatal hepatitis may have a transient severe retardation of bile excretion. On the other hand, consistently pigmented stools rule against biliary atresia. The finding of bile-stained fluid on duodenal intubation also excludes biliary atresia. Palpation of the liver may find an abnormal size or consistency in patients with extrahepatic biliary atresia, which is less common with neonatal hepatitis.

Imaging techniques are generally not helpful, but ultrasonography should be carried out early, as it may detect a choledochal cyst or another unsuspected cause of cholestasis associated with dilatation of the biliary tract.

Hepatobiliary scintigraphy using imidodiacetic acid analogues has been used by some clinicians to differentiate biliary atresia from neonatal hepatitis. In biliary atresia, hepatocyte function is intact and uptake of the agent is unimpaired, but excretion into the intestine is absent; whereas in patients with neonatal hepatitis, uptake is sluggish, but excretion into the biliary tract and intestine eventually occurs. Oral administration of phenobarbital (5 mg/kg/day) for 5 days prior to the study enhances biliary excretion of the isotope in patients with neonatal hepatitis.

Liver biopsy provides the most reliable discriminatory evidence. In **biliary atresia,** there are bile ductular proliferation, the presence of bile plugs, and portal or perilobular edema and fibrosis, with the basic hepatic lobular architecture intact. In **neonatal hepatitis,** on the other hand, there is severe, diffuse hepatocellular disease, with distortion of lobular architecture, marked infiltration with inflammatory cells, and focal hepatocellular necrosis; the bile ductules show little alteration. Giant cell transformation is found in infants with either condition and has no diagnostic specificity.

Histologic changes similar to those in idiopathic neonatal hepatitis occur in a variety of diseases, including α_1-antitrypsin deficiency, galactosemia, and various forms of intrahepatic bile duct hypoplasia. In the last, the paucity of intrahepatic bile ductules may be detected on liver biopsy even within first few weeks of life. Later biopsies in such patients will reveal a more characteristic pattern of bile ductular hypoplasia.

Management of Patients With Suspected Biliary Atresia. In infants in whom clinical features and liver biopsy suggest biliary obstruction, exploratory laparotomy and direct cholangiography should be done to determine the presence and site of obstruction. For patients in whom a **correctable lesion** is present, direct drainage can be accomplished. When no correctable lesion is found, examination of frozen sections obtained from the transected porta hepatis can detect the presence of biliary epithelium and determine the size of the residual bile ducts. In some instances, the finding that the biliary tract is patent but of diminished caliber will suggest that the cholestasis is due to extrahepatic biliary **hypoplasia** or to markedly diminished flow owing to intrahepatic disease. In these cases, transection of or further dissection into the porta hepatis should be avoided.

For patients in whom **no correctable lesion** is found, the hepatoportoenterostomy of Kasai can be carried out in selected cases. The rationale for this operation is that minute bile duct remnants, representing residual channels, may be present in the fibrous tissue of the porta hepatis; such channels may be in direct continuity with the intrahepatic ductule system. In such instances, transection of the porta hepatis with anastomosis of bowel mucosa to the proximal surface of the transection may allow drainage. If flow is not rapidly established within the first months of life, progressive obliteration will ensue. If microscopic channels of patency greater than 150 µ in diameter are found, postoperative establishment of bile flow is likely.

Some patients with extrahepatic biliary atresia, even of the "noncorrectable" type, will derive long-term benefits from such interventions as the Kasai procedure. In most, however, a degree of hepatic dysfunction persists. Patients with extrahepatic biliary atresia usually have persistent inflammation of the **intrahepatic** biliary tree, which suggests that extrahepatic biliary atresia reflects a dynamic process involving the entire hepatobiliary system and which may account for the ultimate development of complications such as portal hypertension. The short-term benefit of hepatoportoenterostomy is that it may sustain the child's growth until a successful liver transplantation can be done.

Management of Chronic Cholestasis

With any form of neonatal cholestasis, whether the primary disease is idiopathic neonatal hepatitis, intrahepatic bile duct hypoplasia, or extrahepatic biliary atresia, if the operation is only partially successful, patients are at increased risk for chronic complications (Fig. 12–24). These reflect varying degrees of residual hepatic functional capacity and are due directly or indirectly to diminished bile flow:

1. Any substance normally excreted into bile is retained in the liver, with subsequent accumulation in tissue and in serum. Involved substances include bile acids, bilirubin, cholesterol, and trace elements.

2. Decreased delivery of bile acids to the proximal intestine leads to inadequate solubilization and malabsorption of dietary long-chain triglycerides and fat soluble vitamins.

3. Impairment of hepatic metabolic function may alter hormonal balance and utilization of nutrients.

4. Progressive liver damage may lead to biliary cirrhosis, portal hypertension, and liver failure.

The management of such patients (Table 12–19) is empirical, and the best guide is careful monitoring. At present, no therapy is known to be effective in halting the progression of cholestasis or in preventing further hepatocellular damage and cirrhosis.

A major concern is growth failure, which is related in part to malabsorption and malnutrition due to ineffective digestion and absorption of dietary fat. Use of a medium-chain triglyceride-containing formula may improve caloric balance.

With chronic cholestasis and prolonged survival, children with hepatobiliary disease may develop deficiencies of the fat soluble vitamins (A, D, E, and K). Inadequate absorption of fat and fat-soluble vitamins may be exacerbated by administration of the bile-acid binder, cholestyramine. Rickets is common.

A degenerative neuromuscular syndrome is found with chronic deficiency of vitamin E; affected children develop progressive areflexia, cerebellar ataxia, ophthalmoplegia, and decreased vibratory sensation. Specific morphologic lesions have been found in the central nervous system, peripheral nerves, and muscles. These lesions resemble those found in animals with vitamin E deficiency and are potentially reversible in young children (i.e., those <3–4 yr old). The deficiency might be prevented by the oral administration of large doses (up to 1000 IU/day) of vitamin E; patients unable to absorb sufficient quantities may require administration of vitamin E (dl-α-tocopherol) intramuscularly. Serum levels may be monitored as a guide to efficacy; affected children will have low serum vitamin E concentrations, increased hydrogen peroxide hemolysis, and low ratios of serum vitamin E to total serum lipids (<0.6 mg/g for children under age 12 yr, and <0.8 mg/g for older patients).

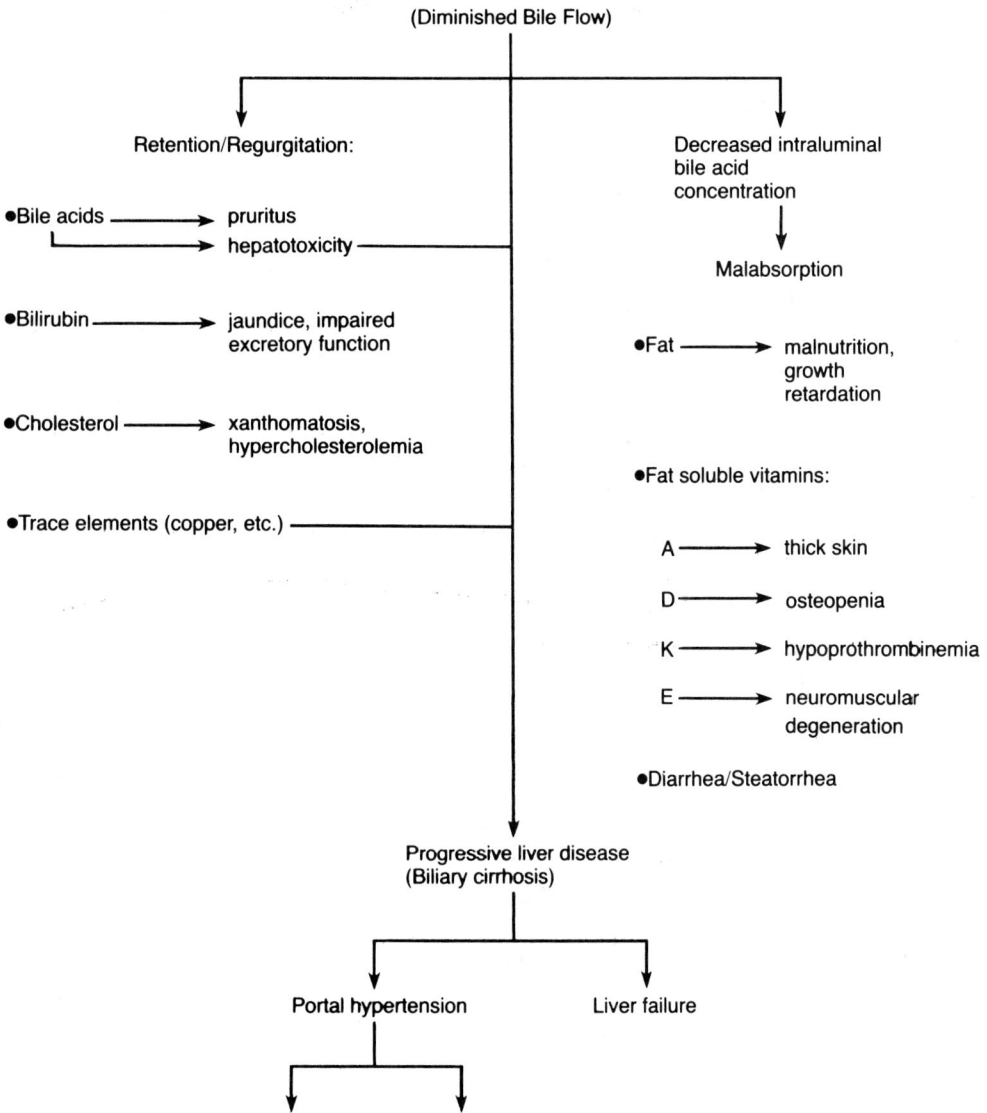

Figure 12–24. Consequences of cholestasis. Clinical consequences of prolonged cholestasis are due to (1) retention by the liver of all substances normally excreted in bile with subsequent regurgitation into serum and tissue; (2) a reduction in bile acid delivery to the proximal intestine; and (3) progressive liver damage. (Reproduced with permission from Balistreri WF: Neonatal cholestasis. *In* Lebenthal E (Ed): Textbook of Gastroenterology and Nutrition. New York, Raven Press, 1982.)

Table 12–19. Suggested Medical Management of Persistent Cholestasis

Clinical Impairment	Management
1. Malnutrition due to malabsorption of dietary long-chain triglyceride (LCT)	Replace with dietary formula or supplements containing medium chain triglycerides (MCT)
2. Fat soluble vitamin malabsorption	
a. Vitamin A deficiency (night blindness, thick skin)	Replace with *10,000–15,000 IU/day* as Aquasol A
b. Vitamin E deficiency (neuromuscular degeneration)	Replace with *50–400 IU/day* as oral α-tocopherol (may require parenteral administration)
c. Vitamin D deficiency (metabolic bone disease)	Replace with *5000–8000 IU/day* of D_2 or *3–5 μg/kg/day* of 25-hydroxycholecalciferol
d. Vitamin K deficiency (hypoprothrombinemia)	Replace with 2.5–5.0 mg every other day as water soluble derivative of menadione
3. Micronutrient deficiency	Calcium/phosphate/zinc supplementation
4. Deficiency of water soluble vitamins	Supplement with twice the recommended daily allowance
5. Retention of biliary constituents such as bile acids and cholesterol (itch/xanthomata)	Administer choleretics (phenobarbital 5–10 mg/kg/day) or bile acid binders (cholestyramine 8–16 g/day)
6. Progressive liver disease:	
a. Portal hypertension (variceal bleeding, ascites, hypersplenism)	a. Interim management (control bleeding; salt restriction)
b. End stage liver disease (liver failure)	b. Transplantation

Serum vitamin A concentrations can usually be maintained at normal levels in patients with chronic cholestasis who received oral supplementation of vitamin A esters. It is essential to monitor the vitamin A status in such patients.

Pruritus is a particularly troublesome complication of chronic cholestasis, often with the appearance of xanthomata. Both features seem to be related to the accumulation of cholesterol and bile acids in serum and in tissues. To enhance the elimination of these retained compounds is difficult when bile ducts are obstructed, but if there is any degree of bile duct patency, administration of phenobarbital (3–5 mg/kg/day) and cholestyramine (8–16 g/day) may increase bile flow or interrupt the enterohepatic circulation of bile acids and thereby decrease the xanthomata and ameliorate the pruritus. Cholestyramine resin is unpalatable and may have such side effects as constipation, hyperchloremia, and exacerbation of fat soluble vitamin deficiency.

In patients with portal hypertension, variceal hemorrhage and the development of hypersplenism is common. However, episodes of gastrointestinal hemorrhage in patients who have chronic liver disease may be due not to esophageal varices but to gastritis or peptic ulcer disease. Because the managements of these various complications differ, differentiation perhaps via endoscopy is necessary before starting treatment.

Initially patients with variceal hemorrhage should have their stomachs gavaged with iced solutions. If the bleeding does not cease, vasopressin, a nonselective vasoconstrictive agent, is administered intravenously. This short-acting drug reduces portal pressure by decreasing splanchnic flow. The dose is 0.3 U/kg body weight (up to 20 U) as a bolus diluted in 2 mL/kg of 5% dextrose over a 10–20 min period. This dose can be repeated at hourly intervals or given via continuous infu-

sion (0.2–0.4 $U/1.73 \, m^2/min$) for 12–24 hr. In rare instances, such as in the presence of massive hemorrhage, the Sengstaken-Blakemore (pediatric) tube may be used to provide balloon tamponade; successful venous compression at the gastroesophageal junction can often be attained without inflating the esophageal balloon. Massive pulmonary aspiration, suffocation, damage to the esophageal mucosa, and esophageal rupture are complications of this modality.

Control of variceal hemorrhage by various surgical procedures offers temporary relief. Repeated sclerotherapy of the bleeding varix may be successful but usually is a temporizing procedure, and a more definitive operation may be required. Shunting procedures, carried out in patients with cirrhosis may cause deterioration in hepatic function and may precipitate the development of encephalopathy. Shunting is technically difficult in young children owing to the small caliber of veins. Moreover, shunting procedures render subsequent liver transplantation more difficult. A high mortality is associated with shunts carried out as emergency procedures. Prophylactic portocaval anastomoses do not alter long-term survival of patients with cirrhosis. Transthoracic ligation of esophageal varices has been used in children as a temporizing procedure.

In patients with **ascites,** initial management consists of dietary salt restriction; sodium intake is limited to 0.5 g (approximately 1–2 mEq/kg/day). It is not necessary to restrict fluid intake in patients with adequate renal output. Diuresis may be maintained by the use of agents such as thiazides, furosemide, and ethacrynic acid, alone or in combination with spironolactone (3–5 mg/kg/day in four doses). Protein intake should be limited in order to minimize the potential for hepatic encephalopathy. Follow-up includes dietary counseling and monitoring of serum and urinary electrolyte concentrations.

In patients with advanced chronic cholestasis, liver transplantation may have a success rate as high as 70%. If the operation is technically feasible, it will prolong life and may correct the metabolic error in such diseases as α₁-antitrypsin deficiency, tyrosinemia, or Wilson disease. Success depends on adequate intraoperative, preoperative, and postoperative care, and on use of cyclosporin as an immunosuppressive agent. Scarcity of donors of small livers severely limits the application of liver transplantation for infants and children.

Prognosis

The prognosis for infants with biliary atresia has been discussed above. For patients with idiopathic neonatal hepatitis, the variable prognosis may reflect the heterogeneity of the disease. In sporadic cases, 60–70% will recover with no evidence of hepatic structural or functional impairment. Approximately 5–10% will have persisting fibrosis or inflammation, and a smaller percentage will have more severe liver disease, such as cirrhosis. Overall mortality rate is 20–30%. Death of infants usually occurs early in the course of the illness, owing to hemorrhage or sepsis. Of infants with idiopathic neonatal hepatitis of the **familial** variety, only 20–30% will recover; 10–15% will develop chronic liver disease with cirrhosis. Mortality is 50–60%.

12.75 CHOLESTASIS IN THE OLDER CHILD

Acute viral hepatitis accounts for the majority of cases of cholestasis after the neonatal period. Other causes include obstruction due to cholelithiasis, abdominal tumors or enlarged lymph nodes, or hepatic inflammation due to drug ingestion. Many of the conditions causing neonatal cholestasis may also cause cholestasis in older patients. An adolescent with conjugated hyperbilirubinemia should be evaluated for acute and chronic hepatitis, α₁-antitrypsin deficiency, Wilson

Table 12–20. Inborn Errors of Metabolism Manifest as Hepatobiliary Dysfunction

Disorders of carbohydrate metabolism
  Disorders of **galactose** metabolism
    Galactosemia (Sec. 7.19)
    Galactokinase deficiency (Sec. 7.19)
    Epimerase deficiency (Sec. 7.19)
  Disorders of fructose metabolism
    Hereditary fructose intolerance (Sec. 7.19)
    F-1,6 DP deficiency (Sec. 7.20)
    Essential fructosuria (Sec. 7.20)
  Glycogen storage diseases:
    Type I (Sec. 7.21)
      Von Gierke (Ia)
      Type Ib
    Type III (Cori/Forbes) (Sec. 7.21)
    Type IV (Andersen) (Sec. 7.21)
    Type VI (Hers) (Sec. 7.21)
Disorders of amino acid/protein metabolism
  Disorders of **tyrosine** (Sec. 7.3) metabolism
    Transient
      Neonatal
      Associated with severe liver disease (e.g., cirrhosis)
    Nontransient
      Hereditary tyrosinemia (type I)
      Tyrosinemia, type II
        Richner-Hanhart
        "Medes Case"
        Atypical forms
          Endo
          Giardi
        "Hawkinsinuria"
  Inherited **urea cycle** enzyme defects (Sec. 7.13)
    CPS deficiency
    OTC deficiency (X-linked dominant)
    Citrullinemia
    Argininosuccinic aciduria
    Argininemia
    N-AGS deficiency
Disorders of **lipid** metabolism
  Wolman disease (Sec. 7.34)
  Cholesterol ester storage disease (Sec. 7.34)
  Gaucher disease (Sec. 7.29)
Disorders of **bile acid** metabolism
  Cerebrotendinous xanthomatosis (Sec. 7.46)
  "Eyssen" syndrome
  Zellweger syndrome (cerebrohepatorenal) (Sec. 7.54)
Disorders of **metal** metabolism
  Wilson disease (Sec. 12.77)
  Hepatic copper overload (Sec. 12.77)
  Indian childhood cirrhosis (Sec. 12.78)
  Menkes (steely-hair) (Sec. 7.54)
  Idiopathic hemochromatosis (Sec. 7.57)
  Neonatal iron storage disease
Disorders of **bilirubin** metabolism
  Crigler-Najjar (Sec. 8.44 and 12.76)
    Type I
    Type II—Arias
    Dubin-Johnson (Sec. 12.76)
    Rotor (Sec. 12.76)
Miscellaneous
  Alpha₁-antitrypsin deficiency (Sec. 12.79 and 13.87)
  Cystic fibrosis (Sec. 13.97)
  Erythropoietic protoporphyria (EEP) (Sec. 7.55)

Table 12–21. Clinical Manifestations that Suggest the Possibility of Metabolic Disease

Jaundice, hepatomegaly (± splenomegaly), fulminant hepatic failure
Hypoglycemia, organic acidemia, hyperammonemia, bleeding (coagulopathy)
Recurrent vomiting, failure-to-thrive, short stature, dysmorphic features
Developmental delay/psychomotor retardation, hypotonia, progressive neuromuscular deterioration, seizures
Cardiac dysfunction/failure, unusual odors, rickets, cataracts

disease, liver disease associated with inflammatory bowel disease, and for the syndromes of intrahepatic bile duct hypoplasia or paucity described above. Management will be similar to that proposed for neonatal cholestasis (Table 12–19).

12.76 METABOLIC DISEASES OF THE LIVER

Also see Chapter 7.

Because the liver plays a central role in synthetic, degradative, and regulatory pathways involving carbohydrate, protein, lipid, trace elements, and vitamin metabolism, there are many metabolic abnormalities or specific enzyme deficiencies that affect the liver primarily or secondarily (Table 12–20). Liver disease may arise when absence of an enzyme produces a block in a metabolic pathway, when unmetabolized substrate accumulates proximal to a block, when deficiency develops of an essential substance produced distal to an aberrant chemical reaction, and/or when synthesis of an abnormal metabolite occurs. The spectrum of pathologic changes includes: (1) *hepatocyte injury*, with subsequent failure of other metabolic functions, often eventuating in cirrhosis or liver tumors or both; (2) *storage* of lipid, glycogen, or other products; and (3) absence of structural change despite profound metabolic effects, as with urea cycle defects. The clinical manifestations of metabolic diseases of the liver mimic infections, intoxications, and hematologic and immunologic diseases (Table 12–21). Further clues are provided by family history of a similar illness or by the observation that the onset of symptoms was closely associated with a change in dietary habits (e.g., initiation of ingestion of fructose). In most cases, clinical and laboratory evidence will guide evaluation. Liver biopsy offers morphologic study and will permit enzyme assays, as well as quantitative and qualitative assays of various other constituents. Such studies require cooperation of experienced laboratories and careful attention to collection and handling of specimens.

WILLIAM F. BALISTRERI

Inherited Deficient Conjugation of Bilirubin (Familial Nonhemolytic Unconjugated Hyperbilirubinemia)

Hepatic glucuronyl transferase activity (Sec. 8.44) is deficient in two genetically and functionally distinct disorders. Type I, which is rarer and more severe than type II, has been reported in about 100 patients.

Crigler-Najjar Syndrome (Type I Glucuronyl Transferase Deficiency). This form is inherited as an autosomal recessive trait. Parents of affected children have partial defects (about 50% of normal) in conjugation by hepatic enzyme assay or by measurement of glucuronide formation, but their serum bilirubin concentrations are normal.

Clinical Manifestations. Severe unconjugated hyperbilirubinemia develops in the homozygous infant during the first 3 days of life, and without treatment serum concentrations of 25–35 mg/dL are reached during the first month. Kernicterus (Sec. 8.45) usually occurs in the early neonatal period, but some treated infants have survived childhood without clinical sequelae. Stools are pale yellow. Persistence of unconjugated hyperbilirubinemia at levels above 20 mg/dL after the first week of life in the absence of hemolysis should suggest the syndrome.

Diagnosis. In the bile, bilirubin concentration is less than 10 mg/dL compared with normal concentrations of 50–100 mg/dL, and there is no bilirubin glucuronide. Definitive diagnosis is established by measuring hepatic glucuronyl transferase activity in a liver specimen obtained by a closed biopsy; open biopsy should be avoided, since surgery and anesthesia may precipitate kernicterus. Identification of the heterozygous state in the parents is also strongly suggestive of the diagnosis. Differential diagnosis is discussed in Sec. 8.44. Type II disease may be distinguished from type I by the marked decline in serum bilirubin level that occurs in type II disease after 1 wk of treatment with phenobarbital.

Treatment. Serum bilirubin concentration should be kept below 20 mg/dL for at least the first 2–4 wk of life; in low birthweight infants the levels should be kept lower. This usually requires repeated exchange transfusions and phototherapy (Sec. 8.44, 8.45 and 8.47). Because the risk of kernicterus persists into adult life, although the serum bilirubin levels required to produce brain injury beyond the neonatal period are considerably higher (usually above 35 mg/dL), phototherapy is generally continued throughout the early years of life. In older infants and children phototherapy is used mainly during sleep in order not to interfere with normal activities. However, despite the administration of increasing intensities of light for longer periods, the serum bilirubin decrement response to phototherapy decreases with age. Prompt treatment of intercurrent infections, febrile episodes, and other types of illness may help prevent the later development of kernicterus, which may occur at bilirubin levels of 45–55 mg/dL. All type I patients have eventually developed severe kernicterus by young adulthood, despite vigorous continuous management which maintained neurologic normality during childhood.

Glucuronyl Transferase Deficiency Type II. This autosomal dominant disease with marked variability of penetrance may present in a manner similar to type I syndrome, or it may be a less severe disorder, occasionally even without neonatal manifestations.

Clinical Manifestations. When this disorder presents in the neonatal period, there is usually unconjugated hyperbilirubinemia during the first 3 days of life; serum bilirubin concentrations may be in a range compatible with physiologic jaundice or may be at pathologic levels. Characteristically, the concentrations remain elevated into and after the 3rd wk of life, persisting in a range of 1.5–22 mg/dL; concentrations in the lower part of this range may create uncertainty as to whether chronic hyperbilirubinemia is present. The onset of kernicterus is unusual. Stool color is normal and the infants are without clinical signs or symptoms of disease. There is no evidence of hemolysis.

Diagnosis. Definitive diagnosis requires testing of the infant and the parents for the capacity to form glucuronides of bilirubin or other test substances. The former requires in vitro measurement of enzymatic activity in a percutaneous liver biopsy. The latter requires administration of substances conjugated as glucuronides, such as menthol or salicylamide, and their measurement in urine; this test is less specific and less accurate but safer than the biopsy. The levels of conjugation are very low and not distinguishable from those found in type I syndrome. In type II syndrome, one of the parents should have a defect in conjugation; jaundice may be minimal to severe. Abnormalities in other family members may support the diagnosis. Bile bilirubin concentration is nearly normal in type II syndrome. Jaundiced infants and young children having type II syndrome respond readily to 5 mg/kg/24 hr of oral phenobarbital with a decrease in serum bilirubin concentration to 2–3 mg/dL within 7–10 days. Those with type I syndrome do not respond.

Treatment. Long-term reduction in serum bilirubin levels can be achieved with chronic administration of phenobarbital at 5 mg/kg/24 hr. The cosmetic and psychosocial benefit should be weighed against the risks of an effective dose of the drug, since there is no long-term risk of kernicterus in the absence of hemolytic disease.

Pregnancy. Pregnancy in the patient with type I syndrome or a severe form of type II syndrome may present a special risk of neurologic manifestations due to increased serum bilirubin concentrations and altered albumin binding.

Inherited Conjugated Hyperbilirubinemia

In inherited conjugated hyperbilirubinemias, which are autosomal recessive disorders characterized by mild jaundice, the transfer of bilirubin and other organic anions from liver to bile is defective. Chronic mild conjugated hyperbilirubinemia is usually detected during adolescence or early adulthood, but may occur as early as the 2nd year of life. Routine liver function tests are normal. Jaundice may be exacerbated with infection, pregnancy, oral contraceptives, alcohol, or surgery. There is usually no morbidity, and life expectancy is normal; but these disorders may initially present difficult problems in the differential diagnosis of more serious diseases.

Dubin-Johnson Syndrome. The defect is in porphyrin metabolism or excretion with more than 90% of the normal total urinary coproporphyrin excretion occurring as a coproporphyrin I isomer. Plasma bile acid and bile acid excretion are normal, but sulfabromophthalein retention is abnormal. Roentgenography of the gallbladder is also abnormal. The liver cells contain black pigment similar to melanin.

Rotor Syndrome. These patients have an additional deficiency in organic anion uptake. Total urinary coproporphyrin excretion is elevated with a relative increase in the amount of the coproporphyrin I isomer. The gallbladder is normal by roentgenography, and there is no black pigment in liver cells. Sulfabromophthalein is often abnormal.

RICHARD E. BEHRMAN

Berk PD, Wolkoff AW, Berlin NI: Inborn errors of bilirubin metabolism. Med Clin N Am 59:803, 1975.
Israel JB, Arias IM: Inheritable disorders of bilirubin metabolism. Adv Intern Med 21:34, 1975.
Wolkoff AW, Cohen L, Arias IM: The inheritance of Dubin-Johnson syndrome. N Engl J Med 288:113, 1973.
Wolkoff AW, Wolpert E, Pascasio F: Rotor's syndrome: A distinct inheritable pathophysiologic entity. Am J Med 60:173, 1976.

Wilson Disease

Wilson disease (hepatolenticular degeneration) is an autosomal recessive disorder characterized by degenerative changes in the brain, cirrhosis, and Kayser-Fleischer rings in the cornea (Sec. 21.21). Incidence is 1:500,000–100,000 births. It is fatal if untreated; but specific, effective treatment is available. Rapid diagnostic investigation of the possibility of Wilson disease in a patient presenting with any form of liver disease not only will facilitate early institution of management of Wilson disease and related genetic counseling but also will allow appropriate treatment of non-Wilson liver disease once copper toxicosis is ruled out.

Pathogenesis. Defective copper excretion leads to accumulation of copper in the liver. It may be that mutation in a controller gene perpetuates the fetal mode of copper metabolism; alternatively, defective copper excretion may be due to an abnormal metallothionein or to a specific lysosomal defect.

Fetal and neonatal liver normally contain relatively high concentrations of sulfur-rich copper-binding protein (metallothionein) and of copper; serum ceruloplasmin and copper levels are relatively low. The control mechanisms responsible for copper homeostasis in older children reach maturity by 2 yr of age; the wilsonian trait may be expressed after this time, but Wilson disease is not clinically manifest before the age of 5 yr.

Altered incorporation of copper into hepatic proteins such as ceruloplasmin is associated with diffuse accumulation of copper in the cytosol of hepatocytes. Later, as liver cells are overloaded, copper is distributed to other tissues, to which it is toxic, primarily as a potent inhibitor of enzymatic processes. Ionic copper inhibits pyruvate oxidase in brain and adenosine triphosphatase in membranes, leading to decreased ATP-phosphocreatine and potassium content of tissue. The glycolytic pathway and microsomal membrane ATPases are inhibited.

Clinical Manifestations. Copper enters the circulation in a non–ceruloplasmin-bound form and accumulates in various organs. Manifestations are variable, with a tendency to familial patterns. The younger the patient, the more likely hepatic involvement will be the predominant manifestation. After the age of 20 yr, neurologic symptoms predominate. Forms of hepatic disease include asymptomatic hepatomegaly (with or without splenomegaly), subacute or chronic hepatitis, or fulminant hepatic failure. Cryptogenic cirrhosis, portal hypertension, ascites, edema, esophageal bleeding, or other effects of hepatic dysfunction (delayed puberty, amenorrhea, or coagulation defects, etc.) may be results of Wilson disease.

Neurologic and psychiatric disorders may develop insidiously or precipitously, with intention tremor, dysarthria, dystonia, deterioration in school performance, or behavioral changes. Kayser-Fleischer rings may be absent in young patients with only liver disease but are always present in patients with neurologic symptoms. Hemolysis may be an initial manifestation, possibly related to the release of large amounts of copper from damaged hepatocytes. During hemolytic episodes urinary copper excretion and serum copper levels (non–ceruloplasmin-bound) are extraordinarily elevated. Manifestations of Fanconi syndrome and progressive renal failure with alterations in tubular transport of amino acids, glucose, and uric acid may be present. Unusual manifestations include arthritis and endocrinopathies such as hypoparathyroidism.

Pathology. All grades of hepatic injury occur, with fatty change, ballooned hepatocytes, glycogen granules, minimal inflammation, and enlarged Kupffer cells. The lesion may be indistinguishable from that of chronic active hepatitis. Ultrastructural changes include large, dense mitochondria with altered smooth endoplasmic reticulum.

Diagnosis. The clinical suspicion is confirmed by study of indices of copper metabolism. Children and teenagers with unexplained acute or chronic liver disease, neurologic symptoms of unknown cause, acute hemolysis, psychiatric illnesses, behavioral changes, Fanconi syndrome, or unexplained bone disease need to have the possibility of Wilson disease considered.

The best screening test is to measure the serum ceruloplasmin level. The vast majority of patients with Wilson disease will have ceruloplasmin levels below 10 μg/dL. Serum copper may be elevated in early Wilson disease, and urinary copper excretion (usually less than 40 μg/day) is increased to greater than 100 μg/day, and often up to 1000 μg or more per day. In equivocal cases the response of urinary copper output to chelation may be of diagnostic help; following a 1 g oral dose of D-penicillamine, affected patients will excrete 1200 to 2000 μg/day.

Liver biopsy is of value for examination of the histology and to measure the copper content (normally <10 μg/g dry weight); in Wilson disease hepatic copper content exceeds 250 μg/g dry weight. In healthy heterozygotes, levels may be intermediate.

Family members of proven cases deserve screening for presymptomatic Wilson disease. Screening includes ceruloplasmin levels, urinary copper excretion, and sometimes liver biopsy.

Treatment. The administration of copper-chelating agents leads to rapid excretion of excess deposited copper. A major attempt should be made to restrict copper intake to less than 1 mg/day. Foods such as liver, shellfish, nuts, and chocolate are to be avoided. If the copper content of the water exceeds 0.1 mg/L, it may be necessary to demineralize the water. Chelation therapy is currently best managed with oral administration of penicillamine (β, β-dimethylcysteine) in a dose of 1.0 g/day in two doses before meals for adults, and 0.5–0.75 g/day for patients less than 10 yr old. In response to D-penicillamine, urinary copper excretion will markedly increase, and there may be slow clinical improvement. Urinary copper levels may become normal with continued administration of D-penicillamine, with marked improvement in hepatic and neurologic function and the disappearance of Kayser-Fleischer rings. Toxic effects of penicillamine are uncommon, and consist of hypersensitivity reactions, interaction with collagen and elastin, deficiency of other elements such as zinc, as well as aplastic anemia and nephrosis. Because penicillamine is an antimetabolite of vitamin B₆, additional amounts of this vitamin are necessary.

Prognosis. Untreated patients with Wilson disease will die from the hepatic, neurologic, renal, or hematologic complications. The prognosis in patients receiving prompt and continuous D-penicillamine is variable and dependent on the time of initiation of and the individual responsiveness to chelation. In asymptomatic siblings of affected patients the expression of the disease can be prevented by early institution of chelation therapy.

12.77 Hepatic Copper Overload Syndrome

Recent studies have identified in American children a form of cirrhosis apparently associated with a genetic disturbance in copper metabolism. This syndrome differs from Wilson disease in its earlier onset; affected children develop progressive lethargy, abdominal distention, and jaundice and die before 6 yr of age. The hepatic histopathology resembles that of Indian childhood cirrhosis.

12.78 Indian Childhood Cirrhosis

Indian childhood cirrhosis is a fatal familial disorder that occurs predominantly in rural India in middle income Hindu families. It has been reported also in the Middle East, in West Africa, and in Central America. It affects children of both sexes, with onset usually at 1–3 yr of age. Hepatomegaly is often the first sign; fever, anorexia, and jaundice occur. There is in most cases rapid evolution to cirrhosis and liver failure. Serum immunoglobulin levels and hepatic copper concentrations are markedly elevated. No effective therapy is known.

It has been suggested that excessive dietary copper may play a role in etiology, owing to the use of copper and brass in cooking and for storage of water and milk. The early introduction of copper-contaminated milk into infant diets may explain the epidemiologic features. There may be a predisposing inherited susceptibility.

12.79 Alpha₁-Antitrypsin Deficiency

See also Sec. 13.87

A small percentage of individuals homozygous for a deficiency of the major serum protease inhibitor, α₁-antitrypsin, have neonatal cholestasis and later childhood cirrhosis. Alpha₁-antitrypsin, a glycoprotein synthesized by the liver, accounts for 80% of the serum α₁-globulin fraction. Alpha₁-antitrypsin is present in more than 20 different codominant alleles, only a few of which are associated with defective enzyme. The most common allele of the protease inhibitor (Pi) system is M, and the normal phenotype is PiMM. The Z allele predisposes to clinical deficiency; patients with liver disease are usually PiZZ and have serum α₁-antitrypsin levels less than 2.0 mg/mL (to approximately 10–20% of normal). The incidence of the PiZZ genotype is estimated at 1:2000–

4000. Intermediate phenotypes PiMS, PiMZ, and PiSZ are not definitively associated with liver disease. Of all PiZZ persons, less than 20% will develop neonatal cholestasis. These patients are indistinguishable from other infants with "idiopathic" neonatal hepatitis, of whom they constitute approximately 5–10%.

In affected patients the course of liver disease is highly variable. Jaundice, acholic stools, and hepatomegaly are present during the 1st wk of life, but the jaundice usually clears during the 2nd–4th mo. There may follow complete resolution, persistent liver disease, or the development of cirrhosis. In older children, there may appear chronic liver disease or cirrhosis, with evidence of portal hypertension.

The fact that liver disease is not universal suggests a complex pathogenesis. The liver disease may be secondary to retention of the α_1-antitrypsin in the liver or to decreased availability of a protease inhibitor that prevents tissue injury.

The diagnosis is best made by determination of α_1-antitrypsin (Pi) phenotype and confirmed by biopsy. PAS-positive diastase-resistant intracytoplasmic globules are seen in periportal hepatocytes. Immunofluorescence and immunocytochemical studies have shown this material to be antigenically related to α_1-antitrypsin. It has been suggested that abnormal biosynthesis of the protein or defective glycosylation may interfere with excretion of the product from the rough endoplasmic reticulum into the extracellular space. Electron microscopy shows amorphous deposits (glycoprotein) within dilated rough endoplasmic reticulum. The pattern of neonatal liver injury may be highly variable. There is hepatocellular damage with giant cell transformation, minimal inflammation, and bile stasis. Varying degrees of portal fibrosis with biliary duct proliferation occur.

Liver transplantation has been curative. There is no other effective therapy as yet, but replacement therapy may become possible.

12.80 INFECTIOUS DISORDERS OF THE LIVER

Viral Hepatitis. This primary viral infection of the liver has been shown to be caused by any of at least five specific hepatotrophic viruses. These include, in addition to hepatitis A virus (HAV) or hepatitis B virus (HBV), the delta agent and at least two types of non-A, non-B hepatitis viruses (Sec. 11.76). Other viruses that cause hepatic inflammation as part of a generalized illness include syphilis (Sec. 11.51), toxoplasmosis (Sec. 11.107), gonococcus (Sec. 11.22), cytomegalovirus (Sec. 11.68), herpes simplex virus (Sec. 11.65), varicella (Sec. 11.66), Epstein-Barr (Sec. 11.69), rubella (Sec. 11.62), echoviruses (Sec. 11.77), yellow fever (Sec. 11.80), dengue (Sec. 11.82), and coxsackie virus B (Sec. 11.77). CMV infection may be transmitted by blood transfusion; the affected patient will typically have fever, lethargy, splenomegaly, and anemia with atypical mononuclear cells in the blood smear 3–6 wk following transfusion. Approximately one quarter of patients infected in this manner will develop clinical evidence of hepatitis. This syndrome was originally identified in patients following heart surgery and was termed "postperfusion syndrome," but exposure to smaller volumes of blood can presumably transmit CMV infection. CMV may also appear as an opportunistic infection in immunocompromised patients such as those undergoing renal, bone marrow, or hepatic transplantation.

Infectious Mononucleosis. This infection is accompanied by hepatic enlargement in 10–15% of uncomplicated cases; there may also be hepatic tenderness. Serum bilirubin levels may be mildly elevated in up to one third of patients with mononucleosis. Jaundice develops in about 5% of patients during the 2nd wk of the illness; it usually lasts 5–7 days. Epstein-Barr virus may rarely be the cause of transfusion-related hepatitis; outbreaks in hemodialysis units have been related to this virus.

Liver Abscess. This is a common association of bacterial infections of the liver. Hepatic abscesses occur in infants in association with sepsis, umbilical vein infection, or vessel cannulation. Beyond infancy, hepatic abscesses occur most commonly in immunosuppressed patients. Of a large series of hepatic abscesses, 40% were found in patients with chronic granulomatous disease, and 20% in otherwise immunosuppressed patients. Pyogenic hepatic abscesses may arise from (1) the portal circulation in patients with pylephlebitis or intra-abdominal sepsis (appendicitis, inflammatory bowel disease); (2) generalized sepsis; (3) cholangitis associated with biliary tract obstruction, as by gallstones, in inflammatory bowel disease, and with choledochal cysts; (4) systemic spread from an intra-abdominal infection or contiguous spread (which usually produces large abscesses); and (5) cryptogenic biliary tract infections. Small abscesses (microabscesses) are most commonly secondary to bacteremia. Implicated organisms include predominantly *Staphylococcus aureus*, *Escherichia coli*, *Salmonella*, and on occasion anaerobic organisms. Symptoms are nonspecific and may suggest systemic infection. There may be fever and pain in the right upper quadrant, and the liver may be tender to percussion. Jaundice is uncommon; serum aminotransferase and alkaline phosphatase activities may be mildly elevated. The erythrocyte sedimentation rate is high, and there is a leukocytosis. Blood cultures are usually positive. Roentgenographic study of the chest may show elevation of the right hemidiaphragm with decreased mobility. Ultrasonography or gallium scans or both may indicate the site of the abscess. In most instances, treatment will require surgical drainage and the administration of antibiotics. *Entamoeba histolytica* may also cause hepatic abscesses in symptomatic or asymptomatic patients with amebic infection of the gastrointestinal tract (Sec. 11.101).

12.81 LIVER DISEASE ASSOCIATED WITH SYSTEMIC DISORDERS

Hepatobiliary disease may complicate ulcerative colitis (Sec. 12.42) *and Crohn disease* (Sec. 12.43). Both the manifestations and the severity vary. Fatty liver, pericholangitis, drug-induced injury, chronic hepatitis, portal fibrosis, cirrhosis, hepatic abscesses, infarction, portal vein thrombosis, sclerosing cholangitis, carcinoma of the biliary tract, and cholelithiasis have all been associated. These complications are more likely to occur in patients with other extraintestinal complications, but there is no correlation with the severity of the inflammatory bowel disease. The etiology of abnormalities in liver function in patients with ulcerative colitis or Crohn disease is unknown. Total colectomy has been beneficial in management of hepatobiliary complications in some patients with ulcerative colitis.

Extensive fatty change in the liver has been found, especially in patients with inflammatory bowel disease who are severely malnourished or chronically incapacitated. Most patients have no symptoms; they have only hepatomegaly as a sign. The chemical abnormalities are mild. The fatty infiltration will usually subside with therapy.

Pericholangitis may be difficult to distinguish from chronic hepatitis in patients with inflammatory bowel disease. The patients may be asymptomatic or have jaundice, pruritus, or abdominal pain. Elevation of alkaline phosphatase or 5'-nucleotidase activities is almost universal. This complication can occur any time in the course of inflammatory bowel disease. The prognosis appears to be favorable; progression to cirrhosis, however, has been reported. There has been no consistent beneficial response to various medications, such as corticosteroids.

Sclerosing cholangitis or fibrosing inflammation of various segments of the bile ducts may lead to obliteration of the duct lumen. The clinical and biochemical picture is that of cholestasis, often with intermittent attacks of acute cholangitis (fever, jaundice, right upper quandrant pain, anorexia, weight loss, and pruritus), followed by portal hypertension. This complication is associated with ulcerative colitis, and rarely with Crohn disease. *Primary sclerosing cholangitis* (*not* associated with inflammatory bowel disease) is rare in children. In either instance, endoscopic retrograde cholangiopancreatography (ERCP) will reveal beading and irregularity of the intrahepatic and extrahepatic bile ducts. Treatment is aimed at improving biliary drainage and attempting to halt the progression of the obliterative process. Symptomatic treatment is required for such complications as pruritus, malnutrition, and infection. There is no definitive treatment; administration of corticosteroids or D-penicillamine has produced inconsistent results. The course is usually progressive to a fatal outcome.

Bacterial sepsis (Sec. 8.59 and 11.12) may be complicated by liver disease. The most frequently associated organisms are *Escherichia coli*, *Klebsiella pneumoniae*, and *Pseudomonas aeruginosa*. It is postulated that bacterial endotoxin directly inhibits bile formation by altering the bile canalicular membrane. Clinical manifestations may be subtle and difficult to differentiate from other causes of neonatal cholestasis. There is an elevation in the serum bilirubin level, usually predominantly in the conjugated fraction. Serum alkaline phosphatase and aminotransferase activities may be elevated. Liver biopsy will show intrahepatic cholestasis with little or no hepatocyte necrosis. Kupffer cell hyperplasia and an increase in inflammatory cells are also common.

Hepatic congestion and injury may occur as a complication of severe *chronic or acute congestive failure* (Sec. 14.80) or *cyanotic heart disease* (Sec. 14.14–14.34). Hepatic dysfunction derives from hypoxemia, systemic venous congestion, and low cardiac output. Hepatic manifestations of left and right heart failure are similar. With decreased cardiac output, there is decreased hepatic blood flow and centrizonal hypoxia. Hepatic necrosis leads to lactic acidosis, elevated aminotransferase activities, jaundice, prolonged partial thromboplastin time, and possibly hypoglycemia. With right heart failure, increases in right atrial and hepatic venous pressures lead to centrizonal sinusoidal distention that presents a barrier to oxygen diffusion. Hemorrhage, pressure atrophy, and necrosis follow. Jaundice and tender hepatomegaly occur. Ascites may also occur with chronic right-sided congestive heart failure. In patients with shock liver, elevated aminotransferase activities may return rapidly to normal when perfusion and cardiac function improve. A syndrome of fulminant hepatic failure may occur, particularly in patients with aortic coarctation.

Histologic abnormalities in the liver are not infrequent at postmortem examinations of patients with congenital heart disease. The abnormalities are similar to those found in adults with congestive heart failure: subcapsular hemorrhage, midzonal hepatic necrosis, and prominent centrilobular necrosis. Hepatic necrosis may be seen in patients with hypoplastic left heart syndrome.

The patient with **sickle cell anemia** (Sec. 15.18) or **sickle cell–thalassemia** (Sec. 15.23) may have hepatic dysfunction owing to acute or chronic viral-associated hepatitis, iron overload, hepatic crises related to severe intrahepatic cholestasis, and ischemic necrosis. In addition, cholelithiasis and a benign form of extreme hyperbilirubinemia have been noted. Hepatic sickle cell crisis or "sickle hepatopathy" may produce intense right upper quadrant pain, fever, leukocytosis, right upper quadrant tenderness, and jaundice. Bilirubin levels may be markedly elevated, alkaline phosphatase activities only moderately elevated.

On occasion, children with sickle cell disease develop bilirubin levels exceeding 20 mg/dL; these levels are unaccompanied by severe pain or fever. There is no change in hematocrit or reticulocyte count nor any association with a hemolytic crisis. The clinical course is benign.

The most common metabolic complication of **total parenteral nutrition** (TPN) in premature infants is the development of liver dysfunction. Cholestasis is the most severe form and is potentially fatal. It is the major factor limiting effective use of TPN (Sec. 8.17).

In *low birthweight infants*, the incidence of TPN-associated cholestasis is inversely correlated with birthweight. It will develop with TPN in nearly half of infants with birthweights less than 1000 g, in 20% of those 1000–1500 g, and in 5–10% of those 1500–2000 g. The incidence of cholestasis also correlates with the duration of TPN, with onset usually after 2 wk. Respiratory distress, acidosis, hypoxia, and sepsis seem to enhance the likelihood and severity of cholestasis. Associated illness, the exclusion of enteral intake, and the nature of the underlying disorder that necessitates TPN may also affect the incidence. Sepsis, abdominal surgery, and necrotizing enterocolitis may predispose to a particularly severe inflammatory and fibrotic lesion of the liver.

The onset is usually insidious, with progressive jaundice and hepatic enlargement or splenomegaly. In low birthweight infants, the onset of jaundice may overlap the phase of physiologic unconjugated hyperbilirubinemia. Any icteric infant who has received TPN for more than 1 wk should have all bilirubin determinations fractionated. Cholestasis is frequently first detected through routine monitoring of infants receiving TPN. A slow progression of abnormalities is found in biochemical measurements of hepatic function. Serum bile acid concentrations may increase. Rises in serum aminotransferase activities may be a late finding. An elevation in serum alkaline phosphatase activity may be due to rickets, a common complication of TPN in low birthweight infants.

In addition to cholestasis, biliary complications of intravenous nutrition include cholelithiasis and the development of biliary sludge, associated with thick, inspissated gallbladder contents. These may be asymptomatic.

An effort must be made to differentiate TPN-associated hepatic dysfunction from benign causes of hepatomegaly, such as the deposition of glycogen or fat, which is common with TPN and with which serum bilirubin and bile acid levels will remain within the normal range. Consideration of other causes of cholestasis is also appropriate. The group in which TPN-associated cholestasis most frequently occurs (i.e., infants in the neonatal intensive care unit), frequently receives blood transfusions or drugs. Therefore, hepatic disease related to viral hepatitis or drug-induced liver disease is a consideration.

The most striking histologic finding in TPN-associated liver disease is canalicular cholestasis, which may begin after less than 2 wk of TPN. Bile duct proliferation may resemble that in biliary atresia. Portal fibrosis is a late finding. Progression of injury to cirrhosis has occurred in a few infants. Milder changes may be reversible with discontinuation of TPN and the initiation of oral feedings.

The pathogenesis of TPN-associated cholestasis is most likely multifactorial. The infant is of low birthweight, is receiving nothing by mouth, may have significant gastrointestinal disease, and often has other systemic complications. In normal newborns there is also a phase of impaired hepatic excretory function ("Physiologic cholestasis") in early infancy. The administered nutrient solution has potential toxicity and may have a specific deficiency. The omission of oral feedings and the absence of intraluminal nutrients blunt the output of the gastrointestinal hormones, which are normal stimulants to bile flow and to development of the hepatobiliary system. Potential hepatotoxins include bacterial endotoxins, specific amino acids or metabolic or degradation products, or copper or manganese; the last two are particularly hepatotoxic. The roles of specific deficiencies (of taurine, essential fatty acids, amino acid, carnitine, or vitamin E) need to be investigated.

The goal in management of the infant with TPN-associated cholestasis is to avoid progressive liver injury. It has been shown that with the administration of oral feedings gradual resolution of the liver disease occurs. The initiation of oral feedings of small volume or the infusion of nutrients by continuous nasogastric drip may enhance biliary flow and intestinal motility. This effect may occur even when the enteral intake does not provide the total caloric needs. Improved solutions that meet the specific needs of the neonate may prevent deficiencies and avoid toxicities. In the decision to continue TPN, one must weigh the risk of further hepatic injury against the risk of malnutrition.

In *older children*, TPN-associated liver dysfunction is less common and less severe than in infants, but biochemical abnormalities are not uncommon in older patients who are maintained on TPN for prolonged periods of time, either at home or in the hospital. Patients with chronic intestinal disease, which may be complicated by infection or bacterial overgrowth, are particularly susceptible to hepatic dysfunction. In most such patients, partial enteral alimentation reverses the abnormalities. It may be necessary at any age, when alkaline phosphatase or aminotransferase activities are elevated, to evaluate the underlying liver disease by liver biopsy. Hepatic steatosis without cholestasis is often the only abnormality.

Hepatic dysfunction is common in patients who have undergone **bone marrow transplantation.** Its genesis is multifactorial and may be related to (1) infections (viral, bacterial, or fungal), drugs, parenteral nutrition, chemotherapy, or radiation; (2) veno-occlusive disease (VOD); or (3) graft-versus-host disease (GVHD); or to any combination of these. Candidates for bone marrow transplantation have often had pre-existing liver disease such as viral hepatitis, drug-related injury, or malignant infiltration. Percutaneous liver biopsy in such patients may show extensive bile duct injury in GVHD, viral inclusions in CMV disease, or the characteristic endothelial lesion in VOD, but the histologic distinction is often unclear. This presents a dilemma, since treatment of one suspected complication (such as initiation of immunosuppressive therapy for GVHD) may have a deleterious effect if the symptoms are due to another (such as fungal infection).

Veno-occlusive disease (VOD) of the liver usually has its onset 1–3 wk following bone marrow transplantation but may appear up to 6 wk afterward. The most characteristic presentation is onset of rapid weight gain, with ascites, hepatomegaly, right upper quadrant pain, jaundice, and oliguria. Hepatic encephalopathy and fulminant hepatic failure may follow. Less severe forms may be characterized by jaundice and ascites with a slow resolution; a mild form of VOD has histologic changes as the sole manifestation. The diagnosis rests on the exclusion of other diseases, such as congestive cardiomyopathy, constrictive pericarditis, and venous thrombosis (Budd-Chiari syndrome).

Pathologic changes in patients with VOD are best demonstrated using special (trichrome) stains to highlight the central veins. An early lesion is concentric narrowing of the lumina of small central veins, owing to edema in the subendothelial zone. There is a dense, wavy continuous band of collagen in the central veins and centrilobular hemorrhagic necrosis. The lesions may be patchy. The venular changes may progress to complete obliteration. The cause of VOD following bone marrow transplantation is not clear; it may be related to ionizing radiation or to antineoplastic drugs, or both. Risk factors for VOD include high-dose conditioning regimens, leukemia, advanced age, and pre-existing liver disease.

Budd-Chiari syndrome involves occlusion of the inferior vena cava or hepatic veins and tributaries; it may be caused by obstruction due to a web, mass, or thrombus. The disease has rarely been noted in children, however, a number of associated diseases may increase the risk. These include trauma, coagulopathies, sickle cell anemia, leukemia, polycythemia vera, hepatic abscesses, irradiation, and GVHD. The syndrome is to be regarded as distinct from VOD, which affects the centrilobular and sublobular hepatic veins, sparing the larger veins; it is not associated with thrombosis.

Graft-versus-host disease (GVHD) of the liver may be acute or chronic and is generally concomitant with GVHD in other target organs (Sec. 10.21). Cholestasis and hepatic injury of varying degrees occur; there may be hepatic tenderness, dark urine, acholic stools, itching, and anorexia. There are parallel rises in serum bilirubin level and alkaline phosphatase activity; AST elevation is less striking. GVHD is characterized histologically by degeneration and loss of small bile ducts and sparse inflammation, along with cholestasis.

Hepatic involvement in patients with **collagen vascular disease** is uncommon. It has been noted especially in patients with systemic lupus erythematosus. Reactive hepatitis, chronic hepatitis, steatosis, and hepatic infarction have also been described. The association of hepatic injury with drug therapy, such as salicylate use, must be differentiated.

12.82 REYE SYNDROME

See also Sec. 21.24.

Since the initial description in 1963, Reye syndrome (acute encephalopathy and fatty degeneration of the viscera) has received a great deal of attention owing to (1) a marked increase in reported incidence, which reflects growing recognition of its clinical features; (2) the potential for high morbidity; (3) a substantial research interest; and (4) evidence of a link between the disease and intake of aspirin.

Epidemiology. Case reports of Reye syndrome were sporadic until 1974, when nearly 400 cases were reported in the United States, with a mortality rate of over 40%. More recent data indicate a higher incidence and lower case fatality rate, owing perhaps to recognition of milder cases. The incidence is increased in direct temporal and geographic relationship to viral epidemics, especially those due to influenza B and varicella. Influenza A may also be associated, but less strongly.

The peak incidence is at about 6 yr of age, with most cases in the 4–12 yr old range. There is no gender difference in incidence, but rural and suburban populations appear to be more frequently affected than urban. The question remains whether Reye syndrome is a new disease or whether affected children have been heretofore classified as having disorders such as "postviral encephalopathy." It is very likely that mild cases are missed and recover without event. In any case, Reye syndrome may be the most common potentially lethal virus-associated encephalopathy in the United States.

Clinical Manifestations. The illness follows a stereotypic biphasic course. It usually occurs in a previously healthy child. A prodromal febrile illness, an upper respiratory tract infection (in 90% of the cases), or chickenpox (in 5–7%) is followed by an interval in which the child has seemingly recovered. The abrupt onset of protracted vomiting then occurs, usually within 5–7 days after the onset of the viral illness. Delirium and stupor may occur simultaneously or within a few hours after the onset of vomiting. Neurologic symptoms may rapidly progress to seizures, coma, and death; focal neurologic signs are absent. There is a slight to moderate liver enlargement with abnormalities of hepatic function; the patient remains anicteric. Cerebrospinal fluid is normal except for elevated pressure.

Diagnosis. The clinical features are best reflected in the system of clinical staging that has been proposed (Table 12–22); grades I through III represent mild to moderate illness, grades IV and V severe illness. The majority of affected children will have mild illness without progression.

There is explosive release from liver and muscle of such enzymes as aminotransferases, creatine kinase (CPK), and lactic dehydrogenase (LDH). The activity of the mitochondrial enzyme serum glutamate dehydrogenase (GDH) is greatly increased. Patients not in coma who have a 3-fold or higher elevation in serum ammonia level are more likely to progress to coma, as are patients who have hypoprothrombinemia unresponsive to vitamin K. Hyperaminoacidemia occurs, involving glutamine, alanine, and lysine. Increased concentrations of free fatty acids in plasma may contribute to depression of the central nervous system. In younger patients, there may be hypoglycemia.

Pathology. The striking and characteristic gross pathologic feature of Reye syndrome is a yellow to white liver, reflective of a high content of triglyceride. Light microscopy shows a uniform foaminess of liver cell cytoplasm with microvesicular fatty accumulation, which may be concealed in routine preparations. The fat stain of a frozen section readily displays the striking histologic abnormality. Triglyceride is distributed throughout the lobule in a monotonous, small droplet pattern affecting each cell. Histochemical study finds reduced activity of mitochondrial enzymes such as succinic acid dehydrogenase, while cytosolic enzyme activity is normal. Electron microscopic (EM) changes include a unique alteration of mitochondrial morphology: a slight rarification of the matrix occurs, with pleomorphism, swelling, and reduction in the number of mitochondria. Glycogen depletion may be noted, and the mitochondria may assume ameboid forms. Mitochondrial injury is uniformly severe; postmortem, the lesion resembles that seen with uncoupled respiration. During recovery, mitochondria divide, budding and branching forms appear, and the matrix and mitochondrial dense bodies rapidly return to normal (in 3–4 days). Liver biopsy is not essential for clinical diagnosis, but the information gained is crucial in precise definition of the syndrome. Biopsy should be carried out in atypical or severe cases in order to rule out other disorders, such as metabolic or toxic liver disease, especially in patients under 1 yr of age. Histologic examination of brain tissue has revealed a similar pattern of injury. Grossly, there is marked edema. Light microscopy reveals an absence of necrosis or inflammation; EM changes include edematous myelin sheaths, and neuronal mitochondria show the unique ultrastructural changes seen in liver.

Table 12–22. Clinical Staging of Reye Syndrome

Grade	Symptoms at Time of Admission
I	Usually quiet, **lethargic** and sleepy, vomiting, laboratory evidence of liver dysfunction
II	Deep lethargy, **confusion**, delirium, combative, hyperventilation, hyperreflexic
III	Obtunded, **light coma**, ± seizures, decorticate rigidity, intact pupillary light reaction
IV	Seizures, deepening coma, **decerebrate rigidity**, loss of oculocephalic reflexes, fixed pupils
V	Coma, loss of deep tendon reflexes, respiratory arrest, fixed dilated pupils, **flaccidity/decerebrate** (intermittent); isoelectric EEG

Pathogenesis. The major site of injury is the mitochondrion. The activities of hepatic intramitochondrial enzymes, including ornithine transcarbamylase (OTC), carbamylphosphate synthetase (CPS), and pyruvate dehydrogenase, are reduced, often to less than half their normal values. Hyperammonemia may result from decreases in the activities of OTC and CPS. Cytosolic enzyme activities are normal.

The reasons for mitochondrial dysfunction are unknown. Speculation must consider epidemiologic features (virus-related, age-related, individual susceptibility) and the possible concomitant influence of a toxin to which a viral infection may sensitize the host. No toxic factor has as yet been conclusively identified, but studies from three geographic areas have suggested an etiologic link between Reye syndrome and use of aspirin. Under what circumstances aspirin may serve as a cofactor (or comitochondrial toxin) in a susceptible host during a viral infection remains to be determined. Until the issue is resolved, it will be prudent to avoid use of aspirin as an antipyretic in patients with influenza or varicella.

Treatment. Successful management of Reye syndrome requires (1) early recognition of mild cases and (2) control of increased intracranial pressure (ICP) secondary to cerebral edema, which is the major lethal factor.

Early diagnosis may be aided by a high level of clinical suspicion and by assessment of hepatic function in suspected cases. Marked elevation of aminotransferase activities, prolongation of prothrombin time, and elevation of the serum ammonia level above 125–150 µg/dL will suggest the diagnosis. It is imperative that cerebral edema be identified and counteracted and that aerobic metabolism be maintained. Cerebral vasoconstriction can be induced without further impairment of perfusion. There is as yet no consensus regarding efficacy of several proposed methods of management.

Management will vary with the severity of the illness. Whereas observation alone may suffice in patients with grade 1 severity, more aggressive therapy will be needed in patients with more severe neurologic deterioration. All patients should initially receive glucose (10–15%) intravenously, since glycogen depletion is common. In patients with cerebral edema, the amount of fluid administered should be restricted to approximately 1500 mL/m²/day. Attempts should be made to maintain relative hypothermia.

In more severely ill, comatose patients, endotracheal intubation will permit adequate oxygenation; hyperventilation will induce hypocarbia, which will decrease cerebral blood flow by cerebral vasoconstriction. Close monitoring of ICP by means of devices emplaced in the epidural, subdural, or subarachnoid space or in the lateral ventricles will assist in decisions regarding management (see also Sec. 5.39). Stimulation of the patient should be minimized, since procedures such as suctioning may generate increases in ICP.

An indwelling arterial line will permit continuous assessment of cerebral perfusion pressure. Osmotherapy (mannitol 0.5–1.0 g/kg every 4–6 hr) should be used to maintain a serum osmolality of 300–320 mOsm/L and to induce cerebral dehydration; the ICP should be held to less than 20 mm Hg and the cerebral perfusion pressure to greater than 50 mm Hg. Pressure monitoring provides an effective guide to therapy with osmotic diuretics and may decrease renal complications due to hyperosmolarity. Use of pentobarbital (2.5 mg/kg) to maintain a serum barbiturate level of 20–30 µg/mL may have a protective effect on the central nervous system by decreasing cerebral metabolic demands, decreasing cerebral blood flow, and causing cerebral vasoconstriction. Pancuronium bromide has been used with the hope of decreasing cerebral blood volume through muscular relaxation and increased peripheral blood pooling.

Controlled trials are needed to establish the merits of various therapeutic regimens. In some patients in whom cerebral edema has not been controlled by the above procedures decompressive craniotomy has been done in hope of avoiding cerebral herniation. Success of this drastic procedure may depend on its timing in patients with rapidly evolving illness. Use of techniques such as portable radionuclide imaging to assess cerebral blood flow may provide guidance in the future.

Prognosis. The duration of disordered cerebral function during the acute stage of illness is the best predictor of eventual outcome. In patients with grade 1 disease, recovery is rapid and complete. In patients with more severe disease there may be subsequent subtle neuropsychologic defects noted (in intelligence, school achievement, visual-motor integration, and concept formation).

WILLIAM F. BALISTRERI

12.83 CHRONIC HEPATITIS

Chronic hepatitis is defined as a continuing hepatic inflammatory process lasting 6 mo or more. The severity is variable; the affected child may have only biochemical evidence of liver dysfunction, may have stigmata of chronic liver disease, or may present in hepatic failure.

Chronic hepatitis can be caused by persistent viral infection, drugs, or unknown factors. Approximately 15–20% of cases are associated with hepatitis B infection (Sec. 11.76); in this group of patients unusually severe disease may be caused by superimposed infection with the delta agent (a defective RNA virus that is dependent on replicating hepatitis B virus). Chronic hepatitis may also follow 30–50% of non-A–non-B forms of viral hepatitis. Patients receiving blood products or who have had massive transfusions are at increased risk. Hepatitis A virus does not cause chronic hepatitis. Drugs commonly used in children that may cause chronic liver injury include isoniazid, methyldopa, nitrofurantoin, dantrolene, and the sulfonamides.

In most cases, the cause of chronic hepatitis is unknown; in many, an autoimmune mechanism is suggested by the finding of antinuclear and anti–smooth muscle antibodies in serum and by multisystem involvement (including rashes, arthropathy, thyroiditis, and Coombs-positive hemolytic anemia). Histologic features have defined two major subdivisions of chronic hepatitis: *chronic persistent hepatitis* and *chronic active hepatitis*. The pathogenesis of each morphologic form is uncertain, but the criteria defining them predict a benign, self-limited course for chronic persistent hepatitis and a progressive course potentially leading to cirrhosis for chronic active hepatitis. Both forms are to be distinguished from unresolved or prolonged acute viral hepatitis in which clinical and biochemical abnormalities last 2–3 mo; liver biopsy in such cases shows predominantly single cell necrosis in the lobule, with minimal portal and lobular inflammation.

Chronic Persistent Hepatitis

Chronic persistent hepatitis is a generally benign inflammatory process of the liver. It most commonly follows acute hepatitis due to hepatitis B virus or to the viruses causing non-A–non-B hepatitis.

Pathology. The lobular architecture is always normal. Inflammation is limited to portal triads, and no significant fibrosis or cirrhosis is found.

Clinical Manifestations. Most patients with chronic persistent hepatitis are asymptomatic or have nonspecific complaints such as fatigue or anorexia. Some patients have minimal hepatomegaly or slight right upper quadrant tenderness. Historical features and physical stigmata of drug abuse should be sought in the adolescent.

There are mild to moderate elevations of serum aminotransferase activities and normal or only slightly increased serum bilirubin concentrations (predominantly of the direct-reacting fraction). Serum alkaline phosphatase (hepatic) activity, albumin level, and prothrombin time are normal. Serum globulin and IgG fraction concentrations are normal or only slightly increased. Tests for anti–smooth muscle and antinuclear antibodies have negative results. As many as one third of patients will be hepatitis B surface antigen (HBsAg) positive.

Diagnosis. There is considerable clinical and laboratory overlap between the variants of chronic hepatitis; accordingly, liver biopsy is essential to the diagnosis of chronic persistent hepatitis. Differential diagnosis should include biliary tract disease and the pericholangitis associated with inflammatory bowel disease.

Treatment and Prognosis. There is no specific treatment for chronic persistent hepatitis. The prognosis is good. Persistent carriers of HBsAg remain at increased risk for hepatocellular carcinoma.

Chronic Active Hepatitis

Chronic active hepatitis is characterized by unresolving inflammation, necrosis, and fibrosis, with the possibility of progression to cirrhosis and liver failure.

Etiology. Chronic active hepatitis may be caused by chronic infection with hepatitis B virus (15–20% of cases). Most patients, however, have no evidence of viral infection, drug, or metabolic liver injury as a cause for their liver disease. Some cases are presumably initiated by infection with a virus causing non-A–non-B hepatitis; in others, clinical features strongly suggest an autoimmune mechanism.

Pathology. The histologic features common to untreated cases include (1) inflammatory infiltrates, consisting of lymphocytes and plasma cells, which expand portal areas and often penetrate the lobule; (2) moderate to severe "piecemeal" necrosis of hepatocytes extending outward from the limiting plate; and (3) variable necrosis, fibrosis, and zones of parenchymal collapse spanning neighboring portal triads or between a portal triad and central vein (bridging necrosis). Distortion of hepatic architecture may be severe; cirrhosis may be found in children at the time of diagnosis.

Clinical Manifestations. The clinical features and course of chronic active hepatitis are extremely variable. Some patients develop chronic active hepatitis following a well-defined episode of hepatitis B infection or post-transfusion non-A–non-B hepatitis; and in 25–30% of patients, particularly children, the illness may mimic acute viral hepatitis. In the majority of patients, however, the onset is insidious. About half of the patients are less than 20 yr of age; most HBsAg-negative patients are female. Patients may be asymptomatic or have fatigue, malaise, behavioral changes, anorexia, and amenorrhea, sometimes for many months before jaundice or stigmata of chronic liver disease are recognized. Extrahepatic manifestations may include arthritis, vasculitis, and nephritis in HBsAg-positive patients, presumably secondary to deposition of hepatitis B antigen-antibody immune complexes. Thyroiditis, Coombs-positive anemia, arthritis, and rash are common in patients with the autoimmune or "lupoid" variety of chronic active hepatitis. Some patients' initial clinical features may reflect cirrhosis (ascites, bleeding esophageal varices, or hepatic encephalopathy).

There is usually mild to moderate jaundice. Spider telangiectasias and palmar erythema may be present. The liver is often tender and slightly enlarged but may not be felt in patients with cirrhosis. The spleen is commonly enlarged. Edema and ascites may be present in advanced cases. Evidence of involvement of other organ systems may be found. Classic features of autoimmune hepatitis (including cushingoid appearance, acne, hirsutism, and striae) occur in a minority of patients.

Laboratory studies reveal moderate elevation (usually less than 1000 IU/L) of serum aminotransferase activities. Serum bilirubin concentrations (predominantly the direct reacting fraction) are commonly 2–10 mg/dL. Serum alkaline phosphatase activity is normal to slightly increased. Serum gamma-globulin levels show marked polyclonal elevations in most patients but may be normal to only slightly increased in HBsAg-positive patients. Hypoalbuminemia is common. The prothrombin time is prolonged, most often as a result of vitamin K deficiency but also as a reflection of impaired hepatocellular function. A normochromic, normocytic anemia, leukopenia, and thrombocytopenia are present and usually become more severe with evolution of portal hypertension and hypersplenism. Evidence of hepatitis B infection (HBsAg, anti-HBc, and HBeAg) may be found. LE cells and autoantibodies may be detected, including antinuclear, smooth muscle, and mitochondrial antibodies.

Diagnosis. The diagnosis of chronic active hepatitis is established by liver biopsy. The differential diagnosis should include α_1-antitrypsin deficiency (Sec. 12.79) and Wilson disease (Sec. 12.76). Chronic active hepatitis may occur in patients with inflammatory bowel disease, but liver dysfunction in such patients is more commonly due to pericholangitis or sclerosing cholangitis.

Treatment. Controlled studies of the drug treatment of chronic active hepatitis have been conducted only in adults, but several retrospective studies in children and adolescents suggest that they respond similarly to immunosuppressive therapy. It is clear that corticosteroid therapy, with or without low doses of azathioprine, improves the clinical, biochemical, and histologic features in most patients with chronic active hepatitis and prolongs survival in most patients with severe disease. Chronic hepatitis B, on the other hand, usually responds poorly to steroid therapy, and recent studies suggest an increased frequency of complications, a higher death rate, and enhanced viral replication in steroid-treated patients. Chronic non-A–non-B hepatitis following blood transfusion has a fluctuating clinical and biochemical course that often improves spontaneously; here the role of drug therapy is uncertain. In severe chronic active hepatitis, after exclusion of HBsAg-positive and transfusion-related cases, the course and response to drug therapy appear to be similar whether or not autoimmune features are present.

The goal of treatment is to suppress or eliminate hepatic inflammation with minimal side effects. Prednisone is given at an initial dose of 1–2 mg/kg/day and continued until aminotransferase values return to a level twice the upper limit of normal. The dose should then be lowered in 5 mg decrements over a 4–6 wk period, until a maintenance dose of less than 20 mg/day is achieved. In patients who respond poorly, who develop severe side effects, or who cannot be maintained on low dose steroids, azathioprine (1.5 mg/kg/day, up to 50 mg/day) may be added, with frequent monitoring for bone marrow suppression. Alternate-day corticosteroid therapy should be used with great caution. In adults, this form of treatment produced improvement or even normalization of serum aminotransferase activities, but histologic resolution did not occur.

Histologic progress should be assessed by liver biopsy 6 mo–1 yr after initiation of treatment, as normal results of biochemical tests during therapy do not ensure histologic resolution. Disappearance of symptoms and biochemical abnormalities, and either resolution of the necroinflammatory process on biopsy or at least improvement to a pattern of chronic persistent hepatitis, justify an attempt at gradual discontinuation of medication.

Prognosis. Treatment of chronic active hepatitis will significantly improve survival in the majority of HBsAg-negative patients. Over 75% of patients can be expected to respond to therapy. In patients meeting the criteria for withdrawal of treatment, 50% can be successfully weaned from medication; in the other 50%, relapse occurs after a variable period of time, but this will usually respond to re-treatment. Progression to cirrhosis can occur, despite a good response to drug therapy and prolongation of life.

12.84 DRUG- AND TOXIN-INDUCED LIVER INJURY

The liver is the main site of drug metabolism and is particularly susceptible to structural and functional injury following ingestion, parenteral administration, or inhalation of chemical agents, drugs, or environmental toxins. The possibility of drug use or toxin exposure at home or in the parental workplace should be explored for every child with liver dysfunction. More drugs with hepatotoxic potential become available each year for use in children. The clinical spectrum of illness may vary from asymptomatic biochemical abnormalities of liver function to fulminant failure. Children may be more or less susceptible than adults to hepatotoxic effects; for example, liver injury after the use of the anesthetic halothane is rare in children, whereas most cases of fatal hepatotoxicity associated with sodium valproate have been reported in children. In some cases, immaturity of hepatic drug metabolic pathways may prevent degradation of a toxic agent; under other circumstances, the same immaturity might limit formation of toxic metabolites.

Chemical hepatotoxicity may be (1) *predictable* or *intrinsic*, or (2) *idiosyncratic* (Table 12–23). *Predictable* hepatotoxicity implies a high incidence of hepatic injury in exposed individuals, with dose-dependency. The agents involved may damage the hepatocyte directly through alteration of membrane lipids (peroxidation) or through denaturation of proteins; such agents include carbon tetrachloride and trichloroethylene. Indirect injury may occur through interference with metabolic pathways essential for cell integrity or through distortion of cellular constituents by covalent binding of a reactive metabolite; examples include the liver injury produced by acetaminophen or by antimetabolites such as methotrexate or 6-mercaptopurine.

Idiosyncratic hepatotoxicity is infrequent and unpredictable. The likelihood of injury is not dose-dependent and may occur at any time during exposure to the agent. An idiosyncratic reaction may be immunologically mediated as a result of prior sensitization (hypersensitivity); extrahepatic manifestations of hypersensitivity may include fever, rash, arthralgia, and eosinophilia. Duration of exposure before reaction is generally 1–4 wk, with prompt recurrence of injury on re-exposure. Idiosyncratic drug reactions in certain patients may reflect aberrant pathways for drug metabolism, with production of toxic intermediates (isoniazid and sodium valproate may cause liver damage through this mechanism). Duration of drug usage prior to liver injury is variable (weeks to 1 yr or more), and the response to re-exposure may be delayed.

The pathologic spectrum of drug-induced liver disease is extremely wide, rarely specific, and may mimic other liver diseases. The only histologic abnormalities may be nonspecific reactive hepatitis (aspirin), fat accumulation (tetracycline), or cholestasis (chlorpromazine). Features of acute (isoniazid) or chronic (methyldopa) hepatitis may be present. Massive zonal necrosis may be caused by some agents (including acetaminophen and carbon tetrachloride); other agents produce vascular lesions, such as hepatic vein thrombosis (oral contraceptives), veno-occlusive disease (antineoplastic drugs), and peliosis hepatis (anabolic steroids). Hepatic adenoma, carcinoma, and focal nodular hyperplasia have been associated with oral contraceptives and androgens.

Symptoms may be mild and nonspecific, such as fever and malaise; and signs of liver dysfunction may be confused with those of the underlying disorder. The differential diagnosis

Table 12–23. Drug- and Toxin-Induced Liver Injury

Category	Incidence	Experimental Reproducibility	Dose Dependency	Mechanism	Histologic Lesion	Example
Predictable						
Direct	high	+	+	Direct damage to membrane cell protein	Necrosis	Carbon tetrachloride
Indirect						
cytotoxic	high	+	+	Interfere with metabolic pathway	Necrosis, steatosis	Acetaminophen, ethanol
cholestatic	high	+	+	Interfere with bile excretory mechanisms	Cholestasis	Androgens
Idiosyncratic						
Hypersensitivity	low	−	−	Immunologic	Necrosis, cholestasis	Phenytoin
Metabolic abnormality	low	−	−	Hepatotoxic metabolites	Necrosis ± cholestasis ± steatosis	Isoniazid, halothane, valproic acid

After Zimmerman M: Hepatotoxicity, The Adverse Effects of Drugs and Other Chemicals on the Liver. New York, Appleton-Century-Crofts, 1979.

should include acute and chronic viral hepatitis, biliary tract disease, septicemia, ischemic and hypoxic liver injury, malignant infiltration, and inherited metabolic liver disease.

The laboratory features of drug- or toxin-related liver disease are extremely variable. Hepatocyte damage may lead to elevations of serum aminotransferase activities and serum bilirubin levels, and to impaired synthetic function as evidenced by decreased serum coagulation factors and albumin. Hyperammonemia may occur with liver failure or with selective inhibition of the urea cycle (sodium valproate). Toxicologic screening of blood and urine specimens may aid detection of drug or toxin exposure. Percutaneous liver biopsy may be necessary to distinguish drug injury from complications of an underlying disorder or from intercurrent infection.

Slight elevation of serum aminotransferase activities (generally less than two to three times normal) may occur during therapy with drugs capable of inducing microsomal pathways for drug metabolism. Liver biopsy reveals proliferation of smooth endoplasmic reticulum but no significant liver injury. Liver test abnormalities often resolve with continued drug therapy.

Treatment of drug- or toxin-related liver injury is largely supportive. Contact with the offending agent should be avoided.

The prognosis of drug- or toxin-induced liver injury depends on its type and severity. Injury is usually completely reversible when the hepatotoxic factor is withdrawn. The mortality of submassive hepatic necrosis with fulminant liver failure may, however, exceed 50%. With continued use of certain drugs, such as methotrexate, effects of hepatoxicity may progress insidiously to cirrhosis. Neoplasia may follow long-term androgen therapy. Rechallenge with a drug suspected of having caused previous liver injury is rarely justified and may result in fatal hepatic necrosis.

12.85 FULMINANT HEPATIC FAILURE

Fulminant hepatic failure is a clinical syndrome resulting from massive necrosis of hepatocytes or from severe functional impairment of hepatocytes in a patient who may or may not have had pre-existing liver disease. The disorder usually evolves over a period of less than 8 wk. Synthetic, excretory, and detoxifying functions of the liver are all severely impaired, with hepatic encephalopathy an essential diagnostic criterion.

Etiology. Fulminant hepatic failure is most commonly a complication of viral hepatitis (A, B, or non-A–non-B). Over 50% of patients with fulminant viral hepatitis are hepatitis B surface antigen (HBsAg) positive. An unusually high risk of fulminant hepatic failure occurs in young people who have combined infections with the hepatitis B virus and the delta agent. Epstein-Barr virus, herpes simplex virus, and enterovirus infections may produce fulminant hepatitis in children.

A variety of hepatotoxic drugs and chemicals may also cause fulminant hepatic failure. Predictable liver injury may occur after exposure to carbon tetrachloride or after acetaminophen overdose. Idiosyncratic damage may follow use of drugs such as halothane or sodium valproate. Ischemia and hypoxia resulting from hepatic vascular occlusion, congestive heart failure, cyanotic congenital heart disease, or circulatory shock may produce liver failure. Metabolic disorders associated with hepatic failure include Wilson disease, acute fatty liver of pregnancy, galactosemia, hereditary tyrosinemia, and hereditary fructose intolerance.

Pathology. Liver biopsy usually reveals massive necrosis of hepatocytes, patchy or confluent. Multilobular or bridging necrosis may be associated with collapse of the reticulin framework of the liver. A zonal pattern of necrosis may be observed with certain insults (e.g., centrilobular damage is associated with acetaminophen hepatotoxicity or with circulatory shock). Hepatocytes may also show swelling and vacuolation; formation of acidophilic bodies may be prominent in viral hepatitis. A mixed inflammatory cell infiltrate is usually present. Evidence of severe hepatocyte dysfunction rather than cell necrosis may occasionally be the predominant histologic finding (e.g., microvesicular fatty infiltrate of hepatocytes is observed in Reye syndrome and in tetracycline toxicity).

Pathogenesis. The mechanisms that lead to fulminant hepatic failure are poorly understood. It is unknown why only about 1–2% of patients with viral hepatitis develop liver failure. Massive destruction of hepatocytes may represent both a direct cytotoxic effect of the virus and an immune response to the viral antigens. Formation of hepatotoxic metabolites that bind covalently to macromolecular cell constituents is involved in the liver injury produced by drugs such as acetaminophen and isoniazid; fulminant hepatic failure may follow depletion of intracellular substrates involved in detoxification, particularly glutathione. Whatever the initial cause of hepatocyte injury, a variety of factors may contribute to the pathogenesis of liver failure, including impaired hepatocyte regeneration, altered parenchymal perfusion, endotoxemia, and decreased hepatic reticuloendothelial function.

Clinical Manifestations. Fulminant hepatic failure may complicate previously known acute liver disease or be the presenting feature of liver disease. Progressive jaundice, fetor hepaticus, fever, anorexia, vomiting, and abdominal pain are common. A rapid decrease in liver size without clinical improvement is an ominous sign. A hemorrhagic diathesis and ascites may develop. Patients should be closely observed for hepatic encephalopathy, which is initially characterized by minor disturbances of consciousness or motor function. Irritability, poor feeding, and a change in sleep rhythm may be the only findings in infants; asterixis may be demonstrable in older children. The patient may rapidly progress to deeper stages of coma in which extensor responses and decerebrate and decorticate posturing appear. Respirations are usually increased early, but respiratory failure may occur in stage IV coma.

Laboratory Findings. Serum direct and indirect bilirubin levels and serum aminotransferase activities may be markedly elevated but do not correlate well with the severity of the illness. Serum aminotransferase activities may decrease as the patient worsens clinically. The blood ammonia concentration is usually increased. Prothrombin time is always prolonged and often does not improve after parenteral administration of vitamin K. Hypoglycemia can occur, particularly in infants. Electrolyte and acid-base disturbances are common.

Treatment. Management of fulminant hepatic failure is supportive. No therapy is known to reverse hepatocyte injury or to promote hepatic regeneration.

The infant or child with advanced hepatic coma should be treated in an intensive care unit where continuous monitoring of vital functions is possible. Endotracheal intubation may be required to prevent aspiration and facilitate pulmonary toilet. Mechanical ventilation and supplemental oxygen are often necessary in advanced coma. Electrolyte and glucose solutions should be administered intravenously to maintain urine output, to correct or prevent hypoglycemia, and to maintain normal serum potassium concentrations. Hyponatremia is common but is usually dilutional and not a result of sodium depletion. Parenteral supplementation with calcium, phosphorus, and magnesium may be required. Coagulopathy should be treated with parenteral administration of vitamin K and may require fresh-frozen plasma; disseminated intravascular coagulation may also occur. Prophylactic use of antacids or H_2 receptor blockers or both should be considered because of the high risk of gastrointestinal bleeding. Hypovolemia should be avoided and treated with cautious infusions of fluids and blood products. Renal dysfunction may occur from dehydration, from acute tubular necrosis, or from functional renal failure (hepatorenal syndrome). The patient should be closely followed for infection, including sepsis, pneumonia, peritonitis, and urinary tract infections. Cerebral edema is an extremely serious complication that responds poorly to such measures as corticosteroid administration and osmotic diuresis.

The pathogenesis of hepatic encephalopathy remains unclear, but likely factors include enteric production of ammonia and other toxins. Gastrointestinal hemorrhage, infection, constipation, sedatives, electrolyte imbalance, and hypovolemia may act as precipitating factors and should be identified and corrected. Protein intake should be restricted or eliminated. The gut should be purged with several enemas. Lactulose should be given every 2–4 hr orally or by nasogastric tube in doses (10–50 mL) sufficient to cause diarrhea. The dose is then adjusted to produce several acidic, loose bowel movements daily. Lactulose syrup diluted with 1–3 volumes of water may also be given as a retention enema every 6 hr. Lactulose, a nonabsorbable disaccharide, is metabolized to organic acids by colonic bacteria; it probably lowers blood ammonia levels through decreasing microbial ammonia production and through trapping of ammonia in acidic intestinal contents.

Controlled trials have shown a worsened outcome of fulminant hepatic failure in patients treated with corticosteroids. Exchange transfusion, cross circulation with a human volunteer or baboon, and hemoperfusion through charcoal or polyacrylonitrile membranes are not of proven benefit.

Prognosis. In patients who progress to stage IV coma, prognosis is poor. A major complication such as sepsis, severe hemorrhage, or renal failure reduces the chance for survival. Severe coagulopathy (factor VII level less than 8% of normal) is associated with a poor prognosis. The prognosis for children may be somewhat better than for adults, but mortality exceeds 60–70%. Several studies indicate that patients who recover from fulminant hepatic failure do not usually develop cirrhosis or chronic liver disease. Orthotopic liver transplantation may be life-saving in patients who reach advanced stages of hepatic coma.

12.86 CYSTIC DISEASES OF THE BILIARY TRACT AND LIVER

Cystic lesions of liver parenchyma or of the biliary system may be recognized initially during infancy and childhood. Their classification is not yet satisfactory. Pathologic features may be found in common among several of these disorders, but different patterns of inheritance indicate that their etiology is heterogeneous.

Choledochal Cysts. A congenital saccular dilatation of the common bile duct is the most common form of choledochal cyst. Diffuse fusiform cysts, small localized dilatations, or diverticula also occur. Dilatation of the intraduodenal portion of the common duct (choledochocele) may be a variant. Dilatation of the intrahepatic bile ducts may be associated with choledochal cyst.

The pathogenesis of choledochal cysts remains uncertain. Some reports have suggested that junction of the common bile duct and the pancreatic duct before their entry into the sphincter of Oddi may allow reflux of pancreatic enzymes into the common bile duct, causing inflammation, localized weakness, and dilatation of the duct. Other possibilities are that choledochal cysts represent malformations of the common duct or occur as part of the disease spectrum that includes neonatal hepatitis and biliary atresia.

Approximately 75% of cases appear during childhood. The classic triad of abdominal pain, jaundice, and mass occurs in only one third of patients. Features of acute cholangitis (including fever, right upper quadrant tenderness, jaundice, and leukocytosis) may be present. The diagnosis may be best made by ultrasonography.

The treatment of choice is primary excision of the cyst and a Roux-en-Y choledochojejunostomy. Simple drainage into the small bowel is less satisfactory owing to a risk for development of carcinoma in the residual cystic tissue. The postoperative course may be complicated by recurrent cholangitis or stricture at the anastomotic site.

Cystic Dilatation of the Intrahepatic Bile Ducts (Caroli Disease). Congenital, saccular dilatation may affect multiple segments of the intrahepatic bile ducts; the dilated ducts are lined by cuboidal epithelium and are in continuity with the main duct system, which is usually normal. There is a marked predisposition to ascending cholangitis and calculus formation within the abnormal bile ducts. Choledochal cysts, features of congenital hepatic fibrosis, and renal tubular ectasia may be associated. The disorder is not thought to be familial.

Affected patients usually develop symptoms of acute cholangitis as children or young adults. Fever, abdominal pain, mild jaundice, and pruritus occur; and a slightly enlarged, tender liver is palpable. Elevated alkaline phosphatase activity, direct-reacting bilirubin levels, and leukocytosis may be observed during episodes of acute infection. Ultrasonography shows the dilated intrahepatic ducts, but definitive diagnosis and extent of disease must be determined by percutaneous transhepatic cholangiography.

Cholangitis and sepsis are treated with appropriate antibiotics. Calculi may require surgery. Partial hepatectomy may be curative in rare cases, when disease is confined to a single lobe. The prognosis is otherwise guarded, largely owing to difficulties in controlling cholangitis and biliary lithiasis.

Congenital Hepatic Fibrosis. This is an autosomal-recessive disorder characterized pathologically by diffuse periportal and perilobular fibrosis in broad bands that contain distorted bile duct-like structures and that often compress or incorporate central or sublobular veins. The duct-like structures may become dilated to the point of microcyst formation but do not communicate with the biliary tract. Irregularly shaped islands of liver parenchyma contain normal-appearing hepatocytes. Caroli disease and choledochal cysts have been associated (see above). About 75% of patients have renal disease, such as renal tubular ectasia, nephronophthisis, or childhood polycystic disease.

The disorder usually has its clinical onset in childhood, with hepatosplenomegaly or with bleeding secondary to portal hypertension. Cholangitis may occur in patients who have associated abnormalities of bile ducts.

Serum aminotransferase activities and bilirubin levels are usually normal; serum alkaline phosphatase activity may be slightly elevated. The serum albumin level and prothrombin time are normal. Liver biopsy is essential for diagnosis.

Treatment of this disorder should focus on control of bleeding from esophageal varices. Infrequent mild bleeding episodes may be managed by endoscopic sclerotherapy of the varices. Following more severe hemorrhage, portacaval anastomosis may bring relief of portal hypertension. The prognosis may be greatly improved by a shunting procedure, but survival in some patients may be limited by renal failure.

A **solitary liver cyst** (nonparasitic) occurs rarely in childhood. Abdominal distention and pain may be present, and poorly defined right upper quadrant mass may be palpable. These benign lesions are best left undisturbed unless they compress adjacent structures or a complication occurs, such as hemorrhage into the cyst.

Adult-type polycystic disease of the kidney is associated with multiple cysts of the liver. This disorder is autosomal dominant, with a high degree of penetrance. The cysts probably arise from defective development of intrahepatic bile ducts. The liver may be normal-sized or markedly enlarged. Most of the affected children are asymptomatic; the prognosis is determined by the severity of the cystic renal disease.

Childhood polycystic disease of the kidneys and liver is inherited as an autosomal recessive trait. Death from renal failure is common within the first weeks or months of life in infants whose kidneys are massively enlarged with cysts. The liver lesion in these patients consists of a striking increase in the number of bile ducts, which are irregularly dilated in all portal areas; mild to moderate portal fibrosis is present.

Portal hypertension may arise in infants who survive the 1st yr. In older children, dilatation of bile ducts is less prominent, but the portal fibrosis is much more severe. The hepatic lesion at this stage may be indistinguishable from that of congenital hepatic fibrosis.

Variable abnormalities of bile ducts (irregular dilatation, proliferation, cysts) and portal fibrosis may be associated with Meckel syndrome, with trisomy 17-18, with tuberous sclerosis, and with asphyxiating thoracic dystrophy.

12.87 DISEASES OF THE GALLBLADDER

Anomalies. The gallbladder is congenitally absent in about 0.1% of the population. Hypoplasia or absence of the gallbladder may be associated with extrahepatic biliary atresia or cystic fibrosis. Duplication of the gallbladder occurs rarely.

Acute Hydrops. Acute noncalculous, noninflammatory distention of the gallbladder may occur in infants and children. The disorder may complicate acute infections including scarlet fever, leptospirosis, and Kawasaki disease, but the cause is often not identified. Hydrops of the gallbladder may also develop in patients receiving long-term parenteral nutrition, presumably as a result of gallbladder stasis during the period of enteral fasting.

Affected patients usually have right upper quadrant pain with a palpable mass. Fever and jaundice may be present. Ultrasonography may help in establishing the diagnosis. Acute hydrops is usually treated by cholecystostomy and drainage. At laparotomy, a large, edematous gallbladder is found that contains white, yellow, or green bile. Obstruction of the cystic duct by mesenteric adenopathy is occasionally observed. Cholecystectomy is required if the gallbladder is gangrenous. Pathologic examination of the gallbladder wall shows edema and mild inflammation. Cultures of bile are usually sterile.

Acute acalculous cholecystitis is uncommon in children and is usually caused by infection. Reported pathogens include streptococci (groups A and B) and gram-negative organisms, particularly *Salmonella*. Parasitic infestation with ascaris or *Giardia lamblia* may be found. Acalculous cholecystitis may rarely follow abdominal trauma or be associated with a systemic vasculitis, such as periarteritis nodosa. It has been reported in association with Kawasaki disease.

Clinical features include right upper quadrant or epigastric pain, nausea, vomiting, fever, and sometimes jaundice. Right upper quadrant guarding and tenderness are present. Ultrasonography discloses an enlarged, thick-walled gallbladder, without calculi. Serum alkaline phosphatase activity and direct-reacting bilirubin levels are elevated. Leukocytosis is usual.

The diagnosis is confirmed at laparotomy. Cholecystectomy and treatment of the systemic infection are required.

Cholelithiasis is relatively rare in otherwise healthy children, occurring more commonly in patients with a variety of predisposing disorders. The frequencies of pigmented and of cholesterol gallstones in children are approximately equal.

The most important clinical feature is recurrent abdominal pain, which is often colicky and localized to the right upper quadrant. The older child may have intolerance for fatty foods. Acute cholecystitis may be the first manifestation, with fever, pain in the right upper quadrant, and often a palpable mass. Pain may radiate to an area just below the right scapula. A plain roentgenogram of the abdomen may reveal opaque calculi, but radiolucent (cholesterol) stones will not be visualized. Accordingly, ultrasonography is the method of choice for gallstone detection. Cholecystectomy is usually curative; operative cholangiography should be done at the time of surgery to exclude common duct calculi.

Patients with hemolytic disease (including sickle cell anemia, the thalassemias, and red cell enzymopathies) and Wilson disease are at increased risk for pigmented cholelithiasis. Increasing numbers of sick premature infants are being found to have gallstones; their management is often complicated by such factors as bowel resection, necrotizing enterocolitis, prolonged parenteral nutrition without enteral feeding, cholestasis, frequent blood transfusions, and use of diuretics.

Cholesterol cholelithiasis in children most frequently affects obese adolescent girls. Cholesterol gallstones are found also in children with disturbances of the enterohepatic circulation of bile acids, including patients with ileal disease and bile acid malabsorption, such as those with ileal resection, ileal Crohn disease, and cystic fibrosis. Chronic cholestasis increases the risk for cholesterol gallstones.

Cholesterol gallstone formation seems to result from an excess of cholesterol in relation to the cholesterol-carrying capacity of micelles in bile. Supersaturation of bile with cholesterol leading to crystal and stone formation could result from decreased bile acid or from an increased cholesterol concentration in bile. Other initiating factors that may be important in stone formation include gallbladder stasis or the presence in bile of abnormal mucoproteins or bile pigments that may serve as a nidus for cholesterol crystallization.

FREDERICK J. SUCHY

Development of Hepatic Structure And Function

Structural Morphogenesis

Andres JM, Mathis RK, Walker WA: Liver disease in infants: Part I and II: Developmental hepatology and mechanisms of liver dysfunction. J Pediatr 90:686, 964, 1977.
Rudolph AM: Hepatic and ductus venosus blood flows during fetal life. Hepatology 3:254, 1983.

Ultrastructure of the Hepatocyte

Jones AL, Schmucker DL: Current concept of liver structure as related to function. Gastroenterology 73:833, 1977.
Jones AL, Schmucker DL, Renston RH, et al: The architecture of bile secretion: A morphological perspective of physiology. Dig Dis Sci 25:609, 1980.

Functional Development

Greengard O: Enzymic differentiation of human liver: Comparison with the rat model. Pediatr Res 11:669, 1977.
Henning SJ: Postnatal development: Coordination of feeding, digestion, and metabolism. Am J Physiol 241:G199, 1981.
Soyka LF, Redmond GP (eds): Drug Metabolism in the Immature Human. Raven Press, New York, 1981.

Hepatic Excretory Function

Balistreri WF, Heubi JE, Suchy FJ: Immaturity of the enterohepatic circulation in early life: Factors predisposing to "physiologic" maldigestion and cholestasis. J Pediatr Gastroenterol Nutr 2:346, 1983.
Blitzer BL, Boyer JL: Cellular mechanisms of bile formation. Gastroenterology 82:346, 1982.
Balistreri WF: The enterohepatic circulation of bile acids in early life. In: Neonatal Cholestasis: Causes, Syndromes, Therapies. Report of the 87th Ross Conference on Pediatric Research—Neonatal Cholestasis. Columbus, OH, Ross Laboratories, 1984, pp 38–47.

Pathologic Alterations Manifest as Liver Disease

Tumors

Ishak KG, Glunz PR: Hepatoblastoma and hepatocarcinoma in infancy and childhood: Report of 47 cases. Cancer 20:396, 1967.
Smuckler EA: The biochemical basis of acute liver cell injury. In: Good RA, Day SB, Yunis JJ (eds): Molecular Pathology. Springfield, IL, Charles C Thomas, 1975, p 490.

Manifestations of Hepatic Disease

Bichet DG, Van Putten VJ, Schrier RW: Potential role of increased sympathetic activity in impaired sodium and water excretion in cirrhosis. N Engl J Med 307:1552, 1982.
Carroll BA, Oppenheimer DA, Muller HH: High-frequency realtime ultrasound of the neonatal biliary system. Radiology 145:437, 1982.
Reiff MI, Osborn LM: Clinical estimation of liver size in newborn infants. Pediatrics 71:46, 1983.

Biochemical Evaluation of the Patient with Possible Hepatic Dysfunction

Balistreri WF: Age-related alterations in hepatic structure and function. In: Children Are Different, 3rd ed, Columbus, OH, Ross Laboratories, 1985.
Berger PE, Kuhn JP: Computed tomography of the hepatobiliary system in infancy and childhood. Radiol Clin North Am 19:431, 1981.

Ferrucci JT, Adson MA, Mueller PR, et al: Advances in the radiology of jaundice: A symposium and review. Am J Roentgenol 141:1, 1983.
Riddlesberger MM Jr: Diagnostic imaging of the hepatobiliary system in infants and children. J Pediatr Gastroenterol Nutr 3:653, 1984.

Specific Diseases of the Liver

Neonatal Cholestasis

Alagille D, Odievre M, Gautier M, et al: Hepatic ductular hypoplasia associated with characteristic facies, vertebral malformation, retarded physical, mental and sexual development and cardiac murmur. J Pediatr 86:63, 1975.
Altman RP: The portoenterostomy procedure for biliary atresia: A 5-year experience. Ann Surg 188:351, 1978.
Alvarez F, Bernard O, Brunelle F, et al: Portal obstruction in children. I. Clinical investigation and hemorrhage risk. Portal obstruction in children. II. Results of surgical portosystemic shunts. J Pediatr 103:696, 703, 1983.
Back P: Phenobarbital-induced alterations of bile acid metabolism in cases of intrahepatic cholestasis. Klin Wochenschr 60:541, 1982.
Balistreri WF: The effects of liver disease on nutrition and growth. In: Cohen SA (ed): The Underweight Child. Norwalk CT, Appleton-Century-Crofts, 1986, pp 121–130.
Balistreri WF: Neonatal cholestasis—medical progress. J Pediatr 106:171, 1985.
Brough AJ, Bernstein J: Conjugated hyperbilirubinemia in early infancy: A reassessment of liver biopsy. Hum Pathol 5:507, 1974.
Danks DM, Campbell PE, Jack I, et al: Studies of the aetiology of neonatal hepatitis and biliary atresia. Arch Dis Child 52:360, 1977.
Danks DM, Campbell PE, Smith AL, et al: Prognosis of babies with neonatal hepatitis. Arch Dis Child 52:368, 1977.
Drop SLS, Colle E, Guyda HJ: Hyperbilirubinaemia and idiopathic hypopituitarism in the newborn period. Acta Paediatr Scand 68:277, 1979.
Fonkalsrud EW: Shunt operations for portal hypertension in children. J Pediatr 103:741, 1983.
Howard ER, Stamatakis JD, Mowat AP: Management of esophageal varices in children by injection sclerotherapy. J Pediatr Surg 19:2, 1984.
Hyams JS, Leichtner AM, Schwartz AN: Recent advances in diagnosis and treatment of gastrointestinal hemorrhage in infants and children. J Pediatr 106:1, 1985.
Kasai M: Treatment of biliary atresia with special reference to hepatic portoenterostomy and its modifications. Prog Pediatr Surg 6:5, 1974.
Kasai M, Watanabe I, Ohi R: Follow-up studies of long-term survivors after hepatic portoenterostomy for "non-correctable" biliary atresia. J Pediatr Surg 10:173, 1975.
LaBrecque DR, Mitros FA, Nathan RJ, et al: Four generations of arteriohepatic dysplasia. Hepatology 4:467, 1982.
Landing BH: Consideration of the pathogenesis of neonatal hepatitis, biliary atresia, and choledochal cyst: The concept of infantile obstructive cholangiopathy. Prog Pediatr Surg 6:113, 1974.
Morecki R, Glaser JH, Cho S, et al: Biliary atresia and reovirus 3 infection. N Engl J Med 307:481, 1982.
Mowat AP, Psacharopoulos HT, Williams R: Extrahepatic biliary atresia versus neonatal hepatitis: Review of 137 prospectively investigated infants. Arch Dis Child 51:763, 1976.
Rosenblum JL, Keating JP, Prensky AL, et al: A progressive neurologic syndrome in children with chronic liver disease. N Engl J Med 304:503, 1981.
Starzl TE: Portal vein thrombosis and portal diversion. J Pediatr 103:741, 1983.
Weber A, Tuchweber B, Yousef I, et al: Severe familial cholestasis in North American Indian children: A clinical model of microfilament dysfunction? Gastroenterology 81:653, 1981.

Transplantation

Iwatsuki S, Shaw BW Jr, Starzl TE: Liver transplantation for biliary atresia. World J Surg 8:51, 1984.
Starzl TE, Iwatsuki S, Van Thiel DH, et al: Evolution of liver transplantation. Hepatology 2:614, 1982.
Zitelli BJ, Gartner JC, Malatack JJ, et al: Hepatic homograft survival in pediatric orthotopic liver transplantation with cyclosporine and steroids. Transplan Proc 15(Suppl 1):2592, 1983.

Metabolic Diseases of the Liver

Heymans HSA, Schutgens RBH, Tan R, et al: Severe plasmalogen deficiency in tissues of infants without peroxisomes (Zellweger syndrome). Nature 306:69, 1983.
Lefkowitch JH, Honig CL, King ME, et al: Hepatic copper overload and features of Indian childhood cirrhosis in an American sibship. N Engl J Med 307:271, 1982.
McCullough AJ, Fleming CR, Thistle JL, et al: Diagnosis of Wilson's Disease presenting as fulminant hepatic failure. Gastroenterology 84:161, 1983.
Moser AE, Singh I, Brown FR, et al: The cerebrohepatorenal (Zellweger) syndrome: Increased levels and impaired degradation of very-long-chain fatty acids and their use in prenatal diagnosis. N Engl J Med 310:1141, 1984.
Nebbia G, Hadchouel M, Odievre M, et al: Early assessment of evolution of liver disease associated with α-1-antitrypsin deficiency in childhood. J Pediatr 102:661, 1983.

Sveger T: Liver diseases in alpha-1-antitrypsin deficiency detected by screening of 200,000 infants. N Engl J Med 294:1316, 1976.

Tanner MS, Kantarjian AK, Bhave SA, et al: Early introduction of copper-contaminated animal milk feeds as a possible cause of Indian childhood cirrhosis. Lancet 2:992, 1983.

Werlin SL, Grand RJ, Perman JA, et al: Diagnostic dilemmas of Wilson's disease: Diagnosis and treatment. Pediatrics 62:47, 1978.

Miscellaneous

Jones EA, Schafer DF, Ferenci P, et al: The neurobiology of hepatic encephalopathy. Hepatology 4:1235, 1984.

Levy M, Wexler MJ: Salt and water balance in liver disease. Hosp Pract 19:57, 1984.

Oldham KT, Guice KS, Kaufman RA, et al: Blunt hepatic injury and elevated hepatic enzymes: A clinical correlation in children. J Pediatr Surg 19:457, 1984.

Spivak W: A case of primary sclerosing cholangitis in childhood. Gastroenterology 82:129, 1982.

Infections

Balistreri WF: Viral Hepatitis: Implications to Pediatric Practice. In: Barnes LA (ed): Advances in Pediatrics, Vol 32, 1985, pp 287–320.

Chusid MJ: Pyogenic hepatic abscess in infancy and childhood. Pediatrics 62:554, 1978.

Dresler S, Linder D: Non-cirrhotic portal fibrosis following neonatal cytomegalo-cytomegalic inclusion disease. J Pediatr 93:887, 1978.

Gitlin N, Visveshwara, Kassel SH, et al: Fulminant neonatal hepatic necrosis associated with echovirus type II infection. West J Med 138:260, 1983.

Hanshaw JB, Betts RF, Simon G, et al: Acquired cytomegalovirus infection: Association with hepatomegaly and abnormal liver function tests. N Engl J Med 272:602, 1965.

Howard CR, Ellis DS, Simpson DIH: Exotic viruses in the liver. Semin Liver Dis 5:361, 1984.

Pelletier LL, Bores DM, Roning DA, et al: Disseminated intravascular coagulation and hepatic necrosis. Complications of infectious mononucleosis. JAMA 235:1144, 1976.

Prince AM, Szmuness W, Millin SJ, et al: A serologic study of cytomegalovirus infections associated with blood transfusions. N Engl J Med 284:1125, 1971.

Liver Disease Associated with Systemic Disease

Balistreri WF, Novak DA, Farrell MK: Bile acid metabolism, total parenteral nutrition, and cholestasis. In: Lebenthal E (ed): Total Parenteral Nutrition in Children: Indications, Complications, and Pathophysiologic Considerations. New York, Raven Press, 1986, pp 319–334.

Bernstein J, Chang C-H, Brough AJ, et al: Conjugated hyperbilirubinemia in infancy associated with parenteral alimentation. J Pediatr 90:361, 1977.

Buchanan GR, Glader BE: Benign course of extreme hyperbilirubinemia in sickle cell anemia: Analysis of six cases. J Pediatr 91:21, 1977.

Cohen JA, Kaplan MM: Left-sided heart failure presenting as hepatitis. Gastroenterology 74:583, 1978.

Kern F: Hepatobiliary disorders in inflammatory bowel disease. In: Popper H, Schaffner F (eds): Progress in Liver Diseases, Vol 5. New York, Grune & Stratton, 1976, p 575.

Klion FM, Weiner MJ, Schaffner F: Cholestasis in sickle cell anemia. Am J Med 37:829, 1964.

Merritt RJ: Hyperalimentation in liver disease. In: Neonatal Cholestasis: Causes, Syndromes, Therapies. Report of the 87th Ross Conference on Pediatric Research—Neonatal Cholestasis, Columbus, OH, Ross Laboratories, 1984.

Sinatra F: Does total parenteral nutrition produce cholestasis? In: Neonatal Cholestasis: Causes, Syndromes, Therapies. Report of the 87th Ross Conference on Pediatric Research—Neonatal Cholestasis. Columbus, OH, Ross Laboratories, 1984.

Weinberg AG, Bolande RP: The liver in congenital heart disease. Am J Dis Child 119:390, 1970.

Wiesner RH, LaRusso NF: Clinicopathologic features of the syndrome of primary sclerosing cholangitis. Gastroenterology 79:200, 1980.

Veno-occlusive Disease/Graft-Versus-Host Disease

McDonald GB, Sharma P, Matthews DE, et al: Venocclusive disease of the liver after bone marrow transplantation: Diagnosis, incidence, and predisposing factors. Hepatology 4:116, 1984.

Sale GE, Shulman HM: Liver disease after marrow transplantation. In: Sale GE, Shulman HM (eds): The Pathology of Bone Marrow Transplantation. Year Book Medical Publishers, Chicago, 1984.

Snover DC, Weisdorf SA, Ramsay NK, et al: Hepatic graft versus host disease: A study of the predictive value of liver biopsy in diagnosis. Hepatology 4:123, 1984.

Reye Syndrome

Corey L, Rubin RJ, Hattwick MAW, et al: A nationwide outbreak of Reye's syndrome: Its epidemiologic relationship to influenza B. Am J Med 61:615, 1976.

Hall S, Bellman M: Reye's syndrome in the British Isles: First annual report of the joint British Paediatric Association and Communicable Disease Surveillance Centre surveillance scheme. Br Med J 288:548, 1984.

LaMontagne JR: Summary of a workshop on disease mechanisms and prospects for prevention of Reye's syndrome. J Infect Dis 148:943, 1983.

Lichtenstein PK, Heubi JE, Daugherty CC, et al: Grade I Reye's Syndrome: A frequent cause of vomiting and liver dysfunction after varicella and upper-respiratory-tract infection. N Engl J Med 309:133, 1983.

Reye RDK, Morgan G, Baral J: Encephalopathy and fatty degeneration of the viscera: A disease entity in childhood. Lancet 2:749, 1963.

Shaywitz BA, Rothstein P, Venes JL: Monitoring and management of increased intracranial pressure in Reye syndrome: Results in 29 children. Pediatrics 66:198, 1980.

Chronic Active Hepatitis

Arasu TS, Wyllie R, Hatch TF, et al: Management of chronic aggressive hepatitis in children and adolescents. J Pediatr 95:514, 1979.

Boyer JL: Chronic hepatitis—a perspective on classification and determinants of prognosis. Gastroenterology 70:1161, 1976.

Czaja AJ, Wolf AM, Baggenstoss AM: Laboratory assessment of severe chronic active hepatitis during and after corticosteroid therapy: Correlation of serum transaminase and gamma globulin levels with histologic features. Gastroenterology 80:687, 1981.

Czaja AJ: Current problems in the diagnosis and management of chronic active hepatitis. Mayo Clin Proc 56:311, 1981.

Kirk AP, Jain S, Popock S, et al: Late results of the Royal Free Hospital prospective controlled trial of prednisone therapy in hepatitis B surface antigen negative chronic active hepatitis. Gut 21:78, 1980.

Wright EC, Seeff LB, Berk PD, et al: Treatment of chronic active hepatitis. An analysis of three controlled trials. Gastroenterology 73:1422, 1977.

Drug-Induced Liver Disease

Zimmerman M: Hepatotoxicity, The Adverse Effects of Drugs and Other Chemicals on the Liver. New York, Appleton-Century-Crofts, 1979.

Fulminant Failure

Dymock IW, Tucker JS, Woolf IL, et al: Coagulation studies as a prognostic index in acute liver failure. Br J Haematol 29:385, 1975.

Gazzard BG, Portman B, Muray-Lyon IM, et al: Causes of death in fulminant hepatic failure and relationship to quantitative histological assessment of parenchymal damage. Q J Med 176:615, 1975.

Horney JT, Galambos JT. The liver during and after fulminant hepatitis. Gastroenterology 73:639, 1977.

Mathiesen LR, Skinoj P, Nielsen JO, et al: Hepatitis type A, B, and non-A and non-B in fulminant hepatitis. Gut 21:72, 1980.

Psacharopoulos HT, Mowat AP, Davies M, et al: Fulminant hepatic failure in childhood: An analysis of 31 cases. Arch Dis Child 55:252, 1980.

Wilkinson SP, Blendis LM, Williams R: Frequency and type of renal and electrolyte disorders in fulminant hepatic failure. Br Med J 1:186, 1974.

Anatomic/Cystic Malformations

Alvarez F, Bernardo O, Brunelle F, et al: Congenital hepatic fibrosis in children. J Pediatr 99:370, 1981.

Barlow B, Tabor E, Blome WA, et al: Choledochal cyst: A review of 19 cases. J Pediatr 89:934, 1976.

Blyth H, Ockenden BG: Polycystic diseases of kidney and liver presenting in childhood. J Med Genet 81:357, 1971.

Landing BH, Wells TR, Claireaux AE: Morphometric analysis of liver lesions in cystic diseases of childhood. Human Pathol II (Suppl):549, 1980.

Murray-Lyon IM, Shikim KB, Law LW, et al: Non-obstructive dilatation of the intrahepatic biliary tree with cholangitis. Q J Med 41:477, 1972.

Gallbladder Disease

Glenn F: Acute Acalculous cholecystitis. Ann Surg 189:458, 1979.

Lachman BSD, Lazerson J, Starshak RJ, et al: The prevalence of cholelithiasis in sickle cell disease as diagnosed by ultrasound and cholecystography. Pediatrics 64:601, 1979.

Ney J, Arvin A, Ariagno R: Hydrops of the gallbladder. Am J Dis Child 134:892, 1980.

Peevy KJ, Wiseman HJ: Gallbladder distention in septic neonates. Arch Dis Child 57:75, 1982.

Roslyn JJ, Rih HA, Mann LL, et al: Gallbladder disease in patients on long-term parenteral nutrition. Gastroenterology 84:148, 1983.

Takiff H, Fonkalsrud E: Gallbladder disease in childhood. Am J Dis Child 138:565, 1984.

12.88 PORTAL HYPERTENSION AND VARICES

Etiology. Extrahepatic portal venous obstruction causes 50–70% of portal hypertension in children, but in about two thirds of cases no specific cause can be found. In many patients it develops gradually after birth; umbilical vein catheterization and infusion are associated in about one third of such cases. Lymphatic spread of infection from the umbilicus to the ductus venosus may cause portal vein thrombosis. Sludging of venous flow at the time of normal closure of the umbilical vein and ductus venosus is another suggested mechanism. In older children, abdominal trauma, pancreatitis, and tumors or inflammatory masses adjacent to the portal vein have occasionally led to portal hypertension. In Gaucher disease, arteriovenous fistulas may develop in the spleen, resulting in portal hypertension. Rarely in children, hepatic vein thrombosis (Budd-Chiari syndrome) causes raised portal venous pressure.

Cirrhosis may also cause portal hypertension; the intrahepatic scarring and collapse distort hepatic vasculature and raise vascular resistance (Sec. 12.72). Most survivors of surgically corrected biliary atresia and all nonoperated cases develop portal hypertension. Many of the remaining known causes of childhood cirrhosis are insidious in onset and often do not progress to portal hypertension until relatively late in childhood. Examples of these conditions are α_1-antitrypsin deficiency, Wilson disease, cystic fibrosis, trypsinemia, and chronic active hepatitis. Congenital hepatic fibrosis may also lead to portal hypertension. The portal pressure may also rise following right hepatic lobectomy as the entire portal flow encounters greater resistance from the reduced vascular bed.

Pathology. The liver is normal in patients with extrahepatic portal obstruction. Some portal blood does reach the liver through collateral channels in the suspensory ligaments, the diaphragmatic veins, and hepatorenal and hepatocolic veins. With intrahepatic obstruction there is no portal flow to the liver other than via the partially obstructed portal vein. A cavernomatous transformation of the portal vein is encountered in some children, with the normal vein being replaced by a number of thin-walled tortuous veins. Whether this is the result or the cause of the portal obstruction is unknown, but the portal venous pressure exceeds the pressure within the inferior vena cava by at least 150 mm of saline. Portal-systemic shunts develop and lead to dilatation and varicosities in otherwise unimportant veins. Such anastomoses are found in the region of the esophagogastric junction, the retroperitoneal veins, the internal hemorrhoidal plexus in the distal rectum, and around the ligamentum teres at the umbilicus. The varicosities in the lower esophagus and cardia of the stomach are especially prone to erosion with consequent massive hemorrhage. Hypersplenism may complicate the picture in any patient with portal obstruction.

Clinical Manifestations. Massive hematemesis is usually the initial symptom of portal hypertension in children. The blood passed per rectum will vary from bright red with severe bleeding to melena. The underlying disease determines the age at which symptoms begin; younger infants tend to present with ascites first rather than hematemesis. There may be jaundice if the obstruction is hepatic. A cluster of diverging, dilated veins with centrifugal flow from the umbilicus (the caput medusae) may develop. Internal anal hemorrhoids are uncommon in children.

Diagnosis. Roentgenographic demonstration of varicosities in the esophagus is relatively noninvasive and usually accurate; a barium paste is used that adheres to the esophageal mucous membrane. In children, peptic ulcer disease rarely coexists with portal hypertension. The varicosities have an unmistakable appearance when visualized directly by fiberoptic gastroesophagoscopy. Liver function should be evaluated. The portal vein may be demonstrated by retrograde umbilical vein catheterization, splenoportography, or selective angiography. Splenoportography also allows the measurement of splenic pulp and portal pressures and indicates the flow within the splenic and portal veins. Selective angiography does not demonstrate the portal vein as well as splenoportography, but it allows assessment of the size of the superior mesenteric vein. If the bleeding is not from varices, this investigation may demonstrate sites of hemorrhage not associated with portal hypertension, e.g., traumatic hemobilia. It may also be useful therapeutically as a means of introducing vasopressor substances selectively into the portal system.

Treatment. Hematemesis from esophageal varices in children usually stops spontaneously without measures other than blood transfusion. A nasogastric tube should be inserted as a guide to the amount and rate of hemorrhage and is *not* contraindicated by a risk of precipitating or aggravating hemorrhage from varices. In many patients the bleeding is from varices at the cardia of the stomach and not the esophagus. A central venous pressure measurement may be helpful in assessing the rate of blood volume replacement required. Vital functions must be measured frequently, including pH, arterial oxygen saturation, and electrolytes. Incipient hepatic failure from cirrhosis made worse by hemorrhage is rarely seen in children. Patients who have cirrhosis will require terminal care unless hepatic transplantation is anticipated; Wilson disease is an exception. Intravenous and local administration of *posterior pituitary extract* may be of use by causing splanchnic vasoconstriction with diminished blood flow to the bleeding varices. Cooling the stomach is probably of no value. If bleeding persists, the passage of the triple lumen Sengstaken-Blakemore tube to produce balloon tamponade may be required. In many instances only the distal gastric balloon needs to be inflated and with traction on the tube, bleeding is controlled; bleeding often recurs on deflation of the balloon(s).

It is rarely necessary to operate upon pediatric patients with portal hypertension as an emergency to stop bleeding. Two types of procedures are currently employed: those that attack the varices directly and those that divert portal blood to the systemic circulation (Sec. 12.72).

There are many methods of diverting portal blood flow to the systemic circulation. Splenorenal shunts offer excellent means of controlling portal hypertension in children. Siguira has reported good results from a thoracoabdominal operation in which as many as 80 varicose veins or their tributaries are ligated within the thorax; the esophagus is transected and then anastomosed to interrupt intramural varicosities; and within the abdomen veins related to the upper stomach are all ligated. The Siguira procedure may be preferable to shunt operations, as it causes no increase in likelihood of subsequent encephalopathy.

BARRY SHANDLING

Aoyama K, Myers NA: Extrahepatic portal hypertension: The significance of variceal hemorrhage. Aust Paediatr J 18:17, 1982.
Eckhauser FE, Appelman HD, Knol JA, et al: Noncirrhotic portal hypertension: Differing patterns of disease in children and adults. Surgery 94:721, 1983.
Fonkalsrud EW: Long term results following surgical management of portal hypertension in children. Z Kinderchir 33:57, 1982.
Fonkalsrud EW: Surgical management of portal hypertension in childhood. Arch Surg 115:1042, 1980.
Howard ER, Stamatakis JJ, Mowat AP: Management of esophageal varices in children by injection sclerotherapy. J Pediatr Surg 19:2, 1984.
Superina RA, Weber JL, Shandling B: A modified Siguira operation for bleeding varices in children. J Pediatr Surg 18:794, 1983.

12.89 PERITONEUM AND ALLIED STRUCTURES

MALFORMATIONS OF THE PERITONEUM

Congenital peritoneal bands may be responsible for intestinal obstruction; numerous other anomalies may occur in the course of the development of the peritoneum but are rarely of clinical importance. Intra-abdominal herniations infrequently occur through ring-like formations produced by anomalous peritoneal bands. Absence of the omentum or its duplication occurs rarely. Omental cysts and torsion are unusual causes of acute abdominal crises.

ASCITES

The term "ascites" indicates an accumulation of fluid in the peritoneal cavity, but it is usually applied to accumulations of serous fluid. Renal, especially nephrotic, and cardiac conditions are most often responsible for ascites. It may be secondary to chronic adhesive pericarditis, or part of a polyserositis in Pick syndrome. Other causes include obstruction of the portal circulation, due to hepatic cirrhosis (Sec. 12.72) or to enlarged lymph nodes, tumors, thrombosis, chronic tuberculous peritonitis, rheumatic peritonitis, or obstruction of the splenic vein.

The abdomen is distended; when distention is great, there is flattening or pouting of the umbilicus. Fluctuation can be detected on palpation; a wave-like impulse is obtained by sharp tapping on one-side of the abdomen while the other hand is placed on the opposite side and an assistant's hand compresses the abdomen in the midline; shifting percussion dullness can often be shown.

Ascites must be differentiated from other conditions that cause distention of the abdomen, which may include gaseous distention of the intestine; fecal distention as occurs with megacolon; tumor masses, including cysts of the mesentery; acute or chronic peritonitis; peritoneal hemorrhage; extreme distention of the bladder; and simple obesity.

The course, prognosis, and treatment of ascites depend entirely on the cause.

CHYLOUS ASCITES

The accumulation of chyle as ascites is uncommon; this form of ascites may occur at any age of childhood and is occasionally congenital. Chylous ascites is caused by an anomaly, injury, or obstruction of the thoracic duct within its abdominal portion. In the case of anomalies the condition is present at birth or shortly thereafter. Chylothorax may be associated (Sec. 13.103). Obstructions may be produced by enlarged lymph nodes or neoplasms. The fluid has the appearance of milk because of its high fat content. In chronic peritonitis, peritoneal fluid may have a somewhat similar color from degeneration of inflammatory products.

The accumulation of chyle can be reduced in some infants by providing a low fat diet containing medium-chain triglycerides which are absorbed directly into the portal circulation. Since there is considerable loss of protein in this fluid, high protein diets should be prescribed and parenteral nutrition supplementation may be indicated. Paracentesis is indicated for respiratory distress due to abdominal distention, but the efficacy of repetitive paracentesis is unknown. It may take several months for medical management to be effective. Abdominal exploration may be justified to search for the site of the leak if a trial of dietary management is unsuccessful.

Grescom NT, Colodny AH, Rosenberg HK: Diagnostic aspects of neonatal ascites: Report of 27 cases. Am J Roentgenol 128:961, 1977.
Unger SW, Chandler JG: Chylous ascites in infants and children. Surgery 93:455, 1983.

PERITONITIS

Acute infections of the peritoneum are arbitrarily designated as *primary* when their origin is outside the abdominal cavity and infection is blood- or lymph-borne. The infection is termed *secondary* when it occurs through extension from or rupture of an intra-abdominal viscus or of an abscess.

Peritonitis in the neonatal period may arise from a transplacental in utero infection; more frequently it is the result of infection acquired during or shortly after birth. It may be a manifestation of septicemia, a direct extension from an umbilical infection or from perforation of the intestine, or, rarely, the sequel of a ruptured appendix. Meconium peritonitis is described in Sec. 8.42.

ACUTE PRIMARY PERITONITIS

Etiology and Epidemiology. Primary peritonitis is a bacterial infection of the peritoneal cavity without a demonstrable intra-abdominal source. The incidence of this entity is decreasing, presumably owing to wide use of effective antimicrobial therapy, but it continues to occur in children with ascites secondary to nephrosis or cirrhosis and, occasionally, in otherwise healthy children. Pneumococci and group A streptococci are the predominant pathogens, with gram-negative bacteria also often involved (*E. coli*). The genders are equally affected; most cases occur before 6 yr of age.

Clinical Manifestations. The onset may be insidious or rapid and is characterized by fever, abdominal pain, and vomiting. Diarrhea is common and extreme prostration may occur. The child may appear toxic or anxious. In very ill patients, especially young infants, the temperature may be normal or subnormal. The pulse may be rapid, small, and compressible, and the respirations rapid and shallow because of the pain that abdominal respiration produces. There is usually distention of the abdomen, moderate diffuse tenderness, and a doughy resistance. Examination often reveals signs of active nephrosis or cirrhosis, including ascites. Palpation may demonstrate rebound tenderness and rigidity. Bowel sounds are hypoactive or absent.

Diagnosis and Treatment. Laboratory studies reveal leukocytosis with 85–95% polymorphonuclear cells. Proteinuria is present in children with active nephrosis. Roentgenographic examination of the abdomen reveals dilatation of the large and small intestines, with edema of the small intestinal wall producing an increased distance between adjacent loops of gas-filled small bowel. In most cases the clinical presentation is indistinguishable from that of appendicitis, with or without perforation; accordingly, the diagnosis of primary peritonitis can be made only at laparotomy. In a child with active nephrosis or cirrhosis, however, whose physical findings are compatible with diffuse peritonitis, an attempt should be made to establish the diagnosis of primary peritonitis by evaluation of peritoneal fluid obtained with a short-beveled needle. Cytologic and chemical analyses of the exudate are helpful. Infected ascitic fluid usually contains an elevated protein concentration and more than 300 leukocytes/mm^3, more than 25% of which are polymorphonuclear. Microscopic examination of Gram-stained ascitic fluid characteristically reveals a single species of gram-positive or, less often, gram-negative bacteria; in this situation initial intravenous antibiotic therapy with clindamycin or ampicillin and gentamicin is indicated, with subsequent changes in antibiotics dependent upon sensitivity testing. Although resolution of all signs and symptoms characteristically occurs within 48 hr, parenteral antibiotic therapy should be continued for a minimum of 7 days. Surgical exploration is indicated if after 48 hr of parenteral antibiotic therapy either the child's clinical condition fails to improve or the physical findings persist and show localization.

Golden GT, Shaw A: Primary peritonitis. Surg Gynecol Obstet 133:513, 1973.
Speck WT, Dresdale SA, MacMillan RW: Primary peritonitis and the nephrotic syndrome. Am J Surg 127:267, 1974.

ACUTE SECONDARY PERITONITIS

This type of peritonitis is most often due to the entry of enteric bacteria into the peritoneal cavity through a necrotic defect in the wall of the intestines or other viscus as a result of obstruction and infarction. In children, peritonitis is most often associated with appendicitis but may occur with intussusception, volvulus, incarcerated hernias, or rupture of a Meckel diverticulum. Peritonitis may also occur as a complication of intestinal mucosal disease, including peptic ulcers, ulcerative colitis, and pseudomembranous enterocolitis. Peritonitis in the neonatal period most often occurs as a complication of necrotizing enterocolitis but may be associated with meconium ileus or spontaneous rupture of the stomach or intestines. The bacteria involved are the normal aerobic and anaerobic flora of the gastrointestinal tract.

Clinical Manifestations. The early clinical manifestations of secondary peritonitis reflect the underlying disease process. Fever, diffuse abdominal pain, nausea, and vomiting are characteristic. Signs of peritoneal inflammation include rebound tenderness, abdominal wall rigidity, and hypoactive or absent bowel sounds. These early findings may be followed by signs and symptoms of shock due to the loss of large quantities of protein-rich fluid from the vascular compartment into the peritoneal cavity and bowel lumen, with associated intravascular volume depletion.

The manifestations of shock from a ruptured viscus or the early symptoms of acute appendicitis may merge with those of peritonitis and may be followed by an increasing toxemia, as evidenced by greater restlessness and irritability, by a higher temperature, often 39.5° C or more (103–105° F), by an increase in the pulse rate, and, at times, by chills or convulsions. In extreme situations, and especially in early infancy, the temperature may be normal or subnormal. Constipation is marked, owing to paralytic ileus.

Laboratory studies reveal blood leukocyte counts in excess of 12,000/mm³ with a predominance of polymorphonuclear forms. Roentgenograms of the abdomen may reveal free air in the peritoneal cavity, evidence of ileus or obstruction, peritoneal fluid, and obliteration of the psoas shadow.

Treatment. The main principle of therapy is to stabilize the patient by correcting fluid and electrolyte deficiencies with parenteral fluids, by alleviating intestinal obstruction with nasal suction, and by controlling the peritoneal infection with broad-spectrum antibiotics. Numerous antibiotic regimens have been advocated depending on the presence or absence of previous illness. In the absence of previous chemotherapy, a regimen consisting of clindamycin or ampicillin and gentamicin is indicated. Surgery should be performed to repair any damaged viscus at the earliest time after the patient is stabilized and antibiotic therapy is initiated. Cultures taken during surgery will determine whether a change in the antibiotic regimen is indicated.

ACUTE SECONDARY LOCALIZED PERITONITIS
(Peritoneal Abscess)

Etiology. A single localized pyogenic abscess, most often secondary to perforation of an inflamed appendix, is somewhat less common in children than in adults. The poor ability of young children to localize peritoneal infection of appendiceal origin has been attributed to lower general resistance and to a relatively smaller omentum. Localized peritoneal abscesses occur most often in the appendiceal region, but may occur at any site, originating from various sources; or appendiceal infections may gravitate to other areas, notably the pelvis. An abscess in the subdiaphragmatic area may originate from an appendiceal or other intra-abdominal infection or, rarely, from an empyema. Diagnostic ultrasonography or CT scan may be helpful in locating an abscess.

Clinical Manifestations. The general symptoms of *peritoneal abscess* are continued fever or its recurrence, poor appetite, and vomiting following ingestion of food. The white blood cell count is increased, with a predominance of polymorphonuclear cells. With *appendiceal abscess*, there is tenderness in the right lower quadrant, often with a palpable mass.

A *pelvic abscess* is suggested by abdominal distention, rectal tenesmus with or without the passage of small stools containing mucus, or bladder irritability. Rectal examination may reveal a tender mass anteriorly.

A *subphrenic abscess* is evidenced by physical signs at the base of the lung, usually on the right, due to elevation of the diaphragm and frequently to the presence of pleural fluid. The diagnosis can often be established roentgenographically. If the infection is on the right side, the diaphragm is elevated and the liver depressed; there is frequently a pocket of air just below the diaphragm, resulting from gas produced by bacteria.

Liver and *suprarenal abscesses* are uncommon in childhood. In the newborn, liver abscess has been associated with umbilical vein catheterization.

Treatment. The abscess should be drained and appropriate antibiotic therapy provided. Initial broad-spectrum coverage with clindamycin and gentamicin should be modified, if indicated, by the results of sensitivity tests of the bacteria obtained from cultures. If the appendix cannot be removed at the initial operation, appendectomy should be done subsequently within 3 mo.

TUBERCULOUS PERITONITIS

See Sec. 11.46.

INGUINAL HERNIA

See Sec. 12.65.

HYDROCELE

See Sec. 17.45.

EPIGASTRIC HERNIA

Epigastric hernias occur in the midline between the umbilicus and the lower end of the sternum. They are uncommon and, except for their location, are similar to umbilical hernias. They may become acutely painful and tender when a bit of preperitoneal fat becomes incarcerated. They should be repaired surgically.

INCISIONAL HERNIA

Postoperative hernias should be repaired as soon as the local condition of the wound and the general condition of the child warrant it. Incisional hernias tend to enlarge and may also become incarcerated.

DIAPHRAGMATIC HERNIA

Diaphragmatic hernias may be congenital or acquired. Acquired hernias are usually traumatic in origin and are not considered here. Congenital herniation of abdominal contents into the thoracic cavity may be responsible for serious respiratory distress, usually constituting a medical-surgical emergency in the immediate neonatal period. Infrequently, when little or no respiratory embarrassment occurs, the hernia may not be detected until later in infancy or childhood. The delayed presentation of a right diaphragmatic hernia should be suspected in an infant with group B streptococcal infection or signs of atelectasis, pleural effusion, or pneumonia whose condition deteriorates. The frequency of major congenital anomalies is increased in infants with diaphragmatic hernia.

In addition to herniation through a defect in the diaphragm (see below), there may be partial herniation of the stomach through the esophageal hiatus (Sec. 12.20), phrenic paralysis with displacement of abdominal contents upward but not herniated, and eventration of the diaphragm. *Eventration is not a herniation* but is also an upward displacement of abdominal contents into an outpouching or saclike structure of the diaphragm resulting from a weakness or absence of diaphragmatic musculature without an abnormal opening. The clinical manifestations of an eventration may simulate those of a diaphragmatic hernia. Complete absence of the diaphragm is rare.

Etiology. Herniation occurs most often in the posterolateral segments of the diaphragm, much more often on the left than on the right side. The defect represents failure of the pleuroperitoneal canal to close completely during embryonic development (foramen of Bochdalek). Much less frequently the herniation is in the anterior portion of the diaphragm in the retrosternal area, representing failure of midline fusion of the two anlagen of the diaphragm with elements of the pericardium (foramen of Morgagni). With this defect there may be herniation of intestine into the pericardial sac or, conversely, ectopia cordis with displacement of the heart into the peritoneal cavity. Umbilical defects are commonly associated with herniation through the foramen of Morgagni.

Pathology. Protrusion of the abdominal viscera through a diaphragmatic hernia into the thoracic cavity occurs in varying degrees. In severe cases the stomach and a large part of the intestines and even, in rare instances, the spleen, liver, and kidneys displace the lungs and heart. Incomplete rotation of the cecum, umbilical defects, and duodenal constricting bands may be associated. The lung on the affected side is compressed and often hypoplastic with a decreased number of airways and blood vessels and diminished total lung volume. An increased muscularity of small pulmonary arteries may contribute to increased pulmonary resistance and hypertension. Hypoplasia of the contralateral lung has also been observed.

Clinical Manifestations. Severe respiratory distress, including dyspnea and cyanosis, is frequently present from birth. If

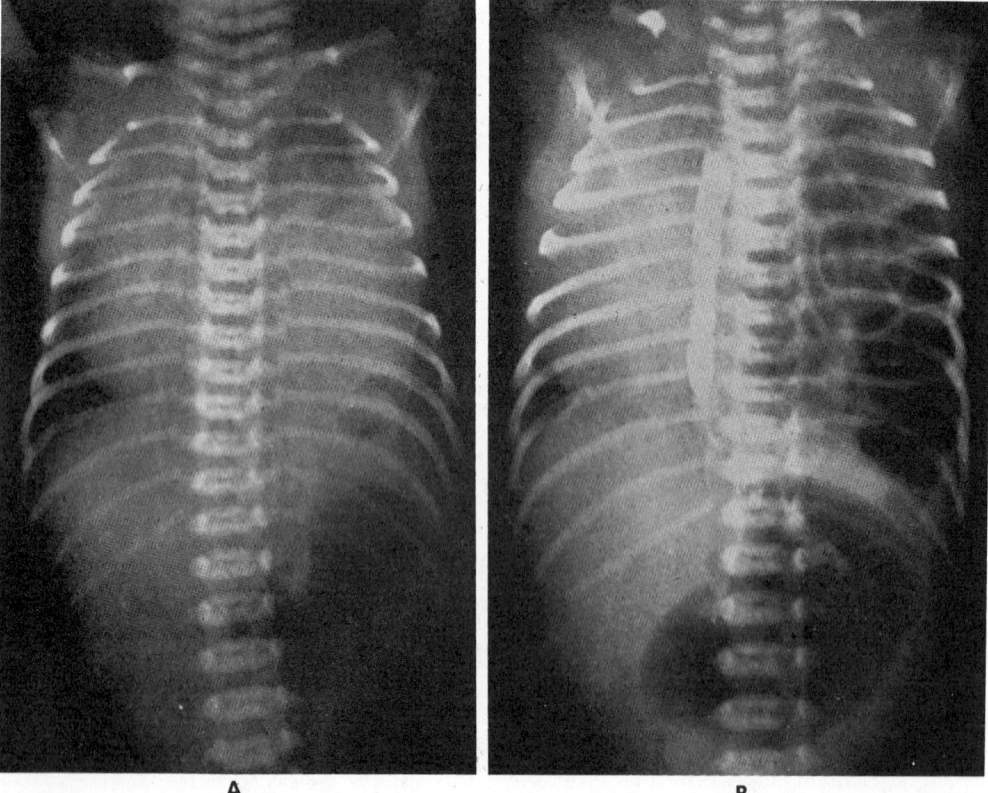

A   **B**

Figure 12–25. Congenital diaphragmatic hernia. *A*, Film exposed shortly after birth: distortion of shadow of left leaf of diaphragm with huge, masslike density in left hemithorax displacing heart to right. *B*, Film exposed about 20 min after *A*. As the result of swallowed air, coils of air-filled small bowel are now demonstrated in the left hemithorax. The esophagus is outlined by swallowed contrast material. Operative correction was attempted because of extreme dyspnea. Infant died 5.5 hr after birth.

symptoms are not present at birth, they may appear at any time during the neonatal period or later. These include vomiting, severe colicky pain, discomfort after eating, and constipation as well as dyspnea. Symptoms and signs of acute intestinal obstruction may occur at any time. Infrequently, there are no symptoms and the condition may be discovered by chance roentgenographic examination.

Findings on physical examination depend on the degree of displacement of abdominal contents into the thoracic cavity. When there is extensive displacement in the newborn infant, the abdomen is usually small and scaphoid in contour; the infant is cyanotic and has obvious respiratory retractions. If the respiratory embarrassment is not relieved, shock and rapidly progressive hypoxia occur. In contrast, in mildly affected patients there may be no or only minimal respiratory distress and no digestive disturbance.

The percussion note over the part of the thorax containing the stomach and intestines may be more tympanic or duller than usual, and the breath sounds absent, decreased, or increased. Occasionally, sounds of intestinal peristaltic movements can be heard over the chest.

The diagnosis is usually established by roentgenographic examination (Fig. 12–25), often without the aid of contrast medium, or, if such is needed, air injected into the stomach may be sufficient. Characteristically, in the neonatal period there are fluid and air-filled loops of intestine in the chest which simulate cysts. The mediastinum is displaced toward the unaffected side, usually the right. Occasionally, in the case of cystic adenomatoid malformations of the lung or congenital lobar emphysema, it may be necessary to use contrast material to demonstrate that the stomach and intestines are in the abdominal cavity.

Treatment. Resuscitation of the newborn is mandatory prior to reduction of the hernia and closure of the diaphragmatic defect. As soon as the diagnosis is suspected, the newborn infant should be positioned with head and thorax higher than the abdomen and feet to facilitate the downward displacement of the abdominal organs. Nasogastric intubation with intermittent suction will decrease entrapment of air and fluid within the herniated viscera and lessen the degree of ventilatory compromise. Positive pressure ventilation, if needed, should be administered cautiously through an endotracheal tube, since pneumothorax may result, owing to the uneven distribution of intrapulmonary pressures in lungs affected by compression atelectasis or pulmonary hypoplasia. Arterial blood gas measurements, including pH, should be obtained preoperatively and metabolic and respiratory acidosis corrected with appropriate intravenous solutions.

Emergency and definitive surgical correction is indicated. A subcostal incision provides excellent exposure of the diaphragm, and the herniated contents can be reduced into the peritoneal cavity after the pressures in the pleural and peritoneal cavities are equalized. Severely affected infants diagnosed within the first 24–72 hr of life have a mortality rate of about 50%. Most infants who do not require surgery early for respiratory distress survive. Low Apgar scores (<6) and acidosis (pH <7.2) are associated with high mortality. Pulmonary hypertension *with persistence of fetal circulation* syndrome is a serious complication in the postoperative period, which requires careful fluid and respiratory management (Sec. 14.12). It is often associated with difficulty in expanding a hypoplastic ipsilateral lung. Forceful attempts to inflate the lung may cause a pneumothorax.

Survivors generally can participate in normal activities through their teenage years, although they may have abnormal results on lung function studies.

RICHARD E. BEHRMAN

Freyschuss U, Lännergren K, Frenckner B: Lung function after repair of congenital diaphragmatic hernia. Acta Pediatr Scand 73:589, 1985.

Geggel RL, Murphy JD, Langleben D, et al: Congenital diaphragmatic hernia: Arterial structural changes and persistent pulmonary hypertension after surgical repair. J Pediatr 107:457, 1985.

Harris MC, Moskowitz WB, Engle WD, et al: Group B streptococcal septicemia and delayed-onset diaphragmatic hernia: A new clinical association. Am J Dis Child 135:723, 1981.

Naeye RL, Shochat SJ, Whitman V, et al: Unsuspected pulmonary vascular abnormalities associated with diaphragmatic hernia. Pediatrics 58:902, 1976.

Reid IS and Hutcherson RJ: Long term follow up of patients with congenital diaphragmatic hernia. J Pediatr Surg 11:939, 1976.

Ruff SJ, Campbell JR, Harrison MW, et al: Pediatric diaphragmatic hernias: 11 year experience. Am J Surg 139:641, 1980.

13

THE RESPIRATORY SYSTEM

13.1 DEVELOPMENT OF THE LUNG

The development of the respiratory system begins early in fetal life and continues long after birth. Large increases occur in: the diameter and lengths of airways; the number and size of bronchioles and alveoli; and the size, dimensions, and rigidity of the chest wall. Significant changes also occur in the support and composition of the lining and walls of the airways and alveoli. In addition, the rate of respiration slows, and the tidal volume and minute volume of ventilation increase as the infant matures into an adult. Yet after the newborn period the normal arterial pressures of oxygen and carbon dioxide in infants and children are the same as in adults. Knowledge about the developing respiratory system is important for recognizing and understanding age-related disease patterns and in providing effective therapy (see also Chapter 8).

13.2 PRENATAL DEVELOPMENT

The embryonic period of fetal development occurs during the first 5 wk after conception, when the primitive lung bud evaginates from the cervical region of the endodermal tube. Dichotomous, asymmetric bronchial branching continues until the number of branches of the conducting airways found in the adult is reached by the end of the 16th fetal wk, completing the pseudoglandular phase. Subsequent conducting airway growth occurs by increase in size and length but not in numbers. The canalicular phase, 16–26 wk, is characterized by the further development and vascularization of the future respiratory portions of the lung. The final phase, the terminal sac period, ends at birth when the respiratory unit consists of three orders of respiratory bronchioles, a generation of transitional ducts, and terminal clusters of alveolar sacs. Fewer than 70 million primitive alveoli are present at birth.

13.3 POSTNATAL DEVELOPMENT

With postnatal growth, alveolar ducts branch off the third respiratory bronchioles. This is followed by development of the atrium, alveolar sacs, and alveoli. The total number of adult alveoli (200–600 million) is probably attained before adolescence. Further growth occurs by increase in alveolar diameter from 100 to 200μ in older children to 200 to 300μ in adults.

Types I and II alveolar cells increase after the 24th–26th wk of gestation, making respiration possible. However, sustained inflation of the lung after the first breath requires surfactant, which is usually not present in adequate amounts before the 32nd wk of gestation.

The cartilage, mucous glands, goblet cells, and ciliated cells of conducting airways are present at birth. Cartilage appears only in trachea and bronchi (in airways down to about 1 mm in diameter). The glands and goblet cells, also, are not normally present in bronchioles. Tracheobronchial mucous secretion probably occurs at a normal rate at birth, although minor alterations of the mucous glycoproteins and a deficiency of lysozyme secretion occur in premature infant airways. Smooth muscle is present throughout the lung at birth and increases with growth, especially around the peripheral airways. Consequently, bronchospasm can occur even in a young infant. Elastic tissue becomes more abundant with age and is the predominant connective tissue in the peripheral part of the lung.

The conducting airways are proportionately larger than the respiratory portion of the lung in the infant and child compared with the adult. The diameter of the trachea doubles at about 15 yr, that of the bronchi at 6 yr. After an increase in diameter of 40% by 2 yr, the bronchioles grow slowly and in adult life are twice the diameter of those existing at birth.

Airway resistance is higher in the newborn and in the young child than in the adult, and the resistance of peripheral airways forms a higher proportion of total airway resistance in children under 5 yr of age. The small conducting airways of the infant are more easily obstructed at the larynx and beyond by inflammation, foreign body, or mucous secretion than in the adult. The maximal inspiratory pressures generated by the infant or child approximate those of the adult, but the chest wall and supporting structures of the infants are softer so that chest wall retraction during respiratory distress is greater in infants than in older patients.

The right lung has three lobes; the upper and middle are separated by a minor fissure and the middle and lower by a major one. On the left, one major fissure creates only two lobes, the upper and lower. The left upper lobe has a lingular segment corresponding to the right middle lobe. Throughout life the right main stem bronchus is shorter and wider and has a smaller angle of origin from the trachea compared with the left main stem bronchus.

The pulmonary circulation serves the respiratory function and the bronchial arteries are the principal source of nutrient supply to the bronchial tree. The bronchial system drains mainly into the pulmonary venous system. These two circulations anastomose through the capillaries at the level of the respiratory bronchioles. The time of development of the main branches of the pulmonary artery and vein roughly parallels bronchial growth in utero.

The pulmonary artery has two sets of branches. One "conventional" set accompanies the airways. The "supernumerary" branches constitute an important source of collateral blood flow. Muscular arteries are not more distal than the terminal bronchiole at birth, but by 4 mo of age they reach

854

the level of the respiratory bronchioles; by 3 yr of age they extend to the alveolar ducts; and by 10 yr of age they are found in the alveolar regions.

The lymphatics are present at birth. Cross communications between the right and left lung exist at the hilar level, where nodes exist at branches of bronchi; other nodes occur within the lung parenchyma.

Nerves from the vagi and sympathetics form anterior and posterior plexuses at the lung hila and supply the bronchi and blood vessels.

Although the body surface area and the number of respiratory airways and alveoli increase about 10-fold from birth to adult life, the air-tissue gas exchange surface area increases by a factor greater than 20-fold. The cylindrical shape of the newborn chest with its relatively horizontal ribs changes during the first several years because of greater transverse growth of the chest wall resulting in the ribs being positioned lower anteriorly than posteriorly, which adds rigidity to the thorax of older children.

The normal spontaneous respiratory rate is usually that which requires the least work of breathing by the respiratory muscles and is optimately efficient for the individual. The respiratory frequency decreases as body size increases; the normal resting infant rate of about 40/min decreases to about 12/min in the adult.

Muscles of Respiration

The diaphragm is the most important muscle of respiration. With increasing effort the intercostal, sternocleidomastoid, spinal, neck, and abdominal wall muscles also are used. Normal exhalation results from the elastic recoil of the lung when the inspiratory muscles are relaxed. During forced exhalation, contraction of the abdominal muscles forces the diaphragm upward, and the internal intercostal muscles decrease the thoracic volume. Innervation of the diaphragm is bilateral from the third, fourth, and fifth cervical segments through the phrenic nerves. In older children, during inspiration the diaphragm moves downward and the rib margins move upward and outward; in infants the compliant rib cage and horizontal ribs may cause subcostal retractions rather than rib elevation.

Hinshaw HC, Murray JF (eds): Diseases of the Chest. Philadelphia, WB Saunders, 1980.
Kendig EL (ed): Disorders of the Respiratory Tract in Children. Philadelphia, WB Saunders, 1983.
Lough MD, Doershuk CF, Stern RC (eds): Pediatric Respiratory Therapy. Chicago, Year Book Medical Publishers, 1986.
Scarpelli M (ed): Pulmonary Physiology of the Fetus, Newborn, and Child. Philadelphia, Lea & Febiger, 1975.
Tisi GM: Pulmonary Physiology in Clinical Medicine. Baltimore, Williams & Wilkins, 1980.

13.4 RESPIRATORY ANATOMY, PHYSIOLOGY, AND PATHOPHYSIOLOGY

13.5 AIRWAY OBSTRUCTION

Narrowing of the airway lumen may result from (1) the presence of intraluminal material (secretions, tumor, or foreign matter), (2) mural thickening (edema and hypertrophy of glands or muscle), (3) contraction of the bronchial smooth muscle (spasm), and (4) extrinsic compression. These factors rarely occur in isolation except in very acute situations, and all impair the normal mechanisms of tracheobronchial hygiene and interfere with air flow.

Since resistance to air flow is inversely proportional to the fourth power of the radius of a tube, small decreases in the lumen of bronchioles or bronchi or in the laryngeal area may significantly decrease airflow. Even a small degree of airflow obstruction can lead to clinical manifestations of obstruction in young children. It is not surprising then that wheezing is a common reason for hospitalizing infants and toddlers.

In partial airway obstruction, the flow of air and drainage of bronchial secretions still take place but are impaired. In complete obstruction, neither airflow nor drainage of the secretions can occur; complete obstruction of a lobar bronchus leads to lobar atelectasis after the residual gas diffuses into the pulmonary circulation.

Partial airway obstruction can be divided into two types, depending on the degree of narrowing of the bronchial lumen and on the nature of the pathologic process producing it. In *bypass valve obstruction* the lumen is narrowed; though resistance to flow is increased, air can still flow in during inspiration and out during expiration. With *check valve obstruction* air entry is possible, but during expiration the lumen is completely occluded so that escape of air is trapped behind (distal to) the point of obstruction. In bypass valve obstruction, air trapping is a result of the changes in the diameter of the airways' lumen: during inspiration the chest enlarges, creating negative intrathoracic pressure and causing enlargement of the lungs and bronchial tree and widening of the bronchial lumen; during expiration the increase in intratho-

racic pressure causes narrowing of the lumen. If expiration is forceful and a positive pressure is produced, this narrowing and air trapping will be even more marked. Thus, alveolar overdistention may occur with either type of partial obstruction but especially with the check valve type.

High Airway Obstruction. This occurs above the level of the secondary bronchi and in general *interferes more with inspiration than expiration.* If obstruction is complete and above the bifurcation of the trachea, asphyxia and death result. Partial obstruction may result in intense dyspnea. A small increase in respiratory rate and a marked increase in respiratory effort may occur, particularly in inspiration, producing a harsh, low-pitched inspiratory sound called *stridor.* Increased inspiratory effort results in more negative intrathoracic pressure and retraction of the skin and muscles over the suprasternal notch, the supraclavicular space, and the intercostal spaces. Violent contraction of the diaphragm often pulls in the ribs at the site of attachment of the diaphragm (subcostal retractions).

Coughing is a mechanism for removing a nonfixed high airway obstruction, but the depth and effectiveness of the cough are often limited by the poor inspiratory air flow. During high obstruction, the air that is expelled by coughing flows through a narrowed large tube, producing a characteristic sound; if the obstruction is adjacent to the larynx, the cough is croupy or barking; if the obstruction is in the trachea or major bronchi, the cough is brassy. In most cases of high obstruction the cough is nonproductive.

Low Airway Obstruction. Peripheral obstructive lesions are generally diffuse in their distribution and primarily involve airways less than 3 mm in diameter. The lumen of these bronchi and bronchioles can be narrowed by spasm of their encircling smooth muscle, accumulation of secretions, edema of the mucous membrane, extrinsic compression, or any combination of these. With complete obstruction, patchy areas of atelectasis occur. Rarely are such atelectatic changes sufficient to produce obvious clinical manifestations.

Though peripheral obstructive lesions interfere with inspiration, *the primary manifestations are expiratory.* Expiration is prolonged. The passage of air through bronchi narrowed by compression changes from a laminar flow to a turbulent flow resulting in the *wheezing* expiratory sound. The excursion of the chest is diminished, and less air flow is heard on auscultation. In most cases accumulation of secretions and inflammation result in a cough that is usually hacking, ineffective, and repetitive.

The marked increase in airway resistance during exhalation rapidly results in overinflation. The chest is held in an inflated position with an increased anteroposterior (AP) diameter and spreading of the intercostal spaces. Percussion over the chest elicits hyper-resonance; depression of the diaphragm can be detected by percussion over the back.

If the obstruction is marked, the accessory muscles of respiration are used. Although inspiratory retractions and use of accessory inspiratory muscles may be prominent, expiration is even more labored. Bulging of soft tissues above the clavicle or between the ribs and violent contraction of the abdominal muscles are often obvious. If ventilation is severely impaired, dyspnea results, often with associated orthopnea. In most cases the individual is limited in exercise tolerance and, with severe obstruction, may need to sit or lie, concentrating solely on breathing. Cyanosis indicates severe peripheral obstruction and impending death.

Chest roentgenogram reveals increased radiolucency from hyperinflation. Coarse bronchovascular markings may be associated with accumulated secretions, hypertrophied mucous glands, inflammation and edema of the bronchial walls, or peribronchial infiltrates. The increased AP diameter, depression of the diaphragm, and narrow, elongated heart shadow indicate the overinflation of the lungs.

13.6 RESPIRATORY FUNCTION AND MECHANISMS OF DEFENSE

The *upper airway* includes the nose, paranasal sinuses, and pharynx; the *lower airway* consists of the remainder of the system from the larynx peripherally. The nose has a relatively large surface area lined with a richly vascular, ciliated epithelium, and by the time the air column reaches the bifurcation of the trachea, up to 75% of the warming and humidification of the inspired air has occurred. During exhalation, heat and moisture are removed from the air stream. Gross filtering of particles larger than 10–15 μm is achieved by the coarse hairs at the nasal orifices, and most inhaled particles larger than 5 μm are impacted on the nasal surface.

Because the larynx is relatively narrow and ringed with cartilage, it is relatively susceptible to obstruction in young children, particularly by inflammation, since the resultant swelling of tissues rapidly encroaches on the lumen and produces inspiratory stridor.

The trachea and bronchi are lined with pseudostratified, ciliated, columnar epithelium and occasional goblet cells. Mucous glands occupy approximately one third the thickness of the airway wall and for the most part lie between the epithelial surface and the cartilage. The trachea is supported by incomplete rings of cartilage with a muscular membrane posteriorly. Irregular plates of cartilage support the bronchi, especially at bifurcations. These diminish and finally disappear in the smallest bronchi. The goblet cells and principally the submucosal glands secrete the mucous layer, which is 2–5 μm in depth and rests on the tips of the cilia. Each ciliated cell has about 275 cilia; movement results from action by microtubules within each cilium. The cilia beat within a periciliary fluid layer at about 1000 beats/min, moving the mucous blanket toward the pharynx at a rate of approximately 10 mm/min in the trachea. In the respiratory portion of the lung the surface cells gradually become cuboidal and then flat; ciliated cells and goblet cells ordinarily are absent.

The final 25% of the warming and humidifying of the inspired air stream occurs in the trachea and large bronchi. Failure of humidification permits dry air to reach more distal airways. Particles 1–5 μm in size precipitate out on the tracheobronchial mucous blanket so that only particles of 1 μm or less reach the respiratory bronchioles and airspaces, where some may deposit and many will be exhaled.

Respiratory tract secretions are primarily derived from mucous (glycoproteins) and serous cells of the submucosal glands that empty onto the surface epithelium; from goblet cells and Clara cells, the special secreting cells in the surface epithelium of bronchi and bronchioles, respectively; from transudation from the vascular space; and from alveolar fluid, which contributes most of the phospholipid found in tracheobronchial mucus. This mucus is about 95% water.

Beyond infancy, collateral alveolar ventilation can increasingly occur with development of the pores of Kohn between alveoli, which provide a means for gas to pass from one lobule to another, perhaps even between segments of lung. Bronchiolar-alveolar communications, known as the canals of Lambert, are also found. These anatomic connections may be helpful in preventing or delaying atelectasis

The defenses of the respiratory system that protect the lung include the filtering of particles, the warming and humidification of inspired air, and the absorption of noxious fumes and gases by the vascular upper airway. The temporary cessation of breathing, reflexly shallow breathing, laryngospasm, or even bronchospasm limits the depth and amount of penetration of foreign matter. Spasm or decreased breathing can provide only brief protection. Aspiration of food, secretions, and foreign bodies are prevented by swallowing and closure of the epiglottis. The respiratory tract distal to the larynx is normally sterile.

Clearance of Particles. Particles deposited in conducting airways are cleared within hours by the mucociliary mechanism, while clearance of those reaching the alveoli may take several days to months. The latter may be phagocytized by alveolar macrophages and removed from lungs by the mucociliary system or carried into the interstitium for clearance by the lymphocytes into regional nodes or the blood. Some particles penetrate into the interstitium without phagocytosis. Mucociliary clearance may be aided by cough, which provides an effective means by propelling excess mucus up the airways at pressures of up to 300 mm Hg and at flows of up to 5–6 L/sec. Mucus raised by the cough mechanism is usually swallowed by young children but may be expectorated.

Defense Against Microbial Agents. Phagocytosis and mucociliary clearance may not be sufficient protection from living agents, such as bacteria and viruses. Additional factors include cellular killing of organisms and immune responses to assist in the phagocytosis-killing process. Alveolar and interstitial macrophages, derived from monocytes, are an essential component of the defense system of the lung. The engulfment and killing of living particles by these macrophages may be enhanced by opsonins or by small lymphocytes. The principal antibody in respiratory secretions is secretory immunoglobulin A (IgA), which is produced by plasma cells in the submucosa of the airways. Two molecules of IgA combine with a polypeptide (secretory component) produced by the respiratory epithelium to yield secretory IgA, which is highly resistant to digestion by proteolytic enzymes released after lysis of bacteria and dead cells. IgA can neutralize certain viruses and toxins and help in the lysis of bacteria. IgA may also prevent antigenic substances from penetrating the epithelial surfaces. Pulmonary secretory IgA reaches adult levels in the first month of life. IgG and IgM are also found in the secretions when lung inflammation occurs.

Lysozyme, lactoferrin, and interferon may also play a defense role in respiratory secretions. In addition a small fraction of the antibodies of the respiratory surface is made up of immunoglobulin E (IgE), which plays an important role in allergic reactions (Sec. 10.42).

Impaired Defense Mechanisms. The phagocytic ability of alveolar macrophages and, in most cases, the mucociliary mechanism can be impaired by ethanol ingestion, cigarette smoke, hypoxemia, starvation, chilling, corticosteroids, nitrogen dioxide, ozone, increased oxygen concentration, narcotics, and some anesthetic gases. The antibacterial killing capacity of the macrophages can be decreased by acidosis, azotemia, and recent acute viral infections, especially rubeola

and influenza. Beryllium and asbestos, organic dust from cotton and sugar cane, and gases such as sulfur, nitrogen dioxide, ozone, chlorine, ammonia, and cigarette smoke are toxic to epithelial cells.

Mucociliary clearance can be reduced by hypothermia, hyperthermia, morphine, codeine, and hypothyroidism. Inhalation of dry gas by mouthbreathing during periods of nasal obstruction, after placement of a tracheostomy, or during use of poorly humidified oxygen results in drying of the mucous membrane and slowing of the ciliary beat. Cold air may irritate the tracheobronchial tree.

Damage to the respiratory epithelium may be reversible with rhinitis, sinusitis, bronchitis, bronchiolitis, acute respiratory infections associated with high levels of air pollution, and the epithelial shedding that can occur in asthma, or with some irritants, bronchospasm, edema, congestion, and perhaps mild surface ulceration. However, severe ulceration, bronchiectasis, bronchiolectasis, squamous cell metaplasia, and fibrosis represent serious injury and permanent impairment of the normal clearance mechanism. Other events that can adversely affect the lung include hyperventilation, alveolar hypoxia, pulmonary thromboembolism, pulmonary edema, hypersensitivity reactions, and certain drugs such as salicylates.

13.7 METABOLIC FUNCTIONS OF THE LUNG

The lung contains more than 40 separate cell types. Among these heterogeneous cells, the type I and II pneumocytes, alveolar macrophage, and Clara cell are unique to the lung. The lung can synthesize lipids and proteins, including glycoproteins, secretory antibodies, interferon, proteolytic and fibrinolytic enzymes and activators, collagen, and elastin. Tissue factors such as thromboplastin are found in higher concentration in the lung than in any other organ. Megakaryocytes are concentrated in the lung.

Since the lung has the only capillary bed through which the entire blood flow must pass in the normal state, the pulmonary capillary circulation is ideally positioned to control circulating vasoactive hormones. Angiotensin II, up to 50 times more active than its precursor, is converted from angiotensin I during one passage through the pulmonary circulation. Other vasoactive materials, including serotonin, bradykinin, ATP, and prostaglandins E_1, E_2, and F_2, are almost completely removed or inactivated by one passage through the pulmonary circulation, while others, such as epinephrine, prostaglandin A_1 and A_2, angiotensin II, and vasopressin, may be minimally affected. Norepinephrine and histamine are taken up to a moderate degree. Failure of inactivation or periodic release of substances such as serotonin, bradykinin,

histamine, slow reacting substance of anaphylaxis (SRS-A), eosinophil chemotactic factor, platelet aggregation factor, endocrine substances, etc., may be important in the pathogenesis of some pulmonary disease or as a mediator of secondary effects.

Fishman AP: Non-respiratory functions of the lung. Chest 72:84, 1977
Fishman AP, Pietra GG: Handling of bioactive materials by the lung. N Engl J Med 291:884, 1974.
Green, GM: In defense of the lung. Am Rev Resp Dis 102:691, 1970.
Kendig EL (ed): Disorders of the Respiratory Tract in Children. Philadelphia, WB Saunders, 1983.
Loosli CG, Potter EL: Pre- and post-natal development of the respiratory portion of the human lung. Am Rev Resp Dis 80 (suppl):5, 1959.
Lough MD, Doershuk CF, Stern RC (eds): Pediatric Respiratory Therapy. Chicago, Year Book Medical Publishers, 1986.
Polgar, G, Weng, TR: The functional development of the respiratory system. Am Rev Resp Dis 120:625, 1979.
Proctor DF: The upper airways. I. Nasal physiology and defense of the lungs. Am Rev Resp Dis 115:97, 1977.
Said SI: The lung as a metabolic organ. N Engl J Med 279:1330, 1968.
Said SI: The lung in relation to vasoactive hormones. Fed Proc 32:1972, 1973.
Scarpelli M (ed): Pulmonary Physiology of the Fetus, Newborn and Child. Philadelphia, Lea & Febiger, 1975.
Thurlbeck WM: Postnatal growth and development of the lung. Am Rev Resp Dis 111:803, 1975.

13.8 PULMONARY FUNCTION

See also Sec. 13.19.

Ventilation. Normally, ventilation maintains arterial oxygen, carbon dioxide, and pH within the normal range at the least level of work. The alveolar-capillary membrane is so thin that usually there is no discernible difference in oxygen tension between the alveolar gas and pulmonary venous blood or in arterial or alveolar carbon dioxide tensions. At sea level the oxygen tension of ambient, relatively dry air is about 150 mm Hg; this is reduced to 100–105 mm Hg in the alveolus, in part because CO_2 and water vapor are also present (Fig. 13–1). The normal pressure of oxygen in the aorta (PaO_2) at sea level is 90–100 mm Hg, while that for carbon dioxide ($PaCO_2$) is about 38–42 mm Hg. The slight further drop in

pO_2 (4–5 mm Hg) observed between alveoli and arterial blood is due to diffusion and shunting from the bronchial arterial circulation and coronary venous blood. Hypoventilation (or hypercapnia) is defined as a $PaCO_2$ greater than 45 mm Hg and hyperventilation (hypocapnia) as a $PaCO_2$ less than 35 mm Hg.

Ventilation-Perfusion. For the lung as a whole, the ratio of alveolar ventilation at rest ($\dot{V}_A$ = 4 L/min) to pulmonary perfusion (Q = 5 L/min) is 0.8. However, the pattern of ventilated air does not uniformly follow the pattern of distribution of blood flow through the lung. In the erect position the lung apices are underventilated with respect to their volume and are underperfused to an even greater extent (high

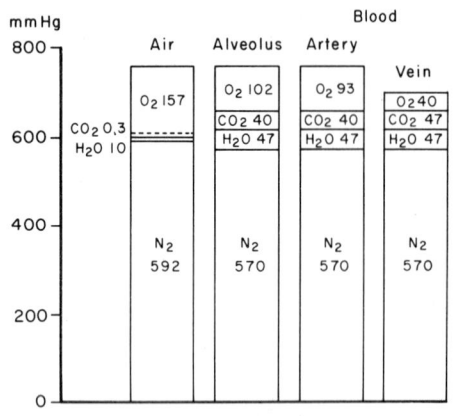

Figure 13–1. Partial pressures of oxygen, carbon dioxide, water vapor, and nitrogen in ambient air and in the body at sea level, where ambient pressure = 760 mm Hg.

$\dot{V}_A/\dot{Q}$) than the lung bases, which receive proportionately more blood flow than ventilated air (low $\dot{V}_A/\dot{Q}$). With disease this matching may be sufficiently deranged so that regional imbalances lead to an early decrease in arterial oxygen tension. In contrast minimal overall alveolar hyperventilation can maintain the carbon dioxide tension at normal levels or lower until much later in the disease process because of the greater ease of diffusion of carbon dioxide across the alveolus.

Causes of Hypoxemia. Ventilation-perfusion abnormalities are the most frequent cause of arterial hypoxemia. Shunts (intracardiac or intrapulmonary), diffusion problems, and primary hypoventilation (e.g., due to central nervous system depression, upper airway obstruction, or neuromuscular problems) also cause arterial hypoxemia. Primary hypoventilation also results in a parallel hypercapnia; however, the other three causes of hypoxemia result in hypercapnia only late in disease, when overall alveolar ventilation is reduced to the extent that CO_2 retention (greater than 45–50 mm Hg) occurs.

Lung Volumes. The standard terminology for various subdivisions of lung volume is diagrammed in Fig. 13–2.

Most lung subdivisions are measured from the resting end-tidal midposition where the retractive lung forces are balanced by the thoracic forces which tend to expand the chest and lungs. The volume of gas remaining in the lungs at this point is the functional residual capacity (FRC), which consists of the expiratory reserve volume (ERV) plus the residual volume (RV) that always remains in normal lungs. The FRC is normally 50% of the total lung capacity (TLC), and the RV is normally about 25% of the TLC and increases somewhat with age. In an average adult the tidal volume is about 500 mL. Approximately two thirds of each tidal volume enters the alveoli and one third remains in the conducting airways per breath (the anatomic dead space).

The volume changes and certain flow rates are measured by using a spirometer or a system that integrates flow through a flowmeter or pneumotachometer. FRC is measured by a closed circuit helium dilution method, by an open circuit nitrogen washout method, or by use of the total body plethysmograph to measure the volume of thoracic gas (V_{TG}). RV and TLC are calculated from the spirometer data and the FRC; for example, RV = FRC − ERV and TLC = FRC + IC (inspiratory capacity). The lung volumes are affected by changes in position and by disease.

Pulmonary function tests do not usually result in an etiologic diagnosis except, perhaps, when a response to a bronchodilator suggests a reversible airways problem consistent with bronchospasm and bronchial asthma. Rather, they permit recognition of two main patterns of pulmonary involvement. The *obstruction* pattern, which is encountered most often in childhood diseases, includes loss of vital capacity, principally ERV, while the FRC increases. The combined effect of these changes is a greater increase in RV than in FRC. TLC is usually somewhat increased in obstructive disease, but the RV/TLC ratio will be increased even more. Flow rates are generally decreased. Bronchiolitis, bronchial asthma, and cystic fibrosis are the most common conditions that produce a pattern of airways obstruction in children.

The *restriction* pattern includes a decrease in VC and TLC while the flow rates remain relatively unimpaired until VC and TLC fall below approximately 50% of predicted normal. The slight decrease of RV results in an apparent increase in the RV/TLC ratio, suggesting obstruction. When the TLC is decreased, no attempt should be made to interpret the RV/TLC ratio. Any condition causing stiffening of the chest or lungs, deformity of the spine, abnormality of the respiratory muscles, neurologic impairment of the diaphragm or other respiratory muscles, or anything acting to decrease the volume of the lungs (tumor, hydrothorax, pneumothorax) will produce a restrictive type of abnormality. Kyphoscoliosis and neuromuscular conditions are the most commonly encountered causes of a restrictive abnormality in childhood. Some conditions, such as cystic fibrosis, advanced tuberculosis, and asthmatic bronchitis, may have a combination of both obstructive and restrictive elements.

The lung volumes and capacities increase with body growth and in the normal child can best be related to body size. There is a relatively wide range of normal for lung volumes and capacities—up to ± 20%; results from test to test in the same individual can vary by as much as 5%.

Mechanics of Respiration. The mechanical factors in lung expansion include (1) the flow-resistive or dynamic properties, which include airway resistance and tissue viscous resistance and which combine to make up total pulmonary resistance; and (2) the elastic or static properties, expressed as compliance. Determining the dynamic forces requires both flow and pressure change measurements; determining the static properties requires both volume and pressure change measurements.

Flow rate measurements can be used to assess flow resistance since not all portions of the lung expand or retract at the same rate. Flow resistance is monitored inferentially by determining fractional portions of the forced expiratory vol-

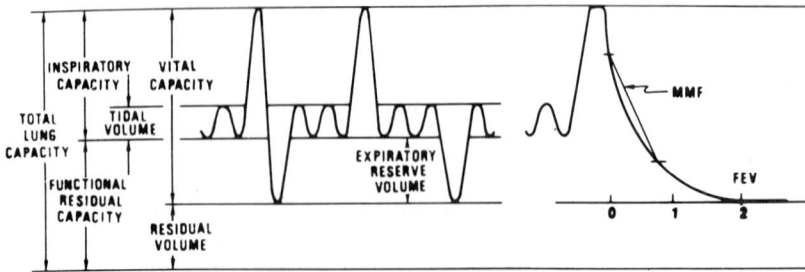

Figure 13–2. Lung volumes and forced vital capacity. MMF = maximal midexpiratory flow rate, i.e., mean flow rate calculated over mid–one half of forced expiratory curve. FEV = forced expiratory volume in a given time, such as 1 sec. Air is almost completely expelled within 3 sec in normal lungs, but emptying is delayed with obstruction. (From Doershuk CF Lough MD, *In* Lough MD, Doershuk CF, Stern RC (eds): Pediatric Respiratory Therapy. Courtesy Year Book Medical Publishers, Chicago, 1974.)

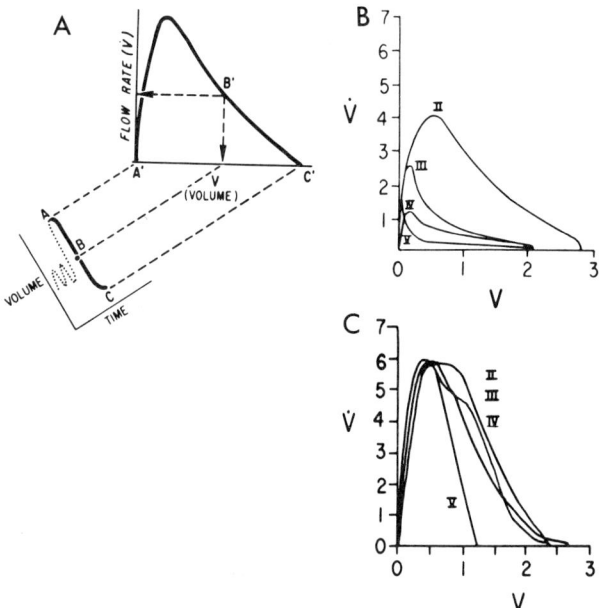

Figure 13–3. *A*, A standard spirogram (points A, B, and C) is compared with the expiratory flow-volume (FV) curve in a normal subject. In the FV curve, expiration proceeds from peak lung inflation at A' along A'B' to the forced expiratory position at C'. Flow rate at a given lung volume may be determined by drawing a tangent at any point in the spirogram. Such measurements are subject to error. By contrast, the flow rate at the same lung volume can be read directly at point B on the FV curve. ($\dot{V}$, flow rate in liters/sec; V, expiratory volume in liters from the total lung capacity.) *B*, Flow-volume curves in obstructive lung disease. Four classes of obstructive disease of increasing severity are shown. The curves in classes III, IV, and V were selected from patients of the same sex and height who had approximately the same forced vital capacities. As obstructive disease becomes more severe, the curve becomes more convex to the volume axis. A universal finding in class V is a sudden drop in flow soon after the onset of expiration. This phenomenon occurs even at low intrathoracic driving pressures. *C*, The flow-volume curve in pulmonary parenchymal fibrosis is characterized by a high peak flow rate and small forced vital capacity. In class V, with marked decrease in vital capacity, the high, peaked curve is distinctive. (From Lord GP, et al: Am J Med 46:73, 1969. Courtesy American Journal of Medicine.)

ume (FEV), expiratory flow rates from the maximal expiratory flow volume (MEFV) curve (Sec. 13–19 and Fig. 13-3), and maximal breathing capacity (MBC) or maximal voluntary ventilation (MVV). These tests are dependent upon the size or overinflation of the lung and are not specific measures of resistance since compliance also enters into the results. The mean flow rate in liters/second calculated over the middle half of the forced expiratory volume achieved is useful early in the course of obstructive disease.

The determinants of **airway resistance** (R_{AW}) during the usually predominant laminar flow that occurs in the airways during tidal breathing are the viscosity of gas and the length and radius of the bronchi and bronchioles. R_{AW} is inversely related to lung volume since airway caliber is affected by increases and decreases in lung size. Although the smallest airways offer the highest resistance, the tremendous increase in total cross sectional area of the airways toward the periphery means that the peripheral airways contribute less than 20% of the airway resistance, and it is thought that peripheral R_{AW} plays a prominent role in children only up to age 4–5 yr. Considerable peripheral airways disease thus may be present before significant alterations in R_{AW} are apparent.

The elastic characteristic of the respiratory system, **compliance**, is expressed as volume/centimeters of H_2O pressure. Since determination of pressure change requires a balloon positioned in the esophagus, compliance is not frequently measured during childhood. The lungs of infants are less compliant than those of older children and young adults, but when the effect of lung size at FRC is considered (specific compliance), no differences are observed. In disease states, altered lung elasticity and surface characteristics, areas of atelectasis or consolidation, or increased airway resistance will alter the pressure-volume characteristics of the lung.

Work of Breathing. This work meets the energy requirements to overcome inertia, surface active forces, air flow and elastic resistance, and tissue viscous resistance. In general, the rate and depth of breathing are adjusted so that alveolar ventilation is maintained at a minimum of total respiratory work. At all ages it appears that approximately 1% of the total basal metabolism is normally expended on the work of breathing.

Diffusion. Oxygen and carbon dioxide diffusion depends upon the thickness of the alveolar-capillary membrane, capillary transit time, uptake of oxygen by the blood, and total surface area of the capillary bed in relation to that of the alveolar membrane. Because of its high diffusing capacity (20 times greater than that of oxygen), carbon dioxide levels are rarely abnormal in diffusion problems. When the inspired oxygen percentage is reduced to 14%, arterial hypoxemia is increased in a diffusion problem, but it can be corrected when 100% oxygen is breathed. Measuring the pulmonary diffusing capacity (D_L) using carbon monoxide can provide a useful index of pulmonary structure and function. Primary diffusion defects are rare in children but are seen in conditions resulting in diffuse interstitial fibrosis.

Arterial Blood Gases. In primary hypoventilation, such as central nervous system depression or muscle paralysis, a decrease in arterial pO_2 will be paralleled by an increase in $PaCO_2$. Diffusion abnormalities, shunt problems, and especially the ventilation-perfusion inequalities occurring in conditions such as bronchial asthma, bronchiolitis, and cystic fibrosis also result in arterial hypoxemia. A decrease in PaO_2 is the earliest observation, usually accompanied by a *decrease* in $PaCO_2$ due to the overall increase in ventilation. When the condition deteriorates to overall alveolar hypoventilation, the $PaCO_2$ returns toward normal. Subsequently, CO_2 retention greater than 45–50 mm Hg indicates respiratory failure.

Acute respiratory failure results in the elevation of $PaCO_2$ and decrease in pH; the bicarbonate (HCO_3^-) remains normal. When the kidneys have had 1–2 days to compensate by retaining HCO_3^-, the pH is restored toward normal and compensated respiratory acidosis results. When improved ventilation reduces the carbon dioxide, there is a slow fall in HCO_3^-, resulting in metabolic alkalosis (Sec. 5.12) for several days.

CARL F. DOERSHUK

Briscoe WA, Dubois AB: The relationship between airway resistance, airway conductance, and lung volume in subjects of different ages and body size. J Clin Invest 37:1279, 1958.

DeMuth GR, Howatt WF, Hill G: The growth of lung function. Pediatrics 35:162, 1965.

Doershuk CF, Lough MD: Pulmonary function testing and interpretation. In: Lough MD, Doershuk CF, Stern RC (eds): Pediatric Respiratory Therapy. 3rd ed. Chicago, Year Book Medical Publishers, 1986.

Lord GP, et al: Flow-volume curves in lung disease. Am J Med 46:73, 1969.

Shapiro BA, Harrison RA: Clinical Application of Blood Gases. Chicago, Year Book Medical Publishers, 1982.

West JB: Respiratory Physiology. Baltimore, Williams & Wilkins, 1985.

13.9 REGULATION OF RESPIRATION

While knowledge of mechanisms regulating respiration has greatly expanded in recent years, many fundamental physiologic questions remain unanswered. The pediatrician needs to understand the basic principles of respiratory control, as they are the key to a smooth transition from fetal to neonatal life, especially in the preterm infant. Beyond the neonatal period, disordered respiratory control has been most commonly implicated in the sudden infant death syndrome (Sec. 26.1). Maturation has a major influence on the various components of respiratory regulation during early infancy (Fig. 13–4).

Central Mechanisms. The generation of rhythmic respiratory activity and the integration of input from peripheral receptors occur in the brain stem, involving neurons in at least two areas on the ventrolateral surface of the medulla as well as the pons. In the medulla, there are also axonal interconnections between a wide variety of contralateral and ipsilateral respiratory neurons, allowing for complex integration of sensory input and respiratory motor output. It is hypothesized that a central generator of inspiratory activity continually integrates input from chemoreceptors and mechanoreceptors until an "off-switch" mechanism is triggered, which may itself be modulated by inputs from other areas of the brain and peripheral receptors.

As gestation advances, fetal respiratory activity occurs, until it becomes present (although episodic) 30–60% of the time. Fetal breathing movements are influenced by such external stimuli as maternal plasma glucose concentration and occur predominantly during the postnatal equivalent of active (or rapid eye movement) sleep. After birth, neonatal breathing patterns are also very sensitive to external stimuli (which may produce apnea in preterm infants) and change in sleep state.

Chemical Control. The change in ventilation in response to increased levels of inspired carbon dioxide or to alterations in inspired oxygen measures the chemical responsiveness of respiratory control mechanisms. The response of the respiratory muscles to a chemical stimulus is initiated by afferent information derived from peripheral and/or central chemoreceptors. The peripheral receptors are situated in the carotid and aortic bodies, while the central receptors are probably located on the ventrolateral surface of the medulla, which is thought to be the primary site at which a hypercapneic stimulus is sensed, although transient and more rapid changes in CO_2 will largely be sensed peripherally. CO_2 sensitivity has been defined as the slope of the line describing minute ventilation (corrected for body weight) versus alveolar pCO_2, usually obtained from at least two steady state levels. The preterm infant's CO_2 sensitivity is decreased compared with that of the term infant. This may be the result of immaturity in some component of the chemical control mechanism, or of a mechanical inability on the part of the respiratory muscles of the chest wall to generate an appropriate ventilatory response. The premature infant's response increases with either advancing gestational or postnatal age. CO_2 sensitivity is decreased in apneic preterm infants, although a clear cause-and-effect relationship is not established.

When challenged with a hypoxic stimulus, both term and preterm neonates respond with a brief increase in minute ventilation over the first minute, followed within 2–3 min by a fall in minute ventilation, sometimes to less than the resting level. After 7–8 days postnatal age, hyperventilation can be sustained as in the older infant and child. The early neonatal response may be due to initial peripheral chemoreceptor stimulation followed by an overriding depression of the respiratory center as a result of hypoxemia. Postulated mechanisms for this ventilatory depression include release of endorphins, a hypoxia-induced increase in cerebral blood flow, or a vagally mediated inhibitory mechanism. It is speculated that the failure of preterm infants to maintain hyperventilation in response to sustained hypoxemia may destabilize respiratory control and aggravate apneic episodes.

Mechanoreceptor Reflexes. In 1968 Hering and Breuer reported that distension of the lungs of anaesthetized animals prolonged expiration and decreased respiratory frequency and that this inhibitory reflex response could be abolished by section of the vagus nerve. The afferent limb of this reflex arc originates in slowly adapting pulmonary stretch receptors, and fibers in the vagus nerve carry the stretch receptor input to the medulla. The efferent limb of the reflex arc travels within the phrenic nerve to the diaphragm. The *Hering-Breuer reflex* may be readily elicited in newborn infants, although it is difficult to elicit later in life. Abrupt lung inflation results in an initial gasp (also known as *Head's reflex*) followed by an apnea of variable duration, which may result from vagal inhibition of inspiration and/or prolongation of expiration due to the Hering-Breuer inflation reflex. Similarly, airway occlusion at end expiration prolongs the subsequent inspiratory effort owing to a decrease in inspiratory inhibition in the absence of lung inflation. Chest wall distortion may trigger an intercostal inhibitory reflex that originates in intercostal muscle spindles, resulting in shortening of inspiration. However, compression or distortion of the underlying lung could also shorten inspiration via vagally mediated irritant or deflation reflexes. Reflexes from the larger airways, bronchioles, alveoli, and intercostal muscles may thus all influence the length and depth of inspiration and expiration during normal breathing and may also influence the maintenance of an appropriate resting lung volume. In newborn infants, the activity of these reflexes appears enhanced, possibly owing to immature chemical control mechanisms or the paucity of central dendritic interconnections.

Respiratory Muscles. Effective ventilation requires coordinated interaction between the respiratory muscles of the chest wall (including diaphragm and abdomen) and those of the upper airway (including pharynx and larynx) under various conditions of altered respiratory drive. In infants, a specific

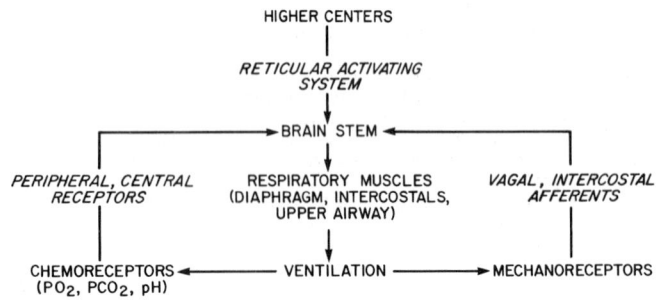

Figure 13–4. An overview of major factors influencing respiratory control mechanisms.

sequential pattern of nerve and muscle activation occurs so that some upper airway muscles contract prior to and during the early part of inspiratory flow: the genioglossus muscle contracts, moving the tongue forward, which prevents pharyngeal obstruction; the vocal cords abduct, reducing inspiratory laryngeal resistance. Laryngeal muscles also modulate expiratory flow and so may influence lung volume. Imbalance of pharyngeal and diaphragmatic activities or their responses to chemo- or mechanoreceptor stimulation may contribute to obstructive apnea in infants and children. Sleep state influences respiratory muscle behavior, as evidenced by the asynchronous (out of phase, paradoxical) chest wall movements in infants during active sleep, which is probably secondary to decreased intercostal muscle activity. This may precipitate diaphragmatic fatigue, increasing vulnerability to apnea during active sleep.

Disordered Respiratory Regulation. The central neurologic mechanisms that predispose infants to *apnea* are not completely understood (also see Sec. 8.31). Incomplete development of brain dendritic synapses may explain the observation that breathing patterns of premature infants in the sleep state are very sensitive to external stimuli and change. An example of the importance of peripheral input is seen in the variety of stimuli that may trigger apnea in premature infants. Apnea appears to be a final common response of the immature respiratory control center to stimuli considerably less potent in an older child or adult.

Apnea is typically defined as a pause in breathing of variable duration (usually <10–15 sec), often associated with cyanosis and/or bradycardia. It is distinguished from periodic breathing, in which the infant exhibits regularly recurring 10–15 sec cycles of respiration interrupted by respiratory pauses at least 3 sec in duration; the pauses are not associated with significant bradycardia and are not pathologically significant. Simultaneous measurements of respiratory movements and air flow have demonstrated that pharyngeal obstruction is common during apnea in preterm and term infants both during and beyond the neonatal period. Such obstructive apneas may be readily misinterpreted as isolated bradycardia by standard impedance monitoring techniques. In older children hypertrophied tonsils or adenoids may precipitate episodes of upper airway obstruction and apnea. Other disorders of respiratory regulation rarely manifest in childhood. Congenital central hypoventilation syndrome (Ondine's curse) is discussed in Sec. 13.110. Patients with familial dysautonomia (Riley-Day syndrome) appear less responsive than normal to changes in pCO_2 and pO_2, presumably owing to a defect in central or peripheral chemoreceptor function (Sec. 21.29). In the obesity-hypoventilation (Pickwickian) syndrome, any defect in chemical drive is compounded by the increased work of breathing secondary to chest wall obesity and abdominal distention (Sec. 13.21 and 13.109).

RICHARD J. MARTIN

Carlo WA, Martin RJ: Regulation of respiratory muscles in infants and children. *In:* Milner ADP, Martin RJ (eds): Pediatric Respiratory Medicine. London, Butterworths, 1985.

Guilleminault C, McQuitty J, Ariagno RL, et al: Congenital central alveolar hypoventilation syndrome in six infants. Pediatrics 70:684, 1982.

Miller, MJ, Martin RJ, Carlo WA: Apnea: A disorder of respiratory control in neonates. *In:* Cherniack NS, Edelman NH (eds): Contemporary Issues in Pulmonary Diseases. New York, Churchill-Livingstone, 1985.

Rigatto H: Control of ventilation in the newborn. Ann Rev Physiol 46:661, 1984.

13.10 DIAGNOSTIC PROCEDURES IN PULMONARY MEDICINE

13.11 RADIOGRAPHIC TECHNIQUES

See also Sec. 5.55.

An appropriate, properly performed and interpreted roentgenogram can be one of the most useful diagnostic tools, but applying faulty technique or interpretation can make it confusing or misleading. To minimize radiation exposure, proper collimation and gonadal shielding should be used, and films must be limited to the area of clinical concern. Roentgenograms should be taken with equipment in the radiology department whenever possible rather than with portable equipment. The area of greatest interest should generally be placed closest to the film, with the patient properly positioned and, if necessary, gently immobilized. Exposure time should be short to minimize motion artifact, particularly for infants.

Chest Roentgenograms. A posterior-anterior and a lateral view, upright and at full inspiration, should be obtained in most circumstances. Films taken during expiration are often misinterpreted, but comparing expiratory and inspiratory films may reveal a mediastinal shift, helpful in evaluating bronchial obstruction (as with foreign body). Decubitus films are indicated if pleural fluid is suspected. Recumbent films may be difficult to interpret in the presence of free fluid, either within the pleural space or in a cavity. Oblique views may be helpful evaluating the hilum and the area behind the heart, while the apices are best seen in a lordotic view.

Computed Tomography. The technique of computed tomography (CT) can be useful in delineating internal structures and their relationships in greater detail than standard roentgenograms can, but it is more expensive and involves higher radiation exposure than plain films and should be used only when necessary. Because relatively long exposures are required, sedation may be needed.

Upper Airway Films. A lateral view of the neck can yield invaluable information about upper airway obstruction and particularly about the conditions of the retropharyngeal space, supraglottic area, and subglottic space (the latter should also be viewed in a posterior-anterior projection). Knowing the phase of respiration during which the film was taken is often essential for accurate interpretation. Patients with suspected obstruction must not be sent unattended to the radiology department.

Xerography. This gives exceptionally good soft tissue detail but requires much higher doses of radiation (especially to the thyroid) and should not be used routinely.

Sinus, Nasal Films. Roentgenographic examination of the sinuses is indicated when sinus disease is suspected. Because of the small size and slow development of the frontal and maxillary sinus cavities in children, transillumination is not as successful in documenting sinus disease as are roentgenograms. The need for examining the nasal passages in children is unusual and occurs most often when the neonate presents with obstruction or when tumor or occult foreign body is suspected.

Fluoroscopy. Fluoroscopy is especially useful for evaluating stridor and abnormal movement of the diaphragm or mediastinum. Many procedures, such as needle aspiration or biopsy of a peripheral lesion, are also best accomplished with the aid of fluoroscopy. Video tape recording, which does not increase radiation exposure, may allow detailed study, through "replay" capability, during a brief exposure to fluoroscopy.

Contrast Studies. *Barium Swallow.* This study is indicated in evaluating patients with recurrent pneumonia, persistent coughs of undetermined etiology, and stridor or persistent wheezing. It should be done with fluoroscopy and spot films. In the search for an "H" type of tracheoesophageal fistula, a simple barium swallow is often inadequate; the barium may have to be injected through catheters placed at several locations in the esophagus. If esophageal atresia is suspected, no more than 0.5 mL of barium should be injected into the esophagus through a soft catheter, carefully avoiding aspiration into the trachea. Many authorities do not recommend contrast studies when esophageal atresia is suspected.

Bronchograms. Smaller bronchi may be delineated by instilling a contrast material directly into the airway. In small children bronchograms are usually performed through an endotracheal tube under general anesthesia. In older children and adults sedation and topical anesthesia may be sufficient. The smallest amount of contrast material necessary to coat (not fill) the airways is placed into the airways with a catheter passed transnasally, through the endotracheal tube or through a fiberoptic bronchoscope. The procedure should be performed with fluoroscopy so that the contrast material can be placed selectively in the areas and in the quantity desired. In general, bronchograms are indicated only when pulmonary surgery may be considered. Specific indications include recurrent hemoptysis, recurrent pneumonia in the same area, chronic productive cough with persistent localized physical findings, and previously demonstrated bronchiectasis unresponsive to therapy.

Pulmonary Arteriograms. These studies allow detailed evaluation of the pulmonary vasculature and are helpful in diagnosing congenital anomalies, such as lobar agenesis, unilateral hyperlucent lung, and vascular rings, and are sometimes useful in evaluating solid or cystic lesions.

Aortograms. Thoracic aortograms demonstrate the systemic (bronchial) pulmonary circulation, especially in suspected pulmonary sequestration. Although most hemoptysis is from the bronchial arteries, bronchial arteriography is seldom helpful in diagnosing or treating intrapulmonary bleeding in children.

Pneumoperitoneum, Pneumothorax. In selected situations, such as in the evaluation of diaphragmatic eventration, it may be advantageous to inject a small amount of air into the pleural or peritoneal cavity, outlining the limits of the diaphragm or pleural surfaces by air contrast. Rapidly absorbed, the air causes no functional impairment.

Radionuclide Lung Scans. The usual scan uses intravenous injection of material (macroaggregated human serum albumin) that will be trapped in the pulmonary capillary bed. The distribution of radioactivity, proportional to *pulmonary capillary blood flow*, is useful in evaluating pulmonary embolism and congenital cardiovascular and pulmonary defects. Acute changes in the distribution of pulmonary perfusion may reflect alterations of pulmonary ventilation.

The distribution of *pulmonary ventilation* may be determined by scanning following the inhalation of a radioactive gas such as xenon-133. After the intravenous injection of xenon-133 dissolved in saline, both pulmonary perfusion and ventilation can be evaluated by continuous recording of the rate of appearance and disappearance of the xenon over the lung. Appearance of xenon early after injection is a measure of perfusion, while the rate of washout during breathing is a measure of ventilation.

13.12 ENDOSCOPY

Laryngoscopy. Inspection of the glottis is often necessary in evaluating stridor and local abnormalities. In infants and small children, direct laryngoscopy is usually necessary and requires general anesthesia. While useful in older children and adults, indirect (mirror) laryngoscopy is rarely possible in infants. Direct laryngoscopy can now also be done with topical anesthesia and mild sedation by passing a small flexible fiberoptic bronchoscope through the nose, allowing the glottis to be seen without the anatomic distortion that a laryngoscope blade sometimes introduces. This newer technique is also more comfortable for the patient and is especially useful for evaluating the dynamics of the larynx and upper airway.

Bronchoscopy. Indications for bronchoscopy include the evaluation of recurrent pneumonia or atelectasis, the possible presence of foreign bodies, unexplained and persistent wheezes and infiltrates, hemoptysis, and suspected congenital anomalies or mass lesions. The bronchoscope is used for visual examination, for biopsy of mass lesions or for transbronchial lung biopsy, and for aspiration of secretions for culture and microscopic examination. Therapeutic applications include removal of foreign bodies and mucus plugs, as well as bronchial toilet and bronchopulmonary lavage. An open tube bronchoscope should be used for patients with massive pulmonary bleeding, for removal of foreign bodies, or for other operative procedures. The advantages of small flexible fiberoptic bronchoscopes include ease of insertion, greater peripheral range, a lower incidence of complications, and the elimination of the need for general anesthesia.

Complications of bronchoscopy depend on the instrument used and on the procedure performed. Transient hypoxia, cardiac arrhythmias, laryngospasm, and bronchospasm are most common, and infection, bleeding, pneumomediastinum, or pneumothorax may occur. After open tube bronchoscopy, the patient must be carefully observed for airway obstruction resulting from trauma to the subglottic space, a much less common occurrence after use of a flexible bronchoscope because of the instrument's relatively small size. Postbronchoscopy croup is treated with oxygen, mist, vasoconstrictor aerosols (racemic epinephrine), and corticosteroids as necessary.

13.13 THORACENTESIS

For diagnostic or therapeutic purposes, fluid may be removed from the pleural space by needle puncture. The site of puncture is chosen to maximize the yield of fluid and minimize the risk. The procedure is usually performed while the patient is in a sitting position. First, local anesthetic is injected using a 1.5 inch, 22 gauge needle passed just *above* the rib margin to avoid the neurovascular bundle. The pleura may be identified by "touch" or by withdrawing an initial volume of pleural fluid. Then a larger needle is inserted to the same depth through the inferior aspect of the intercostal space. It is often advantageous to pass a plastic catheter through the needle into the pleural space, then withdraw the needle. This allows the operator to move both catheter and patient, thereby often collecting more fluid and reducing the possibility of puncture or laceration of the lung. Generally, as much fluid as possible should be withdrawn, and following the procedure, an *upright* chest roentgenogram obtained.

Complications of thoracentesis include infection, pneumothorax, and bleeding. Thoracentesis on the right may be complicated by puncture or laceration of the capsule of the liver, and on the left, by that of the capsule of the spleen. Specimens obtained should always be cultured, examined microscopically for evidence of bacterial infection, and evaluated for total protein and total and differential cell counts. Lactic acid dehydrogenase, glucose, cholesterol, and amylase determinations may also be useful. If malignancy is suspected, cytologic examination is imperative.

Transudates result from mechanical factors influencing the rate of formation or reabsorption of pleural fluid and generally require no further diagnostic evaluation. *Exudates* result from inflammation or other disease of the pleural surface and underlying lung and require a more complete diagnostic evaluation. In general, transudates have a total protein of less than 3 g/dL or a ratio of pleural protein to serum protein under 0.5, a total leukocyte count of fewer than 2000 with a predominance of mononuclear cells, and low lactic acid dehydrogenase levels. Exudates have high protein levels and a predominance of polymorphonuclear cells (although malignant or tuberculous effusions may have a higher percentage of mononuclear cells). Tuberculous effusions may have low glucose and high cholesterol content.

13.14 PERCUTANEOUS LUNG TAP

Using a technique very similar to that for thoracentesis, a percutaneous lung tap is the most direct method of obtaining bacteriologic specimens from the pulmonary parenchyma and is the only technique other than open lung biopsy not associated with at least some risk of contamination by oral flora. After local anesthesia a 20 or 22 gauge, 1.5 inch needle attached to a 10 mL syringe containing approximately 1 mL of nonbacteriostatic sterile saline is inserted using aseptic technique through the inferior aspect of an intercostal space in the area of interest. The needle is rapidly advanced into the lung, the saline injected and reaspirated, and the needle withdrawn, all performed as quickly as possible. This procedure usually yields a few drops of fluid from the lung, which should be cultured and examined microscopically.

Major indications for a lung tap are roentgenographic infiltrates of undetermined etiology, especially those unresponsive to therapy in immunosuppressed patients who are susceptible to unusual organisms. Complications are the same as for thoracentesis, but the incidence of pneumothorax is higher and somewhat dependent on the nature of the underlying disease process. In patients with poor pulmonary compliance, as with pneumocystis pneumonia, the rate may approach 30%, with 5% requiring chest tubes.

13.15 LUNG BIOPSY

Lung biopsy may be the only way to establish a diagnosis, especially in protracted, noninfectious disease. In infants and small children an open surgical biopsy is the procedure of choice, and in expert hands it is associated with an extremely low morbidity. As well as assuring that an adequate specimen can be obtained, the surgeon can inspect the lung surface and choose the site of biopsy. In older patients transbronchial biopsies can be performed using flexible forceps through an endotracheal tube or a bronchoscope, usually with fluoroscopic guidance. This technique is most appropriate when there are diffuse lung diseases such as pneumocystis pneumonia. However, because of the small specimens obtained, the diagnosis may be more easily missed than with an open biopsy.

13.16 TRANSILLUMINATION OF THE CHEST WALL

In infants up to at least 6 mo of age, a pneumothorax may often be diagnosed by transillumination of the chest wall using a fiberoptic light probe. Free air in the pleural space often results in an unusually large halo of light in the skin surrounding the probe. This test is unreliable in older patients or in those with subcutaneous emphysema.

13.17 MICROBIOLOGY

The specific diagnosis of infection in the lower respiratory tract depends on the proper handling of an adequate specimen obtained in an appropriate fashion. Nasopharyngeal or throat cultures are often used but may not correlate with cultures obtained by more direct techniques. Sputum specimens are preferred and are often obtained from patients who do not expectorate by deep throat swab immediately after coughing. Specimens also may be obtained directly from the tracheobronchial tree by nasotracheal aspiration (usually heavily contaminated), by transtracheal aspiration through the cricothyroid membrane (useful in adults and adolescents but hazardous in children), and in infants and children by a sterile catheter inserted into the trachea either during direct laryngoscopy or through an endotracheal tube. A percutaneous lung tap or an open biopsy is the only way to obtain a specimen free of oral flora.

Examination of Secretions. A specimen obtained by direct expectoration is usually assumed to be of tracheobronchial origin, but often it is not. The presence of alveolar macrophages—large, mononuclear cells—is the hallmark of tracheobronchial secretions. Both nasopharyngeal and tracheobronchial secretions may contain ciliated epithelial cells, which are more commonly found in sputum. Nasopharyngeal and oral secretions often contain large numbers of squamous epithelial cells. Sputum may contain both ciliated and squamous epithelial cells.

During sleep, mucociliary transport continually brings tracheobronchial secretions to the pharynx, where they are swallowed. An early morning gastric aspirate will often contain material from the tracheobronchial tract that is suitable for smear and culture for acid-fast bacilli.

The absence of polymorphonuclear leukocytes in a Wright-stained smear of sputum containing adequate numbers of macrophages is significant evidence against a bacterial infectious process in the lower respiratory tract, assuming the patient has normal neutrophil counts and function. Eosinophils suggest allergic disease. Iron stains may reveal hemosiderin granules within macrophages, suggesting pulmonary hemosiderosis. Specimens should also be examined by Gram stain. Squamous epithelial cells are usually covered with bacteria, which should be ignored. Bacteria within or near macrophages and neutrophils are more significant. Viral pneumonia may be accompanied by intranuclear or cytoplasmic inclusion bodies visible on Wright-stained smears, and fungal forms may be identifiable on Gram stains.

Sweat Testing

See Sec. 13.97.

13.18 BLOOD GAS ANALYSIS

An arterial blood gas analysis is probably the single most useful test of pulmonary function. If multiple samples are to be drawn over a relatively short time, an indwelling arterial line may be placed; constant perfusion with heparinized saline (1 unit/mL, 3–5 mL/hr) may prevent thrombus formation.

Arterial punctures are painful, often resulting in hyperventilation unless local anesthesia is used. The artery should be entered with a 21 or 23 gauge straight or scalp vein needle at an angle of approximately 45°. The blood specimen is best collected anaerobically in a heparinized glass syringe containing only enough heparin solution to displace the air from the syringe. The syringe should be sealed, placed in ice, and carried to the laboratory for immediate analysis.

Arterialized capillary blood may be used if tissue perfusion is good and if great care is taken in collecting and handling the specimen. Under ideal conditions arterialized capillary blood correlates well with arterial samples. Local vasodilation is produced in the finger, the heel, or the ear lobe by warming or by applying nitroglycerin or nicotinic acid cream. When the site has become flushed, blood is collected into a capillary tube from a free-flowing stab wound.

A pulse *oximeter* can continually measure peripheral oxygen saturation and usually correlates well with simultaneous arterial saturation. *Transcutaneous oxygen electrodes* can continuously monitor oxygen and carbon dioxide tension if tissue perfusion is adequate. *End-tidal pCO₂* usually correlates well with arterial pCO₂ unless there is a very uneven distribution of ventilation.

Venous pCO₂ averages 6–8 mm Hg higher than arterial pCO₂, and pH is slightly lower. Such samples are more useful in managing chronic acid-base disturbances than in managing acute respiratory disease.

13.19 PULMONARY FUNCTION TESTING

See also Sec. 13.8.

Ventilation, perfusion, and gas exchange may all be quantified, but in clinical practice measurements of ventilation are the most commonly performed "pulmonary function test."

Measurement of Ventilatory Function. A spirometer is used to measure vital capacity (VC) and its subdivisions and expiratory (or inspiratory) flow rates (Figs. 13–2 and 13–3). Volume displacement *spirometers* record changes in the volume of gas the subject breathes into and out of a closed container. Electronic spirometers integrate flow through a pneumotachometer to determine volume. Peak flow rates are measured with either an electronic spirometer or a special peak flow meter. A body *plethysmograph* measures functional residual capacity (FRC), from which are calculated (with spirometric data) the total lung capacity (TLC) and residual volume (RV). The plethysmograph is an airtight box in which the subject sits, holding a closed shutter apparatus in his or her mouth; pressure changes within the box and those at the mouth are measured while breathing against the mouthpiece. *Gas dilution tests*, which are less useful in children, can also measure FRC by allowing the subject to breathe to equilibrium into a closed volume initially containing a known concentration of marker gas (usually helium). A simple *manometer* can measure the maximal inspiratory and expiratory force a subject generates, normally at least 30 cm H₂O, which is useful in evaluating the neuromuscular component of ventilation. Expected normal values for VC, FRC, TLC, and RV are obtained from prediction equations based on body height.

Flow rates measured by spirometry usually include the volume expired in the first second (FEV₁) and the maximal midexpiratory flow rate (MMEF). More information results from a maximal expiratory flow-volume curve (MEFV), in which expiratory flow rate is plotted against expired lung volume (expressed in terms of either VC or TLC). Flow rates at lung volumes less than about 75% VC are relatively independent of effort. Expiratory flow rates at low lung volumes (less than 50% VC) are influenced much more by small airways than are flow rates at high lung volumes (FEV₁). The flow rate at 25% VC ($\dot{V}_{25}$) is a useful index of small airway function. Low flow rates at high lung volumes associated with normal flow at low lung volumes suggest upper airway obstruction.

Airway resistance (R_{AW}) is measured in a plethysmograph and is expressed as cm H₂O/L/sec. Alternatively, the reciprocal of R_{AW}, *airway conductance* (G_{AW}), may be used. Because airway resistance measurements vary with the lung volume at which they are taken, it is convenient to use specific airway resis-

tance, SR_{AW} ($SR_{AW} = R_{AW} \times$ lung volume), which is nearly constant in subjects older than 6 yr (normally less than 7 sec/cm H₂O).

Measurement of Gas Exchange. The *diffusing capacity for carbon monoxide* (D_LCO) is measured by rebreathing from a container having a known initial concentration of CO or by using a single breath technique. Decreases in D_LCO reflect decreases in effective alveolar capillary surface area or decreases in diffusibility of the gas across the alveolar-capillary membrane. This test is rarely used in pediatrics because primary diffusion abnormalities are unusual in children. *Regional gas exchange* may be conveniently estimated with the perfusion/ventilation xenon scan (Sec. 13.11). Determining *arterial blood gases* will also disclose the effectiveness of alveolar gas exchange.

Measurement of Perfusion. Pulmonary blood flow may be measured by cardiac catheterization or by a technique employing the uptake of nitrous oxide. The distribution of blood flow may be studied in a pulmonary arteriogram or with radioisotope scans.

Other Tests of Lung Function. Other available tests measure compliance, distribution of ventilation, dead space, elastic recoil, and closing volume. Pulmonary function tests performed before and after exercise may be useful in detecting exercise-induced bronchospasm. Sufficient exercise should be performed to elevate the pulse to 160–170/min for 5–6 min. Testing should be done 10 min after the end of the exercise period. There is poor correlation between the objective results of exercise testing and the subjective evaluation of exercise tolerance by patient or parent.

Clinical Use of Pulmonary Function Testing. Pulmonary function testing, while rarely resulting in an etiologic diagnosis, is helpful in defining the type of process (e.g., obstruction, restriction) and the degree of functional impairment in following the course and treatment of disease, and in estimating the prognosis. It is also useful in preoperative evaluation and in confirmation of functional impairment in patients having subjective complaints but a normal physical examination. In most patients with obstructive disease, a repeat test after administering a bronchodilator is warranted.

Most tests require some cooperation and understanding by the subject, and interpretation is greatly facilitated if the test conditions and the subject's behavior during the test are known. Accurate testing of children aged 3–6 yr requires great patience by the physician and training of the subject, while most children aged 6 yr or older can be tested reliably without excessive difficulty. Infants and young children may be studied by gas dilution and plethysmographic methods for measurement of FRC and R_{AW}, but sedation may be required.

ROBERT E. WOOD

Hughes WT, Buescher ES: Pediatric Procedures. 2nd ed. Philadelphia, WB Saunders, 1980.

Kendig EL, Chernick V: Disorders of the Respiratory Tract in Children. 4th ed. Philadelphia, WB Saunders, 1983.

Klein JO: Diagnostic lung puncture in the pneumonias of infants and children. Pediatrics 44:456, 1969.

Sackner MA (ed): Diagnostic Techniques in Pulmonary Disease. New York, Marcel Dekker, 1980.

Sperber M: Computerized Tomography of the Lung: Normal Anatomy and Most Common Disorders. Mount Kisco NY, Futra Publishing Co., 1984.

Wood RE: Spelunking in the pediatric airways: Explorations with the flexible bronchoscope. Pediatr Clin North Am 31:785, 1984.

13.20 DISEASES OF THE RESPIRATORY SYSTEM

GENERAL CONSIDERATIONS

The patterns of respiratory tract disease in childhood are modified by age, sex, race, season, geography, and environmental and socioeconomic conditions. Intrauterine acquisition of viral infections, such as cytomegalovirus and herpes simplex virus, may result in neonatal pneumonia; cytomegalovirus, *Ureaplasma*, *Chlamydia trachomatis*, or group B streptococcal respiratory infection may be acquired during descent through the birth canal; immediately after birth, tuberculosis can be transmitted to the newborn, presenting after several weeks of life as a severe pneumonitis. Lung immaturity and other events related to the perinatal period predispose to hyaline membrane disease. Beyond the newborn period a lack of antibodies against common viral pathogens results in an increased incidence of respiratory tract infections that peaks at 1 yr of age. Pneumococcal lobar pneumonia is uncommon in small children, and pneumonia due to mycoplasmal infection is uncommon during the first 3–4 yr of life. The incidence of respiratory tract infection also peaks during the first 2–3 school years because of increased exposure to respiratory infections against which children have not yet developed specific immunity.

The anatomic distribution of respiratory tract disease may also change with age. Group A β-hemolytic streptococcal infections are commonly located in the nasopharynx in young children but in the tonsillar and lower pharyngeal areas of older children. A relatively short and open eustachian tube in infants and young children allows easy access of pharyngeal organisms to the middle ear cavity and is in part responsible for the higher incidence of otitis media in this group. The small size of bronchial and bronchiolar lumina in the first year of life is an important determinant in the incidence of bronchiolitis from respiratory syncytial and other virus infections. Aspiration during the first year of life most often causes lung changes in the upper lobes because during the feeding and postfeeding periods, the infant is usually recumbent; thereafter most aspirations take place when children are upright, and the lung changes occur most often in the lower lobes.

The incidence or severity of respiratory tract disease based on sex varies very little: lower respiratory tract infections are slightly more common in boys than in girls under 6 yr of age; thereafter the infection rates are equal. Noninfectious pulmonary diseases of children usually have an equal sex incidence, except for rare sex-linked recessive disorders such as chronic granulomatous disease. However, lung disease often progresses more rapidly and median survival is shorter in females with cystic fibrosis.

Cystic fibrosis largely affects Caucasians, especially those of central and northern European extraction; its incidence in blacks in the United States is approximately 10% of that in whites and is even less in Orientals. Lung infections and infarctions associated with sickle cell disease occur almost exclusively in black populations.

Seasonal variations in the incidence of respiratory tract infections and bronchial asthma are clinically important. The most common viral pathogens appear in epidemics during the winter and spring months, while mycoplasma infections occur more commonly in autumn and early winter. Pollen-related asthma symptoms occur most often in the spring, summer, and early fall; symptoms due to house dust and mold are more common when children are confined to the house during the cold weather; infection-related asthma also occurs more frequently during the cold weather months.

Certain fungal respiratory tract infections, such as coccidioidomycosis and histoplasmosis, have well-defined geographic distributions in the United States, but the incidence of common viral, mycoplasmal, and bacterial infections varies little with geographic location. At high altitudes, hypoxemia and cor pulmonale may play an earlier or more prominent role in the natural history of chronic lung disease, as in cystic fibrosis. Children living in homes in which their mother or both parents smoke have more frequent respiratory tract infections. In addition, areas with high levels of air pollution predispose to frequent respiratory tract infections and episodes of asthma.

Although the frequency is not different, the severity of lower respiratory tract illness is generally less in middle class than in lower class families, which may reflect differences in nutritional status or availability of medical care.

Finally, health disorders in other systems may influence the severity of acute respiratory tract diseases. For example, respiratory syncytial virus infections are particularly severe, not infrequently fatal, in small children with cyanotic congenital heart disease.

THOMAS F. BOAT
CARL F. DOERSHUK
ROBERT C. STERN

Chretien J, Holland, W, Macklem P, et al: Acute respiratory infections in children. N Engl J Med 310:982, 1984.
Denny FW, Clyde WA, Collier AM, et al: The longitudinal approach to the pathogenesis of respiratory disease. Rev Infect Dis 1:1007:1013, 1979.
Glezen WP, Denny FW: Epidemiology of acute lower respiratory disease in children. N Engl J Med 288:498–505, 1973.
Stagno S, Brasfield DM, Brown MB, et al: Infant pneumonitis with cytomegalovirus, chylamydia, pneumocystitis, and ureaplasma: A prospective study. Pediatrics 68:322–329, 1981.
Wood RE, Boat TF, Doershuk CF: Cystic fibrosis: State of the art. Am Rev Respir Dis 113:833, 1976.

13.21 ACUTE RESPIRATORY FAILURE

Acute respiratory failure may be defined as the development of hypercapnia during an acute illness.

Etiology. Frequently, acute respiratory failure occurs in patients who are known to have mild to moderately severe chronic pulmonary disease with normal arterial carbon dioxide tension. During an intercurrent acute illness (e.g., influenza), such a patient may deteriorate rapidly and develop hypercapnia. Previously well children also may develop acute respiratory failure as a result of pneumonia, epiglottitis or other cause of upper airway obstruction, status asthmaticus, aspiration (including near-drowning), and certain poisonings. Patients with cystic fibrosis or severe scoliosis often develop acute respiratory failure following surgery. Acute central nervous system disease may cause respiratory failure by interfering with the central control of breathing. Severe muscle disease and thoracic abnormalities may result in respiratory failure because of inadequate alveolar ventilation. Occasionally, congenital heart lesions with large right-to-left shunts cause respiratory failure when pulmonary perfusion is too low to allow adequate excretion of carbon dioxide.

Clinical Manifestations. The patient is hyperpneic and cyanotic and may use the accessory muscles of respiration; most will sit up and lean forward to improve leverage for the accessory muscles and to allow easy diaphragmatic movement. Symptoms and signs of the underlying disease are also present. Hypercapnia may cause central depression accompanied by impaired consciousness and confusion. A $PaCO_2$ of over 40 mm Hg suggests the possibility of developing acute respiratory failure, and a $PaCO_2$ of 50 mm Hg or higher suggests it is imminent. Most patients with acute hypercapnia also have a PaO_2 below 55 mm Hg in room air, suggesting

Table 13–1. **Data for Determining Inside Diameter and Length of Pediatric Endotracheal Tubes**

Age	French Size	Internal Diameter (mm)	Oral Length (cm)	Nasal Length (cm)	15 mm Adapter (mm Internal Diameter)
Premature	14–16	3.0–3.5	8	11	3
Newborn–14 days	16	3.5	8.5	13	4
2–24 wk	16–18	3.5–4.0	10	15	4
6–12 mo	18–20	4.0–4.5	12	16	4–5
12–18 mo	20–22	4.5–5.0	13	16	5
18–24 mo	22–24	5.0–5.5	14	17	5–6
2–4 yr	24–26	5.5–6.0	15	18	6
4–7 yr	26–28	6.0–6.5	16	19	6–7
7–10 yr	28–30	6.5–7.0	17	21	7
10–12 yr	30–32	7.0–7.5	20	23–25	7–8

that the oxygen content of the blood may be inadequate to meet the normal needs of the vital organs. Furthermore, at $PaCO_2$ levels above 54 mm Hg, diaphragmatic function may be impaired, accelerating the patient's decline.

Acute hypoxemia and hypercapnia result in dilatation of the cerebral blood vessels and increased blood flow, often accompanied by severe headache. The sudden increased work of the accessory muscles of breathing may result in severe lower back pain. Although moderate to severe hypercapnia can cause peripheral vasodilatation, mild to moderate hypoxemia can cause peripheral vasoconstriction, and the patient may complain of cold extremities. Other symptoms of hypoxia include restlessness, dizziness, and impaired thought.

Treatment. Patients with early respiratory failure should receive maximum therapy aimed at relieving the underlying disease. Recent reports indicating that theophylline improves diaphragmatic strength suggest that this agent may be useful in treating respiratory failure in patients with chronic obstructive pulmonary disease. If these measures fail to reduce arterial carbon dioxide, mechanical ventilation with control of the airway is needed. If the patient is apneic or gasping, 100% oxygen is administered by bag and mask, followed immediately by endotracheal intubation (Table 13–1). When there is less urgency and there is reason to believe that several days of mechanical assistance will be required, nasotracheal intubation is preferable. Immediately following intubation, chest auscultation is important to ensure that the tube is not obstructing one of the main stem bronchi and that there is adequate air exchange. A chest roentgenogram should be obtained to confirm proper tube placement. Patients with upper airway obstruction may not require any treatment other than intubation. For most intubated children, continuous positive airway pressure (CPAP) is useful to prevent alveolar collapse.

The goal of therapy is to achieve adequate oxygen saturation and normal arterial carbon dioxide tension using the least pressure and lowest possible concentration of inspired oxygen (FiO_2). Once artificial ventilation is undertaken, the patient must be monitored closely, by both clinical and arterial blood gas determinations, to ensure adequate ventilation. An indwelling arterial catheter is very helpful (Sec. 13.18). Maintaining adequate tissue oxygenation is of paramount importance since devastating effects of transient severe hypoxemia may persist after restoration of pulmonary function; restoration usually requires maintaining a PaO_2 of at least 45–50 mm Hg but preferably of 50–55 mm Hg. On the other hand, as the patient improves, the inspired oxygen concentration should be decreased as rapidly as possible to reduce the risks of oxygen toxicity. The risk of direct oxygen toxicity to the airways, although demonstrable at FiO_2 levels above 40%, is markedly increased at FiO_2 levels between 70 and 100%. For some patients who have very severe hypoxemia, but who can

be expected to recover quickly, extracorporeal membrane oxygenation has been suggested, although it is still an experimental procedure.

Bedside measurements of tidal volume, vital capacity, and negative inspiratory force are very helpful in predicting when the patient has a good chance of successful extubation. Ventilator assistance is then terminated and the patient extubated. Children having acute respiratory failure should be managed in a pediatric intensive care unit (Sec. 5.39).

Prognosis. Survival should be expected in previously normal children who develop respiratory failure with an acute illness. When acute respiratory failure is superimposed upon underlying chronic illness, the prognosis is related to the nature of the chronic illness and the severity and duration of the acute process. Many of these patients regain their previous status.

Downes JJ, Fulgencio T, Raphaely RC: Acute respiratory failure in infants and children. Pediatr Clin North Am 19:423, 1972.

Juan G, Calverleg P, Talamo C, et al: Effect of carbon dioxide on diaphragmatic function in human beings. New Engl J Med 310:879, 1984.

Kumar A, Falke KJ, Geffin B, et al: Continuous positive pressure ventilation in acute respiratory failure. Effects on hemodynamics and lung function. N Engl J Med 283:1430, 1970.

Murciano D, Aubier M, Lecocquic Y, et al: Effects of theophylline on diaphragmatic strength and fatigue in patients with chronic obstructive pulmonary disease. New Engl J Med 311:349, 1984.

Nicodemus HF: Respiratory failure and airway management in congenital cardiovascular diseases. Clin Pediatr 12:259, 1964.

Rogers RM, Juers JA: Physiologic considerations in the treatment of acute respiratory failure. Basics of RD 3 (No 4):1, 1975.

13.22 IATROGENIC AND DRUG-INDUCED PULMONARY DISEASE

Any patient having had mechanical manipulation of the airway, mechanical ventilation, or prolonged drug therapy who then develops chronic respiratory symptoms or recurrent respiratory infection may have an iatrogenic disease. Prolonged use of high oxygen concentrations and pressure ventilators can cause bronchopulmonary dysplasia (Sec. 8.32). Overtransfusion or excessive doses of plasma expanders may cause pulmonary edema. Anesthetic gases may have direct pulmonary toxicity, and atelectasis may occur as a result of both anesthetic agents and decreased deep breathing and coughing secondary to postoperative pain. Prolonged intubation has resulted in tracheal granulomas and other sequelae. Anticoagulant therapy has resulted in hemoptysis; mineral oil can result in lipoid pneumonia (Sec. 13.71).

Cancer Therapy

Treatment programs based on multiple drug protocols combined with radiation therapy are used frequently in the common childhood malignancies. The increased survival time, together with the increasing total dose of many chemotherapeutic agents and radiation, has been associated with a variety of pulmonary complications (Chapter 16).

Radiation injury probably is mediated primarily by two pathophysiologic mechanisms: First, the radiation may stimulate inflammation, which ultimately leads to progressive fibrosis. Second, in children radiation has a profound long-term retarding effect on the growth of pulmonary parenchyma. Occasionally, scoliosis occurs as a result of radiation, and this may further compromise pulmonary status. Radiation-induced reduction in chest wall growth also may secondarily limit growth of the lung. Since children rarely receive extensive thoracic radiation without chemotherapy, the effects of each may be difficult to distinguish. Doxorubicin and dactinomycin may potentiate or reactivate radiation toxicity.

Oncologic chemotherapeutic drugs may cause progressive pulmonary disease and limit lung size even when used without radiation. Pulmonary complications have occurred following administration of bleomycin, cyclophosphamide, busulfan, methotrexate, semustine, carmustine (BCNU), zinostatin, mitomycin, chlorambucil, and procarbazine. Bleomycin, whose toxicity is increased by oxygen administration, causes pulmonary disease in 40% of patients. But pulmonary toxicity rarely results from 6-mercaptopurine, and vincristine and 5-fluorouracil have been reported to cause pulmonary injury only in patients receiving other drugs with known pulmonary toxicity. Symptoms usually begin after a prolonged period of therapy and even after a toxic drug has been discontinued. There appears to be a total dose-risk relationship for bleomycin and busulfan but not for methotrexate. Early symptoms include dry cough, dyspnea, and, occasionally, fever. Physical findings include cyanosis, tachypnea, and rales. Pulmonary function testing reveals decreased diffusing capacity for carbon monoxide, evidence of restriction, and hypoxemia. Chest roentgenograms show linear interstitial densities in most cases, but a fine nodular pattern or an alveolar filling process has also been reported. Lung tissue shows fibrosis, interstitial infiltrates, and abnormal alveolar epithelial cells. In the case of busulfan, bizarre type II pneumocytes are a common finding. These drugs also may predispose the patient to developing a new pulmonary malignancy.

Diagnosis. The principal problem is to differentiate chemotherapy-induced pulmonary disease from a pneumonia or *Pneumocystis carinii* infestation and, more rarely, from diffuse tumor infiltration. Bronchoscopy and lung biopsy may be needed for definitive diagnosis.

Treatment and Course. The natural history of the pulmonary lesion is unknown. In critically ill patients treatment with antibiotics and trimethoprim-sulfamethoxazole may be justified on an empiric basis even when lung injury from chemotherapy is strongly suspected. Patients occasionally recover even if the suspected drug is continued, but some patients have died from respiratory failure even though chemotherapy was promptly discontinued when pulmonary symptoms appeared. Adrenal corticosteroids have been used with varying success. Supportive treatment with oxygen and mechanical ventilation may be necessary.

Other Drug-Induced Pulmonary Disease

Nitrofurantoin can cause an acute or chronic pulmonary complication. The most common acute reaction is characterized by fever, dyspnea, cough, and, occasionally, chest pain and cyanosis. Eosinophilia may occur transiently. Histologic findings include eosinophilia, proteinaceous edema in the air spaces, and perivasculitis. Chronic pulmonary fibrosis also occurs with prolonged treatment. Dyspnea on exertion and nonproductive cough are the most prominent symptoms. Pulmonary function testing reveals restriction and decreased carbon monoxide diffusing capacity, and the chest roentgenogram shows a diffuse interstitial pattern. Patients usually improve following discontinuation of nitrofurantoin treatment. Corticosteroids have been advocated, but there is little evidence for their effectiveness.

Gold therapy (*chrysotherapy*) of rheumatoid arthritis results in interstitial fibrosis with dyspnea and rales. The pulmonary symptoms may be ascribed to rheumatoid lung disease. Discontinuation of gold treatments is indicated, after which some amelioration of symptoms can be expected. The pathogenesis may involve a drug-induced defect in cell-mediated immunity.

Although chronic *alcohol abuse* may have its onset during adolescence, its pulmonary sequelae (airway obstruction, decreased diffusion capacity, and alteration of ventilation-perfusion adjustment secondary to cirrhosis) will not usually be seen until adult years. The acute pulmonary toxicity of alcohol includes depression of ciliary motion (at high ethanol levels) and of pulmonary macrophage function and interference with production of surfactant. Although these changes usually do not result in clinical pulmonary problems in otherwise healthy individuals, children with chronic pulmonary disease may be at increased risk from infection.

Aspirin intolerance may be associated with nasal polyps and asthma. Pulmonary fibrosis has been reported to result from chronic use of *penicillamine* and *methysergide*. When given to patients receiving leukocyte transfusion, Amphotericin B may cause severe, occasionally fatal, pulmonary toxicity.

A rare but potentially fatal toxicity, particularly for patients with pre-existing severe pulmonary disease, is produced by the *aminoglycosides* and *polymyxin* groups of antibiotics (including colistin), which can cause neuromuscular blockade and paralysis of the diaphragm and of other muscles of respiration.

ROBERT C. STERN

Baptist G, Andrews JI: Pulmonary toxicity of antineoplastic drugs. JAMA 246:1449, 1981.

Epler GR, Snider GL, Gaensler EA, et al: Bronchiolitis and bronchitis in connective tissue disease: A possible relationship to the use of penicillamine. JAMA 242:528, 1979.

Heinemann HO: Alcohol and the lung: A brief review. Am J Med 63:81, 1977.

Jacoby I: Drug-induced pulmonary disease: Confusion with infections of the lungs. Inf Dis Pract 1:1, 1978.

McCormick J, Cole S, Lahirir B, et al: Pneumonitis caused by gold salt therapy: Evidence for the role of cell-mediated immunity in its pathogenesis. Am Rev Resp Dis 122:145, 1980.

Rachelefsky GS, Coulson A, Siegel SC, et al: Aspirin intolerance in chronic childhood asthma: Detected by oral challenge. Pediatrics 56:443, 1975.

Sostman HD, Matthay RA, Putman CE: Cytotoxic drug-induced lung disease. Am J Med 62:608, 1977.

Webster DG, Robichaud KJ, Pizzo PA, et al: Lethal pulmonary reactions associated with the combined use of amphotericin B and leucocyte transfusions. N Engl J Med 304:1185, 1981.

Weiss RB, Muggia FM: Cytotoxic drug-induced pulmonary disease: Update 1980. Am J Med 68:259, 1980.

Winterbauer RH, Wilske KR, Wheelis RF: Diffuse pulmonary injury associated with gold treatment. N Engl J Med 294:919, 1976.

Wohl MEB, Griscom NT, Traggis DG, et al: Effects of therapeutic irradiation delivered in early childhood upon subsequent lung function. Pediatrics 55:507, 1975.

13.23 UPPER RESPIRATORY TRACT

The nose provides initial warming and humidification of inspired air. In the anterior nares turbulent air flow and coarse hairs enhance the deposition of large particulate matter; the remaining nasal airways filter out particles as small as 6 μm in diameter. In the turbinate region the air flow becomes laminar and the air stream is narrowed; thus particle deposition, warming, and humidification are enhanced. Nasal passages contribute as much as 50% of the total resistance of normal breathing. Nasal flaring, a sign of respiratory distress, reduces the resistance to inspiratory flow of air through the nose and may improve ventilation.

The nasal mucosa is more vascular, especially in the turbinate region, than that of the lower airways; however, the surface epithelium is similar, with ciliated cells, goblet cells, submucosal glands, and a covering blanket of mucus. Mucus flows toward the nasopharynx, where the air stream widens, the epithelium becomes squamous, and secretions are wiped away by swallowing; replacement of the mucous layers occurs about every 10 min. In addition to mucous glycoproteins, which provide viscoelastic properties, the nasal secretions contain lysozyme and secretory IgA, both of which have antimicrobial activity.

The *paranasal sinuses* develop as a group of air spaces in the bones of the face. They are lined with ciliated, mucus-secreting epithelium, and their ostia drain into the middle and superior meatuses of the nose. Development of the sinuses occurs largely after birth, with the maxillary sinuses being earliest and the ethmoid sinuses being roentgenographically visible by 1–2 yr of age. The frontal sinuses usually begin their ascent into the frontal bone by the second year but, along with the sphenoid sinuses, are not readily visible roentgenographically until 5–6 yr of age or later. Growth of the sinuses, which may be unequal from side to side, continues through adolescence. Thickening of the epithelial lining and a diffuse haziness detected by roentgenogram suggest sinusitis, which can occur alone or in association with other conditions such as cystic fibrosis, ciliary dysmotility syndromes or immunoglobulin deficiency.

The adenoids on the posterior nasopharyngeal wall and the tonsils at the base of the tongue are directly in line with the mucociliary flow and the air stream, enhancing their protective capabilities. The eustachian tubes, also lined with mucus-secreting, ciliated epithelium, enter the nasopharynx on the lateral walls.

Children and adults breathe through their nose unless nasal obstruction interferes, but most newborns are not obligatory nasal breathers.

13.24 CONGENITAL DISORDERS OF THE NOSE

Congenital structural nasal abnormalities are uncommon compared with acquired malformations. Occasionally, nasal bones are congenitally absent so that the bridge of the nose fails to develop, resulting in nasal hypoplasia. Congenital absence of the nose, complete or partial duplication, or a single centrally placed nostril occasionally occur but usually as a part of malformation syndromes incompatible with life. Rarely, supernumerary teeth may be found in the nose, or teeth may grow into it from the maxilla.

On occasion, nasal bones are sufficiently malformed to produce severe narrowing of the nasal passages. Often such narrowing is associated with a high and narrow hard palate, which is frequently associated with Down syndrome. Children with these defects may have more severe obstruction to

airflow during infections of the upper airways and are more susceptible to the development of chronic or recurrent hypoventilation. Rarely, the alae nasi may be sufficiently thin and poorly supported to result in inspiratory obstruction.

Hypertelorism is a common defect resulting from overdevelopment of the lesser wings of the sphenoid. The most prominent physical manifestation is widening of the base of the nose with the eyes widely separated. Diagnosis requires accurate measurement of interpupillary distance.

Choanal atresia, the most common congenital anomaly of the nose, consists of a unilateral or bilateral bony or membranous septum between the nose and the pharynx. There is a strong familial tendency, and nearly 50% of infants so affected have other congenital anomalies. Since newborn infants have a variable ability to breath through their mouths, the obstruction does not produce the same symptoms in every infant. When only one side is affected, the infant usually does not have severe symptoms at birth and may be asymptomatic for a prolonged period, often until the first respiratory infection, when the diagnosis may be suggested by unilateral nasal discharge or disproportionately severe nasal obstruction.

Infants with bilateral choanal atresia who have difficulty with mouth breathing will make vigorous attempts to inspire, often suck in their lips, and will develop cyanosis. Distressed children then cry (which relieves the cyanosis) and become more calm, only to repeat the cycle after closing their mouths. Those who are able to mouth-breathe at once will experience difficulty when sucking and swallowing, becoming cyanotic when they attempt to nurse. Persistent mouth breathing and cyanosis when the mouth is closed (which is relieved when the infant cries) are additional manifestations.

Diagnosis is established by the inability to pass a firm catheter through each nostril 3–4 cm into the nasopharynx. Occasionally, instilling contrast material and obtaining roentgenograms in the supine position may be necessary to show the area of obstruction. Alternatively, obstruction can be confirmed by direct visualization using fiberoptic rhinoscopy.

Treatment consists of promptly providing an oral airway or maintaining the mouth in an open position. Passage of an orogastric tube is often sufficient to prevent the complete opposition of tongue and soft palate and ensure an open airway. Other techniques use a feeding nipple with large holes at the tip. Once an oral airway is established, the infant can be fed by gavage until breathing and eating without the assisted airway is learned, usually in 2–3 wk. Tracheostomy is rarely indicated. Subsequently, elective operative correction can be done weeks or months later in patients who adapt well to the obstruction. Immediate surgical correction for bilateral choanal atresia is seldom needed. Operative correction of unilateral obstruction should be deferred until infection is controlled and the infant's condition is satisfactory.

Congenital defects of the nasal septum, such as *perforation* or *deviation*, are rare. Perforation can be developmental or secondary to infection, such as syphilis or tuberculosis, and to trauma. Septal deviation can be congenital but more commonly results from trauma and may, in rare instances of obstruction, require surgical correction; it is best deferred until 14–15 yr of age to avoid external deformities of the nose. Abnormal formation of the nasal bones is infrequent unless other malformations are also present, such as cleft lip or palate. *Encephalocele* protruding through a defect in the cribriform plate into the nasal cavity is a rare anomaly that must be differentiated from polyps and tumors of extracranial origin. Poor development of the paranasal sinuses is associated with recurrent or chronic upper airway infection in Down syndrome.

13.25 ACQUIRED DISORDERS OF THE NOSE

Foreign Body

Food, crayons, small toys, erasers, paper wads, beads, beans, stones, and other foreign bodies are frequently introduced into the nose by children. Initial symptoms are local obstruction, sneezing, relatively mild discomfort, and, rarely, pain. Irritation results in mucosal swelling, and, because some foreign bodies are hygroscopic and increase in size as water is absorbed, signs of local obstruction and discomfort may increase with time. Infection usually follows and gives rise to a purulent, malodorous, or bloody discharge. Tetanus is a rare complication in nonimmunized children, as is toxic shock syndrome from surgical packings (Sec. 11.18). *Unilateral nasal discharge and obstruction should suggest the presence of a foreign body*, which can often be seen upon examination with a speculum. The object is usually situated anteriorly at first, but through unskilled attempts at removal it may be forced deeper into the nose. Removal should be carried out promptly to minimize the danger of aspiration and to prevent local tissue necrosis. Usually it can be performed with topical anesthesia, using either forceps or nasal suction. Infection usually clears promptly upon removal of the object, and generally no further therapy is necessary.

Epistaxis

Nosebleeds are rare in infancy, are common in childhood, and decrease in incidence after puberty. Epistaxis, when it does occur, is often transient and not very severe; the bleeding often stops spontaneously or with minimal pressure. These isolated episodes of bleeding require no diagnostic evaluation or specific treatment. However, some children develop recurrent epistaxis with mild or moderate bleeding.

Etiology. Trauma, including picking the nose and foreign bodies, is the most common cause. There is frequently a family history of childhood epistaxis, and susceptibility is increased during respiratory infections and in the winter months when dry air irritates the nasal mucosa, resulting in formation of fissures and crusting. Epistaxis is also associated with adenoidal hypertrophy, allergic rhinitis, sinusitis, polyps, and a variety of acute infections. Diseases with paroxysmal and forceful cough, such as cystic fibrosis, may also foster epistaxis. Severe bleeding may be encountered with congenital vascular abnormalities, such as telangiectasias or varicosities, and in children with thrombocytopenia, deficiency of clotting factors, hypertension, renal failure, or venous congestion. Adolescent girls may have epistaxis at the time of menarche.

Clinical Manifestions. Epistaxis usually occurs without warning, with blood flowing slowly but freely from one nostril or occasionally both. In children with nasal lesions, bleeding may follow physical exercise. When bleeding occurs at night, the blood may be swallowed and may become apparent only when the child vomits or passes blood in his stools. The source of the bleeding is usually the vascular plexus on the anterior septum (Kiesselbach plexus) or the mucosa of the anterior portions of the turbinates.

Treatment. Most nosebleeds stop spontaneously in a few minutes. The nares should be compressed and the child kept as quiet as possible, in an erect position until hemostasis, with the head tilted forward to avoid blood trickling posteriorly into the pharynx. If these measures do not stop the bleeding, local application of a solution of epinephrine (1:1000) with or without topical thrombin may, on occasion, be useful. If bleeding persists, an anterior nasal pack should be inserted; if bleeding originates in the posterior nares, combined anterior and postchoanal packing is necessary. After bleeding has been controlled, and if a bleeding site is identified, its obliteration by cautery with silver nitrate may prevent further difficulties.

In patients with severe or repeated epistaxis, blood transfusions may be necessary. Otolaryngologic evaluation is indicated for these children and for those with bilateral bleeding or with hemorrhage that does not arise from the Kiesselbach plexus. Replacement of deficient clotting factors may be required for patients who have an underlying hematologic disorder (Sec. 15.44–15.46). If a patient lives in a dry environment, a room humidifier may prevent epistaxis.

13.26 INFECTIONS OF THE UPPER RESPIRATORY TRACT

General Considerations. Upper respiratory tract infections are those primarily affecting the structures of the respiratory tract above the larynx, but most respiratory illnesses affect both the upper and lower portions of the tract simultaneously or sequentially. Pathophysiologic features include inflammatory infiltrates and edema of the mucosa, vascular congestion, increased mucus secretion, and alterations of ciliary structure and function.

Many different microorganisms (chiefly viruses) are capable of causing primary upper respiratory tract disease. The same organism may cause inapparent infection or clinical symptoms of differing severity and extent in accordance with such host factors as age, sex, previous contact with the agent, allergy, nutritional status, and the like. For example, among different members of the same family a single virus may simultaneously produce typical colds in the parents, bronchiolitis in the infant, croup in a somewhat older child, pharyngitis in another, and a subclinical infection in another.

Etiology. Most acute respiratory tract infections are caused by viruses and mycoplasma. An exception is acute epiglottitis. Streptococci and the diphtheria organisms are the major bacterial agents capable of causing primary pharyngeal disease; even in cases of acute tonsillopharyngitis, most illnesses are of nonbacterial origin. Though considerable overlapping exists, some microorganisms are more likely to produce a given respiratory syndrome than others, and certain agents have a greater tendency than others to produce severe disease. Some viruses (e.g., rubeola) may be associated with varying amounts of upper and lower respiratory tract symptomatology as part of a general clinical picture involving other organ systems.

The **respiratory syncytial virus** (RSV) is the principal single cause of bronchiolitis, accounting for about one third of all cases. It is a common cause of pneumonia, croup, and bronchitis, as well as of undifferentiated febrile disease of the upper respiratory tract (Sec. 11.73).

The **parainfluenza viruses** account for the majority of cases of the croup syndrome, but may also produce bronchitis, bronchiolitis, and febrile upper respiratory tract disease (Sec. 11.72). The **influenza viruses** do not play a large part in the various respiratory syndromes except during epidemics. In infants and children, influenza viruses account for more disease of the upper than of the lower respiratory tract.

The **adenoviruses** account for fewer than 10% of respiratory illnesses, many of which are mild or asymptomatic. Pharyngitis and pharyngoconjunctival fever are the most common clinical manifestations in children. However, adenoviruses occasionally cause severe lower respiratory tract infection (Sec. 11.74).

The **rhinoviruses** and **coronaviruses** usually produce symptoms limited to the upper tract, most commonly the nose, and account for a significant proportion of the "common cold" syndromes (Sec. 11.75 and 13.27).

Coxsackieviruses A and B produce primarily disease of the nasopharynx (Sec. 11.77). **Mycoplasma** can produce both upper and lower respiratory tract illness, including bronchiolitis, pneumonia, bronchitis, pharyngotonsillitis, myringitis, and otitis media (Sec. 11.60).

THOMAS F. BOAT
CARL F. DOERSHUK
ROBERT C. STERN
ALFRED D. HEGGIE

Carlo WA, Martin RJ, Bruce EN, et al: Alae nasi activation (nasal flaring) decreases nasal resistance in preterm infants. Pediatrics 72:338, 1983.

Carson JL, Collier AM, and Hu SS: Acquired ciliary defects in nasal epithelium of children with acute viral upper respiratory infections. N Engl J Med 312:463–468, 1985.

13.27 ACUTE NASOPHARYNGITIS
(Upper Respiratory Tract Infection; URI; the "Common Cold")

Acute nasopharyngitis is the most common infectious condition of children, but its significance depends primarily upon the relative frequency with which complications occur. In children this syndrome is more extensive than in adults, often involving the paranasal sinuses and middle ear as well as the nasopharynx.

Etiology. The illness is caused by more than 150 serologically different viral agents. The principal agents are rhinoviruses (Sec. 11.75). The period of infectivity lasts from a few hours prior to the appearance of symptoms to 1–2 days after the illness has appeared. Group A streptococci are the principal bacterial cause of acute nasopharyngitis. *Corynebacterium diphtheriae, Mycoplasma pneumoniae, Neisseria meningitidis* and *N. gonorrhoeae* are also primary infectious agents. *Haemophilus influenzae, Streptococcus pneumoniae,* and *Staphylococcus aureus* may infect upper respiratory tract tissues secondarily and are responsible for complications in the sinuses, ears, mastoids, lymph nodes, and lungs. *Mycoplasma pneumoniae* infections may localize to the nasopharynx and in these instances are difficult to distinguish from viral nasopharyngitis.

Epidemiology. Susceptibility to agents causing acute nasopharyngitis is universal, but for poorly understood reasons it varies in the same person from time to time. Although infections occur throughout the year, in the Northern Hemisphere there are peaks of occurrence in September about the time school opens, in late January, and toward the end of April. Children average five to eight infections a year, the highest number occurring during the first 2 yr of life. The frequency of acute nasopharyngitis varies directly with the number of exposures, and in nursery schools and day care centers may be virtually epidemic. Susceptibility may be increased by poor nutrition and purulent complications by malnutrition.

Pathology. The first changes are edema and vasodilatation in the submucosa. A mononuclear cell infiltrate follows, which, within 1–2 days, becomes polymorphonuclear. Structural and functional changes of cilia result in compromised mucus clearance. In moderate to severe infection, the superficial epithelial cells separate and slough. There is profuse production of mucus, at first thin, later thicker and usually purulent.

Clinical Manifestations. Colds are more severe in young children than in older children and adults. In general, children 3 mo–3 yr have fever early in the course of infection, occasionally a few hours before localizing signs appear. Younger infants are usually afebrile, and older children may have low grade fevers. Purulent complications occur with more frequency and severity at younger ages. Persistent sinusitis, however, is more common in older children, occurring rarely in infants.

The initial manifestations in infants older than 3 mo of age are the sudden onset of fever, irritability, restlessness, and sneezing. Nasal discharge begins within a few hours, quickly leading to nasal obstruction, which may interfere with nursing; in small infants having a greater dependency on nose breathing, signs of moderate respiratory distress may occur. During the first 2–3 days the eardrums are usually congested and fluid may be noted behind the drum, whether or not purulent otitis media subsequently occurs. A few infants may vomit and some have diarrhea. The febrile phase lasts from a few hours to 3 days; fever may recur with purulent complications.

In older children the initial symptoms are dryness and irritation in the nose and not infrequently in the pharynx. These are followed within a few hours by sneezing, chilly sensations, muscular aches, a thin nasal discharge, and sometimes coughing. Headache, malaise, anorexia, and low grade fever may be present. Within a day the secretions usually become thicker, and eventually purulent. The discharge is irritating, particularly during the purulent phase. Nasal obstruction leads to mouth breathing, and this, through drying of the mucous membranes of the throat, increases the sensation of soreness. In most cases, the acute phase lasts 2–4 days.

Differential Diagnosis. The initial manifestations of measles and pertussis—and, to a lesser extent, of poliomyelitis, hepatitis, and mumps—are those of nasopharyngitis. A persistent nasal discharge, particularly if it is bloody, suggests a foreign body or diphtheria and, in the first week of life, choanal atresia or congenital syphilis.

Allergic rhinitis (Sec. 10.47) differs from infectious rhinitis in that it is not accompanied by fever: its nasal discharge does not usually become purulent, and it is usually combined with persistent sneezing and itching of the eyes and nose. The nasal mucous membranes in allergic rhinitis are usually pale rather than inflamed, and nasal smears will often contain many eosinophils rather than the polymorphonuclear leukocytes associated with infection. In allergic rhinitis, antihistamines may produce rapid and relatively complete disappearance of signs and symptoms; in infectious rhinitis, they produce little consistent effect.

Drug abuse, especially with cocaine and marijuana, should also be considered in older children and adolescents.

Complications. These result from the bacterial invasion of the paranasal sinuses and other portions of the respiratory tract. The cervical lymph nodes may also become involved and occasionally suppurate. Mastoiditis, peritonsillar cellulitis, or periorbital cellulitis may occur. The most common complication is otitis media, seen in up to 25% of small infants. Although it may occur early in the course of a cold, it usually appears after the acute phase of nasopharyngitis. Thus, otitis media should be suspected if fever recurs. Most viral infections of the upper respiratory tract also involve the lower respiratory tract, and in many cases pulmonary function diminishes even though lower respiratory tract symptoms are inconspicuous or absent. On the other hand, typical laryngotracheobronchitis, bronchiolitis, or pneumonia may develop during the course of acute nasopharyngitis. Viral nasopharyngitis also is a frequent trigger for asthma symptoms in children with reactive airways.

Prevention. Effective vaccines are not available. Neither gamma globulin nor vitamin C reduces the frequency or severity of infections, and their use is not recommended.

Because of the ubiquity of the common cold, it is impossible to isolate children from this condition. However, since in the very young infant complications may be relatively serious, some attempt should be made to protect infants from contact with potentially infected persons.

Treatment. There is no specific therapy. Antibiotics do not affect the course of the illness or reduce the incidence of bacterial complications. Bed rest is generally recommended, but there is no evidence that it shortens the course of the illness or affects the outcome. Acetaminophen is usually helpful in reducing irritability, aching, and malaise for the first 1–2 days of infections, but excessive use should be avoided. Aspirin given to a child with influenza virus infection increases the risk of developing Reye syndrome and is not recommended for children having respiratory tract symptoms.

Most of the distress is due to nasal obstruction. Attempts should be made to relieve this condition if it interferes with sleep or with fluid or food ingestion. Nasal instillation of medications may be an effective method for relieving nasal obstruction. In infants, instillation of sterile saline may assist with physical removal of excessive mucus. Phenylephrine (0.125–0.25%) is widely used in the United States. More potent, longer acting nose drops, while useful to adults, tend to be irritating and occasionally are hyperexcitative or sedative to infants. Nose drops in oily vehicles should be avoided because they are readily aspirated. The addition of antibiotics, corticosteroids, or antihistamines to nose drops increases their expense and adds nothing to their effectiveness.

Nose drops are best administered 15–20 min before feeding and at bedtime. While the child is supine with the neck extended, 1–2 drops are instilled in each nostril. Since this will often produce shrinkage of only the anterior mucous membranes, 1–2 drops can be instilled 5–10 min later. Introducing nasal decongestants by cotton-tipped applicators is not recommended. Older children can use a nasal spray but only under supervision, since such applications tend to be overused. In general, no medication instilled into the nose should be used for more than 4–5 days; after this time any drug may produce chemical irritation and induce nasal congestion, mimicking acute nasopharyngitis.

Nasal obstruction is difficult to treat in infants. Suction with a soft bulb syringe is occasionally essential to clear the nasal passage sufficiently to permit the young infant to nurse. The best drainage can usually be achieved by placing the infant in the prone position, if this does not further compromise respirations. A highly humidified environment provided by an efficient vaporizer prevents drying of secretions and often appears to provide substantial benefit.

Orally administered decongestants are also widely used for shrinkage of engorged nasal mucosa and relief of obstruction. Pseudoephedrine reduces nasal resistance in older children and adults with upper respiratory tract infection; studies in infants and young children have not been reported. Many preparations combine antihistamines and adrenergic agonists. The former have been found effective in some and ineffective in other studies for relief of nasal congestion in children with acute nasopharyngitis. There is no evidence that these drugs prevent otitis media.

Most children with acute nasopharyngitis have decreased appetite, but compelling them to eat serves no purpose. Fluids of the child's choice should be offered at frequent intervals. Transient constipation is common but does not require treatment since it rapidly disappears when the child returns to a normal diet.

RICHARD E. BEHRMAN

Howard JC, Kantner TR, Lilienfield LS, et al: Effectiveness of antihistamines in the symptomatic management of the common cold. JAMA 242:2414, 1979.

Miller JZ, Nance WE, Norton JA, et al: Therapeutic effect of vitamin C. A co-twin control study. JAMA 237:248, 1977.

Schmitt BD: Fever in childhood. Pediatrics 74:929, 1984.

Walson PD: Coughs and colds. Pediatrics 74:937, 1984.

13.28 ACUTE PHARYNGITIS

This term refers to all acute infections of the pharynx, including tonsillitis and pharyngotonsillitis. The presence or absence of tonsils does not affect the susceptibility, the frequency, or the course or complications of the illness. Pharyngeal involvement is part of most upper respiratory tract infections and is also found with various acute generalized infections (Chapter 11). However, in the strict sense "acute pharyngitis" refers to conditions in which the principal involvement is in the throat. The disease is uncommon under 1 yr of age. The incidence then increases to a peak from 4–7 yr but continues throughout later childhood and adult life. In diphtheria (Sec. 11.23), herpangina (Sec. 11.77), adenovirus infection (Sec. 11.74), and infectious mononucleosis (Sec. 11.69) pharyngeal involvement may be prominent.

Etiology. Acute pharyngitis, whether febrile or not, is generally caused by viruses (Sec. 11.71). Group A beta-hemolytic streptococcus (Sec. 11.16) is the only common bacterial causative agent, and, except during epidemics, it accounts for probably fewer than 15% of cases. Other bacteria may proliferate during acute viral infections and may therefore be cultured in large numbers from the pharynx of an affected person. Pharyngeal gonococcal infection may occur secondary to fellatio.

Clinical Manifestations. These differ somewhat, depending on whether streptococci or viruses are the cause. There is, however, much overlapping of signs and symptoms, and it is often impossible to clinically distinguish one form of pharyngitis from another.

Viral pharyngitis is generally considered a disease of relatively gradual onset, which usually has as early signs fever, malaise, and anorexia with moderate throat pain. Sore throat may be present initially but more commonly begins a day or so after onset of symptoms, reaching its peak by the 2nd–3rd day. Hoarseness, cough, and rhinitis are also common. Even at its peak, pharyngeal inflammation may be relatively slight, but on occasion it is severe, and small ulcers may form on the soft palate and the posterior pharyngeal wall. Exudates may appear on lymphoid follicles of the palate and tonsils and be indistinguishable from those encountered with streptococcal disease. The cervical lymph nodes are often moderately enlarged and firm and may or may not be tender. Laryngeal involvement is common, but the trachea, bronchi, and lungs are usually not sources of symptoms. White blood cell counts range from 6000 to above 30,000, an elevated count (16,000–18,000) of predominantly polymorphonuclear cells being common in the early phase of illness. Leukocyte counts are of little value in differentiating viral from bacterial disease. The entire illness may last less than 24 hr and usually does not persist more than 5 days. Significant complications are rare.

Streptococcal pharyngitis in a child over 2 yr often begins with complaints of headache, abdominal pain, and vomiting. These symptoms may be associated with a fever as high as 40° C (104° F); occasionally a temperature elevation is not noted for 12 hr or so. Hours after the initial complaints, the throat may become sore, and in approximately one third of patients tonsillar enlargement, exudation, and pharyngeal erythema are found. The degree of pharyngeal pain is inconstant and may vary from slight to severe, making swallowing difficult. Two thirds of patients may have only mild erythema, with no enlargement of the tonsils and with no exudate. Anterior cervical lymphadenopathy usually occurs early, and the nodes are often tender. Fever may continue for 1–4 days; in very severe cases the child may remain ill for as long as 2 wk. The physical findings most likely to be associated with streptococcal disease are diffuse redness of the tonsils and tonsillar pillars, with a petechial mottling of the soft palate, whether or not lymphadenitis or follicular exudations are found. These features, although common in streptococcal pharyngitis, are not diagnostic and occur with some frequency in viral pharyngitis.

Conjunctivitis, rhinitis, cough, and hoarseness rarely occur with proven streptococcal pharyngitis, and the presence of two or more of these signs or symptoms suggests the diagnosis of viral infection.

The term **streptococcosis** refers to systemic variations in the presentation of acute streptococcal infections, believed to be related to earlier infection with the beta-hemolytic streptococcus. In infants they may take the form of an acute, usually mild episode lasting less than 1 wk and characterized by variable fever (under 39° C [102° F]), mucoserous nasal discharge, and pharyngeal infection. Usually children 6 mo–3 yr of age are most severely ill. Coryza with postnasal discharge, diffusely reddened pharynx, fever, vomiting, and loss of appetite occurs early. For a few days there is usually fever of 38–39.5° C (100–103° F), which continues irregularly for 4–8 wk, gradually becoming normal. Within a few days of onset, cervical nodes begin to enlarge and become tender; the course of the adenopathy typically parallels that of the fever. Focal complications are common.

Diagnosis. Diagnosis can be made by rapid detection method for streptococcal antigens or by culture after pharyngeal swabbing. Rapid detection methods are very specific but may miss 10–15% of culture-proven infections. Therefore, antigen-negative throat swabs from children with compatible clinical features should also be cultured.

A syndrome of purulent nasal discharge, pharyngitis, and fever may also be associated with positive pharyngeal cultures for pneumococci or *H. influenzae*. Although this syndrome is probably a complication of viral pharyngitis, some of these patients respond to antibiotics.

When a membranous exudate is present on the tonsils, diphtheria should be considered. The membranous exudate of infectious mononucleosis may resemble that found in the streptococcal infection and the partially immunized child with a diphtheritic infection. Herpangina (Sec. 11.77) is not usually associated with tonsillar exudates, but rather with many vesiculoulcerative lesions on the anterior pillars, fauces, and soft palate.

Agranulocytosis is often first manifested by symptoms of acute pharyngitis. The tonsils and posterior pharyngeal wall may be covered by a yellowish or dirty white exudate. The mucous membranes under this exudate will usually become necrotic, and ulceration will extend into the mouth and involve the tongue. The lesions are very painful and dysphagia is severe. Enlargement of cervical lymph nodes commonly occurs, as do mucosal hemorrhages.

Children and adolescents who smoke tobacco or marijuana excessively may develop pharyngeal inflammation and sore throat. Allergic rhinitis with a nonpurulent postnasal discharge may also cause a sore throat. Gonococcal pharyngeal infections are usually asymptomatic.

Pharyngoconjunctival fever is discussed in Sec. 11.74.

Complications. With viral infections the complication rate is low, although purulent bacterial otitis media may occur. In debilitated children both viral and streptococcal infections may lead to large, chronic ulcers in the pharynx. With streptococcal disease, peritonsillar abscess occasionally occurs, as do sinusitis, otitis media, and, rarely, meningitis. Acute glomerulonephritis (Sec. 17.5) and rheumatic fever (Sec. 10.87) may follow streptococcal infections. However, the incidence of rheumatic fever has declined nearly 30-fold over the last 20–25 yr, and fear of this complication is no longer a dominant factor in decisions about treatment.

Mesenteric adenitis is occasionally associated with pharyngitis of either viral or bacterial origin. This may result in abdominal pain with or without vomiting which may closely simulate appendicitis.

Treatment. Since even exudative tonsillitis is usually of viral origin, for which there is no specific therapy, the use of antibiotics should be guided by the results of antigen detection tests or cultures, unless there are strong clinical and epidemiologic grounds to suspect a streptococcal infection. Streptococcal pharyngitis is best treated orally with penicillin (125–250 mg of penicillin V three times daily for 10 days). This usually produces prompt clinical response with defervescence within 24 hr and shortens the course of illness by an average of 1.5 days. Erythromycin is a satisfactory alternative if the patient is allergic to penicillin, but erythromycin resistance of group A streptococcal organisms has been documented in the United States.

Most children prefer to remain in bed during the acute phase of the disease. When throat pain is severe, acetaminophen or aspirin is often helpful. Gargling with warm saline solution offers some symptomatic relief for throat pain in children old enough to cooperate; in younger children the inhalation of steam occasionally produces similar effects. Because of pain on swallowing, cool bland liquids such as ginger ale are usually more acceptable than solids or hot foods. No attempt should be made to force the child to eat.

The child with a streptococcal infection is noninfectious to others within a few hours after penicillin therapy has begun. Reculturing is not necessary if symptoms abate. Some children continue to harbor group A streptococcus after adequate treatment. If a carrier state is detected retreatment with a single additional course of penicillin is recommended. Addition of rifampin 20 mg/kg/day in a single dose for the last 4 days of therapy virtually assures elimination of the organism. However, most carriers have no symptoms or complication and become culture negative after a number of weeks. A few children require antibiotic prophylaxis against streptococcal disease, such as those with past history of rheumatic fever (Sec. 10.87).

Breese BB: A simple scorecard for the tentative diagnosis of streptococcal pharyngitis. Am J Dis Child 131:514, 1977.
Kim KS, Kaplan EL: Association of penicillin tolerance with failure to eradicate group A streptococci from patients with pharyngitis. J Pediatr 107:681, 1985.
Rowe RT, Stone RT: Streptococcal pharyngitis in children. Clin Pediatr 16:933, 1977.
Schwartz RH, Wientzen RL, Grundfart KM: Sore throat in adolescents. Pediatr Infect Dis 1:443, 1982.

13.29 ACUTE UVULITIS

Infections of the uvula are infrequent. They are characterized by fever, pain with swallowing, and drooling. Occasionally there are no symptoms or signs referrable to the pharynx. Most cases are due to group A streptococcus or *Haemophilus influenzae* type b, often in association with tonsillitis and acute epiglottis, respectively. However, isolated uvulitis has been reported. In general streptococcal uvulitis tends to occur in older children (>5 years), while that caused by *H. influenzae* occurs before 5 yr of age. In suspected cases blood cultures as well as cultures of the uvula and pharynx are indicated. Young children should be examined carefully for evidence of airway obstruction and treated, initially with ampicillin and chloramphenicol administered intravenously. Older children can be treated as indicated for streptococcal pharyngitis.

13.30 CHRONIC RHINITIS AND NASOPHARYNGITIS

The child with persistent or recurring upper respiratory tract infection with or without associated chronic bronchial involvement cannot be placed in any one category; each must be studied to determine, if possible, the most important etiologic or pathophysiologic factors.

Children should recover completely after acute respiratory infections and should appear healthy between episodes. In the chronic cases the child seems to recover from one acute attack only to enter another, or there is more or less persistent rhinitis and cough and a general failure to do well. Such patterns may reflect familial or individual susceptibility or repeated exposure to respiratory infection either within the home or in a day care school setting.

Chronic Rhinitis. Chronic nasal discharge, with or without acute exacerbations, may reflect an underlying disturbance, such as nasal polyps, chronic sinusitis, chronically infected adenoids, cystic fibrosis, dysmotile cilia syndrome, allergy, foreign bodies, deviated septum, various congenital malformations, nasal diphtheria, or syphilis. In addition, the possibility of a chronic debilitating infection or some nutritional, immunologic, or metabolic (as of the thyroid) deficiency must be considered.

Clinical Manifestations. Symptoms vary, but chronic nasal discharge is common to all cases. In the persistent cases the odor may be foul, and there may be excoriation of the anterior nares and upper lip. Bloody discharge is common in syphilitic and diphtheritic lesions and with foreign bodies but may also occur in other conditions, especially if there is persistent nose picking. Disturbances of taste and smell are frequent. During exacerbations or superimposed infections, fever is common but is otherwise usually absent.

Persistent *allergic rhinitis* is relatively common and may be seasonal (Sec. 10.47). The mucous membrane tends to be pale; the soft tissues are swollen and resistant to pressure.

Chronic rhinitis also may result from prolonged or excessive use of topical nasal decongestants (rhinitis medicamentosa).

Atrophic rhinitis is uncommon and usually associated with some general debilitating condition, or it may be a sequel to long-continued nasal infection. The sense of smell is impaired. There may be little or no discharge but considerable crusting and a sense of dryness in the nose and throat. In some instances there is a profuse, excessively foul nasal discharge (**ozena**).

Treatment. The frequent application to the nares and upper lip of a lanolin, silicone, or petrolatum-base ointment protects against skin excoriation.

In addition, providing humidified air in cold weather may prevent ongoing nasal mucosal damage and foster clearing of the chronic inflammatory state. Otherwise, treatment is directed toward the underlying disturbance. Foci of infection in sinuses, ears, adenoids, or tonsils should be eradicated, and either allergens should be removed from the environment or the patient desensitized. Attention should be given to nutritional status, rest, and prevention of exposure to new infections. Although mucosa-shrinking solutions such as phenylephrine and related compounds may provide symptomatic relief, they may also cause further damage. Local antibiotics should be avoided, but systemic administration may be indicated in selected cases.

Chronic Pharyngitis. Chronic pharyngitis is rare and occurs secondarily to chronic infections of the sinuses, adenoids, or tonsils, although on occasion there is no evidence of infection other than hypertrophied lymphoid tissue on the posterior pharyngeal wall and on the base of the tongue. The latter type of involvement occurs with frequency only in children whose faucial tonsils have been removed; some of these children may also have infected tonsillar tags.

Clinical Manifestations. There are likely to be repeated acute exacerbations; in the intervals there are complaints of throat discomfort such as dryness and raspy irritation. Frequent efforts to clear the throat and the presence of an irritative cough are common. The mucous membrane is usually inflamed, though on occasion it is pale, and the blood vessels are prominent. The pharyngeal wall is frequently covered with a mucopurulent secretion, and the lymphoid tissue is often hypertrophied and has a pebbled appearance.

Treatment. This should be directed toward any disturbance in the sinuses, nose (deformities), adenoids, and tonsils. Attention should also be given to the general nutrition and hygiene of the child.

13.31 RETROPHARYNGEAL ABSCESS

During early childhood the potential space between the posterior pharyngeal wall and the prevertebral fascia contains several small lymph nodes that usually disappear during the 3rd–4th year of life. The lymphatic channels that communicate with these nodes drain portions of the nasopharynx as well as the posterior nasal passages. With purulent infections of these areas the nodes may become infected; this may, in turn, progress to breakdown of the nodes and to suppuration.

Etiology. Retropharyngeal abscess may be a complication of bacterial pharyngitis. Less commonly, it occurs after extension of infection from vertebral osteomyelitis or by wound infection following a penetrating injury of the posterior pharynx. *Staphylococcus aureus* and group A hemolytic streptococci are the most common pathogens.

Clinical Manifestations. The patient usually has a history of an acute nasopharyngitis or pharyngitis, and the clinical features of the earlier illness may still be present. There is generally an abrupt onset of high fever with difficulty in swallowing, refusal of feeding, severe distress with throat pain, hyperextension of the head, and noisy, often gurgling respirations. Respirations become increasingly labored, and secretions accumulate in the mouth and cause drooling due to the difficulty in swallowing.

A bulge in the posterior pharyngeal wall is usually apparent. Sometimes the abscess is located in an area of the nasopharynx where it may cause nasal obstruction and a bulging forward of the soft palate. A digital examination to determine whether the abscess is fluctuant must be performed with the patient in the Trendelenburg position and with provision for adequate suction in case the abscess ruptures. Retropharyngeal abscesses may not be detectable by simple inspection. However, a lateral roentgenogram of the nasopharynx or neck will reveal the retropharyngeal mass; when abscess is present, the retropharyngeal soft tissue is more than one-half the width of the adjacent vertebral bodies when the patient's neck is extended.

If left untreated, the abscess may rupture into the pharynx spontaneously, resulting in aspiration of pus. It may also dissect laterally and present externally on the side of the neck or burrow into the esophagus, mediastinum, or auditory canal. Sudden death may occur with aspiration, if the abscess presses on the larynx, or with erosion into major blood vessels.

Differential Diagnosis. Pressure on the larynx may result in stridor, making retropharyngeal abscess one of the differential diagnostic possibilities in patients with high fever and croup. Many patients have hyperextension of the neck, which may be mistaken for meningismus. Nonfluctuant lymphadenitis may produce a tender bulge in the retropharyngeal space. Tuberculous caries of the cervical spine may on occasion produce a lateral retropharyngeal abscess; considerable rigidity of the neck and other signs of spinal involvement are usually present.

Treatment. If the abscess is recognized in the prefluctuant stage, intensive treatment with parenteral penicillin G (100,000–250,000 units/kg/24 hr) and/or a semisynthetic penicillin (to cover penicillinase-producing *Staphylococcus aureus*) may prevent suppuration and abscess formation. Analgesic drugs may be needed for pain. When fluctuance is present, the abscess should be incised and antibiotics started; the operation is best performed under general anesthesia. Before incision, the mass should be aspirated to see whether retropharyngeal hemorrhage may not also be present from erosion of blood vessels. If no blood is obtained, an incision is made where the abscess is pointing, and the pus is carefully aspirated. If there is serious bleeding, ligation of the carotid artery may be necessary. If properly treated, the prognosis is good.

13.32 LATERAL PHARYNGEAL ABSCESS

This condition occurs later in childhood than does a retropharyngeal abscess. The process is usually so extensive that the entire pharyngeal wall, including the tonsil, the soft palate, and the uvula, is displaced medially.

The patient usually has high fever, appears acutely ill, and complains of severe pain and difficulty in swallowing. The bulge in the lateral pharyngeal wall is obvious. Cervical adenitis is usually present and nuchal rigidity due to muscular spasm is common.

Treatment is identical to that of retropharyngeal abscess.

13.33 PERITONSILLAR AND RETROTONSILLAR ABSCESSES

Both peritonsillar and retrotonsillar abscesses are uncommon in childhood. The tonsil is usually the site from which the process develops. The abscesses are almost always caused by group A beta-hemolytic streptococci, rarely by *S. aureus* or *H. influenzae*.

Clinical Manifestations. The abscesses are usually preceded by an attack of acute pharyngotonsillitis. There may be an afebrile interval of several days, or the fever of the primary infection may not subside. The patient complains of severe throat pain, has progressive difficulty in opening the mouth because of spasm of the pterygoid muscles, and often refuses to swallow or speak. Occasionally, there is sufficient spasm of the homolateral muscles of the neck to produce torticollis. The fever may be septic and reach 40.5° C (105° F). The affected tonsillar area is markedly swollen and inflamed; the uvula is displaced to the opposite side. In untreated patients the abscess becomes fluctuant within a few days and usually points in the region of the anterior faucial pillar. If the abscess is not incised, spontaneous rupture will occur.

Treatment. See *retropharyngeal abscess* (above). Subsequent attacks of peritonsillar abscess should be prevented by removal of the tonsils 3–4 wk after inflammation has subsided.

13.34 SINUSITIS

See also Sec. 13.23.

Starting in infancy, the maxillary antrums and the anterior and posterior ethmoid cells are usually of sufficient size to harbor infection. The frontal sinus is rarely a site of significant infection until the 6th–10th yr. When there is severe ethmoidal disease in the first few years of life, the development and pneumatization of the frontal sinuses may be curtailed or even completely prevented. The sphenoidal sinus usually does not assume clinical significance until the 3rd–5th yr of life.

The paranasal sinuses are probably involved in an exudative process in practically all acute nasal infections, but, as a rule, the sinus involvement does not persist after the nasal infection has subsided unless there has been a pre-existing sinus infection. The incidence of both acute and chronic sinus infections increases in the latter part of childhood. Unrecognized allergic factors, poor sinus drainage such as might occur with septal deviation, associated hereditary conditions, and environmental factors may increase the possibility of sinus infection.

Acute Purulent Sinusitis

In addition to involvement of the sinuses during acute nasal infections, there may be acute empyema of one or more sinuses, signs or symptoms of which often appear 3–5 days following the acute rhinitis.

Clinical Manifestations. Acute purulent sinusitis presents with fever, localized pain or a sense of fullness, localized tenderness to pressure or direct percussion, headache, and, at times, edema over the affected sinus. Sinus headaches, infrequent in children ≤ 5 years of age, may assist in localization. In sphenoidal sinusitis the headache may be in the suboccipital region; in anterior ethmoidal sinusitis, in the region of the temples and over the eyes; and in posterior ethmoidal sinusitis, over the distribution of the trigeminal nerve, especially over the mastoid area. In maxillary sinusitis there may be aching or tenderness on tapping of the underlying teeth. None of these symptoms clearly distinguishes acute sinusitis from acute nasopharyngitis. Sinusitis should be suspected if a "cold" seems more severe than usual (fever >39° C, periorbital edema, facial pain) or if the "cold" lingers for more than 10 days. Unless the sinal ostia are obstructed, there is a purulent discharge that can be observed directly through a nasoscope. Pus in the middle meatus suggests involvement of the maxillary, frontal, or anterior ethmoid sinuses; pus in the superior meatus suggests involvement of the sphenoid or posterior ethmoid cells. Postnasal discharge may result in sore throat or persistent cough, especially at night.

In acute ethmoiditis, especially in infants and small children, periorbital cellulitis with edema of the soft tissues and redness of the skin is a common manifestation.

Diagnosis. Transillumination of maxillary (light source in the mouth) or of frontal (light source under the medial border of the supraorbital ridge) sinuses may be helpful in older children. Roentgenography is often used but may be misinterpreted. The most diagnostic findings are air-fluid levels and complete opacification. Mucosa width of 4 mm or greater in children also correlates with the presence of bacteria in sinuses. However, interpretation of sinus roentgenograms of infants under 12 mo of age is particularly difficult. CT scans are sensitive indicators of sinus disease but are rarely needed to delineate sinusitis. In children it is not necessary initially to puncture a sinus to establish a diagnosis. However, antral puncture is the only reliable means of gathering material for bacterial culture. Indications for sinus aspiration include unresponsiveness to therapy, sinus disease in immunocompromised hosts, or life-threatening complications. Organisms usually recovered in children include *S. pneumoniae*, *B. catarrhalis*, and nontypable *H. influenzae*. Direct smear of the secretions usually reveals mostly neutrophils but may aid in detecting associated allergy if many eosinophils are present. Nasal swab cultures do not correlate well with cultures of sinus aspirates. Complications are epidural or subdural abscess, meningitis, cavernous sinus thrombosis, optic neuritis, periorbital or orbital cellulitis and abscess, and osteomyelitis.

Treatment. Treatment consists primarily of effective antimicrobial therapy. Ampicillin (100 mg/kg/24 hr) is a reasonable initial choice. In areas where *H. influenzae* and *B. catarrhalis* produce β-lactamase or for treatment failures, trimethoprim-sulfamethoxazole or cefaclor may be prescribed. Decongestants and antihistamines are not helpful. Sinus drainage and irrigation is reserved for patients who fail usual therapy, who have intraorbital or intracranial complications, or who experience intense pain.

Chronic Sinusitis

Chronic infection of the paranasal sinuses should suggest the possibility of a local or generalized disturbance that facilitates persistence of the infection. Search should be made for nasal deformities, polyps, or infected and hypertrophied adenoids that might cause obstruction, for infected teeth as a source of maxillary sinusitis, for a sinus polyp or mucocele, and for such general disturbances as allergy, cystic fibrosis, and dyskinetic cilia. Chronic or recurrent sinusitis also is common in patients with absence of secretory antibodies and in other immunodeficiency states.

Clinical Manifestations. Symptoms of chronic sinusitis vary considerably but frequently are not prominent. Fever, when present, is low grade. Malaise, easy fatigability, and anorexia may occur. Nasal discharge, which may be bilateral or unilateral, varies from day to day and during the day. Frequently there is sufficient swelling of the middle turbinates to cause substantial nasal obstruction. Postnasal discharge is common and, in the absence of infected adenoids or acute upper respiratory tract infection, is virtually diagnostic. When there is an associated watery nasal discharge or sneezing, the possibility of allergic rhinitis must be considered.

Any of the complications of acute sinusitis may occur with chronic sinusitis. The term *sinobronchitis* is occasionally used to designate the relationship between sinus and lower respiratory tract symptoms; children with this condition may have reactive airways, cystic fibrosis, immunodeficiency, or dyskinetic cilia as the underlying disease.

Treatment. In addition to the organisms recovered during acute sinusitis, alpha-hemolytic streptococci, *S. aureus*, and anaerobes are frequently found on culture of antral aspirates. In general, appropriate antimicrobials should be given for up to 6 wks. Antihistamines and decongestants are often used in addition, especially if there are associated allergic manifestations. Surgical drainage is frequently required.

In cystic fibrosis, panopacification of sinuses is nearly always present but symptomatic disease is unusual. In the absence of symptoms, treatment of sinus disease is not indicated.

Locally obstructive nasal deformities should be corrected, if possible, and infected or hypertrophic adenoid tissue should be removed.

13.35 NASAL POLYPS

Etiology. Nasal polyps are benign pedunculated tumors formed from edematous, usually chronically inflamed nasal mucosa. They usually originate in the upper turbinates and from the maxillary and ethmoid sinus ostia. Occasionally, they appear within the maxillary antrum. Very large or multiple polyps may completely obstruct the nasal passage.

Cystic fibrosis is probably the most common childhood cause of nasal polyposis; as many as 25% of patients develop polyps. Every child with nasal polyposis should be tested for cystic fibrosis, even in the absence of typical respiratory and digestive symptoms. Nasal polyposis is also associated with chronic sinusitis of other etiologies, chronic allergic rhinitis, and asthma.

Clinical Manifestations. Obstruction of nasal passages with nasal phonation and mouth breathing is prominent. Profuse mucoid or mucopurulent rhinorrhea may also result. Examination of the nasal passages shows glistening, gray, grape-like masses squeezed between the nasal turbinates and the septum. Polyps can be readily distinguished from the well-vascularized turbinate tissue, which is pink or red. Prolonged presence of polyps may widen the bridge of the nose and erode adjacent osseous structures.

Treatment. Local or systemic decongestants are not usually effective in shrinking the polyps. Similarly, corticosteroid nose sprays are not usually helpful, although a trial is warranted in recurrent cases. Polyps should be removed surgically if complete obstruction, uncontrolled rhinorrhea, or deformity of the nose appears. If the underlying pathogenic mechanism cannot be eliminated (e.g., cystic fibrosis), the polyps may soon return. Antihistamines may be helpful in delaying recurrence due to allergic causes.

13.36 TONSILS AND ADENOIDS

The term tonsils is used in its commonly accepted sense of indicating the two faucial tonsils; the term adenoids refers to the pharyngeal tonsil. The tonsils and adenoids are part of the lymphoid tissues that circle the pharynx and are known collectively as *Waldeyer ring*. This consists of the lymphoid tissue on the base of the tongue (lingual tonsil), the two faucial tonsils, the adenoids (pharyngeal tonsil), and the lymphoid tissue on the posterior pharyngeal wall. This tissue serves as a defense against infection, but it may become a site of acute or chronic infection.

The principal disturbances of the tonsils and adenoids are infection and hypertrophy. The latter is usually temporary and secondary to infection. The most important issue is if and when they are to be removed. Though both tonsils and adenoids are often removed at the same operation, separate tonsillectomy or adenoidectomy may be indicated, especially in children under 4–5 yr of age. Tonsillar disturbances are uncommon in infancy.

Neoplasms of the tonsils are rare, although papilloma, lipoma, angioma, teratoma, fibroma, plasmocytoma, and lymphosarcoma have been reported.

Acute infections of the tonsils are considered as acute pharyngitis and are discussed in Sec. 13.28.

Chronic Tonsillitis
(Chronically Hypertrophic and Infected Tonsils)

The management of tonsillitis is of special concern because of its frequency and because tonsils are potentially important to the normal development of the immune system.

Clinical Manifestations. These vary considerably; the significant features are recurrent or persistent sore throat and obstruction to swallowing or breathing, most often due to hypertrophied adenoids. There may be a sense of dryness and irritation in the throat, and the breath may be offensive. Constitutional symptoms are not prominent. Rarely, hypertrophied tonsils and adenoids obstructing the upper airway are associated with respiratory distress, chronic hypoxemia, and the development of pulmonary hypertension.

Indications for Tonsillectomy. Parents often wrongly attribute frequent respiratory infections, allergic bronchitis, mouth breathing, recurrent purulent or serous otitis, poor appetite, failure to gain weight, or recurrent or chronic fever to chronic tonsillitis. Tonsillectomy and adenoidectomy do not decrease the incidence of these problems during childhood. For children with recurrent throat infections (seven in the past year or five in each of the past 2 years), tonsillectomy decreases the number of throat infections in the subsequent 2 years, as compared with no tonsillectomy. However, many children who have not had tonsillectomy also have a decline in the number of throat infections. Until better means are available to identify those children who will truly benefit from tonsillectomy and adenoidectomy, it seems prudent to avoid surgery in most cases.

Decision for removal of tonsils should be based on symptoms and signs directly related to hypertrophy, obstruction, and chronic infection in the tonsils and related structures. *Most hypertrophic tonsils actually are normal in size; the misinterpretation results from failure to appreciate that normally tonsils are relatively larger during childhood than in later years.*

Tonsils may virtually meet in the midline in some children who are asymptomatic; tonsils of average size are projected toward the midline when the child is gagged and may be interpreted as being hypertrophic. Alternatively, infection does not always produce hypertrophy, and chronically infected tonsils may be small and embedded behind the faucial pillars. There is no certain way to directly demonstrate whether tonsils are harboring chronic infection. The consistency or size of the tonsils and the presence of cheesy material within the crypts are not reliable guides. Persistent hyperemia of the anterior pillars is a more reliable sign, and enlargement of the cervical lymph nodes is supporting evidence. Persistent enlargement of the node just below and slightly in front of the angle of the jaw is especially significant. Hypertrophy sufficient to obstruct swallowing or breathing is readily detectable; such tonsils practically meet in the midline when the throat is examined without gagging the patient. However, before tonsillectomy is recommended, it should be ascertained that the hypertrophy is chronic and not the result of a recent acute infection. Tonsils can increase in size greatly during an acute infection and recede after its subsidence.

Peritonsillar (and retrotonsillar) abscess is the only definite indication for tonsillectomy. Tonsillectomy is of no value in the prevention or treatment of acute or chronic sinusitis, chronic otitis media, and middle ear deafness. There is also no evidence to indicate that the removal of tonsils is justified for infections in the lower respiratory tract. No systemic disturbance in itself is an indication for tonsillectomy.

Tonsillectomy in Relation to Age of Child. When, on rare occasions, it seems advisable to recommend tonsillectomy for a child 2–3 yr of age, every attempt should be made to postpone the operation. Frequently when the operation is postponed for reasons of age, the apparent need disappears within the next year or so. In the first few years of life the indications for adenoidectomy, though infrequent, are present more often than those for tonsillectomy. Neither procedure should be performed as a prophylaxis against the "common cold" at any age.

Tonsillectomy in Relation to Active Infection. Tonsillectomy should be postponed until 2–3 wk after subsidence of an infection, except in rare instances of acute respiratory obstruction with pulmonary artery hypertension and cor pulmonale.

Complications of Tonsillectomy. The mean duration of postoperative sore throat is 5 days. Minor hemorrhage, postoperative throat infection, or anesthetic complications occur in more than 10% of procedures. Severe hemorrhage or life-threatening complications occasionally occur and are another reason for carefully assessing the indications for surgical intervention. Pulmonary edema also not infrequently occurs after relief of upper airway obstruction with tonsillectomy and/or adenoidectomy. Therefore, this therapy should be reserved for those settings in which postsurgical respiratory failure can be dealt with effectively.

Adenoidal Hypertrophy
(Hypertrophy of Pharyngeal Tonsil; "Adenoids")

Disturbances of the nasopharyngeal lymphoid tissue (adenoids) tend to parallel those of the faucial tonsils. Hypertrophy and infection may occur separately but often occur together; infection is usually primary. The soft adenoid structure, which is normally widespread in the nasopharynx, especially on the posterior wall and the roof, undergoes hypertrophy, and masses of varying size are formed. These masses may almost fill the vault of the nasopharynx, interfere with the passage of air through the nose, and obstruct the eustachian tubes.

Clinical Manifestations. Mouth breathing and persistent rhinitis are the most characteristic symptoms. Mouth breathing may be present only during sleep, especially when the child lies supine, when snoring is also likely to occur. With

severe adenoid hypertrophy the mouth is kept open during the day as well, and the mucous membranes of the mouth and lips are dry. Chronic nasopharyngitis may be constantly present or recur frequently. The voice is altered with a nasal, muffled quality. The breath is offensive, and taste and smell are impaired. A harassing cough may be present, especially at night, resulting from drainage of pus into the lower pharynx or irritation of the larynx by inspired air which has not been warmed and moistened by passage through the nose. Impaired hearing is common. Chronic otitis media may be associated with infected, hypertrophied adenoids and blockage of the eustachian tube orifices.

A small number of young children with marked adenoidal (also tonsillar) enlargement are unable to mouth-breathe during sleep. They snort and snore loudly and often display signs of respiratory distress, such as intercostal retractions and nasal flaring. These children are at risk for respiratory insufficiency (hypoxemia, hypercapnia, acidosis) during sleep. Apneic spells may result, and some of these children develop pulmonary arterial hypertension and, ultimately, cor pulmonale. Lymphoid tissue enlargement of the upper airway with consequent cor pulmonale has been related to cow's milk hypersensitivity in a number of preschool-aged children. Very obese children (e.g., Prader-Willi syndrome) and children with a large or posteriorly placed tongue (e.g., Pierre Robin syndrome) may also develop upper airway obstruction in sleep, mimicking the adenoidal hypertrophy syndrome.

Diagnosis. During the first few years of life, the size of adenoids can be assessed by digital palpation. Indirect visualization with a pharyngeal mirror is possible in older, cooperative children. Alternatively, the fiberoptic bronchoscope can be used for visualization of the nasopharynx. Lateral pharyngeal roentgenograms are also helpful for detecting nasopharyngeal air column obliteration. The presence of adenoid hypertrophy can be suspected from such symptoms as mouth breathing, snoring, and persistent rhinitis with or without chronic otitis media.

An adenoid tissue abscess is uncommon but may be a cause of protracted fever. Identification and drainage of the abscess have been achieved by digital expression.

Treatment. Adenoidectomy may be indicated for symptoms such as persistent mouth breathing, nasal speech, adenoid facies, repeated attacks of otitis media (especially when accompanied by a conductive hearing loss), deafness, and persistent or recurring nasopharyngitis when these seem to be related to infected hypertrophied adenoid tissue. Tonsillectomy should not be routinely done for such problems. Chronic serous otitis media may improve after adenoidectomy in some patients. The same precautions for complete removal and control of bleeding points as in tonsillectomy should be observed.

THOMAS F. BOAT
CARL F. DOERSHUK
ROBERT C. STERN
ALFRED D. HEGGIE

Boat TF, Polmar SH, Whitman V, et al: Hyperreactivity to cow milk in young children with pulmonary hemosiderosis and cor pulmonale secondary to nasopharyngeal obstruction. J Pediatr 87:23, 1975.

Brook I: Bacteriologic features of chronic sinusitis in children. JAMA 246:967, 1981.

Bye CE, Cooper J, Empey DW, et al: Effects of pseudoephedrine and triprolidine, alone and in combination, on symptoms of the common cold. Br Med J 2:189–190, 1980.

Carson JL, Collier AM, HSS: Acquired ciliary defects in nasal epithelium of children with acute viral upper respiratory infections. N Engl J Med 312:463, 1985.

Collier AM, Pimmel RL, Hasselblad V, et al: Spirometric changes in normal children with upper respiratory infections. Am Rev Respir Dis 177:47, 1978.

Denny FW, Clyde WA: Acute respiratory tract infections: An overview: Pediatr 17:1026, 1983.

Dingle JH, Badger GF, Jordan WS: Illness in the Home. A Study of 25,000 Illnesses in a Group of Cleveland Families. Cleveland, Press of Western Reserve University, 1964, p 129.

Fox JP, Cooney MK, Hall CE: The Seattle virus watch. V. Epidemiologic observation of rhinovirus infections. Am J Epidemiol 101:122, 1975.

Gerber MA, Spadaccini LJ, Wright LL, et al: Latex agglutination tests for rapid identification of group A streptococci directly from throat swabs. J Pediat 105:702, 1984.

Greenwald HM, Messeloff CR: retropharyngeal abcess in infants and children. Am J Med Sci 177:767, 1929.

Hendley JO, Wenzel RP, Gwaltney JM: Transmission of rhinovirus colds by self-inoculation. N Engl J Med 288:1361, 1973.

Johnson F: Bleeding factors and tonsils and adenoid surgery. Arch Otolaryngol 86:584, 1967.

Kovatch AL, Wald ER, Ledesma-Medina J, et al: Maxillary sinus radiographs in children with non-respiratory complaints. Pediatrics 73:306, 1984.

Li K, Kiernon S, Wald ER, et al: Isolated uvulitis due to *Haemophilus influenzae* type b. Pediatrics 74:1054, 1984.

Paradise JL, Bluestone CD, Backman RZ, et al: History of recurrent sore throat as an indication for tonsillectomy. N Engl J Med 298:410, 1978.

Paradise JL, Bluestone CD, Backman RZ, et al: Efficacy of tonsillectomy for recurrent throat infection in severely affected children. N Engl J Med 310:674–683, 1984.

Stern RC, Boat TF, Wood RE, et al: Treatment and prognosis of nasal polyps in cystic fibrosis. Am J Dis Child 136:1067–1070, 1982.

Wald ER: Acute sinusitis in children. Pediatr Infect Dis 2:61–68, 1983.

Wald ER, Reilly JS, Casselbrant M, et al: Treatment of acute maxillary sinusitis in childhood: A comparative study of amoxicillin and cefaclor. J Pediatr 104:297, 1984.

13.37 THE EAR

Diseases of the ear are among the most frequently encountered morbid conditions of childhood. The ability to recognize their presence, the adequate knowledge of the most efficacious treatment, and the skills to prevent complications and sequelae are imperative for every physician caring for children.

Clinical Manifestations. Eight prominent signs and symptoms are associated primarily with diseases of the ear and temporal bone:

(1) **Otalgia** is most commonly associated with inflammation of the external and middle ear but may also arise from involvement of the temporomandibular joint, teeth, or pharynx. In young infants, pulling at the ear or general irritability, especially when either is associated with fever, may be the only sign of ear pain.

(2) Purulent **otorrhea** is a sign of otitis externa, otitis media with perforation of the tympanic membrane, or both. Bloody discharge may be associated with acute or chronic inflammation, trauma, neoplasm, or blood dyscrasias. Clear drainage suggests either a perforation of the drum with a serous middle ear effusion or a cerebrospinal fluid otorrhea draining through a defect in the external auditory canal or through the tympanic membrane from the middle ear.

(3) **Hearing loss** results from disease of either the external or middle ear (conductive hearing loss) or from pathology in the inner ear, retrocochlea, or central auditory pathways (sensorineural hearing loss).

(4) **Swelling** about the ear is most commonly the result of inflammation (e.g., external otitis, perichondritis, or mastoiditis), trauma (hematoma), or, on rare occasions, neoplasm.

(5) **Vertigo** is not a common complaint in children, but may sometimes be present. The most frequent cause is eustachian tube–middle-ear disease, but vertigo may also be due to labyrinthitis; perilymphatic fistula between the inner and middle ear from a congenital defect, trauma, or cholesteatoma; vestibular neuronitis; benign paroxysmal positional vertigo; Meniere disease; or disease of the central nervous system. Older children may describe a feeling of spinning or turning, while younger children may manifest the disequilibrium only by falling, stumbling, or clumsiness.

(6) Unidirectional, horizontal, or jerk **nystagmus,** usually associated with vertigo, is vestibular in origin.

(7) **Tinnitus,** though infrequently described by children, is common, especially in patients with eustachian tube–middle-ear disease or with conductive or sensorineural hearing loss.

(8) **Facial paralysis** is an infrequent but frightening condition for both child and parents. When due to disease within the temporal bone in children, it most commonly occurs as a complication of acute or chronic otitis media, but it may also be idiopathic (Bell palsy) or be the result of temporal bone fracture or neoplasm; on rare occasions it may be due to herpes zoster oticus. Other conditions associated with ear disease may also be present, e.g., symptoms of upper respiratory allergy associated with otitis media.

Diagnosis. Adequately examining the entire child, paying special attention to the head and neck, can reveal a condition that may predispose to or be associated with ear disease. The facial appearance and the character of speech may be important clues to an abnormality of the ear. Many of the craniofacial anomalies, e.g., mandibulofacial dysostosis (Treacher Collins syndrome) and trisomy 21 (Down syndrome), are associated with disorders of the ear. Mouth breathing and hyponasality may indicate intranasal or postnasal obstruction; hypernasality is a sign of velopharyngeal insufficiency. Examining the oropharyngeal cavity may uncover an overt cleft palate or a submucous cleft, both of which predispose to otitis media with effusion. A bifid uvula is also associated with an increased incidence of middle-ear disease. Examination may also reveal posterior nasal or pharyngeal inflammation and discharge. Polyposis, severe deviation of the nasal septum, or a nasopharyngeal tumor may also be associated with otitis media.

Examining the ear itself is the most critical assessment. The auricle and external auditory meatus should be examined first, since the presence or absence of signs of infection in these areas may aid later in the differential diagnosis or evaluation of complications of otitis media. For instance, eczematoid external otitis may result from acute otitis media with discharge, or inflammation of the postauricular area may indicate a periosteitis or subperiosteal abscess extending from the mastoid air cells.

Next, the otoscopic examination, the most important part of physical assessment, is undertaken. However, before adequate visualization of the external canal and tympanic membrane is possible, obstructing cerumen must be removed from the canal, either by using an otoscope having a surgical head and a wire loop or a blunt cerumen curette or by gently irrigating the canal with warm water. Absence of cerumen and inflammation of the ear canal indicate external otitis. The external canal of the newborn is filled with vernix caseosa, which disappears shortly after birth.

The tympanic membrane and its mobility is properly assessed by using the *pneumatic otoscope;* assessing the light reflex is of limited value. The normal tympanic membrane is in the neutral position; a drum that is bulging is a condition that may be due to increased middle-ear air pressure, to an effusion within the middle ear, or to both; the visualization of the malleus handle and short process is obscured by a bulging drum. Retraction of the tympanic membrane usually indicates the presence of middle-ear negative pressure, but it may also result from previous disease and subsequent fixation of the ossicles and ligaments. When retraction is present, the short process of the malleus is prominent and the long process is foreshortened.

The normal tympanic membrane has a ground glass appearance; a blue or yellow color usually indicates a middle-ear effusion. A red membrane alone may not indicate pathology, since the blood vessels of the drum head may be engorged as the result of crying, sneezing, or blowing the nose. The normal tympanic membrane is also translucent, allowing the observer to look through it to visualize the middle-ear landmarks—incudostapedial joint, promontory, round-window niche, and frequently the chorda tympani nerve. If a middle-ear effusion is present medial to a translucent drum, an air-fluid level or bubbles of air mixed with the fluid may be visible. Inability to visualize the middle-ear structures indicates opacification of the drum, usually due to thickening of the tympanic membrane, to a middle-ear effusion, or to both.

Abnormal middle-ear pressure is reflected in the pattern of tympanic membrane mobility when first positive and then negative pressure is applied to the external canal using a pneumatic otoscope. Pressure is applied by first obtaining an adequate seal between the external auditory canal and the ear speculum, then applying slight pressure on the rubber bulb (positive pressure), and then releasing the bulb (negative pressure). Abnormal pressure (positive or negative) or liquid within the middle ear can markedly restrict the movement of the eardrum; when the middle-ear–mastoid cavity is completely filled with liquid, there will be no movement.

Aspiration of the middle ear is the definitive method of verifying the presence and type of a middle-ear effusion. Diagnostic tympanocentesis is performed by inserting, through the inferior portion of the tympanic membrane, an 18-gauge spinal needle attached to a syringe. Alcohol cleansing and culturing of the ear canal should precede tympanocentesis and culture of the middle-ear aspirate. The canal culture helps to determine whether cultured organisms are contaminants from the external canal or pathogens from the middle ear.

Tympanometry with an electroacoustic impedance bridge can help to identify middle-ear effusions, disarticulation or fixation of the ossicular chain, and other pathology not definitively diagnosable with an otoscope. Tympanometry is also useful when the otoscopic diagnosis is equivocal or difficult to obtain and is valuable in screening for otitis media with effusion. *Audiometry* measures hearing. Usually, in patients older than 2–3 yr of age, behavioral audiometry, which is a subjective assessment of hearing, is possible; in the young infant or in children who are difficult to test, objective audiometry is necessary (e.g., auditory brain stem response audiometry) (Sec. 2.67). *Roentgenographic assessment* of the ear and temporal bone is frequently helpful. When the tympanic membrane is not intact (as a result of perforation or insertion of a tympanostomy tube), *assessment of the ventilatory function of the eustachian tube* by pressure-flow studies may be an additional diagnostic aid. *Assessment of labyrinthine function* is essential in evaluation of a child with a vestibular disorder (Sec. 21.2).

13.38 CONGENITAL MALFORMATIONS

The external and middle ear, which are derived from the 1st and 2nd branchial arches and grooves, continue to grow through puberty, but the inner ear, which develops from the otocyst, reaches adult size and shape by the middle of fetal development. Malformed external and middle ears may be associated with serious renal anomalies, mandibulofacial dysostosis, and many other craniofacial malformations. Severely deformed external and middle ears may also be associated with malformations of the inner ear.

Severe malformations of the external ear are rare, but minor deformities are common. A pitlike cutaneous depression just in front of the helix and above the tragus may represent a **cyst** or an epidermis-lined **fistulous tract;** these are common but do not require surgical removal unless they become recurrently infected. Accessory **skin tags** on narrow **pedicles** may be removed by ligation, but if the pedicle is broad-based or contains cartilage, the defect should be corrected surgically. The unusually prominent or **"lop" ear** results from lack of bending of the cartilage that creates the antihelix; it may be improved cosmetically by otoplasty after the auricle has sufficiently developed (at about the age of 5 yr). Microtia includes cases of rudimentary auricles that, besides being abnormally small in size, are often more anterior and inferior in placement than normal auricles. Rarely the auricle may be totally absent **(anotia).**

Congenital stenosis or **atresia of the external auditory canal** may be associated with malformation of the auricle and middle ear. Audiometric, tympanometric, and roentgenographic assessments are essential in diagnosing and managing these conditions. Reconstructive middle-ear surgery for atresia is restricted to patients (1) above 5 yr of age, (2) with bilateral deformities or unilateral lesions in which there is a deformity only of the middle-ear ossicles, resulting in a significant conductive hearing loss, (3) with significant bilateral conductive hearing loss, (4) with roentgenographic evidence of an adequate middle-ear cleft and mastoid, and (5) with a normally positioned facial nerve. A **congenital perilymphatic fistula** of the oval or round window membrane may present as a rapid onset, a fluctuating, or a progressive sensorineural hearing loss with or without vertigo and should be repaired to prevent possible spread of infection from the middle ear to the labyrinth, hearing loss, or both.

Congenital malformations of the inner ear are rare but usually result in severe sensorineural hearing loss. The bony deformities are frequently associated with central nervous system malformations.

Congenital cholesteatoma, a congenital rest of epithelial tissue, may appear as a white cystlike structure medial to or within an intact tympanic membrane. It is unrelated to infections of the middle ear and should be promptly removed since it will invariably enlarge, causing irreversible structural change.

INFLAMMATORY DISEASES

13.39 EXTERNAL OTITIS

In the infant, the outer two thirds of the ear canal is cartilaginous and the inner one third bony, whereas in the older child and adult only the outer one third is cartilaginous. The highly viscid secretions of the sebaceous glands and the watery, pigmented secretions of the apocrine glands in the outer portion of the canal combine with exfoliated surface cells of the skin to form a protective, waxy, water-repellent coating. The normal flora of the external canal consists of *Staphylococcus epidermidis, Corynebacterium* (diphtheroids), *Micrococcus* sp., and occasionally *Staphylococcus aureus* and *Streptococcus viridans.* Excessive wetness (swimming, bathing, or increased environmental humidity) or dryness (previous infection, dermatoses, or insufficient cerumen) and trauma (digital or foreign body) make the skin of the canal vulnerable to infection by endogenous bacteria or virulent exogenous bacteria.

Etiology. External otitis is most commonly caused by *Pseudomonas aeruginosa, Enterobacter aerogenes, Proteus mirabilis, Klebsiella pneumoniae,* streptococci and *S. epidermidis,* and fungi such as *Candida* and *Aspergillus.* The condition known as "swimmer's ear" results from loss of protective cerumen and chronic irritation and maceration from excessive moisture in the canal; *Pseudomonas* sp. is the most commonly isolated bacterium. Herpesvirus hominis and varicella-zoster may also cause external otitis.

Clinical Manifestations. The predominant symptom is ear pain, accentuated by manipulation of the pinna and especially by pressure on the tragus. The severity of the pain and tenderness may be disproportionate to the degree of inflammation since the skin of the external ear canal is attached to the perichondrium and periosteum. Itching is a frequent precursor of pain and is usually characteristic of chronic inflammation of the canal. Conductive hearing loss may occur as a result of edema of the skin and tympanic membrane, serous or purulent secretions, or the progressive meatal skin thickening associated with longstanding external otitis. Edema of the canal, erythema, and greenish otorrhea are prominent signs of the acute disease.

Frequently, the canal is so tender and swollen that the entire ear canal and tympanic membrane cannot be adequately visualized, in which instance complete otoscopic examination should be delayed until the acute swelling subsides. If the tympanic membrane can be visualized, it may be either normal or opaque in appearance, and mobility of the drum may be normal or, when the drum is thickened, reduced in response to positive and negative pressure.

Periauricular edema and fever often result from a combined infection with *Pseudomonas* sp. and *Streptococcus pyogenes* or from *S. aureus*. When there is such secondary infection, lymphadenitis, with tender nodes anterior to the tragus or in the postauricular region, may also occur.

Differential Diagnosis. Diffuse external otitis may be confused with furunculosis, otitis media, and mastoiditis. A furuncle usually causes a localized swelling of the canal limited to one quadrant, whereas external otitis is associated with concentric swelling. In otitis media, the eardrum may be perforated, severely retracted, or bulging and immobile, and hearing is usually impaired. Pain on manipulation of the auricle and lymphadenitis are not features of middle-ear disease. In some patients with external otitis, the periauricular edema is so extensive that the auricle is pushed forward, creating a condition that may be confused with acute mastoiditis and a subperiosteal abscess; however, in mastoiditis the postauricular fold is obliterated, while in external otitis the fold is maintained. When the edema over the mastoid process is due to mastoiditis, there is also usually a history of otitis media and hearing loss, and tenderness is noted over the mastoid antrum or tip and not upon movement of the auricle as in external otitis. Sagging of the posterior external canal wall may also occur with acute mastoiditis.

Treatment. Topical otic preparations containing neomycin (active against gram-positive organisms and also against some gram-negative organisms, notably *Proteus* sp.) with either colistin or polymyxin (active against gram-negative bacilli, notably *Pseudomonas* sp.) and corticosteroids are effective in treating most forms of acute diffuse external otitis. If canal edema is marked, a cotton or selvedged-gauze wick should be inserted into the outer third of the ear canal and the medication applied to the wick as frequently as possible for 24–48 hr; the wick can be removed after these applications and the otic medication instilled 3–4 times a day. Acetic acid preparations (2%), with or without corticosteroids, or half-strength Burow solution (aluminum acetate, 1:20) are probably equally effective. When the pain is severe, analgesics (salicylates, codeine) and dry heat may be necessary.

As the inflammatory process subsides, cleaning the canal with cotton-tipped applications or, more effectively, irrigating with 2% acetic acid to remove the debris will enhance the effectiveness of the topical medications. In subacute and chronic infections, periodic cleansing of the canal is essential. In severe, acute, diffuse external otitis associated with fever

and lymphadenitis from which bacteria have been cultured, oral and, on occasion, parenteral antibiotics are indicated; the choice of drug depends upon the antibiotic susceptibility of the organism. A fungal infection (otomycosis) of the external auditory canal may be treated by applying metacresol acetate. Preventing external otitis may be necessary for individuals susceptible to recurrences, especially children who swim frequently. The most effective prophylaxis is instillation of dilute alcohol or acetic acid immediately following swimming or bathing.

Furunculosis is due to *S. aureus* and is seen only in the hair-containing outer third of the ear canal. It is treated with incision and drainage and systemic penicillin or one of the penicillinase-resistant penicillins, depending upon the antibiotic susceptibility of the organism.

Acute cellulitis of the auricle and external auditory canal is usually caused by *S. pyogenes*, occasionally by *S. aureus*. The skin is red, hot, and indurated without a sharply defined border. Fever may be present with little or no exudate in the canal. Parenteral administration of penicillin G or a penicillinase-resistant penicillin is the therapy of choice.

Dermatoses (seborrheic, contact, infectious eczematoid, atopic, or neurodermatoid) are common causes of inflammation of the external canal and can be precursors of acute diffuse external otitis due to scratching and the introduction of infecting organisms. *Seborrheic dermatitis* is characterized by greasy scales that flake and crumble as they are detached from the epidermis; associated changes in the scalp, forehead, cheeks, brow, postauricular areas, and the concha are usual. *Contact dermatitis* may be caused by topical otic medications such as neomycin, polymyxin, and colistin, which may produce erythema, vesiculation, edema, and weeping. Poison ivy, oak, and sumac may also produce contact dermatitis. *Infectious eczematoid dermatitis* is caused by a purulent infection of the external canal, middle ear, or mastoid; the purulent drainage infects the skin of the canal, auricle, or both. The lesion is weeping, erythematous, or crusted. *Atopic dermatitis* occurs in children with familial or personal histories of allergy; the auricle, particularly the postauricular fold, becomes thickened, scaly, and excoriated. *Neurodermatitis* is recognized by the intense itching and erythematous, thickened epidermis localized to the concha and orifice of the meatus. Treatment of these dermatoses depends on the type but should include application of the aural medication described for external otitis, elimination of the source of infection or contactant when identified, and management of any underlying dermatologic problem.

Herpes simplex may appear as vesicles on the auricle and lips, which eventually become encrusted and dry up, and may be confused with impetigo. Topical application of a 10% solution of carbamide peroxide in anhydrous glycerol is symptomatically helpful.

Herpes zoster oticus (Ramsay Hunt syndrome) is a vesicular eruption on the posterior canal wall accompanied by facial paralysis. Spontaneous recovery is usual.

Bullous myringitis is commonly associated with an acute upper respiratory infection. The ear is very painful, and there are hemorrhagic or serous blebs on the membrane. The disease is difficult to differentiate from acute otitis media since early in the course of acute otitis the drum may appear to have bullae. The organisms involved are probably the same as those causing acute otitis media. Treatment consists of antibiotic therapy of the type usually given for acute otitis media. Incision of the bullae, although not necessary, will promptly relieve the pain.

13.40 OTITIS MEDIA

Inflammation of the middle ear, or otitis media, is the most prevalent disease of childhood after respiratory tract infections. The complications and sequelae of acute otitis media and otitis media with effusion represent significant health hazards for children. Acute otitis media is usually suppurative or purulent, but serous effusions may also have an acute onset. There are many terms for otitis media with effusion, such as serous, secretory, catarrhal, mucoid, nonsuppurative, or allergic otitis media.

Epidemiology and Pathogenesis. Infants and young children are at highest risk for otitis media; incidence rates are 15–20%, with peaks occurring from 6–36 mo and 4–6 yr of age. Children who develop otitis media in the first years of life have an increased risk of recurrent acute or chronic disease. A study of 2565 children followed during their first 3 years found that only 29% of infants failed to develop at least one attack of otitis media, whereas about 33% had three or more episodes. In addition, after the first episode, 40% of children had a middle-ear effusion that persisted for 4 wk and 10% had an effusion that was still present at 3 mo. The incidence of the disease tends to decrease as a function of age after the age of 6 yr. The incidence is high in males, lower socioeconomic groups, Alaskan natives, American Indians, and children with cleft palate and other craniofacial anomalies, and is higher in whites than in blacks. The incidence is also increased in winter and early spring.

The eustachian tube protects the middle ear from nasopharyngeal secretions, provides drainage into the nasopharynx of secretions produced within the middle ear, and permits equilibration of air pressure with atmospheric pressure in the middle ear. Mechanical or functional obstruction of the eustachian tube can result in middle-ear effusion. Intrinsic mechanical obstruction can result from infection or allergy and extrinsic obstruction from obstructive adenoids or nasopharyngeal tumors. Persistent collapse of the eustachian tube during swallowing can result in functional obstruction related to decreased tubal stiffness, an inefficient active opening mechanism, or both. Functional obstruction is common in infants and younger children because the amount and stiffness of the cartilage support of the tube are less than that in older children and adults; marked age differences in the craniofacial base render the tensor veli palatini muscle (the only active opener of the tube) less efficient prior to puberty. All infants with unrepaired palatal clefts have chronic otitis media with effusion due to functional obstruction of the eustachian tube.

Eustachian tube obstruction results in negative middle-ear pressure and, if persisitent, in a sterile transudative middle-ear effusion. Drainage of the effusion is inhibited by impaired mucociliary transport and by sustained negative pressure. When the eustachian tube is mechanically not totally obstructed, contamination of the middle-ear space from nasopharyngeal secretions may occur by reflux (especially when the tympanic membrane has a perforation or when a tympanostomy tube is present), by aspiration (from high negative middle-ear pressure), or by insufflation during crying, nose blowing, sneezing, and swallowing when the nose is obstructed. Rapid alterations in ambient pressure or barotrauma during deep water diving or flying can also result in acute middle-ear effusion that may be hemorrhagic.

Acute Otitis Media

Clinical Manifestations. In the usual course, a child suffering an upper respiratory infection for several days suddenly develops otalgia, fever, and hearing loss. Examination with the pneumatic otoscope reveals a hyperemic, opaque, bulging tympanic membrane of poor mobility; purulent otorrhea may be present, but earache and fever are not invariably present. Children with diminished or absent mobility and opacification of the tympanic membrane should be suspected of having bacterial otitis media with effusion. Any child with a "fever

of undetermined origin" must also be evaluated for a middle-ear infection.

Diagnosis. When the diagnosis of acute otitis media is in doubt or identification of the causative agent is desirable, aspiration of the middle ear should be performed. Tympanocentesis should also be considered for children who are seriously ill or who appear toxic; for children who unsatisfactorily respond to antibiotic therapy; for an onset of otitis media in a patient receiving antibiotic agents; for patients developing suppurative, intratemporal, or intracranial complications; and for otitis in the newborn, the very young infant, or the immunologically deficient patient, in each of whom unusual organisms may cause infection.

Treatment. Therapy depends upon the bacterial cause of the disease and the results of sensitivity testing. *S. pneumoniae* has been cultured from at least 30% of the effusions and is the most common causative agent in all age groups; *Haemophilus influenzae* and *Branhamella catarrhalis* are each isolated in about 20% of cases; group A beta-hemolytic streptococcus and *S. aureus* account for about 5%. In about 25% of cases the effusion is sterile. In neonates approximately 20% of effusions may contain gram-negative enteric bacilli. Since the causative organism is rarely known before therapy begins, oral ampicillin, 50–100 mg/kg/24 hr in four divided doses for 10 days, is recommended, since it is usually effective against the most commonly encountered bacteria. Amoxicillin, 40 mg/kg/24 hr, is equally effective and can be given in three divided doses. An increasing percentage of *H. influenzae* and *B. catarrhalis* strains have become beta-lactamase producing and therefore ampicillin-resistant. When a resistant organism is cultured from a middle-ear aspirate or when the patient fails to improve clinically after initial ampicillin or amoxicillin treatment (probably because of an ampicillin-resistant bacterium) and if a tympanocentesis/myringotomy is not performed, the initial antimicrobial should be changed. Appropriate choices may be erythromycin (50 mg/kg/24 hr) combined with a sulfonamide (100 mg/kg/24 of triple sulfonamides or 150 mg/kg/24 hr of sulfisoxazole) in four divided doses, trimethoprim-sulfamethoxazole (8 and 40 mg/kg/24 hr) in two divided doses, cefaclor (40 mg/kg/24) in three divided doses, or amoxicillin–K clavulanate (40 mg/kg/24 hr) in three divided doses. If the patient is allergic to the penicillins, the combination of oral erythromycin and triple sulfonamides or sulfisoxazole is an alternative. The combination of trimethoprim and sulfamethoxazole also can be given initially to penicillin-sensitive individuals, but its effectiveness in treating acute otitis media due to *S. pyogenes* is uncertain.

Additional supportive therapy, including analgesics, antipyretics, and local heat, is usually helpful. Meperidine hydrochloride may also be required for sedation. An oral decongestant, pseudoephedrine hydrochloride, may relieve some nasal congestion, and antihistamines may help patients with known or suspected nasal allergy. However, the efficacy of antihistamines and decongestants in the treatment of acute otitis media has not been proved.

If the patient continues to have appreciable pain or fever or both after 24–48 hr, tympanocentesis and myringotomy should be performed as diagnostic and therapeutic procedures; identification of the organism(s) is recommended at this stage, but when a diagnostic aspiration is not performed, an antimicrobial agent(s) effective against the resistant organisms prevalent in the community should be administered.

In patients with unusually severe earache, myringotomy may be performed initially to provide immediate relief. When therapeutic drainage is required, a myringotomy knife should be used and the incision should be large enough to allow for adequate drainage of the middle ear.

All patients should be re-evaluated approximately 2 wk after the institution of treatment, at which time there should be some otoscopic evidence of resolution such as decrease in inflammation and return of mobility of the tympanic membrane. Periodic follow-up is indicated for patients who have had recurrent episodes. If the middle-ear fluid is persistent, the patient should be treated as described below.

Persistent Middle-Ear Effusion

If the middle-ear effusion persists after the initial 10–14 days of antimicrobial therapy for acute otitis media, one or more of the following options may help to resolve it during the next, subacute phase: (1) a course of an antimicrobial agent different from the initial one (the new antimicrobial agent may be effective against an organism resistant to the previous one); (2) a topical or systemic nasal decongestant, antihistamine, or a combination of these drugs; (3) topical corticosteroids; and (4) eustachian tube–middle-ear inflation. None of these have been demonstrated to be effective in randomized, controlled trials. Many clinicians do not treat children who have asymptomatic (except for hearing loss) middle-ear effusion still present after 2 wk, but rather re-examine the child 6 wk later, i.e., 2 mo after the initial visit, at which time most patients are effusion-free. Treatment with another antimicrobial, such as cefaclor, trimethoprim-sulfamethoxazole, erythromycin-sulfisoxazole, or amoxicillin–K clavulanate, which are effective against resistant bacteria, may be indicated if the child has any signs or symptoms of persistent infection, such as otalgia, or if, in the community, such organisms have been isolated from subacute effusions.

Recurrent Acute Otitis Media

Some children develop recurrent acute episodes of otitis media with almost every respiratory tract infection, have more or less dramatic symptoms, respond well to therapy, and have fewer episodes with advancing age. Others have persistent middle-ear effusion and suffer recurrent episodes of acute otitis media superimposed on the chronic disorder. The child with recurrent acute otitis media that completely clears between episodes may be managed as previously outlined, but if the bouts are frequent and close together, further evaluation similar to that described for patients having chronic otitis media with effusion is indicated. In many of these children the underlying cause is not evident, but prophylactic antibiotics (a daily dose of amoxicillin or sulfonamides) appear to be effective. Myringotomy and ventilating tubes may also be effective but should be reserved for patients in whom antimicrobial prophylaxis fails to prevent recurrent acute otitis media or in whom chemoprophylaxis is not desirable, because of allergy to the penicillins and the sulfonamides. The preventive efficacies of chemoprophylaxis, myringotomy with tympanotomy tube insertion, hyposensitization, and adenoidectomy are not established. However, immunization with the polyvalent pneumococcal vaccine may be effective when administered to patients above 2 yr of age.

Otitis Media with Effusion

Otitis media with effusion is a middle-ear effusion lacking clinical manifestations of acute infection, such as otalgia and fever. The duration (not the severity) of the effusion can be divided into acute (less than 3 wk), subacute (3 wk–3 mo), and chronic (greater than 3 mo). The effusions may be serous (thin), mucoid (thick), or purulent.

Clinical Manifestations. Frequently either a retracted or convex tympanic membrane is seen. The membrane is usually opaque, but when it is translucent, an air-fluid level or air bubbles may be seen and an amber or sometimes bluish fluid may be apparent in the middle ear. The mobility of the eardrum is almost always impaired. Occasionally, even when there is little effusion, the tympanic membrane is retracted and its mobility impaired, usually because of negative middle-ear air pressure, which, when extreme, is termed "atelectasis of the tympanic membrane." The auditory acuity is usually decreased, and, although systemic symptoms are usually absent, there may be behavioral disturbances due to the child's inability to communicate adequately. A feeling of fullness in the ear, tinnitus, and even vertigo may be present. Some patients, even with thick middle-ear effusions, can hear fairly well; tympanometry is more reliable than audiometry.

Treatment. Treatment may not be indicated since little is known about the possible complications and sequelae associated with this condition and since most of these effusions resolve spontaneously. However, although the significance of hearing loss is uncertain, such a loss may impair cognitive and language development and result in disturbances in psychosocial adjustment. Because of these uncertainties, some clinicians believe treatment is indicated under certain conditions. For example, treatment may be indicated for a child with bilateral chronic middle-ear effusions and a marked hearing loss, although treatment may not be indicated for a child having a unilateral, asymptomatic otitis media with effusion and having only a mild hearing loss without serious secondary changes in the tympanic membrane. Other conditions, in addition to conductive or sensorineural hearing loss, that need to be considered include: (1) occurrence of otitis media with effusion in young infants who are unable to communicate about their symptoms and may have suppurative disease; (2) an associated purulent upper respiratory tract infection; (3) vertigo; (4) alterations of the tympanic membrane such as severe atelectasis, especially a deep retraction pocket in the posterosuperior quadrant, the pars flaccida, or both; (5) middle-ear changes such as adhesive otitis or ossicular involvement; (6) when the effusion persists for 2 to 3 mo or longer; and (7) when the episodes frequently recur, resulting in an accumulation of an excessive amount of effusion over many months.

None of the proposed treatments have been shown to be effective in adequate clinical trials. An orally administered combination of a *decongestant and antihistamine* may be effective in adolescents or children in whom there is evidence of upper respiratory allergy, but it has been shown to be ineffective in infants and children with acute, subacute, and chronic otitis media with effusion. The efficacy of *topical intranasal and systemic corticosteroid therapy* is unproven, and the risks of corticosteroid therapy generally outweigh the possible benefits. However, even though the efficacy of immunotherapy and allergy control is not established for children with evidence of upper respiratory allergy, this method of management seems reasonable for those who have frequent recurrent otitis media with effusion. *Inflation of the eustachian tube,* using the method of Politzer or employing the Valsalva maneuver, may be helpful in enhancing drainage of a thin (serous) middle-ear effusion into the nasopharynx, but its efficacy has not been evaluated.

A trial of antibiotics may be the most appropriate treatment in those children who have not recently received antibiotics. Since bacteria similar to those found in acute otitis media have been isolated from a significant proportion of middle-ear aspirates in children with otitis media with effusion, the antibiotic chosen and duration of treatment should be the same as recommended for acute otitis media. If the effusion is chronic and unresponsive to this therapy, a trial with an antimicrobial agent effective against ampicillin-resistant bacteria is recommended.

If the effusion persists for 3 mo or longer or if there have been frequent recurrences of episodes of acute otitis media, the patient requires further evaluation for respiratory allergy, adenoid tissue obstructing the nose and nasopharynx, an immunologic disorder (if other organs are involved), or abnormalities such as submucous cleft palate or a tumor of the nasopharynx.

For patients in whom medical management (including a trial with an appropriate antibiotic) has failed, *myringotomy and aspiration* of the middle-ear fluid is indicated if the effusion has persisted for 3 mo; inserting a *ventilation or tympanostomy tube* may also allow the middle-ear mucous membrane to return to normal and prevent subsequent accumulation of effusion. Myringotomy and insertion of ventilation tubes may also be helpful in patients with atelectasis of the tympanic membrane when pain, hearing loss, vertigo, or tinnitus is present. Ventilation tubes may prevent permanent structural damage and cholesteatoma if a deep retraction pocket develops in the posterosuperior quadrant or in the attic (pars flaccida) portion of the tympanic membrane. The efficacy of ventilation tubes in these various circumstances, however, is not proven. Furthermore, troublesome otorrhea occasionally develops after the insertion of tubes and can usually be treated successfully with ear drops containing neomycin, polymyxin, or colistin with hydrocortisone. Since these medications may be ototoxic, some physicians use systemic antibiotics without the aural drops.

In selected cases *allergic hyposensitization and adenoidectomy* may be beneficial; the efficacy of these has not been fully assessed. *Tonsillectomy* has not been shown to alter the course of otitis.

Complications and Sequelae of Otitis Media

The intracranial suppurative complications of otitis media are relatively uncommon except in neglected cases. However, complications occurring within the aural cavity and adjacent structures of the temporal bone are more common and include hearing loss, perforation of the tympanic membrane with or without suppuration, acquired cholesteatoma, mastoiditis, petrositis, adhesive otitis media, tympanosclerosis, ossicular discontinuity, facial paralysis, and labyrinthitis.

Hearing loss, the most prevalent complication and morbid outcome of otitis media, may be caused by one or more of the intratemporal complications. To a varying degree, fluctuating or persistent loss of hearing is usually associated with acute or chronic middle-ear effusions or, in the absence of an effusion, with high negative pressure within the middle ear. The audiogram usually reveals a mild to moderate conductive loss. However, there may be a sensorineural component, generally attributed to the effect of increased tension and stiffness of the round window membrane. This hearing loss is usually reversible with resolution of the effusion, but permanent conductive hearing loss can result from irreversible changes secondary to recurrent acute or chronic inflammation, e.g., adhesive otitis, tympanosclerosis, or ossicular discontinuity. Irreparable sensorineural loss may also occur, presumably as the result of spread of infection through the round or oval window membrane. Although persistent or episodic conductive hearing loss may result in impairment of cognitive, language, and emotional development of children, the degree and duration of the hearing loss required to produce such deficits are unknown (Sec. 2.67).

Perforation of the tympanic membrane most frequently occurs when the central portion of the eardrum spontaneously ruptures during an episode of acute otitis media. If persistent purulent otorrhea follows, a culture should be obtained, if possible from the middle ear, and appropriate antibiotics administered. Healing of the tympanic membrane frequently follows cessation of the suppurative process. A central perforation that fails to heal spontaneously despite a dry middle ear and good eustachian tube function may be closed with a graft, tympanoplasty. However, if the otorrhea persists or if the drainage seems to be coming from an apparent posterosuperior or attic (pars flaccida) defect, then a cholesteatoma should be suspected. Aural polyps, which appear as red friable masses, may protrude through one of these defects, indicating the presence of a cholesteatoma.

Chronic suppurative otitis media with mastoiditis may also be associated with a perforation or a cholesteatoma. The purulent discharge may be persistent or episodic; the most common pathogenic organisms are the gram-negative bacilli, e.g., *P. aeruginosa, Bacillus proteus,* and *S. aureus.* Oral or parenteral antimicrobial therapy is indicated; tympanomastoidectomy is required if medical treatment is unsuccessful or if a cholesteatoma is present.

Acquired cholesteatoma is a saclike structure within the middle ear that is lined by keratinized, stratified, squamous epithelium and that contains desquamated epithelium or keratin. White, shiny, greasy debris accompanied by a foul-smelling discharge may be observed. Tympanomastoid surgery is indicated, and if it is delayed, the disease can invade and destroy other structures of the temporal bone and spread to the intracranial cavity.

Mastoiditis or inflammation of the mastoid air cell system frequently accompanies acute otitis media and otitis media with effusion. Roentgenographic examination reveals a cloudy mastoid. The process is usually reversible and the effusion resolves with appropriate medical management. Occasionally, a severe acute otitis media is accompanied by mastoiditis in which there is pain, tenderness, edema, and erythema of the postauricular area. The mastoid periostitis stage, in which the pinna is displaced inferiorly and anteriorly and the posterosuperior canal wall may be swollen or sagging, requires immediate tympanocentesis, myringotomy, and systemic ampicillin; subsequently antibiotics should be adjusted according to the susceptibility of the organism. If the condition progresses to the stage of rarefying osteitis, the infectious process may break through the cortex of the mastoid to form a subperiosteal abscess. The infection may also break through the mastoid tip into the neck (Bezold abscess) or fistulize into the external ear canal. When osteitis is present, mastoid surgery is required to prevent further intratemporal or intracranial complications.

Petrositis may result from acute or chronic infections of the pneumatized apical and perilabyrinthine cells of the temporal bone. The triad of otitis media, paralysis of the external rectus muscle, and pain in the homolateral orbit or retro-orbital area with headache constitutes petrous apicitis, i.e., *Gradenigo syndrome.*

Adhesive otitis is the result of healing following chronic inflammation of the middle ear. The mucous membrane is thickened by proliferation of fibrous tissue, which frequently impairs the movement of the ossicles and thus results in an irreversible conductive hearing loss. **Tympanosclerosis** is a complication of chronic middle-ear inflammation characterized by whitish plaques in the tympanic membrane and nodular deposits in the submucosal layers of the middle ear. There is hyalinization with deposition of calcium and phosphate crystals, and conductive hearing loss may result from the ossicles imbedding in the deposits. Prevention is the only successful means of controlling this disease and adhesive otitis media.

Ossicular discontinuity is the result of rarefying osteitis secondary to chronic middle-ear inflammation. The long process of the incus is commonly involved, but the crural arch of the stapes, the body of the incus, or the manubrium of the malleus may also be eroded. The conductive hearing loss that frequently results can be corrected surgically.

Facial paralysis may occur during an episode of acute otitis media because of exposure of the facial nerve from a congenital bony dehiscence within the middle ear. When it occurs as an isolated complication, a myringotomy should be performed and parenteral antibiotics administered. The paralysis will usually improve rapidly without further surgery (i.e., facial nerve decompression). Mastoidectomy is not indicated unless mastoid osteitis is present. However, immediate surgical intervention is indicated when a facial paralysis develops in a child who has chronic suppurative otitis media with or without cholesteatoma.

Suppurative labyrinthitis may occur during an episode of acute otitis media from the direct invasion of bacteria through the round or oval windows. When chronic otitis media is present, the infection may penetrate the windows or enter through a fistula of the bony horizontal semicircular canal. There may be vertigo, nystagmus, tinnitus, hearing loss, nausea, and vomiting. Treatment consists of intensive parenteral antibiotic therapy, but labyrinthectomy may be indicated to prevent spread to the intracranial cavity.

The **intracranial suppurative complications** of acute and chronic otitis media are meningitis, focal encephalitis, brain abscess, sinus thrombophlebitis, extradural abscess, subdural abscess, and otitic hydrocephalus. These complications occur more often in association with chronic suppurative otitis and mastoiditis, with or without cholesteatoma, than with acute otitis media. Infection spreads from the middle ear and mastoid to the intracranial structures through vascular channels (osteothrombophlebitis), by direct extension (osteitis), or through preformed pathways such as round window, previous skull fracture, and congenital or surgically acquired bony dehiscences. Any child having acute or chronic otitis media who develops one or more of the following signs or symptoms, especially while receiving medical treatment, should be suspected of having a suppurative intracranial complication: persistent headache, severe otalgia, fever, nausea, vomiting, stiff neck, focal seizures, ataxia, blurred vision, hemiplegia, intention tremor, papilledema, diplopia, pastpointing, dysdiadochokinesia, aphasia, or hemianopsia. Conversely, children having intracranial infection (recurrent meningitis or brain abscess) should be evaluated for middle ear–mastoid disease.

INNER EAR

The inner ear may be affected by viral or bacterial infections. Congenital rubella, cytomegalovirus, and mumps are causes of severe sensorineural deafness. Labyrinthitis may be a complication of acute or chronic otitis media and mastoiditis but also may follow bacterial meningitis as a result of organisms entering the labyrinth through the internal auditory meatus, endolymphatic duct, vascular channel, or perilymphatic duct.

13.41 TRAUMATIC INJURIES OF THE EAR AND TEMPORAL BONE

Auricle and External Auditory Canal

Hematoma, or accumulation of blood between the perichondrium and the cartilage, may follow trauma to the pinna. Immediate needle aspiration or, when the hematoma is extensive, incision and drainage and a pressure dressing are necessary to prevent perichondritis, which can result in a **cauliflower ear** deformity. **Frostbite** of the auricle should be managed by rapidly rewarming the exposed pinna with warm irrigation or warm compresses. **Foreign bodies** in the external canal are common in childhood; removal can usually be accomplished without general anesthesia: (1) if the child is informed of the procedure (if old enough to understand it); (2) if the child is properly restrained; (3) when an adequate headlight or surgical head otoscope is used for visualizing the object; and (4) when an alligator forceps, wire loop, or blunt cerumen curette is used, depending on the shape of the object. Irrigation is sometimes helpful. General anesthesia

and the otomicroscope are necessary for the more difficult foreign bodies, especially those deeply imbedded in the canal just lateral to the tympanic membrane. Following removal of the external canal foreign body, the tympanic membrane should be carefully inspected for possible traumatic perforation or for a pre-existing middle-ear effusion. If the foreign body has resulted in acute inflammation of the canal, treatment as described for acute diffuse external otitis should be instituted.

Tympanic Membrane and Middle Ear

Traumatic perforation of the tympanic membrane usually occurs as the result of either a sudden external compression (e.g., a slap) or penetration by a foreign object (e.g., a stick or cotton-tipped applicator). The perforation may be either linear or stellate and is most frequently in the anterior portion of the pars tensa when it is caused by compression; it may be in any quadrant of the tympanic membrane when caused by a foreign object. Spontaneous healing usually occurs, but if the drum does not heal within 2–3 mo, tympanoplastic surgery is indicated. Systemic antibiotics and topical otic medications are not required unless suppurative otorrhea is present. However, otorrhea may occur at any time during periods of upper respiratory tract infection, since the middle-ear air cushion is lost, permitting reflux of nasopharyngeal secretions into the middle-ear cavity. Perforations resulting from penetrating foreign bodies are less likely to heal than those caused by compression. Implantation of epithelium from a traumatic perforation can result in a cholesteatoma.

Immediate surgical exploration is indicated if the injury is accompanied by one or more of the following: vertigo, nystagmus, severe tinnitus, moderate to severe hearing loss, or cerebrospinal fluid otorrhea. Exploratory tympanotomy is necessary to inspect the ossicles, especially the stapes, that may have been dislocated.

Perilymphatic fistula may occur following sudden barotrauma or increase in cerebrospinal fluid pressure. This condition is probably more common than generally appreciated and should always be suspected in a child who develops a sudden or fluctuating sensorineural hearing loss, vertigo, or both, following physical exertion, deep water diving, flying in an airplane, playing a wind instrument, or any other activity that suddenly increases the pressures within the middle ear or the intracranial-labyrinthine system. Characteristically, the leak is at either the oval or the round window, which may be congenitally abnormal; immediate repair of the fistula is essential, since the hearing loss may become irreversible.

Temporal Bone Fractures

Children are particularly prone to basilar skull fractures, which usually involve the temporal bone. Most temporal bone fractures are longitudinal and are commonly manifested by bleeding from a laceration of the external canal and tympanic membrane or, if the drum is intact, by a hemotympanum; by conductive hearing loss resulting from the laceration of the tympanic membrane, hemotympanum, or ossicular injury; by delayed onset of facial paralysis (which usually improves spontaneously); and by temporary cerebrospinal fluid otorrhea. Transverse fractures of the temporal bone have a graver prognosis than longitudinal fractures and are associated with immediate facial paralysis, which may not improve without surgical intervention; severe sensorineural hearing loss, vertigo, nystagmus, tinnitus, nausea, and vomiting associated with complete loss of cochlear and vestibular function; hemotympanum and, rarely, external canal bleeding; and cerebrospinal otorrhea, seen either in the external auditory canal or behind the tympanic membrane, which may come through the nose via the eustachian tube.

Vigorous removal of external auditory canal blood clots, tympanocentesis, and application of otic preparations are not indicated, but prophylactic parenteral administration of antibiotics when cerebrospinal otorrhea is present has been advocated. Surgical intervention is reserved for children who require tympanoplastic repair of the perforated tympanic membrane (that fails to heal spontaneously), who have suffered dislocation of the ossicular chain, or who need decompression of the facial nerve. Sensorineural hearing loss can also occur following a blow to the head without an obvious fracture of the temporal bone (labyrinthine concussion).

Acoustic trauma results from exposure to high intensity sound (e.g., fireworks, gunfire, rock music) and is manifested by a depression at 4000 Hz on the audiometric examination. The loss may be temporary but may become permanent if the noise exposure is chronic. Avoiding chronic exposure to loud noise and protecting the ear against unavoidable exposure are preventive.

13.42 TUMORS OF THE EAR AND TEMPORAL BONE

Benign tumors of the external canal include osteoma and monostotic and polyostotic fibrous dysplasia. Osteomas present as bony masses in the canal and require removal only if hearing is impaired or external otitis results. *Eosinophilic granuloma* of the middle ear should be suspected when there are otalgia, otorrhea, hearing loss, and roentgenographic findings of a sharply delineated destructive lesion of the temporal bone. *Rhabdomyosarcoma* originating in the middle ear should be considered when there is either bleeding from the ear or otorrhea associated with paralysis of the facial nerve. *Reticulum cell sarcoma* and *leukemia* may also present in the middle ear. Although primary neoplasms of the middle ear are relatively uncommon, the initial signs and symptoms of the more common nasopharyngeal neoplasms (e.g., angiofibroma, rhabdomyosarcoma, epidermoid carcinoma) may be associated with the insidious onset of a chronic otitis media with effusion.

13.43 DISEASES OF THE BONY LABYRINTH

Otosclerosis, an autosomal dominant disease, can cause a fixation of the stapes, resulting in progressive hearing loss in older children and teenagers. A hearing aid may be necessary. Corrective surgery is more successful and permanent in adults than in children. *Osteogenesis imperfecta* may involve both the middle and inner ears. If the hearing loss is severe enough, a hearing aid is a preferable alternative to surgical correction of the fixed stapes, since the disease is progressive. *Osteoporosis* may involve the middle ear, resulting in a moderate to severe hearing loss. A hearing aid may be necessary for rehabilitation.

CHARLES D. BLUESTONE

Special References

American Academy of Otolaryngology, Self-Instruction Package from the Committee on Continuing Education in Otolaryngology. Neely JB: Treatment of the Uncomplicated Aural Cholesteatoma (Keratoma), 1977; Part I, Aural Complications (1978); Part II, Intracranial Complications (1979), Rochester, Minn.

Basser LS: Benign paroxysmal vertigo of childhood (a variety of vestibular neuronitis). Brain 87:141, 1964.

Bergstrom L, Hemenway WG, Downs MP: A high risk registry to find congenital deafness. Otolaryngol Clin North Am 4:369, 1971.

Bluestone CD, Cantekin EI: Eustachian tube dysfunction. *In*: English GM (ed): Otolaryngology, Vol 1. Hagerstown, Md., Harper Row, 1980.

Cantekin EI, Mandel EM, Bluestone CD, et al: Lack of efficacy of a decongestant-antihistamine combination for otitis media with effusion ("secretory" otitis media) in children. N Engl J Med 308:297–301, 1983.

Fria TJ: The Auditory Brainstem Response: Background and Clinical Applications. Monographs in Contemporary Audiology, Educational Publications Division, Maico Hearing Instruments, Minneapolis, Minn., Vol 2, No 2, 1980.

Gates G: Vertigo in children. EENT 59:358, 1980.

Gower, D, McGuirt, WF: Intracranial complications of acute and chronic infectious ear disease; A problem still with us. Laryngoscope 93:1028, 1983.

Grundfast KM, Bluestone CD: Sudden or fluctuating hearing loss and vertigo in children due to perilymph fistula. Ann Otol Rhinol Laryngol 87:761, 1978.

Harford ER, Bess FH, Bluestone CD, et al: Use of acoustic impedance measurement in screening for middle ear disease in children. Ann Otol Rhinol Laryngol 87:288, 1978.

Hicks TW, Wright JW, Wright JW: Cerebrospinal fluid otorrhea. Laryngoscope, suppl 25, 90:1, 1980.

Holm VA, Kunze LH: Effect of chronic otitis media on language and speech development. Pediatrics 43:833, 1969.

Hough JVD, Stuart WD: Middle ear injuries in skull trauma. Laryngoscope 78:899, 1968.

Howie VM, Ploussard JH: The "in vivo sensitivity test"—Bacteriology of middle ear exudate. Pediatrics 44:940, 1969.

Jahn AJ, Snell GE: Otogenic intracranial complications. J Otolaryngol 9:184, 1980.

Konigsmark BW: Hereditary deafness in man. N Engl J Med 281:713, 744, 827, 1969.

Kovatch AL, Wald ER, Michaels RH: β-Lactamase-producing *Branhamella catarrhalis* causing otitis media in children. J. Pediatr. 102:261–264, 1983.

Linthicum FH: Evaluation of the child with sensorineural hearing impairment. Otolaryngol Clin North Am 8:69, 1975.

Makishima K, Sobel SF, Snow JB: Histopathologic correlates of otoneurologic manifestations following head trauma. Laryngoscope 86:1303, 1976.

Manning JT, Adour K: Facial paralysis in children—Diagnosis and treatment. Pediatrics 49:102, 1972.

Mills, RP, Cherry, JR: Subjective tinnitus in children with otological disorders. Int J Pediatr Otorhinolaryngol 7:21–27, 1984.

Paparella MM, Oda M, Hiraida F, et al: Pathology of sensorineural hearing loss in otitis media. Ann Otol Rhinol Laryngol 81:632, 1972.

Paparella MM, Winter LE: Sensorineural deafness in childhood. Trans AAOO 72:782, 1968.

Paradise JL, Smith C, Bluestone CD: Tympanometric detection of middle ear effusion in infants and young children. Pediatrics 58:198, 1976.

Perrin JM, Charney E, MacWhinney JB Jr, et al: Sulfisoxazole chemoprophylaxis for recurrent otitis media. A double-blind crossover study in pediatric practice. N Engl J Med 291:667, 1974.

Powers WH, Britton BH: Nonotogenic otalgia: Diagnosis and treatment. Am J Otolaryngol 2:97, 1980.

Proctor C: Diagnosis, prevention and treatment of hereditary sensorineural hearing loss. Laryngoscope 87:suppl 7, 1977.

Pulez JL, Freedman HM: Management of congenital middle ear abnormalities. Laryngoscope 88:420, 1978.

Riding KH, Bluestone CD, Michaels RH, et al: Microbiology of recurrent and chronic otitis media with effusion. J Pediatr 93:739, 1978.

Rodriguez WJ, Schwartz RH, Khan WN, et al: Erythromycin-sulfisoxazole for persistent acute otitis media due to ampicillin-resistant *Haemophilus influenzae*. Pediatr Infect Dis 2:27–29, 1983.

Sarno CN, Clemis JD: A workable approach to the identification of neonatal hearing impairment. Laryngoscope 90:1313, 1980.

Schiff M, Poliquin JF, Catanzaro A, et al: Tympanosclerosis. Ann Otol Rhinol Laryngol suppl 70, 89:1, 1980.

Schuknecht HF: Mondini dysplasia: A clinical and pathological study. Ann Otol Rhinol Laryngol suppl 65, 89:1, 1980.

Shurin PA, Marchant CD, Kim CH et al: Emergence of beta-lactamase-producing strains of *Branhamella catarrhalis* as important agents of acute otitis media. Pediatr Infect Dis 2:34–38, 1983.

Simmons FB: Patterns of deafness in newborns. Laryngoscope 90:448, 1980.

Suehiro S, Sando I: Congenital anomalies of the inner ear. Ann Otol Rhinol Laryngol suppl 59, 88:1, 1979.

Valvassori GE, Buckingham RA: Tomography and Cross Sections of the Ear. Philadelphia, WB Saunders, 1975.

General References

Bluestone CD: Recent advances in the pathogenesis, diagnosis, and management of otitis media. Pediatr Clin North Am 28:727, 1981.

Bluestone CD: Otitis media in children: To treat or not to treat? N Engl J Med 306:1399–1404, 1982.

Bluestone CD, Klein JD: Controversies in antimicrobial agents for otitis media. Pediatr Ann 13:361, 1984.

Bluestone CD, Klein JD, Paradise JL, et al: Workshop on effects of otitis media on the child. Pediatrics 71:639, 1983.

Bluestone CD, Stool SE (eds): Pediatric Otolaryngology, Philadelphia, WB Saunders, 1983, Chapters 6–22.

Hanson DG, Ulvestad RF (eds): Otitis media and child development: Speech, language, and education. Ann Otol Rhinol Laryngol 88:suppl 60, 1979.

Northern JL, Downes MP: Hearing in Children, Ed 2. Baltimore, Williams & Wilkins, 1978.

Paparella MM, Shumrick DA: The ear. In Otolaryngology, Vol II. Ed 2. Philadelphia, WB Saunders, 1980.

Schuknecht HE: Pathology of the Ear. Cambridge, Mass., Harvard University Press, 1974.

Senturia NH, Marcus MD, Lucente FE (eds): Diseases of the External Ear: An Otologic-Dermatologic Manual. Ed 2. New York, Grune and Stratton, 1980.

Shambaugh GE Jr, Glasscock ME III: Surgery of the Ear. Ed. 3. Philadelphia, WB Saunders, 1980.

Stool SF, Bluestone CD: Studies in otitis media: Pittsburgh Otitis Media Research Center Progress Report. Ann Otol Rhinol Laryngol [suppl] 92:107, 1983.

13.44 LOWER RESPIRATORY TRACT

CONGENITAL ANOMALIES

13.45 CONGENITAL LARYNGEAL ANOMALIES

Complete **atresia of the larynx** is incompatible with life; only rarely can an infant in whom the diagnosis is made at birth be saved by an immediate tracheostomy. Subsequent successful surgical restoration of an adequate upper airway has not been reported. Patients with laryngeal atresia often have other congenital defects that also may be incompatible with life. **Laryngeal webs** are uncommon, occasionally familial, defects resulting from incomplete separation of the fetal mesenchyme between the two sides of the larynx. Most webs occur between the vocal cords. Immediate diagnosis of a complete or nearly complete web is essential to prevent asphyxiation of the newborn. Respiratory distress with severe stridor may be present, and the cry weak and abnormal in character. Often the obstruction is not complete, and there is only mild stridor and dyspnea. Direct laryngoscopy is required for prompt diagnosis and treatment. Lysis with a carbon dioxide laser is frequently successful, but surgery is occasionally necessary. Thin supraglottic webs can also be incised, but infants with thicker subglottic or intralaryngeal webs require initial incision, excision, and subsequent dilations, which may be unsuccessful because of reformation of the web. An external approach to divide and excise the web with insertion of silicone or metal is often required. Many surgically treated patients need a tracheostomy for a prolonged period thereafter.

Laryngotracheoesophageal cleft is a very rare congenital lesion in which there is a long connection between the airway and the esophagus, sometimes extending to the level of the carina. The lesion is due to failure of dorsal fusion of the cricoid, which normally is completed by the 8th wk of gestation. Other anomalies, including unilateral pulmonary hypoplasia, may be present. Symptoms of chronic aspiration, gagging during feeding, and pneumonia suggest H-type tracheoesophageal fistula, but the clinical manifestations are usually more severe and associated with abnormalities in voice. Diagnosis is extremely difficult, but careful roentgenographic studies of swallowing will show aspiration of contrast material into the trachea indicating the need for endoscopic examination of the airway and perhaps the esophagus. Successful repair has been reported but requires multiple procedures and prolonged tracheostomy.

13.46 CONGENITAL LARYNGEAL STRIDOR
(Laryngomalacia and Tracheomalacia)

Stridor persisting or appearing after the first few days of life usually results from disturbances in or adjacent to the larynx. The most common of these, **laryngomalacia** and **tracheomalacia,** are congenital deformities or flabbiness of the epiglottis and supraglottic aperture and weakness of the airway walls, leading to collapse and some airway obstruction with inspiration. Laryngomalacia is the most common congenital laryngeal abnormality. Males are affected twice as often as females. The embryologic origin of the defect is unknown.

Clinical Manifestations. Noisy, crowing respiratory sounds, usually associated with inspiration, are relatively common during the neonatal period and the first year of life. Stridor, usually present from birth, may not appear until 2 mo in some patients. Symptoms can be intermittent and are worse when the infant lies on his or her back. Some infants merely have noisy breathing, whereas others have a laryngeal "crow," hoarseness or aphonia, dyspnea, and inspiratory retractions in the supraclavicular, intercostal, and subcostal space. When retractions are severe, thoracic deformity may result. Infants with severe dyspnea may have difficulty nursing, resulting in undernutrition and poor weight gain. Substantial stridor may persist for several months to a year after birth, occasionally becoming slightly worse in the first few months of life and then gradually disappearing with growth and development of the airway.

Diagnosis. Laryngomalacia can usually be diagnosed by direct laryngoscopy. In the first few days of life, distinguishing between a congenital laryngeal disturbance and neonatal tetany or laryngeal edema secondary to trauma or aspiration at birth may be difficult. The differential diagnosis includes malformations of the laryngeal cartilages or vocal cords, intraluminal webs, generalized severe chondromalacia of the larynx and trachea, tumors of the larynx, mucus retention cysts, branchial cleft cysts, thyroglossal duct remnants, hypoplasia of the mandible, macroglossia, hemangioma, lymphangioma, Pierre Robin syndrome, congenital goiters, and vascular anomalies.

Treatment. Usually no specific therapy is indicated; the condition resolves spontaneously, though there may be difficulty in feeding. In one review, only 4 of 1415 patients required tracheostomy. Although laryngomalacia usually has resolved by 18 mo of age, some degree of inspiratory obstruction may persist later in childhood. Parents should be reassured about the ultimate resolution and counseled to provide slow, careful feedings. A small nipple or dropper or, infrequently, gavage may be required. Most patients seem more comfortable or less noisy lying prone. Severe symptoms may require nasotracheal intubation or, rarely, tracheostomy.

Other Anomalies. Bifid epiglottis, resulting from cleavage of two thirds or more of the epiglottis, is a rare condition that may not compromise swallowing. It usually does require treatment, however, and is associated with other laryngeal anomalies and with polydactyly. Total absence of the epiglottis is extremely rare. Laryngeal cysts and laryngoceles are occasionally seen; treatment with endoscopic "unroofing" is usually successful.

Burroughs N, Leape LL: Laryngotracheoesophageal cleft; Report of a case successfully treated and review of the literature. Pediatrics 53:516, 1974.

Landing BH: State of the art: Congenital malformations and genetic diseases of the respiratory tract. Am Rev Respir Dis 120:151, 1979.

McGill TJI, Healy BG: Congenital and acquired lesions of the infant larynx. Clin Pediatr 17:584, 1978.

McSwiney PF, Cavanagh NPC, Languth P: Outcome in congenital stridor (laryngomalacia). Arch Dis Child 52:215, 1977.

Novak RW: Laryngotracheoesophageal cleft and unilateral pulmonary hypoplasia in twins. Pediatrics 67:732, 1981.
Smith GJ, Cooper DM: Laryngomalacia and inspiratory obstruction in later childhood. Arch Dis Child 56:345, 1981.
Smith RJH, Catlin FI: Congenital anomalies of the larynx. Am J Dis Child 138:35, 1984.

TRACHEOESOPHAGEAL FISTULA

The majority of tracheoesophageal fistulas are associated with esophageal stenosis and become symptomatic in the newborn period (Sec. 12.17). Occasionally, a patient with an H-type fistula presents at a later age with a long history of problems "handling mucus," respiratory symptoms after feeding (particularly with fluid), and recurrent pneumonia.

Children whose tracheoesophageal fistulae are surgically repaired have a high incidence of abnormal pulmonary function test scores later in childhood. Bronchial hyperreactivity is the most common finding, but restrictive disease also occurs. These abnormalities may result from continuing aspiration. Alternatively, these children may have recurrent infection, due in part to impaired mucociliary clearance related to the presence of squamous epithelium in the trachea.

VASCULAR RING

Abnormal configuration of the great vessels, often including remnants of normally lost branchial arteries, can cause extrinsic pressure on the trachea and compromise respiration (Sec. 14.65).

13.47 AGENESIS/HYPOPLASIA OF THE LUNG

Bilateral pulmonary agenesis or hypoplasia is rare and incompatible with life; the latter is usually associated with anencephaly, diaphragmatic hernias, urinary tract abnormalities, deformities of the thoracic spine and rib cage (thoracic dystrophy), renal anomalies, right heart malformations, and pleural effusions. Unilateral agenesis or hypoplasia may have few symptoms and nonspecific findings, resulting in only one third of the cases being diagnosed during life. In unilateral agenesis the entire pulmonary parenchyma and supporting structures and airways are absent below the level of the carina. In pulmonary hypoplasia there is a small unexpandable lung. Persistent fetal circulation is often present when pulmonary hypoplasia presents in the newborn period (Sec. 14.12).

There is no specific treatment. Supportive measures including mechanical ventilation and supplemental oxygen may allow sufficient pulmonary parenchymal development to permit survival (25% of the infants in one series). Older patients should be given antibiotics for pulmonary infection and receive yearly influenza vaccine. Prognosis in those patients who survive infancy is extremely variable and largely dependent on the presence of associated anomalies. Death may occur from overwhelming pulmonary infection or from complications of pulmonary hypertension associated with congenital heart disease.

Maltz DL, Nadas AS: Agenesis of the lung. Presentation of eight new cases and review of the literature. Pediatrics 42:175, 1968.
Milligan DWA, Levison H: Lung function in children following repair of tracheoesophageal fistula. J Pediatr 95:24, 1979.
Page DV, Stocker JT: Anomalies associated with pulmonary hypoplasia. Am Rev Respir Dis 125:216, 1982.
Swischuk LE, Richardson CF, Nichols MM, et al: Primary pulmonary hypoplasia in the neonate. J Pediatr 95:573, 1979.

LOBAR EMPHYSEMA

See Sec. 13.86.

13.48 PULMONARY SEQUESTRATION

A mass of nonfunctioning embryonic and cystic pulmonary tissue that receives its entire blood supply from the systemic circulation is known as a sequestration. Although most sequestrations do not communicate with functional airways, this is not always the case. Both intralobar and extralobar sequestration arise through the same pathoembryologic mechanism as a remnant of a diverticular outgrowth of the esophagus. Gastric or pancreatic tissue may also be found within the sequestration.

Intralobar sequestration is generally found in a lower lobe. Patients so affected usually present with infection. In older patients hemoptysis is fairly common. Chest roentgenogram, during a period when there is no active infection, reveals a mass lesion; an air-fluid level may be present. During infection the margins of the lesion may be blurred. There is no difference in the incidence of this lesion in each lung. Treatment is surgical removal of the lesion, a procedure that usually requires excision of the entire involved lobe. Occasionally, a segmental resection will suffice.

Extralobar sequestration is much more common on the left. This lesion is strongly associated with diaphragmatic hernia. Many of these patients are asymptomatic when the mass is discovered by routine chest roentgenogram taken for another reason. Other patients present with respiratory symptoms or heart failure. Surgical resection of the involved area is recommended.

Physical findings in patients with sequestration include an area of dullness to percussion and decreased breath sounds over the lesion. During infection rales may also be present. A continuous or purely systolic murmur may be heard over the back. If routine chest roentgenograms are consistent with the diagnosis, other procedures are indicated prior to surgical intervention. Bronchography reveals a mass of intrathoracic tissue without connection to the airways. Aortography should be performed in these patients, since this procedure allows definitive diagnosis by demonstrating systemic blood supply from an anomalous aortic artery. Identifying the blood supply prior to surgery avoids inadvertently severing this systemic artery, which has accounted for much of the intraoperative mortality in the past.

Case Records of the Massachusetts General Hospital: Case 18–1981. N Engl J Med 304:1090, 1981.
Gottrup F, Lund C: Intralobar pulmonary sequestration: A report of 12 cases. Scand J Resp Dis 59:21, 1978.
Iwai K, Shindo G, Hajikano J, et al: Intralobar pulmonary sequestration, with special reference to developmental pathology. Am Rev Resp Dis 107:911, 1973.
Pryce DM: Lower accessory pulmonary artery with intralobar sequestration of lung: Report of seven cases. J Pathol Bacteriol 58:547, 1946.
Telander RL, Lennox C, Sieber W: Sequestration of the lung in children. Mayo Clin Proc 51:578, 1976.

13.49 BRONCHOGENIC CYSTS

These cysts are originally lined with ciliated epithelium and usually occur close to a midline structure (e.g., trachea, esophagus, carina). Once infected, the ciliated epithelium may be lost, and accurate pathologic diagnosis is then impossible. Cysts are rarely demonstrable at birth. Later, some cysts become symptomatic either by becoming infected or by enlarging in size and compromising the function of an adjacent airway. Fever, chest pain, and productive cough are the most common presenting symptoms. Chest roentgenogram reveals the cyst, which may contain an air fluid level. Treatment for symptomatic cysts is surgical excision following appropriate antibiotic management. An asymptomatic cyst discovered incidentally by chest roentgenogram taken for another reason may not require treatment.

13.50 BRONCHOBILIARY FISTULA

This rare anomaly usually presents life-threatening problems during early infancy but, occasionally, diagnosis has been delayed until after 2 yr of age. It consists of a fistulous connection between the right middle lobe bronchus and the left hepatic ductal system. All patients have recurrent severe bronchopulmonary infection and atelectasis starting in early infancy. Definitive diagnosis requires endoscopy and bronchography or exploratory surgery. Treatment is surgical excision of the entire intrathoracic portion of the fistula. Bronchobiliary communications also occur as acquired lesions resulting from hepatic disease complicated by infection.

Pappas SC, Sasaki A, Minuk GY: Bronchobiliary fistula presenting as cough with yellow sputum. N Engl J Med 307:1027, 1982.
Weitzman JJ, Cohen SR, Woods LO Jr, et al: Congenital bronchobiliary fistula. J Pediatr 73:329, 1958.

13.51 CONGENITAL PULMONARY LYMPHANGIECTASIS

This disease, characterized by greatly dilated lymphatic ducts throughout the lung, is usually symptomatic with dyspnea and cyanosis in the newborn. Chest roentgenograms reveal both punctate and reticular densities. Respiration is compromised because of the space-occupying nature of the lesion and, possibly, because pulmonary compliance is reduced, increasing the work of breathing. Two forms of the disease—one in which the abnormality is limited to the lung and one in which the pulmonary lymphangiectasis is secondary to pulmonary venous obstruction—are always symptomatic in the neonatal period. Familial occurrence of the first type has been reported. A third form, in which the pulmonary lymphangiectasis is part of a generalized disease involving other organ systems (e.g., intestine), is associated with milder pulmonary disease and survival to midchildhood and beyond. Definitive diagnosis requires lung biopsy. There is no specific treatment.

Felman AH, Rhatigan RM, Pierson KK: Pulmonary lymphangiectasis. Am J Roent 116:548, 1972.
Noonan JA, Walters LR, Reeves JT: Congenital pulmonary lymphangiectasia. Am J Dis Child 120:314, 1970.
Scott-Emuakpor AB, Warren ST, Kapur S, et al: Familial occurrence of congenital pulmonary lymphangiectasis. Am J Dis Child 135:532, 1981.

13.52 CYSTIC ADENOMATOID MALFORMATION

In this disease a single lobe of one lung, which is enlarged and often cystic, compresses the remainder of the ipsilateral lung, causing a shift of the mediastinum and compression of the other lung. There is slight male predominance. The lesion may result from an embryologic insult before the 50th day of gestation. The involved lobe contains many glandular structures and very few areas of normal lung. Cysts are common but not universally present. The majority of patients become symptomatic and die in the newborn period, although a few survive after emergency surgery. Other patients may be asymptomatic until midchildhood, when brief episodes of recurrent or persistent pulmonary infection or relatively acute chest pain occur. Breath sounds may be diminished with mediastinal shift away from the lesion on physical examination. Chest roentgenograms reveal a cystic mass with mediastinal shift. Occasionally, an air-fluid level suggests a lung abscess. The lesion may be confused with diaphragmatic hernia in the newborn. Surgical excision of the affected lobe is indicated. After surgery, long-term survival into infancy and even later into childhood has been reported, but these patients may be at increased risk for developing primary pulmonary neoplasms.

Hartman GE, Shochat SJ: Primary pulmonary neoplasms of childhood: A review. Ann Thorac Surg 36:108, 1983.
Moncrieff MW, Cameron AH, Astley R, et al: Congenital cystic adenomatoid malformation of the lung. Thorax 24:476, 1969.
Stocker JT, Madewell JE, Drake RM: Congenital cystic adenomatoid malformation of the lung: Classification and morphologic spectrum. Hum Pathol 8:155, 1977.

ACQUIRED DISEASE

ACUTE INFECTIONS OF THE LARYNX AND TRACHEA

General Considerations. Acute infections of the larynx and trachea are of great importance in infants and small children because their airway is smaller, predisposing it to a relatively greater narrowing than is produced by the same degree of inflammation in an older child.

Croup is a generic term encompassing a heterogeneous group of relatively acute infectious conditions characterized by a peculiarly brassy ("croupy") cough, which may or may not be accompanied by inspiratory stridor, hoarseness, and signs of respiratory distress due to varying degrees of laryngeal obstruction. When there is sufficient involvement of the larynx to produce symptoms, the laryngeal part of the clinical picture is likely to overshadow other manifestations.

The infection in infants and small children is rarely limited to a single area of the respiratory tract, but usually rather affects in varying degrees the larynx, trachea, bronchi, and even the upper respiratory portion. Thus, although an exact classification of these infections is not possible, identification of several clinical varieties is justified:

Acute diphtheritic laryngitis (Sec. 11.23).
Infectious croup (acute nondiphtheritic infections)
Epiglottitis
Laryngitis
Laryngotracheobronchitis
Spasmodic laryngitis
Bacterial tracheitis

13.53 INFECTIOUS CROUP
(Acute Nondiphtheritic Infections)

Etiology and Epidemiology. Viral agents account for nearly all croup except that associated with diphtheria, bacterial tracheitis, and acute epiglottitis. The parainfluenza viruses account for approximately three quarters of all cases, with the adenoviruses, respiratory syncytial, influenza, and measles viruses causing most of the remaining cases for which a viral agent can be identified. In one study, *Mycoplasma pneumoniae* was recovered from 3.6% of patients who had croup. Although *H. influenzae* type b is almost always the cause of acute epiglottitis, the group A streptococcus, the pneumococcus, and the staphylococcus are occasionally implicated. Viral epiglottitis is extremely rare, but a milder and superficially similar picture from inflammation of the supraglottic area is probably caused by viruses.

The majority of patients having viral croup are between the ages of 3 mo and 5 yr, whereas croup due to *H. influenzae* and *C. diphtheriae* is more common from 3–7 yr of age. The incidence of croup is higher in males, and it occurs most commonly during the cold season of the year. Approximately 15% of patients have a strong family history of croup, and laryngitis tends to recur in the same child.

Clinical Manifestations. With progressive compromise of the upper airway, a characteristic sequence of symptoms and signs occurs. At first, there is only a mild brassy cough with intermittent respiratory stridor; the latter is sometimes preceded by 1–2 days of mild upper respiratory symptoms. As obstruction increases, stridor becomes continuous and is associated with nasal flaring and suprasternal, infrasternal, and intercostal retractions. Agitation and crying greatly aggravate the symptoms and signs, and the child prefers to sit up in bed or be held upright.

With further compromise of the airway, air hunger and restlessness occur briefly and then are superseded by severe hypoxemia and weakness, accompanied by decreased air exchange and stridor, increasing pulse, and eventual death from hypoventilation. Most patients with croup progress only as far as stridor and slight dyspnea, then start recovery within a few hours. In the hypoxic child who may be cyanotic, pale, or obtunded, any manipulation of the pharynx, including use of a tongue depressor, may result in sudden cardiorespiratory arrest. This examination, therefore, should be deferred and oxygen administered until transfer to a hospital, where optimal management of the airway and shock is possible.

Acute Epiglottis. This dramatic, potentially lethal condition usually occurs in children 2–7 yr old. It is characterized by a fulminating course of fever, sore throat, dyspnea, rapidly progressive respiratory obstruction, and prostration. Within a matter of hours, epiglottitis may progress to complete obstruction of the airway and death unless adequate treatment is administered. With adequate treatment the illness rarely lasts more than 2–3 days. Respiratory distress is frequently the first manifestation. Often the child, particularly the younger patient, is apparently well at bedtime but awakens later in the evening with a high fever, aphonia, drooling, and moderate to severe respiratory distress with stridor. Usually no other family members are ill with acute upper respiratory disease. The older child often complains initially of sore throat and dysphagia. Severe respiratory distress may ensue within minutes or hours of the onset, with inspiratory stridor, hoarseness, brassy cough, irritability, and restlessness. Drooling and dysphagia are common. The young child may assume a position of hyperextension of the neck, although other signs of meningeal irritation are absent. The older child may prefer a sitting position, leaning forward, with mouth open and tongue somewhat protruding. Some children may progress rapidly to a shocklike state characterized by pallor, cyanosis, and impaired consciousness.

Physical examination may disclose moderate to severe respiratory distress with inspiratory and sometimes expiratory stridor, flaring of the alae nasi, and inspiratory retractions of the suprasternal notch, supraclavicular and intercostal spaces, and subcostal area. The pharynx may be inflamed, and there may be an abundance of mucus and saliva, which may also result in rhonchi. With progression, stridor and breath sounds may be diminished as the patient tires. A brief period of air hunger with restlessness and agitation may be followed by rapidly increasing cyanosis, coma, and death. Alternatively, the child may have only mild hoarseness and a large, shiny, cherry-red epiglottis brought into view when the posterior portion of the tongue is properly depressed.

The diagnosis requires depressing the tongue to see a large, swollen cherry-red epiglottis. Laryngoscopy reveals intense inflammation of the epiglottis and surrounding area: arytenoids and arytenoepiglottic folds, vocal cords, and subglottic regions. If the diagnosis is probable on other clinical grounds, direct viewing of the epiglottis in a seriously ill child should be deferred until complete cardiorespiratory support is available and definitive treatment can be carried out since some patients may have reflex laryngospasm and acute complete obstruction, aspiration of secretions, and cardiorespiratory arrest following examination of the pharynx. If epiglottis is thought to be a reasonable possibility, however remote, in a patient with croup, the patient should have a lateral roentgenogram of the nasopharynx and upper airway prior to physical examination of the pharynx (Fig. 13–5). If a roentgenogram shows a normal epiglottis or if the patient is

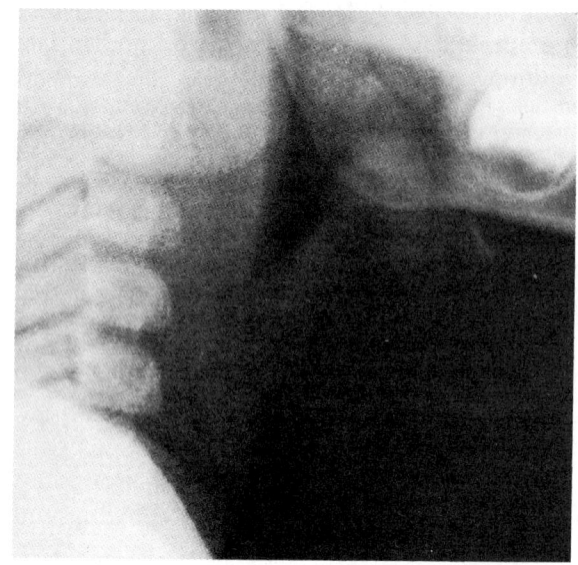

Figure 13–5. Epiglottitis. Lateral roentgenogram of upper airway reveals swollen epiglottis.

unlikely to have croup by history and other physical findings, examination of the epiglottis may be performed when appropriate equipment and personnel are present to control the airway and provide ventilatory support. Patients with suspected epiglottis should be accompanied by a physician and intubation equipment at all times, including the trip to and from the radiology department.

Establishing an airway by either nasotracheal intubation or tracheostomy is indicated in the face of clear evidence of epiglottitis even though the degree of apparent respiratory distress may not seem severe when the patient is initially evaluated. Fulminant pulmonary edema may be associated with acute airway obstruction. The duration of intubation depends upon the clinical course of the patient and the duration of epiglottic swelling, as determined by frequent examination using direct laryngoscopy. In general, children with acute epiglottitis are intubated for 2 to 3 days. Bacteremia is present in a majority of patients; therefore, parenteral antibiotic therapy including ampicillin and chloramphenicol should be instituted promptly. Concomitant infection is unusual, but meningitis, pneumonia, cervical adenitis, and otitis media may occur.

After epiglottitis, subjects develop high serum antibody titers against *H. influenzae* type b, whereas postmeningitic children do not. This development may be a function of their older age, but recent evidence indicates that erythrocyte marker antigens differ significantly in the two groups of patients.

Acute Infectious Laryngitis. Laryngitis is a common illness; except for diphtheria nearly all cases are caused by viruses. The onset is usually characterized by an upper respiratory tract infection during which sore throat, cough, and croup appear. The illness is generally mild; respiratory distress is unusual except in the young infant. In severe cases, however, hoarseness is marked, and the patient may present severe inspiratory stridor, retractions, dyspnea, and restlessness. As the process progresses, air hunger and fatigue become evident, and the child alternates between periods of agitation and exhaustion. Physical examination is usually not remarkable except for evidence of pharyngeal inflammation and, with respiratory distress, evidence of high respiratory obstruction. Inflammatory edema of the vocal cords and subglottic tissue may be demonstrated laryngoscopically. The principal site of obstruction is usually the subglottic area.

Acute Laryngotracheobronchitis. This most common form of croup is caused primarily by viruses. Secondary bacterial infection is rare. Most patients have an upper respiratory tract infection for several days before the brassy cough, inspiratory stridor, and respiratory distress become apparent. As the infection extends downward involving the bronchi and bronchioles, respiratory difficulty increases and the expiratory phase of respiration also becomes labored and prolonged. The child often appears extremely restless and frightened. The temperature may be only slightly elevated or as high as 39–40° C (102–104° F). There are usually bilaterally diminished breath sounds, rhonchi, and scattered rales. Symptoms are characteristically worse at night and often recur with decreasing intensity for several days. Children are usually not seriously ill and often have associated rhinitis, conjunctivitis, or both. Other family members may have mild respiratory illness. Occasionally, the pattern of severe laryngotracheobronchitis may be difficult to distinguish from epiglottitis despite the usually more explosive onset and rapid course of the latter; it also requires similar precautions. Roentgenographic examination of the nasopharynx and upper airway may be helpful. The duration of illness ranges from several days to several weeks, and recurrences are frequent from 3–6 yr of age, decreasing with growth of the airway.

Acute Spasmodic Laryngitis. Spasmodic croup most often occurs in children 1–3 yr of age and is clinically similar to acute laryngotracheobronchitis except that findings of infection in the patient and family are frequent absent. The etiology is viral in most instances, but allergic and psychologic factors are important in some cases. The anxious and excitable child is more prone to this syndrome, and in some instances there is a familial predisposition.

Occurring most frequently in the evening or night, spasmodic croup begins with a sudden onset that is usually preceded by mild to moderate coryza and hoarseness. The child awakens with a characteristic barking, metallic cough, noisy inspiration, and respiratory distress and appears anxious and frightened. Breathing is slow and labored, the pulse accelerated, and the skin cool and moist. The patient is usually afebrile. Dyspnea is aggravated by excitement, and there may be intermittent episodes of cyanosis. Usually the severity of the symptoms diminishes within several hours, and the following day the patient often appears well except for slight hoarseness and cough. Similar, but usually less severe, attacks without extreme respiratory distress may occur for another night or two, eventually concluding in complete recovery. Such episodes often recur several times.

Differential Diagnosis. These four syndromes must be distinguished from one another and from a variety of other entities that may present upper airway obstruction. Bacterial tracheitis is the most important differential diagnostic consideration (Sec. 13.54). *Diphtheritic croup* (Sec. 11.23) is usually preceded by an upper respiratory tract infection for several days; symptoms develop more slowly, although respiratory obstruction may occur suddenly; a serous or serosanguineous nasal discharge is occasionally present; and pharyngeal examination reveals the typical gray-white membrane. *Measles croup* almost always coincides with the full manifestations of systemic disease (Sec. 11.61), and the course may be fulminant.

Sudden onset of respiratory obstruction may be due to *aspiration of a foreign body.* The child is generally 6 mo–2 yr of age. Choking coughing occurs suddenly, usually without signs of inflammation. A *retropharyngeal abscess* may also present as respiratory obstruction; palpation of the posterior pharyngeal wall usually reveals a fluctuant mass. Roentgenographic examination of the upper airway and chest is essential in evaluating these possibilities as well as possible causes of *extrinsic compression* of the airway, such as a hematoma from trauma and *intraluminal obstruction* from masses, e.g., cysts or tumors.

Croup is also occasionally associated with *angioedema* of the subglottic areas as part of anaphylaxis and generalized allergic reactions, edema following *endotracheal intubation* for general anesthesia or respiratory failure, *hypocalcemic tetany, infectious mononucleosis,* trauma, and tumors or malformations of the larynx. A croupy cough may be an early sign of *asthma.* Psychogenic stridor can also occur.

Complications. Complications occur in approximately 15% of patients with viral croup. The most common one is extension of the infectious process to involve other regions of the respiratory tract, such as the middle ear, the terminal bronchioles, or the pulmonary parenchyma. Interstitial pneumonia may occur, but it is difficult to distinguish from patchy areas of atelectasis secondary to obstruction. Bronchopneumonia is unusual unless aspiration of stomach contents has occurred during a period of severe respiratory distress. Secondary bacterial pneumonias are rarely found; suppurative tracheobronchitis is an occasional complication of laryngotracheobronchitis (Sec. 13.61).

Pneumonia, cervical lymphadenitis, otitis, and, rarely, meningitis and septic arthritis may occur during the course of epiglottitis. Mediastinal emphysema and pneumothorax are the most common complications of tracheotomy.

Prognosis. In general, the length of hospitalization and the mortality increase as the infection extends to involve a greater portion of the respiratory tract—except in epiglottitis, in which the localized infection itself may prove fatal. Most deaths from croup are due to laryngeal obstruction or to the complications of tracheotomy. Untreated epiglottitis has a mortality rate of up to 25% in some series, but if the diagnosis is made and appropriate treatment initiated before the patient is moribund, the prognosis is excellent. The outcome of acute laryngotracheobronchitis, laryngitis, and spasmodic croup is also excellent. As a group, children who need to be hospitalized for croup have a somewhat increased bronchial reactivity compared with normal children when tested several years later. The differences, while statistically significant, are small and their functional importance is unclear.

Treatment. Therapy for infectious croup consists primarily of maintaining or providing for adequate respiratory exchange and depends in part on the primary location of the disease and its cause. In the bacterial forms antibiotic therapy is also important.

Sleeping with a humidifier near the bedside, but out of reach, is thought by some to reduce the likelihood of development of spasmodic croup in children known to be susceptible to it.

Most afebrile children with *acute spasmodic croup* or febrile patients with mild *laryngotracheobronchitis* can usually be safely and effectively managed at home. Use of steam from a hot shower or bath in a closed bathroom, hot steam from a vaporizer, or "cold steam" from a nebulizer (which has a safety advantage) often terminates acute laryngeal spasm and respiratory distress within minutes. The same effect has been noted by many parents as they take their child out into the cold night air on the way to the physician's office. Induction of vomiting, either by coughing or by syrup of ipecac, may also break the laryngeal spasm. However, although vomiting occasionally appears to break the laryngeal spasm, there is no objective evidence for the effectiveness of ipecac, and respiratory distress may be complicated by vomiting.

Once laryngeal spasm has been broken, its return may sometimes be prevented by use of warm or cool humidification near the child's bed until the cough has subsided, usually after 2–3 days.

Children with croup and temperatures over 39° C (102.2° F) should be hospitalized if there are any of the following: actual or strongly suspected epiglottitis, progressive stridor, respiratory distress, hypoxia, restlessness, cyanosis, pallor, depressed sensorium, or high fever in a toxic-appearing child. In all instances the decision for hospitalization is made because of the need for reliable observation and relatively safe tracheotomy or nasotracheal intubation, should either of these become necessary.

At home or in the hospital, the croup patient should be watched carefully for intensification of symptoms of respiratory obstruction. The hospitalized child is usually placed in an atmosphere of high cold humidity to lessen irritation and drying of secretions. Frequent or continuous monitoring of the respiratory rate is essential, as a rapid and rising rate may be the first sign of hypoxia and approaching total respiratory obstruction. The patient should be disturbed as little as possible; with moderate to severe respiratory distress, parenteral fluids should be given to lessen physical exertion and vomiting with its potential for aspiration. Sedatives are usually contraindicated since restlessness is used as one of the principal clinical indices of the severity of obstruction and the need for tracheotomy or nasotracheal intubation. Oxygen should be used to alleviate hypoxia and apprehension but, since it reduces cyanosis, which is an indication for tracheotomy or nasotracheal intubation, these patients must be observed particularly closely. Expectorants, bronchodilating agents, and antihistamines are not helpful. Opiates are contraindicated because they may depress respirations and dry secretions.

Laryngotracheobronchitis and *spasmodic croup* do not respond to antibiotics, and antibiotics are not indicated to prevent suprainfection. The use of corticosteroids remains controversial; unequivocal efficacy is unproved. Nonurgent tests should be delayed in view of increased symptoms associated with agitation and anxiety. Racemic epinephrine by aerosol (2.25% solution diluted 1:8 with water in doses of 2–4 mL over 15 min) with or without positive pressure may result in transient relief of symptoms; usually close observation and repeated treatments are necessary. Rarely, there is sufficient obstruction to warrant tracheotomy or nasotracheal intubation.

Epiglottitis, if diagnosed by inspection of the epiglottis or by roentgenographic examination (Fig. 13–5) or if strongly suspected clinically in a severely ill child, should be treated immediately with an **artificial airway;** untreated patients have a substantial mortality even when observed in the hospital with appropriate intubation equipment nearby. **Ampicillin** (200 mg/kg/24 hr) and **chloramphenicol** (50 mg/kg/24 hr) should be given parenterally pending culture and susceptibility reports because of the increasing possibility of ampicillin-resistant strains of *H. influenzae* type b. Cefuroxime (100 mg/kg/24 hr for 7–10 days) may also be effective. All patients should receive **oxygen** en route to the operating room unless it is contraindicated by the increased agitation caused by the mask. Racemic epinephrine and corticosteroids are ineffective, do not avert the need for an artificial airway, and may dangerously delay definitive treatment. After insertion of the artificial airway, the patient should improve immediately, respiratory distress and cyanosis should disappear and normal or near-normal blood gases return. Patients usually fall asleep. The epiglottitis resolves after a few days of antibiotics, and the patient can be weaned from the tracheostomy or nasotracheal tube; antibiotics should be continued for 7–10 days.

Acute laryngeal swelling on an allergic basis responds to epinephrine (1:1000 dilution in dosage of 0.01 mL/kg to a maximum of 0.3 mL/dose) administered subcutaneously, and isoproterenol (1:200 dilution in dosage of 0.01 mL/kg to a maximum of 0.3 mL/dose) by aerosol. Following recovery, the patient and parents should be instructed in emergency administration of these drugs at home. Corticosteroids are frequently required (50–100 mg of hydrocortisone every 6 hr).

Reactive mucosal swelling, severe stridor, and respiratory distress unresponsive to mist therapy may follow *endotracheal intubation* for general anesthesia in children. Intermittent use of racemic epinephrine aerosols or, occasionally, corticosteroids may be helpful.

TRACHEOTOMY AND NASOTRACHEAL INTUBATION. With the introduction of routine tracheotomy for epiglottitis, mortality dropped to almost zero. Nasotracheal intubation has also been reported to be very effective in hospitals having special interest in and appropriate facilities for the care of intubated children. Both procedures should always be done in an operating room if time permits; prior intubation and general anesthesia greatly facilitate doing a tracheotomy without complications.

Tracheotomy or nasotracheal intubation is required for patients with epiglottitis, but it is required only for those with severe laryngotracheobronchitis and for those with spasmodic croup or laryngitis who have increasing signs of respiratory failure secondary to obstruction despite appropriate treatment. Severe forms of laryngotracheobronchitis that required tracheotomy in a high proportion of patients have been reported during severe measles and influenza A virus epidemics. Assessing the need for these procedures requires experience and judgment, since they should not be delayed until cyanosis and extreme restlessness have developed; a pulse rate over 150/min and rising, and an elevated pCO_2, especially in a tiring child, are indications of impending respiratory failure.

The tracheostomy or nasotracheal tube must remain in place until edema and spasm have subsided and the patient is able to handle secretions satisfactorily. They should always be removed as soon as possible, usually within a few days. Adequate resolution of epiglottis inflammation that has been accurately visualized by fiberoptic laryngoscopy may permit much more rapid extubation, often within 24 hours. There is some evidence that hydrocortisone (50–100 mg/24 hr) and racemic epinephrine may be useful to facilitate extubation or to treat croup associated with extubation.

Epiglottitis

Battaglia JD, Lockhart CH: Management of acute epiglottitis by nasotracheal intubation. Am J Dis Child 120:334, 1975.
Cohen SR, Chai J: Epiglottitis: Twenty-year study with tracheostomy. Ann Otol Rhinol Laryngol 87:1, 1978.
Margolis CZ, Ingram DL, Meyer JH: Routine tracheotomy in *Hemophilus influenzae* type b epiglottitis. J Pediatr 81:1150, 1972.
Molteni RA: Epiglottitis: Incidence of extraepiglottic infection: Report of 72 cases and review of the literature. Pediatrics 58:526, 1976.
Nussbaum E: Fiberoptic laryngoscopy as a guide to tracheal extubation in acute epiglottitis. J Pediatrics 102:269, 1983.
Peltola H: C-reactive protein in rapid differentiation of acute epiglottitis from spasmodic croup and acute laryngotracheitis: A preliminary report. J Pediatr 102:713, 1983.
Rapkin RH: The diagnosis of epiglottitis: Simplicity and reliability of radiographs of the neck in differential diagnosis of the croup syndrome. J Pediatr 80:96, 1975.

Laryngotracheobronchitis

Denny FW, Murphy TF, Clyde WA Jr, et al: Croup: An 11 year study in a pediatric practice. Pediatrics 71:871, 1984.
Gurwitz D, Corey M, Levison H: Pulmonary function and bronchial reactivity in children after croup. Am Rev Respir Dis 122:95, 1980.
Koren G, Frand M, Barzilay Z, et al: Corticosteroid treatment of laryngotracheitis in spasmodic croup in children. Am J Dis Child 137:941, 1983.
Leipzig B, Oski FA, Cummings CW, et al: A prospective randomized study to determine the efficacy of steroids in treatment of croup. J Pediatr 94:194, 1979.
Singer OP, Wilson WJ: Laryngotracheobronchitis: 2 years' experience with racemic epinephrine. Can Med Assoc J 115:132, 1976.
Smith MS: Acute psychogenic stridor in an adolescent athlete treated with hypnosis. Pediatrics 72:247, 1983.
Tunnessen WW Jr, Feinstein AR: The steroid-croup controversy: An analytic review of methodologic problems. J Pediatr 96:751, 1980.

13.54 BACTERIAL TRACHEITIS

Bacterial tracheitis, an acute bacterial infection of the upper airway, does not involve the epiglottis but, like epiglottitis and croup, is capable of causing life-threatening airway obstruction. *Staphylococcus aureus* is the most commonly isolated pathogen. Most patients are less than 3 yrs of age, although older children have occasionally been affected. Bacterial tracheitis often follows a viral respiratory infection. Parainfluenza virus type 1 can often be isolated. Initial series indicate that it is substantially less common than viral croup but at least as common as epiglottitis. There are no clear sex differences in incidence or severity.

Clinical Manifestations. Typically, the child develops a brassy cough, apparently as part of a viral upper respiratory infection, perhaps following typical croup. High fever and "toxicity" then occur and are associated with gradually worsening inspiratory stridor. Usual treatment for croup (i.e., mist, intravenous fluid, aerosolized racemic epinephrine) is ineffective. Intubation or tracheostomy is usually necessary. The major pathology appears to be mucosal swelling at the level of the cricoid cartilage, complicated by copious thick, purulent secretions. Suctioning these secretions, although occasionally affording temporary relief, usually does not sufficiently obviate the need for an artificial airway.

Diagnosis. This is based on evidence of bacterial upper airway disease (which includes moderate leukocytosis with many band forms, high fever, and purulent airway secretions) and an absence of the classic findings of epiglottitis (which include radiologic demonstration of a swollen epiglottis, sudden catastrophic onset/rapid progression of symptoms, and typical direct laryngoscopic findings of abnormal epiglottis).

Treatment. Appropriate antimicrobial therapy, which usually includes antistaphylococcal agents, should be instituted in any patient with croup whose course at all suggests bacterial tracheitis. When bacterial tracheitis is diagnosed by direct laryngoscopy or strongly suspected on clinical grounds, an artificial airway is usually indicated. Oxygen should be administered if necessary.

Complications. Chest roentgenograms often show patchy infiltrates and may show focal densities. Subglottic narrowing can also often be demonstrated roentgenographically. When airway management is not optimal, cardiorespiratory arrest can occur.

Prognosis. The prognosis for well-treated patients is excellent. Most patients become afebrile within 2–3 days of instituting appropriate antimicrobial therapy. With decrease in mucosal edema and purulent secretions, extubation can be accomplished. Mean duration of hospitalization was 12 days in one series.

Denneny JC III, Handler SD: Membranous laryngotracheobronchitis. Pediatrics 70:705, 1982.
Jones R, Santos JI, Overall JC: Bacterial tracheitis. JAMA 242:721, 1979.
Liston Sl, Gehrz RC, Siegel LG, et al: Bacterial tracheitis. Am J Dis Child 137:764, 1983.

13.55 FOREIGN BODIES IN THE LARYNX, TRACHEA, AND BRONCHI

The air passages of children are frequent sites for the lodgment of foreign bodies; the carelessness of adults is occasionally an important contributing factor. The symptoms and physical findings produced by foreign bodies depend upon their nature, location, and the degree of obstruction of the air passage. A sharp or irritating object lodged in the larynx produces severe edema and later suppurative perichondritis, whereas an obstructive object in the bronchus produces atelectasis and later bronchiectasis, pulmonary abscess, or empyema.

The vast majority of foreign bodies aspirated into the respiratory tract are probably expelled immediately by reflex cough and never require medical attention. However, if an object too large to be eliminated by mucociliary clearance is aspirated and is not expelled by coughing, respiratory symptoms inevitably result. A large foreign body that can occlude the upper airway completely is an immediate threat to life. Smaller objects that lodge in one of the main stem or lobar bronchi cause more chronic and usually less severe symptoms.

After the initial symptoms, which may have been forgotten, there is often a symptom-free interval that may last from hours to weeks. On occasion, dysphagia may occur from the swelling that results from a foreign body in the region of the larynx, and foreign bodies in the upper esophagus may cause symptoms referable to the air passages by compression or by the overflow of food or secretions into the larynx. Occasionally, a foreign body is not diagnosed until it is revealed by pathologic examination of a lobe that has been removed because of chronic bronchiectasis.

Laryngeal Foreign Body

Clinical Manifestations. A laryngeal foreign body causes hoarseness, a cough that soon becomes croupy, and aphonia. Hemoptysis, dyspnea with wheezing, and cyanosis may occur. Obstruction resulting from the foreign body or the combination of it and the inflammatory reaction may prove fatal if the signs of high respiratory tract obstruction are not promptly recognized and appropriate treatment given. Hot dogs are one of the most common causes of fatal aspirations.

Diagnosis. Roentgenographic and direct laryngoscopic examinations reveal the presence of a foreign body in the larynx (Fig. 13–6). An opaque foreign body in the neck will be clearly demonstrated on a lateral roentgenogram. When it is lodged anteriorly, it is obviously in the larynx; when it is behind the

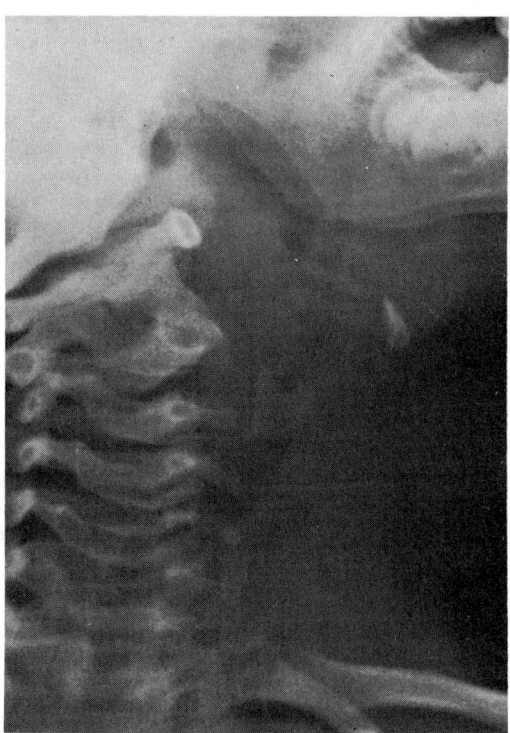

Figure 13–6. Foreign body (fragment of sea shell) in larynx of a 2 yr old child treated for "croup" 6 days before the object was suspected. Fortunately tracheotomy was not required despite the presence of moderately severe laryngeal edema.

soft tissue shadows of the larynx, it is in the hypopharynx or the cervical esophagus. The plane in which the foreign body lies is another differential point in its localization. If it lies in the sagittal plane, it is probably in the larynx. If it is in the coronal plane, it is probably in the esophagus. Even if the foreign body is not opaque, indirect evidence of its presence may be seen on the roentgenogram. Films should always be taken from both the lateral and the anteroposterior projections. In some instances administering a small amount of opaque material may be helpful. Direct laryngoscopy will confirm the diagnosis and provide access for instrumental removal of the foreign body. When there is a severe degree of dyspnea, it may be advisable to do a tracheotomy before the laryngoscopic examination.

Tracheal Foreign Body

Though a tracheal foreign body may be responsible for cough, hoarseness, dyspnea, and cyanosis, the characteristic signs are the asthmatoid wheeze and the audible slap and palpable thud produced by momentary expiratory impaction at the subglottic level. The diagnosis may occasionally be made from the symptoms, physical signs, and roentgenogram of the chest, but in most instances a definite diagnosis can be made only by bronchoscopy.

Bronchial Foreign Body

Clinical Manifestations. The initial symptoms are usually similar to those of foreign bodies in the larynx or trachea. Cough, blood-streaked sputum, and metallic taste with metallic foreign bodies also may be produced by bronchial foreign bodies. The degree of obstruction and the stage in which the patient is seen are the determining factors in the symptomatology as well as in the pathologic changes. A nonobstructive, nonirritating foreign body may produce few symptoms even after a prolonged time in the lung. An obstructive foreign body quickly produces symptoms and signs and pathologic changes. When there is only a slight (bypass valve) obstruction that allows passage of air or fluid in both directions with

only slight interference, a wheeze is noted. When obstruction is of greater degree, obstructive emphysema or obstructive atelectasis is produced; if either is allowed to persist, chronic bronchopulmonary disease may develop.

Most often, the object is aspirated into the right lung. There is usually an immediate episode of choking, gagging, and paroxysmal coughing, which may lead to medical consultation. If this acute episode does not occur or is missed, or if its importance is underestimated by the parents, a relatively long latent period may pass with only occasional cough or slight wheezing; then the patient may develop recurrent lobar pneumonia or intractable "asthma," often with bilateral wheezing and many episodes of "status asthmaticus." Occasionally, chronic wheezing starts immediately after the aspiration. Rarely, a foreign body will present with hemoptysis, occasionally months or years later. History may reveal a forgotten episode of choking while eating or while playing with small objects. Older siblings (3–6 yr old) may have supplied the aspirated object. Physical examination may reveal a tracheal shift. Breath sounds are decreased on the side of the obstruction, but this sign may not be obvious if there is diffuse wheezing.

When both main bronchi are obstructed, there may be severe dyspnea and even asphyxia. If the foreign body is vegetal, e.g., a peanut, a severe condition known as *vegetal* or *arachidic bronchitis* will result. This is characterized by cough, a septic type of fever, and dyspnea. Chronic suppuration may occur when a bronchial foreign body has been present for a long time.

Diagnosis. The possibility of a foreign body must be considered in acute or chronic pulmonary lesions whether or not there is a history of a foreign body accident. The physical signs of bronchial obstruction from foreign bodies include limited expansion, decreased vocal fremitus, impaired (atelectasis) or hyperresonant (overinflation) percussion note, and diminished breath sounds distal to the foreign body. When there is complete obstruction, with a "drowned lung" or with atelectasis, there is absence of vocal resonance and vocal fremitus, which may lead to an erroneous diagnosis of empyema. Varying degrees of tympany may be noted over areas

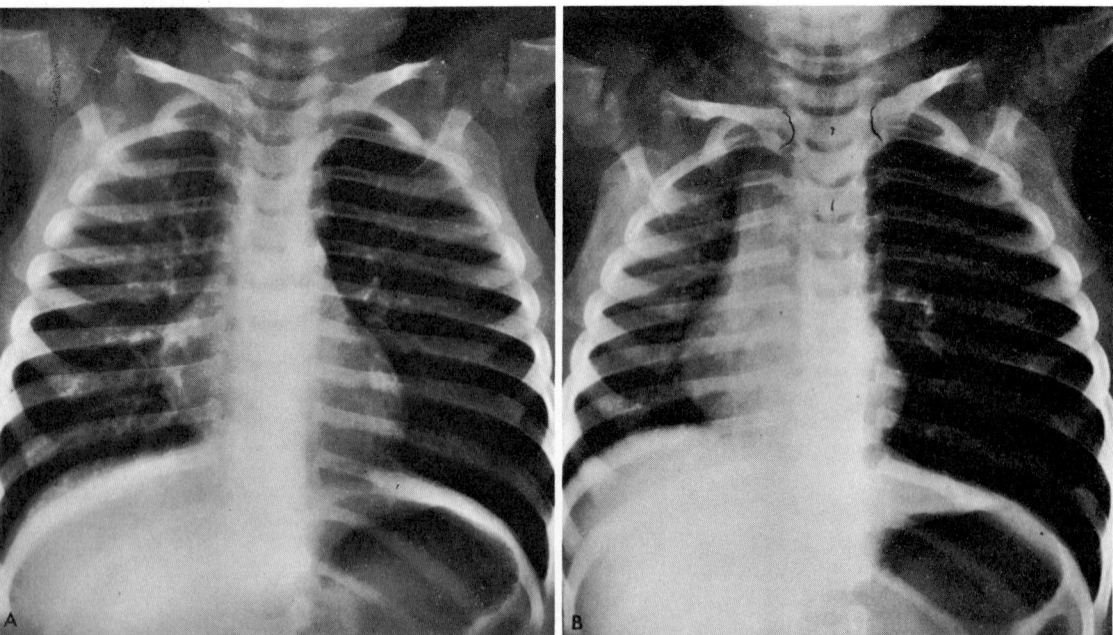

Figure 13–7. Obstructive emphysema (overinflation) due to peanut fragment in left main bronchus. Inspiratory film (*A*) appears relatively normal except for slight mediastinal shift to the right. In expiration (*B*) the left lung remains overaerated (check valve mechanism), and mediastinum moves far to the right.

of obstructive emphysema. Rales are more likely on the uninvaded side than on the invaded one.

If an obstructing object causes complete obstruction in the expiratory phase but allows air to pass in the inspiratory phase, air will enter the distal portion of the lung on inspiration but little or none will escape during expiration (*check valve*). This produces obstructive overinflation (Fig. 13–7). Complete blockage of the bronchus due to the object itself or in combination with the inflammatory swelling of the bronchial mucosa results in a *stop valve* obstruction, and the air in the distal portion of the lung is soon absorbed, leaving an area of atelectasis (Fig. 13–8).

In check valve obstruction, the obstructive emphysema makes it possible to localize a bronchial foreign body by fluoroscopy. The obstructed lung remains expanded during expiration, while the heart and the mediastinum shift to the opposite side as the unobstructed lung empties. The diaphragm is low, flattened, and fixed on the obstructed side; its excursion is free and exaggerated on the unobstructed side. The differences between the lungs are much more evident on expiration than on inspiration. With complete obstruction of the bronchus producing obstructive atelectasis, the heart and the mediastinum are drawn toward the obstructed side and remain there during both phases of respiration. The diaphragm on the obstructed side remains high, while that on the unobstructed side moves normally. Films taken at the end of inspiration and of expiration will show only a slight difference resulting from the filling and emptying of the unobstructed lung. Even extensive roentgenographic procedures may not completely rule out the presence of a foreign body.

Prognosis. Foreign bodies lodged in the air passages are almost invariably fatal if not removed. However, almost all can be removed safely by a skilled bronchoscopist, and almost all patients recover completely after removal.

Prevention. Foreign body aspiration can be prevented by keeping small objects out of reach of children who are too young to obey restrictions; by not giving small pieces of candy, nuts, or similar food to children too young to chew them; and by not giving toys containing small or loosely attached parts to children who are still putting such objects into their mouths. Beads, button boxes, and coins should not be given to toddlers as playthings. Safety pins should always be closed and not left near a baby or in reach of small children. Balloons are also underestimated as potential foreign bodies.

Treatment. Endoscopy and removal of the foreign body under direct vision should be performed as soon as possible. Rarely a thoracotomy is necessary to "milk" the object into a position where it can be removed by bronchoscopy. Occasionally, especially with long duration vegetal foreign bodies, lobectomy may be necessary. Biplane fluoroscopy may be helpful when opaque foreign bodies are lodged in peripheral bronchi. Treatment with pulmonary physiotherapy and bronchodilators is not recommended because of the risk of impacting a dislodged foreign body at the subglottic area, which may result in acute asphyxia, and because a delay in instituting endoscopy may increase morbidity. Treating complications is important to obtaining a good outcome. Secondary infections should be treated with appropriate antibiotics. The outcome of the aspiration of a *large foreign body* that may be immediately life-threatening depends on proper and prompt action taken at the scene of the accident.

Emergency treatment of local upper airway obstruction, as described below, is part of the "basic rescuer course" in cardiopulmonary resuscitation (CPR) of the American Heart Association (Sec. 5.40). These procedures are used only for children who are aphonic and not breathing. The recommendations for treating infants and young children differ slightly from those for treating teenagers and adults. The repetitive use of four back blows and four chest thrusts is recommended. Abdominal thrusts should not be used. The back blows are delivered while holding the infant with the head lower than the trunk. Four blows are delivered with the heel of the hand between the scapulae. The purpose of this maneuver is to loosen the foreign body. After the back blows, the patient is turned and four chest thrusts are delivered using the same technique and hand positioning as is used for closed cardiac compression (i.e., over the midsternum for infants and slightly lower for older children). This maneuver increases intrathoracic pressure, which may cause expulsion of the foreign body. Blind finger sweeps (as recommended for unconscious adult victims) should not be used in infants and young children. Instead, after the administration of the four chest thrusts, the mouth should be opened and a visualized foreign body grasped and removed. Following each sequence of back blows, chest thrusts, and visual attempt to remove foreign body, rescue breathing should be attempted for the unconscious patient. If unsuccessful, the sequence described above is repeated. Although there is controversy concerning the precise technique to be used in total upper airway obstruction by a foreign body, pediatricians should provide up-to-date information in these techniques to parents and should urge parents to expect that their babysitters (including teenagers) are familiar with the symptoms and emergency treatment of foreign body aspiration.

Baker SP, Fisher RS: Childhood asphyxiation by choking or suffocation. JAMA 244:1343, 1980.

Blazer S, Naveh Y, Friedman A: Foreign body in the airway: A review of 200 cases. Am Rev Dis Child 134:68, 1980.

Blumhagen JD, Weisenberg RL, Brooks JG, et al: Endotracheal foreign bodies: Difficulties in diagnosis. Clin Pediatr 19:480, 1980.

Committee on Accident and Poison Prevention: First aid for the choking child. Pediatrics 67:744, 1981.

Gann DS: Emergency management of the obstructed airway. JAMA 243:1141, 1980.

Greensher J, Mofenson HC: Emergency treatment of the chocking child. Pediatrics 70:110, 1982.

Hollinger PH, Andrews AH Jr, Anison GC: Pulmonary complications due to endobronchial foreign bodies. Ill Med J 93:19, 1948.

Law D, Kosloske AM: Management of tracheobronchial foreign bodies in children: A reevaluation of postural drainage and bronchoscopy. Pediatrics 58:362, 1976.

Rothman BF, Boeckman CR: Foreign bodies in the larynx and tracheobronchial tree in children. Ann Otol Rhinol Laryngol 89:434, 1980.

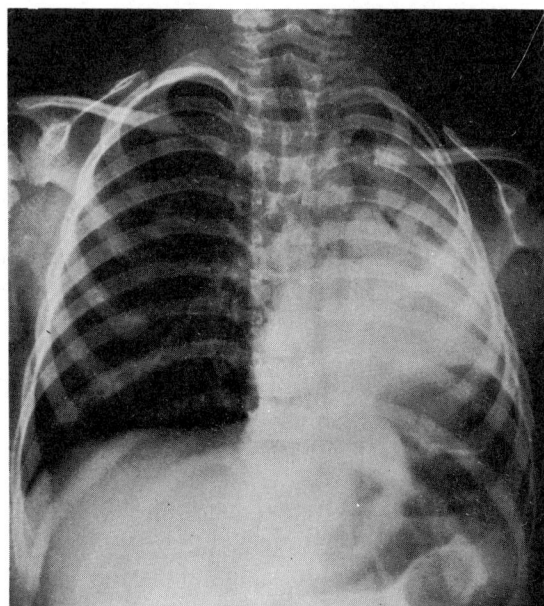

Figure 13–8. Foreign body lodged in left main bronchus, producing atelectasis of left lung. Note that the heart is drawn completely into the left side of the chest.

13.56 TRAUMA TO THE LARYNX

Birth Trauma. Laryngeal injury during birth is not infrequent and may result in dislocation of the cricothyroid or cricoarytenoid articulations. Hoarseness and at times wheezing or fluttering respiratory sounds are heard. The diagnosis is made by direct laryngoscopic examination. Treatment by direct laryngoscopic manipulations, using a laryngeal dilator, may occasionally be effective, but tracheotomy should be done when there is evidence of hypoxia.

Unilateral or bilateral *recurrent laryngeal nerve paralysis* may also be produced by birth trauma, especially during forceps delivery. Bilateral paralysis is often associated with central nervous system disease. When only one cord is paralyzed, there may be only hoarseness and slight stridor without dyspnea. Unilateral paralysis is usually on the left. In bilateral paralysis there is dyspnea with stridor. In both unilateral and bilateral vocal cord paralysis, chronic aspiration can lead to recurrent pneumonia. Direct laryngoscopic examination establishes the diagnosis. Tracheotomy is usually necessary for bilateral paralysis. The older child may wear a valvular cannula, or a laryngoplasty with lateral fixation of one vocal cord may be done to improve the airway and permit decannulation if breathing through the larynx has not improved spontaneously.

Postnatal Trauma. Any trauma, such as that brought about by a fall against a hard object, may produce acute or chronic stenosis of the larynx, as may high tracheotomy and prolonged intubation. Clinically important laryngeal injury is rare in children. Penetrating injuries are usually obvious and require treatment by an otolaryngologic surgeon. Serious nonpenetrating injuries may be deceptive since substantial edema and even a compressing hematoma may give surprisingly few external clues. Laryngeal fracture should be suspected in patients who have hoarseness, hemoptysis, and/or subcutaneous emphysema following neck trauma. Laryngoscopy and, occasionally, surgical exploration may be indicated in patients having relatively normal physical findings but whose history is compatible with substantial blunt neck trauma. Most patients with serious laryngeal or upper tracheal injuries require tracheostomy as part of their management; if there are signs of high obstruction, the need may be urgent. The normal voice is frequently not recovered. Similarly, severe thermal injury (e.g., following accidental inhalation of steam or smoke) is often best managed with tracheostomy.

Acute *overuse of the voice* (e.g., prolonged screaming at a concert or athletic event) may cause transient hoarseness. With cessation of this stress, the voice returns to normal without other treatment. The roles of resting the voice (whispering or no use of speech at all) or mist in accelerating recovery are not clear. Acute laryngitis is fairly common in older children during mild viral respiratory infections; spontaneous recovery is the rule, and the importance of steam and other therapeutic maneuvers is unknown. Occasionally, a teenager may develop chronic laryngitis from heavy cigarette smoking. The differential diagnosis of persistent hoarse voice includes vocal ("singer's" or "screamer's") nodules, papillomas, and serious tumors such as rhabdomyosarcoma. A laryngeal abscess is a rare cause of persistent hoarseness. These masses are diagnosed by laryngoscopy and may require surgical treatment, which may be followed by voice training. Otolaryngologic consultation is indicated for any child with unexplained continuous hoarseness longer than 1 wk.

13.57 ACUTE LARYNGEAL STENOSIS

Acute stenosis may result from any acute infection responsible for edema of the subglottic region or epiglottis and arytenoids; from inflammation secondary to the inspiration of a vegetal foreign body, and especially after instrumentation for the removal of such an object; from edema of an allergic reaction; or from a foreign body lodged in the larynx. Treatment consists of immediate provision of an airway by intubation or tracheotomy, followed by appropriate medical therapy.

13.58 CHRONIC LARYNGEAL STENOSIS

This is a frequent sequela of high tracheotomy in which damage of the first tracheal ring or cricoid cartilage results in perichondritis and subsequent overgrowth of cartilage or fibrous tissue. Chronic stenosis may also result from laryngeal diphtheria, syphilis, tuberculosis, radiation burns, and external trauma. The most common etiology at present, however, is neonatal intubation. Congenital laryngeal stenosis may be transmitted as an autosomal dominant trait in some patients. The clinical manifestations may include dyspnea with audible stridor and suprasternal, supraclavicular, and intercostal retractions, or may be limited to inability to decannulate a patient's tracheostomy or remove a laryngeal tube. The diagnosis is made by direct laryngoscopy, palpation of the larynx, and roentgenographic examination. Scarring and stenosis usually develop in the subglottic region, occasionally with necrosis of cartilage.

Milder cases can be treated by replacing the tracheostomy cannula with a smaller one and closure of this tube, at first partial and then complete, with a cork, thus re-educating the patient to mouthbreathe and permitting the removal of the cannula. If this method is unsuccessful, dilation through a direct laryngoscope may help but should not be done too frequently. In some patients external surgery with or without the use of an indwelling mold may be necessary. The prognosis for eventual cure is good, but treatment may require months or years.

Fearon B: Acute airway obstruction. *In*: Ferguson CF, Kendig EL Jr (eds): Disorders of the Respiratory Tract, Vol 2, Pediatric Otolaryngology. Philadelphia, WB Saunders, 1972.
Landing BH: State of the art: Congenital malformations and genetic diseases of the respiratory tract. Am Rev Respir Dis 120:151, 1979.
McGill TJI, Healy GB: Congenital and acquired lesions of the infant larynx. Clin Pediatr 17:584, 1978.
Proctor DF: The upper airways: II. The larynx and trachea. Am Rev Resp Dis 115:315, 1977.

13.59 NEOPLASMS OF THE LARYNX

Papilloma is the most common tumor of the larynx in childhood; it rarely becomes malignant and often disappears after puberty. The pink, warty tumors may grow profusely from any portion of the larynx, though usually from the vocal cords. This disease is caused by the human papillomavirus. When maternal vaginal condyloma is present, material containing this virus may be aspirated during delivery, producing disease in a small fraction of exposed infants.

The initial symptom is hoarseness, but dyspnea is likely if the condition is allowed to persist. Asphyxia has occurred. Direct laryngoscopy accomplishes both diagnosis (confirmed histologically) and treatment, as the papilloma can be easily removed by forceps. Care should be taken not to damage normal tissue. Cure usually occurs, although at first rapid recurrence is common. Tracheostomy may be required because of recurrences and the threat of aspiration. Cryosurgery and laser surgery have been advocated as alternative or adjuvant therapy. Radical excision and radiation are contraindicated. Patients with laryngobronchial papillomatosis who fail to respond to usual treatment may improve after receiving systemic bleomycin.

Vocal nodules or small tumors may occur in children at the junction of the anterior and middle thirds of the cords. They are usually bilateral and produce slight hoarseness. Spontaneous regression may occur if strenuous use of the voice is avoided. They may be removed under direct laryngoscopic view or treated with laser.

Mehta P, Herold N: Regression of juvenile laryngobronchial papillomatosis with systemic bleomycin therapy. J Pediatr 97:479, 1980.
Steinberg BM, Topp WC, Schneider PS, et al: Laryngeal papilloma virus infection during clinical remission. N Engl J Med 308:1261, 1983.

13.60 TRACHEAL AMYLOIDOSIS

Primary amyloidosis (Sec. 26.2) of the trachea is an extremely rare but potentially treatable lesion. Symptoms are caused by gradual reduction in the tracheal lumen secondary to progressive deposition of amyloid. Cough, dyspnea, and wheezing occur early in the course of the disease. Recurrent infection and hemoptysis are late complications. Expiratory wheezing, cough, and signs of respiratory distress may be present. Chest roentgenogram may be normal. Diagnosis is made by bronchoscopy, which reveals a narrowed tracheal lumen with friable tissue lining the airways; biopsy allows confirmation of the diagnosis. Treatment is repeated bronchoscopy for removal of amyloid until an adequate airway is restored, but improvement may be only temporary, and repeated bronchoscopic treatments are often necessary.

Gottlieb LS, Gold WM: Primary tracheobronchial amyloidosis. Am Rev Respir Dis 105:425, 1972.
Prowse CG: Amyloidosis of the lower respiratory tract. Thorax 13:308, 1958.

13.61 ACUTE BRONCHITIS

Though the diagnosis of "acute bronchitis" is frequently made, this condition may not exist in children as an isolated clinical entity. Rather, bronchitis occurs in association with a number of other conditions of the upper and lower respiratory tracts, and the trachea is nearly always involved. Bronchiolitis ("capillary bronchitis") is an entirely different illness (Sec. 13.64).

Asthmatic bronchitis is a form of asthma that is often confused with acute bronchitis. With a variety of upper respiratory tract infections, some children have bronchial spasm and exudation similar to signs in older children with asthma.

Acute tracheobronchitis is most commonly found in association with an upper respiratory tract infection such as nasopharyngitis but is also associated with influenza, pertussis, measles, typhoid fever (and other salmonelloses), diphtheria, and scarlet fever. An acute, primary, undifferentiated tracheobronchitis also occurs, most commonly in older children and adolescents. It is likely that, except for the bacterial diseases mentioned, acute tracheobronchitis is of viral origin. Pneumococci, staphylococci, *H. influenzae*, and various hemolytic streptococci may be isolated from the sputum, but their presence does not imply a bacterial origin, and antibiotic therapy does not appreciably alter the course of the illness. Some children appear to be far more susceptible to acute tracheobronchitis than others. The reasons are unknown, but allergy, climate, air pollution, and chronic infections of the upper respiratory tract, particularly sinusitis, may be contributing factors.

The syndrome *bronchiolitis obliterans* may begin with an episode of acute bronchitis, bronchiolitis, or bronchopneumonia and then progress over several weeks to severe chronic pulmonary disease characterized by bronchiolar and bronchial obliteration and bronchiectasis.

Clinical Manifestations. Acute bronchitis is usually preceded by a viral upper respiratory infection. Secondary bacterial infection with *S. pneumoniae* or *Haemophilus influenzae* may occur. Typically, the child presents a frequent, dry, hacking, unproductive cough of relatively gradual onset,

beginning 3–4 days after the appearance of rhinitis. Low substernal discomfort or burning anterior chest pain is often present and may be aggravated by coughing. As the illness progresses, the patient may be bothered by whistling sounds during respiration (probably rhonchi), soreness of the chest, and occasionally shortness of breath. Coughing paroxysms or gagging on secretions is occasionally associated with vomiting. Within several days the cough becomes productive, and the sputum changes from clear to purulent. Usually within 5–10 days the mucus thins and the cough gradually disappears. The considerable malaise often associated with the illness may continue for 1 wk or more after acute symptoms have subsided.

Physical findings vary with the age of the patient and the stage of the disease. Initially, the child is usually afebrile or has low grade fever, and there are signs of nasopharyngitis, conjunctival infection, and rhinitis. Later, auscultation reveals roughening of breath sounds, coarse and fine moist rales, and rhonchi which may be high pitched, resembling the wheezing of asthma.

In otherwise healthy children complications are few, but in undernourished children or those in poor health, otitis, sinusitis, and pneumonia are common.

Treatment. There is no specific therapy; most patients recover uneventfully without any treatment. In small infants pulmonary drainage is facilitated by frequent shifts in position. Older children are more comfortable in high humidity, but there is no evidence that this shortens the duration of illness. Irritating and paroxysmal coughing may cause considerable distress and interfere with sleep. Although suppression of cough may increase the possibility of suppuration, judicious use of cough suppressants (including codeine) may be appropriate for symptomatic relief. Antihistamines, which dry secretions, should not be used, and expectorants are not helpful. Antibiotics do not shorten the duration of the viral illness or decrease the incidence of bacterial complications, although the fact that patients with recurrent episodes may occasionally improve with such treatment suggests that some secondary bacterial infection is present.

Children with repeated attacks of acute bronchitis should be carefully evaluated for the possibility of respiratory tract anomalies, foreign bodies, bronchiectasis, immune deficiency, tuberculosis, allergy, sinusitis, tonsillitis, adenoiditis, and cystic fibrosis.

13.62 CHRONIC BRONCHITIS

Although adult chronic bronchitis is defined as 3 or more months of productive cough each year for 2 or more consecutive years, there is no such accepted standard for children. In fact, it is doubted whether it exists in children as an isolated clinical entity, and it should rarely be accepted as a final diagnosis. A chronic or frequently recurring productive cough usually indicates an underlying pulmonary or systemic disease; affected patients should be evaluated for immune deficiencies, anatomic abnormalities, allergic disorders, environmental disease, upper airway infection with postnasal discharge, cystic fibrosis, immotile cilia syndrome, and bronchiectasis. Cough and wheezing are common, often suggesting an allergic basis. Rarely, bronchial irritation may be secondary to the chronic inhalation of dust or noxious fumes. Tobacco and/or marijuana smoking is obviously pertinent historical information. Teenagers should be similarly questioned about industrial fume or automobile exhaust exposure at school or work.

Air Pollution and Cigarette Smoking. There is a significant association between high levels of air pollution and an elevated incidence of chronic pulmonary disease including bronchitis, but a direct causal relationship has not been established. Air pollutants also aggravate pre-existent pulmonary disease and decrease pulmonary function in exercising children and teenagers. Children and their parents should be advised of these relationships.

An increased incidence and exacerbations of bronchitis and other forms of acute and chronic lung disease are associated with cigarette smoking. In addition, there is increased morbidity from respiratory infections in teenagers who smoke, as reflected in school and work absences as well as in functional and pathologic evidence of small airway abnormalities. For example, cigarette smoking is a risk factor for the severity of influenza in young men. Smoking parents, and especially those whose children have chronic lung disease, should be advised that they are subjecting their children's lungs to significant amounts of "secondhand" cigarette smoke in the home; they should be urged to stop smoking.

The Committee on Genetics and Environmental Hazards of the American Academy of Pediatrics has noted that tobacco smoking is one of the most important "sources of environmental contamination and a significant threat to the health of children." It urges physicians to support legislation that would prohibit smoking in public places frequented by children, "particularly in hospitals and other health facilities."

Clinical Manifestations. The chief symptom is cough, with or without expectoration. The child will usually also complain of chest soreness; characteristically these signs and symptoms are worse at night; wheezing may also be prominent, and physical findings are similar to those of acute bronchitis.

Course and Prognosis. Both the course and the prognosis depend upon appropriate management or eradication of any underlying illness. Complications will be those of the underlying illness.

Treatment. When an underlying cause for chronic bronchitis is found, this should receive appropriate management. Allergic management may be helpful on occasion even when no underlying cause can be discovered. Autogenous vaccines or inhalation of antibiotics is not effective.

Committee on Genetics and Environmental Hazards: The environmental consequences of tobacco smoking: Implications for public policy that affect the health of children. Pediatrics 70:314, 1982.
Doctors could dissuade youth from smoking. Pediatr News 4:24, 1970.
Doyle NC: The facts about second hand cigarette smoke. American Lung Association Bulletin, Mar 1974.
Goldsmith JR: Health effects of air pollution. Basics Resp Dis 4:1, 1975.
Kark JD, Lebiush M, Rannon L: Cigarette smoking as a risk factor for epidemic A(H$_1$N$_1$) influenza in young men. N Engl J Med 307:1042, 1982.
Lebowitz MD, Bendheim P, Cristea G, et al: The effect of air pollution and weather on lung function in exercising children and adolescents. Am Rev Resp Dis 109:262, 1974.
Matsukura S, Taminato T, Kitano, N, et al: Effects of environmental tobacco smoke on urinary cotinine excretion in nonsmokers: Evidence for passive smoking. N Engl J Med 311:828, 1984.
Niewoehner DE, Kleineman J, Rice DB: Pathologic changes in the peripheral airways of young cigarette smokers. N Engl J Med 291:755, 1974.
Sheppard D: Adverse pulmonary effects of air pollution. Immunol Allergy Pract 6:25, 1984.
Taussig LM, Smith SM, Blumenfeld R: Chronic bronchitis in childhood: What is it? Pediatrics 67:1, 1981.
White JR, Froeb HF: Small-airways dysfunction in nonsmokers chronically exposed to tobacco smoke. N Engl J Med 203:720, 1980.

13.63 IMMOTILE CILIA SYNDROME
(Dyskinetic Cilia Syndrome; Kartagener Syndrome)

In the respiratory tract the majority of the lining mucosal cells are ciliated (about 275 cilia per cell). Each cilium is anchored to the apical cytoplasm by a basal body and contains two central and nine peripheral microtubules that traverse its entire length and that are loosely bound to one another by radial spokes. It is the movement of these microtubules with relation to the others that causes the typical 1000 cycle/min beat of the cilia. The chemical basis for this movement involves an ATPase located within the cilia and visible ultrastructurally as dynein arms.

Kartagener initially described a group of patients all of whom had situs inversus, chronic sinusitis, and chronic bronchitis with bronchiectasis. Situs inversus is also seen commonly in men with infertility secondary to sperm immotility. These observations led Afzelius to postulate that these patients have a generalized disorder of ciliary motility, some of them lacking the ATPase-containing dynein arms necessary for ciliary movement. The disease appears to be transmitted as an autosomal recessive with an incidence of about 1:20,000 persons.

Clinical Manifestations. The symptoms of this disease reflect the wide distribution of cilia throughout the body. Relentless ciliary activity of embryonal tissues may be responsible for the characteristic direction of the rotation of the intestine. Impairment of ciliary movement and thus of intestinal rotation could produce situs inversus, a very common but not universal finding in the immotile cilia syndrome. Absence of ciliary clearance from the middle ears, eustachian tubes, and sinus cavities results in an increased incidence and greater severity of chronic otitis media and sinusitis in childhood. Sterility resulting from inadequate spermatozoal movement is almost always present, but motile spermatozoa have been demonstrated in a patient totally lacking dynein arms on his respiratory ciliated cells. Abnormal mucociliary clearance in children results in chronic bronchitis, usually without bronchiectasis, which is a relatively late complication. Wheezing is common, perhaps due in part to inadequate clearance of antigen from the airways. Although symptoms are often present in early childhood, they may be delayed in some patients until after age 20 yr.

Diagnosis. The disease should be suspected in children who have chronic sinusitis and otitis media in addition to bronchitis. If such a patient has situs inversus, the diagnosis is a virtual certainty, but definitive testing (see below) should be done. Chronic wheezing, a family history of bronchiectasis in young adults, and/or male infertility are important additional clinical support for this diagnosis.

Decreased ciliary movement may be observed at bronchoscopy. Another preliminary screening test involves examining a suspension of scrapings from the nasal mucosa above the first turbinate by light microscope for evaluation of ciliary activity. Absence of ciliary activity on more than two occasions when the patient does not have an acute upper respiratory infection suggests the need for more definitive testing. However, this technique is plagued by both false positive and false negative results. At present, diagnosis still depends on electron microscopic examination of cilia, obtained either by brushing or biopsy of the trachea at bronchoscopy or by nasal mucosal biopsy. Spermatozoa can also be examined in older patients. Absence of dynein arms is probably the most common form of the disease, but other morphologic abnormalities having the same phenotypic expression (i.e., decreased or absent ciliary movement) are also possible.

Treatment. Treatment is symptomatic and includes close medical supervision with early and aggressive antibiotic treatment of pulmonary infection, chest physiotherapy, and bronchodilators. Early infection involves the pneumococcus and *Haemophilus* organisms primarily. Treatment of serous otitis and sinusitis is also important.

Prognosis. The average life expectancy is unknown, although normal life spans have been reported; however, there is considerable morbidity due to bronchiectasis and other problems. The effects of early aggressive therapy are unknown. The dangers of smoking and of exposure to industrial fumes should be explained to the patient and appropriate vocational guidance supplied.

Afzellius B: A human syndrome caused by immotile cilia. Science 193:317, 1976.
Eliasson R, Mossberg B, Camner P, Afzelius BA: The immotile cilia syndorme. N Engl J Med 297:1, 1977.

Fischer TJ, McAdams JA, Entis GN, Cotton R, Ghory JE, Ausdenmoore RW: Middle ear ciliary defect in Kartagener's syndrome. Pediatrics 62:443, 1978.

Johnson MS, McCormick JR, Gillies CG, et al: Kartagener's syndrome with motile spermatozoa. N Engl J Med 307:1131, 1982.

Pedersen H, Mygind N: Absence of axonemal arms in nasal mucosa cilia in Kartagener's syndrome. Nature 262:494, 1976.

Rooklin AR, McGeady SJ, Mikaelian DO, Soriano RZ, Mansmann HC: The immotile cilia syndrome: A cause of recurrent pulmonary disease in children. Pediatrics 66:526, 1980.

Sturgess JM, Chao J, Wong J, Aspin N, Turner JAP: Cilia with defective radial spokes: A cause of human respiratory disease. N Engl J Med 300:53, 1979.

13.64 ACUTE BRONCHIOLITIS

Acute bronchiolitis is a common disease of the lower respiratory tract of infants resulting from inflammatory obstruction of the small airways. It occurs during the first 2 yr of life, with a peak incidence at approximately 6 mo of age, and in many localities is the most frequent cause of hospitalization of infants. The incidence is highest during the winter and early spring months. The illness occurs both sporadically and epidemically.

Etiology and Epidemiology. Acute bronchiolitis is a viral illness. The respiratory syncytial virus is the causative agent in over 50% of cases (Sec. 11.73); the parainfluenza 3 virus, mycoplasma, some adenoviruses, and occasionally other viruses produce the remaining cases. Adenovirus may be associated with long-term complications, including bronchiolitis obliterans and unilateral hyperlucent lung syndrome (Swyer-James syndrome). There is no firm evidence that bacteria cause bronchiolitis. Occasionally, bacterial bronchopneumonia may be confused clinically with bronchiolitis.

The source of the viral infection is usually a family member with minor respiratory illness. Older children and adults tolerate bronchiolar edema better than infants and thus do not develop the clinical picture of bronchiolitis even when the smaller airways of their respiratory tract are infected by the virus.

Pathophysiology. Acute bronchiolitis is characterized by bronchiolar obstruction due to edema and accumulation of mucus and cellular debris and by invasion of the smaller radicles of the bronchial tree by virus. Since resistance to airflow in a tube is inversely related to the fourth power of the radius, even minor thickening of the bronchiolar wall in infants may produce a profound effect on airflow. Airway resistance in the small air passages is increased during both the inspiratory and expiratory phases, but since the radius of an airway is smaller during expiration, the resulting ball valve respiratory obstruction leads to early air trapping and overinflation. Atelectasis may occur when obstruction becomes complete and trapped air is absorbed.

The pathologic process impaires the normal exchange of gases in the lung. Diminished ventilation results in hypoxemia, which may occur early in the course. Carbon dioxide retention (hypercapnia) usually does not occur except in severely affected patients. Generally, the higher the respiratory rate, the lower the arterial oxygen tension. Hypercapnia is usually not found until respirations exceed 60/min; it then increases in proportion to the tachypnea.

Clinical Manifestations. Most affected infants have a history of exposure to older children or adults with minor respiratory diseases within the week preceding onset of illness. The infant is first noted to have a mild upper respiratory tract infection with serous nasal discharge and sneezing. These symptoms usually last several days and may be accompanied by fever of 38.5 to 39° C (101–102° F) and diminished appetite. There is then the gradual development of respiratory distress characterized by paroxysmal wheezy cough, dyspnea, and irritability. Bottle feeding may be particularly difficult since the rapid respiratory rate may not permit time for sucking and swallowing. In mild cases symptoms disappear

in 1–3 days. On occasion, in the more severely affected patients, symptoms may develop within several hours, and the course is protracted. Other systemic manifestations, such as vomiting and diarrhea, are usually absent. The infant is commonly afebrile, has only a low grade fever, or may be hypothermic.

Examination reveals a tachypneic infant, often in extreme distress. Respirations range from 60–80/min; severe air hunger and cyanosis may be present. There is flaring of the alae nasi, and use of the accessory muscles of respiration results in intercostal and subcostal retractions, which are shallow because of the persistent distention of the lungs by the trapped air. The liver and the spleen may be palpable several centimeters below the costal margins as a result of depression of the diaphragm due to overinflation. Widespread fine rales may be heard at the end of inspiration and in early expiration. The expiratory phase of breathing is prolonged, and wheezes are usually audible. In the most severe cases, breath sounds are barely audible when bronchiolitic obstruction is nearly complete.

Roentgenographic examination reveals hyperinflation of the lungs and an increased anteroposterior diameter on lateral view. Scattered areas of consolidation are found in about one third of patients and are due either to atelectasis secondary to obstruction or to inflammation of the alveoli. Early bacterial pneumonia cannot be excluded on radiographic grounds alone.

The white blood cell and differential counts are usually within normal limits. Lymphopenia, commonly associated with many viral illnesses, is usually not found. Nasopharyngeal cultures reveal normal flora. Virus may be demonstrated in nasopharyngeal secretions by immunofluorescence, in a rise in blood antibody titers, or in culture.

Differential Diagnosis. The condition most commonly confused with acute bronchiolitis is bronchial asthma. Asthma occurs uncommonly in the first year of life, but frequently after this period. The presence of one or more of the following favors the diagnosis of asthma: a family history of asthma, repeated attacks in the same infant, sudden onset without preceding infection, markedly prolonged expiration, eosinophilia, and an immediate favorable response to the administration of a single small dose of epinephrine (0.01 mL/kg of 1:1000 dilution subcutaneously). Repeated attacks represent an important differential point: fewer than 5% of recurrent attacks of clinical bronchiolitis have viral infections as a cause. Other entities that may be confused with acute bronchiolitis are congestive heart failure, foreign body in the trachea, pertussis, organic phosphorus poisoning, cystic fibrosis, and bacterial bronchopneumonias associated with generalized obstructive emphysema.

Course and Prognosis. The most critical phase of illness occurs during the first 48–72 hr after the onset of cough and dyspnea. During this period the infant appears desperately ill, apneic spells occur in the very small infant, and respiratory acidosis is likely to be noted. After the critical period improvement occurs rapidly and often dramatically. Recovery is complete in a few days. The case fatality rate is below 1%; death may result from prolonged apneic spells, severe uncompensated respiratory acidosis, or profound dehydration secondary to loss of water vapor from tachypnea and the inability to drink fluids. Infants with such complications as congenital heart disease or cystic fibrosis have a higher mortality. Bacterial complications, such as bronchopneumonia or otitis media, are uncommon. Cardiac failure during bronchiolitis is rare.

A significant proportion of infants with bronchiolitis have hyperreactive airways during later childhood, but the relation of these two entities, if any, is not understood. Similarly, the suggestion in some recent studies that even a single episode of bronchiolitis may result in very long term small airway abnormality requires further investigation.

Treatment. Infants with respiratory distress should be hospitalized, but only supportive treatment is indicated. The patient is commonly placed in an atmosphere of cold, humidified oxygen to relieve hypoxemia and reduce insensible water loss from tachypnea; this treatment relieves the dyspnea and cyanosis and allays anxiety and restlessness. Sedatives should be avoided whenever possible because of potential depression of respiration. The infant is usually more comfortable sitting at a 30–40° angle or with head and chest slightly elevated so that the neck is somewhat extended. Oral intake must often be supplemented or replaced by parenteral fluids to offset the dehydrating effect of tachypnea. In the event of respiratory acidosis, electrolyte balance and pH should be adjusted by suitable intravenous solutions.

Ribavirin (Virazole), an antiviral agent, is effective in reducing the severity of bronchiolitis due to RSV infection when administered early in the course of the illness. Its use is indicated in children under 2 yr of age who have severe infection documented by fluorescent antibodies or culture or strongly suspected on epidemiologic grounds and whose hospitalization is likely to exceed 3 days. It should also be given to patients with milder bronchiolitis due to RSV infection who have underlying severe chronic illness due to cardiac disease (particularly cyanotic congenital heart disease), pulmonary disease, or immunodeficiency disease. The drug is administered by continuous inhalation as a small particle mist (Small Particle Aerosol Generator—"SPAG-II" unit) for 12–20 hr/24 hr for 3–5 days. It is contraindicated for patients on ventilators because of the risk of mechanical interference with ventilator function, such as blockage of the expiratory port filter.

Antibiotics have no therapeutic value unless there is secondary bacterial pneumonia. The low incidence of bacterial complications is not made lower by antibiotic therapy. Corticosteroids are not beneficial and may, under certain conditions, be harmful. On the other hand, corticosteroids have not been evaluated in patients with severe adenovirus bronchiolitis in whom long term severe sequelae (necrotizing lesions) might be more likely. Bronchodilating drugs, although they may increase restlessness, are frequently used empirically, at least for a single dose trial. Epinephrine or other alpha-adrenergic agents have a theoretical basis for use, but have not been adequately tested. Because the obstruction occurs at the bronchiolar level, tracheostomy is not beneficial and involves substantial risks which are not justified in these acutely ill infants. Occasional patients may progress rapidly to respiratory failure requiring ventilatory assistance.

Becroft DMO: Bronchiolitis obliterans, bronchiectasis and other sequelae of adenovirus type 21 infection in young children. J Clin Pathol 24:72, 1971.
Hall CB, McBride JT, Walsh EE, et al: Aerosolized ribavirin treatment of infants with respiratory syncytial viral infection: a randomized double blind study. N Engl J Med 308:1443, 1983.
Henderson FW, Clyde WA, Collier AM, et al: The etiologic and epidemiologic spectrum of bronchiolitis in pediatric practice. J Pediatr 95:183, 1979.
Hogg JC, Williams J, Richardson JB, et al: Age as a factor in the distribution of lower-airway conductance and in the pathologic anatomy of obstructive lung disease. N Engl J Med 282:1283, 1970.
McConnochie KM, Roghmann KJ: Bronchiolitis as a possible cause of wheezing in childhood: New evidence. Pediatrics 74:1, 1984.
Outwater K, Crone RK: Management of respiratory failure in infants with acute viral bronchiolitis. Am J Dis Child 138:1071, 1984.
Wohl MEB, Chemick V: State of the art: Bronchiolitis. Am Rev Resp Dis 118:759, 1978.

13.65 BRONCHIOLITIS OBLITERANS

In this disease, the bronchioles and occasionally some of the smaller bronchi are partially or completely obliterated by nodular masses, which are found on histologic examination to contain granulation and fibrotic tissue. In adults some cases

can be clearly related to inhalation of the oxides of nitrogen or other chemicals. The syndrome has also been associated with connective tissue diseases, and some drugs (e.g., penicillamine) have also been reported to precipitate it. In children most cases can be temporally related to pulmonary infection; measles, influenza, adenoviral infection, mycoplasma pneumonia, and pertussis have all been reported to precede its development.

Initially, cough, respiratory distress, and, possibly, cyanosis occur and may be followed by a brief period of apparent improvement. The disease then progresses as reflected by increasing dyspnea, cough, sputum production, and wheezing. The pattern may resemble bronchitis, bronchiolitis, or pneumonia. The chest roentgenogram often suggests miliary tuberculosis. A more nonspecific diffuse infiltrate also may be seen. Bronchography shows obstruction of the bronchioles, with little or no contrast material reaching the periphery of the lung. The disease can then be confirmed by lung biopsy.

There is no specific treatment. Since the pathology suggests a progressive fibrotic picture which could theoretically be delayed by corticosteroid treatment, these agents are almost universally used, but there are no data as to their efficacy. Some patients deteriorate rapidly and die within weeks of the onset of initial symptoms; others run a much more chronic course; and a few may go on to develop the unilateral hyperlucent lung syndrome (Sec. 13.86).

Azizirad H, Polgar G, Borns PF,. et al: Bronchiolitis obliterans. Clin Pediatr 14:572, 1975.
Becroft DMO: Bronchiolitis obliterans, bronchiectasis and other sequelae of adenovirus type 21 infection in young chilren. J Clin Pathol 24:72, 1971.
Epler GR, Colby TV: The spectrum of bronchiolitis obliterans. Chest 83:161, 1983.
Wohl MEB, Chernick V: State of the art: Bronchiolitis. Am Rev Respir Dis 118:759, 1978.

BRONCHIAL ASTHMA

See Sec. 10.48.

PNEUMONIA

The various clinical forms of pneumonia are often classified by their anatomic distribution—lobar, lobular, interstitial, bronchopneumonia—or by the agents that cause them, such as viral, bacterial, or aspiration pneumonia (see Chapter 11). Many of the etiologically unclassified infections which occur in infancy are probably of viral origin. Most bacterial infections are susceptible to antimicrobial therapy, whereas viral infections usually are not.

Certain lesions are commonly produced by specific causative agents. For example, the pneumococcus produces an inflammatory mucosal lesion and an alveolar exudate, usually without destruction of mucosal cells or extensive involvement of interstitial tissues. The gross lesion is a consolidation of all or part of a lobe in the lobar variety or of scattered lobules in the bronchopneumonic variety. Pneumococcal pneumonia characteristically assumes a lobar pattern in older children and young adults, but lobar consolidation is less typical in young children. In contrast, viral agents, *H. influenzae*, and certain strains of the viridans group of streptococci invade or destroy the mucous membrane and may produce principally bronchiolitis, peribronchiolitis, and interstitial lesions. Both staphylococcus and *Klebsiella* tend to destroy tissue and to produce multiple small abscesses.

The following classification is helpful in considering pneumonias in children:

    I. Bacterial Infections
       Pneumococcus (also Sec. 11.19)
       Streptococcus (also Sec. 8.66 and 11.16)

Staphylococcus (also Sec. 8.60 and 11.17)
Haemophilus influenzae (also Sec. 11.20)
Klebsiella
Pseudomas aeruginosa (also Sec. 11.30)
Tubercle bacillus (Sec. 11.46)
II. VIRAL OR PROBABLE VIRAL INFECTIONS
Interstitial pneumonitis and bronchiolitis (e.g., respiratory syncytial virus, adenovirus, etc., in Sec. 13.64 and Chapter 11)
Giant cell pneumonia (also Sec. 11.61)
Influenza (Sec. 11.71)
III. OTHER INFECTIONS
Pneumocystis carinii pneumonia (also Sec. 11.11)
Q fever (Sec. 11.92)
Mycoplasma pneumoniae pneumonia (Sec. 11.60)
Treponema pallidum (Sec. 11.49)
Nocardiosis (Sec. 11.45)
Actinomycosis (Sec. 11.44)
Chlamydia (Sec. 11.57)
Ornithosis (Sec. 11.58)
Psittacosis (Sec. 11.58)
IV. MYCOTIC INFECTIONS
Aspergillosis (Sec. 11.97)
Coccidioidomycosis (Sec. 11.98)
Histoplasmosis (Sec. 11.99)
Blastomycosis (Sec. 11.93)
Mucormycosis (Sec. 11.95)
Sporotrichosis (Sec. 11.96)
Thrush (also Sec. 12.9)
V. ASPIRATION OF:
Amniotic contents (also Sec. 8.34 and 8.35)
Food and/or gastric acid (also Sec. 12.21)
Foreign bodies (also Sec. 13.55)
Zinc stearate
Dust
Hydrocarbons
Lipoid substances
VI. LOEFFLER SYNDROME (also Sec. 11.110–11.112, 11.115, and 11.125)
VII. HYPOSTATIC PNEUMONIA (also Sec. 28.6)
VIII. DRUG/RADIATION PNEUMONIA (Sec. 5.55 and Chapter 16)
IX. HYPERSENSITIVITY PNEUMONITIS (also Sec. 10.44)

13.66 BACTERIAL PNEUMONIA

General Considerations. Primary infection of the parenchyma of the lung (pneumonia) is much less common than secondary bacterial infection complicating the acute viral bronchitis that occurs during minor upper respiratory infection. Bacterial pneumonia during childhood and recurrent pneumonia in the absence of an underlying chronic illness, such as cystic fibrosis or immunologic deficiency, is quite unusual. In infants and young children with infection of the lower respiratory tract, signs and symptoms of pulmonary involvement are often nonspecific or surprisingly few. Accordingly, roentgenographic evidence of pneumonia is frequently found in infants who clinically appear to have only upper respiratory tract infections or only tachypnea and fever without physical findings, suggesting pulmonary involvement.

The most common event disturbing the defense mechanisms of the lung (Sec. 13.6) is a viral infection that alters the properties of normal secretions, inhibits phagocytosis, modifies the bacterial flora, and may temporarily disrupt the normal epithelial layer of the respiratory passages. A viral respiratory disease often precedes the development of bacterial pneumonia by a few days.

Children with defects in defense mechanisms or in the chain of events involved in recovery from infection experience recurrent pneumonias or fail to resolve the disease completely. These defects occur with abnormalities of antibody production (agammaglobulinemia), cystic fibrosis, cleft palate, congenital bronchiectasis, immotile cilia syndrome, tracheoesophageal fistula, abnormalities of the polymorphonuclear leukocytes, neutropenia, increased pulmonary blood flow, deficient gag reflex, and so forth. Among iatrogenic factors promoting pulmonary infection are trauma, anesthesia, and aspiration.

Pneumococcal Pneumonia

Though the incidence of pneumococcal pneumonia has declined over the last several decades, the pneumococcus (*Streptococcus pneumoniae*) is still the most common bacterial pathogen, accounting for over 90% of childhood bacterial pneumonia. See also Sec. 11.19.

Epidemiology. Pneumococcal pneumonia most commonly occurs in late winter and early spring, when respiratory infections are at their peak; types 14, 1, 6, and 19 are most frequent. Asymptomatic carriers of pathogenic types of pneumococci play a more important role in their dissemination than do patients ill with pneumonia. In childhood the highest attack rates occur during the first 4 yr of life. The disease is usually sporadic. However, when high carrier rates of pathogenic types occur in a relatively closed community (e.g., orphanages, nurseries, schools), widespread viral disease of the respiratory tract may be followed by an epidemic of pneumococcal pneumonia. Upon recovery, type-specific antibody not only protects the person from reinfection but also renders him or her less likely to become a carrier of that specific serotype of organism.

Pathology and Pathogenesis. Pneumococcal organisms are probably aspirated into the periphery of the lung from the upper airway or nasopharynx. Initially, a reactive edema occurs that supports proliferation of the organisms and aids in their spread into adjacent portions of the lung. The involved lobe undergoes early consolidation, a stage of *red hepatization*, with polymorphonuclear leukocytes, fibrin, red blood cells, edema fluid, and pneumococci filling the alveoli. This passes into the *gray hepatization* stage, characterized by the deposition of fibrin over the pleural surfaces and the presence of fibrin and polymorphonuclear leukocytes in the alveolar spaces where phagocytosis is rapidly taking place. With *resolution*, increasing numbers of macrophages appear in the alveolar spaces, the neutrophils degenerate, and the fibrin threads and remaining bacteria are digested and disappear. In untreated cases a clinical crisis occurs about the 7th day of illness, and resolution and re-expansion require an additional 1–3 wk. Antibiotics given in the first several days of illness interrupt the course, and the characteristic stages are not seen.

Usually one or more lobes, or parts of lobes, are involved, leaving the remaining bronchopulmonary system uninvolved. However, this pattern of lobar pneumonia is often not present in infants who may have a more patchy and diffuse disease that follows a bronchial distribution and that is characterized by many limited areas of consolidation around the smaller airways. Permanent injury is rare.

Clinical Manifestations. The classic history of a shaking chill followed by a high fever, cough, and chest pain described in adults with pneumococcal pneumonia may be seen in older children, but it is rarely observed in infants and young children, in whom the clinical pattern is considerably more variable.

Infants. A mild upper respiratory tract infection characterized by stuffy nose, fretfulness, and diminished appetite usually precedes the onset of pneumococcal pneumonia in infants. This mild illness of several days' duration ends with abrupt onset of fever of 39° C or higher, restlessness, apprehension, and respiratory distress. The patient appears ill with moderate to severe air hunger and often cyanosis. The respiratory distress is manifest by grunting, flaring of the alae nasi, retractions of the supraclavicular, intercostal, and subcostal areas, tachypnea, and tachycardia. Cough is unusual initially but may occur later.

Physical examination of the chest is often unrevealing. Dullness is usually localized to one lobe. Auscultation may reveal diminished breath sounds and fine, crackling rales on the affected side, but these findings are less common than in older children. On the opposite side, breath sounds may be exaggerated and almost tubular in nature. On percussion, if dullness is found in young infants, the presence of pleural effusion or empyema should be suspected. Abdominal distention may be prominent, reflecting gastric distention due to swallowed air or to ileus; it may suggest an acute surgical emergency. The liver may seem enlarged because of downward displacement of the right diaphragm or superimposed congestive heart failure. Nuchal rigidity without meningeal infection (meningismus) may also be prominent, especially with involvement of the right upper lobe. Physical findings in the lung usually change little during the course of illness, although moist rales may become audible during resolution.

Children and Teenagers. The signs and symptoms are similar to those of adults. After a brief, mild, upper respiratory infection there is often onset of a shaking chill followed by fever as high as 40.5° C. This is accompanied by drowsiness with intermittent periods of restlessness, rapid respirations, a dry, hacking, unproductive cough, anxiety, and occasionally delirium. There may be circumoral cyanosis, and many children are noted to be splinting on the affected side to minimize pleuritic pain and improve ventilation; they may lie on their side with knees drawn up to the chest. Abnormal chest findings include retractions, flaring of alae nasi, dullness, diminished tactile and vocal fremitus, diminished breath sounds, and fine and crackling rales on the affected side. On the first day of illness, dullness over the affected lobe is usually not evident, and the suppression of breath sounds on the affected side may lead to misinterpretation of the exaggerated breath sounds in the opposite lung as tubular breathing.

The physical findings undergo change during the course of illness. Classic signs of consolidation are noted on the 2nd–3rd day of illness and are characterized by dullness, increased fremitus, tubular breath sounds, and the disappearance of rales. As resolution occurs, moist rales are heard, and the signs of consolidation disappear. The initial dry, hacking cough loosens and becomes productive of large amounts of blood-tinged mucous material.

The development of a pleural effusion or empyema may cause a visible lag in respiration on the affected side, with exaggerated excursion on the opposite side. Examination usually reveals dullness over the area of the effusion, with diminished fremitus and breath sounds. Tubular breathing is often noted immediately above the fluid level and on the unaffected side.

Laboratory Findings. The white blood cell count is usually elevated to 15,000–40,000 cells/mm³, with a preponderance of polymorphonuclear cells. White blood cell counts below 5000/mm³ are often associated with a grave prognosis. The hemoglobin value is usually normal or only slightly diminished. Arterial blood samples usually show hypoxemia without hypercapnia.

In most patients pneumococci can be isolated from the nasopharyngeal secretions, but this finding cannot be considered proof of a causative relation; the isolation of pneumococci should be attempted from secretions obtained upon deep coughing, from gentle tracheal aspiration, from blood, or from pleural fluid obtained at thoracentesis. Bacteremia is found in about 30% of patients having pneumococcal pneumonia. Counterimmunoelectrophoresis or latex agglutination of blood, pleural fluid, and/or urine may be helpful in establishing the diagnosis.

Roentgenographic Findings. The roentgenographic changes do not always correspond to the clinical observations.

Consolidation may be demonstrated by roentgenography before it is detectable by physical examination, and resolution of the infiltrate may not be complete until several weeks after the child is clinically well. Lobar consolidation is not as common in infants and young children as in the older child. Pleural reaction with the presence of fluid is not uncommon; it may be seen early in the course of illness and, even in the untreated patient, is not necessarily indicative of developing empyema. It is extremely important that roentgenographic demonstration of complete resolution be obtained 3–4 wk after disappearance of all symptoms. Persistence of infiltrate suggests an underlying process, such as a foreign body or immunologic deficiency. If clinical reponse is slow, serial roentgenograms are indicated.

Differential Diagnosis. Pneumococcal pneumonia cannot be differentiated from other bacterial and viral pneumonias without appropriate microbiologic studies. Conditions possibly confused with pneumonia are bronchiolitis, allergic bronchitis, congestive heart failure, acute exacerbations of bronchiectasis, aspiration of a foreign body, sequestered lobe, atelectasis, pulmonary abscess, and endotracheal tuberculosis with secondary bacterial pneumonia.

An older child with right lower lobe pneumonia may have diaphragmatic irritation with pain referred to the right lower quadrant of the abdomen. Since ileus may accompany pneumonia, right lower quadrant pain and absent bowel sounds may be misinterpreted as acute appendicitis.

When meningismus is severe and presents opisthotonos or positive Kernig and Brudzinski signs, it can be differentiated from meningitis only by examining the spinal fluid.

Complications. With the use of antibiotic therapy, complications of bacterial pneumonia have become unusual. Although concomitant pneumococci infection in other locations (e.g., otitis media) may be present prior to the onset of the symptoms of pneumonia, metastatic infection after the initiation of antibiotic treatment is infrequent. Empyema and lung abscess are uncommon. Empyema results from extension of infection to the pleural surfaces and occurs most commonly in the young infant who has received medical attention late in the course of illness or who has been inadequately treated. Persistent pneumatoceles may also occur and usually do not require treatment.

Prognosis. In the preantibiotic era the mortality rate in infants and small children ranged from 20–50% and in older children from 3–5%. Furthermore, the incidence of chronic empyema with altered pulmonary function was relatively high. With appropriate antibiotic therapy instituted early in the course of the illness, the mortality rate during infancy and childhood is now less than 1%, and long-term morbidity is corresponding low.

Treatment. The *drug of choice* is penicillin because most pneumococci are exquisitely sensitive to it. The recent emergence of penicillin-resistant pneumococci in certain areas of the world suggests that alternative antibiotic therapy may be indicated, pending the results of antibiotic sensitivity testing. In infants and young children, initial therapy should be parenteral penicillin G in a dosage of 50,000 units/kg/24 hr. In older children a single intramuscular injection of procaine penicillin, 600,000 units, followed by oral penicillin, is usually adequate outpatient treatment. If the child is not vomiting, initial therapy with oral penicillin V (50,000 units/kg/24 hr) may be appropriate, particularly for older children. In patients allergic to penicillin, a cephalosporin may be used, such as cefazolin (50 mg/kg/24 hr) or cefuroxime (100 mg/kg/24 hr). Treatment is given for 7–10 days in uncomplicated cases.

The majority of older children with pneumococcal pneumonia can be treated at home; the *decision to hospitalize* depends on the severity of illness, the physical adequacy of the home, and the ability of the family to supply good nursing care. Pneumonia in the young infant is best treated in the hospital since fluids and antibiotics may have to be administered intravenously. Furthermore, the course of illness in young infants is more variable and complications more common. Patients with pneumonia associated with pleural effusion or empyema should also be hospitalized. Liberal oral intake of *fluids* and the administration of aspirin for high fever are the principal adjuncts to therapy. *Oxygen* administered promptly to patients with significant respiratory distress will greatly reduce the need for sedatives and analgesics; it should be given before the patient becomes cyanotic.

Polyvalent pneumococcal polysaccharide vaccine (containing antigen of many but not all pathogenic pneumococci) has proved efficacious in certain patient populations such as patients with sickle cell anemia. Unfortunately, young children may not respond well to one or more components of the vaccine; its routine use in healthy children is not indicated.

Streptococcal Pneumonia

Group A streptococci most commonly cause disease limited to the upper respiratory tract, but the organisms may spread to other areas of the body, including the lower respiratory tract. Streptococcal pneumonia and tracheobronchitis are uncommon, but certain viral infections, particularly the exanthems and epidemic influenza, predispose to these diseases, which are most frequently encountered in children 3–5 yr of age and very rarely in infants. Group B streptococcal pneumonia is discussed in Sec. 8.66 and 11.16.

Pathology. Streptococcal infections of the lower respiratory tract result in tracheitis, bronchitis, or interstitial pneumonia. Lobar pneumonia is uncommon. Lesions consist of necrosis of the tracheobronchial mucosa with the formation of ragged ulcers and large amounts of exudate, edema, and localized hemorrhage. The process may extend to the interalveolar septa and involve lymphatic vessels. Infection may spread by way of the lymphatics to the mediastinal and hilar lymph nodes or may proceed in a retrograde direction in occluded vessels and reach the pleural surfaces. Pleurisy is relatively common; the effusion is often large and serous, occasionally serosanguineous, or thinly purulent, with less fibrin than the exudate of pneumococcal pneumonia.

Clinical Manifestations. The signs and symptoms of streptoccal pneumonia are similar to those of pneumococcal pneumonia. The onset may be sudden, characterized by high fever, chills, signs of respiratory distress, and, at times, extreme prostration. However, it may occasionally be more insidious, which is often the case with *H. influenzae* pneumonia, and the child will appear only mildly ill with cough and low grade fever. If an exanthem or influenza precedes the pneumonia, the onset may be seen only as an increasingly severe clinical course of the viral illness. The clinical findings may be less impressive than the disseminated intersitial infiltration noted on roentgenogram. Pleurisy, which commonly occurs, may be evidenced by clinical findings and pleural effusion.

Laboratory Manifestations. Leukocytosis occurs as in pneumococcal pneumonia. A rise in serum antistreptolysin titer is supportive diagnostic evidence. The disease may be suspected if large amounts of group A β-hemolytic streptococci are isolated from throat swab, nasopharyngeal secretions, bronchial washings, or sputum, but definitive diagnosis rests on recovery of the organism from pleural fluid, blood, or lung aspirate. Bacteremia occurs in about 10% of patients.

Chest roentgenograms usually show diffuse bronchopneumonia, often with a large pleural effusion. Occasionally, there is hilar adenopathy. Final roentgenographic resolution should be demonstrated but may not be complete for up to 10 wk.

Differential Diagnosis. The clinical course and roentgenographic findings of streptococcal pneumonia with purulent pleurisy are often similar to those of staphylococcal pneumonia. Pneumatoceles may occur in both conditions. The roentgenographic changes of uncomplicated streptococcal pneumonia may be indistinguishable from other interstitial pneumonitides, including those caused by *Mycoplasma pneumoniae.*

Complications. Bacterial complications and long-term morbidity are common in the untreated patient but rare after antibiotic treatment is begun. Empyema occurs in 20% of children, and occasionally septic foci develop in other areas, such as the bones or joints; otherwise extension of the disease is uncommon. Acute glomerulonephritis occurs rarely.

Treatment. The drug of choice is penicillin G (100,000 units/kg/24 hr). Parenteral penicillin is used initiially, and a 2–3 wk course may be completed orally after clinical improvement has begun in the hospital. If empyema develops, a thoracentesis should be performed for diagnostic purposes and for removal of fluid. On occasion, repeated thoracentesis or closed drainage with indwelling chest tubes may be required if the fluid reaccumulates. Intrathoracic administration of antibiotics or enzymes to liquefy pus or dissolve fibrin is ineffective.

Staphylococcal Pneumonia

Pneumonia caused by *Staphylococcus aureus* is a serious and rapidly progressive infection that, unless recognized early and treated appropriately, is associated with prolonged morbidity and high mortality. It occurs less frequently than pneumococcal or viral pneumonia and is more common in infants than in children (Sec. 8.60 and 8.67).

Epidemiology. The majority of cases occur from October to May, and, as with other bacterial pneumonias, staphylococcal pneumonia is frequently preceded by a viral upper respiratory tract infection. Although it may occur at any age, 30% of all patients are under 3 mo of age and 70% under 1 yr. Boys are affected more commonly than girls.

Although *S. aureus* is commonly found on normal skin and mucous membranes, serious disease is comparatively rare. Nearly 90% of normal infants become nasal carriers in the neonatal period. This declines to about 20% during the first 2 yr of life and then rises to the adult rate of 30–50% by age 4–6 yr.

The occurrence of nursery epidemics of staphylococcal disease is usually associated with specific pathologic strains that are commonly resistant to many antibiotics. Even during these outbreaks most of the colonized infants and hospital personnel or family contacts remain free of disease, although they may serve to spread the infection to others. The infant may exhibit disease within a few days after colonization or not until weeks later. Viral respiratory infections may play a significant role in promoting dissemination of the staphylococcus among infants and in converting colonization to disease.

Pathogenicity and Pathology. *Staphylococcus aureus* produces a variety of toxins and enzymes, such as hemolysin, leukocidin, staphylokinase, and coagulase. Coagulase interacts with a plasma factor to produce an active principle that converts fibrinogen to fibrin, thereby causing clot formation. A good correlation exists between coagulase production and virulence; coagulase-negative staphylococci rarely produce serious disease.

Staphylococci cause confluent bronchopneumonia that is often unilateral or more prominent on one side than the other and is characterized by the presence of extensive areas of hemorrhagic necrosis and irregular areas of cavitation. The pleural surface is usually covered by a thick layer of fibrinopurulent exudate. Multiple abscesses occur, containing clusters of staphylococci, leukocytes, erythrocytes, and necrotic debris. Rupture of a small subpleural abscess may result in a pyopneumothorax, which in turn may erode into a bronchus, producing a bronchopleural fistula. Septic thrombi may form in pulmonary veins in regions of extensive destruction and inflammation.

Clinical Manifestations. Most commonly, the patient is an infant under 1 yr of age, often with a history of staphylococcal skin lesions in him- or herself or in a family member and with signs and symptoms of an upper or lower respiratory tract infection for several days to a week. Abruptly, the infant's condition changes, with the onset of high fever, cough, and evidence of respiratory distress. Signs and symptoms include tachypnea, grunting respirations, sternal and subcostal retractions, nasal flaring, cyanosis, and anxiety. If left undisturbed, the infant is lethargic but upon arousal is irritable and appears toxic. Severe dyspnea and a shocklike state may be present. Some infants have associated gastrointestinal disturbances characterized by vomitimg, anorexia, diarrhea, and abdominal distention secondary to a paralytic ileus. A rapid progression of symptoms is characteristic.

Physical findings depend on the stage of pneumonia. Early in the course of illness diminished breath sounds, scattered rales, and rhonchi are commonly heard over the affected lung. With the development of effusion, empyema, or pyopneumothorax, dullness on percussion is noted, and breath sounds and vocal fremitus are markedly diminished. A lag in respiratory excursion often occurs on the affected side. Physical examination may, however, be misleading, particularly in the young infant with meager findings disproportionate to the degree of tachypnea.

Laboratory Manifestations. In the older infant and child a leukocytosis of 20,000 or more cells/mm³ usually occurs, with the increase primarily among the polymorphonuclear cells; in the young infant the white blood cell count may remain within the normal range. As in other forms of bacterial infection, a count below 5000 cells/mm³ is a poor prognostic sign. Mild to moderate anemia is common.

Material for diagnostic cultures should be obtained by tracheal aspiration or pleural tap; Gram stain frequently reveals gram-positive cocci. The finding of staphylococci in the nasopharynx is of no diagnostic value, but blood culture may be positive. Pleural fluid reveals an exudate with polymorphonuclear cell counts ranging from 300–100,000/mm³, protein above 2.5 g/dL, and low glucose level relative to the blood level.

Roentgenographic Manifestations. Most patients with staphylococcal pneumonia have roentgenographic evidence of nonspecific bronchopenumonia early in the illness. The infiltrate may soon become patchy and limited in extent or be dense and homogeneous and involve an entire lobe or hemithorax. The right lung alone is involved in about 65% of cases; bilateral involvement occurs in fewer than 20% of patients. A pleural effusion or empyema will be noted during the course in most patients; pyopneumothorax occurs in about 25%. Pneumatoceles of varying size are common.

Though no roentgenographic change can be considered diagnostic, progression over a few hours from bronchopneumonia to effusion or pyopneumothorax with or without pneumatoceles is highly suggestive of staphylococcal pneumonia. Chest films should be obtained at frequent intervals if the diagnosis is suspected. Clinical improvement usually precedes roentgenographic clearing by days or weeks, and pneumatoceles may persist in an asymptomatic patient for months.

Differential Diagnosis. Recognizing early staphyloccocal pneumonia in the infant is often difficult. Abrupt onset and rapid progression of symptoms of pneumonia should be considered to be due to staphylococci until proved otherwise. A history of furunculosis, a preceding viral upper respiratory tract infection, a recent hospital admission, or maternal breast abscess should also alert the physician to the possibility of

this diagnosis. Other bacterial pneumonias that cause empyema or pneumatoceles and thus may be readily confused with staphylococcal disease include streptococcal, *Klebsiella*, *H. influenzae*, and pneumococcal pneumonias and primary tuberculous pneumonia with cavitation. Occasionally, the aspiration of a nonradiopaque foreign body followed by pulmonary abscesses may lead to a similar clinical and radiologic picture.

Complications. Since empyema, pyopneumothorax, and pneumatoceles are so commonly seen with staphylococcal pneumonia, they are considered part of the natural course of the illness and not complications. Septic lesions outside the respiratory tract occur rarely except in the young infant, in whom staphylococcal pericarditis, meningitis, osteomyelitis, and multiple metastatic abscesses in soft tissue may occur. Metastatic infection after the initiation of appropriate antibiotic therapy is rare.

Prognosis. Survival has improved substantially with present-day management, but mortality still ranges from 10–30% and varies with the length of illness prior to hospitalization, age of patient, adequacy of therapy, and the presence of other illness or complications. Children who do not have underlying disease have an excellent prognosis for complete recovery, including normal growth and development, normal pulmonary function, and no increased susceptibility to pulmonary infections. The course is usually prolonged, with hospitalizations of from 6–10 wk. All infants with staphylococcal pneumonia should be tested for cystic fibrosis and screened for immunodeficiency disease.

Treatment. Therapy consists of appropriate antibiotics and drainage of collections of pus. The infant should be given oxygen and placed in a semireclining position to relieve cyanosis and anxiety. During the acute phase intravenous hydration and nutrition are indicated, and if the patient is severely anemic, blood transfusion may be beneficial. Assisted ventilation may occasionally be needed.

A *semisynthetic, penicillinase-resistant penicillin* should be administered intravenously immediately after culture while reports are pending (e.g., methicillin, 200 mg/kg/24 hr). Patients receiving these drugs should be closely monitored for possible nephrotoxicity. If the cultures subsequently demonstrate an organism sensitive to penicillin G, then this agent should be used in dosages of 100,000 units/kg/24 hr instead of the initial drug. Some advise initially administering both drugs until the antibiotic sensitivity is known, at which time one can be discontinued. There is no evidence that this practice increases the efficacy of treatment, but it may increase the frequency of adverse reactions. In patients allergic to penicillin, a cephalosporin may be used, such as cefazolin, 50 mg/kg/24 hr. From 3–4 wk of therapy is usually adequate, but the clinical response may indicate a need for longer therapy.

Although patients with staphylococcal pneumonia may occasionally recover completely without *chest tube* drainage, it is recommended even if only a small effusion or empyema is present in order to reduce the chance of bronchopleural fistula and the necessity for repeated pleural taps. Generally, pus reaccumulates so rapidly and becomes so viscous or loculated that closed drainage with a chest tube of the largest possible caliber is required. The appearance of pyopneumothorax is another indication for immediate insertion of a catheter into the pleural space. It is often necessary to use several chest tubes when loculation occurs. Once the infant begins to improve and the lung has re-expanded, the tubes may be removed, even if they are still draining small amounts of pus; in general, tubes should not remain in the chest more than 5–7 days.

Instillation of antibiotics or enzymes into the chest cavity has no beneficial effect and is associated with an increased incidence of pneumothorax and systemic toxic reactions.

Ammann AJ, Addiego J, Wara DW, et al: Polyvalent pneumococcal-polysaccharide immunization of patients with sickle-cell anemia and patients with splenectomy. N Engl J Med 297:897, 1977.

Broome CV, Facklam RR, Fraser DV: Pneumococcal disease after pneumococcal vaccine. N Engl J Med 303:549, 1980.

Ceruti E, Contreras J, Neira M: Staphyloccocal pneumonia in childhood. Long-term follow-up including pulmonary function studies. Am J Dis Child 122:386, 1971.

Honig PJ, Pasquariello PS Jr, Stool SE: H. influenzae pneumonia in infants and children. J Pediatr 83:215, 1973.

Jay SJ, Johanson WG Jr, Pierce AK: The radiographic resolution of Streptococcus pneumonia. N Engl J Med 293:798, 1975.

Klein JO, Mortimer EA: Use of pneumococcal vaccine in children. Pediatrics 61:31, 1978.

Michaels RH, Poziviak CS: Countercurrent immunoelectrophoresis for the diagnosis of pneumococcal pneumonia in children. J Pediatr 88:72, 1975.

Rebban AW, Edwards HE: Staphylococcal pneumonia. Review of 329 cases. Can Med Assoc J 82:513, 1960.

Pneumonias Caused by Gram-Negative Organisms

A small percentage of pneumonias of infants and children after the neonatal period are caused by gram-negative organisms. However, the number has been increasing in recent years, perhaps because of the widespread use of antibiotics, the contamination of hospital equipment, the increasing use of immunosuppressive agents in the treatment of malignant disorders, and the increasing survival of children with chronic pulmonary disease such as cystic fibrosis. The organisms most commonly encountered are *H. influenzae* type b (Sec. 11.20), *Klebsiella pneumoniae* and *Pseudomonas aeruginosa* (Sec. 11.30). The morbidity and mortality rates of these infections are high as a result of the pathogenicity of the bacteria and the altered host resistance in many of these patients (Sec. 11.11).

Haemophilus influenzae Pneumonia. *Haemophilus influenzae* type b is a frequent cause of serious bacterial infection in infants and children. Nasopharyngeal infection precedes almost all clinical varieties of localized *H. influenzae* disease, such as otitis media, epiglottitis, pneumonia, and meningitis. Pneumonia is second in frequency only to meningitis in children with invasive *H. influenzae* disease; most cases occur during winter and spring.

Haemophilus influenzae pneumonias are usually lobar in distribution, but there is no characteristic chest roentgenogram. Segmental infiltrates, single or multiple lobe involvement, pleural effusion, and pneumatoceles occur. Disseminated pulmonary disease and bronchopneumonia have also been described. Males are affected slightly more often than females. Pathologically, involved areas show a polymorphonuclear or lymphocytic inflammatory reaction with extensive destruction of the epithelium of smaller airways, interstitial inflammation, and marked, often hemorrhagic, edema.

Although the *clinical manifestations* may be difficult to distinguish clinically from those of pneumococcal pneumonia, *H. influenzae* pneumonia is more often insidious in onset, and the course is usually prolonged over several weeks. Many patients are already receiving treatment for otitis media at the time of diagnosis. Although chloramphenicol and ampicillin (see below) are recommended for treatment of *H. influenzae* pneumonia, a clinical response to penicillin G is common and does not exclude this diagnosis. Cough is almost always present but may not be productive, and the patient is febrile and often tachypneic with nasal flaring and retractions. There may be localized dullness to percussion and rales and tubular breath sounds; pleural fluid is often present on roentgenogram in the young infant.

The *diagnosis* is established by isolating the organism from the blood, particularly in the young infant, from pleural fluid, or from lung aspirate. There is usually moderate leukocytosis with a relative lymphopenia. Counterimmunoelectrophoresis or latex agglutination tests on tracheal secretions, blood, urine, and pleural fluid may also establish an early diagnosis. If atelectasis is present, bronchoscopy may be indicated to rule out a foreign body.

Complications are frequent, particularly in the young infant, and include bacteremia, pericarditis, cellulitis, empyema, meningitis, and pyarthrosis. Meningitis occurred in 15% of the younger patients in one study; examination of cerebrospinal fluid should be strongly considered when pneumonia due to *H. influenzae* is diagnosed.

Treatment consists of the same symptomatic and supportive measures utilized in pneumococcal and staphylococcal pneumonias. When *H. influenzae* is suspected as the causative agent, chloramphenicol (100 mg/kg/24 hr) should be included in the initial antibiotic therapy until it is known whether the organism produces penicillinase; if the strain is sensitive, ampicillin (200 mg/kg/24 hr) alone may be administered. The child should be hospitalized and both drugs administered intravenously. Cefuroxime (100 mg/kg/24 hr for 7–10 days) may also be effective. Effusion and pyarthrosis may require drainage. Needle thoracentesis is often adequate for effusion drainage, but the procedure may occasionally have to be repeated. Closed chest drainage may be required if purulent pleural fluid is present, but open drainage is infrequently needed. If the initial response to chloramphenicol is good, oral treatment can be instituted to complete a 10–14 day course. Roentgenographic demonstration of complete resolution should be obtained 2–4 wk later; complete resolution may require a prolonged period.

Klebsiella pneumoniae (Friedländer Bacillus) Pneumonia. This organism, found in the respiratory and gastrointestinal tracts of approximately 5% of normal persons, causes pneumonia in debilitated or immunosuppressed patients and frequently occurs as a secondary invader in the lungs of patients with chronic bronchiectasis, influenza, or tuberculosis. Primary *K. pneumoniae* infection is unusual in infants and young children; it may occur, rarely, in nursery epidemics or as a sporadic case in neonates. During epidemics, many infants will carry the organism in their nasopharynges without signs of clinical illness; only an occasional baby will have severe disease. Contaminated fomites, including nursery equipment, and humidification apparatus are the primary source of nosocomial infection with the organism.

Pneumonia due to *K. pneumoniae* may be difficult to distinguish clinically from pneumonia due to other causes. In nursery epidemics, diarrhea and vomiting may be the presenting symptoms; the onset of respiratory difficulty is often abrupt. The disease may have a fulminant course characterized by copious, thick, purulent secretion and the formation of pulmonary abscesses and cavitations. A lobar infiltrate with bulging fissures on roentgenogram is suggestive of the diagnosis (Fig. 13–9). Complications are common and include bacteremia, empyema, and residual parenchymal damage. The fatality rate in sporadic cases is about 50%, but it is lower during epidemics.

Isolation of the organism from purulent tracheal secretions, blood, or lung aspirate establishes the diagnosis. Supportive treatment is similar to that of other bacterial pneumonias; drainage of empyema and abscesses may be necessary. Kanamycin (15–20 mg/kg/24 hr, intramuscularly every 8 hr for 10–14 days) is the agent of choice; however, gentamicin may be employed initially if local sensitivity testing indicates a high degree of kanamycin resistance among *Klebsiella* isolates. In older children and adults the cephalosporins have also proved efficacious in treating these infections.

Pseudomonas aeruginosa Pneumonia. (Sec. 11.30). *Pseudomonas aeruginosa* produces a severe, progressive, usually fatal, necrotizing bronchopneumonia that is rarely a primary infection of the lung but occurs with chronic debilitating illnesses,

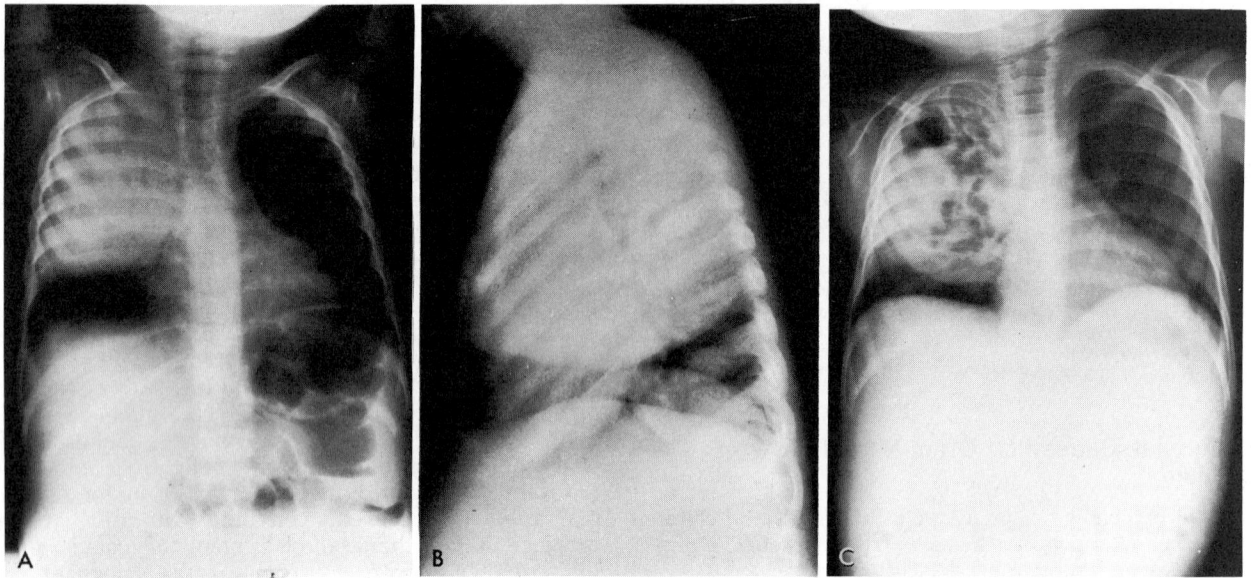

Figure 13–9. *Klebsiella* pneumonia in an 8 mo old infant admitted with complaints of cough, fever, and dyspnea. Roentgenograms (*A, B*) demonstrated pulmonary consolidation with characteristic bulging of fissure. Multiple pneumatoceles and abscesses appeared within 48 hr (*C*). Recovery occurred with kanamycin therapy.

such as cystic fibrosis and malignant disorders; with altered immunologic function; during prolonged antibiotic therapy; and in premature infants exposed to contaminated hospital equipment. In cystic fibrosis a fulminant course is uncommon. Ticarcillin administered alone or in combination with an aminoglycoside represents the most effective therapy.

Ginsburg CM, Howard JB, Nelson JD: Report of 65 cases of *Haemophilus influenzae* b pneumonia. Pediatrics 64:283, 1979.
Jacobs NM, Harris VJ: Acute *Haemophilus* pneumonia in childhood. Am J Dis Child 133:603, 1979.
Morgan HR: The enteric bacteria. *In*: Dubos R, Hirsch J (eds): Bacterial and Mycotic infections of Man. Ed 4. Philadelphia, JB Lippincott, 1965.
Thaler MM: *Klebsiella:Aerobacter* pneumonia in infants. Pediatrics 30:206, 1962.

13.67 PNEUMONIAS OF VIRAL ORIGIN

Etiology. Many viruses cause lower respiratory tract disease in children, principally bronchiolitis and interstitial lesions. The type and severity of the illness are influenced by several factors including age, sex, season of the year, and crowding. Viral pneumonia is most commonly caused by respiratory syncytial virus (Sec. 11.73), one of the parainfluenza viruses (Sec. 11.72), adenovirus (Sec. 11.74), or enterovirus (Sec. 11.77). Less commonly, rhinovirus (Sec. 11.75), influenza virus (Sec. 11.71), herpes simplex virus (Sec. 11.65), and others have also been recovered from children with pneumonia. Local epidemics may skew incidence figures for a given year or location. Respiratory syncytial virus causes a more serious disease during infancy, when it is the agent most commonly recovered.

Clinical Manifestations. Most viral pneumonias are preceded by several days of respiratory symptoms, including rhinitis and cough. Often, other family members are ill. Although cough and fever are prominent, temperatures are generally lower than in bacterial pneumonia. Dyspnea with retractions and nasal flaring is more common in younger children and infants. Physical examination may be surprisingly unrevealing although rales are present late in the illness. Wheezing, apparently related to virus-specific IgE, is frequently present with respiratory syncytial virus pneumonia. The viral pneumonias cannot be definitely differentiated from

mycoplasmal disease on purely clinical grounds and may, on occasion, be difficult to distinguish from bacterial pneumonias.

Diagnosis. The chest roentgenogram is characterized by a diffuse infiltrate, especially in the perihilar areas. In some patients, transient lobar infiltrates may also be present or even dominate the picture. Hyperinflation is common. Effusion may occur. Serologic studies may allow retrospective diagnosis by demonstrating a rise in antibody titer. Respiratory viruses, including parainfluenza virus, respiratory syncytial virus, and, less commonly, adenovirus, are occasionally found in asymptomatic children. The white blood cell count is usually under 20,000/mm³. Platelets may occasionally be slightly depressed.

Treatment. There is no specific treatment. Many patients are given antibiotic agents initially if bacterial pneumonia is suspected. Failure to respond to antibiotic treatment is additional evidence for viral etiology. Usually, only minimal supportive measures are required, although some patients need hospitalization for intravenous fluids, oxygen, or even assisted ventilation. There may be some benefit from continuous treatment with aerosolized ribavirin if RVS infection is documented (Sec. 13.64).

Prognosis. The vast majority of children with viral pneumonia recover uneventfully and have no sequelae, although the course may be prolonged, especially in infants. There is mounting evidence, however, that some patients, particularly infants, may develop bronchiolitis obliterans, unilateral hyperlucent lung, or other complications following a single episode of viral pneumonia. Adenovirus, especially types 1, 3, 4, 7, and 21, seems to be the most dangerous agent in this regard, and it also has been reported to cause a fatal acute fulminant pneumonia. Continuing roentgenographic abnormality for 6–12 mo is not unusual. In one series bronchiectasis was present in 27% of infant survivors of adenovirus (type 7) pneumonia.

Mycoplasma Pneumonia
(Primary Atypical Pneumonia)

See Sec. 11.60.

Giant Cell Pneumonia
(Hecht Pneumonia)

This interstitial pneumonitis is uncommon in infancy and childhood. A definitive diagnosis depends on histologic demonstration of characteristic multinuclear giant cells with intranuclear and intracytoplasmic inclusion bodies in the lung. Also present are a mononuclear infiltrate, squamous metaplasia of the bronchial and bronchiolar epithelium, proliferation of the alveolar lining cells, and the occasional occurrence of giant cells in organs other than the lungs. Patients often develop giant cell pneumonia after measles (Sec. 11.61). Rubeola virus has also been recovered from the lung tissue of patients with giant cell pneumonia who had no clinical evidence of measles or had leukemia complicated by measles infection. The giant cell formation seen in Hecht pneumonia and in cystic fibrosis is not, on the other hand, a histologic feature of the pneumonia commonly encountered with clinical measles. In the former group the process of giant cell formation originates in or near terminal bronchioles or alveoli, whereas in the latter the origin is bronchial. Hecht pneumonia may also follow immunization with attenuated measles vaccine in children who have leukemia or lymphomas and in patients with deficiency of cell-mediated immunity.

Clinically, patients with giant cell pneumonia have moderate to severe respiratory distress manifested principally by tachypnea and dyspnea. Inspiratory and early expiratory rales and musical sounds are heard, but dullness is rarely present. Some patients continue to excrete rubeolar virus from the upper respiratory tract for weeks after the onset of illness. Roentgenographically, there are usually generalized, patchy infiltrates with areas of overinflation.

The course of illness may be several weeks; clinical improvement may occur days to weeks prior to roentgenographic improvement. Occasionally, bacterial superinfection may occur. The mortality rate is high, particularly in patients with debilitating diseases such as leukemia, cystic fibrosis, and immunologic deficiency states. Treatment is symptomatic; gamma globulin is of no value.

Glezen WP, Denny FW: Epidemiology of acute lower respiratory disease in children. N Engl J Med 288:498, 1973.

Henderson FW, Collier AM, Clyde WA, et al: Respiratory-syncytial-virus infections, reinfections and immunity: A prospective, longitudinal study in young children. N Engl J Med 300:530, 1979.

Itall CB, McBride JT, Walsh EF, et al: Aerosolized ribavirin treatment of infants with respiratory syncytial viral infection. N Engl J Med 308:1443, 1983.

James AG, Lang WR, Liang AY, et al: Adenovirus type 21 bronchopneumonia in infants and young children. J Pediatr 95:530, 1979.

Malatzky AJ, Cooney MK, Luce R, et al: Epidemiology of viral and mycoplasmal agents associated with childhood lower respiratory illness in a civilian population. J Pediatr 78:407, 1971.

Similä S, Linna O, Lanning P: Chronic lung damage caused by adenovirus type 7: A ten-year follow-up study. Chest 80:127, 1981.

Welliver RC, Wong DT, Sun M: The development of respiratory syncytial virus-specific IgE and the release of histamine in nasopharyngeal secretions after infection. N Engl J Med 305:841, 1981.

PNEUMONIAS OF MISCELLANEOUS CAUSES

13.68 *Pneumocystis carinii* Pneumonia
(Interstitial Plasma Cell Pneumonia)

Epidemiology. *Pneumocystis carinii* organisms, ubiquitous protozoans, are found only in the peripheral respiratory airways of humans and of a variety of other animals, including rodents. In the human, infection is associated with immunosuppressed or chronic debilitated states or with prematurity or severe neonatal illness (Sec. 11.11). Most cases in the United States occur in patients with primary immunodeficiency diseases or with immunosuppression induced by ma-

lignancy or its treatment. As the treatment of malignancy has become more sophisticated and patients survive longer, the incidence of this complication has increased. In one series 4% of over 1200 children with malignancies had proven pulmonary pneumocystis infestation.

Pathogenesis and Pathology. In newborn infants an incompletely developed immunologic responsiveness and exposure to a humidified atmosphere contaminated with the parasite may interact synergistically to produce sporadic or epidemic disease in the nursery. In some infants intensive treatment of a respiratory tract infection with antibiotics may produce activation of a latent pneumocystic infection. Infants with cytomegalic inclusion disease or children with lymphoreticular malignancies treated with cytotoxic agents, corticosteroids, or prolonged antibiotic therapy are particularly susceptible to *P. carinii* pneumonia. Infection produces a characteristic intraalveolar exudate of lacelike appearance that contains histiocytes, lymphocytes, plasma cells, and cysts. Plasma cells are diminished or absent in agammaglobulinemia and hypogammaglobulinemia. The alveolar septa show varying degrees of edema, inflammation, and fibrosis.

Clinical Manifestations. Onset in infants is usually at 3–5 wk of life, and it may be seen at any age in patients with immune deficiency syndromes or acquired temporary or permanent loss of host resistance. In infants the disease usually begins insidiously with cough and proceeds over a period of 1–4 wk to be characterized by low grade fever, tachypnea, and severe respiratory distress. Nasal flaring, cyanosis, and suprasternal, infrasternal, and intercostal retractions usually occur, but rales may be absent or few. In older children the onset is more abrupt with fever, tachypnea, and cough followed rapidly by retractions, nasal flaring, and cyanosis. Rales are not usually present. Fever and cough, particularly in infants, also may be absent. There is a relative paucity of pulmonary findings for the severity of distress.

The roentgenogram characteristically consists of hyperexpanded lung fields, a generalized granular pattern, and bilateral pulmonary infiltrates that originate at the hilus, extend peripherally, and eventually create a nearly solid appearance. Overaeration is most pronounced in the periphery. Arterial oxygen is reduced, but hypercapnia is uncommon.

Pneumocystis carinii pneumonia usually lasts from 3–6 wk but may continue over many months.

Diagnosis. Definitive diagnosis is made by demonstrating the presence of the organism in the lung by appropriate staining of tracheal or lung aspirates, bronchial washing, or lung biopsies; sputum samples or tonsillar smears may occasionally be satisfactory. A complement fixation test may show conversion after 2–3 wk if the patient's immune system is sufficiently functional. The presence of pneumocystis antigen in 15% of patients with cancer but without pneumonitis suggests that the disease is not always an acute severe illness.

Treatment. Untreated, the disease is often fatal; patients with cellular immune deficiency or extensive malignancy usually die within 3 wk of onset of the typical roentgenographic features. *Trimethoprim* (20 mg/kg/24 hr) and *sulfamethoxazole* (100 mg/kg/24 hr) are the treatment of choice. Treatment with *pentamidine isothionate* (4 mg/kg/24 hr intramuscularly for 2 wk) has allowed over 50% of patients to recover even without restoration of immunocompetence; serious side effects of this drug include azotemia. Pentamidine may be effective despite prior unsuccessful treatment with trimethoprim-sulfamethoxazole. In very ill patients, supplemental oxygen with or without ventilator assistance may be needed. Children over 6 yr of age may recover completely from pneumocystis pneumonia within 6 mo of treatment.

Preventive treatment with trimethoprim (5 mg/kg/24 hr) and sulfamethoxazole (20 mg/kg/24 hr) may be useful in children who are at high risk for this disease.

Harris RE, McCallister JA, Allen SA, et al: Prevention of pneumocystis pneumonia. Am J Dis Child 134:35, 1980.

Hughes WT: Current concepts. *Pneumocystis carinii* pneumonia. N Engl J Med 297:1381, 197.

Hughes WT, Price RA, Kim HK, et al.: *Pneumocystis carinii* pneumonitis in children with malignancies. J Pediatr 82:404, 1973.

Sanyal SK, Mariencheck WC, Hughes WT: Course of pulmonary dysfunction in children surviving *Pneumocystis carinii* pneumonitis. Am Rev Respir Dis 124:161, 1981.

Siegel SE, Wolff LJ, Baehner RL, et al: Treatment of *Pneumocystis carinii* pneumonitis. Am J Dis Child 138:1051, 1984.

Mycotic Pulmonary Infections

See also Sec. 11.93–11.99.

Thrush Pneumonia
(Pulmonary Candidosis)

Pulmonary infections with *Candida albicans* are rare in children despite the relatively high incidence of oral thrush (Sec. 12.9) in infancy. This fact has been attributed to a natural resistance of columnar epithelium to invasion by the fungus. In 17 infants under 8 wk of age, all of whom had respiratory distress, about half had oral thrush, but there was no clinical or roentgenographic characteristic to suggest it as the cause of pulmonary infection. Amphotericin B and 5-fluorocytosine, although toxic, are the only effective therapeutic agents.

Emanuel B, Lieberman AD, Glodin M, et al: Pulmonary candidiasis in the neonatal period. J Pediatr 61:44, 1962.

13.69 Aspiration Pneumonia

See also Sec. 8.34 and 8.35.

Aspiration of Food and Vomitus. Infants with obstructive lesions, such as tracheoesophageal fistula and duodenal obstruction, weak and debilitated infants and children with no obstructive lesions, patients with familial dysautonomia, and patients with impaired consciousness may aspirate, or regurgitate and then aspirate, an amount of food and vomitus sufficient to cause a chemical pneumonia. Aspiration may rarely be an immediate cause of death by asphyxiation. More frequently, following aspiration of gastric contents, there is a relatively brief latent period before the onset of signs and symptoms of pneumonia. Over 90% of patients have symptoms within 1 hr, and almost all patients have symptoms within 2 hr. Fever, tachypnea, and cough are common. Apnea and shock also occur.

Physical examination reveals diffuse rales and wheezing, and many patients are cyanotic. Chest roentgenograms reveal alveolar and, occasionally, reticular infiltrates that may be localized but often are more extensive and frequently are bilateral. The irritated mucous membrane may also subsequently become the site for bacterial invasion and pneumonia.

Prophylaxis is of the greatest importance. Care should be taken to avoid amounts of feedings that will overdistend the stomach, especially in infants who are fed by gavage. After being fed, the infant should be placed on the abdomen or right side. When the infant is supine, the head should not be lower than the rest of the body. While the infant is lying face down, however, drainage from the lungs may be materially aided by lowering the head of the bed.

Immediate suctioning of the airway and administering oxygen are indicated for aspiration. Endotracheal intubation with suctioning and mechanical ventilation is often required in severe cases. Although prophylactic use of antibiotics and corticosteroids is advocated by some for patients who have aspirated gastric contents, evidence of their benefit is lacking. Some data suggest that corticosteroid treatment may predispose the patient to pneumonia due to gram-negative organisms.

Prognosis depends partly on the severity of aspiration and partly on the underlying disease. The majority of patients demonstrate clearing of infiltrates within 2 wk; mortality before clearing of aspiration infiltrates is about 25%. Over half the patients develop a secondary infection with either gram-positive or gram-negative organisms, including *Proteus, Pseudomonas, Escherichia coli,* and *Klebsiella.* Mixed infections are common. Anaerobic organisms can often be recovered from transtracheal cultures and may also play a role in the pneumonia.

Brook I, Finegold SM: Bacteriology of aspiration pneumonia in children. Pediatrics 65:1115, 1980.

Bynium LJ, Pierce AK: Pulmonary aspiration of gastric contents. Am Rev Resp Dis 114:1129, 1976.

Wolfe JE, Bone RC, Ruth WE: Effects of corticosteroids in the treatment of patients with gastric aspiration. Am J Med 83:719, 1977.

Aspiration of Baby Powder. Aspiration pneumonia resulting from inhalation of zinc stearate baby powder has become rare since the use of baby powder has decreased and since the containers still being used are now made better to control the outflow of powder. Severe respiratory distress almost immediately follows inhalation. Generalized obstructive emphysema with an expiratory type of dyspnea occurs as a result of an inflammatory reaction caused by the zinc stearate powder. Following inhalation, it is almost immediately drawn into the finer bronchioles because of its extreme lightness; for this reason bronchoscopic aspiration is useful, if at all, only to remove the secretions that may subsequently accumulate in the larger air passages. Immediate treatment is oxygen therapy in an atmosphere of high humidity.

The commonly used dusting (baby) powders today contain magnesium silicate (and other silicates), and some contain calcium undecylenate. Although not as dangerous as zinc stearate, these powders can also cause serious aspiration pneumonitis. Furthermore, talc is chemically related to asbestos, and "talcum powder" may contain microscopic asbestos particles, which may have a potential to cause malignancy. Systemic corticosteroid treatment appeared useful in one patient having severe dyspnea after aspirating talc.

Hughes WT, Kalmer T: Massive talc aspiration. Am J Dis Child 111:653, 1966.

Mofenson HC, Greensher J, DiTomasso A, et al: Baby powder—A hazard! Pediatrics 68:265, 1981.

Pneumonitis from Other Chemicals. Many chemicals, particularly if inhaled in high concentrations, may cause an inflammatory reaction consisting of edema and cellular infiltrations and acute respiratory distress. Prolonged exposure to lower concentrations of these same agents or other chemicals may cause chronic interstitial pneumonitis characterized by granuloma formation. For example, shellac, polyvinylpyrrolidone (found in hair spray), gum arabic, beryllium, mercury vapors, and chlorine may cause this reaction. Corticosteroids may reduce the inflammatory reaction and prevent fibrosis.

13.70 Hydrocarbon Pneumonia

Etiology. Hydrocarbons, such as furniture polish, kerosene, charcoal lighter fluid, and gasoline, are occasionally accidentally ingested by young children, causing a secondary pneumonitis. Gasoline may be aspirated by teenagers attempting to siphon gasoline (Sec. 28.6).

Pathogenesis. Although some controversy persists over how hydrocarbons reach the lungs, they probably are aspirated during swallowing, vomiting, or gastric lavage. The low viscosity of hydrocarbons allows them to flow from the hypopharynx into the larynx. Therefore, gastric lavage after the ingestion of hydrocarbons is usually contraindicated. Hydrocarbons may interact with pulmonary surfactant, resulting in alveolar collapse. Alveolar macrophages may also be injured. The pulmonary changes observed in animals after hydrocarbon aspiration are edema, inflammation, and hemorrhage.

Clinical Manifestations. Coughing and vomiting follow ingestion almost immediately. Within hours there may be a temperature elevation (38–40° C), and the child may be drowsy or comatose. However, with less extensive aspiration the onset of pulmonary symptoms and inflammation may be delayed 12–24 hr. The pulmonary findings may include dyspnea, diminished resonance on percussion, suppressed or tubular breath sounds, and rales. Pneumonic involvement is disclosed more frequently by roentgenographic examination than by physical findings. Occasionally, roentgenograms may show minimal changes a few hours after ingestion only to progress rapidly after that time with extensive infiltrates. In spite of what may be a stormy clinical course, which averages 2–5 days, recovery occurs in most instances.

Complications. Pneumothorax, subcutaneous emphysema of the chest wall, and pleural effusion, including empyema, have occurred. After the first week, pneumatoceles may develop in areas of extensive consolidation. There may be secondary infection with bacteria or viruses.

Treatment. All patients should be observed closely for 6 hr, even if they are asymptomatic when first seen. Symptoms and lung infiltrates may be delayed. Observation may be done at home if parents are instructed to bring the child to the hospital for any respiratory symptom. A child who is symptomatic when first seen or who becomes symptomatic during the next 6 hr should be admitted. If the history suggests a large amount of ingested material or the agent is particularly toxic (e.g., furniture polish), the child should be admitted for observation. No pulmonary therapy is indicated prior to symptoms.

Following ingestion of small to moderate amounts of hydrocarbons, induction of vomiting or gastric lavage is contraindicated because of the risk of aspiration, especially if several hours have elapsed. If a large volume of hydrocarbon is thought to be in the stomach, nasogastric suction performed with great care to avoid aspiration may be necessary to reduce the other dangers of hydrocarbon poisoning, including central nervous system toxicity. The risk of aspiration during gastric lavage or suctioning can be minimized if an endotracheal tube with a balloon cuff can be inserted without inducing vomiting prior to lavage. If there is dyspnea or cyanosis or if chemical pneumonitis develops, supportive measures including oxygen, physiotherapy, and, if necessary, continuous positive airway pressure or other forms of ventilatory assistance are important components of therapy. A cathartic is usually indicated.

The routine use of antibiotics is not recommended; the occurrence of secondary infection of the affected lung can usually be readily detected by the reappearance of fever on the 3rd–5th day following ingestion and can then be suitably treated with penicillin G and tobramycin. Corticosteroids have no beneficial effect on the course of the illness and may, on occasion, be harmful. Pneumatoceles, when they occur, rarely rupture and do not require treatment. Parents must be reminded to keep cleaning fluids and kerosene in locked cabinets out of reach of children or out of the home.

Prognosis. Although most children survive without complications or sequelae, some progress rapidly to respiratory failure and death. Prognosis depends on a variety of factors, including the volume of the ingestion or aspiration, the specific agent involved, and the adequacy of medical care. In one series, only 39 of 950 patients developed symptoms; 4 required assisted ventilation and 2 died. Long-term pulmonary function studies several years later are inconclusive, but if lasting damage does occur, the small airways seem to be at greatest risk.

Anas N, Vanthaya N, Ginsburg CM: Criteria for hospitalizing children who have ingested products containing hydrocarbons. JAMA 246:840, 1981.
Bergeson PS, Hales SW, Lustgarten MD, et al: Pneumatoceles following hydrocarbon ingestion. Report of three cases and review of the literature. Am J Dis Child 129:49, 1975.
Bratton L, Haddow J: Ingestion of charcoal lighter fluid. J Pediatr 87:633, 1975.
Brown J III, Burke B, Dajani AS: Experimental kerosene pneumonia: Evaluation of some therapeutic regimens. J Pediatr 84:396, 1974.
Guruntz D, Kattan M, Levison H, et al: Pulmonary function abnormalities in asymptomatic children after hydrocarbon pneumonitis. Pediatrics 62:789, 1978.
Nouri LA, Sordelli DO, Cerquetti C, et al: Pumonary clearance of *Staphylococcus aureus* and plasma angiotensin-converting enzyme activity in hydrocarbon pneumonitis. Pediatr Res 17:657, 1983.

13.71 Lipoid Pneumonia

Lipoid pneumonia is a chronic, interstitial, proliferative inflammation resulting from aspiration of lipoid material; it occurs principally in debilitated infants.

Pathogenesis. Factors that may be responsible for aspiration of oil include (1) intranasal instillation of medicated oils; (2) any condition that interferes with swallowing, such as cleft palate, debilitation, or a horizontal position during feeding; and (3) forced feeding, and especially the administration of cod liver oil, castor oil, or mineral oil to crying children.

The severity of the pulmonary reaction depends upon the kind of oil inhaled. Vegetable oils, such as olive, cottonseed, and sesame, are generally the least irritating and produce no inflammation; however, chaulmoogra, also a vegetable oil, produces extensive damage. Animal oils, owing to their high fatty acid content, are the most damaging. Milk aspirated by debilitated infants is one example; cod liver oil also belongs in this category. Liquid petrolatum is chemically inert and not as irritative as some of the other oils but does act as a foreign body. Excessive use of lip gloss can also cause pneumonitis in teenagers.

The reaction within the lung begins as an interstitial proliferative inflammation, and there may be an exudative pneumonia. In the second stage there is diffuse, chronic, proliferative fibrosis and sometimes superimposed acute infectious bronchopneumonia. In the third stage there are multiple localized nodules, tumor-like paraffinomas. There are numerous macrophages in the involved areas, with giant cell formation of the foreign body type. The lipoid substance is both intracellular and extracellular. The oil-laden cells may be carried to the hilar lymph nodes.

Clinical Manifestations. There are no characteristic signs or symptoms; a cough is most common, and in severe cases there may be dyspnea. Unless there is superimposed infection, there is usually no fever or physical sign, although with extensive involvement there may be some impairment to percussion and change in voice and breath sounds. Secondary bronchopneumonic infections are common.

The roentgenographic appearance is characteristic. With mild involvement there is an increase in the density and extent of the hilar shadows. With increasing involvement there is greater density of the perihilar shadows, which widen in all directions (Fig. 13–10). Pulmonary changes may be limited to the right lung, and in the infant who is recumbent most of the time, the changes may be mainly in the right upper lobe.

Prognosis. The prognosis is guarded. It depends upon the extent of pulmonary damage, the discontinuation of oil inhalation, the general condition of the patient, and the avoidance of intercurrent infections.

Prevention. Intranasal medications in an oily vehicle should not be used. Concentrated preparations of vitamins A and D in water-miscible vehicles should be substituted for cod liver oil. Administration of mineral oil and castor oil should be avoided. Infants who regurgitate or vomit frequently should be placed on their abdomens to lessen the likelihood of aspiration.

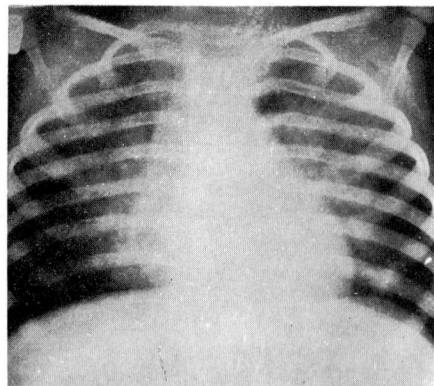

Figure 13–10. Roentgenogram showing increased density radiating from the hilus of each lung in an infant 13 mo of age after intranasal application of liquid petrolatum 3 times a day for 5 mo.

Treatment. There is no specific therapy other than elimination of further exposure. The infant's position should be changed frequently to lessen the chances of hydrostatic pneumonia.

Bection DL, Lowe JE, Falleta JM: Lipoid pneumonia in an adolescent girl secondary to use of lip gloss. J Pediatrics 105:421, 1984.

13.72 Silo Filler's Disease

This rare, acute interstitial pneumonia occurs following the inhalation of nitrogen dioxide, a gas generally encountered only in freshly filled silos. Cough and dyspnea occur immediately after exposure. An asymptomatic phase of several days follows, but then the patient suddenly experiences chills and fever associated with progressive cough, dyspnea, and cyanosis. There are rales throughout both lung fields and widespread pulmonary infiltration on roentgenogram. The interalveolar septa are widened, edematous, and filled with accumulated mononuclear cells and fibroblasts, and the epithelium is hyperplastic. The disease usually progresses rapidly to death. Corticosteroids have been used, but there is no known effective treatment.

13.73 Paraquat Lung

Paraquat, a dipyridylium compound used as a weed killer, is highly toxic, causing death from respiratory failure a few days to weeks after ingestion. The pulmonary lesion is secondary to systemic absorption through the gastrointestinal tract or skin and consists of proliferative bronchiolitis, alveolitis, hemorrhage causing intra-alveolar hyaline membranes and fibrosis. Gas exchange is impaired. It is a corrosive that also causes painful lesions of the mouth and esophagus, renal tubular damage, azotemia, and hematuria. Renal damage may result in prolongation of toxic blood levels, during which time fibroblasts proliferate, filling the terminal air spaces. There is no treatment except for general supportive measures. Oxygen may increase pulmonary toxicity. Increased incidence may be due to large scale use of paraquat in attempts to kill marijuana plants.

Copland GM, Kolin A, Shulman HS: Fatal pulmonary intra-alveolar fibrosis after paraquat ingestion. N Engl Med 291:290, 1974.

13.74 Hypersensitivity to Inhaled Materials

Repeated inhalation of organic dusts may result in chronic pneumonitis that progressively worsens with continued exposure to the antigen. Although the syndrome is most common in adults, it has been reported frequently in children.

Unlike those of asthma, the symptoms of this hypersensitivity syndrome are almost entirely unrelated to bronchospasm (Sec. 10.44). Symptoms may result from inhalation of small particles from moldy hay (farmer's lung), maple bark (maple bark stripper's disease), sugar cane fiber (bagassosis), redwood tree bark, pigeon droppings and feathers (pigeon breeder's disease), cheese, desiccated pituitary powder, dusty output from air conditioners, and a fungus or mold associated with the specific material to which the patient is exposed.

Clinical Manifestations. The signs and symptoms are similar in all of these diseases. Within several hours following exposure cough, dyspnea, chest pain, and sometimes fever occur with few physical findings, though occasional wheezes and moist rales may be audible. Roentgenograms may show minimal emphysema but are usually normal. If no further exposure occurs, the symptoms abate over a period of several days; but if contact with the responsible antigen continues, symptoms progress to severe dyspnea and cyanosis associated with diffuse, fine, interstitial or nodular densities, and peripheral alveolar infiltrates on chest roentgenogram and occasionally irreversible loss of pulmonary function. The disease should be suspected in children with relatively mild symptoms including cough, fever, and occasional dyspnea, particularly if bronchopneumonia persists despite appropriate treatment with antibiotics.

Pathology. Histologically, the infiltrate consists of subacute granulomatous inflammation with accumulation of plasma cells, lymphocytes, epithelioid cells, and giant cells of the Langhans type. With continued exposure, inflammatory lesions may be replaced by fibrosis.

Diagnosis. There may be moderate to marked leukocytosis, particularly with acute attacks, elevated serum immunoglobulins (IgG, IgM, and IgA fractions), and a primary restrictive pattern on pulmonary function tests. Arterial blood gas analysis reveals moderate or marked hypoxemia, usually without hypercapnia. Skin testing with the suspected antigen may cause a vigorous delayed hypersensitivity response and is especially useful if an Arthus reaction can be demonstrated histologically by skin biopsy of the test site. Demonstration of a serum precipitin to a given antigen is frequently encountered in apparently well persons and thus is not diagnostic. Lung biopsy reveals a diffuse fibrotic or granulomatous response. If the antigen is available in purified form, an inhalation challenge may be diagnostic.

Treatment. Optimal therapy requires the complete elimination of exposure to the suspected (or proven) antigen, which includes thoroughly cleaning the home after the source(s) of antigen has been eliminated. The administration of adrenal corticosteroids (e.g., prednisone in initial dosage of 1–1.5 mg/kg/24) usually results in prompt remission of symptoms; continued use for 1–6 mo may prevent the subsequent development of pulmonary fibrosis in cases of chronic exposure. Corticosteroid therapy may be slowly tapered down following evidence of recovery of lung function or following several weeks without exposure to a known antigen. If hypersensitivity pneumonitis is strongly suspected but the antigen remains unknown, long-term use of corticosteroid therapy, perhaps on an alternate day regimen, may be indicated. The patient should be cautioned that re-exposure to the antigen is extremely dangerous even long after apparent complete recovery. Even if treatment is optimal and the exposure is eliminated, some fatalities occur, and a substantial percentage of patients do not completely regain their previous pulmonary status.

Allen DH, Williams GV, Woolcock AJ: Bird breeder's hypersensitivity pneumonitis. Progress studies of lung function after cessation of exposure to the provoking antigen. Am Rev Resp Dis 114:555, 1976.
Cunningham AS, Fink JN, Schlueter DP: Childhood hypersensitivity pneumonitis due to dove antigen. Pediatrics 58:436, 1976.

Katz RM, Knicker WT: Infantile hypersensitivity pneumonitis as a reaction to organic antigen. N Engl J Med 288:233, 1973.

Keith HH, Holsclaw DS, Donsky EH: Pigeon breeder's disease in children: A family study. Chest 79:107, 1981.

Stiehm ER, Reed CE, Tooley WH: Pigeon breeder's lung in children. Pediatrics 39:904, 1967.

13.75 Pulmonary Aspergillosis

See Sec. 10.47 and 11.97.

A variety of species of the fungal genus *Aspergillus* are potentially pathogenic for man. The spectrum of pulmonary manifestations is great and depends upon the nature of the exposure and the condition of the host. A hypersensitivity reaction with bronchospasm is most common. The majority of these cases of *allergic bronchopulmonary aspergillosis* have occurred in children with chronic pulmonary diseases. In some patients the immunologic response that results in allergic aspergillosis appears to be genetically determined. *Aspergillomas* (fungus balls) typically occur in an ectatic bronchus or old tuberculous cavity. Affected patients are generally asymptomatic. There have been, however, isolated case reports of parenchymal invasion by aspergillus in normal children, but *invasive aspergillosis* generally occurs in immunosuppressed patients, and any organ may be involved.

Clinical Manifestations. Allergic aspergillosis should be suspected in an immunosuppressed or chronically ill child who presents relatively acute onset of cough, wheezing, and low grade fever. The cough may be productive, and, occasionally, brown plugs are expectorated that on microscopic examination contain hyphae. Aspergillus can be recovered from this material on culture.

Many patients have multiple precipitin lines on diffusion of serum against aspergillus antigen. The immediate skin test reaction is often strongly positive, and a type III hypersensitivity (Arthus) reaction can usually be demonstrated after skin testing. Chest roentgenograms show transient, occasionally extensive, infiltrates. Peripheral eosinophilia occurs in almost every patient. Serum levels of immunoglobulin E are elevated, and specific immunoglobulin E antibody to aspergillus has been demonstrated. Aspergillus organisms are frequently recovered from cultures of respiratory tract secretions of patients with chronic pulmonary disease who do not have symptoms of allergic aspergillosis. The recovery of these organisms without typical symptoms and serologic evidence of hypersensitivity is not an indication for treatment.

Treatment. Therapy should be directed at eradicating the organism. Unfortunately, the best approach to treatment is not clear. Systemic amphotericin B (0.5–1.0 mg/kg/24 hr intravenously) or 5-fluorocytosine (50–150 mg/kg/24 hr) may be effective. Aerosolized amophotericin or direct instillation of amphotericin into the trachea also has been recommended, but correct dosage is not established. Symptomatic treatment with systemic and aerosolized bronchodilators and corticosteroids may also often be necessary (Sec. 10.48). Disodium cromoglycate is not useful.

Aspergillomas may respond to specific antifungal chemotherapy. However, surgical resection with local instillation of amphotericin is considered the treatment of choice. The prognosis, whatever the treatment, depends heavily on the underlying chronic illness. Invasive aspergillosis may be so fulminant that antifungal chemotherapy is not efficacious. Treatment generally consists of amphotericin B combined with 5-fluorocytosine. Treatment should be continued for 2–3 wk.

Bardana EJ, Sobti KL, Cianciulli FD, et al: Aspergillus antibody in patients with cystic fibrosis. Am J Dis Child 129:1164, 1975.

Berger I, Phillips WL, Shenker IR: Pulmonary aspergillosis in childhood. Clin Pediatr 11:178, 1972.

Graves TS, Fink JN, Patterson, R, et al: A familial occurrence of allergic bronchopulmonary aspergillosis. Ann Intern Med 91:378, 1979.

Katz RM, Kniker WT: Infantile hypersensitivity pneumonitis as a reaction to organic antigens. N Engl J Med 288:233, 1973.

Slavin RG, Laird TS, Cherry JD: Allergic bronchopulmonary aspergillosis in a child. J Pediatr 78:416, 1970.

Strelling MK, Rhaney K, Simmons DAR, et al: Fatal acute pulmonary aspergillosis in two children of one family. Arch Dis Child 41:34, 1966.

Varkey B, Rose HD: Pulmonary aspergilloma: A rational approach to treatment. Am J Med 61:626, 1976.

13.76 Loeffler Syndrome
(Eosinophilic Pneumonia)

This syndrome is characterized by widespread transitory pulmonary infiltrations, which roentgenographically vary in size but may resemble those of miliary tuberculosis, and by a blood eosinophilia that may be as high as 70%. The clinical course is usually not severe and ranges from a few days to several months. There are usually paroxysmal attacks of coughing, dyspnea, pleurisy, and little or no fever. There may be associated hepatomegaly, especially in infants and young children, and biopsy sections of the liver have revealed multiple focal areas of necrosis, granuloma formation, and eosinophilic infiltration. These children have hyperglobulinemia, presumably as the result of hepatic dysfunction and in response to parasitic invasion of tissue. Autopsy studies have revealed evidences of eosinophilic infiltrations in the lungs and in other organs. Localized pneumonic consolidation with an associated eosinophilia may occur.

Loeffler syndrome may be an unusual allergic manifestation of a variety of antigens and not a distinct clinical entity. In children it is most often a manifestation of helminthic infections. Perhaps the most common pathogen in this country is the larva of the dog ascarid, *Toxocara canis*, and less often of the cat ascarid, *Toxocara cati* (Sec. 11.115). Other roundworms may also be responsible for the syndrome; these include *Ascaris lumbricoides* (usually responsible for transient pulmonary lesions), *Strongyloides stercoralis*, and hookworms (Sec. 11.110–11.112). So-called tropical eosinophilia may be manifest as Loeffler syndrome and is probably caused by a number of different helminths. Paragonimiasis caused by a lung fluke (Sec. 11.125) may produce the syndrome as well as extrapulmonary manifestations. A drug reaction may also result in this syndrome; aspirin, penicillin, sulfonamides, and imipramine are among those implicated.

Beaver P: Wandering nematodes as a cause of disability and disease. Am J Trop Med Hyg 6:433, 1967.

Leitch AG: Pulmonary eosinophilia. Basics Respir Dis 7 (No 5):1, 1979.

Zuelzer WW, Apt L: Disseminated visceral lesions associated with extreme eosinophilia: Pathologic and clinical observations on a syndrome of young children. Am J Dis Child 78:153, 1948.

13.77 Pulmonary Involvement in Collagen Diseases

Pulmonary manifestations are rarely the dominant feature of periarteritis, systemic lupus erythematosus, scleroderma, polymyositis, or dermatomyositis. However, recurrent infection and progression to bronchiectasis may occur in scleroderma. Although rare, pulmonary involvement may precede joint symptoms in juvenile rheumatoid arthritis. In one series, pulmonary disease occurred in 40% of children having mixed connective tissue. Diffusion abnormalities are common when the lungs are involved by this group of diseases. Hemoptysis may occur. Pleural effusions and pleuritic pain are fairly common in systemic lupus. Corticosteroid treatment may ameliorate some of these problems. Patients who are chronically immunosuppressed as a part of the therapy of these diseases are at risk to develop *Pneumocystis carinii* pneumonia.

Rheumatic pneumonia is a usually fatal, but rare, complication of acute rheumatic fever, characterized clinically by extensive pulmonary consolidation and rapidly progressive functional deterioration and pathologically by alveolar exudate, inflammatory interstitial infiltrates, and necrotizing arteritis. Physical findings are unexpectedly minimal; frequently there are no rales. Chest roentgenograms reveal transient areas of infiltrate that resemble pulmonary edema. There is no specific treatment; these patients do not respond to corticosteroids, to treatment of congestive heart failure with diuretics and digitalis, or to the antibiotic treatment of presumed infection. If the lesion is diagnosed by lung biopsy, treatment with immunosuppressive agents theoretically may be of value but has not been reported to be effective.

Lovell D, Lindsley C, Langston C: Lymphoid interstitial pneumonia in juvenile rheumatoid arthritis. J Pediatr 105:947, 1984.
Oetgen WJ, Boice JA, Lawless OJ: Mixed connective tissue disease in children and adolescents. Pediatrics 67:333, 1981.
Park S, Nyhan WL: Fatal pulmonary involvement in dermatomyositis. Am J Dis Child 129:723, 1975.
Rajani KB, Aschbacher LV, Kinney TR: Pulmonary hemorrhage and systemic lupus erythematosus. J Pediatr 93:810, 1978.
Serlin SP, Rmisza ME, Gay JH: Rheumatic pneumonia: The need for a new approach. Pediatrics 56:1075, 1975.

13.78 Desquamative Interstitial Pneumonitis

This disease of unknown etiology is characterized pathologically by massive proliferation and desquamation of alveolar cells and thickening of the alveolar walls. The degree of desquamation is far greater than the degree of alveolar wall thickening. In most children there is a history of preceding upper respiratory infection, although the relationship of the desquamative pneumonitis to this infection of probable viral origin has not been firmly established. Two infants were identified in whom desquamative interstitial pneumonitis and congenital rubella were associated. Circulating immune complexes and alveolar deposition of IgG and complement suggest an immune basis for the disease.

Clinical Manifestations. Symptoms usually develop slowly. As alveolar function is compromised, tachypnea and dyspnea occur; as the disease progresses, there is a nonproductive cough, anorexia, and weight loss. Cyanosis eventually results; clubbing is not a constant feature, and fever is unusual. Physical findings include tachypnea, nasal flaring, and, occasionally, fine rales. Use of the accessory muscles of respiration is not as prominent as one would expect in obstructive diseases exhibiting an equal amount of hypoxemia.

Laboratory Manifestations. Chest roentgenograms reveal a diffuse, hazy, ground glass appearance, particularly at the lung bases, along with poorly defined hilar densities. Viral and bacteriologic cultures and acute and convalescent sera analyses are not helpful diagnostically. Arterial blood samples show hypoxemia; most patients seek medical care prior to the advent of hypercapnia. Definitive diagnosis requires open lung biopsy.

Treatment. Patients with desquamative interstitial pneumonitis often recover without specific treatment. Those suspected of having the disease can occasionally be simply observed if their respiratory symptoms are not too severe. With worsening pulmonary status or rapid deterioration shown on the chest roentgenogram, open lung biopsy is important to establish a definitive diagnosis. These patients usually respond to corticosteroid therapy with rapid resolution of symptoms and gradual improvement on roentgenogram. Occasional corticosteroid-resistant patients are reported, and a variety of other treatments, including immunosuppression, have been proposed; corticosteroid therapy may be less effective in familial cases. Supportive treatment including supplemental oxygen is often necessary. Corticosteroid therapy without lung biopsy diagnosis is hazardous; chronic viral pneumonitis can present with a

similar clinical picture and may be worsened by corticosteroid depression of host defenses. Relapses are reported when therapy is prematurely stopped.

Bonner A, Wilmett RW, Dinwiddle R, et al: Desquamative interstitial pneumonia and antigen-antibody complexes in two infants with congenital rubella. Pediatrics 72:835, 1983.
Dreisin RB, Schwartz MI, Theofilopoulus AN, et al: Circulating immune complexes in the idiopathic interstitial pneumonias. N Engl J Med 298:353, 1978.
Stillwell PC, Norris DG, O'Connell EJ, et al.: Desquamative interstitial pneumonitis in children. Chest 77:155, 1980.
Tal A, Maer E, Bar-Ziv J, et al: Fatal desquamative interstitial pneumonitis in three infant siblings. J Pediatr 104:873, 1984.

13.79 Hypostatic Pneumonia

Hypostatic pneumonia occurs after prolonged passive pulmonary congestion and may occur in any marasmic state. Lying for a long time in one position favors its development. There is dependent congestion, edema, and pneumonia. The symptoms are not characteristic. There is neither dyspnea nor fever unless these symptoms are secondary to another disorder. The physical signs are principally slight dullness on percussion, feeble respiratory sounds, and the presence of moist rales. Hypostatic congestion is usually a terminal event. There is no specific treatment. Prophylaxis is of the greatest importance; the position of any immobile patient should be changed frequently.

13.80 RESPIRATORY BURNS AND SMOKE INHALATION

Thermal and chemical injury to the lung, systemic toxicity of inhaled gases—particularly carbon monoxide—and asphyxia are important causes of morbidity and mortality in children who have been exposed to fire and should be considered in the initial treatment whether or not there are surface burns. Excessive heat may injure the respiratory mucosa, especially above the trachea. A variety of noxious gases may be generated by fires, including oxides of sulfur and nitrogen, hydrochloric acid, acetaldehyde, corrosive acids and alkalis, and carbon monoxide. Fine particles of soot carried deep within the lung may cause thermal burns or have toxic gases adsorbed on them.

Although there is usually a history of being trapped in a smoke-filled room or evidence of superficial burns around the face or singed nasal vibrissae, serious respiratory damage may occur in the absence of any of these. Exposure to steam greatly increases the chance that respiratory thermal injury has occurred. The onset of clinical manifestations of respiratory distress may be immediate or delayed several hours. Roentgenographic changes may be delayed from hours to days.

Signs of central nervous system injury from hypoxia due to asphyxia may vary from irritability to depression. Carbon monoxide poisoning may be mild (<20% HbCO) with slight dyspnea and decreased visual acuity and higher cerebral functions; moderate (20–40% HbCO) with irritability, nausea, dimness of vision, impaired judgment, and rapid fatigue; or severe (40–60% HbCO), producing confusion, hallucination, ataxia, collapse, and coma.

Direct measurement of carboxyhemoglobin (HbCO) is important for diagnosis and prognosis, as it reflects the degree of tissue hypoxia caused by the combination of carbon monoxide and hemoglobin and the change in the shape and position of the oxygen dissociation curve. PaO_2 may be normal and the oxyhemoglobin saturation values misleading because HbCO is not detected by the usual tests of saturation. Thermal injury may lead to edema, exudate, and necrosis, and to desquamation of tissue, obstruction, and atelectasis. Respiratory insufficiency may occur from asphyxia, carbon monoxide poisoning, airway obstruction due to edema and necrotic material in the airways, or bronchoconstriction.

Children who have been in fires should be hospitalized for at least 24 hr for careful observation. If carbon monoxide poisoning is suspected, humidified 100% oxygen should be administered.

After thermal injury, respiratory complications follow a fairly predictable timetable. From *1–12 hr after exposure* acute respiratory distress secondary to bronchospasm, laryngeal edema, and/or lung consolidation may occur. Laryngeal obstruction, characterized by a prolonged inspiratory phase and virtually absent breath sounds, is uncommon; endotracheal intubation followed by tracheostomy is necessary in these patients. Bronchospasm, characterized by wheezing and prolonged expiration, reponds best to a large intravenous bolus of corticosteroid. Usual bronchodilator treatment is ineffective. Lung consolidation is an ominous development; in one series, 80% of affected patients died within 36 hr. Pulmonary edema occurs usually *6–72 hr after exposure*. Although fluid overload may account for some of these cases, the majority are directly due to the injury itself. Treatment includes fluid restriction and diuretics. Ventilatory assistance may be required. Cervical eschar formation and constriction of the airway may occur *60–120 hr after exposure* in patients with circumferential full-thickness burns of the neck; treatment consists of vertical division of the burn crust and immediate endotracheal intubation. Bronchopneumonia may complicate the patient's course, especially following the 4th day. At first *Staphylococcus aureus* is the most common pathogen, but by the 8th day *Pseudomonas aeruginosa* and *Klebsiella pneumoniae* are the dominant organisms recovered. Treatment includes encouraging cough, nasotracheal suctioning, and, on occasion, bronchoscopic suctioning. Specific antibiotic treatment based on culture results is important. Early and continuous use of intravenous corticosteroids contributes to a poor prognosis in these patients. Respiratory therapy equipment is the source of the infecting organisms in some patients.

Children with respiratory burns account for the vast majority of fatalities following survival of exposure to fire (Sec. 5.28). Careful observation and specific therapy as complications develop are extremely important. Supportive care, including postural draining and encouragement of cough, are important.

The importance of strategically placed smoke detectors should be presented to families as part of well-child care.

Mellins RB, Park S: Respiratory complications of smoke inhalation in victims of fires. J Pediatr 87:1, 1975.

Pietak SP, Delahaye DJ: Airway obstruction following smoke inhalation. Can Med Assoc J 115:329, 1978.

Stone HH: Pulmonary burns in children. J Pediatr 14:48, 1979.

13.81 PULMONARY HEMOSIDEROSIS

The term "pulmonary hemosiderosis" is used to describe a number of rare conditions characterized by an abnormal accumulation of hemosiderin in the lungs. Hemosiderin deposits follow diffuse alveolar hemorrhage and may occur either as a primary disease of the lungs or as secondary to cardiac or systemic vascular disease. In children, primary hemosiderosis occurs more frequently than the secondary varieties. There are four types of primary pulmonary hemosiderosis: an idiopathic form, a form associated with cow's milk hypersensitivity (Heiner syndrome), a form occurring in association with myocarditis, and a form associated with progressive glomerulonephritis (Goodpasture syndrome). Three types of secondary pulmonary hemosiderosis are recognized: one occurs with mitral stenosis and chronic left ventricular failure of any cause; one is associated with collagen diseases; and one with hemorrhagic diseases.

Idiopathic Primary Pulmonary Hemosiderosis. The cause of this illness is unknown. Although the rarely reported familial incidence suggests a possible genetic basis for some cases, other explanations, such as an environmental toxin, may also play a role. In one study, insecticides were suspected. Onset usually occurs in childhood, rarely later than early adult life. Most of the clinical features are related to blood in the alveoli and to the effects of chronic blood loss. Symptoms are those of recurrent or chronic pulmonary disease and include cough, hemoptysis, dyspnea, wheezing, and occasional cyanosis associated with fatigue and pallor. The cough may be productive of bloody sputum, or the infant or child may simply vomit large quantities of blood. During acute attacks, which usually last 2–4 days, the child may be febrile.

The usual clinical features of fever, tachycardia, tachypnea, leukocytosis, respiratory distress, and abnormal roentgenographic findings may suggest bacterial pneumonia, and only prolonged follow-up will reveal the correct diagnosis. In some children, however, the early manifestations of illness are related to chronic iron deficiency anemia, which is often refractory to therapy, and the characteristic pulmonary symptoms do not appear until much later. Paradoxically, the child may have severe pulmonary manifestations without roentgenographic abnormalities, or the roentgenographic picture may be abnormal before pulmonary symptoms have occurred.

The anemia is typically microcytic and hypochromic; serum iron concentrations are low, and there may be elevations in bilirubin, urobilinogen, and reticulocyte count. The stool usually contains occult blood, presumably swallowed. Hemosiderin can usually be demonstrated in macrophages in smears of sputum or material obtained from tracheal or gastric aspirates. Roentgenographic changes range from minimal infiltrates resembling pneumonia to massive pulmonary involvement with secondary atelectasis, emphysema, and hilar lymphadenopathy. The findings may suggest tuberculosis or pulmonary edema, and significant changes may be seen from day to day. Open lung biopsy may be required to establish the diagnosis by histologic demonstration of intra-alveolar hemorrhage, large numbers of hemosiderin-laden macrophages, alveolar epithelial hyperplasia, interstitial fibrosis, and sclerosis of small vessels. Closed needle biopsy has been followed by serious complications.

Approximately half the patients die within 1–5 yr, usually from acute pulmonary hemorrhage and progressive respiratory failure. A milk-free diet is indicated, pending analysis of serum for precipitins, and also serves as a diagnostic test for cow's milk–related pulmonary hemosiderosis. Corticosteroids (prednisone, 1 mg/kg/24 hr) may produce remission in some patients and be of no benefit to others. Maintenance corticosteroid therapy has been used between attacks with variable results. Immunosuppressant drugs and deferoxamine have not been adequately evaluated.

Primary Pulmonary Hemosiderosis with Hypersensitivity to Cow's Milk (Heiner Syndrome). Children affected with this syndrome have the typical picture of idiopathic hemosiderosis, unusually high serum titers of precipitins to multiple constituents of cow's milk, and positive intradermal skin tests to various cow's milk proteins. They may also have chronic rhinitis, recurrent otitis media, gastrointestinal symptoms, and growth retardation. The symptoms improve when cow's milk is removed from the diet and return with its reintroduction. Some patients fail to improve at all on a milk-free diet, and others without multiple serum precipitins have improved. Some of these patients with high titers of milk precipitins and pulmonary hemosiderosis develop cor pulmonale secondary to hypertrophied nasopharyngeal lymphoid tissue. These patients should also have a tonsilloadenoidectomy. In general, patients with hemosiderosis and precipitins to cow's milk have a better prognosis than do those with other forms of the disease, and they may eventually lose their sensitivity to milk. Corticosteroids may be useful, at least during acute bleeding episodes.

Primary Pulmonary Hemosiderosis with Myocarditis. Some patients have varying degrees of inflammation of the myocardium associated with pulmonary hemosiderosis, and, if significant myocardial disease is present when pulmonary symptoms are first noted, it may be impossible to determine whether the hemosiderosis is a primary or secondary phenomenon. The clinical picture does not differ from that of the idiopathic disease except that the heart may be enlarged and there may be electrocardiographic signs compatible with myocarditis.

Primary Pulmonary Hemosiderosis with Glomerulonephritis (Goodpasture Syndrome). This is a disease primarily of young adult males and is rarely observed in children. Initially, the presentation of the disease may be similar to idiopathic pulmonary hemosiderosis with hemoptysis and iron deficiency anemia, but careful study at the time of the initial attack will usually reveal a proliferative or membranous glomerulonephritis. Patients most often have progressive renal disease with hypertension and eventual renal failure and death. The pulmonary disease has improved following bilateral nephrectomy in a few patients but not in others.

Secondary Pulmonary Hemosiderosis. Heart disease producing a chronic increase in pulmonary capillary pressure, such as mitral stenosis, can lead to intrapulmonary hemorrhage and secondary hemosiderosis. Collagen vascular diseases may present clinical manifestations of pulmonary hemosiderosis. Occasionally, the vascular changes of polyarteritis are initially limited to the lungs. Other diseases, such as rheumatoid arthritis, may also produce pulmonary hemosiderosis as an effect of generalized diffuse vasculitis. A few patients with anaphylactoid purpura or thrombocytopenic purpura have similarly had hemosiderosis secondary to intrapulmonary hemorrhage.

Beckerman RC, Taussig LM, Pinnas JL: Familial idiopathic hemosiderosis. Am J Dis Child 133:609, 1979.
Boat TF, Polmar SH, Whitman V, et al: Hyperreactivity to cow milk in young children with pulmonary hemosiderosis and cor pulmonale secondary to nasopharyngeal obstruction. J Pediatr 87:23, 1973.
Case Records of the Massachusetts General Hospital (case 30–1979). N Engl J Med 301:201, 1979.
Cassimos CD, Chryssanthopoulos C, Panagiotidou C: Epidemiologic observations in idiopathic pulmonary hemosiderosis. J Pediatr 102:698, 1983.
Heiner DC, Sears JW, Kniker WT: Multiple precipitins to cow's milk in chronic respiratory disease. A syndrome including poor growth, gastrointestinal symptoms, evidence of allergy, iron deficiency anemia and pulmonary hemosiderosis. Am J Dis Child 103:634, 1962.

13.82 PULMONARY ALVEOLAR PROTEINOSIS

In children pulmonary alveolar proteinosis is a rare disease of unknown etiology. Occasionally there are families with two affected children, suggesting an underlying genetic basis.

Clinical Manifestations. The first symptoms are usually cough and dyspnea. Fever is present in about a third of the patients. Most clinical findings result from hypoxia and include weakness, fatigue, weight loss, and cyanosis. Physical findings are relatively few unless hypoxia is severe, but roentgenogrpahic changes generally are characteristic and consist of a fine, diffuse infiltrate radiating from the hilus to the periphery, often in a "butterfly" distribution (Fig. 13–11). Some patients demonstrate bilateral lower lobe infiltrates, while others initially show nodular densities progressing to complete lobar consolidaiton. Pulmonary function testing reveals a restrictive pattern, and arterial blood gases show marked hypoxemia, usually with normal CO_2 tensions. Serum

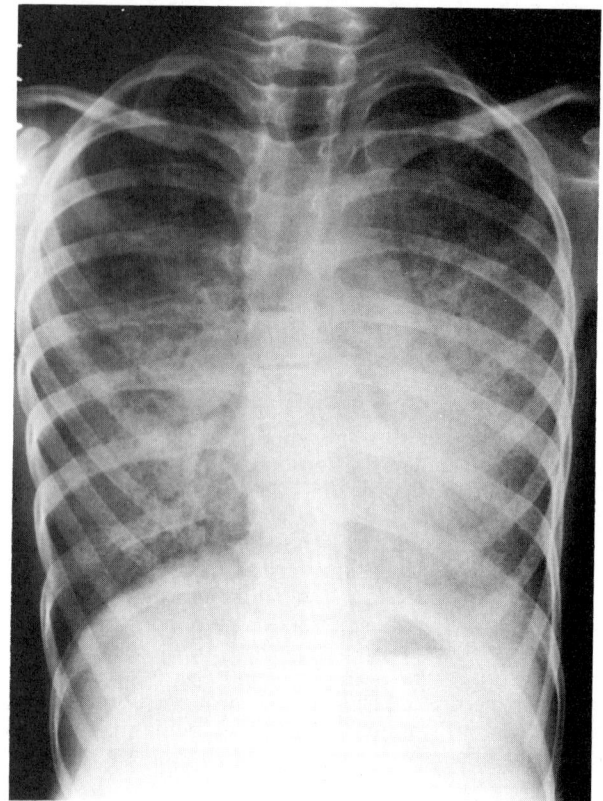

Figure 13–11. Alveolar proteinosis. PA view of chest shows diffuse alveolar infiltrate.

IgA is frequently low and other immunologic abnormalities are relatively common.

The diagnosis of pulmonary alveolar proteinosis must be confirmed by biopsy, although a sputum examination revealing a large amount of PAS-positive material with few or no inflammatory cells is suggestive of the disease. An amorphous lipid-protein complex progressively accumulates in the alveoli, but whether this material accumulates because of an accelerated rate of transport from the serum or because of defective clearance is unknown. Tissue sections show alveoli distended by fine, granular, eosinophilic material which stains positively with PAS stain.

Various immunologic deficiency states, including thymic alymphoplasia, have been found in some children with this disease. Not surprisingly, therefore, various fungal and bacterial superinfections also may be associated with the disease.

No effective treatment exists. Corticosteroids do not alter the relentless, progressive course of the illness. Aerosols with *N*-acetylcysteine or proteolytic enzymes have been reported effective, but the mainstay of treatment is repeated pulmonary lavage to clear out the alveoli. As techniques such as the use of the fiberoptic bronchoscope are improved, lavage can be accomplished without anesthesia and may often produce transient dramatic improvement; eventually, reaccumulation forces another series of lavages. Bacterial infection usually plays a relatively minor role in the progression of symptoms, and antibiotic therapy should be used conservatively. However, fatal fungal infections, as well as other opportunistic pathogens (including pneumocystis), have been reported. Survival has improved greatly with the introduction of modern bronchoscopic techniques. The adult form of pulmonary alveolar proteinosis has a much more favorable prognosis.

Case Records of the Massachusetts General Hospital (case 19–1983). N Engl J Med 308:1147, 1983.
Mazyck EM, Bonner JT, Herd HM, et al: Pulmonary lavage for childhood pulmonary alveolar proteinosis. J Pediatr 80:839, 1972.

Rosen SH, Castelman B, Liebow AA: Pulmonary alveolar proteinosis. N Engl J Med 258:1123, 1958.
Webster JR, Battifora H, Furrey C, et al: Pulmonary alveolar proteinosis in two siblings with decreased immunoglobulin A. Am J Med 69:786, 1980.
Wilkinson RH, Blanc WA, Hagstrom JWC: Pulmonary alveolar proteinosis in three infants. Pediatrics 41:510, 1968.

13.83 IDIOPATHIC DIFFUSE INTERSTITIAL FIBROSIS OF THE LUNG
(Hamman-Rich Syndrome)

This is a rare, chronic, usually fatal disorder of unknown origin, ordinarily observed in adults but occasionally in infants and children. The disease has been hypothesized to result from an uncontrolled inflammatory process following an otherwise minor insult to the lower respiratory tract. Alveolar macrophages, perhaps stimulated by immune complexes, may play a pivotal role by releasing chemotactic factors. The clinical pattern is characterized by progressive pulmonary insufficiency resulting from interstitial fibrosis and alveolar-capillary block.

Onset is usually insidious, with dyspnea initially occurring only with exercise but later present even at rest. A dry cough is frequent and may be productive of blood. The patient is usually afebrile. As the disease progresses, anorexia, weight loss, and fatigability occur, and finally cyanosis, clubbing of the fingers, cor pulmonale, and evidence of right-sided cardiac failure. Usually the lungs are clear on auscultation, but occasionally rales are present. Most children die of respiratory failure following one of the frequent intercurrent pulmonary infections. Serial roentgenograms show progressive widespread granular or reticular mottling or small nodular densities. Hypoxemia may be present and increase with exercise. There is no increase in airway resistance, and vital capacity, compliance, and diffusion capacity are decreased. Bronchoalveolar lavage fluid contains many inflammatory cells and relatively large numbers of mast cells. Gallium-67 scans are usually positive, with the abnormality restricted to the lungs.

The pulmonary pathology is variable. During the early stage of the disease, fibrosis is usually not present, but there is cellular infiltration of the walls of the alveoli, alveolar ducts, and peribronchial tissue by lymphocytes, plasma cells, and occasionally eosinophils. This usually progresses to extensive and diffuse proliferation of fibrous tissue throughout all the lobes of the lung and is associated with organization of intraalveolar exudate.

Corticosteroids may give some symptomatic relief but do not alter the progression of the disease or improve pulmonary function. Other therapy is also symptomatic. Immunosuppressant drugs have been used with benefit in some adults.

Bradley CA: Diffuse interstitial fibrosis of the lungs in children. J Pediatr 48:422, 1956.
Brown CH, Turner-Warwick M: The treatment of cyptogenic fibrosing alveolitis with immunosuppressant drugs. Quart J Med 40:289, 1971.
Crystal RG, Bitterman PB, Rennard SI, et al: Interstitial lung disease of unknown cause: Disorders characterized by inflammation of the lower respiratory tract. N Engl J Med 310:154, 1984.
Ivemark BI, Wallgren CG: Diffuse interstitial pulmonary fibrosis (Hamman-Rich syndrome) in an infant. Report of a case with histologic and respiratory studies. Acta Paediatr 51(Suppl 135):97, 1962.
Rubin EH, Lubliner R: The Hamman-Rich syndrome: Review of the literature and analysis of 15 cases. Medicine 36:397, 1957.

13.84 PULMONARY ALVEOLAR MICROLITHIASIS

This rare disease of unknown etiology often has its onset during childhood, but the clinical manifestations may be delayed until later years. It is characterized by widely disseminated intraalveolar calculi, which create a characteristic pattern on the roentgenogram (Fig. 13–12). Frequently, the

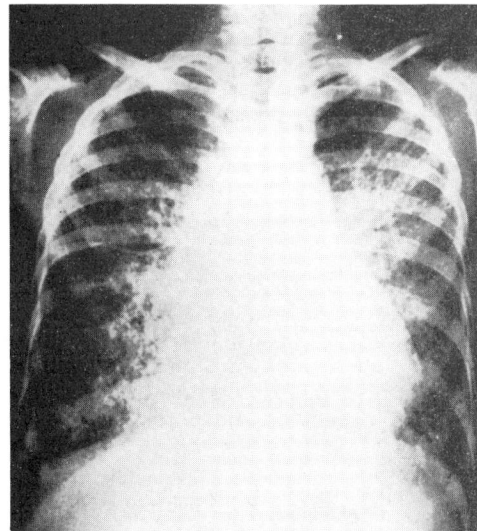

Figure 13–12. Roentgenogram of chest of a 7 yr old boy with pulmonary alveolar microlithiasis. (From Clark RB III, Johnson FC: Pediatrics 28:650, 1961.)

disease is recognized when the roentgenogram is taken for an unrelated illness or when symptoms are still minimal. Definitive diagnosis requires lung biopsy.

The familial incidence strongly suggests a genetic basis, but no specific metabolic abnormalities have been identified. Serum calcium and phosphorus are normal. No treatment is available, and patients eventually die during the middle years of adulthood of slowly progressive cardiorespiratory failure, often with superimposed infection. Bronchopulmonary lavage is ineffective. Following diagnosis, other family members should be screened by chest roentgenograms, and parents should be counseled that future children are also at risk to develop the disease. These children require prompt treatment of respiratory infection and should be advised about the dangers of smoking and exposure to industrial fumes. Immunization to measles and pertussis should be completed and yearly influenza vaccine given.

Caffrey PR, Altman RS: Pulmonary alveolar microlithiasis occurring in premature twins. J Pediatr 66:758, 1965.
Kino T, Kohara Y, Tsuji S: Pulmonary alveolar microlithiasis: A report in two young sisters. Am Rev Resp Dis 105:105, 1972.
Palombini BC, da Silva Porto N, Wallace CU: Bronchopulmonary lavage in alveolar microlithiasis. Chest 80:242, 1981.
Prakash UBS, Barham SS, Rosenow EC III, et al: Pulmonary alveolar microlithiasis: A review including ultrastructural and pulmonary function studies. Mayo Clin Proc 58:290, 1983.

EOSINOPHILIC GRANULOMA OF THE LUNG

See Sec. 26.5.

13.85 ATELECTASIS

Congenital atelectasis and hyaline membrane disease are discussed in Sec. 8.30 and 8.32.

Acquired Atelectasis

Etiology. Atelectasis, the imperfect expansion or the collapse of air-bearing tissue of the lung, is relatively common in infants and children. Collapse may be produced by any factor that completely obstructs the intake of air into the alveolar sacs and persists sufficiently long to permit absorption of alveolar air into the bloodstream. In general, the causes may be divided into three groups: (1) external pressure directly upon the pulmonary parenchyma or a bronchus or bronchiole, (2) intrabronchial or intrabronchiolar obstruction, and (3) any factor responsible for a continuously decreased amplitude of respiratory excursion or for respiratory paralysis. Bronchoconstriction and increased bronchosecretion due to allergy or other stimuli including embolus and chest wall trauma may also be contributing factors. Exudate formation may be responsible for atelectasis as in patients with cystic fibrosis.

EXTERNAL PRESSURE

External factors may be operative in one of two ways: either direct interference with expansion of lungs (pleural effusion, pneumothorax, intrathoracic tumors, diaphragmatic hernia) or external compression of a bronchus completely obstructing ingress of air (enlarged lymph node, tumors, cardiac enlargement).

INTRABRONCHIAL OR INTRABRONCHIOLAR OBSTRUCTION

See also Sec. 13.55.

Complete intraluminal obstruction of a bronchus may be produced by a foreign body; by a neoplasm; by granulomatous tissue, as in tuberculosis; or by secretions (including mucous plugs), as with cystic fibrosis, bronchiectasis, pulmonary abscess, allergy, chronic bronchitis, or acute laryngotracheobronchitis.

Obstruction of one or more bronchioles in a given area may be produced by any of the conditions mentioned, but widespread bronchiolar obstruction is most often produced by bronchiolitis or interstitial pneumonitis and by asthma. Generalized obstructive overinflation is the initial result of such bronchiolar obstructions, but as the pathologic changes progress, some of the bronchioles may become completely obstructed, and there are then interspersed small areas of atelectasis and emphysema. Patchy atelectasis is relatively common in acute bronchiolitis or asthma and is probably always present in advanced chronic diffuse infections, such as the pulmonary infection associated with cystic fibrosis.

REDUCED AMPLITUDE OF RESPIRATORY EXCURSION OR RESPIRATORY PARALYSIS

This may result from: (1) interference with the movements of the thoracic cage (neuromuscular abnormalities as in cerebral palsy, poliomyelitis, spinal muscular atrophy, myasthenia gravis; osseous deformities caused by rickets, scoliosis, kyphosis, scleroderma, overly restrictive casts, and surgical dressings); (2) defective movement of the diaphragm (paralysis of phrenic nerve, increased abdominal pressure); or (3) voluntary restriction of respiratory effort because of postoperative pain.

Pathology. The atelectatic areas are airless, congested, deep red, firm in consistency, and depressed below the neighboring healthy or emphysematous lung.

Clinical Manifestations. Symptoms vary with the cause and extent of the atelectasis. A small area is likely to be asymptomatic. When a large area of the lung becomes atelectatic, especially when it does so suddenly, dyspnea accompanied by rapid shallow respirations, tachycardia, and often cyanosis occurs. If the obstruction is removed, the symptoms disappear rapidly. Even atelectasis of an entire lobe may not be responsible for changes in the percussion note because there is compensatory expansion of the adjacent lung tissue. Breath and voice sounds are decreased or absent over extensive atelectatic areas.

Diagnosis. The diagnosis can usually be established by roentgenographic examination (Fig. 13–13). Small areas may be indistinguishable from pneumonic consolidations, but those that involve as many as several lobules of a lobe can

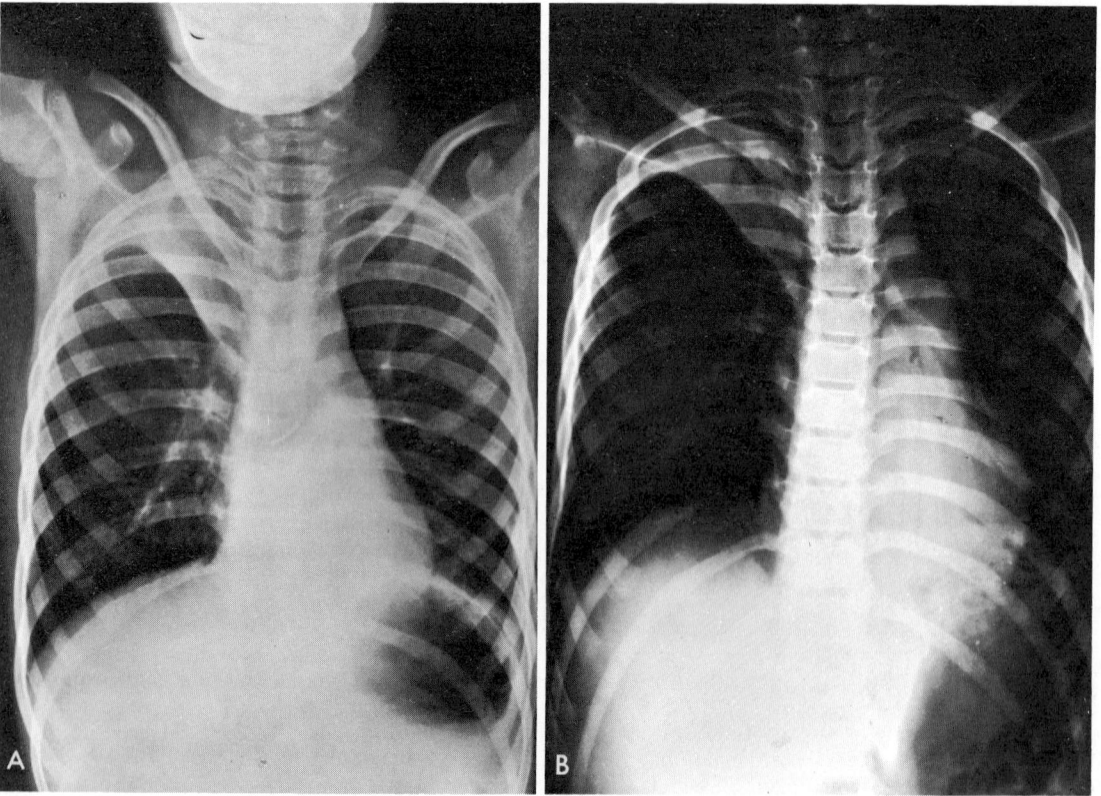

Figure 13–13. Atelectasis that occurred postoperatively and disappeared spontaneously. *A,* The right upper lobe and the left lower lobe are collapsed. The atelectasis of the left lower lobe is demonstrated on the overpenetrated film *(B).*

usually be identified by the contraction of the area. Bronchoscopic examination will reveal a collapsed main bronchus when the obstruction is at the tracheobronchial junction and may also disclose the nature of the obstruction.

Prognosis. If the obstruction disappears spontaneously or is removed, the atelectasis usually disappears unless secondary infection has occurred. The atelectatic area is more susceptible to infection because mucociliary clearance is impaired and cough is ineffective. In persistent cases bronchiectasis is a frequent complication and pulmonary abscess an occasional one.

Treatment. *Bronchoscopic examination* is immediately indicated if atelectasis is the result of a foreign body or any other bronchial obstruction that may be relieved. It is also indicated when an isolated area of atelectasis persists for several weeks. Usually, it is advisable to suction the orifice of the involved bronchus; occasionally, a **mucous plug** can be removed, with prompt re-expansion. If no anatomic basis for atelectasis is found and no material can be obtained by suctioning, the introduction of a small amount of saline followed by suctioning will allow recovery of bronchial secretions for culture and, possibly, for cytologic examination. Frequent *changes in the child's position and deep breathing* may be beneficial. *Oxygen* therapy is indicated when there is dyspnea. Morphine and atropine are contraindicated.

If the atelectasis is unchanged or only partially helped by bronchoscopy, *postural drainage* and, occasionally, *antibiotics* are indicated. In some situations, such as asthma, *bronchodilator* and, possibly, *corticosteroid* treatment may accelerate clearing of the atelectasis. Intermittent positive pressure breathing, incentive inspirometry, and blow bottles have been recommended, but their efficacy remains unproved.

Repeated bronchoscopies may be needed. Postural drainage should be continued at home. *Lobectomy* should not be considered unless chronic infection poses a threat to the remainder of the lung, bronchiectasis is demonstrated by bronchography, or systemic symptoms, such as anorexia or fatigue, are persistent. Occasionally, the atelectatic area becomes completely fibrosed; in this case no further treatment is needed.

Massive Pulmonary Atelectasis

Massive collapse of one or both lungs is most often a postoperative complication but occasionally results from other causes, such as trauma, asthma, pneumonia, tension pneumothorax, the aspiration of foreign material (either a solid object large enough to obstruct a main stem bronchus or liquids such as water or blood), or paralysis, as in diphtheria or poliomyelitis. Massive atelectasis is usually produced by a combination of factors: immobilization or decreased use of the diaphragm and the respiratory muscles, obstruction of the bronchial tree, and abolition of the cough reflex.

Clinical Manifestations. The onset in postoperative cases usually occurs within 24 hr after operation but may not occur for several days, with dyspnea, cyanosis, and tachycardia. The child is extremely anxious and, if old enough, complains of chest pain. Prostration is likely. The temperature may be as high as 39.5–40°C (103-104° F).

The physical signs are characteristic. The chest appears flat on the affected side, where there is also decreased respiratory excursion, dullness to percussion, and feeble or absent breath and voice sounds. Lower lobes are more frequently involved than upper ones. The heart and the mediastinum are displaced toward the affected side. Roentgenograms show the collapsed lung, elevation of the diaphragm, narrowing of the intercostal spaces, and displacement of the mediastinal structures and heart toward the affected side (Fig. 13–14).

Prognosis. Bilateral massive collapse is usually rapidly fatal, although prompt bronchoscopic aspiration and artificial respiration may be lifesaving. In the unilateral cases the prognosis is usually good.

Prevention. Prophylaxis is of the greatest importance. The incidence of postoperative atelectasis can be reduced by adequate ventilation during anesthesia. After operation the child's position in bed should be changed frequently, and collections of secretions in the oropharynx should be aspirated; when consciousness returns, the child should be encouraged to breathe deeply. Incentive inspirometers may be useful. Tight thoracic or abdominal binders should be avoided.

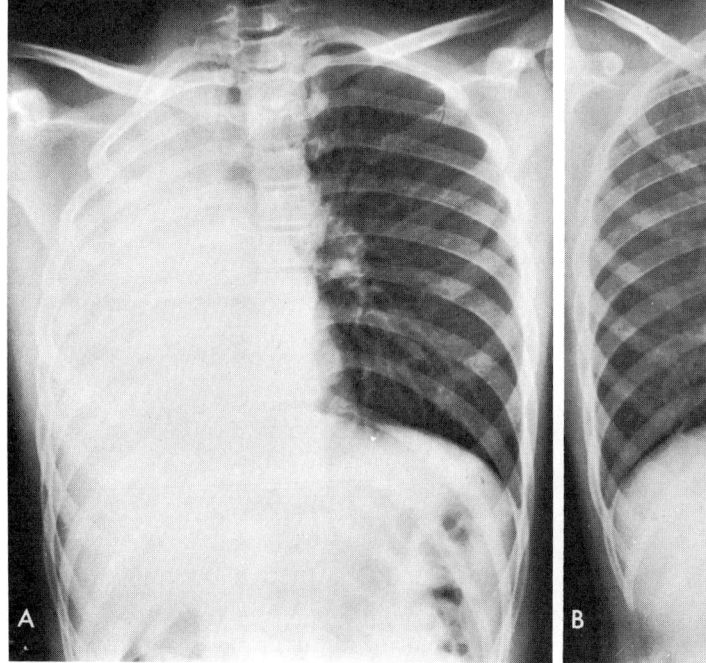
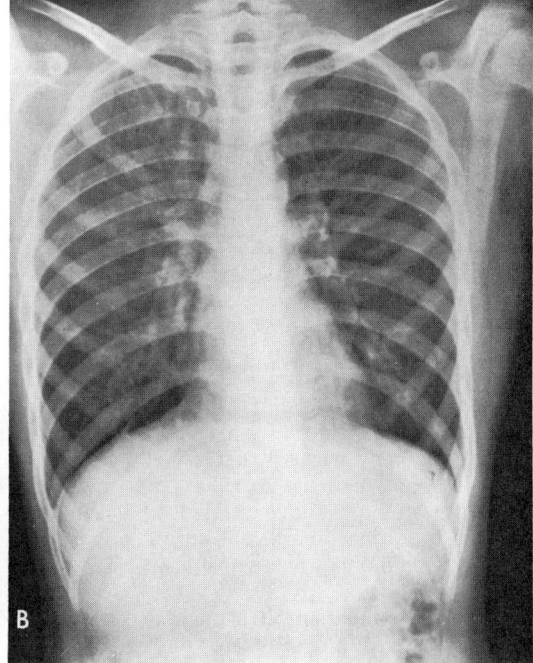

Figure 13–14. *A,* Massive atelectasis of the right lung. The patient is asthmatic. The heart and the other mediastinal structures are shifted to the right during the atelectatic phase. *B,* Comparison study after reaeration following bronchoscopic removal of a mucous plug from the right stem bronchus.

Treatment. When there is bilateral atelectasis, broncho-scopic aspiration should be performed immediately. When there is only unilateral atelectasis, the child should be placed on the unaffected side; forced coughing or crying while the child is lying on the unaffected side may also be helpful, as is positive pressure ventilation, but when these measures are unsuccessful, bronchoscopic aspiration should be performed.

Relapses are not infrequent, and the child should be kept under constant observation.

13.86 EMPHYSEMA AND OVERINFLATION

Pulmonary emphysema is a distention with irreversible rupture of the alveoli. It may be generalized or localized and involve part or all of a lung. Overinflation is a reversible distention without alveolar rupture.

Compensatory overinflation may be either acute or chronic. It occurs in normally functioning pulmonary tissue when for any reason a sizable portion of the lung is partially or completely airless, as may occur with pneumonia, atelectasis, empyema, and pneumothorax.

Obstructive overinflation results from partial obstruction of a bronchus or bronchiole, when getting air out of the alveoli becomes more difficult than getting it in; there is a gradual accumulation of air distal to the obstruction, the so-called bypass or check valve type of obstruction (Sec 13.5 and 13.55).

Localized Obstructive Overinflation

When a bypass type of obstruction partially occludes the main stem bronchus, the entire lobe becomes overinflated; only individual lobules are affected when the obstruction is that of a secondary bronchus. Localized obstructions that may be responsible for overinflation include foreign bodies and the inflammatory reaction to them, intrabronchial tuberculosis or tuberculosis of the tracheobronchial lymph nodes, and intrabronchial or mediastinal tumors. When most or all of a lobe is involved, the percussion note will be hyper-resonant over the area and the breath sounds decreased in intensity. The distended lung may extend across the mediastinum into the opposite hemithorax. Fluoroscopically, during expiration the overinflated area does not decrease in size, and the heart and the mediastinum shift to the opposite side.

Unilateral hyperlucent lung may occur in association with a variety of cardiac and pulmonary diseases of children, but in some patients it occurs without easily demonstrable underlying active disease. Over half the cases follow one or more episodes of pneumonia; in several patients a rising titer to adenovirus has been documented. Patients may present signs and symptoms of pneumonia, but some are discovered only when a chest roentgenogram is taken for an unrelated reason. A few patients have hemoptysis initially. Physical findings may include hyper-resonance and decreased breath sounds over the involved area. Chest roentgenogram reveals unilateral hyperlucency and an apparently small lung with the mediastinum shifted toward the more abnormal lung. Some patients will show mediastinal shift away from the lesion with expiration. Bronchiectasis may be demonstrated on bronchography. There is markedly decreased perfusion on the affected side. In some patients previous chest roentgeno-grams have been normal or have shown only an acute pneumonia, suggesting that hyperlucent lung is an acquired lesion. No specific treatment is known; it may become less symptomatic with time.

Congenital obstructive lobar emphysema may cause severe respiratory distress in early infancy. Familial occurrence has been reported. Symptoms usually become apparent in the neonatal period but may be delayed for as long as 5–6 mo in 5% of the patients. Occasional patients remain undiagnosed

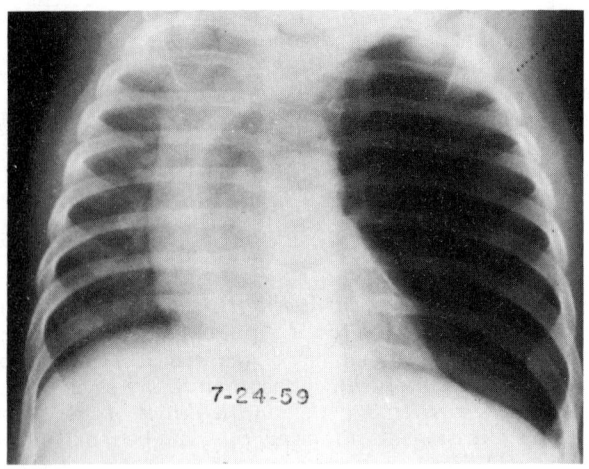

Figure 13–15. Congenital left upper lobe emphysema. Note extension of emphysematous lobe into left lower lobe and its displacement of the mediastinum toward the right.

until school age or beyond. A part, but usually all, of a lobe may be involved; the left upper lobe is most often affected. In some instances the obstruction is not demonstrable, but it is assumed to be produced by a check valve type of mechanism. Such obstructions have been attributed to defective or overly compliant cartilage in the bronchi, mucosal folds that create a valve-like obstruction, bronchial stenosis, and external compression by aberrant vessels or tumors. A radiolucent lobe and a mediastinal shift are often present on roentgeno-graphic examination. When the distention is considerable, the emphysematous lung compresses the unaffected lung below or above it and the opposite lung by extending across the mediastinum (Fig. 13–15). Immediate surgery and excision of the lobe may be lifesaving when cyanosis and severe respiratory distress are present, but some patients have responded to medical treatment.

Overinflation of all three lobes of the right lung has been produced by anomalous location of the left pulmonary artery, which partially constricts the right main bronchus. A number of neonates have developed lobar overinflation while being treated for hyaline membrane disease with assisted ventilation, suggesting an acquired etiology. Medical management, sometimes with selective intubation, has occasionally been successful and lobectomy avoided.

Cumming GR, Macpherson RI, Chernick V: unilateral hyperlucent lung syndrome in children. J Pediatr 78:250, 1971.

Dickman GL, Short BL, Krauss DR: Selective bronchial intubation in the management of unilateral pulmonary interstitial emphysema. Am J Dis Child 131:365, 1977.

Eigen H, Lemen RJ, Waring WW: Congenital lobar emphysema: Long-term evaluation of surgically and conservatively treated children. Am Rev Respir Dis 116:823, 1976.

McBride JT, Wohl MEB, Strieder D, et al: Lung growth and airway function after lobectomy in infancy for congenital lobar emphysema J Clin Invest 66:962, 1980.

McKenzie SA, Allison DJ, Singh MP, et al: Unilateral hyperlucent lung: The case for investigation. Thorax 35:745, 1980.

Shannon DC, Todres ID, Moylan FMB: Infantile lobar hyperinflation: Expectant treatment. Pediatrics 59:1012, 1977.

Wall MA, Eisenberg JD, Campbell JR: Congenital lobar emphysema in a mother and daughter. Pediatrics 70:131, 1982.

Generalized Obstructive Overinflation

Acute overinflation of the lung depends upon widespread involvement of the bronchioles and is reversible. It occurs more commonly in infants than in children and may be secondary to a number of clinical conditions, including res-piratory infections associated with cystic fibrosis of the pan-

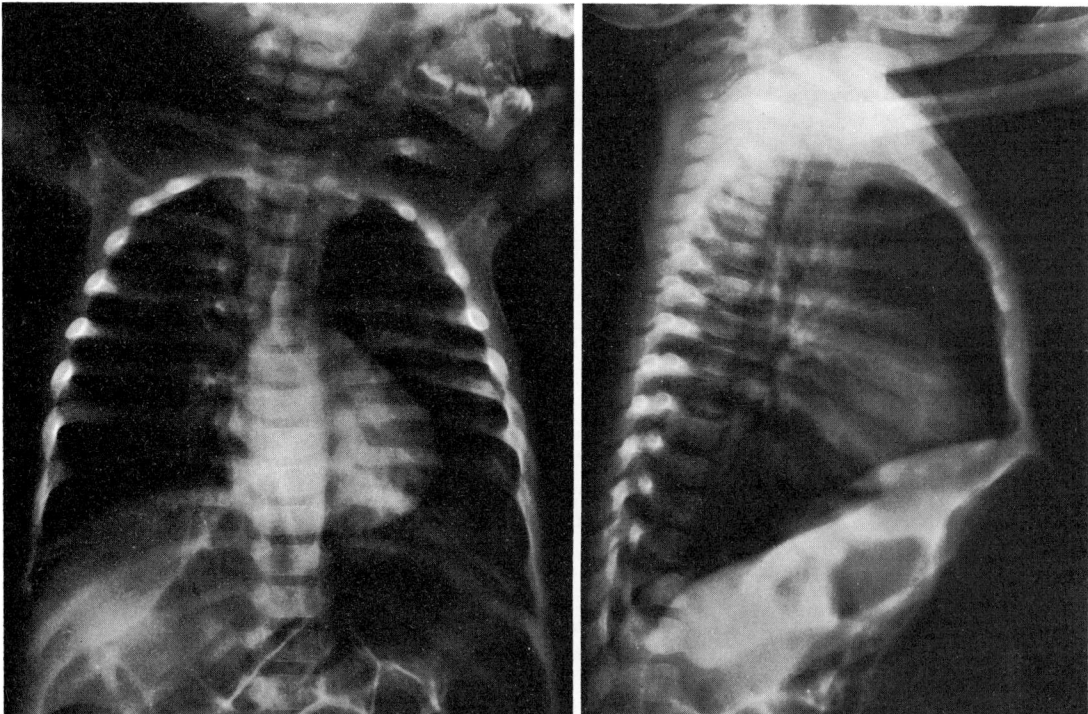

Figure 13–16. Generalized obstructive emphysema (overinflation): dorsal projections of thorax in inspiratory and expiratory phases of respiration. Notice the relative failure of the lungs to empty in the expiratory phase. The left lung is less obstructed than the right (empties to a greater degree in the expiratory phase). This difference between the lungs is not apparent from a study of the diaphragm, which moves very little during respiration; it is evident, however, in the upper portions of the left lung space.

creas, acute bronchiolitis, interstitial pneumonitis, atypical forms of acute laryngotracheobronchitis, aspiration of zinc stearate powder, chronic passive congestion secondary to a congenital cardiac lesion, and miliary tuberculosis. Asthma is a relatively frequent cause in older children but an uncommon one in infants.

Pathology. In chronic overinflation many of the alveoli are ruptured and communicate with one another, producing distended saccules. Air may also enter the interstitial tissue (*interstitial emphysema*), resulting in pneumomediastinum and pneumothorax (Sec. 8.37).

Clinical Manifestations. Generalized obstructive overinflation is characterized by an expiratory type of dyspnea. The lungs become increasingly overdistended, and the chest remains expanded during expiration. An increased respiratory rate and decreased respiratory excursions are due to the overdistention of the pulmonary alveoli and their inability to be emptied normally through the narrowed bronchioles. Air hunger is responsible for forced respiratory movements, and overaction of the accessory muscles of respiration results in retractions at the suprasternal notch, the supraclavicular spaces, the lower margin of the thorax, and the intercostal spaces. There is scarcely any reduction in size of the overdistended chest during expiration, in contrast to the flattened chest during both inspiration and expiration when there is laryngeal obstruction. There is no hoarseness or stridor as with laryngeal obstruction. Cyanosis is common in the severe cases. The percussion note is hyper-resonant, and on auscultation the inspiratory phase is usually less prominent than the expiratory phase, which is prolonged and roughened. Fine or medium rales may be present.

Roentgenographic and fluoroscopic examinations of the chest are a great help in establishing the diagnosis. Both leaves of the diaphragm are low and flattened, the ribs are farther apart than usual, and the lung fields are less dense

(Fig. 13–16). The movement of the diaphragm is restricted, best demonstrated by fluoroscopic examination. The normal "doming" of the diaphragm during expiration is decreased, and the excursion of the low, flattened diaphragm in the severe cases is barely discernible. Retention of air in the lungs during expiration is also increased by a paradoxical increase in the horizontal diameters of the chest during this phase.

Bullous Emphysema

Bullous emphysematous blebs or cysts (**pneumatoceles**) result from overdistention and rupture of alveoli during birth or shortly thereafter, or they may be sequelae of pneumonia and of other infections. They have been observed in tuberculous lesions while the patient was being treated with specific antibacterial therapy. These emphysematous areas presumably result from rupture of distended alveoli so that a single or multiloculated cavity is formed. The cysts may become large (Fig. 13–9C) and may contain some fluid; an air-fluid level may be demonstrated on the roentgenogram. They must be differentiated from pulmonary abscesses. In most instances the cysts disappear spontaneously within a few months, although they may persist for a year or more.

There is almost never any indication for aspiration or surgery unless there is severe respiratory and cardiac embarrassment.

Subcutaneous Emphysema

This occurs whenever free air finds its way into the subcutaneous tissue. It may be a complication of fracture of the orbit permitting free air to escape from the nasal sinuses. In the neck and thorax, subcutaneous emphysema may follow tracheotomy, deep ulcerations in the pharyngeal region, esophageal wounds, or any perforating lesion of the larynx or trachea. It is an occasional complication of thoracentesis, of asthma, or of abdominal surgery. Air may also be formed in the subcutaneous tissues by gas-producing bacteria.

The problem is usually self-limited and requires no specific treatment. Resolution occurs by resorption of subcutaneous air following elimination of its source. Rarely, dangerous compression of the trachea by air in the surrounding soft tissue requires surgical intervention.

Kress MB, Finklestein AH: Giant bullous emphysema occurring in tuberculosis in childhood. Pediatrics 30:269, 1962.
Nelson WE, Smith LW: Generalized obstructive emphysema in infants. J Pediatr 26:36, 1945.
Victoria MS, Steiner P, Rao M: Persistent pneumatoceles in children. Chest 79:359, 1981.

13.87 Alpha₁-Antitrypsin Deficiency and Emphysema

Homozygous deficiency of alpha₁-antitrypsin characterized by the early onset of severe panacinar emphysema is a rare cause of pulmonary disease in children. Alpha₁-antitrypsin and other serum antiproteases are thought to be important in the inactivation of proteolytic enzymes released from dead bacteria or leukocytes in the lung. Deficiency leads to accumulation of these enzymes, proteolytic destruction of pulmonary tissue, and development of emphysema. The concentration of proteases (e.g., elastase) in the patients' leukocytes may also be an important factor in determining the severity of clinical pulmonary disease with a given level of alpha₁-antitrypsin.

The type and concentration of alpha₁-antitrypsin are inherited as a series of codominant alleles; the inferred genotype is referred to as the "pi-type." Normal persons are pi-type MM. Type ZZ and, to a lesser extent, other abnormal pi-types such as SZ have been associated with early onset emphysema and a characteristic form of infantile cirrhosis (Sec. 12.79).

Most patients who have pi-type ZZ have had little or no detectable pulmonary disease during childhood. A few have had very early onset of chronic pulmonary symptoms, including dyspnea, wheezing, and cough, and panacinar emphysema has been documented by lung biopsy. Physical examination may reveal growth failure, an increased anteroposterior diameter of the chest with a hyper-resonant percussion note, rales if there is active infection, and clubbing. Severe emphysema may depress the liver and spleen, making them more easily palpable. Chest roentgenograms reveals overinflation with depressed diaphragms. Serum has a low trypsin inhibitory capacity, and immunoassay confirms the low level of alpha₁-antitrypsin.

Augmentation of alpha₁-antitrypsin synthesis in the liver is theoretically possible, even in patients with severe deficiency. Danazol, an analog of testosterone, has this effect, but its clinical efficacy is unknown. The efficacy of intravenous administration of large amounts of alpha₁-antitrypsin is also unknown. Pending the establishment of a specific treatment, efforts to minimize the presence of proteases in the lung are important. Thus prompt use of antibiotics is indicated for pulmonary infection, and postural drainage may be useful. Influenza vaccine should be administered yearly. The same measures are probably also indicated for other members of the family found to be pi-type ZZ even if they are asymptomatic. Persons with the MZ pi-type do not have an increased risk for developing pulmonary disease. The clinical significance of the SZ pi-type is unknown, but a similar treatment seems reasonable. All persons with low levels of serum antiprotease should be warned that the eventual development of emphysema may be partially related to environmental factors, including exposure to industrial fumes and cigarette smoking.

Bruce RM, Cohen BH, Diamond EL, et al: Collaborative study to assess risk of lung disease in Pi MZ phenotype subjects. Am Rev Respir Dis 130:366, 1984.
Gadek JE, Crystal RG: Experience with replacement therapy in the destructive lung disease associated with severe alpha₁-antitrypsin deficiency. Am Rev Respir Dis 127 (pt 2):545, 1983.
Kidokoro Y, Kravis TC, Moser KM, et al: Relationship of leukocyte elastase concentration to severity of emphysema in homozygous alpha₁-antitrypsin deficient persons. Am Rev Resp Dis 115:793, 1977.
National Institutes of Health: Intravenous replacement therapy for patients with severe α₁ antitrypsin deficiency. JAMA 248:1693, 1982.
Sveger T: Prospective study of children with α₁-antitrypsin deficiency: Eight-year-old follow-up. J Pediatr 104:91, 1984.

13.88 PULMONARY EDEMA

Etiology. Pulmonary edema results from the transudation of fluid from the pulmonary capillaries into the alveolar spaces and the bronchioles. It is usually associated with circulatory or neurocirculatory collapse and consequently is often a terminal event in a variety of diseases. Though pulmonary edema may vary in severity, even in its mildest stages it is an ominous finding. It is a common manifestation of left ventricular failure, the edema resulting from a rise in pulmonary venous pressure, or it may be due to hypervolemia from too rapid or too large an intravenous infusion. It may also be a manifestation of acute or chronic nephritis or, rarely, of pneumonic and other infections with substantial degrees of toxicity. Poisoning by such substances as barbiturates, morphine, epinephrine, and alcohol may be responsible for the development of pulmonary edema, as may the inhalation of toxic gases, such as illuminating gas, ammonia, and nitrogen dioxide, or the ingestion and consequent aspiration of highly volatile hydrocarbons, such as lighter fluid. (Also see Adult Respiratory Distress Syndrome, Sec. 5.41 and 13.89.)

Clinical Manifestations. The onset is variable but rapid in most instances. The child often complains of difficulty in breathing or a sense of oppression or pain in the chest. Cough is usually present and often produces a frothy, pink-tinged sputum. There is tachypnea, and the pulse is rapid and feeble. The child is usually very pale and may be cyanotic. On physical examination, dullness to percussion and moist, bubbly rales are heard in the lower portions of the chest. Chest roentgenogram shows a diffuse perihilar infiltrate (butterfly distribution). Occasionally, one lung is more affected than the other. If the pulmonary edema is superimposed on another pulmonary process (e.g., pneumococcal pneumonia, left heart failure in cystic fibrosis), the clinical and roentgenographic findings of the primary illness may obscure those of pulmonary edema.

Treatment. Treatment is directed at the primary disease causing the pulmonary edema. Administering oxygen is often useful in relieving some of the chest pain and when possible is best accomplished by intermittent positive pressure. Dyspnea can often be relieved by morphine sulfate, in a dosage of 0.1 mg/kg, and oxygen. Antifoaming agents and atropine are not useful. If pulmonary edema is secondary to excessive parenteral administration of fluids or blood or to cardiac failure, administration of diuretics, e.g., furosemide (1 mg/kg), digitalization, or bronchodilators, the application of tourniquets or inflated blood pressure cuffs to the extremities, or the withdrawal of blood may be lifesaving.

High Altitude Pulmonary Edema

This disease characteristically affects children and adolescents at altitudes above 2700 meters (8860 ft). The pathogenesis is unknown. Cough, shortness of breath, vomiting, and chest pain are the most common symptoms and occur within hours of high altitude exposure. Not all persons are affected, and even affected persons may not develop symptoms after every exposure. Chest roentgenogram reveals bilateral patchy pulmonary infiltrates. Oxygen is indicated. Bed rest, diuretics, antibiotics, and corticosteroids have been used, but their efficacy has not been established. Recovery usually occurs within 48 hr, and further residence at high altitude is then tolerated without symptoms. The disease may recur, however, following return to high altitude after even a brief visit to lower levels.

Scoggin CH, Hyers TM, Reeves JT, et al: High-altitude pulmonary edema in the children and young adults of Leadville, Colorado. N Engl J Med 297:1269, 1977.

Spring CL, Rackow EC, Fein IA, et al: The spectrum of pulmonary edema; Differentiation of cardiogenic, intermediate, and noncardiogenic forms of pulmonary edema. Am Rev Respir Dis 124:716, 1981.

13.89 Adult Respiratory Distress Syndrome (ARDS)

Noncardiogenic pulmonary edema may occur in previously healthy persons after an acute massive pulmonary injury. Although the original insult may vary considerably, the subsequent clinical course and pathology is fairly uniform. Reports of children with this syndrome have been increasing.

The etiology of ARDS may be a primary pulmonary event (e.g., inhalation of certain toxic fumes or massive aspiration) or a systemic condition (e.g., shock), but the common feature is diffuse alveolar injury. Pathologic findings include congestion, atelectasis, hyaline membranes, and fibrosis. The final common pathophysiologic pathway may involve activation of the complement system and subsequent neutrophil-aggregation induced by C5a. Aggregated neutrophils release a variety of substances, including proteases and toxic oxygen radicals; the oxygen radicals inactivate the antiproteases, and the unopposed proteases then damage the lung. Pulmonary intravascular coagulation may also play a role.

Respiratory distress occurs with tachypnea, marked use of the accessory muscles of respiration, and severe hypoxemia with little or no hypercapnia. Chest roentgenograms show interstitial infiltrates early in the course and alveolar infiltrates later. The diagnosis is based on clinical findings, historical data, and exclusion of primary pulmonary disease.

Treatment is supportive and includes continuous positive pressure ventilation with positive end-expiratory pressure, supplemental oxygen, avoidance of fluid overload, treatment of infection, and maintenance of nutrition. Parenteral alimentation is often necessary. Avoiding extrapulmonary organ failure is extremely important, since pulmonary status often markedly worsens in the presence of renal or hepatic failure or central nervous system dysfunction. Specific therapy, based on pathophysiology, is not yet available. Controlled studies of corticosteroids have not been reported.

The prognosis is guarded. In children, reported mortality ranges from 28 to 94%. The incidence of long-term pulmonary sequelae in surviving children has not been reported.

Lyrene RK, Truog WE: Adult respiratory distress syndrome in a pediatric intensive care unit: Predisposing conditions, clinical course and outcome. Pediatrics 67:790, 1981.

Petty TL: Adult respiratory distress syndrome: definition and historical perspective. Clin Chest Med 3:3, 1982.

Pfenninger J, Gerber A, Tschappeler H, et al: Adult respiratory distress syndrome in children. J Pediatr 101:352, 1982.

Rinaldo JE, Rogers RM: Adult respiratory-distress syndrome: Changing concepts of lung injury and repair. New Engl J Med 306:900, 1982.

Tate RM Repine JE: Neutrophils and the adult respiratory distress syndrome. Am Rev Respir Dis 128:552, 1983.

13.90 PULMONARY EMBOLISM AND INFARCTION

Pulmonary embolism is rare in infants and children and most often arises from thrombi in the femoral and pelvic veins, usually as a postoperative complication. Scoliosis surgery, in particular, may predispose to deep vein thrombosis and pulmonary embolization. Pulmonary emboli are not uncommon following spinal cord injury and in severe burns. Embolization may also occur following prolonged inactivity or as a complication of intravenous infusions. Intrapulmonary thrombosis also may occur in sickle cell anemia; the subsequent infarction is often difficult to differentiate from pneumonia. Fat emboli are most likely to be derived from fractured bones; on occasion they stem from necrotic tissue in the bone marrow of patients with sickle cell disease. Multiple pulmonary infarcts resulting from small emboli may be associated with severe dehydration in diarrheal disease, cyanotic heart disease, bacterial endocarditis, ventriculoatrial shunts for the treatment of hydrocephalus, and longstanding nutritional deficiencies.

Clinical Manifestations. The clinical pattern often suggests pneumonia, and the diagnosis is usually made at autopsy. Emboli carrying bacteria may be responsible for multiple pulmonary abscesses. In addition to the classic physical findings of phlebothrombosis and thrombophlebitis, radio-labeled fibrinogen, impedance plethysmography, Doppler ultrasound, and contrast venography may help define the presence and extent of deep venous thromboses.

Embolism of the pulmonary artery or its larger branches produces a variable clinical picture. Dyspnea is common, although often transient; pain and collapse are often absent. If present, pain is usually substernal, but it may be pleural and may radiate to the shoulder. Though there are often no physical signs, if the infarct is sufficiently large, there may be impaired resonance and a pleural friction rub. Breath sounds may be distant or absent, and there may be moist rales. Expectorated material, which may be profuse, often contains blood. Large emboli can cause acute right heart failure by raising pulmonary arterial pressure. However, infarction often does not occur and the classic triad of pleuritic chest pain, hemoptysis, and infiltrate is usually absent in pulmonary embolism. The case fatality rate is high, but recovery may occur even when the area of infarction is relatively large. Secondary infection may result in abscess formation.

Chest roentgenograms, although useful in ruling out other treatable causes of the patient's symptoms (e.g., pneumothorax), are often normal and rarely diagnostic. In critically ill patients in whom definitive diagnosis is urgent, pulmonary perfusion studies, ventilation scintiphotography, and pulmonary angiogram should be considered; only angiography gives unequivocal evidence of embolism, but its risk must be weighed against the risk of therapy. In children who are not gravely ill, empiric low dose heparin therapy in "probable pulmonary embolism" may be preferable to angiography.

Exchange transfusion should precede bronchoscopy in patients with sickle cell anemia; otherwise, massive, potentially fatal pulmonary thrombosis may occur.

Chronic showers of emboli from **ventriculoatrial shunts** may cause gradual obliteration of the pulmonary vascular bed and eventually pulmonary hypertension. Clinical findings are those of pulmonary hypertension and may include accentuation of the pulmonic component of the second heart sound and the development of pulmonary or tricuspid insufficiency. In severe cases, exercise intolerance and right-sided heart failure occur, indicating that substantial compromise of lung function has already taken place. Serial electrocardiograms that show increasing right ventricular hypertrophy may give an early clue to continuing chronic embolization. Diagnosis may be confirmed by right heart catheterization and determination of pulmonary arterial blood pressure. If chronic embolization is suspected, the shunt should be removed.

Treatment. Massive embolization of the larger branches of the pulmonary artery is a medical emergency. The initial objective in management is to support cardiovascular function and to prevent circulatory collapse and pulmonary insufficiency through cardiotonic drugs, oxygen, and ventilatory assistance. After stabilization and definitive diagnosis, efforts should be made to prevent further embolization. Recurrent pulmonary emboli arising in patients with deep vein thrombosis may be prevented by immediate anticoagulation with intravenous heparin given by continuous infusion or intermittently (50–100 units/kg given every 4 hr) to maintain the clotting time at 1.5 times the baseline level just prior to the next dose. Heparinization is usually followed by chronic oral anticoagulation with one of the coumarin drugs (sodium warfarin or bishydroxycoumarin). Anticoagulation is usually discontinued after 6 mo. The use of thrombolytic agents remains controversial.

Bromberg PA: Pulmonary aspects of sickle cell anemia. Arch Intern Med 133:652, 1974.

Friedman S, Zita-Gozum C, Chatten J: Pulmonary vascular changes complicating ventriculovascular shunting for hydrocephalus. J Pediatr 64:305, 1964.

Moser KM: Diagnosis and management of pulmonary embolism. Hosp Pract 15:57, 1980.

Sharma GVRK, Burleson VA, Sasahara AA: Effect of thrombolytic therapy on pulmonary-capillary blood volume in patients with pulmonary embolism. New Engl J Med 303:842, 1980.

Uden A: Thromboembolic complications following scoliosis surgery in Scandinavia. Acta Orthrop Scand 50:175, 1979.

PULMONARY SUPPURATION

13.91 Bronchiectasis

Bronchiectasis refers to dilatation of the bronchi associated with inflammatory destruction of bronchial and peribronchial tissue, accumulation of exudative material in dependent bronchi, and, in some instances, distention of dependent bronchi.

Etiology. Some patients may have *congenital bronchiectasis* possibly due to an arrest in bronchial development leading to cyst formation and the destruction of the bronchial wall when the cysts become infected. Alternatively, there may be defective development of the bronchial cartilaginous supports. Tracheobronchomegaly is a rare congenital condition in which the distal trachea and main bronchi are grossly dilated; a similar condition may be associated with recurrent pneumonia.

The majority of instances of bronchiectasis are acquired after birth, usually resulting from chronic pulmonary infection, but the mechanisms involved are poorly understood. Obstruction of the bronchial tree followed by infection is one likely cause. Measles, pertussis, and pneumonia are rare causes of bronchiectasis. Cystic fibrosis is the most common underlying disease in children with generalized bronchial involvement. Other predisposing factors include aspiration of a foreign body, often a nonopaque one, enlarged bronchopulmonary nodes due to tuberculosis, recurrent and chronic lung infections, sarcoidosis, neoplasm, lung abscess, localized cysts, emphysema with compression of the other lung parenchyma, allergy, asthma, and, rarely, extreme forms of pectus excavatum or scoliosis. Patients with immune deficiency syndromes may have bronchiectasis, usually after repeated attacks of bacterial pneumonia and bronchitis. Recurrent aspiration pneumonitis in familial dysautonomia frequently leads to bronchiectasis. The immotile cilia syndrome (Sec. 13.63) results in chronic pulmonary infection which eventually leads to bronchiectasis. Gastroesophageal reflux with chronic aspiration may be a cause of bronchiectasis.

Reversible bronchiectasis or pseudobronchiectasis occurs commonly after pertussis as well as with lobar and interstitial pneumonias. Shortly after or during these illnesses the bronchi may appear cylindrically dilated on bronchography, but if these studies are repeated months later, the changes have disappeared.

Pathology. The first destructive change is a loss of ciliated epithelium, which is regenerated as cuboidal and squamous epithelium. Concurrently the elastic tissue within the bronchial walls disappears and thickening occurs, due to interstitial edema, fibrosis, and round cell infiltration. In adjacent parenchymal and peribronchial tissue, multiple abscesses may develop, and there usually is characteristic obstructive endarteritis of the small pulmonary vessels. Generally, bronchiectasis follows a segmental distribution, except in cystic fibrosis. The right middle lobe segments, the basal segments of the lower lobes, and the lingular segments of the left upper lobe are most frequently affected. The right lower lobe is commonly involved in aspiration of a foreign body, whereas the right middle lobe is most frequently affected by hilar lymphadenopathy.

Clinical Manifestations. In symptomatic cases cough is invariably present and produces copious mucopurulent sputum during acute respiratory infections. The sputum is generally swallowed by young children. Physical activity or change in position, particularly while reclining, will often initiate a bout of coughing.

Recurring infections of the lower respiratory tract are common; they tend to persist and are difficult to control. Anorexia, irritability, and poor weight gain are also common. Fever is much less common. Later in the course, during acute exacerbations, hemoptysis may occur, varying in severity from blood streaked sputum to exsanguinating hemorrhage. Bronchiectasis characteristically follows an intermittently improving and relapsing course.

Physical findings are absent or few. Clubbing of the fingers may be present if the patient has been symptomatic for over 1 yr. Moist or musical rales may be heard or elicited by cough; during acute exacerbations physical signs of atelectasis or diffuse pneumonitis are often present. The usual roentgen examination is never pathognomonic, although mediastinal lymph nodes, radiopaque foreign bodies, and bronchovascular marking near the hilus of the lung may be suggestive. Atelectasis is relatively common.

With extensive bronchiectasis there is persistent dyspnea, and physical development is retarded. Ventilatory and diffusion studies may reveal more widespread or severe pulmonary involvement than suspected otherwise.

Every patient with suspected or proved bronchiectasis should be evaluated for sinusitis, immotile cilia, agammaglobulinemia, tuberculosis, asthma or other respiratory allergy, and cystic fibrosis. If such a diagnosis cannot be made, these patients should have bronchoscopy to exclude bronchial stenosis, strictures, tumors, and foreign bodies, and then bronchography to document the bronchiectasis and determine its extent and severity. A familial deficiency of bronchial cartilage has also been proposed as an explanation of some cases of bronchiectasis in childhood and may be suggested by marked dilatation of the 2nd–4th order bronchi during inspiration and apparent collapse during expiration. Bronchoscopic washings and sputum samples should be cultured for routine pathogens, mycobacteria, and fungi, and a tuberculin skin test should be done.

The **middle lobe syndrome** may occur, which consists of subacute or chronic pneumonitis, bronchial obstruction, and atelectasis, and is generally caused by extrinsic compression of the middle lobe bronchus by hilar nodes, followed by peribronchitis and chronic infection. Bronchiectasis may result. On occasion this syndrome is related to asthma or congenital anomalies of the bronchi.

Young syndrome is characterized by sinusitis and bronchiectasis, often symptomatic in childhood, and by azoospermia, not detectable until later, when semen analysis can be done. Clubbing is rarely seen. Some patients develop azoospermia after a period of fertility. Urologic procedures to reestablish fertility later have been disappointing. The severity of pulmonary symptoms seems to ameliorate during adolescence or young adult life.

Therapy. Treatment includes elimination of all foci of respiratory infection, effective postural drainage, and, when indicated, antibiotic therapy. Postural drainage must be carried out intensively as long as secretions are being formed and is one of the most important aspects of management.

Systemic antibiotic therapy is usually administered only during acute exacerbations in courses of 5–7 days to 2 wk. Patients with cystic fibrosis require more prolonged therapy (Sec. 13.97). Prolonged treatment for most other patients, however, increases the risks of acquiring resistant flora and of drug reactions. The appropriate drug is selected on the basis of the antibiotic susceptibility of bacteria isolated from sputum or at bronchoscopy. If cultures contain only normal flora, antibiotics should not be used. Administering antibiotics by aerosol inhalation immediately following appropriate postural drainage may also be helpful but should not be continued for excessively long periods of time, since this encourages the establishment of a drug-resistant bacterial flora. *Pseudomonas* is particularly troublesome.

When localized severe disease progresses despite adequate medical management, segmental or lobar resection should be considered, even though the long-term results are often discouraging. Some patients with lobar bronchiectasis, especially those with the right middle lobe syndrome, do very well postlobectomy. Surgery may also be indicated when an intrinsic anatomic obstruction of the bronchus is found or when suppurative lesions exist due to aspiration of fragmented foreign bodies, especially such vegetal objects as grass fibers or fragments of peanut which elude bronchoscopic removal.

Becroft DMO: Bronchiolitis obliterans, bronchiectasis and other sequelae of adenovirus type 21 infection. J Clin Pathol 24:72, 1971.

Clark NS: Bronchiectasis in childhood. Br Med J 1:80, 1963.

Davis PB, Hubbard VS, McCoy K, et al: Familial bronchiectasis. J Pediatr 102:177, 1983.

Dees SC, Spock A: Right middle lobe syndrome in children. JAMA 197:8, 1966.

Field CE: Bronchiectasis: Third report of a follow-up study of medical and surgical cases from childhood. Arch Dis Child 44:551, 1969.

Handelsman DJ, Conway AJ, Boylan LM, et al: Young's syndrome: Obstructive azoospermia and chronic sinopulmonary infections. N Engl J Med 310:3, 1984.

Mitchell RE, Bury RG: Congenital bronchiectasis due to deficiency of bronchial cartilage (Williams-Campbell syndrome): Case report. J Pediatr 87:230, 1975.

Williams H, O'Reilly RN: Bronchiectasis in children: Its multiple clinical and pathological aspects. Arch Dis Child 34:192, 1959.

13.92 Pulmonary Abscess

A lung abscess is a suppurative process resulting in destruction of the pulmonary parenchyma and formation of a cavity containing purulent material. In children they most often result from the *aspiration of infected material* when the local defense mechanisms are overwhelmed by a large number of virulent microorganisms or compromised by such factors as alcohol, drug abuse, recent surgery (particularly tonsillectomy or adenoidectomy), or systemic disease. Aspirated material containing bacteria that are normal inhabitants of the naso- and oropharynx reaches the most dependent portions of the lung. Thus, the posterior segments of the upper lobes and the superior segments of the lower lobes are most frequently involved, and anaerobic bacteria including bacteroides, *Fusobacterium*, and anaerobic streptococci are commonly isolated. Occasionally *pneumonia* caused by aerobic pyogenic microorganisms (*Staphylococcus aureus* and *Klebsiella*) or *bronchial obstruction* due to a tumor or foreign body may be complicated by abscess formation. *Metastatic lung abscess* secondary to septic emboli from right-sided bacterial endocarditis and septic thrombophlebitis is uncommon in children. Rare causes also include amebic abscess of the lung and infections with *Nocardia*, actinomyces, and mycobacteria.

Pathology. Lung abscesses occur when pulmonary parenchyma becomes obstructed, infected, and then suppurative and necrotic. Initial inflammatory changes are followed by suppuration and thrombosis of the local blood vessels, which result in necrosis and liquefaction. Granulation tissue forms around the periphery of the abscess and may succeed in walling off the area, but more commonly the abscess ruptures into a bronchus. Contents of the abscess may then be coughed up or aspirated into other parts of the pulmonary tree with additional abscess formation. Sputum is usually fetid. Peripheral abscesses may involve the adjacent pleura, with development of an associated pleural effusion. Abscesses may rupture into the pleural cavity and produce empyema.

Clinical Manifestations. The onset is generally insidious, with fever, malaise, anorexia, and weight loss. Cough, often associated with hemoptysis and producing copious amounts of foul-smelling or purulent sputum, is characteristic about 10 days after the onset in untreated patients. Lung abscess secondary to staphylococcal and *Klebsiella* pneumonia produces the acute signs and symptoms described for bacterial pneumonia. There may be respiratory distress, spiking fevers, chest pain, and marked leukocytosis. The diagnosis is generally made by roentgenographic examination when a cavity with or without a fluid level surrounded by alveolar infiltration is demonstrated. Gram stain of the sputum may reveal numerous polymorphonuclear leukocytes and findings consistent with anaerobic microorganisms, such as pleomorphic, slender, gram-negative bacilli (bacteroides, *Fusobacterium*); gram-negative rods with tapered ends (*Fusobacterium*); large gram-positive bacilli (clostridium); and tiny to small cocci (anaerobic streptococci). Sputum cultures characteristically yield a mixture of anaerobic bacteria.

Treatment. If a predominant aerobic organism is identified, appropriate antibiotic therapy is initiated. However, if lung abscess is secondary to aspiration and the Gram stain is compatible with anaerobic bacteria, treatment with penicillin (100,000 U/kg/24 hr) for an extended period of time (4–6 wk) is the treatment of choice pending the results of anaerobic sputum culture. This drug is effective even in patients infected with penicillin-resistant strains of *Bacteroides fragilis*. Alternative treatment in children allergic to penicillin is chloramphenicol. Experience with clindamycin and metronidazole in children is limited. Appropriate investigation for dental disease should be done in older children and adolescents.

Serial chest roentgenograms show gradual diminution in the size of the abscess cavity over a period of several weeks or months. Most patients are afebrile within 1 wk of institution of appropriate antibiotic therapy. Delayed closure is common. Bronchoscopy is indicated only to identify and remove a foreign body. The routine use of bronchoscopy to facilitate drainage or to obtain culture material is controversial. Chest tube drainage is necessary if empyema occurs. Surgical drainage of a lung abscess is almost never indicated, and resection should be considered only in children with recurrent hemoptysis, a bronchopleural fistula, repeated episodes of infection, or suspicion of malignancy.

The overall prognosis for complete recovery from primary lung abscess is excellent. In patients with secondary lung abscess, the prognosis heavily depends on the underlying disease.

Asher MI, Spier S, Beland M, et al: Primary lung abscess in childhood. Am J Dis Child 136:491, 1982.

Bartlett JG, Gorbach SL, Tally FP et al: Bacteriology and treatment of primary lung abscess. Am Rev Respir Dis 109:510, 1974.

Brook I, Finegold JM: Bacteriology and therapy of lung abscess in children. J Pediatr 94:10, 1979.

Levine MM, Ashman R, Heald F: Anaerobic (putrid) lung abscess in adolescence. Am J Dis Child 130:77, 1976.

13.93 Pulmonary Gangrene

Gangrene of the lung is extremely rare but occasionally follows measles and is seen in persons with severe immunologic deficits. The onset is usually sudden and is associated with early pulmonary hemorrhage; there is rapid development of pneumothorax and putrid empyema, and death may occur quickly. Treatment consists of adequate pleural drainage and intensive antibiotic therapy.

13.94 HERNIA OF LUNG

Protrusion of the lung beyond its normal thoracic boundaries may be a complication of pulmonary disease in which there is frequent coughing with generation of high intrathoracic pressure, such as cystic fibrosis or asthma, or may result from a congenital weakness of the suprapleural membrane or the musculature of the neck. Over half of congenital lung hernias and almost all acquired lung hernias are cervical. Paravertebral or parasternal hernias are usually due to rib anomalies. The presenting complaint is usually the presence of a mass in the neck while straining or coughing. Occasionally, transient pain is noted in the region of the hernia. Physical examination is normal except during a Valsalva maneuver when a soft bulge is noted in the neck. In most cases no treatment is necessary. Occasionally a surgical procedure is justified for cosmetic purposes. In patients with severe chronic pulmonary disease in whom coughing is present daily and cough suppression is contraindicated, permanent surgical correction may not be achieved.

Bronsther B, Coryllos E, Epstein B, et al: Lung hernias in children. J Pediatr Surg 3:544, 1968.
Jones JG: Cervical hernia of the lung. J Pediatr 76:122, 1970.

13.95 PULMONARY NEOPLASMS

Metastatic lesions, such as Wilms tumor, osteogenic sarcoma, and hepatoblastoma, are the most common forms of pulmonary malignancy in childhood (Chapters 16 and 17). A great variety of primary tumors have been reported, but all are extremely rare. Fewer than 250 cases, including 150 malignancies, have been reported in English-language journals. Bronchial adenoma are the most common. A high incidence of "inflammatory pseudotumors" clouds the statistics. Patients with symptoms, or with roentgenographic or other laboratory findings suggesting pulmonary malignancy, should be searched carefully for a tumor at another site before surgical excision is done. Pulmonary tumors may present with fever, hemoptysis, wheezing, cough, pleural effusion, chest pain, dyspnea, or recurrent or persistent pneumonia or atelectasis. Isolated primary lesions and isolated metastatic lesions discovered long after the primary tumor has been removed are best treated by excision. Prognosis is variable and depends on the type of tumor involved.

ROBERT C. STERN

Case records of the Massachusetts General Hospital (Case 4–1976). N Engl J Med 294:210, 1976.
Emory WB, Mitchell WT Jr, Hatch HB Jr: Mucous gland adenoma of the bronchus. Am Rev Resp Dis 108:1407, 1973.
Hartman GE, Shochat SJ: Primary pulmonary neoplasms of childhood: A review. Am Thorac Surg 36:108, 1983.
Wellons HA Jr, Eggleston P, Golden GT, Allen MS: Bronchial adenoma in childhood: Two case reports and review of the literature. Am J Dis Child 130:301, 1976.

13.96 AN APPROACH TO RECURRENT OR PERSISTENT LOWER RESPIRATORY TRACT SYMPTOMS IN CHILDREN

Respiratory tract symptoms such as cough, wheeze, and stridor may occur frequently or persist for long periods of time in a substantial number of children; in others there may be persistent and recurring lung infiltrates with or without

symptoms. Determining the cause of these chronic findings can be very difficult since symptoms may be due to a rapid succession of unrelated acute respiratory tract infections or to a single pathophysiologic process, and there is a paucity of easily performed, specific diagnostic tests for many acute and chronic respiratory conditions. Pressure from the affected child's family for a quick remedy because of concern over symptoms related to breathing may complicate diagnostic and therapeutic efforts.

A systematic approach to the diagnosis and treatment of these children consists of: (1) determining whether the symptom is the manifestation of a minor problem or a life-threatening process; (2) establishing or hypothesizing the most likely underlying pathogenic mechanism; (3) selecting the simplest effective therapy for the underlying process, which may often be only symptomatic therapy; and (4) carefully evaluating the effect of therapy to verify the correctness of the diagnosis and to determine whether additional therapy is required.

Judging the Seriousness of Chronic Respiratory Complaints

Clinical manifestations suggesting that a respiratory tract illness may be life-threatening or associated with the potential for chronic disability are listed in Table 13–2. If none of these are detected, the chronic respiratory process is usually benign. Active, well nourished, and appropriately growing infants who present with intermittent noisy breathing but no other physical or laboratory abnormalities require only symptomatic treatment and parental reassurance. Initially benign-appearing but persistent symptoms occasionally may be the harbinger of a serious lower respiratory tract problem and, conversely, a few children (e.g., with infection-related asthma) may have acute recurrent life-threatening episodes but few or no symptoms in the interval. Repeated examinations over an extended period of time, both when the child appears healthy and when the child is symptomatic, may be required.

Differential Diagnostic Features

Recurrent or Persistent Cough. Cough is a reflex response of the lower respiratory tract to stimulation of irritant or cough receptors in the tracheobronchial mucosa. A common cause in children, presenting without other respiratory tract signs and symptoms, is reactive airways (asthma). Since cough receptors also reside in the pharynx, stomach, and external auditory canal, the source of a persistent cough may need to be sought beyond the respiratory tract. Specific lower respiratory stimuli include excessive secretions, aspirated foreign material, inhaled dust particles or noxious gases, and an inflammatory response to infectious agents or allergic processes. Some of the conditions responsible for chronic cough are listed in Table 13–3.

Some characteristics of cough that may aid in distinguishing its origin are presented in Table 13–4. Additional information may include: (1) a history of atopic conditions (asthma,

Table 13–2. Evidence of Serious Chronic Lower Respiratory Tract Disease in Children

Persistent fever
Restriction of activity
Failure to grow
Failure to gain weight appropriately
Clubbing of the digits
Persistent tachypnea and labored ventilation
Persistent hyperinflation
Substantial hypoxia
Roentgenographic infiltrates
Persistent pulmonary function abnormalities

Table 13–3. Differential Diagnosis of Recurrent and Persistent Cough in Children

Recurrent cough
  Increased bronchial reactivity, including asthma
  Drainage from upper airways
  Occasional aspiration (as in pharyngeal incoordination)
  Frequently recurring respiratory tract infections
  Idiopathic pulmonary hemosiderosis
Persistent cough
  Postinfection hypersensitivity of cough receptors
  Reactive airways disease (asthma)
  Asthmatic bronchitis
  Bronchitis, tracheitis due to chronic infection, smoking (in older children)
  Bronchiectasis, including cystic fibrosis, dysmotile cilia syndrome
  Foreign body aspiration
  Recurrent aspiration due to pharyngeal incompetence, tracheolaryngoesophageal cleft, tracheoesophageal fistula, gastroesophageal reflux
  Pertussis syndrome
  Extrinsic compression of the tracheobronchial tract (vascular ring, neoplasm, lymph node, lung cyst)
  Tracheomalacia
  Endobronchial or endotracheal tumors
  Endobronchial tuberculosis
  Habit cough
  Hypersensitivity pneumonitis
  Fungal infections
  Inhaled irritants, including tobacco smoke

eczema, urticaria, allergic rhinitis), a seasonal or environmental variation in frequency or intensity of cough, and a strong family history of atopic conditions, all suggesting an allergic etiology; (2) symptoms of malabsorption or family history indicative of cystic fibrosis; (3) symptoms related to feeding, suggesting aspiration; (4) a choking episode, suggesting foreign body aspiration; and (5) a smoking history in older children and adolescents.

Considerable information pertaining to the etiology of chronic cough can be obtained at *physical examination*. Posterior pharyngeal drainage coupled with a nighttime cough suggests chronic upper airway disease. An overinflated chest suggests chronic airway obstruction, as in asthma or cystic fibrosis. An expiratory wheeze strongly suggests asthma or asthmatic bronchitis, but may also be consistent with a diagnosis of cystic fibrosis, vascular ring, aspiration of foreign material, or

Table 13–4. Characteristics of a Chronic Cough and Their Etiologic Significance

Type of Cough	Likely Responsible Condition
Loose (discontinuous), productive	Bronchitis, asthmatic bronchitis, cystic fibrosis, other bronchiectasis
Brassy	Tracheitis, habit cough
Croupy	Laryngitis
Paroxysmal (with or without gagging and vomiting)	Cystic fibrosis, pertussis syndrome, foreign body
Staccato	Chlamydia pneumonitis
Nocturnal	Upper and/or lower respiratory tract allergic reaction, sinusitis
Most severe on awakening in morning	Cystic fibrosis, other bronchiectasis, chronic bronchitis
With vigorous exercise	Exercise-induced asthma, cystic fibrosis, other bronchiectasis
Disappears with sleep	Habit cough, mild hypersecretory states as in cystic fibrosis and asthma

pulmonary hemosiderosis. Careful auscultation during forced expiration may reveal expiratory wheezes that are otherwise undetectable and that are the only indication of underlying reactive airways. Coarse crackles suggest bronchiectasis, including cystic fibrosis, but may also attend an acute or subacute exacerbation of asthma. Clubbing of the digits is seen in most patients with bronchiectasis, but in only a few with other respiratory conditions with chronic cough. Tracheal deviation suggests foreign body aspiration or a mediastinal mass.

It is essential to allow sufficient examination time to observe whether a spontaneous cough is present. If not spontaneous, most children by 4–5 yr of age will cough on request. Asking the child to repeatedly take a maximal breath and forcefully exhale usually induces a cough reflex. Children who cough as often as several times a minute with regularity are likely to have a habit (tic) cough. If the cough is loose, every effort should be made to obtain sputum; most older children can comply. It is sometimes possible to pick up small bits of sputum with a throat swab quickly placed into the lower pharynx while the child coughs with the tongue protruding. Clear mucoid sputum is most often associated with an allergic reaction or asthmatic bronchitis. Cloudy (purulent) sputum suggests a respiratory tract infection, but may also reflect increased cellularity (eosinophilia) due to an asthmatic process. Very purulent sputum is characteristic of bronchiectasis. Malodorous expectorations suggest anerobic infection of the lungs. In cystic fibrosis the sputum, even when purulent, is rarely foul smelling.

Laboratory tests may help to evaluate a chronic cough. Only sputum specimens containing alveolar macrophages should be used for studying lower respiratory tract processes. Sputum eosinophilia suggests asthma, asthmatic bronchitis, or hypersensitivity reactions of lung, while a polymorphonuclear cell response suggests infection; if sputum is unavailable, the presence of eosinophilia in nasal secretions also suggests atopic disease. If most of the cells in sputum are macrophages, postinfectious hypersensitivity of cough receptors should be suspected. Sputum macrophages can be stained for hemosiderin content, diagnostic of pulmonary hemosiderosis, or for lipid content, which suggests but is not specific for repeated aspiration. Children whose coughs persist longer than 6 wk should have a sweat chloride test. Sputum culture is helpful but not specific since throat flora may contaminate the sample.

Hematologic assessment may reveal anemia that is the result of pulmonary hemosiderosis, eosinophilia that accompanies asthma and other hypersensitivity reactions of the lung, or a deficiency of polymorphonuclear leukocytes or lymphocytes, indicating a phagocytic or immune deficiency state. Infiltrates on chest roentgenogram may suggest cystic fibrosis, bronchiectasis, foreign body, hypersensitivity pneumonitis, or tuberculosis. When asthma equivalent cough is suspected, a trial of bronchodilator therapy may be diagnostic. After the initial evaluation, especially if the cough does not respond to initial therapeutic efforts, more specific diagnostic procedures may be indicated, including an immunologic or allergic evaluation, paranasal sinus roentgenograms, esophagograms, special microbiologic studies, evaluation of ciliary morphology and function, and bronchoscopy.

Recurrent or Persistent Wheeze. Wheezing is a relatively frequent and particularly troublesome manifestation of obstructive lower respiratory tract disease in children. The site of obstruction may be anywhere from the intrathoracic trachea to the small bronchi or large bronchioles. Children under 2–3 yr of age are especially prone to wheezing, because bronchospasm, mucosal edema, and accumulation of excessive secretions have a relatively greater obstructive effect on their smaller airways. Isolated episodes of acute wheezing, such as may occur with bronchiolitis, are not uncommon, but wheezing which recurs or persists for longer than 4 wk suggests other diagnoses (Table 13–5). Most recurrent or persistent wheezing in children is the result of reactive airways disease.

Frequently recurring or persistent wheezing starting at or soon after birth suggests a variety of other diagnoses, including congenital structural abnormalities involving the lower respiratory tract. Wheezing that attends cystic fibrosis is most common in the first year of life. Sudden onset of severe wheezing in a previously healthy child should suggest foreign body aspiration.

Repeated examination may be required to verify a history of wheezing in a child with episodic symptoms and should be directed toward assessing air movement, ventilatory adequacy, and evidence of chronic lung disease, such as fixed overinflation of the chest, growth failure, and digital clubbing. Clubbing suggests chronic lung infection and is rarely prominent in uncomplicated asthma. Tracheal deviation from foreign body aspiration should be sought. It is essential to rule out wheezing secondary to congestive heart failure. Allergic rhinitis, urticaria, eczema, or evidence of ichthyosis vulgaris suggests asthma or asthmatic bronchitis. The nose should be examined for polyps, which may be present in either allergic conditions or cystic fibrosis.

Sputum eosinophilia, elevated serum IgE levels, and response to bronchodilators suggest allergic reactions.

Frequently Recurring or Persistent Stridor. Stridor, a harsh, medium-pitched, inspiratory sound associated with obstruction of the laryngeal area or the extrathoracic trachea, is often accompanied by a croupy cough and hoarse voice. Stridor is most commonly observed in children with croup; foreign bodies and trauma may also cause acute stridor. However, a small number of children develop recurrent stridor or have persistent stridor from the first day or weeks of life (Table 13–6). Most congenital anomalies of large airways that produce stridor become symptomatic soon after birth. Increase of stridor when a child is supine suggests laryngomalacia or tracheomalacia. An accompanying history of hoarseness or aphonia suggests involvement of the vocal cords.

Table 13–5. Causes of Recurrent or Persistent Wheezing in Children

Reactive airways disease
    Asthma
    Exercise-induced asthma
    Salicylate-induced asthma and nasal polyposis
    Asthmatic bronchitis
    Other hypersensitivity reactions:
        Hypersensitivity pneumonitis
        Tropical eosinophilia
        Visceral larva migrans
        Allergic aspergillosis
Aspiration
    Foreign body
    Food, saliva, gastric contents
    Laryngotracheoesophageal cleft
    Tracheoesophageal fistula, H-type
    Pharyngeal incoordination or neuromuscular weakness
Cystic fibrosis
Immotile cilia syndrome
Cardiac failure
Bronchiolitis obliterans
Extrinsic compression of airways
    Vascular ring
    Enlarged lymph node
    Mediastinal tumor
    Lung cysts
Tracheobronchomalacia
Endobronchial masses
Gastroesophageal reflux
Pulmonary hemosiderosis
Sequelae of bronchopulmonary dysplasia

Table 13–6. Causes of Recurrent or Persistent Stridor in Children

Recurrent	Persistent
Allergic croup	Laryngeal obstruction
Respiratory infections in a child with otherwise asymptomatic anatomic narrowing of the large airways	Laryngomalacia
	Papillomas, other tumors
	Cysts and laryngoceles
Laryngomalacia	Laryngeal webs
	Bilateral abductor paralysis of the cords
	Foreign body
	Tracheobronchial disease
	Tracheomalacia
	Subglottic tracheal webs
	Endotracheal, endobronchial tumors
	Subglottic tracheal stenosis
	Congenital
	Acquired
	Extrinsic masses
	Mediastinal masses
	Vascular ring
	Lobar emphysema
	Bronchogenic cysts
	Thyroid enlargement
	Esophageal foreign body
	Tracheoesophageal fistulas
	Other
	Macroglossia, Pierre Robin syndrome
	Cri du chat syndrome
	Hysterical stridor

Physical examination for recurrent or persistent stridor is usually unrewarding, although changes of its severity and intensity due to changes of body position should be assessed. Anteroposterior and lateral roentgenograms of the laryngeal and tracheal areas may demonstrate focal narrowing of the air column or extrinsic pressure on the tracheobronchial airways. Occasionally a specific lesion, such as a laryngocele, can be identified, but in most cases direct observation is necessary for diagnosis. Undistorted views of the larynx are best obtained with a fiberoptic bronchoscope positioned in the pharynx.

Recurrent and Persistent Lung Infiltrates. Roentgenographic lung infiltrates due to acute pneumonia usually resolve within 1–3 wk, but a substantial number of children, particularly infants, fail to clear infiltrates within a 4 wk period. They may be either febrile or afebrile and may present a wide range of respiratory symptoms and signs. Recurring infiltrates present a diagnostic challenge (Table 13–7).

Symptoms associated with chronic lung infiltrates during the first several weeks of life (but not related to neonatal respiratory distress syndrome) suggest infection acquired in utero or during descent through the birth canal. Early appearance of chronic infiltrates may also be associated with cystic fibrosis or congenital anomalies, which result in aspiration or airway obstruction. A history of recurrent infiltrates, wheezing, and cough may reflect asthma, even in the first year of life.

One uncommon but characteristic syndrome appearing in the first year of life with recurrent lung infiltrates is pulmonary hemosiderosis related to cow's milk hypersensitivity. Children with a history of bronchopulmonary dysplasia frequently have episodes of respiratory distress attended by wheezing and new lung infiltrates. Recurrent pneumonia in a child with frequent otitis media, nasopharyngitis, adenitis, or dermatologic manifestations suggests an immunodeficiency state, complement deficiency, or phagocytic defect. A history of paroxysmal coughing in an infant suggests pertussis syndrome or cystic fibrosis. Persistent infiltrates, especially with

Table 13–7. Diseases Associated with Recurrent or Persistent Lung Infiltrates Beyond the Neonatal Period

Recurrent or migrating infiltrates
  *Asthma
  *Chronic aspiration
   Hypersensitivity pneumonitis
  *Pulmonary hemosiderosis
   Foreign body
  *Immunodeficiency, phagocytic deficiency
   Sickle cell disease
  *Cystic fibrosis
Persistent infiltrates
  *Congenital infection
       Cytomegalovirus
       Rubella
       Syphilis
   Acquired infection
     *Cytomegalovirus
     *Tuberculosis
     *Chlamydia
     *Other viruses
     *Mycoplasma, ureaplasma
     *Pertussis
      Fungal organisms
     *Pneumocystis carinii
      Inadequately treated bacterial infection
   Congenital anomalies
     *Lung cysts
      Pulmonary sequestration
      Bronchial stenosis
      Vascular ring
      Congenital heart disease with large left to right shunt
   Aspiration
     *Pharyngeal incompetence (e.g., cleft palate)
     *Laryngotracheoesophageal cleft

  *Tracheoesophageal fistula
  *Gastroesophageal reflux
   Foreign body
   Lipid aspiration
Immunodeficiency, phagocytic deficiency
  *Humoral, cellular, combined immunodeficiency states
  *Chronic granulomatous disease and related phagocytic defects
  *Complement deficiency states
Allergy-hypersensitivity
  *Pulmonary hemosiderosis (cow's milk–related, other)
   Asthma
   Hypersensitivity pneumonitis (allergic alveolitis)
*Cystic fibrosis
 Immotile cilia syndrome (Kartagener), deficiency of bronchial cartilage, right middle lobe syndrome, other bronchiectasis
 Sarcoidosis
 Neoplasms (primary, metastatic)
*Interstitial pneumonitis and fibrosis
    Usual (Hamman-Rich)
    Desquamative
 Alveolar proteinosis
*Pulmonary lymphangiectasia
 α_1-Antitrypsin deficiency
 Drug-induced, radiation-induced inflammation and fibrosis
 Collagen-vascular diseases
 Eosinophilic pneumonias
 Visceral larva migrans
 Histiocytosis
 Leukemia

*Conditions that often cause chronic lung infiltrates in infants.

loss of volume, in a toddler should suggest foreign body aspiration.

Overinflation and infiltrates suggest cystic fibrosis or chronic asthma. A "silent chest" with infiltrates should arouse suspicion of alveolar proteinosis, *Pneumocystis carinii* infection, desquamative intersititial pneumonitis, or tumors. Growth should be carefully assessed to determine whether the lung process has had systemic effects, indicating substantial severity and chronicity as in cystic fibrosis or alveolar proteinosis. Cataracts, retinopathy, or microcephaly suggest in utero infection. Chronic rhinorrhea may be associated with atopic disease, cow's milk intolerance, cystic fibrosis, or congenital syphilis. The absence of tonsils and cervical lymph nodes suggests a combined immunodeficiency state.

Diagnostic studies should be done selectively, based on information obtained from history and physical examination and on a thorough understanding of conditions listed in Table 13–7. Cytologic evaluation of bronchial secretions may be helpful. In patients unresponsive to antibiotics, needle aspiration of the involved area may demonstrate a pathogenic organism. Bronchography, as a rule, is most helpful in identifying surgically approachable focal bronchiectasis and should not be undertaken for routine evaluation of chronic lung infiltrates. Bronchoscopy is indicated for detecting foreign bodies, congenital or acquired anomalies of the tracheobronchial tract, and obstruction by endobronchial or extrinsic masses. In addition, bronchoscopy provides access to secretions which can be studied cytologically and microbiologically. If all appropriate studies have been completed and the condition remains undiagnosed, open lung biopsy may yield a definitive diagnosis.

Optimal medical or surgical treatment of chronic lung infiltrates frequently depends on a specific diagnosis, but chronic conditions may be self-limiting, e.g., severe and prolonged viral infections in infants; in these instances symptomatic therapy may maintain adequate lung function until spontaneous improvement occurs. Helpful measures include inhalation and physical therapy for excessive secretions, antibiotics for secondary bacterial infections, supplementary oxygen for hypoxemia, and maintenance of adequate nutrition. Because the lung of a young child has remarkable recuperative potential, normal lung function may ultimately be achieved with treatment despite the severity of pulmonary insult occurring during infancy.

THOMAS F. BOAT

Cloutier MM, Loughlin GM: Chronic cough in children: A manifestation of airway hyperreactivity. Pediatrics 67:6, 1981.

Cohlan SQ and Stone SM: The cough and the bedsheet. Pediatrics 74:11–15, 1984.

Danus O, Casar C, Larrain A, et al: Esophageal reflux—an unrecognized cause of recurrent obstructive bronchitis in children. J Pediatr 89:220, 1976.

Eigen H: The clinical evaluation of chronic cough. Pediatr Clin N Am 29:57–68, 1982.

Eliasson R, Mossberg B, Camner P, et al: The immotile cilia syndrome. N Engl J Med 297:1, 1977.

Irwin RS, Rosen MJ, Braman SS: Cough: A comprehensive review. Arch Intern Med 137;1186–1191, 1977.

Stagno S, Brasfield DM, Brown MB, et al: Infant pneumonitis associated with cytomegalovirus, chlamydia, pneumocystis, and ureaplasma: A prospective study. Pediatrics 68:322, 1981.

Wood RE, Boat TF, Doershuk CF: State of the art: Cystic fibrosis. Am Rev Respir Dis 113:833, 1976.

13.97 CYSTIC FIBROSIS

Cystic fibrosis is a multisystem disorder of children and adults, characterized chiefly by chronic obstruction and infection of airways and by maldigestion and its consequences. It is the most common life-threatening genetic trait in the Caucasian population. Dysfunction of exocrine glands is the predominant pathogenetic mechanism and is responsible for a broad, variable, and sometimes confusing array of presenting manifestations and subsequent complications. However, the basic defect is unknown.

Cystic fibrosis is the major cause of severe chronic lung disease of children and is responsible for most exocrine pancreatic insufficiency during early life. It is also responsible for many cases of nasal polyposis, pansinusitis, rectal prolapse, and insulin dependent hyperglycemia. In addition, cystic fibrosis may present as failure to thrive and occasionally as cirrhosis or other forms of hepatic dysfunction. Therefore, this disorder enters into the differential diagnosis of many pediatric conditions.

History. Medieval German folk literature noted a relationship between salty-tasting skin and early death. However, it was not until 1938 that Anderson provided a comprehensive pathologic and clinical description of exocrine pancreatic insufficiency in early childhood associated with severe chronic respiratory tract symptoms, and used the term cystic fibrosis of the pancreas. Farber noted that inspissation of secretions obstructing gland ducts and acini of many organs, including the pancreas, intestinal tract, biliary system airways, and salivary glands, was a general pathologic feature. He suggested that diminished clearance of mucus was the common pathophysiologic event and in 1945 proposed the name mucoviscidosis. In 1953, DiSant'Agnese, investigating salt depletion in children with cystic fibrosis during a summertime heat wave, astutely concluded that excessive loss of salt must occur via the sweat, and documented that sodium and chloride levels in sweat are elevated in virtually all individuals with cystic fibrosis. Measurement of chloride concentrations in sweat subsequently became the standard diagnostic test for this disorder. The report of comprehensive and aggressive approaches to the care of patients by Matthews in 1964 has been accompanied by a steadily increasing longevity despite the failure to identify the underlying abnormality.

Epidemiology. Cystic fibrosis occurs in approximately 1:2000 and 1:17,000 live births in white and black populations of the United States, respectively. The estimated incidence worldwide varies from 1:620 in a confined population with Dutch ancestry in southwest Africa to 1:90,000 in an Oriental population of Hawaii. Generally, the cystic fibrosis gene is most prevalent in Northern and Central Europeans and individuals who derive from these areas.

Cystic fibrosis is most probably inherited as an autosomal recessive trait. Current evidence suggests a single mutant allele. Linkage studies have localized the cystic fibrosis gene to the long arm of chromosome 7. This approach can be used within some families to identify carriers or make antenatal diagnosis. Work is in process to isolate the gene and characterize its product.

In Caucasian populations, 4–5% of individuals are carriers of the cystic fibrosis gene and have no clinical stigmata of disease. There is no test which reliably identifies heterozygotes for genetic counseling.

Pathogenesis. The basic defect in cystic fibrosis has not been identified. Although *cystic fibrosis mucins* may be more highly sulfated than normal and interact more avidly with lipids, the relationship of these differences to altered behavior of mucus is unclear. There is currently little direct evidence that uninfected cystic fibrosis mucus has abnormal rheologic properties.

While basal rates of mucus secretion are appropriate in cultured cystic fibrosis airways and intestinal epithelium, the regulation of secretion in vivo may be disturbed. Patients with cystic fibrosis are hyperresponsive to cholinergic and α-adrenergic drugs and are hyporesponsive to β-adrenergic stimulation, perhaps owing to a disturbance of coupling of the β-adrenergic receptor to adenylate cyclase, a membrane enzyme that generates the intracellular messenger, cyclic AMP. In addition, the blood of patients contains unidentified mucus-stimulating substances.

Mucus secretions in cystic fibrosis are relatively deficient in water. Inadequate secretion of water may explain the inspissation of secretions in airways and plugging of gland ducts. Studies of patients who have some residual pancreatic function indicate that water and bicarbonate secretion are more severely disturbed than enzyme secretion. Water movement across exocrine epithelium is linked to electrolyte transport. It is likely that inadequate hydration of secretions is related to abnormal transport of sodium and chloride.

The most consistent pathophysiologic observation in cystic fibrosis is *elevation of chloride and sodium levels in sweat*, which may be related to the transport properties of the epithelium. For example, elevated bioelectrical potential differences across respiratory epithelium could be explained by the findings of increased reabsorption of sodium from liquids at the lumenal surface through amiloride-sensitive pathways or of decreased chloride permeability of respiratory and sweat duct epithelium. There is evidence for chloride channels in respiratory epithelial cells of patients, which suggests that the cystic fibrosis defect resides in a mechanism regulating the flow of ions through these channels. There is also an elevation of calcium content of epithelial cells and fibroblasts, and the relationship between calcium, sodium, and chloride transport and mucus inspissation in cystic fibrosis is not understood.

Infection, especially with S. *aureus* and P. *aeruginosa*, plays a major, but secondary, role in the pathogenesis of lung disease in cystic fibrosis. Infection is confined to the lung, and humoral and cellular immunity, including complement activity, are generally normal, although functional deficits may occur in cellular immunity and in the alternative pathway of complement as infection progresses to an advanced stage. Pulmonary alveolar macrophages display normal phagocytic properties unless exposed to cystic fibrosis serum from individuals who have been infected with *Pseudomonas*. A predisposition to bacterial colonization of airways may reflect delayed mucociliary clearance, which has been documented in some patients with cystic fibrosis, or it may be the result of an unrecognized biochemical disturbance at the epithelial cell surface favoring bacterial adherence.

Some have claimed that the syndrome of cystic fibrosis, including growth failure, chronic obstructive respiratory tract disease, and sweat electrolyte abnormalities, can be attributed to *fatty acid deficiency*. However, patients with cystic fibrosis who retain exocrine pancreatic function do not develop fatty acid deficiency. The 10–15% of individuals with cystic fibrosis and substantial pancreatic function have statistically lower sweat chloride values and delayed onset of chronic lung disease. However, preservation of pancreatic function does not preclude development of the typical features.

A number of circulating "CF factors" have been described, including those that disrupt ciliary motility, inhibit debrancher enzyme, and stimulate the release of mucus. Only the last of these appears to relate directly to the pathogenesis of cystic fibrosis. None of these factors has been isolated or completely characterized, and the assay systems employed do not yield consistent results from one laboratory to the next.

Cultured fibroblasts from patients with cystic fibrosis, when compared with control cells, have a number of abnormalities.

However, it is not clear that the basic defect in cystic fibrosis is directly expressed in fibroblasts.

Pathology. Striking changes are characteristically observed in the organs which secrete mucus. Eccrine sweat glands and parotid salivary glands, including ducts, are not involved pathologically in spite of abnormalities in the electrolyte content of their secretory product.

The *lung* usually has a normal macroscopic and nearly normal microscopic appearance at birth. Duct lumens of submucosal glands in large airways are enlarged at or soon after birth, suggesting difficulty with passage of secretions even before the appearance of chronic infection. With the development of symptoms, goblet cell hyperplasia and gland hypertrophy with extensive intraluminal accumulation of mucus occur in the bronchial airways secondary to infection. The hypersecretory state is, in part, a response to proteinases released by bacteria and phagocytic cells. Acute and chronic peribronchiolar inflammatory cell infiltrations occur (bronchiolitis), followed by plugging of small airways with inspissated secretions as goblet cell metaplasia of bronchiolar epithelium develops. Bronchiolar stenosis is a frequent consequence. Infection leads to destruction of the airway walls, creating bronchiolectasis and bronchiectasis. Bronchiectatic cysts and abscesses are prominent features of advanced pulmonary disease. Squamous metaplasia of ciliated epithelium may occur. As the airways involvement advances, peribronchial inflammatory disease becomes more extensive and areas of fibrosis develop. Bronchitis and bronchiolitis are potentially reversible with treatment but subsequent changes are essentially irreversible.

Distention of air spaces is an early finding but little alveolar wall destruction (emphysema) is observed. Areas of segmental or even lobar pneumonitis may attend acute exacerbations of pulmonary disease. Bronchiectatic cysts often develop, especially in the upper lobes, and their rupture is responsible for most episodes of pneumothorax. Bronchiectasis results in the development of a rich vascular network in peribronchial granulation, which shunts blood from bronchial to pulmonary arteries, compounding the problem of uneven ventilation-perfusion distribution. Bronchial arteries enlarge and become tortuous.

The *paranasal sinuses* are uniformly filled with secretions and the lining contains hyperplastic and hypertrophied secretory elements.

The *pancreas* is usually small, occasionally cystic, and often difficult to find at postmortem examination. The extent of involvement is variable at birth. In infants, the acini and ducts often are distended and filled with eosinophilic material. In 85–90% of patients the lesion progresses to complete or nearly complete disruption of acini and replacement of exocrine pancreas with fibrous tissue and fat. Infrequently, foci of calcification may be seen on roentgenograms of the abdomen. The islets of Langerhans contain a normal number of β cells, although they may begin to show architectural disruption by fibrous tissue during the second decade of life.

The *intestinal tract* shows only minimal changes. Esophageal and duodenal glands are often distended with mucus secretions. Concretions may form in the appendiceal lumen or cecum. Rectal biopsies uniformly show dilated crypt lumina.

Focal biliary cirrhosis secondary to blockage of intrahepatic bile ducts is uncommon in early life, although it is responsible for occasional cases of prolonged neonatal jaundice. This lesion becomes more prevalent and extensive with age and is found in 25% or more of patients at postmortem. Infrequently this process proceeds to symptomatic multilobular biliary cirrhosis that has a distinctive pattern of large irregular nodules and contracted bands of fibrous tissue. In addition, approximately 30% of patients have fatty infiltration of the liver, in spite of apparently adequate nutrition. At autopsy,

hepatic congestion secondary to cor pulmonale is frequently observed. The gallbladder may be hypoplastic and filled with mucoid material and not infrequently contains stones. The epithelial lining often displays extensive mucous metaplasia. Atresia of the cystic duct has been observed.

Mucus-secreting *salivary glands* are usually enlarged and display focal plugging and dilatation of ducts.

Glands of the uterine cervix are distended with mucus and copious amounts of mucus collect in the cervical canal. Endocervicitis may be more prevalent in teenagers and young women. In more than 95% of males, the body and tail of the epididymis, the vas deferens, and the seminal vesicles are obliterated or atretic.

Clinical Manifestations. Expression of the cystic fibrosis gene defect results in highly variable involvement of the lung, pancreas, and other organs.

Lung Disease. Cough is the most constant symptom of pulmonary involvement. At first the cough may be dry and hacking, but eventually it becomes loose and then productive. In older patients, the cough is most prominent on arising in the morning or after activity. Expectorated mucus is usually purulent and if green may indicate colonization by P. *aeruginosa.* Some patients remain asymptomatic for long periods of time or seem to have only prolonged acute respiratory infections. Others develop a chronic cough within the first months of life and/or repeatedly develop pneumonia. Extensive bronchiolitis is attended by wheezing, a not infrequent symptom during the first years of life. As lung disease progresses, exercise intolerance, shortness of breath, and failure to gain weight or grow are noted. Exacerbations of lung symptoms eventually require hospitalization for effective treatment. Finally, respiratory failure, cor pulmonale, and death supervene.

Early physical findings include increased anteroposterior diameter of the chest, generalized hyper-resonance, scattered or localized coarse or fine crackles, and digital clubbing. High-pitched expiratory rhonchi may be heard, especially in young children. Cyanosis is a late sign. Common pulmonary complications include atelectasis, hemoptysis, pneumothorax, and cor pulmonale, which usually appear in the 2nd or 3rd decade of life.

Even though roentgenographically the paranasal sinuses are virtually always opacified, acute sinusitis is infrequent. Nasal obstruction and rhinorrhea are common, due either to inflamed, swollen mucous membranes or in some cases to nasal polyposis.

Intestinal Tract. In nearly 10% of newborn infants with cystic fibrosis, the ileum is completely obstructed by meconium (meconium ileus); abdominal distention, emesis, and failure to pass meconium appear within the first 24–48 hr of life (Sec. 8.42). Abdominal roentgenograms (Fig. 13–17) show dilated loops of bowel with air fluid levels and frequently a collection of granular, "ground glass" material in the lower central abdomen. Rarely, meconium peritonitis results from intrauterine rupture of the bowel wall and can be detected roentgenographically by the presence of peritoneal or scrotal calcifications. Meconium plug syndrome may occur more commonly in infants with cystic fibrosis than in other infants. Ileal obstruction with fecal material (meconium ileus equivalent) occasionally occurs in older patients, causing cramping abdominal pain and abdominal distention.

More than 85% of children show evidence of maldigestion due to exocrine pancreatic insufficiency. Symptoms include frequent, bulky, greasy stools and failure to gain weight even when food intake appears to be large. Characteristically, stools contain readily visible droplets of fat. A protuberant abdomen, decreased muscle mass, poor growth, and delayed maturation are typical physical signs. Excessive flatus may be a problem.

Less common gastrointestinal manifestations include intus-

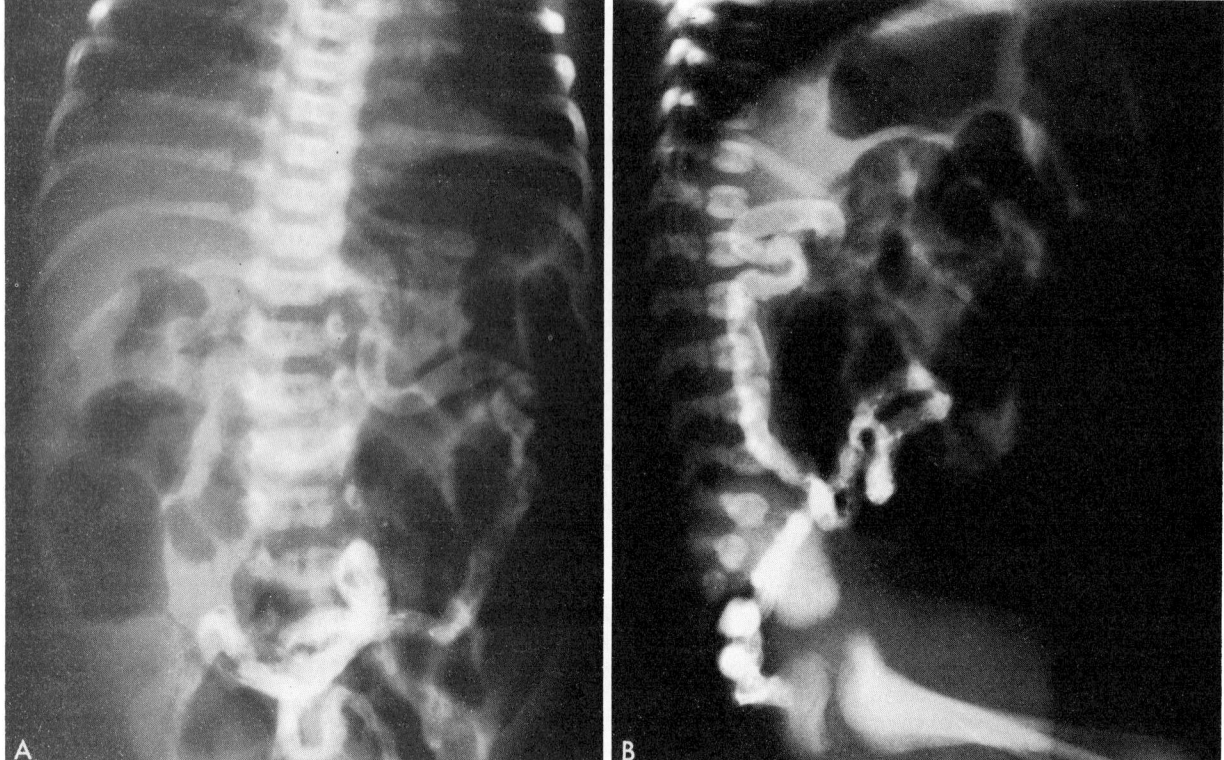

Figure 13–17. *A, B,* Contrast enema in a newborn infant with abdominal distention and failure to pass meconium. Note the small diameter of the sigmoid and ascending colon and dilated, air-filled loops of small intestine. Several air-fluid levels in small bowel are seen on the upright lateral view.

susception, fecal impaction of the cecum or appendix with an asymptomatic right lower quadrant mass, and epigastic pain due to duodenal inflammation. Rectal prolapse is relatively frequent. Occasionally, hypoproteinemia with anasarca appears in infancy, especially if children are fed non–protein-enriched formulas such as soy-base preparations. Hypoproteinemia may be accompanied by hemolytic anemia. Deficiency of fat-soluble vitamins is occasionally symptomatic. For example, hypoprothrombinemia due to vitamin K deficiency may result in a bleeding diathesis. Rarely, clinical manifestations of other vitamin deficiencies occur.

Biliary Tract. Biliary cirrhosis becomes symptomatic in only 2–3% of patients. Manifestations may include icterus, ascites, hematemesis from esophageal varices, and evidence of hypersplenism. Biliary colic secondary to cholelithiasis may occur in the second decade of life.

Pancreas. In addition to exocrine pancreatic insufficiency, evidence for hyperglycemia and glucosuria including polyuria and weight loss may appear, especially after 10 yr of age. In most cases, ketoacidosis does not occur, but eye and other diabetic complications occur in patients living 10 yr or more after onset of hyperglycemia. Recurrent acute pancreatitis occasionally occurs in those adolescents and young adults who have residual exocrine pancreatic function and may be exacerbated by diet and/or tetracycline.

Genitourinary Tract. Sexual development is often delayed, but only by an average of 2 yr. More than 95% of males are azoospermic because of failure of development of wolffian duct structures, but sexual function is generally unimpaired. The incidence of inguinal hernia, hydrocele, and undescended testicle is higher than expected. Adolescent females may experience secondary amenorrhea, especially with exacerbations of pulmonary disease. Cervicitis and accumulation of tenacious mucus in the cervical canal have been noted. The female fertility rate is probably lower than expected. Preg-

nancy is generally tolerated well by women with good pulmonary function but may cause progression of pulmonary disease and even death in those with moderate or advanced lung problems.

Sweat Glands. Excessive loss of salt in the sweat predisposes young children to salt depletion episodes, especially during the time of gastroenteritis associated with vomiting and/or diarrhea and during warm weather. These children present with hypochloremic alkalosis. Frequently, parents note salt "frosting" of the skin or a salty taste when they kiss the child.

Diagnosis. The diagnosis of cystic fibrosis should be based on a positive quantitative sweat test in conjunction with one or more of the following: typical chronic obstructive pulmonary disease, documented exocrine pancreatic insufficiency, or a positive family history. In rare instances, the sweat test may be in the intermediate range (40–60 mEq/L), and a normal range sweat test has been reported in several patients thought to have typical clinical manifestations of cystic fibrosis.

Sweat Testing. The sweat test, using pilocarpine iontophoresis to collect sweat and chemical analysis of its chloride content, is the best diagnostic test (Table 13–8). The procedure requires care and accuracy. A 3 milliamp electric current is used to carry pilocarpine into the skin of the forearm and locally stimulate the sweat glands. After washing the arm with distilled water, sweat is collected on filter paper or gauze which has been placed on the stimulated skin and covered to prevent evaporation. After 30-60 min, the filter paper is removed, weighed, and eluted in distilled water. A chloridometer is recommended for the analysis of chloride in these samples. The amount of sweat collected should be measured and reported. For reliable results, at least 50 and preferably 100 mg of sweat should be collected. In infants, it may be necessary to use the upper back to obtain enough sweat. Reliable testing may be difficult in the first few weeks of life

Table 13–8. Indications for Sweat Testing*

Pulmonary	Gastrointestinal
Chronic or productive cough	Meconium ileus, meconium plug
Recurrent or chronic pneumonia	syndrome
or infiltrates	Steatorrhea, malabsorption
Recurrent bronchiolitis	Rectal prolapse
Atelectasis	Childhood cirrhosis, portal
Hemoptysis	hypertension, bleeding
Infection with *Pseudomonas*	esophageal varices
(mucoid)	Hypoprothrombinemia beyond
Staphylococcal pneumonia	newborn period
Other	
Family history of cystic fibrosis	
Failure to thrive	
Salty taste when kissed	
Nasal polyps	
Heat prostration with	
unexplained hypochloremic	
alkalosis	
Pansinusitis	
Aspermia in mature males	

*Individuals with cystic fibrosis may initially present with any of these signs or symptoms.

owing to low sweat rates. Positive tests should be confirmed; negative tests should be repeated if suspicion of the diagnosis remains.

Up to approximately 20 yr of age more than 60 mEq/L of chloride in sweat is diagnostic of cystic fibrosis when one or more other criteria are present. Values between 40 and 60 mEq/L suggest cystic fibrosis and have been reported in cases with typical involvement. In healthy adults, the sweat chloride values increase so that a level up to 80 mEq/L may be normal. Chloride concentrations in sweat are somewhat lower in individuals who retain exocrine pancreatic function but remain within the diagnostic range.

Other conditions associated with elevated concentrations of sweat electrolytes include untreated adrenal insufficiency, ectodermal dysplasia, hereditary nephrogenic diabetes insipidus, glucose 6-phosphatase deficiency, hypothyroidism, hypoparathyroidism, familial cholestasis, pancreatitis, mucopolysaccharidoses, fucosidosis, and malnutrition. Most of these conditions can be easily distinguished from cystic fibrosis by clinical criteria.

Pancreatic Function. It is important to document exocrine pancreatic insufficiency. Qualitative stool fat evaluation may be suggestive, but a 3 day collection with controlled fat intake is required for documentation of steatorrhea. Duodenal intubation and the pancreozymin-secretin stimulation may help in diagnosis of borderline cases but should not be used routinely. Quantitation of trypsin and chymotrypsin activity in a fresh stool sample is an easy and fairly reliable test to screen for pancreatic insufficiency. Measurement of blood immunoreactive trypsin is being evaluated for use in diagnosis and screening. Pancreatic stool or serum isoamylase is either absent or markedly diminished in patients with pancreatic insufficiency. Urinary excretion of oral para-amino benzoic acid (PABA) correlates with other measures of exocrine pancreatic insufficiency.

Radiology. Radiologic findings may suggest the diagnosis. Generalized hyperinflation by chest roentgenogram occurs early and may be overlooked in the absence of infiltrates or streaky markings. Bronchial thickening and plugging, especially in the upper lobes, and irregular hyperinflation are frequently encountered as symptoms develop. More diffuse patchy areas of atelectasis and infiltration, hilar adenopathy, and more hyperinflation with depression of the diaphragms, anterior bowing of the sternum, and increased anterior-posterior diameter of the chest are common with moderate to advanced disease. Segmental or lobar atelectasis, cyst forma-

tion, extensive bronchiectasis and infiltrates, pneumothorax, dilated pulmonary artery segments, and/or cardiac enlargement all indicate advanced involvement. Bronchoscopy and bronchograms are not required for diagnostic evaluation. Typical progression of changes is shown in Fig. 13–18.

In older children with cystic fibrosis, roentgenograms of the paranasal sinuses reveal diffuse pansinusitis and failure of frontal sinus development in almost all cases.

Pulmonary Function. Pulmonary function studies are not obtained reliably until 4–6 yr of age, by which time most undiagnosed patients will show the typical pattern of obstructive pulmonary involvement (Sec. 13.18–13.19). Decrease in the mid-maximal flow rate is an early functional change in many cases. The earliest involvement occurs in the peripheral airways, affecting the distribution of ventilation and increasing the alveolar-arterial oxygen difference. The finding of obstructive airway disease unresponsive or only minimally responsive to a bronchodilator is consistent with the diagnosis of cystic fibrosis. Subsequent testing once or twice yearly, or more often if needed, can be used to evaluate the effect of therapy and the course of the pulmonary involvement. An increasing number of patients are reaching adolescent or adult life with normal routine tests and without evidence of overinflation. Although there is great variability among these patients in the degree of overinflation they develop, in general those patients who have more normal chest roentgenogram scores during the first year of treatment tend to develop less overinflation and do better clinically.

Screening—Heterozygote Detection—Prenatal Diagnosis. There is no widely accepted routine screening test for cystic fibrosis. The evaluations of meconium for albumin content and of blood for immunoreactive trypsin miss patients without pancreatic function, and there is a moderately frequent occurrence of false-positive results. DNA analysis techniques can detect sibling heterozygotes or fetuses with cystic fibrosis when both parents and their affected child are also available for testing.

Treatment. The treatment plan should be comprehensive and individualized. At the time of diagnosis most individuals have some pulmonary involvement.

General Approach to Care. Because of the serious prognosis, a period of hospitalization for accurate diagnosis, overall baseline assessment, initiation of treatment, optimal clearing of the pulmonary involvement, and education of the patient and parents is recommended. The patient is hospitalized for as long as is necessary to control the pulmonary involvement and achieve steady weight gain. Follow-up outpatient visits are scheduled every 4-8 wk because many aspects of the condition require careful monitoring. The interval history and physical examination should be obtained at such visits. A sputum sample or, if that is not available, a deep throat swab taken during or after a forced cough is obtained for culture and antibiotic susceptibility studies. Even asymptomatic patients may produce sputum after forced exhalations or pharyngeal stimulation with a swab. Since progressive and irreversible loss of pulmonary function from low grade infection can occur very gradually, without acute symptoms, emphasis is placed on the pulmonary history. Changes in cough frequency and/or productivity, the appearance of nocturnal cough, or onset of paroxysmal cough with or without vomiting or hemoptysis indicates exacerbation of pulmonary infection. The appearance of crackles, irritability, decreased activity, decreased appetite, and failure to gain weight also may reflect increased pulmonary infection. All suggest the need for altered or increased antibiotic and physical therapy. Immunoprophylaxis against rubeola, pertussis, and influenza is recommended. When specific medical, financial, school, emotional or other problems are encountered, a nurse, therapist, social worker, dietitian, psychologist, or other special-

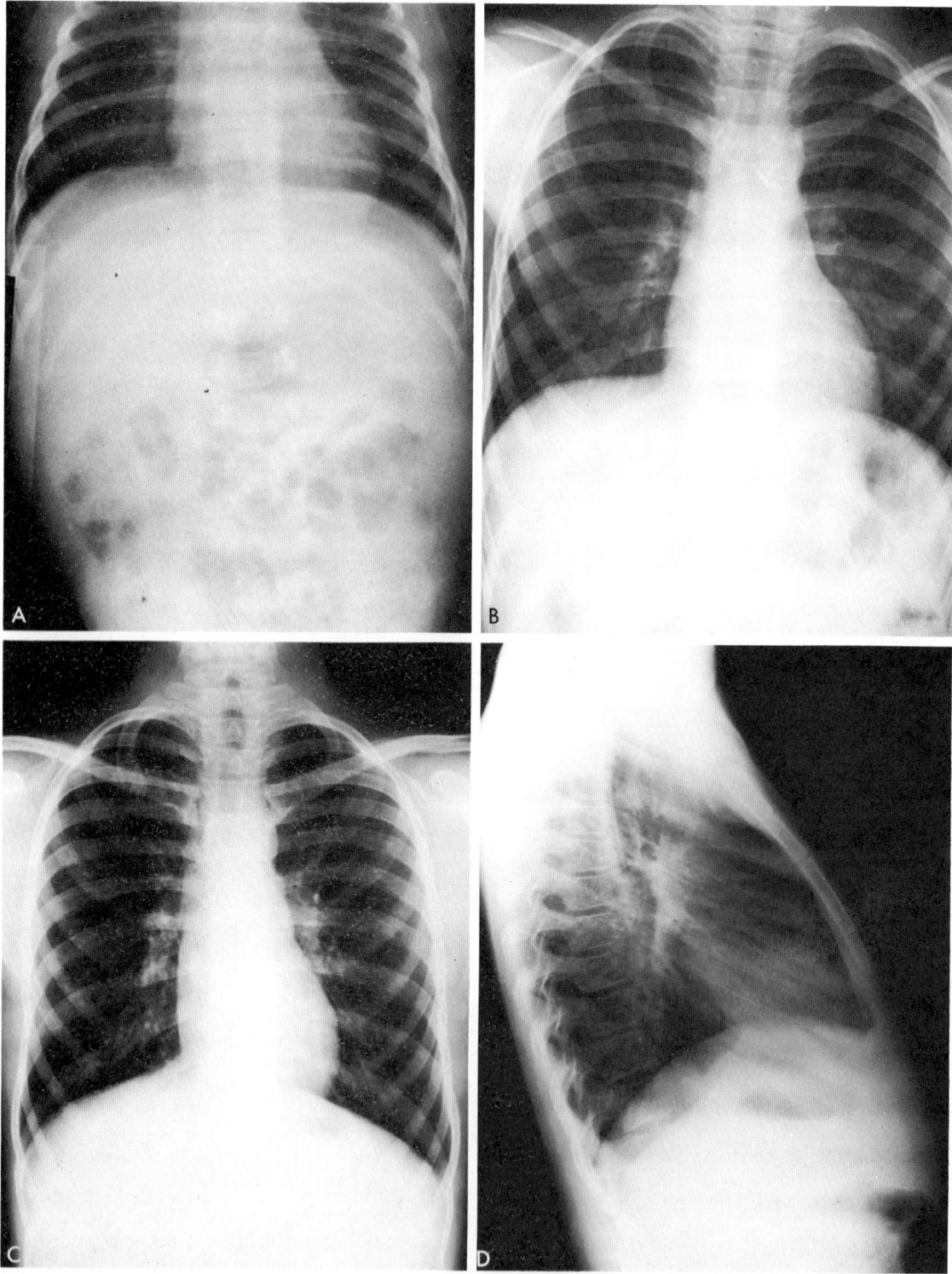

Figure 13–18. Roentgenographic progression of cystic fibrosis lung disease from diagnosis in infant to 17 yr of age. *A,* Admitted with cough and wheezing at 2 mo of age. Note the mild increase in bronchovascular markings especially in the upper lobe areas. *B,* At age 4 yr cough was minimal. Mild increase in bronchovascular markings was present with some improvement in the upper lobes. The wheeze never recurred. *C, D,* At age 13 yr, there was minimal cough and occasional sputum production. The bronchovascular markings were generally further increased with early bronchiectatic changes in the right upper lobe. The lateral view does not suggest overinflation.

Illustration continued on opposite page

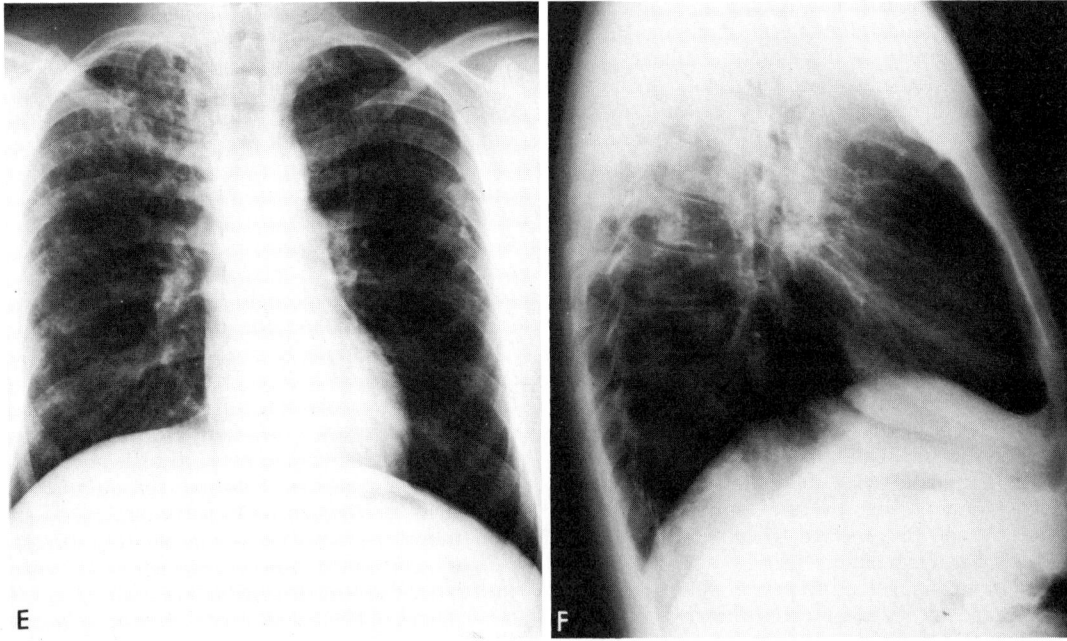

Figure 13–18 *Continued E, F*, Age 18 yr. During adolescence, cough and sputum production increased even though outpatient antibiotic therapy was intensified. Small volume hemoptysis, occasional paroxysms of cough, and weight loss as well as increased nodular infiltrates (especially in the right upper lobe and hyperinflation, as seen on the lateral view) led to the 1st hospitalization since infancy. Height and weight were maintained in the 25th–50th percentile.

ists should participate in the care program until the problem is under control. Considerable understanding, education, and encouragement are required of the patient and parents to maintain an adequate level of home care.

The goal of therapy is to maintain a stable condition for long periods of time. This can be accomplished for the majority of patients by interval evaluation and adjustments of the home treatment program. However, some patients never reach a stable condition but have episodic acute or low grade chronic lung infection (usually with *Pseudomonas aeruginosa*) that progresses. For these patients, rehospitalization for 2 wk or more of intensive inhalation and physical therapy and intravenous antibiotics is indicated. Such admissions may be required infrequently or as often as every 2–3 mo. Significant improvement in pulmonary function and the patient's well-being is usually achieved. Colonization with *Pseudomonas cepacia* and subsequent infection has been associated with increased morbidity and in some cases rapid pulmonary deterioration and death.

The basic daily care program varies depending on the age of the patient, degree of pulmonary involvement, other system involvement, and time available for therapy. The major components of this care are digestive therapy and pulmonary therapy.

Pulmonary Therapy. This is empirical and/or symptomatic. The objective is to clear secretions from airways and to control infection. There is a divergence of opinion about various aspects of therapy. However, the effectiveness of the overall approach to therapy, including close supervision, continuity of care, aggressive intervention, and an optimistic outlook, is more important than minor variations in the use of individual measures. When an individual patient is not doing well, every potentially useful aspect of therapy should be evaluated. Because of the large numbers of medications used, iatrogenic symptoms are frequent and deserve full consideration.

INTERMITTENT AEROSOL THERAPY. Intermittent aerosol therapy (5–10 min duration) is used to deliver medications and/or water to the lower respiratory tract. It is given before and/or after segmental postural drainage. Intermittent positive pres-

sure breathing does not improve delivery of the aerosol and may aggravate the obstructive lesion. The basic aerosol solution consists of 2 mL of 0.125% phenylephrine in 10% USP propylene glycol or of 0.45% saline and is administered 2–4 times daily, usually before chest physiotherapy. In patients with hyperreactive airways, isoetharine or isoproterenol can be added. When secretions are very thick and difficult to clear, a mucolytic agent such as N-acetylcysteine may be useful. Two mL of 20% N-acetylcysteine in 2 mL of basic aerosol solution can be used prior to postural drainage. Because of the potential for irritation of or injury to respiratory epithelium, the duration of use should be limited to 3–5 days.

When the bacteria are resistant to oral antibiotics or when the infection is difficult to control at home, aerosolized antibiotics administered after postural drainage may reduce symptoms, especially those referable to tracheitis or bronchitis. Twenty to 80 mg of colistimethate, gentamicin, or tobramycin in 2 mL of saline has been used 2–4 times daily in home therapy and also in the hospital in conjunction with intravenous therapy. Carbenicillin (1 g) and ticarcillin (0.5 g) have also been used in aerosol. Sensitization or resistance to antibiotics may occur as a result of this use, but are surprisingly infrequent.

A small compressor that drives an aerosol nebulizer is useful for home nebulization therapy. Daily cleaning of the nebulizer should be followed by rinsing and air drying. As soon as the patient can reliably breathe through the mouth and not through the nose, mouth-breathing inhalation therapy should be encouraged with occasional breath-holding following deep inspiration in an effort to increase deposition. The patient's position should not restrict diaphragmatic breathing during aerosol therapy. Nebulization therapy can provoke irritation or intolerance; if either is suspected, the therapy should be discontinued.

MIST INHALATION THERAPY. When thick or copious secretions are difficult to mobilize, some patients benefit from direct inhalation from an ultrasonic nebulizer for 10–20 min prior to postural drainage; one fourth isotonic saline solution is usually well tolerated. Mist tent therapy used overnight to enhance humidification and deposit water droplets in the lower respiratory tract may be beneficial for selected patients. Either a pneumatic-type nebulizer or an ultrasonic nebulizer can be used to generate mist with a mean particle size of 1–2 microns. Ultrasonic units are quiet and have a large water output. They are more difficult to maintain and more easily contaminated by *Pseudomonas*. A relatively small tent should be used to achieve a relatively dense mist. For ultrasonic units, the solutions most commonly nebulized are 5% USP propylene glycol by volume in distilled water, a one fourth isotonic saline solution, or distilled water. In pneumatic units, 10% USP propylene glycol by volume in distilled water is used. The solution should be sterile and free from organic matter to minimize bacterial growth. Nebulizers should be washed every other day with A-33 or 2% acetic acid solution followed by rinsing and thorough drying. Gas sterilization is preferable in the hospital.

CHEST PHYSICAL THERAPY. This therapy is most effective when used in conjunction with inhalation and antibiotic therapy. Postural drainage therapy can be initiated even in the young infant. When old enough to cooperate, children are encouraged to extend exhalations using pursed-lip breathing to prevent airway collapse and to permit better emptying of the lungs. Because localized mucous plugging has been described even in patients with little or no clinical evidence of active pulmonary infection and because early mucous plugging occurs in small airways where relatively slow mass air movement is unlikely to dislodge plugs during deep breathing or cough, a minimum of one aerosol treatment followed by 20–30 min of postural drainage is recommended daily for every patient. Young infants with pulmonary symptoms receive this therapy 3–4 times a day. Flare-ups of the pulmonary infection or periods of acute respiratory illness require additional treatment periods. Although infants and children can be treated effectively on the lap, the use of a tilt board or folding therapy table facilitates this treatment for older individuals. Effective coughing should be encouraged after each segment is clapped. For those positions which are quite productive, the clapping and vibrating should be repeated. Older individuals are encouraged in self-therapy, which can be facilitated by the use of a mechanical percussor or vibrator. On occasion, chest physical therapy may contribute to hemoptysis and may need to be discontinued or modified temporarily. Physical activity, forced deep breathing, and ventilatory maneuvers such as forced expiration or use of positive expiratory pressure may result in expectoration of mucus or improved pulmonary function and may be used as adjunct therapy. A regular program of exercise maintains a feeling of general well-being.

ANTIBIOTIC THERAPY. The goal of antibiotic therapy is to reduce the intensity of pulmonary infection and to minimize or delay the inflammatory reaction and progressive lung damage. While some organisms such as S. *aureus* can be eradicated temporarily from sputum, others such as *P. aeruginosa* are rarely eliminated, even for short periods. Differentiation of colonization from infection is a recurring problem, and the usual guidelines for acute infections such as fever, tachypnea, or chest pain are often absent. Consequently, all aspects of the patient's history and examination must be utilized to guide the frequency and duration of antibiotic therapy. Antibiotic treatment varies from intermittent short courses of one antibiotic to continuous treatment with one or more antibiotics for weeks at a time. Dosages are often two to three times the amount recommended for minor infections because patients having cystic fibrosis have proportionately more lean body mass and higher clearance rates for many antibiotics than do other individuals. In addition, it is difficult to achieve effective drug levels of many antimicrobials in respiratory tract secretions.

Outpatient Antibiotic Therapy. Many patients require at least 2 wk of some antibiotic therapy during each 6–8 wk interval. Indications include the presence of symptoms and identification of pathogenic organisms in respiratory tract cultures, e.g., S. *aureus*, *P. aeruginosa*, pneumococcus, and H. *influenzae*. When acute symptoms develop, initial antibiotic selection should include appropriate therapy for all these organisms. Treatment usually should be continued for 2 wk or more after the symptoms have abated. If improvement is not observed in 5–7 days, the antibiotic therapy should be adjusted. If symptoms reappear after successful therapy, the course of antibiotic therapy should be repeated. Some recommend continuous semisynthetic penicillin therapy in full dosage from the time of diagnosis in an effort to prevent or minimize staphylococcal infection. Low-dosage, continuous antibiotic therapy is not recommended because achievement of adequate airway levels is difficult and because *Pseudomonas* and other organisms tend to develop resistance.

Whenever possible, the choice of antimicrobials should be guided by in vitro sensitivity testing. Often sulfisoxazole or trimethoprim-sulfamethoxazole are the only agents that appear effective. Chloramphenicol succinate can be extremely valuable in cases in which symptoms are uncontrolled by other agents. These agents may be effective even when the cultured organisms are not sensitive in vitro. Tetracyclines should be avoided in children under 9 yr of age. Young children may be colonized with *Pseudomonas* relatively early. If they seem to be doing well clinically, antibiotic therapy should be directed at the other organisms that are present. However, if symptoms are not controlled, *Pseudomonas* should be treated.

Inpatient Antibiotic Therapy. For the patient who has progressive or unrelenting symptoms or signs despite intensive home measures, hospitalization for intravenous antibiotic therapy is indicated. Although many patients improve within 7 days, it is usually advisable to extend the hospital treatment period to at least 14 days. Permanent intravenous access can now be provided for long-term therapy in the hospital or at home.

Antibiotics should be selected on the bases of sputum culture and susceptibility studies. A combination of ticarcillin, 200–400 mg/kg/24 hr, or carbenicillin, 300–800 mg/kg/24 hr, administered every 4 hr, and tobramycin or gentamicin is frequently used against *Pseudomonas*. In cases with resistance to ticarcillin or carbenicillin, treatment with piperacillin or azlocillin has been effective. The aminoglycosides have a relatively short half-life in many patients with cystic fibrosis. The initial dose is 8-10 mg/kg/24 hr, generally given every 8 hr. After blood levels have been determined, the total daily dose should be adjusted to minimize the risk of toxicity. Trough levels should be kept below 2.0 mg/L. New drugs for resistant *Pseudomonas* infections include ceftazidime and imipenem. Frequently an antistaphylococcal antibiotic is added even if the organism is not cultured, especially in children having hemoptysis or a poor response. Changes in therapy should be guided by culture results and by lack of improvement. In patients who do not improve, heart failure, hyperreactive airways, *Aspergillus fumigatus* or mycobacteria, or other rare pulmonary infectious agents should be considered.

BRONCHODILATOR THERAPY. Reversible airway obstruction occurs in up to one third of patients with cystic fibrosis, sometimes in conjunction with frank asthma or acute bronchopulmonary aspergillosis. Reversible obstruction is suggested by improvement of 15% or more in flow rates or indices of hyperinflation after inhalation of a bronchodilator aerosol. Treatment may include regular use of bronchodilator aerosol, oral sympathomimetic agents, and/or sustained-release oral theophylline, with the dosage adjusted after blood levels are obtained. In some cases aerosol or systemic corticosteroid therapy is required, at least briefly. The safety and effectiveness of this therapeutic approach are being examined in a large multicenter study.

ENDOSCOPY AND LAVAGE. Treatment of obstructive airways disease sometimes includes tracheobronchial suctioning or lavage, especially if atelectasis or mucoid impaction is present. Bronchopulmonary lavage may be performed by the instillation of small volumes of saline or mucolytic agent through a fiberoptic bronchoscope or by the introduction of several liters of solution through a Carlens double lumen tube under general anesthesia. Antibiotics (usually gentamicin or tobramycin) may also be directly instilled at lavage, transiently achieving a much higher endobronchial concentration than can be obtained using intravenous therapy. There is no evidence for sustained benefit from endoscopic or lavage procedures.

EXPECTORANTS. Systemic drugs, such as iodides and glyceryl guaiacolate, are not effective in physically removing secretions from the respiratory tract.

Treatment of Pulmonary Complications. A number of pulmonary complications require extra attention or special measures.

ATELECTASIS. Lobar atelectasis occurs relatively infrequently; it may be asymptomatic and noted only at the time of routine chest roentgenogram. Aggressive intravenous therapy with antibiotics and increased chest physical therapy directed at the affected lobe may be effective. If there is no improvement in 7–10 days, bronchoscopy may be indicated for possible removal of a mucous plug. If the atelectasis does not resolve, the patient should be discharged with continued intensive home therapy to the involved lobe, since the atelectasis may resolve over a period of weeks or months. Even if the lobe does not expand, it may not be a source of symptomatic infection. However, lobectomy should be considered if the patient has progressive difficulty from fever, anorexia, unrelenting cough, or sputum production. Lobectomy should be performed only after a period of hospitalization for intensive therapy to improve the status of all remaining portions of the lung.

HEMOPTYSIS. With increasing numbers of older patients, hemoptysis has become a relatively frequent complication. When small amounts (~20 mL) of blood are lost, postural drainage should be continued and the antibiotic regimen reviewed to be certain that coverage is adequate. When the hemoptysis is persistent or increases in severity, hospital admission is indicated. Massive hemoptysis, defined as total blood loss of 250 mL or more within a 24 hr period, requires close monitoring, including a fresh sputum culture and a blood sample for cross-match. Intravenous antibiotic therapy should be instituted. Chest physical therapy is often discontinued until 12–24 hr after the last bleeding episode and then gradually reinstituted. Patients should receive vitamin K in the event that they have or may develop an abnormal prothrombin time. During hemoptysis the patient may require a great deal of reassurance that the bleeding will stop. Hemoptysis may be aggravated in the recumbent position and may require a semi-erect sitting position. Blood transfusion is not indicated unless there is hypotension or the hematocrit is significantly reduced. Ticarcillin may interfere with platelet function and may aggravate hemoptysis. Bronchoscopy has been used in an effort to localize the site of bleeding. However, usually no bleeding site is found. Lobectomy should be avoided if possible because functioning lung must be preserved and because it is difficult to be certain of the bleeding site. Bronchial artery catheterization and embolization can be useful to control persistent, significant hemoptysis.

PNEUMOTHORAX. (Also see Sec. 13.99). This is encountered with increasing frequency, especially in older patients, and may be life threatening. The episode may be asymptomatic but is often attended by chest and shoulder pain, shortness

of breath, or hemoptysis. Even mild symptoms should be taken seriously and a chest roentgenogram obtained. If the pneumothorax is smaller than 5–10%, the patient is admitted to the hospital and observed. A pneumothorax greater than 10% or under tension requires rapid, definitive treatment. Because of frequent delayed closure of the air leak and a high rate of recurrence when closed thoracotomy treatment alone is performed, an open thoracotomy through a small incision with plication of blebs, apical pleural stripping, and basal pleural abrasion is recommended after the first occurrence and within 24 hr of the diagnosis. This procedure is well tolerated even in cases of advanced lung disease. Intravenous antibiotics are begun on admission. The thoracotomy tube is removed as soon as possible, usually by the 2nd or 3rd postoperative day. The patient then can be mobilized and full postural drainage therapy resumed. Recurrences, intraoperative complications, and deaths are extremely rare as a result of this procedure. Closed thoracotomy in conjunction with a sclerosing agent continues to be used by some specialists. Rarely, bilateral simultaneous pneumothorax is encountered; in this case, control of the air leak must be achieved rapidly, at least on one side. Both sides can be treated surgically through a split-sternum approach.

ALLERGIC ASPERGILLOSIS. This complication may present with wheezing, increased cough, shortness of breath, and/or marked hyperinflation on pulmonary function testing (also see Sec. 11.97 and 13.75). In some patients there are new, focal infiltrates on chest roentgenogram. The presence of brown sputum, recovery of *Aspergillus* from the sputum, several serum precipitin bands to *Aspergillus fumigatus* extract, or the presence of eosinophils in fresh sputum samples supports the diagnosis. The IgE level may be high or within normal limits. Treatment is directed at controlling bronchospasm with bronchodilators. In most cases systemic corticosteroid therapy and, possibly, aerosol corticosteroid should also be used. This is usually a self-limited illness and will subside with several weeks of therapy. For refractory cases, aerosolized amphotericin B or systemic 5-fluorocytosine may be required.

HYPERTROPHIC OSTEOARTHROPATHY. This complication causes elevation of the periosteum of the distal portions of long bones and bone pain, edema, and joint effusions. Acetaminophen or ibuprofen may provide relief. Control of lung infection may be most helpful. Some medications may aggravate symptoms.

ACUTE RESPIRATORY FAILURE. Acute respiratory failure (Sec. 13.21) rarely occurs and is usually the result of a severe viral illness such as influenza. Since patients with this complication usually regain their previous status, intensive therapy is indicated. In addition to the aerosol, postural drainage, and intravenous antibiotic treatment, oxygen is required to raise the arterial pO_2 above 50 mm Hg. A rising pCO_2 may require intermittent positive pressure breathing or ventilatory assistance. Endotracheal or bronchoscopic suction may be necessary and can be repeated daily. Right heart failure may occur. Recovery is often slow and does not begin until after the acute illness has subsided. Intensive intravenous antibiotic therapy and postural drainage should be continued for 1–2 wk after the patient has regained baseline status.

CHRONIC RESPIRATORY FAILURE. Patients develop chronic respiratory failure either as a result of incomplete recovery from an acute exacerbation or from prolonged slow deterioration. Although this can occur at any age, it is more frequently seen in adolescent and adult patients. Because a longstanding arterial pO_2 of less than 45–50 mm Hg promotes the development of right heart failure, these patients usually benefit from low-flow oxygen therapy to raise the arterial pO_2 to 50–55 mm Hg. Increasing hypercapnia may prevent the use of optimal FiO_2. These patients do not benefit from continuous ventilator assistance or tracheostomy. Most patients will improve somewhat with intensive antibiotic and pulmonary therapy measures and can be discharged again from the hospital after gradual weaning from supplemental oxygen. In some cases it is necessary to provide low-flow oxygen therapy at home. These patients nearly always display cor pulmonale, should be maintained on a reduced salt intake, and should be watched for edema, increasing shortness of breath, or fatigue. Rehospitalization for intensive care may result in further slow improvement.

RIGHT HEART FAILURE. Some patients develop right heart failure as the result of a complication such as an acute viral infection or pneumothorax. Individuals with longstanding, advanced pulmonary disease, especially those with severe hypoxemia (PaO_2 below 50 mm Hg), often develop chronic right heart failure. Some combination of cyanosis, increased shortness of breath, increased liver size with tender margin, ankle edema, jugular venous distention, an unusual weight gain, increased heart size by chest roentgenogram, and/or evidence for right heart enlargement by electrocardiogram or echocardiography helps to confirm the diagnosis. Furosemide, 1 mg/kg administered intravenously, may result in a good diuresis and confirm the suspicion of fluid retention. Repeated doses may be required at 24–48 hr intervals in the initial period to reduce fluid accumulation and accompanying symptoms. Concomitant use of spironolactone or triamterene may protect against potassium depletion and facilitate long-term diuresis. Digitalis is not effective in pure right-sided failure, but it may be useful when there is associated left-sided failure. The arterial pO_2 should be maintained above 50 mm Hg if at all possible. Loss of respiratory drive may occur during the initial phases of oxygen therapy, and serial arterial blood gases or noninvasive monitoring is required to assure the continuation of adequate respiration. Intensive pulmonary therapy including intravenous antibiotics is most important. Initially the salt intake should be limited to 2 g sodium/day; carbenicillin may be hazardous because of its relatively high sodium content. Fluid overload should be avoided. No clear-cut long-term benefit from tolazoline has been demonstrated. In the past, cardiac failure usually meant death within 1–2 mo. In recent years the prognosis has been improving, and a number of older patients have survived 3–5 yr or longer after an initial episode of cardiac failure.

Gastrointestinal Therapy. Up to 85–90% of patients require digestive therapy, which includes diet adjustment, pancreatic enzyme replacement, and vitamin supplements.

DIET. In the past, a low fat, high protein and caloric diet was generally recommended. With the advent of the microsphere enzyme product, the fat intake is decreased only for symptoms, e.g., cramps or frequent, oily stools. A good protein source is required. When young infants with cystic fibrosis who present with wheezing respirations are fed soy protein formula, they do not utilize this protein well and may develop hypoproteinemia and anasarca within 4 wk unless pancreatic enzyme supplements are prescribed.

PANCREATIC ENZYME REPLACEMENT. Extracts of animal pancreas given with ingested food reduce but do not fully correct stool fat and nitrogen losses. Adjustment of enzyme dosage and product should be individualized for each patient. The introduction of pH-sensitive enteric-coated enzyme microspheres (Pancrease, Cotazym-S) has been a major advance in patient care. One to 3 capsules/meal is sufficient for most patients; infants may need only one-third or one-half capsule or may do better with pancreatin powder (Cotazym). The microsphere preparations usually are sufficiently effective to permit a liberal diet, which may include homogenized milk. Some patients or parents who handle the enzymes develop episodes of rhinitis, watery eyes, or bronchospasm on repeated administration of hog pancreatin extracts, a problem that is less frequent with the use of coated microspheres. Enzyme preparations containing bile salts are infrequently needed. The dose of enzymes required usually increases with age initially, but some teenagers and young adults may later have a decrease in their requirement. Enzyme replacement therapy is best distributed throughout the meal but may be sufficiently effective when taken either right after or in some cases just before eating.

VITAMIN SUPPLEMENTATION. Because pancreatic insufficiency results in malabsorption of fat-soluble vitamins (A, D, E, and K), vitamin supplementation is recommended. Vitamins A and D can be supplied by one of several multivitamin preparations. Vitamin E deficiency is usually corrected with daily doses of 100–200 units. Vitamin K is needed only sporadically: in the newborn period, and during periods of hemoptysis, intense antimicrobial therapy, or surgery. The usual dose is 5 mg orally given daily or every other day. Those with cheilosis may benefit from extra riboflavin (5–10 mg daily), from additional B vitamins, or from local corticosteroid-antifungal applications.

NUTRITIONAL SUPPLEMENTATION. If pancreatic replacement therapy is used and enough calories are provided, nutrition should be adequate unless the cachexia of chronic pulmonary infection intervenes. Anorexia secondary to pulmonary infection cannot be consciously overcome by the patient; attempts to force the consumption of more calories will be unsuccessful and lead to unnecessary emotional upset. However, some children, especially teenagers, fail to eat properly, and efforts to increase caloric intake will result in weight gain. Medium chain triglycerides (MCT) are more readily absorbed without digestion than long chain triglycerides and provide a ready source of calories, but most patients find them unpalatable. Supplemental feedings by overnight nasogastric or gastrostomy tube or hyperalimentation by intravenous infusion have been used during acute illness or for patients unable to maintain their weight.

MECONIUM ILEUS (Sec. 8.42). When meconium ileus is suspected, a nasogastric tube is placed for suction and the infant is hydrated and prepared for surgery. However, in some cases Gastrografin enemas with reflux of contrast material into the ileum have resulted in passage of a meconium plug and clearing of the obstruction. Use of this hypertonic solution requires careful replacement of water losses into the bowel. Patients with an atretic segment of the ileum require resection and anastomosis. Individuals who survive surgery generally have a prognosis similar to that of other patients. Infants with meconium ileus should be treated as having cystic fibrosis until adequate sweat testing can be carried out, usually after 1–2 wk of life.

MECONIUM ILEUS EQUIVALENT, INTUSSUSCEPTION, AND OTHER CAUSES OF ABDOMINAL PAIN. Despite appropriate pancreatic enzyme replacement, some patients accumulate fecal material in the terminal portion of the ileum and in the cecum, which may result in intermittent or complete obstruction (meconium ileus equivalent). For intermittent obstruction, pancreatic enzyme replacement should be continued or even increased and laxative and/or stool softeners (milk of magnesia, Colace, mineral oil) given. Increased fluid intake is also recommended. When there is complete obstruction, a Gastrografin enema, accompanied by large amounts of intravenous fluids, can be therapeutic. If the enema reaches the terminal ileum, this hypertonic material will draw water into the bowel and loosen the inspissated fecal material. Intussusception and volvulus also must be considered in the differential diagnosis. Intussusception, usually ileocolic, occurs at any age and often follows a 1–2 day history of "constipation." If an intussusception is present, it often can be both diagnosed and reduced by a Gastrografin enema. If a nonreducible intussusception or a volvulus is present, a laparotomy is required. Repeated episodes of intussusception may be an indication for cecectomy. Once or twice daily dosages of mineral oil (1 tablespoon) given well before bedtime may prevent repeated episodes of meconium ileus equivalent.

Chronic appendicitis with or without periappendiceal abscess occurs occasionally in patients on long-term antibiotic therapy and may present with recurrent or persistent abdominal pain. Lack of acid buffering in the duodenum appears to promote duodenitis and ulcer formation in some children. Esophagitis and bile reflux into the stomach are being seen more frequently in older patients.

RECTAL PROLAPSE. This occurs frequently in infants with cystic fibrosis and less commonly in older children. It is usually related to steatorrhea, malnutrition, and repetitive cough. The prolapsed rectum usually can be replaced manually by continuous gentle pressure with the patient in the knee-chest position. Sedation may be helpful. To prevent an immediate recurrence, the buttocks can be taped closed. Adequate pancreatin replacement, decreased fat and roughage in the diet, and control of pulmonary infection result in improvement. An infrequent patient may continue to have rectal prolapse and require surgery (a rectal sling of Silastic placed around the rectum just below the skin).

BILIARY CIRRHOSIS. Portal hypertension with esophageal varices, hypersplenism, and/or ascites is the most common complication of biliary cirrhosis (see Sec. 12.72). The acute management of bleeding esophageal varices includes nasogastric suction and cold saline lavage. Intravenous or celiac artery infusion of Pitressin may be of help. The efficacy of sclerotherapy of varices in cystic fibrosis is not established. Significant bleeding is an indication for portal-systemic shunting. Splenectomy and splenorenal anastomosis decrease portal pressure and also effectively treat hypersplenism. Portacaval anastomosis may also be used. The management of ascites is discussed in Sec. 12.74.

Obstructive jaundice occurs infrequently in newborns with cystic fibrosis and requires no specific therapy. Rarely, biliary cirrhosis proceeds to hepatocellular failure, which should be treated as in other patients with hepatic failure (Sec. 12.74, 12.85 and 12.88).

PANCREATITIS. Pancreatitis usually occurs in patients with preservation of some exocrine pancreatic function and is usually precipitated by fatty meals, alcohol ingestion, or tetracycline therapy. Serum amylase and lipase levels may remain elevated for long periods of time. Treatment is discussed in Sec. 12.69.

HYPERGLYCEMIA. Onset can occur at any age and is not related to the severity of the disease; ketoacidosis is rarely encountered. If blood glucose levels are only moderately elevated and urine glucose losses are small, no treatment is necessary. With more marked elevation and polyuria insulin treatment should be instituted. Oral antidiabetic agents are usually not effective. Exocrine pancreatic insufficiency and malabsorption make strict dietary control of hyperglycemia virtually impossible. The development of significant hyperglycemia does not appear to change the prognosis significantly.

Other Therapy. NASAL POLYPS. These occur in 15–20% of cystic fibrosis patients and in some become a recurrent problem. Corticosteroid and decongestant nasal sprays occasionally provide relief. Allergy skin testing and hyposensitization may be helpful in those with allergic symptoms. When the polyps completely obstruct the nasal airway or rhinorrhea becomes constant, surgical removal is indicated; polyps may recur promptly after removal but frequently do not grow to the point of obstruction for long periods. Patients with many recurrences inexplicably may stop developing polyps.

SALT DEPLETION. Sweat salt losses can be high on hot summer days. Infants and, less frequently, older patients may present with hyponatremic hypochloremic dehydration. Children should have free access to salt, and precautions against overdressing infants in hot weather should be observed.

MATURATION. Delayed sexual maturation, often associated with short stature, occurs fairly frequently. Although many have severe pulmonary infection and/or poor nutrition, delayed puberty also occurs in patients with otherwise mild disease and is not well explained. Adolescents with cystic fibrosis should receive specific counseling concerning sexual development and potential reproductive problems through their developing years.

SURGERY. Minor surgical procedures, including dental work, should be performed under local anesthesia if possible. Patients with good or excellent pulmonary status can tolerate general anesthesia without any intensive pulmonary measures prior to the surgery. Those having moderate or severe pulmonary infection are usually better off with a 1–2 wk course of intensive antibiotic treatment prior to surgery. If this is impossible, prompt intravenous antibiotic therapy is indicated once it is recognized that major surgery will be required. An aerosol and postural drainage treatment immediately prior to the anesthesia and surgery is advisable. Total anesthesia time should be kept to a minimum. After induction, tracheal suctioning is useful and should be repeated at least at the end of the operation. Patients having severe disease require frequent monitoring of their blood gases and may require ventilatory assistance in the immediate postoperative period.

After major surgery, cough should be encouraged and postural drainage treatments should be reinstituted as soon as possible, usually within 24 hr, and gradually intensified until full treatments are completed. For those with significant pulmonary involvement, intravenous antibiotics are continued for a minimum of 14 postoperative days. Early ambulation and intermittent deep breathing are important, and an incentive spirometer can also be helpful. Following open thoracotomy for treatment of pneumothorax or lobectomy, the chest tube is the greatest single obstacle to effective pulmonary therapy and should be removed as soon as possible so that full postural drainage therapy can resume.

Prognosis. Cystic fibrosis remains a life-limiting disorder, although survival has improved dramatically during the past 30 yr. Occasionally infants with severe lung disease succumb, but most children survive this difficult period and are relatively healthy into adolescence or adulthood. However, the slow progression of lung disease eventually reaches disabling proportions. National life table data now indicate a median cumulative survival of approximately 20 yr. Male survival is somewhat better than female for reasons that are not readily apparent. Survival beyond 20 years of treatment exceeds 90% at some centers if cystic fibrosis is diagnosed and treatment began before substantial lung damage, as assessed by chest roentgenogram, has occurred.

For the most part, children with cystic fibrosis have good school attendance records and can be unrestricted in their activities. A high percentage eventually attend and graduate from college. Most find satisfactory employment and an increasing number marry.

With increasing life span, a new set of psychosocial considerations has emerged, including dependence-independence issues, self-care, peer relationships, sterility, educational and vocational planning, financial burdens, and psychologic reactions to anxiety. Many of these issues are best addressed during childhood and early adolescence, prior to the onset of psychosocial dysfunction. With appropriate medical and psychosocial support, children and adolescents with cystic fibrosis generally cope well. Achievement of an independent and productive adulthood is a realistic goal for many.

CARL F. DOERSHUK
THOMAS F. BOAT

Auerbach HS, Williams M, Kirkpatrick JA, et al: Alternate-day prednisone reduces morbidity and improves function in cystic fibrosis. Lancet 2:686, 1985.

Bijman J, Quinton PM. Influence of abnormal Cl⁻ impermeability on sweating in cystic fibrosis. Am J Physiol 247(Cell Physiol 16):C3, 1984.

Chase HP, Long MA, and Lavin MH: Cystic fibrosis and malnutrition. J Pediatr 95:337, 1979.

Clay MM, Pavia D, Newman SP, et al: Assessment of jet nebulisers for lung aerosol therapy. Lancet 2:592, 1983.

Cowen L, Corey M, Simmons R, et al: Growing older with cystic fibrosis: Psychologic adjustment of patients more than 16 years old. Psychosom Med 45:363, 1984.

Davis PB, diSant'Agnese PA: Assisted ventilation for patients with cystic fibrosis. JAMA 239:1851, 1978.

Denning CR, Huang NN, Cuasay LR, et al: Cooperative study comparing three methods of performing sweat tests to diagnose cystic fibrosis. Pediatrics 66:752, 1980.

Desmond KJ, Schwenk F, Thomas E, et al: Immediate and long-term effects of chest physiotherapy in patients with cystic fibrosis. J Pediatr 103:538, 1983.

Doershuk CF, Reyes AL, Regan A, et al: Anesthesia for cystic fibrosis patients. Anesth Anal 51:413, 1972.

Esterly JR, Oppenheimer EH: Cystic fibrosis of the pancreas: Structural changes in peripheral airways. Thorax 23:670, 1968.

Knowles M, Gatzy J., Boucher R.: Relative ion permeability of normal and cystic fibrosis nasal epithelium. J Clin Invest 71:1410, 1983.

Levine SB, and Stern RC: Sexual function in cystic fibrosis: Relationship to overall health status and pulmonary disease severity in 30 married patients. Chest 81:422, 1982.

Lloyd-Still JD (ed): Textbook of Cystic Fibrosis. Bristol, England, John Wright, 1983.

Matthews LW, and Drotar D: Cystic fibrosis—A challenging long-term chronic disease. Pediatr Clin North Am 31:133, 1984.

Orenstein DM, Boat TF, Stern RC, et al: The effect of early diagnosis and treatment in cystic fibrosis; A seven-year study of 16 sibling pairs. Am J Dis Child 131:973, 1977.

Rodman H, Doershuk CF, Roland J: The interaction of 2 diseases: Diabetes mellitus and cystic fibrosis. Medicine 65:389, 1986.

Stern RC, Boat TF, Abramowsky CF, et al: Intermediate range sweat chloride concentration and pseudomonas bronchitis: A cystic fibrosis variant with preservation of exocrine pancreatic function. JAMA 239:2676, 1978.

Stern RC, Boat TF, Doershuk CF, et al: Course of ninety-five patients with cystic fibrosis. J Pediatr 89:406, 1976.

Stern RC, Boat TF, Matthews LW, et al: Treatment and prognosis of massive hemoptysis in cystic fibrosis. Am Rev Respir Dis 117:825, 1978.

Stern RC, Borkat G, Hirschfeld SS, et al: Heart failure in cystic fibrosis: Treatment and prognosis of cor pulmonale with failure of the right side of the heart. Am J Dis Child 134:267, 1980.

Stowe SM, Boat TF, Mendelsohn H, et al: Open thoracotomy for pneumothorax in cystic fibrosis. Am Rev Respir Dis 111:611, 1975.

Taussig L (ed): Cystic Fibrosis. New York, Thieme-Stratton, 1984.

Tecklin J: Bronchial hygiene in respiratory physical therapy. In: Lough MD, Doershuk CF, Stern RC (eds): Pediatric Respiratory Therapy. Chicago, Year-book Medical Publishers, 1986.

Thomassen MJ, Demko C, Doershuk CF, et al: Pseudomonas cepacia: Decrease in colonization in patients with cystic fibrosis. Am Rev Respir Dis 134:669, 1986.

Thomassen MJ, Demko C, Doershuk CF: Cystic fibrosis: A review of pulmonary infections and interventions. Pediatric Pulmonology, in press, 1986.

Welsh MJ, Liedtke CM: Chloride and potassium channels in cystic fibrosis airway epithelia. Nature 322:467, 1986.

White R, Woodward S, Leppart M, et al: A closely linked genetic marker for cystic fibrosis. Nature 318:382, 1985.

Wood RE: Prognosis in Cystic Fibrosis. In: Taussig LM (ed): Cystic Fibrosis. New York, Thieme-Stratton, 1984.

Wood RE, Boat TF, and Doershuk CF: State of the art: Cystic fibrosis. Am Rev Respir Dis 113:833, 1976.

DISEASES OF THE PLEURA

13.98 PLEURISY

The most common cause of pleural effusion in children is pneumococcal pneumonia, and metastatic intrathoracic malignancy is the second. Tuberculous effusion has become much less common with improved screening procedures and chemotherapy. A variety of other diseases, including lupus erythematosus, aspiration pneumonitis, uremia, and rheumatoid arthritis, account for the remainder of the cases. Males and females are equally affected. The incidence of effusion is probably lower for infants with lobar pneumococcal pneumonia than for older children.

Inflammatory processes in the pleura are usually divided into three general types: dry or plastic, serofibrinous or serosanguineous, and purulent pleurisy or empyema.

Dry or Plastic Pleurisy

This may be associated with acute bacterial pulmonary infections or may develop during the course of an acute upper respiratory tract illness. The condition also is associated with tuberculosis and with mesenchymal diseases, such as rheumatic fever.

Pathology. The process is usually limited to the visceral pleura. There are usually small amounts of yellow serous fluid and adhesions between the pleural surfaces. In tuberculosis the adhesions develop rapidly and the pleura is often thickened. Occasionally fibrin deposition and adhesions may be sufficiently severe to produce a fibrothorax that markedly inhibits the excursions of the lung.

Clinical Manifestations. Signs and symptoms are often overshadowed by the primary disease. The principal symptom is pain, which is exaggerated by deep breathing, coughing, and straining. Occasionally, pleural pain is described as a dull ache, which is less likely to vary with breathing. Often the pain is localized over the chest wall and referred to the shoulder or the back. Pain with breathing is responsible for grunting and guarding of respirations, the child often lying on the affected side in an attempt to decrease respiratory excursions. Early in the illness a leathery, rough, to-and-fro friction rub may be audible, but this usually disappears rapidly. Occasionally, increased dullness on percussion and suppressed breath sounds are heard when the layer of exudate is thick. Pleurisy may also be asymptomatic and detected only on roentgenography; a diffuse haziness at the pleural surface or a dense, sharply demarcated shadow may be noted. The latter finding may be indistinguishable from small amounts of pleural exudate. Chronic pleurisy is occasionally encountered with such conditions as atelectasis, pulmonary abscess, mesenchymal diseases, and tuberculosis.

Differential Diagnosis. Plastic pleurisy must be distinguished from other diseases, such as epidemic pleurodynia or trauma to the rib cage, particularly fracture of a rib, and from lesions of the dorsal root ganglia, tumors of the spinal cord, herpes zoster, gallbladder disease, and trichinosis. Even if evidence of pleural fluid is not found on physical or roentgenographic examination, a pleural tap in suspected cases will often result in the recovery of a small amount of exudate, which, when cultured, will usually reveal the underlying bacterial cause in cases associated with an acute pneumonia. When pleurisy and pneumonia continue for more than 2 wk, tuberculosis should be considered.

Treatment. Therapy should be aimed at the underlying disease. When pneumonia is present, neither immobilization of the chest with adhesive plaster nor therapy with drugs capable of suppressing the cough reflex is indicated. If pneumonia is not present or is under good therapeutic control, strapping of the chest to restrict expansion may afford relief from pain.

Serofibrinous Pleurisy

This is most commonly associated with infections of the lung or with inflammatory conditions of the abdomen or mediastinum. Less commonly it is found with such mesenchymal diseases as lupus erythematosus, periarteritis, or rheumatic fever. On occasion it is seen with primary or metastatic neoplasms of the lung, pleura, or mediastinum; tumors are, however, more commonly associated with a hemorrhagic pleurisy.

Clinical Manifestations. Since serofibrinous pleurisy is often preceded by the plastic type, the early signs and symptoms may be those of the latter illness. As fluid accumulates, pleuritic pain may disappear and the patient becomes asymptomatic (so long as the effusion remains small), or there may be only the signs and symptoms of the underlying disease. If a large amount of fluid collects, there may be cough, dyspnea, retractions, tachypnea, orthopnea, or cyanosis. Physical findings depend to some degree on the amount of effusion. Dullness to flatness may be found on percussion. There is a decrease or absence of breath sounds, a diminution in tactile fremitus, a shift of the mediastinum away from the affected side, and, on occasion, fullness of the intercostal spaces. If the fluid is not loculated, these signs may shift with changes in position. In infants, physical signs are less definite; sometimes, instead of decreased or absent breath sounds, bronchial breathing will be heard. If extensive pneumonia is present, rales and rhonchi may also be audible. Friction rubs are usually present only during the early or late plastic stage. The process is usually unilateral.

Roentgenographic examination shows a more or less homogeneous density obliterating the normal markings of the underlying lung. Small effusions may cause only obliteration of the costophrenic or cardiophrenic angles or a widening of the interlobar septa. Examination should be performed both in the supine and in the upright positions to demonstrate a shift of the effusion with change in position; the decubitus position may also be helpful. Ultrasound examinations may be useful.

Differential Diagnosis. Thoracentesis should be done when pleural fluid is present or is suspected unless the effusion is very small and the patient has a classic lobar pneumococcal pneumonia. Examining fluid is essential to identify acute bacterial infections and may disclose tubercle bacilli. Furthermore, thoracentesis can differentiate between serofibrinous pleurisy, empyema, hydrothorax, hemothorax, and chylothorax. In hydrothorax the fluid has a specific gravity below 1.015, and only a few mesothelial cells rather than leukocytes. Chylothorax and hemothorax usually have fluid distinctive in appearance; differentiating serofibrinous from purulent pleurisy is impossible without bacterial examination of the fluid. The fluid of serofibrinous pleurisy is clear or slightly cloudy and contains relatively few white cells and, occasionally, some red cells. Protein levels greater than 3 g/dL indicate an exudate and are likely to be associated with an infectious process. Similarly, pleural fluid lactic dehydrogenase values higher than 200 IU/L suggest an exudate. Serofibrinous fluid may rapidly become purulent.

Course. Unless the fluid becomes purulent, it usually disappears relatively rapidly, particularly with bacterial pneumonias. It persists somewhat longer with tuberculosis and mesenchymal diseases and may remain or recur for a long time with neoplasms. As the effusion is absorbed, adhesions usually develop between the two layers of the pleura, but usually little or no functional impairment results. Pleural thickening may develop and is occasionally mistaken for small quantities of fluid or for pulmonary infiltrates. Pleural thickening may persist for a long time. In general, however, the process disappears, leaving no residua.

Treatment. Therapy is that of the underlying diseases. When a diagnostic thoracentesis is done, as much fluid as possible should be removed for therapeutic purposes. If the underlying disease is adequately treated, further drainage is usually unnecessary, but if sufficient fluid reaccumulates to embarrass the patient's respiration, repeated thoracentesis or chest tube drainage should be performed. In older children with parapneumonic effusion, tube thoracostomy is probably necessary if the pleural fluid pH is below 7.20 or the pleural fluid glucose is below 50 mg/dL. If the fluid is clearly purulent (see below), tube drainage is usually indicated. Systemic acidosis reduces the usefulness of pleural fluid pH measure-

ments. Patients with pleural effusions may need analgesia, particularly after thoracentesis or insertion of chest tube. Those with acute pneumonia often need supplemental oxygen in addition to antibiotic treatment.

Gryminski J, Kralowka P, Lypacewicz G: The diagnosis of pleural effusion by ultrasonic and radiologic techniques. Chest 70:1, 1976.
Light RW, Girard WM, Jenkinson SG, et al: Parapneumonic effusions. Am J Med 69:507, 1980.
Wolfe WG, Spock A, Bradford WD: Pleural fluids in infants and children. Am Rev Resp Dis 98:1027, 1968.

Purulent Pleurisy
(Empyema)

An accumulation of pus in the pleural spaces is most often associated with pneumonia due to staphylococci, less frequently with pneumococci (especially types 1 and 3) and *H. influenzae*. The relative incidence of *H. influenzae* empyema may have increased recently. In pediatric practice empyema is most frequently encountered in infants (Sec. 8.67) and preschool children. The disease also may be produced by rupture of a lung abscess into the pleural space, by contamination introduced from trauma or thoracic surgery, or, rarely, by mediastinitis or by the extension of intra-abdominal abscesses.

Pathology. Most commonly, purulent pleurisy is an extensive process consisting of a series of loculated areas involving a large portion of one or both pleural cavities. Thickening of the parietal pleura occurs. If the pus is not drained, it may dissect through the pleura into lung parenchyma, producing bronchopleural fistulas and pyopneumothorax, or into the abdominal cavity. Pockets of loculated pus may eventually develop into thick-walled abscess cavities, or, as the exudate organizes, the lung may collapse and become surrounded by a thick, inelastic envelope.

Clinical Manifestations. The initial signs and symptoms are primarily those of bacterial pneumonia. Patients treated inadequately or with inappropriate antibiotic agents may have an interval of a few days between the clinical pneumonic phase and the evidence of empyema. Most patients are febrile. In infants, there may only be a moderate exacerbation of respiratory distress. The older child is apt to appear more toxic and in greater respiratory difficulty. Physical and roentgenographic findings may be identical to those described for serofibrinous pleurisy and the two conditions differentiated only by thoracentesis, which should always be performed when empyema is suspected. (See Serofibrinous Pleurisy, above.) Roentgenographically, finding no shift of fluid with change of position indicates a loculated empyema. The maximum amount of pus obtainable should be withdrawn. The appearance of pus produced by different organisms is not distinctive; cultures must always be obtained and Gram-stained smears examined for the presence of microorganisms. Blood cultures have a high yield (62% in one series), but latex agglutination or counterimmunoelectrophoresis may also be useful. Leukocytosis and an elevated sedimentation rate may occur.

Complications. With staphylococcal infections, bronchopleural fistulas and pyopneumothorax commonly develop. Other local complications include purulent pericarditis, pulmonary abscesses, peritonitis secondary to rupture through the diaphragm and osteomyelitis of the ribs. Septic complications such as meningitis, arthritis, and osteomyelitis may also occur. With staphylococcal empyema, septicemia occurs infrequently; it is often encountered in *H. influenzae* and pneumococcal infections.

Treatment. If pus is obtained by thoracentesis, closed drainage should be instituted immediately and controlled either by an underwater seal or by continuous suction. A catheter with the largest possible internal diameter should be inserted into the site where accumulation of pus is suspected; sometimes several tubes are required to drain loculated areas. Closed drainage is usually necessary only for 1 wk or so, even though small amounts of material will continue to drain after this time, probably in response to the presence of the tube in the pleural cavity. Chest tubes that are no longer draining should be removed. When it is time to withdraw it, the entire tube should be removed all at once.

Instilling fibrinolytic agents or proteolytic enzymes into the pleural cavity commonly produces severe systemic reactions in small children and does not promote drainage. Antibiotics should not be instilled into the pleural cavity since they do not improve results obtained with systemic antibiotic therapy alone and are associated with local reactions. Controlling empyema by multiple aspirations of the pleural cavity rather than by closed continuous drainage should not be attempted.

Systemic antibiotic therapy is required; the selection of the antibiotic should be based on the in vitro sensitivities of the responsible organism. Infant staphylococcal empyema is best treated by parenteral routes with methicillin or, when applicable, with penicillin G. Pneumococcal infection usually responds to pencillin, and *H. influenzae* to ampicillin or chloramphenicol. With staphylococcal infections, resolution of the process is very slow, and systemic antibiotic therapy is required for 3–4 wk. Clinical response in nonstaphylococcal empyema is also often slow, even with optimal treatment; little improvement may occur for up to 2 wk. In patients with inadequately treated empyema, extensive fibrinous changes may take place over the surface of the collapsed lungs, but decortication procedures are rarely indicated. If pneumatoceles form, no attempt should be made to treat them surgically or by aspiration, unless they reach sufficient size to embarrass respiration or become secondarily infected. The long-term clinical prognosis for adequately treated empyema is excellent, but follow-up pulmonary function studies suggest that some restrictive disease is not uncommon.

Bechamps GJ, Lynn HB, Wenzl JE: Empyema in children. Mayo Clin Proc 45:43, 1970.
McLaughlin FJ, Goldmann DA, Rosenbaum DM, et al: Empyema in children: Clinical course and long-term follow-up. Pediatrics 73:587, 1984.
Murphy D, Lockhart CH, Todd JK: Pneumococcal empyema. Am J Dis Child 134:659, 1980.
Ravitch MM, Fein R: The changing picture of pneumonia and empyema in infants and children. A review of the experience at the Harriet Lane Home from 1934 through 1958. JAMA 175:1039, 1961.
Riley HD Jr, Bracken EC: Empyema due to *Hemophilus influenzae* in infants and children. Am J Dis Child 110:24, 1965.
Siegel JD, Gartner JC, Michaels RH: Pneumococcal empyema in childhood. Am J Dis Child 132:1094, 1978.

13.99 PNEUMOTHORAX

Pneumothorax in the neonatal period is discussed in Sec. 8.37. In infant staphylococcal pneumonia, the incidence of pneumothorax is relatively high, but aside from the accidental introduction of air into the pleural cavity during thoracentesis, pneumothorax is uncommon during childhood. Pneumothorax may occur in pneumonia, usually in connection with empyema; it may also be secondary to pulmonary abscess, gangrene, infarct, rupture of a cyst or an emphysematous bleb (as in asthma), foreign bodies in the lung, and external thoracic trauma or surgical procedures. It is found in about 5% of hospitalized asthmatic children and usually resolves without treatment. Pneumothorax is a serious complication in cystic fibrosis (Sec. 13.97). In association with mediastinal emphysema it may be a complication of tracheotomy. Spontaneous pneumothorax occasionally occurs in teenagers and young adults, most frequently in males. Families have been described in which many members have had spontaneous

pneumothoraces with onset ranging from birth to adulthood. Patients with collagen synthesis defects such as Ehlers-Danlos disease and Marfan syndrome are also unusually prone to develop pneumothorax. Pneumothorax may also occur after acupuncture treatment. *Catamenial pneumothorax* can result from passage of intra-abdominal air through diaphragmatic defects; therefore, when thoracotomy is performed for recurrent pneumothorax of unknown etiology, examination of the diaphragm may be appropriate.

Pneumothorax may be associated with a serous effusion (*hydropneumothorax*) or a purulent effusion (*pyopneumothorax*). Bilateral pneumothorax is rare.

Clinical Manifestations. The onset is usually abrupt and the severity of symptoms may depend upon the extent of the lung collapse and the amount of preexisting lung disease. Extensive pneumothorax may involve pain, dyspnea, and cyanosis. In infancy, symptoms and physical signs may be difficult to recognize. If the pneumothorax is only moderate in extent, there may be little displacement of intrathoracic organs and few or no symptoms. The severity of pain usually does not directly reflect the extent of the collapse.

Usually respiratory distress, retractions, and markedly decreased breath sounds over the involved lung are present. The percussion note over the involved area is tympanitic. Larynx, trachea, and heart may be shifted toward the unaffected side. When fluid is present, there is usually a sharply limited area of tympany above a level of flatness to percussion. It is important to determine whether the pneumothorax is under tension (*tension pneumothorax*) since this will limit expansion of the contralateral lung and may compromise cardiovascular function. The presence of amphoric breathing or, when fluid is present in the pleural cavity, of gurgling sounds synchronous with respirations suggests an open fistula connecting with air-bearing tissues. Confirmatory evidence is provided when the pneumothorax fills rapidly after it has been aspirated. The diagnosis can usually be established by roentgenographic examination (Fig. 13–19).

Differential Diagnosis. Pneumothorax must be differentiated from localized or generalized emphysema, from an extensive emphysematous bleb, from large pulmonary cavities or other cystic formations, from diaphragmatic hernia, and from gaseous distention of the stomach; in most instances, a chest roentgenogram will differentiate them. Expiratory views accentuate the contrast between lung markings and the clear area of the pneumothorax. In the case of diaphragmatic hernia, however, a small amount of barium may be necessary to demonstrate that a portion of the gastrointestinal tract is in the thoracic cavity.

Treatment. Therapy varies with the extent of the collapse and the nature and severity of the underlying disease. A small or even moderately sized pneumothorax in an otherwise normal child may resolve without specific treatment usually within 1 wk or so. A small (less than 5%) pneumothorax complicating asthma may also spontaneously resolve. Administering 100% oxygen may hasten resolution by increasing the nitrogen pressure gradient between the pleural air and the blood. Patients with chronic hypoxemia should be monitored closely during administration of supplemental oxygen. Pleural pain deserves analgesic treatment. Codeine may be justified, but its respiratory depressant effect should be considered. Occasionally, morphine or meperidine is needed. If there is more than 5% collapse or if the pneumothorax is recurrent or under tension, definitive treatment is necessary. Pneumothoraces complicating cystic fibrosis frequently recur, and definitive treatment may be justified with the first episode even with less than 5% collapse.

Closed thoracotomy (simple insertion of a chest tube) and drainage of the trapped air through a catheter, the external opening of which is kept in a dependent position under

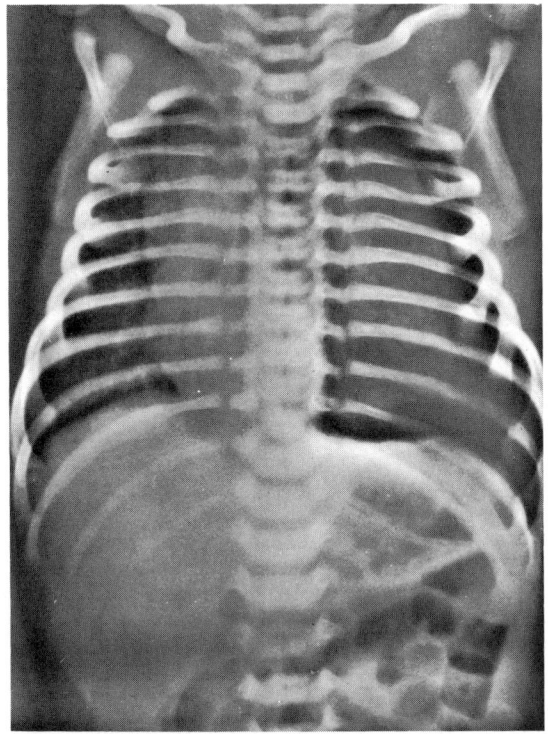

Figure 13–19. Pneumothorax in a newborn infant. The air in the left pleural cavity has partially collapsed the left lung, shifting the heart and mediastinal structures to the right.

water, will be adequate to re-expand the lung in almost all patients. To prevent recurrences when there have already been many pneumothoraces, inducing the formation of strong adhesions between the lung and chest wall by a sclerosing procedure may be indicated, for example, by the introduction of tetracycline or silver nitrate into the pleural space (chemical pleurodesis). Open thoracotomy through a limited incision, with plication of blebs, closure of fistula, stripping of the pleura (usually in the apical lung where the surgeon has direct vision), and basilar pleural abrasion is also an effective treatment for recurring pneumothorax. Postoperative pain is comparable to chemical pleurodesis with silver nitrate, but the chest tube can usually be removed within 24–48 hr, as opposed to the usual 72 hr minimum for closed thoracotomy and pleurodesis.

Treatment of the underlying pulmonary disease should begin on admission. When open thoracotomy is planned for cystic fibrosis patients, it should be done as soon as possible after the patient is admitted, since the patient's condition may gradually deteriorate because the chest tube interferes with postural drainage and physical activity.

Bernhard WF, Malcolm JA, Berry RW, et al: A study of the pathogenesis and management of spontaneous pneumothorax. Dis Chest 42:403, 1962.
Stem H, Toole AL, Merino M: Catamenial pneumothorax. Chest 78:480, 1980.
Wilson WG, Aylsworth: Familial spontaneous pneumothorax. Pediatrics 64:172, 1979.
Youmans CR Jr, Williams RD, McMinn MR, et al: Surgical management of spontaneous pneumothorax by bleb ligation and pleural dry sponge abrasion. Am J Surg 120:644, 1970.

13.100 PNEUMOMEDIASTINUM

Pneumomediastinum usually results from alveolar rupture during the course of an acute or chronic pulmonary disease. However, a diverse group of nonrespiratory entities can also cause pneumomediastinum, and in some of these the lung is not the source of the air. For example, pneumomediastinum has been reported following dental extractions, pneumoencephalography, obstetric delivery, diabetes mellitus with ketoacidosis, acupuncture, and acute gastroenteritis. Pneumomediastinum can also result from esophageal perforation and penetrating chest trauma. Occasionally no underlying cause is found; in an apparently normal child the pneumomediastinum can present as chest pain associated with subcutaneous air.

Following intrapulmonary alveolar rupture, air can dissect through the perivascular sheaths and other soft tissue planes toward the hilum and enter the mediastinum. Pneumomediastinum is rarely a major problem in older children since the mediastinum can be depressurized by escape of air into the neck or abdomen. In the newborn, however, the rate at which air can leave the mediastinum is quite limited, and pneumomediastinum can lead to dangerous cardiovascular compromise or to pneumothorax (Sec. 8.37). Acute asthma is the most common cause of pneumomediastinum in older children and teenagers. Simultaneous pneumothorax is unusual in these patients.

The principal symptom of pneumomediastinum is transient stabbing pains in the chest that may radiate to the neck. However, isolated abdominal pain and sore throat also occur. The patient may complain of dyspnea, but it is difficult to know if this is really a separate symptom or if it is related to the chest pain. Pneumomediastinum is often difficult to detect by physical examination alone. Subcutaneous emphysema, if present, is virtually diagnostic. Although cardiac dullness may be decreased, many of these patients are chronically overinflated, and it is unlikely that the clinician will be sure of this finding. A mediastinal "crunch" is occasionally present but is easily confused with a friction rub. By chest roentgenogram the cardiac border, highlighted by the mediastinal air, is more distinct than normal, and on the lateral projection the posterior mediastinal structures are also clearly defined. Subcutaneous air, seen roentgenographically, confirms the pneumomediastinum.

Treatment is directed primarily at the underlying obstructive pulmonary disease. Analgesics are occasionally needed for chest pain. Rarely, subcutaneous empyema can cause sufficient tracheal compression to justify tracheotomy; the tracheotomy also decompresses the mediastinum.

Church JA, Richards W: Air leak syndromes as complications of respiratory disease in infancy and childhood. Ann Allergy 39:393, 1977.
Girard DE, Carlson V, Natelson EA, Fred HL: Pneumomediastinum in diabetic ketoacidosis: Comments on mechanism, incidence, and management. Chest 60:455, 1971.
Munsell WP: Pneumomediastinum: A report of 28 cases and review of the literature. JAMA 202:689, 1967.
Sandler CM, Libshitz HI, Marks G: Pneumoperitoneum, pneumomediastinum and pneumopericardium following dental extraction. Radiology 115:539, 1975.
Sturtz GS: Spontaneous mediastinal emphysema. Pediatrics 74:431, 1984.
Tsai FY, Lee KF: Pneumopericardium and pneumomediastinum Rare complications of pneumoencephalography. Radiology 112:95, 1974.

13.101 HYDROTHORAX

In hydrothorax the fluid is noninflammatory and has a lower specific gravity (1.015) than that of a serofibrinous exudate. It contains less protein and fewer cells and is usually associated with an accumulation of fluid in other parts of the body, such as the peritoneal cavity and the subcutaneous tissues. Hydrothorax is most often associated with cardiac or renal disease, although on occasion it may be a manifestation of severe nutritional edema, and, rarely, may result from venous obstruction by neoplasms, enlarged lymph nodes, or adhesions. Hydrothorax is usually bilateral in renal disease and in nutritional edema and may be in myocardial disease, although in this instance it may be limited to the right side or greater on the right than on the left side. The physical signs are those described under Serofibrinous Pleurisy, but in hydrothorax there is more rapid shifting of the level of dullness with changes of position. The treatment is that of the primary disorder; aspiration may be necessary when pressure symptoms are notable.

Berger HW, Rammohan G, Neff MS, et al: Uremic pleural effusion. A study in 14 patients on chronic dialysis. Ann Intern Med 82:362, 1975.

13.102 HEMOTHORAX

Extensive bleeding into the pleural cavity may result from erosion of a blood vessel in association with such inflammatory processes as tuberculosis and empyema, but it is rare in children. Hemothorax may complicate a variety of congenital anomalies, including sequestration, patent ductus, and pulmonary arteriovenous malformation. It is also an occasional manifestation of intrathoracic neoplasms and blood dyscrasias and bleeding diatheses, and may be the result of thoracic trauma, including surgical procedures. Rupture of an aneurysm is not likely during childhood. Hemothorax also occurs spontaneously, both in neonates and in older children. When a pleural hemorrhage occurs in association with a pneumothorax, it is termed *hemopneumothorax*. The diagnosis of a hemothorax can be made only by thoracentesis. In every instance an effort must be made to determine and treat the cause. Surgical intervention may be required to control active bleeding, and transfusion is necessary when loss of blood is excessive. Inadequate removal of blood in extensive hemothorax may lead to substantial restrictive disease secondary to deposition and organization of fibrin. A decortication procedure may then be necessary.

Block LF: Pleural disease. Basics Respir Dis 6 (May 1978): 1, 1978.
Fleisher GR, Fichman KR, Honig PJ: Hemothorax in a child: An unusual cause of chest pain. Clin Pediatr 17:300, 1978.
Kilman JS, Charnock E: Thoracic trauma in infancy and childhood. J Trauma 9:863, 1969.

13.103 CHYLOTHORAX

Chylothorax results from the escape of chyle from the thoracic duct into the thoracic cavity. The incidence has increased as cardiac surgery is performed on more complex congenital abnormalities; about 50% of these cases are now operative complications resulting from rupture of the thoracic duct. Most of the remainder are associated with traumatic chest injury or with primary or metastatic intrathoracic malignancy as a result of the pressure of enlarged lymph nodes or tumor. A variety of even less common causes are known and include lymphangiomatosis, restrictive pulmonary diseases, thrombosis of the duct or the subclavian vein, and congenital anomalies of the duct system. Chylothorax can occur in child abuse. In some patients and especially in newborns, no specific etiology is identified. Chylothorax is rarely bilateral, usually being on the left side.

The symptoms and signs are those related to the presence of fluid in the thoracic cavity. The diagnosis is established when thoracentesis demonstrates a chylous effusion, a milky fluid containing fat, protein, lymphocytes, and other constituents of chyle. In newborn infants who have not yet been fed, the fluid may be clear. A pseudochylous milky fluid has been reported in cases of serous effusion, in which the fatty material was thought to arise from degenerative changes within the fluid and not to be due to the presence of lymph. This type of fluid may be distinguished from one containing chyle by shaking it with alkalis or ether; the fluid containing chyle tends to become clear. A more definitive test is the quantitation of fluid triglyceride (elevated in chylous fluid) and fluid cholesterol (which may be elevated in chronic serous effusions).

Spontaneous recovery has occurred in over half of the reported cases in infants under 1 yr of age. Repeated aspirations may be required to relieve the symptoms of pressure. However, chyle reaccumulates quickly, and repeated thoracenteses may cause considerable loss of calories and protein as well as large numbers of lymphocytes. Immunodeficiencies including hypogammaglobulinemia and abnormal cell-mediated immune responses have been reported associated with repeated thoracenteses for chylothorax. Attempts to prevent these problems by intravenous infusion of pleural contents are technically difficult and dangerous and of doubtful benefit. Despite large losses of T lymphocytes, clinical problems of infection are uncommon, but these patients should be protected from potentially dangerous viruses, including cytomegalovirus and live virus vaccines.

Treatment should begin in most cases with a brief period of observation on a low fat (or medium chain triglyceride), high protein diet. For most patients, bed rest, salt restriction, diuresis, and digitalis are also indicated. The total caloric intake should be above the average requirement, and several times the daily requirements of the various vitamins, especially the fat-soluble vitamins A and D, should be added. If fluid continues to reaccumulate over 1–2 wk, a more aggressive attempt to locate and ligate the thoracic duct may be indicated. Many successful ligations have now been reported in patients with nontraumatic chylothoraces.

Berberich FR, Bernstein ID, Ochs HD, et al: Lymphangiomatosis with chylothorax. J Pediatr 87:941, 1975.
Green HG: Child abuse presenting as chylothorax. Pediatrics 66:620, 1980.
Kirkland I: Chylothorax in infancy and childhood. A method of treatment. Arch Dis Child 40:186, 1965.
Macfarlane JR, Holman CW: Chylothorax. Am Rev Respir Dis 105:287, 1972.
McWilliams BC, Fan LL, Murphy SA: Transient T-cell depression in postoperative chylothorax. J Pediatr 99:595, 1981.
Van Aerde J, Campbell AN, Smyth JA, et al: Spontaneous chylothorax in newborns. Am J Dis Child 138:961, 1984.

NEUROMUSCULAR AND SKELETAL DISEASES AFFECTING PULMONARY FUNCTION

13.104 PECTUS EXCAVATUM

Pectus excavatum ("funnel chest") is usually an isolated skeletal anomaly. Its incidence is higher in patients with upper airway obstruction, and spontaneous resolution or successful treatment has sometimes resulted in amelioration or disappearance of the pectus deformity. This midline narrowing of the thoracic cavity may result in demonstrable restrictive pulmonary disease, but clinical consequences of this restriction are unclear. Exercise testing has suggested a link between pectus excavatum and exercise limitation in some patients. Pectus excavatum may be associated with segmental bronchomalacia, especially involving the left main stem bronchus. In some patients, cardiac function may be adversely affected. Surgical correction of this lesion is not beneficial for the vast majority of patients, although for some patients with extreme deformity operative intervention may be indicated for functional or cosmetic reasons (Sec. 23.7).

Beiser GD, Epstein SE, Stampfer M, et al: Impairment of cardiac function in patients with pectus excavatum, with improvement after operative correction. N Engl J Med 287:267, 1972.
Castile RG, Staats BA, Westbrook PR: Symptomatic pectus deformities of the chest. Am Rev Respir Dis 126:564, 1982.
Fan L, Murphy S: Pectus excavatum from chronic upper airway obstruction. Am J Dis Child 135:550, 1981.
Godfrey S: Association between pectus excavatum and segmental bronchomalacia. J Pediatr 96:649, 1980.
Orzaleski MM, Cook CD: Pulmonary function in children with pectus excavatum. J Pediatr 66:898, 1965.

13.105 ASPHYXIATING THORACIC DYSTROPHY

Thoracic dystrophy is one manifestation of a generalized abnormality of skeletal growth and usually causes life-threatening respiratory difficulties in the newborn period or early infancy. Some patients with less severe disease have survived into their school years. The disease is an autosomal recessive defect. A variety of associated congenital malformations have been reported. Most patients have respiratory distress or infection before 1 yr of age. Older children are occasionally brought to the physician when parents note abnormality in the appearance of the chest. Physical examination reveals constriction of the thorax and, usually, short extremities. There is no specific treatment. Progressive renal failure occurs frequently among older children with this disease. Respiratory infections should be treated promptly with antibiotics and, perhaps, physical therapy. Influenza vaccine should be administered yearly.

Hanissian AS, Riggs WW, Thomas DA: Infantile thoracic dystrophy—Variant of the Ellis–van Creveld syndrome. J Pediatr 71:855, 1967.
Herdman RC, Langer LO: Thoracic asphyxiant dystrophy and renal disease. Am J Dis Child 116:192, 1968.
Oberklaid F, Dantes DM, Mayne V, et al: Asphyxiating thoracic dysplasia. Clinical, radiological, and pathological information on 10 patients. Arch Dis Child 52:758, 1977.

13.106 RIB ANOMALIES

The absence or malformation of 1–2 ribs usually has no substantial effect on pulmonary function and does not require treatment. Absence of multiple ribs is associated with vertebral anomalies and, ultimately, scoliosis. In addition, a portion of lung can herniate through the defect in the chest wall; these hernias are most frequent at the level of the first to fifth ribs and are usually anterior. The lung may present as a soft, easily reducible, usually nontender swelling. Minor abnormalities of muscle caused by loss of their normal attachments are also associated with this lesion. Most rib anomalies are discovered as incidental findings on chest roentgenograms obtained as part of a work-up for another illness. When the defect is large and associated with lung hernia, rib splitting and strutting techniques can provide both functional and cosmetic improvement.

Bronsther B, Coryllos E, Epstein B, et al: Lung hernias in children. J Pediatr Surg 3:544, 1968.
Rickham PP: Lung hernia secondary to congenital absence of ribs. Arch Dis Child 34:14, 1959.

13.107 NEUROMUSCULAR DISEASES WITH HYPOVENTILATION

A variety of acute (e.g., poliomyelitis, Guillain-Barré syndrome, spinal cord injury) and chronic (e.g., muscular dystrophy, progressive spinal muscular atrophy, myasthenia gravis) neuromuscular diseases can cause respiratory problems. (See Chapter 22.)

Clinical Manifestations. Alveolar hypoventilation with hypoxemia and respiratory failure is easily recognized, and the need for emergency measures, including artificial ventilation, is obvious. Arterial blood gas determinations and lung volume measurements confirm its presence and are necessary for proper management. Some of these patients cannot handle secretions and may need a cuffed endotracheal tube or tracheostomy.

Chronic, slowly progressive, neuromuscular weakness is more likely to cause the insidious onset of respiratory abnormalities that may ultimately become incapacitating and often life-limiting. With progression of weakness the patients cannot generate sufficient intrathoracic pressure for effective coughing, or they cannot hold the glottis closed well enough to allow sufficient pressure build-up in the lung. In addition, although tidal volumes may continue to be normal, the progressive decrease in vital capacity also compromises the effectiveness of the cough. Multiple minor episodes of aspiration occur as laryngeal muscles become weaker. Finally, with loss of adequate sigh and decreased ability of the diaphragm to prevent compromise of the thoracic volume by the abdominal organs, patchy microscopic atelectasis occurs accompanied by a ventilation perfusion abnormality and hypoxemia. Microscopic atelectasis also appears to be the major cause of decreased lung compliance in these patients. Recurrent or chronic infection then results and further restricts vital capacity. The increased viscosity of infected secretions also aggravates already impaired mucociliary clearance. Progressive loss of pulmonary tissue from the fibrosis associated with chronic infection and the chronic and worsening hypoxemia eventually may lead to pulmonary arterial hypertension and, ultimately, to right heart failure. Finally, weakness of the pharyngeal and laryngeal muscles may result in obstruction when soft tissue, normally retracted away during inspiration, partially occludes the upper airway.

Treatment. All patients with chronic or progressive muscular weakness require close surveillance for, and early treatment of, respiratory complications. Prompt antibiotic treatment of upper respiratory infections is indicated. Most patients intermittently require physical therapy, including postural drainage with chest percussion, and parents should be instructed in these techniques; postural drainage is often effective when used throughout each acute respiratory illness. In some patients, an artificial cough can be accomplished by application of sudden external pressure to the thorax. Influenza vaccine should be administered yearly. Pneumococcal vaccine may be indicated.

A permanent tracheostomy to allow better access to the airway for suctioning can be very helpful. A small tracheostomy can be plugged when suctioning is not being performed, allowing the patient to breathe and talk around the tube. A standard tracheostomy may alleviate upper airway obstruction and is useful in carefully selected patients. Patients with substantial diaphragmatic weakness may benefit from a mechanical rocking bed to reduce alveolar collapse. Intermittent positive pressure breathing has also been proposed for this purpose. Once pulmonary hypertension and overt right heart failure are present, the prognosis is grave, and treatment with supplemental oxygen and other symptomatic measures allows only temporary improvement. Tolazoline is not effective. Respirator management may be appropriate for some patients whose respiratory failure is likely to be temporary, e.g., in myasthenia gravis.

Bergofsky EH: State of the art: Respiratory failure in disorders of the thoracic cage. Am Rev Resp Dis 119:643, 1979.
DeTroyer A, Deisser P: The effects of intermittent positive pressure breathing on patients with respiratory muscle weakness. Am Rev Respir Dis 124:132, 1981.
Gracey DR, Diverhe MB, Howard FM Jr.: Mechanical ventilation for respiratory failure in myasthenia gravis: Two-year experience with 22 patients. Mayo Clin Proc 58:597, 1983.
Greenberg M, Edmonds J: Chronic respiratory problems in neuromyopathic disorders. The nature and management. Pediatr Clin North Am 21:927, 1974.

13.108 KYPHOSCOLIOSIS

Scoliosis, including idiopathic adolescent scoliosis, is discussed in Sec. 23.5. Mild or moderately severe scoliosis does not usually restrict the chest cage enough to seriously affect pulmonary function. Severe scoliosis, however, can dangerously impair function and may be associated with respiratory failure, cor pulmonale, or both. In addition to their restrictive lesion, these patients may also have a diffusion abnormality that aggravates hypoxemia. Minor respiratory infections may be life threatening. There is an age-related worsening of pulmonary function, but acute respiratory failure, although rare, does occur below 20 yr of age. Many of these patients can be managed without mechanical ventilation, and the intermediate term prognosis is good. Even patients with moderate scoliosis may have unexpected severe pulmonary problems immediately after fusion procedures because pain and use of a body cast restrict and interfere with coughing. Patients with severe scoliosis, especially males, may have abnormalities of breathing during sleep, and the resultant periods of hypoxemia may contribute to the eventual development of pulmonary hypertension.

Patients in these categories should be treated as if they had life-threatening pulmonary disease. Influenza vaccine should be given yearly. Careful pulmonary function evaluation is essential prior to elective surgical procedures, especially before fusion. If pulmonary function is marginal (e.g., vital capacity of less than 40–50% of predicted), the patient should receive instruction in, and get experience with, positive pressure breathing prior to surgery. The possibility that the patient may awake on assisted ventilation with an endotracheal tube should be discussed prior to surgery. If possible the patient should actually see the mechanical ventilator and understand how and why it might be used. For patients with marginal pulmonary function, careful postoperative monitoring of blood gases is essential. An occasional patient with extremely severe restrictive disease should have a tracheostomy prior to surgery. Scoliosis surgery may predispose to deep venous thrombosis and pulmonary embolus.

Kafer ER: Idiopathic scoliosis: Gas exchange and the age dependence of arterial blood gases. J Clin Invest 48:825, 1976.
Libby DM, Briscoe WA, Boyce B, et al: Acute respiratory failure in scoliosis or kyphosis: prolonged survival and treatment. Am J Med 73:532, 1982.
Mezon BL, West P, Israels J, et al: Sleep breathing abnormalities in kyphoscoliosis. Am Rev Resp Dis 122:617, 1980.
Uden A: Thromboembolic complications following scoliosis surgery in Scandinavia. Acta Orthop Scand 50:175, 1979.
Weber B, Smith JP, Briscoe WA, et al: Pulmonary function in asymptomatic adolescent with idiopathic scoliosis. Am Rev Resp Dis 111:389, 1975.

13.109 OBESITY

Extreme obesity occasionally causes respiratory embarrassment with somnolence, dyspnea, cyanosis, and, possibly, right heart failure. Chest and diaphragmatic excursions are limited, resulting in rapid shallow breathing; alveolar ventilation is also decreased, resulting in hypoxemia. Ventilation-perfusion abnormalities also contribute to arterial desaturation. Obstructive sleep apnea dominates the clinical picture in many patients. Some of these patients appear to have a diminished ventilatory response to hypoxic drive. In the *Prader-Willi syndrome*, an abnormal ventilatory response to carbon dioxide has been demonstrated in family members who are otherwise normal, suggesting that the abnormal

ventilatory control adds to the respiratory problems caused by the obesity rather than results from them.

Weight loss is the primary goal of treatment and, if successful, it alone will reduce the pulmonary problems. Some children with hypoventilation and right heart failure secondary to the extreme obesity of Prader-Willi syndrome may benefit from treatment with progesterone. Continuous positive airway pressure administered by nasal prongs may help obese patients with obstructive sleep apnea.

Lopata M, Önal E: Mass loading, sleep apnea, and the pathogenesis of obesity hyperventilation. Am Rev Respir Dis 126:640, 1982.
Orenstein DM, Boat TF, Owens RP, et al: The obesity hypoventilation syndrome in children with the Prader-Willi syndrome: A possible role for familial decreased response to carbon dioxide. J Pediatr 67:765, 1980.
Orenstein DM, Boat TF, Stern RC, et al: Progesterone treatment of the obesity hypoventilation syndrome in a child. J Pediatr 90:477, 1977.
Wilhoit SC, Brown ED, Suratt PM: Treatment of obstructive sleep apnea with continuous nasal airflow delivered through nasal prongs. Chest 85:170, 1984.
Zwillick CW, Sutton FD, Pierson DJ, et al: Decreased hypoxic ventilatory drive in the obesity-hypoventilation syndrome. Am J Med 49:343, 1975.

13.110 PRIMARY FAILURE OF RESPIRATORY REGULATION
(Ondine's Curse)

Primary failure of central nervous system regulation of breathing may also occur in nonobese persons but has been infrequently reported in children. The principal abnormality in these patients is an insensitivity to hypercapnia. Hypoventilation, which occurs more severely or exclusively during sleep, is a serious threat to life. Suggested therapeutic measures include bilateral phrenic nerve pacing or tracheostomy in conjunction with assisted ventilation during sleep. Although preliminary success has been reported with both these approaches, the long-term prognosis is unknown.

Deonna T, Arczynska W, Torrado A: Congenital failure of automatic ventilation (Ondine's curse). J Pediatr 84:710, 1974.
Hyland RH, Jones NL, Powles ACP, et al: Primary alveolar hypoventilation treated with nocturnal electrophrenic respiration. Am Rev Respir Dis 117:165, 1978.
Shannon DC, Marsland EW, Gould JB, et al: Central hypoventilation during quiet sleep in two infants. Pediatrics 57:342, 1976.

13.111 COUGH SYNCOPE

Cough syncope has been infrequently reported in children. During a coughing paroxysm in which high intrathoracic pressures are generated, venous obstruction, characterized by redness of the face, is followed by decreased venous return and, ultimately, decreased cardiac output, which results in transient cerebral hypoxia and syncope. Convulsive movements and incontinence are rare. Recovery generally occurs within 10 sec to 2 min. Asthma is the most frequent precipitating disease. There is no specific treatment.

ROBERT C. STERN

Katz RM: Cough syncope in children with asthma. J Pediatr 77:48, 1970.

14

THE CARDIOVASCULAR SYSTEM

EVALUATION OF THE CARDIOVASCULAR SYSTEM

14.1 HISTORY AND PHYSICAL EXAMINATION

The importance of the history and physical examination cannot be overemphasized in the evaluation of infants and children with suspected cardiovascular disorders. After this assessment, patients may require further laboratory evaluation and eventual treatment, or the family may be reassured that no significant problem exists.

There are a number of areas of special interest in taking a *history* for a potential cardiac abnormality. Cyanosis is often overlooked by parents; it may be considered merely a "deep coloring," a normal individual variation. Blueness during exercise is more often noted as an abnormal finding by observant parents. Eliciting a history of fatigue in an older child requires specific questions about activity including stair climbing, walking various distances, bicycle riding, etc.; information should also be obtained regarding more severe manifestations such as orthopnea and nocturnal dyspnea. The history obtained from the parents of a young infant, however, should focus on the feeding process. The baby with congestive heart failure will often take less volume per feeding, become dyspneic while sucking, and perhaps perspire profusely. After falling into an exhausted sleep, the baby, inadequately fed, will awaken for the next feeding after a brief period of time. This cycle continues around the clock and must be carefully differentiated from colic or other feeding disorders.

Physical examination begins with an assessment of growth and development. Cardiac failure results in failure to thrive manifested by poor weight gain; length remains relatively unaffected. An infant with severe congestive heart failure usually appears to be long and undernourished in contrast to an infant with cyanotic heart disease unaccompanied by cardiac decompensation, who may display normal height and weight. Failure to thrive, tachypnea, liver and spleen enlargement, pulmonary rales, and peripheral edema in a baby who appears to be ill are the major clinical manifestations of heart failure. Mild cyanosis may be too subtle for early detection, and clubbing of the fingers and toes is not usually manifested until late in the first year of life even in the presence of severe arterial oxygen desaturation. Blueness is best observed over the nail beds, lips, and mucous membranes. Circumoral cyanosis or blueness about the forehead may be the result of prominent venous plexuses in these areas rather than decreased arterial oxygen saturation.

The *cardiac rate* of newborn infants is rapid and subject to wide fluctuations (Table 14–1). The average rate ranges from 120 to 140 beats/min and may increase to 170 or more during crying and activity or drop to 70–90 during sleep. As the child grows older, the average pulse rate becomes slower, as low as 40/min in athletic adolescents. Persistent tachycardia (over 200/min in neonates, 150/min in infants, or 120/min in older children), bradycardia, or irregular heartbeat other than sinus arrhythmia may require investigation to exclude pathologic arrhythmias.

Careful evaluation of the *character of the pulses* is an important early step in physical diagnosis of congenital heart disease. A wide pulse pressure with bounding pulses may suggest an aortic runoff lesion such as patent ductus arteriosus, aortic insufficiency, an arterial-venous communication, or increased cardiac output secondary to anemia, anxiety, or conditions associated with increased catecholamine secretion. Diminished pulses are associated with heart failure, pericardial tamponade, or cardiomyopathy.

The *blood pressure* should be measured in the arms as well as in the legs, the latter on at least one occasion to be certain that coarctation of the aorta is not overlooked. Palpation of decreased femoral and/or dorsalis pedis pulses is not reliable to diagnose coarctation. In older children a mercury sphygmomanometer with a cuff that covers approximately two thirds of the upper arm or leg may be utilized for measurement. A cuff that is too small will invariably result in falsely high readings, while a cuff that is somewhat too large will record slightly decreased pressures. Three, 5, 7, 12, and 18 cm cuffs should be available to accommodate the large spectrum of pediatric patient sizes. The 1st Korotkoff sounds indicate the systolic pressure. As the cuff pressure is slowly decreased, the sounds usually become muffled before they disappear. The diastolic pressure may be recorded when the sounds are muffled (preferred) as well as when they disappear; the former is usually higher and the latter lower than the true diastolic pressure. For lower extremity blood pressure determination the stethoscope is placed over the popliteal artery. Ordinarily, the pressure recorded in the legs with the cuff technique is about 10 mm Hg higher than in the arms.

In infants the blood pressure can be obtained by auscultation, by palpation, or by the *flush method*. The last is most feasible in a restless infant. A cuff of appropriate size is placed around the upper arm or thigh. The distal limb is squeezed and the cuff rapidly inflated so that blanching is noted. The cuff is then gradually deflated. At the point at which the limb flushes, the blood pressure reading obtained corresponds to

Table 14–1. **Pulse Rates at Rest**

Age	Lower Limits of Normal		Average		Upper Limits of Normal	
Newborn	70/min		125/min		190/min	
1–11 mo	80		120		160	
2 yr	80		110		130	
4 yr	80		100		120	
6 yr	75		100		115	
8 yr	70		90		110	
10 yr	70		90		110	
	Girls	*Boys*	*Girls*	*Boys*	*Girls*	*Boys*
12 yr	70	65	90	85	110	105
14 yr	65	60	85	80	105	100
16 yr	60	55	80	75	100	95
18 yr	55	50	75	70	95	90

a systolic value slightly below what would be found by the direct arterial or auscultatory methods. Also available are ultrasonic (Doppler) devices, which provide accurate measurements in infants as well as children.

The blood pressure varies with the age of the child and is closely related to height and weight. Significant increases occur during adolescence, and there are many temporary variations before the more stable levels of adult life are attained. Exercise, excitement, coughing, and straining may raise the systolic pressures of children as much as 40–50 mm above their usual levels. Variability of blood pressure among children of approximately the same age and body build should be expected, and serial measurements should always be obtained in the evaluation of a patient with hypertension (Figs. 14–1 and 14–2).

In cooperative children, inspection of the regular venous pulse wave provides information about the *venous pressure* and right atrial pressure. The veins should be inspected with the patient sitting at a 90° angle. Under these conditions the external jugular vein should not be visible above the clavicles unless there is elevation of venous pressure. Increased venous pressure transmitted to the internal jugular vein may appear as venous pulsations without visible distention; such pulsation does not occur in normal children reclining at an angle of 45°.

The normal *jugular phlebogram* or direct tracings from the superior vena cava show three positive components corresponding to each cardiac cycle; they are termed "a," "c," and "v," respectively (Fig. 14–3). The "a" wave is synchronous with atrial systole, the "v" wave with atrial diastole, and the "c" wave with early ventricular systole. Since the great veins are in direct communication with the right atrium, changes of pressure and volume of the chamber are transmitted to the veins. For example:

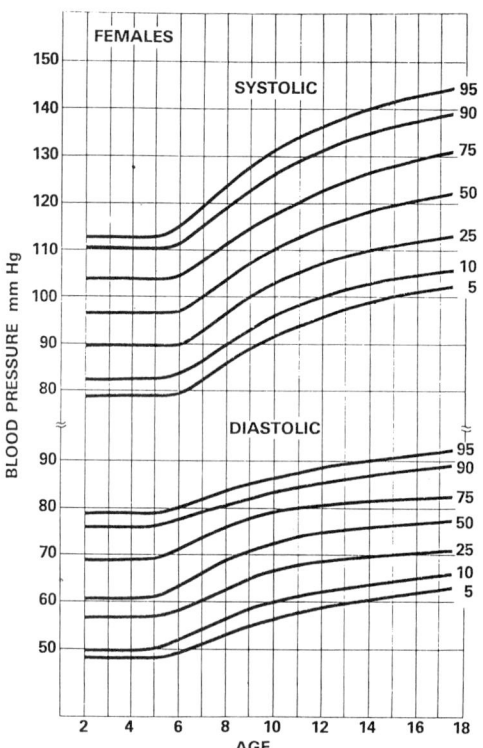

Figure 14–2. Percentiles of blood pressure in seated females. (From Report of the Task Force on Blood Pressure Control in Children, National Heart, Lung, and Blood Institute. Pediatrics (Suppl) 59:803, 1977. Copyright American Academy of Pediatrics.)

1. In congestive cardiac failure the increased right atrial pressure is transmitted to the cervical veins. The main pulsation at the upper part of distribution of these veins occurs in late diastole.

2. Cardiac compression by pericardial effusion or constriction increases the jugular pressure, but the amplitude of venous pulsation is small.

3. In relatively severe pulmonary stenosis the right ventricular diastolic pressure may be elevated. Emptying of the right atrium depends upon a systolic pressure in excess of the right ventricular diastolic pressure. A conspicuous presystolic "a" wave is present under these conditions. Similar "a" waves may be detected in patients with pulmonary stenosis and right ventricular hypertrophy with a normal right ventricular end-diastolic pressure; the mechanism of the "a" wave is due to a decreased distensibility of the right ventricle during diastole.

4. A presystolic "a" wave may be present in tricuspid stenosis or atresia, and the transmission of this wave to the inferior vena cava and hepatic veins produces presystolic hepatic pulsations.

5. In tricuspid insufficiency some of the right ventricular systolic pressure is transmitted to the right atrium and results in large, conspicuous venous pulsations which correspond to ventricular systole and produce a fusion of the "c" and "v" waves.

6. In complete heart block the occurrence of cervical venous pulsations depends on the position of the tricuspid valve at the time of atrial systole. If the right atrium contracts when the tricuspid valve is closed, a large venous pulsation will occur.

7. In superior vena caval obstruction the jugular venous pressure is increased, but the veins do not pulsate.

Cardiac Examination. The heart should be examined in a systematic manner concentrating on the meaning of each

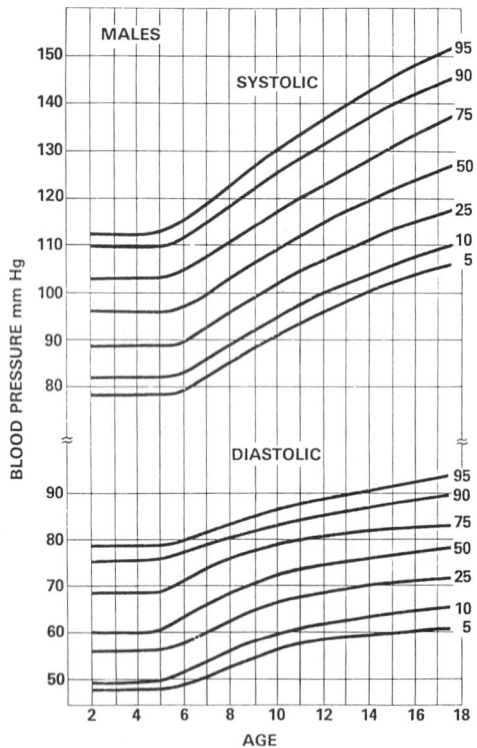

Figure 14–1. Percentiles of blood pressure in seated males. (From Report of the Task Force on Blood Pressure Control in Children, National Heart, Lung, and Blood Institute. Pediatrics (Suppl). 59:803, 1987. Copyright American Academy of Pediatrics.)

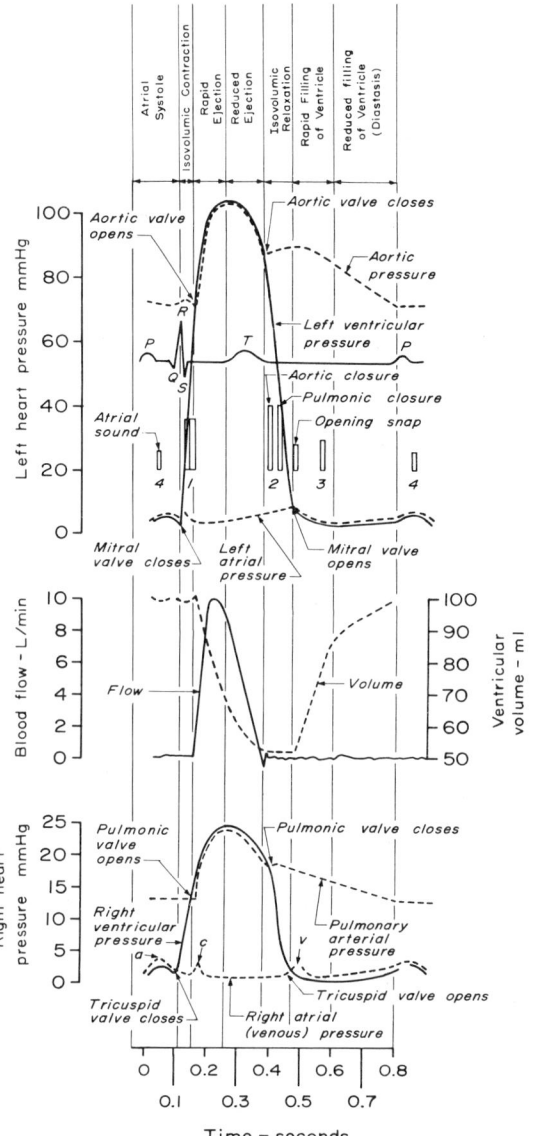

Figure 14–3. Idealized diagram of temporal events of a cardiac cycle.

Auscultation is an art that can be improved upon with practice and determination. The diaphragm of the stethoscope is placed firmly on the chest for high-pitched sounds; a lightly placed bell is optimal for low-pitched sounds. The physician should listen for one component at a time, concentrating initially on the characteristics of the individual heart sound and, later, on the murmurs. He or she must listen for the special characteristics of each heart sound and murmur. The 1st heart sound is caused by the closure of the atrioventricular valve (mitral and tricuspid); the 2nd sound is due to closure of the semilunar valves. During inspiration and increased filling of the right heart, right ventricular ejection time increases and pulmonary valve closure is delayed; the variable normal splitting is thus related to respirations (Fig. 14–4). The 1st heart sound is best heard at the apex, while the 2nd sound should be evaluated at the left upper sternal border. The patient should be supine, lying quietly, and breathing normally. The 2nd sound is split just beyond the height of inspiration and closes with expiration. The presence of splitting is more important than the intensity. The latter varies according to the age of the patient, the thickness of the chest wall, and the cardiac output. The presence of a normally split 2nd sound is strong evidence against the diagnosis of an atrial septal defect, defects associated with pulmonary artery hypertension, severe pulmonary valve stenosis, and numerous other conditions.

The 3rd heart sound is best heard with the bell at the apex in mid diastole (Fig. 14–5). A 4th sound, occurring in conjunction with atrial contraction, may be heard just prior to the 1st heart sound in late diastole. The 3rd sound may be normal in an adolescent with a relatively slow heart rate, but in a patient with the clinical signs of congestive heart failure and tachycardia it may be heard as a gallop rhythm and may merge with a 4th heart sound. A **gallop** rhythm is attributed to poor compliance of the ventricle with an exaggeration of the normal 3rd sound associated with ventricular filling.

Ejection clicks, which are heard in early systole, are related to dilatation of or hypertension in the aorta and pulmonary artery. They are heard so close to the 1st heart sound that they may be mistaken for a split 1st sound. Aortic systolic clicks are best heard at the left lower sternal border and are constant. They occur in conditions in which the aorta is dilated (e.g., aortic stenosis, tetralogy of Fallot, truncus arteriosus). Pulmonary ejection clicks associated with pulmonary stenosis are best heard at the left midsternal border and vary with respiration, disappearing with inspiration. A midsystolic click heard at the apex preceding a late systolic murmur suggests prolapse of the mitral valve.

Murmurs should be described as to their intensity, pitch, timing (systolic or diastolic), area of maximal intensity, and transmission. **Systolic murmurs** are classified as ejection, pansystolic, or late systolic according to the timing of the

manifestation. Much can be learned prior to auscultation. A **precordial bulge** to the left of the sternum with increased precordial activity suggests cardiac enlargement. A **substernal thrust** indicates the presence of right ventricular enlargement; an **apical heave** is noted with left ventricular hypertrophy. Both manifestations may be present. A **hyperdynamic precordium** suggests a volume load like that found with a large left to right shunt. In contrast, a silent precordium with a barely detectable apical impulse suggests pericardial effusion or severe cardiomyopathy. The relationship of the apex beat to the midclavicular line with the child prone is also helpful in the estimation of cardiac size; the apex beat moves laterally with enlargement of the left ventricle. **Thrills** are palpable murmurs, which should always correlate with areas of maximum intensity of the auscultatory murmurs. It is important to palpate the suprasternal notch and neck for **aortic bruits,** which may indicate the presence of aortic stenosis or, when less prominent, pulmonary stenosis. Rough lower sternal border and apical systolic thrills are characteristic of ventricular septal defect and mitral insufficiency, respectively. Diastolic thrills are palpable in the presence of atrioventricular valvular stenosis. The timing and localization of thrills should be carefully noted.

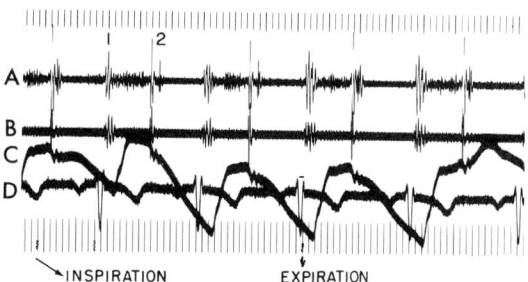

Figure 14–4. Physiologic splitting of 2nd heart sound in a 5 yr old child with an innocent systolic murmur. Tracings from above are (A) phonocardiogram at pulmonary area, (B) phonocardiogram at apex, (C) carotid pulse, (D) electrocardiogram. Time lines 0.04 sec. 1, First heart sound; 2, 2nd heart sound.

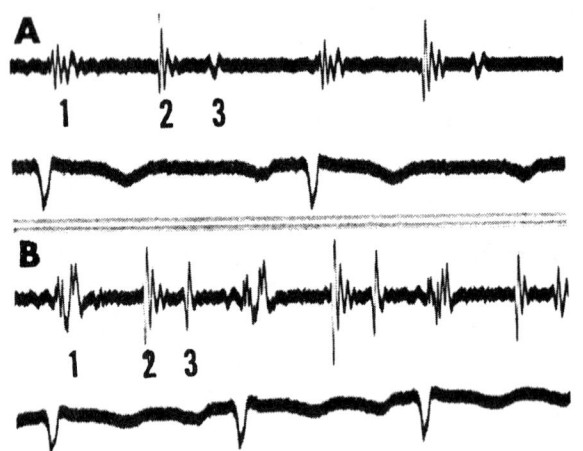

Figure 14–5. *A*, Phonocardiogram at pulmonary area. *B*, Phonocardiogram apex. Numbers indicate heart sounds.

murmur in relation to the 1st and 2nd heart sounds. Ejection systolic murmurs start after a well heard 1st heart sound, increase in intensity, peak, and then decrease in intensity; they usually end before the 2nd sound. However, in patients with severe aortic or pulmonary stenosis, the murmur may extend beyond the 1st component of the 2nd sound, thus obscuring it. Pansystolic murmurs begin almost simultaneously with the 1st heart sound and continue throughout systole, on occasion becoming gradually decrescendo. In general, significant ejection murmurs imply increased flow or stenoses across a semilunar valve, whereas pansystolic murmurs are heard with ventricular septal defects or A-V valve (mitral or tricuspid) insufficiency. A "continuous murmur" is a systolic murmur that continues or "spills" into diastole, and indicates continuous flow such as in the presence of a patent ductus arteriosus. This should be differentiated from a to and fro murmur, which indicates that the systolic component of the murmur ends at or before the 2nd sound and the diastolic murmur begins after semilunar valve closure (e.g., aortic stenosis with insufficiency). A late systolic murmur is a bruit that begins well beyond the 1st heart sound and continues until the end of systole. Such murmurs may be heard after a midsystolic click in the presence of mitral valve prolapse.

Several types of **diastolic murmurs** can be identified:

1. A high-pitched blowing diastolic murmur along the left sternal border beginning with S2 is associated with aortic insufficiency or, if pulmonary pressure is high, pulmonary valve insufficiency.

2. Early, short, lower pitched protodiastolic murmurs along the left mid and upper sternal border are heard with pulmonary valvular insufficiency. These murmurs are typically noted after surgical repair of the pulmonary outflow tract in defects such as tetralogy of Fallot.

3. An early diastolic murmur at the left mid and lower sternal border may be due to increased blood flow across the tricuspid valve such as occurs with atrial septal defect, or less often, stenosis of this valve.

4. Rumbling mid-diastolic murmurs at the apex follow the 3rd heart sound and are due to increased left ventricular flow in conditions with large right to left shunts or with mitral insufficiency.

5. A long diastolic rumbling murmur at the apex, accentuated at the end of diastole (presystolic), indicates anatomic mitral stenosis.

Many murmurs are not associated with significant hemodynamic abnormalities. These are referred to as functional, "normal," insignificant, or innocent (preferred). During routine random auscultation, over 30% of children may have an *innocent murmur*; this percentage increases when auscultation

is carried out under nonbasal circumstances (high cardiac output due to fever, infection, anxiety, etc.). The most common innocent murmur is a medium-pitched, vibratory, relatively short systolic ejection murmur which is heard best along the left lower and midsternal border and has no significant radiation to the apex, base, or back. The short systolic ejection murmurs at the base and the continuous sound of a venous hum are other examples of common but insignificant bruits heard in childhood.

The common innocent murmur is heard most frequently from 3 to 7 yr. The murmur occurs during ejection and is musical, frequently sounding like the vibration of a tuning fork; it is brief in duration, may be attenuated in the sitting position, and is intensified by fever, excitement, or exercise. Innocent pulmonic murmurs are also common in children and adolescents and originate from the normal turbulence during ejection into the pulmonary artery. They are high-pitched, blowing, brief, early systolic murmurs, grades 1–3 (on a scale of 6) in intensity, and best detected in the 2nd left parasternal space with the patient in the supine position. The **venous hum** is another example of a common insignificant bruit heard during childhood. This is produced by turbulence of blood in the jugular venous system; it has no pathologic significance and may be heard in the neck or anterior portion of the upper chest. It consists of a soft humming sound heard in both systole and diastole and can be exaggerated or made to disappear by varying the position of the head or can be decreased by lightly compressing the jugular venous system in the neck. These simple maneuvers are sufficient to differentiate a venous hum from the murmurs produced by organic cardiovascular disease, particularly patent ductus arteriosus.

The lack of significance of an innocent murmur should be discussed with the parents. It is important to offer complete reassurance because lingering doubts about the importance of a cardiac murmur may have profound effects on child-rearing practices, most often in the form of overprotectiveness. An underlying fear that a cardiac abnormality is present may negatively affect a child's self-image and subtly influence personality development. The physician should explain that the innocent murmur is simply a "noise" and does not indicate the presence of a significant cardiac defect. When asked, "Will it go away?" the best response is to state that since the murmur has no meaning, it doesn't matter whether it "goes away" or not. However, with growth, innocent murmurs are less well heard, and may disappear completely.

At times, additional studies may be indicated to rule out a congenital heart defect, but "routine" ECG, x-ray, and/or ultrasound examination for well children with innocent murmurs should be avoided.

14.2 ROENTGENOGRAPHIC EXAMINATION

The chest roentgenogram provides information about cardiac size and shape as well as other features that directly relate to the status of the cardiovascular system. Variations are due to differences in body build, the phase of respiration or cardiac cycle, abnormalities of the thoracic cage, position of the diaphragm, or pulmonary disease.

The most frequently used measurement of cardiac size is the maximal width of the cardiac shadow in a midinspiration posteroanterior film: a vertical line is drawn down the middle of the sternal shadow, and perpendicular lines are drawn from the sternal line to the extreme right and left borders of the heart; the sum of the lengths of these lines is the *maximal cardiac width*. The *maximal chest width* is obtained by drawing a horizontal line between the right and left inner borders of the rib cage at the level of the top of the right diaphragm.

When the cardiac width is more than half the maximal chest width, the heart is usually enlarged. Cardiac size should be evaluated only when the film is taken during inspiration with the patient in an upright position. Diagnosis of "cardiac enlargement" on expiratory or prone films is a common cause of unnecessary referrals and laboratory studies.

The *cardiothoracic ratio* is a *less* useful index of cardiac enlargement in infancy than in subsequent years because the horizontal position of the heart may increase the ratio to more than half in the absence of true enlargement. Furthermore, the thymus may overlap not only the base of the heart, but virtually the entire mediastinum, thus obscuring the true cardiac silhouette.

The lateral chest roentgenogram may be helpful in infancy, as well as in diagnosing older children with pectus excavatum or other conditions resulting in a narrow anteroposterior chest dimension. In these situations the heart may appear quite small in the lateral view, suggesting that the apparent enlargement in the posteroanterior projection was due to either a thymic image, or flattening of the cardiac chambers as a result of a structural chest abnormality.

In the posteroanterior view, the left border of the cardiac shadow consists of three convex shadows produced from above downward by the aortic knob, the main and left pulmonary arteries, and the left ventricle, respectively (Fig. 14–6). In cases of moderate to marked left atrial enlargement the atrium may project between the pulmonary artery and the left ventricle. The outflow tract of the right ventricle or the pulmonary conus does not contribute to the shadows formed by the left border of the heart (Fig. 14–6). The aortic knob is not as easily seen in infants and children as in adults. However, the side of the aortic arch (left or right) often can be inferred as being opposite to the side of the midline from where the air-filled trachea is visualized. Three structures also contribute to the right border of the cardiac silhouette; from above downward they are the superior vena cava, the ascending aorta, and the right atrium.

Interpretation of atrial or ventricular enlargement in infants by roentgenographic means is difficult, especially in the presence of a large thymic image. Abnormal roentgenographic findings should be complemented by an electrocardiogram, which is a more sensitive and accurate index of ventricular hypertrophy.

Enlargement of cardiac chambers or major arteries and veins results in prominence of areas where these structures are normally outlined on the chest roentgenogram. It is also important to assess the degree of pulmonary vascularity as represented by the intrapulmonary shadows. Angiocardiographic studies have shown that the hilar shadows are mainly vascular. Pulmonary overcirculation is usually associated with left to right shunts, and undercirculation with stenosis or atresia of the outflow tract of the right ventricle or of the pulmonary valve.

The esophagus is closely related to the great vessels, and visualization with barium helps to delineate these structures in selected situations such as coarctation of the aorta and vascular ring. However, echocardiographic examination best defines specific intracardiac chamber enlargement. Thus, routine esophagograms and fluoroscopy are not necessary for the evaluation of most cardiac abnormalities.

14.3 THE ELECTROCARDIOGRAM (ECG)

Changes in cardiac anatomy and hemodynamics soon after birth are reflected in the evolution of the electrocardiogram of the neonate. Since vascular resistances in the pulmonary and systemic circulations are nearly equal in the fetus at term, the intrauterine work of the heart results in virtually equal

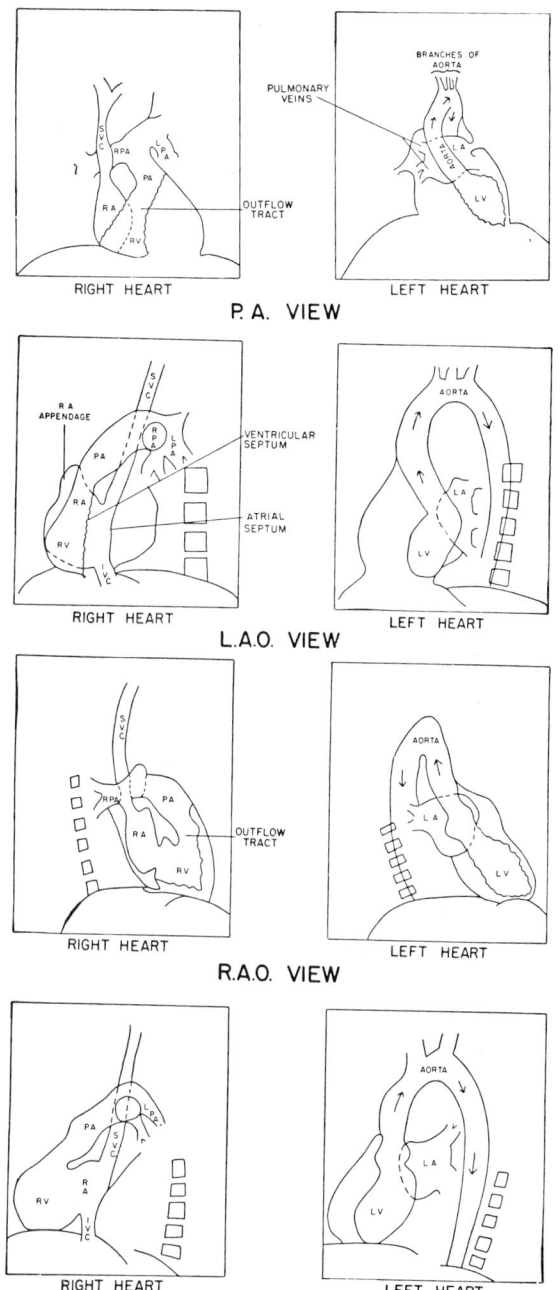

Figure 14–6. Idealized diagrams showing normal position of the cardiac chambers and great blood vessels. P. A., posteroanterior; L.A.O., left anterior oblique; R.A.O., right anterior oblique; SVC, superior vena cava; RA, right atrium; RV, right ventricle; PA, pulmonary artery; RPA, right pulmonary artery; LPA, left pulmonary artery; LA, left atrium; LV, left ventricle; IVC, inferior vena cava. (Adapted and redrawn from Dotter and Steinberg: Radiology, 53:513, 1949.)

mass of both the right and left ventricles. After birth, systemic vascular resistance rises when the placental circulation is eliminated, and pulmonary vascular resistance falls when the lungs expand. These changes are effected over a period of hours or days.

The electrocardiogram demonstrates these anatomic and hemodynamic features principally by changes in the QRS and T wave morphology. It is *essential* that a 13 lead ECG be carried out in pediatric patients, including lead V_3R or V_4R. These right precordial leads are extremely important in the evaluation of right ventricular hypertrophy in childhood. On occasion, lead VI is positioned too far leftward to accurately reflect right ventricular forces, and may display the usual R/S

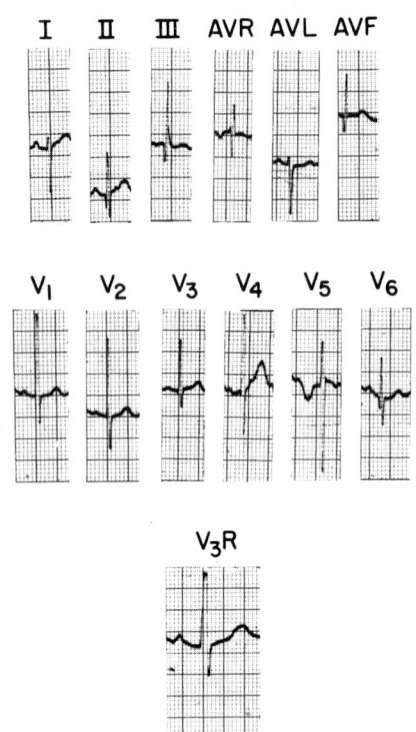

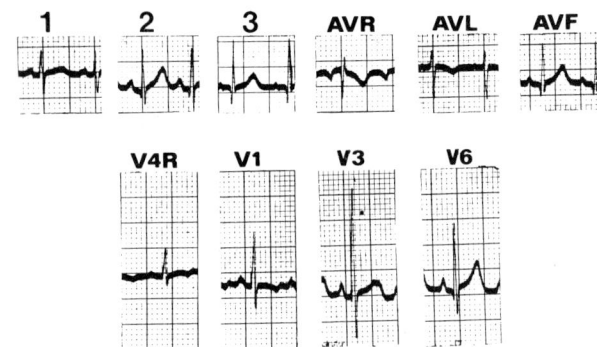

Figure 14–8. Electrocardiogram of a normal infant. Note the tall R and small S waves in V₄R and V₁, and the inverted T wave in these leads. There is also a dominant R wave in V₆.

Figure 14–7. Electrocardiogram in a normal neonate less than 24 hr of age. Note the dominant R wave and upright T waves in leads V₃R and V₁. (V₃R paper speed = 50 mm/sec.)

pattern of a midprecordial lead. At the same time V₃R or V₄R may reflect a dominant R or S pattern, which is important diagnostically. During the first days of life right axis deviation, large R waves, and upright T waves in the right precordial leads (V₃R or V₄R and V₁) are seen (Fig. 14–7). When pulmonary resistance decreases and right ventricular pressure reaches its normal level, the right precordial T waves become negative. In the great majority of instances this occurs within the first 48 hr of life, and if upright T waves persist in leads V₄R and/or VI beyond 1 wk, this represents an abnormal finding.

In the frontal plane leads of the standard ECG, the mean QRS axis in the newborn normally lies in the range of +110 to +180°. The right-sided chest leads reveal a larger positive (R) than negative (S) wave and may do so for months or years since the right ventricle remains relatively thick throughout infancy. Furthermore, owing to proximity, the voltage recorded by the right precordial leads is influenced to a greater extent by right ventricular depolarization. Left-sided leads (V₅ and V₆) also reflect right-sided dominance in the early neonatal period when the RS ratio may be less than 1. However, since left precordial leads are in direct proximity to the left ventricle, a dominant R wave reflecting left ventricular forces quickly becomes evident within the first few days of life (Fig. 14–8). Over the years, the QRS axis gradually shifts leftward and right ventricular forces slowly regress. As the left ventricle becomes dominant, the ECG evolves to the characteristic pattern of the older child (Fig. 14–9), and finally the typical adult electrocardiogram emerges (Fig. 14–10).

With the growth of the infant there is slow regression of right ventricular dominance and an increase in left ventricular forces. Leads V₁ and V₄R will display a prominent R wave until 6 mo–8 yr of age. The majority of children will have an RS ratio greater than 1 in lead V₄R until they are 4 yr of age. The T waves are inverted in V₄R, V₁, V₂, and V₃ during infancy and may remain so into the middle of the 2nd decade of life and beyond. The process of right ventricular thinning and

left ventricular growth are best reflected in the QRS-T pattern over the right precordial leads. The diagnosis of right or left ventricular hypertrophy can be made only with an understanding of the normal states of these chambers at various ages until adulthood is reached.

Ventricular hypertrophy may result in increased voltage in the R and S waves in the chest leads. However, the height of these deflections is governed by the proximity of the exploring electrode to the surface of the heart, and by the sequence of electrical activation through the ventricles, resulting in variable degrees of cancellation of forces, as well as by hypertrophy of the myocardium. Since the chest wall in infants and children as well as in adolescents may be relatively thin, the diagnosis of ventricular hypertrophy should not be based on voltage changes alone in the entire pediatric age range.

The diagnosis of pathologic right ventricular hypertrophy is difficult in the first week of life, since physiologic right ventricular hypertrophy is a normal finding. Serial tracings are often necessary to determine whether marked right axis deviation and potentially abnormal right precordial forces or T waves, or both, will persist (Fig. 14–11). An adult ECG pattern seen in a neonate suggests left ventricular enlargement (Fig. 14–10). The premature infant, however, may display a more "mature" ECG than his or her full term counterpart (Fig. 14–12) as a result of lower pulmonary resistance secondary to underdevelopment of the medial muscular layer of the pulmonary arterioles. Thus, the electrocardiogram may simulate that of the older child with left ventricular dominance manifested by a more mature R wave progression across the precordium (qR in V₆, R/S ratio in V₄R, and V₁ equal to or less than 1). Some premature infants display a pattern of generalized low voltage across the precordium.

The P Wave. Tall, narrow, and spiked P waves are seen in congenital pulmonary stenosis, Ebstein anomaly of the tricuspid valve, tricuspid atresia, and sometimes cor pulmonale. These abnormal waves are due to right atrial hypertrophy and/or dilatation, are usually taller than 2.5 mm, and are most obvious in standard lead II and leads V₄R, V₃R, and V₁ (Fig. 14–13A). Similar waves are sometimes seen in thyrotoxicosis.

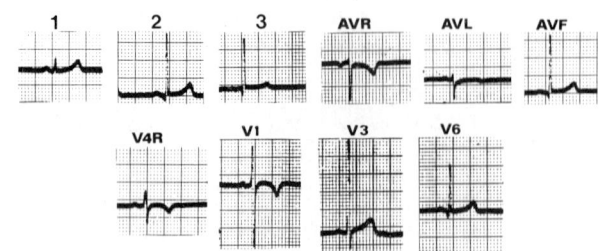

Figure 14–9. Electrocardiogram of a normal child. Note the relatively tall R waves and inversion of the T waves in V₄R and V₁.

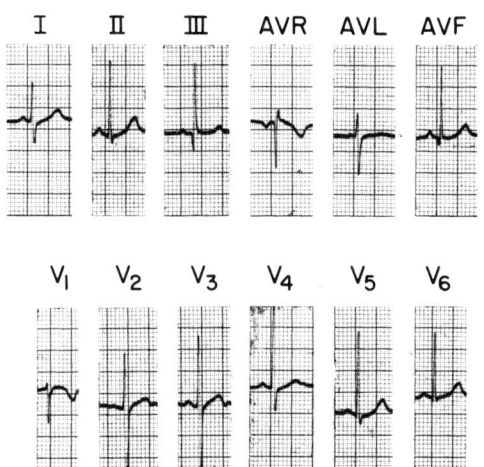

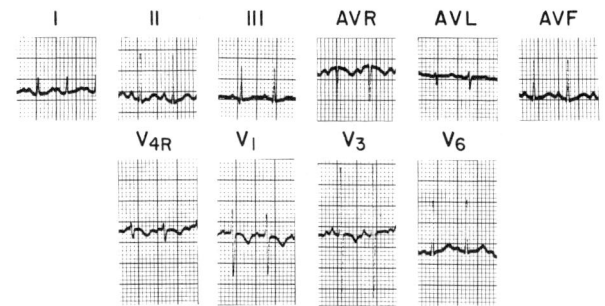

Figure 14–12. Electrocardiogram of premature infant (weight 2 kg and age 5 wk at time of tracing). The cardiovascular system was clinically normal. Left ventricular dominance is manifest by R wave progression across the chest simulating tracings obtained from older children. Compare with tracing from normal fullterm infant, Figure 14–8.

Figure 14–10. Normal adult electrocardiogram. Note the dominant S wave in lead V_1. This pattern in an infant would indicate the presence of left ventricular hypertrophy.

Widened P waves, commonly bifid, indicate left atrial enlargement (Fig. 14–13B). They are seen in some patients with large ventricular septal defects, with communications between the aorta and pulmonary circulation, and with severe mitral stenosis. Flat P waves may be found in hyperkalemia.

With normal position of the atriae and sinus rhythm, the P wave should be upright in leads I and AVF. With atrial inversion (situs inversus), the P wave may be inverted in lead I. Inverted P waves in leads II and AVF are seen in nodal or junctional rhythms regardless of atrial position.

Right Ventricular Hypertrophy. Right ventricular surface leads of infants and children differ from those of adults, and tracings of the right side of the chest (V_4R or V_3R) are essential. In infants with **right ventricular hypertrophy** the following changes may occur singly or in combination (Fig. 14–11): (1) a qR pattern in the right ventricular surface leads; (2) a positive T wave in leads $V_{3-4}R$ through V_3 after the first 48 hr of life; (3) a monophasic R wave in $V_{3-4}R$ and/or V_1; (4) rsR' in right precordial leads often with a tall secondary R wave (this pattern is frequently associated with volume overload and hypertrophy of the right ventricular outflow track as typically seen in atrial septal defect); (5) age-related voltage criteria in $V_{3-4}R$ and $V_1(R)$, and/or $V_{6-7}(S)$; (6) marked right axis deviation (>120°); (7) a complete reversal of the normal adult precordial RS pattern; and (8) right atrial enlargement. At least two of these changes should be present to support a diagnosis of right ventricular hypertrophy. In general, if a pattern of right ventricular hypertrophy in the newborn and young infant persists or even becomes more prominent into early childhood, abnormal right ventricular hypertrophy is present. In contrast, the small infant who displays the pattern of a

"normal" electrocardiogram for an older child may have left ventricular hypertrophy.

Abnormal hemodynamics can be correlated with abnormal electrocardiographic patterns. Obstruction to right ventricular and pulmonary flow (e.g., pulmonary stenosis) is associated with a systolic overload pattern characterized by tall pure R waves in the right precordial leads. In these leads the T wave is initially upright and later becomes inverted. In contrast, diastolic overload of the right ventricle (e.g., with atrial septal defect) is characterized by an rsR' pattern and right ventricular conduction delay (Fig. 14–14). However, these patterns, although useful, may simply reflect the severity of right ventricular hypertrophy rather than serve as specific indicators of increased preload (diastolic) or afterload (systolic). For example, patients with mild to moderate pulmonary stenosis (systolic overload) often exhibit an rsR' in the right precordial leads.

The following features indicate the presence of **left ventricular hypertrophy** (Fig. 14–15): (1) depression of the S-T segments and inversion of T waves and left precordial surface leads (V_5, V_6, and V_7), a left ventricular strain pattern; these findings suggest the presence of a severe lesion and significant myocardial abnormality; (2) increase in magnitude of initial forces to the right (i.e., deep Q in left precordial leads); (3) voltage criteria in V_3R and $V_1(S)$ and/or $V_6(R)$. It is important to emphasize that evaluation of ventricular hypertrophy should not be based on voltage criteria alone. The concepts of systolic and diastolic overload, although not always consistent, are also useful in evaluating left ventricular enlargement. Severe systolic overload of the left ventricles is suggested by straightening of the S-T segments and inverted T waves over the left precordial leads; diastolic overload may result in tall R waves, a large Q wave, and normal T waves over the left precordium.

Bundle Branch Block. Complete right bundle branch block may occur as a congenital finding or be acquired after open

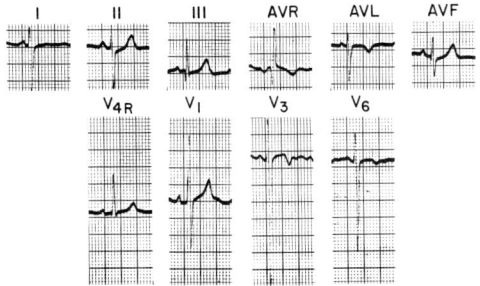

Figure 14–11. Electrocardiogram and vectorcardiogram of infant with right ventricular hypertrophy (tetralogy of Fallot). Note the tall R waves in the right precordium and deep S waves in V_6. The positive T waves in V_4R and V_1 are also characteristic of right ventricular hypertrophy.

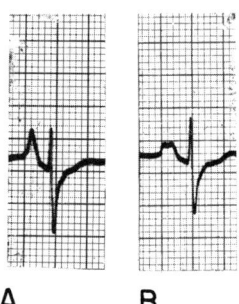

A   B

Figure 14–13. Atrial enlargement. A, Peaked narrow P waves characteristic of right atrial enlargement. B, Wide bifid M-shaped P waves typical of left atrial enlargement.

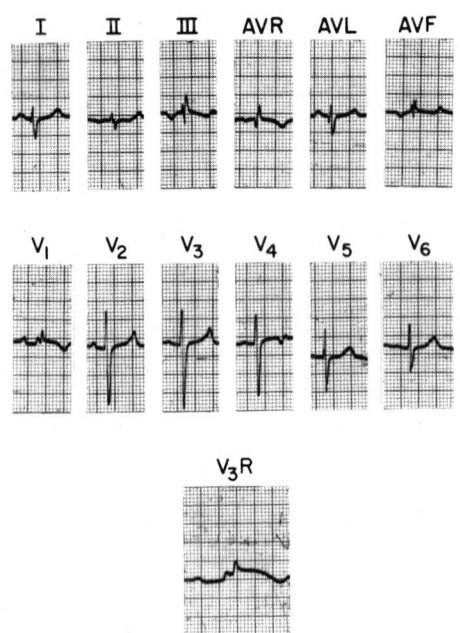

Figure 14–14. Electrocardiogram showing right ventricular conduction delay characterized by an rsR' pattern in V₁ and a deep S wave in V₆ (V₃R paper speed = 50 mm/sec.)

heart surgery, especially when a right ventriculotomy has been carried out. Congenital left bundle branch block is rare; this pattern is occasionally seen with cardiomyopathy.

The Q-T Interval. The duration of the Q-T interval varies with the cardiac rate; a corrected Q-T interval can be calculated by dividing the measured Q-T interval by the square root of the cycle length of the R-R interval. The normal Q-TC should be less than 0.45 sec. It is often lengthened in children with hypokalemia and hypocalcemia; in the former instance a U wave may be noted at the end of the T wave (Figs. 14–16 and 14–17). Prolonged Q-T intervals (Fig. 14–18) may be seen in children who are at risk for ventricular arrhythmias and sudden death (Jervell and Lange-Nielsen syndrome with hearing loss or Romano-Ward syndrome).

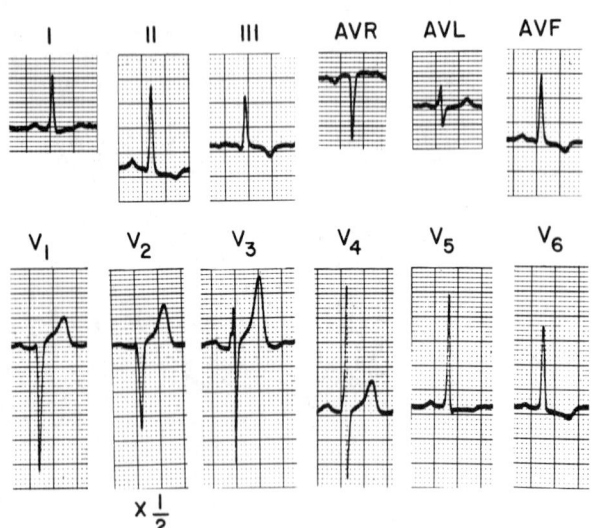

Figure 14–15. Electrocardiogram showing left ventricular hypertrophy in a 12 yr old child with aortic stenosis. Note the deep S wave in V₁–V₃ and tall R in V₅. Also, T wave inversion is present in II, III, AVF and V₆.

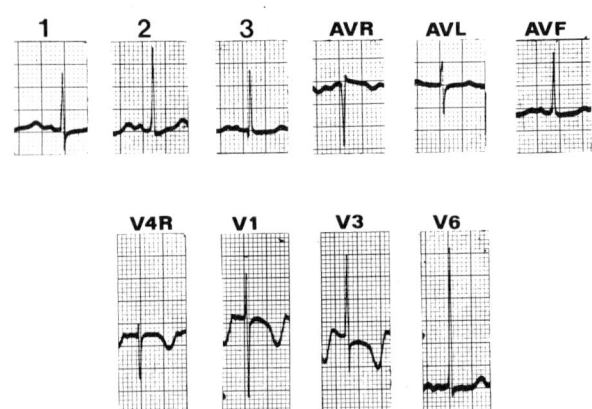

Figure 14–16. Electrocardiogram in hypocalcemia and hypokalemia (serum calcium 1.8 mEq/L; serum potassium 2.2 mEq/L at time of tracing). Note prolongation of electrical systole owing to long S-TU segment. This graph also shows left ventricular hypertrophy.

S-T Segment and T Wave Abnormalities. Elevation of the S-T segment in normal teenagers is attributed to early repolarization of the heart. In generalized pericarditis, superficial epicardial involvement may cause elevation of the S-T segment followed by abnormal T wave inversion as healing progresses. Administration of digitalis is associated with sagging of the S-T segment and abnormal inversion of the T wave. Depression of the S-T segment may also occur in any condition that produces myocardial damage, e.g., anemia, carbon monoxide poisoning, endocardial fibroelastosis, aberrant origin of the left coronary artery from the pulmonary artery, glycogen storage disease of the heart, myocardial tumors, and gargoylism. Aberrant origin of the left coronary artery from the pulmonary artery may lead to changes indistinguishable from those of acute myocardial infarction in adults. Similar changes may occur in patients with other rare abnormalities of the coronary arteries and with cardiomyopathy without anatomic abnormalities of the coronary arteries.

In any form of carditis simple inversion of the T wave may occur. Hypothyroidism may produce flat or inverted T waves in association with generalized low voltage. In hyperkalemia the T waves are commonly of high voltage and are tent-shaped (Fig. 14–19).

14.4 VECTORCARDIOGRAPHIC DISPLAY

The spread of depolarization and repolarization through the ventricles is a succession of innumerable instantaneous

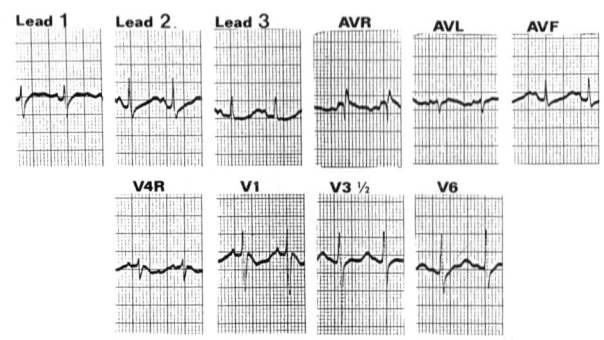

Figure 14–17. Electrocardiogram in hypokalemia (serum potassium 2.7 mEq/L; serum calcium 4.8 mEq/L at time of tracing). Note the prolongation of electrical systole as evidenced by a widened TU wave; also depression of the S-T segment in V₄R, V₁, and V₆.

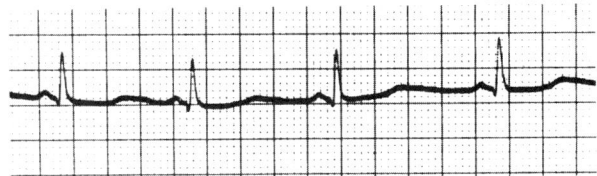

Figure 14–18. Prolonged Q-T intervals.

electrical forces. The average of these forces determines a direction of electrical depolarization beginning with the ventricular septum and spreading to the free wall of the myocardium over both ventricles. The recording of the average direction, magnitude, and orientation of the individual vectors in a single curve constitutes the vectorcardiographic loop. The P wave and T waves are similarly inscribed. Reference lead systems have been devised to record the vectorcardiogram in three planes: horizontal, sagittal, and frontal. Furthermore, distorting factors of proximity, resistivity, and variations in thorax size are "corrected" by the lead systems currently used. Analysis of vectorcardiograms is helpful in supplemental evaluation and understanding of the scalar electrocardiogram.

14.5 HEMATOLOGIC DATA

Evaluation of hematologic findings as part of the assessment of the cardiovascular system should be carried out with an awareness of the normal variations in infancy (Sec. 15.1–15.2). Persistent polycythemia after the first month of life is frequently noted in patients with right to left shunts and cyanosis. Patients with marked polycythemia have a delicate balance between intravascular thrombosis and a bleeding diathesis; this abnormal hemostasis should be recognized and treated prior to any surgical procedure. The most frequent abnormalities are accelerated fibrinolysis, thrombocytopenia, abnormal clot retraction, hypofibrinogenemia, prolonged prothrombin time, and prolonged partial thromboplastin time or thromboplastin generation time. These abnormalities occur singly or in combination and may be related to the severity of the polycythemia. Abnormal coagulation may be related to the effects of hypoxia and polycythemia on platelet production and consumption combined with the effects of chronic liver dysfunction on procoagulants and fibrinolysis.

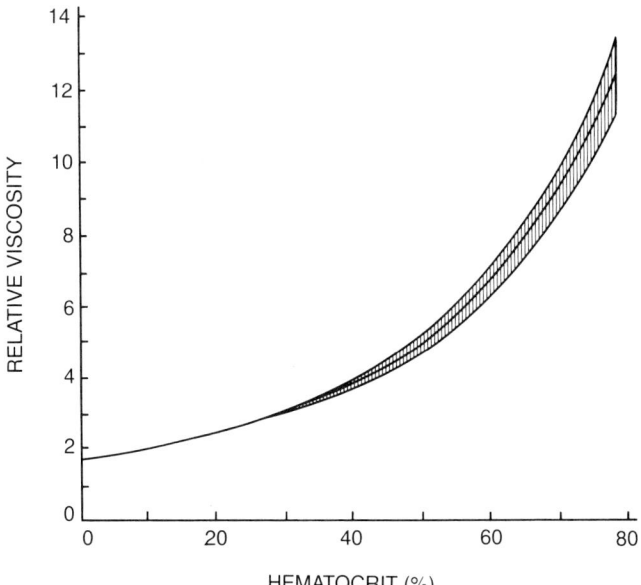

Figure 14–20. Relative viscosity of blood (blood/water viscosity) related to hematocrit. (Adapted from Chien S, Usami S, Skalak R: Blood flow in small tubes. *In*: Handbook of Physiology. Sec 2, The Cardiovascular System. Vol 4. Baltimore, Williams & Wilkins, 1984.)

The preparation of cyanotic polycythemic patients for elective surgery such as dental extraction includes evaluation for and treatment of abnormal coagulation. Accelerated fibrinolysis has been suppressed with epsilon-aminocaproic acid. Thrombocytopenia and hypofibrinogenemia may be improved by phlebotomies.

Because of high viscosity of polycythemic blood (Hct >65%), patients having cyanotic congenital heart disease are at risk to develop vascular thrombosis, especially of cerebral veins (Fig. 14–20). Polycythemic infants with iron deficiency are at even greater risk for cerebrovascular accidents, probably because thrombosis is enhanced by a decrease in velocity of blood flow as well as by altered deformability of the red cells.

Cyanotic patients should have frequent Hgb and Hct determinations. Increasing polycythemia, often associated with headache, fatigue, and/or dyspnea, is an indication for palliative or corrective surgical intervention. Among cyanotic patients with inoperable conditions, phlebotomy may be required to treat individuals whose Hct has risen to the 65–70% level or above, regardless of symptoms. This procedure is not without risk, especially in polycythemic patients with extreme elevation of pulmonary vascular resistance. Because these patients do not tolerate wide fluctuations in circulating blood volume, the phlebotomy should be performed in the same way as an exchange transfusion; blood is replaced with fresh frozen plasma or albumin. Initially, these patients require frequent phlebotomies (often weekly) until the hematocrit is more or less stabilized at the desired level (±60%). Subsequently, phlebotomies may be necessary at only 3–5 wk intervals.

Iron deficiency anemia is poorly tolerated by cyanotic patients with right to left shunts, especially by infants and toddlers. Such children are more susceptible to hypercyanotic spells. Iron therapy produces improvement, but surgical treatment of the cardiac anomaly is often required.

14.6 ECHOCARDIOGRAPHY

Echocardiography (ultrasonography) is an extremely important technique in the diagnosis of congenital and acquired cardiac disease in infants and children (see also Sec. 5.55).

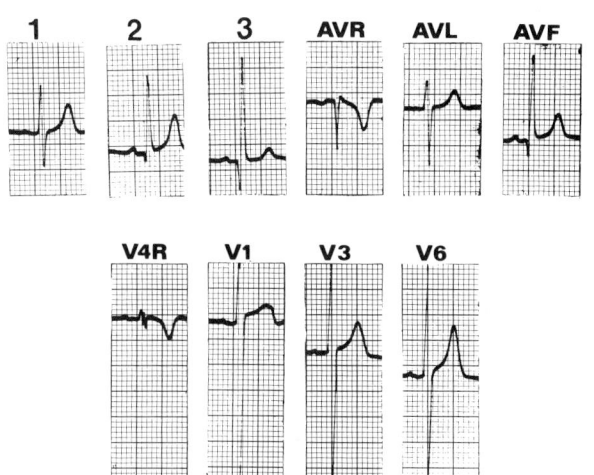

Figure 14–19. Electrocardiogram in hyperkalemia (serum potassium 6.5 mEq/L; serum calcium 5.1 mEq/L). Note the tall, tent-shaped T waves, especially in leads I, II, and V_6.

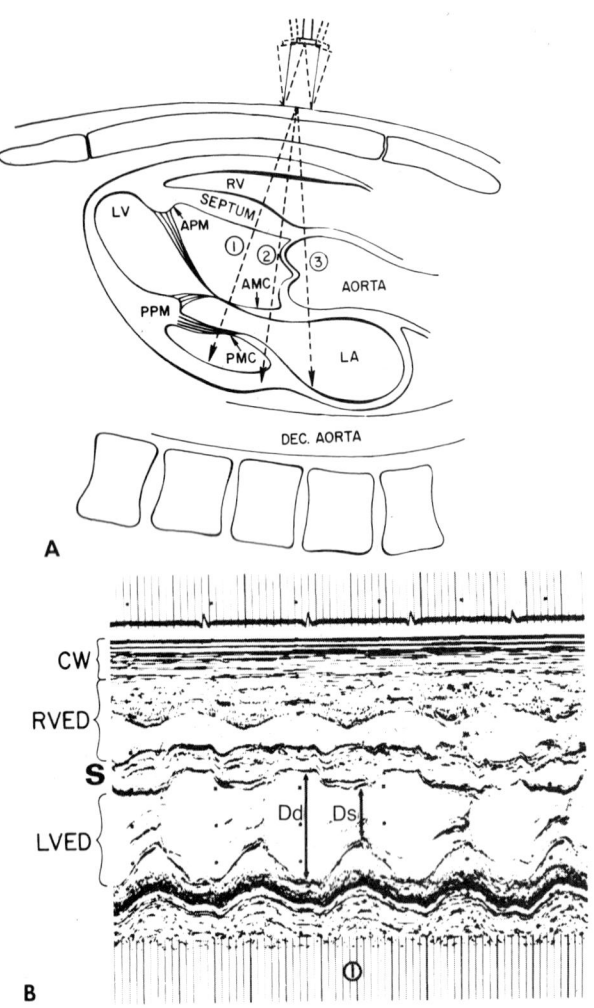

Figure 14–21. Normal echocardiograms. *A*, Diagram of sagittal section of heart showing structures traversed by echo beam in positions (1), (2), and (3). AMC, anterior mitral cusp; APM, anterior papillary muscle; Dec. aorta, descending aorta; LA, left atrium; LV, left ventricle; PMC, posterior mitral cusp; PPM, posterior papillary muscle; RV, right ventricle. *B*, Echocardiogram from transducer position (1); this is the best view to evaluate interventricular septum (S) and for measurement of right ventricular dimension (RVED) as well as of the left ventricular dimension (LVED) in end diastole, (Dd) and end systole (Ds). CW, chest wall. *C*, Normal septal aortic and mitral aortic relationships obtained when transducer is swept from positions (1) through (3) of A. A, aortic valve; LA, left atrium; LV, left ventricle; MV, mitral valve; RV, right ventricle; S, interventricular septum. Note continuity of anterior mitral leaflet with posterior wall of aorta and of the ventricular septum with anterior wall of aorta.

Furthermore, it can be used to evaluate cardiac performance in a variety of circumstances, such as cardiac effects of drug toxicity, where there are secondary influences on myocardial function.

The ultrasound display on an oscilloscope appears as dots. The horizontal axis of the oscilloscope relates to time, the vertical axis to the depth of tissues. The dots that are moving in the vertical axis because of cardiac contractions are swept across the oscilloscope to produce the motion mode (*M-mode*). The method is used to define the presence or absence of individual anatomic structures and their relationships to one another (Figs. 14–21 and 14–22) and to evaluate cardiac function (Table 14–2). The development of cross section or *two-dimensional echocardiography* has greatly enhanced the ability to visualize spatial relationships of the cardiac structure (Fig. 14–23). With this technique the image of the contracting heart is displayed in two dimensions by means of a number of different views which emphasize individual structures (valves, septa, hypertrophied muscle, etc.). Two-dimensional echocardiographic studies display images similar to those seen by angiocardiogram, and they are interpreted in much the same manner (Fig. 14–23). Motion mode and two-dimensional echocardiography complement each other. The former is most important for indirectly evaluating cardiac function, whereas the latter allows specific visualization of structures and spatial relationships.

Doppler echocardiography is an adaptation of ultrasound that identifies flow rather than morphology. It displays flow in the cardiac chambers and vascular channels based on the change in frequency imparted to a sound wave by the move-

Table 14–2. Echographic Measurement of Cardiovascular Performance

1. Per cent shortening $= \dfrac{\text{LVED} - \text{LVES}}{\text{LVED}} \times 100$ (see Fig. 14–21A)

   LVED = left ventricular end-diastolic dimension; LVES = left ventricular end-systolic dimension. (Normal, 28–38%.)

2. Mean VCF $= \dfrac{\text{LVED} - \text{LVES}}{\text{LVED} \times \text{ET}}$

   VCF = mean velocity of circumferential fiber shortening (expressed as circumference [circ] per second); LVED and LVES as in (1) above; ET = ejection time. (*Normal values:* neonates, 1.51 ± 0.04 (SE) circ/sec; children (5–15 yr), 1.34 ± 0.03 (SE) circ/sec.)

3. Systolic time intervals (a) $\dfrac{\text{LPEP}}{\text{LVET}}$ (normal range is 0.3–0.39; average, 0.35). LPEP = left ventricular pre-ejection period. LVET = left ventricular ejection time. (b) $\dfrac{\text{RPEP}}{\text{RVET}}$

   (normal range is 0.16–0.30; average, 0.24). These ratios are indirect indices of changes in afterload, preload, contractility, and electromechanical delay.

4. Isovolumic contraction (ICT) (Fig. 14–22) may be derived from the following regression equation: ICT = 53 − 0.22 × heart rate (SE ± 7.3). ICT is increased in left ventricular myocardial disease and decreased in aortic runoff (e.g., patent ductus arteriosus).

5. Right and left ventricular outflow obstruction may be quantitated by Doppler estimation of the velocity of blood flow (V) across the stenotic segment. The peak systolic ejection gradient (PSEG) = 4V².

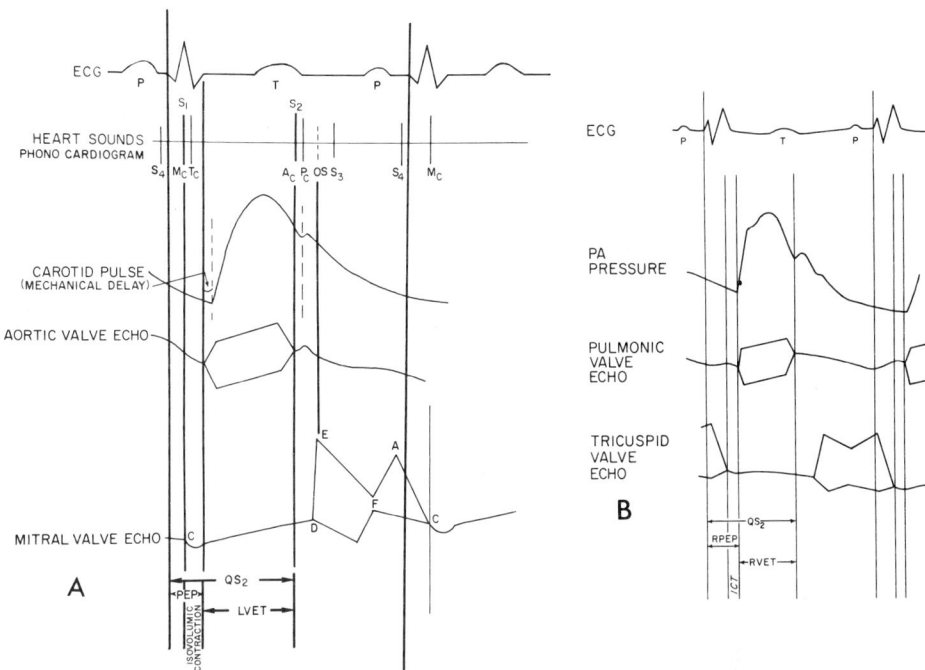

Figure 14–22. Temporal events of cardiac cycle determined by echocardiography. *A*, Left heart. *B*, Right heart. Ac, aortic valve closure; ECG, electrocardiogram; LVET, left ventricular ejection time; Mc, mitral valve closure; OS, opening snap; Pc, pulmonary valve closure; PEP, pre-ejection period; QS$_2$, total electromechanical systole; RVET, right ventricular ejection time; S$_1$, S$_2$, S$_3$, and S$_4$, 1st, 2nd, 3rd, and 4th heart sounds, respectively; Tc, tricuspid valve closure.

ment of red blood cells. The speed and direction of blood flow in the line of the echo beam changes the reference frequency produced by a transducer. The data generated by Doppler are displayed as a "frequency shift," which can be translated into volumetric, i.e., L/min, or barometric, i.e., mm Hg, values. Volumetric data permit noninvasive estimation of systemic and pulmonary blood flow. Barometric data allow estimation of gradients across semilunar and atrioventricular valves. The directional quality of Doppler identifies abnormalities in blood flow that are frequently encountered in the pediatric population (Fig. 14–24).

Used along with other clinical and/or laboratory methods, echocardiography facilitates a more rigorous selection process for cardiac catheterization and helps to improve the timing of hemodynamic studies. An increasing number of patients with various lesions such as ASD can now be operated upon without presurgical invasive studies based on the results of echocardiographic and Doppler testing. Echocardiography has also proved useful in the evaluation of congestive heart failure, pericardial fluid accumulation, atrial or ventricular septal defects, cardiac valve problems, vegetations due to infective endocarditis, intracardiac tumor or hematoma, cardiotoxic agents, and ductus arteriosus in premature infants. It also can monitor the results of surgical or medical intervention.

Contrast Echocardiography. The rapid injection of fluid (e.g., the patient's blood, saline, or other media) produces microbubbles at the site of injection; these are harmless to the patient and travel in a bolus, from the site of injection in a vein or right atrium, through the chambers of the heart. This bolus is manifested by a cloud of echoes, which can be visualized by both M-mode and two-dimensional echocardiograms. The technique has great value in revealing flow patterns through various structures and in detecting intravascular shunts in the preoperative and immediate postoperative periods (Fig. 14–25).

14.7 EXERCISE TESTING

The normal cardiorespiratory system adapts to the extensive demands of exercise with a several-fold increase in oxygen

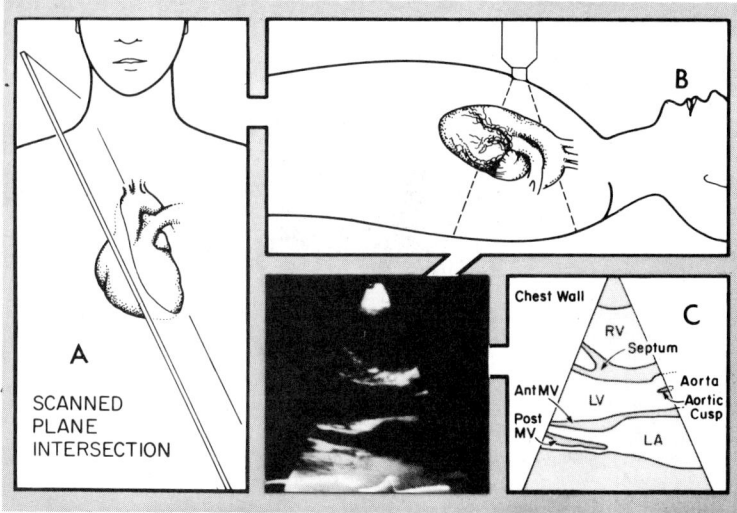

Figure 14–23. *A*, Plane of long axis of heart examined by mechanical sector scanning. *B*, Position of transducer on chest. *C*, One selected frame from a real-time study and idealized diagram of this frame. Ant MV, anterior mitral leaflet; LA, left atrium; LV, left ventricle; Post MV, posterior mitral leaflet; RV, right ventricle.

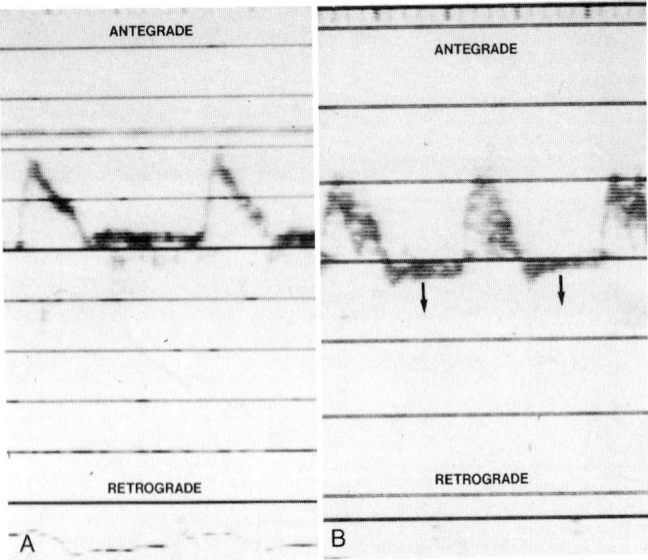

Figure 14–24. Patent ductus arteriosus. A, Doppler flow in the proximal descending aorta of normal infant demonstrating the normal antegrade systolic and diastolic flow. B, Doppler flow configuration in infant with patent ductus arteriosus reveals antegrade systolic but retrograde diastolic flow (arrows).

consumption and cardiac output. Since there is a large reserve capacity for exercise, significant abnormalities of cardiovascular performance may exist without symptoms at rest or during ordinary activities. Generally, patients are evaluated in a resting state during which significant abnormalities of cardiac function may not be appreciated or, if detected, their implications about the quality of life may not be recognized. Permission for children with cardiovascular disease to participate in various forms of physical activity is frequently based on subjective criteria. Exercise testing plays an important role in evaluating symptoms, quantitating the severity of cardiac abnormalities, and assisting in the management of these patients.

Exercise studies are usually performed on a graded treadmill apparatus utilizing timed intervals of increasing grade and speed (Bruce protocol). Many laboratories now have the capacity to measure cardiac output and pulmonary function noninvasively during exercise.

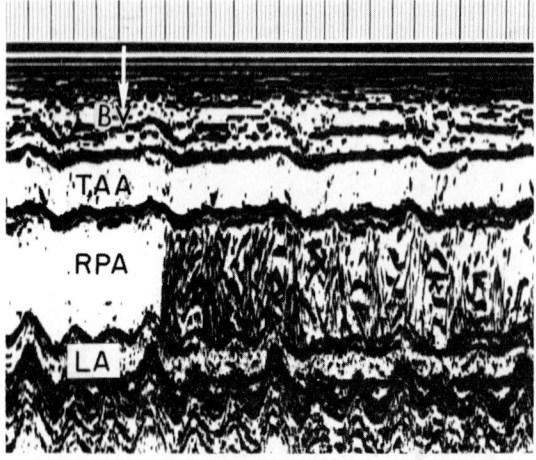

Figure 14–25. Contrast echocardiogram obtained after injection of 1 ml of blood in inferior vena cava of 3 day old infant with aortic atresia. Moment of injection indicated by arrow. Transducer in suprasternal notch identifies the small transverse aortic arch (TAA), the large right pulmonary artery (RPA) filled with a cloud of echocontrast soon after injection, and the small left atrium (LA). Time lines 40 msec.

As the child grows, the capacity for work increases with body size and skeletal muscle mass. All indices of cardiopulmonary function, however, do not increase in a uniform manner. A major response to exercise is an increase in cardiac output, principally as a result of increased heart rate, but stroke volume, systemic venous return, and pulse pressure are also increased. Systemic vascular resistance is greatly decreased as the blood vessels in working muscle dilate as a response to increasing metabolic demands. As the child becomes older and larger, the response of the heart rate to exercise remains prominent, but the cardiac output increases because of growing cardiac volume capacity and hence stroke volume. The responses to dynamic exercise are not dependent only on age. For any given body surface area, boys have a larger stroke volume than size-matched girls. This increase is mediated by posture as well as by sex. Augmentation of stroke volume with upright, dynamic exercise is facilitated by the pumping action of working muscles that overcomes the static effect of gravity and increases systemic venous return.

Dynamic exercise testing defines not only endurance and exercise capacity, but also the effect of such exercise on myocardial blood flow and cardiac rhythm. In normal children an electrocardiogram during exercise shows a decrease in the R-R interval (increased heart rate) commensurate with the level of exercise. Significant S-T segmental depression reflects abnormalities in myocardial perfusion. Subendocardial ischemia commonly occurs during exercise in children with hypertrophied left ventricles. The exercise electrocardiogram is considered abnormal if S-T segmental depression is equal to or greater than 2 mm and extends for at least 0.06 sec after the J point (onset of S-T segment) in conjunction with a horizontal, upward, or downward sloping S-T segment.

Provocation of rhythm disturbances during an exercise study is an important method for evaluating selected patients with known or suspected rhythm disorders. The effect of pharmacologic management can also be tested in this manner.

Conditions in which exercise testing may be helpful include (1) left ventricular outflow obstruction, such as valvular, subvalvular, and supravalvular aortic stenosis, hypertrophic cardiomyopathy, and coarctation of the aorta; (2) chronic volume overload of the left or right ventricles, such as atrioventricular or semilunar valve incompetence and left to right shunts; (3) arrhythmias; and (4) hypertension.

A physician should be present during the exercise test to supervise its performance, and adequate emergency equipment must be immediately available (e.g., defibrillator, medications, IV fluids, etc.). Indications for termination of a study are (1) failure or inadequacy of the electrocardiographic monitoring; (2) onset of serious arrhythmias, such as ventricular or supraventricular tachycardia; (3) premature beats (more than 25% of beats) precipitated or aggravated by exercise; (4) development of heart block; (5) precipitation of pain, headache, dizziness, or syncope; (6) S-T segmental depression or elevation of 3 mm or more; (7) inappropriate hypertension (systolic pressure >230 mm Hg or diastolic pressure >120 mm Hg); (8) inappropriate fall of blood pressure; (9) development of cutaneous vascular insufficiency (e.g., pallor); or (10) severe fatigue.

14.8 RADIONUCLIDE STUDIES

Pediatric nuclear cardiology is useful in several areas:
1. *Radionuclide angiography* to detect and quantify shunts (Fig. 14–26) and to analyze the distribution of blood flow to each lung.
2. *Gated blood pool scanning* to calculate hemodynamic measurements including cardiac output, left and right ventricular ejection fractions, and stroke volume ratios. The latter calcu-

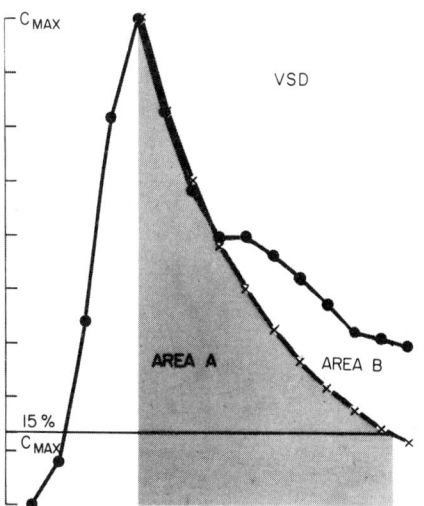

Figure 14–26. Estimation of left to right shunt from a pulmonary time activity curve obtained after injection of a bolus of technetium-99m. The method uses a Stewart-Hamilton extrapolation of the downslope of the curve. On the vertical axis is the course of radionuclide material from the area of interest in the lung. On the horizontal axis is time measured in sec. The line joined by dots represents the time activity curve of a patient with a ventricular septal defect. In the presence of a left to right shunt the exponential decline is interrupted by early recirculation. The line joined by X's represents the idealized exponential decline in the absence of shunting and is extrapolated to a minimum value of 15% of the maximal radionuclide count (C_{max}). Thus the region beyond the peak is divided into two areas: A and B. From the ratio of area B to area A, an approximation of the shunt size can be made. Gamma function fitting of the pulmonary activity curve can be used as an alternative method for shunt estimation.

lation allows quantification of valvular regurgitation and can be assessed both at rest and during exercise. Gated blood pool scanning is also used to detect regional wall motion abnormalities.

3. *Thallium imaging* for the evaluation of perfusion of cardiac muscle mass in order to detect myocardial infarction and/or ischemia.

These methods are the results of the development of gamma computer systems, short lived radionuclides, and portable equipment that can be taken to the bedside of a seriously ill patient. Radionuclide techniques impose little discomfort on the patient, and radiation exposure is low when compared with that of angiocardiography. Serial studies are thus possible when required for patient management. Radionuclide angiographic techniques provide quantitative physiologic data that cannot be obtained at cardiac catheterization, but do not provide visualization of fine anatomic detail.

14.9 CARDIAC CATHETERIZATION

Cardiac catheterization remains a major tool of the pediatric cardiologist in the diagnosis of congenital heart disease. With this technique the various chambers of the heart, great vessels, and veins are entered and blood samples obtained for measuring oxygen saturation. Pressures are measured and contrast and indicator materials may be injected as required. Cardiac catheterization is essentially a presurgical diagnostic test and should be utilized only when there is a reasonable expectation that an operation will be required. Its use for purposes of reassurance when the clinical picture clearly indicates that no significant heart disease is present should be avoided. Although the risks are low, cardiac catheterization involves risk for the patient and should not be used without an opportunity for benefit. In many instances echocardiographic and radio-

nuclide studies may be used in lieu of multiple cardiac catheterizations in individual patients who require careful monitoring of their hemodynamic status.

Cardiac catheterization should be carried out with the patient in a basal state; this is often not possible with children. Children are routinely sedated during these studies, but deep anesthesia is avoided if possible since depression of cardiovascular function by various anesthetic agents may distort the calculations of hemodynamic measurements, including cardiac output, pulmonary and systemic resistance, and shunt ratios.

If cardiac catheterization is performed on a critically ill infant having congenital heart disease, a surgical team should be alerted in the event that an operation is required immediately afterward. The complication rate of cardiac catheterization and angiography is greatest among critically ill infants; they must be studied in a thermally neutral environment and treated quickly for hypothermia, acidemia, or excess blood loss. Development of soft, flow-directed balloon-tipped catheters has greatly decreased the frequency of complications from catheter manipulation, such as severe arrhythmias, cardiac perforations, and intramyocardial injection of contrast material.

In most instances catheterization involves both the left and right heart. The catheter is passed into the heart under

Table 14–3. Normal Values and Formulas for Determination of Hemodynamics in Cardiac Catheterization

1. Cardiac index 3.0–5.0 L/min/m²
2. Arteriovenous oxygen difference 4.5 ± 0.7 mL/dL
3. Oxygen consumption 140–160 mL/m²/min
4. Arterial oxygen saturation 94–100%
5. Difference in oxygen content between venae cavae and right atrium <1.9 vol %
6. Difference in oxygen content between right atrium and right ventricle <0.9 vol %
7. Difference in oxygen content between right ventricle and pulmonary artery <0.5 vol %
8. Normal mean left atrial pressure 4–8 mm Hg
9. Pulmonary arteriolar resistance 50–150 dyne sec cm⁻⁵ (1 unit = 80 dynes)
10. Cardiac output mL/min =
$$\frac{O_2 \text{ intake (mL/min)}}{\left\{\begin{array}{l} O_2 \text{ content of arterial blood (vols \%)} \\ \text{minus } O_2 \text{ content of mixed venous blood} \end{array}\right\}} \times 100$$
11. Cardiac index = cardiac output (L/min)/m² of body surface area
12. Pulmonary artery flow =
$$\frac{O_2 \text{ intake (mL/min)}}{\left\{\begin{array}{l} O_2 \text{ content of pulmonary venous blood (vols \%)} \\ \text{minus } O_2 \text{ content of pulmonary arterial blood (vols \%)} \end{array}\right\}} \times 100$$
If a pulmonary venous sample is not available, it is assumed to be saturated to 95% of capacity
13. Systemic flow =
$$\frac{O_2 \text{ intake (mL/min)}}{\left\{\begin{array}{l} \text{systemic arterial } O_2 \text{ content (vols \%)} \\ \text{minus arterial venous } O_2 \text{ content (vols \%)} \end{array}\right\}} \times 100$$
14. Effective pulmonary artery flow =
$$\frac{O_2 \text{ intake (mL/min)}}{\left\{\begin{array}{l} \text{pulmonary venous } O_2 \text{ content (vols \%)} \\ \text{minus mixed venous } O_2 \text{ content (vols \%)} \end{array}\right\}} \times 100$$
15. Total left to right shunt = pulmonary artery flow minus effective pulmonary artery flow
16. Total right to left shunt = systemic flow minus effective pulmonary artery flow
17. Pulmonary arteriolar resistance $R = \dfrac{PA - PC}{PF}$

Where R = pulmonary arteriolar resistance (resistance units)
PA = mean pulmonary artery pressure in mm Hg
PC = mean pulmonary "capillary" pressure in mm Hg
PF = pulmonary flow in L/min/m²

fluoroscopic guidance via a percutaneous entry point in the femoral vein. The left heart is usually entered by passing the catheter across the former foramen ovale to the left atrium and left ventricle. The left heart is also catheterized by passing the catheter retrograde through the femoral artery and the aorta and across the aortic valve. The catheter is manipulated through abnormal intracardiac defects or into malpositioned great vessels. Complete hemodynamics can be calculated (Table 14–3) through data obtained at catheterization: cardiac output, intracardiac shunts, and systemic and pulmonary resistances. The normal circulatory dynamics are depicted in Figure 14–27.

Indicator Dilution and Appearance Techniques. If a bolus of indicator material is injected intravenously or into the right side of the heart, it traverses the pulmonary circulation and enters the left side of the heart and then the arterial circulation. This indicator material may then be detected in the arterial blood. A continuous record of the circulation of indicator in normal subjects shows two peaks (Fig. 14–28). The time between the instant of injection and the detection of the indicator in arterial blood is known as the appearance time and is a measure of circulation time. The 1st peak of the indicator curve is due to the passage of indicator past the arterial detectors, the 2nd, to recirculation through the systemic arterial and venous systems, the pulmonary circulation, and reappearance in the arterial tree. If the concentration of circulating indicator is known, cardiac output can be computed.

Localization of intracardiac and extracardiac shunts may be facilitated by these methods. Curves obtained after the injection of indicator at or upstream from the site of a **right to left shunt** show a short appearance time because of the escape of indicator across the defect (Fig. 14–28). In the presence of **left to right shunts** some of the indicator has a normal transit time to the detection site while the remaining indicator recirculates through the lungs in a prolonged transit time. Curves recorded from systemic arterial blood have normal appearance times, reduced peak concentrations, and prolonged disappearance times (Fig. 14–28).

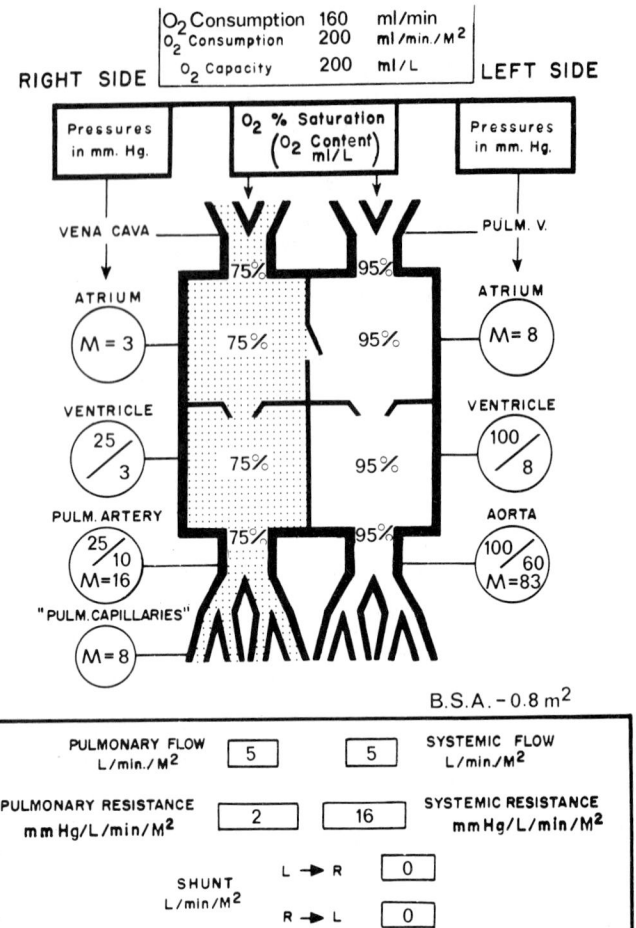

Figure 14–27. Diagram of normal circulatory dynamics with pressures, oxygen contents, and per cent of saturations. (Modified from Nadas AS, Fyler DC: Pediatric Cardiology. 3rd ed. Philadelphia, WB Saunders, 1972.)

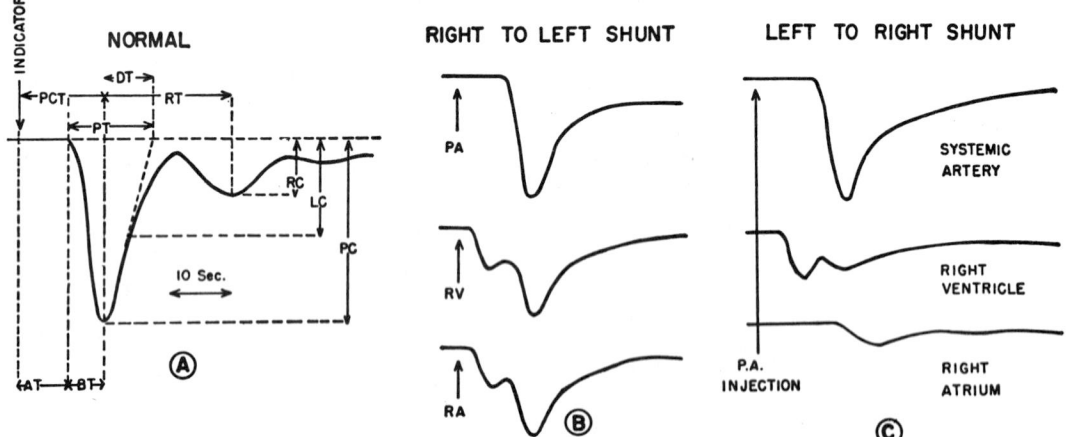

Figure 14–28. Idealized diagrams of indicator dilution curves. A, Normal curve showing time and concentration components. Instant of indicator injection in right side of heart shown by arrow at top left. Curve obtained from indicator detector in a systemic artery. AT, appearance time; BT, build-up time; DT, disappearance time; LC, least concentration; PC, peak concentration; PCT, peak concentration time; PT, passage time; RC, maximal recirculation concentration; RT, recirculation time. Extrapolation of declining slope of concentration is easier if the curve is plotted on a logarithmic scale. Cardiac output may be computed by the formula $\dfrac{601}{c(PT)}$ where 1 = amount of indicator, c = mean concentration of indicator, PT = passage time. B, Localization of *right to left shunt*. Instant of injection of indicator shown by arrows. Example illustrates shunt at ventricular levels. Site of injection: PA, pulmonary artery; RA, right atrium; RV, right ventricle. Indicator detector in systemic artery in all instances. PA injection (i.e., downstream from shunt level) shows normal appearance time. RV and RA injections (i.e., at and upstream from shunt level) show early appearance times. C, Localization of *left to right shunt*. Example illustrates shunt at ventricular level. Indicator injected into distal pulmonary artery (PA) in all instances. In upper tracing indicator detector is in a systemic artery, and curve shows prolonged disappearance time. Middle curve is from indicator detected in right ventricle and shows an early appearance time because of ventricular septal defect. Right atrial curve shows normal appearance time.

The *thermodilution method* for measuring cardiac output is the most commonly used indicator dilution technique. A known change in heat content of the blood is induced at one point in the circulation (usually the right atrium or inferior vena cava), and the resultant change in temperature is detected at a point downstream (usually the pulmonary artery). The injectate is iced or room temperature saline. This method is used to measure cardiac output in the catheterization laboratory in patients without shunts (e.g., aortic stenosis or coarctation of the aorta). When combined with the dye dilution technique, it can also be used to measure the volume of regurgitant flow across diseased mitral or aortic valves. Monitoring the cardiac output by the thermodilution method is also useful in managing critically ill infants and children in an intensive care setting after cardiac surgery or in the presence of shock.

Angiocardiography. The great blood vessels and individual cardiac chambers may be seen by selective angiocardiography, i.e., injection of contrast material into specific cardiac chambers or great vessels. This method allows identification of specific abnormalities without interference from the superimposed shadows of normal chambers. Photofluorography with image intensification has made possible simultaneous cardiac catheterization and selective angiocardiography. The preferred method is a combination of photofluorography with closed-circuit television to monitor the fluoroscopic screen and allow visualization of the cardiac silhouette and the cardiac catheter. After the cardiac catheter is introduced into the chamber to be studied, a small amount of contrast medium is rapidly injected and moving pictures are exposed at 60 frames/sec. Biplane cineangiocardiography allows detailed evaluation of specific cardiac chambers and blood vessels in two planes with the injection of a single bolus of contrast material. Various angle views are utilized to best display anatomic features in individual lesions. These techniques require sophisticated radiographic equipment including special tables and flexibly placed x-ray units.

The rapid injection of contrast medium under pressure into the circulation is not without risks, and each injection should be carefully planned. Contrast agents consist of hypertonic solutions containing organic iodides which can cause complications including nausea, a generalized burning sensation, central nervous system symptoms, and allergic rashes. Intramyocardial injection is generally avoided by careful placement of the catheter prior to injection. Hypertonicity of the contrast media may result in transient myocardial depression and a drop in blood pressure, and soon afterward tachycardia, an increase in cardiac output, and a shift of interstitial fluid into the circulation.

"Idealized" diagrams of the normal angiocardiogram are shown in Figure 14–6. The indications for this study are outlined under the individual congenital lesions.

General

Adams FH, Emmanouilides GC: Moss' Heart Disease in Infants, Children and Adolescents. 3rd ed. Baltimore, Williams & Wilkins, 1983.
Dickerman JD, Lucey JF: Smith's The Critically Ill Child: Diagnosis and Medical Management. Philadelphia, WB Saunders, 1985.
Friedman WF, Lesch M, Sonnenblick EH: Neonatal Heart Disease. New York, Grune & Stratton, 1973.
Keith JD, Rowe RD, Vlad P (eds): Heart Disease in Infancy and Childhood. 3rd ed. New York, Macmillan, 1978.
Nadas AS, Fyler DC: Pediatric Cardiology. 3rd ed. Philadelphia, WB Saunders, 1979.
Rudolph AM: Congenital Diseases of the Heart. Chicago, Year Book Medical Publishers, 1974.
Stark J, DeLeval M (eds): Surgery for Congenital Heart Defects in Infants. New York, Grune & Stratton, 1983.

Cardiac Sounds and Phonocardiography

Baragan J, Fernandez F, Thiron JM, et al (eds): Dynamic Auscultation and Phonocardiography. Bowie, MD, Charles Press Publishers, 1979.

Leatham A: Systolic murmurs. Circulation 17:601, 1958.
Mills P, Craige E: Echophonocardiography. Prog Cardiovasc Dis 20:337, 1978.

Electrocardiogram and Vectorcardiogram

Ellison RC, Restieaux NJ: Vectorcardiography in Congenital Heart Disease. Philadelphia, WB Saunders, 1972.
Garson A: The Electrocardiogram in Infants and Children: A Systematic Approach. Philadelphia, Lea & Febiger, 1983.
Guntheroth WG: Pediatric Electrocardiography. Philadelphia, WB Saunders, 1965.
Lipman BF, Massey EF: Clinical Scalar Electrocardiography. Chicago, Year Book Medical Publishers, 1984.

Echocardiography

Alverson DC, Eldridge M, Dillon T, et al: Noninvasive pulse Doppler determination of cardiac output in neonates and children. J Pediatr 101:46, 1982.
Baker ML, Dalrymple GV: Biologic effects of diagnostic ultrasound: A review. Radiology 126:479, 1978.
Berman W Jr: Pulsed Doppler Ultrasound in Clinical Pediatrics. Mt. Kisco, NY, Futura, 1983.
Bleifeld W, Effert S, Hanrath P, et al: Evaluation of Cardiac Function by Echocardiography. Berlin, Springer-Verlag, 1980.
Feigenbaum H: Echocardiography. 3rd ed. Philadelphia, Lea & Febiger, 1981.
Hatle L, Angelsen B: Doppler Ultrasound in Cardiology, Physical Principles and Clinical Applications. Philadelphia, Lea & Febiger, 1985.
Kleinman CS, Hobbins CC, Lynch DC, et al: The use of fetal echocardiography in the diagnosis and management of antenatal arrythmias. M J Cardiol 47:457, 1981.
Meyer RA: Pediatric Echocardiography. Philadelphia, Lea & Febiger, 1977.
Silverman N, Snyder A: Two-Dimensional Echocardiography in Congenital Heart Disease. Norwalk, CT, Appleton-Century-Crofts, 1982.
Tajik AJ, Seward JB, Hagler DJ, et al: Two-dimensional real-time imaging of the heart and great vessels: Technique, image orientation, structure identification and validation. Mayo Clin Proc 53:271, 1978.
Williams RG: Echocardiographic Diagnosis of Congenital Heart Disease. Boston, Little, Brown, 1977.

Exercise Testing

Astrand P, Rodahl K: Textbook of Work Physiology. New York, McGraw-Hill, 1970.
Cumming GR, Everatt D, Hastman L: Bruce treadmill test in children: Normal values in a clinical population. Am J Cardiol 41:69, 1978.
Fortuin NJ, Weiss JL: Exercise stress testing. Circulation 56:700, 1977.
Godfrey S: Exercise Testing in Children. Philadelphia, WB Saunders, 1974.
James FW, Glueck CJ, Fallat RW, et al: Maximal exercise stress testing in normal and hyperlipidemic children. Atherosclerosis 25:85, 1976.
James FW, Kaplan S, Glueck CJ, et al: Responses of normal children and young adults to controlled bicycle exercise. Circulation 61:902, 1980.
Riopel DA, Taylor AB, Hohn AR: Blood pressure, heart rate, pressure-rate product and electrographic changes in healthy children during treadmill exercise. Am J Cardiol 44:697, 1979.
Rozanski JJ, Dimich I, Steinfeld L, et al: Maximal exercise stress testing in evaluation of arrhythmias in children: Results and reproducibility. Am J Cardiol 42:951, 1979.
Truccone NJ, Steeg CN, Dell R, et al: Comparison of the cardiocirculatory effects of exercise and isoproterenol in children with pulmonary or aortic valve stenosis. Circulation 56:79, 1977.

Nuclear Medicine

Bodenheimer MM, Banka VS, Helfant RH: Nuclear cardiology. Radionuclide angiographic assessment of left ventricular contraction: Uses, limitations, and future directions. Am J Cardiol 45:661, 1980.
Friedman WF, Sahn DJ, Hirschklau MS: A review: Newer, noninvasive cardiac diagnostic methods. Pediatr Res 11:190, 1977.
Hurwitz RA: Quantitation of aortic and mitral regurgitation in the pediatric population: Evaluation by radionuclide angiography. Am J Cardiol 51:252, 1983.
Parrish MD, Graham TP Jr, Bender HW, et al: Radionuclide angiographic evaluation of right and left ventricular function during exercise after repair of transposition of the great arteries. Circulation 67:178, 1983.
Slutsky R, Karliner J, Ricci D, et al: Left ventricular volumes calculated by gated equilibrium angiography: A new method. Circulation 60:556, 1979.
Treves S, Fogl R, Lang P: Radionuclide angiography in congenital heart disease. Am J Cardiol 46:1247, 1980.
Willerson JT (ed): Nuclear Cardiology. Philadelphia, FA Davis, 1979.

Cardiac Catheterization

Bargeron LM, Elliot LP, Soto B, et al: Axial cineangiography in congenital heart disease. Circulation 56:1075, 1977.
Braunwald E, Swan HJC: Cooperative Study on Cardiac Catheterization. Am Heart Assoc Monograph No 20, New York, 1968.

Freed MD, Keane JF: Cardiac output measured by thermodilution in infants and children. J Pediatr 92:39, 1978.

Freedom RM, Culham JAG, Moes CAF: Angiocardiography of Congenital Heart Disease. New York, Macmillan, 1984.

Graham TP Jr: Advances in invasive cardiac diagnosis and management. Pediatr Clin North Am 25:707, 1978.

Kan JS, White RI, Mitchell SE, et al: Percutaneous balloon valvuloplasty: New method for treating congenital pulmonary valve stenosis. N Engl J Med 307:538, 1982.

Kan JS, White RI, Mitchell SE, et al: Treatment of restenosis of coarctation by percutaneous transluminal angioplasty. Circulation 68:1087, 1983.

Lock JE, Castaneda-Zuniga WR, Bass JL, et al: Balloon dilation angioplasty of hypoplastic and stenotic pulmonary arteries. Circulation 67:962, 1983.

Martin EC, Olson AP, Steeg CN, et al: Radiation exposure to the pediatric patient during cardiac catheterization and angiography. Circulation 64:153, 1981.

Rashkind WJ: Transcatheter treatment of congenital heart disease. Circulation 67:711, 1983.

Rushmer RF: Cardiovascular Dynamics. 4th ed. Philadelphia, WB Saunders, 1976.

Schwartz DC, Kaplan S: Cardiac catheterization and selective angiography in infants with a new flow-directed catheter. Cath Cardiovasc Diag 1:59, 1975.

Stanger P, Heymann MA, Tarnoff H, et al: Complications of cardiac catheterization of neonates, infants, and children: A three year study. Circulation 50:595, 1974.

Walls JT, Lababidi Z, Curtis JJ, et al: Assessment of percutaneous balloon pulmonary and aortic valvuloplasty. J Thorac Cardiovasc Surg 88:352, 1984.

Wood EH: Diagnostic applications of indicator dilution technics in congenital heart disease. Circ Res 10:531, 1962.

Yang SS, Bentivoglio LG, Maranhao V, et al: From Cardiac Catheterization Data to Hemodynamic Parameters. 2nd ed. Philadelphia, FA Davis, 1978.

14.10 FETAL AND NEONATAL CIRCULATION

Fetal Circulation. Much of the information concerning fetal circulation has been derived from animal studies. Although there may be some species differences, the human fetal circulation and its adjustments after birth are probably similar to those of animals. Oxygenated blood from the placenta flows to the fetus through the umbilical vein at an average rate of 175 mL/kg with a pressure close to 12 mm Hg and a pO_2 of about 35 mm Hg. Approximately 50% of the umbilical venous blood bypasses the liver and flows through the ductus venosus into the inferior vena cava, where it mixes with the remainder of the venous return from the caudal part of the body and enters the right atrium from the inferior vena cava. Most of this blood preferentially passes across the foramen ovale to the left atrium, flows into the left ventricle, and is ejected into the ascending aorta. The coronary and cerebral arteries and those of the upper extremities are thus perfused with blood having a higher pO_2 than that perfusing other parts of the body, except for the liver. The superior vena caval blood, which is considerably less oxygenated, traverses the tricuspid valve and flows primarily to the right ventricle and pulmonary arterial trunk. The major portion of this blood (which has a pO_2 of 19–22 mm Hg) bypasses the lungs and flows through the ductus arteriosus into the descending aorta to perfuse the caudal part of the body as well as the placenta via the umbilical arteries. The effective fetal cardiac output, i.e., the sum of the left ventricular output and the ductal flow, amounts to about 220 mL/kg/min. Approximately 65% of this blood returns to the placenta; the remaining 35% perfuses the fetal organs and tissues (Fig. 14–29A).

Since the fetal ventricles work in parallel rather than in series, the distribution of their ejected blood depends on resistance and flow and the fact that the large ductus arteriosus equalizes aortic and pulmonary arterial pressures. Approximately 10% of the right ventricular output flows to the lungs via the pulmonary arteries, and 90% enters the descending aorta via the ductus arteriosus (Fig. 14–29B). This occurs primarily because pulmonary vascular resistance in the fetus is considerably higher than systemic resistance, which is predominantly influenced by the low resistance placental vascular bed. Left ventricular output consists of a mixture of venous return from the inferior vena cava, foramen ovale, and left atrium, as well as the minimal pulmonary venous return. Right ventricular output is approximately 50% greater than left ventricular, and thus the right ventricle is dominant during fetal life.

Neonatal Circulation. At birth the fetal circulation must immediately adapt to extrauterine life as gas exchange is transferred from the placenta to the lung. Some of these changes are virtually instantaneous with the first breath, and others are affected over hours or days. After an initial fall in systemic blood pressure, there is a progressive rise. The heart rate slows as a result of a baroreceptor response to an increase in systemic vascular resistance when the placental circulation is eliminated. The average central aortic pressure in the neonate is 75/50 mm Hg. With the onset of ventilation a marked increase in pulmonary blood flow occurs because of the dilatative effect of oxygen on the pulmonary arteriolar bed. Pulmonary venous return and consequently left ventricular output are thus increased. In the normal neonate, ductal closure and fall of pulmonary vascular resistance result in a fall of pulmonary arterial and right ventricular pressures. The major decline of pressure from the high fetal levels to the low "adult" levels in the human infant at sea level usually occurs within the first 2–3 days but may be prolonged for 7 days or more.

Significant differences between the neonatal circulation and that of older infants may be summarized as follows: (1) right to left shunting may persist across the patent foramen ovale; (2) in the presence of cardiopulmonary disease, continued patency of the ductus arteriosus may allow left to right, right to left, or bidirectional shunting; (3) the neonatal pulmonary vasculature constricts more vigorously in response to hypoxemia, hypercapnia, and acidosis; (4) the muscular mass of the left and right ventricles is almost equal; (5) the neonate has more tolerance to hypoxemia; and (6) newborn infants at rest have a relatively high oxygen consumption, which is associated with their relatively high cardiac output. A high percentage of fetal hemoglobin may interfere with delivery of oxygen to the tissues since there is reduced binding of 2,3-diphosphoglycerate in fetal hemoglobin. Under these conditions an increased cardiac output would be required for adequate delivery of oxygen to the tissues.

The foramen ovale is functionally closed by the 3rd month of life, though it is possible to pass a probe through the overlapping flaps in 25% of adults. Functional closure of the ductus arteriosus is usually complete by 10–15 hr in the normal neonate. During the periods of adjustment there are rarely physical signs of patency of these structures. However, in premature newborn infants an evanescent systolic murmur with late accentuation or a continuous murmur may be audible, and in the context of the respiratory distress syndrome the patent ductus arteriosus may be of clinical importance (Sec. 14.46).

The normal ductus arteriosus differs morphologically from the adjoining aorta and pulmonary artery in that the ductus has a significant amount of circularly arranged smooth muscle in its medial layer. Ductal patency during fetal life may be due to an active mechanism produced by circulating or local prostaglandin. In the neonate, oxygen is the most important factor controlling ductal closure. When the pO_2 of the blood passing through the ductus reaches about 50 mm Hg, the ductal wall constricts; the mechanisms by which oxygen

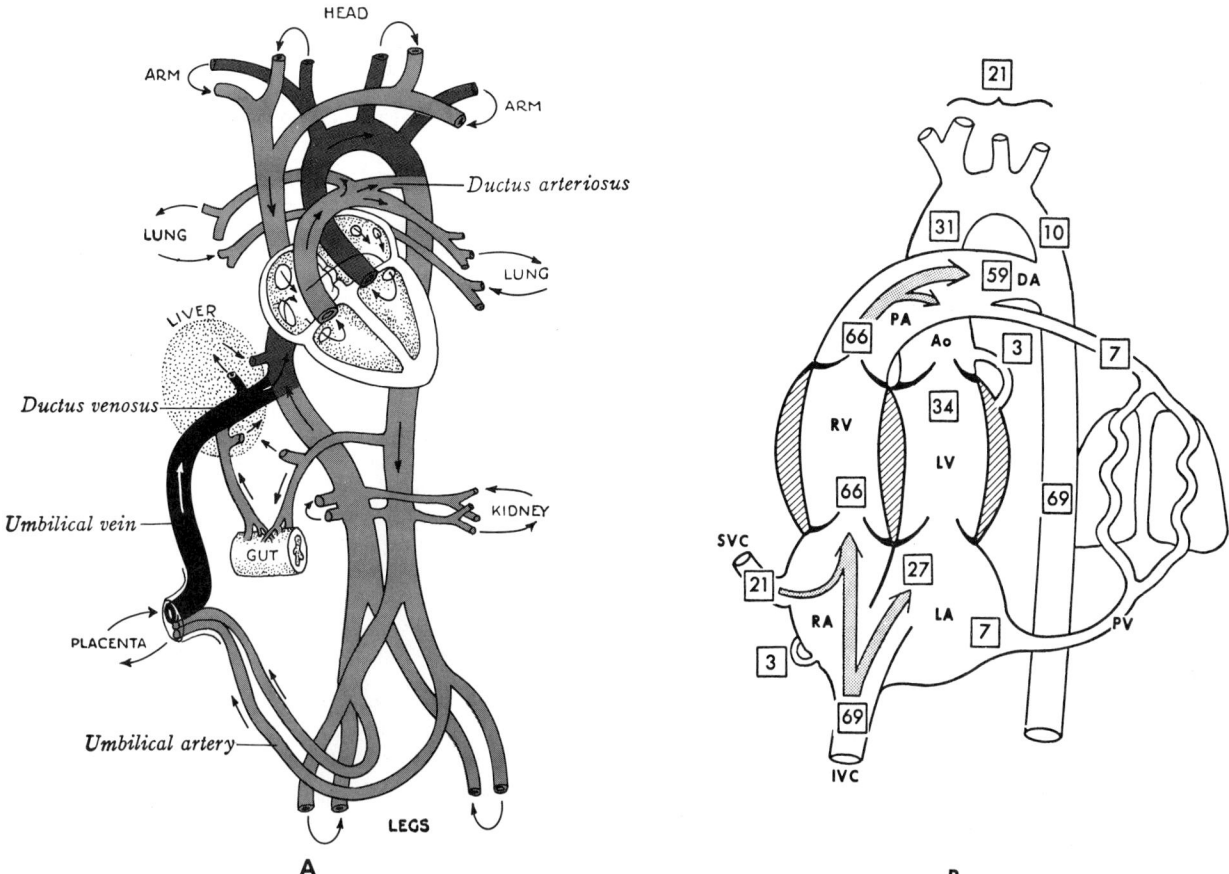

Figure 14–29. *A*, Plan of the human circulation before birth (partly after Dawes). Black shading indicates more oxygenated blood, and arrows indicate the direction of flow (Arey). *B*, Percentages of combined ventricular output that return to the fetal heart, that are ejected by each ventricle, and that flow through the main vascular channels. Figures are those obtained from study of late-gestation lambs. (From Rudolph AM: Congenital Diseases of the Heart. Chicago, Year Book Medical Publishers, 1974.)

activates ductal constriction are not completely understood. The effects of oxygen on the ductal smooth muscle could be direct or mediated by vasoactive substances such as acetylcholine or bradykinin. Gestational age also appears to play a role; the ductus of the premature infant is less responsive to oxygen, even though its musculature is developed (Sec. 8.30).

THE CRITICALLY ILL NEONATE WITH CYANOSIS AND RESPIRATORY DISTRESS

The severely ill infant with cardiorespiratory distress and cyanosis presents a diagnostic challenge. Cyanosis on a cardiac basis occurs secondary to right to left intracardiac or intraductal shunting. The neonate with primary pulmonary disease will be cyanotic on the basis of ventilation-perfusion inequalities or hypoventilation. In addition, the baby with severe central nervous system disease or upper airway obstruction will be cyanotic secondary to hypoventilation.

Cardiac Disease. Congenital heart disease is responsible for cyanosis when obstruction to right ventricular outflow causes intracardiac right to left shunting or when complex anatomic defects, unassociated with pulmonary stenosis, cause admixture of pulmonary and systemic venous return in the heart. In addition, right to left shunts across the foramen ovale and ductus arteriosus due to pulmonary vascular obstruction also occur in neonates (Sec. 14.12).

Central Nervous System Disease. Irregular shallow breathing, secondary to central nervous system depression, results in reduced alveolar ventilation and an abnormally low alveolar oxygen tension. Arterial pCO_2 is elevated. Intracranial hemorrhage accounts for most cases of this type of cyanosis.

Pulmonary Disease. Upper airway obstructions result in cyanosis by the same basic mechanism responsible for central nervous system cyanosis, e.g., alveolar hypoventilation due to reduced pulmonary ventilation. Obstruction may occur from the nares to the carina (Sec. 13.5).

Intrapulmonary diseases such as hyaline membrane disease, atelectasis, and pneumonitis cause inflammation, collapse, and fluid accumulation in alveoli which result in incompletely oxygenated blood in the systemic circulation.

Rarely, a cyanotic infant may have methemoglobinemia resulting in arterial desaturation (Sec. 7.56).

Successful *initial evaluation of the cyanotic infant* lies in careful observation of the infant's breathing pattern. Weak or irregular respiration is often associated with a weak sucking reflex and a central nervous system problem. Convulsions and general depression strongly suggest a central nervous system etiology. The infant with primary cardiac or pulmonary disease, on the other hand, displays vigorous or labored respirations with tachypnea. The differential diagnosis between pulmonary and cardiac cyanosis may be difficult, especially within the first days of life. The baby with congenital heart disease will not raise arterial pO_2 (PaO_2) significantly during administration of 100% oxygen (hyperoxia test), while patients with pulmonary disease will have an increased response as ventilation-perfusion inequalities are overcome by oxygen administration. The infant with only a central nervous system disorder will completely normalize PaO_2 during artificial ventilation. If the PaO$_2$ rises above 150 torr during 100% oxygen administration, an anatomic shunt can generally be excluded.

A significant heart murmur suggests a cardiac basis for cyanosis. However, several of the more severe cardiac defects do not manifest a murmur. The chest roentgenogram may be helpful in the differentiation of pulmonary from cardiac disease and, in the latter, will indicate whether pulmonary blood flow is increased, normal, or decreased. This distinction is important in the differentiation of various congenital heart lesions which cause cyanosis in the neonate.

In recent years two-dimensional echocardiography has become the definitive noninvasive test to determine whether congenital heart disease is present. The information obtained by this technique is essential in avoiding an unnecessary cardiac catheterization and angiography in the absence of a cardiac defect as well as in making a specific diagnosis when congenital heart disease is present.

14.11 NEONATAL PULMONARY HYPERTENSION

Pulmonary hypertension persists in the newborn under a variety of different circumstances and as a result of a number of different underlying mechanisms. Pulmonary arterial pressure is the product of pulmonary blood flow and pulmonary vascular resistance (P = R × F). There are very few conditions in which increased pulmonary blood flow is an important component of pulmonary artery hypertension in the newborn; therefore, the key pathophysiologic element is almost always elevated pulmonary vascular resistance. Pulmonary vasoconstriction and hypertension following hypoxemia can result in right to left patent foramen ovale and ductus arteriosus shunting in what appears to be a primary syndrome (persistent fetal circulation). In addition, pulmonary hypertension may be a secondary feature of a variety of cardiac and pulmonary diseases.

The numerous disease entities that result in pulmonary hypertension should be classified on the basis of anatomic and physiologic causes in order to formulate a rational approach to diagnosis and management (Table 14–4). The term **persistent pulmonary hypertension** is applied to all of these causes but is not a specific diagnosis.

Pulmonary venous hypertension may occur in infants having a variety of congenital defects that cause pulmonary venous obstruction in the first few days of life. These include stenosis of the pulmonary veins, cor triatriatum, congenital mitral stenosis, and supravalvular webs. Infants with left ventricular failure because of a well defined cardiac lesion also have

Table 14–4. Persistent Pulmonary Hypertension in the Newborn Infant: Clinical Classification

Pulmonary venous hypertension
  Pulmonary venous, left atrial, mitral obstruction
  Left ventricular failure; cardiac lesion present
  Transient left ventricular dysfunction (H)
Functional obstruction of pulmonary vascular bed
  Hyperviscosity (H)
Pulmonary vascular constriction (with or without increased pulmonary
    vascular smooth muscle)
  Persistence of the fetal circulation (PFC syndrome) (H)
  Secondary to pulmonary disease (H)
  Premature ductal closure
Decreased pulmonary vascular bed
  Pulmonary hypoplasia, congenital
  Pulmonary hypoplasia, secondary
Systemic right ventricle or single ventricle without pulmonary stenosis
  Cardiac lesions

Hypoxia (H) implicated in etiology of pulmonary vasoconstriction.

pulmonary artery hypertension. Coarctation of the aorta, aortic valve disease, and cardiomyopathy (such as endocardial fibroelastosis) are included in this group. Infants with transient left ventricular dysfunction secondary to hypoxia also have congestive heart failure and pulmonary artery hypertension.

Hyperviscosity syndrome occurs in patients with polycythemia, which may be due to maternal-fetal or fetal-fetal transfusion or may be secondary to perinatal hypoxemia.

The patient with *pulmonary vascular constriction* (with or without increased pulmonary vascular smooth muscle) and no parenchymal pulmonary disease or cardiac lesion should be diagnosed as having *persistence of the fetal circulation*. However, infants with both a pulmonary vascular constrictive component and pulmonary parenchymal disease, although also having an oxygenation defect induced in part by hypoxemia, should be classified according to the basic disease entity, e.g., meconium aspiration with pulmonary vascular constriction and right to left shunting.

A *decreased pulmonary vascular bed* leads to elevated pulmonary resistance and persistent pulmonary hypertension of the newborn. This may occur with *congenital pulmonary hypoplasia* but is also seen secondary to *diaphragmatic hernia*, space-occupying *intrathoracic masses*, and other diseases. Once hypoxia occurs in these patients, the resulting pulmonary vascular constriction may add to the pulmonary resistance and exacerbate the cyanosis.

Infants with *systemic right ventricles* or *single ventricles* as a result of complex congenital heart lesions without pulmonary stenosis have pulmonary hypertension. Such infants also develop medial muscular hypertrophy of small pulmonary vessels.

Perinatal hypoxemia associated with anatomic and physiologic abnormalities results in persistent pulmonary hypertension of mixed etiologies. For example, infants with diaphragmatic hernia have ipsilateral pulmonary hypoplasia and contralateral pulmonary vasoconstriction, both of which contribute to high pulmonary resistance, hypertension, and right to left shunting. Some preterm infants with severe respiratory distress syndrome may also be cyanotic on the basis of pulmonary vasoconstriction, pulmonary hypertension, and right to left ductus arteriosus and foramen ovale shunting in the first few days of life. Later in the neonatal period ventilation-perfusion inequalities result in cyanosis, and large ductal left to right shunting may occur as pulmonary resistance falls.

14.12 PERSISTENCE OF THE FETAL CIRCULATION (PFC)

In this condition the hemodynamics of fetal life are maintained, in part, after birth; the pulmonary vascular bed remains constricted, and the blood entering the right heart shunts away from the lungs into the systemic vascular bed via the foramen ovale and ductus arteriosus. The etiology for persistent constriction of the pulmonary vascular bed is not always known, but in many cases the clinical pattern strongly implicates perinatal hypoxemia.

Pathophysiology. Table 14–5 outlines the relevant multiple effects of perinatal hypoxemia in the newborn that result in the clinical manifestations of the PFC syndrome. Hypoxemia and acidemia lead to pulmonary arteriolar constriction and hypertension, perhaps in the presence of increased pulmonary vascular smooth muscle. However, hypoxemia may also lead to left or right ventricular dysfunction and transient cardiac failure. These manifestations may occur together in various combinations accounting for the variable clinical presentations. Some infants with PFC have echocardiographic

Table 14–5. **Cardiopulmonary Effects of Perinatal Hypoxemia**

Effect	Physiologic Manifestations	Pulmonary Artery Hypertension (PAH)	Disease
Pulmonary arteriolar constriction	PAH ↓ PaO$_2$ R → L shunt (PFO and PDA) ↑ Hct ↓ Glucose ↓ Ca^{++}	+	PFC syndrome (persistent fetal circulation)
LV dysfunction	LV Failure	+	Transient LV myocardial ischemia syndrome
RV dysfunction	RV failure	−	Transient RV myocardial dysfunction (tricuspid insufficiency syndrome)
Combination of above effects	All of above (with CNS, renal, GI manifestations)	+	The asphyxiated newborn

Any or all may occur with concomitant cardiac or pulmonary parenchymal disease.

findings of left ventricular dysfunction with large hearts and congested lung fields; others have clear lung fields but large right ventricles and physical signs of tricuspid insufficiency. In the most severely hypoxic infants many of these manifestations are present along with central nervous system, renal, and gastrointestinal effects of asphyxia. Any or all of these effects may be superimposed on concomitant cardiac or pulmonary parenchymal disease.

Clinical Manifestations. The typical patient is a full-term infant who is observed to be cyanotic virtually from birth with varying degrees of respiratory distress. In approximately 80% of patients there is a history consistent with perinatal hypoxemia. Apgar scores are often low, and resuscitative measures may have been required. Physical examination may also reveal a murmur at the left sternal border consistent with tricuspid regurgitation. An unusually high hematocrit should suggest hyperviscosity as a basis for elevated pulmonary vascular resistance. The electrocardiogram, similar to those of many patients with congenital heart disease, shows right ventricular hypertrophy which is physiologic for age. Cardiac size and pulmonary vascularity on roentgenograms of the chest are not diagnostic. Echocardiographically, the right ventricular pre-ejection period/right ventricular ejection time ratios are consistent with pulmonary artery arterial hypertension but are not specific for PFC syndrome. Administration of oxygen does not initially improve the arterial oxygen saturation significantly in most cases; lack of improvement indicates the presence of true right to left shunt and does not differentiate PFC from cyanotic heart disease.

Mortality is significant, 10–30%. Most survivors improve steadily over a few days and are normal by the end of the first week of life.

Differential Diagnosis. Since this syndrome results in true right to left shunt, the hemodynamics are similar to those in infants having cyanotic heart disease, and the differential diagnosis includes (1) severe left heart failure, (2) obstruction of the mitral valve within the left atrium or of the pulmonary veins, and (3) marked pulmonary vascular constriction secondary to a recognized pathologic process. The major differential diagnosis among congenital cardiac lesions is transposition of the great arteries. In both this condition and PFC, the patient is most often a term infant who is markedly cyanotic, does not have a striking murmur, and has a nondiagnostic electrocardiogram and chest roentgenogram. Echocardiography is very helpful in establishing a diagnosis.

In infants with pulmonary disease or central nervous disturbances the oxygenation defect is due to hypoventilation or ventilation-perfusion inequality, and these infants can usually be differentiated from those with PFC of the primary type on the basis of the clinical features and arterial blood gas analysis in response to oxygen administration. However, PFC may be responsible for a component of cyanosis in a number of entities.

Treatment. The major goal of therapy is to keep the infant well oxygenated until the natural course of the illness leads to spontaneous improvement. Oxygen administration and mechanical ventilation should be utilized as indicated by blood gas measurement. Hyperventilation has been used in managing this group of patients. The hemoglobin should be followed carefully and severe polycythemia treated with appropriate exchanges of blood for plasma (Sec. 8.48). Sodium bicarbonate is administered for metabolic acidosis. Many infants will have severe hypoglycemia or hypocalcemia, which should be corrected.

The vasodilator *tolazoline* has been used for treating PFC syndrome and is successful in some cases; pulmonary vascular dilatation may be minimal in the most severely ill infants. When effective, the administration of this agent acutely increases pulmonary blood flow and raises arterial pO$_2$. Pulmonary arterial pressure may remain elevated initially, but with improved oxygenation falls toward normal levels. However, even when tolazoline is injected directly into the pulmonary artery, there is a marked systemic effect. The lowering of systemic resistance may result in low systemic blood pressure and shock. The drug should be given carefully, first as a bolus (0.5–1.0 mg/kg) over a period of about 1 min, followed by an infusion of 2–5 mg/kg/hr. Monitoring arterial pressure is essential, and adequate blood volume must be maintained. The infant should also be carefully observed for spontaneous gastrointestinal hemorrhage, which has been noted during tolazoline therapy.

The principles of treating PFC also apply to managing neonates with persistent pulmonary hypertension due to other etiologies when a pulmonary vasoconstrictive element is present (e.g., aspiration, pneumonitis, diaphragmatic hernia, etc.).

14.13 MYOCARDIAL DYSFUNCTION SYNDROMES

Syndromes of transient left ventricular dysfunction as well as right ventricular dysfunction with tricuspid insufficiency may occur secondary to perinatal asphyxia. Pulmonary arteriolar constriction with right to left atrial and ductal shunting as a result of hypoxia may or may not accompany these syndromes. For the most part the myocardial dysfunction is completely reversible, and most infants recover completely. However, in the presence of overwhelming asphyxia and multi-organ failure, the prognosis may be poor. Treatment should include oxygen administration, and ventilation when required. It is rarely necessary or advisable to administer digoxin to such patients, but diuretics may be helpful. The major thrust of therapy is the normalization of arterial oxygen content and reversal of acidosis.

CONGENITAL HEART DISEASE

Incidence. Congenital heart disease occurs in approximately 8/1000 live births. Among infants born with cardiac defects there is a spectrum of severity; about 2–3/1000 infants with congenital heart disease will be symptomatic in the first year of life. Since palliative and corrective surgical techniques have evolved, the percentage of individuals who survive with various lesions has changed over the years; complex, severe defects later in childhood now account for a larger number of patients. Table 14–6 summarizes the incidence of specific congenital defects in different age groups.

Most congenital defects are well tolerated during fetal life. It is only after the maternal circulation is eliminated and the cardiovascular system independently sustained that the impact of an anatomic and subsequent hemodynamic abnormality becomes apparent. The infant's circulation continues to change after birth, and later changes have a hemodynamic impact on cardiac lesions. For example, as pulmonary vascular resistance falls over the first weeks of life, left to right shunts become more apparent. The relative significance of various defects also changes with growth; the large ventricular septal defect may become a relatively small communication later. Aortic or pulmonary valve stenosis which is relatively mild may become worse if the orifice of the valve does not grow with the patient. The physician should be aware of both the spectrum of severity for the various malformations and their evolution with time.

Etiology. The cause of congenital heart disease is rarely known in individual cases. Multifactorial inheritance patterns are responsible for most lesions; single gene syndromes are rare (Sec. 6.1). Several chromosomal abnormalities are associated with severe congenital heart disease, but these represent fewer than 5% of the total. In most instances there is a combination of genetic and environmental influences.

With some exceptions, environmental influences during pregnancy have rarely been found to explain congenital cardiac defects in humans. Pregnant women who contract German measles in the first 2 mo of pregnancy may give birth to infants with cardiac lesions, including patent ductus arteriosus, branch pulmonary stenosis, and less often other defects. Seasonal variations have also been described.

Associated noncardiac malformations are common, especially in the context of certain syndromes (Table 14–7); Turner syndrome, Noonan disease, Marfan syndrome, Ellis–van Creveld syndrome, and numerous other less common multisystem diseases have congenital heart disease as a major or minor component of a spectrum of anomalies. Renal anomalies, cleft palate, and abnormalities of the arm and hand may occur with associated cardiac lesions. Congenital heart disease was observed in about 10% of children with the thalidomide syndrome; folic acid antagonists are also cardiovascular teratogens. Maternal therapy with anticonvulsant agents, especially diphenylhydantoin and trimethadione, is associated with a relatively high incidence of congenital heart disease. Dextroamphetamine, lithium chloride, alcohol, progesterone/estrogen, and warfarin are also potential teratogenic agents. Overexposure of the pregnant woman to radiation is potentially teratogenic and has caused congenital heart disease.

Genetic Counseling. Parents who have a child with congenital heart disease require counseling regarding the incidence of a cardiac malformation in subsequent children (Sec. 6.30). With the exception of syndromes due to single gene mutation, most congenital heart disease is the result of a multifactorial inheritance pattern which results in a low risk of recurrence. There is approximately a 1% incidence of congenital heart disease in the normal population, and this incidence increases to 2–6% for a second pregnancy following the birth of a child with congenital heart disease, depending on the type of lesion in the first child. When two siblings have congenital heart disease the risk for a third affected child may reach 20–30%. In general, when a second child is found to have congenital heart disease it will tend to be similar to the lesion that was discovered in the first instance. However, the degree of severity may be disparate, and associated defects may be variable.

The incidence figures for infants born to mothers who have congenital heart disease are similar to those for siblings. However, most often the question is whether a woman with congenital heart disease, either unoperated or operated, will be able to carry a fetus to term. The major factor in determining this is the mother's cardiovascular status. The increased hemodynamic burden on a patient with marginal cardiac function may result in significantly increased risk to the mother as well as to the fetus. The incidence of spontaneous abortion in the presence of severe congenital heart disease is high, especially when the patient is cyanotic. It is important to discuss various methods of birth control with affected young women.

Table 14–6. Incidence of Congenital Cardiac Disease

Defect	%
Ventricular septal defect	28.3
Atrial septal/AV canal defects	10.3
Pulmonary stenosis	9.9
Patent ductus arteriosus	9.8
Tetralogy of Fallot	9.7
Aortic stenosis	7.1
Coarctation of the aorta	5.1
Transposition of the great arteries	4.9

The defects listed above, in order of decreasing frequency, comprise 85% of congenital heart disease. Among the remainder, the diagnoses include: hypoplastic left heart syndromes, total anomalous pulmonary vein drainage, tricuspid atresia, truncus arteriosus, and other rare defects. Bicuspid aortic valve is the most common congenital abnormality, but is included in the table only in the context of aortic stenosis.

Adapted from Keith JD, Rowe RD, Vlad P: Heart Disease in Infancy and Childhood, 3rd ed. Macmillan, New York, 1978, Chap. 1.

Table 14–7. **Cardiovascular Involvement in Various Syndromes**

Chromosomal Abnormalities
Autosomal Chromosomal Abnormalities

Trisomies		Deletions	
Trisomy 21	VSD, ECD, ASD	4p –	VSD, AS, PDA
Trisomy 18	VSD, PDA, PS	5p – (Cri du chat)	VSD, PDA, ASD
Trisomy 13	VSD, DORV, PDA, ASD	13q –	VSD
		18q –	VSD

Sex Chromosomes

XXXXY	PDA, ASD	Turner XO	Coarct, AS, ASD

Heritable and Possible Heritable Syndromes and Disorders

Apert	VSD
Carpenter	PDA
Cockayne	Atherosclerosis
Congenital hypertrophic subaortic stenosis	Obstructive cardiomyopathy
Conradi	VSD, PDA
Crouzon	PDA, Coarct
Cutis laxa	Pulmonary hypertension, PA stenosis
Ellis–van Creveld	Single atrium (other defects in 30%)
Familial deafness	Occasionally arrhythmia, sudden death
Familial dwarfism and nevi	Cardiomyopathy
Familial elfin facies, mental retardation, infantile hypercalcemia	Supravalvular AS, PA branch stenosis
Forney	MI
Holt-Oram	ASD (other defects common)
Jervell and Lange-Nielsen	Prolonged Q-T, sudden death
Kartagener	Dextrocardia
Laurence-Moon-Biedl	Variable, including T of F
Leopard (lentiginosis)	PS, + Q-T interval
Mucolipidosis III	Aortic valve disease
Neurofibromatosis	PS, Pheo, Coarct
Neurologic and muscular diseases:	
Friedreich ataxia	Cardiomyopathy
Muscular dystrophy	Cardiomyopathy
Refsum	Arrhythmia, sudden death
Riley-Day	Episodic hypertension, postural hypotension
Noonan	PS, ASD, cardiomyopathy
Progeria	Accelerated atherosclerosis
Rendu-Osler-Weber	Arteriovenous fistula (lung, liver, mucous membranes)
Romano-Ward	+ Q-T interval, sudden death
Rubinstein-Taybi	PDA
Scimitar	Hypoplasia of right ventricle, anomalous PV return to IVC
Seckel	VSD, PDA
Smith-Lemli-Opitz	VSD, PDA
Thrombocytopenia and absent radius (TAR)	ASD, T of F
Treacher Collins	VSD, ASD, PDA
Tuberous sclerosis	Myocardial rhabdomyoma
von Hippel–Lindau	Hemangiomas, pheochromocytomas
Weill-Marchesani	PDA
Werner	Vascular sclerosis, cardiomyopathy

Inborn Errors of Metabolism

Alcaptonuria	Atherosclerosis, valvular disease
Homocystinuria	Pulmonary arterial and aortic dilatation, intravascular thrombosis, flushing of skin
Pompe disease	Glycogen storage disease of heart

Connective Tissue Disorders

Arterial calcification of infancy	Calcinosis of coronary arteries
Ehlers-Danlos	Arterial dilatation
Hurler-Hunter	Multivalvular and coronary artery disease
Marfan	Aortic dilatation with aortic incompetence, mitral incompetence, dilatation of PA
Morquio-Ulrich	Aortic incompetence
Osteogenesis imperfecta	Aortic incompetence
Pseudoxanthoma elasticum	Peripheral arterial disease
Scheie	Aortic incompetence

AS = aortic stenosis	IVC = inferior vena cava	PS = pulmonic stenosis
ASD = atrial septal defect	MI = mitral insufficiency	Pheo = pheochromocytoma
Coarct = coarctation	Q-T = Q-T interval of electrocardiogram	PV = pulmonary valve
DORV = double-outlet right ventricle	PA = pulmonary artery	T of F = tetralogy of Fallot
ECD = endocardial cushion defect	PDA = patent ductus arteriosus	VSD = ventricular septal defect

CONGENITAL CARDIAC DISEASE WITH CYANOSIS
(Dominant Right to Left Shunt)

14.14 TETRALOGY OF FALLOT

Tetralogy of Fallot classically consists of the combination of (1) obstruction to right ventricular outflow (pulmonary stenosis), (2) ventricular septal defect, (3) dextroposition of the aorta, and (4) right ventricular hypertrophy. Obstruction to pulmonary arterial flow is usually at the right ventricular infundibulum and pulmonary valve. The pulmonary arterial trunk may be smaller than usual, and there may be branch stenosis. Complete obstruction of right ventricular outflow with ventricular septal defect is also classified as an extreme form of tetralogy of Fallot.

Pathology. The pulmonary valve may have a small ring, is often bicuspid, and, occasionally, is the only site of stenosis. Hypertrophy of the crista supraventricularis contributes to the infundibular stenosis and results in an infundibular chamber of variable size and contour. When the right ventricular outflow tract is completely obstructed (pulmonary atresia), the anatomy of the pulmonary arteries is extremely variable; on occasion, pulmonary blood flow is supplied by collateral vessels from the aorta. The ventricular septal defect is large, just below the aortic valve, and related to the posterior and right aortic cusps. The normal continuity of the mitral and aortic valves is maintained. The aorta arches to the right in about 20% of instances; the aortic root is large and overrides the ventricular septal defect to a varying degree.

Pathophysiology. Systemic venous return to the right atrium and right ventricle is normal. When the right ventricle contracts in the presence of marked pulmonary stenosis, blood is shunted across the ventricular septal defect into the aorta. Persistent arterial desaturation and cyanosis result. The pulmonary blood flow, when severely restricted by the obstruction to right ventricular outflow, may be supplemented by bronchial collateral circulation and occasionally by a patent ductus arteriosus. The peak systolic and diastolic pressures in each ventricle are similar at the systemic level, since a large pressure gradient is measured across the obstructed ventricular outflow tract, and pulmonary artery pressure is lower than normal. When obstruction to right ventricular outflow is moderate and there is a balanced shunt across the ventricular septal defect, the patient may not be visibly cyanotic (acyanotic or "pink" tetralogy of Fallot).

Clinical Manifestations. *Cyanosis,* one of the most obvious manifestations of tetralogy, may not be present at birth. Right ventricular outflow obstruction may not yet be severe, and the infant may present with a large left to right shunt and even congestive heart failure. However, with time there is increasing hypertrophy of the infundibulum, and as the child grows, the obstruction is further exaggerated. Later in the first year cyanosis occurs, most prominently on the mucous membranes of the lips and mouth and in the fingernails and toenails. In severe cases, cyanosis is noted immediately in the neonatal period. Older children having extreme cyanosis, with a dusky blue skin surface, gray sclerae with engorged blood vessels (suggesting mild conjunctivitis), and clubbing of the fingers and toes, are rarely seen, since surgical repair of tetralogy is most often carried out in early childhood.

Dyspnea occurs on exertion. Infants and toddlers will play actively for a short time and then sit or lie down. Older children may be able to walk a block or so before stopping to rest. Characteristically, children assume a *squatting* position for the relief of dyspnea due to physical effort; the child is usually able to resume physical activity within a few minutes. These findings occur most often in patients with significant cyanosis at rest.

Paroxysmal hypercyanotic attacks (hypoxic or "blue" spells) are a particular problem during the first 2 yr of life. The infant becomes hyperpneic and restless, cyanosis increases, gasping respirations ensue, and syncope may follow. The spell occurs most frequently in the morning. Temporary disappearance or decrease in intensity of the systolic murmur is usual. The spells may last from a few minutes to a few hours but are rarely fatal. Short episodes are followed by generalized weakness and sleep. Severe spells may progress to unconsciousness and, occasionally, to convulsions or hemiparesis. The onset is usually spontaneous and unpredictable. The spells are associated with a reduction of an already compromised pulmonary blood flow, which when prolonged results in hypoxia and metabolic acidosis. The disappearance or attenuation of the systolic murmur and reduction of arterial oxygen saturation and pulmonary arterial pressure suggest that blue spells are associated with a further increase in resistance at the right ventricular outflow tract, transient decrease in systemic resistance, or both. In the presence of decreased pulmonary blood flow the right to left shunt is increased. The resultant arterial hypoxia, metabolic acidosis, and increased pCO_2 further stimulate the respiratory mechanism and the hyperpnea persists. Infants who are only mildly cyanotic at rest are often more prone to develop hypoxic spells, since they have not developed the homeostatic mechanisms to tolerate rapid lowering of arterial oxygen saturation.

Depending on the frequency and severity of hypercyanotic attacks, one or more of the following procedures should be instituted in sequence: (1) placement of the infant on the abdomen in the knee-chest position, making certain that there is no constricting clothing; (2) administration of oxygen; and (3) injection of morphine subcutaneously in a dose not in excess of 0.1 mg/kg. Since metabolic acidosis develops when the arterial pO_2 is below 40 mm Hg, rapid correction (within several minutes) is necessary if the spell is unusually severe and there is lack of response to the foregoing therapy. This may be accomplished with intravenous administration of sodium bicarbonate. Recovery from the spell is rapid once the pH has returned to normal. Repeated blood pH measurements may be necessary because rapid recurrence of acidosis may occur.

Beta-adrenergic inhibition by intravenous administration of propranolol (0.1 to a maximum of 0.2 mg/kg) has been used successfully in some patients with severe spells, especially spells accompanied by tachycardia. Drugs that increase systemic vascular resistance, such as intravenous methoxamine and phenylephrine, will decrease the right to left shunt and thus improve the symptoms; but their use has been limited and should not be allowed to delay needed surgery.

It is important to emphasize that calming the infant, while holding the child in a knee-chest position over the shoulder, may abort progression of an early spell. Premature attempts to obtain blood may cause further agitation and be counterproductive.

Growth and development may be delayed in severe untreated tetralogy of Fallot. Stature and nutritional status are usually below averages for age, and muscles and subcutaneous tissues are flabby and soft. Puberty is delayed.

The *pulse* is usually normal, as are the venous and arterial pressures. The left anterior hemithorax may bulge anteriorly. The heart is usually normal in size, and there is a substernal right ventricular impulse. In 50% of cases a *systolic thrill* is felt along the left sternal border in the 3rd and 4th parasternal spaces.

The *systolic murmur* is frequently loud and harsh; it may be transmitted widely, but is most intense at the left sternal border. The murmur may be either ejection or pansystolic

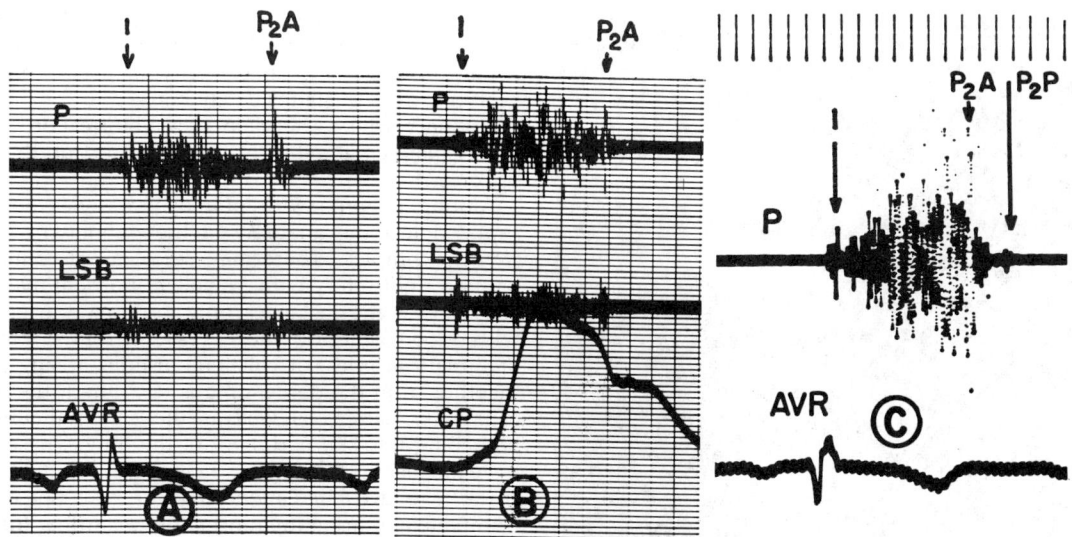

Figure 14-30. Phonocardiograms illustrating the variability of auscultatory findings in cyanotic tetralogy of Fallot. AVR, electrocardiogram; CP, carotid pulse; LSB, left sternal border; P, pulmonary area; P₂A, aortic component of 2nd heart sound; P₂P, pulmonic component of 2nd heart sound; 1, 1st heart sound. The systolic murmur may be early (A), or when long (B) or accentuated in late systole (C), it ends at P₂A. The 2nd heart sound is single, owing to aortic valve closure (A and B) or split with a delayed soft pulmonic component (C). Time lines 0.04 sec.

(Fig. 14-30) and may be preceded by a click. The systolic murmur is due to turbulence over the right ventricular outflow tract and tends to be less prominent with severe obstruction and large right to left shunts. The 2nd heart sound is single and is produced by closure of the aortic valve. Infrequently, the systolic murmur is followed by a diastolic murmur; this continuous murmur may be audible in any part of the chest, anteriorly or posteriorly; it is produced by enlarged bronchial collateral vessels or rarely by persistence of a patent ductus arteriosus. This finding is more frequent with pulmonary atresia.

Diagnosis. *Roentgenographically,* the typical configuration as seen in the anteroposterior view consists of a narrow base, concavity of the left border in the area usually occupied by the pulmonary artery, and normal heart size. The rounded apical shadow situated rather high above the diaphragm is produced chiefly by the hypertrophied right ventricle. The cardiac silhouette has been likened to that of a wooden shoe (**coeur en sabot**) (Fig. 14-31). In the lateral projection the

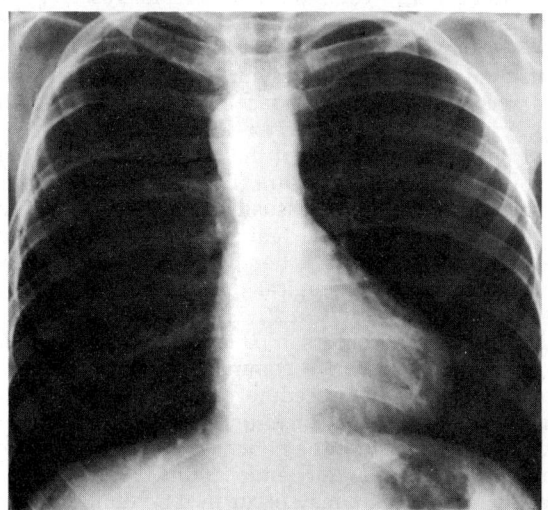

Figure 14-31. Roentgenogram of an 8 yr old boy with tetralogy of Fallot. Note the normal heart size, some elevation of the cardiac apex, concavity in the region of the main pulmonary artery, right aortic arch, and diminished pulmonary vascularity.

anterior encroachment by the hypertrophied right ventricle is usually seen. The hilar areas and lung fields are relatively clear, because of diminished pulmonary blood flow and/or small size of the pulmonary arteries.

The aorta is usually large, and its position may be important diagnostically. In about 20% of instances the aorta arches to the right instead of to the left; this may result in an indentation of the leftward positioned air-filled tracheobronchial shadow in the anteroposterior view or may be confirmed by displacement of the barium-filled esophagus to the left. In the left oblique view a right aortic arch may indent the esophagus.

Variations from the typical roentgenographic picture include poststenotic dilatation of the pulmonary artery, which suggests valvular pulmonary stenosis. Occasionally, pulmonary vascularity is made prominent by collateral bronchial circulation that radiates from the hilus of the lungs.

The *electrocardiogram* reveals right axis deviation and evidence of right ventricular hypertrophy. The latter, without which the diagnosis of tetralogy of Fallot is unlikely, is found in the right precordial chest leads where the configuration of the QRS complex is Rs, R, qR, qRs, rsR', or RS. In these leads the T wave may be positive, further evidence of right ventricular hypertrophy. The P wave is tall and peaked or sometimes bifid (Fig. 14-11).

Two-dimensional echocardiography is often helpful in establishing this diagnosis (Fig. 14-32).

Cardiac catheterization and angiocardiography elucidate anatomic abnormalities and exclude other defects which may mimic the tetralogy of Fallot, especially double outlet right ventricle with pulmonary stenosis and arterial transposition with pulmonary stenosis.

Cardiac catheterization reveals systolic hypertension in the right ventricle equal to systemic pressure, with a marked decrease in pressure as the catheter enters the pulmonary artery or, in some cases, the infundibular chamber beyond the obstruction.

The mean pulmonary arterial pressure is commonly 5-10 mm Hg; the right atrial pressure is usually normal. The aorta may be easily entered from the right ventricle through the ventricular septal defect. The level of arterial oxygen saturation depends on the magnitude of the right to left shunt; at rest it is usually 75-85% in a moderately cyanotic patient. Samples of blood from the venae cavae, right atrium, right

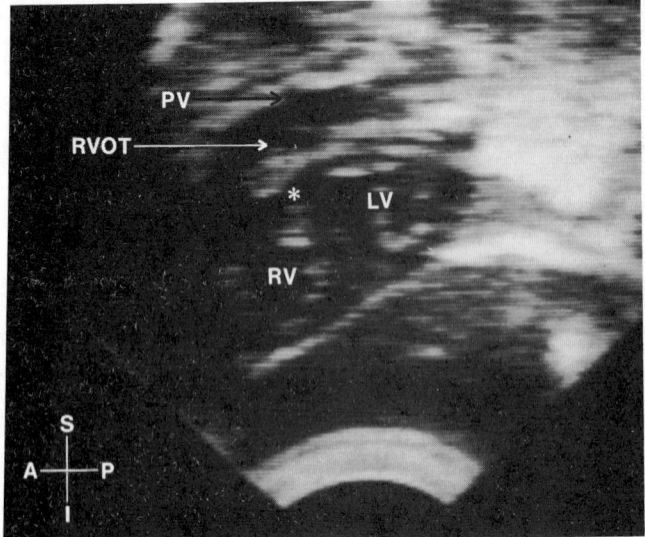

Figure 14–32. Tetralogy of Fallot. This short axis subxiphoid two-dimensional echocardiographic projection demonstrates the anterior/superior displacement of the outflow ventricular septum resulting in stenosis of the subpulmonic right ventricular outflow tract and associated anterior ventricular septal defect. LV, left ventricle; PV, pulmonary valve; RV, right ventricle; RVOT, right ventricular outflow tract; A, anterior; P, posterior; S, superior; I, inferior; asterisk, interventricular septal defect.

ventricle, and pulmonary artery are frequently similar in oxygen content, indicating an absence of a left to right shunt.

Selective right ventriculography best demonstrates the anatomy of tetralogy of Fallot. The contrast medium outlines the heavily trabeculated right ventricle. The infundibular stenosis varies in length, width, contour, and distensibility (Fig. 14–33). An infundibular chamber may also be demonstrated. The pulmonary valve may be normal, but frequently the leaflets are thickened and domed, and the valve ring is small. Nearly

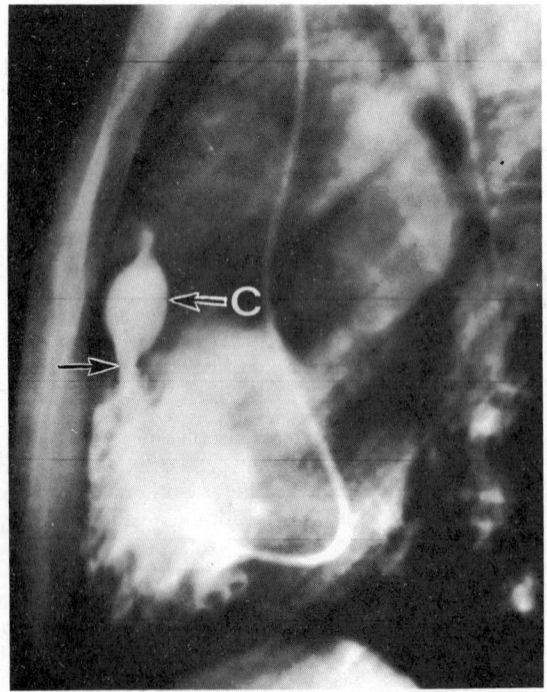

Figure 14–33. Lateral view of selective right ventriculogram in patient with tetralogy of Fallot. Arrow points to infundibular stenosis which is below the infundibular chamber (C).

simultaneous opacification of the aorta and pulmonary artery is usual. The size of the pulmonary trunk varies considerably. In severe cases it is small or hypoplastic, and localized or multiple areas of stenosis may be seen in the branches of the pulmonary artery, especially at the bifurcation. The subaortic ventricular septal defect is usually large, and the aorta is well opacified.

Among patients with pulmonary atresia and ventricular septal defect the anatomy of the pulmonary vessels is extremely complex. There may be a central confluence of the left and right artery with a smaller or absent main pulmonary artery. In some instances only peripheral arteries are seen, with blood entering these vessels from a patent ductus, mammary arteries, or collateral arteries arising separately or together from the descending aorta. Often, there are parallel collateral arteries, as well as the true pulmonary arteries, branching into the periphery of the lung. These vessels may have long stenotic segments as they arise from the descending aorta. The two circulations may or may not communicate. Complete and accurate information regarding the anatomy of the pulmonary arteries is very important in evaluating these children as surgical candidates.

Left ventriculography demonstrates the size of the ventricle, the position of the ventricular septal defect, and the overriding aorta; it also confirms mitral-aortic continuity and rules out double outlet right ventricle. *Aortography* or *coronary arteriography* will outline the course of the coronary arteries. In a few instances an aberrant major coronary artery crosses over the right ventricular outflow tract; this artery must be preserved during repair.

Complications. *Cerebral thromboses*, usually occurring in the cerebral veins or dural sinuses and occasionally in the cerebral arteries, are more common in the presence of extreme polycythemia. They may also be precipitated by dehydration. *Cerebral ischemia* occurs most often in patients under the age of 2 yr. These patients may have iron deficiency anemia, frequently with hemoglobin and hematocrit levels in the normal range. Therapy consists of adequate hydration and supportive measures. Phlebotomy and volume replacement with fresh frozen plasma are indicated in the extremely polycythemic patient. Heparin is of little value since it does not influence blood viscosity and may not prevent extension of venous thrombosis; it is contraindicated in hemorrhagic cerebral infarction. Physical therapy to the affected extremities should be instituted as early as possible.

Brain abscess is less common than cerebral vascular events. Patients are usually over the age of 2 yr. The onset of the illness is often insidious with low grade fever. In some patients there is acute onset of symptoms, which may develop after a recent history of headache, nausea, and vomiting. Epileptiform seizures may occur; localized neurologic signs depend on the site and size of the abscess and the presence of increased intracranial pressure. The sedimentation rate and white blood cell count are usually elevated. Computed tomography and radionuclide brain scans have facilitated diagnosis. Massive antibiotic therapy may help to keep the infection localized, but surgical drainage of the abscess is almost always necessary (Sec. 21.23).

Bacterial endocarditis occurs in patients who have not undergone operation but is more common in children who have had a palliative shunt procedure during infancy. Antibiotic prophylaxis is essential prior to and after dental and certain surgical procedures since the patient is at risk for developing bacteremia and subsequently endocarditis (Sec. 14.74).

Congestive heart failure may occur in the young infant with pulmonary atresia and large collateral blood flow. This almost invariably regresses during the first months of life, and the patient becomes cyanotic with decreased pulmonary blood flow. Heart failure is not a feature in the usual patient with tetralogy.

Associated Cardiovascular Anomalies. An associated patent ductus arteriosus may be present. Associated defects in the atrial septum are occasionally seen. Absence of the pulmonary valve produces a distinct syndrome; cyanosis may be mild, the heart is large and hyperdynamic, and loud to and fro murmurs are present. Aneurysmal dilatation of the pulmonary artery often produces wheezing respiration and recurrent pneumonitis from bronchial compression. This syndrome may be lethal in the neonatal period but improves spontaneously in survivors.

Absence of a pulmonary artery should be suspected if the roentgenographic appearance of the pulmonary vasculature differs on the two sides; generally, because the left pulmonary artery is absent, the right lung appears more vascularized. Absence of a pulmonary artery will often be associated with hypoplasia of the affected lung. It may be difficult to differentiate absence of the left pulmonary artery from severe stenosis or late occlusion. It is important to recognize absence of a pulmonary artery prior to the creation of an anastomosis between the systemic circulation and the single remaining pulmonary artery since occlusion of the latter during operation seriously compromises the already reduced pulmonary blood flow. Right aortic arch occurs in approximately 20% of cases of tetralogy of Fallot, and other anomalies of the pulmonary artery and aortic arch may also be seen. Multiple ventricular septal defects occasionally are present and must be diagnosed prior to corrective surgery. Tetralogy may occur with atrioventricular canal, often associated with Down syndrome.

Treatment. Although tetralogy of Fallot often presents insidiously during the first year with gradually increasing cyanosis, there are patients with severe tetralogy who require medical treatment and palliative surgical intervention in the neonatal period. Therapy is aimed at providing an immediate increase in pulmonary blood flow to prevent the sequela of severe hypoxia. The infant should be transported to a medical center adequately equipped to evaluate and treat neonates under optimal conditions. It is critical that oxygenation and normal body temperature be maintained during the transfer. Prolonged, severe hypoxia may lead to shock, respiratory failure, and intractable acidosis and will significantly reduce the chances of survival after cardiac catheterization and surgery, even when surgically amenable lesions are present. Infants with markedly reduced pulmonary blood flow deteriorate rapidly because the ductus arteriosus does not stay sufficiently patent to provide adequate pulmonary blood flow after birth. The administration of prostaglandin E_1, a potent and specific relaxant of ductal smooth muscle, causes dilatation of the ductus arteriosus and allows adequate pulmonary blood flow to occur until a surgical procedure can be carried out in neonates with severe tetralogy of Fallot and other lesions which benefit from ductal patency. This agent is administered intravenously when the clinical diagnosis is made and continued through cardiac catheterization and surgery. Postoperatively, the infusion may be continued to augment the palliative shunt or forward flow through a surgical valvulotomy. However, it is not used for long-term therapy.

Infants with tetralogy of Fallot who are stable and awaiting surgical intervention require careful observation. The prevention or prompt treatment of dehydration is important to avoid hemoconcentration and possible thrombotic episodes. Paroxysmal dyspneic attacks in infancy may be precipitated by a relative iron deficiency; iron therapy may decrease their frequency and also improve exercise tolerance and general well-being. The hematocrit should be maintained at 55–65%. Oral propranolol (1 mg/kg every 6 hr) has been used to decrease the frequency and severity of dyspneic spells, but it is preferable to go ahead with surgical treatment if spells occur.

In general, infants presenting with symptoms and severe cyanosis in the first months of life have marked obstruction of the right ventricular outflow tract or pulmonary atresia. In such infants a systemic to pulmonary artery shunt procedure is carried out to augment pulmonary artery blood flow; it is hoped that not only will hypoxemia be allayed, but the growth of small pulmonary vessels will be augmented. Corrective open heart surgery in early infancy is rarely advisable in such patients. For infants who can be maintained until later in the first year of life, open correction is a reasonable primary alternative when the usual single high ventricular septal defect is present, pulmonary arteries are of sufficient size, and no other complicating great vessel abnormalities are present. In general, older patients should have open heart correction of the defect regardless of whether an earlier palliative shunt procedure was carried out.

The **Blalock-Taussig** shunt is the most useful shunt procedure and is created by anastomosis of a subclavian artery to the homolateral branch of the pulmonary artery. This operation was previously impractical for the neonate because of technical problems in achieving an unobstructed connection. However, with the advent of microvascular surgery, the operation can now be successfully performed in these infants. Recently, a modified procedure has been effective utilizing a polyfluorotetraethylene (Teflon) conduit side to side from the subclavian to pulmonary artery. Less frequently performed procedures are side to side anastomosis of the ascending aorta and right pulmonary artery (Waterson) and anastomosis of the upper descending aorta and left pulmonary artery (Potts); these procedures have a higher frequency of complicating congestive heart failure and late onset pulmonary hypertension as well as greater technical difficulties in closing the shunt during subsequent corrective surgery. Small conduits directly from the aorta to the pulmonary artery have been utilized for early palliation.

Usually, the postoperative course of patients with a successful shunt procedure is relatively uneventful. However, postoperative complications following a thoracotomy, such as chylothorax, diaphragmatic paralysis, and Horner syndrome, may occur. *Chylothorax* may require repeated thoracocentesis and, on occasion, reoperation in order to ligate the thoracic duct. *Diaphragmatic paralysis* due to injury to the recurrent laryngeal nerve may result in a more difficult postoperative course. More prolonged respiratory support and vigorous physical therapy may be required, but diaphragmatic function will return in 1–2 mo unless the nerve was completely divided. *Horner syndrome* is usually temporary and does not require treatment. Postoperative *cardiac failure* may be due to the large size of the anastomosis; its treatment is described in Sec. 14.80. Vascular problems are rarely seen in the upper extremity supplied by the subclavian artery used for the anastomosis.

After a successful shunt procedure, cyanosis diminishes. The development of a machinery-type murmur after the operation indicates a functioning anastomosis. However, this may not be heard for several days after surgery. The duration of symptomatic relief is variable. As the child grows, more pulmonary blood flow is needed and the shunt may eventually become inadequate. If the anatomy is such that a corrective operation can be carried out, then it should be undertaken. However, if it is not possible or if the first shunt lasts only a brief period in a small infant, a second anastomosis may be required on the opposite side. Infective endocarditis is a threat in any patient with a systemic to pulmonary artery shunt; appropriate prophylactic measures should be taken (Sec. 14.74).

Corrective surgical therapy consists of relief of the obstruction to the right ventricular outflow tract and closure of the ventricular septal defect by direct vision intracardiac surgery with a pump oxygenator. When there is a previously established systemic to pulmonary shunt, it must be obliterated prior to cardiotomy. The surgical risk of **total correction** is currently under 10%. Factors that have contributed to increasing success of this approach include optimal total body perfusion, adequate myocardial protection during bypass, relief of right ventricular outflow obstruction, prevention of air embolism, and meticulous postoperative care. The presence of a previous Blalock-Taussig anastomosis does not increase the operative risk. Increased bleeding in the immediate postoperative period is common in polycythemic patients but should not seriously affect the outcome. The operative risks are higher in small infants because more complicated anatomy is likely to be encountered.

Prognosis. After successful total correction patients are generally asymptomatic and able to lead unrestricted lives. The long-term effects of isolated, surgically induced pulmonary valvular incompetence are unknown, but this lesion is common when a right ventricular outflow patch is utilized and is generally well tolerated. Patients with marked pulmonary valve insufficiency have moderate to marked cardiac enlargement. A patient having severe residual gradient across the right ventricular outflow tract may require reoperation, but mild to moderate obstruction is virtually always present and does not require reintervention.

Follow-up of patients 5–20 yr after operation indicates that the marked improvement in symptomatology is generally maintained. However, even asymptomatic patients have working capacities, maximal heart rates, and cardiac outputs that are lower than those of controls. These abnormal findings may be less frequent when surgery is undertaken at an early age.

Conduction disturbances are also frequent after operation. The atrioventricular node and the bundle of His and its divisions are in close proximity to the ventricular septal defect and may be injured during surgery. Permanent complete heart block following surgery is now rare. When present, it should be treated by placement of a permanently implanted pacemaker. Bifascicular block, due to injury to the anterior fascicle of the left bundle (manifested as postoperative left axis deviation) and of the right bundle (manifested as complete right bundle branch block), occurs in about 10% of patients; the long-term significance is uncertain, but in most instances there are no clinical manifestations. The additional finding of transient complete heart block in the immediate postoperative period, however, appears to be associated with an increased incidence of late onset complete heart block and sudden death. However, unexpected cardiac arrest rarely occurs many years after surgery in patients without postoperative bifascicular block or transient complete heart block.

A number of children will display frequent premature ventricular beats following repair of tetralogy of Fallot. Usually these are benign and nonprogressive. However, 24 hr monitoring studies should be done to be certain that short episodes of ventricular tachycardia are not occurring even when the patient is asymptomatic. In addition, exercise studies may be useful in bringing out cardiac arrhythmias which are not apparent at rest. In the absence of more complex ventricular arrhythmias or severe residual hemodynamic abnormalities, prophylactic antiarrhythmia therapy often is not required. If it is decided that ventricular ectopy requires treatment, quinidine, propranolol, dilantin, or combinations of these agents are most often used.

14.15 PULMONARY ATRESIA WITH VENTRICULAR SEPTAL DEFECT

This condition is an extreme form of tetralogy of Fallot. The pulmonary valve is atretic, rudimentary, or absent, and the pulmonary trunk is atretic or hypoplastic. The entire ventricular output is ejected into the aorta. Pulmonary blood flow is dependent on a patent ductus arteriosus and/or bronchial collaterals.

Clinical Manifestations. These are similar to those of tetralogy but usually with earlier and more severe manifestations; cyanosis usually appears within a few days after birth in contrast to later in the first year; the systolic murmur is absent or soft; the 1st heart sound is frequently followed by an ejection click; the 2nd sound at the base is moderately loud and single; and continuous murmurs of a patent ductus arteriosus or bronchial collateral flow may be heard over the entire precordium, anteriorly and posteriorly.

The presentation of these infants in the neonatal period is variable. Some patients have congestive heart failure due to increased pulmonary blood flow via collateral vessels; others are severely cyanotic and require urgent prostaglandin E_1 infusion and palliative surgical intervention; and some infants have adequate pulmonary blood flow and can be managed like patients with uncomplicated less severe tetralogy.

The *roentgenogram* will reveal a small or enlarged heart, depending on pulmonary blood flow, a concavity at the position of the pulmonary arterial segment, and often the reticular pattern of bronchial collateral flow. The *electrocardiogram* shows right ventricular hypertrophy. The *echocardiogram* identifies the aortic override and the thick right ventricular wall but not the pulmonary valve. At cardiac catheterization, *right ventriculography* reveals a large aorta, opacified immediately by passage of the contrast medium through the septal defect, and no dye entering the lungs through the right ventricular outflow tract. The pathway of pulmonary blood flow from the aorta to the lungs is also demonstrated.

Treatment. Systemic-pulmonary artery anastomosis may be indicated for the patient with pulmonary arteries of reasonable size. An open heart bypass from the right ventricle directly to the pulmonary artery, either by "unroofing" the outflow tract or by implanting a conduit, has been utilized in some patients. There is controversy as to whether this type of bypass may stimulate the growth of the pulmonary arteries better than a standard shunt operation. The pulmonary arteries must be of adequate size to allow the patient to become a candidate for future open heart repair, which would include closure of the ventricular septal defect and a conduit from the right ventricle to the pulmonary artery (Fig. 14–34). Previous systemic to pulmonary anastomoses are eliminated. Conduit replacement must be expected later in life, perhaps as early as 5 yr postoperatively. Some patients have malformations of the primary divisions of the pulmonary arteries in the form of hypoplasia, multiple branch stenoses, absence of a pulmonary artery, and large bronchial collaterals. These vessels are difficult to reconstruct surgically even after early anastomotic procedures.

Acquired total atresia of the right ventricular outflow tract may occur after a systemic-pulmonary anastomosis for tetralogy of Fallot. The systolic murmur due to pulmonary stenosis is attenuated or disappears. The completeness of obstruction can be confirmed by right ventriculography. Corrective surgery of the right ventricular outflow tract is similar to that utilized for tetralogy of Fallot.

14.16 PULMONARY ATRESIA WITH INTACT VENTRICULAR SEPTUM

In this anomaly the pulmonary valve leaflets are completely fused and the right ventricular outflow tract is atretic. Since there is no egress of blood from the right ventricle, right atrial blood is shunted into the left atrium via the foramen ovale, mixes with pulmonary venous blood, and enters the left ventricle. The combined left and right ventricular output is pumped by the left ventricle into the aorta. Pulmonary blood flow occurs via a patent ductus arteriosus. In addition, among the great majority of patients who have small right ventricular cavities, sinusoidal channels within the right ventricle may

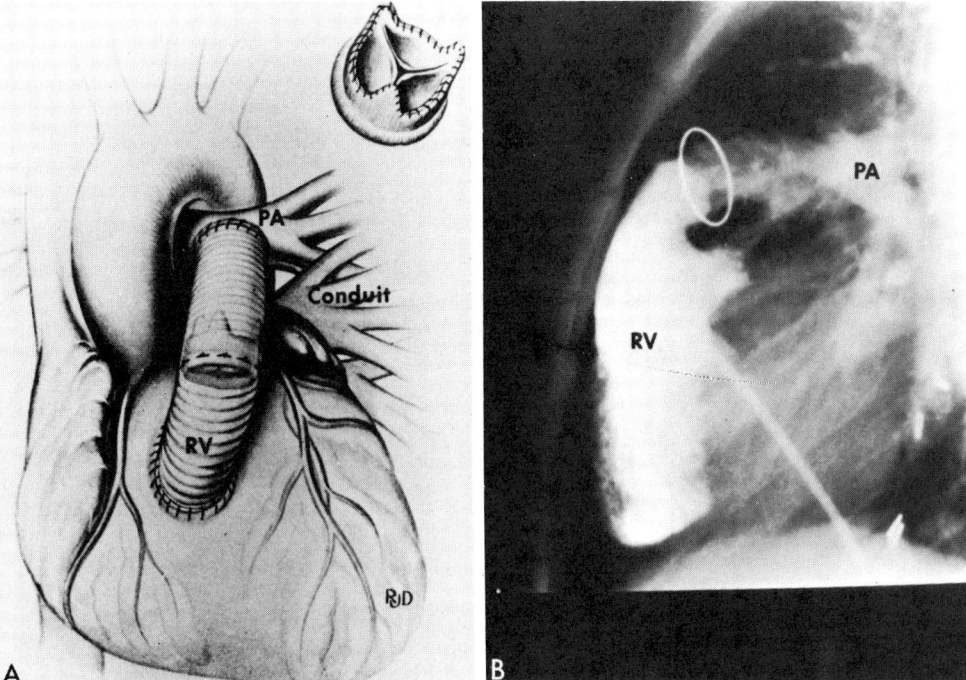

Figure 14–34. *A*, Artist's sketch of valve-containing conduit utilized in repair of pulmonary atresia. The porcine valve is portrayed in the inset. *B*, A right ventricular angiogram (lateral view) in a patient with pulmonary atresia and ventricular septal defect after repair with a valve-containing conduit. Non-valved conduits or aortic homografts are also utilized for this type of repair.

communicate directly to the coronary arterial circulation, resulting in blood flow retrograde to the aorta. Patients with intermediate-sized or large ventricular cavities may have tricuspid insufficiency which serves to decompress the right ventricle.

Clinical Manifestations. As the ductus arteriosus closes in the first days of life, infants with pulmonary atresia and intact ventricular septum become markedly cyanotic. Untreated, most patients die within the first week of life. Physical examination reveals severe cyanosis and respiratory distress. The 2nd heart sound is single, and most often there are no murmurs.

The *electrocardiogram* is helpful in that the frontal QRS axis almost always lies between 0 and +90°. The tall, spiked P waves indicate right atrial enlargement. The electrocardiogram is consistent with left ventricular dominance or hypertrophy; right ventricular forces are markedly decreased in the majority of patients with small right ventricles. Occasionally, with large right ventricular cavities, right ventricular hypertrophy is seen. The chest *roentgenogram* shows the heart to be variable in size with markedly decreased pulmonary vascularity. The two-dimensional *echocardiogram* is useful in helping to estimate the right ventricular dimensions and the size of the tricuspid

valve. *Cardiac catheterization* demonstrates right atrial and ventricular hypertension. Ventriculography reveals the size of the ventricular cavity, the atretic right ventricular outflow tract, the degree of tricuspid regurgitation, and the intramyocardial sinusoids filling the coronary vessel.

Treatment. The prognosis for this lesion has improved with urgent medical and surgical management. Infusion of prostaglandin E_1 is usually effective in keeping the ductus open prior to intervention (Sec. 14.14), thus reducing hypoxemia and acidemia prior to surgery. Pulmonary valvotomy is carried out to relieve outflow obstruction whenever possible, but in order to preserve adequate pulmonary blood flow, a systemic-pulmonary arterial anastomosis is done during the same procedure. Some groups have reported success by unroofing the outflow tract and patch grafting. The aim of surgery is to encourage growth in the right ventricular chamber by allowing forward flow, while utilizing the shunt to provide adequate pulmonary blood flow. Later, when possible, a more extensive valvotomy is carried out and the shunt is taken down (Fig. 14–35). If the right ventricular chamber is minuscule, a Fontan procedure (Sec. 14.17) may be utilized to allow blood to flow to the pulmonary artery directly from the right atrium.

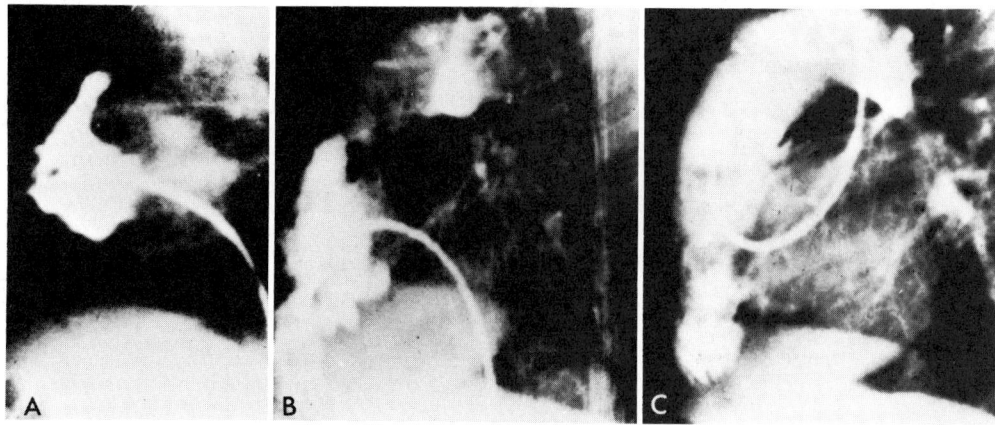

Figure 14–35. Growth of right ventricle in pulmonary atresia and intact ventricular septum (lateral views). *A*, Right ventricular angiogram prior to surgery at 2 days of life. Note the small ventricular chamber and atretic pulmonary outflow tract. The pulmonary artery is not visualized. *B*, At age 2 yr, after valvotomy and systemic pulmonary artery shunt. Normal-sized pulmonary artery fills across narrow outflow tract. The right ventricle is larger, but is trabeculated and hypertrophied. *C*, Normal right ventricle after repair at age 6 yr.

14.17 TRICUSPID ATRESIA

In tricuspid atresia there is no outlet from the right atrium to the right ventricle, and the entire systemic venous return enters the left heart by means of the foramen ovale. Pulmonary blood flow depends on the size of the ventricular septal defect and/or patent ductus arteriosus, the only means by which the pulmonary circulation is perfused. The inflow portion of the right ventricle is always missing in these patients, but the outflow portion is of variable size. If the ventricular septum is intact, the right ventricle is completely hypoplastic and pulmonary atresia is present. Most patients with tricuspid atresia present in the early months of life with decreased pulmonary blood flow and cyanosis. Rarely, a large ventricular septal defect in the absence of right ventricular outflow obstruction can lead to high pulmonary flow and early congestive heart failure.

Clinical Manifestations. Cyanosis, polycythemia, easy fatigability, exertional dyspnea, and occasional hypoxic episodes occur as a result of compromised pulmonary blood flow. The majority of patients have pansystolic murmurs audible along the left sternal border; the 2nd heart sound is single.

Roentgenographic studies show pulmonary undercirculation. Left axis deviation and left ventricular hypertrophy are almost invariably present on the *electrocardiogram* except when there is transposition of the great arteries. In the right precordial leads the normally prominent R wave is replaced by rS complex. The left precordial leads show a qR complex followed by a normal flat diphasic or inverted T wave. RV_6 is normal or tall, and SV_1 generally deep. The P waves are usually biphasic with the initial component tall and spiked in lead II. The *two-dimensional echocardiogram* reveals the absence of a tricuspid valve, the small right ventricle, and the large left ventricle and aorta.

Cardiac catheterization shows normal or slightly elevated right atrial pressure with a prominent "a" wave. If the right ventricle is entered through the ventricular septal defect, the pressure is low, reflecting the restrictive nature of the ventricular communication in most patients. With right atrial angiography there is immediate opacification of the left atrium from the right atrium followed by left ventricular filling and visualization of the aorta (Fig. 14–36). Absence of direct flow to the right ventricle results in a filling defect between the

right atrium and the left ventricle, but a small right ventricle usually is opacified later via a ventricular septal defect. Rarely, the pulmonary arteries are filled only through a patent ductus arteriosus. The presence or absence of associated transposition of the great vessels and pulmonary stenosis is demonstrated by selective left ventriculography.

Treatment. Symptomatic neonates require a surgical shunt procedure to increase pulmonary blood flow. In severe cases adequate pulmonary blood flow may be provided by maintaining ductal patency with infusion of prostaglandin. The Blalock-Taussig procedure (or its variations) is the preferred anastomosis. Patients with tricuspid atresia may remain stable for many years. Eventually, left ventricular dysfunction may occur, since it is this chamber which must provide blood flow to both the pulmonary and systemic circulation. In older patients the Glenn anastomosis (right superior vena cava to right pulmonary artery) has been utilized to provide more physiologic blood flow of unoxygenated systemic venous blood directly to the lungs. This type of shunt does not increase the volume work of the left ventricle.

The Fontan operation is the preferred approach to later surgical management. This procedure is carried out by anastomosing the right atrium to the pulmonary artery either directly or through a conduit insertion. The atrial septal defect or foramen ovale is closed. If the right ventricle is of adequate size, a modification of this procedure may be utilized in which a valve-containing conduit is placed between the right atrium and right ventricle closing the ventricular and atrial septal defects (Fig. 14–37). A 4-chambered, 4-valved heart is thus produced. Early evaluation of patients who have undergone Fontan procedures has been encouraging, and the long-term results of these types of anastomoses appear to be better than the results of systemic-pulmonary artery shunts.

14.18 ORIGIN OF BOTH GREAT VESSELS FROM THE RIGHT VENTRICLE (DOUBLE-OUTLET RIGHT VENTRICLE), WITH PULMONARY STENOSIS

This anomaly is characterized by the aorta and pulmonary artery arising from the right ventricle; the only outlet for the left ventricle is the ventricular septal defect. The aortic and mitral valves are not in continuity, and the ventricular septal defect is inferior to the crista supraventricularis. The physiology among patients with pulmonary stenosis is similar to that which occurs with tetralogy of Fallot. The history, physical examination, electrocardiogram, and roentgenograms are as described in Sec. 14.14. The two-dimensional echocardiograph demonstrates the anatomy and demonstrates the double-outlet right ventricle and mitral-aortic valve discontinuity. Selective angiocardiography shows that the aortic and pulmonary valves lie in the same horizontal body plane and that the anteriorly displaced aorta arises exclusively from the right ventricle. Surgical correction consists of creating an intraventricular channel so that the left ventricle ejects blood through the ventricular septal defect into the aorta. The pulmonary obstruction is relieved with or without a valved conduit. In small infants palliation with an aortic pulmonary shunt provides symptomatic improvement. (See Sec. 14.38.)

14.19 D-TRANSPOSITION OF THE GREAT ARTERIES (TGA)

In this anomaly the aorta arises from the right ventricle and the pulmonary artery from the left ventricle. The systemic veins normally return to the right atrium, and the pulmonary

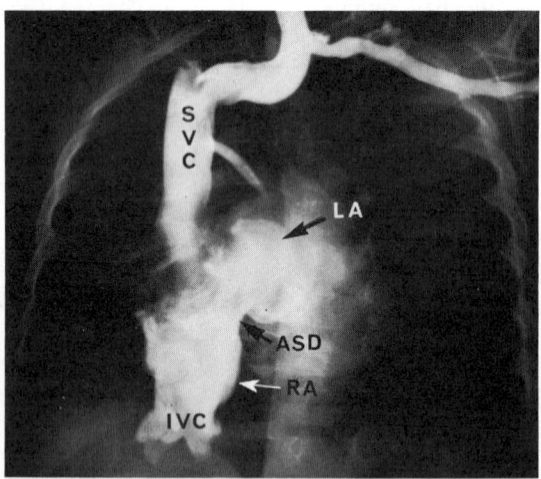

Figure 14–36. Angiocardiogram demonstrates the course of the circulation in tricuspid atresia with underdeveloped right ventricle. Systemic venous blood flows from the right to the left atrium. Absence of right ventricular opacification is due to tricuspid atresia. ASD, interatrial communication through atrial septal defect; IVC, inferior vena cava; LA, left atrium; RA, right atrium; SVC, superior vena cava.

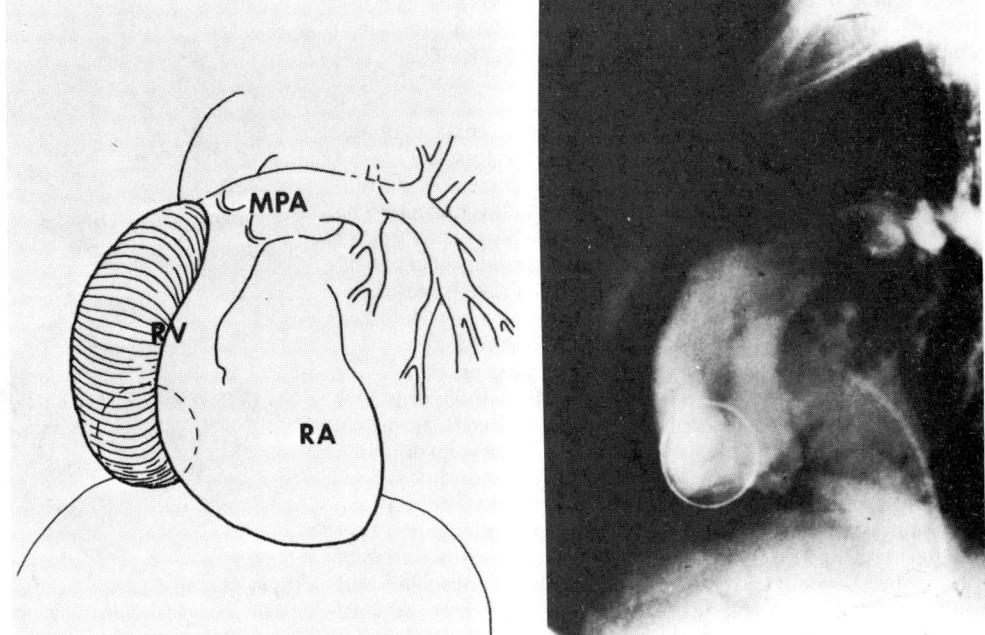

Figure 14–37. Modified Fontan operation, left lateral view. MPA, main pulmonary artery; RV, right ventricle; RA, right atrium.

veins to the left atrium. The atrial-ventricular relationships are normal (concordant). The desaturated blood from the right heart inappropriately passes to the aorta, whereas the oxygenated pulmonary venous blood is returned to the lungs. Thus, the systemic and pulmonary circulation consists of two parallel circuits. The two independent circuits allow survival because the foramen ovale remains patent (with or without an associated ductus arteriosus or ventricular septal defect) to permit some mixture of blood (Fig. 14–38A). TGA has accounted for the majority of deaths in infants under the age of 1 yr with cyanotic congenital heart disease. The anomaly occurs predominantly in males.

The aorta is usually anterior and to the right of the pulmonary trunk. The pulmonary valve is continuous with the mitral valve. Defects of the ventricular septum occur in about 50% of cases. Generally, the right coronary artery arises above the posterior sinus of Valsalva, the left, above the left sinus.

(The right coronary artery normally arises above the right sinus.) The clinical presentation and hemodynamics vary in relation to the presence or absence of associated defects.

14.20 D-TRANSPOSITION OF THE GREAT ARTERIES (TGA) WITH INTACT VENTRICULAR SEPTUM

This anomaly is also referred to as simple transposition of the great arteries or isolated TGA. Prior to birth, oxygenation of the fetus is normal, but after birth the minimal mixing of the systemic and pulmonary blood at the atrial level via the patent foramen ovale is insufficient, and severe hypoxemia ensues within the first few days or weeks of life.

Clinical Manifestations. Cyanosis and tachypnea are most often recognized within the first hours or days of life. Untreated, the vast majority of these infants would not survive

Figure 14–38. *A,* In transposition of the great arteries the circulation is in parallel. Mixing of the pulmonary and systemic circulation must occur in order to sustain life. The diagram shows bidirectional shunting at the atrial level. *B,* After intra-atrial repair (Mustard procedure), systemic venous return is routed to the left ventricle and pulmonary artery, and pulmonary venous blood reaches the systemic circulation via the right ventricle. AO, aorta; PA, pulmonary artery; LV, left ventricle; RV, right ventricle; IVC, inferior vena cava; SVC, superior vena cava; LA, left atrium; RA, right atrium.

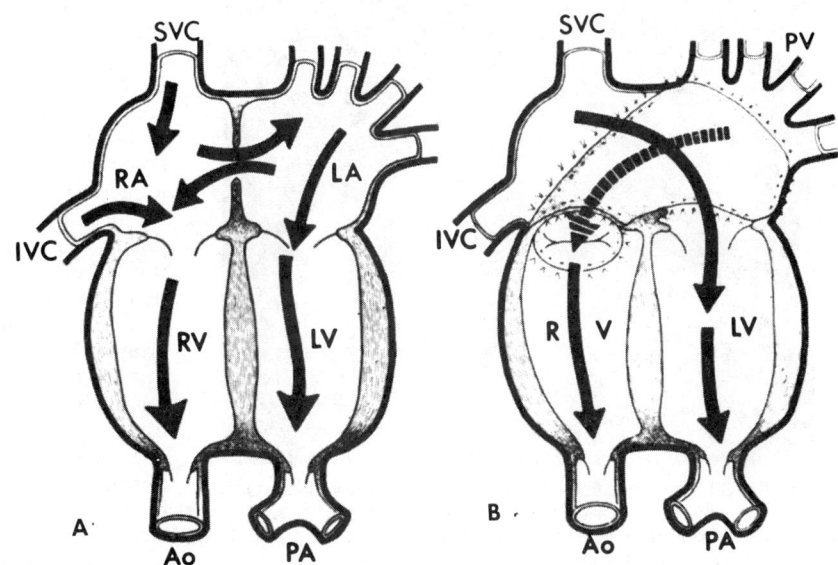

the neonatal period. Hypoxemia is usually severe, but congestive heart failure is not a feature. This condition is a medical
emergency in the neonate, and only early diagnosis and
appropriate intervention can avert the sequelae of prolonged
severe hypoxemia.

Diagnosis. The *electrocardiogram* shows normal neonatal
right-sided dominance. *Roentgenograms* of the chest may show
cardiomegaly, a narrow cardiac waist, and increased pulmonary blood flow, but in most cases is virtually normal. The
arterial pO_2 value is low and does not rise appreciably after
the patient breathes 80–100% oxygen. *Echocardiography* is useful in confirming the diagnosis of isolated TGA. In addition,
the size of the intra-atrial communication can be visualized
by apical and subxiphoid two-dimensional scanning.

Cardiac catheterization shows right ventricular pressure to be
systemic, since this ventricle is supporting the peripheral
circulation. The catheter enters the aorta directly from the
right ventricle; it also passes across the foramen ovale or an
atrial septal defect into the left heart chambers and occasionally into the pulmonary artery. The blood in the left ventricle
and pulmonary artery has a higher oxygen content than that
in the aorta. The degree of arterial desaturation is variable,
but is most often extremely low. The left ventricular and
pulmonary arterial pressures are usually less than 50% of
systemic pressures. *Right ventriculography* demonstrates the
origin of the anteriorly placed aorta from the right ventricle,
the intact ventricular septum, the closure of the ductus arteriosus, and the transposed great arteries; the aortic valve is
anterior and superior to the pulmonary valve. The aortic
origin of the coronary arteries is also shown. *Left ventriculography* shows that the pulmonary artery arises exclusively from
the left ventricle and that the ventricular septum is intact (Fig.
14–39).

Treatment. Prior to the initiation of specific therapy and
during transfer to a neonatal cardiac center, particular attention must be paid to maintaining normal body temperature;
hypothermia intensifies the metabolic acidosis resulting from
hypoxemia. Prompt correction of acidosis and hypoglycemia
is essential.

After the diagnosis is established by two-dimensional echocardiography, the infant is taken immediately to the cardiac
catheterization laboratory. If echocardiography is not diagnostic, appropriate angiographic study should be carried out
to confirm the diagnosis of transposition of the great arteries.
A Rashkind balloon atrial septostomy (Fig. 14–40) is then

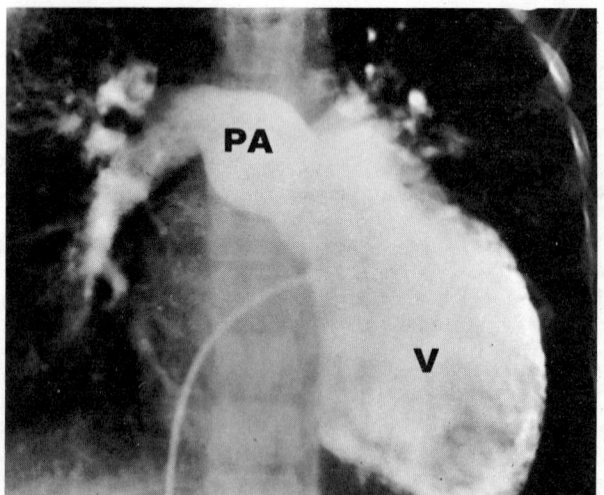

Figure 14–39. Transposition of great vessels. Injection of contrast
medium into a smooth-walled posterior (left) ventricle. The pulmonary
artery (PA) arises exclusively from the posterior ventricle (V), and the
interventricular septum is intact. (Anteroposterior view.)

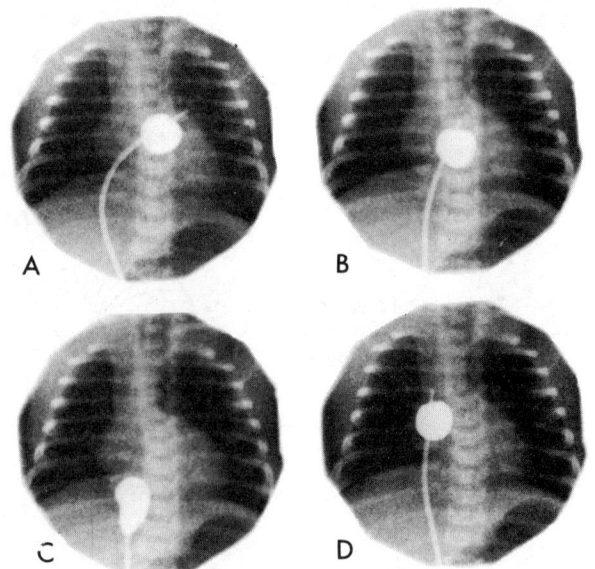

Figure 14–40. Balloon septostomy (Rashkind). Four frames from a
continuous cinema that show the creation of an atrial septal defect in
a hypoxemic newborn infant with transposition of the great arteries
and intact ventricular septum. *A*, Balloon inflated in left atrium. *B*,
Catheter is jerked suddenly so that balloon ruptures the foramen ovale.
C, Balloon in inferior vena cava. *D*, Catheter advanced to right atrium
to deflate balloon. Time from *A* to *C* less than 1 sec.

performed with as little delay as possible. Following this
procedure, a rise in PaO_2 to 35–50 torr suggests that an
adequate communication has been established which will
result in improved mixing of the systemic and pulmonary
venous return. In addition, elimination of the usual presep-
tostomy pressure gradient across the atrial septum suggests
that a large atrial communication has been established. Patients with transposition of the great arteries with associated
anomalies should also undergo balloon septostomy. Some of
the blood of these patients does not mix well at the ventricular
level even in the presence of communications, and others
may benefit by decompression of the left atrium to alleviate
the early pulmonary symptoms of left heart failure. Surgical
methods (Blalock-Hanlon, Baffes, Sterling-Edwards operations) for increasing atrial mixing have been available for
many years, but the balloon septostomy technique has replaced these procedures.

Some infants are so severely cyanotic and acidotic that
management is required prior to the catheterization study. In
this situation prostaglandin E_1 should be infused in order to
maintain ductal patency or reopen a ductus arteriosus that is
in the process of closing (dosage 0.05 to 0.10 μg/kg/min). This
will improve arterial oxygenation. Acidosis should be corrected simultaneously by infusion of sodium bicarbonate. In
some instances prostaglandin administration should be prolonged even after balloon septostomy, until PaO_2 becomes
stable at an acceptable level. However, infusion of prostaglandin E_1 is rarely necessary for more than a few days, and if
the patient appears to be prostaglandin-dependent, surgical
management should be initiated.

In most instances, the infant with transposition of the great
arteries improves noticeably after balloon septostomy. The
infant is less cyanotic and begins to feed well. Although
relatively severe cyanosis may still be noted with crying,
higher arterial blood oxygen levels will reflect the infant's
improved status. Blood pH should consistently remain within
normal limits, and metabolic acidosis should no longer be
present. In some cases PaO_2 begins to fall within hours after
what appears to be a successful septostomy. Reballooning or
surgical alternatives are not necessarily indicated on the basis

of a low PaO_2 alone, even in the range of 20–30 torr, if the baby continues to feed and gain weight and blood pH remains normal. However, in some instances there is little improvement in the infant's condition despite what appears to be a successful septostomy, and immediate intervention is obviously warranted. Echocardiographic studies may indicate that an inadequate atrial communication has been established. Even when a large communication is present, pulmonary and systemic venous blood may tend to follow their original channels to their respective ventricles without adequate mixing at the atrial level. Under these circumstances, a second balloon procedure is rarely helpful, especially if the infant is past the first month of life. Usually the Mustard or Senning operation is performed immediately, rather than a Blalock-Hanlon operation.

Patients with transposition of the great arteries with intact ventricular septum or only a very small ventricular septal defect can be discharged within a few days after successful septostomy, on no medications. Digoxin, diuretics, or antiarrhythmic agents are rarely required. However, close follow-up of these patients is necessary. Anemia is a serious problem which can lead to major central nervous system complications secondary to cerebral ischemia. Hemoglobin levels of 11–13 g/dL represent significant anemia in patients with cyanotic heart disease. Occasionally central nervous system complications occur as the result of severe neonatal hypoxemia even with apparently optimal management. Failure to thrive due to chronic hypoxemia, extremely severe cyanosis, marked polycythemia, or early central nervous symptomatology are urgent indications for further management. The majority of patients, however, will remain stable, and elective surgery can be done on a scheduled basis.

The Mustard or Senning operation performed at any age after initial balloon septostomy is the surgical treatment of choice for infants with transposition of the great arteries and intact ventricular septum. These procedures reverse blood flow patterns at the atrial level, allowing systemic venous blood to reach the lungs via the left atrium and ventricle, and pulmonary-venous blood to cross over to the right atrium, right ventricle, and aorta (Fig. 14–38B). Elective surgery is usually done at 4–9 mo of age, since an older infant is somewhat larger and clinically stable, and thus a better surgical candidate than a desperately ill cyanotic infant. Concerns regarding development of pulmonary vascular obstructive disease preclude delays beyond this age range. Accelerated arteriolar vascular changes of the irreversible intimal type have been documented by the age of 1 yr in infants having transposition of the great arteries with intact ventricular septum, although this complication is even more likely when a large ventricular septal defect is present.

Symptomatic improvement after the intra-atrial repair operations is dramatic with disappearance of cyanosis and marked increase in effort tolerance, but careful follow-up is necessary because of potential complications. Arrhythmias are common and are primarily atrial in origin; they consist of junctional rhythm, bradytachyrhythmia, paroxysmal atrial tachycardia, and atrial flutter. The vast majority of patients have slow junctional rhythms which are well tolerated. Recurrence of cyanosis may be due to defects in the baffle with resultant bidirectional atrial shunting. Obstruction by the baffle may interfere with entry of blood into the atria from the superior and inferior vena cava, from the pulmonary veins, or from both. Left ventricular outflow tract obstruction, of either the fixed or the dynamic type, may be encountered. Reoperation may be required for these problems. Postsurgical right ventricular dysfunction is the most worrisome complication.

In recent years, an arterial switch operation has been devised for the surgical correction of transposition of the great arteries. This involves switching the great arteries above the semilunar valves and transplanting the coronary vessels (Jatene procedure). The indications and timing for this procedure vary widely among medical centers throughout the world, and for patients with transposition of the great arteries without a significant ventricular septal defect, the atrial corrective operations remain the treatment of choice in most hospitals. Although the Mustard and Senning operations are not without early risk or late complications, they are effective and in the United States have an overall survival rate in the range of 80–95%.

Some centers have begun to initiate the switch operation in the first 10–14 days of life while left ventricular pressures remain high or in two stages, with a pulmonary banding done initially in order to raise left ventricular pressure to the degree that hypertrophy is stimulated. Thus, the left ventricle is "prepared" for the role of systemic ventricle, which is not otherwise possible for a thin-walled ventricle that has been acting as a low pressure pulmonary ventricle beyond the first days of life. After the first 2 wk of life the left ventricular pressure is too low to contemplate direct switching of the great arteries.

14.21 TRANSPOSITION OF THE GREAT ARTERIES WITH VENTRICULAR SEPTAL DEFECT

If the septal defect is small, the clinical manifestations, laboratory findings, and treatment are similar to those described above. Many of the small defects close spontaneously.

When the ventricular septal defect is large and nonrestrictive to ventricular ejection, significant mixing of blood often occurs and the *clinical manifestations* are dominated by signs of congestive cardiac failure. The onset of cyanosis may be subtle and frequently delayed, and its intensity is variable. With careful observation, cyanosis can usually be recognized within the first month of life, but in some infants several months elapse before it is apparent. The hypoxemia is usually associated with polycythemia but less prominently than in patients with an intact septum. The heart is significantly enlarged. The murmur is pansystolic and generally indistinguishable from that produced by a large ventricular septal defect with normally related arteries. The *electrocardiogram* shows prominent P waves, isolated right ventricular hypertrophy, or biventricular hypertrophy. Usually, the QRS axis is to the right, but sometimes it is normal or even to the left. Occasionally, isolated dominance of the left ventricle is present. The cardiomegaly, narrow cardiac waist, and significant pulmonary vascularity are demonstrated *roentgenographically*. Pulmonary blood flow can also be assessed by *echocardiography*. (Increased flows are associated with enlargement of the left atrium and ventricle.) The diagnosis is confirmed by *cardiac catheterization* and angiocardiography. Right and left ventriculography indicates the presence of arterial transposition and demonstrates the site and size of the ventricular septal defect. The catheter may cross the ventricular septum from the right ventricle and enter the pulmonary artery. Peak systolic pressures are equal in the two ventricles, the aorta, and the pulmonary artery. The ventricular end diastolic pressures are elevated in the presence of cardiac failure. The left atrial pressure may be much higher than right atrial pressure.

At the time of cardiac catheterization a balloon septostomy is performed to decompress the left atrium even in cases in which adequate mixing is occurring at the ventricular level. Surgical therapy is advised within the first 7–8 mo of life, since congestive heart failure and failure to thrive are difficult to manage and pulmonary vascular disease develops rapidly. Patients with this combination of defects almost always also require maintenance digitalis and diuretic therapy.

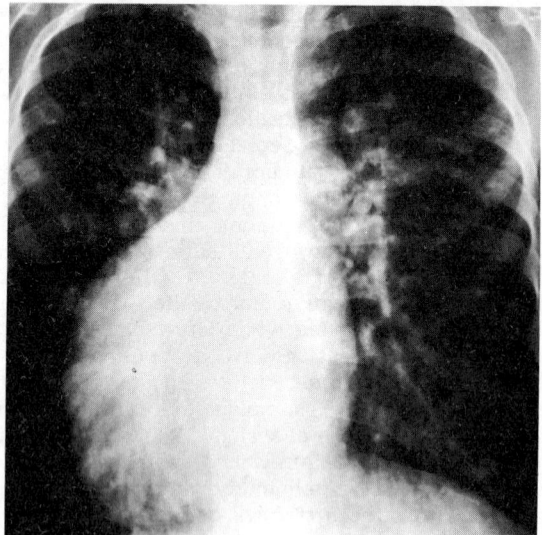

Figure 14–41. Roentgenogram in complete transposition of the great arteries with ventricular septal defect and pulmonary vascular disease, showing cardiomegaly, large proximal pulmonary vessels, and a narrow cardiac base.

Without treatment, *prognosis* is poor; the majority of patients succumb in the first year of life because of congestive cardiac failure, hypoxemia, and pulmonary hypertension. In the past, some survived infancy with medical therapy and without surgical intervention. The clinical picture and treatment of these patients are almost identical to those described in Eisenmenger syndrome (Sec. 14.29) with a large ventricular septal defect (Fig. 14–41). *Surgical palliation* with a Mustard operation has been successful in relieving the hypoxemia of intensely cyanotic patients, but the pulmonary vascular disease is not affected.

The early surgical experience has been with pulmonary artery banding, with or without atrial septectomy, during infancy followed by debanding and correction after the age of about 1 yr. Direct early repair without initial banding has also been advocated. The method of repair consists of intra-atrial correction of venous return (Mustard or Senning procedure) and patch closure of the ventricular septal defect. Mortality remains high. Another approach to correction is placement of an intraventricular patch so that the left ventricle ejects into the aorta through the ventricular septal defect, and establishment of right ventricular-pulmonary artery continuity with a valved or non-valved prosthesis (Rastelli). This procedure is done later in childhood after an initial pulmonary artery banding; there is little experience with this procedure performed on infants.

The switch operation with patch closure of the ventricular septal defect appears to be the best option for patients with transposition of the great arteries and ventricular septal defect. These infants can be operated upon at a few months of age without pulmonary artery banding since the left ventricular pressure is elevated because of the ventricular septal defect; sufficient hypertrophy is present so that the left ventricle can assume the afterload responsibilities of the systemic ventricle. Early results indicate that the mortality rates are lower than for the other approaches, and preliminary follow-up information is encouraging regarding long-term survival with good cardiac function.

14.22 TRANSPOSITION OF THE GREAT ARTERIES WITH A LARGE PATENT DUCTUS ARTERIOSUS

In the neonate with transposition of the great arteries a large patent ductus arteriosus may be of benefit. Persistent patency beyond the first weeks of life, however, aggravates the situation since the dominant flow across the duct runs from aorta to pulmonary artery, further increasing the pulmonary blood flow. This clinical picture is dominated by signs of congestive cardiac failure; cyanosis may not be obvious. Balloon atrial septostomy is done in the neonatal period, but most of these infants remain in uncontrollable congestive cardiac failure and will require early surgical closure of the duct and an intra-atrial correction or a switch operation.

14.23 TRANSPOSITION OF THE GREAT ARTERIES WITH VENTRICULAR SEPTAL DEFECT AND PULMONARY STENOSIS

This combination of anomalies may mimic tetralogy of Fallot. The site of obstruction is either valvular or subvalvular; the latter type may be acquired after successful atrial septostomy or pulmonary arterial banding.

The onset of *clinical manifestations* varies from soon after birth to infancy and includes cyanosis, hypercyanotic (paroxysmal dyspneic) episodes, decreased exercise tolerance, and poor physical development. The manifestations are similar to those described under tetralogy of Fallot. The cyanosis is usually more intense, however, and the heart may be enlarged. The pulmonary vasculature as seen on *roentgenogram* is normal or somewhat diminished but in most instances is relatively normal. The *electrocardiogram* usually shows right axis deviation, right and left ventricular hypertrophy, and sometimes tall, spiked P waves. *Echocardiography* is useful in sequential evaluation of the degree and progression of the left ventricular outflow obstruction.

Cardiac catheterization shows that the pulmonary arterial pressure is low and as in all patients with transposition, the oxygen saturation exceeds that of the aorta. Selective right and left ventriculography demonstrates the origin of the aorta from the right ventricle, the origin of the pulmonary artery from the left ventricle, the ventricular septal defect, and the pulmonary stenosis.

The preferred *treatment* in hypoxemic infants is establishment of a systemic-pulmonary arterial shunt after neonatal balloon atrial septostomy. The patient can then be followed clinically until 5–6 yr of age when a Rastelli operation is the preferable corrective procedure. However, a second shunt operation may be required as an interim measure. This approach has been successful in the majority of cases. Surgical correction by the Mustard operation with simultaneous closure of the ventricular septal defect and relief of left ventricular outflow obstruction may be an alternative when the position of the ventricular septal defect is not suitable for a Rastelli operation.

14.24 TRANSPOSITION OF THE GREAT ARTERIES WITH TRICUSPID ATRESIA

If arterial transposition is associated with tricuspid atresia and pulmonary stenosis, the clinical presentation is similar to that described for tricuspid atresia in Sec. 14.17. If pulmonary stenosis is absent, however, and pulmonary flow excessive, cyanosis is mild. Tachypnea, feeding difficulties, poor weight gain, recurrent respiratory infections, and heart failure are the usual manifestations. Increased venous pressure may result in presystolic pulsations of a large liver and a prominent "a" wave in the jugular venous pulse. Cardiac enlargement is moderate to marked. Systolic ejection murmurs of varying intensity are usual, and the 2nd heart sound is loud and single. Although the electrocardiogram may show prominent P waves, left axis deviation, and left ventricular hypertrophy, more patients will have right axis deviation than when tricuspid atresia is associated with normal great arteries. Cardiac enlargement and increased pulmonary vascularity is present on roentgenogram. The diagnosis can be made by two-dimensional echocardiography. Selective left ventriculography delineates a large left ventricle, arterial transposition, and the relative sizes of the pulmonary artery and aorta. The prognosis may be poor when the aorta is hypoplastic and pulmonary flow torrential. Surgical palliation is achieved with pulmonary arterial banding, which is most effective when the aortic root is near normal in size. Variations of the Fontan concept (right atrium–pulmonary artery connection) may be utilized in selected patients. In essence, the management problems associated with this abnormality are those encountered in patients with single ventricle.

14.25 TOTAL ANOMALOUS PULMONARY VENOUS RETURN

Abnormal development of the pulmonary veins may result in anomalous partial (Sec. 14.44) or complete drainage into the systemic venous circulation. The abnormal point of entry may be the right atrium, the superior or inferior vena cava or one of their major tributaries, or a persistent left superior vena cava which opens into the coronary sinus. The pulmonary veins may join a common trunk which enters the venous circulation below the diaphragm (portal vein, ductus venosus, or inferior vena cava). An associated atrial septal defect is often present; at least a patent foramen ovale is required to sustain life.

Pathology. In *total anomalous pulmonary venous return* there is no direct pulmonary venous connection into the left atrium, and all of the blood returning to the heart (the systemic and pulmonary venous blood) returns to the right atrium. Some of the blood passes into the right ventricle and pulmonary artery, and the remainder passes through an atrial septal defect or patent foramen ovale to the left atrium.

Usually, the pulmonary veins form a single trunk before entering the systemic venous circulation and join the systemic venous return through supra-cardiac, intra-cardiac, or infra-cardiac connections. The sites of its drainage include: left superior vena cava (40%), coronary sinus (20%), and right superior vena cava (10%). The remainder enter the right

atrium directly, below the diaphragm through the portal system, or through mixed connections.

Clinical Manifestations. Three types of clinical patterns are seen. Some infants present in the neonatal period with severe obstruction to venous return. This is most prevalent in the infradiaphragmatic group. Cyanosis is prominent, and there is severe tachypnea. There may be no murmurs present on physical examination.

Another group of patients also with congestive heart failure in early life, but in these infants a large left to right shunt is present; obstruction to pulmonary venous return is only mild or moderate. Since pulmonary artery hypertension is present, the infants will be severely ill. Systolic murmurs along the left sternal border are audible, and there may be a gallop rhythm. A continuous murmur is occasionally heard along the left upper sternal border over the pulmonary area. Cyanosis is mild.

The third group of patients with total anomalous venous return are those in whom pulmonary venous obstruction is not present. In this situation, which is the least common, there is a large left to right shunt, but pulmonary hypertension is absent and the patients are unlikely to be symptomatic during infancy or early childhood. Cyanosis is absent.

Diagnosis. The *electrocardiogram* demonstrates right ventricular hypertrophy (usually a qR pattern in V_4R and V_1, and the P waves are frequently tall and spiked). *Roentgenograms* are pathognomonic in older children if the pulmonary veins enter the innominate vein and persistent left superior vena cava (Fig. 14–42). There is a large supracardiac shadow with a **figure 8** or **snowman** appearance. The supracardiac shadow is produced by the dilated left superior vena cava, left innominate vein, and right superior vena cava. However, this appearance is not helpful for diagnosis in early infancy because of superimposition of the thymic image or because the pulmonary veins may drain elsewhere. In most cases of total anomalous pulmonary venous return, the heart is enlarged, the pulmonary artery and right ventricle are prominent, and the pulmonary vascularity is increased. In neonates having severe cyanosis due to marked venous obstruction (usually infradiaphragmatic), the chest roentgenograms reveal pul-

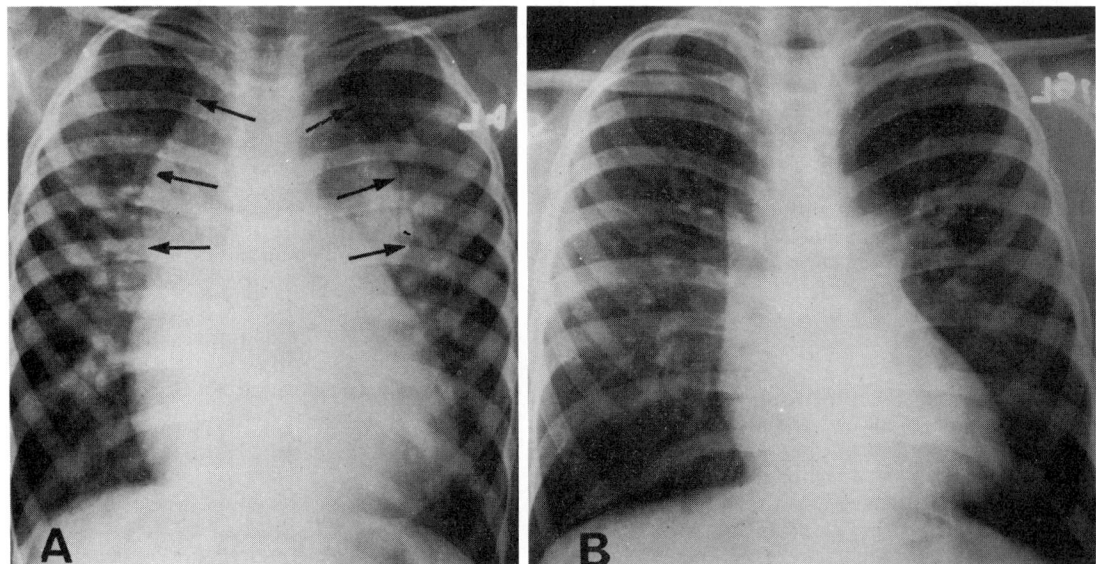

Figure 14–42. Roentgenograms in total anomalous pulmonary venous return to the left superior vena cava. *A,* Preoperative. Arrows point to the supracardiac shadow, which produces the snowman or figure 8 configuration. Cardiomegaly and increased pulmonary vascularity are evident. *B,* Postoperative, showing decrease in size of the heart and supracardiac shadow.

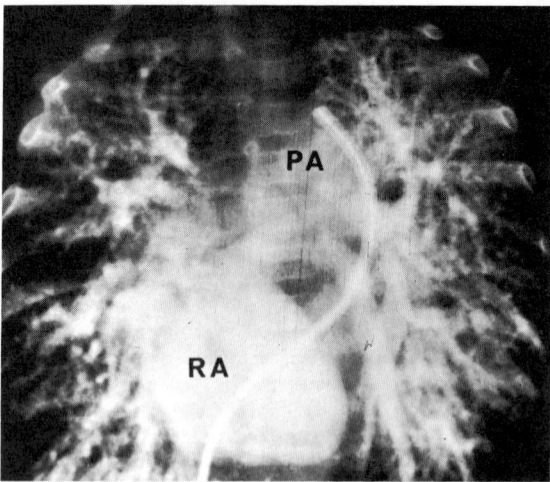

Figure 14–43. Total anomalous pulmonary venous return to the coronary sinus. Injection of contrast medium into the pulmonary artery (PA) opacifies the pulmonary arterial tree. The contrast medium returns to the coronary sinus, which drains into the densely opacified right atrium (RA).

monary edema with a small heart and thus commonly cause confusion with the respiratory distress syndrome.

The *echocardiogram* reflects the right ventricular overload and usually identifies the pattern of pulmonary venous connections.

Cardiac catheterization shows that the oxygen saturations of blood in both atria, both ventricles, and the aorta are more or less similar and higher than the peripheral systemic venous blood proximal to the entry of the pulmonary venous trunk. In older patients the pulmonary arterial and right ventricular pressures may be only moderately elevated, but in infancy pulmonary hypertension is usual. *Selective pulmonary arteriography* shows the anatomy of the pulmonary veins and their point of entry into the systemic venous circulation (Fig. 14–43).

Without treatment, the prognosis for the great majority of patients with total anomalous pulmonary venous return is poor, and survival beyond infancy is unusual in the presence of pulmonary hypertension. Death is due to congestive heart failure. Patients who survive beyond 2 yr of age are those who do not have pulmonary arterial hypertension, and they may remain asymptomatic for many years.

Surgical correction of total anomalous pulmonary venous return during infancy is indicated. The common pulmonary venous trunk is anastomosed to the left atrium, the atrial septal defect is closed, and the connection to the systemic venous circuit is interrupted. The surgical results have been good, even for critically ill neonates. If the postoperative hemodynamics are normal, the prognosis appears to be excellent. Delay of surgical treatment for symptomatic infants with this lesion is not warranted.

14.26 EBSTEIN DISEASE

This anomaly consists of downward displacement of an abnormal tricuspid valve into the right ventricle. The anterior cusp of the valve retains some attachment to the valve ring, but the other leaflets are attached to the wall of the right ventricle. The latter chamber is divided into two parts by the abnormal valve; the first is continuous with the cavity of the right atrium; the second consists of thin-walled ventricular myocardium. The right atrium is huge, and the tricuspid valve may or may not be competent. The effective output from the right side of the heart is decreased because of the

poor functioning small right ventricle and subtle obstruction produced by the large, sail-like, anterior tricuspid leaflet. Variable amounts of right to left shunting occur at the atrial level via the foramen ovale, resulting in mild to severe cyanosis.

Clinical Manifestations. The severity of symptoms depends on the degree of displacement of the tricuspid valve. In many patients, symptoms are mild and the only complaint is fatigue. Cardiac dysrhythmias are frequent, the most common being numerous extrasystoles or attacks of paroxysmal tachycardia, usually supraventricular. A right to left shunt through the foramen ovale is responsible for cyanosis and polycythemia. The venous pressure is normal or increased if there is associated tricuspid insufficiency. On palpation, the precordium is quiet. A systolic murmur is audible over most of the anterior left side of the chest. Gallop rhythm is common as is a scratchy diastolic murmur at the left sternal border. This murmur is superficial and may mimic a pericardial friction rub.

Although some patients may be asymptomatic until well into adult life, newborn infants with Ebstein disease may present with cyanosis, massive cardiomegaly, and long systolic murmurs. Death may occur as a result of cardiac failure and hypoxemia. However, spontaneous improvement occurs rapidly in many symptomatic neonates as pulmonary vascular resistance falls normally and pulmonary blood flow increases.

Diagnosis. The *electrocardiogram* usually shows right bundle branch block without increased right precordial voltage, normal or tall and broad P waves, and normal or prolonged P-R interval. Sometimes the pattern of the Wolff-Parkinson-White syndrome is present.

On *roentgenographic examination* the heart size varies from normal to massive cardiomegaly because of great enlargement of the right atrium and ventricle. The intrapulmonary vasculature is normal or decreased, and the aorta is small.

Echocardiography shows delayed closure and an increased amplitude of the tricuspid valve. Abnormal septal motion, retardation of the E-F slope of the tricuspid valve, and a dilated right atrium is also seen. The atrialized portion of the right ventricle and the abnormal tricuspid valve can be visualized with two-dimensional ultrasound.

Cardiac catheterization and selective angiocardiography confirm the presence of a large right atrium and abnormal tricuspid valve. A right to left shunt at the atrial level, if present, will be demonstrated. The right atrial pressure may be normal, but is often somewhat elevated along with the right ventricular diastolic pressure. There is a significant risk of arrhythmia during catheterization and angiographic studies.

Prognosis. This is extremely variable, depending on where the patient falls within the broad spectrum of severity seen with this defect. Many patients survive into adult life.

Treatment. Control of hypoxemia and supraventricular dysrhythmias is of primary importance. Surgical treatment is seldom necessary in childhood and should be considered only in extreme situations. In deeply cyanotic patients, anastomosis of the superior vena cava to the right pulmonary artery (Glenn) has resulted in symptomatic improvement. Repair or replacement of the abnormal tricuspid valve with closure of the atrial septal defect can be carried out when absolutely necessary in the older child, but the results of such surgery are inconsistent.

14.27 TRUNCUS ARTERIOSUS

In this anomaly a single arterial trunk arises from the ventricular portion of the heart and supplies the systemic, pulmonary, and coronary circulations. A ventricular septal defect is always present, and the number of semilunar valve cusps in the single truncal valve varies from two to six. The pulmonary arteries arise from the ascending portion of the truncus proximal to the origin of the innominate artery as a single vessel or as two separate arteries. When the pulmonary arteries are apparently absent and pulmonary blood flow is derived from collateral arteries, there is nevertheless usually a remnant of a pulmonary artery present. This condition is classified as pulmonary atresia with ventricular septal defect (Sec. 14.15), but is occasionally referred to as pseudotruncus.

Hemodynamics. Both ventricles are at systemic pressure ejecting blood into the truncus. When the pulmonary vascular resistance is relatively normal, the blood flow to the lungs is greatly increased, the arteriovenous oxygen difference is small, and cyanosis is minimal or absent. If the pulmonary resistance increases, the pulmonary blood flow decreases and cyanosis becomes more apparent. The truncal valve is occasionally incomplete.

Clinical Manifestations. These vary with age, depending on pulmonary vascular resistance. In the majority of infants, pulmonary blood flow is torrential and the clinical picture is dominated by dyspnea, fatigue, heart failure, recurrent respiratory infections, poor physical development, and often death in infancy. Cyanosis is minimal or absent. The runoff of blood from the truncus to the pulmonary circulation may result in a wide pulse pressure. This may be further exaggerated by truncal valve insufficiency. The heart is usually enlarged, and the precordium is hyperdynamic. A systolic ejection murmur, sometimes accompanied by a thrill, is usually audible along the left sternal border. The murmur is frequently preceded by an ejection click. In the presence of truncal valve insufficiency, a high-pitched protodiastolic murmur is heard. The 2nd heart sound is loud and generally single, though it may be split. A mid-diastolic apical rumbling murmur is audible. In older children with restricted pulmonary blood flow secondary to the development of pulmonary vascular obstructive disease, progressive cyanosis, polycythemia, and clubbing develop.

Diagnosis. The *electrocardiogram* is variable and shows right, left, or combined ventricular hypertrophy. There is considerable variation in the roentgenographic appearance of the chest. Cardiac enlargement is due to prominence of both ventricles. The truncus may produce a prominent shadow which follows the normal course of the ascending aorta and aortic knob; it arches to the right in almost 50% of patients. Sometimes a high bulge, left of the aortic knob, is produced by the main or left pulmonary artery. The pulmonary vascularity is increased in the presence of normal pulmonary resistance. *Echocardiography* demonstrates the large, overriding, and usually anterior truncal artery.

The diagnosis is confirmed by *cardiac catheterization* and by selective right ventriculography. The catheter may enter the pulmonary arteries from the truncus. A left to right shunt is demonstrated at the ventricular level, and the systolic pressures in both ventricles and the truncus are similar. Selective angiocardiography reveals the large truncus arteriosus and the origin of the pulmonary arteries. Injection of contrast medium into the truncus just above the truncal valve allows assessment of the competence of this valve.

Prognosis. Without surgery, many of the patients succumb during the 1st or 2nd yr of life. If pulmonary blood flow is restricted by development of pulmonary vascular disease, the patient may survive into adulthood.

Treatment. Open heart repair of truncus arteriosus has been accomplished in infants and older children. The ventricular septal defect is closed, the pulmonary arteries are divided from the truncus, and continuity is established between the right ventricle and the pulmonary arteries with a conduit. Immediate surgical results among survivors have been excellent, but the conduit must be replaced as the child grows.

The other option is banding of the pulmonary arteries followed by surgical correction in later years; morbidity and mortality associated with banding, however, are high, and most centers prefer early repair. In older patients with pulmonary vascular obstruction, surgical treatment is contraindicated.

14.28 SINGLE VENTRICLE
(Double-Inlet Ventricle)

With a single ventricle, both atria empty through a common valve or two separate atrioventricular valves into a single ventricular chamber, of left, right, or indeterminate ventricular anatomic characteristics, from which the aorta and pulmonary artery arise. Associated cardiac anomalies are usual and vary considerably. Transposition of the great arteries and rudimentary outlet chamber are present in the vast majority of patients. Pulmonary stenosis or atresia is common.

Clinical Manifestations. The clinical picture is variable, depending on the associated intracardiac anomalies and hemodynamics in the individual patient. If a single ventricle is associated with pulmonary stenosis, cyanosis is present in infancy and increases in intensity during childhood, when clubbing and polycythemia also appear. Dyspnea and fatigue are frequent, cardiomegaly is mild or moderate, a left parasternal lift is palpable, and a systolic thrill is common. The systolic ejection murmur is usually loud; an ejection click may be audible, and the 2nd heart sound is single and loud. When a single ventricle is associated with an unobstructed pulmonary outflow tract, pulmonary blood flow is torrential. These patients present in early infancy with tachypnea, dyspnea, poor physical development, recurrent pulmonary infections, and congestive heart failure. Cyanosis is only mild or moderate. Cardiomegaly is generally marked, and a left parasternal lift is palpable. The systolic ejection murmur is generally not intense, and the 2nd heart sound is loud and closely split. A 3rd heart sound is common and may be followed by a short mid-diastolic murmur. The development of pulmonary vascular disease in patients who have not been operated upon may restrict pulmonary blood flow so that cyanosis increases in intensity, heart size decreases, and signs of cardiac failure appear to improve.

Diagnosis. The *electrocardiogram* is nonspecific. P waves are normal, spiked, or bifid. The precordial lead pattern suggests right ventricular hypertrophy, combined ventricular hypertrophy, or sometimes left ventricular dominance. The initial QRS forces are usually to the left and anterior. *Roentgenographic examination* confirms the degree of cardiomegaly. The rudimentary systemic outflow chamber may produce a bulge on the upper left border of the cardiac silhouette in the posteroanterior projection. In the absence of pulmonary stenosis, pulmonary vasculature is increased with prominence of the major branches of the pulmonary artery. Attenuation of the size of the peripheral pulmonary arteries occurs in the presence of obstructive pulmonary vascular disease. Absence of the ventricular septum is the principal *echographic* sign. The details of the atrioventricular valve anatomy are best delineated echocardiographically.

At *cardiac catheterization* the arterial oxygen saturation is decreased in the presence of severe pulmonary stenosis or obstructive pulmonary hypertension but is near normal when pulmonary blood flow is increased. The pressure in the ventricular chamber is high; a gradient may be demonstrated across the entrance to the rudimentary outflow tract, and/or between the outflow chamber and the pulmonary artery in the presence of pulmonary stenosis. Severe pulmonary hypertension is present in the absence of pulmonary stenosis. Selective ventriculography is diagnostic and demonstrates the single ventricle and the anatomic relationships of the pulmonary artery and aorta.

Prognosis. Some patients succumb during infancy from congestive heart failure. Others may survive to adolescence and early adult life but finally succumb to the effects of pulmonary hypertension secondary to pulmonary vascular disease. Patients with moderate pulmonary stenosis have the best prognosis, since pulmonary blood flow, although restricted, is still adequate.

Treatment. If pulmonary stenosis is severe, a systemic-pulmonary arterial anastomosis is indicated. Pulmonary artery banding is advised for patients with a large pulmonary flow to control heart failure and to prevent progressive pulmonary vascular disease. Definitive repair has been accomplished in selected patients by inserting an artificial septum in single ventricles with two atrioventricular valves. However, at most centers the Fontan operation is the treatment of choice for children whose pulmonary pressure and resistance are low, either because of associated pulmonary stenosis or after pulmonary artery banding in infancy.

14.29 EISENMENGER SYNDROME

The term Eisenmenger syndrome refers to patients with reversed or bidirectional shunt through a ventricular or septal defect as a result of pulmonary vascular obstructive disease. This physiologic abnormality also can occur with atrial septal defect, atrioventricular canal, patent ductus arteriosus, or other communication between the aorta and pulmonary artery. Pulmonary vascular disease with isolated atrial septal defect is rare and does not occur until late in adulthood. In normal neonates, within a few weeks the structure of the pulmonary arteriole changes to that of the adult with a thin wall and a large lumen, and the pulmonary vascular resistance falls to normal adult levels. In the Eisenmenger syndrome the pulmonary vascular resistance either remains high or, after having decreased during early infancy, rises thereafter because of increased shear stress on pulmonary arterioles. This phenomenon is primarily the result of prolonged elevated pulmonary pressure, and results in severe obliterative intimal lesions in these vessels. In the Eisenmenger syndrome, pulmonary hypertension is thought to be the result of high pulmonary resistance (pulmonary vascular disease) rather than the result of markedly increased pulmonary blood flow (hyperkinetic pulmonary hypertension).

Clinical Manifestations. Symptoms usually do not occur until the 2nd or 3rd decade of life, although less often a more fulminant course is seen. Many patients survive for decades with minimal symptoms. Irreversible pulmonary vascular obstruction results in high pulmonary vascular resistance. Intra- or extracardiac communications which normally would shunt left to right allow right to left shunting as pulmonary resistance exceeds systemic resistance. Cyanosis becomes apparent, and dyspnea, fatigue, and tendency toward dysrhythmias begin to occur. In the late stages of the disease, heart failure, chest pain, syncope, and hemoptysis may be seen. Physical examination reveals a right ventricular heave and a loud, narrowly split 2nd heart sound. Only a soft ejection systolic murmur is audible along the left sternal border. Pulmonary artery pulsation may be palpable at the left upper sternal border. The degree of cyanosis depends on the stage of the disease. Functional incompetence of the pulmonary valve may result in a blowing diastolic murmur along the left sternal border (Graham Steell murmur).

Diagnosis. Cyanotic patients have various degrees of polycythemia. *Roentgenographically,* the heart varies in size from normal to greatly enlarged; the latter occurs late in the course of the disease (Fig. 14–44). The main pulmonary artery is

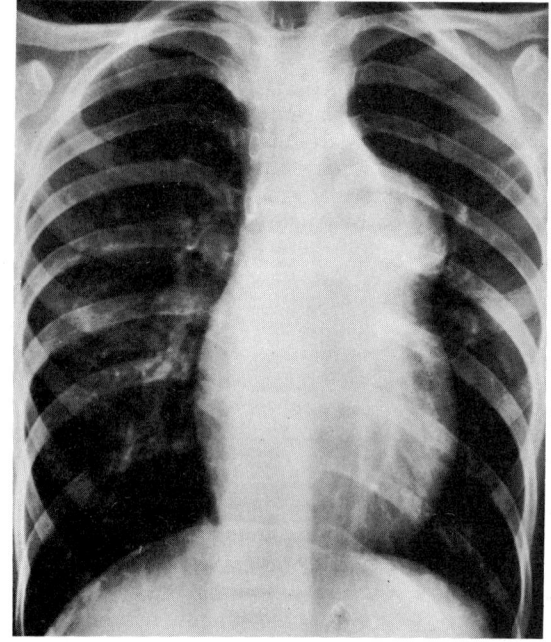

Figure 14–44. Roentgenogram in Eisenmenger syndrome due to a patent ductus arteriosus. The heart size is normal, the pulmonary artery segment is dilated, and the pulmonary vascularity is normal or slightly increased.

prominent. The pulmonary vessels are enlarged in the hilar areas and diminish in caliber in the peripheral branches. The right ventricle and atrium are prominent. The *electrocardiogram* shows marked right ventricular hypertrophy. The P wave may be tall and spiked. The *echocardiogram* shows a thick-walled right ventricle and demonstrates a communication between the systemic and pulmonary circulation. The right side systolic time interval shows a significant increase in the ratio of pre-ejection period to ejection time because of the increased pulmonary vascular resistance.

Cardiac catheterization usually shows a bidirectional shunt at the site of the defect. The systolic pressures are usually equal in the systemic and pulmonary circulations. The pulmonary capillary wedge pressure is normal, ruling out a left heart obstructive lesion as an explanation for the pulmonary artery hypertension. The arterial oxygen saturation is decreased, reflecting the right to left shunt. Selective angiocardiography can locate the site of the shunt, but these studies are avoided in these patients because of increased risk with contrast media injection.

Treatment. The best management of patients who are at risk of developing late pulmonary vascular disease is *prevention* by surgical elimination of large intracardiac or great vessel communications during infancy. Medical treatment of the Eisenmenger syndrome is entirely symptomatic. Older children and adolescents with significant polycythemia may be improved by cautious, repeated venesections with volume replacement.

14.30 HYPOPLASTIC LEFT HEART SYNDROME

The term hypoplastic left heart syndrome is used to describe a closely related group of anomalies that include underdevelopment of the left side of the heart, e.g., atresia of the aortic or mitral orifices, and hypoplasia of the ascending aorta. The left ventricle is small and nonfunctional; the right ventricle

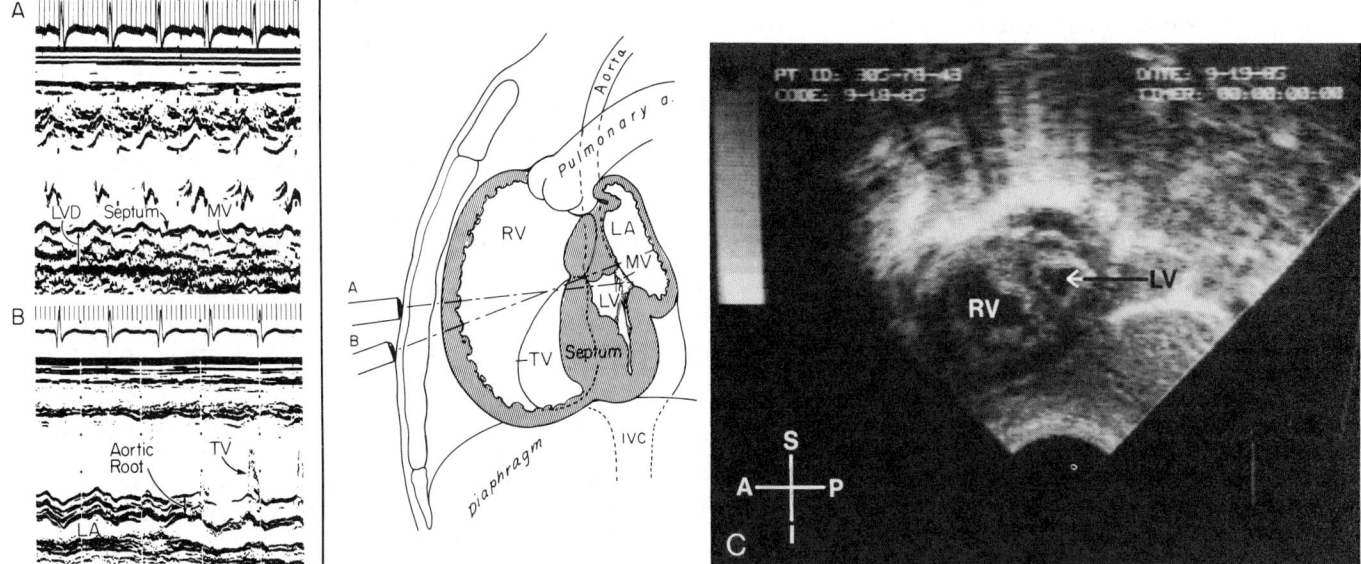

Figure 14–45. Echocardiogram from neonate with aortic valve atresia. Idealized diagram on right shows the small left ventricle and aorta. Echogram *A* (from transducer position *A*) shows minute left ventricular dimension (LVD) containing a small mitral valve (MV). Echogram *B* shows a small aortic root and left atrium. *C*, Subxiphoid ventricular short axis two-dimensional echocardiographic projection demonstrates thick-walled, hypoplastic left ventricle in patient with aortic atresia and severe mitral stenosis. LV, left ventricular cavity; RV, right ventricular cavity.

maintains both pulmonary and systemic circulations. Pulmonary venous blood passes through an atrial defect or dilated foramen ovale from the left to the right side of the heart, where it mixes with systemic venous blood. When the ventricular septum is intact, which is almost always the case, all the right ventricular blood is ejected to the pulmonary arteries; the systemic circulation is supplied via the ductus arteriosus. With a ventricular septal defect and a patent but small aortic orifice, right ventricular blood is ejected to the small left ventricle and ascending aorta as well as to the pulmonary artery. The major hemodynamic abnormalities are inadequate maintenance of the systemic circulation and pulmonary venous hypertension.

Clinical Manifestations. Signs of heart failure appear within the first few weeks of life and include dyspnea, hepatomegaly, and low cardiac output. All peripheral pulses are weak or absent. Although cyanosis may not be obvious in the first 48 hr of life, a grayish blue color of the skin is soon apparent. Cardiac enlargement is usual, with a palpable right ventricular parasternal lift. A nondescript systolic murmur is usually present.

Diagnosis. *Roentgenographically*, the heart is variable in size in the first days of life, but cardiomegaly develops rapidly and is associated with increased pulmonary vascularity. The *electrocardiogram* may show only the normal right ventricular dominance initially, but later P waves become prominent and right ventricular hypertrophy is usual.

The *echocardiogram* is diagnostic (Fig. 14–45). There is absence or gross distortion of the normal mitral valve, absent or small aortic root, a small left atrium and posterior ventricle, a large right atrium and anterior ventricle, and an easily identifiable tricuspid valve. The size of the atrial communication by which pulmonary venous blood leaves the left atrium is assessed. Contrast echocardiography with the transducer in the suprasternal notch identifies the small transverse aortic arch and left atrium. These findings are so characteristic that the diagnosis of aortic atresia can be made without cardiac catheterization. The hypoplastic ascending aorta is best demonstrated by aortography, which also shows the coronary arterial system.

Prognosis. Patients virtually always succumb from this anomaly during the first months of life, usually during the first week.

Treatment. Medical treatment has little to offer, and few patients have had attempts at surgical palliation. Recently, a surgical procedure has been developed in which the left atrium is decompressed by atrial septectomy, the hypoplastic ascending aorta and pulmonary artery are anastomosed, the distal main pulmonary artery is isolated, and pulmonary blood flow is provided by a Blalock shunt. At a second stage, a Fontan operation is performed. The mortality for this operation, when attempted, has been high, but there have been a few survivors beyond the second stage of the procedure. Cardiac transplantation has been successfully accomplished in a few infants with hypoplastic left heart syndrome.

14.31 ABNORMAL POSITIONS OF THE HEART: DEXTROCARDIA AND LEVOCARDIA

An approach to the classification and diagnosis of abnormal cardiac position has been suggested by Van Praagh et al. *Atrial localization* is facilitated by roentgenographic demonstration of the position of the abdominal organs and of the tracheal bifurcation for recognition of the situs of the right and left bronchi. Atrial situs is related to the visceral situs; if the viscera are in normal position, the atria have a normal position. Abdominal situs inversus is associated with the left atrium to the right and right atrium to the left. If the abdominal situs cannot be determined, as with a centrally located liver and asplenia or rudimentary spleen, atrial localization is difficult. *Localization of the ventricles and great arteries* depends on the direction of development of the embryonic cardiac loop. Initial protrusion to the right (d-loop) carries the future right ventricle to the right, and the left ventricle remains on the left. Protrusion to the left (l-loop) carries the future right ventricle to the left, and the left ventricle is on the right. With each type of loop the relations of the great arteries may be normal or transposed. Echocardiographic and angiographic studies demonstrate the atrioventricular and ventriculoarterial relationships. The clinical manifestations of abnormal cardiac position are dominated by the associated cardiovascular anomalies.

Dextrocardia without situs inversus and **levocardia with situs inversus** are virtually always complicated by severe malformations that include various combinations of single ventricle, arterial transposition, pulmonary stenosis, ventricular and atrial septal defects, complete atrioventricular canal, anomalous pulmonary venous return, tricuspid atresia, and pulmonary arterial hypoplasia or atresia. When abdominal heterotaxia is present, the cardiac anomalies associated with polysplenia (left isomerism or bilateral left-sidedness) or asplenia (right isomerism or bilateral right-sidedness) are virtually always complex. Surveys of older children and adults indicate that dextrocardia with situs inversus and with normally related great arteries (so-called mirror-image dextrocardia) is most often associated with a functionally normal heart, although congenital heart disease of a less severe nature is common.

Abnormalities of the lung, diaphragm, and thoracic cage may result in displacement of the heart to the right, mimicking dextrocardia. Hypoplasia of a lung may be accompanied by anomalous pulmonary venous return from that lung. The *electrocardiogram* is difficult to interpret in the presence of lesions with discordant atrial, ventricular, and great vessel anatomy. Diagnosis requires detailed echocardiographic, hemodynamic, and angiographic studies.

Prognosis and treatment of patients with one of the positional anomalies is determined by the underlying defects. Cyanotic infants with pulmonic stenosis and ventricular septal defect as a part of the malformation improve after systemic to pulmonary artery shunts. Atrial septectomy, pulmonary artery banding, repair of associated coarctation of the aorta, and Fontan operations are utilized as indicated, depending on the anatomy and physiology. Multiple procedures are often required. Less complex lesions such as atrial or ventricular septal defect and tetralogy of Fallot can be repaired successfully.

14.32 PULMONARY ARTERIOVENOUS FISTULA

Fistulous vascular communications in the lungs may be large and localized or multiple, scattered, and small. The most common form of this unusual condition is the Rendu-Osler-Weber syndrome (hereditary hemorrhagic telangiectasia), which is also manifested by angiomas of the nasal and buccal mucous membranes, gastrointestinal tract, or liver. A direct communication between the pulmonary artery and left atrium is extremely rare.

Venous blood in the pulmonary artery is shunted through the fistula into the pulmonary vein without exposure to alveolar air, enters the left heart, and results in systemic arterial unsaturation. The shunt across the fistula is at low pressure and resistance so that pulmonary arterial pressure is normal; cardiomegaly and heart failure are not present.

The clinical picture depends on the magnitude of shunt. Dyspnea, cyanosis, clubbing, and polycythemia occur with large fistulas. Hemoptysis is rare, but may be massive. Features of the Rendu-Osler-Weber syndrome occur in about 50% of patients (or other members of their families) and include recurrent epistaxis and gastrointestinal bleeding. Transitory dizziness, diplopia, aphasia, motor weakness, or convulsions may result from cerebral thrombosis, abscess, or paradoxic emboli. Soft systolic or continuous murmurs may be audible over the site of the fistula.

The *electrocardiogram* is normal. *Roentgenographic examination* of the chest (Fig. 14–46A) may show opacities produced by large fistulas; multiple small fistulas may be visualized by fluoroscopy (abnormal pulsations) or tomography. Selective *pulmonary arteriography* demonstrates the site, extent, and distribution of the fistulas (Fig. 14–46B).

Excision of solitary or localized lesions by lobectomy or wedge resection results in complete disappearance of symptoms. However, in most instances fistulas are so widespread that surgery is not possible. If there is a direct communication between the pulmonary artery and left atrium, it can be obliterated by division and suture.

14.33 ECTOPIA CORDIS

In the most common thoracic form of ectopia cordis the sternum is split and the heart protrudes outside the chest. In others the heart protrudes through the diaphragm into the abdominal cavity or may be situated in the neck. Associated intracardiac anomalies are common. Death occurs in the first days of life in the majority of instances, usually from infection, cardiac failure, or hypoxemia. Surgical therapy for neonates without overwhelmingly severe cardiac anomalies consists of covering the heart with skin without compromising venous

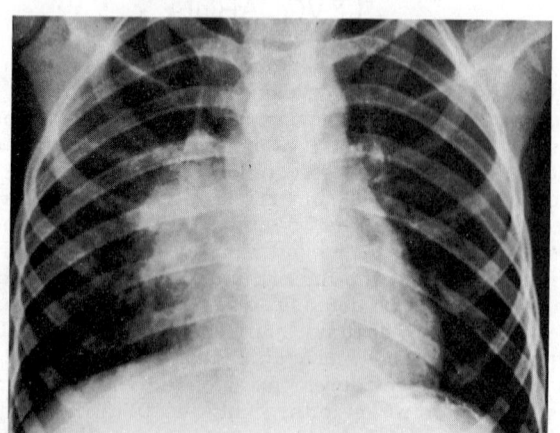
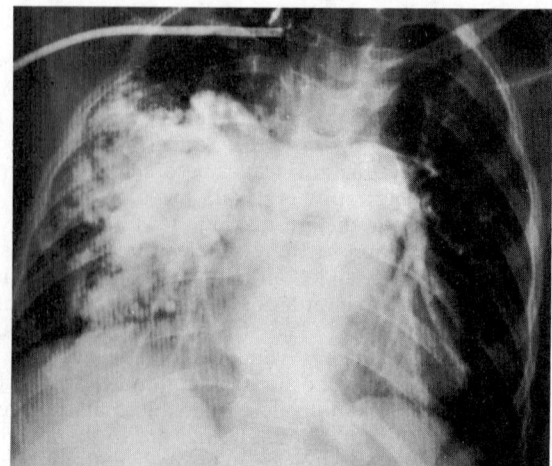

Figure 14–46. *A*, Roentgenogram of patient with pulmonary arteriovenous fistula, showing a localized increase in pulmonary vascularity in the right lung. *B*, Angiocardiogram showing contrast medium delineating the extent of the fistula in the right lung.

return or ventricular ejection. Palliation of associated defects is also often necessary. Occasional patients with the abdominal type have survived to adulthood.

14.34 DIVERTICULUM OF THE LEFT VENTRICLE

In this rare anomaly a diverticulum of the left ventricle protrudes into the epigastrium. The lesion may be isolated or associated with complex cardiovascular anomalies. A pulsating mass is visible and palpable in the epigastrium. Systolic or systolic-diastolic murmurs produced by blood flow in and out of the diverticulum may be audible over the lower sternum and the mass. The *electrocardiogram* shows a pattern of complete or incomplete left bundle branch block. *Roentgenograms* of the chest may or may not show the mass. Associated abnormalities include defects of the sternum, abdominal wall, diaphragm, and pericardium. Surgical treatment of the diverticulum and associated cardiac defects can be utilized in selected cases.

CONGENITAL HEART DISEASE WITH LITTLE OR NO CYANOSIS

14.35 VENTRICULAR SEPTAL DEFECTS (VSD)

Ventricular septal defect is the most common cardiac malformation, accounting for 25% of congenital heart disease. The majority of defects are of the membranous type in a posteroinferior position, anterior to the septal leaflet of the tricuspid valve. Defects between the crista supraventricularis and the papillary muscle of the conus may be associated with pulmonary stenosis and the other manifestations of tetralogy of Fallot. Defects superior to the crista supraventricularis are less common; they are found just beneath the pulmonary valve and may impinge on an aortic sinus, causing aortic insufficiency. Defects in the midportion or apical region of the ventricular septum or apical area are muscular in type and may be single or multiple.

Pathophysiology. If the defect is small, the cardiac chambers and pulmonary vascular bed are normal. Large defects produce more significant left to right shunts and result in left ventricular volume overload as well as right ventricular and pulmonary artery hypertension. The left atrium and ventricle are enlarged because of the large left to right shunt. The pulmonary arterial trunk is large. After birth, in the presence of a large VSD, pulmonary resistance may remain higher than in a normal infant and left to right shunt may be limited. However, within a few weeks there is relatively normal involution of muscular media of the small pulmonary arteries and arterioles. A large left to right shunt ensues, and clinical symptoms become apparent. In some patients with large VSD, medial thickness remains present and, with time, intimal arteriolar pathologic changes occur; this group of patients will eventually shunt right to left and can be characterized as having the Eisenmenger syndrome (Sec. 14.29). However, the great majority of patients with large VSD have a massive left to right shunt. Progressive increases in pulmonary resistance are rarely seen in the present era when prolonged pulmonary hypertension is prevented by early surgical intervention for large VSD.

Hemodynamics. The magnitude of the left to right shunt is determined by the size of the defect and the degree of pulmonary vascular resistance compared to systemic resistance. In most instances, pulmonary resistance is only slightly elevated, and the major contribution to pulmonary hypertension is the extremely large blood flow through the right heart and pulmonary artery. When a small communication is present, the defect is restrictive and right ventricular pressure is normal.

Clinical Manifestations. These vary according to the size of the defect and the pulmonary blood flow and pressure. Small defects with trivial left to right shunts and normal pulmonary arterial pressures are the most common. The patients are asymptomatic, and the cardiac lesion is usually found during routine physical examination. Characteristically, there is a loud, harsh, or blowing left parasternal pansystolic murmur, heard best over the lower left sternal border and frequently accompanied by a thrill (Fig. 14–47). In a few instances the murmur ends well before the 2nd sound, presumably because of closure of the defect during late systole. The left to right shunt is limited in the neonate, and therefore systolic murmur may not be audible during the 1st days of life. In premature infants the murmur may be heard early since pulmonary vascular resistance appears to decrease more rapidly. *Roentgenograms* are usually normal, although minimal cardiomegaly and borderline increase in pulmonary vasculature may be observed. The *electrocardiogram* is usually normal but may suggest left ventricular hypertrophy.

Large defects with excessive pulmonary blood flow and pulmonary hypertension are responsible for dyspnea, feeding difficulties, poor growth, profuse perspiration, recurrent pulmonary infections, and cardiac failure in early infancy. Cyanosis is absent, but duskiness is sometimes noted during infections or crying. In the absence of heart failure, arterial and venous pulses are normal. Prominence of the left precordium and sternum is common, as are cardiomegaly, a palpable parasternal lift, an apical thrust, and a systolic thrill. The systolic murmur may be similar to that of smaller defects, but the sound of pulmonary valvular closure is louder, and the

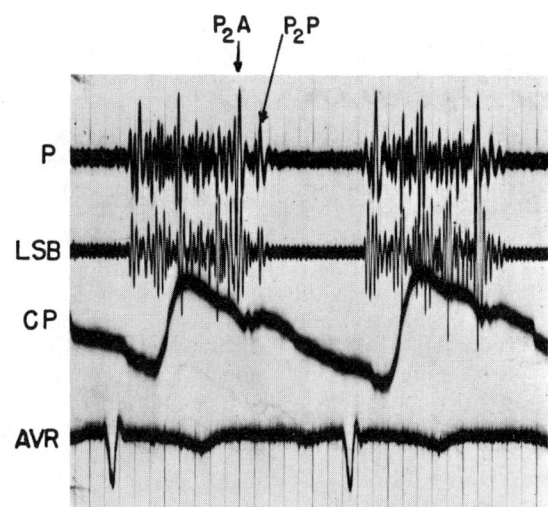

Figure 14–47. Phonocardiograms (P, pulmonary area; LSB, left sternal border) to illustrate auscultatory findings in moderate-sized ventricular septal defect with normal pulmonary arterial pressure. Long pansystolic murmur is evident. AVR, electrocardiogram; CP, carotid pulse; P_2A, aortic components of 2nd sound; P_2P, pulmonary component of 2nd sound.

2nd sound may be virtually single. The presence of a short apical mid-diastolic rumble is caused by increased blood flow across the mitral valve, and indicates an appreciable left to right shunt. *Roentgenographically,* gross cardiomegaly is present with prominence of both ventricles, the left atrium, and pulmonary artery. The *electrocardiogram* shows biventricular hypertrophy; P waves may be notched or peaked. The *two-dimensional echocardiogram* shows volume overload of the left atrium and ventricle; the extent of their increased dimensions reflects the size of the left to right shunt. The position and size of the VSD can be visualized.

Diagnosis. The effects of a VSD on the circulation may be documented by cardiac catheterization. However, this diagnostic procedure is not required when it is clear that an isolated small defect is present. Since oxygenated blood passes across the defect from the left ventricle, blood from the right ventricle is higher in oxygen content than that from the right atrium; this increase is occasionally apparent only in pulmonary arterial blood. Small shunts may not result in a detectable increase in oxygen saturation in the right ventricle, but may be demonstrated by indicator dilution tests (Fig. 14–28). Small defects are associated with normal right heart pressure and pulmonary vascular resistance. Pulmonary blood flow in patients with large defects associated with equal pulmonary and systemic pressures may be more than three times the systemic flow. Pulmonary vascular resistance is only minimally elevated in these patients. The location and number of ventricular defects are demonstrated by left ventriculography. Contrast medium passes across the defect(s) to opacify the right ventricle and pulmonary artery.

Prognosis and Complications. The natural course of VSD includes the following:

1. A significant number (30–50%) of small defects close spontaneously, most frequently during the first year of life. It is less common for moderate or large defects to close spontaneously, although even defects large enough to result in heart failure may become smaller and even rarely close completely.

2. A large number of children remain asymptomatic without evidence of increase in heart size, pulmonary arterial pressure, or resistance.

3. Infective endocarditis occurs in fewer than 1%.

4. A significant number of infants with large defects have repeated episodes of respiratory infection and congestive heart failure.

5. Pulmonary hypertension occurs as a result of high pulmonary blood flow. A few patients will develop elevated pulmonary vascular resistance with time if the defect is not repaired.

6. A small number acquire pulmonary stenosis, which protects the pulmonary circulation from the long-term effects of pulmonary hypertension. In these patients the clinical picture changes from VSD with large left to right shunt to VSD with pulmonary stenosis, and a diminished left to right shunt, a balanced shunt, or a right to left shunt (Sec. 14.14).

Treatment. Parents should be reassured of the benign nature of the small defect, and the child should be encouraged to live a normal life. Surgical repair is not recommended. As a protection against infective endocarditis the integrity of primary and permanent teeth should be carefully maintained; antibiotic prophylaxis should be provided for dental surgery, tonsillectomy, adenoidectomy, and other oropharyngeal surgical procedures as well as for instrumentation of the genitourinary and lower intestinal tracts.

The medical management of infants with a large VSD is primarily aimed at the control of congestive cardiac failure. These patients may show signs of repeated or chronic pulmonary disease and often fail to thrive. If early treatment is successful, the shunt may diminish in size with spontaneous improvement, especially during the first year of life. Since surgical closure can be carried out at low risk in most patients, medical management should not be pursued in symptomatic infants after an unsuccessful trial. Furthermore, pulmonary vascular disease is prevented when surgery is performed in the first 2 yr of life. Thus, the large defects associated with pulmonary hypertension should be closed even electively early in the second year of life. Surgical complications resulting in long-term problems (e.g., heart block) are extremely rare. Early correction is advised in infants with moderate to high elevation of pulmonary artery pressures and large left to right shunts who have failed to respond to maximal medical therapy. The patient's age and size are not prohibitive factors, since successful surgery can be performed on infants.

After obliteration of the left to right shunt the hyperdynamic heart becomes quiet, cardiac size decreases toward normal (Fig. 14–48), thrills and murmurs are abolished, and pulmonary artery hypertension regresses. The patient's clinical status improves markedly. The infant begins to thrive, and cardiac medications are no longer required. In some instances after successful operation, systolic ejection murmurs of low intensity persist for months. The long-term prognosis after surgery is excellent.

14.36 VENTRICULAR SEPTAL DEFECT WITH AORTIC INSUFFICIENCY

In this syndrome the VSD is complicated by prolapse of the aortic valve and aortic insufficiency. It accounts for approximately 5% of patients with ventricular septal defect; a considerably larger incidence is reported among Japanese children. The septal defect, which is small or moderate in size, is usually anterior and subpulmonary (outlet septum); in some cases the VSD is infracristal. The right or less often the noncoronary cusp prolapses into the defect. The VSD may be partially or even completely closed in this manner. Aortic insufficiency is most often not recognized until later in the first decade of life or beyond. Early congestive heart failure secondary to a large left to right shunt rarely occurs, but without operation, severe aortic insufficiency and left ventricular failure may ensue. The physical signs of aortic insufficiency (diastolic murmur and wide pulse pressure) are added to those of VSD. This entity should not be confused with patent ductus arteriosus or other defects associated with aortic runoff.

The *clinical manifestations* vary widely, from trivial aortic regurgitation and small left to right shunt in the asymptomatic child to the symptomatic adolescent with florid aortic incompetence, congestive cardiac failure, angina pectoris, and massive cardiomegaly. Patients having a significant aortic incompetence urgently require surgical intervention to prevent irreversible left ventricular dysfunction. Repair of the aortic valve may be possible only with a prosthesis, but every attempt should be made to achieve a competent valve by means of valvuloplasty. The degree to which aortic insufficiency is affected by closure of the septal defect alone early in the course of the disease is questionable. The asymptomatic child with a small VSD and mild aortic insufficiency should be observed carefully for progression of severity of the insufficiency.

14.37 VENTRICULAR SEPTAL DEFECT WITH LEFT VENTRICULAR–RIGHT ATRIAL SHUNT

Ventricular defects may be associated with an abnormal septal leaflet of the tricuspid valve. During left ventricular systole, arterialized blood is ejected through the defect into the right atrium. The physical signs are those of VSD. Cardiac catheterization reveals a left to right shunt at the atrial level

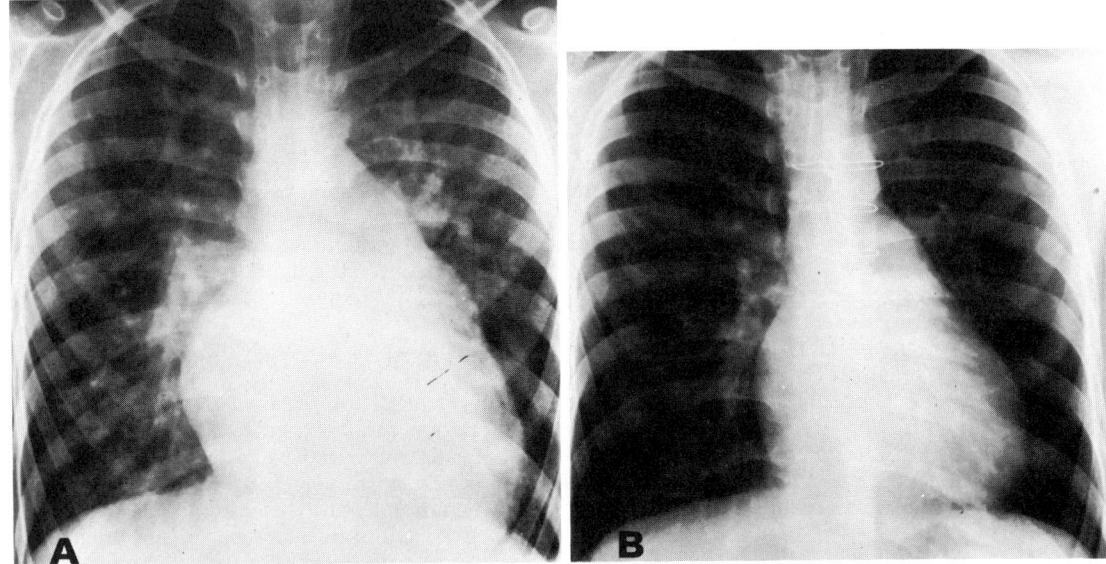

Figure 14–48. *A*, Preoperative roentgenogram in ventricular septal defect with large left to right shunt and pulmonary hypertension. Significant cardiomegaly, prominence of the pulmonary arterial trunk, and pulmonary overcirculation are evident. *B*, Three years after surgical closure of defect. There is marked decrease in heart size, and the pulmonary vasculature is normal.

and may result in the misdiagnosis of atrial septal defect. The diagnosis may be confirmed by left ventriculography; the right atrium opacifies immediately after delivery of contrast medium to the left ventricle. Treatment is surgical closure of the ventricular defect. An isolated left ventricular–right atrial shunt is a rare anomaly.

14.38 DOUBLE-OUTLET RIGHT VENTRICLE
(Origin of Both Great Arteries from the Right Ventricle)

In this anomaly both the aorta and the pulmonary artery arise from the right ventricle (Sec. 14.18). The only outlet from the left ventricle is a ventricular septal defect. The clinical picture closely simulates that of an uncomplicated VSD with a large left to right shunt and pulmonary hypertension. The *electrocardiogram* usually shows a left superior axis and biventricular hypertrophy. *Echocardiography* is diagnostic, showing the right ventricular origin of both great vessels and their anteroposterior relationship as well as the position of the VSD. The condition may also be diagnosed by *left ventricular angiogram*, which demonstrates the commitment of the VSD to one or both of the great arteries. The size of the outlet from the left ventricle confirms mitral-aortic discontinuity and shows the high position of the aortic valve which is at the same level as the pulmonary valve. It is important to differentiate this condition from simple VSD. Surgical correction is accomplished by an intraventricular repair which funnels the ejection of left ventricular blood via the VSD into the aorta without obstructing right ventricular outflow. Pulmonary artery banding may be required in infancy, followed by surgical correction during the preschool years. Natural pulmonary stenosis is common.

In **double outlet right ventricle with transposition of the great arteries** the VSD is supracristal and subpulmonary **(Taussig-Bing complex)** or related to both pulmonary and aortic valves (doubly committed). These patients develop cyanosis early in life and have poor physical development, pulmonary hypertension, and cardiac failure. Cardiomegaly is usual, and there is a parasternal ejection systolic murmur, sometimes preceded by an ejection click and a loud closure

of the pulmonary valve. Left-sided obstructive lesions are frequently associated; these include aortic coarctation, interruption of the aortic arch, and a small VSD which is restrictive to left ventricular ejection. The *electrocardiogram* shows right axis deviation and right, left, or biventricular hypertrophy. The *roentgenogram* documents the cardiomegaly, the large left atrium, and prominence of the pulmonary trunk and vasculature. The anatomic features of the anomaly and associated abnormalities are best demonstrated by a combination of echocardiography and selective right and left ventriculography. Palliation by pulmonary artery banding in infancy will permit surgical correction at a later age, which may be accomplished by a Rastelli procedure (Sec. 14.21) or by closure of the VSD incorporating the pulmonary outflow tract into the left ventricle, coupled with a Mustard or Senning procedure.

14.39 L-TRANSPOSITION OF THE GREAT ARTERIES
(Corrected Transposition)

This malformation consists of discordant atrial-ventricular relationships (ventricular inversion) and transposition of the great arteries. Systemic blood is returned to a normal right atrium, from which it passes through a bicuspid atrioventricular valve into a right-sided ventricle that has the architecture and smooth wall appearance of the normal left ventricle. The venous blood is then ejected via the transposed pulmonary artery into the lungs. Pulmonary venous blood returns to a normal left atrium, passes through a tricuspid valve into a left-sided ventricle, which has the internal structure of a normal right ventricle, and is then ejected into the transposed aorta. The pulmonary artery lies in a medial position and the ascending aorta lies to the left and lateral, almost in the same horizontal plane. The double inversion of atrioventricular and ventriculoarterial relationships results in desaturated right atrial blood reaching the lungs, and pulmonary venous blood appropriately flowing to the aorta. Thus, the circulation is "corrected." Without other defects, the hemodynamics would be normal. However, in almost every instance associated anomalies coexist; most common are VSD, abnormalities of the left atrioventricular valve (tricuspid), pulmonary valvular and/or subvalvular stenosis, and atrioventricular conduction disturbances (complete heart block).

Symptoms and signs are determined by the associated lesions. Posteroanterior chest *roentgenograms* may suggest the abnormal position of the great arteries; the ascending aorta occupies the upper left border of the cardiac silhouette and has a straight profile. In addition to atrioventricular conduction disturbances, *electrocardiograms* may show abnormal P waves; absent QV_6; initial Q waves in leads III, aVR, aVF, and V_1; and upright T waves across the precordium.

Surgical treatment of the associated anomalies, most often the VSD, is complicated by the position of the bundle of His, which can be injured at the time of surgery, causing heart block. Identification of the usual course of the bundle in corrected transposition (superior to the defect) has been accomplished by mapping of the conduction system at surgery. This has been an important step in eliminating this sequela in those patients who were initially in sinus rhythm.

14.40 OTHER DEFECTS ASSOCIATED WITH VENTRICULAR SEPTAL DEFECT

Patent Ductus Arteriosus (PDA). In most infants with large ventricular septal defects and PDA the signs of the VSD dominate; the murmur of the patent ductus is inaudible. In such cases the passage of the cardiac catheter from the pulmonary artery through the ductus and into the descending aorta is diagnostic (as is the aortic angiogram). In addition, two-dimensional echocardiographic and Doppler studies can suggest the presence of the patent ductus. The ventricular defect and the patent ductus are closed during the same operation. When these lesions coexist, an unsuspected PDA may complicate the cardiopulmonary bypass procedure for repair of the VSD.

Multiple Ventricular Septal Defects. In some instances there are multiple defects involving the ventricular septum. Generally, these patients have signs of a large left to right shunt and pulmonary hypertension in infancy. Multiple defects cannot be detected clinically, and small muscular defects are not easily recognized by two-dimensional echocardiography. A left ventricular angiogram in the left anterior oblique view shows the septum in profile and permits identification of the number and location of the defects. Observation of the entire ventricular septum is indicated during open cardiotomy to ensure that all defects have been closed. A surgical approach from the left ventricle has been utilized for apical muscular defects because the smooth nontrabecular left septal surface allows defects to be more easily identified. However, this approach may increase the complications after surgery. In the presence of multiple defects in an infant who requires intervention, pulmonary artery banding may be more prudent (with debanding and closure of the VSD later in childhood).

Atrial Septal Defect. In patients with a ventricular defect and an ostium secundum atrial defect the physical signs are usually dominated by the ventricular defect. The clinical picture is similar to that of moderate-sized or large VSD. This combination of defects may result in congestive heart failure in infancy and should be suspected during cardiac catheterization if left to right shunts are demonstrated at both the atrial and ventricular levels. During atriotomy for closure of ventricular defects the atrial septum is easily explored; if both defects are present, they can be repaired during the same procedure.

Coarctation of the Aorta. Most infants with congestive failure in the presence of coarctation (Sec. 14.56) also have a ventricular septal defect.

14.41 ATRIAL SEPTAL DEFECT

An isolated patent foramen ovale is of no clinical significance and is not considered to be an atrial septal defect. However, if right atrial pressure is increased secondary to another defect (e.g., pulmonary stenosis or atresia, tricuspid abnormalities, right ventricular dysfunction), venous blood may be shunted across the patent foramen ovale into the left atrium with resultant cyanosis. Because of the anatomic structure of a patent foramen ovale, blood cannot be shunted from the left atrium to the right atrium. An isolated patent foramen ovale does not require treatment.

14.42 OSTIUM SECUNDUM DEFECT

This defect in the region of the fossa ovalis is associated with normal atrioventricular valves at birth. Late myxomatous changes in the mitral valve have been described, but this is only rarely an important clinical consideration. The defects may be multiple, and in symptomatic older children openings of 2 cm or more in diameter are not unusual. Large defects may extend inferiorly toward the inferior vena cava and ostium of the coronary sinus, superiorly toward the superior vena cava, or posteriorly.

Hemodynamics. A considerable shunt of oxygenated blood flows from the left to the right atrium. This blood is added to the usual venous return to the right atrium and is pumped by the right ventricle to the lungs. Pulmonary blood flow is usually 2–4 times systemic flow. The principal factor that determines the direction of shunt is the diastolic compliance of the chambers of the right heart. The paucity of symptoms in infants with atrial septal defects is related to the structure of the right ventricle in early life when its muscular wall is thick and less compliant, thus limiting the left to right shunt. As the infant becomes older, the right ventricular wall becomes thinner as a result of its lower pressure generating requirements, and the left to right shunt across the atrial defect increases. The large blood flow through the right side of the heart results in enlargement of the right atrium and ventricle and dilatation of the pulmonary artery. Despite the large pulmonary blood flow, the pulmonary arterial pressure remains normal, since pulmonary vascular resistance remains extremely low. The left ventricle and aorta are normal in size. Cyanosis is extremely rare, seen only occasionally in adults with the complicating features of pulmonary vascular disease.

Clinical Manifestations. A child with an ostium secundum defect is most often asymptomatic, and the lesion may be discovered inadvertently during a physical examination. Even an extremely large ASD (secundum) rarely produces heart failure in childhood; in older children varying degrees of exercise intolerance may be noted. In older infants and children the physical findings are often characteristic, but require careful attention.

The pulses are normal. A right ventricular systolic lift is usually palpable from the left sternal border to the midclavicular line. The systolic murmur is of the ejection type, is medium pitched, is seldom accompanied by a thrill, and is best heard at the left mid and upper sternal border. It is produced by the increased flow across the right ventricular outflow tract into the pulmonary artery. The murmur is preceded by a loud 1st heart sound and sometimes by a pulmonic ejection click. In most patients the 2nd heart sound at the upper left sternal edge is widely split and fixed in all phases of respiration. This auscultatory finding is characteristic (Fig. 14–49) and is due to constantly increased right ventricular diastolic volume and prolonged ejection time. A short early diastolic murmur produced by the high blood flow across the tricuspid valve often is audible at the lower left

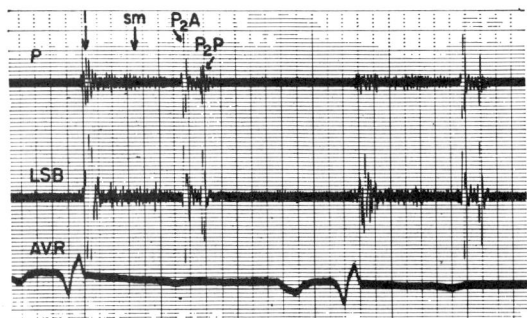

Figure 14–49. Phonocardiograms (P, pulmonary area; LSB, left sternal border) to illustrate auscultatory findings in ostium secundum atrial septal defect. AVR, electrocardiogram; P_2A, aortic component of 2nd sound; P_2P, pulmonary component of 2nd sound; sm, systolic murmur; 1, 1st heart sound. Note wide splitting of 2nd sound. This splitting persisted in all phases of respiration. Time lines 0.04 sec.

sternal border. This finding, which may be subtle, is an excellent diagnostic sign.

Diagnosis. *Roentgenograms* show varying degrees of enlargement of the right ventricle and atrium; the left ventricle and aorta are small. The pulmonary artery is large, and the pulmonary vascularity increased. These signs vary and may not be conspicuous in mild cases. Cardiac enlargement is often best appreciated on the lateral view, since the right ventricle protrudes anteriorly with increased volume.

The *electrocardiogram* shows diastolic overload of the right ventricle with right axis deviation or a normal axis, and right ventricular conduction delay (usually rsR' in right precordial leads); the presence of an ASD is unusual in the absence of right ventricular conduction delay.

The *echocardiogram* shows findings characteristic of right ventricular volume overload, including increased right ventricular end-diastolic dimension and abnormal motion of the ventricular septum. The normal septum moves posteriorly during systole and anteriorly during diastole. With right ventricular overload and normal pulmonary vascular resistance, the septal motion is reversed, i.e., anterior movement in systole, or the motion is intermediate so that the septum remains straight. The location and size of the atrial defect are readily appreciated. In many centers, patients with classic features of ASD secundum, including echocardiographic identification of a well-defined defect, are not catheterized prior to surgical closure.

The diagnosis may be confirmed by *cardiac catheterization.* The oxygen content of blood from the right atrium is much higher than that from the superior vena cava. This feature is not diagnostic since it may occur with anomalous pulmonary venous return to the right atrium, with ventricular septal defect and tricuspid insufficiency, with ventricular septal defects associated with left ventricular–right atrial shunts, and with aortic–right atrial communications (e.g., ruptured sinus of Valsalva). The physical signs produced by the latter three anomalies generally differ greatly from those of atrial septal defects, and their presence can usually be confirmed by selective angiocardiography. Occasionally, mixing of blood is incomplete in the right atrium, and the principal site of shunt appears to be at the ventricular level when this is not the case.

The catheter often enters the left atrium from the right atrium. Indicator dilution curves may be used to demonstrate the site of the left to right shunt and the presence of anomalous pulmonary veins. Streaming of inferior vena caval blood across the defect to the left atrium may occur with uncomplicated atrial septal defects. This small right to left shunt may be demonstrated by indicator dilution curves but rarely results in significant arterial unsaturation or cyanosis. The pressures

in the right side of the heart are usually normal, but small to moderate pressure gradients may be measured across the right ventricular outflow. In the absence of associated organic pulmonary stenosis they are probably due to functional stenosis related to excessive blood flow. The pulmonary arteriolar resistance is almost always normal or lower than normal. The shunt is variable depending on the size of the defect, but it may be considerable (as high as 20 L/min/m²).

Prognosis and Complications. Secundum atrial septal defects are well tolerated during childhood; symptoms usually appear in the 3rd decade or later. Pulmonary hypertension, atrial dysrhythmias, tricuspid or mitral incompetence, and heart failure are late manifestations. Infective endocarditis is extremely rare.

Secundum atrial septal defects are usually isolated, although they may be associated with partial anomalous pulmonary venous return, pulmonary valvular stenosis, ventricular septal defect, pulmonary arterial branch stenosis, and persistent left superior vena cava, as well as mitral valve insufficiency.

Treatment. Closure is carried out at open-heart surgery. The mortality rate from surgery is less than 1%, and surgery is advised even for asymptomatic patients prior to entry into school. It is preferred during childhood because the surgical mortality and morbidity are greater in adulthood when late signs are present. Eliminating the increased risks of pregnancy is another important reason to intervene early in females. Mild symptoms with exercise, and submaximal physical performance during sports activities are also prevented by early elective repair.

The results after operation in children with large shunts are excellent. Symptoms disappear rapidly, and physical development frequently appears enhanced. The heart size decreases to normal, and the electrocardiogram shows decreased right ventricular forces. Late arrhythmias are less frequent and of lesser importance in patients who have had early repair.

14.43 SINUS VENOSUS DEFECT

The defect is situated in the upper part of the atrial septum in close relation to the entry of the superior vena cava. One or more pulmonary veins (usually from the right lung) drain anomalously into the superior vena cava. Sometimes the superior vena cava straddles the defect; some systemic venous blood then enters the left atrium. The abnormal hemodynamics are similar to those of secundum atrial septal defect, e.g., a volume overload of the right ventricle. The clinical picture, electrocardiogram, and roentgenogram are also similar to those of secundum atrial septal defect. The diagnosis is often made by two-dimensional echocardiography. If cardiac catheterization is carried out, the catheter may enter a pulmonary vein from the superior vena cava. Anatomic correction usually requires the insertion of a patch to close the defect while incorporating the entry of anomalous veins into the left atrium; surgical results are generally excellent.

14.44 PARTIAL ANOMALOUS PULMONARY VENOUS RETURN

A varying number of pulmonary veins may enter the systemic venous circulation or the right atrium and produce a left to right shunt of oxygenated blood, which may be further augmented if there is an associated atrial septal defect. Partial anomalous pulmonary venous return usually involves some or all of the veins from only one lung, more often the right. An associated atrial septal defect usually is of the sinus venosus type (Sec. 14.43). The history, physical signs, electrocardiogram, and roentgenographic findings are indistinguishable from those of atrial septal defect (ostium secundum).

Occasionally, an anomalous vein draining into the inferior vena cava is visible roentgenographically as a crescentic shadow of vascular density along the right border of the cardiac silhouette (scimitar syndrome); an atrial septal defect is usually not present. The finding of a sinus venosus atrial septal defect by echocardiography is often accompanied by the identification or suspicion of associated partial anomalous pulmonary venous return. See Sec. 14.25 for discussion of *total anomalous pulmonary venous return.*

During *cardiac catheterization* the catheter may enter the anomalous pulmonary vein from the superior vena cava or right atrium and may traverse the associated atrial septal defect. Frequently, the oxygen content and saturation of the caval and right atrial blood are indistinguishable from those associated with atrial septal defect. The presence of anomalous pulmonary veins may be demonstrated by *selective pulmonary arteriography.*

The prognosis is excellent, similar to that for atrial septal defect (ostium secundum). When a large left to right shunt is present, surgical repair is carried out during cardiopulmonary bypass. The associated atrial septal defect should be closed in such a way as to direct the pulmonary venous return to the left atrium. A single anomalous pulmonary vein without an atrial communication may be difficult to redirect to the left atrium and may be left unoperated.

14.45 OSTIUM PRIMUM DEFECT AND COMMON ATRIOVENTRICULAR CANAL
(Endocardial Cushion Defects)

These abnormalities are grouped together because they represent a spectrum of a basic embryologic abnormality, a deficiency of the endocardial cushions and atrioventricular septum.

The *ostium primum defect* is situated in the lower portion of the atrial septum and overlies the mitral and tricuspid valves. In the majority of instances there is a cleft in the anterior leaflet of the mitral valve. The tricuspid valve is usually functionally normal, although some abnormality of the septal leaflet is present. The ventricular septum is intact.

Common atrioventricular canal (atrioventricular septal defect) consists of a contiguous interatrial and interventricular defect with markedly abnormal atrioventricular valves. The valve, virtually single and common to both ventricles, consists of an anterior and a posterior leaflet related to the ventricular septum with a lateral leaflet in each ventricle. The lesion is common among children with Down syndrome and may occur with pulmonary stenosis (Sec. 14.14 and 14.50).

Transitional varieties of these defects also occur. They include ostium primum defects with clefts in the anterior mitral and septal tricuspid valve leaflets, mild ventricular septal deficiencies, and, less commonly, ostium primum defects with normal atrioventricular valves. In some patients, the atrial septum is intact, but the ventricular septal defect simulates that found in common atrioventricular canal. These defects are also associated with deformities of the atrioventricular valves.

Hemodynamics. The basic abnormality is the combination of a left to right shunt across the atrial defect with mitral incompetence. The shunt is usually moderate to large. The degree of mitral incompetence is ordinarily mild to moderate. Pulmonary arterial pressures are usually normal or only mildly increased.

In *common atrioventricular canal* the left to right shunt is both transatrial and transventricular. Pulmonary hypertension and increased pulmonary vascular resistance are common. Atrioventricular valvular incompetence results in regurgitation of blood from the ventricles to both atria. Some right to left shunting occurs at both atrial and ventricular levels. Although it is usually small in volume, there may be significant arterial

unsaturation. Progressive pulmonary vascular disease will increase the right to left shunt so that more severe cyanosis may develop.

Clinical Manifestations. Many children with *ostium primum defect* are asymptomatic, and the anomaly is discovered during a general physical examination. In patients with moderate shunts and trivial mitral incompetence, the physical signs are similar to those of atrial defect of the secundum type, but with an additional apical systolic murmur.

A history of effort intolerance, easy fatigability, and recurrent pneumonitis may be obtained, especially in infants with large left to right shunts and severe mitral incompetence. In these patients cardiac enlargement is moderate or marked and the precordium is hyperdynamic. The auscultatory signs produced by the left to right shunt include a normal or accentuated 1st sound, wide, fixed splitting of the 2nd sound, a pulmonary ejection systolic murmur sometimes preceded by a click, and a low-pitched early diastolic murmur at the lower left sternal edge and/or apex. Mitral incompetence may be manifested by an apical pansystolic murmur which radiates to the left axilla.

With *common atrioventricular canal*, congestive heart failure and intercurrent pulmonary infection usually appear in infancy. During these episodes minimal cyanosis may be evident. The neck veins are prominent, liver is enlarged, and the infant shows signs of failure to thrive. Cardiac enlargement is moderate to marked, and a systolic thrill is frequently palpable. The 1st heart sound is normal or accentuated and is followed by a widely distributed, harsh systolic murmur. The 2nd heart sound is widely split if pulmonary flow is massive. A low-pitched early diastolic murmur is audible at the lower left sternal edge, and a pulmonic systolic ejection murmur is produced by the large pulmonary flow. The apical pansystolic murmur of mitral insufficiency may also be present.

Diagnosis. *Roentgenograms* of children with endocardial cushion defects confirm the cardiac enlargement due to prominence of both ventricles and the right atrium. The pulmonary artery is large, and pulmonary vascularity is increased.

The *electrocardiograms* of children with endocardial cushion defects are distinctive. The principal abnormalities are (1) superior orientation of the mean frontal QRS axis with left axis deviation to the left or right upper quadrant; (2) counterclockwise inscription of the superiorly oriented QRS vector loop; (3) signs of biventricular hypertrophy or isolated right ventricular hypertrophy; (4) right ventricular conduction delay (VSR' in leads V_3R and V_1); (5) normal or tall P waves; and (6) occasional prolongation of the P-R interval (Fig. 14-50).

The *echocardiogram* is characteristic and shows signs of right ventricular enlargement with encroachment of the mitral valve echo on the left ventricular outflow; this corresponds to the angiographic "goose-neck" deformity. In the common atrioventricular canal, the ventricular septal echo is also deficient and the atrioventricular valve abnormalities are readily appreciated (Fig. 14-51).

Cardiac catheterization and *angiocardiography* confirm the diagnosis. These studies demonstrate the magnitude of the left to right shunt, the severity of pulmonary hypertension, the degree of elevation of pulmonary vascular resistance, and the severity of incompetence of the atrioventricular valve. The shunt is usually demonstrable at the atrial level; in some patients, increased oxygen saturations are noted only in the right ventricle, because of streaming of blood across the primum defect just proximal to the tricuspid valve. The arterial oxygen saturation is normal or mildly reduced unless severe pulmonary hypertension is present. In these patients larger right to left shunt may be demonstrable. Children with ostium primum defects usually have normal or only moderate elevation of the pulmonary arterial pressure. On the other hand,

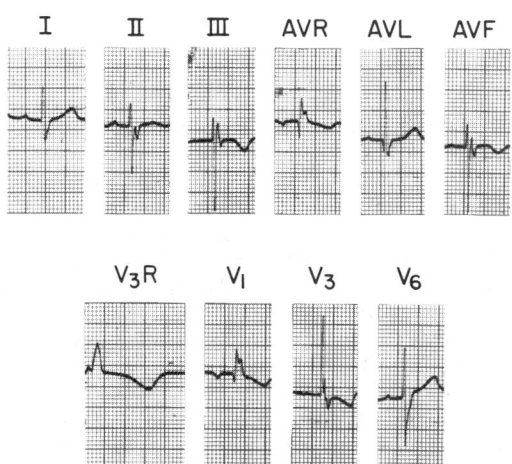

Figure 14–50. Electrocardiogram from a child with atrioventricular canal. Note the QRS axis of −60°, and the RV conduction delay; RSR' in V_1 and V_3R. (V_3R paper speed = 50 mm/sec.)

common atrioventricular canal is associated with right ventricular and pulmonary hypertension as well as with an increase in pulmonary vascular resistance in older patients. The cardiac catheter readily enters the chambers of the left side of the heart from the right side, especially if there is a common atrioventricular canal.

Selective left ventriculography is extremely helpful in diagnosis of endocardial cushion defects. The deformity of the mitral or common atrioventricular valve and the distortion of the outflow of the left ventricle, the goose-neck deformity, are demonstrated. The abnormal anterior leaflet of the mitral valve is serrated, and mitral incompetence is noted, usually with regurgitation of blood to both the left and right atria.

Prognosis. The prognosis for endocardial cushion defects depends on the magnitude of the left to right shunt, the degree of pulmonary vascular resistance, and the severity of mitral incompetence. Death from congestive cardiac failure during infancy is common with common atrioventricular canal not treated by operation. Patients who survive without surgery are likely to develop pulmonary vascular obstructive disease. Most patients with ostium primum defects are asymptomatic or have only minor, nonprogressive symptoms until they reach the 3rd–4th decade of life, similar to the course of patients with secundum defects.

Treatment. Ostium primum defects are approached surgically from an incision in the right atrium. The cleft in the mitral valve is located through the atrial defect and is repaired by direct suture. The defect in the atrial septum is usually closed by insertion of a patch prosthesis. The surgical mortality rate for primum defects is low. Surgical treatment for common atrioventricular canal is more difficult, especially in infants with congestive cardiac failure and pulmonary hypertension. Pulmonary arterial banding has been successful as early palliation in severely ill infants with dominant shunts at the ventricular level. However, successful open heart correction of these defects can be accomplished even in infancy. The atrial and ventricular defects are closed and atrioventricular valves reconstructed. Prosthetic valves are rarely required.

14.46 PATENT DUCTUS ARTERIOSUS (PDA)

During fetal life most of the pulmonary arterial blood is shunted through the ductus arteriosus into the aorta (Sec. 14.10). Functional closure of the ductus normally occurs soon after birth, but if the ductus remains patent when pulmonary vascular resistance falls, aortic blood is shunted into the pulmonary artery. The aortic end of the ductus is just distal to the origin of the left subclavian artery, and the ductus enters the pulmonary artery at its bifurcation. PDA is one of the most common congenital cardiovascular anomalies associated with maternal rubella during early pregnancy.

When a term infant is found to have a PDA, there is deficiency of both the mucoid endothelial layer and the muscular media of the ductus. The premature infant with a patent ductus, however, has a normal structural anatomy; patency is the result of immaturity. Thus a PDA in a term infant will rarely close spontaneously, while in the premature baby, in whom early pharmacologic or surgical intervention was not required, spontaneous closure occurs in most instances.

Hemodynamics. As a result of the higher aortic pressure, blood flow through the ductus goes from the aorta to the pulmonary artery. The extent of shunt depends on the size of the ductus and the pulmonary vascular resistance. In extreme cases 50–65% of the left ventricular output may be shunted through the ductus to the pulmonary circulation. The pressures within the pulmonary artery, the right ventricle, and the right atrium are normal if the PDA is small, but they may be elevated moderately or even to systemic levels with large communications (Sec. 14.11). There is a wide pulse pressure due to runoff of blood into the pulmonary artery during diastole. The total blood volume is increased.

Clinical Manifestations. There are usually no symptoms with a small ductus. A large defect will result in left ventricular

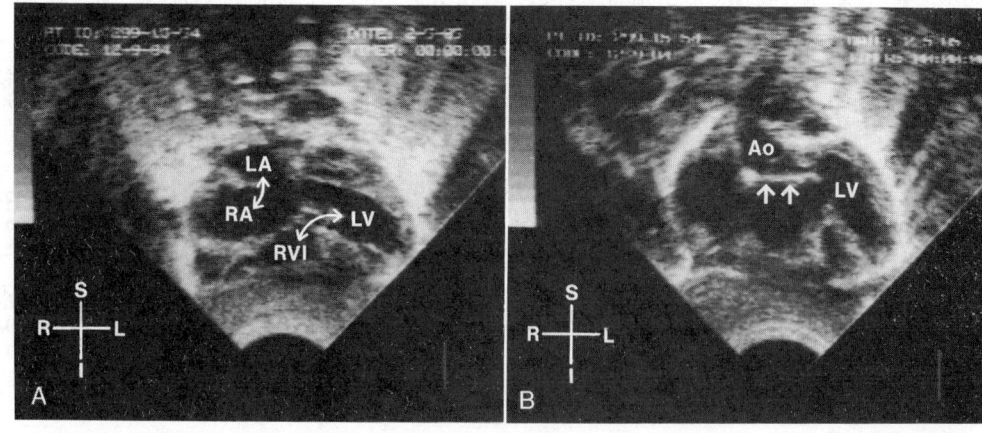

Figure 14–51. Common atrioventricular defect. *A*, Four chamber view demonstrating both interatrial and interventricular septal defect contributing to the large central communication of this lesion (*arrows*). *B*, Left ventricular long axis projection demonstrating the typical goose neck deformity created by the anterior leaflet of the mitral valve (*arrows*). RA, right atrium; LA, left atrium; RVI, right ventricular inflow; LV, left ventricle; R, right; L, left; S, superior; I, inferior; Ao, aorta.

failure similar to that in infants with large VSD and pulmonary hypertension. Retardation of physical growth may be a major manifestation in infants with large shunts.

A large PDA will result in striking physical signs attributable to the wide pulse pressure, most prominently water-hammer arterial pulsations. The heart is normal in size when the ductus is small but moderately or grossly enlarged in cases with a large communication. The apical impulse is normal or left ventricular and, with cardiac enlargement, is heaving. A thrill, maximal in the 2nd left interspace, is often present and may radiate toward the left clavicle, down the left sternal border, or toward the apex. It is usually systolic in time, often extends into diastole, and, in some instances, may be palpated throughout the cardiac cycle. The classic murmur has been variously described as being like machinery, a humming top, a millwheel, or rolling thunder in quality. It begins soon after onset of the 1st sound, reaches maximum intensity at the end of systole, and wanes in late diastole. It may be localized to the 2nd left intercostal space or radiate down the left sternal border or to the left clavicle. The murmur is harsh and uneven with a "clicky" quality. When there is increased pulmonary resistance, the murmur is only systolic in time. In patients with a large left to right shunt a low-pitched mitral diastolic murmur may be audible, due to the large blood flow across the mitral valve.

If the left to right shunt is small, the *electrocardiogram* is normal; if the ductus is large, left ventricular or biventricular hypertrophy is present. The diagnosis of uncomplicated PDA is untenable when isolated right ventricular hypertrophy is noted.

Roentgenographic studies commonly show a prominent pulmonary artery with increased intrapulmonary vascular markings. The cardiac size depends on the degree of left to right shunt; it may be normal, or moderately to grossly enlarged. The chambers involved are the left atrium and ventricle. The aortic knob is normal or prominent and pulsates vigorously.

The *echocardiogram* is normal if the ductus is small. Left atrial and ventricular dimensions are increased, and isovolumic contraction time is decreased with large shunts. Scanning from the suprasternal notch allows visualization of the ductus. The aortic runoff in diastole can be identified by Doppler examination.

The clinical pattern is sufficiently distinctive to allow an accurate diagnosis in the majority of patients. In patients with atypical findings, or when associated cardiac lesions are suspected, hemodynamic studies may be indicated.

Cardiac catheterization reveals normal or increased pressures in the right ventricle and pulmonary artery. The presence of oxygenated blood in the pulmonary artery confirms a left to right shunt. Samples of blood from the venae cavae, right atrium, and right ventricle have normal oxygen contents. The catheter may pass through the ductus into the descending aorta. Injection of contrast medium into the ascending aorta shows opacification of the pulmonary artery from the aorta and identifies the ductus.

Differential Diagnosis. The diagnosis of uncomplicated PDA is usually not difficult. However, there are other conditions that, in the absence of cyanosis, produce systolic and diastolic murmurs in the pulmonic area and must be differentiated.

The characteristics of a *venous hum* are described in Sec. 14.1. An *aorticopulmonary septal defect* may be clinically indistinguishable from a patent ductus, although in most cases the murmur is only systolic and is loudest at the right upper sternal border rather than at the left. Similarly, a *sinus of Valsalva that has ruptured into the right side of the heart or pulmonary artery, coronary arteriovenous fistulas,* and an *aberrant left coronary artery with massive collaterals from the right coronary* display the dynamics of an arteriovenous fistula with a ma-

chinery murmur and a wide pulse pressure. Sometimes the murmur is not maximal in the pulmonary area but is heard along the lower left sternal border. *Truncus arteriosus* with torrential pulmonary flow also has an "aortic runoff" physiology. *Pulmonary branch stenosis* is associated with systolic and diastolic murmurs, but the pulse pressure is normal. *Peripheral arteriovenous fistula* also results in a wide pulse pressure, but the distinctive murmur of a PDA is not present.

Ventricular septal defect with aortic insufficiency and *combined rheumatic aortic and mitral insufficiency* may be confused with PDA, but the murmurs should be differentiated by their to and fro rather than continuous timing. The combination of a large VSD and a PDA results in findings more like those in isolated VSD (Sec. 14.35).

Prognosis and Complications. Patients with a small PDA may live a normal span with little or no cardiac symptoms; however, a sufficient number have clinically manifest complications to make it clear that the lesion is not innocuous. Spontaneous closure of the ductus after infancy is extremely rare.

Congestive cardiac failure most often occurs in early infancy in the presence of a large ductus, but may occur late in life with a moderate-sized communication. The chronic left ventricular volume load is less well tolerated with aging.

Infective endarteritis may be seen at any age. Pulmonary and/or systemic emboli may occur. Treatment with appropriately selected antibiotics should be followed by surgical closure of the ductus after apparent cure of the infective process.

Rare complications include aneurysmal dilatation of the pulmonary artery or the ductus, calcification of the ductus, noninfective thrombosis of the ductus with embolization, and paradoxic emboli. Pulmonary hypertension (Eisenmenger syndrome) can occur in patients with large PDA who do not undergo surgical treatment.

Treatment. Irrespective of age, patients with PDA require surgical closure of the duct. If congestive cardiac failure develops, surgical treatment should not be postponed too long after adequate medical therapy has been instituted, even if some signs of failure persist.

Because the case fatality rate with surgical treatment is less than 1% and the risk without it is greater, ligation and division of the ductus are indicated in the asymptomatic patient, preferably at 1 or 2 yr of age. Pulmonary hypertension is not a contraindication to operation at any age if it can be demonstrated that the shunt goes from aorta to pulmonary artery and is not reversed as a result of severe pulmonary vascular obstructive disease.

Surgical closure is achieved by ligation and division. After closure, symptoms of frank or incipient cardiac failure rapidly disappear. There is usually immediate improvement in physical development of the infant who had failed to thrive. The pulse and blood pressure return to normal, and the machinery murmur disappears. A functional systolic murmur over the pulmonary area may occasionally persist; it may represent turbulence in a persistently dilated pulmonary artery. The roentgenographic signs of cardiac enlargement and pulmonary overcirculation also disappear (Fig. 14–52), and the electrocardiogram becomes normal. Pulmonary hypertension, if present preoperatively, also recedes.

PATENT DUCTUS ARTERIOSUS IN LOW BIRTHWEIGHT INFANTS

See also Sec. 8.17.

Virtually all infants whose birth weight is less than 1750 g have a PDA in the first 24 hr of life. Beyond that time the number of infants with continued patency is greater in the lower birthweight groups. In a significant number of neonates with respiratory distress syndrome clinical symptoms, and

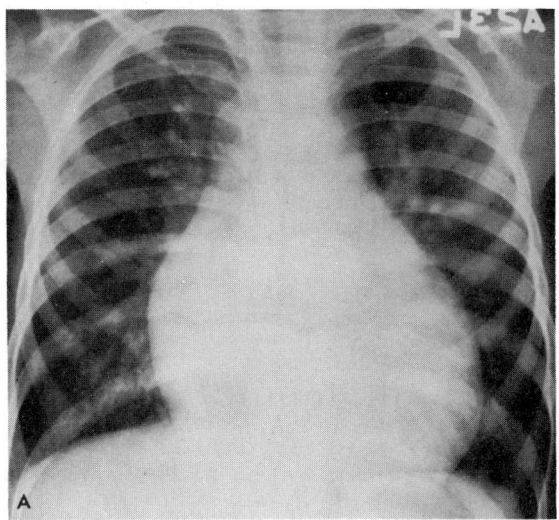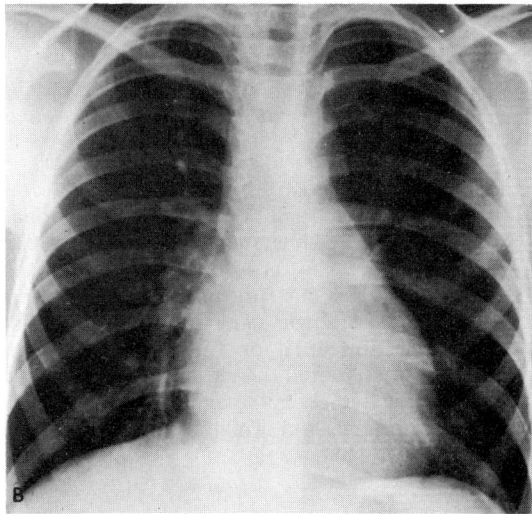

Figure 14–52. Preoperative *(A)* and 3 yr postoperative *(B)* roentgenograms of a child with patent ductus arteriosus. Preoperative roentgenogram shows cardiac enlargement, prominent aorta and pulmonary artery, and increased pulmonary vascularity. The decrease in heart size and degree of pulmonary vasculature is evident in the postoperative roentgenogram.

considerable morbidity and mortality, can be related to the presence of a large left to right shunt via the ductus arteriosus. The clinical features of significant left to right shunting in a preterm infant characteristically appear on the 4th–5th day of life but may be earlier in severe cases. The diagnosis may be made clinically in some instances on the basis of bounding peripheral pulses and a continuous murmur along the infraclavicular region and left upper sternal border. Occasionally, only a systolic murmur or no murmurs may be audible. *Chest roentgenograms* demonstrate pulmonary plethora in the great majority of patients. Cardiac enlargement is observed. *Echocardiography* shows enlargement of the left atrium and left ventricle. Contrast echocardiography with injection of saline into the aortic root, although nonquantitative, may be helpful in establishing the diagnosis. Doppler investigation also can document the presence of a left to right shunt between the aorta and pulmonary artery. These studies are especially important in patients having RDS, whose only manifestation may be the necessity for continued ventilator support after the 3rd–4th day of life, a time when their clinical state should be improving.

In uncomplicated cases the ductus closes spontaneously within the 1st weeks or months of life. When a large symptomatic PDA is present, general treatment may include fluid restriction, correction of anemia, digitalization, and diuretic therapy. Oxygen is administered so that the PaO_2 is kept between 50 and 70 mm Hg. Continuous positive airway pressure (CPAP) and positive pressure ventilation may be required. If medical management fails and the infant cannot be weaned from the ventilator, pharmacologic or surgical closure of the ductus should be carried out.

Delayed closure should be differentiated from patency. The former is to be expected in the premature infant, while the latter occurs as a pathologic entity in a full-term infant. Ductus arteriosus patency is mediated through the prostaglandins, and the ductus arteriosus in preterm infants with respiratory distress syndrome can be constricted and closed by administration of inhibitors of prostaglandin synthesis such as indomethacin (Sec. 8.32). Indomethacin administration early in the course of respiratory distress syndrome associated with large ductal left to right shunts is approximately 80% effective in closing the ductus, thus limiting mortality and morbidity in premature infants with this syndrome. Surgical closure is

a safe and effective backup technique for management when indomethacin is contraindicated or has not been successful.

Untoward effects of indomethacin include oliguria, increases in blood urea nitrogen and serum creatinine, and substantial reduction in urinary sodium concentration. Platelet function may also be altered by indomethacin; the drug should not be used if there is evidence of a coagulation disorder.

14.47 AORTICOPULMONARY SEPTAL DEFECT

This defect consists of a communication between the ascending aorta and main pulmonary artery. The presence of pulmonary and aortic valves and an intact ventricular septum distinguishes this anomaly from truncus arteriosus. Symptoms similar to those of a large ventricular septal defect or of PDA often appear during early infancy and include recurrent pulmonary infections, congestive heart failure, and, occasionally, minimal cyanosis. The defect is usually large and the cardiac murmur is systolic with a mid-diastolic rumble reflecting the increased blood flow across the mitral valve. In the rare instance when the communication is somewhat smaller and pulmonary hypertension is absent, the signs can mimic PDA; a wide pulse pressure, cardiac enlargement, and a continuous right and left upper sternal border systolic murmur may be present. The electrocardiogram shows either left or biventricular hypertrophy. Roentgenographic studies confirm the cardiac enlargement and demonstrate prominence of the pulmonary artery and intrapulmonary vascularity. The echocardiogram shows large volume left heart chambers, and the window can often be delineated.

Cardiac catheterization reveals a left to right shunt at the level of the pulmonary artery as well as hyperkinetic pulmonary hypertension since the defect is almost always large. Selective aortography with injection of contrast medium into the ascending aorta demonstrates the lesion, and manipulation of the catheter from the main pulmonary artery directly to the ascending aorta and brachiocephalic vessels is also diagnostic.

Aorticopulmonary defect is surgically corrected during infancy utilizing cardiopulmonary bypass. If surgery is not carried out in infancy, survivors carry the risk of progressive pulmonary vascular obstructive disease, similar to that of other patients who have intracardiac or great vessel communications and who have pulmonary artery hypertension.

14.48 CORONARY ARTERY FISTULA

A congenital fistula may exist between a coronary artery and an atrium, ventricle (especially the right), or pulmonary artery. Regardless of the recipient chamber, the signs are similar to those of patent ductus arteriosus, although the machinery murmur may be more diffuse. When a *coronary artery empties directly into the right side of the heart*, there is a left to right shunt at the atrial or ventricular level. The involved coronary artery is often dilated or aneurysmal. The anatomic abnormality is demonstrable by injection of contrast medium into the ascending aorta. Treatment consists of surgical abolition of the fistula.

14.49 RUPTURED SINUS OF VALSALVA

When one of the sinuses of Valsalva of the aorta is weakened by congenital or acquired disease, an aneurysm may form and rupture, usually into the right atrium or ventricle. This condition is extremely rare in childhood. The onset is usually sudden. The diagnosis is suspected in a patient who develops acute congestive heart failure, associated with a new loud to and fro murmur. Cardiac catheterization demonstrates the left to right shunt at the atrial or ventricular level. Aortography with injection of contrast medium into the ascending aorta demonstrates the site of aneurysm and rupture. Urgent surgical repair is required.

14.50 PULMONARY VALVE STENOSIS WITH INTACT VENTRICULAR SEPTUM

Various forms of right ventricular outflow obstruction with intact ventricular septum exist. The most common is valvular pulmonary stenosis. In this entity the valve cusps are deformed so that a dome-like obstruction occurs during systole. The cusps are thickened, and there is an eccentric outlet. The ventricular septum is intact. Isolated infundibular stenosis, supravalvular pulmonary stenosis, and branch pulmonary artery stenosis are rarely encountered. In some instances when pulmonary valve stenosis is the dominant lesion, a small associated ventricular septal defect is present, but this problem is better classified as pulmonary stenosis than as tetralogy of Fallot. In addition, pulmonary stenosis and atrial septal defect are occasionally seen as associated defects. The clinical and laboratory findings reflect the dominant lesion, but it is important to make a complete diagnosis.

Hemodynamics. The obstruction to outflow from the right ventricle to the pulmonary artery results in increased systolic pressure and hypertrophy of the right ventricle. The severity of these abnormalities depends on the size of the restricted valvular opening. In severe cases right ventricular pressure may be much higher than systemic systolic pressure, whereas in milder obstruction right ventricular pressure is only mildly or moderately elevated. Pulmonary artery pressure is normal or decreased. Arterial oxygen saturation is normal except in severe cases, when a combination of decreased right ventricular compliance and intra-atrial communication leads to right to left shunting at the atrial level. This is seen most often in the neonate or small infant.

Clinical Manifestations. With mild or moderate stenosis there are usually no symptoms. If the stenosis is severe, there may be exercise intolerance. In infancy, when obstruction is

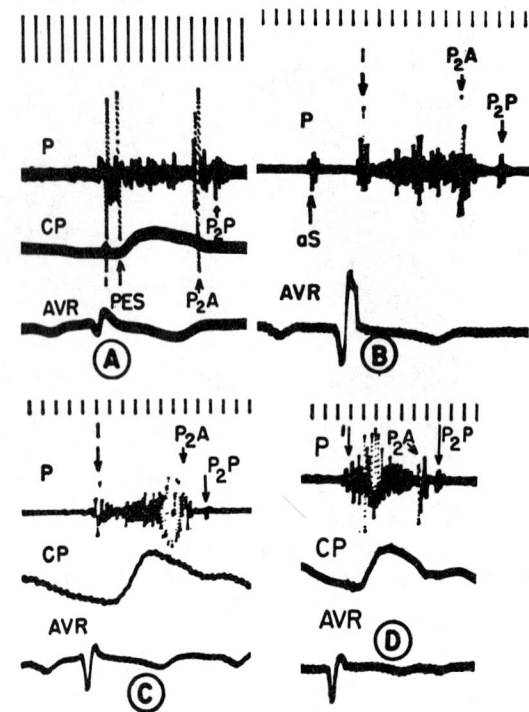

Figure 14–53. Phonocardiograms to illustrate auscultatory findings in valvular pulmonary stenosis of varying severity. AS, atrial sound; AVR, electrocardiogram; CP, carotid pulse; P, pulmonary area; PES, pulmonic ejection sound; P₂A, aortic component of 2nd sound; P₂P, pulmonary component of 2nd sound. Time lines 0.04 sec.
   A, Mild pulmonary stenosis. Ejection sound followed by midsystolic murmur. Second sound split with delayed, diminished pulmonic component. *B, Severe pulmonary stenosis.* Systolic murmur accentuated in late systole and extends beyond P₂A, P₂P delayed and diminished. *C, Severe pulmonary stenosis (preoperative).* Compare with B, *D.* Same patient as in C, 1 wk postoperative. Murmur is now in early systole and midsystole. P₂P more accentuated and closer to P₂A. Compare with A.

critical, there are signs of right ventricular failure and cyanosis. Growth and development are most often normal, and usually older infants and children with pulmonary stenosis appear to be especially well developed and healthy. Pulmonary stenosis with valve dysplasia is the common cardiac abnormality of *Noonan syndrome* (Sec. 19.30).

With mild pulmonary stenosis the venous pressure and pulse are normal. The heart is not enlarged; the apical impulse is normal, and the right ventricle is not palpable. A relatively short pulmonary systolic ejection murmur is maximally audible over the pulmonic area. The murmur is usually preceded by a pulmonic ejection click which is heard best during expiration. The 2nd heart sound is split with a pulmonary element of normal intensity which may be delayed (Fig. 14–53). The *electrocardiogram* is normal or characteristic of mild right ventricular hypertrophy. The only abnormality demonstrable *roentgenographically* is poststenotic dilatation of the pulmonary artery. *Two-dimensional echocardiography* shows a domed valve.

In moderate stenosis the venous pressure may be slightly elevated with an intrinsic "a" wave noted in the jugular pulse. A right ventricular sternal lift may be palpable. The systolic ejection murmur is prolonged later into systole, and a pulmonic ejection sound may or may not be present. The 2nd heart sound is split, with a delayed and diminished pulmonary component which may not be audible. The *electrocardiogram* reveals varying degrees of right ventricular hypertrophy (systolic overload), sometimes with a prominent spiked P wave. *Roentgenographically,* the heart is normal in size or mildly enlarged because of prominence of the right ventricle; intrapulmonary vascularity may be decreased.

In severe stenosis, mild to moderate cyanosis may be noted if there is an interatrial communication. Hepatic enlargement and peripheral edema are observed in the presence of right ventricular failure. Elevation of the venous pressure is common and is due to a large presystolic jugular "a" wave. The heart is moderately or greatly enlarged, and there is a conspicuous sternal and parasternal right ventricular lift which frequently extends to the midclavicular line. A loud systolic ejection murmur, frequently accompanied by a thrill, is maximally audible in the pulmonic area and may radiate widely over the entire precordium into the neck and to the back. The murmur has late systolic accentuation, frequently encompasses the aortic component of the 2nd sound, but is not preceded by an ejection sound. The pulmonary element of the 2nd sound is usually inaudible. The *electrocardiogram* shows gross right ventricular hypertrophy, frequently accompanied by a tall spiked P wave. The *two-dimensional echocardiogram* shows a severe pulmonary valve deformity, an intact ventricular septum, and right ventricular hypertrophy. In the late stages of the disease, dysfunction of the right ventricle is seen. *Roentgenographic studies* confirm the cardiac enlargement and prominence of the right ventricle and atrium. Prominence of the pulmonary artery segment is due to poststenotic dilatation (Fig. 14–54). The intrapulmonary vascularity is decreased. The classic findings of severe pulmonary stenosis are now rarely seen. Critical stenosis is usually encountered in the context of cyanotic heart disease in the neonate.

Cardiac catheterization demonstrates an abrupt gradient of pressure across the pulmonary valve. The pulmonary arterial pressure is normal or low. The right ventricular systolic pressure is 30–50 mm Hg in mild cases; 50–100 mm in moderate cases; and in severe cases higher than the systemic systolic pressure unless cardiac output is low or a significant right to left shunt exists across the atrial septum. In severe and in some moderate cases the right atrial pressure shows a prominent, frequently giant, "a" wave. *Selective right ventriculography* clearly demonstrates the obstruction. The flow of contrast medium through the stenotic valve in ventricular systole produces a jet of dye which fills the dilated pulmonary artery. The abnormal pulmonary valve is visible. Subvalvular hypertrophy which may intensify the obstruction may also be present (Fig. 14–55). This study also indicates whether the ventricular septum is intact.

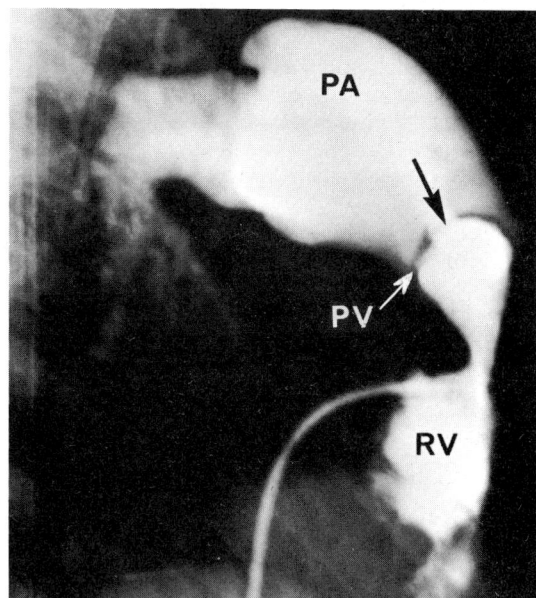

Figure 14–55. Lateral projection of selective right ventriculogram in severe valvular pulmonary stenosis. Black arrow points to jet of contrast medium through minute opening of pulmonary valve. Subvalvular infundibular hypertrophy is also present. PA, poststenotic dilatation of pulmonary artery; PV, thickened pulmonary valve; RV, right ventricle.

Complications. Congestive cardiac failure, the most common complication, occurs only in severe cases and most often during the first month of life. The development of cyanosis from a right to left shunt across a foramen ovale is seen in infancy when stenosis is very severe. Infective endocarditis is not common.

Course and Prognosis. Children with mild or moderate stenosis can lead a normal life, but their progress should be evaluated at regular intervals. Patients who have small gradients rarely show progression, but children having moderate stenosis are more likely to develop a significant gradient. Worsening of obstruction is most often due to the development of secondary subvalvular muscular and fibrous tissue hypertrophy. Progressive electrocardiographic signs of right ventricular hypertrophy indicate increasing obstruction to right ventricular outflow. In severe stenosis the course may abruptly worsen with the development of right ventricular dysfunction and cardiac failure. Infants with severe stenosis require urgent surgical treatment.

Treatment. Patients with moderate or severe isolated pulmonary stenosis require relief of obstruction. Relief of pulmonary valve stenosis is being accomplished by balloon dilatation, which has become the treatment of choice for isolated valvular stenosis in patients in whom surgery would otherwise be indicated. Emergency closed or open valvotomy for the neonate or infant with critical obstruction is required.

Good results should be obtained in the majority of instances. The gradient across the pulmonary valve is reduced or abolished. A pulmonary diastolic murmur due to pulmonary valvular incompetence is to be expected and is not clinically significant.

14.51 INFUNDIBULAR STENOSIS AND DOUBLE RIGHT VENTRICLE

Infundibular stenosis is due to muscular or fibrous obstruction in the outflow tract of the right ventricle. The site of obstruction may be close to the pulmonary valve or well below it; an infundibular chamber may be present between the right ventricular cavity and the pulmonary valve. In a significant number of cases a ventricular septal defect may have been

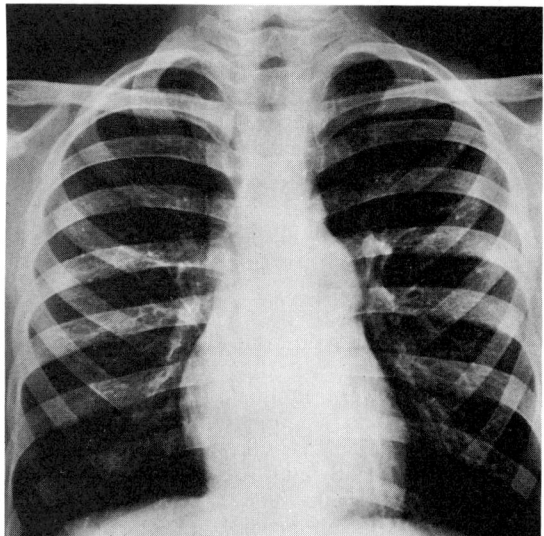

Figure 14–54. Roentgenogram in valvular pulmonary stenosis with normal aortic root. The heart size is within normal limits, but there is poststenotic dilatation of the pulmonary artery.

present initially and later closed spontaneously. When the pulmonary valve is also stenotic, the combined defect is primarily classified as valvular stenosis with secondary infundibular hypertrophy. The *hemodynamics* and *clinical manifestations* of patients with isolated infundibular pulmonary stenosis are similar, for the most part, to those described under simple valvular pulmonary stenosis (Sec. 14.50).

A more common variation of right ventricular outflow obstruction below the pulmonary valve is that of *double right ventricle*. In this condition there is a muscular band in the mid right ventricular region which divides the chamber into two parts and creates obstruction from the inlet portion to the outlet. There is often an associated ventricular septal defect which can close spontaneously. Obstruction is not seen early in life, but may progress rapidly in a similar manner to the progressive infundibular obstruction observed with tetralogy of Fallot.

The diagnosis of isolated right ventricular infundibular stenosis or double chamber right ventricle can be made by echocardiography and/or cardiac catheterization and angiography. When contrast material is injected into the right ventricle the site of the stenosis is demonstrated. The ventricular septum must be evaluated to determine whether an associated ventricular septal defect is present. The prognosis for untreated cases of severe right ventricular outflow obstruction is similar to that for valvular pulmonary stenosis (Sec. 14.50). When obstruction is severe, surgery is indicated. After operation the pressure gradient is abolished or markedly reduced and the outlook is excellent.

14.52 PULMONARY STENOSIS WITH LEFT TO RIGHT SHUNT

Valvular or infundibular pulmonary stenosis, or both, may be associated with a left to right shunt across an atrial septal defect or a ventricular septal defect. The clinical features depend on the degree of stenosis and the magnitude of the left to right shunt.

The presence of a large left to right shunt at the atrial or ventricular level is evidence that the pulmonary stenosis is mild. However, worsening of obstruction will limit the shunt and perhaps even lead to right to left shunting; this more often occurs with VSD. These anomalies are treated by direct vision surgery. Defects in the atrial or ventricular septa are closed, and the pulmonary stenosis is relieved by infundibular resection or pulmonary valvuloplasty as indicated.

14.53 PULMONARY STENOSIS WITH RIGHT TO LEFT SHUNT

See pulmonary valve stenosis with intact ventricular septum (Sec. 14.50) and tetralogy of Fallot (Sec. 14.14).

14.54 PULMONARY ARTERIAL BRANCH STENOSIS

Single or multiple constrictions may occur anywhere along the major branches of the pulmonary artery and may be mild, extensive, localized, or multiple. Frequently, this defect is associated with other types of congenital heart disease, especially pulmonary valvular stenosis, tetralogy of Fallot, patent ductus arteriosus, ventricular septal defect, atrial septal defect, and supravalvular aortic stenosis. A familial tendency has been recognized in some patients with peripheral stenosis. A high incidence has been found in infants with the congenital rubella syndrome. Supravalvular aortic stenosis with pulmo-

nary arterial branch stenosis has also been observed with idiopathic hypercalcemia of infancy (Williams syndrome).

With a mild constriction there is little effect on the pulmonary circulation. With multiple severe constrictions there is an increase in pressure in the right ventricle and in the pulmonary artery proximal to the site of obstruction. When the anomaly is isolated, the diagnosis is suspected by the presence of murmurs in widespread locations over the chest, anteriorly or posteriorly. These murmurs are usually systolic but may be continuous. They are occasionally heard in newborn infants and will eventually disappear, suggesting that mild branch stenosis in this age group may be transient. Most often, the physical signs are dominated by the associated anomaly, e.g., tetralogy of Fallot. If the stenosis is severe, there is electrocardiographic evidence of right ventricular and right atrial hypertrophy.

On roentgenographic examination, cardiomegaly and prominence of the main pulmonary artery are present in severe cases. Generally, the pulmonary vasculature is normal; in some cases small intrapulmonary vascular shadows are seen which may be shown by pulmonary arteriography to be areas of poststenotic dilatation. Pressure gradients across the areas of obstruction are demonstrable by cardiac catheterization. These gradients may not be easily identified if right ventricular outflow obstruction coexists since the pressure in the main pulmonary artery is normal or low in such patients. Severe obstruction of the main pulmonary artery and its primary branches should be relieved during corrective surgery for tetralogy of Fallot or valvular pulmonary stenosis. Multiple peripheral intrapulmonary obstructions are not amenable to surgical management, but most often are mild.

14.55 PULMONARY VALVULAR INSUFFICIENCY

Pulmonary valvular insufficiency most often accompanies other cardiovascular diseases and may be secondary to severe pulmonary hypertension. Incompetence of the valve is an expected result after surgery for right ventricular outflow obstruction, e.g., pulmonary valvotomy and infundibular resection. Isolated congenital incompetence of the pulmonary valve is a rare anomaly. The patient is usually asymptomatic since the incompetence is usually mild.

The prominent physical sign is a diastolic murmur at the upper left sternal border which has a lower pitch than the murmur of aortic insufficiency. Roentgenograms of the chest show prominence of the main pulmonary artery. The electrocardiogram is normal or shows minimal right ventricular hypertrophy. The diagnosis can be confirmed by cardiac catheterization if necessary. There is a low pulmonary arterial diastolic pressure. Selective pulmonary arteriography shows the incompetent valve but is difficult to evaluate, since the catheter crossing the valve results in some iatrogenic insufficiency during the injection. Isolated pulmonary valvular incompetence is usually well tolerated and does not require surgical treatment.

Absence of the pulmonary valve is usually associated with ventricular septal defect, often in the context of tetralogy of Fallot (Sec. 14.14). In infancy, the pulmonary arteries become widely dilated and compress the bronchi, thus causing recurrent episodes of wheezing, pulmonary collapse, and pneumonitis. Florid pulmonary valvular incompetence may not be well tolerated, and death may occur from a combination of bronchial compression, hypoxemia, and heart failure. In older patients a valved conduit may be inserted at the time of correction of the ventricular defect and the infundibular stenosis.

14.56 COARCTATION OF THE AORTA

Constrictions of varying length may occur at any point from the arch to the bifurcation of the aorta, but 98% occur just below the origin of the left subclavian artery at the origin of the ductus arteriosus. The anomaly occurs twice as often in males as in females. Coarctation of the aorta may be a feature of Turner (XO) syndrome (Sec. 19.34) and is associated with bicuspid aortic valve in over 70% of patients. Mitral valve abnormalities and subaortic stenosis also are not uncommon.

Pathology. Coarctation of the aorta occurs in the form of a preductal segmental tubular hypoplasia or as a more discrete juxtaductal obstruction. Often, both components are present. It is postulated that coarctation is initiated in the presence of a cardiac abnormality that results in decreased antegrade aortic blood flow (e.g., bicuspid aortic valve) and proportionately increased flow through the pulmonary artery and ductus arteriosus. A contraductal shelf-like structure bifurcates ductal blood flow retrograde into the left subclavian and antegrade to the descending aorta (Fig. 14–56). Antegrade aortic flow supplies the innominate, left carotid, and vertebral arteries, but when very little blood reaches the aortic isthmus proximal to the left subclavian artery, isthmic tubular hypoplasia results. Occasionally, severely hypoplastic segments of the aortic isthmus may become completely atretic, resulting in an interrupted arch with the left subclavian artery arising either proximal or distal to the interruption. The nature of the coarctation lesion depends on the ultimate flow across the aortic isthmus proximal to the left carotid artery. If the segment remains patent but narrow, then the "infantile" type of coarctation occurs, usually with right to left ductal flow to the descending aorta and almost invariably with an associated ventricular septal defect. If antegrade aortic flow becomes normal after birth, isthmic narrowing will not be prominent, and the most common type of discrete coarctation will occur.

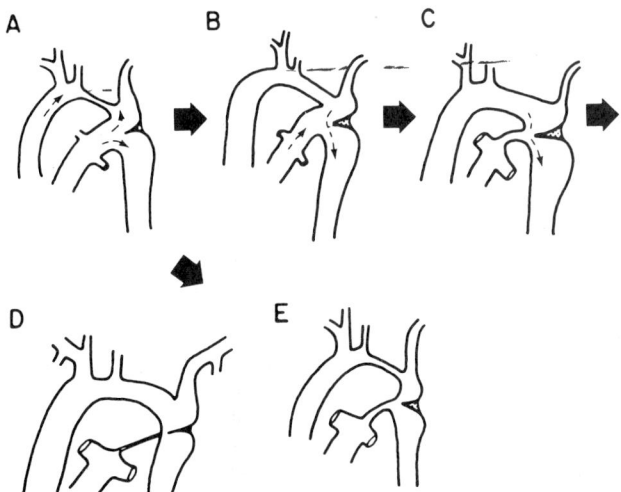

Figure 14–56. Metamorphosis of coarctation. *A,* Fetal prototype. No flow obstruction. *B,* Late gestation. Aortic ventricle increases output and dilates hypoplastic segment. Antegrade aortic flow bypass shell via ductal orifice. *C,* Neonate. Ductal constriction initiates obstruction by removing bypass and increasing antegrade arch flow. *D,* Mature juxtaductal stenosis. Bypass completely obliterated; intimal hypoplasia on edge of shell aggravates stenosis. Collaterals develop. *E,* Infantile type fetal prototype persists. Intracardiac left heart obstruction precludes an increase in antegrade aortic before or after birth. Both isthmal hypoplasia and contraductal shelf are present. Lower body flow often depends on patency of the ductus. (Modified from Gersony WM: Coarctation of the aorta. *In:* Adams FH, Emmanouilides GC: Moss' Heart Disease in Infants, Children, and Adolescents. 3rd ed. Baltimore, Williams & Wilkins, 1983.)

The blood pressure is elevated in the vessels that arise proximal to the coarctation; the blood pressure as well as pulse pressure below the constriction is lower. Hypertension is not due to the mechanical obstruction alone, but almost certainly involves renal mechanisms. Coarctation of the aorta usually results in the development of extensive collateral circulation, chiefly from the branches of the subclavian, the superior intercostal, and the internal mammary arteries. The thoracic and subscapular branches of the axillary artery may also enlarge as collateral channels. These vessels unite with the intercostal branches of the descending aorta and inferior epigastric branches of the femoral artery to create a channel for arterial blood to bypass the area of coarctation. The vessels contributing to the collateral circulation may become markedly enlarged and tortuous by early adulthood.

Coarctation of the aorta recognized after infancy rarely is associated with significant symptomatology. An occasional child will complain about weakness and/or pain in the legs after exercise, but in the great majority of instances, even patients with severe coarctation will be asymptomatic.

Clinical Manifestations. The classic sign of coarctation of the aorta is disparity in pulsations and blood pressures of the arms and legs. The femoral, popliteal, posterior tibial, and dorsalis pedis pulsations are weak and delayed or absent in contrast with the bounding pulses of the arms and carotid vessels. In normal persons the systolic blood pressure in the legs obtained by the cuff method is 10–20 mm Hg higher than that in the arms. In coarctation of the aorta the blood pressure in the legs is lower than that in the arms; frequently, it cannot be obtained. There is also a more prominent rise of systemic blood pressure in response to exercise.

This differential in blood pressures is very common in patients over 1 yr of age, about 90% of whom have systolic hypertension in the upper extremity greater than the 95th percentile for age. In one study mean upper extremity blood pressure was 145 ± 12 mm Hg; lower extremity blood pressure, when it could be obtained, was 70 ± 10 mm Hg. Although absent femoral and pedal pulses are the hallmark of the disease, in only 40% of patients were the femoral pulses completely absent. Weakly palpable femoral pulses with a pulse lag were evident in 44%; in 16% the pulses were characterized as normal. Palpable pedal pulses were noted in 23% of the patients.

It is essential to determine the blood pressure in each arm; a significant difference between the right and left arms suggests involvement of the left subclavian artery in the area of coarctation.

A short systolic murmur is often heard along the left sternal border at the 3rd and 4th intercostal spaces. The murmur is well transmitted to the back and neck. An interscapular systolic murmur over the region of the coarctation is quite characteristic. Often, the typical murmur of mild aortic stenosis can be heard in the 3rd right intercostal space and an apical systolic ejection click is also common. The latter findings suggest that an aortic valve deformity is present in addition to coarctation; occasionally a significant degree of obstruction across the aortic valve is also present. Among patients with well developed collateral blood flow, systolic or continuous murmurs may be heard over the left and right chest laterally and posteriorly.

Diagnosis. The findings on *roentgenographic examination* depend on the age of the patient and on the effects of hypertension and collateral circulation. In infancy there are usually no changes except cardiac enlargement if congestive cardiac failure is present. During childhood the findings are not striking unless the left ventricle is prominent. After the 1st decade the heart tends to be mildly or moderately enlarged because of left ventricular prominence. The enlarged left subclavian artery commonly produces a prominent shadow in the left

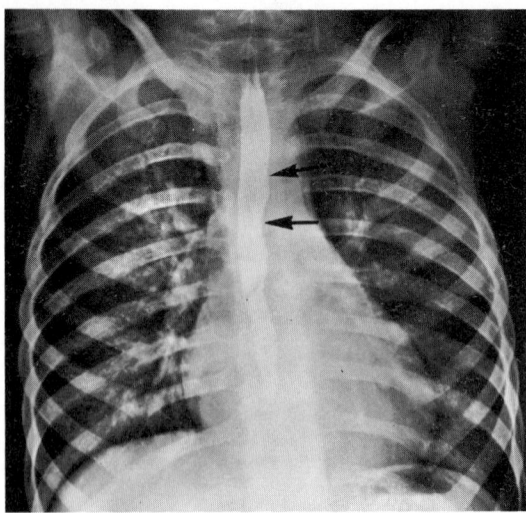

Figure 14–57. Roentgenogram of a 6 yr old boy with coarctation of the aorta. The barium-filled esophagus shows indentations produced by the aortic knob and left subclavian artery (upper arrow) and poststenotic dilatation (lower arrow). These two indentations produce the E sign. The left ventricle is prominent; there is no evidence of notching of the ribs.

superior mediastinum. Notching of the inferior border of the ribs from pressure erosion by enlarged collateral vessels is common by late childhood except in the upper and lower 2–3 ribs. In the majority of instances there is an area of poststenotic dilatation of the descending aorta. This may be demonstrated by displacement of the barium-filled esophagus and by discontinuity of the lateral margin of the aorta below the arch (Fig. 14–57).

The *electrocardiogram* is usually normal in young children but reveals evidences of left ventricular hypertrophy in older patients. Neonates and infants will display right ventricular dominance.

Most often, the diagnosis can be made simply by careful evaluation of the pulse in all major accessible peripheral arteries and by comparative blood pressure determinations in the arms and legs. The segment of coarctation can be visualized by two-dimensional *echographic scanning;* associated anomalies of the aortic valve can also be demonstrated. *Cardiac catheterization* with selective left ventriculography and aortography is especially important in selected cases with additional anomalies, and as a means of visualizing collateral blood flow.

Associated Abnormalities. Abnormalities of the aortic valve are present in a majority of patients. Bicuspid aortic valves are common but usually do not produce signs unless stenosis is significant. The association of patent ductus arteriosus and coarctation of the aorta is also common. Ventricular and atrial septal defects may be suspected by signs of left to right shunt. Mitral valve abnormalities are also occasionally seen, as is subvalvular aortic stenosis.

Severe neurologic damage or even death rarely may occur from associated cerebrovascular disease. Subarachnoid or intracerebral hemorrhage may result from rupture of congenital aneurysms in the circle of Willis, of other vessels with defective elastic and medial tissue, or of normal vessels; these accidents are secondary to the hypertensive state. Abnormalities of the subclavian arteries may include involvement of the left subclavian artery in the area of coarctation, stenosis of the orifice of the left subclavian artery, and anomalous origin of the right subclavian artery.

Prognosis and Complications. Untreated, the great majority of patients with coarctation of the aorta would succumb between the ages of 20 and 40 yr; some live well into middle life without serious handicap. The common serious complications are related to the hypertensive state, which may result in premature coronary artery disease, congestive cardiac failure, or intracranial hemorrhage. Heart failure may be related to complicating anomalies, especially in infancy. Infective endocarditis or endarteritis is a significant complication in adults. Aneurysms of the descending aorta or of the enlarged collateral vessels are not unusual.

Treatment. Patients with significant coarctation of the aorta should be treated surgically. The optimal age for operation is 2–4 yr; the mortality rate at this age is less than 1%. After the 2nd decade the operation may be less successful because of decreased left ventricular function and degenerative changes. Nevertheless, if cardiac reserve is sufficient, satisfactory repair is possible well into mid adult life. Associated valvular lesions increase the hazards of surgery.

The operation of choice is excision of the area of coarctation and primary anastomosis. A subclavian turndown procedure, which incorporates the subclavian artery into the wall of the repaired coarctation, has been utilized in the younger age group. This vertical incision may be less often associated with recoarctation compared to horizontal resection and end-to-end anastomosis in this age group. Rarely, if the length of aortic constriction precludes primary anastomosis, Dacron grafts may be utilized.

After operation there is striking increase in the amplitude of pulsations in the femoral artery and dorsalis pedis and arterial tibial pulses. However, in the immediate postoperative course, "rebound" hypertension is common and may require medical management. Usually hypertension gradually subsides. Residual murmurs are common and may be due to associated cardiac anomalies, to flow across the repaired area, and/or to collateral blood flow. Repair of coarctation in the 2nd decade of life or beyond may be associated with a higher incidence of premature cardiovascular disease, even in the absence of residual cardiac abnormalities. There may be recurrence or early onset of adult hypertension, which has occurred even in patients with adequately resected coarctation. However, most follow-up studies involve young adults who were operated on several decades earlier, and the excellence of the original repair has not been documented. Most centers now advocate repair of coarctation early in the 1st decade of life in an attempt to decrease the incidence of premature cardiovascular disease during adult life. In patients with normal blood pressure following repair at 3–4 yr of age, late hypertension, early atherosclerosis, and dissecting aneurysm, all of which have been reported in the older age group, should be less likely to occur.

Although restenosis in older patients who had an adequate coarctectomy is extremely rare, a significant number of infants with end-to-end anastomoses carried out urgently in the first months of life require revision later in childhood. Balloon dilatation of restenosis has been successfully carried out, but concerns about aneurysm formation must contraindicate the use of this technique for relief of native (unoperated) coarctation. It remains to be seen whether follow-up of patients who had subclavian turndown procedures in this age group will show that restenosis is much less likely. All patients should be followed carefully for an indefinite period after repair of coarctation of the aorta.

14.57 THE POSTCOARCTECTOMY SYNDROME

Postoperative mesenteric arteritis may be associated with hypertension and abdominal pain in the immediate postoperative period. The pain varies in severity and may be associated with anorexia, nausea, vomiting, leukocytosis, and even signs of small bowel obstruction. Relief is usually obtained with antihypertensive drugs and intestinal decompression; corticosteroids may help to alleviate the symptoms and thus avoid surgical exploration for bowel obstruction. This syndrome has been seen much less frequently in recent years.

14.58 COARCTATION IN INFANCY

Coarctation occurs in infancy associated with other cardiovascular anomalies, including patent ductus arteriosus, ventricular septal defect, severe aortic valvular disease, transposition of the great arteries, and variations of single ventricle. Severe coarctation may also be associated with endocardial sclerosis and mitral valve disease. The clinical pattern in this age group depends on the effects of the associated malformations as well as of the coarctation itself. Both anatomic and physiologic classifications have been utilized to describe all existing abnormalities and their contributions to the clinical manifestations of coarctation in infancy. These depend on the site and length of coarctation, the site of the aortic opening of the ductus, and the size of the aorta proximal to the coarctation. The direction of blood flow across the ductus depends on position, severity of obstruction at the site of the coarctation, and pulmonary vascular resistance. Virtually all coarctations are juxtaductal rather than in the pre- and postductal positions.

In infants with severe hypoplasia of the aortic isthmus or interruption of the aortic arch, right ventricular blood is ejected through the ductus to the descending aorta. Systemic flow to the lower body is dependent on right ventricular output. In this situation femoral pulses are palpable, and differential blood pressures are not helpful in the diagnosis. Such infants will have severe pulmonary hypertension and high pulmonary vascular resistance. Cyanosis, failure to thrive, and heart failure are prominent. Because the descending aorta is supplied with venous blood, differential cyanosis may be noted, but this is rarely a conspicuous sign. The heart is large, and there is a systolic murmur heard along the left sternal border with a loud 2nd heart sound. The electrocardiogram shows right ventricular hypertrophy, and the chest roentgenogram shows cardiac enlargement and prominent vascularity. In coarctation with a large right to left shunt across the ductus arteriosus the prognosis may be poor, but some cases respond well to medical management and surgical excision of the coarctation. On the other hand, the occasional infant with coarctation and a large left to right shunt through the ductus arteriosus has a much better outlook. In some of these infants, surgical repair may be delayed if response to digitalization and diuretic therapy is good.

Coarctation of the aorta associated with severe mitral and aortic valve disease may have to be considered within the context of hypoplastic left heart syndrome. Such patients have a long segment narrow arch with or without isolated coarctation at the site of the entrance of the ductus into the aorta. Coarctation of the aorta with transposition of the great arteries or single ventricle may be repaired alone or in combination with other palliative measures.

14.59 COARCTATION WITH VENTRICULAR SEPTAL DEFECT IN INFANCY

Isolated coarctation of the aorta is rarely a cause of congestive heart failure during infancy. However, coarctation in the presence of ventricular septal defect results in both increased preload and afterload on the left ventricle, and patients with this combination of defects will present in the first month of life, often with intractable cardiac failure. The clinical picture is that of a seriously ill infant with tachypnea, failure to thrive, and typical findings of heart failure. Often, there is not a marked difference in blood pressures between the upper and lower extremities since cardiac output may be low. These infants present earlier in a more severely ill state than those with either ventricular septal defect or coarctation alone. Although medical management may be helpful initially, early surgery is necessary. In the majority of cases coarctation is the major anomaly causing the severe symptoms, and resection of the coarcted segment will result in marked improvement. Some centers do not band the pulmonary artery, and a number of patients will improve sufficiently so that further surgery is not required during infancy. Later repair of the ventricular septal defect is carried out in other patients. However, if there is difficulty in managing the infant after surgery, open repair of the ventricular septal defect is done in infancy. When it is determined that a complicated ventricular septal defect is present (multiple, muscular), pulmonary artery banding can be done at the time of coarctation repair to avoid infant open heart surgery for complex ventricular septal abnormalities.

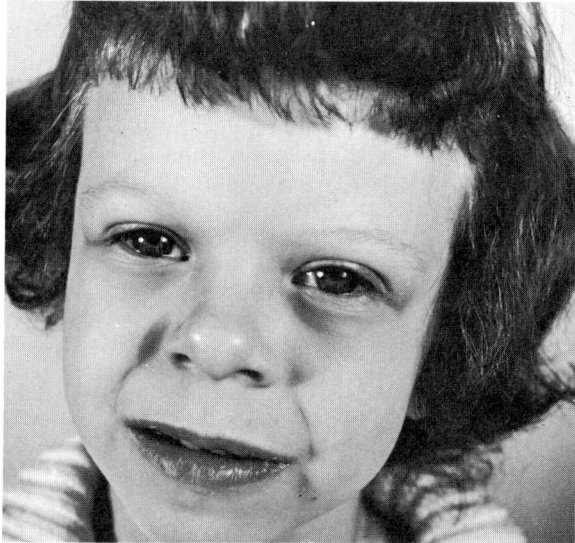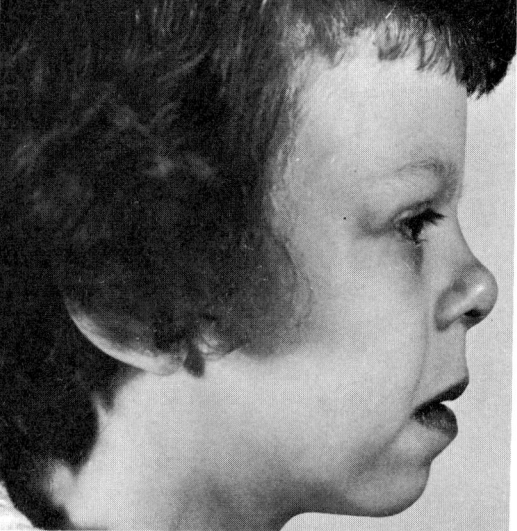

Figure 14–58. Patient with documented hypercalcemia during infancy who had supravalvular aortic stenosis relieved surgically at 8. The upper lip is prominent, the bridge of the nose is flat, the nose is short and upturned, and hypertelorism is present.

14.60 CONGENITAL AORTIC STENOSIS

Congenital aortic stenosis accounts for about 5% of cardiac malformations recognized in childhood, but an abnormality of the aortic valve (bicuspid) is the most common congenital heart lesion identified in adults. Stenosis is more common in males (3:1).

In the majority of instances, aortic stenosis is valvular, the leaflets are thickened, and most often the commissures fused to varying degrees. *Subvalvular (subaortic) stenosis* with a discrete fibrous or muscular obstruction to the left ventricular outflow below the aortic valves is also an important form of left ventricular outflow obstruction. *Supravalvular aortic stenosis*, a less common type, may be sporadic, familial, or associated with a syndrome of mental retardation and an elfin facies (full face, broad forehead, flattened bridge of nose, long upper lip, and rounded cheeks). Stenoses of other arteries may also be present. This syndrome (Williams syndrome) (Fig. 14–58) is associated with idiopathic hypercalcemia of infancy (Sec. 23.55).

Clinical Manifestations. Symptomatology among patients with aortic stenosis depends on the severity of the obstruction. Aortic stenosis presents in early infancy with severe left ventricular failure. However, most children with critical aortic stenosis will remain asymptomatic and display a normal growth and development pattern. The murmur is usually discovered during routine physical examination. It is rare to see an older child with severe obstruction to left ventricular outflow with fatigue, angina, dizziness, or syncope. Sudden death has been reported with aortic stenosis but usually occurs in patients with severe left ventricular outflow obstruction manifested by electrocardiographic changes and a large gradient across the aortic valve, in whom surgical relief has been delayed.

The pulse is usually normal but may have a small volume when obstruction is critical. The heart size and apical impulse are normal when stenosis is mild or moderate. In severe cases the heart may be enlarged with a left ventricular apical thrust. A rough systolic ejection murmur, usually accompanied by a suprasternal notch thrill, is audible maximally at the right upper sternal border and radiates to the neck and down the left sternal border. In patients with subvalvular stenosis, the murmur may be maximal along the left sternal border or even at the apex. In valvular aortic stenosis the murmur is usually preceded by an aortic ejection click best heard at the apex and left sternal edge (Fig. 14–59). Clicks are unusual in discrete subaortic stenosis. A diastolic murmur indicative of mild aortic insufficiency is often present when the obstruction is subvalvular, or in patients with a bicuspid aortic valve. Occasionally, an apical mid-diastolic rumbling murmur is audible even in the presence of a normal mitral valve. The normal splitting of the 2nd heart sound is present in mild cases. In patients with severe obstruction, aortic valve closure is diminished, or, rarely in children, the 2nd sound may be split paradoxically. A prominent 4th heart sound may be audible when the obstruction is severe.

Diagnosis. The diagnosis should be made by physical examination. Generally, a loud murmur accompanied by a right upper sternal border thrill indicates the presence of significant obstruction. If the pressure gradient across the aortic valve is small, the *electrocardiogram* is likely to be normal. The ECG may also be normal with severe obstruction, but evidence of left ventricular hypertrophy and strain are often present if severe stenosis is longstanding. *Roentgenograms* frequently show a prominent ascending aorta, but the aortic knob is normal. Heart size is usually normal. Valvular calcification has been noted in older children. *Echocardiography* identifies the anomaly and helps evaluate both the site and the severity of obstruction. Anatomic echographic M-mode

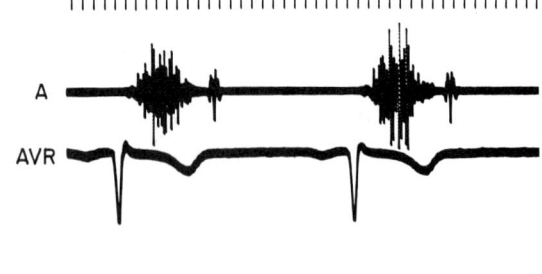

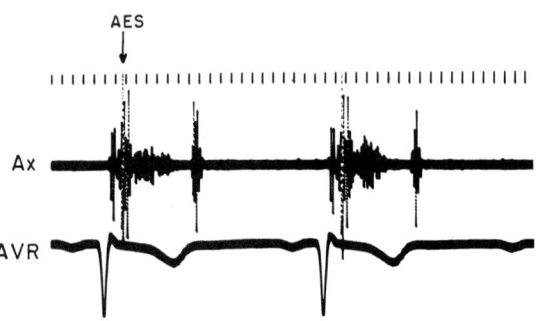

Figure 14–59. Phonocardiogram to illustrate auscultatory findings in congenital aortic valvular stenosis. At the aortic area the systolic murmur is ejection in type. At the apex the systolic murmur is initiated by an aortic ejection sound. *A*, aortic area; *AES*, aortic ejection sound; *AVR*, electrocardiogram; *Ax*, apex.

features include multiple diastolic echoes of the aortic valve, eccentric aortic valve closure, and increased thickness of the ventricular septum and the free wall of the left ventricle. Two-dimensional studies visualize the domed stenotic aortic valve or subvalvular obstruction. In the absence of left ventricular failure the shortening fraction of the left ventricle is increased since the ventricle is hypercontractile. Peak systolic left ventricular outflow gradients that exceed 45 mm Hg are usually associated with shortening fractions greater than 40%.

Graded exercise testing is useful in evaluating the severity of left ventricular outflow obstruction in older children. As the severity of the gradient increases, working capacity decreases, systolic blood pressure fails to rise adequately, diastolic blood pressure may rise, and S-T segmental depression can occur. Since patients with severe aortic stenosis may deny symptoms and have normal electrocardiograms and chest roentgenograms, serial echocardiograms and graded exercise tests are valuable in determining the timing of cardiac catheterization.

Left cardiac catheterization demonstrates the magnitude of pressure gradient from the left ventricle to the aorta. The site of obstruction is best identified by selective left ventriculography. The aortic pressure curve is abnormal if obstruction is severe; an early-appearing anacrotic notch, a slow, prolonged, and delayed systolic upstroke, a narrow pulse pressure, and a delayed dicrotic notch are noted. In patients with severe obstruction and decreased left ventricular compliance, the left atrial pressure is increased.

Prognosis. The prognosis is good in the majority of children having mild to moderate aortic stenosis. In a small number of patients having a severe obstruction, sudden death has occurred. In such instances there is usually evidence of gross left ventricular hypertrophy. Neonates having critical aortic stenosis who die from congestive heart failure frequently have endocardial fibroelastosis of the left ventricle.

Treatment. Surgery is indicated for patients having severe obstruction in order to prevent progressive left ventricular dysfunction secondary to severe afterload requirements. Aortic valvular stenosis is usually treated by open valvotomy. Late calcification is likely to occur, and reoperation will often be required, usually resulting in valve replacement. Discrete subaortic stenosis can usually be resected without damage to the aortic valve, the anterior leaflet of the mitral valve, or the conduction system. Relief of supravalvular stenosis can be achieved if the area of obstruction is discrete and is not associated with a hypoplastic aorta. Surgery is not indicated in the absence of definitive evidence of left ventricular hypertrophy or of a significant gradient across the aortic valve. The definition of a "significant gradient" is difficult, but it is generally agreed that surgery should be advised when the peak systolic gradient between the left ventricle and aorta exceeds 60 mm Hg at rest with a normal cardiac output. Balloon dilatation is now being utilized for valvular aortic stenosis and is the treatment of choice at an increasing number of centers.

Careful follow-up is essential since recurrence of ventricular obstruction later in life is common. Electrocardiographic signs of left ventricular hypertrophy, deterioration of echocardiographic indices of left ventricular function, and recurrence of signs during graded exercise are compatible with severe restenosis.

There may be some danger in allowing patients with significant aortic stenosis to participate in active competitive sports, but otherwise they should lead normal lives. The status of each patient should be reviewed annually and intervention advised if progression of signs is definite. Prophylaxis against infective endocarditis is essential.

14.61 CONGENITAL MITRAL STENOSIS

This relatively rare anomaly can be isolated or associated with other defects, the most common being patent ductus arteriosus, aortic stenosis, and coarctation of the aorta. The mitral valve is funnel shaped, with thickened leaflets and chordae tendineae that are shortened and deformed.

Symptoms usually appear within the first 2 yr. The infants are underdeveloped and usually have obvious dyspnea secondary to congestive heart failure; cyanosis and pallor are common. Heart enlargement due to dilatation and hypertrophy of the right ventricle and left atrium is common. Most patients have rumbling diastolic murmurs followed by a loud 1st sound, but the auscultatory findings may be relatively obscure. The 2nd sound is loud and split. An opening snap of the mitral valve may be present. The *electrocardiogram* reveals right ventricular hypertrophy with normal, bifid, or spiked P waves. *Roentgenograms* usually show left atrial and right ventricular enlargement and pulmonary congestion. The *echocardiogram* is characteristic, showing thickened mitral valve leaflets, diminished E-F slope, and an enlarged left atrium with a normal or small left ventricle. Two-dimensional examinations in the short axis show a significant reduction of the mitral valve orifice in diastole; the size of the mitral valve orifice can be measured. At *cardiac catheterization* there is an increase in right ventricular, pulmonary arterial, and pulmonary capillary wedge pressures. Associated anomalies such as patent ductus arteriosus may be demonstrated. *Angiocardiography* may show delayed emptying of the left atrium, and the small mitral orifice.

The prognosis is usually poor; the majority of children succumb during the first 2 yr of life. The results of surgical treatment have been variable; a mitral valve prosthesis is required.

14.62 CONGENITAL MITRAL INSUFFICIENCY

This anomaly may be isolated or associated with patent ductus arteriosus, coarctation of the aorta, ventricular septal defect, corrected transposition of the great vessels, anomalous origin of the left coronary artery from the pulmonary artery, endocardial fibroelastosis, or Marfan syndrome. Mitral incompetence is an integral part of endocardial cushion defects.

In isolated mitral insufficiency the mitral valve annulus is usually dilated; the chordae tendineae are short and may insert anomalously; and the valve leaflets are deformed. Endocardial sclerosis of varying degree is present in severe cases. When mitral incompetence is clinically significant, the left atrium enlarges to accommodate the regurgitant flow and the left ventricle becomes hypertrophied and dilated. Pulmonary venous pressure is increased and ultimately results in pulmonary hypertension and right ventricular hypertrophy and dilatation. Mild lesions produce no symptoms; the only abnormal sign is the murmur of mitral incompetence. However, severe regurgitation results in symptoms that can appear at any age. These include poor physical development, frequent respiratory infections, fatigue on exertion, and episodes of pulmonary edema or congestive heart failure. The typical apical pansystolic murmur of mitral insufficiency is present with the associated apical mid-diastolic rumbling murmur of increased diastolic flow across the mitral valve. The pulmonary component of the 2nd heart sound is accentuated in the presence of pulmonary hypertension. The *electrocardiogram* usually shows bifid P waves, signs of left ventricular hypertrophy, and sometimes signs of right ventricular hypertrophy. *Roentgenographic examination* shows enlargement of the left atrium, which at times is massive. The left ventricle is prominent, and the pulmonary vascularity is normal or prominent. *Echocardiograms* demonstrate the enlarged left atrium and ventricle. Although motion of the mitral valve is excessive with a steep E-F slope, this sign is not diagnostic.

Cardiac catheterization shows an elevated left atrial pressure measured either directly via a patent foramen ovale or by means of pulmonary capillary wedge pressure. Pulmonary artery hypertension of varying severity may be present. Selective left ventriculography reveals the presence of mitral regurgitation. *Mitral valvuloplasty* has resulted in striking improvement in symptoms and heart size, but in some patients installation of a prosthetic mechanical mitral valve may be necessary. Prior to surgery, associated anomalies must be identified. In children beyond 3–4 yr it may be difficult to exclude rheumatic fever as the cause of mitral insufficiency.

14.63 MITRAL VALVE PROLAPSE

This distinctive syndrome results from an abnormal mitral valve mechanism that causes billowing of one or both mitral leaflets, especially the posterior cusp, into the left atrium toward the end of systole. The abnormality is almost always congenital but may not be recognized until adolescence or adulthood. The syndrome is more common in girls and may affect siblings. The dominant abnormal signs are auscultatory. The apical murmur is late systolic in timing and may be preceded by a click, but these signs vary in the same patient so that at times only the click is audible. In the standing position the click appears earlier in systole and the murmur is longer. Arrhythmias, primarily unifocal or multifocal premature ventricular contractions, may occur.

The *electrocardiogram* is usually normal, but may show diphasic T waves, especially in leads II, III, VF, and V_6; the T wave abnormalities may vary in the same patient. The *chest roentgenogram* is normal. The *echocardiogram* shows a characteristic posterior movement of the posterior mitral leaflet during mid or late systole or pansystolic prolapse of both anterior and posterior mitral leaflets. These M-mode echographic findings must be interpreted cautiously since the appearance of minimal mitral prolapse may be a normal variant. Two-dimensional real-time echocardiography appears to be more accurate; both the free edge and the body of the mitral leaflets move posteriorly in systole toward the left atrium. The lesion is not progressive in childhood, and specific therapy is not indicated. The patient may be at risk to develop infective endocarditis. Antibiotic prophylaxis is recommended during surgery and dental procedures (see Table 14–10).

14.64 PULMONARY VENOUS HYPERTENSION

A variety of lesions may result in chronic pulmonary venous hypertension, which when extreme may be followed by pulmonary arterial hypertension and right heart failure. These lesions include congenital mitral stenosis, mitral insufficiency, some varieties of total anomalous pulmonary venous return, left atrial myxomas, cor triatriatum (stenosis of the common pulmonary vein), individual pulmonary venous stenosis, and supravalvular mitral ring or web. In these conditions early symptoms can be confused with chronic pulmonary disease as there may be no specific cardiac findings on physical examination. However, subtle signs of pulmonary hypertension may be present. The *electrocardiogram* shows right ventricular hypertrophy with spiked P waves. *Roentgenographic studies* show cardiac enlargement and prominence of pulmonary veins, the right ventricle and atrium, and the main pulmonary artery; the left atrium is normal in size or only slightly enlarged. *Echocardiograms* may demonstrate a left atrial myxoma, cor triatriatum, or a mitral valve abnormality. *Cardiac catheterization* excludes the presence of a shunt and demonstrates pulmonary hypertension with an elevated pulmonary arterial wedge pressure. The left atrial pressure is normal if the lesion is proximal. Selective pulmonary arteriography may delineate the anatomic lesion. It is important to recognize this clinical pattern since cor triatriatum, left atrial myxoma, and supravalvular mitral webs are successfully managed surgically.

14.65 ANOMALIES OF THE AORTIC ARCH

Right Aortic Arch. In this abnormality the aorta curves to the right, and, if it descends on the right side of the vertebral column, it is usually associated with other cardiac malformations. It is found in about 20% of cases of tetralogy of Fallot and is common in truncus arteriosus. A right aortic arch without another anomaly is not associated with symptoms. Right aortic arch can be visualized on roentgenograms. The trachea is deviated to the left of the midline rather than to the right as in the presence of a normal left arch. The barium-filled esophagus is indented on its right border at the level of the aortic arch.

Vascular Rings. Congenital abnormalities of the aortic arch and its major branches result in the formation of vascular rings around the trachea and esophagus with varying degrees of compression. The following are the more common anomalies: (1) double aortic arch (Figs. 14–60 and 14–61), (2) right aortic arch with left ligamentum arteriosum, (3) anomalous innominate artery arising further to the left on the arch than usual, (4) anomalous left carotid artery arising further to the right than usual and passing anterior to the trachea, and (5) anomalous left pulmonary artery (vascular sling). In the latter anomaly, the abnormal vessel arises from an elongated main pulmonary artery or from the right pulmonary artery. It courses between and compresses the trachea and esophagus.

If the vascular ring produces compression of the trachea and esophagus, symptoms are frequently present during infancy. Wheezing respirations tend to be chronic and are aggravated by crying, feeding, and flexion of the neck. Extension of the neck tends to relieve the noisy respiration. Vomiting is frequent. There may be a brassy cough, and pneumonia is common. Sudden death from aspiration is a threat. Roentgenographic examination of the barium-filled esophagus and aortography identify the anomaly (Fig. 14–61). An aberrant right subclavian artery is commonly seen but does not cause compression of the trachea.

Surgery is advised for symptomatic patients who have roentgenographic evidence of tracheal compression. The anterior vessel is usually divided in patients with double aortic arch (Fig. 14–60). Compression produced by a right aortic arch and left ligamentum arteriosum is relieved by division of the latter. Anomalous innominate or carotid arteries cannot be divided; the tracheal compression is relieved by attaching the adventitia of these vessels to the sternum. Anomalous left pulmonary artery is corrected during cardiopulmonary bypass by division at its origin and reanastomosis to the main pulmonary artery after it has been brought in front of the trachea. In this condition, severe tracheomalacia may be present and result in a poor prognosis.

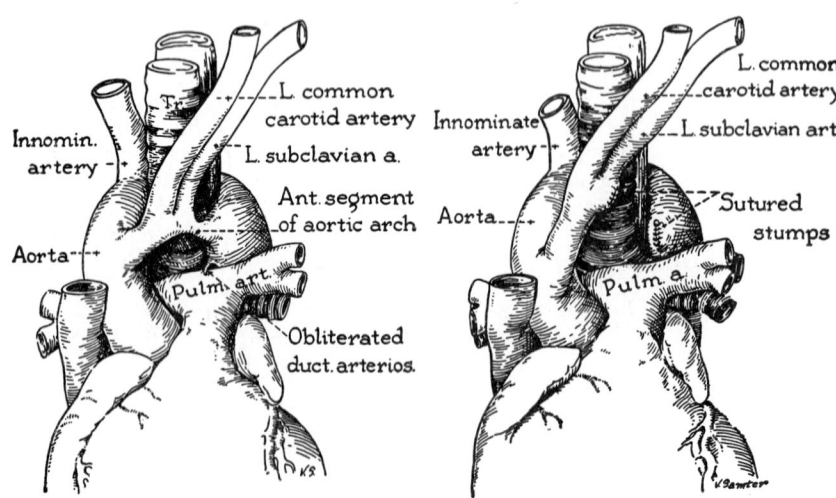

Figure 14–60. Double aortic arch. *A,* Small anterior segment of double aortic arch (most common type). *B,* Operative procedure for release of vascular ring.

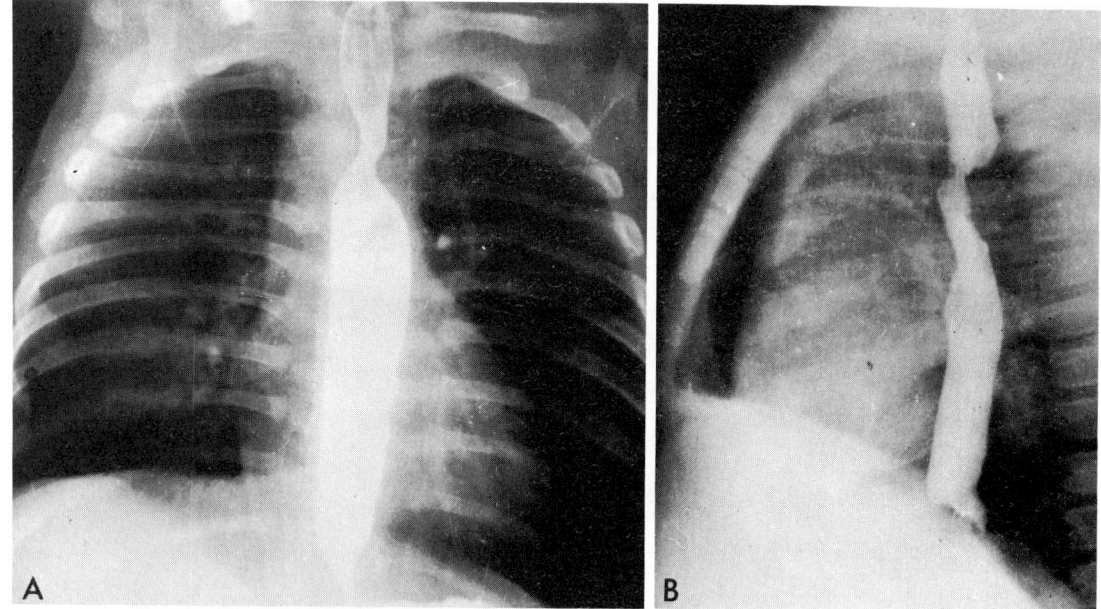

Figure 14–61. Double aortic arch in an infant aged 5 mo. A, Anteroposterior view. The barium-filled esophagus is constricted on both sides. B, Lateral view. The esophagus is displaced forward. The anterior arch was the smaller and was divided at operation. (Courtesy of Drs. Eugene Saenger, Frederick Silverman, and Edward McGrath.)

14.66 ANOMALOUS ORIGIN OF CORONARY ARTERIES

Anomalous Origin of the Left Coronary Artery from the Pulmonary Artery. In this anomaly the blood supply to the left ventricular myocardium is compromised. Soon after birth, as the pulmonary arterial pressure falls, the perfusion pressure to the left coronary artery becomes inadequate; myocardial infarction and fibrosis may result. In some instances interarterial collateral anastomoses develop between the right and left coronary arteries. Blood flow in the left coronary artery is then reversed, and it empties into the pulmonary artery. The left ventricle becomes dilated and performance is decreased as a result of myocardial injury. Mitral incompetence is a frequent complication secondary to infarction of papillary muscle. Localized aneurysms may also develop in the left ventricle.

Evidence of congestive heart failure becomes apparent within the first few months of life and is often precipitated by respiratory infection. Recurrent attacks of discomfort, restlessness, irritability, sweating, dyspnea, and pallor with or without mild cyanosis could be interpreted as due to angina pectoris. Cardiac enlargement is moderate to massive. Gallop rhythm is common. If present, murmurs may be of the nonspecific, ejection type or may be regurgitant because of mitral incompetence. Older patients with abundant intercoronary anastomoses may have continuous murmurs and little or no left ventricular dysfunction.

Roentgenographic examination confirms the cardiomegaly, but the contour and pulsations are not specific unless there is a complicating ventricular aneurysm. The *electrocardiogram* resembles the pattern described in lateral wall myocardial infarction in adults. A QR pattern followed by inverted T waves is seen in leads I and aVL. The left ventricular surface leads (V_5 and V_6) may also show deep Q waves and exhibit elevated S-T segments and inverted T waves (Fig. 14–62). *Two-dimensional echocardiography* may suggest the diagnosis but is not always reliable. *Aortography* is diagnostic; there is immediate opacification of only the right coronary artery. Generally, this

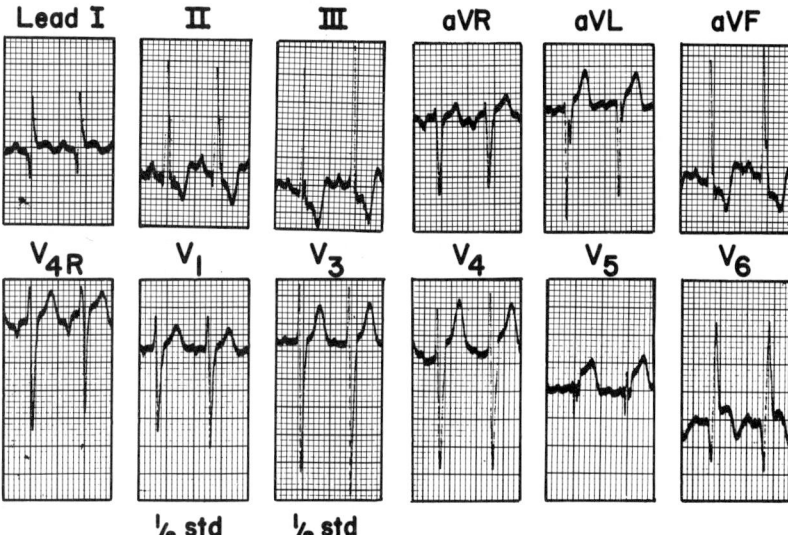

Figure 14–62. Electrocardiogram of a 3 mo old child with anomalous origin of the left coronary artery from the pulmonary artery. Lateral myocardial infarction is present as evidenced by abnormally large and wide Q waves in leads 1, V_5 and V_6, elevated S-T segment in V_5 and V_6, and inversion of TV_6.

vessel is large and tortuous. After filling of the intercoronary anastomoses, the left coronary artery and the pulmonary artery are in turn opacified. Selective pulmonary arteriography may opacify the anomalous left coronary artery. Selective left ventriculography in the infantile type reveals a dilated left ventricle which empties poorly.

Usually death from heart failure occurs within the first 6 mo. Those who survive usually have abundant intercoronary anastomoses.

Treatment is not standardized. In older patients the anomalous left coronary artery can be detached from the pulmonary artery and attached to the ascending aorta to establish normal arterial perfusion. The seriously ill infant who does not respond to anticongestive measures presents a difficult therapeutic problem. Ligation of the anomalous left coronary artery at its origin may be carried out to prevent runoff from the coronary circuit and possibly to increase myocardial perfusion by collateral circulation. This operation, however, is of variable effectiveness, and attempts to transplant the anomalous artery in infancy may be warranted.

Anomalous Origin of the Right Coronary Artery from the Pulmonary Artery. This unusual anomaly rarely produces signs or symptoms in infancy or early childhood.

14.67 PRIMARY PULMONARY HYPERTENSION

Primary pulmonary hypertension is a disease of unknown origin characterized by hypertension of the lesser circulation and right-sided heart failure. It may occur at any age. A genetic component may be present. Pulmonary hypertension is associated with precapillary obstruction of the pulmonary vascular bed due to hyperplasia of the muscular and elastic tissues and to the thickened intima of the small pulmonary arteries and arterioles. Atherosclerotic changes may be found in the larger pulmonary arteries. Other causes of pulmonary heart disease (chronic cor pulmonale) are absent, and there is no evidence of emphysema, pancreatic fibrosis, or kyphoscoliosis. Recurrent pulmonary emboli may produce the same clinical picture, but this disease is rare in childhood. Severe pulmonary hypertension may result from myriads of minute microemboli from an indwelling intravascular catheter inserted for hyperalimentation. Primary pulmonary hypertension must also be differentiated from elevated pulmonary pressure resulting from persistent obstruction of the upper airway (e.g., gross enlargement of the tonsils and adenoids), liver disease, or chronic pulmonary parenchymal disease.

Hemodynamics. Pulmonary hypertension places an afterload burden on the right ventricle, which results in right ventricular hypertrophy. Dilatation of the pulmonary artery is present and pulmonary valve insufficiency may occur. At the late stages cardiac output is decreased.

Clinical Manifestations. The predominant symptoms include effort intolerance and fatigability; occasionally, there is precordial chest pain, dizziness, or syncope. Peripheral cyanosis may be present and is associated with cold extremities; in the late stages of the disease the patient may have a gray appearance associated with low cardiac output. Arterial oxygen saturation is normal. If right-sided heart failure has supervened, the jugular venous pressure is elevated and hepatomegaly and edema are present. Jugular venous "a" waves are present, and when there is functional tricuspid insufficiency, a conspicuous jugular "cv" wave and systolic hepatic pulsations are manifest. The heart is moderately enlarged, and there is a right ventricular heave. The 1st heart sound is often followed by a pulmonic ejection click. The systolic murmur is soft and short and is sometimes followed

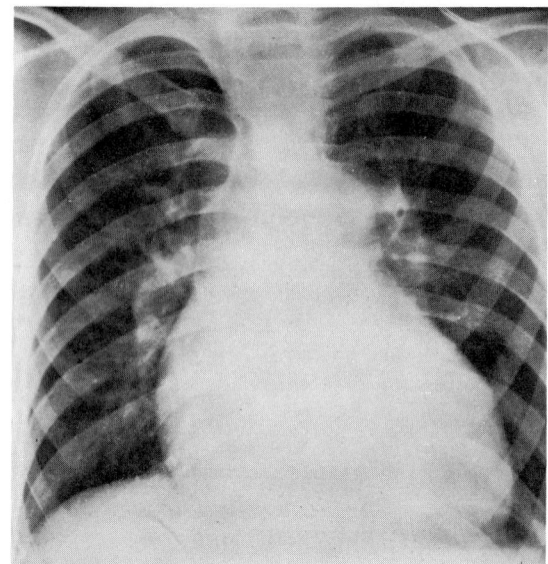

Figure 14–63. Roentgenogram in primary pulmonary hypertension; note the moderate cardiac enlargement, dilatation of the pulmonary artery, and relative pulmonary undervascularity in the outer two thirds of the lung fields.

by a blowing diastolic murmur due to pulmonary incompetence. The 2nd heart sound is closely split, loud, and sometimes booming; it is frequently palpable. A presystolic gallop rhythm may be audible down the left sternal border.

Roentgenograms reveal a prominent pulmonary artery and right ventricle (Fig. 14–63). The pulmonary vascularity in the hilar areas may be prominent and contrast with the peripheral lung fields, which are clear. The *electrocardiogram* shows right ventricular hypertrophy with spiked P waves.

Diagnosis. At cardiac catheterization this condition must be differentiated from Eisenmenger syndrome (Sec. 14.29) associated with a communication between the left and right heart or great arteries, as well as from left-sided obstructive lesions which result in pulmonary venous hypertension (Sec. 14.64). In the latter conditions the pulmonary arterial wedge pressure is significantly elevated. The risks of cardiac catheterization may be high in severely ill patients with primary pulmonary hypertension, and syncope or death may occur after pulmonary artery angiography (which should rarely be done in the most severely ill individuals). The presence of pulmonary artery hypertension with a normal pulmonary capillary wedge pressure is diagnostic.

Prognosis. Primary pulmonary hypertension is progressive, and most often there is no specific treatment. Recently, some success has been reported in infants or young children with significant pulmonary vasoreactivity with the use of calcium blocking agents. The terminal event most often is sudden in a patient with low cardiac output and is related to a lethal arrhythmia.

14.68 MARFAN SYNDROME: CARDIOVASCULAR MANIFESTATIONS

Cardiac complications occur with Marfan syndrome (Sec. 23.43) secondary to the elastic tissue disorder. Dilatation of the aorta may be noted at any age, beginning at the aortic valve and usually confined to the ascending portion and arch. The valve ring is stretched, and aortic insufficiency may ensue. Left ventricular failure occurs with or without angina pectoris. Dissecting aneurysm of the aorta with medial cystic necrosis may be the terminal event. Cardiac symptoms may occur as early as the 5th yr of life but frequently do not appear until adult life. Mitral insufficiency is even more common than aortic involvement and results from redundant cusps and chordae tendineae. Infective endocarditis may be a complication. Other congenital cardiac malformations have occasionally been reported. Surgery may be beneficial in some cases.

14.69 PRINCIPLES OF TREATMENT OF CONGENITAL HEART DISEASE

The majority of patients having mild congenital heart disease require no treatment. Parents and the child should be made aware that a normal life is expected and that no restriction of the child's activities is necessary. Overprotective parents may use the presence of a mild congenital lesion or even a functional heart murmur as a means to excessively control the child's activities. Although he or she may not express fears overtly, the child may become quite anxious regarding early death or debilitation, especially when an adult member of the family develops symptomatic heart disease. The family may have an unexpressed fear of sudden death, and the rarity of this manifestation should be emphasized in discussions directed at improving their understanding of the child's congenital heart defect. The difference between congenital heart disease and degenerative coronary disease in adults should be outlined. General health maintenance, including a well balanced diet, prevention of anemia, and the usual immunization program, should be encouraged.

Even patients with moderate to severe heart disease need not be markedly restricted in physical activities. Physical education should be modified appropriately to the child's capacity to participate. Rough, competitive sports should be discouraged. Patients with severe heart disease with decreased exercise tolerance will tend to limit their own activities. Transportation to school may be helpful so that fatigue will not interfere with classroom activities. Dyspnea, headache, and fatigability in cyanotic patients may be a sign of increasing hypoxemia and may require some limitation of activities among those for whom specific medical or surgical treatment is not available.

Bacterial infections should be treated vigorously, but the presence of congenital heart disease is not an appropriate reason to utilize antibiotics indiscriminately. Prophylaxis against infective endocarditis should be carried out during extensive dental procedures, during instrumentation of the urinary tract, and prior to lower gastrointestinal manipulation. Treatment of iron deficiency anemia is especially important in cyanotic patients who will improve their exercise tolerance and general well being with adequate hemoglobin levels. On the other hand, these patients should also be carefully observed for polycythemia. Cyanotic patients should avoid situations in which dehydration may occur. High altitudes and sudden changes in thermal environment should also be avoided. Venisection with volume replacement should be carried out at intervals in the presence of severe polycythemia (Hct > 65%) in inoperable patients. Patients with severe congenital heart disease or a history of rhythm disturbance should be carefully monitored during anesthesia for even routine surgical procedures. Women should be counseled on the dangers of child-bearing and the use of contraceptives and tubal ligation. Pregnancy is an especially high risk for patients having chronic cyanosis and/or pulmonary artery hypertension and rarely results in normal delivery at term. However, women with mild to moderate heart disease and many of those who have had corrective surgery can have normal pregnancies.

The treatment for congestive heart failure is described in Sec. 14.80, for paroxysmal hypercyanotic attacks in Sec. 14.14, and for cardiac arrhythmias in Sec. 14.70. Appropriate surgical procedures for specific cardiac lesions are discussed in the relevant sections of this chapter.

Recently, *cardiac transplantation* has been more frequently used for children and adolescents. This extreme measure may be indicated for patients in whom all medical and surgical therapy has been exhausted, and in whom the great veins and arteries are of sufficient size and in an acceptable position so that a donor heart can be implanted. In addition, pulmonary arterial vascular disease should not be present. Most pediatric candidates for cardiac transplantation have cardiomyopathy with chronic congestive heart failure and extremely poor myocardial performance. Although the long-term prognosis is unknown, some patients are living on an immunosuppressive regimen (cyclosporin) 2 years or more after transplantation. The quality of life for most has been acceptable, and it appears that for selected patients with no other options, this mode of therapy may become an acceptable alternative.

The Postoperative Period (Sec. 5.49). After successful open heart surgery, the postoperative course depends on numerous factors. The type of congenital defect operated upon, the age and condition of the patient prior to surgery, the events in the operating room, and the quality of the postoperative care will influence the patient's course following surgery. Many patients will have a benign postoperative period without complications, but others may be in a precarious state for hours or days after the operation.

Postoperative care should be initiated in the intensive care unit by a staff experienced with the unique problems encountered after open heart surgery (Sec. 5.39). A femoral arterial catheter is inserted prior to open heart surgery to allow direct arterial pressure measurements and arterial samplings for blood gas determinations. A second catheter positioned in the inferior vena cava via the saphenous or femoral vein is used for measuring central venous pressure. Left atrial or pulmonary artery catheters are often also utilized as are pacing wires on the atrium and ventricle.

Functional failures in one system may cause profound physiologic and biochemical changes in another. Respiratory insufficiency, for example, will lead to hypoxia, acidosis, and hypercarbia, which in turn will compromise cardiac and renal function. The latter problems cannot be managed successfully until adequate ventilation is re-established. Thus, it is essential that the primary source of each postoperative problem be identified and treated.

Respiratory failure is probably the major postoperative complication encountered after open heart surgery. Cardiopulmonary bypass carried out in the presence of pulmonary congestion results in decreased lung compliance, copious tracheal and bronchial secretions, atelectasis, and increased breathing efforts. Since fatigue and subsequently hypoventilation and acidosis may rapidly ensue, mechanical positive pressure endotracheal ventilation is instituted immediately following open heart surgery. This is continued for a minimum of several hours in relatively stable patients and up to 2–3 days or more in severely ill patients, especially infants.

Cardiac rhythm disorders must be diagnosed quickly since a prolonged untreated arrhythmia may add a severe hemodynamic burden to the heart in the critical early postoperative period. Injury to the heart's conduction system during surgery can cause postoperative *complete heart block*. This rare complication is treated with surgically placed pacing wires which are later removed. Occasionally, heart block will become permanent, requiring insertion of an implanted pacemaker, but in most instances this rhythm pattern is transient, and only temporary pacing wires are needed. *Tachyarrhythmias* are more often a problem in postoperative patients.

The *electrocardiogram* should be monitored continuously during the postoperative period. A change in the heart rate may be the first indication of a serious complication, such as hemorrhage, hypothermia, hypoventilation, or congestive heart failure.

Congestive heart failure following cardiac surgery may be secondary to respiratory failure, serious arrhythmias, myocardial injury, blood loss, hypervolemia, or significant residual hemodynamic abnormality. Specific treatment related to etiology should be instituted. Isoproterenol, dopamine, dobutamine, digoxin, and nitroprusside are the cardioactive agents most often used in patients with myocardial dysfunction in the early postoperative period; diuretic therapy is also often required (Sec. 5.7).

Acidosis secondary to low cardiac output, renal failure, or hypovolemia must be prevented or promptly corrected. An arterial pH below 7.30 may result in a decrease in cardiac output with increase in lactic acid production and may be the forerunner of a series of arrhythmias or cardiac arrest.

Kidney function may be compromised by congestive heart failure and further impaired by prolonged cardiopulmonary bypass. Persistent anuria or oliguria indicates poor cardiac function, hypokalemia, and/or acute renal failure. Blood and fluid replacement and/or a cardiotonic regimen will rapidly re-establish normal urine flow in patients with hypovolemia or cardiac failure, but renal failure secondary to tubular injury may require peritoneal dialysis.

The *postcardiotomy syndrome* may occur toward the end of the first postoperative week or sometimes be delayed until weeks or months after operation. This febrile illness is characterized by pericarditis and pleurisy, which in most instances is self-limiting and associated with a benign course. When pericardial fluid accumulates, the potential danger of cardiac tamponade should be recognized. Symptomatic patients usually respond to salicylates or indomethacin and bed rest. A prolonged illness or late recurrences are not unusual.

Hemolysis of probable mechanical origin is rarely seen after repair of endocardial cushion defects or the insertion of an artificial prosthetic valve. It occurs secondarily to unusual turbulence of blood at increased pressure. Reoperation may be necessary in patients with severe and progressive hemolysis who require frequent blood transfusions, but in most instances the problem slowly regresses.

Infection. Sepsis with infective endocarditis is an infrequent complication but can be difficult to manage, especially when prosthetic patches or valves are used (Sec. 14.74).

Prognosis. Patients who have had palliative procedures for extremely complex heart disease may lead limited but productive lives. Such patients require careful follow-up and various restrictions depending on the severity of their disease. The great majority of congenital heart defects can be corrected by open heart surgery; in most patients cardiac dynamics are improved and symptoms disappear. Some patients may develop late complications or require reoperation. Children who have undergone repair of complex cardiac lesions should be followed closely with appropriate laboratory tests (e.g., Holter monitors, exercise studies, echocardiograms, radionuclide studies, and, when indicated, cardiac catheterizations). The need for special studies should be decided upon after careful clinical evaluation, electrocardiogram, and chest roentgenogram. After successful repair of simple lesions with no evidence of residual abnormalities, such as patent ductus arteriosus, atrial septal defect, or valvular pulmonary stenosis, patients require very few specific follow-up studies, and should be encouraged to lead active and full lives.

The Neonatal Circulation

Dawes GS: Fetal and Neonatal Physiology. Chicago, Year Book Medical Publishers, 1968.
Freed MD, Heymann MA, Lewis AB, et al: Prostaglandin E in infants with ductus arteriosus–dependent congenital heart disease. Circulation 64:899, 1981.
Friedman WF: The intrinsic physiologic properties of the developing heart. Prog Cardiovasc Dis 15:87, 1972.
Gersony WM, Duc GV, Sinclair JC: "PFC" syndrome (persistence of the fetal circulation). Circulation 40:111, 1969.
Gersony WM, Peckham GJ, Ellison RC, et al: Effects of indomethacin in premature infants with patent ductus arteriosus: Results of a national collaborative study. J Pediatr 102:895, 1983.

Incidence and Etiology

Dennis NR, Warren J: Risks to offspring of patients with some common congenital heart defects. J Med Genet 18:8, 1981.
Fyler DC, Buckley LP, Hellenbrand WE, et al: Report of the New England Regional Infant Cardiac Program. Pediatrics 65(Suppl):377, 1980.
Hoffman JIE, Christianson R: Congenital heart disease in a cohort of 19,502 births with long-term follow-up. Am J Cardiol 42:641, 1978.
Michels VV, Ricardi VM: Congenital heart defects. In: Emery AEH, Rimoin DL (eds): Principles and Practice of Medical Genetics. Edinburgh, New York, Churchill Livingstone, 1983, pp 945–955.
Mitchell SC, Karones SB, Berendes HW: Congenital heart disease in 56,109 births: Incidence and natural history. Circulation 43:323, 1971.
Nadas A, Ellison R, Weidman W: Report from the joint study on the natural history of congenital heart defects. Circulation 56(2):Suppl 1, Aug, 1977.
Noonan JA: Syndromes associated with cardiac defects. Cardiovasc Clin 11:97, 1980.
Nora JJ: Etiologic factors in congenital heart diseases. Pediatr Clin North Am 18:1059, 1971.
Whittemore R, Hobbins JC, Engle MA: Pregnancy and its outcome in women with and without surgical treatment of congenital heart disease. Am J Cardiol 50:641, 1982.

Tetralogy of Fallot and Pulmonary Atresia

Anderson RH, Allwork SP, Ho SY, et al: Surgical anatomy of tetralogy of Fallot. J Thorac Cardiovasc Surg 81:887, 1981.
Barratt-Boyes BG, Neutze MJ: Primary repair of tetralogy of Fallot in infancy using profound hypothermia with circulatory arrest and limited cardiopulmonary bypass. Ann Surg 178:406, 1974.
Dabizzi RP, Caprioli G, Aiazzi L, et al: Distribution and anomalies of coronary arteries in tetralogy of Fallot. Circulation 61:95, 1980.
Garson A, Nihill MR, McNamara DG, et al: Status of the adult and adolescent after repair of tetralogy of Fallot. Circulation 59:1232, 1976.
Gersony WM, Batthany S, Bowman FO Jr, et al: Late followup of patients evaluated hemodynamically after total correction of tetralogy of Fallot. J Thorac Cardiovasc Surg 66:209, 1973.
Guntheroth WG, Morgan BC: Physiologic studies of paroxysmal hyperpnea in cyanotic congenital heart disease. Circulation 31:70, 1965.
Kirklin JW, Blackstone EH, Kirklin JK, et al: Surgical results and protocols in the spectrum of tetralogy of Fallot. Ann Surg 198:251, 1983.
Kirklin JW, Karp RB: The Tetralogy of Fallot: From a Surgical Viewpoint. Philadelphia, WB Saunders, 1970.
Malm JR, Bowman FO Jr, Hayes CJ, et al: Results of surgical treatment of pulmonary atresia with intact ventricular septum. In: Advances in Cardiology. Vol II. Basel, Karger, 1974.
Rocchinl AP: Hemodynamic abnormalities in response to supine exercise in patients after operative correction of tetralogy of Fallot after early childhood. Am J Cardiol 48:325, 1981.

Transposition of the Great Arteries

Allwork SP, Bentall HH, Becker AE, et al: Congenitally corrected transposition of the great arteries: Morphologic study of 32 cases. Am J Cardiol 38:910, 1976.
Duncan WJ, Freedom RM, Rowe RD, et al: Echocardiographic features before and after the Jatene procedure (anatomical correction) for transposition of the great vessels. Am Heart J 102:227, 1981.
Freedom RM, Culham JA, Olley PM, et al: Anatomical correction of transposi-

tion of the great arteries: Pre- and postoperative cardiac catheterization with angiocardiography in five patients. Circulation 63:905, 1981.

Gillette PC, Kugler JD, Gutgesell HP, et al: Mechanisms of cardiac arrhythmias after the Mustard operation for transposition of the great arteries. Am J Cardiol 45:1225, 1980.

Hayes CJ, Gersony WM: Arrhythmias after the Mustard operation for transposition of the great arteries: A long term study. J Am Coll Cardiol 7:133, 1986.

Hagler D, Ritter D, Mair D, et al: Clinical angiographic and hemodynamic assessment of late results after Mustard operation. Circulation 57:1214, 1978.

Mustard WT, Keith JD, Trusler GA, et al: The surgical management of transposition of the great vessels. J Thorac Cardiovasc Surg 48:593, 1965.

Rashkind WJ, Miller WW: Creation of an atrial septal defect without thoracotomy: A palliative approach to complete transposition of the great vessels. JAMA 196:991, 1966.

Rastelli GC, McGoon DC, Wallace RB: Anatomic correction of transposition of the great arteries with ventricular septal defect and subpulmonary stenosis. J Thorac Cardiovasc Surg 58:545, 1969.

Westerman GR, Lang P, Castenada AR, et al: Corrected transposition and repair of associated intracardiac defects. Circulation 66:I–197, 1982.

Wilcox BR, Ho SY, Macartney FJ, et al: Surgical anatomy of double-outlet right ventricle with situs solitus and atrioventricular concordance. J Thorac Cardiovasc Surg 82:405, 1981.

Yacoub M, Bernhard A, Lange P, et al: Clinical and hemodynamic results of the two-state anatomic correction of simple transposition of the great arteries. Circulation 62(Suppl):190, 1980.

Pulmonary Vascular Disease

Friedman WF, Heiferman M: Clinical problems of pulmonary vascular disease. Am J Cardiol 56:31, 1982.

Heath D, Edwards JE: The pathology of hypertensive pulmonary vascular disease. Circulation 18:533, 1958.

Hoffman JIE, Rudolph AM, Heymann MA: Pulmonary vascular disease with congenital heart lesions: Pathologic features and causes. Circulation 64:873, 1981.

Wood P: Pulmonary hypertension. Mod Conc Cardiovasc Dis 28:513, 1959.

Tricuspid Atresia

Bowman FO Jr, Malm JR, Hayes CJ, et al: Physiological approach to surgery for tricuspid atresia. Circulation 58(Suppl):83, 1978.

Fontan F, Deville C, Quaegebeur J, et al: Repair of tricuspid atresia in 100 patients. J Thorac Cardiovasc Surg 85:647, 1983.

Gale AW, Danielson GK, McGoon DC, et al: Fontan procedure for tricuspid atresia. Circulation 62:91, 1980.

Ebstein Disease

Danielson GK, Fuster A: Surgical repair of Ebstein's anomaly. Ann Surg 196:499, 1982.

Genton E, Blount SG: The spectrum of Ebstein's anomaly. Am Heart J 73:395, 1967.

Kumar AE, Fyler DC, Miettinen OS, et al: Ebstein's anomaly. Am J Cardiol 28:84, 1971.

Zuberbuhler JR, Allwork SP, Anderson RH: The spectrum of Ebstein's anomaly of the tricuspid valve. J Thorac Cardiovasc Surg 77:202, 1979.

Atrial Septal Defect and Atrioventricular Canal

Cohn LH, Morrow AG, Braunwald E: Operative treatment of atrial septal defect: Clinical and haemodynamic assessments in 175 patients. Br Heart J 29:725, 1967.

Evans JR, Rowe RD, Keith JD: Clinical diagnosis of atrial septal defect in children. Am J Med 30:345, 1961.

Mair DD, McGoon DC: Surgical correction of atrioventricular canal during the first year of life. Am J Cardiol 40:66, 1977.

Rastelli GC, Kirklin JW, Titus JL: Anatomic observations on complete form of persistent common atrioventricular canal, with special reference to atrioventricular valves. Proc Mayo Clin 41:296, 1966.

Wallace RB, McGoon DC, Danielson GK: Complete atrioventricular canal. Repair and results. Adv Cardiol 11:26, 1974.

Ventricular Septal Defect

Edwards JE: The pathology of ventricular septal defect. Semin Radiol 1:2, 1966.

Kirklin J: Current status of corrective surgery for ventricular septal defect. In: Rowe RD, Kidd BSL (eds): The Child with Congenital Heart Disease after Surgery. Mt. Kisco, NY, Futura, 1976.

Levin AR, Spach MS, Canent RV Jr, et al: Intracardiac pressure-flow dynamics in isolated ventricular septal defects. Circulation 35:430, 1967.

Ritter DG, Feldt RH, Weidman WH, et al: Ventricular septal defect. Circulation 32(Suppl 3):42, 1965.

Sigman JM, Perry BL, Behrendt DM, et al: Ventricular septal defect: Results after repair in infancy. Am J Cardiol 39:66, 1977.

Tatsuno K, Konno S, Ando M, et al: Pathogenetic mechanisms of prolapsing

aortic valve and aortic regurgitation associated with ventricular septal defect. Anatomical, angiographic, and surgical considerations. Circulation 48:1028, 1973.

Weidman WH, Blount SG Jr, DuShane JW, et al: Clinical course in ventricular septal defect. Circulation 56:156, 1977.

Weidman WH, Gersony WM, Nugent EW, et al: Indirect assessment of severity in ventricular septal defect. Circulation 56(Suppl):24, 1977.

Pulmonary Stenosis with Normal Aortic Root

Abrahams DG, Wood PH: Pulmonary stenosis with normal aortic root. Br Heart J 13:519, 1951.

Ellison RC, Freedom RM, Keane JF, et al: Indirect assessment of severity in pulmonary stenosis. Circulation 56(Suppl):14, 1977.

Leatham A, Weitzman D: Auscultatory and phonocardiographic signs of pulmonary stenosis. Br Heart J 19:303, 1957.

Nugent EW, Freedom RM, Nora JJ, et al: Clinical course in pulmonary stenosis. Circulation 56(Suppl):38, 1977.

Total Anomalous Pulmonary Venous Return

Cooley DA, Hallman GL, Leachman RD: Total anomalous pulmonary venous drainage. Correction with the use of cardiopulmonary bypass in 62 cases. J Thorac Cardiovasc Surg 51:88, 1966.

Delisle G, Masahiko A, Calder AL, et al: Total anomalous pulmonary venous connection: Report of 93 autopsied cases with emphasis on diagnostic and surgical considerations. Am Heart J 91:99, 1976.

Duff DG, Nihill MR, McNamara DG: Infradiaphragmatic total anomalous pulmonary venous return. Review of clinical and pathological findings and results of operation in 28 cases. Br Heart J 39:619, 1977.

Gersony WM, Bowman FO Jr, Steeg CN, et al: The management of total anomalous pulmonary venous drainage in early infancy. Circulation 43:1, 1971.

Turley K, Tucker WY, Ullyot DJ, et al: Total anomalous pulmonary venous connection in infancy: Influence of age and type of lesion. Am J Cardiol 45:92, 1980.

Whight CM, Barratt-Boyes BG, Calder AL, et al: Total anomalous pulmonary venous connection. Long-term results following repair in infancy. J Thorac Cardiovasc Surg 75:52, 1978.

Aortic Stenosis

Doyle EF, Arumugham P, Lara E, et al: Sudden death in young patients with congenital aortic stenosis. Pediatrics 53:481, 1974.

Edmunds LH, Wagner HR, Heyman MA: Aortic valvulotomy in neonates. Circulation 61:421, 1980.

Freedom RM, Dische MR, Rowe RD: Pathologic anatomy of subaortic stenosis and atresia in the first year of life. Am J Cardiol 39:1035, 1977.

Friedman WF, Pappelbaum SJ: Indications for hemodynamic evaluation and surgery in congenital aortic stenosis. Pediatr Clin North Am 18:1207, 1971.

Kelly DT, Wulfsberg E, Rowe RD: Discrete subaortic stenosis. Circulation 46:309, 1972.

McCue CM, Spicuzza TJ, Robertson LW, et al: Familial supravalvular aortic stenosis. J Pediatr 73:889, 1968.

Sandor GG, Olley PM, Trusler GA, et al: Long-term follow-up of patients after valvotomy for congenital valvular aortic stenosis in children: A clinical and actuarial follow-up. J Thorac Cardiovasc Surg 80:171, 1980.

Wagner HR, Ellison RC, Keane JF, et al: Clinical course in aortic stenosis. Circulation 56(Suppl):47, 1977.

Wagner HR, Weidman WH, Ellison RC, et al: Indirect assessment of severity in aortic stenosis. Circulation 56(Suppl):20, 1977.

Mitral Valve Anomalies

Barlow JB, Bosman CK: Aneurysmal protrusion of the posterior leaflet of the mitral valve. Am Heart J 71:166, 1966.

Bisset GS, Schwartz DC, Meyer RA, et al: Clinical spectrum and long-term follow-up of isolated mitral valve prolapse in 119 children. Circulation 62:423, 1980.

Daoud G, Kaplan S, Perrin EV, et al: Congenital mitral stenosis. Circulation 27:185, 1963.

John S, Krishnaswami S, Jairaj PS, et al: The profile and surgical management of mitral stenosis in young patients. J Thorac Cardiovasc Surg 69:631, 1975.

Reed GE, Pooley RW, Moggio RA: Durability of measured mitral annuloplasty: Seventeen year study. J Thorac Cardiovasc Surg 79:321, 1980.

Sahn DJ, Allen HD, Goldberg SJ, et al: Mitral valve prolapse in children. A problem defined by real-time cross-sectional echocardiography. Circulation 53:651, 1976.

Dextrocardia and Levocardia

Liberthson RR, Hastreiter AR, Sinha SN, et al: Levocardia with visceral heterotaxy–isolated levocardia: Pathologic anatomy and its clinical implications. Am Heart J 85:40, 1973.

Van Praagh R: Malposition of the heart. In: Moss AJ, Adams FH (eds): Heart Disease in Infants, Children and Adolescents. Baltimore, Williams & Wilkins, 1968.

Principles of Treatment

Benzing G, Kaplan S: Late complications of cardiac surgery. Pediatr Clin North Am 18:1225, 1971.

Engle MA, Zabriskie JB, Seuterfit LB, et al: Viral illness and post-pericardiotomy syndrome: A prospective study in children. Circulation 62:1151, 1980.

Gersony WM, Krongrad E: Evaluation and management of patients after surgical repair of congenital heart disease. Progr Cardiovasc Dis 18:39, 1975. Also *In*: Rosenthal EH, Sonnenblick EH, Lesch M (eds): Postoperative Congenital Heart Disease. New York, Grune & Stratton, 1975, p 145.

14.70 DISTURBANCES OF RATE AND RHYTHM OF THE HEART

Childhood cardiac rhythm disturbances are recognized more often now than in the past because diagnostic methods have improved. There are also more surgical survivors than previously after repair of congenital heart disease who may be prone to rhythm disturbances.

The major risk of a cardiac rhythm disorder is that of severe tachycardia or bradycardia leading to decreased cardiac output, a more severe arrhythmia, syncope, or sudden death. When there is ectopic cardiac activity, the major issue is whether the particular rhythm disturbance noted may be prone to deteriorate into a life-threatening tachyarrhythmia or bradyarrhythmia. Some rhythm abnormalities, such as single premature atrial and ventricular beats, are common among children without heart disease and in the great majority of instances do not pose a risk.

An increasing number of pharmacologic agents are available for treating significant rhythm disturbances in children. Problems with frequency of administration, compliance, side effects, and variable responses still remain, and selection of an appropriate agent involves a great deal of empiricism. However, most rhythm disturbances can be reliably controlled with a single agent. Surgical intervention to eliminate bypass tracts associated with pre-excitation syndromes or unusually electrically active areas in the heart is available for infrequent refractory abnormalities. Also, implanted pacemakers have become more reliable and less prone to technical failure than in the past. Implanted defibrillators are now available for use in high-risk patients with sudden onset ventricular tachycardia or fibrillation.

Sinus arrhythmia represents a physiologic variation in impulse discharges from within the sinus node related to respirations. There is slowing during expiration and acceleration during inspiration. Occasionally, if the sinus rate becomes slow enough there will be an escape beat from the atrioventricular junctional region (Fig. 14–64). Irregularities of sinus rhythm are commonly seen in premature infants, especially bradycardia associated with periodic apnea. Sinus arrhythmia is exaggerated during convalescence from febrile illness and by drugs which increase vagal tone, such as digitalis; it is usually abolished by exercise or by atropine. Some children have great variation in rate during sinus arrhythmia, which should not be confused with a significant rhythm disorder.

Sinus bradycardia is due to slow discharge of impulses from the sinus node. The normal resting sinus rate decreases during childhood, and the lower limit at a given rate is determined empirically. In general, a sinus rate under 90/min in neonates and under 60/min thereafter is considered to be sinus bradycardia. Sinus bradycardia is commonly seen in athletes. In healthy individuals it is without significance. Sinus bradycardia may occur in systemic disease, e.g., myxedema, and will resolve when the disorder is under control. It must be differentiated from sinoatrial and A-V blocks. Children with sinus bradycardia will significantly increase their heart rate with exercise to well over 100/min, whereas patients with A-V block are unable to do so. *Low birthweight infants* display great variation in sinus rate. Sinus bradycardia is common and may be associated with junctional escape beats. Prema-

ture atrial contractions are frequent. These rhythm changes, especially bradycardia, appear more commonly during sleep and are not associated with symptoms. No therapy is necessary.

Wandering atrial pacemaker (Fig. 14–65) is defined as an intermittent shift in the pacemaker of the heart from the sinus node to another part of the atrium. This is common in childhood and usually represents a normal variant.

Extrasystoles are produced by the discharge of an ectopic focus that may be situated anywhere in atrial, junctional, or ventricular tissue. In the majority of instances extrasystoles are of no clinical or prognostic significance. Under certain circumstances premature beats may be due to organic heart disease (inflammatory, ischemic, fibrotic, etc.). Drug toxicity, especially with digitalis, may also produce extrasystoles.

Premature atrial complexes are not uncommon in childhood, even in the absence of cardiac disease. Depending on the degree of prematurity and the preceding cycle length, some premature atrial complexes result in a normal QRS configuration. In other instances they may be conducted to the ventricle while the specialized ventricular conducting system is partially refractory and result in an abnormal QRS configuration (Fig. 14–66), which then must be distinguished from premature ventricular systoles. Careful scrutiny of the electrocardiogram for a premature P wave, preceding the QRS, that has a different contour from sinus P waves is essential for diagnosis.

Premature ventricular complexes (PVC's) may arise in any region of the ventricles. They are characterized by premature, widened, bizarre QRS complexes which are not preceded by a P wave (Fig. 14–67). When they have identical contours, they are classified as unifocal in origin. When PVC's vary in contour, they are designated as multifocal.

Extrasystoles are usually followed by a compensatory pause as they interfere with the next sinus beat. In the majority of instances extrasystoles disappear during the tachycardia of exercise. If they remain or become exaggerated during exercise, the arrhythmia may have greater significance. Extrasystoles produce a smaller stroke and pulse volume than normal and, if very premature, may not be audible with a stethoscope or palpable at the radial pulse. Extrasystoles may assume a definite rhythm, e.g., alternating with normal beats (pulsus bigeminus) or occurring after 2 normal beats (pulsus trigeminus). The following criteria are indications for further investigation of PVC's, which could require suppressive therapy: (1) sequential ventricular depolarizations without intervening sinus beats, (2) multiform origin, (3) increased ventricular ectopia with exercise, (4) R on T phenomenon (premature ventricular depolarization occurs on the T wave of the preceding beat), (5) significantly increased ectopy during exercise, (6) presence of underlying heart disease, and (7) unusual patient awareness of beats associated with marked anxiety.

Most patients are unaware of premature contractions, although some may be aware of a "skipped beat" or a sudden "turnover" or "tickle" over the precordium. This is due to the increased cardiac output from the normal beat following a compensatory pause. Anxiety, a febrile illness, or ingestion of various drugs or stimulants causes premature ventricular

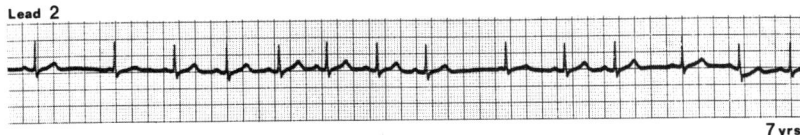

Figure 14–64. Sinus arrhythmia with junctional escape beat: note the variation in P-P interval with little change in P morphology or P-R interval. When the sinus rate is slow enough the atrioventricular junction takes over, producing escape beats. This rhythm is normal.

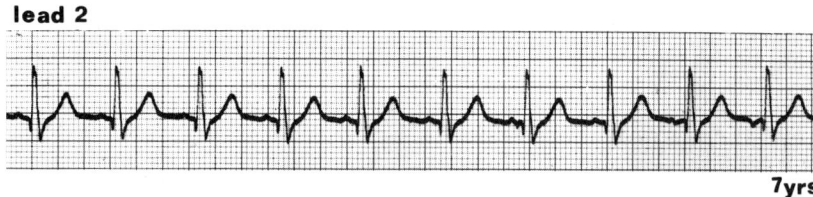

Figure 14–65. Wandering atrial pacemaker: note the change in P wave configuration in the 7th, 9th, and 10th beats. The 7th P wave may represent a fusion between the sinus P and the ectopic atrial pacemaker seen in the 10th beat.

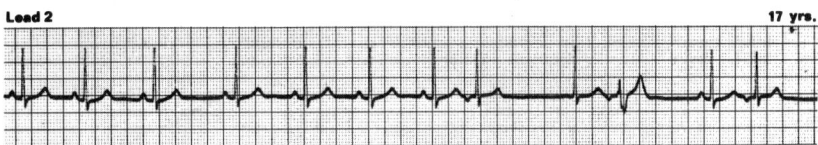

Figure 14–66. Premature atrial contraction (PAC): QRS complexes, the 8th, 10th, and final, in this strip are preceded by a P wave that is inverted, denoting an ectopic origin of atrial depolarization. Note that the 8th and final QRS complexes resemble those of sinus origin, whereas the 10th is aberrantly conducted. This is a function of the preceding cycle length that influences the refractory period of the bundle branches. Note that the pause after the PAC is longer than 2 P-P intervals, implying that the premature atrial depolarization has invaded and discharged the sinus node, and reset it, so that it fires later.

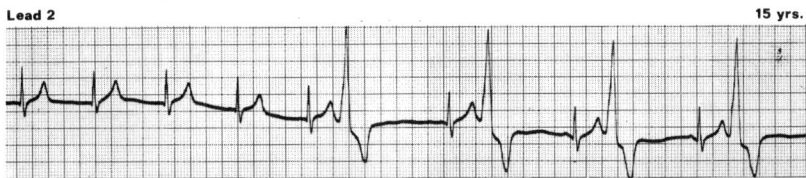

Figure 14–67. Premature ventricular contractions (PVC) induced by hyperventilation: note that the premature beat is wide and has a completely different morphology from that of the sinus beat. The premature beat is not preceded by a P wave, and the pause following it is fully compensatory, i.e., the P-P interval containing the PVC equals 2 sinus cycles; this indicates that the sinus mechanism has not been disturbed by the premature beats.

beats. The basis of therapy for benign PVC's is convincing reassurance that the arrhythmia is not the result of structural heart disease; sedatives or suppressive agents may be used in selected cases.

14.71 TACHYARRHYTHMIAS

SUPRAVENTRICULAR TACHYARRHYTHMIAS

Paroxysmal Atrial Tachycardia (PAT). Re-entry within the A-V node is the most common mechanism of paroxysmal atrial tachycardia. The tachycardia is initiated by a premature atrial beat which is conducted through a tract within the A-V node. The ventricular response induces an atrial echo beat via a retrograde tract within the A-V node which in turn is transmitted back to the ventricle and so on.

In older children paroxysmal atrial tachycardia is characterized by abrupt onset and cessation; the attack may be precipitated by an acute infection. If an attack is not witnessed, its occurrence may be elicited by an accurate history. Attacks may last only a few seconds or may persist for hours, seldom for more than 2–3 days. The cardiac rate usually exceeds 180/min and occasionally may be as rapid as 300/min. The only complaint may be awareness of the rapid cardiac rate. Many children tolerate these episodes extremely well, and it is unlikely that short paroxysms are a danger to life. If the rate is exceptionally rapid or if the attack is prolonged, precordial discomfort and congestive cardiac failure may supervene.

In young infants, the diagnosis may be more obscure since the cardiac rate at this age is normally rapid and increases greatly with crying. A baby having PAT may present with congestive heart failure, if the precipitating severe tachycardia was not recognized for a long time. A persistent tachycardia during quiet periods or sleep suggests the diagnosis. The cardiac rate during paroxysms is frequently in the range of 200–300/min. If the attack lasts 6–24 hr or more, the infant becomes acutely ill, has an ashen color, and is restless and irritable. Tachypnea and hepatomegaly are the prominent signs of cardiac failure, and there may be fever and leukocytosis. Intrauterine tachycardia can cause severe cardiac failure and be responsible for hydrops fetalis (Fig. 14–68).

Treatment. Vagal stimulation by a simple procedure, such as unilateral carotid sinus massage, may abort the attack. This approach is usually ineffective in infants, but placement of an ice bag over the face has been quite effective. Older children may be taught vagotonic maneuvers to abolish the paroxysm, such as straining, the Valsalva maneuver, breath-holding, drinking ice water, or the adoption of a particular posture. When these measures fail and the child is symptomatic enough to warrant treatment, several alternatives are available. In urgent situations when congestive heart failure has occurred, electrical cardioversion is recommended as initial management. Pharmacotherapy should be considered as the initial approach under other circumstances. Digoxin has been the mainstay of therapy for patients with supraventricular tachycardia. Conduction is slowed within the A-V node and the re-entrant circuit is interrupted. Digoxin is effective in 95% of instances but often requires several hours to take effect. In neonates, digoxin therapy should be instituted even if the paroxysm has been abolished by vagal stimulation since the recurrence rate is high; therapy should be maintained for 3–6 mo or longer.

Other drugs that have been used to abolish the paroxysms include infusions of phenylephrine (Neo-Synephrine) or edrophonium (Tensilon) and oral administration of quinidine sulfate or propranolol. Calcium channel blockers have also been used in the initial treatment of paroxysmal supraventricular tachyarrhythmias in infants and children. When verapamil (Isoptin, Cordan) is administered intravenously 92–96% of infants and children can be converted to normal sinus rhythm within 5 min of an initial 0.1–0.2 mg/kg dose. No side effects are experienced by patients whose supraventricular tachycardias are due to re-entrant mechanisms. For maintenance therapy digoxin remains the treatment of choice for most patients.

In most instances of paroxysmal atrial tachycardia there is no underlying structural cardiac disease. If cardiac failure occurs during prolonged tachycardia in an infant with a normal heart, cardiac function rapidly returns to normal after sinus rhythm is reinstituted.

Between attacks some children may exhibit the electrocardiographic changes of the *Wolff-Parkinson-White (pre-excitation) syndrome:* short P-R interval and slow upstroke of the QRS (delta wave) (Fig. 14–69). Although most often present in a normal heart, this syndrome may also be associated with Ebstein anomaly, corrected transposition (ventricular inversion), and cardiomyopathy. The syndrome causes a predilec-

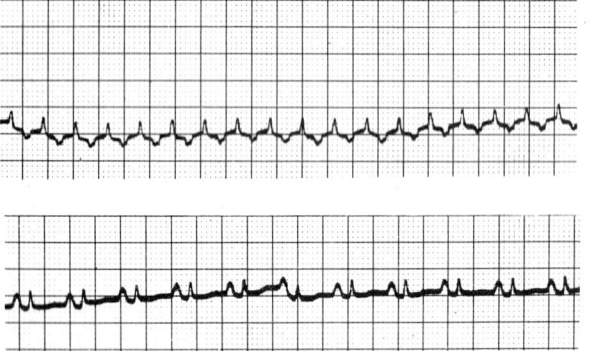

Figure 14–68. Upper tracing shows paroxysmal supraventricular tachycardia ("pat") with a ventricular rate of 230/min. The lower tracing shows sinus rhythm after D-C cardioversion. Note that during the tachycardia, the T wave is deformed by an inverted, presumably retrograde, P wave. The QRS morphology is unchanged during the tachycardia. Low voltage is due to peripheral edema in a 1 day old infant who had intrauterine tachycardia and hydrops fetalis.

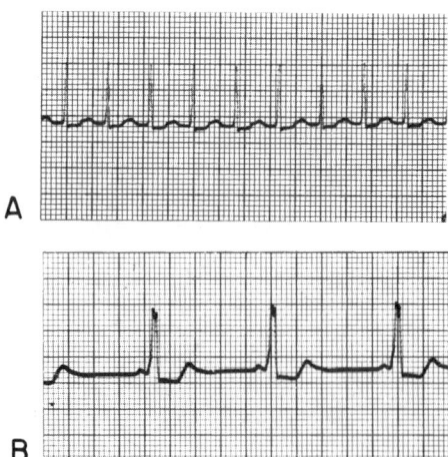

Figure 14–69. *A,* PAT in a child with Wolff-Parkinson-White (WPW) syndrome. Note the normal QRS complexes during the tachycardia. *B,* Later the typical features of WPW are apparent (short P-R interval, delta wave, and wide QRS).

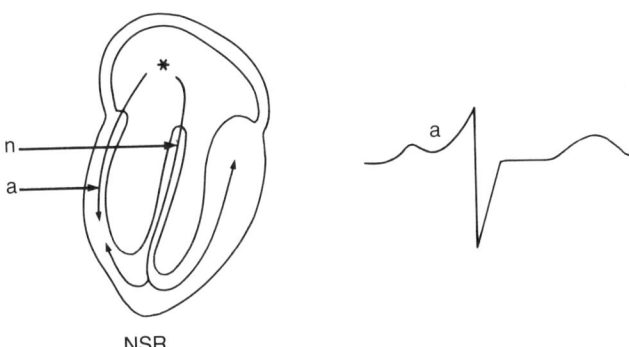

NSR

Figure 14–70. Schematic representation of the heart with a right-sided anomolous pathway. The asterisk indicates the initiation of the sinus beat. The arrows indicate the direction and spread of excitation. The electrocardiographic complex shown represents a fusion beat which combines activation over the normal (n) and accessory (a) pathways. The latter inscribes the delta wave.

tion for a re-entrant tachycardia. The anatomic substrate comprising the re-entrant circuit is the A-V node and an accessory pre-excitation pathway, a muscular bridge connecting atrium to ventricle on the right or left lateral cardiac border or within the ventricular septum (Fig. 14–70). During sinus rhythm the impulse is carried over both the A-V node and the accessory pathway; it produces some degree of fusion of the two depolarization fronts that results in an abnormal QRS. During tachycardia an impulse is usually carried antero-gradely over the A-V node, resulting in a normal QRS complex, and in retrograde fashion through the accessory pathway, reaching the atrium and perpetuating the tachycardia. Only after cessation of the tachycardia are the typical features of Wolff-Parkinson-White syndrome recognized (Fig. 14–69). Increasing numbers of cases are reported in which an accessory pathway can conduct only retrogradely and thus is responsible for cases of PAT in which the diagnosis cannot be made from the standard ECG. This situation is indistinguishable from other supraventricular tachycardias because conduction occurs anterograde only over the A-V node and can be diagnosed only by invasive electrophysiologic studies. When rapid antegrade conduction occurs through the pre-excitation pathway during tachycardia and the retrograde re-entry pathway to the atrium is via the A-V node, the potential for more serious arrhythmias is greater, especially should atrial fibrillation occur. Digoxin or verapamil should not be used for treatment, procainamide or quinidine may be used. Surgical excision of bypass tracts can be successfully carried out in selected patients.

Ectopic atrial tachycardia is an uncommon tachycardia in childhood. It is characterized by a variable rate (seldom greater than 200), identifiable P waves with abnormal frontal plane axis, and chronicity in either a sustained or intermittent tachycardia. It is usually more difficult to control pharmacologically than the more common paroxysmal tachycardias. Suppression of the ectopic atrial focus is difficult; therapy should, therefore, be directed to slowing atrioventricular conduction with digitalis or propranolol rather than relying on drugs that suppress atrial automaticity, such as quinidine and disopyramide. In some cases no treatment is necessary.

Chaotic or multifocal atrial tachycardia is characterized by two or more ectopic P waves with two or more different ectopic P-P cycles, frequent blocked P waves, and varying P-R intervals of conducted beats. This arrhythmia usually occurs in the absence of cardiac disease and usually terminates spontaneously after weeks or months. If the patient is asymptomatic, no treatment is necessary. Digitalis may be used to control the ventricular rate.

Accelerated junctional tachycardia is an arrhythmia in which the junctional rate exceeds that of the sinus node so that atrioventricular dissociation results. This arrhythmia is most often recognized in the early postoperative period following cardiac surgery, and may be difficult to control. It often disappears spontaneously without specific treatment. Junctional tachycardia may be a sign of digitalis intoxication, and when this occurs, the drug should be discontinued.

Atrial flutter is a regular or regularly irregular tachycardia due to atrial activity at a rate of 250–400/min. These contractions may be due to a circus movement in the atria and produced by an irritable focus in the atrial muscle similar to that responsible for paroxysmal atrial tachycardia and atrial extrasystoles. Because the atrioventricular node cannot transmit such rapid impulses, there is virtually always some degree of A-V block, and the ventricles respond to every 2nd–4th atrial beat. Occasionally, the response will be variable and the rhythm will appear irregular.

Atrial flutter is rare in children without heart disease. It may occur during acute infectious diseases, but is most often seen in patients with large stretched atria, such as those associated with longstanding mitral or tricuspid insufficiency. Atrial flutter also can occur after palliative or corrective intra-atrial surgery, e.g., for transposition of the great arteries, ostium secundum defect, or total anomalous pulmonary venous return. As with supraventricular tachycardia, uncontrolled atrial flutter may precipitate congestive cardiac failure. Carotid sinus pressure usually produces a temporary slowing of the cardiac rate. The diagnosis is confirmed by electrocardiography which demonstrates the rapid and regular atrial flutter or "f" waves. Digitalis slows the ventricular response in atrial flutter by prolonging conduction time through the A-V node. Occasionally, the rhythm will then convert to atrial fibrillation. After full digitalization, quinidine may be added to convert to sinus rhythm. However, atrial flutter usually converts immediately to sinus rhythm by cardioversion, and this has become the treatment of choice.

Atrial fibrillation is produced by a mechanism similar to that causing atrial flutter; the atrial excitation is irregularly irregular and more rapid (300–500/min) (Fig. 14–71). The arrhythmia occurs most frequently in older children with rheumatic mitral valve disease. It also is seen rarely as a complication of atrial septal defect, after intra-atrial surgery (e.g., Mustard operation), and with left atrial enlargement secondary to left atrioventricular valve incompetence. The rhythm is most often the result of chronically stretched atrial myocardium. The best initial treatment is digitalization, which restores the ventricular rate to normal, although the atrial fibrillation persists. Normal sinus rhythm may then be restored with quinidine sulfate or electrical cardioversion. However, reinstitution of sinus rhythm may not be possible in the patient whose atrial fibrillation is associated with florid atrio-

Figure 14–71. Atrial fibrillation, characterized by absence of P waves; presence of fibrillatory waves, which are grossly irregular, rapid undulations; and an irregular ventricular response. Fibrillatory waves may not be visible in all leads and should be carefully sought in every tracing with irregular R-R intervals. (The coexisting qR in V₁ is diagnostic of right ventricular hypertrophy in this patient with Eisenmenger syndrome.)

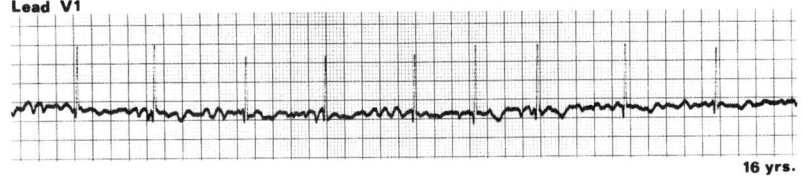

Lead V1

16 yrs.

Table 14–8. **Diagnosis of Tachyarrhythmias**

| | Heart Rate/Minute | Electrocardiographic Findings | | |
		P Wave	QRS Duration	Regularity
Sinus tachycardia	<225	Always present Normal axis	Normal	Rate varies with respiration
Atrial tachycardia	180–320	Present—50% Superior axis common	Normal or prolonged (RBBB pattern)	Regular
Atrial fibrillation	120–180	Fibrillatory waves	Normal or prolonged (RBBB pattern)	Irregularly irregular
Atrial flutter	Atrial: 250–400 Ventricular response variable: 100–320	Sawtoothed flutter waves	Normal or prolonged (RBBB pattern)	Regular ventricular response (e.g., 2:1, 3:1, 3:2, etc.)
Ventricular tachycardia	120–240	Absent	Usually prolonged	Slightly irregular

RBBB = right bundle branch block

ventricular valve disease and cardiomegaly. In such cases, chronic therapy with digitalis is usually required.

VENTRICULAR TACHYARRHYTHMIAS

Ventricular tachycardia is more common than had been thought in the past, but is less often seen than supraventricular tachycardia. It may be associated with myocarditis, develop many years after intraventricular surgery, or occur without obvious organic heart disease. It must be distinguished from supraventricular tachycardia with aberrancy or rapid conduction over an accessory pathway. The presence of capture and fusion beats confirms the diagnosis. In the absence of these features, diagnosis is more difficult. Right precordial and/or esophageal leads may be helpful in identifying P waves. Although some children tolerate rapid ventricular rates for many hours, unless this arrhythmia has been established as a benign disturbance, it should be promptly treated because hypotension and ventricular fibrillation may result. Lidocaine and cardioversion are methods of choice for rapid treatment. Quinidine, procainamide, and propranolol are most useful for chronic therapy.

Ventricular fibrillation results in death unless an effective ventricular beat is restored. A thump on the chest sometimes restores sinus rhythm. Usually external cardiac massage with artificial ventilation and electrical defibrillation is necessary. Recently, implanted defibrillators have been inserted in selected patients who have demonstrated refractoriness to preventive therapy.

Differential Diagnosis of Tachyarrhythmias. It is important from the standpoint of prognosis and treatment to accurately identify the type of tachyarrhythmia that is present (Table 14–8). Often the diagnosis is clear on a clinical and electrocardiographic basis, but in some instances differential diagnosis may be difficult.

First, it should be determined whether the patient is actually in sinus tachycardia. Time for treating an infection, acute anemia, or other illness which results in sinus tachycardia may be lost while a tachyarrhythmia is being considered, wrongly diagnosed, or even treated. Heart rates greater than 225/min are too rapid for sinus tachycardia, but rates in the 140–220 range could signify either an arrhythmia or sinus tachycardia. Ventricular tachycardia is almost invariably slower than supraventricular tachycardia.

Second, the configuration of the P waves should be evaluated. Although it is possible to have a supraventricular tachycardia with P waves of normal configuration (upright in leads I, II, and AVF), in most instances P waves will be abnormal. In many cases of supraventricular tachycardia with rapid ventricular response, the P wave will not be visible on the standard electrocardiogram, and it may be necessary to obtain Lewis-Golub leads (exploring right chest electrodes) or an esophageal lead to identify obscure P waves. The distinctive saw-toothed atrial waves produced by atrial flutter are best recognized in lead V_1. During atrial fibrillation atrial activity is represented by a chaotic baseline. During ventricular tachycardia the P wave is either absent or noted to be out of phase with the QRS deflections.

Third, an extremely narrow QRS suggests that the rhythm comes from either the supraventricular area or the region of the A-V node. However, prolonged QRS duration may be seen with a QRS aberrancy in the face of a supraventricular tachycardia as well as with ventricular arrhythmias. In the former the QRS morphology is almost always of the right bundle branch block type.

Finally, the rhythmicity should be determined. In sinus tachycardia the rate will vary every few seconds and will gradually slow with vagotonic maneuvers only to speed up again when they are discontinued. Atrial tachycardia is extremely regular, except at the onset or just prior to ending, whereas ventricular tachycardia displays slight beat-to-beat variations. Either atrial flutter will be regular or, with block, the ventricular response will consistently be some multiple of the interval between the flutter waves. In atrial fibrillation the ventricular response will be irregularly irregular.

14.72 BRADYARRHYTHMIAS
(Heart Block)

Sinus arrest and sinoatrial block may cause a sudden pause in the heart beat. The former is presumed to be due to failure of impulse formation within the sinus node, the latter, to a block between the sinus impulse and the surrounding atrium. These arrhythmias are rare in childhood except as manifestations of digitalis intoxication or in patients who have had extensive atrial surgery.

Atrioventricular block may be divided into *1st degree block*, in which the P-R interval is prolonged but all of the atrial impulses are conducted to the ventricle; *2nd degree block*, in which some impulses are not conducted to the ventricle; and *3rd degree block* (complete heart block), in which no impulses

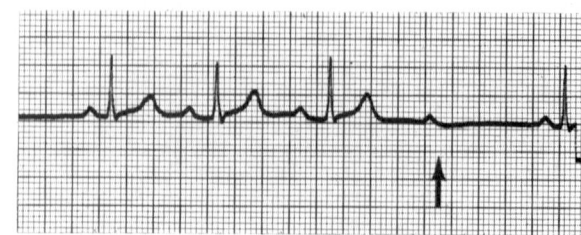

Figure 14–72. Wenckebach phenomenon (Mobitz I). The P-R interval gradually lengthens until the 4th P wave in the cycle is not conducted to the ventricle (arrow). The ensuing P-R interval is once again normal.

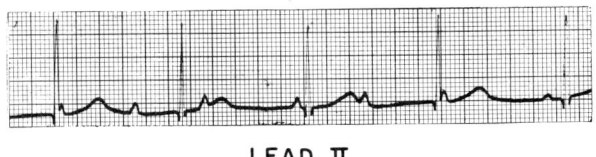

LEAD II

Figure 14–73. Complete atrioventricular block: the ventricular rate is regular at 53/min. The atrial rate varied from 65–95/min (probably sinus arrhythmia) The QRS morphology is normal, which is usual in congenital A-V block.

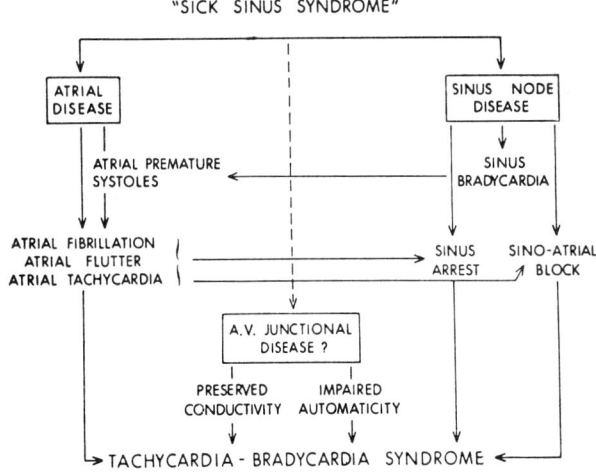

Figure 14–74. Factors resulting in the sick-sinus syndrome. (Kaplan BM, Langendorf R, Lev M., et al: Am J Cardiol 31:497, 1973. Reproduced by permission of Technical Publishing Company.)

from the atria reach the ventricles. In a variant of 2nd degree block, known as the *Wenckebach type* (also called Mobitz type I), the P-P interval remains constant, the P-R interval increases until a P wave is not conducted, and, in the cycle following the pause, the P-R is again shorter (Fig. 14–72). In Mobitz II, occasional atrial beats are not conducted to the ventricle; this conduction defect has more potential to cause syncope, and may be progressive.

Congenital complete atrioventricular block in children is probably the result of a congenital defect in the main stem of the bundle of His. The arrhythmia is occasionally suspected in the fetus. In an international study of almost 600 patients about 70% had no other evidence of heart disease. At greatest risk were infants with associated congenital heart disease who, in the first weeks of life, were in congestive cardiac failure, with atrial rates exceeding 150/min and ventricular rates less than 55. The most frequently associated cardiac malformations were "corrected" transposition of the great arteries (ventricular inversion), single ventricle, and patent ductus arteriosus. Isolated ventricular septal defect was seldom associated with complete heart block.

In older children with otherwise normal hearts the condition is commonly asymptomatic, although attacks of syncope may occur. The peripheral pulse is of the water-hammer type as a result of the large ventricular stroke volume and the peripheral vasodilatation; the systolic blood pressure is elevated. Jugular venous pulsations occur irregularly and may be large when the atrium contracts against a closed tricuspid valve (cannon wave). The 1st cardiac sound has varying intensity. Exercise and atropine produce an acceleration of 10–20 beats/min or more in the child. Systolic murmurs are frequent along the left sternal border, and apical mid-diastolic murmurs are not unusual. Heart block in itself results in cardiac enlargement.

The diagnosis is confirmed by electrocardiogram; the P waves and QRS complexes have no constant relation (Fig. 14–73). The QRS duration may be prolonged or may be normal if the heart beat is initiated high in the His bundle.

The prognosis for congenital heart block is usually favorable; patients who have been observed to the age of 30–40 yr have lived normally active lives. However, some patients have episodes of dizziness with or without syncope (Stokes-Adams attacks); this complication requires the implantation of a permanent cardiac pacemaker. Acquired heart block is a rare complication of cardiac surgery (Sec. 14.69).

14.73 SICK-SINUS SYNDROME

The sick-sinus syndrome is the result of abnormalities in the sinus node and/or atrial conduction pathways as outlined in Fig. 14–74. This syndrome may occur in the absence of congenital heart disease and has been reported in siblings, but is most commonly seen after surgical correction of congenital heart defects, especially the Mustard procedure for transposition of the great arteries. Clinical presentation depends on the heart rate. Most patients remain asymptomatic without treatment. Dizziness and syncope can occur during periods of marked sinus slowing with failure of junctional escape (Fig. 14–75). Supraventricular tachycardias may alternate with bradycardia (bradycardia-tachycardia syndrome) causing palpitations, exercise intolerance, and/or dizziness. Treatment must be individualized. In general, aside from digitalis, drug therapy to control tachyarrhythmia (e.g., propranolol, quinidine, procainamide) may suppress sinus and atrial ventricular nodal function to the degree that sympto-

Figure 14–75. Sick-sinus syndrome with bradytachycardia: note the bursts of supraventricular tachycardia, probably multifocal in origin, followed by long periods of sinus arrest and by sinus bradycardia.

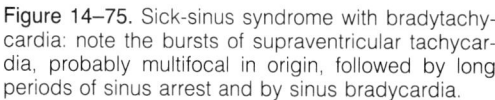
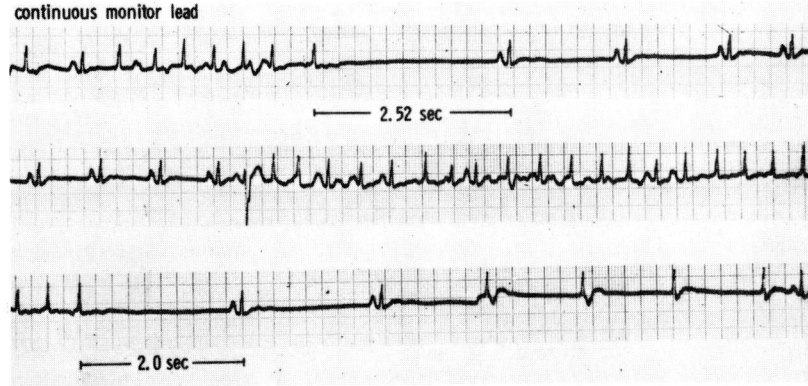

matic bradycardia may be produced. Therefore, an insertion of a demand ventricular pacemaker in conjunction with drug therapy is necessary for symptomatic patients.

Benson DW Jr, Smith WM, Dunnigan A, et al: Mechanisms of regular, wide QRS tachycardia in infants and children. Am J Cardiol 49:1778, 1982.

Bigger JT Jr: Anti-arrhythmic treatment: An overview. Am J Cardiol 53:9A, 1984.

Bigger JT Jr, Goldmeyer BN: The mechanism of supraventricular tachycardia. Circulation 42:673, 1970.

Gallagher JJ, Pritchett ELC, Sealy WC, Kassell J, Wallace AG: The pre-excitation syndromes. Prog Cardiovasc Dis 20:285, 1978.

Garson A, Gillette PC, McNamara DG: Supraventricular tachycardia in children: Clinical features, response to treatment and long-term follow-up in 217 patients. J Pediatr 98:875, 1981.

Gillette PC, Garson A: Pediatric Cardiac Dysrhythmias. New York, Grune & Stratton, 1981.

Gillette PC, Garson A, Kugler JD: Wolff-Parkinson-White syndrome in children: Electrophysiologic and pharmacologic characteristics. Circulation 60:1487, 1979.

Gillette PC, Shannon C: Cardiac pacing in children. Cardiovasc Clin 14:209, 1983.

Gillette PC, Shannon C, Blair H, et al: Transvenous pacing in pediatric patients. Am Heart J 105:843, 1983.

Greenwood RD, Rosenthal A, Sloss LJ, et al: Sick sinus syndrome after surgery for congenital heart disease. Circulation 52:208, 1975.

Hayes CJ, Gersony WM: Arrhythmias after the Mustard operation for transposition of the great arteries: A long-term study. J Am Coll Cardiol 7:133, 1986.

Michaelson M, Engle MA: International cooperative study of congenital complete heart block. In: Engle MA (ed): Cardiovascular Clinics: Pediatric Cardiology. Philadelphia, FA Davis, 1972.

Pickoff AS, Zies L, Ferrer PL, et al: High-dose propranolol therapy in the management of supraventricular tachycardia. J Pediatr 94:144, 1979.

Porter CJ, Gillette PC, Garson A Jr, et al: Effects of verapamil on supraventricular tachycardia in children. Am J Cardiol 48:487, 1981.

Porter CJ, Gillette PC, McNamara DG: Twenty-four hour ambulatory ECG's in the detection and management of cardiac dysrhythmias in infants and children. Pediatr Cardiol 1:203, 1980.

Roberts NK, Gelband H: Cardiac Arrhythmias in the Neonate, Infant and Child. New York, Appleton-Century-Crofts, 1977.

Rocchini AP, Chun PO, Dick M: Ventricular tachycardia in children. Am J Cardiol 47:1091, 1981.

Wit AL, Rosen MR: Pathophysiologic mechanisms of cardiac arrhythmias. Am Heart J 106:798, 1983.

14.74 INFECTIVE ENDOCARDITIS

The term infective endocarditis includes the entities referred to as acute and subacute bacterial endocarditis (Sec. 11.16–11.18) as well as infections of nonbacterial endocarditis such as those caused by viruses, fungi, and other agents. The disease remains a significant cause of morbidity and mortality among children and adolescents despite the advances in the management and prophylaxis of the disease with antimicrobial agents. The inability to eradicate infective endocarditis by prevention or early treatment stems from several factors: the nature of the infecting organism has changed over the years; physicians, dentists, and the public are not sufficiently aware of the threat of infective endocarditis and the preventive measures available; diagnosis may be difficult when delayed; and special risk groups have emerged which include an increasing number of narcotics abusers, survivors of cardiac surgery, and patients with lower resistance to infection who require intravascular catheters. Brain abscess, which is rarely seen among patients with cyanotic heart disease, is virtually never associated with endocarditis.

Etiology. *Streptococcus viridans* is responsible for approximately 50% of cases of infective endocarditis. Staphylococcal endocarditis has become more common over the past 2 decades and is now responsible for almost one third of the cases. Other organisms cause endocarditis less frequently, and in approximately 10% of cases blood cultures are negative. No relationship exists between the infecting organism and the type of congenital defect, duration of the illness, or age of the child. However, staphylococcal endocarditis is more common in patients who do not have underlying heart disease.

Epidemiology. Infective endocarditis is most often a complication of congenital or rheumatic heart disease but can also occur in children who do not have a cardiac malformation. In developed countries, congenital heart disease is the overwhelming predisposing factor. The disease is extremely rare in infancy.

Patients with a lesion that is associated with a high velocity of blood injected into a chamber or vessel are most susceptible to the infection. Vegetation is usually formed at the site of the endocardial or intimal erosion that results from the turbulent flow. Thus, children with ventricular septal defect, left-sided valvular disease, and systemic-pulmonary arterial communications are at the highest risk for developing infective endocarditis, while a very low incidence is reported in secundum atrial septal defect, a lesion characterized by low velocity flow across the interatrial defect. The postoperative pediatric patient with a palliative systemic to pulmonary artery shunt is most at risk for infective endocarditis. However, children who have had valve replacement and valve conduit repairs are also at high risk.

In approximately 30% of patients with infective endocarditis a predisposing factor is recognized. A surgical or dental procedure can be implicated in approximately two thirds of the cases in which the potential source of bacteremia is identified. Furthermore, poor dental hygiene in children with cyanotic heart disease results in a greater risk for contamination of blood and eventually of the endocardium. The occurrence of endocarditis directly following cardiac catheterization or heart surgery is relatively low. However, on the basis of frequency of the performance of these procedures, they are frequent antecedent events.

Clinical Manifestations. The early symptoms and signs are usually mild, especially when *Streptococcus viridans* is the infecting organism. Prolonged fever, without other manifestations (except occasionally weight loss), persisting for as long as several months may often be the only medical history that can be elicited. Alternatively, the onset may be acute and severe, with high, intermittent fever and prostration. Usually, however, the onset and course vary within a range between these two extremes. The symptoms are usually nonspecific and consist of low-grade fever with afternoon elevations, fatigue, myalgia, arthralgia, headache, and at times chills, nausea, and vomiting. Depending on the virulence of the agent the clinical findings may include signs of embolization and changes in the cardiac examination. Splenomegaly is relatively common, and petechiae may occur. New or changing heart murmurs are common, especially when there is destruction of valves and when there is associated congestive heart failure.

Serious neurologic complications, such as emboli, cerebral abscesses, mycotic aneurysms, and hemorrhage, that are manifested by meningismus, increased intracranial pressure, altered sensorium, and focal neurologic signs are most often associated with staphylococcal disease.

Myocardial abscesses may also occur with staphylococcal disease and may rupture into the pericardium. Pulmonary and other systemic emboli are infrequent except with fungal disease. Many of the classic skin manifestations develop late in the course of the disease; hence, they are seldom seen in the appropriately treated patient. These are *Osler nodes* (tender pea-sized intradermal nodules in the pads of the fingers and toes), *Janeway lesions* (painless small erythematous or hemorrhagic lesions on the palms and soles), and *splinter hemorrhages* (linear lesions beneath the nails). These lesions probably represent vasculitis produced by circulating antigen-antibody complexes.

The identification of infective endocarditis will most often be based on a high index of suspicion in the evaluation of an infection in a child with an underlying contributory factor.

Laboratory Data. *The critical information for appropriate treatment of infective endocarditis is obtained from blood cultures.* All other laboratory data are secondary in importance. Mild to moderate leukocytosis can be expected; the erythrocyte sedimentation rate is commonly elevated, and a mild hemolytic anemia (hemoglobin value seldom <9 g/dL) is not unusual. Microscopic hematuria, when present, is usually a manifestation of immune complex glomerulonephritis. Autoantibodies may develop as the disease progresses, and rheumatoid factors (antiglobulins), the Kahn reaction, and/or cryoglobulins may be demonstrable at times.

Blood cultures must be obtained as promptly as possible in each child in whom infective endocarditis is a diagnostic possibility. These must be drawn even if the child feels well and has no other physical findings. Three separate blood collections should be obtained after careful preparation of the phlebotomy site.

Contamination presents a special problem since bacteria found on the skin may themselves cause infective endocarditis. The timing of collections is not important because bacteremia can be expected to be relatively constant. In 90% of cases of endocarditis the etiologic agent is recovered from the first two blood cultures. Therefore, further blood drawings may be deferred for 2–3 days until the results of the initial cultures are known.

Echocardiography has been utilized to document the presence and specific location of vegetations, but this modality is not always helpful in the early stages of the disease. The effects of mitral and aortic valvular incompetence on left ventricular performance can also be evaluated by ultrasound techniques.

Prognosis and Complications. In the preantibiotic era infective endocarditis was a fatal disease. After a marked improvement in the 1950's the percentage of survivals continues to increase but at a slow rate. Mortality remains at 20–25%. Complications occur in 50–60% of children with documented infective endocarditis; the most common is cardiac failure due to vegetations involving the aortic or mitral valve. Myocardial abscesses and toxic myocarditis may also lead to congestive heart failure but without characteristic changes in auscultatory findings.

Table 14–9. **Treatment of Infective Endocarditis**

Etiologic Agent	Drug	Dosage	Route	Duration of Therapy
Streptococcus viridans	Penicillin G	300,000 units/kg/24 hr every 4 hr or up to 20 million units*	IV	4–6 wk†
	+ Streptomycin‡	30 mg/kg/24 hr every 12 hr	IM	2 wk
Streptococcus faecalis	Penicillin G or	300,000 units/kg/24 hr every 4 hr or up to 20 million units*	IV	6 wk
	Ampicillin +	200 mg/kg/24 hr every 4 hr	IV	6 wk
	Gentamicin	4–6 mg/kg/24 hr every 8–12 hr	IV	6 wk
Staphylococcus aureus Penicillin sensitive	Penicillin G	300,000 units/kg/24 hr every 4 hr or up to 20 million units*	IV	6–8 wk
Penicillin resistant	Oxacillin or Nafcillin or Methicillin§ +	200 mg/kg/24 hr every 4–6 hr	IV	6–8 wk
	Rifampin‖ or	10 mg/kg/24 hr every 12 hr—not to exceed 600 mg/24 hr	PO	6–8 wk
	Gentamicin†	4–6 mg/kg/24 hr every 8–12 hr	IV	2 wk
Methicillin resistant	Vancomycin +	50 mg/kg/24 hr every 6 hr	IV	6–8 wk
	Rifampin‖	10 mg/kg/24 hr every 12 hr—not to exceed 600 mg/24 hr	PO	6–8 wk
Unknown agent	Penicillin G +	300,000 units/kg/24 hr every 4 hr or up to 20 million units*	IV	6–8 wk
	Oxacillin +	200 mg/kg/24 hr every 4–6 hr	IV	6–8 wk
	Gentamicin or	4–6 mg/kg/24 hr every 8–12 hr	IV	6–8 wk
	Gentamicin + Vancomycin	See above dosages		

*For relatively resistant organisms.

†With sensitive organisms and appropriate monitoring, 2 wk IV therapy which may be completed by PO penicillin for 2–4 wk; dosage is dependent on serum bacterial levels.

‡Addition of aminoglycoside advocated by some centers.

§Least preferred.

‖Addition of rifampin advocated by some centers.

IV = intravenous; IM = intramuscular; PO = oral.

Superimposed on left heart or aortic lesions, systemic emboli, often with central nervous system manifestations, are a major threat in patients with infective endocarditis. Pulmonary emboli may occur in children with ventricular septal defect or tetralogy of Fallot, although massive life-threatening pulmonary embolization is extremely rare. Mycotic aneurysms, ruptured sinus of Valsalva, obstructive valve disease secondary to large vegetations, acquired ventricular septal defect, and heart block as a result of involvement of the specialized conduction system have all been reported as a result of infective endocarditis.

Treatment. Antibiotic therapy should be instituted immediately on diagnosis of infective endocarditis. When virulent organisms are responsible, small delays may result in progressive endocardial damage and a greater likelihood of severe complications. The choice of antibiotics, method of administration, and length of treatment are outlined in Table 14–9. High serum bactericidal levels must be maintained long enough to eradicate organisms that are growing in relatively inaccessible avascular vegetations. From 5 to 20 times the minimum in vitro inhibiting concentration must be produced at the site of infection to destroy bacteria growing at the core of these lesions. Several weeks are required for a vegetation to organize completely; thus, therapy must be continued through this period so that recrudescence can be avoided. A total of 4–6 wk of treatment is recommended, with serumcidal levels by tube dilution of at least 1:8 prior to administration of a subsequent dose of antibiotic. Depending on the clinical and laboratory responses, antibiotic therapy may require modification, and in some instances more prolonged treatment is required. With highly sensitive *Streptococcus viridans* infections, shortened regimens including oral penicillin have been recommended.

Bed rest should be instituted and should be extended if congestive heart failure occurs. Similarly, digitalis, restriction of sodium, and diuretic therapy should be utilized when indicated.

Surgical intervention during the course of infective endocarditis is an integral part of management in cases in which severe aortic or mitral valve involvement leads to intractable heart failure. Rarely, a mycotic aneurysm or a rupture of an aortic sinus requires emergency operation. Although antibiotic therapy should be administered for as long as possible prior to surgical intervention, active infection is not a contraindication if the patient is critically ill as a result of severe hemodynamic deterioration from infective endocarditis. Removal of vegetations and, in some instances, valve replacement may be lifesaving, and sustained antibiotic administration will most often prevent reinfection. Successful late surgical intervention has been reported in children with infective endocarditis who have been unresponsive to treatment and in patients who have shown evidence of continued embolic phenomena. Replacement of infected prosthetic valves carries a higher risk but is necessary in refractory cases.

Fungal endocarditis is difficult to manage and most often has a poor prognosis regardless of treatment. It has been encountered after cardiac surgery in severely debilitated patients, or in the immunosuppressed patient. The drug of choice is amphotericin B, but surgery to excise infected tissue is occasionally attempted with limited success.

Prevention. Antimicrobial prophylaxis prior to and after various procedures, including tooth extractions and other forms of dental manipulation, reduces the incidence of infective endocarditis in susceptible patients. However, proper general dental care and oral hygiene is most important in decreasing the risk of infective endocarditis in susceptible individuals. Vigorous treatment of sepsis and local infections

and careful asepsis during cardiac surgery and catheterization will also reduce the incidence of infective endocarditis.

Recommendations for specific antibiotic regimens for prevention of infective endocarditis under various circumstances are listed in Table 14–10.

Table 14–10. Recommendations for Prevention of Bacterial Endocarditis

Dental Procedures and Surgery of the Upper Respiratory Tract

1. For most patients: Oral Penicillin	**Adults:** 2.0 g of penicillin V 1 hr prior to procedure and then 1.0 g 6 hr after initial dose. **Children less than 60 pounds:** 1.0 g of penicillin V 1 hr prior to procedure and then 500 mg 6 hr after initial dose.
2. For those *allergic to penicillin* (may also be selected for those receiving oral penicillin as continuous rheumatic fever prophylaxis): Erythromycin	**Adults:** 1.0 g orally 1 hr prior to procedure and then 500 mg 6 hr after initial dose. **Children:** 20 mg/kg orally 1 hr prior to procedure and then 10 mg/kg 6 hr after intial dose.
3. For those patients at *higher risk* of infective endocarditis (especially those with prosthetic heart valves) who are not allergic to penicillin: Ampicillin plus Gentamicin	**Adults:** Amicillin 1.0–2.0 g plus gentamicin 1.5 mg/kg IM or IV, both given 30 min before procedure; then penicillin V 1.0 g orally 6 hr after initial dose. **Children:** Timing of doses is same as for adults. Dosages are ampicillin 50 mg/kg and gentamicin 2.0 mg/kg.
4. For *higher risk* patients (especially those with prosthetic heart valves) who are *allergic to penicillin:* Vancomycin	**Adults:** Vancomycin 1 g IV over 60 min, begun 60 min before procedure; no repeat dose is necessary. **Children:** Vancomycin 20 mg/kg IV over 60 min, begun 60 min before procedure; no repeat dose is necessary.

Gastrointestinal and Genitourinary Tract Surgery and Instrumentation

1. For most patients: Ampicillin plus Gentamicin	**Adults:** 2.0 g ampicillin IM or IV plus gentamicin 1.5 mg/kg IM or IV given 30 min before procedure. May repeat once 8 hr later. **Children:** Same timing of medications as adult schedule. Dosages are ampicillin 50 mg/kg and gentamicin 2.0 mg/kg.
2. For patients *allergic to penicillin:* Vancomycin plus Gentamicin	**Adults:** 1.0 g vancomycin IV given over 60 min plus 1.5 mg/kg gentamicin IM or IV, each given 60 min before procedure. Doses may be repeated once 8–12 hr later. **Children:** Timing as above. Doses are vancomycin 20 mg/kg and gentamicin 2.0 mg/kg.
3. Oral regimen for minor or repetitive procedures in low risk patients: Amoxicillin	**Adults:** 3.0 g amoxicillin 1 hr before procedure and 1.5 g 6 hr after initial dose. **Children:** Same timing of doses. 50 mg/kg initial dose and 25 mg/kg follow-up dose.

Note: In patients with compromised renal function, it may be necessary to modify or omit the second dose of antibiotics. Intramuscular injections may be contraindicated in patients receiving anticoagulants. Children's doses should not exceed adult doses.

Adapted from A Statement for Health Professionals by the Committee on Rheumatic Fever and Infective Endocarditis. Prevention of Bacterial Endocarditis. *Circulation* 70:1123A, 1984; also excerpted in *J Am Dent Assoc* 110:98, 1985.

14.75 RHEUMATIC HEART DISEASE

Rheumatic involvement of the valves and endocardium is the most important manifestation of rheumatic fever (Sec. 10.87). The lesions begin as small verrucae composed of fibrin and blood cells along the borders of one of the heart valves; the mitral valve is affected most often. The aortic valve is next in frequency; right heart manifestations are rare. As the inflammation subsides, the verrucae tend to disappear and leave scar tissue. With a repeated attack of rheumatic fever, new verrucae form near the previous ones, and the mural endocardium and chordae tendineae become involved.

Clinical Patterns of Valvular Disease. *Mitral Insufficiency.* This is the result of structural changes that usually include some loss of valvular substance and shortening and thickening of the chordae tendineae. During acute rheumatic fever with severe cardiac involvement, congestive heart failure is most often due to a combination of the mechanical effects of severe mitral insufficiency coupled with inflammatory disease which may involve the pericardium, myocardium, endocardium, and epicardium. Because of the high volume load and inflammatory process the left ventricle becomes large and inefficient. The left atrium dilates as blood regurgitates into this chamber. Increased left atrial pressure results in pulmonary congestion and symptoms of left heart failure. In patients with severe chronic mitral insufficiency the pulmonary artery pressure becomes elevated, and enlargement of the right ventricle and atrium and subsequent right heart failure will occur. However, in most cases mitral insufficiency is mild or moderate. Even in those patients in whom incompetence is severe at the onset, there is spontaneous improvement with time. The resultant chronic lesion is most often mild or moderate in severity, and the patient will be asymptomatic. Over half of patients with mitral insufficiency during an acute attack will no longer have the murmur of mitral involvement 1 yr later.

The principal physical signs of mitral insufficiency include a heaving apical left ventricular precordial impulse with a pansystolic murmur at the apex radiating to the axilla and the sternal edge. A mid-diastolic rumble at the apex suggests severe insufficiency. There is rarely a midsystolic ejection click as seen in patients with nonrheumatic mitral valve prolapse. In a young child with mitral insufficiency and no history suggestive of acute rheumatic fever, the differential diagnosis between a congenitally abnormal valve and rheumatic mitral involvement on the basis of the physical examination may be impossible. With severe mitral insufficiency, signs of chronic congestive heart failure, including fatigue, weight gain, weakness, and dyspnea on exertion, may be noted. The heart is enlarged with an apical systolic thrill. The 1st heart sound is normal; the 2nd heart sound may be accentuated if pulmonary hypertension is present. A 3rd heart sound is prominent. In addition to the pansystolic murmur a short diastolic rumble follows the 3rd sound; it is due to increased blood flow from the left atrium across the mitral valve as a result of the massive insufficiency. This murmur is associated with mitral incompetence and does not mean that mechanical mitral stenosis is present. The latter lesion takes many years to develop and is characterized by a diastolic murmur of greater length with presystolic accentuation.

The *electrocardiogram* and *roentgenograms* are normal if the lesion is mild. With more severe insufficiency the electrocardiogram shows prominent bifid P waves, signs of left ventricular hypertrophy, and sometimes associated right ventricular hypertrophy. Roentgenographically, there is prominence of the left atrium and ventricle. When pulmonary hypertension or congestive heart failure supervenes, the pulmonary artery segment and right heart chambers are prominent. Signs of pulmonary venous hypertension may also be evident. Calci-

fication of the mitral valve is rare in children. *Echocardiography* shows enlargement of the left atrium and ventricle. The signs of classic mitral valve prolapse are usually absent, but differentiation between these conditions may not always be possible.

Cardiac catheterization and *left ventriculography* are considered *only* if there is rapid progression of the disease and surgical treatment is contemplated. The cardiac output is normal or decreased in severe lesions. The left atrial pressure is frequently but not always increased. The pulse curve of the left atrium shows a steep rise in early systole to the peak of the "v" wave and is followed by a rapid "y" descent. A diastolic gradient may be measured across the mitral valve even in the absence of mitral stenosis. The left ventricular end-diastolic pressure rises during exercise or in the presence of left ventricular failure. Left ventriculography results in opacification of the left atrium. The degree of opacification is used as a qualitative assessment of the severity of incompetence.

COMPLICATIONS. Severe mitral incompetence may result in cardiac failure that may be precipitated by progression of the rheumatic process, the onset of atrial fibrillation with rapid ventricular response, or infective endocarditis. After many years, the effects of chronic mitral insufficiency may become manifest without a new event. Right-sided heart failure may be accompanied by tricuspid or pulmonary valve incompetence. Occasional atrial or ventricular extrasystoles are well tolerated. Atrial fibrillation is more common when mitral incompetence is associated with a large left atrium.

TREATMENT. In the majority of patients with mitral insufficiency, prophylaxis against recurrences of rheumatic fever is all that is required since the lesions are mild and well tolerated (Sec. 10.87). The treatment of complicating heart failure, dysrhythmias, and infective endocarditis is described elsewhere in this chapter. Surgical treatment is indicated in patients who, despite adequate medical therapy, suffer from recurrent episodes of heart failure, extreme dyspnea with moderate activity, and progressive cardiomegaly, often with pulmonary hypertension. Although annuloplasty gives good results in some children and adolescents, valve replacement may be required. Many children with murmurs suggestive of mitral insufficiency lose all evidence of cardiac disease after some years. Activity should not be restricted in children having mild mitral incompetence.

Mitral Stenosis. Congenital mitral stenosis has been described in Sec. 14.61.

Mitral stenosis of rheumatic origin results from fibrosis of the mitral ring, commissural adhesions, and contracture of the valve leaflets, chordae, and papillary muscles over a significant period of time. It usually takes 10 yr or more for the lesion to become fully established, although the process may occasionally be accelerated. Rheumatic mitral stenosis is seldom encountered prior to adolescence, and usually is not recognized until adult life.

Mitral stenosis of critical degree exists if the valvular orifice is reduced to 25% or less of the expected normal. Such reductions result in increased pressure and hypertrophy of the left atrium. The increased pressure causes pulmonary venous hypertension, increased pulmonary vascular resistance, and pulmonary hypertension. Right ventricular and atrial dilatation and hypertrophy ensue and are followed by right-sided heart failure.

Generally, there is a good correlation between symptoms and severity of obstruction. Patients with mild lesions are asymptomatic. More severe degrees of obstruction are associated with effort intolerance and dyspnea. Critical lesions can result in orthopnea, paroxysmal nocturnal dyspnea, and

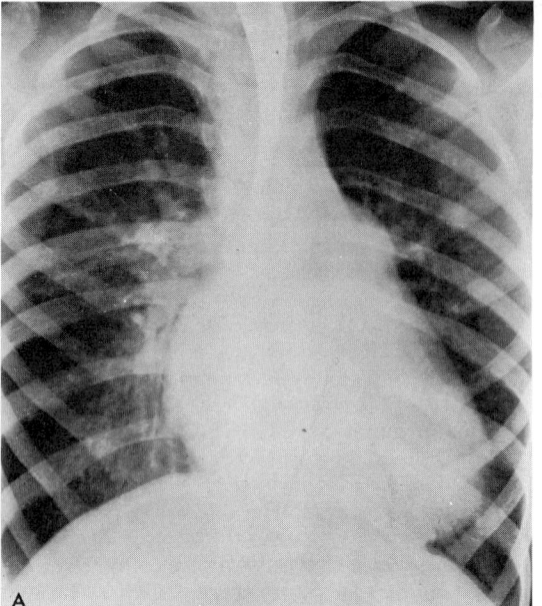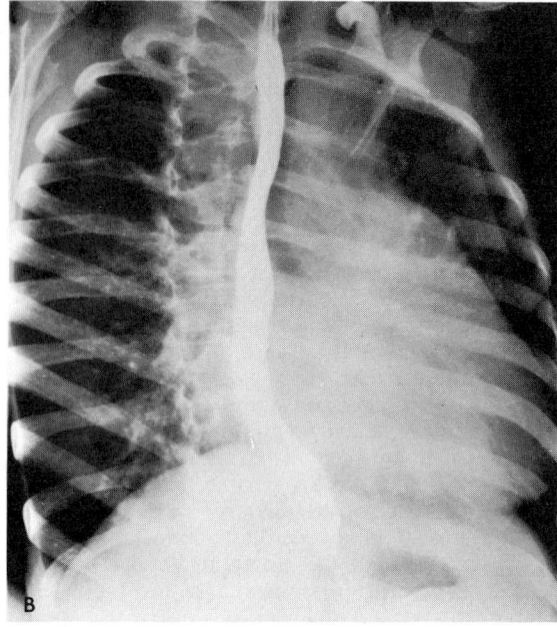

Figure 14–76. Roentgenograms in isolated rheumatic mitral stenosis. *A*, Posteroanterior view showing cardiomegaly and prominent main pulmonary artery. Vascular shadows in lungs are due to prominent pulmonary arteries and veins. *B*, Right anterior oblique view showing indentation of esophagus by large left atrium. This patient required valvotomy at age 8 yr.

overt pulmonary edema. These symptoms may be precipitated by uncontrolled tachycardia, atrial fibrillation, or pulmonary infections. Congestive heart failure is usually associated with moderate or severe pulmonary hypertension. Right ventricular dilatation may result in functional tricuspid incompetence, hepatomegaly, ascites, and edema. Hemoptysis due to ruptured bronchial or pleurohilar veins and, occasionally, pulmonary infarction may occur. Blood-streaked sputum occurs during episodes of pulmonary edema. With chronic severe mitral stenosis cyanosis and a malar flush are noted.

The jugular venous pressure is increased in the presence of congestive heart failure, tricuspid valve disease, or severe pulmonary hypertension. The heart size is normal with minimal disease. Moderate cardiomegaly is usual with severe mitral stenosis and sinus rhythm, but cardiac enlargement can be great, especially when atrial fibrillation and heart failure supervene. The apical impulse is brief and tapping, and a parasternal right ventricular lift is palpable when pulmonary pressure is high. The principal auscultatory findings are a loud 1st heart sound, an opening snap of the mitral valve, and a long, low-pitched, rumbling mitral diastolic murmur with presystolic accentuation. The mitral diastolic murmur may be absent in the presence of congestive heart failure. A systolic murmur due to tricuspid incompetence may be audible. In the presence of pulmonary hypertension, pulmonary valvular closure is accentuated. An early diastolic murmur may be due to associated aortic incompetence or pulmonary valvular incompetence (Graham Steell murmur).

Electrocardiograms and *roentgenograms* are normal if the lesion is mild; as severity increases, there are prominent and notched P waves and varying degrees of right ventricular hypertrophy. Atrial fibrillation is a common late manifestation. Moderate or severe lesions are associated with roentgenographic signs of left atrial enlargement, prominence of the pulmonary artery and right heart chambers, and a normal or small aorta and left ventricle (Fig. 14–76); there may be calcifications noted in the region of the mitral valve. Severe obstruction is associated with a redistribution of pulmonary blood flow so that the apices of the lung have a greater perfusion (i.e., reverse of

normal). Septal lines at the costophrenic angles may also be present. *Echocardiography* shows distinct narrowing of the mitral orifice during diastole and left atrial enlargement. *Cardiac catheterization* quantitates the diastolic gradient across the mitral valve and the degree of pulmonary hypertension.

TREATMENT. Surgical treatment is undertaken when there are clinical signs and hemodynamic evidence of severe obstruction, but prior to the severe manifestations outlined earlier. Since extreme valvular distortion and calcification are rare, mitral valvotomy generally yields good results in rheumatic mitral stenosis; valve replacement should be avoided unless absolutely necessary.

Aortic Insufficiency. In chronic rheumatic aortic insufficiency, sclerosis of the aortic valves results in distortion and retraction of the cusps. Regurgitation of blood results in a volume overload with dilatation and hypertrophy of the left ventricle. *Combined mitral and aortic insufficiency are more common than aortic involvement alone.* Left ventricular failure may eventually occur.

Symptoms are unusual except in gross aortic incompetence. The large stroke volume and forceful left ventricular contractions may result in palpitations. Excessive sweating and heat intolerance are related to vasodilatation. Dyspnea on effort progresses to orthopnea and pulmonary edema. Angina pectoris may occur during heavy exertion. In adolescents with severe incompetence, nocturnal attacks with nightmares, sweating, tachycardia, chest pain, and hypertension may occur. In the United States it is rare to encounter patients with the classic clinical picture of florid mitral or aortic disease.

Because of the reflux of blood through the aortic valve during diastole, the pulse pressure is wide with bounding peripheral pulses. The systolic blood pressure is elevated, the diastolic lowered.

In severe aortic insufficiency, the heart is enlarged and there is a left ventricular apical heave. There may be a diastolic thrill. The typical murmur begins immediately with the 2nd heart sound and continues until late in diastole. The murmur is heard over the upper and middle left sternal border with radiation to the apex and to the aortic area. Characteristically, it has a hollow, high-pitched blowing quality. Generally, the murmur is more easily audible in full expiration, with the diaphragm of the stethoscope placed firmly on the chest and the patient leaning forward. Occasionally, it may be louder in the recumbent position. A systolic ejection murmur sometimes preceded by a click is frequent and is produced by the large stroke volume. An apical presystolic murmur (Austin Flint) resembling that of mitral stenosis is sometimes heard.

The *echocardiogram* shows a large left ventricle and diastolic mitral valve flutter or oscillation. The two-dimensional echocardiogram shows the abnormal aortic valve, and Doppler studies demonstrate aortic runoff.

Roentgenograms show prominence and exaggerated pulsations of the left ventricle and aorta. The *electrocardiogram* may be normal but in advanced cases reveals signs of left ventricular hypertrophy and strain with prominent P waves.

Cardiac catheterization is seldom necessary and is undertaken only when surgery is contemplated because of a progressive lesion. The degree of elevation of left ventricular end-diastolic, left atrial, and pulmonary arterial pressures is established, and ascending aortography demonstrates the regurgitant flow across the aortic valve into the left ventricle.

Mild and moderate lesions are well tolerated. Many adolescents with severe regurgitation are symptom-free and tolerate advanced lesions into the 3rd–4th decades. Unlike mitral incompetence, aortic insufficiency does not regress. Patients with combined lesions at the time of acute rheumatic fever may have only aortic involvement 1–2 yr later. Surgical intervention should be carried out well in advance of the onset of congestive heart failure, pulmonary edema, or angina, when there are signs of decreasing myocardial performance, such as early symptoms, ST-T wave changes on the ECG or decreasing left ventricular ejection fraction.

Treatment in most cases consists of prophylaxis against the recurrence of acute rheumatic fever and occurrence of infective endocarditis as well as encouragement to lead as active and normal a life as possible. Surgical treatment (usually valve replacement) is undertaken when there is progressive cardiomegaly and early signs of left ventricular dysfunction.

Tricuspid Valvular Disease. Primary tricuspid involvement is rare following rheumatic fever. *Tricuspid insufficiency* secondary to right ventricular dilatation resulting from severe left-sided lesions can occur in patients with severe cases in whom surgery is not carried out. The signs produced by tricuspid insufficiency include prominent pulsations of the jugular veins with a "c-v" wave, systolic pulsations of the liver, and blowing systolic murmur in the 4th and 5th left parasternal spaces that increases in intensity during inspiration. Concomitant signs of mitral or aortic valve disease, with or without atrial fibrillation, are frequent. Signs of tricuspid incompetence decrease or disappear when heart failure produced by the left-sided lesions is successfully treated. However, tricuspid valvuloplasty may be required in some cases.

Pulmonary Valvular Disease. Pulmonary insufficiency occurs on a functional basis secondary to pulmonary hypertension or dilatation of the pulmonary artery. This is a late finding with severe mitral stenosis (Graham Steell murmur). The murmur is similar to that of aortic insufficiency, but the peripheral arterial signs are absent.

Arnett EN, Roberts WC: Prosthetic valve endocarditis. Am J Cardiol 38:281, 1976.

Bisno SL, Dismukes WE, Durack DT, et al: Treatment of infective endocarditis due to viridans streptococci. Circulation 63:730A, 1981.

Durack DT, Kaplan EL, Bisno AL: Apparent failures of endocarditis prophylaxis. JAMA 250:2318, 1983.

Gersony WM, Hayes CJ: Bacterial endocarditis in patients with pulmonary stenosis, aortic stenosis, or ventricular septal defect. Circulation 56(Suppl):84, 1977.

Gersony WM, Hordof AH: Infective endocarditis and diseases of the pericardium. Pediatr Clin North Am 25:831, 1978.

Johnson DH, Rosenthal A, Nadas A: A forty-year review of bacterial endocarditis in infancy and childhood. Circulation 51:581, 1975.

Kaplan EL, Rich H, Gersony WM, et al: A collaborative study of endocarditis in the 1970's. Circulation 59:327, 1979.

Shulman ST, Amren DP, Bisno AL, et al: Prevention of bacterial endocarditis: A statement for health professionals by the Committee on Rheumatic Fever and Infective Endocarditis of the Council on Cardiovascular Disease in the Young. Circulation 70:1123A, 1984.

Weinstein L, Schlesinger JJ: Pathoanatomic, pathophysiologic and clinical correlation in endocarditis. N Engl J Med 291:832, 1122, 1974.

Wilson WR, Nichols DR, Thompson RL, et al: Infective endocarditis: Therapeutic considerations. Am Heart J 100:689, 1980.

14.76 DISEASES OF THE MYOCARDIUM

14.77 CONDITIONS CAUSING MYOCARDIAL DAMAGE

The status of the myocardium is a critical factor in the prognosis of cardiac disease. If, in spite of congenital cardiac malformations, acquired valvular disease, or arrhythmias, the myocardium is still able to provide satisfactory circulation of blood, the child will be able to maintain adequate nutrition, growth, and activity. In addition to injury resulting from chronic volume and/or pressure load, the myocardium may be directly affected by infections, mesenchymal diseases, endocrine disorders, metabolic and nutritional diseases, neuromuscular diseases, blood diseases, tumors, hypertension, and congenital anomalies.

Bacterial Infections. In **diphtheria** (Sec. 11.23) the toxin of the bacillus may produce peripheral circulatory failure or toxic myocarditis. Peripheral circulatory failure occurs within the first 2 wk of the disease and is associated with a rapid, thready pulse; cold, pale, and clammy skin; and hypotension. In addition to therapy for diphtheria, treatment for cardiogenic shock is essential. This disease is especially prone to affect the conduction system.

Toxic myocarditis is characterized by the development of atrioventricular block, bundle branch block, or extrasystoles. Congestive cardiac failure occurs later and is associated with cardiac enlargement and gallop rhythm. In addition to the arrhythmia, the electrocardiogram shows S-T segment depression and T wave inversion in most leads. The immediate prognosis is grave (about 50% mortality). Treatment includes strict bed rest until all signs of myocarditis have disappeared and management of arrhythmias, including cardiac pacing. Digitalis is reserved for patients with frank congestive heart failure but must be used with care because of the possibility of increased sensitivity.

In **typhoid fever** (Sec. 11.27), toxic myocarditis may be inferred if there is electrocardiographic evidence of T wave inversion in most leads. This sign may be transient, however, and by itself is of no clinical significance. Cardiac failure is rare, and peripheral circulatory failure is no longer common.

In **other bacterial infections,** circulatory involvement is manifested as peripheral circulatory collapse or toxic myocarditis. Toxic myocarditis as evidenced by tachycardia, gallop rhythm, and cardiac enlargement may complicate pneumonia, infective endocarditis, and septicemia. The prognosis depends on control of the primary infection.

Rickettsial Diseases. Rocky Mountain spotted fever (Sec. 11.89), in particular, may be complicated by hypotension and peripheral vascular collapse. This complication has been attributed to the general vasculitis characteristic of the disease, but acute myocarditis may be a contributing factor.

Viral Infections. A viral etiology has been implicated in many patients with acute myocarditis. The viral agents include among others those of coxsackievirus A and B, echovirus, rubella, varicella, and influenzal infections. However, in many instances in which a viral infection is suspected, a virus cannot be identified. Acute myocarditis may occur in conjunction with diseases of other systems, especially of the central nervous system.

The clinical spectrum of viral myocarditis varies widely from that of a rapidly fatal disorder, especially in the newborn infant, to that of a mild disease with apparent complete recovery. Between these two extremes is a range of clinical patterns; a chronic course characterized by cardiomegaly with mitral incompetence that progresses to chronic congestive cardiac failure is not unusual.

Parasitic and Fungal Infections. Lesions in the myocardium have been described in association with *histoplasmosis, coccidioidomycosis, toxoplasmosis,* and *trichinosis.* In these conditions the cardiac lesion seldom produces clinical signs of myocarditis. *Actinomycosis* may involve the pericardium and myocardium by direct contiguity to, for example, a pulmonary abscess. *Hydatid cysts* of the pericardium may be found on routine roentgenograms of the chest and usually produce symptoms only when they rupture. *Schistosomiasis* may produce pulmonary hypertension and cor pulmonale. *Cruz trypanosomiasis* (Chagas disease) may produce acute or subacute myocarditis and sudden death.

Mucocutaneous Lymph Node Syndrome (Kawasaki Disease). See Sec. 10.67. Arteritis disease initially involves small arterioles, but in the 2nd and 3rd week of illness medium-sized arteries become inflamed and aneurysmal dilatation of the coronary arteries may occur. During the healing phase alternate areas of coronary dilatation and stenosis may result and have led to myocardial infarction and death.

Nonspecific ST-T wave changes may occur early in the course of the disease. Two-dimensional echocardiography is helpful in diagnosing coronary aneurysms, especially in the proximal vessels. Coronary angiography is reserved for patients in whom there is a high degree of suspicion that the aneurysms will be clinically significant. A few patients have required coronary artery bypass surgery. The long-term effects of extensive coronary artery involvement has yet to be determined. The administration of intravenous gamma globulin during the acute phase of the disease may have a preventive effect on coronary involvement.

Mesenchymal Diseases. *Rheumatic carditis* is described in Sec. 14.75, and the cardiovascular manifestations of *rheumatoid arthritis, disseminated lupus erythematosus, periarteritis nodosa, dermatomyositis,* and *scleroderma* are described in Chapter 10.

Endocrine Disorders. *Hyperthyroidism* (Sec. 19.15) produces tachycardia, vasodilatation, wide pulse pressure, cardiac enlargement, and, rarely, atrial fibrillation. *Cretinism* seldom produces gross cardiac involvement, but the electrocardiogram is characterized by bradycardia, low voltage of all complexes—especially of the P and T waves, left axis deviation, and prolonged electrical systole. These signs may disappear within 1 mo after initiation of adequate thyroid therapy.

Metabolic and Nutritional Diseases. Among vitamin deficiency diseases, *beriberi* (Sec. 3.23) causes the most conspicuous cardiac damage. In patients with malnutrition the deficiencies are often multiple, and it is difficult to separate the cardiac lesion of one nutritional disease from that of another. (See Blood Diseases below and Sec. 15.11.)

Neuromuscular Diseases. Heart disease is common in *Friedreich ataxia.* In most instances cardiac symptoms are less intense than the neurologic component (Sec. 21.20), which limits physical activities. In some patients effort intolerance, chest pain, and heart failure have been the presenting symptoms. These are due to primary myocardial disease that chiefly affects the left ventricle and results in congestive or obstructive cardiomyopathy. The electrocardiogram shows generalized T wave inversion or signs of left ventricular hypertrophy. Arrhythmias may also occur and consist of atrial tachycardia or fibrillation or extrasystoles. Varying degrees of cardiomegaly, left ventricular prominence, and pulmonary congestion are demonstrable roentgenographically.

In *progressive muscular dystrophy* (Sec. 22.6) 50% of children have postmortem evidence of myocardial involvement similar to that of the striated muscle. Cardiac symptoms, however, are not common, but the electrocardiogram is frequently abnormal and may reveal tachycardia, abnormalities of the P waves, short P-R interval, and abnormal Q and T waves. Minimal evidence of right or left ventricular hypertrophy also may be noted, and some patients have congestive heart failure.

Blood Diseases. In infants and children anemia is the most common blood disease associated with cardiac involvement. Although cardiac output increases when the hemoglobin is below about 7 g/dL, cardiac enlargement in infants with or without congestive heart failure occurs only with an extreme reduction in hemoglobin, to 3–4 g or less. The heart rate is rapid, the pulse pressure widened, and the venous pressure increased. A systolic murmur at the apex and/or along the left sternal border is usual; diastolic murmurs may occur in the same areas, and gallop rhythm is common. The electrocardiographic changes include depressed S-T segments and flat T waves. Occasionally, only minimal signs and symptoms are present when extreme states of anemia have developed gradually.

Treatment is directed toward the cause of the anemia. If blood transfusions are indicated in the presence of cardiomegaly or cardiac failure, small volumes (4–5 mL/kg) of packed cells should be administered. (See Sec. 15.11 and 15.34–15.36.) Often, it is more prudent to use exchange transfusion to avoid an acute increase in blood volume.

Glycogen Storage Disease. Cardiac as well as skeletal muscle is affected in the generalized form of glycogen storage disease known as Type II or Pompe disease (Sec. 7.21). Cardiomegaly is massive, but murmurs are insignificant. Pulmonary atelectasis with secondary infection is common and is related to compression by the large heart. The *electrocardiogram* is characteristic and shows prominent P waves, short P-R interval, massive QRS voltage, signs of isolated left or biventricular hypertrophy, and intraventricular conduction defects. *Roentgenograms* confirm the striking cardiomegaly with prominence of the left ventricle. The prognosis is poor.

Hurler Syndrome (Sec. 7.24). The lesion in the heart and great vessels is the same as that in the connective tissue elsewhere in the body. The most pronounced lesions are found in the valves and coronary arteries, but abnormalities in the pericardium and aorta are not uncommon. The heart may be moderately enlarged, with electrocardiographic signs of left ventricular hypertrophy. Cardiac murmurs may result from incompetence and stenosis of the mitral and aortic valves. Sometimes the pulmonary and tricuspid valves are also involved. Coronary arterial disease may result in angina and perhaps explain the frequent occurrence of sudden death. The prognosis is poor.

Calcinosis of the Coronary Arteries. This is a rare disease of infancy. The coronary arteries are tortuous and calcareous, and the ventricles, especially the left, are hypertrophied. Other blood vessels may be similarly involved. The onset of cardiac failure is sudden; death usually occurs in infancy.

Adriamycin (Doxorubicin Hydrochloride) Cardiotoxicity. Severe, dose-dependent cardiomyopathy occurs in about 30% of patients when the total cumulative dose of Adriamycin exceeds 550 mg/m^2. Cardiomegaly is due principally to left ventricular and left atrial enlargement. If congestive cardiac failure develops, the case fatality rate is 30–50%. T wave flattening or inversion is nonspecific evidence of cardiac involvement; early cardiac changes may be detected by serial echocardiograms which show progressive decrease in myocardial contractility, even in asymptomatic patients. The child's condition may remain clinically stable for many years.

14.78 ENDOCARDIAL FIBROELASTOSIS (EFE)

This condition has been called fetal endocarditis, endocardial fibrosis, prenatal fibroelastosis, elastic tissue hyperplasia, and endocardial sclerosis.

It is classified into two general types: primary and secondary. In *primary EFE* there is no apparent predisposing valvular lesion or other congenital abnormality. Genetic forms have been described. In the *secondary* type severe congenital heart disease of the left-sided obstructive type (e.g., aortic stenosis or atresia, forms of hypoplastic left heart, and severe coarctation of the aorta) is present. In secondary EFE the ventricular cavity is often contracted, whereas in the primary disease a dilated left ventricular chamber is seen in the infant. However, in young adults a primary contracted type of EFE has been observed.

No etiology for primary EFE has been established; possibilities include inflammation or infection before or after birth, maldevelopment, and inadequate blood supply to the endocardium. The endocardial changes could also be secondary to myocardial disease which, resulting in cardiac dilatation and in stretching of the endocardium, initiates fibroelastic proliferation. The disease has occurred in siblings.

Pathologically, there is a white, opaque fibroelastic thickening of the endocardium, virtually always in the left ventricle, which frequently obscures the trabeculation of the inner surfaces of the cardiac chamber. The lesion may spread to involve the valves. Microscopically, the lesion consists of a fibroelastic thickening of the endocardium and may result in subendocardial degeneration or necrosis of muscle with vacuolation of muscle fibers. The involved valve leaflets are characterized by a myxomatous proliferation with an increase in collagenous elements.

The *clinical manifestations* are variable. Infants, usually less than 6 mo of age, who apparently have been in good health develop severe congestive cardiac failure, often precipitated by a respiratory infection. The prognosis is poor unless there is a significant response to therapy for cardiac failure. Other infants have similar milder symptoms with periods of remission. Affected infants may manifest some dyspnea, refusal to feed, failure to gain weight adequately, and recurrent pulmonary infections. Chronic congestive cardiac failure can be controlled for some time by digitalis and diuretics. Most patients eventually succumb. Infants in whom valvular lesions or associated congenital cardiovascular defects are predominant expire in the first months of life.

During episodes of congestive cardiac failure the infant with primary EFE is acutely ill with dyspnea, cough, and anorexia. The jugular venous pressure is elevated, the liver greatly enlarged, and edema of the extremities, sacral area, or face may be present. Pulmonary rales and rhonchi are due to intercurrent pulmonary infection and congestion. The heart is moderately or greatly enlarged and has a normal or left ventricular impulse. Murmurs of mitral incompetence are frequent.

Roentgenograms confirm the cardiac enlargement (Fig. 14–77). There may be signs of intercurrent pulmonary infection or edema. The *electrocardiogram* is abnormal, with changes indicative of left atrial and ventricular hypertrophy with

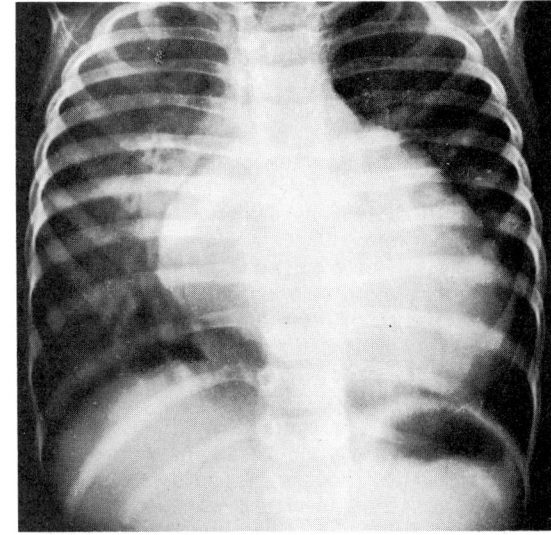

Figure 14–77. Roentgenogram of a 7 mo old girl with endocardial fibroelastosis. Note enlargement of the heart, without a distinctive contour and clear lung fields.

strain. The *echocardiogram* shows a dilated, poorly functioning left ventricle.

The short-term *prognosis* has improved because of the availability of potent diuretics and peripheral vasodilator therapy. In patients who have survived with clinical findings and a course suggestive of primary EFE, the clinical diagnosis is inferential, since it is not possible to be certain that the original cardiac involvement was that of EFE or of another myocardial disease.

Treatment is directed toward alleviation of congestive cardiac failure and prevention of intercurrent infections.

14.79 CARDIOMYOPATHY

Heart muscle disease of unknown origin can be classified into hypertrophic, congestive, and restrictive.

Hypertrophic Cardiomyopathy. This condition is also known as *idiopathic hypertrophic subaortic stenosis* and *asymmetric septal hypertrophy.* Massive ventricular hypertrophy with principal involvement of the ventricular septum characterizes the disease, but all portions of the left ventricle and sometimes of the right are affected. Varying degrees of myocardial fibrosis are also present. The mitral valve is displaced anteriorly by the hypertrophy of papillary muscle, and the left ventricular cavity is distorted by the massive generalized hypertrophy. Microscopically, patchy areas of abnormally thick and short muscle fibers are arranged in circular collections and interspersed among normal as well as hypertrophied muscle fibers. Electron microscopy shows disarray of myofibrils and myofilaments.

Hemodynamics. The hypertrophic, fibrosed, stiff muscle has a decreased distensibility so that there is resistance to left ventricular filling, but systolic pumping function remains good until late in the course of the disease. Obstruction to left ventricular outflow may develop due to apposition of the abnormally placed anterior mitral leaflet against the hypertrophied septum. Peak systolic pressure gradients across the left ventricular outflow may be constantly or intermittently present or may be absent. Varying degrees of mitral valve regurgitation are common.

Epidemiology. The disease has been recognized in all age groups, even in neonates, and may occur in many members of the same family, although overt manifestations are present in only about one third of affected individuals discovered through a screening process. Familial studies, using echocardiographic evidence of disproportionate ventricular septal hypertrophy, suggest that in some patients disease is transmitted in an autosomal dominant pattern with a high degree of penetrance.

Often hypertrophic cardiomyopathy occurring in a child is not typical of the adult disease, although clinically and dynamically the disease seems similar. In childhood, there is a greater tendency for right ventricular outflow obstruction to occur; the disease may be more diffuse through the left ventricular muscularity, as opposed to being restricted more or less to the ventricular septum; and a pure disease form with autosomal dominant inheritance is less often seen.

Clinical Manifestations. Many children are asymptomatic and are first evaluated only because of a heart murmur. In others the clinical pattern is dominated by weakness, fatigue, dyspnea on effort, palpitations, angina pectoris, dizziness, and syncope. There is risk of sudden death even in asymptomatic children. The pulse is brisk because of the early systolic ejection of blood from the ventricle. There is a prominent left ventricular lift and double apical impulse. The 1st and 2nd heart sounds are usually normal. The rarity of systolic ejection clicks helps to differentiate valvular aortic stenosis. A 3rd sound is not common, but a 4th sound may be audible. The systolic murmur is ejection in type and of medium intensity; it is heard maximally at the left sternal edge and apex. The *electrocardiogram* shows left ventricular hypertrophy with or without S-T segment depression and T wave inversion. The Wolff-Parkinson-White syndrome and other intraventricular conduction defects may be present. *Roentgenograms* show mild cardiomegaly with prominence of the left ventricle. The ascending aorta and aortic knob are usually normal. The *echocardiogram* shows asymmetric ventricular septal hypertrophy, systolic anterior motion of the anterior leaflet of the mitral valve, and premature closure of the aortic valve.

At *cardiac catheterization,* left ventricular outflow obstruction may or may not be present. When a systolic gradient is present, its severity may be variable even during a relatively short study. The obstruction may be intensified by digitalis glycosides, isoproterenol, amyl nitrite, and nitroglycerin. The gradient may increase shortly after exercise is discontinued, during the Valsalva maneuver, or during assumption of the erect position. Left ventriculography shows encroachment on the left ventricular cavity by the hypertrophied muscle, especially by the interventricular septum. During systole the anterior mitral leaflet is drawn into the left ventricular outflow tract. Mitral regurgitation is common. It is extremely important to rule out a discrete obstruction with secondary muscular hypertrophy in patients with left ventricular outflow gradients.

The prognosis is unpredictable, especially in the asymptomatic patient.

Treatment. There is no standardized therapy. Competitive sports and strenuous physical activity should be discouraged. Digitalis is not appropriate, and in most patients is contraindicated. Brisk diuresis or the infusion of isoproterenol should also be avoided. Beta-adrenergic blocking agents (propranolol) and calcium blocking agents (verapamil) have been used with apparent success in decreasing the degree of outflow obstruction, but obliteration of an LV-AO gradient does not necessarily affect prognosis. Surgical ventricular septal myotomy or resection of the left ventricular outflow tract has been successfully accomplished in some patients, especially in those with disabling angina or syncope and in some with severe obstruction at rest (a gradient exceeding 70 mm Hg).

Congestive Cardiomyopathy. This condition is characterized by massive cardiomegaly as a result of the extensive dilatation of the ventricles, especially the left. Associated ventricular hypertrophy is mild to moderate. The etiology is unknown and is probably multifactorial; a remote history of viral disease in some patients suggests that the disease may be a sequel of a previous myocarditis. Myocardial performance is poor as evidenced by reduced stroke volume, low ejection fraction, and increased systolic and diastolic volumes. All age groups are affected, even infants. Usually the onset is insidious, but sometimes symptoms of congestive cardiac failure occur suddenly. Irritability, anorexia, cough due to pulmonary congestion, and dyspnea with mild exertion are common. When the disease is fully established, the skin is cool and pale, the arterial pulse volume is decreased, the pulse pressure is reduced, and tachycardia is present. Jugular venous pressure is increased, and hepatomegaly and edema are common. The heart is enlarged, and pansystolic murmurs of mitral and tricuspid incompetence are present. A gallop rhythm is audible in the presence of severe congestive heart failure.

The *electrocardiogram* shows a combination of atrial enlargement, varying degrees of left ventricular hypertrophy, and nonspecific T wave abnormalities. The *roentgenogram* confirms the cardiomegaly; and pulmonary congestion and pleural effusions may be present. The *echocardiogram* shows the inordinate dilatation of the left ventricle and poor contractions. A relatively enlarged left atrium and displaced mitral valve are noted.

The course of the disease is usually downhill. Vigorous treatment for heart failure may result in remissions, but relapses are common, and in time patients tend to become resistant to therapy. The prognosis is poor. Cardiac transplantation has been utilized successfully in this group of patients as well as in patients with other forms of cardiomyopathy. Complications include arrhythmias (premature atrial and ventricular complexes and later atrial fibrillation) and systemic emboli from intracardiac thrombi.

Restrictive Cardiomyopathy. Poor ventricular compliance is the major abnormality and in this type of cardiomyopathy is responsible for inadequate filling of the ventricular cavities during diastole. This results in a clinical pattern which closely simulates that of constrictive pericarditis. In its full-blown form restrictive cardiomyopathy results in dyspnea, edema, ascites, hepatomegaly, increased venous pressure, and pulmonary congestion. The heart is mildly or moderately enlarged, and murmurs are nonspecific. The electrocardiogram shows prominent P waves, often normal QRS voltage, S-T segment depression, and T wave inversion. Roentgenographic examination shows slight or moderate cardiomegaly. Differential diagnosis from constrictive pericarditis is important since the latter can be treated surgically with dramatic success. The prognosis for restrictive cardiomyopathy is generally poor. Treatment is directed toward relief of edema with diuretics, and calcium blocking agents may be used to increase diastolic compliance.

14.80 CONGESTIVE HEART FAILURE

Heart failure is that state in which the heart cannot produce the cardiac output required to sustain the metabolic needs of the body without evoking certain compensatory mechanisms (cardiac reserve). As these mechanisms become ineffective, increasingly severe clinical manifestations result.

Cardiac output can be calculated as the product of heart rate and stroke volume (HR × SV). There are several types of pathophysiologic derangements that, when sufficiently severe, compromise stroke volume and thus lead to cardiac decompensation. These include *afterload* (pressure work), *preload* (volume work), and *myocardial* abnormalities. In addition, *tachyarrhythmias* shorten the diastolic time interval for filling

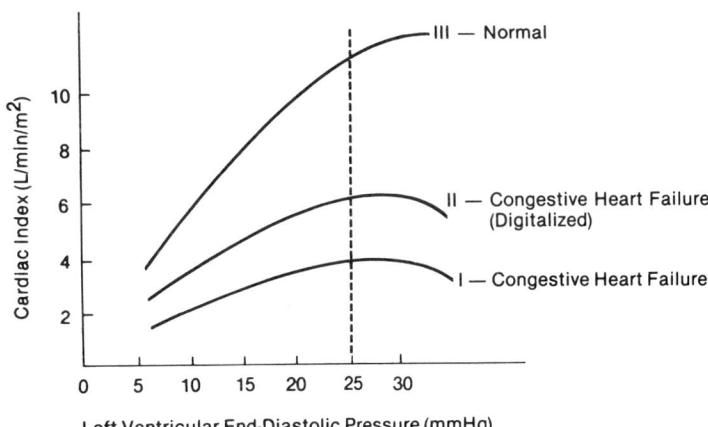

Figure 14–78. As the left ventricular end-diastolic pressure (LVED) increases, cardiac index increases, even in the presence of congestive heart failure, until a critical level of LVED is reached. Adding an inotropic agent (digoxin) shifts the curve from I to II. (From Gersony WT, Steep CN: *In* Dickerman JD, Lucey JF [eds]: Smith's The Critically Ill Child: Diagnosis and Medical Management. 3rd ed. Philadelphia, WB Saunders, 1984.)

of the ventricles, compromising stroke volume and cardiac output.

Pathophysiology. The heart can be viewed as a pump whose output is directly proportional to its filling volume. As end-diastolic volume increases, the healthy heart will increase cardiac output in a linear fashion until a maximum is reached (Frank-Starling principle) and cardiac output can no longer be augmented (Fig. 14–78). The increased stroke volume obtained in this manner is due to increased myocardial contractility associated with stretching of muscle fibers, but also requires increased wall tension and increased myocardial oxygen. Hearts functioning under various types of stress will produce different types of Frank-Starling curves (Fig. 14–78). Cardiac muscle whose contractility is compromised will require greater dilatation to produce increased stroke volume, but will not achieve the cardiac output of the normal myocardium. If a cardiac chamber is already dilated because of a lesion causing an increased preload (e.g., left to right shunt, valve insufficiency, anemia, etc.), there will be little room for further dilatation and augmentation of cardiac output. The presence of lesions that result in severe afterloads will also markedly compromise the usual Frank-Starling relationships between filling volume and cardiac output.

High output failure is the development of signs and symptoms of congestive heart failure when there is no basic abnormality in myocardial function and the cardiac output is greater than normal. It is caused by conditions such as profound anemia, severe hyperthyroidism, and large systemic arteriovenous fistulae. These diseases reduce peripheral vascular resistance and cardiac afterload and increase myocardial contractility. Heart "failure" results when the demands for cardiac output exceed the ability of the heart to respond. Chronic severe high output failure may eventually result in a decrease in myocardial performance as the metabolic requirements of the myocardium itself are not met.

Clinical Manifestations. The clinical manifestations of congestive heart failure depend on the degree of cardiac reserve under various conditions. A critically ill infant or child who has exhausted his compensatory mechanisms to the point where he can no longer achieve sufficient cardiac output to meet the basal metabolic needs of the body will be symptomatic at rest. Other patients may be comfortable when quiet, but are incapable of increasing cardiac output in response to even mild activity without developing significant symptoms. On the other hand it may take rather vigorous exercise to compromise cardiac function in children who have less severe heart disease.

A thorough history is extremely important both in making the diagnosis of heart failure and in evaluating the possible causes. Parents who are observing their infant on a daily basis may not recognize subtle changes that have occurred over the course of days or weeks. Cyanosis may be considered merely "a deep coloring" and not recognized as an abnormal finding. The history obtained from the parents of a young infant should focus on the feeding process. The infant having congestive heart failure will often take less volume per feeding, become dyspneic while sucking, and perhaps perspire profusely. After falling into an exhausted sleep, the infant, inadequately fed, will soon awake for the next feeding. This cycle continues around the clock and must be carefully differentiated from colic or other feeding disorders. Eliciting a history of fatigue in an older child requires specific questions about activity, including stair climbing, walking various distances, bicycle riding, etc. Inquiry should also be made regarding orthopnea and nocturnal dyspnea.

In children the signs and symptoms of congestive heart failure are similar to those in adults. These include fatigue, effort intolerance, anorexia, abdominal pain, and cough. Dyspnea is a reflection of pulmonary congestion. Elevation of systemic venous pressure may be gauged by clinical assessment of the jugular venous pressure, and liver enlargement. Orthopnea and basal rales may be present; edema is usually discernible in dependent portions of the body, or anasarca may be present. Cardiomegaly is invariably noted. Gallop rhythm is common; other auscultatory findings are those produced by the basic lesion.

In infants congestive heart failure may be more difficult to identify. Prominent manifestations include tachypnea, feeding difficulties, poor weight gain, excessive perspiration, irritability, weak cry, and noisy, labored respiration with costal and subcostal retractions as well as flaring of the alae nasi and sternal retractions. Pulmonary congestion may be indistinguishable from signs and symptoms of bronchiolitis. Pneumonitis with or without atelectasis of part of the lung is common. Hepatomegaly nearly always occurs, and cardiomegaly is invariably present. In spite of pronounced tachycardia, gallop rhythm can frequently be recognized. The other auscultatory signs are those produced by the cardiac lesion that resulted in heart failure. Clinical assessment of the jugular venous pressure in infants may be difficult because of the shortness of the neck and the difficulty of observing a relaxed state. Edema, especially in infants, is frequently not clinically detectable; when present, the edema may be generalized, involving the eyelids as well as the sacrum, legs, and feet.

Laboratory Data. *Roentgenograms of the chest* show cardiac enlargement. The pulmonary vascularity is variable depending on the etiology of the heart failure. Infants and children having large left to right shunts will have exaggeration of the pulmonary arterial vessels to the periphery of the lung fields, whereas patients having cardiomyopathy may have a relatively normal pulmonary vascular bed early in the course of their disease. Fluffy pulmonary markings suggestive of venous congestion and acute pulmonary edema are usually not seen in childhood except in the most extreme circumstances.

The diagnosis of specific chamber enlargement by *electrocardiography* may be helpful in assessing the etiology of congestive heart failure, but does not establish the diagnosis. Left and/or right ventricular ischemic changes may correlate well with clinical and other noninvasive parameters of ventricular function. Low voltage QRS morphology with ST-T wave abnormalities may suggest myocardial inflammatory disease, and can also be seen with pericarditis. The electrocardiogram is the best tool for evaluating rhythm disorders as a cause of cardiac failure.

Echocardiographic techniques to determine the relationship between end-systolic and end-diastolic diameters (shortening fraction) are useful in assessing ventricular function. The normal shortening fraction should be 28–36%, compared with the normal ejection fraction of 55–65% measured by angiography. The pre-ejection/ejection period ratio (PEP/EP) should be less than 40%. A long pre-ejection time with a very short ejection time usually denotes myocardial failure. *Radionuclide studies* are also useful, since the ejection fraction can be determined by injecting a radioisotope (e.g., technetium-99m) into a vein and measuring end-diastolic volume and systolic volume by counts over the ventricles.

Arterial Blood Gases and Electrolytes. Arterial oxygen levels may be decreased when ventilation/perfusion inequalities occur secondary to pulmonary edema. When heart failure is severe, mild respiratory acidemia may be present. Infants with severe heart failure and decreased cardiac output will demonstrate metabolic acidemia. In contrast, infants with marked tachypnea associated with decreased pulmonary compliance secondary to interstitial congestion without alveolar edema, may have mild respiratory alkalosis.

Infants with congestive heart failure often display hyponatremia owing to water retention. Although serum sodium is low, total body sodium is increased. An abnormal steady state is reached in which relatively more water is retained.

Treatment. The underlying cause of cardiac failure must be removed or alleviated if possible. If the etiology is a congenital cardiovascular anomaly amenable to surgery, medical treatment is indicated for a time before the surgical procedure, and should usually be continued in the immediate postoperative period. For many patients with cardiomyopathies only medical management can be provided unless cardiac transplantation is indicated.

General Measures. Strict bed rest is rarely necessary except in extreme cases, but it is important that the child rest often and sleep adequately. Most patients feel better in a semiupright position, and an infant chair is advisable for infants with chronic congestive heart failure. When patients are responding to treatment, restrictions on activities should be within the context of the patient's ability to be relatively active.

For patients with pulmonary edema, bed rest, positive pressure ventilation, and morphine (0.05 mg/kg) may be required along with other drug therapy. In extreme situations, beta agonists such as isoproterenol, dopamine, and dobutamine along with peripheral vasodilators (e.g., nitroprusside, captopril) may be required in an intensive care setting.

Digitalis. Digoxin is the digitalis glycoside used most often in the pediatric patient. The half-life of 36 hr is long enough to allow daily or twice daily administration, and short enough to limit toxic effects from overdosage. Digoxin is absorbed by the gastrointestinal tract. When taken with or after meals the rate of absorption may be somewhat retarded, but the amount of digoxin absorbed is almost always unchanged. Following oral administration, approximately 60–85% of digoxin is absorbed. Absorption is greater for the elixir than for tablets. The peak effect for oral digoxin is approximately 2–6 hr; an initial effect can be seen as early as 30 min after administration. When the drug is administered intravenously the initial effect is seen in 15–30 min and the peak effect occurs at 1–4 hr. The drug crosses the placenta, and therefore the fetus can be treated via administration to the mother. Digoxin is eliminated by the kidney and the rate of excretion is proportional to the glomerular filtration rate. After intravenous administration, 50–70% is excreted unchanged in the urine. The half-life of digoxin is 1–2 days in children who have normal renal function, but is 6 days in patients with renal shutdown, who must utilize slower hepatic excretion pathways.

Rapid digitalization of infants and children in congestive heart failure may be carried out intravenously. The dose depends on the patient's age (Table 14–11), and various regimens are utilized. The recommended schedule is to give one third of the total digitalizing dose immediately and the succeeding two doses 8–16 hr later. In cases of profound congestive failure, more rapid digitalization using narrower intervals and a larger initial loading dose may be required. The electrocardiogram must be closely monitored and rhythm strips obtained prior to each of the three digitalizing doses.

Table 14–11. Dosage of Drugs Commonly Used for the Treatment of Congestive Heart Failure

Drug	Dosage
Digoxin	
Digitalization (PO) (3 doses q 8 hr)	Premature 0.02–0.025 mg/kg
	Neonate (≤ 1 mo) 0.03–0.04 mg/kg
	Infant or child 0.04–0.06 mg/kg
	Adolescent or adult 1.0–1.5 mg in divided doses
Digitalization (IV) (Timing of dosage variable, depending on clinical indications)	75% of PO dose
Maintenance	¼–⅓ of digitalizing dose, divided q 12 hr
Furosemide	
IV	1–2 mg/dose, prn
PO	1–4 mg/kg/24 hr, qd, bid, or qid
Chlorothiazide (PO)	20–50 mg/kg/24 hr, bid, or qid
Spironolactone (PO)	2–3 mg/kg/24 hr, bid
Beta-Agonists (IV)	
Isoproterenol	0.01–0.5 µg/kg/min
Dopamine	2–20 µg/kg/min
Dobutamine	2–20 µg/kg/min
Afterload reducing agents	
Nitroprusside (IV)	0.5–8 µg/kg/min
Hydralazine	
IV	0.5 mg/kg
PO	0.5–7.5 mg/kg/24 hr, tid
Prazosin (PO)	
Starting dose	0.2–0.4 mg/kg/24 hr or 1–3 mg/24 hr, qid
Chronic dose	6–15 mg/24 hr, qid
Captopril (PO)	0.5–6 mg/kg/24 hr, qid

Digoxin should be discontinued if a new rhythm disturbance is noted. A prolongation of the PR interval is not in itself an indication to withhold digitalis, but a delay in administering the next dose or a reduction in the dosage should be considered depending on the patient's clinical status. Serum digoxin determination is helpful when digitalis toxicity is suspected. ST segments or T wave changes are commonly noted with digitalis administration and should not affect the digitalization regimen. Baseline serum electrolyte levels should be measured prior to and after digitalization.

Maintenance digitalis therapy is started approximately 12 hr after full digitalization. The daily dosage is divided in two and given at 12 hr intervals for more consistent blood levels and more flexibility in case of toxicity. The dosage is one quarter to one third of the full digitalizing dose. For patients who are initially digitalized intravenously, maintenance digoxin can be given orally once oral feedings are tolerated. Since absorption from the gastrointestinal tract is less certain, the oral maintenance dose is approximately 25% higher than when digoxin is utilized parenterally (Table 14–11). The normal daily dosage of digoxin for older children (>5 yr of age) should not exceed the usual adult dose of 0.2–0.5 mg/24 hr.

Patients who are not critically ill may be digitalized initially using the oral regimen (Table 14–11), and in most instances digitalization should be completed within 24 hr. When slow digitalization is acceptable, initiation of a maintenance digoxin schedule without loading dosage will achieve full digitalization in 7–10 days. This often can be carried out on an outpatient basis.

If an infant improves significantly on digitalis over a period of a few months and the need for the drug appears to be lessening (e.g., a ventricular septal defect that is becoming smaller), dosage is not increased as the child gains weight. If the clinical status warrants, the drug is eventually discontinued.

If there are questions as to the effectiveness and/or toxicity of digitalis, plasma digoxin levels should be measured. Blood should be drawn at least 4 hr after the last dose so that tissue/plasma equilibration has occurred. A normal blood level in an infant is approximately 2–4 ng/mL and in older children 1–2 ng/mL. Exceeding this level will not generally add significantly to the management of congestive failure.

Measurement of *serum digoxin levels* is useful under three circumstances: (1) when a standard dose of digoxin is not having beneficial therapeutic effects; (2) when an unknown amount of digoxin has been administered or ingested accidentally; and (3) when a toxic response is suspected. In this third situation, *elevated serum digoxin levels are not in themselves diagnostic of toxicity but must be interpreted as an adjunct to other clinical and electrocardiographic findings.* A finding of toxicity is primarily based on rhythm and conduction disturbances; nausea and vomiting are not frequent in the pediatric patient. Hypokalemia and hypercalcemia, cardiac inflammation, and prematurity may potentiate digoxin toxicity. A cardiac arrhythmia that develops in a child with congestive heart failure who is taking digitalis also may be related to cardiac disease rather than to the drug. However, *any form of arrhythmia occurring following the institution of digitalis therapy must be considered to be drug related until proven otherwise.* Succeeding dosage should be withheld until the question is resolved.

Diet. Infants having congestive heart failure are calorically deprived due to increased metabolic requirements and decreased caloric intake. Increasing daily calories is an important aspect of their management. Often as other therapeutic measures take effect, the child will have an improved appetite. However, increasing calories per ounce of feeding may occasionally be beneficial, e.g., using formulas containing 24 calories per ounce. Some infants will not tolerate increased concentration of calories because of gastrointestinal disturbances, particularly diarrhea. These formulas may also provide too large a solute load for compromised kidneys, which may then fail to maintain adequate sodium and water balance.

Severely ill infants in congestive heart failure may lack sufficient strength for effective sucking because of extreme fatigue, rapid respirations, and generalized weakness. Nasogastric feedings may be helpful. When congestive heart failure continues unabated, however, an increased caloric diet will frequently be of no avail. Indeed, continued malnutrition may be an important factor in the decision to undertake early surgical intervention in patients who have an operable congenital heart lesion.

The use of very low sodium formulas in the routine management of infants with congestive heart failure is not recommended, since these preparations are often poorly tolerated and thus, although sodium intake is decreased, caloric needs are less well met than with standard formulas. The use of more potent diuretic agents allows more palatable standard formulas to be utilized for nutrition while controlling salt and water balance by chronic diuretic administration. Some infants and children can be managed with "no added salt" diets and abstinence from foods containing large amounts of sodium. A strict extremely low sodium diet is rarely required.

Diuretics. Diuretic agents interfere with reabsorption of water and sodium by the kidneys, which results in the reduction of circulating blood volume and thereby reduces ventricular filling pressures. These agents are most often used in conjunction with digitalis therapy in patients with severe congestive heart failure.

Furosemide is the most commonly used diuretic in patients with cardiac failure. It inhibits the reabsorption of sodium and chloride, not only in the distal tubules but also in the loop of Henle. Patients requiring acute diuresis should be given intravenous or intramuscular furosemide at an initial dose of 1–2 mg/kg. This often results in rapid diuresis and prompt improvement in clinical status, particularly if symptoms of pulmonary congestion are present. Chronic furosemide therapy is then prescribed at a dose of 1–4 mg/kg/24 hr or every other day, usually as a single morning oral dose. Careful monitoring of electrolytes is necessary with long-term diuretic therapy, since there may be significant loss of potassium. Potassium chloride supplementation and/or spironolactone may be administered in conjunction with chronic diuretic therapy to preserve potassium. Spironolactone is given orally in divided doses of 2–3 mg/kg/24 hr in order to enhance potassium retention and inhibit aldosterone. When furosemide is administered every other day, dietary potassium supplementation may be adequate to maintain normal serum potassium levels. Chronic administration of furosemide may cause contraction of the extracellular fluid compartment resulting in a "contraction alkalosis" (Sec. 5.12). When this occurs, the medication should be discontinued and acetazolamide, a carbonic anhydrase inhibitor, substituted until the metabolic disturbance has been corrected.

Chlorothiazide is occasionally used for diuresis in children with less severe chronic congestive heart failure. It is less immediate in action and less potent than furosemide, and it affects the reabsorption of electrolytes only in the renal tubules. The usual dose is 20–50 mg/kg/24 hr or every other day in divided doses. Potassium supplementation may also be utilized concurrently with this diuretic agent.

Afterload Reducing Agents. A group of drugs are available that reduce ventricular afterload by decreasing peripheral vascular resistance, thereby improving myocardial contractility. Some of these agents also decrease systemic venous tone, significantly reducing preload. Afterload reducers are of greatest benefit to children with congestive heart failure secondary to a cardiomyopathy, but they are also effective in patients with severe mitral regurgitation or aortic insufficiency. Congestive heart failure secondary to left to right shunts or stenotic lesions is less often treated with afterload reducing agents. This therapy has not been used often in the management of large left to right shunts because of uncertain effects on pulmonary vascular resistance. If heart failure is the result of a fixed obstructive cardiac lesion, peripheral vasodilatation beyond the site of stenosis will not significantly affect total ventricular afterload. Afterload reducing agents are most often used in conjunction with other anticongestive drugs, such as digoxin and diuretics. In pediatrics, these drugs are rarely first line therapeutic modalities, but are added to treatment in specific situations when decreasing peripheral vascular resistance will add significantly to optimal management. Only a few afterload reducing agents have been used extensively in children (Table 14–11).

Nitroprusside directly dilates arterial and venous vessels and is a potent intravenous medication that should be administered only in an intensive care setting. Peripheral arterial vasodilatation and afterload reduction is the major effect, but venodilatation causing a decrease in venous return is also beneficial to the patient on the basis of preload reduction. Blood pressure must be continuously monitored by means of an intra-arterial line, since sudden hypotension can occur with overdosage. Nitroprusside is contraindicated when hypotension pre-exists. As the drug is metabolized, small amounts of circulating cyanide are produced, which are detoxified in the liver to thiocyanate, that is excreted in the urine. However, when high doses of nitroprusside are administered for several days, toxic symptoms related to thiocyanide poisoning may occur, such as fatigue, nausea, disorientation, and muscular spasm. If nitroprusside use is prolonged, blood thiocyanate levels should be monitored; values of 5–10 μg/dL are consistent with clinical symptoms of toxicity. Nitroprusside should be utilized only in the most critically ill patients and for as short a period of time as possible.

Hydralazine is a direct arteriolar smooth muscle relaxant and has virtually no effects on preload. Therefore, it is occasionally administered together with a venodilating agent such as a nitrate derivative. The usual oral dose of hydralazine is 0.5–7.5 mg/kg/24 hr in three divided doses. In some cases it may be advantageous to evaluate the acute effects of intravenous hydralazine; if increased cardiac output, decreased peripheral vascular resistance, and decreased left ventricular filling pressure are observed, then chronic oral therapy is instituted. Many patients require increasing dosage with time in order to maintain the peripheral dilating effects (tachyphylaxis).

Adverse reactions with hydralazine include headache, palpitations, nausea, and vomiting. In addition, systemic lupus erythematosus occasionally occurs after administration of large doses of hydralazine over prolonged periods; these manifestations are reversible when the drug is discontinued.

Prazosin is a postsynaptic alpha-adrenergic blocking agent that affects the arterial and venous systems and thereby reduces both preload and afterload. Cardiac output increases and there is a decrease in systemic venous return. This agent is especially beneficial when cardiomyopathy or left heart valve disease is associated with pulmonary edema. The usual starting dose for children is 0.2–0.4 mg/kg/24 hr in four divided doses. Total daily dosage of 6–15 mg may be given to the adolescent patient. However, increasing the dosage beyond 20 mg/24 hr does not significantly increase efficacy.

Adverse reactions to prazosin include dizziness, drowsiness, and palpitations. There also may be excessive postural hypotension with syncope, so monitoring of blood pressure is mandatory. In most instances side effects completely disappear when dosage is reduced.

Captopril is an orally active angiotensin-coverting-enzyme inhibitor that produces marked arterial dilatation by blocking the production of angiotensin II, resulting in significant afterload reduction. Venodilatation and consequent preload re-

duction has also been reported. This agent also interferes with aldosterone production and thereby also helps control salt and water retention. The oral dose is 0.5–6 mg/kg/24 hr given in 2–4 divided doses. Some patients who initially do not show significant improvement on captopril have clinical benefits when the drug is administered on a long-term basis. However, the converse occurs in some patients.

The adverse reactions to captopril include hypotension and its sequelae (e.g., syncope, weakness, and dizziness). A maculopapular pruritic rash is encountered in 5–8% of patients, but the drug may be continued since the rash often disappears spontaneously with time. Neutropenia and proteinuria have also been reported.

Beta Agonists. *Isoproterenol*, an intravenous preparation used for treating low cardiac output, has central and peripheral beta-adrenergic effects, and therefore both enhances myocardial contractility and reduces cardiac afterload. The drug is administered in an intensive care setting where the dose is titrated between 0.01 and 0.5 μg/kg/min depending on the heart rate response. Continuous determinations of arterial blood pressure and heart rate are mandatory, and measuring cardiac output at the bedside also may be helpful in assessing drug efficacy. Since isoproterenol has a marked chronotropic effect, it should not be used in patients who have significant tachycardia. Children receiving isoproterenol must be carefully monitored for atrial or ventricular premature depolarizations, as they may lead to supraventricular or ventricular tachycardia. As the patient's clinical condition improves, the drug is gradually tapered, usually over 1–2 days. Often, as isoproterenol treatment is withdrawn, digoxin therapy is added for continued inotropic effect.

Dopamine is an effective beta-adrenergic agent which is less chronotropic and arrhythmogenic than isoproterenol. In addition, it is a selective renal vasodilator, particularly useful in patients with the compromised kidney function that is often associated with low cardiac output. At a dose of 2–10 μg/kg/min, dopamine results in both inotropism and peripheral vasodilatation. However, if the dose must be increased beyond 10 μg/kg/min, peripheral alpha-adrenergic effects may result in vasoconstriction rather than in dilatation.

Dobutamine, a derivitive of dopamine, is used to treat low cardiac output. It has the advantage of causing direct inotropic effects without dose-related variations in peripheral vascular resistance. Dobutamine can be used as an effective substitute for high-dose dopamine therapy in order to avoid vasoconstrictive effects, and it is unlikely to cause cardiac rhythm disturbances even at maximal dosage. The usual dose is similar to that of dopamine (2–20 μg/kg/min).

14.81 CARDIOGENIC SHOCK

See also Sec 5.41.

Cardiogenic shock may occur as a complication of (1) severe cardiac dysfunction, often following surgery; (2) septicemia; (3) severe burns; (4) immunologic disease; (5) hemorrhage or dehydration; (6) severe debilitation; and (7) acute central nervous system disorders. It is characterized by low cardiac output and hypotension resulting in inadequate tissue perfusion.

Treatment is aimed at reinstitution of adequate cardiac output and peripheral perfusion to prevent the untoward effects of prolonged ischemia to vital organs as well as management of the underlying cause. Under physiologic conditions, the cardiac output is most reliably increased by increasing heart rate with positive chronotropic agents such as isoproterenol and epinephrine. However, in the presence of marked tachycardia a further increase in heart rate will not increase and may decrease cardiac output by decreasing

Table 14-12. Treatment of Cardiogenic Shock

Goal—to improve peripheral perfusion by increasing cardiac output

Cardiac output = Heart rate × stroke volume

	Preload	Determinants of Stroke Volume Contractility	Afterload
Parameters measured	CVP, PCWP	CO, BP	CO, BP
Abnormal physiologic manifestations	Low CVP and/or PCWP ↓ CO ↓ BP	Elevation of CVP and/or PCWP ↓ CO ↓ BP	Elevation of CVP and/or PCWP ↓ CO → ↑ BP
Treatment to improve cardiac output	Volume expansion Plasma Whole blood	Catecholamines Isoproterenol, 0.05–2 μg/kg/min Dopamine, 5–20 μg/kg/min Dobutamine, 2.5–20 μg/kg/min	Vasodilatation Nitroprusside, 0.5–8 μg/kg/min Hydralazine, 0.5 mg/kg

CVP = Central venous pressure   ↓ = Decreased
PCWP = Pulmonary capillary wedge pressure   → = Normal
CO = Cardiac output   ↑ = Increased
BP = Blood pressure

diastolic filling time. Cardiac output may also be increased by increasing stroke volume. If fluid administration is increased, the Starling mechanism results in increased stroke volume by increasing central venous pressure and ventricular filling pressure (preload). When central venous pressure is low, infusion of volume will reliably increase cardiac output. Optimal filling pressure is variable and depends on a number of extracardiac factors including ventilatory support with high positive end-expiratory pressure, peak inspiratory pressure, and intra-abdominal pressure. The increased pressure necessary to fill relatively noncompliant right ventricles should also be considered, particularly after open heart surgery. If incremental fluid administration does not result in improved cardiac output, abnormal myocardial contractility and/or high afterload must be implicated as the cause of low cardiac output.

Myocardial contractility will improve when treatment of the basic cause of shock is instituted, hypoxia eliminated, and acidosis corrected. However, isoproterenol, dopamine, epinephrine, and dobutamine are catecholamines which will also improve cardiac contractility, increase heart rate, and ultimately increase cardiac output. The major differences among these agents lie in their effects on the peripheral vascular bed. *Isoproterenol* has pure beta-adrenergic action and will decrease peripheral vascular resistance throughout the therapeutic dosage range. *Dopamine* has no significant peripheral beta effects on vascular resistance at dosage of 2–10 μg/kg/min. However, at higher doses (>10 μg/kg/min) it causes significant dose-dependent increases in systemic vascular resistance via alpha receptors similar to those seen with norepinephrine. Dopamine also has specific effects on the renal vascular system and increases renal blood flow out of proportion to other vascular beds at doses <10 μg/kg/min. At high doses dopamine may cause an increase in pulmonary vascular resistance, particularly in patients with extremely reactive pulmonary vascular circulations. *Epinephrine* will also cause a dose-dependent increase in systemic vascular resistance via the alpha-adrenergic receptors. All of these agents may cause tachycardias and, particularly in the presence of hypoxia and/or acidosis, may be arrhythmogenic. A major advantage of the catecholamines is their very short half-lives; therefore, positive inotropic effects are virtually immediate, and untoward effects can be reversed quickly by discontinuation of the drug. *Dobutamine* has "pure" central beta effects similar to those of isoproterenol with fewer peripheral vascular effects than the other catecholamines at equivalent therapeutic doses. Along with dopamine, dobutamine has less chronotropic effect than isoproterenol and is more advantageous when a marked tachycardia is present prior to initiation of an inotropic agent. These drugs may be used in various combinations.

The use of cardiac glycosides to treat acute low cardiac output states should be avoided. Digoxin has a slower effect than the catecholamines, even with intravenous administration. In addition, adverse effects may result from larger doses, and toxicity is less predictable, depending on myocardial and serum potassium and calcium levels. Since it is quite common for patients with cardiovascular shock to have compromised renal perfusion, the administration of digoxin may result in high persistent blood levels because it is excreted in the kidneys. When digoxin is required for such patients, a lower dosage scale should be used and serum digoxin levels frequently monitored.

Patients with cardiogenic shock may have a marked increase in systemic vascular resistance resulting in high afterload and poor peripheral perfusion. If high systemic vascular resistance is persistent and the administration of positive inotropic agents alone does not improve tissue perfusion, the use of afterload reducing agents may be appropriate, e.g., nitroprusside used in combination with dopamine.

Sequential evaluation and management of cardiovascular shock is mandatory (Sec. 5.41). Table 14–12 outlines the treatment of acute cardiac circulatory failure under most circumstances. The treatment of infants and children with low cardiac output following cardiac surgery depends on the nature of the operative procedure and the patient's status after surgery (Sec. 14.69).

Awan NA, Miller RR, Mason DT: Comparison of effects of nitroprusside and prazosin on left ventricular function and the peripheral circulation in chronic refractory congestive heart failure. Circulation 57:152, 1978.

Benzing G III, Helmsworth JA, Schreiber JT, et al: Nitroprusside after open-heart surgery. Circulation 54:467, 1976.

Black-Schaffer B: Infantile endocardial fibroelastosis: A suggested etiology. Arch Pathol 63:281, 1957.

Chatterjee K, Parmley WW: The role of vasodilator therapy in heart failure. Prog Cardiovasc Dis 19:301, 1977.

Dickerman JD, Lucey JF: Smith's The Critically Ill Child. 3rd ed. Philadelphia, WB Saunders, 1985.

Doering W: Quinidine-digoxin interaction: Pharmacokinetics, underlying mechanism and clinical implications. N Engl J Med 301:401, 1979.

Dungan WT, Doherty JE, Harvey C, et al: Tritiated digoxin XVIII. Studies in infants and children. Circulation 46:983, 1972.

Goodwin JF: Prospects and predictions for the cardiomyopathies. Circulation 50:210, 1974.

Greenwood RD, Nadas AS, Fyler DC: The clinical course of primary myocardial disease in infants and children. Am Heart J 92:549, 1976.

Harris LC, Nghiem QX: Cardiomyopathies in infants and children. Prog Cardiovasc Dis 25:255, 1972.

Hayes CJ, Butler VP Jr, Gersony WM: Serum digoxin studies in infants and children. Pediatrics 52:561, 1973.

Hernandez A, Burton RM, Pagtakhan RD, et al: Pharmacodynamics of ³H-digoxin in infants. Pediatrics 44:418, 1969.

Lang D, von Bernuth G: Serum concentration and serum half-life of digoxin in premature and mature infants. Pediatrics 59:902, 1977.

Loggie JMH, Kleinman LI, VanMaanen EF: Renal function and diuretic therapy in infants and children. J Pediatr 86:485, 657, 825, 1975.

14.82 DISEASES OF THE PERICARDIUM

Major diseases that involve the pericardium include bacterial, tuberculous, fungal, and parasitic infections; acute rheumatic fever; rheumatoid arthritis; systemic lupus erythematosus; uremia; radiation injury; thalassemia; trauma; pericardial cysts; congenital malformations; postpericardiotomy syndrome; and chronic constrictive disease. In some instances the involvement of the pericardium is only one manifestation of a more generalized illness, and the prominence of the pericardial component will vary depending on the disease entity.

Hemodynamics. Pericardial inflammation results in an accumulation of fluid in the pericardial space. The fluid varies according to the etiology of the pericarditis and may be serous, fibrinous, purulent, or hemorrhagic. Cardiac tamponade occurs when the amount of pericardial fluid reaches a level that compromises cardiac function. In a healthy child there is 10–15 mL of fluid in the pericardial space, whereas in an adolescent with pericarditis an excess of 1000 mL of fluid may accumulate. For every small increment of fluid the pericardial pressure rises slowly, but once a critical level is reached, there is a rapid rise in pressure culminating in severe cardiac compression. Inhibition of ventricular filling during diastole, elevated systemic and pulmonary venous pressures, and, if untreated, eventual compromised cardiac output and shock occur.

Clinical Manifestations. The first symptom of pericardial disease is often precordial pain. The major complaint is a sharp, stabbing sensation of the left shoulder; the chest, shoulder, and back pain which occurs may be exaggerated by lying and relieved by sitting, especially leaning forward. Since there is no sensory innervation of the pericardium, the pain is probably referred pain from diaphragmatic and pleural irritation. Cough and fever may also occur. The presence of symptoms or signs associated with other organs and systems depends on the basic etiology of the pericarditis.

On physical examination, many of the findings relate to the degree of fluid accumulation in the pericardial sac. The presence of a friction rub is helpful but may be a late sign in acute pericarditis, becoming apparent only after the effusion is reduced. Narrow pulses, quiet precordium, distant heart sounds, neck vein distention, and a paradoxical pulse suggest significant fluid accumulation.

Greater than 20 mm Hg of *paradoxical pulse* in a child with pericarditis is a reliable indicator of the presence of cardiac tamponade; 10–20 mm Hg change is equivocal. There is normally a slight decrease in systolic arterial pressure during inspiration. With cardiac tamponade this normal phenomenon is exaggerated, probably because of decreased left heart filling with the inspiratory phase of respiration. In order to determine the degree of pulsus paradoxus, one first measures the exact systolic blood pressure during normal expiration. The manometer is then slowly allowed to fall. The point when the systolic pressure is heard equally well during inspiration and expiration is then recorded. The difference between the two determinations represents the degree of paradox. Significant pulsus paradoxus may also be present with severe dyspnea of any origin and is not infrequent in patients who have emphysema or asthma or who are being ventilated with a positive pressure respirator. In these patients the paradoxical pulse is due to a marked increase in intrathoracic pressure. Determination of the etiology of paradoxical pulse in a child on a ventilator after cardiac surgery may therefore be difficult to assess.

Laboratory Data. The specific findings depend on the underlying disease. The effects of pericarditis on the *electrocardiogram* are multiple. Low voltage of the QRS complexes results from a damping effect of pericardial fluid. Pressure on the myocardium by fluid or exudate produces a current of injury that results in mild elevation of S-T segments. Generalized T wave inversion occurs as a consequence of associated myocardial inflammation. The S-T segment and T wave changes with pericarditis are more generalized than those seen with myocardial infarction, and the S-T segment elevations tend to precede the T wave changes. There may be an interval when the ECG is in a transitional phase and appears to be normal. This may occur during the acute phase of the illness prior to diagnosis. In some instances clear cut abnormalities are never identified.

A relatively large pericardial effusion must be present to cause an enlarged cardiac shadow with the usual "water-bottle" configuration on *chest roentgenogram* (Fig. 14–79). In most instances the lung fields are clear. With constrictive disease the heart is relatively small and calcification may be present.

The *echocardiogram* is a sensitive technique for evaluating the size and progression of pericardial effusions. Normally, the pericardium is closely adherent to the epicardium, and the two layers can be only narrowly separated by the ultrasound beam. In patients with pericardial effusion a clear echo-free space is recorded between the epicardium and pericardium. A posterior effusion is recorded behind the left ventricular epicardium and ends at the junction of the left ventricle and left atrium. An anterior effusion will be recorded between the chest wall and the anterior right ventricular wall. The presence of both an anterior and posterior effusion generally indicates that a large collection of fluid is present. False positives are rare in the hands of experienced echocardiographers.

Differential Diagnosis. *Viral and Acute Benign Pericarditis.* These entities are considered synonymous since most episodes of acute benign pericarditis follow or coincide with viral illness. Viruses recognized to cause pericarditis include coxsackievirus B, influenza, echovirus, and adenovirus. The pathogenesis is unclear but may be related to a hypersensitivity reaction to a viral disease. However, pericardial inflammation is not necessarily the precursor of a generalized inflammatory process. Most cases are mild, and recovery occurs within several weeks.

Only symptomatic therapy is indicated. In rare instances the patient will be severely ill, and cardiac tamponade may ensue. There are also patients in whom a chronic relapsing illness occurs. The differential diagnosis between these patients and those with collagen vascular disease may be difficult. These patients respond dramatically to corticosteroids or indomethacin; milder forms may be controlled with aspirin. The clinical course may vary from months to 1–2 yr, during which time the patients are dependent on drug therapy for suppression of the pericarditis. Ultimately, the patients improve and the prognosis is good.

The clinical differential diagnosis between acute pericarditis and myocarditis may be difficult. Indeed, in patients with pericarditis there is usually a myocardial inflammatory component, and the reverse is also true. However, management of these conditions is quite different; anti-inflammatory treatment and urgent response to cardiac tamponade are appropriate in the former, and therapy for congestive heart failure is required in the latter. The echocardiogram is useful in the differential diagnosis as it will demonstrate large pericardial effusions and can also indicate the presence of myocardial dysfunction.

Purulent Pericarditis. This is most often associated with bacterial infections such as pneumonia, epiglottitis, meningi-

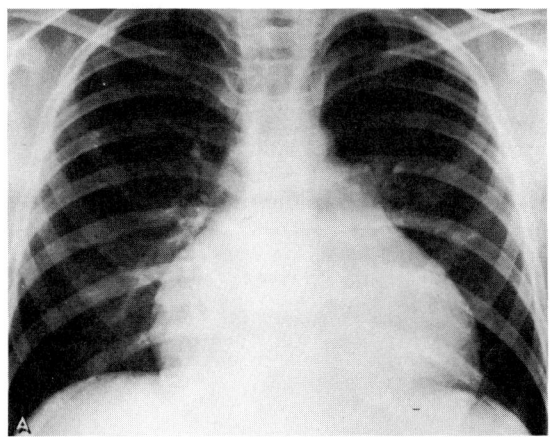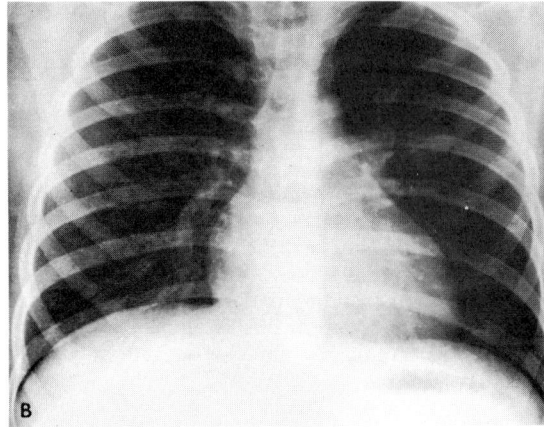

Figure 14–79. Roentgenograms in acute nonspecific pericarditis. *A*, Increase in cardiopericardial shadow due to pericardial effusion. *B*, One month later after complete recovery.

tis, or osteomyelitis. There may be signs and symptoms of the primary infection. Once the purulent process is established, the course is fulminant, terminated by acute cardiac tamponade and death. Open pericardial drainage is mandatory, along with appropriate intravenous antibiotics. Although closed pericardial aspiration provides exudate for diagnostic purposes and may be lifesaving in the face of severe cardiac compression, it should not be considered final therapy. Without open drainage, tamponade will recur because with large effusions only a small reaccumulation of pericardial fluid may markedly increase intrapericardial pressure. Open pericardial drainage has significantly increased survival in patients with this disease. Rarely, with infections that are identified extremely early and with pericardial fluid that is more of a transudate than an exudate, multiple pericardial taps and antibiotic therapy have been successful; in the vast majority of cases, this approach should not be considered. The most common organisms implicated in purulent pericarditis are *Staphylococcus aureus*, *Haemophilus influenzae* type b, and *Neisseria meningitidis*. (For treatment, see Sec. 11.17, 11.20, and 11.21, respectively.) Tuberculous pericarditis rarely occurs in children outside of underdeveloped countries. Extensive treatment with antituberculous chemotherapy is required (Sec. 11.46), and late constriction may occur.

Acute Rheumatic Fever. Pericarditis occurs in acute rheumatic fever as a component of pancarditis (Sec. 10.87 and 14.75). Rheumatic pericarditis is associated with acute valvulitis, and a murmur of mitral and/or aortic regurgitation will be audible. Pericarditis and other manifestations of acute rheumatic pancarditis respond to therapy with steroids. Cardiac tamponade is extremely rare.

Rheumatoid Arthritis. Pericarditis is not an uncommon manifestation of rheumatoid arthritis in children (Sec. 10.58). Rarely, pericarditis may be the only manifestation of rheumatoid arthritis and precede the onset of arthritis by months or even years. Differentiation of rheumatoid pericarditis from that seen with other collagen vascular disease, particularly lupus erythematosus, may be difficult. Treatment consists of steroids or salicylates, which may be needed on a long-term basis to suppress the disease process.

Uremia. Uremic pericarditis only occurs in the presence of prolonged severe renal failure and results from chemical irritation of the pericardium secondary to the metabolic abnormalities. In most instances it is an incidental part of end-stage chronic renal disease. However, with the advent of chronic hemodialysis, uremic pericarditis has been recognized as a more chronic problem, culminating in cardiac tamponade. Pericardial effusion has also been implicated in the etiology of recurrent hypotension during hemodialysis. If adequate relief of uremic pericarditis does not occur with hemodialysis, pericardiectomy is recommended.

Neoplastic Disease. Neoplastic pericardial effusion is seen in patients with Hodgkin disease, lymphosarcoma, and leukemia and results from direct neoplastic invasion of the pericardium. Cardiac tamponade may occur late in the course of the illness. Rarely, pericardial infiltration is the initial manifestation of neoplastic disease, and the diagnosis can be made by examination of the pericardial fluid for neoplastic cells.

Patients with malignancy may also develop pericarditis as a result of radiation therapy to the mediastinum. This manifestation may be related to the radiation dose and to the technique utilized.

Postpericardiotomy Syndrome. Postpericardiotomy syndrome is characterized by fever, chest pain, pleural and pericardial effusion, and fluid retention (Sec. 14.69). It is seen 1–2 wk following open heart surgery in approximately 15% of postoperative patients. The syndrome is a nonspecific hypersensitivity reaction to trauma to the pericardium and epicardial surface of the heart. High titers of anti-heart antibody are reported to correlate with clinical signs of the syndrome.

In most patients, postpericardiotomy syndrome is a relatively short illness, and affected children will generally respond well to anti-inflammatory therapy with aspirin. Corticosteroids are very rarely needed. Treatment is maintained for 1–3 mo, but recurrences may be seen as long as 1 yr postoperatively and require reinstitution of therapy.

Constrictive Pericarditis. This disease represents a special problem in terms of both the clinical picture and the differential diagnosis. Predisposing pericardial diseases include purulent pericarditis, tuberculous pericarditis, acute benign or viral pericarditis, mediastinal irradiation for intrathoracic malignancy, neoplastic invasion of the pericardium, and trauma. In most instances constriction occurs months or years after the initial insult, but occasionally it may be an acute, rapidly progressive process. Constrictive pericarditis most often occurs without a preceding illness or generalized systemic disease.

The *clinical manifestations* occur as a result of impairment of diastolic ventricular filling, compromise of myocardial contractility, and resultant depression of cardiac function. Hepatomegaly and ascites may be out of proportion to the other signs and symptoms and thus suggest chronic liver disease. However, liver function studies are only mildly abnormal, and careful physical examination reveals other sometimes subtle findings of constriction including neck vein distention, narrow pulses, quiet precordium, distant heart sounds, faint pericardial friction rub, and paradoxical pulse. Typical findings become apparent gradually and thus may be easily overlooked. The auscultatory presence of an early pericardial knock and the appearance of calcification of the pericardium on chest roentgenogram are the more obvious manifestations. Protein-losing enteropathy with hypoproteinemia and lymphopenia may be seen in association with constriction.

Constrictive pericarditis may be difficult to distinguish from chronic restrictive cardiomyopathy. Impaired myocardial function occurs with both conditions. However, the myocardial disease of constrictive pericarditis is almost always reversible with pericardiectomy. At times, a definite diagnosis can be made only by exploratory thoracotomy and direct examination of the pericardium.

Radical pericardiectomy with decortication of the pericardium over a wide area of the heart, including the systemic and pulmonary veins, is the only therapy for constrictive pericarditis. In most patients surgical intervention elicits a rapid response characterized by increased cardiac output and prompt diuresis. The long-term prognosis is usually excellent.

Benzing G III, Kaplan S: Purulent pericarditis. Am J Dis Child 106:289, 1963.
Gersony WM, Hordof AH: Infective endocarditis and diseases of the pericardium. Pediatr Clin North Am 25:831, 1978.
Gersony WM, McCracken GH: Purulent pericarditis in infancy. Pediatrics 40:224, 1967.

14.83 DISEASES OF THE BLOOD VESSELS

14.84 ANEURYSMS AND FISTULAS

Aneurysms are not common in children and occur most frequently in the aorta in association with coarctation of the aorta, patent ductus arteriosus, and Marfan syndrome and in intracranial vessels (Sec. 21.25). They may also occur secondary to an infected embolus; infection contiguous to a blood vessel; trauma; congenital abnormalities of structure, especially of the medial coat; and arteritis, e.g., polyarteritis nodosa (Sec. 10.65) and Takayasu arteritis (Sec. 10.69). Aneurysm of the coronary arteries, rarely with thrombosis and myocardial infarction, may complicate the mucocutaneous lymph node syndrome (Sec. 10.67 and 14.77).

Arteriovenous fistulas may be limited to small cavernous hemangiomas or may be extensive (Sec. 21.25 and 24.7). The most common sites in infants and children are intracranial, hepatic, and pulmonary sites and the extremities. They have also been described in other parts of the body, especially in vessels in or near the thoracic wall. The fistulas, though usually congenital, may follow trauma or be a manifestation of hereditary hemorrhagic telangiectasia (Rendu-Osler-Weber syndrome).

Cardiovascular manifestations occur only in association with large communications when arterial blood flows into a low pressure venous system, increasing local venous pressure and decreasing arterial flow beyond the fistula. Systemic arterial resistance falls because of the runoff of blood through the fistula. Compensatory mechanisms include tachycardia and increased stroke volume so that cardiac output rises. Blood volume is also increased. Cardiac failure may develop with large arteriovenous fistulas.

The clinical manifestations of arteriovenous fistulas depend on the size of the shunt across the fistula. In extensive fistulas, left ventricular hypertrophy and dilatation, a widened pulse pressure, and congestive heart failure occur. Arteriograms after injection of contrast material into an artery proximal to the fistula confirm the diagnosis.

Large *intracranial arteriovenous fistulas* most often occur in the newborn infant in association with a vein of Galen malformation. The large intracranial left to right shunt results in congestive heart failure secondary to the demand for extremely high cardiac output. Patients with smaller communications may not have cardiovascular manifestations, but later develop hydrocephalus (Sec. 21.12) or seizure disorders (Sec. 21.7). The newborn infant with a large symptomatic intracranial arteriovenous fistula has a grave prognosis; some will survive with medical management but are subject to later complications due to the intracranial mass. Older patients with more diffuse intracranial arteriovenous malformations may be recognized on the basis of intracranial calcification and a high cardiac output, without frank cardiac failure.

Hepatic arteriovenous fistulas may be localized or generalized in the liver. The fistula may be located between the hepatic artery and ductus venosus or portal vein. Congenital hemorrhagic telangiectasia may also be associated. Large arteriovenous fistulas are associated with a large cardiac output and heart failure. Hepatomegaly is usual, and systolic or continuous murmurs may be audible over the liver.

Peripheral arteriovenous fistulas usually involve the extremities. These lesions are associated with disfigurement, swelling of the extremity, and visible hemangiomas. Since only a small minority result in large arterial runoff, cardiac failure is not common.

Treatment. Surgical removal of a large arteriovenous fistula is often not possible, especially in the most severe cases with large arterial runoffs, such as intracranial and hepatic types. Medical management of congestive heart failure is initially helpful in the neonate with these conditions; with time the size of the shunt may diminish and symptoms spontaneously regress. Hemangiomas of the liver often completely disappear with time. This abnormality is occasionally treated by steroid administration and/or local radiation; the beneficial effects of this management are not established but this approach may be worth a trial. Individual patients display marked variations in clinical course without treatment. Surgical removal of a large fistula may be attempted in the presence of severe cardiac failure and the lack of improvement with medical treatment. However, surgical treatment may be unsuccessful when the lesion is extensive and diffuse or is located in a position where adjoining tissue may be injured during the surgery or related procedures, e.g., extubation.

14.85 COLD INJURY

See also Neonatal Cold Injury, Sec. 8.54.

Frostbite. Frostbite may occur especially in the face or extremities from exposure to cold. Cellular injury is due to intravascular thrombosis or ice crystal formation in the tissues. The skin initially becomes red and then pale or, rarely, cyanotic as the arterioles remain in spasm in an effort to preserve body heat. During thawing, hyperemia occurs, and blisters may form on the skin. Gangrene may occur if early relief is not obtained.

Treatment consists of rapidly rewarming the skin of the affected area that is still white. Analgesics are usually necessary. Massage of the **damaged area or** rubbing with snow or ice is contraindicated. Other therapeutic measures which have yielded equivocal results include anticoagulants (especially heparin), low molecular weight dextran, and sympathectomy. Meticulous local care to the injured area is essential. Recovery of an extremity from severe frostbite can be striking and, in the absence of infection, amputation or excision of tissue should be postponed as long as possible to make certain that it is necessary.

Chilblains (Pernio). This form of cold injury, presumably vascular in origin, consists of a (sometimes blistering) localized erythema which itches, may be painful, and frequently results in swelling and in scabbing ulcerations of the affected areas. The mechanism is unknown, but it is probably related to prolonged constriction of peripheral arterioles, which is manifested by pallor and coldness of the subsequently affected areas during cold, particularly damp, weather.

The tops of the ears and tips of the fingers and toes are most frequently affected; the exposed legs of girls wearing skirts and no stockings may also be affected. Without further exposure the lesions usually clear in 1–2 wk but may persist longer.

Avoiding prolonged chilling or protecting susceptible areas with woolen caps, gloves, and stockings can be preventive. Therapeutic measures include dermal corticosteroid preparations for itching and antibiotics for infection.

14.86 EMBOLISM

Emboli, consisting of bacteria and fibrinous material, usually arise from mural thrombi or vegetations in the heart or large blood vessels, as, for example, in infective endocarditis. Within weeks after bacteriologic cure of infective endocarditis, sterile embolization to major vessels may rarely occur; this does not necessarily indicate reactivation of infection. Other rarer causes of emboli include fat (secondary to trauma) and foreign material such as air introduced accidentally into the vascular system during therapeutic procedures. Large systemic emboli are common in patients with left atrial myxomas. In patients with atrial or ventricular septal defects associated with complex heart disease, emboli arising in the systemic venous system may pass across the defect and enter the systemic arterial system (*paradoxic embolus*). In patients with cardiomyopathy, emboli may arise from thrombi in the left atrium or ventricle.

When emboli lodge in an artery, the blood flow through the vessel is compromised. If the collateral circulation is inadequate, necrosis or gangrene supervenes; if the collateral circulation is adequate, the emboli may be silent.

The manifestations of arterial emboli depend on their location: e.g., an embolus to the middle cerebral artery may result in hemiparesis; an embolus to the femoral artery may result in ischemia with or without gangrene in the leg. If the emboli are infected, an abscess may form locally.

Treatment consists of eradicating the source of the emboli, e.g., infective endocarditis, and increasing the collateral circulation to the affected area. Embolectomy, sympathectomy, or amputation may be indicated in specific instances.

Pulmonary embolism is not as frequent in children as in adults. Thrombosis of the calf veins with secondary pulmonary embolism is rare in children. Pulmonary emboli may arise secondary to infective endocarditis in patients with a left to right shunt and have also occurred in association with ventriculocardiovascular shunts for hydrocephalus. Occasionally, pulmonary embolism is seen in older children with chronic rheumatic heart disease and atrial fibrillation. Multiple small pulmonary emboli are described in Sec. 14.67.

14.87 THROMBOSIS

Arterial thrombosis in children may occur with severe polycythemia secondary to cyanotic congenital heart disease. Prevention of this complication is the major reason for venisection with volume replacement in such patients (Sec. 14.69). A frequent site for such thrombi is the brain, but they may occur anywhere in the body. They may be precipitated by dehydration.

Venous thrombosis may occur in veins used for prolonged intravenous therapy or in an area surrounding an infective process. The inflammation in the vein (*phlebitis*) is usually local; the thrombi seldom give rise to emboli.

Any severe illness associated with intense dehydration may be complicated by venous thrombosis. This complication is relatively frequent in infants with severe diarrhea or septicemia and in children with cyanotic congenital heart disease and polycythemia who become dehydrated. The common sites for thrombosis are the sagittal sinus of the brain (Sec. 21.25) and the renal vein with extension into the inferior vena cava (Sec. 17.19).

WELTON M. GERSONY

14.88 SYSTEMIC HYPERTENSION

Systemic hypertension, a sign of underlying pathophysiology, is recognized more commonly in adults (in about 15–20% of the adult population) than in children and adolescents. Untreated essential or primary hypertension increases the risk of myocardial infarction, stroke, and renal failure in affected individuals. In order to increase early detection of hypertension, blood pressure measurement should be a part of the periodic physical examination of children.

Definition. Blood pressure is a product of peripheral vascular resistance and cardiac output. Since systemic blood pressure gradually increases with age and correlates with height and weight throughout childhood and adolescence, reference standards (Figs. 14–1 and 14–2) are necessary in order to interpret values obtained during physical examinations. Measuring blood pressure in the young requires attention to cuff size and the emotional state of the patient (Sec. 14.1). The bladder of the pressure cuff should encircle the upper arm and cover at least two thirds of the length of the arm. Although the systolic pressure is indicated by the appearance of the 1st Korotkoff sound, the true diastolic pressure probably lies between the muffling and the disappearance of sound as the cuff pressure is decreased. Doppler technique may be used satisfactorily in infants and young children. Patients must be calm, seated or supine, for accurate measurements to be obtained. Repeated measurements are necessary after the patient becomes accustomed to the procedure since hypertension is never diagnosed on the basis of a single blood pressure reading. Pressure that is consistently above the 95th percentile for age is abnormal and requires further evaluation.

Etiology and Pathophysiology. An increase in cardiac output or peripheral resistance results in an increase in blood pressure. When the cause of the increase in pressure can be explained by an associated disease, the hypertension is referred to as secondary; primary or essential hypertension implies that no known underlying disease is present. However, it is recognized that many factors, such as heredity, salt intake, stress, and obesity, may play a role in the development of essential hypertension.

There is accumulating evidence that precursors of *essential hypertension,* although usually not manifest until adolescence or adulthood, are present in the young. Children with pressure above the 90th percentile for age are likely to become adults with elevated pressure. Erythrocyte sodium transport, free-calcium concentration in platelets, urine kallikrein excretion, and sympathetic nervous system activity are being evaluated as possible markers for subsequent essential hypertension. Since essential hypertension is probably not a single entity, it is likely that several pathogenic mechanisms are involved. Categorization of essential hypertension according to the level of plasma renin activity (high, normal, low) has been useful in understanding the pathophysiology and developing treatment regimens in adults; similar large studies have not been conducted in adolescents with primary hypertension. There is evidence, however, that some affected adolescents progress from a high cardiac output, normal systemic vascular resistance state to the adult pattern of normal cardiac output with elevated systemic vascular resistance. Black adults with hypertension have greater elevations in peripheral resistance, whereas hypertensive white adults show predominantly an increase in cardiac output.

Secondary hypertension is more common than essential hypertension in infants and children. Both transient and chronic hypertension may accompany diseases as listed in Tables 14–13 and 14–14. The etiology of hypertension varies with age. For example, elevated pressure in the newborn is most often associated with high umbilical artery catheterization and renal artery obstruction. Hypertension during childhood is also usually secondary, but primary hypertension occurs with increasing frequency in later childhood and adolescence. The level of blood pressure is also helpful in distinguishing secondary from primary hypertension; in general, adolescents

Table 14–13. Conditions Associated with Transient or Intermittent Hypertension in Children

Renal
Acute poststreptococcal glomerulonephritis
Anaphylactoid purpura with nephritis
Hemolytic-uremic syndrome
Acute tubular necrosis
After renal transplant (immediate and during episodes of rejection)
After blood transfusion in patients with azotemia
Hypervolemia
After surgical procedures on genitourinary tract
Pyelonephritis
Renal trauma
Leukemic infiltration of kidney

Central and Autonomic Nervous System
Increased intracranial pressure
Guillain-Barré syndrome
Burns
Familial dysautonomia
Stevens-Johnson syndrome
Porphyria

Drugs and Poisons
Oral contraceptives
Sympathomimetic agents
Amphetamines
Phenycyclidine
Cocaine
Corticosteroids and ACTH
Licorice (glycyrrhizinic acid)
Lead, mercury, cadmium, thallium
Antihypertensive withdrawal (clonidine, methyldopa, propranolol)
Vitamin D intoxication

Miscellaneous
Pre-eclampsia
Fractures of long bones
Hypercalcemia
Postcoarctation repair
White cell transfusion

Table 14–14. Conditions Associated with Chronic Hypertension in Children

Renal
Chronic pyelonephritis
Chronic glomerulonephritis (including that due to collagen vascular disease)
Hydronephrosis
Congenital dysplastic kidney
Multicystic kidney
Solitary renal cyst
Vesicoureteral reflux
Segmental hypoplasia (Ask-Upmark kidney)
Ureteral obstruction
Renal tumors
Renal trauma
Rejection damage following transplantation
Postirradiation damage

Vascular
Coarctation of thoracic or abdominal aorta
Renal artery lesions (stenosis, fibromuscular dysplasia, thrombosis, aneurysm)
Umbilical artery catheterization
Neurofibromatosis (intrinsic or extrinsic narrowing of vascular lumen)
Renal vein thrombosis
Vasculitis
Arteriovenous shunt

Endocrine
Hyperthyroidism
Hyperparathyroidism
Congenital adrenal hyperplasia (11β-hydroxylase and 17-hydroxylase defect)
Cushing syndrome
Primary aldosteronism
Dexamethasone-suppressible hyperaldosteronism
Pheochromocytoma
Other neural crest tumors (neuroblastoma, ganglioneuroblastoma, ganglioneuroma)

Central Nervous System
Intracranial mass
Hemorrhage
Residual following brain injury

Essential Hypertension
Low renin
Normal renin
High renin

with essential hypertension have diastolic pressures at or slightly above the 95th percentile for age.

Approximately 75–80% of children with secondary hypertension have a renal abnormality. Pyelonephritis occurs in 25–50% of these patients and is often related to an obstructive lesion of the urinary tract. This hypertension may be associated with sodium retention, renin secretion, or a decrease in bradykinin production. A proportion of children with pyelonephritis do not develop hypertension until they become azotemic. Other children, however, demonstrated elevated blood pressure during an episode of acute pyelonephritis; the infection may simply unmask essential hypertension.

Other renal parenchymal lesions associated with hypertension include acute and chronic glomerulonephritis, congenital lesions, tumors, and trauma. The reduced glomerular filtration rate of nephritis results in salt and water accumulation, whereas mass lesions (cysts, solid tumors, hematoma) may impair perfusion of portions of the kidney and stimulate renin production by the juxtaglomerular apparatus. There is also evidence that both Wilms tumor and juxtaglomerular cell tumor (hemangiopericytoma) secrete renin or a pressor substance without feedback control.

Renovascular lesions result in hypertension through stimulation of the renin-angiotensin-aldosterone system. Renin is a proteolytic enzyme secreted by juxtaglomerular cells that converts the alpha-2 globulin, angiotensinogen, to angiotensin I. Renin production is affected to some extent by the sympathetic nervous system, renal blood flow, prostaglandin synthesis and urine/plasma sodium concentration. Angiotensin I, a decapeptide, possesses little physiologic activity and is rapidly converted to angiotensin II by converting enzyme, which is present in high concentration in the pulmonary vascular bed. Angiotensin II is a potent vasoconstrictor and also stimulates aldosterone secretion; both effects lead to increase in blood pressure.

Although probably not the primary cause of hypertension in patients with coarctation of the aorta, activation of the renin-angiotensin system may contribute to the postoperative hypertension frequently seen in those patients. Intracranial hemorrhage may occur because of elevated pressure in the cerebral vessels and associated congenital aneurysms in the circle of Willis.

Endocrinopathies linked with hypertension involve the thyroid, parathyroid, and adrenal glands. Systolic hypertension and tachycardia are common in hyperthyroidism, but diastolic pressure is usually not elevated. Hypercalcemia, whether secondary to hyperparathyroidism or other causes, often results in mild elevation in pressure because of an increase in vascular tone. Adrenocortical disorders may produce hypertension if there is an increased mineralocorticoid effect due to increase in active precursors, aldosterone, or cortisol.

Catecholamine-secreting tumors give rise to hypertension because of the cardiac and vascular effects of epinephrine and norepinephrine. Children with pheochromocytoma usually have sustained hypertension (Sec. 19.27). The tumor may be unilateral or bilateral and may arise in the adrenal medulla or in other chromaffin cells. Approximately 5% of patients with neurofibromatosis will develop pheochromocytoma. Hypertension is much less frequent with other neural crest tumors, but may occur owing to catecholamine secretion or to interference with renal perfusion.

Excess catecholamines appear to play a role in intermittently elevating blood pressure in patients with Guillain-Barré syndrome, poliomyelitis, burns, and Stevens-Johnson syndrome. Autonomic instability is suggested by episodic increases in urinary excretion of catecholamine metabolites. Sympathetic outflow from the central nervous system is also affected by intracranial lesions.

A number of therapeutic agents, drugs of abuse, and toxins may increase blood pressure. Oral contraceptives are a common cause of hypertension in adolescent females. Although as many as 15% of patients who take oral contraceptives may develop hypertension, it is unknown whether the incidence can be reduced through the use of low-estrogen preparations. The pathogenesis of the elevated blood pressure may be due to stimulation of the renin-angiotensin system, or to a direct effect of estrogen on salt and water retention. Sympathomimetic agents used as nasal decongestants, appetite suppressants, and stimulants for attention deficit disorder produce peripheral vasoconstriction and varying degrees of cardiac stimulation. Both phencyclidine and cocaine cause a rapid rise in blood pressure that may be lethal. Licorice, not licorice flavoring, contains glycyrrhizinic acid, which acts similarly to aldosterone on the distal tubule.

Clinical Manifestations. Pre-adolescents and adolescents with primary hypertension rarely have clinical evidence of disease until the blood pressure elevation is detected, usually at the time of a routine examination or during an athletic pre-participation physical evaluation. In addition to having a mild elevation in pressure, many affected individuals are somewhat overweight. Blood pressure is often at the highest level while the patient is supine.

The pressure in children with secondary hypertension may be only a few millimeters above the 95th percentile for age or

may be markedly elevated. Unless the pressure has been sustained (diastolic > 120 mm Hg) or is rising rapidly, hypertension usually will not produce symptoms. Therefore clinical manifestations of the underlying disease, such as growth failure in children with chronic renal disease, most frequently draw attention to the blood pressure. With substantial elevation, however, headache, dizziness, changes in vision, and seizures may occur. Hypertensive encephalopathy is suggested by the presence of vomiting, temperature elevation, ataxia, stupor, and seizures. Regardless of the cause of the hypertension, cardiac and renal function deteriorate in the face of marked increases in blood pressure.

Young children and infants with unexplained heart failure or seizures should have their blood pressure measured. Such patients often cannot communicate symptoms such as headache, and their behavior may not be considered abnormal until the complications of hypertension are present. Often, in retrospect, after blood pressure has been lowered, parents of hypertensive infants will comment that their child had been increasingly irritable before the hypertension was recognized.

Specific manifestations of the diseases associated with hypertension (Tables 14–13 and 14–14) are discussed in their respective sections. Routinely measuring blood pressure in infants, children, and adolescents will result in identification of affected patients before symptoms of hypertension develop.

Diagnosis. Essential hypertension is suggested by the patient's age, level of blood pressure, obesity, and paucity of signs and symptoms of underlying disease. It is uncommon to make this diagnosis in children younger than 10 yr of age. Before a patient is diagnosed as hypertensive, several recordings of blood pressure should be obtained. If the pressure is only mildly elevated on first visit, measurement on two or three occasions over the ensuing weeks may reveal that the initial elevation was related to apprehension; such patients, however, need annual evaluation, since they may subsequently develop sustained hypertension. Excess body weight is associated with essential hypertension; except with disorders of the adrenal cortex, patients with secondary hypertension are rarely obese. Heredity is also a strong determinant of blood pressure; therefore an adolescent with mild elevation of pressure and a family history of essential hypertension rarely needs evaluation for underlying disease. Adolescents suspected of having essential hypertension require regular measurement of blood pressure to determine the course of the elevation over time. If the pressure continues to rise over several weeks or months of observation, additional diagnostic studies are indicated.

If age, level of blood pressure, or symptomatology suggests that secondary hypertension is likely, the initial focus should be the urinary tract. Screening tests should include complete blood count, urinalysis, serum electrolytes, blood urea nitrogen, serum creatinine, and uric acid. Urine culture should be obtained even if the sediment is unremarkable. Chest roentgenography and electrocardiography are helpful in assessing cardiac response to the elevated pressure.

Renal imaging is discussed in Sec. 5.55. Radionuclide scan is helpful in distinguishing variation in perfusion of the two kidneys. Renal angiography can demonstrate lesions in the main arteries or in the segmental branches; at angiography, venous blood samples should be collected from both renal veins and the inferior vena cava for assay of plasma renin activity.

Peripheral plasma renin activity is a useful screening test for both renovascular and renal parenchymal disease. Normal values gradually decrease with age and vary between laboratories. A suppressed value suggests excess mineralocorticoid effect, and an elevated value indicates renal or renovascular involvement.

Course and Prognosis. The natural history of essential hypertension that is first detected during adolescence is unknown; a large number of such patients will probably continue to have essential hypertension as adults. Collaborative studies have shown the value of drug therapy in reducing cardiovascular, renal, and central nervous system complications of uncontrolled hypertension in adults. Although similar studies are not available for children with essential hypertension, survival is probably improved in children who are adequately treated for secondary hypertension.

Prognosis for secondary hypertension, however, is primarily determined by the nature of the underlying disease and its responsiveness to specific therapy. For example, survival in patients with underlying chronic renal diseases is now greatly improved by aggressive dialysis and transplant programs. Renal vein renin activity may help predict prognosis in patients with hyperreninemic hypertension (e.g., renovascular disease). A discrepancy in renin secretion between the two kidneys of more than 1.5:1 suggests that the kidney producing the higher level is primarily responsible for the hypertension. Surgical correction of the lesion on the involved side yields a high probability of marked improvement or resolution of the hypertension.

Treatment. Both pharmacologic and nonpharmacologic methods are available for affecting elevated blood pressure. Nonpharmacologic regimens may be appropriate for managing essential hypertension, but rarely are such measures efficacious when used alone in secondary hypertension. Small reductions in blood pressure can be achieved with weight loss and restriction of salt intake. Similar changes in pressure have been noted as a result of aerobic exercise programs, relaxation training, and biofeedback. Reduction of blood pressure without the use of drugs requires a high level of motivation but also provides substantial patient satisfaction.

A large number of pharmacologic agents are available for hypertensive emergencies and for chronic therapy (Table 14–15). Rapid reduction in blood pressure is best achieved with an intravenously administered vasodilator. Such agents act quickly and do not have central nervous system side effects, which can interfere with assessment of the severely hypertensive patient. Hydralazine has had widespread use in children with moderate hypertension. Marked elevation in pressure and impending encephalopathy should be treated with intravenous diazoxide or sodium nitroprusside infusion. Such patients also benefit from the diuretic effect of intravenously administered furosemide. Several calcium channel blocking drugs, especially diltiazem and nifedipine, are being evaluated as antihypertensive agents for use in acute and chronic conditions; they act on the peripheral vasculature to reduce peripheral resistance.

An understanding of the underlying pathophysiology will help direct the choice of an agent for long-term use. Excessive activity of the renin-angiotensin-aldosterone system may be controlled by the use of a beta-blocking drug (propranolol) for suppression of renin secretion, a converting enzyme inhibitor (captopril) for inhibition of angiotensin II production, or an angiotensin II blocking agent (saralasin). Spironolactone opposes the distal tubular effect of aldosterone. Alpha blocking agents (phentolamine, phenoxybenzamine) are useful in patients with neural crest tumors and high levels of circulating catecholamines. In such patients, beta blocking drugs are also needed to control cardiac rate. Patients in whom the underlying physiology is not understood may be successfully managed with agents that affect the sympathetic nervous system through various mechanisms (reserpine, alpha methyldopa, clonidine); such patients may, however, require combination therapy.

The basic principle of combination antihypertensive therapy is the use of drugs with different sites or mechanisms of action. For example, a patient with chronic renal disease may eventually require a diuretic, a sympatholytic agent, and a vasodilator. Often a thiazide diuretic is the initial therapy, but as the disease progresses, either propranolol, methyldopa, or clonidine may be needed. For further reduction in pressure, the addition of hydralazine may be necessary. Obviously, with complex regimens compliance is a frequent problem. Drug calendars, parental supervision, and close patient-physician communication help to assure that the medications are taken.

ALBERT W. PRUITT

Berenson GS, Cresanta JL, Webber LS: High blood pressure in the young. Ann Rev Med 35:535, 1984.
Gruskin AB, Perlman SA, Baluarte HJ, et al: Primary hypertension in the adolescent: Facts and unresolved issues. *In:* Loggie JMH, Horan MJ, Gruskin AB, et al (eds): NHLBI Workshop on Juvenile Hypertension. New York, Biomedical Information Corporation, 1984, p 305.
Haber E: Renin inhibitors. N Engl J Med 311:1631, 1984.
Lauer RM, Anderson AR, Beaglehole R, et al: Factors related to tracking of blood pressure in children. Hypertension 6:307, 1984.
Oparil S, Haber E: The renin-angiotensin system. N Engl J Med 291:389, 1974.
Pruitt AW: Pharmacologic approach to the management of childhood hypertension. Pediatr Clin North Am 28:135, 1981.
Report of the Task Force on Blood Pressure Control in Children. Pediatrics 59(Suppl):797, 1977.

14.89 TUMORS OF THE HEART

Tumors of the heart are rare in infancy and childhood, and approximately three fourths of them are benign. Clinical manifestations are variable but depend primarily upon the location of the tumor, and to a lesser extent upon the histologic type.

The most common benign cardiac tumors in children are rhabdomyomas, fibromas, and myxomas. *Rhabdomyomas* usually present as multiple nodules embedded in chamber walls, producing mechanical obstruction or arrhythmias and at times resulting in fetal or neonatal death. Rhabdomyomas may be familial, and are often found in association with cerebral lesions of tuberous sclerosis and adenomas of the sebaceous glands. Incessant ventricular tachycardia in an infant less than 2 yr of age should raise suspicion of an endocardial or epicardial rhabdomyoma or Purkinje cell tumor. *Fibromas* are usually solitary encapsulated nodules, located in the ventricles, which are easily removed by surgery. *Myxomas* develop in intracavitary locations, most frequently in the left atrium.

These tumors are usually pedunculated masses that attach to the interatrial septum, protrude into the atrial chamber, and, by their position relative to the mitral valve, cause intermittent obstruction and a clinical picture consistent with mitral stenosis. A myxoma should be considered in the presence of fainting spells, a changing character to the murmur, or evidence of systemic embolization. Treatment consists of surgical excision, which must include all of the base of the tumor to prevent recurrence. Other benign tumors include *papillomas*, which are attached to valve leaflets and may present in the neonate; *lipomas*, which are situated in ventricular walls; and *mesotheliomas*, which may involve the atrioventricular node and cause abnormalities of electrical conduction, including complete heart block.

Primary malignant cardiac tumors in children are almost exclusively *sarcomas*. These tumors are usually located in the right side of the heart, in the atrial septum, right atrial wall, or root of the pulmonary artery. They may extend either into

Table 14–15. **Antihypertensive Drugs**

Drug	Mechanism of Action	Dosage Range	Route	Duration	Side Effects
Vasodilators					
Hydralazine	Relax arteriolar smooth muscle	0.4–0.8 mg/kg/dose	IV	2–4 hr	Tachycardia, nausea
		0.75 mg/kg/24 hr and increase to max 200 mg/24 hr	PO	8–12 hr	Drug induced lupus
Diazoxide	Relax smooth muscle	2–5 mg/kg/dose	IV	6–24 hr	Tachycardia, hypotension, hyperglycemia
Nitroprusside	Dilatation of arterioles and venules	0.5–8.0 μg/kg/min	IV	With infusion	Thiocyanate production, hypothyroidism
Minoxidil	Arteriolar dilatation	0.2–1.0 mg/kg/24 hr max 50 mg/24 hr	PO	12–24 hr	Hypertrichosis, pericardial effusion
Adrenergic blockade					
Phentolamine	Alpha-receptor blockade	0.1 mg/kg/dose max 5 mg	IV	1 hr	Reflex tachycardia
Phenoxybenzamine	Alpha-receptor blockade	2–5 mg/24 hr	PO	6–12 hr	Tachycardia may progress to arrhythmia
Prazosin	Alpha-receptor blockade	1 mg initial dose, may increase to 15 mg/24 hr	PO	8–12 hr	First dose orthostatic hypotension
Propranolol	Beta-receptor blockade	0.025–0.1 mg/kg/dose	IV	6–8 hr	Bronchospasm, bradycardia
		0.25–1.0 mg/kg/dose	PO		
Sympatholytic agents					
Reserpine	Depletion of catecholamines	0.02–0.07 mg/kg/dose	IM	6–8 hr	Sedation, depression, gastric bleeding, nasal congestion
Methyldopa	Decrease sympathetic tone	10 mg/kg/24 hr and increase	PO	6–8 hr	Sedation, hepatic dysfunction, positive Coombs reaction
Clonidine	Alpha-2 agonist in CNS	3–5 μg/kg/dose	PO	6–8 hr	Sedation, constipation, rebound hypertension
Renin-angiotension					
Captopril	Converting enzyme inhibition of angiotensin II synthesis	0.3 mg/kg/24 hr and increase to max 2 mg/kg/24 hr	PO	8 hr	Proteinuria, neutropenia, rash, dysgeusia
Saralasin	Angiotensin II blocker	Constant or increasing infusion rate	IV		Transient pressor response
Diuretic agents					
Hydrochlorothiazide	Diuresis	1–2 mg/kg/24 hr	PO	12–24 hr	Hypokalemia
Furosemide	Diuresis	1 mg/kg/dose	IV	4–6 hr	Hypokalemia, alkalosis
		2 mg/kg/dose	PO	4–6 hr	
Spironolactone	Aldosterone antagonist	1.5–3 mg/kg/24 hr	PO	12–24 hr	Gynecomastia, rash, menstrual irregularity

the adjacent chamber to cause obstruction to blood flow, or into the pericardial cavity to produce effusion or tamponade.

Finally, the heart may be involved in the metastatic dissemination of a noncardiac malignancy, such as leukemia or lymphoma.

A cardiac tumor should be considered in every infant or child who presents with an unexplained murmur, arrhythmia, or congestive failure, and in particular should be considered as a possible cause of persistent ventricular tachycardia in small infants. Conduction system involvement can be assessed by electrocardiography. Noninvasive evaluation has been enhanced by two-dimensional echocardiography, which may provide excellent visualization of the location and extent of the tumor. Cardiac catheterization, including pressure measurement and angiography, provides important information about the severity of intracardiac obstruction.

Surgical intervention is directed toward complete removal of the tumor, relief of obstruction, and control of arrhythmia. Long-term outcome depends upon the type of tumor, early diagnosis, and completeness of surgical removal.

THOMAS A. RIEMENSCHNEIDER

Bini RM, Westaby S, Bargeron LM Jr, et al: Investigation and management of primary cardiac tumors in infants and children. J Am Coll Cardiol 2:351, 1983.

Fine G: Primary tumors of the pericardium and heart. Cardiovasc Clin 5:208, 1973.

Garson A Jr, Gillette PC, Titus JL, et al: Surgical treatment of ventricular tachycardia in infants. N Engl J Med 310:1443, 1984.

Longino LA, Meeker IA Jr: Primary cardiac tumors in infancy. J Pediatr 43:724, 1953.

Whorton CM: Primary malignant tumors of the heart. Report of a case. Cancer 2:245, 1949.

15

DISEASES OF THE BLOOD

DEVELOPMENT OF THE HEMATOPOIETIC SYSTEM

During early evolution when the cells of the aquatic protozoan had direct access to the surrounding sea water, exchange of gas and nutrients was easily effected by simple diffusion. As multicellular and terrestrial organisms evolved, the vascular system and hemic fluid developed. Blood probably originated as a simple saline solution similar to sea water, cellular components with specialized functions coming later. Among the functions of blood cells are transport of respiratory gases, hemostasis, and phagocytosis and other defense mechanisms. Advanced organisms have separate lines of blood cells, each with specialized functions.

Blood formation in the human embryo can be recognized as early as the 3rd wk after conception. Large, primitive hematopoietic elements are then widely scattered through mesodermal tissues, intimately associated with developing vascular channels. By 2 mo active hematopoiesis is established in the liver, which is the main site of blood formation during the middle portion of fetal life. After about 6 mo hematopoiesis shifts gradually to the medullary spaces, and by birth most blood formation normally takes place in bone marrow.

Active hematopoietic tissue (red marrow) fills the medullary spaces of the bones of infants. During childhood fatty tissue (yellow marrow) gradually replaces hematopoietic tissue in the long bones, active blood formation in the older child and adult being concentrated in ribs, sternum, vertebrae, pelvis, skull, clavicles, and scapulas. The yellow marrow of the extremities can resume active hematopoiesis in response to certain severe hematologic stresses.

Study of the bone marrow provides valuable information for evaluating many hematologic diseases. *Marrow aspiration* is safe and technically simple. Although the marrow aspirate represents only a minute sample of the entire hematopoietic tissue, in most instances there is a striking uniformity of aspirates taken simultaneously from multiple sites. In the infant the preferred sites for aspiration are the proximal tibia and posterior iliac crest. In older children the posterior iliac crest provides a large marrow-bearing space that is not near major blood vessels or vital organs. *Marrow biopsy* using special instruments (e.g., the Jamshidi needle) permits more accurate assessment of marrow cellularity than is possible through simple aspiration. Biopsy is also useful for detecting focal involvement of marrow in metastatic or granulomatous processes. Table 15–1 lists the types and proportions of cells that occur in marrow of normal infants and children.

15.1 THE RED CELLS

Synthesis of red cells requires a constant supply of amino acids, iron, certain vitamins, and other trace nutrients. Production of red cells is regulated by a specific hormone—erythropoietin. The prohormone of erythropoietin is produced in the epithelial cells of the glomerular tuft; a serum factor activates it to biologically active erythropoietin. The process is stimulated by decreases in tissue oxygenation. The principal action of erythropoietin is to induce differentiation of stem cells into an erythrocytic sequence. The early erythroid-committed progenitor cells then undergo successive cellular division. Studies of bone marrow in tissue culture have added to understanding of red cell development. After culture of small mononuclear, lymphocyte-like marrow cells in semisolid media for 5–6 days, small numbers of erythropoietin-sensitive precursors form recognizable clusters of red cells called colony-forming units, erythroid (CFUe). At 12–14 days larger burst-forming erythroid units (BFUe) appear, which are believed to be the most primitive committed erythroid precursors (no longer erythropoietin sensitive). Cellular differentiation as the red cell attains maturity includes condensation and extrusion of the nucleus and production of hemoglobin. Ninety per cent of the dry weight of the mature red cell is hemoglobin.

15.2 HEMOGLOBIN

The combustion that is essential to life requires that tissues receive a constant supply of oxygen. The evolutionary development of oxygen-carrying proteins, the hemoglobins, has increased the capacity of blood to give fluid transport to this

Table 15–1. **Differential Counts of Bone Marrow During Infancy and Childhood**

Age	Blasts %	Promyelocytes %	Myelocytes and Metamyelocytes %	Bands and Polymorpho-nuclears %	Eosinophils %	Lymphocytes %	Nucleated Red Blood Cells %	Myeloid/ Erythroid (M:E) Ratio
Birth	1	2	5	40	1	10	40	1.2/1
7 days	1	2	10	40	1	20	25	2.1/1
6 mo–2 yr	0.5	0.5	8	30	1	40	20	2.0/1
6 yr	1	2	15	35	1	25	20	2.7/1
12 yr	1	2	20	40	1	15	20	3.2/1
Adult	1	2	21	44	2	10	20	3.5/1

gas. Further, the combination of oxygen with and its dissociation from hemoglobin are accomplished without expenditure of metabolic energy.

Hemoglobin is a complex protein consisting of iron-containing heme groups and the protein moiety, globin. A dynamic interaction between heme and globin gives hemoglobin its unique properties in the reversible transport of oxygen. The hemoglobin molecule is a tetramer made up of two pairs of polypeptide chains, each chain having a heme group attached. The polypeptide chains of various hemoglobins are of chemically different types. For example, the major hemoglobin of the normal adult (Hgb A) is made up of alpha (α) and beta (β) polypeptide chains, one pair of each. Hgb A can therefore be represented as $\alpha_2\beta_2$. Alpha and beta chains differ in both the number and sequence of amino acids, and their synthesis is directed by separate genes.

Within the red cells of the embryo, fetus, child, and adult, six different hemoglobins may normally be detected: the embryonic hemoglobins, Gower 1, Gower 2, and Portland; the fetal hemoglobin, Hgb F; and the adult hemoglobins, Hgb A and A_2. The electrophoretic mobilities of hemoglobins vary with their chemical structures. The compositions of the polypeptide chains of human hemoglobins are listed in Table 15–2. The time of appearance and quantitative relationships among the hemoglobins are determined by complex developmental processes. The relationships are depicted in Figure 15–1. Two sets of genes for α polypeptide chains are located on human chromosome 16. β, γ, and δ genes are closely linked on chromosome 11.

Embryonic Hemoglobins. The blood of early human embryos contains two slowly migrating hemoglobins, Gower 1 and Gower 2, and Hgb Portland, which has Hgb F–like mobility. The zeta (ζ) chains of Hgb Portland and Gower 1 are structurally quite similar to α chains. Both Gower hemoglobins contain a unique type of polypeptide chain, the epsilon (ε) chain. Hgb Gower 1 has the structure $\zeta_2\epsilon_2$ and Gower 2, $\alpha_2\epsilon_2$. Hgb Portland has the structure $\zeta_2\gamma_2$. In embryos of 4–8 wk gestation the Gower hemoglobins predominate, but by the 3rd mo they have disappeared.

Fetal Hemoglobin. Hgb F contains gamma polypeptide chains in place of the beta chains of Hgb A, and can be represented as $\alpha_2\gamma_2$. Its resistance to denaturation by strong alkali is usually used in its quantitation. After the 8th gestational wk Hgb F is the predominant hemoglobin; in the 6 mo old fetus it constitutes 90% of the total hemoglobin. Then a gradual decline occurs so that at birth Hgb F averages 70% of the total. Synthesis of Hgb F decreases rapidly postnatally, and by 6–12 mo of age only a trace is present. Less than 2.0% can be detected by alkali denaturation in older children and adults. Hgb F is heterogeneous because of two types of γ chains, whose synthesis is directed by two sets of genes. The chains differ at position #136 in the presence of either a

glycine (Gγ) or an alanine (Aγ) residue. In the newborn the relative proportion or ratio of Gγ to Aγ chain is 3:1.

Adult Hemoglobins. Some Hgb A ($\alpha_2\beta_2$) can be detected in even the smallest embryos. Accordingly, it is possible as early as 16–20 wk gestation to make a prenatal diagnosis of major β chain hemoglobinopathies, such as sickle cell anemia and thalassemia major. By the 6th mo of gestation there is about 5–10% of Hgb A present. A steady increase follows so that at term Hgb A averages 30%. By 6–12 mo of age the normal adult hemoglobin pattern appears. The minor adult hemoglobin component Hgb A_2 contains delta (δ) chains and has the structure of $\alpha_2\delta_2$. It is seen only when significant amounts of Hgb A are also present. At birth less than 1.0% of Hgb A_2 is seen, but by 12 mo of age the normal level of 2.0–3.4% is attained. Throughout life the normal ratio of Hgb A to A_2 is about 30:1.

Normal Relationships Among the Hemoglobins. During fetal life and early childhood the rates of synthesis of gamma and beta chains and the amounts of Hgb A and Hgb F are inversely related. This relationship has been attributed to a "switch mechanism" similar to genetic regulatory mechanisms in bacteria, but the genetic, biologic, and developmental processes that direct a switchover from predominantly γ-chain synthesis in utero to predominantly β-chain synthesis after birth are unclear. It is not certain whether the mechanisms involve selective genetic inhibition or facilitation. It has been shown that differential selection and amplified production of red cell precursors derived from BFUe result in considerable HbF production. This may be the basis for the increased levels of HbF that occur in many anemias when there is severe erythropoietic stress. Alternative explanations involve more basic genetic regulators in the DNA sequences that flank the hemoglobin gene complexes.

Alterations of the Hemoglobins by Disease. Since hemoglobins containing epsilon chains are normally present only very early in intrauterine life, they are largely of theoretic

Table 15–2. The Normal Human Hemoglobins

Hemoglobin Name	Formula	Comment
Gower 1	$\zeta_2\epsilon_2$	Major embryonic hemoglobins
Gower 2	$\alpha_2\epsilon_2$	Not present after 3rd mo of gestation
Portland	$\zeta_2\gamma_2$	
Fetal (γG)	$\alpha_2\gamma_2^{136\ glycine}$	Predominant hemoglobin throughout fetal life, alkali-resistant
(γA)	$\alpha_2\gamma_2^{136\ alanine}$	
A_1	$\alpha_2\beta_2$	Major adult hemoglobin
A_2	$\alpha_2\delta_2$	Detectable postnatally

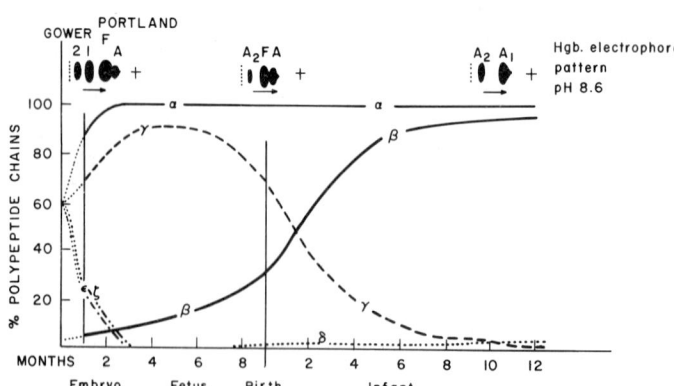

Figure 15–1. Proportions of the various human hemoglobin polypeptide chains through early life. The hemoglobin electrophoretic pattern typical for each period is also shown. (Modified from Pearson HA: J Pediatr 69:466, 1966.)

interest. Small amounts of the Gower hemoglobins have been detectable in a few newborn infants wih 13–15 trisomy. Increased levels of Hgb Portland have been found in cord blood of stillborn infants with homozygous α-thalassemia.

Levels of fetal hemoglobin may be influenced by a variety of factors. In persons heterozygous for β-thalassemia (β-thalassemia trait) the postpartum decrease of Hgb F is retarded; about 50% of such persons have elevated levels of Hgb F (more than 2.0%) in later life. In homozygous thalassemia (Cooley anemia) and in hereditary persistence of fetal hemoglobin, large amounts of Hgb F are characteristically found. In patients with major β-chain hemoglobinopathies (Hgb SS, SC, and so on) Hgb F is usually increased, particularly during childhood. Finally, moderate elevations of Hgb F may be seen in many diseases accompanied by hematologic stress, such as hemolytic anemias, leukemia, and aplastic anemia, because of a minor population of red cells that contains increased amounts of Hgb F, as can be demonstrated by the acid-elution staining technique of Kleihauer and Betke. Tetramers of γ chains (γ_4 or Hgb Bart) or β chains (β_4, Hgb H) may be seen in α-thalassemia syndromes.

The normal adult level of Hgb A_2 (2.4–3.4%) is seldom altered. Levels of Hgb A_2 exceeding 3.4% are found in most persons with the β-thalassemia trait and in those with megaloblastic anemias secondary to vitamin B_{12} and folic acid deficiency. Decreased Hgb A_2 levels are found in iron deficiency anemia and α-thalassemia.

15.3 METABOLISM OF THE RED CELL

The nucleated red cells in bone marrow participate in a variety of metabolic functions, including active protein synthesis. After extrusion of the nucleus much of this metabolic capacity is lost, including ability to synthesize proteins. Loss of the nucleus makes the red cell a better vessel for oxygen transport, but it imposes upon the red cell a finite life span, for the cell cannot replace or repair its vital enzymatic proteins. The mature red cell contains more than 40 enzymes. Many of these are essential for cellular viability, but genetically determined deficiencies of others, such as catalase, do not interfere with normal survival.

The mature red cell is not metabolically inert. It has no mitochondria, however, and ATP generation cannot occur by oxidative phosphorylation in Krebs cycle reactions. Rather, glucose is utilized and lactic acid produced mostly by anaerobic glycolysis (Embden-Meyerhof pathway); about 10% of glucose is metabolized oxidatively through the pentose phosphate pathway. At least five functions for ATP generated by glucose metabolism are essential to normal cell viability: (1) *Maintenance of electrolyte gradients.* The principal intracellular cation of the red cell is potassium, while that in plasma is sodium. Reversal of the constant tendency for sodium to enter the red cell and concomitantly for potassium to leak out, with preservation of normal ionic gradients, is accomplished by an energy (ATP)-dependent membrane mechanism, the cation pump. When the cation pump fails, sodium and water enter the red cell, causing it to swell and ultimately to hemolyze. Energy is also utilized to maintain low intracellular levels of calcium ion. (2) *Initiation of energy production.* ATP is required for the initial reaction of glycolysis involving phosphorylation of glucose to glucose-6-phosphate. (3) *Maintenance of red cell membrane and shape.* Energy is required to maintain the complex phospholipid structure of the red cell membrane. Maintenance of the biconcave shape is probably also energy-dependent. (4) *Maintenance of heme iron in the reduced (ferrous) form.* Oxidative potentials within the red cell may cause oxidation of the iron of hemoglobin. Hemoglobin containing ferric iron (methemoglobin) is ineffective in oxygen transport. Moreover, if peroxides and other oxidant substances are not inactivated, hemoglobin may be denatured and precipitated. Cells containing such denatured hemoglobin (Heinz bodies) are rapidly removed from the circulation. Protection of the red cell from the effects of oxidation ultimately depends upon NADPH and NADH. These compounds are continually regenerated by activities of the glycolytic pathway and pentose shunt. In many genetically determined deficiencies of glycolytic and pentose pathway enzymes, hemolytic states occur because the energy necessary to perform these vital functions cannot be generated. (5) *Maintenance of the levels of organic phosphates such as 2,3-diphosphoglycerate (2,3-DPG) and ATP within the red cells.* These compounds interact with hemoglobin and have profound effects upon oxygen affinity.

THE ANEMIAS

Anemia is defined as a reduction of the red cell volume or hemoglobin concentration below the range of values occurring in healthy persons. Table 15–3 lists the means and ranges for hemoglobin and hematocrit values by age groups of well nourished children. Recent extensive studies of American children suggest that there may be racial differences in hemo-globin levels. Black children have levels that average about 0.5 g/dL lower than those of white and Oriental children of comparable age and socioeconomic status, possibly in part because of the relatively high incidence of α-thalassemia and nutritional anemias in blacks.

Although reduction in amount of circulating hemoglobin

Table 15–3. **Hematologic Values During Infancy and Childhood**

	Hemoglobin g/DL		Hematocrit %		Reticulocytes %	Leukocytes WBC/mm³		Differential Counts					
								Neutrophils %		Lymphocytes %	Eosinophils %	Monocytes %	Nucleated Red Cells/ 100 WBC
Age	Mean	Range	Mean	Range	Mean	Mean	Range	Mean	Range	Mean*	Mean	Mean	
Cord blood	16.8	13.7–20.1	55	45–65	5.0	18,000	(9–30,000)	61	(40–80)	31	2	6	7.0 (3–10)
2 wk	16.5	13.0–20.0	50	42–66	1.0	12,000	(5–21,000)	40		48	3	9	0
3 mo	12.0	9.5–14.5	36	31–41	1.0	12,000	(6–18,000)	30		63	2	5	0
6 mo–6 yr	12.0	10.5–14.0	37	33–42	1.0	10,000	(6–15,000)	45		48	2	5	0
7–12 yr	13.0	11.0–16.0	38	34–40	1.0	8000	(4500–13,500)	55		38	2	5	0
Adult													
Female	14	12.0–16.0	42	37–47	1.6	7500	(5–10,000)	55	(35–70)	35	3	7	0
Male	16	14.0–18.0	47	42–52									

*Relatively wide range.

decreases the oxygen-carrying capacity of the blood, few physiologic disturbances occur until the hemoglobin level falls below 7–8 g/dL. Below this level pallor becomes evident in skin and mucous membranes. Physiologic adjustments to anemia include tachycardia, increased cardiac output, a shift in the dissociation curve, which makes oxygen more readily available to the tissues, and a deviation of blood flow toward vital organs and tissues. In response to anemia or hypoxia the concentration of 2,3-DPG increases within the red cell. The resultant "shift to the right" of the oxygen dissociation curve, by reducing the affinity of hemoglobin for oxygen, results in more complete transfer of oxygen to the tissues. The same shift may also occur at high altitude in response to a decrease in oxygen content of inspired air. When moderately severe anemia develops slowly, surprisingly few symptoms or objective findings may be evident, but weakness, tachypnea, shortness of breath on exertion, tachycardia, cardiac dilatation, and congestive heart failure ultimately result from increasingly severe anemia, regardless of its cause.

Anemia is not a specific entity but an indication of an underlying pathologic process or disease. A useful physiologic (erythrokinetic) classification of the anemias of childhood divides them into two large groups: (1) those resulting primarily from decreased production of red cells or hemoglobin, and (2) those in which increased destruction or loss of red cells is the predominant mechanism. In Table 15–4 the important anemias of childhood are classified by these criteria. In addition, a morphologic classification is often used, the red cells being characterized by their mean corpuscular volume (MCV) as microcytic (MCV <75 fL), macrocytic (MCV >100 fL), or normocytic (75–100 fL). In every case of significant anemia it is essential to describe the morphologic characteristics of the red cells, to determine the relative importance of defective red cell production and of cell destruction in the genesis of the anemia, and, when possible, to identify the basic etiologic process.

ANEMIAS RESULTING FROM INADEQUATE PRODUCTION OF RED CELLS

These anemias result when the bone marrow is unable to produce sufficient numbers of new red cells to replace those removed from the circulation. A slight reduction in the red cell life span may be present, but generally this is insufficient to cause anemia if hematopoiesis is adequate. Low reticulocyte counts are observed in most anemias of this group.

15.4 CONGENITAL PURE RED CELL ANEMIA

(Congenital Hypoplastic Anemia; Diamond-Blackfan Syndrome)

This rare condition usually becomes symptomatic in early infancy. The most characteristic diagnostic feature is a deficiency of red cell precursors in an otherwise normally cellular bone marrow.

Etiology. A genetic basis is suggested by instances of familial occurrence. Males and females are affected in equal numbers. An ill-defined abnormality of tryptophan metabolism has been reported in some patients. Adenosine deaminase (ADA) activity has been reported to be increased in the red cells of patients with this disorder but not in other types of hypoplastic anemia. A consistent finding is low numbers of CFUe and BFUe in the bone marrow. High levels of erythropoietin are present in serum and urine.

Clinical Manifestations. About half of affected infants appear pale even in the first new days of life, but hematopoiesis

must be generally adequate in fetal life. Profound anemia usually becomes evident by 2–6 mo of age, occasionally somewhat later. Unless blood transfusions are given, the anemia progresses to heart failure and death. The liver and spleen are not enlarged initially. Some cases of pure red cell anemia have been associated with congenital anomalies, including triphalangeal thumbs; others have had the Turner syndrome phenotype with normal karyotypes.

Laboratory Data. The red blood cells are normochromic and macrocytic. Assay of red cell enzymes reveals a pattern characteristic of a "young" erythrocyte population. The level of Hgb F is increased for age; in more chronic cases the fetal membrane antigen i is found on the red cells. Thrombocytosis and occasionally neutropenia may also be present initially. The most important feature is the lack of erythropoietic activity in blood and bone marrow despite high levels of erythropoietin. Reticulocytes are diminished even when the anemia is severe. Red cell precursors are markedly reduced in the marrow, and myeloid-erythroid ratios are 10–200:1. In

Table 15–4. Classification of the Anemias*

Anemias resulting primarily from inadequate production of red cells or hemoglobin
  Decreased numbers of red cell precursors in the marrow
    "Pure red cell" anemias
      Congenital pure red cell anemia
      Acquired pure red cell anemias (e.g., TEC)
  Inadequate production despite normal numbers of red cell precursors
    Anemia of infection, inflammation, and cancer
    Anemia of chronic renal disease
    Congenital dyserythropoietic anemias
  Deficiency of specific factors
    Megaloblastic anemias
      Folic acid deficiency or malabsorption
      Vitamin B_{12} deficiency, malabsorption, or transport
      Orotic aciduria
    Microcytic anemias
      Iron deficiency
      Pyridoxine-responsive and X-linked hypochromic anemias
      Lead poisoning
      Thalassemia trait
Hemolytic anemias
  Intrinsic abnormalities of the red cell
    "Structural" defects
      Hereditary spherocytosis
      Hemolytic elliptocytosis
      Paroxysmal nocturnal hemoglobinuria
      Pyropyknocytosis
    Enzymatic defects (nonspherocytic hemolytic anemias)
      Enzymes of glycolytic pathway; pyruvate kinase, hexokinase, and others
      Enzymes of the pentose phosphate pathway and glutathione complex
    Defects in synthesis of hemoglobin
      Hgbs S, C, D, E, etc., alone and in combination
      Thalassemia
  Extrinsic (extracellular) abnormalities
    Immunologic disorders
      Passively acquired antibodies (hemolytic disease of the newborn)
        Rh isoimmunization
        A or B isoimmunization
        Other blood group families
      Active antibody formation
        Idiopathic autoimmune hemolytic anemia; cold agglutinin diseases
        Symptomatic—lupus, lymphoma
        Drug-induced
    Nonimmunologic disorders
      Toxic from drugs, chemicals
      Infections—malaria, clostridium

*See also anemia in pancytopenias and leukemia.

some cases a few pronormoblasts may be present but not more mature forms. A normal complement of other marrow elements is usually present. Serum iron levels are elevated, with a decrease in the iron-binding capacity. Red cell survival is normal. Bone marrow culture shows markedly reduced numbers of CFUe and BFUe. In a few cases incubation of the marrow cells with T cell antibodies prior to culture has restored normal red cell maturation in vitro.

Differential Diagnosis. Congenital hypoplastic anemia must be differentiated from other anemias in which blood shows low reticulocyte counts. The anemia of the convalescent phase of hemolytic disease of the newborn may, on occasion, be associated with markedly reduced erythropoiesis. This terminates spontaneously at 5–8 wk of age, whereas congenital hypoplastic anemia is not usually recognized before this time. Aplastic crises characterized by reticulocytopenia and by decreased numbers of red cell precursors may complicate various types of hemolytic disease. Recent studies relate these transient episodes of "aplastic crisis" to parvovirus-like infections (Sec. 15.5).

The syndrome of transient erythroblastopenia may be differentiated from Diamond-Blackfan syndrome by its relatively late onset and by biochemical differences in the red cells (Sec. 15.6).

Prognosis. Unless corticosteroid therapy produces remission of hypoplastic anemia, survival depends upon blood transfusions. By late childhood affected children may have had 100 or more transfusions, and hemosiderosis is an inevitable consequence. The liver and spleen enlarge, and secondary hypersplenism with leukopenia and thrombocytopenia may occur. Growth retardation is usual, and puberty may not occur. Diabetes mellitus due to hemosiderosis is common.

Death usually occurs in the 2nd decade. Chronic congestive heart failure due to ischemic and siderotic myocardial disease is a common terminal event.

Treatment. When anemia becomes severe, blood transfusions must be given. Corticosteroid therapy is frequently beneficial if begun early; the mechanism of its effect is unknown. Relatively large doses, 2–4 mg/kg, of prednisone or its equivalent are administered initially. Red cell precursors appear in bone marrow 1–3 wk after therapy is begun, and then a brisk peripheral reticulocytosis occurs. The hemoglobin may reach normal levels in 4–6 wk. The dose of corticosteroid may then be reduced gradually until the lowest effective dose is found. This is often a very small amount, such as 2.5 mg/24 hr of prednisone or less, which may produce no adverse side effects or growth suppression. Intermittent administration every other day or for 3–4 consecutive days each week may also be effective. Therapy should be discontinued periodically to determine whether the child is still dependent upon steroids, since many responsive cases ultimately outgrow the dependence on steroid therapy.

About 10–15% of patients do not respond to corticosteroid therapy, and transfusions at intervals of 4–8 wk are necessary to sustain life. Other therapies, including hematinics, cobalt, and testosterone, have had no beneficial effect. Reports of late responses to immunosuppressive therapy need further evaluation before this can be recommended, but this might be considered in refractory cases with abnormal T-cell function. Splenectomy is usually of no value but may decrease the need for transfusion if hypersplenism or isoimmunization has developed. Since spontaneous remission occasionally occurs, children refractory to corticosteroid therapy should be maintained as long as possible by transfusions, preferably of freshly drawn, packed red cells. The use of chelating agents to induce excretion of excess iron is discussed with thalassemia major (Sec. 15.25). The role of bone marrow transplantation is undefined at the present time.

15.5 ACQUIRED PURE RED CELL ANEMIAS

A number of forms of acquired anemia with reticulocytopenia and reduced red cell precursors in the marrow have been described. The causes of most of them are uncertain. In some cases in adults remission has followed removal of a tumor of the thymus. Association with thymoma has been reported in a child. In other cases an erythropoietin-inhibiting antibody, antibodies to erythroblasts, or inhibitors of heme synthesis have been found in plasma. The presence of a complement-dependent antibody cytotoxic for erythroblasts in some adults has suggested their need for immunosuppressive therapy. The acquired pure red cell anemias may respond to therapy with corticosteroids, and a trial is indicated in any chronic case. Immunosuppressive therapy with cyclophosphamide or azathioprine may be given a trial if corticosteroids are ineffective.

Large doses of chloramphenicol inhibit erythropoiesis. Reticulocytopenia, erythroid hypoplasia, and vacuolated pronormoblasts in the marrow are reversible effects of this drug (Sec. 15.32).

Episodes of acute failure of erythropoiesis may follow a variety of viral infections. During these episodes a marked reduction in circulating reticulocytes ($<0.1\%$) and an elevation of the serum iron level occur. Bone marrow aspiration shows markedly reduced numbers of erythrocytic precursors. These episodes are self limited, last only 10–14 days, and are of no consequence to a child with a normal red cell survival. In a patient with a shortened red cell survival, however, profound anemia may ensue; this is the basis of the so-called *aplastic crises* of some hemolytic anemias (Sec. 15.12).

15.6 TRANSIENT ERYTHROBLASTOPENIA OF CHILDHOOD (TEC)

This increasingly recognized syndrome of severe aregenerative anemia involves previously normal children, 6 mo–5 yr of age, who slowly develop anemia with reticulocytopenia and decreased numbers of red cell precursors in the bone marrow. Serum iron and iron saturation are increased. The level of Hgb F is normal, and the profile of red cell enzymes is consistent with an "old" red cell population. MCV is normal. Activity of red cell adenosine deaminase is normal. Marrow culture studies suggest varying pathogenetic mechanisms: in some cases, a serum inhibitor of erythroid stem cells; in others, abnormalities of erythroid stem cells either in number or in responsiveness to erythropoietin. It is likely that this is an autoimmune disease directed at the primitive red cell precursors rather than at the mature red cell. Spontaneous remission occurs; corticosteroid therapy is not necessary or indicated. Transfusions may be necessary until recovery occurs.

15.7 ANEMIAS OF CHRONIC INFECTION, INFLAMMATION, AND RENAL DISEASE

Anemia complicates a number of chronic systemic diseases associated with infection, inflammation, or tissue breakdown. Examples of such conditions include chronic pyogenic infections such as bronchiectasis and osteomyelitis; chronic inflammatory processes such as rheumatic fever, rheumatoid arthritis, and ulcerative colitis; and advanced renal disease. Despite diverse underlying causes the erythrokinetic abnormalities are similar. Red cell life span is moderately decreased, reflecting increased red cell destruction by a hyperactive reticuloendothelial system. This increased hemolysis is less important, however, than a relative failure of bone marrow response, reflecting both hypoactivity of marrow and an erythropoietin production inadequate for the degree of anemia. Further, there are abnormalities of iron metabolism, including defective iron release from the tissues into the plasma. In renal failure accumulation of toxic nondialyzable substances in the blood can directly inhibit erythropoiesis.

Clinical Manifestations. Few symptoms are attributable to the usually moderate degree of anemia present; the important symptoms and signs are those of the underlying disease.

Laboratory Data. Hemoglobin concentrations usually range from 6–9 g/dL. The anemia is usually normochromic and normocytic; occasionally, modest hypochromia and microcytosis are observed. Reticulocyte counts are normal or low, and leukocytosis is common. Free erythrocyte protoporphyrin (FEP) levels are moderately elevated (>35 μg/dL whole blood). Serum iron is low, averaging 30 μg/dL; there is, however, no increase in total iron-binding capacity as in iron deficiency (average 200 μg/mL). This pattern of serum iron and iron-binding protein is a regular and valuable diagnostic feature. Serum ferritin is often elevated. The bone marrow has normal cellularity; the red cell precursors are adequate, and granulocytic hyperplasia may be present. Increased hemosiderin can often be seen in marrow. A frequent clinical challenge is to identify iron deficiency in the patient with an inflammatory disease. Such patients may have normal levels of serum ferritin, which are inappropriately low in the presence of an inflammatory process. A trial of iron therapy may be needed to resolve the issue.

Treatment and Prognosis. Since these anemias are secondary to other disease processes, they do not respond to iron or hematinics unless there is concomitant deficiency. Transfusions raise the hemoglobin concentration only temporarily and are rarely indicated. If the underlying systemic disease can be controlled, the anemia is spontaneously corrected.

15.8 CONGENITAL DYSERYTHROPOIETIC ANEMIAS

These rare normocytic or macrocytic anemias display multinuclearity and abnormal chromatin patterns in red cell precursors. Four types have been distinguished, with considerable variation within each type and overlap among them. Type I (about 15% of cases) is defined by binuclearity of erythroblasts and megaloblastic morphology. Type II (more than 60% of cases) has erythroblastic multinuclearity and a positive acidified serum (Ham) test, but only with some normal serum added. Red cells in Type II are strongly agglutinated by anti-i antibody. Types I and II appear to be inherited as autosomal recessive traits. Type III (about 15% of cases) has pronounced multinuclearity and huge red cell precursors in marrow. It appears to be inherited as an autosomal dominant trait. Type IV is rare; it resembles Type II morphologically but does not have associated serologic abnormalities. In all types there are variable degrees of anemia (sometimes only in adults), ineffective erythropoiesis, and abnormal utilization of iron. Findings of chronic hemolysis, such as intermittent jaundice, gallstones, and splenomegaly, are common. There is no treatment other than blood transfusion for anemia. Splenectomy has been advocated for patients with anemia severe enough to require chronic transfusions.

15.9 PHYSIOLOGIC ANEMIA OF INFANCY

The normal newborn has higher hemoglobin and hematocrit levels than older children and adults. Within the 1st wk of life a progressive decline in hemoglobin level begins, which persists for approximately 6–8 wk. This decline is generally referred to as a physiologic anemia of infancy. The term is a misnomer, for at its nadir the hemoglobin level in the full-term infant rarely falls below 9 g/dL.

Several factors are operative. First, there is abrupt cessation of erythropoiesis with onset of respiration when arterial oxygen saturation rises from 45 toward 95%. Concomitantly, the high fetal levels of erythropoietin drop to undetectable levels. A shortened survival of the fetal red cell also contributes to the development of physiologic anemia. Further, the sizable expansion of blood volume that accompanies rapid weight gain during the first 3 mo of life creates a situation which has aptly been described as "bleeding into the circulation." When the hemoglobin level has fallen to 9–11 g/dL at 2–3 mo of age, erythropoiesis resumes. This "anemia" should be viewed as a physiologic adaptation to extrauterine life.

The premature infant also develops a physiologic anemia; the same factors are operative as in term infants, but they are exaggerated. The decline in hemoglobin level is both more extreme and more rapid. Minimal hemoglobin levels of 7–9 g/dL commonly occur by 3–6 wk of age, and, in very small premature infants, levels may be even lower.

The difference between term and premature infants is not due to their relative abilities to secrete erythropoietin but may rather be due to lower respiratory quotients and metabolic rates in premature infants. Further, when premature infants are transfused with adult blood containing Hgb A, the shift of the oxygen dissociation curve due to Hgb A facilitates delivery of oxygen to the tissues. Accordingly, the definition of anemia and the need for transfusion in the premature infant must be based not only upon hemoglobin level but also upon oxygen requirements and the affinity of the infant's circulating hemoglobin for oxygen.

The marginal erythropoietic equilibrium responsible for physiologic anemia can aggravate processes associated with increased hemolysis such as congenital hemolytic states which may be associated with severe anemia in the early wk of life.

Dietary factors may also aggravate physiologic anemia. Deficiencies of folic acid or vitamin E superimposed upon the physiologic process may result in more severe anemia.

In premature infants vitamin E has an important role in red cell stability. Such infants are born with a small reserve of vitamin E and frequently become deficient, with serum vitamin E levels falling to less than 0.5 mg/L during the first months of life. If the diet contains a high proportion of polyunsaturated fatty acids (as in many proprietary formulas), and especially if an iron supplement is given, hemolytic anemia, thrombocytosis, and edema may occur. Red cells include many bizarre acanthocytes (burr cells). Vitamin E prophylaxis, 5 mg/24 hr, should be considered for the small premature infant, with therapeutic doses (50 mg) indicated for established deficiency. The composition of most proprietary formulas is such that hemolysis does not occur even when iron supplementation at a concentration of 10–12 mg/qt is used. Larger doses of medicinal iron are not indicated in the newborn; they may not only provoke hemolysis but also predispose to serious infections, particularly if parenteral iron preparations are used. In patients with malabsorption of fat, vitamin E deficiency may lead to significant hemolytic anemia, as occurs in cystic fibrosis.

Infantile pyknocytosis, a self-limited hemolytic process with large numbers of acanthocytes in blood, probably represents vitamin E deficiency.

Unless there has been significant perinatal blood loss, iron deficiency should not be considered as a cause of anemia in the first 3 mo of life.

Treatment. As a developmental process, physiologic anemia usually requires no therapy other than seeing that the diet of the infant contains the essential nutrients for normal hematopoiesis, especially folic acid and vitamin E. A premature infant who is feeding well and growing normally rarely needs transfusion. Occasionally, very low hemoglobin levels (<7 g/dL) or complicating medical conditions requiring frequent blood samples for testing may necessitate small transfusions of packed red blood cells. If so, only enough blood should be given to raise the hemoglobin level to about 9 g/dL. Larger transfusions may delay spontaneous recovery by suppressing normal erythropoiesis. Neither iron nor any other hematinic substance has any effect upon physiologic anemia.

15.10 MEGALOBLASTIC ANEMIAS

The megaloblastic anemias all have in common certain diagnostic abnormalities of red cell morphology and maturation. The red cells at every stage of development are larger than normal and have a peculiar open, finely dispersed arrangement of nuclear chromatin and an asynchrony between the maturation of nucleus and cytoplasm. Megaloblastic tissues have an increased amount of RNA in proportion to DNA. Megaloblastic morphology may be seen in a number of conditions; almost all instances in children result from a deficiency of folic acid, of vitamin B_{12}, or of both. Both substances are cofactors required in synthesis of nucleoproteins. Megaloblastic anemias are uncommon in the United States.

Folic Acid Deficiencies

Megaloblastic Anemia of Infancy. This disease is caused by a deficient intake or absorption of folic acid. Dietary deficiency is usually compounded by rapid growth or infection, which may increase folic acid requirements. The normal daily requirement is small, estimated at 20–50 µg/24 hr. Human and cow milks provide adequate amounts of folic acid. Goat milk is clearly deficient; folic acid supplementation must be given when it is the main food. Unless supplemented, powdered milk may also be a poor source of folic acid. Ascorbic acid deficiency probably impairs the availability of dietary folic acid conjugates.

CLINICAL MANIFESTATIONS. Mild megaloblastic anemia has been reported in very low birth weight infants and routine folic acid supplementation advised. Megaloblastic anemia has its peak incidence at 4–7 mo of age, somewhat earlier than iron deficiency anemia. Besides having the usual features of severe anemia, affected infants are irritable, fail to gain weight adequately, and have chronic diarrhea. Thrombocytopenic hemorrhages occur in advanced cases. Concomitant signs and symptoms of scurvy may be present. Folic acid deficiency may accompany kwashiorkor or marasmus.

LABORATORY DATA. The anemia is progressive. The red blood cell count is disproportionately lower than the hematocrit; accordingly, the anemia is macrocytic (MCV >100 fL). Variations in red cell shape and size are common (Fig. 15–2B). The reticulocyte count is low, but nucleated red cells demonstrating megaloblastic morphology are often seen in the blood. Neutropenia and thrombocytopenia may be present. The neutrophils are large, with hypersegmented nuclei; more than 5% of neutrophils will have five or more nuclear segments. Normal serum folic acid levels are 5–20 ng/mL; deficiency is accompanied by levels of less than 3 ng/mL. Levels of red cell folate are a better indicator of chronic deficiency. The normal red cell folate level is 150–600 ng/mL of packed cells. Levels of iron and vitamin B_{12} in serum are normal or elevated. Formiminoglutamic acid is excreted in the urine, especially after an oral dose of histidine. Serum activity of lactic acid dehydrogenase (LDH) is markedly elevated. The bone marrow is hypercellular because of erythroid hyperplasia. Megaloblastic changes are prominent, though some normal red cell precursors may also be found. Large, abnormal neutrophilic forms (giant metamyelocytes) with cytoplasmic vacuolization are seen as well as hypersegmentation of the nuclei of megakaryocytes.

TREATMENT. Initially, folic acid may be administered parenterally in a dose of 2–5 mg/24 hr. Since a hematologic response can be expected within 72 hr, transfusions are indicated only when the anemia is severe or the child is very ill. Folic acid therapy should be continued for 3–4 wk. Satisfactory responses have been obtained with doses of folic acid as low as 50 µg/24 hr. These "physiologic" doses have no effect on primary vitamin B_{12} deficiencies; a therapeutic test using such low amounts may be used, therefore, to differentiate between primary folic acid and vitamin B_{12} deficiencies. If juvenile pernicious anemia may be present or if the anemia recurs after therapy, the prolonged use of folic acid should be avoided, since in pernicious anemia folic acid may produce a partial response of anemia without benefiting the neurologic abnormalities. If signs of scurvy are present, therapeutic doses of ascorbic acid should be given. Antibiotic therapy should be used for superimposed bacterial infection.

Megaloblastic Anemia of Pregnancy. Folate requirements increase markedly during pregnancy, in part to meet fetal needs. Decreases in serum and red cell folate levels occur in as many as 25% of pregnant women at term and may be aggravated by infection. Folate supplementation, 1 mg/day, is often advocated, particularly during the last trimester.

Folic Acid Deficiency of Malabsorption Syndromes. Folic acid is absorbed throughout the small intestine, and diffuse inflammatory or degenerative disease of the intestine may reduce intestinal polyglutamate deconjugase activity as well as markedly impair absorption. Celiac disease, chronic infectious enteritis, and enteroenteric fistulas may lead to folic acid deficiency and megaloblastic anemia. Measurement of serum folate is widely used to assess small intestinal absorptive functions in malabsorptive disorders. Oral folic acid supplements of 1 mg/day may be indicated in these states. (See also Chapter 12.)

Congenital Defect of Folic Acid Absorption. A specific congenital defect in the intestinal absorption of folic acid and an associated inability to transfer folate from the plasma to the central nervous system have been associated with megaloblastic anemia, convulsions, mental retardation, and cerebral calcifications. Treatment with oral folic acid, 15–50 mg/24 hr, was necessary to maintain normal hematologic values.

Folic Acid Deficiency Complicating Hemolytic Anemias. It is possible that chronic hemolytic processes may increase the requirement for folic acid, probably more often in adults than in children. Frank megaloblastic erythropoiesis may lead to more severe anemia and increased need for transfusion. The bone marrow should be examined for megaloblastic changes if there is an unexplained worsening of chronic anemia or increased transfusion requirements in chronic hemolytic states. Continuous folic acid supplementation is not ordinarily necessary for such patients if their diets are normal, at least during childhood.

Folic Acid Deficiency Associated with Anticonvulsants and Other Drugs. Many patients have low serum levels of folic acid during therapy with certain anticonvulsant drugs (e.g., phenytoin, primidone, or phenobarbital), but they usually have no anemia or symptoms. Frank megaloblastic anemia is rare and responds to folic aid therapy even if administration of the offending drug is continued. Malabsorption of folic acid induced by anticonvulsant drugs is the probable mechanism; displacement by the drug of folate from its serum carrier has also been suggested. Megaloblastic anemia, probably due to folic acid malabsorption, has been seen in users of oral contraceptives.

A number of drugs have antifolic acid activity as their primary pharmacologic effect and will regularly produce megaloblastic anemia. Methotrexate and aminopterin prevent the utilization of folic acid by inhibiting its enzymatic reduction to active coenzymatic forms. Pyrimethamine (Daraprim),

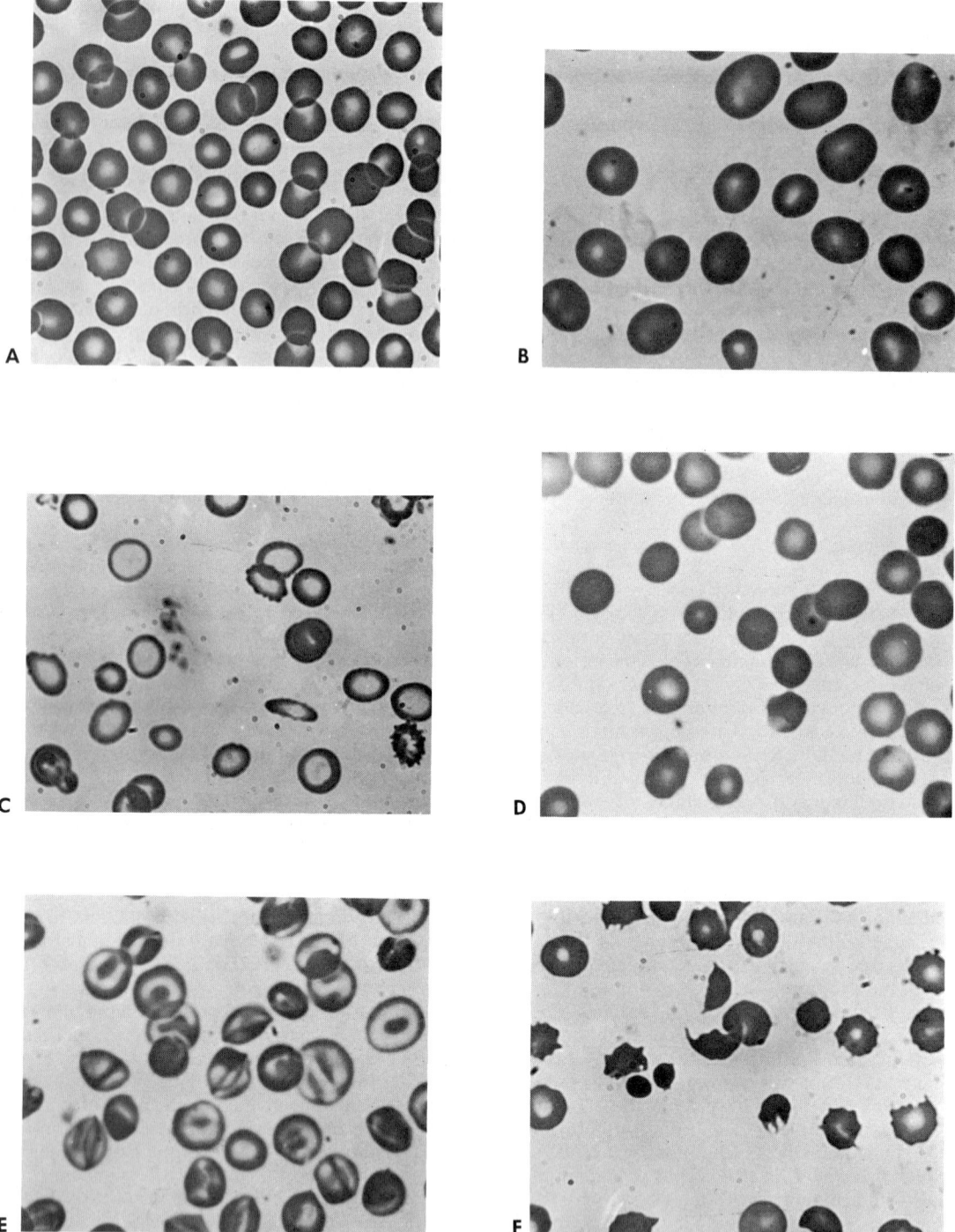

Figure 15–2. Morphologic abnormalities of the red cell. *A,* Normal. *B,* Macrocytes (folic acid deficiency). *C,* Hypochromic microcytes (iron deficiency). *D,* Spherocytes (hereditary spherocytosis). *E,* Target cells (Hgb CC disease). *F,* Schizocytes (hemolytic-uremic syndrome).

which is used in the therapy of toxoplasmosis, may induce folic acid deficiency and megaloblastic anemia. Trimethoprim-sulfamethoxazole, which is also being increasingly used for the treatment of urinary infections and pneumonia due to *Pneumocystis carinii,* also may cause megaloblastic anemia.

Congenital Dihydrofolate Reductase Deficiency. This has been reported in several patients who were unable to form biologically active tetrahydrofolate and developed severe megaloblastic anemia in early infancy. These patients were successfully treated with large doses of folic acid or tetrahydrofolic acid.

Deficiency of methylene tetrahydrofolate reductase has been described in some patients with homocystinuria who had no hematologic abnormalities.

Vitamin B$_{12}$ Deficiencies

In order to be absorbed, dietary vitamin B$_{12}$ must combine with a glycoprotein (intrinsic factor) secreted by the parietal cells of the gastric fundus. The B$_{12}$–intrinsic factor complex passes to the terminal ileum, where specific absorptive sites exist. In the presence of intrinsic factor and ionic calcium, vitamin B_{12} traverses the intestinal mucosa and enters the blood. Vitamin B_{12} deficiency may therefore result from: (1) inadequate intake, (2) lack of secretion of intrinsic factor by the stomach, (3) consumption or inhibition of the B_{12}–intrinsic factor complex, or (4) abnormalities involving the receptor sites in the terminal ileum.

Because vitamin B_{12} is present in many foods, dietary deficiency is rare. It may be seen in extreme dietary restriction ("vegans") in which no milk, eggs, or animal products are consumed. B_{12} deficiency is not commonly seen in kwashiorkor or infantile marasmus. Instances have been reported in breast-fed infants whose mothers had deficient diets or pernicious anemia. Since vitamin B_{12} is so ubiquitous, most cases of deficiency stem from failure to absorb the vitamin.

Juvenile Pernicious Anemia (Congenital Pernicious Anemia). This rare disease is due to inability to secrete gastric intrinsic factor. It differs from the typical disease in adults in that the stomach secretes acid normally and is histologically normal. Consanguinity is common in parents of affected children and suggests mendelian recessive inheritance.

CLINICAL MANIFESTATIONS. The symptoms of juvenile pernicious anemia become prominent at 9 mo–10 yr of age. This interval is consistent with exhaustion of the stores of vitamin B_{12} acquired in utero. As the anemia becomes severe, irritability, anorexia, and listlessness occur. The tongue is smooth, red, and painful. Neurologic manifestations include ataxia, paresthesias, hyporeflexia, Babinski responses, clonus, and coma.

LABORATORY DATA. The anemia is macrocytic, with prominent macro-ovalocytosis of the red cells. The neutrophils are large and hypersegmented. In advanced cases neutropenia and thrombocytopenia are seen. Serum vitamin B_{12} levels are below 100 pg/mL. Concentrations of serum iron and serum folic acid are normal or elevated. Serum LDH activity is markedly increased, primarily because of the first and second heat-stable isoenzymes. Moderate elevations (2–3 mg/dL) of serum bilirubin may be seen. Serum iron levels are elevated. Excessive excretion of methylmalonic acid in the urine is a reliable and sensitive index of vitamin B_{12} deficiency. In contrast to many adult cases, serum antibodies directed against parietal cells or intrinsic factor cannot be detected in children. Gastric acidity may be reduced initially but returns to normal when vitamin B_{12} therapy is instituted. Biopsy reveals a normal gastric mucosa, but intrinsic factor activity is absent in gastric secretion.

Absorption of vitamin B_{12} is usually assessed by the Schilling test. When a normal person ingests a small amount of vitamin B_{12} into which ^{57}Co or ^{60}Co has been incorporated, the radioactive vitamin combines with the intrinsic factor in the stomach secretions and passes to the terminal ileum, where absorption occurs. Since the absorbed vitamin is bound to blood proteins and tissues, none is normally excreted in the urine. If a large (1000 µg) dose of *nonradioactive* vitamin B_{12} is then injected parenterally ("flushing dose"), from 10–30% of the previously absorbed radioactive vitamin will appear in the urine. Patients with pernicious anemia excrete 2% or less under these conditions. That malabsorption of vitamin B_{12} is due to lack of intrinsic factor can be confirmed through a modification of the standard Schilling test: 30 mg of intrinsic factor is administered along with the radioactive vitamin. If absence of intrinsic factor is the basis of the B_{12} malabsorption, normal amounts of radioactive vitamin should now be absorbed and flushed out. On the other hand, when vitamin B_{12} malabsorption is due to disease of ileal receptor sites or other intestinal causes, no improvement in absorption will be seen with intrinsic factor. The Schilling test result will remain abnormal in pernicious anemia even when therapy has completely reversed hematologic and neurologic manifestations of the disease.

TREATMENT. A prompt hematologic response follows parenteral administration of vitamin B_{12}. The physiologic requirement for vitamin B_{12} is 1–5 µg/24 hr, and hematologic responses have been observed with these small doses. If there is evidence of neurologic involvement, 1 mg should be injected intramuscularly daily for at least 2 wk. Maintenance therapy will be necessary throughout the patient's life; monthly intramuscular administration of 1 mg of vitamin B_{12} is sufficient. Attempts at oral therapy are contraindicated.

Transcobalamin Deficiency. The two major vitamin B_{12} binding proteins in the plasma are transcobalamins I and II. Transcobalamin II is the principal transport vehicle for vitamin B_{12}; a congenital deficiency is inherited as an autosomal recessive condition, with failure to absorb and transport vitamin B_{12}. Severe megaloblastic anemia occurs in early infancy; therapy requires massive parenteral doses of vitamin B_{12}.

Vitamin B_{12} Deficiency in Older children. In some cases of vitamin B_{12} malabsorption in late childhood atrophy of the gastric mucosa and achlorhydria have been seen; in others the stomach is normal. Malabsorption of vitamin B_{12} may also occur in combination with a familial syndrome of cutaneous candidosis, hypoparathyroidism, and other endocrine deficiencies; the serum contains antibodies against intrinsic factor and parietal cells; an abnormal Schilling test result is corrected by addition of exogenous intrinsic factor. Vitamin B_{12} should be administered parenterally regularly to these patients to prevent the development of megaloblastic anemia. A case of megaloblastic anemia with a structurally abnormal intrinsic factor has been reported.

Vitamin B_{12} Malabsorption Due to Intestinal Causes. A few cases have been reported of familial occurrence of a specific intestinal defect in the absorption of vitamin B_{12}, in some instances associated with proteinuria (Imerslund syndrome); histology of the stomach is normal, and intrinsic factor and acid are present in gastric secretions.

Surgical resection of the terminal ileum or such inflammatory diseases as regional enteritis or tuberculosis may also impair absorption of vitamin B_{12}. When the terminal ileum has been removed, lifelong parenteral administration should be considered if the Schilling test indicates that vitamin B_{12} is not absorbed. An overgrowth of intestinal bacteria within diverticula or duplications of the small intestine may cause vitamin B_{12} deficiency by consumption of or competition for the vitamin or by splitting of its complex with intrinsic factor. In these cases hematologic response may follow broad spectrum antibiotic therapy. Similar mechanisms may operate when the fish tapeworm *Diphyllobothrium latum* infests the upper small intestine. When megaloblastic anemia occurs in these situations, the serum vitamin B_{12} level is low, the gastric juice contains intrinsic factor, and the abnormal Schilling test result is not corrected by addition of exogenous intrinsic factor.

Rare Megaloblastic Anemias

Orotic aciduria is a genetically determined defect in pyrimidine biosynthesis associated with a severe megaloblastic anemia, neutropenia, and crystalluria due to excretion of orotic acid. Physical and mental retardation may be frequently present. The anemia is refractory to vitamin B_{12} or folic acid, but responds promptly to administration of the nucleic acid precursor, uridine, or yeast. The basic defect appears to be a deficiency of orotate phosphoribosyl transferase and orotidine-5-phosphate decarboxylase, which involves many tissues. Inheritance is autosomal recessive. Megaloblastic anemia can also occur in the Lesch-Nyhan syndrome, in which regeneration of purine nucleotides is blocked.

Two instances of thiamine responsive and thiamine dependent megaloblastic anemia have been reported. Administration of thiamine, 100 mg/24 hr, produced a brisk reticulocyte response and a sustained increase in hemoglobin level. Sensorineural deafness and diabetes mellitus were associated. The pathogenesis of this disorder is unclear.

MICROCYTIC ANEMIAS

15.11 IRON DEFICIENCY ANEMIA

Anemia due to lack of sufficient iron for synthesis of hemoglobin is by far the most common hematologic disease of infancy and childhood. Its frequency is related to certain basic aspects of iron metabolism and nutrition. The body of the newborn infant contains about 0.5 g of iron, whereas adult content is estimated at 5.0 g. In order to make up this 4.5 g discrepancy, an average of 0.8 mg of iron must be absorbed each day during the 1st 15 yr of life. In addition to this growth requirement a small amount is necessary to balance normal losses through excretion of iron. Accordingly, to maintain positive iron balance in childhood, 0.8–1.5 mg of iron must be absorbed each day. Since less than 10% of dietary iron is absorbed, a diet containing 8–15 mg of iron is necessary for optimal nutrition. Absorption of iron from human milk is much more efficient than from cow milk; breast-fed infants may, therefore, require less from other foods. During the 1st years of life, because relatively small quantities of iron-rich foods are taken, it is often difficult to attain these amounts. For this reason the diet should include such foods as infant cereals or cow milk formulas that have been fortified with iron. At best, the infant is in a precarious situation with respect to iron. Should the diet become inadequate or external blood loss occur, anemia ensues rapidly.

Etiology. Most of the iron of the newborn is contained in the circulating hemoglobin. Low birth weight and significant perinatal hemorrhage are associated with decreases in neonatal hemoglobin mass and stores of iron. As the high hemoglobin concentration of the newborn falls during the first 2–3 mo of life, considerable iron is reclaimed and stored (Sec. 15.9). These reclaimed stores are usually sufficient for blood formation for the first 6–9 mo of life; transplacental iron stores are exhausted by the time the birth weight approximately triples. In low birth weight infants or with perinatal blood loss, stored iron may be depleted earlier, and dietary sources become of paramount importance. Anemia due solely to inadequate dietary iron is unusual during the first 4–6 mo, but becomes common from 9–24 mo of age. Thereafter, it is relatively infrequent. The usual dietary pattern observed in infants with iron deficiency anemia is the consumption of large amounts of milk and of carbohydrates unsupplemented with iron.

Blood loss must be considered a possible cause in every case of iron deficiency anemia, particularly in the older child. Chronic iron deficiency anemia from occult bleeding may be due to a lesion of the gastrointestinal tract, such as peptic ulcer, Meckel diverticulum, polyp, or hemangioma. In some geographic areas hookworm infestation is an important cause.

As many as one third of infants with severe iron deficiency in the United States have chronic intestinal blood loss induced by exposure to a heat labile protein in whole cow milk (Wilson, Lahey, and Heiner); loss of 1–7 mL of blood in the stools each day can be shown not to be influenced by iron replacement or transfusion but to be prevented either by reducing the quantity of whole cow milk to 1 pint/day or less or by using heated or evaporated milk or a milk substitute. This gastrointestinal reaction is not related to enzymatic abnormalities in the mucosa, such as lactase deficiency, or to typical "milk allergy." Characteristically, involved infants develop

anemia that is more severe and occurs earlier than would be expected simply from inadequate intake of iron.

Histologic abnormalities of the mucosa of the gastrointestinal tract are present in advanced iron deficiency anemia. The morphologic changes may be a direct manifestation of tissue deficiency of iron.

Clinical Manifestations. Pallor is the most important clue to iron deficiency. In mild to moderate iron deficiency (hemoglobin levels of 6–10 g/dL) compensatory mechanisms, including increased levels of 2,3-DPG and a shift of the oxygen dissociation curve, may be so effective that few symptoms of anemia are noted. When the hemoglobin level falls below 5.0 g/dL, irritability and anorexia are prominent. Tachycardia and cardiac dilatation occur, and systolic murmurs are often present.

The spleen is palpably enlarged in 10–15% of cases, and in longstanding cases widening of the diploë of the skull similar to that seen in congenital hemolytic anemias may occur. These changes resolve slowly with adequate replacement therapy. The child with iron deficiency anemia may be obese, or underweight with other evidences of undernutrition. Pica is sometimes prominent. The irritability and anorexia characteristic of advanced cases may reflect deficiency in tissue iron, for with iron therapy striking improvement in behavior frequently occurs before significant hematologic improvement.

Monoamine oxidase (MAO), an iron-dependent enzyme, plays a crucial role in neurochemical reactions in the central nervous system. MAO can also be measured in platelets. Iron deficiency produces decreases in the activities of enzymes such as catalase and cytochromes. Catalase and peroxidase contain iron, but their biologic essentiality is not well established. It is not possible to measure easily and accurately in vivo the iron in the enzymatic compartment, and yet this is perhaps the most vital area of iron metabolism. In the past the intracellular enzyme iron component was held to be tenaciously maintained even in the face of marked depletion in the other iron compartments, including in severe anemia, but this view is being questioned.

Iron deficiency may also have effects on neurologic and intellectual function. A number of reports suggest that iron deficiency anemia and even iron deficiency without significant anemia affect attention span, alertness, and learning of both infants and adolescents.

Laboratory Data. In progressive iron deficiency a sequence of biochemical and hematologic events occurs (Table 15–5). First, the tissue iron stores represented by liver and bone marrow hemosiderin disappear. It is possible to measure in the serum small amounts of ferritin, the iron-storage protein of the tissues. The level of serum ferritin provides a relatively accurate estimate of body iron stores. During infancy and childhood the mean level of serum ferritin is 35 ng/mL. Levels less than 10 ng/mL accompany iron deficiency. Next, there is a decrease in serum iron to less than 30 μg/dL, the iron-

Table 15–5. Sequence of Changes in Iron Deficiency Anemia

1. Decrease in iron stores; decrease in hemosiderin content of liver and bone marrow
2. Decrease in levels of serum ferritin to less than 10 ng/mL
3. Decrease in level of serum iron; increase in total iron-binding capacity; fall in per cent of saturation to less than 15%
4. Increase in levels of free erythrocyte protoporphyrins (FEP)
5. Anemia; progressive hypochromia and microcytosis
6. Decrease in activity of intracellular enzymes containing iron*

*Depletion of the enzyme compartment of iron is listed as the final stage of iron deficiency, but certain iron-containing enzymes may be significantly and functionally decreased even when the degree of anemia is relatively mild.

Table 15–6. Mean Corpuscular Volume in Children

Age	MCV (fL) Mean (Range)
Birth	119 (110–128)
6–24 mo	77 (70–85)
2–6 yr	81 (75–90)
6–12 yr	85 (78–95)
Adult	90 (80–100)

After Koerper MA, Mentzer WC, Brecher G, et al: J Pediatr 89:580, 1976.

binding capacity of the serum increases to more than 350 μg/dL, and the per cent saturation falls below 15%. At a level of transferrin saturation of 10–15%, availability of iron becomes rate limiting for hemoglobin synthesis, and a moderate accumulation of the heme precursors called free erythrocyte protoporphyrins (FEP) results. Normal FEP levels are 1.9 ± 0.4 μg/g Hgb (<35 μg/dL whole blood); a characteristic level in iron deficiency is 10.9 ± 6.2 μg/g Hgb (>50 μg/dL whole blood).

As the deficiency progresses, the red cells become smaller than normal and their hemoglobin content decreases. The morphologic characteristics of red cells are best quantified by determination of mean corpuscular volume (MCV) and mean corpuscular hemoglobin (MCH). Developmental changes in MCV require utilization of age-related standards for diagnosis of microcytosis (see Table 15–6). With increasing severity the red cells become deformed and misshapen and present characteristic microcytosis, hypochromia, and poikilocytosis (Fig. 15–2C), without which a diagnosis of significant iron deficiency anemia is untenable. The reticulocyte count is normal or minimally elevated; nucleated red cells may occasionally be seen in the peripheral blood. White blood cell counts are normal. Thrombocytosis, sometimes of a striking degree (600,000–1,000,000/mm³) may occur, or, in a few cases, significant thrombocytopenia. The mechanisms of these platelet abnormalities is not clear; they appear to be a direct consequence of iron deficiency, and they return to normal with iron therapy. The bone marrow is hypercellular with erythroid hyperplasia. The normoblasts have scanty, fragmented cytoplasm with poor hemoglobinization. Leukocytes and megakaryocytes are normal. Hemosiderin cannot be demonstrated in marrow specimens by the Prussian blue staining techniques. In about a third of cases occult blood can be detected in the stools.

Differential Diagnosis. Iron deficiency must be differentiated from other hypochromic microcytic anemias. In lead poisoning the red cells are morphologically similar, but coarse basophilic stippling of the red cells is prominent. Very marked elevations of blood lead, free erythrocyte protoporphyrins, and urinary coproporphyrins are seen. Many cases of lead poisoning have concomitant iron deficiency. The blood changes of the β-thalassemia trait resemble those of iron deficiency, but characteristic elevations in the levels of Hgb A₂ and Hgb F are usually present, which do not occur in iron deficiency. Alpha-thalassemia trait occurs in about 3% of blacks and in many Southeast Asian peoples. The diagnosis requires complicated tests after the newborn period; the diagnosis can be assumed when a case of familial hypochromic microcytic anemia with normal levels of Hgb A₂ is refractory to iron therapy. In the newborn period infants with α-thalassemia trait have 3–5% Bart hemoglobin (Sec. 15.2). Thalassemia major with its pronounced erythroblastosis and hemolytic component should present no diagnostic confusion. The red cell morphology of chronic inflammation and infection, though usually normochromic, may be microcytic, but in these conditions both serum iron and iron-binding capacity are reduced, and serum ferritin levels are normal or elevated.

Treatment. The regular response of iron deficiency anemia to adequate amounts of iron is an important diagnostic as well as therapeutic feature. Oral administration of simple ferrous salts (sulfate, gluconate, fumarate) provides inexpensive and satisfactory therapy. There is no evidence that addition of any trace metal, vitamin, or other hematinic substance significantly increases the response to simple ferrous salts. On the other hand, absorption of some iron chelates may be suboptimal. For routine clinical use the physican should familiarize himself with an inexpensive preparation of one of the simple ferrous compounds. The therapeutic dose should be calculated in terms of elemental iron; ferrous sulfate is 20% and ferrous gluconate is 10–12% elemental iron by weight. A daily total of 6 mg/kg of elemental iron in three divided doses provides an optimal amount of iron for the stimulated bone marrow to utilize. Doses of elemental iron in excess of 6 mg/kg/24 hr do not result in a more rapid hematologic response. Better absorption may result when medicinal iron is given between meals. Ingestion of large amounts of milk may significantly decrease absorption of iron. Intolerance to oral iron is extremely rare; malasorption of oral iron is more frequently suspected than proved. A parenteral iron preparation (iron-dextran) is an effective, form of iron, safe when given in a properly calculated dose, but the response to parenteral iron is no more rapid or complete than that obtained with proper oral administration of iron; in most cases the indication for parenteral iron therapy is a social one (to ensure compliance).

While adequate iron medication is given, the family must be educated about the patient's diet, and the consumption of milk should be limited to a reasonable quantity, preferably to 500 mL (1 pt)/day or less. This reduction has a dual effect: the amount of iron-rich foods in the diet is increased, and gastrointestinal blood loss from intolerance to cow's milk proteins is prevented. When the re-education of child and parent is not successful, parenteral iron medication may be indicated. Iron deficiency can be prevented in high risk populations by providing iron-fortified formula or cereals during infancy.

The expected clinical and hematologic responses to iron therapy are described in Table 15–7.

Within 72–96 hr after administration of iron to the anemic child peripheral reticulocytosis is seen. The height of this response is inversely proportional to the severity of the anemia. Reticulocytosis is followed by a rise in the hemoglobin level, which may increase as much as 0.5 g/dL/24 hr. Iron medication should be continued for 4–6 wk after blood values are normal. Failures of iron therapy occur when the child does not receive the prescribed medication, when it is given in a form that is poorly absorbed, or when there is continuing unrecognized blood loss. An incorrect original diagnosis of iron deficiency anemia may be revealed by therapeutic failure of iron medication.

Since a rapid hematologic response can be confidently predicted in typical iron deficiency, blood transfusion is indicated only when the anemia is very severe or when superimposed infection may interfere with the response. It is not

Table 15–7. Responses to Iron Therapy in Iron Deficiency Anemia

12–24 hr:	Replacement of intracellular iron enzymes; subjective improvement; decreased irritability; increased appetite
36–48 hr:	Initial bone marrow response; erythroid hyperplasia
48–72 hr:	Reticulocytosis, peaking at 5–7 days
4–30 days:	Increase in hemoglobin level
1–3 mo:	Repletion of stores

necessary to attempt rapid correction of severe anemia by transfusion and may be dangerous because of associated hypervolemia and cardiac dilatation. Packed or sedimented red cells, which are relatively fresh or preserved in CPD anticoagulant to assure normal oxygen-hemoglobin affinity, should be administered slowly in an amount sufficient to raise the hemoglobin to a safe level at which the response to iron therapy can be awaited. In general, severely anemic children with hemoglobins under 4 g/dL should be given only 2–3 mL/kg of packed cells at any one time. If there is evidence of frank congestive heart failure, a modified exchange transfusion employing fresh packed red cells should be considered. Furosemide may also be administered. Digitalis is usually unnecessary.

Sideroblastic Anemias

The sideroblastic anemias are a heterogeneous group of hypochromic microcytic anemias whose basic defects may be abnormalities of iron or heme metabolism. Serum iron levels are increased. In the bone marrow ringed sideroblasts are found; these are nucleated red cells with a perinuclear collar of coarse hemosiderin granules that represent iron-laden mitochondria.

A form of sideroblastic anemia transmitted as an X-linked recessive trait becomes symptomatic by late childhood. Splenomegaly is usually present. FEP levels are not elevated. In some cases an enzymatic deficiency of ALA synthetase has been postulated. A syndrome of refractory sideroblastic anemia with vacuolization of marrow precursor cells and exocrine pancreatic dysfunction has been reported. Acquired sideroblastic anemias occur in adults with a variety of inflammatory and malignant processes or with alcoholism.

Some cases of sideroblastic anemia are partially responsive to pyridoxine (vitamin B_6) given in doses of 200–500 mg/24 hr, though abnormalities of tryptophan metabolism may not occur and other findings of B_6 deficiency are not observed.

Lead Poisoning

See also Chapter 28.

Lead interferes with iron utilization and hemoglobin synthesis so that a hypochromic microcytic anemia is a prominent finding in chronic lead poisoning. The red cells are hypochromic and microcytic, with coarse basophilic stippling. Examination of the red cells with the ultraviolet microscope reveals intense fluorescence due to markedly increased levels of red cell porphyrins. Blood levels of FEP in excess of 150 μg/dL of blood, and urinary excretion of large amounts of coproporphyrins are regularly seen in chronic lead poisoning.

Rare Types of Hypochromic Microcytic Anemia

Isolated cases are known of hypochromic microcytic anemia with other abnormalities of iron metabolism; some cases have had defects in iron mobilization or reutilization. Congenital absence of the iron-binding protein (atransferrinemia) is associated with severe hypochromic anemia requiring life-long transfusions. Iron is absorbed normally and is deposited in the visceral organs rather than in bone marrow.

Several patients have had refractory hypochromic anemia associated with lymphatic tumors or lymphoid hyperplasia. Correction of the anemia followed removal of the abnormal lymphatic tissue in these cases.

See also Thalassemia, Sec. 15.23.

15.12 HEMOLYTIC ANEMIAS

The fundamental basis of the hemolytic anemias is a shortened survivial time of the red blood cells. Red blood cells normally spend 100–120 days in the circulation; about 1% of red cells (senescent ones) are removed from the blood each day and are replaced by an equal number of new cells released from the bone marrow.

In response to a shortened survival of red cells, the activity of bone marrow increases, and the reticulocyte count exceeds 2%. Sustained reticulocytosis in conjunction with an unchanging hemoglobin level is presumptive evidence of a hemolytic disorder. Hyperplasia of the erythropoietic marrow elements occurs, with lowering or reversal of the myeloid-erythroid ratio from the normal ranges of 2:1 to 4:1. In the chronic hemolytic processes of childhood, hypertrophy of the marrow may expand the medullary spaces, producing striking roentgenographic changes, particularly in the skull, metacarpals, and phalanges.

Elevations of unconjugated (indirect) bilirubin may accompany many hemolytic states, but overt jaundice is unusual if hepatic function is not impaired. Accelerated destruction of red cells increases the biliary excretion of heme pigments, which can be quantitated by measurement of fecal urobilinogen. Pigmented gallstones composed of calcium bilirubinate may be formed as early as the 4th yr of life. A chronic hemolytic process should be considered possible in any case of pigmentary cholelithiasis in childhood, but only about 15% of cases of gallstones in children are a consequence of hemolytic anemia. Plasma concentrations of hemoglobin increase in hemolytic anemias, and the free hemoglobin combines irreversibly with specific binding proteins (haptoglobins). The large haptoglobin-hemoglobin complex is cleared from the circulation by reticuloendo-

thelial activity. Normal levels of serum haptoglobin are 20–200 mg/dL. In severe hemolytic states the loss of haptoglobin exceeds the synthetic capacity of the liver, and serum haptoglobin is decreased or absent. The level of hemopexin, another plasma protein that binds hemoglobin, is also reduced in hemolytic states. Catabolism of hemoglobin results in formation of carbon monoxide, and quantitation of CO in blood or expired air can provide a dynamic indicator of hemolysis. The assay is difficult, however, and not often used.

Besides these indirect indicators of hemolysis, isotopic techniques can estimate red cell survival directly. Sodium chromate ($Na_2{}^{51}CrO_4$) and diisofluorophosphate ($DF^{32}P$) are the radioactive compounds most often used as red cell "tags." After injection of ^{51}Cr-tagged red cells, blood radioactivity normally decreases to 50% of its initial level in 25–35 days (^{51}Cr T½ or half-life). A shortened red cell survival is likely when the ^{51}Cr T½ is reduced below 20 days. $DF^{32}P$ is expensive and more difficult to count but permits an actual measurement of red cell survival. In practice it is rarely necessary to use these techniques.

The stimulated normal bone marrow can ordinarily increase its output 6–8-fold; accordingly, red cell survival can theoretically be reduced to 15–20 days without producing anemia, but in childhood chronic hemolysis usually results in some degree of anemia. Patients with hemolytic anemias of whatever type may have transient episodes of bone marrow failure. These aplastic crises are characterized by reticulocytopenia and markedly decreased numbers of red cell precursors in the marrow. Occasionally, huge abnormal erythroid precursors ("gigantoblasts") are seen. Profound and life-threatening anemia may develop quickly because the shortened red cell survival is no longer even partially compensated. These episodes of acute marrow failure are self-limited and last 10–14 days. Aplastic crises appear to be associated usually with parvovirus infection and may occur within a few days in several affected members of a family. They constitute a potentially serious, life-threatening complication of any chronic hemolytic process.

The hemolytic anemias may be generally divided into two large classes: (1) those with premature destruction due to intrinsic abnormalities of the red cell, and (2) those due to noxious extraerythrocytic factors. Table 15–4 lists the important hemolytic anemias of childhood. In hemolytic states associated with intrinsic defects red cell survival is short in normal persons receiving transfusions of the patient's red cells as well as in patients themselves. In contrast, red cells from patients with anemias due to extrinsic factors survive normally in healthy recipients.

HEMOLYTIC ANEMIAS DUE TO INTRINSIC ABNORMALITIES OF THE RED CELL

15.13 HEREDITARY SPHEROCYTOSIS

(Congenital Hemolytic Anemia; Congenital Acholuric Jaundice)

This is the most common of the hereditary hemolytic states in which there is no abnormality of hemoglobin. The classic features are a congenital and familial hemolytic process associated with splenomegaly and with red cells that are spherical in shape. Cases have been reported in most ethnic groups, but the disease is most common among persons of northern European origin.

Etiology. Hereditary spherocytosis is transmitted as an autosomal dominant trait; about 25% of cases are sporadic and presumably represent new mutations. The basic defect is thought to be an abnormality of the spectrin of the red cell membrane. Affected cells are unduly permeable to sodium and acquire the characteristic spherocytic shape because of loss of membrane function and increases in volume. An increased intracellular concentration of sodium is believed to lead to an increased utilization of ATP to drive the "cation pump." Premature senescence and destruction are thought to result from metabolic overwork and loss of red cell membrane.

The spleen is intimately involved in the hemolytic process. The splenic circulation imposes a metabolic environment that is stressful to spherocytic cells, and repeated passages through this unfavorable environment result in their sequestration and destruction. The spherocyte is relatively rigid and passes with difficulty through the minute apertures between the splenic cords and sinuses. The hemolytic process abates after splenectomy, though the biochemical and morphologic abnormalities persist.

Clinical Manifestations. The disease has its onset in infancy and may present in the neonatal period with anemia and hyperbilirubinemia severe enough to require phototherapy or exchange transfusions. The anemia varies considerably in severity during infancy and childhood but tends to be similar within families. Some patients with relatively severe anemia during the first 6–8 mo of life show more satisfactory compensation thereafter. Slight jaundice is usually present. Moderate expansion of the marrow cavity of the skull may occur, but to a lesser extent than in thalassemia or other hemoglobinopathies. After infancy the spleen is almost always palpably enlarged. Pigmentary gallstones have been reported as early as 4–5 yr of age, but they usually do not develop until late childhood or adolescence. Approximately 50% of unsplenectomized patients will ultimately form gallstones. Aplastic

crises associated with parvovirus infections are the most serious complications during childhood.

Laboratory Data. Evidences of hemolysis include reticulocytosis, anemia, and hyperbilirubinemia. The hemoglobin level usually ranges from 6–10 g/dL and the reticulocyte count from 5–20%, averaging 10%. The characteristic spherocytic red cell is smaller than the normal erythrocyte and lacks the central pallor of the biconcave disk (Fig. 15–2D). This morphologic change may be subtle, and only a relatively small proportion of the cells may be spherocytic. There is erythroid hyperplasia in marrow, but the red cell precursors are not spherocytic. There are no abnormal hemoglobins.

The abnormality of the red cell membrane can be demonstrated by osmotic fragility studies. When red cells are placed in hypotonic saline solutions, water and sodium enter the cells, causing them to swell. The normal red cell of biconcave shape can increase its volume, but the spherical cell already has the maximal volume for its surface area. Imbibition of small amounts of water causes the spherocyte to rupture. In 10–20% of cases of hereditary spherocytosis the abnormality may be demonstrated only if the blood is incubated at 37° C for 24 hr before determining osmotic fragility. The autohemolysis test is also useful. When normal blood is incubated under sterile conditions for 48 hr at 37° C, fewer than 5% of the red cells hemolyze. Red cells of patients with hereditary spherocytosis have markedly increased rates of autohemolysis (15–45%). Abnormal autohemolysis can be corrected by the addition of small amounts of glucose to the blood before incubation.

Differential Diagnosis. Hereditary spherocytosis must be differentiated from other congenital hemolytic states. The family history, blood smear, and studies of osmotic fragility and autohemolysis are of most diagnostic value. Acquired spherocytosis of the red cells is seen in autoimmune hemolytic anemias; here the spherocytosis is more noticeable than in hereditary spherocytosis, and the Coombs test result is usually positive. It may be difficult to differentiate hereditary spherocytosis in the newborn infant from hemolytic disease due to A or B incompatibility when an appropriate blood group incompatibility is coincidentally present. A period of observation may be necessary to clarify the diagnosis. Acquired spherocytosis may follow thermal injury to red cells during extensive burns.

Treatment. Splenectomy invariably produces a clinical cure. Splenectomy should be deferred whenever possible until the patient is 5–6 yr of age or older. If anemia is severe enough to impair growth or if aplastic crises are frequent, the operation may be considered earlier; an extended period of observation will be indicated before splenectomy can be justified in infancy. Splenectomy prevents gallstones and eliminates the threat of aplastic crises. Hemochromatosis and hepatic failure have occurred in adults with hereditary spherocytosis who have not had splenectomy. After splenectomy, jaundice and reticulocytosis rapidly disappear, and the hemoglobin level attains the normal range, though the spherocytosis and osmotic fragility become more pronounced. Thrombocytosis may occur in the immediate postoperative period, but anticoagulation therapy is not routinely indicated. Overwhelming sepsis after splenectomy is not a frequent threat to older patients, but after splenectomy the febrile child should be carefully evaluated and therapy initiated on the presumption of life-threatening infection. Polyvalent pneumococcal vaccine should be given prior to splenectomy. Prophylactic penicillin therapy afterward is advocated by many authorities (Sec. 15.59).

15.14 HEREDITARY ELLIPTOCYTOSIS

Oval or elliptical shape of red cells occurs as a benign, dominantly inherited morphologic curiosity in about 1 in 2000

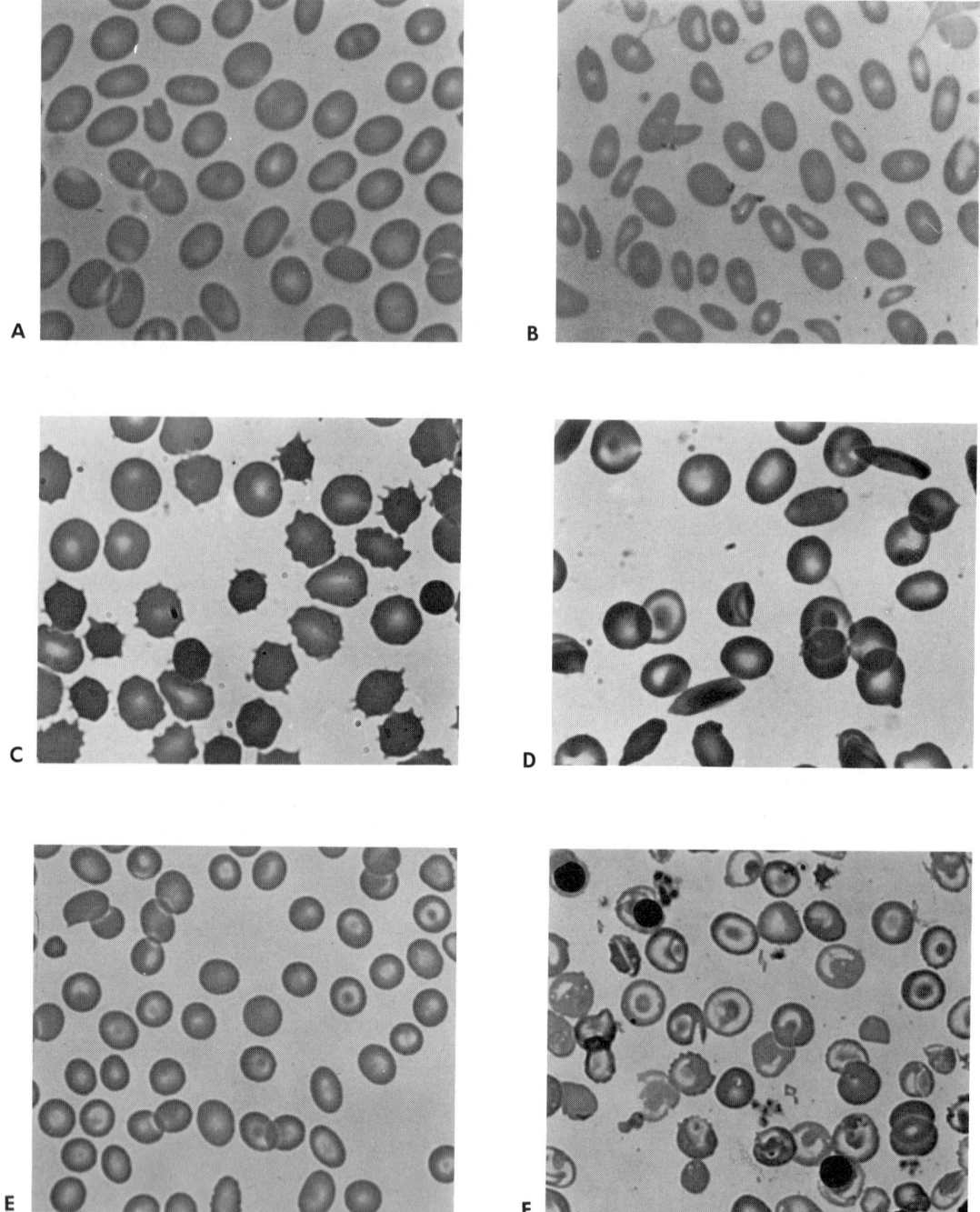

Figure 15–3. Morphologic abnormalities of the red cell. *A*, Elliptocytes (hereditary ellipcytosis). *B*, Bizarre elliptocytes (hemolytic elliptocytosis). *C*, Acanthocytes (abetalipoproteinemia). *D*, Sickle cells (Hgb SS disease). *E*, Thalassemia trait. *F*, Thalassemia major.

persons (Fig. 15–3*A*). Elliptocytes may be seen in other conditions, such as thalassemia and iron deficiency anemia, but in these they are far fewer in number than in hereditary elliptocytosis. Hemolysis is usually mild or absent, but about 10% of patients have a significant hemolytic anemia.

Etiology. Family studies of affected children usually reveal one parent with elliptocytosis without hemolysis, while the other parent is normal. A few cases may have represented homozygous inheritance. The gene for elliptocytosis is sometimes linked with the Rh locus. No biochemical abnormality of the red cell has been defined; a primary membrane abnormality involving spectrin is postulated. Recent reports suggest a relationship between hemolytic elliptocytosis and some cases of pyropoikilocytosis.

Clinical Manifestations. Hemolytic elliptocytosis may produce neonatal jaundice even though characteristic elliptocytosis may not be evident at that time; the blood of the affected newborn may show bizarre poikilocytes and pyknocytes. The usual features of a chronic hemolytic process are seen later as anemia, jaundice, splenomegaly, and osseous changes. Cholelithiasis may occur in later childhood, and aplastic crises have been reported.

Laboratory Data. The morphology of the red blood cells is the most important diagnostic feature (Fig. 15–3*B*). Elliptical cells are prominent, but in cases with overt hemolysis many bizarre poikilocytes, microcytes, and spherocytes are also present. The reticulocyte count is increased. Erythroid hyperplasia is present in the bone marrow, but red cell precursors are not elliptical. There is no abnormal hemoglobin. The genes for abnormal hemoglobin, thalassemia, or G-6-PD deficiency do not interact with the gene for elliptocytosis to produce more severe disease.

Treatment. Splenectomy decreases the hemolytic component of this disease, although some degree of hemolysis may continue. It should be considered if there is significant chronic hemolysis. The red cell morphology is not corrected by the operation, and may become more abnormal after splenectomy.

15.15 OTHER STRUCTURAL DEFECTS

Paroxysmal Nocturnal Hemoglobinuria. Paroxysmal nocturnal hemoglobinuria is a rare chronic anemia with prominent intravascular hemolysis. The hemolysis is characteristically worse during sleep, and nocturnal and morning hemoglobinuria is a classic finding. The disease is not congenital; it results from an ill-defined acquired dysplastic defect of the red cell membrane that renders it susceptible to hemolysis by serum complement. In addition to chronic hemolysis, there may be thrombocytopenia and/or leukopenia. Pyogenic infection, thrombosis, and thromboembolic phenomena are serious complications. Abdominal, back, and head pain may be prominent complaints. Some cases have been associated with hypoplastic or aplastic pancytopenia. The diagnosis of either disorder may precede the other. The diagnosis is established by a positive result in the acid serum (Ham) or thrombin tests. The sucrose lysis test is also useful. Markedly reduced levels of red cell acetylcholinesterase activity are found. Splenectomy is not indicated. Prolonged anticoagulation therapy may be of benefit when thromboses occur. Since there is chronic loss of iron in the urine, iron therapy may be necessary. Bone marrow transplantation has been successful in some cases.

Hereditary Stomatocytosis. Hereditary stomatocytosis is a rare condition in which the red cells are swollen and cup shaped; on stained smears they present a mouthlike slit in place of the usual circular area of central pallor. There may be hemolytic anemia. Extreme permeability of the red cell membrane to cations has been observed. Splenectomy is not consistently effective but may be indicated in patients with severe hemolysis. Acquired stomatocytosis may be seen in several conditions, especially liver disease.

Acanthocytosis. This rare defect of lipid metabolism is characterized by malabsorption, neuromuscular abnormalities, and retinitis pigmentosa. The distorted red cells have sharp projections (Fig. 15–3C), but there is usually no significant hemolytic anemia. The morphologic changes presumably result from decreased levels of cholesterol and betalipoprotein in the serum. (See Abetalipoproteinemia in Sec. 7.48, 12.49, and 21.20.)

Pyropoikilocytosis. This rare, recessively transmitted, hemolytic anemia is characterized by bizarre fragmented and poikilocytic red cells and spherocytes that have reduced thermal stability. Osmotic fragility is abnormal. In some families there may be an association between pyropoikilocytosis and elliptocytosis. Splenectomy may be helpful; the morphologic abnormalities are more pronounced after the operation.

HEMOLYTIC ANEMIAS DUE TO ENZYMATIC DEFECTS OF THE RED CELLS

Within a group of diseases known collectively as congenital nonspherocytic hemolytic anemias because they lack spherocytosis and have normal osmotic fragility, the quantitation of various red cell enzymes has permitted the identification of a number of specific entities. Abnormal enzymes have been found in the major pathways of glucose catabolism, the anaerobic Embden-Meyerhof pathway and the oxidative pentose phosphate shunt. Disorders involving G-6-PD affect more than 100 million people throughout the world; patients with pyruvate kinase deficiency probably number in the thousands; all of the other reported red cell enzyme deficiencies probably affect only a few hundred individuals.

Biochemical criteria suggested for diagnosis of these diseases include demonstration of a markedly reduced level of enzyme activity in the patient's red cells by specific assay. In addition, there should be increases in glycolytic intermediates that precede the enzyme block and reduced levels of substances dependent upon the enzyme for formation. Assays for G-6-PD and pyruvate kinase are widely available; some research laboratories are able to quantitate all glycolytic enzymes and intermediate compounds.

15.16 PYRUVATE KINASE DEFICIENCY

A congenital hemolytic anemia occurs in persons homozygous for an autosomal recessive gene that causes either a marked reduction in red cell content of pyruvate kinase or production of an abnormal enzyme with decreased activity. Generation of ATP within the red cell is impaired, and low levels of ATP, pyruvate, and NAD are seen. Concentrations of 2,3-DPG are increased. As a consequence of decreased ATP, potassium leaks from the red cell at a markedly increased rate and the cell's life span is considerably reduced.

Clinical Manifestations and Laboratory Data. The clinical manifestations vary from a severe, congenital hemolytic process to a mild, well-compensated one noted first in adulthood. Jaundice and anemia may occur in the neonatal period, and kernicterus has been reported. The later severity of the hemolytic component varies from patient to patient, but pallor, jaundice, and splenomegaly are usually present. A severe form of the disease has a relatively high frequency among the Amish of the midwestern United States.

Macrocytosis and polychromatophilia reflect the elevated reticulocyte count. Spherocytes are uncommon, but a few spiculated pyknocytes are usually present. Nonincubated osmotic fragility is normal. Autohemolysis is moderately or markedly increased, but addition of glucose does not regularly correct the abnormality as it does in hereditary spherocytosis.

Diagnosis rests upon demonstration of marked reductions of pyruvate kinase (PK) activity in the red cells. Other red cell enzyme activities are normal or elevated. There are no abnormalities of hemoglobin. The white blood cells have normal PK activity and must be excluded from hemolysates used to measure PK activity. Heterozygous carriers usually have moderately reduced levels of PK activity.

Treatment. Exchange transfusions may be indicated for hyperbilirubinemia in the newborn. Transfusions of packed red cells are necessary for severe anemia or for aplastic crises. If the anemia is consistently severe or if frequent transfusions are required, splenectomy should be performed after 5–6 yr of age. Although not curative, the operation may be followed by higher hemoglobin levels and by strikingly high (30–60%) reticulocyte counts. Deaths due to overwhelming pneumococcal sepsis have followed splenectomy (Sec. 15.59).

DEFICIENCIES OF OTHER GLYCOLYTIC ENZYMES

Congenital nonspherocytic anemias may stem from defects in hexokinase, glucose phosphate isomerase, phosphofructo-kinase, glyceraldehyde 3-phosphate dehydrogenase, triose phosphate isomerase, aldolase, and 2,3-diphosphoglycerate kinase and mutase; these defects are transmitted as autosomal recessive traits. Phosphoglycerate kinase deficiency due to an X-linked defect has been reported in a mentally retarded boy. In homozygous triose phosphate isomerase deficiency, progressive neurologic dysfunction, mental retardation, and cardiac abnormalities occur in infants who live to more than a few months of age.

In these conditions the red cell morphology is not strikingly abnormal except for polychromasia and macrocytosis. Non-incubated osmotic fragility is normal. Splenectomy has been of variable benefit and is indicated when the hemolytic process is severe.

In addition to these glycolytic enzymopathies, rare cases of hemolytic anemia due to pyrimidine-5′ nucleotidase or ATPase have been reported as well as deficiencies of other red cell enzymes (lactic hydrogenase, methemoglobin reductase, catalase, and others) without hemolysis.

DEFICIENCIES OF ENZYMES OF THE PENTOSE PHOSPHATE PATHWAY AND RELATED COMPOUNDS

The most important function of the pentose pathway, through which about 10% of the glucose utilized by the red cell passes, is to provide the NADPH or reduced triphospho-pyridine nucleotide (TPNH) necessary for conversion of oxidized to reduced glutathione. This is essential for the physiologic inactivation of oxidant compounds, such as hydrogen peroxide, that accumulate within the red cell. If glutathione or any of the compounds or enzymes necessary for maintaining it in the reduced state are decreased, hemoglobin may become denatured and precipitated into red cell inclusions called *Heinz bodies*. Once Heinz bodies have formed, the red cell is rapidly removed from the circulation; an acute hemolytic process may result from damage to the red cell membrane by the precipitated hemoglobin and the action of the spleen.

15.17 GLUCOSE-6-PHOSPHATE DEHYDROGENASE (G-6-PD) DEFICIENCY

G-6-PD deficiency, the most important disease in this group, is responsible for two clinical syndromes: an episodic hemolytic anemia induced by infections or certain drugs and a spontaneous chronic nonspherocytic hemolytic anemia. The deficiency is due to inheritance of any of a large number of abnormal alleles of the gene responsible for the synthesis of the G-6-PD molecule. The normal enzyme found in most populations is designated G-6-PD B⁺. A normal variant designated G-6-PD A⁺ is common in American blacks. Nearly 100 distinct enzyme variants of G-6-PD have been found associated with a wide spectrum of hemolytic disease.

Drug-Induced Hemolytic Anemia Associated with G-6-PD Deficiency

(Primaquine Sensitivity)

Synthesis of red cell G-6-PD is determined by genes borne on the X chromosome. Diseases involving this enzyme occur, therefore, more frequently in males than in females. About 13% of American black males and 2% of black females have a mutant enzyme (G-6-PD A⁻) that results in a deficiency of red cell G-6-PD activity (to 5–15% or less of normal). Italians, Greeks, and other Mediterranean, Middle Eastern, African,

and Oriental ethnic groups also have high frequencies ranging from 5–40% of a variant designated G-6-PD B⁻ (G-6-PD Mediterranean). The G-6-PD activity of the homozygous female or the heterozygous male is <5% of normal. The heterozygous female has an intermediate enzymatic activity and, as an example of random X chromosome inactivation (Lyon hypothesis), has two populations of red cells; one is normal, the other deficient in G-6-PD activity. The heterozygous female does not, however, have clinical hemolysis after exposure to oxidant drugs.

There is considerable variation in the defect among various racial groups; the defect in blacks is less severe than in affected whites. In blacks, the electrophoretically distinct enzyme variant is unstable in vivo, and its activity is decreased in the older red cells in the circulation. The activity of red cells containing the white variant enzyme (G-6-PD B⁻) is very low, often under 1% of normal. A third common mutant enzyme with markedly reduced activity (G-6-PD Canton) occurs in about 5% of Chinese. A number of other rare enzyme variants have been associated with drug-induced hemolysis. The basic defect appears to be production of an unstable enzyme that becomes inactive much more rapidly than normal.

In the usual pattern of G-6-PD deficiency no evidence of hemolysis is apparent until 48–96 hr after the patient has ingested a substance that has oxidant properties. Drugs that have these properties include antipyretics, sulfonamides, antimalarials, and naphthaquinolones. The fava bean, a Mediterranean dietary staple, is also particularly potent, producing an acute and severe hemolytic syndrome called "favism." The degree of hemolysis varies with the agent, the amount ingested, and the severity of the enzyme deficiency in the patient. In severe cases hemoglobinuria and jaundice result, and the hemoglobin concentration may decrease 60–70%. Death may occur as a consequence of severe hemolysis. Even if administration of the responsible drug is continued, recovery is the rule, with evidence of a compensated hemolytic process. Infection may result in hemolysis. This defect is an important cause of neonatal hyperbilirubinemia and kernicterus in Greek and Chinese newborn infants with the G-6-PD B⁻ and Canton variants. Significant hemolysis may occur even when no exposure to drugs can be documented. In the G-6-PD A⁻ variant the hemolytic process after drug exposure is usually self-limited and mild because the younger red cells in the circulation have nearly normal enzyme activity and resist hemolytic destruction. In black newborns spontaneous hemolysis may occur in premature, but not term, infants with G-6-PD deficiency. When a pregnant woman ingests drugs such as sulfonamides or naphthalene, they may be transmitted to her G-6-PD-deficient fetus, and hemolytic anemia and jaundice may ensue after birth.

Laboratory Data. Hemoglobinemia and hemoglobinuria are manifested in severe acute cases, with falls in hemoglobin of 2–10 g/dL. Unstained or supravital preparations of red cells reveal Heinz bodies, which are not visible on Wright-stained blood smears. Because cells containing these inclusions are rapidly removed from the circulation, they are not seen after the first 3–4 days of illness. Recovery is heralded by reticulocytosis and an increase in hemoglobin concentration.

Diagnosis. Diagnosis depends upon direct or indirect demonstration of reduced G-6-PD activity in red cells. By direct measurement, enzyme activity in affected persons is 10% of normal or less, and the reduction of enzyme is more extreme in whites and Orientals than in blacks. Satisfactory screening tests are based upon decoloration of methylene blue and upon reduction of methemoglobin. Immediately after a hemolytic episode reticulocytes and young red cells predominate. These young cells have significantly higher enzyme activity than older cells; testing may, therefore, have to be deferred for a few weeks before a diagnostically low level of enzyme can be shown. The diagnosis can be suspected when the G-6-PD activity is within the low normal range in the presence of a high reticulocyte count. G-6-PD variants can also be detected by electrophoretic analysis.

Treatment. Prevention of hemolysis constitutes the most important therapeutic measure. When possible, males belonging to ethnic groups in which there is a significant incidence of G-6-PD deficiency (Greeks, southern Italians, Sephardic Jews, Filipinos, southern Chinese, blacks, and Thais) should be tested for the defect before drugs are given that are known to be oxidant. When hemolysis has occurred, supportive therapy may include blood transfusions. Spontaneous recovery is the rule.

Other Hemolytic Anemias Associated with Deficiencies of G-6-PD and Related Substances

Rare instances of chronic hemolytic anemia have been associated with profound deficiencies of G-6-PD due to enzyme variants particularly defective in quantity, activity, or stability. Occasionally and unaccountably, persons with G-6-PD B⁻ (Mediterranean) enzyme deficiency have chronic hemolysis; the condition is X-linked recessive and has affected many males of northern European origin. Chronic hemolytic anemia is maintained, and worsening of the hemolytic process may follow ingestion of oxidant drugs. Splenectomy is of little value. A mild, chronic nonspherocytic anemia has also been reported in association with a genetically determined deficiency of red cell glutathione. 6-Phosphogluconate dehydrogenase deficiency has been associated with drug hemolysis. Hyperbilirubinemia has been related to a deficiency of glutathione peroxidase in several newborn infants.

HEMOLYTIC ANEMIAS DUE TO HEMOGLOBINOPATHIES

The molecular and biochemical characteristics of the hemoglobins are remarkably well known. The genes of their component polypeptide chains have been located on chromosomes 11 and 16, and the actual genes have been isolated and their DNA sequences determined. Alpha and beta chains consist of about 150 amino acids, and the precise sequence of these amino acids in the peptide chains has been defined. It is possible to identify and locate precisely the single amino acid substitutions that result in abnormal hemoglobins.

The clinically important abnormal hemoglobin syndromes result from single amino acid substitutions in the α or β chains of adult hemoglobin. Many hemoglobin variants have been described; only a few of them are relatively prevalent. Hemoglobin variants are usually identified by electrophoresis.

15.18 SICKLE CELL HEMOGLOBINOPATHIES

The sickle cell hemoglobinopathies are superb models of molecular disease, from the levels of gene structure and action to the ultimate clinical syndrome in the patient. The basic defect resides in a mutant, autosomal gene that causes valine to be substituted for glutamic acid in the No. 6 position of a beta polypeptide chain ($\alpha_2\beta_2^{6val}$). This minor substitution has profound physiochemical consequences: deoxygenation now results in a change that facilitates stacking of deoxygenated sickle hemoglobin molecules into monofilaments; these aggregate into elongated crystals, distorting the red cell membrane and ultimately forming the sickled cell.

It is possible to make a diagnosis of sickle cell anemia as early as 16–20 wk of gestation. Fetal blood from aspiration of the placenta or of a fetal vein is incubated with ^{14}C-leucine to assess polypeptide chain synthesis by reticulocytes. In fetuses destined to have sickle cell anemia only α, γ, and β^s polypeptide chains are synthesized. Techniques using recombinant DNA and endonuclease restriction enzymes have shown that the DNA segment bearing a Hgb S gene often differs from the segment bearing a Hgb A gene; this finding may permit the diagnosis of sickle cell anemia using fibroblasts from amniotic fluid. Biopsy of trophoblastic tissue may obtain sufficient fetal tissue for diagnosis as early as 10–12 wk of gestation. The possibilities of prenatal diagnosis may help in genetic counseling for the hemoglobinopathies.

SICKLE CELL TRAIT

Heterozygous occurrence of the sickle gene usually has a benign clinical course. About 8% of American blacks have the trait; there is a much higher incidence in parts of Africa. Typical cases also occur in other ethnic groups from Mediterranean and Mid- and Near-Eastern areas. Possession of a sickle gene is believed to confer a degree of resistance to falciparum malaria. The individual red cells of persons with the trait contain a mixture of normal and sickle hemoglobins (Hgb A and Hgb S). The Hgb S proportion varies from 35–45%. With these low proportions of Hgb S, sickling does not occur under physiologic conditions. Rarely, severe hypoxia resulting from shock or from flying at high altitudes in unpressurized aircraft may produce vaso-occlusive phenomena. Spontaneous hematuria, usually from the left kidney, and mild hyposthenuria may also occur; but anemia, hemolysis, or other clinical abnormalities are not attributable to the uncomplicated sickle trait. The sickle cell trait does not affect longevity. Carriers should avoid situations in which hypoxia may occur, but do not need otherwise to modify their life or activities.

SICKLE CELL ANEMIA

Sickle cell anemia is a severe, chronic hemolytic anemia occurring in persons homozygous for the sickle gene. The clinical course is marked by episodes of pain due to occlusion of small blood vessels by spontaneously sickled red cells. These have traditionally been called "crises." Crises are of several varieties, however, and the "crisis" is not a specific diagnostic entity.

Clinical Manifestations. Manifestations of sickle cell disease do not usually appear until the latter part of the 1st yr of life. The large amounts of Hgb F present in the red cells of young infants obscure the detection of small amounts of nonfetal hemoglobins. Use of specialized techniques such as agar gel electrophoresis at acid pH or microcolumn chromatography is necessary for precise diagnosis in early life. Coincidentally with the postnatal decrease in Hgb F, the concentration of Hgb S rises. Intravascular sickling and evidences of a hemolytic process are present by 6–8 wk of age, but clinical symptoms are unusual before 5–6 mo.

The painful or *vaso-occlusive crises*, the most frequent variety, with distal ischemia and infarction, may be precipitated by infections or may develop spontaneously in any or in many parts of the body. Symmetric, painful swelling of the hands and feet (hand-foot syndrome or sickle cell dactylitis) caused by infarction in the small bones of the extremities may be the initial manifestation of sickle cell anemia in infancy. Striking bony destruction with periosteal reaction may be observed roentgenographically (Fig. 15–4). In older patients the large joints and surrounding parts become painful and swollen. Severe abdominal pains resembling those of an acute surgical condition of the abdomen often accompany infarction in abdominal structures. Strokes due to cerebral occlusion are serious and, if not immediately fatal, may leave hemiplegias.

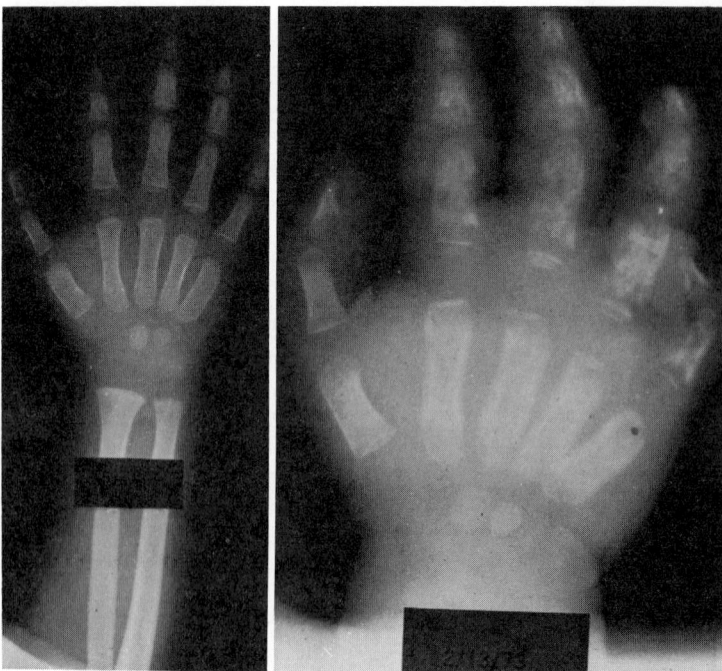

Figure 15–4. Roentgenograms of an infant with sickle cell anemia. The bones at the onset of the episode (*left*) are normal. Two weeks later destructive lesions and periosteal reaction are evident.

Extensive pulmonary infarction is difficult to differentiate from pneumonia. Vaso-occlusive crises are not associated with pronounced changes in the usual hematologic picture.

A second type of crisis, seen only in the young patient, is the so-called *sequestration crisis*. For unknown reasons large amounts of blood become acutely pooled in the liver and the spleen. The spleen becomes massively enlarged, and signs of circulatory collapse develop rapidly. If the patient is supported by hydration and by blood transfusion, much of the sequestered blood is remobilized. This sort of episode is a frequent cause of death in the infant with sickle cell disease and occurs in older patients with sickle cell variants in whom splenomegaly persists into later life.

The third well-characterized type of crisis is the *aplastic crisis* previously described (Sec. 15.5).

Hyperhemolytic crises are unusual but may result when a person with homozygous sickle cell disease, who coincidentally has G-6-PD deficiency, ingests an oxidant drug. They may also be precipitated by infection.

In addition to the acute crises, a wide variety of clinical signs and symptoms result from severe hemolytic anemia and chronic vaso-occlusive disease. Progressive impairment of liver function contributes to the visible jaundice these patients regularly demonstrate. Gallstones have occurred in patients as young as 3 yr of age. Central nervous system infarctions, manifested as "strokes," occur in 5–10% of children and may leave permanent sequelae such as hemiplegia. Renal function is progressively impaired by diffuse glomerular and tubular fibrosis; hyposthenuria and polyuria are regularly present. Renal papillary necrosis and the nephrotic syndrome may occasionally occur.

The spleen is initially considerably enlarged, but the clinically enlarged spleen has markedly reduced phagocytic and reticuloendothelial functions, and there is functional hyposplenism. Later, because of repeated episodes of infarction, the spleen becomes small and fibrotic and is rarely palpably enlarged after 5–6 yr of age. Episodes of severe pulmonary involvement due to infarction occur with or without infection.

Persons with sickle cell anemia have a markedly increased susceptibility to pneumococcal meningitis and septicemia, like patients after splenectomy, especially in the 1st years of life.

As many as 30% of children with sickle cell anemia develop sepsis and meningitis during the first 5 yr of life; mortality is as high as 25%. The increased risk stems from the functional hyposplenia and a deficiency of serum opsonins against pneumococci. A striking susceptibility to *Salmonella* osteomyelitis is also present.

By mid-childhood most patients are underweight, and puberty is delayed, particularly in males. Chronic leg ulcers are common in adolescent and early adult life.

Laboratory Data. Hemoglobin concentrations range from 5–9 g/dL. A peripheral blood smear usually contains irreversibly sickled cells (Fig. 15–3D). Spontaneous sickling in capillary blood smears almost always indicates classic homozygous sickle cell disease; it is not observed with the trait and is infrequently present with the sickle cell variants. Target cells and poikilocytes are seen. The reticulocyte count ranges from 5–15%, and nucleated red cells and Howell-Jolly bodies are usually present. The total white blood cell count is elevated to 12,000–20,000/mm³ with a predominance of neutrophils. The platelet count is increased; the sedimentation rate is slow. Other changes include abnormal liver function test results, hyperbilirubinemia and diffuse hypergammaglobulinemia. The bone marrow is markedly hyperplastic and shows erythroid predominance. Roentgenograms show expanded marrow spaces and osteoporosis.

Studies of the red cells and hemoglobin are essential to the diagnosis. A rapid, simple test for the presence of Hgb S is the sickle cell preparation, in which red cells are deoxygenated or exposed to reducing agents such as sodium metabisulfite. Virtually 100% of the red cells can be induced to sickle in both sickle disease and sickle trait, but sickling is more rapid and extreme in the disease than with the trait. Under 100% of sickling occurs only after transfusion or during early infancy. Rapid solubility tests are also available for detection of the presence of Hgb S in red cells, utilizing the principle that reduced Hgb S is insoluble and precipitates into a turbid solution. Neither sickling nor solubility tests are definitive, both giving false positive and false negative test results. Electrophoretic examination of hemoglobin is conclusive. After infancy the red cells of patients with sickle cell anemia contain approximately 90% Hgb S, 2–10% Hgb F, and a normal amount of Hgb A$_2$. No Hgb A is present. Each parent has the sickle cell trait or one of the sickle variants (HbSC, S-thal, etc.).

Differential Diagnosis. Sickle cell disease may be associated with a wide variety of signs and symptoms. Painful joints, with the heart murmurs of anemia, may suggest acute rheumatic fever or rheumtoid arthritis. Pneumonia, osteomyelitia, and leukemia are occasionally difficult to differentiate. The varied signs and symptoms of sickle cell anemia make it important to perform electrophoretic studies on black patients.

Treatment. No therapy is necessary except during acute episodes. Administration of extra quantities of vitamins or of hematinics is of no proven value, though some centers prescribe folic acid supplements. Iron therapy is not indicated unless iron deficiency can be proved. No pharmacologic treatment of the painful crisis has proved safe or of consistent value, including the use of intravenous infusions of urea and of oral cyanate. Analgesics such as codeine and phenothiazines usually suffice for the discomfort and pain. Regular administration of narcotics should be avoided to prevent addiction. Dehydration and acidosis should be vigorously corrected by the intravenous route. Complicating bacterial infections require appropriate antibiotic therapy. Blood transfusions are not necessary for the usual painful crises but are indicated for prolonged or extreme pain, for extensive involvement of lungs or central nervous system, in preparation for general anesthesia, and during the latter part of pregnancy. Transfusions of packed red cells are given to dilute the patient's red cells with normal ones. When the proportion of Hgb SS red cells can be reduced to less than 40% by transfusions, vaso-occlusive symptoms will generally abate. Partial exchange transfusion can rapidly lower the number of sickling cells. Transfusions are essential in sequestration and aplastic episodes. Splenectomy is not indicated unless sequestration crises have been recurrent or hypersplenism is present.

15.19 OTHER HEMOGLOBINOPATHIES

Hemoglobin C ($\alpha_2\beta_2^{6\ lys}$). Hemoglobin C occurs in about 2% of American Blacks. In the heterozygous state (Hgb AC) no anemia or disease is present, but increased numbers of target cells are seen in the peripheral blood. In the homozygous person (Hgb CC disease) a moderately severe hemolytic anemia with hemoglobin levels from 8–11 g/dL, a reticulocytosis of 5–10%, and splenomegaly are regularly observed. The peripheral blood contains striking numbers of target cells and spherocytes (Fig. 15–2E).

Hemoglobin D. The hemoglobin Ds include several varieties of abnormal hemoglobin with electrophoretic mobilities similar to those of Hgb S, but with different biochemical and physical properties. Sickling does not occur in Hgb D syndromes. The homozygous state (Hgb DD) is characterized by a mild hemolytic anemia with splenomegaly.

Hemoglobin E ($\alpha_2\beta_2^{26\ lys}$). Hemoglobin E is prevalent in persons from Southeast Asia, particularly Thailand and Cambodia. Homozygous Hgb E disease is characterized by a hemolytic anemia, with prominent target cells, microcytosis, and moderate to severe splenomegaly.

Hemoglobin SC Disease. When the genes for both Hgb S and Hgb C are present in the same person, a moderately severe anemia with splenomegaly results. There are vaso-occlusive episodes, but these are usually less frequent and milder than those of sickle cell disease. Aseptic necrosis of the femoral head is an occasional complication, and severe retinal damage also occurs. The hemoglobin concentration averages 9–10 g/dL. Target cells are numerous, but irreversibly sickled cells are usually not present in the blood. Hemoglobin electrophoresis reveals a nearly equal mixture of Hgb S and Hgb C, with slight elevation of Hgb F. Hgb SC disease does not usually affect growth and is compatible with extended survival into adult life. Aplastic and sequestration crises are potential threats to life.

15.20 UNSTABLE HEMOGLOBINS

For at least 50 varieties of abnormal hemoglobin, amino acid substitutions in either α or β chains cause molecular instability leading to denaturation and precipitation of hemoglobin within the red cell. The precipitated hemoglobin attaches to the red cell membrane, damaging the cell. These chronic hemolytic processes are characterized by Heinz bodies and sometimes by excretion of dark brown urine containing dipyrrolic compounds, especially pronounced after splenectomy. These anemias are transmitted as autosomal dominant states. Each variant is usually assigned the name of its city of origin (Hgb Zürich, Köln, Santa Ana, Bristol, etc.).

Hemolysis is usually evident 3–6 mo after birth with β variants. The severity ranges from a compensated mild anemia to a severe hemolytic process. Mean corpuscular hemoglobin concentration is characteristically reduced. Jaundice and splenomegaly are regularly found. The abnormal hemoglobin accounts for 30–40% of the total. It may or may not be detected by electrophoresis, but heating of hemolysate at 50° C for 1 hr results in a heavy precipitate of the abnormal hemoglobin, whereas normal hemoglobin is not affected. Unstable hemoglobins may also be demonstrated by adding fresh hemolysate to a 17% buffered solution of isopropanol. Heinz bodies may be produced by incubation of whole blood for 48 hr prior to supravital staining with brilliant cresyl blue, and appear in markedly increased numbers following splenectomy. In some variants (Hgb Zürich, Hgb Toronto) severe hemolysis is precipitated by ingestion of sulfonamides. Splenectomy appears sometimes to improve patients with moderately severe disease, but those with severe hemolysis derive little benefit.

15.21 HEMOGLOBINS CAUSING CYANOSIS (Hgb M)

A group of five abnormal hemoglobins designated as the hemoglobin Ms are associated with dominantly transmitted familial cyanosis due to the production of methemoglobinemia. Because the characteristic amino acid substitutions are strategically located near the attachments of heme groups, internal oxidation of heme iron to the trivalent (ferric) form occurs. The Hgb M diseases are characterized by cyanosis and mild polycythemia. With Hgb M variants resulting from β chain substitutions, such as Hgb M Saskatoon, cyanosis is not seen until 4–6 mo of age, whereas in α chain variants, such as Hgb M Boston, cyanosis is congenital. Hgb M disease has often been mistaken for cyanotic congenital heart disease.

Methemoglobinemias due to Hgb M can be distinguished from other forms of methemoglobinemia by characteristic changes in the spectral absorption patterns of hemoglobin solutions and by normal levels of methemoglobin reductase (diaphorase). (See Sec 7.56) Electrophoresis can demonstrate and quantitate the abnormal hemoglobin. No therapy is indicated; specifically, use of methylene blue or ascorbic acid is of no benefit.

15.22 HEMOGLOBINS WITH ALTERED OXYGEN AFFINITY

More than 20 abnormal hemoglobins have a marked increase in their affinity for oxygen, as indicated by a shift to the left of the oxygen dissociation curve and a low P_{50} (12–18 torr). Because of the increased affinity for hemoglobin there is decreased release of oxygen to the tissues, leading to tissue hypoxia. This causes increased production of erythropoietin and secondary polycythemia. Most of these variants can be demonstrated electrophoretically (Sec. 15.2). Examples include Hgbs Chesapeake, Rainier, and Malmo.

Six hemoglobin variants with markedly reduced affinity for oxygen have been reported. These are associated with familial chronic cyanosis or "pseudoanemia." The oxygen dissociation curve is shifted to the right, with P_{50} values greater than 30 torr. Examples include Hgbs Kansas and Providence.

15.23 THALASSEMIA

The thalassemias are a heterogeneous group of heritable hypochromic anemias of varying degrees of severity. Various genetic defects include abnormalities of messenger RNA processing, deletion of genetic material, and changes in DNA sequence. These result in a deficient quantity of mRNA, which leads to deficient synthesis of hemoglobin polypeptide chains. More than 30 distinct mutations leading to thalassemia phenotype have been described. Different types of thalassemia with different clinical and biochemical manifestations are associated with defects in each polypeptide chain (α,β, γ, δ). In contrast to the hemoglobinopathies, no basic chemical abnormality of hemoglobin species lies behind the thalassemias, although alterations in the amounts of Hgb A_2 and Hgb F may be seen. Tetrameric forms, such as Hgb H (β_4) and Hgb Bart (γ_4), may be found in certain types of α-thalassemia (see below). Polypeptide chain synthesis may be totally absent, as in the β^0 type of β-thalassemia, or only partially deficient (β^+ type).

The most common genetic variety of thalassemia involves impaired production of beta chains (β-thalassemia). The gene is prevalent in ethnic groups from areas around the Mediterranean Sea, especially in Italy, in Greece, on the Mediterranean islands, and in the mid-Eastern Arab countries. Foci of high prevalence exist also in India and Southeast Asia. From 3–8% of Americans of Italian or Greek ancestry and 0.5% of black Americans carry a gene for β-thalassemia. The incidence of β-thalassemia in most non-Mediterranean peoples is very low, but typical cases occur in many racial groups. Like the sickle cell gene, that of thalassemia appears to be associated with increased resistance to malaria, which may account for its incidence and geographic distribution. Most cases can be clinically classified as thalassemia major or minor, to correspond in general with homozygous or heterozygous genotype.

15.24 THALASSEMIA MINOR
(β-Thalassemia Trait)

Heterozygous β-thalassemia is associated with mild anemia. The hemoglobin concentration averages 2–3 g/dL lower than age-related normal values. The red cells are hypochromic and microcytic, with poikilocytosis, ovalocytosis, and often coarse basophilic stippling (Fig. 15–3E). Target cells are present but usually not prominent, and not specific for thalassemia. The mean corpuscular volume (MCV) is low, averaging 65 fL. Mean corpuscular hemoglobin (MCH) is also low (< 26 pg). A mild decrease in red cell survival can be shown, but overt signs of hemolysis are usually absent. The serum iron level is normal or elevated.

Persons with thalassemia trait are often misdiagnosed as having iron deficiency anemia and may be inappropriately treated with iron for extended periods of time. More than 90% of persons with β-thalassemia trait have diagnostic elevations of Hgb A_2 of 3.4–7.0%. About 50% of these persons also have slight elevations of Hgb F, from 2–6%. In a small

number of otherwise typical cases, normal levels of Hgb A_2 with Hgb F levels ranging from 5–15% are found (the so-called high fetal or β-δ-thalassemia variant). Rarely, a person with thalassemia trait may be hematologically normal (a "silent carrier"). The Lepore hemoglobin is a molecular variant that represents a combination of β and δ chains. Individuals heterozygous for Lepore hemoglobin have clinical and hematologic features of thalassemia minor.

Other than being mistaken for iron deficiency anemia, the most important implication of thalassemia trait is genetic. When both mother and father have thalassemia trait, each pregnancy carries a 25% risk of thalassemia major. Fetal blood sampling permits prenatal diagnosis of thalassemia major. A small sample of fetal blood obtained at 16–20 wk of gestation by fetoscopy with aspiration from a placental vein is incubated with ^{14}C leucine, and the synthesis of α, β, and γ chains can be quantitated. Fetuses having homozygous β-thalassemia will demonstrate a marked reduction of β-chain synthesis. Endonuclease restriction enzyme analysis of DNA from amniotic fluid fibroblasts also permits diagnosis of affected fetuses and has become the method of choice for prenatal diagnosis. Trophoblastic biopsy permits diagnosis as early as 10–12 wk of gestation.

15.25 THALASSEMIA MAJOR
(Cooley Anemia)

Homozygous β-thalassemia usually becomes symptomatic as a severe, progressive hemolytic anemia during the second 6 mo of life. Regular blood transfusions are necessary to prevent profound weakness and cardiac decompensation due to anemia. Without transfusion life expectancy is only a few years. In untreated cases or cases receiving infrequent transfusions at times of severe anemia, hypertrophy of erythropoietic tissue occurs in medullary and extramedullary locations. The bones become thin, and pathologic fractures may occur. Massive expansion of the marrow of the face and skull (Figs. 15–5 and 15–6) produces a typical facies. Pallor, hemosiderosis, and jaundice combine to produce a greenish-

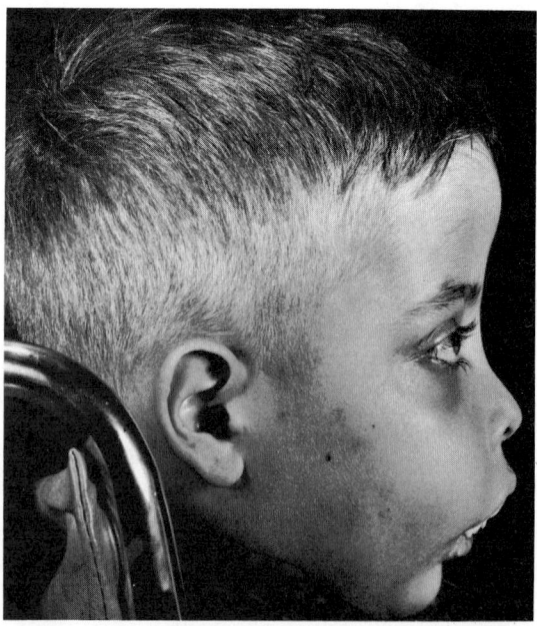

Figure 15–5. Appearance of patient with undertransfused thalassemia major (Cooley anemia). Note the maxillary hyperplasia and resulting dental abnormality. These severe cosmetic changes should be preventable by hypertransfusion.

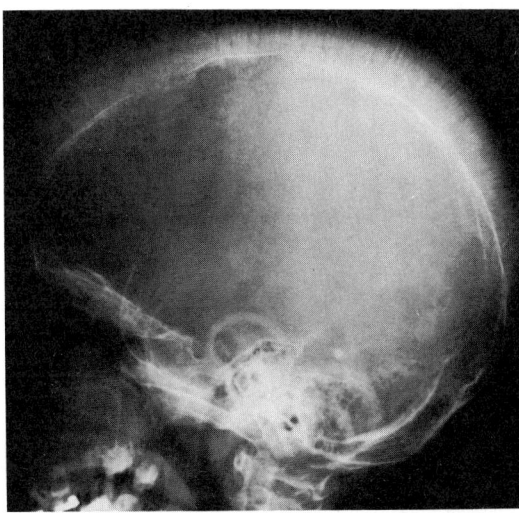

Figure 15–6. Roentgenogram of skull, showing overgrowth of the maxilla with opacification of the sinuses. The diploic spaces are widened, with prominent vertical trabeculae (hair on end).

brown complexion. The spleen and liver are enlarged by extramedullary hematopoiesis and hemosiderosis. In older patients the spleen may become so enlarged that it causes mechanical discomfort and secondary hypersplenism. Growth is impaired in older children; puberty rarely occurs, owing to endocrine abnormalities. Diabetes mellitus due to pancreatic siderosis occurs often. Cardiac complications such as pericarditis and chronic congestive failure due to myocardial siderosis are common terminal events. In transfusion-dependent patients death usually occurs during the 2nd decade; only a few patients have survived to their 30's.

Laboratory Data. The red cell changes of thalassemia major are extreme. In addition to severe hypochromia and microcytosis (Fig. 15–3F), many bizarre, fragmented poikilocytes and target cells are present. Large numbers of nucleated red cells circulate, especially after splenectomy. Intraerythrocytic precipitations thought to represent excess alpha chains are also seen after splenectomy. In the usual case the hemoglobin level falls progressively to less than 5 g/dL unless transfusions are given. About 10% of patients with homozygous thalassemia can maintain hemoglobin levels of 6–8 g/dL without transfusions (thalassemia intermedia). The unconjugated serum bilirubin level is elevated. The serum iron level is high, with saturation of iron-binding capacity. LDH activities are also very high, reflecting ineffective erythropoiesis. A striking biochemical feature is large amounts of fetal hemoglobin in the red cells. The level of Hgb F exceeds 70% during the early years of life but tends to decline with increasing age. Quantitation of fetal hemoglobin is imprecise because of frequent transfusions. Hemoglobin A_2 level is usually under 3%, but the ratio of Hgb A_2 to Hgb A is markedly increased. Dipyrrolic compounds render the urine dark brown, especially after splenectomy.

Treatment. Transfusions are given to maintain the hemoglobin level above 10 g/dL. This "hypertransfusion" has striking clinical benefit: it permits normal activity with comfort, prevents progressive marrow expansion and cosmetic problems associated with facial bone changes, and minimizes cardiac dilatation and osteoporosis. Transfusions of 15 mL/kg of packed cells are usually necessary every 4–5 wk. Even more vigorous transfusional programs ("supertransfusion") have been advocated to keep the hemoglobin level above 12 g/dL and completely suppress erythropoiesis.

Careful cross-matching should be performed to forestall isoimmunization and prevent transfusion reactions. The use of packed red blood cells that are relatively fresh (less than 1 wk in CPD anticoagulant) is desirable. Even with meticulous care, febrile reactions to transfusions are common. These may be minimized with the use of erythrocytes reconstituted from frozen blood, or leukocyte-poor red cell preparations, and by the administration of salicylates before transfusions.

Hemosiderosis is an inevitable consequence of prolonged transfusion therapy because each 500 mL of blood delivers to the tissues about 200 mg of iron that cannot be excreted by physiologic means. The usual causes of death appear to be a consequence of myocardial siderosis. It may be possible to reduce this lethal iron burden by means of iron-chelating agents. The most promising of these is deferoxamine, which must be given parenterally. A single daily intramuscular injection usually does not remove the average daily amount of iron delivered by transfusions. The efficiency of deferoxamine in removing iron can be markedly enhanced if 1.5–2.0 g of the drug is administered subcutaneously over an 8–12 hr period using a compact battery-driven pump, during sleep, 5–6 nights/wk. In most patients over 7 yr old a "negative" iron balance is possible. Such chronic chelation programs may alter the poor prognosis of this disease, if compliance with the demanding regimen can be obtained.

Liberal transfusion therapy prevents massive splenomegaly due to extramedullary erythropoiesis. Splenectomy is often necessary because of the size of the organ or because of secondary hypersplenism, but it has no effect on the basic hematologic disease. In some patients who have had splenectomy, severe, overwhelming sepsis may develop. For this reason the operation should be performed only for significant indications and should be deferred as long as possible. The most important indication for splenectomy is an increased need for transfusions, indicating an element of hypersplenism. A transfusion requirement exceeding 180–200 mL/kg of packed red cells per year is usually evidence of "hypersplenism" and may be an indication for considering splenectomy. Immunization with pneumococcal polysaccharide vaccine is indicated and prophylactic penicillin therapy is advocated by some authorities (Sec. 15.59).

15.26 OTHER THALASSEMIC SYNDROMES

THALASSEMIA INTERMEDIA

This term is often assigned to patients with thalassemia syndromes intermediate in severity between major and minor. Jaundice and moderate splenomegaly are present, and the hemoglobin level is 7–8 g/dL. Transfusions are not regularly necessary to prevent severe anemia, but transfusion therapy may prevent marked cosmetic and other osseous abnormalities. Even without regular blood transfusions these patients absorb large amounts of iron, and hemosiderosis may occur. Tea, which markedly reduces iron absorption, has been advocated with meals. Splenectomy is often necessary.

These patients are heterogeneous: Some are apparently homozygous; others are double heterozygotes for thalassemia genes with genes for other thalassemia variants, such as βδ or Lepore traits.

HEMOGLOBIN S-β-THALASSEMIA

Combination of a thalassemia gene with that of an abnormal β-chain hemoglobin results in clinical disease more severe than with either trait alone. Hgb S-thalassemia is a moderately severe hemolytic anemia with mild to moderate vaso-occlusive symptoms and significant splenomegaly. With the B+-thalassemia gene, the hemoglobin electrophoretic pattern shows a predominance of Hgb S, ranging from 60–80%, the remainder being Hgb F and Hgb A. When the β⁰-thalassemia gene is present, no Hgb A can be detected in some instances, and the electrophoretic pattern is like that of sickle cell disease. In sickle cell anemia, however, the red cells are normocytic, whereas in Hgb S-thalassemia they are microcytic, with an MCV under 75 fL. In such instances family studies will usually reveal one parent to have thalassemia trait and the other the sickle cell trait.

HEMOGLOBIN C-β-THALASSEMIA AND D-β-THALASSEMIA

Hemoglobin C-β-thalassemia and hemoglobin D-β-thalassemia are mild hemolytic anemias with significant splenomegaly. Hemoglobin electrophoresis reveals that the abnormal hemoglobin, C or D, constitutes more than 60% of the total.

HEMOGLOBIN E-β-THALASSEMIA

Both Hgb E and β-thalassemia are very prevalent in Southeast Asian peoples. The immigration from this area into the United States has made Hgb E-β-thalassemia much more common here. The disease resembles thalassemia major; only Hgbs E and F are present.

ALPHA-THALASSEMIA

A group of diseases especially prevalent in Southeast Asia and in China results from genetic deletions, with genetically determined blocks in α-chain synthesis (α-thalassemia). Understanding of α-thalassemia syndromes is difficult because their genetic basis is complex. There are four α-chain genes. In Orientals four distinct thalassemia syndromes are noted: the silent carrier, α-thalassemia trait, Hgb H disease, and fetal hydrops. These result from increasing numbers of α-thalassemia gene deletions, from 1–4. No specific alterations in the proportions of the minor hemoglobins A_2 or F are seen in the first two states. Special techniques may reveal traces of hemoglobin tetramers lacking alpha chains. These are Hgbs H (β_4) and Bart (γ_4). In the newborn period 3–6% of Hgb Bart is found in the blood of persons with α-thalassemia trait. It does not persist after 6 mo, except occasionally in trace amounts. The most severe form of α-thalassemia, associated with deletion of four α-thalassemia genes, produces the clinical picture of hydrops fetalis. In these cases the predominant hemoglobin is Bart (γ_4). This variant has abnormal oxygen dissociation properties that make oxygen unavailable to the tissues under physiologic conditions.

α-Thalassemia is also involved in Hgb H syndromes. These moderately severe anemias resemble Cooley anemia but are characterized by an unstable hemoglobin component (Hgb H or β_4). In blacks, Hgb H disease is very rare, and the fact that fetal hydrops syndrome has not been reported indicates that in blacks α-thalassemia genes have a different arrangement on the chromosome from that occurring in Oriental and Mediterranean peoples. The combination of α-thalassemia with genes for β-chain hemoglobin abnormalities or β-thalassemia results in hematologic diseases that are no more severe than with either trait alone.

HEREDITARY PERSISTENCE OF HIGH FETAL HEMOGLOBIN

This condition is associated with high levels of normal fetal hemoglobin but with no other abnormalities. It is thought to result from genetic deletions that result in inability to convert from γ-chain to β-chain synthesis at the time of birth. The trait occurs most frequently in blacks, Italians, and Greeks. In the heterozygous person the level of Hgb F is 15–30%. In blacks the proportion of Hgb F is higher than that in Mediterraneans. There is an even distribution of fetal hemoglobin through the red cell population, in contrast to the thalassemias, in which Hgb F content shows variation from cell to cell. Patients with homozygosity for the high fetal Hgb gene have been observed; their hemoglobin was completely Hgb

F, but no significant anemia or manifestations of hematologic disease were found. When both the high fetal gene and the sickle genes are present in the same person, hematologic manifestations are very mild. Only Hgbs S and F are found; the electrophoretic pattern resembles that of sickle cell anemia. The even distribution of a large amount of Hgb F through the red cell population prevents sickling.

HEMOLYTIC ANEMIAS DUE TO ABNORMALITIES OF THE RED CELL PRODUCED BY EXTRINSIC FACTORS

A number of agents with capacity to damage red blood cells may lead to their premature destruction. Among the most clearly defined are antibodies associated with immune hemolytic anemias. These antibodies, directed against specific intrinsic antigens, so damage the red cell that viability is compromised and rapid destruction ensues in the reticuloendothelial tissues of the spleen and liver. The hallmark of this group of diseases is a positive result of the Coombs test, which detects a coating of immunoglobulin or components of complement on the red cell surface. The most important immune hemolytic disorder in pediatric practice is hemolytic disease of the newborn (erythroblastosis fetalis), caused by transplacental transfer of maternal antibody active against the red cells of the fetus (Sec. 8.47).

15.27 AUTOIMMUNE HEMOLYTIC ANEMIAS ASSOCIATED WITH "WARM" ANTIBODIES

In the autoimmune hemolytic anemias, abnormal antibodies directed against red cells are produced by the patient. The pathogenic mechanisms are uncertain. One theory postulates autonomous proliferation of a forbidden clone of immunologically competent cells that do not recognize self-antigens. Alternative explanations suggest that drugs or infectious agents in some way alter the red cell membrane so that it becomes "foreign" or antigenic to the host.

Autoimmune hemolytic anemias associated with an underlying disease process such as lymphoma, lupus erythematosus, or immunodeficiency are said to be secondary or symptomatic. In other instances (idiopathic) no underlying cause can be found. In as many as 20% of cases of immune hemolysis, drugs may be implicated. A number of drugs, such as penicillin and cephalosporins, attach to the red cell membrane, changing antigenicity and evoking production of antibodies directed against the red cell–drug complex. Other drugs, such as phenacetin and quinidine, form immune complexes that become attached to the red cell, causing its destruction. Alpha-methyldopa produces an autoimmune hemolytic process by unknown mechanisms.

Clinical Manifestations. Autoimmune hemolytic anemias occur in two general clinical patterns. The first is an acute transient type that occurs predominantly in infants and younger children and is frequently preceded by an infection, usually respiratory. The onset is acute, with prostration, pallor, jaundice, pyrexia, and hemoglobinuria. The spleen is usually markedly enlarged. Underlying systemic disorders are unusual in this group. A consistent response to corticosteroid therapy, low mortality, and full recovery within 3 mo are characteristic of the acute form.

The second type pursues a prolonged and chronic course. Hemolysis continues for many months or years. Abnormalities involving other blood elements are common, and the response to corticosteroids is variable and inconsistent. Mortality is about 10%, often attributable to an underlying systemic disease.

Laboratory Data. In many cases the anemia is profound, with hemoglobin levels under 6 g/dL. Considerable spherocytosis and polychromasia are present. More than 50% of the circulating red cells may be reticulocytes, and nucleated red cells are usually present. In some cases an initially low reticulocyte count may reflect a process so acute that the bone marrow has not yet had time to respond. Leukocytosis is common. The platelet count is usually normal; occasionally, there is a concomitant immune thrombocytopenic purpura (*Evans syndrome*). The prognosis of Evans syndrome is poor; many cases become chronic.

The direct Coombs test result is strongly positive, and free antibody can sometimes be demonstrated in the serum. These antibodies are active at 37° C ("warm" antibodies) and belong to the IgG class. They do not require complement for activity and may not produce agglutination in vitro. Antibodies from the serum and those eluted from the red cells react with red cells of many persons besides the patient. They have often been regarded as nonspecific panagglutinins, but careful studies have revealed many to have specificity for certain red cell antigens, usually those of the Rh system. A number of such antibodies have had anti-e(hr") specificity. Since more than 95% of the population have the red cell e antigen, the antibody might be considered a panagglutinin unless careful tests are performed. In other cases antibodies specific for the ubiquitous antigen LW are found. Sometimes spontaneous agglutination of the patient's own red cells occurs in all testing sera so that the patient may be mistakenly blood-typed as group AB Rh-positive. In many cases only complement is found on the red cells, chiefly the C3 and C4 components. A "broad spectrum" Coombs serum must be used to detect complement-coated red cells. In 80% of acute transient cases only complement-type positive Coombs tests are found, whereas in the chronic variety an IgG or mixed type of Coombs response occurs in over 80% of cases. Occasionally, the Coombs test is negative because of the limited sensitivity of the Coombs reaction. A minimum of 250–500 molecules of IgG is necessary on the red cell membrane to produce a positive reaction. Special tests are required to detect the antibody in cases of "Coombs test negative" autoimmune hemolytic anemia.

Treatment. Transfusions are usually of only transient benefit but may be required by the severity of the anemia. It may be extremely difficult to find compatible blood; blood in which the red cells give the least positive in vitro reaction by the Coombs technique should be chosen. Sometimes it is necessary to give blood that is "incompatible" as judged by the cross-match. Failure to transfuse a profoundly anemic infant may lead to serious morbidity and even death.

Prednisone or its equivalent should be administered in a dose of 2.5 mg/kg/24 hr. In some cases with severe hemolysis doses up to 6 mg/kg/24 hr of prednisone may be required in order to reduce the rate of hemolysis. Treatment should be continued until the evidence of hemolysis decreases, and then the dose is gradually reduced. If relapse occurs, resumption of full dosage may be necessary. The disease tends to remit spontaneously within a few weeks or months. The Coombs test result may remain positive even after hemolysis has subsided. When hemolytic anemia remains severe despite corticosteroid therapy or if very large doses are necessary to maintain a reasonable hemoglobin level, splenectomy may be beneficial. Immunosuppressive agents have been of some benefit in chronic cases refractory to conventional therapy.

Course and Prognosis. The acute variety of idiopathic autoimmune hemolytic disease in childhood may be severe, but is self-limited. The disease may be fulminating; severe cases have been refractory to corticosteroids, immunosuppressive agents, splenectomy, and thymectomy. In immune hemolytic anemia secondary to lymphoma or lupus erythematosus the status of the basic disease determines the prognosis.

15.28 AUTOIMMUNE HEMOLYTIC ANEMIAS ASSOCIATED WITH "COLD" ANTIBODIES

Red cell antibodies that are more active at low body temperatures have been called "cold." They are of the IgM class and require complement for activity.

Cold Agglutinin Disease. Cold antibodies may be present in low levels in normal blood. Following viral infections or mycoplasmal pneumonia, the levels may increase considerably, and occasionally enormous increases may occur, titers of 1/30,000 or greater being recorded. The antibody has specificity for the I antigen and reacts poorly with human cord blood cells possessing the i antigen. Spontaneous agglutination and rouleaux formation are seen on the blood smear.

When very high titers of cold antibodies are present, severe episodes of intravascular hemolysis with hemoglobinemia and hemoglobinuria may follow exposure of the patient to cold.

Occasionally, patients with infectious mononucleosis develop acute immunohemolytic anemia. The antibodies in these cases have anti-i specificity.

Paroxysmal Cold Hemoglobinuria. This form of hemolytic anemia is associated with a specific type of cold antibody, the Donath-Landsteiner hemolysin, which has anti-P specificity. About one third of cases are associated with either congenital or acquired syphilis. Transfusions are given for severe anemia. Chilling of the patient should be avoided.

15.29 HEMOLYTIC ANEMIAS OF INTOXICATIONS AND INFECTIONS

In sufficiently large doses arsenic and phenylhydrazine produce hemolysis.

Hemolytic anemias may complicate a variety of infections. Direct red cell damage by microorganisms or their toxins may be the basis of hemolysis observed in septicemia. Actual parasitism of the red cell occurs in malaria and bartonellosis.

General

Miller DR, Bachner RE, McMillan O: Blood Diseases of Infancy and Childhood. Ed 5. St. Louis, CV Mosby, 1984.
Nathan DG, Oski FA: Hematology of Infancy and Childhood. 4th ed. Philadelphia, WB Saunders, 1986.
Oski FA, Naiman, JL: Hematologic Problems of the Newborn. 3rd ed. Philadelphia, WB Saunders, 1982.
Wintrobe MD: Clinical Hematology. 8th ed. Philadelphia, Lea and Febiger, 1981.

The Red Cells

Harris JW, Kellermeyer RW: The Red Cell. 2nd ed. Cambridge, Mass., Harvard University Press, 1970.

Pure Red Cell Anemias

Alter BP: Childhood red cell aplasia. Am J Pediatr Hematol 2:121, 1980.
Diamond LK, Wang WS, Alter BP: Congenital hypoplastic anemia. Adv Pediatr 22:349, 1976.
Glader B, Backer K, Diamond LK: Elevated erythrocyte adenosine deaminase activity in congenital hypoplastic anemia. N Engl J Med 309:1486, 1983.
Nathan DG, Clarke BJ, et al: Erythroid precursors in congenital hypoplastic (Diamond-Blackfan) anemia. J Clin Invest 61:489, 1978.
Wang WC, Mentzer WC: Differentiation of transient erythroblastopenia of childhood from congenital hypoplastic anemia. J Pediatr 88:784, 1976.

Anemias of Chronic Infections, Inflammation, and Renal Disease

Cartwright GE: The anemia of chronic disorders. Semin Hematol 3:351, 1966.
Douglas SW, Adamson JW: The anemia of chronic disorders: Studies of marrow regulation and iron metabolism. Blood 45:55, 1975.
Koerper MA, Stempel DA, Dallmar PR: Anemia in patients with juvenile rheumatoid arthritis. J Pediatr 91:878, 1978.

Physiologic Anemia of Infancy

O'Brien RT, Pearson HA: Physiologic anemia of infancy. J Pediatr 79:132, 1971.
Stockman JA, Graeber JE, Clark DA, et al: Anemia of prematurity: Determinants of the erythropoietin response. J Pediatr 105:786, 1984.
Williams ML, Shott RJ, O'Neal PL, et al: Role of dietary iron and fat in vitamin E deficiency of infancy. N Engl J Med 292:887, 1975.

Megaloblastic Anemias

Haggard ME, Lockhart LH: Megaloblastic anemia and orotic aciduria: an hereditary disorder of pyrimidine metabolism responsive to uridine. Am J Dis Child 113:733, 1967.
Hakami N, Neiman PE: Neonatal megaloblastic anemia due to inherited transcobalamin II deficiency in two siblings. N Engl J Med 285:1163, 1971.
Heisil MA, Siegel SE, Falk RE, et al: Congenital pernicious anemia: report of seven patients with study of an extended family. J Pediatr 105:564, 1984.
Higgenbottom MC, Swertman L, Nyhan WL: A syndrome of methylmalonic aciduria, homocystinuria megaloblastic anemia and neurologic abnormalities in a vitamin B_{12} deficient breast fed infant of a strict vegetarian. New Engl J Med 299:317, 1978.
Hoffbrand AV: Megaloblastic anaemia. Clin Haematol 5:52, 1976.
Lampkin BC, Shore NA, Chadwick D: Megaloblastic anemia of infancy secondary to maternal pernicious anemia. N Engl J Med 274:1168, 1966.
Vrana MB, Carvalho RJ: Thiamine responsive megaloblastic anemia. Sensorineural deafness and diabetes mellitus: A new syndrome. J Pediatr 93:235, 1978.

Microcytic Anemia

Dallman PR, Siimes MA, Stekel A: Iron deficiency in infancy and childhood. Am J Clin Nutr 33:86, 1980.
Oski FA, Honig AS, Helu B: Effect of iron therapy on behavior performance in nonanemic, nondeficient infants. Pediatr 71:877, 1983.
Reeves JD, Vichinsky E, Addiego J Jr; et al: Iron deficiency in health and disease. Adv Pediatr 30:281, 1983.
Siimes MA, Addiego JE Jr, Dallman PR: Ferritin in serum: Diagnosis of iron deficiency and iron overload in infants and children. Blood 43:581, 1974.
Wilson JF, Lahey ME, Heiner DC: Studies on iron metabolism. V. Further observations on cow's milk induced gastrointestinal bleeding. J Pediatr 84:355, 1974.

Hemolytic Anemias

Dacie JV: The Haemolytic Anemias. 3rd ed. New York, Grune and Stratton, 1985.

Hereditary Spherocytosis

Bellingham AJ, Prankerd TAJ: Hereditary spherocytosis. Clin Haematol 4:139, 1975.
Kelleher JH, Lerban NLC, Mortimer PP: Human serum "parvovirus": A specific cause of aplastic crisis in children with hereditary spherocytosis. J Pediatr 102:722, 1983.
Kruger HC, Burgert EO: Hereditary spherocytosis in 100 children. Mayo Clin Proc 41:921, 1966.
Trucco JT, Brown AK: Neonatal manifestations of hereditary spherocytosis. Am J Dis Child 113:263, 1967.
Valentine WN: The molecular lesion of hereditary spherocytosis: A continuing enigma. Blood 49:241, 1977.

Hereditary Elliptocytosis

Austin RF, Desforges JF: Hereditary elliptocytosis: An unusual presentation of hemolysis in the newborn associated with transient morphologic abnormalities. Pediatrics 44:196, 1969.
Jensson O, Jonasson T, Olafsson O: Hereditary elliptocytosis in Iceland. Br J Haematol 13:884, 1967.
Pearson HA: The genetic basis of hereditary elliptocytosis with hemolysis. Blood 32:972, 1968.

Paroxysmal Nocturnal Hemoglobinuria

Dacie JV, Lewis SM: Paroxysmal noctural hemoglobinuria: Clinical manifestations, hematology and nature of the disease. Ser Haematol 5:3, 1972.

Miller DR, Baehner RL, Diamond LK: Paroxysmal nocturnal hemoglobinuria in childhood and adolescence, Pediatrics 39:675, 1967.

Hereditary Stomatocytosis

Mentzer WC, Smith WB, Goldstone J, et al: Hereditary stomatocytosis: Membrane and metabolism studies. Blood 46:659, 1975.

Enzymatic Defects of the Red Cell

Beutler E: Abnormalities of the hexose monophosphate shunt. Semin Hematol 8:311, 1971.
Gilman PA: Hemolysis in the newborn resulting from deficiencies of red blood cell enzymes: Diagnosis and management. J Pediatr 84:625, 1974.
Jaffe ER: Hereditary hemolytic disorders and enzymatic deficiencies of human erythrocytes. Blood 35:116, 1970.
Tanaka KR, Paglia DE: Deficiency of pyruvate kinase. Semin Hematol 8:367, 1971.

Autoimmune Hemolytic Anemia

Buchanan GR, Boxer LA, Nathan DG: The acute and transient nature of idiopathic immune hemoytic anemia in childhood. J Pediatr 88:780, 1976.
Dacie JV, Worlledge SM: Autoimmune hemolytic anemias. Prog Hematol 6:82, 1969.
Garratty G, Petz LD: Drug induced immune hemolytic anemia. Am J Med 58:398, 1975.
Habibi B, Homberg JC, Schaison G, et al: Autoimmune hemolytic anemia in children. Am J Med 56:61, 1974.
Zuelzer WW, Mastrangelo R, Shulberg CS, et al: Autoimmune hemolytic anemia; natural history and viral-immunologic interactions in childhood. Am J Med 49:80, 1970.

Hemoglobinopathies

Bunn HF, Forgt BG, Ranney HM: Hemoglobinopathies. Major Probl Int Med 13:1, 1977.
Chang JC, Kan YW: A sensitive new prenatal test for sickle cell anemia. N Engl J Med 307:30, 1982.
Charach S, Lubin B, Reid CD (eds.): Management and Therapy of Sickle Cell Disease. Washington, DC: U.S. Dept of Health & Human Services. NIH Pub No 84–2117, Sept 1984.
Davis JR, Vichinsky EP, Lubin BL: Current treatment of sickle cell disease. Curr Probl Pediatr 10:1, 1980.
Goosens M, Dumey Y, Kaplan L: Prenatal diagnosis of sickle cell anemia in the first trimester of pregnancy. N Engl J Med 309:831, 1983.
O'Brien RT, McIntosh S, Aspnes GT, et al: Prospective study of sickle cell anemia in infancy. J Pediatr 89:205, 1976.
Pearson HA: Sickle cell disease crises and their management. In: Dickerman J and Lucey J (eds.): The Critically Ill Child. 3rd ed. Philadelphia, WB Saunders 1985.
Pearson HA, Spencer RP, Cornelius EA: Functional asplenia in sickle cell anemia. N Engl J Med 281:293, 1969.
Pirastu M, Kan YW, Cao A: Prenatal diagnosis of β-thalassemia. N Engl J Med 309:284, 1983.
Powers DR: Natural history of sickle cell disease—the first ten years. Semin Hematol 12:267, 1975.
Serjeant GR: Sickle Cell Disease. Oxford, Oxford U. Press, 1985.

Thalassemia

Alter BP: Prenatal diagnosis of hemoglobinopathies and other hematologic diseases. J Pediatr 95:701, 1979.
Cerami, A: "Proper" use of desferrioxamine. N Engl J Med 294:1456, 1976.
Orkin SH, Nathan DG: Current Concepts: The Thalassemias. N Engl J Med 295:710, 1976.
Pearson HA, O'Brien RT: Management of thalassemia major. Semin Hematol 12:255, 1975.
Problems of Cooley's anemia. Ann NY Acad Sci 119:371, 1964; 165:1, 1969; 232:1, 1974; 344:1, 1980; 445:1, 1985.
Wetherall DJ, Clegg JB: The Thalassemia Syndromes. Ed 2. London, Blackwell Scientific Publications, 1972.

15.30 POLYCYTHEMIA
(Erythrocytosis)

Polycythemia exists when the red cell count, the hemoglobin and hematocrit levels, and the total red cell volume significantly exceed the upper limits of normal. In the older child the levels of hemoglobin and hematocrit that can be considered to represent polycythemia are 16 g/dL and 55%, respectively, corresponding to a total red cell mass exceeding 35 mL/kg. A decrease in plasma volume, such as occurs in acute dehydration and burns, may result in disproportionately high levels of hemoglobin and hematocrit, but these situations are more accurately designated hemoconcentration than relative polycythemia. The volume of red cell mass is not increased; expansion of the plasma voume or rehydration restores the hematocrit to normal levels.

Measurement of the total red cell volume by radioisotopic techniques is essential in the differential diagnosis of polycythemia. True polycythemia is characterized by increases of both the total red cell and total blood volumes.

SECONDARY POLYCYTHEMIA

Polycythemia may be present in any clinical situation associated with chronic arterial oxygen desaturation. Hypoxia of the kidney results in increased production of erythropoietin, which stimulates increased production of red cells and ultimately results in an expanded red cell mass. Cardiovascular defects involving right to left shunts and pulmonary diseases interfering with proper oxygenation are the most common causes of secondary polycythemia. Examples of such conditions are cyanotic congenital heart disease, emphysema, and bronchiectasis. Clinical findings usually include cyanosis, hyperemia of sclerae and mucous membranes, and clubbing of the fingers. The red blood cell count and hemoglobin and hematocrit values are all increased. The oxygen saturation of arterial blood is decreased. In children with cardiac lesions causing severe cyanosis, as the hematocrit rises above 65%, symptoms of hyperviscosity may require phlebotomy. On the other hand, such children may also have iron deficiency (as indicated by microcytosis and relatively low hemoglobin levels); the risk of intracranial thrombosis has been reported to be increased by such anemia, and iron therapy is indicated. Living at high altitudes also causes a secondary polycythemia; the hemoglobin level increases about 4% for each rise of 1000 meters in altitude.

More subtle forms of hypoxia may also cause polycythemia. Congenital methemoglobinemia due to a deficiency of NADH-reactive diaphorase may cause familial cyanosis and polycythemia. This condition is transmitted as an autosomal recessive. Dominantly transmitted cyanosis and polycythemia may be associated with the hemoglobins that have altered oxygen affinity (Sec. 15.22). Transient benign polycythemia is said to occur in otherwise healthy adolescents; this syndrome has not been studied sufficiently to determine its frequency or cause. In several families benign polycythemias seem to have been transmitted as dominant or recessive conditions, the bases of which are not known.

Polycythemia has also been associated with renal tumors and cysts and with vascular tumors of the cerebellum when these tumors have secreted erythropoietin.

When the hematocrit exceeds 65–70% there is a marked increase in blood viscosity, and periodic phlebotomies may be done, blood being replaced with plasma or saline solution.

POLYCYTHEMIA RUBRA VERA
(Erythremia)

This disorder, characterized by polycythemia, leukocytosis, thrombocytosis, and hyperplasia of the bone marrow, has been reported in only a few children. High leukocyte alkaline phosphatase activities and elevated serum vitamin B_{12} levels are characteristic. In contrast to those of normal persons, in vitro cultures of erythroid precursors of affected persons do not require added erythropoietin to stimulate growth.

PLETHORA OF THE NEWBORN

High levels of hemoglobin and hematocrit are usual in the newborn infant. The range of normal hemoglobin at birth is 14.7–21 g/dL, and the hematocrit 45–65%. The blood volume of normal term newborns is 70–100 mL/kg, and the red cell volume 40–60 mL/kg. Occasionally, findings in newborn infants significantly exceed these ranges. Some plethoric infants have convulsions, respiratory distress, tachycardia, congestive heart failure, and hyperbilirubinemia. Hypoglycemia and hypocalcemia may contribute to morbidity. Monozygotic twins with placental vascular anastomosis may have unequal distribution of the circulation so that one twin is born with anemia and hypovolemia while the other twin is plethoric. On rare occasions maternofetal transfusion or congenital adrenal hyperplasia may be associated with neonatal polycythemia. Neonatal polycythemia has also been reported to have increased frequency in the Down and Beckwith syndromes and with intrauterine growth retardation in newborn infants small for gestational age. In most instances no cause can be discovered. When these infants have symptomatic difficulties, such as tachypnea, congestive heart failure, hypoglycemia, or jaundice, phlebotomy in aliquots of 10–15 mL/kg replaced with equal volumes of plasma or normal saline may be indicated to reduce red cell mass and hyperviscosity. (See also Sec. 8.48.)

THE PANCYTOPENIAS

Aplasia of bone marrow, or replacement of its hematopoietic elements by other tissue, results in profound depression of all the formed elements of the blood. The clinical manifestations that result are anemia, thrombocytopenic hemorrhage, and decreased resistance to infection because of neutropenia. The pancytopenias have traditionally been classifed with the anemias, but the consequences of the thrombocytopenia and the neutropenia are much more striking and serious than the anemias. The pancytopenias may be constitutional and genetically determined, may be acquired as a result of damage to the marrow by a variety of chemical or other agents, including viruses, or may result from invasion by abnormal tissue. In these conditions underproduction of blood cells is due to hypocellularity or replacement of marrow. Examination of an adequate sample of marrow obtained by needle or surgical biopsy is essential to diagnosis.

15.31 CONSTITUTIONAL APLASTIC PANCYTOPENIA
(Fanconi Syndrome)

The constitutional aplastic anemias are familial disorders, believed to be inherited as autosomal recessive conditions with variable penetrance, whose expression may be modified by other genetic and environmental factors. About two thirds of affected children have evident congenital anomalies; especially common are microcephaly, microphthalmia, and absence of the radii and thumbs (Fig. 15–7); abnormalities of heart and kidney are also relatively common. Short stature is found in more than two thirds of cases, as is generalized hyperpigmentation of the skin. Some affected children have no serious anatomic defects.

Pancytopenia is not usually present at birth or during early

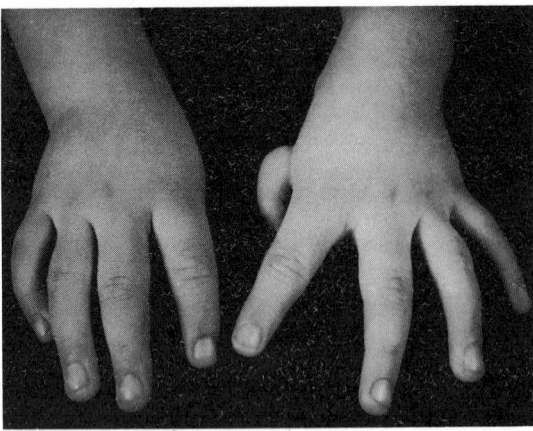

Figure 15–7. Hands of a child with constitutional aplastic pancytopenia. The thumb is absent on the right and rudimentary on the left.

infancy. The clinical onset occurs from 1½–22 yr, with an average of 6–8 yr. Bruising due to thrombocytopenia is noted first, followed by progressively severe anemia and leukopenia.

Laboratory Data. Severe pancytopenia is evident in peripheral blood. The red cells are macrocytic, with MCV of 95–105 fL. The bone marrow is strikingly hypocellular, with depression of all cell types and an increase in fatty tissue. Reticulum, plasma, and mast cells are prominent. A surgical or needle biopsy of the bone marrow is useful as an adjunct to aspiration, for it provides a large specimen in which to judge cellularity. There is an increase in the percentage of Hgb F of 5–15%, which may antedate development of marrow aplasia and cytopenia. A patchy distribution of Hgb F within each cell is shown by Kleihauer-Betke preparations. In vitro cultures of bone marrow show decreased numbers of precursors of both erythroid and granulocytic series. Chromosomal studies of blood lymphocytes reveal an abnormally high percentage (10–70%) of chromatid breaks, gaps, rearrangements, exchanges, and endoreduplications (changes seen in fewer than 10% of chromosomes of normal individuals); these changes, too, precede frank pancytopenia. The same changes are seen in tissue fibroblast cultures and offer the possibility of prenatal diagnosis by amniocentesis (not yet reported).

Treatment. In addition to symptomatic treatment with blood transfusions and antibiotics, therapy with androgenic steroids is beneficial. Testosterone propionate is given as sublingual tablets in a dose of 1–2 mg/kg/24 hr to a maximum of 60 mg/24 hr. Alternatively, 400–600 mg may be given as an intramuscular injection every 4 wk. Synthetic androgen derivatives such as oxymetholone and stanozolol are also effective. Relatively small doses of corticosteroids, such as 5–10 mg of prednisone or its equivalent, are also given to reduce the tendency to bruising and bleeding and to retard acceleration of bone age. In a majority of instances a hematologic response becomes evident within 2–4 mo. The marrow develops greater cellularity, and the hemoglobin rises. The response of the neutrophils is usually less complete, and platelets may show only moderate increases in numbers. When the hemoglobin has reached normal levels, it is sometimes possible to reduce the dose of androgen, but if the drug is too rapidly or drastically decreased, relapse occurs. Most patients require continuous therapy to maintain hematologic response, and many ultimately become refractory to androgen therapy.

These effective doses of androgen regularly produce signs and symptoms of masculinization, including acne, hirsutism, deepening of the voice, and enlargement of the penis or clitoris. Synthetic androgen derivatives have fewer of these side effects, but some degree of masculinization is probably inevitable. Some of the testosterone preparations have hepatic

toxicity. Prior to the advent of testosterone therapy these patients usually died during late childhood of hemorrhage, infection, or the complications of multiple transfusions. Hemorrhagic cysts of the liver (peliosis hepatis) and malignant hepatomas occur with increased frequency in patients receiving prolonged treatment with large doses of oral synthetic androgens. Bone marrow transplantation can be considered when a histocompatible sibling is available. Acute myelogenous leukemia (AML) develops in 5–10% of patients with Fanconi anemia, and their close relatives are at increased risk of AML.

Fanconi anemia must be differentiated from *dyskeratosis congenita*, a rare form of ectodermal dysplasia. Cutaneous hyperpigmentation, pancytopenia, and short stature occur in both conditions. Skeletal and renal anomalies do not regularly occur in dyskeratosis congenita.

15.32 ACQUIRED APLASTIC PANCYTOPENIAS

A number of physical, chemical, and infectious agents may severely damage the bone marrow and lead to severe pancytopenia. Some of these agents will produce marrow aplasia in any person who is exposed to them in a sufficient dose. Such obligate marrow depressants include ionizing radiation; chemotherapeutic drugs, such as nitrogen mustard, 6-mercaptopurine, and methotrexate; and certain organic solvents, especially benzene. A second group of agents produces aplastic pancytopenia only in a small (often remarkably small) number of persons exposed to them. In these persons the adverse hematologic reactions must reflect idiosyncrasies. The drug most frequently associated with aplastic pancytopenia is chloramphenicol. It has been estimated that only 1 in 24,000–60,000 patients taking chloramphenicol suffers marrow aplasia, but this drug has been involved in more than 50% of drug-related aplastic pancytopenias. Other drugs associated with appreciable incidences of marrow aplasia are sulfonamides, phenylbutazone, and certain anticonvulsants. Severe infections may also produce severe marrow damage, but it is often difficult to decide whether the infection represents cause or effect. Some cases of marrow aplasia have followed instances of apparent infectious hepatitis, and it has been reported to follow infectious mononucleosis or appear as a complication of pregnancy. In about 50% of cases of aplastic pancytopenia no history of exposure to toxins or other agents can be elicited; these cases are usually called idiopathic, but the possibility of an environmental factor cannot be excluded.

Clinical and Laboratory Data. Hemorrhage secondary to thrombocytopenia is usually the first clinical manifestation. The signs and symptoms of anemia and neutropenia become apparent later. The spleen and lymph nodes are not enlarged. Profound decreases in red cells, platelets, and neutrophils are observed. The marrow aspirate is scanty; the particles are fatty, and lymphocytes, plasma cells, and reticulum cells predominate. Culture of bone marrow reveals decreased numbers of progenitor stem cells of the erythroid and granulocytic series. Chromosome configuration is normal. Levels of Hgb F may be above 2%; earlier reports that elevated levels of Hgb F indicate a good prognosis are not confirmed. T lymphocyte suppressor cells active against both erythroid and granulocytic colony growth have been found in some patients.

Treatment. The patient must immediately be removed from contact with any potentially toxic drugs or agents. When the onset of the disease is acute, with massive hemorrhage and serious sepsis, aggressive therapy with platelet concentrates and antibiotics is necessary; choice of antibiotic should be based upon bacterial culture and sensitivity tests. Even with the best of supportive therapy the prognosis of severe aplastic pancytopenia is grave. As many as two thirds of patients succumb within 6 mo of diagnosis, and fewer than 10–20% recover. Reports of success with androgen and corticosteroid therapy in acquired aplastic pancytopenia have not been confirmed by more recent studies. Other forms of therapy are of dubious value.

Controlled studies indicate that when an HLA compatible sibling is available as a donor, bone marrow transplantation is effective. Siblings of patients with severe pancytopenia who have markedly hypocellular bone marrows should be examined for both HLA and MLC compatibility. If compatibility between patient and sibling is established, bone marrow transplantation, after suitable immunosuppression, can be considered. About 50% of transplanted patients will accept the donor marrow and have restoration of normal peripheral blood values. Graft-versus-host disease is common and may be severe.

Occurrence of hematologic improvement in severe aplastic pancytopenia after unsuccessful marrow transplantation and intense immunosuppressive therapy indicates that some patients may have an immunologic basis for their bone marrow depression. Criteria identifying patients who should be treated with immunosuppressive therapy alone have not been defined, but successful treatment with anti-thymocyte globulin (ATG), anti-lymphocyte globulin (ALG), or high dose dexamethasone is being increasingly reported.

Course. Unless marrow engraftment is possible or the patient responds to immunotherapy, approximately a third of patients die quickly as a result of hemorrhage and infection. *Pseudomonas* and staphylococcal septicemias are common causes of death. The remaining two thirds of children have a subacute clinical course. In some of these androgen therapy may be beneficial. Half of this group ultimately recover completely; the other half have a chronic course, many succumbing to sepsis and hemorrhage months or years after onset. Leukemia and paroxysmal nocturnal hemoglobinuria have developed in some children after recovery from aplastic pancytopenia.

15.33 PANCYTOPENIA DUE TO MARROW REPLACEMENT

Diffuse replacement of bone marrow by nonhematopoietic tissue results in peripheral pancytopenia. *Neuroblastoma* is the childhood tumor that most frequently metastasizes to the bone marrow. *Osteopetrosis* is frequently associated with anemia and thrombocytopenia because of marrow obliteration; an element of hypersplenism may also be present. In these diseases the red cell morphology is frequently abnormal, showing teardrop forms and ovalocytes. Nucleated red cells are noted in the blood. Bone marrow transplantation has been used successfully in a small number of patients with severe osteopetrosis. *Acute leukemia* occasionally presents pancytopenia with a reticular appearance of the initially aspirated marrow. Adequate sampling or biopsy of the marrow from other sites will usually provide the correct diagnosis. A short trial of corticosteroid therapy that results in rapid return of the blood counts to normal favors a diagnosis of leukemia.

Myelofibrosis has occurred in a few infants and children, presenting as severe anemia with abnormal forms (teardrops, ovalocytes), nucleated red cells, and high white blood cell counts (leukoerythroblastic anemia), and with enlarged liver and spleen due to extramedullary erythropoiesis.

TRANSFUSIONS*

The most important indications for transfusions are to restore blood volume and treat shock following acute blood loss and to provide red cells for maintenance of the blood hemoglobin level. An individual component of blood, such as red cells, platelets, plasma, or specific plasma proteins, may often be used effectively in place of whole blood.

15.34 INDICATIONS FOR TRANSFUSION

Acute Hemorrhage

The signs and symptoms accompanying hemorrhage vary with the magnitude and rapidity of the blood loss. When 15–20% or more of the circulating blood volume is acutely lost, tachycardia, hypotension, and shock may develop, accompanied by weakness, restlessness, and syncope. Immediately after acute hemorrhage the hemoglobin or hematocrit level may be deceptively high, but hemodilution soon reduces this to a value reflecting the magnitude of the blood loss. Thrombocytosis and neutrophilia occur within a few hours and reticulocytosis within a few days of an acute bleeding episode. The most common causes of severe acute hemorrhage are trauma and gastrointestinal bleeding from peptic ulcers, Meckel diverticulum, and esophageal varices. In patients with defects of the hemostatic mechanism, exsanguinating hemorrhage may occur from nosebleeds or gastritis.

Severe bleeding in the perinatal period may result in the clinical picture of asphyxia pallida. Pallor, shock, tachycardia, and low venous pressures are seen. External hemorrhage may occur from the umbilicus or the gastrointestinal tract. The fetus may bleed before and during birth into the maternal circulation, and fetofetal transfusions may occur between identical twins.

Laboratory Data. The anemia of acute blood loss is usually normochromic and normocytic. Depending upon the duration of the hemorrhage and timing of the tests, compensatory reticulocytosis and normoblastemia may be seen. In the newborn infant with hemorrhage, the Coombs test result is generally negative and the level of serum bilirubin low. With loss of blood from fetus to mother, maternal blood will contain a minor population of red cells that contain Hgb F (Kleihauer-Betke technique).

Treatment. When possible, local measures to control the hemorrhage should be taken. Whole blood transfusions should be given to restore blood volume and treat shock; 20 mL/kg of blood should be administered initially. The need for additional blood will be determined by the clinical response and by physical and laboratory findings. Plasma or plasma expanders may be used to sustain the patient in shock until blood can be made available, but if the blood loss has been great, red cell replacement will be necessary.

Chronic Anemias

With anemias that develop slowly and stabilize at hemoglobin levels of 6–9 g/dL, the patient may have remarkably few symptoms, and transfusions are not routinely indicated. When such anemias result from deficiency of a specific factor, such as folic acid or iron, a rapid response will follow replacement therapy. Transfusion is indicated only if the anemia is profound or if infections or other complications are present. No firm rule can be made as to the hemoglobin level at which transfusion is recommended. Some children with iron deficiency anemia may have hemoglobin levels of 4–5 g/

---

*See Sec 8.47 for Exchange Transfusion.

dL with few signs of clinical or cardiorespiratory distress. A reasonable estimate of the effect of transfusion of packed red cells is that the increase in hematocrit (%) will equal the mL/kg of packed cells given. For example, if 5 mL/kg of packed cells is given, the recipient's hematocrit will rise about 5%. The formula assumes a recipient blood volume of about 75 mL/kg and a hematocrit of about 75% for packed red cells.

In progressive refractory anemias such as thalassemia major and pure red cell anemias, transfusions are necessary to sustain life. Packed red cells, especially leukocyte-poor or glycerol-frozen preparations, are preferred for control of such chronic anemias because they reduce the frequency of febrile reactions secondary to development of leukoagglutinins. The maximal dose of packed red cells to be given in one transfusion is 15 mL/kg; if signs suggestive of incipient congestive heart failure are present, considerably smaller amounts should be used. In extreme anemia with secondary heart failure, multiple small transfusions of 2–4 mL/kg of packed red cells may be helpful, and the simultaneous use of furosemide may be considered. If frank congestive heart failure is present, exchange transfusion should be considered, replacing the patient's blood isovolumetrically with packed red cells. Digitalis is of limited value.

15.35 USE OF BLOOD FRACTIONS
Platelet Transfusions

Platelets may be transfused to attain temporary hemostasis in some patients with thrombocytopenic hemorrhage. The life span of transfused platelets is normally 9–10 days. Although administration of fresh whole blood produces inconsequential rises in the recipient's platelet count, clinical hemorrhage may be controlled. Use of platelet-rich plasma or platelet concentrates prepared from fresh blood drawn in plastic equipment permits attainment of more nearly normal platelet counts. It is desirable to use platelets that are ABO and Rh compatible, but it is frequently impossible to do so. Infusion of platelet concentrates from incompatible donors rarely produces problems, but since these concentrates contain red cells, those from Rh-positive donors should not be given to Rh-negative recipients. Transfusion of platelets that are HLA compatible does not readily evoke isoimmunization and results in more satisfactory platelet survival. Platelet transfusions are temporarily beneficial in thrombocytopenias due to inadequate production, such as hypoplastic pancytopenia and leukemia, but are useless or of only transient value in states characterized by peripheral hyperdestruction of platelets such as idiopathic thrombocytopenic purpura. In addition, isoantibodies to platelet antigens are frequently formed after transfusions of platelets from multiple donors. With successive platelet transfusions, decreasing therapeutic responses are noted. Transfusion of one unit of platelet concentrate can be expected to produce an increment in platelet count of about 100,000/mm³ in the newborn and about 10,000 mm³ in the adult.

Granulocyte Transfusions

Because of the brief intravascular life span and low concentration of granulocytes in normal blood, transfusions of normal whole blood have no practical value in supplying white blood cells. Transient clinical and hematologic benefit in neutropenias has been reported from use of donor blood from patients with chronic granulocytic leukemia who have very high total white blood cell counts. Extraction of large numbers of polymorphonuclear leukocytes from normal donors can be accomplished with continuous-flow blood separators employing differential centrifugation or nylon fiber filter systems. Double-flow plasmapheresis and continuous flow centrifugation techniques are also used to harvest large numbers of granulocytes from single donors. Administration of granulocytes lowers mortality in profoundly leukopenic patients with gram-negative sepsis, and is used in management of febrile and infected patients with severe potentially self-limited neutropenia resulting from cancer chemotherapy or bone marrow transplantation. Granulocyte transfusions have been recommended for treatment of septic newborns who have neutropenia and depletion of granulocyte reserves (Sec. 8.59).

Plasma and Plasma Concentrates

In acute dehydration, when the plasma volume is decreased but the red cell mass is adequate, plasma can be used effectively to expand the blood volume and to restore circulation and renal blood flow. The usual dose of plasma is 10 mL/kg. The use of fresh plasma and of concentrates of plasma such as factor VIII and fibrinogen preparations for bleeding disorders is described elsewhere. The usual gamma globulin preparations cannot be administered intravenously because they form large reactive aggregates that produce hypotension and shock, but special preparations of gamma globulin that can be safely and effectively administered intravenously are now available.

15.36 SPECIAL CONSIDERATIONS
Choice of Blood for Transfusion

Storage of blood at 4° C results in a decrease in red cell viability that is proportional to the length of storage time. When blood is given for acute hemorrhage, this is of no consequence, but for children who must receive transfusions repeatedly the blood selected should be as fresh as possible.

A citrate-phosphate-dextrose (CPD) mixture has supplanted ACD as the standard anticoagulant because it better maintains red cell viability and function.

Blood for transfusion should be of the same blood group (O, A, B, or AB) as the recipient's. The donor red cells should always be tested for compatibility with the recipient's plasma (major cross-match) by the Coombs technique. Compatibility for the Rh antigens between donor and recipient is desirable. Rh-negative (d/d) persons should never receive Rh-positive blood; the reverse is permissible. Considerable battlefield experience indicates that the use of so-called universal donor blood (group O Rh-negative blood with a low titer of anti-A and anti-B isohemagglutinins) is safe, but with adequate modern blood banking facilities this is rarely necessary except in an emergency.

Risks of Blood Transfusion

Although modern technology has made blood transfusion a generally safe procedure, a definite risk is involved. Transfusions should be given, therefore, only when the benefit to the patient exceeds the inherent danger of the procedure. It has been estimated that 1 of every 2000 persons receiving a blood transfusion has a severe reaction as a result of the immediate procedure or its consequences. Problems may arise from:

Clerical Errors. The mislabeling or faulty identification of containers may lead to a patient's receiving the wrong blood. If a type O patient receives type A or B blood, fatal intravascular hemolysis may occur.

Red Cell Isoimmunization. In almost every blood transfusion the donor red cells have some antigen factor that the recipient does not possess. Many such factors are poor antigens, but some evoke intense antibody formation, the immunized persons being at increased risk if another transfusion is given.

Hepatitis. (See Sec. 11.76 and 12.80.) A small proportion of the normal population are asymptomatic carriers of agents for serum hepatitis. In the United States the routine screening of blood for HB$_s$Ag prior to transfusion has significantly reduced the risk for transfusion-related hepatitis B, but only about one third of donors who can transmit serum hepatitis have demonstrable hepatitis B–associated antigen (Australia antigen, HB$_s$Ag) in their blood. Currently, the most common cause of transfusional hepatitis is designated non A–non-B (see Sec. 11.76); it has a variable incubation period and is usually clinically mild. It seems to be fairly common and is often manifested by elevated levels of AST (SGOT) and ALT (SGPT). There is no reliable way to detect all carriers or to inactivate the agent in blood, the risk in pooled plasma being proportional to the number of donors to the pool. Use of frozen red blood cells is believed to reduce the risk of hepatitis. Syphilis, malaria, toxoplasmosis, and cytomegalovirus infection can also be transmitted by blood transfusion.

Acquired Immunodeficiency Syndrome (AIDS). AIDS was first reported in homosexual men and intravenous drug users. Later, cases were found among recipients of blood transfusions and hemophiliacs who had received factor VIII concentrate. The cause of AIDS is human T cell lymphotropic virus, type III (HTLV-III). (See Sec. 10.23 and 11.11.)

In the spring of 1985 blood banks in the United States began testing all donor blood for antibodies against HTLV-III, using an enzyme-linked immunosorbent assay (ELISA) that is believed to identify almost all potentially infectious blood. This procedure, with the exclusion of high risk persons from the donor population, should markedly reduce the risk of contracting this disease through transfusions.

Cytomegalovirus (CMV) Infection. Severe transfusion-transmitted CMV infections characterized by pneumonia, hepatitis, thrombocytopenia, and hemolytic anemia have been described in premature infants receiving blood from CMV-seropositive donors. Use of seronegative donors markedly reduces the incidence of this disease (see Sec. 8.68 and 11.68).

White Cell, Platelet, and Plasma Protein Immunization. White cells, platelets, and some of the serum proteins have polymorphic antigens; multiple transfusions may be associated with development of antibodies against these components.

Circulatory Overload. Patients with chronic anemia have expanded plasma volume and increased cardiac output, infusion of blood or plasma may precipitate congestive heart failure; rapid administration of large volumes of blood should be avoided.

Depletion of Labile Substances. Storage of blood is associated with loss of platelets and decreasing activities of the labile coagulation factors, such as factor VIII, 75% of which is lost after 7 days of storage. When massive or exchange transfusions of stored blood are given, a complex disturbance of hemostasis may ensue. Use of fresh blood will avoid these complications. As a general rule, when multiple transfusions are given in a short period of time, every 4th unit of blood should be fresh. Reconstitution of packed red cells with fresh frozen plasma is also effective. Acute citrate toxicity may occur.

Iron Overload. Each 500 mL of blood contains about 200 mg of iron. Patients with refractory anemias who need frequent transfusion ultimately have hemosiderosis. Iron deposited in skin, liver, spleen, and other organs may interfere with normal function (Sec. 15.4).

Reactions to Blood Transfusion

Allergic Reactions. These are associated with 1–2% of transfusions. The most common manifestation is urticaria with itching; occasionally, wheezing and arthralgia occur. The mechanism of these reactions is not certain, but they may be due to allergenic substances or to antibodies in the donor plasma. The development of urticaria alone does not necessitate discontinuing the transfusion; therapy with antihistamines or corticosteroids is effective in treating or preventing this type of reaction.

Febrile Reactions. The use of disposable plastic equipment has eliminated most external pyrogenic substances. Sensitization to white cell antigens may produce febrile reactions characterized by shaking chills and an increase in temperature of 1–2° C (2–4° F) beginning during or shortly after the transfusion and lasting only a few hours. The use of washed, leukocyte-poor packed cells excluding the buffy coat, and liberal dosage of salicylates may reduce these reactions. Use of reconstituted frozen red cells may greatly ameliorate severe febrile reactions. Rarely, a unit of blood may be contaminated with bacteria. Severe febrile reactions, shock, and death may occur if infected blood is transfused. Because it is difficult to differentiate febrile from hemolytic reactions, blood transfusions must be promptly discontinued if fever and chills occur during their administration.

Hemolytic Transfusion Reactions. Hemolytic reactions result in massive intravascular destruction of red cells, manifested clinically by fever, chills, headache, and back pain. These symptoms do not appear when the patient is anesthetized. In severe reactions, shock and acute renal failure may ensue. Hemoglobinemia and hemoglobinuria are usually observed. When a hemolytic reaction is suspected, the transfusion should be *terminated immediately*. Diagnosis is proved by reexamining the blood types of donor cells and of the recipient, repeating the cross-match, and examining plasma and urine for free hemoglobin. A diuresis should be established by fluid therapy and administration of mannitol. The patient generally survives the initial acute episode; if a period of renal failure can be adequately managed, recovery is the rule.

Polycythemia

Michael AF Jr, Mauer AM: Maternal-fetal transfusion as a cause of plethora in the neonatal period. Pediatrics 28:458, 1961.
Naeye R: Human intrauterine parabiotic syndrome and its complications. N Engl J Med 268:804, 1963.
Natelson EA, Lynch EC: Polycythemia vera in childhood. Am J Dis Child 122:241, 1971.
Ramamurthy RS, Brans YW: Neonatal polycythemia. 1. Criteria for diagnosis and therapy. Pediatrics 68:168, 1981.
Weinberger MM, Oleinick A: Congenital marrow dysfunction in Down's syndrome. J Pediatrics 77:273, 1970.

The Pancytopenias

Alter BP, Potter NU: Classification and aetiology of the aplastic anemias. Clin Haematol 7:431, 1978.
Beard MEJ: Fanconi anemia. Congenital disorders of erythropoiesis. Ciba Foundation Symposium No 37 (new series). New York, Elsevier, Excerpta Medica, North-Holland, 1976.
Bloom GE, Warner S, Gerald PS, et al: Chromosome abnormalities in constitutional aplastic anemia. N Engl J Med 274:8, 1966.
Camitta BM, Thomas ED, Nathan DG: Severe aplastic anemia: A prospective study of the effect of early marrow transplantation on acute mortality. Blood 48:63, 1976.
Williams DM, Lynch RE, Cartwright GE: Drug induced aplastic anemia. Semin Hematol 10:195, 1973.

Transfusions

Bove JR: Practical Blood Transfusion. 3rd ed. Boston, Little, Brown, 1986.
Bucholz DM: Pediatric transfusion therapy. J Pediatr 84:1, 1974.
Champlain R, Ho W, Gale RP: Antithymocyte globulin treatment in patients with aplastic anemia. N Engl J Med 308:113, 1983.
Christiansen RD, Rothstern G, Anstall HB: Granulocyte transfusions in neonates with bacterial infection, neutropenia, and depletion of mature marrow neutrophils. Pediatrics 70:1, 1982.
Gordon-Smith EC: Treatment of aplastic anemias. Hosp Pract 20:69, 1985.
Herzig RH, Herzig GP, Graw RG, et al: Successful granulocyte transfusion therapy for gram-negative septicemia. N Engl J Med 296:701, 1977.
Landesman SH, Gruzburg HM, Weiss, SH: The AIDS epidemic. N Engl J Med 312:521, 1985.

Mollison PL: Blood Transfusion in Clinical Medicine. 7th ed. London, Blackwell, 1983.

Race RR, Sanger R: Blood Groups in Man. 6th ed. London, Blackwell Scientific Publishers, 1975.

Storb R: Bone marrow transplantation for severe aplastic anemia. Semin. Hematol 21:27, 1984.

Yeager AS, Grumet FC, Hafleigh EB: Prevention of transfusion acquired cytomegalovirus infections in newborn infants. J Pediatr 98:281, 1981.

DISORDERS OF THE LEUKOCYTES

The leukocytes of the blood and their precursors in the bone marrow are easily studied, enumerated, and classified. The most important leukocyte functions are concerned with resistance to infection and disposal of products of cellular breakdown. Because characteristic changes occur in many diseases, the white blood cell and differential counts are important as general screening tests. Normal values are listed in Table 15–3.

The leukocytes are divided into two major classes: the granulocytes, consisting of neutrophils, eosinophils, and basophils, and the nongranulated lymphocytes and monocytes. White cells have cellular antigens different from those of the erythrocyte.

15.37 TYPES OF LEUKOCYTES

Neutrophils. Neutrophils are the predominating type of granulocyte. The nuclei of these cells have 1–5 segments and are called polymorphonuclear leukocytes. They have ameboid motility, chemotaxis, and the capacity for active phagocytosis. Wright stain gives their fine cytoplasmic granules a light purple (neutrophilic) color. These granules are lysosomes and contain digestive enzymes of several sorts, including proteases, cathepsins, and lysozymes. When bacteria or other particles are ingested by neutrophils, degranulation occurs as the enzymes of the granules are discharged into a vacuole formed about the ingested material. The phagocytic process is associated with a burst of metabolic activity and a considerable increase in oxygen consumption. The metabolic burst is associated with hydrogen peroxide formation and a marked increase in activity of the pentose phosphate pathway of glucose metabolism. Aberrations of the biochemistry of phagocytosis and intracellular digestion may result in markedly impaired resistance to disease.

The neutrophils occupy definable compartments or pools within the body. The *mitotic compartment* consists of myeloblasts, promyelocytes, and myelocytes of the bone marrow. The *maturation compartment* consists of metamyelocytes and band forms, which are relatively completely differentiated and have lost the capacity to divide but still reside within the marrow. The *marrow storage compartment* consists of a rapidly mobilizable reserve of mature neutrophils. It has been estimated that it takes 6–11 days for a cell to pass through the stages of differentiation from a myeloblast to a mature neutrophil emerging into the peripheral blood.

The neutrophils of the blood exist in two exchangeable pools of approximately equal size. The *circulating granulocytic compartment* is in equilibrium with a *marginal compartment* consisting of neutrophils sequestered in small blood vessels. Vigorous exercise or injection of epinephrine causes the marginal pool to be mobilized into the circulation. The half time of granulocytes within the circulation is 6–9 hr, after which they enter the *tissue pool*, where they carry out their primary function of phagocytosis. Little is known of their survival in the tissues.

The intramedullary mitotic and maturation compartments are generally estimated by examining bone marrow. Hypertrophy of the neutrophilic series is reflected in alterations of the ratio between myeloid and erythroid elements (M/E ratio). With chronic inflammatory processes the usual M/E ratio of 2–4:1 may be increased to 5–10:1. Adequacy of the marrow

storage compartment can be estimated from changes in the blood leukocyte count after intravenous injection of extracts of bacterial endotoxin or the steroid compound etiocholanolone. Normally a 2–4 fold increase in the numbers of circulating neutrophils results from such stimulated release of cells from the marrow storage compartment. In states of marrow hypoplasia or failure no increase occurs. Radioisotopic techniques can estimate the time required for maturation and release of neutrophils from the marrow or the rate of turnover of neutrophils in the blood.

Neutrophil formation and regulation can be assessed by the culture of cells in semisolid agar gel. Normal bone marow contains a small number of colony-forming cells or units (CFU). In tissue culture, CFU form aggregates of granulocytes under stimulation of a hormone-like glycoprotein, which has been designated colony-stimulating factor (CSF) and is elaborated by blood monocytes or tissue macrophages. Measurements of CFU and CSF are being used increasingly in the study of diseases involving neutrophils, along with assessments of neutrophil mobility and chemotaxis. The Rebuck skin window method may be used to study leukocyte migration and motility in vivo.

Eosinophils. Eosinophils are characterized by large coarse granules of a prominent red color with Romanowsky stains and by a nucleus with one or two segments. They normally account for fewer than 5% of circulating leukocytes. Eosinophil counts are depressed by high levels of adrenocortical hormones and increased in parasitic and allergic disorders. Eosinophilia may also accompany Hodgkin disease, and mild eosinophilia may be seen during convalescence from viral infections. The most pronounced eosinophilia encountered in the United States accompanies invasion of the tissues by parasitic helminths, in such diseases as visceral larva migrans and trichinosis. Familial, and presumptively genetic, eosinophilia has been described.

Basophils. These leukocytes are distinguished by coarse, deep blue granules that fill the cytoplasm and obscure the nucleus. They contain large amounts of heparin and histamine. They normally account for under 1% of the circulating leukocytes. Increases occur in chronic myelogenous leukemia and in generalized mast cell disease.

Lymphocytes. Lymphocytes constitute 30–60% of the blood leukocytes. Most are small cells measuring 9 μ in diameter, with a round, dark, blue-black nucleus and scanty blue cytoplasm. Other lymphocytes, probably younger forms, have more abundant blue cytoplasm. Lymphocytes are actively motile, but not phagocytic. The lymphocytes can be characterized as T or B lymphocytes on the basis of physical and immunologic properties (Chapter 10.) Marked lymphocytosis is characteristic of pertussis and the syndrome of infectious lymphocytosis. In infectious mononucleosis atypical lymphocytes characteristically appear in large numbers. Thymic alymphoplasia is associated with profound lymphopenia and immunoglobulin deficiency.

Monocytes. These large phagocytic cells are characterized by a large lobulated nucleus and an abundant gray cytoplasm containing fine azurophilic granules. They normally account for 1–5% of the circulating leukocytes; they are increased in such diseases as tuberculosis, systemic mycosis, bacterial endocarditis, and certain protozoan infections. Monocytes spend about 8 hr in the circulation before entering the tissues, where they become alveolar macrophages, Kupffer cells, and other tissue macrophages.

QUANTITATIVE DISORDERS OF THE NEUTROPHILS

Absolute neutrophil counts vary widely in normal subjects. The relative proportion of neutrophils and lymphocytes in the blood varies with age (Table 15–1). Neutrophils predominate at birth but decrease rapidly in the first few days of life. During infancy they constitute 20–30% of the circulating leukocytes. Parity between neutrophils and lymphocytes occurs by about 5 yr of age, but the approximately 70% predominance of neutrophils characteristic of the adult is not attained until puberty. In normal healthy children, therefore, from 20–70% of the total circulating white blood cells may be neutrophils. In absolute terms they number 2500–6000/mm³. Levels exceeding this range are designated neutrophilia or polymorphonuclear leukocytosis.

15.38 NEUTROPHILIA

Neutrophilia accompanies a wide variety of localized and generalized pyogenic infections as well as some noninfectious inflammatory processes. Both the total white blood cell count and the proportion of neutrophils increase. In addition, larger numbers of nonsegmented (band) neutrophils and even a greater number of cells that are more immature (metamyelocytes and myelocytes) may be seen ("shift to the left"). In general, younger children demonstrate more pronounced responses to infections than adults and manifest higher white cell counts with greater numbers of immature forms. When the total white cell count exceeds 40,000/mm³, a "leukemoid" blood picture is said to be present. A presumptive cause is usually evident for leukemoid reactions, such as infection, intoxication, and the like, but occasionally the blood picture may be difficult to differentiate from chronic myelogenous leukemia. The neutrophils in leukemoid reactions have elevated levels of alkaline phosphatase activity, whereas this enzyme is low in chronic myelocytic leukemia. The neutrophilia of infection or inflammation is accompanied by increased activity and hypertrophy of the entire neutrophilic series. On the other hand, the transient neutrophilia accompanying acute stress reflects shifts of previously formed neutrophils between circulating and marginal pools rather than actual increased production and is not accompanied by changes in marrow.

15.39 NEUTROPENIA

Neutropenia is a reduction below normal of the numbers of circulating neutrophils. This occurs in a substantial number of congenital and acquired diseases and results from either underproduction or peripheral hyperdestruction of neutrophils. When the absolute neutrophil count is under 1500/mm³, and especially under 500/mm³, the patient becomes unusually susceptible to bacterial infections, especially to those of the skin and respiratory tract. Buccal and rectal ulcerations are also frequently associated.

Infantile Lethal Agranulocytosis. This familial, probably autosomal recessive, disease is characterized by the onset in early infancy of recurrent, severe pyogenic infections, especially of the skin and the lung. The basic defect is unknown. Neutrophils are totally absent in the blood or present in reduced numbers (<300/mm³); absolute monocytosis and eosinophilia are present. The platelets are normal, and primary anemia is absent. The bone marrow contains markedly decreased numbers of mature neutrophilic precursors. The neutrophilic series is represented by abnormally vacuolated promyelocytes and myelocytes. CFU and CSF are usually normal. Lymphocyes and plasmacytes are prominent. Erythrocytic and megakaryocytic elements are normal.

There has been no effective therapy. Hematinics, corticosteroids, and splenectomy produce no beneficial effect. Bone marrow transplantation may offer a cure. Antibiotics may be of temporary value, but death frequently occurs during infancy or the first years of life as a result of overwhelming sepsis. Bone marrow transplantation may be considered.

Transitory Neutropenia of the Newborn. Neutrophilia is characteristic of the immediate postnatal period, but with severe infections, such as cytomegalic inclusion disease, toxoplasmosis, or bacterial sepsis, striking neutropenia may occur. Granulocyte transfusions have been advocated for neutropenic newborns with bacterial sepsis (Sec. 15.35). Newborn infants have been described with familial neutropenia and bacterial infections; in some cases the mother has also been neutropenic, suggesting transmission of a humoral inhibitor or antibody from mother to infant. Maternal isoimmunization to fetal neutrophil antigens is analogous to Rh sensitization. Bacterial infections usually respond to vigorous antibiotic therapy. The duration of neutropenia is variable, but usually lasts 2–4 wk.

Chronic Neutropenias. This group of diseases usually produces relatively mild clinical manifestations and is differentiated from the preceding disorder by its relative mildness and sporadic occurrence. The child experiences recurrent pneumonia, skin infections, and mouth ulcerations. Because of the paucity of granulocytes at sites of inflammation, the usual indications of infection, including pus, may be minimal. The white blood cell count is decreased, and there is a striking paucity of neutrophils; absolute neutrophil counts range from 0–1000/mm³. There is usually no anemia, and the platelets are normal. Compensatory monocytosis and eosinophilia are usually present. Serum protein studies demonstrate diffuse hypergammaglobulinemia. In the bone marrow there is often maturation arrest at the myelocyte or metamyelocyte stage as well as plasmacytosis, but no alteration of the erythrocytic and megakaryocytic elements. Some affected patients appear able to mobilize a neutrophilic response in case of major pyogenic infection.

Infections can be controlled by appropriate antibiotic therapy. Attempts to stimulate granulopoiesis with corticosteroids or other therapy are usually ineffectual. Several cases of congenital neutropenia have paradoxically responded to administration of chloramphenicol. Affected children tend to improve with age, and some undergo total remissions in late childhood. Familial patterns of occurrence have suggested both autosomal dominant and recessive transmission, and some cases appear to be sporadic. Bone marrow cultures from children with chronic neutropenia have revealed no consistent pattern; assay for colony-stimulating factor (CSF) is usually positive. Neutropenia may occur in patients with various immunodeficiencies. Immunoglobulin determinations are indicated.

Acquired Neutropenia. Decrease in the total white blood cell count and concomitant neutropenia occur in many viral infections, particularly roseola infantum, rubella, rubeola, and influenza. This is the most common type of neutropenia seen in children. Neutropenia is also characteristic of typhoid and paratyphoid infections and brucellosis. In severe pyogenic infections the observation of neutropenia is an ominous prognostic sign, often indicating the overwhelming nature of the disease. In some cases of rheumatoid arthritis and lupus erythematosus, neutropenia occurs; its pathogenesis in these diseases is uncertain but may represent peripheral sequestration or hyperutilization.

Acquired neutropenia may have an autoimmune basis.

Serologic assays for antineutrophil antibodies may be positive. In some such cases therapy with corticosteroids has been effective in increasing circulating neutrophil numbers. Children with the syndrome of the autoimmune neutropenia of early childhood have severe neutropenia (counts <300/mm³) that is usually discovered coincidently during mild infections. Neutropenia persists for 6–24 months and then undergoes spontaneous remission. Administration of intravenous gamma globulin (400 mg/kg) has rapidly, but transiently, restored the neutrophil count to normal.

A few cases of acquired infantile copper deficiency have had profound neutropenia and osseous abnormalities. Serum copper levels were very low, and hematologic responses occurred with oral copper therapy.

Neutropenia results from marrow insufficiency in leukemia, aplastic pancytopenia, and disseminated neoplasms such as neuroblastoma. In advanced megaloblastic anemia due to deficiency of vitamin B_{12} or folic acid, neutropenia regularly occurs, possibly because of ineffective leukopoiesis. On the other hand, an enlarged spleen may filter or sequester large numbers of neutrophils from the circulation. Ionizing radiation and such drugs or chemicals as nitrogen mustard, methotrexate, and benzene regularly cause marrow depression and neutropenia in any person receiving them in sufficient amounts.

Cyclic Neutropenia. This ill-defined disease is characterized by periodic episodes of fever and oral ulcerations, with profound neutropenia. Onset usually occurs by 10 yr of age. Neutropenia persists for 5–10 days, after which the white blood cell count returns to normal and symptoms abate. Such episodes occur in cycles, generally of 19–21 days but ranging from 14–30 days. Bone marrow during periods of neutropenia shows diminished numbers of neutrophilic precursors or maturation arrest. Between episodes blood and marrow are normal. Monocytosis may precede the drop in neutrophil count. Therapy is symptomatic, with antibiotics for bacterial infections. The course is usually benign, but catastrophic complications, including intestinal perforations and peritonitis, may occur. A similar disorder, genetically determined, occurs in the gray collie dog.

Pancreatic Insufficiency and Neutropenia
(Bodian-Shwachman Syndrome)

This is a familial syndrome of severe, chronic neutropenia, with pancreatic insufficiency due to atrophy and fatty replacement (Sec. 12.68 and 13.97). It can be diffentiated from cystic fibrosis by the normal electrolyte levels in sweat and the absence of pulmonary disease. The blood count and smear reveal decreased numbers of neutrophils and occasionally thrombocytopenia and anemia. Bone marrow is markedly hypocellular. Roentgenograms reveal metaphyseal dysostosis in some cases. The most prominent symptoms are related to pancreatic insufficiency, which produces malabsorption, diarrhea, and growth failure. This is to be differentiated from a syndrome of refractory sideroblastic anemia with vacuolated marrow precursors and fibrosis of the exocrine pancreas.

No therapy has been effective in improving the hematologic abnormalities; pancreatic enzyme replacements ameliorate the malabsorption.

15.40 DRUG-INDUCED NEUTROPENIA
(Malignant Agranulocytosis)

This syndrome is characterized by a profound reduction of neutrophils in the blood and of their precursors in the bone marrow, accompanied by severe systemic infection. It is usually self-limited but occasionally lethal.

Etiology. The drugs or agents that produce this condition do so in relatively small numbers of patients, so that idiosyncrasies seem partly responsible. In some instances, such as in neutropenia associated with aminopyrine, an immunologic basis is probable. This drug acts as a hapten in combination with a protein of the neutrophil, forming an antigenic complex that stimulates formation of a leukocidal antibody. Recently, the drug most frequently producing neutropenia has been the aminopyrine derivative, dipyrone (Pyralgin); the use of this potentially dangerous drug for its symptomatic effect on fever is inappropriate. Neutropenia following the use of phenothiazines has been attributed to a toxic inhibition of nucleic acid synthesis. Administration of semisynthetic penicillins (oxacillin, methicillin) may in large doses produce agranulocytosis after 3–4 wk. Recovery occurs promptly when the drug is discontinued. Other drugs associated with a significant incidence of neutropenia include thiourea derivatives and sulfonamides. In many cases of neutropenia no cause can be discovered.

Clinical Manifestations. An abrupt onset with a racking chill often occurs in aminopyrine-induced neutropenia. In other cases the onset may be insidious. The fever is septic, with frequent high spikes. Ulcerations of the mouth and rectum, cutaneous infections, and pneumonia are common, but purulent exudates are not formed so that the usual physical findings of pyogenic infections may not occur. Death results from overwhelming sepsis in the first week of the disease in about 20% of cases unless antibiotic therapy can control bacterial infections. Intestinal perforations may occur.

Laboratory Data. The total white blood cell count is reduced. Neutrophils are reduced (<1000/mm³), but compensatory monocytosis and eosinophilia are frequently present. There is no anemia or thrombocytopenia. Bone marrow changes depend upon the stage of illness. At the height of the disease the marrow is cellular, with normal numbers of erythroid precursors and megakaryocytes, but neutrophilic precursors are reduced. Of the nucleated cells 5–20% may be plasma cells. Recovery is presaged by a return of granulopoiesis in the marrow, which proceeds as a surge of maturation through the several stages of development. Bone marrow examination in this early recovery stage may be misinterpreted as showing a maturation arrest. Some 4–5 days after the return of precursors to the marrow, mature neutrophils reappear in the blood, and prompt defervescence and clinical improvement usually ensue.

Treatment. The most important therapeutic measure is immediate discontinuation of any medications that may be causative. Infection should be treated with therapeutic doses of antibiotics, the choice of which should be determined by cultures and sensitivity studies; when feasible, bactericidal antibiotics should be used. Prophylactic use of antibiotics is not indicated. Corticosteroid therapy is not of significant value. Once a patient has acquired neutropenia after administration of a specific drug, that drug or closely related agents should not be administered again. White blood cell transfusions have been used for support during periods of profound neutropenia.

15.41 INHERITED ABNORMALITIES OF THE LEUKOCYTES

Ninety per cent of the neutrophils in the blood of normal persons have 2–4 segments. Only about 5% are unsegmented (bands), and fewer than 5% have 5 or more segments. An increase in unsegmented forms, or shift to the left, usually indicates infection or inflammation, whereas hypersegmentation, or shift to the right, most commonly occurs in megaloblastic anemias due to folic acid or vitamin B$_{12}$ deficiency.

Hereditary Hyposegmentation (Pelger-Huet Anomaly). This defect of neutrophil segmentation is inherited as an autosomal dominant trait. In heterozygous persons more than 90% of circulating neutrophils and eosinophils either are unsegmented or have only two lobes. Their phagocytic capacity is normal, and no predisposition to infection is associated. The homozygous state may be lethal.

Hereditary Hypersegmentation (Undritz Anomaly). This rare condition, inherited as an autosomal dominant trait, is characterized by predominance of neutrophils with 4 and 5 or more segments. No adverse clinical effects are associated.

May-Hegglin Anomaly. This rare, dominantly transmitted anomaly involves the neutrophils and platelets. A majority of the neutrophils contain irregular blue cytoplasmic inclusions similar to Döhle bodies. Döhle bodies consist of precipitated ribosomal material and are usually observed in patients with severe systemic infections. In patients with the May-Hegglin anomaly no infection need be present. There are abnormally large platelets and, at times, thrombocytopenia. The thrombocytopenia responds to splenectomy.

Alder Anomaly. In this condition, which is probably transmitted as an autosomal recessive trait, the neutrophilic granulations are larger and stain much more prominently than normal ones. The granules are distinctly lavender or blue and are thus easily differentiated from eosinophils. A small proportion of patients with mucopolysaccharidoses may show somewhat similar granulations in their neutrophils (Reilly bodies) or, more commonly, metachromic granules in the cytoplasm of lymphocytes (Mitwoch bodies).

15.42 QUALITATIVE ABNORMALITIES OF THE NEUTROPHILS

A number of syndromes with intracellular defects of the neutrophils display increased susceptibility to infections despite adequate numbers of these cells in the circulation.

Chronic Granulomatous Disease (CGD). This disease is characterized by a metabolic defect (deficiency of NADPH-oxidase activity) which results in failure of intracellular killing of certain types of bacteria following their phagocytosis by neutrophils (Sec. 10.31).

Myeloperoxidase Deficiency. A few patients with increased susceptibility to pyogenic infections have defective and delayed intracellular killing of bacteria owing to a defect of the enzyme myeloperoxidase (Sec 10.33).

G-6-PD Deficiency. Blacks and most whites with G-6-PD deficiency (Sec. 15.17) have normal levels or only moderate decreases of leukocyte G-6-PD, but a few persons have been reported to have 1% WBC G-6-PD activity with lifelong susceptibility to recurrent infections, resembling chronic granulomatous disease (Sec. 10.34).

Chédiak-Higashi Disease. See Sec. 10.32.

Job Syndrome. This apt term describes patients with recurrent severe cold staphylococcal abscesses of the skin. Levels of serum IgE are markedly elevated and neutrophil chemotaxis is depressed. See Sec. 10.37.

Disorders of Leukocyte Chemotaxis. Migration of leukocytes to areas of inflammation and infection depends in part upon the complement system; accordingly, in congenital or acquired deficiency of any of several components of complement, impaired chemotaxis may result in infection. Isolated defects in chemotaxis due to cellular abnormalities have also been described (lazy leukocyte syndrome). See Sec. 10.37.

General

Davidson WM: Inherited variations in leukocytes. Br Med Bull 17:190, 1961.
Robinson WA, Mangalik A: The kinetics and regulation of granulopoiesis. Semin Hematol 12:7, 1975.

Neutropenia

Adam E, Pearson HA: Chloramphenicol-responsive congenital neutropenia. N Engl J Med 309:1039, 1983.
Al-Rashed R, Spangler J: Neonatal copper deficiency. N Engl J Med 285:841, 1971.
Boxer LA, Greenberg MS, Boxer GJ: Autoimmune neutropenia in children. N Engl J Med 293:748, 1975.
Leventhal JM, Silken AB: Oxacillin-induced neutropenia in children. J Pediatr 89:769, 1976.
Pearson HA, Lobel JF, Kocoshis SA, et al: A new syndrome of refractory sideroblastic anemia with vacuolization of marrow precursors and exocrine pancreatic dysfunction. J Pediatr 95:976, 1979.
Pincus SH, Boxer LA, Slossel TP: Chronic neutropenia in childhood. Am J Med 61:849, 1976.
Shwachman H, Diamond LK, Oski FA, et al: The syndrome of pancreatic insufficiency and bone marrow dysfunction. J Pediatr 65:645, 1964.

Qualitative Abnormalities

Baehner RL: Microbe ingestion and killing by neutrophils: Normal mechanisms and abnormalities. Clin Haematol 4:609, 1975.
Miller ME: Pathology of chemotaxis and random mobility. Semin Hematol 12:59, 1975.
Quie PG: Pathology of bactericidal power of neutrophils. Semin Hematol 12:143, 1975.

HEMORRHAGIC DISEASES

The blood is in dynamic equilibrium between fluidity and coagulation. This balance must be precisely maintained to assure that exsanguination does not follow trivial trauma or that spontaneous thrombosis does not occur. The hemostatic mechanism is complex: it involves local reactions of the blood vessels, the several activities of the platelet, and the interactions of specific coagulation factors that circulate in the blood. The vascular endothelium is the primary barrier against hemorrhage. When small blood vessels are transected, active vasoconstriction and local tissue pressure control minute areas of bleeding even without mobilization of the coagulation process, but the platelet is essential for maintenance of small blood vessels and of their endothelial stability. Hemostatic defects due to abnormalities of the vessels are manifested by small intracutaneous hemorrhages and petechiae. Hemorrhagic states related to the platelets and the soluble coagulation proteins are more dramatic and urgent.

15.43 SCHEMA OF COAGULATION

The classic schema of coagulation has pictured coagulation as proceeding in three phases: in phase I a hypothetical substance called thromboplastin is formed by interaction of plasma, platelets, and tissue juice; in phase II prothrombin is converted to thrombin in the presence of thromboplastin and calcium; and in phase III soluble fibrinogen is converted by thrombin into the visible fibrin clot. This simple scheme, involving only six substances, has been expanded; a dozen factors have now been defined, but retention of the concept of a basic three-phase reaction has considerable merit. Table 15–8 lists the currently recognized coagulation factors and their common synonyms. A comprehensive schema of coagulation is depicted in Fig 15–8.

In phase I, in addition to an increased number of factors, intrinsic and extrinsic systems have been recognized. The

Table 15–8. **The Coagulation Factors**

International Numbers	Synonyms	Comment
I	Fibrinogen	Number rarely used—congenital deficiency known (afibrinogenemia)
II	Prothrombin	Number rarely used—congenital deficiency known
III	Thromboplastin	No specific factor identified
IV	Calcium	Number rarely used
V	Labile factor, proaccelerin	Congenital deficiency known (parahemophilia, Owren disease)
VI	Activated labile factor, accelerin	No longer differentiated from factor V
VII	Stable factor, SPCA, proconvertin	Congenital deficiency known
VIII	Antihemophilic factor (AHF) or globulin (AHG)	Hemophilia A (classic hemophilia) results from congenital deficiency
IX	Christmas factor, plasma thromboplastin component (PTC)	Hemophilia B results from congenital deficiency
X	Stuart-Prower factor	Congenital deficiency known
XI	Plasma thromboplastin antecedent, PTA	Congenital deficiency known
XII	Hageman factor	No clinical symptoms associated with congenital deficiency
XIII	Fibrin stabilizing factor	Congenital deficiency known

intrinsic mechanism involves the successive enzymatic conversion of the inactive forms of factors XII, XI, and IX. Activated factor IX interacts with factor VIII, platelet factor 3, and calcium to activate factor X. Activated factor X interacts with factor V in generation of a plasma activity called prothrombinase that converts prothrombin to thrombin. The extrinsic mechanism involves the conversion of inactive factor VII to its active state by a substance (thromboplastin) derived from tissue fluid. In the extrinsic system active factor VII directly activates factor X.

Phase II of coagulation is concerned with the enzymatic cleavage of inactive prothrombin into smaller molecules, one of which is active thrombin. This step requires factor II as substrate as well as active factor X, factor V, and calcium.

Finally, in phase III thrombin splits four small peptides from the fibrinogen molecule, uncovering reactive sites in the fibrin monomer. These monomers then spontaneously poly-merize, both side to side and end to end, to form fibrin. Factor XIII facilitates lateral bonding by specific peptide cross-links between fibrin strands to form a stable three-dimensional clot. The coagulation mechanism interacts with other systems such as the kallikrein and fibrinolytic systems.

TESTS FOR EVALUATION OF THE HEMOSTATIC MECHANISM

Laboratory tests are of considerable value in the diagnosis of hemorrhagic disorders, but the importance of the history, including the family history, and of the physical examination cannot be overemphasized. Significant congenital defects are almost invariably associated with histories of easy bruising or prolonged bleeding after minor injury.

The platelet count, tourniquet test, and bleeding time are used to assess the integrity of hemostasis in small blood vessels. The *tourniquet test* is performed by inflating a blood pressure cuff to a point midway between the systolic and diastolic pressures for 5 min. Normally, this stress results in fewer than five petechiae on an area of skin on the forearm 2.5 cm square. A greater number of petechiae indicates thrombocytopenia, abnormally functioning platelets, or increased fragility or dysfunction of the small blood vessels. The *Ivy bleeding time* also assesses the vascular and platelet phases of hemostasis. A blood pressure cuff is applied to the arm and inflated to 40 mm Hg, and a stab incision 2 mm long and deep is made using a scalpel blade or utilizing a template. At 30-sec intervals drops of blood are blotted from the margin of the incision. Normally blood flow stops within 4–8 min. A *platelet count* or estimation is essential in the evaluation of any patient suspected of having a hemostatic disorder. When the platelet count is under 40,000/mm^3, those tests that rely upon platelet function, such as the bleeding time and tourniquet test, usually give abnormal results. Platelet function tests include measurement of clot retraction, glass bead adhesion (Salzman test), and platelet aggregation.

The *whole blood clotting time* is a crude but useful testing of the entire coagulation mechanism. The interval for a firm blood clot to form in a glass test tube is normally 8–12 min; if a careful three-tube technique is used, the upper limit of normal is 15–19 min. Normal clotting times may accompany fairly severe defects. Capillary tube clotting time is unreliable.

The three phases of coagulation can be individually assessed by simple, reliable tests. In any hemorrhagic state the adequacy of phase III should be ascertained first. Unless adequate fibrinogen is present, the blood is incoagulable, and the other laboratory tests in which the formation of a visible clot is the end-point must give abnormal results. Phase III can be evaluated by the *thrombin time*, the time required for plasma to clot after the addition of bovine thrombin. The normal throm-

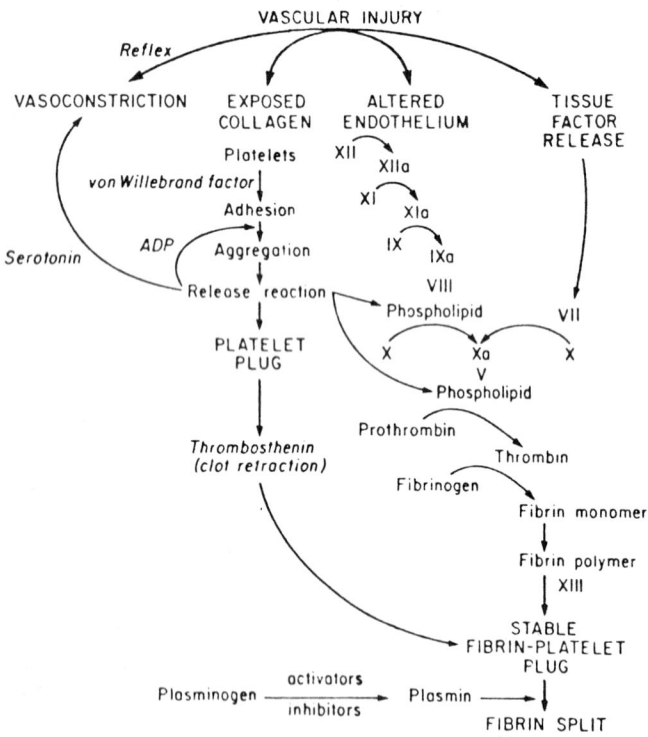

Figure 15–8. Diagrammatic representation of the hemostatic mechanism. (From Nathan DG, Oski FA: Hematology of Infancy and Childhood. 2nd ed. Philadelphia, WB Saunders, 1981.)

bin time is 15–20 sec. Prolongation indicates hypofibrinogenemia or a circulating anticoagulant. Fibrinogen can be measured also by chemical or immunologic methods.

Phase II as a whole is assessed by the *prothrombin time*, the time taken for plasma to clot after the addition of thromboplastin and calcium. Normal prothrombin time is 12–14 sec. If phase III is intact, a prolonged prothrombin time indicates a deficiency involving factors II, V, VII, or X, alone or in combination. Specific assays for all these factors are available. The level of ionized calcium must be below 2.5 mg/dL (1.25 mmol/L) in order to impair blood coagulation.

Phase I, the most complex part of the coagulation mechanism, can be evaluated by several tests. The *activated partial thromboplastin time* (PTT) is the time required for clotting of plasma that has been activated by incubation with kaolin when calcium and platelets, or a lipid substitute for platelets (partial thromboplastin), are added. The normal partial thromboplastin time is 25–40 sec. The PTT is a simple, inexpensive, and reliable way to assess the adequacy of factors XII, XI, IX, and VII. The *prothrombin consumption time* is a standard prothrombin determination performed on serum instead of plasma. Because prothrombin is used up during coagulation, the serum normally contains little prothrombin and the serum prothrombin time is prolonged to 35 sec or more. Deficiencies of the phase I factors are associated with poor utilization of prothrombin. If the serum prothrombin time does not differ significantly from that obtained with plasma, deficiency of one of the phase I factors is likely.

The *thromboplastin generation* test is the most sensitive of all the tests of phase I. The thromboplastic activity of an incubated mixture of plasma, serum, and platelet substrate is estimated at regular intervals. A deficiency of any of the phase I factors will be reflected in an abnormal generation test result. This test can be modified to quantitate precisely factors VIII and IX.

There is considerable difference in sensitivity among these tests. For example, a plasma level of factor VIII that is only 1–2% of normal is sufficient for a normal clotting time. A level of factor VIII at 3–5% of normal produces a normal prothrombin consumption test. Results of PTT and thromboplastin generation tests become abnormal when the factor VIII level is 15–20% of normal or less.

If the PTT, prothrombin consumption, or thromboplastin generation test results are abnormal, the way in which they can be corrected identifies the specific deficiency. Normal plasma adsorbed with barium sulfate retains factors VIII and XI. Normal serum contains factors IX and XI. Accordingly, if an abnormal test result can be rectified by adsorbed plasma but not by serum, factor VIII deficiency is proved. If an abnormal result is corrected by serum but not by adsorbed plasma, factor IX deficiency is present. If both serum and plasma are corrective, factor XI deficiency may be present.

COAGULATION DISORDERS

15.44 PHASE I DISORDERS—THE HEMOPHILIAS

The hemophilias are the most common and serious of the congenital coagulation disorders. They are associated with genetically determined deficiencies of factors VIII, IX, or XI.

Factor VIII Deficiency
(Classic Hemophilia; Hemophilia A; Antihemophilic Factor (AHF) Deficiency)

About 80% of cases of hemophilia are caused by a gene carried on the X chromosome that results in a profound depression of the level of factor VIII (AHF) activity in the plasma. The factor VIII molecule has two components: a high molecular weight portion designated VIIIag, which contains von Willebrand factor and an antigenic determinant, and a second low molecular weight portion designated VIIIc, containing the procoagulant or clotting activity. Specific antibodies have been made against both portions of the molecule. It is possible, therefore, to measure the concentrations of VIIIag and VIIIc in plasma; in the normal person their ratio is unity.

In the patient with severe classic hemophilia the VIIIag level in the blood is normal, but the level of VIIIc is reduced to 0–5% of normal. The disease is usually transmitted by asymptomatic female carriers to affected sons. A carrier state is characterized by a normal level of VIIIag antigen, while the VIIIc is reduced by 50–60%. These findings now identify the carrier female with accuracy and permit reliable genetic counseling in most instances.

In 80% of cases the family history is positive. Sporadic cases may represent new mutations and tend to be severe. The clinical severity depends upon the level of factor VIII in the plasma, severe cases having 0–1% of the normal activity, moderate cases 1–5%, and mild cases 6–30%. The degree of severity tends to be consistent within a given family.

Clinical Manifestations. Since factor VIII does not cross the placenta, a bleeding tendency may be evident in the neonatal period. Hematomas after injections and bleeding from circumcision are common, but many affected newborns exhibit no clinical abnormalities. As ambulation begins, excessive bruising occurs. Large intramuscular hematomas result from minor trauma. A relatively minor traumatic laceration, as of the tongue or lip, which bleeds persistently for hours or days, is frequently the event that leads to diagnosis. Ninety per cent of patients with severe disease have had clear clinical evidence of increased bleeding by 3–4 yr of age.

The hallmark of hemophilia is hemarthrosis. Hemorrhages into the elbows, knees, and ankles cause pain and swelling and limit movement of the joint; these may be induced by relatively minor trauma but often appear to be spontaneous. Repeated hemorrhages may produce degenerative changes, with osteoporosis, muscle atrophy, and, ultimately, a fixed, unusable joint. Spontaneous hematuria is a troublesome but not usually serious complication. Intracranial hemorrhage and bleeding into the neck constitute life-threatening emergencies.

Patients with factor VIII activities greater than 6% may not have severe spontaneous symptoms. These patients with "mild hemophilia" may experience only prolonged bleeding following tooth extractions, surgery, or injury.

Laboratory Data. The only significant laboratory abnormalities occur in coagulation tests and reflect serious deficiency of factor VIII. The partial thromboplastin time (PTT) is greatly prolonged. Prothrombin consumption is so markedly impaired that the serum and plasma prothrombin times may be similar. The thromboplastin generation test result is grossly abnormal. The abnormal tests can be corrected by fresh normal plasma adsorbed with barium sulfate but not by serum. In less severe cases only the PTT and thromboplastin generation test result may be abnormal.

Treatment. Prevention of trauma is an important aspect of care for the hemophilic child. During early life the crib and the playpen should be padded, and the child should be carefully supervised while learning to walk. As he becomes older, physical activities that do not entail a risk of trauma should be encouraged. It is important that a course between overprotection and permissiveness be followed. Aspirin and other drugs that affect platelet function may provoke severe hemorrhage and must be strictly avoided by hemophilic patients. Because the child with severe hemophilia will be exposed to blood products throughout his life, he should be immunized against hepatitis B (HB). The vaccine may be given as early as 3–6 mo of age (Sec. 11.76).

When bleeding episodes occur, replacement therapy is essential to prevent pain, disability, or life-threatening hemorrhage. The aim of therapy is to increase factor VIII activity in the plasma to a level securing hemostasis. Currently, this can be done only by the intravenous infusion of fresh plasma or plasma concentrates (fresh or fresh-frozen plasma in a dose of 10–15 mL/kg every 12 hr). This regimen maintains a plasma level from 10–25% of normal. Because of danger of circulatory overload no more than 30 mL/kg of plasma should be administered in a 24-hr period.

Therapy of the hemophilic patient has been considerably facilitated by the development of factor VIII concentrates; these permit fairly precise estimation of the dosage necessary to attain hemostatic levels. By definition, 1 mL of normal plasma contains 1 unit of factor VIII. Because the plasma volume is about 45 mL/kg, it is necessary to infuse 45 units/kg of factor VIII to increase its level in the hemophilic recipient from 0–100%. A dose of 25–50 units/kg of factor VIII is usually given to raise the recipient's level to 50–100% of normal. Because the half-life of factor VIII in the plasma is about 8–12 hr, repeated infusions can be given as necessary to maintain a desired level of activity.

Several factor VIII concentrates are available. The most inexpensive of these is cryoprecipitate, which can be prepared in the blood bank from fresh plasma. The yield from 250 mL of fresh plasma is one bag of cryoprecipitate, which usually contains 75–125 units of factor VIII; there may, however, be marked variability in the content of bags. One bag of cryoprecipitate/5 kg of body weight will raise the recipient's level to about 50% of normal. Because cryoprecipitate is produced from single units of whole blood, the risk of blood-borne diseases such as hepatitis B and acquired immunodeficiency syndrome (AIDS) (Secs. 10.23 and 11.11) is much less than when concentrates prepared from large plasma pools are used. Some authorities recommend using cryoprecipitates in younger children. Currently used AHF concentrates are tested to exclude the presence of HBV and HIV (AIDS). Heating the concentrates may decrease the risk even further.

Commercial preparations containing large amounts of relatively pure factor VIII are also available. These are dispensed as lyophilized powders in bottles of 250–500 units that can be reconstituted just prior to use; they have tremendous utility and convenience. Their potency and relatively low protein content permit rapid restoration of normal hemostatic levels with very small volumes.

Commercial factor VIII concentrates also contain anti-A and anti-B isohemagglutinins; when massive amounts of them are given to persons of blood group A or B, hemolysis may occur. Hyperfibrinogenemia due to the fibrinogen content of the concentrations may also result.

When the hemophilic child has significant bleeding, replacement therapy should be given promptly. Local measures should include application of cold and pressure, but these should not substitute for adequate replacement therapy. For ordinary hemarthroses, it is necessary to raise the factor VIII level to about 50% and to maintain it at least above 5% for 48–72 hr. A single infusion of 20–30 units/kg of factor VIII concentrate suffices, permitting the "one shot" therapy of ordinary bleeding episodes. Immobilization is indicated initially, but passive exercise should be started within 48 hr to prevent joint stiffness and fibrosis. The need for aspiration of blood from the joint is controversial. When the skin overlying the joint is very tense because therapy has been delayed, aspiration of blood, after adequate factor VIII has been given, may provide relief of pain. Replacement therapy is the most important part of management of hemarthrosis, since equally good results have been obtained by some who routinely practice joint aspiration and by others who do not. Aggressive replacement therapy with factor VIII and careful orthopedic management of hemarthroses can prevent much severe deformity and crippling, which are now much less common than in the past.

When hemorrhage occurs in vital areas such as the brain or neck or when major surgery is contemplated, intensive therapy using factor VIII concentrates is indicated to maintain the plasma level above 75% for 2 wk; a continuous infusion of factor VIII in a dose of 2 units/kg/hr can maintain a steady level of 50%. Epsilon-aminocaproic acid, 100 mg/kg every 6 hr, may be indicated, in conjunction with replacement therapy, for mucous membrane hemorrhage and dental extraction. Venipunctures should be performed only from superficial veins; aspiration from femoral or internal jugular veins is hazardous and has led to some deaths. There is compelling evidence that early treatment with factor VIII concentrates will reduce disability and deformity as well as the amount and duration of replacement treatment necessary for bleeding episodes. Parents, or the older patient himself, can be trained to give intravenous infusions of concentrates at home, with substantial decreases in hospitalization, morbidity, and risk of blood-transmitted diseases.

The major obstacles to home treatment have been the unavailability and cost of concentrates and the reluctance of some health insurance programs to underwrite this kind of treatment. Home treatment with periodic assessment and counsel from the physician represents optimal or ideal management for the hemophilic child and family, and this enlightened management may permit the present generation of hemophilic children to enter adult life without major physical or psychologic crippling. On the other hand, some long term complications may result from modern therapy. Abnormalities of hepatic enzyme activities are found in 50% of patients. Instances of chronic active hepatitis and cirrhosis have occurred. A high proportion of patients now have antibodies against HB, and many have antibodies against the AIDS agent (HTLV-III). These findings are the basis for recommending active immunization against HB. Hypertension and renal disease with hematuria occur in many adult patients; their causes have not been defined. Recent reports indicate that in mild and moderate hemophilia circulating factor VIII activity increases after administration of desmopressin (DDAVP) or danazol. These agents are not effective in severe hemophilia but may be useful in treating moderate bleeding episodes in patients who have mild disease.

Factor VIII Inhibitors. Five–10% of patients with hemophilia become refractory to factor VIII therapy because a circulating inhibitor or antibody develops. The development of inhibitors is not related to the number of plasma transfusions, and replacement therapy should not be withheld in hope of avoiding this. These inhibitors are IgG globulins and are specifically active against factor VIII. The inhibitors may be of low titer and transient or of extremely higher titer and very persistent. The "Bethesda unit" of inhibition is the amount of inhibitory activity in 1 mL of plasma that reduces the factor VIII level in 1 mL of normal plasma from 1 to 0.5 unit. It is virtually impossible to overpower a high titer inhibitor, but when hemorrhage occurs, massive doses of factor VIII concentrates or exchange transfusions with fresh blood should be given and may be of temporary benefit. Such replacement therapy should be limited to life-threatening hemorrhage. Immunosuppressive therapy has been of no value.

Another attempt at therapy of the hemophilic child who has developed a factor VIII inhibitor has used certain factor IX concentrates (Konyne, Proplex), which apparently contain small amounts of activated factor VII and other coagulants. These activated coagulants enter the coagulation cascade distal to the level of factor VIII (Fig. 15–8) and so bypass the effects of the inhibitor. However, the activities, of various preparations and even of different lots of the same preparation vary markedly.

Prenatal Diagnosis. Each male fetus of a mother who carries hemophilia has a 50% risk of having the disease. Prenatal diagnosis is possible through examination of the blood of the (male) fetus, which can be obtained at fetoscopy at 20–22 wk of gestation. Fetal plasma is assayed for VIIIag and VIIIc; as in the older patient, a VIIIag level markedly higher than the VIIIc level will identify an affected male. It has recently become possible to identify a fetus with hemophilia by examining DNA polymorphisms in amniotic fluid fibroblasts. Trophoblastic biopsy in fetuses at risk may permit the diagnosis of hemophilia as early as 10–12 wk of gestation.

Factor IX Deficiency
(Christmas disease; Hemophilia B)

About 15% of cases of hemophilia are due to a genetically determined deficiency of factor IX. This disease is clinically indistinguishable from factor VIII deficiency and is also transmitted as an X-linked recessive trait. The disease has a wide range of clinical severity, which in general corresponds to the level of factor IX in the serum.

Laboratory Data. The partial thromboplastin time (PTT), prothrombin consumption, and thromboplastin generation test results are usually abnormal. These in vitro abnormalities can be corrected by normal serum but not by absorbed normal plasma.

Treatment. Replacement therapy is accomplished by infusions of plasma. Ten to 15 mL/kg should be given every 12–24 hr during bleeding episodes. The response to fresh or fresh-frozen plasma is superior to that obtained with stored plasma; cryoprecipitate and factor VIII concentrates are of no value.

Commercial concentrates containing factors II, VII, IX, and X (Konyne, Proplex) have excellent levels of factor IX—about 250 units/bottle—and can be given in dosage similar to that outlined for factor VIII. Because the half-life of factor IX is about 24 hr, administration may be less frequent. Some of the commercial concentrates are contaminated with the agent for serum hepatitis; they must be used with caution, particularly in patients with liver disease. Episodes of thrombosis have occurred following use of these concentrates, especially in postoperative patients, presumably because they contain coagulants.

Factor XI Deficiency
(Plasma Thromboplastin Antecedent [PTA] Deficiency; Hemophilia C)

This usually mild bleeding disorder is inherited as an autosomal dominant or completely recessive trait. Typical cases are seen in both sexes. The usual clinical manifestations are mild, including nosebleeds; excessive hemorrhage and hemarthroses are rare. The PTT, prothrombin consumption, and thromboplastin generation test results are abnormal in the more severe cases. Adsorbed normal plasma and serum correct the deficiency. Plasma therapy in a dose of 10–15 mL/kg every 12–24 hr should be given for significant clinical hemorrhage.

Factor XII Deficiency
(Hageman Factor Deficiency)

Homozygous occurrence of an autosomal gene results in a profound deficiency of factor XII. Despite markedly abnormal test results of the 1st phase of coagulation (PTT and clotting times), affected persons have no clinical abnormalities of bleeding; in fact, some patients have a thrombotic tendency.

Von Willebrand Disease
(Vascular Hemophilia)

This dominantly inherited disease is complex and variable in its chemical manifestations. It is characterized by a vascular abnormality which prolongs bleeding time and by decreased levels of factor VIII. In contrast to classic hemophilia, there is no discrepancy between the levels of VIIIc and VIIIag; in von Willebrand disease both are depressed. The platelets in von Willebrand disease have decreased adhesiveness, and they do not aggregate when the antibiotic ristocetin is added to platelet-rich plasma, unlike platelets from normal individuals. This platelet defect is attributed to deficiency of a plasma factor necessary for normal platelet functioning (VW factor).

Clinical manifestations are nosebleeds, bleeding from the gums, menorrhagia, prolonged oozing from cuts, and increased bleeding after trauma or surgery. The bleeding time is usually prolonged. Fresh plasma infusions result in increases in factor VIII activity which are sustained for several days because of de novo synthesis, but they have an inconsistent effect on the bleeding time. Cryoprecipitate corrects the prolonged bleeding time and is probably the preferred form of replacement therapy for hemorrhage or of preparation for surgery. The recommended dose is 3–4 bags of cryoprecipitate/10 kg of body weight every 12 hr for 2 days and then 2 bags/10 kg/24 hr for 4–6 days. DDAVP may also be used as in hemophilia (Sec 15.44).

15.45 PHASE II DISORDERS

Factors II, V, VII, and X are involved in the 2nd phase of coagulation and are designated the *prothrombin complex.* The factors are produced in the liver, and all except factor V require vitamin K for normal synthesis. The vitamin is necessary for the α-carboxylation of glutamic acid residues, which converts inactive precursors of factors II and VII into their active forms. Gamma carboxylation permits interaction with Ca^{++}. The laboratory diagnosis of these deficiencies depends upon a prolonged prothrombin time. Significant bleeding does not usually occur until the prothrombin time exceeds 20–25 sec, corresponding to a level of 10–15% of normal.

Genetically determined congenital deficiencies of factors II, V, and VII have been described, the most common of which is factor V deficiency (parahemophilia, Owren disease). The clinical manifestations of these deficiencies are mucocutaneous hemorrhages, bleeding into tissues, and hemorrhages after injury. Hemarthroses occur infrequently. These deficiencies are refractory to vitamin K therapy, and fresh plasma should be administered for active hemorrhage.

Hemorrhagic Disease of the Newborn

Hemorrhagic disease of the newborn is a self-limited bleeding disorder resulting from a deficiency of the coagulation factors dependent upon vitamin K. Whether hepatic immaturity may also contribute to the genesis of hemorrhagic disease of the newborn has been questioned.

The levels of factors II, VII, IX, and X are about 50% of normal in umbilical cord blood and decline rapidly to reach a nadir at 48–72 hr of life. In 0.25–0.5% of infants the decline is so extreme that severe hemorrhage may result. Thereafter the levels of these factors slowly increase but remain below adult values for several weeks. The increase results from absorption of vitamin K from the diet. Cow's milk contains a good level of vitamin K. Breast milk, on the other hand, has quite low levels, and symptomatic hemorrhagic disease of the newborn is much more common in breast-fed than in formula-fed infants unless vitamin K prophylaxis is given.

Clinical Manifestations. In most instances hemorrhagic manifestations become evident on the 2nd–3rd day of life.

Melena, bleeding from the navel, and hematuria are frequent signs of the disorder. The most serious complications are intracranial hemorrhagic and hypovolemic shock.

Treatment. Prophylactic administration of vitamin K_1 to the newborn prevents the postnatal decline of the factors of the prothrombin complex and virtually eliminates hemorrhagic disease of the newborn. Preparations of vitamin K_1 are indicated, for they do not have the hemolytic effect of large doses of synthetic vitamin K analogues. Vitamin K given to the prepartal mother may be beneficial, but a therapeutic effect is more certain if the drug is administered to the infant. As little as 25 μg of vitamin K prevents the postnatal decline of the prothrombin complex; the currently recommended dose of 1 mg of vitamin K_1 is safe and effective, given parenterally or orally. Larger doses do not increase the therapeutic effect.

In overt hemorrhagic disease 1 mg of vitamin K_1 should be given by intravenous or intramuscular injection. Clinical hemorrhage usually stops within 2 hr. If intracranial or other serious hemorrhage has occurred, an infusion of 10–15 mL/kg of fresh plasma will immediately correct the hemostatic defects. Profound anemia and shock may be corrected by infusions of fresh blood.

Premature infants may experience a complex hemorrhagic state involving several coagulation factors as well as platelet abnormalities. Vitamin K therapy is ineffective in correcting the abnormalities because of hepatic immaturity. Fresh plasma infusions are indicated if significant hemorrhage occurs.

Vitamin K deficiency rarely occurs after the neonatal period, though "late" hemorrhagic disease has been reported in the Far East, especially Japan, in children who are breast fed. Intestinal malabsorption of fats and prolonged administration of broad spectrum antibiotics may result in vitamin deficiency, and cystic fibrosis and biliary atresia may be complicated by disorders of the prothrombin complex. Prophylactic administration of water-soluble vitamin K is indicated in these situations. In the past certain formulas based on meats or hydrolysates of protein were low in vitamin K, but this deficiency has been corrected. In advanced liver disease, synthesis of the factors of the prothrombin complex may be compromised by hepatocellular damage. Vitamin K therapy is not often effective in correcting the disorders if advanced liver disease is present. The anticoagulant properties of dicumarol and related anticoagulants depend on interference with activation of factors II, VII, and X. Vitamin K_1 is a specific antidote.

15.46 PHASE III DISORDERS

Congenital Afibrinogenemia. This rare hemorrhagic disorder is due to an autosomal recessive gene. Despite totally incoagulable blood these patients usually do not have severe spontaneous hemorrhages or hemarthroses, but trauma or surgery may be followed by severe bleeding. Therapy with 100 mg/kg of concentrated fibrinogen provides a hemostatic plasma level. Since the plasma half-life of fibrinogen is 5 days, frequent infusions are not necessary. A high risk of homologous serum hepatitis attends use of fibrinogen concentrates. Cryoprecipitate also contains fibrinogen and may be used effectively for therapy.

Congenital Dysfibrinogenemias. A number of abnormal fibrinogens with defective function may be associated with mild bleeding states. Inheritance is dominant. The thrombin time is prolonged, but chemical or immunologic methods reveal normal levels of fibrinogen.

Factor XIII Deficiency (Fibrin-Stabilizing Factor Deficiency). Deficiency of factor XIII has its onset most often in infancy, with bleeding after separation of the umbilical cord stump. Gastrointestinal, intracranial, and intra-articular hemorrhages have been the most common clinical manifestations.

Routine coagulation studies are normal. Factor XIII deficiency is diagnosed by finding an abnormal solubility of the clot in 5 M urea solution and a short euglobulin lysis time.

Abildgaard CF: Current concepts in the management of hemophilia. Semin Hematol 12:223, 1975.
Abildgaard CF, Button M, Harrison J: Prothrombin complex concentrate (Konyne) in the treatment of hemophilic patients with factor VIII inhibitors. J Pediatr 88:200, 1976.
Aledort LM: Current concepts in diagnosis and management of hemophilia. Hosp Pract 17:77, 1982.
Baehner RL, Strauss HS: Hemophilia in the first year of life. N Engl J Med 275:524, 1966.
Bleyer WA, Hakami N, Shepard TH: The development of hemostasis in the human fetus and newborn infant. J Pediatr 75:838, 1971.
DeForges JF: AIDS and preventative treatment in hemophilia. N Engl J Med 308:94, 1983.
Glader BE, Buchanan GR: The bleeding neonate. In: Smith CA (ed): The Critically Ill Child—Diagnosis and Management. 2nd ed. Philadelphia, WB Saunders, 1977.
Hathaway WE: The bleeding newborn. Semin Hematol 12:175, 1975.
Hilgartner MW: Hemophilic arthropathy. Adv Pediatr 21:139, 1974.
Lane PA, Hathaway WE: Vitamin K in infancy. J Pediatr 106:351, 1985.
Perkins HA: Correction of the hemostatic defects of von Willebrand's disease. Blood 30:375, 1967.
Sutherland JM, Glueck H, Gliser G: Hemorrhagic disease of the newborn. Am J Dis Child 113:524, 1967.
Wanier AI, Lusha JM: DDAVP: Useful alternative to blood components in moderate hemophilia A and von Willebrand's Disease. J Pediatr 102:228, 1983.

THE PURPURAS

The purpuras are a group of diseases in which small hemorrhages occur into the superficial layers of the skin, producing areas of purple discoloration. Minute extravasations of blood about the small vessels are recognized as petechiae; more extensive hemorrhages cause ecchymoses. Bleeding may also occur from the mucous membranes and into other organs and tissues. The purpuras may be classified into two general groups according to platelet count. In *thrombocytopenic purpuras* the platelet count is reduced below 40,000/mm³, and hemorrhages are due to this quantitative deficiency. In *nonthrombocytopenic purpuras* bleeding results from defects in the small blood vessels or from defective platelet function despite their adequate numbers.

Platelets are non-nucleated, cellular fragments produced by the megakaryocytes of the bone marrow. The large size of the megakaryocyte reflects its polyploidy. As the megakaryocyte reaches maturity, fragmentation of the cytoplasm occurs and large numbers of platelets are liberated. They have a life span in the circulation of 7–10 days. The platelet has a number of intrinsic antigens, which are distinct from those of the red blood cell; some are shared by the leukocytes.

The platelets are intimately involved in both the vascular and the clotting aspects of hemostasis. They are necessary for integrity of the vascular endothelium; when small blood vessels are transected, platelets accumulate at the site of injury, forming a hemostatic plug. Platelet adhesion is initiated by contact with extravascular components such as collagen. Release of thromboxane (a prostaglandin derivative) and endogenous ADP causes firm aggregation. Serotonin and histamine liberated during these processes increase local vasoconstriction. Platelets have a phospholipid with partial thromboplastin activity, which makes an important contribution to coagulation. They also transport other blood coagulation factors through adsorption to the platelet surface. Finally, the platelet is necessary for normal clot retraction.

The *normal platelet count* is 150,000–400,000/mm³. Counts below this range indicate thrombocytopenia, due either to inadequate production or to excessive destruction or removal of platelets. Inadequate production is almost always due to marrow dysfunction, with decreases in the number of megakaryocytes. By contrast, in the thrombocytopenias due to increased destruction, the megakaryocytes are quantitatively normal or increased. The hypomegakaryocytic thrombocytopenias result from aplasia of the marrow or from its infiltration by abnormal or neoplastic tissue. Because of the grave prognosis of such disorders bone marrow aspiration is indicated in every case of significant unexplained thrombocytopenia. Bone marrow aspiration can usually be performed without serious bleeding even in patients with severe thrombocytopenia, since thromboplastins in tissue juice will usually effect hemostasis.

15.47 NONTHROMBOCYTOPENIC PURPURAS

PURPURA ASSOCIATED WITH NORMAL NUMBERS OF PLATELETS

The most common nonthrombocytopenic purpura is *anaphylactoid purpura*, or *Henoch-Schönlein syndrome* (Sec. 10.64), an acute inflammatory process of unknown origin involving the small blood vessels of the skin, joints, gut, and kidney. The striking centrifugal distribution of the rash and involvement of the legs and buttocks are characteristic, particularly when combined with arthritis, nephritis, or gastrointestinal bleeding. The petechiae must be differentiated from those of early meningococcemia or septicemia due to other microorganisms. Septic emboli cause the petechiae observed in bacterial endocarditis. Toxic vasculitis may produce a hemorrhagic rash as a reaction to drugs such as arsenicals and iodides. Similar findings may occur during viral or rickettsial infections.

In *thrombasthenias*, or thrombocytopathic purpuras, quantitatively normal platelets have defective function. Abnormal function is reflected in petechiae and excessive bleeding. The abnormality of platelet function may also be revealed by defective clot retraction or by failure of the patient's platelets to support normal thromboplastin generation. Platelets in these diseases may be much larger than normal and have other abnormal morphology. A number of other congenital disorders of platelet function have been described, some with associated somatic defects; these have been summarized by Weiss.

DRUG-INDUCED ABNORMALITIES OF PLATELET AGGREGATION

Some drugs produce an irreversible reduction of prostaglandin synthesis within the platelet by inhibition of cyclooxygenase enzymes. This action prevents release of endogenous ADP and the prostaglandin derivative thromboxane, which are essential for platelet aggregation. This abnormality can be demonstrated most easily with a platelet aggregometer, by which an ablation of the so-called secondary wave of platelet aggregation can be demonstrated. The most important drug having this effect is aspirin. The effect is not dose-related. Abnormal platelet aggregation can be demonstrated in adults within 1 hr of ingestion of as little as 300 mg of aspirin. This abnormality persists for 4–6 days, until the platelets which have been exposed to the drug have been replaced. Under usual circumstances the effects of these drugs produce no clinical problems, though prolongation of the bleeding time is frequently seen. If, however, the patient has an underlying bleeding disorder such as hemophilia or undergoes a surgical operation, severe hemorrhage may occur. Aspirin or other drugs that inhibit platelet aggregation are contraindicated in these circumstances and should be replaced with other agents such as acetaminophen when indicated. Aspirin may have transplacental effects on platelet function in the newborn, producing neonatal hemorrhage; maternal aspirin consumption should be avoided during the last trimester of pregnancy. Transfusions of normal platelets are indicated if serious hemorrhage follows administration of aspirin.

15.48 THROMBOCYTOPENIC PURPURAS

Idiopathic Thrombocytopenic Purpura (ITP)

Acute idiopathic thrombocytopenic purpura (ITP), the most common of the thrombocytopenic purpuras of childhood, is associated with petechiae, mucocutaneous bleeding, and, occasionally, hemorrhages into tissues. There is a profound deficiency of circulating platelets despite adequate numbers of megakaryocytes in the marrow.

Etiology. The disease often appears to be related to sensitization by viral infections, for in about 70% of cases there is an antecedent disease such as rubella, rubeola, or viral respiratory infection. The interval between infection and onset of purpura averages 2 wk. By analogy with the disease seen in adults, it seems likely that an immune mechanism is the basis for the thrombocytopenia. Platelet antibodies can be detected in some acute cases. Increased amounts of IgG have been found bound to platelets and may represent immune complexes adsorbed on the platelet surface. No consistently reliable test yet exists for serologic diagnosis of ITP.

Clinical Manifestations. The onset is frequently acute. Bruising and a generalized petechial rash occur 1–4 wk after a viral infection or without antecedent illness. The bleeding is typically asymmetrical and may be most prominent over the legs. Hemorrhages in mucous membranes may be prominent, with hemorrhagic bullae of the gums and lips. Nosebleeds may be severe and difficult to control. The most serious complication is intracranial hemorrhage, which occurs in fewer than 1% of cases. The liver, spleen, and lymph nodes are not enlarged. Except for the signs of bleeding the patient appears clinically well. The acute phase of the disease associated with spontaneous hemorrhages lasts for only 1–2 wk. Thrombocytopenia may persist, but spontaneous mucocutaneous hemorrhages subside. In some instances the onset is more insidious, with moderate bruising and few petechiae.

Laboratory Data. The platelet count is reduced below 20,000/mm³. The few platelets observed on blood smear are large in size (megathrombocytes) and reflect increased marrow production. Those tests that depend upon platelet function such as the tourniquet test and bleeding time and clot retraction give abnormal results. The white blood cell count is normal, and anemia is not present unless significant blood loss has occurred.

Bone marrow aspiration reveals normal granulocytic and erythrocytic series and frequently modest eosinophilia. Normal or increased numbers of megakaryocytes are seen. Some of the latter are immature, with deep basophilic cytoplasm; platelet budding may be scanty, but there is no pathognomonic or diagnostic megakaryocyte morphology. The changes seen reflect increased megakaryocytic turnover.

Differential Diagnosis. Idiopathic thrombocytopenic purpura must be differentiated by marrow examination from aplastic or infiltrative processes of the bone marrow. Marrow aplasia or replacement is unlikely if the physicial examination is normal and the blood count is normal except for thrombocytopenia. On occasion, however, failure to perform a marrow examination may lead to diagnostic error and delay institution of correct therapy. Significant enlargment of the spleen will suggest primary liver disease with congestive splenomegaly, lipidosis, or reticuloendotheliosis. Thrombocytopenic purpura may be an initial manifestation of systemic lupus erythematosus or lymphoma, but this sequence is unusual in young children; in adolescents the possibility is greater, and serologic studies for systemic lupus erythematosus are indicted. Genetically determined thrombocytopenias must be considered in infants (particularly males) found to have low platelet counts.

Treatment. Idiopathic thrombocytopenic purpura has an excellent prognosis even when no specific therapy is given. Seventy-five per cent of patients recover completely within 3 mo, most within 8 wk. Severe spontaneous hemorrhages and intracranial bleeding are usually confined to the initial phase of the disease. After the initial acute phase, spontaneous manifestations tend to subside. Nine–12 mo after the onset about 90% of affected children have regained normal platelet counts, and relapses are unusual.

Fresh blood or platelet concentrates are of no value or are of transient benefit because transfused platelets survive only briefly, but they should be administered when life-threatening hemorrhage occurs.

When the disease is mild and hemorrhages of the retina or mucous membranes are not present, no specific therapy may be indicated. The affected child should be protected from falls or trauma. Bacterial infections should be treated with appropriate antibiotics. Vitamins K and C have no therapeutic effect.

Infusions of plasma and, more recently, intravenous gamma globulin have been found to be followed by sustained rises of platelet count. Large doses of intravenous gamma globulin (400 mg/kg for 4 days) will result in remission of many cases of acute and occasional cases of chronic ITP.

Corticosteroid therapy is of great value; though it has not decreased the number of chronic cases, it does reduce the severity and shorten the duration of the initial phase. In more severe cases therapy with a corticosteroid, such as prednisone in a dose of 1–2 mg/kg/day or its equivalent, is indicated. The necessity for corticosteroid therapy in mild cases has been debated, though the platelet count returns to a hemostatic level more rapidly with such therapy. If the hemorrhagic manifestations are severe or if intracranial hemorrhage is suspected because of headache, meningismus, or other neurologic signs, larger doses of prednisone (5–10 mg/kg/day) should *be used initially.* This therapy is continued until the platelet count is normal or for 3 wk, whichever comes first. At this point, steroid therapy should be discontinued even if the platelet count remains low. Prolonged corticosteroid theapy is not indicated and may depress the bone marrow, in addition to producing cushingoid changes and growth failure. If thrombocytopenia persists for 4–6 mo, a second short course of corticosteroid therapy may be given. At the present time whether the initial therapy of choice in acute ITP should be no therapy, intravenous gamma globulin, or corticosteroids is being reassessed. Splenectomy should be reserved for chronic cases, defined by thrombocytopenia persistent for more than 1 yr, and for the severe ones that do not respond to corticosteroids. Considerable improvement can be expected in most instances. Only about 2% of cases of idiopathic thrombocytopenia purpura in children tend to be chronic and refractory. In these chronic cases therapy with immunosuppressive drugs (azathioprine, vincristine) may be attempted.

Other Thrombocytopenic Purpuras

Drug-Induced Thrombocytopenias. A number of drugs may be associated with immune thrombocytopenia. Quinidine and apronalide (Sedormid) function as haptens that combine with proteins on the platelet surface and stimulate antibody formation. Administration of these drugs to sensitized persons is followed by severe thrombocytopenia. This syndrome is unusual in pediatric practice because the responsible drugs are rarely prescribed. In any case of thrombocytopenia, however, a careful search for any drug exposure should be made and the patient removed from contact with potential offenders.

Wiskott-Aldrich Syndrome and Other Inherited Thrombocytopenias. The Wiskott-Aldrich syndrome consists of eczema, thrombocytopenic hemorrhage, and increased susceptibility to infection due to an immunologic defect that is transmitted as an X-linked recessive trait (see Sec. 10.18). The bone marrow contains a normal number of megakaryocytes, but many have bizarre nuclear morphology. Homologous platelets survive normally when transfused into these patients, but autologous platelets have a shortened life span and are small in size. Wiskott-Aldrich syndrome may represent an unusual circumstance in which thrombocytopenia results from abnormal platelet formation or release despite quantitatively adequate numbers of megakaryocytes. Splenectomy has often been followed by overwhelming sepsis and death, but significant improvement in thrombocytopenia occurs after splenectomy. Prophylactic use of penicillin is probably essential postsplenectomy. A number of patients with Wiskott-Aldrich syndrome have developed lymphoreticular malignancies. A few cases have been reported to benefit from administration of transfer factor or from bone marrow transplantation.

A number of other types of inherited thrombocytopenias have been described. Some are X-linked, and some have autosomal transmission. Responses to therapy, including splenectomy, have usually been disappointing. The inordinately high mortality of young males splenectomized for presumed idiopathic thrombocytopenic purpura suggests that, even without other stigmata, X-linked thrombocytopenia may represent a variant of Wiskott-Aldrich syndrome. Thus, the young thrombocytopenic male must be carefully studied before a diagnosis of ITP is made. A platelet survival study is indicated in such patients.

Thrombopoietin Deficiency. A few patients have had chronic thrombocytopenia attributed to deficiency of a megakaryocyte maturation factor contained in normal plasma. Plasma infusions repeatedly produced a sustained rise in the platelet count. In somewhat similar cases episodic thrombocytopenia and microangiopathic hemolysis have been reversed by infusions of plasma.

Thrombocytopenia with Cavernous Hemangioma (Kasabach-Merritt Syndrome). Some infants with large cavernous hemangiomas of the trunk, extremities, or abdominal viscera have severe thrombocytopenia and other evidence of intravascular coagulation. Histologic and isotopic studies indicate that platelets are trapped and destroyed within the extensive vascular bed of the tumor. The peripheral blood shows thrombocytopenia and red cell fragments, and the bone marrow contains adequate numbers of megakaryocytes. Spontaneous thrombosis within the tumor may lead to obliteration of the vascular channels and spontaneous recovery; radiation therapy in a single dose of 600–800 rad may accelerate this process, but repeated courses may be necessary. When anatomically feasible, external compression or total excision may be attempted, but surgery may be associated with uncontrollable hemorrhage. Corticosteroids may hasten involution and warrant trial, especially in the young infant. Splenectomy is unnecessary and contraindicated.

Neonatal Thrombocytopenia

Thrombocytopenia of the newborn may reflect diseases primary in the infant's hematopoietic system or may be due to transfer of abnormal factors from the mother.

Thrombocytopenias may occur in a variety of fetal and neonatal infections and may be responsible for serious spontaneous bleeding. These include viral infections (especially rubella and cytomegalic inclusion disease); protozoal infections such as toxoplasmosis; syphilis; and bacterial infections, especially those caused by gram-negative bacilli. Hemolysis is usually also present in infants with prominent anemia and jaundice. The liver and spleen are considerably enlarged. The bone marrow changes are variable, but reduced numbers of megakaryocytes may be seen.

Immune Neonatal Thrombocytopenia. About 30% of infants born of mothers with active idiopathic thrombocytopenic purpura have in the neonatal period thrombocytopenia due to transplacental transfer of antiplatelet antibodies. Rarely, infants with neonatal disease have been born of mothers with past histories of idiopathic thrombocytopenic purpura who have normal platelet counts and whose disease has been inactive for many years. Petechiae are not present initially but appear in a generalized distribution within a few minutes after birth. Bleeding from bowel or kidney and intracranial hemorrhage may occur. In mild cases there may be few abnormal findings. Hepatosplenomegaly is not present. The duration of the thrombocytopenia is 2–3 mo. Therapy is not strikingly successful, but fresh blood, exchange transfusions, or platelet transfusions may be temporary value in arresting acute bleeding. Corticosteroid therapy has not been proved beneficial but can be used when thrombocytopenia is severe (platelet counts below 20,000/mm³). Because of the self-limited nature of the disease, splenectomy is contraindicated. Corticosteroid therapy given to the mother 1 wk prior to delivery or administration of intravenous gamma globulin to the mother late in pregnancy may reduce the severity of disease in the infant.

When the fetus has platelet antigens that the mother does not have, isoimmunization may occur. If maternal antibodies to fetal platelet antigens reach a sufficiently high titer, enough may cross the placenta to produce thrombocytopenia in the fetus. The disease may be familial, and first-born infants are frequently affected. The clinical signs include petechiae and other hemorrhagic manifestations. By use of sensitive tests involving complement fixation, antiplatelet antibodies can be demonstrated in about 50% of cases. The PLA-1 antigen is most frequently involved. Exchange transfusion is temporarily effective in stopping bleeding. If compatible platelets can be obtained (these are most easily procured by preparing washed platelet concentrates from the mother), they offer specific effective therapy. Infants born of successive pregnancies may be affected. Elective cesarean section has been advocated to spare the infant's head the trauma of delivery.

When the mother has drug-induced thrombocytopenia, both antibody and drug may cross the placenta and cause neonatal thrombocytopenia. Corticosteroid therapy and especially exchange transfusions should be considered when bleeding manifestations are severe.

Congenital Hypoplastic Thrombocytopenia with Associated Malformations (Thrombocytopenia Absent Radius [TAR] Syndrome). Severe thrombocytopenia associated with aplasia of radii and thumbs and cardiac and renal anomalies occurs as a familial condition. Severe hemorrhagic manifestations are evident in the first days of life. Hemoglobin levels are normal; leukocytosis and even leukemoid reactions have been found in some cases. Megakaryocytes are absent from the bone marrow.

The anomalies in this disease are similar to those observed in Fanconi pancytopenia, in which the hematologic abnormalities are not usually observed until the 3rd–4th yr of life. In this disorder chromosomes do not show the abnormalities found in Fanconi syndrome. No infants with congenital hypoplastic thrombocytopenia have been reported to develop full blown Fanconi syndrome, nor have both conditions been observed in the same family.

15.49 THROMBOCYTOSIS
(Thrombocythemia)

Platelet counts in excess of 750,000/mm³ may be designated as thrombocytosis. Markedly elevated counts may accompany hemorrhage, iron deficiency anemia, hemolytic anemias, and primary myeloproliferative disorders. Acute and chronic inflammatory states may be accompanied by elevated platelet counts. Platelet counts exceeding 600,000/mm³ are regularly observed in Kawasaki disease. Persons with asplenia and children with sickle cell anemia often have somewhat elevated platelet counts. After splenectomy for idiopathic thrombocytopenic purpura or hemolytic anemia the platelet count often rises precipitously and may exceed 1,000,000/mm³ 10–14 days postoperatively. In general, no specific therapy such as anticoagulation is necessary, for thrombosis is extremely rare. The use of aspirin (or dipyridamole), which inhibits platelet function, may be considered if there are factors predisposing to thrombosis.

A case of primary thrombocytosis associated with thrombotic episodes and myocardial infarction has been described.

Canales ML, Mauer AM: Sex-linked hereditary thrombocytopenia as a variant of Wiskott-Aldrich syndrome. N Engl J Med 277:899, 1967.
Glader BE, Buchanan GR: The bleeding neonate. In: Smith CA (ed): The Critically Ill Child—Diagnosis and Management. Ed 2. Philadelphia WB Saunders, 1977.
Hall J, Levin J, Kuhn J, et al: Thrombocytopenia with absent radius (TAR). Medicine 48:411, 1969.
Imbach P, Barundune S, d'Apuzzo V: High dose gamma globulin for idiopathic thrombocytopenic purpura. Lancet 1:1228, 1981.
Karpatkin M, Pargesh F, Karpatkin S: Platelet counts in infants of women with autoimmune thrombocytopenia: Effect of steroid administration to the mother. N Engl J Med 305:936, 1981.
Karpatkin S: Autoimmune thrombocytopenic purpura. Blood 56:329, 1980.
Lightsey AL, Koenig HM: Platelet associated immunoglobulin G in childhood idiopathic thrombocytopenic purpura. J Pediatr 94:20, 1979.
Lum LG, Tubergen DG, Corash L, et al: Splenectomy in the management of thrombocytopenia of the Wiskott-Aldrich Syndrome. N Engl J Med 302:892, 1980.
McIntosh S, Pearson HA: Isoimmune neonatal purpura. J Pediatr 82:1020, 1973.
Sartorius JA: Steroid therapy of acute idiopathic thrombocytopenia purpura in children: Pulmonary results of a randomized cooperative study. Am J Pediatr Hem Oncol 6:165, 1984.
Sills RH: Thrombotic thrombocytopenia purpura. Am J Pediatr Hem Oncol 6:425, 1984.
Simons SM, Main CA, Yarsh HM, et al: Idiopathic thrombocytopenic purpura in children. J Pediatr 87:16, 1975.
Spach MA, Howell DA, Harris JS: Myocardial infarction with multiple thrombosis in a child with primary thrombocytosis. Pediatrics 31:268, 1963.
Weiss HJ: Platelet physiology and abnormalities of platelet function. N Engl J Med 293:531, 1975.
Zinkham WH, Osborn JE, Medearis DN Jr: Blood and bone marrow findings in congenital rubella. J Pediatr 67:985, 1965.

15.50 DISSEMINATED INTRAVASCULAR COAGULATION
(Consumption Coagulopathy)

Consumption coagulopathy is a unifying concept linking a large group of conditions associated with disseminated intravascular coagulation (DIC). Consequences of this process include widespread intravascular deposition of fibrin and may lead to tissue ischemia and necrosis, a generalized hemorrhagic state, and hemolytic anemia.

Etiology. A number of pathologic processes may incite episodes of disseminated intravascular coagulation, including hypoxia, acidosis, tissue necrosis, endotoxic shock, and endothelial damage. Accordingly, it is not surprising that a large number of diseases have been reported associated with disseminated intravascular coagulation. These include incompatible blood transfusions, cyanotic congenital heart diseases, sepsis (especially gram-negative), rickettsial infections, snakebite, purpura fulminans, giant hemangioma, malignancies, acute promyelocytic leukemia, and many other conditions.

Clinical Manifestations. Disseminated intravascular coagulation most frequently accompanies a severe systemic disease process. Bleeding frequently first occurs from sites of venipuncture or surgical incision, with associated petechiae and purpura. Tissue thrombosis may involve many organs and may be most spectacular as infarction of large areas of skin and subcutaneous tissue or of kidneys. Anemia due to hemolysis may develop rapidly.

Laboratory Data. There is no well defined sequence of events. The labile coagulation factors (II, V, and VIII), fibrinogen, and platelets may be consumed by the ongoing intravascular clotting process, with prolongation of the prothrombin, partial thromboplastin, and thrombin times. Platelet count may be profoundly depressed. Blood contains fragmented burr and helmet-shaped red cells (schizocytes), changes referred to as microangiopathic. In addition, because the fibrinolytic mechanism is activated, fibrin split products (FSP) appear in the blood.

Treatment. The most important component of therapy is control or reversal of the process that initiated disseminated intravascular coagulation. Infection, shock, acidosis, and hypoxia must be treated promptly and vigorously. If the underlying problem can be controlled, bleeding quickly ceases, and there is improvement of the abnormal laboratory findings.

Infusions of platelets and fresh-frozen plasma may be considered as replacement therapy to support the child until the underlying disease can be controlled. The use of heparin in disseminated intravascular coagulation has become restricted because there is increasing evidence that it does not alter mortality or prognosis. Most authorities restrict its use to situations in which there is actual widespread thrombosis, as in purpura fulminans. If heparin is to be used, it should be given in doses of 100 units (1 mg)/kg intravenously every 4–6 hr. In the bleeding sick neonate with disseminated intravascular coagulation, exchange transfusion with fresh blood may be considered.

15.51 THROMBOPHLEBITIS

Symptomatic thrombophlebitis is uncommon in children. The most common precipitating factor is trauma of the lower extremities or pelvis. Stasis from immobilization increases the risk. Increased frequency of spontaneous thrombophlebitis has been reported in pregnancy, with the use of oral contraceptive agents and in the nephrotic syndrome. Management commonly involves manipulation of the clotting mechanism.

Massive deep thrombophlebitis involving an entire lower extremity produces diffuse edema, pain, and cyanosis. Thrombophlebitis of the deep veins of the lower leg is accompanied by calf pain elicited by sharp dorsiflexion of the foot (Homan sign). A deep painful cordlike mass can sometimes be felt. When necessary, diagnosis can be corroborated by venography.

Venous thrombosis of the deep leg veins should be treated with bed rest, elevation of the leg, and heat. Heparin should be administered intravenously in a dose of 50–100 units/kg every 4 hr. Alternatively, continuous intravenous therapy can be accomplished by an initial injection of 50–75 units/kg of heparin to be followed in 2 hr by constant infusion of 10–20 units/kg/hr. The partial thromboplastin time should be maintained at 60–80 sec (twice its normal value). When the process appears to be resolving, the patient can be maintained with oral anticoagulation with sodium warfarin. The adolescent or young adult should receive a loading dose of 10 mg of warfarin (2.5–5.0 mg for smaller children). Daily dose is 1–5 mg, but adequacy of dosage should be assessed frequently by determinations of prothrombin time, which should be maintained

between 20 and 30 sec. Therapy should be continued for 3–6 mo.

Pulmonary embolism may occur as a complication of deep vein thrombophlebitis; signs vary with the magnitude of the infarct. Chest roentgenogram and radionuclide perfusion studies are useful in diagnosis. Long-term anticoagulation is necessary.

Congenital deficiency of antithrombin III, an autosomal dominant trait, is associated with recurrent episodes of deep vein thrombosis and pulmonary embolism. Standard coagulation tests are normal, but antithrombin III levels are 25–50% of normal in affected individuals. Chronic therapy with warfarin has been suggested.

Bennet B, Mackie M, Douglas AS: Familial thrombosis due to antithrombin III deficiency: An extensive family study. Thromb Haemost 38:78, 1977.

15.52 THE FIBRINOLYTIC MECHANISM

Fibrinolysis, the process of dissolution of the clot, is a complex and essential physiologic mechanism. It comprises a number of fairly well defined factors, the most important of which involves a fibrinolytic enzyme called plasmin and its inactive precursor plasminogen. Thrombin and a urokinase found in urine are particularly potent converters of inactive plasminogen to its active enzymatic form. The fibrinolytic system is activated at the same time that coagulation occurs, with the result that in disease associated with diffuse intravascular coagulation, increased fibrinolytic activity of the plasma and fibrin degradation products (fibrin split products, FSP) is also often found in the circulation. Increased fibrinolytic activity is demonstrated in the test tube by spontaneous dissolution of the clot on incubation of clotted blood or by a shortened euglobulin lysis time. Rarely, spontaneous fibrinolytic states may be associated with hemorrhagic symptoms. It may be difficult to differentiate these primary fibrinolytic states from consumption coagulopathies, in which fibrinolysis is a secondary phenomenon. In consumption coagulopathies factors I, II, V, and VIII and platelets are usually decreased, whereas in fibrinolytic states platelets are usually normal and the other factors inconstantly affected. Treatment with epsilon-aminocaproic acid (EACA) may be of value in fibrinolytic states, but it is not indicated in consumption coagulopathies.

15.53 HEMOLYTIC-UREMIC SYNDROME

See also Sec. 17.13.

This acute disease of infancy and early childhood usually follows an episode of acute gastroenteritis. Shortly thereafter, signs and symptoms of hemolytic anemia, thrombocytopenia, and glomerulonephritis develop. Bilateral renal cortical necrosis may occur, and case fatality rates as high as 30% have been reported. Its sometimes epidemic occurrence suggests that an infectious agent may be involved.

Laboratory Data. The hemolytic anemia is associated with characteristically bizarre red cell morphology. Many of the red cells are contracted and distorted, with prominence of spherocytes, burr cells, and helmet-shaped forms (Fig. 15-2F). A depressed platelet count despite normal numbers of megakaryocytes in marrow indicates excessive peripheral destruction. Tests of the coagulation mechanism are usually normal. Protein, red cells, and casts are present in the urinary sediment, and grave renal damage is reflected in oliguria and azotemia.

Treatment. For management of uremia and anuria see Sec. 17.13. Transfusions are indicated for severe anemia. Corticosteroid and heparin therapy do not appear to affect survival or prognosis.

15.54 THROMBOTIC THROMBOCYTOPENIC PURPURA

This rare and serious disease has many similarities to the hemolytic-uremic syndrome. Diffuse embolism and thrombosis of the small blood vessels of the brain are evidenced by shifting neurologic signs such as aphasias, blindness, and convulsions. The prognosis is grave. Laboratory findings include thrombocytopenia and a hemolytic anemia associated with distorted and fragmented red cells microangiopathy. Plasmapheresis and plasma or intravenous gamma globulin infusions are effective in 60–70% of cases. Corticosteroids and splenectomy are reserved for refractory cases.

15.55 PURPURA FULMINANS

Purpura fulminans is an unusual disease that typically occurs in the convalescent phase of a bacterial or viral infection. Diffuse symmetrical hemorrhages occur, with prominent inflammatory vasculitis and necrosis of skin and subcutaneous tissues, particularly involving the buttocks and lower extremities. Systemic toxicity may be extreme, and mortality is high. In nonfatal cases large areas of gangrenous skin and muscle may slough, leaving areas requiring plastic surgical repair. The platelet count is normal or low. Fragmented red cells may be seen on blood smear. The levels of consumable coagulation factors, especially of fibrinogen, are decreased. Replacement therapy with fibrinogen and fresh plasma transfusions and high doses of corticosteroids have appeared to be helpful on occasion. Intravenous administration of heparin, 50–100 units/kg (0.5–1 mg/kg) every 4–6 hr or the use of dextran infusions may arrest the progression of the cutaneous lesions and correct the coagulation defects.

Allen DM: Heparin therapy of purpura fulminans. Pediatrics 32:211, 1966.
Corrigan JJ, Jordan CM: Heparin therapy in septicemia with disseminated intravascular coagulation. N Engl J Med 283:778, 1970.
Corrigan JJ, Kiemat JF: Effect of heparin in experimental gram-negative septicemia. J Infect Dis 131:138, 1975.
Hathaway WE: Disseminated intravenous coagulation. In Smith CA (ed): The Critically Ill Child. 2nd ed. Philadelphia, WB Saunders, 1977.
Liberman E: Hemolytic uremic syndrome. J Pediatr 80:1, 1972.

15.56 THE SPLEEN

The spleen has excited speculation since antiquity. Pliny believed it to be the seat of mirth and laughter; Galen pronounced it an organ full of mystery. No unique cells or tissues occur within the spleen, but the particular arrangements and anatomic relations within it are responsible for unique functions. The spleen is a large mass of lymphoid and phagocytic reticuloendothelial cells with a complex network of tortuous capillaries and fenestrated sinusoids. These impart the important properties of a biologic filter.

Functions. A number of functions can be assigned to the spleen, some of which are germane to hematologic processes and diseases.

Reservoir Function. In lower animals the spleen is a contractile organ because considerable smooth muscle is present in the capsule and trabeculae. In humans little muscle is present, and the reservoir function is normally not very great. The spleen does release both factor VIII and platelets following infusion of epinephrine. The normal spleen contains only about 25 mL of blood, but when the spleen enlarges for any reason, its content of blood increases. The sequestration crisis of sickle cell states is an exaggeration of reservoir function.

Hematopoiesis. The spleen is a site of active blood formation during fetal life, but by about 6 mo of gestation hematopoiesis disappears unless a condition such as hemolytic disease of the newborn is present. In a few exceptional diseases such as thalassemia and osteopetrosis, hematopoiesis persists or is resumed postnatally. The stimulus for this is not known.

"Culling." This term has been used to describe the ability of the spleen by virtue of its unique circulation and structure to remove damaged or abnormal blood cells from the circulation. This function is clearly demonstrated by the fact that red cells and platelets lightly coated by antibodies are selectively sequestered and destroyed by the spleen. The spleen's activity in destroying spherocytes is another example of culling.

"Pitting." The spleen has the ability to remove or "pit" intracytoplasmic inclusions such as Howell-Jolly bodies or siderotic granules from within the red cell without destroying the cell. The blood of a person with no spleen contains relatively large numbers of these intracellular inclusions.

Destruction of Old Red Cells. The spleen is probably the principal site of destruction of senescent red cells. This function is easily assumed by other portions of the reticuloendothelial system, however, and red cell life span is not significantly increased in the absence of spleen.

Membrane Effect. The normal spleen is postulated to have an ill-defined effect on the red cell membrane. When the spleen is absent, red cells are flatter and thinner than normal, increased numbers of target cells are seen, and osmotic fragility is decreased. Examination of red blood cells by the technique of interference phase contrast microscopy shows membrane indentations resembling craters in 20% or more of the cells of asplenic persons. Fewer than 1% of the red cells of individuals with normal spleen have these depressions or "pocks," which may be small vesicles.

Filtering and Immunologic Functions. Because of the intimate relation of the circulating blood with lymphoid and reticuloendothelial elements within the spleen, this organ plays an important role in primary defense against bacteria that gain access to the circulation. The spleen is especially vital in the immature and nonimmune person, for it constitutes the primary site of clearance of organisms such as pneumococci in the absence of specific antibody. The spleen has a relatively minor role in overall antibody formation so long as the antigen is administered by intramuscular or subcutaneous routes, but the spleen is essential to antibody formation in response to small doses of particulate intravenous antigens.

The spleen participates in a major way in synthesis of IgM, properdin, and "tuftsin," a phagocytosis-promoting tetrapeptide. Levels of these humoral factors are depressed in the splenectomized child.

Hormonal Function. It has been postulated that the spleen produces a hormonal substance ("splenin") that exerts an effect on bone marrow activity. There is little evidence for such a hormone, and "hypersplenism" is better explained on the basis of excessive filtering or culling activities. The spleen can be functionally inactive despite clinical enlargement, as in young children with sickle cell anemia (functional hyposplenism).

Clinical Examination. Careful and gentle palpation of the relaxed abdomen provides reliable information about the size of the spleen. The tip can be felt at the left costal margin in 5–10% of normal children and in a higher proportion of children with viral infections. The spleen must be increased to two to three times average size before it can be regularly

Table 15–9. Some Causes of Splenomegaly in Children

I. *Hematologic diseases*
   Hemolytic anemias—due to extramedullary hematopoiesis and
      reticuloendothelial hyperplasia
   A. Congenital and acquired hemolytic anemias
   B. Hemoglobinopathies and thalassemia
II. *Infections*
   A. Bacterial: septicemias; typhoid; endocarditis
   B. Viral: Epstein-Barr, cytomegalovirus, etc.
   C. Protozoal: malaria, toxoplasmosis
III. *Congestive splenomegaly*
   A. Secondary to portal or splenic vein obstruction
   B. Secondary to intrahepatic disease—cirrhosis
   C. Chronic congestive heart failure
IV. *Infiltrations*
   A. Lipidoses—Niemann-Pick, Gaucher diseases
   B. Nonlipid reticuloendothelioses
V. *Cysts*
   A. Congenital—epidermoid cysts
   B. Acquired—pseudocysts
VI. *Neoplasms*
   A. Leukemia and lymphosarcoma
   B. Hodgkin disease
   C. Hemangioma and lymphangioma
VII. *Miscellaneous*
   A. Rheumatoid arthritis (Still disease)
   B. Lupus erythematosus

felt on physical examination. Lesser degrees of enlargement can be detected radiographically. An enlarged spleen must be differentiated from other masses in the left upper quadrant. Useful physical characteristics that aid in identifying the spleen include concealment of its upper margin by the rib cage, the presence of a palpable notch, and the absence of overlying bowel. When it is impossible to be certain of the identity of a mass, isotopic scanning studies are of value. Short-lived isotopes such as technetium-99m (^{99m}Tc) may be used to label gelatin sulfur colloid particles. Injected intravenously, this radioactive colloid is rapidly cleared by reticuloendothelial elements in the liver, spleen, and, to a lesser extent, bone marrow; scanning permits definition of the size and configuration of spleen and liver. This technique has proved of great value in demonstrating anatomic abnormalities of the spleen; it is noninvasive and involves a very low radiation exposure.

The spleen has vascular, lymphatic, and reticuloendothelial components; pathologic processes involving any of these may produce splenomegaly. Table 15–9 lists important causes of splenic enlargement.

15.57 CONGESTIVE SPLENOMEGALY
(Banti Syndrome)

The venous outflow from the spleen may be obstructed within the liver or in the portal or splenic veins (Sec. 12.88). This vascular obstruction produces congestion and ultimately splenomegaly. Liver diseases associated with parenchymal inflammation, fibrosis, and vascular constriction include postnecrotic cirrhosis, galactosemia, Wilson disease, cystic fibrosis, biliary atresia, α_1-antitrypsin deficiency, and microcystic disease of liver and kidney. Septic omphalitis, either primary or following umbilical vein cannulation, may progress to portal vein thrombophlebitis and thrombosis. Rarely, congenital or acquired anomalies of the splenic or portal veins may cause obstruction and secondary splenomegaly. In some areas of the world schistosomiasis and malaria are important causes of splenomegaly.

Clinical Manifestations. Observation or palpation of an enlarged spleen may be the initial indication of the disease process. The enlarged spleen may filter out and destroy excessive numbers of blood cells and platelets and thus cause thrombocytopenic hemorrhage and anemia. In response to portal vein obstruction, collateral circulation develops through the short gastric, esophageal, superficial abdominal, and hemorrhoidal veins. In some cases massive hemorrhage from ruptured esophageal varices is the 1st clinical manifestation of congestive splenomegaly.

Laboratory Data. Pancytopenia of varying degree is seen. The bone marrow shows active hematopoiesis with abundant megakaryocytes. Liver function tests may indicate hepatocellular disease. It is possible to measure portal venous pressure, and injection of radiopaque dyes into the spleen permits radiologic visualization of the splenic and portal veins. This should usually be done under direct vision, for percutaneous needling may lacerate the splenic capsule. In cases of hepatic fibrosis and cirrhosis, ^{99m}Tc scan may show a contracted liver with massive splenomegaly.

Treatment. The site of obstruction must be determined. If only the splenic vein is involved, splenectomy is curative. In cases in which the portal vein is extensively involved or in which intrahepatic obstruction is present, splenectomy will correct pancytopenia but will not relieve portal hypertension. On the other hand, because generalized bleeding or infection rarely results from thrombocytopenia or neutropenia, these hematologic findings do not mandate splenectomy. Portacaval anastomosis, which in general is preferred to splenorenal shunting in the young child, is indicated when portal hypertension is clearly shown or when repeated episodes of life-threatening hemorrhage have occurred. Successful relief of portal hypertension may result in decrease in splenic size and improvement of pancytopenia. It may also result in metabolic complications, especially hyperammonemia.

15.58 ANOMALIES AND TRAUMA

Splenic Cysts. Cysts of the spleen are of two general types: epidermoid cysts are lined with stratified columnar epithelium, and pseudocysts, presumably of post-traumatic or postinfarction origin, have no epithelial lining and are filled with necrotic material and blood. Diagnosis is suggested by an asymptomatic smooth mass in the left upper quadrant, displacing the stomach medially. Isotopic scans with ^{99m}Tc gelatin colloid indicate that the cystic mass is within the substance of the spleen. Ultrasonography and computed tomography (CT scan) effectively demonstrate splenic cysts.

Accessory Spleens. Multiple and accessory spleens are not uncommon. Of 1413 children subjected to splenectomy 229 (16%) had 1 or more accessory spleens (145 had only 1; 10 had 5 or more). Accessory spleens are usually located close to the hilum or adjacent to the tail of the pancreas. A congenital syndrome of polysplenism is characterized by left-sided visceral isomerism and cardiac defects. Affected children have a high rate of intrahepatic biliary atresia.

Congenital Absence of the Spleen. Absence of the spleen occurs as part of an unusual group of anomalies, including complex abnormalities of the heart and great vessels with severe cyanotic congenital heart disease. Apparent dextrocardia and varying degrees of heterotopia of the abdominal viscera are seen (Ivemark syndrome). The condition can be suspected from examination of the blood: target cells, increased numbers of spherocytes, intraerythrocytic inclusions (such as Howell-Jolly and Heinz bodies), and hemosiderin granules are easily demonstrated. The incidence of overwhelming sepsis is increased in congenital asplenia.

Hypersplenism. Hypersplenism is not a specific diagnosis but rather a descriptive term for a clinical complex that includes (1) depression of one or more of the cellular elements of the blood; (2) active formation of that element in the bone marrow; (3) an enlarged spleen, which may be due to a large number of causes (Table 15–9); and (4) correction of the hematologic abnormalities by splenectomy. A diagnosis of primary hypersplenism is difficult to establish; other causes of splenomegaly with secondary pancytopenia must be excluded.

Functional Hyposplenia. Occasionally, anatomically enlarged spleens may be devoid of reticuloendothelial system (RES) activity. This has been most clearly demonstrated in infants and young children with sickle cell anemia. In the great majority of these children, after 6–18 mo of age ^{99m}Tc scan fails to demonstrate RES activity of the anatomically enlarged organ. Howell-Jolly and Heinz bodies are seen in the blood. Young children with sickle cell anemia are 600 times more likely to develop pneumococcal meningitis and sepsis than their normal peers, and this propensity to infection is, in part, due to defective splenic function. Functional hyposplenia can be temporarily reversed with transfusion of normal red blood cells; after years, autoinfarction ultimately reduces the spleen to a siderofibrotic nubbin.

Rupture of the Spleen. Traumatic injury of the spleen may result from a hard, direct blow to the left flank or left side of the abdomen, such as may occur during automobile accidents or contact sports. If the tear in the splenic capsule is small, the symptoms may be moderate and include left upper quadrant or left shoulder pain and signs of peritoneal irritation due to blood. In more extreme cases shock may develop rapidly. When the spleen is pathologically enlarged, rupture may occur after relatively minor trauma. This occurs in the newborn infant with hemolytic disease and in the older child with infectious mononucleosis. Radionuclide and CT scanning are valuable in demonstrating lacerations and hematomas of the spleen.

Laparotomy and splenectomy are indicated when rupture leads to severe intra-abdominal bleeding and hypotension, but splenectomy is not always mandatory for splenic laceration. In the child, bleeding from the lacerated splenic surface often stops spontaneously. If the child's vital signs are stable or controlled with relatively small amounts of blood transfusion (< 25 mL/kg) during the first 48 hr after splenic injury, nonoperative management may be safely attempted. This observational period requires a surgeon in attendance who can act rapidly if deterioration occurs. Serial examinations of the spleen with ^{aa}MTC scans, ultrasonography, or computed tomography are needed to show that the splenic lesion is not expanding. The child should be watched carefully in the hospital for 10–14 days and maintained on restricted activities for several months. Late rupture or splenic pseudocysts have not been observed; scans have shown complete healing of the lesion.

Nonoperative management is not indicated if other abdominal organs are damaged or if severe shock develops. If laparotomy is necessary, it may be possible to repair the damaged spleen or to leave some splenic tissue in situ (see below).

Splenosis. Heterotopic autotransplantations of splenic tissue onto the surface of the peritoneum, with its subsequent growth, occur frequently after splenic injury requiring splenectomy. Changes in the circulating red blood cells (Howell-Jolly bodies, membrane craters) are not found in affected patients. ^{99m}Tc spleen scans show extrahepatic uptake of the radionuclide by small masses of regenerated splenic tissue, that may be to some degree protective against severe bacterial infections. The degree of protection may vary, however, with the amount of splenic tissue and its arterial blood supply; death from overwhelming infection has occurred in patients with splenosis.

15.59 SPLENECTOMY

Removal of the spleen is a common operation performed for a variety of indications. Primary surgical indications include (1) rupture of the spleen; (2) removal of tumors, cysts, or vascular anomalies involving the spleen; (3) need for adequate surgical exposure of the left upper portion of the abdomen; (4) certain shunting procedures; (5) relief of mechanical distress due to massive enlargement in thalassemia major or Gaucher disease; and (6) need for staging procedures for Hodgkin disease and other lymphoreticular malignancies (Sec. 16.8 and 16.9).

Hematologic indications include (1) congenital hemolytic states, such as hereditary spherocytosis and elliptocytosis, and some cases of nonspherocytic anemias, such as pyruvate kinase deficiency; (2) autoimmune hemolytic anemia when chronic and refractory to corticosteroid therapy; (3) chronic idiopathic thrombocytopenia purpura (ITP); and (4) hypersplenism.

Overwhelming Sepsis Following Splenectomy. Removal of the spleen alters host resistance, and overwhelming and often fatal meningitis and septicemia are seen with increased frequency in asplenic persons. The risks vary with the reasons for which splenectomy was done and especially with the age of the patient.

The risk of overwhelming sepsis is low (0.5–1%) when splenectomy is done for traumatic rupture, hereditary spherocytosis, or idiopathic thrombocytopenic purpura. A higher incidence of infection is seen when the indication is thalassemia major, histiocytosis, or lipidosis. The risk is high when there is an underlying disease that in itself has a predisposition to infection, such as the Wiskott-Aldrich syndrome. The risk is higher in all categories for younger infants and children. Sepsis has occurred at all ages and regardless of the indication for splenectomy or the interval after the operation. Severe infections after splenectomy (usually meningitis and septicemia) are characterized by an acute and fulminating course, death often occurring within 12–24 hr after onset of symptoms. In more than 60% of cases, pneumococci are the responsible agents; *Haemophilus influenzae* and meningococci are responsible for a smaller number of infections. Because of this risk splenectomy should be performed only for clear indications, and when possible the operation should be deferred until after 5–6 yr of age or even longer if the condition of the patient is well compensated. Prophylactic use of penicillin has been advocated for the young child after splenectomy, and many centers use this routinely. There are no adequately controlled studies assessing effectiveness of such management.

Immunization with polyvalent capsular polysaccharide antigens of pneumococci, *H. influenzae*, and meningococci probably reduces the frequency of postsplenectomy infection but is generally ineffective before 18–24 mo.

In any case, patients whose spleens have been removed should know that splenectomy carries a risk of development at any time of a life-threatening infection, and that any febrile illness calls for immediate medical evaluation.

Crosby WH: Normal functions of the spleen relative to red blood cells; A review. Blood 14:399, 1959.

Eraklis AJ, Filler RM: Splenectomy in childhood: A review of 1413 cases. J Pediatr Surg 7:382, 1972.

Likhite VV: Immunological impairment and susceptibility to infection after splenectomy. JAMA 236:1376, 1976.

Medical Letter: Prevention of serious infections after splenectomy. Med Let 19:2, 1977.

Pearson HA: The born again spleen. N Engl J Med 298:1373, 1978.

Pearson HA: Splenectomy, its risk and role. Hosp Pract Aug 1980, p 85.

Pearson HA, Spencer RP, Cornelius E: Functional asplenia in sickly cell anemia. N Engl J Med 281:923, 1969.

Pearson HA, Spencer RP, Touloukian R: The binary spleen: A radioisotopic scan sign of splenic pseudocyst. J Pediatr 77:216, 1970.

Sherman R: Perspective in management of trauma to the spleen. J Trauma 20:1, 1980.

Singer DB: Post-splenectomy sepsis. Perspect Pediatr Pathol 1:3, 1973.

15.60 THE LYMPHATIC SYSTEM

The lymphatic system includes the free lymphocytes of the blood and lymph as well as organized lymphatic structures such as lymph nodes, spleen, Peyer patches, appendix, and tonsils. The origin of lymphocytes is uncertain; some are believed to originate or be modified in the embryonic thymus, from which their progenitors migrate to populate other lymphatic tissues. Others may arise from the lymphoid areas of the gastrointestinal tract, tonsillar area, or appendix.

The lymph vessels start as small capillaries between the cells of all organs except the brain and the heart. Small lymphatic capillaries join to form progressively larger channels that drain the extremities, trunk, and head. The largest of the lymphatic vessels is the thoracic duct, which discharges most of the central return of body lymph into the left subclavian vein.

The lymph channels are characteristically interrupted by lymph nodes. These structures are networks of dilated sinusoids lined by reticuloendothelial elements and surrounded by masses of actively proliferating lymphocytes. The lymph nodes are located in groups, through which the lymphatic drainage of well defined anatomic areas passes. The lymph nodes function as protective barriers to the spread of infections. They also filter particulate antigens, and the lymphocytes and plasma cells within lymph nodes actively participate in antibody formation.

The superficial lymph nodes are evaluated by palpation. Small nodes can normally be felt in the neck, axillae, and groin. Roentgenograms of the chest assess enlargement of the mediastinal lymph nodes. Lymphangiography permits evaluation of the size and structure of the pelvic and retroperitoneal lymph nodes.

The lymph is a clear fluid. It has a protein content intermediate between that of interstitial fluid and plasma, and it contains a substantial number of small lymphocytes.

15.61 DISEASES OF THE LYMPH VESSELS

Acute Lymphangitis. This is an inflammation of the lymphatics draining an area of acute infection, usually bacterial. It is manifested as red painful streaks radiating proximally from the infected site. Painful swelling of the regional nodes is also usually present.

Lymphedema. Lymphedema is a diffuse, permanent, pitting edema due to obstruction of the lymph drainage of an area, usually an extremity. Congenital lymphedema occurs in Milroy disease and as part of the syndrome of gonadal dysgenesis. Acquired lymphedema may result from inflammatory processes or from surgical or radiologic obliteration of lymph nodes or lymph channels.

15.62 DISEASES OF THE LYMPH NODES

Enlargement of the lymph nodes occurs in response to a wide variety of infectious, inflammatory, and neoplastic processes. Enlargement of a single node or group of nodes is most frequently due to an infection in the area it drains. Generalized lymphadenopathy occurs in many acute infections, especially rubella, rubeola, typhoid, tularemia, and infectious mononucleosis. Leukemia, lymphoma, and reticuloendotheliosis are sometimes accompanied by striking degrees of lymph node enlargement. Malignant tumors such as neuroblastoma sometimes metastasize to lymph nodes, and large numbers of lipid bearing histiocytes may be present in the lymph nodes of Gaucher disease and other lipidoses.

Acute Lymphadenitis. As a result of cellulitis or other infections, bacteria and toxins and other byproducts of acute inflammation are carried in the lymph to regional lymph nodes where an acute inflammatory process occurs. Bacteria may cause abscess formation. Acute cervical adenitis secondary to acute pharyngitis and inguinal lymphadenopathy resulting from infections of the lower extremity are common. The involved nodes become swollen and painful, and the overlying skin is hot and red. The primary infectious process is usually obvious, but the site of inoculation may not be apparent, as in cat-scratch disease. Mediastinal lymphadenitis secondary to pulmonary infections may produce obstructive symptoms and cough. Mesenteric lymphadenopathy may, on occasion, be associated with crampy abdominal pain simulating appendicitis.

Treatment. Antibiotic therapy that is appropriate for the primary infection will benefit the lymphadenitis. When suppuration occurs, needle aspiration or surgical drainage is necessary.

Chronic Lymphadenitis. Chronic infection or inflammation is frequently associated with hyperplasia of the lymph nodes. Tuberculous infections regularly result in regional lymphadenopathy. Scrofula, or chronic cervical lymphadenopathy, may be secondary to infection of the nasopharynx with bovine tuberculosis. This organism is uncommon in the United States, where chronic lymphadenopathy is more often due to infection by atypical acid-fast organisms. The organisms are trapped in the nodes, where granuloma and caseous necrosis occur. Affected nodes are hard, nontender, and frequently matted to adjacent tissues. Biopsy may be necessary to differentiate chronic infections from malignant processes.

HOWARD A. PEARSON

16

NEOPLASMS AND NEOPLASM-LIKE STRUCTURES

16.1 GENERAL CONSIDERATIONS

In the United States, cancer causes more deaths than any other disease of children between the ages of 1 and 15 yr. The incidence rate of malignant tumors in children under 15 yr of age is estimated to be 130/million/yr for the years 1977–1980. The death rate, however, for malignant neoplasms in children during this same period was only about one third the incidence. Mortality rates range from virtually none for thyroid cancer to almost 100% for patients over the age of 1 yr who have disseminated neuroblastoma. Incidence and mortality rates for some of the more common cancers are shown in Table 16–1. It should be emphasized that some of the favorable rates reflect improvements in therapy over the past several decades and that a child in whom possible cancer is diagnosed should be referred as soon as possible to a center where appropriate treatment will be available. There is evidence that for most tumors prognosis improves if the patient is enrolled in a study protocol.

In most instances, the development of cancer probably involves environmental as well as host factors. In adults, of those cancers that occur primarily in organs exposed directly to the environment, from 60–90% are estimated to be caused by environmental carcinogens. Not all those who work outdoors in strong sunlight will get skin cancer, however, nor will all those who smoke develop lung cancer; accordingly, even with these agents there are probably important host factors. In children, moreover, the common cancers tend to occur in tissues that are not exposed directly to the environment, such as hematopoietic, nervous, and supportive connective tissues.

ENVIRONMENTAL FACTORS

Ionizing Radiation. Increases in the incidence of acute lymphocytic leukemia, acute myeloid leukemia, and chronic granulocytic leukemia followed exposure of children to the atomic bombs in Hiroshima and Nagasaki. A linear relationship was found between the radiation dose and the frequency of leukemia. The type of leukemia and the rate at which it developed were related to the age of the individual at the time of exposure. The increases in acute lymphatic and chronic granulocytic leukemia were most dramatic in the younger children, whereas acute myelogenous leukemia was seen with increasing frequency among the older children. Leukemia developed after a relatively short incubation, with a peak rate of occurrence 5 years after exposure. Only recently have investigators found an increased incidence of breast cancer in those exposed who were under 20 yr old at the time. We can conclude that critical environmental events may cause cancers with long latency periods and that these cancers under normal circumstances may be more difficult to discover than after so dramatic an event as massive exposure to atomic radiation.

The use of radiation therapy for nonmalignant conditions is now generally abandoned, since it was shown to be asso-

ciated with the development of malignancy. Examples include the increased incidence of thyroid cancer after external irradiation to the head and neck (once given for a variety of benign conditions, such as enlarged thymus, enlarged tonsils, or tinea capitis). Before 1955 significant doses of radiation were administered during fluoroscopy in hospitals or physicians' offices, and even in shoe stores to measure children's feet. Such exposures are now sharply curtailed or eliminated. Either causally or coincidentally, leukemia mortality rates for children under the age of 5 yr dropped substantially during the early 1960's, when chemotherapy was not yet producing the cures that it is today.

Exposure in utero of the fetus to diagnostic x-rays has been associated with a risk ratio of about 1.5 for development of a childhood tumor; but, although an as yet unexplained relationship exists, the facts that there was no increase in such cancer among children exposed in utero to the atomic bomb and that animal models do not indicate any supersensitivity of the fetus to radiation oncogenesis suggest that the relationship is probably not causal.

Solar Radiation. Sunlight may cause cancer of the skin, but this does not usually occur in young individuals unless they have a genetic predisposition, such as xeroderma pigmentosum or another congenital defect in DNA repair.

Asbestos. Investigation of a cluster of cases of mesothelioma among adults in South Africa has found that, although only a few worked with asbestos, most had as children lived near open pits where asbestos was mined and some had played on the refuse dumps. Moreover, asbestos carried home on the father's workclothes has been found to cause mesothelioma 3–4 decades later in the wife or children. Children exposed to asbestos in their homes or neighborhoods may be especially prone to the carcinogenicity of cigarette smoking, since asbestos potentiates the capacity of cigarette smoking to cause lung cancer in adults. Mesotheliomas that occur in persons under 20 yr old, however, are apparently not due to asbestos and are histologically unlike those produced by this agent.

Table 16–1. **Incidence and Mortality Rates/Million/Year for Childhood Cancer in the US (1977–1980)**

	Incidence	Mortality Rate
All forms	130.0	44.9
Acute lymphocytic leukemia	29.4	9.4
Brain and CNS	26.1	8.7
Neuroblastoma and ganglioneuroblastoma	10.4	NA*
Soft tissue sarcoma	9.4	4.2
Wilms tumor	8.1	1.8
Non-Hodgkin lymphoma	8.0	3.4
Hodgkin lymphoma	7.0	0.5
Acute granulocytic leukemia	4.8	2.6

*Coding of death did not permit same classification as incidence group. Heise HW, Myers MH, Miller RW et al: National Cancer Institute Report. J Pediatr (submitted).

Drugs. Intrauterine exposure to *diethylstilbestrol* carries an increased risk of clear cell adenocarcinoma of the vagina in daughters of women given this drug. In addition, exposed children of both sexes commonly have malformations of the genital tract (see also Sec. 18.4). DES is currently the only proven human transplacental carcinogen known, although two cases of neuroblastoma have been reported in infants with fetal *hydantoin* syndrome, and another in a child with fetal *alcohol* syndrome.

Immunosuppressive agents administered following renal or other transplantation have been associated with an increased incidence of malignancy (and, particularly, of non-Hodgkin lymphoma [reticulum cell sarcoma]). Since the types of tumors that occur in immunosuppressed individuals do not have the same relative incidence as tumors that occur in other children, this effect cannot be merely a breakdown in immune surveillance against cancer; there must be other mechanisms at work.

Treatment of aplastic anemia (especially of the Fanconi type) with *anabolic androgenic steroids* has led to various liver tumors: hepatocellular carcinoma, hepatoma, or hepatic adenoma. The underlying condition may enhance the induction of liver neoplasia by these drugs, for such neoplasms have not been reported in athletes who use these androgens to build up muscles; such athletes, however, may well be at risk.

Chemotherapy for malignancy may result in second neoplasms, with a cumulative risk as high as 12% at 25 yr.

Diet. There is an unexplained association between high fat intake, obesity, and the development of cancers of breast, colon, and uterus in adults. Speculation is rife as to whether dietary manipulation may prevent the development of cancer in later life, with emphasis on the possible prevention of colon cancer through a diet high in vegetable fiber. No convincing clinical data support such ideas at present.

VIRUSES

RNA Viruses. There is convincing evidence for both vertical and horizontal transmission in animals of lymphatic leukemia and lymphoma associated with type c RNA viruses; and retroviruses also cause leukemia/lymphoma in cats and cows, with horizontal transmission. A type of T-cell leukemia in humans has been associated with a retrovirus (human T-cell leukemia virus [HTLV 1]). This form of leukemia is endemic on two islands in southern Japan and also occurs in the Caribbean and sporadically elsewhere, including the United States and Israel. The youngest case so far reported was 17 yr old at the time of diagnosis; some cases are known to have had latency periods of over 20 yr.

DNA Viruses. The Epstein-Barr (EB) virus is implicated in the development of infectious mononucleosis as well as in African Burkitt lymphoma and lymphoepithelioma. In the United States, however, about 80% of cases of Burkitt lymphoma are not associated with EB virus. EB virus infection in vitro leads to "immortalization" of B cell lines. It is postulated that uncontrolled proliferation of B cells that have been neoplastically transformed by EB virus is an important factor in the development of Burkitt lymphoma, particularly in Africa. It is not clear how EB virus infection is related to the chromosomal changes in Burkitt lymphoma that are described below.

Papova Viruses. This family of viruses is known to cause warts and papillomas in a variety of tissues. Subtypes of the virus appear to have strong tissue tropisms. Types 6 and 11 are found in the lesions of laryngeal papillomatosis as well as condyloma acuminata. Although these viral lesions rarely become spontaneously malignant, they can frequently be converted to squamous cell carcinomas by the action of a secondary carcinogen such as cigarette smoke or therapeutic irradiation. Subtypes 16 and 18 of the papova viruses seem to be the most likely etiologic agents in carcinoma of the uterine cervix.

GENETIC MECHANISMS

Genetic Deletion and Malignancy. Observations of the characteristics of sporadic and genetically determined tumors have led to a hypothesis that malignant transformation of a cell occurs by a two-step process. For example, about half the offspring of patients surviving the heritable form of retinoblastoma will also have the disease, which is often bilateral and multicentric and occurs soon after birth. In patients with the sporadic form of retinoblastoma the time of appearance is later and the tumors unilateral. It is therefore postulated that retinoblast transformation requires (at least) two gene changes (the "two-hit" hypothesis of Knudson). In heritable cases, it is argued, the first gene change is present in all cells, including germ cells; transformation requires a second gene change in a retinoblast already carrying the first "hit." In sporadic cases, both "hits" presumably develop as chance events in the same retinoblasts. Recent laboratory data are consistent with this hypothesis. Some years ago certain patients with retinoblastoma and an associated syndrome of mental retardation and microcephaly were found to have a deletion of chromosome 13 (13q- syndrome). Since then, sensitive gene mapping techniques have related all forms of retinoblastoma to some abnormality of chromosome 13. The tumors studied have shown submicroscopic deletions in chromosome 13 even when the constitutional karyotype from the same patient is normal. It is now postulated that the first "hit" is a deletion on chromosome 13, which may be systemic (as in the 13q-syndrome) or localized. The second (or later) events which constitute the second "hit" are variable, and the molecular mechanisms of tumorigenesis are unknown.

A similar pattern occurs with Wilms tumor. The association of aniridia with Wilms tumor led to identification of a deletion on chromosome 11. Gene mapping studies have shown that many Wilms tumors are homozygous for products of chromosome 11, whereas surrounding normal host tissue is heterozygous. Somehow the genetic deletion has set the stage for development of malignancy.

Oncogenes and Malignancy. Oncogenes are DNA sequences that when applied to an appropriate target, such as the NIH 3T3 tissue culture cell line, will cause a transformed focus. Originally, oncogenes were identified as that portion of the genome of a retrovirus that led to malignant transformation, as distinct from the portion responsible for viral replication. The first oncogene studied was the *src* gene, which enables the Rous sarcoma virus to induce sarcomas in vivo and to transform chicken fibroblasts in monolayer culture. The *src* gene is now known to encode the structure of a tyrosine kinase. It is not a unique viral genome at all; instead, it stems from a closely related gene that is an integral part of the normal genome of the chicken. That is, the cellular genome contains a gene that can exhibit strong transforming properties when properly activated. This antecedent gene is termed a *proto-oncogene*. Two dozen cellular proto-oncogenes have been discovered to date through the study of retrovirus and the use of gene transfer techniques. At least five distinct mechanisms may result in their conversion to active oncogenes. Activation of an oncogene within the cell is probably only one component of a multistep process leading to the creation of a tumor cell.

The juxtaposition of the oncogene *myc* and immunoglobulin domains following chromosomal translocation appears to result in deregulation of the *myc* gene as part of the development of Burkitt lymphoma.

CLINICAL ASSOCIATIONS

Associations between underlying genetic disorders and malignancy are listed in Table 16–2. In addition to these specific associations, there appear to be certain families in which cancer is common. Hodgkin disease, brain tumors, and Ewing sarcoma have been reported in siblings more often than would likely occur by chance alone. Patients with soft tissue sarcomas often have primary relatives with brain tumors; breast cancer at a young age in the mother is also reported.

In the case of children with tumors, it is important to look for familial associations, either with malignancy or with any congenital syndrome or abnormality. Syndromes such as neurofibromatosis or hemihypertrophy may not become obvious until the patient is 5–10 yr old, and may not be recognizable at the time the diagnosis of tumor is made in the child. Accordingly, in some situations it may be important to examine the parents as well as the child. Awareness of these associations may protect the parents as well; for example, one should make sure that the mother of a child with a soft tissue sarcoma knows how to perform breast self-examination.

There are as yet no rules that will help prevent the development of cancer in childhood, but pediatricians can help to avoid cancers in adults. They should counsel patients about the avoidance of smoking and obesity, for example, and do Pap smears regularly in teenage girls who are sexually active.

Table 16–2. **Conditions Associated with an Increased Risk of Malignant Neoplasia During Childhood**

Condition	Associated Neoplasm
Congenital anomalies	
Hemihypertrophy	Wilms tumor, hepatoma, adrenocortical carcinoma
Sporadic aniridia	Wilms tumor
Renal dysplasia	Wilms tumor
Visceral cytomegaly syndrome (Beckwith-Wiedemann syndrome)	Wilms tumor, hepatoma, adrenocortical carcinoma
Gonadal dysgenesis	Gonadal cancer
DNA repair defects	
Xeroderma pigmentosum	Skin cancer
Ataxia-telangiectasia	Lymphoma, leukemia
Immunodeficiency states	
Congenital X-linked immunodeficiency	Lymphoma, leukemia
Severe combined immunodeficiency	Lymphoma, leukemia
IgM deficiency	Lymphoma
Wiskott-Aldrich syndrome	Lymphoma
Chromosomal anomalies	
Down syndrome	Leukemia
Klinefelter syndrome	Breast cancer
Fanconi anemia	Leukemia, hepatoma
Bloom syndrome	Leukemia
11p− syndrome	Wilms tumor
13q− syndrome	Retinoblastoma
Miscellaneous genetic diseases	
Neurofibromatosis	Fibrosarcoma, schwannoma, pheochromocytoma Neurosarcoma, rhabdomyosarcoma, brain tumors
von Hippel–Lindau syndrome	Pheochromocytoma
Multiple endocrine adenomatosis I (Wermer syndrome)	Schwannoma
Multiple endocrine adenomatosis II (Sipple syndrome)	Thyroid carcinoma, pheochromocytoma
Familial polyposis	Carcinoma of the colon

16.2 PRINCIPLES OF DIAGNOSIS

Since only about one child in 10,000 will develop cancer each year, it is unusual for a general physician in practice to encounter a child with cancer. Physicians must, therefore, be alert to the possible occurrence of a rare but important disease. The diagnosis of cancer is too frequently overlooked while studies for infection or collagen disease or both are pursued in detail. Atypical courses of what appear to be common childhood conditions, prolonged (over 3–4 wk) and unexplained pain or fever, or unexplained (and especially growing) masses, particularly when these are associated with weight loss, should initiate prompt and appropriate studies.

Delays in diagnosis are a particular problem in certain clinical situations. Tumors of the nasopharynx or middle ear may mimic infection; prolonged unexplained ear pain, nasal discharge, retropharyngeal swelling, or trismus should be investigated, therefore, as possibly due to malignancy. Cervical lymph node enlargement is common in children with infection, but it is also common in children with Hodgkin and non-Hodgkin lymphoma. Persistent or progressively enlarging nodes, which are often nonpainful, can be the hallmark of lymphoma and should lead to consideration of biopsy. Osteosarcoma and Ewing sarcoma usually occur during the 2nd decade of life, a time associated with physical activity. The cardinal symptom is localized and persistent pain, which the patient often associates with an episode of trauma. Such persistent pain should be investigated radiologically. The early symptoms of leukemia may also be nonspecific: low grade fever, or bone or joint pain. Careful attention to blood counts in such patients, with particular sensitivity to the development of normocytic anemia or mild thrombocytopenia, may help to determine when bone marrow should be examined, even if leukemic blast forms are not seen in the blood smear.

When a malignant neoplasm is suspected, the immediate goal is to determine its nature and extent. A tentative diagnosis can be inferred from such clinical features as the presenting symptoms, location of the tumor, and age of the child. Figure 16–1 shows the incidence of primary sites of tumor by age at the time of diagnosis. From this it can be seen, for example, that an abdominal mass is much more likely to be a neuroblastoma or Wilms tumor in a young child than in a child over the age of 10 yr.

It is usually appropriate to make a relatively thorough search for metastatic disease before obtaining a biopsy for confirmation of the diagnosis. If the surgeon knows the likelihood of disseminated disease, he or she can exercise better judgment in choosing between an attempt at complete resection and a more limited diagnostic biopsy. The studies appropriate for this preoperative review depend on the tentative diagnosis and will be discussed for each specific tumor. A number of noninvasive techniques are useful in the search for metastases. The invasive procedure most often used before surgery is examination of bone marrow by aspiration or biopsy or both.

At the time of diagnosis, it is critical that the extent of disease be accurately defined; this delineation is called "staging." A system of staging must be designed for each tumor and will depend on the experience that has been gained in relating the extent of disease at the time of diagnosis to the subsequent clinical course. Staging will help determine prognosis and treatment plan. Specific staging systems will be described for each tumor type, as appropriate.

At the core of the initial diagnostic studies of any tumor is the examination of its histologic character. The initial specimen of tumor tissue should be obtained under conditions that allow for the full range of pathologic studies that may be necessary to identify the tumor accurately; in some tumors, such as lymphoma, these studies may require fresh tissue for

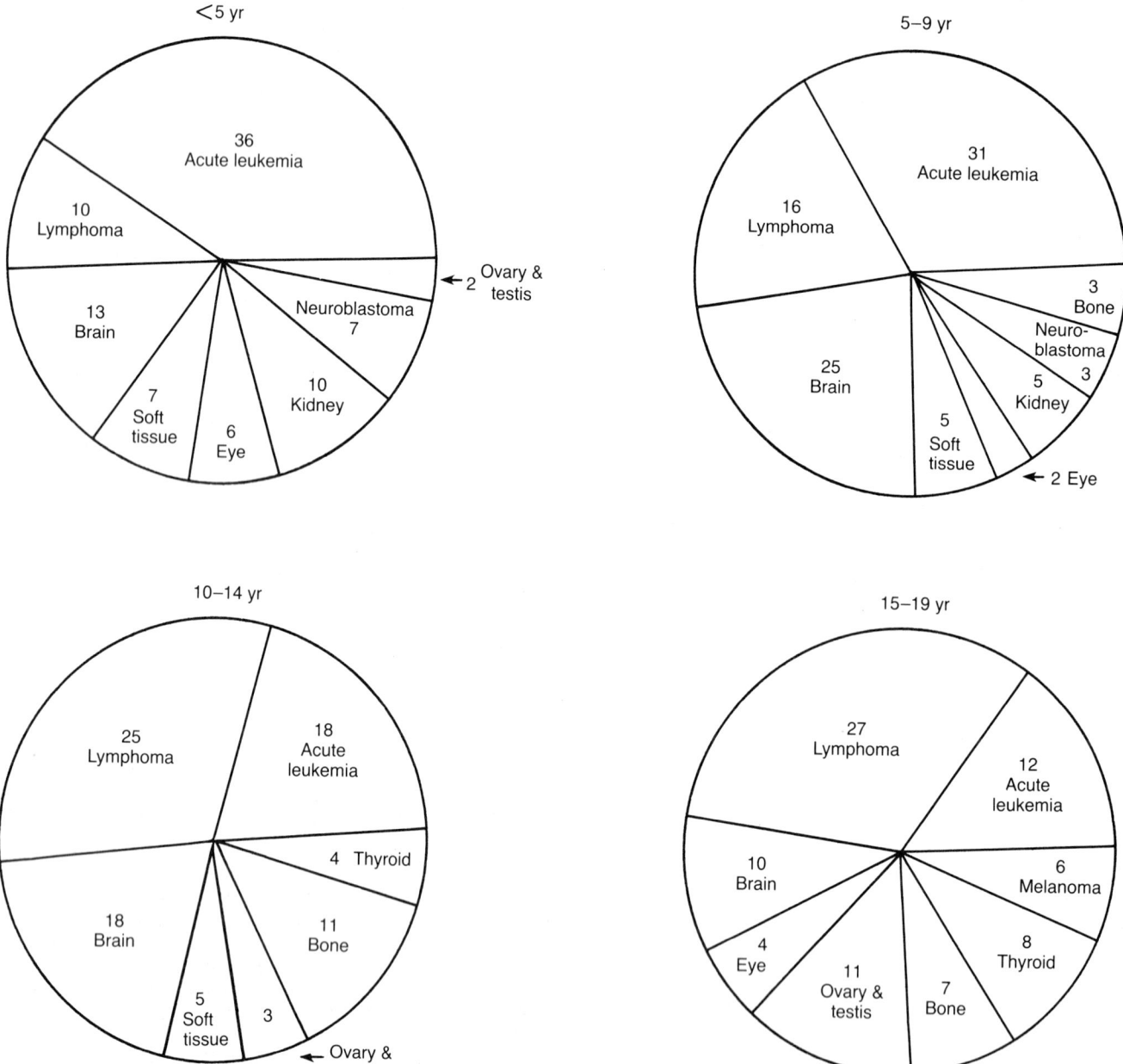

Figure 16–1. Percent of primary tumors by site of origin at differing ages at diagnosis. Incidence of neuroblastoma estimated from site of origin. (Adapted from National Cancer Institute Monograph No. 57. SEER Program.)

antigen marker or other studies such as electron microscopy. The results of these studies may take time to become available, and it is often impossible immediately after surgery to discuss diagnosis in detail with a family.

The surgeon must search carefully at biopsy, excision, or exploration for evidences of regional dissemination to lymph node groups or to adjacent organs. If an attempt is made to remove the whole tumor or the organ containing the tumor, the pathologist will need to examine carefully the margins of resection to make sure that no microscopic residual tumor remains. The planning for subsequent treatment of the patient rests on this cornerstone of initial diagnostic studies; the planning must be done by physicians trained and experienced in the care of children with cancer.

16.3 PRINCIPLES OF TREATMENT

General. Treatment of the child with cancer has two aspects: the specific and the supportive. For specific therapy the physician can offer surgical removal, irradiation, and chemotherapy. The majority of tumors in childhood have spread beyond the site of origin at the time of diagnosis and are not, therefore, amenable to complete surgical removal or to destruction by local irradiation alone. In most children with cancer, all three modalities will be necessary. The goal of all forms of treatment is the same: to remove or destroy as much tumor as possible, with the least damage to normal cells.

The patient's prognosis varies with the type of tumor and the extent of disease at the time of diagnosis as well as upon the adequacy of treatment. The best chance for cure exists during the initial course of treatment, which should be optimized; accordingly, patients should be referred early to an appropriate specialized center. Major advances have been made in the treatment of childhood malignancy in the past three decades and at least half of patients diagnosed today will be cured. These advances have been made as a result of

the participation by patients and their physicians in clinical research programs. Some of the discoveries, such as the importance of sanctuary therapy for the central nervous system in acute leukemia, have been made at individual institutions, while others, such as the curability of patients with stage I Wilms tumor through short-term chemotherapy without radiotherapy have been made by collaborative groups of investigators. Not all patients and families may wish to participate in clinical experiments, but further progress will not be made without assessment of new treatments in a systematic fashion, and because there are such small numbers of patients with any single diagnosis, progress may well require that a patient be entered into a collaborative study directed by a protocol or treatment plan from one of the cooperative Clinical Cancer Research groups.

Chemotherapy. Drugs for treatment of cancer are selected from several classes of agents, including hormones, antimetabolites, antibiotics, plant alkaloids, and alkylating agents (Table 16–3). New agents with apparent antitumor activity can be identified in a number of ways. The effects of these agents are studied in animals for their efficacy in suppressing tumor growth and for toxicity. The few agents of promise are then studied in humans. The initial (phase I) studies are carried out to assess the toxicity of the new compounds. They are usually performed in adults with tumors for which there is no available therapy, who have given their informed consent to the procedure. The starting doses of a new drug to be tested are small, the dose increasing to the point of tolerance as the study progresses. With the maximum tolerated dose determined, the drug is then studied (phase II) in patients with a wide variety of tumors to determine its range of effectiveness. For those tumors found to be responsive to the drug, further trials are designed (phase III) in which the agent is incorporated into schedules with other active drugs and new and old regimens are compared for effectiveness.

Bone Marrow Transplantation. Early experiments with marrow transplantation involved patients in florid relapse of

Table 16–3 **Cancer Chemotherapeutic Agents**

Drug	Major Mode of Action	Important Toxicities
Methotrexate	Inhibits tetrahydrofolate synthesis	Marrow suppression, mucosal and gut ulceration, liver damage, leukoencephalopathy*
5-Fluorouracil	Inhibits thymidine synthetase	Marrow suppression, mucosal and gut ulceration
6-Mercaptopurine	Inhibits purine biosynthesis	Marrow suppression, mucosal and gut ulceration, liver damage
Cytosine arabinoside	Inhibits initiation of DNA synthesis and DNA polymerase	Marrow suppression, mucosal and gut ulceration, liver damage, febrile reaction
Alkylating agents (nitrogen mustard, cyclophosphamide, phenylalanine mustard, chlorambucil, and the nitrosoureas)	Alkylation of DNA and RNA	Marrow suppression, immunosuppression, hemorrhagic cystitis (cyclophosphamide), sterility in males
Procarbazine	Inhibits DNA and RNA synthesis	Marrow suppression, mucosal and gut ulceration, CNS toxicity
Bleomycin	DNA strand scission	Pulmonary fibrosis*
Actinomycin D	Inhibits DNA-dependent RNA synthesis	Marrow depression, mucosal and gut ulceration, radiosensitization
Anthracyclines (doxorubicin, daunomycin)	Complex with DNA	Marrow suppression, radiosensitization, myocardial damage,* mucosal and gut ulceration
Plant alkaloids (vincristine and vinblastine)	Microtubule disruption with metaphase block	Marrow suppression, paresthesias, loss of deep tendon reflexes, paresis, abdominal and jaw pain, constipation, inappropriate ADH secretion
Asparaginase	Induces asparagine deficiency, inhibits protein synthesis	Chills, fever, anaphylactic reactions, liver dysfunction, pancreatitis,* hyperglycemia, immunosuppression
Epipodophyllotoxins (VM-26, VP-16)	Premitotic cell cycle delay	Myelosuppression, vomiting, fever, chills, hypotension, anaphylaxis

*Dose related, potentially irreversible.

leukemia, and the death rate after transplantation was high. Patients are now undergoing transplantation while in remission; the death rate from infection in the immediate post-transplantation period is much lower, and it appears that 40–60% of patients may show long-term survival. In general, the younger the patient, the more favorable the response may be. A number of centers now use or recommend transplantation of allogeneic or syngeneic bone marrow for patients with acute myeloblastic leukemia in first remission or for acute lymphoblastic leukemia in a second or subsequent remission.

There has as yet been no definitive comparison between the best available chemotherapy (which is continually improving) and marrow transplantation. The survival curves of groups of patients given chemotherapy alone take their origin from the day of first treatment and reflect the outcomes of patients who have failed to achieve remission or who have died during introduction. On the other hand, the marrow transplant curves measure survival from the time of transplantation. To be eligible for marrow transplantation, a patient must already have achieved remission with induction chemotherapy. Such survival curves cannot, therefore, be directly compared.

Current methods of allogeneic bone marrow transplantation require an HLA-matched sibling as donor (see Sec. 10.57). As family size has tended to decrease, so has the proportion of patients for whom a match is available, since there is only one chance in four that any sibling will be appropriate. Studies are under way to determine whether minor degrees of HLA mismatch or better immunosuppression will allow the use of donors other than HLA-matched siblings.

Graft-versus-host disease (GVHD) and interstitial pneumonitis remain serious post-transplantation problems. GVHD occurs less often in younger patients, and newer agents such as cyclosporin are decreasing its incidence (see also Sec. 10.21). Chronic GVHD can remain a problem, however, and can lead to serious disfigurement (e.g., with a scleroderma-like skin picture as well as more debilitating conditions). Leukemic relapse also limits the proportion of patients achieving long-term disease control. Patients with GVHD appear to have a lesser likelihood of relapse (graft-versus-leukemia effect); accordingly, reducing the incidence and severity of GVHD may increase the likelihood of relapse.

A number of investigators are exploring the possibility of **autologous bone marrow transplantation.** After the patient's own bone marrow is harvested, doses of radiation or chemotherapy are administered that would ordinarily be lethal owing to marrow toxicity. The autologous marrow is then reinfused so that the marrow can be repopulated. GVHD is generally not a problem in this situation, as long as meticulous care is taken to irradiate all blood products administered at the time of marrow harvest, as well as during the support period after marrow reinfusion. A problem with this procedure is that the marrow must be kept viable more than 24–48 hr through special techniques. The marrow is usually cryopreserved in dimethylsulfoxide (DMSO), which prevents ice crystals from forming, and DMSO will be reinfused with the marrow and excreted through the lungs (with a garlic odor), and may have toxicities of its own (specifically cataract formation). Moreover, there may be tumor cells in the harvested marrow that are reinfused after irradiation or drug therapy. A variety of techniques to circumvent this are under trial: first, the patient should be in remission at the time of harvest for autotransplantation; and second, cytoxan derivatives, which appear to kill tumor cells and spare marrow stem cells, have been used to purge bone marrow in vitro, as have specific monoclonal antibodies (e.g., against T cells). Another problem, which is shared with allogeneic transplantation, is that the intensive treatment, which sets the stage for autologous transplantation, may be insufficient to eradicate the disease.

Active investigation is under way now in the use of autologous transplantation in acute myelogenous leukemia, non-Hodgkin lymphoma, neuroblastoma, Ewing sarcoma, and other solid tumors in which effective chemotherapy is available but hematopoietic toxicity may be dose-limiting. Unfortunately, when higher doses of antitumor agents are not restricted by hematopoietic toxicity, toxic effects on other organs are likely to appear. There has been some success in relapsed non-Hodgkin lymphoma with combination chemotherapy as preparation for autotransplantation. L-Phenylalanine mustard appears to be a promising agent in both neuroblastoma and Ewing sarcoma.

Complications. Complications of therapy include metabolic disorders, bone marrow suppression, and immunosuppression. Patients with a large tumor load may have been breaking down tumor cells for some time before the diagnosis is made. Their renal function may be impaired from tubular precipitates of uric acid crystals. Before initiating therapy, therefore, the serum levels of uric acid and creatinine should be measured in all patients, adequate hydration should be assured, and allopurinol (a xanthine oxidase inhibitor) should be given, if necessary, to bring the uric acid level to within the normal range. This problem arises particularly with hematopoietic tumors, but may occur with other large tumors (e.g., neuroblastoma). If proper attention is not given and the metabolic "tumor lysis syndrome" ensues, phosphates and potassium will be released into the circulation in large quantities as further cell lysis takes place, and symptomatic hypocalcemia and hyperkalemia may develop.

All chemotherapeutic regimens are capable of producing *bone marrow suppression,* and tumors that invade and replace bone marrow can also result in pancytopenia. Anemia can be corrected by blood transfusions of packed red blood cells. Thrombocytopenia can be corrected by platelet infusions. Granulocytopenia poses a risk of serious bacterial infections when the granulocyte count is less than $500/mm^3$. Febrile granulocytopenic patients should have appropriate cultures obtained and receive antimicrobial therapy, usually with a penicillinase-resistant penicillin and an aminoglycoside to give broad antibacterial coverage until the granulocyte count rises. Granulocyte transfusions are toxic and currently are rarely used.

Immunosuppression of variable degree is a consequence of some tumors and of some treatment regimens. Viruses normally of low pathogenicity can then produce serious disease. Patients should not be given vaccines containing live virus. Patients on chemotherapy who are exposed to varicella should receive varicella zoster immune globulin and, if severe clinical disease develops, should be hospitalized and treated with acyclovir. An attenuated varicella vaccine is being developed that appears to be safe at present for use in patients with leukemia on chemotherapy. Fungal infections are common, particularly with *Candida* species. Opportunistic organisms such as *Pneumocystis carinii* can produce fatal disease. If severe degrees of immunosuppression are anticipated, prophylactic treatment against pneumonitis due to *P. carinii* should be given with trimethoprim/sulfamethoxazole. See also Sec. 11.11.

Nutrition. It is not uncommon for patients undergoing cancer therapy to lose 10% or more of body weight. Malnutrition may become a particular problem in patients undergoing radiotherapy to the head and neck, or with intensive chemotherapy and total body irradiation for marrow transplantation. Such patients may require parenteral hyperalimentation. There is no evidence, however, that hyperalimentation improves a patient's chances of responding to therapy, and anxious parents should be reassured that they need not be concerned if the child's appetite is poor.

Emotional Support. A foremost consideration should be psychologic and emotional support for patient and family. An honest examination of the facts is the best policy in dealing both with child and parents. In practice, the child should be told all that he or she can understand and would find useful to know or wishes to know. Special problems, such as the need for amputation of a limb or of loss of hair during chemotherapy must be anticipated and fully discussed. Explanations may have to be repeated several times before distraught family members feel they really understand what is being said.

Whenever possible, the child should remain in school and with classmates. Since most treatment regimens are intensive, most of the patients will miss considerable schooling in the first year or two after diagnosis, even if they are eventually cured. Tutoring should be encouraged so that they do not fall behind academically. Parents, patients, siblings, and medical staff will need help in expressing feelings of anxiety, depression, guilt, and anger (Sec. 2.71).

Late Sequelae. Late consequences of therapy may result in serious morbidity. Successful surgical removal of a tumor may require the sacrifice of important functional structures. Following amputation of a leg for bone tumor, for example, careful attention must be given to rehabilitation with a functional prosthesis.

Irradiation may produce irreversible damage to organs, the symptoms and degree of limitation depending on the organ involved and the severity of injury. These may not become fully obvious until the patient is fully grown, when it may be noted that irradiated and nonirradiated areas or extremities are markedly asymmetric. Irradiation of endocrine organs can cause abnormalities in function. Hypothyroidism and sterility commonly follow thyroid and gonadal irradiation, and neurologic dysfunction may follow cranial irradiation.

Chemotherapy also carries the risk of irreversible damage to organs. Of particular concern are the leukoencephalopathy that follows high-dose methotrexate therapy, sterility in the male after therapy with alkylating agents, myocardial damage with anthracyclines, pulmonary fibrosis after bleomycin, and pancreatitis after asparaginase; all of these may be dose-related and are poorly, if at all, reversible. Appropriate studies must be done before these medicines are administered, in order to ensure that dangerous damage to organs has not already occurred.

Another late effect is the occurrence of *second cancers* in patients successfully cured of a first. The risk appears to be cumulative at about 0.5%/yr, up to 12% for patients who are 25 years beyond their treatment. Patients who have been treated for childhood cancer should be examined yearly and carefully assessed for the late effects of therapy.

16.4 THE LEUKEMIAS

The leukemias are the most common form of childhood cancer. They account for about one third of new cases of cancer diagnosed each year. The acute lymphocytic leukemias make up about 76% of cases, with a peak in incidence around the age of 4 yr. Acute nonlymphocytic leukemia accounts for about another 20%, with incidence increasing with age into late adulthood. Chronic myelogenous leukemia and other leukemias difficult to classify account for the remainder. Chronic lymphocytic leukemia is essentially never seen in childhood.

Leukemia occurs in 42.1/million white and 24.3/million black children/yr. The difference is due chiefly to the lower incidence of acute lymphocytic leukemia among black children. The acute lymphocytic leukemia (ALL) of childhood was the first form of disseminated cancer to respond completely to chemotherapy. It is, therefore, an important model upon which concepts of chemotherapy in other malignancies have been developed.

The general clinical features of the leukemias are similar, since all involve a severe disruption of bone marrow function. Specific clinical and laboratory features differ, however, and there are considerable differences in the responses to therapy and prognosis.

16.5 ACUTE LYMPHOCYTIC LEUKEMIA (ALL)

ALL occurs slightly more frequently in boys than in girls. Several reports of clusters of acute leukemia in children have suggested some common environmental factor in etiology, but careful statistical analyses have not supported this possibility. Lymphoid leukemias do occur more often than expected in patients with immunodeficiency, chromosomal abnormalities (such as Down syndrome), and ataxia-telangiectasis.

Pathology. Patients with ALL are subclassified according to the morphologic and immunologic features of their blast cells as well as by their clinical presentation. Definitive diagnosis must be made on examination of a bone marrow aspirate. The variability in cytologic appearance of the blast cells is so great, even within a single specimen, that no completely satisfactory system has yet been devised for differentiation of the various forms of ALL by cytologic appearance alone. A French-American-British (FAB) working group has devised a classification based on the appearance of bone marrow leukemia cells at the time of diagnosis. Three cytologic types are identified: L-1 lymphoblasts are predominantly small with little cytoplasm; L-2 cells tend to be larger and have greater amounts of cytoplasm, irregular nuclear membranes, and more prominent nucleoli; and L-3 cells have characteristic cytoplasmic vacuolization. L-3 morphology is uncommon and usually associated with blast cells having surface immunoglobulin (in B-cell ALL).

Cytochemical characteristics that identify blast cells of ALL are the absence of peroxidase positive and Sudan black positive granules in the cytoplasm, negative nonspecific esterase reaction, and the frequent appearance of clumps of periodic acid–Schiff (PAS) positive material.

The most useful classification of subtypes of ALL depends on cell membrane markers. It is first determined whether the cells represent a malignant proliferation of T (thymus-derived) lymphocytes, by using monoclonal antibody against the sheep erythrocyte receptor or other T-cell antigens. Within the subclass of T cells, monoclonal antibodies can be used further to determine whether the abnormal cell arises from early or late stages of T-cell maturation. If the cells are not T cells, they are then screened with fluorescein-tagged anti-immunoglobulin reagents. If immunoglobulin is detected on the cell surface (sIg), the cell is considered a mature B (bone marrow-derived) cell. If immunoglobulin is found in the cytoplasm (cIg), the cell is considered a B-cell precursor, or PreB cell. The largest group of leukemic patients have lymphoblasts that do not react with any of the above reagents; they are said to have "null cell" leukemia. They have been thought to represent an even earlier stage in B-cell maturation than the PreB cell for two reasons: first, almost all of them show immunoglobulin gene rearrangement, suggesting an attempt of their cells to mature along the B-cell pathway; and second, the majority of them have the common ALL antigen (cALLa) and the immune-associated (Ia) antigen, both of which are lost with T-cell maturation. Some leukemias in both the null and the PreB class do not possess cALLa. They represent a minority of the leukemias found in older children but virtually all the leukemias that have their onset before 6 mo of age. The subtypes of ALL with their relative incidences are shown in Table 16–4, along with certain clinical characteristics.

Table 16–4. Incidence of the Subtypes of ALL in a Single Study, with Incidence of Some Clinical Features at the Time of Diagnosis

Subtype	Number of Patients	(%)	Age (median)	WBC × 10³ (median)	% Male	% Having a Mediastinal Mass
T (T+)	44	(14)	7.4 yr	61.2	67.1	38.2
B (sIg+)	2	(0.6)				
PreB (cIg+)	56	(18)	4.7 yr	12.2	54.8	1.2
Early PreB (T−, sIg−, cIg−)	209	(67)	4.4 yr	12.4	56.5	1.0

Adapted from Pullen JD, Boyett JM, Crist WM, et al.: Pediatric Oncology Group utilization of immunologic markers in the designation of acute lymphocytic leukemia subgroups: Influence on treatment response. Ann NY Acad Sci 428:26, 1983.

Another biologic marker with potential usefulness is the increased terminal desoxynucleotidyltransferase activity found in cells of null-, preB-, and T-cell ALL. Since this enzyme is present only rarely in normal non-T lymphocytes, it may prove useful in identifying leukemic cells in difficult diagnostic situations; e.g., it may help to distinguish early CNS relapse from aseptic meningitis.

Patients with leukemia almost always have disseminated disease at the time of diagnosis, with marrow involvement at all sites and with leukemic blast cells in blood. Spleen, liver, and lymph nodes are also usually involved. Accordingly, there is no staging system like those developed for solid tumors.

Clinical Manifestations. Children with ALL present a fairly consistent clinical onset. About two thirds of them will have had signs and symptoms of their disease for less than 6 wk at the time of diagnosis. The first symptoms are usually nonspecific; there may be a history of a viral respiratory infection or exanthem from which the child has not appeared to recover fully. Frequent early manifestations are anorexia, irritability, and lethargy. Progressive failure of bone marrow function leads to pallor, bleeding, and fever, which are usually the features that precipitate diagnostic studies.

On initial examination most of the patients are pale, and about half have petechiae or mucous membrane bleeding. About a quarter have fever, which can sometimes be ascribed to a specific cause, such as respiratory infection. Lymphadenopathy is occasionally prominent, and splenomegaly (usually less than 6 cm below the costal margin) can be demonstrated in about two thirds of patients. Hepatomegaly is less common. out one third of patients have bone tenderness, owing to periosteal invasion and subperiosteal hemorrhage. Bone pain and arthralgia are important presenting complaints in about one quarter of patients. Rarely, signs of increasing intracranial pressure such as headache and vomiting may indicate leukemic meningeal involvement. Children with T-cell ALL are likely to be older, are more often male, and more often have a mediastinal mass; these features do not distinguish between children with PreB and those with null-cell ALL (Table 16–4).

Diagnosis. On initial examination most patients will have anemia; only about 25% will have hemoglobin levels below 6 g/dL. Most patients will also have thrombocytopenia, but as many as 25% may have platelet counts greater than 100,000/mm³. A significant proportion of patients will have white/blood cell counts less than 3000/mm³, and about 20% will have counts greater than 50,000/mm³. The diagnosis of leukemia can be suspected on the finding of blast cells on blood smear, but the definitive study is examination of bone marrow, which in almost all patients will be found to be completely replaced by leukemic lymphoblasts. Occasionally, patients in whom an aspirated specimen is hypocellular will require a needle biopsy of the bone marrow to demonstrate the leukemic replacement.

A chest roentgenogram should be made to determine if there is a mediastinal mass, as is frequently the case in patients with T-cell ALL. Bone roentgenograms may show altered medullary trabeculae, cortical defects, or subepiphyseal bone resorption, but these findings have no clinical or prognostic significance. Cerebrospinal fluid should be examined for leukemic cells. Early central nervous system involvement has important prognostic implications. Uric acid level and renal function should be determined before treatment is started (See Sec. 16.3).

Differential Diagnosis. The diagnosis of ALL is usually easily made once the possibility of ALL has been considered, but thinking of the diagnosis may be delayed for a child who has been sick and febrile with adenopathy for several weeks. The diseases to be considered in the differential diagnosis are those also associated with bone marrow failure. Bone marrow infiltration by other malignant cells can occasionally produce pancytopenia. In children the tumors capable of producing marrow replacement are neuroblastoma, rhabdomyosarcoma, Ewing sarcoma, and retinoblastoma. Usually these tumors are found in clumps scattered throughout normal marrow tissue, but occasionally there may be complete replacement of marrow. In such patients there is usually evidence of a primary tumor in some other site.

The bone marrow failure of ALL needs to be distinguished from the nonmalignant marrow failure associated with aplastic anemia or myelofibrosis. Patients with ALL who have marked leukopenia sometimes have no evidence of blast cells either on a blood smear or in aspirated marrow, the hypoplastic marrow resembling that of aplastic anemia. Examination of an adequate bone marrow biopsy will usually resolve any uncertainty. Occasionally, a patient who presents with aplastic marrow will develop frank leukemia a few weeks later.

Infectious mononucleosis should rarely be confused with ALL despite their somewhat similar clinical pictures. Careful examination of the blood smear should permit identification of the typical cells of infectious mononucleosis. If doubt remains, a bone marrow aspirate will demonstrate a normal cell population.

Treatment. The treatment of ALL varies with the clinical risk features. A patient at standard risk at the time of diagnosis is more than 2 yr old and less than 10, has a white blood cell count under 100,000/mm³, a normal mediastinum on chest roentgenogram, no evidence of leukemic central nervous system involvement, and blast cells that do not have B- or T-cell features. The basic components of a treatment program for such an individual include initial induction therapy until the bone marrow no longer shows leukemic cells, prophylactic treatment to the central nervous system, and a continuation of systemic treatment for 2.5–3 yr. A sample plan is outlined in Table 16–5.

A combination of prednisone and vincristine can be expected to produce remission in about 95% of children with standard-risk ALL. For almost all such patients remission is achieved within 4 wk. For the residual 5–10% of patients, another 2 wk of therapy should be given. Once remission has been achieved, these two drugs should be followed by another

Table 16–5. An Effective Treatment Regimen for Standard-Risk ALL

Remission induction (4–6 wk)
 Vincristine 1.5 mg/m^2 (max 2 mg) iv/wk
 Prednisone 40 mg/m^2 (max 60 mg) po/day

Followed by
 Asparaginase (*E. coli*) 6000 U/m^2/day daily iv × 14 days

Intrathecal treatment
 Triple therapy: Methotrexate 15 mg/m^2 (max 15 mg)
          Hydrocortisone 15 mg/m^2 (max 15 mg)
          Cytosine arabinoside 30 mg/m^2 (max 30 mg)
 Wkly × 6 during induction, and then every 8 wk for the first yr

Systemic continuation treatment
 6-mercaptopurine 50 mg/m^2/day po
 Methotrexate 20 mg/m^2/week po

With reinforcement
 Vincristine 1.5 mg/m^2 (maximum 2 mg) IV every 8 wk
 Prednisone 40 mg/m^2/day po × 28 days every 16 wk

agent, such as asparaginase. There is evidence that this will prolong the remission. Systemic continuation therapy should be given for 2.5–3 yr.

In more than 50% of patients who have not received prophylactic treatment of the CNS this body system will be the site of initial relapse. Evidence indicates that leukemic cells are present in the meninges at the time of diagnosis and that their survival is due to the lower drug concentrations achieved in the cerebrospinal fluid. Therapeutic invasion of this sanctuary area was first achieved through cranial irradiation; this therapy has been found, however, to produce late effects on school performance and behavior, particularly in younger children. For the standard-risk patient, intrathecal chemotherapy alone is thought to be sufficient therapy for clinically inapparent CNS involvement.

The response of patients with T-cell ALL to treatment is at present unsatisfactory. A regimen similar to that for standard-risk ALL will often achieve an initial remission, but most patients with T-cell ALL will relapse within 2 yr. More intensive multidrug regimens are being explored by the Cooperative Treatment Groups, and there is interest in bone marrow transplantation for this group of patients. Investigators are trying to take advantage of characteristics of T cells that set them apart from other lymphocytes, in order to target specific therapy. Anti–T-cell monoclonal antibodies are being used to purge autologous marrow before reinfusion, and the adenosine deaminase inhibitor deoxycoformycin may provide specific biochemical therapy for T-cell disease.

The few patients with L-3 morphology and surface immunoglobulin have the worst prognosis. They are best treated according to regimens designed for B-cell lymphoma and are considered candidates for early marrow transplantation.

In most centers, bone marrow is examined at regular intervals to see whether remission is continuing. If bone marrow relapse should occur, particularly after the patient has completed continuation therapy, intensive retreatment with a combination such as cytosine arabinoside and the epipodophyllotoxin VM 26, will achieve some cures.

When relapse occurs in both standard and high risk patients, it is often in an extramedullary site. The most important sites are the CNS and the testes. The common early manifestations of CNS leukemia are due to increasing intracranial pressure. Vomiting, headache, papilledema, and lethargy occur with increasing severity. These symptoms may also occur as part of a chemical meningitis secondary to intrathecal therapy, and this must be considered in the differential diagnosis. Convulsions and isolated cranial nerve palsies (such as of the 6th and 7th nerves) may also be manifestations of CNS leukemia. Hypothalamic involvement is rare but must

be suspected if excessive weight gain or behavioral disturbances occur. In almost all patients with leukemia involving the CNS, spinal fluid pressure is elevated and the fluid shows a pleocytosis due to leukemic cells. When the cell count is not increased, leukemic cells may be found in smears of spinal fluid specimens after centrifugation.

If CNS relapse occurs after preventive CNS therapy and during hematologic remission, the patient should be given intrathecal methotrexate 15 mg/m^2 (maximum 15 mg) weekly for 4–6 wk after the cells have disappeared. Craniospinal irradiation should then be given. In addition, the patient's systemic treatment should be intensified. Preventive CNS therapy should be repeated in all patients in whom relapses have occurred in the bone marrow or in other extramedullary sites.

Testicular size should be assessed as part of the routine examination of all patients with leukemia, to make sure the size is appropriate for age. Testicular relapse generally produces painless swelling of one or both testicles, of which the patient may not be aware. Diagnosis should be confirmed by biopsy. Treatment should include irradiation of the gonads (2000 rad), but since a number of patients show involvement of retroperitoneal lymph nodes at the time of testicular relapse, systemic therapy should be reinforced, for patients still on treatment, or reinstituted for those off treatment. CNS preventive therapy should be repeated as well.

Prognosis. Unfavorable prognostic features for patients with ALL include onset at age less than 2 yr or more than 10 yr of age, with a white cell count over 100,000/mm^3, or with a mediastinal mass. The significance of these clinical signs was established before the subtypes of ALL were known; the latter now permit clearer delineation of prognosis.

Null-cell ALL has the most favorable prognosis. Around 95% of affected patients will enter remission, and about 75% will still be in remission 5 yr after the start of therapy. A cure may be achieved in the majority of patients with this form of ALL. PreB-cell ALL has a somewhat less promising prognosis. About 95% of patients will achieve remission, but only about 60% will still be in remission after 5 yr. Patients whose cells lack cALLa may have a poor prognosis; almost all patients in whom ALL is diagnosed at less than 1 yr of age have cALLa-negative leukemia. T-cell leukemia is curable in only a minority of patients; B-cell leukemia is rarely cured with current therapy.

16.6 ACUTE NONLYMPHOCYTIC LEUKEMIA (ANLL)

ANLL accounts for about 20% of cases of leukemia in children. It is more common in older children and occurs with equal frequency in boys and girls. ANLL characteristically occurs in children having such predisposing conditions as Fanconi anemia and Bloom syndrome, in which there is excessive chromosomal breakage, or as a second tumor after cancer chemotherapy.

Pathology. The subtypes of ANLL shown in Table 16–6 are distinguished in the FAB system by differences in cytomorphology in Wright-stained smears of blood and bone marrow. The degree to which the predominant cell resembles a normal cell of bone marrow provides the designation of type. In the most common type the leukemic cells resemble myeloblasts or myelomonoblasts. The proportion of cell types resembling myeloblasts or monoblasts in the admixture makes the distinction between these two subtypes, which account for 90% of all ANLL.

Although there are cytologic differences, the clinical presentations and responses to therapy are similar for subtypes, with one exception: when the predominant cell resembles a promyelocyte (M3), there is increased risk that bleeding as-

Table 16–6. Subtypes of Nonlymphocytic Leukemia

Type	
Acute nonlymphocytic leukemia (ANLL)	*FAB classification*
Myeloblastic, no maturation	M1
Myeloblastic, some maturation	M2
Hypergranular promyelocytic	M3
Myelomonocytic	M4
Monocytic	M5
Erythroleukemia	M6
Chronic myelocytic leukemia (CML)	
Adult form	
Chronic phase	
Blast crisis	
Juvenile form	
Congenital leukemia	

sociated with disseminated intravascular coagulation will occur during the course of an early response to therapy. This M3 subtype occurs in about 5% of patients with ANLL.

Clinical Manifestations. The duration of symptoms and signs before the diagnosis is made in patients with ANLL is usually brief, 50% of patients having less than 6 wk of illness. In a few patients, however, the history may indicate a probable onset up to 12 mo before definitive presentation; in such patients the usual complaints are fatigue and recurrent infections. Worsening symptoms or signs during the 2 wk immediately before diagnosis are likely to include pallor, fever, active bleeding, bone pain, gastrointestinal distress, or severe infection. It is not possible to distinguish between ALL and ANLL on the basis of prediagnostic findings. A finding relatively specific for ANLL, however, is gingival swelling due to infiltration of leukemic cells.

The initial physical findings do not differ greatly from those in patients with ALL. The liver and spleen are enlarged in 60% of patients; marked hepatosplenomegaly occurs in only 10–15%. In 20% there may be marked lymphadenopathy. A few patients may initially have joint pain mimicking arthritis or a localized tumor mass (chloroma) that may produce such findings as proptosis or neurologic manifestations of CNS leukemia.

Diagnosis. The variability of initial leukocyte and platelet counts is similar to that in patients with ALL. Initial hemoglobin levels range from markedly decreased to normal, most patients having levels from 5–10 g/dL. The suspected diagnosis is confirmed by examination of the blood smear and bone marrow. In patients in whom the cytology is consistent with acute promyelocytic leukemia, coagulation studies must be done at the time of diagnosis to detect any acceleration of intravascular coagulation and to provide baseline values for evaluation of the subsequent clinical course.

The same considerations for differential diagnosis of ALL apply to ANLL. Additionally, there may be megaloblastic features in the bone marrow in ANLL that may superficially mimic those of folic acid or vitamin B_{12} deficiency. The experienced cytologist can easily distinguish ANLL by the more striking defects in maturation, the greater degree of atypical morphology, and the greater proportion of blast cells seen in this disease.

Sometimes children with ANLL have a long antecedent period of progressive marrow failure. In this early phase the proportion of blast cells may be so small that the diagnosis of leukemia cannot be confirmed. Sometimes the diagnosis can be facilitated by the demonstration that there are clones of bone marrow cells having aneuploid karyotypes. In such patients the course of progressive marrow failure may be hastened rather than reversed by chemotherapy; accordingly, a period of observation is the best current management, there being no indication that early treatment is of benefit.

In most cases, standard Wright- or Giemsa-stained blood and bone marrow smears are adequate to differentiate between the two characteristic types of blast cells. Histochemical stains are also useful. The cells in ANLL are usually positive for peroxidase and Sudan B black stains; and when their cytoplasm is positive for the periodic acid–Schiff (PAS) stain, the reaction is diffuse rather than aggregated or clumped as in ALL. In monoblastic leukemia the cytoplasm will be positive with the nonspecific esterase stain.

Monoclonal antibodies are now being developed that detect membrane antigens associated with discrete phases of maturation of myeloid cells. These help to identify myeloid leukemia cells as being mature or less mature (i.e., as stem cell phenotypes). Monoclonal antibodies can be particularly helpful in patients in whom histologic diagnosis is confusing. Even with these aids there are a few patients whose leukemia cells show no definite markers and others who will be seen to have definite markers of two cell lines (e.g., myeloid surface antigens and immunoglobulin gene rearrangement). It is not clear at present how such patients should be treated.

Treatment. Treatment of ANLL is improving with the availability of new drugs, and particularly with improvement in supportive care. Presumably because the myeloid leukemia cell closely resembles the normal myeloid stem cell, successful induction therapy seems to require a period of marrow aplasia. A regimen employing cystosine arabinoside 100 mg/m² by continuous intravenous infusion for 7 days, with intravenous daunorubicin 30 mg/m² day for 3 days, should achieve remission in 70% or more of the patients. In patients with promyelocytic leukemia, heparin should be given during induction to prevent fatal hemorrhage from disseminated intravascular coagulation. Maintenance therapy is generally given with rotating combinations of several agents for a period of up to 2 yr. One should expect that at least 50% of those who achieve remission will remain in remission when therapy is stopped. The central nervous system is an important site of relapse in ANLL, as in ALL. Following initial spinal taps for evaluation of CNS disease, prophylactic chemotherapy is administered in a fashion similar to that recommended for ALL. The use of bone marrow transplantation after the patient has achieved an initial remission is being studied. Children have longer remissions and survival than do adults, both with chemotherapy alone and after marrow transplantation; it is important, therefore, that experimental and control groups be matched for age.

Prognosis. The prognosis for patients with ANLL has improved; 30–40% of children can be expected to be cured with chemotherapy alone. Studies done principally in adults, in whom the disease is more common, tend to show that patients with membrane markers consistent with "stem cell phenotype" will be less likely to do well than those with a mature cell phenotype. The immunologic phenotypes have not correlated well with histologic appearance.

16.7 CHRONIC MYELOCYTIC LEUKEMIA (CML)

The adult type of CML accounts for only 3% of cases of leukemia in children. The age of maximal incidence in children is 10–12 yr. This condition has been seen with increased frequency in individuals exposed to radiation of the atomic bombs.

Pathology. In CML there are increased numbers of differentiating myeloid cells in blood and bone marrow. Splenomegaly is a prominent finding. Levels of vitamin B_{12} in serum and of fetal hemoglobin in erythrocytes will be elevated, whereas leukocyte alkaline phosphatase activity will be absent. If the pathognomonic Ph¹ chromosome is present, the diagnosis of CML is established; but some patients who have all the features of the clinical syndrome lack the Ph[1] chromosome (Ph[1]-negative CML), and a few patients who have the clinical syndrome of ALL have the Ph[1] chromosome in their leukemic blast cells (Ph[1]-positive ALL).

Clinical Features. The onset of symptoms is generally insidious. The diagnosis may not be suspected until splenomegaly or an abnormal blood count is found on routine examination. The spleen may become firm and enlarge as far as into the pelvis.

Diagnosis. Laboratory abnormalities are usually confined initially to the white blood cell count, which may be greater than 100,000/mm³, with all forms of myeloid cells seen in the blood smear. There are no characteristic morphologic abnormalities of the cells, but eosinophilia and basophilia are usually present and may be striking. The bone marrow is hypercellular, with normal myeloid cells in all stages of differentiation, and megakaryocytes may be increased in number. Initially, the platelet count is usually normal or increased. Anemia may or may not be present, and nucleated red cells may be seen. Laboratory abnormalities are noted above. Examination of bone marrow, with chromosome studies, is essential for diagnosis.

Treatment. There is as yet no treatment that will reverse the underlying disease process in CML, although intensive chemotherapy in adults has demonstrated that normal stem cells do exist in affected patients. Therapy should be aimed at preserving these stem cells in the hope that new treatments will soon be developed. The white blood cell count should probably be kept below 100,000/mm³, in order to avoid increased blood viscosity and cerebrovascular accidents. For this purpose, hydroxyurea (Litalir), which does not damage stem cells is preferred to busulfan (Myleran), which does. Splenic radiation may be used if the enlarged spleen is causing severe discomfort. Allogenic bone marrow transplantation may be effective early in the disease, and some responses to interferon have been seen.

The terminal phase of this disease is characterized by a gradual increase in the number of myeloblasts in the blood (blast crisis) and by the development of anemia and thrombocytopenia. With the onset of a blast crisis, which may be myeloid or lymphoid, the treatment program is changed to that for acute leukemia. Median survival from time of diagnosis is about 3 yr.

Juvenile chronic myelocytic leukemia occasionally affects patients, usually under the age of 2 yr, who have histories of eczematoid rash, lymphadenopathy, and recurrent bacterial infections, with moderate enlargement of liver and some splenomegaly. They have an elevated white cell count with a blood smear similar to that found in CML, although monocytosis is often more prominent. The proportion of fetal hemoglobin ranges from 30–70%. The serum vitamin B₁₂ level is elevated, but leukocyte alkaline phosphatase is usually detectable. The Ph[1] chromosome is not present. Such patients share some of the features of CML, and this form has been called juvenile CML, but this terminology probably reflects our poor understanding of the pathogenesis of this disease. Treatment with single agents or with combination chemotherapy regimens employed for acute myelogenous leukemia has not been very successful.

Sometimes an **infant with an underlying chromosomal abnormality,** and particularly trisomy-21, may be born with hepatosplenomegaly, a high white blood cell count with immature myeloid forms, and thrombocytopenia. It is unclear whether this "congenital leukemia" truly represents a leukemic process. Affected patients should be treated with supportive platelet transfusions only if needed for bleeding, and/or with single agent chemotherapy only if needed to control the white count, in order to see whether they will have spontaneous remission during the first few weeks of their disease.

LYMPHOMA

(See Sec. 10.1–10.3 and 15.60 for related discussion of the immune and lymphatic systems.)

Lymphoma, the third most common cancer in children in the United States, affects 13.2/million children/yr. The rates are similar for white and black children. The two broad categories of lymphoma, Hodgkin disease and non-Hodgkin lymphoma, have such different clinical manifestations, treatment, and prognosis that they will be considered separately.

16.8 HODGKIN DISEASE

Incidence. This tumor rarely occurs before the age of 5 yr, the incidence increasing steadily thereafter to a peak at 15–34 yr of age; a second peak occurs after the age of 50. The condition is almost twice as common in boys as in girls. No definitive causal factors are known, but occurrence in like-sex siblings has suggested a virus of low virulence and infectivity. Hodgkin disease appears to arise in T-dependent areas of lymphoid tissue. The central histologic feature is the Reed-Sternberg cell (Fig. 16–2). This cell is thought to originate from an antigen-presenting cell of the mononuclear phagocyte-reticulum cell lineage, perhaps from the interdigitating reticulum cell.

Pathology. There are four histologic subtypes of Hodgkin disease, each with special clinical features and implications for prognosis. In the *lymphocyte predominant* variety, almost all of the cells appear to be mature lymphocytes or a mixture of lymphocytes and benign histiocytes, with only an occasional Reed-Sternberg cell. This type affects 10–20% of patients and has the best prognosis.

The *nodular sclerosing* variety, the most common form, affects about 50% of patients. Broad bands of collagen divide the involved lymph node into nodular cellular areas. A special cytologic feature is clear spaces surrounding "lacunar cells," which are variants of the Reed-Sternberg cell. Because of the amount of collagen, the radiographic appearance of these lesions (particularly in the mediastinum) may be slow to return to normal, even when the patient is responding to therapy.

Hodgkin disease of *mixed cellularity* is the second most common form and affects 40–50% of patients. It is characterized by accumulations of lymphocytes, plasma cells, eosinophils, histiocytes, malignant reticular cells, and Reed-Stern-

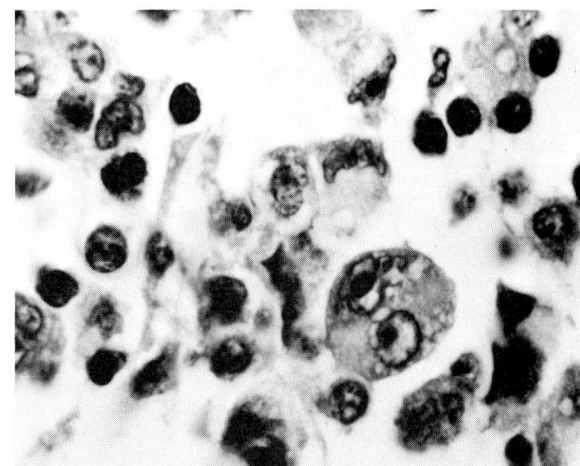

Figure 16–2. A Reed-Sternberg cell, which contains 2 nuclei, each with a prominent nucleolus and distinct nuclear membrane. The cytoplasm of this cell is relatively abundant. Other cells present are lymphocytes, plasma cells, and tissue mononuclear cells. This appearance in a lymph node is diagnostic of Hodgkin disease.

berg cells. Foci of necrosis may be present. This form is more likely to involve extranodal areas at the time of diagnosis.

The least common and least favorable form of the disease is the *lymphocyte depletion* variety, which affects fewer than 10% of patients. Numerous bizarre malignant reticular cells are found, with Reed-Sternberg cells and relatively few lymphocytes. There may also be varying degrees of partly hyalinized fibrosis with a paucity of cells, mostly of reticular and Reed-Sternberg types.

Hodgkin disease arises in lymph nodes in almost all instances; extranodal primary sites occur in fewer than 1% of patients. The manner of spread suggests direct anatomic extension. Adjacent lymph node areas are the first site of spread in the majority of patients, presumably as the result of spread along adjacent lymphoid channels. These observations have provided the basis for radiotherapy regimens. When the disease is no longer confined to lymph nodes, the more common sites of extranodal involvement are spleen, liver, lung, bone, and bone marrow.

For determining prognosis and for planning treatment, anatomic staging should be done at the time of diagnosis (Table 16–7). This will often involve exploratory laparotomy to establish the extent of intra-abdominal disease. In addition, patients should be assigned to an A or B category in accordance with the absence or presence, respectively, of systemic symptoms such as night sweats, fever, or recent weight loss of more than 10% of body weight.

Clinical Manifestations. The most common presenting finding is enlarged cervical lymph nodes. Occasionally, nodes of the supraclavicular, axillary, or inguinal areas may be the site of primary involvement. The enlargement is firm, nontender, and usually discrete, involving single or multiple lymph nodes. It is generally first noted by the patient or parents. Characteristically, no regional inflammation can be found to explain the lymphadenopathy. Mediastinal lymph node enlargement is common and may produce a cough, usually nonproductive, or symptoms of tracheal or bronchial compression. It may be found on a chest roentgenogram taken for an unrelated purpose. In younger children, mediastinal lymph node involvement may be difficult to distinguish from a large, normal thymus. Computed tomography (CT scan) of the mediastinum may reveal differences in texture from thymus.

Usually the patient has few, if any, systemic manifestations at the time of diagnosis. Typical symptoms would include night sweats, unexplained fever, weight loss, lethargy, easy fatigability, and anorexia. Pruritus is an unusual early complaint; alone it does not place the patient in a B category.

Extranodal involvement is unusual at the time of diagnosis, but may occur with progression of the disease. Lung involve-

ment may be represented roentgenographically by diffuse fluffy exudates, difficult to distinguish from disseminated fungal infection. Fever and tachypnea are usual, and pulmonary insufficiency may develop. If pulmonary involvement is suspected, the lesions should be biopsied first, since establishment of this diagnosis will identify stage IV, and a staging laparotomy will not be required.

Liver involvement is associated early with signs of intrahepatic biliary obstructive disease. With progression, signs of hepatocellular disease may develop. Bone marrow involvement may result in neutropenia, thrombocytopenia, and anemia. Extradural tumor masses in the spinal canal can cause progressive cord compression. A variety of immune disorders may occur, such as immunohemolytic anemia, immunothrombocytopenia, or the nephrotic syndrome.

Cellular immunity is impaired in Hodgkin disease as a consequence both of the disease and of its treatment. Affected patients are at increased risk of the infections characteristic of immunosuppressed patients. Varicella-zoster infections occur in up to one third of the patients and should be treated with *acyclovir* if severe; fungal infections such as cryptococcosis, histoplasmosis, and candidosis, may also become disseminated. Once the spleen has been removed, sepsis with encapsulated bacteria (such as *Streptococcus pneumoniae* or *Haemophilus influenzae*) may be lethal.

Diagnosis. Hodgkin disease should be suspected in the patient with persistent unexplained lymphadenopathy. The disease is more common in older children and adolescents, when infectious cervical lymphadenopathy is common. If a careful history and physical examination find no evidence that an underlying inflammatory process is responsible for the enlarged nodes and if the lymphadenopathy is persistent, then biopsy is warranted. In a significant percentage of patients, there will be a history of relatively recent antecedent, serologically proven infectious mononucleosis; accordingly, enlarged nodes that fail to regress after infectious mononucleosis should also be considered for biopsy. Before biopsy of a cervical node, a chest roentgenogram should explore the possibility of mediastinal involvement and examine the patency of the airway. The blood counts are generally not helpful; characteristic changes in the white blood cell count include a neutrophilic leukocytosis, lymphopenia, and sometimes eosinophilia and monocytosis. Anemia and thrombocytopenia occur only in patients with disseminated disease. The erythrocyte sedimentation rate may be increased, and in some patients the serum copper level is elevated. Since Hodgkin disease is a disease of the reticuloendothelial system, and the proteins that affect copper assays are made in the reticuloendothelial system, they may be useful, albeit nonspecific, markers of disease activity to follow.

When the diagnosis is made, staging should be done in order to establish the extent of the disease. Most patients first present evidence of lymph node enlargement above the diaphragm. A roentgenogram and CT scan of the chest should be performed. Sometimes disease will be seen on the latter when the former appears normal. In addition, CT can evaluate the extent of pericardial and chest wall involvement, which may affect prognosis. Liver function tests are unreliable indicators of hepatic disease, and the size of the spleen correlates poorly with splenic involvement.

Lymphangiography is generally accurate in indicating lymph node involvement below the level of the second lumbar vertebra, but above that level involved lymph nodes may not be filled with contrast materials. CT scans of the abdomen may indicate node enlargement but not the nature of the underlying process. Accordingly, for most patients, unless there is definite evidence of systemic spread, a staging laparotomy is indicated to determine with certainty the presence or absence of infradiaphragmatic disease. At laparotomy the spleen is removed, the liver is biopsied, and samples are

Table 16–7 Ann Arbor Staging System for Hodgkin Disease*

Stage I	Involvement of a single lymph node region or of a single extralymphatic organ or site
Stage II	Involvement of two or more lymphoid regions on the same side of the diaphragm; or localized involvement of an extralymphatic organ or site and of one or more lymph node regions on the same side of the diaphragm
Stage III	Involvement of lymph node regions on both sides of the diaphragm, which may be accompanied by localized involvement of an extralymphatic organ or site or by splenic involvement
Stage IV	Diffuse or disseminated involvement of one or more extralymphatic organs or tissues, with or without associated lymph node enlargement

*Patients are further categorized as A or B, based on the absence or presence, respectively, of systemic symptoms.

taken of nodes from all accessible areas. In addition, if radiotherapy to the pelvis is contemplated in a female, the ovaries should be moved to an area away from the radiation field, e.g., tucked behind the uterus in the midline. Bone marrow biopsies may be done to determine possible marrow involvement. In about one third of affected children, the stage of disease assigned from clinical findings will be revised when the anatomic findings are known.

Treatment. Both radiation therapy and chemotherapy are highly effective in the treatment of Hodgkin disease. Many patients have a good chance of long-term disease control or of cure, and the goal of current treatment regimens is to achieve cure with as little morbidity and toxicity as possible. For localized (stage I or IIA) disease in patients who have achieved their full growth, radiation alone to standard fields with doses of 3500–4000 rad may be the treatment of choice. Up to 50% of such patients, however, will have recurrences and will require combination chemotherapy. Regimens of chemotherapy either with nitrogen mustard, vincristine (Oncovin), procarbazine, and prednisone (MOPP) or with doxorubicin (Adriamycin), bleomycin, vinblastine, and dacarbazine (ABVD) can produce long disease-free periods for patients with advanced Hodgkin disease. A usual course of therapy would consist of six cycles of either of these treatments and would take about 6 mo. For patients with advanced disease or with disease that has recurred after radiotherapy, it may be that 1 yr of alternating courses of these non–cross-resistant chemotherapy combinations represents the best possible therapy. Questions such as which patients should be treated initially with chemotherapy, who should receive radiation and in what doses, and how toxic these treatments are to the growing child are still under investigation.

Prognosis. With current treatment more than 90% of patients with Hodgkin disease achieve a complete initial clinical remission. The likelihood of prolonged remission or cure is related primarily to the stage at diagnosis. Most patients with disease in stages I and II will be cured, as will around 75% of those in stage III if treated with both chemotherapy and radiation, and at least 50% of those in stage IV if treated with intensive chemotherapy.

The longer survival of patients has created more concern about the complications of treatment. The complications of irradiation depend on the site. Irradiation of upper body node areas may lead to restriction of lung capacity, to cardiac involvement, or to late hypothyroidism. In the younger child the growth of the vertebral column can be affected. Irradiation of the ovaries in the female patient may induce sterility or premature menopause or both, and irradiation of growing breast buds may prevent their development. With chemotherapy, there may also be late pulmonary (bleomycin) and cardiac (doxorubicin) toxicity. MOPP may produce sterility in the male.

One to two per cent of patients who have had splenectomy at staging laparotomy may develop overwhelming sepsis with *S. pneumoniae* or *H. influenzae*. These patients should be given pneumococcal vaccines around the time of laparotomy and receive long-term prophylactic penicillin. Abdominal adhesions may follow laparotomy, particularly in patients whose abdomens have been irradiated. A second malignancy (most frequently acute leukemia in patients who have received chemotherapy) occurs with an incidence, currently, of about 0.5%/yr after treatment.

16.9 NON-HODGKIN LYMPHOMA

Non-Hodgkin lymphoma, which designates a heterogenous group of solid lymphoid tumors, is more common than Hodgkin disease in young children, and affects boys about three times as frequently as it does girls. Both congenital and acquired immunodeficiencies predispose to the development of this type of lymphoma. Children with infantile X-linked agammaglobulinemia or severe combined immunodeficiency have about a 5% incidence of malignancy, usually lymphoma, and children with Wiskott-Aldrich syndrome and ataxia-telangiectasia a 10% or greater incidence. The incidence of lymphomas is increased also in immunosuppressed patients after renal transplantation.

A form of lymphoma in American patients resembles the Burkitt lymphoma of African children; the cells carry surface immunoglobulins, are derived from B lymphocytes (as in the African form of the disease), and show the chromosomal translocations described in Sec. 16–1. Unlike the African form, the American lymphoma does not have a nearly universal association with the Epstein-Barr virus.

Pathology. The classification of non-Hodgkin lymphomas is under continual revision. Children, more often than adults, tend to have the diffuse, more rapidly growing forms. A recent classification divides lymphomas into low, intermediate, and high grades. The majority of childhood lymphomas fall into the high grade category.

As new techniques identify subpopulations of normal lymphocytes, non-Hodgkin lymphomas are being reclassified in accordance with the stage in differentiation of lymphocytes that each represents. Table 16–8 shows a striking association between mediastinal primary site and T-cell origin of the tumor, and between abdominal primary site and B-cell origin. The series shown includes only patients from whom enough material was obtained to do immunologic typing, and underrepresents nodal primaries. In general, immunologic type and histologic type are correlated; T-cell tumors usually have lymphoblastic histology, whereas undifferentiated, Burkitt, and "histiocytic" lymphomas are of B-cell origin. When it can be done, immunologic subtyping is important, since optimal therapies vary with subtype.

Since children tend to have the more high grade tumors that do not spread in an orderly fashion and that disseminate readily, staging systems applicable to adults may not apply to children. A system devised for non-Hodgkin lymphoma in childhood is shown in Table 16–9.

Clinical Manifestations. The clinical features of lymphoma depend on the site of primary tumor and the extent of local and distant disease. The tumor commonly presents in the head and neck region as a painless, unexplained swelling of cervical or supraclavicular lymph nodes. The growth may be rapid, significant increases occurring within 1–2 wk. There may also be periods of regression. The nodes are generally nontender and firm, discrete in the early phases of growth, but often confluent later. Other nodal areas such as axilla, ileocecal region, or groin may also be primary sites of tumor.

Lymphoma of the chest generally arises in the anterior mediastinum, and the presenting feature may be cough or progressive dyspnea owing to compression of the airway or to pleural effusion, which may contain lymphoma cells. Obstruction of the superior vena cava may occur.

Table 16–8. Distribution of Cases of Non-Hodgkin Lymphoma in Childhood, According to Site of Primary Tumor and Cell-Marker Phenotype

Primary Site	T Cell	B Cell	Non-T, Non-B	Totals
Mediastinal	50	0	0	50
Abdominal	0	44	1	45
Nodal	7	2	1	10
Skin	1	0	4	5
Other	0	4	2	6
Totals	58	50	8	116

From Bernard A, Murphy SB, Melvin S, et al: Non-T, non-B lymphomas are rare in childhood and associated with cutaneous tumor. Blood 59:549, 1982.

Table 16–9. A Staging System for Non-Hodgkin Lymphoma in Childhood

Stage I
A single tumor (extranodal) or single anatomic area (nodal), with the exclusion of mediastinum or abdomen.

Stage II
A single tumor (extranodal) with regional node involvement.
Two or more nodal areas on the same side of the diaphragm.
Two single (extranodal) tumors with or without regional node involvement on the same side of the diaphragm.
A primary gastrointestinal tract tumor, usually in the ileocecal area, with or without involvement of associated mesenteric nodes only.

Stage III
Two single tumors (extranodal) on opposite sides of the diaphragm.
Two or more nodal areas above and below the diaphragm.
Any primary intrathoracic tumor (mediastinal, pleural, thymic).
Any extensive primary intra-abdominal disease.

Stage IV
Any of the above, with initial involvement of CNS and/or bone marrow at time of diagnosis.

From Murphy SB: Prognostic features and obstacles to cure of childhood non-Hodgkin's lymphoma. Sem Oncol 4:265, 1977.

Abdominal lymphoma occurs most frequently in the ileocecal region, presenting possibly as an abdominal mass, as intestinal obstruction, or as intussusception. There may be associated ascites.

Lymphoma of bone produces local or diffuse bone pain and usually represents dissemination from some other primary site.

Along with findings related to the local tumor, there may be manifestations of systemic dissemination. Meningeal involvement may present signs of increased intracranial pressure, or there may be direct extension of tumor to involve cranial nerves or produce spinal cord compression. Bone marrow may be involved. If more than 25% of the marrow cells are lymphoblasts, the patient is arbitrarily classified as having T-cell leukemia. Systemic symptoms of fever and weight loss are not uncommon. Occasionally, particularly in patients with immunodeficiency, primary intracerebral lymphoma may present as a mass lesion.

Treatment. After biopsy, surgery has a role principally for the excision of localized lymphoma of the bowel. Because of the systemic nature of this tumor and its propensity for hematogenous dissemination, all patients require chemotherapy. Before therapy is started, renal function and serum uric acid levels should be determined (Sec. 16.3) and administration of allopurinol begun. If airway obstruction is severe, corticosteroid medication should be given as an emergency measure; irradiation can also be used but will not act more quickly. An attempt should be made to obtain a tissue diagnosis before any therapy is started.

Recommended therapy now depends on the site of origin of the tumor, as well as the degree of dissemination. For localized nodal disease treatment similar to that for acute lymphoblastic leukemia (see Table 16–5), but lasting only 1 yr, currently represents the treatment of choice. For patients with a Burkitt lymphoma histology, regimens relying on high dose methotrexate and cytoxan should be employed. In general, these tumors of B-cell origin grow rapidly and will recur quickly if they are going to do so. For this reason therapy is intensive but is usually not given for more than 1 yr.

For primary intrathoracic tumors, a more intensive, 10-drug regimen gives the best chance of cure. Particularly with lymphomas of T-cell origin, some form of preventive CNS therapy (chemotherapy or irradiation or both) should be given, and maintenance continued for up to 1 yr.

Prognosis. With current treatment, perhaps 90% of patients with stage I and II disease can expect to be cured, as can about 50% of those with stage III and IV disease. Once tumor has spread to the bone marrow and undergone "leukemic conversion", the prognosis is worse. In patients who have had relapses, there has been some success in the use of intensive chemotherapy followed by autologous bone marrow reinfusion or identical-twin marrow transplantation.

16.10 HISTIOCYTOSES

A group of diseases characterized by proliferation of cells of the monocyte/macrophage line have been traditionally referred to as histiocytoses or reticuloendothelioses. Their nature is not known. Careful attention to clinical features and histologic characteristics permits sufficient definition to guide treatment and determine prognosis. It should be remembered that "histiocytic lymphoma" is thought to represent malignant proliferation of B cells (see Sec. 16.9).

Histiocytosis X. This term encompasses three sporadic illnesses, once thought to be distinct but now believed to be expressions of the same fundamental pathologic process: Hand-Schüller-Christian disease, Letterer-Siwe disease, and eosinophilic granuloma of bone. These are also called reticuloendothelioses. They are discussed in Sec. 26.5.

Familial Histiocytosis. A condition clinically and histologically identical to histiocytosis of the sporadic form has been reported in monozygotic twins and in nontwin siblings, with both X-linked recessive and autosomal recessive patterns of inheritance. The relationship between familial and sporadic forms is unknown (see above). There are no clinical distinctions.

Histiocytic Medullary Reticulosis. This is a rapidly progressive illness. Clinical features include fever, hepatosplenomegaly, liver failure, lymphadenopathy, and pancytopenia. The bone marrow contains marked erythrophagocytosis; other tissues are markedly infiltrated with histiocytes, and erythrophagocytosis is seen there also. This tends to be a disease of adults and older children. Although it is often fatal, responses to cyclophosphamide, doxorubicin, vincristine, and prednisone have been reported.

Sinus Histiocytosis. In this benign form of histiocytosis, the clinical manifestations are massive lymphadenopathy, particularly of the cervical region, fever, and moderate leukocytosis. Mediastinal lymph nodes may also be massively enlarged, but there is minimal, if any, enlargement of liver and spleen. The characteristic histologic pattern in lymph nodes involves dilatation of the subcapsular and medullary sinuses with benign-appearing macrophages that frequently contain phagocytosed lymphocytes. This accumulation of macrophages may totally efface lymph node architecture. Bone marrow aspirate or biopsy will generally show an increased number of macrophages. Most patients have an onset in the first decade of life; the condition affects boys and girls with the same frequency.

The disease resembles an atypical inflammatory response, but no etiologic agent has been defined. Reversible alterations in cellular immunity have been reported, but the relationship of these to the fundamental process is unknown. The clinical course may run for months, with gradual resolution of the lymphadenopathy. No therapy is indicated.

NEOPLASMS OF NERVOUS TISSUE ORIGIN

Tumors of the central nervous system are discussed in Sec. 21.22. Other tumors arise from the primitive neural crest cells that form the adrenal medulla and sympathetic nervous system. In children, these tumors are represented almost exclusively by neuroblastoma and its benign variant, ganglioneuroma.

16.11. NEUROBLASTOMA

Neuroblastoma in children under the age of 15 yr occurs at a rate of about 1/100,000/yr. It is slightly more common in white children than in black and slightly more common in boys than in girls. The median age at the time of diagnosis is around 2 yr; about 75% of cases are diagnosed before the age of 5 yr. Occasionally, cases occur in older children or adults. Familial occurrence is known, including in identical twins, but this tumor seems generally to be sporadic. Deletions in chromosome 1 are commonly found in tumor tissue.

Neuroblastoma has a uniquely high rate of spontaneous regression. Neuroblastoma in situ is related to the nodular clusters of neuroblasts normally found in the adrenal glands of fetuses and in about 1/200 neonates at autopsy; this frequency is far above the incidence of clinical neuroblastoma. It is believed that most of these small tumors disappear spontaneously. Spontaneous regression of clinically apparent disease after birth also occurs, particularly in patients under the age of 1 yr who have stage I or stage IVS disease (see below and Table 16–10). Although the reasons for this spontaneous regression are unknown, proposed possibilities include an immunologic response to the tumor and the response to some normal growth factor as yet undefined. Some have questioned whether stage IVS neuroblastoma in infancy represents a true malignancy, despite its dissemination. Hyperdiploid tumor cells of clonal origin have been reported in infants with stage IVS neuroblastoma, possibly indicating true malignancy rather than benign hyperplasia.

Pathology. Neuroblastoma is usually a firm, gray mass. Hemorrhage into this vascular neoplasm commonly imparts a variegated maroon color, often with necrosis and calcification. The degree of cell differentiation in neuroblastoma is variable. Most tumors consist of primitive neuroblastoma cells with little evidence of differentiation. Some tumors have admixtures of cells with larger amounts of cytoplasm, cytoplasmic processes, rosettes with central fibrillar material, and mature ganglion cells. Electron microscopy reveals distinctive features: peripheral dendritic processes containing longitudinally oriented microtubules; and small, spherical, membrane-bound granules with electron-dense cores, which represent cytoplasmic accumulation of catecholamines (neurosecretory granules). With treatment, serial biopsy specimens may contain increasing proportions of mature ganglion cells, and "maturation" of the tumor to a ganglioneuroma may take place at some sites; this does not, however, indicate an improved prognosis.

The tumor may arise in any site where neural crest cells are present. The sympathetic chain extends from the posterior cranial fossa to the coccyx. About 70% of the tumors arise in the abdomen, half of these in the adrenal gland. Another 20% arise in the thorax, usually in the posterior mediastinum, and the remainder arise elsewhere. In some children with widely disseminated tumor, the initial site cannot be defined.

Neuroblastoma may extend to surrounding tissue by local invasion or to regional lymph nodes via lymphatics. Extension of a paravertebral lesion into the spinal canal may produce spinal cord compression. Hematogenous spread most frequently involves liver, bone marrow, and skeleton. Metastases to the orbits not uncommonly result in proptosis; those to the dura, in signs of increasing intracranial pressure (including split sutures). Metastases to the brain are rare.

Two staging systems are currently in use for neuroblastoma (Table 16–10). A special designation (stage IVS) is reserved

Table 16–10. Neuroblastoma Staging Systems

Evans Stages	Pediatric Oncology Group Stages
Stage I Tumor confined to organ or structure of origin.	**Stage A** Complete gross resection of primary tumor with or without microscopic residual; intracavitary lymph nodes, not adherent to and removed with primary,* histologically free of tumor; if primary in abdomen or pelvis, liver histologically free of tumor.
Stage II Tumor extending in continuity beyond organ or structure of origin but not crossing the midline; regional nodes on homolateral side may be involved.	
Stage III Tumor extending in continuity beyond the midline; regional nodes may be involved bilaterally; bilateral extension of midline disease.	**Stage B** Grossly unresected primary tumor; nodes and liver same as stage A.
Stage IV Remote disease involving skeleton, organs, soft tissue, distant nodes, and so on.	**Stage C** Complete or incomplete resection of primary; intracavitary nodes not adherent to primary histologically positive for tumor; liver as in stage A.
Stage IVS Patients who would otherwise be stage I or II, i.e., with small and/or resectable primary tumor; but who have remote disease confined only to one or more of the following sites: liver, skin or bone marrow (not bone).	**Stage D** Any dissemination of disease beyond intracavitary nodes—e.g., to extracavitary nodes, liver, skin, bone marrow, bone.

*Nodes adherent to or within tumor resection may be positive for tumor without upstaging patient to stage C.

for patients with small or unidentifiable primary tumors in whom remote involvement is confined to liver, skin, or bone marrow. Almost all such patients are under the age of 6 mo. Their skin nodules may have a firm, purplish "blueberry muffin" appearance. Patients with this form of neuroblastoma generally have a good prognosis with minimal or no therapy.

Clinical Manifestations. No tumor has such polymorphic symptoms as neuroblastoma, owing to the numerous sites for primary tumor, as well as to the patterns of widespread metastases. Moreover, some symptoms arise out of tumor-associated metabolic disturbances. The primary tumor is usually in the abdomen and presents as a firm, irregular, and nontender mass. Since the primary tumor is often in the adrenal, the mass is usually in the upper abdomen. Hemorrhage into the enlarging tumor is common and may produce pallor or even hypotension. With metastasis to the liver, hepatic enlargement and occasionally ascites occur. Severe ascites may result in respiratory embarrassment, and surgical decompression may be required. Bony metastases can produce pain and tenderness, generally manifested in the young child as extreme irritability.

Patients with primary tumors outside the abdomen are often not as sick at presentation. Thoracic masses are often discovered unexpectedly on chest roentgenogram. Occasionally, a large upper thoracic mass will give rise to respiratory distress. Tumors in the head and neck may be palpable or may result in Horner syndrome. Tumors in the pelvis may produce problems in defecation or urination. A rectal examination should be performed at least once in any patient with such symptoms. Neuroblastoma can develop either intraspinally or extraspinally or can extend in dumb-bell fashion between intervertebral foramina to cause cord compression, with back tenderness, sphincter dysfunction, and gait disturbance. A primary tumor in the nasopharynx (esthesioneuroblastoma) usually presents unilateral epistaxis or occlusion of nasal passageways.

Other symptom complexes accompany neuroblastoma. An encephalopathy involving the cerebellum produces a syndrome (opsomyoclonus) characterized by progressive ataxia and titubation of the head, myoclonic jerks, and chaotic conjugate jerking movements of the eyes (opsoclonus), with progressive dementia. The cause of this syndrome is not known. Severe diarrhea with atonic bowel and extreme loss of potassium may occur as an effect of overproduction of vasoactive intestinal peptide (VIP) and may disappear rapidly with resection of the primary tumor. Hypertension is relatively rare in patients with neuroblastoma; it is much more common in those with pheochromocytoma. Episodes of unexplained flushing and sweating are often reported, however, in patients with neuroblastoma and have even been reported in mothers of infants with the tumor in utero. Table 16–11 shows the reported incidence of these syndromes in one series of patients with neuroblastoma. The systemic syndromes occurred in patients with all stages of disease, and do not necessarily reflect disseminated disease or poor prognosis.

Diagnosis. Initial studies are determined by the site of origin and the evidence of dissemination. For abdominal tumors, computed tomography (CT scan) with oral or intravenous enhancement is probably the most helpful study. Conventional radiographic evaluation of adrenal neuroblastoma includes the abdominal roentgenogram and excretory urography. Helpful findings include calcification, or displacement of the renal collecting system or of the ureter. The relationship of the tumor to adjacent retroperitoneal organs (particularly the great vessels) is usually inadequately assessed by these methods, however, and such determinations may be critical in deciding whether the tumor is resectable or not and in planning the initial surgical procedure. On CT scan neuroblastomas generally have mixed tissue density indicating both solid and cystic components. The cystic areas are either hemorrhage or necrotic tumor. Calcification, sometimes not appreciated on a plain x-ray film, is found on CT scan in as many as 80% of neuroblastomas. If there has been significant hemorrhage into the tumor, this calcification may have a ring configuration difficult to distinguish from that of traumatic adrenal hemorrhage. Metastases may also be appreciated on the CT scan of organs such as liver or skeleton. Posterior mediastinal or paraspinal tumors are usually revealed by chest roentgenography. Widening of intervertebral foramina may help in detection of intraspinal extension of tumor. Metrizamide myelography along with CT may be required to define fully the extent of intraspinal extension of disease.

Bone scan is also useful in detecting primary tumor and in defining the extent of metastatic disease. Sixty per cent of patients will show primary tumor uptake of technetium diphosphonate. Metastatic lesions will be detected on bone scan but are sometimes difficult to identify because they often occur symmetrically at epiphyseal plates, e.g., in the proximal

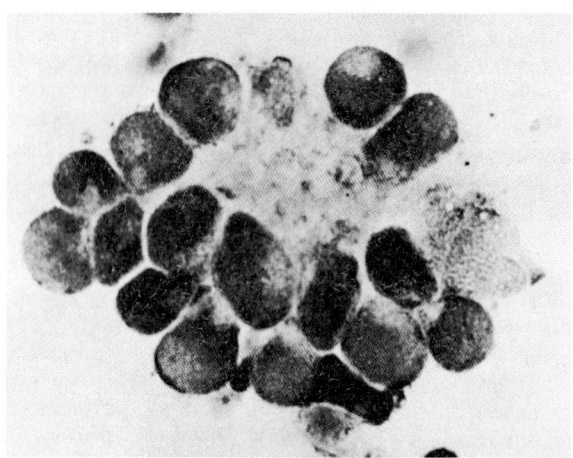

Figure 16–3. Neuroblastoma cells aspirated from the bone marrow. Clumps of cells often contain 3 or more cells without evidence of rosette formation. Rosettes of cells surrounding an inner mass of fibrillary material are characteristic of neuroblastoma.

humerus. Plain roentgenograms of symptomatic areas may help define the extent of metastatic disease.

Bone marrow aspiration or biopsy should be performed for staging in all patients. It may reveal infiltrating tumor cells in clumps (Fig. 16–3) or complete replacement of the marrow with sheets of tumor cells indistinguishable from those of acute lymphoblastic leukemia. Pancytopenia may result from marrow involvement.

A specific diagnostic feature is the elevated levels of catecholamines in urine. Increased amounts of dopa, dopamine, norepinephrine, normetanephrine, homovanillic acid (HVA), or vanillylmandelic acid (VMA) are found in about 90% of patients. The use of paper chromatography to identify VMA and HVA in 24-hour collections of urine may be confounded by medications or by dietary substances such as bananas, nuts, chocolate, and vanilla. A method involving gas chromatography and mass spectrography ("mass fragmentography") has greater precision and sensitivity; is free of diet and drug interference; measures all end-products of metabolism of dopamine, norepinephrine, and epinephrine; and requires only a few milliliters of urine.

Definitive diagnosis depends on the histologic characteristics of tumor obtained at excision or diagnostic biopsy. The above studies to demonstrate the site of primary tumor and the degree of dissemination should be done before surgery. For some patients with widely disseminated disease, a limited diagnostic biopsy of a superficial lesion or a bone marrow aspiration will be sufficient, particularly when accompanied by elevated catecholamine levels in the urine.

Treatment. For localized tumor, complete surgical resection gives the best chance for cure. For unresectable regional disease, the surgeon should establish the degree and nature of the local extension. Biopsies of lymph nodes draining the tumor area should be obtained; and for tumors primarily in the abdomen, liver biopsy specimens should be examined for microscopic involvement. For cases in which metastatic disease has already occurred, the value of an attempt at resection of the primary tumor has not been established. For patients with disseminated disease who have shown a response to chemotherapy, attempts have been made later to resect the primary tumor; the value of this second look for therapy has not been established, but a significant percentage of patients thought to be tumor free by clinical restaging have been discovered at the time of such surgery to have residual disease and to require further therapy.

Most neuroblastomas are radiosensitive; irradiation may be used for local symptomatic relief of disseminated tumor or

Table 16–11. **Frequency of Symptoms at Time of Diagnosis in 127 Cases of Neuroblastoma**

| Symptoms | Stage | | | | | |
	I	II	III	IV	IVS	Total
Opsomyoclonus	1	6	0	2	0	9
Diarrhea	2	0	3	1	1	7
Intraspinal extension	0	4	4	1	0	9
Hypertension	1	0	0	3	1	5
Total	7	28	17	56	10	12

From Rosen EM, Cassady JR, Frantz DN, et al: Neuroblastoma: The Joint Center for Radiation Therapy/Dana Farber Cancer Institute Children's Hospital Experience. J Clin Oncol 2:719, 1984.

for reduction in size of tumor masses. The use of total body irradiation or extensive radiation to treat systemic disease has been generally disappointing.

Because disseminated disease is common at the time of diagnosis of this tumor, chemotherapy is the mainstay of treatment. A regimen incorporating cytoxan and doxorubicin has been shown to induce remission in about 50% of patients. The combination of cisplatinum and the epipodophyllotoxin, VM 26, is also active. A number of other combinations have also been tried, with short-term responses. Bone marrow transplantation is now being assessed in patients with disseminated disease in first remission. Autologous marrow is reinfused after purging with cyclophosphamide derivatives to remove possible contaminating tumor cells; allogeneic marrow transplantation is also being studied.

Patients whose tumors are identified as pure ganglioneuroma should not receive chemotherapy or radiation if the tumors have been resected and probably not even if total resection was impossible.

Prognosis. The success of treatment in neuroblastoma is heavily dependent on age and stage. The older the patient and the more widespread the disease, the worse the prognosis. Patients whose tumors can be completely resected may do well with surgery alone. Local irradiation may be employed if there are small amounts of residual tumor. Patients with stage III and IV disease generally receive chemotherapy. Patients under the age of 1 yr may tolerate chemotherapy less well but are more likely than older patients to have a successful response to chemotherapy, particularly if their tumors are hyperdiploid.

Table 16–12 shows the results in a single institution of various regimens. The long-term survival of less than 10% for patients over the age of 1 yr with stage IV disease at the time of diagnosis illustrates the poor prognosis in this large group of patients. Marrow transplantation in remission may achieve closer to 25% long-term survival. The excellent prognosis of stage IVS patients is seen. Unless tumors in these patients seem likely to be lethal through interference with function of vital organs, they should probably not be treated but rather observed for the first few months after diagnosis to see whether spontaneous remission will occur.

Pathologists debate whether signs of histologic maturation are a significant prognostic factor. In the next few years, a new histologic grading system will be assessed that considers mitotic index and the degree and pattern of stromal infiltration into the tumor, in addition to histologic maturation. Among patients under the age of 1 yr, hyperdiploid tumors respond better to therapy than do diploid tumors.

16.12 PHEOCHROMOCYTOMA

Pheochromocytoma is a tumor of the sympathetic nervous system, rare in children and more benign than neuroblastoma. This metabolically active tumor is discussed in Sec. 19.27.

Table 16–12. Neuroblastoma: Treatment Results by Stage and Age

	Age at Diagnosis		2 Yr Survivors/Total
Evans Stage	<1 yr	>1 yr	(%)
I	5/5*	2/2	7/7 (100)
II	9/9	17/19	26/28 (93)
III	8/9	5/8	13/17 (76)
IV	9/10	4/46	13/56 (23)
IVS	6/7	3/3	9/10 (90)

*Number of disease-free survivors at 2 yr/Total number of patients in age group at given stage. Follow-up of 2–12 yr.

From Rosen EM, Cassady JR, Frantz CN, et al: Neuroblastoma: The Joint Center for Radiation Therapy/Dana Farber Cancer Institute Children's Hospital Experience. J Clin Oncol 2:719, 1984.

NEOPLASMS OF THE KIDNEY

16.13 WILMS TUMOR

Wilms tumor accounts for almost all renal neoplasms in childhood. It occurs with approximately equal frequency in both sexes and in all races, with an annual incidence of 7.8/million children under the age of 15 yr.

An important feature of Wilms tumor is its association with congenital anomalies. The most common associations are with genitourinary anomalies (4.4%), hemihypertrophy (2.9%), and sporadic aniridia (1.1%). Wilms tumor has developed in children of parents with hemihypertrophy and in siblings of children with hemihypertrophy. Hemihypertrophy may often not become obvious until the time of the adolescent growth spurt; accordingly, a child with asymmetric growth following treatment for Wilms tumor may have hemihypertrophy rather than a complication of therapy.

A deletion in chromosome 11 was first noted in families of children with the aniridia-Wilms syndrome. It is consistently present at a submicroscopic level in cells of most Wilms tumors, even when the constitutional chromosomal composition is normal (see Sec. 16.1).

As with retinoblastoma (Sec. 16.20), the familial form of Wilms tumor is more likely to be bilateral than the sporadic form. Moreover, patients with bilateral or familial disease also have a higher incidence of congenital anomalies, and their tumor may develop at an earlier age. It is estimated that a child of a patient with bilateral or familial Wilms tumor has a 30% risk of developing the tumor.

Pathology. The classic Wilms tumor is a solitary growth that may occur in any part of either kidney. It is sharply demarcated and variably encapsulated. Small areas of hemorrhage are common. The tumors usually distort the renal outline, the residual normal kidney often being compressed into a thin rim around the tumor (Fig. 16–4A and B).

The microscopic appearance in patients with favorable histology generally includes both epithelial and stromal elements (Fig 16–5). There are three "unfavorable" histologic patterns; these are found in 10% of cases of Wilms tumor but are responsible for 60% of the deaths. *Anaplasia* involves marked variation in nuclear size with abnormal mitotic figures. It tends to occur in older patients. The *rhabdoid* tumor has cells with fibrillar eosinophilic inclusions; the presence of true striated muscle, however, excludes the diagnosis of rhabdoid Wilms tumor. This tumor type is found most often in very young patients. *Clear cell sarcoma* of the kidney is characterized by a spindle cell pattern with a striking vasocentric arrangement. This tumor is predominant in males and is most likely to metastasize to bone.

The staging system most frequently used is that of the National Wilms Tumor Study (NWTS) Group. Stage I tumors are limited to the kidney and can be completely excised with capsular surface intact. The stage II tumor extends beyond the kidney but can be completely excised. In stage III, there is residual nonhematogenous extension of tumor, confined to the abdomen following surgery. Stage IV indicates hematogenous metastases, which most frequently involve the lung. Five to ten per cent of Wilms tumors will be bilateral, and survival will be related to prognosis for the most severely involved kidney. (Stage V designates bilateral renal involvement, which is usually concordant in time). The relative incidence of stages I–IV and survival rates are shown in Table 16–13.

Clinical Manifestations. The median age at time of diagnosis of Wilms tumor is about 3 yr. The most frequent sign is an abdominal mass, which is often asymptomatic. The mass is generally smooth and firm and rarely crosses the midline. Masses vary greatly in size at the time of discovery; mean diameter in one series of cases was 11 cm. Masses are often

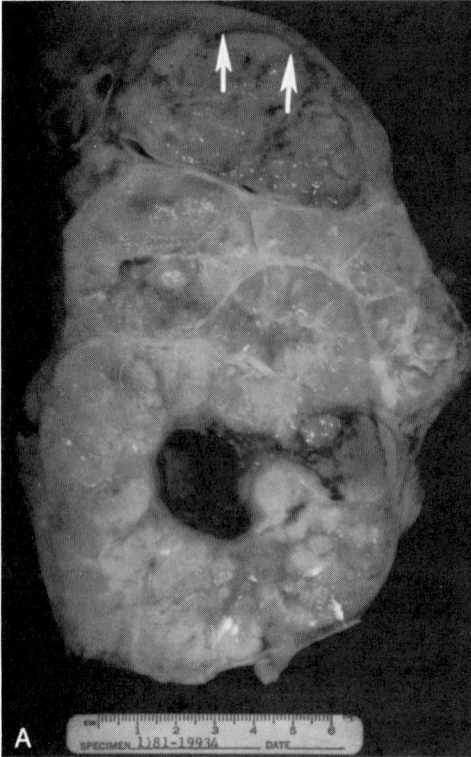

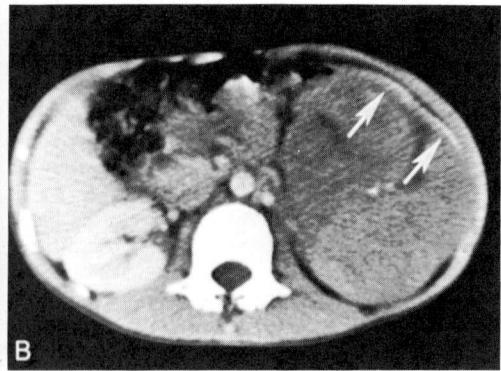

Figure 16–4. Wilms tumor. *A*, Gross specimen. A large mass compressing small rim of normal renal tissue. *B*, CT scan of kidney. A rim of compressed normal tissue represents the residual normal renal parenchyma.

discovered on routine examination, or by parents. About half of affected children may have additional symptoms of abdominal pain or vomiting or both. In general, patients with Wilms tumor are slightly older and appear less ill than those whose abdominal mass will prove to be neuroblastoma.

Hypertension has been reported in as many as 60% of patients. Hypertension results from renal ischemia, usually owing to pressure of the tumor on the renal artery. It may be sufficiently severe and prolonged to produce congestive cardiac failure.

Diagnosis. The diagnosis of Wilms tumor must be suspected in any young child with an abdominal mass. In 10–25% of patients, microscopic or gross hematuria may be the only indication that the tumor is renal. Intravenous pyelography may indicate that the mass is intrarenal. The major differential diagnostic consideration may be neuroblastoma. Computed tomography (CT) is generally most helpful. On CT studies without enhancement, the usual Wilms tumors arise from kidney as inhomogeneous masses with areas of low density indicating necrosis. Areas of hemorrhage and small focal calcifications are generally less common and less prominent than in neuroblastoma. After injection of a contrast medium, slight enhancement of tumors is noted. There is often a sharp demarcation between the tumor and normal parenchyma, correlated with a pseudocapsule, and persistent ellipsoid areas of increased attenuation corresponding to the compressed uninvolved renal parenchyma (see Fig. 16–4*B*). The primary clinical usefulness of CT in Wilms tumor is to establish the intrarenal origin of the tumor, which rules out neuroblastoma; to detect multiple masses; to determine the extent of tumor, including great vessel involvement; and to evaluate the opposite kidney. The major problems in differential diagnosis are hydronephrosis, renal cysts, and mesoblastic nephroma or other renal malignancies such as renal cell carcinoma, sarcoma, and lymphoma.

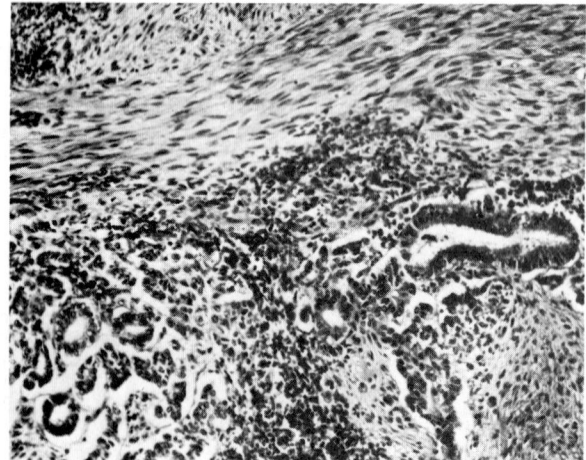

Figure 16–5. The histologic features of Wilms tumor. The epithelial component is respresented by the round oval tumor tubules; an elongated tumor tubule is also present. The mesodermal component is representec by the band of aligned nuclei across the photomicrograph.

Table 16–13. **Survival by Stage and Histology at Time of Diagnosis in National Wilms Tumor Study 3 (NWTS 3)**

Stage	Number of Patients	Percent of Total	Percent Having 2 Yr RFS*
I	371	28%	89–92%
II	377	28%	83–93%
III	383	29%	75–87%
IV +UH	198	15%	66–72%
Total	1329	100%	

*RFS = Relapse free survival at 2 yr, range indicates differences between experimental treatment arms. UH = Unfavorable histology.

Adapted from D'Angio GJ, Evans AE, Breslow N, et al: Results of the third National Wilms' tumor study (NWTS 3): A preliminary report. Proc AACR 25:183, 1984.

Pulmonary metastases will be evident on roentgenograms in 10–15% of patients at the time of diagnosis, which is more common than in neuroblastoma. CT scan of the chest is useful, particularly to visualize the portions of the lung below the level of the dome of the diaphragm (Fig. 16–6). In a patient in whom hepatic metastases are suspected, radionuclide scan of the liver may be performed. Evaluation of bone and bone marrow should be done only after surgery and only if the patient has a tumor with unfavorable histology or has persistent pain.

Certain rare paraneoplastic syndromes may be associated with Wilms tumor. The neoplasm may produce erythropoietin, leading to polycythemia; and secondary hypercalcemia has been reported.

Treatment. The usual immediate treatment is surgical removal of the kidney containing the tumor even if pulmonary metastases are present. At the time of operation careful inspection should be made of the other kidney to exclude the possibility of bilateral tumor and of the liver for possible metastasis. The retroperitoneal lymph nodes and renal vein should be examined for involvement. Every attempt should be made to remove the tumor without spillage, but since postoperative chemotherapy and radiation are capable of destroying residual tumor, life-threatening attempts to remove every bit of tumor should not be undertaken.

Wilms tumor is sensitive both to chemotherapy and to radiotherapy. The logical and systematic treatment of this tumor has been greatly advanced by the formation in 1969 of the NWTS group of participating institutions. Prior to that time, virtually all patients received postoperative radiation and various single-agent chemotherapies. The NWTS group has shown that combination chemotherapy with vincristine and actinomycin is clearly superior to single-agent therapy in patients with localized disease, and that doxorubicin is a significant addition to the treatment of patients with advanced disease. In addition, the NWTS group has shown that postoperative radiotherapy is not necessary for patients with stage I disease, for whom a short postoperative course (6 mo or less) of combination chemotherapy appears to suffice. They are currently investigating the best dose and field for postoperative radiation in patients with stage II and III disease who also receive chemotherapy. For patients with stage IV disease, radiotherapy and combination chemotherapy with three or four drugs for 15 mo is recommended.

Preoperative therapy is not recommended for patients with unilateral disease, but it may be the treatment of choice for patients with bilateral disease so that shrinkage of primary tumors can allow partial nephrectomy with salvage of the greatest amount of residual normal kidney. For patients with bilateral disease, bilateral nephrectomy with secondary renal transplantation has usually not been effective.

Prognosis. In general, prognosis is better in children positively diagnosed before the age of 2 yr and whose Wilms tumor weighs less than 250 g. The most significant prognostic variables, however, are histology and stage (Table 16–13). Any recurrence of disease carries a poor prognosis.

Pulmonary involvement has not been studied systematically. Pulmonary lesions amenable to surgery at the time of recurrence should probably be resected.

16.14 OTHER RENAL NEOPLASMS

Nephroblastomatosis. One or more independent foci of malformation or benign neoplasia or both may accompany Wilms tumors in at least one third of patients. This condition is generally called the nephroblastomatosis complex; its pathologic features include the presence grossly of multicentric tumor-like lesions and microscopically of metanephric elements matured beyond the 36th wk of gestation. All patients with bilateral Wilms tumor have manifestations of nephroblastomatosis, and the finding of these blastomatous components in one kidney is an indication for careful inspection of the contralateral kidney. The incidence of development of an asynchronous second Wilms tumor in patients with unilateral and nephroblastomatous tumor was once thought to be as high as 60%, but it is declining, perhaps owing to a chemo-preventive effect, since all patients now receive combination chemotherapy at the time of the diagnosis of the initial tumor. Patients with nephroblastomatosis should be followed carefully with CT scans.

Mesoblastic Nephroma. Congenital mesoblastic nephroma is a massive, firm, infiltrative, solitary renal mass, grossly and microscopically resembling a leiomyoma or a low grade leiomyosarcoma with trapped nephrons. The infiltrative margins are difficult to delineate histologically from normal or dysplastic renal stroma. By electron microscopy, the cells are fibroblasts or myofibroblasts. This tumor accounts for the majority of congenital renal tumors. Male preponderance has been noted, as well as renin production. The tumor is generally thought to be benign, for which surgical removal represents adequate therapy. Occasionally a patient may have a very cellular tumor that more closely resembles a clear cell sarcoma, and such patients may show local recurrence and even metastatic disease; they should receive chemotherapy and irradiation.

Renal Cell Carcinoma. This tumor is rare in the first decade of life, but occurs occasionally in teenagers. The initial findings are an abdominal mass and hematuria. The microscopic appearance and clinical course are similar to those found in adults with this neoplasm. Complete surgical resection may result in cure but the prognosis is grim in patients with postoperative residual disease. The tumor is radiosensitive.

SOFT TISSUE SARCOMAS

Soft tissue sarcomas have an annual incidence of 8.4 per million white children under the age of 15 yr and about half that incidence in black children. Rhabdomyosarcoma accounts for more than half of these tumors (Table 16–14).

16.15 RHABDOMYOSARCOMA

There appears to be a bimodal curve for incidence of rhabdomyosarcoma. An early peak occurs before 5 yr of age, with tumors of the neck, head, prostate, bladder, and vagina (in females) common; a later peak occurs around 15–19 yr of age, with involvement of the genitourinary tract (particularly of testes or paratesticular tissue in males). There is a slight predominance of male patients.

There appears to be a familial aggregation of rhabdomyosarcoma with other sarcomas. Rhabdomyosarcoma may com-

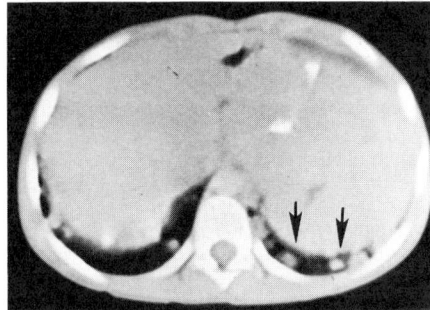

Figure 16–6. Wilms tumor. CT scan of chest showing metastatic lesions below the dome of diaphragm which would be difficult to visualize on plain radiograph.

Table 16–14. **Soft Tissue Sarcomas**

Tissue of Origin	Tumor	Natural History
Primitive Mesenchyme	Malignant mesenchymoma	May occur as a congenital tumor. Usually involves extremities or retroperitoneum. Characterized by rapid growth and frequent recurrence. Lung, brain, liver, and lymph nodes are the most frequent sites of metastases.
Connective Tissues Adipose	Liposarcoma	Rare in children. Generally develops in a previous lipoma, with rapid growth, occasionally with systemic symptoms (e.g., fever). Metastases relatively common in adults, less so in children. Outcome correlated with the degree of cellular differentiation.
Fibrous	Fibrosarcoma	May occur as a congenital tumor. Patients under 5 yr old (i.e., with infantile form) have a better survival rate (metastases in 7.5%) than patients over 15 yr old (metastases in 50%; local recurrence rate 40%). Extremities the most common site. Primary lesion occasionally related to prior irradiation.
	Dermatofibrosarcoma protuberans	Slow-growing tumor, especially likely on trunk, scalp, or face. Usually progresses from skin nodule to pedunculated tumor over years, but (rarely) can grow rapidly. High frequency of local recurrence. Tumor spread is usually to subcutaneous tissue, muscle, and bone; metastasis predominantly to lung and brain.
	Fibromatoses (fibrous hamartoma, fibrosis colli, infant and juvenile aponeurotic fibroma, congenital generalized fibromatosis, infantile digital fibroma	Locally invasive; only rarely metastatic. An exception: congenital generalized fibromatosis (CGF), which usually has visceral involvement and a poor prognosis. Prognosis generally good for these tumors, but local recurrence rate is high (90%).
	Malignant fibrous histiocytosis	Rare before the fourth decade; the most common soft tissue sarcoma of late adult life. Typically on the extremities (especially the thigh) and in the retroperitoneum, arising from deep fascia or muscle. Local recurrence rate is 44%. Prognosis is related to the size and the initial depth of the tumor (i.e., whether fascia or deeper structures are involved).
	Epithelioid sarcoma	Slow-growing, locally infiltrating tumor; usually presents as painful nodules on extremity (especially on forearm or hand or in popliteal area). The nodules frequently have ulcerated overlying skin. High rate of local recurrence. The most frequent metastases are to lung, lymph nodes, and skin.
Vascular Tissue Lymphatic	Lymphangiosarcoma	Very rare tumor, presenting predominantly in the extremities, sometimes decades following congenital or acquired lymphedema. Rapidly progressive, with metastases to the chest wall or pleura.
Blood	Angiosarcoma	Rapidly progressive, highly fatal tumor, predominantly involving extremities, liver, and head and neck regions. Has been associated with exposure to Thorotrast and vinyl chloride. May occur in children 1 yr old. Metastasizes to liver, bone, and adrenal gland.
	Hemangiopericytoma	May occur as a tumor. Most frequent primary sites are extremities and trunk. High rate of local recurrence (50%); metastases may occur late (10 yr), usually to lung, brain, and liver.
	Juvenile angiofibroma	The primary site is the nasopharynx. Does not metastasize, but is locally invasive.
Supportive Tissue Synovium	Synovial cell sarcoma	Rare; occurs mainly between ages of 20–40 yr. Predominantly involves the extremities (80–90%), especially the knee, foot, and hand. Metastases common to lung, bone, and lymph nodes. Characterized by local recurrence and late relapse (even 10–15 yr after diagnosis).
Fascia	Alveolar soft part sarcoma	Generally slow-growing; most common primary site the thigh or abdominal wall. High rate of local recurrence and metastasis, generally late and especially to lung, bone, and brain. Occurs in children as young as 3 yr old.
Mesothelioma	Malignant mesothelioma	Rare in children. Associated with exposure to asbestos in adults. The most common primary sites are the pleura and peritoneum. Rapidly progressive, with extensive local spread and metastases.
Muscle Tissue Aponeurotic	Desmoid	Rare in children: median age of onset 23 yr, most commonly in abdominal wall or shoulder girdle. Generally presents as a fixed, sometimes painful mass. Tumors may be exacerbated by estrogens or during the postpartum period.
Smooth	Leiomyosarcoma	Rare in children; has been observed in neonates. The gastrointestinal, genitourinary, and respiratory tracts represent the most common sites. Major sites of metastases: liver, regional nodes, lungs, peritoneum, and pancreas.
Striated	Rhabdomyosarcoma	See Sec. 16.15.

Modified from page 1330, P.A.: Rhabdomyosarcoma and other soft tissue sarcomas. *In* Levine, AS (ed): Cancer in the Young. New York, Masson Publishing, 1982, pp 615–632.

plicate neurofibromatosis. In addition, patients with rhabdomyosarcoma are often found in "cancer families," in which there is a high incidence of brain tumors and breast cancer at an early age, particularly when such occurs in parents.

Pathology. Rhabdomyosarcoma is thought to arise from the same embryonic mesenchyme as striated skeletal muscle. It can occur anywhere in the body. In general, rhabdomyosarcoma and the other soft tissue sarcomas belong to the group of tumors often called "small round cell tumors" on light microscopy; they include Ewing sarcoma, neuroblastoma, and lymphoma. Definitive diagnosis of a pathologic specimen may require additional studies such as electron microscopy to distinguish characteristic features. There are four recognized histologic subtypes of rhabdomyosarcoma. The *embryonal* type accounts for about 60% of the tumors. The botryoid type (also called sarcoma botryoides) is a variant of the embryonal form in which the tumor cells and an edematous stroma project into a body cavity like a bunch of grapes; it accounts for 6% of the total and is commonly seen in the vagina, uterus, bladder, nasopharynx, and middle ear. The *alveolar* type accounts for about 20% of cases. The tumor cells tend to grow in cores that often have cleft-like spaces resembling alveoli. It is found most often in trunk and extremities, primarily in older children, and carries the poorest prognosis. The *pleomorphic* type (adult form) is rare in childhood (1% of cases). About 20% of patients are considered to have *undifferentiated* tumor. New classification schemes that might have prognostic significance are under consideration by the Intergroup Rhabdomyosarcoma Study (IRS).

The most commonly used staging system is that of the IRS. Group I is localized disease, completely removable, with regional nodes not involved. Group II represents grossly resected tumor with regional nodes involved or microscopic residual disease. Group III indicates gross residual disease, and group IV distant metastatic disease at the time of diagnosis. The first IRS study found only 13% of patients in group I.

Clinical Features. The most common presenting feature is a mass, which may be painful. Origin in the nasopharynx may be associated with nasal congestion, mouth breathing, epistaxis, and difficulty with swallowing and chewing. Regional extension into the cranium may produce cranial nerve paralysis, blindness, and signs of increasing intracranial pressure, with headache and vomiting. When the tumor develops in the face or cheek there may be swelling, pain, trismus, and, as extension occurs, paralysis of cranial nerves. In the neck region the original finding may be progressive swelling, with neurologic symptoms following regional extension. In the orbit there may be proptosis, periorbital edema, ptosis, change in visual acuity, and local pain. When the tumor arises in the middle ear, the early signs are usually pain, loss of hearing, chronic otorrhea, or a tumor mass in the ear canal; extensions of the tumor produce cranial nerve paralysis and signs of an intracranial mass on the involved side. With tumor of the larynx there may be an unremitting croupy cough and progressive stridor. Since most of these signs and symptoms are also associated with common problems of the head and neck area, the clinician must be alert to the possibility of tumor.

Rhabdomyosarcoma of the trunk or extremities appears as a tumor, not uncommonly first noticed after trauma and for a time regarded as a hematoma. When the tumor shows little change in size or even grows at a time when a hematoma should be resolving, the true diagnosis should be suspected. Involvement of the genitourinary tract may produce hematuria, obstruction of the lower urinary tract, recurrent urinary tract infections, incontinence, or a mass detectable on abdominal or rectal examination. Involvement of the paratesticular tissues usually presents a rapidly growing mass in the scrotum. Vaginal rhabdomyosarcoma may present as a grape-like mass of tumor tissue bulging through the vaginal orifice (sarcoma botryoides) and may cause symptoms relating to the urinary tract or to the large bowel. Vaginal bleeding or obstruction of the urethra or the rectum may occur. Similar findings may occur when the tumor arises in the uterus.

With tumors in any location there may be early dissemination, and the presenting symptoms can be bone pain or the respiratory distress of pulmonary metastases. Extensive bone involvement may produce symptomatic hypercalcemia. In patients with disseminated tumor, it is sometimes difficult to identify the primary lesions.

Diagnosis. The early diagnosis of rhabdomyosarcoma requires an alert physician. Often several months elapse between first symptoms and biopsy.

Diagnostic procedures are determined in large degree by the area of involvement. In the head and neck area, roentgenograms should be examined for evidence of the tumor mass and for indications of bony erosion. CT scans should be used as well to check for intracranial extension and to look for bony involvement at the base of skull, which is difficult to visualize roentgenographically. For abdominal tumors, ultrasound examinations and CT with oral and intravenous contrast media can help delineate the tumor mass. Cystourethrograms are useful for tumors in the bladder. Before a patient has definitive surgery, a full skeletal metastatic survey should be done as well as radionuclide scans of the skeleton. A chest roentgenogram study should be obtained, followed by CT if the roentgenogram is negative, and bone marrow should be examined. These studies should be evaluated before any surgical procedure so that the extent of proposed surgery can be defined. The most essential element of the diagnostic workup is the examination of tumor tissue.

Treatment. Rhabdomyosarcoma is rarely completely resectable. Tumor margins should be carefully defined and an appropriate search for metastatic disease (e.g., to nodes or liver or both) should be made at the time of initial surgery, even if this is only a biopsy. The treatment program for each patient must be designed according to the location and stage of the tumor. Some patients are being given chemotherapy prior to surgery in the hope that vital organs, particularly in the genitourinary tract, might be preserved and in order to reduce the amount of surgery required. In group I tumor, complete local excision is followed by chemotherapy to reduce the likelihood of subsequent metastatic disease. For groups II and III, surgery should be followed by a regimen involving local irradiation and systemic chemotherapy. The treatment of group IV rhabdomyosarcoma relies principally on systemic chemotherapy. Intrathecal therapy is generally given to patients with primary disease in parameningeal sites (nasopharynx, nasal cavity, paranasal sinuses, middle ear, mastoid, or pterygopalatine or infratemporal fossae).

Prognosis. Of patients with resectable tumor, 80–90% have prolonged tumor-free survival. In addition, unresectable tumor localized at certain favorable sites (such as orbit) has a high likelihood of cure. About two thirds of patients with incompletely resected regional tumor will also achieve long-term disease-free survival. Patients with disseminated disease have a poor prognosis; only about half will achieve remission and less than half of these will be cured. Older children have a worse prognosis than younger ones and have a greater frequency of lesions of the extremities and of alveolar histology.

16.16 OTHER SOFT TISSUE SARCOMAS

Subtypes of soft tissue sarcoma can be identified with the normal tissues from which each appears to have arisen (Table 16–14). Some grow aggressively, others relatively slowly. In most patients, the sarcomas appear as masses. Here again, it is critical to determine the extent of disease prior to surgery, particularly with respect to bony or pulmonary metastases. For a number of these tumors, radical surgical excision offers the only chance of cure. Perhaps for no other group of tumors is it so important to have the tissues reviewed carefully by an experienced pathologist, both for definition of the specific type of tumor and for an assessment of its malignant or benign nature. Post-operative chemotherapy is indicated for high grade tumors with prominent mitotic activity, regardless of tumor size or resectability.

NEOPLASMS OF BONE

Bone tumors have an annual incidence in white children of 5.6/million and in black children 4.8/million. Osteosarcoma, the most common malignant bone tumor, is twice as common in white children as Ewing tumor. Ewing tumor almost never occurs among black children. Bone tumors tend to occur in adolescents, rather than in younger children. Rare bone tumors include chondrosarcomas and fibrosarcomas.

16.17 OSTEOSARCOMA

Bone growth and the occurrence of osteosarcoma seem to be correlated. Onset is most common during the adolescent growth spurt. The mean age at the time of diagnosis is 15 yr. During the first 13 yr of life, boys and girls have the same incidence of osteosarcoma, but older boys have an increasing rate whereas girls reach a plateau. One study found children with osteosarcoma to be taller at the time of diagnosis than control children with other cancers; it also found that osteosarcoma occurs more commonly in giant breeds of dogs (e.g., Great Danes). Osteosarcoma occurs most commonly in long bones at the metaphyseal ends, the points of most active growth and reconstruction. The most common primary site is the distal femur; the proximal humerus and proximal tibia are also common sites. Osteosarcoma can arise in any bone.

Children with bilateral retinoblastoma have an increased incidence of osteosarcoma. In past years osteosarcoma developed most often in the field of irradiation, but it is being increasingly reported in bones that were not included in the radiation portal and as multifocal disease. The gene associated with retinoblastoma may predispose to osteosarcoma as well.

Certain diseases of bone, some genetically determined, may also predispose to osteosarcoma. These include multiple osteochondromatosis (Ollier disease), which may also be found with hemangiomas (Maffucci syndrome); multiple hereditary exostoses; osteogenesis imperfecta; and Paget disease. Osteosarcoma is occasionally familial. It occurs also as a secondary tumor in the treated bone of long-term survivors of Ewing tumor; latency period ranges from 4 to over 20 yr.

Pathology. Osteosarcoma has been defined as a primary malignant bone tumor, the neoplastic cells of which produce osteoid. The classic osteosarcoma arises within the medullary canal of the shaft and may break through the cortex of the bone of origin to form a soft tissue mass which can achieve considerable size. The tumor may also extend along the medullary cavity. The tumor may have osteosarcomatous, chondrosarcomatous, and fibrosarcomatous differentiation within a single lesion. A characteristic section is shown in Fig. 16–7. Osteosarcoma has some important subclassifications. *Parosteal* osteogenic sarcoma is a well-differentiated, extramedullary tumor of low metastatic potential. Surgical resection alone is often considered adequate therapy. In contrast, a similarly located lesion, *periosteal* osteogenic sarcoma, is histologically a much more pleomorphic lesion that behaves more aggressively clinically. *Telangiectatic* osteosarcoma

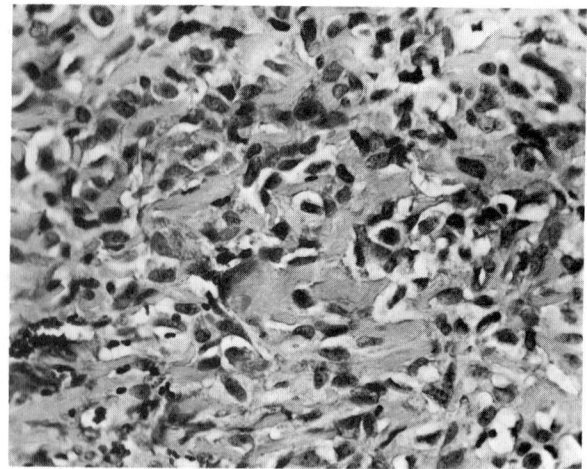

Figure 16–7. The diagnostic histologic features of osteosarcoma. The nuclei are of various sizes, and chromatin densities; most have a dark chromatin appearance. The cells are intimately involved with the background amorphous material, which is osteoid.

is a bloody, cystic lesion that produces no new bone radiographically and may be confused with aneurysmal bone cyst. Prognosis may be poor.

Osteosarcoma may appear simultaneously in many sites, with a predominantly osteoblastic pattern (multifocal sclerosing osteosarcoma).

Clinical Manifestations. The most common initial finding is pain at the site of the tumor. The patient and family usually ascribe this pain to trauma. Later, limitation of motion and a palpable or visible tumor may develop. With involvement of bones of the legs or pelvis, there may be limping or alterations of gait. Later manifestations are tenderness and local erythema and hyperthermia. The most common site of metastasis is the lungs; early pulmonary involvement is usually asymptomatic, but more extensive disease may produce respiratory embarrassment. Pleural effusion and pneumothorax can occur. Other sites of metastasis include other bones, hilar lymph nodes, and central nervous system.

Diagnosis. Persistent unexplained bone pain, particularly when associated with a palpable mass, requires roentgenographic examination of that bone. A typical lesion is shown in Fig. 16–8. Sclerosis of bone and periosteal new bone formation are common. Prior to initial surgery, minimal staging should include a radionuclide scan to look for metastatic bony lesions and a roentgenographic study (Fig. 16–9) and CT scan of the chest. CT scan of the chest will detect more lesions than will be seen on roentgenogram and is particularly important in the patient for whom the latter is negative. On the other hand, about half the additional nodules defined by CT in a series of adult patients proved at thoracotomy to be benign granulomas or pleura-based lymph nodes.

CT scan with contrast enhancement of the affected extremity can help to define the extent of medullary involvement and will assist in surgical planning. If a limb salvage procedure is contemplated, arteriography will be performed to see whether it is possible to preserve function distal to the resected tumor. Serum alkaline phosphatase activity may be increased, and this may serve as a marker to follow the effect of therapy. Confirmation of the diagnosis must be made by histologic examination through open biopsy of the lesion.

Treatment. For the patient with no evident metastatic disease, the recommended treatment is amputation of the affected extremity or wide local excision of a flat bone when feasible. Amputation should be defined by medullary involvement on CT scan. In the prechemotherapy era, amputation alone yielded a 5 yr survival rate of about 17%. The usual

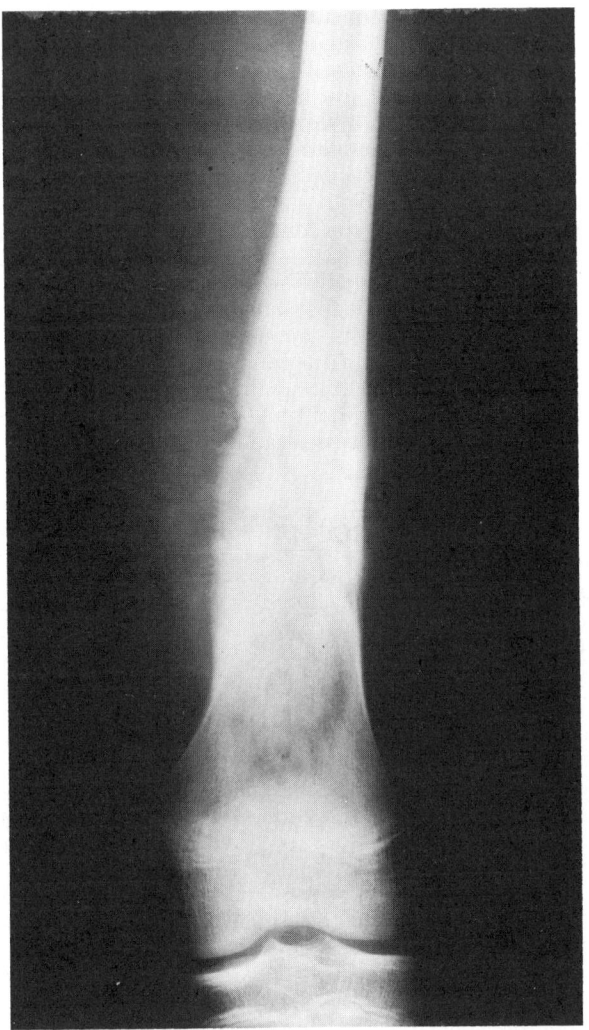

Figure 16–8. Osteosarcoma of the distal portion of the femur. The tumor has broken through the cortex; calcification of the tumor is seen in the surrounding soft tissues.

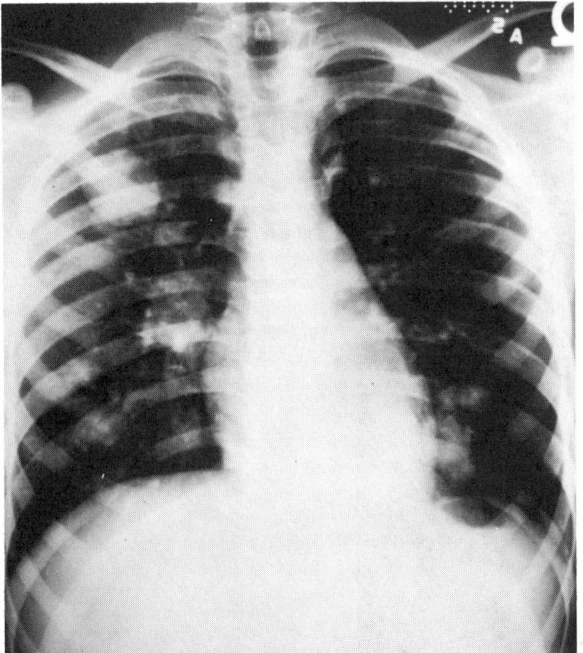

Figure 16–9. Multiple metastatic nodules of osteosarcoma.

cause of death was pulmonary metastases, which developed within 2 yr in patients who had no obvious pulmonary metastases at the time of diagnosis. The thought that pulmonary micrometastases present at the time of diagnosis might account for this phenomenon has led to uncontrolled small studies with single agent chemotherapy. Administration of high doses of methotrexate or doxorubicin has produced a disease-free survival rate of about 40%. A trial using multiple agents (high-dose methotrexate, bleomycin, cyclophosphamide, dactinomycin, doxorubicin, and platinum) appears to have produced a disease-free survival rate closer to 80%. On the other hand, one series of patients treated with surgery alone had a disease-free survival rate as high as 40%. A recent randomized concurrent controlled trial by the Pediatric Oncology Group has compared the multiple chemotherapy regimen with surgery alone. The results indicate that complex, intensive chemotherapy is the postoperative treatment of choice for osteosarcoma. Osteosarcoma is not radiosensitive.

For patients with resectable pulmonary metastatic disease, surgery is recommended, since in this situation there is about a 20% disease-free survival rate with surgery alone. It is usual, however, that a patient in whom only a few lesions are seen on conventional roentgenograms will have more visible on CT and even more seen at the time of surgery.

Attempts have been made to preserve the involved extremity through preoperative chemotherapy followed by resection of the involved bone and insertion of an internal prosthesis. Selection of this approach requires careful assessment of the relative functional capacity of a limb with an internal prosthesis, which will be much less strong than a normal limb. In general, the more active the patient, the more likely he or she is to do well with amputation rather than an internal prosthesis. The internal prosthesis may be most attractive for the upper extremity, where the hand of the involved arm may be preserved and where weight bearing is not required.

Careful rehabilitation must follow amputation. Affected patients are likely to experience postoperative phantom limb pain. They are likely to have first postoperative swelling and later shrinkage of the residual stump, which will require multiple fittings of a prosthesis. Long-term psychologic support should be available.

Prognosis. Prognosis is best with low grade tumors such as parosteal osteosarcoma. With surgery alone about 20% of patients with the classic form of osteosarcoma will have long-term survival. The survival rate after intensive chemotherapy is not yet known but will be at least 50%. Some cases of long-term survival have followed resection of metastatic pulmonary disease, but none have occurred in patients with diffuse pulmonary metastases or metastatic disease to bone.

16.18 EWING SARCOMA

Ewing sarcoma is a round-cell tumor of bone of later childhood and adolescence. It is more common in males than in females, and is rarely seen in blacks either in the United States or in Africa. Familial cases have been described. There is no evidence that radiation exposure is important in the etiology.

Pathology. Histologically, Ewing tumor is composed of uniform small round cells with scanty cytoplasm and little or no surrounding stroma. The presence of glycogen, as indicated by the periodic acid–Schiff reaction, helps differentiate this tumor from neuroblastoma. The cell of origin for this tumor is uncertain.

The tumor may arise either in long bones of the extremities or in flat bones of the head and trunk. As with osteosarcoma, the most commonly involved long bone is the femur. The most commonly involved flat bone is the pelvis. Extraskeletal neoplasms histologically resembling Ewing sarcoma have been described, most frequently arising in the soft tissues of the lower extremity and paravertebral regions. Their relationship to Ewing sarcoma of bone is uncertain. Metastatic disease most frequently involves lungs and bone, occasionally bone marrow and central nervous system, and is present in up to one third of patients at the time of diagnosis.

Clinical Manifestations. The primary symptom is pain, which may be accompanied by fever and tenderness. The degree of soft tissue involvement varies but may be massive. The two conditions most often mistaken clinically for Ewing sarcoma are eosinophilic granuloma and osteomyelitis. Occasionally, there may even be periods of improvement in symptoms of a Ewing sarcoma with antibiotic therapy. A clinician confronted with the diagnosis of osteomyelitis should always consider Ewing sarcoma when bacterial cultures are negative. Typical roentgenographic features are seen in Figure 16–10.

Diagnosis. Ewing sarcoma may be suspected from clinical history and roentgenographic features; confirmation requires surgical biopsy. Differentiation from infection may be difficult unless pulmonary metastatic disease is present. This tumor may be difficult to distinguish on biopsy from the other small round-cell tumors of childhood. Evaluation by an experienced pathologist is critical.

Once the diagnosis is made, patients should be screened for metastases to the lung by roentgenography and CT scan, to the bones by radionuclide bone scan, and to the bone marrow by biopsy (so that an adequate tissue specimen is obtained). The extent of the primary lesion can be most precisely defined by CT scan, which will be helpful in following response to therapy.

Treatment. In general, amputation is not recommended in patients with Ewing sarcoma, since the tumor is sensitive both to radiation and to chemotherapy. Pathologic fracture may occur through bone, either as a result of tumor destruction or at a biopsy site. This may heal poorly during radiotherapy and chemotherapy and may cause pain. Patients should be cautioned against vigorous weight bearing on an involved bone during therapy.

High-dose irradiation of the primary tumor site and combination chemotherapy are recommended. The optimal dose and field of radiation are currently under investigation. Problems with high-dose radiation include failure of bone growth, fibrosis, and development of secondary osteosarcomas.

Ewing sarcoma that is clinically localized at the time of diagnosis develops into systemic disease with high frequency. All patients should, therefore, receive chemotherapy. Active agents are vincristine, cyclophosphamide, dactinomycin, and doxorubicin. It is probable that a four-drug regimen combining these agents will give the longest disease-free period after initiation of therapy.

Prognosis. A poor prognosis is associated with metastatic disease at the time of diagnosis and a proximal primary site; primary tumors in pelvis, humerus, or rib carry a worse prognosis than those in distal long bones. Recent trials with combinations of drugs and irradiation indicate that 40–60% of patients who present without metastatic disease will be free of tumor at 3 yr. Late relapses can occur.

16.19 CHONDROSARCOMA

This tumor of bone is rare in children and is usually seen during the second decade. It occurs with equal frequency in boys and girls and is associated with Ollier disease and Maffucci syndrome (Sec. 23.15). Exposure to ionizing radiation is an etiologic factor in some patients.

The histologic picture is that of malignant formation of cartilage. The tumor may arise in any bone but is most common in the pelvis. It occurs in flat bones of the trunk as well as in long bones of the extremities. It can metastasize to lung and bone, but the usual form of spread is local extension to contiguous normal tissues, with recurrence following surgical removal.

Clinical features are local pain and tumor mass. Diagnosis can be suspected from the roentgenogram of the area; it must be confirmed by biopsy. Histologic examination requires care, since osteosarcoma can have a large chondrosarcomatous component. The prognosis for these two tumors is quite different as to likelihood of metastatic disease. Treatment is surgical removal of the tumor or amputation if an extremity is involved. Chondrosarcoma is relatively radioresistant. Ow-

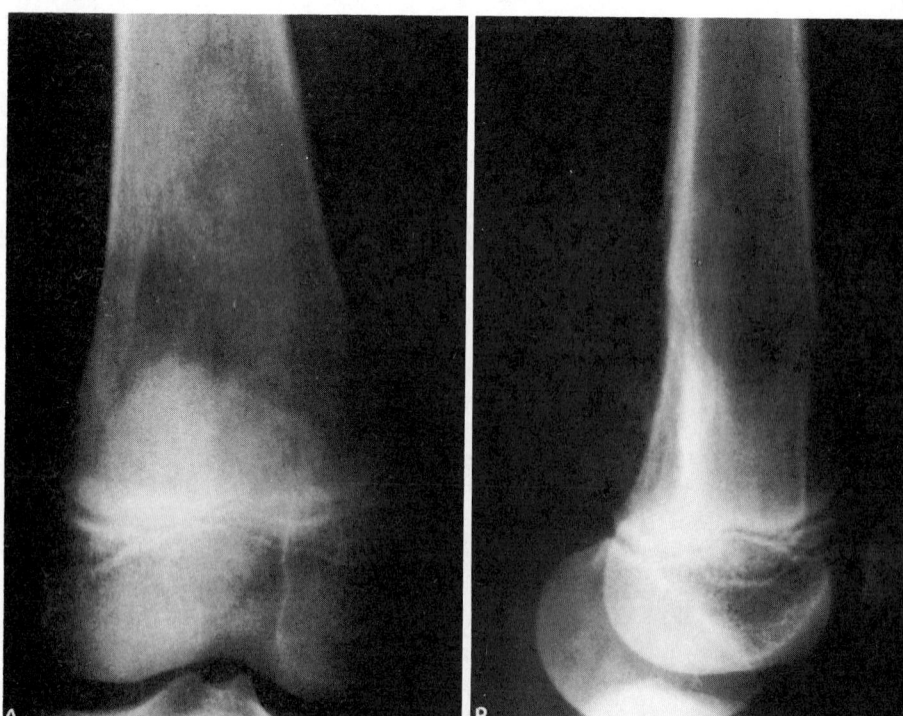

Figure 16–10. Anterior and lateral views of the distal femur of a patient with Ewing sarcoma. The lateral view shows the destruction of cortex, with growth of tumor into the surrounding soft tissues. With time, progressive calcification of periosteum lifted away from the bone may lead to a typical "sunburst" appearance.

ing to its rarity, the effect of chemotherapy has not been adequately evaluated.

16.20 RETINOBLASTOMA

This tumor has an annual incidence of 3.4/million children, similar for black and white children. The average ages at time of diagnosis are 8 mo for bilateral tumors and 26 mo for unilateral tumors. About 30% of patients with retinoblastoma have bilateral involvement; they have a dominantly inherited predisposition to retinoblastoma. About 10–20% of patients with unilateral disease also have the genetic predisposition. The retinoblastoma locus was discovered to be on chromosome 13 when a group of patients with growth delay, mental retardation and a characteristic facies, and a deletion on the long arm of that chromosome (13q− syndrome) were found to have retinoblastoma as well. Genetic mapping techniques (Sec. 16.1) have shown that the cells of most retinoblastoma tumors have submicroscopic deletions of chromosome 13. The retinoblastoma gene also carries increased risk of other tumors; about 1% of the survivors of the hereditary form of retinoblastoma will develop osteosarcoma at around 10 yr of age. Such osteosarcomas may occur either at a site irradiated for treatment for retinoblastoma or at a nonirradiated site and are often multifocal. A "trilateral" retinoblastoma syndrome has been reported in patients who have shown bilateral ocular disease as well as pineal tumors.

Pathology. Retinoblastoma usually develops in the posterior portion of the retina. It consists of small, closely packed, round, malignant cells with scanty cytoplasm. Occasionally, rosette formation occurs, which is thought to be an abortive attempt at formation of rods and cones. Retinoblastoma may appear as a single tumor in the retina but typically arises in multiple foci. When it arises in the internal nuclear layers of the retina, it grows forward into the vitreous cavity. This endophytic growth is easily seen with the ophthalmoscope, whereas if the tumor is exophytic (arising in the external nuclear layer and growing into the subretinal space, with detachment of the retina), the diagnosis is more difficult, because the tumor is hidden. Tumor fragments may break off from endophytic tumors and float free in the vitreous to seed unaffected parts of the retina. These vitreous seeds are associated with large tumors (usually more than 5 disc diameters) and a poor prognosis. Extension of retinoblastoma into the choroid usually occurs with massive tumors and may indicate a propensity for hematogenous metastases. Extension of tumor through the lamina cribrosa and down the optic nerve may lead to involvement of the central nervous system.

Since these tumors rarely metastasize, the primary concern at the time of diagnosis is generally to preserve useful vision. Accordingly, staging of these tumors is in accord with the extent of disease within the eye (Table 16–15).

Clinical Manifestations. This tumor usually presents with leukokoria, an asymptomatic patient being discovered to have a yellowish white reflex in the pupil owing to tumor behind the lens. Other presenting findings can be loss of vision, sometimes reflected as a squint in the affected eye, or with more advanced tumor, complaints of pain, pupillary irregularity, or hyphema. With far advanced tumor, there may be proptosis, signs of increasing intracranial pressure, or bone pain associated with metastatic disease.

More than 80% of patients with the hereditary bilateral form have tumors involving both eyes at the time of diagnosis. Delay in involvement of the second eye rarely exceeds 18 mo. In many patients with the familial form of the disease, the retinoblastoma will be discovered on a routine funduscopic examination made under anesthesia, performed because a parent or sibling has had the disease.

Table 16–15. Staging for Retinoblastoma

Group I
Solitary or multiple tumors, <4 disc diameters in size, at or behind the equator.

Group II
Solitary or multiple tumors, 4–10 disc diameters in size, at or behind the equator.

Group III
Any lesion anterior to the equator.
Solitary tumors >10 disc diameters, behind the equator.

Group IV
Multiple tumors; some >10 disc diameters, any lesion extending anterior to the ora serrata.

Group V
Massive tumors involving over half the retina.
Vitreous seeding.

After Ellsworth RM: The practical management of retinoblastoma. Trans Am Ophthalmol Soc 67:462, 1969.

Diagnosis. The finding of leukokoria must be followed by a careful funduscopic examination, which will usually necessitate anesthesia in children. In about 75% of patients roentgenography will show calcification within the globe. CT scan of the orbits should be performed to evaluate the intraorbital extent of tumor and also to see whether optic nerve or bony structures are involved. Other causes of leukokoria include retinal detachment, persistent hyperplastic primary vitreous, nematode endophthalmitis (usually visceral larva migrans), bacterial panendophthalmitis, cataract, coloboma of the choroid, and the retinopathy of prematurity. These conditions can be differentiated by an experienced ophthalmologist.

Additional studies to search for metastatic disease should include a skeletal survey, radionuclide bone scan, CT scan of the head with contrast, and examination of the spinal fluid and bone marrow for tumor cells. Elevated plasma levels of carcinoembryonic antigen and alpha-fetoprotein are frequently found at the time of diagnosis; they fall to normal levels after removal of the tumor. Their subsequent rise may indicate recurrence of tumor.

Treatment. The standard treatment for unilateral disease is enucleation of the eye. If the tumors are so small that it is felt that useful vision might be preserved after irradiation (e.g., group I, II, or III), then irradiation might be preferred. It is rare to see unilateral disease with tumors so small that useful vision can be preserved in the involved eye.

For patients with bilateral disease attempts should be made to salvage useful vision in at least one eye with radiotherapy. This can be administered bilaterally from the outset, since an eye that appears more involved may also have a more dramatic response. On the other hand, if an eye is so heavily involved that no useful vision remains, or if painful glaucoma has developed as a complication, then that eye should be enucleated. When enucleation is done, an attempt should be made to resect as much of the optic nerve as possible (10 mm or more). In addition, radiation therapy to the orbit should be considered if regional extraocular extension of the tumor has been found at the time of enucleation. Radiation therapy will require daily sedation of the patient and perhaps daily anesthesia.

There is no definite role for chemotherapy in patients whose tumor is localized to the globe. If there is gross or microscopic residual disease in the orbit after enucleation, then chemotherapy (probably with cytoxan and doxorubicin) should be considered along with radiotherapy. Widespread metastatic disease will respond to chemotherapy, but cure is most unlikely.

Prognosis. In groups I–IV the survival rate is 100%. In group V survival is at least 85%. Less than 10% of patients have extraglobal extension of disease at the time of presentation. No cures have been reported in patients who have had massive orbital disease or extensive optic nerve involvement when first seen, since intracranial spread and distant metastases have already occurred. If microscopic examination finds tumor in the periglobal tissues of the optic nerve, there is about a 30% chance of long-term survival with irradiation and chemotherapy.

16.21 GASTROINTESTINAL NEOPLASMS

(See also Sec. 12.64.)

The incidence of tumors arising in the gastrointestinal tract is much lower in children than in adults. A malignant lesion in the oral cavity in the very young is likely to be sarcomatous.

Salivary Gland Tumors. Most enlargements of the salivary glands result from such benign causes as inflammation or the formation of mucocoeles. About two thirds of tumors involving the salivary glands are benign, such as hemangiomas, hamartomas, or the mixed tumor of salivary glands (pleomorphic adenoma).

Mixed tumors are rare during the first decade; they are occasionally seen during the second decade and are evenly distributed between boys and girls. The gland most often involved is the parotid, and the most frequent presenting manifestation is a mass in the area. The mass is usually hard, movable, and nontender. Facial nerve paralysis may occur. Treatment is excision of the tumor. The prognosis for control of the disease is excellent; recurrences may necessitate a second surgical procedure.

Mucoepidermoid carcinoma is the malignant tumor of salivary glands. It is found primarily during the second decade of life and most frequently involves the parotid gland, usually as a hard, nontender mass. Metastases to regional lymph nodes are unusual, but once they have occurred the prognosis is poor. Treatment is excision; if this is complete, the prognosis is excellent. Local recurrence may necessitate a second surgical procedure.

Nasopharyngeal Carcinoma (Lymphoepithelioma). In adults this tumor is most common in the Far East and North Africa, where it occurs in familial clusters. There is high frequency of association with Epstein-Barr virus. In the United States it occurs in or after the second decade of life. Black children in the southern United States have four to seven times the incidence of whites. Male predominance is observed in adults but not in children. The histologic appearance is that of undifferentiated carcinoma.

The most frequent early finding is cervical adenopathy, usually unilateral and frequently tender. Other early symptoms and signs are trismus, epistaxis, sore throat, and difficulty swallowing. There may be weight loss due to dysphagia.

Diagnosis is usually made through biopsy of a cervical node. On careful examination, including CT scan, it is possible to find the primary tumor in the nasopharynx in the majority of affected children. If the tumor has not metastasized, multiple biopsies of the nasopharynx may be required to obtain appropriate tissue. Extension occurs locally to the base of the skull and to the soft tissues surrounding the nasopharynx. Regional lymph node metastases are common, and there may be hematogenous spread to bone (detectable on radionuclide scan) and to lung.

The primary therapy is irradiation of the involved areas of the nasopharynx. This will result in cure in up to 50% of patients. Experience with chemotherapy is limited; the tumor responds to cyclophosphamide and doxorubicin.

Carcinoma of the Stomach. This form of gastrointestinal cancer has been rarely reported in children. The usual symptoms are caused by a mass; bleeding and gastric obstruction have also occurred.

Malignant lesions affecting the stomach are more often lymphomas or soft tissue sarcomas. If the lesion is a true carcinoma, resection is the treatment of choice.

Pancreatic Carcinoma. This tumor is extremely rare in children. The usual site of origin is the head of the pancreas, and the initial clinical findings are those of upper abdominal mass, weight loss, and pain. Obstruction to the common bile duct may lead to obstructive jaundice. Treatment is resection where possible, and prognosis is poor.

Pancreatoblastoma is an exocrine tumor that behaves as a benign lesion located in the head of the pancreas. Since it is encapsulated and does not communicate with the pancreatic ducts, it can be removed without interfering with pancreatic function. The symptoms in these patients generally are those of an abdominal mass. The prognosis is favorable after resection of these tumors; it is important, therefore, that they be differentiated from pancreatic carcinoma.

Beta-cell endocrine tumors are generally seen in the form of *nesidioblastosis* or diffuse islet cell malformation or dysplasia (Sec. 20.7). Diagnosis is based on the finding of hypoglycemia followed by the demonstration that there are high serum levels of insulin even at low glucose levels, confirming the autonomous behavior of islet cells. Pancreatectomy is the treatment of choice.

Colonic Polyps. The juvenile or retention polyp constitutes about 85% of all polypoid lesions found in the colon and rectum of children. Bright red rectal bleeding is the most common presenting sign or symptom, occurring in almost all cases. Polyps occur most commonly between 3 and 5 yr of age. Most can be removed through a sigmoidoscope. A new polyp will develop in about 25% of cases. This is not a premalignant lesion, but there is an entity of multiple juvenile polyposis that does not have a benign connotation. Adenomatous polyps may coexist with these lesions, but true adenomatous polyps of the colon in children are rare except as part of familial polyposis or Gardner syndrome.

Adenocarcinoma of the Colon and Rectum. Adenocarcinoma of the colon and rectum represents less than 1% of all the malignant tumors that occur in children but has been described in a child as young as 9 mo of age. Affected patients may present bloody stools or melena. Abdominal pain (which may be colicky), anorexia, and weight loss are common. An abdominal mass may be found, and there may be liver enlargement due to metastases. The diagnosis can be confirmed by barium enema or direct endoscopic examination or both. Radionuclide or CT scans of liver and spleen will help detect hepatic metastases. The tumor is rarely confined to the mucosa at the time of diagnosis; it has usually extended through the serosa with involvement of the regional lymph nodes. Other metastases can occur within the abdominal cavity, commonly to the liver. Late hematogenous dissemination may occur. Predisposing conditions are familial multiple polyposis, ulcerative colitis, regional enteritis, and the Peutz-Jeghers syndrome. For most patients with these conditions regular endoscopic examination and occasionally prophylactic colectomy are recommended.

16.22 NEOPLASMS OF THE LIVER

Two kinds of primary liver cancer occur in children: hepatoblastoma and hepatocellular carcinoma (hepatoma).

Epidemiology. Hepatoblastoma is the more common; it is seen almost exclusively in children under the age of 3 yr. Boys predominate in a ratio of 1.5:1. Hepatocellular carcinoma shows two age peaks, one before the age of 4 yr and the other between the ages of 12 and 15 yr. This tumor predominates in boys by a ratio of 1.3:1.

The congenital defects associated with hepatic malignancy are similar to those that occur in patients with Wilms tumor and adrenocortical neoplasms and include congenital hemihypertrophy and extensive hemangiomas. Hepatic tumor and Wilms tumor have occurred in the same patient, which indicates that similar mechanisms may be involved in the predisposition to all three neoplasms. Hepatoblastoma and hepatocellular carcinoma have been reported in siblings.

The occurrence of hepatic carcinoma with cirrhosis is much rarer in children than in adults; on the other hand, the cirrhosis of malnutrition and the biliary cirrhosis secondary to biliary atresia or giant cell hepatitis are associated with an increased incidence of primary malignant tumors of the liver. In addition, hepatic tumors develop in patients with Fanconi anemia who have been treated with androgens. Patients with the chronic form of hereditary tyrosinemia who survive beyond the age of 2 yr have about a 40% risk of developing hepatocellular carcinoma.

Pathology. Hepatoblastoma may consist entirely of cells with an epithelial appearance, or there may be an admixture of mesenchymal components. Gland-like structures may be seen. The individual cells are poorly differentiated. In the mixed type of tumor mesenchymal components and areas of primitive osteoid tissue may be seen. The hepatocellular carcinoma consists of well-differentiated large polygonal cells with highly eosinophilic cytoplasm. The cells form hepatic cord-like structures surrounded by sinusoidal vessels. Foci of extramedullary erythropoiesis are found in both tumors.

In both forms of hepatic cancer the right lobe is more commonly involved than the left. In about half the patients, however, the tumor involves both lobes or is multicentric. The most frequent site of metastasis is the lungs; local extension within the abdomen is also common. Less often, the central nervous system may be the site of metastasis.

Clinical Manifestations. The most frequent finding is an upper abdominal mass with abdominal enlargement. Pain is present in only 15–20% of the patients at the time of diagnosis; anorexia and weight loss occur with the same frequency. Even less common initial complaints are vomiting and jaundice. Rarely, there may be virilization in affected boys, owing to production of gonadotropin by the tumor.

Diagnosis. The major diagnostic problem is the differentiation of hepatic enlargement due to primary tumor from that caused by other diseases, benign or malignant. A careful search should be made for another primary site of tumor, which will most frequently be neuroblastoma. Infantile hemangioendotheliomas and cavernous hemangiomas can enlarge the liver and a careful survey for other hemangiomas should be made. Metabolic storage diseases may also simulate hepatic tumor.

Results of laboratory studies of liver function are most often normal. About 20% of patients may have increases in bilirubin levels or in transaminase activities. Most patients will have increased serum levels of alpha-fetoprotein, and this is a useful marker to follow after surgery.

The roentgenogram of the abdomen will demonstrate hepatic enlargement; in about 30% of patients, calcification will be seen within the tumor. In about 10% of patients pulmonary metastases will be present at the time of diagnosis, and abdominal and chest CT are indicated for initial staging. Angiography is particularly valuable in providing the surgeon with an indication of the blood supply of the tumor, which will determine its resectability. Radionuclide scan of the liver will indicate tumor. Final diagnosis depends on histologic examination.

Treatment. The only effective treatment is surgical resection. In only about one third of patients are the size and location of the tumor at the time of diagnosis such that complete excision can be attempted. Rapid regeneration of the liver occurs within 4–6 wk after surgery and it is at about this time that the postoperative baseline CT and liver scan should be obtained. The tumor is relatively radioresistant. Various chemotherapeutic agents have a temporarily beneficial effect in metastatic disease, but there is no definitive chemotherapy.

Prognosis. The prognosis for patients with hepatic tumors is poor. Overall survival in hepatoblastoma is 35%, in hepatocellular carcinoma only 13%. The survivors are exclusively patients who have had complete surgical excision of the tumor. Less than complete excision is always associated with local recurrence and eventual death.

16.23 GONADAL AND GERM CELL NEOPLASMS

Epidemiology. Gonadal and germ cell tumors are uncommon in children, although sacrococcygeal teratoma is the most common solid tumor in newborns (1:40,000 live births). Most reports indicate a female preponderance. The age incidence for both ovarian and testicular tumors peaks before the age of 2 yr, with a second increase in rate beginning after the age of 6 yr for ovarian tumors and after the age of 14 yr for testicular tumors. Patients with cryptorchid testes have a 50 times greater risk of malignant testicular tumors. Of the tumors that occur in cryptorchid males, 20% arise in the descended testis. Gonadal dysgenesis is the consistent underlying clinical feature of patients who develop gonadoblastoma (Sec. 19.34).

Pathology. The germ cell tumors are an interrelated group of malignancies expressing the multipotential characteristics of differentiation of the cells from which they arise. These relationships are expressed graphically in Figure 16–11. The mixtures of different cell types that may occur in the same tumor confirms their interrelationship.

Germ cell tumors occur most commonly in the gonads but may appear in such sites as the retroperitoneum, mediastinum, sacrococcygeum, and central nervous system. These tumors in extragonadal sites are thought to represent aberrancies in the migration of germ cells from the yolk sac into the developing fetus.

Differentiation may occur in the direction of extra-embryonic tissues, resulting in choriocarcinoma or yolk sac carcinoma (endodermal sinus tumor).

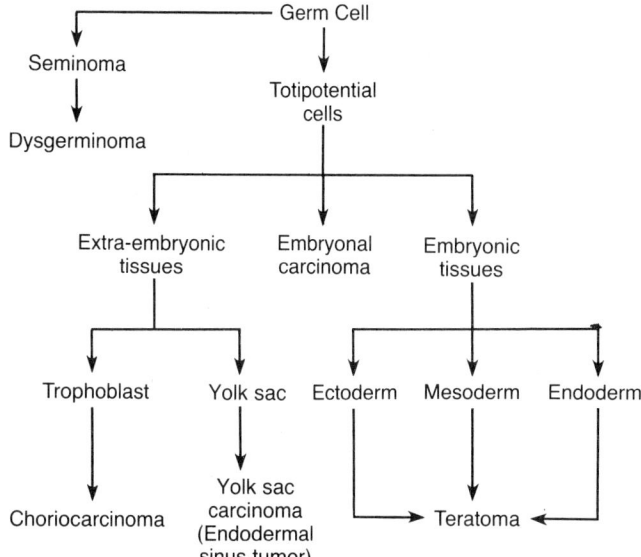

Figure 16–11. Tumors of germ cell origin. (Adapted from Pierce GB, Abell MR: Pathol Annu 5:27, 1970.)

Choriocarcinoma is a component of both gonadal and extragonadal germ-cell neoplasms. It occurs after puberty in the testicle, but both before and after puberty in the ovary. Choriocarcinoma is not commonly the predominant pattern of the tumor. There is frequently hemorrhagic necrosis. Masses of cytotrophoblast are overlain by caps of syncytiotrophoblastic giant cells. Choriocarcinoma may also be gestational (arising in the placenta), and there are rare cases reported of infants developing widespread choriocarcinoma from maternal placental disease. The *yolk sac carcinoma (endodermal sinus tumor)* has histologic features resembling the endodermal sinuses of the placenta. A pattern of differentiation predominantly in the direction of embryonic tissues leads to *teratomas* or *teratocarcinomas*, which have elements of all three germ layers. The malignant component of a teratocarcinoma is usually an embryonal carcinoma.

Seminoma of the testicle occurs almost exclusively during the second decade of life and later. The tissue is cellular, histologically, with clear cells aggregated in lobules and separated by fibrous stroma. *Dysgerminoma*, the ovarian counterpart, frequently occurs prior to puberty; the cells are morphologically and histochemically identical to primordial germ cells. These tumors metastasize to regional lymph nodes, with hematogenous dissemination to lung and bone. Metastasis from ovarian tumors may also be found within the peritoneal cavity, either by implantation, often with accompanying ascites, or by regional extension.

Just as the primary tumor may contain a mixture of histologic elements, metastatic tumor is generally also mixed; occasionally, a representation purely of one cell type may be found.

Clinical Manifestations. During the 1st yr of life, the usual initial sign of a testicular tumor is a mass in the scrotum, sometimes found at birth. Delays in diagnosis arise when the mass is initially considered a hydrocele, and hydrocele may accompany these tumors. They are usually not painful at first, nor are there signs of inflammation. An initial finding of metastatic disease is uncommon. In older boys, a gradual swelling of the involved testicle is usually noted over some weeks, and pain and tenderness are found in more than half the cases. Clinical complications of metastasis to retroperitoneal lymph nodes or to lungs may be the initial findings in some patients. Gynecomastia may occur as an effect of chorionic gonadotropin. In a few patients the early clinical findings may be those of disseminated cancer, such as weight loss, anorexia, and lethargy.

With ovarian tumors the most common initial symptoms are pain, nausea, and vomiting. Some patients have no symptoms, an abdominal mass or abdominal fullness being noted incidentally. An acute onset of abdominal pain may occur in patients who have ovarian torsion; in such patients, the findings may simulate an inflammatory process, such as appendicitis. Germ-cell tumors of the ovary seldom make their initial appearance through signs of metastatic disease. Of all ovarian germ-cell tumors 95% are benign cystic teratomas, but an inverse relationship exists between age and likelihood of malignancy, with 84% of germ-cell tumors being malignant in girls less than 10 yr old.

Sacrococcygeal teratoma or teratocarcinoma is usually detected during infancy and frequently at the time of birth. The most common finding is a mass in the area of the sacrum and buttocks. The incidence of malignancy is 10% in tumors diagnosed at less than 2 mo of age, and increases to 50–70% for tumors diagnosed after this age. Additional symptoms and signs result if the growing mass causes obstruction of the rectum or urinary tract. Associated clinical features include congenital anomalies involving the lower vertebrae, genitourinary system, or anorectum.

Initial clinical features of patients with germ-cell tumors arising in other extragonadal sites depend on the location of the primary tumor. In the abdomen, tumors will usually present as masses. In the chest there may be respiratory symptoms. Intracranial tumors will present as mass lesions.

Diagnosis. The chief diagnostic aid is careful examination. Testicular tumors are solid and usually opaque to transillumination (although they may be accompanied by hydrocele). Testicular size can be estimated via ultrasonography or CT scan. Abdominal pain, nausea, and vomiting in a girl may be severe enough to warrant ultrasound evaluation of the ovaries.

A sacrococcygeal tumor in early infancy should immediately suggest teratoma. Other masses found in the same area include meningoceles, chordomas, duplications of the rectum, neurogenic tumors, lipoma, rhabdomyosarcoma, and hemangioma. At times, masses in the area may be confused with perirectal abscess. When the bulk of the tumor is intrapelvic, only constipation and anuria may ensue, as symptoms of obstruction. A rectal examination should always be done for an infant with such symptoms. Germ-cell tumors in other extragonadal sites cannot in most cases be identified until excision or biopsy has been done and the histologic character established.

All patients suspected of having germ-cell tumors should have roentgenograms and CT scans of the chest and radionuclide scans of bone to detect any metastatic disease. CT scan of the abdomen in boys with testicular tumors may demonstrate retroperitoneal lymph node metastasis. Serum levels of alpha-fetoprotein and chorionic gonadotrophin should be measured. The levels of these two biologic markers prior to treatment may be useful in subsequent evaluation of the effectiveness of therapy.

Treatment. Therapy depends primarily on prompt recognition and surgical removal of the tumor. Dysgerminoma and seminoma are highly radiosensitive. Even when no metastatic disease is found, malignant germ-cell tumors should receive combination chemotherapy, because it is likely that inapparent dissemination has already occurred. The optimal regimen of chemotherapy is still uncertain. Cisplatin, bleomycin, and vinblastine (Velban) are most commonly used, and are highly successful in adult patients.

Prognosis. Prognosis rests mainly on the extent of disease at the time of diagnosis. It is important, therefore, that germ-cell tumors be suspected as early as possible. In general, the finding of extraembryonal elements in a germ-cell tumor denotes a poor prognosis. It is difficult to assess results of treatment, because only a small number of patients have been treated in any consistent manner; treatment should be planned, however, with the assumption that early intervention and adjuvant chemotherapy provide reasonable expectation for long-term disease-free survival.

Other tumors of the gonads are uncommon in children. *Sertoli tumors* of the testicle are usually benign and arise from sustentacular cells originating from the primitive gonadal mesenchyme. Occasionally, endocrine activity can occur, with sexual precocity or gynecomastia. The tumor is most likely to occur during the 1st or 2nd yr of life. Treatment is surgical removal.

Almost half of ovarian tumors are *benign ovarian cysts*. These cysts may be found incidentally at laparotomy for other purposes or on physical examination of an otherwise well child. Occasionally, torsion of the involved ovary can cause acute abdominal pain, nausea, and vomiting. Other ovarian tumors are quite uncommon. The *granulosa-theca cell tumor* is thought to arise in cells of ovarian stromal origin; it is usually associated with precocious puberty and a mass in the lower abdomen. The tumor is only rarely malignant, and its removal alleviates the endocrine abnormality. *Cystadenocarcinoma* of the ovary is even more uncommon and cannot be differentiated by clinical manifestations from other malignant ovarian tumors. *Hemangiomas* may involve the ovary (Sec. 24.7). Occasionally, ovarian enlargement will be the first manifestation of *lymphoma*.

Gonadoblastomas are found exclusively in patients with gonadal dysgenesis. Of affected patients, 80% are phenotypic females, usually with evidence of virilization. The others are phenotypic males, usually with such abnormalities as cryptorchidism, hypospadias, or female internal or secondary sex organs. The gonadoblastoma is regarded as a cancer in situ from which germinomas may develop. The tumor may be bilateral; it presents as a growing mass with the added features of virilization in some female patients. Histologic examination shows an intimate mixture of germ cells and elements resembling immature granulosa or Sertoli cells, with or without Leydig cells or lutein-type cells. The tumor should be removed along with the other abnormal gonad (and the uterus if one is present), since the other gonad may undergo malignant degeneration. Prolonged exogenous hormone administration may be required in such patients for development of secondary sexual characteristics, and secondary uterine cancer may occur under these circumstances.

16.24 MISCELLANEOUS CARCINOMAS

ADENOCARCINOMA OF THE VAGINA AND CERVIX

This tumor, once extremely rare, has become more common as the result of intrauterine exposure to diethylstilbestrol. Other genitourinary anomalies occur in affected patients (Sec. 18.4).

CARCINOMA OF THE THYROID

Thyroid cancer is discussed in Sec. 19.16. It occurs in increased incidence in patients who have had irradiation to the head and neck in childhood. Spontaneous thyroid cancer is more common in girls than in boys and is most likely to be papillary and to grow slowly. Medullary carcinoma of the thyroid may occur sporadically or in a familial pattern; in its familial form, it is associated with Marfan-like habitus, pheochromocytoma, hyperparathyroidism, and mucosal neuromas (Sec. 19.16).

CARCINOMA OF THE ADRENAL GLAND

Adrenocortical carcinoma is quite rare. It may occur at any age during childhood but is more common during the first few years. The tumor may be associated with hemangiomas of the skin, hemihypertrophy, urinary tract anomalies, and astrocytomas. Girls predominate among patients with this tumor. The usual presenting symptoms are secondary to the endocrine function of the cancer. Affected children present signs of adrenal hyperfunction (Sec. 19.25), which may include Cushing syndrome (Sec. 19.24), virilization (Sec. 19.23), feminization (Sec. 19.26), or a combination of these.

CARCINOMA OF THE BREAST

Unilateral or bilateral enlargement of the breast is almost never a cause to consider cancer in children. Prepubertal enlargement is almost always related to growth of normal glandular tissue, owing either to an excessively sensitive end organ or to inappropriately early production of stimulatory hormones. The adolescent or postpubertal female breast mass is also likely to be a benign lesion. *Fibroadenoma* is the most common such lesion. It is usually a unilateral, isolated, rubbery, mobile mass that ranges from less than 1 cm up to 8 cm in size. It grows slowly and may have been known to the patient for several months. Bilateral or multiple tumors (fibroadenomatosis) occur but only in a minority of patients. Before considering biopsy, all breast masses in adolescents should be observed through at least one complete menstrual cycle, to see whether they show an increase in size and tenderness at the time of menstruation (which would be more consistent with a benign lesion).

Breast cancer in adolescents is extremely rare. The tumors tend to be fairly well differentiated and slow growing; most are localized in the breast, and axillary metastases have occasionally been found. The tumors are usually circumscribed, firm, and painless. Biopsy is essential before surgery is undertaken. With removal the prognosis has been reported excellent, although local recurrences may arise.

CANCER OF THE SKIN

Cancer of the skin is rare in children (Sec. 24.32). *Malignant melanoma* may occur during the first two decades, with clinical behavior much like that in adults. It usually appears as a rapidly growing, easily traumatized, ulcerated lesion that is darkly pigmented or has changed in color. It may be found on any part of the body. Certain conditions such as *giant hairy cell nevus syndrome* or *dysplastic nevus syndrome* will predispose to the development of melanoma. Because malignant melanoma is rare in children, an excisional biopsy of a suspected lesion is indicated initially. If malignancy is found, then wide local resection is indicated, which may necessitate skin grafting. Regional lymph nodes should be carefully examined; if they are enlarged, then a lymph node dissection also should be done. For patients with metastatic disease, good clinical responses may be obtained with doxorubicin and cyclophosphamide.

Xeroderma pigmentosum is an autosomal recessive condition in which there is a defective mechanism for DNA repair. When the affected person is exposed to sunlight, the ultraviolet radiation produces breaks in DNA, which provides an opportunity for mutant malignant growth. The skin is the organ of primary involvement. Multiple skin cancers appear in the exposed areas. Surgical resection of the tumors is necessary, and affected children must be protected as much as possible from sunlight. The *nevoid basal cell carcinoma syndrome* (basal cell nevus syndrome) is discussed in Sec. 24.32.

MISCELLANEOUS BENIGN TUMORS

A variety of benign tumors in infants and children present problems in differential diagnosis; many will also require treatment. Some can be life-threatening, although histologically benign.

16.25 BENIGN TUMORS AND TUMOR-LIKE PROCESSES IN BONE

A number of benign processes in bone must be recognized by the clinician and distinguished from malignant tumors in order to avoid tragic consequences of overtreatment. Some of them may be reactions to trauma, but the putative trauma usually cannot be identified. Others appear to be hamartomas, or true overgrowths of normal tissue in situ. Still other lesions, less well understood, are considered to be benign neoplasia, with perhaps the potential for malignancy.

Osteoid osteoma occurs with moderate frequency in adolescents, especially in boys; it usually involves the femur or tibia, much less frequently the spine, humerus, or phalanges. The cardinal clinical feature is pain, dull at first and accentuated by weight-bearing, typically more severe at night, and relieved by aspirin. After weeks or months of increasing pain there may be localized tenderness, but signs of inflammation are unusual. The roentgenogram is diagnostic, disclosing a sharply demarcated radiolucent nidus of osteoid tissue surrounded by sclerotic bone. There may be calcification of the osteoid within the nidus. Treatment is surgical: the nidus must be completely removed to prevent recurrence. A related tumor is the *osteoblastoma*, which tends to be larger and to have little or no sclerosis. It involves the spine more commonly than does osteoid osteoma.

Fibrous (benign) cortical defects are eccentric in location and presumably arise from the periosteum to erode the cortex from without. They have been estimated to occur in as many as 53% of boys and 31% of girls, most commonly from 4–8 yr of age. They may persist into adolescence and even into early adult life. They are found always in the metaphyses of cylindrical bones, usually near the knees. The radiographic picture is characteristic. They are asymptomatic and heal spontaneously. Their recognition is important lest they be mistaken for malignant lesions.

Nonossifying fibroma or *fibroxanthoma* is most common in late childhood and early adolescence and may be related to the fibrous cortical defect. About half of all cases are found incidentally in roentgenograms made for other purposes. There are often no symptoms, but chronic bone pain may occur. A pathologic fracture may be the first sign. The ends of the shafts of the long bones of the lower limbs are most commonly involved. The roentgenographic picture of a rarefied scalloped lesion is so characteristic that biopsy for histologic confirmation may not be required. Treatment often is not required, spontaneous cure being expected after months or years. Curettage or other interventions may be required for weakened or fractured bones.

Osteochondroma (cartilaginous exostosis) is the solitary lesion that corresponds to those of osteochondromatosis (hereditary multiple exostoses, Sec. 23.35). Osteochondroma occurs in any bone formed in cartilage, most often near the ends of femur or tibia at the knee. Growth appears in childhood and early adolescence and ceases with closure of the neighboring epiphyseal plates, at which time ossification of its cartilaginous cap may occur. A mass may be present, or pain if there is a fracture. The roentgenographic features are characteristic; some lesions are pedunculated, others sessile. Reactivation of growth occurs spontaneously on rare occasions, sometimes after a fracture; such lesions should be considered malignant until proved otherwise by excisional biopsy. Lesions should be removed prophylactically when possible, particularly if there are symptoms.

Enchondroma is the solitary lesion that corresponds to those of multiple enchondromatosis (Ollier disease, Sec. 23.14). It is less common than osteochondroma and is most likely to involve metacarpals, metatarsals, and phalanges. Enchondromas appear as deforming masses or become apparent when they induce pathologic fractures. Roentgenograms show circumscribed areas of rarefied bone with thinning and often bulging of the cortex and stippled calcification. Lesions in the hands or feet are benign; those in the large long bones, in any diaphysis, or in membranous bone have malignant potential and may be difficult to separate histologically from malignant lesions. Treatment is curettage of clearly benign lesions or wide excision of doubtful ones.

Solitary (unicameral) cysts fall somewhere between dysplasias and true tumors. These common lesions begin close to the epiphyseal plate and appear to migrate toward the diaphysis with growth of bone. The cavity is unilocular or multilocular and contains fluid or blood. The origin of the cysts is unknown; they have been attributed to traumatic hematomas. Symptoms may be absent or scant; the cysts may first declare themselves because of pathologic fracture. The roentgenographic appearance consists of an area of rarefaction, often pseudoloculated, that does not cross the epiphyseal plate.

These lesions may resolve spontaneously. Those in the upper extremity sometimes need no therapy; those of the lower extremity are at greater risk of fracture and should usually be treated with curettage or excision.

16.26 HEMANGIOMA

This tumor is among the most common neoplasms found in infants and children. Most occur in the skin and do not achieve great size (Sec. 24.7).

In a few children, large, rapidly growing hemangiomas can produce serious or life-threatening complications or grotesque deformity, especially in the area of the head and neck or on an extremity. Most such hemangiomas become evident before the age of 6 mo. They are evenly distributed between boys and girls. Their natural history is unpredictable. Usually there is rapid growth during the 1st and 2nd yr of life, followed by slow regression. Hemangiomas in the head and neck area can be unsightly and may progressively distort normal structures. Growth of these tumors may produce airway obstruction, pressure necrosis of surrounding structures, difficult feeding, and obstruction of the ear canal. The tumors may become secondarily infected through the ulceration of overlying skin. If arteriovenous communications of sufficient size develop, congestive cardiac failure may ensue.

Treatment of large tumors by resection is frequently difficult because of extensive involvement, and complete removal may be impossible. In some patients the administration of prednisone may suppress tumor growth, and regression may occur. Stopping the treatment may be followed by regrowth of tumor.

Hemangioma of the liver most frequently becomes evident before the age of 6 mo. Histologically, hemangioendothelioma is much more common than are cavernous hemangiomas. The initial symptoms may be jaundice, vomiting, or diarrhea, or, in some infants, increases in abdominal size without symptoms. The hemangioma is sometimes found when routine examination discloses an enlarged liver. Arteriovenous fistulas may lead to congestive cardiac failure. Roentgenograms of the abdomen show an enlarged liver and occasionally calcification in the tumor. Radionuclide and computed tomographic scans of liver and spleen will show the defect in hepatic tissue; hepatic angiograms will show an abnormal vascular pattern. Initial treatment with prednisone is recommended. If hemangioma of the liver is confined to a single lobe, surgical resection may be possible.

In some patients with large, cavernous hemangiomas, hemolysis and intralesional clotting may produce thrombocytopenia and hypofibrinogenemia with clinical symptoms. The anemia is not easily corrected by transfusion because of the ongoing red cell destruction, and a hemorrhagic diathesis may be impossible to correct by the transfusion of platelets and plasma clotting factors (Sec. 15.48).

16.27 LYMPHANGIOMA (CYSTIC HYGROMA)

Lymphangiomas are found in the head and neck region in about three fourths of cases. Like hemangiomas they appear early in life, with almost all evident by the age of 3 yr, and some have been diagnosed antenatally on maternal sonography. The embryonic origin of lymphangiomas is uncertain; it is not known whether they are malformations, benign neoplasms, or hamartomas. They may present as unilocular or multicystic masses, with thin, often-transparent walls. The contents of the cysts are straw colored. Histologically, the lining of the cystic areas is one or two cells thick, with varying amounts of intervening fibrous stroma.

Cystic hygroma is compressible and feels cystic. The tumors

are not tender or painful. There may be some thinning of the overlying skin. There is no erythema unless the lesion becomes infected. Unlike hemangiomas, these lesions do not regress spontaneously, and they should be resected as soon as possible. Planning for surgery involves evaluation of the extent of disease. Roentgenograms and CT scans will demonstrate intrathoracic extension in at least 10% of patients, and the tumor as it grows may result in tracheal compression and respiratory embarrassment. The tongue may also be involved and enlarged in some patients. Complete surgical excision, which is required for cure, may involve extensive dissection, with reconstructive surgery if vital structures are involved.

16.28 THYMOMA

Thymoma is rare in children, occurring with equal frequency in boys and girls. This anterior mediastinal tumor may be found in an asymptomatic person on routine chest roentgenogram. With growth of the tumor, there may be progressive compression of surrounding tissues, with the development of cough, dyspnea, dysphagia, and even superior vena cava compression.

A number of paraneoplastic syndromes have occurred with thymoma, including myasthenia gravis, hypogammaglobulinemia, and pure red cell aplasia. It is thought that these disorders may arise as a result of imbalances in immune regulation (e.g., enhanced production of suppressor lymphocytes by the tumor).

The tumor extends locally and rarely metastasizes outside the thorax. The treatment of choice is complete surgical excision. The tumor is radiosensitive, and recurrent disease will respond to chemotherapy with agents such as doxorubicin, cyclophosphamide, and cisplatin.

16.29 SPLENIC CYSTS

Splenic cysts can produce an enlarged spleen, which may suggest a malignant neoplasm. Any such mass should be investigated by abdominal ultrasonography or CT scan to establish its nature and exactly which organ is involved.

BRIGID G. LEVENTHAL

General Considerations

Doolittle RF, Hunkapiller MW, Hood LE, et al: Simian sarcoma virus onc gene, V-sis, is derived from the gene (or genes) encoding a platelet derived growth factor. Science 22KL:275, 1983.
Gilbert F: Retinoblastoma and recessive alleles in tumorigenesis. Nature 305:761, 1983.
Knudson AG: Mutation and cancer: Statistical study of retinoblastoma. Proc Nat Acad Sci USA 68:820, 1971.
Land H, Parada LF, Weinberg RA: Cellular oncogenes and multistep carcinogenesis. Science 222:771, 1983.
Leder P, Battey J, Lenoir G, et al: Translocations among antibody genes in human cancer. Science 222:765, 1983.
Miller RW: Environmental causes of cancer in childhood. Adv Pediatr 25:97, 1978.
Popovic M, Wong-Staal F, Sarin PS, et al: Biology of human T cell leukemia/lymphoma in vivo and in vitro. Adv Viral Oncol 4:45, 1984.
Solomon E: Recessive mutation in etiology of Wilms' tumor. Nature 309:111, 1984.
Yunis JJ: The chromosomal basis of human neoplasia. Science 21:227, 1983.

Bone Marrow Transplantation as Therapy

August CS, Serota FT, Koch PA, et al: Treatment of advanced neuroblastoma with supralethal chemotherapy, radiation and allogeneic or autologous marrow reconstitution. J Clin Oncol 2:609, 1984.
Begg CB, McGlave PB, Bennett JM, et al: A critical comparison of allogeneic bone marrow transplantation and conventional chemotherapy as treatment for acute nonlymphocytic leukemia. J Clin Oncol 2:369, 1984.
Fefer A, Cheever MA, Thomas ED, et al: Bone marrow transplantation for refractory acute leukemia in 34 patients with identical twins. Blood 57:421, 1981.

Jansen J, Falkenburg JHF, Stepan DE et al: Removal of neoplastic cells from autologous bone marrow grafts with monoclonal antibodies. Sem Hematol 21:164, 1984.
Johnson FL, Thomas ED, Clark BS, et al: A comparison of marrow transplantation with chemotherapy for children with acute lymphoblastic leukemia in second or subsequent remission. N Engl J Med 305:846, 1981.
Kaizer H, Chow HS: Autologous bone marrow transplantation (ABMT) in the treatment of cancer. Cancer Invest 2:203, 1984.
Krivit W, Ramsay NKC, Woods W, et al: Bone marrow transplantation in pediatrics. Adv Pediatr 30:549, 1983.
O'Reilly RJ: Allogeneic bone marrow transplantation: Current status and future directions. Blood 62:941, 1983.
Weiden PL, Sullivan KM, Flournoy N, et al: Antileukemic effect of chronic graft versus host disease. Contribution to improved survival after allogeneic marrow transplantation. N Engl J Med 304:1529, 1981.

Acute Lymphocytic Leukemia (ALL)

Crist WM, Boyett JM, Roper M, et al: Pre B cell leukemia responds poorly to treatment: A Pediatric Oncology Group study. Blood 63:407, 1984.
Freeman AI, Weinberg V, Brecher ML, et al: Comparison of intermediate-dose methotrexate with cranial irradiation for the post-induction treatment of acute lymphocytic leukemia in children. N Engl J Med 308:477, 484, 1983.
Pullen DJ, Boyett JM, Crist WM, et al: Pediatric Oncology Group utilization of immunologic markers in the designation of acute lymphocytic leukemia subgroups: Influence on treatment response. Ann NY Acad Sci 428:26, 1983.
Roper M, Crist WM, Metzgar R, et al: Monoclonal antibody characterization of surface antigens in childhood T cell lymphoid malignancies. Blood 61:830, 1983.

Acute Nonlymphocytic Leukemia (ANLL)

Lampkin BC, Woods W, Strauss R, et al: Current status of the end treatment of acute non lymphocytic leukemia in children (report of the ANLL strategy group of the Children's Cancer Study Group). Blood 61:215, 1983.
Steuber P, Ruymann F, Culbert S, et al: A Pediatric Oncology Group study: Comparison of two induction regimens for acute myelogenous leukemia. Blood 72:208A, 1983.
Weinstein HJ, Mayer RJ, Rosenthal DS, et al: Chemotherapy for acute myelogenous leukemia in children and adults. VAPA update. Blood 62:315, 1983.
Yates J, Glidewell O, Wiernik P, et al: Cytosine arabinoside plus daunorubicin or adriamycin for therapy of acute myelocytic leukemia. A CALGB study. Blood 60:454, 1982.

Chronic Myelocytic Leukemia (CML)

Koeffler HP, Golde DW: Chronic myelogenous leukemia: New concepts. N Engl J Med 304:1210, 1269, 1981.
Phillips GL, Herzig GP: Intensive chemotherapy, total body irradiation, and autologous marrow transplantation for chronic granulocytic leukemia: Blast phase. Report of four additional cases. J Clin Oncol 2:379, 1984.

Hodgkin Disease

Boyle-Weissberger C, Lemercier N, Teiller F, et al: Hodgkin's disease in children: Results of therapy in a mixed group of 178 clinically and pathologically staged patients over 13 years. Cancer 54:215, 1984.
Chilcote RR, Baehner RL, Hammond D: Septicemia and meningitis in children splenectomized for Hodgkin's disease. N Engl J Med 295:798, 1976.
DeVita VT Jr, Simon RM, Hubbard SM, et al: Curability of advanced Hodgkin's disease with chemotherapy. Long term follow up of MOPP treated patients at the National Cancer Institute. Ann Int Med 92:57, 1980.
Grufferman S, Delzell E: Epidemiology of Hodgkin's disease. Epidemiol Rev 6:76, 1984.
Kadin M: Possible origins of the Reed Sternberg cell from an interdigitating reticulum cell. Cancer Treat Rep 66:601, 1982.
Kaplan HS: Hodgkin's Disease. Harvard University Press, Cambridge, MA, 1980.
Rostock R, Siegelman S, Lenhard R: Thoracic CT scanning for mediastinal Hodgkin's disease. Int J Radiation Oncol 9:1451, 1983.
Russell KL, Donaldson SS, Cox RS, et al: Childhood Hodgkin's disease: Patterns of relapse. J Clin Oncol 2:80, 1984.
Santoro A, Bonadonna G, Bonfante V, et al: Alternating drug combinations in the treatment of advanced Hodgkin's disease. N Engl J Med 306:770, 1982.

Non-Hodgkin Lymphoma

Bernard A, Murphy SB, Melvin S, et al: Non-T, non-B lymphomas are rare in childhood and associated with cutaneous tumor. Blood 59:549, 1982.
Jenkin RDT, Anderson JR, Chilcote R, et al: Pediatric non Hodgkin's lymphomas: The Children's Cancer Study Group experience—an interim report. In: Rosenberg S, Kaplan H (eds): Malignant lymphomas: etiology, immunology, pathology, treatment. New York, Academic Press, 1982, pp 591–601.
Murphy SB: Prognostic features and obstacles to cure of childhood non-Hodgkin's lymphoma. Sem Oncol 4:265, 1977.
Murphy SB, Melvin SL, Mauer AM: Correlation of tumor cell kinetic studies

with surface marker results in childhood non Hodgkin's lymphoma. Cancer Res 39:1534, 1979.

The Non-Hodgkin's Lymphoma Pathologic Classification Project: National Cancer Institute sponsored study of classifications of non-Hodgkin's lymphomas: Summary and description of a working formulation for clinical usage. Cancer 49:2112, 1982.

Neuroblastoma

Beckwith JB, Martin RF: Observations on the histopathology of neuroblastoma. J Pediatr Surg 3:106, 1968.

Groncy P, Finkelstein JZ: Neuroblastoma. Pediatr Ann 7:73, 1978.

Hayes FA, Green AA, Mauer AM: Correlation of cell kinetics and clinical response to chemotherapy in disseminated neuroblastoma. Cancer Res 37:3766, 1977.

Look AT, Hayes FA, Nitschke R, et al: Cellular DNA content as a predictor of response to chemotherapy in infants with unresectable neuroblastoma. N Engl J Med 211:231, 1984.

Rosen EM, Cassady JR, Frantz DN, et al: Neuroblastoma: The Joint Center for Radiation Therapy/Dana Farber Cancer Institute Children's Hospital Experience. J Clin Oncol 2:719, 1984.

Shimada H, Chatten J, Newton WA Jr, et al: Histopathologic prognostic factors in neuroblastic tumors: Definition of subtypes of ganglioneuroblastoma and an age-linked classification of neuroblastomas. J Nat Cancer Inst 73:405, 1984.

Wilms Tumor

Beckwith JB, Palmer NF: Histopathology and prognosis of Wilms' tumor: Results from the First National Wilms' Tumor Study. Cancer 41:1937, 1978.

Bolande RP: Congenital mesoblastic nephroma. Arch Pathol Lab Med 98:357, 1974.

Bove KE, McAdams AJ: The nephroblastomatosis complex and relationship to Wilms' tumor; a clinico pathologic treatise. Per Pediatr Pathol 3:185, 1976.

D'Angio GJ, Evans AE, Breslow N, et al: The treatment of Wilms' tumor: Results of the National Wilms' Tumor Study. Cancer 38:633, 1976.

D'Angio GJ, Evans AE, Breslow N, et al: The treatment of Wilms' tumor: Results of the Second National Wilms' Tumor Study. Cancer 47:2302, 1981.

Fishman EK, Hartmen DS, Goldman SM, et al: The CT appearance of Wilms' tumor. J Comput Assist Tomog 7:659, 1983.

Soft Tissue Sarcomas

Hays DM, Raney RB, Lawrence W Jr, et al: Bladder and prostatic tumors in the Intergroup Rhabdomyosarcoma Study (IRS-1). Cancer 50:1472, 1982.

Pizzo PA: Rhabdomyosarcoma and other soft tissue sarcomas. In Levine, AS (ed): Cancer in the Young. Masson Publishing, 1982, pp 615–632.

Sarcomas of soft tissue and bone in childhood. NCI Monograph 56. United States Government Printing Office, 1981.

Osteosarcoma

Carter SF: The dilemma of adjuvant chemotherapy for osteogenic sarcoma. Cancer Clin Trials 3:29, 1980.

Dahlin DC, Unni KK: Osteosarcoma of bone and its important recognizable varieties. Am J Surg Pathol 1:61, 1977.

Goorin AM, Delorey MJ, Lack EE, et al: Prognostic significance of complete surgical resection of pulmonary metastases in patients with osteosarcoma: Analysis of 32 patients. J Clin Oncol 2:425, 1984.

Link MP, Goorin AM, Miser AW, et al: The effect of adjuvant chemotherapy on relapse-free survival in patients with osteosarcoma of the extremity. N Engl J Med 314:1600, 1986.

Rosen G, Nienberg A: Preoperative chemotherapy for osteogenic sarcoma: Selection of postoperative adjuvant chemotherapy based on the response of primary tumor to preoperative chemotherapy. Cancer 49:1221, 1982.

Schaner EG, Chang AE, Doppman JL, et al: Comparison of computed and conventional whole lung tomography in detecting pulmonary nodules. A prospective radiologic-pathologic study. Am J Roentgenol 131:51, 1978.

Ewing Sarcoma

Askin FB, Rosai J, Sibley RK, et al: Malignant small cell tumor of the thoracopulmonary region in childhood: A distinctive clinicopathologic entity of uncertain histogenesis. Cancer 43:2438, 1979.

Freeman CR, Geldhill R, Chevalier LM, et al: Osteogenic sarcoma following treatment with megavoltage radiation and chemotherapy for bone tumors in children. Med Pediatr Oncol 3:375, 1980.

Hayes FA, Thompson EI, Hustu HO, et al: The response of Ewing's sarcoma to sequential cyclophosphamide and adriamycin induction therapy. J Clin Oncol 1:45, 1983.

Rosen G, Caparros B, Nirenberg A, et al: Ewing's sarcoma: Ten years' experience with adjuvant chemotherapy. Cancer 47:2204, 1981.

Soule EH, Newton W Jr, Moon TE, et al: Extraskeletal Ewing's sarcoma: A preliminary study of 26 cases encountered in the Intergroup Rhabdomyosarcoma Study. Cancer 42:259, 1978.

Gastrointestinal Neoplasms

Horie A, Yano Y, Kotto Y, et al: Morphogenesis of pancreatoblastoma, infantile carcinoma of the pancreas: Report of two cases. Cancer 39:247, 1977.

Krolls SO, Trodahl JN, Boyers RC: Salivary gland lesions in children—a survey of 430 cases. Cancer 30:459, 1972.

Pratt CB, Rivera G, Shanks E, et al: Colorectal carcinoma in adolescents: Implications regarding etiology. Cancer 40:2464, 1977.

Rich RH, Dehner LP, Okinaga K, et al: Surgical management of islet cell adenoma in infancy. Surgery 84:519, 1978.

Siegel SE, Hays DM, Romansky, S, et al: Carcinoma of the stomach in childhood. Cancer 38:1781, 1976.

Taxy JB: Adenocarcinoma of the pancreas in childhood. Cancer 37:1508, 1976.

Toccalino H, Guastavino E, DePinni F, et al: Juvenile polyps of the rectum and colon. Acta Pediatr Scan 62:337, 1973.

Neoplasms of the Liver

Exelby PR, Filler RM, Grosfeld JL: Liver tumors in children in the particular reference to hepatoblastoma and hepatocellular carcinoma. American Academy of Pediatrics Surgical Survey—1974. J Pediatr Surg 10:329, 1975.

Evans AE, Land VJ, Newton WA, et al: Combination chemotherapy (vincristine, adriamycin, cyclophosphamide, and 5-fluorouracil) in the treatment of children with malignant hepatomas. Cancer 50:821, 1982.

Vawter G: Hepatoblastoma: A clinical and pathologic study of 54 cases. Am J Surg Pathol 6:693, 1982.

Wineberg AG, Finegold MJ: Primary hepatic tumors of childhood. Hum Pathol 14:512, 1983.

Gonadal and Germ Cell Neoplasms

Hogan JM, Johnson DE: The etiology of testicular tumors. In Johnson DE (ed): Testicular Tumors. 2nd ed. Flushing, NY, Medical Examination Publishing Co, 1976.

Witzleben CL, Bruninga G: Infantile choriocarcinoma: A characteristic syndrome. J Pediatr 73:378, 1968.

Woodruff JD, Protos P, Peterson WF: Ovarian teratomas. Relationship of histologic and oncogenic factors to prognosis. Am J Obstet Gynecol 102:702, 1968.

Miscellaneous Carcinomas

Dudgeon DL: Pediatric breast lesions. Contemp Pediatr (in press).

Hayes FA, Green AA: Malignant melanoma in childhood: Clinical cause and response to chemotherapy. J Clin Oncol 2:1229, 1984.

Herbst AL, Scully RE: Adenocarcinoma of the vagina in adolescence. Cancer 25:745, 1970.

Leape LL, Miller HH, Graze K, et al: Total thyroidectomy for occult familial medullary carcinoma of the thyroid in children. J Pediatr Surg 11:831, 1976.

Oberman HA, Stephens PJ: Carcinoma of the breast in childhood. Cancer 30:470, 1972.

Stewart DR, Jones PH, Jolleys A: Carcinoma of the adrenal gland in children. J Pediatr Surg 9:59, 1974.

17

THE URINARY SYSTEM

NEPHROLOGIC DISEASES

17.1 THE ANATOMY OF THE GLOMERULUS

The kidneys lie in the retroperitoneal space slightly above the level of the umbilicus and range in length and weight, respectively, from approximately 6 cm and 24 g in the full-term newborn to 12 cm or more and 150 g in the adult. The kidney (Fig. 17–1) has an outer layer, the *cortex*, which contains the glomeruli, proximal and distal convoluted tubules, and collecting ducts, and an inner layer, the *medulla*, which contains the straight portions of the tubules, the loops of Henle, the vasa recta, and the terminal collecting ducts (Fig. 17–2).

The blood supply to each kidney usually consists of a main renal artery that arises from the aorta; multiple renal arteries are not uncommon. The main artery divides into segmental branches within the medulla and these into interlobar arteries that pass through the medulla to the junction of the cortex and medulla. At this point, the interlobar arteries branch to form the arcuate arteries which run parallel to the surface of the kidney. Interlobular arteries originate from the arcuate arteries and give rise to the afferent arterioles of the glomeruli. Specialized muscle cells in the wall of the afferent arteriole, in combination with the lacis cells and that portion of the distal tubule (macula densa) that is adjacent to the glomerulus, form the juxtaglomerular apparatus that controls the secretion of renin. The afferent arteriole divides into the glomerular capillary network, which then merges into the efferent arteriole (Fig. 17–3). The efferent arterioles of glomeruli next to the medulla (juxtamedullary glomeruli) are larger than those in the outer cortex and provide the blood supply (vasa recta) to the tubules and medulla.

Each kidney contains approximately one million nephrons (glomeruli and associated tubules). In humans, formation of nephrons is complete at birth, but functional maturation does not occur until later. As no new nephrons can be formed after birth, progressive loss of nephrons may lead to renal insufficiency.

The glomerular network of specialized capillaries serves as the filtering mechanism of the kidney. The glomerular capillaries are lined by endothelial cells (Fig. 17–4) having very thin cytoplasm that contains many holes (fenestrations). The glomerular basement membrane forms a continuous layer between the endothelial and mesangial cells on one side and the epithelial cells on the other. The membrane has three layers: (1) a central electron-dense lamina densa, (2) the lamina rara interna, which lies between the lamina densa and the endothelial cells, and (3) the lamina rara externa, which lies between the lamina densa and the epithelial cells. The visceral epithelial cells cover the capillary and project cytoplasmic "foot processes," which come in contact with the lamina rara externa. Between the foot processes are spaces or filtration slits. The mesangium (mesangial cells and matrix) lies between the glomerular capillaries on the endothelial cell side of the basement membrane and forms the medial part of the capillary wall. The mesangium may serve as a supporting structure for the glomerular capillaries and probably plays a role in the removal of macromolecules (such as immune complexes) from the glomerulus, either through intracellular phagocytosis or by transport through intercellular channels to the juxtaglomerular region. The Bowman capsule, which surrounds the glomerulus, is composed of (1) a basement membrane, which is continuous with the basement membranes of the glomerular capillaries and the proximal tubules, and (2) the parietal epithelial cells, which are continuous with the visceral epithelial cells.

17.2 GLOMERULAR FILTRATION

As the blood passes through the glomerular capillaries, the plasma is filtered through the glomerular capillary walls. The ultrafiltrate, which is cell-free, contains all the substances in the plasma (electrolytes, glucose, phosphate, urea, creatinine, peptides, low molecular weight proteins) except proteins (like albumin and the globulins) having a molecular weight exceeding 68,000. The filtrate is collected in Bowman space and enters the tubules, where its composition is modified in accordance with body needs until it leaves the kidney as urine.

Glomerular filtration is the net result of opposing forces across the capillary wall. The force for ultrafiltration (glomerular capillary hydrostatic pressure) stems from the systemic arterial pressure, as modified by the tone of the afferent and efferent arterioles. The major force opposing ultrafiltration is the glomerular capillary oncotic pressure which is created by the gradient between the high concentration of plasma proteins within the capillary and the almost protein-free ultrafiltrate in Bowman space. Filtration may be modified by the rate of glomerular plasma flow, the hydrostatic pressure within Bowman space, and the permeability of the glomerular capillary wall. The permeability, as measured by the ultrafiltration coefficient (K_f), is the product of the water permeability of the

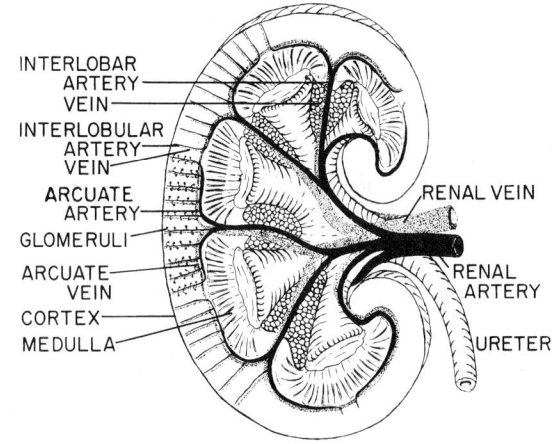

Figure 17–1. Gross morphology of the renal circulation. (From Pitts RF: Physiology of the Kidney and Body Fluids. 3rd ed. Chicago, Year Book Medical Publishers, 1974. Used by permission.)

1111

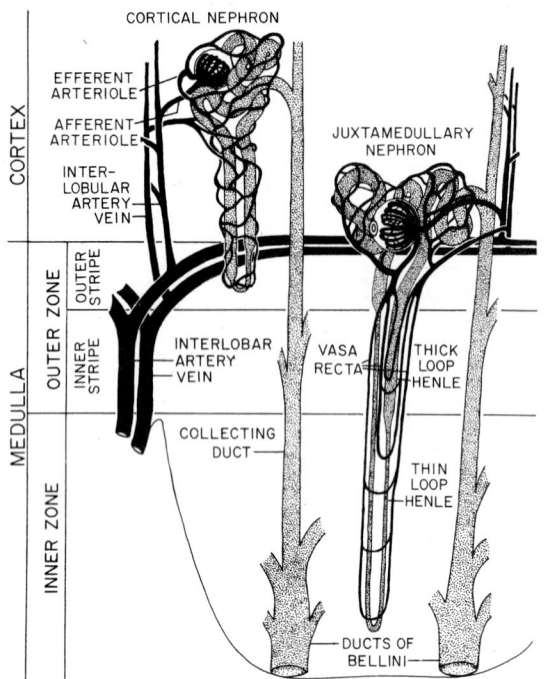

Figure 17–2. Comparison of the blood supplies of cortical and juxtamedullary nephrons. (From Pitts RF: Physiology of the Kidney and Body Fluids. 3rd ed. Chicago, Year Book Medical Publishers, 1974. Used by permission.)

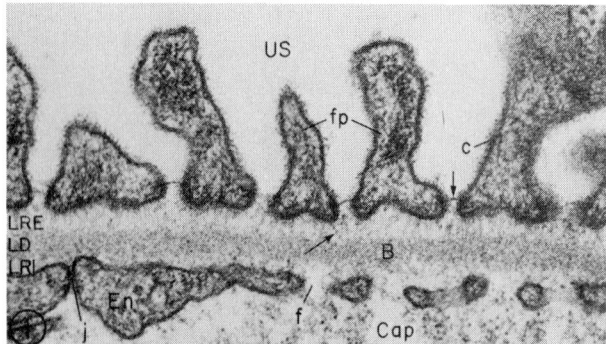

Figure 17–4. Electron micrograph of the normal glomerular capillary (Cap) wall demonstrating the endothelium (En) with its fenestrations (f), the glomerular basement membrane (B) with its central dense layer, the lamina densa (LD) and adjoining lamina rara interna (LRI) and externa (LRE; *long arrow*), and the epithelial cell foot processes (fp) with their thick cell coat (c). The glomerular filtrate passes through the endothelial fenestrae, crosses the basement membrane, and passes through the filtration slits (*short arrow*) between the epithelial cell foot processes to reach the urinary space (US). (× 60,000.) (From Farquhar MG, Kanwar YS: Functional organization of the glomerulus: state of the science in 1979. *In* Cummings NB, Michael AF, Wilson CB [eds]: Immune Mechanisms in Renal Disease. New York, Plenum, 1982. Reprinted by permission.)

membrane and the total glomerular capillary surface area available for filtration.

Although glomerular filtration begins around the 9th week of fetal life, kidney function does not appear necessary for normal intrauterine homeostasis, the placenta serving as the major excretory organ. Following birth, the rate of glomerular filtration increases until growth ceases toward the end of the 2nd decade of life (Fig. 17–5). To facilitate the comparison of the glomerular filtration rates (GFR) of children and adults, the rate is standardized to the surface area (1.73 m²) of a 70 kg adult. It should be noted (Fig. 17–6) that even after correcting for surface area the glomerular filtration rate of the child does not approximate adult values until the third year of life.

The glomerular filtration rate may be estimated by measurement of the serum creatinine level (Fig. 17–7). Creatinine

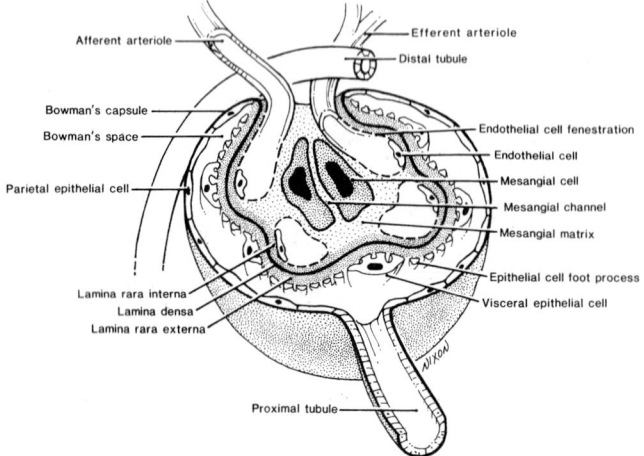

Figure 17–3. Schematic depiction of the glomerulus and surrounding structures.

is derived from muscle metabolism. Its production is relatively constant and its excretion is primarily through glomerular filtration (although tubular secretion may become important in renal insufficiency). In contrast to the concentration of blood urea nitrogen, the serum creatinine level is minimally influenced by factors (nitrogen balance, state of hydration) other than glomerular function. The serum creatinine is of value in estimating the glomerular filtration rate in the steady state only (e.g., a patient very shortly after the onset of acute renal failure and cessation of urine output may have a normal creatinine level but no effective renal function). The value of the serum creatinine is further compromised by the fact that its level does not rise above normal until the filtration rate falls below 70% of normal.

The precise measurement of the glomerular filtration rate is accomplished by quantitating the "clearance" of a substance that is freely filtered across the capillary wall and that is neither reabsorbed nor secreted by the tubules. The clearance (C_s) of such a substance(s) is that volume of plasma which, when completely "cleared" of the contained substance, would yield a quantity of that substance equal to that excreted in the urine over a specified time. The clearance is represented by the following formula:

$$C_s(mL/min) = \frac{U_s(mg/mL)V(mL/min)}{P_s(mg/mL)}$$

where C_s equals the clearance of substance s, U_s reflects the urinary concentration of s, V represents the urinary flow rate, and P_s equals the plasma concentration of s. To correct the clearance for body surface area, the formula is:

$$\text{Corrected clearance} = C_s(mL/min) \times \frac{1.73}{\text{Patient's surface area (m}^2)}$$

The glomerular filtration rate is optimally measured by the clearance of inulin, a fructose polymer having a molecular weight of approximately 5000. Because the inulin clearance technique is cumbersome, the glomerular filtration rate is commonly estimated by the clearance of endogenous creatinine. When the glomerular filtration rate is relatively normal, the creatinine clearance closely approximates the inulin clearance. However, as the glomerular filtration rate declines, an increasing proportion of the total creatinine in the urine is

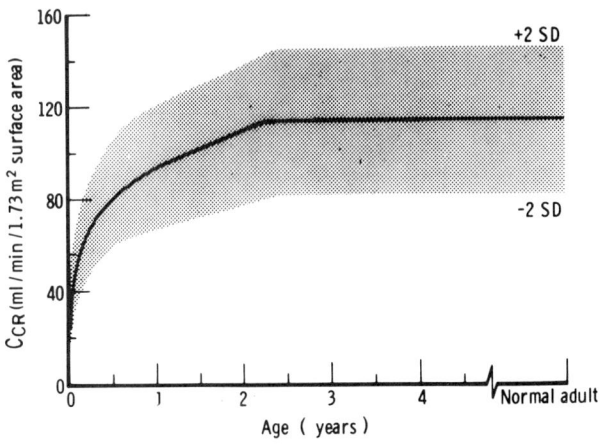

Figure 17–5. Actual glomerular filtration rate (GFR) from birth to 14 years of age. (From McCrory WW: Developmental Nephrology. Cambridge, Harvard University Press, 1972. Reprinted by permission.)

1 = average 6 mos - 1 yr
2 = average 1 - 3 yrs
3 = average 3 - 8 yrs
4 = average 8 - 11 yrs
5 = average 11 - 14 yrs

Average normal adult male

Figure 17–6. Changes in the normal value of the glomerular filtration rate, as measured by the creatinine clearance (C_{CR}), when standardized to mL/min/1.73m² of body surface area. The solid line depicts the mean value and the shaded area includes two standard deviations. (From McCrory WW: Developmental Nephrology. Cambridge, Harvard University Press, 1972. Reprinted by permission.)

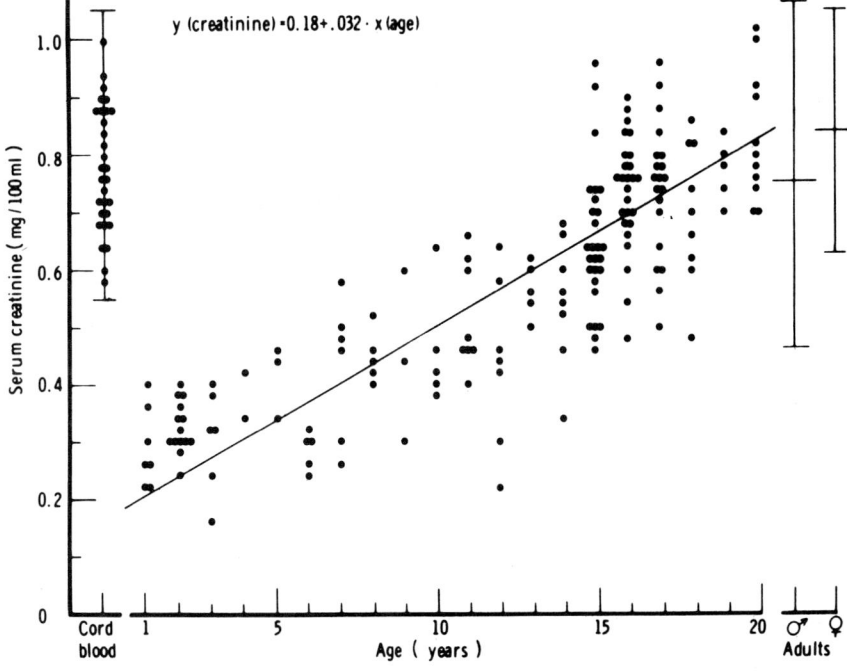

Figure 17–7. The serum creatinine in relation to age. (From McCrory WW: Developmental Nephrology. Cambridge, Harvard University Press, 1972. Reprinted by permission.)

y (creatinine) = 0.18 + .032 · x (age)

secreted by tubules, with the result that the creatinine clearance progressively overestimates the actual filtration rate. There is little merit, therefore, in measuring creatinine clearance when serum creatinine levels exceed 2.0 mg/dL; changes in renal function can then be monitored by the serum creatinine concentration.

The absence of plasma proteins larger than the size of albumin from the glomerular filtrate confirms the effectiveness of the glomerular capillary wall as a filtration barrier. Major factors restricting the filtration of these and other macromolecules include their size and their ionic charge.

Clearance studies of macromolecules in animals have shown no restriction to the filtration of molecules up to the size of inulin (molecular weight 5000). As size increases further, filtration diminishes progressively, approaching zero for substances the size of albumin (molecular weight 68,000). Morphologic studies suggest that the size-selective filtration barrier resides within the glomerular basement membrane.

The endothelial cell, basement membrane, and epithelial cell of the glomerular capillary wall possess strong negative ionic charges. These anionic charges are a consequence of two negatively charged moieties: proteoglycans (heparan sulfate) and glycoproteins containing sialic acid. Proteins in the blood have a relatively low isoelectric point and carry a net negative charge. Consequently, they are repelled by the negatively charged sites in the glomerular capillary wall, thus restricting filtration.

Brenner BM, Bohrer MP, Baylis C, et al: Determinants of glomerular permselectivity: Insights derived from observations in vivo. Kidney Int 12:229, 1977.
Brenner BM, Hostetter TH, Humes HD: Glomerular permselectivity: Barrier function based on discrimination of molecular size and charge. Am J Physiol 234:F455, 1978.
Farquhar MG: The primary glomerular filtration barrier—basement membrane or epithelial slits? Kidney Int 8:197, 1975.
McCrory WW: Developmental Nephrology. Cambridge, MA, Harvard University Press, 1972.
Michael AF, Keane WF, Raij L, et al: The glomerular mesangium. Kidney Int 17:141, 1980.
Renkin EM, Robinson RR: Glomerular filtration. N Engl J Med 290:785, 1974.
Venkatachalam MA, Rennke HG: The structural and molecular basis of glomerular filtration. Circ Res 43:337, 1978.

CONDITIONS PARTICULARLY ASSOCIATED WITH HEMATURIA

Hematuria may be gross (visible to the naked eye) or microscopic (detected only by dipstick or microscopic examination of the urine sediment). Gross hematuria may originate from the kidney, in which case it is generally brown or cola-colored and may contain red blood cell casts, or from the lower urinary tract (bladder and urethra), in which case the urine has a red to pink color and may contain clots. Gross hematuria may be associated with edema, hypertension, and renal insufficiency. This constellation of findings is typical of "the acute nephritic syndrome" and is frequently seen in patients having postinfectious (e.g., poststreptococcal) glomerulonephritis, systemic lupus erythematosus, membranoproliferative glomerulonephritis, anaphylactoid purpura, and rapidly progressive glomerulonephritis. The urine may be colored by pigments other than blood (Table 17–1).

In children, microscopic hematuria is most commonly discovered at periodic health examinations, by dipstick or by microscopic examination of the urine sediment. As the quantitation of blood (actually hemoglobin) on dipsticks is not precise, results should be interpreted as negative (negative or trace readings) or positive (small, medium, and large readings). A positive dipstick test for blood calls for a urinalysis. Microscopic hematuria is defined as more than five red blood cells per high power field in the sediment from 10 mL of centrifuged freshly voided urine.

Asymptomatic microscopic hematuria is found in 0.5–2.0% of school aged children, but whether screening for isolated microscopic hematuria can discover occult renal disease is unclear. In view of this uncertainty and its cost, screening urinalysis with microscopic examination of sediment for hematuria or pyuria seems unwarranted in asymptomatic children. On the other hand, a dipstick can detect blood or protein inexpensively, suggesting that this evaluation should be included in health maintenance routines.

Causes of hematuria are listed in Table 17–2. Children with

Table 17–1. Urinary Hues

Dark Yellow
  Concentrated urine
  Bile pigments

Red
  Blood (red cells or hemoglobin)
  Myoglobin
  Porphyrins
  Beets
  Blackberries
  Red food coloring
  Phenolphthalein
  Urates
  Pyridium

Dark Brown or Black
  Blood
  Homogentisic acid

Table 17–2. Causes of Hematuria in Children

 I. Glomerular Diseases
    A. Recurrent gross hematuria syndrome
       1. IgA nephropathy - Berger
       2. Idiopathic hematuria
       3. Alport syndrome
    B. Acute poststreptococcal glomerulonephritis
    C. Membranous glomerulopathy
    D. Systemic lupus erythematosus
    E. Membranoproliferative glomerulonephritis
    F. Nephritis of chronic infection
    G. Rapidly progressive glomerulonephritis - Crescents
    H. Goodpasture disease
    I. Anaphylactoid purpura Henoch - Schönlein
    J. Hemolytic-uremic syndrome

 II. Infection
    A. Bacterial
    B. Tuberculosis
    C. Viral

 III. Hematologic
    A. Coagulopathies
    B. Thrombocytopenia
    C. Sickle cell disease
    D. Renal vein thrombosis

 IV. Stones and Hypercalciuria

 V. Anatomic Abnormalities
    A. Congenital anomalies
    B. Trauma
    C. Polycystic kidneys
    D. Vascular abnormalities
    E. Tumors

 VI. Exercise

 VII. Drugs

gross hematuria should be hospitalized for evaluation because of the increased likelihood of finding hypertension and renal failure. Tradition suggests that children having persistent microscopic hematuria (more than five red blood cells per high power field on three urinalyses at monthly intervals) should have further outpatient evaluation. The cost-effectiveness of such evaluation remains to be determined.

17.3 GLOMERULAR DISEASES

Pathogenesis. Glomerular injury may be the result of immunologic, inherited (presumably biochemical), or coagulation disorders. Immunologic injury is the most common cause and results in "glomerulonephritis," which is both a generic term for several diseases and a histopathologic term signifying inflammation of the glomerular capillaries. Evidence that glomerulonephritis is caused by immunologic injury includes: (1) morphologic and immunopathologic similarities to experimental immune-mediated glomerulonephritis; (2) the demonstration of immune reactants (immunoglobulin and complement components) in glomeruli; and (3) abnormalities in serum complement and the finding of autoantibodies (e.g., anti–glomerular basement membrane) in some of these diseases. There appear to be two major mechanisms of immunologic injury: (1) localization of circulating antigen-antibody immune complexes; and (2) interaction of antibody with local antigen in situ. In the latter circumstance, the antigen may be a normal component of the glomerulus (e.g., the noncollagenous domain [NC-1] of type IV collagen, which is the putative antigen in human anti–glomerular basement membrane nephritis) or an antigen that has been planted in the glomerulus.

In immune complex–mediated diseases, antibody is produced against and combines with an antigen that is usually unrelated to the kidney. The immune complexes accumulate in glomeruli and activate the complement system, leading to immune injury. Experimental studies suggest that the complexes may be formed in the circulation and deposited in the kidney. The best-studied model, acute serum sickness in the rabbit, is produced by a single intravenous injection of bovine albumin. Within 1 wk after injection, the rabbit produces antibody against bovine albumin, while the antigen remains in the blood in high concentration. As antibody enters the circulation, it forms immune complexes with antigen. While the amount of antigen in the circulation exceeds that of antibody (antigen excess), the complexes formed are small, remain soluble in the circulation, and are deposited in glomeruli. The processes involved in glomerular localization are not well understood but include attributes of the complex (concentration, charge, size), characteristics of the glomerulus (mesangial trapping, negatively charged capillary wall), hydrodynamic forces, and the influence of various mediators (angiotensin II, prostaglandins).

With deposition of immune complexes in glomeruli, rabbits develop an acute proliferative glomerulonephritis. Immunofluorescence microscopy demonstrates granular ("lumpy-bumpy") deposits containing immunoglobulin and complement in the glomerular capillary wall. Electron microscopic studies show these deposits to be on the epithelial side of the glomerular basement membrane (GBM) and in the mesangium. Over the next few days, as additional antibody enters the circulation, the antigen is ultimately removed from the circulation and the glomerulonephritis subsides. In the rabbit, complement does not participate in the capillary injury, which is largely related to influx of macrophages. In other animal models, complement does play a role in capillary injury.

A unique form of immune complex nephritis (Heymann nephritis) occurs in rats following intraperitoneal injections of an extract of rat kidney. Antibodies are produced against antigens residing in the brush border of the proximal tubules. A nephrotic syndrome develops with a histologic picture similar to that of human membranous glomerulopathy. Early studies presumed that Heymann nephritis resulted from glomerular deposition of circulating immune complexes, but more recent studies have shown that the proximal tubular antigen is found also in pits on the membrane of glomerular epithelial cell foot processes, suggesting that the immune complexes actually form within the glomerular capillary wall. Such in situ immune complex formation may be created also by intravenous administration of positively charged antigens. These adhere to negative charges in the capillary wall (sites of heparan sulfate proteoglycan), where antibodies complex to the fixed antigen. At present, no clear human analogue exists for in situ complex formation, although it may occur in membranous and poststreptococcal glomerulonephritis.

Another example of in situ antigen-antibody interaction is anti–glomerular basement membrane (anti-GBM) antibody disease, in which antibody reacts with antigen(s) of the GBM. The antibody to GBM may be produced either in an animal species other than the one in which the disease will be produced (heterologous antibody) or in the host animal itself (autoantibodies) by immunization with GBM preparations. When rats are given an intravenous injection of antiglomerular basement membrane antibody made in rabbits, the disease process evolves in two phases. In the initial or heterologous phase, rabbit antibody attaches to the rat glomerular basement membrane immediately after injection, fixing complement, and producing a mild glomerulonephritis with infiltration of polymorphonuclear leukocytes. The second or autologous phase begins a week later. This phase is due to the production by the host (rat) of antibody to the rabbit antibody fixed to the GBM. Fixation of host antibody to rabbit antibody also activates the complement and coagulation systems, producing a severe glomerulonephritis with crescent formation and infiltration of macrophages into the glomerulus. Immunopathologic studies reveal linear deposition of immunoglobulin and complement on the GBM, similar to that seen in Goodpasture disease and certain types of rapidly progressive glomerulonephritis. The severity of the second (autologous) phase can be markedly reduced if the animal is given anticoagulant therapy at the time of injection of the anti–glomerular basement membrane antibody.

The inflammatory reaction that follows immunologic injury results from activation of one or more biochemical mediation systems (Fig. 17–8). Perhaps the most important of these is the complement system, which has two initiating sequences: (1) the classic pathway, which is activated by antigen-antibody immune complexes, and (2) the alternative or properdin pathway, which is activated by polysaccharides and endotoxin. These pathways converge at C3; from that point on, for both, the same sequence leads to lysis of cell membranes. The major noxious products of complement activation are produced after activation of C3 and include anaphylatoxin (which stimulates contractile proteins within vascular walls and increases vascular permeability), and chemotactic factors (C5a) that direct neutrophils and perhaps macrophages to the site of complement activation, where the cells release substances that damage vascular cells and basement membranes.

The coagulation system may be activated directly, following endothelial cell injury which bares the thrombogenic subendothelial layer (initiating the coagulation cascade), or indirectly, following complement activation (Fig. 17–8). Fibrin deposits may occur within glomerular capillaries or within Bowman space in crescents. Activation of the coagulation process may activate the kinin system, which also produces chemotactic and anaphylatoxin-like factors.

Pathology. The glomerulus may be injured by several

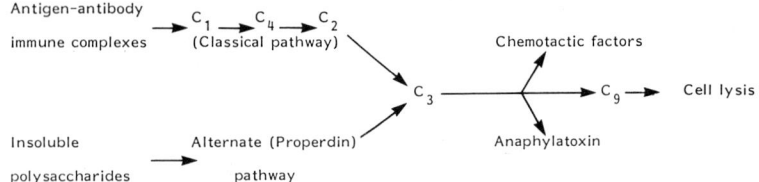

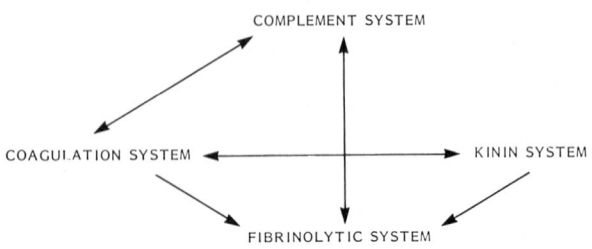

Figure 17–8. Interrelationships between activation of the complement, coagulation, fibrinolytic, and kinin systems.

mechanisms but has only a limited number of histopathologic responses; accordingly, different disease states may produce similar microscopic changes.

Proliferation of glomerular cells occurs in most forms of glomerulonephritis and may be generalized, involving all glomeruli, or focal, involving only some glomeruli while sparing others. Within a single glomerulus, proliferation may be diffuse, involving all parts of the glomerulus, or segmental, involving only some areas but not others. Proliferation commonly involves the endothelial and mesangial cells and is frequently associated with an increase in the mesangial matrix. Immunofluorescent and electron microscopic studies indicate that mesangial proliferation may result from immune complex deposition within the mesangium. The resultant increase in cell size and number in mesangial matrix may increase glomerular size and narrow the lumina of glomerular capillaries, leading to renal insufficiency.

Crescent formation in Bowman space (capsule) is a result of proliferation of parietal epithelial cells. Crescents develop in several forms of glomerulonephritis (termed "rapidly progressive") and are thought to be a response to fibrin deposited in Bowman space. New crescents contain fibrin, the proliferating epithelial cells of Bowman space, basement membrane-like material produced by these cells, and macrophages that may play a role in the genesis of glomerular injury. In days to weeks, the crescent is invaded by connective tissue (fibroepithelial crescent); this generally results in glomerular obsolescence. Crescent formation is frequently associated with glomerular cell death (necrosis). The necrotic glomerulus has a characteristic eosinophilic appearance with hematoxylin and eosin stain and usually contains nuclear remnants. Crescent formation is usually associated with generalized proliferation of the mesangial cells and with either immune complex or anti-GBM antibody deposition in the glomerular capillary wall.

In addition to proliferation, certain forms of acute glomerulonephritis show glomerular exudation of blood cells, most commonly neutrophils; eosinophils, basophils, and mononuclear cells may be seen in lesser numbers. The thickened appearance of glomerular basement membrane may result from a true increase in the width of the membrane (as seen in membranous glomerulopathy), from massive deposition of immune complexes which have staining characteristics similar to the membrane (as seen in systemic lupus erythematosus), or from the interposition of mesangial cells and matrix into the subendothelial space between the endothelial cells and the membrane. The latter may give the basement membrane a "split" appearance, as seen in type I membranoproliferative glomerulonephritis and other diseases.

Sclerosis refers to the presence of scar tissue within the glomerulus. Occasionally, pathologists will use this term to refer to an increase in mesangial matrix.

17.4 RECURRENT GROSS HEMATURIA OR PERSISTENT MICROSCOPIC HEMATURIA

In patients having a syndrome of recurrent gross hematuria (RGH), recurrent episodes of generally painless hematuria occur (mild flank pain may be felt). The gross hematuria usually develops 1–2 days after the onset of a presumably viral upper respiratory infection. This short latent period between the onset of infection and appearance of hematuria contrasts with the 7–14 day latent period seen in children developing acute poststreptococcal glomerulonephritis. Patients with RGH do not usually have such manifestations of the acute nephritic syndrome as edema, hypertension, or

Table 17–3. **Evaluation of the Child with Hematuria**

Step 1: Studies Performed in All Patients
  Complete blood count
  Urine culture
  Serum creatinine level
  24-hr urine collection for:
    creatinine
    protein
    calcium
  Serum C_3 level
  Intravenous pyelography

Step 2: Studies Performed in Selected Patients
  DNase B titer or Streptozyme test if hematuria less than 6 mo
    duration
  Skin or throat cultures when appropriate
  ANA titer
  Coagulation studies/platelet count when suggested by history
  Sickle cell screen in all black patients
  Voiding cystourethrography with infection, or when a lower tract
    lesion is suspected

Step 3: Invasive Procedures
  Renal biopsy indicated for:
  1. Persistent high-grade microscopic hematuria
  2. Microscopic hematuria plus any of the following:
     a. diminished renal function
     b. proteinuria exceeding 150 mg/24 hr
     c. hypertension
  3. Second episode of gross hematuria

  Cystoscopy indicated for:
    pink to red hematuria, dysuria, and sterile urine culture

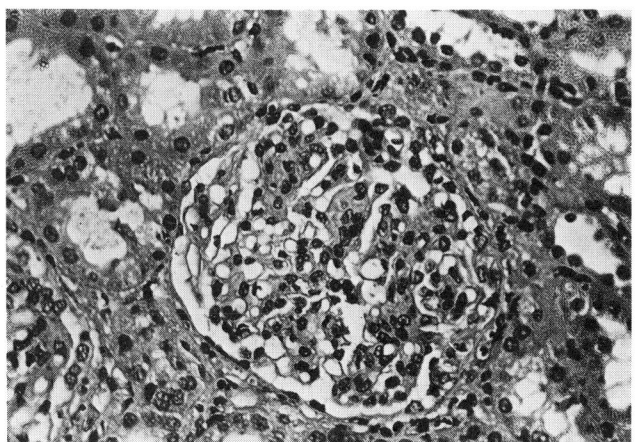

Figure 17–9. Light microscopy of IgA nephropathy demonstrating segmental mesangial proliferation and increased matrix. (× 180.)

renal insufficiency. Other patients have persistent microscopic hematuria without episodes of gross hematuria.

Patients having a first episode of gross hematuria are hospitalized and evaluated for other causes of hematuria (Table 17–3). In patients with RGH, routine radiographic and laboratory studies will fail to reveal a cause of hematuria. The gross hematuria resolves over 1–2 wk, but microscopic hematuria usually persists. Later, with another respiratory infection there is a recurrence of gross hematuria. Renal biopsy is indicated after the second episode, to determine the nature of any underlying disease, which will most frequently be IgA nephropathy, idiopathic hematuria, or familial nephritis (Alport syndrome).

IgA Nephropathy (Berger nephropathy). In 1967, Berger and his associates described a group of patients who, in the absence of any systemic disease such as systemic lupus erythematosus or anaphylactoid purpura, had glomerulonephritis with IgA as the predominant immunoglobulin in mesangial deposits.

Pathology and Pathogenesis. By light microscopy, most kidney biopsies reveal focal and segmental mesangial proliferation and increased matrix (Fig. 17–9). Some show generalized mesangial proliferation, occasionally associated with crescent formation and scarring. IgA is the predominant immunoglobulin deposited in the mesangium (Fig. 17–10),

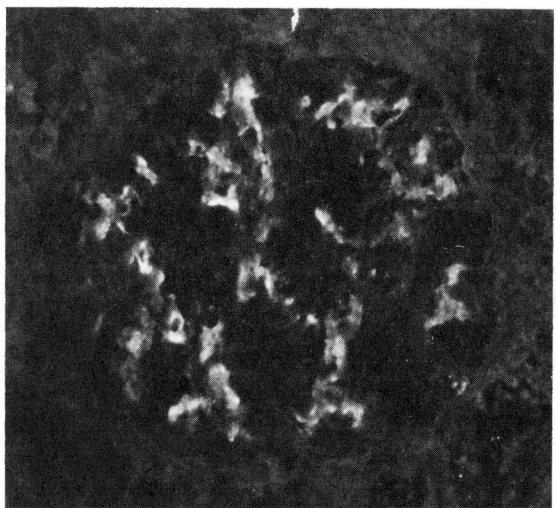

Figure 17–10. Immunofluorescence microscopy of the biopsy from a child having recurrent episodes of gross hematuria demonstrating mesangial deposition of IgA. (× 250.)

but lesser amounts of IgG, IgM, C3, and properdin are common. Electron microscopic studies confirm these findings.

Most evidence points to an immune complex etiology for IgA nephropathy. If the patient with IgA nephropathy has a kidney transplantation, the nephropathy commonly recurs in the transplanted kidney, indicating the systemic nature of this disorder.

Clinical and Laboratory Features. IgA nephropathy is more common in males than in females (2:1). Patients either present with an episode of gross hematuria or are found to have microscopic hematuria on routine examination. While the gross hematuria lasts, renal function usually remains relatively normal and proteinuria minimal (less than 1 g/day). Normal serum levels of C3 in IgA nephropathy help to distinguish this disorder from poststreptococcal glomerulonephritis.

Prognosis and Treatment. IgA nephropathy does not lead to significant kidney damage in most patients. Treatment is supportive and activity need not be restricted. Neither the number of episodes of gross hematuria nor the persistence of microscopic hematuria between episodes correlates with the likelihood of progressive disease. Progressive disease develops in 20% of patients, in whom a poor prognosis is associated with hypertension, diminished renal function, and/or proteinuria exceeding 1 g/day between episodes of gross hematuria, or with histologic evidence of diffuse glomerulonephritis with crescents and scarring. No effective treatment is known for patients with progressive IgA nephropathy.

Idiopathic Hematuria. Within the clinical spectrum of recurrent episodes of gross hematuria, *idiopathic hematuria* is defined histologically by normal findings on light and immunofluorescence microscopy. In some patients, electron microscopy demonstrates marked thinning of the glomerular basement membrane, but the membrane width may be normal in others.

Idiopathic hematuria has an excellent prognosis, but long-term follow-up is required to exclude Alport syndrome. Both disorders may be familial and Alport syndrome may have minimal light microscopic changes, negative immunofluorescence, and thin basement membranes. In patients presumed to have idiopathic hematuria, the development of decreased renal function, proteinuria, or hypertension calls for a second renal biopsy.

Alport Syndrome. This is the most common of several types of hereditary nephritis. There is marked variability in clinical presentation, natural history, histologic abnormalities, and genetic patterns.

Pathology. Kidney biopsies obtained during the first decade of life may show few changes by light microscopy. Later, the glomeruli may develop mesangial proliferation and capillary wall thickening, leading to progressive glomerular sclerosis. Tubular atrophy, interstitial inflammation and fibrosis, and foam cells (nonspecific lipid-laden tubular or interstitial cells) develop if the disease progresses. Immunopathologic studies are usually negative.

In most patients, electron microscopic studies have revealed thickening, thinning, splitting, and layering of the basement membranes of the glomeruli (Fig. 17–11) and tubules, but these lesions are not specific for Alport syndrome and may be absent in certain families that have the typical clinical manifestations of the syndrome.

Clinical Manifestations. Patients with Alport syndrome most commonly present with asymptomatic microscopic hematuria, but recurrent episodes of gross hematuria are not uncommon. In those with microscopic hematuria the development of proteinuria indicates the need for a kidney biopsy, which establishes the diagnosis.

Besides kidney involvement, a minority of patients have sensorineural hearing loss, which may begin in the high frequency range but progresses to involve the speech range and results in deafness. About 10% of patients suffer eye

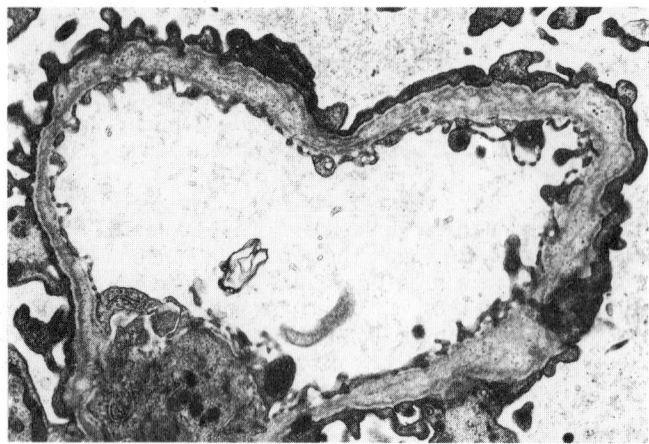

Figure 17–11. Electron micrograph of the biopsy from a child with Alport syndrome, depicting thickening, thinning, splitting, and layering of the glomerular basement membrane. (× 16,250.) (From Yum M, Bergstein JM: Basement membrane nephropathy. Hum Pathol 14:996, 1983. Used by permission.)

abnormalities, the most frequent of which are cataracts, keratoconus, and spherophakia.

Genetics. The inheritance of Alport syndrome best fits an autosomal dominant disorder, but this fails to explain the more severe clinical course in males than in females and the fact that in some kindreds inheritance has been reported to be X-linked dominant. Up to 20% of patients with Alport syndrome have no family history of renal disease; this suggests a high spontaneous mutation rate for the abnormal gene. The nature of the inherited defect is unknown; it may be related to composition of membrane collagen.

Complications. If renal function deteriorates, hypertension, urinary tract infections, and the manifestations of chronic renal failure may appear.

Prevention. Genetic counseling involving the entire family may limit propagation of the genetic abnormality.

Prognosis and Treatment. Males with Alport syndrome commonly develop end-stage renal failure in the second or third decade of life, occasionally in association with hearing loss. There is no specific therapy, but such patients are good candidates for dialysis and kidney transplantation. The development of anti–glomerular basement membrane nephritis in the transplanted kidneys of some patients with Alport syndrome suggests that the glomerular basement membrane of their native kidneys lacks a nephritogenic antigen. Females usually have a normal life span (for this reason, more mothers than fathers transmit the disease to their children) and only subclinical hearing loss.

IgA Nephropathy

Clarkson AR, Woodroffe AJ, Bannister KM, et al: The syndrome of IgA nephropathy. Clin Nephrol 21:7, 1984.
Hogg RJ, Silva F, Walker P, et al: A multicenter study of IgA nephropathy in children. Kidney Int 22:643, 1982.
Kher KK, Makker SP, Moorthy B: IgA nephropathy (Berger's disease)—a clinicopathologic study in children. Int J Pediatr Nephrol 4:11, 1983.

Idiopathic Hematuria

Piel CF, Biava CG, Goodman JR: Glomerular basement membrane attenuation in familial nephritis and "benign" hematuria. J Pediatr 101:358, 1982.
Tina L, Jenis E, Jose P, et al: The glomerular basement membrane in benign familial hematuria. Clin Nephrol 17:1, 1982.
Yoshikawa N, White RHR, Cameron AH: Familial hematuria: Clinico-pathological correlations. Clin.Nephrol 17:172, 1982.
Yum M, Bergstein JM: Basement membrane nephropathy: A new classification for Alport's syndrome and asymptomatic hematuria based on ultrastructural findings. Hum Pathol 14:996, 1983.

Alport Syndrome

Bernstein J, Kissane JM: Hereditary nephritis. *In:* Edelmann CM (ed): Pediatric Kidney Disease. Boston, Little, Brown, 1978, p 571.
Grunfeld, J-P: The clinical spectrum of hereditary nephritis. Kidney Int 27:83, 1985.
Habib R, Gubler MC, Hinglais N, et al: Alport's Syndrome: Experience at Hopital Necker. Kidney Int 21:S-20, 1982.
O'Neill WM, Atkin CL, Bloomer HA: Hereditary nephritis: A re-examination of its clinical and genetic features. Ann Intern Med 88:176, 1978.

17.5 ACUTE POSTSTREPTOCOCCAL GLOMERULONEPHRITIS

This disease is the classic example of the acute nephritic syndrome: the sudden onset of gross hematuria, edema, hypertension, and renal insufficiency. It was formerly the most common cause of gross hematuria in children, but its frequency has so declined over the past decade that IgA nephropathy now seems to be the most common cause of gross hematuria.

Etiology and Epidemiology. Acute poststreptococcal glomerulonephritis follows infection of the throat or skin with certain "nephritogenic" strains of group A beta-hemolytic streptococci. The factors that allow only certain strains of streptococci to be "nephritogenic" remain unclear. During cold weather poststreptococcal glomerulonephritis commonly follows streptococcal pharyngitis, whereas during warm weather the glomerulonephritis generally follows streptococcal skin infections or pyoderma. Epidemics of nephritis have been described in association with both throat (serotype 12) and skin (serotype 49) infections, but the disease is now most commonly sporadic.

Pathology. As in most forms of acute glomerulonephritis, the kidneys appear symmetrically enlarged. By light microscopy, all glomeruli appear enlarged and relatively bloodless and show diffuse mesangial cell proliferation with an increase in mesangial matrix (Fig. 17–12). Polymorphonuclear leukocytes are common in glomeruli during the early stage of the disease. Crescents and interstitial inflammation may be seen in severe cases. These changes are not specific for poststreptococcal glomerulonephritis.

Immunofluorescence microscopy reveals lumpy-bumpy deposits of immunoglobulin and complement on the glomerular basement membranes and in the mesangium. By electron microscopy, electron-dense deposits or "humps" are observed on the epithelial side of the glomerular basement membrane (Fig. 17–13).

Pathogenesis. Although morphologic studies and a depres-

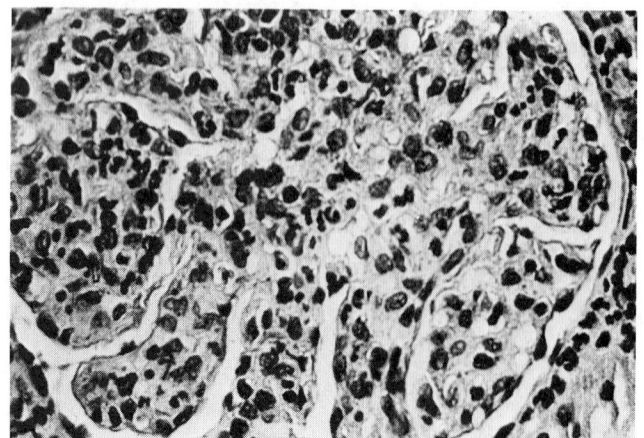

Figure 17–12. Glomerulus from a patient having poststreptococcal glomerulonephritis, appearing enlarged and relatively bloodless and showing mesangial proliferation and exudation of neutrophils. (× 400.)

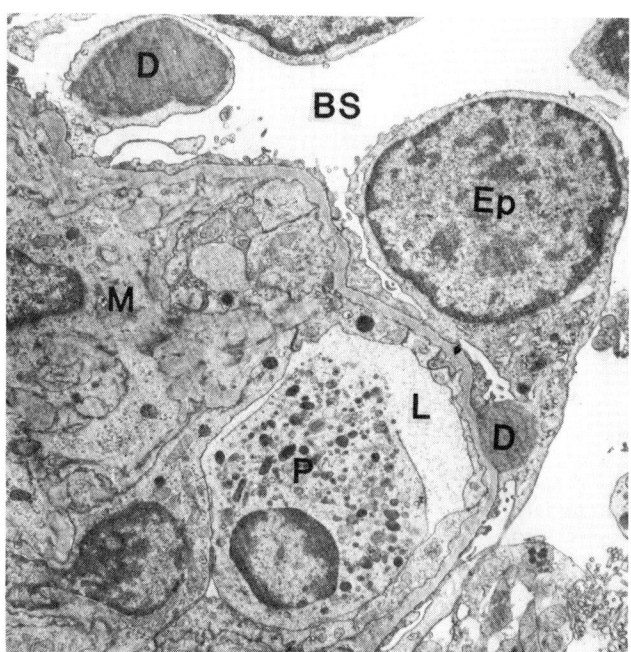

Figure 17–13. Electron micrograph in poststreptococcal glomerulone-phritis, demonstrating electron-dense deposits (D) on the epithelial cell (EP) side of the glomerular basement membrane. A polymorpho-nuclear leukocyte (P) is present within the lumen (L) of the capillary. BS, Bowman's space; M, mesangium.

sion in the serum complement (C3) level strongly suggest that poststreptococcal glomerulonephritis is mediated by immune complexes, the precise mechanisms whereby nephritogenic streptococci induce complex formation remain to be determined. Despite clinical and histologic similarities to acute serum sickness in the rabbit, the finding of circulating immune complexes in poststreptococcal glomerulonephritis is not uniform and complement activation is primarily through the alternative rather than the classic (immune complex–activated) pathway.

Clinical Manifestations. Poststreptococcal glomerulonephritis is most common in children but rare before the age of 3 yr. One to 2 wk after an antecedent streptococcal infection, the typical patient develops an acute nephritic syndrome. The severity of renal involvement may vary from asymptomatic microscopic hematuria with normal renal function to acute renal failure. Depending on the severity of renal involvement, patients may develop varying degrees of edema, hypertension, and oliguria. An encephalopathy or congestive heart failure or both may also develop. The edema is usually the result of salt and water retention, but a nephrotic syndrome may occur. Nonspecific symptoms such as malaise, lethargy, abdominal or flank pain, and fever are common. The acute phase generally resolves within 1 mo following onset, but urinary abnormalities may persist for more than 1 yr.

Diagnosis. Urinalysis demonstrates red blood cells, frequently in association with red blood cell casts and proteinuria; polymorphonuclear leukocytes are not uncommon. A mild normochromic anemia may be present owing to hemodilution and low grade hemolysis. The serum C3 level is usually reduced.

Confirmation of the diagnosis requires clear evidence of invasive streptococcal infection. Thus, positive throat cultures may support the diagnosis or may simply represent the carrier state. To document streptococcal infection properly, an elevated antibody titer to streptococcal antigen(s) should be confirmed. Although most commonly obtained, determination of the ASO titer may not be helpful because it rarely rises

after streptococcal skin infections. The best single antibody titer to measure is that to the DNase B antigen. An alternative is the Streptozyme test (Wampole Laboratories, Stamford, CT), a slide agglutination procedure that detects antibodies to streptolysin O, DNase B, hyaluronidase, streptokinase, and NADase.

In the child with an acute nephritic syndrome, evidence of recent streptococcal infection, and a low C3 level, the clinical diagnosis of poststreptococcal glomerulonephritis is warranted and renal biopsy ordinarily is not indicated. It is important, however, to exclude systemic lupus erythematosus and an acute exacerbation of chronic glomerulonephritis. Considerations for renal biopsy would include the development of acute renal failure or nephrotic syndrome, the absence of evidence for streptococcal infection, the absence of hypocomplementemia, or the persistence of marked hematuria or proteinuria or both, diminished renal function, or a low C3 level for more than 3 mo after onset.

The differential diagnosis of poststreptococcal glomerulonephritis includes many of the causes of hematuria listed in Table 17–2. Acute glomerulonephritis may also follow infection with coagulase-positive and -negative staphylococci, *Streptococcus pneumoniae*, and certain viruses.

Complications. The complications are those of acute renal failure, and include volume overload, circulatory congestion, hypertension, hyperkalemia, hyperphosphatemia, hypocalcemia, acidosis, seizures, and uremia.

Prevention. Early systemic antibiotic therapy of streptococcal throat and skin infections will reduce but not eliminate the risk of glomerulonephritis. Family members of patients with acute glomerulonephritis should be cultured for group A beta-hemolytic streptococci and treated if culture-positive.

Treatment. As there is no specific therapy for acute poststreptococcal glomerulonephritis, the management is that of acute renal failure (Sec. 17.35). Although a 10-day course of systemic antibiotic therapy, generally with penicillin, is recommended to limit the spread of the nephritogenic organisms, there is no evidence that antibiotic therapy affects the natural history of glomerulonephritis. Activity need not be restricted except during the acute phase of the disease when the complications of acute renal failure may be present, since activity has no detrimental effect on healing.

Prognosis. Complete recovery occurs in more than 95% of children with acute poststreptococcal glomerulonephritis. There is no evidence that progression to chronic glomerulonephritis occurs. Infrequently, however, the acute phase may be very severe and lead to glomerular hyalinization and chronic renal insufficiency. Mortality in the acute stage can be avoided by appropriate management of the acute renal or cardiac failure. Recurrences are extremely rare.

Heptinstall RH: Pathology of the Kidney. 3rd ed. Boston, Little, Brown, 1983.
Lange K, Seligson G, Cronin W: Evidence for the in situ origin of poststreptococcal glomerulonephritis: Glomerular localization of endostreptosin and the clinical significance of the subsequent antibody response. Clin Nephrol 19:3, 1983.
Travis LB: Acute postinfectious glomerulonephritis. *In*: Edelmann CM (ed): Pediatric Kidney Disease. Boston, Little, Brown, 1978, p. 611.

17.6 MEMBRANOUS GLOMERULOPATHY (GLOMERULONEPHRITIS)

Membranous glomerulopathy is the most common cause of nephrotic syndrome in adults, but it is uncommon in childhood and a rare cause of hematuria.

Pathology. By light microscopy, the glomeruli show diffuse thickening of the glomerular basement membranes, without significant proliferative changes (Fig. 17–14). The thickening is presumably due to the production of membrane-like material by the visceral epithelial cells in response to immune complexes deposited on the epithelial side of the membrane.

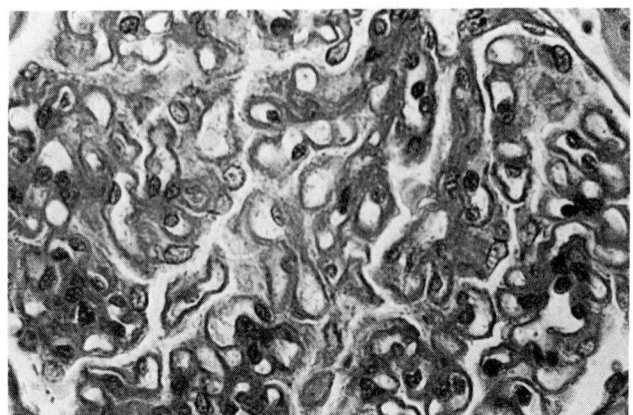

Figure 17–14. Glomerulus from a patient having membranous glomerulopathy, demonstrating diffuse thickening of the glomerular basement membrane in the absence of cellular proliferation. (× 400.)

This new material may, in certain areas, appear as "spikes" on the epithelial side of the basement membrane. Immunofluorescent microscopy demonstrates granular deposits of IgG and C3, which electron microscopy shows to be located on the epithelial side of the membrane.

Pathogenesis. Morphologic studies suggest that membranous glomerulopathy is an immune complex–mediated disease, but the mechanism of complex formation and the nature of the antigen within the complexes remains unknown in most patients. Despite close clinical and histologic similarities to the experimental Heymann nephritis, attempts to demonstrate proximal tubular antigen in the deposits have been largely unsuccessful.

Clinical Manifestations. In children, membranous glomerulopathy is most common in the second decade of life. The disease usually presents as nephrotic syndrome. However, almost all patients have microscopic hematuria and occasional patients suffer gross hematuria. The blood pressure and C3 levels are normal.

Diagnosis. The diagnosis is confirmed by kidney biopsy. The usual indications for biopsy include the presentation of nephrotic syndrome in a child more than 8 yr old or the presence of unexplained hematuria and proteinuria.

Membranous glomerulopathy may occasionally be seen in association with systemic lupus erythematosus, cancer, gold or penicillamine therapy, and syphilis and hepatitis B virus infections. These conditions should be considered in patients having membranous disease, since elimination of the presumed stimulus might lead to resolution of the glomerulopathy. Patients with membranous glomerulopathy are at increased risk of renal vein thrombosis.

Treatment. Fortunately, membranous glomerulopathy resolves spontaneously in the majority of children, although some may have persistent proteinuria. The nephrotic state is best controlled with salt restriction and diuretic agents. Studies in adults suggest that intermittent prednisone therapy may retard the progressive renal insufficiency observed in some patients.

Habib R, Kleinknecht C, Gubler MC, et al: Membranous glomerulopathy in children. *In:* Edelmann CM (ed): Pediatric Kidney Disease. Boston, Little, Brown, 1978, p 646.

Kleinknecht C, Levy M, Gagnadoux MF, et al: Membranous glomerulonephritis with extra-renal disorders in children. Medicine 58:219, 1979.

Latham P, Poucell S, Koresaar A, et al: Idiopathic membranous glomerulopathy in Canadian children: A clinicopathologic study. J Pediatr 101:682, 1982.

Ramirez F, Brouhard BH, Travis LB, et al: Idiopathic membranous nephropathy in children. J Pediatr 101:677, 1982.

17.7 SYSTEMIC LUPUS ERYTHEMATOSUS

This systemic disease is characterized by fever, weight loss, rash, hematologic abnormalities, arthritis, and involvement of the heart, lungs, central nervous system, and kidneys. The nonrenal manifestations are discussed in Sec. 10.61. Kidney disease is one of the most common manifestations of lupus in childhood and may occasionally be the only manifestation.

Pathogenesis and Pathology. Studies in a mouse (NZB/NZW) strain and in humans suggest that the clinical manifestations of lupus are mediated by immune complexes, which are formed in the circulation and deposited in various organs. Recent studies have revealed aberrations in both B-cell and T-cell function.

Of the several classifications of lupus nephritis, that offered by the World Health Organization (WHO), which uses light, immunofluorescent, and electron microscopy, is most accepted. In patients with WHO class I nephritis, no histologic abnormalities are detected. In WHO class II (also called mesangial lupus nephritis), some glomeruli have mesangial deposits containing immunoglobulin and complement; light microscopy may be normal (class II-A) or show focal and segmental mesangial hypercellularity and increased matrix (class II-B).

WHO class III (also called focal proliferative lupus nephritis) shows mesangial deposits in almost all glomeruli, and subendothelial deposits (between the endothelial cells and glomerular basement membrane) in some. In addition to focal and segmental mesangial proliferation, occasional glomeruli show capillary wall necrosis and crescent formation.

WHO class IV (also called diffuse proliferative lupus nephritis) is the most common and most severe form of lupus nephritis. All glomeruli contain massive mesangial and subendothelial deposits of immunoglobulin and complement. By light microscopy, all glomeruli show mesangial proliferation. The capillary walls are frequently thickened (owing to subendothelial deposits), creating the "wire-loop" lesion, and commonly show necrosis, crescent formation, and scarring.

WHO class V (also called membranous lupus nephritis) is the least common form of lupus nephritis; it resembles idiopathic membranous glomerulopathy histologically, except for mild to moderate mesangial proliferation.

Transformation of the histologic lesion from one class to another (usually to a more severe class) is common, especially in inadequately treated patients.

Clinical Manifestations. The large majority of children with systemic lupus are adolescent girls who present with evidence of systemic disease, leading to the ultimate diagnosis. The clinical findings in patients having the milder forms (all class II, some class III) of lupus nephritis include hematuria, normal renal function, and proteinuria of less than 1 g/day. Some patients with class III and all with class IV nephritis have hematuria and proteinuria, with reduced renal function, nephrotic syndrome, or acute renal failure. In some patients with proliferative glomerulonephritis, the finding of normal urinary sediment obscures the renal involvement. Patients with class V nephritis commonly have a nephrotic syndrome.

Diagnosis. The diagnosis of lupus is suggested by the detection of circulating antinuclear antibodies and is confirmed by demonstrating that these antibodies react with native (double-stranded) DNA. In most patients with active disease, C3 and C4 levels are depressed. In view of the lack of clear correlation between the clinical manifestations and the severity of the renal involvement, renal biopsy should be done in all patients with lupus. The findings will guide the selection of immunosuppressive therapy.

Treatment. Immunosuppressive therapy in lupus nephritis aims at clinical and serologic remission (normalization of the anti-DNA, C3, and C4 levels). Therapy is initiated in all patients with prednisone, 60 mg/m²/day, divided into three or four doses. In patients having more severe forms of nephritis (some class III, all class IV), azathioprine is added in a once daily dosage of 2–3 mg/kg. After serologic remission is obtained after 1–2 mo, the dose of prednisone is reduced to 60 mg/m² taken every other day as a single morning dose, being certain that the serologic studies remain normal and renal function stable while the dose is reduced. After a varying period of time, the dose may then be further reduced by 5 mg decrements to 30 mg/m², so long as serologic studies remain normal and renal function stable. The dose of azathioprine may be reduced gradually, while serology and renal function are monitored, and discontinued after 1 yr.

Prognosis. Aggressive immunosuppressive therapy has dramatically improved the prognosis of lupus in childhood; but the disease is controlled, not cured. The risk of relapse, as well as the side effects of chronic immunosuppressive therapy, persists; of special concern are the effects of corticosteroids in teen-aged girls. Patients with lupus should be managed in conjunction with specialists in medical centers where both medical and psychologic support can be given to both patients and their families.

Balow JE, Austin HA, Muenz LR, et al: Effect of treatment on the evolution of renal abnormalities in lupus nephritis. N Engl J Med 311:491, 1984.

Fish AJ, Blau EB, Westberg NG, et al: Systemic lupus erythematosus within the first two decades of life. Am J Med 62:99, 1977.

Grishman E, Gerber MA, Churg J: Pattern of renal injury in systemic lupus erythematosus: Light and immunofluorescence microscopic observations. Am J Kidney Dis 2:135, 1982.

Jarrett MP, Sablay LB, Walter L, et al: The effect of continuous normalization of serum hemolytic complement on the course of lupus nephritis. Am J Med 70:1067, 1981.

Lee HS, Mujais SK, Kasinath BS, et al: Course of renal pathology in patients with systemic lupus erythematosus. Am J Med 77:612, 1984.

17.8 MEMBRANOPROLIFERATIVE (MESANGIOCAPILLARY) GLOMERULONEPHRITIS

The term "chronic glomerulonephritis" implies continuing glomerular injury, such as frequently leads to glomerular destruction and end-stage renal failure. Membranoproliferative glomerulonephritis is the most common cause of chronic glomerulonephritis in older children and young adults.

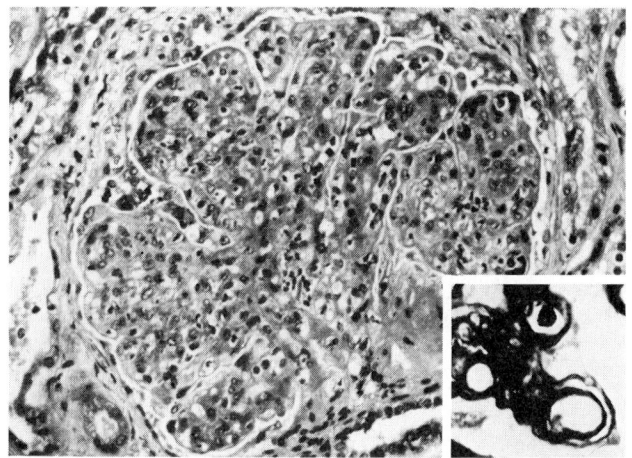

Figure 17–15. Glomerulus from a patient having Type I membranoproliferative glomerulonephritis, demonstrating an accentuated lobular pattern, a generalized increase in mesangial cells and matrix, and "splitting" of the glomerular capillary wall (inset). (× 250.) (From Kim Y, Michael AF: Idiopathic membranoproliferative glomerulonephritis. Reproduced, with permission, from the Annual Review of Medicine, Vol 31. © 1980 by Annual Reviews, Inc.)

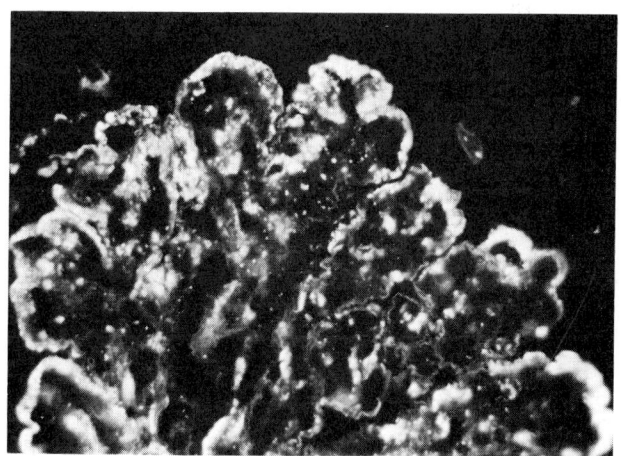

Figure 17–16. Immunofluorescence microscopy in Type I membranoproliferative glomerulonephritis, demonstrating granular deposition of C3 along the glomerular basement membranes and in the mesangium. (× 610.) (From Kim Y, Michael AF: Idiopathic membranoproliferative glomerulonephritis. Reproduced, with permission, from the Annual Review of Medicine, Vol 31. © 1980 by Annual Reviews, Inc.)

Pathology and Pathogenesis. Membranoproliferative glomerulonephritis was initially distinguished from other forms of chronic glomerulonephritis by the finding of hypocomplementemia, in some patients the result of an antibody (called C3 nephritic factor) that activates the alternative complement pathway. Not all patients have hypocomplementemia. Three histologic types are described.

Type I membranoproliferative glomerulonephritis is the most common form; the glomeruli reveal an accentuation of the lobular pattern, owing to a generalized increase in mesangial cells and matrix (Fig. 17–15). The glomerular capillary walls appear thickened and, in some areas, duplicated or split, owing to interposition of mesangial cytoplasm and matrix between the endothelial cells and glomerular basement membrane. Crescents may be present; when detected in a high percentage of glomeruli, they indicate a poor prognosis. Immunofluorescent microscopy reveals C3 and lesser amounts of immunoglobulin in the mesangium and along the peripheral capillary walls in a lobular pattern (Fig. 17–16), and electron microscopy confirms the presence of immune complex–like deposits in the mesangial and subendothelial regions.

In type II disease, the mesangial changes are less prominent than in type I. The capillary walls demonstrate irregular ribbon-like thickening, owing to dense deposits. Splitting of the membrane is rare, but crescents are common. By electron microscopy, the dense deposits are seen as thickenings of glomerular basement membrane in the region of but distinct from the lamina densa. The deposits are also found in Bowman capsule, mesangium, and tubular basement membranes; their composition is unknown. Immunofluorescent studies show C3, usually with minimal immunoglobulin, along the margin of the dense deposit material.

In type III disease, the light and immunofluorescent microscopic findings resemble those found in type I disease. Electron microscopy reveals contiguous subepithelial and subendothelial deposits, associated with disruption and layering of the lamina densa portion of the basement membrane.

Clinical Manifestations. Membranoproliferative glomerulonephritis is most common in the second decade of life. The majority of patients present with mild nephrotic syndrome, others with gross hematuria or asymptomatic microscopic hematuria and proteinuria. Renal function may be normal to depressed. Hypertension is common. The serum C3 complement level may be decreased.

Diagnosis and Differential Diagnosis. The diagnosis of membranoproliferative glomerulonephritis is made by renal biopsy. Indications for biopsy include onset of nephrotic syndrome in a child more than 8 yr old, or persistent microscopic hematuria and proteinuria.

Both membranoproliferative glomerulonephritis and poststreptococcal glomerulonephritis may present gross hematuria, low C3 levels, and elevated antistreptococcal antibody titers (coincidental in patients with membranoproliferative disease); their natural histories will distinguish between the two. Patients with poststreptococcal glomerulonephritis will improve dramatically within 2 mo of onset, whereas in children having membranoproliferative glomerulonephritis, persistent clinical manifestations will lead to kidney biopsy.

Prognosis and Treatment. The outlook for all types of membranoproliferative disease is poor. Complete recovery has been reported, but most patients with type II and many patients with types I and III progress to end-stage renal failure. Types I and II membranoproliferative glomerulonephritis have been found to recur in patients with kidney transplants, suggesting the presence of systemic disorder.

No definitive therapy exists, but stabilization of the clinical course has been reported in some patients receiving long-term alternate-day prednisone therapy and in others treated with inhibitors of platelet function.

Cameron JS, Turner DR, Heaton J, et al: Idiopathic mesangiocapillary glomerulonephritis. Am J Med 74:175, 1983.
Donadio JV Jr, Anderson CF, Mitchell JC, et al: Membranoproliferative glomerulonephritis. A prospective clinical trial of platelet-inhibitor therapy. N Engl J Med 310:1421, 1984.
Habib R, Gubler MC, Loirat C, et al: Dense deposit disease: A variant of membranoproliferative glomerulonephritis. Kidney Int 7:204, 1975.
Kim Y, Michael AF: Idiopathic membranoproliferative glomerulonephritis. Ann Rev Med 31:273, 1980.
McEnery PT, McAdams AJ, West CD: Membranoproliferative glomerulonephritis: Improved survival with alternate day prednisone. Clin Nephrol 13:117, 1980.
Strife CF, Jackson EC, McAdams AJ: Type III membranoproliferative glomerulonephritis: Long-term clinical and morphologic evaluation. Clin Nephrol 21:323, 1984.

17.9 GLOMERULONEPHRITIS OF CHRONIC INFECTION

Occurrence of glomerulonephritis has been recognized during the course of various chronic infections, including subacute bacterial endocarditis (*Streptococcus viridans* and other organisms), infected ventriculoatrial shunts for hydrocephalus (*Staphylococcus albus*), syphilis, hepatitis B, candidosis, and malaria. In each condition, the infecting organism has low virulence, and the host is chronically seeded with foreign antigen. In the presence of high levels of circulating antigen, the host's antibody response leads to formation of immune complexes, which deposit in the kidneys and initiate the glomerulonephritis.

The histopathologic findings may resemble poststreptococcal, membranous, or membranoproliferative glomerulonephritis. The clinical manifestations are generally those of an acute nephritic or nephrotic syndrome. The C3 level is frequently depressed.

Eradication of the infection before severe glomerular injury occurs usually results in resolution of the glomerulonephritis. Progression to end-stage renal failure has been described.

Arze RS, Rashid H, Morley R, et al: Shunt nephritis: Report of two cases and review of the literature. Clin Nephrol 19:48, 1983.
Chesney RW, O'Regan S, Guyda HJ, et al: Candida endocrinopathy syndrome with membranoproliferative glomerulonephritis: Demonstration of glomerular candida antigen. Clin Nephrol 5:232, 1976.
Collins AB, Bhan AK, Dienstag JL, et al: Hepatitis B immune complex glomerulonephritis: Simultaneous glomerular deposition of hepatitis B surface and e antigens. Clin Immunol Immunopathol 26:137, 1983.

Hendrickse RG, Adeniyi A: Quartan malarial nephrotic syndrome in children. Kidney Int 16:64, 1979.
Kim Y, Michael AF: Infection and nephritis. In Edelmann CM (ed): Pediatric Kidney Disease. Boston, Little, Brown, 1978, p 828.
Neugarten J, Baldwin DS: Glomerulonephritis in bacterial endocarditis. Am J Med 77:297, 1984.
O'Regan S, Fong JSC, de Chadarevian JP, et al: Treponemal antigens in congenital and acquired syphilitic nephritis. Ann Intern Med 85:325, 1976.

17.10 RAPIDLY PROGRESSIVE (CRESCENTIC) GLOMERULONEPHRITIS

The term "rapidly progressive" describes the clinical course of several forms of glomerulonephritis whose unifying abnormality is the presence of crescents in the majority of glomeruli. The natural history in most forms is rapid progression to end-stage renal failure.

Classification. Crescents may be found in several well-defined types of glomerulonephritis, such as poststreptococcal, lupus, membranoproliferative, and the glomerulonephritides of Goodpasture disease or anaphylactoid purpura. In these diseases, the typical findings on light, immunofluorescent, and electron microscopic examinations are maintained despite crescent formation, and these histologic findings, in conjunction with appropriate laboratory studies, should reveal the underlying disease. After these recognized forms of glomerulonephritis are excluded, an idiopathic variety of rapidly progressive disease remains.

Pathology and Pathogenesis. Crescents are found on the inside of Bowman capsule and are composed of the proliferating epithelial cells of the capsule, and of fibrin, basement membrane–like material, and macrophages (Fig. 17–17). The stimulus for crescent formation is presumed to be the deposition of fibrin in Bowman space, probably as a result of necrosis or disruption of the glomerular capillary wall.

In many patients having the idiopathic variety of rapidly progressive disease, no evidence for immunologic mechanisms can be detected; others have antibodies against glomerular basement membrane or deposits of immune complexes on capillary walls. The C3 level is normal.

Clinical Manifestations. The majority of patients develop acute renal failure, often after an acute nephritic or nephrotic episode. Progression to end-stage renal failure follows within weeks to months after onset.

Diagnosis and Differential Diagnosis. Appropriate serologic studies (ANA, C3, anti-DNase B titers) should be obtained to search for defined types of glomerulonephritis. The diagnosis is confirmed by kidney biopsy.

Prognosis and Treatment. Children having rapidly progres-

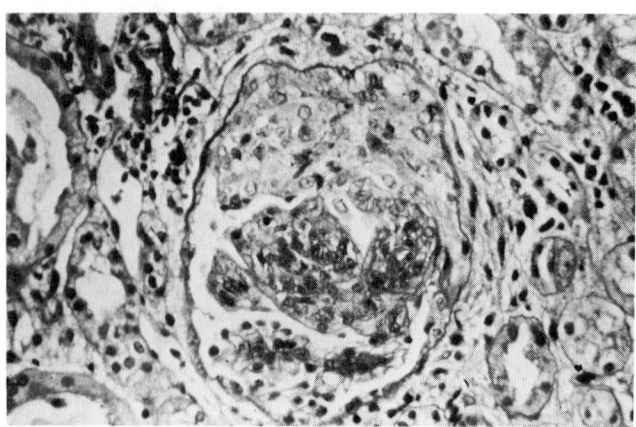

Figure 17–17. Light micrograph of biopsy specimen from a child with anaphylactoid purpura glomerulonephritis, demonstrating a crescent overlying the glomerulus. (× 180.)

sive disease associated with poststreptococcal glomerulonephritis may recover spontaneously. We have had success in treating the rapidly progressive nephritis of lupus and of anaphylactoid purpura with prednisone and azathioprine. The prognosis is poor for the remaining types of rapidly progressive glomerulonephritis, although a few patients have been reported to improve with therapy combining immunosuppressive agents, anticoagulants, and plasmapheresis.

Couser WG: Idiopathic rapidly progressive glomerulonephritis. Am J Nephrol 2:57, 1982.

Miller MN, Baumal R, Poucell S, et al: Incidence and prognostic importance of glomerular crescents in renal diseases of childhood. Am J Nephrol 4:244, 1984.

Neild GH, Cameron JS, Ogg CS, et al: Rapidly progressive glomerulonephritis with extensive glomerular crescent formation. Q J Med 52:395, 1983.

17.11 GOODPASTURE DISEASE

Goodpasture disease (pulmonary hemorrhage and glomerulonephritis associated with antibodies against lung and against glomerular basement membrane) should be distinguished from Goodpasture syndrome (a clinical picture of pulmonary hemorrhage and glomerulonephritis that may be seen with several disorders, including systemic lupus erythematosus, anaphylactoid purpura, polyarteritis nodosa, and Wegener granulomatosis). In some patients, anti–glomerular basement membrane nephritis occurs without pulmonary hemorrhage, as one form of rapidly progressive glomerulonephritis. (See also Sec. 10.79.)

Pathology. In most patients, the changes on light microscopy resemble those of rapidly progressive glomerulonephritis; immunoflourescent microscopy shows a continuous linear pattern of IgG along the glomerular basement membrane, typical of anti–glomerular basement membrane antibody (Fig. 17–18).

Clinical Manifestations. Goodpasture disease is extremely rare in childhood. Hemoptysis is usually the presenting complaint, and pulmonary hemorrhage is a potential cause of death. In days to weeks, hematuria, proteinuria, and progressive renal failure develop. The C3 level is normal.

Diagnosis. The diagnosis is suggested by kidney biopsy. Other diseases that may show linear glomerular basement membrane staining for IgG are excluded when serum is found to contain anti–glomerular basement membrane antibody.

Prognosis and Treatment. Patients who survive the pulmonary hemorrhage commonly progress to end-stage renal failure. No definitive therapy exists; some patients have

improved following combined immunosuppression and plasmapheresis.

Briggs WA, Johnson JP, Teichman S, et al: Antiglomerular basement membrane antibody-mediated glomerulonephritis and Goodpasture's syndrome. Medicine 58:348, 1979.

Herman PG, Balikian JP, Seltzer SE, et al: The pulmonary-renal syndrome. Am J Roentgenol 130:1141, 1978.

Simpson IJ, Doak PB, Williams LC, et al: Plasma exchange in Goodpasture's syndrome. Am J Nephrol 2:301, 1982.

17.12 ANAPHYLACTOID (HENOCH-SCHÖNLEIN) PURPURA GLOMERULONEPHRITIS

Anaphylactoid purpura is the most common form of systemic vasculitis in children. It is presumably an immune complex–mediated disease, but the precise etiology is unclear.

Pathology. Anaphylactoid purpura is a vasculitis of the smallest blood vessels. Perivascular accumulation of white blood cells may be seen in several organs, and in the majority of patients with renal involvement, there are focal and segmental increases in mesangial cells and matrix. A minority of patients show generalized mesangial changes, and rare patients will have diffuse necrotizing glomerulitis with crescent formation.

Immunofluorescent microscopy reveals mesangial deposits of IgA, frequently in association with IgG, C3, and fibrin. The predominant deposition of IgA suggests a relationship to IgA nephropathy. Electron microscopy confirms the presence of mesangial deposits and may also reveal deposits along the capillary wall in the subendothelial space.

Clinical Manifestations. The typical patient presents with an urticarial and/or purpuric rash on the buttocks and lower extremities, arthritis or arthralgias, and abdominal pain. Evidence for renal involvement is usually detected within 1 mo of onset but may appear later.

Clinical evidence of kidney disease develops in approximately 50% of patients. A large majority suffer only mild renal involvement, characterized by hematuria, preserved renal function, and proteinuria of less than 2 g/24 hr. Patients with severe kidney involvement have diminished renal function and heavy proteinuria and frequently a nephrotic syndrome.

Diagnosis. The disease is usually defined by the clinical constellation of the typical rash and abdominal and joint complaints, with normal platelet count and C3 level and absence of antinuclear antibodies in serum.

Renal involvement is usually mild and kidney biopsy rarely necessary. Indications for biopsy include diminished renal function, proteinuria exceeding 2 g/24 hr, or development of a nephrotic syndrome.

Prognosis and Treatment. In most patients, the clinical manifestations resolve completely over several months, although microscopic hematuria may persist for more than 1 yr. With severe renal involvement, especially when biopsy shows the morphologic picture of rapidly progressive glomerulonephritis, the ultimate prognosis is extremely poor. No form of therapy is reliably effective in patients having severe renal involvement, but we have seen dramatic improvement in some such patients following treatment with prednisone and azathioprine.

Allen DM, Diamond LK, Howell DA: Anaphylactoid purpura in children (Schönlein-Henoch syndrome). Am J Dis Child 99:833, 1960.

Meadow SR, Glasgow EF, White RHR, et al: Schönlein-Henoch nephritis. Q J Med 4:241, 1972.

Meadow SR: The prognosis of Henoch-Schönlein nephritis. Clin Nephrol 9:87, 1978.

Sinniah R, Feng PH, Chen BTM: Henoch-Schönlein syndrome: A clinical and morphological study of renal biopsies. Clin Nephrol 9:219, 1978.

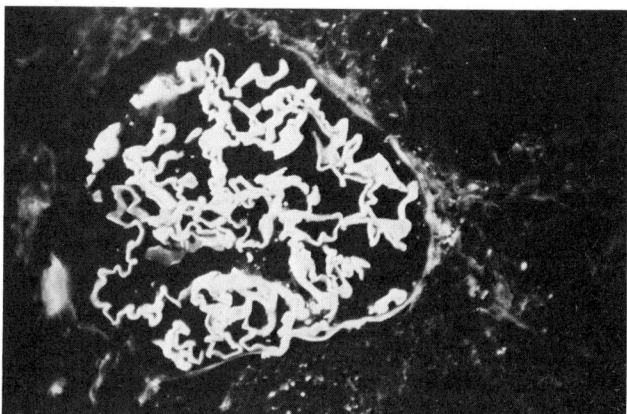

Figure 17–18. Immunofluorescence micrograph demonstrating the continuous linear staining of IgG along the glomerular basement membrane, as found in diseases mediated by anti–glomerular basement membrane antibody. (× 250.)

17.13 HEMOLYTIC-UREMIC SYNDROME

The hemolytic-uremic syndrome is the most common cause of acute renal failure in young children. It was initially felt to be a renal disorder with secondary hematologic manifestations, but recent studies indicate that the syndrome should be regarded as a systemic disease.

Etiology. The precise etiology of the disease is unknown. It has been associated with bacterial (*Shigella, Salmonella, E. coli, Streptococcus pneumoniae*), *Bartonella*, and viral (Coxsackie, ECHO, influenza, varicella, Epstein-Barr) infections and with endotoxemia. It has been reported also to follow use of oral contraceptives and pyran copolymer, an inducer of interferon. In addition, a hemolytic-uremic type of disorder has been reported to be associated with systemic lupus erythematosus, malignant hypertension, pre-eclampsia, postpartum renal failure, and radiation nephritis. Recent studies of pathogenesis have implicated the absence of a plasma factor that stimulates endothelial cell prostacyclin production. There are several reports of occurrence in more than one member of a family, but the role of genetic factors in predisposition to the disease is unknown.

Pathology. The initial changes in the glomeruli include thickening of the capillary walls, narrowing of the capillary lumina, and widening of the mesangium. Electron microscopy shows these changes to be the result of subendothelial and mesangial deposition of a granular, amorphous material of unknown origin. Fibrin thrombi can be found in glomerular capillaries and arterioles and may lead to cortical necrosis.

Severely involved glomeruli progress to partial or total sclerosis; severe vascular involvement may render others obsolescent from ischemia. In these severely involved small arteries and arterioles, concentric intimal proliferation leads to vascular occlusion.

Pathogenesis. The primary event in pathogenesis of the syndrome appears to be endothelial cell injury. Capillary and arteriolar endothelial injury in the kidney leads to localized clotting. Evidence for disseminated intravascular coagulation is commonly lacking. The microangiopathic anemia results from mechanical damage to the red blood cells as they pass through the altered vasculature. Thrombocytopenia is due to intrarenal platelet adhesion and/or damage. Damaged red cells and platelets are removed from circulation by the liver and spleen.

Clinical Manifestations. The syndrome is most common in children under the age of 4 yr. The onset is usually preceded by gastroenteritis (fever, vomiting, diarrhea) or, less commonly, by an upper respiratory infection. This is followed in 5–10 days by the sudden onset of pallor, irritability, weakness, lethargy, and oliguria. Physical examination may reveal dehydration, edema, petechiae, hepatosplenomegaly, and marked irritability.

Diagnosis and Differential Diagnosis. The diagnosis of the syndrome is supported by the findings of a microangiopathic hemolytic anemia, thrombocytopenia, and acute renal failure. The hemoglobin is commonly in the range of 5–9 g/dL. The blood film reveals helmet cells, burr cells, and fragmented red blood cells (Fig. 17–19). Plasma hemoglobin levels are elevated and plasma haptoglobin levels diminished. The reticulocyte count is moderately elevated; Coombs test is negative. The white blood cell count may rise to 30,000/mm³. Thrombocytopenia (20,000–100,000/mm³) occurs in more than 90% of patients. Findings on urinalysis are surprisingly mild and usually consist of low grade microscopic hematuria and proteinuria. Partial thromboplastin time and prothrombin time are usually normal; their prolongation is more commonly due to vitamin K deficiency than to disseminated intravascular coagulation. The severity of the renal involvement, and the complications thereof, vary from mild renal insufficiency to acute renal failure requiring dialysis.

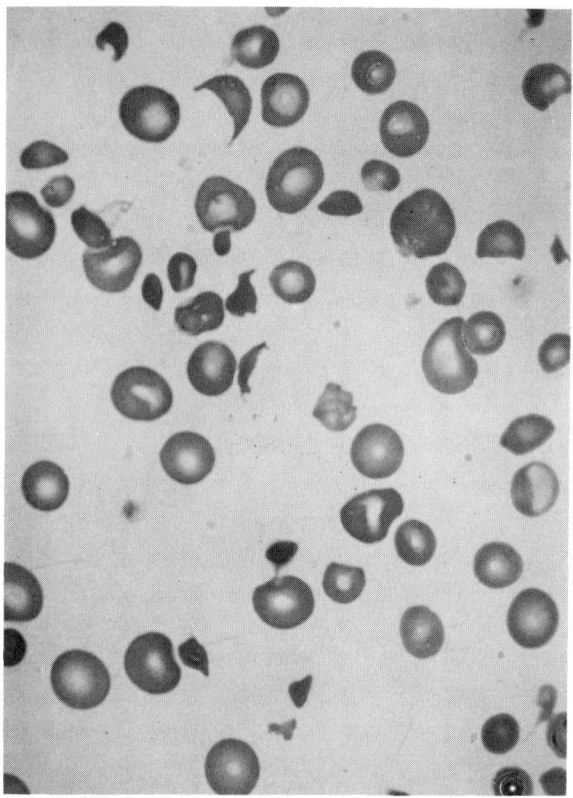

Figure 17–19. Blood film from a patient with the hemolytic-uremic syndrome, demonstrating the bizarre shapes of the fragmented red cells. (× 1000.)

The sudden onset of acute renal failure in a child should always call this entity to mind. The typical history, clinical picture, and laboratory findings confirm the diagnosis in most patients. Other causes of acute renal failure, especially those that can be associated with a microangiopathic anemia (lupus, malignant hypertension), should be excluded. Except in the rare patient who suffers prolonged renal failure (more than 2 wk) or who fails to develop thrombocytopenia, a renal biopsy is rarely indicated; it cannot be performed in the thrombocytopenic patient.

Patients suffering bilateral renal vein thrombosis (Sec. 17.15) may be difficult to distinguish from those with the hemolytic-uremic syndrome. Both disorders may be preceded by gastroenteritis, and in both the children may present dehydration, pallor, and evidence of microangiopathic hemolytic anemia, thrombocytopenia, and acute renal failure. The marked enlargement of kidneys of the child with renal vein thrombosis helps to distinguish the disorders, but angiography may be necessary in obscure cases.

Complications. Complications may include anemia, acidosis, hyperkalemia, fluid overload, congestive heart failure, hypertension, and uremia. In addition, extrarenal involvement may include central nervous system manifestations (irritability, seizures, coma), colitis (melena, perforation), diabetes mellitus, and rhabdomyolysis. The pathogenesis of these complications is unknown; they seem likely to be the result of intravascular thrombosis.

Prognosis and Treatment. With aggressive management of the acute renal failure, more than 90% of patients survive the acute phase and the majority of these recover normal renal function. It has been difficult to evaluate the results of therapy. Corticosteroids appear to be of no value, and experience with platelet inhibitors is so far inconclusive. The treatment has mostly involved anticoagulants, primarily heparin. Analysis of the results fails to demonstrate beneficial effects in the majority of patients, who in any case lack evidence of active hypercoagulation. Fibrinolytic therapy to dissolve intrarenal thrombi would have theoretical benefit, but the risks seem to outweigh the potential gains. Plasmapheresis or the administration of fresh-frozen plasma, or both, has been recommended in hopes of replacing a missing plasma stimulator of prostacyclin production, but results do not as yet permit interpretation.

Currently, we believe that careful medical management of the hematologic and renal manifestations, in conjunction with early and frequent peritoneal dialysis, offers the best chance of recovery from the acute phase. Long-term observation is necessary to watch for late development of hypertension or chronic kidney disease. Recurrence of the disease is quite rare.

Andreoli SP, Bergstein JM: Development of insulin-dependent diabetes mellitus during the hemolytic-uremic syndrome. J Pediatr 100:541, 1982.
Andreoli SP, Bergstein JM: Acute rhabdomyolysis associated with the hemolytic-uremic syndrome. J Pediatr 103:78, 1983.
Bergstein JM, Kuederli U, Bang NU: Plasma inhibitor of glomerular fibrinolysis in the hemolytic-uremic syndrome. Am J Med 73:322, 1982.
Gianantonio CA, Vitacco M, Mendilaharzu F, et al: The hemolytic-uremic syndrome. Nephron 11:174, 1973.
Goldstein MH, Churg J, Strauss L, et al: Hemolytic-uremic syndrome. Nephron 23:263, 1979.
Kaplan BS, Thomson PD, de Chadarevian JP: The hemolytic uremic syndrome. Pediatr Clin North Am 23:761, 1976.
Remuzzi G, Misiani R, Marchesi D, et al: Treatment of the hemolytic uremic syndrome with plasma. Clin Nephrol 12:279, 1979.
Riella MC, George CRP, Hickman RO, et al: Renal microangiopathy of the hemolytic-uremic syndrome in childhood. Nephron 17:188, 1976.

17.14 INFECTION AS A CAUSE OF HEMATURIA

Gross or microscopic hematuria may be associated with bacterial, mycobacterial, or viral infections of the urinary tract (Sec. 17.38). Why the same organism may cause hematuria in one patient with cystitis and not in another is unclear; the occurrence of hematuria may be related to the depth and severity of the inflammatory reaction within the bladder wall.

Urethritis may present gross or microscopic hematuria, usually in conjunction with urgency and urethral discomfort. Urinalysis reveals red blood cells and pyuria. Urine cultures occasionally reveal bacteria, *Ureaplasma*, or *Chlamydia*, but are usually negative. A history of trauma should be sought. The disorder frequently resolves spontaneously. Treatment can be considered with a 10 day course of tetracycline, with a urinary analgesic (phenazopyridine hydrochloride) given for relief of pain. If conservative management fails, cystoscopy may be required to determine the nature of any underlying abnormality.

17.15 HEMATOLOGIC DISEASES CAUSING HEMATURIA

COAGULOPATHIES AND THROMBOCYTOPENIA

Gross or microscopic hematuria may be associated with inherited or acquired disorders of coagulation (e.g., with hemophilias or with disseminated intravascular coagulation or with thrombocytopenia of any cause). In these cases, however, hematuria is almost never the presenting complaint, but usually develops after other manifestations. (See Sec. 15.43–15.50).

SICKLE CELL NEPHROPATHY

Gross or microscopic hematuria may be seen in children with sickle cell disease or trait. The hematuria presumably results from sickling in the relatively hypoxic, acidic, hypertonic renal medulla, with vascular stasis, diminished blood flow, ischemia, papillary necrosis, and interstitial fibrosis. Additional clinical manifestations of sickle cell nephropathy may include a urinary concentrating defect, renal tubular acidosis, and, rarely, a nephrotic syndrome that morphologically resembles membranoproliferative glomerulonephritis. The hematuria resolves spontaneously in the majority of patients. (See Sec. 15.18)

Alleyne GAO, Van Eps LWS, Addae SK, et al: The kidney in sickle cell anemia. Kidney Int 7:371, 1975.
Buckalew VM, Someren A: Renal manifestations of sickle cell disease. Arch Intern Med 133:660, 1974.
McInnes BK: The management of hematuria associated with sickle hemoglobinopathies. J Urol 124:171, 1980.

RENAL VEIN THROMBOSIS

Epidemiology. Renal vein thrombosis seems to occur in two distinct patterns. In newborns and infants, the disease is commonly associated with asphyxia, dehydration, shock, and sepsis; it occurs rarely in infants of diabetic mothers. After infancy, the disease is more commonly associated with the nephrotic syndrome (most frequently with membranous nephropathy), with cyanotic heart disease, and with the use of angiographic contrast agents.

Pathogenesis. The disease presumably begins in the intrarenal venous radicles, with both antegrade and retrograde spread. The main renal vein may escape involvement. Thrombus formation is presumably mediated by endothelial cell injury (by hypoxia, endotoxin, or contrast media) in conjunction with diminished vascular blood flow, which may be due to hypovolemia (shock, sepsis, dehydration, or nephrotic syndrome), or to the intravascular sludging of blood that results from polycythemia.

Clinical Manifestations. The development of renal vein thrombosis in infants is usually heralded by the sudden onset of gross hematuria and unilateral or bilateral flank masses. Older children commonly present with gross or microscopic hematuria and flank pain. The disease is more frequently unilateral than bilateral; bilateral involvement results in acute renal failure.

Diagnosis. The diagnosis is suggested by the development of hematuria and flank masses in a patient with predisposing clinical factors. Most patients will also have a microangiopathic hemolytic anemia and thrombocytopenia. Ultrasonography will show marked enlargement, whereas radionuclide studies reveal little or no renal function in involved kidneys. Venacavography of the inferior vena cava may be necessary to confirm the diagnosis in occult cases, but contrast studies should generally be avoided in order to minimize the risk of further vascular damage.

Differential Diagnosis. The differential diagnosis includes other causes of hematuria (especially the hemolytic-uremic syndrome) or renal enlargement (hydronephrosis, cystic disease, Wilms tumor, abscess, hematoma).

Treatment. For unilateral renal vein thrombosis, treatment is supportive and involves correction of fluid and electrolyte abnormalities and treatment of infection. Prophylactic anticoagulation to prevent thrombosis in the remaining kidney is unwarranted, except perhaps in patients with disseminated intravascular coagulation.

Since bilateral renal vein thrombosis frequently leads to chronic renal failure, consideration should be given to use of such measures as thrombectomy or the systemic use of fibrinolytic agents.

Prognosis. In infants, the thrombosed kidney undergoes progressive atrophy, ultimately leaving a small scarred kidney. Nephrectomy should not be performed in the acute phase, and later only if hypertension or chronic infection develops. In older children, the involved kidney may recover function, especially if the thrombosis was associated with nephrotic syndrome or cyanotic heart disease.

Arneil GC, MacDonald AM, Murphy AV, et al: Renal venous thrombosis. Clin Nephrol 1:119, 1973.
Baum NH, Moriel E, Carlton CE Jr: Renal vein thrombosis. J Urol 119:443, 1978.
Belman AB: Renal vein thrombosis in infancy and childhood. Clin Pediatr 15:1033, 1976.
Llach F, Papper S, Massry SG: The clinical spectrum of renal vein thrombosis: Acute and chronic. Am J Med 69:819, 1980.
Rowe JM, Rasmussen RL, Mader SL, et al: Successful thrombolytic therapy in two patients with renal vein thrombosis. Am J Med 77:111, 1984.

17.16 ANATOMIC ABNORMALITIES ASSOCIATED WITH HEMATURIA

CONGENITAL ANOMALIES

Gross or microscopic hematuria may be associated with almost any type of malformation of the urinary tract. The sudden onset of usually painless gross hematuria after minor trauma to the flank is frequently associated with ureteropelvic junction obstruction or cystic kidneys.

TRAUMA

Blunt or penetrating injury to the abdomen may injure the kidney. Gross or microscopic hematuria, flank pain, and abdominal rigidity may occur; associated injuries may be present. Urethral trauma may result from crushing-type injury, frequently associated with a fractured pelvis, or from direct injury by a foreign object. The injury is suspected when gross blood appears at the external meatus.

Levitt SB: Urologic trauma in childhood. In Edelmann CM (ed): Pediatric Kidney Disease. Boston, Little, Brown, 1978, p 1145.
Mendez R: Renal trauma. J Urol 118:698, 1977.

17.17 INFANTILE POLYCYSTIC DISEASE

This rare autosomal recessive disorder may not be detected until after infancy. Besides cysts in the kidneys, cysts may be found also in the liver, with significant liver disease.

Pathology. Both kidneys are markedly enlarged and grossly show innumerable cysts throughout the cortex and medulla. Microscopic studies show the "cysts" to be dilatations of the collecting ducts. The interstitium and remainder of the tubules may be normal at birth, but development of interstitial fibrosis and tubular atrophy may lead to renal failure.

The majority of patients also have cysts in the liver. In severe cases, the cysts in the liver may be associated with cirrhosis, portal hypertension, and death from ruptured esophageal varices. When the severity of hepatic manifestations exceeds that of renal involvement, the disorder is called *congenital hepatic fibrosis*. Whether infantile polycystic disease and congenital hepatic fibrosis are the opposite ends of the spectrum of a single disorder or distinct autosomal recessive disorders with similar manifestations remains to be determined.

Clinical Manifestations. The typical patient has bilateral flank masses at birth. The disorder may be associated with oligohydramnios, owing to inadequate formation of urine by the fetus. The oligohydramnios may produce Potter syndrome (flat nose, recessed chin, epicanthal folds, low-set abnormal ears, limb abnormalities), as a result of compression of the fetus, and pulmonary hypoplasia. The pulmonary hypoplasia may produce neonatal respiratory distress, with spontaneous pneumothorax. (The association of developmental disorders of the lungs and kidneys is sufficiently frequent to warrant ultrasonic evaluation of the kidneys in all neonates suffering spontaneous pneumothorax.) Gross or microscopic hematuria

and hypertension (which may be severe) are common. Renal function may be normal or diminished, depending on the severity of the renal malformation. Rarely, patients beyond infancy may first present with a nephrogenic diabetes insipidus–like state, renal insufficiency, or hypertension.

Diagnosis. The diagnosis is suggested by the clinical manifestations. Since ultrasonic evaluation of the kidneys may fail to define the cysts, intravenous pyelography should be done. A satisfactory pyelogram will reveal opacification of the dilated collecting ducts. Because these ducts run from cortex to medulla, they will appear as radial streaks similar to the spokes of a wheel. But radiographic studies are rarely able to confirm the diagnosis; it is our practice, therefore, in questionable instances, to perform open surgical biopsy of the liver and right kidney toward the end of the 1st yr of life, to confirm the diagnosis and to permit genetic counseling.

The differential diagnosis includes other causes of bilateral renal enlargement, such as multicystic dysplasia, hydronephrosis, Wilms tumor, and renal vein thrombosis.

Treatment. The treatment is supportive, including careful management of the hypertension.

Prognosis. Children with severe renal involvement may die in the neonatal period of pulmonary or renal insufficiency. Survivors may live for several years before developing renal insufficiency. During this period, the kidneys shrink in size and the hypertension becomes less severe. When renal failure develops, dialysis and kidney transplantation should be considered. In patients having hepatic fibrosis, cirrhosis may lead to portal hypertension, for which the prognosis is poor.

Alvarez F, Bernard O, Brunelle F, et al: Congenital hepatic fibrosis in children. J Pediatr 99:370, 1981.
Bernstein J: Polycystic disease. In Edelmann CM (ed): Pediatric Kidney Disease. Boston, Little, Brown, 1978, p 557.
Blyth H, Ockenden BG: Polycystic disease of kidneys and liver presenting in childhood. J Med Genet 8:257, 1971.
Landing BH, Wells TR, Claireaux AE: Morphometric analysis of liver lesions in cystic diseases of childhood. Hum Pathol 11:549, 1980.
Lieberman E, Salinas-Madrigal L, Gwinn JL, et al: Infantile polycystic disease of the kidneys and liver. Medicine 50:277, 1971.

Adult Polycystic Disease

This autosomal dominant disorder is a common cause of end-stage renal failure in adults but is rarely encountered in childhood. In affected adults, both kidneys are enlarged and show cortical and medullary cysts that are primarily dilated tubules. The disease commonly presents in the fourth or fifth decade of life with gross or microscopic hematuria, bilateral flank pain or masses, or both, and hypertension. Associated abnormalities may include hepatic cysts of no clinical significance and aneurysms of the cerebral circulation that may result in intracranial hemorrhage. Children with the disease may present with unilateral or bilateral flank masses. Hypertension may develop. The cysts are frequently demonstrable by ultrasonography, intravenous pyelography, or computed tomography (CT scan). In conjunction with the clinical manifestations and family history, radiographic studies usually confirm the diagnosis. In occult cases, especially those lacking a family history of the disease (the disease has a high spontaneous mutation rate), open renal biopsy may be necessary to confirm the diagnosis. Treatment is supportive. End-stage renal failure frequently develops by the sixth or seventh decade.

Chevalier RL, Garland TA, Buschi AJ: The neonate with adult-type autosomal dominant polycystic kidney disease. Int J Pediatr Nephrol 2:73, 1981.
Kaplan BS, Rabin I, Nogrady MG, et al: Autosomal dominant polycystic renal disease in children. J Pediatr 90:782, 1977.
Kaye C, Lewy PR: Congenital appearance of adult-type (autosomal dominant) polycystic kidney disease. J Pediatr 85:807, 1974.
Shokeir MHK: Expression of "adult" polycystic renal disease in the fetus and newborn. Clin Genet 14:61, 1978.

17.18 KIDNEY STONES AND HYPERCALCIURIA

Kidney stones in children usually result from chronic infection or the excessive urinary excretion of calcium, uric acid, or cystine. Presenting complaints may include abdominal or flank pain, gross or microscopic hematuria, or symptoms of urinary tract infection.

Hypercalciuria may be associated with asymptomatic gross or microscopic hematuria in the absence of hypercalcemia and stone formation. The mechanism of such hematuria is unknown. A screening test for hypercalciuria may be performed on a random urine specimen by measuring the concentrations of calcium and creatinine. A calcium to creatinine ratio exceeding 0.20 is presumptive evidence of hypercalciuria. The diagnosis is confirmed by finding in a 24 hr urine collection a calcium content of more than 4 mg/kg of body weight. Treatment with a low dose of chlorothiazide (10–20 mg/kg/day) will reduce the urinary calcium excretion to normal and eliminate the hematuria in most patients, presumably reducing the risk of stone formation. The need or effectiveness of long-term diuretic therapy has not been fully evaluated.

Hymes LC, Warshaw BL: Idiopathic hypercalciuria. Am J Dis Child 138:176, 1984.
Kalia A, Travis LB, Brouhard BH: The association of idiopathic hypercalciuria and asymptomatic gross hematuria in children. J Pediatr 99:716, 1981.
Moore ES: Hypercalciuria in children. Contr Nephrol 27:20, 1981.
Stapleton FB, Rog S, Noe HN, et al: Hypercalciuria in children with hematuria. N Engl J Med 310:1345, 1984.

17.19 VASCULAR ABNORMALITIES

Hemangiomas and arteriovenous malformations of the kidneys and lower urinary tract are extremely rare causes of hematuria. They usually present gross hematuria and the passage of blood clots. Renal colic may develop if the upper tract is involved. The diagnosis is confirmed by angiography.

17.20 TUMORS

Kidney tumors in children (Wilms tumor is most common) rarely have hematuria as the first sign; a flank mass is most common (see Sec. 16.13). Extrarenal tumors, such as the leukemias, lymphomas, or neuroblastoma, may cause hematuria, by direct infiltration of the kidney or by infiltration of the bone marrow, with resulting thrombocytopenia.

17.21 EXERCISE HEMATURIA

Gross or microscopic hematuria may follow vigorous exercise. Exercise hematuria is rare in females and can be associated with dysuria. The color of the urine may vary from red to black; myoglobinuria should be excluded. Blood clots may be present in the urine. Findings on urine culture, intravenous pyelography, voiding cystourethrography, and cystoscopy are normal in most patients. This seems to be a benign condition, and the hematuria generally resolves within 48 hr after cessation of exercise. The absence of red blood cell casts or of evidence of renal disease, and the presence of dysuria and blood clots in some patients, suggest that the source of bleeding lies in the lower urinary tract.

Bailey RR, Dann E, Gillies AHB, et al: What the urine contains following athletic competition. N Z Med J 83:309, 1976.
Fred HL, Natelson EA: Grossly bloody urine of runners. South Med J 70:1394, 1977.
Siegel AJ, Hennekens CH, Solomon HS, et al: Exercise-related hematuria. JAMA 241:391, 1979.

17.22 DRUGS

Gross or microscopic hematuria has been associated with use of various medications. Mechanisms include alterations in the coagulation system (heparin, warfarin, aspirin), tubular damage (penicillins, sulfonamides), and hemorrhagic cystitis (cyclophosphamide).

Northway JD: Hematuria in children. J Pediatr 78:381, 1971.

17.23 EVALUATION OF THE CHILD WITH HEMATURIA

A thorough history and physical examination may give clues to the etiology of hematuria. For example, a history of recent upper respiratory, skin, or gastrointestinal infection might suggest acute glomerulonephritis or the hemolytic-uremic syndrome. Frequency, dysuria, and unexplained fevers suggest urinary tract infection. A flank mass may indicate hydronephrosis, cystic disease, renal vein thrombosis, or tumor. Recurrent episodes of gross hematuria suggest IgA nephropathy, idiopathic hematuria, Alport syndrome, or hypercalciuria. Rash and joint pains point toward anaphylactoid purpura or lupus. A history of trauma, of bleeding difficulties, of drug usage, or of kidney disease or high blood pressure in other family members could be useful.

Laboratory evaluation of the child having hematuria is done in steps, beginning with the studies most likely to reveal the etiology (Table 17–3). Depending on the results of the initial group of tests, additional studies may be indicated.

The finding of certain hematologic abnormalities may narrow the differential diagnosis. Anemia may be dilutional (the result of fluid overload in acute renal failure), hemolytic (hemolytic-uremic syndrome, systemic lupus erythematosus), or the result of blood loss (pulmonary hemorrhage in Goodpasture disease, melena in anaphylactoid purpura, hemolytic-uremic syndrome). Confirmation of a hemolytic state (elevated reticulocyte count and plasma hemoglobin level, with depressed plasma haptoglobin level) indicates additional studies. Observation of the blood film may reveal a microangiopathic process as seen in the hemolytic-uremic syndrome, renal vein thrombosis, vasculitis, and systemic lupus erythematosus. In the last, the presence of autoantibodies may result in a positive Coombs test, ANA, leukopenia, and multisystem disease. All black children with hematuria should be screened for sickle hemoglobin, even in the absence of anemia. Thrombocytopenia may result from decreased platelet production (malignancies) or increased platelet consumption (lupus, idiopathic thrombocytopenic purpura, hemolytic-uremic syndrome, renal vein thrombosis). The best screening test for a bleeding diathesis, however, is a good history; coagulation studies or platelet counts are not routinely obtained unless personal or family history suggests a bleeding tendency.

Urine culture evaluates the possibility of urinary tract infection. Optimally, a timed urine specimen is also collected to measure the creatinine clearance, protein and calcium excretion. If this is not possible, then determination of the serum creatinine, urine protein by dipstick, and calcium:creatinine ratio in a random urine specimen are adequate.

The serum C3 level is determined in all patients, since a low level narrows the differential diagnosis to certain forms of glomerulonephritis: poststreptococcal, lupus, membranoproliferative, and chronic infection. When the hematuria is of less than 6 months' duration, serologic evidence for streptococcal infection should be sought. Throat or skin infections should be cultured for streptococci. An ANA titer should be obtained as a test for lupus.

If the above studies do not yield the diagnosis, intravenous pyelography should be carried out to exclude structural abnormalities. Cystography is done only in patients with infection or in patients in whom a lesion of the lower tract is suspected.

The studies in steps 1 and 2, as presented in Table 17–3, will frequently reveal the etiology of the hematuria. In some patients, however, results of all these studies will be normal and no cause for the hematuria will be found. In such patients, despite the lack of a diagnosis, no further studies need be performed. The parents should be reassured that the child does not at present have evidence of urinary tract disease. Because it remains possible, however, that significant renal disease (e.g., IgA nephropathy, Alport syndrome) may be present, the child with persistent microscopic hematuria should have long-term follow-up, with an annual re-evaluation consisting of history, physical examination, blood pressure determination, urinalysis, creatinine clearance, and determination of protein level in a 24 hr specimen.

Renal biopsy may not yield a definitive diagnosis in children with unexplained microscopic hematuria and no other laboratory abnormalities. The finding of normal histology can be reassuring to the family and physician, however, since it excludes the most serious kidney diseases and reduces the need for close surveillance of the child. Biopsy is indicated in children with persistent microscopic hematuria associated with decreased renal function, proteinuria, or hypertension; in those children having one or more episodes of unexplained gross hematuria; and in those with persistent high grade microscopic hematuria.

Cystoscopy is not part of the routine evaluation of hematuria in children. We have found cystoscopy most helpful in patients having bright red hematuria, dysuria, and sterile urine cultures. In boys, cystoscopy frequently reveals a hemorrhagic lesion in the urethra, probably the result of local trauma. Although neoplasms of the lower urinary tract rarely present as asymptomatic gross hematuria in children, debate persists regarding the need for cystoscopy to exclude the remote possibility of a tumor.

17.24 CONDITIONS PARTICULARLY ASSOCIATED WITH PROTEINURIA

Protein may be found in the urine of healthy children. Estimates vary, but a reasonable upper limit of normal protein excretion in healthy children is 150 mg/24 hr. Approximately half of this protein derives from the plasma, albumin representing the largest fraction (less than 30 mg/day). The remainder of normal urinary protein is Tamm-Horsfall protein, a mucoprotein of unknown function produced in the distal tubule.

Proteinuria is commonly detected by the dipstick test. Dipsticks detect primarily albuminuria and are less sensitive (and may miss) other forms of proteinuria (e.g., low molecular weight proteins, Bence Jones protein, gamma globulins). The depth of color of the dipstick reaction increases in a semi-quantitative manner with increasing urinary protein concentrations. Owing to their high sensitivity, dipsticks may detect amounts of protein in the urine that are within normal limits. Because the dipstick reaction cannot accurately measure protein excretion, persistent proteinuria should be quantitated by a more precise method (sulfosalicylic acid) in a timed (preferably 24 hr) urine collection. False-positive test results for proteinuria may be found with both the dipstick test (highly concentrated urine, gross hematuria, contamination with chlorhexidine or benzalkonium, pH over 8.0, phenazopyridine therapy) and the sulfosalicylic acid method (radiographic contrast media, penicillin or cephalosporin therapy, tolbutamide, sulfonamides).

17.25 NONPATHOLOGIC PROTEINURIA

Proteinuria in excess of 150 mg/day may be divided into two categories (Table 17–4). In the first category, nonpathologic proteinuria, the excessive protein excretion is apparently not the result of a disease state. The level of proteinuria in this category is generally less than 1000 mg/day and is never associated with edema.

POSTURAL (ORTHOSTATIC) PROTEINURIA

Children with this disorder excrete normal or slightly increased amounts of protein in the supine position. In the upright position, the amount of protein in the urine may increase 10-fold or more. The proteinuria is usually discovered at routine urinalysis; its etiology is unknown. Hematuria is absent and the creatinine clearance and C3 complement level are normal. Renal biopsy (not part of the evaluation) is normal or shows mild nonspecific alterations.

In the child having asymptomatic low grade proteinuria, a study for postural proteinuria should be performed. At bedtime, the child goes to bed without voiding. After 30 min supine, the child voids in this position. This urine is discarded

Table 17–4. **Classification of Proteinuria**

I. Nonpathologic Proteinuria < 1g/day
   A. Postural (orthostatic)
   B. Febrile
   C. Exercise

II. Pathologic Proteinuria
   A. Tubular usually < 1 gm/day
      1. *Hereditary*
         Cystinosis
         Wilson disease
         Lowe syndrome
         Proximal renal tubular acidosis
         Galactosemia
      2. *Acquired*
         Analgesic abuse
         Vitamin D intoxication
         Hypokalemia
         Antibiotics
         Interstitial nephritis
         Acute tubular necrosis
         Sarcoidosis
         Cystic diseases
         Homograft rejection
         Penicillamine
         Heavy metal poisoning (mercury, gold, lead, bismuth, cadmium, chromium, copper)
   B. Glomerular
      1. Persistent asymptomatic
      2. Nephrotic syndrome > 2 gm/day
         a. Idiopathic nephrotic syndrome
            Minimal change
            Mesangial proliferation
            Focal sclerosis
         b. Glomerulonephritis
         c. Tumors
         d. Drugs
         e. Congenital

but the time of voiding is recorded as the beginning of the supine collection. The child is then given a large glass of liquid and allowed to sleep. In the morning, the child again voids supine before rising; this ends the supine collection and begins the upright collection, which is terminated at bedtime. The child may have normal daily activities, avoiding the supine position. The protein excretion is measured in the two urine collections, and for each collection the result is calculated as mg of protein excreted per min. A finding of essentially normal protein excretion in the supine collection and increased protein excretion in the upright collection establishes the proteinuria as orthostatic.

Studies in adults suggest that postural proteinuria is a benign process, but similar data are not available for children. Accordingly, long-term follow-up of children is necessary (unless the proteinuria resolves) in order to monitor the patient for evidence of renal disease (hematuria, hypertension, diminished renal function, or proteinuria exceeding 1 g/24 hr).

Springberg PD, Garrett LE Jr, Thompson AL, et al: Fixed and reproducible orthostatic proteinuria: Results of a 20-year follow-up study. Ann Intern Med 97:516, 1982.

FEBRILE PROTEINURIA

Transient proteinuria may be found in patients having fever in excess of 38.3° C (101° F). The mechanism of proteinuria associated with fever is unknown. The proteinuria does not exceed +2 on the dipstick and may be considered benign if it resolves when the fever abates.

Jensen H, Henriksen K: Proteinuria in non-renal infectious disease. Acta Med Scand 196:75, 1974.
Marks MI, McLaine PN, Drummond KN: Proteinuria in children with febrile illnesses. Arch Dis Child 45:250, 1970.

EXERCISE PROTEINURIA

Proteinuria, like hematuria, may follow vigorous exercise. The level rarely exceeds +2 on the dipstick. The disorder can be considered benign if the proteinuria resolves after 48 hr of rest.

Campanacci L, Faccini L, Englaro E, et al: Exercise-induced proteinuria. Contr Nephrol 26:31, 1981.

17.26 PATHOLOGIC PROTEINURIA

The second category of proteinuria may result from glomerular or tubular disorders.

TUBULAR PROTEINURIA

Healthy individuals filter large amounts of proteins of lower molecular weight than albumin (e.g., lysozyme, light chains of immunoglobulin, β_2-microglobulin, insulin, growth hormone); these are normally reabsorbed in the proximal tubule. Injury to the proximal tubules results in diminished reabsorptive capacity and the loss of these low molecular weight proteins in the urine; such proteinuria rarely exceeds 1 g/24 hr; it is not associated with edema. Tubular proteinuria (Table 17–4) may be seen in acquired and inherited disorders and may be associated with other defects of proximal tubular function, such as glucosuria, phosphaturia, bicarbonate wasting, and aminoaciduria. Tubular proteinuria rarely presents a diagnostic dilemma because the underlying disease is usually detected before the proteinuria. Asymptomatic patients having persistent proteinuria generally have glomerular rather than tubular proteinuria. In occult cases, glomerular and tubular proteinuria can be distinguished by electrophoresis of the urine. In tubular proteinuria, the low molecular weight proteins migrate primarily in the alpha and beta regions and little or no albumin is detected, whereas in glomerular proteinuria the major protein is albumin.

Alt JM, Von der Heyde D, Assel E, et al: Characteristics of protein excretion in glomerular and tubular disease. Contr Nephrol 24:115, 1981.
Maack T, Johnson V, Kau ST, et al: Renal filtration, transport, and metabolism of low-molecular-weight proteins: A review. Kidney Int 16:251, 1979.

GLOMERULAR PROTEINURIA

The most common cause of proteinuria is increased permeability of the glomerular capillary wall. The amount of glomerular proteinuria may range from less than 1 to more than 30 g/24 hr. Glomerular proteinuria may be termed selective (loss of plasma proteins of molecular weight up to and including albumin) or nonselective (loss of albumin and of larger molecular weight proteins such as IgG). Most forms of glomerulonephritis are accompanied by nonselective proteinuria. Selective proteinuria is seen primarily in minimal-change nephrosis and in that disease, the finding of selective proteinuria increases the likelihood of corticosteroid responsiveness. The determination of urinary protein selectivity is generally of little clinical value, owing to considerable overlap of selectivities among various forms of renal disease.

PERSISTENT ASYMPTOMATIC PROTEINURIA

Persistent asymptomatic proteinuria is defined as proteinuria in an apparently healthy child that occurs without hematuria and that persists for 3 mo. The prevalence in school aged children may be as high as 6%. The amount of proteinuria is usually less than 2 g/24 hr; it is never associated with edema. Causes include postural proteinuria, membranous and membranoproliferative glomerulonephritis, pyelonephritis, hereditary nephritis, developmental anomalies, and "benign" proteinuria.

Evaluation of the child having persistent asymptomatic proteinuria should include urine culture; measurement of creatinine clearance, 24 hr protein excretion, serum albumin, and C_3 complement levels; and intravenous pyelography. In patients with low grade proteinuria in whom findings are normal, renal biopsy may not be indicated because evidence for a progressive disease is rarely found. Such patients should have an annual re-evaluation consisting of physical examination and blood pressure determination, urinalysis, creatinine clearance, and 24 hr protein excretion. Indications for renal biopsy include persistent asymptomatic proteinuria in excess of 1000 mg/24 hr or the development of hematuria, hypertension, or diminished renal function.

Dodge WF, West EF, Smith EH, et al: Proteinuria and hematuria in school-age children: Epidemiology and early natural history. J Pediatr 88:327, 1976.
McLaine PN, Drummond KN: Benign persistent asymptomatic proteinuria in childhood. Pediatrics 46:548, 1970.
Vehaskari VM, Rapola J: Isolated proteinuria: Analysis of a school-age population. J Pediatr 101:661, 1982.
Yoshikawa N, Uehara S, Yamana K., et al: Clinicopathological correlations of persistent asymptomatic proteinuria in children. Nephron 25:127, 1980.

17.27 THE NEPHROTIC SYNDROME (NEPHROSIS)

The nephrotic syndrome is characterized by proteinuria, hypoproteinemia, edema, and hyperlipidemia.

Etiology. The large majority (90%) of children with nephrosis have some form of the idiopathic nephrotic syndrome;

minimal-change disease is found in approximately 85%, mesangial proliferation in 5%, and focal sclerosis in 10%. In the remaining 10% of children with nephrosis, the nephrotic syndrome is mediated by some form of glomerulonephritis, membranous and membranoproliferative being most common.

Pathophysiology. The underlying pathogenetic abnormality in nephrosis is proteinuria, which results from an increase in glomerular capillary wall permeability. The mechanism of this increase in permeability is unknown but may be related, at least in part, to loss of negatively charged glycoproteins within the capillary wall. In the nephrotic state, the protein loss generally exceeds 2 g/day and is composed primarily of albumin; the hypoproteinemia is fundamentally a "hypoalbuminemia." In general, edema appears when the serum albumin level falls below 2.5 g/dL.

The mechanism of edema formation in nephrosis is incompletely understood. It seems likely that the edema is initiated by the development of hypoalbuminemia, the result of urinary protein loss. The hypoalbuminemia leads to a decrease in the plasma oncotic pressure, which permits the transudation of fluid from the intravascular compartment to the interstitial space. The reduction in intravascular volume decreases renal perfusion pressure, activating the renin-angiotensin-aldosterone system, which stimulates distal tubular reabsorption of sodium. The reduced intravascular volume also stimulates the release of antidiuretic hormone, which enhances the reabsorption of water in the collecting duct. Because of the decreased plasma oncotic pressure, the reabsorbed sodium and water are lost into the interstitial space, exacerbating the edema. That other factors may also play a role in the formation of the edema is indicated by the observations that some patients with nephrotic syndrome have normal or increased intravascular volume and normal to diminished plasma levels of renin and aldosterone. Hypothetical explanations include an intrarenal defect in sodium and water excretion or the presence of a circulating agent that increases capillary wall permeability throughout the body, as well as in the kidneys.

In the nephrotic state, almost all serum lipid (cholesterol, triglycerides) and lipoprotein levels are elevated. Two factors offer at least partial explanation: (1) the hypoproteinemia stimulates generalized protein synthesis in the liver, including the lipoproteins; and (2) lipid catabolism is diminished, owing to reduced plasma levels of lipoprotein lipase, the major enzyme system that removes lipids from the plasma. Whether lipoprotein lipase is lost in the urine is unclear.

Dorhout Mees EJ, Geers AB, Koomans HA: Blood volume and sodium retention in the nephrotic syndrome: A controversial pathophysiological concept. Nephron 36:201, 1984.

Meltzer JI, Keim HJ, Laragh JH: Nephrotic syndrome: Vasoconstriction and hypervolemic types indicated by renin-sodium profiling. Ann Intern Med 91:688, 1979.

Melvin T, Sibley R, Michael A: Nephrotic syndrome. In Tune B, Mendoza S, Brenner B, Stein J (eds): Pediatric Nephrology. New York, Churchill Livingstone, 1984, p 191.

Michaeli J, Bar-on H, Shafrir E: Lipoprotein profiles in a heterogeneous group of patients with nephrotic syndrome. Israel J Med Sci 17:1001, 1981.

Oetliker OH, Mordasini R, Lutschg J, et al: Lipoprotein metabolism in nephrotic syndrome in childhood. Pediatr Res 14:64, 1980.

Strauss J, Freundlich M, Zilleruelo G: Nephrotic edema: Etiopathogenic and therapeutic considerations. Nephron 38:78, 1984.

Usberti M, Federico S, Meccariello S, et al: Role of plasma vasopressin in the impairment of water excretion in nephrotic syndrome. Kidney Int 25:422, 1984.

IDIOPATHIC NEPHROTIC SYNDROME

This syndrome accounts for approximately 90% of nephrosis in childhood. Occasional reports that one of the three histologic types has been transformed into another type suggest that this syndrome may be a single disorder with varying histologic features. It seems more likely, however, that the syndrome represents several diseases having similar clinical manifestations. The resolution of this issue awaits the discovery of the pathogenetic factors. The syndrome has been reported in certain families with a frequency that appears to be increased over the expected, but it does not appear to be inherited.

Etiology. The cause of the syndrome remains unknown. Early success in controlling nephrosis with "immunosuppressive" drugs suggested that the disease was mediated by immunologic mechanisms, but evidence for classical mechanisms of immunologic injury has been lacking, and it now seems clear that "immunosuppressive" drugs have many effects other than suppression of antibody formation. A few patients have evidence supporting IgE mediation of the disease, but increasing evidence suggests that the syndrome may result from an abnormality in thymus-derived (T-cell) lymphocyte function, perhaps through the production of a factor that increases vascular permeability.

Pathology. Idiopathic nephrotic syndrome occurs in three morphologic patterns. In minimal-change disease (85%), the glomeruli appear normal or show a minimal increase in mesangial cells and matrix. Findings on immunofluorescent microscopic studies are typically negative. Electron microscopy reveals retraction of the epithelial cell foot processes. More than 95% of children having minimal-change disease respond to corticosteroid therapy.

The mesangial proliferative group (5%) is characterized by a diffuse increase in mesangial cells and matrix. The frequency of mesangial deposits containing IgM and C3 by immunofluorescence is not different from that observed in minimal change disease. Approximately 50–60% of patients with this histologic lesion will respond to corticosteroid therapy.

In biopsies from patients having the focal sclerosis lesion (10%), the majority of glomeruli appear normal or manifest mesangial proliferation. Others, especially those close to the medulla (juxtamedullary), show segmental scarring in one or more lobules (Fig. 17–20). The disease is frequently progressive, ultimately involving all glomeruli, and leads to end-stage renal failure in most patients. Approximately 20% of such patients respond to prednisone or cytotoxic therapy or both. The disease may recur in a transplanted kidney.

Clinical Manifestations. The idiopathic nephrotic syndrome is more common in boys than in girls (2:1) and most commonly appears between the ages of 2 and 6 yr. It has been reported as early as the last half of the 1st yr of life and is not uncommon in adults. The initial episode and subsequent relapses may follow an apparent viral upper respiratory infection. The disease usually presents as edema, which is initially noted around the eyes and in the lower extremities,

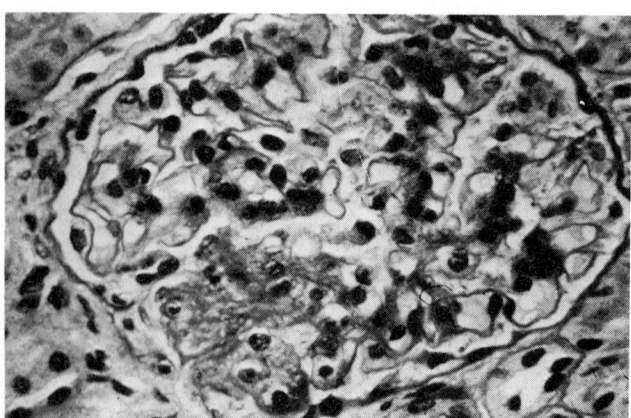

Figure 17–20. Glomerulus from a patient having corticosteroid-resistant nephrotic syndrome, showing mesangial hypercellularity and an area of sclerosis in the lower portion. (× 250.)

where it is "pitting" in nature. With time, the edema becomes generalized and may be associated with weight gain, the development of ascites and/or pleural effusions, and declining urine output. The edema accumulates in dependent sites and appears to shift from the face and back to the abdomen, perineum, and legs as the day progresses. Anorexia, abdominal pain, and diarrhea are common; hypertension is uncommon.

Diagnosis. Urinalysis reveals +3 or +4 proteinuria; microscopic hematuria may be present, but gross hematuria is rare. Renal function may be normal or reduced. The low creatinine clearance is due to diminished renal perfusion resulting from contraction of the intravascular volume and will return to normal when intravascular volume is restored. Protein excretion exceeds 2 g/24 hr. The serum cholesterol and triglyceride levels are elevated, the serum albumin level is generally less than 2.0 g/dL, and the total serum calcium level is diminished, owing to a reduction in the albumin-bound fraction. The C3 level is normal.

Children with onset of nephrotic syndrome during the first 8 yr of life are likely to have steroid-responsive minimal-change disease, and corticosteroid therapy should be initiated without renal biopsy. Minimal-change disease remains common in children presenting with nephrosis above the age of 8 yr, but membranous and membranoproliferative glomerulonephritis become increasingly common; renal biopsy is recommended in this group to establish a firm diagnosis prior to considering therapy.

Complications. Infection is the major complication of nephrosis; it results from increased susceptibility to bacterial infections during relapse. Proposed explanations include decreased immunoglobulin levels, the edema fluid acting as a culture medium, protein deficiency, decreased bactericidal activity of the leukocytes, "immunosuppressive" therapy, decreased perfusion of the spleen owing to hypovolemia, and loss in the urine of a complement factor (properdin factor B) that opsonizes certain bacteria. For reasons that are unclear, peritonitis is the most frequent type of infection; sepsis, pneumonia, cellulitis, and urinary tract infections may also be seen. *Streptococcus pneumoniae* is the most common organism causing peritonitis; gram-negative bacteria are also encountered. Fever and physical findings may be minimal in the presence of corticosteroid therapy. Accordingly, a high index of suspicion, prompt evaluation (including cultures of blood and peritoneal fluid), and the early initiation of therapy that covers both gram-positive and gram-negative organisms are critical to prevention of life-threatening illness. When in remission, all patients having nephrosis should receive a single injection of polyvalent pneumococcal vaccine.

Additional complications may include an increased tendency to arterial and venous thrombosis (owing at least in part to elevated plasma levels of certain coagulation factors and inhibitors of fibrinolysis, decreased plasma level of antithrombin III, and increased platelet aggregation), deficiencies of coagulation factors IX, XI, and XII, and reduced serum levels of vitamin D.

Treatment. The child may be hospitalized with the first episode of nephrosis for diagnostic, educational, and therapeutic purposes. When edema develops, sodium intake is reduced by the initiation of a "no added salt diet." The mother is advised to cook without salt, to hide the salt shaker, and to avoid serving obviously salty foods. Salt restriction is terminated when the edema resolves. Unless the edema is severe, fluid intake is not restricted but need not be encouraged. The child may attend school and participate in physical activities as tolerated. Until corticosteroid-induced diuresis begins, mild to moderate edema can be managed at home with chlorothiazide, 10–40 mg/kg/24 hr, in two divided doses. If hypokalemia develops, spironolactone (3–5 mg/kg/24 hr divided into four doses) may be added. If the edema becomes

severe, resulting in respiratory distress from massive pleural effusions and ascites or in severe scrotal edema, the child should be hospitalized. Sodium restriction should be continued, but further reduction in intake is rarely effective in controlling edema. The swollen scrotum is elevated with pillows to enhance the removal of fluid by gravity. In the past, severe edema was treated with intravenous administration of albumin, followed in some patients by an intravenous dose of furosemide. This type of therapy has now been supplanted by the oral administration of furosemide (1–2 mg/kg every 4 hr) in conjunction with metolazone (0.2–0.4 mg/kg/24 hr in two divided doses); the latter diuretic may act in both proximal and distal tubules. When using this potent combination, electrolyte levels and renal function must be closely monitored. In some instances of severe edema, intravenous administration of 25% human albumin (1 g/kg/24 hr) may be necessary, but the effect is usually transient and volume overload with hypertension and heart failure must be avoided.

After the diagnosis is confirmed by the appropriate laboratory studies, the pathophysiology and treatment of nephrosis is reviewed with the family to enhance their understanding of the child's disease. Remission is then induced by administration of prednisone, the least expensive corticosteroid, at a dosage of 60 mg/m²/24 hr (maximum daily dose 60 mg), divided into three or four doses over the day. Divided-dose rather than single-dose therapy is used because some patients who fail to respond to a single daily dose will respond to divided doses. The time needed for response to prednisone averages about 2 wk, response being defined as the urine becoming free of protein. If the child continues to have proteinuria (2 + or greater) after 1 mo of continuous, daily, divided-dose prednisone, the nephrosis is termed "steroid-resistant" and renal biopsy is indicated to determine the precise etiology of the disease.

Five days after the urine becomes free of protein, the dose of prednisone is changed to 60 mg/m² (maximum dose 60 mg) taken every other day as a single dose with breakfast. This alternate-day regimen is continued for 3–6 mo. The purpose of alternate-day therapy is to maintain the remission using a relatively nontoxic dose of prednisone, thus avoiding frequent relapses of the disease and the cumulative toxicity of frequent courses of daily administration of corticosteroids. After such a period of alternate-day therapy, the prednisone may be discontinued abruptly. Adequate experience indicates that there has been sufficient recovery of pituitary-adrenal axis function that the patient is not at risk for adrenal insufficiency after abrupt withdrawal of the alternate-day prednisone. On the other hand, for up to 1 yr after completing corticosteroid therapy, the child will require corticosteroid supplementation for severe illness or surgery.

Each relapse of the nephrosis is treated in a similar manner. A relapse is defined as the recurrence of edema and not simply of proteinuria, since many children with this condition will have intermittent proteinuria that resolves spontaneously. A small number of patients who respond to daily, divided-dose therapy will have relapses shortly after switching to or after terminating alternate-day therapy. Such patients are termed "steroid-dependent."

If there are repeated relapses and especially if the child suffers severe corticosteroid toxicity (cushingoid appearance, hypertension, growth failure), then cyclophosphamide therapy should be considered. Cyclophosphamide has been shown to prolong the duration of remission and to prevent relapses in children with frequently relapsing nephrotic syndrome. The potential side effects of the drug (leukopenia, disseminated varicella infection, hemorrhagic cystitis, alopecia, sterility) should be reviewed with the family. A renal biopsy is recommended to confirm the diagnosis prior to initiating such therapy. The dose of cyclophosphamide is 3 mg/kg/24 hr as a single dose, for a total duration of 8 wk. Alternate-day prednisone therapy is often continued during the course of cyclophosphamide administration. During cyclophosphamide therapy, the white count must be monitored weekly and the drug withheld if the count falls below 5000/mm³.

Prognosis. The large majority of children having steroid-responsive nephrosis will have repeated relapses until the disease resolves itself spontaneously toward the end of the second decade of life. It is important to indicate to the family that the child will have no residual renal dysfunction, that the disease is generally not hereditary, and that the child (in the absence of cyclophosphamide or chlorambucil therapy) will remain fertile. To minimize the psychologic effects of the nephrosis, we emphasize that when in remission, the child is normal and may have unrestricted diet and activity. While the child is in remission, it is generally unnecessary to test the urine for protein.

Arbeitsgemeinschaft fur Pediatrische Nephrologie: Alternate-day prednisone is more effective than intermittent prednisone in frequently relapsing nephrotic syndrome. Eur J Pediatr 135:229, 1981.

Arbus GS, Poucell S, Bacheyie GS, et al: Focal segmental glomerulosclerosis with idiopathic nephrotic syndrome: Three types of clinical response. J Pediatr 101:40, 1982.

Arnold WC: Efficacy of metolazone and furosemide in children with furosemide-resistant edema. Pediatrics 74:872, 1984.

Baluarte HJ, Hiner L, Gruskin AB: Chlorambucil dosage in frequently relapsing nephrotic syndrome: A controlled clinical trial. J Pediatr 92:295, 1978.

Cameron JS, Turner DR, Ogg CS, et al: The long-term prognosis of patients with focal segmental glomerulosclerosis. Clin Nephrol 10:213, 1978.

Chesney RW, Hamstra A, Rose P, et al: Vitamin D and parathyroid hormone status in children with the nephrotic syndrome and chronic mild glomerulonephritis. Int J Pediatr Nephrol 5:1, 1984.

Chiu J, McLaine PN, Drummond KN: A controlled prospective study of cyclophosphamide in relapsing, corticosteroid-responsive, minimal-lesion nephrotic syndrome in childhood. J Pediatr 82:607, 1973.

Churg J, Habib R, White RHR: Pathology of the nephrotic syndrome in children. Lancet 1:1299, 1970.

Geary DF, Farine M, Thorner D, et al: Response to cyclophosphamide in steroid-resistant focal segmental glomerulosclerosis: A reappraisal. Clin Nephrol 22:109, 1984.

Habib R: Focal glomerular sclerosis. Kidney Int 4:355, 1973.

International Study of Kidney Disease in Children: Minimal change nephrotic syndrome in children: Deaths during the first 5 to 15 years' observation. Pediatrics 73:497, 1984.

Ji-Yun Y, Melvin T, Sibley R, et al: No evidence for a specific role for IgM in mesangial proliferation of idiopathic nephrotic syndrome. Kidney Int 25:100, 1984.

Krensky AM, Ingelfinger JR, Grupe WE: Peritonitis in childhood nephrotic syndrome. Am J Dis Child 136:732, 1982.

McCrory WW, Shibuya M, Wen-Hsiung L, et al: Therapeutic and toxic effects observed with different dosage programs of cyclophosphamide in treatment of steroid-responsive but frequently relapsing nephrotic syndrome. J Pediatr 82:614, 1973.

Melvin T, Sibley R, Michael A: Nephrotic Syndrome. In Tune B, Mendoza S, Brenner B, Stein J (eds): Pediatric Nephrology. New York, Churchill-Livingston, 1984, p 191.

Pardo V, Riesgo I, Zilleruelo G, et al: The clinical significance of mesangial IgM deposits and mesangial hypercellularity in minimal change nephrotic syndrome. Am J Kidney Dis 3:264, 1984.

Remuzzi G, Mecca G, Marchesi D, et al: Platelet hyperaggregability and the nephrotic syndrome. Thromb Res 16:345, 1979.

Trompeter RS, Lloyd BW, Hicks J, et al: Long-term outcome for children with minimal-change nephrotic syndrome. Lancet 1:368, 1985.

White RHR, Glasgow EF, Mills RJ: Clinicopathological study of nephrotic syndrome in childhood. Lancet 1:1353, 1970.

Williams SA, Makker SP, Ingelfinger JR, et al: Long-term evaluation of chlorambucil plus prednisone in the idiopathic nephrotic syndrome of childhood. N Engl J Med 302:929, 1980.

GLOMERULONEPHRITIS

Nephrotic syndrome may develop during the course of any type of glomerulonephritis but is most common in association with membranous, membranoproliferative, poststreptococcal, lupus, chronic infection (including malaria and schistosomiasis), and anaphylactoid purpura glomerulonephritis. Although the development of a secondary nephrotic syndrome may indicate severe glomerular disease, the nephrotic syndrome frequently resolves if the nephritis improves.

Andrade ZA, Rocha H: Schistosomal glomerulopathy. Kidney Int 16:23, 1979.

Boonpucknavig V, Sitprija V: Renal disease in acute Plasmodium falciparum infection in man. Kidney Int 16:44, 1979.

Hendrickse RG, Adeniyi A: Quartan malarial nephrotic syndrome in children. Kidney Int 16:64, 1979.

TUMORS

See also Sec. 16.8–16.9.

Nephrotic syndrome has been associated with several extrarenal neoplasms. In patients having solid tumors, such as carcinomas, the glomerular changes resemble membranous glomerulopathy. The renal involvement is presumably mediated by immune complexes composed of tumor antigens and tumor-specific antibodies. In lymphomas (especially Hodgkin disease), minimal-change disease is most commonly found; proliferative lesions have also been described. In patients having the minimal-change lesion, the nephrosis may develop before or after the malignancy is detected, may resolve as the tumor regresses, and may return if the tumor recurs. The mechanism of the nephrosis is unknown; it has been proposed that the tumor produces a lymphokine that increases glomerular capillary wall permeability.

Eagen J, Lewis EJ: Glomerulopathies of neoplasia. Kidney Int 11:297, 1977.

Kaplan BS, Klassen J, Gault MH: Glomerular injury in patients with neoplasia. Ann Rev Med 27:117, 1976.

DRUGS

Nephrotic syndrome has developed during therapy with several types of drugs and chemicals. The histologic picture may resemble membranous glomerulopathy (penicillamine, gold, mercury compounds), minimal-change disease (probenecid, ethosuximide, methimazole, lithium), or proliferative glomerulonephritis (procainamide, chlorpropamide, mephenytoin, trimethadione, paramethadione).

CONGENITAL NEPHROTIC SYNDROME

Nephrotic syndrome is rare during the 1st yr of life. Causes of nephrosis developing during the first 6 mo of life include the congenital nephrotic syndrome, congenital infection (syphilis, toxoplasmosis, cytomegalovirus), and diffuse mesangial sclerosis of unknown etiology. Nephrosis developing during the last half of the 1st yr is most commonly associated with the idiopathic nephrotic syndrome or drugs.

The congenital nephrotic syndrome (Finnish type) is an autosomal recessive disorder that is most common in populations of Scandinavian descent. The major pathologic feature in some patients is dilatation of the proximal convoluted tubules (microcystic disease) but this is variable even within the same kindred. The glomeruli show mesangial proliferation and sclerosis. The pathogenesis of the syndrome is unknown; a reduction in the number of heparan sulfate–rich anionic sites has been demonstrated in the glomerular basement membrane. Although proteinuria is present at birth, the nephrotic syndrome becomes apparent within the first 3 mo of life. Additional clinical features include prematurity, an enlarged placenta, respiratory distress, and separation of the cranial sutures. The clinical course is one of persistent edema and recurrent infections. Death due to infection or renal failure is likely by the age of 5 yr. Corticosteroid and immunosuppressive agents are of no value. Treatment is supportive, with the ultimate goal of kidney transplantation. In families at risk, antenatal diagnosis is possible by measuring the amniotic fluid alpha-fetoprotein level prior to 20 wk gestation.

Aula P, Rapola J, Karjalainen O, et al: Prenatal diagnosis of congenital nephrosis in 23 high-risk families. Am J Dis Child 132:984, 1978.

Hoyer JR, Anderson CE: Congenital nephrotic syndrome. Clin Perinatol 8:333, 1981.

Kaplan BS, Bureau MA, Drummond KN: The nephrotic syndrome in the first year of life: Is a pathologic classification possible: J Pediatr 85:615, 1974.

Mahan JD, Mauer SM, Sibley RK, et al: Congenital nephrotic syndrome: Evolution of medical management and results of renal transplantation. J Pediatr 105:549, 1984.

Shahin B, Papadopoulou ZL, Jenis EH: Congenital nephrotic syndrome associated with congenital toxoplasmosis. J. Pediatr 85:366, 1974.

Vernier RL, Klein DJ, Sisson SP, et al: Heparan sulfate-rich anionic sites in the human glomerular basement membrane. N Engl J Med 309:1001, 1983.

17.28 TUBULAR DISORDERS

TUBULAR FUNCTION

Except for reduced protein levels, the ultrafiltrate of blood that enters the proximal tubule is similar to plasma. Body homeostasis is maintained by tubular reabsorption of salts and water.

Sodium. After the first year of life, the tubules have the reabsorptive capacity to lower the urinary sodium concentration to 1 mEq/L. Approximately 65% of filtered sodium is isotonically reabsorbed in the proximal tubule. Glucose and amino acids are also reabsorbed in the proximal tubule in conjunction with sodium transport. An additional 25% of filtered sodium is reabsorbed from the ascending limb of the loop of Henle in association with the active transport of chloride. The remainder of sodium reabsorption is accomplished in the distal tubule and collecting duct, mediated in part by aldosterone. Sodium excretion is closely related to the extracellular fluid volume and may be modified by factors that regulate the extracellular fluid volume.

Potassium. Essentially all of the filtered potassium is reabsorbed, primarily in the proximal tubules. The potassium excreted is derived from distal tubular and collecting duct potassium secretion, as modifed by the pH of the extracellular fluid, by aldosterone, and by the urinary flow rate and sodium concentration.

Calcium. Approximately 98% of filtered calcium is reabsorbed by the tubules. Proximal tubular reabsorption (65% of the filtered load) is linked to sodium reabsorption. Calcium reabsorption is enhanced by parathyroid hormone and reduction of the extracellular fluid volume.

Phosphate. The majority of the filtered phosphate is reabsorbed in the proximal tubule. Reabsorption is inhibited by parathyroid hormone.

Magnesium. About 25% of filtered magnesium is reabsorbed in the proximal tubule; the major site of magnesium reabsorption and the principal moderator of magnesium excretion is the thick ascending limb of Henle.

Acidification and Concentrating Mechanisms. These are discussed in the sections on renal tubular acidosis and nephrogenic diabetes insipidus (Sec. 17.29 and 17.30).

Maturation of Tubular Function. At birth and for several months thereafter, tubular functional capabilities are at less than adult levels. Tubular function is adequate for healthy infants, but limitations may contribute to fluid and electrolyte abnormalities in sick infants.

Maximal urinary concentrating capacity in the healthy full-term newborn is 600–700 mOsm/kg H_2O. This reduction in concentrating capacity in comparison with older children and adults (who can concentrate to more than 1000 mOsm/kg H_2O) is related to reduced glomerular filtration rate, to tubular cell immaturity, to reduced nephron length, to reduced medullary solute gradient owing to increased medullary blood flow and low urea production, and to diminished tubular responsiveness to antidiuretic hormone. Although the ability of newborn infants to dilute the urine is comparable to that of adults, their capacity to excrete a water load is diminished, owing to the reduced glomerular filtration rate. The capacity of the neonate to excrete sodium, potassium, hydrogen ion, and phosphate is also limited, owing in part to the low glomerular filtration rate and/or immaturity of tubular function.

McCrory WW: Developmental Nephrology. Cambridge, Harvard University Press, 1972.

Spitzer A: Renal physiology and functional development. In Edelmann CM (ed): Pediatric Kidney Disease. Boston, Little, Brown, 1978, p 25.

TUBULAR DISEASES

Renal tubular disorders may be functional or anatomic. Functional disorders involve defects in the function of tubular cells, are relatively rare, may be inherited or acquired, and are initially associated with normal renal function. Certain of these disorders may be associated with the development of progressive renal damage. Anatomic disorders involve the structure of the tubules, as in the cystic diseases.

17.29 RENAL TUBULAR ACIDOSIS   Pg 184

Renal tubular acidosis (RTA) is a clinical state of systemic hyperchloremic acidosis resulting from impaired urinary acidification. Three types exist: distal RTA (type I), proximal RTA (type II), and mineralocorticoid deficiency (type IV). A proposed type III has been found to be a variant of type I.

Normal Urinary Acidification. After the first few months of life, approximately 85% of the filtered bicarbonate is reabsorbed in the proximal tubules, but in prematures and neonates, such reabsorption of bicarbonate is transiently reduced, and bicarbonate wasting results when the serum bicarbonate level exceeds 20–22 mEq/L. The proximal tubular reabsorption of bicarbonate involves the secretion of hydrogen ion into the tubular lumen in exchange for sodium (Sec. 5.12). The hydrogen ion combines with filtered bicarbonate to form carbonic acid which, under the influence of carbonic anhydrase, dissociates into carbon dioxide and water. The carbon dioxide diffuses into the proximal tubular cells where, under the influence of carbonic anhydrase, it is reconverted to carbonic acid. The carbonic acid dissociates to yield a hydrogen ion that is again secreted to absorb additional bicarbonate, and to yield also a bicarbonate ion that enters the peritubular capillary. The remaining 15% of filtered bicarbonate is reabsorbed in the distal tubule. The normal kidney reabsorbs all filtered bicarbonate, but this does not make the urine acid. Acidification of the urine is mediated by distal tubular secretion of hydrogen ion (which is in part mineralocorticoid-dependent) and of ammonia (which forms ammonium ion in an acid urine).

Proximal Renal Tubular Acidosis

Pathogenesis. Proximal RTA results from reduced proximal tubular reabsorption of bicarbonate, presumably owing to deficient carbonic anhydrase production. Rather than reabsorbing the normal 85% of filtered bicarbonate, the proximal tubules in this condition may reabsorb only 60%, thus presenting the distal tubules with 40% rather than the usual 15%

Table 17–5. **Classification of Renal Tubular Acidosis**

II Proximal	I Distal	IV Mineralocorticoid Deficiency*
Isolated	Isolated	Adrenal Disorders (↓A, ↑R)
Sporadic	Sporadic	Addison disease
Hereditary	Hereditary	Congenital hyperplasia
Fanconi syndrome	Secondary	Primary hypoaldosteronism
Primary	Interstitial nephritis	Hyporeninemic Hypoaldosteronism (↓A, ↓R)
Secondary	Obstructive	Obstruction
Inherited	Pyelonephritis	Pyelonephritis
Cystinosis	Transplant rejection	Interstitial nephritis
Lowe syndrome	Sickle cell nephropathy	Diabetes mellitus
Galactosemia	Lupus nephritis	Nephrosclerosis
Hereditary fructose intolerance	Ehlers-Danlos syndrome	Glomerulonephritis
Tyrosinemia	Nephrocalcinosis	Pseudohypoaldosteronism (↑A, ↑R)
Wilson disease	Hepatic cirrhosis	
Medullary cystic disease	Elliptocytosis	
Acquired	Medullary sponge kidney	
Heavy metals	Toxins	
Outdated tetracycline	Amphotericin B	
Proteinuria	Lithium	
Interstitial nephritis	Toluene	
Hyperparathyroidism		
Vitamin D deficiency rickets		

*A signifies aldosterone; R signifies renin.

of the filtered load. Because the distal tubules can, at a maximum, reabsorb only 15% of the normal filtered load of bicarbonate, up to 25% may be lost in the urine. Proximal RTA is generally more severe than distal RTA, since complete loss of the distal bicarbonate recovery mechanism (which is rare) would waste only 15% of filtered bicarbonate. With urinary bicarbonate loss, the serum bicarbonate level falls until it reaches a level (bicarbonate threshold) at which bicarbonate wasting ceases. At this level (15–18 mEq/L), the quantity of filtered bicarbonate is reduced to an amount that can be totally reabsorbed by the tubules. Because distal tubular acidification mechanisms remain intact, the urine may then be acidified (pH less than 5.5). Flooding the distal tubule with sodium bicarbonate stimulates sodium reabsorption in exchange for potassium, leading to hypokalemia. Contraction of the extracellular fluid volume (as a result of the loss of sodium bicarbonate) stimulates chloride reabsorption (resulting in hyperchloremia) and aldosterone secretion (enhancing potassium loss).

Proximal RTA (Table 17–5) may occur as an isolated disorder not associated with other diseases or with other abnormalities of proximal tubular function. Isolated proximal RTA may be transient or persistent, sporadic or inherited (usually autosomal dominant). Proximal RTA may also occur as part of a generalized defect in proximal tubular transport (Fanconi syndrome), characterized by glucosuria, phosphaturia, aminoaciduria, and proximal RTA. A primary form of Fanconi syndrome, also not associated with other disease states, has been reported to show both autosomal dominant and recessive modes of inheritance. Secondary Fanconi syndrome may develop during the course of several inherited or acquired disease states. Inherited forms include the following.

Cystinosis. (See Sec. 7.5.) This autosomal recessive defect may present either during the first 3 yr of life (nephropathic form) or later (juvenile form). In the nephropathic variety, initial clinical manifestations may include polyuria and polydipsia (concentrating defect), fever (dehydration), growth retardation, rickets, blond hair and fair skin (diminished pigmentation), and photophobia. The diagnosis is suggested when cystine crystals are observed in the corneas with use of the slit-lamp and is confirmed by demonstration of an elevated cystine content of leukocytes. Intracellular accumulation of cystine in the kidney leads to progressive renal damage, resulting in end-stage renal failure by the end of the first decade. No therapy is known to prevent intracellular cystine accumulation; a clinical trial with cysteamine is currently in progress. The juvenile form of the disease presents later in life; it has the same but less severe clinical manifestations but may also progress to renal failure.

Lowe Syndrome. This X-linked disorder is associated with mental retardation, hypotonia, cataracts, glaucoma, and generalized proximal tubular dysfunction. The underlying metabolic defect is unknown (Sec. 23.59).

Galactosemia. (See Sec. 7.19.) The renal manifestations of this disorder result from prolonged galactose accumulation in the proximal tubules.

Hereditary Fructose Intolerance. (See Sec. 7.19.) This autosomal recessive deficiency of fructose 1-phosphate aldolase leads to proximal tubular dysfunction.

Tyrosinemia. Generalized proximal tubular dysfunction is common in hereditary tyrosinemia (Sec. 7.3).

Wilson Disease. The clinical manifestations of this autosomal recessive disorder include proximal tubular dysfunction; it is discussed in Sec. 12.77 and 21.21.

Medullary Cystic Disease. This disorder is inherited as an autosomal dominant trait, whereas a similar disorder, juvenile nephronophthisis, is inherited as an autosomal recessive trait. Whether these are separate disorders or the same disorder with variable inheritance is uncertain. Children more commonly have the recessive form, whereas the dominant form is more common in adults. The major pathologic finding is cysts in the medulla. As the "cysts" seem to be dilatations of the distal tubules and collecting ducts, some may also be found in the renal cortex. Progressive interstitial inflammation and fibrosis lead to glomerular sclerosis, cortical atrophy, and renal insufficiency. Some children suffer no clinical problems until reaching end-stage renal failure. Others show manifestations of tubular dysfunction such as polyuria and polydipsia (concentrating defect), sodium wasting, and proximal RTA. Red or blond hair is common. Urinalysis may be normal or show minimal abnormalities. Radiographic studies show small, poorly functioning kidneys. The diagnosis is confirmed by biopsy or at nephrectomy, if either is warranted in preparation for transplantation.

Causes of Acquired Fanconi Syndrome. These include tubular toxins such as heavy metals (lead, mercury, cadmium, uranium), outdated tetracycline, proteinuric states (myeloma, nephrotic syndrome), and interstitial nephritis. Excessive parathyroid hormone secretion (primary and secondary hyperparathyroidism, vitamin D deficient rickets) may also cause proximal RTA, presumably by inhibition of carbonic anhydrase.

Distal Renal Tubular Acidosis

Pathogenesis. The genesis of distal RTA is best explained as a deficiency of hydrogen ion secretion by the distal tubule and collecting duct, although other mechanisms may also be involved. The lack of secreted hydrogen ion reduces the formation of carbonic acid and then carbon dioxide in the tubular lumen. The loss of bicarbonate in the urine is usually less than 5% of the filtered load. Owing to the nature of the defect, the pH of the urine cannot be reduced below 5.8 despite severe systemic acidosis. Loss of sodium bicarbonate results in hyperchloremia and hypokalemia. The hypokalemia is less severe than that found in proximal RTA because less bicarbonate is wasted. Nephrocalcinosis may be present.

Distal RTA may occur as an isolated condition not associated with any other disorder; as such it may be sporadic or inherited as an autosomal dominant or recessive trait. Secondary distal RTA may develop during the course of several diseases and intoxications involving the distal tubules and collecting ducts (Table 17–5).

Medullary Sponge Kidney. This noninherited disorder is characterized by cystic dilatation of the terminal portions of the collecting ducts as they enter the renal pyramids. Although renal function and life span are typically normal, the disorder may be complicated by pyelonephritis, hypercalciuria, nephrocalcinosis, nephrolithiasis, impaired concentrating capacity, and distal RTA.

Mineralocorticoid Deficiency

Pathogenesis. This form of RTA results from inadequate production of or reduced distal tubular responsiveness to aldosterone. The lack of aldosterone effect impairs the establishment across the tubular cell membrane of an electrochemical gradient (with negative electrical potential in the tubular lumen) favorable to hydrogen ion secretion. The excretion of ammonium ion is also reduced. In the absence of aldosterone-mediated sodium reabsorption, hyperkalemia develops. The net effect is a hyperkalemic, hyperchloremic acidosis. The systemic acidosis may render the urine pH acid (less than 5.5).

Mineralocorticoid-deficiency RTA may result from diseases of the adrenal gland (Addison disease, congenital adrenal hyperplasia, primary hypoaldosteronism) in which aldosterone production is deficient. In these disorders, renal function is normal, urinary sodium wasting is common, and the plasma renin level is elevated. Hyporeninemic hypoaldosteronism is a form of RTA that may result from kidney diseases associated with interstitial damage and destruction of the juxtaglomerular apparatus; it may also be observed with volume expansion and prostaglandin inhibition. In these conditions, plasma levels of renin and, as a result, of aldosterone are reduced; renal function may be compromised. Rarely, type IV RTA may be the result of distal tubular unresponsiveness to aldosterone (pseudohypoaldosteronism); plasma renin and aldosterone levels are elevated, renal function is usually normal, and salt wasting is the rule. In adults, this form of RTA may be observed in patients with medullary disease and renal insufficiency.

Clinical Management of RTA

Clinical Manifestations. Children having isolated forms of proximal or distal RTA commonly present with growth failure toward the end of the first year of life. Gastrointestinal symptoms are common. Children having secondary forms of proximal or distal RTA may present in a similar fashion or with complaints unique to their fundamental disease. Mineralocorticoid deficiency is usually found as an underlying feature of a primary kidney disease.

Distal RTA is complicated by hypercalciuria, which may lead to nephrocalcinosis, nephrolithiasis, and renal parenchymal destruction. The causes of the hypercalciuria are unknown; potential mechanisms include bone breakdown to release calcium carbonate (the carbonate to be converted to bicarbonate in an attempt to control the acidosis) and diminished levels of urinary citrate (which chelates calcium).

Diagnosis. Before considering the diagnosis of RTA, other causes of systemic acidosis such as diarrhea, lactic acidosis, diabetes mellitus, and renal failure should be excluded. The biochemical features of proximal and distal RTA include low serum bicarbonate and potassium levels in association with hyperchloremia. In mineralocorticoid-deficiency RTA, systemic acidosis is associated with hyperkalemia.

Patients suspected of having proximal or distal RTA should be evaluated by comparing the pH (by pH meter) of a first morning urine specimen (collected under mineral oil to prevent the loss of carbon dioxide) with simultaneous measurements of serum electrolytes. In patients who have substantial systemic acidosis (serum bicarbonate less than 16 mEq/L), a urine pH of less than 5.5 supports the diagnosis of proximal RTA, whereas patients with distal RTA will have a urine pH of 5.8 or greater. In patients having mild acidosis (serum bicarbonate 17–20 mEq/L), ammonium chloride loading may be required to distinguish between the two types. In occult cases, measurement of the fractional excretion of bicarbonate after raising the serum bicarbonate to normal by intravenous infusion of bicarbonate should be considered. If proximal RTA is detected, then other defects of proximal tubular function should be sought (glucosuria, phosphaturia, aminoaciduria). When any form of RTA is confirmed, potential underlying causes (Table 17–5) should be investigated.

Treatment. The goals of therapy are correction of the acidosis and maintenance of normal serum bicarbonate and potassium levels. Most patients' conditions can be corrected with oral therapy; in infants having severe acidosis and hypokalemia, intravenous therapy may be required initially. The least expensive and easiest alkalinizing solution for oral use is Shohl solution (Bicitra*) containing 1 mEq/mL of sodium as sodium citrate. For patients requiring potassium supplementation, potassium citrate can be added (Polycitra*), to form a solution that contains 1 mEq/mL each of sodium and potassium and 2 mEq/mL of bicarbonate equivalent. Sodium bicarbonate tablets (325 and 650 mg) may be used in older patients. Patients having mineralocorticoid-deficiency RTA may also require diuretics and/or polystyrene sulfonate resin (Kayexalate, Breon Laboratories, New York) to reduce the serum potassium level to normal.

Prognosis. Isolated proximal RTA, although initially more severe than the distal variety, may resolve over the first decade of life. Isolated distal RTA seems to be a lifelong disease; in some instances, renal failure may develop; the prognosis is excellent, however, if the disease is recognized and therapy initiated prior to the development of nephrocalcinosis. A continuing need for alkali therapy and for lifelong monitoring of clinical status is the rule.

Mineralocorticoid-deficiency RTA most frequently results from obstructive uropathy and usually resolves within 12 mo after correction of the obstruction. In other secondary forms of RTA, the ultimate prognosis may depend on the severity of the primary disorder.

---

*Willen Drug Company, Baltimore, MD.

Brodehl J: The Fanconi syndrome. *In* Edelmann CM (ed): Pediatric Kidney Disease. Boston, Little, Brown, 1978, p 955.

Burke JR, Inglis JA, Craswell PW, et al: Juvenile nephronophthisis and medullary cystic disease—the same disease (report of a large family with medullary cystic disease associated with gout and epilepsy). Clin Nephrol 18:1, 1982.

Chan JCM: Renal tubular acidosis. J Pediatr 102:327, 1983.

Chesney RW: Etiology and pathogenesis of the Fanconi syndrome. Mineral Electrolyte Metab 4:303, 1980.

Kurtzman NA: Acquired distal renal tubular acidosis. Kidney Int 24:807, 1983.

McSherry E, Morris RC Jr: Attainment and maintenance of normal stature with alkali therapy in infants and children with classic renal tubular acidosis. J Clin Invest 61:509, 1978.

O'Neil M, Breslau NA, Pak CYC: Metabolic evaluation of nephrolithiasis in patients with medullary sponge kidney. Am Med Assoc J 245:1233, 1981.

Rodriguez-Soriano J, Vallo A, Castillo G, et al: Natural history of distal renal tubular acidosis treated since infancy. J Pediatr 101:669, 1982.

Schneider JA, Schulman JD: Cystinosis: A review. Metabolism 26:817, 1977.

Sebastian A, Hulter HN, Kurtz I, et al: Disorders of distal nephron function. Am J Med 72:289, 1982.

Steele BT, Lirenman DS, Beattie CW: Nephronophthisis. Am J Med 68:531, 1980.

Yudkoff M, Foreman JW, Segal S: Effects of cysteamine therapy in nephropathic cystinosis. N Engl J Med 304:141, 1981.

17.30 Nephrogenic Diabetes Insipidus

In this disorder, the kidney fails to respond to antidiuretic hormone despite elevated blood levels of antidiuretic hormone.

Etiology. Primary nephrogenic diabetes insipidus is a rare inherited disease characterized by complete tubular unresponsiveness to antidiuretic hormone in males and partial unresponsiveness in females. Partial or complete nephrogenic diabetes insipidus (secondary) may also be associated with disorders that (1) result in loss of the medullary concentrating gradient (acute or chronic renal failure, obstructive and postobstructive uropathy, vesicoureteral reflux, cystic diseases, interstitial nephritis, osmotic diuresis, nephrocalcinosis); or (2) diminish the effect of antidiuretic hormone on the tubules (hypokalemia, hypercalcemia, lithium, and demeclocycline therapy).

Pathogenesis. Concentration of the urine is dependent on the establishment of a hypertonic renal medulla and the permeability of the distal tubules and collecting ducts to water. The hypertonicity of the medulla is established by a countercurrent mechanism linked to reabsorption of sodium and urea. The permeability of the collecting ducts is regulated by antidiuretic hormone, release of which from the neurohypophysis is triggered by monitors of intravascular volume that reside in the heart, large arteries, kidney, liver, and brain. In the kidney, the hormone acts to increase the permeability of the distal tubules and collecting ducts to water by means of a cyclic adenosine monophosphate–dependent mechanism. This permits water to flow by passive diffusion from the tubule into the hypertonic medullary interstitium of the kidney.

In primary nephrogenic diabetes insipidus, the distal tubule fails to respond normally to antidiuretic hormone, whether endogenous or exogenous. In secondary forms of nephrogenic diabetes insipidus, the hypertonic medullary gradient may be diminished owing to a solute diuresis or inability of tubules to reabsorb sodium chloride and urea. Alternatively, the secondary form may result from induced tubular unresponsiveness to the hormone.

Clinical Manifestations. Males with primary nephrogenic diabetes insipidus have dramatic history of polyuria and polydipsia in infancy, often with episodes of hypernatremic dehydration. Females with the primary defect have milder symptoms that may not be detected until later in life. Patients having secondary forms of the disease present with hypernatremia during the course of their primary disorder.

Diagnosis. The diagnosis of primary nephrogenic diabetes insipidus is suspected on clinical history, often with a positive family history in males. Laboratory findings include hypernatremia and dilute urine. If the serum osmolality at initial study exceeds 295 mOsm/kg H_2O and concurrent urine osmolality is less than this value, then a dehydration test to establish the diagnosis is unnecessary. The diagnosis is confirmed by administering an intramuscular injection of 0.1–0.2 units/kg of aqueous vasopressin and measuring the serum and urine osmolality each hour for 4 hr. If the ratio of urine-to-plasma osmolality remains less than 1.0, the patient has nephrogenic diabetes insipidus. If the ratio becomes greater than 1.0, then central diabetes insipidus is suggested, but psychogenic polydipsia must be excluded. Patients with initial serum osmolality levels less than 295 mOsm/kg H_2O should be fasted (during the day rather than overnight) until serum osmolality exceeds 295 mOsm/kg H_2O; vasopressin is then given as before. The withholding of fluids should be terminated if body weight declines by as much as 3%. In patients suspected of primary nephrogenic diabetes insipidus, appropriate biochemical and radiographic studies should be done to exclude secondary causes.

Complications. As originally described, primary nephrogenic diabetes insipidus was associated with mental retardation. Retardation now seems more likely the result of repeated episodes of hypertonic dehydration than the consequence of the disease itself. Growth retardation is uniformly present in males with the primary disorder but is usually absent in females. Growth failure was originally thought to result from inadequate caloric intake owing to excessive fluid intake, but it now seems that growth failure is intrinsic to the homozygous state. Dilatation of the urinary collecting system may result from excessive urine production. Accordingly, the anatomy of the urinary tract should be examined for evidence of hydronephrosis every few years by renal scan (intravenous pyelography may not visualize the collecting systems when there is rapid flow of large volumes of dilute urine).

Treatment. The keys to treatment include the provision of adequate fluid and caloric intake and reduction of the urinary solute load. These are accomplished by restricting the intake of a low sodium formula (SMA, Wyeth Laboratories, Philadelphia, PA; Similac PM 60/40, Ross Laboratories, Columbus, OH) to only that which is necessary to supply optimal caloric intake for growth. The remainder of the daily fluid requirement (as determined by the maintenance of a normal serum sodium level) is administered as water or fruit juice. The parents should be cautioned that until the child can obtain free access to water, fluids should be offered every 1–2 hr during the day and 3 times during the night. Once the child becomes old enough to obtain free access to water, the intact thirst mechanism will provide the appropriate stimulus for fluid intake.

In patients with the primary disorder, the urinary volume can be dramatically reduced by diuretic therapy. This paradoxical response results because sodium depletion seems to enhance proximal tubular reabsorption of sodium and water. Less water, therefore, is presented to the defective portion of the tubules. Chlorothiazide (20–40 mg/kg/day in divided doses) in conjunction with moderate salt restriction may significantly reduce the need for fluid intake and the frequency of voiding. The patient should be monitored for the development of hypokalemia. This type of therapy is of no value for secondary forms of the disease.

Prognosis. Primary nephrogenic diabetes insipidus is a lifelong disease with a good prognosis if hypernatremic dehydration can be avoided. Genetic counseling should be provided for the family. The prognosis of secondary forms of the disease will depend on the nature of the primary disorder. The syndrome may resolve after correction of obstructive lesions.

Berl T, Anderson RJ, McDonald KM, et al: Clinical disorders of water metabolism. Kidney Int 10:117, 1976.

Gibbons MD, Koontz WW Jr: Obstructive uropathy and nephrogenic diabetes insipidus in infants. J Urol 122:556, 1979.

Hodjatilt, Salcedo Jr: Polyuria in children: Clinical evaluation and differential diagnosis. J Urol 121:223, 1979.

Jamison RL, Oliver RE: Disorders of urinary concentration. Am J Med 72:308, 1982.

Shapiro SR, Woerner S, Adelman RD, et al: Diabetes insipidus and hydronephrosis. J Urol 119:715, 1978.

Skorecki KL, Brenner BM: Body fluid homeostasis in man. Am J Med 70:77, 1981.

17.31 BARTTER SYNDROME

This rare form of renal potassium wasting is characterized by hypokalemia, normal blood pressure, vascular insensitivity to pressor agents, and elevated plasma concentrations of renin and aldosterone. In certain families, the disorder may be inherited as an autosomal recessive trait.

Pathology. Generalized hyperplasia of the juxtaglomerular apparatus, the site of renin production, is observed in most patients with the syndrome. The renal parenchyma is otherwise normal in most patients; a few have shown nonspecific glomerular disease or interstitial disease or both.

Pathogenesis. The etiology is unknown. Currently, the disorder is best explained as a primary defect in chloride reabsorption in the ascending limb of the loop of Henle. The resultant decrease in sodium chloride reabsorption in this portion of the loop will reduce medullary hypertonicity, perhaps explaining the concentrating defect. The defect in chloride reabsorption presents extra sodium chloride to the distal tubule where sodium is reabsorbed in exchange for potassium; the result is urinary potassium wasting. The induced hypokalemia stimulates the synthesis of prostaglandins (which may account for the vascular insensitivity to pressor agents and the defect in platelet aggregation); these, in turn, activate the renin-angiotensin-aldosterone system by increasing renin release and by stimulating aldosterone synthesis. The latter exacerbates renal potassium wasting.

Clinical Manifestations. Young children typically present growth failure, muscle weakness, constipation, polyuria, and dehydration due to urinary salt and water loss. Older children have muscle weakness and/or cramps and carpopedal spasms.

Diagnosis. The diagnosis is suggested by the finding of hypokalemia; the serum potassium level is usually less than 2.5 mEq/L. Supportive findings include normal blood pressure; defective platelet aggregation; hypochloremia; metabolic alkalosis; elevated plasma levels of renin, aldosterone, and prostaglandin E_2; and high urinary levels of potassium and chloride. Some patients may also have hypercalciuria, hyperuricemia, hypomagnesemia, and urinary sodium-wasting. The diagnosis is confirmed by the histologic demonstration of hyperplasia of the juxtaglomerular apparatus, but this abnormality is not found in all patients and is most frequently absent in young children.

Bartter syndrome must be differentiated from licorice abuse, laxative or diuretic use, persistent vomiting or diarrhea, pyelonephritis, and diabetes insipidus. Several of these (laxative use, vomiting, diarrhea, diabetes insipidus) are associated with hypovolemia, which results in a low urinary chloride level; whereas Bartter syndrome is associated with an elevated level.

Treatment. The goals of therapy are to supply adequate nutrition and to maintain the serum potassium level above 3.5 mEq/L. Therapy is initiated with oral potassium chloride supplementation, increasing the dose until the serum potassium level reaches 3.5 mEq/L or the dosage reaches 250 mEq/day. A reasonably well-tolerated potassium preparation is K-Lyte/Cl (Mead Johnson Company, Evansville IN), flavored effervescent tablets containing 25 or 50 mEq of potassium chloride. Sodium chloride supplementation may also be required in small children. If the serum potassium level remains below 3.5 mEq/L after reaching a dose of 250 mEq/day of potassium chloride, then triamterene, 5–10 mg/kg/day in divided doses, should be added. If this fails to resolve the hypokalemia, then indomethacin, 3–5 mg/kg/day divided into three doses, should be given. The use of indomethacin is generally avoided or minimized because of gastrointestinal complications.

Prognosis. The long-term prognosis of Bartter syndrome is uncertain. Many patients remain well, but some (especially those with glomerular or interstitial abnormalities) progress to renal insufficiency. Despite severe growth retardation in infancy, normal stature is ultimately obtained. The suggestion that mental retardation occurs in patients who have severe disease in the 1st yr of life remains to be confirmed.

Bartter FC: On the pathogenesis of Bartter's syndrome. Mineral Electrolyte Metab 3:61, 1980.

Chan JCM: Bartter's syndrome. Nephron 26:155, 1980.

Dunn MJ: Prostaglandins and Bartter's syndrome. Kidney Int 19:86, 1981.

Gill JR Jr: Bartter's syndrome. Ann Rev Med 31:405, 1980.

Robson WL, Arbus GS, Balfe JW: Bartter's syndrome. Am J Dis Child 133:636, 1979.

Simopoulos AP: Growth characteristics in patients with Bartter's syndrome. Nephron 23:130, 1979.

Stoff JS, Stemerman M, Steer M, et al: A defect in platelet aggregation in Bartter's syndrome. Am J Med 68:171, 1980.

17.32 INTERSTITIAL NEPHRITIS

Interstitial nephritis is a histopathologic term signifying inflammation between the glomeruli in the areas surrounding the tubules (the interstitium). Acute and chronic forms are recognized, depending on the nature of the inflammatory infiltrate and the presence or absence of edema and fibrosis. Tubular damage is generally present; glomerular changes may be minimal. Common causes of interstitial nephritis in children are listed in Table 17–6.

Table 17–6. **Causes of Interstitial Nephritis**

Acute	Chronic
Drugs	*Drugs*
Penicillin derivatives	Analgesics
Sulfonamides	Lithium
Cotrimoxazole	
Rifampin	*Infections*
Phenytoin	Pyelonephritis
Thiazides	
Furosemide	*Disease-Associated*
Allopurinol	Vesicoureteral reflux
Cimetidine	Nephrocalcinosis
Amphotericin B	Prolonged hypokalemia
	Oxalate nephropathy
Infections	Heavy metals
Streptococcal	Radiation
Pyelonephritis	Obstructive uropathy
Toxoplasmosis	Medullary cystic disease
Diphtheria	
Brucellosis	
Leptospirosis	
Mononucleosis	
Cytomegalovirus	
Disease-Associated	
Sarcoidosis	
Glomerulonephritis	
Transplant rejection	
Idiopathic	

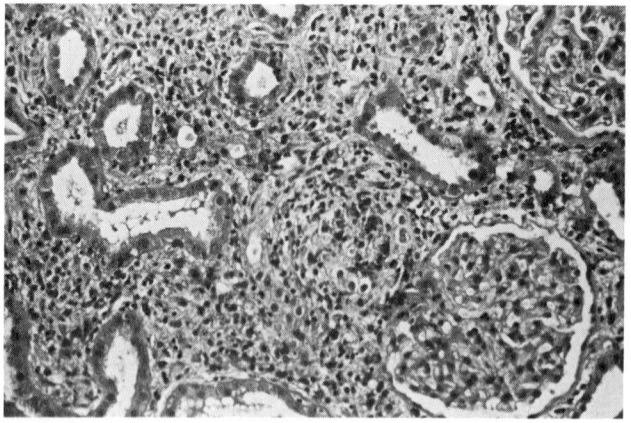

Figure 17–21. Biopsy from a patient having acute interstitial nephritis. The tubules are widely separated by edema and an intense inflammatory infiltrate containing lymphocytes, plasma cells, eosinophils, and neutrophils. The glomeruli are preserved. (× 80.)

ACUTE INTERSTITIAL NEPHRITIS

Pathology. Whatever the cause of interstitial disease, the interstitial infiltrate is composed of lymphocytes, plasma cells, eosinophils, and occasional neutrophils (Fig. 17–21). The tubules are separated by edema and may show degeneration or frank necrosis. Unless the interstitial nephritis is associated with glomerulonephritis, the glomeruli are normal.

Pathogenesis. The genesis of acute interstitial nephritis is poorly understood. When it is due to drug ingestion, failure of the amount of drug administered to correlate with incidence of the syndrome suggests a hypersensitivity reaction. For methicillin, an immunologic mechanism has been suggested in several instances by the finding of anti–tubular basement membrane antibodies. Whether infections cause interstitial inflammation by direct invasion or by other mechanisms remains unclear. In certain forms of glomerulonephritis, tubular basement membrane deposition of immune complexes (lupus, membranoproliferative) or of anti–basement membrane antibodies (Goodpasture, membranous) may initiate the inflammatory reaction. In sarcoidosis and transplant rejection, cell-mediated mechanisms may play a role.

Clinical Manifestations. In hospitalized patients, drugs are the most common cause of acute interstitial nephritis. After a week or so of drug therapy, patients typically present fever and a maculopapular skin rash. Urine output may be normal or diminished. Increased numbers of eosinophils may be detected in the blood or urine or both. Acute renal failure or generalized tubular dysfunction or both may result. Other forms of acute interstitial nephritis present a clinical picture resembling acute glomerulonephritis or acute renal failure, along with manifestations of the initiating disorder.

Diagnosis. The diagnosis is confirmed by renal biopsy, although it may not be suspected prior to the biopsy. The differential diagnosis includes other causes of acute nephritis or renal failure.

Prevention. The development of drug-related interstitial nephritis may be reduced by using alternative therapeutic agents when possible (e.g., the substitution of nafcillin for methicillin).

Treatment and Prognosis. Following appropriate management of the acute renal failure, withdrawal of possible inciting agents, and treatment of precipitating infection, the acute interstitial nephritis may resolve completely, but residual renal dysfunction is not uncommon. In patients suffering severe histologic injury and renal failure, high-dose corticosteroid therapy may bring dramatic improvement.

CHRONIC INTERSTITIAL NEPHRITIS

Pathology. In chronic interstitial nephritis, the inflammatory infiltrate consists of lymphocytes and plasma cells. The edema of the acute form is replaced by interstitial fibrosis. Tubular dilatation and atrophy are widespread. The glomeruli show partial or total sclerosis, presumably as a result of ischemia.

Clinical Manifestations. In children, chronic interstitial nephritis usually develops in association with an occult structural abnormality of the kidneys or lower urinary tract (cystic disease, obstruction, reflux). The presenting clinical manifestations may be those of chronic renal failure (nausea, vomiting, pallor, headache, fatigue, hypertension, growth failure) or manifestations of the underlying disorder (urinary tract infection, flank mass).

Diagnosis. The diagnosis is suggested by the presence of chronic renal insufficiency in association with a known cause of the disorder; renal biopsy is not usually indicated.

Treatment and Prognosis. The natural history of chronic interstitial nephritis is progression to end-stage renal failure. Whether elimination of infection and/or correction of reflux or obstruction will alter this progression is unclear. In adults, avoidance of analgesics (phenacetin) and lithium prior to the development of end-stage renal failure may result in improvement in renal function.

Ellis D, Fried WA, Yunis EJ, et al: Acute interstitial nephritis in children: A report of 13 cases and review of the literature. Pediatrics 67:862, 1981.
Galpin JE, Shinaberger JH, Stanley TM, et al: Acute interstitial nephritis due to methicillin. Am J Med 65:756, 1978.
Kincaid-Smith P: Analgesic abuse and the kidney. Kidney Int 17:250, 1980.
Linton AL, Clark WF, Driedger AA, et al: Acute interstitial nephritis due to drugs. Ann Intern Med 93:735, 1980.
Papper S: Interstitial nephritis. Contr Nephrol 23:204, 1980.
Rudnick MR, Bash CP, Elfenbein IB, et al: Cimetidine-induced acute renal failure. Ann Intern Med 96:180, 1982.

17.33 TOXIC NEPHROPATHIES

Medications, diagnostic agents (iodinated radiographic contrast media), and chemicals may alter the kidneys directly (through reduction of renal blood flow, acute tubular necrosis, intratubular obstruction) or indirectly (through induction of an allergic or hypersensitivity reaction in the vessels or interstitium). Commonly nephrotoxic agents and their clinical manifestations are listed in Table 17–7. Nephrotoxicity is frequently reversible if the noxious agent is removed.

Useful agents should not be withheld because of potential nephrotoxicity, but preventive measures may reduce the risks of nephrotoxicity: (1) in patients with pre-existing renal disease, substitution of ultrasonography or isotopic scans for studies using contrast media; (2) substitution of non-nephrotoxic agents for nephrotoxic agents if possible; (3) use of the lowest effective dose of the agent in conjunction with monitoring of the blood level; (4) reduction of the dose in patients with renal insufficiency; (5) avoidance of simultaneous use of several nephrotoxic agents.

Bennett WM: Aminoglycoside nephrotoxicity. Mineral Electrolyte Metab 6:277, 1981.
Bennett WM, Plamp C, Porter CA: Drug-related syndromes in clinical nephrology. Ann Intern Med 87:582, 1977.
Berkseth RO, Kjellstrand CM: Radiologic contrast-induced nephropathy. Med Clin North Am 68:351, 1984.
Clive DM, Stoff JS: Renal syndromes associated with nonsteroidal anti-inflammatory drugs. N Engl J Med 310:563, 1984.
Fer MF, McKinney TD, Richardson RL, et al: Cancer and the kidney: renal complications of neoplasms. Am J Med 71:704, 1981.
Ozols RF, Corden BJ, Jacob J, et al: High-dose cisplatin in hypertonic saline. Ann Intern Med 100:19, 1984.
Porter GA, Bennett WM: Nephrotoxic acute renal failure due to common drugs. Am J Physiol 241:F1, 1981.
Roxe DM: Toxic nephropathy from diagnostic and therapeutic agents. Am J Med 69:759, 1980.
Wedeen RP: Occupational renal disease. Am J Kidney Dis 3:241, 1984.

Table 17-7. **Nephrotoxic Compounds***

Nephrotic Syndrome		Renal Vasculitis with or without Glomerular Capillary Involvement	
Gold salts	Perchlorate	Hydralazine	Any of the numerous other
Mercurial diuretics	Probenecid	Isoniazid	drugs that may cause a
Mercury compounds	Tolbutamide	Sulfonamides	hypersensitivity reaction
Paramethadione	Trimethadione		
Penicillamine		**Nephrocalcinosis or Nephrolithiasis**	
		Allopurinol	Methoxyflurane
Nephrogenic Diabetes Insipidus		Ethylene glycol	Vitamin D
Amphotericin B	Methoxyflurane		
Demeclocycline	Propoxyphene	**Miscellaneous Renal Manifestations Including Proteinuria, Hematuria, Oliguria, Tubular Necrosis, and Renal Failure**	
Lithium carbonate		Arsenic	Iron
		Bacitracin	Kanamycin
Fanconi Syndrome		Cadmium	Mercury salts
Cadmium	Nitrobenzene	Carbon tetrachloride	Neomycin
Gentamicin	Outdated tetracycline	Cephaloridine	Pentamidine
Lead	Salicylate	Cephalothin	Poisonous mushrooms
Lysol	Uranium	Colistin	Polymyxin B
Mercury		Copper	Streptomycin
		Ethylene glycol	Sulfonamides
Renal Tubular Acidosis		Gentamicin	Tetrachlorethylene
Lithium salts		Gold salts	Vancomycin
Toluene sniffing		Indomethacin	Viomycin
Interstitial Nephritis with or without Papillary Necrosis			
Amidopyrine	Phenacetin		
p-Aminosalicylate	Phenylbutazone		
Bunamiodyl	Salicylate		
(papillary necrosis only)	Sulfonamides		
Penicillins			
(especially methicillin)			

*The agents are grouped according to the principal site of injury or manifestations. (Dr. Sean O'Regan assisted in the preparation of this table.)

17.34 KIDNEY PROBLEMS IN THE NEWBORN INFANT

Almost all premature and full-term infants void within the first 24 hr after birth. If an infant has not voided by the end of the first day of life, a search should be initiated for underlying anatomic abnormalities.

The urine of the healthy neonate may have a pH from 5–7 and an osmolality of 60–600 mOsm/kg H_2O. It usually has many epithelial cells and may contain an occasional red blood cell. White blood cells should be absent, and the culture should be sterile. Trace amounts of glucose and protein may be found on dipstick testing.

Some kidney disorders of the newborn (obstructive disorders, cystic diseases, renal vein thrombosis (Sec. 8.56), congenital nephrotic syndrome) are discussed in other sections. This section considers the remaining disorders particular to the newborn.

RENAL DYSGENESIS

Aplasia. Aplasia (agenesis) of the kidney may be unilateral or bilateral. When bilateral, oligohydramnios is followed by absence of urine production. Prematurity and spontaneous pneumothorax are common. Oligohydramnios causes compression of the fetus, resulting in Potter syndrome (flat nose; recessed chin; epicanthal folds; folded, flattened low-set ears; limb abnormalities; and pulmonary hypoplasia). Death occurs within the 1st mo of life, owing to uremia or pulmonary insufficiency. The disorder may be familial; ultrasonographic screening of parents and siblings should be considered to detect asymptomatic malformations.

Unilateral aplasia occurs in approximately 1/1000 live births, more commonly in males than in females, with the left kidney more commonly missing. The remaining kidney is usually normal and shows compensatory hypertrophy. Life expectancy in such patients is probably normal. In some patients with unilateral aplasia, the remaining kidney is hypoplastic or dysplastic and can be associated with developmental abnormalities of the upper and lower urinary tract, heart, gastrointestinal tract, nervous system, bones, and Müllerian duct system.

Hypoplasia. This term signifies small kidneys having a reduction in the number of nephrons. Hypoplasia does not appear to be inherited; it may be unilateral or bilateral. When unilateral, the hypoplasia may involve the entire kidney or portions thereof. In the latter case (segmental hypoplasia or Ask-Upmark kidney), transverse scars may run from cortex to medulla. Unilateral hypoplasia of either type is one of the more common causes of hypertension in the first decade of life.

Bilateral hypoplasia usually presents with the manifestations of chronic renal failure and is a leading cause of end-stage renal failure during the first decade of life. A history of polyuria and polydipsia is common. Urinalysis may be normal. A rare form of bilateral hypoplasia is called *oligomeganephronia*, in which the number of nephrons is markedly reduced but those present are markedly hypertrophied.

Dysplasia. This term indicates altered structural differentiation of the fetal kidney such that it contains cysts, abnormal ducts, undifferentiated mesenchyme, and/or nonrenal elements (such as cartilage).

Dysplasia may result from *intrauterine obstruction* of the urinary tract (prune-belly syndrome, ureterocele, urethral valves, ureteropelvic junction, and so on). Such dysplasia is bilateral and frequently leads to end-stage renal failure.

Another form of the disorder is *multicystic dysplasia*. This may be unilateral or bilateral and is commonly associated with developmental anomalies of the lower tracts. In the unilateral form, the patient presents with a nonfunctioning flank mass that appears histologically to be a mass of cysts containing little or no identifiable renal tissue. The mass is usually removed. Bilateral multicystic dysplasia is associated with chronic renal failure; severe cases may show Potter syndrome.

Arant BS Jr, Sotelo-Avila C, Bernstein J: Segmental "hypoplasia" of the kidney (Ask-Upmark). J Pediatr 95:931, 1979.

Ashkenazi S, Merlob P, Stark H, et al: Renal anomalies in neonates with spontaneous pneumothorax—incidence and evaluation. Int J Pediatr Nephrol 4:25, 1983.

Carter JE, Lirenman DS: Bilateral renal hypoplasia with oligomeganephronia. Am J Dis Child 120:537, 1970.

Clark DA: Times of first void and first stool in 500 newborns. Pediatrics 60:457, 1977.

Kissane JM: Congenital malformations. In: Heptinstall RH (ed): Pathology of the Kidney. Boston, Little, Brown, 1983, p 83.

Moore ES, Galvez MB: Delayed micturition in the newborn. J Pediatr 80:867, 1972.

Roodhooft AM, Birnholz JC, Holmes CB: Familial nature of congenital absence and severe dysgenesis of both kidneys. N Engl J Med 310:1341, 1984.

Thomas IT, Smith DW: Oligohydramnios, cause of the nonrenal features of Potter's syndrome, including pulmonary hypoplasia. J Pediatr 84:811, 1974.

CORTICAL NECROSIS

Renal cortical (and frequently medullary) necrosis seems to represent a final common result of several types of renal injury. It usually involves both kidneys and may be patchy or involve the entire cortex.

Etiology. In the newborn, cortical necrosis develops after dehydration, asphyxia, shock, disseminated intravascular coagulation, or renal vein thrombosis. After the newborn period, cortical necrosis most commonly develops with the hemolytic-uremic syndrome.

Pathology. Involved portions of the cortex show infarction, with congestion of the glomeruli, thrombosis of the arterioles, and necrosis of the tubules.

Pathogenesis. Cortical necrosis seems to develop when endothelial cell injury occurs in conjunction with diminished renal cortical blood flow. Toxins that presumably develop during shock or sepsis (endotoxin) may injure the endothelial cells and initiate intrarenal coagulation, leading to thrombosis and cortical necrosis.

Clinical Manifestations. Cortical necrosis commonly presents as acute renal failure developing in infants having the above-mentioned predisposing causes. The kidneys are frequently enlarged. Urine output is diminished and may show gross hematuria.

Diagnosis. The diagnosis is supported by the detection on ultrasonography of enlarged, nonobstructed kidneys, which on isotopic renal scan show little or no renal blood flow or function. The differential diagnosis includes other causes of renal failure (Table 17–8).

Treatment and Prognosis. Therapy is supportive and involves correction of dehydration, asphyxia, and shock and treatment of sepsis. The prognosis depends on the amount of surviving renal cortex.

Anand SK, Northway JD, Smith JA: Neonatal renal papillary and cortical necrosis. Am J Dis Child 131:773, 1977.

Bernstein J: Renal cortical and medullary necrosis. In: Edelmann CM (ed): Pediatric Kidney Disease. Boston, Little, Brown, 1978, p 1105.

Chevalier RL, Campbell F, Brenbridge ANAG: Prognostic factors in neonatal acute renal failure. Pediatrics 74:265, 1984.

Dauber IM, Krauss AN, Symchych PS, et al: Renal failure following perinatal anoxia. J Pediatr 88:851, 1976.

Guignard JP, Torrado A, Mazouni SM, et al: Renal function in respiratory distress syndrome. J Pediatr 88:845, 1976.

Reimold EW, Don TD, Worthen HG: Renal failure during the first year of life. Pediatrics 59:987, 1977.

Rodriguez-Soriano J, Vallo A, Bilbao F, et al: Different functional characteristics of residual nephrons in infantile vs adult diffuse cortical necrosis. Int J Pediatr Nephrol 3:71, 1982.

URINARY TRACT INFECTION IN THE NEWBORN

This subject is reviewed in depth in Sec. 8.62. A few points specific to the newborn are worth emphasizing. Infection is more common in males than in females. It is usually caused

Table 17–8. Causes of Acute Renal Failure in the Newborn

Renal dysgenesis	Hemorrhage
Obstructive uropathy	Sepsis
Renovascular accidents	Anoxia
Congenital heart disease	Shock
Dehydration	Renal vein thrombosis

by a gram-negative organism; the route of infection is bacteremia or by ascent of the urethra. The most frequent signs and symptoms (fever, jaundice, weight loss, irritability, cyanosis, vomiting, diarrhea) do not indicate that the site of the infection is in the urinary tract.

The diagnosis is suspected on detection of pyuria and bacteriuria and confirmed by quantitative culture of urine obtained by catheterization or bladder aspiration. The results of a culture of urine collected in a bag are significant only if the specimen is sterile. The growth of organisms from a bag collection is uninterpretable, as the bags are easily contaminated. Blood cultures should also be obtained.

Therapy should be initiated with intravenous administration of antibiotics of broad coverage, such as ampicillin and gentamicin. The antibiotic agents may be changed if tests of bacterial sensitivities indicate. If blood cultures are positive, then parenteral therapy should be continued for 10 days. If blood cultures are sterile after 5 days, then intravenous therapy may be changed to oral.

All neonates suffering a urinary tract infection should have a thorough radiographic evaluation of the upper urinary tract (ultrasonography, renal scan, or intravenous pyelography) and lower urinary tract (voiding cystourethrogram), to exclude underlying anatomic abnormalities (present in 50%).

RENAL FAILURE

17.35 ACUTE RENAL FAILURE

Acute renal failure develops when renal function is diminished to the point at which body fluid homeostasis can no longer be maintained. Although oliguria (daily urine volume less than 400 mL/m^2) is common, the urine volume may approximate normal (nonoliguric renal failure) in certain types of acute renal failure (aminoglycoside nephrotoxicity). To monitor renal function, it is important to use biochemical studies (BUN, creatinine) as well as measurement of urine volume.

Etiology. The causes of acute failure are listed in Table 17–9. In the first category (prerenal), decreased perfusion of the kidney results in decreased renal function; the second category includes diseases of the kidney, while the third is composed primarily of obstructive disorders.

Pathogenesis. *Prerenal causes* of acute renal failure produce decreased renal perfusion through decreases in the total or "effective" circulating blood volume. Evidence of kidney damage is absent. Diminished intravascular volume leads to a fall in cardiac output and an increase in renal arteriolar resistance, causing a decline in renal cortical blood flow and glomerular filtration rate. If, within a certain time, the underlying cause of the hypoperfusion is reversed, then renal function may return to normal. If hypoperfusion persists beyond this critical point, then renal parenchymal damage may develop.

Renal causes of acute renal failure include the rapidly progressive forms of several types of glomerulonephritis (Table 17–9) that are common causes of acute renal failure in older children. Activation of the coagulation system within the kidney, resulting in small vessel thrombosis, may lead to

Table 17–9. Causes of Acute Renal Failure

I. Prerenal	II. Renal	III. Postrenal

A. Hypovolemia
  1. Hemorrhage
  2. Gastrointestinal losses
  3. Hypoproteinemia
  4. Burns
  5. Renal or adrenal disease with salt wasting
  6. Hepatorenal syndrome
B. Hypotension
  1. Septicemia
  2. Disseminated intravascular coagulation
  3. Hypothermia
  4. Hemorrhage
  5. Heart failure
C. Hypoxia
  1. Pneumonia
  2. Aortic clamping
  3. Respiratory distress syndrome
	A. Glomerulonephritis
	  1. Poststreptococcal
	  2. Lupus erythematosus
	  3. Membranoproliferative
	  4. Idiopathic rapid progressive
	  5. Anaphylactoid purpura
	B. Localized intravascular coagulation
	  1. Renal vein thrombosis
	  2. Cortical necrosis
	  3. Hemolytic-uremic syndrome
	C. Acute tubular necrosis
	  1. Heavy metals
	  2. Chemicals
	  3. Drugs
	  4. Hemoglobin, myoglobin
	  5. Shock
	  6. Ischemia
	D. Acute interstitial nephritis
	  1. Infection
	  2. Drugs
	E. Tumors
	  1. Renal parenchymal infiltration
	  2. Uric acid nephropathy
	F. Developmental abnormalities
	  1. Cystic disease
	  2. Hypoplasia-dysplasia
	G. Hereditary nephritis
		A. Obstructive uropathy
		  1. Ureteropelvic junction
		  2. Ureterocele
		  3. Urethral valves
		  4. Tumor
		B. Vesicoureteral reflux
		C. Acquired
		  1. Stones
		  2. Blood clot

acute renal failure. The hemolytic-uremic syndrome is the most common cause of acute renal failure in toddlers.

The term "acute tubular necrosis" originally described a syndrome of acute renal failure in the absence of arterial or glomerular lesions. The proposed mechanism of the renal failure was necrosis of the tubular cells. Certain agents (heavy metals, chemicals) may indeed cause renal failure by producing tubular cell necrosis, but significant histologic changes are absent in kidneys from patients having other forms of "acute tubular necrosis." The precise mechanism of renal failure in these patients is unknown. Proposed mechanisms include alterations in intrarenal hemodynamics, tubular obstruction, and passive backflow of the glomerular filtrate across injured tubular cells into the peritubular capillaries.

Acute interstitial nephritis is an increasingly common cause of acute renal failure and is usually the result of a hypersensitivity reaction to a therapeutic agent. Tumors may produce acute renal failure by infiltration of the kidney or by obstruction of the tubules by uric acid crystals (Sec. 16.4–16.7).

Developmental abnormalities and hereditary nephritis may be associated with acute renal failure. Inability to conserve sodium and water is common in patients having these disorders, but losses are usually compensated by increased oral intake. If oral intake is compromised (vomiting) and/or extrarenal salt and water loss develops (diarrhea), then these, in conjunction with the obligate urinary salt and water losses, may lead to intravascular volume contraction and renal failure.

Postrenal causes of acute renal failure include obstructions of the urinary tract. With two functioning kidneys, ureteral obstruction must be bilateral to produce renal failure. It is important to recognize that dilatation of the upper collecting system may not occur until several days after acute ureteral obstruction.

Clinical Manifestations. The presenting signs and symptoms may be dominated or modified by the precipitating disease. Clinical findings related to the renal failure include pallor (anemia), diminished urine output, edema (salt and water overload), hypertension, vomiting, and lethargy (uremic encephalopathy).

Diagnosis. A careful history may aid in defining the cause of renal failure. Vomiting, diarrhea, and fever suggest dehydration and prerenal azotemia, but these may also precede development of the hemolytic-uremic syndrome or renal vein thrombosis. Antecedent skin or throat infection suggests poststreptococcal glomerulonephritis. Rash may be found in systemic lupus erythematosus or anaphylactoid purpura. A history of exposure to chemicals and medications should be sought. Flank masses suggest renal vein thrombosis, tumors, cystic disease, or obstruction.

Laboratory abnormalities may include anemia (with the rare exception of blood loss, the anemia is usually dilutional or hemolytic, as seen in lupus, renal vein thrombosis, and the hemolytic-uremic syndrome); leukopenia (lupus); thrombocytopenia (lupus, renal vein thrombosis, hemolytic-uremic syndrome); hyponatremia (dilutional); hyperkalemia; acidosis; elevated serum concentrations of BUN, creatinine, uric acid, and phosphate (diminished renal function); and hypocalcemia (hyperphosphatemia). The serum C3 level may be depressed (poststreptococcal, lupus, or membranoproliferative glomerulonephritis), and antibodies may be detected in the serum to streptococcal (poststreptococcal glomerulonephritis), nuclear (lupus), or basement membrane (Goodpasture disease) antigens. Chest roentgenography may reveal cardiomegaly and pulmonary congestion (fluid overload). In all patients presenting in acute renal failure, the possibility of obstruction (which, if detected, is quickly reversed by percutaneous nephrostomy) should be immediately assessed by obtaining a plain roentgenogram study of the abdomen, renal ultrasonography, and a radionuclide scan; retrograde pyelography may occasionally be needed, to detect occult obstructions. Renal biopsy may ultimately be required, to determine the precise cause of renal failure.

Treatment. In children with *hypovolemia*, the need for volume replacement may be critical. The initial physical examination of the patient should include a careful assessment of the state of hydration. In some oliguric patients, it may be impossible to distinguish whether oliguria is due to hypoperfusion (hypovolemia) or impending acute tubular necrosis.

Evaluation of the urine may prove helpful in this regard. In patients with hypovolemia, the urine is concentrated (urine osmolality exceeds 500 mOsm/kg H_2O), its sodium content is usually less than 20 mEq/L, and the fractional excretion of sodium (urine/plasma sodium concentration divided by the urine/plasma creatinine concentration × 100) is usually less than 1%. By contrast, in patients with tubular necrosis, the urine is dilute (osmolality less than 350 mOsm/kg H_2O), the sodium concentration usually exceeds 40 mEq/L, and the fractional excretion of sodium usually exceeds 1%.

If hypovolemia is detected, intravascular volume should be expanded by the intravenous administration of isotonic saline, 20 mL/kg, over 30 min. In the absence of blood loss or hypoproteinemia, colloid-containing solutions are not required for volume expansion. Following this infusion, the dehydrated patient will generally void within 2 hr. Failure to do so indicates a thorough re-evaluation of the patient. Catheterization of the bladder and determination of the central venous pressure may be helpful. If clinical and laboratory evaluations show that the patient is adequately hydrated, then aggressive diuretic therapy may be considered.

In patients with *impending renal failure* the value of diuretics in preventing development of anuria remains controversial. It seems clear that diuretics have no value in patients with established anuria. In some oliguric patients, furosemide or mannitol or both may increase the rate of urine production. These agents act by altering tubular function, but it should be recognized that the increase in urine flow does not represent an improvement in renal function nor will it affect the natural history of the disease that precipitated the renal failure. On the other hand, enhancement of urine output may be of value in the management of hyperkalemia and fluid overload.

The pharmacodynamics of furosemide in renal failure are such that the urinary response (which is a function of the dose and blood level obtained) may be delayed for several hours. In the oliguric patient who lacks clinical and laboratory evidence of hypovolemia (and who may have already failed to respond to volume expansion), furosemide may be administered as a single intravenous dose of 2 mg/kg at the rate of 4 mg/per min (to avoid ototoxicity); if no response occurs, a second dose of 10 mg/kg may be given. If no increase in urine production is obtained following this dose, then further furosemide therapy is contraindicated. A single intravenous dose of 0.5 g/kg of mannitol may be given over 30 min in addition to or in place of furosemide. Regardless of the response, no additional mannitol should be given, owing to the risk of toxicity.

Fluid restriction will be essential for the patient who fails to obtain adequate urine output following volume expansion or the administration of diuretics. The degree of fluid restriction will depend upon the state of hydration. For the patient with oliguria or anuria having a relatively normal intravascular volume, fluid administration should be limited to 400 mL/m²/ 24 hr (insensible losses) plus an amount of fluid equal to the urine output for that day. On the other hand, markedly hypervolemic patients may require almost total fluid restriction; omitting the replacement of insensible fluid losses and urine output will aid in diminishing the expanded intravascular volume. Access to the vascular space should be maintained; this is best obtained using an infusion pump at the slowest possible rate. In general, glucose-containing solutions (10–30%) without electrolytes are used as maintenance fluids. The composition of the fluid may be modified in accordance with the state of electrolyte balance. Except in the overhydrated patient, extrarenal (blood, gastrointestinal tract) fluid losses should be replaced, milliliter for milliliter, with appropriate fluids.

In acute renal failure, rapid development of *hyperkalemia* (serum level greater than 6 mEq/L) may lead to cardiac arrhythmia and death. *The patient should receive no potassium-containing fluid, foods, or medications until adequate renal function is re-established.* The earliest electrocardiographic change seen in patients with developing hyperkalemia is the appearance of tall, peaked T waves. This may be followed by ST-segment depression, prolongation of the P-R and widening of the QRS intervals, ventricular fibrillation, and cardiac arrest.

In children with acute renal failure, procedures to deplete body potassium are initiated when the serum potassium rises to 5.5 mEq/L. To miminize the rate at which the serum potassium rises, all solutions given to the patient should contain high concentrations of glucose. Sodium polystyrene sulfonate resin (Kayexalate), 1 g/kg, should be given orally or by retention enema. This material exchanges sodium for potassium. For best results, the resin should be given orally, suspended in 2 mL/kg of 70% sorbitol. Sorbitol produces an osmotic diarrhea, which will increase fluid and electrolyte losses (the usual patient in renal failure is hypervolemic with increased total body sodium and potassium levels), as well as enhance the movement of the resin through the gastrointestinal tract. Since 70% sorbitol is locally irritating to the rectum, the concentration should be reduced to 20% and the volume increased to 10 mL/kg when it is given by enema. Resin therapy may be repeated every 2 hrs, the frequency being limited primarily by the risk of sodium overload.

If the serum potassium rises above 7 mEq/L, emergency measures in addition to Kayexalate must be initiated. The following agents should be given sequentially:

1. Calcium gluconate 10% solution, 0.5 mL/kg intravenously, over 10 min. The heart rate must be closely monitored during the infusion; a fall in rate of 20 beats/min requires stopping the infusion until the pulse returns to the preinfusion rate.

2. Sodium bicarbonate 7.5% solution, 3 mEq/kg intravenously. Possible complications include volume expansion, hypertension, and tetany.

3. Glucose 50% solution, 1 mL/kg, with regular insulin, 1 unit/5 g of glucose, given intravenously over 1 hr. The patient should be monitored closely for hypoglycemia.

Calcium gluconate does not lower the serum potassium but counteracts the potassium-induced increase in myocardial irritability. Bicarbonate lowers serum potassium; the mechanism is not clearly defined. The effect of glucose and insulin is to shift potassium from the extracellar to the intracellular compartment. The duration of action of these emergency measures is just a few hours. Persistent hyperkalemia, therefore, especially in patients requiring the emergency measures, should be managed by dialysis.

Moderate *acidosis* is common in renal failure as a result of inadequate excretion of hydrogen ion and ammonia but it rarely requires treatment. Severe acidosis (arterial pH less than 7.15, serum bicarbonate less than 8 mEq/L) may cause depression of respiratory drive and increased myocardial irritability and requires treatment. Because of the risks involved in the rapid infusion of alkali, we choose to correct the acidosis only partially by the intravenous route, generally giving enough bicarbonate to raise the arterial pH to 7.20 (which approximates a serum bicarbonate level of 12 mEq/L). The correction formula is:

$$\text{mEq NaHCO}_3 \text{ required} = 0.3 \times \text{weight (kg)} \times (12 - \text{serum bicarbonate [mEq/L]})$$

The remainder of the correction, which should be accomplished only after normalization of the serum calcium and phosporus, may be made by the oral administration of sodium bicarbonate tablets or sodium citrate solution.

In addition to the risks involved in administration of intravenous bicarbonate that have been noted, correction of acidosis with intravenous bicarbonate may precipitate tetany. In patients with renal failure, an inability to excrete phosphorus leads to hyperphosphatemia and a reciprocal hypocalcemia. Acidosis prevents the development of tetany by increasing the ionized fraction of the total calcium. Rapid correction of acidosis will reduce the ionized calcium concentration, resulting in tetany.

Hypocalcemia is treated by lowering the serum phosphorus. Unless tetany develops, calcium is not given intravenously, in order to avoid reaching a calcium × phosphorus product (mg/dL × mg/dL) of 70 in the serum, the point at which calcium salts are deposited in tissue. To lower the serum phosphorus, a phosphate-binding gel is given by mouth, increasing fecal phosphate excretion; a common agent is Amphogel (aluminum hydroxide). The initial dose is imprecise (1–3 mL/kg/24 hr divided into four doses); the total daily dose should be gradually increased until the serum phosphorus level falls to normal.

Hyponatremia is commonly the result of administration of excessive amounts of hypotonic fluids to the oliguric-anuric patient. Correction may be accomplished by fluid restriction. Patients whose serum sodium levels fall below 120 mEq/L seem to be at increased risk for developing cerebral edema and central nervous system hemorrhage. In the absence of dehydration, water restriction is essential. When the serum sodium falls below 120 mEq/L, it may be elevated to 125 mEq/L by the intravenous infusion of hypertonic (3%) sodium chloride, using the following formula:

$$\text{mEq NaCl required} = 0.6 \times \text{weight (kg)} \times (125 - \text{serum sodium [mEq/L]})$$

The risks of administration of hypertonic saline include volume expansion, hypertension, and congestive heart failure; if these occur, they may be treated by dialysis.

Hypertension may result from the primary disease process or expansion of the extracellular fluid volume or both. In patients with renal failure and hypertension, salt and water restriction is critical.

In children with severe hypertension, the drug of choice is diazoxide. This potent vasodilator must be given by rapid (less than 10 sec) intravenous injection at a dose of 5 mg/kg (maximum dose 300 mg). A fall in blood pressure is usually seen within 10 to 20 min; if that following the first injection is insufficient, a second injection may be given 30 min later. As most hypertensive patients in renal failure are volume-overloaded, and as diazoxide can promote sodium retention, concomitant injection of furosemide, if it had not been previously administered, should be considered. For less severe hypertension, control of extracellular volume expansion (salt and water restriction, furosemide), and use of beta-blockers (e.g., propranolol) and vasodilators (e.g., apresoline) are generally effective.

Seizures may be the result of the primary disease process (e.g., systemic lupus erythematosus), hyponatremia (water intoxication), hypocalcemia (tetany), hypertension, or the uremic state itself. If possible, therapy should be directed toward the precipitating cause.

We have found that some of the usual anticonvulsant agents (paraldehyde, phenobarbital, phenytoin) are of limited effectiveness in uremia. Diazepam seems to be the most effective agent in controlling seizures. It should be remembered that its metabolic products are excreted in the urine and may accumulate in patients with renal insufficiency.

Except in the presence of hemolysis (e.g., hemolytic-uremic syndrome, lupus) or bleeding, the *anemia* of acute renal failure is generally mild (hemoglobin 9–10 g/dL), is primarily the result of volume expansion (hemodilution), and does not require transfusion. Blood loss from active bleeding should be replaced appropriately.

In patients with hemolytic anemia or prolonged renal failure, if hemoglobin levels fall below 7 g/dL, blood should be given. In the hypervolemic patient, blood transfusion carries the risk of further volume expansion, which may produce hypertension, congestive heart failure, and pulmonary edema. Slow (4–6 hr) transfusion with fresh (to minimize the amount of potassium administered) packed red blood cells will diminish the risk of hypervolemia. In the presence of severe hypervolemia, anemia should be corrected during dialysis.

The diet of most previously healthy and well-nourished children who suddenly develop acute renal failure should be restricted initially to fats and carbohydrates (gum drops and jelly beans), given the likelihood that the acute renal failure will resolve or respond to therapy within a reasonably brief period of time. Restrictions of sodium, potassium, and water administration have already been mentioned. If renal failure persists beyond 7 days, then an expanded oral diet for renal failure or parenteral hyperalimentation with essential amino acids should be considered.

Indications for *dialysis* in acute renal failure may comprise various combinations of the following factors: acidosis, electrolyte abnormalities, central nervous system disturbances, hypertension, fluid overload, and congestive heart failure. It appears that the early initiation of dialysis has significantly improved the survival in children with acute renal failure.

In certain patients with acute renal failure, careful medical management may minimize complications and delay the need for dialysis; other patients will eventually require dialysis for the uremic state itself. The life-threatening complications of uremia are hemorrhage, pericarditis, and central nervous system dysfunction; their precise causes are unknown. The risk of developing these complications correlates more closely with the level of BUN than with that of creatinine.

Prognosis. The prognosis for recovery of renal function depends on the disorder that precipitated the renal failure. In general, recovery of function is likely following renal failure resulting from prerenal causes, the hemolytic-uremic syndrome, acute tubular necrosis, acute interstitial nephritis, or uric acid nephropathy. On the other hand, recovery of renal function is unusual when renal failure results from most types of rapidly progressive glomerulonephritis, bilateral renal vein thrombosis, or bilateral cortical necrosis.

Arbeit LA, Weinstein SW: Acute tubular necrosis. Med Clin North Am 65:147, 1981.
Chesney RW, Kaplan BS, Freedom RM, et al: Acute renal failure: An important complication of cardiac surgery in infants. J. Pediatr 87:381, 1975.
Diamond JR, Yoburn DC: Nonoliguric acute renal failure. Arch Intern Med 142:1882, 1982.
Epstein M: Pathogenesis of renal sodium handling in cirrhosis. Am J Nephrol 3:297, 1983.
Hodson EM, Kjellstrand CM, Mauer SM: Acute renal failure in infants and children: Outcome of 53 patients requiring hemodialysis treatment. J Pediatr 93:756, 1978.
Honda N: Acute renal failure and rhabdomyolysis. Kidney Int 23:888, 1983.
Kjellstrand CM, Pru CE, Jahnke WK, et al: Acute renal failure. In Drukker W, Parsons FM, Maher JF (eds): Replacement of Renal Function by Dialysis. Boston, Martinus Nijhoff, 1983, p 536.
Miller TR, Anderson RJ, Linas SL, et al: Urinary diagnostic indices in acute renal failure. Ann Intern Med 89:47, 1978.
Steiner RW: Interpreting the fractional excretion of sodium. Am J Med 77:669, 1984.

17.36 CHRONIC RENAL FAILURE

Etiology. The etiology of chronic renal failure in childhood seems to correlate closely with the age of the patient at the time when the renal failure is first detected. Chronic renal failure in children under the age of 5 yr is commonly the result of anatomic abnormalities (hypoplasia, dysplasia, obstruction, malformations), whereas after 5 yr of age, acquired glomerular diseases (glomerulonephritis, hemolytic-uremic

THE URINARY SYSTEM: NEPHROLOGIC DISEASES

syndrome) or hereditary disorders (Alport syndrome, cystic disease) predominate.

Pathogenesis. Regardless of the cause of kidney damage, it appears that once a critical level of renal functional deterioration is reached, progression to end-stage renal failure is inevitable. The precise mechanisms resulting in progressive functional deterioration are unclear, but factors that may play important roles include ongoing immunologic injury; hemodynamically mediated hyperfiltration in surviving glomeruli; dietary protein and phosphorus intake; persistent proteinuria; and systemic hypertension.

Ongoing deposition of immune complexes or anti–glomerular basement antibodies in the glomerulus may result in persistent glomerular inflammation that leads to eventual scarring.

Hyperfiltration injury may be an important final common pathway of ultimate glomerular destruction, independent of the initiating mechanism of renal injury. Once nephrons are lost for any reason, the remaining nephrons undergo structural and functional hypertrophy mediated, at least in part, by an increase in glomerular blood flow. The increased blood flow increases the driving force for glomerular filtration in the surviving nephrons. This beneficial "hyperfiltration" in surviving glomeruli, which serves to preserve renal function, may also damage these glomeruli by mechanisms that are not understood. Potential mechanisms of damage include the direct effect of the elevated hydrostatic pressure on the integrity of the capillary wall, the resultant increase in the passage of proteins across the capillary wall, or both. Ultimately, this leads to changes in the mesangium and epithelial cells with the development of glomerular sclerosis. As sclerosis advances, the remaining nephrons suffer an increasing excretory burden, resulting in a vicious cycle of increasing glomerular blood flow and hyperfiltration.

Experimental models of chronic renal insufficiency have found that a high protein diet accelerates the development of renal failure, perhaps by means of afferent arteriolar dilatation and hyperperfusion injury. Conversely, a low protein diet diminishes the rate of functional deterioration. Recent studies of humans confirm that in normal individuals the glomerular filtration rate correlates directly with protein intake, and preliminary studies suggest that restriction of dietary protein may reduce the rate of functional deterioration in chronic renal insufficiency.

Some controversial studies in animal models have suggested that dietary phosphorus restriction preserves renal function in chronic renal insufficiency. Whether this beneficial effect is due to the prevention of calcium-phosphate salt deposition in the blood vessels and tissues or to suppression of secretion of parathyroid hormone, a potential nephrotoxin, is unclear.

Persistent proteinuria and/or systemic hypertension from any cause may directly damage the glomerular capillary wall, leading to glomerular sclerosis and initiation of hyperfiltration injury.

As renal function begins to deteriorate, compensatory mechanisms develop in remaining nephrons to maintain a normal internal environment. When the glomerular filtration rate falls below 20% of normal, however, a complex constellation of clinical, biochemical, and metabolic abnormalities develop that together constitute the uremic state. The pathophysiologic manifestations of the uremic state are listed in Table 17–10.

Clinical Manifestations. In patients developing chronic renal failure from glomerular or hereditary diseases, the renal disease is usually detected because of clinical manifestations apparent prior to the onset of renal insufficiency. The development of renal failure may be insidious, however, in patients having anatomic abnormalities, and their presenting complaints may be nonspecific (headache, fatigue, lethargy, anorexia, vomiting, polydipsia, polyuria, growth failure). Physical examination occasionally may be surprisingly unrewarding, but most patients with chronic renal failure appear pale and weak and have high blood pressure. Patients having

Table 17–10. Pathophysiology of Chronic Renal Failure

Manifestation	Mechanisms
Accumulation of nitrogenous waste products (azotemia)	Decline in glomerular filtration rate
Acidosis	Urinary bicarbonate wasting Decreased ammonia excretion Decreased acid excretion
Sodium wasting	Solute diuresis Tubular damage Functional tubular adaption for sodium excretion
Sodium retention	Nephrotic syndrome Congestive heart failure Anuria Excessive salt intake
Urinary concentrating defect	Nephron loss Solute diuresis Increased medullary blood flow
Hyperkalemia	Decline in glomerular filtration rate Acidosis Excessive potassium intake
Renal osteodystrophy	Decreased intestinal calcium absorption Impaired production of 1,25-dihydroxy-vitamin D by the kidneys Hypocalcemia and hyperphosphatemia Secondary hyperparathyroidism
Growth retardation	Protein-calorie deficiency Renal osteodystrophy Acidosis Unknown factors
Anemia	Decreased erythropoietin production Low grade hemolysis Bleeding Inadequate iron intake Inadequate folic acid intake
Bleeding tendency	Thrombocytopenia Defective platelet function
Infection	Defective granulocyte function Impaired cellular immune functions
Neurologic (fatigue, poor concentration, headache, drowsiness, loss of memory, slurred speech, muscle weakness and cramps, seizures, coma, peripheral neuropathy)	Unknown
Gastrointestinal ulceration	Gastric acid hypersecretion
Hypertension	Sodium and water overload Excessive renin production
Hypertriglyceridemia	Diminished plasma lipoprotein lipase activity
Pericarditis and cardiomyopathy	Unknown
Glucose intolerance	Tissue insulin resistance

anatomic abnormalities, in whom the renal failure has developed slowly over several years, may also have growth retardation and rickets.

Treatment. The management of the child having chronic renal failure requires close monitoring of the patient's clinical (physical examination and blood pressure) and laboratory status. Blood studies to be followed routinely include the hemoglobin (anemia), electrolytes (hyponatremia, hyperkalemia, acidosis), BUN and creatinine (nitrogen accumulation and level of renal function), calcium and phosphorus levels, and alkaline phosphatase activity (hypocalcemia, hyperphosphatemia, osteodystrophy). Periodic examination of parathyroid hormone levels and roentgenogram studies of bone may be of value in detecting early evidence of osteodystrophy. Chest roentgenography and echocardiography may be helpful in assessing cardiac function. Nutritional status may be monitored by periodic evaluation of the serum albumin, zinc, transferrin, folic acid, and iron levels. Optimally, the patient should be managed in conjunction with a medical center capable of supplying medical, nursing, social service, and nutritional support as the patient progresses to end-stage renal failure.

Diet in Chronic Renal Failure

In children with renal insufficiency, the growth rate diminishes when the glomerular filtration rate falls below 50% of normal. The precise cause of growth failure is unknown; a major factor is inadequate caloric intake (less than 70% of recommended dietary allowance). The optimal caloric intake in renal insufficiency is unknown, but an attempt should be made to equal or exceed (in patients with growth failure) the recommended daily caloric allowance for age. Caloric intake can be enhanced by adding to the diet unrestricted amounts of carbohydrate (sugar, jam, honey, glucose polymers*) and fat (medium chain triglycerides oil†), as tolerated by the patient.

When BUN exceeds approximately 80 mg/dL, patients may develop nausea, vomiting, and anorexia. These symptoms result from the accumulation of nitrogenous waste products and can be relieved by restricting dietary protein intake. Because children in renal failure continue to require adequate protein intake for growth, protein is provided at the level of 1.5 g/kg/24 hr and should consist of proteins of high biologic value that are metabolized primarily to usable amino acids rather than to nitrogenous wastes. The proteins of highest such biologic value are those of eggs and milk, followed by meat, fish, and fowl. Because cow's milk contains a high concentration of phosphate, moderate restriction or the use of a formula containing a reduced amount of phosphate (Similac PM 60/40, Ross Laboratories), sometimes in conjunction with an oral phosphate binder (see subsequent section on renal osteodystrophy), may be indicated.

Owing to inadequate intake, children with renal insufficiency may become deficient in water-soluble vitamins. These should be routinely supplied, using preparations such as Berocca tablets (Roche Laboratories, Nutley NJ 07110). Zinc and iron supplements should be added only after deficiencies are confirmed. Supplementation with fat-soluble vitamins A, E, and K is not required.

Water and Electrolyte Management in Chronic Renal Failure

Until the development of end-stage renal failure requires the initiation of dialysis, water restriction is rarely necessary

*Polycose, Ross Laboratories, Columbus, OH 43216.
†MCT Oil, Mead Johnson and Company, Evansville IN 47721.

in children with renal insufficiency, since water needs are regulated by the thirst center in the brain.

Most children with renal insufficiency will maintain normal sodium balance with the sodium intake derived from an appropriate diet. Some patients whose renal insufficiency is a consequence of anatomic abnormalities may waste sodium in the urine and require dietary salt supplementation. On the other hand, patients with high blood pressure, edema, or congestive heart failure may require sodium restriction, sometimes in conjunction with aggressive furosemide therapy (1–4 mg/kg/day).

In most children with renal insufficiency, potassium balance will be maintained until renal function deteriorates to the level at which dialysis is initiated. Hyperkalemia may develop in patients having only moderate renal insufficiency, however, as a result of excessive dietary potassium intake, the development of severe acidosis, or aldosterone deficiency (destruction of the juxtaglomerular apparatus). The hyperkalemia may be controlled by reducing dietary potassium intake and adding oral alkalinizing agents and/or Kayexalate (Breon Laboratories, New York, NY 10016), an oral resin that (in 1 g/kg/dose) binds to and removes potassium from the intestine.

Acidosis in Chronic Renal Failure

Acidosis develops in almost all children with renal insufficiency and need not be treated unless the serum bicarbonate falls below 20 mEq/L. Either Bicitra (1 mL equals 1 mEq of base) or sodium bicarbonate tablets (325 and 650 mg; 325 mg equals 4 mEq of base) may be used to raise the serum bicarbonate above 20 mEq/L.

Renal Osteodystrophy

Renal osteodystrophy commonly develops in association with hyperphosphatemia, hypocalcemia, and elevation of the serum alkaline phosphatase activity. In general, serum phosphorus levels rise when the glomerular filtration rate falls below 30% of normal. Hyperphosphatemia lowers the serum calcium level because of their reciprocal solubility relationship; secondary hyperparathyroidism results. Hyperphosphatemia may be controlled by enhancing fecal excretion by using oral aluminum hydroxide, an antacid that coincidentally also binds phosphate in the intestinal tract. The usual dosage range is 1–4 tsp (ALternaGEL, Stuart Pharmaceuticals, Wilmington, DE 19897) or tablets (Alu-Tab, Riker Laboratories, Northridge, CA 91326) with each meal. Because aluminum may be absorbed from the gastrointestinal tract, especially in small children, and lead to aluminum poisoning (dementia, osteomalacia), aluminum compounds should be used cautiously, with periodic monitoring of the serum aluminum level. Calcium carbonate suspension (Titralac, 3M Company, St. Paul, MN 55144) is an alternative phosphate-binder.

Hypocalcemia may result from hyperphosphatemia, inadequate dietary intake, and decreased calcium absorption caused by a deficiency in the active form (1,25-dihydroxycholecalciferol) of vitamin D. If the serum calcium remains low after correction of the serum phosphorus, then oral calcium supplements (Neo-Calglucon Syrup, Dorsey Pharmaceuticals, East Hanover, NJ 07936; Os-Cal Tablets, Marion Laboratories, Kansas City, MO 64371) at a dose of 500–1000 mg/day can be administered.

Vitamin D is converted to its active form (1,25-dihydroxycholecalciferol) by 1-hydroxylation in the kidney. With severe kidney destruction, insufficient conversion results in vitamin D deficiency. Vitamin D therapy is indicated (1) in patients having persistent hypocalcemia despite reduction of the serum phosphorus below 6.0 mg/dL and the addition of oral calcium supplements; and (2) in patients with osteodystrophy, as indicated by elevated serum alkaline phosphatase activities and radiographic evidence of rickets. Therapy may be initiated with 1 capsule (0.25 μg) per day of the active form of dihydroxy vitamin D (Rocaltrol, Roche Laboratories, Nutley, NJ 07110) or 0.05–0.20 mg/day of dihydrotachysterol solution (DHT Oral Solution, Roxane Laboratories, Columbus, OH 43216), which is metabolized to its active form in the liver. The dose of vitamin D is progressively increased until the serum calcium level and alkaline phosphatase activity are normal and radiographic healing of the rickets is seen. The dose of vitamin D should then be reduced to the initial level.

Anemia in Chronic Renal Failure

Anemia is common in chronic renal failure and is primarily the result of inadequate erythropoietin production by the failing kidneys, but inadequate dietary intake of iron and folic acid should not be overlooked. In most patients, the hemoglobin level will stabilize in the range of 6–9 g/dL; transfusion therapy is not indicated, as this would further suppress erythropoietin production. If the hemoglobin falls below 6 g/dL, 10 mL/kg of packed red blood cells should be administered cautiously (the small volume reduces the risk of circulatory overload).

Hypertension in Chronic Renal Failure

Hypertensive emergencies should be treated with intravenous administration of diazoxide (Hyperstat, Schering Corporation, Kenilworth, NJ 07033). The dose is 5 mg/kg, up to a maximum of 300 mg; it is given within 10 sec by manual injection. When severe hypertension is associated with circulatory overload, 5 mg/kg of furosemide may also be administered at the rate of 4 mg/min. Sodium nitroprusside should be used with great caution in renal insufficiency, owing to the possible accumulation of toxic thiocyanate.

The treatment of sustained hypertension may include a combination of salt restriction (2–3 g/day), furosemide (1–4 mg/kg/day), propranolol (Inderal, Ayerst Laboratories, New York, NY 10017; 1–4 mg/kg/day), and hydralazine (Apresoline, CIBA Pharmaceutical Company, Summit, NJ 07901; 1–5 mg/kg/day). Newer agents, such as minoxidil and captopril, should be used only in patients whose blood pressure is inadequately controlled with the above measures and should be administered with the guidance of a pediatric nephrologist.

Drug Dosage in Chronic Renal Failure

As many drugs are excreted by the kidneys, their administration to patients with renal insufficiency must be altered to maximize effectiveness and minimize the risk of toxicity. The principles of and guidelines for prescribing medications for patients in renal failure are summarized by Bennett and associates. As these recommendations are primarily obtained from data derived from adults, further modifications of dose levels and careful monitoring of blood levels (when available) may be necessary in children.

17.37 END-STAGE RENAL FAILURE

In the treatment of end-stage renal failure in children, the ultimate goal is a successful kidney transplant. Both cadaver and living-related donors have been used extensively as sources for the organ graft. In centers using predominantly living-related donors, when the patient's serum creatinine is progressively increasing and is in the range of 5–6 mg/dL, the patient and his or her family (parents and siblings over the age of 18 yr) are generally typed for histocompatibility antigens. At that point, the physicians, nurses, and social workers

Table 17–11. Value of Continuous Ambulatory Peritoneal Dialysis (CAPD)

Advantages	Disadvantages
Rapid training	Catheter malfunction
Technical simplicity (no machines)	Infection
Greater mobility	Poor appetite
Minimal dietary restriction	Poor body image
Feel better than hemodialysis patients	Parental "burnout"
Steady state chemistries	(emotional
Can live far from medical center	exhaustion)
Cheaper than hemodialysis	Elevated serum lipids
Improved growth rate	
Fewer blood transfusions	

begin a thorough education program for the family regarding both dialysis and transplantation. If there is a willing, compatible potential donor in the family, the person undergoes a complete medical evaluation prior to confirmation as the donor.

Dialysis is generally initiated when the patient's creatinine level approaches 10 mg/dL, depending on the patient's clinical status, the results of other laboratory studies, and the availability of a kidney donor. If no family donor is available, after beginning dialysis, the patient is placed on a waiting list for a cadaver kidney. Children are usually hospitalized for initiation of dialysis. If, in preparation for transplantation, bilateral nephrectomies are required (for severe hypertension, vesicoureteral reflux, or chronic pyelonephritis), these may be done at this time.

Until recently, hemodialysis was the standard technique for chronic dialysis in children, and the use of long-term indwelling subclavian vein catheters and arteriovenous fistulas created at the wrist has greatly simplified access to the vascular system for hemodialysis. The more recent development of Continuous Ambulatory Peritoneal Dialysis (CAPD), however, has revolutionized chronic dialysis in children, and the majority of children now use this technique.

In CAPD, dialysis across the peritoneal membrane removes excess body water through an osmotic gradient created by the glucose concentration in the dialysate; wastes are removed by diffusion from the peritoneal capillaries into the dialysate. CAPD is not as efficient as hemodialysis, but the fact that it is continuous around the clock (as contrasted with 12–18 hr/wk for hemodialysis) permits the maintenance of satisfactory levels of BUN and creatinine.

Access to the peritoneal cavity is achieved by inserting a soft Tenckhoff catheter through a midline infraumbilical incision; the catheter is brought out through the skin by means of a subcutaneous tunnel and connected to an extension tube that has a spike for insertion into the dialysis bag.

The parents (and patient, if more than 10–12 yr old) are then taught the techniques of spiking the bags of dialysate, allowing the dialysate to run in and dwell in the peritoneal cavity for the prescribed period of time, draining the dialysate back into the dialysate bag, and replacing the used bag of dialysate with a fresh one. Because the advantages of CAPD seem to far outweigh the risks (Table 17–11), CAPD appears to be the optimal form of chronic dialysis for most children.

The success rate for kidney transplants in children over the age of 5 yr approximates that for adults, and successful grafts have been performed in children as small as 5 kg. Ongoing research into better and less toxic means to prevent graft rejection should improve these statistics. Psychologic aspects of care of these children are discussed in Sec. 2.53 and 2.70.

JERRY MICHAEL BERGSTEIN
ALFRED F. MICHAEL

Andreoli SP, Bergstein JM, Sherrard DJ: Aluminum intoxication for aluminum-containing phosphate binders in children with azotemia not undergoing dialysis. N Engl J Med 310:1079, 1984.

Baldwin DS: Chronic glomerulonephritis: Nonimmunologic mechanisms of progressive glomerular damage. Kidney Int 21:109, 1982.

Baum M, Powell D, Calvin S, et al: Continuous ambulatory peritoneal dialysis in children. N Engl J Med 307:1537, 1982.

Bennett WM, Aronoff GR, Morrison G, et al: Drug prescribing in renal failure: Dosing guidelines for adults. Am J Kidney Dis 3:155, 1983.

Brenner BM: Hemodynamically mediated glomerular injury and the progressive nature of kidney disease. Kidney Int 23:647, 1983.

Coburn JW: Renal osteodystrophy. Kidney Int 17:677, 1980.

Defronzo RA, Smith D, Alvestrand A: Insulin action in uremia. Kidney Int 24:S-102, 1983.

Deykin D: Uremic bleeding. Kidney Int 24:698, 1983.

Fisher JW: Mechanism of the anemia of chronic renal failure. Nephron 25:106, 1980.

Klahr S, Buerkert J, Purkerson ML: Role of dietary factors in the progression of chronic renal disease. Kidney Int 24:579, 1983.

Levey AS, Harrington JT: Continuous peritoneal dialysis for chronic renal failure. Medicine 61:330, 1982.

Mooradian AD, Morley JE: Endocrine dysfunction in chronic renal failure. Arch Intern Med 144:351, 1984.

Morrison G, Murray TG: Electrolyte, acid-base, and fluid homeostasis in chronic renal failure. Med Clin North Am 65:429, 1981.

Nevins TE, Kjellstrand CM: Hemodialysis for children—a review. Int J Pediatr Nephrol 4:155, 1983.

Norman ME, Mazur AT, Borden S, et al: Early diagnosis of juvenile renal osteodystrophy. J Pediatr 97:226, 1980.

Novello AC, Fine RN: Renal transplantation in children—a review. Int J Pediatr Nephrol 3:87, 1982.

Raskin NH, Fishman RA: Neurologic disorders in renal failure. N Engl J Med 294:143, 204, 1976.

Renfrew R, Buselmeier TJ, Kjellstrand CM: Pericarditis and renal failure. Ann Rev Med 31:345, 1980.

Rotundo A, Nevins TE, Lipton M, et al: Progressive encephalopathy in children with chronic renal insufficiency in infancy. Kidney Int 21:486, 1982.

Weidmann P, Beretta-Piccoli C: Chronic renal failure and hypertension. Handbook of Hypertension 2:80, 1983.

UROLOGIC DISORDERS IN INFANTS AND CHILDREN

17.38 URINARY TRACT INFECTIONS

Symptoms suggestive of urinary tract infection are common in children, but the importance of urinary tract infection in childhood has been both exaggerated and understated. These biases have resulted in aggressive diagnostic and therapeutic measures for trivial conditions and in neglect of serious disorders.

Prevalence and Etiology. The prevalence of urinary infections varies markedly with sex and age. Symptomatic urinary tract infections occur in about 1.4/1000 newborn infants, with a slight male preponderance. Thereafter, infections are much more common in females. Symptomatic and asymptomatic urinary tract infections occur in 1.2–1.9% of school-aged females and are most common in the 7–11 yr old age group (2.5%). Infections are quite rare in males of similar age.

Urinary tract infections are caused mainly by colonic bacteria. In females 75–90% of all infections are caused by *Escherichia coli*, followed by *Klebsiella* and *Proteus*. Some series report that in males over 1 yr of age, *Proteus* is as common as *E. coli*; others report a preponderance of gram-positive organisms in males. *Staphylococcus albus* is a proven pathogen in both sexes. Viral infections may also occur.

Pathogenesis and Pathology. In the neonatal period bacteria reach the urinary tract via the blood stream, whereas later in life they ascend the urinary tract from below. Individual differences in susceptibility to urinary tract infections may be explained by such host factors as production of urethral and cervical antibodies (IgA), and other factors that influence bacterial adherence to the epithelium of the introitus and the urethra. Once the organisms gain entrance to the bladder, the severity of the infection may reflect the virulence of the bacteria and such anatomic factors as vesicoureteral reflux, obstruction, urinary stasis, and the presence of calculi. With urinary stasis, bacteria have increased opportunity to multiply, since urine is an excellent culture medium. In addition, vesical overdistension decreases the blood flow to the bladder wall and may decrease the bladder's natural resistance to infection.

Acute bacterial cystitis is characterized by mucosal congestion and edema, occasionally with petechiae and hemorrhage. The inflammatory reaction causes hyperactivity of the detrusor muscle and a decrease in the functional capacity of the bladder. These changes may precipitate vesicoureteral reflux, particularly when the vesicoureteral junction is already ab-

normally developed. Chronic or frequently recurrent infections may cause changes of *cystitis cystica* in the bladder wall, with characteristic endoscopic and histologic appearances.

Bacteria can reach the kidney from the bladder by way of established vesicoureteral reflux or through transient reflux precipitated by the inflammation of the bladder wall. (Patients with the P1 blood group can develop ascending recurrent pyelonephritis in the absence of vesicoureteral reflux, because *E. coli* binds specifically to the P1 antigens on the epithelial cell surface.) *Acute pyelonephritis* leads to enlargement of the kidney, owing to edema and acute inflammatory infiltrates in the medulla and pelvis. If untreated, these changes may lead to the formation of renal microabscesses, which may become confluent. Acute pyelonephritis is always more severe when obstruction is present. These changes may result in the development of renal scars, with the histologic findings commonly known as chronic pyelonephritis; however, prompt treatment of the infection can result in complete healing.

Histologically, *chronic pyelonephritis* is often difficult to distinguish from other causes of renal scarring such as medullary cystic disease, ischemia, irradiation, analgesic abuse, and others. The scars can be focal or diffuse. The characteristic finding in chronic pyelonephritis is a cortical scar with an underlying calyceal deformity (Fig. 17–22). Microscopically, the lesions are patchy with glomerular fibrosis, interstitial chronic inflammation, and fibrosis and atrophy of the tubules. Local conditions of the renal medulla such as high osmolality, which interferes with phagocytic activity of leukocytes, make this region of the kidney more susceptible to infections than the cortex.

Such renal scars are found also in children with vesicoureteral reflux who have no history of urinary tract infection; for this reason some investigators prefer the term "reflux nephropathy" to "chronic pyelonephritis." In any case, 90% of children with lesions of chronic pyelonephritis have vesicoureteral reflux. Reflux nephropathy or chronic pyelonephritis is the most common cause of arterial hypertension in children; some of the vascular and glomerular changes may be secondary to hypertension rather than to the inflammatory process. In experimental animals reflux nephropathy occurs only in areas of the kidney where the renal papillae allow reflux of urine from the calyx to the collecting tubules (intrarenal reflux) (Fig. 17–23), which is facilitated by the anatomic configuration of the flat papillae present in the compound calyces; conical papillae usually present in simple calyces help

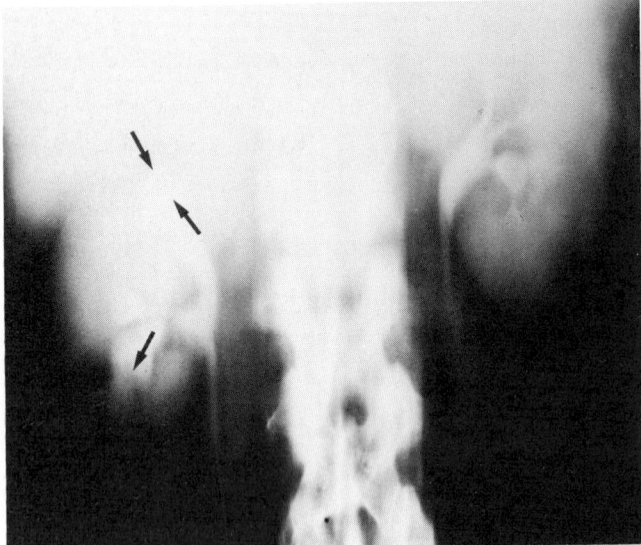

Figure 17–22. Chronic pyelonephritis. Tomographic cut made during intravenous urography, showing characteristic changes of chronic pyelonephritis on the right side. Note the smaller size of the right kidney, the clubbing of the calyces, particularly those of the upper and lower poles, and the marked thinning of the cortex in the poles of the kidney. The left kidney is normal.

to prevent the occurrence of intrarenal reflux. Autoimmune responses to Tamm-Horsfall protein may also play a role in the development and progression of the pyelonephritic scar.

In addition to the inflammatory changes just described, infection by urea-splitting organisms such as *Proteus* can lead to stone formation. The ammonia derived from urea produces a strongly alkaline urine in which calcium phosphate and triple calcium magnesium and ammonium phosphate can precipitate. The calculi act as foreign bodies and help perpetuate the infection. With ureteral obstruction, renal infection can rapidly lead to septicemia, pyonephrosis, and the formation of renal and perirenal abscesses.

Xanthogranulomatous pyelonephritis is a distinct histologic type of renal infection characterized by granulomatous inflammation with giant cells and foamy histiocytes. It may present clinically as a renal mass or an acute or chronic infection. Renal calculi, obstruction, and infection with *Proteus* or *E. coli* contribute to the development of this rare lesion, which usually requires nephrectomy.

Clinical Manifestations. Asymptomatic bacteriuria is common; in most cases either there have been symptoms suggestive of urinary tract infection or there will be. The clinical manifestations often fail to indicate clearly whether the infection is confined to the bladder or involves the kidneys as well. In infancy, fever, weight loss, failure to thrive, nausea, vomiting, diarrhea, and jaundice are common. In children with fever of unknown origin, cultures of urine should be obtained to exclude urinary tract infection. Later in childhood, urinary frequency, pain during micturition, urinary incontinence associated with urgency, bedwetting in a previously dry child, abdominal pain, and foul-smelling urine are common symptoms. Chronic or frequently recurrent cystitis is often responsible for daytime incontinence and other manifestations of bladder instability, which may persist even after the urine has become sterile (Sec. 17.43).

Hematuria is occasionally observed as a sign of hemorrhagic cystitis caused by *E. coli*. In acute pyelonephritis, fever, chills, and flank or abdominal pain and tenderness are common. The kidney may be enlarged. Children with chronic pyelonephritis are often asymptomatic. Arterial hypertension is commonly associated with renal scars. Reflux nephropathy,

commonly attributed to the combination of vesicoureteral reflux and infection, is responsible for up to 15% of cases of end-stage renal failure in children. Sepsis is common in infants and older children with infection and urinary tract obstruction. Hyperammonemia with central nervous system manifestations is a rare complication of urinary tract infections due to *Proteus* and associated with urinary stasis or obstruction.

Laboratory Studies. The diagnosis of urinary tract infections depends on the culture of bacteria from the urine. The finding of any bacteria in urine obtained from the bladder or renal pelvis is indicative of infection. An accurate diagnosis may be difficult to establish, owing to the frequent contamination of voided specimens or to prior treatment of the patient with antibiotics.

In toilet-trained children, a midstream urine culture obtained after cleansing the urethral meatus with a povidone-iodine solution and rinsing with sterile water or saline is usually satisfactory. In females the labia should be spread manually to avoid contamination of the urine or contact with the skin. In uncircumcised males the prepuce must be retracted; if the prepuce is not retractable, this method of urine collection is not reliable. Skillful nurses can help the child's mother to obtain these specimens. For midstream voided specimens the colony count is often used to differentiate between infected and contaminated specimens. Cultures indicating more than 10^5 colonies/mL of a single organism are more than 90% specific for urinary tract infections. It should be recognized, however, that lower colony counts in infected patients may be due to overhydration, to recent bladder emptying, or to antibiotic therapy; such counts do not rule out infection.

In infants and both male and female young children, the application of an adhesive, sealed, sterile collection bag after disinfection of the skin of the genitalia can be useful, particularly if a sterile culture results. The specificity of these cultures is much lower than that of a midstream specimen. When greater assurance as to the possibility of infection is needed, a catheterized specimen must be obtained. Proper skin preparation and good technique of catheterization are important. The use of a 5F polyethylene feeding tube in infants or of an 8F tube with proper lubrication in older children minimizes the chance of urethral trauma and contamination. Catheterization shortly after spontaneous voiding

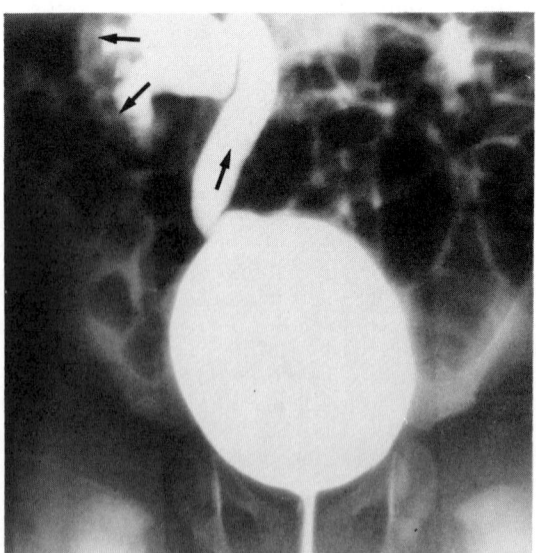

Figure 17–23. Intrarenal reflux. Retrograde cystogram in a young infant male with a past history of a urinary tract infection. Note right vesicoureteral reflux with ureteral dilatation, with opacification of the renal parenchyma representing intrarenal reflux.

produces a measure of the residual urine in the bladder and helps assess problems related to bladder emptying. In theory, the normal flora of the distal urethra may be a source of false-positive culture results, but in practice the finding of any colonies grown from bladder urine should be considered as indicating infection.

In infant males and in uncircumcised older boys, the use of a suprapubic puncture of the full bladder with a 25- or 22-gauge needle yields reliable results. With the child properly hydrated (when the bladder can be percussed or palpated), the skin is disinfected and a puncture performed 1 finger-breadth above the pubis in the midline. A syringe is used to aspirate as the needle is inserted. One or 2 mL of urine is sufficient for culture. The urine specimen for bacterial culture should be kept refrigerated until the culture is plated to avoid bacterial overgrowth. False-negative findings on urine culture may result from unrecognized antibiotic treatment, dilution from overhydration, or contamination of the specimen with the antiseptic solution.

A urinalysis should be obtained from the same specimen as that cultured. Pyuria (leukocytes in the urine) suggests infection, but infection can occur in the absence of pyuria; accordingly, this finding is more confirmatory than diagnostic. Conversely, pyuria can be present without urinary tract infections. Microscopic hematuria is common in acute cystitis. Casts in the urinary sediment suggest renal involvement. *Proteus* infections consistently produce an alkaline pH.

With acute renal infection, leukocytosis and neutrophilia are common. Unfortunately, in children such tests to differentiate upper from lower urinary tract infections as the detection of antibody-coated bacteria, response to single-dose antibiotic therapy, and other immunologic and biochemical tests are unreliable. Inability to concentrate the urine is a common but unreliable finding in acute and chronic pyelonephritis. In 30% of infants with renal infections the serum creatinine level is transiently elevated. Since sepsis is common in renal infections, particularly in infants and with obstruction, blood cultures should be obtained during febrile infections.

Imaging Studies. The indications for imaging studies in children with urinary tract infection vary to some degree with the experience of the physician (see Sec. 5.55). During acute febrile infection, renal ultrasonography should be obtained to rule out hydronephrosis and renal or perirenal abscesses; other indications for this study are when the response to antibiotic therapy is not prompt, when the child is severely ill and toxic, and when the serum creatinine level is elevated. Approximately 3 wk after treatment of the acute infection all children should have voiding cystourethrography to assess reflux. Some physicians would restrict such studies to all males and to females under 5 yr of age who have an initial infection; older females would be studied at the time of a second infection. We prefer the former approach, since reflux will be found in 25% of all children under the age of 10 yr who have had symptomatic or asymptomatic bacteriuria; it is more frequently observed in children under 3 yr of age. If it is available, radioisotopic voiding cystourethrography can be used in females; this technique is sensitive and exposes the ovaries to 50- to 100-fold less radiation than would conventional voiding cystourethrography with intermittent fluoroscopic control. In males radiographic definition of the urethra is important; accordingly, radiographic voiding cystourethrography with fluoroscopic control is recommended for the initial workup. Renal ultrasonography may also be carried out as part of the initial workup in order to exclude obstruction and to determine kidney size.

If vesicoureteral reflux is present, intravenous pyelography with nephrotomography should be obtained to evaluate kidney size and detect possible calyceal blunting, ureteral dilatation, and renal scarring. In Europe, 2,3-dimercaptosuccinic acid (DMS) scans are commonly used to detect renal scars but involve significant radiation exposure to the kidneys. Further evaluation of children with infections and reflux or obstructive uropathy will be discussed in other sections.

The frequently performed cystoscopies and measurements of urethral caliber advocated for girls in the past contribute nothing to the therapeutic decisions to be made in children with normal findings on radiographic study or with primary reflux. Narrowing of the female urethra was once postulated to be a contributing factor in the development of urinary tract infections, but the urethras of girls with recurrent urinary tract infections are not narrower than those of girls without infections.

Differential Diagnosis. Inflammations of the external genitalia, vulvitis, and vaginitis caused by yeast, pinworms, and other agents may be accompanied by symptoms mimicking cystitis. Viral and chemical cystitis must be distinguished from bacterial cystitis on the basis of history and results of urine culture. Radiographically, the hypoplastic or dysplastic kidney or a small kidney secondary to a vascular accident may appear similar to a kidney with chronic pyelonephritis. With the latter, however, vesicoureteral reflux is usually present.

Acute hemorrhagic cystitis is frequently caused by *E. coli*; it has been attributed also to adenovirus types 11 and 21. Adenovirus cystitis is more frequent in males; it is self-limiting, with hematuria lasting approximately 4 days. *Eosinophilic cystitis* is a rare form of cystitis of obscure origin that occasionally has been found in children. Usual symptoms are those of cystitis with hematuria, ureteral dilatation, and filling defects in the bladder caused by masses that consist histologically of inflammatory infiltrates with eosinophils.

Treatment. Acute cystitis should be treated promptly to prevent its possible progression to pyelonephritis. If the symptoms are severe, a specimen of bladder urine is obtained for culture and treatment is started immediately. If the symptoms are mild or the diagnosis doubtful, treatment can be delayed until the results of culture are known and the culture can be repeated if the results are uncertain. For example, if midstream culture grew between 10^4 and 10^5 colonies of a gram-negative organism, a second culture may be obtained by catheterization or suprapubic aspiration before treatment is initiated. If treatment is initiated before the results of a culture and sensitivities are available, a 7–10 day course of therapy with short-acting sulfonamide such as sulfisoxazole (100–125 mg/kg/24 hr in 4 divided doses) will be effective against most strains of *E. coli*. Nitrofurantoin (5–7 mg/kg/24 hr in 3–4 divided doses) is also very effective and has the advantage of being active against *Klebsiella-Enterobacter* organisms. Amoxicillin (50 mg/kg/24 hr) is also effective as initial treatment but has no clear advantages over the sulfonamides or nitrofurantoin.

In acute febrile infections suggestive of pyelonephritis, the use of broad-spectrum antibiotics capable of reaching significant tissue levels is preferable. Cefadroxil (40–60 mg/kg/24 hr orally) or cefaclor (20 mg/kg/24 hr orally) is useful, but if the child is acutely ill, parenteral treatment with cefamandole (100 mg/kg/24 hr) or with an aminoglycoside such as gentamicin (1.0–1.5 mg/kg/24 hr in 3 divided doses) is preferable. The potential ototoxicity and nephrotoxicity of aminoglycosides should be considered, and serum creatinine levels must be obtained prior to initiating treatment as well as daily thereafter so long as treatment continues. Treatment with aminoglycosides is particularly effective against *Pseudomonas*, and alkalinization of urine with sodium bicarbonate increases their effectiveness in the urinary tract. The combination of sulfamethoxazole and trimethoprim (Cotrim, Bactrim, Septra), either orally or intravenously, is effective against a variety of gram-negative organisms other than *Pseudomonas*. The oral dosage is 20 mg/kg/24 hr for sulfamethoxazole and 4 mg/kg/24 hr for trimethoprim, given in 2 divided doses. Penicillin G is often effective against *Proteus* infections.

A urine culture should be obtained a week after the termination of treatment of any urinary tract infection to assure that the urine remains sterile. Given the tendency of urinary tract infections to recur even in the absence of predisposing anatomic factors, follow-up urine cultures should be obtained at 3 mo intervals for 1–2 yr even when the child is asymptomatic. If recurrences are frequent, prophylaxis against reinfection, using either sulfamethoxazole-trimethoprim combination or nitrofurantoin at one-third the normal therapeutic dose once a day, is often effective. It is important, however, to obtain periodic urine cultures if the child is receiving prolonged prophylactic treatment, in order to rule out asymptomatic infections caused by resistant organisms. Antibacterial prophylaxis is also indicated for as long as vesicoureteral reflux persists (Sec. 17.39), or when recurrent cystitis causes such symptoms as incontinence, frequency, and urgency of urination, which are perpetuated by frequent reinfections. Other indications for long-term prophylaxis (neurogenic bladder, urinary tract stasis and obstruction, reflux, and calculi) are discussed below. The prolonged use of any chemotherapeutic agent should be monitored for evidence of toxicity (anemia, leukopenia, and so on). Broad-spectrum antibiotics are usually ineffective for prophylaxis, since the colonic bacteria likely to be responsible for reinfections quickly become resistant to these agents.

The long-term prognosis for urinary tract infections is usually excellent, provided prompt and adequate treatment is instituted when the diagnosis is established. The prompt treatment of acute bacterial pyelonephritis in animals has prevented the development of renal scars. Notwithstanding this usually favorable long-term outcome, children with recurrent urinary tract infections often present difficult and frustrating problems in treatment and prophylaxis. The main consequences of chronic renal damage caused by pyelonephritis are arterial hypertension and renal insufficiency; when they are found they should be treated appropriately. Some children with urinary tract infections void infrequently and many also have severe constipation. Counseling of parents to try to establish more normal patterns of voiding and defecation may be helpful in controlling recurrences.

Children with renal or perirenal abscesses or with infections in obstructed urinary tracts require surgical or percutaneous drainage in addition to antibiotic therapy and other supportive measures.

17.39 VESICOURETERAL REFLUX

Reflux of urine from the bladder to the ureter and renal pelvis results from incompetence of the valvular mechanism at the ureterovesical junction that normally allows passage of urine only from the ureter to the bladder. Reflux can be harmful to the kidneys because (1) it exposes the renal pelvis (which has a normal pressure of less than 10 mm Hg) to the much higher vesical pressures produced during voiding; and (2) it facilitates the passage of bacteria from the bladder to the kidneys. Accordingly, reflux can result in dilatation of the ureter and upper collecting systems as well as the development of renal scars, particularly in association with urinary tract infections. Reflux of urine from the intrarenal collecting system to the collecting tubules also plays an important role in the development of renal scars (Sec. 17.38). Massive reflux into dilated ureters also prevents complete bladder emptying, inasmuch as urine "voided" into the upper collecting system rapidly returns to the bladder, with development of progressive bladder dilatation, as in the megaureter-megacystic syndrome (Fig. 17–24). Reflux nephropathy accounts for 15–20%

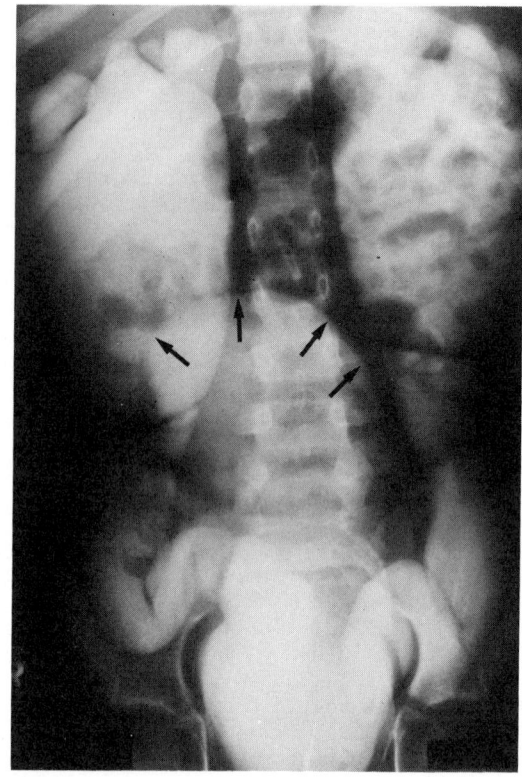

Figure 17–24. Excretory urogram in a male with megaureter-megacystic syndrome. Note the massive ureteral dilatation due to high grade vesicoureteral reflux. The bladder is very distended, reaching the level of the third lumbar vertebra. There was no urethral obstruction or neurogenic dysfunction.

of all end-stage renal failure in children and young adults and is an important cause of hypertension in children.

Classification. Primary vesicoureteral reflux results from a congenital anomaly of the ureterovesical junction in which the intramural ureteral tunnel is short, the ureteral orifice is placed in a lateral and cephalad direction, and the trigone is underdeveloped. This shortening of the intramural tunnel decreases the efficiency of the valvular mechanism. The degree of vesicoureteral reflux varies with the degree of malformation of the orifice (Fig. 17–25). A wide spectrum of anomalies may be associated (Table 17–12).

With duplication of the ureters and ureterocele, the ureterocele obstructs the upper collecting system, and there is often reflux to the ureter of the lower collecting system and occasionally to the contralateral side. In duplicated systems, reflux is more common in the lower ureter, which enters the bladder higher and more laterally and has a less competent valve.

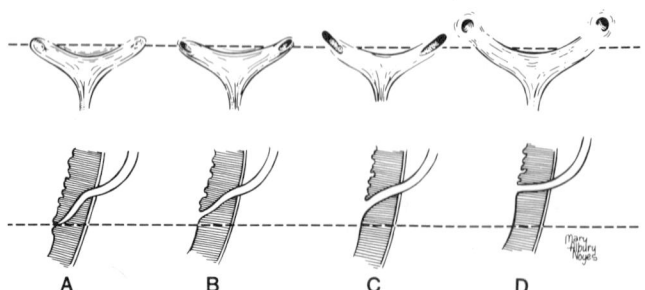

Figure 17–25. Normal and abnormal configuration of the ureteral orifices. Shown from left to right, progressive lateral displacement of the ureteral orifices and shortening of the intramural tunnels. *Top:* Endoscopic appearance. *Bottom:* Sagittal view through the intramural ureter.

Table 17–12. **Classification of Vesicoureteral Reflux**

Type	Cause
1. Primary	Congenital incompetence of the valvular mechanism of the vesicoureteral junction
2. Primary associated with other malformations of the ureterovesical junction	Ureteral duplication Ureterocele with duplication Ureteral ectopia Paraureteral diverticula
3. Secondary to increased intravesical pressure	Neurogenic bladder Non-neurogenic bladder dysfunction Bladder outlet obstruction
4. Secondary to inflammatory processes	Severe bacterial cystitis Foreign bodies Vesical calculi Clinical cystitis
5. Secondary to surgical procedures involving the ureterovesical junction	

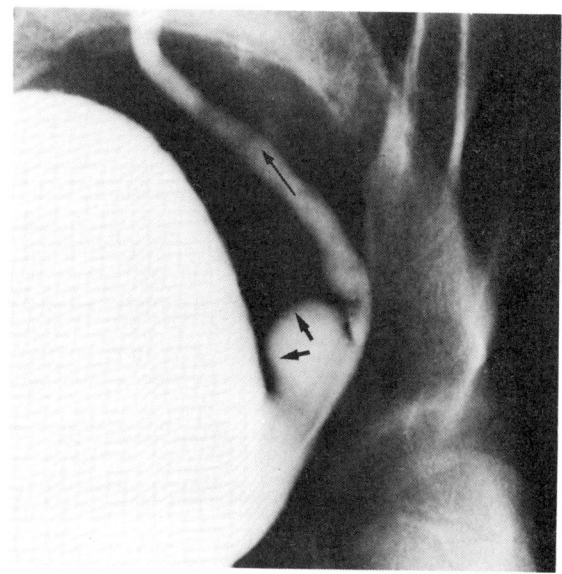

Figure 17–27. Reflux and bladder diverticulum. Voiding cystourethrogram demonstrates left vesicoureteral reflux and a paraureteral diverticulum.

Reflux is always present when the ureter enters a diverticulum (Figs. 17–26 and 17–27).

In cases of congenital neurogenic bladder, such as myelomeningocele and sacral agenesis, reflux is present in one third of the cases at birth and develops eventually in more than half of affected children. Reflux is seen in more than half of cases of posterior urethral valves. Both clinically and experimentally, reflux with increased intravesical pressures (as in bladder outlet obstruction and vesical dysfunction) has severe consequences for the kidney, even in the absence of infection. Reflux is classified into five grades according to its severity and the degree of ureteral dilatation and calyceal deformity, as depicted in Fig. 17–28. This grading of reflux has prognostic and therapeutic significance.

Natural History. In children with reflux the incidence of renal scarring or reflux nephropathy increases with the grade of reflux. Intrarenal reflux seems to increase the risk of scarring. In grades I and II reflux in patients who have no ureteral dilatation, the anatomy of the vesicoureteral region tends to be nearly normal, and in about 80% of cases reflux will cease spontaneously with maturation of the child. With greater degrees of ureteral dilatation and of abnormality of the vesicoureteral junction, the chances of spontaneous disappearance decrease.

Presentation. In the majority of children, reflux is discovered during an evaluation for urinary tract infection. In other children, voiding cystourethrography is part of an evaluation of voiding dysfunction, renal insufficiency, hypertension, or other suspected pathology of the urinary tract.

Differential Diagnosis. The distinction between primary and secondary reflux is usually easy to make on the basis of history and radiographs. In the case of the child who has reflux, infection, and voiding dysfunction, it may be difficult to determine whether the voiding dysfunction is secondary to infection or the cause of reflux that predisposes to infection. Urodynamic studies of the lower urinary tract (Sec. 17.43) may be necessary in such cases.

Evaluation. Once reflux is diagnosed, graded, and determined to be primary, secondary to other malformations of the vesicoureteral junction, or secondary to inflammatory processes or increased intravesical pressure, it is important then to know the renal size and whether scars are present; intravenous pyelography and tomography are appropriate studies. Blood pressure and baseline creatinine clearance should also be measured. In patients with primary reflux, the degree of abnormality of the intramural tunnel can be pre-

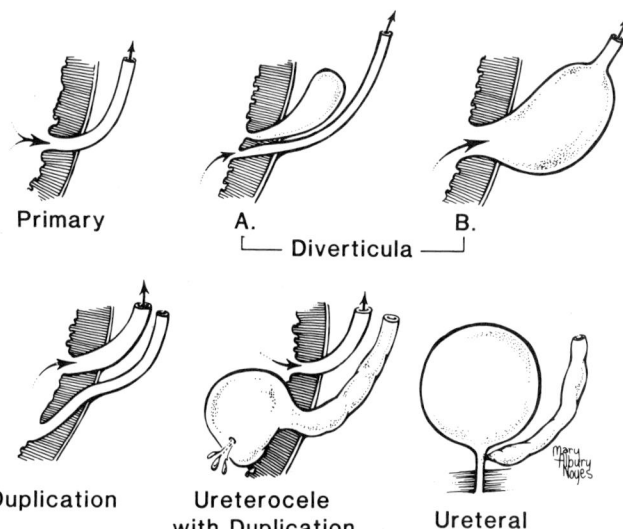

Figure 17–26. Various anatomical defects of the ureterovesical junction associated with vesicoureteral reflux.

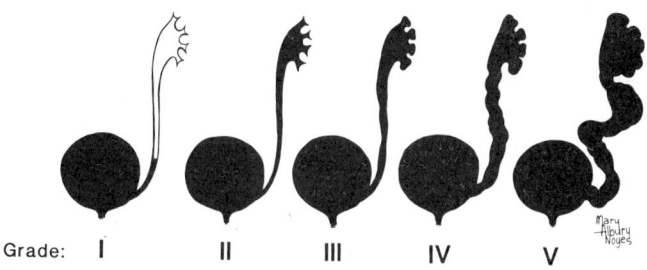

Grade: I   II   III   IV   V

Figure 17–28. Grading of vesicoureteral reflux. Grade I: reflux into a nondilated distal ureter. Grade II: reflux into the upper collecting system without dilatation. Grade III: reflux into dilated ureter and/or blunting of calyceal fornices. Grade IV: reflux into a grossly dilated ureter. Grade V: massive reflux, with ureteral dilatation and tortuosity and effacement of the calyceal details.

dicted from the grade of reflux. Accordingly, when anomalies of the urethra or bladder and associated anomalies of the vesicoureteral junction can be ruled out radiographically, cystoscopy is of doubtful value in determining the prognosis or choosing between surgical and medical treatment.

Treatment. The treatment of *primary reflux* and that associated with complete duplication of the ureters can be considered together. In grades I and II reflux the likelihood of spontaneous resolution is great, and a period of expectant treatment is warranted, during which the child must be protected from infection by administration of an antibacterial medication such as sulfamethoxazole-trimethroprim combination or nitrofurantoin (Sec. 17.38). At the beginning of treatment, urine cultures are obtained at monthly intervals; when the efficacy of prophylaxis has been established, cultures can be obtained at 3 mo intervals.

Since asymptomatic bacteriuria and reflux can be harmful, it is important to culture the urine even in the absence of symptoms. Using a radionuclide, voiding cystourethrography is obtained at yearly intervals, with limited intravenous pyelography approximately every other year to assess the possibility of new scars and to evaluate renal growth. When a radiographic study indicates spontaneous cessation of the reflux, another study made in 3–6 mo should confirm this before antibacterial therapy is discontinued, since reflux is occasionally intermittent. Grade II reflux seldom needs surgical correction, but if antibacterial prophylaxis fails to keep the urine consistently sterile, surgery is indicated.

In cases of grade III reflux, it is appropriate to repeat voiding cystourethrography after 6 mo of treatment to ensure that the degree of reflux has not been underestimated. It also may be necessary to have yearly intravenous pyelography, since several months may elapse between an episode of renal infection and appearance of radiologic changes indicating resultant renal scars. More than 50% of children with grade III reflux may ultimately need surgical treatment.

In grades IV and V reflux (that is, reflux associated with significant ureteral dilatation and upper urinary tract changes), spontaneous cessation is unlikely and early surgical treatment is indicated after a brief period of prophylaxis and confirmation of the persistence of the reflux. Surgical treatment is particularly indicated for the infant and young child, because the risk of renal scarring is higher in children less than 5 yr of age.

Secondary reflux associated with duplications can be treated exactly as primary reflux. When a periureteral diverticulum is present, spontaneous cessation of reflux is significantly less likely, and early surgical treatment is therefore indicated. For a large bladder diverticulum, surgical treatment is necessary to improve bladder emptying. Reflux secondary to severe cystitis, such as that which may accompany foreign bodies or chemical irritation, will usually cease once the primary cause of the cystitis is removed. Iatrogenic reflux usually requires surgical treatment. The treatment of reflux in cases of ureteroceles, posterior urethral valves, and neurogenic bladder will be discussed later.

The results of surgical treatment of reflux are usually excellent. On the other hand, most past series reporting up to 95% or greater success included many cases of low grade reflux, which is now known seldom to need corrective surgery. Antireflux operations involving dilated ureters carry a lower success rate, but with one or more reoperations success is usually achieved.

Complications of antireflux surgery include persistence of reflux and obstruction of the distal ureter. Careful follow-up of patients after surgery is therefore required. When only unilateral reflux has been demonstrated, bilateral correction of reflux is usually unnecessary. Reflux may appear transiently on the opposite side after surgery, but it usually ceases spontaneously.

17.40 OBSTRUCTIONS OF THE URINARY TRACT

Obstructive lesions of the urinary tract occur at any level from the urethral meatus to the calyceal infundibula. In children, obstruction can be congenital (anatomical) or caused by trauma, neoplasia, calculi, inflammatory processes, or surgical procedures. The pathophysiologic effects of obstruction depend on its level, extent of involvement, age of onset, and acute or chronic nature. In childhood most obstructive lesions are congenital, and may therefore be present during fetal life.

A partial list of obstructive lesions is given in Table 17–13. High grade ureteral obstruction of early onset in fetal life results in renal dysplasia, ranging from the multicystic kidney, usually associated with ureteral or pelvic atresia (Fig. 17–29), to various degrees of histologic renal cortical dysplasia seen

Table 17–13. **Types and Causes of Urinary Tract Obstruction**

Location	Cause
Infundibula	Congenital Calculi Inflammatory (tuberculosis) Traumatic Postsurgical Neoplastic
Renal Pelvis	Congenital (infundibulopelvic stenosis) Inflammatory (tuberculosis) Calculi Neoplasia (Wilms tumor, neuroblastoma)
Ureteropelvic Junction	Congenital stenosis Calculi Neoplasia Inflammatory Postsurgical Traumatic

Ureter	Congenital obstructive megaureter
	Ureteral ectopia
	Ureterocele
	Retrocaval ureter
	Ureteral fibroepithelial polyps
	Ureteral valves
	Calculi
	Postsurgical
	Extrinsic compression
	  Neoplasia (neuroblastoma, lymphoma, and other retroperitoneal or pelvic tumors)
	  Inflammatory (Crohn disease, chronic granulomatous disease)
	  Hematoma, urinoma
	  Lymphocele
	  Retroperitoneal fibrosis

Bladder Outlet and Urethra	Neurogenic bladder dysfunction (functional obstruction) Posterior urethral valves Anterior urethral valves Diverticula Urethral strictures (congenital, traumatic, or iatrogenic) Urethral atresia Ectopic ureterocele Meatal stenosis (males) Calculi Foreign bodies Phimosis Extrinsic compression by tumors Urogenital sinus anomalies

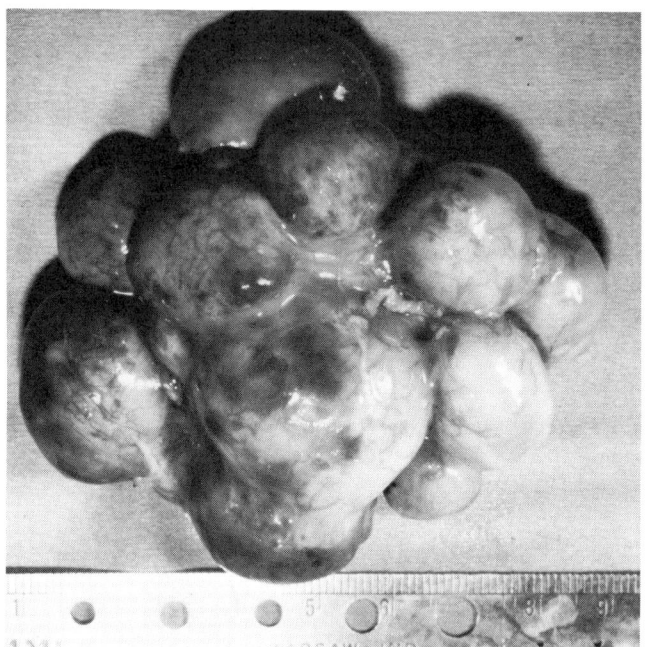

Figure 17–29. Surgical specimen of a multicystic dysplastic kidney associated with ureteral atresia.

with less severe obstruction. Chronic ureteral obstruction in late fetal life or after birth results in hypertrophy and later dilatation of the ureter and upper collecting system, with alterations of renal parenchyma ranging from minimal tubular changes to dilatation of Bowman space, glomerular atrophy, and interstitial fibrosis. After birth, infections often complicate obstruction and may increase renal damage.

Urethral obstruction in the fetus can result in a patent urachus, which serves to decompress the bladder. More commonly there is urethral dilatation above the obstruction and hypertrophy of the detrusor muscle. The ureters are dilated because of impeded drainage into the obstructed bladder, owing to high intravesical pressure and to obstruction of the intramural portion of the ureter by the hypertrophied detrusor muscle. Vesicoureteral reflux commonly complicates congenital urethral obstruction. Urinary extravasation sometimes occurs in children with congenital obstruction when urine under pressure leaks out of the intrarenal collecting system, usually through ruptured calyceal fornices, into the subcapsular or perirenal spaces (urinomas) or into the peritoneal cavity (urinary ascites). Bilateral ureteral obstruction or urethral obstruction may cause oligohydramnios and pulmonary hypoplasia. The immediate prognosis for newborns with severe obstructive uropathy is often more closely related to the degree of pulmonary insufficiency than to the degree of renal damage.

In high grade urethral obstruction or bilateral ureteral obstruction there is renal failure. The urinary output may be low, normal, or increased because of tubular dysfunction with decreased concentrating ability. Renal function usually recovers completely following relief of a brief acute obstruction. The potential for recovery of renal function in chronic (including all congenital) cases depends on the degree of dysplasia or irreversible renal damage. In renal failure with obstructive uropathy both the concentrating ability and the ability of the tubules to excrete hydrogen ions are decreased. Accordingly, infants with renal failure secondary to obstruction may, after relief of obstruction, continue to have polyuria, dilute urine, and chronic acidosis with normal serum creatinine levels.

Hypertrophy and dilatation in the bladder and collecting systems persist long after correction of the obstruction and

are often irreversible. Following relief of obstruction in the uremic child, postobstructive diuresis may ensue. This is usually transient and due to the combination of tubular dysfunction and an osmotic diuresis caused by high blood levels of urea.

Diagnosis. Urinary tract obstructions are often silent, and advanced lesions (particularly unilateral ones) can be found in children without symptoms. In the newborn a palpable abdominal mass is most commonly a hydronephrotic kidney. With infravesical obstructive lesions the bladder as well as the kidneys may be palpably enlarged. A patent urachus should suggest urethral obstruction. Ascites in the newborn may be caused by intraperitoneal urinary extravasation (see above). Prune-belly syndrome (abdominal muscle deficiency and undescended testes) is often accompanied by massive dilatation of the bladder and ureters and occasionally by infravesical obstruction.

Urinary tract obstruction may be diagnosed prenatally by ultrasonography. In such cases further ultrasonography and, if indicated, a more complete evaluation should be undertaken in the neonatal period. Oligohydramnios and various degrees of pulmonary hypoplasia accompany the more severe cases of urethral or bilateral ureteral obstruction.

Infection and sepsis may be the first indications of an obstructive lesion of the urinary tract. The combination of infection and obstruction poses a serious threat to infants and children and usually requires parenteral administration of antibiotics and drainage of the obstructed kidney. For this reason renal ultrasonography should be performed for all children during the acute stage of febrile urinary tract infections. Obstructive renal insufficiency can manifest itself by failure to thrive, vomiting, diarrhea, or other nonspecific signs and symptoms. In older children infravesical obstruction can be associated with overflow urinary incontinence or a poor urinary stream. Acute ureteral obstruction causes flank or abdominal pain and there may be nausea and vomiting. Chronic ureteral obstruction can be silent or cause vague abdominal or typical flank pain with increased fluid intake.

Imaging Studies. Intravenous urography is the standard method for diagnosis of obstruction. The preliminary radiography of the abdomen should be inspected for calculi, spinal abnormalities, or an abnormal intestinal gas pattern. In infravesical obstruction, the bladder wall is irregular or trabeculated because of detrusor hypertrophy. A postvoiding film may show residual bladder urine. In ureteral obstruction there is dilatation of the collecting system above the obstruction and blunting of the calyces. Concentration of the radiopaque medium on the obstructed side is decreased, and there may be delayed appearance of the dye in the collecting system with progressive increase in dye concentration at the point of obstruction when delayed radiographs are obtained. In high grade obstruction the dye may remain in the collecting system after 24 hr.

Urinary extravasation can be detected in the early or delayed films of a urographic study. When intermittent obstruction is suspected, intravenous urography during an acute episode of pain is often the most valuable diagnostic study. Renal ultrasonography is valuable mainly as a screening test in patients with acute infections and in the newborn with suspected hydronephrosis. It may also be of value for follow-up after treatment. In acute ureteral obstruction, the dilatation of the collecting system may be minimal and ultrasonography misleading.

A dilated collecting system seen in an intravenous urogram does not always indicate obstruction. Following correction of chronic obstructive lesions or with the presence of megacalycosis or nonobstructed megaureters, dilatation may occur without obstruction. In these cases injection of furosemide during intravenous pyelography may show increased dilatation of the collecting system (indicative of obstruction) or show complete washout of the dye (interpreted as demonstrating dilatation without obstruction). Unfortunately, this diuresis urography seldom yields clear-cut results, and its usefulness is limited.

A radioisotopic renogram with the injection of diuretics (diuretic renogram) can be more useful. With obstruction, the radioisotope lingers in the collecting system and the excretion time is prolonged. If after injection of furosemide the radioisotope remains in the renal pelvis, the test indicates obstruction. The four patterns commonly obtained in the diuresis renogram in patients with normal, dilated nonobstructed, or obstructed collecting systems are shown in Fig. 17–30. Diuresis renograms should be interpreted with care, since both false-positive and false-negative results may occur.

Pressure Flow Studies. The most accurate way to establish the diagnosis of obstruction of the upper collecting systems in equivocal cases is by performing pressure flow studies, as described by Whitaker. Percutaneous access is gained to the renal pelvis, using a 22-gauge needle; the collecting system is then perfused with radiopaque dye at a measured flow rate, usually 10 mL/min. The pressures in the renal pelvis and the bladder are monitored during this infusion, and pressure differences exceeding 20 cm of water indicate obstruction. This test can be done under sedation in infants and older children but requires general anesthesia for immobilization in toddlers. In experienced hands, this test is accurate and has negligible risk of complications. Antegrade pyelography is obtained at the same time, which provides excellent delineation of the anatomy of the collecting system (Fig. 17–31).

Voiding Cystourethrography. In all cases of ureteral dilatation voiding cystourethrography should be obtained to rule out vesicoureteral reflux as a possible cause of the dilatation. The voiding cystourethrogram is also necessary to rule out urethral obstruction, particularly in cases of posterior urethral valves. In infravesical obstruction in infants the bladder may be palpable because of chronic distention and incomplete emptying. In older children the urinary flow rate can be measured in a simple noninvasive way with a urinary flow meter, and decreased flow in the presence of normal bladder contraction is diagnostic of infravesical obstruction. When the urethra cannot be catheterized to obtain a voiding cystourethrogram, one must suspect a urethral stricture or an obstruc-

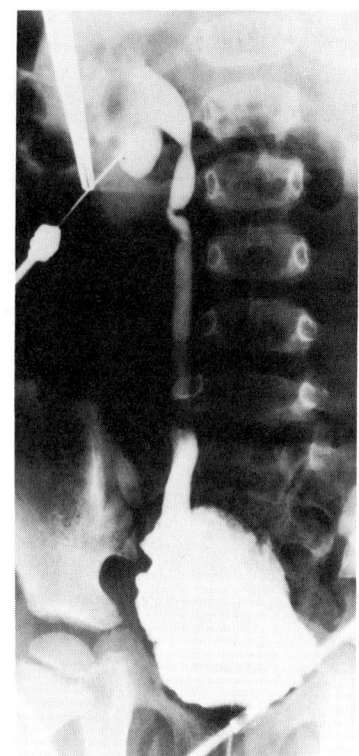

Figure 17–31. Percutaneous antegrade pyelogram made at the time of a Whitaker test with a 22-gauge needle.

tive urethral lesion other than valves. Retrograde urethrography with dye injected into the urethral meatus will help delineate the anatomy of the urethral obstruction.

SPECIFIC TYPES OF URINARY TRACT OBSTRUCTION

Hydrocalycosis. This term refers to a localized dilatation of the calyx caused by obstruction of its infundibulum. Such obstruction can be developmental in origin or secondary to inflammatory processes (particularly tuberculosis, now rarely seen). In congenital obstructions due to stenosis or extrinsic vascular compressions, the presenting symptom is usually pain which can be relieved by surgical correction of the obstruction. The diagnosis of infundibular obstruction is usually established by intravenous urography.

Obstruction of the Ureteropelvic Junction. This is the most common obstructive lesion in childhood and is caused most often by congenital stenosis of the ureteropelvic junction. Ureteral kinks, fibrous bands, and apparently aberrant vessels are usually secondary phenomena caused by dilatation of the pelvis above the obstruction. Ureteropelvic junction obstruction most commonly presents as: (1) maternal ultrasonography revealing fetal hydronephrosis; (2) a palpable renal mass in a newborn; (3) abdominal, flank, or back pain; (4) a febrile urinary tract infection; or (5) hematuria after minimal trauma. Twenty percent of obstructions are bilateral.

The diagnosis is established by intravenous urography (Fig. 17–32). When the kidneys function poorly and are not visualized on the delayed postinjection radiographs, renal ultrasonography will show hydronephrosis. Retrograde pyelography on the operating table will establish the point of obstruction. In the differential diagnosis the following entities should be considered: (1) megacalycosis, a congenital nonobstructive dilatation of the calyces without pelvic or ureteric dilatation; (2) vesicoureteral reflux with marked dilatation and kinking of the ureter (voiding cystourethrography should be

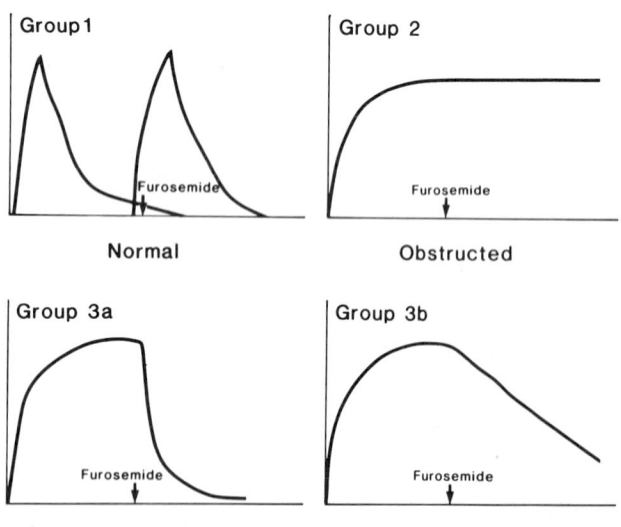

Figure 17–30. Patterns commonly observed in diuresis renography. Group I—normal; group 2—obstructed; group 3a—stasis without obstruction (75%) or with compensated obstruction (25%); group 3b—partial obstruction (40%) or stasis without obstruction (60%). (From Gonzalez R, Chiou R-K: J Urol 133:646, 1985.)

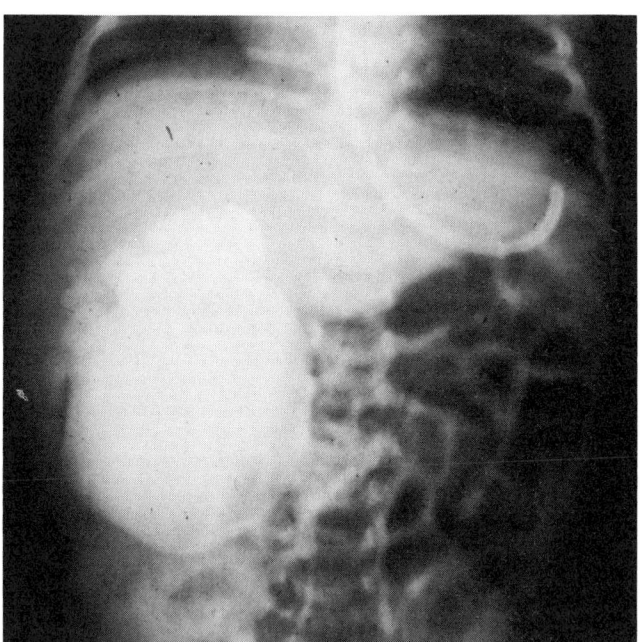

Figure 17–32. Ureteropelvic junction obstruction. Excretory urogram on a newborn, showing dilatation of the right renal pelvis and blunting of the calyces characteristic of a ureteropelvic junction obstruction.

done on all patients with suspected ureteropelvic junction obstruction); and (3) midureteral or distal ureteral obstructions when the ureter is not well visualized on the urogram.

In the neonate with a renal mass, ureteropelvic junction obstruction must be distinguished from multicystic renal dysplasia, solid renal tumors, and renal vein thrombosis. The clinical picture and imaging studies will help establish an accurate diagnosis. A multicystic dysplastic kidney may mimic a ureteropelvic junction obstruction on ultrasonography but invariably shows no function on the radioisotopic renogram. Treatment consists of surgical excision of the obstructed ureteropelvic junction with reanastomosis of the ureter and renal pelvis. The success rate of pyeloplasties is high, but postoperative ultrasonography and intravenous urography often show persistent dilatation of the calyces. Diuresis renography is useful for the longitudinal follow-up of these patients.

Midureteral Obstruction. Congenital ureteral stenosis or ureteral valves can sometimes occur in the midureter. A retrocaval ureter can be partially obstructed; such circumcaval ureters are invariably on the right side and represent anomalous development of the vena cava, with persistence of the ventral infrarenal subcardinal veins. Excretory urography shows the right ureter to be medially deviated at the level of the 3rd lumbar vertebra (Fig. 17–33). Surgical treatment is needed only when obstruction is present. Retroperitoneal tumors, fibrosis caused by surgical procedures, inflammatory processes (as in chronic granulomatous disease), and radiation therapy can cause acquired midureteral obstruction.

Ureteral Ectopia. An ectopic ureteral orifice can be located anywhere along the path of migration of the mesonephric duct. The ectopic ureter may drain a single collecting system but more commonly it belongs to the upper moiety of a duplicated collecting system. The ureteral orifice of the upper collecting system is always caudal to that of the lower collecting system. In males, ectopic ureters are usually single; may enter the bladder neck, the urethra above the external sphincter, the seminal vesicle, or the vas deferens; and are commonly associated with high grade obstruction and symptoms of urinary tract infection or epididymitis. When the contralateral

side is normal, nephroureterectomy is usually indicated. When single ectopic ureters are bilateral, or in the rare unilateral cases when the function of the involved kidney is good, the ectopic ureter should be reimplanted.

In females ureteral ectopia is usually associated with duplication. When the ureter of the upper collecting system enters the bladder neck or the urethra at or above the level of the sphincter there is obstruction, and treatment consists of an upper pole nephroureterectomy. When the ureter enters the vestibule, vagina, or uterus, the most common presenting complaint is urinary incontinence or vaginal discharge. In either case the diagnosis is established by careful inspection of the urogram, renal ultrasonography, and endoscopy. Although obstructed, the collecting system drained by a duplicated ectopic ureter may be very small and difficult to detect even after careful inspection of the intravenous urogram. A high degree of suspicion is always necessary to establish this diagnosis. In bilateral simple ectopic ureters in the female there is usually bladder hypoplasia in addition to ureteral obstruction; such cases are difficult to manage.

Ureterocele. Ureterocele is a congenital cystic dilatation of the distal ureter that protrudes into the bladder and has a pinpoint ureteral orifice. Its embryogenesis remains uncertain. Ureteroceles are more common in females than in males. *Simple ureteroceles* are associated with nonduplicated collecting systems, and the orifice is in the expected location in the bladder. They are usually discovered during an investigation for a urinary tract infection. Intravenous pyelography reveals varying degrees of ureteral and calyceal dilatation, and there is a round filling defect in the bladder (Fig. 17–34). In delayed films the cystic dilatation of the ureter may be clearly visible and full of contrast material. Transurethral incision of the ureterocele effectively relieves the obstruction, but it may

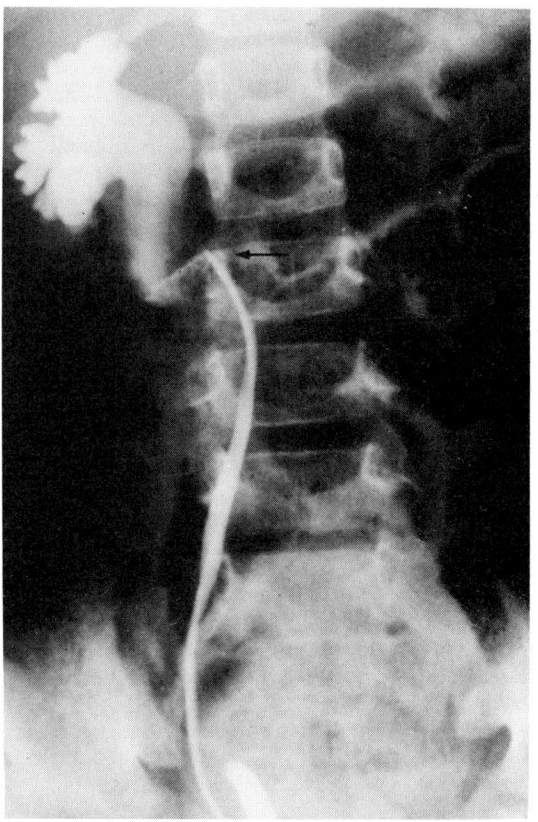

Figure 17–33. Circumcaval ureter. Retrograde pyelogram showing medial deviation of a dilated upper ureter to the level of the 3rd lumbar vertebra, characteristic of a circumcaval ureter.

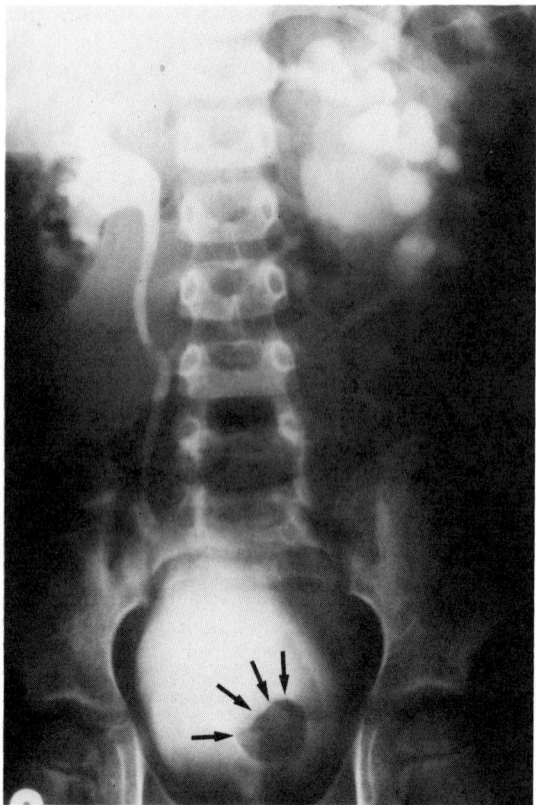

Figure 17–34. Simple intravesical ureterocele. Excretory urogram showing left hydronephrosis and a round filling defect on the left side of the bladder corresponding to a simple ureterocele causing left ureteral obstruction.

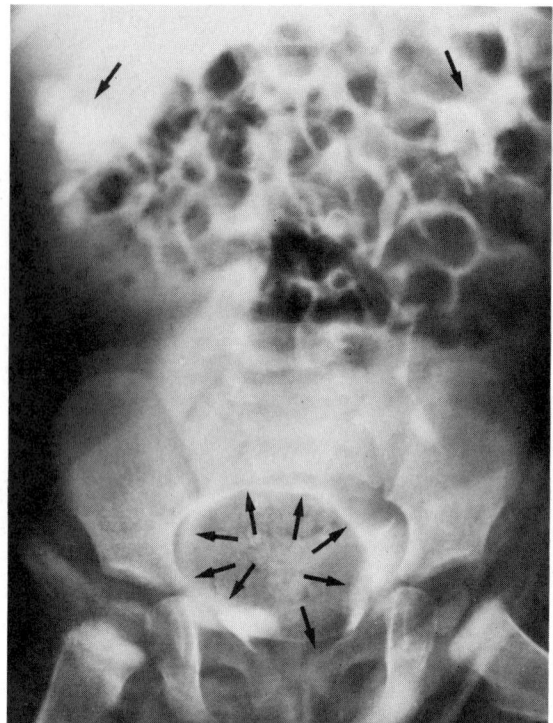

Figure 17–35. Bilateral ectopic ureteroceles. Excretory urogram of a 1 yr old girl with a history of febrile urinary tract infections. The large filling defect in the bladder represents bilateral ectopic ureteroceles. The visualized portion of the upper urinary tracts reveals only the lower moiety of the duplicated kidneys, with characteristic drooping lily configuration. The upper moieties drained by the ureters involved in the ureteroceles function poorly and are not opacified. The majority of cases of ectopic ureteroceles are unilateral.

result in vesicoureteral reflux necessitating ureteral reimplantation later. Some prefer open excision of the ureterocele and reimplantation as the initial form of treatment. Small, simple ureteroceles incidentally discovered without upper tract dilatation may not require treatment. In questionable cases diuresis renography and pressure flow studies (see above) are useful.

More commonly, ureteroceles are associated with ureteral duplication. The ureter involved with the ureterocele drains the upper renal moiety, which frequently functions poorly or is dysplastic because of congenital obstruction. The more cephalad ureter drains the lower renal moiety and frequently refluxes. These *ectopic ureteroceles* may extend submucosally into the posterior urethra. Affected children also present with urinary tract infections. Rarely, large ectopic ureteroceles may cause bladder outlet obstruction and retention of urine; and in females the ureterocele may prolapse from the urethral meatus. Reflux to the ipsilateral lower segment ureter is common. Contralateral reflux is usually present when the bladder neck is obstructed. Both simple and ectopic ureteroceles can be bilateral. Intravenous pyelography usually shows a large filling defect in the bladder corresponding to the ureterocele and characteristic findings of duplication of the collecting systems (poor or absent function of the upper collecting system and total displacement of the lower collecting system) (Fig. 17–35).

Treatment of ectopic ureteroceles is the excision of the upper collecting system, involving partial nephrectomy and ureterectomy. When the ectopic ureterocele is small and there is low grade or no reflux in the ipsilateral duplicated ureter, the decompressed ureterocele need not be excised and usually will cause no further problems. Large ureteroceles, however, or those with high grade reflux to the ipsilateral lower ureter

are best treated by excision of the ureterocele and reimplantation of the remaining ureter, plus partial upper moiety nephroureterectomy. This can usually be accomplished in a single operation. In the treatment of an acutely ill, septic infant with an obstructing ureterocele, drainage of the involved collecting system may be necessary, either transureterally or (preferably) by percutaneous nephrostomy of the upper collecting system.

Megaureter. This term refers generally to the dilated ureter. A classification of megaureters is given in Table 17–14. In this section, primary obstructed and nonrefluxing nonobstructed megaureters will be discussed. Megaureters are usually discovered through intravenous urography done for urinary tract infections, hematuria, or abdominal pain. A careful history, physical examination, and voiding cystourethrography will help rule out causes of secondary megaureters and refluxing

Table 17–14. **International Classification of Megaureters***

	Primary	Secondary
Obstructed	Intrinsic ureteral obstruction	Associated with urethral obstruction or extrinsic lesions
Refluxing	Reflux is only abnormality	Associated with bladder outlet obstruction or neurogenic bladder
Nonrefluxing, nonobstructed	Idiopathic ureteral dilatation	Associated with polyuria (diabetes insipidus) or infection

*King, LR: Ureter and ureterovesical junction. In: Kelalis PP, King LR, Belman AB (eds): Clinical Pediatric Urology. Philadelphia, WB Saunders, 1985, p 486.

megaureters as well as the prune-belly syndrome. Primary obstructed megaureters and nonobstructed megaureters probably represent opposite extremes of a spectrum of the same anomaly.

Radiographically, the distal ureter is more dilated in its distal segment and tapers abruptly at or above the junction of the bladder (Fig. 17–36). The lesion may be unilateral or bilateral. When the upper collecting system shows dilatation and calyceal blunting, the diagnosis of obstruction is clear. In other cases, however, pressure flow studies (Whitaker, see above) are necessary to differentiate between obstructed and nonobstructed megaureters. The former require surgical treatment, with tapering and reimplantation of the ureter. The results of surgical reconstruction are usually good but the prognosis depends on pre-existing renal function and whether complications develop.

Prune-Belly Syndrome. This syndrome, also called abdominal muscle deficiency syndrome or Eagle-Barrett syndrome, occurs in approximately 1 in 40,000 births. The characteristic association of deficient abdominal muscles, undescended testes, and urinary tract abnormalities probably results from severe urethral obstruction in fetal life (Fig. 17–37). Oligohydramnios and pulmonary dysplasia are frequent complications in the perinatal period. Many affected infants are stillborn. Urinary tract abnormalities include massive dilatation of the ureters and upper tracts, and a very large bladder, with a patent urachus or a urachal diverticulum. There may be vesicoureteral reflux. The prostatic urethra is usually dilated and the prostate is hypoplastic. The anterior urethra may be dilated, resulting in a megalourethra. Rarely, there is urethral stenosis or atresia. The kidneys usually show various degrees of dysplasia, and the testes are usually intra-abdominal. There often is malrotation of the bowel with a universal mesentery. Cardiac abnormalities occur in 10% of cases, and over 50% have abnormalities of the musculoskeletal system, including limb abnormalities and scoliosis. Only about 3% of patients with prune-belly syndrome are females.

In the majority of patients there is no demonstrable obstruction of the urinary tract at the time of birth, and treatment is symptomatic for urinary tract infections. In a minority of cases obstruction of the ureters or urethra can be demonstrated or suspected, and temporary drainage procedures such as pye-

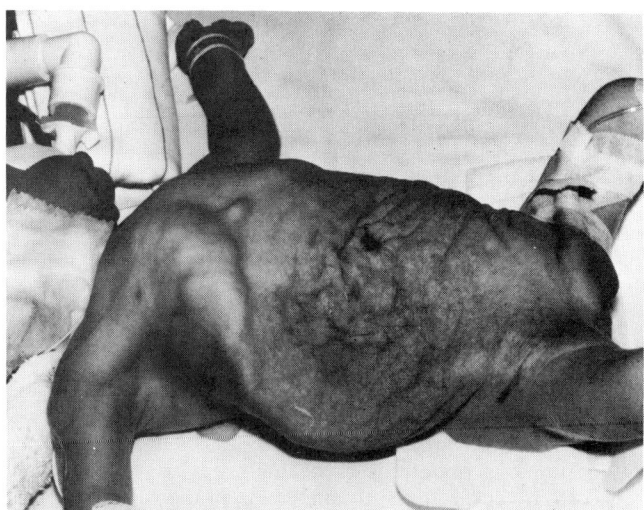

Figure 17–37. Eagle-Barrett syndrome. Photograph of a 1600-gm newborn with the prune-belly syndrome. Note the lack of tonicity of the abdominal wall and the wrinkled appearance of the skin.

lostomies or vesicostomies may help to preserve renal function until the child is old enough for reconstructive surgery. Some children with prune-belly syndrome have been found to have classic or atypical posterior urethral valves. Urinary tract infections are frequent and should be treated promptly. Antibacterial prophylaxis is often necessary. Correction of the undescended testis by orchidopexy in these children can be quite difficult and is best accomplished in the 1st yr of life. The prognosis ultimately depends on the degree of pulmonary and renal dysplasia.

Bladder Neck Obstruction. Bladder neck obstruction is usually secondary to ectopic ureteroceles, bladder calculi, or tumors of the prostate (rhabdomyosarcoma). The manifestations include difficulty voiding, urinary retention, urinary tract infection, and bladder distension with overflow incontinence. Apparent bladder neck obstruction is common in cases of posterior urethral valves, but it seldom has any functional significance. Primary bladder neck obstruction is exceptional in males and, according to current thinking, probably never occurs in females. Functional bladder neck obstruction can also result from nonrelaxation of the bladder neck in neurogenic bladder dysfunction.

Posterior Urethral Valves. The most common type of urethral valves are located in the posterior urethra. They are sail-shaped membranes that arise from the verumontanum in males and extend distally and attach to the anterolateral walls of the urethra. Valves are congenitally abnormal structures of unclear embryologic origin, and cause varying degrees of obstruction. The prostatic urethra dilates and the detrusor muscle hypertrophies. There may be vesicoureteral reflux or distal ureteral obstruction resulting from a chronically distended bladder or bladder muscle hypertrophy. The renal changes range from mild hydronephrosis to severe dysplasia; their severity probably depends on the severity of the obstruction and the time of its onset in fetal life. As in other cases of obstruction or renal dysplasia, there may be oligohydramnios and pulmonary hypoplasia.

With increasing frequency, posterior urethral valves are being discovered prenatally when maternal ultrasonography reveals bilateral hydronephrosis, a dilated bladder, and, if the obstruction is severe, oligohydramnios. In the male neonate posterior urethral valves are suspected when there is a palpably distended bladder and the urinary stream is weak. If the obstruction is severe and goes unrecognized during the neonatal period, infants will present later in life with failure to

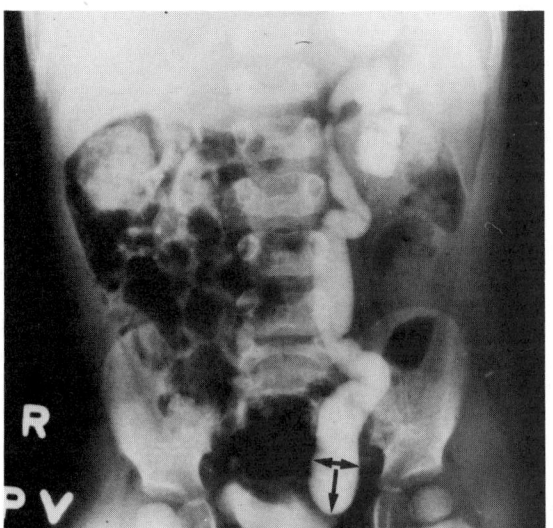

Figure 17–36. Obstructed megaureter. Excretory urogram in a girl with a history of a febrile urinary tract infection. The right side is normal. The left side reveals hydroureteronephrosis with predominant dilatation of the distal ureter. Note the characteristic appearance of the distal ureter. There was no vesicoureteral reflux. The diagnosis of obstruction was confirmed by pressure-flow studies.

thrive due to uremia or sepsis caused by infection in the obstructed urinary tract. With lesser degrees of obstruction children present later in life with difficulty in maintaining urinary continence during the daytime or with urinary tract infections. The diagnosis is established by voiding cystoure-thrography (Fig. 17–38).

Vesicoureteral reflux is present in two thirds of cases and may be unilateral or bilateral. The prognosis for renal function is worse when reflux is present. Once the diagnosis is established, renal function and the anatomy of the upper urinary tract should be carefully evaluated. In the healthy neonate, a small polyethylene feeding tube (5F or 8F) is inserted in the bladder and left indwelling for several days. If the serum creatinine level remains normal or returns to normal, treatment is by primary ablation of the valves through a trans-urethral approach or by temporary vesicostomy. If the urethral caliber is insufficient for transurethral ablation, temporary vesicostomy is preferred, to be followed by closure of the vesicostomy and transurethral ablation of the valves at a later date when the growth of the child allows urethral instrumentation.

If the serum creatinine level remains high or increases despite bladder drainage by a small catheter, secondary ureteral obstruction, irreversible renal damage, or renal dysplasia should be suspected. In such cases upper tract drainage by cutaneous pyelostomy or high ureterostomy is necessary. If renal function does not improve, the child should have reconstructive surgery at a relatively early age to prevent infections and restore bladder function before the need for renal transplantation arises. If renal function improves between the ages of 6 mo and 1 yr, the ureters are re-evaluated by pressure flow studies. Distal obstruction caused by hypertrophy of the detrusor muscle may reverse spontaneously; if it persists, however, the child should have ablation of the valves, closure of the pyelostomies, and correction of the distal ureteral obstruction.

Infants presenting later in life with uremia without infection should be evaluated and treated following identical guidelines. In the septic and uremic infant, lifesaving measures must include prompt correction of the electrolyte imbalance and control of the infection by appropriate antibiotics. Drainage of the upper tracts by percutaneous nephrostomy and hemodialysis are frequently required. After the patient's condition becomes stable, step-by-step evaluation and treatment can be undertaken. Prolonged use of intubated nephrostomy drainage is inconvenient for the parents, introduces infection, and is generally detrimental to renal function.

Most children presenting with incontinence can be treated by primary valve ablation. When vesicoureteral reflux is present, expectant treatment and suppressive doses of anti-bacterial drugs are advisable; however, if reflux persists more than 1 yr after ablation of the valves and if the function of the involved kidney warrants it, surgical correction should be undertaken.

There is some degree of urinary incontinence in up to 50% of children after treatment of posterior urethral valves. Assuming there has been no surgical damage to the sphincter, the dilatation of the prostatic urethra, poor bladder compliance, and polyuria from renal damage are all important factors that contribute to incontinence. Urinary incontinence usually improves with age, particularly after puberty. The prognosis in the newborn is related to the degree of pulmonary hypoplasia and potential for recovery of renal function. Severely affected infants are often stillborn. Of those who survive the neonatal period, approximately one third will retain some degree of renal insuffiency and many will eventually require renal transplantation.

Urethral Strictures. Urethral strictures *in males* are rarely congenital. They usually result from urethral trauma, either iatrogenic (catheterization, endoscopic procedures, or previous urethral reconstruction) or accidental (straddling injuries or pelvic fractures). Because these lesions develop gradually, the decrease in force of the urinary stream is seldom noticed by the child or his parents. More commonly, the obstruction causes symptoms of bladder instability, hematuria, or dysuria. Catheterization of the bladder is usually impossible. The diagnosis is made by a voiding film obtained during intravenous urography; retrograde urethrography and endoscopy are confirmatory. Endoscopic treatment of short strictures by dilatation or internal urethrotomy is usually successful. Longer strictures surrounded by periurethral fibrosis often require urethroplasty. Repeated endoscopic procedures should generally be avoided, since they may cause additional urethral damage.

In females true urethral strictures are exceptional, since the female urethra is protected from trauma, particularly in childhood. Until recently it was thought that urethral ring commonly caused obstruction of the female urethra and urinary tract infection, and that affected girls benefited from urethral dilatation. The diagnosis was suspected when a "spinning top" deformity of the urethra was found in the voiding cystourethrogram and was confirmed by urethral calibration. Treatment for this condition invariably included antibiotic therapy, and adequately controlled studies were not done. Moreover, other studies have found no correlation between the radiologic appearance of the urethra in the voiding cysto-urethrogram and the urethral caliber and no significant difference in urethral caliber between females with recurrent cystitis and normal age-matched controls. This area remains somewhat controversial, but we hold that endoscopy and urethral dilatation are seldom justified solely by the radiologic appearance of the urethra or by a history of recurrent urinary tract infections.

Anterior Urethral Valves and Urethral Diverticula in the Male. *Anterior urethral valves* are usually associated with congenital urethral diverticulum. They are considerably rarer than valves of the posterior urethra, but they may cause similar symptoms and have identical effects on the urinary tract. The

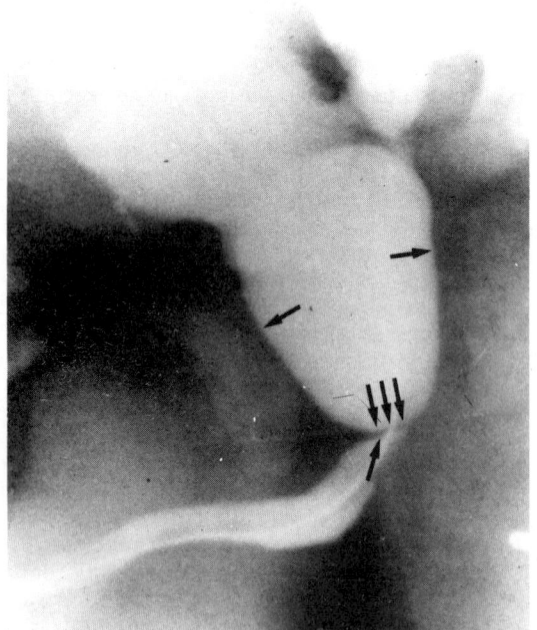

Figure 17–38. Posterior urethral valves. Voiding cystourethrogram in an infant with posterior urethral valves. Note the dilatation of the prostatic urethra and the transverse linear filling defect corresponding to the valves.

diagnosis is established on voiding cystourethrography. *Urethral diverticula* are discovered on voiding cystourethrography, often during evaluation for hematuria or urinary tract infections. Many diverticula are believed to arise from dilatations of Cowper glands and ducts. Small diverticula require no treatment; larger ones are usually managed endoscopically.

Fusiform dilatation of the urethra or megalourethra may result from underdevelopment of the corpus spongiosum and support structures of the urethra. This is commonly associated with the prune-belly syndrome.

Male Urethral Meatal Stenosis. Congenital stenosis of the urethral meatus in the male is rare. It has in the past probably been overdiagnosed, and unrelated conditions, such as nocturnal enuresis, have been blamed on presumed meatal stenosis. True urethral meatal stenosis (a meatus less than 8F in boys under 4 yr old or less than 10F in prepubertal boys over the age of 10) usually results from inflammation associated with ammoniacal dermatitis of the glans following neonatal circumcision. Children with hypospadias rarely may have stenosis of the urethral meatus. The treatment of symptomatic urethral meatal stenosis is by a meatoplasty with careful follow-up to avoid reapproximation of the edges of the enlarged meatus.

17.41 OTHER DISORDERS AND ANOMALIES OF THE BLADDER

BLADDER EXSTROPHY

Exstrophy of the urinary bladder occurs about once in every 10,000–40,000 births. It is more common in boys than in girls. The severity ranges from a small cutaneous fistula in the abdominal wall or simple epispadias to complete exstrophy of the cloaca involving exposure of the entire hindgut and the bladder.

These anomalies result when the mesoderm fails to invade the cephalad extension of the cloacal membrane; the extent of this failure determines the degree of the anomaly. In classic bladder exstrophy (Fig. 17–39), the bladder protrudes from the abdominal wall and its mucosa is exposed. The umbilicus is displaced downward, the pubic rami are widely separated in the midline, and the recti muscles are separated. In males there is complete epispadias with a wide and shallow scrotum.

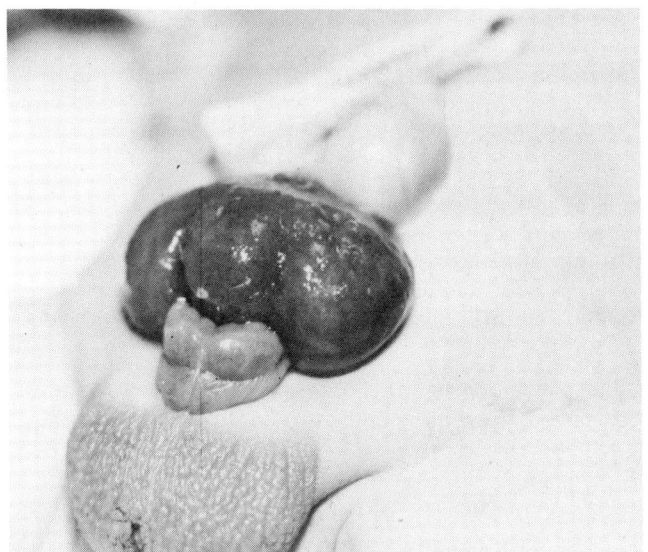

Figure 17–39. Classical bladder exstrophy. The bladder is exposed in the midline, the umbilical cord is caudally displaced, the penis is epispadiac, and the scrotum is broad.

Undescended testes and inguinal hernias are common. Females also have epispadias, with duplication of the clitoris and wide separation of the labia. The anus is displaced anteriorly in both sexes, and there may be rectal prolapse. The consequences of untreated bladder exstrophy are total urinary incontinence and increased incidence of bladder cancer, usually adenocarcinoma. The genital deformities produce sexual disability in both sexes, but particularly in the male. The wide separation of the pubic rami causes a characteristic broad-based gait but no significant disability.

Treatment for bladder exstrophy should start at birth. The bladder should be covered with a Silastic shield or another appropriate plastic dressing that will prevent desiccation of the bladder mucosa but allow urinary drainage. Application of gauze or vaseline-gauze to the bladder mucosa is to be avoided. The infant should then be transferred promptly to a center equipped for the treatment of such anomalies.

Closure of the exstrophied bladder is the preferred treatment, ideally performed during the first 48 hr of life before permanent changes in the bladder wall are established. At this time the flexibility of the pelvic joints allows precise reconstruction of the bladder and prostatic urethra in the male, with approximation of the pubic rami and reconstruction of the abdominal wall without the iliac osteostomies that are often required in the older child. This treatment can be applied to more than three fourths of infants with classic bladder exstrophy. Treatment should be deferred in certain exceptional circumstances when surgery would be excessively risky or complex, such as when the bladder is extremely small or there are upper tract changes, or when there are complex genital anomalies such as complete duplication of the penis.

The purpose of the initial operation is the precise closure of the bladder and prostatic urethra in the male, elongation of the urethral plate and penis, and closure of the abdominal wall. Postoperatively, the infant's upper urinary tract is watched closely for the possible development of hydronephrosis and infection. The majority of such infants have vesicoureteral reflux and should receive antibiotics. When the child is between 1 and 2 yr old, the resulting epispadias is repaired, to create an anterior urethra and correct the malformation of the penis. At about 3 yr of age, most children will have total incontinence, and bladder neck reconstruction with bilateral ureteral reimplantation is undertaken.

This plan of treatment has yielded less than 15% deterioration of the upper urinary tract and over 70% continence in some centers. This continence rate reflects not only the successful reconstruction but also the quality and size of the bladder. It appears that children who have reconstructive surgery as newborns have a greater chance for obtaining a normally functioning bladder. Children whose sphincters cannot be successfully reconstructed should have artificial sphincters implanted. If the cause of incontinence is a small bladder capacity, an augmentation cystoplasty using a segment of the large bowel will help obtain continence. The exceptional children whose anomaly cannot be reconstructed can have a urinary diversion by means of a sigmoid urinary conduit with an abdominal stoma. Ureterosigmoidostomy has been popular in the past and is still employed in some centers; it is attractive because it avoids the need for external urinary diversion. This operation, however, carries a significant risk of chronic pyelonephritis, of upper urinary tract damage, of electrolyte imbalance resulting from absorption of hydrogen ion and chloride in the intestine, and of colonic carcinoma after a long latency period.

Other Exstrophy Anomalies

The more complex cases of *cloacal exstrophy* may have severe abnormalities of the colon and the rectum and often have a short bowel syndrome. Mortality in infancy is high for such patients, but some can undergo genital reconstruction and others can be helped with permanent urinary diversions and colostomies. Because genital reconstruction in males with cloacal exstrophy is extremely difficult, most authors recommend assigning female gender to such infants.

Epispadias is in the spectrum of exstrophy anomalies. Distal epispadias should be repaired by reconstructing the urethra and the penis. The more severe cases of epispadias also have separation of the pubic rami and urinary incontinence. Such children require surgical reconstructions analogous to those of the second and third stages of management of patients with classic bladder exstrophy.

BLADDER DIVERTICULA

Bladder diverticula usually occur at the ureterovesical junction and are associated with vesicoureteral reflux (see Fig. 17–26). Congenital diverticula in other locations also occur. Bladder diverticula are also commonly associated with distal urethral obstruction or neurogenic bladder dysfunction. Small diverticula require no treatment other than that of the primary disease, whereas large diverticula may contribute to inefficient voiding, residual urine, urinary stasis, and urinary tract infections and should be excised.

URACHAL ANOMALIES

Urachal abnormalities are more common in males than in females. A patent urachus can occur as an isolated anomaly, and should be corrected surgically, or may be associated with prune-belly syndrome. Other anomalies related to the urachus are cysts and bladder diverticula and umbilical sinus; these should be excised.

17.42 NEUROGENIC BLADDER

Neurogenic bladder dysfunction in children is often congenital and may result from myelomeningocele, lipomeningocele, sacral agenesis, or other spinal abnormalities. Acquired diseases and traumatic lesions of the spinal cord are less frequent. Cerebral palsy, central nervous system tumors and their treatment, and pelvic operations such as repair of imperforate anus or excision of a sacrococcygeal teratoma can result in abnormal innervation of the bladder and the sphincters. The two most important consequences of neurogenic bladder dysfunction are upper tract deterioration and urinary incontinence.

Renal damage is the result of lack of coordination between the contraction of the detrusor muscle and the relaxation of the sphincter, normally a function located in the brain stem. This dyssynergia results in functional obstruction of the bladder outlet leading to high intravesical pressures, bladder muscle hypertrophy and trabeculation, vesicoureteral reflux, and rapid deterioration of the upper tracts. Infection often compounds the problem. For example, vesicoureteral reflux is present in 30% of neonates with myelomeningocele and develops later in life in another 20%. Reflux secondary to neurogenic bladder has much more severe consequences than primary reflux. However, not all children with myelomeningocele (or any other neurologic anomaly) have similar patterns of lower tract dysfunction, so that its occurrence cannot be predicted accurately from the neurologic examination or radiographic appearance of the spine. Accordingly, accurate urodynamic studies (by cystometrography and sphincter electromyography) and radiologic evaluation of the urinary tract are required in every case. If the bladder is atonic or the sphincters denervated, bladder pressure tends to be low, and vesicoureteral reflux is unlikely to develop even when bladder emptying is incomplete.

Urinary incontinence in the child with neurogenic bladder can result from total or partial denervation of the sphincter, from bladder hyper-reflexia or poor bladder compliance, from chronic urinary retention, or from a combination of factors. The treatment of children with neurogenic bladder aims at protecting the upper urinary tracts and eventually providing continence. Supravesical diversion, once commonly performed to achieve these goals, yielded unsatisfactory long-term results and is now seldom employed. The neonate with low intravesical pressures and no vesicoureteral reflux can be treated expectantly with follow-up renal ultrasonography to detect possible development of hydronephrosis and radioisotopic cystography for the early detection of reflux. Occasionally, limited intravenous pyelography is needed as well. Recurrent urinary tract infections may require prolonged antibiotic prophylaxis (Sec. 17.38). Urodynamic studies should be repeated at 6 mo of age to detect possible neurologic changes following repair of the myelomeningocele.

When reflux is present or there are elevated intravesical pressures (indicative of high risk for developing reflux), treatment with antibacterial prophylaxis, intermittent catheterization, and often anticholinergic drugs (oxybutynin up to 0.4 mg/kg/24 hr in 2 divided doses) will cure the reflux in up to 40% of patients without ureteral dilatation (grades I and II). Children with more severe reflux require corrective surgery followed by intermittent catheterization and anticholinergic drugs. When intermittent catheterization is impossible, as may be the case in male neonates and small infants, when there are urethral abnormalities that preclude catheterization, or when anticholinergics are not well tolerated, a temporary cutaneous vesicostomy provides effective, temporary bladder decompression. Failure of these methods to relieve intravesical pressures is an indication for augmentation enterocystoplasty and intermittent catheterization. Attempts to denervate the bladder to control bladder hypertonicity have yielded unsatisfactory long-term results.

The treatment of incontinence should be tailored to the individual case. If the sphincter tone is sufficient and the bladder has adequate compliance, intermittent catheterization every 4 hr is usually successful in keeping the child dry. Anticholinergic drugs are sometimes needed to relax the bladder and enhance continence. Most children 7 or 8 yr old who have adequate manual dexterity, can learn the technique of intermittent self-catheterization. Bacteriuria is seen in up to 50% of children using intermittent self-catheterization, but it seldom causes symptoms. In the absence of reflux, there seems to be little cause for concern. Antibacterial prophylaxis can often be effective in keeping the urine sterile while intermittent catheterization is used.

When the bladder capacity and compliance are adequate but the urethral resistance is low, implantation of an artificial sphincter is usually successful. This sphincter consists of an inflatable cuff that is placed around the bladder neck, a pressure-regulating balloon implanted in the extraperitoneal space, and a pumping mechanism that is implanted in the scrotum of males and in the labia of females. On rare occasions, bladder augmentation by enterocystoplasty alone or in combination with other means to increase outlet resistance is necessary, along with intermittent catheterization. With the treatment as outlined above and lifelong follow-up, urinary diversion can be avoided in most cases, children can reach a satisfactory degree of continence, and the chances of upper tract deterioration are low.

17.43 VOIDING DYSFUNCTION
Nocturnal Enuresis

Enuresis is the occurrence of involuntary voiding at an age when volitional control of micturition is expected. *Nocturnal enuresis* without overt daytime voiding symptoms affects up to 20% of children at the age of 5 yr; it ceases spontaneously in approximately 15% of the involved children every year thereafter. Its frequency among adults is probably less than 1%. The cause of nocturnal enuresis is not precisely known but appears to involve delayed maturation of the cortical mechanisms that allow voluntary control of the micturition reflex. The disorder can be primary (when the child never has a period of night-time continence) or secondary (developing in a formerly "dry" child following some emotionally disruptive event). Nocturnal enuresis is 3 times more common in males than in females, and there is often a family history of bedwetting.

The child with nocturnal enuresis should be examined carefully for neurologic and spinal abnormalities. A careful history should be obtained especially with respect to fluid intake and urinary output. Children with diabetes insipidus, diabetes mellitus, and chronic renal disease may have high obligatory urinary output and a compensatory polydipsia. A complete examination should include palpation of the abdomen and rectal examination after voiding, to assess the possibility of a chronically distended bladder. If possible, the child should be watched during micturition to observe the force and quality of the urinary stream; measurement of the urinary flow rate helps rule out obstructive lesions. Bacteriuria has increased frequency in enuretic girls and, if found, should be investigated and treated (Sec. 17.38), though this will not always lead to resolution of bedwetting. Urinalysis should be obtained after an overnight fast and evaluated for specific gravity or osmolality or both in order to exclude polyuria as a cause of frequency and incontinence and to ascertain that the concentrating ability is normal. The absence of glycosuria should be confirmed. Urine culture should be done routinely. If there are no daytime symptoms and if the physical examination, urinalysis, and culture are normal, then further evaluation for urinary tract pathology is not warranted, even in older children.

The best approach to treatment is to assure parents that the problem is self-limited and to eliminate punitive measures that may adversely affect the psychologic development of the child. Fluid restriction, midnight awakening to void, or systems of reward and punishment are usually unsuccessful. Treatment with imipramine, which decreases the frequency of voiding and alters the sleep pattern, may produce dry nights, but enuresis usually recurs when this therapy is discontinued; considering the potential hazards of this treatment, its use is rarely justified except in an older child whose self-esteem is being eroded. Treatment with vasopressin analogues, such as desamino-D-arginine vasopressin, a drug that drastically reduces urine output during the night, also decreases the frequency of enuresis by 50%, but the beneficial results do not outlast the treatment period, and long-term side effects have not been investigated. Treatment by conditioning with an alarm that wakes the child when voiding occurs can succeed in converting nocturnal enuresis to nocturia, but this requires a considerable degree of commitment by both child and parents.

Non-neurogenic Voiding Dysfunction

Voiding dysfunction not related to neurologic abnormalities or dysfunction is common in children. The child with an uninhibited bladder usually exhibits urinary frequency, urgency, and episodes of diurnal urinary incontinence with or without bladder pain. Such symptoms are seen also in about 15% of children with nocturnal enuresis, but sometimes the daytime symptoms predominate and certainly always have greater psychosocial consequences, particularly in school' age children. In females, a history of recurrent urinary tract infection is common, but incontinence may persist long after infections are brought under control. It is not clear in these cases if the voiding dysfunction is a sequel of the infections or if the voiding dysfunction disposes to recurrent infections. In other female cases and usually in male cases, there is no antecedent history of infection and the cause of uninhibited bladder is obscure. Many authors attribute it to a delayed maturation of the neurologic mechanisms that modulate the spinal micturition reflex. Bladder outlet obstructions result in detrusor hyper-reflexia and also can lead to uninhibited bladder contractions.

In the evaluation of affected children, a careful history helps rule out the possibility of previous urinary tract infections. The physical examination is directed at detecting neurologic abnormalities and residual urine after voiding. Urinalysis and urine culture rule out infection and causes of polyuria. Examination of the urinary flow rate by visual inspection of the urinary stream or, ideally, with a uroflowmeter helps rule out gross urethral obstruction. Abdominal ultrasonography excludes hydronephrosis and gross bladder abnormalities and confirms the completeness of bladder emptying. In males, voiding cystourethrography is usually necessary to rule out bladder or urethral abnormalities. If the evaluation rules out significant urinary tract pathology, a therapeutic trial with oxybutynin or other anticholinergic drugs is warranted and often effective. The treatment is usually prolonged and should be interrupted periodically to determine its continued need. If there is a history of cystitis but no other abnormalities such as vesicoureteral reflux that require additional evaluation and treatment, prophylactic antibacterial agents help prevent recurrence of infection which can exacerbate bladder instability. Children not responding to this simple treatment should be evaluated endoscopically and urodynamically to rule out other possible forms of bladder or sphincter dysfunction.

Non-neurogenic Neurogenic Bladder

This is a more serious but less common disorder involving failure of the external sphincter to relax during voiding, in children without neurologic abnormalities. Children with this syndrome, also called non-neurogenic detrusor/sphincter dyssynergia, exhibit daytime and night-time wetting. There is usually a history of urinary tract infections and constipation, with or without encopresis. Evaluation of affected children usually reveals vesicoureteral reflux, a trabeculated bladder, and decreased urinary flow rate with an intermittent pattern. The pathogenesis of this syndrome appears to involve problems during toilet training, since the syndrome is not seen in children before the age when voluntary micturition occurs. The treatment is usually difficult and requires appropriate treatment of the reflux with antibacterial prophylaxis. Behavioral modification and encouragement of relaxation during voiding are sometimes useful. Biofeedback has been used successfully in older children to teach relaxation of the external sphincter. Some investigators have recommended intermittent catheterization and anticholinergic drugs to decrease intravesical pressures; others have administered diazepam to facilitate relaxation of the external sphincter. These children require long-term treatment and careful follow-up, since severe renal damage is likely to occur.

Infrequent Voiding

Infrequent voiding is a common disorder of micturition usually associated with urinary tract infections. Affected children, usually girls, void only twice a day rather than the normal three to five times. With bladder overdistension and prolonged retention of urine, growth of bacteria leads to recurrent urinary tract infections. Some such children are

Table 17–15. **Urinary Incontinence in Childhood**

With Complete Bladder Emptying:	
Ectopic ureter and fistulas	Neurogenic
Sphincter failure (with total or partial incontinence)	Traumatic
	Iatrogenic
Urgency Incontinence:	
Detrusor hyperactivity is caused by inflammation, neurogenic dysfunction, or detrusor instability secondary to functional or mechanical obstruction	Cystitis
	Unstable bladder
	Neurogenic bladder
	Hyperreflexia
	Bladder outlet obstruction
	Noncompliant bladder, neurogenic or non-neurogenic
	Detrusor sphincter dyssynergia, neurogenic or non-neurogenic
With Incomplete Bladder Emptying:	
Overflow incontinence (incomplete bladder emptying may be due to decompensated obstruction or paralysis of the detrusor muscle)	Bladder outlet obstruction (e.g., posterior urethral valves)
	Neurogenic detrusor areflexia
	Detrusor sphincter dyssynergia, neurogenic or non-neurogenic
	Behavioral
Other:	
Combination of above	Multiple factors

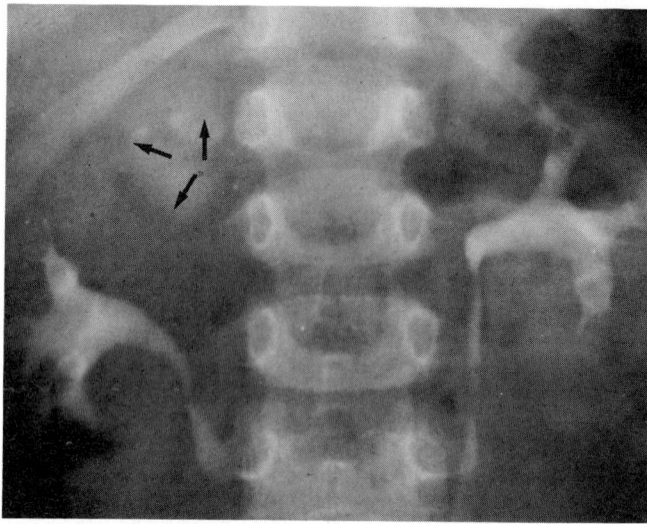

Figure 17–40. Duplication of the right collecting system with ectopic ureter. Excretory urogram in a female presenting with a normal voiding pattern and constant urinary dribbling. The left kidney is normal and the right side, well visualized, is the lower collecting system of a duplicated kidney. On the upper pole opposite the first and second vertebral bodies, note accumulation of contrast material corresponding to a poorly functioning upper pole drained by a ureter opening in the vestibule.

constipated. There is sometimes a family history of infrequent voiding. Some of these children also have occasional episodes of incontinence due to overflow or urgency. The etiology of this disorder appears to be behavioral. When the children have urinary tract infections, the treatment is by antibacterial prophylaxis, and encouragement of frequent voiding and of complete emptying of the bladder by double voiding until a normal pattern of micturition is re-established.

Table 17–15 lists other causes of urinary incontinence. *Ureteral ectopia*, usually associated with a duplicated collecting system in girls, can produce urinary incontinence characterized by constant dribbling of urine during day and night, in addition to a normal voiding pattern. Sometimes the urine production from the renal segment drained by the ectopic ureter is small and urinary drainage is confused with watery vaginal discharge. Children with a history of vaginal discharge or incontinence and an abnormal voiding pattern require careful study. The ectopic orifice is usually difficult to find. On intravenous urography, one may suspect duplication of the collecting system (Fig. 17–40), but the upper collecting system drained by the ectopic ureter usually has poor or very delayed function. Ultrasonography and CT scan of the kidneys help rule out subtle duplication that may not be discovered on intravenous urography. Examination under anesthesia for an ectopic ureteral orifice in the vestibule or the vagina is often necessary (Fig. 17–41). The treatment in these cases is by partial nephroureterectomy, removing the involved segment of the duplicated kidney and the ureter down to the pelvic brim.

17.44 OTHER DISEASES AND ANOMALIES OF THE PENIS AND URETHRA

Hypospadias. Hypospadias occurs in approximately 1 of 500 newborns. In the mildest cases the urethral meatus opens on the ventral aspect of the glans, there are various degrees of malformation of the glans, and the prepuce is defective ventrally with the appearance of a dorsal hood. With increasing degrees of severity the penis is curved ventrally (chordee)

and the penile urethra is progressively shorter (Fig. 17–42), but the distance between the meatus and the glans may not increase significantly until the chordee is corrected. It is misleading, therefore, to classify hypospadias solely on the basis of the location of the meatus. In some cases, the meatus is at the penoscrotal junction; and in extreme cases, the

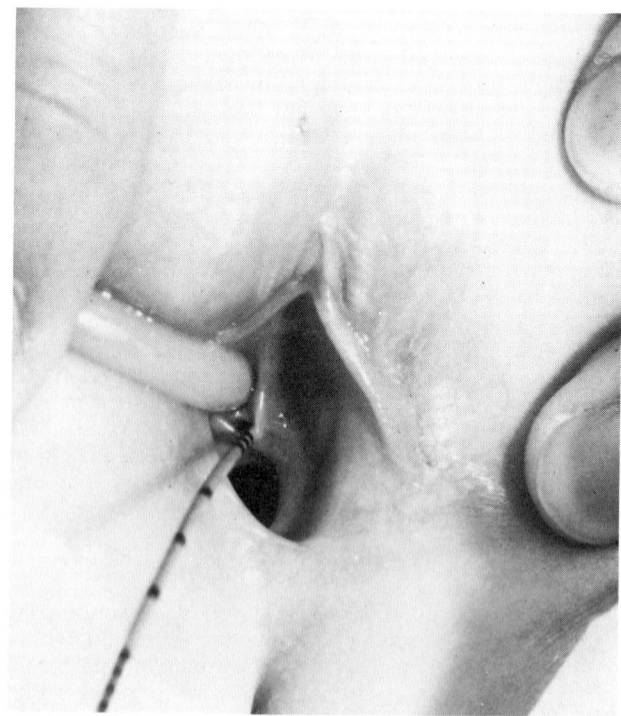

Figure 17–41. Ectopic ureter. The photograph shows an ectopic ureter entering the vestibule next to the urethral meatus. The thin ureteral catheter with transverse marks has been introduced into this ectopic ureter. This girl had a normal voiding pattern and constant urinary dribbling.

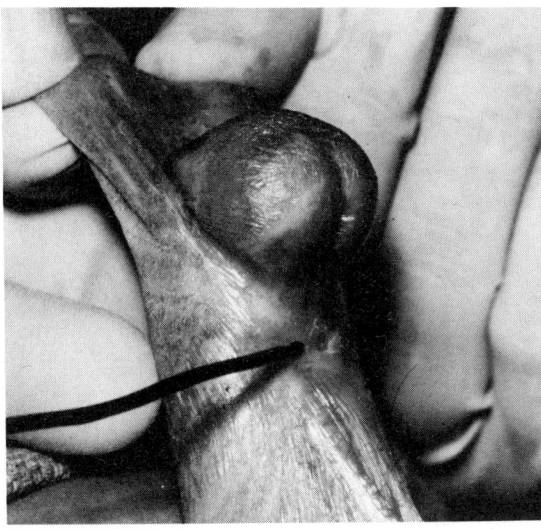

Figure 17–42. Distal hypospadias. Note the urethral meatus in the subcoronal position and the incomplete or hooded prepuce. There was no ventral curvature of the penis in this case.

urethra opens in the perineum, the scrotum is bifid and sometimes extends to the dorsal base of the penis (scrotal transposition), and the chordee is extreme (Fig. 17–43). In such cases, there is usually a dorsal urethral diverticulum opening at the level at the verumontanum, representing a vestige of müllerian structures. In variant cases ventral curvature of the penis occurs without a hypospadiac urethral meatus. In these cases, the prepuce is usually hooded and the corpus spongiosum may be underdeveloped.

Testes are undescended in 10% of boys with hypospadias. Inguinal hernias are also common. In the newborn period the differential diagnosis of severe penoscrotal and perineal hypospadias with undescended testes should include other forms of ambiguous genitalia, particularly masculinization of females (congenital adrenal hyperplasia). The incidence of other anomalies of the genitourinary tract in boys with hypospadias is low, and with the probable exception of the more severe cases of perineal hypospadias, radiographic studies of the urinary tract are not justified.

The treatment of hypospadias starts in the newborn period.

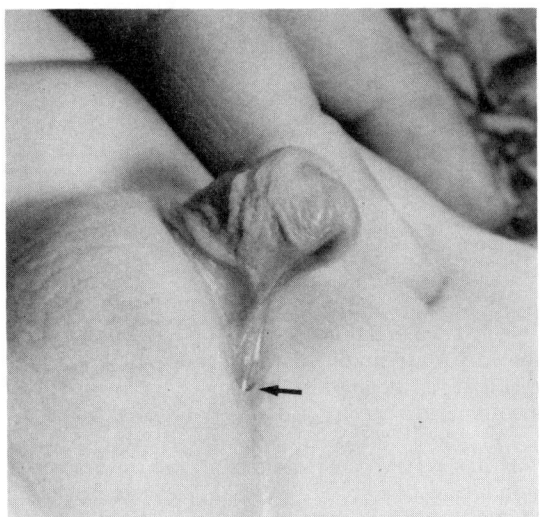

Figure 17–43. Severe perineoscrotal hypospadias. Note the ventral curvature and the underdeveloped ventral surface of the penis, the hooded prepuce, and the urethral meatus in the midline of the bifid scrotum. This child had palpable gonads and a normal chromosome pattern.

Routine circumcisions should be avoided, since the foreskin is often essential for repair later in life. Mild cases of hypospadias are usually repaired for cosmetic reasons alone, but with increasing severity, repair becomes essential in order to allow the child to void standing, to allow future normal sexual function, and to avoid psychologic consequences of having malformed external genitalia. The ideal age for repair is somewhat controversial; the current trend is to operate before the age of 18 mo. Most of these anomalies can now be repaired in a single operation with minimal hospitalization; accordingly, emotional trauma is less likely or severe now than with the older techniques. We prefer to do these repairs before the child is toilet trained and, if possible, during the 1st yr of life. Repair of hypospadias is a technically demanding operation and should be performed by surgeons with extensive experience.

Agenesis and Micropenis. *Agenesis* of the penis is rare and usually associated with anorectal and renal anomalies. If the child is viable, rearing as a female is recommended, with later genital reconstruction.

The length of the normal newborn penis is 3.5 ± 0.7 cm. *Micropenis* results from primary or secondary testicular failure during fetal life after morphogenesis is complete. Secondary congenital testicular failure is seen in anencephaly, pituitary agenesis, and Kallmann, Noonan, Prader-Willi and other syndromes. Other cases may be due to the presence of rudimentary testes, dwarfism, or maternal hormone administrations. Treatment options include a trial of hormonal stimulation, or rearing as female, with later genital reconstruction.

Phimosis and Paraphimosis. In 90% of uncircumcised males the prepuce becomes retractable by the age of 3 yr. Inability to retract the prepuce before this age is therefore not pathologic and not an indication for circumcision. *Phimosis* is the inability to retract the prepuce at an age when it should normally be retractable. Phimosis can be congenital or a sequel of inflammation. True phimosis usually requires surgical enlargement of the phimotic ring or circumcision. Accumulation of smegma under the infantile prepuce is not pathologic and does not require surgical treatment.

Paraphimosis occurs when a phimotic prepuce is retracted behind the coronal sulcus and this retraction cannot be reduced. This causes venous stasis distal to the corona, with edema leading to severe pain and inability to reduce the foreskin. If discovered early, the condition can be treated by reduction of the foreskin with appropriate lubrication, while the child is under heavy sedation or a short-acting general anesthetic. In some cases, circumcision is required.

Circumcision. There are no medical indications for routine neonatal circumcision. In the United States, circumcision is usually performed for cultural reasons, or because some believe that the circumcised penis is more hygienic and may be less prone to disease later in life. Both beliefs lack firm scientific foundation. Routine neonatal circumcision carries a very small but real risk of potentially serious complications, including sepsis, amputation of the distal part of the glans, removal of an excessive amount of foreskin, and the occurrence of urethrocutaneous fistulas.

Urethral Prolapse. Urethral prolapse is encountered predominantly in black females who exhibit vulvar bleeding (Fig. 17–44). Surgical excision and reapproximation of the mucosal edges is curative.

17.45 DISORDERS AND ANOMALIES OF THE SCROTAL CONTENTS

UNDESCENDED TESTES

Undescended and Ectopic Testes. Failure to find one or both testes in the scrotum may indicate any of a variety of

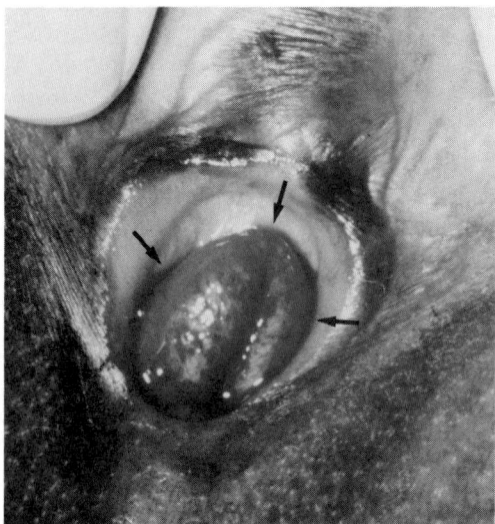

Figure 17–44. Urethral prolapse in a 4 yr old black girl who had blood spotting of her underwear.

congenital or acquired conditions, including true undescended testes, ectopic or maldescended testes, retractile testes, and absent testes.

True undescended testes and *maldescended or ectopic* testes can be differentiated from each other only by surgical exploration, and both conditions usually are referred to as cryptorchidism or hidden testes. The true undescended testis is found along the normal path of descent and the processus vaginalis is usually patent. The ectopic testis has completed its descent through the inguinal canal but ends up in a subcutaneous location other than the scrotum, the most common being a point lateral to the external inguinal ring, below the subcutaneous fascia. Cryptorchidism is present in 0.7% of children after 1 yr of age and in adults. The incidence is higher in full-term newborns (3.4%) and increases with prematurity (to 17% in infants with birthweights between 2000 and 2500 g and to 100% in those under 900 g). This reflects the fact that testicular descent from the inguinal canal into the scrotum takes place in the 7th mo of gestation. Spontaneous testicular descent does not occur after the age of 1 yr.

The consequences of cryptorchidism include infertility in adulthood, tumor development in the undescended testes, associated hernias, torsion of the cryptorchid testis, and the possible psychologic effects of an empty scrotum. Cryptorchidism is bilateral in up to 30% of cases. Infertility is the rule in adults with untreated bilateral cryptorchidism, and of those treated in childhood less than one third will be fertile. Infertility is common also (up to 50%) in adults with a history of unilateral cryptorchidism, suggesting that the contralateral testis is congenitally abnormal or that it has been damaged by an undetermined mechanism related to contralateral cryptorchidism.

The undescended testis is often histologically normal at birth, but failure of development and atrophy are detectable by the end of the 1st yr of life, and by the end of the 2nd yr the number of germ cells in the affected testis is severely reduced. Recent reports indicate that surgical correction at an early age results in a greater probability of fertility in adulthood. The patient with cryptorchidism has a 20 to 44% increase in risk of developing a malignant testicular tumor in the third or fourth decade of life. Patients with untreated intra-abdominal cryptorchidism or those who underwent surgical correction during or after puberty are at greatest risk. Some studies have suggested that although surgical correction of the cryptorchidism did not change the overall risk of malignant transformation, very few cases of tumors have been reported in patients whose operations were performed before the age of 8 yr. Carcinoma in situ is occasionally discovered when the testis is biopsied at the time of orchiopexy or during evaluation for infertility later in life; its significance is unclear. The most common tumor developing in undescended testes is the seminoma (60%); in contrast, seminomas represent only 30% of tumors occurring in normally descended testes.

Indirect inguinal hernias always accompany true undescended testes and are common with ectopic testes. Torsion and infarction of the undescended testis can occur because of excessive mobility of such testes. The treatment of the unilateral cryptorchid testis is best undertaken early in the 2nd yr of life. Most testes located extra-abdominally can be brought down to the scrotum and the associated hernia corrected with an operation (orchidopexy). This can often be performed without hospitalization. When the testis is not palpable, ultrasonography is used to determine its location. In the majority of cases, orchiopexy of the intra-abdominal testis located immediately inside the internal inguinal ring offers little difficulty, but orchidectomy should be considered in the more difficult cases or when the testis appears to be severely atrophied. Testicular prostheses are available for older children and adolescents when the absence of the gonad in the scrotum may have an undesirable psychologic effect.

Treatment of bilateral undescended testes is identical to the treatment of unilateral undescended testes when the testes are palpable. When testes are not palpable, however, differential diagnosis must be made from absent testes by measuring serum testosterone levels before and after stimulation with human chorionic gonadotropin (hCG). If the testosterone level rises, an abdominal exploration and orchiopexy should be undertaken. A negative response does not rule out the possible existence of intra-abdominal testicular tissue. An attempt is made to preserve these gonads for hormonal production after puberty; the likelihood of preserving fertility is very low.

Hormonal treatment with hCG or luteinizing hormone releasing hormone (LH-RH) has not replaced surgical treatment of cryptorchidism. Most authors agree that hormonal stimulation, which induces an early pseudopuberty, succeeds only in bringing down retractile testes (see below). Some authors believe that preoperative treatment with hCG facilitates surgery.

Retractile Testes. These testes retract into the inguinal canal in response to an exaggerated cremasteric reflex. The cremasteric reflex is weak or absent at birth. Consequently, when testes that were palpable at birth become nonpalpable later, retractile testes should be suspected. Retractile testes can be brought down by careful palpation when the child is relaxed in a warm room, and scrotal examination is facilitated if the child is in a squatting position. Often more than one examination is required to establish the diagnosis. The retractile testis adopts a permanent scrotal position during puberty and has none of the complications commonly associated with the true undescended or ectopic testis.

Absent Testes. Approximately 20% of nonpalpable testes are absent. Congenital absence of the testis is possible, but it is quite rare and should be associated with some degree of feminization of the internal organs on the ipsilateral side. More commonly, the testis appears to have vanished some time after the differentiation of the internal and external genitalia has occurred. This vanishing of the testis is usually attributed to a vascular accident that has taken place prenatally or after birth but was not recognized clinically. At exploration, the spermatic vessels and the vas deferens end blindly, usually somewhere in the inguinal region or in the scrotum. Since this condition is analogous to testicular torsion, some authors advocate fixation of the contralateral testis to prevent torsion from occurring in the remaining gonad. In these cases, placement of a testicular prosthesis can be considered as well.

TORSION OF THE TESTIS OR APPENDICES

This uncommon condition requires prompt diagnosis and treatment if the gonad is to survive. Testicular torsion accounts for approximately 40% of all cases of acute scrotal pain and swelling and for the majority of such cases in patients less than 6 yr old. It is caused by an abnormal fixation of the testis to the scrotal envelope. Under normal conditions, the testis is partially covered on its anterior portion by the tunica vaginalis, a serosal membrane derived from the processus vaginalis of the peritoneum. When the tunica vaginalis covers not only the testis but also the epididymis and the distal part of the spermatic cord, the testis is allowed to rotate freely within this serosal space and torsion can occur (bell clapper deformity). This abnormality of the tunica vaginalis is often bilateral.

Testicular torsion produces acute pain and swelling of the scrotum. On examination, the scrotum is swollen, very tender, and often difficult to examine. The cremasteric reflex is absent. The condition can be differentiated from an incarcerated hernia because swelling in the inguinal area is often absent. The differential diagnosis includes torsion of one of the testicular or epididymal appendices (embryologic vestiges), which usually causes less swelling and pain; occasionally a blue dot is observed above the testis and there is tenderness in this area. Often, however, differentiation can be made only at the time of surgical exploration. Torsion of the appendices is more common between the ages of 7–12 yr.

In children over 13 yr old, the differential diagnosis should include *epididymitis*. In epididymitis, the urinalysis is often abnormal, and there may be an antecedent history of sexual activity or urinary tract infection. Epididymitis is, of course, the most common cause of acute scrotal pain and swelling in patients over 18 yr of age. Nevertheless, we should keep in mind that in the prepubertal or adolescent boy with acute painful and swollen testes, testicular torsion is present until proven otherwise. The accuracy of ultrasonography, Doppler examination, and isotopic scans in differentiating testicular torsion from other conditions is uncertain, and this diagnostic measure often delays unnecessarily a surgical procedure that can salvage the gonad.

The optimal treatment is prompt surgical exploration. If the testis is explored within 6 hr of torsion, up to 90% of the gonads will survive after detorsion and fixation to the scrotum. Survival decreases rapidly with a greater than 6 hr delay, and such cases usually require orchidectomy. It is probably unwise not to remove a necrotic testis if torsion is confirmed. The contralateral testis should be fixed to the scrotum to prevent future torsion. If torsion of the appendices or epididymis is found, surgical removal of the necrotic appendix will result in cure.

In cases of *neonatal torsion* the mechanism for torsion appears to be different, in that abnormal fixation of the testis to the scrotum is not necessarily present. These torsions are usually extravaginal, as the entire testis and tunica vaginalis rotate within the lax subcutaneous tissue of the scrotum. This type of torsion can occur in utero or be present at birth. Salvage of testes with neonatal torsion is extremely rare. Many authors recommend exploration to remove the necrotic testis and to fix the contralateral side, since there have been some reports of torsion involving the remaining testis later.

VARICOCELE

Dilatation of the pampiniform venous plexus results from valvular incompetence of the spermatic vein. Varicoceles occur predominantly on the left side, are bilateral in 10% of cases, and rarely involve the right side only. Rarely seen before the age of 10 yr, varicoceles are present in 15% of adult males. In some cases, varicoceles cause male subfertility with decreased sperm concentration or motility. Varicoceles are also associated with decrease in size of and characteristic testicular histologic changes in the involved testis.

A large varicocele can be painful, particularly during strenuous physical activity. In the standing position, venous varicosities can be palpated along the spermatic cord. This venous distension increases with the Valsalva maneuver and collapses with recumbency. A fixed varicocele is suggestive of a retroperitoneal tumor. Surgical treatment by ligation of the internal spermatic vein is sometimes required in adolescents to relieve pain or, when there is disparity in testicular size, to allow normal development of the testis. The effect of early surgical correction of variococeles on future fertility is unknown.

HYDROCELE

Hydrocele is an accumulation of fluid in the tunica vaginalis. When the amount of fluid varies with time, communication with the peritoneal cavity is certain. Small hydroceles can disappear by the age of 1 yr, but larger ones often persist and require surgical treatment. Communicating hydroceles should be treated as indirect inguinal hernias.

EPIDIDYMITIS

Acute inflammation of the epididymis presents acute scrotal pain and swelling; it is rare before puberty and should raise the question of a congenital abnormality of the wolffian duct, such as an ectopic ureter entering the vas. After puberty, epididymitis becomes progressively more common and is the principal cause of acute painful scrotal swelling in young adults. Urinalysis usually reveals pyuria. Epididymitis can be bacterial, but often the organism remains undetermined. Treatment is by bed rest and antibiotics. Differentiation from torsion can be very difficult, and in children surgical exploration is usually required.

17.46 TRAUMA TO THE GENITOURINARY TRACT

Accidental injuries to the genitourinary tract in children are usually the result of blunt trauma from falls, athletic activities, or motor vehicle accidents. In childhood, genitourinary trauma is exceeded in frequency only by trauma to the skeleton and the central nervous system. In more than half of the cases there are also major injuries to the brain, spinal cord, skeleton, lungs, or other intraperitoneal organs. In cases of isolated renal injury, particularly following minor trauma, a pre-existent anomaly such as a horseshoe kidney, renal ectopia, hydronephrosis, or tumor should be suspected. Hematuria, bleeding through the urethral meatus, a flank mass, fractured lower ribs or lumbar transverse processes, or a perineal or scrotal hematoma suggests a major injury to the genitourinary tract in a child with trauma. In lesions involving the renal pedicle, hematuria is often absent.

Evaluation of the patient starts as soon as an adequate airway has been established and the patient is hemodynamically stable. The bladder should be catheterized in all cases except when there is bleeding from the urethral meatus, an indication of urethral injury. Straddling injuries are usually associated with trauma to the bulbous urethra. Rupture of the membranous urethra occurs in 3% of cases of pelvic fractures. Passing the catheter in the presence of a urethral injury may increase the extent of the damage and convert a partial tear to a total disruption. Instead, a retrograde urethrogram should be performed by injecting a radiopaque medium into the urethral meatus. Oblique radiographs will demonstrate the extent of the injury and whether urethral continuity is preserved or has been disrupted. Treatment is by suprapubic cystostomy drainage until the hematoma is reabsorbed, followed by urethroplasty when necessary to correct a resulting stricture. Erectile impotence, urethral stricture, and urinary incontinence are the major complications of rupture of the membranous urethra.

When the bladder can be catheterized, cystography is performed by infusing radiopaque medium through the catheter by gravity. If possible, flat and oblique views are obtained; a radiograph is also obtained after the bladder is drained. Bladder ruptures can be intraperitoneal or extraperitoneal. All intraperitoneal ruptures require surgical repair. Minor extraperitoneal near-ruptures might be treated by catheter drainage but generally require surgical treatment as well.

Intravenous urography is next done, to evaluate the kidneys. Complete absence of function of the one kidney without contralateral compensatory hypertrophy (indicative of congenital absence) should be regarded as an indication of major injury to the renal pedicle. Renal angiography should be done immediately before surgical exploration.

Renal injuries are usually classified as minor and major. *Minor renal injuries* include contusion of the renal parenchyma and shallow cortical lacerations not involving the collecting system. The majority of renal injuries fall into this category and can be treated nonoperatively with bed rest and supportive measures. *Major renal injuries* include deep lacerations involving the collecting system, the shattered kidney, and renal pedicle injuries. After the bladder is evaluated by cystography, intravenous pyelography is obtained; in some cases, this can be done intraoperatively when immediate surgical exploration is required for related life-threatening conditions. The observation of prompt function of both kidneys without extravasation usually excludes major renal injury. When findings on intravenous urography are not diagnostic, however, computed tomography is the ideal method for evaluating these lesions and has largely replaced angiography. Computed tomography appears to define better the extent of injury and also allows evaluation of other intra-abdominal organs.

Major renal injuries may require surgical treatment either during the course of an exploration for other intra-abdominal injuries or as management of the renal injury per se to control bleeding or significant urinary extravasation. Besides loss of renal parenchyma, the main long-term complication of renal injury is arterial hypertension. Children who sustain renal injuries should have periodic measurement of the blood pressure for approximately 1 yr following injury. All penetrating injuries of the kidneys should be surgically explored.

Ureteral injuries are usually iatrogenic. Injuries of the ureter by blunt or penetrating trauma require immediate surgical attention.

Testicular injuries are relatively uncommon in children because of the small size of the testes and their great mobility. Such injuries usually result from athletic activities. Prompt surgical treatment of testicular injuries increases the testicular salvage rate.

17.47 URINARY LITHIASIS

Urinary lithiasis in children is very common in some parts of the world but rare in the United States. The wide geographic variations in the incidence of lithiasis in childhood appear related to climatic, dietary, and socioeconomic factors. These factors also influence the location of the calculi; primary bladder stones are common in developing countries, whereas upper tract stones predominate in the United States (except in children with pre-existing bladder diseases such as neuro-

logic dysfunction, obstruction, or previous surgical procedures).

Children with urolithiasis almost always have either gross or microscopic hematuria. In order of frequency, abdominal pain, flank or back pain, and symptoms of urinary tract infection follow. When the diagnosis of urolithiasis is suspected, a plain radiograph of the abdomen will detect radiopaque stones, mainly those containing calcium. Cystine stones and infectious stones (composed of struvite) may be faintly radiopaque. Radiolucent stones (uric acid, 2,8-dihydroxyadenine and xanthine calculi) can be detected by abdominal ultrasonography or as filling defects found in the upper collecting system or bladder on intravenous urography or on computed tomography of the abdomen. When lithiasis is diagnosed, a complete functional and radiographic evaluation of the urinary tract is made, to rule out stasis, obstruction, or infection as predisposing factors. One fourth of children with urinary calculi have vesicoureteral reflux. The best insight into the etiology of lithiasis in a given patient is the complete chemical and crystallographic analysis of the stone (as obtained by spontaneous passage, or surgical or endoscopic extraction).

A metabolic evaluation for the most common predisposing factors should be undertaken as well, keeping in mind that structural, infectious, and metabolic factors often coexist. The basic laboratory studies required are listed in Table 17–16.

The causes of urolithiasis are multiple, and a complete listing is given in Table 17–17. Here we shall discuss some of the more frequently encountered types of calculi.

Calcium Stones. The most common urinary calculi in children in the United States are made of calcium oxalate. Cases in which no metabolic explanation for the stone formation is found are referred to as *idiopathic urolithiasis*. Hypercalciuria often leads to the formation of calcium oxalate stones and may be associated with hypercalcemia (due to hyperparathyroidism, sarcoidosis, immobilization, hypervitaminosis D, or idiopathic causes, and so on) but more often is an isolated phenomenon. Normocalcemic hypercalciuria may result from administration of furosemide (which often leads to stone formation in neonates), or from uncontrolled distal renal tubular acidosis, total parental alimentation, or alkalosis. In most cases, however, hypercalciuria leading to stone disease is idiopathic and may result from a renal tubular calcium "leak" which causes usually mild, secondary compensatory hyperparathyroidism and intestinal hyperabsorption of calcium. Another type of isolated hypercalciuria is related to

Table 17–16. Laboratory Tests Suggested to Evaluate Urolithiasis

Serum
  Calcium
  Phosphorus
  Uric acid
  Electrolytes and acid-base balance
  Creatinine
  Alkaline phosphatase

Urine
  Urinalysis
  Urine culture
  Urinary pH
  Calcium/creatinine ratio
  Spot test for cystinuria
  24 hr collection for:
    creatinine clearance
    calcium
    phosphorus
    oxalate
    uric acid
    dibasic amino acids (if cystine spot test is positive)

Table 17–17. Classification of Urolithiasis

Renal Tubular Syndromes
Renal tubular acidosis
Distal defect, type I
Carbonic anhydrase inhibitors
Cystinuria
Glycinuria

Enzyme Disorders
Primary hyperoxaluria
Type I, glycolic aciduria
Type II, L-glyceric aciduria
Xanthinuria
Metabolic (enzymatic) hyperuricosuria
2,8-dihydroxyadeninuria

Hypercalcemic States
Primary hyperparathyroidism
Sarcoidosis
Hypervitaminosis D
Milk-alkali syndrome
Neoplasms
Cushing's syndrome
Hyperthyroidism
Idiopathic infantile hypercalcemia
Immobilization

Uric Acid Lithiasis and Related Disorders
Hereditary metabolic hyperuricosuria
Hereditary renal hypouricemia
2,8-dihydroxyadeninuria
Myeloproliferative disorders
Low urine output states

Nephrolithiasis and Intestinal Disease
Acquired hyperoxaluria
Uric acid lithiasis

Idiopathic Renal Lithiasis

Infected Urolithiasis and Urinary Stasis

Endemic Calculi

Nephrocalcinosis

From Malek RS: Urolithiasis. In: Kelalis PP, King LR, Belman AB (eds): Clinical Pediatric Urology. Philadelphia, WB Saunders, 1985.

primary intestinal hyperabsorption of calcium, which increases the filtered load of calcium and causes parathyroid inhibition.

The precise cause of these disorders remains unclear. Children with hypercalciuria sometimes have recurrent episodes of gross hematuria and flank pain years before the first stone is detected; accordingly, the workup of children with recurrent gross hematuria should include the measurement of urinary calcium. Upper limits of normal are 4 mg/kg/24 hr or a urinary calcium/creatinine ratio greater than 0.25 mg/mg. A detailed metabolic workup to differentiate the various types of hypercalciuria has been described by Pak. Despite careful evaluation, there remains a group of children who are stone-formers, in whom neither metabolic nor anatomic abnormalities can be detected. Calculi of calcium oxalate can also occur in children in whom small bowel disease and malabsorption lead to excessive reabsorption of oxalate in the colon (intestinal hyperoxaluria). Renal stone formation and nephrocalcinosis in primary hyperoxaluria (type 1 or 2) usually begins before the age of 4–5 yr and often runs a progressive course leading to renal failure.

Cystinuria. This inborn error of transport of the dibasic amino acids (cystine, ornithine, arginine, and lysine) results in excessive urinary excretion of these products. The only known complication of this familial disease is the formation of calculi, owing to the low solubility of cystine. The sulfur content of cystine gives these stones their faint radiopaque appearance.

Struvite Stones. Urinary tract infections caused by urea-splitting organisms (such as *Proteus* and occasionally *Klebsiella*, *E. coli*, *Pseudomonas*, and others) cause urinary alkalinization and excessive production of ammonia which can lead to the precipitation of magnesium ammonium phosphate (struvite) and calcium phosphate. The stones act as foreign bodies, causing obstruction and perpetuating infection. Patients with struvite stones may also have metabolic abnormalities that predispose to stone formation.

Uric Acid Stones. Calculi containing uric acid represent less than 5% of all cases of lithiasis in children in this country but are more common in less developed areas of the world. Hyperuricosuria with or without hyperuricemia is the common underlying factor in most cases. The stones are radiolucent. The diagnosis should be suspected when there is a persistently acid urine and urate crystalluria. Hyperuricosuria may result from various inborn errors of purine metabolism that lead to overproduction of uric acid, the end product of purine metabolism in humans. Children with the Lesch-Nyhan syndrome and patients with glucose-6-phosphatase deficiency (G-6-PD) form urate calculi as well. In children with short bowel syndrome, and particularly in those with ileostomies, chronic dehydration and acidosis are sometimes complicated by uric acid lithiasis. One of the most common causes of uric acid lithiasis is the rapid turnover of purine with some tumors and myeloproliferative diseases. The risk of uric acid lithiasis is especially great when treatment of these diseases causes rapid breakdown of nucleoproteins. Uric acid calculi or "slush" can fill the entire upper collecting system and cause renal failure and even anuria. In addition, urates also are present within calcium-containing stones. In these cases more than one predisposing factor for stone formation may exist. A related disorder only recently recognized is *2,8-dihydroxyadenine lithiasis*, which results from a deficiency in adenine phosphoribosyltransferase. The stones are radiolucent and can be differentiated from uric acid calculi by mass spectrometry but not by routine chemical analysis. In contrast to uric acid, which is very soluble in alkaline urine, the solubility of 2,8-dihydroxyadenine changes little within physiologic pH ranges.

Treatment. The treatment of urinary lithiasis is approached from two perspectives. One aspect is the treatment of the underlying metabolic disorder, infections or predisposing anatomic factors; the other is the treatment of complications associated with the stone itself, principally obstruction and infection. The simplest and most effective measure to prevent recurrence in all forms of lithiasis is to maintain an adequate state of hydration and diuresis 24 hr a day, in order to keep the urine dilute and to diminish the likelihood of precipitation of stone ingredients. Alterations of the urine pH can also prevent recurrence of calculi. Cystine is much more soluble when the urinary pH is over 7.5, and alkalinization of urine with sodium bicarbonate or sodium citrate is effective. Recurrence of uric acid lithiasis may likewise be prevented by keeping the urinary pH above 7.5; indeed, hydration, urinary alkalinization, and measures directed at reducing uric acid excretion can cause dissolution of uric acid calculi. Acidification impairs the growth of struvite stones but this cannot be achieved in practice so long as the stone or an infection by urea-splitting organisms is present. Whenever possible, and if simple measures fail, specific therapy for any underlying metabolic disorder should be used. Thiazides appear to be effective in controlling primary renal hypercalciuria, but their effectiveness in the treatment of calcium oxalate stones caused by primary hypercalciuria remains debatable. Treatment of renal tubular acidosis controls recurrence of stone disease or nephrocalcinosis. Allopurinol is an inhibitor of xanthinoxidase and is effective in reducing the production both of uric acid and of 2,8-dihydroxyadenine, and can help control recurrence of both types of stones. Rarely, excessive urinary excretion of xanthine with stone formation has been reported during treatment with allopurinol. D-Penicillamine is a chelating agent that binds to cysteine or hemicystine, increasing the solubility of the product. Although poorly tolerated by many patients, it has been reported to be effective in dissolving cystine stones and in preventing recurrences when hydration and urinary alkalinization fail. N-acetylcysteine appears to have low toxicity and may be effective in controlling cystinuria, but long-term experience with it is lacking. Other specific therapies that have been used for the treatment of lithiasis include the use of cellulose phosphate to bind calcium in the intestine in cases of primary absorptive hypercalciuria. Poor compliance with treatment and poor tolerance of the medication are significant drawbacks to its use. Pyridoxine has been used in some cases of hyperoxaluria. Salts of phosphate, citrate, magnesium, and other compounds directed at increasing the solubility of calcium oxalate and other stone ingredients in the urine are used in some centers, with varying success.

Surgical treatment of stone disease has been widespread in the past. Stones must be removed when they cause obstruction of the collecting system, pain, or bleeding, or if they are a factor in perpetuating infections. All struvite stones should be removed, because these carry a significant risk of renal parenchymal destruction and of renal or perirenal abscess formation. Newer modalities of stone removal, both endoscopically and by percutaneous access to the kidney, have been applied on a limited scale in children. The extracorporeal lithotriptor promises to allow the nonsurgical disintegration of most cases of renal lithiasis.

RICARDO GONZALEZ
ALFRED MICHAEL

Urinary Tract Infections

Bergstrom T, Larson H, Lincoln K, et al: Studies of urinary tract infections in infancy and childhood: Eighty consecutive patients with neonatal infection. Fetal Neonat Med 80:858, 1972.
Burbige KA, Retik AB, Colodny AH, et al: Urinary tract infection in boys. J Urol 132:54, 1984.
Gillenwater YJ, Harrison RB, Kunin CM: Natural history of bacteriuria in school girls. A long term case control study. New Engl J Med 301:396, 1979.
Gonzalez R, Sheldon CA: Septic obstruction and uremia in the newborn. Urol Clin North Am 9(2):297, 1982.
Govan DE, Fair WR, Fredland GW: Management of children with UTI. Urology 6:275, 1975.
Hodson J, Kincaid-Smith P: Reflux Nephropathy. New York, Masson Publishing, 1979.
Kunin CM: Emergence of bacteriuria, proteinuria and symptomatic urinary tract infections among a population of school girls followed for 7 years. Pediatrics 41:968, 1968.
Longberg H, Hanson LA, Jacobsson B, et al: Correlation of P blood group, vesicoureteral reflux and bacterial attachment in patients with recurrent pyelonephritis.
Mayrer AR, Miniter P, Andriole VT: Immunopathogenesis of chronic pyelonephritis. Am J Med 75:59, 1983.
Newcastle Asymptomatic Bacteriuria Research Group: Asymptomatic bacteriuria in school children in Newcastle upon Tyne. Arch Dis Child 50:90, 1975.
Sheldon CA, Gonzalez R: Differentiation of upper and lower urinary tract infections. How and when? Med Clin North Am 68(2):321, 1984.
Sibley RK, Rosai J: Urinary tract. In: Rosai J (ed): Ackerman's Surgical Pathology. St Louis, CV Mosby, 1981.
Sinha B, Gonzalez R: Hyperammonemia in boys with obstructive ureterocele and proteus infection. J Urol 131:1, 1984.
Stamey TA: Pathogenesis and Treatment of Urinary Tract Infections. Baltimore, Williams & Wilkins, 1980.

Vesicoureteral Reflux

Bauer SB, Willscher MK, Ammuto PJ, et al: Longterm results of antireflux surgery in children. In: Hodson J, Kinkaid-Smith P (eds): Reflux Nephropathy. New York, Masson Publishing, 1979, Chap 20.
Chantler C, Donckerwolcke RA, Brunner FP, et al: Combined report on regular dialysis and transplantation in children in Europe, 1978. Proceedings of the European Dialysis and Transplant Association 16:76, 1979.
Edwards D, Normand ICS, Prescod N, et al: Disappearance of vesicoureteric reflux during longterm prophylaxis of urinary tract infection in children. Br Med J 2:285, 1977.

Jenkins GR, Nol N: Familial vesicoureteral reflux: A prospective study. J Urol 128:774, 1982.
Koff SA, Murtagh DS: Uninhibited bladder in children: Effect of treatment on recurrent urinary tract infection and on vesicoureteral reflux resolution. J Urol 130:1138, 1983.
Nasrallah PF, Nava S, Crawford J: Clinical application of nuclear cystography. J Urol 128:550, 1982.
Rance CP, Arbus GS, Balfe JW, et al: Persistent systemic hypertension in infants and children. Pediatr Clin North Am 21(4):801, 1974.
Ransley PG: Intrarenal reflux: Anatomical, dynamic and radiological studies. Urol Res 5:61, 1977.
Report of the International Reflux Committee: Special article: Medical versus surgical treatment of primary vesicoureteral reflux. Pediatrics 67:392, 1981.
Stephens FD: Cystoscopic appearances of the ureteric orifices associated with reflux nephropathy. In: Hodson J, Kinkaid-Smith P (eds): Reflux: Nephropathy. New York, Masson Publishing, 1979, Chap 12.

Obstruction

Churchill BM, Krueger RP, Fleischer MH, et al: Complications of posterior urethral valve surgery and their prevention. Urol Clin North Am 10(3):519, 1983.
Gonzalez R, Chiou RK: The diagnosis of upper urinary tract obstruction in children: Comparison of diuresis renography and pressure flow studies. J Urol 133:1, 1985.
Gonzalez R, Lapointe S, Sheldon CA, et al: Undiversion in children with chronic renal failure. J Pediatr Surg 19:632, 1984.
Hendren WH: Posterior urethral valves in boys. A broad clinical spectrum. J Urol 106:298, 1971.
Immergut M, Notman GE: The urethral course of female children with recurrent urinary tract infection. J Urol 99:189, 1965.
Kaplan GW, Sammons TA, King LR: Blind comparison of dilatation urethrotomy and medication alone in the treatment of infection in girls. J Urol 109:917, 1973.
Kelalis PP: Ureteropelvic junction. In: Kelalis PK, King LR, Belman AB (eds): Clinical Pediatric Urology. Philadelphia, WB Saunders, 1985, Chap 16.
Kramer SA: Current status of fetal intervention for congenital hydronephrosis. J Urol 130:641, 1983.
Kroovand RL, Perlmutter AD: A one stage surgical approach to ectopic ureterocele. J Urol 122:367, 1979.
Lapointe S, Gonzalez R: Acute and chronic urinary tract obstruction: Pathophysiology, diagnosis and management. In: Mandel A (ed): Clinical Nephrology. Philadelphia, Lea & Febiger, in press.
Lockhart JL, Singer AM, Glenn JF: Congenital megaureter. J Urol 122:310, 1979.
Sullivan M, Halpern L, Hodges CV: Extravesical ureteral ectopia. Urology 11:577, 1978.
Whitaker RH: Percutaneous upper urinary tract dynamics in equivocal obstruction. Urol Radiol 2:187, 1981.
Williams DI, Whitaker RH, Barratt TM, et al: Urethral valves. Br J Urol 45:200, 1973.
Woodhouse CRJ, Kellett JS, Williams DI: Minimal surgical interference in prune belly syndrome. Br J Urol 51:475, 1979.

Other Diseases and Anomalies of the Bladder

Exstrophy

Arap S, Giron DM, Menezes de Goes G: Initial results of the complete reconstruction of bladder exstrophy. Urol Clin North Am 7(2):477, 1980.
Jeffs RD: Exstrophy and cloacal exstrophy. Urol Clin North Am 5(1):127, 1978.
Sheldon CA, McKinley R, Hartig P, et al: Carcinoma at the site of the ureterosigmoidostomy. J Dis Colon Rectum 26:55, 1983.

Bladder Diverticula

Johnston JH: Vesical diverticula without urinary obstruction in childhood. J Urol 84:535, 1960.

Urachal Anomalies

Bauer SB, Retik AB: Urachal and related umbilical disorders. Urol Clin North Am 5:195, 1978.

Neurogenic Bladder

Bauer SB: Urodynamic evaluation and neuromuscular dysfunction. In: Kelalis PK, King LR, Belman AB (eds): Clinical Pediatric Urology. Philadelphia, WB Saunders, 1985.
Gonzalez R, Sheldon CA: Artificial sphincters in children with neurogenic bladders. Long term results. J Urol 128:1270, 1982.
Kaplan WE, Firlit CF: Management of reflux in myelodysplastic child. J Urol 129:1195, 1983.
Kass EJ, Koff SA, Biokno AC: Fate of vesicoureteral reflux in children with neuropathic bladders managed by intermittent catheterization. J Urol 125:63, 1981.
Lapides J, Diokno AC, Lowe BS: Follow-up on unsterile intermittent self catheterization. J Urol 111:184, 1974.

Sidi AA, Dykstra DD, Gonzalez R: The value of urodynamic testing in the management of neonates with myelodysplasia. A prospective study. J Urol 135:90, 1986.

Sidi AA, Peng W, Gonzalez R: Vesicoureteral reflux in children with myelodysplasia: Natural history and results of treatment. J Urol 136:329, 1986.

Enuresis and Voiding Dysfunction

Allen TD: The non-neurogenic neurogenic bladder. J Urol 117:232, 1977.

Bauer SB, Retik AB, Colodny AH, et al: The unstable bladder in childhood. Urol Clin North Am 7(2):321, 1980.

Mikkelsen EJ, Rappaport JL: Enuresis: Psychopathology, sleep stage and drug response. Urol Clin North Am 7(2):361, 1980.

Pedersen PS, Hejl M, Kjoller SS: Desamino-D-arginine vasopressin in childhood. Nocturnal enuresis. J Urol 133:65, 1985.

Perlmuter AD: Enuresis. In: Kelalis, PP, King LR, Belman AB (eds): Clinical Pediatric Urology. Philadelphia, WB Saunders, 1985, p 311.

Other Diseases and Anomalies of the Penis and Urethra

Hypospadias

Bauer SB, Retik AB, Colodny AH: Genetic aspects of hypospadias. Urol Clin North Am 8:559, 1981.

Johnston JH: Abnormalities of the penis. In: Williams DI, Johnston JH (eds): Paediatric Urology. London, Butterworth Scientific, 1982, p 435.

Kaplan GW: Complications of circumcision. Urol Clin North Am 10(13):543, 1983.

Rozenman J, Hertz M, Boichis H: Radiological findings of the urinary tract in hypospadias. A report of 770 cases. Clin Radiol 30:471, 1979.

Section on Urology, American Academy of Pediatrics: The timing of elective surgery on the genitalia of male children with particular reference to undescended testes and hypospadias. Pediatrics 56:479, 1975.

Wallerstein E: Circumcision: The uniquely American medical enigma. Urol Clin North Am 12(1):123, 1985.

Diseases and Anomalies of the Scrotal Contents

Bartsch G, Frank ST, Marberger H: Testicular torsion: Late results with special regard to fertility and endocrine function. J Urol 124:375, 1980.

Farrington GH: The position and retractability of the normal testes in childhood with reference to the diagnosis and treatment of cryptorchidism. J Pediatr Surg 3:353, 1968.

Fonkalsrud EW, Menzel W (eds): The Undescended Testes. Chicago, Year Book Medical Publishers, 1981.

Gonzalez R: Outpatient orchidopexy in children. In: Kaye KW (ed): Outpatient Urologic Surgery. Philadelphia, Lea & Febiger, 1985.

Heinz HA, Voggenthaler J, Weissbach L: Histologic findings in testes with varicocele during childhood and their therapeutic consequences. Eur J Pediatr 133:139, 1980.

Martin DC: Malignancy on the cryptorchid testes. Urol Clin North Am 9:371, 1982.

Papadotos C, Moutsouris C: Bilateral testicular torsion in the newborn. J Pediatr Surg 71:249, 1967.

Sarer CG: The descent of the testes. Arch Dis Child 39:605, 1964.

Trauma

Brower P, Paul J, Brosman SA: Urinary tract abnormalities presenting as a result of shunt abdominal trauma. J Trauma 18:719, 1978.

Burrington JD: Childhood trauma. In: Holder TM, Ashcroft KLW (eds): Pediatric Surgery. Philadelphia, WB Saunders, 1980, p 149.

Cass AS: Blunt renal trauma in children. J Trauma 23:123, 1983.

Pinhas ML, Gonzales ET: Genitourinary trauma in children. Urol Clin North Am 12:53, 1985.

Urinary Lithiasis

Churchill DN, Malone CM, Nolan MH, et al: Pediatric urolithiasis in the 1970s. J Urol 123:233, 1980.

Hulbert JC, Reddy PK, Gonzalez R, et al: Percutaneous nephrostolithotomy. An alternative approach to the management of pediatric calculous disease. Pediatrics 76:610, 1985.

Malek RS: Urolithiasis. In: Kelalis PP, King LR, Belman BA (eds): Clinical Pediatric Urology. Philadelphia, WB Saunders, 1985, p 1093.

Noe HN, Stapleton FB, Roxy S III: Potential surgical implications of hematuria in children. J Urol 132:737, 1984.

Pak CYC: The spectrum and pathogenesis of hypercalciuria. Urol Clin North Am 8:245, 1981.

Sinno K, Boyce WH, Resnick MI: Childhood urolithiasis. J Urol 121:662, 1979.

Stapleton FB, Rog S, Noe HN, et al: Hypercalciuria in children with hematuria. N Engl J Med 310:1345, 1984.

18

PEDIATRIC GYNECOLOGY

Pediatric gynecology is defined by certain problems unique to the female infant, child, or adolescent. Some of these problems are uncommon and require the attention of specialists. Others are relatively common; and some reflect the community's increased awareness of and concern with sexual activity, sexually transmitted diseases, sex education, and sexual abuse. For discussion of problems particular to adolescents, see Chapter 9.

EXAMINATION OF THE GENITALIA

Complete gynecologic assessment of children includes a general history and physical examination, assessment of general growth and development, evaluation of sexual maturity (Sec. 2.30 and 9.7), examination of the genitalia, and the pelvic examination. An understanding of the child's stage of psychologic and cognitive development as well as her current emotional state is essential to creation of an appropriate relationship during the examination and subsequently. For example, a toddler being examined after traumatic sexual abuse may be fearful of pain when placed in an uncomfortable position, while being unaware of the sexual connotation of the examination, whereas an adolescent girl requires sensitive concern for her sexual consciousness and her possible feelings of invasion of privacy.

Position. The pelvic examination in the young child is best performed in the position that is most comfortable for her. Restraint is rarely required if the child is appropriately informed prior to and during the examination. The lithotomy position used for adolescents and adults is not well received by most young children. A modified frog-leg position with hips flexed and feet on the table is better received. This position may be obtained with the patient's cooperation by asking her to sit on the table, flex her knees, and grasp her ankles, followed by allowing her legs to fall open. For the anxious child this position may also be achieved while she sits on her mother's lap. Some advocate the knee-chest position; the abdomen faces the table and weight is supported on bent knees separated by 15–20 cm (6–8 in), with the child's head resting on her hands and turned to one side. This position permits good eye contact with physician, parent, or assistant and helps to overcome the child's anxiety and fear. It also permits a good view of the labia, hymen, vagina, and sometimes cervix without instrumentation.

With either the lithotomy or frog-leg position a successful examination requires diminishing anxiety with relaxation. For adolescents, the lithotomy position with adequate draping is essential, especially if instruments are to be used. Many authorities recommend that the adolescent girl's mother not be present during the examination. The privacy of adolescents should be respected, especially when their sexual activities are being discussed, but the presence of mother or friend may be comforting during the pelvic examination. The patient's preferences should be discussed with her and honored; such discussion should include topics to be addressed as well as the method and extent of physical examination. Many male physicians prefer to have a female assistant present, but it is desirable to give the patient the option of deciding whether that would be helpful. Some children of any age are best examined without the mother in attendance; these decisions are best made by a physician familiar with past and current parent-child interactions, in the context of the purposes of the examination.

Specimens. Specimens for microscopic examination, wet preparations, Papanicolaou smears, assessment of estrogen effect, and culture can be obtained using simple equipment. Dry cotton swabs should not be used to obtain specimens since the twisting motion necessary to insert such a swab may be very painful. A nasopharyngeal swab moistened with saline may be used to obtain cultures. Vaginal secretions can be secured also with a small, soft plastic eye dropper using gentle suction. A small, soft plastic tube can be inserted through very small hymenal openings, and injection of 1–2 mL of sterile saline may facilitate aspiration. Care should be taken not to dilute the specimen so as to make culturing difficult.

Instrumentation. For most purposes adequate illumination of the external genitalia and vagina can be obtained using an ordinary otoscope head without a speculum, but this will not be sufficient for a more detailed examination nor for visualization of the cervix. The Cameron-Miller or Huffman-Huber fiberoptic vaginoscopes are easy to use with young children, but they are expensive; their cylindrical specula of varying lengths are easy to insert and permit good visualization. Less costly alternatives are veterinary otoscopic specula, which come in lengths up to 7 cm and in diameters up to 7 mm and which fit on Welch-Allyn otoscopes.

For older, virginal girls a Huffman-Graves virginal bivalved speculum may be used; for sexually active nulliparous girls the medium-sized Pederson vaginal speculum (4.5 in long, 1 in wide) is most appropriate. The Graves speculum is 3.75 in long and 1.375 in wide, with a duck-bill appearance; although wider than the Huffman-Graves instrument, it is well tolerated by sexually active adolescents. Some feel that this instrument is best reserved for those patients who have had a vaginal delivery. Metal specula should be adequately warmed, lubricated with water, and inserted at a 45° angle, using a gentle rotary movement.

The Mini-Examination in Young Children. In young children *inspection* is one of the most useful components of the genital examination. Adequate illumination, comfortable positioning, and cooperation are essential. *Superficial palpation* of the labia and vagina is best done by depressing the perineum on either side of the labia with both thumbs or by gently pulling the labia apart. In the knee-chest position little manipulation may be required; simply holding the buttocks apart and pressing laterally and slightly upward will provide good visualization. *Bimanual vaginal examination* is usually not possible; when it is possible, it is often not indicated. An alternative examination that involves placing the little or index finger in the rectum and palpating the abdomen with the other hand can provide considerable information regarding the uterus, any masses, or vaginal foreign bodies. To feel the adnexa of young girls and early adolescents is very difficult.

18.1 DEVELOPMENTAL DISABILITIES PRESENTING IN THE NEWBORN PERIOD

The external genitalia of the newborn infant girl must be carefully examined. Virilization of the female fetus in utero may lead to development of *ambiguous genitalia* (Sec. 2.24). The most common cause is congenital adrenal hyperplasia (Sec. 19.23). Chromosomal dysgeneses and a variety of developmental hormonal defects may lead to discrepancies among the external and internal genitalia and chromosomal sex. Early recognition of ambiguous genitalia is important for treatment and for establishment of sexual identity (Sec. 2.24 and 19.23).

Imperforate hymen is generally not identified until menarche when the patient may have amenorrhea, abdominal pain, and lower abdominal swelling, with or without a bulging introitus. Occasionally, in the newborn period bulging of the imperforate hymen is due to accumulation of vaginal secretions from the estrogenized vagina. The volume of such secretions is generally small; they may contain blood as the result of endometrial slough in response to withdrawal of maternal estrogens. Excision of the membrane is the treatment of choice; other defects are rarely associated.

Congenital absence of the vagina is usually not discovered in the newborn period. In the first several months of life many infant girls develop *adhesions of the labia* (labial agglutination) as a result of recurrent or continuous irritation and inflammation. This may suggest absence of the vagina, but the distinctive feature is a markedly translucent midline raphe at the site of adhesion. Local application of an estrogen cream and good hygiene, with elimination of irritation, will reverse the adhesion. This may become a recurrent problem that is resolved at puberty with the onset of endogenous estrogen stimulation. Rarely, urinary retention and infection behind the adhesions require immediate separation of the labia. This can be accomplished with use of a well lubricated probe or cotton swab, followed by application of an estrogen cream to maintain the separation.

18.2 INFECTIONS OF THE FEMALE GENITALIA

Vulvovaginitis is the most common gynecologic problem of children and adolescents. It has numerous causes, both infectious and noninfectious. The physiologic state of the vagina is the most important determinant of vaginal flora.

Vaginal Physiology. At birth, under the influence of maternal estrogens, the vagina is hypertrophied, with numerous layers of glycogen-containing, stratified squamous epithelium. The pH is 5.5–7.0. This normal state results in the thick milky-white discharge seen during the first 3 wk of life, which rapidly diminishes as estrogen stimulation ceases. From about 3 wk of age until just before menarche, the vaginal mucosa is relatively atrophic, lacks glycogen, and has a neutral to alkaline pH (6.5–7.4).

Clinical Features. The complaints of the child with vulvovaginitis will vary with age. The young child may rub or scratch the genitalia and cry with voiding or defecation; the older child will describe itching and pain. The occurrence and nature of any vaginal discharge are variable, and discharge is frequently not the first sign of vaginitis. Specific inquiry should be made about foreign bodies, which are commonly overlooked. The older girl may have a retained tampon or other paper product used as a substitute for a menstrual pad. Contact irritants include soaps, perfumes, feminine hygiene sprays, and clothing. The common use of synthetic fabrics and tight clothing (such as leotards) has increased the incidence of this problem. Both cloth and paper diapers can serve as irritants. Soaps and disinfectants used in washing cloth diapers should be evaluated and a mild detergent substituted. Paper diapers frequently contain perfumes and other chemicals. Tight-fitting paper diapers may lead to diaper dermatitis and vaginitis. Administration of an antibiotic for several weeks may alter vaginal flora, allowing colonization by organisms (such as *Candida*) that are more commonly seen in postmenarchal women. A family history of diabetes mellitus, of pinworms or other parasites, or of skin problems such as eczema, atopic dermatitis, psoriasis, or seborrhea, may accompany, aggravate, or trigger vulvovaginitis.

The clinical manifestations may reflect involvement primarily of the skin and vulva or be the result of a true vulvovaginitis; there is considerable overlap between these two categories. Table 18–1 shows the most common skin disorders affecting the external genitalia, often only as a component of a generalized skin disorder. In the perineal area of young children, secondary infection of such disorders may result from contamination with urine and stool and make diagnosis difficult. Table 18–2 presents the most common viral infections and parasitic infestations of the perineum; these affect primarily the skin of the external genitalia.

Table 18–1. Common Skin Disorders Affecting the Genitalia

	Age of Onset	Symptoms/Involved Areas	Appearance	Management
Seborrhea	Commonly <3 mos; may occur at any age	Pruritus, frequent secondary infection; in folds of diaper area, between labia minora, and labia majora; often seborrhea elsewhere	Elevated, red lesions with yellow, greasy scales	Hydrocortisone cream 1%; treat secondary infection
Psoriasis	Any age	Usually associated with disease elsewhere; pruritus	Variable-sized, sharply demarcated, erythematous plaques, with silver scale on flat surface	Hydrocortisone cream 1%; Burow soaks if acute and exudative
Atopic dermatitis	Any age	Common on surface areas in contact with offending agent; pruritus; secondary infection	Erythema; vesicles may be excoriated and exudative	Remove causative agent (clothes, diapers, perfumes); Burow soaks if exudative; hydrocortisone cream 1%; treat secondary infection
Lichen sclerosus	Any age; generally improves at puberty	Vulva and labia; chronic, severe pruritus	White parchment appearance of vulva; fissuring; easily traumatized	Hydrocortisone cream 1%; testosterone 2% in petrolatum if severe

Table 18–2. **Common Infections Affecting Vulvar Area**

Condition /Agent	Menarchial Pre	Menarchial Post	Source	Symptoms	Diagnosis	Management
Herpes Herpes simplex virus, type 2 primarily	±	+ +	Maternal contamination Venereal	Small vesicles on erythematous base; pruritus; ulcerations; may have systemic symptoms (fever, lymphadenopathy); dysuria	Inspection; scraping-multinucleated giant cells seen with Wright stain in scrapings of lesions	Acyclovir 5% ointment, 6 times/day for 7 days; local anesthetic; light therapy
Pediculosis pubis; *Phthirus pubis* ("crab lice")	–	+	Venereal or close contact	Pruritus	Inspection (lice, or eggs [nits] attached to hair follicle)	Gamma benzene hexachloride 1% (Kwell)
Molluscum contagiosum (DNA virus of poxvirus group)	±	+	Venereal or close contact	Pruritus; autoinoculation; may become secondarily infected	2–4 mm flesh-colored papules, with central umbilication containing a "cheesy" plug	Spontaneous regression; may be curetted or cauterized
Scabies (mite; *Sarcoptes scabiei*)	+	+	Close physical contact	Pruritus; erythematous papules with wavy burrows; family members or sexual partners affected	Scrapings or skin biopsy to visualize mite	Wash clothing and bedding; gamma benzene hexachloride 1% (Kwell), or crotamiton (Eurax)
Condylomata acuminatum (papova-papilloma virus)	±	+	Venereal or close contact	Dry, warty lesions on skin of labia, perineum and vestibule; associated with irritating vaginal discharge	Inspection	Podophyllin (25%) in tincture of benzoin at 1–2 wk intervals (not in pregnancy or young child); freezing; cauterization

Herpes simplex infection has become one of the most prevalent sexually transmitted diseases among adolescents and adults. Acyclovir ointment is an effective treatment for symptomatic genital herpes and may be used in young children and adolescents. The oral form of this antiviral agent may be used in the treatment of primary herpes infection.

Table 18–3 summarizes the most common causes and management of vulvovaginitis. The sexually transmitted diseases of adolescents are discussed in Sec. 9.9.

18.3 NEOPLASMS

The incidence of gynecologic neoplasms in infancy and childhood is not accurately known; all types are rare. Consolidated reporting has been instituted only for tumors in diethylstilbestrol (DES)-exposed females. Routine gynecologic examination of otherwise normal young girls and adolescents for detection of neoplasm prior to menarche and sexual activity is neither indicated nor cost-effective. Pelvic examination should be limited to those patients who have unusual genital lesions, abnormal genital bleeding, vaginal discharge, tissue protruding from the vagina, unexplained abdominal swelling or masses, or abnormalities of growth.

The most common gynecologic neoplasms of children are of ovarian origin and generally present as abdominal masses. These tumors are highly malignant, and intensive investigation with tissue diagnosis is necessary to plan treatment and to preserve ovarian function. Rarely, the vagina or vulva may be the site of a benign or malignant lesion in childhood. Benign lesions include mesonephric duct cysts, paraurethral cysts, and simple inclusion cysts. The most common malignant lesion of the vagina is the clear-cell adenocarcinoma associated with DES exposure in utero, discussed in Sec. 18.4 (see also Sec. 16.24). Sarcoma botryoides is discussed in Sec. 18.5.

18.4 DIETHYLSTILBESTROL (DES)-EXPOSED FEMALES

The association between intrauterine exposure to DES and clear-cell adenocarcinoma was first identified in 1971, when a relationship was established between such exposure and the occurrence of vaginal adenosis and later malignancy.

The incidence of adenosis (the finding in vaginal scrapings of mucinous columnar cells or metaplastic squamous cells, or both, with or without mucinous droplets) varies from 20 to 90%, depending on (1) whether adenosis is defined to include cervical as well as vaginal abnormalities; (2) time of DES exposure in utero (more frequent if given prior to 18th wk of gestation); (3) length and dose of exposure; and (4) method of selection of exposed subjects (with rates lowest in those identified by retrospective review of medical records and highest in self-referred women). Women exposed to DES in utero are at increased risk for vaginal adenosis and development of clear-cell adenocarcinoma; they are not at increased risk for squamous cell carcinoma.

Management of girls or women exposed to DES in utero starts with a complete history, including evaluation of prenatal records. All exposed women should have pelvic examination by an experienced gynecologist after menarche or by the age of 14 yr. This should include meticulous inspection and palpation of the entire vagina, collection of cytologic samples from the vagina and cervix, iodine staining (half-strength Lugol solution) of the vagina, colposcopy, and direct biopsy of any suspicious lesions. Subsequent, similar examinations should be made every 1–2 yr unless an abnormality is found. Treatment of clear-cell adenocarcinoma is with vaginectomy, hysterectomy, and lymphadenectomy. Survival rates are 80% overall and 90% in those identified with stage 1 disease. Ovarian function is generally preserved. Therapies combining surgery, radiation, and chemotherapy are being evaluated.

It is suspected that affected women may have increased

Table 18–3. **Etiology of Vulvovaginitis**

Condition /Agent	Menarchial Pre	Menarchial Post	Source	Symptoms	Diagnosis	Management
Nonspecific vaginitis (*Gardnerella* vaginitis) Gram-negative bacilli	±	+	Normal flora; potentially pathogenic Venereal	Few symptoms; gray-white, thick discharge; fishy odor	On wet preparation: "clue cells" (epithelial cells with organisms adherent to surface); KOH releases amines causing fishy odor; culture on colistin/ nalidixic acid agar (CNA)	Metronidazole 500 mg bid orally for 5 days; treat asymptomatic male consort
Trichomoniasis (flagellated parasite)	±	+	Maternal colonization in newborn / Venereal (male symptomatic)	Asymptomatic to severe / Profuse watery, frothy, yellow-green discharge	On wet preparation: flagellated organisms among WBC's	Metronidazole: 250 mg tid, orally, for 1 wk *or* 2 g in single dose; contraindicated in pregnancy; treat asymptomatic male consort
Candidosis (Candida albicans)	±	+ +	Secondary to diabetes mellitus, antibiotics, skin disease, oral contraceptives, obesity; not venereal	Pruritus; thick cheesy discharge; red, edematous vulva	KOH preparation: spores and hyphae Culture on Nickerson or Sabouraud agar	Sitz baths; miconazole vaginal cream or suppositories, at bedtime for 7 days; nystatin (for child, cream applied to vulva; for adolescent, suppositories, twice a day for 14 days); hydrocortisone cream for severe symptoms and erythema; nystatin, orally, if recurrent; clotrimazole vaginal cream or suppositories, at bedtime for 7–14 days; topical gentian violet
Pinworms (*Enterobius vermicularis*)	+ +	±	Poor hygiene (spread from anus)	Pruritus; erythema	Visualization of ova in cellophane tape preparation	Mebendazole (Vermox) 1 tablet, orally
Foreign body (FB)	+ +	+	Foreign body (tampon)	Foul-smelling discharge; secondary bacterial infection	Physical examination; x-ray examination for opaque FB	Removal of FB

rates of miscarriage, premature births, infertility, and menstrual irregularities. Since administration of this drug to pregnant women did not cease until 1972, there are exposed teenage children who will continue to need discovery and evaluation.

In males exposed to DES in utero, abnormalities may include an increased incidence of hypoplastic testes, epididymal cysts, testicular capsular induration, urologic abnormalities such as microphallus, cryptorchidism, meatal stenosis, and alterations in sperm production, with or without infertility. No increased risk for neoplasms has been demonstrated, but studies so far are inconclusive; longer-term follow-up is necessary.

18.5 PREPUBERTAL VAGINAL BLEEDING

Conditions associated with vaginal bleeding in girls include estrogen withdrawal in the newborn, severe vulvovaginitis, foreign bodies, and genital neoplasms. Certain others deserve special comment.

Trauma is common in young girls and is often associated with straddle injuries. Sexual abuse is discussed below. If not extensive, simple tears of the vagina and vulva heal readily without scarring and require only supportive and symptomatic treatment including cold compresses, local anesthetics, and antibiotic creams for superficial infections. If bleeding is persistent or if the trauma is known to be more extensive, with or without visible signs, a complete vaginal examination must be carried out, under anesthesia if necessary. Puncture or other penetrating wounds are of particular concern, since rectal perforation and urethral or bladder injuries are possible; if these are suspected, appropriate investigation must be made.

Urethral prolapse may occur in prepubertal girls, because the adequacy of the supporting tissue of the distal urethra is in part dependent on estrogen effect (Sec. 17.44). Prolapse occurs most commonly with straining that leads to increased intraabdominal pressure, such as may occur with temper tantrums; but it may occur spontaneously. Irritation and excoriation, with bleeding of the friable mucosa, may be mistaken for vaginal bleeding. Usually the prolapse is self-limited and repair is rarely necessary. The diagnosis may be made by passing a urinary catheter into the bladder. Associated urologic anomalies or complications are rare.

Precocious puberty is true menstrual bleeding at an unexpectedly early age. Problems associated with early menarche are discussed in Sec. 9.10 and Sec. 19.6.

Sarcoma botryoides (Sec. 16.24) arises from the upper vagina and cervix; the first sign is generally a bloody vaginal discharge. This lesion is highly malignant; survival is rare. Any diagnosis of vaginal polyps in the young child requires that sarcoma botryoides be specifically ruled out. Radical surgery of vagina, cervix, and uterus may be required. Radiation and chemotherapy are being evaluated.

Billmire ME, Farrell MK, Dine MS, et al: A simplified procedure for pediatric vaginal examination. Use of veterinary otoscope specula. Pediatrics 65:823, 1980.

Chacko MR, Lovchik J: *Chlamydia trachomatis* infection in sexually active adolescents: prevalence and risk factors. Pediatrics 73 (6):836, 1984.

Cowell CA (ed): Symposium on pediatric and adolescent gynecology. Pediatr Clin North Am 28:245, 1981.

Emans SJ, Goldstein DP: Pediatric and Adolescent Gynecology. Boston, Little, Brown, 1977.

Emans SJ, Goldstein DP: The gynecologic examination of the pre-pubertal child with vulvovaginitis. Pediatrics 65:758, 1980.

Eschenbach DA: Epidemiology and diagnosis of acute pelvic inflammatory disease. Obstet Gynecol 55 (Suppl):142, 1980.

Hammerschlag MR, Alpert S, Rosner I, et al: Microbiology of the vagina in children: Normal and potentially pathogenic organisms. Pediatrics 62:57, 1978.

Herbst AL: Clear cell adenocarcinoma and the current status of DES-exposed females. Cancer 48 (Suppl):484, 1981.

Herbst AL, Hubby MM, Blough RR, et al: A comparison of pregnancy experience in DES-exposed and DES-unexposed daughters. J Reprod Med 24:62, 1980.

Herbst AL, Scully RE, Robboy SJ, et al: Complications of prenatal therapy with diethylstilbestrol. Pediatrics 62:1151, 1978.

Jacobs AH (ed): Symposium on pediatric dermatology. Pediatr Clin North Am 25:189, 1978.

Robboy SJ, Szyfelbein WM, Goellner JR, et al: Dysplasia and cytologic findings in 4589 young women enrolled in diethyl-adenosis (DESAD) project. Am J Obstet Gynecol 140:579, 1981.

Shafer MB, Irwin CE, Sweet RL, et al: Acute salpingitis in the adolescent female. J Pediatr 100:339, 1982.

Singleton AF: Vaginal discharge in children and adolescents. Clin Pediatr 19:799, 1980.

Stillman, RJ: In utero exposure to diethylstilbestrol: Adverse effects on the reproductive tract and reproductive performance in male and female offspring. Am J Obstet Gynecol 142 (7):905, 1982.

Wald, ER: Gynecologic Infections in the Pediatric Age Group. Pediatr Infect Dis May–June (Suppl):3:510, 1984.

18.6 SEXUAL MISUSE OF CHILDREN AND ADOLESCENTS

See also Sec. 2.57–2.59.

Sexual misuse is being identified and addressed with increasing frequency. Its legal definitions include child molestation, incest, and rape. The well-being of the misused child depends on appropriate inquiry, treatment, and adequate follow-up by an understanding and skillful physician. Childhood victims of sexual misuse have a median age of 11 yr, but significant numbers of episodes occur as early as the 1st yr of life. Girls are abused more often, but it is estimated that one out of four girls and one out of five boys will be molested by the age of 18 yr. Family members, close relatives, neighbors, and friends account for 30–50% of all incidents; 80% of children know their attackers. Incestuous relationships particularly frequently involve stepfathers. One study found that 17% of young women with stepfathers had been abused by them, as opposed to only 2% by biologic fathers. These figures may become more alarming with the increase in divorce (with the potential for subsequent remarriage and/or live-in male companions). Incest often starts before adolescence and may continue throughout this period, with severe psychologic disturbances associated. Sexual abuse occurs in all socioeconomic and ethnic groups. The physician must maintain a high level of suspicion if these problems are to be identified. Over 30% of reported cases of rape involve adolescent victims; some victims sustain significant genital and/or other physical injury, but in most cases injuries are relatively minor.

Many large medical centers and community agencies have developed multidisciplinary teams and programs to address problems of sexual abuse or rape, both as a service to the individual patient and as a community resource for education and awareness. The major issues to be addressed by such programs include preparation of the misused or abused child and family and preparation of the physician for the interview, examination, and follow-up of any problem. Management must be guided by assessment of the child's level of cognitive development with respect to such factors as capacities for concrete or formal thinking processes and for factual and logical construction of events with regard to facts and the timing of events. This understanding of the child's cognitive level allows the physician to plan the interview, to decide whether use of such aids as anatomically correct dolls is appropriate, etc. The family must be helped to feel comfortable and to be able to support the child. Considerable time may need to be spent in gaining rapport with the child or adolescent.

In the case of children or adolescents believed to have been the victims of sexual misuse or violence (rape) a thorough general physical examination must be done, during which police should not be present. Bruises should be looked for, particularly in areas where they commonly occur following forcible abuse or rape: around the mouth (often to prevent the child from screaming), neck, lips, etc. Significant bruising may not appear immediately after injury; re-examination in 24 hr may be important. An evaluation of sex maturity rating (Tanner) and menstrual history will help determine the likelihood of pregnancy. Careful examination must be made of the perineum in girls and of the genitalia and rectum in boys. A decision as to the need for pelvic examination should be based on (a) the possibility of injury; (b) the possibility of sexually transmitted disease; and (c) the acuteness of the episode. This decision should be made only after careful consideration of the benefits and risks for each patient.

Laboratory examinations should include (1) cultures for gonorrhea and *Chlamydia trachomatis* from appropriate sites (urethra; vagina in prepubertal girls, cervix in postpubertal; anal canal or rectum in accordance with history or physical findings; oropharynx); (2) a screening test for syphilis; (3) examination of a preparation of vaginal fluid in isotonic saline for spermatozoa and *Trichomonas*; and (4) testing for pregnancy when the sex maturity rating indicates it. Microscopic examination of material obtained from mouth, urethra, and rectum can be helpful. The need for particular specimens for medicolegal use should be reviewed according to local regulations and the details of each case. Such specimens may include blood and semen for typing; clothing specimens for examination; vaginal fluid or other specimens for detection of prostatic acid phosphatase or the p30 glycoprotein of semen; fingernails; hair (including that combed from the pubic hair of the adolescent); and photographs.

Medical prophylaxis or treatment of sexually transmitted disease should be considered (Sec. 9.9), as should the prevention of pregnancy. A 7–10 day course of tetracycline or doxycycline therapy is effective against gonorrhea, chlamydia, or incubating syphilis, but should not be used in pregnant patients, those in whom poor compliance with a regimen is anticipated, or in children younger than 8 yr. In these latter cases, single oral doses of ampicillin or amoxicillin, given with probenecid, may be adequate treatment for uncomplicated gonorrhea of the lower genital tract but not for anorectal or pharyngeal gonorrhea. Tests for cure should always be obtained after 14 days of treatment. Prophylaxis against pregnancy should be considered in consultation with the patient and her parents. If exposure occurred within the preceding 72 hr, pregnancy may be prevented using estrogen therapy alone. An alternative is oral administration of the contraceptive Ovral, 2 pills at time of initial examination and 2 pills 12 hr later. Antiemetics may be needed. It should be understood in advance that after such therapy is initiated, if a pregnancy then occurred, its termination would be strongly recommended. Patients require follow-up to re-examine medical and psychologic issues, and to re-evaluate the possibilities of sexually transmitted disease or of pregnancy.

Other management issues to be addressed include possible need for hospitalization when examination under anesthesia is required, when internal injury is suspected, when the child is too anxious to go home, when there is danger in returning home, or when there is risk of psychologic decompensation. Social intervention must be arranged through local social service agencies, abuse hot lines, etc., and a report of child abuse or rape must be made to the police or to another appropriate public agency. In the case of sexual abuse or misuse, especially within a household, it must be determined whether other family members (e.g., siblings) also should be physically examined, to confirm abuse or misuse or to judge whether they too are at risk.

Mental health counseling by professionals who are experienced and comfortable in dealing with these problems is an important element in crisis intervention in cases such as these and should be afforded all victims and their families. The need for long-term counseling should be assessed; such intervention may involve individual, family, or group therapy.

Rape involves more than physical assault; a "rape trauma syndrome," as described by Burgess and Holmstrom, includes two phases of psychologic adaptation: (1) an acute phase of disorganization, and (2) a long-term phase of reorganization. Adolescent rape victims are particularly likely to feel chronic anxieties, and a sense of lasting injury and invasion, with loss of self-esteem.

I. BRUCE GORDON

Anglin T: Personal communication, 1985.

Burgess AW, Holmstrom LL: Rape trauma syndrome. Am J Psychiatry 131:981, 1974.

DeJong AR, Hervada AR, Emmett GA, et al: Epidemiologic variations in childhood sexual abuse. Child Abuse and Neglect 7:155, 1983.

Finkelhor D: Sexually Victimized Children. New York, Macmillan, The Free Press, 1981.

Graves MCB, Sensabaugh GF, Blake ET, et al: Post coital detection of a male specific semen protein. N Engl J Med 312:338, 1985.

Russell DEH: The prevalence and seriousness of incestuous abuse: Stepfathers vs biological fathers. Child Abuse and Neglect 8:15, 1984.

19

THE ENDOCRINE SYSTEM

19.1 DISORDERS OF THE HYPOTHALAMUS AND PITUITARY GLAND

The hypothalamus and pituitary gland consist of seven or more functional units working in concert to maintain endocrine homeostasis. Many conditions formerly classified as pituitary have a hypothalamic origin, and advances in isolation and synthesis of hypothalamic hormones have permitted more precise delineation of endocrinologic conditions. New techniques help differentiate between hypopituitary and hypothalamic aberrations, with new therapeutic approaches available.

The pituitary gland is attached by a stalk to the median eminence of the brain and consists of a posterior lobe (neurohypophysis) and an anterior lobe. The differing connections of each lobe to the hypothalamus reflect their different embryologic origins. The posterior lobe is derived from the infundibulum of the diencephalon; it has direct neural connections via a large tract of fibers with neurons in the supraoptic and paraventricular nuclei of the anterior hypothalamus. The anterior lobe develops from ectoderm of the stomadeum (Rathke pouch) and is controlled by hypothalamic secretions. The endings of some hypothalamic nerve fibers liberate neurohormones into the capillaries of the median eminence, from which they are carried by portal vessels to the pituitary gland. Accordingly, the median eminence is the final common pathway of all releasing factors. Fetal rests of the original connection of the Rathke pouch with the primitive oral cavity may persist in postnatal life; tumors developing from such rests, known as craniopharyngiomas, are the most common tumors arising in this region during childhood.

Function. *Anterior Lobe.* The anterior pituitary has at least six different types of secretory cells, which synthesize and secrete a variety of protein hormones. These hormones act either on other endocrine glands or directly on certain body cells to affect almost every organ. The pituitary gland itself is under the control of hypothalamic secretions, each of which regulates specific pituitary cells. Hypothalamic secretions are of two types: releasing hormones, which release pituitary hormones; and inhibitory hormones, which inhibit such secretion. These pituitary hormones that lack feedback control from the product of a target gland (growth hormone, prolactin, and melanocyte-stimulating hormone) are controlled by hypothalamic inhibitors and stimulators. Only stimulators are known for corticotropin, thyrotropin, luteinizing hormone, and follicle-stimulating hormone; inhibition is effected by target gland hormones (corticosteroids, thyroxine, and sex steroids).

Growth hormone (hGH) is a protein with 191 amino acids; its gene is located on chromosome 17. Growth hormone is closely related to chorionic somatomammotropin (85% homology) and more distantly related to prolactin (26% homology). Unlike other pituitary hormones, hGH is relatively species-specific; only primate growth hormone is effective in humans. Growth hormone used in the past to treat hGH-deficient children was obtained from human pituitaries collected at autopsy; hGH is now being made by recombinant DNA technology.

Hypothalamic growth hormone–releasing factor (GRF) has been isolated from two different pancreatic tumors. One of these preparations was designated GRF-44-NH$_2$, the other GRF-40-NH$_2$; the former appears to be identical to the human hypothalamic hormone. Both peptides have been synthesized and are undergoing clinical trials as tests for pituitary function and for possible therapeutic indications. The growth hormone–inhibiting hormone is known as *somatostatin*. It is found in the hypothalamus, where it has a physiologic role in growth hormone secretion, and is also widely distributed in the central nervous system outside the hypothalamus. Evidence suggests that it is a secretory product of neurons and acts as a neurotransmitter or neuromodulator. It also occurs in defined populations of epithelial cells (D cells), in the pancreatic islets, and in the gut, where it is regulated by paracrine (side-by-side) secretion. Somatostatin-secreting pancreatic tumors (somatostatinomas) have been reported in adults. Somatostatin is a 14–amino acid peptide but 28–amino acid and larger prohormone forms are known. A long-acting analogue 45 times more active than somatostatin is being used experimentally in therapy of acromegaly.

A deficiency of growth hormone results in dwarfism, an excess in gigantism or acromegaly. Growth hormone has direct regulatory effects on protein, carbohydrate, and lipid metabolism in many tissues and organs. Its nitrogen-retaining, calciuric-phosphaturic, and insulinotropic effects are mediated indirectly through formation of *somatomedins* or *insulin-like growth factors*. It is now known that somatomedin C and insulin-like growth factor I (IGF I) are identical single-chain proteins with 70 amino acids coded for by a gene on chromosome 12. Insulin-like growth factor II (IGF II) is a single-chain protein with 67 amino acids coded for by a gene on the short arm of chromosome 11. Both IGF I and IGF II are homologous to proinsulin in structure. Somatomedins appear to be synthesized in liver and kidney, and circulate in plasma bound to carrier proteins. Growth hormone–deficient children have low levels of IGF I (somatomedin C) that return to normal during treatment with hGH. Defects in this class of potent insulin-like substances are now known to account for some types of growth disorders. Somatomedin C levels can be measured by radioimmunoassay; levels are normally quite low before 6 yr of age and rise markedly during puberty. IGF II appears to be induced by placental lactogen during prenatal development; its function is unknown.

Secretion of growth hormone is pulsatile; levels in normal healthy children are quite low for much of the day and are indistinguishable from those in hGH-deficient patients. In growing children there are five to nine discrete pulses every 24 hr. After 3–6 mo of age the most consistent pulses occur 45–90 min after onset of sleep. Because basal levels are low and secretion is pulsatile, evaluation of children for growth hormone deficiency is difficult, and provocative tests are often indicated for definitive diagnosis. Studies with DNA probes are delineating various defects in hGH synthesis.

Human *prolactin* is composed of 199 amino acid residues;

its gene is located on chromosome 6. The only established role for prolactin is the initiation and maintenance of lactation. Stimulation of the nipple is a potent stimulus to prolactin secretion. Mean serum levels in children and in fasting adults of both sexes are about 5–20 ng/mL. Elevated levels occur in full-term neonates and during pregnancy. Concentrations in amniotic fluid are 10–100 times the levels in maternal or fetal serum; the major source of amniotic prolactin appears to be the decidua.

A prolactin-inhibiting factor (PIF) and a prolactin-releasing factor (PRF) have been proposed. The PIF peptide has been isolated and found to reside within the precursor protein for gonadotropin-releasing hormone. Administration of thyrotropin-releasing factor (TRH) increases prolactin levels, but its physiologic role is unknown. Dopamine decreases secretion of prolactin. No definitive tests can as yet separate hyperplasia from tumors of the lactotrophs.

Prolactin is pathologically elevated with section of the pituitary stalk, in certain pituitary tumors, and in a variety of hypothalamic disorders. Elevated levels of both thyrotropin (TSH) and prolactin occur in primary hypothyroidism, presumably in response to elevated levels of TRH (see below).

TSH consists of two glycoprotein chains linked by hydrogen bonding. The α chain is identical to that found in follicle-stimulating hormone (FSH), luteinizing hormone (LH), and human chorionic gonadotropin (hCG). The β chain is unique in each of these hormones and confers specificity. The gene for the α chain has been mapped on chromosome 6, that for the β chain of TSH on chromosome 1, and those for the β chains for LH and hCG on chromosome 19. TSH increases iodine uptake, iodide clearance from the plasma, iodotyrosine and iodothyronine formation, thyroglobulin proteolysis, and release of thyroxine and triiodothyronine from the thyroid. Deficiency results in inactivity and atrophy of the thyroid, and excess results in hypertrophy and hyperplasia. Radioimmunoassay for TSH in serum aids in the study of clinical problems.

TRH was the first hypothalamic hormone to be isolated, characterized, and synthesized; it is a tripeptide ([pyro] Glu-His-Pro-NH$_2$). Thyroxine and triiodothyronine inhibit TSH secretion by blocking the action of TRH upon the pituitary cell. TRH also stimulates the release of prolactin, in males as well as in females. Synthetic TRH is useful for testing pituitary reserves of TSH and prolactin. Through such studies it is possible to discriminate between the hypothalamic and pituitary origins of many disorders.

Corticotropin (ACTH) is derived by proteolytic cleavage from a large precursor glycoprotein product of the pituitary gland called *pre-opiomelanocortin* (POMC). Cleavage of POMC yields both ACTH (a single, unbranched glycoprotein chain of 39 amino acids) and β-lipotropin (β-LPH) (a 91-amino acid glycoprotein). Further cleavage of ACTH and β-LPH in the pituitary yields yet other hormonal products. Thus, α-melanocyte–stimulating hormone (α-MSH) is identical to the first 13 amino acids of ACTH but has no corticotropin activity; cleavage of β-LPH results in neurotropic peptides with morphinomimetic activity (fragment 61–91 is β-endorphin); and β-melanocyte–stimulating hormone (β-MSH) consists of a 17–amino acid fragment of β-LPH.

Corticotropin acts primarily on the adrenal gland; it produces changes in structure, chemical composition, enzymatic activity, and release of corticosteroid hormones. ACTH release has a diurnal rhythm; it is lowest between 10 P.M.–2 A.M. with peak levels reached about 8 A.M. Levels of β-LPH and of β-endorphin are elevated in endocrine disorders with increased ACTH. It appears that ACTH, rather than MSH, is the principal pigmentary hormone in humans.

Secretion of ACTH is regulated by corticotropin-releasing factor (CRF), a 41–amino acid residue. CRF has been synthe-

sized; it appears to be particularly useful in differentiation of different forms of Cushing syndrome. Vasopressin and the catecholamines may also participate in regulating secretion of ACTH in basal and stress-related states.

Gonadotropic hormones include two glycoproteins: LH and FSH. Each has an α subunit and a β subunit. The α subunits of these two hormones and of TSH are identical; specificity of hormone action resides in the β subunit, which is different for each of the three. Receptors for FSH on the ovarian granulosa cells and on testicular Sertoli cells mediate FSH stimulation of follicular development in the ovary and of gametogenesis in the testis. On binding to specific receptors on ovarian theca cells and testicular Leydig cells, LH promotes luteinization of the ovary and Leydig cell function of the testis. Both LH and FSH activate adenyl cyclase. Highly specific and sensitive radioimmunoassays for FSH and LH can measure levels in the plasma of prepubertal children.

Hypothalamic control of gonadotropic hormones has long been known, and separate releasing hormones for FSH and LH were once anticipated. Luteinizing hormone–releasing hormone (LH-RH), a decapeptide, has been isolated, synthesized, and widely used in clinical studies. Since it leads to the release of both LH and FSH, it is now proposed that there may be only one gonadotropin-releasing hormone. In addition to sex steroids, the gonads produce *inhibin*, a protein that selectively inhibits release of FSH.

Posterior Lobe. The posterior lobe of the pituitary is part of a functional unit (the neurohypophysis) that consists of (1) the neurons of the supraoptic and paraventricular nuclei of the hypothalamus; (2) neuronal axons, which form the pituitary stalk; and (3) neuronal terminals, either in the median eminence or in the posterior lobe.

The neurohypophysis is the source of *arginine vasopressin* (AVP, the antidiuretic hormone) and of *oxytocin*; both are octapeptides, differing in only two amino acids. These hormones are produced by neurosecretion in the hypothalamic nuclei. The neurons of the supraoptic and paraventricular nuclei also synthesize specific *neurophysins* during the biosynthesis of vasopressin and oxytocin. These are transported to nerve terminals in the posterior pituitary, where they are released together with oxytocin or vasopressin. Radioimmunoassays of the neurophysins provide a direct index of vasopressin and oxytocin levels in plasma. The concentration of arginine vasopressin in umbilical cord plasma appears to be a sensitive indicator of fetal stress.

Vasopressin has a short half-life and responds very quickly to changes in hydration. It changes the permeability of the renal tubular cell membrane via cyclic AMP. Vasopressin and oxytocin are thought to be synthesized in separate and specific cells. A synthetic analogue, desmopressin, is resistant to peptidases and has a prolonged half-life. Small amounts administered intranasally are effective in therapy of patients with diabetes insipidus.

19.2 HYPOPITUITARISM

Here we shall discuss only those hypopituitary states associated with deficiency of growth hormone (Table 19–1). Affected children have usually been referred to as pituitary dwarfs, a designation best avoided. Isolated deficiencies of thyrotropin, corticotropin, and gonadotropin are discussed later.

Etiology. *Congenital Defects.* Aplasia or hypoplasia of the pituitary is rare. Developmental abnormalities of the pituitary are associated with such defects as anencephaly, holoprosencephaly (cyclopia, cebocephaly, orbital hypotelorism), and septo-optic dysplasia (de Morsier syndrome). In *Hall-Pallister syndrome* absence of pituitary gland is associated with hypo-

Table 19–1. Etiologic Classification of Hypopituitarism: Pituitary and/or Hypothalamic Dysfunction

Developmental defects
  Anencephaly
  Holoprosencephaly (cyclopia, cebocephaly, orbital hypotelorism)
  Midfacial anomalies (e.g., hypertelorism)
  Basal encephalocele
  Septo-optic dysplasia (de Morsier syndrome)
  Cleft lip and palate
  Solitary maxillary central incisor
  Hall-Pallister syndrome (hypothalamic hamartoblastoma, imperforate anus, polydactyly)
  Rieger syndrome
  Fanconi syndrome
Genetic defects of LGH or GRF
  Isolated hGH deficiency
    Autosomal recessive–type I
      Type 1A–deletion of gene for GH
      Type 1B
    Autosomal dominant–type II
    X-linked–type III
  Multiple pituitary deficiencies
    Autosomal recessive–type I
    X-linked–type III
Destructive lesions
  Trauma
    Perinatal (trauma, anoxia, hemorrhagic infarction)
    Basal skull fractures
    Child abuse
  Infiltrative lesions
    Tumors
      Histocytosis X
      Craniopharyngioma
      Hypothalamic tumors
      Germinoma
      Optic glioma
      Pituitary adenomas
    Sarcoidosis
    Hemochromatosis
    Tuberculosis
    Toxoplasmosis
  Irradiation (CNS, eyes, middle ears)
    Empty sella with enlarged sella
  Surgery
    Removal of pharyngeal pituitary
    Surgery for craniopharyngioma and other tumors
  Vascular
    Infarctions (e.g., hemoglobinopathy)
    Aneurysm
    Autoimmune hypophysitis
Unresponsiveness to growth hormone
  Insulin-like growth factor I deficiency
    Laron syndrome
    African pygmy
  Bioinactive growth hormone
Other functional deficiency
  Hypothyroidism
  Psychosocial deprivation

thalamic hamartoblastoma, postaxial polydactyly, nail dysplasia, bifid epiglottis, imperforate anus, and anomalies of the heart, lungs, and kidneys; most patients die neonatally, but in at least one instance neonatal hypopituitarism was recognized, CT scan revealed the hypothalamic tumor, and surgical removal was successful at 1 yr of age. In the neonate, symptoms of hypopituitarism with postaxial polydactyly and bifid epiglottis should suggest this diagnosis. Hypoplasia of the pituitary with anencephaly has long been known, but recent observations reveal a large residuum of normal pituitary function and suggest that hypoplasia may be secondary to the hypothalamic defect. With hypothalamic-releasing hormones it is possible to determine whether defects in pituitary function reside in the pituitary or in the hypothalamus. Many of these conditions are lethal early in life, but partial defects may occur in siblings. A child has been reported with isolated deficiency of growth hormone and mild hypotelorism who had two siblings with holoprosencephaly with hypopituitarism. Deficiency of growth hormone occurs in 4% of all patients with *cleft lip* or *cleft palate* and in 32% of those who have short stature. Midfacial anomalies or the finding of a *solitary maxillary central incisor* will indicate high likelihood of growth hormone deficiency.

Optic nerve hypoplasia, bilateral or unilateral, is often associated with hypopituitarism. When it is also associated with absence of the septum pellucidum, the condition is known as *septo-optic dysplasia.* The fundus exhibits hypoplastic discs with typical double rims and sparse retinal vessels. Endocrine abnormalities are extremely variable. Hormonal deficiency most often involves growth hormone alone, but multiple pituitary deficiencies, including diabetes insipidus, may occur. The defect resides primarily in the hypothalamus. Delay in linear growth may begin as early as 3 mo of age or may not be observed before 3–4 yr of age. Affected newborns often have apnea, hypotonia and seizures, prolonged jaundice, hypoglycemia without hyperinsulinism, and (in males) microphallus. The condition is usually sporadic but has been reported in first cousins. The cause is unknown but young maternal age and nulliparity are strongly associated.

Aplasia of the pituitary without abnormalities of the brain or skull is very rare, but affected infants are being increasingly recognized because hypoglycemia occurs early and in males there is microphallus. Some have had evidence of the neonatal hepatitis syndrome, but the relationship of hypopituitarism is obscure. The condition has been reported in siblings of both sexes, and consanguinity has been noted in two families; autosomal recessive inheritance is suggested. Studies in some children have placed the defect in the hypothalamus. This may be a heterogeneous group of disorders.

In *empty-sella syndrome* a deficient sellar diaphragm leads to herniation of the suprasellar subarachnoid space into the sella turcica, with remodeling of the sella and flattening of the pituitary gland. It may follow surgery or radiation therapy or be idiopathic. Of 17 cases reported in children, significant hypopituitarism was present in 5. Empty-sella with an enlarged sella and hypopituitarism has been observed in siblings.

Hypogammaglobulinemia has been associated with isolated growth hormone deficiency in one family as an X-linked trait. The relationship between the two disorders is not clear.

Other syndromes in which short stature is a prominent feature may be associated with deficiency of growth hormone; for example, occasionally patients with Turner, Fanconi, Russell-Silver, Rieger, Williams or the CHARGE syndrome have been found to have hypopituitarism.

Destructive Lesions. Any lesion which damages the anterior pituitary or hypothalamus may cause cessation of growth. Since such lesions are not selective, multiple hormonal deficiencies are usually observed. The most common lesion responsible for this condition is the craniopharyngioma; central nervous system germinoma and other hypothalamic tumors, tuberculosis, sarcoidosis, toxoplasmosis, and aneurysms may also cause hypothalamic-hypophyseal destruction. These lesions are frequently associated with roentgenographic changes in the skull. Besides diabetes insipidus, deficiency of growth hormone and other pituitary hormones may occur in children with histiocytosis, especially if treated with cranial irradiation. Enlargement of the sella or deformation or destruction of the clinoid processes usually indicates a tumor. Intrasellar or suprasellar calcifications usually indicate a craniopharyngioma. Trauma, including child abuse, traction at delivery, anoxia, and hemorrhagic infarction may also damage the pituitary, its stalk, or the hypothalamus.

Irradiation for tumors of the central nervous system, eyes, and middle ears may cause hypothalamic-pituitary damage. Children with acute lymphocytic leukemia who receive prophylactic cranial irradiation have decreased rates of growth, and in many instances hypopituitarism has appeared many years after cancer therapy. Deficiency of growth hormone is the most common defect, but deficiencies of TSH, ACTH, and gonadotropins may also occur. The latent period may be long between irradiation and onset of clinical manifestations.

Idiopathic Hypopituitarism. In the majority of patients with hypopituitarism, there is no demonstrable lesion of the pituitary or hypothalamus; and in most, the functional defect is hypothalamic rather than pituitary. The deficiency may be of growth hormone only or of multiple hormones. The condition is most often sporadic. Association with breech birth, forceps delivery, and intrapartum and maternal bleeding suggest that birth trauma and anoxia may be pathogenic factors in some instances.

In 5–10% of cases the deficiency is familial. Analysis of pedigrees and endocrine studies have delineated autosomal recessive (type I), autosomal dominant (type II), and X-linked (type III) forms of isolated growth-hormone deficiency, as well as autosomal recessive (type I) and X-linked (type II) forms of multiple pituitary deficiencies (hGH, TSH, LH, FSH). The locus of defect in these disorders is now being intensively investigated through DNA probes and testing of patients with GRF.

Type I (autosomal recessive) isolated hGH deficiency (IGHD) has been subdivided into two subtypes. Patients with type IA IGHD have no response of hGH to provocative stimuli; the gene for hGH is known to be absent. These patients develop antibodies to exogenous hGH, presumably because it acts as a foreign protein in a patient who has never been exposed to endogenous hGH. Most patients become refractory to treatment with hGH and growth ceases, but there is some phenotypic heterogeneity. Patients with type IB IGHD produce small amounts of growth hormone to provocative stimuli and respond well to exogenous hGH. The genes coding for growth hormone are present and normal in structure. A brisk response to GRF suggests that the defect in type IB IGHD is a genetic deficiency of GRF.

The nature of the defect in type II IGHD (autosomal dominant) is uncertain. In type III IGHD (X-linked) the defect is unknown, but does not involve the growth hormone gene. Patients with multiple pituitary deficiencies would not be expected to have a defect in the growth hormone gene but rather to have hypothalamic defects.

Unresponsiveness to Growth Hormone. Children with *Laron syndrome* have all the clinical findings of those with hypopituitarism, but plasma levels of biologically active growth hormone are elevated, whereas those of somatomedin C are low. These patients fail to grow, and levels of somatomedin C do not increase after administration of hGH. The defect appears to be failure of generation of somatomedin C in response to growth hormone. The disorder has been reported primarily in Jewish families of Oriental origin, but cases have been reported sporadically in other ethnic groups; it appears to be an autosomal recessive defect. The molecular defect is unknown.

African pygmies in the rain forest of Equatorial Africa resemble patients with deficiency of growth hormone but have normal levels of growth hormone and do not respond to large doses of hGH. Pygmies appear to have a primary deficiency in IGF I (somatomedin C).

Clinical Manifestations. *In Patients Without Demonstrable Lesions of the Pituitary.* The hypopituitary child is usually of normal size and weight at birth. In about half of affected children the retardation of growth is noticed by 1 yr of age. In others there may be regular but slow growth in height, with the increments always below those of coevals, or periods of lack of growth may alternate with short spurts of growth. Delayed closure of the epiphyses permits growth beyond the age when normal persons cease to grow.

Infants with congenital defects of the pituitary or hypothalamus usually present such neonatal emergencies as apnea, cyanosis, or severe hypoglycemia. Microphallus in the male is an important diagnostic clue. Deficiency of growth hormone may be accompanied by hypoadrenalism and hypothyroidism, and clinical manifestations of hypopituitarism evolve more rapidly than in the usual hypopituitary child.

The head is round and the face short and broad. The frontal bone is prominent and the bridge of the nose depressed and saddle-shaped. The nose is small, and the nasolabial folds are well developed. The eyes are somewhat bulging. The mandible and the chin are underdeveloped and infantile, and the teeth, which erupt late, are frequently crowded. The neck is short and the larynx small. The voice is high-pitched and remains high after puberty. The extremities are well proportioned, with small hands and feet. The genitalia are usually underdeveloped for the child's age, and sexual maturation may be delayed or absent. Facial, axillary, and pubic hair is usually absent; the hair of the scalp is fine. Symptomatic hypoglycemia, usually after fasting, occurs in 10–15% of children with panhypopituitarism as well as with isolated growth hormone deficiency. Intelligence is usually normal. Affected children may become shy and retiring.

In Patients with Demonstrable Lesions of the Pituitary. The child is normal initially, and manifestations similar to those seen in idiopathic pituitary growth failure gradually appear and progress. When complete or almost complete destruction of the pituitary gland occurs, severe manifestations of pituitary insufficiency are present. Atrophy of the adrenal cortex, thyroid, and gonads results in loss of weight, asthenia, sensitivity to cold, mental torpor, and absence of sweating. Sexual maturation fails to take place or regresses if already present. Thus, there may be atrophy of the gonads and genital tract with amenorrhea and loss of pubic and axillary hair. There is a tendency to hypoglycemia and coma. Growth ceases. Diabetes insipidus may be present early but tends to improve spontaneously with progressive destruction of the anterior pituitary.

If the lesion is an expanding tumor, symptoms such as headache, vomiting, visual disturbances, pathologic sleep, decreased school performance, seizures, polyuria, and growth failure may be present. Growth failure frequently antedates the neurologic signs and symptoms, especially in patients with craniopharyngiomas, but symptoms of hormonal deficit account for only 10% of presenting complaints. In other patients the neurologic manifestations may precede the endocrinologic, or evidence of pituitary insufficiency may first appear after surgical intervention. In children with craniopharyngiomas visual field defects, optic atrophy, papilledema, and cranial nerve palsy are common.

Laboratory Data. The diagnosis of growth hormone deficiency rests upon demonstration of absent or subnormal reserve of pituitary hGH. Random serum levels of growth hormone over 10 ng/mL exclude growth hormone deficiency, but lower levels must be studied further. Exercise is a benign and physiologic stimulus to growth hormone release; in most normal children elevated levels of growth hormone will be found after 20 min of strenuous exercise. Levels of growth hormone are also elevated 45–90 min after onset of sleep. If only low levels are found under these conditions, provocative tests for growth hormone release are required to verify a deficiency and to identify those children who will not respond to treatment with growth hormone. The usual provocative agents are L-dopa, insulin, and arginine, and tests with each may be required. Finding levels below 7–10 ng/mL after two provocative tests establishes the diagnosis of growth hormone deficiency. Great care must be taken in the administration of insulin to patients with hypopituitarism because of their decreased ability to overcome hypoglycemia. At greatest risk are thin children under 5 yr of age, particularly if they exhibit low levels of glucose when fasting. Levels of somatomedin C are increasingly used to indicate hGH deficiency. Diagnostic use of measurements of somatomedin C requires comparison with age- and sex-matched controls. In healthy children, levels gradually increase from birth to peak levels at puberty with peak levels 2 yr earlier in girls than in boys. In growth hormone-deficient children levels are very low but rise significantly within 16–28 hr of hGH administration in the majority of patients. Before 10 yr of age, a single level of somatomedin C cannot usually discriminate between children with hypopituitarism and healthy children; nor does a lack of rise in somatomedin level after growth hormone administration predict the response to long-term therapy with hGH.

Decreased growth hormone responses may also occur in children with primary hypothyroidism or with emotional deprivation, but in these conditions correction of the underlying disorder restores growth hormone levels to normal.

Once hGH deficiency is established, it is necessary to examine the functions of the remainder of the pituitary-hypothalamic axis. When there is deficiency of thyrotropin, serum levels of thyroxine and TSH are low. A normal rise in TSH and prolactin following stimulation with TRH places the defect in the hypothalamus, whereas absence of response localizes the defect in the pituitary. In most patients with idiopathic multiple anterior pituitary hormone deficiency, normal responses to TRH indicate that the deficiency is primary in the hypothalamus and secondary in the pituitary. An elevated random level of plasma prolactin in the hypopituitary patient is also strong evidence that there is a defect in the hypothalamus rather than in the pituitary. Some children with craniopharyngioma have elevated levels of prolactin before surgery, whereas after surgery they have prolactin deficiency due to pituitary damage.

Decreased urinary corticosteroid and plasma cortisol levels indicate deficiency of corticotropin. Insulin-induced hypoglycemia provokes a rise in cortisol levels by stimulating ACTH release; measurements of cortisol levels, therefore, during the provocative test for growth hormone with insulin provide information concerning corticotropin reserve. Serum FSH and LH levels may be decreased even below the ordinarily low prepubertal levels, but gonadotropin deficiency cannot be excluded until after the child has gone through puberty. Antidiuretic hormone deficiency may be established by appropriate studies.

Studies of children with hypopituitarism who have been given the recently synthesized growth hormone-releasing factor (GRF) have found a rise of growth hormone levels of variable magnitude in the majority, which provides further evidence that in most cases the defect is hypothalamic rather than pituitary. A single failure of response to GRF does not exclude a hypothalamic defect. GRF is currently an investigational agent in the United States.

Roentgenographic Examination. The long bones are slender and poor in minerals, the centers of ossification appear late, and the epiphyseal clefts remain open. The fontanels may remain open beyond the 2nd yr and intersutural wormian bones may be found. The sella turcica may be abnormally small, but a normal sellar volume does not exclude the diagnosis. Roentgenograms of the skull are most helpful when there is a destructive or space-occupying lesion causing hypopituitarism. In patients with nausea, vomiting, loss of vision, headache, or increase in circumference of the head evidence of increased intracranial pressure may be found. Enlargement of the sella, especially ballooning with erosion and calcifications within or above the sella, may be detected. CT scan is indicated in all patients with hypopituitarism.

Differential Diagnosis. The causes of growth disorders are legion; only those that most closely mimic hypopituitarism are considered here.

Responses of growth hormone secretion to pharmacologic stimuli do not mimic the physiologic pulsatile secretion of growth hormone. It is now clear that some children with short stature and decreased growth velocity who are not found to be growth hormone deficient when studied by the usual growth hormone provocative tests, will, when levels of growth hormone are measured every 20 min for a 24 hr period, show a marked deficiency of pulsatile secretion or of 24 hr integrated concentration; this condition has been called *growth hormone neurosecretory dysfunction*. Treatment of such patients with hGH often results in increased growth velocity. Since such studies are neither generally available nor practical, more effective tests and criteria need to be developed for the diagnosis of this group of growth hormone–deficient patients.

A small number of children with decreased growth velocity have normal levels of immunoreactive growth hormone but deficient levels by radioreceptor assay and an abnormal ratio of the two levels. Levels of somatomedin C may be low or normal. Treatment with growth hormone may result in normalization of growth rate and in increase in somatomedin levels. In one such patient the circulating growth hormone was an abnormal polymer with low bioactivity. Many other theoretical defects of growth hormone structure resulting in *bioinactive growth hormone* are possible; this cause of hypopituitarism may be more frequent than heretofore recognized.

A small number of otherwise normal children are short (more than 3 SD below the mean for age) and grow 5 cm or less per yr but have normal levels of growth hormone in response to provocative tests. Surprisingly, a significant percentage of such children have increased rates of growth when treated with growth hormone in doses comparable to those used to treat hypopituitary children. Plasma levels of somatomedin in these patients may be normal or low and the response of somatomedin to growth hormone after 4–10 daily injections does not predict the response to later growth with prolonged treatment. No long-term results are available, and it is not known whether the final height of this group of patients will be improved. There are no methods that predict reliably which of these children will respond to growth hormone. Since treatment of otherwise normal short children without proven hypopituitarism is still undergoing experimental trials, this use of growth hormone should be restricted at present.

Constitutional growth delay is one of the most frequent growth problems encountered by the pediatrician. Length and weight of affected children are normal at birth, with growth normal for the first 4–12 mo of life. Growth then decelerates to near or below the 3rd percentile for height and weight. By 2–3 yr of age, growth resumes at a normal rate of 5 cm/yr or more. Studies of growth hormone secretion and other studies are within normal limits. Osseous maturation is consistent with height-age rather than chronologic age. Detailed questioning will uncover other family members (frequently one or both of the parents) with histories of short stature in childhood, delayed puberty, and eventual normal stature. The prognosis for these children to achieve normal adult height is excellent. Boys with unusual degrees of delayed puberty may occasionally require a short course of testosterone therapy to initiate puberty. The cause for this variant of normal growth is unknown. Constitutional growth delay can be differentiated from *genetic short stature* by the level of skeletal maturation, which is consistent with chronologic age in the latter condition. Genetic short stature will usually be found in other family members. Results of studies of growth, however, are normal.

Primary hypothyroidism is usually easily distinguished on clinical grounds. Responses to growth hormone provocative tests may be subnormal, however, and enlargement of the sella may be present. Elevated levels of TSH clearly establish the diagnosis, and these secondary changes disappear following treatment with thyroid hormone.

Turner syndrome must always be considered in short girls. When this is associated with the usual characteristic congenital deformities, the diagnosis is not difficult, but in other instances there may be few characteristic findings other than shortness of stature. Chromosomal analysis is necessary to establish the diagnosis. Girls aged 9–20 yr who have Turner syndrome have decreased episodic secretion of growth hormone, but its contribution to the short stature is not known. Treatment of girls with Turner syndrome with hGH is currently undergoing clinical trials.

Emotional deprivation is an important cause of retardation of growth and mimics hypopituitarism. The condition is known as psychosocial dwarfism, deprivation dwarfism, or reversible hyposomatotropism. The mechanisms whereby sensory and emotional deprivation interferes with growth are not fully understood. Functional hypopituitarism is indicated by low levels of somatomedin, by inadequate responses of growth hormone to provocative stimuli, by decreased pituitary responses to metyrapone stimulation, and perhaps by delayed puberty. Appropriate history and careful observations reveal disturbed mother-child or family relations and provide clues to diagnosis. Proof may be difficult to establish because the adults responsible often hide from professionals the true situation in the family and the children rarely divulge their plight. Emotionally deprived children frequently have perverted or voracious appetites, enuresis, encopresis, insomnia, crying spasms, and sudden tantrums. They may be excessively passive or aggressive and are borderline or dull-normal in intelligence. When child-rearing practices are altered or when the child is removed from the domicile of abuse, the rate of growth improves significantly. During this period of catch-up growth, separation of the cranial sutures and other evidence of pseudotumor cerebri may occur; these should not be mistaken for signs of a mass lesion.

The *Silver-Russell syndrome* is characterized by short stature, frontal bossing, small triangular facies, sparse subcutaneous tissue, shortened and incurved 5th fingers, and, in many cases, asymmetry. Affected children have low birthweights for gestational age. Growth hormone levels are usually normal, but five affected patients have had growth hormone deficiencies, one due to a craniopharyngioma and four idiopathic.

Prognosis. With the expanding supply of hGH, prognosis for achievement of an acceptable height is excellent, provided diagnosis is established early and treatment is not delayed. Patients with defects in growth hormone responsiveness, such as those with Laron syndrome, and patients who develop high titers of antibodies, such as those with Type IA (autosomal recessive) isolated growth hormone deficiency, have a less satisfactory outlook; prognosis for these patients may change when IGF I is synthesized and becomes available for trial.

Treatment. In patients with demonstrable organic lesions treatment should be directed to the underlying disease process. Evaluation of pituitary function is indicated after surgery and/or irradiation.

Treatment with growth hormone should begin as early as possible; younger children respond better than older ones, and long-term expectations are better. The recommended dose of hGH is 0.1–0.2 unit/kg, three times a week, administered intramuscularly or subcutaneously. Therapy should be continuous until there is no further response, a point usually concomitant with closure of the epiphyses. If the effect of therapy wanes, the dose should be increased. Almost half of treated patients develop antibodies to hGH, but less than 5% become resistant to therapy. With the prospect of an unlimited supply of hGH manufactured by recombinant DNA technology, intensive investigations are in progress to determine the full spectrum of short children who may benefit from treatment with hGH.

Replacement should also be directed at other hormonal deficiencies when present. In TSH-deficient subjects, thyroid hormone is given in full-replacement doses; in corticotropin-deficient patients the dose of hydrocortisone should not exceed 10–15 mg/m²/day. In patients with deficiency of gonadotropins, gonadal steroids are given when the bone-age reaches the age when puberty usually takes place. For infants with microphallus one or two 3-mo courses of monthly intramuscular injections of 25 mg of testosterone enanthate may bring the penis to normal size without inordinate effect on osseous maturation.

In the high percentage of hypopituitary children with deficiency of growth hormone–releasing factor (GRF), administration of GRF may prove useful in treatment. Pulsatile administration of this agent every 3 hr for 6 mo resulted in satisfactory acceleration of growth in two children.

19.3 DIABETES INSIPIDUS
(Arginine Vasopressin Deficiency)

Diabetes insipidus, characterized by polyuria and polydipsia, results from lack of the antidiuretic hormone, arginine vasopressin. Destruction of the supraoptic and paraventricular nuclei or division of the supraoptic-hypophyseal tract above the median eminence results in permanent diabetes insipidus. Transection of the tract below the median eminence or removal of just the posterior lobe may result in transitory polyuria, but in this case arginine vasopressin released into the median eminence prevents occurrence of diabetes insipidus. Vasopressin acts directly on the distal tubules and collecting ducts of the kidney to facilitate reabsorption of water. Vasopressin deficiency may be total or partial with varying degrees of polydipsia and polyuria.

Etiology. Any lesion which damages the neurohypophyseal unit may result in diabetes insipidus. Tumors of the suprasellar and chiasmatic regions, particularly craniopharygiomas (Fig. 19–1), optic gliomas, and germinomas, are common causes; the symptoms of increased intracranial pressure may accompany those of diabetes insipidus or may follow years later. Approximately 25–50% of patients with histiocytosis have diabetes insipidus as a consequence of histiocytic infiltration of the hypothalamus and pituitary. Deficiency of growth hormone is found in most patients with reticuloendothelioses who manifest diabetes insipidus. Encephalitis, sarcoidosis, tuberculosis, actinomycosis, and leukemia are occasional causes. Injuries to the head, especially basal skull fractures, may produce diabetes insipidus immediately or after a delay of several mo. Operative procedures near the pituitary or hypothalamus may result in transitory or permanent diabetes insipidus.

In a minority of instances diabetes insipidus is hereditary. Autosomal dominant and X-linked recessive forms occur; affected males with either type are indistinguishable. In the genetic forms of the disorder there is marked reduction in neurosecretory cells of the supraoptic and paraventricular nuclei. In the Brattleboro strain of rat, diabetes insipidus is transmitted as an autosomal recessive trait; the neurosecretory cells are normal or hypertrophied; thus, the basic defect is in the synthesis of the peptide hormone.

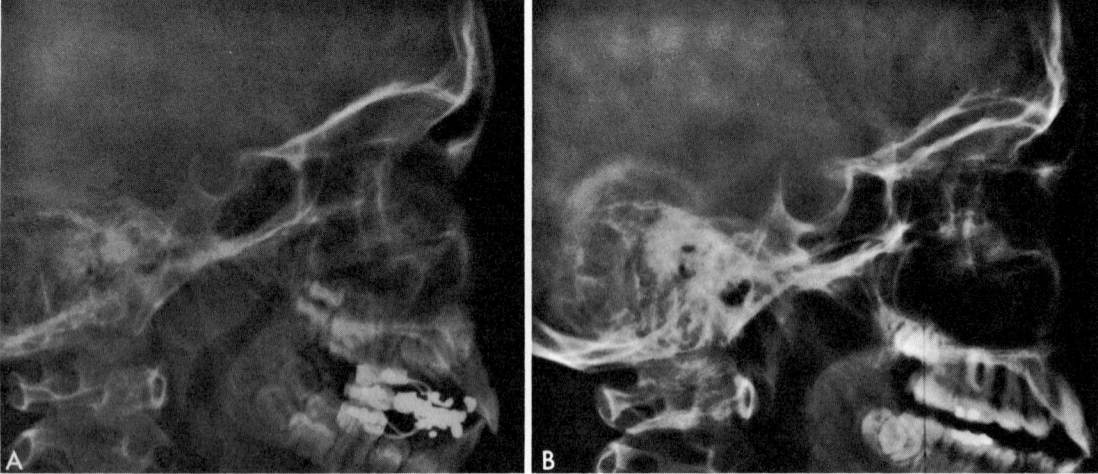

Figure 19–1. *A*, Roentgenograph of skull of 9 yr old boy with polydipsia, polyuria, nocturia, and enuresis. Urine specific gravity was 1.016 after water deprivation. Growth was normal, and the sella turcica was considered roentgenographically to be at upper limit of normal, but was probably enlarged. Over the ensuing 6 mo the symptoms of diabetes insipidus abated. *B*, The patient returned at 14 yr of age because of growth failure and delay in sexual maturation. Studies revealed a deficiency of growth hormone, gonadotropins, corticotropin, and thyrotropin. Note enlargement and thinning of the sella turcica but absence of intrasellar or suprasellar calcification. Neurologic and ophthalmologic examinations were normal. There was exacerbation of diabetes insipidus with administration of hydrocortisone and thyroxine. At surgery a large craniopharyngioma was found.

Diabetes insipidus is associated with diabetes mellitus, optic atrophy, and sensorineural deafness in *Wolfram syndrome*. The order of appearance of the various components varies. Pathologic studies suggest that a systemic degenerative process involves the optic nerve, supraoptic and paraventricular nuclei, and 8th cranial nerve. Incomplete forms of the syndrome may occur in patients or in their siblings; an autosomal recessive mode of inheritance is likely. Diabetes insipidus occasionally accompanies *septo-optic dysplasia*.

Diabetes insipidus has been reported in the newborn infant following asphyxia, intraventricular hemorrhage, intravascular coagulopathy, *Listeria monocytogenes* sepsis, and group B beta-hemolytic streptococcal meningitis.

In many instances, the cause of diabetes insipidus cannot be found initially, but only about 20% of affected patients will eventually be classified as idiopathic. In over half of all patients with intracranial tumors clinical or neuroradiologic signs (or both) are not manifest until 1 yr after diagnosis of diabetes insipidus, and in 25% the delay is as long as 4 yr. Periodic re-evaluation is required for at least 4 yr before the entity can be called "idiopathic." In 50% of children with idiopathic diabetes insipidus, the condition appears to have an autoimmune basis, since antibodies reacting with vasopressin-synthesizing cells have been found. Diabetes insipidus is being increasingly recognized as a terminal event in brain dead individuals.

Clinical Manifestations. Polydipsia and polyuria are the outstanding symptoms of diabetes insipidus. In families with the hereditary disorder the polyuria is often noted in early infancy. The infant cries excessively and will not be satisfied with additional milk but is quieted with water. Hyperthermia, rapid loss of weight, and collapse are common in infancy. Vomiting, constipation, and growth failure may be observed. Dehydration in early infancy may result in brain damage and mental impairment. In vasopressin deficiency there is wide variability in manifestations. Severity tends to increase with age, some affected members being asymptomatic until adolescence. Many affected families accept polydipsia and polyuria as a family habit and do not seek medical attention or may even prefer the symptoms to injections of vasopressin.

In a child who has acquired bladder control, enuresis may be the first symptom. The excessive thirst is disturbing and interferes with play, learning, and sleep. Children with diabetes insipidus do not perspire; their skin is dry and pale. Anorexia is common; there is a preference for carbohydrates.

Other signs and symptoms depend on the primary lesion; for example, patients with tumors in the region of the hypothalamus may have disturbance of growth, progressive cachexia or obesity, hyperpyrexia, sleep disturbance, sexual precocity, or emotional disorders. Lesions initially causing diabetes insipidus may eventually destroy the anterior pituitary; in such instances the diabetes insipidus tends to become milder or disappear completely.

Laboratory Data. The daily volume of urine may be 4–10 or more liters. The urine is pale or colorless; the specific gravity varies from 1.001–1.005, with a corresponding osmolality of 50–200 mOsm/kg water. During periods of severe dehydration the specific gravity may rise to 1.010 and the osmolality to 300. Other renal function studies are normal. Serum osmolality is normal with adequate hydration. During water deprivation tests patients must be closely observed to prevent surreptitious intake of water on the one hand and to avoid severe and rapid development of dehydration on the other. In patients with severe deficiency a 3 hr period of dehydration leads to elevation of plasma osmolality, while urine osmolality characteristically remains below plasma levels. Administration of desmopressin or vasopressin quickly raises urine osmolality. When the polyuria is mild and the deficiency incomplete, urine osmolality may exceed that of plasma and the response to vasopressin is attenuated.

Radioimmunoassay for vasopressin is available but usually is not essential for diagnosis. Plasma levels consistently below 0.5 pg/mL indicate severe neurogenic diabetes insipidus. Vasopressin levels that are subnormal for the concomitant hyperosmolality indicate partial neurogenic diabetes insipidus. The assay is particularly useful in distinguishing partial diabetes insipidus from primary polydipsia.

Roentgenograms of the skull may reveal evidence of an intracranial tumor such as calcifications, enlargement of the sella turcica, erosion of the clinoid processes, or increased width of the suture lines. Roentgenograms of the skull or other bones in patients with the reticuloendothelioses may reveal areas of rarefaction. CT scan of the head is indicated.

Differential Diagnosis. Polydipsia, polyuria, and impaired concentration are common in patients with hypercalcemia or potassium deficiency. In the male infant nephrogenic diabetes insipidus must be differentiated from inherited or acquired vasopressin deficiency; failure of response to exogenous vasopressin or desmopressin is a critical differential criterion.

Compulsive water drinking (*psychogenic polydipsia*) is rare but may easily be confused with diabetes insipidus. Affected persons are usually able to produce a concentrated urine when fluids are withheld. Occasionally, however, diagnosis is difficult because prolonged polydipsia lowers the maximal urinary concentrations achievable following dehydration or even following infusion of hypertonic saline solution. As a rule, a urine osmolality greater after dehydration than after administration of vasopressin alone indicates the ability to secrete vasopressin. On the other hand, if administration of vasopressin produces a urinary osmolality substantially higher than dehydration alone, vasopressin secretion is deficient. This rule seems to apply no matter how low or high urinary concentration may be.

Defects in urinary concentrations also occur in a variety of chronic renal disorders. Familial nephronophthisis, in particular, can mimic diabetes insipidus. Elevated plasma levels of urea and creatinine, anemia, and isotonic rather than hypotonic urine are characteristics of primary renal disease.

Adipsia, an impairment of thirst center function as a result of osmoreceptor dysfunction, is being increasingly recognized in patients with diabetes insipidus and central nervous system tumors; adipsia seriously complicates the management of problems of water balance.

Prognosis. When diabetes insipidus is diagnosed the underlying process must be determined. Diabetes insipidus itself rarely threatens life, but it may signify a serious underlying condition. It may be only transitory following trauma or surgical intervention in the region of the hypothalamus or pituitary. In some patients with reticuloendothelioses spontaneous remission occurs, whereas in others diabetes insipidus may be the only residuum long after remission of the primary condition. Amelioration of clinical diabetes insipidus may herald the development of anterior pituitary insufficiency. The prognosis of patients with brain tumors depends upon the site of the lesion and upon the type of neoplastic cell.

Treatment. The causative factor deserves first consideration in the treatment. Patients with uncomplicated diabetes insipidus may go untreated for years with only the inconvenience of polyuria and polydipsia so long as they have an intact thirst mechanism and are allowed free access to water.

The drug of choice is desmopressin (1-desamino-8-D-arginine vasopressin; DDAVP), a highly effective analogue of vasopressin. It is administered intranasally in a dose of 1.25–15 μg, once or twice daily, for either complete or partial vasopressin deficiency. The duration of action varies from 6–24 hr; accordingly, the dose must be individualized. Patients and parents should be instructed in the use of the nasal catheter to deliver the accurately measured dose. To avoid water retention, it is important that a dosage schedule be found that allows patients to revert to mild polyuria before the next dose is due. Advantages of desmopressin therapy over other types of treatment are ease of administration, long duration of action, absence of pressor activity, rarity of induced hyponatremia, and virtual lack of adverse effects. Its cost is 2–4 times that of other agents but its efficacy and safety are superior.

Great care must be taken in patients with diabetes insipidus who are comatose, undergoing surgery, or receiving intravenous fluids for any reason. Regardless of the form of therapy, any effective dose should be repeated only after its effect has worn off and polyuria recurs. Postoperative diabetes insipidus is often transient; daily reassessment of the need for antidiuretic hormone is necessary after it has been initiated. Desmopressin is also available for parenteral administration; it is useful postoperatively, particularly after transsphenoidal surgery when nasal packing precludes nasal insufflation.

Desmopressin in parenteral form produces transient increases in factor VIII coagulant activity, and its prophylactic use is now recommended before minor surgery or to treat minor bleeding episodes in patients with mild or moderate hemophilia A or von Willebrand disease (see Sec. 15.44). Desmopressin also appears to be useful in the management of some children with enuresis.

Nephrogenic Diabetes Insipidus
(Vasopressin-Insensitive Diabetes Insipidus)

This disorder closely mimics vasopressin deficiency, but levels of the hormone in plasma and urine are normal. Affected patients show no antidiuresis even with large doses of vasopressin, and renal medullary production or release of cyclic AMP is deficient. The disorder occurs primarily in males as an X-linked recessive trait. Heterozygous females are usually asymptomatic but may exhibit a variable defect in concentration, which is probably explained by the Lyon hypothesis of sex-chromosome inactivation. Administration of vasopressin raises cortisol levels, indicating that at least one extrarenal effect of vasopressin is intact. On the other hand, the defect in other tissues is demonstrated by failure of desmopressin to increase factor VIII activity in affected patients.

For further discussion see Sec. 17.30.

19.4 INAPPROPRIATE SECRETION OF ANTIDIURETIC HORMONE
(Hypersecretion of Vasopressin)

The syndrome of inappropriate secretion of antidiuretic hormone (SIADH) is now recognized as one of the most common aberrations of arginine vasopressin (AVP) secretion. In this condition plasma levels of AVP are inappropriately high for the concurrent osmolality of the blood and are not suppressed by further dilution of body fluids.

Etiology. The syndrome is being recognized in an increasing number of clinical conditions, particularly those involving the central nervous system, including meningitis, encephalitis, brain tumor and abscesses, subarachnoid hemorrhage, Guillain-Barré syndrome, head trauma, and after transsphenoidal surgery for pituitary tumors. Pneumonia, tuberculosis, acute intermittent porphyria, cystic fibrosis, perinatal asphyxia, use of positive pressure respirators, and certain drugs such as vincristine and vinblastine also produce the syndrome. The mechanism of the disturbed regulation of vasopressin in these conditions is not fully understood, but in many instances it is clear that there is direct involvement of the hypothalamus. The syndrome has been observed in patients with Ewing sarcoma; with malignant tumors of the pancreas, duodenum, or thymus; and particularly with oat cell carcinoma of the lung. In these instances the tumor presumably synthesizes and secretes vasopressin, the syndrome disappearing when the tumor is removed. In rare instances no cause for the syndrome has been found.

The syndrome has occurred during chlorpropamide therapy for diabetes mellitus, presumably because this drug potentiates vasopressin. Patients with diabetes insipidus treated with various antidiuretic preparations readily develop the syndrome during periods of excessive ingestion of fluids or during intravenous fluid therapy.

Clinical Manifestations. The syndrome is probably most often latent and asymptomatic and forms the basis for the long known observation that serum sodium levels may be unexpectedly low in conditions such as pneumonia, tuberculosis, and meningitis. Careful attention to fluid replacement in patients with conditions known to be associated with the syndrome may prevent the development of symptoms.

The clinical manifestations are attributable to hypotonicity of body fluids and are those of water intoxication. If the serum sodium is not below 120 mEq/L, there may be no symptoms. Early, there is loss of appetite followed by nausea and sometimes vomiting. Irritability and personality changes, including hostility and confusion, may occur. When the serum sodium falls below 110 mEq/L, neurologic abnormalities and/or stupor are common, and convulsive seizures may occur. Skin turgor and blood pressure are normal, and there is no evidence of dehydration.

Serum sodium and chloride concentrations are low, whereas serum bicarbonate usually remains normal. Despite low serum sodium there is continued renal excretion of sodium. The serum is hypo-osmolar, but the urine is less than maximally dilute and its osmolality greater than appropriate for the tonicity of the serum. Hypouricemia is often present, probably owing to increased urate clearance secondary to volume expansion. Concurrence of hypouricemia with hyponatremia is a clue to diagnosis of SIADH and is especially helpful in the neonate. Renal and adrenal functions are normal.

Treatment. Successful treatment of the underlying disorder (meningitis, pneumonia) is followed by spontaneous remission. Immediate management of the hyponatremia consists simply of *restriction of fluids*. Sodium should be made available to replace the sodium loss; hypertonic saline solution is usually of little benefit, however, since even large sodium loads are excreted in the urine. In instances of severe water intoxication, with convulsions or coma, administration of hypertonic saline solution will increase osmolality and control the central nervous system manifestations. In such emergencies administration of furosemide with 300 mL/m² of 1.5% sodium chloride will cause both a rise in sodium levels and a diuresis. Demeclocycline interferes with the action of AVP on the renal tubule. Experience in adults with SIADH indicates that this agent may be useful, but its role in the treatment of children is not established. An 8 yr old child with chronic SIADH has been successfully treated with single daily doses of furosemide.

19.5 HYPERPITUITARISM

Hypersecretion of pituitary hormones is an expected finding in conditions in which deficiency of a target organ gives decreased hormonal feedback, as in primary hypogonadism or hypoadrenalism. In primary hypothyroidism pituitary hyperfunction and hyperplasia can enlarge and erode the sella and on rare occasions increase intracranial pressure. Such changes are not to be confused with primary pituitary tumors; they disappear when the underlying thyroid condition is treated. On the other hand, two patients with congenital hypothyroidism have developed thyrotropic adenomas as adults, following longstanding inadequate treatment for their hypothyroidism.

Primary hypersecretion of pituitary hormones is usually associated with a suspected or proven neoplasm of the pituitary; it is rare in childhood. The principal hormone-secreting tumors are eosinophilic adenoma (growth hormone), basophilic adenoma (ACTH), and chromophobe adenoma (prolactin). There is mounting evidence that these tumors may in some instances be secondary to primary defects in the hypothalamus, with stimulation of the pituitary by hypothalamic releasing factors. Any pituitary tumor may cause pituitary insufficiency by compression of pituitary tissue.

Pituitary Gigantism and Acromegaly

In young persons with open epiphyses, overproduction of growth hormone results in gigantism; in persons with closed epiphyses, acromegaly results. Often some acromegalic features are seen with gigantism, even in children and adolescents; after closure of the epiphyses, the acromegalic features become more prominent.

Etiology. Pituitary gigantism is rare. The cause is most often an eosinophilic adenoma, but gigantism has been observed in a 2.5 yr old boy with a hypothalamic tumor. Two boys with McCune-Albright syndrome and accelerated growth have had functioning pituitary tumors; levels of growth hormone were markedly elevated and were not suppressed by a glucose tolerance test. Because of the rarity of eosinophilic adenoma few children with this tumor have had evaluation of pituitary function by currently available techniques. Tumors in many adults with acromegaly as well as in a 5 yr old child have responded with changes in growth hormone levels to administration of provocative or suppressive agents. These data suggest that in some patients gigantism and acromegaly may begin as a hypothalamic disturbance, resulting in hypertrophy and hyperplasia and, ultimately, in tumors of somatotropic cells.

It now appears that hamartomas of the hypothalamus (gangliocytomas) produce acromegaly in adults by secretion of growth hormone-releasing hormone (GRH); this is additional evidence for a syndrome of hypothalamic acromegaly. Other tumors, particularly in the pancreas, have also produced acromegaly by secretion of large amounts of GRH with resultant hyperplasia of the somatotrophs; GRH was first isolated and characterized from two such pancreatic tumors.

Clinical Manifestations. In most of the recorded cases the abnormal growth became evident at puberty, but the condition has been established as early as 5 yr of age. Giants may grow to a height of 8 ft or more. Acromegaly consists chiefly in enlargement of the distal parts of the body, but manifestations of abnormal growth actually involve all portions. The circumference of the skull increases, the nose becomes broad, and the tongue is often enlarged, with coarsening of the facial features. The mandible grows excessively, and the teeth become separated. The fingers and toes grow chiefly in thickness. There may be dorsal kyphosis. Fatigue and lassitude are early symptoms. Delayed sexual maturation or hypogonadism may occur. Signs of increased intracranial pressure appear later; visual loss may be demonstrable only on careful examination of visual fields.

Laboratory Data. Growth hormone levels are elevated and may occasionally reach 400 ng/mL. Random fluctuations are common, with no increase in secretion during deep sleep. There is usually no suppression of growth hormone levels by the hyperglycemia of a glucose tolerance test. There may be no response, normal responses, or paradoxical responses to various other stimuli. For example, L-dopa may paradoxically decrease growth hormone levels. Administration of thyrotropin-releasing hormone results in increased growth hormone levels in some acromegalics and in a 5 yr old giant resulted in a 3-fold increase in levels of growth hormone. Somatomedin C levels are consistently elevated in acromegaly, in one study ranging from 2.6–21.7 U/mL, with normal levels 0.31–1.4 U/mL. Detailed evaluation of each child is indicated because the results of such studies provide not only insight into pathologic mechanisms but clues to therapy.

Adenomas may compromise other anterior pituitary function through growth or cystic degeneration. Secretion of gonadotropins, thyrotropin (TSH), and/or ACTH may be impaired. Prolactin levels may be elevated; and in 1 instance a tumor was shown to secrete prolactin and growth hormone.

Roentgenograms of the skull may reveal enlargement of the sella turcica and of the paranasal sinuses; CT scans delineate the tumor. Tufting of the phalanges and increased heel pad thickness are common. Osseous maturation is normal.

Differential Diagnosis. In the differential diagnosis hereditary tall stature must be considered; in this condition there is usually abnormal height in 1 or both parents or in close relatives. Such tall persons are well proportioned and free of signs of increased intracranial pressure. Excessive growth during preadolescence in obese children is a temporary state; though such children may become tall, they do not attain the height of giants. Children with precocious puberty are often unusually tall but do not develop into giants since their epiphyses close early and growth ceases prematurely. Patients with tall stature associated with untreated thyrotoxicosis, hypogonadism, or Marfan syndrome are easily distinguished clinically and have normal levels of growth hormone. Gigantism and increased growth hormone levels may occur in some patients with lipodystrophy, but absence of subcutaneous fat is a characteristic finding; there is increasing evidence for disordered hypothalamic function in this condition. Cerebral gigantism, which is far more common than pituitary gigantism, can usually be differentiated on clinical grounds (see below).

Treatment. Treatment is difficult and controversial. If there is increased intracranial pressure, surgical intervention is indicated. In the absence of ocular symptoms such as choked discs and constricted visual fields, irradiation, either conventional or with high energy proton beams, may be effective therapy. Bromocriptine, a long-acting dopamine receptor agonist, has been effective in a 9 yr old boy in whom surgery and irradiation were not successful.

Sotos Syndrome
(Cerebral Gigantism)

This disorder is characterized by rapid growth, but there is no evidence that it is an endocrine disorder. A hypothalamic defect has been suggested as a cause, but none has been demonstrated functionally or at necropsy. Birthweight and length are above the 90th percentile in most affected infants, and macrocrania may be noted. Growth is rapid, and by 1 yr of age affected infants are over the 97th percentile in height. Accelerated growth continues for the first 4–5 yr, and then a normal rate is observed. Puberty usually occurs at the normal time but may occur slightly early. The hands and feet are large, with thickened subcutaneous tissue. The head is large and dolichocephalic, the jaw prominent; there is hypertelorism, and the eyes have an antimongoloid slant. Clumsiness and awkward gait are characteristic, and affected children have great difficulty in sports, in learning to ride a bicycle, and in other tasks requiring coordination. Some degree of mental retardation is present in most patients; in some children, perceptual deficiencies may predominate (Fig. 19–2).

Roentgenograms reveal a large skull, a high orbital roof, a sella of normal size but slightly posterior inclination, and an increased interorbital distance. Osseous maturation is compatible with the patient's height. Growth hormone levels and results of other endocrine studies are usually normal; there are no distinctive laboratory markers for the syndrome. Abnormal electroencephalograms are common; other studies will frequently reveal a dilated ventricular system.

The cause of the disorder is unknown; nor is it clear whether all patients with this syndrome have the same defect. Most cases are sporadic. Familial cases are usually consistent with autosomal dominant inheritance, occasionally with autosomal recessive inheritance. Affected patients may be at increased risk for neoplasia; hepatic carcinoma and Wilms, ovarian, and parotid tumors have been reported.

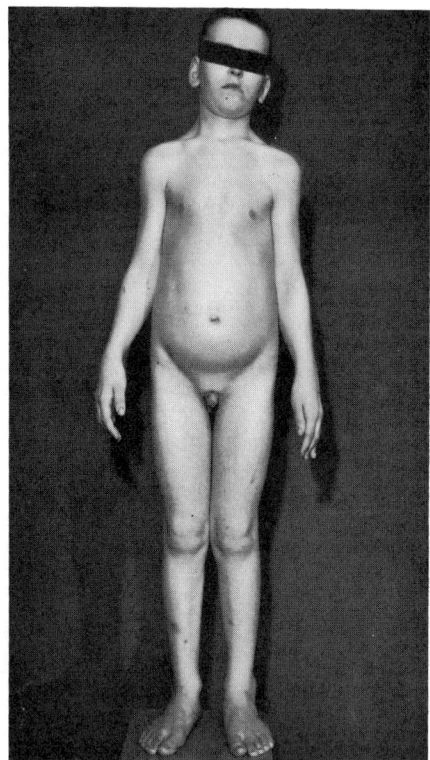

Figure 19–2. Cerebral gigantism in an 8 yr old boy. Height age was 12 yr; bone age, 12 yr; IQ, 60; abnormal electroencephalogram. Note prominence of forehead and jaw and the large hands and feet. Sexual development was consistent with chronologic age. Hormone studies were normal. Adult height was 208 cm (6 ft, 10 in); normal sexual development. He wears size 18 shoes.

Prolactinoma

Prolactin-secreting pituitary adenomas are the most common tumor of the pituitary in adults but are rare in children. Presenting features in children and adolescents include headache, decreased growth rate and delayed puberty, primary or secondary amenorrhea, gynecomastia, galactorrhea, and advanced puberty either singly or in various combinations. Prolactin levels may be moderately or markedly elevated (as high as 5000 ng/mL) and are not appropriately increased by TRH stimulation. Most prolactinomas thus far recognized in children have been large (macroadenomas), have caused the sella to enlarge, and in some instances have caused visual field defects. The mechanism for pubertal delay is probably multifactorial, with possible mechanisms being decreased secretion of growth hormone, of gonadotropic hormones, or of luteinizing hormone–releasing hormone (LH-RH), as well as direct inhibition of gonads by prolactin. Treatment for most children has been surgical resection by transfrontal or transsphenoidal approach. Bromocriptine is highly effective in reducing levels of prolactin and in decreasing tumor size by 50% or more in two thirds of adults. Experience in adults indicates that microadenomas usually do not become macroadenomas and that spontaneous remission of clinical manifestations is common. The management of microadenomas is becoming increasingly conservative.

19.6 PRECOCIOUS PUBERTY

Physiology of Puberty. The hypothalamus, pituitary, and gonads are active and interacting for years before appearance of the secondary sex characteristics associated with puberty. Levels of FSH and LH are low but measurable throughout childhood and rise slowly during the prepubertal years. When LH levels are measured at 20 min intervals, irregular pulsatile secretion may be observed in prepubertal children with further amplification occurring during sleep. Evidence of hypothalamic-pituitary-gonadal interaction prior to puberty is the fact that patients with Turner syndrome or with anorchia have levels of gonadotropins higher than those of normal children of the same age. The prepubertal testis responds to administration of human chorionic gonadotropin with marked increases in testosterone levels. Factors that influence the onset of puberty are being unraveled, but the details remain obscure. Prior to puberty very small amounts of gonadal steroids are able to suppress the hypothalamus and pituitary. With the onset of puberty the hypothalamic "gonadostat" becomes progressively less sensitive to the suppressive effects of sex steroids on gonadotropin secretion. Consequently LH and FSH levels increase and stimulate the gonad, and a new homeostatic level is achieved (gonadarche). This decrease in hypothalamic sensitivity is thought to be important to the onset of puberty. In girls at puberty, a sharp rise in FSH production precedes the increase in plasma estradiol; in boys LH production rises prior to the sharp increase in testosterone. Plasma levels of bioactive LH increase more during puberty than those of immunoreactive LH, indicating qualitative as well as quantitative changes. FSH and LH act synergistically to promote changes in the gonad at puberty.

Other evidence suggests that neither pituitary nor gonadal maturation is involved in the initiation of puberty; for example, pulsed administration of luteinizing hormone-releasing hormone (LH-RH) can induce puberty in the infantile monkey. The factors which activate the dormant hypothalamic mechanism are unknown. It appears that a neuronal oscillator discharging at approximately hourly intervals causes a discharge of LH-RH and in turn LH. Pulsatile discharge of LH is of considerable significance in onset of puberty and in reproductive physiology.

A second critical event occurs in middle or late adolescence, at least in girls, in whom cyclicity and ovulation occur. A positive feedback mechanism develops whereby rising levels of estrogen in midcycle cause a distinct increase (rather than decrease) of LH. Prior to midadolescence this ability of estrogen to release LH is not found. Other changes known to occur at the onset of puberty include an increase in LH release during sleep and increased ability of the pituitary to release LH in response to LH-RH administration.

Adrenal cortical androgens also play a role in pubertal maturation (adrenarche). Levels of dehydroepiandrosterone (DHEA) and its sulfate (DHEA-S) begin to rise before the earliest physical changes of puberty. This increase occurs before those of gonadotropins, testosterone, or estradiol at about 6 yr of age; the rise is more rapid in girls than in boys. DHEA-S is the most abundant adrenal C-19 steroid in blood, but its function is unknown. It has been postulated that an adrenal androgen-stimulating factor other than ACTH initiates adrenarche, but direct evidence is lacking.

Age of onset of puberty is variable and more closely correlated with osseous maturation than with chronologic age (see Sec. 2.9 and Sec. 9.10). In girls the breast bud is usually the first sign of puberty (10–11 yr) and the interval to menarche is usually 2–2.5 yr but may be as long as 6 yr. In the United States about 95% of girls have at least one sign of puberty by 12 yr, and the mean age of menarche is about 12½ yr. Peak height velocity always precedes menarche and is attained about 2 yr earlier in girls than in boys. There are, however, wide variations in the sequence of changes involving growth spurt, breast, pubic hair, and genital development.

Genetic and environmental factors also affect onset of puberty. The drop in menarchal age in the past century is probably due to better nutrition and improved general health. Black girls are significantly more advanced in development of secondary sex characteristics than white girls. Ballet dancers, gymnasts, swimmers, runners, and other girl athletes in whom leanness and strenuous physical activity have coexisted from early childhood frequently exhibit a marked delay in puberty and/or menarche. This observation supports the thesis that there may be a relation between weight and body composition and pubertal maturation.

In boys, growth of the testes is the first sign of puberty (prepubertal testicular volume is 2–4 cc). This is followed by pigmentation and thinning of the scrotum and growth of the penis (Sec. 2.9). Pubic hair then appears. Appearance of axillary hair usually marks the midpoint of puberty. In boys, unlike girls, acceleration of growth begins after puberty is well under way and is maximal from 14–16 yr of age; growth may continue well beyond 18 yr of age.

Precocious puberty is difficult to define because of the marked variation in the age at which puberty begins normally. Onset of secondary sexual characteristics before 8 yr of age in girls and 9 yr in boys may be considered precocious, but these are arbitrary guidelines.

Disorders of Pubertal Development

Precocious pubertal development may be classified as true precocious puberty or precocious pseudopuberty (Table 19–2). True precocious puberty is always isosexual and involves not only precocity of secondary sexual characteristics but also an increase in the size and activity of the gonads. In precocious pseudopuberty some of the secondary sex characteristics appear, but the gonads do not mature and there is no activation of normal pituitary-hypothalamic-gonadal interplay. In this latter group the sex characteristics may be isosexual or heterosexual (see Sec. 19.23, 19.30, and 19.34).

A recently delineated type of precocious puberty has been found to be gonadotropin independent. Affected patients resemble those with true precocious puberty, but the hypothalamic-pituitary axis is not involved in pathogenesis (see below).

19.7 TRUE PRECOCIOUS PUBERTY

In this section we discuss precocious puberty that is initiated either by premature activation of the hypothalamic-pituitary-gonadal axis or by ectopic secretion of human chorionic gonadotropin. Gonadotropin-independent precocious puberty is also included.

Precocious Puberty without Other Pathologic Findings (Constitutional)

In the past, no causative factor could be found to account for precocious puberty in about 80–90% of girls and 50% of boys. Computed tomography (CT) and magnetic resonance imaging (MRI) are lowering the percentages of children in this category. The condition occurs far more frequently in girls and is usually sporadic.

Clinical Manifestations. The clinical course is extremely variable. Affected children may complete sexual maturation rapidly or slowly; manifestations may remain stationary or even regress, only to resume development later. Sexual development may begin at any age. In girls the first sign is development of the breasts; pubic hair may appear simultaneously but more often appears later. Development of the external genitalia, the appearance of axillary hair, and the

Table 19–2. Conditions Causing Precocious Puberty

True precocious puberty (gonadotropin-dependent)
  Idiopathic (constitutional, functional)
  Central nervous system lesion
    Hypothalamic hamartoma, brain tumors, hydrocephalus,
      postencephalitic scars, and so on
  hCG-secreting tumor
    CNS tumors
    Hepatoblastoma
    Mediastinal tumor
      In association with Klinefelter syndrome
    Others
  Prolonged untreated primary hypothyroidism
  Therapy of congenital adrenal hyperplasia
  McCune-Albright syndrome—late
  Administration of gonadotropins
Precocious pseudopuberty (gonadotropin-independent)
  Females
    Isosexual (feminization)
      Ovarian tumors
        Granulosa–theca cell tumor
          Associated with Ollier disease
        Teratoma, chorionepithelioma
        Sex cord tumor with annular tubules (associated with Peutz-
          Jeghers syndrome)
      Autonomous functional cyst of ovary
      McCune-Albright syndrome
      Adrenocortical tumor
      Exogenous estrogen
    Heterosexual (virilization)
      Congenital adrenal hyperplasia
      Adrenocortical tumor
        Testosterone-secreting tumor
      Androblastoma (arrhenoblastoma)
      Androgen-producing teratoma
      Exogenous androgen
  Males
    Isosexual (masculinization)
      Primary Leydig cell hyperplasia
        Sporadic
        Male-limited autosomal dominant
        Tuberous sclerosis
      Congenital adrenal hyperplasia
      Adrenocortical tumor
      Leydig cell tumor
      Teratoma (containing adenocortical tissue)
      Exogenous androgen
    Heterosexual (feminization)
      Adrenocortical tumor
      Exogenous estrogen
      Sertoli cell tumor
        Sex cord tumor with annular tubules (associated with Peutz-
          Jeghers syndrome)
Partial precocious puberty
  Premature adrenarche
  Premature thelarche
  Premature menarche

onset of menstruation follow. The early menstrual cycles may be more irregular than with normal puberty. Menarche has been observed within the 1st yr of life. The initial cycles are usually anovulatory, but pregnancy has been reported as early as 5.5 yr of age (Fig. 19–3).

In boys enlargement of the penis and testes, appearance of pubic hair, acne, and frequent erections occur. The voice deepens, and linear growth is accelerated. Spermatogenesis has been observed as early as 5–6 yr of age, and nocturnal emissions may occur. Testicular biopsies have shown all elements of the testes to be stimulated. If the precocity is complete, various degrees of spermatogenesis are present; even if it is incomplete, the interstitial cells are present.

In both girls and boys height, weight, and osseous maturation are advanced. The increased rate of ossification results in early closure of epiphyses so that ultimate stature is less than it would have been otherwise. Without treatment, approximately one third of patients do not achieve a height of 152 cm (5 ft) as adults. Dental age and mental development are usually compatible with chronologic age.

Laboratory Data. Levels of plasma FSH and LH may be elevated for the age of the patient. In as many as 50% of patients, however, there is overlap with levels in normal children of the same age. Serial determinations often reveal well-defined pulsatile secretion of gonadotropins, especially during sleep, with LH secretion predominating. After administration of LH-RH, a brisk response occurs, similar in degree to that in normal puberty. Markedly elevated LH levels should suggest the presence of a human chorionic gonadotropin (hCG)–secreting tumor since most assays for LH cross-react with hCG.

Plasma testosterone (in boys) and estradiol (in girls) are usually elevated to levels consistent with the stage of puberty and osseous maturation. Like normal pubertal girls, girls with idiopathic precocious puberty may have wide fluctuations of levels of estrogens. Urinary 17-ketosteroids may be normal or only slightly elevated. Osseous maturation is advanced and consistent with the stage of pubertal development. Electroencephalographic abnormalities in many patients suggest a primary cerebral disturbance.

Differential Diagnosis. In girls, lesions of the central nervous system, tumors of the ovaries, feminizing adrenocortical tumors, McCune-Albright syndrome, and exogenous sources of estrogens must be considered in the differential diagnosis. A carefully obtained history, a complete physical examination, and appropriate laboratory studies usually resolve the diagnosis. Examination by ultrasonography may be indicated to outline the ovaries. Computed tomography and/or MRI is indicated to rule out intracranial lesions.

In boys, gonadotropin-independent precocious puberty, cerebral lesions, adrenogenital syndrome, Leydig cell tumor, and gonadotropin-producing hepatoma must be considered diagnostic possibilities. In the *adrenogenital syndrome* the testes are small relative to the degree of sexual maturation. A *Leydig cell tumor* can usually be detected on physical examination, and a *hepatoma* usually causes hepatomegaly. A family history of sexual precocity in males suggests gonadotropin-independent precocious puberty.

When there is no evidence of a cerebral lesion, even on CT scan or MRI, the child must be carefully and repeatedly observed for several yr before the possibility of an intracranial lesion can be excluded.

Treatment. Treatment consists of administration of an analogue of LH-RH that is more potent, has a longer duration of action than native LH-RH, and suppresses pulsatile discharge of gonadotropins, because to maintain sustained release of gonadotropin pituitary gonadotropic cells require intermittent periods of absence of stimulation by LH-RH.

Within 1 wk of onset of therapy basal plasma levels of gonadotropins and their response to LH-RH decrease; within 2 wks plasma levels of estradiol in girls and of testosterone in boys decrease. In the ensuing months one observes decrease in the size of the breasts and uterus (ultrasonographically), regression of pubic hair, and cessation of menses in girls who have had menarche. In boys, testicular volume, pubic hair, and aggressive behavior decrease. Growth velocity and skeletal maturation also decelerate.

When therapy is discontinued, there is immediate return of manifestations of sexual precocity, and good suppression occurs when therapy is resumed. The agent has only been used for about 6 yr and is still investigational in the United States, but it appears to be safe and effective; its use has required daily subcutaneous injections, but recent experiences with monthly depot injections and with intranasal therapy appear promising.

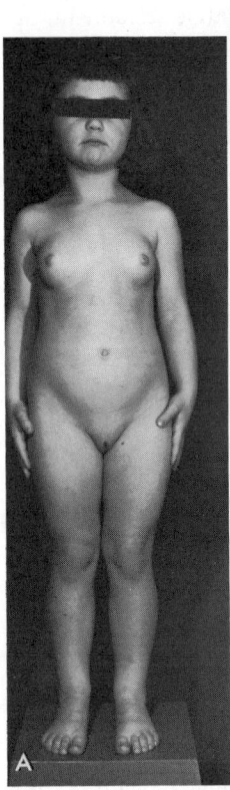
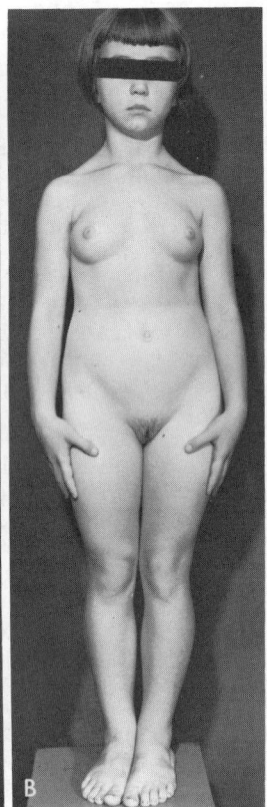
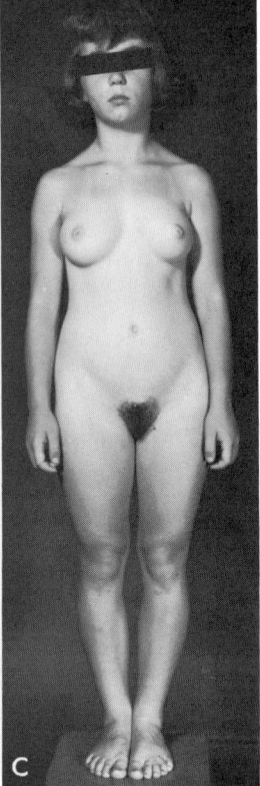

Figure 19–3. Idiopathic precocious puberty. Patient at (*A*) 3¹¹⁄₁₂, (*B*) at 5⁸⁄₁₂, and (*C*) at 8½ yr of age. Breast development and vaginal bleeding began at 2½ yr of age. Osseous age was 7½ yr at 3¹¹⁄₁₂ and 14 yr at 8 yr of age. Repeated estrogen assays varied between normal prepubertal and adult female levels. Urinary gonadotropins were not demonstrable until the child was 5 yr of age. Intelligence and dental age were normal for chronologic age. Growth was completed at 10 yr; ultimate height was 142 cm (56 in).

Precocious Puberty Resulting from Organic Brain Lesions

Etiology. A wide variety of lesions of the central nervous system have been associated with sexual precocity. Postencephalitic scars, tuberculous meningoencephalitis, hydrocephalus, tuberous sclerosis, and severe head trauma have each, on occasion, been etiologic factors. Optic gliomas, astrocytomas, ependymonas, and neurofibromas may cause sexual precocity. How these lesions activate hypothalamic mechanisms that initiate puberty is unknown, but they usually involve the hypothalamus by scarring, invasion, or pressure.

With the advent of CT scan and MRI, *hypothalamic hamartoma* is being increasingly recognized as a cause of true precocious puberty (Fig. 19–4). These congenital malformations consist

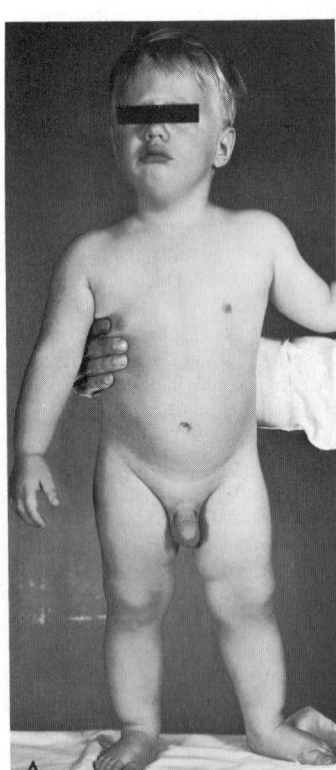
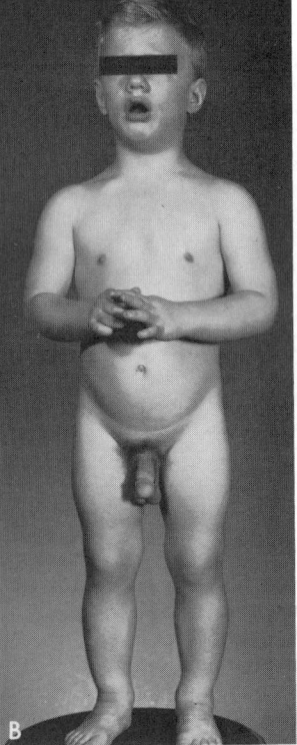

Figure 19–4. Precocious puberty with central nervous system lesion. Photographs at (*A*) 1.5 and (*B*) 2.5 yr of age. Accelerated growth, muscular development, osseous maturation, and testicular development were consistent with the degree of secondary sexual maturation. Urinary gonadotropins were repeatedly negative, 17-ketosteroids usually 2–3 mg/24 hr. In early infancy he began having frequent spells of rapid, purposeless motion; later in life he had episodes of uncontrollable laughing with ocular movements. At 7 yr he exhibited emotional lability, aggressive behavior, and destructive tendencies. Although a hypothalamic hamartoma had been suspected, it was not established until computed tomography became available, when the patient was 23 yr of age. Epiphyses fused at 9 yr of age; final height was 142 cm (56 inches). At 24 yr of age he developed an embryonal cell carcinoma of the retroperitoneum.

of ectopically located neural tissue resembling nerve cells of the tuber cinereum. These lesions are small, grow slowly or remain static in size, and are occasionally connected to the tuber cinereum by a stalk. Evidence suggests that these lesions autonomously release LH-RH into vessels that communicate with the portal blood system.

Most tumors in the pineal region are *germinomas* (atypical teratomas, ectopic pinealomas); true tumors of the pineal are very rare. Germinomas are germ cell tumors. They may be confined to the pineal or to the suprasellar region, or they may occur in both locations. These tumors may cause precocious puberty in boys by secreting hCG, which stimulates the Leydig cells of the testes. An intracranial hCG-secreting germinoma found in a prepubertal girl did not cause precocious puberty, because FSH was not present.

Clinical Manifestations. Some of these tumors grow slowly and produce no signs other than precocious puberty. Neuroendocrine manifestations may be present for 1–2 yr before tumors can be detected radiologically. Other hypothalamic signs or symptoms such as diabetes insipidus, adipsia, hyperthermia, obesity, cachexia, and unnatural crying or laughing (gelastic seizures) should suggest the possibility of an intracranial lesion.

The sexual precocity is always isosexual and the endocrine patterns are those found in children without demonstrable organic lesions. Measurement of levels of hCG may be indicated; serum/spinal fluid ratios of hCG may be helpful in localizing the tumor in the central nervous system when CT scans are normal. About 40% of boys, but only 10% of girls, with true precocious puberty have an intracranial tumor; accordingly, the diagnosis of idiopathic precocious puberty can be made with less confidence in boys than in girls. Rapidly progressive sexual precocity in very young children or gelastic epilepsy suggests the likelihood of a hamartoma of the tuber cinereum. CT scan and/or MRI is indicated in all children with true precocious puberty.

Treatment. Therapy depends on the nature and location of the lesion. Hypothalamic hamartomata that are pedunculated may be surgically removed; otherwise, their effects are best treated with an LH-RH analogue, as described for true precocious puberty with organic lesions. Other untreatable lesions, such as trauma, may also be treated in this fashion. Some tumors, such as germinomas, are extremely sensitive to irradiation.

SYNDROME OF PRECOCIOUS PUBERTY AND HYPOTHYROIDISM

In children with untreated hypothyroidism, onset of puberty is usually delayed until epiphyseal maturation has reached 12–13 yr of age. Precocious puberty in a child with untreated hypothyroidism and a prepubertal bone age presents, therefore, a striking appearance and an unexpected association. The phenomenon appears to be not uncommon. Among 54 carefully studied children with primary hypothyroidism, half had varying degrees of isosexual development in advance of their osseous maturation.

Affected patients have usually had severe hypothyroidism of long duration, with the usual manifestations including retardation of growth and of osseous maturation. The causes of the hypothyroidism include lymphocytic thyroiditis, thyroidectomy, and overtreatment with antithyroid drugs.

A preponderance of the reported instances involved girls, probably reflecting the higher incidence of hypothyroidism in females. A significant number have also had Down syndrome; this observation probably relates to the delay in recognition of hypothyroidism in children with Down syndrome. Sexual maturation usually includes breast development in girls and testicular enlargement in boys. Adrenarchal changes of puberty are mild with sparse or absent pubic and axillary hair. Menstrual bleeding is a common feature, even in girls with minimal breast development. Enlargement of the sella turcica, galactorrhea, excessive pigmentation, and papilledema present in some.

Plasma levels of TSH are markedly elevated. LH, FSH, and prolactin levels are also elevated for reasons as yet unknown. Presumably, thyrotropin-releasing factor is markedly elevated, but in normal individuals it does not cause release of LH and FSH. Whatever the derangement, hypothalamic-pituitary regulating mechanisms rapidly return to normal upon treatment with thyroid hormone.

GONADOTROPIN-SECRETING TUMORS

Hepatic Tumors. Twenty-five instances of isosexual precocious puberty associated with hepatoblastoma or hepatoma have been recorded. All have involved males, the age of onset varying from 4 mo–8 yr, the average being 2 yr. An enlarged liver or mass in the upper quadrant should suggest the diagnosis. Testicular histology reveals interstitial cell hyperplasia and absence of spermatogenesis. The tumor cells produce chorionic gonadotropin (hCG), which stimulates precocious maturation of the testes. Plasma levels of hCG and alpha-fetoprotein are usually markedly elevated; they serve as useful markers for following the effects of therapy. Plasma levels of testosterone are elevated, FSH levels are low, and LH levels are high because the radioimmunoassay cross-reacts with hCG. Treatment for these tumors is the same as for other carcinomas of the liver; survival is usually less than 1 yr from time of diagnosis. One patient has survived disease free for over 5 yr.

Other Tumors. Chorionic gonadotropin-secreting choriocarcinomas, teratocarcinomas, or teratomas (also called ectopic pinealomas or atypical teratomas) may also cause precocious puberty. These tumors may be located in the central nervous system, mediastinum, or gonads. They are much more common in boys with precocious puberty (21/100) than in girls (1/100). Ten affected boys with mediastinal tumors and precocious puberty had small testes leading to diagnosis of Klinefelter syndrome. Why extragonad tumors (particularly mediastinal) occur more frequently than gonadal tumors in Klinefelter syndrome is not known. Affected patients often have very marked elevation of hCG and alpha-fetoprotein. FSH is suppressed, but LH levels appear elevated because of cross-reactivity with hCG assay.

PRECOCIOUS PSEUDOPUBERTY

The adrenal causes of pseudopuberty are discussed in Sec. 19.23 and the gonadal causes in Sec. 19.32 and 19.37.

Precocious Puberty with Polyostotic Fibrous Dysplasia and Abnormal Pigmentation
(McCune-Albright Syndrome)

The association of fibrous dysplasia of the skeletal system with patchy cutaneous pigmentation and endocrine dysfunction is referred to as McCune-Albright syndrome. The most common endocrine disturbance is sexual precocity; hyperthyroidism or Cushing syndrome may also occur. The condition affects many more girls than boys. For many years the disorder was presumed to originate in the hypothalamus, but data now suggest that endocrine disorders in this syndrome result from autonomous hyperfunction of the peripheral target glands. For example, the hyperthyroidism in this condition is not hypothalamic in origin since TSH is suppressed. The hyperthyroidism differs from Graves disease in that the goi-

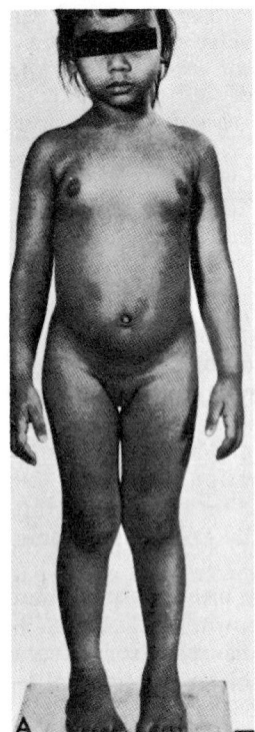 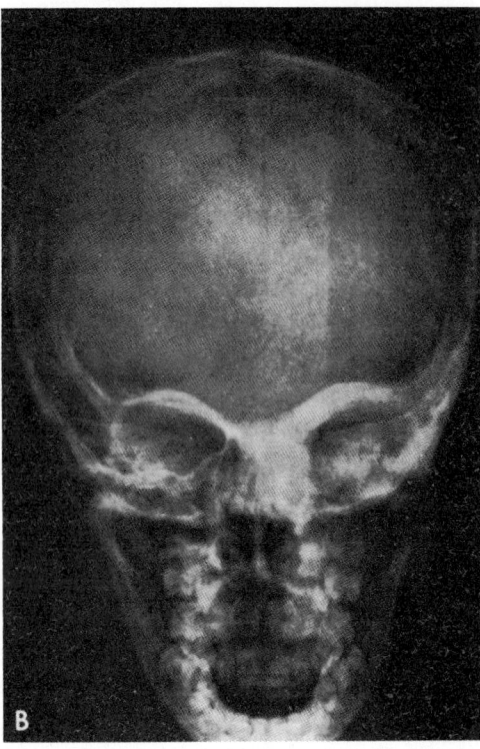

Figure 19–5. Precocious puberty associated with polyostotic fibrous dysplasia (McCune-Albright syndrome) in a girl 4.5 yr of age; at this time her height age and osseous age were normal. Menarche occurred at 4 yr. *A*, Note bilateral breast development, hyperpigmented spots on abdomen, and prominence on left side of face. *B*, Roentgenograms revealed fibrous dysplasia in the distal end of the left ulna and the thickening of the bones about the left orbit and the maxillary portion of the frontal bones shown here.

ters tend to be multinodular and there is an equal distribution between males and females. In the instances of jassociated Cushing syndrome the lesions were bilateral nodular adrenocortical hyperplasia; in one case the plasma levels of ACTH were low. Most girls have suppressed or normal prepubertal levels of LH and FSH, normal prepubertal nocturnal rises in LH and FSH, minimal response of LH level to LH-RH stimulation, and resistance to treatment with a long-acting agonist of LH-RH. Estradiol levels vary from normal to markedly elevated (> 900 pg/mL) and may be cyclic, even while the patient is receiving treatment with an LH-RH agonist. In many affected girls ultrasonography finds ovarian cysts; levels of estradiol may correlate with the size of the cyst. A few patients with evidence of true precocious puberty were older when studied, suggesting that early pseudopuberty may have activated the hypothalamic-pituitary unit (Fig. 19–5).

The average age of menarche in affected girls is about 3 yr, but vaginal bleeding has occurred as early as 4 mo of age and secondary sex characteristics at 6 mo. The Cushing syndrome has occurred in early infancy, antedating the sexual precocity. The onset of hyperthyroidism occurs in most instances from 3–12 yr, although it has occurred as early as 9 mo. Gigantism and acromegaly may occur with or without precocious puberty. In two boys, markedly elevated levels of growth hormone were not suppressed during a glucose tolerance test; a functioning pituitary chromophobe adenoma was found in one, an eosinophilic adenoma in the other.

All patients must be thoroughly investigated. Functioning ovarian cysts often disappear spontaneously; surgical excision is rarely indicated. Long acting analogues of LH-RH are ineffective as treatment. Early reports of treatment with testolactone, an aromatase inhibitor, are encouraging. Cushing syndrome requires adrenalectomy; hyperthyroidism is treated as in any other patient with Graves disease. Prognosis is favorable for longevity, but deformities may result from the bony lesions and repeated pathologic fractures. The osseous lesions become static in adult life.

PRIMARY LEYDIG CELL HYPERPLASIA
Gonadotropin-Independent Precocious Puberty

This form of precocious puberty in boys has been categorized separately from true precocious puberty. Affected patients have prepubertal baseline levels of LH, absence of pubertal pattern of pulsatile secretion of LH, absence of a pubertal response to LH-RH, and absence of detectable hCG; yet testosterone levels are markedly elevated to the same range as in boys with true precocious puberty. Testicular biopsies show the normal changes of pubertal or adult men, including maturation of the seminiferous tubules. It is clear that the sexual precocity is not initiated by hypothalamic-pituitary activation. The nature of the testicular defect that results in activation of Leydig cell function is unknown. The disorder is genetically determined and transmitted through affected males and unaffected female carriers in a male-limited autosomal dominant pattern. It is now known that a dozen or so previously described pedigrees with male-limited autosomal dominant sexual precocity represent this condition. Affected adult males have relatively normal hypothalamic-pituitary-gonadal function and manifest normal fertility. Affected boys are indistinguishable clinically from children with centrally mediated puberty, except for a somewhat earlier age of onset. A family history of sexual precocity in males is a clue to diagnosis.

Treatment. Because the condition is not centrally mediated, LH-RH agonists have no effect on this type of puberty. Early reports suggest that ketoconazole, an antifungal drug that inhibits C 17–20 lyase and testosterone synthesis, is effective in the management of this disorder.

19.8 INCOMPLETE (PARTIAL) PRECOCIOUS DEVELOPMENT

Isolated manifestations of precocity without development of other signs of puberty are not unusual; development of the breasts and growth of sexual hair are the two most common.

Premature Thelarche. This term applies to girls with isolated development of breasts before 8 yr of age without other evidence of precocious puberty. It most often appears in the first 2 yr of life and in about one third of affected infants is present at birth and persists. The breast development may fluctuate in degree and may be asymmetric or may involve only 1 breast. The breast development regresses within 2 yr in 50% of infants; it may persist unchanged 5 yr or longer. Growth and osseous maturation are usually normal but may be slightly advanced; menarche occurs at the usual time. The condition is usually sporadic, rarely familial.

Plasma levels of FSH and LH are usually within normal limits, but basal levels of FSH and their response to LH-RH stimulation are greater than in normal controls. Plasma levels of estradiol are usually normal but may be slightly elevated. These findings suggest the presence of a mild defect in the hypothalamic-pituitary-ovarian axis in some patients. Occasionally, solitary follicular cysts that resolve spontaneously have accounted for the condition.

Premature thelarche is a benign condition, but it may be the first sign of true or of pseudoprecocious puberty. It may also be caused by medications and other exogenous exposure to estrogens (see below). An "epidemic" of premature thelarche in Puerto Rico was suspected to have been due to contamination of food with estrogens but was not proved. In addition to a detailed history, plasma levels of FSH, LH, and estradiol should be obtained. Pelvic ultrasonography may be indicated in some instances. Continued observation is important.

Premature Adrenarche. This term applies to the appearance of sexual hair before the age of 8 yr in girls or 9 yr in boys without other evidence of maturation. It is much more frequent in girls than in boys and may occur more frequently in black girls than in others. Hair appears first on the labia majora; in young children it progresses slowly to the pubic region and finally appears in the axilla. Adult-type axillary odor is common. Affected children are slightly advanced in height and osseous maturation.

Plasma levels of gonadotropins and gonadal steroids are normal; levels of dehydroepiandrosterone sulfate are elevated. This condition results from premature activation of the adrenal cortex (adrenarche) quite apart from activation of the gonads (gonadarche). Premature adrenarche is a benign condition but must be differentiated from early true precocious puberty (in boys) and from adrenal cortical tumors and adrenal hyperplasia (in both girls and boys). Measurements of 17-hydroxyprogesterone, androstenedione, and testosterone are indicated.

Premature Menarche. Isolated menses without other evidence of sexual development occurs less frequently than premature thelarche or premature adrenarche. The majority of affected girls have only one to three episodes of bleeding; puberty occurs at the usual time and menstrual cycles are normal. Plasma levels of gonadotropins are normal but estradiol levels may be elevated, probably owing to bursts of ovarian activity. Occasional patients are found to have ovarian follicular cysts by ultrasonography. Vaginal causes of bleeding such as vulvovaginitis, foreign body, urethral prolapse, and sarcoma botryoides must be ruled out by careful physical examination.

19.9 MEDICATIONAL PRECOCITY

A variety of medicaments can induce the appearance of secondary sexual characteristics which may be confused with precocious puberty. A careful history to explore the possibility of accidental exposure to or ingestion of sex hormones is of paramount importance. Precocious pseudopuberty has occurred in both boys and girls from the accidental ingestion of estrogens (including contraceptive pills) and from the administration of anabolic steroids. Estrogens in cosmetics, hair creams, and breast augmentation creams have caused breast development in girls and gynecomastia in boys; estrogens are readily absorbed through the skin. Contamination of vitamin tablets by sex hormones has been reported to cause precocious pseudopuberty. A recent "epidemic" of premature thelarche and precocious pseudopuberty in Puerto Rico has been attributed to contamination of meats, particularly chicken, with estrogens used in animal husbandry. Ultrasonography in affected children revealed ovarian enlargement or ovarian cysts or both in 50% and uterine enlargement in 35%; gonadotropin levels were normal but estrogens elevated in about 33%. Exogenous estrogens may produce an intense, dark brown color in the areola of the breasts which is not usually seen in endogenous types of precocity. The precocious changes disappear after cessation of exposure to the hormones.

General

Kaplan SA: Clinical Pediatric and Adolescent Endocrinology. Philadelphia, WB Saunders, 1982.
Wilson JD, Foster DW (eds): Williams Textbook of Endocrinology. 7th ed. Philadelphia, WB Saunders, 1985.

Hypopituitarism

Asa SL, Bilbao JM, Kovacs K, et al: Lymphocytic hypophysitis of pregnancy resulting in hypopituitarism: A distinct clinicopathologic entity. Ann Intern Med 95:166, 1981.
Bala RM, Lopatka J, Leung A, et al: Serum immunoreactive somatomedin levels in normal adults, pregnant women at term, children at various ages, and children with constitutionally delayed growth. J Clin Endocrinol Metab 52:508, 1981.
Blethen SL, Welden VV: Hypopituitarism and septo-optic "dysplasia" in first cousins. Am J Med Genet 21:123, 1985.
Costin G, Murphree AL: Hypothalamic-pituitary function in children with optic nerve hypoplasia. Am J Dis Child 139:249, 1985.
Dean HJ, Bishop A, Winter JSD: Growth hormone deficiency in patients with histiocytosis. J Pediatr 109:615, 1986.
Draznin M, Steeling MW, Johanson AJ: Silver-Russell syndrome and craniopharyngioma. J Pediatr 96:887, 1970.
Ellyin F, Khatir AH, Singh SP: Hypothalamic-pituitary functions in patients with transsphenoidal encephalocele and midfacial anomalies. J Clin Endocrinol Metab 51:854, 1980.
Fleisher TA, White RM, Broder S, et al: X-linked hypogammaglobulinemia and isolated growth hormone deficiency. N Engl J Med 302:1429, 1980.
Frasier SD: Human pituitary growth hormone (hGH) therapy in growth hormone deficiency. Endocrinol Rev 4:155, 1983.
Gertner JM, Genel M, Gianfredi SP, et al: Prospective clinical trial of human growth hormone in short children without growth hormone deficiency. J Pediatr 104:172, 1984.
Golde DW, Bersch N, Kaplan SA, et al: Peripheral unresponsiveness to human growth hormone in Laron dwarfism. N Engl J Med 303:1156, 1980.
Hall JG, Pallister PD, Carren SK, et al: Congenital hypothalamic hamartoblastoma, hypopituitarism, imperforate anus, and postaxial polydactyly—a new syndrome? Part 1: Clinical, causal and pathogenetic considerations. Am J Med Genet 7:47, 1980.
Hanna CE, Krainz PL, Skeels MR, et al: Detection of congenital hypopituitary hypothyroidism: Ten year experience in The Northwest Regional Screening Program. J Pediatr 109:959, 1986.
Herman SP, Baggenstoss AM, Clothier MD: Liver dysfunction and histologic abnormalities in neonatal hypopituitarism. J Pediatr 87:892, 1975.
Jacobs LS, Sneid DS, Garland JT, et al: Receptor-active growth hormone in Laron dwarfism. J Clin Endocrinol Metab 42:403, 1976.
Johanson AJ, Morris GL: A single growth hormone determination to rule out growth hormone deficiency. Pediatrics 59:467, 1977.
Johnson JD, et al: Hypoplasia of the anterior pituitary and neonatal hypoglycemia. J Pediatr 82:634, 1973.
Klachko DM, Winder N, Burns TW, et al: Traumatic hypopituitarism occurring before puberty: Survival 35 years untreated. J Clin Endocrinol Metab 28:1768, 1968.
LaFranchi SH, Lippe BM, Kaplan SA: Hypoglycemia during testing for growth hormone deficiency. J Pediatr 90:244, 1977.
Lovinger RD, Kaplan SL, Grumbach MM: Congenital hypopituitarism associated with neonatal hypoglycemia and microphallus: Four cases secondary to hypothalamic hormone deficiencies. J Pediatr 87:1171, 1975.
Margalith D, Tze WJ, Jan JE: Congenital optic nerve hypoplasia with hypothalamic-pituitary dysplasia. Am J Dis Child 139:361, 1985.

Merimee JT, Zapf J, Froesch ER: Insulin-like growth factors (IGF's) in pygmies and subjects with the pygmy trait: Characterization of the metabolic actions of IGF I and IGF II in man. J Clin Endocrinol Metab 55:1081, 1982.

Miller WL, Kaplan SL, Grumbach MM: Child abuse as a cause of post-traumatic hypopituitarism. N Engl J Med 302:724, 1980.

Money J: The syndrome of abuse dwarfism (psychosocial) or reversible hyposomatotropism. Am J Dis Child 131:508, 1977.

Nishi Y, Aihara K, Usui T, et al: Isolated growth hormone deficiency type 1 A in a Japanese family. J Pediatr 104:885, 1984.

O'Dwyer JA, Newton TH, Hoyt WF: Radiologic features of septo-optic dysplasia (deMorsier syndrome). Am J Neuroradiol 1:443, 1980.

Rapaport EB, Ulstrom RA, Gorlin RJ, et al: Solitary maxillary central incisor and short stature. J Pediatr 91:924, 1977.

Richards GE, et al: Delayed onset of hypopituitarism: Sequelae of therapeutic irradiation of the central nervous system, eye and middle ear tumors. J Pediatr 89:553, 1976.

Rivarola MA, Phillips JA III, Migeon CJ, et al: Phenotypic heterogeneity in familial isolated growth hormone deficiency Type 1-A. J Clin Endocrinol Metab 59:34, 1984.

Rogol AD, Blizzard RM, Foley TP, et al: Growth hormone releasing hormone and growth hormone: genetic studies in familial growth hormone deficiency. Pediatr Res 19:489, 1985.

Rogol AD, Blizzard RM, Johnson AJ, et al: Growth hormone release in response to human pancreatic tumor growth hormone-releasing hormone-40 in children with short stature. J Clin Endocrinol Metab 59:580, 1984.

Rudman D, Davis GT, Priest JH, et al: Prevalence of growth hormone deficiency in children with cleft lip or palate. J Pediatr 93:378, 1978.

Rudman D, Kutner MH, Blackston RD, et al: Children with normal-variant short stature: Treatment with human growth hormone for six months. N Engl J Med 305:123, 1981.

Schriock EA, Lustig RH, Rosenthal SM, et al: Effect of growth hormone (GR)-releasing hormone (GRH) on plasma GH in relation to magnitude and duration of GH deficiency in 26 children and adults with isolated GH deficiency or multiple pituitary hormone deficiencies: Evidence for hypothalamic GRH deficiency. J Clin Endocrinol Metab 58:1083, 1984.

Shalet SM, Beardwell CG, Twomey JA, et al: Endocrine function following the treatment of acute leukemia in childhood. J Pediatr 90:920, 1977.

Sklar CA, Grumbach MM, Kaplan SL, Conte FA: Hormonal and metabolic abnormalities associated with central nervous system germinoma in children and adolescents and effect of therapy: Report of 10 patients. J Clin Endocrinol Metab 52:9, 1981.

Tanner JM, Lejarraga H, Cameron N: The natural history of the Silver-Russell syndrome: A longitudinal study of thirty-nine cases. Pediatr Res 9:611, 1975.

Thomasett MJ, Conte FA, Kaplan SL, Grumbach MM: Endocrine and neurologic outcome in childhood craniopharyngioma: Review of effect of treatment in 42 patients. J Pediatr 97:728, 1980.

Thorner MO, Reschke J, Chitwood J, et al: Acceleration of growth in two children treated with human growth hormone-releasing factor. N Engl J Med 312:4, 1985.

Valenta LJ, Siegel MB, Lesniak MA, et al: Pituitary dwarfism in a patient with circulating abnormal growth hormone polymers. N Engl J Med 312:214, 1985.

Van Vliet G, Styne DM, Kaplan SL, et al: Growth hormone treatment for short stature. N Engl J Med 309:1016, 1983.

White MC, Chahal P, Banks L, et al: Familial hypopituitarism associated with an enlarged pituitary fossa and an empty sella. Clin Endocrinol 24:63, 1986.

Wilkinson IA, Duck SC, Gager WE, et al: Empty-sella syndrome. Occurrence in childhood. Am J Dis Child 136:245, 1982.

Zadik Z, Chalew SA, Raiti S, et al: Do short children secrete insufficient growth hormone? Pediatr 76:355, 1985.

Hyperpituitarism

AvRuskin TW, Sau K, Tang S, et al: Childhood acromegaly: Successful therapy with conventional radiation and effects of chlorpromazine on growth hormone and prolactin secretin. J Clin Endocrinol Metab 37:380, 1973.

Bale AE, Drum A, Perry DM, et al: Familial Sotos syndrome (cerebral gigantism): Craniofacial and psychological characteristics. Am J Med Genet 20:613, 1985.

Clemmons DR, Van Wyk JJ, Ridgway EC, et al: Evaluation of acromegaly by radioimmunoassay of somatomedin-C. N Engl J Med 301:1138, 1979.

Costin G, Fefferman RA, Kogut MD: Hypothalamic gigantism. J Pediatr 83:419, 1973.

Dodge PR, Holmes SJ, Sotos JF: Cerebral gigantism. Devel Med Child Neurol 25:248, 1983.

Guyda H, Robert F, Colle E, et al: Histologic, ultrastructural and hormonal characterization of a pituitary tumor secreting both HGH and prolactin. J Clin Endocrinol Metab 36:531, 1973.

Lightner ES, Winter JSD: Treatment of juvenile acromegaly with bromocriptine. J Pediatr 98:494, 1981.

Liuzzi A, Dellabonzana D, Oppizzi G, et al: Low doses of dopamine agonists in the long-term treatment of macroprolactinomas. N Engl J Med 313:656, 1985.

Lucas C: Diagnostic and developmental aspects of prolactin adenomas in children. Arch Fr Pediatr 37:79, 1980.

Patton ML, Woolf PD: Hyperprolactinemia and delayed puberty: A report of three cases and their response to therapy. Pediatr 71:572, 1983.

Sack J, Friedman E, Tadmor R, et al: Growth and puberty arrest due to prolactinoma. Acta Paediatr Scand 73:863, 1984.

Sadeghi-Nejad A, Wolfsdorf JI, Biller BJ, et al: Hyperprolactinemia causing primary amenorrhea. J Pediatr 99:802, 1981.

Spense JH, Trias EP, Raiti S: Acromegaly in a 9½ year old boy. Am J Dis Child 123:504, 1972.

Whitaker MD, Scheithaver BW, Hayles AB, et al: The hypothalamus and pituitary in cerebral gigantism. A clinico-pathologic and immunocytochemical study. Am J Dis Child 139:679, 1985.

Diabetes Insipidus

Adams JM, Kenny JD, Rudolph AJ: Central diabetes insipidus following intraventricular hemorrhage. J Pediatr 88:292, 1976.

Assadi FK, John EG: Hypouricemia in neonates with syndrome of inappropriate secretion of antidiuretic hormone. Pediatr Res 19:424, 1985.

Bode HH, Harley BM, Crawford JD: Restoration of normal drinking behavior by chlorpropamide in patients with hypodipsia and diabetes insipidus. Am J Med 51:304, 1971.

Braverman LE, Mancini JP, McGoldrick DM: Hereditary idiopathic diabetes insipidus. A case report with autopsy findings. Ann Intern Med 63:503, 1965.

Coggins CH, Leaf A: Diabetes insipidus. Am J Med 42:807, 1967.

Czernichow P, Pomerade R, Basmaciogullari A, et al: Diabetes insipidus in children. III. Anterior pituitary dysfunction in idiopathic types. J Pediatr 106:41, 1985.

Friedman AL, Segar WE: Antidiuretic hormone excess. J Pediatr 94:521, 1979.

Hays RM: Antidiuretic hormone. N Engl J Med 295:659, 1976.

Hendricks SA, Lippe B, Kaplan SA, et al: Differential diagnosis of diabetes insipidus: Use of DDAVP to terminate the seven-hour water deprivation test. J Pediatr 98:244, 1981.

Khare SK: Neurohypophyseal dysfunction following perinatal asphyxia. J Pediatr 90:628, 1977.

Kohn B, Norman ME, Feldman H, et al: Hysterical polydipsia (compulsive water drinking). Am J Dis Child 130:210, 1976.

Lee WP, Lippe B, LaFranchi SH, et al: Vasopressin analogue DDAVP in the treatment of diabetes insipidus. Am J Dis Child 130:166, 1976.

Linshaw MA, Sey M, DiGeorge AM, et al: A potential danger of oral chlorpropamide therapy: Impaired excretion of a water load. J Clin Endocrinol Metab 34:562, 1972.

Miller M, Moses AM: Urinary antidiuretic hormone in polyuric disorders and in appropriate ADH syndrome. Ann Intern Med 77:715, 1972.

Richardson DW, Robinson AG: Desmopressin. Ann Intern Med 103:228, 1985.

Richman RA, Post EM, Notman DD, et al: Simplifying the diagnosis of diabetes insipidus in children. Am J Dis Child 135:839, 1981.

Sklar C, Fertig A, David R: Chronic syndrome of inappropriate secretion of antidiuretic hormone in childhood. Am J Dis Child 139:733, 1985.

Toth EL, Bowen PA, Crockford PM: Hereditary central diabetes insipidus: Plasma levels of antidiuretic hormone in a family with a possible osomoreceptor defect. Canad Med Assoc J 131:1237, 1984.

Zerbe RL, Robertson GL: A comparison of plasma vasopressin with a standard direct test in the differential diagnosis of polyuria. N Engl J Med 305:1539, 1981.

Precocious Puberty

Barnes ND, Hayles AB, Ryan RJ: Sexual maturation in juvenile hypothyroidism. Mayo Clin Proc 48:849, 1973.

Bidlingmair F, Butenandt O, Knorr D: Plasma gonadotropins and estrogens in girls with precocious puberty. Pediatr Res 17:91, 1977.

Bullough VL: Age at menarche: A misunderstanding. Science 213:365, 1981.

Clements JA, Reyes FI, Winter JSD, et al: Studies on human sexual development. IV. Fetal pituitary and serum, and amniotic fluid concentrations of prolactin. J Clin Endocrinol Metab 44:408, 1977.

Comite F, Pescovitz OH, Rieth KG, et al: Luteinizing hormone-releasing hormone analog treatment of boys with hypothalamic hamartoma and true precocious puberty. J Clin Endocrinol Metab 59:888, 1984.

Comite F, Shawker TH, Pescovitz OH, et al: Cyclical ovarian function resistent to treatment with an analogue of luteinizing hormone releasing hormone in McCune-Albright syndrome. N Engl J Med 311:1032, 1984.

Conte FA, Grumbach MM, Kaplan SL, et al: Correlation of luteinizing hormone-releasing factor-induced luteinizing hormone and follicle-stimulating hormone release from infancy to 19 years with the changing pattern of gonadotropin secretion in agonadal patients: Relation to the restraint of puberty. J Clin Endocrinol Metab 50:163, 1980.

Curatola P, Cusmai R, Finocchi G, et al: Gelastic epilepsy and true precocious puberty due to hypothalamic hamartoma. Devel Med Child Neurol 26:509, 1984.

Danon M, Robboy SJ, Sully R, et al: Cushing syndrome, sexual precocity and polyostotic fibrous dysplasia in infancy. J Pediatr 87:817, 1975.

DiGeorge AM: Albright syndrome: Is it coming of age? J Pediatr 87:1018, 1975.

Feuillan P, Foster CM, Pescovitz OH, et al: Treatment of precocious puberty in the McCune Albright syndrome with the aromatase inhibitor testolactone. N Engl J Med 315:115, 1986.

Foster CM, Ross JR, Shawker T, et al: Absence of pubertal gonadotropin secretion in girls with McCune-Albright syndrome. J Clin Endocrinol Metab 58:1161, 1984.

Frisch RE, Wyshak G, Vincent L: Delayed menarche and amenorrhea in ballet dancers. N Engl J Med 303:17, 1980.

Harlan WR, Grillo GP, Cornoni-Huntley J, Leaverton PE: Secondary sex characteristics of boys 12–17 years of age. J Pediatr 95:293, 1979.

Harlan WR, Harlan EA, Grillo GP: Secondary sex characteristics of girls 12 to 17 years of age: The US Health Examination Survey. J Pediatr 96:1074, 1980.

Hertz R: Accidental ingestion of estrogens by children. Pediatrics 21:203, 1958.

Holland FJ, Fishman L, Bailey JD, et al: Ketoconazole in the management of precocious puberty not responsive to LH-RH-analogue therapy. N Engl J Med 312:1023, 1985.

Ilicke A, Prager Lewin R, Kauli R, et al: Premature thelarche—Natural history and sex hormone secretion in 68 girls. Acta Paediatr Scand 73:756, 1984.

Jenner MR, Kelch KP, Kaplan SL, et al: Plasma estradiol in prepubertal children, pubertal females, and in precocious puberty, premature thelarche, hypogonadism, and in a child with a feminizing ovarian tumor. J Clin Endocrinol 34:521, 1972.

Kulin HE, Reiter EO: Gonadotropins during childhood and adolescence: A review. Pediatrics 51:260, 1973.

Lee PA, Xenakis T, Winer J, et al: Puberty in girls: Correlation of serum levels of gonadotropins, prolactin, androgens, estrogens, and progestins with physical changes. J Clin Endocrinol Metab 42:775, 1976.

Lightner ES, Penny R, Frasier SD: Pituitary adenoma in McCune-Albright syndrome: Follow-up information. J Pediatr 89:159, 1976.

Lin TH, LePage ME, Henzl M, et al: Intranasal nafarelin: An LH-RH analogue treatment of gonadotropin-dependent precocious puberty. J Pediatr 109:954, 1986.

Lippe BM, Edwards MSB, Braunstein GD, et al: A nonmalignant teratoma secreting hCG: Expanding the spectrum of ectopic hormone production. J Pediatr 105:765, 1984.

Lucky AW, Rich BH, Rosenfield RL, et al: LH bioactivity increases more than immunoactivity during puberty. J Pediatr 97:205, 1980.

Mills JL, Stolley PD, Davies J, et al: Premature thelarche. Natural history and etiologic investigation. Am J Dis Child 135:743, 1981.

Nakagawara A, Ikeda K, Tsuneyoshi M, et al: Hepatoblastoma producing alpha-fetoprotein and human chorionic gonadotropin. Cancer 56:1636, 1985.

Pescovitz OH, Comite F, Hench K, et al: The NIH experience with precocious puberty: Diagnostic subgroups and response to short-term luteinizing hormone releasing hormone analogue therapy. J Pediatr 108:47, 1986.

Price RA, Lee PA, Albright AL, et al: Treatment of sexual precocity by removal of a luteinizing hormone-releasing hormone secreting hamartoma. JAMA 251:2247, 1984.

Rieter EO, Fuldauer VG, Root AW: Secretion of the adrenal androgen dehydroepiandrosterone sulfate, during normal infancy, childhood and adolescence in sick infants, and in children with endocrinologic abnormalities. J Pediatr 90:766, 1977.

Romshe CA, Sotos JF: Intracranial human chorionic gonadotropin-secreting tumor with precocious puberty. J Pediatr 86:250, 1975.

Rosenfeld RG, Reitz RE, King AB, Hintz RL: Familial precocious puberty associated with isolated elevation of luteinizing hormone. N Engl J Med 303:859, 1980.

Saenz de Rodriquez CA, Bongiovanni AM, Conde de Bossego L: An epidemic of precocious development in Puerto Rican children. J Pediatr 107:393, 1985.

Schimke RN, Madigan CM, Silver BJ et al: Choriocarcinoma, thyrotoxicosis, and the Klinefelter syndrome. Cancer Genet Cytogenet 9:1, 1983.

Shaul PW, Towbin RB, Chernausek SD: Precocious puberty following severe head trauma. Am J Dis Child 139:467, 1985.

Stanhope R, Adams J, Brook CGD: Fluctuation of breast size in isolated premature thelarche. Acta Paediatr Scand 74:454, 1985.

Stanhope R, Adams J, Brook CGD: The treatment of central precocious puberty using an intranasal LHRH analogue (Buserlin). Clin Endocrinol 22:795, 1985.

Styne DM, Harris DA, Egli CA, et al: Treatment of true precocious puberty with a potent luteinizing hormone-releasing factor agonist: Effect on growth, pelvic sonography and hypothalamic-pituitary gonadal axis. J Clin Endocrinol Metab 61:142, 1985.

Voutilainen R, Perheentupa J, Apter D: Benign premature adrenarche: Clinical features and serum steroid levels. Acta Paediatr Scand 72:707, 1983.

19.10 DISORDERS OF THE THYROID GLAND

The main function of the thyroid gland is to synthesize thyroxine (T_4) and 3,5,3'-triiodothyronine (T_3). The only known physiologic role of iodine is in the synthesis of these hormones; the estimated requirement is 75–150 μg/day. The daily intake in North America varies from 240 to more than 700 μg. Whatever the chemical form ingested, iodine eventually reaches the thyroid gland as iodide. Thyroid tissue has an avidity for iodine and is able to trap (with a gradient of 100–1), transport, and concentrate it in the follicular lumen for synthesis of thyroid hormone.

Before trapped iodide can react with tyrosine, it must be oxidized; this reaction is catalyzed by thyroidal peroxidase. The thyroid cells also elaborate a specific thyroprotein, a globulin with approximately 120 tyrosine units. Iodination of tyrosine forms monoiodotyrosine and diiodotyrosine; two molecules of diiodotyrosine then couple to form one molecule of T_4, or one molecule of diiodotyrosine and one of monoiodotyrosine to form T_3. It is uncertain whether a coupling enzyme exists. Once formed, hormones are stored as thyroglobulin in the lumen of the follicle (colloid) until ready to be delivered to the body cells. Thyroglobulin (Tg) is a large globular glycoprotein with a molecular weight of about 660,000 and under normal conditions is detectable in the blood of most individuals at nanogram levels. T_4 and T_3 are liberated from thyroglobulin by activation of proteases and peptidases.

The metabolic potency of T_3 is 3–4 times that of T_4. Only 20% of circulating T_3 is secreted by the thyroid; the remainder is produced by deiodination of T_4 in the liver, kidney, and other peripheral tissues by thyroxine-5'-deiodinase. T_3 carries out most of the physiologic actions of the thyroid hormones. T_4 is more abundant, but it binds weakly to nuclear receptors, and most of its physiologic effects occur via conversion to T_3. Reliable methods now measure the level of T_3 directly in blood; its concentration is 1/50 that of T_4. The thyroid hormones increase oxygen consumption, stimulate protein synthesis, influence growth and differentiation, and affect carbohydrate, lipid, and vitamin metabolism. The free hormones enter cells, bind to cytosol receptors specific for T_3 or T_4, and are transported to the mitochondria or the nucleus where they participate in activating transcription.

The circulating thyroid hormones (T_4 and T_3) are firmly bound to thyroxine-binding proteins, of which the major one is thyroxine-binding globulin (TBG); less important are thyroxine-binding prealbumin (TBPA) and albumin. The concentration or binding capacity of TBG is altered in many clinical circumstances; its status must be considered in the interpretation of T_4 or T_3 levels.

The thyroid is regulated by thyroid-stimulating hormone (TSH), a glycoprotein produced and secreted by the anterior pituitary. This hormone activates adenylate cyclase in the thyroid gland to effect release of thyroid hormones. TSH is composed of two noncovalently bound subunits (chains): alpha (hTSH-α) and beta (hTSH-β). The free subunits as well as TSH can be measured in blood by specific radioimmunoassays. TSH synthesis and release are stimulated by thyroid-releasing hormone (TRH), which is synthesized in the hypothalamus and secreted into the pituitary. TRH is found in other parts of the brain besides the hypothalamus, and in many other organs; aside from its endocrine function, it seems to serve as a neurotransmitter. TRH is a simple tripeptide that is available for clinical use. In states of decreased production of thyroid hormone, TSH and presumably TRH are increased. An excess of TRH or of TSH results in hypertrophy and hyperplasia of thyroid cells, increased trapping of iodine, and increased synthesis of thyroid hormones. Exogenous thyroid hormone or increased thyroid hormone synthesis inhibits TSH production.

Further control of the level of circulating thyroid hormones occurs in the periphery. In many nonthyroidal illnesses extrathyroidal production of T_3 decreases; factors which inhibit thyroxine-5'-deiodinase include fasting, chronic malnutrition, acute illness, and certain drugs. Levels of T_3 may be significantly decreased while levels of T_4 and TSH remain normal.

Presumably, the decreased levels of T_3 result in decreased rates of oxygen production, of substrate utilization, and of other catabolic processes.

19.11 THYROID HORMONE STUDIES

Serum Thyroid Hormones. Most other methods to measure T_4 and T_3 have been made obsolete by radioimmunoassay (RIA). Measurements of T_3 (3,5,3'-triiodothyronine) are valuable in the diagnosis of thyroid disorders, particularly in hyperthyroidism. A metabolically inert form of T_3, reverse T_3 (3,3',5'-triiodothyronine), is also present in sera; both T_3 and rT_3 are measurable by radioimmunoassay. Normal levels of T_4, T_3, and rT_3 vary with age; accordingly, age must be considered in interpreting results, particularly in the neonate (see below).

Thyroglobulin (Tg) is present in measurable amounts in the circulation of normal subjects but is absent in the sera of congenitally athyrotic infants. Its production appears to be controlled by TSH. Elevated levels of Tg are found in patients with differentiated carcinoma of the thyroid, where it serves as a useful marker in their post-treatment follow-up.

Thyrotropin (TSH) is readily measured by radioimmunoassay (RIA); its level is one of the most sensitive indicators of primary hypothyroidism. After the neonatal period, normal levels are below 6 μU/mL. TSH secretion can be stimulated by intravenous administration (7 μg/kg) of thyrotropin-releasing hormone (TRH). In normal subjects TRH administration increases baseline levels of TSH within 30 min. In hyperthyroidism there is no rise in serum levels of TSH in response to TRH because the elevated levels of thyroid hormones block the effect of TRH on the pituitary. On the other hand, in patients with even very mild degrees of thyroid failure, administration of TRH results in an exaggerated TSH response. Patients with pituitary or hypothalamic failure have low basal levels of TSH; a normal response to TRH localizes the defect in the hypothalamus.

Fetal and Newborn Thyroid. The fetal hypothalamic-pituitary-thyroid system develops independently of maternal influence. T_4, T_3, and TSH do not cross the mammalian placenta. By 10–12 wk of gestation the fetal thyroid is able to concentrate iodine and to synthesize iodothyronines. By the same time the fetal pituitary contains TSH. Fetal serum T_4 increases progressively from midgestation to approximately 11.5 μg/dL at term. Fetal levels of T_3 are below measurable levels before 30 wk and then gradually rise to about 50 ng/dL at term. Reverse T_3 levels, however, are very high in the fetus (250 ng/dL at 30 wk) and fall to 150 ng/dL at term. Serum levels of TSH peak in the fetus at 20-24 wk to about 15 μU/mL and then gradually decrease to 10 μU/mL at term.

At birth there is an acute release of TSH; peak serum concentrations reach 70 μU/mL in 30 min in full term infants. A rapid decline occurs in the ensuing 24 hr and a more gradual decline within the next 2 days to below 10 μU/mL. The acute increase in TSH produces a dramatic rise in levels of T_3 to approximately 300 ng/dL in about 4 hr. This T_3 seems largely derived from increased peripheral conversion of T_4 to T_3. T_3 levels then decline during the 1st wk of life to levels under 200 ng/dL. rT_3 levels are maintained for 2 wk (200 ng/dL) and fall by 4 wk to around 50 ng/dL.

Serum Thyroxine-Binding Globulin (TBG). The thyroid hormones are transported in plasma bound to TBG, a glycoprotein synthesized in the liver. Estimation of TBG levels is occasionally necessary because TBG is increased or decreased in a variety of clinical situations, with effects on the level of thyroxine. TBG binds about 80% of T_4 and 50% of T_3. TBG levels increase in pregnancy and in the newborn period, and with estrogens (oral contraceptives), perphenazine, heroin,

and clofibrate, and decrease with androgens, anabolic steroids, glucocorticoids, and L-asparaginase. These effects are the results of modulation of hepatic synthesis of TBG. Phenytoin (diphenylhydantoin) is the most common cause of drug-induced abnormality of thyroid function tests. Phenytoin, an inducer of hepatic enzymes, stimulates hepatic degradation of T_4 and accelerates transport of T_4 into tissues. Phenobarbital has a similar effect. Some drugs, particularly phenytoin, also inhibit binding of T_4 and T_3 to TBG. Decreased or increased levels of TBG also occur as genetic traits (see below).

The most commonly used measures of TBG or TBG-binding capacity are variations of the resin triiodothyronine uptake test, RT_3U, a screening test with which to interpret T_4 results; it should never be used as an autonomous test of thyroid function. The product of the serum T_4 concentration and T_3 uptake (thyroxine-resin T_3 index or T_4-RT_3U index) correlates closely with free T_4 concentration in serum. This index increases in hyperthyroidism, decreases in hypothyroidism, and is normal in euthyroid patients with abnormalities in the concentration of TBG. Normal values for the index vary among laboratories since T_4 levels and T_3 uptakes are often determined by a variety of kit methods and calculations and expressions of the index vary also among laboratories. A radioimmunoassay method for TBG is available.

In Vivo Radionuclide Studies. Markedly improved direct tests of thyroid function have made radioiodine uptake studies less useful. The iodine-trapping or concentrating mechanism of the thyroid can be evaluated by the radioactive isotope ^{123}I (half-life 13 hr). Present technology allows doses of radioiodine (0.1–0.5 μCi) that are only a fraction of those formerly used. Technetium (^{99m}Tc) is a particularly useful radioisotope for children since, in contrast to iodine, it is trapped but not organified by the thyroid and has a half-life of only 6 hr. Thyroid scanning may be indicated to detect ectopic thyroid tissue, to evaluate thyroid nodules, and to assess presence of thyroid tissue in questions of thyroid agenesis. These studies should be performed with ^{99m}Tc as pertechnetate since it has the advantages of lower radiation exposure and high quality scintigrams. Use of ^{131}I in children should be limited to those known to have thyroid cancer.

DEFECTS OF THYROXINE-BINDING GLOBULIN

Abnormalities in levels of TBG are not associated with clinical disease and do not require treatment, but they may be sources of confusion in the diagnosis of hypo- or hyperthyroidism.

TBG deficiency occurs as an X-linked dominant disorder. Affected males are euthyroid. TBG is absent or low, T_4 is low, and levels of RT_3U are high. Heterozygous females have intermediate levels of TBG, low-normal levels of T_4 and high normal levels of RT_3U. Homozygous females have not been reported, but an affected 45,X female is known. Absence of TBG from the cord blood of affected males indicates that it does not cross the placenta. A rare instance of total deficiency of TBG in a normal woman established that TBG is not necessary for normal pregnancy.

TBG deficiency is being found through screening programs for neonatal hypothyroidism. It occurs in 1/14,000 neonates. Levels of T_4 in affected infants are usually as low as with congenital hypothyroidism; in contrast to hypothyroidism, however, serum levels of TSH are not elevated. The diagnosis is confirmed by finding low levels of TBG by radioimmunoassay.

There appears to be also an autosomal dominant form of the disorder in which deficiency of TBG is partial.

Elevated TBG is also a harmless X-linked dominant anomaly, occurring in about 1/40,000 persons. It has been recognized primarily in adults, but neonatal screening programs are now uncovering the condition in the neonate. The level of T_4 is elevated, T_3 is variably elevated, TSH is normal, and RT_3U is decreased. The elevated levels of TBG and normal levels of free T_4 confirm the diagnosis. In neonates, levels of T_4 as high as 95 μg/dL have been found, which decrease to 20–30 μg/dL after 2–3 wk. Such high levels of T_4 are thought to be related in part to the normally elevated levels of TBG in neonates during the 1st mo of life, presumably as an effect of maternal estrogens. Affected patients are euthyroid. Family studies may be indicated to alert other affected individuals.

19.12 HYPOTHYROIDISM

Hypothyroidism results from deficient production of thyroid hormone (Table 19–3). The disorder may be manifest very early in life. When symptoms appear after a period of apparently normal thyroid function, the disorder may either be truly "acquired" or only appear so as a result of one of a variety of congenital defects in which the manifestation of the deficiency is delayed. The term "cretinism" is often used synonymously with congenital hypothyroidism but should be avoided.

CONGENITAL HYPOTHYROIDISM

Congenital causes of hypothyroidism may be sporadic or familial, goitrous or nongoitrous. In many instances the de-

Table 19–3. Etiologic Classification of Hypothyroidism

Deficiency of TRH
  Isolated
  Multiple hypothalamic deficiencies (e.g., idiopathic hypopituitarism)
Deficiency of TSH
  Isolated
  Multiple pituitary deficiencies (e.g., craniopharyngioma)
Deficiency of thyroid hormone
  Aplasia, hypoplasia or ectopia of thyroid
    Developmental defects (thyroid dysgenesis)
    Maternal radioiodine
    Maternal autoimmune disease?
  Defective synthesis of thyroid hormone (goitrous hypothyroidism)
    Iodide-trapping defect
    Iodide-organification defects
      Absent peroxidase
      Defective binding of peroxidase
      Inactive bound peroxidase
      Pendred syndrome
    Iodotyrosine coupling defect
    Iodotyrosine deiodination defect
    Thyroglobulin synthesis defect
  Iodine deficiency (endemic cretinism)
  Damage to thyroid gland
    Autoimmune disease (lymphocytic thyroiditis)
    Cystinosis
  Maternal ingestion of medications (neonatal goiter)
    Iodides
    Propylthiouracil, methimazole
  Iatrogenic
    Thyroidectomy
    Drugs (iodides, lithium, cobalt, propylthiouracil, methimazole, para-aminosalicylic acid)
    Neck irradiation (e.g., for Hodgkin disease)
End-organ defect
  TSH unresponsiveness
    Defective TSH receptor
    Defective G unit
    Type I pseudohypoparathyroidism
    Maternal TSH-binding inhibitor
  Thyroid hormone unresponsiveness
    Autosomal recessive
    Autosomal dominant

ficiency of thyroid hormone is severe, and symptoms develop in the early weeks of life. In others, lesser degrees of deficiency occur, and manifestations may be delayed for months or years.

Etiology. *Aplasia and Hypoplasia.* Developmental defects of the thyroid gland (*thyroid dysgenesis*) are the most common causes of congenital hypothyroidism. Neonatal screening programs have screened about 50 million infants, and it is established that 90% of infants with congenital hypothyroidism have thyroid dysgenesis. The incidence is 1/3800–1/4000 infants worldwide, lower in Japan (1/5500) and in American blacks (1/12,000). Radionuclide scans find no thyroid in about one third of affected infants; rudiments of thyroid tissue may be found in the others when sensitive scanning techniques are used. The thyroid rudiment is frequently found in an ectopic location anywhere from the base of the tongue (*lingual thyroid*) to the normal position in the neck. Little is known of the factors which interfere with normal migration and development of the thyroid gland. The disorder is usually sporadic; familial cases have been reported. Twice as many females as males are affected. Congenital hypothyroidism has been reported confined to one of monozygotic twins; this observation suggests that a deleterious factor operated during intrauterine life; occasionally, the onset of hypothyroidism in a twin is delayed. In one of identical twins hypothyroidism associated with an inadequate thyroid in the normal position was diagnosed at 4 mo of age; in the second twin an ectopic thyroid did not lose adequate function until about 4–6 yr of age.

Lingual thyroid represents extreme failure of migration of the thyroid gland; the ectopic tissue may provide adequate amounts of thyroid hormone for many years, or may fail in early childhood. Newborn screening programs usually detect the condition. Hypothyroidism usually follows surgical removal of a lingual thyroid from a euthyroid patient since most such patients have no other thyroid tissue. Lingual thyroid has been associated with thyroglossal duct cysts and with a family history of other thyroid disorders.

For years it has been proposed that passive transplacental transfer of an autoimmune process in the mother might cause congenital hypothyroidism through a thyrosuppressive factor. One study of 104 infants with congenital hypothyroidism found thyroid antimicrosomal antibodies in only one infant, but in 14% of their mothers. A recent study found 50% of mothers of infants with congenital hypothyroidism and 50% of affected infants to have an antibody that blocks TRH-induced thyroid growth. It is possible that such antibodies interfere with development of the fetal thyroid gland. Some women with nongoitrous autoimmune thyroiditis have an *inhibitory immunoglobulin* that can pass the placenta and cause *transient hypothyroidism*; the condition has affected siblings. Such autoimmune perturbations during pregnancy should be evaluated in the search for the etiology of congenital hypothyroidism.

Radioiodine. Administration of radioiodine during pregnancy for treatment of cancer of the thyroid or of hyperthyroidism has been reported to damage the fetal thyroid; in most instances pregnancy was not suspected at the time of administration of ^{131}I. Whenever radioiodine is administered to a woman of child-bearing age, a pregnancy test must be made before a therapeutic dose of ^{131}I is given. The fetal thyroid gland is capable of trapping iodine by 70-75 days. In one instance, ^{131}I was administered to the mother at 14 wk of gestation for treatment of thyroid carcinoma; the athyrotic infant had a tracheal stricture at the site of the thyroid, T_4 and T_3 were undetectable in cord serum, and TSH was markedly elevated (340 μU/mL). This is clear evidence that maternal thyroid hormones do not cross the placenta in significant amounts late in pregnancy. Administration of radioactive iodine to lactating women is also contraindicated since it is readily excreted in milk.

Thyrotropin Deficiency. Deficiency of TSH and hypothyroidism may occur in any of the conditions associated with developmental defects of the pituitary or hypothalamus or in children with idiopathic hypopituitarism (Sec. 19.2). More often in these conditions the deficiency of TSH is secondary to a deficiency of thyrotropin-releasing factor (hypothalamic hypothyroidism). With administration of TRH an increase of TSH indicates a primary hypothalamic defect. TSH-deficient hypothyroidism is found in 1/50,000–1/100,000 infants screened for neonatal hypothyroidism. The majority of those affected have other clinical features of hypopituitarism such as hypoglycemia, microgenitalia, persistent jaundice, and facial anomalies.

Isolated deficiency of TSH is rare and has been reported only about 20 times, mostly in adults. Isolated TSH deficiency might also be primary or secondary to TRH deficiency.

Thyrotropin Unresponsiveness. Congenital nongoitrous hypothyroidism has been reported in two boys of two consanguineous matings who had elevated levels of biologically active TSH and normal ^{131}I uptake. Absence of response to thyrotropin was shown in vivo and in metabolism of thyroid tissue in vitro.

Mild congenital hypothyroidism has been detected in at least five newborn infants who subsequently proved to have *type Ia pseudohypoparathyroidism.* The molecular cause for resistance to TSH in these patients is the generalized impairment of cAMP synthesis caused by deficient activity of guanine nucleotide–binding regulatory unit (Sec. 19.19).

Thyroid Hormone Unresponsiveness. An increasing number of patients are being found who are resistant to the action of endogenous and exogenous T_4 and T_3. Most have a goiter and clearly elevated levels of T_4, T_3, free T_4, and free T_3. These findings have often led to the erroneous diagnosis of Graves disease although the patients are clinically euthyroid. Since the pituitary is also resistant to thyroid hormones, TSH levels are normal or elevated and inappropriate for the levels of T_4 and T_3. Abnormally large doses of T_3 are required to suppress the levels of TSH. Fibroblasts from affected patients have defective receptor affinity for T_3. The resistance to thyroid hormone appears to vary among different tissues and variable expression has been observed within families. Both autosomal recessive and autosomal dominant modes of inheritance have been described, suggesting heterogeneity of the disorder. Usually no treatment is necessary.

Defective Synthesis of Thyroxine. Congenital hypothyroidism may be due to a variety of defects in the biosynthesis of thyroid hormone. The presence of a goiter is the hallmark of these defects, and the condition is termed goitrous hypothyroidism or goitrous cretinism. Goitrous hypothyroidism is detected in 1/30,000–50,000 live births in neonatal screening programs. It is genetically determined and in most instances transmitted in an autosomal recessive manner. The following defects have been identified:

IODIDE-TRAPPING DEFECT. This defect has been reported in 22 patients, many from Japan, and in nine related infants of the Hutterite sect. The condition has been detected in neonatal screening programs. Evidence suggests autosomal recessive inheritance but heterogeneity is likely. Clinical hypothyroidism, with or without a goiter, may develop in the 1st few mo of life. In Japan, however, goiter and hypothyroidism often appear after 10 yr of age, perhaps because of the very high iodine content (often 19 mg/day) of the Japanese diet.

The energy-dependent mechanism for concentrating iodide is defective not only in thyroid but also in the salivary glands. In contrast to all the other defects, the uptakes of radioiodine and pertechnetate are low; saliva/serum ratios of ^{123}I may be required to establish the diagnosis.

IODIDE ORGANIFICATION DEFECT. After iodide is trapped by the thyroid, it is rapidly oxidized by H_2O_2 and thyroid peroxidase and is incorporated into tyrosine. In this defect, iodide is not organified and may be rapidly discharged from the thyroid by administration of perchlorate. Three different organification defects have now been characterized:

1. Complete absence of peroxidase activity in a severe form of goitrous hypothyroidism.

2. Failure of a prosthetic hematin group to bind to thyroidal apoperoxidase in euthyroid goitrous patients.

3. Inactive peroxidase due to an abnormality in its bound state.

Deficient organification also occurs in Pendred syndrome, but peroxidase activity is normal and the biochemical defect unknown.

COUPLING DEFECT. After iodine is incorporated into tyrosine in thyroglobulin to form iodotyrosine, an intramolecular rearrangement occurs, leading to coupling of iodotyrosines to form diiodothyronines. Because this reaction is complex, heterogeneity of defects is likely, but little is known of the biochemical aberrations involved. It has been proposed that errors may involve defects in coupling enzymes or an abnormality in steric configuration.

DEIODINASE DEFECT. Free monoiodotyrosine and diiodotyrosine are normally deiodinated within the thyroid or in peripheral tissues by a deiodinase. The iodine thus liberated is then reused in synthesis of hormone. Patients with iodotyrosine-dehalogenase deficiency have large amounts of monoiodotyrosine and diiodotyrosine in blood and in urine. The constant loss of iodine from the thyroid into the urine leads to hormone deficiency and goiter.

DEFECT OF THYROGLOBULIN SYNTHESIS. Patients with this disorder release from the thyroid into the bloodstream iodinated proteins or polypeptides which are calorigenically inactive. Because thyroglobulin synthesis is complex, this category has diverse etiologies.

Clinical Manifestations. The clinician is becoming increasingly dependent on neonatal screening tests for diagnosis of congenital hypothyroidism. Laboratory errors occur, however, and awareness of early symptoms must be maintained. Congenital hypothyroidism is twice as common in girls as in boys. Prior to neonatal screening programs congenital hypothyroidism was rarely recognized in the newborn since the signs and symptoms are usually not sufficiently developed. It can be suspected and the diagnosis established during the early weeks of life if the initial but less characteristic manifestations are recognized. Hypothyroid infants may be significantly heavier at birth than normal newborn infants, but there is little diagnostic value to this observation. Prolongation of physiologic icterus, owing to delayed maturation of glucuronide conjugation, may be the earliest sign. Feeding difficulties, especially sluggishness, lack of interest, somnolence, and choking spells during nursing, are often present during the 1st mo of life. Respiratory difficulties, due in part to the large tongue, include apneic episodes, noisy respirations, and nasal obstruction. Typical respiratory distress syndrome may also occur. Affected infants cry little, sleep much, have poor appetites, and are generally sluggish. There may be constipation which does not usually respond to treatment. The abdomen is large, and an umbilical hernia is usually present. The temperature is subnormal, often below 35° C (95° F), and the skin, particularly of the extremities, may be cold and mottled. Edema of the genitals and extremities may be present. The pulse is slow; heart murmurs and cardiomegaly are common. Anemia is often present and is refractory to treatment with hematinics. Since symptoms appear gradually, the diagnosis is often delayed.

These manifestations progress; retardation of physical and mental development becomes greater during the following months, and by 3-6 mo of age the clinical picture is fully developed (see Fig. 19–6). When there is only a partial deficiency of thyroid hormone, the symptoms may be milder, the syndrome incomplete, and the onset delayed. Although

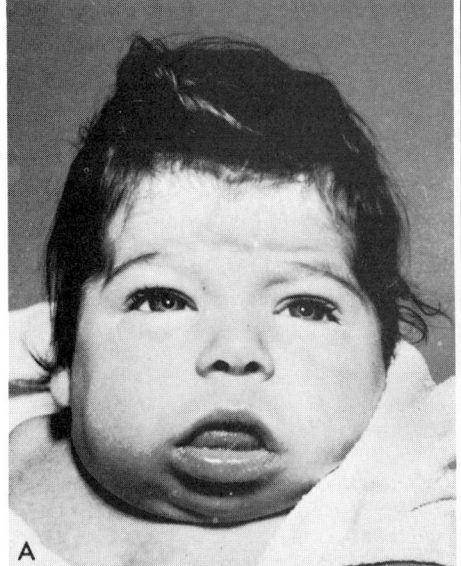
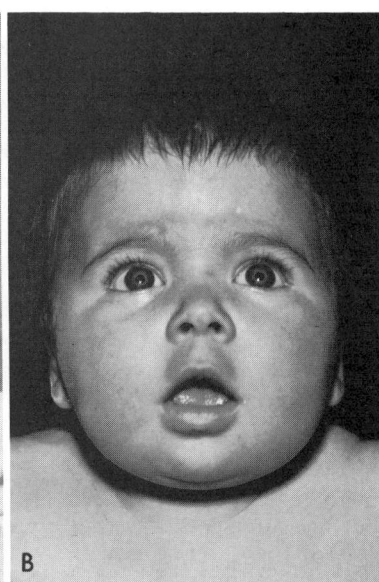

Figure 19–6. Congenital hypothyroidism in an infant 6 mo of age. The infant fed poorly in the neonatal period and was constipated. She had a persistent nasal discharge and a large tongue, was very lethargic, and had no social smile and no head control. *A*, Note puffy face, dull expression, hirsute forehead. Negligible uptake of radioiodine. Osseous development was that of newborn. *B*, Four mo after treatment. Note decreased puffiness of face, decreased hirsutism of forehead, and alert appearance.

breast milk contains significant amounts of thyroid hormones, particularly T_3, it is inadequate to protect the breast-fed infant with congenital hypothyroidism, and it has no effect on neonatal thyroid screening tests.

The child is stunted in growth, the extremities short, with head size normal or even increased. The anterior and posterior fontanels are widely open; observation of this sign at birth may serve as an initial clue for early recognition of congenital hypothyroidism. Only 3% of normal newborn infants have a posterior fontanel larger than 0.5 cm. The eyes appear far apart, and the bridge of the broad nose is depressed. The palpebral fissures are narrow and the eyelids swollen. The mouth is kept open, and the thick and broad tongue protrudes from it. Dentition is delayed. The neck is short and thick, and there may be deposits of fat above the clavicles and between the neck and shoulders. The hands are broad and the fingers short. The skin is dry and scaly, and there is little perspiration. Myxedema manifests itself, particularly in the skin of the eyelids, of the back of the hands, and of the external genitalia. Carotenemia may cause a yellow discoloration of the skin, but the scleras remain white. The scalp is thickened, and the hair is coarse, brittle, and scanty. The hairline reaches far down on the forehead, which usually appears wrinkled, especially when the infant cries.

Development is usually retarded. Hypothyroid infants appear lethargic and are late in sitting and standing. The voice is hoarse, and they do not learn to talk. The degree of physical and mental retardation increases with age. Sexual maturation may be delayed or not take place at all or may occur precociously (Sec. 19.7).

The muscles are usually hypotonic, but in rare instances generalized muscular hypertrophy occurs (*Kocher-Debré-Sémé-laigne syndrome*). Affected children may have an athletic appearance due to pseudohypertrophy, particularly in the calf muscles. Its pathogenesis is unknown; nonspecific histochemical and ultrastructural changes seen on muscle biopsy return to normal with treatment. Boys are more prone to develop the syndrome, which has been observed in siblings born to a consanguineous mating. Affected patients have hypothyroidism of longer duration and severity.

Laboratory Data. Serum levels of T_4 and T_3 are low or borderline. If the defect is primarily in the thyroid, levels of TSH in serum are elevated, commonly to above 100 μU/mL. Most newborn screening programs measure levels of T_4, but the diagnosis is confirmed by assay of TSH, which should always be measured to confirm a diagnosis of primary hypo-

thyroidism at any age. Euthyroid patients with low levels of TBG caused by genetic deficiencies or medications will have low levels of T_4 but will have normal levels of TSH. Hypothyroid patients with low levels of TSH may have pituitary or hypothalamic defects and require study with TRH stimulation. With all these assays, special care must be given to the normal range of values for the age of the patient, particularly in the newborn period.

Retardation of osseous development can be shown roentgenographically at birth in about 60% of congenitally hypothyroid infants and indicates some deprivation of thyroid hormone during intrauterine life. For example, the distal femoral epiphysis, normally present at birth, is often absent (Fig. 19–7A). In untreated patients the discrepancy between chronologic age and osseous development increases. The epiphyses often have multiple foci of ossification (epiphyseal dysgenesis, Fig. 19–7B); deformity ("beaking") of the 12th thoracic or 1st or 2nd lumbar vertebra is common. Roentgenograms of the skull show large fontanels and wide sutures; intersutural (wormian) bones are common. The sella turcica is often enlarged and round; in rare instances there may be erosion and thinning. Delays in formation and eruption of teeth may occur. Cardiac enlargement or pericardial effusion may be present.

Levels of growth hormone and responses to provocative stimuli may be abnormally low in primary hypothyroidism; they return to normal with treatment.

Scintigraphy is indicated to determine whether there is any thyroid tissue; ^{123}I sodium iodide appears to be superior to ^{99m}Tc sodium pertechnetate for this purpose. Measurement of levels of thyroglobulin in plasma is also of value; undetectable levels are associated with absence of thyroid tissue, whereas detectable or low levels are found when thyroid tissue is present. Patients with goitrous hypothyroidism may require extensive evaluation, including radioiodine studies, perchlorate discharge tests, kinetic studies, chromatography, and studies of thyroid tissue if the biochemical nature of the defect is to be determined.

The electrocardiogram may show low voltage P and T waves with diminished amplitude of QRS complexes. The electroencephalogram frequently shows low voltage. In children over 2 yr of age the serum cholesterol level is usually elevated.

Differential Diagnosis. With the careful plotting on growth charts of lengths and heights of all infants and children, deceleration of growth velocity frequently provides the first clue to the diagnosis. Once it has been considered, confirmation is not difficult since direct tests of thyroid function are generally available and reliable. Familiarity with those conditions which affect test results, such as alterations in TBG, is essential.

Prognosis. Without treatment, affected infants become mentally deficient dwarfs. Treatment with thyroid hormone results in normality in linear growth, osseous maturation, and sexual development. Mental development, however, is much less predictable. Thyroid hormone is critical for normal cerebral development in the early postnatal months; hence, the diagnosis must be made early in life and effective treatment initiated promptly in order to minimize irreversible brain damage. In general, the more profound the deprivation of the thyroid hormone early in life, the poorer the prognosis for mental development. With the advent of neonatal screening programs for detection of congenital hypothyroidism, the prognosis for affected infants has improved dramatically. Infants detected on neonatal screening with adequate treatment begun in the 1st mo of life have normal IQ's at 6 yr, but measurements of school performance remain to be assessed. There is no conclusive evidence that treatment of the pregnant woman with huge doses of thyroid hormone to enhance transplacental transfer of protective levels of hormone to the hypothyroid fetus is effective.

When clinical evidence of hypothyroidism is delayed in onset, the outlook for normal mental development is much better; children who acquire hypothyroidism after 2 yr of age and are treated appropriately have a good prognosis for mental development.

Treatment. Whatever the cause of hypothyroidism, replacement therapy with thyroid hormone is indicated and effective. Sodium-L-thyroxine given orally is the drug of choice. It has been estimated that normally 30–50% of circulating thyroxine undergoes peripheral deiodination to become triiodothyronine, most circulating T_3 being derived from T_4 rather than directly from the thyroid gland. Hence, treatment with sodium-L-thyroxine provides both T_4 and T_3. In infants the dose is 6–8 µg/kg. Older children appear to require about 4 µg/kg and may be treated initially with 100–150 µg/24 hr; only rarely is more than 200 µg/24 hr required.

Levels of both T_4 and TSH should be monitored and maintained within the upper half of the normal range (>8 µg/dL), especially during the 1st yr of life. In seven children, 8–13 yr, pseudotumor cerebri developed within the first 4 mo of initiation of thyroid therapy. In older children, after catch-up growth is complete, the growth rate provides an excellent index of adequacy of therapy. Parents should be forewarned of changes in behavior and activity expected with therapy, and special attention must be given to any developmental or neurologic deficits.

JUVENILE HYPOTHYROIDISM
(Acquired Hypothyroidism)

The development of hypothyroidism in a child who was previously euthyroid may be due to a wide variety of defects. A congenitally hypoplastic thyroid gland may furnish amounts of hormone sufficient for the 1st few yr, but the deficiency may become manifest when rapid growth of the body increases demands on the gland. Accordingly, any or all of the etiologic causes of congenital hypothyroidism must be considered. Clinical manifestations of congenital defects may develop as if they were acquired lesions.

Complete or subtotal thyroidectomy for thyrotoxicosis or cancer may result in hypothyroidism, as may removal of an anomalous thyroid when it constitutes the sole source of thyroid hormone. For example, a thyroid ectopically placed at the base of the tongue (lingual thyroid) is often the only thyroid tissue, or the entire thyroid gland may consist of a midline nodule and be mistaken for a thyroglossal duct cyst.

In nephropathic *cystinosis* accumulation of intracellular cystine results in impaired thyroid function with eventual destruction of the gland. Hypothyroidism may be overt, but compensated forms are more frequent and periodic assessment of TSH levels is indicated.

Irradiation to the area of the thyroid that is incidental to the treatment of Hodgkin disease and other malignancies or prior to bone marrow transplantation results in thyroid dysfunction in approximately one third of children and adolescents. These groups of patients require periodic assessment of TSH.

Hypothyroidism associated with a goiter may be caused occasionally by chronic infectious processes or by the protracted ingestion of medications such as iodides or cobalt. Acquired hypothyroidism, however, most often results from *lymphocytic thyroiditis*, which may or may not be associated with a goiter.

The clinical manifestations depend upon the age of the child at onset and upon the extent of dysfunction. The later

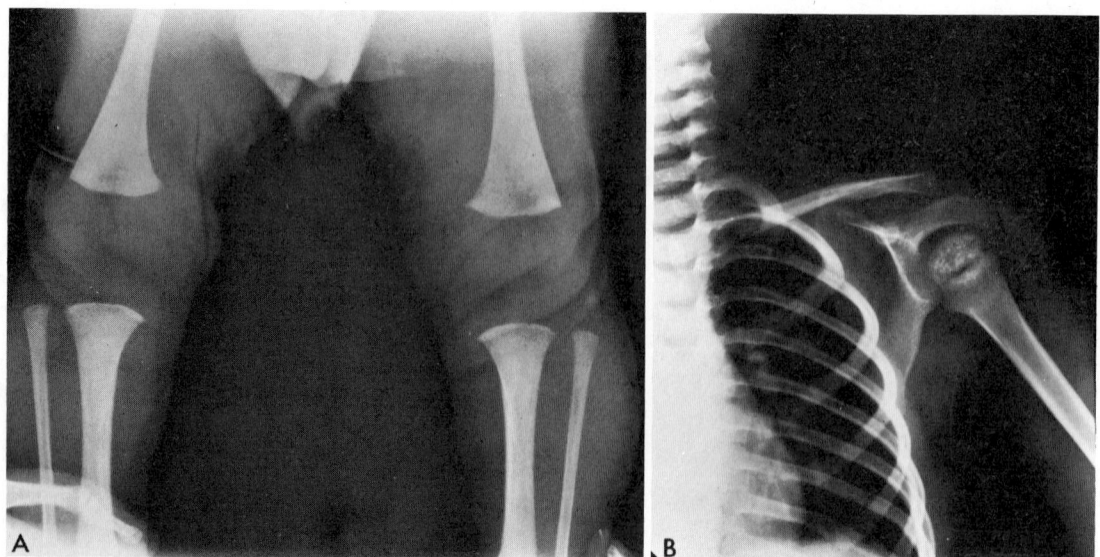

Figure 19–7. Congenital hypothyroidism. *A,* Absence of distal femoral epiphysis in a 3 mo old infant who was born at term. This is evidence for the onset of the hypothyroid state during fetal life. *B,* Epiphyseal dysgenesis in the head of the humerus in a 9 yr old girl who had been inadequately treated with thyroid hormone.

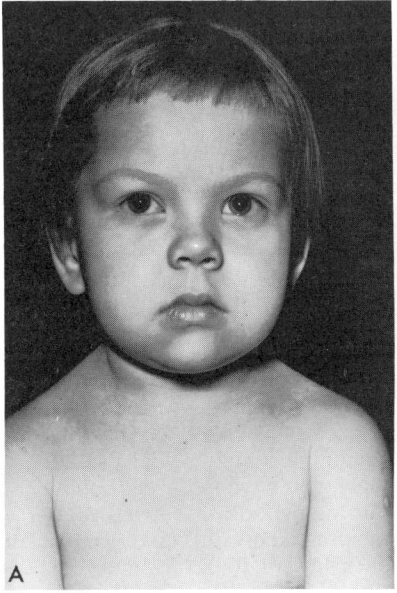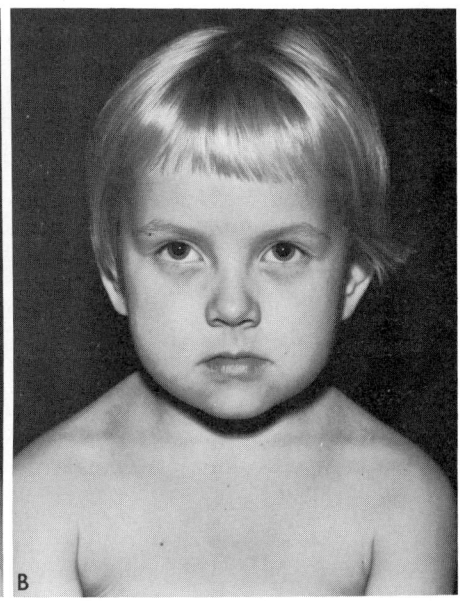

Figure 19–8. *A*, Acquired hypothyroidism in a girl 6 yr of age. She was treated with a wide variety of hematinics for refractory anemia for 3 yr. She had almost complete cessation of growth, constipation, and sluggishness of 3 yr duration. Height age was 3 yr; bone age, 4 yr. She had a sallow complexion and immature facies with a poorly developed nasal bridge. Serum cholesterol, 501 mg/dl.; radioiodine uptake, 7% at 24 hr; PBI, 2.8 μg/dl. *B*, After therapy for 18 mo. Note nasal development, increased luster and decreased pigmentation of hair, and maturation of face. Height age was 5.5 yr; bone age, 7 yr. There was decided improvement in her general condition. Menarche occurred at 14 yr. Ultimate height was 155 cm (61 in). She graduated from high school. She was well controlled with sodium-L-thyroxine daily.

in life hypothyroidism is acquired, the less will be the impairment of growth and development. Nevertheless, myxedematous changes of the skin, constipation, sleepiness, and a mental decline may be manifested at any age. Cessation or retardation of growth in a child whose growth has previously been normal should always alert one to the possibility of hypothyroidism (Fig. 19–8). Obese children are frequently, but usually erroneously, considered to have hypothyroidism. Most obese children are tall and have warm moist skin, a ruddy complexion, and normal thyroid function.

Diagnostic studies and treatment are the same as described for congenital hypothyroidism.

19.13 GOITER

A goiter is an enlargement of the thyroid gland. Persons with enlarged thyroids may have normal function of the gland (*euthyroidism*), thyroid deficiency (*hypothyroidism*), or overproduction of the hormones (*hyperthyroidism*). Goiter may be congenital or acquired, endemic or sporadic.

The goiter often results from increased pituitary secretion of thyrotropic hormone in response to decreased circulating levels of thyroid hormones. Thyroid enlargement may also result from infiltrative processes which may be inflammatory or neoplastic. Goiter in patients with thyrotoxicosis is caused by thyroid-stimulating immunoglobulin (TSI).

CONGENITAL GOITER

Congenital goiter is usually sporadic and may result from the administration of antithyroid drugs and/or iodides during pregnancy for the treatment of thyrotoxicosis. The concomitant administration of thyroid hormone with the goitrogen does not prevent this effect. Iodides are included in many proprietary preparations used to treat asthma; these preparations must be avoided during pregnancy, as they have often been a cause of unexpected congenital goiter. Goitrogenic drugs and iodides cross the placenta and at high doses may interfere with synthesis of thyroid hormone, resulting in goiter and hypothyroidism in the fetus. Even when the infant is clinically euthyroid, there may be retardation of osseous maturation, low levels of T_4, and elevated levels of TSH. Since these effects can occur when the mother takes only 100–200 mg of propylthiouracil/day, all such infants should be carefully

examined. Administration of thyroid hormone to affected infants may be indicated to treat clinical hypothyroidism, to hasten the disappearance of the goiter, and to prevent brain damage. Since the condition is rarely permanent, thyroid hormone may be safely discontinued after several mo.

Enlargement of the thyroid at birth may occasionally be sufficient to cause respiratory distress which interferes with nursing and may even cause death. The head may be maintained in extreme hyperextension. When respiratory obstruction is severe, partial thyroidectomy rather than tracheostomy is indicated (Fig. 19–9).

Goiter is almost always present in the congenitally hyperthyroid infant. These goiters are usually not large; the infant manifests clinical symptoms of hyperthyroidism, and the mother often has a history of Graves disease (Sec. 19.15).

When no causative factor is identifiable, a defect in synthesis of thyroid hormone must be suspected. One in 30,000–50,000 live births is found in neonatal screening programs to have such a defect. Study of this group of infants is complex. If the infant is hypothyroid, it is advisable to treat immediately with thyroid hormone and to postpone more detailed studies for later in life. Since these defects are transmitted by recessive genes, precise diagnosis is important for sound counseling.

Iodine deficiency as a cause of congenital goiters has become rare but persists in isolated endemic areas (see below). More important is the recent recognition that severe iodine deficiency early in pregnancy may cause neurologic damage during fetal development even in the absence of goiter.

When the "goiter" is lobulated, asymmetric, firm, or large to an unusual degree, a teratoma within or in the vicinity of the thyroid must be considered in the differential diagnosis (Sec. 16.23).

ENDEMIC GOITER AND CRETINISM

The association between deficiency of iodine and the prevalence of goiter and/or cretinism has been recognized for over half a century. If there is a moderate deficiency of iodine, the demand can be satisfied by increased efficiency in synthesis of thyroid hormone. Iodine liberated in the tissues is returned rapidly to the gland, which resynthesizes the hormone at a higher rate than normal. This increased activity is achieved by compensatory hypertrophy and hyperplasia, which satisfy the demands of the tissues for thyroid hormone. In geographic areas where deficiency of iodine is severe, decompensation and hypothyroidism may result.

Sea water is rich in iodine, and the iodine content of fish and shellfish is also high. Endemic goiter is rare therefore in populations living along the sea. Iodine is deficient in the water and native foods in the Pacific West and the Great Lakes areas of the United States. Deficiency of dietary iodine is even greater in certain Alpine valleys, the Himalayas, the Andes, the Congo, and the Highlands of Papua New Guinea. In areas such as in the United States, where iodine is provided in foods from other areas and in iodized salt, endemic goiter has disappeared. Iodized salt in the United States contains potassium iodide (100 μg/g) and provides excellent prophylaxis. Further iodine intake in the United States is contributed by iodates used in baking, iodine-containing coloring agents, and iodine-containing disinfectants used in the dairy industry. The recommended daily allowance of iodine for infants is 40–50 μg/dL; this is exceeded 4-fold in breast-fed infants and 10-fold in cow's-milk–fed infants in the United States.

Clinical Manifestations. If the deficiency of iodine is mild, thyroid enlargement does not become noticeable except when there is increased demand for the hormone during periods of rapid growth, as in adolescence and during pregnancy. In regions of moderate iodine deficiency, goiter observed in school children may disappear with maturity and reappear during pregnancy or lactation. Iodine-deficient goiters are more common in girls than in boys. Where iodine deficiency is severe, as in the hyperendemic Highlands of Papua New Guinea, nearly half the population have large goiters, and endemic cretinism is common.

Serum thyroxine levels are often low in endemic goiter, though clinical hypothyroidism is rare. This is true in New Guinea, the Congo, the Himalayas, and South America. Despite low serum levels of thyroid hormone, serum TSH concentrations are often only moderately increased. In such patients circulating levels of T_3 are elevated. Moreover, T_3 levels are also elevated in those patients with normal T_4 levels, indicating a preferential secretion of T_3 by the thyroid in this disease.

Endemic cretinism has been recognized for centuries and only in geographic association with endemic goiter. On the other hand, endemic goiter may occur in the absence of endemic cretinism. Past confusion concerning the pathogenesis of endemic cretinism was caused by including in the term "endemic cretinism" 2 very different but overlapping syndromes.

The "nervous" syndrome is characterized by ataxia, spasticity, deaf-mutism, and mental retardation. These "cretins" may have normal stature and little or no impairment of thyroid function. Recent evidence from Papua New Guinea strongly suggests that in the "nervous" type a deficiency of iodine throughout fetal life has damaged the developing nervous system quite apart from its role in the synthesis of thyroid hormone, the damage occurring in the 1st trimester of pregnancy even before the fetal thyroid has developed.

The "myxedematous" syndrome is characterized by marked delays in growth and sexual development and by mental retardation and myxedema. Neurologic examination is normal, and perceptive deafness is absent. In these patients the iodine deficiency occurred in late fetal life and postnatally. About 25% of the "myxedematous" type have goiters, but enlargement of the gland is minimal. Serum thyroid hormone levels are low, and TSH levels are markedly elevated. Thyroid scans are normal and preclude thyroid dysgenesis. There is marked delay in osseous maturation, which indicates that hypothyroidism appears around birth or during the 1st months of life. It is hypothesized that iodine deficiency in conjunction with an unknown toxic factor (goitrogen in food?) may alter thyroid function during fetal and neonatal life.

The term "endemic cretinism" continues to be used for both syndromes because the geographic distribution of both is the same and because both disappear from the population when iodine prophylaxis is introduced. The frequency of the two types varies among different populations; in Papua New Guinea the "nervous" type occurs almost exclusively, whereas in the Northeastern Congo the "myxedematous" type pre-

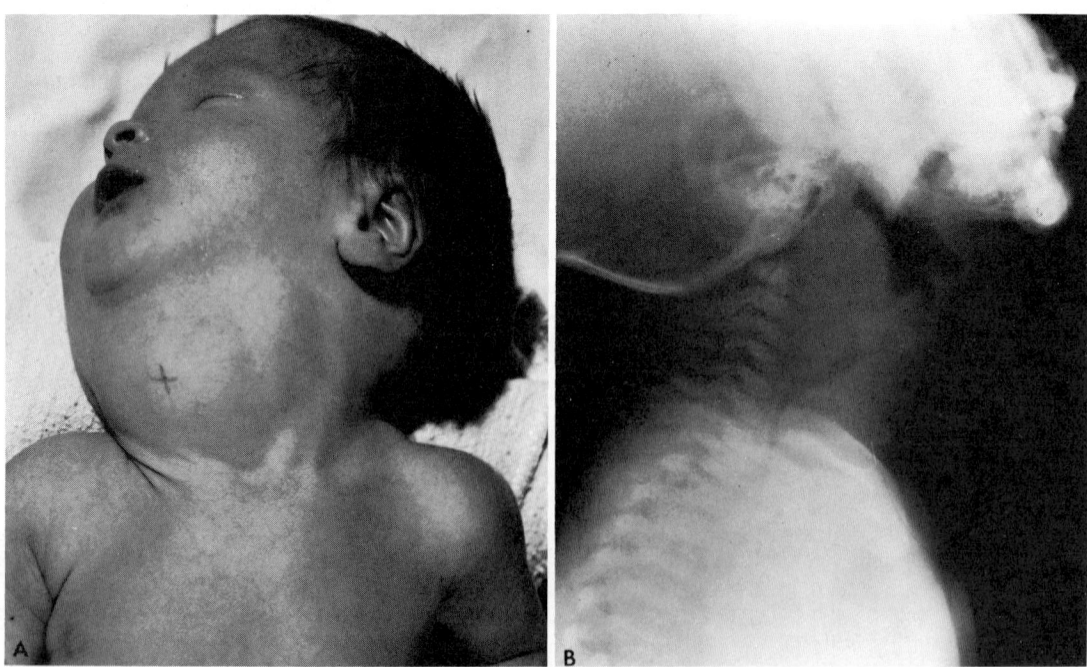

Figure 19–9. Congenital goiter in infancy. *A,* Large congenital goiter in an infant born to a mother with thyrotoxicosis who had been treated with iodides and methimazole during pregnancy. *B,* A 6 wk old infant with increasing respiratory distress and cervical mass since birth. Operation revealed a large goiter which almost completely encircled the trachea. Note anterior deviation and posterior compression of the trachea. Partial thyroidectomy completely relieved the symptoms. No cause for goiter was found. It is apparent why a tracheostomy is not adequate treatment for these infants.

dominates. It has been shown in Papua New Guinea that a single intramuscular injection of iodinated poppy seed oil to women prevents iodine deficiency during future pregnancies for about 5 yr.

SPORADIC GOITER

The term "sporadic goiter" encompasses goiters developing from a variety of causes; patients are usually euthyroid but may be hypothyroid. The most common cause of sporadic goiter is lymphocytic thyroiditis (below). Intrinsic biochemical defects in the synthesis of thyroid hormone are almost always associated with goiter (above); the occurrence of the disorder in siblings, the onset in early life, and the possible association with hypothyroidism (goitrous hypothyroidism) are important clues to diagnosis.

Iodide Goiter. A small percentage of patients treated with iodide preparations for prolonged periods develop goiters. Iodides are commonly included for their expectorant effect in cough medicines and in proprietary mixtures for asthma. The goiter is firm and diffusely enlarged, and in some instances hypothyroidism may develop. In normal subjects acute administration of large doses of iodine inhibits the organification of iodine and the synthesis of thyroid hormone (Wolff-Chaikoff effect). This effect is short-lived and does not lead to hypothyroidism. When iodide administration continues, an autoregulatory mechanism in normal persons limits iodine trapping and thus permits the level of iodide in the thyroid to fall and organification to proceed normally. In patients with iodide-induced goiter this escape does not occur because of an underlying abnormality of biosynthesis of thyroid hormone. Subjects most susceptible to the development of iodide goiter are those with lymphocytic thyroiditis or with a subclinical inborn error in thyroid hormone synthesis as well as those who have been treated with radioactive iodine for thyrotoxicosis.

Lithium carbonate also causes goiters; it is currently widely used as a psychotropic drug. Lithium competes with iodide; the mechanism producing the goiter and/or hypothyroidism is similar to that described above for iodide goiter. Lithium and iodide also act synergistically to produce goiter; their combined use should be avoided.

Amiodarone, a drug used to treat cardiac arrhythmias, can cause thyroid dysfunction with goiter because it is rich in iodine. It is also a potent inhibitor of 5'-deiodinase, preventing conversion of T_4 to T_3. It can cause hypothyroidism, particularly in patients with underlying autoimmune disease; in other patients, it may cause hyperthyroidism.

Simple Goiter (Colloid Goiter). A few children with euthyroid nontoxic goiters have simple goiters, a condition of unknown etiology not associated with hypothyroidism or hyperthyroidism and not caused by inflammation or neoplasia. The condition predominates in girls and has a peak incidence before and during the pubertal years. Histologic examination of the thyroid either is normal or reveals variable follicular size, dense colloid, and flattened epithelium. The goiter may be small or large. It is firm in consistency in half the patients and is occasionally asymmetric or nodular. Levels of TSH are normal or low; scintiscans are normal; thyroid antibodies are absent. Differentiation from lymphocytic thyroiditis may not be possible without a biopsy, but biopsy is ordinarily not indicated. Therapy with thyroid hormone may be indicated to avoid progression to a large multinodular goiter. Untreated patients should be re-evaluated periodically. This condition must be differentiated from lymphocytic thyroiditis (below).

Multinodular Goiter. Rarely, a firm goiter with a lobulated surface and single or multiple palpable nodules is encountered. Areas of cystic change, hemorrhage, and fibrosis may be present. The condition has decreased markedly in inci-

dence with the use of iodine-enriched salt. A mild goitrogenic stimulus, acting over a long time, is thought to be the etiology. Ultrasonography may reveal multiple echo-free and echogenic lesions that are nonfunctioning on scintiscans. Thyroid studies are usually normal, but TSH may be elevated and thyroid antibodies may be present. The condition occurs in children with McCune-Albright syndrome and has been described in three children (including two siblings) with digital anomalies and cystic renal disease. If the nodules are not suppressed with replacement therapy with thyroxine, surgery is indicated because malignancy cannot be readily ruled out.

PENDRED SYNDROME
(Goiter and Congenital Deafness)

This syndrome of congenital deafness and goiter is transmitted in an autosomal recessive fashion and is not to be confused with the deaf-mutism seen in endemic cretinism or with the minor impairment of hearing which may be found in severely hypothyroid persons. It must also be differentiated from the lymphocytic thyroiditis that may be associated with congenital rubella. The hearing loss is usually severe and present at birth, although it may not be recognized until later. It is most pronounced in the higher frequencies, is of the perceptive type, and exhibits recruitment. The goiter generally appears at puberty or later but may be present in early childhood; it may be barely detectable or pronounced. Initially, the goiter is soft and diffuse; it tends to become nodular in adult life. Most affected persons are clinically euthyroid, but hypothyroidism may ensue even during childhood. Affected persons are otherwise normal.

Administration of perchlorate causes a significant discharge of iodide from the thyroid gland, indicating a defect in organification. The biochemical defect is not known. There does not appear to be a deficiency in iodide peroxidase or iodotyrosine synthesis or any defect in binding to apoenzyme. Lifelong treatment with thyroid hormone is indicated to prevent development or progression of the goiter.

INTRATRACHEAL GOITER

One of the many ectopic locations of thyroid tissue is within the trachea. The intraluminal thyroid lies beneath the tracheal mucosa and is frequently continuous with the normally situated extratracheal thyroid. The thyroid tissue is susceptible to goitrous enlargement, which involves the normally situated as well as the ectopic thyroid. When there is obstruction of the airway associated with a goiter, it must be ascertained whether the obstruction is extratracheal or endotracheal. If obstructive manifestations are mild, administration of sodium-L-thyroxine (100–200 μg/24 hr) will usually cause the goiter to decrease in size. When symptoms are severe, surgical removal of the endotracheal goiter is indicated.

19.14 THYROIDITIS

LYMPHOCYTIC THYROIDITIS
(Hashimoto Thyroiditis; Autoimmune Thyroiditis)

Lymphocytic thyroiditis is the most common cause of thyroid disease in children and adolescents and accounts for many of the enlarged thyroids formerly designated "adolescent" or "simple", goiter. It is also the most common cause of juvenile hypothyroidism, with or without goiter. Its incidence may be as high as 1% in schoolchildren.

Etiology. This is a typical organ-specific autoimmune disease. Various abnormalities of suppressor-cytotoxic T-cell ratios have been found, but the basic immunologic defect is unsettled. The condition is characterized histologically by lymphocytic infiltration of the thyroid. Early in the course of the disease there may be only hyperplasia; this is followed by infiltration of lymphocytes and plasma cells between the follicles and by atrophy of the follicles. Lymphoid follicle formation with germinal centers is almost always present; the degree of atrophy and of fibrosis of the follicles varies from mild to moderate.

Clinical Manifestations. The disorder is four to seven times more frequent in girls than in boys. It may occur during the first 3 yr of life but becomes sharply more common after 6 yr of age and reaches a peak incidence during adolescence. The goiter may appear insidiously and vary in size from slight to marked. In the majority of patients the thyroid is diffusely enlarged, firm, and nontender. In about a third of the patients the gland is lobular and may seem to be nodular. Most of the affected children are clinically euthyroid and asymptomatic; some may have symptoms of pressure in the neck. Some children have clinical signs of hypothyroidism, while others who appear clinically euthyroid have laboratory evidence of hypothyroidism. A few children have manifestations suggestive of hyperthyroidism, such as nervousness, irritability, increased sweating, or hyperactivity, but results of laboratory studies are not those of hyperthyroidism. Occasionally, the disorder may coexist with Graves disease. Ophthalmopathy may occur in lymphocytic thyroiditis in the absence of Graves disease.

The clinical course is variable. The goiter may become smaller or disappear spontaneously, or it may persist unchanged for years while the patient remains euthyroid. A significant percentage of patients who are euthyroid initially exhibit hypothyroidism gradually within months or years; thyroiditis is the cause of most instances of nongoitrous juvenile hypothyroidism. Lymphocytic thyroiditis may also occur without symptoms, and in many children persists for many years.

Familial clusters of lymphocytic thyroiditis are common; the incidence in siblings and/or parents of affected children may be as high as 25%. The concurrence within families of cases of lymphocytic thyroiditis, "idiopathic" hypothyroidism, and Graves disease provides cogent evidence for a basic relationship among these three conditions. The disorder has been found associated with many of the other autoimmune disorders more often than expected by chance alone. The association of Addison disease with insulin-dependent diabetes mellitus or autoimmune thyroid disease or both is known as *Schmidt syndrome* or *type II polyglandular autoimmune disease.* Autoimmune thyroid disease also tends to be associated with pernicious anemia, vitiligo, and/or alopecia. Thyroid microsomal antibodies are found in approximately 20% of Caucasian and 4% of black children with diabetes mellitus. Autoimmune thyroid disease has an increased incidence in children with congenital rubella. Lymphocytic thyroiditis is also associated with certain chromosomal aberrations, particularly Turner syndrome and Down syndrome. The pathogenetic mechanisms for these associations is not known.

Since thyroid antibodies cross the placenta, it has been suspected that they may cause fetal thyroid damage and congenital cretinism, but autoimmunity is not a frequent cause of congenital hypothyroidism.

Laboratory Data. The definitive diagnosis can be established by biopsy of the thyroid, but this procedure is rarely indicated for clinical purposes alone. Thyroid function tests are usually normal, though the level of TSH may be slightly or even moderately elevated in some euthyroid individuals. With progressive thyroid failure a decrease in the levels of T_4 is followed by a decrease in levels of T_3 and progressive increases in levels of TSH. The fact that many patients with lymphocytic thyroiditis do not have elevated levels of TSH indicates that the goiter may be caused by the lymphocytic infiltrations and/or thyroid growth-stimulating immunoglobulins. In 50%

of patients thyroid scans reveal irregular and patchy distribution of the radioisotope, and in about 60% or more the administration of perchlorate results in a greater than 10% discharge of iodide from the thyroid gland. The majority of patients with lymphocytic thyroiditis have serum antibody titers to thyroid microsomal antigens, whereas the tanned red blood cell hemagglutination test for thyroid antibodies is positive in fewer than 50%. When both tests are used, approximately 95% of patients with thyroid autoimmunity will be detected. In general, levels in children are lower than those in adults with lymphocytic thyroiditis, and repeated measurements are indicated in questionable instances since titers may increase later in the course of the disease.

Antithyroid antibodies may be found also in almost half the siblings of affected patients and in a significant percentage of the mothers of children with Down syndrome or Turner syndrome without demonstrable thyroid disease. They are also found in 20% of children with diabetes mellitus and in 23% of children with the congenital rubella syndrome.

Treatment. If there is evidence of hypothyroidism, replacement treatment with sodium-L-thyroxine (50–150 μg daily) is indicated. The goiter slowly decreases in size, but antibody levels remain unchanged. Since the disease may be self-limited in some instances, the need for continued therapy requires periodic re-evaluation. Untreated patients should also be periodically checked. Prominent nodules that persist despite suppressive therapy should be examined histologically, as thyroid cancer has occurred in patients with lymphocytic thyroiditis.

OTHER CAUSES OF THYROIDITIS

Specific conditions such as tuberculosis, sarcoidosis, mumps, and cat scratch disease are rare causes of thyroiditis.

Acute suppurative thyroiditis is uncommon; it is usually preceded by a respiratory infection or is secondary to trauma. Abscess formation may occur. Anaerobic organisms, with or without aerobes, are the most common organisms; *Eikenella corrodens* has been reported several times recently. Recurrent episodes and/or the detection of a mixed bacterial flora suggest that the infection arises from a thyroglossal duct remnant. Exquisite tenderness of the gland, swelling, erythema, dysphagia, and limitation of head motion are characteristic findings. Systemic manifestations are often but not invariably absent. Scintigrams of the thyroid often reveal decreased uptake in the affected areas and ultrasonography may show a complex echogenic mass. Thyroid function is usually normal, but thyrotoxicosis due to escape of thyroid hormone has been encountered in a child with suppurative thyroiditis resulting from *Aspergillus.* When suppuration occurs, incision and drainage and administration of antibiotics are indicated.

19.15 HYPERTHYROIDISM

Hyperthyroidism results from excessive secretion of thyroid hormone and, with few exceptions, is due to diffuse toxic goiter (Graves disease) during childhood. Other rare causes of hyperthyroidism which have been observed in children include toxic uninodular goiter (Plummer disease), hyperfunctioning thyroid carcinoma, thyrotoxicosis factitia, and acute suppurative thyroiditis. Hyperthyroidism is common in patients with McCune-Albright syndrome; suppression of plasma TSH indicates that the hyperthyroidism is not hypothalamic in origin. Hyperthyroidism due to excess thyrotropin secretion is rare and in most instances is caused by a TSH-secreting pituitary tumor. One child with thyrotoxicosis and elevated levels of TSH has been reported; since no pituitary tumor was found, disordered hypothalamic-pituitary homeostasis was suggested as the cause. In infants born to mothers with Graves disease hyperthyroidism may occur as a transitory phenomenon or as classic Graves disease during the neonatal period. Choriocarcinoma, hydatidiform mole, and struma ovarii have caused hyperthyroidism in adults but have not as yet been recognized as causes in children.

GRAVES DISEASE

Etiology. There is evidence that immune factors participate in the pathogenesis of Graves disease and may be essential to its initiation. Enlargement of the thymus, splenomegaly, lymphadenopathy, infiltration of the thyroid gland and of retro-ocular tissues with lymphocytes and plasma cells, and peripheral lymphocytosis are common findings in Graves disease.

Patients with this condition produce an immunoglobulin which binds to the receptor for TSH and which, on such binding, stimulates the process which normally is set in motion by TSH. This sequence leads to thyroid autonomy and hyperthyroidism. Graves disease is the only disease known to be caused by an antibody which stimulates endocrine cells. Evidence suggests that the thyroid-stimulating antibodies (TSAb) result from an antigen-specific suppressor cell defect. An association between HLA-DR3 and HLA-B8 is believed to represent linkage between these HLA types and a gene controlling the immune response of thyroid origin.

The ophthalmopathy that occurs in Graves disease does not appear to be caused by TSAb; increasing evidence points to other antibodies specifically affecting retro-orbital tissues.

Other evidence for an autoimmune basis for Graves disease is its coexistence with lymphocytic thyroiditis in the same gland. Like lymphocytic thyroiditis, Graves disease is often associated with other autoimmune disorders such as pernicious anemia, idiopathic adrenal insufficiency, myasthenia gravis, and insulin-dependent diabetes mellitus. Antimicrosomal thyroid autoantibodies and other autoantibodies are frequently found in patients with Graves disease as well as in other members of their families.

Clinical Manifestations. About 5% of all patients with hyperthyroidism are under 15 yr of age; the peak incidence occurs during adolescence. The disease is being increasingly recognized in early infancy apart from the transitory condition which occurs in infants of thyrotoxic mothers (see below); Graves disease has had its onset between 6 wk-2 yr of age in children born to mothers without a history of hyperthyroidism. The incidence is about 5 times higher in girls than in boys.

The clinical course is highly variable but is in general not so fulminant as in many adults. Symptoms develop gradually; the usual interval between onset and diagnosis is 6–12 mo. The earliest signs in children may be emotional disturbances accompanied by motor hyperactivity. They become irritable and excitable and cry easily. Their schoolwork suffers, and their restlessness, which may resemble that of chorea, causes conflicts. Tremor of the fingers can be noticed if the arm is extended. There may be a voracious appetite combined with loss of or no increase in weight. The thyroid is enlarged, palpable, and visible, and bruits may be audible over it. Exophthalmos is noticeable in the majority of patients but is rarely severe. *Graefe sign* (lagging of the upper eyelid as the eye looks downward), *Moebius sign* (impairment of convergence), and *Stellwag sign* (retraction of the upper eyelid and infrequent blinking) may be present. The skin is smooth and flushed, with excessive sweating. Muscular weakness is uncommon but may be so severe as to result in falling spells. Tachycardia, palpitation, dyspnea, and cardiac enlargement and insufficiency cause discomfort and may endanger the patient's life. Atrial fibrillation is a rare complication. Mitral regurgitation, probably resulting from papillary muscle dysfunction, is the cause of the apical systolic murmur present

in some patients. The systolic blood pressure and the pulse pressure are increased. Children with hyperthyroidism are usually tall and their osseous development is advanced for their age.

Thyroid "crisis" or "storm" is a form of hyperthyroidism manifested by an acute onset, hyperthermia, and severe tachycardia and restlessness. There may be rapid progression to delirium, coma, and death. "Apathetic" or "masked" hyperthyroidism is another variety of hyperthyroidism characterized by extreme listlessness, apathy, and cachexia. A combination of both forms may also occur. These symptom complexes are rare in children.

Laboratory Data. Levels of both T_4 and T_3 are usually increased, and TSH is suppressed to unmeasurable levels, even after stimulation with TRH. Radionuclide is rapidly and diffusely concentrated in the enlarged thyroid. In some patients the level of T_4 may be normal and only the level of T_3 elevated, a situation which is termed T_3 *toxicosis.* After treatment of hyperthyroidism the level of T_4 may be low even though the patient is clinically euthyroid. In such patients T_3 levels may be normal. More extensive investigation is rarely necessary if the clinical manifestations are characteristic. For borderline cases evaluation of the response to TRH may be necessary. Elevated levels of thyroid-stimulating immunoglobulin (TSAb) may be found in most patients with newly diagnosed Graves disease; levels appear to correlate with activity of the disorder. Serum levels of thyroglobulin are also increased and remain constant during treatment with antithyroid drugs. A return to normal of thyroglobulin and disappearance of thyroid-stimulating immunoglobulins predict remission of the Graves disease. Antithyroid antibodies are found in most children with Graves disease but are not helpful in predicting remission. Very young children with Graves disease often have advanced skeletal maturation and craniostenosis.

Differential Diagnosis. Diagnosis is rarely difficult once it has been considered. Functional nodules producing hyperthyroidism (Plummer disease) tend to secrete T_3 preferentially and can be detected on radionuclide scanning. Patients with lymphocytic thyroiditis may, on occasion, present manifestations of hyperthyroidism and must be differentiated by appropriate laboratory studies. The clinical pattern of pheochromocytoma may resemble hyperthyroidism, but the elevation of blood pressure is greater, the level of thyroid hormones is within the normal range, and that of catecholamines is elevated. Patients with thyroid hormone unresponsiveness have a goiter and elevated levels of T_4 and T_3 but levels of TSH are normal or elevated, and response to stimulation with TRH is normal. Many patients with this disorder have been erroneously treated for hyperthyroidism.

Treatment. There is no consensus as to the preferred method of treatment. Some prefer subtotal thyroidectomy; others, including ourselves, elect a trial of medical therapy before considering surgery. Most pediatric endocrinologists and radiotherapists avoid the use of radioactive iodine to treat children except for the unusual patient in whom medical treatment is not feasible and operation is contraindicated or refused.

The recommended antithyroid drugs are propylthiouracil and methimazole (Tapazole). These compounds inhibit incorporation of trapped inorganic iodide into organic compounds and propylthiouracil inhibits extrathyroidal conversion of T_4 to T_3. Recent evidence suggests that they may also inhibit synthesis of thyroid autoantibodies and directly affect intrathyroidal autoimmunity. Toxic reactions occur with about equal frequency with both drugs (1–5%). The initial dose of propylthiouracil is 100–150 mg, three times daily, and that of methimazole is 10–15 mg, three times daily. Subsequently, the dose is increased or decreased as indicated. Smaller initial doses should be used in early childhood. Overdosage can lead to a hypothyroid state. Clinical response becomes apparent in 2–3 wk, and adequate control in 1–3 mo. The dose of the medication is then reduced to the minimal level that will maintain the child in a euthyroid state. Careful surveillance is required. Serum levels of T_4 and T_3 should be maintained in the normal range. Rising of serum levels of TSH above 6 µU/mL indicates overtreatment, which will lead to increased size of the goiter.

Drug therapy may be continued for 6 yr or longer since there appears to be a remission rate of about 25% every 2 yr. If a relapse occurs, it will usually appear within 3 mo and almost always within 6 mo after therapy has been discontinued. Therapy may be resumed in case of a relapse. Patients over 13 yr of age, boys, and those with small goiters and modestly elevated T_3 levels appear to have earlier remissions.

The most common toxic reactions are urticarial rashes, leukopenia, fever, arthritis, or arthralgia. Transient leukopenia (total white cell count below 4000/mm³) occurs in 25% of patients; it is asymptomatic, is not a harbinger of agranulocytosis and is usually not a reason to discontinue treatment. More serious reactions such as agranulocytosis, hepatitis, or a lupus-like syndrome are uncommon. These reactions have been noted with both propylthiouracil and methimazole with about the same incidence, but changing from one drug to the other may avert the undesirable effect. A cutaneous vasculitis consisting of intermittent purpuric lesions has been reported in a few children treated with propylthiouracil. It is probably best to treat unusually hypersensitive patients by thyroidectomy.

A beta-adrenergic blocking agent such as propranolol is a useful supplement in management of severely toxic patients. Thyroid hormones potentiate the actions of catecholamines, which include tachycardia, tremor, excessive sweating, lid lag, and stare. These symptoms abate with use of propranolol, which does not, however, alter thyroid function or exophthalmos.

Operation is indicated when adequate cooperation for medical management is not possible or when adequate trial of medical management has failed to result in permanent remission. Subtotal thyroidectomy, a rather safe procedure, is performed only after the patient has been brought to a euthyroid state. This may be accomplished with propylthiouracil or methimazole over 2–3 mo. After a euthyroid state has been attained, 5 drops of a saturated solution of potassium iodide/day are added to the regimen for 2 wk before operation in order to decrease the vascularity of the gland. Complications of surgical treatment are rare and include hypoparathyroidism (transient or permanent) and paralysis of the vocal cords. The incidence of residual or recurrent hyperthyroidism or of hypothyroidism depends upon the extent of the surgery. With extensive thyroidectomy the incidence of recurrence may be low, but that of hypothyroidism may exceed 50%.

The ophthalmopathy remits gradually and usually independently of the hyperthyroidism.

CONGENITAL HYPERTHYROIDISM

When hyperthyroidism has its onset in the newborn period, the condition is usually transitory, remitting within 3 mo. Infants with transient hyperthyroidism have thyroid-stimulating antibody (TSAb) in their circulation, and their mothers have active Graves disease, a history of Graves disease, or, on rare occasions, Hashimoto thyroiditis. The condition is caused by transplacental passage of TSAb; remission of the condition parallels the disappearance of TSAb in the infant. High levels of TSAb in the mother during pregnancy is a good predictor of neonatal thyrotoxicosis. Unlike Graves disease at every other age, the transitory variety affects males as often as females. Occasionally, the condition does not remit but persists for several years or longer. These patients appear

to have typical Graves disease and frequently have impressive family histories of Graves disease. In some infants TSAb transfer from the mother appears to blend with infantile onset of autonomous Graves disease.

The clinical onset is at birth, but if TSH-inhibiting antibodies are also present, symptoms may be delayed several wk. Many of the infants are premature; the majority, but not all, have goiters. The infant is extremely restless, irritable, and hyperactive and appears anxious and unusually alert. The eyes are widely opened and appear exophthalmic. There may be extreme tachycardia and tachypnea, and the temperature is elevated. In severely affected infants there is progression of symptoms; weight loss occurs despite a ravenous appetite, hepatomegaly increases, and jaundice may become manifest. Cardiac decompensation is common, and severe hypertension may occur. The condition usually resolves in 6–12 wk, but the infant may die if therapy is not instituted promptly. The serum level of T_4 is markedly elevated. Advanced bone age, frontal bossing, and cranial synostosis are common, especially in those infants with persistent clinical manifestations of hyperthyroidism. Prognosis for intellectual development is guarded for infants with craniostenosis.

Treatment consists of administration of Lugol solution (1 drop every 8 hr) and propylthiouracil (10 mg every 8 hr). If the thyrotoxic state is severe, parenteral fluid therapy, digitalization, and propranolol (2 mg/kg/24 hr given in three divided doses) may be indicated. When propranolol is used during pregnancy to treat thyrotoxicosis, it crosses the placenta and may cause respiratory depression in the newborn infant. Methimazole passes more readily than propylthiouracil into breast milk. Furthermore, scalp defects (aplasia cutis congenita) have occurred in 17 infants whose mothers were treated during pregnancy with methimazole; this drug should be avoided during pregnancy and breast feeding.

19.16 CARCINOMA OF THE THYROID

Carcinoma of the thyroid is rare in children; only 37 new cases per million people are found annually and about 7% of these occur under 18 yr of age. Unlike other malignancies in childhood, thyroid cancer usually has a very indolent course even after pulmonary metastases have developed. Radiation is known to be an important inducer of thyroid cancer. About 80% of 227 patients were found to have had irradiation to the neck and adjacent areas during infancy for such benign conditions as "enlarged" thymus, hypertrophied tonsils and adenoids, hemangiomas, nevi, acne, eczema, tinea capitis, and "cervical adenitis." Irradiation for thymic enlargement in infancy has been found to carry a 4% risk of thyroid carcinoma and an approximately 30% risk of thyroid nodularity. A study of 735 adults with a history of radiation therapy to the head and neck for benign conditions during childhood found 159 to have palpable nodules. Of 49 patients operated upon because of growth of the nodule despite suppression therapy with thyroxine, 11 were found to have carcinoma. The interval between irradiation and discovery of a tumor has been as long as 40 yr. Exposure to radioactive fallout containing isotopes of iodine (especially ¹³¹I) appears to be a greater risk factor in the child than in the adult.

Girls are affected twice as often as boys. The average age at diagnosis is 9 yr, but the onset may be as early as the 1st yr of life. A painless nodule in the thyroid or in the neck is the usual 1st evidence of disease. Cervical lymph node involvement is usually present at the time of the initial diagnosis and is often bilateral. Any unexplained cervical lymph node enlargement requires examination of the thyroid, which will occasionally have a primary tumor too small to be felt, the diagnosis being made on biopsy of the lymph node. The lungs are the most common site of metastases beyond the neck. There may be no clinical manifestations referable to them; roentgenographically, they appear as diffuse miliary or nodular infiltrations, principally in the basal portions. They may be mistaken for tuberculosis, histoplasmosis, or sarcoidosis. Other sites of metastases include the mediastinum, long bones, skull, and axilla. On rare occasions the carcinoma may be functional and produce symptoms of hyperthyroidism.

Histologically, the carcinomas are usually papillary, follicular, or mixed differentiated tumors. The neoplasm frequently grows slowly and may even remain dormant for years. Undifferentiated neoplasms, however, may have a rapidly fatal course.

A thyroid scan should be performed whenever a thyroid nodule is found. [123]Iodine or ^{99m}Tc pertechnetate is the preferred scanning agent. Most malignant lesions show decreased concentration of radioisotope (are "cold"), but some cold lesions are benign. Serum levels of thyroglobulin (Tg) are often elevated and return to normal after surgical removal of differentiated tumors; this test also permits early detection of metastases. The thyroglobulin levels do not correlate with any histologic characteristics or with malignancy or benignity of thyroid tumors.

Because differentiated thyroid carcinoma is a chronic disease with long survival, optimal therapy is still evolving. There is increasing evidence that papillary carcinoma, the least aggressive type, is effectively treated by subtotal thyroidectomy and suppressive doses of thyroid hormone. Total thyroidectomy and treatment with ^{131}I do not appear to improve prognosis. Many patients with cervical or pulmonary metastases have survived for many years. Pure follicular and mixed papillary and follicular cancers are more aggressive; affected patients may require total thyroidectomy and neck dissection. For any form of therapy, survival or recurrence does not appear different for patients with or without involvement of cervical nodes. Even patients with cervical or pulmonary metastases have survived for many years. The 10-yr cure rate is 80–90%.

Thyroid cancer from irradiation to the head and neck for benign conditions has virtually vanished in children, but it is being increasingly reported as a second neoplasm in children treated for other malignancies. Children who have received irradiation and chemotherapy for leukemia, lymphoma, Hodgkin disease, Wilms and other tumors have developed thyroid cancer or adenomas. Since in some patients the irradiation was not directly to the neck, it is thought that an increased propensity to develop tumors with multimodal therapy is an additional etiologic factor in these patients.

After surgery all patients should be treated with sodium-L-thyroxine in doses sufficient to suppress TSH. Periodic determinations of serum levels of Tg provide an excellent marker for recurrence in patients taking T_4 and are supplanting routine radionuclide scans.

SOLITARY THYROID NODULE

Solitary nodules of the thyroid are uncommon in children. In the past it was estimated that as many as half were carcinoma, but more recent studies indicate about a 15% incidence of malignancy, perhaps because of decreasing exposure of children to irradiation. Children exposed to irradiation have a high incidence of benign adenoma as well as of carcinoma of the thyroid.

Benign disorders which may present as solitary thyroid nodules include benign adenomas (follicular, embryonal, Hurthle cell), lymphocytic thyroiditis, thyroglossal duct cyst, ectopically located normal thyroid tissue, a single median thyroid, agenesis of one of the lateral thyroid lobes with hypertrophy of the contralateral lobe, thyroid cysts, and abscess. Sudden appearance of or rapidly enlarging thyroid

mass may indicate hemorrhage into a benign adenoma. In most instances the child is euthyroid and thyroid function studies are normal. A ^{99m}Tc scan is usually indicated. Ultrasonography is particularly useful in detecting cystic lesions. When lymphocytic thyroiditis is the cause of the nodule, T_4 may be low, TSH may be elevated, and thyroid antibodies are usually present. The scan may reveal a motheaten appearance. Rarely, lymphocytic thyroiditis may be associated with carcinoma of the thyroid.

Some nodules are "cold" on ^{99m}Tc scan, as is the case for carcinoma, but other lesions, such as developmental defects of the thyroid, are usually "hot." In questionable cases one may use suppressive therapy with 0.2–0.3 mg daily of sodium-L-thyroxine. Cold nodules that continue to grow over 4–6 mo or that do not reduce in size by 50% in 1 yr should be surgically explored. Surgery without delay is indicated when the nodule is hard or has grown rapidly, when there is evidence of tracheal or vocal cord involvement, or when there is enlargement of adjacent lymph nodes. All persons with a history of head or neck irradiation should have careful examination of the thyroid at least every 2 yr, indefinitely.

Very rarely, thyroid nodules may be functional, producing hyperthyroidism (Plummer disease). The uptake of radionuclide is concentrated in the nodule ("hot" nodule), and thyroid function studies indicate that the nodule is functioning autonomously. Such nodules are almost always benign. They may secrete T_3 preferentially; hence, T_4 levels may be normal, whereas T_3 levels are elevated (T_3 toxicosis).

A suppressible functioning nodule in a euthyroid child has been reported only once.

MEDULLARY CARCINOMA

This carcinoma of the thyroid arises from the parafollicular cells (C cells) of the thyroid and accounts for about 10% of thyroid malignancies. The tumor is pleomorphic, with sheets of spindle or small cells with eosinophilic granular cytoplasm. Amyloid is invariably deposited in the stroma, and calcification is common. The most common symptom is goiter or a palpable thyroid nodule. In about a third of patients roentgenograms reveal dense, conglomerate, homogeneous calcification in the thyroid. Metastases to regional lymph nodes and to liver are common, and these too may calcify. Death may result, but long survivals are not uncommon.

These tumors arise from the cells which secrete calcitonin; accordingly, circulating levels of calcitonin are consistently elevated. There are no clinically recognizable manifestations of elevated calcitonin levels. These tumors elaborate other specific biochemical markers, particularly histaminase and dopa decarboxylase. In addition, elevated levels of prostaglandins, serotonin, ACTH, and β-endorphin have been detected in tumors and in serum of some patients and have accounted for diarrhea or for Cushing syndrome, both of which are occasionally associated.

When the tumor occurs sporadically, it is usually unicentric in origin and presents a palpable thyroid nodule. But diagnosis of medullary thyroid carcinoma should always lead one to search for associated tumors, pheochromocytoma in particular, and for other affected family members. The tumor is often hereditary, as a component of two distinct autosomal dominant syndromes (see below). In affected families, the tumor is multicentric and often begins as hyperplasia of C cells; all persons at risk require careful investigation. Patients with C-cell hyperplasia or tumors too small to be found by palpation, scintigraphy, or ultrasonography may also have normal basal serum levels of calcitonin; calcitonin-stimulation tests using infusions of calcium or pentagastrin or both are required to detect these occult tumors.

Multiple Endocrine Neoplasia, Type II. In some families medullary carcinoma of the thyroid is associated with pheochromocytoma and parathyroid hyperplasia. This association is also known as Sipple syndrome or multiple endocrine adenomatosis (MEA). Penetrance for the various components of the syndrome is high. When pheochromocytomas are found, they are frequently bilateral and may be multiple. The parathyroid glands may reveal chief-cell hyperplasia or only hypercellularity. Hypercalcemia may be present. The hyperparathyroidism is probably the result of the same genetic defect responsible for the thyroid carcinoma and for the pheochromocytoma; it does not seem to be secondary to the elevated calcitonin level since elevated levels of parathormone have been found in patients with normal levels of calcitonin. A primary defect of the neural crest can account for all the findings in the syndrome.

The distinguishing feature of the entity known as MEN type IIb, MEN-III, or *mucosal neuroma syndrome* is the occurrence of multiple neuromas in addition to medullary carcinoma of the thyroid and pheochromocytoma. The neuromas most often occur on the tongue, buccal mucosa, lips, and conjunctivae. Peripheral neurofibromas and café-au-lait patches may be present, and intestinal ganglioneuromatosis is common. Diffuse ganglioneuromatosis of the submucosal and myenteric plexuses may involve the esophagus as well as the small and large intestines. The patients may be tall, with arachnodactyly and a Marfan-like appearance. Scoliosis, pectus excavatum, pes cavus, and muscular hypotonia are common. The eyelids may be thickened, the lips patulous, the jaw prognathic. Feeding difficulties, poor sucking, diarrhea, constipation, and failure to thrive may begin in infancy or early childhood many years before the appearance of neuromas or endocrine symptoms.

Treatment. Total thyroidectomy is indicated for all children with medullary carcinoma of the thyroid, even for those in whom C-cell hyperplasia is demonstrable only by calcitonin stimulation tests. Recognition of familial forms of this tumor is critical to early diagnosis in patients at risk. Evidence suggests that for MEN-III thyroidectomy must be done very early, as some children already have metastatic disease by 4 yr of age. Monitoring the levels of calcitonin is useful in detecting metastatic lesions and for following the course of the disease after operation.

General

Kaplan SA: Clinical Pediatric and Adolescent Endocrinology. Philadelphia, WB Saunders, 1982.
Wilson JD, Foster DW (eds): Williams Textbook of Endocrinology. 7th ed. Philadelphia, WB Saunders, 1985.

Hypothyroidism

Bachrach LK, Daneman D, Daneman A, et al: Use of ultrasound in childhood thyroid disorders. J Pediatr 103:547, 1983.
Brown RS, Kertiles LP, Rosenfield C, et al: Thyrotropin-receptor autoantibodies in children and young adults with Graves disease. Am J Dis Child 140:238, 1986.
Burrow GN, Dussault JH (eds): Neonatal Thyroid Screening. New York, Raven Press, 1980.
Burt L, Kulin HE: Head circumference in children with short stature secondary to primary hypothyroidism. Pediatrics 59:628, 1977.
Codaocioni JL, Cargyon P, Miche-Bechet M, et al: Congenital hypothyroidism associated with thyrotropin unresponsiveness and thyroid cell membrane alterations. J Clin Endocrinol Metab 50:932, 1980.
Connors MA, Styne DM: Transient neonatal "athyreosis" resulting from thyrotropin-binding inhibiting immunoglobulins. Pediatrics 78:287, 1986.
Cutler AT, Benezra-Obeiter R, Brink SJ: Thyroid function in young children with Down syndrome. Am J Dis Child 140:479, 1986.
Czernichow P, Schlumberger M, Pomarede R, et al: Plasma thyroglobulin measurements help determine the type of thyroid defect in congenital hypothyroidism. J Clin Endocrinol Metab 56:242, 1983.
Dussault JH, Letarte J, Guyda H, et al: Thyroid function in neonatal hypothyroidism. J Pediatr 89:541, 1976.
Dussault JH, Letarte J, Guyda H, et al: Serum thyroid hormone and TSH concentrations in newborn infants with congenital absence of thyroxine-binding globulin. J Pediatr 90:264, 1977.
Dussault JH, Letarte J, Guyda H, et al: Lack of influence of thyroid antibodies on thyroid function in the newborn infant and on a mass screening program for congenital hypothyroidism. J Pediatr 96:385, 1980.

Fisher DA, Klein AH: Thyroid development and disorders of thyroid function in the newborn. N Engl J Med 304:702, 1981.
Franklin R, O'Grady C, Carpenter L: Neonatal thyroid function: Comparison between breast fed and bottle fed infants. J Pediatr 106:124, 1985.
Glorieux J, Dussault JH, Murisette J, et al: Follow-up at ages 5 and 7 on mental development in children with hypothyroidism detected by Quebec Screening Program. J Pediatr 107:913, 1985.
Greig WR, Hendersen AS, Boyle JA, et al: Thyroid dysgenesis in two pairs of monozygotic twins and a mother and child. J Clin Endocrinol Metab 26:1309, 1966.
Gushurst CA, Muehler JA, Green JA, et al: Breast milk iodide: Reassessment in the 1980's. Pediatrics 73:354, 1984.
Heyman S, Crigler JF Jr, Treves S: Congenital hypothyroidism: [123]I thyroidal uptake and scintigraphy. J Pediatr 101:571, 1982.
Kaplan MM, Swartz SL, Larsen PR: Partial peripheral resistance to thyroid hormone. Am J Med 70:1115, 1981.
Levine MA, Jap TS, Hung W: Infantile hypothyroidism in two sibs: An unusual presentation of pseudohypoparathyroidism type Ia. J Pediatr 107:919, 1985.
Martino E, Safran M, Aghini-Lombardi F, et al: Environmental iodine intake and thyroid dysfunction during chronic amiodarone therapy. Ann Intern Med 101:28, 1984.
Menezes-Fereira MM, Eil C, Wortsman J, et al: Decreased nuclear uptake of (^{123}I)triiodo-L-thyronine in fibroblasts from patients with peripheral thyroid hormone resistance. J Clin Endocrinol Metab 59:1081, 1984.
Miyai K, Azukizawa M, Komahara Y: Familial isolated thyrotropin deficiency with cretinism. N Engl J Med 285:1043, 1971.
Moncrief MW, McArthur RG: Hypothyroidism in one of monozygotic twins. Postgrad Med J 44:423, 1968.
Najjar SS: Muscular hypertrophy in hypothyroid children. The Kocher-Debré-Sémélaigne syndrome. J Pediatr 85:236, 1974.
New England Congenital Hypothyroidism Collaborative: Neonatal hypothyroidism screening: Status of patients at 6 years of age. J Pediatr 107:915, 1985.
Refetoff S, DeGroot LJ, Barsano CP: Defective thyroid hormone feedback regulation in the syndrome of peripheral resistance to thyroid hormone. J Clin Endocrinol Metab 51:41, 1980.
Rezvani I, DiGeorge AM: Reassessment of the daily dose of oral thyroxine for replacement therapy in hypothyroid children. J Pediatr 90:291, 1977.
Rezvani I, DiGeorge AM, Cote ML: Primary hypothyroidism in cystinosis. J Pediatr 91:340, 1977.
Sklar CA, Qazi R, David R: Juvenile autoimmune thyroiditis. Hormonal status at presentation and after long-term follow-up. Am J Dis Child 140:877, 1986.
Smith DW, Klein AM, Henderson JR, et al: Congenital hypothyroidism—signs and symptoms in the newborn period. J Pediatr 87:958, 1975.
Smith DW, Popich G: Large fontanels in congenital hypothyroidism: A potential clue toward earlier recognition. J Pediatr 80:753, 1972.
Staffer SS, Hamburger JI: Inadvertent ^{131}I therapy for hypothyroidism in the first trimester of pregnancy. J Nucl Med 17:146, 1976.
van der Gaag RD, Drexhage HA, Dussault JH: Role of maternal immunoglobulin blocking TSH-induced thyroid growth in sporadic forms of congenital hypothyroidism. Lancet 1:246, 1985.
VanDop C, Conte FA, Koch TK, et al: Pseudotumor cerebri associated with initiation of levothyroxine therapy for juvenile hypothyroidism. N Engl J Med 308:1076, 1983.
VanHerle AJ, Vassart G, Dumont JE: Control of thyroglobulin synthesis and secretion. N Engl J Med 301:239, 307, 1979.

Goitrous Cretinism

Burrow GN, Spaulding SW, Alexander NM, et al: Normal peroxidase activity in Pendred's syndrome. J Clin Endocrinol Metab 36:522, 1973.
Couch RM, Dean HJ, Winter JSD: Congenital hypothyroidism caused by defective iodide transport. J Pediatr 106:950, 1985.
Gattereau A, Bernard B, Bellabarba D, et al: Congenital goiter in four euthyroid siblings with glandular and circulating iodoproteins and defective iodothyronine synthesis. J Clin Endocrinol Metab 37:118, 1973.
Goslings BM, et al: Hypothyroidism in an area of endemic goiter and cretinism in central Java, Indonesia. J Clin Endocrinol Metab 44:481, 1977.
Illum P, Kiaer HW, Hvidberg-Hansen J, et al: Fifteen cases of Pendred's syndrome. Congenital deafness and sporadic goiter. Arch Otolaryngol 96:297, 1972.
Lissitzky S, et al: Congenital goiter with impaired thyroglobulin synthesis. J Clin Endocrinol Metab 36:17, 1973.
Riesco G, Bernal J, Sanchez-Franco F: Thyroglobulin defect in a human congenital goiter. J Clin Endocrinol Metab 38:33, 1974.
Savoie JC, Massin JP, Savoie F: Studies of mono- and diiodohistidine. II. Congenital goitrous hypothyroidism with thyroglobulin defect and iodohistidine-rich iodoalbumin production. J Clin Invest 52:116, 1973.
Silva JE, Santelices R, Kishihara M, Schneider A: Low molecular weight thyroglobulin leading to a goiter in a 12-year-old girl. J Clin Endocrinol Metab 58:526, 1984.
Stanbury JB: Familial goiter. In: Stanbury JB, Wyngaarden JB, Fredrickson DS, et al (eds): The Metabolic Basis of Inherited Disease. 5th ed. New York, McGraw-Hill, 1983.
Valenta LJ, Bode H, Vickery AL, et al: Lack of thyroid peroxidase activity as a cause of congenital goitrous hypothyroidism. J Clin Endocrinol Metab 36:830, 1972.

Goiter

Daneman D, Davy T, Mancer K, et al: Association of multinodular goiter, cystic renal disease, and digital anomalies. J Pediatr 107:270, 1985.

Delange F, Ermans AM, Vis HL, et al: Endemic cretinism in Idjwi Island (Kivu Lake, Republic of the Congo). J Clin Endocrinol Metab 34:1059, 1972.

Galina MP, Avnet NL, Fanhorn A: Iodides during pregnancy. An apparent cause of neonatal death. N Engl J Med 267:1124, 1962.

Martin MM, Renato RD: Iodide goiter with hypothyroidism in two newborn infants. J Pediatr 61:94, 1962.

Patel YC, Pharoah POD, Hornabrook RW, et al: Serum triiodothyronine, thyroxine and thyroid-stimulating hormone in endemic goiter: A comparison of goitrous and non-goitrous subjects in New Guinea. J Clin Endocrinol Metab 7:783, 1973.

Pharoah POD, Buttfield IH, Hetzel BS: Neurological damage to the foetus resulting from severe iodine deficiency during pregnancy. Lancet 1:308, 1971.

Ramalingaswami V: Endemic goiter in Southeast Asia. New clothes on an old body. Ann Intern Med 78:277, 1973.

Randolph J, Grunt JA, Vawter GF: The medical and surgical aspects of intratracheal goiter. N Engl J Med 268:457, 1963.

Vichyanond P, Howard CP, Olson LC: *Eikenella corrodens* as a cause of thyroid abscess. Am J Dis Child 137:971, 1983.

Hyperthyroidism

Cheron RG, Kaplan MM, Larsen PR, et al: Neonatal thyroid function after propylthiouracil therapy for maternal Graves' disease. N Engl J Med 304:525, 1981.

Collen RJ, Landaw EM, Kaplan SA, et al: Remission rates of children and adolescents with thyrotoxicosis treated with antithyroid drugs. Pediatrics 65:550, 1980.

Cooper DS: Antithyroid drugs. N Engl J Med 311:1353, 1984.

Daneman D, Howard NJ: Neonatal thyrotoxicosis: Intellectual impairment and craniosynostosis in later years. J Pediatr 97:257, 1980.

Darby CP: Three episodes of spontaneous thyroid storm occurring in a nine year-old child. Pediatrics 30:927, 1962.

Hayles AB: Problems of childhood Graves' disease. Mayo Clin Proc 47:850, 1972.

Hollingsworth DR, Mabry CC: Congenital Graves disease. Am J Dis Child 130:148, 1976.

Hulazun JF, Anst CS, Lukens JN: Thyrotoxicosis associated with Aspergillus thyroiditis in chronic granulomatosis disease. J Pediatr 80:106, 1972.

Kogut MD, Kaplan SA, Collipp PJ, et al: Treatment of hyperthyroidism in children. N Engl J Med 272:217, 1965.

Lightner ES, Allen HD, Laughlin G: Neonatal hyperthyroidism and heart failure. Am J Dis Child 131:68, 1977.

McGregor AM, Peterson MM, McLachlan SM, et al: Carbimazole and the autoimmune response in Graves' disease. N Engl J Med 303:302, 1980.

Mihailovic V, Feller MS, Kourides IA, Utiger RD: Hyperthyroidism due to excess thyrotropin secretion: Follow-up studies. J Clin Endocrinol Metab 50:1135, 1980.

Milham S Jr: Scalp defects in infants of mothers treated for hyperthyroidism with methimazole or carbimazole during pregnancy. Teratology 32:321, 1985.

Perry LW, Hung W: Atrial fibrillation and hyperthyroidism in a 14-year-old boy. J Pediatr 79:668, 1971.

Pompa BH, Cloutier MD, Hayles AB: Thyroid nodule producing T_3 toxicosis in a child. Mayo Clin Proc 48:273, 1973.

Riggs W Jr, Wilroy RS Jr, Etteldorf JN: Neonatal hyperthyroidism with accelerated skeletal maturation, craniosynostosis, and brachydactyly. Radiology 105:621, 1972.

Samuel S, Gilman S, Maurer HS, et al: Hyperthyroidism in an infant with McCune-Albright syndrome: Report of a case with myeloid dysplasia. J Pediatr 80:275, 1972.

Smith CS, Howard NJ: Propranolol in treatment of neonatal thyrotoxicosis. J Pediatr 83:1046, 1973.

Stenszky V, Kozma L, Balazs C, et al: The genetics of Graves disease: HLA and disease susceptibility. J Clin Endocrinol Metab 61:835, 1985.

Viscardi RM, Shea M, Sriwantanakul K, et al: Hyperthyroxinemia in newborns due to excess thyroxine-binding globulin. N Engl J Med 309:897, 1983.

Volpe R, Ehrlich R, Steiner G, et al: Graves' disease in pregnancy years after hypothyroidism with recurrent passive-transfer neonatal Graves' disease in offspring. Therapeutic considerations. Am J Med 77:572, 1984.

Wilroy RS Jr, Etteldorf JN: Familial hypothyroidism including two siblings with neonatal Graves' disease. J Pediatr 78:625, 1971.

Zakarija M, McKenzie JM: Pregnancy-associated changes in the thyroid-stimulating antibody of Graves' disease and the relationship to neonatal hyperthyroidism. J Clin Endocrinol Metab 57:1036, 1983.

Zakarija M, McKenzie JM, Banovic K: Clinical significance of assay of thyroid-stimulating antibody in Graves' disease. Ann Intern Med 93:28, 1980.

Lymphocytic Thyroiditis

Doniach D, Nilsson LR, Roitt IM: Autoimmune thyroiditis in children and adolescents. Acta Pediatr 54:260, 1965.

Greenberg AH, Czernichow P, Hung W, et al: Juvenile chronic lymphocytic thyroiditis: Clinical, laboratory and histologic correlations. J Clin Endocrinol Metab 30:293, 1970.

Goldsmith RE, McAdams AJ, Larsen PR, et al: Familial autoimmune thyroiditis: Maternal-fetal relationship and the role of generalized autoimmunity. J Clin Endocrinol Metab 37:265, 1973.

Hung W, Chandra R, August GP, et al: Clinical, laboratory and histologic observations in euthyroid children and adolescents with goiters. J Pediatr 82:10, 1973.

Lebeouf G, Bongiovanni AM: Thyroiditis in childhood. Adv Pediatr 13:183, 1964.

Loeb PB, Drash AL, Kenny FM: Prevalence of low titer and "negative" antithyroglobulin antibodies in biopsy-proven juvenile Hashimoto's thyroiditis. J Pediatr 82:17, 1973.

Monteleone JA, Danis RK, Tung KSK, et al: Differentiation of chronic lymphocytic thyroiditis and simple goiter in pediatrics. J Pediatr 83:381, 1973.

Rallison ML, Dobyns BM, Keating FR, et al: Occurrence and natural history of chronic lymphocytic thyroiditis in childhood. J Pediatr 86:675, 1975.

Riley WJ, Maclaren NK, Lezotte DC, et al: Thyroid autoimmunity in insulin-dependent diabetes mellitus. The case for routine screening. J Pediatr 98:350, 1981.

Carcinoma of the Thyroid

Ashcroft NW, Van Herle AJ: The comparative value of serum thyroglobulin measurements and iodine I^{131} total body scans in the follow-up of patients treated with differentiated thyroid cancer. Am J Med 71:806, 1981.

Black EG, Cassoni A, Gimlette TMD, et al: Serum thyroglobulin in thyroid cancer. Lancet 2:443, 1981.

Carney JA, Go VLW, Sizemore GW, et al: Alimentary tract ganglioneuromatosis. A major component of the syndrome of multiple endocrine neoplasia, type 2b. N Engl J Med 295:1287, 1976.

Crile Y Jr, Antunez AR, Esselstyn CB, et al: The advantages of subtotal thyroidectomy and suppression of TSH in the primary treatment of papillary carcinoma of the thyroid. Cancer 55:2691, 1985.

Fisher DA: Thyroid nodules in children and their management. J Pediatr 89:866, 1976.

Forsman PJ, Jenkins ME: Medullary carcinoma of the thyroid with Marfan-like body habitus. Pediatrics 52:188, 1973.

Gutjahr P, Spranger J: Thyroidectomy in Type IIb multiple-endocrine-neoplasia syndrome. Lancet 1:1149, 1977.

Hempelmann LH, Hall WJ, Phillips M, et al: Neoplasms in persons treated with x-rays in infancy: Fourth survey in 20 years. J Natl Cancer Inst 55:519, 1975.

Jones BA, Sisson JC: Early diagnosis and thyroidectomy in multiple endocrine neoplasia, type 2b. J Pediatr 102:219, 1983.

Keiser HR, Beaven MA, Doppham J, et al: Sipple's syndrome: Medullary thyroid carcinoma, pheochromocytoma and parathyroid disease. Ann Intern Med 78:561, 1973.

Kirkland RT, Kirkland JL, Rosenberg HS, et al: Solitary thyroid nodules in 30 children and report of a child with a thyroid abscess. Pediatrics 51:85, 1973.

Levin DL, Perlia C, Tashjian AH: Medullary carcinoma of the thyroid gland: The complete syndrome in a child. Pediatrics 52:192, 1973.

Pilch BZ, Kahn R, Ketcham AS, et al: Thyroid cancer after radioactive iodine diagnostic procedures in childhood. Pediatrics 51:898, 1973.

Razack MS, Sako K, Shimaoka K, et al: Radiation-associated thyroid carcinoma. J Surg Oncol 14:287, 1980.

Refetoff S, Harrison J, Karanifilski BT, et al: Continuing occurrence of thyroid carcinoma after irradiation to the neck in infancy and childhood. N Engl J Med 292:171, 1975.

Rojeski MT, Gharib H: Nodular thyroid disease. Evaluation and management. N Engl J Med 313:428, 1985.

Sazmaan NA, Maheshwari YK, Nader S, et al: Impact of therapy for differentiated carcinoma of the thyroid: An analysis of 706 cases. J Clin Endocrinol Metab 56:1131, 1983.

Scott MD, Crawford JD: Solitary thyroid nodules in childhood: Is the incidence of thyroid carcinoma declining? Pediatrics 58:521, 1976.

Stjernholm MR, Freudenborrg JC, Mooney HS, et al: Medullary carcinoma of the thyroid before age 2 years. J Clin Endocrinol Metab 51:252, 1980.

Sussman L, Librik L, Clayton GW: Hyperthyroidism attributable to a hyperfunctioning thyroid carcinoma. J Pediatr 72:208, 1968.

Vane D, King DR, Boles ET Jr: Secondary thyroid neoplasma in pediatric cancer patients: Increased risk with improved survival. J Pediatr Surg 19:855, 1984.

19.17 DISORDERS OF THE PARATHYROID GLANDS

Parathyroid hormone (PTH), vitamin D, and calcitonin are the principal regulators of calcium homeostasis.

Parathyroid Hormone. PTH is an 84 amino acid chain (9500 dalton), but its biologic activity resides in the first 34 residues. In the parathyroid gland a proparathyroid hormone (90 amino acid chain) and a pre-pro-PTH (115 amino acid chain) are synthesized. Pre-pro-PTH is converted to pro-PTH in the endoplasmic reticulum and pro-PTH to PTH in the Golgi apparatus. PTH (1–84) is the major secretory product of the gland, but it is rapidly cleaved, probably in the liver and kidney, into smaller COOH-terminal and NH$_2$-terminal fragments. The 1–34 amino-terminal fragment possesses biologic activity but is poorly immunoreactive. Discrepancies in the results of radioimmunoassays (iPTH) are due in part to the fact that various assays for PTH have differing specificities for species of PTH in serum or plasma which vary in immunologic activities. It is now generally agreed that carboxy-terminal fragments represent 80% of circulating iPTH. Although these fragments are biologically inactive, there is a good correlation of their quantity with hyperparathyroidism.

When serum levels of calcium fall, secretion of PTH increases, and PTH mobilizes calcium by direct enhancement of bone resorption; this effect requires normal levels of 1,25-dihydroxycholecalciferol (1,25-[OH]$_2$-D$_3$). PTH also decreases renal excretion of calcium, but this effect plays a relatively minor role in restoration of normocalcemia. The effects of PTH on bone and kidney are mediated through binding to specific receptors on the membranes of target cells and subsequent activation of the adenylate cyclase system. Cyclic AMP, in turn, binds to specific intracellular receptor proteins which mediate the hormone effect. The most important action of PTH is to increase absorption of calcium from the intestine. This effect is achieved indirectly by activation of 1a-hydroxylase activity, with ensuing increase in the synthesis of 1,25-(OH)$_2$-D$_3$; 1,25-(OH)$_2$-D$_3$ induces synthesis of calcium-binding protein in the intestinal mucosa, with resultant increased absorption of calcium.

Vitamin D. (See Sec. 3.29 and 23.48).

Calcitonin. Calcitonin is a polypeptide of 32 amino acids. Its gene is on chromosome 11p and is tightly linked to that for PTH. In birds, amphibians, and teleost fish calcitonin is synthesized in a discrete structure, the ultimobranchial gland. In mammals this gland has become incorporated into the thyroid gland as the parafollicular or C cells. Although calcitonin was discovered through its hypocalcemic effect, patients with medullary carcinoma of the thyroid (a tumor arising from the parafollicular cells) usually have normal plasma levels of calcium in spite of markedly increased levels of calcitonin.

The physiologic role of calcitonin remains uncertain. Its action appears to be independent of PTH and of vitamin D. Its main biologic effect appears to be the inhibition of bone resorption by decreasing the number and activity of bone-resorbing osteoclasts. This action of calcitonin is the rationale behind its use in treatment of Paget disease. Calcitonin is synthesized also in other organs, such as the gastrointestinal tract, pancreas, brain, and pituitary. In these organs calcitonin is believed to behave as a neurotransmitter to impose a local inhibitory effect on cell function.

19.18 HYPOPARATHYROIDISM

Etiology (Table 19–4). The normal level of PTH in cord blood is low; it doubles by the 6th day to reach a level nearly that of normal infants and children. Hypocalcemia is common from 12–72 hr of life, especially in premature infants, in infants with asphyxia at birth, and in infants of diabetic mothers (*early neonatal hypocalcemia*) (see also Sec. 8.54). After the 2nd–3rd day and during the 1st wk of life, the type of feeding is also a determinant of the level of serum calcium (*late neonatal hypocalcemia*). The role played by the parathyroids in these hypocalcemic infants remains to be clarified though functional immaturity of the parathyroids has often been invoked as pathogenetic. In a group of infants with *transient idiopathic hypocalcemia* (1–8 wk of age) serum levels of parathormone were significantly lower than in normal infants. It is possible that the functional immaturity is a manifestation of a delay in development of the enzymes which convert glandular PTH to secreted PTH; other mechanisms are possible.

Transient hypocalcemia also occurs in infants born to *mothers with hyperparathyroidism*. It appears that the hypocalcemia in such infants results from suppression of the fetal parathyroids by exposure to elevated levels of calcium in maternal serum. Tetany usually develops within 3 wk but may be delayed 1 mo or more; hypocalcemia may persist for weeks or months. When the cause of hypocalcemia in young infants is unknown, their mothers should have measurements of calcium, phosphorus, and parathyroid hormone.

Aplasia of the parathyroid glands is often associated with other developmental defects arising from the 3rd and 4th pharyn-geal pouches (*DiGeorge syndrome*) (see Fig. 19–10 and Sec. 10.13). The most common associations are aplasia of the thymus and congenital heart defects (especially those involving the aorta, such as truncus arteriosus and interruption of the aortic arch). The disorder is usually sporadic, but autosomal dominant and autosomal recessive inheritance have been reported. In other instances deletions of the short arm of chromosome 22 have been associated. The syndrome has occurred in infants of diabetic mothers, in association with the fetal alcohol syndrome, and in infants born to mothers who were inadvertently treated with retinoic acid for acne early in pregnancy. Tetany may have a delayed onset, and the manifestations of thymic deficiency may be attenuated.

Administration of ^{131}I during pregnancy has resulted in hypoparathyroidism as well as in hypothyroidism.

Familial Congenital Hypoparathyroidism. In two large pedigrees this disorder appears to be transmitted by an X-linked recessive gene. Onset of afebrile seizures characteristically occurs from 2 wk–6 mo of age. Familial hypoparathyroidism that has been observed also in both sexes in successive generations suggests autosomal dominant inheritance. The age of onset ranges from infancy to young adulthood. The nature of the defect is not known for either type, and there are no associated congenital defects. Hypocalcemia, hyperphosphatemia, and low levels of immunoreactive PTH occur. Parathyroid antibodies are absent in both types.

Removal or damage of the parathyroid glands may complicate thyroidectomy (*surgical hypoparathyroidism*). Hypoparathyroidism has developed even when the parathyroid glands

Table 19–4. Etiologic Classification of Hypocalcemia

Parathyroid hormone (PTH) deficiency
  Transient hypofunction
    Early neonatal hypocalcemia
    Late neonatal hypocalcemia
    Maternal hyperparathyroidism
    Other
  Congenital aplasia or hypoplasia of parathyroids
    With thymic and other III–IV arch defects (DiGeorge syndrome)
      With Zellweger, Vater, CHARGE syndromes
      With chromosomal abnormalities (especially 22p −)
      With maternal diabetes mellitus, alcoholism, or retinoic acid
        treatment
      With congenital hypothyroidism due to maternal ^{131}I
  Familial hypoparathyroidism
    X-linked
    Autosomal dominant
  Idiopathic hypoparathyroidism
    Autoimmune hypoparathyroiditis
      Isolated
      With Addison disease and/or mucocutaneous candidosis (type
        I autoimmune polyendocrinopathy)
  Surgical removal or damage to parathyroids
  Hemosiderosis (treatment of thalassemia)
  Copper deposition (Wilson disease)
  Inactive parathyroid hormone
    (pseudoidiopathic hypoparathyroidism)
  Parathyroid hormone unresponsiveness
    (pseudohypoparathyroidism)
    Type Ia—reduced G unit
    Type Ib—normal G unit
    Type II—normal cAMP response
Vitamin D deficiency
  Inadequate irradiation (clothing, housing, smog, climate)
  Dietary deficiency
  Malabsorption
    Deficiency of bile salts (liver disease)
    Deficiency of calcium-binding protein (gluten-sensitive
      enteropathy)
    Intestinal bypass operations
  Depletion (bile fistulas)
  Altered metabolism (chronic therapy with phenytoin
    [diphenylhydantoin] and/or phenobarbital)
  Impaired synthesis of 25-(OH)-D_3 (severe hepatic disease)
  Impaired synthesis of 1,25-(OH)$_2$-D_3
    Renal failure
    Renal tubular disease?
    Genetic deficiency of 1α-hydroxylase (vitamin D dependent
      rickets, type I)
    Hypoparathyroidism
  End-organ resistance to 1,25-(OH)$_2$-D_3 (vitamin D dependent
    rickets, type II)
    With alopecia
    Without alopecia
Magnesium deficiency
  Familial hypomagnesemia
  Other malabsorption syndromes
Inorganic phosphate excess
  Poisoning
  Initial therapy of leukemia

have been identified and left undisturbed at the time of operation. This, presumably, is the result of interference with the blood supply or of postoperative edema and fibrosis. Symptoms of tetany may occur abruptly postoperatively and be temporary or permanent. In some instances symptoms develop insidiously and go undetected until months after thyroidectomy. Occasionally, the first evidence of surgical hypoparathyroidism may be the development of cataracts. All patients subjected to thyroidectomy should have the status of parathyroid function carefully monitored.

Deposition in the parathyroid glands of iron pigment (as in thalassemia) or of copper (as in Wilson disease) may produce hypoparathyroidism.

Idiopathic Hypoparathyroidism. The term "idiopathic" should be reserved for the small residuum of children with hypoparathyroidism for which no etiologic mechanism can be defined. The majority of children in whom hypoparathyroidism has an onset after the 1st few yr of life have an autoimmune condition. A much smaller percentage have incomplete forms of DiGeorge syndrome or the autosomal dominant type of familial hypoparathyroidism.

Autoimmune Hypoparathyroidism. An autoimmune mechanism for hypoparathyroidism is strongly suggested by the finding of parathyroid antibodies and by the frequent association with other autoimmune disorders and/or organ-specific antibodies. Autoimmune hypoparathyroidism is usually associated with Addison disease and chronic mucocutaneous candidosis. The association of at least two of these three conditions has been tentatively classified as *polyglandular autoimmune disease, type I.* One third of patients with this syndrome have all three components; two thirds have only two of three conditions. The candidosis almost always precedes the other disorders (70% under 5 yr of age); the hypoparathyroidism (90% after 3 yr of age) usually occurs before the Addison disease (90% after 6 yr of age). In addition, a variety of other disorders occur at variable times; these include alopecia areata or totalis, malabsorption disorder, pernicious anemia, gonadal failure, chronic active hepatitis, autoimmune thyroid disease, and vitiligo. These associations may occur in 10–25% of patients; insulin-independent diabetes and IgA deficiency are much less frequent concomitants.

Affected siblings may have the same or different constellations of disorders (e.g., hypoparathyroidism and Addison disease). No HLA type has been found in excess in these patients. There is a slight predominance of affected females (4:3), but the disorder is thought to have an autosomal recessive mode of inheritance.

Siblings have been observed with nephrosis, nerve deafness, and hypoparathyroidism, a constellation also likely to have an autoimmune basis.

Pseudoidiopathic hypoparathyroidism designates the hypoparathyroidism found in a young adult who had the onset of tetany at 8 yr of age, with all the laboratory findings of idiopathic hypoparathyroidism. He had a normal response to administration of PTH. His serum contained normal to high levels of immunoreactive parathyroid hormone by several assay systems. This patient's endogenous parathyroid hormone appeared to lack biologic effect, possibly because of a defect in conversion of proparathyroid hormone to parathyroid hormone in the gland or a defect in peripheral activation of a secreted, precursor form of PTH.

Clinical Manifestations. There is a spectrum of parathyroid deficiencies with clinical manifestations varying from no symptoms to those of complete and longstanding deficiency. Mild deficiency may be revealed only by appropriate laboratory studies. Muscular pain and cramps are early manifestations; they progress to numbness, stiffness, and tingling of the hands and feet. There may be only positive Chvostek and/or Trousseau signs or laryngeal and carpopedal spasms. Convulsions with loss of consciousness may occur at intervals of days, weeks, or months. These may begin with abdominal pain, followed by tonic rigidity, retraction of the head, and cyanosis. Hypoparathyroidism is frequently mistaken for epilepsy. Headache, vomiting, increased intracranial pressure, and papilledema may be associated with convulsions and may suggest a brain tumor.

The teeth erupt late and irregularly. Enamel formation is irregular, and the teeth may be unusually soft. The skin may be dry and scaly, and the nails of the fingers and toes may have horizontal lines. Manifestations of a wide variety of other disorders which are not direct consequences of parathyroid hormone deficiency may also be seen. Mucocutaneous candidosis, when present, antedates the development of

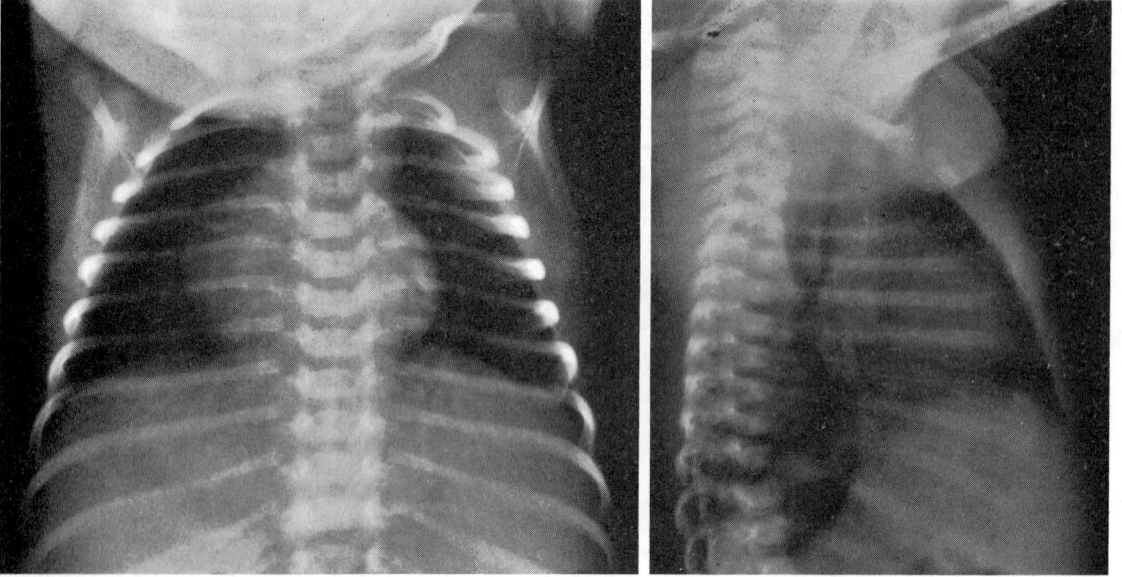

Figure 19–10. Congenital absence of parathyroid glands. Roentgenograms of chest exposed at 6 days of age reveal no evidence of thymus. *A*, The mediasinum is narrow; *B*, the substernal area is radiolucent. (Kirkpatrick JA Jr, DiGeorge AM: Am J Roentgenol 103:32, 1968.)

hypoparathyroidism; the candidal infection most often involves the nails, the oral mucosa, the angles of the mouth, and, less often, the skin.

Cataracts in patients with longstanding untreated disease are a direct consequence of hypoparathyroidism; other ocular disorders such as keratoconjunctivitis may also occur. Manifestations of Addison disease, lymphocytic thyroiditis, pernicious anemia, alopecia areata or totalis, hepatitis, and primary gonadal insufficiency may also be associated with those of hypoparathyroidism.

Permanent physical and mental deterioration occurs if initiation of treatment is long delayed.

Laboratory Data. The serum calcium level is low (5–7 mg/dL) and the phosphorus elevated (7–12 mg/dL). The serum alkaline phosphatase activity is normal or low. The level of magnesium is normal but should always be checked in hypocalcemic patients (see below). Serum levels of PTH and of $1,25\text{-}(OH)_2\text{-}D_3$ are low, even in the presence of hypocalcemia. Roentgenograms of the bones occasionally reveal an increased density limited to the metaphyses, suggestive of heavy metal poisoning, or an increased density of the lamina dura. Roentgenograms or computed tomography of the skull may reveal calcifications in the basal ganglia. There is a prolongation of the Q-T interval on the electrocardiogram, which disappears when the hypocalcemia is corrected. The electroencephalogram usually reveals widespread slow activity; the tracing returns to normal after the serum calcium has been within the normal range for a few weeks unless irreversible brain damage has occurred or unless the parathyroid insufficiency is associated with epilepsy. When hypoparathyroidism occurs concurrently with Addison disease, the serum level of calcium may be normal, but hypocalcemia appears after effective treatment of the adrenal insufficiency.

Treatment. Emergency treatment for tetany consists in intravenous injections of 5–10 mL of a 10% solution of calcium gluconate at the rate of 0.5–1 mL/min. Additionally 1,25-dihydroxycholecalciferol (calcitriol) should be given. The initial dose is 0.25 μg/24 hr; the maintenance dose ranges from 0.01–0.10 μg/kg/24 hr. Calcitriol has a short half-life and should be given in two equal, divided doses; it has the advantages of rapid onset of effect (1–4 days), and rapid reversal of hypercalcemia after discontinuation in the event of overdosage (calcium begins to fall in 3–4 days).

Once normocalcemia has been achieved, one may wish to continue therapy with vitamin D_2, because it is considerably less costly than calcitriol. The usual doses are 0.1–0.5 mg/24 hr in infants and young children. One mg of vitamin D_2 has a biologic activity of 40,000 IU. Older children require 1.25–2.00 mg (50,000–100,000 IU) once daily. Vitamin D_2 has a slow onset of effect, and reversal of hypercalcemia after discontinuation of treatment is markedly delayed; its main advantage is its low cost.

An adequate intake of calcium should be ensured. This can be done by giving supplemental calcium in the form of calcium gluconate or calcium glubionate (Neocalglucon) to provide 800 mg of elemental calcium daily. Foods with a high phosphorus content such as milk, eggs, and cheese should be reduced in the diet.

Clinical evaluation of the patient and frequent determinations of the serum calcium levels are indicated in the early stages of treatment in order to determine the requirement of calcitriol or vitamin D_2. Blood levels of ionized calcium (normal 4.05–5.14 mg/dL) more nearly reflect physiologic adequacy than levels of total calcium. If hypercalcemia occurs, therapy should be discontinued and resumed at a lower dose after the serum calcium level has returned to normal. In cases of long standing, repair of cerebral and dental changes is not likely. Pigmentation, lowering of the blood pressure, or weight loss may indicate adrenal insufficiency, which requires specific treatment.

Differential Diagnosis. *Magnesium deficiency* must be considered in patients with unexplained hypocalcemia. Concentrations of magnesium in serum below 1.5 mg/dL (1.2 mEq/L) are usually abnormal. *Familial hypomagnesemia* with secondary hypocalcemia has been reported in 32 patients, most of whom developed tetany and seizures from 2–4 wk of age. Administration of calcium is ineffective, but administration of magnesium promptly corrects both calcium and magnesium levels. Oral supplements of magnesium are necessary to maintain levels of magnesium in the normal range. The profoundly low levels of magnesium result from a specific defect in intestinal absorption. The disorder has been most frequently diagnosed in boys, but it appears to be caused by an autosomal recessive gene. (See also Sec. 8.54 for treatment.)

Hypomagnesemia also occurs in malabsorption syndromes and has been noted in granulomatous colitis and cystic fibrosis. Therapy with aminoglycosides causes hypomagnesemia by increasing urinary losses. Patients with autoimmune hypoparathyroidism may have concurrent steatorrhea and low magnesium levels.

It is not clear how low levels of magnesium lead to hypocalcemia. Current evidence suggests that hypomagnesemia impairs release of PTH and induces resistance to the effects of the hormone, but other mechanisms also may be operative.

Poisoning with inorganic phosphate leads to hypocalcemia and tetany. Infants poisoned with large doses of inorganic phosphates, either as laxatives or as sodium phosphate enemas, have had sudden onset of tetany, with serum calcium levels below 5 mg/dL and markedly elevated levels of phosphate. Symptoms are quickly relieved by intravenous administration of calcium. The mechanism of the hypocalcemia is not clear.

Hypocalcemia may occur early in the course of treatment of *acute lymphoblastic leukemia*. It is usually associated with hyperphosphatemia (resulting from destruction of lymphoblasts), which is probably the primary cause of hypocalcemia.

Episodic symptomatic hypocalcemia occurs in the *Kenny-Caffey syndrome*, which is characterized by medullary stenosis of the long bones, short stature, and high hyperopia, with onset ranging from the neonatal period to the 4th decade. Recent evidence suggests heterogeneity of the syndrome; idiopathic hypoparathyroidism and abnormal PTH have both been found.

19.19 PSEUDOHYPOPARATHYROIDISM
(Albright Syndrome; Hereditary Osteodystrophy)

In this syndrome, in contrast to the situation in idiopathic hypoparathyroidism, the parathyroid glands are normal or hyperplastic histologically, and they can synthesize and secrete parathyroid hormone. Serum levels of immunoreactive PTH are elevated even when the patient is hypocalcemic. The disorder is caused by a genetic defect in receptor tissues, particularly of the kidney and skeleton. Neither endogenous nor administered parathyroid hormone raises serum levels of calcium or lowers levels of phosphorus.

In most patients with *pseudohypoparathyroidism (PHP),* an infusion of PTH evokes an inadequate increase in levels of cAMP in plasma and urine (type I PHP). Most patients (type Ia PHP) have a 50% decrease in activity of the guanine nucleotide regulatory unit (G-unit), a coupling factor required for hormone-bound receptors to activate adenylate cyclase; a minority of patients (type Ib PHP) have normal G-unit activity. Deficiency of the G-unit appears to be generalized and accounts for the frequent association of PHP with other endocrine disorders involving cAMP activation.

A small group of patients with PHP (type II) have elevated urinary excretion of cAMP, both in the basal state and after stimulation with PTH. It is presumed that the target cells are unable to respond to the cAMP signal.

Type I PHP has been regarded as an X-linked trait, but current evidence supports an autosomal dominant mode of inheritance. Decreased fertility in affected males may account for the rarity of father-to-son transmission, of which several cases are now known, including one with G-unit deficiency in both father and son.

Clinical manifestations vary in severity and in age of onset. They tend to develop gradually, and the diagnosis of PHP has only rarely been suspected during the 1st yr of life. Affected older children have a short, stocky build and a round face. Growth failure may be striking. Brachydactyly with dimpling of the dorsum of the hand is usually present. The 2nd metacarpal is the least often involved. As a result, on occasion, the index finger may be longer than the middle finger. Likewise, the 2nd metatarsal is only rarely affected.

Tetany often is the presenting sign. There may be other skeletal abnormalities such as short and wide phalanges, bowing, exostoses, thickening of the calvaria, and general demineralization of the bones. These patients frequently have calcium deposits and metaplastic bone formation subcutaneously. Mental retardation is common as are calcifications of the basal ganglia and lenticular cataracts.

In some patients with pseudohypoparathyroidism, the resistance to PTH appears to be limited to the kidneys, the bones being normally responsive to the elevated levels of circulating hormone. As a result, in addition to the skeletal changes described above, these patients exhibit subperiosteal resorption, osteitis fibrosa, and, in children, widening and irregularity of the epiphyseal plates. The condition has been termed *pseudohypohyperthyroidism* by some, but *pseudohypoparathyroidism with osteitis fibrosa* appears to be a less confusing designation.

Some patients have the usual anatomic stigmata of pseudohypoparathyroidism but normal serum calcium and phosphorus levels. Their condition has been called pseudopseudohypoparathyroidism. Transition from the normocalcemic to the hypocalcemic form has been observed, however, and some families have normocalcemic and hypocalcemic forms in different members.

Other endocrine disorders associated with type Ia PHP include hypothyroidism and resistance to the metabolic effects of glucagon and gonadotropins. In several instances, the hypothyroidism was detected by neonatal thyroid screening. Each of these abnormalities can be related to deficient synthesis of cAMP.

Serum levels of calcium and phosphorus may be normal, especially in infancy. When hypocalcemia is present, it is usually accompanied by hyperphosphatemia and elevated levels of PTH. Concentrations of 1,25-$(OH)_2$-D_3 are also elevated in early childhood but low levels have been reported in adults.

Clinical hypothyroidism is uncommon but basal levels of TSH are elevated and thyrotropin-releasing hormone-stimulated TSH responses are exaggerated, indicating primary hypothyroidism. In adults, gonadal dysfunction is common, as manifested by sexual immaturity, amenorrhea, oligomenorrhea, and infertility.

Diagnosis rests on the demonstration that no increase in urinary phosphate and cAMP occurs after intravenous infusion of 2 units/kg of bovine parathyroid extract. This test can also be used to reveal latent pseudohypoparathyroidism in persons at genetic risk who have no other signs of the condition.

Treatment is the same as for hypoparathyroidism.

19.20 HYPERPARATHYROIDISM

Excessive production of parathyroid hormone may result from a primary defect of the parathyroid glands such as an adenoma or idiopathic hyperplasia (*primary hyperparathyroidism*).

More often, the increased production of parathyroid hormone is compensatory, usually aimed at correcting hypocalcemic states of diverse origins (*secondary hyperparathyroidism*). In vitamin D deficient rickets and in the malabsorption syndromes, intestinal absorption of calcium is deficient, but hypocalcemia and tetany may be averted by increased activity of the parathyroid glands. In chronic renal disease, hyperphosphatemia and the consequent hypocalcemia result in compensatory hyperparathyroidism with marked increases in serum levels of parathyroid hormone. In some instances, if stimulation of the parathyroids has been sufficiently intense and protracted, the glands may continue to secrete increased

Table 19–5. **Causes of Hypercalcemia**

Parathyroid hormone (PTH) excess
  Primary hyperparathyroidism
    Sporadic—adenoma
    Familial
      Clear cell hyperplasia of infancy (with familial hypocalciuric
        hypercalcemia)
      Clear cell hyperplasia of infancy, sporadic
      Adenoma-hyperplasia (dominant)
      Multiple endocrine neoplasia I (dominant)
      Multiple endocrine neoplasia II (dominant)
  Secondary hyperparathyroidism—post-renal—transplantation
  Transient neonatal hyperparathyroidism—maternal
    hypoparathyroidism
Without PTH excess
  Idiopathic hypercalcemia of infancy (Williams syndrome)
  Familial hypocalciuric hypercalcemia
  Vitamin D excess
  Hypervitaminosis A
  Thyrotoxicosis
  Hypophosphatasia
  Prolonged immobilization
  Subcutaneous fat necrosis
  Malignancy
    Leukemia, lymphoma
    Rhabdomyosarcoma, neuroblastoma, bone tumors
  Granulomatous disease
    Sarcoidosis
    Tuberculosis

levels of PTH for months or years after renal transplantation, with resulting hypercalcemia (Table 19–5). This situation, where there may be some autonomy of the parathyroids, has been called *tertiary hyperparathyroidism.*

Primary hyperparathyroidism is uncommon in children and is usually due to a single *adenoma*. Symptoms generally begin after 10 yr of age.

There have been many kindreds with three or more members with hyperparathyroidism. In such instances of *familial hyperparathyroidism* most of the affected members are adults, but children have been involved in about a third of pedigrees. Some affected patients in these families are asymptomatic and are revealed only by careful study. In some kindreds, in addition to hyperparathyroidism, there is a high frequency of peptic ulcer with islet cell tumors (Zollinger-Ellison syndrome) and prolactin-secreting pituitary adenomas; this constellation is known as multiple endocrine neoplasia, type I (MEN-I). In other families there is an association with medullary carcinoma of the thyroid and pheochromocytoma; this syndrome is known as multiple endocrine neoplasia, type II (MEN-II) (see Sec. 19.16). In familial hyperparathyroidism the adenomas are apt to be multiple, and in some patients the parathyroid may reveal only hyperplasia. Recent studies have identified a new factor in the blood of individuals with MEN-I, which stimulates parathyroid mitogenic activity. Inheritance is autosomal dominant, with a high degree of penetrance.

Another form of familial hyperparathyroidism consists of *clear-cell hyperplasia of the parathyroids in infancy.* The condition has its onset in the early weeks of life and may have a rapidly fatal course if diagnosis is delayed. Its occurrence in siblings and with parental consanguinity in some families suggests autosomal recessive inheritance. Of 23 cases of neonatal primary hyperparathyroidism, 10 have been in kindreds with definite or probable familial hypocalciuric hypercalcemia, an autosomal dominant disorder. It is believed that this form of congenital hyperparathyroidism is caused by homozygosity for this autosomal dominant gene.

Ectopic PTH production has been suggested as an explanation for the hypercalcemia which occurs with various nonendocrine tumors in adults, including those arising in lung,

kidney, cervix, ovary, parotid gland, and reticulum cell sarcoma, but ectopic hyperparathyroidism has not been proved. Hypercalcemia and hypophosphatemia are the usual diagnostic clues. Hypercalcemia without hypophosphatemia frequently occurs in other malignancies, especially carcinoma of the breast. The cause for hypercalcemia in these patients is not known.

Transient neonatal hyperparathyroidism has occurred in a few infants born to mothers with hypoparathyroidism (idiopathic or surgical) or with pseudohypoparathyroidism. In each instance the maternal disorder had been undiagnosed or inadequately treated during pregnancy. The cause of the condition is chronic intrauterine exposure to hypocalcemia with resultant hyperplasia of the fetal parathyroid glands. In the newborn, manifestations involve the bones primarily, and healing occurs between 4–7 mo.

Clinical Manifestations. At all ages the clinical manifestations of hypercalcemia of any cause include muscular weakness, anorexia, nausea, vomiting, constipation, polydipsia, polyuria, loss of weight, and fever. Calcium may be deposited in the renal parenchyma (nephrocalcinosis), with progressively diminished renal function. Renal calculi (noted in 12 of 46 children with adenoma) may produce renal colic and hematuria. Osseous changes may produce pain in the back or extremities, disturbances of gait, deformities, fractures, and tumors. Height may decrease from compression of vertebrae; the patient may become bedridden.

Abdominal pain is occasionally prominent and may be associated with acute pancreatitis. Parathyroid crisis may occur, manifested by serum calcium levels greater than 15 mg/dL and progressive oliguria, azotemia, stupor, and coma. In infants failure to thrive, poor feeding, and hypotonia are common. Mental retardation, convulsions, and blindness may occur as sequelae.

Laboratory Data. The serum calcium is elevated; 39 of 45 children with adenomas had levels over 12 mg/dL. The hypercalcemia is more severe in infants with parathyroid hyperplasia; concentrations from 15–20 mg/dL are common, and values as high as 30 mg/dL have been reported. Ionized (Ca^{++}) calcium levels are often elevated even when total serum calcium is borderline or only slightly elevated. The serum phosphorus level is reduced to about 3 mg/dL or less, and the level of serum magnesium is low. The urine may have a low and fixed specific gravity, and serum levels of nonprotein nitrogen and uric acid may be elevated. In patients with adenomas who have skeletal involvement serum phosphatase is elevated, whereas in infants with hyperplasia the levels of alkaline phosphatase may be normal even when there is extensive involvement of bone.

Serum levels of parathyroid hormone (PTH), as measured by carboxyterminal antisera, are elevated, especially in relation to the level of calcium. Results may vary markedly from one laboratory to another, depending on the antibody used. Calcitonin levels are normal. Acute hypercalcemia can stimulate calcitonin release, but with prolonged hypercalcemia, hypercalcitoninemia does not occur.

The most consistent and characteristic roentgenographic findings are resorption of subperiosteal bone, best seen along the margins of the phalanges of the hands. In the skull there may be gross trabeculation or a granular appearance resulting from focal rarefaction; the lamina dura may be absent. In more advanced disease there may be generalized rarefaction, cysts, tumors, fractures, and deformities. About 10% of patients have roentgenographic signs of rickets. Roentgenograms of the abdomen may reveal renal calculi or nephrocalcinosis.

Differential Diagnosis. *Hypercalcemia* of any origin results in a similar clinical pattern; other causes must be differentiated from hyperparathyroidism. A low serum phosphorus level with hypercalcemia is characteristic of primary hyperparathyroidism; elevated levels of PTH are also diagnostic. Pharmacologic doses of corticosteroids lower the serum calcium level to normal in patients with hypercalcemia from other causes but generally do not affect the calcium level in patients with hyperparathyroidism. Administration of corticosteroids may be useful in differential diagnosis.

Vitamin D intoxication can be excluded by history, by a normal level of serum phosphorus, and by roentgenographic evidence of increased bone density. *Idiopathic hypercalcemia* of infancy may be easily confused with hyperparathyroidism; the serum phosphorus level is normal or slightly elevated, however, and serum levels of PTH and 1,25-$(OH)_2D_3$ are suppressed or normal. A blunted calcitonin response to IV calcium and parathyroid hormone infusions has recently been reported. A deficiency of calcitonin may be the central defect. The increased bone density of idiopathic hypercalcemia contrasts strikingly with the rarefaction of primary hyperparathyroidism. Hypercalcemia is not present during the 1st weeks of life; hypersensitivity to normal doses of vitamin D has been suggested as a possible cause for the condition. Affected infants may have an elfin face, supravalvular aortic stenosis or other cardiac defects, mental retardation, and other abnormalities *(Williams syndrome)*. Hypercalcemia may also occur in infants with *subcutaneous fat necrosis*. PTH and vitamin D metabolite levels are normal; the cause for this condition is unknown. *Phosphate depletion* may be induced by total parenteral nutrition in the neonate; it leads in turn to severe hypercalcemia. *Hypophosphatasia*, especially when severe, is frequently associated with mild to moderate hypercalcemia. The serum phosphorus level is normal; alkaline phosphatase activity is depressed. Roentgenograms of the bones may reveal disappearance of the zone of provisional calcification and lack of calcification of the metaphyseal bone (Table 19–5).

Prolonged immobilization may lead to hypercalcemia and occasionally to decreased renal function, hypertension, and encephalopathy. Hypercalcemia has been associated also with a variety of *malignancies*; 17 cases were identified among 2400 patients with solid tumors. Children with non-Hodgkin lymphoma, rhabdomyosarcoma, and rhabdoid Wilms tumor appear to be preferentially affected. The mediator for the hypercalcemia is not known, as PTH levels are often not elevated. Hypercalcemia occurs in 30–50% of children with *sarcoidosis*, and in other granulomatous diseases. Levels of iPTH are suppressed and levels of 1,25-$(OH)_2$-D_3 elevated. There is substantial evidence that the 1,25-$(OH)_2$-D_3 is produced ectopically. Therapy with prednisone lowers serum levels of 1,25-$(OH)_2$-D_3 to normal and corrects the hypercalcemia. Elevated serum calcium levels have also been observed in patients with *hypervitaminosis A*, in *thyrotoxicosis*, and in malignant disease with *osseous metastases*. Administration of *thiazide diuretics* to hypoparathyroid patients treated with vitamin D can lead to hypercalcemia.

Familial hypocalciuric hypercalcemia (familial benign hypercalcemia) a disorder with autosomal dominant transmission, occurs in children and adults; it may be asymptomatic. The clinical course is mild, the usual renal problems of hyperparathyroidism are absent, and no other endocrine disorders are associated. Parathyroid glands are usually normal, PTH levels are rarely elevated, and subtotal parathyroidectomy does not correct the hypercalcemia. The rate of urinary excretion of calcium is one third that in primary hyperparathyroidism. The basic defect in the condition is unknown; the insensitivity of the kidneys and parathyroid glands to hypercalcemia suggests a generalized insensitivity to calcium ion. Screening of family members is worthwhile; affected persons aware of the diagnosis can avoid inappropriate parathyroid surgery. No treatment is necessary for the condition. Homozygosity

for this autosomal dominant gene is thought to be the cause of most cases of *clear-cell hyperplasia of the parathyroids in infancy* and severe hyperparathyroidism (see above).

Hypercalcemia in patients with *familial pheochromocytoma* is usually due to hyperparathyroidism; however, the reported return to normal of the calcium level in a 12 yr old boy after removal of a pheochromocytoma suggests that the tumor itself may have produced a calcium-affecting factor.

Treatment. Surgical exploration is indicated in all instances. All glands should be carefully inspected; if an adenoma is discovered, it should be removed; only two instances of carcinoma are known in children. If there is only generalized hyperplasia, total parathyroidectomy appears indicated to avoid recurrence of the hypercalcemia. Nests of ectopic parathyroid cells in adipose tissue of the neck or mediastinum may also become hyperplastic and may lead to recurrent hyperparathyroidism *(parathyromatosis)*. The patient should be carefully observed postoperatively for the development of hypocalcemia and tetany; intravenous administration of calcium gluconate may be required for a few days. The serum calcium level then gradually returns to normal, and, under ordinary circumstances, a diet high in calcium and phosphorus needs to be maintained for only several mo after operation.

Arteriography and selective venous sampling with radioimmunoassay of PTH have been used successfully for preoperative localization and for differentiation of a single adenoma from hyperplasia in adults. These procedures are particularly advisable before re-exploration in cases of persistent or recurrent hyperparathyroidism.

Prognosis. The prognosis is good if the disease is recognized early and there is appropriate surgical treatment. When extensive osseous lesions are present, deformities may be permanent; with renal disease the prognosis is less hopeful. A search for other affected family members is indicated.

Barakat AY, D'Albora JB, Martin MM, et al: Familial nephrosis, nerve deafness and hypoparathyroidism. J Pediatr 91:61, 1977.
Berliner BC, Shenker IR, Weinstock MS: Hypercalcemia associated with hypertension due to prolonged immobilization. (An unusual complication of extensive burns.) Pediatrics 49:92, 1972.
Blizzard RM, Chee D, Davis W: The incidence of parathyroid and other antibodies in the sera of patients with idiopathic hypoparathyroidism. Clin Exp Immunol 1:119, 1966.
Brandi ML, Aurbach GD, Fitzpatrick LA, et al.: Parathyroid mitogenic activity in plasma from patients with familial multiple endocrine neoplasia Type I. N Engl J Med 314:1287, 1986.
Bronsky D, Kiamko RT, Moncado R, et al: Intrauterine hyperparathyroidism secondary to maternal hypoparathyroidism. Pediatrics 42:606, 1968.
Culler FL, Jones KL, Deltos LJ: Impaired calcitonin secretion in patients with Williams syndrome. J Pediatr 107:720, 1985.
Daum F, Rosen JF, Boley SJ: Parathyroid adenoma, parathyroid crisis and acute pancreatitis in an adolescent. J Pediatr 83:275, 1973.
Davis RF, Eichner JM, Bleyer WA, et al: Hypocalcemia, hyperphosphatemia, and dehydration following a single hypertonic phosphate enema. J Pediatr 90:484, 1977.
Deftos LJ, Powell D, Parthemore JG, et al: Secretion of calcitonin in hypocalcemic states in man. J Clin Invest 52:3109, 1973.
DiGeorge AM: Congenital absence of the thymus and its immunologic consequences, concurrence with congenital hypoparathyroidism. In: Bergsma D, Good RA (eds): Birth Defects. Original Article Series, No 1, Vol IV. New York, The National Foundation, 1968.
Fanconi S, Fischer JA, Wieland P, et al.: Kenny syndrome: Evidence for idiopathic hypoparathyroidism in two patients and for abnormal parathyroid in one. J Pediatr 109:469, 1986.
Fairney A, Jackson D, Clayton BE: Measurement of serum parathyroid hormone, with particular reference to some infants with hypocalcemia. Arch Dis Child 48:419, 1973.
Fisher F, Skillern PG: Hypercalcemia due to hypervitaminosis A. JAMA 227:1413, 1974.
Fitch N: Albright's hereditary osteodystrophy: A review. Am J Med Genet 11:11, 1982.
Glass EJ, Barr DGD: Transient neonatal hyperparathyroidism secondary to maternal pseudohypoparathyroidism. Arch Dis Child 56:555, 1981.
Goodyer PR, Frank A, Kaplan BS: Observations on the evolution and treatment of idiopathic infantile hypercalcemia. J Pediatr 105:771, 1984.
Green CG, Doershuk CF, Stern RC: Symptomatic hypomagnesemia in cystic fibrosis. J Pediatr 107:425, 1985.

Jacobsen BB, Terslev E, Lund B, Sorensen OH: Neonatal hypocalcemia associated with maternal hyperparathyroidism. Arch Dis Child 53:308, 1978.

Kind HP, Handysides A, Kook SW, et al: Vitamin D therapy in hypoparathyroidism and pseudohypoparathyroidism: Weight-related doses for initiation of therapy and maintenance therapy. J Pediatr 91:1006, 1977.

Law WM Jr, Bollman S, Kumar R, et al: Vitamin D metabolism in familial benign hypercalcemia (hypocalciuric hypercalcemia) differs from that in primary hyperparathyroidism. J Clin Endocrinol Metab 58:744, 1984.

Leblanc A, Caillaud JM, Hartmann O, et al: Hypercalcemia preferentially occurs in unusual forms of childhood non-Hodgkin's lymphoma, rhabdomyosarcoma, and Wilms' tumor. Cancer 54:2132, 1984.

Lee WK, Vargas A, Barnes J, et al: The Kenny-Caffey syndrome: Growth retardation and hypocalcemia in a young boy. Am J Med Genet 14:773, 1983.

Levine MA, Downs RW Jr, Moses AM, et al: Resistance to multiple hormones in patients with pseudohypoparathyroidism. Association with deficient activity of guanine nucleotide regulatory protein. Am J Med 74:545, 1983.

Levitt M, Gessert C, Finberg L: Inorganic phosphate (laxative) poisoning resulting in tetany in an infant. J Pediatr 82:479, 1973.

Lund B, Sorensen OH, Lund B, et al: Vitamin D metabolism in hypoparathyroidism. J Clin Endocrinol Metab 51:606, 1980.

Markowitz ME, Rosen JF, Smith C, et al: 1,25-dihydroxyvitamin D₃-treated hypoparathyroidism: 35 patient years in 10 children. J Clin Endocrinol Metab 55:727, 1982.

Marx SJ, Fraser D, Rapoport A: Familial hypocalciuric hypercalcemia. Mild expression of the gene in heterozygotes and severe expression in homozygotes. Am J Med 78:15, 1985.

Mason RS, Frankel T, Chan YL, et al: Vitamin D conversion by sarcoid lymph node homogenate. Ann Intern Med 100:59, 1984.

Miller RR, Menke JA, Mentser MI: Hypercalcemia associated with phosphate depletion in the neonate. J Pediatr 105:814, 1984.

Neufeld M, Blizzard RM: Polyglandular autoimmune disease. In: Pinchera A, Doniach D, Fenzi GF, Baschiori L (eds): Autoimmune Aspects of Endocrine Disorders. New York, Academic Press, 1980.

Nusynowitz ML, Klein MH: Pseudoidiopathic hypoparathyroidism. Hypoparathyroidism with ineffective parathyroid hormone. Am J Med 55:677, 1973.

Rapaport D, Rubin ZM, Huminer D, et al.: Primary hyperparathyroidism in children. J Pediatr Surg 21:395, 1986.

Reddick RL, Costa JC, Marx SJ: Parathyroid hyperplasia and parathyromatosis. Lancet 1:549, 1977.

Root A, Gruskin A, Reber RM: Serum concentrations of parathyroid hormone in infants, children and adolescents. J Pediatr 85:329, 1974.

Ross AJ III, Cooper A, Attie MF, et al.: Primary hyperparathyroidism in infancy. J Pediatr Surg 21:493, 1986.

Steinmann B, Gnehm HE, Rao VH, et al: Neonatal severe primary hyperparathyroidism and alkaptonuria in a boy to related parents with familial hypocalciuric hypercalcemia. Helv Paediatr Acta 39:171, 1984.

Stromme JH, Steen-Johnson J, Harnaes K, et al: Familial hypomagnesemia—a follow-up examination of three patients after 9 to 12 years of treatment. Pediatr Res 15:1134, 1981.

Swinton NW, Clerkin EP, Flint LD: Hypercalcemia and familial pheochromocytoma. Correction after adrenalectomy. Ann Intern Med 76:455, 1972.

Taylor AB, Stern PH, Bell NH: Abnormal regulation of circulating 25-hydroxyvitamin D in the Williams syndrome. N Engl J Med 306:972, 1982.

Theintz GE, Sizonenko PC, Paunier L: Primary hyperparathyroidism and rickets. A case report and review of the literature. Helv Paediatr Acta 39:509, 1984.

Tsang RC, Venkatararaman P, Ho M, et al: The development of pseudohypoparathyroidism. Involvement of progressively increasing serum parathyroid hormone concentrations, increased 1, 25-dihydroxyvitamin D concentrations, and "migratory" subcutaneous calcifications. Am J Dis Child 138:654, 1984.

Van Dop C, Bourne HR, Neer RM: Father to son transmission of decreased Ns activity in pseudohypoparathyroidism Type Ia. J Clin Endocrinol Metab 59:825, 1984.

Veldhuis JD, Kulin HE, Demers LM, Lambert PW: Infantile hypercalcemia with subcutaneous fat necrosis: Endocrine studies. J Pediatr 95:460, 1979.

Whyte MP, Weldon VV: Idiopathic hypoparathyroidism presenting with seizures during infancy: X-linked recessive inheritance in a large Missouri kindred. J Pediatr 99:608, 1981.

Winter WE, Silverstein JH, MacLaren NK, et al: Autosomal dominant hypoparathyroidism with variable, age-dependent severity. J Pediatr 103:387, 1983.

Young TO, Satzstein EC, Boman DA: Parathyroid carcinoma in a child: Unusual presentation with seizures. J Pediatr Surg 19:194, 1984.

19.21 DISORDERS OF THE ADRENAL GLANDS

The adrenal gland is composed of two endocrine systems, the medullary and the cortical systems. Mesodermal cells contribute to the development of the adrenal cortex, the gonads, and the liver; these three tissues are active in steroid metabolism in the fetus. Adrenals and gonads have in common certain enzymes involved in steroid synthesis, and an inborn defect in one tissue may also involve the other.

At about the 7th wk of gestation the primordium of the adrenal cortex is invaded by sympathetic neural elements. About 1 wk later these cells begin to differentiate into the chromaffin cells capable of synthesizing and storing catecholamines; the methyl transferase which converts norepinephrine to epinephrine develops later.

In a fetus of 2 mo the adrenals are larger than the kidneys, but from the 4th mo the kidneys grow rapidly, becoming about twice as large as the adrenals by the end of the 6th mo. In the full-term infant the adrenal gland is one third the size of the kidney, and the combined weight of both glands is 7–9 g.

The adrenal cortex in the fetus and the newborn infant has two histologically distinct components: an outer portion, the true cortex, and a more central portion, the "fetal cortex." At birth the "fetal" cortex makes up about 80% of the gland. Within a few days it begins to involute, undergoing a 50% reduction by 2 wk of age and disappearing completely by about 6 mo of age.

The true cortex consists of three zones. In the zona glomerulosa, situated beneath the capsule, there is an alveolar arrangement of the cells; in the broader zona fasciculata the columns of cells are radially arranged; in the zona reticularis the cells form a network next to the medulla.

Fetoplacental Unit. Fetal adrenal does not possess the 3β-hydroxysteroid dehydrogenase necessary to form progesterone; it utilizes placental pregnenolone to synthesize cortisol, aldosterone, and particularly dehydroepiandrosterone sulfate (DHEAS). The placenta in turn utilizes the fetal DHEAS to produce estrone and estriol. Estriol is the major estrogen found in maternal urine in pregnancy, especially in the late stages. In instances of fetal adrenal hypoplasia, maternal urinary estriol levels are markedly reduced.

Adrenal Cortex. The adrenal cortex secretes various steroid compounds essential to life. Recent studies indicate that the zona fasciculata and zona glomerulosa behave as two separate glands: ACTH primarily stimulates the zona fasciculata to secrete cortisol and androgens; the zona glomerulosa is involved primarily in synthesis of aldosterone.

Glucocorticoids have a 21-carbon structure and are also referred to as 17-hydroxycorticosteroids or simply as corticosteroids. The principal one is cortisol, also known as compound F or hydrocortisone. Cortisone (compound E) is a metabolite of cortisol. Glucocorticoids are produced by the zona fasciculata.

Glucocorticoids affect the metabolism of most tissues. They attach to specific intracellular receptor proteins which then bind to the cell nucleus to influence RNA and protein synthesis. In many tissues glucocorticoids have a catabolic effect, resulting in increased degradation of protein; primarily affected are muscles, skin, and connective, adipose, and lymphoid tissues. On the other hand, glucocorticoids are anabolic in the liver, where they stimulate a number of enzymes, increase protein and glycogen content, and enhance its capacity for gluconeogenesis. Patients with cortisol excess (e.g., Cushing syndrome) have increased glucose production, whereas those with deficiency of cortisol (Addison disease) have decreased gluconeogenesis, with hypoglycemia. Insulin and androgens have effects antagonistic to glucocorticoids. Some actions of catecholamines and of glucagon are facilitated by glucocorticoids.

The 17-hydroxycorticosteroids are excreted in urine; cortisol itself is also excreted in urine in amounts less than 1% of the adrenal production. Levels of cortisol and of its precursors and metabolites can be measured by radioimmunoassay and by high performance liquid chromatography (HPLC) in biologic fluids and tumor tissues. Levels of cortisol in plasma vary with the time of day; after the 1st few yr of life a circadian rhythm follows that of corticotropin.

Glucocorticoid synthesis is regulated primarily by ACTH, with cortisol exerting negative feedback on ACTH secretion. One of the major regulators of ACTH is corticotropin-releasing factor (CRF), a recently characterized hypothalamic peptide.

Many synthetic analogues of cortisone and hydrocortisone are available. Derivatives with an additional double bond in ring A are known as prednisone and prednisolone. They are four times as potent in anti-inflammatory and carbohydrate activity as the natural steroids but have less effect on salt and water retention. Halogenated derivatives have different effects; 9α-fluorohydrocortisone is approximately 15 times as active as hydrocortisone in anti-inflammatory activity but is more than 20 times as active in salt and water retention. Betamethasone and dexamethasone are approximately 25 times as potent as cortisol and have little effect on the retention of water and electrolytes. These analogues are usually used in pharmacologic doses for their anti-inflammatory or immunosuppressive properties.

Aldosterone, a potent mineralocorticoid, is the 18-aldehyde of corticosterone and is produced primarily in the zona glomerulosa. Its secretion is regulated by activation of the renin-angiotensin system. Renin produced by the juxtaglomerular apparatus of the kidney reacts with renin substrate, an α_2-globulin produced by the liver, to yield the inactive decapeptide, angiotensin. A converting enzyme rapidly changes angiotensin I to the biologically active octapeptide, angiotensin II. Angiotensin II is a pressor agent 50 times more potent than norepinephrine. One of its main functions is to act directly on the adrenal cortex to stimulate the secretion of aldosterone.

In good health and on a normal dietary intake, ACTH plays a minor role in regulation of aldosterone secretion, but under some conditions, as in anephric man, it may have a more significant effect. On the other hand, potassium may be of equal importance to the renin-angiotensin system in the regulation of aldosterone secretion. In studies of aldosterone secretion, dietary potassium and sodium must be rigidly controlled. Aldosterone and renin activity in plasma can be measured by radioimmunoassay.

Sodium deprivation is a potent stimulus to secretion of aldosterone. Changes in intake of sodium result in small changes in blood volume, arterial pressure, and renal blood flow. These changes are sensitively monitored by the juxtaglomerular cells on the renal afferent arterioles, which form the receptor site or volume receptor. Activation of the juxtaglomerular apparatus results in increased output of angiotensin II followed by increased secretion of aldosterone.

The principal action of aldosterone is the maintenance of electrolyte equilibrium, which in turn contributes to the stabilization of blood volume and blood pressure. Aldosterone controls sodium reabsorption (and hence water reabsorption) in the distal tubule of the kidney.

Androgens are produced mainly by the zona fasciculata. Dehydroepiandrosterone and androstenedione are capable of increasing retention of nitrogen, potassium, phosphorus, and sulfate. They promote growth and have androgenic effects which are most conspicuous when adrenal hyperplasia or adrenal tumors induce precocious growth and development of male secondary sex characteristics. The adrenal androgens seem partly responsible for development of axillary and pubic hair in the female.

Dehydroepiandrosterone sulfate (DHEAS) is the most abundant of the C19 steroids in blood and serves as a precursor for dehydroepiandrosterone. The function of these hormones is not fully understood. Levels of DHEAS rise prior to the other hormonal changes of puberty, but the fact that boys and girls have equal levels indicates that DHEAS does not have significant virilizing or feminizing actions. Levels of DHEAS are undetectable in hypopituitarism, low in Addison disease, and elevated in untreated congenital adrenal hyperplasia, in precocious adrenarche, and in sick premature and full-term infants.

Metabolites of adrenal androgens appear in the urine as 17-ketosteroids. Their measurement is a crude index of the production of adrenal androgens in the female. In the male approximately one third of the urinary 17-ketosteroids can be attributed to testicular and two thirds to adrenal androgens. In children under 8–10 yr of age the urinary excretion of these substances is small, but a constant increase is seen throughout adolescence until adult levels are reached. Increased production of adrenal androgens is usually reflected in increased secretion of urinary 17-ketosteroids.

Adrenal Medulla. The principal hormones of the adrenal medulla are the physiologically active catecholamines: dopamine, norepinephrine, and epinephrine. The sequence of their biosynthetic reactions is depicted in Fig. 19–11. Catecholamine synthesis occurs also in the brain, in sympathetic nerve endings, and in chromaffin tissue outside the adrenal medulla. Metabolites of catecholamines are excreted in the urine. The principal ones are 3-methoxy-4-hydroxymandelic acid (VMA), metanephrine, and normetanephrine. Measurement of VMA in urine has been the usual method for detection of functioning tumors of the adrenal medulla; new methods now measure levels of catecholamines directly.

The proportions of epinephrine and norepinephrine in the adrenal vary with age. In early fetal stages there is practically no epinephrine, and even at birth norepinephrine is predominant. In adults norepinephrine makes up only 10–30% of the pressor amines in the medulla. Both epinephrine and norepinephrine raise the mean arterial blood pressure, norepinephrine without changing the cardiac output. By increasing peripheral vascular resistance, norepinephrine increases systolic and diastolic blood pressures with only a slight reduction in the pulse rate. Epinephrine increases the pulse rate and, by decreasing the peripheral vascular resistance, decreases the diastolic pressure. The hyperglycemic and calorigenic effects of norepinephrine are much less pronounced than those of epinephrine.

19.22 ADRENOCORTICAL INSUFFICIENCY

Deficient production of cortisol and/or aldosterone may result from a wide variety of congenital or acquired lesions of the hypothalamus, pituitary, or adrenal cortex (Table 19–6). Depending upon the pathologic lesions, symptoms may be severe or mild, become manifest abruptly or insidiously, begin in infancy or later, and be permanent or temporary.

Etiology. *Corticotropin Deficiency.* Congenital hypoplasia or aplasia of the pituitary is almost always associated with secondary hypoplasia of the adrenals as well as with other hormonal deficiencies. These congenital defects are usually associated with abnormalities of the skull and brain such as anencephaly and holoprosencephaly. Such infants have a considerable residuum of pituitary function, and the hypoplasia of the pituitary is probably secondary to hypothalamic deficiency of corticotropin-releasing factor (CRF). Isolated deficiency of corticotropin has been reported in 8 children including 2 sets of siblings. Idiopathic hypopituitarism and

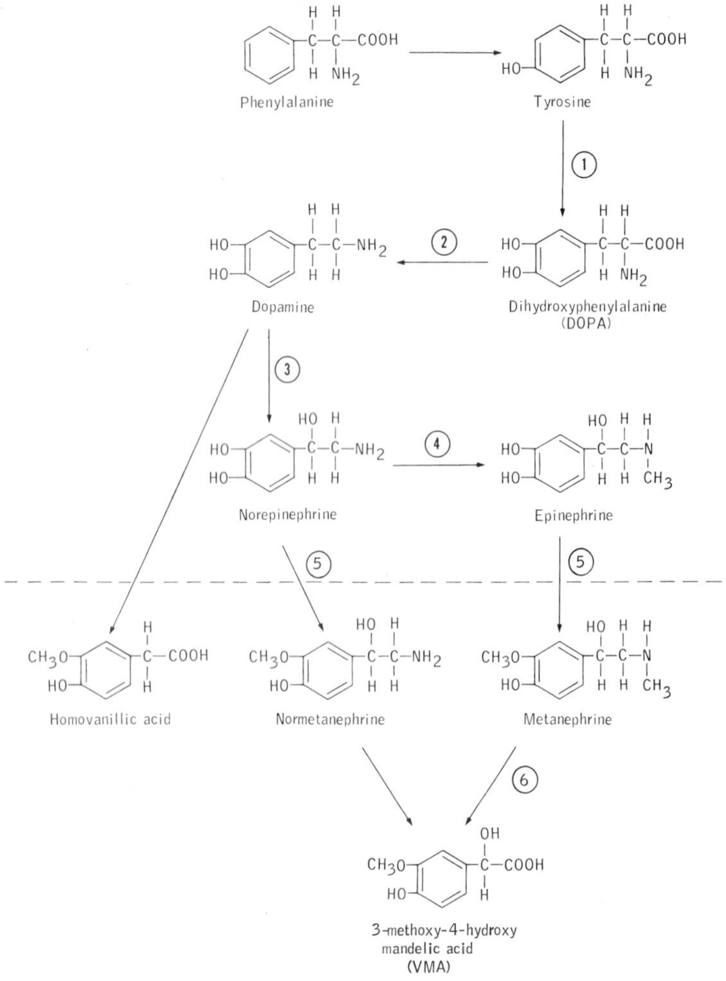

Figure 19–11. Biosynthesis (above dashed line) and metabolism (below dashed line) of the catecholamines: norepinephrine and epinephrine.

1. Tyrosine hydroxylase
2. Dopa decarboxylase
3. Dopamine-β-hydroxylase
4. Phenylethanolamine-N-methyltransferase
5. Catechol-o-methyltransferase
6. Monoamine oxidase

destructive lesions in the area of the pituitary, such as craniopharyngioma, are the most common causes of corticotropin deficiency; the defect is in the hypothalamus in many patients. In rare instances, autoimmune hypophysitis has been the cause of corticotropin deficiency.

Primary Adrenal Aplasia or Hypoplasia. Aplasia and hypoplasia have been noted in the same patient or in siblings. The disorder appears to be a defect of organogenesis, without demonstrable disturbance of pituitary function. Corticotropin is present, and the adrenal defect involves both cortisol and aldosterone. The condition occurs predominantly in males and has been twice observed in half-brothers with different fathers, establishing X-linked inheritance. Much less frequently, both male and female siblings are affected; thus, autosomal recessive inheritance is possible. It is not clear whether sporadic cases are genetically transmitted. In most patients with the X-linked form histologic examination of hypoplastic adrenal cortex reveals disorganization and cytomegaly, findings not present in the adrenals from corticotropin-deficient infants.

Most boys with the X-linked disorder do not spontaneously undergo puberty because of deficiency of gonadotropins. The mechanism is not clear; either failure of fetal adrenal androgens to activate hypothalamic-pituitary secretion of gonadotropins or primary congenital gonadotropin deficiency may be possible. Cryptorchidism is occasionally associated, but the testes respond normally to hCG stimulation.

In three families, siblings with X-linked adrenal hypoplasia have had coexisting glycerol kinase deficiency and psycho-motor retardation. Since the genes for both conditions have recently been mapped at the Xp 21.2 region, an area that also has the gene for Duchenne muscular dystrophy, a subkaryotypic deletion is probable.

Familial Glucocorticoid Deficiency. This form of chronic adrenal insufficiency is characterized by isolated deficiency of glucocorticoids, elevated levels of corticotropin, and normal aldosterone production. The salt-losing manifestations of most other forms of adrenal insufficiency do not occur; instead, patients present primarily with hypoglycemia, seizures, and pigmentation. The disorder affects both sexes equally and appears to be inherited in an autosomal recessive manner. Histologically, there is marked adrenocortical atrophy with relative sparing of the zona glomerulosa. It has been suggested that the unresponsiveness of the adrenal cortex may be due to failure of membrane attachment or to failure of activation of adenyl cyclase by corticotropin, but evidence suggests that the adrenocortical defect may result from a degenerative process. The syndrome may be heterogeneous. Most patients exhibit achalasia of the cardia, deficient tear production, and other autonomic dysfunctions. How these manifestations relate to the adrenal disorder is not clear.

Inborn Defects of Steroidogenesis. The most common causes of adrenocortical insufficiency in infancy are the salt-losing forms of congenital adrenal hyperplasia (Sec. 19.23). About half the infants with the 21-hydroxylase defect, all infants with lipoid adrenal hyperplasia, and most infants with deficiency of 3β-hydroxysteroid dehydrogenase manifest salt-losing symptoms in the newborn period. In these defects

Table 19–6. Etiologic Classification of Adrenocortical Hypofunction

Corticotropin-releasing factor deficiency
  Isolated deficiency
  Multiple deficiencies
    Congenital defects (e.g., anencephaly, septo-optic dysplasia)
    Destructive lesions (e.g., tumor)
    Idiopathic (e.g., idiopathic hypopituitarism)
Corticotropin deficiency
  Isolated
  Multiple deficiencies
    Pituitary hypoplasia or aplasia
    Destructive lesions (e.g., craniopharyngioma)
    Autoimmune hypophysitis
Primary adrenal hypoplasia or aplasia
  X-linked
    Isolated
    With glycerol kinase deficiency
  Autosomal recessive
  Sporadic?
Familial glucocorticoid deficiency
  With autonomic dysfunction
  Without autonomic dysfunction
Inborn defects of steroidogenesis
  Congenital adrenal hyperplasia
    Lipoid adrenal hyperplasia (desmolase defect)
      Severe
      Mild
    3β-Hydroxysteroid dehydrogenase deficiency
      Severe
      Mild
    21-Hydroxylase deficiency
      Classic
        Salt-loser
        Non-salt-loser
      Late onset
  Isolated defects of aldosterone synthesis
    Corticosterone methyl oxidase I
    Corticosterone methyl oxidase II
  Aldosterone unresponsiveness—pseudohypoaldosteronism
  Adrenoleukodystrophy and adrenomyeloneuropathy
  Lysosomal acid lipase deficiency (Wolman syndrome)
Destructive lesions of adrenal cortex
  Granulomatous lesions (e.g., tuberculosis)
Autoimmune adrenalitis (idiopathic Addison disease)
  Isolated
  Associated with hypoparathyroidism and/or mucocutaneous
    candidosis (Type I autoimmune polyglandular syndrome)
  Associated with autoimmune thyroid disease and insulin-
    requiring diabetes (Type II autoimmune polyglandular
    syndrome)
X-linked Addison disease
Neonatal hemorrhage
Acute infection (Waterhouse-Friderichsen syndrome)
Iatrogenic
  Abrupt cessation of exogenous corticosteroids or corticotropin
  Removal of functioning adrenal tumor
  Adrenalectomy for Cushing disease
  Drugs
    Aminoglutethimide
    Mitotane (o,p'-DDD)
    Metyrapone
    Ketoconazole
Fetal adrenal suppression—maternal hypercortisolism
  Endogenous
  Therapeutic

there is a deficiency in the synthesis of both cortisol and aldosterone.

Isolated Deficiency of Aldosterone. This rare disorder is due to a defect in either of two mixed-function oxidases, corticosterone methyl oxidase, type I or type II (CMO I or CMO II) (see Fig. 19–12). Levels of aldosterone and its metabolites are relatively or absolutely low, and levels of plasma renin activity are markedly elevated. In CMO II deficiency levels of 18-hydroxycorticosterone are greatly increased; levels of 17-ketosteroids, cortisol, and pregnanetriol are normal. There is no unusual pigmentation, and clinical manifestations consist primarily of hyponatremia, hyperkalemia, metabolic acidosis in the neonate, failure to thrive in infancy, or retardation of growth during childhood. Some adaptation or compensation occurs, the salt-losing manifestations improving with increasing age. The biosynthetic defect persists, however, and can be demonstrated in adults. The type II defect has been detected in 21 Iranian Jews, in a large North American pedigree, and in other siblings; its inheritance is autosomal recessive. Specific diagnosis depends on measurement of the ratio of 18-hydroxycorticosterone to aldosterone in plasma and/or urine; a markedly elevated ratio was found even on the first day of life in an infant at risk. Treatment consists of administration of enough salt and/or mineralocorticoid to return plasma renin activity to normal.

Pseudohypoaldosteronism. About 70 patients are known to have a salt-losing syndrome despite normal adrenocortical and renal function. Secretion and urinary excretion rates of aldosterone are elevated and remain so after salt supplementation. Administration of DOCA, fluorohydrocortisone or aldosterone does not correct the urinary sodium loss. Elevated renin activity in plasma indicates that the hyperaldosteronism is secondary to hyperactivity of the renin-angiotensin system. Besides distal renal tubules, the defect may involve salivary and sweat glands and colonic mucosal cells. The syndrome appears to be heterogeneous, with generalized target organ involvement inherited in an autosomal recessive fashion, whereas isolated renal unresponsiveness is an autosomal dominant disorder.

Destructive Lesions of Adrenal Cortex. In older children one of the more common causes of adrenal insufficiency is a destructive lesion of the adrenal gland (*Addison disease*). Tuberculosis is no longer the most frequent cause. Histoplasmosis, coccidioidomycosis, torulosis, mycosis fungoides, amyloidosis, and metastatic malignancies have been identified as causative agents in adults but not in children, in whom in most instances "idiopathic atrophy" is noted. The adrenal glands may be so small that they are not visible at autopsy, and only remnants of tissue are found in microscopic sections. Usually, however, the medulla is not destroyed, and there is lymphocytic infiltration in the area of the former cortex and in the medulla. About half of affected patients have antibodies against adrenal tissue, a finding which suggests that the adrenocortical insufficiency results from an *autoimmune adrenalitis.*

Patients with idiopathic Addison disease are exceptionally prone to a variety of other conditions known or believed to be autoimmune in origin. In individuals and families with associated hypoparathyroidism and chronic mucocutaneous candidosis, there is a high association of alopecia, malabsorption, pernicious anemia, gonadal failure, chronic active hepatitis, and vitiligo (type I autoimmune polyglandular syndrome). The candidosis and hypoparathyroidism almost always antedate the Addison disease. These patients do not have any HLA predominance. Another group of patients with Addison disease have a conspicuous association with autoimmune thyroid disease and insulin-dependent diabetes, with a predominance of HLA-DR3 and HLA-DR4 (type II autoimmune polyglandular syndrome).

Adrenoleukodystrophy. In the childhood form of this disorder symptoms usually begin from 3–12 yr of age. Central nervous system manifestations dominate the clinical course and consist of behavioral changes, disturbance of gait, dysarthria, dysphagia, and loss of vision. Eventually seizures, spastic quadriparesis, and decorticate posturing occur. Ap-

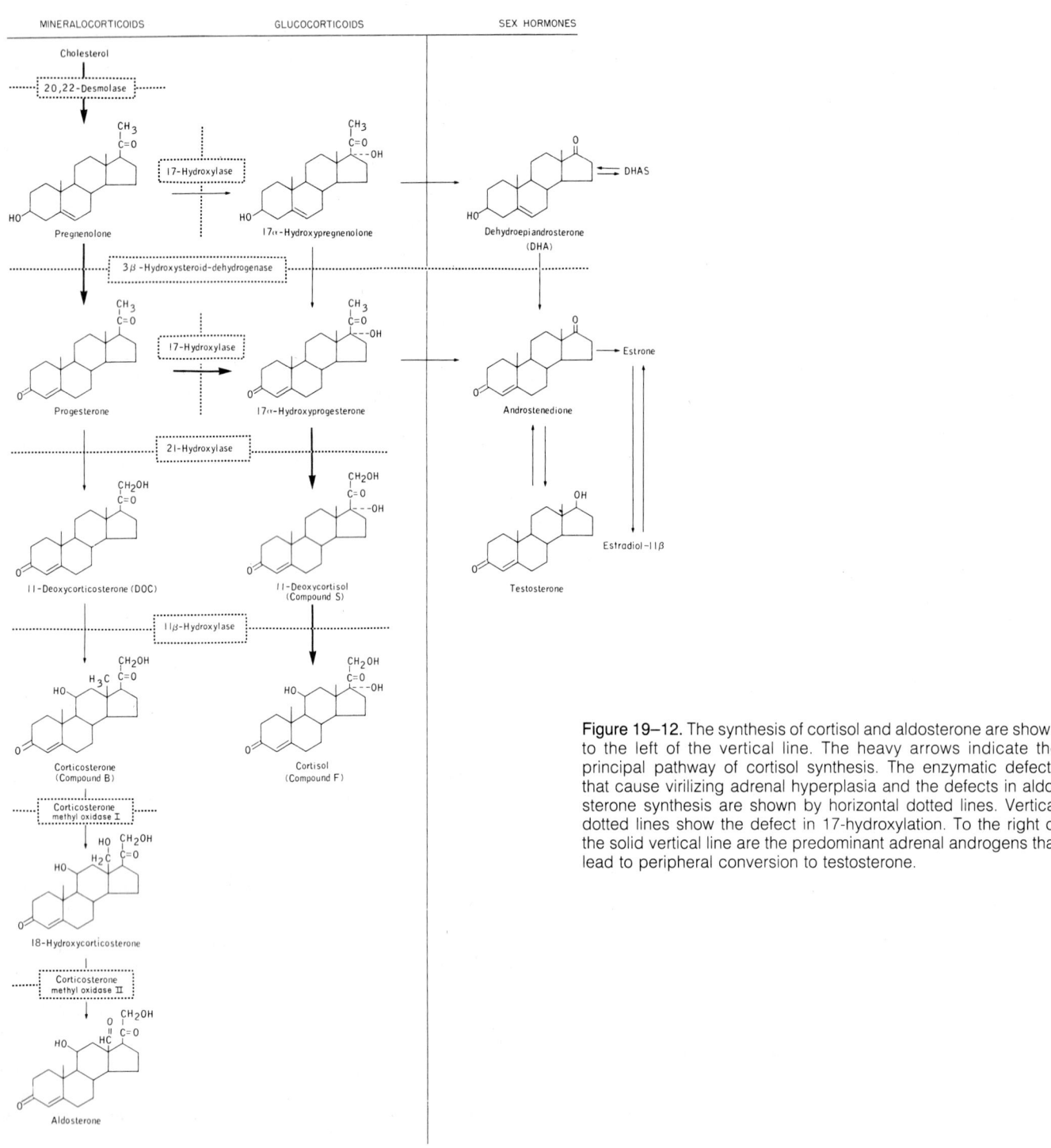

Figure 19–12. The synthesis of cortisol and aldosterone are shown to the left of the vertical line. The heavy arrows indicate the principal pathway of cortisol synthesis. The enzymatic defects that cause virilizing adrenal hyperplasia and the defects in aldosterone synthesis are shown by horizontal dotted lines. Vertical dotted lines show the defect in 17-hydroxylation. To the right of the solid vertical line are the predominant adrenal androgens that lead to peripheral conversion to testosterone.

proximately a third of patients exhibit signs and symptoms of adrenal insufficiency, usually after 4 yr of age. These develop insidiously and may antedate or appear concomitantly with the neurologic manifestations. Reduced adrenal cortical reserve may be demonstrable even in children without clinical manifestations of the disorder.

A relatively mild adult variant is known as *adrenomyeloneuropathy*. Onset is usually after 21 yr of age and is characterized by progressive leg stiffness and paralysis, ataxia, and polyneuropathy. Both types of the disorder have occurred in male siblings. X-linkage is firmly established for both types; the gene is located on the long arm of the X chromosome close to the genes for G-6-PD, color blindness, and hemophilia. It appears that there is a deficiency of a peroxisomal enzyme that oxidizes the very long chain fatty acids, such as C24:0 and C26:0 (hexicosanoic acid). Increased levels of these fatty acids are found in adrenal cortex, cerebral white matter, plasma, cultured fibroblasts, amniotic fluid, and chorionic villus biopsy. Female carriers of the gene can be identified, and prenatal diagnosis has been accomplished.

Hemorrhage into Adrenal Glands. This may occur in the neonatal period as a consequence of difficult labor or of asphyxia. The hemorrhage may be sufficiently extensive to result in death from exsanguination or from hypoadrenalism. Often the hemorrhage is asymptomatic initially and is identified by later calcification of the adrenal. On rare occasions, gradual impairment in function resulting from progressive fibrosis or cystic changes may culminate in adrenocortical insufficiency in infancy or childhood.

Waterhouse-Friderichsen Syndrome. This characteristic state of shock resulting from bacterial infection is usually associated with hemorrhage into the adrenal glands. The syndrome has been recognized most often in patients with fulminating meningococcemia, but it also occurs with septicemia caused by other organisms. The various lesions, including the adrenal hemorrhage, have been attributed to a generalized Shwartzman reaction. The circulatory collapse has been attributed to impaired adrenocortical function, but in most patients blood levels of corticosteroids are appropriately elevated. On the other hand, in some children with hemorrhagic adrenals, serum levels of corticosteroids have been undetectable. It appears that the circulatory collapse results in most instances from severe toxemia, but it may be aggravated by adrenal insufficiency.

Abrupt cessation of administration of corticotropin or a corticosteroid may result in adrenal insufficiency. Symptoms are most likely to occur after these substances have been given in large doses for a long time to patients who are subsequently subjected to stressful situations such as severe infections or surgical procedures.

Drugs. Ketoconazole, an antifungal drug, can cause adrenal insufficiency by inhibiting adrenal enzymes. Rifampicin and anticonvulsive drugs such as phenylhydantoin and phenobarbital reduce the effectiveness and bioavailability of corticosteroid replacement therapy by inducing steroid-metabolizing enzymes in the liver.

Clinical Manifestations. The age of onset of symptoms and the clinical manifestations depend on the specific etiologic factor involved. In patients with adrenal hypoplasia, defects in steroidogenesis, or pseudohypoaldosteronism, symptoms and signs begin shortly after birth and are those of salt loss. Failure to thrive, vomiting, lethargy, anorexia, and dehydration occur; circulatory collapse may be fatal.

In older children with Addison disease the onset is usually more gradual and characterized by muscular weakness, lassitude, anorexia, loss of weight, general wasting, and low blood pressure. Abdominal pain may simulate an acute abdominal process, and there may be an intense craving for salt. If the condition is not recognized and treated, *adrenal*

crisis may supervene. The patient suddenly becomes cyanotic, the skin cold, and the pulse weak and rapid. The blood pressure falls, and respirations are rapid and labored. In the absence of immediate and intensive therapy, the course is rapidly fatal. In patients with inadequately treated chronic adrenal insufficiency, crises may be precipitated by infection, trauma, excessive fatigue, or drugs such as morphine, barbiturates, laxatives, thyroid hormone, or insulin.

Increased pigmentation of the skin should always alert the clinician to the possibility of adrenocortical insufficiency. This manifestation occurs in those conditions in which there are deficiency of cortisol and excessive secretion of corticotropin, as in primary adrenal hypoplasia, familial glucocorticoid deficiency, and Addison disease. Pigmentation may be first apparent on the face and hands and is most intense around the genitalia, umbilicus, axillae, nipples, and joints. Scars and freckles may be especially pigmented. Areas of depigmentation (vitiligo) may be interspersed with dark areas. The exposed areas of the skin are the most intensely affected, and failure of a suntan to disappear may be the first clue to the condition. In the buccal mucosa the pigmentation is usually bluish brown.

The presenting manifestations may be those of hypoglycemia, particularly in the neonate with congenital adrenal hypoplasia. Patients with adrenocortical insufficiency are deficient in gluconeogenic substrates; the hypoglycemia may be associated with ketosis, therefore, and confused with ketotic hypoglycemia (Sec. 20.10).

In young children with familial glucocorticoid deficiency, salt-losing manifestations do not occur, and the symptoms are primarily increased pigmentation and hypoglycemia. Symptoms may begin shortly after birth and almost always by 5 yr of age. Many affected children have had other treatment for seizures before the hypoglycemic cause was recognized.

In patients with deficiency of corticotropin, pigmentation does not occur. Hypoglycemia is the usual presenting manifestation, but salt-losing is uncommon, presumably because of residual ability of the adrenal to secrete aldosterone.

In those conditions known to have a genetic basis it is important to evaluate fully the adrenocortical function of siblings.

Laboratory Data. When salt-losing manifestations are present, the levels of sodium and chloride in the serum are usually low and that of potassium elevated, with increased plasma renin activity. Urinary excretions of sodium and chloride are increased and that of potassium decreased. The nonprotein nitrogen level in plasma is elevated if there is dehydration. Hypoglycemia may be striking or become manifest only after prolonged fasting. The blood eosinophils may be increased in number. When hemorrhage, adrenal cysts, or tuberculosis have been causative factors, roentgenograms of the abdomen may reveal calcifications in the area of the adrenals. Ultrasonography and computed tomography may also be helpful. A small and narrow roentgenographic shadow of the heart reflects hypovolemia. Electrocardiographic changes reflect potassium levels. The electroencephalogram may show a greatly decreased content or absence of low-voltage, fast-frequency waves.

The most definitive test is measurement of plasma levels of cortisol before and after administration of corticotropin; resting levels are low, and no increase occurs after administration of corticotropin. Occasionally, normal resting levels which do not increase after administration of corticotropin indicate an absence of adrenocortical reserve. A low initial level followed by a significant response to corticotropin may indicate adrenal insufficiency secondary to endogenous insufficiency of corticotropin. Levels of corticotropin are elevated in disorders of primary cortisol deficiency and are low when the adrenal insufficiency is secondary to a hypothalamic or pituitary disorder. Testing with corticotropin-releasing hormone may be helpful in localizing the defect.

Measurement of plasma levels of 17-hydroxyprogesterone is necessary in infants suspected of congenital adrenal hyperplasia. Aldosterone secretion is low in salt-losing congenital adrenal hyperplasia, in adrenal hypoplasia, and in Addison disease, but its measurement is rarely needed for diagnosis. Measurement of aldosterone is necessary in infants suspected of isolated defects of aldosterone synthesis (in whom it is low) and in those suspected of pseudohypoaldosteronism (in whom it is usually elevated). In patients with familial glucocorticoid deficiency aldosterone levels are normal and rise appropriately to salt deprivation.

Treatment. Treatment for acute adrenal insufficiency or for crises must be immediate and vigorous. If the cause of adrenal insufficiency has not been established, a blood sample should be obtained prior to therapy for determination of levels of cortisol, 17-hydroxyprogesterone, and adrenal androgens. Intravenous administration of 5% glucose in 0.9% saline solution should be given to correct the hypoglycemia and the sodium loss. Concomitantly, a water-soluble form of hydrocortisone, such as hydrocortisone hemisuccinate, should be given intravenously. High levels are achieved instantaneously, and large doses can be used safely. As much as 25 mg for infants and 75 mg for older children should be given intravenously at 6 hr intervals for the first 24 hr. These doses may be reduced during the next 24 hr if progress is satisfactory. A salt-retaining hormone should be added to maintain electrolyte balance; desoxycorticosterone acetate (DOCA) in oil may be used in doses of 1–5 mg/24 hr intramuscularly. After the first 48 hr, if oral intake is satisfactory, the intravenous fluids may be discontinued and the corticosteroid given orally as cortisol in doses of 5–20 mg at 8 hr intervals. Further reduction can then be accomplished until maintenance levels and a stable clinical situation are achieved. The daily administration of DOCA is continued throughout this period of treatment.

Once the acute manifestations are under control, most patients require chronic replacement therapy for their deficiencies of aldosterone and cortisol. The cortisol may be given orally in daily doses of 5 mg twice daily for infants, and 15 mg twice daily for adolescents. During situations of stress, such as periods of infection or operative procedures, the dose of hydrocortisone should be increased. The daily injections of DOCA can be replaced by fluorohydrocortisone, administered orally in doses of 0.05–0.1 mg/24 hr. Measurements of serum renin activity are useful in monitoring adequacy of mineralocorticoid replacement.

Overdosage with DOCA or fluorohydrocortisone results in hypertension and may lead to cardiac enlargement and edema because of excessive retention of sodium chloride and water; excessive loss of potassium may produce weakness or paralysis.

Patients with primary corticotropin deficiency or with familial glucocorticoid deficiency do not require a salt-retaining hormone since their ability to secrete aldosterone is intact. On the other hand, patients with primary defects in aldosterone synthesis do not require cortisol; a salt-retaining hormone may be required, but in milder forms the addition of salt to the diet is adequate to maintain homeostasis. In patients with pseudohypoaldosteronism administration of salt-retaining hormones does not correct the urinary sodium loss; therapy must consist of supplementation with sodium chloride. The disorder is self-limited and treatment may be discontinued after 1–2 yr. In newborn infants with adrenal hemorrhage vitamins K and C and transfusions with whole blood may be indicated.

Patients with Addison disease must be closely observed for the development of other endocrine disorders. Appropriate counseling is indicated for disorders known to have a genetic basis.

ADRENOCORTICAL HYPERFUNCTION

Four syndromes are attributable to hyperadrenocorticism: the *adrenogenital syndrome, Cushing syndrome, hyperaldosteronism,* and *feminization* (Table 19–7).

19.23 ADRENOGENITAL SYNDROME

The adrenogenital syndrome is produced by congenital adrenal hyperplasia and by virilizing adrenocortical tumors.

Congenital Adrenal Hyperplasia

Pathogenesis. When the adrenogenital syndrome is associated with congenital adrenal hyperplasia, it is caused by an inborn defect in the biosynthesis of adrenal cortisol. Five enzymatic defects are known (Fig. 19–12); virilization is associated with some. The deficiency of cortisol results in increased secretion of corticotropin, which leads in turn to adrenocortical hyperplasia and overproduction of intermediary metabolites. Each defect is inherited as an autosomal recessive trait, and each exhibits severe and mild forms, presumably because of allelic variants.

Deficiency of 21-Hydroxylase accounts for 95% of affected patients. 21-Hydroxylase is a cytochrome P_{450} enzyme. The gene locus is on the short arm of chromosome 6, within the HLA complex, and is closely linked to HLA-B and to the C4A

Table 19–7. Etiologic Classification of Adrenocortical Hyperfunction

Excess androgen (adrenogenital syndrome)
  Congenital adrenal hyperplasia
    21-Hydroxylase defect
    11β-Hydroxylase defect
    3β-Hydroxysteroid dehydrogenase defect (females)
  Tumor
    Carcinoma
  Adenoma—isolated testosterone secretion
Excess cortisol (Cushing syndrome)
  Bilateral adrenal hyperplasia
    Hypersecretion of corticotropin (Cushing disease)
    Ectopic secretion of corticotropin
    Exogenous corticotropin
  Tumor
    Carcinoma
    Adenoma
      Adrenocortical nodular dysplasia
Excess mineralocorticoid (hypertensive hypokalemic syndrome)
  Primary hyperaldosteronism
    Adrenal hyperplasia
      Glucocorticoid suppressible
      Nonsuppressible
    Tumor
      Adenoma
      Carcinoma
  Desoxycorticosterone excess
    Adrenal hyperplasia
      11β-Hydroxylase defect
      17-Hydroxylase defect
    Tumor—carcinoma
Unidentified mineralocorticoid excess
  11β-hydroxysteroid dehydrogenase deficiency
Excess estrogen (adrenal feminization syndrome)
  Carcinoma
  Adenoma
Mixed hypercorticism—tumor

and C4B complement genes. There are two classic forms of the disease: salt-wasting and simple virilizing. When 21-hydroxylase deficiency is complete or severe, it usually results in virilization early in life. The two disease forms tend to have different HLA-B associations: HLA-Bw47 for the salt-wasting type, and HLA-B5 for the simple virilizing type. The classic variant affects approximately 1/5000 births (1/500 among Yupic Eskimos).

The nonclassic variant (also referred to as late onset, attenuated, or cryptic) is a less severe form of 21-hydroxylase deficiency with onset of symptoms usually during or after puberty. This variant is strongly associated with HLA-B14. It appears to be more common than the classic defect, especially among Ashkenazi Jews, Yugoslavs, and Italians.

Deficiency of 11β-Hydroxylase accounts for 5–8% of cases of congenital adrenal hyperplasia; about 100 cases have been reported. In Israel, among Jews of Moroccan or Iranian ancestry, this defect is the most common cause of the syndrome. Classic and mild forms are known. Hypertension, a common but not invariable finding, is absent in the first few years of life. A mild form of the disorder has been detected in normotensive women with normal genitalia who have hirsutism, acne, and menstrual irregularities. Plasma characteristically contains large amounts of 11-deoxycortisol (compound S) and of desoxycorticosterone (DOC). The elevated level of DOC is thought to cause the hypertension and to prevent salt-losing symptoms, although several affected infants have manifested salt wasting in the neonatal period. Unlike 21-hydroxylase, 11β-hydroxylase is not HLA-linked.

Deficiency of 3β-hydroxysteroid dehydrogenase. (3-β-HSD) has been reported in several dozen patients. Salt-wasting is usual. Girls are only slightly virilized at birth; boys are incompletely virilized, with hypospadias. Incomplete defects without salt-losing and/or with normal genitalia have been reported. A variant with onset during or after puberty, with hirsutism and/or primary amenorrhea, also occurs. The hallmark of this defect is marked elevation of the Δ^5 steroids (such as pregnenolone) preceding the enzymatic block (Fig. 19–12). On the other hand, 17-OHP in plasma may be markedly elevated as a consequence of extra-adrenal 3-β-HSD activity. These patients are readily mistaken for those with 21-hydroxylase deficiency, if 17-OHP levels alone are measured in the newborn period. The ratio of Δ^5 to Δ^4 steroids in urine is more than 1, and the plasma Δ^5 androstenediol/testosterone ratio is usually more than 4. The inadequate virilization in males is a consequence of deficiency of 3-β-HSD in the testes.

Lipoid Adrenal Hyperplasia has been reported in 32 patients, 18 of whom were Japanese. Failure of conversion of cholesterol to pregnenolone is due to a defect in the cholesterol side-chain cleavage enzyme $P_{450}SCC$, formerly termed 20,22-desmolase. There is marked accumulation of lipids and cholesterol in the adrenal cortex, with failure of synthesis of any adrenal steroids. The same enzymatic defect is present in the testis, preventing synthesis of testicular hormones. As a consequence, males are phenotypically female and females exhibit no genital abnormality. Salt-losing manifestations are usual, and most patients have died in early infancy. Because adrenal steroid levels are not elevated in this form of adrenal hyperplasia, affected infants are apt to be confused with those with adrenal hypoplasia.

17-Hydroxylase Deficiency has been described in approximately 18 patients. Deficiency of the enzyme leads to decreased synthesis of cortisol and sex steroids. Overproduction of progesterone, 11-deoxycorticosterone (DOC), corticosterone (B), and 18-hydroxycorticosterone leads to hypertension, hypokalemia, and renin-aldosterone suppression (Fig. 19–12). Affected females exhibit absent secondary sexual characteristics and primary amenorrhea. Males present with hypospadias and cryptorchidism, or may be female in form, with inguinal testes. This defect must be considered in the differential diagnosis of male pseudohermaphroditism or of testicular feminization. 17-Hydroxylase deficiency in females must be considered in the differential diagnosis of primary hypogonadism (See Sec. 19.42).

Clinical Manifestations. The majority of patients with congenital adrenal hyperplasia have the defect in 21-hydroxylation and exhibit the classic form of the disease. About 50% of affected patients have the compensated variant of the disorder without salt losing.

Patients Without Salt Losing. In the *male* the main clinical manifestations are those of premature isosexual development. The infant usually appears normal at birth, but signs of sexual and somatic precocity may appear within the first 6 mo of life or develop more gradually, becoming evident at 4–5 yr of age or later. Enlargement of the penis, scrotum, and prostate, appearance of pubic hair, and development of acne and a deep voice are noted. Muscles are well developed, and bone age is advanced for chronologic age. Premature closure of the epiphyses causes growth to stop relatively early, and adult stature is stunted.

The testes are normal in size so that they appear relatively small in contrast to the enlarged penis. Occasionally, ectopic adrenocortical cells in the testes of patients with adrenal hyperplasia become hyperplastic just as the adrenal glands do, producing enlargement of the testes. Spermatogenesis does not take place. Mental development is usually normal, but the abnormal physical development may result in behavioral problems.

In the *female* congenital adrenal hyperplasia results in female pseudohermaphroditism (Fig. 19–13). Since the disorder of steroidogenesis begins early in fetal life, there is almost always evidence of some degree of masculinization at birth. It is manifested by enlargement of the clitoris and varying degrees of labial fusion. The vagina has a common opening with the urethra (urogenital sinus). The clitoris may be so enlarged that it resembles a penis, and, since the urethra opens below this organ, a mistaken diagnosis of hypospadias and cryptorchidism is often made. Occasionally, the urogenital sinus extends to the tip of the phallus, and the genitalia resemble those of a cryptorchid male. The severity of the virilization is in general greater in infants who are salt losers than in those who are not. The internal genital organs are those of a normal female (Fig. 19–14).

After birth the masculinization progresses. Pubic and axillary hair develops prematurely, acne appears, and the voice assumes a masculine quality. Affected girls are tall for their age, and ossification is advanced; they show good muscular development and, in general, have the body build of a boy. Although the internal genitalia are female, breast development and menstruation do not occur unless the excessive production of androgens is suppressed by adequate treatment.

A number of such virilized female pseudohermaphrodites whose condition was not diagnosed until adult life have been erroneously reared as males. These patients have behaved in every way as males, including having sexual intercourse; some have had satisfactory (albeit infertile) marriages.

With the *11-hydroxylase defect* salt-losing manifestations do not occur. Most patients are hypertensive, but several have been normotensive or have had intermittent hypertension only. The disorder has been diagnosed only rarely in early life, but hypertension was not present. Several prepubertal children with this defect presented with gynecomastia. Virilization occurs in all patients and is as severe as with the 21-hydroxylase defect.

Patients with Salt Losing. In patients with salt-losing variant, symptoms begin shortly after birth, with failure to regain birth weight, progressive weight loss, and dehydration. Vom-

\n\n\n

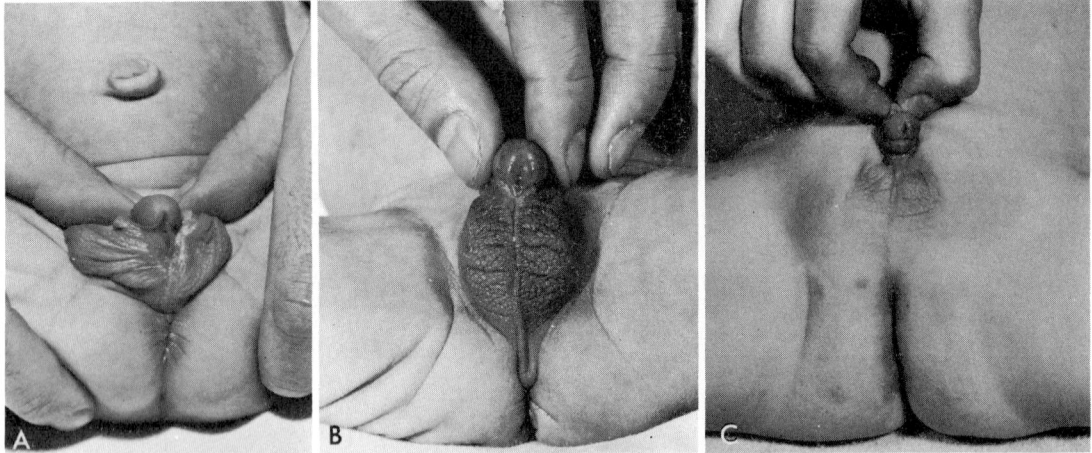

Figure 19–13. Three female pseudohemaphrodites with untreated congenital adrenal hyperplasia. All were erroneously assigned male sex at birth, and each had normal female sex-chromosome complement. Infants *A* and *B* were salt losers and were diagnosed in early infancy. Infant *C* was referred at 1 yr of age because of bilateral cryptorchidism. Note completely penile urethra; such complete degrees of masculinization in females with adrenal hyperplasia are rare; most such infants are salt losers.

iting is prominent, with anorexia. Disturbances in cardiac rate and rhythm may occur, with cyanosis and dyspnea. Without treatment, collapse and death usually occur within a few weeks.

In females virilization of the external genitalia in an infant with the above manifestations directs attention to the correct diagnosis. In the male, on the other hand, the genitalia appear normal, and clinical manifestations are apt to be confused with those of pyloric stenosis, intestinal obstruction, heart disease, cow's milk intolerance, or other causes of failure to thrive.

Familial homogeneity of defect is usually observed for the salt-losing and non–salt-losing forms. Under conditions of stress or sodium deprivation, salt losing may be provoked in compensated patients.

Patients with the *3β-hydroxysteroid dehydrogenase* defect are usually salt losers but less virilized. In the female labial fusion and enlargement of the clitoris may be mild and escape detection; rarely, the genitalia are normal. In the male varying degrees of hypospadias may occur, with or without bifid scrotum and/or cryptorchidism.

Late-Onset 21-Hydroxylase Variant. In this attenuated form the most common manifestation is appearance of varying degrees of hirsutism after onset of normal puberty. Menses may be normal or irregular and dysovulatory. Completely asymptomatic females with the biochemical defect have been ascertained in HLA-identical siblings. Males are always asymptomatic. Differences in sensitivity to androgens may explain the differences in clinical expression of the disorder in sisters. About 75% of patients are HLA-B14, and it has

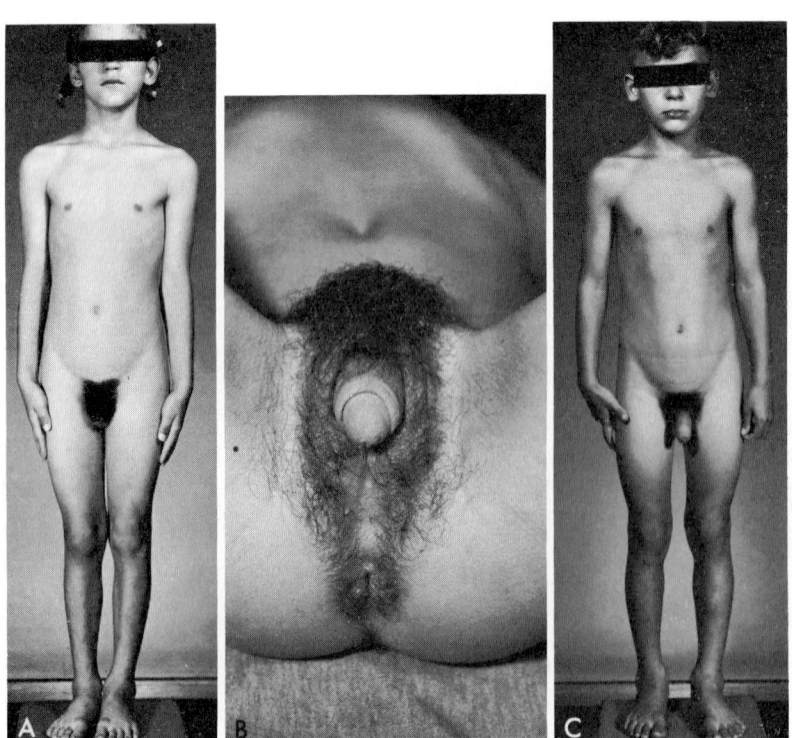

Figure 19–14. *A*, A 6-yr-old girl with congenital virilizing adrenal hyperplasia. Height age, 8.5 yr; bone age, 13 yr; urinary 17-ketosteroids, 50 mg/24 hr. *B*, Note clitoral enlargement and labial fusion. *C*, Five yr old brother of girl in *A* was not considered abnormal by parents. Height age, 8 yr; bone age, 12.5 yr; urinary 17-ketosteroids, 36 mg/24 hr.

been estimated that 6% of North American caucasians are carriers for this gene.

Laboratory Data. Salt losers may have low serum concentrations of sodium and chloride and elevated levels of potassium and nonprotein nitrogen. Plasma levels of renin are elevated. In classic 21-hydroxylase deficiency, plasma levels of progesterone and 17-hydroxyprogesterone (17-OHP) are markedly elevated. Levels of 17-OHP are especially helpful in diagnosis, but they are normally high during the first 2–3 days of life and may range as high as levels found in affected patients; by the 3rd day, however, levels in normal infants fall and those in affected infants rise to clearly diagnostic levels. Blood levels of cortisol are usually low in patients with the salt-losing type but normal in those with the simple virilizing type. A large part of the virilization is caused by increased levels of testosterone; the excess 17-OHP is partially diverted to androstenedione, which is converted to testosterone in the periphery (see Fig. 19–12). Levels of urinary 17-ketosteroids and pregnanetriol are elevated; 24-hour urine collections are often unnecessary, however, since radioimmunoassay permits measurement in plasma of the levels of the steroids involved in all forms of congenital adrenal hyperplasia.

In the late-onset variant of congenital adrenal hyperplasia, basal plasma levels of 17-OHP are not as high as in the classic form and may even be normal. There is, however, a dramatic rise in level 60 min following an intravenous bolus of 0.25 mg of ACTH (1–24).

In patients with the 11-hydroxylase defect, plasma levels of 11-deoxycorticosterone (DOC) and 11-deoxycortisol (compound S) are elevated. Urinary levels of their tetrahydro derivatives (THDOC and THS) are also elevated.

The 3β-hydroxysteroid dehydrogenase defect is characterized by markedly elevated Δ^5 steroids such as pregnenolone. 17-OHP levels are also elevated, however, and the condition may be confused with the 21-hydroxylase defect. It is necessary to determine the ratios of Δ^5 to Δ^4 steroids in plasma and/or urine for definitive diagnosis.

Affected females are chromatin positive and have an XX karyotype; males have a normal XY chromosome constitution. Injection of contrast medium into the urogenital sinus of female pseudohermaphrodites usually demonstrates vagina and uterus. Ultrasonography is also helpful.

Diagnosis. Congenital adrenal hyperplasia in an infant or child should always alert one to the diagnosis in later siblings. The salt-losing form of the disorder must be suspected in any infant who fails to thrive and especially in female infants with ambiguous external genitalia. When virilization occurs postnatally, in either male or female, a virilizing adrenocortical tumor must be considered in the differential diagnosis.

An adrenal tumor may be palpable or suggested on pyelography by displacement of the adjacent kidney. Ultrasonography or CT scans may be necessary if hormonal studies have ruled out congenital adrenal hyperplasia. Urinary 17-ketosteroid excretion is elevated with congenital hyperplasia and with cortical tumors, but very high values favor the diagnosis of neoplasm. High levels of urinary pregnanetriol are highly suggestive of adrenal hyperplasia. Administration of hydrocortisone quickly reduces excretion of urinary 17-ketosteroids to normal levels in patients with congenital adrenal hyperplasia but does not do so in those with a virilizing tumor. Corticosteroids, by inhibiting secretion of corticotropin, reduce the excessive stimulation of the adrenals in patients with hyperplasia, whereas adrenocortical tumors are not subject to pituitary regulation.

In males with virilization interstitial cell tumor of the testis and true precocious puberty must also be considered in differential diagnosis. In true precocious puberty, gonadotropins may be elevated, and 17-hydroxyprogesterone levels in plasma are normal; the testes are usually well developed.

Females with this condition must be differentiated from those with other causes for ambiguity of the external genitalia. Only in this condition are urinary 17-ketosteroids and plasma 17-hydroxyprogesterone levels elevated. Males with 3β-hydroxysteroid dehydrogenase defect may be confused with female pseudohermaphrodites because they lack normal virilization of the external genitalia. These male patients are 46XY and do not have elevated urinary pregnanetriol levels; they are thus easily differentiated from the 46XX female pseudohermaphrodite.

Detection of the heterozygous carrier is often, but not always, possible by measuring the rate of increase of 17-hydroxyprogesterone 60 min after an intravenous bolus injection of 0.25 mg of ACTH (1–24). In families in which there is an affected individual with 21-hydroxylase deficiency, HLA genotyping provides a reliable basis for counseling.

Prenatal Diagnosis and Treatment. Elevated levels of 17-hydroxyprogesterone and Δ^4-androstenedione in amniotic fluid permit prenatal diagnosis by midgestation of infants with 21-hydroxylase deficiency. HLA typing of the fetus and affected siblings permits confirmation of the diagnosis and detection of heterozygotes. Early reports suggest that the genital abnormality in females may be mitigated by administration of dexamethasone to the mother before 9 fetal weeks, even before a fetal diagnosis is possible.

Prenatal diagnosis of 11β-hydroxylase deficiency has been made by demonstrating increased levels of tetrahydro-17-deoxycortisol in amniotic fluid and in maternal urine during pregnancy.

Treatment. Hydrocortisone inhibits excessive production of adrenal androgens and stems the progressive virilization. The maintenance dose may be administered orally as follows: 10–15 mg/24 hr to children under 5 yr of age; 15–20 mg/24 hr to children from 5–12; and 20–30 mg/24 hr after 12 yr of age. These daily doses should be divided into two administrations. Such amounts suppress excessive secretion of androgens without producing undesirable effects. Serial determinations of the urinary levels of 17-ketosteroids and pregnanetriol are helpful but not essential guides to dosage. Concentrations in plasma of 17-hydroxyprogesterone or of androstenedione at 9 A.M. reflect adrenal suppression reliably and may indicate inadequate control earlier than urinary studies. Measurements of growth, bone age, and plasma renin activity also give important indications of adequacy of treatment.

Patients who have disturbances of electrolyte regulation ("salt losers") and elevated plasma renin activity require increased salt intake and mineralocorticoid therapy in addition to hydrocortisone. Dehydrated infants may require 4–8 g of sodium chloride for adequate replacement therapy during the first 24 hr. DOCA, 2–4 mg, should be given daily by intramuscular injection. The blood pressure should be carefully monitored since excessive mineralocorticoid can cause hypertension. Once control has been achieved, maintenance therapy is instituted with fluorohydrocortisone, in once daily doses of 0.05–0.10 mg; the dose should be sufficient to reduce plasma renin activity to normal. This medication is continued indefinitely in salt losers. Non–salt losers also may manifest elevated plasma renin activity and require a mineralocorticoid. With this regimen additional sodium chloride is usually not required, but patients are given free access to salt.

The administration of hydrocortisone must be continued indefinitely in *all* patients. Increased doses are indicated during periods of stress such as infection or surgery or during periods of decreased salt intake for both salt losers and non–salt losers, including those with the 11-hydroxylase defect, since they all have defective adrenal reserve.

The enlarged clitoris of female infants usually requires surgical correction; a good age for this elective surgery is 6–12 mo. Recession of the clitoris is preferred, rather than its removal; the clitoris is freed and repositioned beneath the pubis with preservation of the glans, corporal components, and all neural and vascular elements. Parents should be reassured that it has been established that complete sexual gratification, including orgasm, can be achieved. The menarche occurs at the appropriate age in most girls who have been well controlled. It is not exceptional for adolescents past the age of 16 not to have begun menstruating; such delay is probably related to suboptimal control.

Non-salt losers, particularly males, are frequently not diagnosed until 3–7 yr of age, at which time osseous maturation may be 5 yr or more in advance of chronologic age. Institution of treatment slows growth and osseous maturation to more nearly normal rates in some children; in others, especially if the bone age is 12 yr or more, spontaneous puberty may occur, therapy with hydrocortisone having suppressed production of adrenal androgens and permitted release of pituitary gonadotropins if the appropriate level of hypothalamic maturation is present. This form of superimposed true precocious puberty may now be effectively treated with a luteinizing hormone–releasing hormone analogue.

Males who have had inadequate corticosteroid therapy may develop bilateral testicular tumors, which may or may not regress with increased dosage. The tumors are thought to arise from pluripotential cells present in the testes. Prolonged inadequate adrenal suppression may also result in adenomatous changes in the adrenal gland.

Virilizing Adrenocortical Tumors

Tumors of the adrenal cortex may result in masculinization in girls and pseudoprecocious puberty in boys. Hypertension is common, and manifestations of Cushing syndrome may accompany virilization since these tumors frequently secrete excessive cortisol and mineralocorticoids in addition to androgens.

In males the symptoms are usually the same as those occurring with non-salt-losing congenital adrenal hyperplasia. It is virtually impossible to differentiate the two conditions on clinical grounds. In females virilizing tumors of the adrenal cause masculinization of a previously normal female, whereas congenital hyperplasia is almost always associated with genital abnormalities at birth. Virilization in congenital adrenal hyperplasia may have its onset during childhood. An adrenal adenoma is known to have caused intrauterine clitoral enlargement and mild labial fusion.

Tumors of the adrenal (with or without Cushing syndrome) may be associated with hemihypertrophy, usually during the first few years of life. These tumors are also associated with Beckwith syndrome and other congenital defects, particularly genitourinary tract and central nervous system abnormalities and hamartomatous defects.

Urinary 17-ketosteroids and plasma levels of DHEAS and testosterone are usually increased, often markedly. In four infants with predominantly testosterone-producing adenomas, urinary 17-ketosteroids were normal or near normal. Assay of testosterone production is essential to the investigation of virilized patients. Roentgenographic studies may reveal calcification in the tumor or displacement of a kidney. Ultrasonography and computed tomography are indicated and may detect masses as small as 1.3 cm. Selective venous sampling is rarely any longer indicated.

The treatment is surgical; a transperitoneal approach is usually recommended. Some of these neoplasms are highly malignant and metastasize widely, but cure with regression of the masculinizing features may follow removal of less malignant encapsulated tumors.

A neoplasm of one adrenal may produce atrophy of the other as excessive production of cortical hormones by the tumor suppresses stimulation of the normal gland by ACTH. Consequently, adrenal insufficiency may follow surgical removal of the tumor. This situation can be avoided by giving 100 mg of hydrocortisone daily, starting on the day of operation and continuing for 3–4 days postoperatively. It may also be necessary to give corticotropin concurrently with cortisol to reactivate the atrophied gland. Adequate quantities of water, sodium chloride, and glucose must also be provided. On rare occasions, the tumors are bilateral, and in at least five instances the contralateral adrenal was absent; in such instances replacement therapy must be continued indefinitely.

Tumors that are easily resected and weigh less than 150 g have a good prognosis. If the tumor is large or incompletely removed, prognosis is guarded. Radiotherapy is not generally helpful. Adrenal androgen levels should be measured at monthly intervals to detect recurrences early. Intensive therapy with mitotane (o,p′-DDD), an isomer of DDD, is indicated for inoperable tumors and for recurrences. This agent can induce regression of metastases and of abnormal steroid excretion through suppression of hormonal production in the tumor; only a few long-term survivals are known. In at least eight patients a second primary tumor has developed, the central nervous system being the most frequent site.

19.24 CUSHING SYNDROME

Cushing syndrome, a characteristic pattern of obesity with associated hypertension, is the result of maintenance of abnormally high blood levels of cortisol by hyperfunction of the adrenal cortex.

Etiology. In infants Cushing syndrome is most often caused by a functioning adrenocortical tumor, usually a malignant carcinoma but occasionally a benign adenoma. Over 50% of cortical tumors occur in children 3 yr of age or younger and 85% in children 7 or younger. Patients with cortical tumors often exhibit a mixed form of hypercorticism due to overproduction of such other steroids as androgens, estrogens, and aldosterone.

Primary pigmented nodular adrenocortical disease is being increasingly recognized as a cause of Cushing syndrome in infants and children. The characteristic feature is small (<4 mm) pigmented (black, brown, dark-green, red) adrenal nodules. Several instances have been dominantly inherited or have affected only siblings. In some families, lentigenes, cardiac and cutaneous myxomas, and mammary, testicular, and pituitary tumors may be associated.

In children over 7 yr of age bilateral adrenal hyperplasia (Cushing disease) is usually found. In 1932 Cushing attributed this entity to a basophilic adenoma of the pituitary, but CT scans find such tumors in only 20% of affected children. On the other hand, covert pituitary adenomas (microadenomas) are present in most instances of Cushing disease, and resection of these tumors results in correction of the hypercorticalism. In some children the pituitary tumors become overt after adrenalectomy (Nelson syndrome); these consist principally of chromophobe cells and produce increased levels of β-lipotropin and β-endorphin as well as of ACTH. There are only two reports of ACTH-secreting tumors in infants with Cushing syndrome.

Bilateral hyperplasia of the adrenals may also result from ectopic production of ACTH. In adults a variety of tumors have caused this form of Cushing syndrome, in particular thymoma and bronchogenic carcinoma. Cushing syndrome has been associated with an islet cell carcinoma of the pancreas in four children, with neuroblastoma or ganglioneuroblastoma in several children, with a hemangiopericytoma arising from the cerebral tentorium in a 7 yr old boy, and in two children with Wilms tumors.

Prolonged exogenous administration of corticotropin or hydrocortisone or its analogues results in a clinical pattern identical to the spontaneous disorder and is frequently referred to as cushingoid syndrome.

Clinical Manifestations. Symptoms may begin in the neonatal period and have been recognized in infants under 1 yr of age on at least 35 occasions. Early in life girls outnumber boys 3:1, and adrenocortical tumors (carcinoma, adenoma, and nodular hyperplasia) are the usual causative lesions. The disorder appears to be more severe and the clinical findings more flagrant than later in life. The face is rounded, with cheeks prominent and flushed (moon facies). The chin is doubled, there is a buffalo hump, and generalized obesity is common. Signs of abnormal masculinization, due to the androgen production of tumors, occur frequently; accordingly, there may be hypertrichosis on the face and trunk, pubic hair, acne, deepening of the voice, and, in girls, enlargement of the clitoris. Growth is impaired, length falling below the 3rd percentile, except when significant virilization produces normal or even accelerated growth. Hypertension is common and may lead to heart failure. An increased susceptibility to infection may lead to fatal sepsis. Infants with Cushing syndrome, despite a robust appearance, are generally very fragile. Occasionally, the condition is associated with hemihypertrophy or other congenital defects.

In older children bilateral hyperplasia of the adrenals is the most common lesion, and the sex incidence is equal. In addition to obesity, short stature is a common presenting feature. Gradual onset of obesity and deceleration or cessation of growth may be the only early manifestations. Purplish striae on the hips, abdomen, and thighs are common. Pubertal development may be delayed, or amenorrhea may occur in girls past menarche. Weakness, headache, deterioration in schoolwork, and emotional lability may be prominent. Hypertension is usual. Renal stones have occurred both in older children and in infants.

Laboratory Data. Polycythemia, lymphopenia, and eosinopenia are common. The glucose tolerance test may be diabetic despite elevated levels of insulin. Levels of serum electrolytes are usually normal, but potassium may be decreased.

Cortisol levels in blood are usually elevated, but these may fluctuate widely from day to day, and repeated determinations may be required to establish the diagnosis. In most patients with Cushing syndrome, the normal diurnal rhythm in levels of plasma cortisol is abolished; measurements of the levels at 8 A.M. and 8 P.M. may be useful except in children under 3 yr of age, in whom the circadian rhythm is not always established. Urinary excretion of 17-hydroxycorticosteroids is increased (>5 mg/m^2/24 hr). Urinary 17-ketosteroids may be increased, particularly in virilized patients; very high levels usually indicate adrenal carcinoma. Children and adolescents with Cushing disease usually have normal levels of DHEAS and DHEA.

Special studies are frequently necessary to establish the definitive diagnosis or to differentiate hyperplasia from tumor. The low-dose dexamethasone suppression test will suppress urinary excretion of corticosteroids in normal healthy children but not in those with Cushing syndrome. This steroid (20 μg/kg/body weight/24 hr) is given in four equal doses each day for 2 days. Urinary 17-hydroxycorticosteroids in normal children decrease to less than 1.5 mg/m^2/24 hr. The same test with a larger dose (80 μg/kg/24 hr) will suppress the adrenals in children with Cushing disease due to bilateral adrenal hyperplasia but not in those with adrenocortical tumors or ectopic secretion of ACTH. The reliability of the test is improved when free cortisol excretion is measured rather than 17-OHCS.

Corticotropin-releasing factor is also of value in differentiating patients with functioning pituitary adenomas (Cushing disease) from other causes of Cushing syndrome. Patients with Cushing disease respond to CRF with normal or increased concentrations of ACTH and cortisol; other causes of Cushing syndrome usually fail to respond. At this time, CRF is still an investigational agent and not generally available.

Osseous maturation is usually moderately retarded but may be normal; in virilized children the bone age is apt to be advanced. Osteoporosis is common and is most evident in roentgenograms of the spine. Pathologic fractures may be noted. Sellar tomography is indicated, though the pituitary sella is usually normal. The growth hormone response to hypoglycemia may be impaired but usually returns to normal when the hypercortisolism is corrected. Diminution of muscle mass and increased deposition of adipose tissue may be noted in roentgenograms of the extremities. The thymic shadow is absent because excessive cortisol produces involution. Adrenal tumors occasionally have calcifications and frequently displace the kidney on the affected side. Computed tomography and ultrasonography are helpful in diagnosis and localization of tumors.

Differential Diagnosis. Cushing syndrome is frequently suspected in children with obesity, particularly when striae and hypertension are present. Differential diagnosis is complicated by the fact that elevated urinary concentrations of corticosteroids are frequently secondary to obesity itself. Children with simple obesity are usually tall, whereas those with Cushing syndrome are short or decelerating in growth rate. The excretion of urinary corticosteroids is rapidly suppressed by oral administration of low doses of dexamethasone in persons with uncomplicated obesity.

Treatment. If the lesion is benign cortical adenoma, unilateral adrenalectomy is indicated. Such adenomas are occasionally bilateral; then the treatment of choice is subtotal adrenalectomy. In either instance an excellent therapeutic result is achieved by removal of the tumor. Adrenocortical carcinomas, on the other hand, frequently metastasize, especially to the liver and lungs, and the prognosis may be unfavorable in spite of removal of the primary lesion. Rarely, the tumors are bilateral and require total adrenalectomy. It is often impossible to differentiate benign and malignant tumors by histologic appearance alone.

The management of bilateral adrenal hyperplasia (Cushing disease) is still unsettled. Total adrenalectomy has been most widely used but has fallen into disfavor. Current treatment is increasingly directed at the pituitary. Pituitary irradiation appears to induce remission in children and is advocated by some as the initial treatment. Hypopituitarism and behavioral changes may be sequelae of this form of treatment. The most promising new approach is transsphenoidal pituitary microsurgery, even in those patients in whom no adenoma is demonstrable. In the hands of an experienced neurosurgeon, selective adenomectomy has low morbidity and a good remission rate.

Cyproheptadine, a centrally acting serotonin antagonist that blocks ACTH release, has been used to treat Cushing disease in adults; remissions are usually not sustained after discontinuation of therapy. A child with Cushing disease treated with this agent has had a 3 yr remission after cessation of therapy; further therapeutic trials are needed.

In some patients after adrenalectomy, enlargement of the sella occurs and chromophobe adenomas appear, even with adequate replacement therapy with cortisol. Slight increase in pigmentation may occur after adrenalectomy and is of no clinical import, but intense melanosis is generally a harbinger of a pituitary tumor (*Nelson syndrome*). Large doses of hydrocortisone pre- and postoperatively have been recommended to avert possibly too rapid withdrawal of endogenous cortisol.

Management of patients undergoing adrenalectomy requires adequate pre- and postoperative replacement therapy with a corticosteroid. Tumors which produce corticosteroids usually lead to atrophy of the normal adrenal tissue, and replacement with both cortisol and corticotropin may be required. Patients with adrenal hyperplasia must be carefully watched after adrenalectomy for the development of pituitary tumor. Periodic examination of the pituitary fossa and of the ocular system is indicated. Postoperative complications have included sepsis, pancreatitis, thrombosis, poor wound healing, and sudden collapse, particularly in infants with Cushing syndrome. Substantial catch-up growth occurs, but adult height is often compromised.

19.25 EXCESS MINERALOCORTICOID SECRETION

The principal mineralocorticoid secreted by the adrenal is aldosterone. Increased secretion may result from a primary defect of the adrenal (primary hyperaldosteronism) or from factors which activate the renin-angiotensin system (secondary hyperaldosteronism). Patients with primary hyperaldosteronism usually have hypertension or hypokalemia; those with secondary hyperaldosteronism do not.

Desoxycorticosterone is a precursor of aldosterone, with only about one thirtieth the sodium-retaining potency of aldosterone (see Fig. 19–12). Overproduction of desoxycorticosterone occurs with two distinct defects of adrenal steroidogenesis: the first defect involves 11-hydroxylation, which also leads to androgen excess and presents clinically as the hypertensive form of congenital adrenal hyperplasia (see above); the second involves 17-hydroxylation, producing hypogonadism in the female and male pseudohermaphroditism in the male since the synthesis of androgens and estrogens as well as of cortisol is impaired.

Etiology. Primary hyperaldosteronism is rare in children. Ten children (3½–18 yr) are known to have had *aldosterone-secreting adenomas*; nine were female and one male.

In older children hyperaldosteronism is associated with *bilateral hyperplasia* of the zona glomerulosa. The cause is idiopathic. Recently an aldosterone-stimulating factor has been found to be elevated in serum of adults with idiopathic hyperaldosteronism, but it is not yet clear whether this factor is the cause for the condition.

A subgroup of children with bilateral hyperplasia of the zona glomerulosa respond to treatment with glucocorticoids (*glucocorticoid-suppressible hyperaldosteronism*). This has been reported in five kindreds, with an autosomal dominant mode of transmission. When the diagnosis is established in a proband, family members at risk should be investigated for this easily treated cause of hypertension.

Clinical Manifestations. Some affected children have no symptoms, the diagnosis being established after incidental discovery of moderate hypertension. Others have severe hypertension (up to 240/150 mm Hg), with headache, dizziness, and visual disturbances. Chronic hypokalemia may lead to "clear cell nephrosis," polyuria, nocturia, enuresis, and polydipsia. Muscle weakness and discomfort, tetany, intermittent paralysis, fatigue, and growth failure have been noted.

Laboratory Studies. Hypertension, hypokalemia, and suppressed plasma renin activity are the hallmarks of hyperaldosteronism. The serum pH, carbon dioxide content, and sodium concentrations may be elevated and the serum chloride and magnesium levels decreased. Serum levels of calcium are normal, even in children who manifest tetany. The urine is neutral or alkaline. Plasma and urine levels of aldosterone are increased and plasma levels of renin persistently low.

Differential Diagnosis. After establishing the diagnosis of primary aldosteronism, it is necessary to determine the etiology. All children should have a therapeutic trial with dexamethasone before invasive studies are done. Daily administration of 0.25 mg every 6 hr results in marked suppression of aldosterone and disappearance of hypertension in those patients with the glucocorticoid-suppressible variant of hyperaldosteronism. If there is no response to dexamethasone, computed tomography (CT scan) may help find an adrenal adenoma, but the tumors are often quite small and there is little experience with this diagnostic study in this condition.

If CT scans are normal, adrenal vein catheterization is indicated. High concentrations of aldosterone are found in only one adrenal vein when an adenoma is present and in both when bilateral hyperplasia is the cause. If adrenal vein catheterization is not successful, exploratory laparotomy may be required to establish the diagnosis.

Hyperaldosteronism occurs in many other conditions in which it is a normal homeostatic response. In such *secondary hyperaldosteronism*, serum renin activity is high or rises with a low salt diet, whereas in primary hyperaldosteronism the renin-angiotensin system is suppressed. Increased aldosterone secretion occurs in edematous disorders with reduced effective volume, such as nephrotic syndrome, congestive cardiac failure, and cirrhosis of the liver. Increased secretion of aldosterone also occurs in conditions in which compromise of renal perfusion results in increased secretion of renin, such as in stenosis of the renal artery. Wilms tumor and juxtaglomerular cell tumors may also secrete renin and cause secondary hyperaldosteronism.

In *pseudohypoaldosteronism* the increased levels of aldosterone are due to a defect in mineralocorticoid receptors, with ensuing activation of the renin-angiotensin system (Sec. 19.27).

Bartter syndrome is also characterized by hypokalemic alkalosis, hypochloremia, and hyperaldosteronism. The blood pressure is normal, however, and secretion of renin is increased. Growth failure is the usual presenting complaint. Renal biopsy reveals hyperplasia of the juxtaglomerular apparatus. Urinary excretion of prostaglandin $F_{1\alpha}$ has been demonstrated, and it has been suggested that this mediates the hyperreninemia. Drugs that reduce prostaglandin levels (such as indomethacin) correct the aldosterone, renin, and prostaglandin abnormalities but do not completely correct the hypokalemia.

11β-hydroxysteroid dehydrogenase deficiency is characterized by low levels of aldosterone and renin, with hypokalemia and hypertension (*low renin hypertension*). Onset is in early childhood with polyuria, polydipsia, failure to thrive, severe hypertension, and hypokalemia. Strokes have occurred in young children. A defect involving the terminal metabolism of cortisol to cortisone has been identified resulting in a high tetrahydrocortisol to tetrahydrocortisone ratio in urinary steroid excretion. It is not clear how this defect accounts for the clinical manifestations; an unidentified mineralocorticoid or a known steroid acting as a mineralocorticoid appears to be at the basis of the syndrome. The condition has been reported in one set of siblings and is thought to have a genetic basis. Spironolactone and triamterene have been used for treatment.

Treatment. Glucocorticoid-suppressible hyperaldosteronism is managed by daily administration of dexamethasone. Bilateral adrenal hyperplasia which does not respond to this therapy requires bilateral adrenalectomy; the results are excellent, but adrenal replacement therapy is required. Removal of an aldosterone-secreting adenoma results in a cure.

Treatment of secondary hyperaldosteronism is directed to the specific causative disorder.

19.26 FEMINIZING ADRENAL TUMORS

Adrenocortical tumors have been associated in nine boys with excessive production of estrogens and heterosexual precocious puberty. Gynecomastia was the initial manifestation, appearing from 6 mo–7 yr of age. Growth and development were otherwise normal, or concomitant virilization was sometimes evidenced by acne, deep voice, phallic enlargement, and advanced osseous maturation. The testes were not enlarged. Hypertension is common in affected adults but has not been observed in children. Levels of estrogens in plasma and urine are markedly elevated, and urinary 17-ketosteroids may be abnormally high. Tumors may be either carcinomas or benign adenomas and may be calcified on roentgenography. Gynecomastia regresses after removal of the tumor, and hormone values return to normal.

Estrogen-secreting adrenocortical tumors have been reported in 12 girls ranging in age from 6 mo–10 yr. The majority of the tumors were adenomas, some of which also elaborated androgens (with virilization) and/or mineralocorticoids (with hypertension). In addition to elevated plasma and urinary levels of estrogens, there were usually elevated levels of 17-ketosteroids in urine and of Δ^5 adrenal steroids (DHEA and DHEAS) in plasma. Plasma gonadotropin levels are suppressed and gonadotropin-releasing hormone (Gn-RH) stimulation does not elicit a response. Intravenous pyelography, ultrasonography, and/or computed tomography may localize the tumor.

19.27 EXCESSIVE SECRETION OF CATECHOLAMINES

PHEOCHROMOCYTOMA

The pheochromocytoma, a catecholamine-secreting tumor, arises from the chromaffin cells. The most common site of origin is the adrenal medulla; tumors may develop, however, anywhere along the abdominal sympathetic chain and are particularly apt to be located near the aorta at the level of the inferior mesenteric artery or at its bifurcation. They also appear in the periadrenal area, the urinary bladder or ureteral walls, the thoracic cavity, and the cervical region. Fewer than 5% of reported instances have occurred in children. Tumors vary from about 1–10 cm in diameter; they are found more often on the right side than on the left. In 20% of affected children the adrenal tumors are bilateral, and in 30% tumors are found in both the adrenal and extra-adrenal areas or only in an extra-adrenal area.

Pheochromocytoma is frequently inherited as an autosomal dominant trait. In affected families the ages of patients at the time of diagnosis have varied from the 1st–5th decade of life; more than half the patients have had multiple tumors.

Pheochromocytoma is frequently associated with other syndromes or tumors. Approximately 5% of patients with pheochromocytoma have neurofibromatosis. Sporadic as well as familial instances of pheochromocytoma have been noted in patients with von Hippel–Lindau disease. Kinships have been reported in which some affected members also have asymptomatic islet cell adenomas and some with pheochromocytoma are asymptomatic despite elevated urinary concentrations of catecholamines.

Pheochromocytoma also may coexist with medullary carcinoma of the thyroid; this association is known as *Sipple syndrome*. Of patients with these two tumors, some also have parathyroid disease *(multiple endocrine neoplasia, type II)*; others have *mucosal neuromas (multiple endocrine neoplasia, type IIb or type III)* (Sec. 19.16). Mucosal neuromas appear early in life and affect primarily the tongue and lips; they may also affect the gingival, buccal, or conjunctival mucosa. *Ganglioneuromatosis* of the alimentary tract is often a major component of the syndrome, leading to constipation or diarrhea before other manifestations appear.

These syndromes are all inherited in an autosomal dominant fashion, with highly variable expression.

Clinical Manifestations. These result from excessive secretion of epinephrine and norepinephrine; the clinical picture varies with quantitative variations in their secretion. All patients have hypertension at some time. The hypertension is usually sustained, but it may often be *paroxysmal*. Paroxysms should particularly suggest pheochromocytoma as a diagnostic possibility. When there are paroxysms of hypertension,

the attacks are usually infrequent at first but become more frequent and eventually give way to a continuous hypertensive state. Between attacks of hypertension the patient may be free of symptoms. During attacks the patient complains of headache and palpitation; and pallor, vomiting, and sweating also occur. Convulsions and other manifestations of hypertensive encephalopathy may occur. In severe cases precordial pains radiate into the arms, and pulmonary edema and cardiac and hepatic enlargement may develop. The child has a good appetite but because of hypermetabolism does not gain weight, and severe cachexia may develop. Polyuria and polydipsia can be sufficiently severe to suggest diabetes insipidus. Growth failure may be striking. The blood pressure may range from 180–260 systolic and 120–210 diastolic, and the heart may be enlarged. Ophthalmoscopic examination may reveal papilledema, hemorrhages, exudate, and arterial constriction.

Laboratory Data. The urine contains protein, a few casts, and occasionally glucose. Gross hematuria suggests that the tumor is in the bladder wall. Polycythemia is occasionally noted.

The most direct and specific test is the demonstration of increased basal plasma levels or excretion of catecholamines. Pheochromocytomas produce both norepinephrine and epinephrine; norepinephrine in plasma is derived, however, from both the adrenal gland and adrenergic nerve endings, whereas epinephrine is derived primarily from the adrenal. In affected children the predominant catecholamine is norepinephrine, and total urinary catecholamine excretion usually exceeds 300 µg/24 hr. The concentrations of catecholamines in urine are directly related to those in the tumor. Urinary excretion of VMA (3-methoxy-4-hydroxymandelic acid), the major metabolite of epinephrine and norepinephrine, and of metanephrine (see Fig. 19–11) is also increased. Measurement of plasma catecholamines in the resting, supine state (by radioenzymatic assay) may replace urinary studies. Excretion of catecholamine metabolites may be similar in children with neuroblastoma and with pheochromocytoma, but levels are usually higher with pheochromocytoma. Daily urinary excretion of these compounds by unaffected children increases with age; and vanilla-containing foods and fruits can produce falsely elevated levels of VMA. Certain drugs interfere with fluorometric determinations of catecholamines.

Plasma renin levels may be elevated secondary to reduced renal cortical blood flow.

Differential Diagnosis. The various causes of hypertension in children must be considered, such as renal or renovascular disease, coarctation of the aorta, acrodynia, thallium intoxication, hyperthyroidism, Cushing syndrome, 11β-hydroxylase and 17-hydroxylase deficiency, primary aldosteronism, adrenal cortical tumors, and essential hypertension. A nonfunctioning kidney may result from compression of a ureter or of a renal artery by a pheochromocytoma. Paroxysmal hypertension may be associated with familial dysautonomia. Urinary excretion of VMA is low in familial dysautonomia because of a defect in release rather than in synthesis of catecholamines. Cerebral disorders, diabetes insipidus, diabetes mellitus, and hyperthyroidism must also be considered in the differential diagnosis. Hypertension in patients with neurofibromatosis may be caused by renal vascular involvement as well as by concurrent pheochromocytoma.

Neuroblastoma, ganglioneuroblastoma, and ganglioneuroma frequently produce catecholamines. Secreting neurogenic tumors commonly produce hypertension, excessive sweating, flushing, pallor, rash, polyuria, and polydipsia. Diarrhea also may be associated with these tumors, particularly with ganglioneuroma, and at times may be sufficiently persistent to suggest the "celiac syndrome."

Management. Computed tomography is the method of

choice to localize these tumors. Venous catheterization with sampling of blood at different levels for catecholamine determinations is now only rarely necessary to localize the tumor. A new radiopharmaceutical agent, ^{131}I-metaiodobenzylguanidine, offers hope for more reliable localization of pheochromocytomas. Since these tumors are often multiple, especially in children, a thorough transabdominal exploration of all the usual sites offers the best chance of finding all of them. Removal of the tumor(s) results in cure. Although these tumors often appear malignant histologically, only rarely has malignancy been unequivocally established, as demonstrated by the metastasis to lymph nodes of hormonally active chromaffin cells. The operation is not without danger because an extreme rise of blood pressure may result from massive discharge of hormone during operative manipulation. Shock from a precipitous drop of blood pressure during operation or within the first 48 hr postoperatively is also a danger. These risks can be lessened by alpha- and beta-adrenergic blockade preoperatively, by careful monitoring during surgery, and by continuous postoperative surveillance. The urinary excretion of catecholamines should be determined after operation as a measure of the completeness of the surgical removal. Prolonged follow-up is indicated since functioning tumors at other sites may become manifest many years after the initial operation. Examination of relatives of affected patients may reveal other persons harboring unsuspected tumors. In one family with 10 affected individuals the highest blood pressures and urinary concentrations of catecholamines were found in the children, whereas some of the affected adults were normotensive and had only moderately elevated urinary concentrations of catecholamines and VMA.

OTHER CATECHOLAMINE-SECRETING NEURAL TUMORS

Excessive elaboration of catecholamines is not exclusive to pheochromocytomas but frequently occurs with other neurogenic tumors (neuroblastoma, ganglioneuroblastoma, and, less frequently, ganglioneuroma). Consequently, many of the systemic manifestations characteristic of pheochromocytoma may be seen in patients with other tumors of neural origin. Hypertension, excessive sweating, flushing, pallor, rash, polyuria, and polydipsia are the most common findings. *Chronic diarrhea* occurs with other manifestations or may be the only symptom. It occurs in approximately 8% of patients with these tumors but only rarely in patients with pheochromocytoma. The diarrhea is voluminous, may result in severe electrolyte depletion, and is intractable to treatment; it ceases abruptly with removal of the tumor. Diarrhea is more apt to be associated with ganglioneuroma and ganglioneuroblastoma, but it may occur with neuroblastoma. Increased levels of *vasoactive intestinal peptide* (VIP) are present in the tumor and/or plasma. This peptide is a potent stimulator of water and electrolyte secretion and stimulates adenylate cyclase production in the mucosa of the small intestine.

Benign adrenal cortical hyperplasia with Cushing disease has been observed in children with these neural tumors; the secretion of an ACTH-like hormone by the tumor is a likely but not proven explanation. An 18 mo old girl has been reported to have a ganglioneuroblastoma as well as an adrenocortical adenoma in each adrenal.

Many patients with these tumors have increased excretion of dopa, dopamine, norepinephrine, normetanephrine, homovanillic acid, and vanillylmandelic acid (VMA). Patients with pheochromocytoma usually excrete only epinephrine, norepinephrine, their methoxy analogues, and VMA (see Fig. 19–11). Elevated excretion of homovanillic acid generally indicates malignant pheochromocytoma or other malignant neural tumors, but it has been noted also with benign pheo-

chromocytoma. Biochemical differentiation between neuroblastomas, ganglioneuroblastomas, and benign ganglioneuromas is not possible. Serial determinations of VMA and catecholamines, and particularly of norepinephrine and dopamine, help in detecting recurrences and in assessing the effectiveness of therapy in the postoperative evaluation of children whose VMA levels were elevated prior to treatment. Excretion of these compounds returns to normal if the tumor is completely removed.

Screening tests for VMA excretion may detect neuroblastoma. A mass screening program has been initiated in Japan; examination of 6 mo old infants uncovered 1/17,621 with neuroblastoma.

19.28 CALCIFICATION WITHIN THE ADRENAL

Calcification within the adrenal glands may occur in a wide variety of situations, some serious and others of no obvious consequence. Adrenal calcifications are often detected as incidental findings in roentgenographic studies of the abdomen in infants and children. One may elicit a history of anoxia or trauma at birth. Hemorrhage into the adrenal at or immediately after birth is probably the common factor that leads to subsequent calcification. Though it is advisable to assess the adrenocortical reserve of such patients, there is rarely any functional disorder.

Neuroblastomas, ganglioneuromas, cortical carcinomas, pheochromocytomas, and cysts of the adrenal gland may be responsible for calcifications, particularly if hemorrhage has occurred within the tumor. Calcification in such lesions is almost always unilateral.

The most common infection associated with calcifications within the adrenal is tuberculosis, and the patient usually has the clinical manifestations of Addison disease. Calcifications may also develop in the adrenal glands of children who recover from the Waterhouse-Friderichsen syndrome; such patients are usually asymptomatic.

Infants with *Wolman syndrome*, a rare lipid disorder due to deficiency of lysosomal acid lipase, have extensive bilateral calcifications of the adrenal glands (Sec. 7.34).

General

Kaplan SA: Clinical Pediatric and Adolescent Endocrinology. Philadelphia, WB Saunders, 1982.
Wilson JD, Foster DW (eds): Williams Textbook of Endocrinology. 7th ed. Philadelphia, WB Saunders, 1985.

Adrenal Cortical Insufficiency

Armanini D, Kuhnle U, Strasser T, et al: Aldosterone-receptor deficiency in pseudohypoaldosteronism. N Engl J Med 313:1178, 1985.
Arulananthan K, Dwyer JM, Genel M: Evidence for defective immunoregulation in the syndrome of familial candidiasis endocrinopathy. N Engl J Med 300:165, 1979.
Bartley JA, Miller DK, Hayford JT, et al: Concordance of X-linked glycerol kinase deficiency with X-linked congenital adrenal hypoplasia. Lancet 2:733, 1982.
Blizzard RM, Kyle M: Studies of the adrenal antigens and antibodies in Addison's disease. J Clin Invest 42:1653, 1963.
Carey DE: Isolated ACTH deficiency in childhood: Lack of response to corticotropin-releasing hormone alone and in combination with arginine vasopressin. J Pediatr 107:925, 1985.
Carney JA, Hruska LS, Beauchamp GD, et al: Dominant inheritance of the complex of myxomas, spotty pigmentation, and endocrine overactivity. Mayo Clinic Proc 61:165, 1986.
Chitayat D, Spirer Z, Ayalon D, et al: Pseudohypoaldosteronism in a female infant and his family: Diversity of clinical expression and mode of inheritance. Acta Paediatr Scand 74:619, 1985.
Hay ID: Pubertal failure in congenital adrenocortical hypoplasia. Lancet 2:1035, 1977.
Hintz RL, Menking M, Sotos JF: Familial holoprosencephaly with endocrine dysgenesis. J Pediatr 72:81, 1968.

Kaplowitz PB, Carpenter R, Newsome NH, et al.: Cushing syndrome resulting from primary pigmented nodular adrenocortical hyperplasia. Am J Dis Child 140:1072, 1986.

Kelch RP, Kaplan SL, Biglieri EG, et al: Hereditary adrenocortical unresponsiveness to adrenocorticotropic hormone. J Pediatr 81:726, 1972.

Kirkland RT, Kirkland JL, Johnson CM, et al: Congenital lipoid adrenal hyperplasia in an eight-year-old phenotypic female. J Clin Endocrinol Metab 36:488, 1973.

Kreines K, DeVaux WD: Neonatal adrenal insufficiency associated with maternal Cushing syndrome. Pediatrics 47:516, 1971.

Kruse K, Sippell WG, Schnakenburg KV: Hypogonadism in congenital adrenal hypoplasia: Evidence for a hypothalamic origin. J Clin Endocrinol Metab 58:12, 1984.

Migeon CJ, Kenny FM, Hung W, et al: Study of adrenal function in children with meningitis. Pediatrics 40:163, 1967.

Mittelstaedt CA, Volberg FM, Merten DF, et al: Sonographic diagnosis of neonatal adrenal hemorrhage. Radiology 131:453, 1979.

Moser HW, Moser AB, Powers JM, et al: The prenatal diagnosis of adrenoleukodystrophy. Demonstration of increased hexacosanic acid levels in cultured amniocytes and fetal gland. Pediatr Res 16:171, 1982.

Moser HW, Moser AE, Singh J, et al: Adrenoleukodystrophy: Survey of 303 cases: Biochemistry, diagnosis, and therapy. Ann Neurol 16:628, 1984.

Moshang T, Rosenfield RL, Bongiovanni AM, et al: Familial glucocorticoid insufficiency. J Pediatr 82:821, 1973.

Rosler A: The natural history of salt-wasting disorders of adrenal and renal origin. J Clin Endocrinol Metab 59:689, 1984.

Savage MO, Jefferson IG, Dillon MJ, et al: Pseudohypoaldosteronism: Severe salt wasting in infancy caused by generalized mineralocorticoid unresponsiveness. J Pediatr 101:239, 1982.

Sperling MA, Wolfsen AR, Fisher DA: Congenital adrenal hypoplasia: An isolated defect of organogenesis. J Pediatr 82:444, 1973.

Ulick S, Eberlein WR, Bliffeld AR, et al: Evidence for an aldosterone biosynthetic defect in congenital adrenal hyperplasia. J Clin Endocrinol Metab 51:1346, 1980.

Veldhuis JD, Kulin HE, Santen RJ, et al: Inborn error in the terminal steps of aldosterone biosynthesis. Corticosterone methyl oxidase Type II deficiency in a North American pedigree. N Engl J Med 303:117, 1980.

Veldhuis JD, Kulen HE, Wilson TE, et al: Detection of isolated aldosterone deficiency in the neonate. J Pediatr 102:83, 1983.

Adrenal Cortical Hyperfunction

Aronin N, Krieger DT: Sustained remission of Nelson's syndrome after stopping cyproheptadine treatment. N Engl J Med 302:453, 1980.

Bergstrand CG, Nilsson KO: Treatment of Cushing's disease in children. Acta Paediatr Scand 71:1, 1982.

Bryer-Ash M, Wilson DM, Tune BM, et al: Hypertension caused by an aldosterone-secreting adenoma. Occurrence in a 7-year-old child. Am J Dis Child 138:673, 1984.

Burr IM, Sullivan J, Graham T, et al: A testosterone-secreting tumour of the adrenal producing virilization in a female infant. Lancet 2:643, 1973.

Cara JF, Moshang T Jr, Bongiovanni AM, et al: Elevated 17-hydroxyprogesterone and testosterone in a newborn with 3-beta-hydroxysteroid dehydrogenase deficiency. N Engl J Med 313:618, 1985.

Carey RM, Sen S, Dolan LM, et al: Idiopathic hyperaldosteronism. A possible role for aldosterone-stimulating factor. N Engl J Med 313:94, 1984.

Chrousos GP, Schuermeyer TH, Doppman J, et al: Clinical applications of corticotropin-releasing factor. Ann Intern Med 102:344, 1985.

Comite F, Schiebinger RJ, Alertson BD, et al: Isosexual precocious pseudopuberty secondary to a feminizing adrenal tumor. J Clin Endocrinol Metab 58:435, 1984.

Couch RM, Smail PJ, Dean HJ, et al: Prolonged remission of Cushing disease with cyproheptadine. J Pediatr 104:906, 1984.

Dahms WT, Gray G, Vrana M, et al: Adrenocortical adenoma and ganglioneuroblastoma in a child. Am J Dis Child 125:608, 1973.

D'Armiento M, Reda G, Kater C, et al: 17 α-hydroxylase deficiency: Mineralocorticoid hormone profiles in an affected family. J Clin Endocrinol Metab 56:597, 1983.

David M, Forest MG: Prenatal treatment of congenital adrenal hyperplasia resulting from 21-hydroxylase deficiency. J Pediatr 105:799, 1984.

Duck SC: Acceptable linear growth in congenital adrenal hyperplasia. J Pediatr 97:93, 1980.

Franco-Saenz R, Antonipillai I, Tan SY, et al: Cortisol production by testicular tumors in a patient with congenital adrenal hyperplasia (21-hydroxylase deficiency). J Clin Endocrinol Metab 53:85, 1981.

Fraumeni JF Jr, Miller RW: Adrenocortical neoplasms with hemihypertrophy, brain tumors, and other disorders. J Pediatr 70:129, 1967.

Ganguly A, Grim CE, Bergstein J, et al: Genetic and pathophysiologic studies of a new kindred with glucocorticoid-suppressible hyperaldosteronism manifest in three generations. J Clin Endocrinol Metab 53:1040, 1981.

Grim CE, McBryde AC, Glenn JF, et al: Childhood primary aldosteronism with bilateral adrenocortical hyperplasia. Plasma renin activity as an aid to diagnosis. J Pediatr 71:377, 1967.

Gullner HG, Cerletti C, Bartter FC, et al: Prostacycline overproduction in Bartter's syndrome. Lancet 2:767, 1979.

Hodgkinson DJ, Telander RL, Sheps SG, et al: Extra-adrenal intrathoracic functioning paraganglioma (pheochromocytoma) in childhood. Mayo Clin Proc 55:271, 1980.

Holler W, Scholz S, Knon D, et al: Genetic differences between the salt-wasting simple virilizing and nonclassical types of congenital adrenal hyperplasia. J Clin Endocrinol Metab 60:757, 1985.

Howard CP, Takahashi H, Hayles AB: Feminizing adrenal adenoma in a boy. Case report and literature review. Mayo Clin Proc 52:354, 1977.

Jennings AS, Liddle TW, Orth DN: Results of treating childhood Cushing's disease with pituitary irradiation. N Engl J Med 297:957, 1977.

Kershnar AK, Borut D, Kogut MD, et al: Studies on a phenotypic female with 17-α-hydroxylase deficiency. J Pediatr 89:395, 1976.

Kutten F, Couillin P, Girard F, et al: Late onset adrenal hyperplasia in hirsutism. N Engl J Med 313:224, 1985.

Lee PDK, Winter RJ, Green OC: Virilizing adrenocortical tumors in childhood: Eight cases and a review of the literature. Pediatr 76:437, 1985.

LeFevre M, Gerard-Marchant R, Gubler JP, et al: Adrenal cortical carcinoma in children: 42 patients treated from 1958 to 1980 at Villejuif. Cancer Treat Res 17:265, 1983.

Levy SR, Val Wynne C Jr, Lorentz WB Jr: Cushing's syndrome in infancy secondary to pituitary adenoma. Am J Dis Child 136:605, 1982.

McArthur RG, Bahn RC, Hayles AB: Primary adrenocortical nodular dysplasia as a cause of Cushing's syndrome in infants and children. Mayo Clin Proc 57:58, 1982.

McArthur RG, Bloutier MD, Hayles AB, et al: Cushing's disease in children. Findings in 13 cases. Mayo Clin Proc 47:379, 1972.

McArthur RG, Hayles AB, Salassa RM: Childhood Cushing disease: Results of bilateral adrenalectomy. J Pediatr 95:214, 1979.

Modlinger RS, Nicolis GL, Krakoff LR, et al: Some observations on the pathogenesis of Bartter's syndrome. N Engl J Med 289:1022, 1973.

Mosier HD Jr, Smith FG, Schultz MA: Failure of catch-up growth after Cushing's syndrome in childhood. Am J Dis Child 124:251, 1972.

New MI, Lorenzen F, Lerner AJ, et al: Genotyping steroid 21-hydroxylase deficiency: Hormonal reference data. J Clin Endocrinol Metab 57:320, 1983.

Pang S, Levine LS, Stoner E, et al: Nonsalt-losing congenital adrenal hyperplasia due to 3β-hydroxysteroid dehydrogenase deficiency with normal glomerulosa function. J Clin Endocrinol Metab 56:808, 1983.

Pang S, Pollack MS, Loo M, et al: Pitfalls of prenatal diagnosis of 21-hydroxylase deficiency congenital adrenal hyperplasia. J Clin Endocrinol Metab 61:89, 1985.

Pescovitz OH, Comite F, Cassorla F, et al: True precocious puberty complicating congenital adrenal hyperplasia: Treatment with a luteinizing hormone-releasing hormone analog. J Clin Endocrinol Metab 58:857, 1984.

Pombo M, Alvez F, Varela-Cives R, et al: Ectopic production of ACTH by Wilms' tumor. Hormone Res 16:160, 1982.

Raiti S, Grant DB, Williams DI, et al: Cushing's syndrome in childhood: Postoperative management. Arch Dis Child 47:597, 1972.

Rosler A, Leiberman E, Rosenmann A, et al: Prenatal diagnosis of 11β-hydroxylase deficiency congenital adrenal hyperplasia. J Clin Endocrinol Metab 49:546, 1979.

Schackleton CHL, Rodriquez J, Arteago E, et al: Congenital 11β-hydroxysteroid dehydrogenase deficiency associated with juvenile hypertension: Corticosteroid metabolite profiles of four patients and their families. Clin Endocrinol 22:701, 1985.

Solomon JL, Schoen EJ: Juvenile Cushing syndrome manifested primarily by growth failure. Am J Dis Child 130:200, 1976.

Streetan DHP, Faas FH, Elders MJ, et al: Hypercortisolism in childhood: Shortcomings of conventional diagnostic criteria. Pediatrics 56:797, 1975.

Sultan C, Descomps B, Garandeau P, et al: Pubertal gynecomastia due to an estrogen-producing adrenal adenoma. J Pediatr 95:744, 1979.

Styne DM, Grumbach MM, Kaplan SL, et al: Treatment of Cushing's disease in childhood and adolescence by transphenoidal microadenomectomy. N Engl J Med 310:889, 1984.

Styne DM, Isaac R, Miller WL, et al: Endocrine, histological and biochemical studies of adrenocorticotropin-producing islet cell carcinoma of the pancreas in childhood with characterization of propiomelanocortin. J Clin Endocrinol Metab 57:723, 1983.

Zachman M, Tassinari D, Prader A: Clinical and biochemical variability of congenital adrenal hyperplasia due to 11β-hydroxylase deficiency. A study of 25 patients. J Clin Endocrinol Metab 56:222, 1983.

Zancan L, Zacchello F, Mantero F: Indomethacin for Bartter's syndrome. Lancet 2:1334, 1976.

Pheochromocytoma and Other Neural Tumors

El Shafie M, Samuel D, Klippel CH, et al: Intractable diarrhea in children with VIP-secreting ganglioneuroblastoma. J Pediatr Surg 18:34, 1983.

Gitlow SE, Bertani LM, Greenwood SM, et al: Benign pheochromocytoma associated with elevated excretion of homovanillic acid. J Pediatr 81:1112, 1972.

Kaufman BH, Telander RL, VanHeerden JA, et al: Pheochromocytoma in the pediatric age group: Current status. J Pediatr Surg 18:879, 1983.

Keiser HR, Beauen MA, Doppman J, et al: Sipple's syndrome: Medullary thyroid carcinoma, pheochromocytoma, and parathyroid disease. Ann Intern Med 78:561, 1973.

Kogut MD, Kaplan SA: Systemic manifestations of neurogenic tumors. J Pediatr 60:697, 1962.

Phillips AF, McMurty RJ, Taubman J: Malignant pheochromocytoma in childhood. Am J Dis Child 130:1252, 1976.

Sawada T, Hirayama M, Nakata T, et al: Mass screening for neuroblastoma in infants in Japan. Interim report of a mass screening study group. Lancet 2:271, 1984.

Schimke RN, Hartman WH, Prout TE, et al: Syndrome of bilateral pheochromocytoma, medullary thyroid carcinoma and multiple neuromas. A possible regulatory defect in the differentiation of chromaffin tissue. N Engl J Med 279:1, 1968.

Sisson JC, Frager MS, Valk TW, et al: Scintigraphic localization of pheochromocytoma. N Engl J Med 305:12, 1981.

Smith AA, Dancis J: Catecholamine release in familial dysautonomia. N Engl J Med 277:61, 1967.

Stackpole RH, Melicow MM, Uson AC: Pheochromocytoma in children. Report of 9 cases and review of the first 100 published cases with follow-up studies. J Pediatr 63:315, 1963.

Voorhess ML: Urinary catecholamine excretion by healthy children. I. Daily excretion of dopamine, norepinephrine, epinephrine and 3-methoxy-4-hydroxymandelic acid. Pediatris 39:252, 1967.

Voorhess ML: Neuroblastoma-pheochromocytoma: Products and pathogenesis. Ann NY Acad Sci 230:187, 1974.

Wise KS, Gibson JA: Von Hippel-Lindau's disease and pheochromocytoma. Br Med J 1:441, 1971.

Adrenal Calcification

Crocker AC, Vawter GF, Neuhauser EBO, et al: Wolman's disease: Three new patients with recently described lipidosis. Pediatrics 35:627, 1965.

Hill EE, Williams JA: Massive adrenal haemorrhage in the newborn. Arch Dis Child 34:178, 1959.

Jarvis JL, Seaman WB: Idiopathic adrenal calcification in infants and children. Am J Roentgenol 82:510, 1959.

Stevenson J, MacGregor AM, Connelly P: Calcification of the adrenal glands in young children. A report of three cases with a review of the literature. Arch Dis Child 36:316, 1961.

19.29 DISORDERS OF THE GONADS

Maturation in Boys. The main hormonal product of the testis is testosterone. It is produced in the Leydig cells, which have many enzymes in common with cells of the adrenal cortex. Defects have now been described for each of the steps in biosynthesis of testosterone (see Fig. 19–18). Because testosterone is important to normal virilization of the XY fetus, each of these defects has produced some degree of male pseudohermaphroditism. Defects in synthesis of testosterone become more clearly evident at puberty when normal masculinization fails to occur. These defects are all genetic and almost surely all autosomal recessive.

Within specific target cells, testosterone is converted by 5α-reductase to dihydrotestosterone, another potent androgen (see Fig. 19–18). There appears to be differential binding of these two androgens in different cells, with differences in functional activity. In the male fetus at the critical time of masculinization (8–12 wk) these two androgens appear to have distinct and separate functions. Patients with deficiency of 5α-reductase clearly demonstrate that testosterone is necessary for wolffian differentiation, whereas dihydrotestosterone is necessary for masculinization of the external genitalia. Evidence from these same patients suggests that growth of facial hair and prostate may also depend on dihydrotestosterone.

In prepubertal boys and girls the plasma levels of testosterone are at the same low levels. The level of testosterone rises sharply in boys during puberty, particularly in stage 3 (generally after 12 yr of age). The size of the testis increases slightly from 6–12 yr of age, before testosterone levels rise; thereafter, growth of the testis is markedly accelerated. Pubic hair growth, acne, voice change, and axillary hair growth correlate with the rising levels of testosterone. Estradiol and adrenal androgens also increase during puberty. In the early stages of puberty a nocturnal rise of plasma testosterone occurs 40–80 min after onset of sleep because of a slightly earlier sharp rise in the level of LH.

The ability of prepubertal testis to secrete testosterone can be assessed by administration of chorionic gonadotropin (hCG), which stimulates the testis in a manner analogous to luteinizing hormone (LH). After administration of hCG for 1–3 days, levels of testosterone rise in all stages of puberty.

Progressive maturation of the testis occurs under the influence of gradually rising levels of gonadotropins. The normally low levels of follicle-stimulating hormone (FSH) and LH begin to rise slowly around the age of 6–8 yr; there is slight growth of the testis during this period. A sharper rise in the levels of FSH and LH occurs at the onset of puberty. Plasma levels of FSH increase only to midpuberty, whereas plasma levels of LH continue to rise until about 17 yr of age. The somatic changes of puberty and the rising levels of testosterone correlate best with the levels of LH.

The hormonal changes described above are initiated by maturation of the hypothalamus. The first hormonal sign of puberty is the pulsatile secretion of gonadotropins during sleep, which is caused by pulsatile release of luteinizing hormone–releasing hormone (LH-RH). Another physiologic change at puberty is a decreasing sensitivity of the hypothalamus to the negative feedback effects of the sex steroids. Increasing sensitivity of the pituitary to LH-RH also occurs. Administration of LH-RH to the prepubertal child results in a smaller release of LH than occurs when it is administered during puberty. Thus, puberty and gonadal maturation are associated with stepwise maturation, first in the hypothalamus, then in the pituitary, and lastly in the gonad.

Clinical patterns of pubertal changes vary widely. In 95% of boys enlargement of the genitalia begins between 9½–13½ yr, reaching maturity from 13–17 yr. In a small minority of normal boys puberty begins after 15 yr of age. In 50% of boys pubic hair is present by 11 yr of age, and by 13–17½ yr it is equivalent in amount to that of normal adult females. In some boys pubertal development is completed in less than 2 yr, whereas in others it may take longer than 4½ yr. The adolescent growth spurt occurs later in boys than in girls at corresponding levels of sexual maturation; for example, the peak velocity of change in height is not attained in boys until the genitalia are well developed, whereas in girls the growth rate is usually at its maximum when the nipple and areola have developed but before there is any other significant breast development.

Maturation in Girls. The most important estrogens produced by the ovary are estradiol-17β (E_2) and estrone (E_1); estriol is a metabolic product of these two, and all three estrogens may be found in the urine of mature females. Estrogens also arise from androgens, both in the adrenal and in the testis; the pathway for this conversion is shown in Fig. 19–15. This conversion explains why in certain types of male pseudohermaphroditism feminization occurs at puberty; in 17β-hydroxysteroid dehydrogenase deficiency, for example, the enzymatic block results in markedly increased secretion of androstenedione, which is converted in the peripheral tissues to estradiol and estrone; these estrogens, in addition to that directly secreted by the testis, result in normal breast development. The ovary also synthesizes progesterone, a progestational steroid; adrenal cortex and testis also synthesize progesterone as a precursor for other adrenal and testicular hormones.

Plasma levels of estradiol increase slowly but steadily with advancing sexual maturation and correlate well with clinical evaluation of pubertal development, skeletal age, and rising levels of FSH. Levels of LH do not rise until secondary sexual characteristics are well developed. Estrogens, like androgens, inhibit secretion of both LH and FSH (negative feedback). In

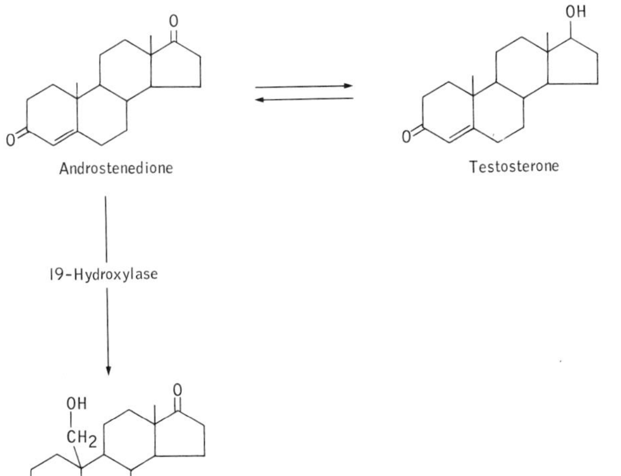

Figure 19–15. Conversion of androgens to estrogens.

females estrogens also provoke the surge of LH secretion that occurs in the midmenstrual cycle. The capacity for this positive feedback is another maturational milestone of puberty. The average age at menarche in American girls is 12½–13 yr, but the range of "normal" is wide, and 1–2% of "normal" girls have not menstruated by 16 yr of age. Menarche generally correlates closely with skeletal age.

Diagnostic Aids. Rapid advances in understanding the hypothalamic-pituitary-gonadal interactions involved with puberty and in the clinical diagnosis of aberrations of pubertal development have been made possible by markedly improved assays for pituitary and gonadal hormones that can be measured in small amounts of blood. With LH-RH it is also possible to differentiate between primary pituitary and hypothalamic defects in hypogonadotropic patients.

Therapeutic Aids. Naturally occurring estrogens administered orally are rapidly destroyed by gastrointestinal and liver enzymes; accordingly, they are usually given as conjugates or esters. The most widely used oral preparations are equine conjugated estrogens (e.g., Premarin) and ethinyl estradiol. Androgens are generally injected as long acting esters (enanthate, cyclopentylpropionate, or phenylacetate) because of their potency and steady response. Oral preparations, such as methyltestosterone or fluoxymesterone, do not produce as potent an androgenic response.

HYPOFUNCTION OF THE TESTES

Testicular hypofunction may be primary in the testis (primary hypogonadism) or secondary to deficiency of pituitary gonadotropic hormones (secondary hypogonadism). Patients with primary hypogonadism have elevated levels of gonadotropin (hypergonadotropic); those with secondary hypogonadism have low or absent levels (hypogonadotropic).

19.30 HYPERGONADOTROPIC HYPOGONADISM IN THE MALE
(Primary Hypogonadism)

Only those conditions of decreased androgen production that occur in males who were normally virilized during intrauterine life will be discussed here. Defects of androgen production involving the fetal testis and resulting in male pseudohermaphroditism are discussed in Sec. 19.42.

Etiology. *Congenital anorchia* is found in a few boys with bilateral cryptorchidism who are otherwise normal. In this condition it is presumed that a noxious factor damaged the fetal testes of the chromosomal male some time after sexual differentiation had taken place. When testicular function fails before the 7th–14th wk of fetal life, normal male somatic differentiation does not take place and an intersex results.

A syndrome of *rudimentary testes* has been described in which the testes are exceedingly small; it appears to be inherited as an autosomal or X-linked recessive trait. The etiology is unknown. *Atrophy* of the testes may follow damage to the vascular supply as a result of unskillful manipulation of the testes during surgical procedures for correction of cryptorchidism or as a result of bilateral torsion of the testes. *Acute orchitis* in pubertal or adult males with mumps may also damage the testes; usually, only the reproductive function of the testes is impaired. The routine immunization of all prepubertal males with mumps vaccine should prevent this complication.

Testicular damage is a frequent sequela of *chemotherapy* and of *radiotherapy* for cancer. The frequency and extent of damage depend on the agent used, total dosage, duration of therapy, and post-therapy interval of observation. Another important variable is age at therapy; germ cells are less vulnerable in prepubertal than in intrapubertal and postpubertal boys. Evidence suggests that testicular function recovers in some individuals 2–4 yr after discontinuation of treatment. Because of these variables, reports of frequency and degree of testicular damage are often conflicting. Testicular function should be carefully evaluated in adolescents who have prolonged survival after multimodal treatment for cancer in childhood. Replacement therapy with testosterone and/or counseling concerning fertility may be indicated.

In *germinal cell aplasia (Del Castillo syndrome)* sexual maturation occurs normally, Leydig cells are normal, and testosterone secretion is normal. The testes are small, however, and the seminiferous tubules are small and devoid of germ cells. Azoospermia and infertility are the rule. The disorder has affected brothers, but the mode of transmission is not clear. FSH levels are elevated, LH levels normal. These findings support the hypothesis that the germ cells produce a specific inhibitor of FSH, now termed inhibin.

The term "hypogonadism" has been widely used to describe aspects of children with a variety of syndromes of multiple malformations. It often refers simply to cryptorchidism, a small phallus, or a scrotal anomaly. For many of these syndromes little is known concerning the function of the testes; hyper- or hypogonadotropic hypogonadism has been proved in some instances.

Varying degrees of hypogonadism also occur in a significant percentage of patients with chromosomal aberrations such as Klinefelter syndrome or XX males (see below).

Clinical Manifestations. Primary hypogonadism may be suspected at birth if the testes and penis are abnormally small. The condition often is not noted until puberty is expected and secondary sex characters fail to develop. Facial, pubic, and axillary hair is scant or absent; there is neither acne nor regression of scalp hair, and the voice remains high pitched. The penis and scrotum remain infantile and may be almost obscured by pubic fat; the testes are small or absent. Fat accumulates in the region of the hips and buttocks and sometimes also in the breasts and on the abdomen. The epiphyses close late in life; therefore, extremities are long. The span is several inches longer than the height, and the distance from the symphysis pubis to the soles of the feet is much greater than from the symphysis to the vertex. This clinical state is also known as *eunuchism*, and the proportions of the body are described as "eunuchoid." Many individuals with milder degrees of hypogonadism may be detected only by appropriate studies of the pituitary-adrenal axis.

Diagnosis. Levels of serum FSH and, to a lesser extent, of LH are elevated above age-specific normal values. These elevated levels indicate that even in the prepubertal child there is an active hypothalamic-gonadal feedback relationship. After the age of 11 yr FSH and LH levels rise significantly, reaching the postmenopausal range. Plasma testosterone levels are ordinarily low in normal prepubertal children, rising during puberty to attain adult levels. During puberty these levels correlate better with testicular size and stage of sex maturity (SMR) than with age. In patients with primary hypogonadism, testosterone levels remain low at all ages, and there is an attenuated or no rise following administration of hCG, whereas in normal males at any stage of development hCG produces a significant rise in plasma testosterone.

In the newborn period, levels of gonadotropins and testosterone are normally high. In the hypogonadotropic infant, basal testosterone levels are low and LH levels are elevated for age. Stimulation with gonadotropin hormone-releasing hormone (LH-RH) results in a supranormal LH response; this test may be more reliable than the hCG test as an indicator of Leydig cell failure in the early weeks of life.

Noonan Syndrome

The term Noonan syndrome has been applied to phenotypic males and females who have certain anomalies that occur also in females with Turner syndrome. These boys and girls have normal karyotypes. The disorder is usually sporadic, but affected siblings of the same and of different genders have been reported. Partial expression of the syndrome is often present in 1st degree relatives. Reports of male-to-male transmission suggest an autosomal dominant gene with variable expressivity.

The most common abnormalities are short stature, webbing of the neck, pectus carinatum or pectus excavatum, cubitum valgum, congenital heart disease, and a characteristic facies. Hypertelorism, epicanthus, an antimongoloid palpebral slant, ptosis, micrognathia, and ear abnormalities are common. Other abnormalities such as clinodactyly, hernias, and vertebral anomalies occur less frequently. Developmental delay is common. The cardiac defect is most often pulmonary valvular stenosis or atrial septal defect. Recent reports of a number of children with the Noonan phenotype associated with *neurofibromatosis* suggest a separate disorder. Gonadal defects vary from severe deficiency to apparently normal sexual development. Males frequently have cryptorchidism and small testes; they may be hypogonadal or normal. Puberty may be normal or arrive late or never.

Klinefelter Syndrome

Etiology. Approximately 1/750 newborn males has a 47,XXY chromosome complement. Accordingly, Klinefelter syndrome is slightly more common than Down syndrome. The incidence approximates 1% among the mentally retarded, clustering among patients with IQ's above 50 and among children admitted to psychiatric hospitals or referred to psychiatric clinics. The chromosomal aberration most often results from meiotic nondisjunction of an X chromosome during parental gametogenesis; the extra X chromosome is maternal in origin in 67% and paternal in origin in 33% of patients. Increased maternal age predisposes to meiotic nondisjunction and to this syndrome, but in most instances maternal age is not advanced.

The 47,XXY complement is the most common chromosomal pattern in persons with Klinefelter syndrome; some have mosaic patterns: 46,XY/47,XXY; 46,XY/48,XXYY; 45,X/46,XY/46,XXY; or 46,XX/47,XXY. Rarely, occurrence of more than two X chromosomes may result in Klinefelter variants: 48,XXXY; 49,XXXYY; 49,XXXXY; 50,XXXXYY; 47,XXY/48,XXXY; 47,XXY/49,XXXXY; or 48,XXYY karyotypes. It is noteworthy that even with as many as four X chromosomes, the Y chromosome determines a male phenotype.

Clinical Manifestations. The diagnosis is rarely made prior to puberty because of the paucity or subtleness of clinical manifestations in childhood. Since behavioral or psychiatric disorders may often be apparent long before defects in sexual development, the condition should be considered in all boys with mental retardation as well as in children with psychosocial, learning, or school adjustment problems. Affected children may be anxious, immature, excessively shy, or aggressive; they may engage in antisocial acts. Problems often first become apparent after the child begins school. The patients tend to be tall, slim, and underweight and to have relatively long legs; but body habitus can vary markedly. The testes tend to be small for age, but this sign may become substantially apparent only after puberty, when normal testicular growth fails to occur. The phallus tends to be smaller than average, and cryptorchidism and/or hypospadias may occur in a few patients.

Pubertal development may be delayed. Some degree of androgen deficiency is usually noted, though some patients may undergo almost normal masculinization. About 40% of adults have gynecomastia; they have sparser facial hair, most shaving less than daily. Azoospermia and infertility are usual, though rare instances of fertility are known. Height tends to be increased. There is also an increased incidence of pulmonary disease, varicose veins, and cancer of the breast.

In a prospective study a group of children with 47,XXY karyotypes identified at birth exhibited relatively mild deviations from normal during the first 5 yr of life. None had major physical, intellectual, or emotional disabilities; some were inactive, with poorly organized motor function and mild delay in language acquisition. Whether more serious impairments will develop later in these children is unknown.

In adults with XY/XXY *mosaicism* the features of Klinefelter syndrome are decreased in severity and frequency. Little is known of children with mosaicism, but they may have a better prognosis for virilization, fertility, and psychosocial adjustment. The XXYY *male* phenotype is not distinctively different from that of the XXY patient except that XXYY adults tend to be taller than the average XXY patient.

Klinefelter Variants. When the number of X chromosomes exceeds 2, the clinical manifestations, including the mental retardation and the impairment of virilization, are more severe. The rare 49,XXXXY *variant* is sufficiently distinctive to be detected in childhood. Affected patients are severely retarded, and many have large malformed ears, a short neck, and a typical facies with wide-set eyes which have a mild mongoloid slant; epicanthus, strabismus, a wide, flat upturned nose, and a large open mouth may also be present. The testes are small and may be undescended, the scrotum is hypoplastic, and the penis is very small. Defects suggestive of Down syndrome (such as short incurved terminal 5th phalanges, single palmar creases, and hypotonia) and other skeletal abnormalities (including defects in the carrying angle of the elbows and restricted supination) are common. The most frequent radiographic abnormalities are radioulnar synostosis or dislocation, elongated radius, pseudoepiphyses, scoliosis or kyphosis, coxa valga, and retarded osseous age. Most patients with such extensive changes have a 49,XXXXY chromosome karyotype; the following mosaic patterns have also been observed: 48,XXXY/49,XXXXY (Fig. 19–16); 48,XXXY/49,XXXXY/50,XXXXXY; and 48,XXXY/49,XXXXY/50XXXXYY.

Laboratory Data. The chromosomes should be examined in all patients suspected of Klinefelter syndrome, particularly those attending child guidance, psychiatric, and mental retardation clinics. Prior to 10 yr of age boys with 47,XXY Klinefelter syndrome have normal basal plasma levels of FSH and LH. Response to gonadotropin stimulating hormone and to hCG are also normal. The testes show normal growth early in puberty but by midpuberty testicular growth stops, gonadotropins become elevated, and testosterone levels are slightly low. Elevated levels of estradiol resulting in a high estradiol:testosterone ratio account for the development of gynecomastia during puberty.

Testicular biopsy before puberty may reveal only a deficiency or absence of germinal cells. After puberty the seminiferous tubular membranes are hyalinized, and there is adenomatous clumping of Leydig cells. Azoospermia is characteristic; only rarely is spermatogenesis sufficient to permit fertility.

Treatment. Replacement therapy with long-acting testosterone preparation should begin at 11–12 yr of age. The cyclopentylpropionate ester may be used in a starting dose of 50 mg injected intramuscularly every 3 wk with 50 mg increments

every 6–9 mo until a maintenance dose for adults (250 mg every 3 wk) is achieved. For older boys larger initial doses and increments can achieve more rapid virilization.

XX Males

Approximately 140 males with 46,XX chromosome constitution have been identified; the disorder is thought to occur in 1/20,000 males. Affected individuals have a male phenotype, small testes, a small phallus, and no evidence of ovarian or müllerian duct tissue; they appear, therefore, to be distinct from the XX true hermaphrodite (below). This disorder resembles Klinefelter syndrome, but stature is greater in the latter. The histologic features of the testes are essentially the same in the two conditions. Only about 20% of reported patients have been prepubertal; patients with the condition usually come to medical attention in adult life because of hypogonadism or gynecomastia. About 50% of those detected as children have had hypospadias and/or chordee. Hypergonadotropic hypogonadism occurs secondary to testicular failure.

For two decades it has been theorized that male-determining genes have been translocated from the Y chromosome to the X chromosome during meiosis in the father. The finding of $X_g(a-)$ affected patients with $X_g(a+)$ fathers supported this theory. Recently the genomes of a number of 46,XX males have been found to contain Y-specific DNA sequences by use of several Y-specific probes. It has been well established that the short arms of the Y and X chromosomes pair during meiosis. Among XX males the anomalous X–Y interchange is usually sporadic, most patients having inherited one paternal and one maternal X chromosome. In at least one of the few families with two or more XX males, the same mechanism was operative in each affected member.

XYY Males

The 47,XYY male does not have hypogonadism; his condition is discussed here for easy comparison with the XXY and the XX male syndromes.

Approximately 1/1000 newborn males has an XYY chromosome pattern. Thus far, in a small number of children detected at birth as part of routine screening programs and followed prospectively, no abnormal physical or behavioral characteristics have been detected except for a tendency to tall stature and some problems in motor and language development. When this disorder was first discovered in adults, studies of XYY individuals in mental or penal institutions created a stereotype of affected individuals as having deviant behavior marked by physical aggressiveness and violence. It now appears that the rate at which XYY males are found in mental or penal settings may be as high as 20 times the rate at which they are born, but studies not biased by behavioral ascertainment do not show deviant behavior to be a prominent feature. Recent studies indicate that adults with this karyotype may be relatively impulsive, antisocial, and apt to break the law, but they are not especially aggressive.

The XYY adult has few phenotypic manifestations. He tends to be tall and to have severe nodulocystic acne. Dermatoglyphics do not differ significantly from XY males. In affected persons genital abnormalities have been noted, but cryptic mosaicism, such as X/XYY, is a possibility in these instances. Prolonged P-R intervals on electrocardiography and radioulnar synostosis appear to occur more often than in the general population. No clear-cut endocrine abnormalities have been found. It is not certain why XYY individuals are more apt to be found in mental or penal institutions though it is possible that an abnormality of neural development due to the XYY genotype favors deviant behavior in some persons. The nature and extent of such an association are yet to be determined.

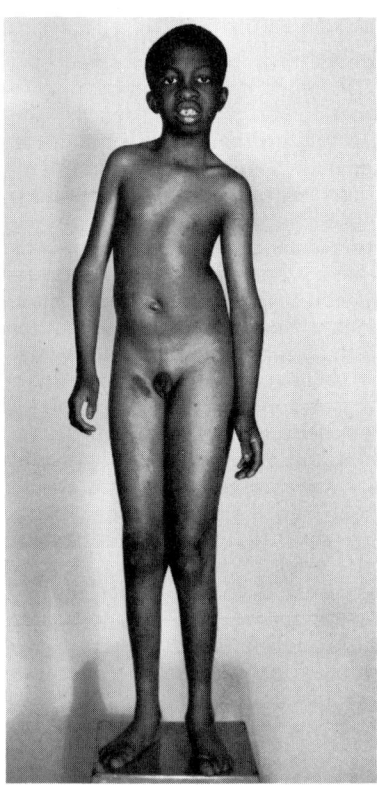

Figure 19–16. A 12 yr old boy with 48,XXXY/49,XXXXY mosaicism, who has prognathism, epicanthal folds, scoliosis, very small testes, severe mental retardation, clinodactyly, and radioulnar synostoses.

This condition poses a serious dilemma for counseling of parents of infants or children discovered to have this sex chromosome complement. The risks for some developmental disability may not be trivial; neither do they appear as dire as earlier thought.

19.31 HYPOGONADOTROPIC HYPOGONADISM IN THE MALE
(Secondary Hypogonadism)

In hypogonadotropic hypogonadism there is deficiency of follicle-stimulating hormone (FSH) and/or of luteinizing hormone (LH). The primary defect may lie in the anterior pituitary or in the hypothalamus as a deficiency of gonadotropin-releasing hormone. The testes are normal but remain in the prepubertal state because stimulation by gonadotropins is lacking. The classification of these disorders is in active evolution.

Etiology. *Hypopituitarism.* Patients with growth hormone deficiency frequently have associated deficiency of one or more of the other pituitary hormones. The most frequently associated deficiency is that of gonadotropin. In patients with organic lesions in or near the pituitary (e.g., craniopharyngiomas), the gonadotropin deficiency is pituitary in origin. On the other hand, in many patients with "idiopathic" or "familial" hypopituitarism, it now appears that the defect lies in the hypothalamus; administration of luteinizing hormone-releasing hormone (LH-RH) to these patients indicates that the pituitary is capable of response. In some patients in whom the rise of FSH and LH in response to acute administration of LH-RH has been impaired or absent, more intensive stimulation produced a response. These findings suggest that the pituitary cells responsible for gonadotropin production can release hormone into the circulation if appropriately stimulated.

Isolated Deficiency of Gonadotropin. When deficiency of gonadotropin occurs as an isolated deficiency, the defect usually involves the hypothalamus rather than the pituitary. *Kallmann syndrome* (hypogonadotropic hypogonadism with *anosmia*) is the most frequent cause of isolated deficiency of gonadotropins. Affected patients fail to develop sexually or exhibit only minimal development at puberty. Inability to smell is present from early childhood, but it is usually not discovered except on direct questioning. Both FSH and LH remain at prepubertal levels in adult life. Agenesis of the olfactory lobes of the brain accounts for the anosmia. No histologic lesion has been defined, but a hypothalamic defect is the cause for the gonadotropin deficiency inasmuch as administration of LH-RH to affected patients produces increases in FSH and LH.

Other somatic defects observed in some patients with Kallmann syndrome include cryptorchidism, choanal abnormalities, and renal abnormalities. Familial occurrences have suggested X-linked, autosomal dominant, and autosomal recessive forms of transmission; genetic heterogeneity is evident. The expression is variable; some kindreds contain anosmic individuals without, as well as others with, hypogonadism; other kindreds contain individuals with only harelip or cleft palate or with only hypogonadism or anosmia. The incidence of hyposmia in affected families is not known; more males than females have been recognized with the syndrome. Spermatogenesis can be induced by treatment with human menopausal gonadotropins (hMG).

Isolated deficiency of LH has been observed in patients with the *fertile eunuch syndrome.* Failure of the Leydig cells to mature at puberty is accompanied by delayed pubertal development. The testes may be normal in size, however, and spermatogenesis may occur. A good response to administration of chorionic gonadotropin reveals the presence of normal Leydig

cell precursors. Serum and urine FSH concentrations are normal, whereas those of LH are undetectable or low. An increase in LH levels follows administration of LH-RH, indicating a hypothalamic defect. Fertility has occasionally been noted, but evidence suggests that testicular androgen is necessary for completely normal spermatogenesis. This rare syndrome has been observed in brothers and in association with Kallmann syndrome.

Biologically inactive LH has been demonstrated in one hypogonadal male born of a consanguineous union who had immunologically active LH of normal molecular weight. The defect may reside in the primary structure of the molecule. Isolated *autoimmune gonadotrope failure* has been observed in two young men with the *polyglandular autoimmune syndrome.*

Other Syndromes. Some syndromes of hypogonadism with gonadotropin deficiency have not yet been evaluated by up-to-date techniques, and the sites of their defects are unknown. In the recessively inherited *Laurence-Moon-Biedl syndrome* hypogonadism occurs in both males and females, but its incidence is unknown. On occasion, the hypogonadism is primary, but there is usually hypothalamic-pituitary dysfunction. Several syndromes of ataxia and hypogonadotropic hypogonadism appear to have distinctive genetic origins. Ichthyosis and male hypogonadism has been described in several families. In 10 males in four generations of one kindred, hypogonadotropic hypogonadism and ichthyosis were associated with anosmia and mild mental retardation. In the *multiple lentigines syndrome*, an autosomal dominant disorder, delayed puberty occurs in about 25% of affected patients. An 18 yr old male with this syndrome and delayed puberty had deficiency of FSH and LH and anosmia, suggesting a hypothalamic defect. The *Prader-Willi syndrome* presents variable hypogonadotropic hypogonadism as well as hypergonadotropic hypogonadism. We have observed hypogonadotropic hypogonadism in *Carpenter syndrome* and in *Lowe syndrome.*

Diagnosis. Constitutional delay of puberty is extremely difficult to differentiate from hypogonadotropic hypogonadism since in both conditions gonadotropin levels remain low after the usual age of puberty. The diagnosis should always be considered if puberty is delayed beyond 16–17 yr of age. The detection of other pituitary deficits, the discovery of anosmia by careful questioning, and the history of hypogonadism in other family members are important clues. Plasma levels of LH and of testosterone during sleep may identify boys with delayed puberty who are on the verge of spontaneous puberty inasmuch as augmentation of LH secretion during sleep has its onset in early puberty. In hypogonadotropic hypogonadism there is no sleep-associated rise in LH secretion. Though they may have blunted gonadotropin responses to LH-RH during the prepubertal years, most children (76–90%) with isolated growth hormone deficiency undergo normal puberty. Accordingly, the response to LH-RH is not a reliable prepubertal indicator of gonadotropin status in children with isolated growth hormone deficiency. In the hypopituitary patient absent or delayed adrenarche, as compared with bone age, usually indicates gonadotropin deficiency. Children with ACTH deficiency are also usually deficient in gonadotropins. Prolactinomas are being increasingly recognized as a cause for delayed puberty.

Treatment. Administration of chorionic gonadotropin induces satisfactory development of secondary sex characters by stimulating the Leydig cells. The recommended dose is 4000–5000 IU three times weekly for 6 wk. After discontinuation of therapy a period of observation for evidence of regression is necessary to establish the diagnosis. If puberty regresses, the patient probably has hypogonadotropic hypogonadism, whereas if puberty continues, the patient has had physiologic delay of maturation. Several such courses may be necessary to exclude the diagnosis of physiologic delay of adolescence. When the diagnosis of secondary hypogonadism is established, maintenance therapy with androgen is initiated. When fertility is desired, it is necessary to stimulate spermatogenesis. The androgen is discontinued and treatment with hCG is begun. Levels of testosterone rise to normal and spermatogenesis usually occurs. In prepubertal patients in whom hypogonadism has been recognized, treatment also with human menopausal gonadotropin is usually required. Long-term intermittent treatment with LH-RH has also been used successfully in a few patients to induce spermatogenesis and fertility.

19.32 PSEUDOPRECOCITY RESULTING FROM TUMORS OF THE TESTES

Functional tumors of the testis are rare causes of sexual pseudoprecocity. Such tumors arise from the Leydig cells, which are sparse before puberty. Tumors derived from them are more common in the adult; about 50 cases in children have been reported, including one member in each of two pairs of identical twins. Leydig cell tumors are usually benign.

The clinical manifestations are those of puberty in the male; onset occurs usually from 4–6 yr of age. Gynecomastia has occurred in five patients. The tumor of the testis can usually be readily felt; the contralateral unaffected testis is normal in size for the age of the patient.

Urinary 17-ketosteroids are only slightly or moderately increased, but testosterone levels are markedly elevated. FSH and LH levels are suppressed and there is no response to LH-RH. Treatment consists of surgical removal of the affected testis. Progression of virilization ceases, and partial reversal of the signs of precocity may occur.

There are few other causes of testicular enlargement to be considered in the differential diagnosis. Rarely, in untreated congenital adrenal hyperplasia, the testes will contain ectopic adrenal cortical cells, which give rise to bilateral testicular enlargement; treatment with corticosteroids suppresses adrenocortical activity, and they return to normal size. Occasionally, adolescents and young adults with inadequately treated congenital adrenal hyperplasia develop bilateral testicular tumors which may be suppressed by corticosteroids; these are thought to arise from pluripotential cells in the testes. In boys with unilateral cryptorchidism, the contralateral testis is about 25% larger than normal for age. The enlargement of the testes which occurs in boys with true precocious puberty is bilateral and symmetrical.

The association of marked enlargement of the testes (macro-orchidism) with mental retardation occurs in the *fragile X syndrome* (Sec. 6.27), in which, after puberty, the testicular size reaches 40–50 cc. Twenty-seven per cent of males in an institution for the retarded who had testicular volumes over 34 cc had the fragile X syndrome. Macro-orchidism has been recognized in individuals as young as 5 mo of age. The penis is normal in size, and there is no evidence of precocious puberty. Hormonal studies and testicular histology are normal. Patients with macro-orchidism who have a fragile site at the terminus of the long arm of the X chromosome (Xq 27 fra) have an associated X-linked mutation. The relationship between chromosomal abnormality and genetic disorder is not understood, but the fragile X serves as a useful marker to study affected families. The identification of affected boys is important to genetic counseling in families where macro-orchidism is associated with X-linked mental retardation.

19.33 GYNECOMASTIA

Gynecomastia, or the occurrence of mammary tissue in the male, is a common condition. It occurs in most newborn males as a result of stimulation by maternal hormones. The effect disappears in a few weeks.

During midpuberty approximately two thirds of boys develop varying degrees of subareolar hyperplasia of the breasts. *Physiologic pubertal gynecomastia* may involve only one breast, and it is not unusual for both breasts to enlarge at disproportionate rates or at different times. Tenderness of the breast is common but transitory. Spontaneous regression may occur within a few mo; it rarely persists longer than 2 yr. Mean concentrations of FSH, LH, prolactin, testosterone, estrone, and estradiol are the same as in boys without gynecomastia. When, however, levels are correlated with stage of puberty, a decreased ratio of testosterone to estradiol is found in boys with gynecomastia. Treatment usually consists of reassurance of the boy and his family of the physiologic and transient nature of the phenomenon. Surgical removal of the breast is rarely indicated; when enlargement is striking and persistent and causes serious emotional disturbance to the patient, removal may be justified.

Occasionally, breast development may mimic female breast development (to Tanner stages 3–5) and fails to regress. *Familial gynecomastia* has occurred in several kindreds as an X-linked or autosomal dominant sex-limited trait. Levels of gonadotropins, testosterone, prolactin, and steroid-binding globulins are normal. Several patients studied in detail had elevated levels of estradiol with evidence of increased peripheral conversion of C_{19}-steroids to estrogens (increased aromatization). The molecular genetic defect is unknown.

In young children with gynecomastia an exogenous source of estrogens must be sought. Either accidental or therapeutic exposure to small amounts of estrogens by inhalation, percutaneous absorption, or ingestion may cause gynecomastia. Increased pigmentation of the nipple and areola should suggest this cause. Gynecomastia may also be caused by exogenously administered androgens.

A number of other pathologic conditions may cause gynecomastia. It has been noted in two children (1 yr and 6 1/2 yr old) with the 11β-hydroxylase–deficient form of congenital virilizing adrenal hyperplasia, probably owing to excessive adrenal production of estrogens. It may be associated with Leydig cell tumors of the testis or with feminizing tumors of the adrenal. A young boy with the *Peutz-Jeghers syndrome* and gynecomastia had a *sex-cord tumor with annular tubules* of the testes. Gynecomastia occurs in Klinefelter syndrome and with other types of testicular failure (hypergonadotropic states). It is a common finding in certain types of male pseudohermaphroditism, particularly in Reifenstein syndrome, in the testicular feminization syndrome, and in patients with the 17β-hydroxysteroid dehydrogenase defect. When gynecomastia is associated with galactorrhea, a prolactinoma should be considered. In adults gynecomastia occurs with liver cirrhosis, with digitalis therapy for congestive heart failure, with bronchogenic carcinoma, with administration of various nonsteroidal therapeutic agents, and with heavy marijuana smoking. Ketoconazole, a new antifungal drug, causes gynecomastia by direct inhibition of testosterone synthesis.

HYPOFUNCTION OF THE OVARIES

Hypofunction of the ovaries may be due to congenital failure of development or to postnatal destruction (primary or hypergonadotropic hypogonadism) or to lack of stimulation by the pituitary (secondary or hypogonadotropic hypogonadism). Many chronic diseases may result in the latter type.

19.34 HYPERGONADOTROPIC HYPOGONADISM IN THE FEMALE
(Primary Hypogonadism)

Diagnosis of hypergonadotropic hypogonadism prior to puberty is possible. Except in the case of Turner syndrome, most affected patients have no prepubertal clinical manifestations.

Turner Syndrome

In 1938 Turner described a syndrome consisting of sexual infantilism, webbed neck, and cubitum valgum in adult females. It was found that such women have elevated levels of urinary gonadotropins and that the gonads consist of rudimentary elongated streaks containing no germinal elements but whorls of connective tissue suggestive of ovarian stroma.

Pathogenesis. In 1959 it was demonstrated that patients with Turner syndrome have a single X chromosome (a 45,X chromosome constitution). The X chromosome is maternal in 77% and paternal in 23% of cases. The occurrence of Turner syndrome is not influenced by maternal age; the mechanism of origin is unknown. A large prospective study found a seasonal pattern, two thirds of births with nondisjunction occurring between May and October.

The 45,X disorder occurs in about 1/3000 live born females and is much less common than Klinefelter syndrome. It appears that over 95% of all 45,X conceptions are aborted; 5–10% of all abortuses are 45,X. Mosaicism (46,XX/45,X) among patients with Turner syndrome is 25%, a proportion higher than with any other aneuploid state, whereas the mosaic Turner constitution is rare among the abortuses; these findings indicate preferential survival for mosaic forms.

Other types of mosaics, such as isochromosome for the long arm, deletion of the short arm, and rings of the X chromosome, are less common.

Primordial germ cells are found in the gonadal ridges of aborted 45,X fetuses up to 3 mo of gestation but disappear thereafter. In the normal fetus the number of germ cells declines rapidly at about 5 mo of gestation and then decreases at a slower rate after birth. In the 45,X patient this normal process may be hastened and exaggerated. The streak gonads usually consist of only connective tissue; rarely, a few germ cells may be found to explain partial sexual maturation.

Clinical Manifestations. In the past the diagnosis was generally first suspected in childhood or at puberty when sexual maturation failed to occur. It is now clear that most 45,X patients are recognizable at birth, because a characteristic edema of the dorsum of the hands and feet and loose skin folds at the nape are present. Significantly low birth weight and short stature are common. Clinical manifestations in childhood include webbing of the neck, a low posterior hairline, small mandible, prominent ears, epicanthic folds, high arched palate, a broad chest presenting the illusion of widely spaced nipples, cubitum valgum, and hyperconvex fingernails. Stature is almost always below the 3rd percentile; the mean adult height is 146.3 ± 5.5 cm. With increasing age, pigmented nevi become more prominent. At the expected age sexual maturation fails to occur. Many patients have minimal manifestations and come to medical attention primarily because of short stature.

Associated defects are common. Coarctation of the aorta occurs in about 15% of patients, isolated nonstenotic bicuspid aortic valve can be detected in about one third of patients by

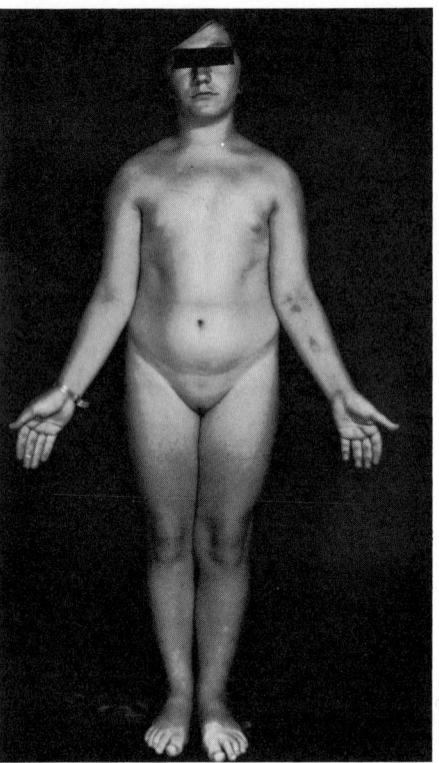

Figure 19–17. Turner syndrome in a 15 yr old girl exhibiting failure of sexual maturation, short stature, cubitus valgus, and a goiter. There is no webbing of the neck. Karyotype revealed 45,X/46,XX chromosome complement, and urinary gonadotropin was over 96 mouse units/24 hr. T_4 was 2.2 μg/dl. Biopsy of the thyroid revealed lymphocytic thyroiditis.

echocardiography, and hypertension of unknown etiology is found in a few patients. A dissecting aortic aneurysm is a rare complication. Approximately half the patients have abnormal urograms, horseshoe kidney and malrotation being the most common anomalies. Recurrent bilateral otitis media is common. Deficits in hearing and in perceptual spatial skills are more common than in the general population.

Goiter should suggest lymphocytic thyroiditis; abdominal pain, tenesmus, or bloody diarrhea may represent inflammatory bowel disease; and recurrent gastrointestinal bleeding may indicate gastrointestinal telangiectasia. Patients with Turner syndrome have a higher than expected incidence of these conditions.

In the *45,X/46,XX mosaic* the abnormalities are attenuated and fewer. The affected newborn usually has no recognizable findings. Webbing of the neck, coarctation of the aorta, and edema of hands and feet are infrequent. Short stature is as frequent as in the 45,X patient and may be the only manifestation (Fig. 19–17).

Sexual maturation fails to occur in both the 45,X and 45,X/46,XX patients; occasional patients with some degree of breast development or even menstruation are likely to be 45,X/46,XX mosaics. Fertility has been reported in seven patients with a 45,X karyotype.

Laboratory Data. Chromosomal analysis should be done in all suspected patients. A minority of girls with the features of Turner syndrome have a Y chromosome; their management differs from that of those who are 45,X or 45,X/46,XX (see below, mixed gonadal dysgenesis).

Plasma levels of gonadotropins, particularly of follicle-stimulating hormone (FSH), are usually elevated above those of age-matched controls, even in infancy. In prepubertal children occasional levels of FSH may not be clearly abnormal because of the overlap with the range of normal values. After 10 yr of age plasma levels are markedly elevated and approximate menopausal levels. At puberty the pulsatile release of FSH and luteinizing hormone (LH) accounts for day-to-day variability in plasma levels. Urinary gonadotropins are clearly elevated after 10–12 yr of age but are less helpful in prepubertal children. Urinary excretion of estrogens and plasma levels of estradiol are very low. Growth hormone secretion in response to provocative stimuli is normal.

Roentgenographic studies may reveal cardiovascular or renal abnormalities. The most common skeletal abnormalities are shortening of the 4th metatarsal and metacarpal bones, epiphyseal dysgenesis in the joints of the knee and elbow, inadequate osseous mineralization, scoliosis, and spina bifida occulta.

A high percentage of patients and other family members have significant titers of antithyroid antibodies. Mild chemical diabetes is present in about one third of patients.

Treatment. Replacement therapy with estrogens is indicated, but there is little consensus as to an optimal age for its initiation. The psychosocial preparedness of the patient to accept therapy must be taken into account. Some endocrinologists have recommended a period of treatment with an anabolic agent to enhance growth before treating with estrogens, but this does not appear to alter adult height. Some recommend deferring therapy with estrogens beyond the mid-teens in order to avoid early closure of epiphyses, but this also appears to have no benefit. Others recommend initiating therapy with very small doses of estrogens (ethinyl estradiol, 100 ng/kg/24 hr) at 9–10 yr of age; it remains to be determined if this will alter final height. In any event, eventually all patients receive estrogen-progesterone cyclic therapy.

At present treatment of the short stature with combined growth hormone and oxandrolone is undergoing clinical trials; short-term growth is accelerated, but the effect on final adult height remains to be determined. Patients who receive adequate continuing psychosocial support have an excellent prognosis for normal lives.

XX Gonadal Dysgenesis

Some phenotypically normal females have gonadal lesions identical to those in 45,X patients but without somatic features of Turner syndrome; their condition is termed "pure gonadal dysgenesis." Some with a 46,XY karyotype are also designated as having the Swyer syndrome, which is discussed below, with male pseudohermaphroditism. Here we discuss only those with the XX chromosome constitution. These two conditions are quite distinct entities; in no instance have XX and XY gonadal dysgenesis been reported in the same family.

The disorder is rarely recognized in children because the external genitalia are normal, no other abnormalities are visible, and growth is normal. At pubertal age sexual maturation fails to take place. Plasma gonadotropin levels are elevated. Delay of epiphyseal fusion results in a eunuchoid habitus.

Affected siblings, parental consanguinity, and failure to uncover mosaicism (even in the streak gonads) all point to autosomal recessive inheritance. It appears that autosomal genes have an important role in the differentiation of normal ovaries. In five families XX gonadal dysgenesis has been associated with sensorineural deafness; there may be distinct genetic forms of this disorder. Tumors of the gonads have not been reported in these patients. Treatment consists of replacement therapy with estrogens.

45,X/46,XY Gonadal Dysgenesis

This condition, *mixed gonadal dysgenesis,* has extreme variability, which may extend from a Turner-like syndrome to a male phenotype with a penile urethra; it is possible to delineate three major clinical phenotypes. Short stature is a major finding in all affected patients.

Some patients have no evidence of masculinization; they have a female phenotype and often the somatic signs of Turner syndrome. The condition is discovered prepubertally when chromosomal studies are made in short girls, or later, when chromosomal studies are made because of failure of sexual maturation. Fallopian tubes and uterus are present. The gonads consist of intra-abdominal undifferentiated streaks; chromosome study of the streak often reveals an XY cell line. The streak gonad differs somewhat from that in Turner syndrome; in addition to wavy connective tissue there are often tubular or cord-like structures, occasional clumps of granulosa cells, and frequently mesonephric or hilus cells. Occasionally, the Y chromosome may be represented by only a fragment (45,X/45,X + fra). Cytogenetic techniques may be inadequate to establish the fragment as a Y chromosome, but application of Y-specific probes may reveal Y-specific DNA sequences in the fragment, thereby establishing its origin.

Some patients have mild virilization manifested only by prepubertal clitorimegaly. Normal müllerian structures are present, but at puberty virilization occurs. These patients usually have an intra-abdominal testis, a contralateral streak gonad, and bilateral fallopian tubes.

Many patients present with frank ambiguity of the genitalia; this is the most frequent phenotype encountered in infants. A testis and vas deferens are found on one side in the labioscrotal fold, and a streak gonad on the contralateral side. Despite the presence of a testis, fallopian tubes are usually present bilaterally. An infantile or rudimentary uterus is almost always present.

Other genotypes and phenotypes, particularly 45,X/46,XY/47,XYYY, have been described. It is not clear why the same genotype (45,X/46,XY) can result in such diverse phenotypes. Variable expression of the Y chromosome is a likely explanation; in some instances, high resolution cytogenetic techniques have revealed abnormalities of the Y chromosome.

Patients with a female phenotype present no problem in gender of rearing. Patients who are only slightly virilized are usually assigned a female gender of rearing before a diagnosis is established. Patients with ambiguity of the genitalia are readily confused with various types of male pseudohermaphroditism. In most instances these patients are best reared as females; the short stature, the ease of genital reconstruction, and the predisposition of the gonad to develop malignancy favor this choice. In some patients followed to adulthood the putative normal testis proved to be dysgenetic with eventual loss of Leydig and Sertoli cell function.

Gonadal tumors, usually gonadoblastomas, occur in about 25% of these patients, particularly in those with the more female phenotypes. These germ cell tumors are preceded by the changes of carcinoma in situ. Accordingly, both gonads should be removed in all patients reared as girls and the undifferentiated gonad should be removed in the few patients reared as males.

XXX, XXXX, and XXXXX Females

XXX Females. The 47,XXX chromosomal constitution is the most frequent X chromosome abnormality in females, occurring in almost 1/1000 live born females. Affected infants are not usually recognized but frequently have minor anomalies, particularly clinodactyly, epicanthal folds, and wide-set eyes. The majority have normal intelligence with an increased tendency to emotional immaturity, speech difficulties, and learning disorders. Sexual maturation occurs at puberty and fertility is usually normal, but there may be an increased incidence of congenital defects in progeny.

XXXX and XXXXX Females. About 17 females with four X and 6 with five X chromosomes have been described. All have been mentally retarded except for one of the 48,XXXX girls. Commonly associated defects are epicanthal folds, hypertelorism, clinodactyly, simian crease, radioulnar synostosis, and congenital heart disease. Sexual maturation is often incomplete and may not occur at all.

Noonan Syndrome

Girls with Noonan syndrome show certain anomalies which also occur in girls with 45,X Turner syndrome, but they have normal 46,XX chromosomes. The most common abnormalities are the same as described for males with Noonan syndrome (Sec. 19.30). The phenotype differs from Turner syndrome in the following respects: (1) Mental retardation is more common; (2) the cardiac defect is most often pulmonary valvular stenosis or atrial septal defect rather than aortic coarctation; and (3) gonadal defects may be present, but normal sexual maturation usually occurs.

Other Ovarian Defects

An increasing number of other young women with no chromosomal abnormality are being found to have "streak" gonads which may contain only occasional germ cells, if any. Gonadotropins are increased. *Cytotoxic drugs* and exposure of the ovaries to radiation for the treatment of malignancy are increasingly frequent causes of ovarian failure. A study of young women with Hodgkin disease found that combination chemotherapy and pelvic irradiation may be more deleterious than either therapy alone. Teenagers are more apt than older women to retain or have recovery of ovarian function after either irradiation or combined chemotherapy; normal pregnancies have occurred after such treatment. Current treatment regimens may result in some ovarian damage in 50% of girls treated for cancer.

Autoimmune ovarian disease occurs predominantly in association with Type I autoimmune polyendocrinopathy syndrome but may occur with other autoimmune disorders or as an isolated event. Affected girls may not develop sexually, or secondary amenorrhea may occur in young women. The ovaries may have lymphocytic infiltration or appear simply as streaks. The majority of affected patients have circulating steroid cell antibodies.

Galactosemia may cause ovarian failure, with primary or secondary amenorrhea the presenting clinical manifestation. Elevated levels of FSH and LH, even early in life, reflect early ovarian failure. Antiovarian antibodies are not found. Ovarian failure may begin during intrauterine life since it has occurred even in girls treated with a galactose-free diet from birth. A galactose-free diet during pregnancy in a woman known to be heterozygous failed to prevent accumulation in cord blood erythrocytes of galactose-1-phosphate; that indicates endogenous production by the fetus.

Ataxia-telangiectasia may be associated with ovarian hypoplasia and elevated gonadotropins; the cause is not known, but it appears to be an integral part of the syndrome.

19.35 HYPOGONADOTROPIC HYPOGONADISM IN THE FEMALE
(Secondary Hypogonadism)

Hypofunction of the ovaries can result from failure to secrete normal levels of gonadotropins. The defect may lie in the anterior pituitary, but as in the male, there is increasing evidence for a hypothalamic defect in most such hypogonadal females.

Etiology. *Hypopituitarism.* Destructive lesions in or near the pituitary almost always result in impaired secretion of gonadotropins as well as of other pituitary hormones. In patients with idiopathic hypopituitarism, however, the defect is usually found in the hypothalamus. In these patients administration of LH-RH results in increased plasma levels of FSH and LH, and administration of thyrotropin-releasing hormone (TRH) provokes a rise in plasma level of thyroid-stimulating hormone (TSH), establishing the integrity of the pituitary gland.

Isolated Deficiency of Gonadotropins. This heterogeneous group of disorders is only now being sorted out with the help of the LH-RH test. Isolated pituitary deficiency of FSH has been documented, but in most patients the pituitary is normal, the defect residing in the hypothalamus.

Several sporadic instances of anosmia with hypogonadotropic hypogonadism have been reported. Anosmic hypogonadal females have also been reported in kindreds with Kallmann syndrome, but hypogonadism more frequently affects the males in these families.

Some autosomal recessive disorders such as the Laurence-Moon-Biedl, multiple lentigines, and Carpenter syndromes also appear in some instances to include gonadotropic hormone deficiency.

Diagnosis. The diagnosis is not difficult in patients with other deficiencies of pituitary tropic hormones. On the other hand, it is difficult to differentiate isolated hypogonadotropic hypogonadism from physiologic delay of puberty. Repeated measurements of FSH and LH, particularly during sleep, may reveal rising levels which herald the onset of puberty.

19.36 POLYCYSTIC OVARIES
(Stein-Leventhal Syndrome)

The classic syndrome is characterized by obesity, hirsutism, and secondary amenorrhea, with bilaterally enlarged polycystic ovaries, but these manifestations may not all be present. Onset is often at puberty or shortly thereafter; menstrual irregularities and hirsutism are the most frequent complaints. In the reproductive years, the condition is a common cause of infertility, owing to anovulation. The enlarged ovaries can often be felt on combined rectal and abdominal palpation, and are always demonstrable by ultrasonography.

The cause of the disorder is unsettled, but evidence is increasing for a hypothalamic defect as the initiating event.

The association of the polycystic ovarian syndrome with *acanthosis nigricans,* insulin resistance, and obesity is being increasingly recognized in young women. All women with acanthosis nigricans should have assessment of ovarian function and glucose tolerance.

Late onset congenital virilizing adrenal hyperplasia may mimic polycystic ovarian disease. Basal levels of 17-hydroxyprogesterone may be normal, and an ACTH stimulation test may be required to reveal the defect.

Bilateral wedge resections of the ovaries result in normal ovulatory menstrual cycles in 70–80% of patients, in some way relieving the suppression of FSH and restoring normal follicular maturation. Success of this therapy is often of short duration; accordingly, surgery may be deferred until the patient wishes to become pregnant. For young girls therapy with clomiphene citrate is probably preferable.

19.37 PSEUDOPRECOCITY DUE TO LESIONS OF THE OVARY

Most of the functioning lesions of the ovary in children are neoplasms. The majority synthesize estrogens; a few synthesize androgens. Infrequently, a lesion produces both estrogens and androgens, or the same lesion may produce estrogenic manifestations in one patient and androgenic in another; for example, the rare androblastoma of the ovary has caused isosexual precocity in some girls, masculinization in others. (See also Sec. 16.23.)

19.38 ESTROGENIC LESIONS OF THE OVARY

These lesions cause isosexual precocious sexual development but account for only a small percentage of all instances of precocity.

Juvenile Granulosa Cell Tumor

In childhood the most common neoplasm of the ovary with estrogenic manifestations is the granulosa-cell tumor. These tumors have distinctive histologic features that differ from those encountered in older women (adult granulosa-cell tumor). Follicles are often irregular, Call-Exner bodies are rare, and luteinization is frequent.

Clinical Manifestations. The tumor has been observed in a newborn infant, and 36 instances are known with sexual precocity at 2 yr of age or less; about half of these tumors have occurred before 10 yr of age. They are almost always unilateral. The breasts become enlarged, rounded, and firm and the nipples prominent. The external genitalia resemble those of a normal girl at puberty, and the uterus is enlarged. A white vaginal discharge is followed by irregular or cyclic menstruation. Ovulation, however, does not occur. The presenting manifestation may be abdominal pain or swelling. Pubic hair is usually absent unless there is mild virilization.

A mass is readily palpable in the lower portion of the abdomen in most patients by the time sexual precocity is evident. The tumor may be small, however, and escape detection even on careful rectal and abdominal examination; such tumors are usually detectable by ultrasonography.

Plasma estradiol levels are markedly elevated; a 9 yr old girl with a granulosa cell tumor had a level of 413 pg/dL, whereas levels in fully mature women or in children with idiopathic precocious puberty are under 100 pg/dL. Plasma levels of gonadotropins are suppressed and do not respond to LH-RH stimulation. Alpha-fetoprotein levels may be elevated. Osseous development is moderately advanced.

The tumor should be removed as soon as the diagnosis is established. Prognosis is excellent since less than 5% of these tumors in children are malignant. Vaginal bleeding immediately after removal of the tumor is common. Signs of precocious puberty abate and may disappear within a few mo after operation. The secretion of estrogens returns to normal.

Sex-cord tumor with annular tubules is a distinctive tumor, thought to arise from granulosa cells, that occurs primarily in patients with Peutz-Jeghers syndrome. In three girls (two siblings) with Peutz-Jeghers syndrome, precocious puberty developed in association with this tumor.

Follicular Cyst

Ovarian cysts are common in childhood, but most are nonfunctioning and hence not feminizing. Follicular cysts are common also in girls with true sexual precocity, in whom the cyst is a secondary event; it is not the cause of sexual precocity, and its removal does not alter the course of sexual precocity. In rare instances, on the other hand, removal of a follicular cyst has resulted in regression of clinical signs of sexual precocity. Such functional cysts are being increasingly recognized as the major cause for sexual precocity in children with McCune-Albright syndrome. Since these cysts function autonomously, gonadotropins are suppressed and estradiol levels

markedly elevated, though they may fluctuate widely and even return spontaneously to normal. Stimulation of these children with luteinizing hormone-releasing hormone (LH-RH) results in a prepubertal type of response rather than the pubertal type response expected in true precocious puberty. Ultrasonography is the method of choice to detect such cysts. Small evanescent cysts are thought to account for some instances of isolated premature menarche or premature thelarche.

19.39 ANDROGENIC LESIONS OF THE OVARY

Virilizing ovarian tumors are rare at all ages but particularly so in prepubertal girls. The *androblastoma (arrhenoblastoma)* has been reported as early as 4 yr of age, but fewer than 2 dozen cases have been reported under 16 yr of age. Other androgen-secreting tumors include lipoid cell tumors and such benign ovarian lesions as ovarian hyperthecosis. The clinical features are the same as for virilizing adrenal tumors and include acne, hirsutism, and clitoral enlargement. These conditions must be given consideration in adolescent girls with hirsutism and secondary amenorrhea. Urinary 17-ketosteroids may be normal or only slightly elevated, but plasma levels of testosterone are usually elevated, and levels of LH are suppressed. In order to differentiate these lesions from adrenal tumors, dexamethasone suppression and chorionic gonadotropin stimulation studies may be necessary. Even such studies, however, may not differentiate among them, and selective venography and venous blood sampling or exploratory laparotomy may be indicated.

Patients with polycystic ovaries usually have elevated plasma levels of LH as well as of testosterone, and they may exhibit excessive response to LH-RH. Wedge resection of the ovary may be beneficial.

19.40 HERMAPHRODITISM
(Intersexuality)

Hermaphroditism in man implies a discrepancy between the morphology of the gonads and of the external genitalia. Many chromosomal aberrations resulting in ambiguity of the external genitalia have been discussed earlier in this section. Here we discuss those conditions of aberrant sexual differentiation that are imposed on the XX or XY genotype (female and male pseudohermaphrodites) (Table 19–8). An increasing number of such conditions are now understood through advances in the understanding of normal sexual differentiation. The category known as true hermaphroditism, with few exceptions, is still a poorly understood heterogeneous group of disorders.

Embryonic Sexual Differentiation. In normal differentiation, the final form of all sexual structures is consistent with normal sex chromosomes (either XX or XY). A 46,XX complement of chromosomes is necessary for the development of normal ovaries. Both the long and the short arms of X chromosomes bear genes for normal ovarian development. An autosomal gene also appears to play a role in normal ovarian organogenesis (see XX gonadal dysgenesis, above). A deletion affecting the short arm of the X chromosome produces the typical somatic anomalies of Turner syndrome.

Development of the male phenotype is more complex. Testicular differentiation is controlled by genes on the short arm of the Y chromosome near the centromere. With few exceptions the finding of testes indicates presence of a Y chromosome; the exceptions (XX males and XX true hermaphrodites) usually have translocations of male-determining genes onto paternal X chromosomes. Histocompatibility Y

Table 19–8. Etiologic Classification of Hermaphroditism

Female pseudohermaphroditism
  Androgen exposure
    Fetal source
      Congenital adrenal hyperplasia
        21-Hydroxylase deficiency
        11β-Hydroxylase deficiency
        3β-Hydroxysteroid dehydrogenase deficiency
      Adrenal tumor?
    Maternal source
      Virilizing tumor
        Ovary
        Adrenal
      Androgenic drugs
      Progestational drugs
  Undetermined origin
    Usually associated with other defects (skeleton, urinary and
      gastrointestinal tracts)
Male pseudohermaphroditism
  Defect in testicular differentiation
    Deletion short arm of Y chromosome
    XY pure gonadal dysgenesis (Swyer syndrome)
    XY gonadal agenesis syndrome
    XY antigen deficiency with camptomelic dysplasia
  Defect in testicular hormones
    Leydig cell aplasia—abnormality of hCG-LH receptor?
    Inborn errors of testosterone synthesis
      Cholesterol 20,22-desmolase deficiency
      3β-Hydroxysteroid dehydrogenase deficiency
      17α-Hydroxylase deficiency
      17,20-Desmolase deficiency
      17β-Hydroxysteroid dehydrogenase deficiency
    Defect in antimüllerian hormone action (uterine hernia
      syndrome)
      Defective synthesis
      Defective response
  Defect in androgen action
    Defect in conversion of testosterone to dihydrotestosterone—
      5α-reductase deficiency
    Testicular feminization syndrome
      Cytosol receptor defect
      Post-receptor defect
    Incomplete testicular feminization
    Reifenstein syndrome (Lubs, Gilbert-Dryfus, Rosewater
      syndromes)
      Decreased cytoplasmic receptor
      Normal cytoplasmic receptor
  Undetermined—male pseudohermaphroditism
    With aniridia
    With Wilms tumor
    With nephrosis or nephritis
True hermaphroditism
  XX
  XY
  XX/XY chimeras
  Familial

(H-Y) antigen, a cell surface component found in cells from males of every mammalian species studied, is required for testicular differentiation and appears to be the primary male-determining factor. The H-Y antigen triggers the initially indifferent gonad to differentiate as a testis, beginning around the 5th–6th wk of intrauterine life. Evidence suggests that a gene on the Y chromosome is the structural gene for H-Y antigen, whereas a gene that regulates the H-Y gene is on the distal end of the short arm of the X chromosome. Less well documented is the hypothesis that H-Y genes are also on the autosomes of normal individuals. The serologic method that has been used to evaluate H-Y antigen is a formidable assay with many technical pitfalls. New assays utilizing monoclonal antibody and an ELISA assay may give this test wider application to clinical problems of hermaphroditism. Assay for the H-Y antigen can detect the effect of the genes of the

Y chromosome even when the Y chromosome cannot be found in the karyotype. In the XX fetus the female phenotype develops simply because there are no male-determining genes or H-Y antigen. The original bipotential gonad in the H-Y negative fetus develops into an ovary but not until about the 12th wk.

In the male fetus, once the indifferent gonad has differentiated into a testis, it begins to produce hormones, and masculinization of the fetus begins at about 8 wk. During this period of masculinization (8–12 wk) the fetal testis secretes two hormones. The first of these is testosterone, as shown

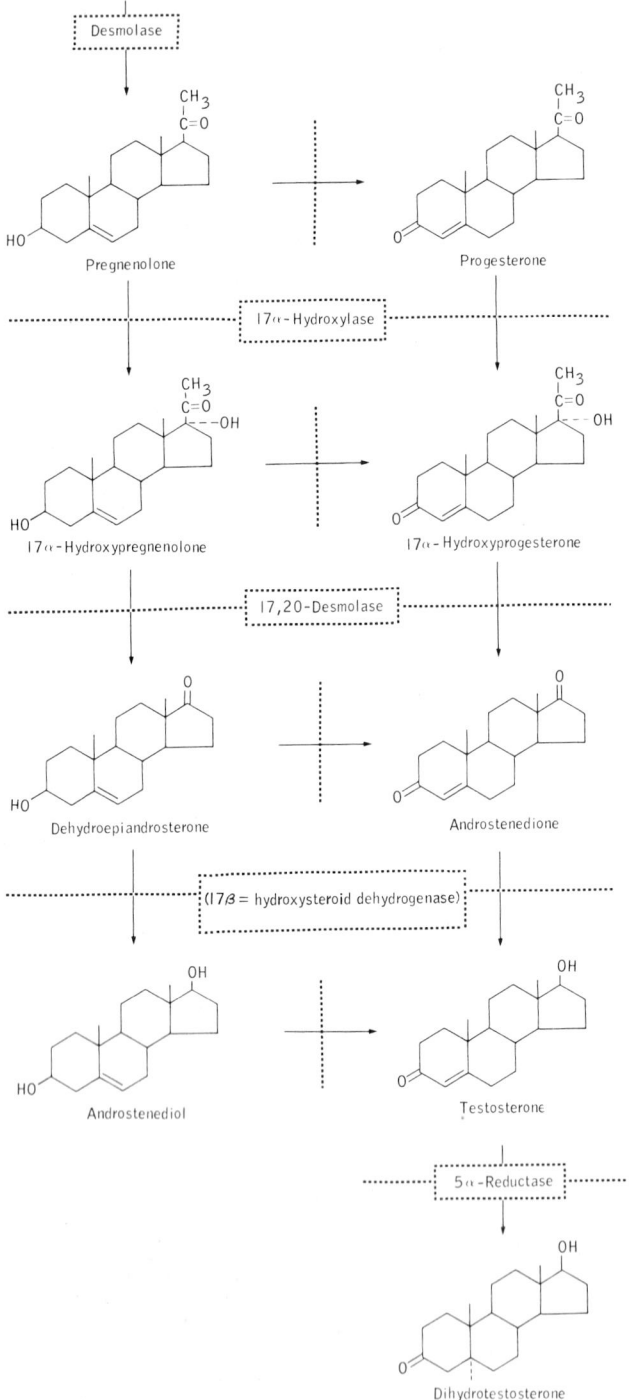

Figure 19–18. Biosynthesis of androgens. Dotted lines indicate enzymatic defects associated with male pseudohermaphroditism. Vertical dotted line indicates defect in 3β-hydroxysteroid dehydrogenase.

indirectly by correlation with cytodifferentiation of the Leydig cells and directly by measurement of testosterone concentration of fetal testes and plasma. Secretion of testosterone during this critical period of differentiation probably occurs in response to placental chorionic gonadotropin (hCG). It appears that testosterone initiates virilization of the wolffian duct into the epididymis, vas deferens, and seminal vesicle. Testosterone is also converted by a 5α-reductase to an active metabolite, dihydrotestosterone, which causes virilization of the urogenital sinus and the external genitalia. A functional androgen receptor, controlled by an X-linked gene, is required for testosterone to give a masculine phenotype to XY individuals. When there is a defect in the synthesis of testosterone, normal masculinization may not occur, even when the testis has H-Y antigen and there are normal androgen receptors. The pathway for testosterone biosynthesis is given in Fig. 19–18, which also indicates the various biosynthetic defects.

The second hormone produced by the fetal testis is the müllerian duct inhibiting factor (MIF); it is a glycoprotein of high molecular weight produced by the Sertoli cells. Though it has its effect only during a short critical period, it is produced from shortly after testicular differentiation until the perinatal period. MIF causes the müllerian ducts to regress; in its absence they persist. It is clear, therefore, that the female phenotype develops independently of the gonads. Normal female differentiation requires that there be no H-Y antigen, no testosterone, and no anti-müllerian hormone; maleness is imposed upon a basically female potential by the hormones of the fetal testis. Defects are now known at each of these steps.

19.41 FEMALE PSEUDOHERMAPHRODITISM

In the female pseudohermaphrodite the genotype is XX and the gonads are ovaries, but the external genitalia are virilized. Since there is no anti-müllerian hormone, uterus, tubes, and ovaries develop. The mechanisms involved in normal female differentiation are considerably less complex than those required for male differentiation, and the varieties and causes of female pseudohermaphroditism are fewer. Most instances result from exposure of the female fetus to excessive androgens during intrauterine life; and the changes consist principally of virilization of the external genitalia (clitoral hypertrophy and labioscrotal fusion).

Congenital Adrenal Hyperplasia. This is by far the most common cause of the condition. Females with the 21-hydroxylase and 11-hydroxylase defects are the most highly virilized, though minimal virilization also occurs with the 3β-hydroxysteroid dehydrogenase defect. Salt-losers tend to have greater degrees of virilization than non-salt-losers. The masculinization may be so intense as to result in a complete penile urethra and may mimic a male with cryptorchidism.

Masculinizing Maternal Tumors. In 18 instances the female fetus has been virilized during fetal life by a maternal androgen-producing tumor. In 4 instances the lesion was a benign adrenal adenoma, but all others were ovarian tumors, particularly androblastomas, luteomas, and Krukenberg tumors. Maternal virilization may be manifested by enlargement of the clitoris, acne, deepening of the voice, decreased lactation, hirsutism, and elevated levels of androgens. In the infant there is enlargement of the clitoris of varying degrees, often with labial fusion. Mothers of children with unexplained female pseudohermaphroditism should have measurements of their own levels of plasma testosterone and DHEAS.

Administration of Androgenic Drugs to Women During Pregnancy. Testosterone and 17-methyltestosterone have been reported to cause female pseudohermaphroditism in some instances. The greatest number of cases, however, have resulted from the use of certain progestational compounds for the treatment of threatened abortion. In recent years most of these progestins have been replaced by nonvirilizing ones.

Infants with female pseudohermaphroditism have been reported for whom no masculinizing agent could be identified. In such instances the disorder is usually associated with other congenital defects, particularly of the urinary and gastrointestinal tracts. No etiologic factors are known.

19.42 MALE PSEUDOHERMAPHRODITISM

In the male pseudohermaphrodite the genotype is XY, but the external genitalia are incompletely virilized, ambiguous, or completely female. When gonads can be found, they are invariably testes; their development may range from rudimentary to normal. Because the process of normal virilization in the fetus is so complex, it is not surprising that there are many varieties of male hermaphroditism.

Defects in Testicular Differentiation

The first step in male differentiation is conversion of the indifferent gonad to a testis. If in the XY fetus there is a deletion of the *short arm of the Y chromosome* and/or deletion of the male-determining genes, male differentiation does not occur. The phenotype is female; müllerian ducts are well developed, but gonads consist of undifferentiated streaks. By contrast, even extreme deletions of the *long arm of the Y chromosome* (Yq−) have been found in normally developed males most of whom are azoospermic and have short stature, indicating that the long arm of the Y chromosome normally has genes that prevent these manifestations. In other syndromes in which the testes fail to differentiate, Y chromosomes are morphologically normal.

Camptomelic dysplasia, a form of short-limbed dysplasia, is probably inherited as an autosomal trait (Sec. 23.21). Many of the affected phenotypic females have an XY karyotype and exhibit sex reversal. Uterus and fallopian tubes are present. The gonads appear grossly to be ovaries; histologically, some resemble dysgenetic testicular tissue, and others more closely resemble the ovaries of the newborn. H-Y antigen was absent in three cases examined. It is postulated that the mutation causing camptomelic dysplasia may also prevent the production of H-Y antigen or prevent its association with the cell surface; hence, normal testicular differentiation may not occur.

XY Pure Gonadal Dysgenesis (Swyer Syndrome). The designation "pure" distinguishes this from forms of gonadal dysgenesis which are of chromosomal origin and associated with somatic anomalies. Affected patients have a female phenotype, including vagina, uterus, and fallopian tubes, but at pubertal age breast development and menarche fail to occur. The gonads consist of almost totally undifferentiated streaks despite the presence of a cytogenetically normal Y chromosome. Although H-Y antigen is demonstrable in most patients, it is postulated that the embryonic gonad has failed to respond to the H-Y antigen for reasons not known. In patients who are H-Y negative it has been suggested that a gene on the short arm of the X chromosome which regulates production of H-Y antigen is mutated. In either case the primitive gonad fails to differentiate and cannot accomplish any testicular function, including suppression of müllerian ducts. There may be hilar cells in the gonad capable of producing some androgens; accordingly, some virilization, such as clitoral enlargement, may occur at the age of puberty. Growth is normal; there are no associated defects. The streak gonads may undergo neoplastic changes, such as gonadoblastomas and dysgerminomas, and even earlier than in the testicular feminization syndrome. The gonads should, therefore, be removed shortly after ascertainment, irrespective of age.

Pure gonadal dysgenesis also occurs in XX individuals (Sec. 19.34).

XY Gonadal Agenesis Syndrome (Embryonic Testicular Regression Syndrome). In this rare syndrome the external genitalia are slightly ambiguous but more nearly female. Hypoplasia of the labia, some degree of labioscrotal fusion, a small clitoris-like phallus, and a perineal urethral opening are present. No uterus, no gonadal tissue, and usually no vagina can be found. At the age of puberty no sexual development occurs, and gonadotropins are elevated. Most patients have been reared as females. In several patients with XY gonadal agenesis in whom no gonads could be found on exploration, significant rises in testosterone followed stimulation with human chorionic gonadotropin, indicating Leydig cell function somewhere. Siblings with the disorder are known.

In this condition it is presumed that testicular tissue was active long enough during fetal life to inhibit development of müllerian ducts but not long enough to develop wolffian ducts. Of 21 or so known instances of the condition, H-Y antigen was studied in two cases and found to be positive. Testicular degeneration seems to occur between the 8th–12th fetal wk. Regression of the testis before the 8th fetal wk results in Swyer syndrome (see above), between the 14th–20th wk of gestation the rudimentary testis syndrome, and after the 20th wk anorchia (see below).

In *bilateral anorchia* testes are absent, but the male phenotype is complete; it is presumed that tissue with fetal testicular function was active during the critical period of genital differentiation but that sometime later it was damaged. Bilateral anorchia in identical twins and unilateral anorchia both in identical twins and in siblings suggest a genetic predisposition. Coexistence of anorchia and the gonadal agenesis syndrome in a sibship is evidence for a relationship between the disorders.

Defects in Testicular Hormones

Five genetic defects have been delineated in the enzymatic synthesis of testosterone by fetal testis, and a defect in Leydig cell differentiation has been described. These defects produce male pseudohermaphroditism through inadequate masculinization of the XY fetus (Fig. 19–18). Since levels of testosterone are normally low prior to puberty, a chorionic gonadotropin stimulation test must be used in children to assess the ability of the testes to synthesize testosterone.

Leydig Cell Aplasia. Ten patients with aplasia or hypoplasia of the Leydig cells have been described. The phenotype is usually female, but there may be mild virilization. Testes, epididymis, and vas are present; uterus and fallopian tubes are absent. There are no secondary sexual changes at puberty; pubic hair may be normal. Plasma levels of testosterone are low and do not respond to hCG; gonadotropins are elevated. The Leydig cells of the testes are absent or markedly deficient. In several cases the defect appeared to involve lack of receptors that permit LH to bind to Leydig cells. In children, hCG stimulation is necessary to differentiate the condition from testicular feminization. Parents of one patient were first cousins; thus, autosomal recessive inheritance is suggested.

20,22-Desmolase Deficiency. This enzyme, now designated $P_{450}SCC$, is required early in the biosynthetic pathway to cleave the cholesterol side chain (Sec. 19.23). In its absence there is inability to synthesize glucocorticoids, mineralocorticoids, and sex steroids. There is marked accumulation of lipids in the adrenal (lipoid adrenal hyperplasia). Affected males have a female phenotype but male genital ducts. Salt-losing manifestations and early adrenal crisis are the presenting manifestations in both genetic males and females. Partial defects with partially virilized males and delayed onset of salt loss have been described.

3β-Hydroxysteroid Dehydrogenase Deficiency. Males with this form of congenital adrenal hyperplasia (Sec. 19.23) have varying degrees of hypospadias, with or without bifid scrotum and cryptorchidism. Affected infants usually develop salt-losing manifestations shortly after birth. Incomplete defects have been reported, and normal pubertal changes have occurred in some boys.

Deficiency of 17-Hydroxylase. Deficiency of this enzyme leads to reduced secretion of gonadal sex steroids and of adrenal cortisol, with secondary overproduction of salt-retaining adrenal steroids (Sec. 19.23). Males with this defect are usually phenotypically females; four patients have shown varying degrees of virilization from labioscrotal fusion to perineal hypospadias and cryptorchidism. Müllerian ducts are absent, indicating that fetal production of müllerian-inhibiting substance is normal. Levels of cortisol and testosterone are low, but there is ACTH-dependent hypersecretion of corticosterone and DOC; the renin-aldosterone axis is suppressed. The blood pressure may be normal early in life, but by the 2nd decade hypertension and hypokalemia are characteristic findings. With failure of androgen production, puberty does not occur. This defect follows autosomal recessive inheritance. Genotypic females have normal fetal sexual development but fail to undergo pubertal changes and develop hypokalemia and hypertension.

Deficiency of Steroid 17,20-Desmolase. This enzyme cleaves the side chain of 17-hydroxypregnenolone and 17-hydroxyprogesterone to form dehydroepiandrosterone and androstenedione (Fig. 19–18). In deficiency states, production of testosterone is decreased or absent. Depending on the degree of enzyme deficiency, the external genitalia in affected children vary from a female phenotype to an undervirilized male with microphallus, bifid scrotum, and perineal hypospadias. The disorder has been reported in 10 XY individuals, including siblings and first cousins, and is probably caused by an autosomal recessive gene.

Diagnostic studies for this condition include measurements of C_{21} and C_{19} steroids and urinary pregnanetriolone before and after adrenal and gonadal stimulation.

Deficiency of 17β-Hydroxysteroid Dehydrogenase. This enzyme, also called 17-ketosteroid reductase, is the last in the biosynthetic pathway to testosterone. Affected XY patients have a female phenotype or ambiguous external genitalia; in one instance a near-normal male phenotype was present. Affected persons reared as females become virilized at puberty and often develop gynecomastia; absence of müllerian ducts precludes menses. A shallow vagina is present. In prepubertal children the defect can be confused with the testicular feminization syndrome, but appropriate studies using hCG stimulation demonstrate the defect in conversion of Δ^4-androstenedione to testosterone (Fig. 19–18). Plasma levels of testosterone are low, those of Δ^4-androstenedione are elevated, and the Δ^4-A:T ratio is markedly elevated after hCG stimulation. Consanguinity of parents in several families and occurrence of affected siblings suggest autosomal recessive transmission. Patients reared as females require removal of testes and replacement therapy with estrogens. Rearing in the male gender is often possible.

Uterine Hernia Syndrome. In this disorder fetal testosterone production is normal and affected males completely virilized. There is, however, a deficiency of testicular müllerian duct inhibiting factor (MIF), with persistence of müllerian ducts. These are usually detected when surgical correction of an inguinal hernia in an otherwise normal male discloses uterus and uterine tubes. The degree of müllerian development is variable and may be asymmetrical. Testicular function, including spermatogenesis, may be normal. The disorder may result from a biosynthetic defect or from end-organ unresponsiveness to anti-müllerian hormone. At least seven sibships have been reported, each with several affected males; these suggest recessive inheritance, either X-linked or autosomal. Treatment consists of removal of as much of the müllerian structures as possible without damage to testis, epididymis, or vas deferens. About 10% of affected patients have developed testicular tumors after puberty.

Defects in Androgen Action

In the following group of disorders fetal synthesis of testosterone is normal, and defective virilization results from inherited abnormalities in androgen action.

5α-Reductase Deficiency. In this disorder decreased production of dihydrotestosterone (DHT) in utero results in severe ambiguity of the external genitalia of the affected male fetus. Biosynthesis and peripheral action of testosterone are normal.

Affected boys have a small phallus, bifid scrotum, urogenital sinus with perineal hypospadias, and a blind vaginal pouch. Testes are in the inguinal canals or labial-scrotal folds and are normal histologically. There are no müllerian structures; the vas deferens, epididymis, and seminal vesicles are present. At puberty, masculinization occurs normally; the phallus enlarges, the testes descend and grow normally, and spermatogenesis occurs. There is no gynecomastia. Beard growth is scanty, acne is absent, the prostate is small, and recession of the temporal hair line fails to occur. The T:DHT ratio is elevated in early infancy and postpubertally or may be demonstrable by hCG stimulation in prepubertal children.

These findings are consistent with studies in animals which show virilization of the wolffian duct to be due to the action of testosterone itself, whereas masculinization of the urogenital sinus and external genitalia depends on the action of dihydrotestosterone during the critical period of fetal masculinization. Growth of facial hair and of the prostate also appears to be dihydrotestosterone dependent. The disorder is inherited as an autosomal recessive but is limited to males; normal homozygous females with normal fertility indicate that in females dihydrotestosterone has no role in sexual differentiation or in ovarian function later in life. In 23 interrelated families in the Dominican Republic, although many of the 38 affected males had been reared as females, most assumed a male gender role coincident with masculinization at puberty. It appears that exposures to testosterone in utero, neonatally, and at puberty contribute to the formation of male gender identity.

Testicular Feminization Syndrome. This is one of the more common and most extreme examples of failure of virilization. These XY patients appear female at birth and are invariably reared accordingly. The external genitalia are female; the vagina ends blindly in a pouch, and the uterus is absent. The gonads are testes which consist largely of seminiferous tubules. They are usually intra-abdominal but may descend into the inguinal canal. At puberty there is normal development of breasts and the habitus is female, but menstruation does not occur and sexual hair is often absent. Psychosexual orientation of such persons is entirely female.

The testes of affected adult patients produce normal male levels of testosterone. Affected patients are able to convert testosterone to 5α-dihydrotestosterone. The absence of androgenic effects is due to a striking resistance to the action of endogenous or exogenous testosterone at the peripheral cellular level. Evidence suggests that there are clinically identical but genetically distinct variants: in some the cytosol receptor for androgen may be absent or structurally abnormal; in others the receptor is normal and the defect presumed to be postre-

ceptor. Failure of normal male differentiation during fetal life reflects the defective response to testicular androgens at that time.

In adults amenorrhea is the usual presenting symptom. Prepubertal children with this disorder are often detected when inguinal masses prove to be testes or when a testis is unexpectedly found during herniorrhaphy in a phenotypic female. Examination of chromosomes is indicated for any female with an inguinal hernia; 1–2% will prove to have this syndrome.

The disorder follows X-linked recessive inheritance, the gene being transmitted by female carriers. About half of all XY offspring are affected, while half of the daughters are carriers. In prepubertal children the condition must be differentiated from other types of XY male pseudohermaphroditism in which there is complete feminization. These include XY pure gonadal dysgenesis (Swyer syndrome), true agonadism, Leydig-cell aplasia, and the testicular 17-ketosteroid reductase defect.

Affected patients should always be reared as females. The testes should be removed since there is about a 2.6% incidence of tumors before the age of 15 yr and about 33% by the age of 50 yr. Some recommend not removing the testes until after completion of secondary sexual development. To relieve parental anxiety and to avoid adverse effects on psychosexual orientation of the child, we recommend that the testes be removed as soon as they are discovered. Replacement therapy with estrogens is then indicated at the age of puberty.

Incomplete Testicular Feminization. In this disorder patients exhibit some degree of masculinization and at birth may have enlargement of the phallus and labioscrotal fusion. The vagina ends blindly, and the uterus is absent. Testes are present in the inguinal canal or in the labioscrotal folds. At puberty, breast development occurs as well as axillary and pubic hair. These patients have lesser degrees of insensitivity to androgen than those with the complete syndrome; the androgen receptor may have low responsiveness or be structurally abnormal. In a family studied by the author the pattern of inheritance is compatible with X-linkage; the "complete" and "incomplete" forms have not been reported in the same family.

Reifenstein Syndrome. This syndrome and other syndromes of defective virilization (described by Lubs and by Gilbert-Dreyfus) are caused by decreased end-organ responsiveness to androgens and are best described as *partial androgen insensitivity*. These patients differ from those in the above section; the phenotype is more male than female. There are marked phenotypic differences in various affected individuals, even within affected families. Severely affected children have perineal hypospadias, a small phallus, and cryptorchidism. Most patients are sufficiently virilized, however, to be considered male at birth. Mildly affected individuals may manifest only microphallus and a bifid scrotum. After puberty there is inadequate masculinization. There is lack of facial hair and voice change. Female escutcheon, azoospermia, and infertility are usual. The disorder is being increasingly recognized in adults with relatively normal male phenotype who have a small phallus, small testes and azoospermia.

In adults plasma levels of testosterone and of dihydrotestosterone are normal or elevated. Levels of LH, and often of FSH, are also elevated. Diagnosis is also possible in the neonatal period when plasma levels of testosterone and LH are elevated. Androgen receptor studies in skin fibroblasts reveal low or normal androgen-binding capacity. There appear to be two variants of the syndrome, as in the case of testicular feminization. The cause of the insensitivity to androgen in patients with normal androgen binding is not known. Inheritance is believed to be X-linked recessive.

Undetermined Causes

Other XY male pseudohermaphrodites display much variability of the external and internal genitalia and varying degrees of phallic and müllerian development. Testes may be histologically normal or rudimentary, or there may only be one. Even the newer techniques may find no recognized cause of pseudohermaphroditism in as many as one third of patients. Some ambiguity of genitalia is associated with a wide variety of chromosomal aberrations, which must always be considered in the differential, the most common being the 45,X/46,XY syndrome (Sec. 19.34). It may be necessary to examine several tissues in order to establish mosaicism. Other complex genetic syndromes, many resulting from single gene mutations, are associated with varying degrees of ambiguity of the genitalia, particularly in the male. For example, XY males with the Smith-Lemli-Opitz syndrome may have external genitalia that are normal, markedly ambiguous, or completely female. These entities must be identified on the basis of the associated extragenital malformations.

Pseudohermaphroditism and Wilms Tumor

Male pseudohermaphroditism has been reported to be associated with glomerulopathy in 22 patients; 12 of these developed Wilms tumor, a triad known as *Drash syndrome*. Such children develop a chronic glomerular or nephrotic syndrome in the first few years of life, progressing rapidly to end-stage renal disease. All cases have been sporadic, and the etiology is thought to be defective embryogenesis of the urogenital ridge.

Male infants with *sporadic aniridia* also often have cryptorchidism and/or hypospadias as well as mental retardation. In at least five instances a gonadoblastoma has arisen in the presumably dysgenetic testis. Most patients with this syndrome have deletions of the short arm of chromosome 11 (11p−), usually involving the 11p 12–13 bands. Wilms tumor occurs in about half of all children with this chromosome abnormality.

19.43 TRUE HERMAPHRODITISM

In true hermaphroditism both ovarian and testicular tissues are present, either in the same or in opposite gonads. The clinical features may include any of those described for the other types of hermaphroditism. The phenotype may be male or female; usually, the external genitalia are ambiguous.

The majority (80%) of true hermaphrodites have a 46,XX karyotype, 10% a 46,XY, and 10% mosaics. Patients with 46,XX/46,XY mosaicism are the best understood of patients with true hermaphroditism. Of 12 reported cases, nine were derived from more than one zygote; that is, they were chimeras (chi 46,XX/46,XY). The presence of both paternal alleles for some blood groups and of both maternal alleles for other blood groups is clear evidence for chimerism. Various mechanisms are possible. In one instance, study of chromosome heteromorphisms established that two different spermatozoa had fertilized an ovum and its second meiotic division polar body, with subsequent fusion of the two zygotes.

There are probably many causes for 46,XX true hermaphroditism. Because many of these patients have been found to have H-Y antigen, it appears that X-Y interchange or Y-autosome translocation has taken place. In 46,XY true hermaphroditism, undetected chimerism or mosaicism are possible causes.

The most frequently encountered gonad in true hermaphroditism is an ovotestis; a testis is the rarest. In ovotestes the ovarian and testicular portions are often arranged end-to-end, permitting clear differentiation. The testicular tissue is often defective in secretion of androgens and of anti-müllerian hormone. The majority of true hermaphrodites are best reared as females, with selective removal of testicular tissue. Fourteen pregnancies with 12 living offspring have been reported in true hermaphrodites reared as females.

Diagnosis and Management

In the neonate ambiguity of the genitalia requires emergency medical attention. Diagnosis depends on a thorough review of the numerous mechanisms which may lead to the condition. Screening tests (examination of sex chromatin or fluorescence of the Y chromosome) must always be supplemented by complete chromosomal analysis. It is important in conditions in which mosaicism is a possibility to establish the chromosomal constitution of tissues other than blood, such as skin or any tissues removed at biopsy or exploration.

For all XX patients a detailed search for the source of virilization should be undertaken. Studies of adrenal hormones, 17-ketosteroids, pregnanetriol, and 17-dehydroxyprogesterone are needed to exclude the common varieties of adrenogenital syndrome. Urethrovaginography or endoscopic examination is indicated to establish whether vagina and/or cervix may exist in patients with ambiguous external genitalia. Ultrasonography is useful in visualizing the ovaries and uterus.

For XY patients it is necessary to determine whether testicular production of androgen is normal. In the prepubertal child determination requires stimulation of the testes with hCG. It may be necessary to verify the ability to convert testosterone to dihydrotestosterone and the ability to bind androgen of fibroblasts grown from biopsy of genital skin. Precise diagnosis is essential to genetic counseling since genes both on autosomes and on the X chromosome are known to cause hermaphroditism. Many XY hermaphrodites are at high risk of gonadal neoplasia; it is important to identify them and to remove the gonads promptly.

Many male pseudohermaphrodites, like boys with hypopituitarism, have a small penis (*microphallus*). A course of 3 monthly intramuscular injections of testosterone (25–50 mg testosterone enanthate) may assist differential diagnosis as well as treatment. The phallus will respond in patients with defects in testosterone synthesis or with hypopituitarism but not in those with complete androgen insensitivity. Such a course of treatment must precede any plan for surgical reconstruction of XY males as anatomic females.

The assignment of sex of rearing should be settled as early in life as possible. The decision is based largely on the possibilities for correction of the ambiguous genitalia and not on the chromosomal constitution. Female pseudohermaphrodites should almost always be reared as females even when highly virilized. Male pseudohermaphrodites who are totally or significantly feminized should also be reared as females. It is more feasible to reconstruct the external genitalia to create a functional female, particularly when a vagina is already present, than to create a functional male phallus. The management of the potential psychologic upheaval that such problems can generate in patient and/or family is of paramount importance and requires physicians with sensitivity and with training and experience in this field. Once the appropriate sex of rearing has been established, parents should be left with no ambiguity in their minds as to the gender of the child.

In some mammals the female exposed to androgens prenatally or in early postnatal life will exhibit aberrant sexual behavior in adult life. Girls who have undergone fetal masculinization from congenital adrenal hyperplasia or from maternal progestin therapy have no such problems in sexual identity, although during childhood they may appear to prefer male playmates and activities over girl playmates and feminine play with dolls in mothering roles.

ANGELO M. DIGEORGE

General

Kaplan SA: Clinical Pediatric and Adolescent Endocrinology. Philadelphia, WB Saunders, 1982.

Wilson JD, Foster DW (ed): Williams Textbook of Endocrinology. 7th ed. Philadelphia, WB Saunders, 1985.

Hypofunction of Testes

Barkam AL, Kelch RP, Marshall JC: Isolated gonadotrope failure in the polyglandular autoimmune failure. N Engl J Med 312:1535, 1985.

Bender B, Fry E, Pennington B, et al: Speech and language development in 41 children with sex chromosome anomalies. Pediatrics 71:262, 1983.

Bender BG, Puck MH, Salbenblatt JA, et al: The development of four unselected 47,XXY boys. Clin Genet 25:435, 1984.

Borgaonkar DS, Mules E, Char F: Do the 48 XXYY males have a characteristic phenotype? Clin Genet 1:272, 1970.

Caldwell PD, Smith DW: The XXY (Klinefelter's) syndrome in childhood: Detection and treatment. J Pediatr 80:250, 1972.

Chaussain JL, Lemerle J, Roger M, et al: Klinefelter syndrome, tumor and sexual precocity. J Pediatr 97:607, 1980.

Dekaban AS, Parks JS, Ross GT: Laurence-Moon syndrome: Evaluation of endocrinological function and phenotypic concordance and report of cases. Med Ann District Columbia 41:687, 1972.

DeLaChapelle A, Schroder J, Murros J, et al: Two XX males in one family and additional observations bearing on the etiology of XX males. Clin Genet 11:91, 1977.

Dunkel L, Perheentupa J, Tapanainen J, et al: Hypergonadotropic hypogonadism in newborn males with primary testicular failure. Acta Pediatr Scand 73:740, 1984.

Dunkel L, Perheentupa J, Virtanen M, et al: Gonadotropin-releasing hormone test and human chorionic gonadotropin test in the diagnosis of gonadotropin deficiency in prepubertal boys. J Pediatr 107:388, 1985.

Evain-Brion D, Gendred D, Bozzola M, et al: Diagnosis of Kallmann's syndrome in early infancy. Acta Paediatr 71:937, 1982.

Ewer RW: Familial monotropic pituitary gonadotropin insufficiency. J Clin Endocrinol 28:783, 1968.

Finkel DM, Phillips JL, Snyder PJ: Stimulation of spermatogenesis by gonadotropins in men with hypogonadotropic hypogonadism. N Engl J Med 313:651, 1985.

Haseltine FP, Genel M, Crawford JD, Breg WR: HY antigen negative patients with testicular tissue and 46,XY karyotype. Hum Genet 57:265, 1981.

Hook EB: Behavioral implications of the human XYY genotype. Science 179:139, 1973.

Karpouzas J, Papaioannov AC: Noonan syndrome in twins. J Pediatr 85:84, 1974.

Leonard MF, Land G, Ruddle FH, et al: Early development of children with abnormalities of the sex chromosomes: A prospective study. Pediatrics 54:208, 1974.

Levy EP, Pashasyan H, Fraser FC, et al: XX and XY Turner phenotypes in a family. Am J Dis Child 120:36, 1970.

Lieblich JM, Rogol AD, White BJ, et al: Syndrome of anosmia with hypogonadotropic hypogonadism (Kallmann syndrome). Clinical and laboratory studies in 23 cases. Am J Med 73:506, 1982.

Matus-Ridley M, Nicosia SV, Meadows AT: Gonadal effects of cancer therapy in boys. Cancer 55:2353, 1985.

Meisner LF, Inhorn SL: Normal male development with Y chromosome long arm deletion (Yq−). J Med Genet 9:373, 1972.

Melman A, Leiter E, Perez JM, et al: The influence of neonatal orchiopexy upon the testis in persistent müllerian duct syndrome. J Urol 125:856, 1981.

Money J, Franzke A, Borgaonkar DS: XYY syndrome, stigmatization, social class, and aggression. South Med J 68:1536, 1975.

Najjar SS, Takla RJ, Nassar VH: The syndrome of rudimentary testes: Occurrence in five siblings. J Pediatr 84:119, 1974.

Neuhauser G, Opitz JM: Autosomal recessive syndrome of cerebellar ataxia and hypogonadotropic hypogonadism. Clin Genet 7:426, 1975.

Nora JJ, Torres FG, Sinha AK, et al: Characteristic cardiovascular anomalies of XO Turner syndrome, XX and XY phenotype and XO/XX Turner mosaic. Am J Cardiol 25:639, 1970.

Partsch CJ, Hermaussen M, Sippell WG: Differentiation of male hypogonadotropic hypogonadism and constitutional delay of puberty by pulsatile administration of gonadotropin-releasing hormone. J Clin Endocrinol Metab 60:1196, 1985.

Philip J, Lundsteen C, Owen D, et al: The frequency of chromosome aberrations in tall men with special reference to 47,XYY and 47,XXY. Am J Hum Genet 28:404, 1976.

Reinfrank RF, Nichold FL: Hypogonadotropic hypogonadism in the Laurence-Moon syndrome. J Clin Endocrinol 24:48, 1964.

Roth JC, Kelch RP, Kaplan SE, et al: FSH and LH response to luteinizing hormone-releasing factor in prepubertal and pubertal children, adult males and patients with hypogonadotropic and hypergonadotropic hypogonadism. J Clin Endocrinol Metab 35:926, 1972.

Salbenblatt JA, Bender BG, Puck MH, et al: Development of eight pubertal males with 47,XXY karyotype. Clin Genet 20:141, 1981.

Salbenblatt JA, Bender BG, Puck MH, et al: Pituitary-gonadal function in Klinefelter syndrome before and during puberty. Pediatr Res 19:82, 1985.

Santen RJ, Paulsen CA: Hypogonadotropic eunuchoidism. I. Clinical study of the mode of inheritance. J Clin Endocrinol Metab 36:47, 1973.

Saunder SE, Corley KP, Hopwood NJ, Kelch RP: Subnormal gonadotropin responses for gonadotropin-releasing hormone persist into puberty in children with isolated growth hormone deficiency. J Clin Endocrinol Metab 53:1186, 1981.

Seyler LE, Arulananthan K, O'Connor CF: Hypergonadotropic-hypogonadism in the Prader-Labhart-Willi syndrome. J Pediatr 94:435, 1979.

Shalet SM, Hann IM, Lendon M, et al: Testicular function after combination chemotherapy in childhood for acute lymphoblastic leukaemia. Arch Dis Child 56:275, 1981.

Sherins RJ, Olweny CLM, Ziegler JL: Gynecomastia and gonadal dysfunction in adolescent boys treated with combination chemotherapy for Hodgkin's disease. N Engl J Med 299:12, 1978.

Swanson SL, Santen RJ, Smith DW: Multiple lentigenes syndrome: New findings of hypogonadotrophism, hyposmia, and unilateral renal agenesis. J Pediatr 78:1037, 1971.

Valentine GH, McClelland MA, Sergovich FR: The growth and development of four XYY infants. Pediatrics 48:853, 1971.

Volpe R, Metzler WS, Johnston MW: Familial hypogonadotropic eunuchoidism with cerebellar ataxia. J Clin Endocrinol Metab 23:107, 1963.

White BJ, Rogol AD, Brown KS, et al: The syndrome of anosmia with hypogonadotropic hypogonadism: A genetic study of 18 new families and a review. Am J Med Genet 15:417, 1983.

Wieland RC, Folk RI, Taylor JN, et al: Studies of male hypogonadism. I. Androgen metabolism in a male with gynecomastia and galactorrhea. J Clin Endocrinol Metab 27:763, 1967.

Williams C, Wieland AG, Zorn EM, et al: Effect of synthetic gonadotropin-releasing hormone (GnRH) in a patient with the "fertile eunuch" syndrome. J Clin Endocrinol Metab 41:176, 1975.

Winter JSD, Faiman C: Serum gonadotropin concentrations in agonadal children and adults. J Clin Endocrinol Metab 35:561, 1972.

Witkin HA, Mednick SA, Schulsinger F, et al: Criminality in XYY and XXY men. Science 193:547, 1976.

Tumors of the Testes

Canty JM, Seaglia HE, Medina M, et al: Inherited congenital normofunctional testicular hyperplasia and mental deficiency. Hum Genet 33:23, 1975.

Carmi R, Meryash DL, Wood J, et al: Fragile-X syndrome ascertained by the presence of macro-orchidism in a 5 month-old infant. Pediatrics 74:883, 1984.

Martin MM, Canary JJ, Balsamo PA: Virilizing tumor of the testis in one twin. J Clin Endocrinol Metab 22:345, 1962.

Nisula BC, Loriaux DL, Sherins RJ, et al: Benign bilateral testicular enlargement. J Clin Endocrinol Metab 38:440, 1974.

Rosenberg T, Gilboay, Golik A, et al: Pseudoprecocious puberty in a young boy due to interstitial cell adenomas of the testis. Helv Paediatr Acta 39:79, 1984.

Turner G, Daniel A, Frost M: X-linked mental retardation, macro-orchidism, and the Xq 27 fragile site. J Pediatr 96:837, 1980.

Turner WR, Derrick FC, Wohltmann W: Leydig cell tumor in identical twin. Urology 7:194, 1976.

Gynecomastia

August GP, Chandra R, Hung W: Prepubertal male gynecomastia. J Pediatr 80:259, 1972.

Berkovitz GD, Guerami A, Brown TR, et al: Familial gynecomastia with increased extraglandular aromatization of plasma carbon$_{19}$-steroids. J Clin Invest 75:1763, 1985.

Goldfine I, Rosenfeld RL, Landau KL: Hyperleydigism: A cause of severe pubertal gynecomastia. J Clin Endocrinol Metab 32:751, 1971.

Laron Z: Breast development induced by methandrostenolone (Dianabol). J Clin Endocrinol Metab 22:450, 1962.

Lee PA: The relationship of concentrations of serum hormones to pubertal gynecomastia. J Pediatr 86:212, 1975.

Maclaren NK, Migeon CJ, Raiti S: Gynecomastia with congenital virilizing adrenal hyperplasia (11β-hydroxylase deficiency). J Pediatr 86:579, 1975.

Nydick M, Bustos J, Dale JH Jr, et al: Gynecomastia in adolescent boys. JAMA 178:449, 1961.

Van Meter QL, Gareis FJ, Hayes JW, et al: Galactorrhea in a 12-year-old boy with a chromophobe adenoma. J Pediatr 90:756, 1977.

Hypofunction of the Ovaries

Allanson JE, Hall JG, VanAllen MI: Noonan phenotype associated with neurofibromatosis. Am J Med Genet 21:457, 1985.

Arulanantham K, Kramer MS, Gryboski J: The association of inflammatory bowel disease and X chromosomal abnormality. Pediatrics 66:63, 1980.

Bender B, Puck M, Salbenblatt J, et al: Cognitive development of unselected girls with complete and partial X monosomy. Pediatrics 73:175, 1984.

Chang RJ, Davidson BJ, Carlson HE, et al: Hypogonadotropic hypogonadism associated with retinitis pigmentosa in a female sibship: Evidence for gonadotropin deficiency. J Clin Endocrinol Metab 53:1179, 1981.

Fryns JP, Kleczkowska A, Petit P, et al: X-chromosome polysomy in the female: Personal experience and review of the literature. Clin Genet 23:341, 1983.

Horning SJ, Hoppe RT, Kaplan HS, et al: Female reproductive potential after treatment for Hodgkin's disease. N Engl J Med 304:1377, 1981.

Kaufman FR, Kogut MD, Donnell GH, et al: Hypergonadotropic hypogonadism in female patients with galactosemia. N Engl J Med 304:994, 1981.

Krasna IH, Lee M, Sciorre L, et al: The importance of surgical evaluation of patients with "Turner-like" sex chromosomal abnormalities. J Pediatr Surg 20:61, 1985.

Magenis RE, Tochen ML, Holalan KP, et al: Turner syndrome resulting from partial deletion of Y chromosome short arm: Localization of male determinants. J Pediatr 105:916, 1984.

McDonough PG, Thi Tho P: The spectrum of 45,X/46,XY gonadal dysgenesis and its implications (a study of 19 patients). Pediatr Adoles Gynecol 1:1, 1973.

Miller MJ, Geffner ME, Lippe BM, et al: Echocardiography reveals a high incidence of bicuspid aortic valve in Turner syndrome. J Pediatr 102:47, 1983.

Moll GW Jr, Rosenfield RL: Plasma free testosterone in the diagnosis of adolescent polycystic ovary syndrome. J Pediatr 102:461, 1983.

Muller J, Shakkeback NE, Ritzen M, et al: Carcinoma in situ of the testis in children with 45,X/46,XY gonadal dysgenesis. J Pediatr 106:431, 1985.

Nicosia SV, Matus-Ridley M, Meadows AT: Gonadal effects of cancer therapy in girls. Cancer 55:2364, 1985.

Polychronakos C, Letarte K, Collu R, et al: Carbohydrate intolerance in children and adolescents with Turner syndrome. J Pediatr 96:1009, 1980.

Raiti S, Moore WV, Van Vliet G, et al: Growth-stimulating effects of human growth therapy in patients with Turner syndrome. J Pediatr 109:944, 1986.

Rosenfeld RG, Hintz RL, Johanson AJ, et al: Methionyl human growth hormone and oxandrolone in Turner syndrome: Preliminary results of a prospective randomized trial. J Pediatr 109:936, 1986.

Ross JL, Long LM, Skeida M, et al: Effect of low doses of estradiol on 6 month growth rates and predicted height in patients with Turner syndrome. J Pediatr 109:950, 1986.

Spitz IM, Diamant Y, Rosen E, et al: Isolated gonadotropin deficiency: A heterogeneous syndrome.N Engl J Med 290:10, 1974.

Sybert VP: Adult height in Turner syndrome with and without androgen therapy. J Pediatr 104:365, 1984.

Tagatz G, Fialkow PJ, Smith D, et al: Hypogonadotropic hypogonadism associated with anosmia in the female. N Engl J Med 282:1326, 1970.

Tulandi T, Kinch RAH: Premature ovarian failure. Obstet Gynecol Survey 36:521, 1981.

Zumoff B, Freeman R, Coupey S, et al: A chronobiologic abnormality in luteinizing hormone secretion in teenage girls with the polycystic-ovary syndrome. N Engl J Med 301:1206, 1983.

Tumors of the Ovary

Ammann AJ, Kaufman S, Gilbert A: Virilizing ovarian tumor in a 2½-year-old girl. J Pediatr 70:782, 1967.

Lack EE, Perez-Atayde AR, Murthy AS, et al: Granulosa theca cell tumors in premenarchal girls: A clinical and pathologic study of ten cases. Cancer 48:1846, 1981.

Solh HM, Azoury RS, Najjar SS: Peutz-Jeghers syndrome associated with precocious puberty. J Pediatr 103:593, 1983.

Tucci JR, Zäh W, Kalderon AE: Endocrine studies in arrhenoblastoma responsive to dexamethasone, ACTH and human chorionic gonadotropin. Am J Med 55:681, 1973.

Young RH, Dickersin GR, Scully RE: Juvenile granulosa cell tumor of the ovary. A clinicopathologic analysis of 125 cases. Am J Surg Pathol 8:575, 1984.

Zaloudek C, Norris HJ: Granulosa cell tumors of the ovary in children: a clinical and pathological study of 32 cases. Am J Surg Pathol 6:513, 1982.

Hermaphroditism

Amrhein JA, Jones Klingensmith G, Walsh PC, et al: Partial androgen insensitivity. The Reifenstein syndrome revisited. N Engl J Med 297:350, 1977.

Armendares S, Buentello L, Frenk S: Two male sibs with uterus and fallopian tubes. A rare, probably inherited disorder. Clin Genet 4:291, 1973.

Benirschke K, Naftolin G, Gittes R, et al: True hermaphroditism and chimerism. Am J Obstet Gynecol 113:449, 1971.

Berkovitz GD, Lee PA, Brown TR, et al: Etiologic evaluation of male pseudohermaphroditism in infancy and childhood. Am J Dis Child 138:755, 1984.

Bernstein R, Koo GC, Wachtel SS: Abnormality of the X chromosome in human 46,XY female siblings with dysgenetic ovaries. Science 207:768, 1980.

Berthezene F, Forest MG, Grimaud JA, et al: Leydig-cell agenesis. A cause of male pseudohermaphroditism. N Engl J Med 295:696, 1976.

Book JA, Eilon B, Halbrecht I, et al: Isochromosome Y (46,X,I (Yq)) and female phenotype. Clin Genet 4:410, 1973.

Bricarelle FD, Fraccaro M, Lindsten J, et al: Sex-reversed XY females with camptomelic dysplasia are H-Y negative. Hum Genet 47:12, 1981.

Brook CGB, Wagner H, et al: Familial occurrence of persistent müllerian structures in otherwise normal males. Br Med J 1:771, 1973.

Burstein S, Grumbach MM, Kaplan SL: Early determination of androgen-responsiveness is important in the management of microphallus. Lancet 2:983, 1979.

Chasalow FI, Blethen SL, Marr HBK, et al: An improved method for evaluating testosterone biosynthetic defects. Pediatr Res 18:759, 1984.

David R, Yoon DJ, Landin L, et al: A syndrome of gonadotropin resistance possibly due to luteinizing hormone receptor defect. J Clin Endocrinol Metab 59:156, 1984.

Dean HJ, Shackleton CHL, Winter JSD: Diagnosis and natural history of 17-hydroxylase deficiency in a newborn male. J Clin Endocrinol Metab 59:513, 1984.

Dewald G, Haymond MW, Spurbeck JL, et al: Origin of chi 46,XX/46,XY chimerism in a true hermaphrodite. Science 207:321, 1980.

Eddy AA, Maver SM: Pseudohermaphroditism, glomerulopathy, and Wilms tumor (Drash syndrome): Frequency in end-stage renal failure. J Pediatr 106:584, 1985.

Eil C, Austin RM, Sesterhenn I, et al: Leydig cell hypoplasia causing male pseudohermaphroditism: Diagnosis 13 years after prepubertal castration. J Clin Endocrinol Metab 58:441, 1984.

Fitch N, Richer CL, Pinsky L, et al: Deletion of the long arm of the Y chromosome and review of Y chromosome abnormalities. Am J Med Genet 20:31, 1985.

Fitzgerald PH, Donald RA, Kirk RL: A true hermaphrodite dispermic chimera with 46,XX and 46,XY karyotypes. Clin Genet 15:89, 1979.

Greene C, Pitts W, Rosenfeld R, et al: Smith-Lemli-Opitz syndrome in two 46,XY infants with female external genitalia. Clin Genet 25:366, 1984.

Griffin JE, Wilson JD: The syndromes of androgen resistance. N Engl J Med 302:198, 1980.

Imperato-McGinley J, Peterson RE, Gautier T, et al: Androgens and the evolution of male gender identity among male pseudohermaphrodites with 5α-reductase deficiency. N Engl J Med 300:1233, 1979.

Imperato-McGinley J, Gautier T, Pichardo M, et al: The diagnosis of 5-α-reductase deficiency in infancy. J Clin Endocrinol Metab 63:1313, 1986.

Josso N, Briard ML: Embryonic testicular regression syndrome: Variable phenotypic expression in siblings. J Pediatr 97:200, 1980.

Kaufman FR, Costin G, Goebelsmann U, et al: Male pseudohermaphroditism due to 17,20-desmolase deficiency. J Clin Endocrinol Metab 57:32, 1983.

Kinoshita K, Shina Y, Bando M, et al: Agonadism with positive H-Y antigen. Clin Genet 26:61, 1984.

Kirkland RT, Kirkland JL, Johnson CM, et al: Congenital lipoid adrenal hyperplasia in an eight-year-old phenotypic female. J Clin Endocrinol Metab 36:488, 1973.

Kohn G, Lasch EE, El Shawwa R, et al: Male pseudohermaphroditism due to 17-β-hydroxysteroid dehydrogenase deficiency (17 β HSD) in a large Arab kinship. Studies on the natural history of the defect. J Pediatr Endocrinol 1:29, 1985.

Manuel M, Katayama KP, Jones HW Jr: Age of occurrence of gonadal tumors in intersex patients with a Y chromosome. Am J Obstet Gynecol 124:293, 1976.

Medina M, Chavez B, Perez-Palacios G: Defective androgen action at the cellular level in the androgen resistance syndromes. I. Differences between the complete and incomplete testicular feminization syndromes. J Clin Endocrinol Metab 53:1243, 1981.

Migeon CJ, Brown TR, Lanes R, et al: A clinical syndrome of mild androgen insensitivity. J Clin Endocrinol Metab 59:672, 1984.

Morerira-Filho CA, Wachtel SS: Study of H-Y antigen in abnormal sex determination with monoclonal antibody and an ELISA. Am J Med Genet 20:525, 1985.

Nagel RA, Lippe BM, Griffin JE: Androgen resistance in the neonate: Use of hormones of hypothalamic-pituitary-gonadal axis for diagnosis. J Pediatr 109:486, 1986.

Nihoul-Fékété C, Lorat-Jacob S, Cachin O, et al: Preservation of gonadal function in true hermaphroditism. J Pediatr Surg 19:50, 1984.

O'Leary TJ, Ooi TC, Miller JD: Virilization of two siblings by maternal androgen-secreting adrenal adenoma. J Pediatr 109:840, 1986.

Page DC, de la Chapelle A, Weissenbach J: Chromosome Y-specific DNA in related human XX males. Nature 315:224, 1985.

Pergament E, Heimler A, Shah P: Testicular feminization and inguinal hernia. Lancet 2:740, 1973.

Peterson RE, Imperato-McGinley K, Gautier T, et al: Male pseudohermaphroditism due to steroid 5α-reductase deficiency. Am J Med 62:170, 1977.

Reyes FI, Winter JJD, Faiman C: Studies on human sexual development. I. Fetal gonadal and adrenal sex steroids. J Clin Endocrinol Metab 37:74, 1973.

Roberts CM, Adams PW, Lilford RJ: Complete steroid 17 alpha hydroxylase deficiency in an XY patient presenting as primary amenorrhea and low body weight. Pediatr Adol Gynecol 3:183, 1985.

Rockhill TA, Schmidt CL: Male pseudohermaphroditism secondary to early fetal testicular regression. Pediatr Adoles Gynecol 3:15, 1985.

Rosenberg HS, Clayton GW, Hsu TC: Familial true hermaphroditism. J Clin Endocrinol Metab 23:203, 1963.

Saenger P: Abnormal sexual differentiation. J Pediatr 104:1, 1984.

Shanfield I, Young RB, Hume DM: True hermaphroditism with XX/XY mosaicism: Report of a case. J Pediatr 83:471, 1973.

Siiteri PK, Wilson JD: Testosterone formation and metabolism during male sexual differentiation in the human embryo. J Clin Endocrinol Metab 38:113, 1974.

Turleau C, de Grouchy J, Dufier JL, et al: Aniridia, male pseudohermaphroditism, gonadoblastoma, mental retardation, and del 11 p13. Hum Genet 57:300, 1981.

Ulloa-Aquirre A, Bassal S, Poo J, et al: Endocrine and biochemical studies in a 46,XY phenotypically male infant with 17-ketoreductase deficiency. J Clin Endocrinol Metab 60:639, 1985.

Wachtel SS, Chervenak FA, Brunner M, et al: Notes on the biology of H-Y antigen. J Pediatr Endocrinol 1:1, 1985.

Wenstrup RJ, Pagon RA: Female pseudohermaphroditism with anorectal, Müllerian duct and urinary tract malformations: Report of four cases. J Pediatr 107:751, 1985.

Wilson JD, Carlson BR, Weaver DD, et al: Endocrine and genetic characterization of cousins with male pseudohermaphroditism: Evidence that the Lubs phenotype can result from a mutation that alters the structure of the androgen receptor. Clin Genet 26:363, 1984.

Wu RH, Boyer RM, Knight R, et al: Endocrine studies in a phenotypic girl with XY gonadal agenesis. J Clin Endocrinol Metab 43:506, 1976.

20

METABOLIC DISORDERS

20.1 DIABETES MELLITUS

Diabetes mellitus, a syndrome of disturbed energy homeostasis, is caused by deficiency of insulin or of its action and is manifested by abnormal metabolism of carbohydrate, protein, and fat. It is the most common endocrine/metabolic disorder of childhood and adolescence with important consequences on physical and emotional development. Individuals affected by insulin-dependent diabetes confront serious burdens that include an absolute daily requirement for exogenous insulin, the necessity of monitoring their own metabolic control, and the constant need for attention to dietary intake. Morbidity and mortality stem from metabolic derangements and from the long-term complications that affect small and large blood vessels, resulting in retinopathy, nephropathy, neuropathy, ischemic heart disease, and arterial obstruction with gangrene of extremities. The acute clinical manifestations are explainable in terms of current knowledge of deviations in secretion and action of insulin; genetic and other etiologic considerations point to autoimmune mechanisms in the genesis of type I diabetes. There is an emerging consensus that the long-term complications are related to metabolic disturbances. These considerations form the current base for therapeutic approaches to this disease.

Classification. Diabetes mellitus is not a single entity, but rather a heterogeneous group of disorders in which there are distinct genetic patterns as well as other etiologic and pathophysiologic mechanisms that lead to impairment of glucose tolerance. Table 20–1 presents a classification system for three major forms of diabetes and several forms of carbohydrate intolerance:

Type I diabetes (juvenile-onset diabetes) is characterized by severe insulinopenia, with dependence on exogenous insulin to prevent ketosis and to preserve life; it is, therefore, also termed **insulin-dependent diabetes mellitus (IDDM).** Occasionally in its natural course there may be preketotic, non–insulin-dependent phases both before and after the initial diagnosis. Although the onset is predominantly in childhood, it may occur at any age. Hence, such terms as juvenile

diabetes, ketosis-prone diabetes, and brittle diabetes should be abandoned in favor of Type I or IDDM. Type I diabetes is distinctive owing to its association with certain HLA antigens, the presence of circulating antibodies to cytoplasmic and cell-surface components of islet cells, lymphocytic infiltration of islets early in the disease, and other autoimmune manifestations. With few exceptions, diabetes in children is insulin-dependent and fits the Type I category.

Type II diabetes (formerly known as adult-onset diabetes, maturity-onset diabetes [MOD], or stable diabetes) is not insulin-dependent and only infrequently results in ketosis; insulin, however, may be required for symptomatic hyperglycemia, and ketosis may develop in some patients during severe infections or other stress.

Serum concentration of insulin may be normal or moderately depressed, but it is usually elevated. In the majority of instances, the onset of non–insulin-dependent diabetes mellitus occurs after age 40, but it may occur at any age. It is rare in childhood, when it may be manifested as abnormal glucose tolerance, usually in obese individuals; the secretion of insulin is adequate, but there is resistance to it. Weight reduction is indicated in affected children as an initial approach. Abnormal carbohydrate tolerance may also occur in children who have a strong family history of Type II diabetes in a pattern suggestive of dominant inheritance; this pattern of diabetes has been termed MODY (maturity-onset diabetes of the young) and may require treatment with insulin. Of importance in this type of diabetes is the lack of association with HLA antigens, autoimmunity, and/or islet-cell antibodies.

The subclass of **secondary diabetes** contains a variety of types of diabetes; for some the etiologic relationship is known. Examples include diabetes secondary to exocrine pancreatic diseases, such as cystic fibrosis; endocrine disorders other than pancreatic ones, e.g., Cushing syndrome; and ingestion of certain drugs or poisons, e.g., the rodenticide Vacor. Certain genetic syndromes, including those with abnormalities of the insulin receptor, also are included in this category.

Table 20–1. **Summary of Classification of Diabetes Mellitus in Children and Adolescents***

Classification	Criteria
Diabetes mellitus	
1. Insulin-dependent (IDDM, Type I)	Typical manifestations: glucosuria, ketonuria, random plasma glucose (PG) >200 mg/dL
2. Non–insulin-dependent (NIDDM, Type II)	FPG >140 mg/dL and 2 hr value >200 mg/dL during OGTT on more than 1 occasion and in absence of precipitating factors
3. Other types	Type I or II criteria in association with certain genetic syndromes (including cystic fibrosis), other disorders, and drugs (see text)
Impaired glucose tolerance (IGT)	FPG <140 mg/dL with 2 hr value >140 mg/dL during OGTT
Gestational diabetes (GDM)	2 or more of following abnormalities during OGTT: FPG >105 mg/dL; 1 hr, >190 mg/dL; 2 hr, >165 mg/dL; 3 hr, >145 mg/dL
Statistical risk classes	
1. Previous abnormality of glucose tolerance	Normal OGTT following a previous abnormal one, spontaneous hyperglycemia or gestational diabetes
2. Potential abnormality of glucose tolerance	Genetic propensity (e.g., identical nondiabetic twin of a diabetic mate); islet-cell antibodies

*Proposed by National Diabetes Data Group (Diabetes 28:1039, 1979) and endorsed by various diabetes associations worldwide.
PG = plasma glucose; FPG = fasting plasma glucose; OGTT = oral glucose tolerance test.

There are no associations with HLA antigens, autoimmunity, or islet cell antibodies among the entities in this category.

For all types of diabetes, many believe that the criterion of a fasting blood glucose level in excess of 140 mg/dL is too stringent because normal children do not exceed a fasting blood glucose value of 120 mg/dL.

TYPE I DIABETES MELLITUS
(Insulin-Dependent Diabetes (IDDM; Juvenile-Onset Diabetes)

Epidemiology. Surveys in the United States indicate that the prevalence of diabetes among school-age children is about 1.9/1000. The frequency is highly correlated with increasing age; the estimated range is 1 case/1430 children at 5 yr of age to 1 case/360 children at 16 yr. Data on prevalence in relation to racial or ethnic backgrounds are incomplete. In the United States blacks are affected less often than whites; various reports have placed the occurrence of insulin-dependent diabetes in American blacks as low as 20–30% or as high as two thirds of the rate in American whites. These observations have implications for genetic counseling (see below). The annual incidence is about 16 new cases per 100,000 children; it is possibly as high as 30 new cases per 100,000 children in some parts of Scandinavia. Males and females are almost equally affected, and there is no apparent correlation with socioeconomic status. Peaks of presentation occur in two age groups: at 5–7 yr of age and at puberty. The first peak corresponds to the time of increased exposure to infectious agents at the beginning of school, and the second peak, to the pubertal growth spurt induced by gonadal steroids, which may antagonize insulin action, and to the emotional stresses of puberty. These possible cause-and-effect relationships remain to be proved. The prevalence and incidence of insulin-dependent diabetes in the United States are similar to those reported in Great Britain, Sweden, and Australia.

Seasonal and long term cyclic variations occur in the incidence of insulin-dependent diabetes mellitus. Newly recognized cases appear with greater frequency in the autumn and winter months; children under 6 yr have an exaggerated variation. In one study the long-term cycle appeared to parallel the incidence of mumps, when allowance was made for a 4 yr time lag. There is an increased incidence of diabetes in children who have had congenital rubella. These associations with viral infections suggest a potential role for viruses as direct or indirect triggering mechanisms in the etiology of diabetes.

Etiology and Pathogenesis. The basic cause of the initial clinical findings in Type I diabetes is the sharply diminished secretion of insulin. Although basal plasma concentrations of insulin may be normal in newly diagnosed patients, insulin production in response to a variety of potent secretagogues is blunted and usually disappears over a period of months to years, rarely exceeding 5 yr. In certain individuals at high risk for development of Type I diabetes, such as the nonaffected identical twin of a diabetic, a progressive decline in insulin secreting capacity has been noted for months to years before the appearance of symptomatic diabetes, which is usually manifest when insulin secreting reserve is ≤ 20% of normal.

The failure of pancreatic beta-cell function in Type I diabetes is incompletely understood, but the possibility of autoimmune destruction of pancreatic islets in predisposed individuals appears to be a major factor. An increased prevalence of IDDM has been noted among persons with such disorders as Addison disease, Hashimoto thyroiditis, and pernicious anemia, in which autoimmune mechanisms are known to be pathogenic. These conditions, as well as Type I diabetes, are known to be frequently associated with certain histocompatibility antigens (HLA), in particular HLA-B8, -DR3, -B/W15,

and -DR4. Located on chromosome number 6, the HLA system is the major histocompatibility complex; it consists of a cluster of genes that code transplantation antigens and plays a central role in immune responses.

Increased susceptibility to a number of diseases has been related to one or more of the identified HLA antigens. The inheritance of HLA-D3 or -D4 antigens appears to confer a 2- to 3-fold increased risk for developing Type I diabetes. When both D3 and D4 are inherited, the relative risk for developing diabetes is increased 7- to 10-fold. A rare genetic type of properdin factor B (BfF1), which is closely linked to the HLA system on chromosome 6, is found in more than 20% of Type I diabetics but in less than 2% of healthy subjects; thus there is a relative risk factor of 15 for those who inherit this genetic marker. Certain blood groups have also been associated with an increased risk of diabetes. Furthermore, there is a heterogeneity in the HLA-D region among individuals with and without diabetes who possess the DR3 or DR4 markers, which suggests a yet to be defined "susceptibility" locus within these markers.

These and other observations, such as the increased incidence in some families, the concordance rates in monozygotic twins, and ethnic and racial differences in prevalence, provide a rational framework for the long-recognized association of Type I diabetes with genetic factors. For example, Type I diabetes among American blacks is associated with the same HLA genes as it is in American whites. Because the ratios of the prevalence of these genes with Type I diabetes in the American black and white populations (about 0.2–0.3:1) are quite similar, it has been proposed that the disease may be transmitted by autosomal dominant inheritance. Genetic models, however, have also been observed that exhibit features of both dominant and recessive inheritance. It has been proposed that if a sibling shares both HLA-D haplotypes with an index case, the risk of Type I diabetes in the sibling is 12 to 20%; with one haplotype, the risk is 5–7%, and with no haplotypes in common the risk is only 1–2%. HLA typing is not recommended, however, for genetic counseling, since no intervention to prevent Type I diabetes is available at this time. In general, for purposes of genetic counseling, it can be safely assumed that for whites the overall recurrence risks to siblings are approximately 6% if the proband is under 10 years of age or 3% if older at the time of diagnosis. The risk to offspring is 2–5%; the risk tends to be in the higher range when the proband is the father. In American blacks, these risks are only one half to two thirds of those in whites.

Factors other than pure inheritance must also be involved in evoking clinical diabetes. For example, D3 or D4 is found in approximately 50% of the general population, and yet the risk for Type I diabetes in these subjects is only one tenth that in an HLA identical sibling of a proband who possesses these two markers. Even non–HLA-identical siblings, or those sharing only one haplotype, have a 6- to 10-fold greater risk of developing Type I diabetes as compared to the normal population. In addition, at least 10% of patients with Type I diabetes do not possess either HLA-D3 or -D4. Most compelling is the fact that the concordance rate among identical twins when one has insulin-dependent diabetes is only 50%, suggesting the participation of environmental triggering factors.

Such triggering factors might include viral infections. In animals, a number of viruses can cause a diabetic syndrome, the appearance and severity of which depend on the genetic strain and immune competence of the species of animal tested. In man, epidemics of mumps, rubella, and coxsackievirus infections have been associated with subsequent increases in the incidence of Type I diabetes among those infected. The viruses may act by directly destroying beta cells, by persisting in these cells as "slow viruses," or by triggering a widespread immune response to various endocrine tissues. The virus may induce initial beta cell damage that results in the presentation of previously masked or altered antigenic determinants. It is also possible that the virus shares some antigenic determinants with those present on beta cells, so that antibodies formed in response to the virus may interact with these shared determinants of beta cells, resulting in their destruction (an example of molecular mimicry). Antecedent stress and exposure to certain chemical toxins have been implicated in the development of Type I diabetes. Histologic examination of pancreatic tissue from patients with Type I diabetes who die from incidental causes has revealed lymphocytic infiltration around the islets of Langerhans. Later, these islets become progressively hyalinized and scarred, a process suggestive of an ongoing inflammatory response, possibly autoimmune in nature.

Considerable evidence now supports an autoimmune basis for the development of Type I diabetes. Some 80–90% of newly diagnosed patients have islet cell antibodies (ICA) directed at cell surface or cytoplasmic determinants in their islet cells; the prevalence of these antibodies decreases with the duration of the established disease. In contrast, after pancreatic transplantation, ICA may reappear in patients whose sera had become negative for ICA prior to transplantation. Taken together, these findings suggest that ICA disappear as the antigens in the form of pancreatic islets are destroyed and then reappear when fresh antigen (transplanted islets) is presented. Studies in identical twins and in family pedigrees demonstrate that the existence of ICA may precede by months to years the appearance of symptomatic Type I diabetes. In vitro, ICA may impair insulin secretion in response to secretagogues and is cytotoxic to islet cells, especially in the presence of complement or T cells from patients with Type I diabetes. There is also some evidence of abnormal T cell function with an alteration in the ratio of suppressor to killer T cells at the onset of the disease. These findings suggest that Type I diabetes, like other autoimmune diseases such as Hashimoto thyroiditis, is a disease of "autoaggression," in which autoantibodies in cooperation with complement, T cells, or other factors induce destruction of the insulin-producing islet cells. Thus, the inheritance of certain genes intimately associated with the HLA system on chromosome 6 appears to confer a predisposition for autoimmune disease, including diabetes, when triggered by an appropriate stimulus such as a virus. Although it is understood that some insulin-dependent diabetic patients have none of the frequently associated HLA antigens, the evidence for an immune basis of islet cell destruction is sufficiently compelling to have fostered several studies of immunosuppressive agents in the treatment of newly diagnosed diabetics.

Pathophysiology. The progressive destruction of beta cells leads to progressive deficiency of insulin, a major anabolic hormone. Its normal secretion in response to feeding is exquisitely modulated by the interplay of neural, hormonal, and substrate-related mechanisms to permit controlled disposition of ingested food as energy for immediate or future use; mobilization of energy during the fasted state depends on low plasma levels of insulin. Thus, in normal metabolism there are regular swings between the postprandial, high-insulin anabolic state and the fasted, low-insulin catabolic state that affect three major tissues: liver, muscle, and adipose tissue (Table 20–2). Type I diabetes mellitus, as it evolves, becomes a permanent low-insulin catabolic state in which feeding will not reverse but rather exaggerate these catabolic processes. The liver is more sensitive than muscle or fat to a given concentration of insulin; i.e., endogenous glucose production from the liver via glycogenolysis and gluconeogenesis can be restrained at insulin concentrations which do not fully augment glucose utilization by peripheral tissues. Conse-

Table 20–2. Influence of Feeding (High Insulin) or of Fasting (Low Insulin) on Some Metabolic Processes in Liver, Muscle, and Adipose Tissue

Insulin is considered to be the major factor governing these metabolic processes. Diabetes mellitus may be viewed as a permanent low-insulin state that, untreated, results in exaggerated fasting.

	High Plasma Insulin (Postprandial State)	Low Plasma Insulin (Fasted State)
Liver:	Glucose uptake	Glucose production
	Glycogen synthesis	Glycogenolysis
	Absence of gluconeogenesis	Gluconeogenesis
	Lipogenesis	Absence of lipogenesis
	Absence of ketogenesis	Ketogenesis
Muscle:	Glucose uptake	Absence of glucose uptake
	Glucose oxidation	Fatty acid and ketone oxidation
	Glycogen synthesis	Glycogenolysis
	Protein synthesis	Proteolysis and amino acid release
Adipose tissue:	Glucose uptake	Absence of glucose uptake
	Lipid synthesis	Lipolysis and fatty acid release
	Triglyceride uptake	Absence of triglyceride uptake

quently, with progressive failure of insulin secretion, the initial manifestation is postprandial hyperglycemia; fasting hyperglycemia indicates excessive endogenous glucose production and is a late manifestation reflecting severe insulin deficiency.

Although insulin deficiency is the primary defect, several secondary changes that involve the stress hormones (epinephrine, cortisol, growth hormone, and glucagon) accelerate and exaggerate the rate and magnitude of metabolic decompensation. Increased plasma concentrations of these counterregulatory hormones magnify metabolic derangements by further impairing insulin secretion (epinephrine), by antagonizing its action (epinephrine, cortisol, growth hormone), and by promoting glycogenolysis, gluconeogenesis, lipolysis, and ketogenesis while decreasing glucose utilization and glucose clearance. With progressive insulin deficiency, excessive glucose production and impairment of its utilization result in hyperglycemia with glucosuria when the renal threshold of approximately 180 mg/dL is exceeded. The resultant osmotic diuresis produces polyuria, urinary losses of electrolytes, dehydration, and compensatory polydipsia. These evolving manifestations, especially dehydration, represent physiologic stress, resulting in hypersecretion of epinephrine, glucagon, cortisol, and growth hormone that accelerate metabolic decompensation. The acute stress of trauma or infection may likewise accelerate metabolic decompensation to ketoacidosis. Hyperosmolality, commonly encountered as a result of progressive hyperglycemia, contributes to the symptomatology, especially to cerebral obtundation. Serum osmolality has important implications in the therapy of diabetic ketoacidosis. It can be estimated by the following formula:

Serum osmolality in mOsm/kg =

$$(\text{Serum Na}^+ \text{ [mEq/L]} + \text{K}^+ \text{ [mEq/L]}) \times 2 + \frac{\text{glucose (mg/dL)}}{18} + \frac{\text{BUN (mg/dL)}}{3}$$

The combination of insulin deficiency and elevated plasma values of the counterregulatory hormones is also responsible for accelerated lipolysis and impaired lipid synthesis, with resulting increased plasma concentrations of total lipids, cholesterol, triglycerides, and free fatty acids. The hormonal interplay of insulin deficiency and excess glucagon shunts the free fatty acids into ketone body formation; the rate of formation of these ketones, principally beta-hydroxybutyrate and acetoacetate, exceeds the capacity for peripheral utilization and for their renal excretion. Accumulation of these ketoacids is a major factor in the development of metabolic acidosis; the compensatory rapid deep breathing is an attempt to excrete excess CO_2 (Kussmaul respiration). Acetone, formed by nonenzymatic conversion of acetoacetate, is responsible for the characteristic fruity odor of the breath. Ketones are excreted in the urine in association with cations and thus further increase losses of water and electrolytes (Table 20–3). With progressive dehydration, acidosis, hyperosmolality, and diminished cerebral oxygen utilization, consciousness becomes impaired, the patient ultimately becoming comatose. Thus, insulin deficiency produces a profound catabolic state—an exaggerated starvation—in which all of the initial clinical features can be explained on the basis of known alterations in intermediary metabolism mediated by insulin deficiency in combination with an excess of the counterregulatory hormones. Because the counterregulatory hormonal changes are secondary, the severity and duration of the symptoms are a reflection of the extent of primary insulinopenia.

Clinical Manifestations. The classic presentation of diabetes in children is a history of **polyuria, polydipsia, polyphagia,** and **weight loss.** The duration of these symptoms varies but is often less than 1 mo. A clue to the existence of polyuria may be enuresis in a previously toilet-trained child. An insidious onset with lethargy, weakness, and weight loss is also quite common. The loss of weight in spite of an increased dietary intake is readily explicable by the following illustration:

The average healthy 10 yr old child has a daily caloric intake of about 2000 kcal, of which approximately 50% are derived from carbohydrate. With the development of diabetes, daily losses of water and glucose may be as much as 5 L and 250 g, respectively. This represents 1000 kcal lost in the urine or 50% of an average daily caloric intake. Therefore, despite the child's compensatory increased intake of food and water, the calories cannot be utilized, excessive caloric losses continue and increasing catabolism and weight loss ensue.

Pyogenic skin infections and, in teenage girls, monilial vaginitis are occasionally present at the time of diagnosis. They are rarely the sole clinical manifestations of diabetes in children, and a carefully taken history will invariably reveal the coexistence of polydipsia and polyuria.

Ketoacidosis is responsible for the initial presentation of many diabetic children. The early manifestations may be relatively mild and consist of vomiting, polyuria, and dehydration. In prolonged and severe cases, Kussmaul respiration is present

Table 20–3. Fluid and Electrolyte Maintenance Requirements and Estimated Losses in Diabetic Ketoacidosis

	Approximate Daily Maintenance Requirements*	Approximate Accumulated Losses†
Water	2000 mL/m²	100 mL/kg (range 60–100 mL/kg)
Sodium	45 mEq/m²	6 mEq/kg (range 5–13 mEq/kg)
Potassium	35 mEq/m²	5 mEq/kg (range 4–6 mEq/kg)
Chloride	30 mEq/m²	4 mEq/kg (range 3–9 mEq/kg)
Phosphate	10 mEq/m²	3 mEq/kg (range 2–5 mEq/kg)

*Maintenance is expressed in surface area to permit uniformity because fluid requirements change as weight increases. See also Sec. 5.27.

†Losses are expressed per unit of body weight since the losses remain relatively constant in relation to total body weight.

and there is an odor of acetone on the breath. Abdominal pain and/or rigidity may mimic appendicitis or pancreatitis. Cerebral obtundation and ultimately coma ensue. Laboratory findings include hyperglycemia, ketonemia, glucosuria, ketonuria, and metabolic acidosis. Leukocytosis is common, and serum amylase may be elevated; serum lipase is usually not elevated. In those with abdominal pain, it should not be assumed that the related physical findings are evidence of a surgical emergency until appropriate fluid, electrolyte, and insulin therapy designed to correct dehydration and acidosis has had sufficient time to be effective; the abdominal manifestations frequently disappear after several hours of such treatment.

Diagnosis. Children in whom the diagnosis of diabetes mellitus must be considered may, for practical purposes, be divided into three general categories: (1) those who have a history suggestive of diabetes, especially polyuria with polydipsia and failure to gain or a loss of weight in spite of a voracious appetite; (2) those who have transient or persistent glycosuria; and (3) those who have clinical manifestations of metabolic acidosis with or without stupor or coma. *In all instances the diagnosis of diabetes mellitus is dependent on the demonstration of hyperglycemia in association with glucosuria with or without ketonuria.* When polyuria and polydipsia are associated, the glucose tolerance test is not needed to support the diagnosis.

Renal glucosuria may be an isolated congenital disorder or a manifestation of the Fanconi syndrome and other renal tubular disorders due to severe heavy metal (e.g., lead) intoxication, ingestion of certain drugs (e.g., outdated tetracycline), or inborn errors (e.g., cystinosis). When vomiting, diarrhea, and/or inadequate intake of food are complicating factors in any of these conditions, starvation ketosis may ensue and simulate diabetic ketoacidosis. The absence of hyperglycemia eliminates the possibility of diabetes. It is also important to recognize that not all urinary sugar is glucose, and infrequently galactosemia, pentosuria, and the fructosurias require consideration as diagnostic possibilities.

The discovery of glucosuria, with or without a mild degree of hyperglycemia, during a hospital admission with which there is an evident or masked emotional upheaval may, but usually does not, herald the existence of diabetes; in most instances the glucosuria is quite transient. Inasmuch as this observation may indicate a limited capacity for insulin secretion, which is unmasked by elevated plasma concentrations of stress hormones, a glucose tolerance test should be done several weeks after recovery to determine the existence of hyperglycemia and the possibility of diabetes; the glucose loading dose should be adjusted for weight.

Screening procedures, such as postprandial blood glucose values or oral glucose tolerance tests, have yielded low detection rates in children, even among those considered at risk, such as siblings of diabetic children. Accordingly, such screening procedures are not recommended in children.

Diabetic ketoacidosis must be differentiated from acidosis and/or coma related to such other causes as hypoglycemia, uremia, gastroenteritis with metabolic acidosis, lactic acidosis, salicylate intoxication, encephalitis, and other intracranial lesions. Diabetic ketoacidosis can be said to exist when there is hyperglycemia (glucose greater than 300 mg/dL), ketonemia (ketones clearly demonstrable in serum at greater than 1:2 dilutions), acidosis (pH less than 7.30; bicarbonate less than 15 mEq/L), glucosuria, and ketonuria in addition to the clinical features described. Precipitating factors, even for the initial presentation, include stress such as trauma, infections, vomiting, and psychologic disturbances. Recurrent episodes of ketoacidosis in established diabetics often represent deliberate errors in recommended insulin dosage or unusual stress responses that indicate severe psychologic disturbances, at times manifested by pleas to be removed from home environments perceived to be stressful or intolerable. Diabetic ketoacidosis also should be distinguished from nonketotic hyperosmolar coma.

Nonketotic hyperosmolar coma is a syndrome characterized by severe hyperglycemia (blood glucose greater than 600 mg/dL); absence of or only slight ketosis; nonketotic acidosis; severe dehydration; depressed sensorium or frank coma; and various neurologic signs that may include grand mal seizures, hyperthermia, hemiparesis, and positive Babinski signs. Respiration is usually shallow, but coexistent metabolic (lactic) acidosis may be manifested by Kussmaul breathing. Serum osmolarity is commonly 350 mOsm/kg or higher. This condition usually occurs in middle-aged or elderly individuals who have "mild" diabetes; among them mortality rates have been as high as 40–70%, possibly in part because of delays in recognition and in initiation of appropriate therapy. In children this condition is infrequent; among reported cases there has been a high incidence of pre-existing neurologic damage. The profound hyperglycemia may develop over a period of days, and, initially, the obligatory osmotic polyuria and dehydration may be partially compensated by increasing fluid intake. With progression, thirst becomes impaired, possibly because of alteration of the hypothalamic thirst center by hyperosmolarity and possibly in some instances because of a pre-existing defect in the hypothalamic osmoregulating mechanism.

The low production of ketones is attributed mainly to the hyperosmolarity, which in vitro blunts the lipolytic effect of epinephrine and the antilipolytic effect of insulin; blunting of lipolysis by the therapeutic use of beta-adrenergic blockers may contribute to the syndrome. Depression of consciousness is closely correlated with the degree of hyperosmolarity; hemoconcentration may predispose to cerebral arterial and venous thromboses.

Treatment is directed at repletion of the vascular volume deficit and correction of the hyperosmolar state (also see management of ketoacidosis). One-half isotonic saline (0.45% NaCl) is administered at a rate estimated to replace 50% of the volume deficit in the first 12 hr and the remainder over the ensuing 24 hr. When the blood glucose concentration approaches 300 mg/dL, the hydrating fluid should be changed to 5% dextrose in 0.2% NaCl. Approximately 20 mEq/L of potassium chloride should be added to each of these fluids to prevent hypokalemia. Serum potassium and plasma glucose concentrations should be monitored at 2 hr intervals for the first 12 hr and at 4 hr intervals for the next 24 hr to permit appropriate dosage adjustments in the administration of potassium and insulin.

Insulin can be given in the continuous intravenous infusion beginning with the 2nd hr of fluid therapy. Inasmuch as blood glucose may decrease dramatically in response to fluid therapy alone, the loading dose should be 0.05 U/kg of regular (fast-acting) insulin followed by 0.05 U/kg/hr of the same insulin, rather than 0.1 U/kg/hr as advocated for diabetic ketoacidosis. During the recovery period, therapy with insulin and diet and monitoring of the patient are as described for patients recovering from diabetic ketoacidosis (see Fluid and Electrolyte Therapy, below, and Table 20–4).

Treatment. The management of insulin-dependent diabetes mellitus may be divided into three phases: that of ketoacidosis; the postacidotic or transition phase for establishment of metabolic control; and the continuing one of long-term guidance of the diabetic child and his or her family. Each of these phases has separate goals, although in practice they merge into a continuum.

Ketoacidosis. The immediate aims of therapy are expansion of intravascular volume, correction of deficits in fluid, electrolyte, and acid-base status, and initiation of insulin therapy to correct intermediary metabolism. Treatment should be instituted as soon as the clinical diagnosis is confirmed by the presence of hyperglycemia and ketonemia. Determinations of blood pH and electrolytes should also be obtained at this time, and an ECG is useful to provide a rapid reference for the existence of hyperkalemia. If sepsis is suspected as a possible precipitating factor, a blood culture should be obtained and the urine examined for bacteria and leukocytes. A flow sheet is essential for the chronologic recording of fluid input (composition and rate), urine output, and insulin administered (dose of bolus injections and/or dose and rate of continuous IV administration) as well as the sequential acid-base electrolyte values of the blood. Catheterization of the bladder is not routinely recommended in children; bag collection or condom drainage permits an assessment of urinary output, but catheterization may be indicated in comatose patients.

FLUID AND ELECTROLYTE THERAPY (Table 20–4). The expansion of reduced intravascular volume and correction of depleted fluid and electrolyte stores are most important in the treatment of diabetic ketoacidosis. It must be stressed, however, that exogenous insulin is essential to arrest further metabolic decompensation and to restore intermediary metabolism.

Dehydration is commonly of the order of 10% and initial fluid therapy can usually be based on this estimate; subsequent adjustments must be related to clinical and laboratory data. The initial hydrating fluid should be isotonic saline (0.9%). Because of the hyperglycemia, hyperosmolality is universal in diabetic ketoacidosis; thus, even 0.9% saline is hypotonic relative to the patient's serum osmolality. A gradual decline in osmolality is desirable; too rapid declines have been implicated in the development of cerebral edema, one of the major complications of therapy in children. For the same reason, the rate of fluid replacement is adjusted to provide only 50–60% of the calculated deficit within the initial 12 hr of therapy; the remaining 40–50% is administered during the following 24 hr. Also, administration of glucose (5% solution in 0.2% NaCl solution) is initiated when the blood glucose concentration approximates 300 mg/dL in order to slow the decline in serum osmolality and to reduce the risk that cerebral edema will develop (Table 20–4). Cerebral edema, if it occurs, usually becomes apparent several hours after therapy has begun and when there are improvements in blood glucose concentration, the acid-base status, and the clinical state of hydration. A previously alert patient may become drowsy, complain of headache, have abnormal neurologic findings including papilledema, progress to coma, and have respiratory arrest with herniation of the brain stem. Recovery may occur with prompt recognition and treatment with intravenous mannitol. Clinically apparent cerebral edema is often fatal, but subclinical cerebral edema is present in many patients during therapy for ketoacidosis.

Administration of potassium (K$^+$) should be started early. Total body potassium may be considerably depleted during acidosis, even when the serum potassium concentration is normal or elevated. Whereas potassium moves from intra- to extracellular sites during acidosis, the reverse occurs during correction of acidosis, particularly when exogenous insulin and glucose are available in the circulation. This shift of potassium back to the intracellular compartment may result in life-threatening hypokalemia. Hence, after the initial fluid replacement with approximately 20 mL/kg of isotonic saline, potassium should be added to subsequent infusates, provided that urinary output is adequate; serum potassium concentration should then be monitored periodically. An ECG provides a rapid assessment of serum potassium concentration; T waves are peaked in hyperkalemia and are low and associated with U waves in hypokalemia. Because the total potassium deficit cannot be replaced within the initial 24 hr of treatment, potassium supplementation should be continued as long as fluids are administered intravenously (Table 20–4).

It is almost inevitable that the patient will receive an excess

Table 20–4. Fluid and Electrolyte Therapy for Diabetic Ketoacidosis

Recommendations for replacement of fluid losses and for maintenance of a 30 kg (surface area 1.0 m²) child with assumed 10% dehydration. Duration of treatment: 36 hours.

REPLACEMENT FLUIDS	Approximate Accumulated Losses with 10% Dehydration	Approximate Requirements for Maintenance (36 hr)	Approximate Totals for Replacement and Maintenance (36 hr)
Water (mL)	3000	2250	5500
Sodium (mEq)	180	65	250
Potassium (mEq)	150	50	200
Chloride (mEq)	120	45	165
Phosphate (mEq)	90	15	100

REPLACEMENT SCHEDULE (continuous intravenous infusion)

Approximate Duration	Fluid (Composition)	Sodium (mEq)	Potassium (mEq)	Chloride (mEq)	Phosphate (mEq)
Hour 1	500 mL of 0.9% NaCl (isotonic saline)	75	—	75	—
Hour 2	500 mL of 0.45% NaCl (0.5 isotonic saline) plus 20 mEq of KCl	35	20	55	—
Hr 3 to 12 (200 mL/hr for 10 hours)	2000 ml of 0.45% NaCl with 30 mEq/L of potassium phosphate	150	60	150	40
Subtotal initial 12 hr	3000 mL	260	80	280	40
Next 24 hr 100 mL/hr	5% glucose in 0.2% NaCl with 40 mEq/L of potassium phosphate	75	100	75	60
Total over 36 hours	5400 mL	335	180	355	100

Note: All replacement values should be halved if dehydration is estimated to be 5%. Maintenance requirements remain the same.

ADDITIONAL GUIDELINES

A **diabetic flow-sheet** with laboratory data appropriately recorded must be maintained in the patient's chart.

Insulin therapy by continuous low-dose intravenous method: Priming dose—bolus injection of 0.1 U/kg of regular insulin IV followed immediately by continuous IV infusion of 0.1 U/kg/hr of regular insulin beginning with 2nd hr.

Directions for making insulin infusion: Add 50 U of regular insulin to 500 mL of isotonic saline. Flush 50 mL through the tubing to saturate insulin binding sites. For 30 kg patient, infuse at rate of 30 mL/hr. When the blood glucose concentration approaches 300 mg/dL, discontinue the insulin infusion and start insulin therapy by subcutaneous injections of 0.2–0.4 U/kg of insulin at intervals of 6 hr.

Bicarbonate therapy: For pH >7.20, no therapy necessary. For pH 7.10–7.20, 40 mEq/m² of bicarbonate over 2 hr; then re-evaluate. For pH <7.10, 80 mEq/m² of bicarbonate over 2 hr; then re-evaluate. New diabetics, <2 yr of age, with diabetic ketoacidosis and 10% dehydration, or any diabetic with pH <7.00, should be managed in an intensive care unit or equivalent setting.

---

of chloride, which may aggravate acidosis; the extent of acidosis, however, can be reduced by substitution of phosphate, which is also significantly depleted in diabetic ketoidosis. Moreover, available phosphate in conjunction with glycolysis is essential for the formation of 2,3-diphosphoglycerate (2,3-DPG), which governs the oxygen dissociation curve. During deficiency of 2,3-DPG, the oxygen dissociation curve is shifted to the left, i.e., more oxygen is retained by hemoglobin and less is available to tissues, a situation that predisposes to lactic acidosis. Acidosis per se tends to shift the oxygen dissociation curve toward the right (Bohr effect) and thus partially "compensates" for 2,3-DPG deficiency. As acidosis resulting from the accumulation of ketones is corrected by the provision of insulin, with or without administration of bicarbonate, the effects of 2,3-DPG deficiency may no longer be "compensated" and the release of oxygen to tissues may again be impaired. Exogenous phosphate, by contributing to the formation of 2,3-DPG, permits the oxygen dissociation curve to shift to the right and thus facilitates release of oxygen to tissues and aids in the correction of acidosis. Furthermore, resistance to insulin action is associated with hypophosphatemia. Hence, we recommend the administration of potassium phosphate (Table 20–4). Since excessive use of phosphate may result in hypocalcemia, serum calcium should be measured periodically. Symptomatic hypocalcemia should be corrected with calcium gluconate.

ALKALI THERAPY. With provision of fluids, electrolytes, glucose, and insulin, metabolic acidosis is usually corrected through the interruption of ketogenesis, the metabolism of ketones to bicarbonate, and the generation of bicarbonate by the distal renal tubule. However, severe acidosis, blood pH 7.1 or less, diminishes respiratory minute volume, may produce hypotension secondary to peripheral vasodilation, impairs myocardial function, and may contribute to insulin resistance. Therefore, treatment with sodium bicarbonate may be indicated.

Since administration of bicarbonate according to the calculated base-deficit overcorrects the acidosis and may result in alkalosis, there are justified concerns about its use in diabetes. Alkalosis, by shifting the oxygen dissociation curve to the left, may diminish the release of oxygen to the tissues and predispose to lactic acidosis. Alkalosis also accelerates the entry of potassium into cells and hence may produce hypokalemia. Perhaps most important, exogenous bicarbonate may worsen cerebral acidosis while the plasma pH is being reduced to normal, because HCO_3^- combines with H^+ and dissociates to CO_2 and H_2O. Inasmuch as bicarbonate passes the blood-brain barrier slowly and CO_2 diffuses freely, cerebral acidosis, and possibly cerebral depression, may be exacerbated.

In light of the above considerations, administration of bicarbonate is recommended only when the pH is 7.2 or lower (Table 20–4). At pH 7.1–7.2, 40 mEq of HCO_3^-/m^2, and below pH 7.1, 80 mEq of HCO_3^-/m^2, should be infused over a period of 2 hr; acid-base status should then be re-evaluated prior to further alkali therapy. Bicarbonate should not be given by bolus infusion, as it may precipitate cardiac arrhythmias.

INSULIN THERAPY. There are in general two methods for insulin therapy of ketoacidosis in current use: the low-dose continuous intravenous method and the one by intermittent bolus injections. The latter has been the standard since the availability of insulin, but is becoming increasingly replaced by the continuous intravenous method.

In the *low-dose continuous intravenous infusion method*, a priming dose of 0.1 U/kg of regular insulin is followed immediately by a constant infusion of 0.1 U/kg/hr (Table 20–4). This method is effective, simple, and physiologically sound and has gained wide acceptance as the preferred method for administering insulin during diabetic ketoacidosis. It provides a constant steady concentration of insulin in plasma that approximates the peak attained in normal individuals during an oral glucose tolerance test. Presumably, the same steady concentration is attained at the cellular level and permits a steady metabolic response without the fluctuations that must occur with intermittent injections of insulin. Concern that the insulin may adhere to glass and tubing has proved to be unfounded, and effective delivery of insulin can be provided without the use of albumin or gelatin added to the infusate. Moreover, the infusion can be provided by gravity drip without the use of a special pump, although such a pump is helpful. We recommend a separate infusion set for insulin that is connected to the infusion line used for fluid and electrolytes so that adjustments in the dosage of each can be made independently. After the amount of insulin for the initial 6–8 hr has been calculated, this quantity is added to a 250 or 500 mL bottle of 0.9% saline (Table 20–4).

When the blood glucose concentration approaches 300 mg/dL, the ongoing potassium requirement is added to 5% glucose in 0.2% saline, and the insulin infusion rate is reduced to 0.05 U/kg/hr; the rate should be periodically adjusted in relation to the blood glucose and acid-base response. Alternatively, the continuous infusion may be discontinued and insulin can be given immediately by subcutaneous injection at a dose of 0.2–0.4 U/kg, and continued at 6–8 hr intervals while the glucose infusion is maintained until the child can fully tolerate food. Subcutaneous injections of regular insulin at doses of 0.2–0.4 U/kg every 6–8 hr before meals should then be continued for 24 hr after the child is eating adequately. The blood glucose level should be monitored before and 2 hr after each meal; the insulin dose is then adjusted to maintain blood glucose concentration in the range of 80–180 mg/dL. The total dose of regular insulin used in this representative day serves as a guide for subsequent insulin treatment with a combination of intermediate- and short-acting insulin as described below. Intermediate-acting insulin can usually be begun within 36 hr after commencing therapy for ketoacidosis.

Insulin can also be administered during diabetic ketoacidosis by *intermittent intramuscular or subcutaneous bolus injections;* a portion of the dose is also usually injected intravenously (Table 20–5). If plasma ketones are only moderately elevated, the recommended doses may be half of those listed. Administration of insulin as the fast-acting form is repeated every 2–4 hr, and blood glucose values and acid-base status are monitored as described for the continuous intravenous insulin method. When the concentration of blood glucose has fallen to approximately 300 mg/dL, subsequent insulin and fluid therapy is the same as that described in the above paragraph.

Ketonemia and ketonuria may persist for a short time despite clinical improvement. The nitroprusside reaction that is routinely used to measure "ketones" reacts with acetoacetate and weakly with acetone but not with beta-hydroxybutyrate. The usual ratio of beta-hydroxybutyrate to acetoacetate is approximately 3:1, but is commonly as much as 8:1 or more in diabetic ketoacidosis. With correction of acidosis, beta-hydroxybutyrate dissociates to acetoacetate, which is identified by the nitroprusside reaction. Hence, persistence of ketonuria for a day or more may not reflect the clinical improvement and should not be interpreted as a poor therapeutic response.

Postacidotic Phase or Transition Period for Establishment of Metabolic Control. Diabetic ketoacidosis is usually corrected within 36–48 hr by the foregoing therapeutic regimens. At this time, the so-called transition period, food and fluids are usually tolerated orally, and insulin can be given by subcutaneous injection. The treatment of the child who presents with classic symptoms of diabetes mellitus associated with hyperglycemia and glucosuria but without ketonuria is comparable to that of the child who has recovered from the ketoacidotic phase. For such children, subcutaneous injections of fast-acting insulin are begun at doses of 0.1–0.25 U/kg every 6–8 hr before meals with simultaneous monitoring of blood glucose concentration and adjustment of the insulin dose for 1–2 days. The initial dose of insulin is lower because these children generally have lower blood glucose concentrations and are more sensitive to insulin than those presenting in diabetic ketoacidosis. One to 2 days of fast-acting insulin therapy are needed to estimate the total daily insulin requirement as a guide to subsequent use of combined intermediate- and short-acting forms.

The aims of management during the transitional period are treatment of any recognized precipitating cause of the diabetic ketoacidosis, such as infection; stabilization of metabolic control by adjustment of insulin dosage; institution of an appropriate nutritional pattern for the child; and education of the parents and patient in the principles of diabetic management. These include techniques of insulin injection, monitoring of blood and urine glucose, monitoring of ketonuria, an understanding of nutritional requirements, recognition of hypoglycemia (insulin shock) and its management, and adjustments of insulin dosage during minor illnesses and for regularly planned exercise. This education is best carried out by the coordinated participation of physician, dietitian, and nurse educator who have special training in diabetes. For newly diagnosed patients, this phase commonly lasts 5 to 10 days; less time may be required for stabilization and re-education of previously diagnosed patients. Ongoing education and adjustment of insulin dosage are continued after discharge from the hospital through patient visits and inquiries by telephone; during this phase, gradual reductions in insulin dosage are frequently required, and the patients should be so advised (see Residual Beta Cell Function, below).

Long-Term Management. *The immediate goals in managing children with Type I diabetes are the provision of adequate nutrition and exogenous insulin in a manner that prevents polydipsia and polyuria (including nocturia), avoids ketoacidosis and severe hypo-*

Table 20–5. Intermittent Insulin Regimen for Diabetic Ketoacidosis

Blood Glucose	Total Insulin Dose	Intravenous Dose	Intramuscular or Subcutaneous Dose	Frequency
>600 mg/dL	1 U/kg	0.5 U/kg	0.5 U/kg	Every 2–4 hr
300–600 mg/dL	0.5 U/kg	0.25 U/kg	0.25 U/kg	Every 2–4 hr
	These doses may be halved if serum ketones are only modestly elevated.			

When blood glucose approaches 300 mg/dL, the intravenous infusion for fluid and electrolyte replacement should contain 5% glucose (see Table 20–4 for rate of administration). Continue subcutaneous injections of insulin at 0.2–0.4 U/kg every 6 hr and monitor blood glucose concentration at the same time. If blood glucose concentration rises, increase the next insulin dose by 50%; if glucose concentration falls, decrease the next insulin dose by 50%. Continue this metabolic regimen for 24 hr after oral intake of fluid and food is established. See text for subsequent management.

glycemia, and permits normal growth and development with an active life pattern. These goals are achievable by most patients and their parents, if they come to understand the principles of the pathophysiology and management of this disease. Ongoing supervision by the physician is essential and should be provided in a manner that avoids undue anxiety and psychologic dependence on the part of the child or parents or a sense of guilt on the part of the parents.

Evidence is emerging that the long-term complications of diabetes are related to the degree of metabolic control. Therefore, long-term management should also aim for as nearly normal metabolism as possible. Completely normal metabolism, however, is not possible by the standard pattern of treatment that consists of 1–2 daily injections of insulin and attention to nutritional intake and exercise. In highly motivated adolescents, however, near-normal metabolism can now be achieved by (1) monitoring blood glucose values at home with appropriate adjustment of insulin dosage 2–3 times a day and with close attention to nutritional intake, or (2) continuous subcutaneous infusion of insulin by a pump worn externally that can be programmed to provide a basal rate of delivery with meal-related increments. For the majority of pediatric patients, however, neither of these newer approaches is available or applicable, and routine management rests on determination of and guidance in respect to insulin dosage, attention to nutritional intake, and exercise.

INSULIN REGIMENS. The diurnal pattern of insulin concentration in the plasma of normal persons is characterized by a basal level on which are superimposed secretory episodes that coincide with intake of food. Each rise in plasma insulin concentration during feeding is synchronous with, and proportional to, the rise in blood glucose. Plasma insulin concentrations, however, do not reflect total insulin secretion. Because insulin is secreted into the portal circulation, its first target organ is the liver, the key organ governing the initial disposal of a glucose load (Table 20–2).

Table 20–6. Common Types of Available Insulin

Product	Form	Strength
*Rapid-Acting**		
Humulin R (Regular)[a]	Human	U-100
Regular Iletin I[a]	Mixed beef and pork	U-100
Regular Iletin II[a]	Pork	U-100, U-500
Regular Iletin II[a]	Beef	U-100
Semilente Iletin I[a]	Mixed beef and pork	U-100
Regular Purified Insulin[b]	Pork	U-100
Semitard Insulin Zinc Susp.[b]	Pork	U-100
Actrapid Regular Insulin[b]	Pork or human	U-100
Velosulin Regular[c]	Pork	U-100
Intermediate-Acting†		
Lente Iletin I[a]	Mixed beef and pork	U-100
Lente Iletin II[a]	Pork or beef	U-100
Humulin N (NPH)[a]	Human	U-100
NPH Iletin I[a]	Mixed beef and pork	U-100
NPH Iletin II[a]	Pork or beef	U-100
Lentard Insulin Zinc Susp.[b]	Mixed beef and pork	U-100
Lente Purified[b]	Beef	U-100
Monotard Insulin Zinc Susp.[b]	Pork or human	U-100
NPH (Isophane) Purified[b]	Beef	U-100
Protaphane (NPH) Insulin[b]	Pork	U-100
Insulatard NPH[c]	Pork	U-100
Mixtard NPH + Regular Insulin[c]	Pork	U-100
Long-Acting‡		
Protamine Zinc Iletin I[a]	Mixed beef and pork	U-100
Protamine Zinc Iletin II[a]	Pork or beef	U-100
Ultralente Iletin I[a]	Mixed beef and pork	U-100
Ultratard Zinc Susp.[b]	Beef	U-100

[a]Lilly.
[b]Squibb-Novo.
[c]Nordisk.

*Onset ½–1 hr, peak effect 2–4 hr, duration 6–8 hr.
†Onset 1–2 hr, peak effect 4–12 hr, duration 24 hr.
‡Onset 4–8 hr, peak effect 14–20 hr, duration 24–36 hr.
Onset and duration can vary from person to person.

Currently available insulins are listed in Table 20–6. Each type (short-acting, intermediate-acting, or long-acting) is available in a concentration of 100 units/mL (U-100); higher concentrations are available for the unusual patient who has high resistance to insulin. Appropriate dilutions can be prepared for younger patients who require lower doses. Refinements in manufacture are now responsible for insulins with distinctly less contamination than formerly by such other pancreatic hormones as proinsulin, glucagon, pancreatic polypeptide, and somatostatin. Antibodies to these and other contaminants have been demonstrated in the sera of insulin-treated diabetics. It is unclear whether the new and more highly purified insulins facilitate metabolic control, but they probably do result in fewer local and systemic allergic reactions, including lipoatrophy and lipohypertrophy. The currently available insulins are extracted from beef and pork pancreas and are marketed separately or as a mixture of the two insulins. Human insulin, synthesized in bacteria via recombinant DNA technology (synthetic) or by chemical modification of pork insulin (semi-synthetic) is also now available for therapy. Human insulin may be less allergenic and less likely to induce antibody formation, but limited data do not indicate any significant advantages over highly purified pork insulin.

Because exogenous insulins are injected subcutaneously rather than directly into the portal vein, their rate of absorption may be variable; and because the dose injected is determined empirically, it lacks the precision of endogenously secreted insulin. It should be apparent that a single injection of intermediate-acting insulin cannot duplicate the pattern of normal insulin secretion, and that periodic excesses of plasma insulin resulting in hypoglycemia and periodic inadequate insulin levels that permit hyperglycemia are virtually inevitable. Even with injections of regular fast-acting insulin prior to each meal, normalization of blood glucose values (euglycemia) is not entirely achieved, although the degree of control is clearly improved. Hence, the regimen of insulin administration selected for the diabetic child must represent a compromise designed to achieve as nearly normal intermediary metabolism as will permit normal growth and development and avoid frequent hypoglycemic reactions and the consequences of unrestrained hyperglycemia.

At the onset of diabetes, or after recovery from ketoacidosis, the total daily dose of insulin is about 0.5–1.0 U/kg; the initial total daily requirement of insulin is estimated from a representative 24 hr period when regular insulin only is administered before each meal during the transition phase. Long-acting insulins are not often used in children. In most instances one of the intermediate insulins is employed, usually combined with a fast-acting (regular) insulin, to achieve an early therapeutic effect. With the single daily dose regimen, approximately two thirds of the total dose is an intermediate-acting insulin (NPH, lente, etc.), and the remainder is regular insulin; the injection is given 30 min before breakfast. The two insulins should always be drawn into the syringe in the same sequence (regular first) so that the residual insulin in the "dead space" is always the same type; thus, greater stability of the patient can be assured when a therapeutic dose is established. Disposable syringes with fine needles, minimal dead space, and easy-to-read calibration for use with U-100 insulin are available. For small children, syringes calibrated to a maximum of 50 units are also available; in some European countries diluted insulins are marketed.

In order to avoid hypoglycemia, the single daily dose of insulin combining intermediate- and short-acting forms is initially calculated on the basis of two thirds of the estimated total daily dose or approximately 0.5 U/kg. Step increases or decreases of 10–15% can then be made daily during the initial phase in hospital until the desired degree of control is achieved. Insulin requirements for the first few days may on occasion be found to be even greater than 1 U/kg/day. The increased amount is apparently necessary for reaccumulation of lost stores of glycogen, protein, and fat. Adjustments in the dose of insulin are made in relation to the blood glucose values monitored before each meal and/or to the urinary glucose. If the predominant hyperglycemia or glucosuria occurs in late morning, then the quick-acting form of insulin is increased by 10–15%. If the predominant hyperglycemia or glucosuria occurs in late afternoon or evening, then the intermediate-acting insulin is increased by 10–15%. Should hypoglycemic reactions occur in mid-morning to noon, the quick-acting form of insulin is reduced by 10–15%, and, if hypoglycemia occurs in late afternoon or evening, the intermediate-acting insulin is decreased by 10–15%. In anticipation of increased exercise upon discharge from the initial hospitalization, the daily dose of insulin should be decreased by 10%.

Although a number of children can be managed with a single daily injection of insulin, many will achieve better control with two daily injections. When there is persistent nocturia and morning glucosuria associated with excessive fasting hyperglycemia in response to a single daily injection of insulin, consideration should be given to dividing the total daily dose into two injections. In this plan two thirds of the daily total dose is given before breakfast and one third before the evening meal; each injection consists of intermediate- and short-acting insulins in proportions of 2:1 to 3:1. For example, assuming a total daily dose of 1 U/kg for a 30 kg child, 14 U of NPH or lente combined with 6 U of regular insulin would be given before breakfast, and 6 U of NPH or lente with 4 U of regular insulin before the evening meal. As with the single daily dose regimen, step increases or decreases, each consisting of 10–15%, should be made to minimize hypoglycemic reactions and undue hyperglycemia, respectively (see above paragraph for guidelines).

Two daily injections of insulin are especially appropriate for infants and children under 5 yr of age, in whom intake of food and extent of activity are not always predictable, and for adolescents, especially during the pubertal growth spurt. Two daily injections may also be more effective when the evening meal is the major one (see Nutritional Management below). With explanation of the rationale, adherence to this twice-daily regimen by patients and parents is usually good. When compliance is not good, we attempt to avoid an attitude of rigidity, particularly with adolescents, in whom there is evidence that 2 daily injections may not always result in better metabolic control than the 1 daily injection. The physician should in all instances attempt to determine what may be in the best interest of the patient. For children who insist on only 1 daily injection of insulin, we adjust the daily dose according to carefully kept records of blood and/or urinary glucose values until the best possible degree of metabolic control is achieved. In this way, it is hoped that confidence in the patient-family-physician relationship is maintained and that a sense of guilt in patient and/or family is avoided.

The *technique for injection of insulin* should be taught to the parents, and to the patient when he or she is ready for it. Injections are given subcutaneously, rotating sites on arms, thighs, buttocks, and abdomen in a regular sequence. An appropriate rotation helps to ensure adequate absorption of insulin, prevent fibrosis, and minimize lipodystrophic changes. With a formalized rotation and the availability of the new purer, single-peak insulins, lipoatrophy and lipohypertrophy are now quite unusual. Younger children may find injections in the abdominal wall difficult or painful. Depending on the physical and psychologic maturity of the child, those over the age of 10–12 yr should be encouraged to administer their own insulin and to monitor their own responses to it. Self-monitoring by the child should be a gradual process in which the child for practical purposes assumes responsibility, always knowing there is consultation available.

Guidelines for adjusting the dose of insulin with exercise, illness, and "brittle" diabetes are provided in greater detail in the following section. It should be stressed, however, that the adolescent growth spurt is regularly associated with an increase in insulin requirements, which may become lower again when puberty is completed.

Hypersensitivity to insulin is uncommon in children. Local skin reactions are characterized by erythema or urticaria, burning, itching, and tenderness within an hour or less after an injection. These reactions usually resolve spontaneously over a period of days but may require a change from mixed beef-pork to pure pork or human insulin, or from NPH to lente insulin because of allergy to protamine in the former; antihistamines may be used if necessary. Generalized reactions with severe urticaria or angioedema are extremely rare and may also spontaneously resolve, but a change in the type of insulin is usually indicated, as noted for local reactions. Desensitization may also be necessary, as may a course of systemic corticosteroid therapy for 1–2 wk. Rarely, insulin resistance develops in response to a local tissue enzyme which destroys injected insulin; some affected patients have benefited from the addition of a protease enzyme inhibitor to the insulin solution; others have required chronic intravenous infusion and are best managed in a hospital with a specialized diabetes unit.

After several months of insulin therapy nearly all patients will have acquired antibodies to insulin. In the majority of instances, they do not interfere with the metabolic response. They may, however, promote instability by creating a reservoir of insulin that may be released at unpredictable times. Rarely, children with antibodies develop true resistance to insulin and require more than 2 U/kg/24 hr. A change to a preparation of pure pork, pure beef, or human insulin usually resolves this problem; in some instances a period of corticosteroid therapy or a course of desensitization may be necessary. Antibodies causing allergy are usually of the IgE class; IgA and IgM antibodies may be responsible for resistance to insulin.

Nutritional Management. Because the word diet may connote restriction and denial and impose a source of anxiety and rebellion on the part of parent and/or patient, we tend to avoid its use and categorize our instructional discussion under such terms as "nutritional requirements" and "meal plans." Actually, there are no special nutritional requirements for the diabetic child other than those for optimal growth and development. Inasmuch, however, as the capacity to secrete insulin in response to the intake of food is negligible in the diabetic child, and since the dose of insulin is predicated on caloric intake, regularity of the eating pattern for the determined insulin regimen becomes paramount. In outlining nutritional requirements for the child on the basis of age, sex, weight, and activity, food preferences including any based on cultural and ethnic backgrounds must be considered. Although general guidelines are usually applicable, the program for each child should be individualized.

Total recommended caloric intake is based on size or surface area and can be obtained from standard tables. The caloric mixture should consist of approximately 55% carbohydrate, 30% fat, and 15% protein. Approximately 70% of the carbohydrate content should be derived from complex carbohydrates such as starch; intake of sucrose and highly refined sugars should be avoided. Complex carbohydrates require prolonged digestion and absorption so that plasma glucose rises slowly, whereas glucose in refined sugars, including those in carbonated beverages, is rapidly absorbed and may cause wide swings in the metabolic pattern; carbonated beverages should therefore be of the sugar-free variety. In the United States the ban on saccharin as an artificial sweetener has been removed pending further evidence of its toxic or teratogenic effect. Although in children there is concern about the potential cumulative effect, available data do not support an association of moderate amounts with bladder cancer. Other non-nutritive sweeteners such as aspartame are used in a variety of products. Sorbitol and xylitol should not be used as artificial sweeteners; they are products of the polyol pathway and are implicated in some of the complications of diabetes.

Diets with high fiber content are useful in improving control of blood glucose in diabetic subjects. Inclusion of about 50 g/day of fiber from foods such as vegetables, especially legumes, whole meal bread, bran cereals, and fruits in the diet of adult diabetics has led to significant reductions in the concentration not only of blood glucose but also of total and low-density lipoprotein (LDL) cholesterol. In addition, small amounts of sucrose consumed with fiber-rich foods such as whole meal bread may have no more glycemic effect than their low-fiber, sugar-free equivalents. The concept of biologic equivalence or of a "glycemic index" of foods is currently under investigation. When completed, these studies may provide a listing of foods with more predictable effects on blood glucose and serum lipid patterns for patients with diabetes than is currently available.

The intake of fat is adjusted so that the polyunsaturated/saturated (P/S) ratio is increased to about 1.2:1.0, in contrast to the estimated American average of 0.3:1.0. Dietary fats derived from animal sources are therefore reduced and are replaced by polyunsaturated fats from vegetable sources. Substitutions of margarine for butter, vegetable oil for animal oils in cooking, and lean cuts of meat, poultry, and fish for fatty meats are advisable. The intake of cholesterol is also reduced by these measures and by limiting the number of egg yolks consumed. There is ample evidence that these simple measures reduce serum LDL cholesterol, a predisposing factor to atherosclerotic disease (Sec. 7.39).

The total daily caloric intake may be divided to provide 20% at breakfast, 20% at lunch, and 30% at dinner, leaving 10% for each of the mid-morning, mid-afternoon, and evening snacks, if they are desired. In older children, the mid-morning snack may be omitted and its caloric equivalent added to the lunch. Special brochures and pamphlets describing the exchanges and sample meal plans for children are usually available from regional diabetes associations; their use should be encouraged as part of the educational process. Meal plans are often based on groups of food exchanges; within each of the lists of exchangeable foods that are principal sources of carbohydrates, proteins, and fats, respectively, there is a wide variety of foods. For practical purposes there are few restrictions so that each child, with the help of the physician and/or dietitian, may select a diet based on personal taste or preferences. Emphasis should be placed on regularity of food intake and especially on the constancy of carbohydrate intake. Occasional excesses for birthdays and other parties are permissible and are tolerated so as not to foster rebellion and stealth in obtaining desired food. Similarly, cakes, doughnuts, and even candies are permissible on special occasions as long as the food exchange value and carbohydrate content are adjusted in the meal plan. Adjustments in meal planning must be made for anticipated vigorous exercise (see below). Above all, adjustments must constantly be made to meet the needs as well as the desires of each child; with experience and coordination between the parent and child and the physician, these can usually be accomplished.

Monitoring. Success in the daily management of the diabetic child can be measured to a considerable extent by the competence acquired by the family, and subsequently by the child, in assuming responsibility for day-to-day "diabetic care." Their initial and ongoing instruction in conjunction with their supervised experience can lead to a sense of confidence in making intermittent adjustments in insulin dosage for dietary deviations, unusual physical activity, and even, for some, minor intercurrent illnesses as well as for otherwise unexplained, repeated hypoglycemic reactions and excessive glucosuria. Within limits such acceptance of responsibility should make them relatively independent, provided that there is ongoing interested supervision and shared responsibility by the physician.

Self-monitoring is essential to such a plan and necessitates a regimen that includes measurements of blood or urinary glucose and at times of ketones; the keeping of a standardized record of the results and of the corresponding data of dietary deviations, unusual physical activity, hypoglycemic reactions, intercurrent illness, the daily dose of insulin, and other items of possible relevance. Many of these records, however, are patently unreliable for a number of reasons. There may be self-delusion, reliance on memory with charting just prior to the visit to the physician, attempts to please the physician and avoid rebuke, as well as reluctance to perform some aspects of the blood or urinary tests. In spite of these deviations, asking patients to keep records does appear to be justified. Initially, following dismissal from the hospital, the parent or patient is apt to be particularly attentive to a prescribed regimen. It is after some months of satisfactory experience that parents or patients tend to become less attentive to detail. When the physician apparently accepts the contrived report, the parent or the child may come to find increasing reasons for nonconformance. If the physician mistrusts the report, it may be justifiable to make independent evaluations (see below); should these data be counter to those in the parent's or child's report, attempts can be made to clarify the situation with them in a manner that will not undermine their confidence. Such situations test the physician's skill in the management of patients with persistent but not confining illness.

The *daily tests for glucosuria* should be performed just prior to each of the three major meals and at the time of the evening snack. This timing is designed to secure an estimate of the effect of the prescribed insulin 3–4 hr after each meal. The preciseness of this estimate is increased if the child voids a half hour or so prior to the test voiding; the initial specimen is discarded. When reliable measurements *consistently* indicate 2% or more glucose in the urine for a given portion of the day, the appropriate dose of the short- or intermediate-acting insulin should be increased by 10–15%. Conversely, when urine is *consistently* free of glucose for any portion of the day, the insulin dose may need to be reduced by 10–15% if hypoglycemic reactions ensue or if the blood glucose concentration, as determined by the glucose oxidase strip, is 60 mg/dL or less. In the absence of symptomatic hypoglycemia and of documented low blood glucose concentrations, absence of glucosuria does not warrant a reduction in insulin dosage; such patients are manifesting desirable metabolic control. Consistent patterns of excessive glucosuria at fixed times in the morning or afternoon are indications for appropriate increases in the morning and/or evening doses, and at times for a change to another type of insulin. When more precise adjustments are deemed necessary, the physician may request a fractional 24 hr collection of urine. The urine should be collected in three fractions: 8:00 AM to 2:00 PM; 2:00 PM to 8:00 PM; and 8:00 PM to 8:00 AM. Assessment of volume and semiquantitative or quantitative glucose values in each sample permits a rational basis for adjusting the respective doses of the rapid and intermediate-acting insulins.

Short-term (daily) *monitoring of blood glucose values* has been distinctly simplified by the availability of "strips" impregnated with glucose oxidase that permit blood glucose measurement from a drop of blood. The blood glucose concentration can be approximated directly by comparison to a color scale or accurately by a portable calibrated reflectance meter. A small spring-loaded device that automates capillary bloodletting in a relatively painless fashion is also commercially available.

Parents and patients should be taught to use these devices and to measure blood glucose 3 to 4 times daily: before breakfast, lunch, and supper and before retiring at night. Initially, in the hospital, the blood glucose measurement should also be performed at 3:00 to 4:00 AM to exclude inappropriate nocturnal hypoglycemia and avoid the Somogyi phenomenon (see below). Ideally, blood glucose should range from approximately 80 mg/dL in the fasting state to 140 mg/dL after meals. In practice, however, a range of 60–240 mg/dL is quite acceptable. Blood glucose measurements that are consistently at or outside these limits, in the absence of an identifiable cause such as exercise or dietary indiscretion, are an indication for a change in the insulin dose. For example, if the fasting blood glucose is high, the evening dose of intermediate insulin is increased by 10–15%; if the noon glucose value exceeds set limits, the dose of the morning regular insulin is increased by 10–15%; if the pre-supper glucose value is high, the morning dose of intermediate-acting insulin is increased by 10–15%; and, if the pre-bedtime glucose measurement is high, the evening dose of regular insulin is increased by 10–15%. Similarly, reductions in the dose of the appropriate insulin type should be made when the respective blood glucose values are consistently below desirable limits.

Daily blood glucose measurements should be continued after discharge from the hospital as long as they are acceptable to the patient. Practical considerations require a reduction in the frequency of blood glucose monitoring at home, as few children tolerate capillary bloodletting 4 times daily for prolonged periods. Consequently, after the initial stabilization period of several weeks, when the routine of insulin administration and meal planning is established, we suggest that home blood glucose monitoring be performed only 2 days/wk, varying the days each week to achieve a representative profile in time. Monitoring of urinary glucose is performed on those days when blood glucose measurements are omitted. Blood glucose measurement, however, should be performed if there are symptoms suggestive of hypoglycemia or if glucosuria persists at 2% or greater. In highly motivated adolescents and young adults who become sufficiently knowledgeable about managing their diabetes, self-monitoring of blood glucose values before and 2 hr after meals, in conjunction with multiple daily injections of insulin, adjusted as necessary, can maintain near-normal glycemia for prolonged times.

A reliable index of long-term glycemic control is provided by *measurement of glycosylated hemoglobin*. Glycohemoglobin (HbA$_{1c}$) represents the fraction of hemoglobin to which glucose is nonenzymatically attached in the blood stream. The formation of HbA$_{1c}$ is a slow reaction that is dependent on the prevailing concentration of blood glucose; it continues irreversibly throughout the red blood cell's life span of approximately 120 days. The higher the blood glucose concentration and the longer the red blood cell's exposure to it, the higher will be the fraction of HbA$_{1c}$, which is expressed as a percentage of total hemoglobin. Since a blood sample at any given time contains a mixture of red blood cells of varying ages, exposed for varying times to varying concentrations of blood glucose, an HbA$_{1c}$ measurement reflects an approximate average of blood glucose concentrations during the preceding 2–3 months. When measured by standardized methods to remove labile forms, the fraction of HbA$_{1c}$ is not influenced by an isolated episode of hyperglycemia. Consequently, as an index of long-term glycemic control a measurement of HbA$_{1c}$ is superior to measurements of glycosuria or of a single blood glucose determination. Periodic measurements of HbA$_{1c}$ may also help to resolve questions relating the degree of metabolic control to subsequent development of complications. Although values of HbA$_{1c}$ may vary according to the method used for its measurement, in normal individuals the HbA$_{1c}$ fraction is usually less than 7%; in diabetics, values of 6–9% represent very good metabolic control, values of 9–12%, fair control, and values above 12%, poor control.

Exercise. Exercise is an integral component of growth and development. No form of exercise, including competitive sports, should be forbidden to the diabetic child, who should not be made to feel different or restricted. Examples of athletes with diabetes who have excelled in national or international sports are not rare. Regular exercise tends to improve glucoregulation by increasing insulin receptors. In patients who are in poor metabolic control, however, vigorous exercise may precipitate ketoacidosis because of the exercise-induced increase in the counter-regulatory hormones.

The major complication of exercise in diabetic patients is hypoglycemic reaction during or within hours after exercise. The principal contributing factor is an increased rate of absorption of insulin from its injection site. If hypoglycemia does not occur with exercise, adjustments in diet or insulin dose are not necessary, and glucoregulation is likely to be improved through the increased utilization of glucose by muscles.

When regularly planned exercise is associated with hypoglycemia, the child and parent, guided by the physician, should be able to develop an appropriate regimen to avoid the reaction. For example, prior to the exercise, one additional carbohydrate unit from the exchange list may be taken by the child, and glucose in the form of orange juice, a carbonated beverage, or candy should be available during and after exercise. In addition, it may be necessary, in some instances, to decrease the dose of insulin prior to the exercise by 10 to 15%. The appropriateness or necessity of these alterations is determined by experience with each child. Prolonged exercise, such as long-distance running, may require reduction of as much as 50% of the usual insulin dose.

Residual Beta Cell Function (So-Called Honeymoon Period). After initial stabilization some 75% of newly diagnosed diabetic children will require a progressive reduction in their daily dose of insulin from approximately 1 U/kg to 0.5 U/kg or less. Recurrent hypoglycemia is the manifestation that prompts a reduction in the insulin dose. A minority of children can even maintain normoglycemia for a time without any administered insulin; this complete remission occurs in less than 5% of diabetics, but even in these patients glucose tolerance tests demonstrate abnormal carbohydrate metabolism. The duration of this "honeymoon" phase is variable; it commonly lasts several weeks or months but may last as long as 1–2 yr. Residual insulin secretion, measured as C-peptide, is present during this remission period and to some extent in virtually all diabetic children in the initial year of their disease; in approximately 20% there will be some C-peptide response even after 5 yr. Stable, well-controlled subjects have higher C-peptide secretion than nonstable subjects, and the required dose of insulin is inversely correlated to the basal or the stimulated C-peptide response.

It is not completely clear why this residual insulin secretion is inadequate to prevent the evolution of diabetes including ketoacidosis, but the reasons presumably relate to stress-provoked secretion of catecholamines that inhibit still further the insulin secretory capacity of the pancreatic beta cells. In any event, the clinical remission phase is limited; with isolated exceptions, insulin-dependent diabetes inevitably recurs. Although opinion varies, our policy is to maintain insulin treatment unless a daily dose of 0.1 U/kg still causes hypoglycemia, in which case we discontinue insulin treatment and periodically test the patient for the re-emergence of glycosuria. The physician may decide to discontinue insulin treatment completely if it appears to be in the patient's best interests to do so. The patient and family, however, should not be led to believe that the disease is "cured" and should continue to examine the child's urine for glucose.

Hypoglycemic Reactions (Insulin Shock). Virtually all diabetic children experience a hypoglycemic reaction at some time during the course of their disease. Hypoglycemia occurs suddenly or over minutes, in contrast to diabetic ketoacidosis, which develops over hours or days. The symptoms and signs are those due to an outpouring of catecholamines, which include pallor, sweating, apprehension, trembling, and tachycardia, and those due to cerebral glucopenia, which include hunger, drowsiness, mental confusion, seizures, and coma. Particular mood and personality changes plus certain abnormal physical patterns may be characteristic for an individual and provide an early clue to the more pronounced reaction. There is some evidence that these symptoms may occur with a sudden drop in blood glucose to levels that do not meet the criterion for hypoglycemia (less than 60 mg/dL) in healthy subjects.

The occurrence of hypoglycemia in a diabetic child indicates too much insulin relative to food intake and energy expenditure. Common causes include the evolution of the "honeymoon" phase (see above), deliberate or accidental errors in insulin dosage, inadequate caloric intake, and strenuous and sustained physical activity in the absence of increased caloric intake.

The most important factor in the management of hypoglycemia is an understanding by patient and family of the symptoms and signs of the reaction, especially of the patient's individual pattern, so that the known precipitating factors can be avoided or compensated for. For the acute episode a carbohydrate-containing snack or drink, such as orange juice or a sugar-containing carbonated beverage or candy (equivalent to 5–10 g of glucose) should be available. Patients, parents, and teachers should also be instructed in the administration of glucagon; 0.5 mg given intramuscularly is particularly useful when the patient is losing consciousness or is vomiting. When exercise is the precipitating factor, definitive preventive measures can be taken (see Exercise, above). Avoiding severe hypoglycemic episodes should be a major objective of treatment; they have been implicated in ultimately provoking epileptic seizures, and an increased frequency of abnormal EEG changes has been observed in diabetics.

The Somogyi Phenomenon, the Dawn Phenomenon, and "Brittle Diabetes." Hypoglycemic episodes, which may be mild and often may be manifested as late nocturnal or early morning sweating, night terrors, and headaches alternating rapidly, within 4–5 hr, with ketosis, hyperglycemia, ketonuria, and excessive glucosuria, should suggest the possibility of the Somogyi phenomenon. This syndrome has been aptly described as "hypoglycemia begetting hyperglycemia" and is believed to be due to an outpouring of counter-regulatory hormones in response to insulin-induced hypoglycemia. The coexistence of this brittle form of diabetes with daily doses of more than 2 U/kg of insulin suggests the presence of this phenomenon and the need to reduce the dose of insulin. The term brittle diabetes implies that control of blood glucose fluctuates widely and rapidly despite frequent adjustments of the dose of insulin.

The Somogyi phenomenon must be distinguished from the "dawn phenomenon," in which early morning elevations of blood glucose concentration occur between 5 and 9 AM without preceding hypoglycemia. The dawn phenomenon occurs even in patients treated by continuous subcutaneous infusion of insulin unless the rate of insulin infusion is increased in the early morning hours. Thus, the dawn phenomenon reflects the waning effects of biologically available insulin, perhaps as a consequence of increased clearance of insulin or other normal physiologic changes that remain to be defined; the normal early morning rise in cortisol is not responsible for this phenomenon. Together, the Somogyi and dawn phenomena are the most common causes of instability or "brittleness" in diabetic children. To distinguish the dawn and Somogyi phenomena, blood glucose concentrations

should be measured at 3, 4, and 7 AM. If blood glucose concentrations are over 80 mg/dL in the first two samples and markedly higher in the third, then the dawn phenomenon is likely; in this case an increase of 10–15% in the evening dose of intermediate insulin may be helpful. It may also be helpful to delay the evening dose of intermediate acting insulin by 2–3 hr so that its delayed peak effect coincides with the anticipated timing of the dawn phenomenon.

On the other hand, if the 3 or 4 AM blood glucose measurement is 60 mg/dL or less followed by rebound hyperglycemia at 7 AM, the Somogyi phenomenon is likely and a reduction of the evening intermediate acting insulin of 10–15% is indicated.

In other patients with brittle diabetes better control is often achieved by a change from 1 to 2 daily injections of insulin and/or by a change from beef-pork mixtures to pure pork or human insulin. The latter may circumvent problems with antibodies that bind insulin. Attention should also be directed to psychologic problems within or without the home that may be bases for deliberate errors in insulin and/or nutritional intake.

Psychologic Aspects. Diabetes in a child affects the lifestyle and interpersonal relationships of the entire family. Feelings of anxiety and guilt are common in parents. Similar feelings, coupled with denial and rejection, are equally common in children, particularly during the rebellious teenage years. No specific personality disorder or psychopathology is characteristic of diabetes; similar feelings are observed in families with other chronic disorders.

In children these feelings find expression in nonadherence to instructions regarding nutritional and insulin therapy and in noncompliance with self-monitoring. Deliberate overdosage with insulin resulting in hypoglycemia, or omission of insulin, often in association with excesses in nutritional intake resulting in ketoacidosis, may be pleas for psychologic help or manipulative events to escape an environment perceived as undesirable or intolerable; occasionally, they may be manifestations of suicidal intent. Frequent admissions to hospital for ketoacidosis or hypoglycemia should arouse suspicion of underlying emotional conflict. Overprotection on the part of parents is common and often is not in the best interest of the patient. Feelings of being different and/or of being alone are common and may be justified in view of the restrictive schedules imposed by requirements to test urine and blood, to administer insulin, and to limit nutritional intake. Furthermore, publicity regarding the likelihood of developing complications and of decreased life span in Type I diabetes must foster anxiety. Unfortunately, misinformation abounds regarding the risks of development of diabetes in siblings or offspring and the dangers of pregnancy in young diabetic women. In turn, even appropriate information often causes further anxiety.

Many, but not all, of these problems can be averted through continued empathic counseling based on correct information and attempts to build attitudes of normality in the patient as a productive and potentially reproductive member of society. Peer discussion groups may be useful in lessening feelings of isolation and frustration by the sharing of common problems. Summer camps for diabetic children afford an excellent opportunity for learning and sharing under expert supervision. Education regarding the pathophysiology of diabetes, insulin dose and technique of administration, nutrition, exercise, and hypoglycemic reactions can be reinforced by medical and paramedical personnel. The presence of numerous peers with similar problems affords new insights for the diabetic child.

The physician managing a child or adolescent with diabetes should be aware of his pivotal role as counselor and advisor and should anticipate the common emotional problems of the patient. When emotional problems are clearly responsible for poor compliance with the medical regimen, referral for psychologic help may be indicated. Such help is often available in pediatric centers where psychologists form part of the management team for diabetic children.

Management during Infections. Systemic and local infections are no more common in diabetic children than in nondiabetic ones. During intercurrent illnesses, either infectious or traumatic, diabetic children nearly always require additional insulin, especially during prolonged serious episodes that necessitate inactivity. In the latter situations, when glucosuria is excessive, a good working rule is to add 10–20% of the total daily dose as regular (short-acting) insulin prior to each meal. Subsequent increases or decreases should then be based on careful monitoring of urinary and blood glucose values.

Patients who are vomiting should nevertheless take some insulin; approximately 50% of the daily dose is a general rule, followed by careful monitoring of urinary or blood glucose with subsequent adjustments of the dose of insulin as indicated. If vomiting continues and the patient cannot tolerate clear liquids, admission to the hospital and administration of intravenous therapy with glucose, electrolytes, and insulin may be indicated.

Management during Surgery. The objectives are the prevention of hypoglycemia during anesthesia, of severe loss of fluids, and of diabetic acidosis. The regimens described below are generally applicable, but vigilance and individual adjustments for each patient are necessary to achieve these goals.

When surgery is elective, the patient should be admitted to the hospital 24 hr prior to surgery; during this time the usual nutritional requirements and insulin dose are provided. Supplemental regular insulin may be given to achieve better control of blood glucose when indicated. On the morning of surgery an infusion of 5% glucose in 0.45% saline solution plus 20 mEq/L of potassium chloride is begun; initially 1 U of regular insulin is added to the infusate for each 4 g of administered glucose. The rate of infusion should provide maintenance fluid requirements plus estimated losses during surgery. The blood glucose concentration should be monitored at periodic intervals before, during, and after surgery; concentrations of approximately 120–150 mg/dL should be the goal, which can be achieved by varying the rate of infusion of the glucose and electrolyte mixture or the amount of insulin added. This regimen may be discontinued when the patient is awake and capable of taking food and fluid orally. Prior to reinstitution of the patient's usual diet, regular insulin may be administered at a dose of 0.25 U/kg at 6 hr intervals; appropriate adjustments in the dose are based on blood or urinary concentrations of glucose.

An equally effective plan that is particularly useful for surgery of short duration is as follows: on the morning of surgery administer one half of the usual morning dose of insulin subcutaneously and initiate intravenous infusion of the electrolyte and glucose solution described in the preceding paragraph, but do not include insulin in it. After surgery regular insulin in a dose of 0.25 U/kg is administered subcutaneously; subsequent doses at intervals of 6 hr are adjusted on the basis of blood glucose concentrations until the patient is ready for his or her usual dietary pattern.

For emergency surgery an intravenous infusion is initiated that provides 5–10% glucose in 0.45% saline solution, 20 mEq of potassium chloride, and 1 U of regular insulin for each 2–4 g of glucose. Blood glucose concentration should be maintained at approximately 120–150 mg/dL. When possible, rehydration and metabolic balance should precede the surgery. After surgery the regimen described above can be instituted.

For minor surgery with local anesthesia the usual insulin and dietary regimens can be maintained. If there should be extensive vomiting, the losses can usually be compensated with glucose solution administered intravenously.

Neurovascular and Other Complications: Relation to Glycemic Control. The increasingly prolonged survival of the diabetic child is associated with an increasing prevalence of complications that affect the microcirculation of the eye (retinopathy), the kidney (nephropathy), and the nerves (neuropathy) as well as the large vessels (atherosclerosis) and the lens (cataracts). Retinopathy is present in 45–60% of insulin-dependent diabetics after 20 yr of known disease and in 20% after 10 yr; lens opacities are present in at least 5% of those under 19 yr of age. Diabetic nephropathy is also common; it is present after 25 yr of insulin-dependent diabetes in about 40% of patients in whom the onset occurred during childhood; it may account for about 50% of deaths in long-term insulin-dependent diabetics.

There is an emerging consensus based on clinical experience and experimental data that strongly suggests an association between glycemic control and the later development of complications. It is not known, however, if this relationship is directly proportional to the degree of hyperglycemia or if there is a set point of average glycemia above which complications develop exponentially or below which complications may be less frequent. In addition, studies implicate some possible biochemical pathways that might be responsible for these complications. For example, the process of glycosylation of erythrocytic hemoglobin, which is directly proportional to the blood glucose concentration, also involves other serum and tissue proteins; it has been implicated in basement membrane thickening in the glomeruli. There is evidence that activation of the polyol pathway and disturbances in myoinositol metabolism are related, respectively, to cataracts and to neuropathy. In humans, typical lesions of diabetic nephropathy develop in normal kidneys within several years after they have been transplanted to diabetics with chronic renal failure. In contrast, the early histologic changes of diabetic nephropathy regress when kidneys of a diabetic are transplanted to a nondiabetic recipient with chronic renal failure. These observations suggest that it is the diabetic environment and not the genetic background that predisposes to these renal changes. Similarly, renal lesions that mimic those of human diabetes develop in animals rendered diabetic, and these changes tend to regress following cure of the diabetes by islet transplantation.

Other complications that have been described in diabetic children include *dwarfism associated with a glycogen-laden, enlarged liver (Mauriac syndrome), osteopenia, and a syndrome of limited joint mobility associated with tight, waxy skin, growth impairment, and maturational delay.* The Mauriac syndrome is clearly related to under-insulinization; it is now rare because of the availability of the longer-acting insulins. The syndrome of limited joint mobility is frequently associated with the early development of diabetic microvascular complications, such as retinopathy and nephropathy, which may appear before the age of 18 yr. None of these complications has been demonstrated in a nondiabetic identical twin, even after 20 yr of recognized diabetes in the insulin-dependent twin. Genetic predisposition to the development of diabetic vascular complications does, however, play a role.

Despite the evidence in experimental animals and suggestive evidence in humans with diabetes, the possible relationship of the degree of glycemic control to these complications in humans remains unproven because none of the available modes of treatment has resulted in sufficiently normal metabolic control to provide an adequate study group. Nevertheless, the substantial evidence for a relationship, in conjunction with improved methods for monitoring glycemic control and for delivery of insulin, justifies a multicenter trial examining the relationship between metabolic control and complications. As long as reduction of these late complications remains a possibility, physicians have the responsibility to maintain as nearly normal metabolism as is compatible with the physical and psychologic limits of each diabetic child. Despite the potential for developing complications, survival for 40 yr and more is feasible; the goal should be to make these years increasingly free of debilitating diabetic-related disease.

Long-Term Outcome. Type I diabetes mellitus increases mortality and morbidity. In one study of 45 children under 12 yr of age at the time of diagnosis, there were 7 deaths within 10–25 yr of diagnosis: 3 were directly attributable to diabetes, and 2 were due to suicide; 3 patients attempted suicide unsuccessfully. Visual, renal, neuropathic, and other complications were relatively frequent. Furthermore, although diabetic children eventually attain a height within the normal adult range, puberty may be delayed, and the final height may be less than the genetic potential.

The recent introduction of portable devices programmed to provide continuous subcutaneous infusion of insulin with meal-related pulses is one approach to the resolution of these long-term problems. In selected individuals, nearly normal patterns of blood glucose and other indices of metabolic control, including HbA_{1c}, have been maintained for several years. This approach, however, should be reserved for highly motivated persons committed to rigorous self-monitoring of blood glucose and alert to potential complications such as infections at the site of needle implantation, and mechanical failure of the infusion device causing hyper- or hypoglycemia.

20.2 IMPAIRED GLUCOSE TOLERANCE AND TYPE II NON–INSULIN-DEPENDENT DIABETES

The term "impaired glucose tolerance" (see Table 20–1) is used to characterize individuals who have a plasma glucose concentration in excess of 140 mg/dL 2 hr after initiation of the standard oral glucose tolerance test but who do not have symptoms of diabetes or fasting hyperglycemia. The indication for an oral glucose tolerance test may be the discovery of isolated or intermittent glucosuria or the occurrence of hyperglycemia during a stressful illness or during corticosteroid therapy. Individuals considered at risk for abnormal glucose metabolism may also need to be tested; these include obese children, those who have symptoms suggestive of reactive postprandial hypoglycemia, and close relatives of known diabetics. An oral glucose tolerance test is not indicated in a child who has characteristic diabetic symptoms and a random blood glucose value in excess of 200 mg/dL.

The term *impaired glucose tolerance* is suggested to replace such terms as asymptomatic diabetes, chemical diabetes, subclinical diabetes, borderline diabetes, or latent diabetes in order to avoid the stigma associated with the term diabetes mellitus, which may influence the choice of vocation, eligibility for health or life insurance, and self-image. Furthermore, although impaired glucose tolerance represents a biochemical intermediate between normal glucose metabolism and that of diabetes, few children with impaired glucose tolerance go on to develop diabetes; estimates range from 0 to 10%. There is disagreement whether the degree of glucose intolerance is useful as a prognostic index of the likelihood of progression, but there is evidence that among the few who do progress, the insulin response during glucose tolerance testing is severely impaired. In the majority of children with impaired glucose tolerance, particularly the obese, insulin responses during oral glucose tolerance tests are higher than the mean of age-adjusted controls; these individuals may have some resistance to the effects of insulin rather than an inability to secrete it.

In normal children the glucose response during an oral glucose tolerance test is similar at all ages. In contrast, plasma insulin responses during the test increase progressively within the age span of about 3–15 yr, so that interpretation of them requires comparison with age-adjusted criteria.

Preparation of the candidate for a glucose tolerance test should be standardized according to currently accepted criteria. These include at least 3 days of a well-balanced diet containing approximately 50% of calories from carbohydrates; fasting from midnight until the time of the test in the morning; and a dose of glucose for the test of 1.75 g/kg but not in excess of 75 g. Plasma samples are obtained prior to ingestion of the glucose and at 1, 2, and 3 hr thereafter. The arbitrarily designated response to the test that identifies "impaired glucose tolerance" is a fasting plasma glucose value < 140 mg/dL and a value at 2 hr > 140 mg/dL. The determination of serum insulin responses during the glucose tolerance test is not necessary in reaching a diagnosis; the magnitude of the response, however, may have prognostic value.

In children with impaired glucose tolerance, but without fasting hyperglycemia, repeated oral glucose tolerance tests are not recommended. The degree of impaired glucose tolerance in such children tends to remain stable or may actually decrease over a period of years, except in patients with markedly subnormal insulin responses. Consequently, apart from reduction in weight for the obese child, no therapy is indicated. In particular, the use of oral hypoglycemic agents should be restricted for investigational studies.

If fasting hyperglycemia and/or characteristic symptoms of diabetes should develop, the affected children will have the characteristics of non–insulin-dependent diabetes (Type II), previously known as adult-onset diabetes (see Table 20–1 and Sec. 20.1 under Classification). Such children may require insulin for control of hyperglycemia although they generally do not develop ketosis in the absence of exogenous insulin therapy and hence, by definition, are not insulin-dependent.

20.3 DISEASES ASSOCIATED WITH DIABETES

Cystic Fibrosis. Because of improvements in the medical care of children with cystic fibrosis, many survive to the late teen and early adult years. In addition to the primary insufficiency of pancreatic exocrine function, there is an increasing incidence of pancreatic endocrine dysfunction manifested as glucose intolerance that progresses occasionally to overt diabetes mellitus. When hyperglycemia develops, the accompanying metabolic derangements are usually mild, and, if insulin therapy becomes necessary, relatively low doses usually suffice for adequate management. Ketoacidosis is uncommon but may occur with progressive deterioration of islet cell function. Treatment with insulin is as outlined for Type I diabetes, but dietary management may be limited by the constraints of the primary disturbance.

Autoimmune Diseases. *Chronic lymphocytic thyroiditis* (Hashimoto thyroiditis) is frequently associated with Type I diabetes in children. As many as 1 in 5 insulin-dependent diabetics may have thyroid antibodies in their serum; the prevalence is 2–20 times greater than that observed in control populations. Only a small proportion of these diabetics, however, develop clinical hypothyroidism; the interval between diagnosis of diabetes and of thyroid disease averages about 5 yr. Periodic palpation of the thyroid gland is indicated in all diabetic children; if the gland feels firm and/or enlarged, serum measurements of thyroid antibodies and thyroid stimulating hormone (TSH) should be obtained. A TSH level of greater than 10 μU/mL indicates existing or incipient thyroid dysfunction that warrants replacement with thyroid hormone. Deceleration in the rate of growth may also be due to thyroid failure and is, in itself, a reason for securing serum measurements of thyroxine and TSH concentrations.

When diabetes and thyroid disease coexist, the possibility of *adrenal insufficiency* should also be considered. It may be heralded by decreasing insulin requirements, increasing pigmentation of the skin and buccal mucosa, salt craving, weakness, asthenia, and postural hypotension, or even frank addisonian crisis as evidence of primary adrenal failure. This syndrome is most unusual in the 1st decade of life, but it may become apparent later.

Circulating antibodies to gastric parietal cells and to intrinsic factor are 2–3 times more common in patients with Type I diabetes than in control subjects. There are good correlations of antibodies to gastric parietal cells with atrophic gastritis and of antibodies to intrinsic factor with malabsorption of vitamin B_{12}. Although the possibility of megaloblastic anemia should be considered in children with Type I diabetes, its occurrence is rare.

A variant of the *multiple endocrine deficiency syndrome* is characterized by Type I diabetes, idiopathic intestinal mucosal atrophy with associated inflammation and severe malabsorption, IgA deficiency, and circulating antibodies to multiple endocrine organs including the thyroid, adrenal, pancreas, parathyroid, and gonads. In addition, nondiabetic family members have an increased frequency of vitiligo, Graves disease, multiple sclerosis, low complement levels, and antibodies to endocrine tissues.

That Type I diabetes may itself be an autoimmune disease has been discussed above.

Acanthosis Nigricans with Insulin Resistance Type A. This syndrome is characterized by acanthosis nigricans especially of the axillae and neck, variable degrees of glucose intolerance including symptomatic diabetes, hirsutism, accelerated growth suggestive of gigantism, and endogenous hyperinsulinemia with severe resistance to exogenous insulin. It occurs predominantly in black females, who commonly present during adolescence for evaluation of menstrual irregularities; many are obese and have laboratory findings suggestive of the polycystic ovary syndrome. The carbohydrate intolerance, hyperinsulinemia, and resistance to exogenous insulin result from a congenitally reduced number of insulin receptors. Weight reduction may ameliorate the carbohydrate intolerance, but exogenous insulin is usually not helpful.

20.4 GENETIC SYNDROMES ASSOCIATED WITH DIABETES MELLITUS

A number of rare genetic syndromes associated with insulin-dependent diabetes mellitus or with carbohydrate intolerance have been described. These syndromes represent a broad spectrum of diseases ranging from premature cellular aging, as in the Werner and Cockayne syndromes, to excessive obesity associated with hyperinsulinism, resistance to insulin action, and carbohydrate intolerance as in the Prader-Willi syndrome. Some of these syndromes are characterized by primary disturbances in the insulin receptor or in antibodies to the insulin receptor without any impairment in insulin secretion. Although rare, these syndromes provide unique models to study the multiple causes of disturbed carbohydrate metabolism from defective insulin secretion or from defective insulin action at the cell receptor or postreceptor step. Some of these syndromes are described in the report of the National Diabetes Data Group.

20.5 TRANSIENT DIABETES MELLITUS OF THE NEWBORN

Onset of persistent insulin-dependent diabetes before the age of 6 mo is most unusual. The syndrome of transient diabetes mellitus in the newborn infant has its onset in the first weeks of life and persists only several weeks to months before spontaneous resolution. It occurs most often in infants who are small for gestational age and is characterized by hyperglycemia and pronounced glycosuria resulting in severe dehydration and at times metabolic acidosis, but with only minimal or no ketonemia or ketonuria. Insulin responses to glucose or tolbutamide are low to absent; basal plasma insulin concentrations, however, are normal. After spontaneous recovery the insulin responses to these same stimuli are brisk and normal. Occurrence of the syndrome in consecutive siblings has been reported. Permanent diabetes is not known to have developed in any affected infant who has recovered from the transient syndrome. This syndrome should be distinguished from *severe hyperglycemia*, which may occur with *hypertonic dehydration*, usually in infants beyond the newborn period; infants with severe hyperglycemia respond promptly to rehydration with a minimal requirement for insulin.

Administration of insulin is mandatory during the active phase of this syndrome. One to 2 U/kg/24 hr of an intermediate-acting insulin in 2 divided doses usually results in dramatic improvement and accelerated growth and gain in weight. Attempts at gradually reducing the dose of insulin may be made as soon as recurrent hypoglycemia becomes manifest or after 2 mo of age. The parents should be assured of the transient nature of the disease and the excellent prognosis.

FUTURE DIRECTIONS

Several avenues of research are being followed to elucidate the etiology of Type I diabetes, to find a "cure," to improve methods of insulin delivery, and to reduce long-term complications.

The evidence that Type I diabetes mellitus is caused by autoimmune destruction of pancreatic beta cells has led investigators to attempt various forms of immunosuppression in newly diagnosed cases in order to preserve residual insulin secreting capacity and to arrest ongoing beta cell destruction; there are promising preliminary results. Transplantation of the whole pancreas has been performed, but except in identical twins success has been limited by problems of rejection and by leakage of pancreatic enzymes. Transplantation of isolated pancreatic islets obviates the problems associated with pancreatic enzymes; culture of islets prior to their transplantation has had limited success in overcoming the problems of rejection between and within species of diabetic animals. Development of portable insulin delivery systems that may be computer-controlled and that could provide insulin in a more physiologic manner shows increasing promise. Devices depending on continuous monitoring of blood glucose with computer-controlled delivery of insulin (closed loop) are too cumbersome for long-term use; their successful use must await the development of an implantable glucose sensor. The portable devices that provide preprogrammed, continuous, subcutaneous delivery of insulin at two rates, constant basal and meal-related increments (open loop), can be adjusted for individual needs and have been used by some patients for several years; blood glucose, serum lipids, hormonal profiles, and glycosylated hemoglobin are maintained within normal ranges.

Human insulin synthesized by recombinant DNA technology or by chemical modification of porcine insulin is available for therapy. Inhibitors of certain enzymes that are believed to participate in the development of diabetic complications are also undergoing clinical trials. These advances justify some optimism toward solving some of the problems of diabetes mellitus.

MARK A. SPERLING

Epidemiology, Etiology, Pathophysiology, and Classification

Cahill GF, McDevitt HO: Insulin dependent diabetes mellitus: The initial lesion. N Engl J Med 304:1454, 1981.

Dobersen MJ, Scharff JE, Ginsberg-Fellner F, et al: Cytotoxic autoantibodies to beta cells in the serum of patients with insulin-dependent diabetes mellitus. N Engl J Med 303:1493, 1980.

Fajans SS, Cloutier MC, Crowther RL: Clinical and etiologic heterogeneity of idiopathic diabetes mellitus. Diabetes 27:1112, 1978.

Fleegler FM, Rogers KD, Drash AL, et al: Age, sex, and season of onset of juvenile diabetes in different geographic areas. Pediatrics 63:374, 1979.

Gamble DR: An epidemiological study of childhood diabetes affecting two or more siblings. Diabetologia 19:341, 1980.

Karam JH, Lewitt PE, Young CW, et al: Insulinopenic diabetes after rodenticide (Vacor) ingestion: A unique model of acquired diabetes in man. Diabetes 29:971, 1980.

LaPorte RE, Fishbein HA, Drash AL, et al: The incidence of insulin dependent diabetes mellitus in Allegheny County, Pennsylvania (1965–1976). Diabetes 30:279, 1981.

Lebovitz HE: Etiology and pathogenesis of diabetes mellitus. Pediatr Clin North Am 31:521, 1984.

National Diabetes Data Group: Classification and diagnosis of diabetes mellitus and other categories of glucose intolerance. Diabetes 28:1039, 1979.

Neufeld M, MacLaren NK, Riley NF, et al: Islet cell and other organ-specific antibodies in US Caucasians and blacks with insulin-dependent diabetes mellitus. Diabetes 29:589, 1980.

Rabinowe SL, Eisenbarth GS: Type I diabetes mellitus: A chronic autoimmune disease? Pediatr Clin North Amer 31:531, 1984.

Rayfield EJ, Seto Y: Viruses and the pathogenesis of diabetes mellitus. Diabetes 28:1126, 1978.

Rosenbloom AL, Kohrman A, Sperling M: Classification and diagnosis of diabetes mellitus in children and adolescents. J Pediatr 98:320, 1981.

Srikanta S, Ganda OP, Jackson RA, et al: Type I diabetes mellitus in monozygotic twins: Chronic progressive beta cell dysfunction. Ann Intern Med 99:320, 1983.

Yoon JW, Austin M, Onodera T, et al: Virus-induced diabetes mellitus: Isolation of a virus from the pancreas of a child with diabetic ketoacidosis. N Engl J Med 300:1173, 1979.

Genetics

Barbosa J, Rich S, Dunsworth T, et al: Linkage disequilibrium between insulin-dependent diabetes and the Kidd blood group Jk^b allele. J Clin Endocrinol Metab 55:193, 1982.

Chern MM, Anderson VE, Barbosa J: Empirical risk for insulin-dependent diabetes (IDD) in sibs. Further definition of genetic heterogeneity. Diabetes 31:1115, 1982.

Cudworth AG, Gorsuch AN, Wolf E, et al: A new look at HLA genetics with particular reference to type I diabetes. Lancet 2:389, 1979.

Gorsuch AN, Spencer KM, Lister J, et al: Can future type I diabetes be predicted? A study in families of affected children. Diabetes 31:862, 1982.

Permutt MA, Chirgwin J, Rotwein P, et al: Insulin gene structure and function: A review of studies using recombinant DNA methodology. Diabetes Care 7:386, 1984.

Raum D, Stein R, Alper CA, et al: Genetic marker for insulin-dependent diabetes mellitus. Lancet 1:1208, 1979.

Rotter JL, Hodge SE: Racial differences in juvenile-type diabetes are consistent with more than one mode of inheritance. Diabetes 29:115, 1980.

Warram JH, Krolewski AS, Gottlieb MS, et al: Differences in risk of insulin-dependent diabetes in offspring of diabetic mothers and diabetic fathers. N Engl J Med 311:149, 1984.

Diabetic Ketoacidosis

Adrogue HJ, Wilson H, Boyd AE III, et al: Plasma acid-base patterns in diabetic ketoacidosis. N Engl J Med 307:1603, 1982.

Duck SC, Weldon VV, Pagliara AS, et al: Cerebral edema complicating therapy for ketoacidosis. Diabetes 25:111, 1976.

Foster DW, McGarry JD: The metabolic derangements and treatment of diabetic ketoacidosis. N Engl J Med 309:159, 1983.

Heber D, Molitch M, Sperling MA: Low-dose continuous insulin therapy for diabetic ketoacidosis: Prospective comparison with "conventional" insulin therapy. Arch Intern Med 137:1377, 1977.

Kaye R: Diabetic ketoacidosis—the bicarbonate controversy. J Pediatr 87:156, 1975.

Keller U, Berger W: Prevention of hypophosphatemia by phosphate infusion during treatment of diabetic ketoacidosis and hyperosmolar coma. Diabetes 29:87, 1980.

Krane EJ, Rockoff MA, Wallman JK, et al: Subclinical brain swelling in children during treatment of diabetic ketoacidosis. N Engl J Med 312:1147, 1985.

Rubin HM, Kramer R, Drash A: Hyperosmolality complicating diabetes mellitus in childhood. J Pediatr 74.177, 1969.

Schade DS, Eaton RP: The temporal relationship between endogenously secreted stress hormones and metabolic decompensation in diabetic man. J Clin Endocrinol Metab 50:131, 1980.

Sperling MA: Diabetic ketoacidosis. Pediatr Clin North Am 31:591, 1984.

Waldhausl W, Kleinberger G, Korn A, et al: Severe hyperglycemia: Effects of rehydration on endocrine derangements and blood glucose concentration. Diabetes 28:577, 1979.

Winegrad AI, Kern EFO, Simmons DA: Cerebral edema in diabetic ketoacidosis. N Engl J Med 312:1184, 1985.

Management of Type I Diabetes in Children

Arky RA: Nutritional therapy for the child and adolescent with type I diabetes mellitus. Ped Clin North Am 31:711, 1984.

Bolli GB, Gerich JE: The "dawn phenomenon"—a common occurrence in both non–insulin-dependent and insulin-dependent diabetes mellitus. N Engl J Med 310:746, 1984.

Bolli GB, Gottesman IS, Campbell PJ, et al: Glucose counterregulation and waning of insulin in the Somogyi phenomenon (posthypoglycemic hyperglycemia). N Engl J Med 311:1214, 1984.

Cerreto MC, Travis LB: Implications of psychological and family factors in the treatment of diabetes. Pediatr Clin North Am 31:689, 1984.

Gale EAM, Kurtz AB, Tattersall RB: In search of the Somogyi effect. Lancet 2:279, 1980.

Goldstein DE, Walker B, Rawlings SS, et al: Hemoglobin A_{1c} levels in children and adolescents with diabetes mellitus. Diabetes Care 3:503, 1980.

Langdon DR, James FD, Sperling MA: Comparison of single and split-dose insulin regimens with 24-hour monitoring. J Pediatr 99:854, 1981.

Rosenbloom AL, Giordano BP: Chronic overtreatment with insulin in children and adolescents. Am J Dis Child 131:881, 1977.

Ross JM: Allergy to insulin. Pediatr Clin North Am 31:675, 1984.

Sonksen PH, Judd SL, Lowy D: Home-monitoring of blood-glucose: Method for improving diabetic control. Lancet 1:729, 1978.

Sperling MA: Insulin biosynthesis and C-peptide. Am J Dis Child 134:1119, 1980.

Stein R, Goldberg N, Kalman F, et al: Exercise and the patient with type I diabetes mellitus. Pediatr Clin North Am 31:665, 1984.

Tamborlane WV, Press CM: Insulin infusion pump treatment of type I diabetes. Pediatr Clin North Am 31:721, 1984.

Witters LA, Ohman JL, Weir GC, et al: Insulin antibodies in the pathogenesis of insulin allergy and resistance. Am J Med 63:703, 1977.

Long-Term Outcome of Childhood Diabetes: Relation of Control to Development of Complications

Abouna GM, Kremer GD, Daddah SK, et al: Reversal of diabetic nephropathy in human cadaveric kidneys after transplantation into non-diabetic recipients. Lancet 2:1274, 1983.

Beyer MM: Diabetic nephropathy. Pediatr Clin North Am 31:635, 1984.

Diabetes Data: U.S. Department of Health, Education and Welfare. Publication No. 78:1468 (NIH), compiled 1977.

Gabbay KH: The sorbitol pathway and complications of diabetes. N Engl J Med 288:831, 1983.

Hostetter TH: Diabetic nephropathy. N Engl J Med 312:642, 1985.

Kirschenbaum DM: Glycosylation of proteins: Its implications in diabetic control and complications. Pediatr Clin North Am 31:611, 1984.

Kroc Collaborative Study Group: Blood glucose control and the evolution of diabetic retinopathy and albuminuria. A preliminary multicenter trial. N Engl J Med 311:365, 1984.

MacGregor M: Juvenile diabetics growing up. Lancet 1:944, 1977.

Mauer SM, Barbosa J, Vernier R, et al: Development of diabetic vascular lesions in normal kidneys transplanted into patients with diabetes mellitus. N Engl J Med 295:916, 1976.

Pax-Guevara AT, Hsu TH, White P: Juvenile diabetes after forty years. Diabetes 24:559, 1976.

Rosenbloom AL: Skeletal and joint manifestations of childhood diabetes. Pediatr Clin North Am 31:569, 1984.

Skyler JS: Complications of diabetes mellitus: Relationship to metabolic dysfunction. Diabetes Care 2:499, 1979.

Steffes MW, Sutherland DER, Goetz FC, et al: Study of kidney and muscle biopsy specimens from identical twins discordant for type I diabetes mellitus. N Engl J Med 312:1282, 1985.

Tamborlane WV, Sherwin RS: Diabetes control and complications: New strategies and insights. J Pediatr 102:805, 1983.

Tattersall RB, Pyke DA: Growth in diabetic children: Studies in identical twins. Lancet 2:1105, 1973.

Unger RH: Meticulous control of diabetes: Benefits, risks, and precautions. Diabetes 31:479, 1982.

White NW, Waltman SR, Krupin T, et al: Reversal of neuropathic and gastrointestinal complications related to diabetes mellitus in adolescents with improved metabolic control. J Pediatr 99:41, 1981.

Diseases and Syndromes Associated with Diabetes

Flier JS, Kahn CR, Roth J: Receptors, antireceptor antibodies and mechanisms of insulin resistance. N Engl J Med 300:1979.

Lippe BM, Sperling MA, Dooley RR: Pancreatic alpha and beta cell functions in cystic fibrosis. J Pediatr 90:751, 1977.

Maccuish AC, Irvine WJ: Autoimmunological aspects of diabetes mellitus. Clin Endocrinol Metab 4:435, 1975.
National Diabetes Data Group: Classification and diagnosis of diabetes mellitus and other categories of glucose intolerance. Diabetes 28:1039, 1979.

Transient Diabetes of the Newborn

Blethen SL, White NH, Santiago JV, et al: Plasma somatomedins, endogenous insulin secretion, and growth in transient neonatal diabetes mellitus. J Clin Endocrinol Metab 52:144, 1981.
Pagliara AS, Karl IE, Kipnis DB: Transient neonatal diabetes: Delayed maturation of the pancreatic beta cell. J Pediatr 82:97, 1973.
Schiff D, Colle E, Stern L: Metabolic and growth patterns in transient neonatal diabetes. N Engl J Med 287:119, 1972.

Future Directions

Assan R, Debray-Sachs M, Laborie C, et al: Metabolic and immunological effects of cyclosporin in recently diagnosed type I diabetes. Lancet 1:67, 1985.
Mecklenburg RS, Benson DA, Benson JW, et al: Acute complications associated with insulin infusion pump therapy. JAMA 252:3265, 1984.
Santiago JV, Clemens AH, Clarke WL, et al: Closed-loop and open-loop devices for blood glucose control in normal and diabetic subjects. Diabetes 28:71, 1978.
Stiller CR, Dupre J, Gent M, et al: Effects of cyclosporine immunosuppression in insulin-dependent diabetes mellitus of recent onset. Science 223:1362, 1984.
Sutherland DER, Goetz FC, Chin PL, et al: Pancreas transplantation. Pediatr Clin North Am 31:735, 1984.
Tamborlane WV, Press CM: Insulin infusion pump treatment of type I diabetes. Pediatr Clin North Am 31:721, 1984.

20.6 HYPOGLYCEMIA

Hypoglycemia is defined as an abnormally low level of blood glucose, the principal and physiologically most important circulating hexose. The normal fasting blood glucose level is lower in infants than in children. Hypoglycemia is especially common in newborn infants, affecting 4/1000 live-born fullterm infants and 16/1000 premature infants. It may occur immediately (within 30 min) after birth, as in infants of diabetic mothers; or it may be delayed (24–48 hr), as in infants who are small for gestational age, in the smaller of discordant twins, and in those infants whose mothers have had hypertensive disease of pregnancy. Hypoglycemia in the neonate may be asymptomatic, mild, and transient, or severe, persistent, and intractable to usual modes of treatment.

In the newborn period it is generally agreed that hypoglycemia exists if glucose levels in plasma fall below 35 mg/dL in the fullterm infant or below 25 mg/dL in the premature infant. After 72 hr of age the plasma glucose level is normally over 45 mg/dL, and in older infants and children fasting levels below 50 mg/dL are considered hypoglycemic.

The diagnosis and management of hypoglycemia in the newborn are discussed in Sec. 8.57.

Physiologic Considerations. Glucose may be derived directly from dietary intake by intestinal absorption, by conversion of other hexoses after absorption (galactose, fructose), by hydrolysis of polyglucose units (maltose, starch, glycogen), or by combinations of these processes (lactose, sucrose). Glucose can also be derived from dietary or endogenous amino acids, but there is no *net* synthesis of glucose from exogenous or endogenous lipids.

Figure 20–1 depicts some of the pathways of glucose metabolism. Although free glucose may passively diffuse through most cell membranes, insulin is required for glucose to enter adipose and muscle cells. A specific glucose transport protein in cell surface membranes has been identified. It is usually taken up from the lumen of the intestinal tract by the mucosal cells, from the lumen of the renal tubules by their epithelial cells, or from the bloodstream by various parenchymal cells using an active process requiring energy. The phosphorylation of glucose requires ATP and either hexokinase(s) or glucokinase. Within the cells, the glucose-6-phosphate may be metabolized or may be hydrolyzed in intestinal, renal tubular, or liver cells to glucose, which is then free to diffuse out of the cells again.

The main routes of metabolism are as follows:

1. The Embden-Meyerhof pathway of anaerobic glycolysis converts the 6-carbon glucose to 3-carbon acids (pyruvic and lactic) with a small release of energy.

2. The pentose-phosphate shunt, initiated by the enzyme glucose-6-phosphate dehydrogenase, yields ribose among other sugars or joins the Embden-Meyerhof scheme at the level of glyceraldehyde-3-phosphate. The reduction of NADP along this pathway is important for a variety of oxido-reductive processes, such as for lipid synthesis and for the maintenance of glutathione in the reduced form.

3. Glucose is also converted to glucose-1-phosphate, which is in equilibrium with galactose-1-phosphate. Glycogen is the form in which glucose units are stored, mainly in the liver, and is in equilibrium with circulating glucose via the pathways depicted.

The ultimate product of glycolysis is pyruvic acid. After the addition of carbon dioxide or after oxidation to acetyl coenzyme A, it enters the citric acid cycle (tricarboxylic acid or Krebs cycle). Acetyl coenzyme A can also be used in the synthesis of fatty acids, cholesterol, and steroid hormones or in the formation of ketone bodies (acetone, acetoacetic acid, and beta-hydroxybutyric acid). The enzymes of the citric acid cycle are found in the mitochondria within the cells where most of the energy of glucose is released and captured in the form of ATP. Many amino acids are in equilibrium with glucose within the citric acid cycle. By transamination or oxidation, glutamic acid is converted to alpha-ketoglutaric acid, aspartic acid to oxaloacetic acid, and alanine to pyruvic acid.

The process of gluconeogenesis involves overcoming the thermodynamically unfavorable reaction that changes pyruvic acid to phosphoenolpyruvic acid (Fig. 20–1) by the transfer of pyruvic acid from the cytosol to the mitochondrion. Once within the mitochondrion, pyruvic acid is converted to either oxaloacetic acid or malic acid, both of which can then diffuse out into the cytosol, where they are in equilibrium with each other. Once in the cytosol, oxaloacetic acid is converted to phosphoenolpyruvic acid by phosphoenol-pyruvate carboxykinase, one of the key rate-limiting enzymes in the gluconeogenic pathway.

Many of the enzyme systems involved in the metabolism of glucose are under hormonal control. Insulin is known to increase the activity of glucokinase in liver and of glycogen synthase in muscle and liver and to suppress key enzymes of gluconeogenesis in liver. In contrast, glucagon and epinephrine act via specific membrane receptors to stimulate the adenyl cyclase system, thereby producing 3′,5′-cyclic AMP and initiating a complex series of integrated reactions. In particular, glycogen degradation by activation of the phosphorylase cascade and glucose synthesis via gluconeogenetic mechanisms are stimulated. The enzymatic sites of action of growth hormone, corticotropin, and glucocorticoids, all of which produce hyperglycemia after prolonged administration, are not yet well defined. One of the effects of glucocorticoids is to promote gluconeogenesis via amino acids. The interaction of hormones and of neural control on enzymatic processes and the availability of substrates in the liver are essential to the mature, fine control of glucose homeostasis. Blood glucose concentration is then dependent upon gastrointestinal or hepatic production of glucose to meet the requirements of

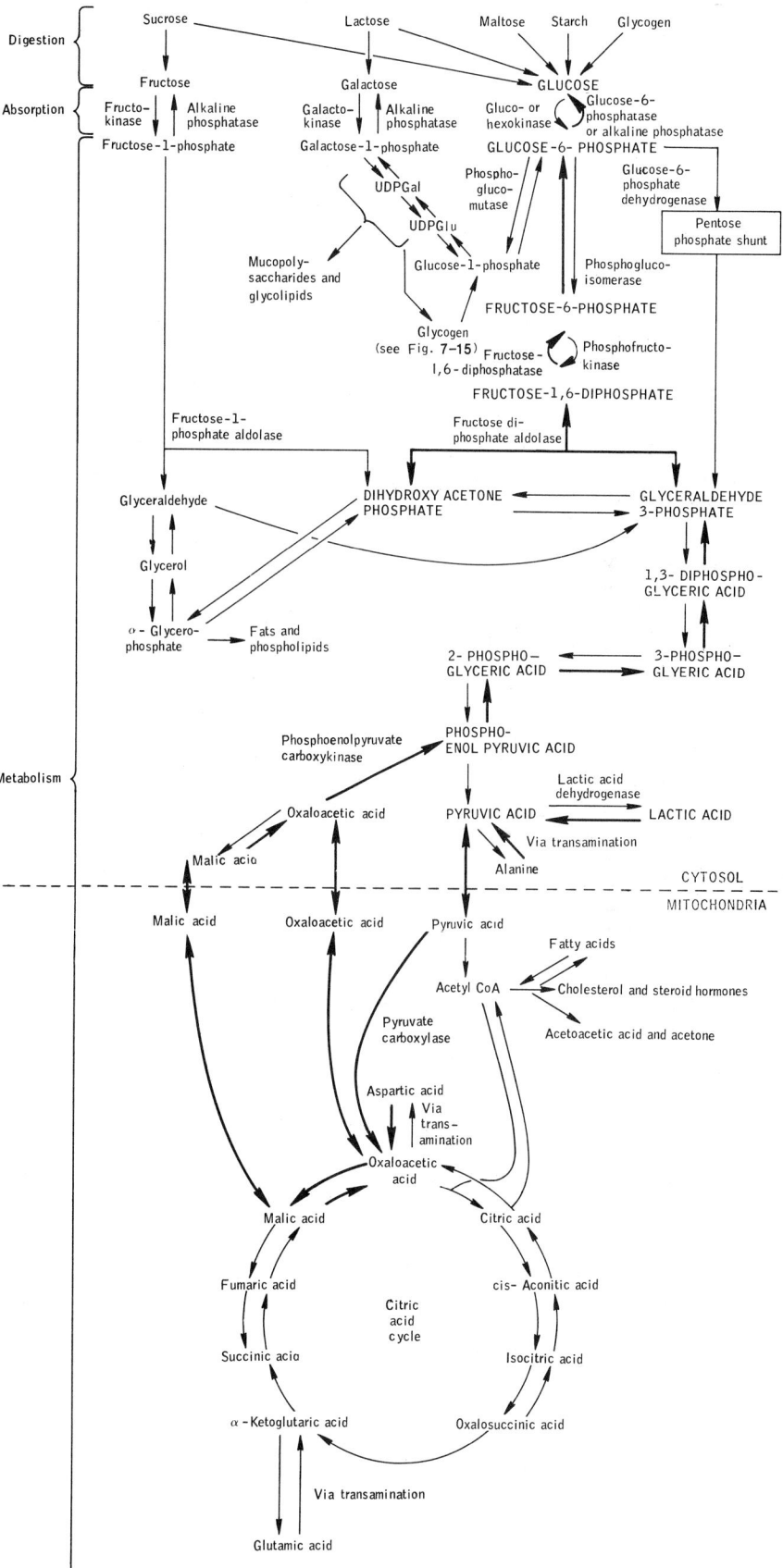

Figure 20–1. The metabolism of glucose. The compounds of the Embden-Meyerhof pathway are indicated in capital letters. The pathway for gluconeogenesis is indicated by heavy arrows.

nervous tissue and blood elements. A low blood glucose level may reflect diminished hepatic production or increased peripheral tissue uptake or some combination of both.

CAUSES OF HYPOGLYCEMIA

There are numerous ways for aberrations of glucose metabolism to lead to hypoglycemia. Defects in the glucose control mechanisms may involve inborn errors of metabolism, alterations of endocrine balance, or exogenous drugs and toxins (Table 20–7). Since hypoglycemia may result from many disorders, and since rational treatment and prognosis depend upon the nature of the specific disorder, it is essential to determine the cause of the hypoglycemia.

20.7 HYPERINSULINISM

When blood glucose falls to hypoglycemic levels, a concomitant fall of insulin to very low levels occurs in patients with normal homeostasis. Levels of insulin greater than 10 μU/mL in the presence of hypoglycemia are abnormal; in some infants even lower levels of insulin may be inappropriate for the degree of hypoglycemia and indicate autonomous secretion of insulin. Many patients with the condition previously called *idiopathic hypoglycemia of infancy* are now known to have hyperinsulinism.

Many children with hyperinsulinism exhibit marked sensitivity to administration of L-leucine with a fall of glucose to hypoglycemic levels. In normal children leucine produces only a small rise in the level of insulin in blood and a concomitant decrease of approximately 10 mg/dL in the level of glucose. Leucine stimulates beta cell secretory activity directly. Patients with islet cell adenoma, islet cell hyperplasia, or nesidioblastosis usually, but not always, exhibit an exaggerated response to leucine. Many of the children diagnosed as having *leucine-sensitive hypoglycemia* in the past probably had nesidioblastosis rather than a discrete diagnostic entity related to leucine.

Islet Cell Adenoma. Functioning beta cell adenoma of the pancreas is a rare lesion. In most instances onset of symptoms occurs after 4 yr of age, but in approximately one third hypoglycemia appears during the neonatal period. Symptoms may be severe and unremitting or may be mild and intermittent. The adenoma is usually solitary but may be multiple or associated with adenomatosis. Four cell types, including beta (insulin), alpha (glucagon), delta (somatostatin), and pp (pancreatic polypeptide), have been identified in varying proportions in islet adenomas. Plasma insulin levels are usually disproportionately elevated relative to glucose levels, indicating autonomous secretion. In adults approximately 10% of beta cell tumors are malignant, but in children malignancy is rarer.

Nesidioblastosis. Hyperinsulinism frequently occurs in the absence of a discrete islet cell adenoma. The pancreatic duct cell is thought to be the primordial cell of the pancreas from which the duct and acinar and islet cells arise when appropriately stimulated (nesidioblast means "islet builder"). Nesidioblastosis may result from inappropriate control of early development of the endocrine pancreas.

The histologic findings consist of diffuse proliferation of islet cells and disorganization throughout the pancreas. These cells vary in size and are found budding from pancreatic duct epithelium; all 4 islet cell types are involved. These cells may be scattered singly or in small clusters throughout the pancreas and occur in association with islets that are normal or have increased cell numbers. A 5-fold increase in total endocrine area is found. Approximately 50–60% of cells are beta cells; the remainder are cells that secrete glucagon, somatostatin, or pancreatic polypeptide. Because nesidioblastosis

Table 20–7. Classification of Hypoglycemias

A. With hyperinsulinism
  1. Islet (beta) cell tumors
  2. Beta cell adenomatosis
  3. Nesidioblastosis
  4. Beta cell hyperplasia
    a. In association with hypopituitarism
    b. Infant of diabetic mother
    c. Infant with erythroblastosis fetalis
    d. Beckwith syndrome
    e. Leprechaunism
    f. Etiology unknown
  5. Teratoma containing pancreatic tissue
  6. Functional beta cell secretory defect
B. With hepatic enzyme deficiencies
  1. Glucose-6-phosphatase
  2. Amylo-1,6-glucosidase
  3. Phosphorylase system
  4. Glycogen synthase
  5. Fructose-1-phosphate aldolase
  6. Fructose-1,6-diphosphatase
  7. Pyruvate carboxylase
  8. Phosphoenolpyruvate carboxykinase deficiency
  9. Galactose-1-phosphate uridyl transferase
  10. Branched chain amino acid abnormalities
  11. Biotin-responsive multiple carboxylase deficiency
C. With endocrine deficiencies
  1. Pituitary
    a. Isolated growth hormone deficiency
    b. Isolated ACTH deficiency
    c. Panhypopituitarism
      (1) With hypoinsulinism
      (2) With hyperinsulinism
  2. Adrenal
    a. Addison disease
    b. Congenital adrenal hypoplasia
    c. Congenital adrenal hyperplasia
    d. Familial glucocorticoid deficiency
    e. Adrenal medullary unresponsiveness
  3. Glucagon deficiency
D. Ketotic hypoglycemia
E. Due to drugs and toxins
  1. Ethyl alcohol
  2. Salicylates
  3. Sulfonylureas
  4. Propranolol
  5. Jamaican vomiting sickness
F. Other
  1. Hepatic damage
    a. Reye syndrome
    b. Leukemia
  2. Malabsorption
  3. Renal glycosuria
  4. Malnutrition
    a. Kwashiorkor
    b. Low phenylalanine diet
  5. Extrapancreatic neoplasms
  6. Carnitine deficiency syndromes

Hypoglycemia in the neonate may be caused by many of the conditions listed above as well as by other less well delineated factors (Sec. 8.57).

might be considered a normal variant of development, it has been suggested that the proliferation of islet cells leading to hyperinsulinism be referred to as nesidiodysplasia.

The hypoglycemia most often begins in the first weeks or months of life and is usually severe and intractable. Other infants may be asymptomatic or only mildly irritable with similar degrees of hypoglycemia. Insulin levels may be only slightly increased in serum, beta cell proliferation may not be increased, and pancreatic insulin content may not be elevated. In such patients, deficiency of glucagon and/or somatostatin secretory cells results in alteration of pancreatic hormone balance and may explain the hypoglycemia. Differentiation of this condition from islet cell adenoma is usually not possible without pathologic examination of the pancreas.

Nesidioblastosis has been reported in siblings in six families, suggesting a recessive mode of inheritance. The condition has also been seen in association with multiple endocrine adenomatosis, an autosomal dominant condition. Heterogeneity of nesidioblastosis seems likely.

Hyperinsulinism in Association with Panhypopituitarism. Patients having this condition usually develop hypoglycemia during the first days of life. In spite of deficiencies of growth hormone, ACTH, and TSH, serum insulin levels are inappropriately elevated for the level of glucose. Hyperplasia of the beta cells occurs in some patients. The hypopituitarism appears to be hypothalamic in origin, but the cause for the hyperinsulinism is obscure. In newborn males with hypoglycemia, microphallus provides an important clinical clue to the syndrome.

Newborn Infants of Diabetic and Gestationally Diabetic Mothers. Hypoglycemia is common but may not be symptomatic (Sec. 8.56).

Other Hypoglycemias. In newborn infants with moderate to severe *erythroblastosis fetalis* clinical manifestations of hypoglycemia and blood glucose levels under 30 mg/dL occur with some frequency (see also Sec. 8.47). Hyperplasia of the pancreatic islets has been observed in many infants dying with this disorder; it is not as marked as that which occurs in infants of diabetic mothers, and eosinophilic infiltrations are usually not present. The insulin content of the pancreas is increased as are insulin levels in blood and urine. The stimulus that leads to the hyperplasia of the islet cells is not known. The condition is ordinarily transitory, but hypoglycemia has been reported in two siblings at 7 and 25 mo of age, presumably as a late sequel of severe erythroblastosis fetalis.

The use of blood containing acid citrate dextrose (ACD) for exchange transfusion of infants having hyperbilirubinemia may lead to hypoglycemia 2–3 hr after completion of the transfusion. The high level of glucose in ACD blood corrects any initial hypoglycemia but causes an increased secretion of insulin, which may subsequently provoke a precipitous fall of blood glucose. Careful monitoring of glucose levels should continue beyond the period of exchange transfusion.

Hyperplasia of the pancreatic islets has also been observed in *Beckwith syndrome* (Sec. 8.57).

Hypoglycemia associated with a marked increase in the size and number of islets has been observed in *leprechaunism (Donohue syndrome)*. A defect in insulin receptors has been found.

Teratomas, especially mediastinal and sacrococcygeal, frequently contain pancreatic tissue. Asymptomatic hypoglycemia and an increased level of insulin were detected in a 5 yr old boy with a mediastinal teratoma. This type of hypoglycemia may occur more often than heretofore suspected.

Most infants with hyperinsulinism do not come to surgery; it is not firmly established, therefore, that increased numbers of beta cells are invariably present in these patients. A deranged homeostatic mechanism leading to increased responsiveness of the islet cells remains a possible cause of hypoglycemia. It is even possible that *functional hyperinsulinism* is a primary defect leading to increased numbers of beta cells (Sec. 8.57).

The most common form of hyperinsulinemic hypoglycemia is that associated with treatment of known Type I, insulin-dependent diabetes mellitus (Sec. 20.1).

20.8 HEPATIC ENZYME DEFICIENCIES

Glycogenoses (Glycogen Storage Diseases). *Deficiency of glucose-6-phosphatase* (type 1a) or glucose-6-phosphate translocase (type 1b) leads to severe hypoglycemia in the fasting state and 4–6 hr after meals. In the liver, this is the most important enzyme complex involved in the release of glucose whether derived from glycogenolysis or via gluconeogenesis. Its deficiency leads to accumulation of glycogen and fat and to hepatomegaly (Sec. 7.21). After even a short period of fasting, rather than yielding a normal release of glucose, the glycogen is metabolized via the Embden-Meyerhof pathway with release of pyruvic and lactic acids (Fig. 20–1). As a consequence, the hypoglycemia is associated with metabolic acidosis. Patients may have levels of glucose that are unmeasurable (< 10 mg/dL) and of lactate as high as 200 mg/dL.

Affected children are not usually mentally retarded or excessively prone to convulsions even at these low concentrations of glucose. Lactate may provide 40–50% of cerebral energy.

When there is *deficiency of debranching enzyme (amylo-1,6-glucosidase)*, glycogen can be degraded only up to branch points in the molecule (Sec. 7.21). The decreased production of glucose from the liver leads to hypoglycemia, but this is largely compensated for by increased gluconeogenesis. Marked hepatomegaly and growth failure are common.

Children with *deficiency of the phosphorylase system* manifest hepatomegaly, mild muscular weakness, growth retardation, and mild hypoglycemia (Sec. 7.21). Glycogen is slightly increased in liver (10% compared with normal <5%) and in muscle (1.5% compared with normal <1%). Considerable degradation of glycogen is possible since injection of glucagon may result in an appropriate rise in the level of blood glucose. This "defect" may be inherited as an X-linked trait; all other hepatic enzymatic defects resulting in hypoglycemia are inherited in autosomal recessive fashion. Heterozygous females may manifest enlargement of the liver in childhood. The signs and symptoms of this disorder disappear at puberty.

In the very rare instances of *deficiency of glycogen synthase* (Sec. 7.21), only small amounts of glycogen can be synthesized in the liver. Severe hypoglycemia occurs after an overnight fast.

Hereditary Fructose Intolerance. The ingestion of fructose leads to abnormally elevated blood levels of fructose (fructosemia) in two conditions: *benign fructosemia*, also known as fructosuria, is an asymptomatic disorder resulting from a deficiency of fructokinase; *hereditary fructose intolerance* is a serious disorder of infancy and an easily treated cause of hypoglycemia (Sec. 7.19).

Affected infants do not exhibit symptoms until fructose or sucrose is added to the diet. The infant then becomes anorexic, vomits, and fails to thrive. Hypoglycemic manifestations include drowsiness during feeding, excessive sweating, pallor, rolling of the eyes, twitching, and convulsions. Jaundice and hepatosplenomegaly develop and may be the presenting manifestations. With reduced fructose intake, growth retardation may be predominant rather than the hypoglycemic symptoms seen after acute ingestion. Renal tubular involvement may result in glycosuria, aminoaciduria, proteinuria, and acidosis. A low blood glucose concentration may be masked by elevated levels of fructose unless the measurement is made by a specific enzymatic analysis, such as the glucose oxidase method. If not recognized and treated, the disorder may be fatal. The development of an aversion to fruits and other fructose-containing foods or to sucrose results in the spontaneous amelioration of symptoms and may account for survival into childhood before recognition of the disorder. The hepatomegaly may persist for many years, but liver function returns to normal.

The mechanism of the hypoglycemia is unknown. The accumulation of fructose-1-phosphate may inhibit hepatic enzymes involved in the release of glucose.

Fructose-1,6-Diphosphatase Deficiency. Hypoglycemia, acidosis, and hepatomegaly are the characteristic hallmarks of this disorder (Sec. 7.20); these findings are also typical of

Type I glycogen storage disease (glucose-6-phosphatase deficiency). Fasting hypoglycemia may be severe or moderate and frequently has its onset in the newborn period. Episodes of dyspnea, tachypnea, and hypotonia may occur, and there is progressive hepatomegaly. Increased plasma levels of lactate, pyruvate, free fatty acids, ketones, alanine, and uric acid are present.

Administering glucagon results in a hyperglycemic response in the fed state but not in the fasting state. Glucose, galactose, maltose, and lactose can be utilized, or stored as glycogen and then metabolized since the glycogenolytic pathway is intact. However, with periods of fasting and depletion of glycogen stores, the gluconeogenic precursors, including alanine, lactate, pyruvate, and glycerol, cannot be converted to glucose. In patients with complete enzymatic deficiency, oral administration of fructose, glycerol, or alanine induces profound hypoglycemia. In several patients with partial deficiency of the enzymatic defect, improved tolerance to these precursors appears to have occurred following oral administration of folic acid.

Pyruvate Carboxylase Deficiency. Severe hypoglycemia with lactic acidosis has been reported in a neonate with deficiency of one of the two enzymatic activities of pyruvate carboxylase normally found in liver (Sec. 7.20).

Mild hypoglycemia has been noted in some patients with *Leigh syndrome (subacute necrotizing encephalomyelopathy)* (Sec. 7.20).

Phosphoenolpyruvate Carboxykinase Deficiency. Severe, persistent neonatal hypoglycemia has been reported in association with an absence of the extramitochondrial form of hepatic phosphoenolpyruvate carboxykinase, a key gluconeogenic enzyme. Similarities to other enzymatic defects of gluconeogenesis include lactic acidosis and hepatomegaly with fatty infiltration.

Galactosemia. Hypoglycemia may occur in the presence of weight loss, jaundice, and evidence of hepatocellular dysfunction following milk ingestion. The absence of galactose-1-phosphate uridyl transferase results in diverse toxic effects due to galactose-1-phosphate or galactitol accumulation. (See also Sec. 7.19.) Removal of all galactose from the diet prevents mental retardation, cataracts, and renal and hepatic dysfunction.

Branched Chain Amino Acid Defects. Fasting hypoglycemia in patients with maple syrup urine disease or in propionic acidemia appears to be related to a defect in gluconeogenesis from amino acids (Sec. 7.7). Multiple carboxylase deficiency (holocarboxylase synthetase deficiency) may also be associated with secondary hypoglycemia, which may be responsive to high concentrations of biotin (Sec. 7.7). A related defect involving hydroxymethylglutaryl–coenzyme A lyase has resulted in severe hypoglycemia and organic acidosis in the newborn.

20.9 ENDOCRINE DEFICIENCIES

Cortisol and growth hormone are two of the principal hormones antagonistic to insulin and are necessary to maintain glucose homeostasis. Symptomatic hypoglycemia, especially after fasting, occurs in 10–20% of patients with *isolated deficiency of growth hormone* or with *panhypopituitarism* (Sec. 19.1–19.2). Prolonged and profound hypoglycemia in the neonatal period may be the first clue to severe hypopituitarism. The hypoglycemia may result from an inadequate supply of endogenous gluconeogenic substrates. For example, concentrations of amino acids 2–4 hr after a meal are markedly reduced. The hepatic gluconeogenic enzyme system is normal. When there is deficiency of both ACTH and growth hormone, replacement therapy with both cortisol and growth hormone is necessary to restore carbohydrate metabolism to

normal. "Ketotic" hypoglycemia has been described in patients with isolated deficiency of ACTH or of growth hormone.

Children with failure to thrive or *maternal deprivation syndrome* (Sec. 5.36) may first be seen with an episode of seizure or coma resulting from severe hypoglycemia. Deficiencies of ACTH, growth hormone, or both have been incriminated, but they probably only aggravate the effects of the already deficient gluconeogenic substrates present in these patients.

Fasting hypoglycemia is a frequent concomitant of *Addison disease* (Sec. 19.22) but is an uncommon presenting manifestation. In *congenital virilizing adrenal hyperplasia* (Sec. 19.23), hypoglycemia has rarely been noted. By contrast, hypoglycemia is frequently the presenting manifestation in the newborn with *congenital adrenal hypoplasia* and in children with *familial glucocorticoid insufficiency* (Sec. 19.22). The increased pigmentation that is almost invariably associated with the latter disorder is an important diagnostic clue.

Adrenal medullary unresponsiveness may be the cause of hypoglycemia in some children. The failure to increase levels of epinephrine in response to hypoglycemia is a concomitant of ketotic hypoglycemia.

Glucagon deficiency has occurred in a newborn with severe, persistent neonatal hypoglycemia. Insulin secretion was normal, while glucagon did not rise in response to intravenous alanine. The infant responded remarkably to exogenous glucagon administration. This disorder may be autosomal recessive.

Hypoglycemia associated with hypopituitarism is discussed in Sec. 19.2).

20.10 KETOTIC HYPOGLYCEMIA

Ketotic hypoglycemia is one of the common causes of hypoglycemia in childhood, accounting for more than 50% of cases. With identification of specific metabolic defects, its frequency appears to be on the decline. Onset usually occurs from 18 mo to 5 yr of age with spontaneous remission by 9–10 yr. Boys are affected twice as often as girls, and low birthweight is a common characteristic of affected children.

Clinical Manifestations. The attacks are episodic, most apt to occur in the morning, and frequently associated with ketonuria. Episodes may be related to periods of illness, vomiting, or deprivation of food. Otherwise, affected children are in good health but tend to be small and thin. Hypoglycemic episodes respond promptly to administration of glucose.

Laboratory Findings. Between attacks, carbohydrate tolerance tests give normal results. Hypoglycemia can be precipitated by a prolonged fast (18–24 hr) or by a low calorie, high fat, low carbohydrate (ketogenic) diet. Ketonuria frequently occurs under these conditions, but is not a specific finding since it may occur in normal children during fasting; moreover, unlike adults, about 20% of normal children have blood glucose levels below 40 mg/dL after a 24 hr fast. Children with ketotic hypoglycemia usually do not respond to administration of glucagon with appropriate rises in blood glucose during either spontaneous or induced episodes of hypoglycemia; by contrast, normal children usually have a >10 mg/dL rise in glucose following administration of glucagon after a 24 hr fast. Failure to respond to glucagon reflects depletion of hepatic glycogen, but it may also be noted occasionally in fasted normal children and is not diagnostic. Between hypoglycemic episodes the normal response to glucagon indicates normal hepatic glycogenolysis. During hypoglycemic episodes or during prolonged fasting, levels of insulin are appropriately low for the level of glucose. Insulin levels are normal after overnight fasting or after glucose tolerance tests made between attacks.

Pathogenesis. The precise mechanism of ketotic hypoglycemia is not known. The underlying defect is probably present at birth but does not become manifest until the child is stressed with caloric deprivation. Some believe this entity represents one end of a spectrum of variability, related to the large relative mass of glucose-requiring tissues (e.g., brain) in the young. Physiologic observations are compatible with the hypothesis that persistent oxidation of glucose occurs with an accelerated adaptation to starvation in which there is a failure of gluconeogenesis, in some circumstances due to deficient substrate. Concentrations of plasma alanine may be abnormally low in these children under basal and fasting conditions; infusions of alanine restore the hypoglycemic blood glucose level to normal without altering concentrations of pyruvate or lactate. The cause for the hypoalaninemia in some of these patients is unknown. Patients with deficiency of pituitary or adrenocortical hormones are also deficient in the same substrate; it is not surprising, therefore, that "ketotic" hypoglycemia has been reported in these conditions. Patients with ketotic hypoglycemia may also have increased excretion of the keto derivatives of branched chain amino acids in urine (Sec. 7.7).

Children with an inability to increase their plasma levels of epinephrine (adrenal medullary hyporesponsiveness) when they are subjected to hypoglycemia develop ketotic hypoglycemia. In normal persons during hypoglycemic episodes excretion of epinephrine in the urine and levels in plasma are increased 5- to 20-fold above euglycemic levels. In children with ketotic hypoglycemia, both urinary excretion and rises in plasma levels of epinephrine are deficient when hypoglycemia is induced either by insulin or by a ketogenic diet. The cause for this effect is not known, nor is it settled whether it is specific for ketotic hypoglycemia or a primary or secondary effect. Many affected children also exhibit a subnormal response of endogenous cortisol level to hypoglycemia. Adrenomedullary and adrenocortical hyporesponsiveness are independent of each other, and it has been suggested that the primary defect may be in the hypothalamus or in delayed maturation of adrenal medullary synthesis of epinephrine.

20.11 DRUGS AND TOXINS

Ingestion of ethyl alcohol precipitates hypoglycemia in normal adults after a fast of 2–3 days, but in persons in whom the gluconeogenic reserve is decreased, the hypoglycemic potential of alcohol occurs after only 12 hr or so of fasting. The hypoglycemia is not mediated by an increase in insulin secretion and is not responsive to glucagon administration. This effect results from suppression of hepatic gluconeogenesis and reduction of hepatic glucose output secondary to changes in the oxidoreductive state associated with the metabolism of ethanol.

Young children are unusually susceptible to alcohol and may develop profound, disabling, and even lethal hypoglycemic coma within 1 hr of drinking a leftover cocktail. There are many reports of children developing hypoglycemia following ingestion of alcoholic beverages or substances containing alcohol; in one case hypoglycemia was induced in a 6 mo old febrile infant by sponging with alcohol. Convulsions are common, and deaths have occurred. The prevalence of this cause of hypoglycemia is much greater than the number of reported cases indicates. Immediate intravenous administration of glucose corrects the condition; relapse is uncommon, and continued administration of glucose is rarely necessary. Hypoglycemia has not been found in infants receiving transplacental ethanol from mothers treated for premature labor, presumably because of the immaturity of the alcohol dehydrogenase system in the fetal liver.

Salicylates and related compounds such as acetaminophen may cause hypoglycemia. This effect is not mediated through increased release of insulin; these drugs may interfere with enzyme systems involved in glucose homeostasis in the liver.

Therapy with sulfonylureas during the last trimester of pregnancy has resulted in life-threatening hypoglycemia in newborn infants within hours of birth. Chlorpropamide, acetohexamide, and tolbutamide have all been incriminated. Sulfonylureas cross the placenta and stimulate secretion of insulin from fetal islets. Intravenous glucose may be required continuously for as long as 4 days. Exchange transfusion has also been an effective treatment.

Propranolol, a beta-adrenergic blocking agent, has caused hypoglycemia in children who have been fasted in preparation for surgery or who have been on diminished oral intakes because of illness. In such instances, tachycardia and sweating may not be manifest because of the effect of the drug.

Jamaican vomiting sickness results from ingestion of "bush tea" made from unripe fruits of the ackee, which is grown in Jamaica. This disorder is characterized by severe vomiting, prostration, drowsiness, convulsions, hypoglycemia, and coma, with blood glucose levels as low as 10 mg/dL. The mortality rate is high, death occurring within 24 hr. There are severe hepatic changes including depletion of liver glycogen and fatty degeneration. The agent responsible is the plant toxin hypoglycin A, an unusual amino acid, the chemical structure of which is α-aminomethylenecyclopropylpropionic acid. Hypoglycin A is a specific inhibitor of isovaleryl CoA dehydrogenase and leads to increased concentrations of isovaleric acid with some features of isovaleric acidemia (Sec. 7.7). Accumulation of branched pentanoic acids may account for the fact that some patients with the illness fail to respond even to massive infusions of glucose.

20.12 OTHER CAUSES OF HYPOGLYCEMIA

Functional Hypoglycemia. Adolescents and adults often are diagnosed as having postprandial hypoglycemia based on such symptoms as sweating, palpitations, irritability, dizziness, tremors, shakiness, fatigue, confusion, hunger, and headache. Since the symptoms may be reproduced during an oral glucose tolerance test with blood glucose levels below 50 mg/dL, the diagnosis is not uncommon. However, many normal individuals may have chemical glucose values in this range and remain asymptomatic, while subjects with more normal glucose responses may be clearly symptomatic. The disorder has recently been renamed "the idiopathic postprandial syndrome."

In a recent study of 19 nondiabetic subjects evaluated for glucose tolerance and hormonal responses, there was a strong relationship between plasma epinephrine response (elevation) and the true glucose nadir. The adrenergic signs and symptoms were thought to be caused by excessive release of catecholamines; however, since they may precede documentation of changes in plasma epinephrine levels, relative neuroglycopenia has been suggested to explain the symptoms.

At present, distribution of meals and avoidance of excessive calories at a single meal appears to be appropriate therapy. Pharmacologic agents are not indicated to suppress the catecholamine responses.

Hepatic Damage. Severe hepatic damage may disturb the metabolism of carbohydrates sufficiently to produce hypoglycemia. Hepatotoxic agents such as phosphorus, halogenated hydrocarbons (carbon tetrachloride), and hydrazine may be responsible for hypoglycemia. Extensive infiltration of the liver by neoplastic cells, fibrous tissue, granulomas, or fat may also lead to hypoglycemia, as may acute and chronic infectious hepatitis in the terminal stages. The mechanisms are not completely understood, but the hypoglycemia probably results from failure to store glycogen, impaired release of glucose into the blood stream, and decreased net synthesis of glucose from amino acids.

Reye syndrome is characterized by encephalopathy and fatty degeneration of the viscera; blood glucose levels below 25–30 mg/dL are common in younger children. Serum insulin levels are normal, and blood glucose levels are not increased by administration of glucagon. The hypoglycemia appears to be secondary to decreased hepatic glucose production; it is easily managed by infusion of glucose, but such treatment appears to have little influence on the outcome (Sec. 12.82).

On rare occasions hypoglycemia occurs in patients with *leukemia*. The cause is unknown; reduced levels of glucose-6-phosphatase in the liver infiltrated by leukemia may play a role.

Impaired Intestinal Absorption of Glucose. Unlike most adults, children and especially infants may exhibit low blood glucose levels when carbohydrate is withheld for 24–48 hr. Fasting is rarely, however, by itself a cause of clinical hypoglycemia; it may be a precipitating factor when other defects that may cause hypoglycemia are present, such as impaired intestinal absorption accompanying chronic diarrhea, celiac disease, or the edematous phase of the nephrotic syndrome. Several specific defects in the intestinal absorption of sugars (Sec. 12.49), such as of glucose and galactose, of sucrose and isomaltose, and of lactose, are characterized by diarrhea, but they do not lead to significant hypoglycemia. Delayed absorption of glucose occurs in hypothyroidism, but this rarely leads to hypoglycemia.

Renal Glycosuria. Glycosuria due to defective tubular reabsorption of glucose occurs in a variety of clinical entities: as an isolated hereditary condition, in combination with glycinuria, in the de Toni–Fanconi syndrome, and in some patients with lead poisoning. It is rare that any of these conditions leads to hypoglycemia.

Other. Mild hypoglycemia is a complication of *kwashiorkor*, in which it may be secondary to impaired gluconeogenesis.

Hypoglycemia has occurred in *phenylketonuric* children when dietary restriction of phenylalanine has been too severe during the course of treatment. In these instances general malnutrition is probably the principal factor causing the hypoglycemia.

Hypoglycemia has been observed repeatedly in association with some *extrapancreatic tumors.* The tumors are usually large mesodermal neoplasms (sarcomas) arising in the abdominal or thoracic cavity. The phenomenon has also been observed in children with Wilms tumor and infants with congenital neuroblastoma. Hypoglycemia due to tumor is probably underdiagnosed since fasting blood glucose levels are not determined routinely in children with tumors; its mechanism is unsettled.

Though the residuum of instances in which no cause for hypoglycemia can be established has decreased markedly in recent years, new pathogenetic causes continue to be discovered. A defect in glycerol metabolism has been found to account for hypoglycemia and ketonuria in a young child. Systemic carnitine deficiency may be associated with severe hypoglycemia (Sec. 7.20). Other reports of unique and bizarre symptom complexes with hypoglycemia suggest that much remains to be learned concerning glucose homeostasis.

20.13 CLINICAL MANIFESTATIONS OF HYPOGLYCEMIA

There is no constant relationship between blood glucose levels and the development or severity of symptoms of hypoglycemia in different patients or even in the same patient at different times. The rate of fall of blood glucose is important; a rapid fall is especially likely to produce symptoms. Even at extremely low blood levels of glucose, children manifest great variability in their responses. Some become conditioned to repeated hypoglycemic episodes or to hypoglycemia of long duration so that they have few or no symptoms, especially children with type I glycogenosis (von Gierke disease).

The symptoms of hypoglycemia are derived chiefly from disturbances of the central nervous system. Neural tissue has little stored carbohydrate and, unlike other tissues, cannot utilize sugars other than glucose; it is therefore dependent upon a continuous and adequate supply of blood glucose to maintain its normal functions. There is evidence that neural tissue can utilize ketones or amino acid as sources of energy; this is thought to occur in children with prolonged hypoglycemia who are asymptomatic.

Hypoglycemic symptoms are protean but often produce more or less characteristic patterns in individual patients. Sweating, pallor, fatigue, hunger, tachycardia, and nervousness occur as a result of excessive secretion of epinephrine in response to the hypoglycemia. Central nervous system dysfunction is manifested by headache, irritability, negativism, alterations in behavior, drowsiness, mental confusion, psychotic behavior, seizures, and coma.

In newborn and young infants recognition and evaluation of symptoms may be difficult. Convulsions are often the first recognized manifestation, but irritability, poor feeding, lethargy, excessive drowsiness, eye-rolling, sweating, and twitching are more common symptoms. Even with very low glucose levels, hypoglycemic symptoms may be absent in the neonate. Young infants with hypoglycemia may manifest cardiomegaly and even heart failure, which remit promptly with elevation of the blood level of glucose.

20.14 DIAGNOSIS OF HYPOGLYCEMIA

The diagnosis of hypoglycemia involves two distinct problems: (1) the detection of hypoglycemia and (2) the determination of its cause. Many children in whom clinical manifestations on one or more occasions suggest hypoglycemia can be demonstrated to be hypoglycemic only under specific conditions. In others, hypoglycemia is readily demonstrated by blood glucose determinations. Once hypoglycemia is established, it is essential to determine the cause. There is no routine approach for the study of patients with manifestations of hypoglycemia; individualization in the choice of diagnostic procedures is essential.

The information obtained from the history and physical examination should be thoroughly evaluated before exhaustive tests of carbohydrate function are undertaken. Since many causes of hypoglycemia are genetically determined, a family history of other affected persons or of consanguinity may be pertinent. The initial episode of hypoglycemia caused by ingestion of alcohol or other toxins can usually be identified by the history. The infant with galactosemia usually has other clinical manifestations to suggest the diagnosis before hypoglycemia is suspected. A history of aversion to fruits and sweets and the occurrence of gastrointestinal manifestations, as well as those of hypoglycemia, following ingestion of foods containing fructose should suggest hereditary fructose intolerance. Aggravation of hypoglycemic symptoms by meals rich in protein suggests leucine sensitivity and hyperinsulinism.

Hepatomegaly should suggest hepatic causes of hypoglycemia. Growth failure directs attention to pituitary hypofunction, whereas manifestations of Addison disease lead to consideration of adrenal hypofunction. The association of large tumors in the thoracic or abdominal cavity with hypoglycemia should suggest appropriate studies. The presence of acidosis points to a deficiency of one of the hepatic enzymes.

Hypoglycemic episodes that follow periods of undereating or of vomiting and that have their onset after 1–2 yr of age are suggestive of ketotic hypoglycemia. Once the acute episode is over, all the usual tolerance tests are normal and it generally requires a period of prolonged fasting (18–24 hr) to provoke hypoglycemia.

One of the most difficult differentials is to distinguish the child with a functioning islet cell tumor. Levels of insulin in other conditions may not be clearly elevated. In the presence of abnormally low glucose levels, however, plasma insulin should normally be suppressed; levels as low as 7–15 μU/mL associated with very low levels of plasma beta-hydroxybutyrate, therefore, may indicate hyperinsulinism. The leucine and tolbutamide tests are useful for detecting states of insulin hypersecretion, and once this is established, trial therapy with diazoxide may be useful for treatment as well as diagnosis. Most patients with functioning beta cell tumors will not respond to diazoxide, and laparotomy is then usually necessary to establish the diagnosis. Somatostatin infusion should suppress insulin, glucagon, and growth hormone secretion. It may be beneficial acutely and during surgery.

Laboratory Data. The most important period of observation is the time of a spontaneous hypoglycemic episode. Ideally, blood should be obtained then to test for plasma glucose, beta-hydroxybutyrate, and specific amino acids as well as for hormones (insulin, glucagon, and growth hormone). An aliquot of plasma should be frozen for additional studies to be determined by the patient's future course. If a defect in amino acid metabolism is suspected, analyses of plasma and urine for amino acids and other organic acids are indicated. Examination of the initial urine for substrates and catecholamines may also be important. However, tests evaluating carbohydrate metabolism (Table 20–8) are usually performed after an overnight fast except in young infants, for whom a 6 hr period is adequate. Occasionally, shorter periods of fasting are indicated if the hypoglycemia is severe. When the expected response to a given test is a lowering of the blood glucose level, the fasting glucose level should be 50 mg/dL or higher to permit a sufficient differential in glucose levels for comparative purposes. The patient should be in a reasonably good nutritional state and free of fever when a test is performed.

Appropriate analytic methods should be used to determine the concentration of glucose. Glucose is measured specifically when glucose oxidase or certain other enzymatic methods are used, whereas methods depending upon reduction are not specific for glucose. Values for serum or plasma levels of glucose are approximately 15% higher than those obtained when whole blood is utilized.

A number of tests are used to study the patient with hypoglycemia. Some are of little value and others of importance only to delineate specific disorders. The appropriate use of these tests is based on a knowledge of carbohydrate metabolism and the purposes for which the tests were designed. Precise diagnosis of some hypoglycemic conditions requires measuring lactate, ketones, growth hormone, or cortisol or assay of specific enzyme activities.

Levels of insulin should be measured in all hypoglycemic patients. The fasting level is rarely above 10 μU/mL. A level above 10 μU/mL in plasma with a blood glucose under 50 mg/dL is abnormal and suggests hyperinsulinism.

The *glucagon tolerance test* is useful to study the ability of the liver to release glucose into the circulation from stored glycogen. (The *epinephrine tolerance test* has been replaced by the safer glucagon test.) Normally, a rise of blood glucose of 25–50 mg/dL should occur within 15–45 minutes. Failure of an adequate response may be due to depletion of liver glycogen by starvation or hepatic disease. It may be necessary to test the patient in both the fed and fasting state. For example, in glucose-6-phosphatase deficiency there is no rise in glucose level following administration of glucagon in either the fasting or fed state, whereas in debrancher deficiency the response is normal postprandially but not after fasting. Children with ketotic hypoglycemia exhibit an inadequate response to glucagon during the hypoglycemic episode or after a 24 hr fast but respond normally between attacks.

The *galactose tolerance test* should not be used for the diagnosis of galactosemia since it may be toxic to the nervous system and may induce severe hypoglycemia; direct assay of uridyl transferase activity is the appropriate diagnostic method. Infusion of galactose provokes a rise in the level of lactate in patients with glucose-6-phosphatase deficiency but not with other conditions.

The *fructose tolerance test* is primarily of use in the detection of hereditary fructose intolerance and of fructose-1,6-diphosphatase deficiency. Administration of fructose to patients results in a decrease of blood glucose to hypoglycemic levels and a rise in the level of blood fructose. In addition, the level of serum inorganic phosphorus is decreased, the concentration of lactic acid is increased, and the insulin level remains

Table 20–8. Tolerance Tests for the Evaluation of Carbohydrate Metabolism

Compound	Route		Time to Obtain Samples (Minutes)	Critical Measurements
L-Alanine	Oral	500 mg/kg	0,30,60,90	Glucose and lactate
	IV	250 mg/kg (as 10% solution in sterile pyrogen-free water)	0,10,20,30,45,60,90	
Glucose	Oral	1.75 g/kg	0,30,60,90,120, 180,240,300	Glucose and insulin
	IV	0.5 g/kg (as 10 to 20% solution over 4 min period)	0,5,10,20,30,40, 50,60	
Galactose	Oral	1.75 g/kg	0,30,60,90,120	Glucose and lactate
Glycerol	Oral	1 g/kg	0,10,20,30,45,60,90,120	Glucose and lactate
Fructose	IV	0.25 g/kg (as 10% solution over 4 min period)	0,10,20,30,45,60,90,120	Glucose, phosphate, lactate, and uric acid
L-Leucine	Oral	150 mg/kg (as 2% solution or slurry)	0,15,30,45,60,90,120	Glucose and insulin
	IV	75 mg/kg (as 2% solution in 0.45% NaCl)	0,10,20,30,45,60,90	
Glucagon	IM	30 μg/kg (1 mg maximum)	0,15,30,45,60,90,120	Glucose and lactate
Tolbutamide	IV	20 mg/kg (1 g maximum) (over 1 min period)	0,5,10,20,30,45, 60,90,120	Glucose and insulin

IV = intravenous; IM = intramuscular.

unchanged. For this test the blood glucose level must be measured by the glucose oxidase method, since the total concentration of reducing sugar remains relatively constant.

The *leucine tolerance test* is used to determine whether this amino acid provokes an exaggerated release of insulin. It is helpful in unmasking hypersecretory states. Normal children exhibit a small but significant rise in concentration of blood insulin and a decrease of approximately 10 mg/dL in concentration of glucose. In some pathologic states a marked rise in level of insulin is accompanied by a profound fall in level of glucose, as in leucine-sensitive hypoglycemia. In other conditions, such as obesity, a marked rise in the level of insulin is associated with only a normal decline in blood glucose concentration.

The *tolbutamide tolerance test* measures the ability of the pancreas to release insulin as determined by the degree and duration of the hypoglycemic response. In normal children the blood glucose level falls about 20–40% within 20–30 min and returns to normal within 60–90 min. In hypoglycemic patients there is an exaggerated response in the increase of insulin level and in the decrease of glucose level. The increase in insulin level is quite rapid and can be easily missed if blood levels are not obtained early. Infants with hyperinsulinism of any etiology may exhibit a profound and prolonged response to tolbutamide.

The *alanine tolerance test* is useful for evaluating gluconeogenesis. In normal individuals who have been suitably fasted and whose hepatic glycogen stores are depleted, administering L-alanine results in an increase in blood levels of glucose. Patients with deficiency of fructose-1,6-diphosphatase do not exhibit a rise in blood glucose; instead, the already elevated level of lactate is increased further.

The *glycerol tolerance test* may be utilized for the same purpose as alanine.

The *rate of glucose infusion to sustain normoglycemia* is important, diagnostically and therapeutically. Rates exceeding 15 mg/kg/min occur in neonatal persistent hypoglycemia.

20.15 TREATMENT OF HYPOGLYCEMIA

During a hypoglycemic attack the child should never be left unattended. The immediate symptoms may be relieved by the administration of glucose, but hypoglycemia of either the organic or functional type may be only temporarily abated by administering glucose and may rebound to hypoglycemic levels as the release of additional insulin is evoked. In such situations frequent feedings of small amounts of carbohydrates are advisable until the patient is stabilized. Infants of diabetic mothers and those with erythroblastosis fetalis ordinarily respond satisfactorily, as do the majority of children with hyperinsulinism. When the cause of hypoglycemia is established, treatment should be related to it.

For some conditions glucagon (1 mg intramuscularly) is usually effective in terminating a hypoglycemic episode. This form of therapy is a useful emergency measure which parents can be trained to use at home. It is *not* effective in the glycogenoses, in other hepatic disease, or in ketotic hypoglycemia. Even when it is effective, it should be followed by the oral administration of sugar in some readily absorbable form acceptable to the child.

Patients with ketotic hypoglycemia respond well to a program of frequent feedings (4–5 meals a day) of a diet high in protein and carbohydrate. During periods of illness and fasting, high carbohydrate liquids should be offered at frequent intervals. Patients with deficiencies of specific hepatic enzymes may require special dietary management to remove offending foodstuffs. Children with pituitary or adrenocortical insufficiency require replacement therapy with the appropriate hormones.

The most difficult patients to manage have been some of those with hyperinsulinism. Diazoxide, a nondiuretic benzothiodiazine, has proved to be an effective agent in controlling hypoglycemia in some of these patients. The drug acts primarily by suppressing insulin release. The usual dose is 10 mg/kg/24 hr (range 5–20 mg/kg/24 hr) given orally in 2 divided doses. The most common side effect is hypertrichosis, particularly of the back, extremities, and face. Once the drug is discontinued, the hypertrichosis disappears. Failure to respond suggests a functioning adenoma or adenomatosis, though there have been occasional patients with proven adenomas who have responded quite satisfactorily to diazoxide. On the other hand, some patients with beta cell hyperplasia or nesidioblastosis have failed to respond. Patients who fail to respond to treatment with diazoxide should be explored for an adenoma. If none is found, a subtotal or near total pancreatectomy will often be helpful in reducing the frequency and severity of hypoglycemic attacks. If hypoglycemia recurs after pancreatectomy, another course of diazoxide is indicated, since the drug may then be effective. The occasional refractory patient may require corticosteroids, repeated attempts at surgical control, or even streptozotocin, a potent diabetogenic antibiotic used primarily to treat carcinoma of the pancreatic islet cells.

A significant number of patients with hyperinsulinism exhibit spontaneous remissions. The hypoglycemic episodes become less frequent and fasting glucose levels gradually rise. Diazoxide may be discontinued and the patient remains asymptomatic. Some such patients still exhibit leucine sensitivity. Patients with ketotic hypoglycemia characteristically experience remission by 10 yr of age.

Brain damage is a frequent concomitant of hypoglycemia. The earlier in life the onset and the more protracted and profound its course, the more likely is brain damage a sequel. It is usually manifested by mental retardation, learning and behavior problems, ataxia, and/or seizures. The electroencephalogram is usually abnormal during hypoglycemic episodes and may remain abnormal between seizures. Even after hypoglycemia is in remission, abnormal EEG tracings and seizures may persist; such normoglycemic seizures require treatment with anticonvulsant agents. Psychologic guidance of the hypoglycemic child and his or her family is of paramount importance.

ROBERT SCHWARTZ

Ampola MG: Metabolic Diseases in Pediatric Practice. Boston, Little, Brown, 1982.

Aynsley-Green A, Polak JM, Bloom SR, et al: Nesidioblastosis of the pancreas: Definition of the syndrome and management of the severe neonatal hyperinsulinemic hypoglycemia. Arch Dis Child 56:496, 1981.

Baker L, Kaye R, Root AW, et al: Diazoxide treatment of idiopathic hypoglycemia of infancy. J Pediatr 71:494, 1967.

Balsam MJ, Baker L, Bishop HC, et al: Beta cell adenoma in a child with hypoglycemia controlled with diazoxide. J Pediatr 80:788, 1972.

Bishop AE, Polak JM, Chesa PG, et al: Decrease of pancreatic somatostatin in neonatal nesidioblastosis. Diabetes 30:122, 1981.

Bord C, Ravazzola M, Pollack A, et al: Neonatal islet cell adenoma: A distinct type of islet cell tumor? Diabetes Care 5:122, 1982.

Chalew SA, McLaughlin JV, Mersey JH, et al: The use of the plasma epinephrine response in the diagnosis of idiopathic postprandial syndrome. JAMA 251:612, 1984.

Chaussain JL: Glycemic response to 24 hour fast in normal children and children with ketotic hypoglycemia. J Pediatr 82:438, 1973.

Christensen NJ: Hypoadrenalinemia during insulin hypoglycemia in children with ketotic hypoglycemia. J Clin Endocrinol Metab 38:107, 1974.

Colle E, Ulstrom RA: Ketotic hypoglycemia. J Pediatr 64:632, 1964.

Collipp PJ: Hypoglycemia and leukemia. Pediatrics 46:788, 1970.

Dahlquist G, Genta J, Hagenfeldt L, et al: Ketotic hypoglycemia in childhood. A clinical trial of several unifying etiological hypotheses. Acta Pediatr Scand 68:649, 1979.

Dahms BB, Landing BH, Blaskovics M, et al: Nesidioblastosis and other islet cell abnormalities in hyperinsulinemic hypoglycemia of childhood. Human Pathol 11:641, 1980.

DiGeorge AM, Auerbach VH, Mabry CC: Leucine-induced hypoglycemia. III. The blood glucose depressant action of leucine in normal individuals. J Pediatr 63:295, 1963.

Ehrlich RM, Martin JM: Tolbutamide tolerance test and plasma-insulin response in children with idiopathic hypoglycemia. J Pediatr 71:485, 1967.

Falorni A, Fracassini F, Mass-Benedetti F, et al: Glucose metabolism, plasma insulin, and growth hormone secretion in newborn infants with erythroblastosis fetalis compared with normal newborns and those born to diabetic mothers. Pediatrics 49:682, 1972.

Fernandes J, Berger R, Smit GPA: Lactate as a cerebral metabolic fuel for glucose-6-phosphatase deficient children. Pediatr Res 18:335, 1984.

Goodall McC, Cragan M, Sidbury J: Decreased epinephrine excretion in idiopathic hypoglycemia. Am J Dis Child 123:569, 1972.

Gould VE, Memoli VA, Dardi LE, et al: Nesidiodysplasia and nesidioblastosis in infancy. Pediatr Pathol 1:7, 1983.

Gruppuso PA, DeLuca F, O'Shea PA, et al: Near-total pancreatectomy for hyperinsulinism. Spontaneous remission of resultant diabetes. Acta Paediatr Scand 74:311, 1985.

Hirsch JH, Loo S, Evans N, et al: Hypoglycemia of infancy and nesidioblastosis. N Engl J Med 296:1323, 1977.

Honicky RE, dePapp EW: Mediastinal teratoma with endocrine function. Am J Dis Child 126:650, 1973.

Hopwood NJ, Forsman PJ, Kenny FM, et al: Hypoglycemia in hypopituitary children. Am J Dis Child 129:918, 1975.

Jaffe R, Hashida Y, Yunis EJ: The endocrine pancreas of the neonate and infant. Perspect Pediatr Pathol 7:137, 1982.

Johnson JD, Hansen RC, Albritton WL, et al: Hypoplasia of the anterior pituitary and neonatal hypoglycemia. J Pediatr 82:634, 1973.

Kerr DS, Stevens MCG, Picon DIM: Estimation of Fasting Glucose Flux in Malnourished and Hypoglycemic Children by Constant Infusion of U-13$_c$ Glucose. Argonne, Ill., Second International Conference on Stable Isotopes, October, 1975.

Kirkland J, Ben-Menachem Y, Akhtar M, et al: Islet cell tumor in a neonate. Diagnosis by selective angiography and histologic findings. Pediatrics 61:790, 1978.

Koffler H, Schubert WK, Hug G: Sporadic hypoglycemia: Abnormal epinephrine response to the ketogenic diet or to insulin. J Pediatr 78:448, 1971.

Kramer JL, Bell MJ, DeSchryver K, et al: Clinical and histological indications for extensive pancreatic resection in nesidioblastosis. Am J Surg 143:116, 1982.

Landau H, Perlman M, Meyer S, et al: Persistent neonatal hypoglycemia due to hyperinsulinism: Medical aspects. Pediatrics 70:440, 1982.

Loridan L, Sadeghi-Nejad A, Senior B: Hypersecretion of insulin after the administration of L-leucine to obese children. J Pediatr 78:53, 1971.

Loutfi AH, Mehrez I, Shahbender S, et al: Hypoglycaemia with Wilms' tumour. Arch Dis Child 39:197, 1964.

McBride JT, McBride MC, Viles PH: Hypoglycemia associated with propranolol. Pediatrics 51:1085, 1973.

Mock DM, Perman JA, Thaler MM, et al: Chronic fructose intoxication after infancy in children with hereditary fructose intolerance. N Engl J Med 309:764, 1983.

Narisawa K, Otomo H, Igarashi Y, et al: Glycogen storage disease type 1b: Microsomal glucose-6-phosphatase system in two patients with different clinical findings. Pediatr Res 17:545, 1983.

Pagliara AS, Karl IE, Haymond M, et al: Hypoglycemia in infants and childhood. J Pediatr 82:365, 1973.

Roe TF, Kogut MD: Idiopathic leucine-sensitive hypoglycemia syndrome: Insulin and glucagon responses and effects of diazoxide. Pediatr Res 16:1, 1982.

Schutgens RBH, Heymans H, Ketel A, et al: Lethal hypoglycemia in a child with a deficiency of 3-hydroxy-3-methylglutaryl-coenzyme A lyase. J Pediatr 94:89, 1979.

Schutt-Aine JC, Drash AL, Kenny FM: Possible relationship between spontaneous hypoglycemia and "maternal deprivation syndrome." J Pediatr 82:809, 1973.

Schwartz JF, Zwiren GT: Islet cell adenomatosis and adenoma in an infant. J Pediatr 79:232, 1971.

Schwartz SS, Rich BH, Lucky AW, et al: Familial nesidioblastosis: Severe neonatal hypoglycemia in two families. J Pediatr 95:44, 1979.

Seltzer HS: Drug-induced hypoglycemia. A review based on 473 cases. Diabetes 21:955, 1972.

Shapiro M, Sincha A, Rosenmann E, et al: Hypoglycemia associated with neonatal neuroblastoma and abnormal responses of serum glucose and free fatty acids to epinephrine injection. Israel J Med Sci 2:705, 1966.

Stanley CA, Baker L: Hyperinsulinism in infancy: Diagnosis by demonstration of abnormal response to fasting hypoglycemia. Pediatrics 57:702, 1976.

Tietze HU, Zurbrugg RP, Zuppinger KA, et al: Occurrence of impaired cortisol regulation in children with hypoglycemia associated with adrenal medullary hyporesponsiveness. J Clin Endocrinol Metab 34:948, 1972.

Van Obberghen-Schilling EE, Rechler MM, Romanus JA, et al: Receptors for insulin-like growth factor I are defective in fibroblasts cultured from a patient with leprechaunism. J Clin Invest 68:1356, 1981.

Vidnes J, Oyasaeter S: Glucagon deficiency causing severe neonatal hypoglycemia in a patient with normal insulin secretion. Pediatr Res 11:943, 1977.

Wapnir RA, Lifshitz F, Sekaran C, et al: Glycerol-induced hypoglycemia: A syndrome associated with multiple liver enzyme deficiencies. Clinical and in vitro studies. Metabolism 31:1057, 1982.

Ware AJ, Burton WC, McGarry JD, et al: Systemic carnitine deficiency. J Pediatr 93:959, 1978.

Yakovac WC, Baker L, Hummeler K: Beta cell nesidioblastosis in idiopathic hypoglycemia of infancy. J Pediatr 79:226, 1971.

21

THE NERVOUS SYSTEM

EVALUATION OF THE CHILD WITH NEUROLOGIC DISEASE

21.1 HISTORY—THE SYMPTOMATOLOGY OF NEUROLOGIC DISORDERS

The neurologic evaluation should include a thorough pediatric history, with special attention to the evolution of the illness, which may provide important clues regarding the category of neurologic disorder. A static disability dating from early infancy suggests a congenital malformation or a lesion acquired in the perinatal period, but even in static brain lesions new symptoms emerge as the brain matures since the expression of a disorder of a particular function cannot become apparent until the age at which that function normally appears. Steady progression of disability with loss of previously acquired functions is seen in degenerative brain diseases, and in chronic encephalitis, uncompensated hydrocephalus, and brain tumors. Arrest of development generally precedes loss of function in progressive brain disease in infancy. Sudden disability followed by gradual improvement is characteristic of cerebral vascular diseases. Episodes of exacerbation followed by partial remission are seen most commonly in the demyelinating diseases. Histories of deterioration in school performance, loss of interest, irritability, and emotional lability are common in children with cerebral dysfunction.

Unsteadiness of gait, limping, stumbling, clumsiness, floppiness, tightness of muscles, and loss of skill in handwriting are all symptoms of motor dysfunction, but the history should never be relied upon for localization of motor disorders. This is accomplished only by neurologic examination.

Because children rarely complain of sensory deficits, these often go unnoticed until they are quite severe. Absence of visual following, random searching eye movements, and a tendency to look directly at bright lights without evidence of discomfort suggest severe visual defects in the infant. In the older child loss of visual acuity manifests itself by a tendency to walk into objects and to hold objects close to the eyes for inspection. Unilateral visual loss is usually asymptomatic even in the school-age child until formal testing of vision is carried out. A lack of response to sounds suggests severe hearing loss in the young child but is easily confused with the inattention of the retarded or autistic child. Partial hearing loss may express itself only as absence of speech or delay in its development, which may also be the presenting complaints in retardation or autism. Repeated injuries of which the child fails to complain suggest loss of pain sensation.

The history is especially important in the diagnosis of paroxysmal disorders of the nervous system, such as seizures, syncope, and paroxysmal vertigo. When such attacks occur at infrequent intervals, decisions regarding diagnostic studies or therapy may have to depend on historical data alone. The events that precede an attack may provide clues. Anxiety, excitement, pain, or crying may commonly precede syncopal attacks but only rarely do they precede seizures. Exposure to unusual sensory stimuli such as flickering lights (e.g., television) may precipitate seizures. The older child who has seizures may describe a warning sensation or aura. The state

of the patient during an attack should be ascertained as completely as possible. Was he or she unconscious, in a state of confusion, or lucid? Were there convulsive movements? If so, were they lateralized? Was there incontinence of urine or feces? Was recovery rapid, or was there a period of sleep or drowsiness? In infancy and early childhood manifestations of seizures may be so slight as not to be mentioned by parents unless specific inquiry is made. This is especially true of infantile myoclonic seizures; the momentary flexion of head, trunk, and arm is often dismissed as a normal startle response or as colic.

Vertigo, the sensation that the environment is turning or tilting, is easily misinterpreted in the young child who is unable to describe this sensation. The outward manifestations of an attack include unsteadiness, vomiting, fright, and unwillingness to move the head, which may be kept rigidly in one position. The child with vertigo remains lucid throughout the attack, in contrast to the child with epilepsy.

The correct diagnosis of headache is largely dependent on a careful history, which should ascertain time of occurrence of head pain, localization, quality (throbbing, dull, sharp, pressing, or band-like), and associated symptoms such as nausea, vomiting, or visual disturbance. Headache that occurs principally after the child arises from bed and is associated with vomiting and drowsiness should suggest the possibility of increased intracranial pressure.

21.2 THE NEUROLOGIC EXAMINATION

A careful neurologic examination is essential for the correct localization of neurologic illness; it is a challenging task in the potentially uncooperative young child. The confidence of the child is secured by being gentle and informal and by making the procedure interesting to the patient. Uncomfortable tests, such as the funduscopic examination and sensory testing, should be postponed to the last portion of the examination. Much can be learned by observing the child playing, walking, or running. A portion of the examination can be carried out with the child sitting comfortably and securely on the mother's lap. Examination of the newborn infant, the child with psychiatric disorder, and the comatose patient presents special problems. The usual neurologic examination should record the following observations.

Assessment of the Child's Mental Status and Behavior

Aspects of behavior that provide important clues are the child's ability to relate to others, level of activity, distractibility, attention span, mood, ability and/or willingness to cooperate with the examination, and appropriateness of responses to various situations.

Speech functions are divided into expressive speech (talking) and receptive speech (understanding). Their evaluation is discussed in Sec. 2.68. Isolated disorders of central speech mechanisms are referred to as *aphasias*. Several types of aphasia can be distinguished. In *expressive (Broca) aphasia* the patient is unable to speak, or speech is sparse and labored in telegraphic style. Understanding of verbal commands is preserved. In *receptive (Wernicke) aphasia* there is loss of comprehension of speech. The patient speaks fluently but with little content and may use empty words such as "that thing," circumlocutions, or made-up words (neologisms). The ability to repeat verbatim is impaired in both types of aphasia. In *global asphasia* both receptive and expressive speech are affected. Aphasia usually implies a lesion in the dominant temporal lobe; in children under the age of 8 yr it is always transient following unilateral temporal lobe lesions, owing to the plasticity of the child's brain, which permits the opposite hemisphere to assume speech functions. Aphasia must be distinguished from speech disorders secondary to hearing loss and from dysarthria, a speech defect resulting from dysfunction of muscles of articulation.

Ability to read is tested by use of graded reading paragraphs. An isolated inability to read in a child of otherwise normal intellectual functions is referred to as *dyslexia*. The neurologic examination should include an assessment of writing, drawing, and copying of shapes. The drawing of a person, for example, tests the ability to control a pencil, to produce recognizable shapes, and to arrange shapes in space in proper proportions. As a rough approximation, a 4 yr old child should be able to draw a figure with four recognizable parts, a 5 yr old with eight recognizable features. Ability to draw shapes can also be tested by having the child copy geometric figures (Sec. 2.61–2.66). In a child with otherwise normal motor functions and with good ability to recognize shapes, inability to draw objects is referred to as *apraxia*. This type of defect is associated with lesions of a parietal lobe. It also occurs as a transient maturational lag in early school aged children with learning disabilities.

Handedness should be noted. Normally, clear preference for one hand in writing, eating, and reaching is established by the age of 3 yr. Delayed development of handedness is found in children with mental slowness and learning disorders. Right-handed children have left cerebral dominance for speech, but the dominant hemisphere cannot be predicted for left-handed children, more than 50% of whom also have speech localization in the left hemisphere. Memory can be tested by giving the child a list of four or five object words to be recalled 5 min later. Testing of arithmetic ability such as counting, addition, and subtraction is helpful in the assessment of children with possible mental slowness, in whom the understanding of abstract mathematical concepts tends to be especially poor. Formal psychologic testing is often helpful.

Motor Examination

The motor examination requires an understanding of the organization of the motor system (Fig. 21–1). Voluntary movements depend on intact neural pathways, including at least two motor neurons, upper and lower. The axons of the upper motor neurons, whose cells of origin are in the motor cortex, form the *pyramidal tract*, which passes via the internal capsule and brain stem to the spinal cord. The pyramidal tract fibers cross to the opposite side in the lower medulla and synapse on anterior horn cells in the spinal cord. The anterior horn cells (lower motor neurons) send their axons via peripheral nerves to muscle. Each lower motor neuron innervates a group of muscle fibers, up to several hundred in some of the large muscles of the extremities. A lower motor neuron and the group of muscle fibers it innervates are a *motor unit*. The basic motor pathway (Fig. 21–1) is influenced by a number of other centers, which as a group are known as the *extrapyramidal motor system*. These include the basal ganglia and the cerebellum. The functions of the extrapyramidal motor system include control of repetitive motor acts and the coordination of movements. In general, lesions of the upper motor neuron or of the extrapyramidal motor system interfere with volun-

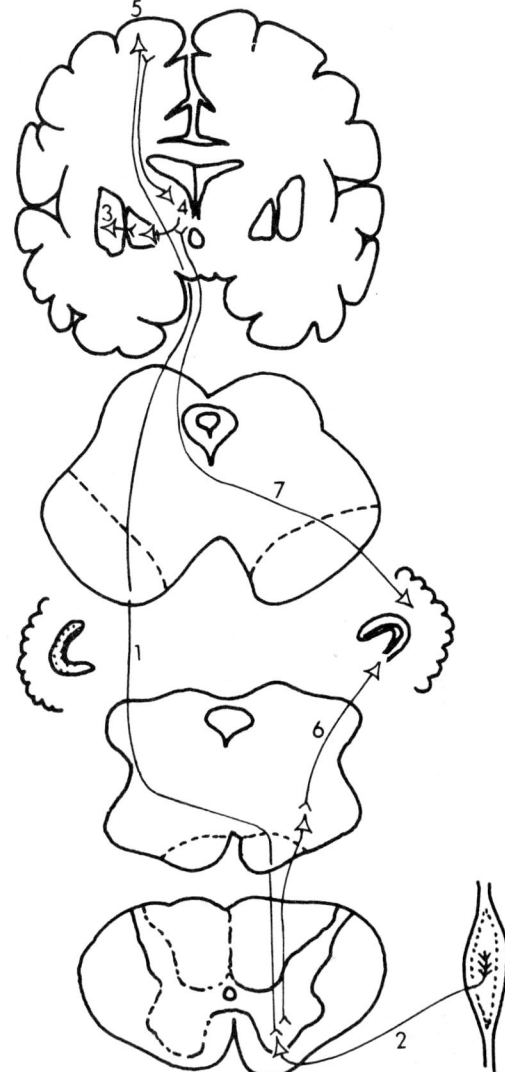

Figure 21–1. Schematic representation of the more important motor pathways. 1, Upper motor neuron. 2, Lower motor neuron. 3, Basal ganglia, which send efferent fibers to the thalamus (4), which in turn influences the motor cortex (5). 6, Descending fibers from cerebellum influencing motor neuron activity in spinal cord. 7, Ascending fibers from cerebellum, which act on motor cortex via the thalamus.

tary motor activities without interrupting involuntary and reflex motor functions. In many instances such lesions result in enhancement of involuntary and reflex motor activity through release from central inhibitory influences. Lesions of the lower motor neuron lead to loss of both voluntary and involuntary motor activities. In addition, the denervation of muscle leads to atrophy and to spontaneous activity (*fibrillation*) of individual muscle fibers. Fibrillations are visible only in the tongue, where they appear as worm-like movements. Coarse, irregular twitches, due to simultaneous contraction of entire motor units (*fasciculations*), are seen primarily in diseases involving the anterior horn cells.

It is usually possible to localize a motor lesion in upper or lower motor neurons or in the extrapyramidal motor system by the following simple clinical tests:

Assessment of Muscle Strength. Strength is tested informally in the younger child. Ability to stand up from the supine position tests back, hip, and proximal leg muscles. Having the child walk on tiptoes and on heels tests the gastrocnemius-soleus and the tibialis anterior, respectively. Shoulder muscles are tested by supporting and/or lifting the child with the examiner's hands in the child's axillae. Intercostal muscles can be assessed by observing spontaneous respirations and by asking the child to blow out a match. In the older child strength is tested separately in individual muscle groups and is graded on a 0–5 scale as follows:

0 = no movement
1 = movement with gravity eliminated
2 = full range against gravity
3 = movement against slight resistance
4 = movement against moderate resistance
5 = normal strength

Muscular weakness occurs with lesions of upper or lower motor neurons but is usually absent in extrapyramidal disorders. Upper motor neuron lesions produce weakness especially in the extensor muscles of the upper limbs and in the flexors of the legs. Diseases of the peripheral nerve result in distal weakness; most muscle diseases primarily affect proximal muscles.

Assessment of Muscle Bulk. Atrophy of muscle is marked in lower motor neuron lesions, less striking in diseases of upper motor neurons. Fasciculations should always be looked for in atrophic muscles since their presence tends to localize the lesion in the anterior horn cells. Both upper and lower motor neuron lesions interfere with growth of the affected extremity. Excessive muscle bulk or muscular hypertrophy is usually due to increased muscular activity. It occurs normally in athletes and abnormally in muscle diseases with myotonia and in the adrenogenital syndrome. Pseudohypertrophy refers to enlargement of muscles that are weak. It is usually due to infiltration of muscle with fat, such as occurs in muscular dystrophy, or to distention of muscle by an abnormal substance, e.g., glycogen in type II glycogenosis (Pompe disease).

Assessment of Muscle Tone. This is estimated by the resistance to passive movement of an extremity. It ranges from atonia and hypotonia to severe rigidity. Diminished muscle tone occurs in lower motor neuron diseases and in some extrapyramidal disorders, especially those of the cerebellum. *Rigidity* is an increase in resistance throughout passive movement of a joint; it occurs in disorders of the basal ganglia. It must be distinguished from *spasticity*, or increased resistance to passive movement which gives way suddenly (*clasp-knife effect*). Spasticity is a sign of upper motor neuron disease.

Tests of Fine Motor Coordination. Impairment of skilled movements is found in disorders of upper motor neurons and in cerebellar diseases. It can be assessed informally by watching the child manipulate toys, control a pencil, or put on clothing. A more formal test consists of rapid alternating supination and pronation of the hands. Irregular and slow performance of this test is seen in children with cerebellar disease, but care must be exercised in interpretation since the adult level of performance is not reached until the midteens. Incoordination of gait (ataxia) is also characteristic of cerebellar lesions. In diseases of a cerebellar hemisphere the patient tends to reel to the side of the lesion. When cerebellar involvement is diffuse or confined to the midline vermis, the child may stagger to either side. Mild degrees of ataxia can be brought out by having the child walk a line with heel to toe or hop on one foot.

Involuntary Movements. These occur principally in diseases of basal ganglia and of the cerebellum. They are brought out by attempts to maintain a given posture or to carry out a skilled motor act. *Tremor* is defined as a rapid, regular, repetitive involuntary movement, usually of the distal extremities. A fine tremor of the outstretched hands is seen in anxiety and in thyrotoxicosis. A similar, somewhat coarser tremor occurs as a benign hereditary trait. A more proximal tremor of outstretched arms and wrists (*wing-beating tremor*) is seen in Wilson disease. Tremor that becomes more marked

on approach to the target is known as *intention tremor*; it is a sign of cerebellar disorder. It can be seen as the young child reaches for a toy. In the older child it is brought out by a test in which the child touches his or her own nose and the examiner's finger alternatively.

Three characteristic disorders of movement—chorea, athetosis, and dystonia—are seen in *disease of the basal ganglia:*

Chorea consists of irregular jerking and writhing movements, often in proximal muscles such as the tongue, face, neck, and shoulder. These may be quite violent and may cause the child to fling the arms or suddenly to drop a held object. Gait is irregular, with sudden lurching to the side; walking may be impossible when chorea is severe. Mild chorea is to be distinguished from *tic,* which is a stereotyped sudden movement, always involving the same muscle group. Tic can be voluntarily inhibited by the patient for a short period of time.

Athetosis is a slow writhing movement, often more marked in the distal extremities, consisting of alternating supination-pronation and flexion-extension of the limbs.

Dystonia is a tendency toward hyperextension of joints, brought out especially when the patient tries to walk. Typically, there is plantar flexion of the feet, hyperextension of the legs, extension and pronation of arms, arching of the back, and extension and rotation of the neck.

All abnormal extrapyramidal movements are accentuated during emotional stress and disappear during sleep. Failure to appreciate these features may lead to the erroneous impression that there is a psychiatric disorder.

Examination of Reflexes. The tendon reflexes are elicited by stretching of a tendon, usually by a quick tap with a reflex hammer. They provide evidence of the intactness of a particular *reflex arc* which includes sensory nerve endings in tendon, sensory nerve fibers, spinal cord, motor neuron, and muscle. The *tendon reflexes* are decreased or absent in disorders of peripheral nerves or muscle and in diseases that affect the spinal cord or brain stem at the level of the reflex arc. The intactness of specific segments of the neuraxis can be assessed as follows:

Neuraxial Segment	Related Reflex
Pons	Jaw jerk
C5–6	Biceps jerk
C5–6	Supinator jerk
C6,7,8	Triceps jerk
L3–4	Knee jerk
S1–2	Ankle jerk

A tense or anxious patient may have difficulty relaxing sufficiently for demonstration of the tendon reflexes. Distraction of the patient by having him or her squeeze hands together may produce the necessary relaxation. Hyperactivity of tendon reflexes, especially when associated with clonus, is a sign of upper motor neuron disease.

Several superficial reflexes are elicited by stroking the skin. The *plantar reflex* is produced by a firm stroke against the lateral aspect of the sole, moving from the heel forward. A normal response consists of flexion of the toes. The abnormal response or *Babinski sign* consists of extension of the great toe, often associated with fanning of the other toes. Beyond the age of 2 yr it indicates pyramidal tract dysfunction. *Abdominal reflexes* consist of contraction of the abdominal muscles following stroking of the overlying skin. Their absence suggests either a lesion of the spinal cord segment that is stimulated (T10–L1) or a central motor lesion. The *cremasteric reflex* consists of ascent of the testis upon stroking the skin of the medial thigh; it is absent in lesions involving the L1–2 segment. The *anal reflex*, elicited by stroking the perianal skin, assesses the lower sacral segments.

Table 21–1 summarizes the clinical abnormalities in various categories of neuromuscular disease.

Table 21–1. **Diseases of the Neuromuscular System**

	Upper Motor Neuron	Basal Ganglia	Cerebellum	Anterior Horn Cells	Peripheral Nerve	Muscle
Strength	Decreased	Normal	Normal	Decreased	Decreased	Decreased
Muscle tone	Spasticity (usually)	Hypotonia or rigidity	Hypotonia	Hypotonia	Hypotonia	Normal or hypotonia
Coordination	Decreased	Decreased	Decreased	Normal	Normal	Normal
Involuntary movements	None	Chorea, athetosis, or dystonia	Intention tremor	Fasciculations	None	None
Tendon reflexes	Hyperactive	Normal	Decreased	Absent or decreased	Absent or decreased	Decreased
Babinski sign	Present	Absent	Absent	Absent	Absent	Absent
Sensory deficit	Usually present	Absent	Absent	Absent	Present	Absent

Sensory Examination

This is necessarily limited in the infant and young child. Response to pain can be tested by observation of withdrawal and of emotional reaction to pinprick. This maneuver tests intactness of peripheral pain fibers and of pain pathways up to the level of the thalamus. In the evaluation of unilateral sensory impairment it has to be remembered that near the midline there is an overlap of innervation from the two sides. A sensory defect which ends abruptly at the midline is due to hysteria or malingering rather than to neurologic disease. Function of the posterior columns in the spinal cord is tested by asking the child to identify direction of passive movement of a joint (*position sense*) and by response to the vibration of a tuning fork placed on a bony prominence such as the lateral malleolus. Intactness of the sensory cortex is determined by sensory discrimination tests, such as identification of objects placed into the hand (*stereognosis*), recognition of numbers drawn onto the skin (*graphesthesia*), or responses to simultaneous stimulation of two points (*two-point discrimination*) and to bilateral simultaneous stimulation.

Examination of Cranial Nerves and Their Central Connections

The cranial nerves innervate eye muscles, facial muscles, and muscles of deglutition, and carry somatosensory fibers from the face and fibers from the special sensory organs. In testing muscles innervated by cranial nerves, the same principles apply as in the extremities: motor abnormalities in muscles supplied by cranial nerves may be due to lower motor neuron, upper motor neuron, or extrapyramidal disorders.

Cranial Nerve I (Olfactory Nerve). Ability to identify odors such as peppermint or coffee is determined for each nostril separately. Chronic rhinitis is the most common cause of *anosmia*.

Cranial Nerve II (Optic Nerve). *Vision* is frequently affected in children with neurologic disease. Techniques for assessment of visual acuity and of visual fields are described in Sec. 25.2. Visual field defects provide important data concerning sites of lesions in the visual pathways. The course of visual pathways from the different retinal areas is indicated schematically in Fig. 21–2.

Homonymous hemianopsia, in which the defect involves the temporal field of one eye and the nasal fields of the opposite eye, is seen in lesions of the optic radiations or of the visual cortex. The cerebral lesion is opposite the side of the field defect. A homonymous upper quadrant defect indicates a lesion in the temporal lobe white matter, through which the optic radiation fibers from the inferior portion of the retina pass on their way to the visual cortex.

Bitemporal hemianopsia implies a lesion in the region of the optic chiasm, due most often in children to craniopharyngioma.

Funduscopic examination is always included in a complete neurologic examination. A pale optic nerve head with sparsity of capillary vessels on the disc indicates optic atrophy. In papilledema the optic disc is hyperemic, the optic cup is obliterated, and the disc may protrude forward into the vitreous. The retinal veins are distended, and venous pulsations are absent. Hemorrhage may be present on the disc or adjacent to it. The appearance of papilledema may be indistinguishable from inflammation of the optic disc or papillitis.

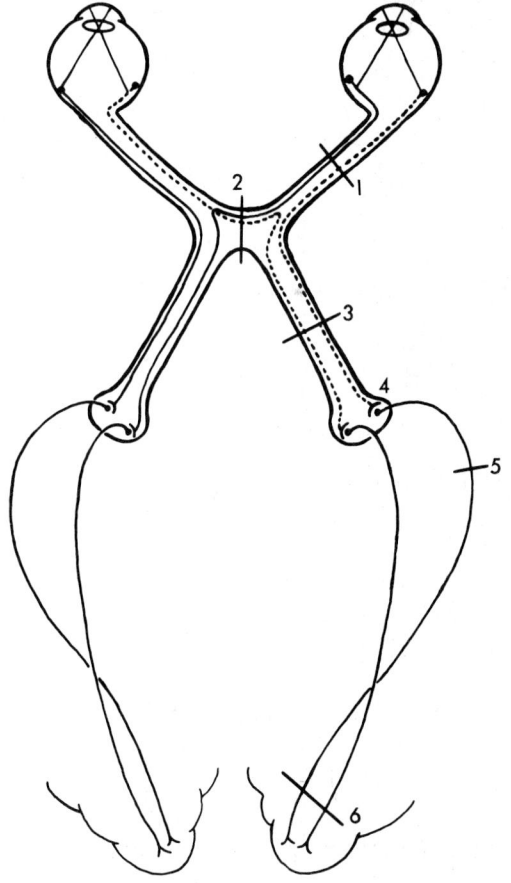

Figure 21–2. Schematic representation of visual pathways. 1, Optic nerve. Lesion in this location causes unilateral visual loss. 2, Optic chiasm. Lesion results in bitemporal hemianopsia because it interrupts fibers to the nasal half of both retinas. 3, Optic tract. Lesion causes homonymous hemianopsia by interrupting temporal fibers on the same side and nasal fibers on the opposite side. 4, Lateral geniculate body. 5, Optic radiation. Fibers are widely separated and partial lesions are common. The fibers from the lower part of the retina pass in the white matter beneath the temporal cortex; thus homonymous upper quadrant anopsia in temporal lobe lesions is frequent. 6, Visual cortex. Lesions may cause partial or complete homonymous hemianopsia.

In papilledema, however, visual acuity tends to be preserved until late, whereas it is lost early in papillitis.

Cranial Nerve III. This nerve carries the pupilloconstrictor fibers and innervates all the extraocular muscles except the lateral rectus and superior oblique. Pupillary asymmetry at rest may be due to unilateral visual loss, a midbrain lesion, 3rd nerve palsy, or a lesion of cervical sympathetic nerves (Horner syndrome, Sec. 21.29). Slight but definite asymmetry of pupillary size is not uncommon, however, in normal children. In unilateral visual loss the pupil on the affected side is dilated and the pupillary reflex diminished or absent when the affected eye is exposed to light; the pupil constricts normally, however, when the opposite (seeing) eye is stimulated (consensual light reflex). In lesions of the 3rd nerve or of its cells of origin in the upper midbrain the pupil of the affected side is dilated, and both direct and consensual light reflexes are lost. Third nerve palsy causes deviation of the eye down and out as a result of unopposed action of the superior oblique and the lateral rectus; there also is ptosis due to paralysis of the voluntary portion of the levator palpebrae.

Cranial Nerve IV. This nerve innervates the superior oblique muscle only. An isolated palsy, which is rare, causes inability to turn the affected eye downward when it is in the adducted position.

Cranial Nerve VI. Palsy of the 6th nerve results in inability to abduct the eye on the affected side. The lesion has to be distinguished from convergent strabismus. In strabismus, eye movements generally are full when each eye is tested alone; the abnormality is evident only when both eyes are open. Patching of the good eye for a time may be necessary before the child becomes able to abduct the squinting eye.

Abnormalities of Eye Movements Secondary to Supranuclear Lesions. Brain stem lesions may result in abnormalities of eye movements because of disruption of the fibers connecting the various oculomotor nuclei. In *internuclear ophthalmoplegia* the patient is unable to adduct either eye during visual following movements, but adduction during convergence is usually preserved. In *skew deviation,* one eye is elevated with respect to the other in all directions of gaze. Lesions of the upper brain stem in the pineal region cause paralysis of upward gaze. Paralysis of conjugate lateral gaze may be due to a lesion in the pons on the same side, but more commonly it is caused by a cortical lesion involving the gaze centers in the frontal or the occipital cortex on the opposite side. With cortical lesions, only voluntary eye movements are affected. Reflex eye turning, such as may be induced by vestibular stimulation, is preserved.

Lesions involving cerebellar and vestibular pathways produce rhythmic jerking of the eyes *(nystagmus)*. Most forms of nystagmus have a slow and a fast component. In nystagmus due to dysfunction of the cerebellum or of cerebellar connections in the brain stem the nystagmus becomes more marked when the eyes are deviated laterally; the slow component is always toward the midline. This type of nystagmus is seen in intoxication with certain drugs such as phenytoin and the barbiturates. It may also occur with structural lesions of the cerebellum or brain stem, and it is often present in children with cerebellar tumors. The nystagmus tends to be coarser and of greater amplitude when the eye is deviated to the side of the tumor.

Nystagmus due to cerebellar or brain stem disorders has to be distinguished from nystagmus caused by labyrinthine dysfunction and from congenital nystagmus. Labyrinthine nystagmus often varies with head position, tends to have a rotary component, is most obvious at rest when the patient is not fixing on any object, and is associated with vertigo and nausea. It occurs acutely following trauma to or inflammation of the labyrinth (labyrinthitis). Congenital nystagmus is pendular at rest, with irregular jerking when the eyes are deviated to the sides. It is usually associated with poor visual acuity and is thought to be due to failure of development of visual fixation in infancy.

Cranial Nerve V. The trigeminal nerve conveys sensation, including touch and pain, from the entire face except for a small area at the angle of the mandible. Its upper (ophthalmic) division is tested by the corneal reflex. The 5th nerve also has a motor component which innervates the muscles of mastication. Unilateral paralysis causes deviation of the jaw to the side of the lesion. The intactness of the segmental arc involving the muscles of mastication is tested by means of the jaw jerk. A brisk jaw jerk or jaw clonus implies a bilateral upper motor neuron lesion.

Cranial Nerve VII. The facial nerve is frequently affected in childhood as a result of congenital anomalies, birth injury, inflammation (Bell palsy), and tumor. It innervates all the facial muscles except the levator palpebrae. Mild weakness is made evident by asking the child to show the teeth; it can be detected in the infant by watching facial movements during crying. The palpebral fissure is larger on the side of the weakness. In addition to motor fibers, the facial nerve carries parasympathetic fibers to the lacrimal and salivary glands and a sensory branch which transmits taste sensation from the anterior two thirds of the tongue. Lacrimation, salivation, and taste are affected only in lesions of the proximal portion of the nerve in its course through the facial canal in the temporal bone. Taste is tested by placing salt or sugar on the outstretched tip of the tongue by means of a cotton applicator and having the patient indicate by head nods which taste sensation is felt. Peripheral facial nerve weakness has to be distinguished from weakness due to a central (corticobulbar) lesion. In weakness of facial muscles due to a central nervous system lesion the upper face is less severely affected, and the patient continues to be able to wrinkle the forehead.

Cranial Nerve VIII. This consists of auditory and vestibular divisions. Hearing can be tested grossly in the young child by observing the response to the noise made by rubbing the fingers together or by crinkling a piece of paper and in the older child by asking for identification of whispered words. Formal audiometry is indicated in any child suspected of hearing or speech disorder since partial deafness, especially for high tones, is easily missed by gross clinical testing. Vestibular dysfunction is rare in childhood but should be suspected in a child with episodic vertigo, staggering, and vomiting, especially when there is associated labyrinthine nystagmus. It can be confirmed by caloric testing with cold water, which normally produces deviation of the eyes to the side of stimulation. A more comfortable test consists of rotation of the child while being held upright under the arms of the examiner. If vestibular functions are intact, ocular deviation toward the direction of rotation will occur.

Cranial Nerves IX and X. Dysfunction of these nerves produces difficulty in swallowing and in phonation. Palatal paralysis can be observed by inspection of the soft palate and uvula when the patient says "ah." The gag reflex is diminished or absent. Secretions pool in the oropharynx, and the patient drools excessively. With unilateral lesions the voice is nasal or hoarse; bilateral lesions cause aphonia and stridor.

Cranial Nerve XI (Spinal Accessory). This nerve innervates the sternocleidomastoid and trapezius muscles. Paralysis causes weakness in head rotation toward the opposite side and in elevation of the shoulder on the affected side.

Cranial Nerve XII (Hypoglossal). Lesions of this nerve produce paralysis of tongue movements and atrophy and fibrillations of the tongue. In unilateral involvement the tongue is deviated to the side of the lesion on attempted protrusion.

Lesions of the 9th, 10th, and 12th cranial nerves have to be distinguished from impairment of swallowing, phonation, and tongue movement resulting from bilateral central nervous system (corticobulbar) disorders. The latter lesions, known collectively as *pseudobulbar palsy*, are manifested by difficulty in swallowing, slurred speech, and impaired control of emotional expression, with inappropriate laughing and crying, and by brisk reflex responses involving the bulbar muscles, including a brisk gag reflex. This type of deficit is common in children with spastic cerebral palsy.

Examination of the Cranium

The neurologic examination includes measurement of head circumference and inspection of the skull for symmetry and shape. Abnormalities of shape, especially those associated with palpable bony ridges, suggest craniosynostosis. Auscultation over the skull or over the eyes may reveal a cranial bruit. This is a normal finding until about the age of 6 yr. Later it suggests the possibility of a cerebral vascular malformation or of increased intracranial pressure. Percussion of the skull gives a sound resembling that of a cracked pot (*Macewen sign*) when the cranial sutures are separated because of increased intracranial pressure.

Examination of the Autonomic Nervous System

A limited number of clinical tests can be used to assess intactness of the autonomic nervous system. These consist of measurement of blood pressure and of body temperature, including diurnal variations. Absence of sweating can be shown by painting a portion of the skin involved with iodine and covering it with starch powder, which fails to turn dark blue in areas of anhidrosis. Parasympathetic function is tested by the *Mecholyl test:* A 2% solution of methacholine (Mecholyl) is instilled into one conjunctival sac; this produces constriction of the pupil in patients with parasympathetic disorders such as familial dysautonomia. Disorders of the parasympathetic innervation of the bladder result in urinary retention and incomplete emptying. The cystometrogram helps to evaluate partial lesions.

21.3 NEUROLOGIC EXAMINATION OF THE INFANT

At birth human neurologic function is largely at a subcortical (brain stem and spinal cord) level. Cortical functions cannot be tested reliably, and even major cerebral defects may go unnoticed. Accordingly, extreme caution is indicated in giving a prognosis as to future intellectual function from neurologic findings in the neonatal period. Measurement of head size can at times give indirect evidence of major cerebral defect. A head circumference more than 3 standard deviations below the normal for gestational age suggests a defect in brain growth that will usually be permanent. Major malformations of the cerebrum can sometimes be detected by transillumination of the skull with a bright flashlight equipped with a soft rubber cuff or with a specially constructed (commercially available) high-intensity transilluminator. A totally darkened room is essential. A light beam applied to the occiput can be seen shining through the globes of the eyes in infants with hydranencephaly. Less marked transillumination is seen with subdural effusions or extreme hydrocephalus. A localized area of increased transillumination, usually unilateral, is found in porencephaly. During the 1st yr of life intracranial pressure can be assessed clinically by palpation of the anterior fontanelle. Normally the fontanelle of the sitting infant is soft and slightly depressed. The fontanelle is tense and bulging in the infant with increased intracranial pressure; it is sunken with dehydration or with destructive brain lesions which lead to low intracranial pressure. Chronic increase in intracranial pressure is manifested by abnormal head enlargement.

Reflexes. Many reflex patterns mediated by brain stem and spinal cord mechanisms are found in the newborn infant and during the 1st months of postnatal life. The responses are stereotyped; they are normally present but may be less brisk in the sleepy or recently fed infant. Absence of reflex responses indicates general depression of central or peripheral motor functions; asymmetric responses suggest focal motor lesions, either peripheral or central. As the infant matures, the neonatal reflexes disappear in a predictable order as voluntary motor functions supersede them. Abnormal persistence of these reflexes is seen in infants with general developmental lag or with central motor lesions; ages of appearance and disappearance of certain of the reflexes are shown in Table 21–2.

The *Moro reflex* (Fig. 21–3) is elicited by placing the infant supine upon the examining table, the head supported by the examiner's hand. The support is withdrawn suddenly, and the head is allowed to fall backward for 10–15 degrees. The reflex consists of extension of the trunk and extension and abduction followed by flexion and adduction of the arms, with less regular participation of the legs. The *stepping reflex* consists of movements of walking which are elicited when the infant is held upright and inclined forward with soles of feet touching a flat surface. The *placing reflex* occurs when the infant is held erect and the dorsum of one foot is drawn along the under edge of a table top. The response consists of flexion followed by extension of the leg that is stimulated.

Several *postural reflexes* can be easily observed in the infant. The *tonic neck reflex* (Fig. 21–3), which is elicited by rapidly turning the head of the supine infant to one side, consists of extension of the arm and leg on the side to which the face is turned and flexion of the limbs on the opposite side (fencing posture). Tonic neck patterns are normally prominent in the 2–4 mo old infant. Their persistence past the age of 6–9 mo occurs with central motor lesions, especially in infants with spastic cerebral palsy. The *neck righting reflex* consists of rotation of the trunk in the direction in which the head of the supine infant is turned. The *Landau reflex* is demonstrated by supporting the infant in the prone position with the examiner's hand beneath the abdomen. A normal response consists of extension of head, trunk, and hips. Flexion of trunk and hips occurs when the examiner flexes the head. The *parachute reflex* consists of extension of arms, hands, and fingers when the infant, suspended in prone position, is suddenly allowed to fall for a short distance onto a soft pad.

Table 21–2. Reflexes of Neonates

Reflex	Age When Reflex Usually Appears	Age When Reflex Is Normally no Longer Obtainable
Moro	Birth	3 mo
Stepping	Birth	6 wk
Placing	Birth	6 wk
Sucking and rooting	Birth	4 mo awake 7 mo asleep
Palmar grasp	Birth	6 mo
Plantar grasp	Birth	10 mo
Adductor spread of knee jerk	Birth	7 mo
Tonic neck	2 mo	6 mo
Neck righting	4–6 mo	24 mo
Landau	3 mo	24 mo
Parachute reaction	9 mo	Persists

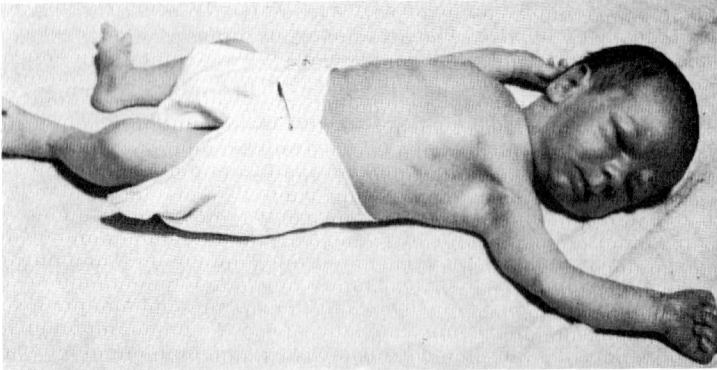

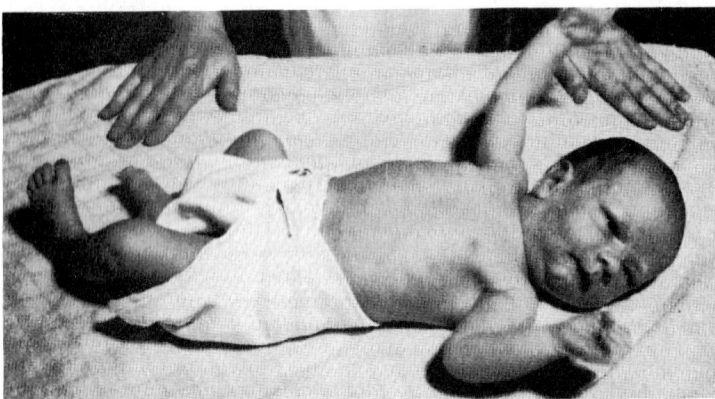

Figure 21–3. Upper photograph shows a spontaneous tonic neck reflex. Lower photograph shows the Moro reflex.

The *sucking reflex* is initiated by stroking the lips. Stroking of the cheek produces the *rooting reflex*, which consists of turning the mouth toward the stimulus. *Grasp reflexes* are elicited by light pressure on the palms or on the soles of the feet. *Tendon reflexes* are generally present in the normal neonate; only the knee jerk may be easily obtainable. Brisk tendon jerks may be normal, and there may be adductor spread of the knee jerk and unsustained ankle clonus. Spontaneous clonus of arms, legs, and feet is seen in infants with cerebral disorders. Absence of tendon reflexes suggests a neuromuscular disorder, such as Werdnig-Hoffmann disease. The *Babinski sign* is not helpful in infancy since either flexion or extension of toes may normally be obtained.

Assessment of Motor Functions. This includes careful observation of spontaneous activity, which should be symmetrical. Consistent fisting of hands with adduction of thumbs is abnormal and suggests a central motor lesion. Maintained opisthotonus is evidence of severe spasticity; it is rarely seen in neonatal meningitis except in the terminal stage but is common in kernicterus and may be seen in other conditions, including congenital toxoplasmosis, maple syrup urine disease, and poisoning, e.g., with the phenothiazines and strychnine. *Scissoring* of legs as a result of increased tone in adductors of the hips is a sign of spasticity. *Diminished muscle tone* is seen in infants with diffuse cerebral dysfunction and in peripheral neuromuscular diseases. Hypotonic infants tend to lie in the frog-leg position, with arms abducted at the shoulders. There is head lag and absence of contraction of shoulder muscles (absent traction response) when the supine infant is pulled to the sitting position. Rapid *tremors* of the limbs (jitteriness) are seen in infants with metabolic disturbances such as hypoglycemia or hypocalcemia and occur also without obvious cause. They must be distinguished from the slower and often focal intermittent clonic movements characteristic of seizure activity in infancy.

The quality of the *infant's cry* can be of diagnostic help. The cry is high-pitched in the infant with increased intracranial pressure, hoarse in cretinism, feeble in the infant with Werdnig-Hoffmann disease, and cat-like in the cri-du-chat syndrome.

Examination of the Cranial Nerves. In the neonate the presence of vision is indicated by blinking in response to a bright light. Visual following can usually be demonstrated in the normal full-term infant; it is one of the few signs of cortical function in the immediate neonatal period. A light or the examiner's face, moved slowly 20–30 cm in from the child's eyes, is an adequate stimulus. Visual following movements of the infant are irregular and poorly sustained. The eyes tend to move conjugately, but intermittent disconjugate eye movements may occur normally. The presence of full lateral eye movements can be ascertained by rotation of the infant's head, which results in deviation of the eyes to the side opposite the rotation (oculocephalic or doll's eye reflex). The pupils of the newborn infant should be approximately equal in size and should respond to bright light. Corneal reflexes are well developed. Funduscopic examination is easily carried out in a dark room with the infant sucking on a nipple. The optic disc is normally pale, with underdevelopment of the fine capillary vessels on the nervehead. Preretinal hemorrhages occur in about 10% of normal neonates. Chorioretinitis may signify congenital toxoplasmosis, cytomegalic inclusion disease, generalized herpes simplex infection, or congenital syphilis. Acute chorioretinitis appears as gray, indistinct retinal masses with pigmented borders. After a few weeks the center of the lesion takes on a white, punched-out appearance.

Gross assessment of hearing is possible. The normal infant startles to a sudden loud noise. Responses to more subtle auditory stimuli consist of changes in spontaneous motor activity. Facial movements are assessed most easily when the child is crying. The neonate has a good gag reflex and well-coordinated swallowing movements. The tongue should be inspected. An atrophic tongue with fibrillations is seen in Werdnig-Hoffmann disease. The tongue is large and may protrude in cretinism, glycogen storage disease, and Beckwith syndrome. The protruding tongue of trisomy 21 is due more to a shallow oropharynx than to large size.

A careful developmental evaluation is part of the neurologic examination of the infant. For developmental milestones see Sec. 2.3.

21.4 NEUROLOGIC EVALUATION OF THE CHILD WITH PSYCHIATRIC DISEASE

Older children and adolescents with psychiatric disorders may have symptoms and signs mimicking neurologic disease. Problems in differential diagnosis arise especially in *conversion disorders* (hysteria). The hysterical patient has often had a variety of previous symptoms. Fairly characteristic ones include a sensation of compression of the throat *(globus hystericus)* and recurrent abdominal pain without abnormal physical findings. Common manifestations easily confused with neurologic dysfunction include hysterical blindness, spasm of convergence, gait disturbance, paralysis, sensory loss, seizures, and urinary retention. The patient tends to report symptoms and disabilities in a matter-of-fact, detached manner, an emotional state referred to as *"la belle indifférence."*

Hysterical blindness can usually be distinguished from true visual loss by the absence of funduscopic abnormality and by preservation of pupillary constriction to light and of optico-kinetic nystagmus. Differentiation from cortical blindness, such as may occur transiently after head injury or cerebral angiography, may be difficult. Hysterical visual field defects tend to be concentric, with general constriction of the fields in both eyes. Characteristically, the absolute size of the visual fields on a screen remains the same no matter at what distance from the screen the field is tested. This type of *"tunnel vision"* cannot be explained on the basis of any organic lesion.

Spasm of convergence tends to be of sudden onset, usually during some traumatic experience such as a difficult school examination. The child complains of blurring vision or double vision, and on examination it is noted that the eyes are disconjugate, both in the adducted position. Reassurance and suggestion usually lead to rapid improvement.

Hysterical gait disturbances usually occur in the form of *astasia abasia*, an inability to stand or to walk, without any evidence of neurologic deficit when the patient is tested in the lying position. The gait is bizarre, with extreme lurching to the sides, requiring exquisite balancing acts to prevent a fall. It has to be distinguished from cerebellar ataxia, in which the patient walks on a wide base and has great difficulty maintaining balance.

Hysterical paralysis is distinguished from true paralysis by presence of normal muscle tone, normal tendon reflexes, and absence of Babinski signs. *Hoover sign* is helpful in unilateral paralysis involving the legs. The examiner places a hand under the heel of the paralyzed leg and then asks the patient to raise the normal leg against resistance. In hysteria forceful raising of the normal leg leads to downward pressure of the "paralyzed" leg against the examiner's hand; no such pressure occurs in true paralysis.

When sensory loss is unilateral, hysterical loss ends exactly at the midline, whereas loss due to an organic lesion is restored about 2.5 cm short of the midline because of overlapping innervation of the midline areas. Anesthesia in glove and stocking distribution is commonly hysterical. In sensory neuropathy the transition from abnormal to normal is more gradual. A useful maneuver is to test repeatedly, each time shifting the point at which testing is begun. As one starts higher, the boundary of the hysterical sensory loss also moves

upward. Occasionally, the child with hysteria can be persuaded to report touches felt as "yes" and ones supposedly not felt as "no" during testing with eyes closed. The anesthetic side may shift from left to right or vice versa when the patient is moved from supine to prone. The *Japanese illusion* may be used to bring out left-right confusion in unilateral anesthesia. The patient is asked to cross arms, oppose the palms, and clasp fingers. The clasped hands are then rotated inward and the arms extended. This maneuver makes it very difficult for the patient to tell right fingers from left.

Hysterical seizures may be difficult to distinguish from epilepsy unless evaluated by an experienced observer. The seizure activity tends to be bizarre, often with rhythmic thrusting and writhing of the trunk. Tongue-biting, apnea, and incontinence are absent. The eyes tend to be held forcibly closed.

Hysterical urinary retention may have to be distinguished from bladder paralysis secondary to spinal cord lesions. The cystometrogram is normal when urinary retention is due to hysteria.

21.5 SPECIAL DIAGNOSTIC PROCEDURES

Lumbar Puncture and Examination of Cerebrospinal Fluid. Lumbar puncture is contraindicated in patients with increased intracranial pressure caused by a space-occupying lesion or with untreated clotting defects. The puncture should not be done through an area of infected skin. If possible, the child should be kept from struggling during the tap; local procaine infiltration is helpful, even in the infant. Infants should be allowed to suck on a pacifier; sedation may be necessary in later childhood. The puncture is made in the lateral recumbent position except in the neonate, for whom the sitting position may be preferable. The neck and back are held flexed by an attendant. Careful cleansing of the skin is essential; drapes are unnecessary. The needle should not be inserted above the L2–3 interspace; L3–4 is the preferred site. A sharp needle with stylet should be used. Omission of the stylet may increase the chance of carrying a fragment of skin into the spinal canal, with formation of a spinal epidermoid tumor. The needle is advanced slowly, exactly in the midline, the tip of the needle pointed slightly cephalad. In the small child it often is not possible to feel the change in resistance that occurs as the dura is penetrated and the subarachnoid space is entered. It is therefore necessary to remove the stylet repeatedly during advance of the needle until the cerebrospinal fluid drips out. A bloody tap usually occurs when the needle is advanced too far.

Cerebrospinal fluid pressure should be measured whenever it is possible to obtain relaxation. The measurement is most accurate when legs and neck are extended prior to the reading. The normal opening pressure (recumbent) ranges from 60–160 mm of water.

The color of the fluid should be compared with that of distilled water against a white background. After the neonatal period *xanthochromia*—a yellow tint—is always abnormal. It may be due to elevation of spinal fluid protein or to accumulation of bilirubin. The latter usually implies recent subarachnoid hemorrhage, but it may also be seen in the absence of central nervous system lesions in patients with hyperbilirubinemia. Fluid that contains more than about 100 leukocytes/mm^3 appears cloudy. Bloody fluid may be due to a traumatic tap or a recent subarachnoid hemorrhage. To discover the origin of the blood, the fluid should be centrifuged and the supernatant inspected; in subarachnoid hemorrhage the supernatant is xanthochromic, and equal amounts of blood are present in successive fractional specimens of fluid. In a bloody tap the supernatant is clear or only faintly yellow, and the amount of blood decreases in successive tubes.

Normal spinal fluid contains no red blood cells and at most 5 leukocytes/mm³, except in the newborn infant, in whom up to 500 red cells and up to 15 leukocytes, including granulocytes, may be insignificant. Later in childhood, predominance of granulocytes most often indicates bacterial infection but is occasionally found in the early phase of acute viral meningitis. Elevation in numbers of lymphocytes is seen in a large variety of illnesses in which meningeal irritation and inflammation are factors.

The protein content of lumbar spinal fluid in childhood normally ranges from 10–30 mg/dL except in the 1st weeks of infancy, when values up to 100 mg/dL are accepted as normal. By the age of 3 mo the protein should be below 30 mg/dL; elevation is usually due to increased permeability of meningeal vessels and occasionally to obstruction of spinal fluid circulation, with decrease in resorption of protein. Elevations in the concentration of protein are seen in many neurologic disorders, including brain and spinal cord tumors, degenerative brain diseases, and inflammatory diseases of the central nervous system or of peripheral nerves.

Elevation in spinal fluid globulin content is detected by immunoelectrophoresis. Normally about 30% of the protein in spinal fluid is represented by globulins. The ratio of IgG to albumin is normally below 0.21; an increased ratio is associated with only a few illnesses, which include multiple sclerosis, subacute sclerosing panencephalitis, neurosyphilis, and postinfectious encephalomyelitis. Measurement of measles antibody titer in spinal fluid is an important diagnostic aid in subacute sclerosing panencephalitis.

The glucose concentration of spinal fluid is normally more than 50% that of blood. It is the ratio between spinal fluid and blood glucose values that is of importance, rather than the absolute value of the former. A low ratio is seen in bacterial meningitis, fungal meningitis, meningeal tumor, and, rarely, aseptic meningitis.

Spinal fluid should always be cultured for bacteria and, when indicated, for fungi, mycobacteria, and viruses. When meningitis is suspected, the fluid is centrifuged and a Gram-stained smear of the sediment examined. An excellent method of spinal fluid preparation for morphologic examination is to add a drop of liquid albumin to an aliquot of spinal fluid and spin the mixture in a cytocentrifuge. The sediment is dried and then stained with Wright stain. Histiocytes and tumor cells as well as normal leukocytes can be readily identified.

Subdural Tap. This procedure is helpful for the diagnosis and treatment of subdural effusion in infancy. The scalp hair must be shaved and strict aseptic precautions observed. The head is firmly held by an attendant. A blunt, short-beveled #20 needle with a stylet is used. The needle is introduced into the lateral angle of the fontanelle or into the coronal suture, *at least 2 cm lateral to the midline;* it is advanced perpendicular to the scalp surface. A popping sensation usually occurs when the dura is penetrated. The needle should be advanced slowly, never more than 1.5 cm from the scalp surface, and the stylet should be removed repeatedly to determine whether a fluid-filled space has been reached. If intracranial pressure is not elevated, it is advisable to hold the head in a somewhat dependent position during the tap so that flow is aided by gravity. Care has to be taken to avoid to-and-fro movements of the needle, which could lead to laceration of the meninges or cerebral cortex.

Subdural fluid is xanthochromic, bloody, or reddish brown in color, depending on the age of the effusion and the amount of admixed blood. The protein content is always elevated, usually above 100 mg/dL. At times, a fairly copious amount of clear fluid with low protein content is obtained. This is subarachnoid fluid, the presence of which is usually of no pathologic significance. In general, the protein content of subarachnoid fluid obtained over the convexities is about twice that obtained from a lumbar tap.

Subdural fluid should be removed slowly, with no more than 15 mL taken from one side in any one tap. Rapid removal of large quantities may cause shock or intracranial hemorrhage from sudden shift of the intracranial structures. Usually both sides need to be tapped, since subdural effusions in infancy are bilateral in 80% of cases. After the tap a pressure dressing is applied and the infant placed in a semi-erect position in an infant seat to diminish the chance of prolonged leakage from the puncture site.

Ventricular Taps. These taps should not be performed by the pediatrician except in cases of life-threatening increase in intracranial pressure when a neurosurgeon is not immediately available. The needle is introduced as for a subdural tap but is inclined slightly forward, toward the nasion. The needle is advanced until ventricular fluid is obtained, usually fewer than 4 cm from the surface when intracranial pressure is elevated because of ventricular obstruction. The procedure carries the risk of intracerebral or ventricular hemorrhage, and it always leads to some damage to cerebral cortex.

Electroencephalography. The electroencephalogram (EEG) records the electrical activity of the cerebral cortex. Normally, fairly regular wave forms predominate. They are classified according to their frequency as delta (1–3/sec), theta (4–7/sec), alpha (8–12/sec), or beta waves (13–20/sec). During maturation the waves gradually become more regular and increase in frequency. In premature infants up to about 36 wk gestational age the electrical activity in cerebral cortex is as yet intermittent, especially during sleep. Asymmetry of the background activity is normal during the 1st yr of life. Theta waves are normally seen during waking periods in the infant and young child. By the age of 10 yr the normal background rhythm in the waking state consists largely of alpha activity posteriorly and of beta waves in frontal areas. Slower waves are normal during sleep. In addition, high voltage slow and sharp waves (K complexes) and regular 12–14/sec waves (sleep spindles) are seen during sleep. They are symmetrically distributed over the central regions. These features disappear during REM ("rapid eye movement") sleep, the stage associated with dreaming, during which the EEG shows low voltage beta activity.

Spike discharges, which may replace or be superimposed on the basic brain waves, indicate a lowered seizure threshold and are an important confirmatory sign in the child with a suspected seizure disorder. Metabolic and inflammatory diseases of cerebral cortex tend to be associated with generalized high voltage slow wave (delta) activity. Focal structural lesions of cerebral cortex, such as brain abscesses or brain tumors, cause localized slow wave activity.

Evoked Potentials. Visual, auditory, and somatosensory evoked potential studies provide information concerning the function of the primary sensory pathways. Brain stem auditory evoked potentials (BAEP) are particularly useful in the pediatric age group. They can be used to determine the threshold at which a sound will produce a response in brain stem auditory pathways, which provides an objective measure of hearing acuity. Evoked potentials also are useful for the detection in afferent pathways of demyelinating and other lesions that tend to increase the latency of evoked responses.

Electromyography. Electromyography is useful in the differential diagnosis of neuromuscular disease. A needle is inserted into the muscle as an electrode to record the electrical activity. Normal muscle is electrically silent at rest. Spontaneous discharges of single muscle fibers at rest (*fibrillation potentials*) indicate denervation. During normal muscular contraction, groups of muscle fibers in a motor unit are activated in unison and generate a *motor unit potential.* Decrease in size of motor unit potentials is seen in primary diseases of muscle. In diseases of peripheral nerves the motor units are decreased in number, but they often are of abnormally large size as a result of collateral innervation of denervated muscle fibers.

Measurements of velocity of nerve conduction are helpful in the confirmation of peripheral nerve disorders. Maximum velocity is decreased in inflammatory and metabolic diseases of peripheral nerves, especially when the myelin sheaths of the nerve fibers are affected.

Muscle Biopsy. This is frequently necessary to establish the diagnosis of a specific neuromuscular disease. Both histochemical and electron microscopic examination of the biopsy tissue may be needed.

Neuroroentgenography. *Skull roentgenograms* can identify intracranial calcifications, craniosynostosis, skull fractures, or bony defects. They may also provide information regarding intracranial pressure. Elevated pressure in the child causes separation of the cranial sutures; if it is longstanding, the posterior clinoid processes are eroded, the sella turcica may be flattened and enlarged, and the convolutional impressions on the inner table of the skull are accentuated and have a "beaten-silver" appearance. This pattern of the skull is not by itself necessarily evidence of increased intracranial pressure or of any abnormality.

Computed tomography (CT scan) is a noninvasive technique for demonstration of intracranial structures. The method uses a computer to detect small variations in tissue density by assembling data from multiple tomographic sections through the head. Brain tissue is clearly distinguishable from cerebrospinal fluid-filled spaces; the technique is therefore well suited for the demonstration of ventricular size, displacements of the ventricular system by mass lesions, and subdural collections of fluid. Edematous brain (e.g., in the area of an infarct or contusion) has lower density than normal brain. Cerebral hemorrhages, calcifications, and some solid tumors are detectable as areas of high density. The resolution of the method is increased if the study is repeated after intravenous infusion of a radiopaque contrast material. Such infusion results in increased density in areas of heightened vascularity such as vascular malformations, the capsule surrounding a brain abscess, and vascular tumors. Computed tomography now is the primary method for the study of space-occupying intracranial lesions. *Magnetic resonance imaging (MRI)* is an alternative method to CT. It detects changes in spin resonance of protons subjected to a strong magnetic field. Tissues that differ in water content can be differentiated. Tomographic sections similar to CT sections are generated through brain or spinal cord. The method has the advantage of high safety, since ionizing radiation is not involved. It provides remarkably clear views of normal brain anatomy in vivo. Early data indicate that it is particularly useful for detection of demyelinating disease and for study of spinal cord lesions.

Cerebral *angiography* remains the definitive test for the study of cerebral vascular disorders, including arteriovenous malformations, arterial occlusions, and venous thrombosis. In the child, the procedure is carried out most easily and safely via an arterial catheter introduced into one of the femoral arteries.

Radionuclide brain scan is of value for detection of certain local brain lesions. A radioactive material, usually involving technetium-99m, is injected intravenously, and radioactivity over the skull is counted after a fixed time interval. The test material tends to accumulate in areas of defective blood-brain barrier, especially in tumors and around brain abscesses. Positive uptakes are also seen with encephalitis and with subdural hematoma. Cerebral infarcts due to vascular occlusion often lead to positive brain scans starting about 1 wk after infarction; reversion to normal occurs in 3–4 wk.

Two-dimensional (B mode) *ultrasonography* of the head can safely and rapidly evaluate ventricular size and detect intracranial hemorrhages or masses in infants with open anterior fontanelles.

Myelography is important in the diagnosis of mass lesions situated in or encroaching upon the spinal cord. Either metrizamide or air is used as contrast material. The injection is made through a lumbar spinal needle when possible. Pantopaque myelography carries some small definite risk of meningeal reaction to the injected material, which may result in incapacitating and occasionally fatal arachnoiditis.

Bachman DS, Hodges FJ III, Freeman JM: Computerized axial tomography in neurologic disorders of children. Pediatrics 59:352, 1977.
Brazelton TB, Scholl ML, Robey JS: Visual responses in the newborn. Pediatrics 37:284, 1966.
Denny-Brown D: Handbook of Neurological Examination and Case Recording. Cambridge, Harvard University Press, 1965.
Dodge PR, Porter P: Demonstration of intracranial pathology by transillumination. Arch Neurol 5:594, 1961.
Fois A: Clinical Electroencephalography in Epilepsy and Related Conditions in Childhood. Springfield, IL, Charles C Thomas, 1963.
Harwood-Nash D, Fitz CR: Neuroradiology in infants and Children. St. Louis, CV Mosby, 1976.
Hurley PJ, Wagner HN: Diagnostic value of brain scanning in children. JAMA 221:877, 1972.
Lorber J, Granger RG: Cerebral cavities following ventricular puncture in infants. Clin Radiol 14:98, 1963.
Norris F: The EMG: A Guide and Atlas for Practical Electromyography. New York, Grune & Stratton, 1963.
Paine RS, Oppe TE: Neurologic Examinations of Children. Clinics in Developmental Medicine, Vol 20–21. London, William Heinemann, Ltd., 1966.
Rumack CM: Perinatal and Infant Brain Imaging: Role of Ultrasound and Computed Tomography. Year Book Medical Publishing Chicago, 1984.
Shaywitz BA: Epidermoid spinal cord tumors and previous lumbar puncture. J Pediatr 80:638, 1972.
Smith FW: NMR imaging in Pediatric practice. Pediatrics 71:852, 1983.
Widell S: On the cerebrospinal fluid in normal children and in patients with acute abacterial meningo-encephalitis. Acta Pediatr Suppl 115, 1958.

21.6 THE COMATOSE CHILD

Clinical Assessment. Evaluation of the comatose child must provide certain critical information as soon as possible: Is circulation adequate? Is the airway patent, with sufficient respiratory exchange? Is intracranial pressure elevated, and, if so, is the elevation great enough to be life-threatening? Is there a focal neurologic sign or deficit that might indicate a localized, surgically remediable brain lesion? Is the coma likely to be due to remediable metabolic disease?

The *vital signs*—pulse, respiration, and blood pressure—evaluate circulation and airway and may give clues to the diagnosis. The pulse is often slow and blood pressure elevated when intracranial pressure is high. Hyperventilation is usually the result of metabolic acidosis, but it may also occur in respiratory alkalosis because of abnormal stimulation of the medullary respiratory center (e.g., in salicylate poisoning, hepatic coma, or Reye syndrome). Periodic breathing and irregular (ataxic) breathing are signs of medullary dysfunction; they often precede complete apnea.

The *pupillary reactions* should be assessed when the patient is first seen and at frequent intervals thereafter. Unilateral dilatation with decrease in the light reflex is usually secondary to 3rd nerve damage by tentorial herniation of the brain (Fig. 21–4); it is often an indication for emergency medical or surgical measures to reduce intracranial pressure. A dilated pupil may also be due to eye trauma, or it may be a transient postictal finding following a major motor seizure. When both pupils are in fixed dilation for more than 5 min, it often (but not invariably) reflects irreversible brain stem damage. The pupils may be unreactive in hypothermia and in reversible coma resulting from poisoning by sedative or atropine-like drugs. Dilated, unreactive pupils may also be due to previous local instillation of mydriatics. Pinpoint pupils are seen in poisoning with opiates, during barbiturate coma, and with pontine lesions.

Eye movements in comatose patients are tested by the *doll's head maneuver*. The head is quickly rotated to one side, then to the other. The eyes normally show conjugate deviation to the side opposite the direction of head rotation. Absence of this response in a comatose patient implies dysfunction of

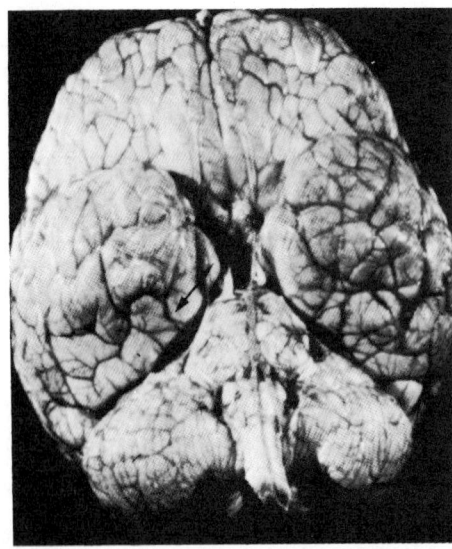

Figure 21–4. Tentorial herniation secondary to diffuse cerebral edema. The arrow points to the portion of temporal lobe that has herniated through the tentorium. A groove, produced by the tentorial edge, is clearly visible. The 3rd nerve is just below and medial to the area of herniation.

brain stem or of oculomotor nerves. Deviation of the eye down and laterally is frequently seen in association with pupillary dilatation in 3rd nerve dysfunction due to tentorial herniation. Sixth nerve palsy is usually due to increased intracranial pressure; it does not carry as ominous a prognosis as does 3rd nerve dysfunction.

Funduscopic examination should be carried out to determine whether papilledema is present. Mydriatics should not be used since they interfere with pupillary reactions that are critical in clinical assessment of the comatose patient. The absence of papilledema does not rule out increased intracranial pressure of recent onset since papilledema takes 24–48 hr to develop. Distention of retinal veins and absence of venous pulsations are early signs of elevated intracranial tension. Preretinal hemorrhages are usually the result of subarachnoid or subdural bleeding.

Assessment of motor functions includes observations of spontaneous activity, posture, and response to noxious stimuli. In deep coma, primitive postural reflex patterns emerge as cortical control over motor functions is lost. In *"decorticate posturing"* the arms are flexed on the chest, hands are fisted, and legs extended. This position is seen in severe, diffuse dysfunction of the cerebral cortex. *"Decerebrate posturing"* is characterized by rigid extension and pronation of arms and extension of legs, often in response to painful stimulation. It is a sign of dysfunction at the level of the midbrain. When decerebrate posturing is unilateral, it is often caused by tentorial herniation, in which case there may be associated contralateral paralysis of the 3rd nerve.

Hemiplegia can be diagnosed even in the deeply comatose patient. The paretic leg lies in external rotation. It moves less than the opposite leg, both spontaneously and in response to pain. The paretic extremity drops more limply when it is picked up and allowed to fall.

Grading of the *stage of coma* is helpful in charting the course of the patient:

Stage I—drowsiness.

Stage II—stupor. The patient can be roused for brief periods, during which he or she may be able to make simple verbal and voluntary motor responses. Stupor may alternate with *delirium*, which is a state of mental confusion and motor excitement.

Stage III—light coma. The patient cannot be roused, even with painful stimuli. He may moan and make semipurposeful avoidance movements.

Stage IV—deep coma. Painful stimuli now fail to produce a response, or they lead to extension and pronation of arms (decerebrate posturing).

Stage V—patient is flaccid and apneic. All brain stem functions are lost. Some spinal reflexes may be preserved.

The Glasgow coma scale provides more detailed information about motor, visual, and verbal responses and is often used in following the course of patients with head injury.

The use of artificial ventilation has made it possible to maintain circulation after all brain function is irreversibly lost. This state has been called *brain death*. The criteria for brain death are as follows: (1) absence of all cerebral function, including pupillary responses, spontaneous respiratory efforts, and all but local spinal reflexes for a period of at least 24 hr; (2) total absence of brain waves on at least two EEG recordings obtained 24 hr apart; (3) certainty that absence of brain functions is secondary to conditions other than drug intoxication or hypothermia. Termination of resuscitative efforts is justified when each of these three conditions has been appropriately determined to have been met.

Differential Diagnosis. Information gained during the examination will usually make it possible to place the patient into one of four categories, depending on whether intracranial pressure is elevated and on whether there are focal neurologic signs. Table 21–3 provides the likely diagnostic possibilities in each category.

Laboratory studies which may be needed include blood sugar, serum electrolytes, blood gases, blood urea nitrogen (BUN), liver function tests, and toxicologic screening. Examination of cerebrospinal fluid (CSF) is usually necessary to rule out bacterial meningitis. Lumbar puncture carries a risk of tentorial herniation in the patient with increased intracranial pressure, especially when a focal brain lesion is present. Neurosurgical consultation should be obtained prior to spinal tap in a child with increased intracranial pressure and focal neurologic signs. Diagnosis of the comatose child with focal signs usually requires computed tomography.

Management. The comatose child requires meticulous attention to respiratory status. The child should not be maintained supine but rather on his or her side or in a semiprone position to minimize the danger of aspiration of saliva or vomitus. Frequent suctioning of secretions is essential. The comatose patient should never be left unattended.

Moderately severe hypoxia may not be clinically evident; accordingly, repeated determinations of blood gas values are necessary. Hyperventilation may lead to respiratory alkalosis, which can be distinguished from metabolic acidosis only by measurement of pH.

Intravenous fluid therapy in the comatose child must be carefully monitored by serial determinations of serum electrolytes. The most common mistake is overhydration, which may result in water intoxication; frequently, the child in coma is unable to cope with what would be a moderate water load at other times. This inability is thought to be the result of dysfunction of the hypothalamus, with inappropriate secretion of antidiuretic hormone (ADH). The affected patient excretes scant quantities of concentrated urine in the face of hypervolemia and hyponatremia. Attention only to urine output may give the erroneous impression that the child is dehydrated. Fatal cerebral edema may result if excess administration of hypotonic solutions is continued. The treatment of inappropriate ADH secretion consists only of fluid restriction until serum electrolyte levels and osmolality return to normal (Sec. 5.30).

Prompt therapeutic intervention may be lifesaving in the comatose patient with marked increase in intracranial pres-

Table 21–3. **Differential Diagnosis of Coma**

No Focal Signs		Focal Signs	
Normal CSF Pressure	*Increased CSF Pressure*	*Normal CSF Pressure*	*Increased CSF Pressure*
Most metabolic encephalopathies	Some metabolic encephalopathies (lead poisoning, water intoxication, Reye syndrome, severe anoxia)	Vascular disease (cerebral artery occlusion)	Trauma (subdural, epidural or intracerebral hemorrhage, cerebral contusion)
Drug intoxication CNS infection (meningitis, encephalitis)	CNS infection (meningitis, encephalitis)	CNS infection (encephalitis)	Brain tumor CNS infection (brain abscess, subdural empyema, encephalitis)
Trauma (concussion)	Trauma (subdural hemorrhage in infants, subarachnoid hemorrhage)	Trauma (cerebral contusion)	
Epilepsy (postictal state)	Brain tumor (midline tumors) Hydrocephalus	Epilepsy (postictal state with Todd paralysis)	Vascular disease (arteriovenous malformation)

sure, especially when evidence of tentorial herniation is present. When increased intracranial pressure is due to hydrocephalus or to ventricular obstruction by tumor, it is relieved most quickly and effectively by ventricular tap. Several medical measures can reduce the increased intracranial pressure caused by brain swelling. Controlled hyperventilation rapidly lowers intracranial pressure through constriction of cerebral vessels. Osmotic diuretics also are useful in emergencies; they lead to decrease in brain volume and to lowering in pressure within minutes of the start of infusion. Mannitol (0.5–2 g/kg) and urea (0.5–1 g/kg) administered rapidly by vein are most effective. An indwelling urinary catheter is needed to prevent overdistention of the bladder by the induced diuresis. The effect of these agents is transient, rarely lasting over 6 hr. Their effectiveness decreases markedly on repeated use. High doses of synthetic corticosteroids are useful for more prolonged control of cerebral edema. Dexamethasone, 0.2–0.4 mg/kg intravenously, followed by 0.1–0.2 mg/kg intramuscularly every 6 hr, is commonly employed. A therapeutic response is usually seen within 6 hr. Stools must be checked for occult blood, and serum electrolytes must be carefully monitored while the child is receiving steroids. The above measures should not replace or delay definitive therapy for the underlying disease when it is available. In the management of severe cerebral edema such as occurs in major head injury and in Reye syndrome, continuous monitoring of intracranial pressure by means of intraventricular catheters or devices implanted in the subdural or subarachnoid spaces is useful.

Adequate nutritional intake must be assured when coma is prolonged. Nasogastric or nasojejunal feeding should be initiated as soon as the acute phase of the illness has subsided. The usual hospital diet mixed in a food blender makes an excellent feeding mixture, which is often tolerated better than many artificial formulas.

Goldberg M: Hyponatremia and the inappropriate secretion of antidiuretic hormone. Am J Med 35:293, 1963.
Guidelines for the determination of death. Report of the Medical Consultants on the Diagnosis of Death to the President's Commission for the Study of Ethical Problems in Medicine and Biomedical and Behavioral Research. JAMA 246:2184, 1981.
Mickell JJ, Reigel DH, Cook DR, et al: Intracranial pressure: Monitoring and normalization therapy in children. Pediatrics 59:606, 1977.
Plum F, Posner JB: The Diagnosis of Stupor and Coma. Ed 2. Philadelphia. FA Davis Co, 1972.
Teasdale G, Jennett B: Assessment of coma and impaired consciousness: A practical scale. Lancet 2:81, 1974.

21.7 THE CHILD WITH A CONVULSIVE DISORDER

Convulsions are among the most common acute and potentially life-threatening events encountered in infants and children. About 5% of children have had one or more convulsions by the time they reach maturity. The range of clinical manifestations is wide, with several syndromes having specific types of seizure as the major symptom. Accurate diagnosis is important, since etiology, therapy, and prognosis differ for the various forms.

Several terms are applied to convulsive disorders. "Seizure" is the least specific and refers to a variety of paroxysmal events thought to represent abnormal electrical activity in cerebral neurons. "Convulsions" are seizures that include motor phenomena, either repetitive (clonic) or maintained (tonic) involuntary contractions of muscles, which may be generalized or confined to specific muscle groups. "Epilepsy"

Table 21–4. **Classifications of Seizures**

ILAE Classification	Other Terminology
I. Partial seizures	
A. Simple partial seizures	
1. With motor signs	Jacksonian seizures or focal motor seizures
2. With somatosensory or special sensory (visual, auditory, olfactory, gustatory, vertiginous) symptoms	Sensory seizures
3. With autonomic symptoms or signs	Abdominal epilepsy or epileptic equivalent
B. Complex partial seizures	Psychomotor or temporal lobe seizures
II. Generalized seizures	
A. Absence seizures	
1. Typical	Petit mal
2. Atypical	Petit mal variant or complex petit mal
B. Myoclonic seizures	Myoclonic seizures
C. Atonic seizures	Akinetic seizures or drop attacks
D. Tonic-clonic seizures	Grand mal, major motor seizures, generalized convulsive seizures

refers to recurrent seizures, either of unknown etiology (idiopathic epilepsy) or due to congenital or acquired brain lesions (symptomatic, organic, or secondary epilepsies).

Several classifications of seizures have been proposed, with a scheme developed by the International League Against Epilepsy [ILAE] coming into increasing use. A short version of this classification, together with previously used terms, is given in Table 21–4.

TYPES OF SEIZURES

Partial seizures affect only one cerebral hemisphere, in part or totally. Consciousness is preserved, but certain cognitive functions may be transiently impaired, such as speech in seizures involving the dominant hemisphere.

Partial seizures with motor signs include several types. Clonic seizure activity may start in a single muscle group (often finger flexors), from where it spreads to contiguous groups (jacksonian march) until an entire side of the body is involved. The patient remains alert, unless seizure activity spreads to the other cerebral hemisphere, in which case the attack eventuates in a generalized tonic-clonic seizure. Seizures with jacksonian march are often due to focal lesions located in the part of the motor cortex in which the first affected movement originates. Focal motor seizures without jacksonian march have less localizing value, especially in the case of seizures including head and eye deviation to one side (versive seizures), which may be due to epileptic discharges in either the ipsilateral or the contralateral cerebral hemisphere. Following a focal motor seizure there often is transient paralysis on the involved side (Todd paralysis), which may last up to about 24 hr. It is especially common in young children. Focal motor seizure activity may rarely be continuous over a period of weeks, months, or even years. This condition is known as epilepsia partialis continua. In children, it is usually a manifestation of chronic focal encephalitis.

Partial seizures with sensory symptoms may produce a transient sensation of pins and needles or of numbness on one side, sometimes with focal onset and a march analogous to jacksonian, but reflecting epileptic discharges in parietal rather than motor cortex. Visual seizures due to occipital lobe involvement are reported as a sensation of flashing white lights. Olfactory seizures may begin as unpleasant odors and become generalized into clonic or tonic-clonic seizures; such "uncinate fits" are often an early manifestation of a temporal lobe tumor. Vertiginous seizures may be difficult to differentiate from other causes of vertigo, including benign paroxysmal vertigo, migraine, and labyrinthitis.

Autonomic seizures consist of transient disturbances in vegetative functions. They include such symptoms and signs as pallor, flushing, headache, tachycardia, dilation of the pupils, abdominal pain, and loss of bladder control. The abdominal pain experienced during an autonomic seizure is poorly localized and is associated with other signs of transient autonomic disturbance. In children, recurrent abdominal pain is usually due to conditions other than seizures. Symptoms and signs of autonomic nervous system stimulation are commonly associated with other seizure types—especially with complex partial seizures.

Complex partial seizures are due to epileptic discharges in the temporal lobes. They have a wide range of clinical manifestations. The patient is confused at the time of the attack, without complete loss of consciousness. The early part of the attack is often remembered. Reported experiences include dreamy states, flashbacks during which prior experiences are recalled in rapid succession, feelings of depersonalization, and the sensation that an event had occurred previously (*déjà vu*) or that something that should be familiar appears totally strange or novel (*jamais vu*). Various illusions may occur, including complex formed visual hallucinations and distortions of perception, such as objects appearing larger (macropsia) or smaller (micropsia), or voices sounding far away and indistinct or unusually loud. In focal seizures involving the dominant temporal lobe, speech is arrested or garbled. Disturbances in mood occur if deep temporal lobe or limbic structures are involved. Fear and anxiety are the most common mood changes. Anger and aggression are less likely and tend to be unprovoked and undirected. Laughing may occur as one component of the attack ("gelastic seizures"). Complex partial seizures usually are accompanied by stereotyped and semipurposeful motor activities (motor automatisms), the most common of which involve movements of the mouth, including chewing and swallowing. Often there also is meaningless repetition of speech sounds. Other automatisms include picking at clothing, walking, and running—the latter often in association with fright or terror. Following a complex partial seizure there may be a period of postictal depression with drowsiness or sleep. After brief attacks normal alertness may be regained almost immediately.

Generalized seizures affect the brain as a whole, including both cerebral hemispheres and often also subcortical structures. They may be generalized from the onset, or focal in onset with secondary generalization. When onset is focal, the seizure may be preceded by symptoms or signs of a partial seizure. When these symptoms are remembered after a seizure, they are referred to as a seizure warning or *aura*. Consciousness is lost during a generalized seizure, but the period of loss may be so short as to be barely noticeable (for example, in generalized myoclonic seizures).

Typical absence seizures (petit mal) are a form of primary generalized seizure consisting of sudden brief arrest of motor activity associated with a blank stare and loss of awareness. Upward deviation of the eyes or rapid eye blinking may occasionally be associated. Postural tone is not affected, and the patient does not fall with the attacks. There is no remembrance of the attack, except for the realization that a short period of time has been lost.

Atypical absence attacks may have associated motor automatisms (such as lip smacking or fumbling with the hands) or autonomic disturbances (including loss of bladder control). Such attacks may be difficult to distinguish clinically from complex partial seizures, and electroencephalographic study is usually needed for definitive identification. At times, atypical absence attacks become almost continuous over periods of hours or days, in which case the child lapses into a constant state of stupor (petit mal status or spike-wave stupor).

Myoclonic seizures consist of sudden, brief shock-like contractions of muscles. They often involve flexor muscles bilaterally. In infants, the sudden flexion movements of the limbs and trunk are referred to as infantile spasms. In older children generalized myoclonic seizures often result in sudden falls (lightning or jackknife seizures). Myoclonic seizures need to be differentiated from myoclonus due to subcortical mechanisms, such as intention or action myoclonus due to disturbances in cerebellar and brain stem functions (often as a sequel to cerebral anoxia). In intention myoclonus voluntary movement of a limb toward a target produces repetitive jerking of muscles. Another form of myoclonus not related to epilepsy is that seen in the infantile polymyoclonus-opsoclonus syndrome (Sec. 21.20). Occasionally, myoclonus confined to one or more adjacent spinal cord segments is due to a focal spinal cord lesion, such as tumor or vascular malformation.

Atonic seizures consist of sudden loss of postural tone and consciousness. They may be very brief, in which case a sudden drop of the head or sudden fall may be the only manifestation. Differentiation from myoclonic seizures may be difficult. More prolonged attacks may begin with a fall, but the patient then remains limp and unresponsive for seconds or minutes. These attacks may mimic syncope and cataplexy. The more prolonged atonic seizures are usually followed by postictal drowsiness, which helps to distinguish them from these other conditions.

Tonic-clonic seizures are the most severe types of seizures and are potentially life-threatening. An attack may start suddenly or be preceded by an aura. The patient loses consciousness and may fall to the floor. The early part of the seizure often consists of sustained contraction of muscles (tonic phase). Respirations are impaired, and the patient becomes cyanotic. The teeth are tightly clenched and the tongue or lip may be bitten. There may be excessive salivation, vomiting, and loss of bladder and bowel control, as indicators of autonomic nervous system involvement. The tonic phase is followed by intermittent muscular contraction (clonic phase). The eyes may jerk upward or to one side. At the end of the seizure the patient relaxes, and normal respirations resume. A period of deep sleep–like postictal depression of variable duration follows. When the patient awakens, he or she often reports severe headache and muscle aches. Prolonged tonic-clonic seizures produce major metabolic disturbances, including hypoxemia, hypercarbia, respiratory acidosis, and lactic acidemia. Partial seizures may represent only a tonic or clonic phase.

In *status epilepticus* repeated tonic-clonic seizures occur without intervening recovery of consciousness. It always represents a medical emergency and may end fatally or with permanent sequelae of anoxic brain damage unless properly treated.

Commission on Classification and Terminology of the International League Against Epilepsy: Proposal for revised clinical and electroencephalographic classification of epileptic seizures. Epilepsia 22:489, 1981.

CONDITIONS HAVING SEIZURES AS MAJOR MANIFESTATIONS

Febrile Convulsions

Definition. Simple febrile convulsions are a form of generalized tonic-clonic seizure seen characteristically in childhood and meeting the following diagnostic criteria: (1) occurrence in infancy or early childhood, usually between ages 6 mo and 5 yr; (2) fever at the time of the attack, usually greater than 38°C; (3) brief duration (always less than 15 min); (4) absence of central nervous system infection; and (5) absence of neurologic abnormalities in the interictal period.

Pathophysiology and Etiology. Febrile convulsions are triggered by a rapid rise in body temperature. The associated increase in metabolic rate of cerebral neurons lowers their seizure threshold. The occurrence of febrile convulsions appears to require also a genetic susceptibility; a history of febrile convulsions is found in parents or siblings in 60–70% of cases.

Incidence. Between 4 and 5% of all children have one or more febrile convulsions. These are especially commonly associated with illnesses that cause high fever late in infancy, such as otitis media and roseola infantum. The convulsion usually occurs early in the illness, during the period of rapid temperature rise and may be the first indication that the child is ill. About 50% of children have no recurrence during subsequent febrile episodes. The occurrence in a child of more than five or six febrile convulsions is unusual. Occasionally, more than one convulsion occurs during a single febrile episode.

Clinical Manifestations. The seizures are generalized tonic-clonic or atonic, without aura. Children who have partial seizures or prolonged generalized seizures with fever are likely to have conditions other than simple febrile convulsions, most commonly idiopathic epilepsy. There is rarely any marked disturbance in respiration. The postictal stupor tends to be brief, and the child has often returned to normal alertness by the time he or she is seen by a physician.

Laboratory Studies and Differential Diagnosis. It is most important that the possibility of central nervous system infections, especially acute bacterial meningitis, be excluded promptly. Examination of the spinal fluid is essential if there is persistent drowsiness, fullness of the anterior fontanel, or nuchal rigidity. The possibility needs to be excluded also of intoxication by medications that may have been used for symptomatic treatment, such as phenothiazines, xanthines, or narcotics. When diarrhea or vomiting is associated, one has to consider electrolyte imbalance, ketotic hypoglycemia, and toxic encephalopathy such as occurs with *Shigella* infection. It may be difficult to differentiate simple febrile convulsions from epilepsy, which frequently has its onset with fever-associated seizures in infancy. Such seizures in children with epilepsy usually fail, however, to fulfill all of the diagnostic criteria for simple febrile convulsions. There is often pre-existing neurologic impairment or developmental delay, the seizures tend to be more prolonged and may have focal aspects, and they tend to occur with fevers that are lower than those seen with simple febrile seizures.

Electroencephalography is of little use for the 1st wk after a seizure, when it is apt to show diffuse postictal slow-wave activity. A tracing obtained after one or more weeks may be of diagnostic help in doubtful cases. In children with simple febrile convulsions results of such a study tend to be normal, whereas epileptiform discharges will be seen in about two thirds of children with idiopathic epilepsy.

Treatment. Antipyretic measures including sponging with tepid water and antipyretic medications such as acetaminophen are indicated to prevent a second seizure during the same illness and to minimize the risk of seizures during subsequent febrile illnesses. Salicylates should be avoided if the fever is due to influenza or varicella, as their use may increase the risk for Reye syndrome.

The use of anticonvulsant drugs for prevention of recurrent febrile seizures is controversial. Limitation of administration of an anticonvulsant such as phenobarbital to the onset of febrile illnesses is ineffective, since a therapeutic blood level cannot usually be achieved by oral administration by the time the child is at greatest risk for convulsions. Continuous treatment has been advocated by some for the period when febrile seizures tend to occur (until the age of about 5 yr). Phenobarbital is most commonly used, a dosage of about 3 mg/kg/day aiming for a blood level between 15 and 20 μg/mL. This regimen decreases the number of subsequent febrile convulsions, but does not eliminate them; its universal adoption would commit about 4% of children to the use of this drug for a period of several years. Since about 50% of children with a single febrile convulsion have no recurrence, even if untreated, at least half of the children would get no possible benefit from this therapy. A more reasonable regimen is the institution of phenobarbital therapy after a second or third febrile seizure, especially if the seizures are triggered by only modest rises in body temperature and if previous seizures have caused respiratory embarrassment. Disadvantages of chronic use of phenobarbital include a high incidence of behavioral effects, most commonly hyperkinesis, and the occasional occurrence of allergic reactions. Other drugs have been advocated, including acetazolamide and sodium valproate. The potential hepatotoxicity of the latter drug, however, makes it undesirable for use in treatment of this essentially benign disorder.

Prognosis. Earlier reports stressed the risk of anoxic brain damage during febrile convulsions, with subsequent intellectual impairment, behavior disturbances, and complex partial seizures. Such an outcome must be considered a rare event in children whose condition fulfills the diagnostic criteria for simple febrile convulsions. Prospective follow-up studies such as the United States Maternal and Infant Health Study indicate a generally good prognosis, irrespective of therapeutic regimen. Seizures independent of fever develop in about 2% of patients, approximately four times the incidence of epilepsy in the general population. The intellectual function of children with a history of febrile convulsions does not differ from that of children without such history.

Ellenberg JH, Nelson KB: Febrile seizures and later intellectual performance. Arch Neurol 35:17, 1878.

Febrile convulsions: A suitable case for treatment. Lancet 72:680, 1980.

Freeman JM: Febrile seizures: A consensus of their significance, evaluation, and treatment. Pediatrics 66:1009, 1976.

Lennox-Buchthal MA: Febrile convulsions. A reappraisal. Electroenceph Clin Neurophysiol 32(Suppl):1, 1973.

Nelson KB, Ellenberg JH: Prognosis in children with febrile seizures. Pediatrics 61:720, 1978.

Wolf, SM, Forsyth A: Behavior disturbance. phenobarbital, and febrile seizures. Pediatrics 61:728, 1978.

Idiopathic Epilepsy

Definition. Idiopathic epilepsy designates a group of conditions in which recurrent seizures occur without definable cause. Several distinct syndromes can be distinguished that differ in clinical manifestations, response to therapy, and prognosis. The diagnosis is often one of exclusion, made after definable causes of seizures have been ruled out.

Pathophysiology. Epileptic seizures reflect abnormal electrical activity in cerebral neurons. During a seizure large numbers of neurons discharge synchronously and at high frequency. The normal balance between excitatory and inhibitory influences on the activity of nerve cells seems to be disrupted. Increasing evidence points to a decrease in inhibitory influences as an important factor in epileptic activity, with the inhibitory neurons that use gamma-aminobutyric acid (GABA) as a neurotransmitter substance being particularly implicated. This concept is well supported in several animal models; in humans, the evidence for a disturbance in function of inhibitory GABAergic neurons is mainly indirect. For example, the anticonvulsant effects of a number of drugs including the benzodiazepines, barbiturates, hydantoins, and valproic acid appear to be mediated via modulation of GABA receptors or of GABA levels in brain. Abnormalities in GABAergic neurons are likely to play a role in epilepsy, but it is unlikely that this system is specifically affected in all types of seizures.

Patients with primary generalized seizures appear to have an increase in excitability of the entire cerebral cortex. Seizures appear to be triggered by afferent stimuli to hyperexcitable cortex from centers in the brain stem reticular formation. In such patients, seizure activity has its onset synchronously in all areas of cerebral cortex. In contrast, partial seizures originate in focal areas of hyperexcitable cerebral cortex; the abnormal neuronal discharges may remain localized to the seizure focus, or there may be secondary generalization. A chronic epileptogenic focus in cerebral cortex may cause abnormal neuronal activity in remote areas, especially in those with which it is directly connected, such as the homologous area in the opposite hemisphere. A so-called mirror focus in such areas may eventually act as an independent site of epileptic discharges. The development of mirror foci is thought to be especially likely in the immature brain.

Predisposition to seizures in humans is often genetically determined. Both polygenic or multifactorial inheritance and dominant inheritance with incomplete penetrance have been suggested. Hereditary factors have been well documented in petit mal epilepsy, in benign focal epilepsy of childhood, and

in photosensitive epilepsy. The incidence of clinical seizure disorder in siblings or offspring of propositi is rarely more than 7–8%, but larger percentages of relatives have abnormal electroencephalographic tracings, especially when these are obtained during childhood, when there is the greatest likelihood of expression of epileptic discharges.

Incidence. Estimates of incidence range from about 2–6/1000, reflecting inaccuracies in assignment of cases to the idiopathic versus the symptomatic category. Use of newer diagnostic methods, and especially of computed tomography, has increased the proportion of cases in which the finding of definable (usually atrophic) brain lesions more accurately classifies them among symptomatic epilepsies.

Clinical Manifestations. Any of the seizure types listed in Table 21–4, either alone or in combination with others, may be manifestations of idiopathic epilepsy. One form of seizure commonly predominates, and several specific syndromes are recognized.

Petit mal epilepsy occurs mainly during the childhood years. An otherwise well child begins to have frequent episodes of blank staring and arrest of activity (typical absence seizures). The frequency of seizures may vary from seldom to several hundred per day. Inattention and decline in school performance may be noted. The problem may be ascribed at first to daydreaming. Stressful situations may precipitate attacks, probably because children with petit mal are very sensitive to hyperventilation. A simple clinical test consists of asking the child to hyperventilate for about 3 min. In children with untreated petit mal an absence seizure is almost always produced by this maneuver. There are usually no other abnormal findings on physical or neurologic examination. Intelligence is usually within the normal range.

In patients with *photosensitive epilepsy*, seizures are precipitated by flickering light. The onset often is in late childhood or adolescence. Typical precipitating stimuli include flickering sunlight encountered while driving beside a row of trees or along a rail fence or the flickering light of a defective television screen. Both myoclonic and tonic-clonic seizures are seen, often with several myoclonic jerks preceding the tonic-clonic convulsion.

Benign focal epilepsy of childhood (sylvian seizures, benign rolandic epilepsy) is seen only in children. The attacks frequently occur during sleep, and many affected children have nocturnal seizures only. Tonic-clonic seizures are seen, but more commonly attacks are partial with motor signs, the most typical being clonic movements of the facial muscles on one side. The children usually awaken during the attack and are able to hear what is said to them but unable to speak. Intelligence is normal and there are no abnormal neurologic signs.

Grand mal epilepsy may have its onset at any age from infancy to early adult life. In the young child, the first convulsions are often triggered by fever (see above). Frequency of seizures varies from several per wk to less than one per yr. It is usually not possible to identify factors that are likely to precipitate attacks. In some instances, seizures may be triggered by such specific activities as reading or exposure to specific sound patterns. Postmenarchal girls may have seizures more frequently during the days just prior to the onset of menses. Nonspecific factors such as fatigue or emotional upheaval are often implicated, but such relationships are difficult to prove.

The child with frequent, prolonged tonic-clonic or grand mal seizures is at risk of anoxic brain damage during the attacks. The risk appears to be greater in younger children. Sequelae include intellectual impairment, behavior changes, and less commonly motor deficits such as ataxia and spasticity.

Laboratory Studies. Electroencephalography (EEG) is the most useful laboratory study for diagnosis and classification

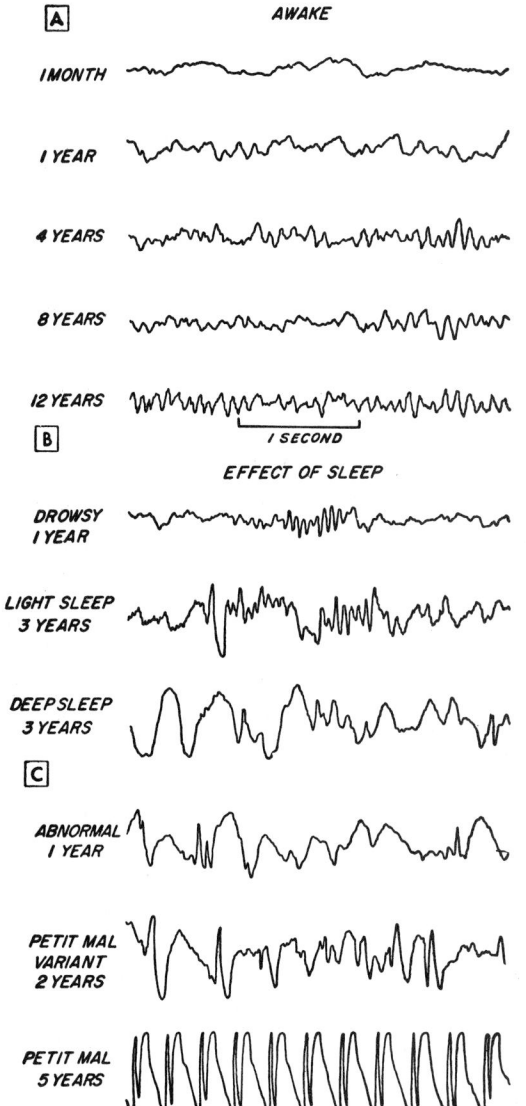

Figure 21–5. Electroencephalograms of infants and children. *A*, Tracings from comparable areas of the scalp illustrating variations with age of electrical activity in the motor cortex; all were secured during a quiet phase just before sleep. *B*, The effects of sleep, variations of patterns in normal children; compare with tracings in *A* and *C*. *C*, Abnormal waves.

of patients with epilepsy. Specific EEG patterns are found in various epileptic syndromes (Fig. 21–5). The EEG in petit mal is characterized by bursts of generalized spike-wave discharges of high voltage at a rate of 3 Hz (3/sec). Bursts lasting more than about 5 sec are accompanied by absence attacks, but shorter bursts have no obvious clinical accompaniments. In photosensitive epilepsy the EEG shows spike or spike-wave discharges in response to repetitive light flashes, most commonly at stimulus rates between 10 and 20 Hz. The EEG in children with sylvian seizures shows single spike or spike-wave discharges in the central and midtemporal areas, localized to one side. The EEG is less characteristic in children with other clinical manifestations of idiopathic epilepsy. In about 30% the interictal record is normal, even when activation procedures are employed, which include hyperventilation, repetitive photic stimulation, and recording during sleep.

Indications for other laboratory tests depend on seizure type and on associated physical and neurologic findings. In the child with typical absence attacks confirmed by a characteristic EEG tracing, there is no need for further diagnostic studies. A CT scan of the head is usually obtained in patients with other types of recurrent seizures, in order to find the occasional patient in whom the seizures are due to brain tumor or cerebrovascular malformation. CT scan also helps to differentiate idiopathic epilepsy from such other conditions as malformations of the brain, tuberous sclerosis, and atrophic brain lesions. The CT scan is normal in children with idiopathic epilepsy except, occasionally, when severe tonic-clonic seizures have produced cerebral atrophy through hypoxia. Rarely, focal areas of low density on CT scan occur as a transient abnormality after prolonged seizures.

Basic blood studies (fasting glucose, calcium, magnesium, and electrolyte measurements) are usually indicated to rule out common metabolic disturbances that may cause seizures. A blood lead level should be obtained in the young child who may be at risk for lead poisoning. Urine amino acid and organic acid analyses are indicated when recurrent seizures and mental retardation coexist.

Differential Diagnosis. The differential diagnosis of idiopathic epilepsy is complex, especially in patients with tonic-clonic seizures and with partial seizures. A partial list of conditions to be considered is provided in Table 21–5. Careful examination of the child will help to exclude many of these. The dermatologic manifestations of the neurocutaneous syndromes are usually obvious, except in the young child with tuberous sclerosis who may have faint hypopigmented macules as the only physical finding, demonstrable only by examination under ultraviolet light. Funduscopic examination may demonstrate papilledema in patients with space-occupying intracranial lesions, chorioretinitis in children with prior intrauterine infections, and phacomata in tuberous sclerosis.

The neurologic examination is normal in children with idiopathic epilepsy, with few exceptions. Neurologic signs such as the Babinski sign, enhanced tendon reflexes, and asymmetry of pupils may occur transiently following a seizure. Patients receiving anticonvulsant medications may have neurologic signs of drug toxicity, such as lethargy, nystagmus, and ataxia.

The differentiation of seizures from pseudoseizures of hysteria or malingering may present special problems during the late childhood and teenage years, especially since both conditions may coexist in the same patient. Forced eye closure and moaning, often seen during pseudoseizures, do not occur during true convulsions. In doubtful cases prolonged EEG recordings are indicated, with careful correlation of clinical and electrical events during seizure episodes.

A number of other paroxysmal disorders may be confused with epilepsy. They include benign paroxysmal vertigo, breath-holding attacks, migraine, vasovagal and cardiac forms of syncope, and narcolepsy. Careful observation and description of the attacks is essential for proper diagnosis. The presence of postictal depression after most types of epileptic seizures is of help in their differentiation from other paroxysmal events.

Treatment. The physician should be thoroughly familiar with the indications and effects of the commonly used anticonvulsant drugs. In addition, proper management includes education of the family and of the child, and attention to any associated emotional and learning disorders.

Chronic Anticonvulsant Drug Therapy. A drug schedule that controls the seizures and at the same time has minimal side effects has to be tailored to the needs of each patient. The choice of drug depends on seizure type and to some extent on the age of the child. Treatment should always begin with a single drug, given at increasing dosage until seizures are controlled or until clinical manifestations of toxicity appear or blood levels near the high end of the recommended therapeutic range are reached. If the first drug fails to control the attacks at therapeutic blood levels, a second drug may be

Table 21–5. **Conditions in Which Recurrent Convulsions Occur Commonly**

Cerebral neoplasms

Cerebral vascular disorders
  Arteriovenous malformations
  Cortical vein thrombosis
  Cerebral artery thrombosis or embolism
  Vasculitis

Cerebral Trauma
  Subdural hematoma (especially child abuse)
  Cerebral contusion or hemorrhage

Neurocutaneous syndromes
  Tuberous sclerosis
  Neurofibromatosis
  Sturge-Weber disease
  Klippel-Trenaunay-Weber syndrome
  Linear sebaceous nevus syndrome
  Incontinentia pigmenti

Cerebral malformations
  Chromosomal anomalies (Down syndrome, fragile X syndrome)
  Agenesis of corpus callosum
  Porencephaly
  Hydrocephalus

Nutritional disorders
  Pyridoxine deficiency

Poisonings
  Lead encephalopathy
  Drug intoxications (phenothiazines, xanthines, amphetamines)

Metabolic disorders
  Hypoglycemia
  Hypocalcemia and hypomagnesemia
  Renal failure
  Water intoxication
  Inborn metabolic errors (especially phenylketonuria, pyridoxine dependency, defects in Krebs urea cycle enzymes, congenital lactic acidemia, propionic acidemia, maple sugar urine disease, Menkes (kinky hair) disease)

Atrophic brain lesions
  Postanoxic
  Post-traumatic
  Postinfectious

Central nervous system infections
  Meningitis
  Encephalitis
  Brain abscess

Degenerative brain diseases
  Gangliosidoses
  Batten disease
  Alper disease
  Familial myoclonus epilepsy

In petit mal ethosuximide is the drug of choice. Significant reduction in seizure frequency occurs at therapeutic blood levels in almost all patients. Occasionally, addition of a second drug, either phenobarbital or acetazolamide, may be necessary. Valproic acid and tridione also are effective, but their potential for serious toxicity probably outweighs their therapeutic benefit in an essentially benign condition such as petit mal.

For drug treatment of the other forms of epilepsy, four major anticonvulsants are available: phenobarbital, phenytoin, carbamazepine, and valproic acid. In preschool children, phenobarbital or one of its derivatives such as mephobarbital or primidone should be used first, since valproic acid has been reported occasionally to cause severe hepatotoxicity in this age group. The cosmetic effects of phenytoin, including development of acromegaloid features, are especially prominent when administration is begun in the young child. Experience with carbamazepine in preschool children is still somewhat limited, and the recommended frequent monitoring of blood counts and liver function tests may be disturbing to the young child. The use of barbiturates is limited in some children by unacceptable behavior changes, especially hyperactivity, even when blood levels are well within the therapeutic range. In that case one of the other three agents needs to be substituted. In the older child or adolescent carbamazepine, phenytoin, or valproic acid may be used as the first drug. In older children there are no major differences in the relative safety of these agents. Phenytoin is the most difficult to regulate of the three, since small changes in dosage may have large effects on blood levels once a therapeutic level is reached. Symptoms of overdosage include nausea, vomiting, drowsiness, deterioration in school performance (pseudodementia), ataxia, and nystagmus. These drugs may be used in combination if one alone fails to control the attacks. It is rarely necessary to combine more than two anticonvulsants, and there is no good evidence that seizure control can be improved by using four or more agents.

Anticonvulsant therapy is usually continued until the patient has been seizure-free for 3–4 yr. A shorter seizure-free interval is acceptable in the young child in whom continuing rapid development of the brain may raise the seizure threshold relatively quickly. The dosage of anticonvulsant drugs should always be lowered gradually over a period of several months. Whether the EEG can help guide the rate of lowering anticonvulsant dosage is not fully answered by available data. Several studies have found little predictive value in the EEG and have concluded that anticonvulsants may be safely discontinued after an appropriate seizure-free interval even when epileptiform discharges persist on the EEG tracing.

Acute Management of Tonic-Clonic Seizures or of Status Epilepticus. This begins with the establishment of an airway and adequate ventilation. Insertion of an oral airway tube, gentle suctioning of the oropharynx, and provision of oxygen by mask are usually sufficient. Tracheal intubation is rarely needed and is likely to be traumatic if attempted during a seizure. The patient is placed on his or her side rather than supine to minimize the risk of aspiration. Anticonvulsant drugs are administered intravenously if emergency equipment is available. Prior to drug injection a sample of blood is withdrawn for measurement of glucose, calcium, electrolyte, and anticonvulsant levels. A rapid infusion of a glucose solution (about 2 mL/kg of 20% dextrose in sterile water) is given if hypoglycemia is a possible or likely cause of seizure.

Diazepam is the drug of choice for control of ongoing convulsive activity in view of its high efficacy, very rapid onset of action, and relative safety. Transient respiratory depression may occur, especially if other CNS depressant drugs have been given previously and if the drug is injected repeatedly. In that case, ventilatory assistance is given by air

added or another one may be tried alone. Monitoring of anticonvulsant blood levels is essential for proper management, both because rates of metabolism and degree of absorption of anticonvulsant drugs vary considerably from patient to patient and to ensure that there is compliance with drug administration. It has to be kept in mind that unless an initial loading dose has been given, steady state blood levels are reached slowly, owing to the long serum half-life of most anticonvulsants (Table 21–6), and that initial failure of a drug to control the seizures may reflect this fact, rather than ineffectiveness of the agent. The frequency of administration depends on the pharmacokinetics of the drug that is used. Twice daily and at most three times daily dosages are sufficient for most of the commonly used anticonvulsants. Some of the properties and toxicities of the most commonly used anticonvulsant drugs are listed in Table 21–6.

Table 21–6. **Properties and Toxic Reactions of Commonly Used Anticonvulsants**

Drug	Serum t½* (hours)	Thera-peutic Blood Level (μg/mL)	Starting Dosage (mg/kg/ Day)	Daily Doses	Days to Attain Steady State Blood Level	How Supplied	Life Threatening Side Effects	Other Side Effects
Pheno-barbital	36–72	10–30	2–3	1 or 2	14–21	Elixir: 4 mg/mL; tablets: 15, 30, 60, and 100 mg	Stevens-Johnson syndrome (rare); blood dyscrasias (rare)	Hyperkinesis; drowsiness; drug rash
Primidone	6–18	5–10	5	2 or 3	4–7	Tablets: 50 and 250 mg; Suspension: 50 mg/mL	Same as phenobarbital	
Phenytoin	15–45	10–20	5–7	2	7–21	Tablet: 50 mg; Capsules: 30 and 100 mg	Stevens-Johnson syndrome (rare); acute hepatic necrosis (rare); blood dyscrasias (rare)	Drug rash (10% in first 2 weeks), gingival hyperplasia, lymphadenopathy, hirsutism, acromegaloid facies, ataxia, nystagmus, vomiting, dystonic reaction, rickets, folate deficiency, embryopathy (fetal hydantoin syndrome) if used during pregnancy
Carbamaz-epine	8–20	5–10	10–15	2 or 3	5–10	Tablets: 100 and 200 mg	Leukopenia, thrombocytopenia, aplastic anemia (rare)	Drowsiness, abdominal distress
Valproic acid	6–14	40–80	10–20	3 or 4	4	Capsules: 250 mg; Syrup: 50 mg/mL	Acute hepatic failure (Reye syndrome–like)	Hyperammonemia, drowsiness, alopecia, abdominal discomfort
Ethosuximide	24–36	40–80	10–20	2	5–8	Capsules: 250 mg; Syrup: 50 mg/mL	Blood dyscrasias (very rare)	Drowsiness, nausea
Clonazepam	20–32	0.015–0.04	0.04–0.05	2	10–14	Tablets: 0.5, 1, and 2 mg	Blood dyscrasias (very rare)	Drowsiness (common)
Aceta-zolamide	4–10	—	10–20	2 or 3	3	Tablets: 125 and 250 mg	Blood dyscrasias (very rare)	Metabolic acidosis, paresthesias, anorexia, weight loss

*t½ = half-life.

bag and face mask until normal respirations resume, usually within 2–3 min. The dosage of diazepam is 0.3 mg/kg body weight up to a total of 10 mg given over a period of 2–3 min. The duration of the anticonvulsant action of single dose of diazepam is only 30–60 min, owing to redistribution of the drug in tissues. It therefore is advisable to administer an anticonvulsant with longer half-life, usually phenobarbital, after the seizure has been brought under control with diazepam, or if the initial injection has failed to control the seizure. The initial dose of phenobarbital is about 10 mg/kg injected intravenously over a period of 2–3 min. Administration of diazepam may be repeated if seizure activity continues more than 10 min after the end of the phenobarbital infusion, or the administration of phenobarbital may be repeated to a total of 20 mg/kg. Another acceptable method is the intravenous administration of 20 mg/kg of phenytoin. This needs to be given slowly over a period of 15–20 min with ECG monitoring since rapid intravenous administration may depress cardiac conduction. In patients who are already receiving these drugs the dosages of phenobarbital and phenytoin need to be lowered in accordance with blood levels found prior to the start of intravenous therapy.

Persistence of status epilepticus for over 30 min despite use of the above measures calls for care by a specialist in anesthesiology or intensive care. A method that is frequently effective is the slow intravenous injection of amobarbital sodium until seizure activity subsides. This requires preparation for im-

mediate tracheal intubation and assisted ventilation if prolonged respiratory depression should occur.

Environmental Therapy of Patients with Chronic Seizure Disorders. This includes education of the family and of the child. The long-term prognosis of idiopathic epilepsy in the child with normal intellect is generally good, and this fact needs to be stressed in view of the apprehension and misinformation that most parents have regarding epilepsy. Excellent educational pamphlets may be obtained through the Epilepsy Foundation of America.

The child with good control of seizures needs a minimum of restrictions. Swimming should be closely supervised, and the child should not be allowed to climb to places where a fall might produce serious injury. All other activities, including sports, should be encouraged. In patients with uncontrolled seizures, more severe restrictions may be needed. The rare patient who has frequent unpredictable falls due to myoclonic or atonic seizures may need constant supervision and may need to wear a helmet to prevent serious head and facial injuries.

Adolescents with convulsive disorders commonly have emotional difficulties, including acting out, withdrawal, and depression. These may reflect feelings of loss of control and shame when attacks have occurred in public, reactions to peers' attitudes about their disorders, and resentment at having to take medications. Group discussions and group therapy frequently help these patients in their attempts to cope with these problems. Depressive reactions may be exacerbated by some of the anticonvulsant drugs, such as primidone. Other drugs (e.g., carbamazepine) have antidepressant actions. The adjustment difficulties of patients with uncontrolled seizures tend to be more severe after the end of the school years and may be exacerbated by job discrimination and by inability to obtain a license to drive a car.

Prognosis. In most of the few prospective long-term follow-up studies, distinction has not been made between patients with idiopathic epilepsy and those with seizures due to definable brain lesions. The prognosis is generally worse in the latter group. Pure petit mal is almost never due to structural lesions. Nearly 80% of children with typical absence seizures have outgrown the attacks by maturity; petit mal persists in about 10% of patients and another 10% develop tonic-clonic seizures, which usually respond well to anticonvulsant therapy.

The prognosis for disappearance of tonic-clonic seizures in children with negative neurologic findings is similar to that in children with petit mal. Risk factors that make it less likely that tonic-clonic seizures will remit include long duration (5 yr or more) between onset and control by drug therapy, onset after the age of 11 yr, subnormal intelligence, abnormal findings on neurologic examination, occurrence of multiple types of seizures, and abnormality of background activity on the interictal EEG. Relapses after withdrawal of medication occur in 10–15% of patients with only a single type of generalized seizures, but in 40–50% of those who have had multiple types of seizure. Patients who have remained seizure-free for more than 5 yr after withdrawal of medication are unlikely to relapse later. The prognosis of patients with focal seizures is discussed below.

Delgado-Escueta AV, Ferrendelli JA, Prince DA: Basic mechanisms of the epilepsies. Ann Neurol 16(Suppl), 1984.
Delgado-Escueta AV, Wasterlain C, Treiman DM, et al: Current concepts in neurology. Management of status epilepticus. N Engl J Med 306:1337, 1982.
Glaser GH: Kindling. Dev Med Child Neurol 25:137, 1983.
Hollowach-Thurston J, Thurston DL, Hixon BB, et al: Prognosis in childhood epilepsy. N Engl J Med 306:831, 1982.
Jeavons PM, Harding GFA: Photosensitive Epilepsy. Clinics in Developmental Medicine No. 56. London, Spastics International Publications, 1975.
Livingston S: Comprehensive Management of Epilepsy in Infancy, Childhood and Adolescence. Springfield, IL, Charles C Thomas, 1972.
Loiseau P, Beaussart M: The seizures of benign childhood epilepsy with Rolandic paroxysmal discharges. Epilepsia (Amst) 14:381, 1973.
Morselli PL, Pippenger CE, Penry JK (eds): Antiepileptic Drug Therapy in Pediatrics. New York, Raven Press, 1983.
Newmark ME, Penry JK: Genetics of Epilepsy. A Review. New York, Raven Press, 1980.
Rumack CM, Guggenheim MA, Fasules JM, et al: Transient positive postictal computed tomographic scan. J Pediatrics 97:263, 1980.
Ware S, Millward-Sadler GH: Acute liver disease associated with sodium valproate. Lancet 2:1110, 1980.

Symptomatic Epilepsy

The symptomatic, secondary, or organic epilepsies are a group of disorders in which seizures are the major clinical manifestation of known disorders or insults to the brain. Events that commonly lead to recurrent seizures include anoxic brain damage, severe head trauma, and central nervous system infections, including meningitis and encephalitis. Epilepsy may develop immediately following such an event or after a time interval of months or years. The delayed onset of seizures appears to be due to the gradual development of glial scars in damaged brain. Neurons in the areas of gliosis are distorted, with altered dendritic morphology. Small inhibitory GABAnergic neurons appear to be especially susceptible to damage, and a predominance in survival of excitatory neurons in such glial scars may be the basis for the development of epileptiform discharges.

Patients with symptomatic epilepsy often have abnormal findings on neurologic examination and significant intellectual deficits, in contrast to those with idiopathic seizures. Findings on CT scan of the brain are often abnormal, with focal or generalized brain atrophy as the most common finding. Several syndromes are recognized in which recurrent seizures are usually due to a definable cause, although the precise cause may not be evident in every case.

Neonatal Seizures

Definition. All types of seizures occurring within the first 2 wk of life are included in this category.

Pathophysiology and Etiology. The threshold for seizures is higher in the newborn infant than later in life; idiopathic epilepsy, therefore, rarely has any clinical expression at this age. On the other hand, seizures are quite common in neonates, owing to major metabolic derangements and to the increased risks of cerebral anoxia, hemorrhage, and infection in the perinatal period. The overall incidence is about 1/200 births. Neonatal seizures tend to be brief because immature neurons are unable to sustain repetitive activity for long periods of time, and to be focal or multifocal because the pathways connecting different cortical regions (e.g., in the corpus callosum) are as yet unmyelinated and do not transmit nerve impulses effectively.

A specific cause for the seizures can be determined in over 70% of cases (Table 21–7). Seizures during the first 24 hr postnatally in full-term infants are due most commonly to intrapartum asphyxia. Intracranial hemorrhage, hypoglycemia, hypocalcemia, congenital anomalies, drug intoxication or withdrawal, central nervous system infections, and inborn metabolic errors are other important causes in the first postnatal days. Infection becomes the most common etiology late in the 1st wk and during the 2nd wk. Seizures in premature infants are due usually to intraventricular and subependymal hemorrhage.

Clinical Manifestations. Neonatal seizures may be classified into several types including multifocal (fragmentary), focal clonic, myoclonic, and tonic attacks. In addition, apnea without any motor component other than limpness may be a manifestation of seizure activity.

The clonic movements of neonatal seizures tend to be slow, at a rate of 1–2/sec and they are often so faint as to be barely noticeable (subtle seizures). Focal jerking of one corner of the mouth or of an eyelid and deviation of the eyes to one side are common. In multifocal attacks seizure activity occurs at multiple sites but is rarely maintained at any one site for more than 1 or 2 min. Clonic seizure activity in the limbs has to be distinguished from tremulousness—a rapid, symmetrical tremor seen in some infants when they are stimulated—and from spontaneous clonus due to hyperactivity of the spinal reflex arc. Spontaneous clonus subsides when stretch on a tendon is removed, which can be accomplished by passive flexion of an extremity. This maneuver fails to affect clonic movements due to a seizure. Tremulousness and spontaneous clonus are signs of increased excitability of the nervous system at subcortical levels. They commonly occur in infants who also have seizures. Apneic seizures are difficult to distinguish from apnea due to dysfunction of the respiratory center in the medulla. Electrophysiologic studies are essential for their diagnosis.

Laboratory Studies. The EEG often helps to confirm the diagnosis but is normal in about one third of cases. Polygraphic studies that include monitoring of EEG, respirations, and heart rate are needed for the diagnosis of apneic seizures. In apnea due to seizure activity spike discharges appear on the EEG just prior to the onset or during the early phase of the apneic episode.

The exclusion of various causes of neonatal seizures requires laboratory investigation; determination of blood glucose, calcium, magnesium, and electrolyte levels is essential, as is examination of the spinal fluid for evidences of infection or

Table 21–7. **Causes and Features of Neonatal Seizures**

Causes	Percent of Total Cases	Time of Onset	Preceding or Associated Conditions
Hypoxic-ischemic encephalopathy	up to 60	1st 24 hr	Perinatal asphyxia
Intracranial hemorrhage	10–15	2nd day or later	Traumatic delivery
Infection	10–20	Usually 3rd day or later	Premature rupture of membranes
Hypoglycemia	8–10	2nd day or later	Small for gestational age, maternal diabetes
Hypocalcemia/hypomagnesemia	10–20	2nd day or later	Low birthweight, perinatal asphyxia
Drug withdrawal	<2	7–14 days	Maternal drug addiction, especially methadone use
Local anesthetic intoxication	<1	1st 6 hr	Local anesthetic use at time of delivery
Inborn errors of metabolism: (pyridoxine dependency, hyperammonemic syndromes, other defects in amino acid or organic acid metabolism)	<1	Anytime, often after start of milk feeding	
Congenital malformations of brain	5–10	Anytime	Multiple developmental anomalies, chromosome defects
Unknown	10–30	Usually 2nd day or later	Includes familial cases

subarachnoid hemorrhage. The possibility of intraventricular and parenchymal brain hemorrhages can be safely assessed by cranial ultrasonography; this should always be performed in the premature infant with seizures. Computed tomography of the head may be needed for diagnosis of cerebral malformations. A careful search for inborn errors of metabolism should be made in infants in whom no cause for the seizures is found on initial study, with screening of urine for amino acids and organic acids, and measurement of blood ammonia and lactate. The possibility of pyridoxine dependency is assessed by intravenous injection of 20–50 mg of pyridoxine during EEG recording; in infants with this syndrome, spike activity in the EEG disappears almost immediately after the administration of pyridoxine.

Treatment. Specific therapy is available for most of the metabolic disorders that cause seizures in neonates. Glucose is given intravenously at a dosage of 10 mL of a 20% solution for control of hypoglycemic seizures. Calcium gluconate is given slowly by vein, up to 6 mL of a 2.5% solution, to correct hypocalcemia. Magnesium sulfate, up to 6 mL of a 2.5% solution, is used for hypomagnesemia. Therapy for the inborn metabolic errors is discussed elsewhere.

Phenobarbital is the drug of choice for the nonspecific control of neonatal seizures. The initial loading dose is about 20 mg/kg, given slowly by vein. The maintenance dosage is 2–3 mg/kg/24 hr. Measurement of phenobarbital blood levels is needed for determination of the exact dosage, as the rate of metabolism varies considerably among infants. Phenytoin has also been recommended, but there is no proof of its effectiveness in neonates, and maintenance of anticonvulsant blood levels is difficult, owing to incomplete and unpredictable absorption of the drug in newborns. Diazepam may be given intravenously as a single dose of 0.3–0.4 mg/kg for ongoing seizure activity that is uncontrollable by phenobarbital.

Prognosis. Of all infants with neonatal seizures, about 20% die during the first 2 postnatal wk, 30% survive with residual damage, and 50% make good recovery. Mental retardation, persistent seizures, and cerebral palsy are the most common sequelae. The outlook varies markedly among the diagnostic categories. It is favorable in infants who have hypocalcemic seizures without other abnormal findings. A dominantly inherited form of benign neonatal seizures affects a few infants

who have a uniformly good outcome. Most infants whose seizures are secondary to subarachnoid hemorrhage also do well. In contrast, only about 50% of infants with hypoglycemic seizures and 20% with postanoxic seizures have a favorable outcome. The outlook is even worse in infants with postnatal seizures due to malformations of the brain, in whom developmental retardation is a universal finding.

The interictal EEG has prognostic significance. Infants whose recordings show generalized absence of cerebral electrical activity and full-term infants with records showing a burst-suppression pattern have a uniformly poor prognosis; and infants with multifocal spike discharges have only a 12% chance of favorable outcome. In contrast, more than 80% of infants with normal EEGs develop normally.

Neonatal seizures usually subside within a few days of onset, even in infants with residual brain damage. Other seizure patterns, such as infantile spasms, may develop later in such infants. The dosage of phenobarbital may be decreased fairly rapidly after the neonatal seizures subside. There is no evidence that recurrence of seizures is more common in infants in whom phenobarbital was discontinued within 2 mo than in infants maintained on long-term therapy.

Herzlinger RA, Kandall SR, Vaughan HG: Neonatal seizures associated with narcotics withdrawal. J Pediatr 91:638, 1977.

Hill A, Volpe JJ: Seizures, hypoxic-ischemic brain damage and IVH in the newborn. Ann Neurol 10:109, 1981.

Painter MJ, Pippenger C, MacDonald H, et al: Phenobarbital and diphenylhydantoin levels in neonates with seizures. J Pediatr 92:315, 1978.

Rose AL, Lombroso CT: Neonatal seizure states. A study of clinical, pathological and electroencephalographic features in 137 full-term babies with a long-term follow-up. Pediatrics 45:404, 1970.

Tibbles JAR: Dominant benign neonatal seizures. Dev Med Child Neurol 22:664, 1980.

Volpe JJ: Neurology of the Newborn. Philadelphia, WB Saunders, 1981, pp 111–137.

Infantile Spasms (Infantile Myoclonic Seizures, West Syndrome)

Definition. Infantile spasms are a form of generalized myoclonic seizures that occur during infancy and that are usually associated with a characteristic EEG pattern (hypsarrhythmia).

Pathophysiology and Etiology. Infantile spasms are a nonspecific reaction of immature cerebral cortex to injury or to abnormalities of growth and development. They may follow cerebral anoxia (especially neonatal asphyxia), cerebral trauma, or brain damage due to meningitis or to intrauterine infections. They may also be due to disturbance of the metabolism of immature neurons (e.g., in phenylketonuria, pyridoxine deficiency or dependency, the cerebral lipidoses, or severe hypoglycemia) or to malformations of the brain such as occur in tuberous sclerosis, the Aicardi syndrome, Down syndrome, and congenital hydrocephalus. Rarely, a focal cerebral lesion such as a brain tumor may lead to infantile spasms. A common factor appears to be failure of development of the normal organization of the electrical activity of the brain. The hypsarrhythmic EEG pattern seen in patients with infantile spasms consists of multifocal high-voltage spike-and-slow-wave activity that resembles the spontaneous activity of isolated slabs of cerebral cortex, suggesting that intracortical and afferent connections may be deficient. Histologic studies of cerebral cortex have shown deficiency in the dendritic arborizations of cortical neurons.

Clinical Manifestations. The age of onset is usually between 3 and 8 mo, but onset as early as the neonatal period and as late as 2 yr has been reported in some cases. About half of the infants have a history of perinatal complications, including neonatal asphyxia, birth trauma, and meningitis. Developmental progress may have been normal until the time of onset of the seizures or there may have been earlier developmental delay. Regression is common in those infants who initially progressed normally. The infants often become less alert visually, and blindness due to ocular disorders may be suspected. The optic fundi and pupillary light reactions are normal, however, indicating that the blindness is due to dysfunction of the central visual pathways or of the visual cortex.

The infantile spasms consist of sudden flexion of the trunk, neck, and limbs, followed by more gradual relaxation. There is some resemblance to the Moro reflex, except that the spasms occur without preceding stimuli. Usually, a flurry of several spasms occur together, each separated from the next by an interval of several seconds. Attacks are most common shortly after arousal from sleep. Extension of limbs rather than flexion occurs in some infants and in some there is an associated vocalization or cry. Upward deviation of the eyes or turning of the head to one side may be seen. In about 30% of patients with infantile spasms other seizure types (including tonic-clonic and focal motor seizures) coexist.

Laboratory Studies. The EEG is essential for confirmation of the diagnosis. It shows a hypsarrhythmic pattern in two thirds or more of the children on initial examination. The remainder show focal epileptiform discharges or (rarely) a normal record. Hypsarrhythmia develops in a majority of these on follow-up study within weeks of onset of infantile spasms.

Computed tomography of the head is useful for differentiation of the various causes of infantile spasms. It is abnormal in about two thirds of patients. The most common finding is cerebral atrophy. Hydrocephalus, cerebral calcifications secondary to either tuberous sclerosis or intrauterine infections, and agenesis of corpus callosum are less common but diagnostically important findings.

Metabolic abnormalities are found in less than 5% of patients. It is important to exclude these, however, as they may respond to or require specific therapies. Fasting blood glucose determination, urine amino acid and organic acid analysis, and a trial of pyridoxine therapy (50 mg/24 hr) are indicated when infantile spasms are of unknown cause.

Treatment. Conventional anticonvulsant drugs are of limited effectiveness. Partial responses occur occasionally to clonazepam or to valproic acid. Much more consistent improvement is found in response to corticotropin (ACTH) or

to corticosteroid hormones, with neither of these clearly established as superior to the other. ACTH is administered intramuscularly in gel form. A commonly used dosage schedule consists of an initial high dose, 40–80 units/day as a single or twice-daily injection, until a response is obtained. The dosage then is tapered gradually for a total duration of treatment of 4–8 wk. Corticosteroids may be given orally for a similar period of time; starting dosages of 2 mg/kg/24 hr for prednisolone or of 0.3 mg/kg/24 hr for dexamethasone have been recommended. A good initial response, with cessation of infantile spasms and normalization of the EEG occurs in over 50% of cases, usually within 1–5 wk after start of treatment. In approximately half of the patients with initial good response, relapses occur after withdrawal of therapy. A second course of treatment may again be effective. Infants with multiple types of seizures need additional long-term therapy with one of the conventional anticonvulsants such as phenobarbital. During the period of steroid therapy the infants require careful observation for bacterial infections, which should be treated promptly with antibiotics. Hypertension is a common side effect but is usually asymptomatic.

Prognosis. Infantile spasms generally remit, either following corticosteroid therapy or spontaneously at a later date, and usually prior to the age of 3 yr. Other seizure types develop later in life in about 50% of patients. Mental retardation has been reported in 80–90% of cases on long-term follow-up and is usually moderate to profound. About 20% of patients die during childhood, with most of the deaths occurring in the severely retarded group. The prognosis is somewhat better in infants with unknown etiology who have normal findings on CT scan. In this group there also is evidence suggestive of better intellectual outcome when corticosteroid therapy has been started promptly after the onset of the infantile spasms.

Hrachovy RA, Frost JD, Kellaway P, et al: Double blind study of ACTH vs. prednisone therapy in infantile spasms. J Pediatr 103:641, 1983.
Lacy JR, Penry JK: Infantile Spasms. New York, Raven Press, 1976.
Snead OC III: ACTH and prednisone in childhood seizure disorders. Neurology 33:966, 1983.
West WJ: On a peculiar form of infantile convulsions. Lancet 1:724, 1841.

The Lennox-Gastaut Syndrome

Definition. The Lennox-Gastaut syndrome is a form of early childhood epilepsy characterized by myoclonic and atypical absence seizures, regression in intellectual functions, and generalized spike-wave discharges on EEG at a rate below that seen in petit mal, usually at about 2/sec.

Clinical Manifestations. These attacks begin somewhat later than infantile spasms, usually between the ages of 2 and 4 yr. A variety of brief seizures are seen, including myoclonic, atonic, and atypical absence. The onset may be sudden in a child who was previously well or may occur in one who may have had a prior history of other forms of seizures or developmental delay, or both. Several hundred attacks may occur in a day, and because these children often fall during a seizure, they are apt to sustain multiple bruises and lacerations of the skin, especially over the face and scalp. Developmental arrest or regression occurs soon after the start of the seizures. Neurologic examination may show signs of cerebellar ataxia but tends to be normal otherwise.

Laboratory Studies and Differential Diagnosis. The EEG is useful for confirmation of the diagnosis. It is always severely abnormal, with frequent bursts of slow spike-wave activity as the most common finding. This may become continuous or nearly so in some patients. CT scan of the head shows abnormal findings—usually diffuse cerebral atrophy—in about 60% of cases.

Specific illnesses with which children may exhibit this pattern of seizures include tuberous sclerosis, cerebral lipidoses (especially Batten disease), and Sanfilipo disease. These should be excluded by careful examination of the eyes and skin and by specific enzyme assays for disorders with known metabolic errors.

Treatment. Response to anticonvulsant drugs tends to be incomplete at best. Clonazepam, valproic acid, acetazolamide, and ethosuximide, either alone or in various combinations, may be effective. In refractory patients, ACTH or corticosteroid hormones may be tried, at dosages identical to those used in the treatment of infantile spasms. Ketogenic diets in which the majority of calories are provided in the form of either dietary fat or medium chain triglycerides are sometimes helpful in patients who fail to respond to drugs.

Prognosis. The outcome in children with Lennox-Gastaut syndrome resembles that in children with infantile spasms. The characteristic seizures and EEG findings usually disappear later in childhood, but there is a high incidence of mental defect that fails to remit. The prognosis is uniformly poor in children who develop this syndrome as a manifestation of a degenerative brain disease.

Gastaut H, Gastaut JL: Computerized transverse axial tomography in epilepsy. Epilepsia 17:325, 1976.
Huttenlocher PR: Ketonemia and seizures: Effects of two ketogenic diets in childhood epilepsy. Pediatr Res 10:536, 1976.
Kurokawa A, Goya N, Fukuyama Y, et al: West syndrome and Lennox-Gastaut syndrome: A survey of natural history. Pediatrics 65:81, 1980.

Psychomotor Epilepsy (Temporal Lobe Epilepsy)

Definition. This is a syndrome in which the occurrence of complex partial seizures is the major symptom.

Etiology. Psychomotor epilepsy is due to abnormality in function of the temporal lobes. There is often an underlying atrophic lesion with formation of a glial scar in the mesial portion of the temporal lobe (mesial temporal sclerosis). This may be unilateral or bilateral. Mesial temporal sclerosis is thought to be due to brain damage sustained during an episode of cerebral anoxia. There is often a history either of perinatal asphyxia or of an anoxic insult later in infancy; for example, an episode of respiratory impairment during a prolonged tonic-clonic seizure. Head trauma, meningitis, encephalitis, tumors, and vascular malformations of the temporal lobe may also lead to this syndrome. The most common type of tumor is a small, benign variety that is sometimes referred to as a hamartoma. In a minority of patients with psychomotor epilepsy the syndrome occurs in the absence of any definable anatomic lesion but with a positive family history in multiple generations, suggesting that this type of seizure may occasionally be a manifestation of idiopathic epilepsy.

Clinical Manifestations. The major finding is the occurrence of complex partial seizures, as described in Sec. 21.7. The onset may be at any time from infancy through adolescence. In the infant and young child, this condition is especially difficult to diagnose, because the child is as yet unable to describe the characteristic mental and perceptual distortions that precede the seizures. Recurrent autonomic disturbances including nausea and vomiting, dreamy states from which the child cannot be roused, and motor automatisms (chewing, swallowing movements, aimless walking) may be early signs. Affected children commonly have behavioral disturbances, including irritability, hyperkinesis, aggressive behavior, temper tantrums, and rapid mood swings. Mild intellectual impairments are common, as is delay in language development. The neurologic examination is usually normal except for fluctuating postictal reflex asymmetries in some patients and, less commonly, visual field defects with superior quadrantanopia in patients with structural lesions in temporal lobes.

Laboratory Studies. The EEG is essential to confirm the diagnosis and also to determine whether seizure activity originates in one or both temporal lobes. The EEG shows unilateral or bilateral spike or slow-wave activity in temporal areas in about 60% of patients. The number of positive studies can be increased somewhat by use of special procedures, including EEG recording after a period of sleep deprivation and use of nasopharyngeal or sphenoidal leads.

Computed tomography of the head is indicated for demonstration of any structural lesion in the temporal lobes.

Treatment. Response to anticonvulsant drugs is often incomplete, especially when there is an underlying structural lesion. Phenytoin, carbamazepine, and primidone are the most effective agents. Addition of valproic acid or ethosuximide occasionally leads to improved seizure control. Attention to the behavioral difficulties that are common in these children is an important aspect of management. Special school placement and involvement in a child guidance program may be needed. In some children, the addition of psychotropic medications such as methylphenidate or one of the phenothiazines is helpful.

Patients in whom medical therapy is unsuccessful should be evaluated for possible surgical removal of an epileptogenic focus. This is best postponed until late childhood or adolescence unless a tumor or vascular malformation of the brain is demonstrated, or unless severe behavioral abnormalities make the child unmanageable. The studies that need to be performed prior to surgery, the selection of patients for surgery, and the actual resection of temporal lobe should be attempted only in centers specialized in this work. The best candidates for surgery are patients who have a unilateral anterior temporal lobe lesion, atrophic or other, and in whom repeated EEG recordings indicate the origin of the epileptiform discharges to be the region of the anatomical lesion.

Prognosis. The outlook is favorable in children with psychomotor epilepsy who have a resectable temporal lobe lesion. About two thirds of patients became seizure-free postoperatively, and in many of these the dosage of anticonvulsant medications can be reduced or discontinued. Behavioral disturbances often improve after surgery. A second group with good prognosis comprises children without evident underlying cause who have normal intellect; seizures remit spontaneously prior to maturity in more than half of this group, and most of the remainder are controllable with medication. Adverse factors include low intelligence, the finding of bilateral temporal lobe lesions, onset prior to the age of 2 yr, and occurrence of additional other seizure types, such as tonic-clonic seizures.

Davidson S, Falconer MA: Outcome of surgery in 40 children with temporal lobe epilepsy. Lancet 1:1260, 1975.
Glaser GH: Limbic epilepsy in childhood. J Nerv Ment Dis 144:391, 1967.
Lindsay J, Glaser G, Richards P, et al: Developmental aspects of focal epilepsies of childhood treated by neurosurgery. Dev Med Child Neurol 26:574, 1984.
Lindsay J, Ounsted C, Richards P: Long-term outcome in children with temporal lobe seizures. I: Social outcome and childhood factors. Dev Med Child Neurol 21:285, 1979.

21.8 PAROXYSMAL DISORDERS OTHER THAN EPILEPSY

HEADACHE

Recurrent head pain is a common, frequently benign symptom late in childhood and in adolescence; in the young child it is unusual and more often indicative of serious underlying disease. Headache may stem from any of the pain-sensitive structures of the head, including all the tissues covering the cranium, the intracranial blood vessels, the cranial nerves that carry sensory fibers (V, IX, X), the upper cervical nerves, and the meninges near the base of the brain. The brain itself, the calvarium, and the meninges overlying the cerebral hemispheres are insensitive to pain.

The following is a useful classification of the various types of headache:

1. *Vascular headache*
   Migraine
   Headache secondary to fever
   Hypertensive headache
2. *Headache related to epilepsy*
3. *Headache secondary to changes in intracranial pressure*
   Brain tumor headache
   Low CSF pressure headache
4. *Tension headache*
5. *Headache related to psychiatric disease*
6. *Headache due to eye strain*
7. *Nasal sinus pain*

Migraine. This is a common cause of vascular headache in children. Its pathogenesis is incompletely understood. The aura preceding the onset of head pain is thought to be due to abnormal constriction of intracranial arteries, with localized transient ischemia of cerebral tissue. The headache itself is secondary to vasodilatation and pulsation of cranial vessels, especially those of the scalp, with stimulation of pain fibers in the vessel walls. Food allergies may trigger the attacks in some patients.

Clinical Manifestations. Over two thirds of affected patients have a positive family history; a dominant pattern of inheritance is suggested in many families. The onset usually occurs late in childhood or in early adolescence. In some instances there is a history of repeated vomiting in infancy or earlier childhood (cyclic vomiting). Classically, an attack of migraine is preceded by an aura, which often consists of transient visual disturbance but which may include a variety of other fleeting neurologic disabilities. The visual aura consists of scintillating scotomas and of zigzag lines ("*fortification phenomena*" or *teichotic scotomata*) which move slowly across the visual field. Within minutes or at most a few hours the aura is followed by throbbing unilateral head pain and by nausea and vomiting. Sleep usually terminates an attack. The frequency of attacks varies greatly even in the same patient; stress appears to increase the number of attacks. Partial forms, in which there is no aura, and atypical attacks with bilateral head pain and without vomiting are probably considerably more common than is the classic migraine described above. A severe form (basilar artery migraine) occurs occasionally, with symptoms of transient disturbance of function in the basilar artery territory, including hemianopsia, vertigo, dysarthria, diplopia, bilateral sensory changes, alternating hemiplegia and, rarely, loss of consciousness.

Differential Diagnosis. The diagnosis of migraine can usually be made from the history in combination with the absence of positive findings on careful funduscopic, physical, and neurologic examination. Fever may produce a similar throbbing head pain secondary to peripheral vasodilatation and increased cerebral blood flow. Hypertension or increased intracranial pressure should always be ruled out. Congenital cerebrovascular malformations are a rare cause of vascular headache. They usually produce an audible cranial bruit over the head or eyes. Basilar artery migraine needs to be distinguished from epilepsy.

Laboratory Studies. These are of little value. Occasionally, it may be necessary to obtain skull and nasal sinus roentgenograms, CT scan, and an electroencephalogram to supplement the clinical evaluation.

Treatment. Therapy is often only partially satisfactory. Vasoconstrictors such as ergotamine and caffeine taken at the very onset of symptoms may abort an attack; a combination of these two agents (Cafergot) is widely used. The dosage in a child over the age of 10 yr is 1 tablet at the first sign of an attack, repeated twice at 30 min intervals if necessary. Simple analgesics, such as aspirin, may be as effective and should be tried first. Maintenance therapy with phenobarbital or with propranolol sometimes prevents attacks but is justifiable only if attacks are frequent and incapacitating. Reassurance that the child has a benign condition is often more helpful than drugs. Potentially dangerous medications such as methysergide and narcotics are to be strictly avoided.

Headache as a Symptom in Epilepsy. Headache may occur as part of the aura preceding a grand mal seizure or as a postictal event. In autonomic seizures headache may be a striking part of the attack itself. Other autonomic disturbances, such as pallor, tachycardia, or pupillary dilatation, are easily overlooked. The concept that headache may be the only manifestation of a seizure is difficult to prove. Finding an abnormal electroencephalogram in a child with recurrent head pain is of little help since abnormal EEG records are common in children with classic migraine, especially at the time of attack.

Headache Secondary to Changes in Intracranial Pressure. This head pain is probably the result of stretching and deformation of cerebral vessels and of meninges. The headache of increased intracranial pressure often occurs following changes in position of the head, such as after arising from sleep. Morning headache in a child should always arouse the suspicion of brain tumor. There may be associated vomiting, often with minimal nausea, followed by a feeling of wellbeing. The location of head pain is a good localizing sign in brain tumor. Headache due to posterior fossa tumor is almost always occipital.

Low pressure headache is usually due to a persistent CSF leak after spinal tap. It may also be seen after traumatic meningeal tears with CSF fistula. The pain appears almost immediately on assumption of the upright position and is relieved by lying down. This type of headache is best treated by bed rest, preferably in the prone position.

Tension Headache. This is thought to be due to persistent contraction of neck and temporalis muscles, leading to localized ischemia of these structures. It is often described as a dull, steady pain, increasing as the day advances, and relieved after sleep. In its classic form it is rarely seen prior to adolescence.

Headache Related to Psychiatric Disease. Headache is a rather common symptom of depression in childhood. This type of headache is described as continuously present, whereas organic head pain is almost always intermittent. The facial expression of the depressed child with headache bespeaks suffering. Speech may be reduced to a whisper. Poor appetite, constipation, and insomnia are frequently associated. Failure to recognize this syndrome often leads to extensive and potentially harmful diagnostic studies.

Eye Strain. Eye strain is often blamed for headache, and glasses are prescribed for relief, but there is little evidence of such an association. Occasionally, prolonged reading by a child with a refractive error may lead to tension headache.

BENIGN PAROXYSMAL VERTIGO IN CHILDHOOD

This syndrome has its onset in young children, usually from 1–4 yr of age. It is thought to be secondary to a disturbance in vestibular function. During a typical attack the child suddenly becomes unsteady on his or her feet, appears frightened, and may clutch at a parent. The older child may report a rotational experience. There is no alteration of consciousness, and after a few minutes the child returns to his or her former state. The condition is self-limited, tending to subside within 2–3 yr. Benign paroxysmal vertigo is often misdiagnosed as epilepsy, with anticonvulsant drugs prescribed unnecessarily. Preservation of normal alertness during the attack is the most important differential point distinguishing this from epilepsy.

Cold water caloric tests may show diminished or absent vestibular response in one or both ears. Audiograms and electroencephalograms are normal. A trial of dimenhydrinate (Dramamine) is indicated for frequent attacks.

Barlow C: Headaches and Migraine in Childhood. Philadelphia, JB Lippincott Co, 1985.
Congdon PJ, Forsythe WI: Migraine in childhood: A study of 300 children. Dev Med Child Neurol 21:209, 1979.
Egger J, Wilson J, Carter CM, et al: Is migraine food allergy? Lancet 2:865, 1983.
Graham JH, et al: Fibrotic disorders associated with methysergide therapy for headache. N Engl J Med 274:360, 1966.
Hockaday JM: Basilar migraine in childhood. Dev Med Child Neurol 21:455, 1979.
Koenigsberger MR, Chutorian AM, Gold AP, et al: Benign paroxysmal vertigo of childhood. Neurology 20:1108, 1970.
Ludvigsson J: Propranolol used in prophylaxis of migraine in children. Acta Neurol Scand 50:109, 1974.
Malmquist CP: Depressions in childhood and adolescence. N Engl J Med 284:955, 1971.
Waters WF: Headache and the eye. Lancet 2:1, 1970.

SLEEP DISORDERS

Narcolepsy and Cataplexy. In patients with narcolepsy, sleep occurs uncontrollably and inappropriately during the daytime. These patients are mentally alert rather than drowsy between attacks of sleep, but such attacks may suddenly interrupt ongoing activities such as a conversation or driving a car. The condition may lead to repeated accidents and to inability to perform in school or on a job. It is uncommon during childhood but has its onset not infrequently during adolescence. In about half of the patients, narcolepsy is associated with cataplexy, a sudden loss of muscle tone and strength that may cause the patient to fall but that is not associated with loss of consciousness. Cataplexy is usually precipitated by an emotional reaction, such as uproarious laughter.

The etiology of narcolepsy and cataplexy is unknown in most cases. There often is a positive family history in a parent or siblings, suggesting that dominant inheritance may play a role. A strong association with the histocompatibility antigen HLA DR2 has been reported. Rarely, narcolepsy has been associated with specific neurologic diseases such as multiple sclerosis, encephalitis, or tumors of the upper midbrain and hypothalamus. A defect in the normal progression of stages of sleep occurs in all patients with narcolepsy, who progress very rapidly from waking to rapid eye movement (REM) sleep. This diagnostic finding can be confirmed by EEG recording of the transition from waking to sleep. The differential diagnosis includes akinetic (atonic) seizures and syncope.

Narcolepsy can be effectively treated with stimulant medications. Methylphenidate is the drug of choice, at a starting dosage of 5 mg, given two or three times daily. Amphetamines have been used also but have a higher incidence of undesirable side effects, especially weight loss and potential for abuse.

Sleep Paralysis. This condition occurs during the transition from waking to sleep or from sleep to waking. There is a transient inability to move, which clears spontaneously. It is sometimes associated with narcolepsy but usually occurs alone as a benign symptom.

Somnambulism. Sleep walking is common in children. It tends to improve with maturation and does not require therapy. There is no association with epilepsy.

Sleep Apnea. Two major types are seen, obstructive and central sleep apnea. Obstructive sleep apnea is accompanied by snoring. Intermittently, the snoring ceases and there are respiratory pauses that may last 30 sec or longer. Sleep provides little rest, and the patient is chronically tired during the daytime. In children, this condition is usually secondary to obstruction of the airway by enlarged tonsils and adenoids. It can be cured by tonsillectomy and adenoidectomy. Patients with untreated severe cases may develop pulmonary hypertension.

Central sleep apnea is due to either immaturity or disease of the respiratory centers in the medulla oblongata. Affected children have repeated apneic episodes lasting 20 sec or longer occurring during sleep, usually with bradycardia. The condition is very common in premature infants; its frequency has been reported to be over 50% in otherwise healthy infants less than 35 wk gestational age. In older infants and children it may be a symptom of several diseases that affect the brain stem, including encephalitis, brain stem tumors, the Arnold-Chiari malformation, and Leigh disease. It is a cause of sudden death and may account for some cases of the sudden infant death syndrome (Sec. 26.1). Patients with central apnea require continuous monitoring of respirations during sleep. Stimulant drugs such as theophylline may prevent the attacks in some patients. Tracheostomy and connection to a ventilator during sleep are required in patients with severe cases.

Sleep apnea needs to be distinguished from nocturnal seizures. Polygraphic recordings during sleep, including EEG, ECG, nasal air flow, and respiratory movements, are important diagnostic aids. They also differentiate between obstructive and central apnea. During episodes of obstructive apnea nasal air flow ceases while respiratory movements continue; both become arrested in central apnea.

Frank Y, Kravath RE, Pollak CP, et al: Obstructive sleep apnea and its therapy: Clinical and polysomnographic manifestations. Pediatrics 71:737, 1983.
Gabriel M, Albani M, Schulte FJ: Apneic spells and sleep states in preterm infants. Pediatrics 57:142, 1976.
Guilleminault C, Dement WC, Passouant P (eds): Narcolepsy. New York, Spectrum Publications, 1976.
Guilleminault C, McQuitty J, Ariagno RL, et al: Congenital central alveolar hypoventilation syndrome in six infants. Pediatrics 70:684, 1982.
Langdon N, van Dam M, Welsh KI: Genetic markers in narcolepsy. Lancet 2:1178, 1984.
Zarcone V: Narcolepsy. N Engl J Med 288:1156, 1973.

SYNCOPE

Syncope, or fainting, is a transient loss of consciousness that occurs secondary to cerebral anoxia or cerebral ischemia. It may be caused by any condition that leads to transient impairment in the supply of oxygen to cerebral neurons. The following is a list of the more common forms of syncope in infants and children:

    Infantile syncope
        Type 1: Breathholding or cyanotic attacks
        Type 2: Pallid attacks
    Vasovagal syncope
    Postural hypotension
    Hyperactive carotid sinus reflex
    Syncope of cardiac origin

Breathholding attacks occur commonly in young children, between the ages of 6 mo and 4 yr (Sec. 2.6). The onset always is with crying. The infant then stops breathing and becomes deeply cyanotic. The limbs become rigidly extended. Prolonged attacks of breathholding produce transient loss of consciousness, and occasionally several convulsive jerks of the extremities. The child then becomes limp, resumes respirations, and after a few seconds returns to full alertness. The typical history of onset with crying and holding of the breath distinguishes breathholding attacks from convulsions. This form of syncope is always benign and always disappears spontaneously prior to school age. Children with this history have a higher incidence of vasovagal syncopal attacks later in childhood.

The second, or *pallid*, type of infantile syncope follows a bump of the head or other sudden minor injury. The child may start to cry but then turns pale and collapses. There is transient apnea and limpness, followed by rapid recovery. These attacks are due to vagal reflex overactivity, which leads to marked, transient bradycardia and circulatory impairment. The typical history and absence of postictal drowsiness help to distinguish these attacks from epilepsy. The EEG is normal and is of diagnostic aid in doubtful cases. The attacks disappear spontaneously prior to school age.

Vasovagal syncope is a condition in which sudden painful stimuli or emotional reactions lead to fainting. Two factors are involved: (1) decreased peripheral vascular resistance; and (2) bradycardia due to increased vagal activity. These lead to hypotension and decreased cerebral perfusion. Obscuration of vision, lightheadedness, nausea, and sweating precede the loss of consciousness. The patient becomes pale and may slump to the floor. The period of loss of awareness is brief and recovery is rapid.

Postural hypotension is common in late childhood and during the adolescent growth spurt. It is due to inadequacy of the vasomotor reflexes that regulate blood pressure in response to changes in position. It follows sudden change from the lying to the standing position, especially on arising in the morning; it may also occur while standing quietly. The symptoms are identical to those of vasovagal syncope. Consciousness is regained rapidly upon assumption of a horizontal position. Similar attacks may occur during voiding in the upright position (micturition syncope).

A *hyperactive carotid sinus reflex* is an uncommon cause of syncope. Pressure over the carotid sinus in the anterior cervical region causes marked bradycardia, followed by hypotension and fainting in susceptible individuals.

Cardiac Syncope. Syncope may be a manifestation of low cardiac output (as in supravalvular aortic stenosis), of severe oxygen unsaturation (as with tetralogy of Fallot), or of cardiac conduction defects (including complete heart block, prolonged Q-T interval, and the Wolff-Parkinson-White syndrome) (Sec. 14.72). The initial syncopal event may be followed by an anoxic seizure when circulation or oxygenation is severely impaired.

Diagnostic Evaluation. The diagnostic evaluation of the patient with a history of fainting includes testing for vasomotor instability. The blood pressure is measured with the patient in the lying and then in the standing position, when postural hypotension is suspected. Pressure over the carotid sinus will reproduce the attack in the hyperactive carotid sinus syndrome. A cardiac evaluation including an ECG is essential when syncope occurs without apparent cause.

Therapy. Treatment of these patients is directed toward avoidance of conditions that may lead to fainting. The person with postural hypotension should arise from bed slowly and should lie or sit down when faintness develops. Pressure over the anterior neck region should be avoided when hyperactivity of the carotid sinus reflex has been demonstrated. A trial of atropine or one of its derivatives may be indicated for frequently recurring type 2 (pallid) infantile syncope.

Braham J, Hertzeanu H, Yahini JH, et al: Reflex cardiac arrest presenting as epilepsy. Ann Neurol 10:277, 1981.
Lombroso CT, Lerman P: Breath holding spells (cyanotic and pallid infantile syncope). Pediatrics 39:563, 1967.

21.9 STATIC AND DEVELOPMENTAL LESIONS OF THE NERVOUS SYSTEM

Most neurologic disabilities in childhood result from congenital malformations or from brain damage in the perinatal period and are usually nonprogressive. Understanding of their etiology is often incomplete, and any classification is at best only partly satisfactory. The following classification is based on presumed time of onset of the defect, on the structures involved, and on etiology when known.

I. **Developmental defects of the nervous system (congenital malformations)**
    A. *Defects of closure of the neural tube*
        Anencephaly
        Encephalocele
        Myelomeningocele and the Arnold-Chiari malformation
        Spina bifida occulta
        Dermal sinus
        Neurenteric cyst
    B. *Defects in the differentiation and growth of the cerebral hemispheres*
        Chromosomal defects (see other sections)
        Morphologic syndromes with mental retardation (see Chapter 6)
        Holoprosencephaly (arrhinencephaly)
        Agenesis of corpus callosum
        Porencephaly and hydranencephaly
        Lissencephaly
        Polymicrogyria
        Microcephaly
        Megalencephaly
    C. *Defects in development of cerebrospinal fluid circulation (congenital hydrocephalus)*
        Aqueductal stenosis
        The Dandy-Walker malformation
        "Communicating" hydrocephalus
    D. *Development defects of brain stem*
        Moebius syndrome

II. **Perinatally acquired cerebral lesions**
    A. *Intrauterine and neonatal infections of the nervous system*
        Congenital syphilis
        Congenital toxoplasmosis
        Cytomegalic inclusion disease
        Neonatal herpesvirus infection
        Other viral encephalitides
        Neonatal bacterial meningitis
    B. *Perinatal anoxic encephalopathy*
    C. *Cerebral trauma incident to birth*
        Intraventricular hemorrhage (not necessarily traumatic, see also Sec. 8.23)
        Intracerebral hemorrhage and cerebral contusion
        Subarachnoid hemorrhage
        Subdural hemorrhage
    D. *Neonatal metabolic encephalopathies*
        Bilirubin encephalopathy (kernicterus)
        Hypoglycemia encephalopathy
        The aminoacidurias
        Cretinism

21.10 DEFECTS OF CLOSURE OF THE NEURAL TUBE

(See Sec. 6.30 for recurrence risks and prenatal diagnosis.) These developmental anomalies are best understood in the context of normal formative stages of the nervous system as indicated in Fig. 21–6. In the human the first evidence of development of neural tissue occurs at about 20 days' gestation, at which time a distinct depression, the neural groove, appears in the dorsal ectoderm of the embryo (Fig. 21–6*A*). This groove quickly deepens, and its two margins become apposed and fuse. This fusion forms the neural tube; it begins near the center of the embryo and progresses cephalad and caudad. By about 23 days' gestation the neural tube is complete, except for an opening at each end, the anterior and posterior neuropores (Fig. 21–6*B*). Failure of closure of the

Figure 21–6. Early developmental stages of the human central nervous system. *A*, Dorsal view of embryo at 20 days of age. The future nervous system is indicated by a midline depression, the neural groove. *B*, 23 days' gestational age. The neural groove has closed dorsally, except for openings at either end (the anterior and posterior neuropores), to form the neural tube. *C*, Cephalic portion of the embryo, 28 days. The cerebral hemispheres are represented by a single midline structure, the prosencephalon. *D*, 36 days' gestational age. Paired lateral ventricles and cerebral hemispheres are formed. The outlines of the ventricular system, including the 3rd ventricle, aqueduct of Sylvius, and 4th ventricle, are discernible.

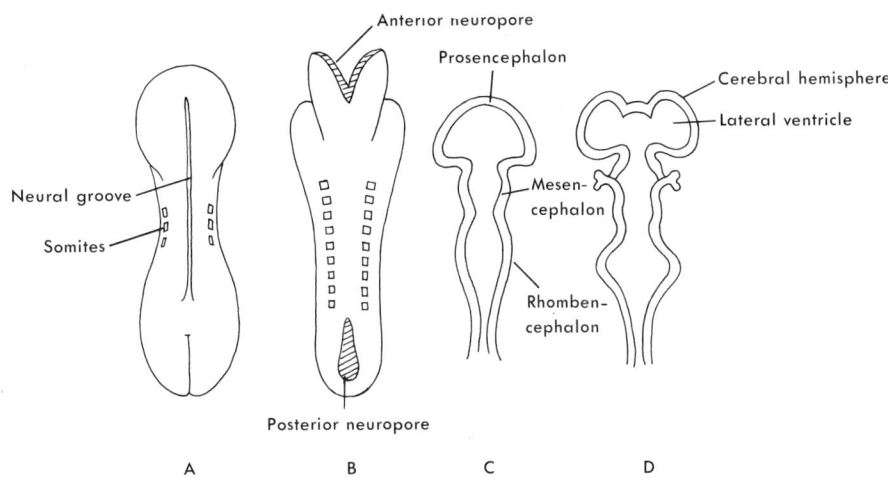

anterior neuropore causes anencephaly and encephalocele; a closure defect of the posterior neuropore leads to spina bifida and meningomyelocele. The term *rachischisis* is used for very extensive spinal closure defects involving most or all of the dorsal, lumbar, and sacral regions.

Anencephaly. Anencephaly is evident immediately at birth; the membranous skull is absent, as well as the cerebral hemispheres. Brain stem and basal nuclei may be well formed and are visible at the base of the skull. Affected infants are stillborn or die within a few days.

Encephalocele. Encephalocele consists of a herniation of brain and meninges through a defect in the skull, resulting in a sac-like structure. When the defect contains only meninges it is referred to as a *cranial meningocele*. About 75% of encephaloceles occur in the occipital area; the remainder are parietal, frontal, or nasopharyngeal.

Encephalocele is usually obvious at birth as a midline skull defect through which a large pedunculated or sessile mass protrudes. Nasopharyngeal encephaloceles may have no externally visible anomaly; the child may have nasal airway obstruction or cleft palate, with the nasal passages containing a smooth, round mass projecting downward, which must be differentiated from nasal polyp. A frontal encephalocele may extend into the orbit and produce proptosis of one eye.

The differentiation of encephalocele from cranial meningocele is made by palpation and transillumination of the mass and by computed tomography. The latter shows associated hydrocephalus in approximately two thirds of infants with encephalocele.

Therapy of encephalocele consists of surgical repair of the defect unless a major associated malformation of the brain is severe enough to preclude the possibility of meaningful survival. The associated hydrocephalus frequently requires a shunt operation. The prognosis is good in cranial meningocele, with normal intellectual and motor function in 60% of affected infants, but infants with occipital encephalocele have only about a 10% chance of normal intelligence.

Spina Bifida with Meningomyelocele. This is a midline defect of skin, vertebral arches, and neural tube, usually in the lumbosacral region. It is one of the most common developmental anomalies of the nervous system; the incidence ranges among population groups from 0.2–4.0/1000 births; the highest incidence is reported in the Welsh and Irish. Little is known about the etiology of meningomyelocele, although it appears to be linked with anencephaly. A woman whose child has had either anencephaly or meningomyelocele has an increased risk of either in subsequent pregnancies (see *Anencephaly* above). Each defect has been observed following administration of aminopterin during the 1st mo of pregnancy.

Meningomyelocele is evident at birth as a skin defect over the back, bordered laterally by bony prominences of the unfused neural arches of the vertebrae. The defect is usually covered by a transparent membrane which may have neural tissue attached to its inner surface. Cerebrospinal fluid leaks from this membrane initially, but soon after birth drying of the membrane tends to decrease its permeability. As cerebrospinal fluid accumulates, the membrane begins to bulge, and it may eventually form a large sac unless surgical closure of the defect is carried out. In almost all cases meningomyelocele is associated with the *Arnold-Chiari malformation* (Fig. 21–7), which consists of maldevelopment and downward displacement into the cervical spinal canal of parts of the cerebellum, 4th ventricle, and medulla oblongata. Other developmental anomalies of neural tissue may coexist, including aqueductal stenosis and arrest of migration of cerebral neurons. Hydrocephalus develops in about 90% of affected children as a result of the Arnold-Chiari malformation or of aqueductal stenosis.

Neurologic assessment of the infant with meningomyelocele should be carried out soon after birth to determine the severity of the functional defect. The upper level of spinal cord dysfunction can usually be detected by observing the response to pinprick over legs and trunk. Functional integrity is present when the sensory stimulus leads to limb movements and to arousal and crying. Stimulus-induced movement of limbs without change in the infant's behavior is of little significance since it may be due to reflexes in spinal cord segments that have no functional connection with higher centers. Defective innervation of bladder is indicated by urinary dribbling, that of the perianal region by a patulous anal sphincter and lack of anal reflex. The denervated limbs are flaccid and areflexic. Deformities such as talipes equinovarus and dislocated hips are often present. The Arnold-Chiari malformation may lead to medullary and lower cranial nerve dysfunction, including difficulty in swallowing, stridor, and atrophy of tongue.

Optimal therapy of meningomyelocele consists of prompt surgical closure of the skin defect, preferably within 48 hr after birth, to prevent meningeal infection. Wide excision of the membranous covering is contraindicated since the membrane may contain functioning neural tissue. After closure of the defect the infant must be carefully observed for development of hydrocephalus, which is treated surgically when indicated. Urinary retention can be managed by repeated catheterizations, done by caretakers for infants and young children, in older children by the patients themselves. Or-

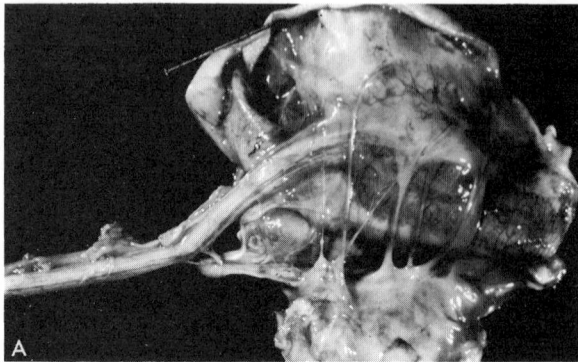
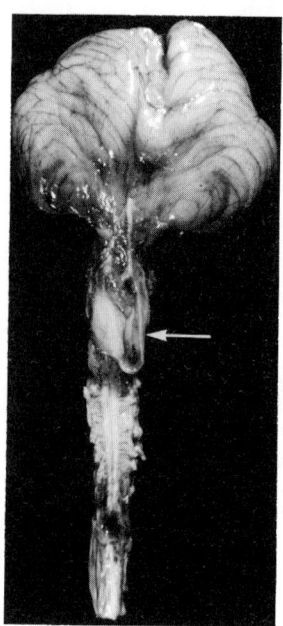

Figure 21–7. Meningomyelocele and Arnold-Chiari malformation. *A,* Characteristic deformity of the spinal cord. The normally formed thoracic spinal cord (left side of figure) gradually becomes flattened; the lumbar cord is represented by a platelike structure which is firmly adherent to the surrounding skin. The lumbar spinal nerves can be seen to emerge from the malformed neural plate. *B,* Arnold-Chiari malformation, same case. The medulla oblongata and 4th ventricle (*arrow*) show marked downward displacement. The malformed cerebellum is visible above.

thopedic procedures sometimes help to correct hip and foot deformities but should be considered only when the child has some chance of useful function of his lower extremities. An organized plan for management by a specialized multidisciplinary clinical group is essential.

The prognosis depends on the extent of the motor deficit at birth, on the status of bladder innervation, and on the nature of any associated cerebral anomalies. For the infant with total paralysis of legs and urinary bladder the outlook is poor even with optimal medical care; most such infants die during early childhood from complications of therapy for hydrocephalus or from chronic renal failure. The remainder are severely restricted by their motor disability, and 50% are mentally retarded. Advanced hydrocephalus at birth also carries a poor prognosis. Children with lesser degrees of involvement may lead successful lives, especially those with spina bifida and meningocele without evidence of neurologic deficit at birth. In severely affected infants deciding whether to carry out operative procedures or to allow the disorder to take its natural course presents serious ethical problems. Without surgery, over 90% of affected infants die in their 1st yr.

Spina Bifida Occulta. This consists of a defect of the vertebral arch with failure of posterior fusion of the vertebral laminae and often with absence of the spinous processes. The anomaly is most common at L5 and S1 levels, but it may affect any portion of the vertebral column. There may be associated anomalies of vertebral bodies, such as hemivertebrae. The overlying skin and subcutaneous tissues may be normal or show abnormal tufts of hair, telangiectasia, or subcutaneous lipoma. Spina bifida occulta is an isolated, insignificant finding in about 20% of all spines examined roentgenographically. A small percentage of affected infants have functionally significant developmental defects of the underlying spinal cord and spinal roots.

As with meningomyelocele, the neurologic deficit may be manifested as motor and sensory disturbances in the lower extremities and/or disturbances of the bladder and bowel sphincters. Unilateral foot deformity and weakness of foot muscles are the most common defects. Smallness of the foot, trophic ulcers, and pes cavus occur. These may be associated with sensory loss, especially in L5 and S1 distribution. Bladder sphincter disturbance is seen in about 25% of infants with neurologic involvement and leads to urinary incontinence,

dribbling, and recurrent urinary infections. It is usually associated with weakness of the anal sphincters and with sensory impairment in the perineal region. The neurologic impairments may gradually worsen, especially during adolescent growth.

The differential diagnosis includes spinal cord tumor, poliomyelitis, developmental defects of the spine such as diastematomyelia, and foot deformities. Diagnostic studies should be limited to roentgenograms of the spine unless there is progressive neurologic impairment. In that case myelography, either with metrizamide or with air is performed to rule out associated surgically remediable defects. Lipoma is especially common; it has been found on surgical exploration in about 40% of children with neurologic impairment associated with spina bifida occulta; a dermoid cyst has been present in about 5%. If these tumors can be removed without damage to neural structures, they should be.

Diastematomyelia. Diastematomyelia is a fissure or cleft of the spinal cord, usually in the lumbar region. The cleft is often transfixed by a bony or fibrous septum which prevents the normal ascent of the spinal cord as the child grows. Tethering of the spinal cord in the vertebral canal may lead to progressive neurologic deficit. Progressive flaccid paraparesis, weakness of one leg, or bladder dysfunction may occur. Frequently associated anomalies include spina bifida with meningomyelocele, spina bifida occulta, dermal sinus, and hemivertebrae. Cutaneous hemangioma, lipoma, or a tuft of hair may overlie the site of the spinal defect.

The diagnosis can often be made by roentgenographic demonstration of a bony spicule in the spinal canal. Myelography further delineates the abnormality. Surgical exploration and resection of the abnormal bone and fibrous tissue is indicated when the lesion is discovered in infancy or in early childhood.

Dermal Sinus. Dermal sinus is a small midline closure defect which is of importance primarily because the sinus may be a route of entry of bacteria into the subarachnoid space and thus lead to recurrent meningitis. It is usually located in the lumbosacral area but may occur at any level of the spine or in the midline of the cranium. Its point of origin on the skin is visible as a dimple, often surrounded by a tuft of hair or by a small hemangioma. The low sacral defects known as *pilonidal dimples or sinuses* usually end blindly without communication with the subarachnoid space and are therefore rarely significant. Sinus tracts above that level should be surgically explored and closed.

Neurenteric Cyst. These rare lesions arise from incorporation of entodermal tissue into developing neural tissue of the early embryo. They consist of epithelium-lined tracts and cysts which protrude into the spinal canal. They are most common in the thoracic and lower cervical regions. Neurologic dysfunction results from compression of the spinal cord by the cystic mass.

The symptoms and signs are those of spinal cord tumor or of infection of the subarachnoid space (sometimes recurrent or chronic meningitis). The diagnosis can occasionally be suspected from examination of an anterior view of the spine, which may show a rounded, midline defect in one of the vertebral bodies through which the neurenteric tract gains entry to the spinal canal. In other cases these lesions have been entirely intraspinal without any associated bony defect. The diagnosis then depends on myelography and on pathologic examination of tissue removed at surgery.

Alter M: Anencephalus, hydrocephalus and spina bifida. Epidemiology with special reference to a survey in Charleston, S.C. Arch Neurol 7:411, 1962.

Caviness VS: The Chiari malformations of the posterior fossa and their relation to hydrocephalus. Develop Med Child Neurol 18:103, 1976.

Holcomb GW Jr, Matson DD: Thoracic neurenteric cyst. Surgery 35:115, 1954.

Ingraham FD: Spina Bifida and Cranium Bifidum. Papers reprinted from the New England Journal of Medicine with addition of a comprehensive bibliography. Boston, Massachusetts Medical Society, 1944.

Laurence KM: The recurrence risk in spina bifida cystica and anencephaly. Develop Med Child Neurol Suppl 13, 1967, p 75.

McLaughlin JF, Shurtleff DB, Lamers JY, et al: Influence of prognosis on decisions regarding the care of newborns with myelodysplasia. N Engl J Med 312:1589, 1985.

McLone DG: Results of treatment of children with myelomeningocele. Clin Neurosurg 30:407, 1983.

Matson DD: Neurosurgery of infancy and Childhood. Springfield, IL, Charles C Thomas, 1969.

Matson DD, Jerva MJ: Recurrent meningitis associated with lumbosacral dermal sinus tracts. J Neurosurg 25:288, 1966.

Sheptak PR, Susen AF: Diastematomyelia. Am J Dis Child 113:210, 1967.

Sieben RL, Hamida MB, Shulman K: Multiple cranial nerve deficits associated with the Arnold-Chiari malformation. Neurology 21:673, 1971.

Swinyard CA: The Child with Spina Bifida. New York, Association for the Aid of Crippled Children, 1971.

Thiersch JB: Therapeutic abortions with a folic acid antagonist, 4-aminopteroylglutamic acid administered by the oral route. Am J Obstet Gynecol 63:1298, 1952.

21.11 DEFECTS IN THE DIFFERENTIATION AND GROWTH OF THE CEREBRAL HEMISPHERES

The future cerebrum makes its appearance as a recognizable structure in the human embryo at about 28 days' gestation, when the anterior end of the neural tube shows a globular expansion, *the prosencephalon* (Fig. 21–6C). Over the next several days the prosencephalon cleaves into two lateral expansions which represent the beginnings of the cerebral hemispheres and of the lateral ventricles (Fig. 21–6D). The walls of the ventricles at this stage are formed by a germinal layer of actively dividing neuroblasts. Newly formed neuroblasts migrate away from the ventricular wall toward the surface of the primitive cerebral hemisphere, where their accumulation leads to formation of the cerebral cortex. The first arrivals form the lower cortical layers, and later arrivals pass them to form the upper layers. Differentiation of neuroblasts leads to formation of neurons and of glial cells. Migrating neuroblasts tend to maintain contact with the ventricular lumen through cellular extensions which steadily increase in length and which eventually make up the axons of the subcortical white matter. Axons crossing from one hemisphere to the other in the future corpus callosum first appear during the 3rd mo of gestation; the formation of the corpus callosum is complete by the 5th mo. About then, the surface of the cerebral cortex begins to show indentations

which are progressively elaborated during the last trimester until at term major cerebral sulci and gyri are clearly delineated.

The brain of the term infant contains the full adult complement of neurons, but its weight is only about one third that of the adult. The postnatal increase in weight is the result of myelination of subcortical white matter, of elaboration of neuronal processes (both dendrites and axons), and of increase in glial cells (Fig. 21–8).

Generally, abnormal influences occurring prior to the 6th mo of gestation tend to affect development of the gross structure of the brain and to diminish total neuronal number. Pathologic influences in the perinatal period tend to have more subtle effects, such as retardation of myelination and decrease in elaboration of dendrites. Loss of brain substance due to destructive lesions in late fetal life or early infancy may occur either alone or in combination with developmental defects.

Holoprosencephaly. Holoprosencephaly is an early developmental defect of brain in which there is failure to form paired cerebral hemispheres. The cerebrum is made up of an unpaired sphere, and the lateral ventricles are represented by a single midline cavity. Usually there is associated *arrhinencephaly*—absence of olfactory bulbs and tracts, cleft lip, and microphthalmia or cyclopia. Occasionally, holoprosencephaly occurs with trisomy 13–15; in other instances the etiology is unknown. Severe mental and motor defects are usually present; affected children rarely survive past infancy.

Agenesis of the Corpus Callosum. In this developmental anomaly the major fiber tracts that connect the two cerebral hemispheres are absent. Rarely, partial agenesis of the corpus callosum is transmitted by X-linked recessive inheritance; most cases are of unknown etiology. *Two clinical syndromes are recognized:* (1) The patient has normal intellectual and motor functions, and the malformation manifests itself only as an inability to transfer information from one cerebral hemisphere to the other. For example, the patient, if right-handed, may have difficulty in naming objects placed in the left hand since this requires transfer of information from right sensory cortex to the speech areas in the left cerebral hemisphere. (2) More commonly, the condition is associated with other developmental defects of the cerebrum, including failure of migration of neurons and hydrocephalus; affected children present in infancy with seizures, developmental retardation, abnormal head enlargement, and, often, hypertelorism. The diagnosis is made by computed tomography.

Porencephaly. Porencephaly is a defect in the cerebral mantle resulting in a cyst-like expansion of the lateral ventricle, which may extend up to the pia arachnoid membrane.

Porencephaly is occasionally due to a primary defect in development of the cerebral mantle, in which case it tends to be bilateral, with replacement of the temporoparietal areas by fluid-filled spaces; affected infants have severe amentia. More commonly, porencephaly is unilateral and is secondary to local damage of the cerebrum during the later fetal or early infantile period. Vascular occlusion, encephalitis, and needle puncture of the brain have been implicated as possible etiologic factors. Depending on the location of the porencephaly, the child may have spastic hemiparesis, hemisensory defects, or homonymous hemianopsia. The skull may expand laterally and be thinner on the side of the porencephaly, apparently as a result of fluid waves set up in the porencephalic cavity by pulsations of the choroid plexus.

Transillumination of the skull is of great value in the diagnosis of porencephaly and should always be performed in infants with unexplained hemiparesis. The differential diagnosis includes chronic subdural effusion, in which skull transillumination is also positive. The differentiation can be made by computed tomography. Shunt surgery may be indicated in rare instances when porencephaly is associated

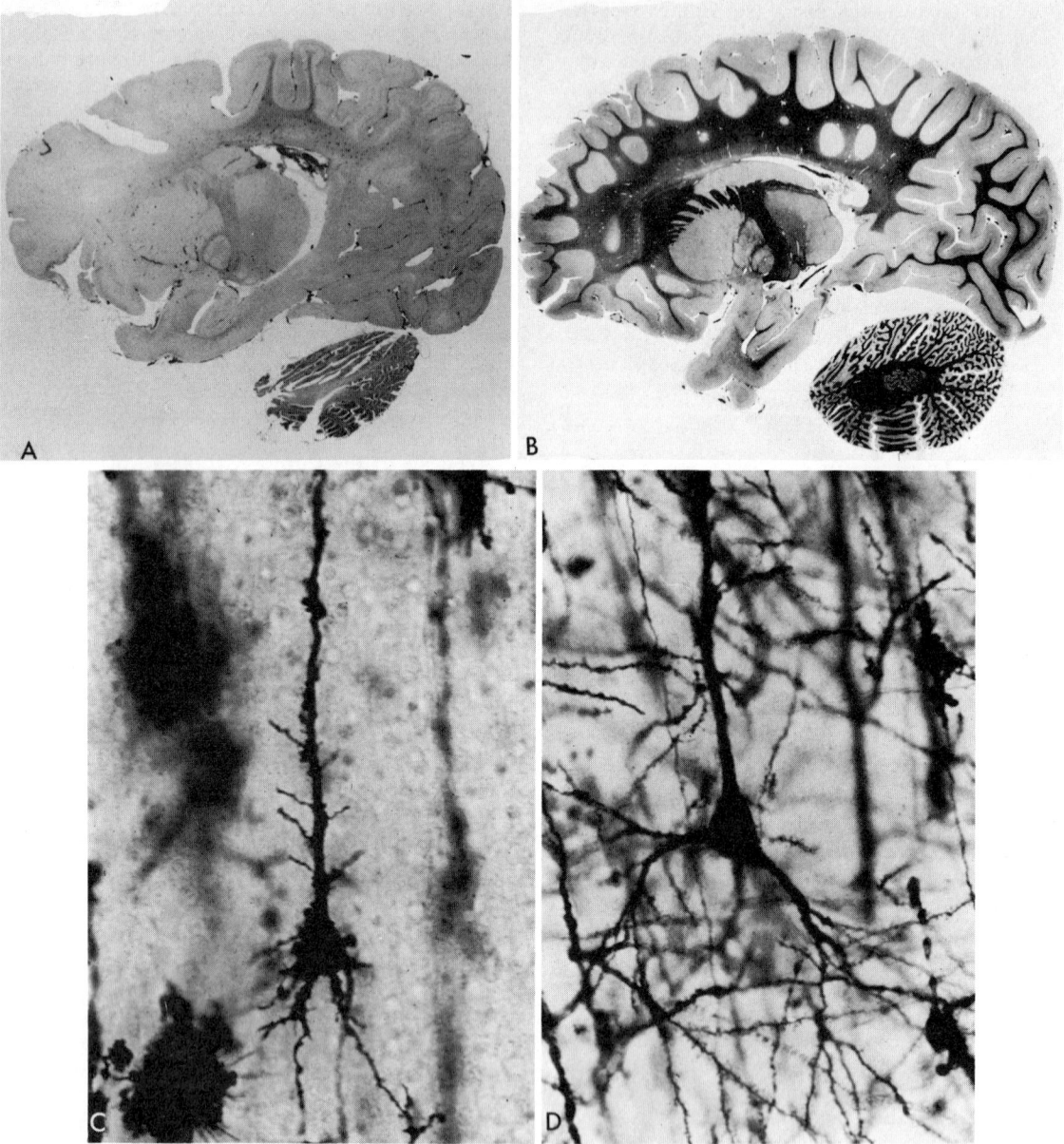

Figure 21–8. *A* and *B*, Sagittal sections of brain stained with myelin stain. *A*, The brain of a newborn shows little myelin in the subcortical white matter. *B*, The brain of a 9 mo old shows extensive myelination, especially in the primary visual, somatosensory, and motor areas. *C* and *D*, Single cortical pyramidal neurons stained by the Golgi method to show dendritic development. *C* is from frontal cortex of a newborn, *D* from the same area in a 4 yr old child, showing marked increase in length and complexity of dendritic branching. (× 100.)

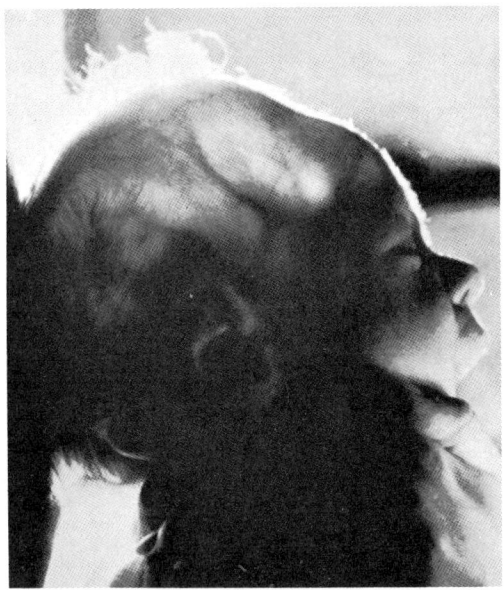

Figure 21–9. Hydranencephaly shown by transillumination.

with abnormal enlargement of the head and progressive motor deficit.

Hydranencephaly. Hydranencephaly is congenital absence of the cerebral hemispheres, which are replaced by a large, fluid-filled cavity. The brain stem and basal ganglia are well formed, and rudiments of frontal and occipital cortex may be present. The etiology is unknown. Failure of development of the cerebral arteries and destruction of brain by severe intrauterine infection have been suggested as possible causes.

The hydranencephalic infant may look remarkably normal at birth. Head size is normal or slightly enlarged. All the normal neonatal reflex patterns may be present. The infant does not have visual following, however, and there is failure of further voluntary motor and intellectual development. Seizures may occur. The diagnosis is suggested by total transillumination of the skull (Fig. 21–9). A similar clinical picture may be seen in advanced congenital hydrocephalus and with extensive bilateral subdural effusions. The diagnosis should be confirmed by cerebral angiography, which shows absence of the major cerebral vessels. Most of the affected infants die within 1 yr, but survival past 3 yr has been reported.

Lissencephaly. In this defect in migration of cerebral neurons, cortical gyri fail to develop. The surface of the cerebral hemispheres is smooth; microscopic examination shows absence of the normal cortical cell layers and persistence of groups of neurons in the subcortical white matter. The clinical picture is that of severe mental retardation. The diagnosis can be made by computed tomography.

Polymicrogyria. Polymicrogyria is another defect in neuronal migration; a great excess of poorly developed cerebral gyri is formed. The abnormality has been associated with intrauterine cytomegaloviral infection, but in most cases the etiology is obscure. Severe mental retardation is always present. The diagnosis is made at autopsy.

Microcephaly. This is a defect in the growth of the brain as a whole, resulting from developmental abnormalities and destructive processes affecting the brain during the fetal and early infancy periods. Head size is more than 3 standard deviations below the normal mean. The more important known causes are listed in Table 21–8.

The microcephalic brain always shows a decrease in weight, which may be as low as 25% of normal. The number and complexity of cortical gyri may be diminished. The frontal lobes are most severely stunted; the cerebellum is often disproportionately large. In microcephaly due to perinatal or postnatal disorders there may be neuronal loss and gliosis in the cerebral cortex.

The most severe microcephaly tends to occur in the recessively inherited form. Affected children have marked backward sloping of the forehead and disproportionately large ears. Motor development is often remarkably good, but mental retardation becomes progressively more evident and is often profound.

The conditions listed in Table 21–8 have to be considered in the differential diagnosis of the microcephalic infant or child. A backward-sloping forehead, large ears, or a history of parental consanguinity suggests the diagnosis of hereditary microcephaly. The possibility that microcephaly may be due to maternal phenylketonuria should always be pursued by appropriate examination of the mother's urine. Skull roentgenograms, lumbar puncture, and serologic tests are useful in the diagnosis of microcephaly secondary to intrauterine infection. Diffuse cerebral calcifications are frequently found in congenital toxoplasmosis; periventricular calcifications are more prevalent in cytomegaloviral disease (Fig. 21–10). The fetal alcohol syndrome has to be considered in a microcephalic child whose mother has a history of alcoholism.

Microcephaly must be distinguished from small head size secondary to synostosis of sagittal and coronal sutures. In craniosynostosis a palpable ridge is present in the region of the prematurely closed suture, and there is evidence of increased intracranial pressure, including papilledema and increase in convolutional markings on skull radiographs.

None of the forms of microcephaly are treatable, but accurate diagnosis is important for genetic counseling, some disorders being hereditary, others clearly sporadic.

Megalencephaly. In this rare developmental defect excessive growth of brain occurs during infancy and is responsible for abnormally rapid enlargement of the head. Brains weighing up to 2800 g have been reported, the excessive weight usually due to overgrowth of glial cells rather than of neurons. Similar excessive growth of brain may occur in Canavan disease, in Hurler syndrome, in Tay-Sachs disease, and in

Table 21–8. **Causes of Microcephaly**

Defects in Brain Development	Intrauterine Infections	Perinatal and Postnatal Disorders
Hereditary (recessive) microcephaly	Congenital rubella	Intrauterine or neonatal anoxia
Mongolism and other autosomal trisomy syndromes	Cytomegaloviral infection	Severe malnutrition in early infancy
Fetal ionizing radiation exposure	Congenital toxoplasmosis	Neonatal herpes virus infection
Maternal phenylketonuria	Congenital syphilis	
Seckel dwarfism		
Cornelia de Lange syndrome		
Rubinstein-Taybi syndrome		
Smith-Lemli-Opitz syndrome		
Fetal alcohol syndrome		

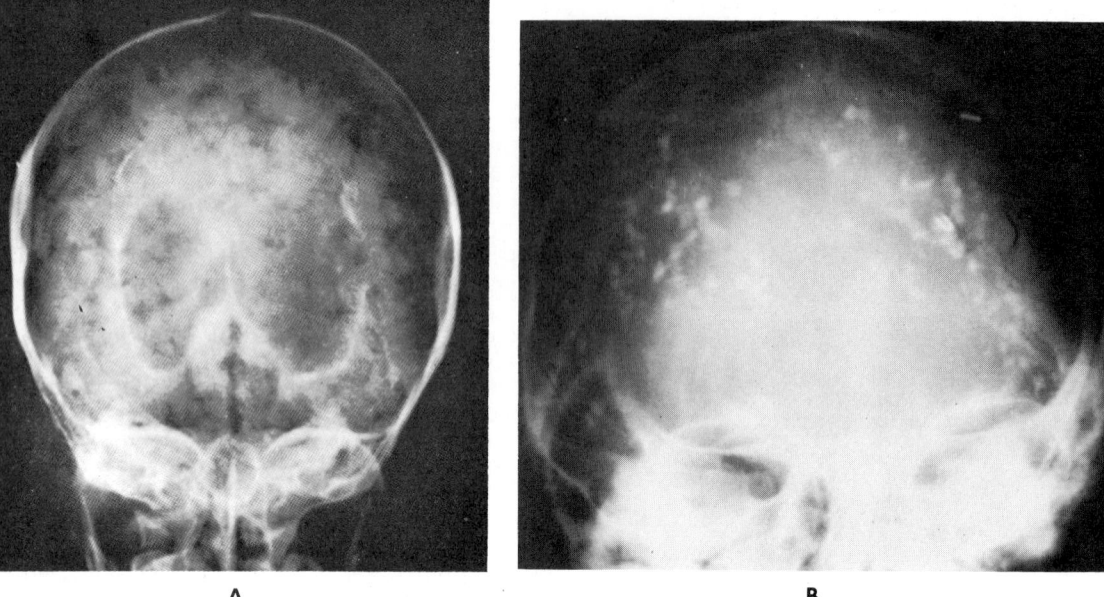

Figure 21–10. *A,* Periventricular calcification and hydrocephalus following cytomegalic inclusion disease in the newborn. *B,* Diffuse intracerebral calcifications following congenital toxoplasmosis.

metachromatic leukodystrophy, but the cause of megalencephaly is often unknown. Affected infants usually have considerable developmental delay. Signs of increased intracranial pressure are absent. Differentiation from hydrocephalus is made by computed tomography. The prognosis is guarded; severe mental deficiency is common.

Baron J, Youngblood L, Siewers MF, et al: The incidence of cytomegaloviruses, herpes simplex, rubella and toxoplasma antibodies in microcephalic, mentally retarded and normocephalic children. Pediatrics 44:932, 1969.

Bishop K, Connolly JM, Carter CH, et al: Holoprosencephaly. J Pediatr 65:406, 1964.

Brent RL: Radiation teratogenesis. Teratology 21:281, 1980.

DeMyer W: Megalencephaly in children. Clinical syndromes, genetic patterns, and differential diagnosis from other causes of megalocephaly. Neurology 22:634, 1972.

Freeman JM, Gold AP: Porencephaly simulating subdural hematoma in childhood. Am J Dis Child 107:327, 1964.

Haberland C, Brunngraber E: Micropolygyria: A histopathological and biochemical study. J Ment Defic Res 16:1, 1972.

Hamby WB, Krauss RF, Beswick WF: Hydranencephaly: Clinical diagnosis. Presentation of seven cases. Pediatrics 6:371, 1950.

Hansen H: Epidemiological considerations on maternal hyperphenylalaninemia. Am J Ment Defic 75:22, 1970.

Jones KL, Smith DW: Recognition of the fetal alcohol syndrome in early infancy. Lancet 2:999, 1973.

Koch FP, Doyle PJ: Agenesis of the corpus callosum. Report of eight cases in infancy. J Pediatr 50:345, 1957.

Lorber J, Granger RG: Cerebral cavities following ventricular puncture in infants. Clin Radiol 14:98, 1963.

Menkes JH, Philippart M, Clark DB: Hereditary partial agenesis of corpus callosum. Arch Neurol 11:198, 1964.

Osburn BI, Silverstein AM, Prendergast RA, et al: Experimental viral-induced congenital encephalopathies. I. Pathology of hydranencephaly and porencephaly caused by bluetongue vaccine virus. Lab Invest 25:197, 1971.

Penrose LS: Microcephaly. Folia Hered Pathol 5:79, 1956.

Yakovlev PI, Wadsworth RC: Schizencephalies. A study of congenital clefts in the cerebral mantle; Clefts with fused lips. J Neuropathol Exp Neurol 5:169, 1946.

Yu JS, O'Halloran MT: Children of mothers with phenylketonuria. Lancet 1:210, 1970.

21.12 HYDROCEPHALUS

Definition. The term "hydrocephalus" is applied to conditions in which enlargement of the ventricular system results from an imbalance between production and absorption of cerebrospinal fluid (CSF). CSF pressure is usually elevated in progressive hydrocephalus, but occasionally it may be normal or nearly so.

Pathophysiology and Etiology. CSF production depends largely on the active transport of ions, especially sodium, across the specialized epithelial membrane of the choroid plexus into the ventricular cavities. Water follows passively to re-establish osmotic equilibrium; the result is the passage of fluid into the cerebral ventricles. This fluid circulates via the aqueduct of Sylvius and the 4th ventricle and gains access to the subarachnoid spaces through the foramina of Luschka and Magendie. It is reabsorbed into the venous circulation from the subarachnoid spaces over the brain, to some extent from those over the spinal cord, and from the ependymal lining of the ventricles. The circulation of CSF is shown schematically in Fig. 21–11.

Hydrocephalus is almost always due to interference with the circulation and absorption of CSF. Rarely, it is due to overproduction of fluid. Excessive fluid production is best documented in papilloma of the choroid plexus, a tumor which actively secretes CSF.

Two anatomic types of hydrocephalus are distinguished: (1) In *obstructive hydrocephalus* there is interference with circulation of CSF within the ventricular system itself. As a result ventricular fluid cannot gain ready access to the subarachnoid spaces. Enlargement of the ventricular system occurs proximal to the site of obstruction. (2) In *communicating hydrocephalus* CSF pathways inside the ventricular system are open and ventricular fluid is able to move freely into the spinal subarachnoid space. Interference with absorption of CSF is due either to occlusion of the subarachnoid cisterns around the brain stem or to obliteration of subarachnoid spaces over the convexities of the brain. The entire ventricular system becomes uniformly distended. A number of congenital and acquired conditions may lead to hydrocephalus (Table 21–9).

Obstructive Hydrocephalus. This is due most commonly to *congenital aqueductal stenosis.* The aqueduct of Sylvius is narrowed or is replaced by multiple small channels or "forks" which end blindly (Fig. 21–12). In a small number of cases aqueductal stenosis is transmitted as an X-linked recessive trait. It may also be a residuum of inflammation in the

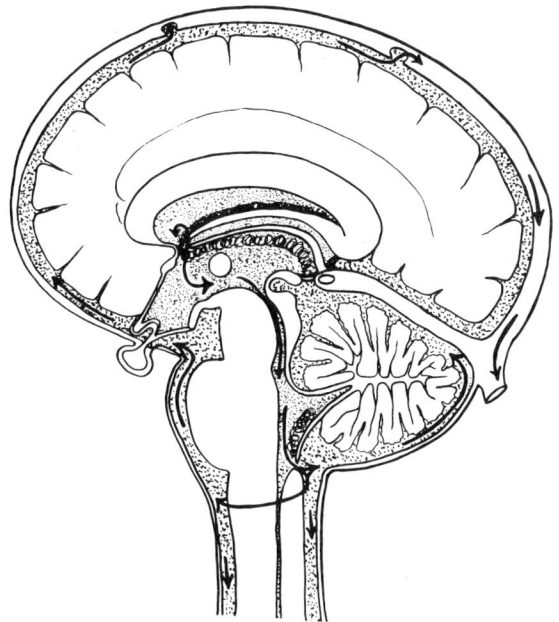

Figure 21-11. Schematic representation of CSF circulation.

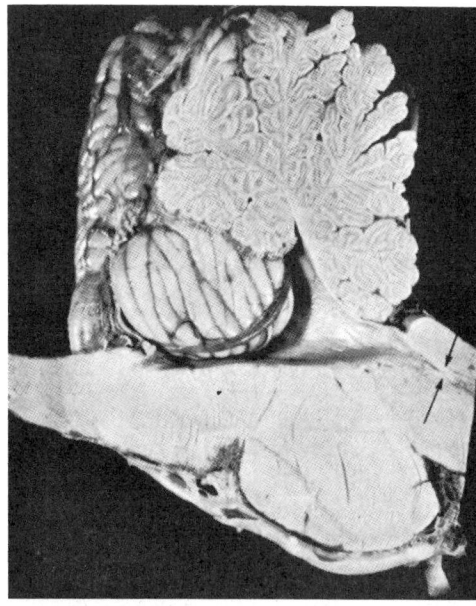

Figure 21-12. Congenital stenosis of aqueduct of Sylvius (*arrows*). Despite severe obstructive hydrocephalus, patient lived to 6th decade as a self-supporting person.

periaqueductal region. Experimental evidence in several animal species implicates fetal viral infection, especially mumps, as an etiologic factor. Occasionally, obstructive hydrocephalus is due to compression of the aqueduct by an extrinsic lesion posterior to the brain stem, such as congenital aneurysm of the vein of Galen or subdural hematoma in the posterior fossa. The latter occurs as a birth injury; the bleeding is secondary to traumatic rupture of veins bridging from the surface of the cerebellum to the transverse sinuses. The diagnosis of posterior fossa subdural hematoma has to be considered in infants who develop hydrocephalus during the 1st postnatal weeks, especially when there is a history of difficult birth. The *Dandy-Walker malformation* is a congenital defect of midline cerebellar structures in which hydrocephalus is caused by atresia of the foramina of Luschka and Magendie. When obstructive hydrocephalus is acquired postnatally, it is often due to brain tumors which compress or extend into the ventricular system. Aqueductal stenosis also may be of postnatal onset and may not become manifest until late in childhood or adolescence.

Communicating Hydrocephalus. Often of unknown etiology, this occurs with the *Arnold-Chiari malformation*, in which it is due to obstruction of subarachnoid pathways around the brain stem by downward displacement of the medulla oblongata and cerebellum. Communicating hydrocephalus may follow bacterial meningitis, toxoplasmosis, cytomegaloviral

infection, and subarachnoid hemorrhage as a result of obliteration of subarachnoid spaces by fibrous tissue reaction to meningeal inflammation or to hemorrhage. Hydrocephalus may complicate *Hurler syndrome* because of fibrous tissue proliferation in the subarachnoid spaces. In *achondroplasia* hydrocephalus is probably due to underdevelopment of the occipital skull, an abnormally small posterior fossa interfering with circulation of CSF in the subarachnoid spaces at the base of the brain. *Vitamin A intoxication* is a rare cause of communicating hydrocephalus; the mechanism is unknown.

Incidence. The incidence of congenital hydrocephalus varies in different populations, especially the hydrocephalus associated with meningomyelocele. The incidence of all other forms of hydrocephalus is nearly 1/1000. Aqueductal stenosis is found in about one third of all hydrocephalic children.

Clinical Manifestations. Signs and symptoms of hydrocephalus depend on the time of onset and on the severity of the imbalance between CSF production and resorptive capacity. Abnormal enlargement of the head is a common feature of congenital hydrocephalus and of hydrocephalus with onset in infancy. In severe cases of congenital hydrocephalus massive enlargement of the head during the fetal period may preclude normal delivery of the infant. In milder forms the head is of normal size at birth but then grows at an excessive rate. Serial measurements of head circumference are essential for early diagnosis and for assessment of rate of progression. The skull is distended in all directions but especially in the frontal area. Occipital expansion is seen in the Dandy-Walker malformation as a result of massive dilatation of the 4th ventricle, which can be demonstrated by occipital transillumination of the skull. Infants with rapidly progressive hydrocephalus have a large, bulging anterior fontanelle and palpable separation of cranial sutures. Apparently normal fontanelle tension does not, however, rule out the diagnosis. Separation of the cranial sutures leads to a resonant note on percussion of the skull (Macewen or "cracked-pot" sign). The scalp skin is thin and shiny, and the scalp veins are often prominent. The cry becomes high-pitched as intracranial pressure rises. In severe infantile hydrocephalus the eyes often appear deviated downward ("setting-sun" sign). Optic atrophy, resulting from compression of the optic nerve and chiasm, occurs in chronic, untreated cases.

Table 21-9. Causes of Hydrocephalus

Obstructive Hydrocephalus	Communicating Hydrocephalus

Aqueductal stenosis
  Congenital
  Acquired (postinfectious)
Midline brain tumors
Vein of Galen malformation
Posterior fossa subdural
  hematoma
Dandy-Walker malformation
	Arnold-Chiari malformation
	Postinfectious (meningitis,
	  toxoplasmosis, cytomegaloviral
	  infection)
	Secondary to subarachnoid
	  hemorrhage
	Secondary to excessive production
	  of CSF (papilloma of choroid
	  plexus)
	Diseases of connective tissue
	  (Hurler syndrome,
	  achondroplasia)
	Vitamin A intoxication

When the onset of hydrocephalus is late in childhood, there may be no appreciable enlargement of the head. Instead, the child has evidence of increased intracranial pressure with chronic papilledema. Spasticity and ataxia affecting the legs more than the arms are common, as is urinary incontinence. Progressive decline in mental activity occurs. Higher cortical functions such as judgment and reasoning tend to be affected disproportionately, while speech, often preserved, results in rather characteristic empty chatter. There is poor correlation between degree of hydrocephalus and intellectual dysfunction. Some children with hugely dilated ventricular systems and thin cerebral mantles have normal intelligence.

Laboratory Studies. Computed tomography reliably and safely differentiates hydrocephalus from other disorders that cause abnormal enlargement of the head and identifies the site of obstruction to CSF flow. The cerebrospinal fluid should be examined in cases of uncertain etiology to rule out chronic meningeal infection as a cause and to determine whether CSF protein is elevated.

Differential Diagnosis. A number of conditions other than hydrocephalus cause abnormal enlargement of the cranial vault in infancy. Megalencephaly mimics hydrocephalus, but signs of increased intracranial pressure are absent in megalencephaly and the mental defect is more profound. Chronic subdural effusion in infancy may lead to head enlargement. The characteristic expansion of the skull occurs in the parietal areas rather than frontally as in hydrocephalus. Transillumination is positive in the frontoparietal regions in chronic subdural effusions but negative in all but extreme cases of hydrocephalus, in which the cortical mantle is virtually absent. Ventricular enlargement follows cerebral atrophy in degenerative and metabolic brain diseases, in which head size is normal or small.

The possibility that hydrocephalus may be secondary to midline brain tumor always has to be considered. Cerebellar, pineal region, and 3rd ventricular tumors are likely to produce head enlargement in the absence of focal neurologic signs. Brain tumor has to be considered especially when enlargement of the head is very rapid in a previously normal infant and when papilledema is present. An underlying cerebral neoplasm can be ruled out by computed tomography with infusion of radiopaque contrast material.

Therapy. The treatment of hydrocephalus has improved in recent years but still presents many formidable problems. The ideal goal is to re-establish equilibrium between CSF production and resorption. Acetazolamide in a dose of 40–75 mg/kg/24 hr diminishes CSF production by about one third and is occasionally effective in mild, slowly progressive hydrocephalus. In most cases, however, shunt operations provide the best treatment for progressive hydrocephalus.

In obstructive hydrocephalus the site of obstruction can sometimes be bypassed. The Torkildsen operation bypasses aqueductal stenosis with a plastic tube that connects one lateral ventricle with the cisterna magna and the spinal subarachnoid spaces; the operation is not successful in infants since these spaces are as yet poorly developed. At present, the most widely used and successful treatments involve shunting of excess fluid into some extracranial body compartment. Ventriculoperitoneal shunts are most commonly used. A one-way valve that closes when ventricular fluid pressure falls below a fixed value is inserted into the tubing to prevent complete drainage of CSF and collapse of the cerebral ventricles. Complications with this type of shunt include bacterial colonization of the shunt (especially with *Staphylococcus albus*), kinking, plugging, or separation of the shunt tubing, and subdural hematoma due to low intracranial pressure. Shunt infection may cause recurrent episodes of septicemia and ventriculitis. In either case, cure of the infection usually requires removal of the shunt in addition to antibiotic therapy. Plugging of the shunt tubing is especially apt to occur when

CSF protein is elevated. Growth of the head, neck, and chest necessitates repeated shunt revisions during early childhood. Ventriculoatrial shunts, which deliver ventricular fluid from a lateral ventricle to the right atrium, are used less commonly now because of higher rates of infection and the complications of pulmonary embolism, superior vena caval occlusion, and nephritis.

Careful initial evaluation is essential to determine whether a shunt operation is needed or spontaneous arrest of hydrocephalus has occurred. In general, a shunt is not indicated in hydrocephalic infants whose head growth has become arrested or is progressing at or below the normal rate. Repeated lumbar punctures rather than shunt surgery appear to be the initial treatment of choice when acute hydrocephalus occurs after subarachnoid hemorrhage or bacterial meningitis.

When a successful shunt has been established, it usually has to be maintained for the life of the patient. Such a child needs careful medical supervision for early detection of evidences of shunt malfunction. Acute shunt failure in the older child causes rapidly progressive increase in intracranial pressure, with headache, vomiting, and stupor, progressing to coma and death unless shunt revision is performed promptly. Chronic shunt malfunction may result in school failure, lethargy, and deterioration of gait. Serial computed tomography or ultrasonography of the head is useful for detection of early shunt failure.

Prognosis. The prognosis of infantile hydrocephalus is significantly improved by shunt operations. Untreated, 50–60% of infants with hydrocephalus succumb to the disorder itself or to intercurrent illnesses. About 40% of survivors are of near-normal intelligence. With good neurosurgical and medical management at least 70% can be expected to live beyond infancy; of these, about 40% will have normal intellect, and about 60% (mainly the children with meningomyelocele) will have significant intellectual and motor handicaps.

Ameli NO: Arrest of development and Dandy-Walker malformation. Brain 89:459, 1966.
Drachman DA, Richardson EP: Aqueductal narrowing, congenital and acquired. Arch Neurol 5:552, 1961.
Foltz EL, Shurtleff DB: Five-year comparative study of hydrocephalus in children with and without operation (113 cases). J Neurosurg 20:1064, 1963.
Gilles F, Shilito J: Infantile hydrocephalus: Retrocerebellar subdural hematoma. J Pediatr 76:529, 1970.
Goldstein GW, et al: Transient hydrocephalus in premature infants: Treatment by lumbar punctures. Lancet 1:512, 1976.
Hagberg B, Naglo AS: The conservative management of infantile hydrocephalus. Acta Paediatr Scand 61:165, 1972.
Hagberg B, Sjorgen I: The chronic brain syndrome of infantile hydrocephalus. Am J Dis Child 112:189, 1966.
Hart MN, Malamud N, Ellis WG: The Dandy-Walker syndrome: A clinical-pathological study of 28 cases. Neurology 22:771, 1972.
Huttenlocher PR: Treatment of hydrocephalus with acetazolamide. Results in 15 cases. J Pediatr 66:1023, 1965.
Ignelzi RJ, Kirsch WM: Follow-up analysis of ventriculoperitoneal and ventriculoatrial shunts for hydrocephalus. J Neurosurg 42:679, 1975.
Laurence KM, Coates S: The natural history of hydrocephalus. Detailed analysis of 182 unoperated cases. Arch Dis Child 37:345, 1962.
Milhorat TH: Hydrocephalus and the Cerebrospinal Fluid. Baltimore, Williams & Wilkins, 1972.
Olsen L, Frykberg T: Complications in the treatment of hydrocephalus in children. Acta Pediatr Scand 72:385, 1983.
Russell DS: Observations on the pathology of hydrocephalus. Special Report No 265. Medical Research Council London, His Majesty's Stationery Office, 1949.
Schick RW, Matson DD: What is arrested hydrocephalus? J Pediatr 58:791, 1961.
Timmons GD, Johnson KP: Aqueductal stenosis and hydrocephalus after mumps encephalitis. N Engl J Med 283:1505, 1970.
Woodard WK, Miller LJ, Legant O: Acute and chronic hypervitaminosis A in a 4 month old infant. J Pediatr 59:260, 1961.

21.13 DEFECTS IN DEVELOPMENT OF THE BRAIN STEM

Moebius Syndrome. In this syndrome, also known as congenital nuclear aplasia, there is absence or maldevelopment of cranial nerve nuclei and of their nerves. The 7th nerves are affected most frequently, but most of the cranial nerves may be involved. The most severely affected children have ptosis, complete ophthalmoplegia, inability to close the eyes, facial immobility, and difficulty with chewing and swallowing. Congenital anomalies often associated include absence of pectoralis muscles and clubfoot deformities. The expressionless face and constant drooling may give the erroneous impression of mental defect. When lid closure is defective, it is important to protect the corneas by use of artificial tears and by taping the eyelids at night. Familial cases have been reported.

Becker-Christensen F, Lund HT: A family with Möbius syndrome. J Pediatr 84:115, 1974.
Hoefnagel D, Biery B: Spasmus nutans. Develop Med Child Neurol 10:32, 1968.
Van Allen MW, Blodi FC: Neurologic aspects of the Moebius syndrome. Neurology 10:249, 1960.

21.14 PERINATALLY ACQUIRED CEREBRAL LESIONS

Damage to the central nervous system in the perinatal period is a major cause of intellectual handicap and of nonprogressive motor disorders. This is related in part to the unusual stresses to the infant incident to birth, in part to the peculiar susceptibility of the immature central nervous system to injury by a variety of agents. Cerebral anoxia, trauma to brain, infection, hyperbilirubinemia, hypoglycemia, hypothyroidism, and the inborn errors of amino acid metabolism are important causes of brain damage in the infant. The reaction of the immature brain to these agents differs markedly from that of the mature central nervous system.

Cerebral anoxia in the infant, in contrast to the older child or adult, frequently causes selective damage to subcortical structures rather than to cortical neurons; this is especially the case in the premature infant, in whom the subcortical white matter is particularly vulnerable. The resulting brain lesion, periventricular leukomalacia, is found frequently at autopsy of premature infants who have had repeated anoxic episodes. The basal ganglia are also susceptible to anoxic damage in the neonate. Pathologically, one finds loss of neurons in basal ganglia and abnormal deposition of myelin to replace them, giving with myelin stains a marbled appearance, "status marmoratus," to the basal ganglia.

Meningeal infection involves cerebritis and cerebral vasculitis much more frequently in the neonate than in the older child, and these account for brain damage in the majority of survivors. Infections with rubella, cytomegalovirus, herpesvirus, coxsackievirus, and toxoplasma are more likely to involve brain in the fetus and neonate than in the older person. The reaction in the nervous system is usually one of widespread necrosis.

Elevation in the blood level of unconjugated bilirubin above 15–20 mg/dL causes damage in selected structures of the neonatal brain, especially the basal ganglia and cranial nerve nuclei in the lower brain stem, including those of the 8th nerve (Sec. 8.44). The most prominent acute, pathologic change is yellow staining of the affected nuclei (*kernicterus*) due to deposition of bilirubin in the damaged tissues. The chronic lesion consists of loss of nerve cells, gliosis, and defective myelination.

Severe neonatal *hypoglycemia* (Sec. 8.57) may cause diffuse necrosis of cortical neurons and damage to cerebellum. These lesions are uncommon, however, and it is generally assumed that the immature brain is less sensitive to damage by hypoglycemia than is the mature one.

Metabolic diseases that lead to cerebral dysfunction by interference with normal developmental events in postnatal brain

include congenital hypothyroidism (cretinism) and the large group of inborn errors of amino acid metabolism, of which phenylketonuria is the most common. Myelination of subcortical white matter and the elaboration of dendrites and of synaptic connections between nerve cells are the two most important developmental events in postnatal brain (see Fig. 21–8). They are most likely to be disturbed in the metabolic encephalopathies. Defective myelination occurs in phenylketonuria and in maple syrup urine disease. In cretinism both the elaboration of cortical dendrites and myelination appear to be inhibited.

In many infants damaged in the perinatal period the paucity of early clinical signs of CNS lesions presents a major problem. The infant may initially appear to improve, cerebral dysfunction becoming manifest only later, as he or she matures. Intellectual handicaps ranging from severe mental defect to mild learning disabilities are common sequelae of neonatal brain damage. In some damaged infants motor deficits predominate, with relative preservation of intellectual functions. (See Cerebral Palsy below.) Seizures may develop, sometimes 1 yr or more after the initial insult. Since the mental and motor manifestations of cerebral damage may not appear until much later, it often is difficult to ascribe them with certainty to specific events; accordingly the causes of static cerebral lesions in many children are unknown or conjectural.

Anderson JM, Milner RDG, Stritch SJ: Effects of neonatal hypoglycemia on the nervous system: A pathological study. J Neurol Neurosurg Psychiatr 30:295, 1967.
Banker BQ, Larroche JC: Periventricular leukomalacia of infancy: A form of neonatal anoxic encephalopathy. Arch Neurol 7:386, 1962.
Berman PH, Banker BQ: Neonatal meningitis. A clinical and pathological study of 29 cases. Pediatrics 38:6, 1966.
Diamond I, et al: Kernicterus: Revised concepts of pathogenesis and management. Pediatrics 38:539, 1966.
Eayres JT, Horn G: The development of cerebral cortex in hypothyroid and starved rats. Anat Rec 121:53, 1955.
Norman RM: État marbré of the corpus striatum following birth injury. J Neurol Neurosurg Psychiatr 10:12, 1947.
Prensky AL, Carr S, Moser HW: Development of myelin in inherited disorders of amino acid metabolism. Arch Neurol 19:552, 1968.
Rosman NP, et al: The effect of thyroid deficiency on myelination of brain. Neurology 22:99, 1972.
Towbin A: Central nervous system damage in the human fetus and newborn infant. Am J Dis Child 119:529, 1970.
Volpe JJ: Neurology of the Newborn. Philadelphia, WB Saunders, 1981.

21.15 CEREBRAL PALSY
(Little Disease)

Cerebral palsy is defined as any nonprogressive central motor deficit dating to events in the prenatal or perinatal periods. It is one of the most common crippling conditions of childhood; almost 300,000 children are affected in the United States alone. It is not a specific disease but a group of disorders of varied causes.

Etiology. The relationship of cerebral palsy to neonatal anoxia was first established by Little in 1843. Recent studies find that more than one third of children with cerebral palsy weighed less than 2500 g at birth. The most likely etiologic event in these infants is cerebral anoxia, often complicated by intraventricular and subependymal hemorrhages (Sec. 8.23); physical trauma to the brain at birth is also a cause, especially in those with spastic hemiplegia. Congenital malformations of brain and cerebral vascular occlusions during fetal life appear to account for a smaller percentage. Kernicterus, an important cause of cerebral palsy prior to the introduction of exchange transfusion for neonatal hyperbilirubinemia, is now relatively uncommon.

Pathology. The most severely disabled children are apt to have widespread cerebral atrophy, often with cavity formation in subcortical white matter. Atrophy of basal ganglia is found when rigidity and extrapyramidal movement disorders were present during life. With hemiplegia, atrophy and gliosis of the opposite cerebral hemisphere often occur, usually confined to the areas supplied by the middle cerebral artery and probably due to arterial occlusion. Porencephaly occurs in some cases. In milder forms of cerebral palsy the brain may appear grossly normal but is often reduced in weight. The sparseness of subcortical white matter suggests that some nerve fibers may have been destroyed by the initial cerebral insult.

Clinical Manifestations. Clinical classification of patients with cerebral palsy is based on the nature of the observed motor deficit. The following classification is useful: (1) *Spastic cerebral palsy* (quadriplegia, paraplegia, hemiplegia, monoplegia); (2) *extrapyramidal cerebral palsy* (choreoathetosis, dystonia); (3) *atonic cerebral palsy* (atonic diplegia, congenital cerebellar ataxia); and (4) *mixed types.*

Spastic Cerebral Palsy. This is the most common type of palsy. Early manifestations are those of reflex hyperexcitability and abnormal persistence of neonatal reflexes. Hyperactivity of the grasp reflex leads to tight fisting of the hands. Tonic neck reflexes are often obligatory and may continue to be present long after the normal age of disappearance. Vertical suspension of the infant leads to extensor postures (arching of the back and rigid extension and adduction and internal rotation of the legs). When hip adduction is marked, it leads to crossing (scissoring) of the legs. The severely spastic infant may have arching of the back and scissoring even at rest. Tendon reflexes are brisk, often with sustained ankle clonus. A persistent Babinski sign is helpful in diagnosis after the age of 2 yr. Spasticity and rigidity become more evident as the child matures and often lead to abnormal postures of limbs and to contractures. Heel cord contractures, limitation in abduction and external rotation of the hips, and limitation in extension and supination of the forearms are common. Pseudobulbar palsy is present when spasticity is bilateral; it accounts for the swallowing difficulties and excessive drooling of affected children.

In *spastic quadriplegia* all four limbs are involved. There is usually associated mental defect. Pseudobulbar palsy is prominent, and convulsions are common. *Diplegia* refers to a motor deficit that affects all four limbs but is much more severe in the lower extremities than in the upper ones. The involvement of hands may be minimal, expressing itself only in clumsiness in grasping and, later in life, in awkwardness of hand movements. Evidence of pseudobulbar palsy may be absent or limited to a brisk jaw jerk. Intelligence is often normal or borderline, but apraxias are common and may lead to difficulties in learning to draw and to form letters. More than 50% of children with diplegia had low birth weights.

In *spastic paraplegia*, a rare form of cerebral palsy, only the lower extremities are affected. The possibility of a spinal cord lesion must always be carefully considered in the child who has spasticity confined to the legs.

Spastic hemiplegia accounts for about one third of children with cerebral palsy. There is often homonymous hemianopsia and a hemisensory deficit on the side of the hemiplegia. The posture of the affected arm is quite characteristic: maintained flexion and pronation of the forearm and flexion of the wrist. The gait of these children is characterized by limping, often with circumduction of the affected leg. The intellectual level tends to be in the low normal range but may be normal or superior, especially in children with small unilateral lesions.

Monoplegia, spastic weakness confined to one limb, is rare. Careful examination will usually disclose an asymmetric diplegia or hemiplegia with one limb more severely affected than the other.

Extrapyramidal Cerebral Palsy. This is manifest as hypotonia in early infancy and by choreoathetoid movements and dystonia later in childhood. Identification is unusual until after the age of 6 mo; abnormal posturing of hands when the

infant attempts to reach for an object is an early sign. When choreoathetosis is associated with deafness, it is almost always the result of kernicterus. The combination of motor handicap and absence of speech function caused by deafness may give an erroneous impression of severe mental retardation; intellectual capacity can be surmised only after prolonged study.

Atonic Diplegia. Atonic diplegia is a diagnostic term designating hypotonia and motor disability due to central nervous system damage. Severe mental defect is common. The tendon reflexes are easily obtainable and may be quite brisk, in contrast to the pattern in hypotonia due to peripheral neuromuscular diseases. Spasticity often develops in later childhood.

Congenital Cerebellar Ataxia. In this rare form of cerebral palsy hypotonia and hypoactive tendon reflexes are present in infancy. Usually by the 2nd yr intention tremor and gait ataxia are present. Nystagmus is uncommon. There may be associated mental defect, usually mild.

Differential Diagnosis. *Spastic cerebral palsy* has to be distinguished from the leukodystrophies. In doubtful cases a spinal tap may provide helpful diagnostic information; spinal fluid protein is almost always elevated in the leukodystrophies but not in cerebral palsy. The possibility that spastic weakness may be due to hydrocephalus or to subdural effusion should be considered whenever head size is large or when signs of increased intracranial pressure are present. Rarely, a slowly growing tumor of a cerebral hemisphere may be confused with the hemiplegic form of cerebral palsy. In brain tumor the disability is always progressive, and signs of increased intracranial pressure are usually present. Spinal cord lesions, including birth injuries to the cervical cord, atlanto-axial dislocation, tumors, and congenital malformations, should be considered when spasticity and weakness are limited to the muscle groups below the neck. Spastic diplegia is sometimes confused with muscular dystrophy; heel cord contractures and weakness of legs occur in both. Spasticity, however, is absent in muscular dystrophy, and the tendon reflexes are normal or reduced. In doubtful and early cases measurement of serum enzymes is helpful, especially of creatine kinase, which is always increased in Duchenne muscular dystrophy. *Atonic diplegia* must be distinguished from neuromuscular diseases of infancy, including Werdnig-Hoffmann disease and benign congenital hypotonia. The mental defect and the preservation of tendon reflexes in atonic diplegia usually make clinical differentiation possible. *Congenital cerebellar ataxia* must be differentiated from a number of slowly progressive cerebellar degenerations. Early, the distinction from ataxia-telangiectasia may be especially difficult; children with this illness are often diagnosed as having cerebral palsy. If more than one child in the same family has a motor deficit, this always suggests a disease other than cerebral palsy; there is no "familial cerebral palsy."

Prognosis. The outlook for the child with cerebral palsy depends largely on the severity of any associated intellectual handicaps. Good adjustment can be made to fairly severe motor deficits as long as intellectual capacity is good. The response of the family to the situation and the availability of adequate educational and therapeutic facilities are of great importance.

Treatment and Prevention. Treatment of the child with cerebral palsy consists of ensuring the fullest physical and social development possible. This is discussed in general terms in Sec. 2.70. In specific terms, treatment consists of early application of stretching exercises to prevent contractures, orthopedic appliances and surgical procedures to improve mobility, and special educational techniques to compensate for motor and intellectual defects insofar as possible.

The prevention of cerebral palsy constitutes a great challenge to the pediatrician. Much has been accomplished in the prevention of kernicterus. Skillful care of low birthweight infants may reduce the incidence of spastic diplegia. Careful attention to the respiratory status of the infant and prompt therapy of apneic episodes appear to be especially important.

Cohen ME, Duffner PK: Prognostic indicators in hemiparetic cerebral palsy. Ann Neurol 9:353, 1981.

Crothers B, Paine R: The Natural History of Cerebral Palsy. Cambridge, Harvard University Press, 1959.

Ford FR: Cerebral birth injuries and their results. Medicine 5:121, 1926.

McDonald AD: The aetiology of spastic diplegia. A synthesis of epidemiological and pathological evidence. Dev Med Child Neurol 6:277, 1964.

Mitchell RG: The prevention of cerebral palsy. Dev Med Child Neurol 13:137, 1971.

Myers RE: Atrophic cortical sclerosis with status marmoratus in the perinatally damaged monkey. Neurology 19:1177, 1969.

Plum P: Aetiology of athetosis with special reference to neonatal asphyxia, idiopathic icterus and ABO-incompatibility. Arch Dis Child 40:376, 1965.

Towbin A: The Pathology of Cerebral Palsy. Springfield, IL, Charles C Thomas, 1960.

Twitchell TE: The neurological examination in infantile cerebral palsy. Dev Med Child Neurol 5:271, 1963.

21.16 THE NEUROCUTANEOUS SYNDROMES

Several distinct neurocutaneous syndromes, also known as phakomatoses or ectodermal dysplasias, present lesions of both skin and central nervous system, often also with ocular and visceral abnormalities.

TUBEROUS SCLEROSIS
(Bourneville Disease)

See also Sec. 24.11.

This disorder, a major cause of mental defect and of intractable convulsions, is inherited as a dominant trait, with wide variation in expression. About 50% of cases appear to be new mutations. The fully developed disease involves numerous organs, including brain, skin, eyes, kidneys, heart, bones, and lungs.

The characteristic cerebral lesions are sclerotic patches (tubers) scattered throughout the cortical gray matter. They consist of collections of astrocytes, neurons, and bizarre giant cells without the cellular organization characteristic of normal cerebral cortex. In addition, glial nodules occur in a periventricular distribution. These lesions, present at birth, gradually enlarge and become calcified. Periventricular tumors consisting of giant cells and blood vessels may form large masses, obstructing the foramina of Monro.

Convulsions are the most common clinical sign of brain involvement and occur in more than 90% of patients. Infantile spasms occur during the 1st yr of life in about one third of cases; grand mal and psychomotor seizures predominate later. Mental defect, varying from mild to severe, is present in 60–70% of patients. Behavior disorders are common, especially hyperactivity and destructiveness. Focal neurologic signs such as hemiparesis are rare except in patients with periventricular giant cell tumors, in which case headache and papilledema related to ventricular obstruction are usually also found.

Adenoma sebaceum is the most characteristic skin lesion of tuberous sclerosis. It consists of small bright red or brownish nodules in a butterfly distribution on the nose and cheeks. Histologically, these lesions consist of a mixture of fibrous tissue and blood vessels. They usually appear between 2 and 5 yr of age, and by late childhood are found in more than 80% of patients. *Hypopigmented macules* on the skin of arms, legs, and trunk are usually present from birth; they may be oval or irregular in outline and a few mm to several cm in diameter. Two or more such skin lesions in an infant strongly suggest the diagnosis of tuberous sclerosis. Other manifestations include slightly raised, indurated areas of skin, usually

over the back (*shagreen patches*), and gingival and periungual fibromas.

Benign tumors made up of a mixture of fibrous tissue, fat, blood vessels, and smooth muscle, often partly cystic, are found in many organs, especially kidneys, heart, liver, spleen, and lungs. Renal tumors are present in about 80% of patients and may cause renal failure by compression of the ureters or renal pelvis. Renal cysts also occur and may produce similar symptoms. Rhabdomyoma of the heart is often asymptomatic but may cause cardiac failure, arrhythmia, and sudden death in early infancy. Small tumor nodules and cystic malformations throughout the lungs may lead to recurrent pneumothorax. About 50% of patients have retinal lesions, visible on funduscopic examination as white or yellow raised areas, often near the edge of the optic disc. These are malformations in the nerve fiber layer of the retina, consisting primarily of glial fibers and malformed retinal neuroglial cells. Such lesions usually do not impair vision.

The *diagnosis* of tuberous sclerosis is based on clinical findings. Demonstration of characteristic calcifications on skull roentgenograms and computed tomography is confirmatory (Fig. 21–13). Abdominal ultrasonography can demonstrate the renal lesions. Roentgenograms of long bones may disclose areas of sclerosis and of rarefaction, especially in metacarpal and metatarsal bones.

The *prognosis* varies. Patients with mild involvement may have full, productive lives. Those with severe mental deficiency may require institutional care. Early death may be due to status epilepticus, brain tumor, renal failure, or tumor of the heart.

Proper *management* includes treatment of seizures and assessment of intellectual function as a guide to an appropriate educational program. Methylphenidate (Ritalin) or dextroamphetamine may be helpful for control of hyperactivity in young children with tuberous sclerosis. Surgical excision is indicated for enlarging tumors, especially those near a foramen of Monro. Genetic counseling is essential. Both parents should be carefully examined for stigmata, including those of skin, retina, and brain (by CT scan of head). Evidence of tuberous sclerosis in one parent suggests a 50% likelihood of

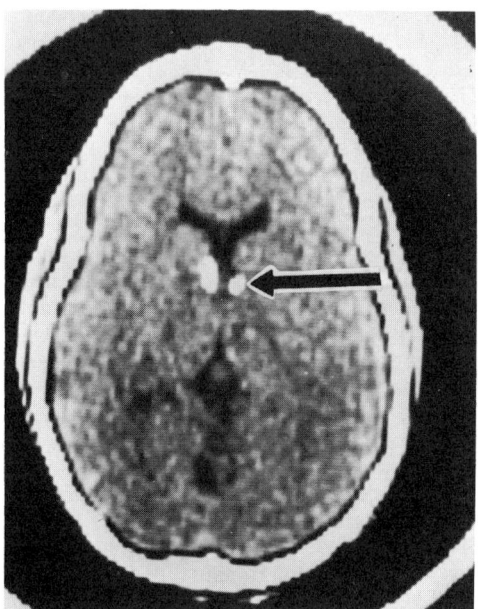

Figure 21–13. Computed tomogram (CT scan) of a 9 yr old girl with hypopigmented skin macules, mental retardation, and history of infantile myoclonic seizures. Two very dense, calcified lesions are seen in a periventricular location, typical of tuberous sclerosis.

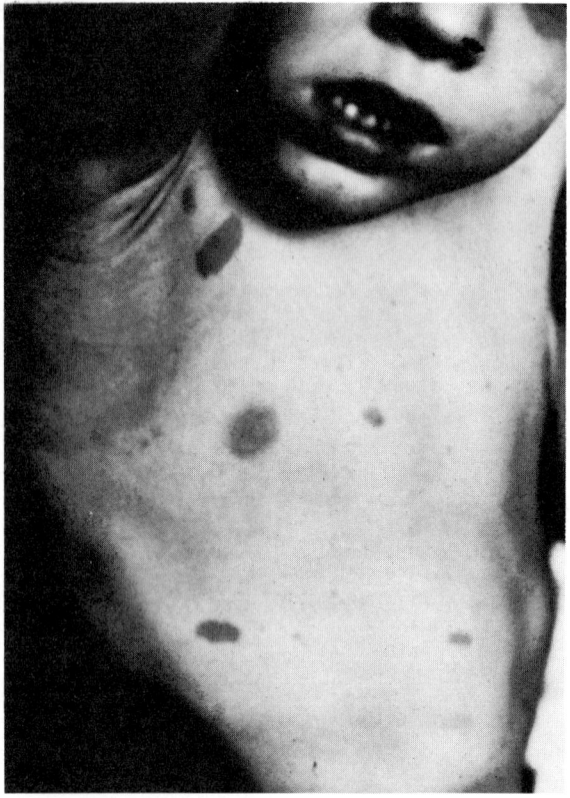

Figure 21-14. Café-au-lait spots in neurofibromatosis.

occurrence in subsequent children; a new mutation can be assumed if both parents are free of stigmata.

NEUROFIBROMATOSIS
(von Recklinghausen Disease)

See also Sec. 24.10.

Neurofibromatosis is transmitted as an autosomal dominant trait, but new mutations are common and have been estimated to account for about 50% of cases. Manifestations are extremely varied. The skin is involved in the great majority of patients. *Café-au-lait spots*, irregularly shaped areas of increased skin pigmentation, are a hallmark of the disease (Fig. 21-14). A few such spots are commonly found in otherwise normal persons, but the presence of more than six that are greater than 1.5 cm in diameter is pathognomonic of neurofibromatosis. In addition, there tends to be freckling, especially in the axillae, and general hyperpigmentation of skin.

Cutaneous and subcutaneous neurofibromas commonly appear in late childhood or in adolescence. These are thought to arise from the Schwann cells of peripheral nerves. The cutaneous tumors tend to form multiple soft pedunculated masses *(molluscum fibrosum)*; the subcutaneous ones are usually felt as soft nodules attached to the larger peripheral nerves. Less common are plexiform neuromas; these large infiltrative tumors cause considerable disfigurement, usually involving the face or an extremity. Sarcomatous degeneration of one or more neurofibromas occurs in about 10% of patients; it is rare in childhood.

Neurofibromas on cranial or spinal nerve roots may lead to a variety of neurologic symptoms. Tumor of the 8th nerve (acoustic neuroma) causes tinnitus, nerve deafness, loss of corneal reflex, vertigo, ataxia, and signs of increased intracranial pressure. Neurofibroma involving a spinal root may be manifested as an extramedullary spinal cord tumor. There is also increased incidence of other types of neural tumors,

such as glioma of the optic nerve and optic chiasm, meningioma, and pheochromocytoma.

A large variety of congenital malformations have been associated, including congenital bowing and pseudarthrosis of the tibia, cysts of long bones, overgrowth of bone and of soft tissue, scoliosis, megalencephaly, and malformation of the greater wing of the sphenoid bone (with pulsating exophthalmos). Mild intellectual impairment is common, but severe mental defect is rare. About 5% of patients have convulsions. Life expectancy is near normal; neural tumors and sarcomas are the principal risks.

The diagnosis of neurofibromatosis is based on the physical findings. Confirmation by biopsy of a subcutaneous nodule may be necessary if cutaneous manifestations are lacking. A careful family history and examination of immediate family members are essential in determining whether the propositus represents a new mutation. The family should be advised that any offspring of a person found to have neurofibromatosis has a 50% chance of inheriting the disorder. Therapy is limited to excision of tumors which produce pain or impairment in function and of rapidly growing masses suspected of malignant transformation.

STURGE-WEBER DISEASE
(Encephalotrigeminal Angiomatosis)

Sturge-Weber disease occurs sporadically without known hereditary factors. The basic lesion is a congenital capillary hemangioma which involves skin of the face and cervical area, mucous membranes, meninges, and choroid, usually unilaterally. The skin angioma (*"nevus flammeus"* or *"port wine stain"*) is in the trigeminal distribution, most commonly in the ophthalmic division, but it may extend over cervical segments. In the meninges the malformation is often confined to the pial vessels in the occipitoparietal areas. Sluggish flow of blood in malformed pial vessels leads to anoxic injury in underlying cerebral cortex. The clinical manifestations of cortical damage include convulsions, mental defect, and hemiparesis or hemianopsia on the side opposite that of the lesion. Subarachnoid hemorrhage rarely occurs. Calcifications in the damaged cortical layers may become visible roentgenographically even in infancy and nearly always by late childhood (Fig. 21-15). They are often curvilinear and double contoured ("railroad track pattern") and are pathognomonic in a child with facial nevus. Angioma in the choroid may lead to buphthalmos in infancy or to glaucoma in childhood.

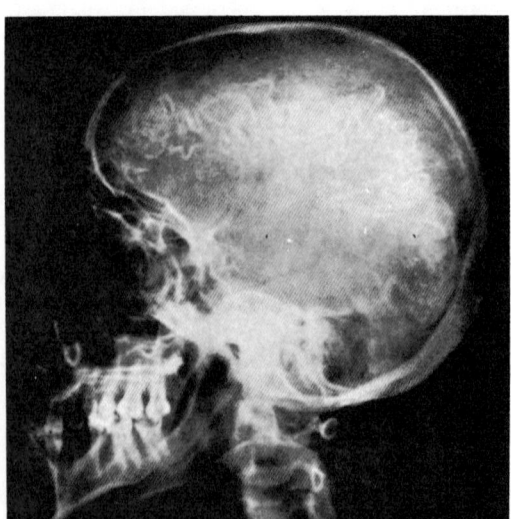

Figure 21-15. Extensive calcification of cerebral cortex in Sturge-Weber disease.

Management of the child with Sturge-Weber disease is determined by clinical manifestations: e.g., anticonvulsant drugs for seizures, physiotherapy for paretic limbs, and periodic eye examination for early detection of glaucoma. Local resection of the cerebral cortical lesion may be indicated when severe convulsions are refractory to medication. A covering cream may be used on the face for cosmetic purposes.

KLIPPEL-TRENAUNAY-WEBER SYNDROME

This syndrome resembles Sturge-Weber disease. A port wine nevus of the skin is always present but tends to be distributed much more extensively over trunk and extremities. Hypertrophy of soft tissue (especially in the face and extremities), glaucoma, digital malformations, and hemangiomas of visceral organs are commonly associated, along with megalencephaly, mental retardation, and seizures.

INCONTINENTIA PIGMENTI ACHROMIANS
(Hypomelanosis of Ito)

Patients with this disorder have characteristic bizarre hypopigmentations of skin in a whorl-like distribution, usually over the chest and abdomen (Sec. 24.11). The hypopigmented areas are usually evident from birth. The CNS is affected in over one half of the patients. Mental retardation and seizures are the most common manifestations.

LINEAR SEBACEOUS NEVUS SYNDROME

This syndrome is associated with CNS dysfunction in about 50% of patients. Infantile spasms (infantile myoclonic seizures), other types of seizures, mental retardation, and hemiparesis have been described.

VON HIPPEL–LINDAU DISEASE

This disorder is often included among the neurocutaneous disorders although the skin is not involved. Retinal angiomas are associated with hemangioblastoma of the cerebellum and less frequently with such other tumors as hemangioma of spinal cord, hypernephroma, and cystadenomas of visceral organs. Dominant inheritance has occurred in several families. Symptoms include visual loss and evidences of cerebellar and spinal cord dysfunction; these do not usually appear until adolescence or later.

Alexander GL, Norman RM: The Sturge-Weber Syndrome. Bristol, John Wright and Sons, 1960.
Cooper JR: Brain tumors in hereditary multiple system hamartomatosis (tuberous sclerosis). J Neurosurg 34:194, 1971.
Crowe FW, Schull WJ, Neel JV: Multiple Neurofibromatosis. Springfield, IL, Charles C Thomas, 1956.
Fienman NL, Yakovac WC: Neurofibromatosis in childhood. J Pediatr 76:339, 1970.
Gold AG, Freeman JM: Depigmented nevi: The earliest sign of tuberous sclerosis. Pediatrics 35:1003, 1965.
Gomez MR (ed): Tuberous Sclerosis. New York, Raven Press, 1979.
Hurwitz S, Braverman IM: White spots in tuberous sclerosis. J Pediatr 77:587, 1970.
Peterman AF, Hayles AB, Dockerty MB, et al: Encephalotrigeminal angiomatosis (Sturge-Weber disease). Clinical study of 35 cases. JAMA 167:2169, 1958.
Pitt MJ, Mosher JF, Ederken J: Abnormal periosteum and bone in neurofibromatosis. Radiology 103:143, 1972.

21.17 DEGENERATIVE BRAIN DISEASES

The outstanding characteristic of these illnesses is progressive loss of previously acquired intellectual, motor, and sensory functions. Most of them are genetically autosomal recessive; specific enzymatic defects have been demonstrated in

some, and enzymatic assays permit identification of carriers (heterozygotes) and intrauterine diagnosis in several. Some cerebral degenerations cannot be specifically categorized. Effective therapy is lacking for most of them.

Classification (see below) usually divides the disorders into those which principally affect cerebral gray matter and those which affect white matter, or reflects, at least in part, the functional systems involved (e.g., basal ganglia and spinocerebellar systems). In the gray matter diseases, dementia and seizures are the predominant early manifestations, whereas deterioration in motor function, manifested by spasticity, hypotonia, or ataxia, is the early sign of degenerations involving white matter. In both varieties the entire nervous system tends eventually to become affected, and the end-stage picture of all the disorders is generally similar: the child becomes helpless, with loss of all intellectual and voluntary motor functions.

I. **Degenerations of cerebral gray matter**
  A. *Neuronal storage* diseases
    1. Ganglioside storage diseases
      Tay-Sachs disease and variants
      Generalized gangliosidosis
    2. Sphingolipid storage other than of gangliosides
      Infantile Gaucher disease
      Niemann-Pick disease
      Farber disease (lipogranulomatosis)
    3. Other neuronal storage diseases
      Late infantile and juvenile cerebromacular degeneration (Bielschowsky, Spielmeyer-Vogt, and Batten)
      Glycogen storage disease of heart, muscle, and central nervous system (Pompe disease)
  B. Degenerations *without neuronal storage*
    Alper disease
    Leigh disease
    Kinky-hair (Menkes) disease
    Subacute sclerosing panencephalitis (SSPE)
II. **Degenerative disorders of cerebral white matter**
  A. The leukodystrophies
    Metachromatic leukodystrophy (sulfatide lipidosis)
    Krabbe disease (cerebroside lipidosis)
    Sudanophilic leukodystrophies
    Canavan disease
  B. Demyelinating diseases
    Schilder disease
    Multiple sclerosis
    Neuromyelitis optica
III. **System degenerations**
  A. Spinocerebellar and cerebellar degenerations
    Friedreich ataxia and its variants
    Ataxia-telangiectasia
    Bassen-Kornzweig syndrome
    Refsum disease
  B. Basal ganglia degenerations
    Wilson disease (hepatolenticular degeneration)
    Dystonia musculorum deformans
    Huntington chorea
    Hallervorden-Spatz disease

21.18 DEGENERATIONS OF CEREBRAL GRAY MATTER

Neuronal Storage Diseases

These diseases are characterized by accumulation of lipid substances in cerebral neurons. In most instances the stored material is a sphingolipid; in some, a ganglioside. Sphingolipids are normal components of all cell membranes; the simplest are made up of the base, sphingosine, and a fatty acid. The resulting compound is referred to as ceramide. More complex sphingolipids have a variety of side chains added to

Table 21–10. **Sphingolipids That Are the Major Storage Materials in the Lipid Storage Diseases**

Disease	Storage Compound
Niemann-Pick disease	Ceramide-p-choline (sphingomyelin)
Infantile Gaucher disease	Ceramide-glucose (glucocerebroside)
Generalized gangliosidosis	Ceramide-glucose-galactose-acetylgalactosamine-galactose (GM_1)*
Juvenile GM_1 gangliosidosis	Sialic acid
Tay-Sachs disease	Ceramide-glucose-galactose-acetylgalactosamine (GM_2)
Sandhoff disease	Sialic acid

*GM_1 also is the major ganglioside found in normal human brain.

the ceramide molecule; several such compounds of ceramide are of particular importance in neuronal storage disease (Table 21–10). Gangliosides are complex sphingolipids that are normally present in high concentration in neurons; their function is unknown. Neuronal lipid storage is due to deficiency of specific enzymes which normally degrade the sphingolipids. In general, the substrate of the defective enzyme is stored in the cells.

The terminology of Svennerholm is generally used to classify the gangliosides. In this system the letter G refers to ganglioside; M, D, or T refers to the number of sialic acid groups (mono-, di-, or trisialic acid), and the subscript (1, 2, or 3) refers to the number of hexosides in the molecule. Tetrahexosides are assigned the number 1; trihexosides, the number 2; dihexosides, the number 3.

Ganglioside Storage Diseases

See also Sec. 7.25–7.26.

The disorders in this group are differentiated on the basis of clinical findings, age of onset, and specific enzyme assays. Each of them follows autosomal recessive transmission. The salient features of the more common ones are summarized in Table 21–11. In each disorder the enzymatic defect affects all body cells, but functional derangement appears to be limited to the central nervous system in all except generalized gangliosidosis, in which visceral and osseous lesions are associated with cerebral degeneration. In each disorder assay of the affected enzyme in white blood cells permits specific diagnosis. Heterozygous carriers of the trait have partial deficiency of the enzyme. Enzyme assay of cultured amniotic fluid cells permits intrauterine diagnosis.

Tay-Sachs Disease. Infantile cerebromacular degeneration is by far the most common of the gangliosidoses. It is most frequently found in children of Eastern European Jewish (Ashkenazi) ancestry; the incidence of the carrier state among Ashkenazi Jews is estimated to be 2.7%, about 10 times higher

than in other population groups. The clinical findings are characteristic. At 2–6 mo of age a previously well infant becomes apathetic and loses interest in his or her surroundings. There is progressive loss of acquired motor functions and of visual ability. An exaggerated startle response to noise (hyperacusis) is an early sign. Progressive spasticity with hyperreflexia and decerebrate posturing, feeding difficulties, and emaciation occur in the late stages of the illness, and the head may become abnormally large. Grand mal, tonic, or myoclonic seizures are seen. The most characteristic feature is the cherry-red spot of the macula, a bright red area in the region of the fovea surrounded by a grayish-white rim (Fig. 21–16). The latter is due to lipid accumulation in retinal ganglion cells. The cherry-red spot may also occur in Niemann-Pick and Sandhoff diseases (Table 21–11).

Routine laboratory examinations are not helpful in the diagnosis. There is virtual absence of the enzyme hexosaminidase A from all body tissues. Measurement of this enzyme in serum, amniotic fluid cells, or white cells has become the definitive diagnostic measure. Deficiency of hexosaminidase A results in marked accumulation of GM_2 ganglioside in all neurons, including those in the peripheral autonomic nervous system. GM_2 gangliosides, which normally make up only 1–3% of total brain gangliosides, account for more than 90% in patients with Tay-Sachs disease. The accumulation of ganglioside is visible by light microscopy as marked ballooning of neurons. By electron microscopy the ganglioside is seen as discrete intracellular concretions with a characteristic lamellar structure. Neuronal degeneration and gliosis are marked in infants who survive for several years.

There is no therapy for Tay-Sachs disease. Death usually occurs prior to the age of 4 yr (although a late-onset form of Tay-Sachs disease has been described, with ataxia and weakness due to anterior horn cell degeneration beginning in childhood or adolescence). Heterozygous carriers in populations known to be at risk can be identified by serum assay of

Table 21–11. **Ganglioside Storage Diseases**

Disease	Enzyme Defect	Age at Onset	Characteristic Physical Features
Tay-Sachs disease (GM_2 gangliosidosis, type 1)	Absence of hexosaminidase A	3–6 mo	Hyperacusis, dementia, seizures, cherry-red spot of macula, blindness, macrocephaly
Sandhoff disease (GM_2 gangliosidosis, type 2)	Absence of hexosaminidase A and B	3–6 mo	Same as Tay-Sachs disease
Juvenile GM_2 gangliosidosis (GM_2 gangliosidosis, type 3)	Partial deficiency of hexosaminidase A	2–6 yr	Dementia, ataxia, spasticity, seizures
Generalized gangliosidosis (GM_1 gangliosidosis, type 1)	Absence of β-galactosidase A, B, and C	In utero or early infancy	Hepatosplenomegaly, Hurler-like features and bone changes, failure of intellectual and motor development
Juvenile GM_1 gangliosidosis (GM_1 gangliosidosis, type 2)	Absence of β-galactosidase B and C	6 mo–2 yr	Spasticity, ataxia, dementia

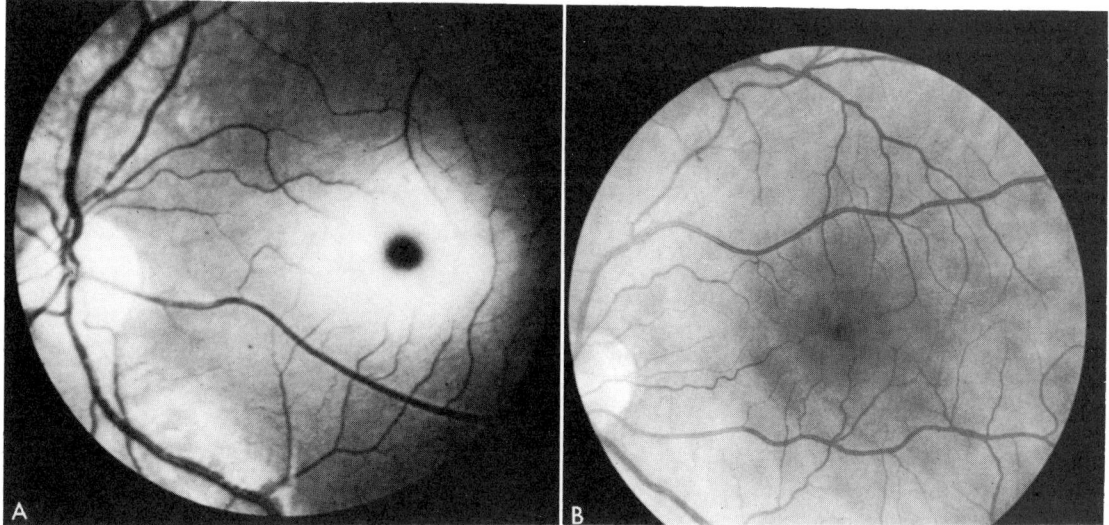

Figure 21–16. *A,* Cherry-red spot of the macula in Tay-Sachs disease. *B,* Normal macula for comparison.

hexosaminidase A. Diagnostic amniocentesis should be offered when both parents are known to be heterozygotes. It should be carried out at about 18 wk gestation, in time for safe termination of pregnancy, if indicated.

Other Ganglioside Storage Diseases. See Table 21–11 and Sec. 7.25–7.26.

Late Infantile and Juvenile Cerebromacular Degenerations (Ceroid Lipofuscinosis)

See also Sec. 7.37.

These disorders are the second most common group of degenerative disorders of cerebral gray matter. Onset is from 1–3 yr of age in the late infantile form *(Bielschowsky syndrome)* and usually from 5–7 yr in the more common juvenile variety *(Spielmeyer-Vogt* or *Batten disease).* It is unknown whether the two represent variants of the same illness or different genetic defects. Transmission of both is autosomal recessive.

Pathologically, neurons are distended with material that has the staining characteristics of lipofuscin. Electron microscopy shows curvilinear and lattice-like neuronal cytoplasmic inclusions. Involvement includes neurons in the anterior horn of the spinal cord and in peripheral autonomic ganglia. Lipofuscin-like material also accumulates in other organs, especially in the thyroid gland and in sweat glands.

The illness often starts with progressive loss of vision. Ophthalmologic changes vary among affected families; they may consist of retinitis pigmentosa, pigmentary degeneration of the macular region, or simple optic atrophy. The electroencephalogram may be abnormal, with diffuse spike-wave activity, long before the onset of neurologic deterioration. Spike-wave discharges in response to photic stimulation at a slow rate (1–2/sec) are a common early finding. Grand mal or myoclonic seizures and dementia may appear 1–3 yr after onset of visual loss. The child becomes hyperactive and irritable. Speech deteriorates, often with a peculiar stammering, slurring, and repetition of words. Cerebellar ataxia, tremor, rigidity, spastic paralysis, and complete dementia appear late. Progression is slow; the later the onset, the slower the course. Some patients survive into adolescence or early adult years.

The diagnosis should be suspected in a child with progressive visual loss, seizures, and mental deterioration. Ganglioside storage disease may present identical clinical findings but can be ruled out by assay of hexosaminidases and beta-galactosidases in white cells. Electron microscopic examination of rectal ganglion cells is useful in diagnosis. Muscle or

sweat glands may show electron-dense bodies similar to those found in neurons.

Aronson SM, Volk BW (eds): Cerebral sphingolipidoses. A Symposium on Tay-Sachs Disease and Allied Disorders. New York, Academic Press, 1962.
Carpenter S, Karpati G, Andermann F: Specific involvement of muscle, nerve and skin in late infantile and juvenile amaurotic idiocy. Neurology 22:170, 1972.
Fawcett JS, Anderman F, Wiglesworth FW, et al: On the natural history of late infantile cerebromacular degeneration. Neurology 16:1130, 1966.
Johnson WG: The clinical spectrum of hexosaminidase deficiency diseases. Neurology 31:1453, 1981.
Landing BH, Silverman FN, et al: Familial neurovisceral lipidosis. Am J Dis Child 108:503, 1964.
Milunsky A, Littlefield JW, et al: Prenatal genetic diagnosis. N Engl J Med 283:1370, 1441, 1498, 1970.
O'Brien JS, Okada S, Chen S, et al: Tay-Sachs disease. Detection of heterozygotes and homozygotes by serum hexosaminidase assay. N Engl J Med 283:15, 1970.
O'Brien JS, Stern MB, Landing BH, et al: Generalized gangliosidosis. Am J Dis Child 109:338, 1965.
Wolfe LS, Kin NM, Baker RR, et al: Identification of retinoyl complexes as the autofluorescent compound of the neuronal storage material in Batten's disease. Science 195:1360, 1977.
Zeman W, Dyken P: Neuronal ceroid-lipo-fuscinosis (Batten's disease): Relationship to amaurotic family idiocy. Pediatrics 44:570, 1969.

Degeneration of Gray Matter Without Neuronal Storage

Poliodystrophy (Alper Disease). Poliodystrophy includes a heterogeneous group of degenerations of cerebral cortex with onset in infancy or early childhood. Pathologic changes in brain are nonspecific; widespread neuronal loss and gliosis occur in cerebral cortex and in cerebellum. The most prominent symptoms are recurrent seizures and dementia. Involvement of siblings may suggest recessive inheritance. Several metabolic errors may be involved. Some cases have lactic acidosis, probably secondary to deficiency of an enzyme in the pyruvate dehydrogenase complex. Others have progressive hepatic cirrhosis. Treatment with corticosteroids or with a ketogenic diet may produce transient clinical improvement in patients with poliodystrophy who have lactic acidosis.

Leigh Disease (Subacute Necrotizing Encephalomyelopathy). This metabolic brain disease leads to widespread cerebral damage, especially in the brain stem. It is autosomal recessive.

Pathologic changes include degeneration of neural structures and capillary proliferation in a characteristic distribution surrounding the 3rd ventricle, the aqueduct of Sylvius, and the 4th ventricle. The lesions are strikingly similar to those of thiamine deficiency (Wernicke) encephalopathy. Leigh disease may be related to an inborn error in thiamine metabolism (Sec. 7.20).

Onset is usually in infancy; the course may be subacute, with vomiting, weight loss, weakness, seizures, and stupor, or more chronic, with developmental arrest, loss of vision, and dementia. Nystagmus and extraocular palsies are common. Both spastic weakness due to upper motor neuron degeneration and flaccidity due to spinal cord and peripheral nerve involvement are seen. Irregular respirations, periodic hyperventilation, and sudden apnea are late manifestations. The course is often one of exacerbations and remissions, a feature that may aid in differentiation from other cerebral degenerations; survival may be for a few weeks or many years. Therapy with massive doses of thiamine has given inconclusive results.

Kinky Hair Disease (Menkes Syndrome). In this sex-linked recessive abnormality in copper metabolism, severe cerebral degeneration and arterial changes lead to death in infancy.

Pathologic changes include widespread cerebral degeneration with loss of cortical neurons; gliosis and cysts replace the most severely damaged areas. Vascular changes include fragmentation of the elastica and intimal thickening. The basic defect appears to consist of excessive binding of copper to certain tissues, including fibroblasts and intestinal mucosa, with a decrease in intestinal mucosa absorption and serum level of copper, which may account for diminished synthesis of ceruloplasmin (see Sec. 7.54).

Inadequate gain in weight and hypothermia are manifest from birth, with unusual susceptibility to sepsis. The scalp hair is initially normal but rapidly becomes sparse and brittle. Microscopically the shaft has a twisted appearance (pili torti). Seborrheic dermatitis is common. Developmental retardation becomes evident within the first few mo of life, and myoclonic seizures may occur. Death usually occurs within the first yr.

Laboratory studies are necessary for definitive diagnosis. Roentgenograms of long bones show changes resembling those of scurvy. Serum copper and ceruloplasmin levels are low. Parenteral copper therapy does not seem to prevent cerebral damage, even when begun in early infancy.

Subacute Sclerosing Panencephalitis (SSPE). This disease is caused by measles virus but is included among the cerebral degenerative disorders because of its chronic course and absence of clinical evidences of infection. The incidence varies with geographic area from 1–4/million; it has decreased following the widespread introduction of measles vaccination (Sec. 11.61).

Changes in brain include perivascular lymphocytic infiltrates, intranuclear viral inclusions in neurons and glial cells, widespread loss of cortical neurons, and gliosis. Measles virus has been grown from cerebral tissue, presumably following entry of measles virus into the brain during acute measles infection, with subsequent chronic intracellular propagation. Cerebral degeneration appears at an average of 7 yr after primary infection.

Clinical manifestations appear from 2–21 yr of age, with peak incidence from 8–14 yr. The first signs are those of progressive decline in higher cerebral functions (especially school failure), subtle personality changes, and emotional lability. Generalized myoclonic jerks, at regular intervals of several sec, are characteristic. Barely noticeable at first, they eventually become so severe that ambulation is hampered. Grand mal seizures also may occur. In the late stages the child becomes demented and is bedridden with generalized rigidity.

Changes in the cerebrospinal fluid include elevated gamma globulin levels and a measurable antibody titer against measles virus. CSF protein concentration and cell count are often normal. The titer of measles antibody in serum is usually above 1:128 by the complement-fixation method. The electroencephalographic pattern is fairly characteristic, consisting of regularly repeated bursts of generalized high-voltage slow wave complexes.

The disease is usually fatal within 2 yr of onset, but rare instances of prolonged spontaneous remission have been reported.

Blackwood W, Buxton PH, Cummings JN, et al: Diffuse cerebral degeneration of infancy (Alper's disease). Arch Dis Child 38:193, 1963.

Danks DM, Campbell PE, Stevens BJ, et al: Menkes' kinky hair syndrome. An inherited defect in copper absorption with widespread effects. Pediatrics 50:188, 1972.

Detels R, Brody JA, McNew J, et al: Further epidemiologic studies of subacute sclerosing panencephalitis. Lancet 2:11, 1973.

Falk RE, Cederbaum SD, Blass JP, et al: Ketonic diet in the management of pyruvate dehydrogenase deficiency. Pediatrics 58:713, 1976.

Goka TJ, Stevenson RE, Hefferan PM, et al: Menkes' disease: A biochemical abnormality in cultured human fibroblasts. Proc Natl Acad Sci USA 73:604, 1976.

Katz M, Rorke LB, Masland WS, et al: Subacute sclerosing panencephalitis: Isolation of a virus encephalitogenic for ferrets. J Infect Dis 121:188, 1970.

Pincus JH: Subacute necrotizing encephalomyelopathy (Leigh's disease): A consideration of clinical features and etiology. Dev Med Child Neurol 14:87, 1972.

Sever JL, Zeman W (eds): Measles virus and subacute sclerosing panencephalitis. Neurology 18 (pt 2):1, 1968.

Shapira Y, Cederbaum SD, Cancilla PA, et al: Familial poliodystrophy, mitochondrial myopathy and lactate acidemia. Neurology 25:614, 1975.

21.19 DEGENERATIVE DISORDERS OF CEREBRAL WHITE MATTER

In most of these diseases there is faulty formation or excessive breakdown of myelin, a major component of cerebral white matter, which consists of proteolipid membranes wrapped around axons in concentric layers. Myelination markedly increases the speed and efficiency of conduction of nerve impulses; it is essential for normal function of the mammalian nervous system. In the human, myelination of axons in subcortical white matter is largely postnatal with maximal formation occurring within the first yr of life. Accordingly, diseases in which there is faulty formation of central myelin tend to have their onset during infancy; they present clinically as arrest of motor development or as progressive disturbances of gait, weakness, spasticity, and ataxia.

Two groups of degenerative diseases involve cerebral white matter. In one, the *leukodystrophies*, enzymatic defects in myelin lipid metabolism lead to excessive tissue deposition of a normal component of myelin lipids or of breakdown products of myelin. The clinical disorders include *metachromatic leukodystrophy* and *Krabbe disease*. In the second group, the *demyelinating diseases*, degeneration of previously normal myelin is caused by an unknown exogenous factor. *Multiple sclerosis, neuromyelitis optica,* and *Schilder disease* belong in this group.

The Leukodystrophies

See also Sec. 7.31 and 7.35.

Metachromatic Leukodystrophy (Sulfatide Lipidosis). This is the most common leukodystrophy in childhood. It is autosomal recessive.

The basic defect in metachromatic leukodystrophy is deficiency of aryl sulfatase A in brain and other tissues. This enzyme normally splits the sulfate group from ceramide-galactose-sulfate or sulfatide, a normal component of myelin lipids. Sulfatide accumulates in white matter and can be identified on light microscopy by metachromatic (reddish-brown) staining with toluidine blue. Similar deposits are found in peripheral nerves. There is diffuse demyelination of white matter tracts throughout the nervous system, most extensive in tracts which myelinate late.

Clinical manifestations usually appear at about 1 yr of age, but onset may occur later. Initially there is a disturbance in gait, and the child may be unable to learn to run or to walk up stairs. Spasticity of limbs, hyperreflexia, and extensor plantar responses are noted early. Though most of the tendon reflexes are brisk, the ankle jerks may be diminished or absent because of involvement of peripheral nerves. Flaccid weakness and atrophy of distal muscles, especially in the lower extremities, occur when peripheral nerve involvement is severe. Eventually the child becomes demented and bedridden. Death usually occurs before the age of 10 yr. Variants with late onset have extrapyramidal motor signs and mental changes as the most common early findings.

Definitive diagnosis depends on finding absent or significantly reduced activity of aryl sulfatase A in one or more body tissues. White blood cells or cultured fibroblasts are suitable for this analysis. A screening test, rapid but unreliable, involves the demonstration of metachromatic material in urinary sediment stained with toluidine blue. Dysfunction of the gallbladder, resulting from storage of sulfatide in its wall, leads to failure of filling on oral cholecystography. Conduction velocity in peripheral motor and sensory nerves is decreased. The concentration of protein in CSF is usually increased, the elevation aiding the differentiation of leukodystrophy from the much larger group of nonprogressive motor deficits classified as cerebral palsy. Magnetic resonance imaging of brain is a sensitive method for demonstration of myelin degeneration in the subcortical white matter. Accurate diagnosis is important for genetic counseling and for prognosis. Intrauterine diagnosis of metachromatic leukodystrophy is possible by measurement of aryl sulfatase A in cultured cells from the amniotic fluid; the test should be offered to prospective parents when both are known to be carriers of the abnormal gene.

Krabbe Disease (Cerebroside Lipidosis, or Globoid Leukodystrophy). This disease is autosomal recessive. The pathologic changes in brain consist of diffuse lack of myelin in white matter and an accumulation of peculiar multinucleated giant cells (globoid cells). The white matter contains an increased ratio of cerebroside (ceramide galactose) to sulfatide (ceramide-galactose-sulfate) but usually no absolute increase in the quantity of cerebroside. These changes are thought to be secondary to a deficiency of galactocerebrosidase activity.

The illness becomes evident in early infancy with progressive rigidity, hyperreflexia, and swallowing difficulties and with failure of normal motor and intellectual development. Peripheral nerve involvement may lead to hypotonia; death usually occurs within 2 yr. The diagnosis is established by assay of galactocerebrosidase in peripheral white blood cells. Spinal fluid protein is increased, and the velocity of peripheral nerve conduction is slowed. Intrauterine diagnosis is possible by enzymatic assay of cultured amniotic fluid cells.

Adrenoleukodystrophy. This disease is X-linked recessive. The pathologic changes in the brain consist of degeneration of the cerebral white matter with accumulation of breakdown products of myelin, especially neutral fats. Macrophages in damaged tissue have characteristic curvilinear inclusions. The adrenal cortex is atrophic, with similar intracellular inclusions.

The basic defect is in metabolism of hexacosanoate, a C26 long-chain fatty acid that is increased in brain, adrenal glands, muscle, cultured fibroblasts, and plasma. Measurement in plasma is used for diagnosis and identification of carriers.

Onset usually occurs toward the end of the 1st decade, with progressive spasticity and dementia and later the increased pigmentation of skin and other evidence of Addison disease. In some cases spinal cord and peripheral nerves are predominantly involved (adrenomyeloneuropathy). A variant with onset in infancy has been described.

Several *other forms of leukodystrophy* are as yet incompletely defined and usually are diagnosable only by postmortem examination of the brain:

Canavan Disease (Spongy Degeneration of the Cerebral White Matter). This condition is autosomal recessive. The characteristic pathologic change is diffuse vacuolization in the deep cortical layers and in subcortical white matter, apparently secondary to excessive accumulation of water in glial cells and in myelin. Clinical manifestations appear in early infancy with poor head control, blindness, optic atrophy, rigidity, hyperreflexia, and progressive macrocephaly. The last may suggest hydrocephalus or subdural effusion. The ventricular system is normal in size, however, or only mildly dilated. Death occurs within 5 yr.

Pelizaeus-Merzbacher Disease. This is an X-linked recessive disease. The onset occurs in infancy, with nystagmus and head nodding, followed by progressive ataxia, spasticity, and choreoathetosis. Progression is slow, with survival into adulthood. Clinical differentiation from cerebral palsy may be difficult.

Austin J: Studies in globoid (Krabbe) leukodystrophy. Arch Neurol 9:207, 1963.

Austin J, Armstrong D, Fouch S, et al: Metachromatic leukodystrophy. Arch Neurol 18:225, 1968.

Banker BQ, Robertson JT, Victor M: Spongy degeneration of the central nervous system in infancy. Neurology 14:981, 1964.

Griffin JW, Goren E, Schaumberg H, et al: Adrenomyeloneuropathy: A probable variant of adrenoleukodystrophy. Neurology 27:1107, 1977.

Leroy JG, Van Elsen AF, Martin JJ, et al: Infantile metachromatic leukodystrophy. Confirmation of a prenatal diagnosis. N Engl J Med 288:1365, 1973.

Moser HW, Moser AE, Singh I, et al: Adrenoleukodystrophy: Survey of 303 cases: Biochemistry: diagnosis and therapy. Ann Neurol 16:628, 1984.

Norman RM, Tingey AH, Harvey PW, et al: Pelizaeus-Merzbacher disease: A form of sudanophilic leucodystrophy. J Neurol Neurosurg Psychiat 29:521, 1966.

Percy AK, Brady RO: Metachromatic leukodystrophy: Diagnosis with sample of venous blood. Science 161:594, 1968.

Suzuki Y, Suzuki K: Krabbe's globoid cell leukodystrophy: Deficiency of galactocerebrosidase in serum, leukocytes, and fibroblasts. Science 171:73, 1971.

Young RSK, Osbakken MD, Alger PM, et al: Magnetic resonance imaging in Leukodystrophies of childhood. Pediatric Neurology 1:15, 1984.

The Demyelinating Diseases

These illnesses, which include *Schilder disease, multiple sclerosis,* and *neuromyelitis optica,* occur sporadically without known genetic factors. It is not clear whether they are separate entities or variants of the same pathologic process. Transitional forms have been described. In all three there is breakdown of myelin in the central nervous system without involvement of myelin of the peripheral nerves. A perivascular lymphocytic inflammatory reaction in the areas of demyelination suggests an autoimmune disorder or a viral infection; conclusive evidence for either is lacking.

Schilder Disease (Diffuse Sclerosis). This disease may occur at any age but is most common in late childhood. Definitive diagnosis is usually possible only at autopsy; there is diffuse demyelination of central white matter with relative sparing of subcortical U fibers. Lipid breakdown products of myelin accumulate in the areas of demyelination. The pathologic picture resembles that of the leukodystrophies. Neurologic findings are extremely varied. Cortical blindness, optic neuritis, spastic hemiplegia, paraparesis, cortical deafness, aphasia, and seizures have been described in the early phase. Late manifestations include dementia and coma. Occasionally, there are signs of increased intracranial pressure, with papilledema secondary to cerebral swelling. The course may be acute, death occurring within a few weeks of onset, or last months or years. Rarely, there is partial remission or a relapsing course. The cerebrospinal fluid may be normal or show an increase in protein and lymphocytes. The differential diagnosis includes brain tumor, viral encephalitis, subacute sclerosing panencephalitis (SSPE), multiple sclerosis, and the leukodystrophies.

Multiple Sclerosis (Disseminated Sclerosis). Multiple sclerosis is a chronic cerebral disorder characterized by remissions and exacerbations and by multifocal lesions. The onset occurs before 15 yr of age in about 1% of cases. Scattered foci of demyelination are found in cerebral white matter, often in a perivenous distribution with associated perivascular lymphocytic infiltrates. Lesions may occur also in brain stem and spinal cord.

In order of frequency, the most common presenting signs in childhood or adolescence are cerebellar ataxia, spastic weakness (often asymmetric), optic neuritis, and diplopia. The optic neuritis tends to be retrobulbar. Loss of vision occurs without funduscopic changes at first. Temporal pallor of the optic discs indicative of optic atrophy develops over weeks or months. The onset may be acute or subacute over several weeks. Recovery from acute episodes may initially be complete or nearly so, but after repeated attacks the patient is left with fixed neurologic deficits, often including spastic paralysis and ataxia. Intellectual functions are preserved until late. The clinical diagnosis is based on (1) the finding of multiple neurologic deficits which cannot be due to a single anatomic lesion and (2) the relapsing course. A definite diagnosis cannot be established at the time of the first attack. Differentiation from hysteria may be difficult initially, especially when visual disturbance occurs without objective eye findings. The spinal fluid may be normal or show an increase in gamma globulin, with a positive first-zone colloidal gold curve. A pleocytosis up to 100 lymphocytes/mm³ may occur during acute exacerbations.

Treatment of acute exacerbations of multiple sclerosis with short courses of ACTH has a slight but statistically significant beneficial effect. ACTH gel is given intramuscularly, 40–80 units/24 hr for 2 wk; the dose is then tapered and discontinued over the subsequent week. Physiotherapy can help patients with spastic weakness. Careful bladder care and therapy of urinary tract infections are essential when spinal cord involvement results in bladder dysfunction. The prognosis is guarded but not hopeless; exacerbations may be infrequent with symptom-free intervals of many years.

Neuromyelitis Optica (Devic Disease). This disorder is probably a variant of multiple sclerosis in which demyelination occurs in the optic nerves and in the spinal cord. The only reason for separation from multiple sclerosis is that there may be a single attack without later exacerbations. A relapsing course with eventual involvement of other white matter tracts is also possible. The illness starts acutely, usually with eye pain followed by loss of vision, which may affect one or both eyes. Funduscopic examination may reveal swelling and hyperemia of the optic disc, distended retinal veins, and peripapillary hemorrhages; in some instances the fundi initially appear normal. The onset of spinal cord involvement is also acute, at times with fever, back pain, and nuchal rigidity. It usually follows the visual loss by several days but may precede it. A level of sensory involvement on the trunk can be demonstrated, usually in the thoracic area. Initially the legs are weak, flaccid, and areflexic, and the plantar responses are absent or flexor. The bladder is distended. After a few days the involved extremities become spastic, the tendon reflexes hyperactive, with clonus at the ankles and a Babinski sign.

The spinal fluid may be normal or show pleocytosis; polymorphonuclear cells may be present initially. Myelography may be necessary to rule out acute compression of the cord, especially by spinal epidural abscess. This study is usually normal in neuromyelitis optica, but partial obstruction at the level of the cord lesion may reflect edema of the spinal cord. Dexamethasone in high doses for a period 5–7 days during the acute illness may help prevent pressure necrosis of the edematous segment of the cord. The prognosis for return of vision is good, but some degree of persistent paraparesis and bladder dysfunction can be expected.

Gall JC Jr, Hayles AB, Siekert RG, et al: Multiple sclerosis in children: Clinical study of 40 cases with onset in childhood. Pediatrics 21:703, 1958.

Kennedy C, Carter S: Relationships of optic neuritis to multiple sclerosis in children. Pediatrics 28:377, 1961.

Low NL, Carter S: Multiple sclerosis in children. Pediatrics 18:24, 1956.

Rose AS, Kuzma JW, Kurtzke JF, et al: Cooperative study in the evaluation of therapy in multiple sclerosis: ACTH vs. placebo—final report. Neurology 20, May, 1970 (Suppl).

Salguero LF, Itsabashi JH, Gutierrez NB: Childhood multiple sclerosis with psychotic manifestations. J Neurol Neurosurg Psychiatr 32:572, 1969.

Suzuki K, Grover WD: Ultrastructural and biochemical studies of Schilder's disease. J Neuropathol Exp Neurol 29:392, 1970.

Walsh FB: Neuromyelitis optica. An anatomical-pathological study of one case. Clinical studies of three additional cases. Bull Johns Hopkins Hosp 56:183, 1935.

21.20 DEGENERATIVE DISEASES OF THE CEREBELLUM AND BASAL GANGLIA

In a number of illnesses spinocerebellar pathways or basal ganglia are selectively involved in degenerative processes. Most are genetically determined; in a few the metabolic error has been defined, but for most the etiology is unknown.

The Spinocerebellar Degenerations

Friedreich Ataxia. This term is applied to a heterogeneous group of disorders which share the onset in late childhood or adolescence of progressive cerebellar and spinal cord dysfunction. Several disorders, such as ataxia-telangiectasia and the Bassen-Kornzweig syndrome, have been clearly separated from Friedreich ataxia; it is likely that others will be, as underlying metabolic disturbances are defined. In most families so-called Friedreich ataxia displays autosomal recessive transmission. A few families with similar abnormalities, but usually somewhat later in onset, have dominant inheritance.

Pathologic changes include degeneration of spinocerebellar, posterior column, and corticospinal tracts. In addition, necrosis and degeneration of cardiac muscle fibers are often present.

The clinical history is that of a progressive gait disturbance, followed by incoordination of the upper limbs. Initially, associated skeletal deformities, including a highly arched foot (pes cavus) (Fig. 21–17), hammer toes, and scoliosis, may attract more attention than the neurologic disabilities. Occasionally, the child presents cardiac failure, with cardiomegaly and arrhythmias. Signs of cerebellar disorder include gait ataxia, dysarthria, intention tremor, and, less commonly, nystagmus. In addition, affected patients usually have evidence of corticospinal tract dysfunction and peripheral neuropathy. The former leads to a Babinski sign, the latter to loss of tendon reflexes and to distal weakness and muscle atrophy.

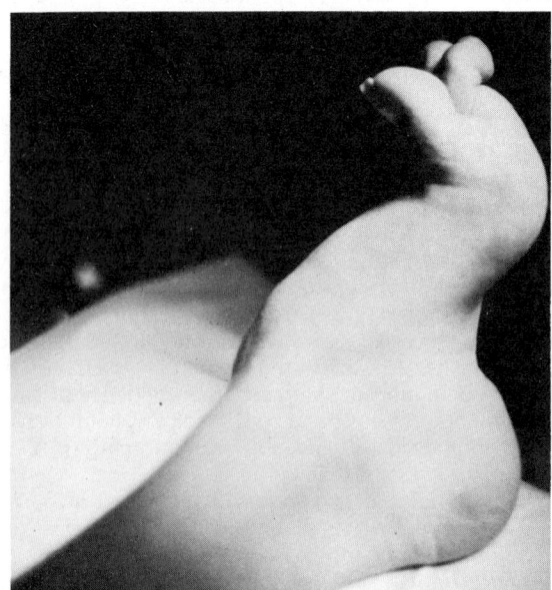

Figure 21–17. Pes cavus in a 12 yr old child with Friedreich ataxia.

The combination of ataxia, Babinski sign, and absent ankle jerks is almost pathognomonic. Sensory loss occurs, especially in the feet, with position and vibration senses most severely affected.

Several related syndromes cannot be clearly separated from Friedreich ataxia. Hyperreflexia and spasticity, rather than areflexia and muscle atrophy, occur in some families. Some patients have onset of areflexic ataxia and pes cavus in infancy, with very slow progression consistent with a normal life span. This condition (*Roussy-Lévy syndrome*) is dominantly inherited.

Diagnosis is almost totally dependent on the clinical findings. Laboratory examinations are negative, except for electrocardiographic changes suggestive of cardiomyopathy, and in some instances slowing of nerve conduction velocity due to peripheral neuropathy. There is no effective treatment. Extensive orthopedic procedures, especially those requiring prolonged confinement to bed, should be avoided. The disease tends to be relentlessly progressive; the gait ataxia usually precludes independent walking by early adult years. Death in childhood is almost always due to myocardial failure.

Ataxia-Telangiectasia. In this complex disorder a specific immunologic dysfunction is associated with progressive cerebellar degeneration, telangiectasis of bulbar conjunctiva and skin, and an increased likelihood of malignancy (especially lymphoma and brain tumor). The disease is autosomal recessive. Affected children have immunologic deficits, including a decrease in delayed hypersensitivity which suggests early thymic dysfunction. It is not known how the immunologic disorder and the cerebellar degeneration are related. Pathologic changes in the nervous system tend to be limited to degeneration in the cerebellum and spinocerebellar tracts.

The *neurologic manifestations* usually begin in infancy. Affected children walk late, always with an ataxic gait. Late in childhood progressive dysarthria, nystagmus, intention tremor, and choreoathetosis appear. Tendon reflexes are diminished or absent. A peculiar abnormality of eye movements is characteristic, the child being unable to move the eyes on command, whereas involuntary movements are retained. The *skin changes*, usually evident by 5 yr of age, consist of telangiectases over the bulbar conjunctiva (Fig. 21–18), along the nasolabial folds, over the external ears, and along flexor creases of the extremities. Clinical evidences of *immunologic deficiency* are variable: some children have severe recurrent sinus, ear, and pulmonary infections from early childhood; some never suffer from increased susceptibility to infection. Tonsillar tissue is diminished or absent; there are usually no palpable lymph nodes. The illness runs a slowly progressive course. The neurologic deficits often lead to scoliosis in late childhood; by early adolescence independent ambulation becomes impossible. Mild dementia is seen during the late stages of the illness. Death usually occurs in adolescence or

in early adulthood as a result of pulmonary failure, infection, or malignancy.

Laboratory findings include, in varying combinations, a decrease or absence of serum IgA and IgE, a decrease in the number of circulating small lymphocytes, and decrease or absence of delayed hypersensitivity reactions to intradermal injection of mumps or of *Candida* antigens. The skin sensitization reaction to dinitrochlorobenzene is usually absent. The serum level of alpha-fetoprotein is often increased. These tests help differentiate the condition from Friedreich ataxia and from the ataxic form of cerebral palsy, which are easily confused with ataxia-telangiectasia during the early stages. Further, a Babinski sign is found in Friedreich ataxia but not in ataxia-telangiectasia. Friedreich ataxia tends to be of later onset and lacks the eye movement abnormalities seen in ataxia-telangiectasia.

Therapy is limited to the prompt treatment of the associated infections; replacement therapy with gamma globulin does not appear to be helpful. See also Sec. 10.19.

Abetalipoproteinemia (Acanthocytosis, Bassen-Kornzweig Syndrome) (Sec. 7.48). In this rare, recessively inherited disease malabsorption of fat and abetalipoproteinemia are associated with progressive cerebellar ataxia and pigmentary degeneration of the retina. Onset occurs in infancy with manifestations of intestinal malabsorption. Slowly progressive ataxia appears later in childhood; retinal degeneration becomes evident during adolescence. The clinical pattern may resemble that of Friedreich ataxia, including the Babinski sign, distal sensory loss, areflexia, scoliosis, and pes cavus.

Low density lipoproteins are absent or markedly reduced in serum; carotene, vitamin A, and cholesterol levels are also low, the last below 60 mg/dL. Lipid droplets (triglycerides) can be seen in intestinal mucosal cells obtained by peroral biopsy. The red blood cells have multiple spiny projections, a feature that accounts for the term acanthocytosis as well as for the low sedimentation rate. The basic defect is unknown. Therapy at present is limited to supplementary administration of the fat-soluble vitamins.

Refsum Syndrome. Refsum syndrome, another rare form of hereditary ataxia, has a known metabolic defect and an effective therapy. The onset is in late childhood or in adolescence, with progressive cerebellar ataxia, distal weakness and sensory loss due to polyneuritis, retinitis pigmentosa, deafness, and ichthyosis. The metabolic abnormality consists of inability to oxidize phytanic acid (3,7,11,15-tetramethylhexadecanoic acid), which accumulates in serum and in body tissues. The CSF protein is elevated. Therapy with a diet low in foods containing phytanic acid (i.e., exclusion of all green vegetables) has resulted in improvement in the neurologic deficit (Sec. 7.36).

Myoclonic Encephalopathy of Childhood (Kinsbourne Syndrome). This is a rare neurologic disorder of unknown etiology that has its onset from 1–3 yr of age. It is characterized by irregular, rapid jerking movements of limbs and trunk (myoclonus) and by similar chaotic, irregular jerking of the eyes (opsoclonus). In addition, gait ataxia, intention tremor, and nystagmus are present. Some cases have been associated with occult neuroblastoma, with removal of the tumor bringing striking improvement in the neurologic state. In children without tumor and in those with inoperable neoplasms, therapy with ACTH or cortisone may induce remissions.

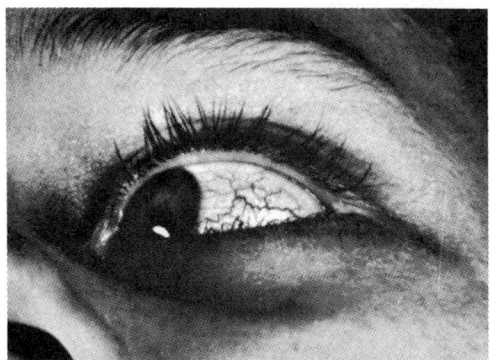

Figure 21–18. Ataxia-telangiectasia. Arterial telangiectasis on bulbar conjunctiva.

Ackroyd RS, Finnegan JA, Green SH: Friedreich's ataxia. A clinical review with neurophysiological and echocardiographic findings. Arch Dis Child 59:217, 1984.

Boder E, Sedgwick RP: Ataxia-telangiectasia: Familial syndrome of progressive cerebellar ataxia, oculocutaneous telangiectasia, and frequent pulmonary infection. Pediatrics 21:526, 1958.

Boyer SH, Chisolm AW, McKusick VA: Cardiac aspects of Friedreich's ataxia. Circulation 25:493, 1962.

Greenfield JC: The Spino-Cerebellar Degenerations. Springfield, IL, Charles C Thomas, 1954.

Herbert PN, Gotto AM, Fredrickson DS: Familial lipoprotein deficiency. *In*: Stanbury JB, Wyngaarden JB, Fredrickson DS (eds): The Metabolic Basis of Inherited Disease. Ed 4. New York, McGraw-Hill, 1978.

Herndon JH Jr, Steinberg D, Uhlendorf BW: Refsum's disease: Defective oxidation of phytanic acid in tissue cultures derived from homozygotes and heterozygotes. N Engl J Med 281:1034, 1969.

Hosking G: Ataxia telangiectasia. Dev Med Child Neurol 24:77, 1982.

Kinsbourne M: Myoclonic encephalopathy of infants. J Neurol Neurosurg Psychiatr 25:271, 1962.

McFarlin DE, Strober W, Waldman TA: Ataxia-telangiectasia. Medicine 51:281, 1972.

Moe PG, Nellhaus G: Infantile polymyoclonus-opsoclonus syndrome and neural crest tumors. Neurology 20:756, 1970.

21.21 Degenerations of the Basal Ganglia

Wilson Disease (Hepatolenticular Degeneration). This is a recessively inherited disorder of copper metabolism which leads to injury of liver and of basal ganglia. Changes in the brain include cavitation, gliosis, and neuronal degeneration in basal ganglia, most severe in the putamen. Similar changes may occur in the cerebral cortex, especially in the frontal lobes. The pathogenesis is not completely understood, but a defect in the synthesis of the copper-carrying protein, ceruloplasmin, explains many of the findings. Decreased protein-binding of serum copper appears to lead to increased leakage of copper into the tissues. Copper poisoning is a plausible explanation for the damage to the liver, basal ganglia, and renal tubules. (See also Sec. 12.77.)

Clinical Manifestations. Clinical onset may occur as subacute or chronic hepatic failure in early childhood. Neurologic abnormalities generally do not appear until later in childhood or in adolescence, but they may precede clinical evidence of liver disease. The diagnosis of Wilson disease should be considered in any child past 8 yr of age who develops a motor disorder or unexplained mental changes. A peculiar flapping tremor of the shoulders and wrists (*wing-beating tremor*) is characteristic but not always present. Instead, there may be dysarthria, choreoathetoid movements, or rigidity. Dysfunction of the bulbar musculature tends to occur early and leads to an immobile grinning facial expression, drooling, and dysarthria. Rarely, there is spasticity, hemiparesis, or a Babinski sign. Wilson disease may present mental changes in the absence of other neurologic changes. Emotional lability, progressive school failure, and frank psychotic states may occur. The most diagnostic physical finding is the *Kayser-Fleischer ring* of the cornea, a greenish yellow rim near the limbus, often most evident superiorly and inferiorly. It is due to deposition of copper in Descemet membrane and occurs only in Wilson disease and in exogenous copper poisoning. It is usually visible; if not, slit lamp examination will reveal it.

Laboratory Data. The diagnosis is confirmed by measurement of serum ceruloplasmin (the copper-carrying protein) and urinary copper excretion. A serum ceruloplasmin level under 50% of normal suggests the diagnosis, but a normal value does not rule it out. Urine copper values are usually above 200 μg/24 hr, as they may also be in hepatic cirrhosis from other causes. Increase in excretion after administration of penicillamine is a helpful diagnostic test in doubtful cases. Serum copper concentrations tend to be lower than normal because of deficiency of the fraction bound to ceruloplasmin. Other laboratory findings include generalized aminoaciduria, low serum concentration of uric acid, and glycosuria (all due to renal tubular damage) and usually chemical evidence of liver disease.

Prognosis. The prognosis of untreated Wilson disease is poor, with a fatal outcome usual by 5 yr after onset. Early treatment, directed at removal of excessive copper stores from tissues, has greatly improved the outlook.

Therapy. Various chelating agents have been used; penicillamine, 1–2 g/24 hr by mouth, is most effective. Allergic reactions, including fever, rash, and leukopenia, are common.

Penicillamine is a pyridoxine antimetabolite, and supplemental pyridoxine should be given during long-term therapy. A diet low in copper is a valuable adjunct to penicillamine therapy. Foods to be avoided include liver, shellfish, nuts, and chocolate.

Dystonia Musculorum Deformans (Torsion Dystonia). Dystonia occurs in a number of static and progressive brain diseases. The static disorders are perinatal brain injuries and postencephalitic syndromes; the progressive ones include Wilson disease, Huntington disease, and several other rare degenerative brain disorders.

The term *dystonia musculorum deformans* (torsion dystonia) is applied to a clinical entity characterized by dystonia as an isolated, genetically determined abnormality. Inheritance may be dominant or recessive, the latter especially among East European (Ashkenazi) Jews. The pathogenesis is obscure, and there are no consistent pathologic lesions in the brain. A biochemical rather than structural lesion of the basal ganglia

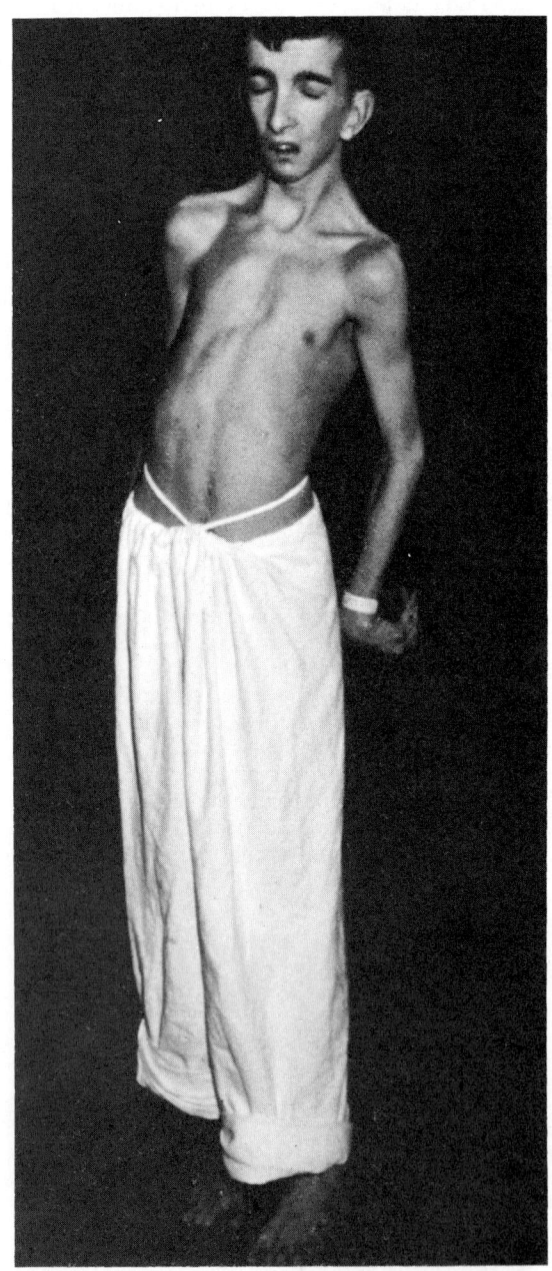

Figure 21–19. Hyperextension of back and abnormal posture of limbs in a patient with dystonia.

appears to be responsible. Torsion dystonia has its onset during childhood or early adolescence in the recessive group, usually somewhat later in families with dominant inheritance. The course is very variable, with progression to severe distortion of the limbs (Fig. 21–19) and incapacitation within a few years of onset in some patients and with stabilization or remission in others. Intelligence is preserved, and there is no evidence of disorder of the pyramidal motor system. Wilson disease should be ruled out by appropriate laboratory tests. There are no other helpful laboratory studies. A few patients with torsion dystonia have responded to therapy with L-dopa; trihexyphenidyl and carbamazepine have occasionally been helpful. Stereotactic thalamotomy produces dramatic but often transient improvement.

Hallervorden-Spatz Disease. This recessively inherited degeneration of basal ganglia is characterized by the deposition of iron in the damaged tissues. Iron metabolism appears normal, however, and the metabolic basis of the disease is unknown. Two variants occur: onset in early childhood (mean age 4 yr), with progressive dystonia, pigmentary degeneration of the retina, and often acanthocytosis; or onset in adolescence, with dystonia, rigidity, and spasticity as major manifestations. Dementia occurs late in the course in both types. There is no effective therapy.

Huntington Disease. This is a dominantly inherited degeneration of the basal ganglia, especially of the caudate nucleus, manifested clinically by dementia, choreiform movements, and irregular, dancing gait. Onset usually occurs in middle age but may occur in childhood, with learning disorders, seizures and rigidity or with chorea. In the latter instance it must be differentiated from Sydenham chorea, from Wilson disease, and from a dominantly inherited *benign chorea* which does not lead to dementia or to marked incapacitation. Usually, the diagnosis of Huntington chorea in childhood is possible only if a parent has the fully developed disease. L-Dopa may cause chorea in an asymptomatic person who is a carrier of the gene for Huntington chorea; this test is unreliable for early diagnosis. At present, there is no effective therapy. Genetic counseling is important.

Byers RK, Dodge JA: Huntington's chorea in children. Neurology 17:587, 1967.
Chun RWM, Daly RF, Mansheim BJ Jr, et al: Benign familial chorea with onset in childhood. JAMA 225:1603, 1973.
Conneally PM: Huntington disease: Genetics and epidemiology. Am J Hum Genet 36:506, 1984.
Denny-Brown D: Hepatolenticular degeneration (Wilson's disease). N Engl J Med 270:1149, 1964.
Dooling EC, Schoene WC, Richardson EP: Hallervorden-Spatz syndrome. Arch Neurol 30:70, 1974.
Eldridge R (ed): Torsion dystonias (dystonia musculorum deformans). Neurology 20(pt 2):1, 1970.
Fahn S: High dosage anticholinergic therapy in dystonia. Neurology 33:1255, 1983.
Goldstein NP, Tauxe WN, McCall JT, et al: Wilson's disease (hepato-lenticular degeneration). Treatment with penicillamine and changes in hepatic trapping of radioactive copper. Arch Neurol 24:391, 1971.
Luckenbach MW, Green WR, Miller NR, et al: Ocular clinicopathologic correlation of Hallervorden-Spatz syndrome with acanthocytosis and pigmentary retinopathy. Am J Ophthalmol 95:369, 1983.
Oliver J, Dewhurst K: Childhood and adolescent forms of Huntington's chorea. J Neurol Neurosurg Psychiatr 32:455, 1969.
O'Reilly S: Problems in Wilson's disease. Neurology 17:137, 1967.
Pincus JH, Chutorian A: Familial benign chorea with intention tremor: A clinical entity. J Pediatr 70:724, 1967.
Sternlieb I, Scheinberg IH: Prevention of Wilson's disease in asymptomatic patients. N Engl J Med 278:352, 1968.
Tu J, Blackwell RQ, Lee PF: DL-Penicillamine as a cause of optic axial neuritis. JAMA 185:83, 1963.
Walshe JM: The physiology of copper in man and its relation to Wilson's disease. Brain 90:149, 1967.

21.22 NEOPLASMS OF THE BRAIN

General Considerations. After leukemias, brain tumors are the most common neoplasms in children. Incidence is highest

during the second half of the 1st decade, but they may occur at any age, including early infancy. The incidences of the various cerebral neoplasms and their locations differ greatly from those observed in adults. Tumors of the cerebellum are most common and account for about 40% of the total. Tumors in other posterior fossa structures, including the brain stem and the 4th ventricle, make up about 15%. Suprasellar lesions, which include craniopharyngiomas, optic pathway gliomas, and gliomas of the hypothalamus, account for another 15%. Tumors of the cerebral hemispheres, the ventricles, and the meninges account for the remainder. In about 80% of neoplasms in children the basic cell is glial. The remainder are craniopharyngiomas, teratomas, hemangiomas, sarcomas, and meningiomas. Metastatic tumors of the brain are rare in childhood.

Most brain tumors occur sporadically and are of unknown cause; several, including teratomas and craniopharyngiomas, result from congenital malformations. An increased incidence of certain intracranial neoplasms is seen in the neurocutaneous syndromes. Irradiation of the brain increases the incidence of cerebral sarcomas.

Clinical Manifestations. The clinical manifestations in childhood are largely those of increased intracranial pressure because the majority of the tumors are in the posterior fossa and midline, where a mass lesion will obstruct CSF circulation. An important exception is the brain stem glioma, which, despite a midline location, rarely leads to increased intracranial pressure.

The manifestations of increased intracranial pressure vary somewhat with age. In infancy there is abnormal enlargement of the head. (Brain tumor should always be considered in the differential diagnosis of hydrocephalus.) Later in childhood marked expansion of the skull is no longer possible, and the increased intracranial pressure produces symptoms by compression of brain, meninges, and cerebral vessels. Headache is a common early symptom, characteristically occurring shortly after the child arises from bed or following changes in head position at other times of day. As pressure rises, headache becomes more severe and prolonged, but it is rarely continuous. The site of the pain has some localizing value; it tends to be suboccipital with posterior fossa tumors and on the side of the lesion in tumors of a cerebral hemisphere. Vomiting is common. It eventually becomes projectile and is characteristically unaccompanied by nausea. It is due to compression of the medulla and is therefore most severe in tumors of the posterior fossa. Drowsiness and stupor are rather late signs and are most likely due to pressure on the midbrain. Compression of vagal nuclei in the medulla leads to slowing of the pulse. Blood pressure is frequently elevated. Papilledema is often present but less likely in early infancy. Several intracranial structures are especially susceptible to damage by increased intracranial pressure. Sixth nerve palsies are common, with blurring of vision and diplopia; damage to optic nerves causes diminished visual acuity and may lead to total blindness. Important shifts of brain substance may occur; inferior portions of cerebellum (the inferior vermis and the cerebellar tonsils) may herniate downward through the foramen magnum, producing the syndrome of *tonsillar herniation*. This is especially likely in patients with posterior fossa tumors. It is manifested by neck stiffness and often by head tilt toward the side of herniation. Respirations become irregular and may suddenly cease because the respiratory centers in the medulla are compromised. Forceful neck flexion must be carefully avoided since it may lead to further compression of the medulla and sudden respiratory arrest. Supratentorial lesions, especially the laterally located ones, may lead to *tentorial herniation*.

The diagnostic study and management of brain tumor present many problems which fall outside the scope of pediatrics. The pediatrician needs to be thoroughly familiar with the presenting symptoms and signs, however, since he or she is likely to be the first to evaluate the child. The differential diagnosis includes some common and benign syndromes, even school phobia. The pediatrician also has a role in the pre- and postoperative care of children with brain tumors, especially those with suprasellar tumors which may lead to severe disorders of fluid and electrolyte balance. A most important role will be to provide support and comfort to parents during the course of a very trying illness.

INFRATENTORIAL NEOPLASMS

Four types of neoplasm are common in the posterior fossa: cerebellar astrocytoma and medulloblastoma are of approximately equal incidence and account for about 65% of the tumors in this location; brain stem gliomas account for about 20% and ependymomas of the 4th ventricle for about 10%. Acoustic neuromas and meningiomas in this area are rare in childhood.

Cerebellar Astrocytoma. This is usually a cystic tumor which tends to arise near the midline but often extends into one cerebellar hemisphere. It may occur at any time in childhood, with highest incidence from 2–8 yr. Signs of increased intracranial pressure appear early and may be the only changes; more commonly, signs of unilateral cerebellar dysfunction are superimposed, including hypotonia and intention tremor on the side of the lesion and nystagmus that is of greater amplitude when the child attempts to look toward the side of the tumor. Gait ataxia may be present, often with a tendency to veer toward one side. Somnolence occurs eventually because the brain stem is compressed. Pressure on vital structures in the brain stem appears to account for peculiar seizure-like states characterized by loss of consciousness with extensor rigidity, neck retraction, dilatation of pupils, and respiratory irregularity, which have been referred to as "cerebellar fits"; such attacks are cause for immediate investigation.

Early diagnosis is aided by computed tomography, which localizes the tumor in the majority of instances. Roentgenograms of the skull may show lateralized thinning and bulging of the occipital bone on the side of the lesion in addition to nonspecific signs of increased intracranial pressure. Rarely, calcifications are visible in the tumor. Vertebral angiography may be needed to localize the tumor in doubtful cases. Therapy requires surgical excision. Expert surgical management results in close to 90% long-term survivals; most of these appear to be cures, though late recurrence is possible. Radiation therapy is used only when a tumor is recurrent or is not completely resectable.

Medulloblastoma. Medulloblastoma is a midline cerebellar tumor made up of undifferentiated small round cells. It grows extremely rapidly, has a tendency to seed along the entire cerebrospinal axis, and is one of the few brain tumors that may metastasize to extraneural tissues. Incidence peaks from 2–6 yr, with boys affected about twice as frequently as girls. It is not possible to differentiate this tumor reliably from cerebellar astrocytoma on the basis of history or clinical examination, though the tumor is particularly likely to be found in a boy who has a history of rapidly progressive signs of increased intracranial pressure. There is often gait ataxia without lateralizing signs. Roentgenograms of the skull show evidence of increased intracranial pressure but no focal abnormalities. The tumor can usually be localized by computed tomography (Fig. 21–20).

Therapy consists of surgical excision of accessible tumor followed by focal radiation to the posterior fossa and low dose radiation to the entire neuraxis. After completion of a course of radiation, chemotherapy may be advisable. A simple and well-tolerated regimen consists of weekly intravenous injections alternately of vincristine and cyclophosphamide, contin-

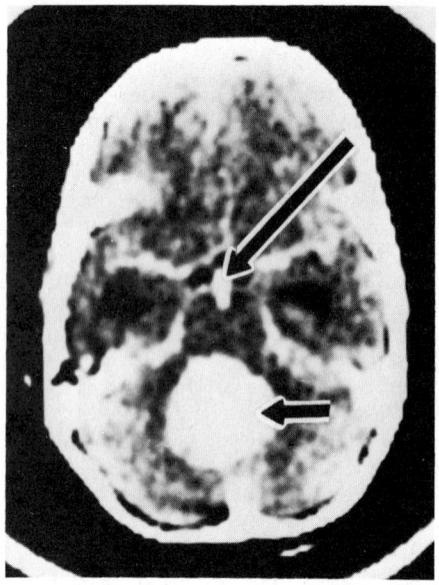

Figure 21–20. Computed tomogram (CT scan) after intravenous infusion of radiopaque material in a 4 yr old girl with morning vomiting, cachexia, and irritability but without positive findings on neurologic or funduscopic examination. A large tumor mass is shown in midline cerebellum (*short arrow*). A smaller, metastatic lesion is seen in the suprasellar cistern (*long arrow*). The temporal horns of the lateral ventricles are enlarged because the 4th ventricle is obstructed by the cerebellar tumor, which proved to be a medulloblastoma.

ued for 12–18 mo. The prognosis of medulloblastoma is hopeless with surgical therapy alone but improves somewhat with the use of combined treatment. A 20–30% cure rate has been achieved with surgery plus radiation. The effects of the addition of chemotherapy are not yet known. The outlook is hopeful if the child has no evidence of recurrence 18 mo after initial surgery.

Ependymoma. Ependymoma in the posterior fossa arises from the ependymal lining of the floor of the 4th ventricle. Upward extension into the ventricle causes early obstruction to CSF flow. The symptoms and signs are those of increased intracranial pressure. Cranial nerve palsies and positive Babinski signs may be present because of infiltration of the brain stem. These tumors may calcify, and the diagnosis can occasionally be made by visualization of calcification in the area of the 4th ventricle on a lateral roentgenogram of the skull. Surgical excision of accessible tumor often results in transient improvement, but surgical removal is rarely possible. Postoperative radiation therapy is given to the posterior fossa. There are few long-term survivors.

Glioma of the Brain Stem. Pontine glioma has its peak incidence from 6–8 yr of age. The clinical history and physical findings are almost pathognomonic. They consist of progressive appearance of multiple bilateral cranial nerve palsies in combination with pyramidal tract signs (hyperreflexia and Babinski sign) and ataxia. Usually, there is no evidence of increased intracranial pressure. All the cranial nerves may be affected, with 6th and 7th nerve palsies being most common. The diagnosis is established by computed tomography, which shows enlargement of the pons and posterior displacement of the 4th ventricle and aqueduct of Sylvius.

The tumors cannot be removed surgically; therapy consists of local radiation. Most patients die within 18 mo of diagnosis; a few long-term survivors have been reported.

SUPRATENTORIAL NEOPLASMS

Craniopharyngioma. Craniopharyngioma is the most common tumor of the sellar and suprasellar regions in childhood.

Its special pediatric interest is due to the numerous problems in management which arise from hypothalamic and pituitary dysfunctions. The tumor arises from squamous epithelial cell rests of the embryonic Rathke pouch. It often has a large cystic component; the growth features are those of a benign neoplasm.

Symptoms may appear at any time during childhood and adolescence and include (1) growth failure, (2) progressive visual loss, and (3) symptoms of increased intracranial pressure. These may occur singly or in any combination. The diagnosis should be considered whenever there is an arrest of linear growth after a period of normal gain in height. Other endocrine abnormalities are rare initially. Diabetes insipidus occurs *preoperatively* in fewer than 10%. Puberty is delayed. The visual impairment classically consists of bitemporal hemianopsia but may consist of asymmetric field defects, unilateral blindness, or bilateral decrease in visual acuity. Funduscopic examination reveals optic atrophy or papilledema. Roentgenograms of the skull show calcifications in a supra- or intrasellar location in about 80% of craniopharyngiomas that present during childhood (Fig. 21–21). The sella turcica may be ballooned or distorted. Bone age is often retarded.

The location of the craniopharyngioma makes therapy a formidable problem. Cure by complete surgical removal requires both unusual surgical skill and meticulous postoperative care. Therapy with cortisone is initiated on the day prior to operation, at a dosage of about 40 mg/m^2/24 hr, and is continued for at least 2 wk postoperatively. Supplementary hydrocortisone is given intravenously during the operation. Postoperatively, fluid intake is carefully matched to output; diabetes insipidus occurs almost invariably and must be controlled by replacement therapy. A marked decrease in urine output often occurs on the 2nd or 3rd postoperative day because of inappropriate release of antidiuretic hormone. It is essential that fluids be restricted during this period to prevent water intoxication and cerebral edema. Serum electrolytes must also be carefully monitored and imbalances corrected. Occasionally, there is persistent hypernatremia due to damage to the hypothalamic thirst-regulating mechanism. A satisfactory result can be achieved in approximately 60% of patients. Aspiration of the tumor cyst followed by radiation of the tumor has been proposed as an alternative method of therapy.

Gliomas of the Optic Pathways. These occur with increased frequency in patients with neurofibromatosis. They present unilateral or bilateral visual loss. Extension of the tumor into the orbit may cause proptosis. Evidences of hypothalamic dysfunction and of increased intracranial pressure appear late. Surgical cure can be achieved when the tumor is confined to one optic nerve; those involving the optic chiasm are inoperable. These lesions progress very slowly, however, and survival without treatment may be as long as 20 yr. Radiation therapy has been advocated.

Hypothalamic Gliomas. These occur mainly in infants, in whom they produce a very characteristic syndrome of emaciation, *the diencephalic syndrome of infancy.* Tumors of the hypothalamus occurring later in childhood usually present as precocious puberty in children who tend to be excessively large for age. They may have increased intracranial pressure due to extension of the tumor into the 3rd ventricle and visual loss due to involvement of the optic chiasm. Various types of tumor are seen, including hamartomas, gliomas, ectopic pinealomas, and teratomas.

TUMORS OF THE CEREBRAL HEMISPHERES

In childhood, tumors of the cerebral hemispheres include astrocytoma, oligodendroglioma, ependymoma, glioblastoma, and sarcoma. The symptoms and signs depend on the location of the tumor and its growth characteristics. Low-grade hemispheral tumors such as astrocytomas or oligodendrogliomas may initially cause convulsions without other abnormalities. These lesions often become partially calcified, a possibility warranting CT scans as part of the study of a child with seizures. As the tumors enlarge, they tend to produce spastic hemiparesis, hemisensory defects, or hemianopsia. Symptoms of increased intracranial pressure appear late. The more malignant tumors, such as the glioblastomas, present with rapidly progressive increase in intracranial pressure and with focal neurologic signs, including hemiparesis, hemianopsia, aphasia, and unilateral choreoathetoid movements. Accurate localization is made by computed tomography and cerebral angiography. Hemispheral tumors in childhood are rarely curable, but partial removal of the more benign types may lead to many years of symptom-free life.

Neoplasms in the Pineal Region. These are uncommon in childhood, but they deserve mention in view of their characteristic clinical presentation. Early compression of the upper midbrain produces pupillary dilatation with diminution in the light reflex and paralysis of upward gaze (*Parinaud syndrome*). Hydrocephalus is due to obstruction of the posterior 3rd ventricle and the aqueduct. The lesions cannot be removed surgically, but palliation can be achieved by a shunt operation followed by radiation.

Developmental tumors (*epidermoids, dermoids,* and *teratomas*) may occur in the pineal region and elsewhere along the midline. Epidermoids contain only stratified squamous epithelium; dermoids have all skin structures, including hair and sebaceous glands; teratomas contain mesodermal and endodermal tissues as well. Occasionally, teratomas may be revealed roentgenographically when bones or teeth are seen in the tumor. These developmental tumors may form large cysts filled with sebaceous secretions and desquamated skin. Complete surgical removal may be possible.

Papillomas of the Choroid Plexus. Papillomas are most common prior to 3 yr of age. They usually arise from choroid plexus of a lateral ventricle. Focal neurologic signs are rare. Increased production of CSF and obstruction to CSF flow by the tumor mass lead to early hydrocephalus. This tumor needs to be considered in the differential diagnosis of any child with hydrocephalus of obscure etiology. Diagnosis is usually apparent on computed tomography. Complete surgical removal is possible and leads to cure of the associated hydrocephalus.

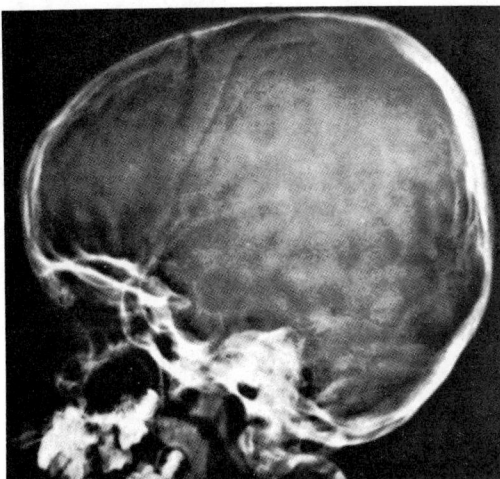

Figure 21–21. Craniopharyngioma in a boy 8 yr of age. Note fluffy suprasellar calcification, enlarged sella turcica, digital markings of skull, and early sutural separation.

PSEUDOTUMOR CEREBRI

As the name implies, this condition produces symptoms and signs that mimic those of brain tumor. The increased intracranial pressure is caused by diffuse cerebral edema.

Pseudotumor cerebri may occur as a complication of hypoparathyroidism, galactosemia, corticosteroid therapy (especially while the dose is being reduced or after it has been discontinued), tetracycline therapy, or high doses of vitamin A. The majority of cases are of obscure etiology; obese adolescent girls are especially apt to acquire this condition.

The clinical presentation includes headache, morning vomiting, papilledema, and sometimes a 6th nerve palsy. Somnolence may occur but is rarely marked. Signs of focal neurologic disease are absent. A child with this combination of symptoms and signs usually requires computed tomography to rule out a focal mass lesion. The diagnosis of pseudotumor cerebri should be suspected in a child with increased intracranial pressure in whom neither a mass lesion nor enlargement of the ventricular system is found. The lateral ventricles may be reduced in size because of compression by the edematous brain. The CSF is normal except for a low protein content in some instances.

The elevation in intracranial pressure may persist for several mo, but it always subsides eventually. The chief danger is damage to optic nerves from chronic compression. No treatment is needed in mild cases. Patients with severe increase in pressure may be helped by repeated removal of CSF via lumbar puncture or by acetazolamide at a dosage of 30–50 mg/kg/24 hr. Corticosteroid therapy is often effective, but relapse may occur when therapy is discontinued. Weight reduction is indicated if the child is obese.

Banna M, Hoare RD, Stanley P, et al: Craniopharyngioma in children. J Pediatr 83:781, 1973.
Bray PF, Carter S, Taveras JM: Brain stem tumors in children. Neurology 8:1, 1958.
Chutorian AM, Schwartz JF, Evans RA, et al: Optic gliomas in children. Neurology 14:83, 1964.
Farwell JR, Dohrmann GJ, Flannery JT: Central nervous system tumors in children. Cancer 40:3123, 1977.
Gareis FJ, Johnson JA: Inanition in infants associated with diencephalic neoplasms. Am J Dis Child 102:349, 1965.
Greer M: Benign intracranial hypertension. Neurology 12:472, 1962; 14:469, 1964; 15:382, 1965.
Kramer S: The value of radiation therapy for pituitary and parapituitary tumors. Can Med Assn J 99:1120, 1968.
Lassman LP, Pearce GW, Gang J: Sensitivity of intracranial gliomas to vincristine sulfate. Lancet 1:296, 1965.
Lysak WR, Svien JH: Long-term follow-up on patients with diagnosis of pseudotumor cerebri. J Neurosurg 25:284, 1966.
Matson DD: Neurosurgery of Infancy and Childhood. Springfield, IL, Charles C Thomas, 1969.
McFarland DR, Horwitz H, Saenger EL, et al: Medulloblastoma—a review of prognosis and survival. Br J Radiol 42:198, 1969.
Rose A, Matson DD: Benign intracranial hypertension in children. Pediatrics 39:227, 1967.
Wilson CB: Medulloblastoma. Current views regarding the tumor and its treatment. Oncology 24:273, 1970.

21.23 INTRACRANIAL MASS LESIONS SECONDARY TO INFECTION

Pyogenic infections may lead to abscess formation within the brain or to effusions or purulent exudates in subdural or epidural spaces. In each of these conditions intracranial pressure is increased by a local mass effect. When signs of infection are absent, differentiation from other conditions that cause increased intracranial pressure may be difficult.

BRAIN ABSCESS

Children with cyanotic congenital heart disease are at increased risk of development of pyogenic abscess of the brain.

This peculiar susceptibility appears to be due to the fact that a right to left shunt eliminates the normal filtering of venous blood by the capillary bed of the lungs. In addition, the hypoxic brain appears to be an especially good culture medium for the anaerobic bacteria that are usually found in such lesions. Somewhat fewer than half of brain abscesses in childhood represent spread from foci of infection in other locations. Some occur by intracranial extension of infection from mastoids, paranasal sinuses, and skull; these were much more common prior to the widespread use of antibiotics. Occasionally brain abscess is metastatic from lung abscess, empyema, or endocarditis. Rarely, it is a complication of bacterial meningitis or of a penetrating injury to the skull. Some affected children have no history of any major preceding infection. The organisms found in brain abscess include microaerophilic or anaerobic streptococci, *Staphylococcus aureus*, pneumococcus, *Proteus, Haemophilus influenzae*, and *H. aphrophilus*.

Clinical signs of infection may be absent throughout the course of the illness. When present, they usually consist of low grade fever and stiffness of the neck. Neurologic signs depend on the location of the abscess. Focal seizures and hemiparesis occur with abscess of a cerebral hemisphere. Temporal lobe abscess, which may complicate mastoiditis, causes aphasia if the dominant side is involved. Cerebellar abscess, also usually secondary to mastoiditis, results in ataxia and nystagmus. Evidence of increased intracranial pressure is almost always present. Headache, vomiting, irritability, and drowsiness may be the presenting symptoms, and papilledema is usually present. The course is usually subacute over a period of weeks. Untreated, the child eventually becomes comatose. Death results from rupture of the abscess with overwhelming meningitis or from tentorial or cerebellar herniation.

Leukocytosis and elevated sedimentation rate may or may not be present. Computed tomography (Fig. 21–22), radionuclide brain scan, and electroencephalography are useful

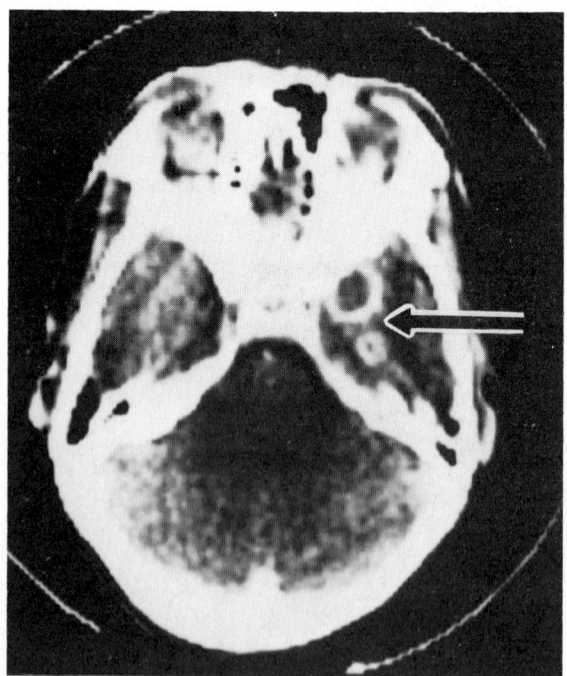

Figure 21–22. Two ring-shaped lesions in the right temporal lobe (*arrow*) in a computed tomogram obtained after intravenous injection of radiopaque material. The patient, an 11 yr old boy, had a history of frontal and sphenoid sinusitis and headache. The appearance of the lesions is typical of brain abscess. Resolution occurred following long-term antibiotic therapy.

initial laboratory tools. The radionuclide scan is almost always positive; it may show a ring-shaped area of increased uptake corresponding to the capsule of the abscess. In supratentorial abscesses the EEG shows a prominent slow-wave focus in the area of the lesion. CSF is of limited diagnostic help, and lumbar puncture should be avoided when intracranial pressure is high. The CSF is sterile unless the abscess has ruptured. The protein content is usually elevated, and white blood cells may be increased, with lymphocytes predominating. A roentgenogram of the chest is essential to look for a suppurative lesion of the lungs.

As soon as a tentative diagnosis of brain abscess is made, broad spectrum intravenous antibiotic therapy should be initiated and maintained for at least 6 wk. Use of osmotic diuretics, such as mannitol, will be important when intracranial pressure is elevated. Surgical drainage of the abscess is performed when there is a large collection of purulent material, and may be an emergency procedure in the comatose child with markedly increased intracranial pressure. Excision of the abscess, including its capsule, is advocated by some neurosurgeons. The most common sequel is the occurrence of seizures, for which continuous anticonvulsant therapy is usually needed.

SUBDURAL AND EPIDURAL EMPYEMA

Collections of pus in the subdural or epidural spaces have become relatively rare. They are usually secondary to frontal sinusitis or to infections of the scalp and skull. The purulent mass compresses the underlying brain. In addition, there is thrombophlebitis of the cortical veins that pass through the infected subdural space; interference with venous drainage leads to severe cerebral swelling. The course is subacute, with fever, severe headache, lethargy, convulsions, and hemiparesis. Papilledema is present, and there may be rapid progression to coma and to tentorial herniation. The differential diagnosis includes brain abscess and cortical vein thrombosis. The diagnosis is confirmed by computed tomography, which shows a low density mass overlying a cerebral hemisphere, with shift of midline structures to the opposite side. Therapy consists of prompt surgical drainage and appropriate antibiotic therapy.

SUBDURAL EFFUSION COMPLICATING MENINGITIS

This disorder is thought to be peculiar to infancy. Incidence peaks from 4–6 mo of age; it is rarely recognized beyond 1 yr. Subdural effusion may be associated with any of the bacterial meningitides but occurs most often following *Haemophilus influenzae* meningitis. It seems probable that there are small collections of fluid in the subdural spaces in most persons with meningitis, the great majority of which are insignificant and resorb spontaneously. The incidence of large collections which require therapy is much smaller and probably less than has been thought to be the case.

The pathogenesis of subdural fluid collections with meningitis is incompletely understood. The arachnoid membrane in the infant is a poor barrier to the spread of infection into the subdural space. Early in the course of meningitis subdural fluid is often purulent and bacteria may be grown from it. After the infection has been controlled, several mechanisms appear to act to maintain and enlarge the fluid collection. As the subdural space becomes expanded, there may be rupture of small bridging veins; hemorrhage into the space is suggested by the fact that the fluid is frequently bloody. Transudation of fluid from inflamed capillary vessels may also be important; the protein content of subdural fluid is that of a transudate of plasma. The formation of large collections of fluid is aided by the distensibility of the skull of the infant.

Longstanding effusions lead to the formation of vascular membranes, which become especially well developed along the outer wall of the subdural space. These membranes are friable, and capillary bleeding may occur from their surface.

It is difficult to identify symptoms that are clearly related to postmeningitic subdural effusions. Convulsions, vomiting, irritability, and persistent drowsiness are also seen in infants with meningitis not complicated by effusion. Physical findings in infants with subdural effusions include persistent fever, a bulging anterior fontanelle, and abnormal head enlargement. The diagnosis is confirmed by transillumination of the skull and by computed tomography. The effusions are bilateral in over two thirds of cases. Treatment is directed toward prevention of large fluid collections, which may damage the brain by compression. It is not necessary to tap small collections which are not associated with increased intracranial pressure. Too many taps may actually worsen the problem by causing bleeding into the subdural spaces. Small collections subside spontaneously. In infants with bulging fontanelle or abnormal head enlargement, subdural taps are repeated every 24–48 hr, always bilaterally if fluid collections have been demonstrated on both sides. If large quantities of high-protein or bloody fluid continue to accumulate after 2 wk of repeated tapping, the subdural spaces should be surgically drained via bilateral burr holes. Surgical excision of subdural membranes has been advocated, but it has not been proved effective.

Berg B, Franklin G, Cuneo R, et al: Nonsurgical cure of brain abscess. Early diagnosis and follow-up computerized tomography. Ann Neurol 3:474, 1978.
Farmer TW, Wise GR: Subdural empyema in infants, children and adults. Neurology 23:254, 1973.
Gitlin D: Pathogenesis of subdural collections of fluid. Pediatrics 16:345, 1955.
Hitchcock E, Andreadis A: Subdural empyema: A review of 29 cases. J Neurol Neurosurg Psychiatr 27:422, 1964.
Liske E, Weikers NJ: Changing aspects of brain abscess. Neurology 14:294, 1964.
Matson DD, Salam M: Brain abscess in congenital heart disease. Pediatrics 27:772, 1961.
McKay RJ Jr, Ingraham FS, Matson DD: Subdural fluid complicating bacterial meningitis. JAMA 152:387, 1953.
Raimondi AJ, Matsumo S, Miller RA: Brain abscess in children with congenital heart disease. J Neurosurg 23:588, 1965.

21.24 ACUTE TOXIC ENCEPHALOPATHY AND REYE SYNDROME

The differential diagnosis of Reye syndrome (Sec. 12.82) includes a number of toxic and metabolic disorders, including drug poisoning (especially with salicylates), hypoglycemic encephalopathy, hepatic coma due to acute hepatitis, and acute water intoxication. When convulsions occur early, the possibility of anoxic brain damage secondary to a seizure has to be considered. Sudden obstruction to CSF flow by an intraventricular tumor may cause a similar clinical picture, as may the occasional case of encephalitis without spinal fluid pleocytosis. Chemical evidence of hepatic dysfunction, including ammonia intoxication, is of great value for the rapid differentiation of Reye syndrome from most other severe, acute encephalopathies. Acute hepatitis can usually be excluded by the absence of jaundice. The liver tends to be small and nonpalpable in the rare cases of fulminant anicteric hepatitis.

Kolata G: Study of Reye's–aspirin link raises concern. Science 227:391, 1985.

21.25 CEREBRAL VASCULAR DISEASES

This group of illnesses falls into two categories: *intracranial hemorrhage* and *vascular occlusion*. Both are characterized by the precipitous onset of signs and symptoms of neurologic dysfunction.

INTRACRANIAL HEMORRHAGE

(See also Sec. 8.23.)

Spontaneous intracranial hemorrhage in childhood usually results from the rupture of a congenital vascular lesion such as an arteriovenous malformation or an arterial aneurysm. Hemorrhage from a vascular malformation or an aneurysm has to be differentiated from intracranial bleeding secondary to blood coagulation defects and from traumatic hemorrhage. Intracranial bleeding occurs occasionally in hemophilia and in idiopathic thrombocytopenia and may be a terminal event in leukemia. Traumatic hemorrhage may be especially difficult to distinguish in the small child with no history of head trauma.

Arteriovenous Malformations (Fistulas). These may occur in any part of the brain; they consist of large arterial feeding vessels, a mass of dilated communicating channels, and large draining veins that carry arterialized blood. The larger malformations may produce symptoms in infancy without hemorrhage. This is especially true of malformations involving the posterior cerebral artery and the great vein of Galen; the arteriovenous shunt may be so large as to cause congestive heart failure and polycythemia. Enormous saccular dilatation of the vein of Galen may also lead to hydrocephalus in infancy by obstruction of the aqueduct of Sylvius. The majority of arteriovenous malformations, however, are clinically silent for a number of years, then suddenly cause symptoms when rupture of one of the communicating vessels leads to subarachnoid and intracerebral hemorrhage.

Sudden severe headache, drowsiness, nuchal rigidity due to subarachnoid hemorrhage, and focal neurologic signs from damage of brain tissue at the site of the hemorrhage are the most common presenting signs. Detection of an intracranial bruit is a helpful confirmatory sign, especially after the age of 4 or 5 yr. With massive intracranial bleeding the child rapidly lapses into coma. Funduscopic examination may show retinal and preretinal hemorrhages. Occasionally, there are repeated episodes of headache and focal convulsions, which probably represent recurrent minor episodes of bleeding.

The diagnosis is confirmed by bloody or xanthochromic cerebrospinal fluid. Cerebral angiography is essential for determination of the exact location and extent of the lesion. Arteriovenous malformations superficially located in the cerebral cortex may be amenable to complete surgical excision. Embolization of the abnormal vessels is the preferred method of treatment in large or deeply situated malformations. Ligation of feeding arteries alone is usually of limited effectiveness.

Intracranial Arterial Aneurysms. The most common aneurysms are due to *congenital malformations* in the media of arterial walls at points of bifurcation (berry aneurysm). The incidence is increased in patients with coarctation of the aorta and with polycystic disease of the kidney. The most common sites are the anterior communicating and anterior cerebral arteries and the terminal branching of the internal carotid artery. Occasionally, aneurysms form at sites of damage to cerebral arteries by infection (*mycotic aneurysms*).

Intracranial arterial aneurysms are rarely diagnosed in childhood. Though the defect is almost always congenital, it is not apt to be manifested until early adult years. Symptoms are mainly those of subarachnoid and intracerebral hemorrhage following rupture. The typical history involves a previously well child who suddenly develops excruciating headache and then lapses into stupor and coma. Nuchal rigidity and preretinal hemorrhage are signs of subarachnoid bleeding. Third nerve palsy is common after rupture of an aneurysm of the carotid artery, hemiparesis after rupture of a middle cerebral artery aneurysm. The CSF is bloody and xanthochromic and

is under increased pressure. Cerebral angiography is needed for definitive diagnosis. Surgical ligation or clipping of the aneurysm is indicated if it is possible. The mortality of unoperated ruptured aneurysms is about 50%. Bleeding may recur many years later in survivors.

CEREBRAL VASCULAR OCCLUSIONS

Occlusive cerebral vascular disorders include arterial occlusions, either thrombotic or embolic, and venous occlusions, which are due to thrombosis or thrombophlebitis in cerebral veins.

Arterial Occlusions (Acute Infantile Hemiplegia). Occlusion of cerebral arteries is uncommon in childhood; it has its peak incidence from 1–3 yr of age. It is due to thrombosis or embolism in a major cerebral artery, usually the internal carotid or middle cerebral. Thrombosis in the extracranial (cervical) portion of the internal carotid artery may be caused by localized vasculitis from spread of tonsillar infection or cervical adenitis or by local trauma, especially from a pencil point or other sharp object pushed into the region of the tonsillar fossa. The cause is less often evident in occlusions of the intracranial vessels. Local arteritis, atherosclerosis, and fibromuscular hyperplasia of the vessel wall have been implicated, often without proof. Thrombocytosis has been associated, but its relationship to the thrombosis is uncertain. Systemic illnesses that may be complicated by cerebral artery occlusions in childhood include sickle cell disease, lupus erythematosus, polyarteritis nodosa, Takayasu arteritis, and cyanotic heart disease. Infants under 2 yr of age with cyanotic congenital heart disease who have both polycythemia and iron deficiency are especially prone to cerebral arterial occlusion. The possibility of cerebral embolus has to be considered in the older child with congenital heart disease.

Recurrent strokes in otherwise healthy children are usually due to *moyamoya disease,* in which there is progressive narrowing and occlusion of the major intracranial vessels, including the internal carotid, middle cerebral, and anterior cerebral arteries. Prominent collateral vessels through the basal ganglia lead to a characteristic appearance on cerebral angiography from which the disease derives its name (Japanese, "a puff of smoke"). The pathologic changes in the affected major cerebral arteries consist of intimal thickening and defects in the elastic lamina. The cause is unknown. The disorder may begin during infancy and early childhood, with most severe changes in the group with early onset.

The clinical manifestations of cerebral vascular occlusion in childhood resemble those of stroke in the adult. In the child there is often a preceding acute febrile illness. The child may be found to be hemiparetic on awakening from sleep. In other instances weakness is progressive over a period of hours. The child may remain lucid; transient aphasia is common when the dominant hemisphere is affected. Convulsions, focal or generalized, frequently occur during the acute phase. There are no signs of increased intracranial pressure, and the CSF remains normal. The diagnosis may be confirmed by cerebral angiography if it is performed early. Recanalization of the occluded vessel occurs rapidly, and arteriography a few wk after the onset may show a normal vascular system. Cerebral angiography is essential for the diagnosis of moyamoya disease.

The differential diagnosis of cerebral arterial occlusion includes postictal (Todd) paralysis when the acute illness is complicated by convulsions. Encephalitis has to be considered but can usually be ruled out if the child remains fairly alert and if there are no inflammatory changes in the CSF.

Therapy is limited to treatment of definable underlying conditions such as infection. Surgical procedures have improved collateral circulation to the brain in some children with moyamoya disease.

The prognosis depends on the size of the cerebral infarct and on the age of the child at the time of the stroke. In children under the age of 8 yr, there can be complete or near-complete recovery from aphasia in left hemisphere infarcts. Almost always there is some residual hemiparesis. Spasticity tends to develop over a period of weeks or months. Recurrent seizures are common, especially following acute hemiplegia in infancy. Many children are left with mild intellectual impairment and behavioral abnormalities.

Venous Occlusions. Thrombosis of cerebral veins occurs principally as a complication of severe dehydration or as an extension of local infection. Several clinical syndromes depend on the site of the venous occlusion.

Sagittal Sinus Thrombosis. This may be a complication of severe dehydration, especially in the infant with diarrhea. Obstruction of the sinus leads to cerebral swelling, which produces signs of increased intracranial pressure, including stupor, coma, and bulging anterior fontanelle. When thrombosis extends into the cortical veins, there may be widespread hemorrhagic infarction of the brain. Seizures and quadriparesis may occur. The clinical diagnosis can rarely be made with certainty. The clinical picture may mimic encephalitis and various metabolic encephalopathies, especially water intoxication in the dehydrated infant who has been rehydrated too rapidly.

Lateral Sinus Thrombosis. This complication of neglected otitis media and mastoiditis has become rare. Obstruction to the sinus results from septic thrombophlebitis. There may be chills and fever, or the onset may be insidious with signs of increased intracranial pressure. Focal neurologic signs are usually absent.

Cavernous Sinus Thrombosis. This follows infection of the face, orbit, or nasal sinuses that spreads via anastomoses from the facial vein to the ophthalmic veins, which drain directly into the cavernous sinus. Pyogenic infections of the nose are a common source. Onset occurs with high fever, drowsiness, and proptosis of the eye on the affected side. Within hours or at most 1–2 days the veins of the lid become distended and chemosis develops. There is paralysis of one or more of the ocular muscles. On funduscopic examination disc margins are blurred and retinal veins engorged. Untreated, the thrombophlebitis spreads to the other side via the circular sinus, and fatal intracranial extension usually follows.

Diagnosis. The diagnosis of cerebral venous thrombosis is based to a large extent on the clinical findings. CSF examination is of little help. CSF pressure is usually elevated; the fluid may be bloody, and it may show white cells and an elevated protein content. Cerebral angiography is of value in localizing the site of obstruction.

Treatment. Treatment of cerebral vein thrombosis consists of appropriate antibiotic therapy if thrombosis is secondary to infection. Localized collections of pus should be drained surgically. Life-threatening increases in intracranial pressure may be treated with mannitol or dexamethasone. Anticoagulant therapy is not indicated; it may worsen hemorrhage into infarcted brain.

Brown P: Septic cavernous thrombosis. Bull Johns Hopkins Hosp 109:68, 1961.

Gold AP, Ransohoff J, Carter S: Vein of Galen malformation. Acta Neurol Scand 8 (Suppl) 1964.

Greer M: Benign intracranial hypertension. 1. Mastoiditis and lateral sinus obstruction. Neurology 12:472, 1962.

Isler W: Acute Hemiplegias and Hemisyndromes in Childhood. Clinics in Developmental Medicine. Nos 41/42. Philadelphia, JB Lippincott, 1971.

Levine OR, Jameson AG, Nelhaus G, et al: Cardiac complications of cerebral arteriovenous fistula in infancy. Pediatrics 30:563, 1962.

Matson DD: Intracranial arterial aneurysms in childhood. J Neurosurg 23:578, 1965.

Pool JL, Potts DG: Aneurysms and Arteriovenous Anomalies of the Brain: Diagnosis and Treatment. New York, Paul B Hoeber, 1965.

Solomon GE, et al: Natural history of acute hemiplegia of childhood. Brain 93:107, 1970.

Suzuki J, Kodama N: Moyamoya disease—a review. Stroke 14:104, 1983.

Tyler HR, Clark DB: Incidence of neurological complications in congenital heart disease. Arch Neurol Psychiatr 77:17, 1957.

21.26 HEAD INJURY

Craniocerebral trauma is a major cause of serious disability and death in childhood. About 200,000 children each year are admitted to United States hospitals for observation and treatment following head injury. A much larger number are managed at home. The decision as to whether a potentially life-threatening head injury requires hospitalization is frequently difficult.

MINOR HEAD TRAUMA

Normally a closed head injury can be assumed to be insignificant when the initial blow to the head is not followed by unconsciousness; the child can usually be followed at home without special diagnostic study. Dizziness, nausea, occasional vomiting, and headache may be seen during the first 24–48 hr after minor head trauma. They are not cause for alarm unless they are accompanied by marked or progressive lethargy. But even after apparently mild head trauma the parents should be instructed to make certain at least once during the first night that the child is rousable and that there has not been a significant drop in heart rate (to 60/min or below) since intracranial hemorrhage, especially into the subdural space, occasionally follows apparently trivial head trauma.

CONCUSSION

With concussion, head injury is immediately followed by a period of unconsciousness. Concussion is not associated with obvious pathologic changes in brain; it is assumed to be due to disturbance in function of the brain stem caused by sudden jarring. After a concussion the patient may have loss of memory for events that preceded the injury (*retrograde amnesia*) or for occurrences after the injury (*antegrade amnesia*). In general, the duration of unconsciousness and the extent of retrograde amnesia correlate well with the severity of injury. Retrograde amnesia diminishes during recovery but never disappears completely.

Concussion implies a significant blow to the head, with sufficient distortion of intracranial structures to make severance of intracranial vessels a possibility. After a concussion the child should be carefully observed for delayed signs of intracranial hemorrhage. A baseline neurologic examination should include a check for pupillary size and reaction to light, funduscopic examination, and assessment of reflexes for symmetry and for the Babinski sign. In the infant, tension of the fontanelle should be assessed and the head size measured. It is advisable to obtain roentgenograms of the skull for skull fractures. Not every child with concussion or even skull fracture needs to be treated in the hospital. Close observation at home may be sufficient if the initial evaluation finds no neurologic abnormality, if the child has regained normal alertness, and if the parents are reliable and responsible.

SKULL FRACTURE

The roentgenographic demonstration of a skull fracture provides important information regarding the site of injury but does not necessarily indicate serious brain injury. The possibility of intracranial hemorrhage must, of course, be assessed. A fracture that crosses the groove for the middle meningeal artery suggests the possibility of epidural hemorrhage. Occipital skull fracture may be associated with posterior fossa hemorrhage (see below). Basal skull fractures may lead to leakage of CSF into the middle ear with bulging of the tympanic membrane and to otorrhea if the tympanic membrane is ruptured. Rhinorrhea due to escape of CSF from the nose occurs with fractures through the cribriform plate. Basal skull fractures may lead to meningitis by spread of organisms from the nose or ear. Prophylactic use of one of the penicillins is justifiable for basal skull fracture. Linear fractures require no specific therapy. Depressed fractures should be elevated surgically unless depression is minimal. Occasionally, surgical closure of dural defects is necessary to control CSF leakage.

Skull fractures in infancy may lead over periods of months or years to progressively enlarging defects of the skull (spreading fractures, leptomeningeal cysts) when meninges are trapped in the fracture line. Large leptomeningeal cysts may need surgical resection.

SEVERE HEAD INJURY

This should be assumed when a child fails to awaken within some minutes after an accident. Structural damage to brain has to be expected in such a patient. This may take the form of *contusion* or bruising of brain, usually either at the site of the blow (coup) or opposite the site (contrecoup). Actual *laceration* of brain tissue and meninges may occur, often with intracerebral, subarachnoid, or subdural hemorrhage. Intracranial pressure may increase rapidly as a result both of hemorrhage and of edema of injured tissue.

The acute management of the child with severe head injury is demanding. Generally, the child is comatose. The first priorities are that the patient have adequate blood pressure, that the airway be patent, and that respirations be well maintained. Movement of the patient should be avoided until it is clear that there are no serious injuries such as fractures of the spine or of other major bones. Prompt neurologic assessment should be carried out as summarized above for the comatose patient. This is repeated at frequent intervals until the patient's condition is stable. Neuroroentgenographic studies and/or neurosurgical intervention may be indicated when coma progressively deepens or when signs of tentorial herniation appear. The medical management of the child who remains comatose following severe head injury is that of coma from any cause. Management of cerebral edema complicating head injury includes use of dexamethasone, intravenous mannitol, and controlled ventilation as indicated. Continuous monitoring of intracranial pressure (via an intraventricular catheter or a pressure transducer inserted into the epidural or subdural space) is a valuable aid to management of critically ill children.

POST-TRAUMATIC SYNDROMES

The brain of the child shows remarkable capacity for recovery from acute injury. Good functional recoveries have been reported in children comatose for over 2 mo. Post-traumatic epilepsy occurs in about 10% of survivors from severe head injury and usually has its onset within 1 yr. The most common residuals are minor changes in behavior and in learning. Headache and dizziness are rather common. Hydrocephalus may follow subarachnoid hemorrhage.

EPIDURAL HEMORRHAGE

This is usually secondary to severance of the middle meningeal artery, most often as a result of a fracture that crosses the artery's groove in the skull. Fracture is less likely in the infant or small child with epidural hemorrhage, in whom bleeding is frequently venous from dural veins. The patient with epidural hemorrhage characteristically awakens from a concussion and after a brief lucid interval lapses into coma again. Signs of tentorial herniation rapidly follow unless therapy is promptly instituted. If the initial injury is severe enough to cause cerebral contusion, the lucid interval is absent and coma progressively deepens. Prompt surgical evacuation of blood from the epidural space is lifesaving.

When epidural hemorrhage is venous in origin, the course is less rapid and is clinically indistinguishable from that of subdural hematoma. Hemorrhage into the epidural space of the posterior fossa may follow trauma to the occiput, with or without fracture. The bleeding originates in the lateral sinus or tributary veins. The child becomes progressively drowsy after a lucid interval. Vomiting and irregular respirations occur early because the brain stem is compressed. Hydrocephalus may follow compression of the aqueduct and 4th ventricle; this lesion is a possibility in infants who develop hydrocephalus following traumatic deliveries.

21.27 SUBDURAL HEMATOMA

Subdural hematoma may be acute or chronic. The latter is most common in infants, in whom it presents special problems.

Acute subdural hematoma is almost always associated with meningeal tears and with contusion and hemorrhage in the underlying brain. The affected child with severe head trauma remains in deep coma and has evidence of progressively increasing intracranial pressure. Prognosis is guarded even when the collection of blood is removed promptly because there is usually severe injury to the brain.

Chronic subdural hematoma in the infant or child involves gradual leakage of blood from torn frontal or parietal cortical veins which traverse the subdural space in their course to the sagittal sinus.

Chronic subdural hematoma in the *infant* occurs with maximum incidence from 2–6 mo of age. About 25% of affected infants have a history of postnatal head injury. There may be no clear history of trauma even when there are distinct evidences of such injuries as fractures of long bones, ribs, and skull (see Sec. 2.57–2.58). The evolution of chronic subdural hematoma in infancy is as follows: the initial clot liquefies, and water moves into the subdural space to maintain osmotic equilibrium. Repeated small hemorrhages occur from rupture of bridging veins, which are put under stress as the subdural space enlarges. The infant's skull expands in response to increasing intracranial pressure. Very large collections of fluid may form. The fluid is initially bloody; it gradually clears and becomes straw-colored, with a high protein content. Chronic subdural effusions become encapsulated by vascular inner and outer membranes. The outer membrane may become quite thick and occasionally calcifies.

Presenting symptoms include vomiting, failure to gain weight, unexplained fever, irritability, drowsiness, and convulsions. Focal neurologic signs are rare; rather, one finds signs of increased intracranial pressure, including a bulging fontanelle and mild head enlargement. Biparietal prominence of the skull is characteristic, in contrast to hydrocephalus, in which the prominence tends to be frontal. Transillumination of the skull is increased after liquefaction of the initial hematoma has occurred. Retinal hemorrhages are found in more than 50% of infants.

The diagnosis is made by subdural tap and by computed tomography (Fig. 21–23). Initial therapy consists of repeated subdural taps, but surgical drainage is frequently required. Shunting of the subdural fluid to the peritoneal cavity may be indicated if other measures fail. The prognosis depends on the severity of cerebral damage that occurred at the time

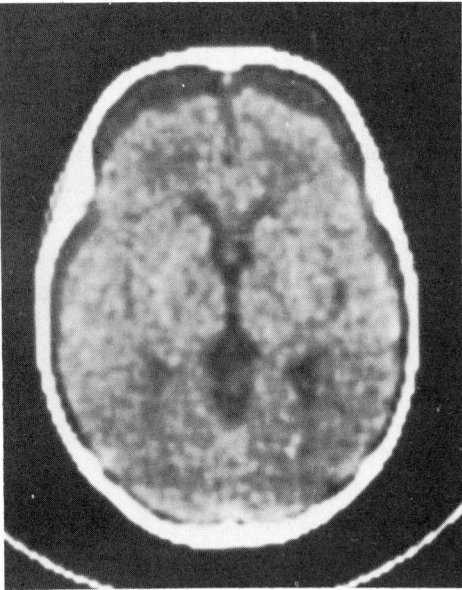

Figure 21–23. Computed tomogram (CT scan) of a 7 mo old boy with a history of lethargy and vomiting and with bilateral retinal hemorrhages on funduscopic examination. Bilateral fluid collections are seen between the inner table of the skull and the brain surface, typical of chronic subdural hematoma.

of the initial trauma and on the size and duration of the subdural effusion at the time therapy was initiated. The outcome is satisfactory in about 60% of patients. Mental defects, convulsions, and quadriparesis are the most common residuals.

The initial injury to a *child* may be minor, often a concussion with apparent initial recovery. Within days or sometimes weeks signs of increased intracranial pressure develop, including headache, vomiting, drowsiness, unsteadiness of gait, and 6th nerve palsy. Hemiparesis and convulsions may occur. Papilledema is usually present. The initial injury may have been forgotten, and the first consideration may be of brain tumor. Coma and signs of tentorial herniation develop in neglected cases. The diagnosis is made by computed tomography, which shows a low density mass between the inner table of the skull and the surface of the brain, with displacement of the ventricular system. Radionuclide scan may show increased uptake in the area of the hematoma. The EEG may show lower amplitude on the affected side, but this finding is not reliable. Surgical evacuation of the chronic subdural hematoma in the older child usually results in cure.

Collins W, Pucci G: Peritoneal drainage of subdural hematomas in infants. J Pediatr 58:682, 1961.
DeVivo DC, Dodge PR: The critically ill child: Diagnosis and management of head injury. Pediatrics 48:129, 1971.
Ingraham FD, Matson DD: Subdural hematoma in infancy. J Pediatr 24:1, 1944.
Mealey J Jr: Pediatric Head Injuries. Springfield, IL, Charles C Thomas, 1968.
Richardson F: Some effects of severe head injury. A follow-up study of children and adolescents after protracted coma. Dev Med Child Neurol 5:471, 1963.
Shulman K, Ransohoff J: Subdural hematoma in children. The fate of children with retained membranes. J Neurosurg 18:175, 1961.
Taveras TM, Ransohoff J: Leptomeningeal cysts of the brain following trauma with erosions of the skull: A study of 7 cases treated by surgery. J Neurosurg 10:233, 1953.
Till K: Subdural hematoma and effusion in infancy. Br Med J 3:400, 1968.

21.28 DISEASES OF THE SPINAL CORD

General Considerations. Diseases of the spinal cord are uncommon in childhood, but their prompt recognition is urgent since early diagnosis and treatment may avoid permanent paraplegia and incontinence.

Compression of the spinal cord produces characteristic symptoms and signs that vary with the location of the spinal lesion. These include localized back tenderness, pain and immobility, scoliosis, and bladder dysfunction, manifested initially as frequency and urgency and later as distention and incontinence. The most common motor manifestation is a disturbance of gait, initially a limp, which may progress to paraplegia. Lesions involving the cervical cord may produce a quadriparesis, usually with muscle atrophy, areflexia, and hypotonia in the upper limbs and hyperreflexia and spasticity in the legs. In general, flaccid weakness and areflexia are found at the level of the lesion, with spasticity below that level. In acute lesions, however, the paralysis is flaccid throughout because of spinal "shock." A sensory level on the trunk identified by pinprick and touch is indicative of spinal cord disease and establishes the approximate site of the lesion. Often the actual lesion is several segments above the upper extent of sensory impairment.

NEOPLASMS OF THE SPINAL CORD

When spinal cord dysfunction evolves in a subacute or chronic manner, it is most often due to a neoplasm. Gliomas, including astrocytomas and ependymomas, are the most common types. Neuroblastoma is next in frequency; it is the most likely cause of spinal cord compression in the infant. In lymphoma the spinal cord may be compressed by tumor masses in the epidural space. Spinal neurofibroma may be associated with generalized neurofibromatosis. Various developmental lesions, including teratoma, lipoma, and neurenteric cysts, account for most of the remaining spinal cord tumors in childhood. Spinal cord compression occurs occasionally with chronic hemolytic anemia as a result of extramedullary hematopoiesis in the extradural space.

Careful neurologic examination of the child with unexplained limp or bladder dysfunction is essential for early diagnosis of spinal tumors. Roentgenograms of the spine may be helpful; with slowly growing tumors, the spinal canal is widened in the area of the lesion and there is bony erosion, especially of the pedicles. Defects of neural arches are found in developmental tumors. The lumbar spinal fluid is xanthochromic and high in protein content when there is obstruction of the spinal subarachnoid space at a higher level. Myelography or magnetic resonance imaging is needed to define the level and extent of the tumor and to determine whether it is extrinsic or intrinsic to the cord.

Intrinsic spinal cord tumors may be difficult to distinguish from *syringomyelia*, a condition of unknown cause producing cavitation in the cord, usually in the cervical area. Atrophy of hand muscles and loss of pain sensation in the upper limbs are the most common clinical findings.

Prompt surgical exploration is indicated in most types of spinal cord tumor. Local irradiation manages cord compression due to lymphoma.

ACUTE SPINAL CORD LESIONS

Spinal cord trauma in childhood is most often the result of breech deliveries, automobile accidents, and diving injuries. It is usually associated with fracture or dislocation of vertebrae. Dislocations are especially common at the C1–2 level with fractures of the odontoid process, at the lower cervical level, and at T12–L1. Complete cord transection at the upper cervical level leads to rapid death from respiratory paralysis. Less severe injury at this level causes quadriparesis and often respiratory embarrassment requiring assisted ventilation. It is very important to avoid movement of such a patient; when absolutely necessary, movement must be accomplished en bloc. If possible, the patient should be kept supine on a firm support. Gentle neck traction is helpful during transportation of the patient with cervical spine injury. Complete loss of function below the level of the lesion lasting over 24 hr is almost always permanent. Surgical exploration of the damaged area, to have any chance of success, must be carried out within the first few hours.

Atlantoaxial (C1–2) dislocation may occur without a clear history of trauma, especially in patients with congenital malformations of the spine or with metabolic bone diseases such as the chondrodystrophies. Flexion of the neck causes compression of the cervical cord in such patients. There is a history of progressive weakness and gait disturbance. Spastic paresis of arms and legs occurs without dysfunction of cranial nerves. The lesion must be differentiated from spastic cerebral palsy and from the leukodystrophies and demyelinating diseases. Therapy consists of reduction of the dislocation by neck traction followed by immobilization of the neck.

Spinal epidural abscess is a localized accumulation of pus in the spinal epidural space, usually posterior to the cord in the thoracic area. It may be acute, usually staphylococcal in origin, or subacute, from extension of tuberculous osteomyelitis of the spine. Exquisite pain and percussion tenderness are present over the abscess, and the spine is held rigidly extended. Signs of spinal cord dysfunction, including paraparesis, loss of bladder and bowel control, and a sensory level on the trunk, evolve rapidly. Systemic evidence of infection may be absent. The diagnosis is occasionally made at lumbar puncture when pus under pressure is obtained before the dura is penetrated. Myelography may be necessary to define spinal cord compression. Spinal epidural abscess represents a neurosurgical emergency; prompt drainage may prevent permanent paraplegia.

Vascular anomalies of the spinal cord include arteriovenous malformations, venous angiomas, and telangiectasia. These lesions may cause sudden spinal cord dysfunction if rupture of a blood vessel leads to hemorrhage into the spinal cord or into the spinal subarachnoid space. Nuchal rigidity occurs when subarachnoid hemorrhage is massive. Recurrent, acute exacerbations and partial remissions are characteristic. The cerebrospinal fluid may be bloody or the protein content elevated. Myelography is usually diagnostic, showing tortuous, dilated vascular channels. At times, the vascular anomaly may be suggested when a port wine stain (nevus flammeus) covers the skin in a segmental distribution corresponding to the level of the vascular malformation. Surgical removal of vascular anomalies of the spinal cord is occasionally successful.

Transverse myelopathy is often misdesignated transverse myelitis. It is a syndrome in which segmental spinal cord dysfunction appears rapidly, usually within hours, without evidence of a compressive lesion or of hemorrhage. In some instances the disorder is secondary to demyelinating disease. In others segmental necrosis of the cord is probably a result of vascular occlusion. Occlusion of the anterior spinal artery is likely when posterior column functions (position and vibration senses) are spared. The onset of transverse myelopathy may follow a mild febrile illness or be sudden in a previously healthy child. Back pain at the site of the lesion is usually present but is much less severe than in spinal epidural abscess. This is followed by paraparesis, a sensory level, and inability to void. The CSF is usually normal, but there may be mild elevation in protein content and in cell count. Myelography may be needed to rule out compressive lesions. Corticosteroid therapy has produced equivocal results. Partial recovery of function is usual.

CHRONIC CARE OF THE PARAPLEGIC CHILD

Children who survive acute spinal cord diseases are frequently left with paraplegia and bladder dysfunction. The paraplegia is initially flaccid, but spasticity develops gradually, often with appearance of painful flexor spasms. These are especially common in paraplegics with decubitus ulcers, as stimulation of pain fibers in the areas of skin breakdown activates flexor reflexes in the severed spinal cord segments. Frequent turning, use of an air mattress, and physiotherapy may prevent both decubitus ulcers and flexor spasms. The urinary bladder of the acutely paraplegic patient is atonic and becomes massively distended unless catheter drainage is instituted. Chronically, the bladder may become spastic with frequent partial reflex emptying. Chronic urinary tract infection from inadequate drainage and calciuria from immobility lead to renal and bladder calculi (Sec. 17.47).

Alexander E Jr, Masland R, Harris C: Anterior dislocation of first cervical vertebra simulating cerebral birth injury in infancy. Am J Dis Child 85:151, 1953.

Matson DD: Neurosurgery of infancy and Childhood. Springfield, IL, Charles C Thomas, 1969.

Paine RS, Byers RK: Transverse myelopathy in childhood. Am J Dis Child 85:151, 1953.

Rand RW, Rand CW: Intraspinal Tumors of Childhood. Springfield, IL, Charles C Thomas, 1960.

Ropper AH, Poskanzer DC: The prognosis of acute and subacute transverse myelopathy. Ann Neurol 4:51, 1978.

Rowland LP, Shapiro JH, Jacobson HG: Neurological syndromes associated with congenital absence of the odontoid process. Arch Neurol Psychiatr 80:286, 1958.

Tarlov IM: Spinal cord injuries—early treatment. Surg Clin North Am 35:2, 1955.

21.29 DISORDERS OF THE AUTONOMIC NERVOUS SYSTEM

The autonomic nervous system provides neural control over a large variety of vegetative functions such as heart rate, blood pressure, temperature regulation, micturition, and intestinal motility. Its two large divisions are sympathetic and parasympathetic; their actions are often but not always antagonistic. The highest level of integration of autonomic functions occurs in the hypothalamus; from there central parasympathetic and sympathetic pathways descend to the brain stem and spinal cord.

Parasympathetic nerve fibers leave the central nervous system via the cranial nerves and the sacral spinal nerves. These fibers synapse in peripheral parasympathetic ganglia, whence peripheral fibers are distributed in turn to visceral organs as follows:

Via	Organ(s) innervated
Cranial III	Sphincter of pupil
VII	Submaxillary and sublingual glands
IX	Parotid gland, esophagus
X	Bronchi, lungs, heart, stomach, pancreas, small intestine, proximal colon
Sacral (S$_2$–S$_4$)	Distal colon, rectum, bladder, external genitalia

Stimulation of parasympathetic nerves releases acetylcholine at the nerve terminals. The actions of this system can be explained entirely in terms of pharmacologic effects of acetylcholine and can be reproduced by administration of such parasympathomimetic drugs as methacholine (Mecholyl) and pilocarpine and blocked by atropine and atropine-like drugs. Parasympathetic effects include constriction of the pupils, salivation, bronchial constriction, slowing of the heart rate, gastric secretion of hydrochloric acid, stimulation of peristalsis, and micturition.

Sympathetic nerve fibers leave the central nervous system only at the spinal level and travel with the thoracic and upper two lumbar spinal nerves. They synapse in peripheral sympathetic ganglia and are distributed to the visceral organs and to blood vessels, hair follicles, sweat glands, and adrenal medulla. Stimulation of the sympathetic nervous system releases norepinephrine at most of the peripheral nerve endings; exceptions are the sweat glands, where the neurohumoral substance is acetylcholine, and the adrenal medulla, where it is epinephrine. Many of the effects of sympathetic nervous system stimulation can be reproduced by administration of norepinephrine or of such sympathomimetic drugs as amphetamine and ephedrine and blocked by adrenergic blocking agents. Effects of sympathetic nervous system stimulation include pupillary dilatation, constriction of blood vessels, acceleration of heart rate, sweating, piloerection, and bronchodilatation.

Autonomic nervous system functions are disturbed in a large number of systemic and neurologic illnesses, among them particularly the following:

1. *Developmental defects*
   Familial dysautonomia (Riley-Day syndrome)
   Congenital sensory neuropathy (Sec. 22.3)
   Hirschsprung disease
2. *Tumors*
   Neuroblastoma
   Ganglioneuroma
   Pheochromocytoma
   Hypothalamic tumor—the diencephalic syndrome of infancy
3. *Poisonings*
   Atropinism
   Botulism
4. *Injuries to autonomic nerves*
   Horner syndrome
   Adie syndrome
5. *Inflammatory disorders of autonomic nerves*
   Autonomic neuropathy
   Postinfectious polyneuritis (Guillain-Barré syndrome)
6. *Other disorders*
   Cushing-Rokitansky ulcer
   Curling ulcer
   Psychophysiologic disorders

FAMILIAL DYSAUTONOMIA

The *Riley-Day syndrome* is a familial, autosomal recessive disturbance in autonomic and peripheral sensory functions. It is most common in Ashkenazi Jews, among whom the frequency of the carrier state is estimated to be about 1%.

Neuropathologic findings are sparse and are confined to the peripheral sensory system. The taste buds (fungiform papillae) of the tongue are absent or decreased in number. The peripheral nerves have a deficit in the number of small unmyelinated fibers, which normally carry pain, temperature, and taste sensations, and of the large myelinated fibers, which carry afferent impulses from muscle spindles. These abnormalities are not always present, and the autonomic nervous system usually has no demonstrable pathologic changes. Disturbed autonomic function is reflected in metabolic abnormalities: the plasma of about 25% of affected children shows no dopamine-beta-hydroxylase, the enzyme which catalyzes the conversion of dopamine to norepinephrine; vanillylmandelic acid (VMA), an excretion product of norepinephrine, is usually diminished in the urine of patients; and homovanillic acid (HVA), a metabolite of dopamine, is increased in urine and in CSF.

Clinical manifestations are prominent in infancy. Swallowing movements are poorly coordinated and therefore lead to gagging, vomiting, and aspiration. Excessive bronchial secretions and repeated aspiration contribute to recurrent bouts of pulmonary infection with eventual chronic pulmonary failure.

Evidence of autonomic disturbances includes excessive salivation and sweating, decrease or absence of tear formation, marked blotching of the skin during excitement, urinary incontinence, labile hypertension and orthostatic hypotension, and defective temperature regulation with periodic fevers. Clinical manifestations of peripheral sensory dysfunction consist of absence of taste sensation, diminished or absent pain sense (leading to repeated skin trauma and to asymptomatic fractures), and absence of corneal sensation (which, with the defect in tear formation, increases the susceptibility to corneal ulceration). Tendon reflexes are diminished or absent, probably as a result of defective formation of afferent fibers of muscle spindles. The central nervous system is usually affected; the manifestations include mental defect, dysarthria, clumsiness, and emotional lability.

Laboratory Data. Chest roentgenograms show atelectasis and pulmonary infiltrates similar to the changes in cystic fibrosis. The Mecholyl test for denervation hypersensitivity of the pupil (a fresh 2% solution of Mecholyl instilled into one conjunctival sac, the other eye serving as a control) is positive: constriction of the pupil appears within 10 min. There is no response to the histamine skin test (0.05 mL of a 1:10,000 solution of histamine injected intradermally), which is normally characterized by a red flare and pain at the injection site. Urinary VMA is decreased; HVA is increased. Slow intravenous infusion of norepinephrine produces an exaggerated pressor response. The hypotensive response to infusion of Mecholyl is increased.

The **differential diagnosis** of familial dysautonomia includes other causes of "failure to thrive" in infancy, chronic pulmonary diseases in childhood, congenital universal indifference to pain, and congenital sensory neuropathy.

Treatment is directed toward control of recurrent respiratory infections, prevention of corneal ulceration by use of artificial tears, and protection from injuries related to lack of pain sensation. Bethanecol (Urecholine) has been used to increase tear formation.

The **prognosis** is poor. Most patients die prior to adulthood, usually from chronic pulmonary failure.

DIENCEPHALIC SYNDROME OF INFANCY

This cause of failure to thrive is usually due to glioma of the anterior hypothalamus, but the same syndrome may also occur with inflammatory or destructive lesions in this region. Affected infants have endocrine and central autonomic disturbances secondary to hypothalamic dysfunction. The most striking clinical findings are extreme emaciation in spite of apparently adequate food intake and a hypermetabolic state with overactivity and "hyperalertness." The autonomic disturbances consist of excessive sweating, easy flushing of the skin, tachycardia, and vomiting. Signs of endocrine abnormality include increased linear growth, advanced bone age, and excessive size of hands and feet. Late in the course enlargement of the head develops, with optic atrophy and visual loss leading to searching nystagmus. Onset may occur at any time from 3 mo–4 yr of age.

Soft tissue roentgenograms of the extremities show complete absence of the normal subcutaneous fat shadow. There may be fasting hypoglycemia. The CSF protein level is increased if there is an underlying hypothalamic tumor. The neoplasm is usually demonstrable by computed tomography. Therapy is often unsatisfactory; long remissions have been induced by radiation directed at the hypothalamic tumor.

INJURY TO AUTONOMIC NERVES

Horner syndrome is due to a lesion of the cervical sympathetic nerve fibers. These fibers are especially prone to injury because of their long intra- and extracranial course. Central sympathetic neurons descend in the lateral medulla and spinal cord to the upper thoracic spinal level. Preganglionic cervical sympathetic fibers then leave the spinal cord in the upper thoracic ventral spinal roots and pass upward in the paravertebral sympathetic chain; the majority of fibers synapse in the superior cervical ganglion and then follow the course of the common carotid artery in the neck. Sudomotor and vasomotor fibers travel in close relation to the external carotid artery to be distributed to the skin over the face; fibers innervating the pupil and the upper eyelid (oculosympathetic fibers) follow the internal carotid and ophthalmic arteries to the orbit. The Horner syndrome may follow lesions involving the medulla oblongata, the cervical or upper thoracic spinal cord, the posterior mediastinum, or the neck; it is usually unilateral. A partial syndrome, involving only the oculosympathetic fibers, occurs with lesions near the internal carotid artery or in the orbit.

Horner syndrome consists of ptosis due to weakness of the levator palpebrae muscle, miosis due to dysfunction of pupillodilator fibers, and absence of sweating over the ipsilateral face. In congenital Horner syndrome, heterochromia iridis results from failure in pigmentation of the iris on the affected side.

Pharmacologic tests may help differentiate Horner syndrome caused by a central nervous system lesion from that caused by a peripheral sympathetic lesion. Instillation of a 4% solution of cocaine into the conjunctival sac normally produces dilatation of the pupil by potentiation of the effect of locally released norepinephrine. This response is absent when Horner syndrome is due to a peripheral sympathetic lesion, whereas it is preserved with lesions involving central pathways. Instillation of a 1:1000 solution of epinephrine normally produces no pupillary reaction but will result in dilatation of the pupil in Horner syndrome caused by a peripheral sympathetic lesion. The results of these tests may be equivocal when the Horner syndrome is incomplete. A search for tumor or other compressive lesion is indicated in any patient who develops Horner syndrome. This should include careful palpation of the neck and of the supraclavicular areas and roentgenograms of the chest and the cervical spine. Horner syndrome per se does not produce significant disability and requires no therapy.

Adie syndrome is a disorder of the parasympathetic innervation of the iris of unknown etiology; it usually first appears in young adults but may occasionally occur in childhood. The affected pupil is large and reacts little or not at all to light but will often react slowly to accommodation. Patients with Adie pupil often have hyporeflexia, especially absence of the knee jerk. Occasionally, there is associated anhidrosis over the trunk. The Adie pupil is hypersensitive to parasympathomimetic agents, and instillation of 2% Mecholyl into the conjunctival sac produces brisk contraction. The Adie syndrome is an essentially benign condition, needing no therapy; its prompt recognition may avert unnecessary studies.

INFLAMMATORY DISORDERS OF AUTONOMIC NERVES

The peripheral autonomic nervous system is occasionally involved in inflammatory diseases of nerve. In postinfectious polyneuritis (Guillain-Barré syndrome), autonomic dysfunction may represent a clinically significant complication. Evidences of autonomic disturbance include postural hypotension, hypertension, unexplained tachycardia, sweating, and urinary retention. Urinary excretion of vanillylmandelic acid (VMA) may be increased.

Cases of *acute autonomic neuropathy* have been reported, with acute onset of diminished pupillary reaction to light, dryness of mouth, hypohidrosis, urinary retention, and vomiting. Recovery is gradual over a period of weeks or months. The condition must be distinguished from atropinism and from botulism.

AUTONOMIC STIMULATION LEADING TO VISCERAL LESIONS

It has long been known that lesions of the central nervous system may induce visceral abnormalities through stimulation of central autonomic pathways. A striking example is the *Cushing-Rokitansky ulcer* of the stomach or duodenum which occurs in children with posterior fossa tumor, often a few days after surgical resection of the neoplasm. Gastric ulceration in these children is probably due to abnormal stimulation of vagal (parasympathetic) nuclei in the medulla, which leads to increased gastric hydrochloric acid secretion. Stress may lead to overactivity of hypothalamic parasympathetic centers with the same result of gastric and duodenal ulceration and hemorrhage. This complication has been observed with special frequency in patients suffering from extensive burns *(Curling ulcer)*.

It has been suggested that less specific stresses of life may be causative factors in the formation of gastric and duodenal ulcers as well as in the etiology of a number of other disorders such as ulcerative colitis, asthma, and essential hypertension. However, proof of cause-effect relationships has been inconclusive (see also Sec. 2.54).

21.30 SPASMUS NUTANS

This disorder of eye movements is peculiar to infancy and is usually first noted from the ages of 4–12 mo. It consists of intermittent rapid pendular nystagmoid movements, often confined to one eye, and, when bilateral, almost always more prominent on one side. About 80% of infants have intermittent head nodding. The etiology is unknown. Insufficient lighting and relative absence of visual stimuli for the infant to fix on have been implicated as possible etiologic factors without convincing evidence. Spontaneous improvement always occurs.

Spasmus nutans has to be distinguished from searching nystagmus due to decreased visual acuity and from hereditary congenital nystagmus. In congenital nystagmus the abnormal movement of the eyes is bilaterally symmetrical, with pendular movements when the eyes are at rest giving way to jerk nystagmus on attempted lateral gaze.

PETER R. HUTTENLOCHER

Aguayo A, Nair P, Bray G: Peripheral nerve abnormalities in the Riley-Day syndrome. Arch Neurol 24:106, 1971.

Axelrod FB, Nachtigall RF, Dancis J: Familial dysautonomia: Diagnosis, pathogenesis and management. Adv Pediatr 21:75, 1974.

Esterly N, Cantoline SJ, Alter BP, et al: Pupillotonia, hyporeflexia and segmental hypohidrosis: Autonomic dysfunction in a child. J Pediatr 73:852, 1968.

Loggie JMH, Van Maanen EF: The autonomic nervous system and some aspects of the use of autonomic drugs in children. J Pediatr 81:205, 432, 1972.

Mitchell PL, Meilman E: The mechanism of hypertension in the Guillain-Barré syndrome. Am J Med 42:986, 1967.

Poznanski AK, Manson G: Radiographic appearance of the soft tissues in the diencephalic syndrome of infancy. Radiology 81:101, 1963.

Riley CM, Moore RH: Familial dysautonomia differentiated from related disorders. Pediatrics 37:435, 1966.

Russell A: A diencephalic syndrome of emaciation in infancy and childhood. Arch Dis Child 26:274, 1951.

Sauer C, Levinsohn MW: Horner's syndrome in childhood. Neurology 26:216, 1976.

Smith AA, Dancis J: Catecholamine release in familial dysautonomia. N Engl J Med 277:61, 1967.

Thomashefsky AJ, Horowitz SJ, Feingold MH: Acute autonomic neuropathy. Neurology 22:251, 1972.

Weinshilboum RM, Axelrod J: Reduced plasma dopamine-hydroxylase activity in familial dysautonomia. N Engl J Med 285:938, 1971.

22

NEUROMUSCULAR DISEASES

22.1 CLASSIFICATION OF NEUROMUSCULAR DISORDERS

Disorders of the peripheral motor and sensory systems are known collectively as the neuromuscular diseases. These illnesses involve one or more of the structures concerned with the segmental spinal reflex arc: the anterior horn cells, motor nerve fibers, neuromuscular junction, muscle, and sensory nerve fibers from muscle and tendons (Fig. 22–1). Interference with this reflex arc leads to depression of tendon reflexes, which is characteristic of all neuromuscular diseases. In addition, weakness and muscle atrophy usually are present.

The following is a useful classification of the more common disorders:

1. *Anterior horn cell diseases*
   Werdnig-Hoffmann disease
   Poliomyelitis (Sec. 11.77)
   Other viral infections (Sec. 11.71)
2. *Polyneuropathies*
   Postinfectious polyneuritis (Guillain-Barré syndrome)
   Diphtheritic polyneuritis (Sec. 11.23)
   Toxic neuropathies (heavy metal poisoning, Sec. 28.12 and 28.15), drug-induced neuropathies, metabolic diseases with polyneuropathy (Table 22–2)
   Hypertrophic interstitial neuritis (Déjérine-Sottas disease)
   Charcot-Marie-Tooth disease (peroneal muscular atrophy)
   Congenital sensory neuropathy
   Congenital indifference to pain
3. *Mononeuropathies*
   Congenital ptosis
   Oculomotor nerve palsy (Tolosa-Hunt syndrome)
   Sixth nerve palsy (Duane syndrome)
   Facial palsy (Bell palsy)
   Erb palsy (Sec. 8.25)
   Peroneal palsy
   Sciatic nerve injury
4. *Diseases of the neuromuscular junction*
   Myasthenia gravis
   Botulism (Sec. 11.39 and 28.2)
5. *Diseases of muscle*
   Inflammatory diseases of muscle
   Polymyositis
   Myositis ossificans

Endocrine or metabolic myopathies
   Hyperthyroid myopathy
   Hypothyroid myopathy
   Corticosteroid myopathy
   Muscle carnitine deficiency
   Systemic carnitine deficiency
Congenital defects of muscle
   Absence of muscle
   Congenital torticollis
   Congenital myopathies (central core disease and nemaline myopathy)
   Mitochondrial myopathies
Myotonia
   Myotonia congenita (Thomsen disease)
Periodic paralyses
   Hyperkalemic form (adynamia episodica hereditaria)
   Hypokalemic form
   Paroxysmal myoglobinuria
   Carnitine palmityltransferase deficiency
   McArdle disease (Sec 7.21)
The muscular dystrophies
   Pseudohypertrophic form (Duchenne)
   Congenital muscular dystrophy
   Facioscapulohumeral form
   Limb-girdle form
   Ocular myopathy
   Myotonic dystrophy

22.2 ANTERIOR HORN CELL DISEASES

The anterior horn cells are selectively affected in poliomyelitis and occasionally in infection with other viruses, including coxsackieviruses and echoviruses. Inherited degeneration of the anterior horn cells occurs primarily in infancy.

Infantile Spinal Muscular Atrophy (Werdnig-Hoffmann Disease). This disease is transmitted as a recessive trait. The primary pathologic change is atrophy of anterior horn cells in the spinal cord and of motor nuclei in the brain stem (Fig. 22–2), with secondary atrophy of motor nerve roots and of muscle.

Onset occurs prior to the age of 2 yr and often in utero. Rare instances of similar illness with onset later in childhood have been described. Early manifestations are weakness and hypotonia of the proximal and distal limb and intercostal and

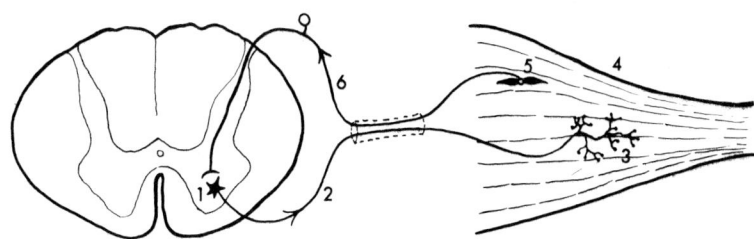

Figure 22–1. Schematic representation of the structures that make up the neuromuscular system. 1 = anterior horn cell; 2 = motor nerve fiber; 3 = motor end-plate on muscle; 4 = muscle; 5 = sensory receptor in muscle (muscle spindle); 6 = sensory nerve fiber.

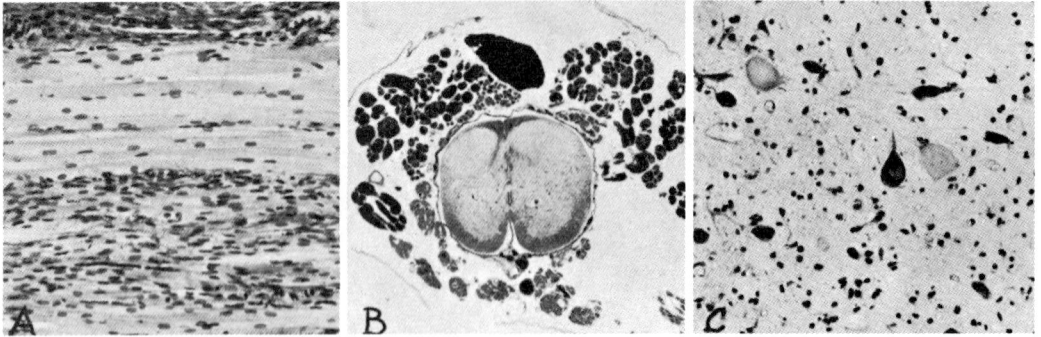

Figure 22–2. Werdnig-Hoffmann disease. *A,* Fascicular atrophy of muscle. *B,* Pallor of ventral roots. *C,* Degenerating motor neurons.

bulbar muscles. The legs tend to lie in a frog-leg position, with hips abducted and knees flexed (Fig. 22–3). The diaphragm is relatively spared; diaphragmatic function in the presence of weakness of the intercostal muscles results in characteristic paradoxic breathing, with inward movement of the chest on inspiration. Extraocular muscles are unaffected. Fibrillations usually are visible in the tongue. Tendon reflexes are almost always absent. Mental development is normal, and the bright look of these infants provides striking contrast to their lack of motor activity. Initially, the infants tend to be obese. In the late stages swallowing becomes impossible. Death results from respiratory failure and from aspiration of food. Infants with onset in utero usually die prior to the age of 2 yr. Those with later onset may survive for some years, occasionally to adulthood.

The *diagnosis* of Werdnig-Hoffman disease is based largely

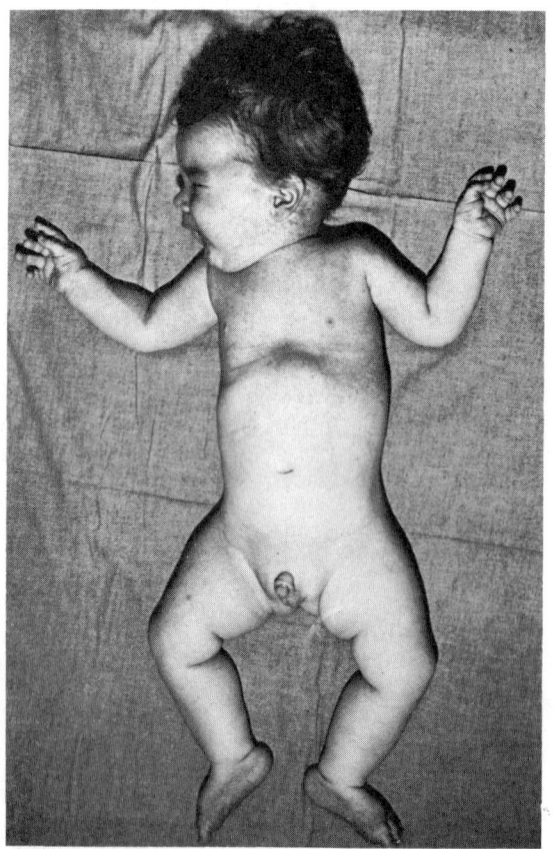

Figure 22–3. Typical posture of the infant with Werdnig-Hoffmann disease.

on the clinical findings. Electromyography often shows evidence of denervation of muscle, including fibrillation potentials and fasciculations. In biopsied muscle, groups of cells are seen in varying states of degeneration; each group represents cells innervated by a single motor neuron. Spinal fluid, nerve conduction measurements, and serum enzyme activities are within normal ranges.

The *differential diagnosis* of Werdnig-Hoffmann disease includes a large number of less common conditions in which hypotonia and weakness occur in infancy. Tlhe term "floppy infant syndrome" is used for this group of disorders (Table 22–1).

Disorders of the central nervous system presenting with hypotonia can usually be differentiated from the peripheral neuromuscular diseases by decreased alertness and visual responsiveness and by the preservation of tendon reflexes. Special studies, including examination of CSF, nerve conduction velocity measurements, serum enzyme determinations, and muscle biopsy, may be needed to distinguish Werdnig-Hoffmann disease from disorders of peripheral nerves or of muscle. A small number of hypotonic infants cannot be placed into the classification of Table 22–1. These infants appear normally alert. Tendon reflexes are depressed but usually not completely absent. Laboratory investigations, including muscle biopsy, are unrevealing. Hypotonia and weakness gradually improve in most of these infants. Such labels as *benign congenital hypotonia* and *amyotonia congenita* have been used; it is unlikely that this group represents a single entity.

Brandt S: Werdnig-Hoffmann's Infantile Progressive Muscular Atrophy. Copenhagen, Ejnar Munksgaard, 1950.
Byers RK, Banker BQ: Infantile muscular atrophy. Arch Neurol 4:140, 1961.
Chambers R, MacDermot V: Polyneuritis as a cause of "amyotonia congenita." Lancet 1:397, 1957.
Dubowitz V: The Floppy Infant. London, William Heinemann, 1969.
Eden AN: Guillain-Barré syndrome in a 6 month old infant. Am J Dis Child 102:224, 1961.
Garvie JM, Woolf AL: Kugelberg-Welander syndrome (hereditary spinal muscular atrophy). Br Med J 1:1458, 1966.
Paine RS: The future of the "floppy infant." A follow-up study of 133 patients. Dev Med Child Neurol 5:115, 1963.
Pickett J, Berg B, Chaplin E, et al: Syndrome of botulism in infancy: Clinical and electrophysiological study. N Engl J Med 295:770, 1976.
Rabe EF: The hypotonic infant. J Pediatr 64:422, 1964.
Walton JN: Amyotonia congenita. A follow-up study. Lancet 1:1023, 1956.

22.3 POLYNEUROPATHIES

Involvement of multiple peripheral nerves is found in many systemic diseases, intoxications, and infections. In addition, there are a number of genetically determined illnesses in which degeneration of peripheral nerves is the primary abnormality. The more common causes of polyneuropathy are listed in Table 22–2.

Table 22–1. Diseases Included in the Diagnostic Term "Floppy Infant Syndrome" and Characterized by Persistent Hypotonia

Central Nervous System Disorders	Spinal Cord Disease	Diseases of Peripheral Nerve	Diseases of the Neuromuscular Junction	Muscle Diseases
Atonic diplegia Congenital cerebellar ataxia Kernicterus Chromosomal defects Oculocerebrorenal syndrome (Lowe) Cerebral lipidoses Prader-Willi syndrome	Spinal cord trauma Werdnig-Hoffmann disease	Polyneuritis (Guillain-Barré syndrome) Familial dysautonomia Congenital sensory neuropathy	Myasthenia gravis Infantile botulism	Congenital muscular dystrophy Myotonic dystrophy Glycogen storage disease of muscle and heart (Pompe) Central core disease Nemaline myopathy Mitochondrial myopathies

The *clinical manifestations of polyneuropathy* include weakness, muscular atrophy, loss of tendon reflexes, and sensory impairment. The distal limbs—feet and hands—are affected first, and there is gradual proximal progression as the disorder becomes more severe. Motor fibers are more severely affected than sensory ones in some polyneuropathies, including lead poisoning, the Guillain-Barré syndrome, and Charcot-Marie-Tooth disease. Gait disturbance with foot drop is an early manifestation in these illnesses. Fairly selective damage to sensory fibers occurs in diabetes mellitus and in some of the genetically determined neuropathies. All types of sensation, including pain, touch, temperature, position, and vibration sense, are impaired, often in a "stocking and glove" distribution. Injured sensory nerve endings may become abnormally sensitive to stimulation, and innocuous stimuli may be interpreted as being painful (hyperpathia), while tingling or "pins and needles" sensations may occur in the absence of stimulation. Loss of sensory and autonomic innervation results in trophic changes in skin and nails and occasionally in loss of toes and fingers. Remarkable recovery from polyneuritis may follow removal of the offending agent because of the capacity of peripheral nerves, in contrast to central neural pathways, to regenerate after injury.

The *pathologic changes* in some peripheral neuropathies consist of patchy loss of the myelin sheath of the nerve fibers (segmental demyelination); in other instances, degeneration of the axons appears to be the primary process. In chronic neuropathies there is often considerable fibrous tissue reaction which may result in palpable enlargement of the affected nerves.

Measurement of nerve conduction velocity is the most helpful diagnostic aid. Decrease in conduction velocity is seen exclusively in disorders of peripheral nerves and is especially striking when demyelination is a prominent pathologic feature. Biopsy of the sural nerve may also be useful in confirming the diagnosis except in predominantly motor neuropathies, in which this sensory nerve may be spared. Neither of these measures, however, provides information regarding the specific cause of the neuropathy. The recognizable toxic and metabolic causes listed in Table 22–2 must, when possible, be identified by toxicologic and other special tests. A careful family history and examination of family members are important for the diagnosis of the genetically determined polyneuropathies. Included in this group are hypertrophic interstitial neuritis, Charcot-Marie-Tooth disease (peroneal muscular atrophy), and several forms of sensory neuropathy.

Guillain-Barré Syndrome (Postinfectious or Idiopathic Polyneuritis). This acute or subacute disease affects nerve roots and peripheral nerves in a diffuse manner. The disorder occurs sporadically at any age from early infancy. It usually follows viral infections; occasional cases occur after immunizations. A variety of viral illnesses, including infectious mononucleosis, mumps, measles, echovirus, coxsackievirus, and influenza viral infections, have been observed prior to the development of Guillain-Barré syndrome. The viral illness, however, has usually run its course by the time the neurologic symptoms appear, and there is no evidence for viral invasion of the nervous system. About 2.5% of cases occur in patients with immune disorders, including lupus erythematosus and rheumatoid arthritis.

Sensitization of lymphocytes to a protein component of myelin has been found in Guillain-Barré syndrome and is likely to be of etiologic importance. Migration of sensitized lymphocytes into peripheral nerves appears to be the earliest pathologic change; myelin breakdown follows. The disease can be reproduced in animals by sensitization to the basic protein of myelin derived from peripheral nerves.

Clinical manifestations appear within about 2 wk after the onset of a viral illness in about two thirds of cases. The remainder have no evidence of prior illness. Pain suggestive of nerve root irritation and paresthesias in the legs and feet are early symptoms; sensory loss is rarely demonstrable. Cranial nerve involvement occurs in over 75% of cases; facial weakness is the most common, may be unilateral, may precede other neurologic findings, and may initially be indistinguishable from Bell palsy. Muscle weakness evolves over a period of 3–21 days, often starting in the legs and spreading to the arms and to the muscles of respiration. The weakness is both proximal and distal and tends to be symmetric. Tendon reflexes are lost, but plantar responses usually remain normal. Muscle tone is diminished. Occasionally, autonomic nerves are involved, in which case there may be urinary retention,

Table 22–2. The More Common Polyneuropathies

Poisoning	Drug Toxicity	Infections	Metabolic Disorders	Degenerative Diseases
Lead Mercury Thallium Arsenic	Vincristine Isoniazid Nitrofuran	Diphtheria Guillain-Barré syndrome Leprosy	Diabetes mellitus Uremia Porphyria Thiamine deficiency Vitamin B_{12} deficiency Refsum disease	Hypertrophic interstitial neuritis Charcot-Marie-Tooth disease Congenital sensory neuropathy Metachromatic leukodystrophy Krabbe disease Leigh disease Spinocerebellar degeneration

postural hypotension, or hypertension. Drowsiness, mental changes, papilledema, and Babinski signs indicative of concurrent involvement of the central nervous system are observed in a small proportion of affected children.

The *diagnosis* is made largely from the clinical manifestations. Spinal fluid changes may be confirmatory; the protein concentration becomes elevated in about 75% of cases, but this finding may not appear until 1–2 wk after the onset of clinical manifestations. CSF protein often remains elevated for several mo, even after clinical improvement is clearly evident. Typically, there are no cells in the CSF, but up to 10 lymphocytes/mm³ have been observed. Nerve conduction is slow in both motor and sensory nerves.

The *differential diagnosis* includes poliomyelitis, polymyositis, spinal cord tumors, transverse myelopathy, and, in the young child, acute cerebellar ataxia. In poliomyelitis, weakness is less symmetric, and the CSF shows an increase in white cells, primarily lymphocytes, usually with a normal protein content. In polymyositis the CSF is normal, but serum enzyme activities (such as creatine kinase and aldolase) are usually elevated, as is the erythrocyte sedimentation rate. Spinal cord tumors and transverse myelopathy may initially cause flaccid weakness and areflexia, but these rapidly give way to spasticity, hyperreflexia, and Babinski signs. A level of sensory loss on the trunk and early and severe impairment of bladder and rectal sphincter functions also aid in differentiating spinal cord lesions from Guillain-Barré syndrome. Cerebellar ataxia presents a problem of differentiation in the young child, when formal testing of strength is not possible and when gait ataxia may be confused with leg weakness.

Respiratory insufficiency secondary to paralysis of intercostal muscles is the most serious complication of the Guillain-Barré syndrome. Patients should be closely observed by serial measurements of vital capacity. Blood gas determinations are necessary if confusion, drowsiness, or tachypnea appears. Tracheal intubation and assisted ventilation should be performed before there is advanced respiratory failure. Recovery has occurred after more than 8 mo of complete ventilatory support. With good supportive treatment, more than 90% of children with Guillain-Barré syndrome recover. Complications of tracheostomy and of respiratory therapy, pneumonia, and cardiac arrhythmia account for the occasional fatal outcome. Recovery is usually complete in children, but it tends to be slow, over a period of up to 2 yr. Physiotherapy may be helpful during the recovery period. Rarely, there is a relapsing course with multiple attacks or a chronic progressive course. Therapy with corticosteroid hormones is probably ineffective in acute cases but may improve the outcome in the chronic form of the disease.

Hypertrophic Interstitial Neuritis (Déjérine-Sottas Disease). This is an uncommon, recessively inherited disease that has its onset in late infancy or early childhood. Motor development may be slow from the start. Later in childhood there is progressive gait disturbance, with foot drop and ataxia caused by loss of position sense. Associated findings include pes cavus and scoliosis. Eventually, but rarely during childhood, the peripheral nerves become palpably enlarged. The disease is slowly progressive and permits a normal life span. The CSF protein content is usually elevated, a finding of some value in differentiation from most other chronic neuropathies and from diseases of muscle.

Charcot-Marie-Tooth Disease. *Peroneal muscular atrophy* is a motor neuropathy that disproportionately affects the nerves to the legs. Inheritance is usually on a dominant basis. Onset occurs during late childhood or adolescence, with pes cavus, foot drop, and peroneal myatrophy. The distal wasting of the legs gives the characteristic "stork leg" appearance. Foot drop leads to a high "steppage" gait. The intrinsic hand muscles are affected eventually. Mild distal sensory impairment may

be present. Progression is slow, and the disease rarely becomes severe enough to preclude ambulation. The CSF is normal.

Congenital Sensory Neuropathy. This recessively inherited abnormality is usually noted in late infancy when the child fails to respond to painful stimuli to the hands or feet. These children tend to bite and otherwise injure their fingers. Ulceration and progressive loss of digits are common. All sensory modalities are affected, with distal limbs involved more severely than proximal. Anhidrosis may be present and may be manifested by recurrent fever. Associated abnormalities include mental retardation, deafness, and retinitis pigmentosa. Absence of the flare response to intradermal injection of 1:10,000 histamine phosphate supports the diagnosis. The differential diagnosis includes hereditary ectodermal dysplasia, Lesch-Nyhan syndrome (Sec. 7.50), infantile autism, the Riley-Day syndrome (Sec. 21.29), and congenital indifference to pain.

Congenital Indifference to Pain. In this rare syndrome absence of appropriate responses to painful stimuli is found as an isolated abnormality. Failure to appreciate pain leads to repeated minor skin trauma and to burns. Acute surgical abdominal disorders and fractures may go undetected for a long time. Other sensory functions are intact. In some patients the condition has been associated with anhidrosis and mental defect. The cause of congenital indifference to pain is unknown. The condition is distinguished from congenital sensory neuropathy by the universal absence of pain sensation and by the preservation of touch, position, vibration, and temperature senses.

Asbury AK, Arnason BG, Adams RD: The inflammatory lesion in idiopathic polyneuritis. Its role in pathogenesis. Medicine 48:173, 1969.
Axelrod FB, Pearson J: Congenital sensory neuropathies. Diagnostic distinction from familial dysautonomia. Am J Dis Child 138:947, 1984.
Baxter DW, Olszewski J: Congenital universal indifference to pain. Brain 83:381, 1960.
Byers RK, Taft LT: Chronic multiple peripheral neuropathy in childhood. Pediatrics 20:517, 1957.
Colan RV, Snead OC, Or SJ, et al: Steroid-responsive polyneuropathy with subacute onset in childhood. J Pediatr 97:374, 1980.
Dyck PJ, Lambert EH: Lower motor and primary sensory neuron diseases with peroneal muscular atrophy. 1. Neurologic, genetic and electrophysiologic findings in hereditary polyneuropathies. Arch Neurol 18:603, 1968.
Gamstorp I: Encephalo-myelo-radiculo-neuropathy: Involvement of the CNS in children with Guillain-Barré-Strohl syndrome. Dev Med Child Neurol 16:654, 1974.
Haymaker W, Kernohan JW: The Landry-Guillain-Barré syndrome. Medicine 28:59, 1949.
Hughes RAC, Newsom-Davis JM, Perkin GD, et al: Controlled trial of prednisolone in acute polyneuropathy. Lancet 2:750, 1978.
Pinsky L, DiGeorge AM: Congenital familial sensory neuropathy with anhidrosis. J Pediatr 68:1, 1966.
Wiederholt WC, Mulder CW, Lambert EH: The Landry-Guillain-Barré-Strohl syndrome or polyradiculo-neuropathy: Historical review, report on 97 patients, and present concepts. Proc Staff Meetings Mayo Clin 39:427, 1964.

22.4 MONONEUROPATHIES

Defects involving single peripheral nerves may be congenital or secondary to inflammation, trauma, or injection of irritant materials.

Congenital Ptosis. Congenital ptosis is probably secondary to faulty innervation of the levator palpebrae muscle. It is often transmitted by dominant inheritance. Drooping of one or both eyelids is noted in the neonatal period and persists throughout life. The ptosis is rarely complete. Occasionally, movements of the jaw will elevate the ptotic eyelid. This finding ("jaw winking" or Marcus Gunn phenomenon) is due to innervation of the levator palpebrae with an admixture of 3rd and 5th cranial nerve fibers.

Congenital ptosis has to be differentiated from myasthenia gravis, brain stem lesions, and ocular myopathy. Surgical

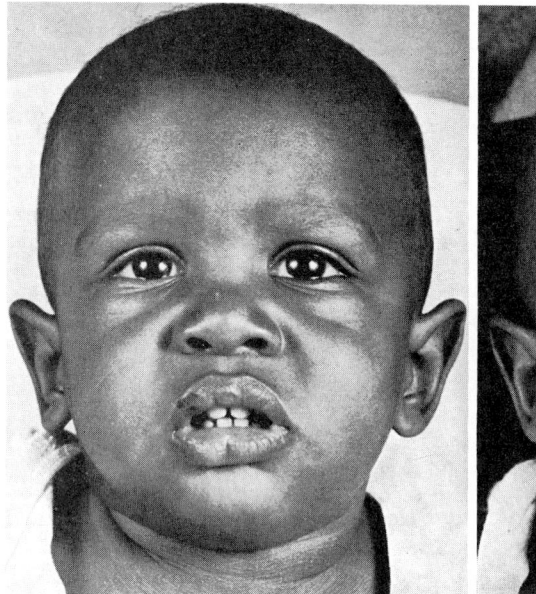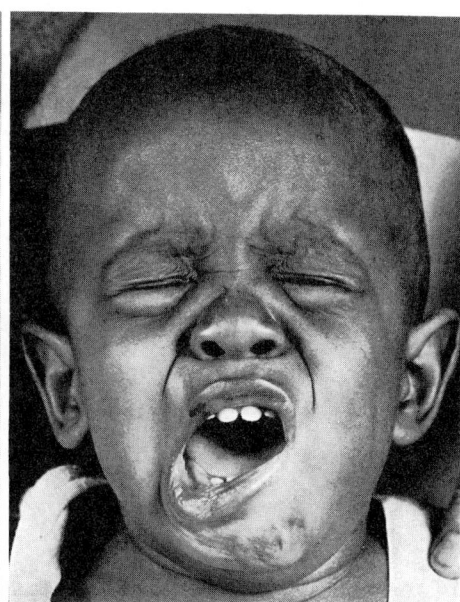

Figure 22–4. Congenital paralysis of left inferior angle of mouth. *A,* At rest, face is symmetrical. *B,* During crying the left labial angle does not depress, and right facial palsy may be misdiagnosed.

correction for cosmetic reasons is indicated when the defect is severe.

Tolosa-Hunt Syndrome. *Oculomotor nerve palsy* consists of painful, unilateral paralysis of one or more oculomotor nerves (usually the 3rd) of unknown etiology. The onset is acute, with retro-orbital pain and diplopia, and usually with ptosis and mydriasis on the affected side. Gradual improvement always occurs, but there may be repeated attacks. Distinction from ophthalmoplegic migraine may be difficult. Aneurysm of the internal carotid artery and parasellar neoplasm have to be excluded by appropriate studies; carotid angiography is usually required. A rapid response to corticosteroids is said to be characteristic.

Sixth Nerve Palsy. This may occur as an isolated congenital anomaly. There is inability to abduct the eye on the affected side. The abducens muscle may be replaced by a fibrous band that also prevents full adduction of the eye. Attempted adduction leads to retraction of the globe (Duane syndrome). The differentiation of congenital 6th nerve palsy from convergent strabismus may be difficult. In strabismus, however, the squinting eye will move fully after a period of patching.

Seventh (Facial) Nerve Palsy. This may be congenital or acquired.

Congenital Facial Nerve Palsy. The palsy is often partial; selective weakness of muscles innervated by the mandibular branch results in paralysis of the lower lip and the angle of the mouth. The unopposed action of the opposite lower facial muscle pulls the mouth toward the normal side (Fig. 22–4). The cosmetic defect tends to be quite mild; other anomalies may be associated.

Bell Palsy. Bell palsy refers to 7th nerve paralysis of sudden onset and usually of obscure etiology. Otitis media and herpes zoster of the geniculate ganglion have been implicated in some instances. The facial weakness appears over a few hr, occasionally with associated pain in the ear on the affected side. The face is pulled toward the normal side; the nasolabial fold on the affected side is flattened, and the child is unable to close the eye. Attempted closure leads to upward deviation of the eye (Bell sign). Loss of taste may occur over the anterior two thirds of the tongue, and there may be hyperacusis due to involvement of the nerve to the stapedius muscle. Occasionally, recurrent attacks of 7th nerve weakness of obscure

etiology are associated with edema of the lips (*Melkersson syndrome*).

The *differential diagnosis* includes tumor of the brain stem or temporal bone, demyelinating disease, basal skull fracture, otitis media, and mastoiditis. Therapy consists of protection of the cornea on the affected side by taping the eye in a closed position or by instillation of artificial tears into the conjunctival sac. ACTH and corticosteroids have been used to reduce inflammatory swelling of the facial nerve; there is some evidence of benefit. The incidence of permanent residual weakness is 10–20%.

Trauma to Peripheral Nerves. Trauma occurs rather frequently at birth (Erb palsy, Sec. 8.25). Later in infancy or childhood peripheral nerves may be injured by pressure such as may occur from an improperly applied cast or restraint or from failure to position the limbs properly in a comatose child. The *peroneal nerve* is most frequently affected, damage leading to foot drop and to sensory impairment over the lateral aspect of the leg and dorsum of the foot. *Radial nerve* injury causes wrist drop. Paralysis of intrinsic hand muscles with claw-hand deformity is characteristic of *ulnar nerve* palsy.

Sciatic nerve injury by faulty intramuscular injection in the buttock is an important cause of mononeuropathy in early childhood. When such injury is severe, there is paralysis of knee flexion and of all movements below the knee as well as anesthesia over the foot and over the lateral aspect of the lower leg.

Pressure neuropathies are usually self-terminating if the nerve is protected from repeated compression. Lacerations of peripheral nerves require surgical suture of the severed nerve ends. Surgical lysis of adhesions has been recommended for postinjection injuries of the sciatic nerve when there is no improvement 3 mo after the injury. Permanent sciatic nerve damage in early childhood results in considerable disability, including arrest of growth of the affected limb.

Adour KK, Wingerd J, Bell DN, et al: Prednisone treatment for idiopathic facial paralysis (Bell's palsy). N Engl J Med 287:1268, 1972.
Gilles FH, French JH: Postinjection sciatic nerve palsies in infants and children. J Pediatr 58:195, 1961.
Hoefnagel D, Penry JK: Partial facial paralysis in young children. N Engl J Med 262:1126, 1963.
Lloyd AVC, Jewitt DE, Still JDL: Facial paralysis in children with hypertension. Arch Dis Child 41:292, 1966.

McHugh HE, Sowden KA, Levitt MN: Facial paralysis and muscle agenesis in the newborn. Arch Otolaryngol 89:157, 1969.
Manning JJ, Adour KK: Facial paralysis in children. Pediatrics 49:102, 1972.
Paine RS: Facial paralysis in children. Pediatrics 19:303, 1957.
Pape KE, Pickering D: Asymmetric crying facies and other congenital anomalies. J Pediatr 81:21, 1972.
Terrence CF, Samaha FJ: The Tolosa-Hunt syndrome (painful ophthalmoplegia) in children. Dev Med Child Neurol 15:506, 1973.

22.5 DISEASES OF THE NEUROMUSCULAR JUNCTION

There are several disorders in which muscular weakness is caused by a defect in neuromuscular transmission. Normal transmission of the nerve impulse to muscle involves three steps: (1) release of acetylcholine at terminal nerve endings; (2) action of acetylcholine at receptor sites in the muscle membrane, leading to depolarization of this membrane; and (3) removal of excess released acetylcholine through hydrolysis by the enzyme cholinesterase. Blockade of neuromuscular transmission may result from interference with any of these steps.

Several toxins, such as those of botulinus and of the tick, act by preventing step 1. Step 2 is blocked by curare. The lesion in myasthenia gravis appears to lie at the muscle receptor sites. Step 3 is prevented by inhibitors of acetylcholinesterase, which include certain organic phosphate insecticides (Sec. 28.16) and drugs such as neostigmine. Poisoning by these substances leads to excessive accumulation of acetylcholine in the synaptic cleft and to paralysis by persistent depolarization of the muscle membrane (depolarized block).

Myasthenia Gravis. Myasthenia gravis is uncommon in childhood, but prompt recognition and proper therapy may be lifesaving. The disorder appears to be secondary to an autoimmune reaction directed against acetylcholine receptors in muscle. Both circulating antibodies and a lymphocyte-mediated immune response to acetylcholine receptors have been identified. Myasthenia can be passively transferred from affected patients to mice by repeated injection of immunoglobulin fractions derived from the patient's serum. Other immunologic disorders may coexist, in particular, thymic hyperplasia, thymoma, and lupus erythematosus. Three myasthenic syndromes occur in childhood: *transient neonatal myasthenia gravis, persistent neonatal myasthenia gravis,* and *juvenile myasthenia gravis.*

Transient Neonatal Myasthenia Gravis. This is seen only in infants whose mothers have myasthenia, and typically just after birth. The disease in the mother may be mild or unrecognized. About 15% of children born to mothers with myasthenia will have this transient disorder. The infant is weak and hypotonic, with poor suck, feeble respiratory effort, and ptosis. Anti–acetylcholine receptor antibodies can be demonstrated in affected neonates and in many asymptomatic infants of myasthenic mothers. Untreated, these infants may die within hours or days or may gradually improve. Respiratory and nutritional support should be provided. Anticholinesterase drugs (see below) are usually effective. Recovery occurs within 2–4 wk.

Persistent Neonatal Myasthenia Gravis. In the neonatal period, symptoms are identical to those of the transient form, but there is no indication of myasthenia in the mother and anti–acetylcholine receptor antibody is absent. Mild disorders may not be recognized for several months. More than one sibling may be affected. This inherited disease persists throughout life. The eyelids and extraocular muscles tend to be most severely affected. Respiratory and nutritional support and anticholinesterase drugs (see below) are indicated.

Juvenile Myasthenia Gravis. Onset usually occurs after the age of 10 yr; girls are affected 6 times as often as boys. Ptosis and double vision due to weakness of extraocular muscles are the most common initial symptoms. Neck, facial, bulbar, and intercostal muscles are also frequently affected. Paralysis of virtually all muscles occurs in the most severe form. A striking feature of the weakness is its amelioration after rest and its exacerbation on repetitive movement. Sudden, life-threatening exacerbations known as *myasthenic crises* may occur during intercurrent infections or during stresses such as minor surgical procedures.

The diagnosis is based on the characteristic distribution of weakness and on the demonstration of progressive weakness after repetitive or sustained muscular contractions. The latter can often be brought out by having the patient maintain upward gaze, which leads to progressively increasing ptosis. Acetylcholine receptor antibody is often present in blood. The diagnosis is confirmed by the response to anticholinesterase drugs. Edrophonium chloride (Tensilon), 0.2 mg/kg intravenously, or neostigmine, 0.04 mg/kg intramuscularly, may be used. Increase in strength after intravenous injection of edrophonium chloride is almost immediate but lasts for less than 5 min. A more prolonged response is obtained with neostigmine. Atropine sulfate, 0.01 mg/kg, should be readily available during the neostigmine test and should be given if the patient develops signs of excessive parasympathetic stimulation, such as abdominal cramps, salivation, or bradycardia. Electrical testing of neuromuscular transmission is a helpful adjunct to diagnosis; there is progressive decrease in muscle response on repetitive stimulation of nerve at low rates. The possible presence of thymoma should be explored.

Anticholinesterase drugs are effective therapeutic agents. Pyridostigmine bromide (Mestinon) is the least toxic. The beginning dose is about 30 mg orally every 4 hr in the older child and 5 mg every 4 hr for the infant. Neostigmine (Prostigmin) or ambenonium chloride (Mytelase) may be used instead of or in addition to pyridostigmine. The dosage of the anticholinesterase drug is gradually increased until the weakness is controlled or until symptoms of parasympathetic stimulation occur such as lacrimation, salivation, vomiting, diarrhea, abdominal cramps, or bradycardia. Further increase in dosage may be dangerous and may actually exacerbate weakness because of excessive accumulation of acetylcholine at the neuromuscular junction (see above). At times it may be difficult to be certain whether increase in weakness is due to worsening of the myasthenia or to overdosage of anticholinesterase drugs. The edrophonium test is helpful in the differentiation; edrophonium will improve myasthenic symptoms but will transiently increase weakness due to excess of anticholinesterase drugs. The parents of a child with myasthenia gravis should be warned of the possibility of sudden exacerbation at times of stress and of the need for immediate medical attention in such an event. If possible, the therapy of severe myasthenia should be supervised by physicians with wide experience in the management of this disease. Intermittent assisted ventilation and tracheostomy may be needed. Thymectomy or corticosteroid therapy may be indicated in intractable, severe myasthenia.

The prognosis of myasthenia gravis in childhood is somewhat better than in later life. With optimal therapy most children can lead near-normal lives. Complete remissions occur in about 25% of affected children.

Appel SH, Almon RR, Levy N: Acetylcholine receptor antibodies in myasthenia gravis. N Engl J Med 293:760, 1975.
Brunner NG, Namba T, Grob D: Corticosteroids in management of severe generalized myasthenia gravis. Neurology 22:603, 1972.
Mackay RI: Congenital myasthenia gravis. Arch Dis Child 26:289, 1951.
Millichap JG, Dodge PR: Diagnosis and treatment of myasthenia gravis in infancy, childhood and adolescence. Neurology 10:1007, 1960.
Richman DP, Patrick J, Arnason BGW: Cellular immunity in myasthenia gravis. N Engl J Med 294:694, 1976.
Roach ES, Buono G, Mclean WT, et al: Early onset myasthenia gravis. J Pediatr 108:193, 1986.
Snead OC, Benton JW, Dwyer D, et al: Juvenile myasthenia gravis. Neurology 30:732, 1980.

Teng P, Osserman KE: Studies in myasthenia gravis: Neonatal and juvenile types. A report of 21 and a review of 188 cases. J Mt Sinai Hosp (NY) 23:711, 1956.

Toyka KV, Drachman DB, Pestronk A, et al: Myasthenia gravis: Passive transfer from man to mouse. Science 190:397, 1975.

22.6 DISEASES OF MUSCLE

Skeletal muscle is affected in a large number of degenerative, metabolic, and inflammatory disorders. Degeneration of muscle fibers occurs in most of these, and, in chronic states, there is often replacement of muscle by fibrous connective tissue and fat. Proximal muscles tend to be affected more severely than distal ones, and lower extremities more than upper. Affected children often have a waddling gait, are unable to run, and have difficulty climbing stairs and standing up from the sitting position. The tendon reflexes are usually depressed in proportion to the degree of weakness. There are no sensory abnormalities.

Measurement of serum enzyme activity, especially that of creatine kinase (CPK), is often a helpful laboratory test in the differential diagnosis of muscle disease. The enzyme, which catalyzes the reaction, phosphocreatine + ADP → creatine + ATP, is present primarily in brain and muscle tissues. Excessive leakage of the enzyme into the extracellular spaces and into blood occurs in several diffuse muscle diseases, especially in the muscular dystrophies. Serum lactic dehydrogenase and glutamic-oxaloacetic transaminase are also often elevated in muscle disease, but the wide distribution of these enzymes in other tissues, including liver, makes these tests less specific. A muscle biopsy is usually needed for the definitive diagnosis of muscle disease.

Inflammatory Diseases of Muscle. Inflammation of muscle occurs in a number of infectious illnesses, especially in trichinosis (Sec. 11.117), toxoplasmosis (Sec. 11.107), and coxsackievirus infections (Sec. 11.77). It also is a component of collagen diseases (Sec. 10.57), including dermatomyositis, lupus erythematosus, polyarteritis nodosa, and rheumatoid arthritis.

Polymyositis. Diffuse inflammation of muscles, as an isolated abnormality of unknown cause, is known as polymyositis. It presents with progressive, principally proximal, muscular weakness and pain. The neck muscles are frequently affected, and the child may have difficulty lifting the head or supporting it in the upright position. Laboratory evidence of inflammation includes elevation of sedimentation rate and of the leukocyte count, but their absence does not rule out the diagnosis. The serum enzymes are usually elevated. Muscle biopsy shows degeneration and attempted regeneration of muscle fibers and lymphocytic infiltration. Differentiation from muscular dystrophy or dermatomyositis may be difficult. Polymyositis may represent a forme fruste of dermatomyositis, but the histologic appearance of muscle differs somewhat in the two conditions. Vasculitis is prominent in dermatomyositis but usually absent in polymyositis. The prognosis is somewhat better in polymyositis. Therapy with a corticosteroid frequently leads to remission, but relapse may occur following withdrawal of the drug.

Myositis Ossificans Progressiva. This is a rare progressive disease of connective tissue and muscle of unknown etiology. It has been described in siblings, including identical twins, and in successive generations. An autosomal dominant pattern of inheritance with variable expression has been suggested. More boys than girls are affected, at a ratio of 2–3:1.

Pathologic changes depend on the age of the lesions. During the early stages localized areas of edema and inflammatory cell infiltrates are found in muscle and tendons. Later, granulation tissue replaces the areas of inflammation and, eventually, sheets of cartilage and of bone are laid down in involved areas.

About 75% of affected children have congenital malformations, most commonly microdactyly and ankylosis of phalanges of the great toes; there may also be small thumbs, polydactyly, incurving of digits, webbing of toes, deformity of the ears, deafness, and absence of teeth. The same anomalies may occur in relatives who do not develop the progressive connective tissue and muscle lesions. Age of onset of these lesions varies from birth to late childhood. A typical lesion evolves through three stages: (1) a localized, often hot and tender doughy swelling of soft tissue may follow mild local trauma; (2) after a few days evidences of inflammation subside, and the affected area becomes indurated; and (3) the lesion becomes ossified. New lesions appear periodically, especially in the cervical and dorsal regions. Torticollis, due to lesions in the sternocleidomastoid, may be the initial feature. Eventually, there is widespread ossification of tendons and fascia. The spine and the joints of the extremities become ankylosed (Fig. 22–5). The masseter and mandibular joints are likely to be affected, and difficulty in chewing results. Spicules of bone may be extruded through the skin. Severe incapacitation and death from respiratory failure often occur in the early adult years; cases of survival to old age have been reported. The incidence of osteosarcoma is increased.

The process may at times remain localized to one area, usually following trauma to soft tissue (*myositis ossificans*

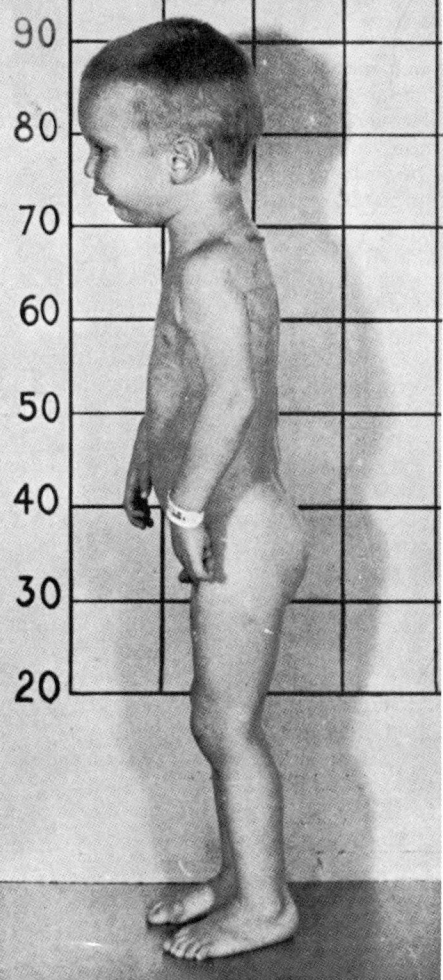

Figure 22–5. Myositis ossificans progressiva. No roentgenographically demonstrable calcification, but typical histologic changes. Note posture and rigidity of neck and back.

circumscripta). Widespread calcification of muscle also may occur in chronic polymyositis and dermatomyositis.

Laboratory studies are of little help in the diagnosis. Serum calcium, phosphate, and alkaline phosphatase values are normal, as are those of creatine kinase and the other serum enzymes. Analysis of the bone in the soft tissues has shown no difference from normal bone.

Therapy is unsatisfactory; corticosteroids and ACTH have been reported to decrease the rate of progression in a few cases. It is doubtful that they have an effect on the eventual outcome.

Endocrine and Metabolic Myopathies. *Hyperthyroid myopathy* is an uncommon complication of thyrotoxicosis. Ptosis, bifacial weakness, and proximal weakness of limb muscles occur. Some of the usual signs of hyperthyroidism may be masked by the weakness, but tachycardia, excessive sweating, and enlargement of the thyroid gland are evident. Tendon reflexes remain brisk, in contrast to those in most other forms of myopathy. The weakness disappears slowly after correction of the hyperthyroidism.

Hypothyroidism in the infant is associated with weakness and hypotonia. In the older child with myxedema, weakness, slowness of muscular contraction and relaxation, and, at times, muscular hypertrophy (Debré-Sémélaigne syndrome) are present. The weakness and hypertrophy may suggest muscular dystrophy.

Corticosteroid myopathy may complicate Cushing disease but occurs more commonly during therapy with high doses of synthetic steroids. Weakness is most marked in hip girdle muscles, leading to a waddling gait and to difficulty in standing and in climbing stairs. Knee jerks are depressed. Muscle wasting may be marked. Myopathic changes seen in muscle tissue are usually mild, even when weakness is profound. Recovery after discontinuance of steroid therapy is slow, requiring months.

Hyperparathyroidism leads to weakness and hyporeflexia that appear to be secondary to hypercalcemia; they are readily reversed after correction of the metabolic abnormality by parathyroidectomy (Sec. 19.20).

Carnitine deficiency (lipid myopathy) results in the accumulation of lipids in muscle and deprives muscle fibers of an important source of energy (Sec. 7.20). Carnitine is an essential component of the system in muscle that transports long chain fatty acids from cytosol to mitochondria for beta oxidation. In at least two disorders carnitine deficiency leads to muscular weakness.

Muscle carnitine deficiency presents progressive, usually proximal weakness during childhood and adolescence. In severe cases there is respiratory paralysis. Weakness may be intermittent at first and associated with myoglobinuria. Serum enzyme values are elevated, including creatine kinase and aldolase. Electromyography shows nonspecific myopathic changes. Muscle biopsy shows excess lipid droplets as the major pathologic change. Muscle but not serum carnitine concentration is decreased. The condition is of importance since it is treatable but easily misdiagnosed as muscular dystrophy. Some patients have responded to therapy with oral carnitine (100 mg/kg/day); in others pharmacologic doses of corticosteroid hormones have been effective.

Systemic carnitine deficiency produces progressive myopathy, including cardiomyopathy, in association with hepatic failure and hepatic encephalopathy. The clinical presentation may resemble Reye syndrome (Sec. 12.82 and 21.24) except for the occurrence of repeated attacks of encephalopathy and for the presence of muscular weakness between attacks. Serum creatine kinase is markedly elevated. Both serum and muscle carnitine concentrations are decreased. The muscle pathology is identical to that in muscle carnitine deficiency. Similar clinical and pathologic changes, including carnitine deficiency,

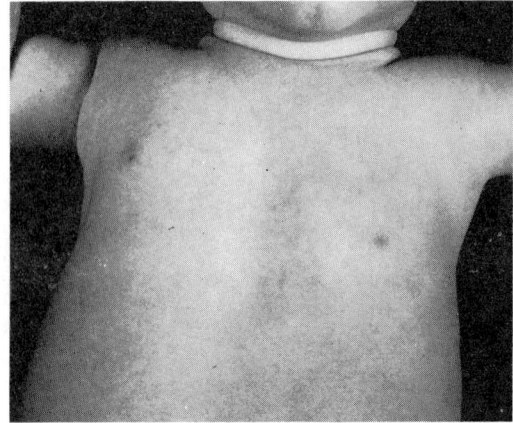

Figure 22–6. Congenital absence of left pectoral muscle. Note absence of anterior axillary fold and low placement of nipple.

may be seen in several disorders of organic acid metabolism, including methylmalonic aciduria and glutaric aciduria ("secondary carnitine deficiency"). Therapy of systemic carnitine deficiency includes a high carbohydrate, low fat diet and supplementary oral carnitine (100 mg/kg/day).

Congenital Defects of Muscle. *Congenital Absence of Muscle.* Failure of muscle development may be widespread, leading to immobility of multiple joints or arthrogryposis multiplex congenita (Sec. 23.44). More commonly, congenital absence is limited to one muscle. Absence of the sternal head of the pectoralis major is a common anomaly (Fig. 22–6), occasionally with syndactyly on the same side (Poland syndrome). Absence of the pectoral muscle is found with increased frequency in children with muscular dystrophy. Congenital absence of abdominal muscles is often associated with anomalies of the urinary tract (Sec. 17.40).

Congenital Torticollis. Torticollis or *wryneck* is due to shortening or contracture of the sternocleidomastoid muscle on 1 side. The head is tilted toward the side of the contracture, and the chin is turned toward the opposite side (Fig. 22–7).

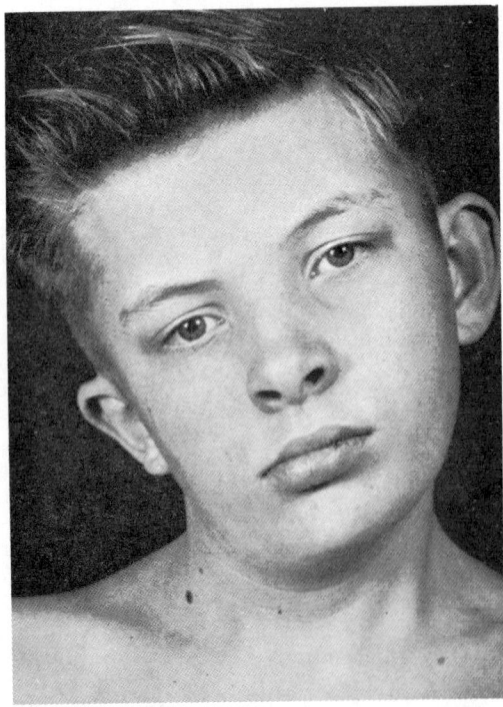

Figure 22–7. Congenital torticollis, untreated until the age of 12 yr. Note wryneck and asymmetry of face.

Considerable resistance is encountered in attempts to correct the deviation. A firm mass may be palpable in the involved muscle. The cause is unclear; birth trauma has long been incriminated, but torticollis has been observed at cesarean section, suggesting a prenatal cause in some cases.

The differential diagnosis of congenital torticollis includes head tilt secondary to malformation of the cervical spine, such as occurs in the Klippel-Feil anomaly, and fracture or dislocation of cervical vertebrae. Roentgenograms of the cervical spine should be obtained to rule these out. In the older child, head tilt may also occur secondary to strabismus, dystonia, posterior fossa or cervical cord tumor, myositis ossificans, cervical adenitis, or hiatus hernia. Most infants with congenital torticollis improve with simple muscle-stretching exercises. Persistent torticollis leads to asymmetric development of the face and skull (Fig. 22–7) and may require surgical section of the affected muscle for a good cosmetic outcome.

Congenital Myopathies. This group includes several rare inherited disorders in which weakness and hypotonia are present from infancy (see Table 22–1). The correct diagnosis of these disorders is important from a prognostic standpoint. In general, the outlook for a normal life span and useful existence is good, in contrast to that of the hypotonic infant with Werdnig-Hoffmann disease or with congenital muscular dystrophy. Identification of the congenital myopathies depends on biopsy of skeletal muscle.

CENTRAL CORE DISEASE. The center of each muscle fiber stains abnormally but homogeneously. Electron microscopy shows a decrease of mitochondria and of sarcoplasmic reticulum in the central portion of the affected fibers.

NEMALINE MYOPATHY. Nemaline myopathy derives its name from the presence of threadlike structures within muscle cells. Electron microscopy indicates that these are the result of abnormalities of the Z bands of myofibrils.

Mitochondrial Myopathies. Several myopathies have been described in which alteration of muscle mitochondria is the most prominent pathologic finding. Mitochondria may be extremely numerous, increased in size, or both. Weakness and hypotonia may be present from infancy or may be progressive later in childhood. Cardiomyopathy, encephalopathy, and lactic acidemia are often associated with these disorders. (See also Kearns-Sayre syndrome, below.)

Myotonia. Myotonia is a symptom of a variety of muscle diseases, including myotonic dystrophy, the hyperkalemic form of familial periodic paralysis, and glycogen storage disease of muscle. It is defined as abnormal slowness in relaxation of muscle following voluntary or induced muscular contraction. Clinically, it is manifested by inability to relax the hand grip and by visible maintained contraction following direct stimulation of a muscle by sharp tap (Fig. 22–8A). The latter is demonstrated by tapping a superficial muscle group such as the tongue or the thenar eminence with a reflex hammer. The presence of myotonia is confirmed by electromyography, which shows persistence of muscle action potentials following relaxation of voluntary contraction (myotonic discharges).

Myotonia Congenita (Thomsen Disease). In this disorder, transmitted by dominant inheritance, myotonia occurs as an isolated finding. It may be manifested in infancy as slow swallowing and gagging due to failure of normal relaxation of oropharyngeal muscles or, later in childhood, as inability to release a firm hand grip. The muscles tend to become stiff when the child first attempts to carry out a motion. This stiffness gradually subsides when the movement is repeated a few times. For example, an affected child may have difficulty initiating the act of walking. The first few steps tend to be slow and awkward. After a few seconds the gait becomes normal, or nearly so. These symptoms are worse during emotional upset and on exposure to cold. Strength is normal,

and muscles are well developed, often unusually large, so that the child has an athletic appearance.

The diagnosis is based on the clinical and electromyographic demonstration of myotonia. Serum enzymes are normal. The only histologic alteration is hypertrophy of muscle fibers.

Differentiation from myotonic dystrophy is based on the absence of muscle weakness or atrophy and on the lack of dystrophic changes in biopsied muscle tissue. Therapy with procainamide or quinidine sulfate lessens the myotonia and is indicated when there is functional impairment. The disorder is benign and may improve with age.

The Periodic Paralyses. In this group of illnesses weakness is intermittent, with complete or nearly complete recovery of strength between attacks. The group includes also muscle phosphorylase deficiency (McArdle disease, Sec. 7.21).

Hyperkalemic Periodic Paralysis. Adynamia episodica hereditaria or paramyotonia is transmitted as a dominant trait, with more severe expression in the male. Onset occurs during early childhood and sometimes in infancy. Rest after strong exertion appears to precipitate paralytic episodes. Weakness develops rapidly and lasts up to a few hours. Legs are most severely affected; respiration is usually spared. Myotonia is common and may persist between attacks. It tends to be most marked in the eyelids, with lid lag on downward gaze (Fig. 22–8B).

During the attack the serum concentration of potassium is often elevated, but repeated measurements in several episodes may be needed to demonstrate it. An oral potassium load of 2–3 g may be used to precipitate an attack but should be given only with monitoring of the ECG. Acetazolamide prevents recurrent paralysis. Severely affected patients eventually develop mild persistent weakness and dystrophic changes in muscle.

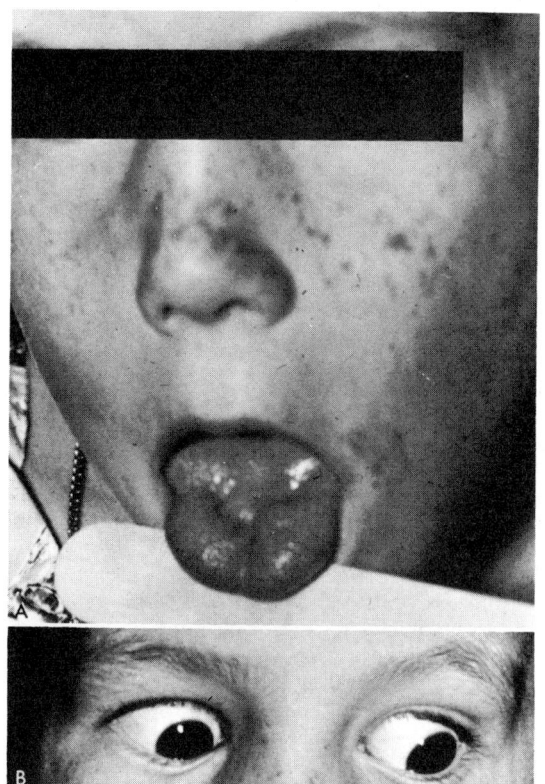

Figure 22–8. *A*, Myotonia following tap of the right tongue with a reflex hammer. *B*, Myotonia of the eyelid in a child with the hyperkalemic form of familial periodic paralysis. The lid remains retracted when the child is asked to look down.

Hypokalemic Periodic Paralysis. *Familial periodic paralysis* also is transmitted in a dominant manner, with symptoms more severe in males. In contrast to the hyperkalemic form, first attacks usually occur in late childhood or early adolescence. Large carbohydrate meals or rest after exertion may precipitate paralysis. Typically, the patient awakens paralyzed on the morning after a day of heavy exercise capped by a large evening meal. During the attack the limbs are flaccid and areflexic. Respiration may be affected. Cardiac arrhythmias may include ventricular premature beats and ventricular tachycardia. An attack may last longer than 24 hr. Serum potassium levels are usually low, 2–3 mEq/L, during the paralytic phase. The basic defect is unknown. Patients with repeated severe attacks develop fixed weakness and dystrophic changes in muscle. Therapy during an attack consists of oral potassium chloride, beginning with a dose of 2–3 g. Acetazolamide reduces the frequency of attacks.

Paroxysmal Myoglobinuria (Idiopathic Myoglobinuria). Idiopathic myoglobinurias are a heterogeneous group of entities in which attacks of paralysis with myoglobinuria occur spontaneously or following strenuous exercise. Dominant and X-linked inheritance have been reported. Affected muscles, often of the calf and thigh, become painful and swollen during an attack. The urine becomes dark red or brown. The myoglobinuria may cause renal tubular necrosis, with death from renal failure.

The diagnosis is confirmed by demonstration of myoglobin in urine. A positive benzidine test in urine free of red cells suggests the presence of myoglobin, especially when a concomitant serum sample is clear (free of hemoglobin). Definite differentiation from hemoglobin is made on spectrophotometry. Paroxysmal myoglobinuria must be distinguished from McArdle disease (Sec. 7.21), from carnitine palmityltransferase deficiency, and from the myoglobinuria that may occur in a normal person following severe unaccustomed exertion or crushing injury of muscle. Myoglobinuria after heavy exertion occurs occasionally in pseudohypertrophic (Duchenne) muscular dystrophy.

Treatment consists of bed rest, assisted ventilation when necessary, and hydration to minimize the danger of renal injury.

Carnitine Palmityltransferase Deficiency. This disorder involves an enzyme system that is essential for the transport of long chain fatty acids to intramitochondrial sites of beta oxidation and ketone production (Sec 7.54). Deficiency of the type II isoenzyme is transmitted as a recessive trait. The defect results in impaired ketogenesis in multiple tissues, including muscle and liver. Clinical onset is usually during childhood or adolescence, with recurrent episodes of muscle pain, weakness, and fever precipitated by prolonged exercise or fasting. Myoglobinuria occurs during the attacks and may lead to renal failure. Fasting hypoglycemia may occur. Between attacks the patients are asymptomatic. The disorder is differentiated from other conditions that cause periodic weakness and myoglobinuria by assay of carnitine palmityltransferase II activity, which is decreased in muscle, liver, leukocytes, and cultured fibroblasts. Therapy with a high carbohydrate, low fat diet prevents recurrent attacks.

The Muscular Dystrophies. The muscular dystrophies are a group of familial disorders in which degeneration of muscle fibers occurs. Classification is based on age of onset, rate of progression, distribution of muscular involvement, and mode of inheritance.

Pseudohypertrophic Muscular Dystrophy. The *childhood* or *Duchenne* form of muscular dystrophy is the most common of this group of muscle diseases; the incidence is about 0.14/1000 children. Its classic form occurs only in boys, with a history of X-linked inheritance in about 50% of propositi. The remainder appear to represent new mutations. Rarely, a disorder clinically identical to Duchenne muscular dystrophy is recessively inherited, with boys and girls equally affected. The diagnosis is rarely made prior to the age of 3 yr. A history of slow motor development with late onset of sitting, walking, and running is usually obtained, however, indicating a much earlier onset. Waddling gait, difficulty in climbing stairs, and hypertrophy of calf muscles are the common presenting findings. Occasionally, muscles other than the calf, including deltoid, brachioradialis, or tongue, are increased in bulk. Early in the disease the hypertrophied muscles have considerable strength, but later the enlarged muscles are often weak (pseudohypertrophy) since much of the increased bulk is due to fatty infiltration. The hypertrophic calf muscles are stronger than the anterior leg muscles; accordingly, toe walking and contracture of the heel cords are common. Weakness of pelvic girdle muscles results in characteristic waddling, lordotic gait, and difficulty in arising from the floor. The child with moderately severe muscular dystrophy demonstrates Gowers sign: in getting up from the floor he first rolls to the prone position, kneels, and then raises himself to standing by pushing with his hands against shins, knees, and thighs (Fig. 22–9). Weakness of shoulder girdle muscles can be brought out by lifting the child by means of hands placed under the axillae. He will slip through the hands rather than support himself by adducting the arms. Eventually the child becomes unable to lift his arms above his head. Profound muscle atrophy occurs in late stages. Ambulation usually becomes impossible by the age of 12 yr, and death occurs prior to 20 yr in 75% of patients. The majority of patients have cardiomyopathy; it is occasionally the cause of sudden death. Instances of X-linked pseudohypertrophic muscular dystrophy occur with onset in late childhood and prolonged survival (Becker muscular dystrophy). The mean IQ of children with Duchenne muscular dystrophy is 80; 25% have frank mental defect.

The *differential diagnosis* of Duchenne muscular dystrophy includes the late infantile form of Werdnig-Hoffmann disease and such diseases of muscle as the endocrine myopathies, carnitine deficiency, glycogen storage disease of muscle, and polymyositis. Occasionally, the presence of heel cord contractures and of toe walking suggests cerebral palsy, but the spasticity and hyperreflexia of cerebral palsy are absent in muscular dystrophy.

The *diagnosis* of Duchenne muscular dystrophy is confirmed by measurement of serum enzymes, by electromyography, and by muscle biopsy. Serum enzyme values, especially of creatine kinase (CPK), often are increased to more than 10 times normal, even in infancy prior to onset of weakness. Electromyography reveals primarily decreases in amplitude and duration of motor unit potentials. Histologic changes include degeneration of muscle fibers, with variation in fiber size and central nuclei and replacement of muscle fibers by fat and connective tissue. The diagnosis can be established at birth by measurement of CPK values; intrauterine diagnosis is not yet possible. Female carriers cannot be identified with certainty, but mild to moderate elevations of serum CPK are found in 60–80% of known carriers; this finding is more likely during childhood than in later life.

There is no effective treatment for muscular dystrophy. Affected children should be kept active and ambulatory as long as possible. Strenuous exercise is to be avoided since it may hasten the breakdown of muscle fibers. Occasionally, surgical lengthening of heel cords may improve ambulation, but prolonged bed rest after orthopedic procedures may hasten muscle atrophy. Genetic counseling is an important aspect of management.

Congenital Muscular Dystrophy. This autosomal recessive disorder is characterized by hypotonia and weakness in infancy and should be considered in the differential diagnosis of the "floppy infant" (Table 22–1). The onset occurs in utero.

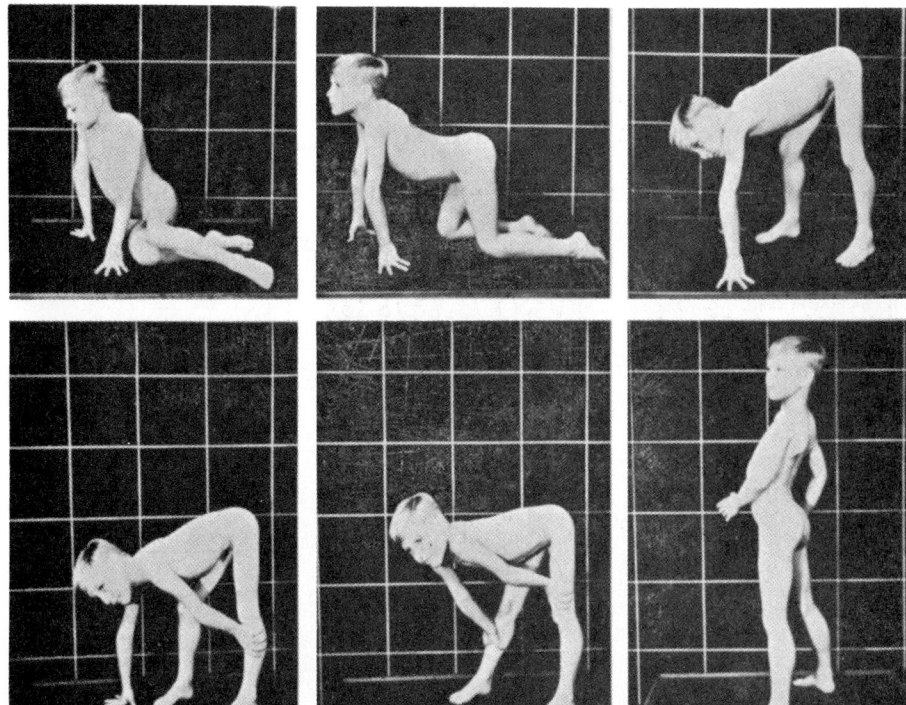

Figure 22–9. A child 7 yr of age with pseudohypertrophic muscular dystrophy, showing characteristic manner of rising from the floor (Gowers sign). The last picture shows the standing position with the severe lordosis.

Occasionally, profound muscle atrophy, contractures, and limitation of joint movements are present at birth. Differentiation from Werdnig-Hoffmann disease is difficult. Fasciculations of the tongue, common in Werdnig-Hoffmann disease, do not occur in congenital muscular dystrophy. The tendon reflexes are depressed but usually not absent. Muscles of respiration, including the diaphragm, are affected. Severely ill infants die of respiratory failure prior to the age of 1 yr; milder forms may have prolonged survival. Serum enzymes are not consistently elevated, although muscle shows dystrophic changes.

Facioscapulohumeral Muscular Dystrophy. This mild form of dystrophy has autosomal dominant transmission. Onset usually occurs in the 2nd decade, with weakness and atrophy of facial and shoulder girdle muscles. The face is expressionless; forceful eye closure and whistling are not possible. The illness progresses slowly and is compatible with a normal life span but cases with early onset and rapid progression occur. The diagnosis is based on the clinical findings and pattern of inheritance. Biopsy of affected muscles shows dystrophic changes. Serum CPK may be normal or mildly elevated.

Limb-Girdle Muscular Dystrophy. This heterogeneous disorder is characterized by slowly progressive muscular dystrophy, usually autosomal recessive. Onset may occur in late childhood, adolescence, or adulthood. The pelvic girdle muscles are most commonly affected.

Ocular Myopathy. This dystrophic process affects principally the extraocular muscles. Onset occurs usually during childhood or adolescence, with progressive ptosis and limitation of eye movements; occasionally, weakness extends to facial and neck muscles. There is no clear inheritance pattern. This disorder must be differentiated from myasthenia gravis and from cranial nerve palsies due to brain stem tumor.

A progressive ophthalmoplegia beginning in childhood or adolescence is associated with atypical pigmentary degeneration of the retina and heart block (*Kearns-Sayre syndrome*). Progressive ataxia, nerve deafness, growth retardation, and delayed sexual maturation are common. Changes in muscle consist of large subsarcolemmal collections of abnormal mitochondria. The disorder is usually sporadic, but a few familial cases have been reported. Sudden death due to the cardiac conduction defect may be prevented by use of a cardiac pacemaker.

Myotonic Dystrophy. Myotonic dystrophy has usually seemed to have its onset in adulthood, but it begins in infancy or childhood with considerable frequency. Transmission is autosomal dominant. Onset in childhood may be more likely when the affected parent is the mother; accordingly, intrauterine factors may influence the severity of expression. Hypotonia and poor sucking ability may be present at birth. Developmental delay is noted later in infancy, as is mental retardation. In early childhood muscle weakness and atrophy are found principally in the facial, jaw, and temporalis muscles; bilateral ptosis is common. Myotonia may be demonstrated by percussion of muscle, by electromyography, or by the child's inability to relax a hand grip (see Myotonia Congenita above). Weakness and atrophy of limb muscles, often distal in distribution, become evident in later childhood and adolescence. Cataracts, baldness, and testicular atrophy are characteristic of the adult form of the disease.

The diagnosis is based on the demonstration of myotonia along with characteristic distribution of weakness, history of dominant inheritance, and findings of dystrophic changes in muscle. The prognosis of the childhood form of the disease must be guarded. Mental defect is usually present, and the muscle weakness is apt to be a major handicap by early adulthood. Treatment with procainamide or quinidine is indicated if the myotonia leads to functional impairment.

PETER R. HUTTENLOCHER

Byers RK, Bergman AB, Joseph MC: Steroid myopathy. Pediatrics 29:26, 1962.
DiMauro S, Bonilla E, Zeviani M, et al: Mitochondrial myopathies. Ann Neurol 17:521, 1985.
Dodge PR, Gamstorp I, Byers RK, et al: Myotonic dystrophy in infancy and childhood. Pediatrics 35:3, 1965.
Dowben RM, Vawter GF, Brandfonbrenner A, et al: Polymyositis and other diseases resembling muscular dystrophy. Arch Intern Med 115:584, 1965.

Dubowitz V: Intellectual impairment in muscular dystrophy. Arch Dis Child 40:296, 1965.

Dubowitz V: Muscle Disorders in Childhood. Philadelphia, WB Saunders, 1978.

Engel WK, Foster JB, Hughes BP, et al: Central core disease—an investigation of a rare muscle cell abnormality. Brain 84:167, 1961.

Favara BE, Vawter GF, Wagner R, et al: Familial paroxysmal rhabdomyolysis in children. Am J Med 42:196, 1967.

Frame B, Heinze EG Jr, Block MA, et al: Myopathy in primary hyperparathyroidism. Ann Intern Med 68:1022, 1968.

Gonatas NK, Shy GM, Godfrey EH: Nemaline myopathy. The origin of nemaline structures. N Engl J Med 274:535, 1966.

Harper PS, Dyken PR: Early-onset dystrophia myotonica. Evidence supporting a maternal environmental factor. Lancet 1:53, 1972.

Illingworth RS: Myositis ossificans progressiva (Munchmeyer disease). Arch Dis Child 46:264, 1971.

Jackson CE, Strehler DA: Limb-girdle muscular dystrophy: Clinical manifestations and detection of preclinical disease. Pediatrics 41:495, 1968.

Kakulas BA, Adams RD: Diseases of Muscle. 4th ed. Philadelphia, Harper & Row, 1985.

Layzer RB, Lovelace RE, Rowland LP: Hyperkalemic periodic paralysis. Arch Neurol 16:455, 1967.

Levitt LP, Rose LI, Dawson DM: Hypokalemic periodic paralysis with arrhythmia. N Engl J Med 286:253, 1972.

McArdle B: Familial periodic paralysis. Br Med Bull 12:226, 1956.

Najjar SS, Nachman HS: Kocher-Debré-Sémélaigne syndrome: Hypothyroidism with muscular "hypertrophy." J Pediatr 66:901, 1965.

Pearson CM: The periodic paralyses: Differential features and pathological observations in permanent myopathic weakness. Brain 87:391, 1964.

Ramsey I: Thyrotoxic muscle disease. Postgrad Med J 44:385, 1968.

Resnick JS, Engel WK, Griggs RC, et al: Acetazolamide prophylaxis in hypokalemic periodic paralysis. N Engl J Med 278:582, 1968.

Smith HL, Amick LD, Johnson WW: Detection of subclinical and carrier states in Duchenne muscular dystrophy. J Pediatr 69:67, 1966.

Thompson CE: Polymyositis in children. Clin Pediatr 7:24, 1968.

Vignos PJ Jr, Bowling GF, Watkins MP: Polymyositis. Effect of corticosteroids on final results. Arch Intern Med 114:263, 1964.

Walton J: Disorders of Voluntary Muscle. 4th ed. Edinburgh, Churchill, Livingstone, 1981.

Zellweger H, Afifi A, McCormick WF, et al: Severe congenital muscular dystrophy. Am J Dis Child 114:591, 1967.

Zundels WS, Tyler FH: The muscular dystrophies. N Engl J Med 273:537, 1965.

23

THE BONES AND JOINTS

ORTHOPEDIC PROBLEMS

Musculoskeletal problems will be presented by anatomic region, by frequency with which they are encountered, and by age groups primarily affected. Neoplasms of bone are discussed in Sec. 16.17–16.19, and infections of bone in Sec. 11.14.

23.1 THE FEET AND TOES

The Infant. The normal infant's foot at birth is proportionately longer and thinner than that of the older child, and the joints of the ankle and foot are very supple. The foot can be dorsiflexed so that the top of the foot touches the tibia anteriorly, plantar flexed so that the dorsum of the forefoot is parallel with the tibia, and inverted or everted in the hindpart 45°. The forefoot should be flexible enough to be moved into 45° of adduction or abduction.

The feet of a newborn infant may appear to be in abnormal positions, but if the feet can be moved through the range of motion described above, there is no need for concern. Such "positional" foot configurations resolve spontaneously.

In-toeing. This common condition may be due to inturning of the forepart of the foot (i.e., metatarsus varus, see below) or inturning of the entire foot (i.e., medial tibial torsion). Both causes are aggravated by sleeping face down or crawling with the feet and toes turned inward. With standing and walking, in-toeing, in which the entire foot turns inward, diminishes. In general, if the amount of in-toeing is greater than 45° at 3 mo, 30° at 9 mo, or 20° at 1 yr, orthopedic evaluation should be considered.

Treatment usually employs some method of holding the feet turned outward during sleeping hours. This can be achieved by pinning or sewing the pajama legs together or by sewing each half of a wristwatch strap to the backs of soft tissues. The most commonly used method is attaching to each of a pair of shoes a bar that is as long as the pelvis is wide. Six–12 mo of treatment is usually satisfactory. Children over 1.5 yr of age often will not tolerate the restrictions of the nighttime footwear and are best left alone until after about the age of 3, when they may again use a night brace.

Out-toeing. Out-toeing may slightly delay walking since standing with the feet externally rotated is unstable. It is usually the entire leg that points outward rather than just the foot. Correction of out-toeing is usually spontaneous but is hastened by exercises. The child's thighs are grasped above the knee, rotated medially, and held at maximum medial rotation for a count of 5. This is repeated 5 times at each diaper change. In addition, the legs of the pajamas can be sewn or pinned together to prevent sleeping in the "frog position."

Metatarsus Varus (Metatarsus Adductus). In the normal foot a line along the middle of the heel should run through the 2nd toe (Fig. 23–1). Many infants are born with the front part of the foot turned inward. If the foot becomes fixed in such a position, proper fit of shoes may be a lifelong problem.

If the forefoot can be abducted past the midline but less than 30° beyond, exercises provided by the parents at each diaper change are usually sufficient treatment. Stretching can

be done by holding the heel in neutral position with the thumb and index finger of one hand while moving the forefoot into abduction with the other hand, where it is held for a count of 5, repeated 5 times. Parents need encouragement to be moderately vigorous with the exercises. Since pushing on the great toe can create hallux valgus, the pressure should be over the 1st metatarsal head. If the forepart of the foot cannot be moved beyond the neutral point, the infant should be referred for orthopedic care. The feet are stretched by manipulation and held with casts, a procedure that is repeated at approximately weekly intervals. Casting is usually followed by the use of outflare shoes until the child is walking.

Clubfoot. This term is used for a number of congenital anomalies of the foot. The most common (about 95% of clubfeet) is an equinovarus deformity. This deformity has three elements: the ankle is in equinus; the subtalar joint is in varus; and the mid and foreparts of the foot are in varus. If this form of clubfoot is not treated, further stiffening occurs in the abnormal position, with secondary changes in osseous development.

Early treatment is critical and should be started within the first hours after birth since the joints of the foot are maximally flexible at that time. The feet are manipulated to the position of maximum correction and held there by casts or adhesive taping. Manipulation and casting are repeated every few days for 1–2 wk and then at 1–2 wk intervals. In the past, emphasis was given to manipulation and casting for the entire course of therapy, and operative treatment was viewed as a mark of failure. Manipulation against very thickened ligaments, however, leads to distortion of the cartilaginous anlage of the bones with permanent damage. If manipulation becomes ineffective, surgical release of the Achilles tendon, capsules of the ankle, subtalar joints, medial ligaments, and joint capsules is required. The age at which surgery is necessary may be as early as 2–3 mo. Parents should be advised early that surgery is often necessary.

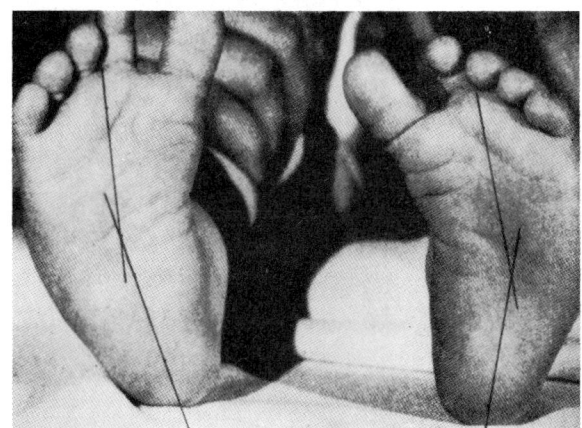

Figure 23–1. Metatarsus varus: A line bisecting the hindpart of the foot should pass through the 2nd toe or between the 2nd and 3rd toes.

1343

By the first year of life a treated clubfoot may look relatively normal. However, the lateral part of the foot will always have excess soft tissue and the calf of that leg will be thinner. Because this disorder tends to recur, orthopedic care is necessary throughout childhood.

Other forms of clubfoot, such as calcaneovalgus, usually present less difficult problems; the principles of treatment are the same.

Vertical Talus (Congenital Rocker-Bottom Foot). This condition is characterized by malposition of the navicular on the neck of the talus. The ankle is held in marked equinus and the forefoot in dorsiflexion; thus the foot has a rocker-bottom shape. Palpation of the sole of the foot reveals a hard mass, the head of the talus. A patient with vertical talus should be referred to the orthopedic surgeon immediately.

Overlapping Toes. Most commonly the 2nd toe is displaced dorsally while the 3rd toe touches the 1st. Though this condition is of concern to parents, it does not result in functional problems and resolves spontaneously with weight bearing. Adhesive tape or a Band-Aid wrapped under the 1st toe, over the 2nd, and under the 3rd may relieve anxiety in some patients.

Extra Toes. These may make it difficult to fit shoes and should be removed. They are often associated with a partial or complete extra metatarsal, which usually causes the major problem with shoes. Since segments of the metatarsals may not be sufficiently ossified to be recognized by roentgenograms in the neonate, resection should be delayed until about 1 yr of age when they are visible. There will be ample time for healing before the child is walking a great deal.

Syndactyly of the Toes. This condition is rarely a problem except cosmetically; separation of such toes is usually unnecessary.

The Toddler. The normal toddler's foot is somewhat chubby and wider than that of the older child. The fat pad on the medial aspect creates a fullness so that the foot appears fat. When the child first stands and walks, the foot may be everted; eversion is accentuated if the child stands with the legs externally rotated. Such an appearance should not be of concern. Only after the child has attained a stable standing and walking pattern does the pediatrician need to be concerned about the configuration of the foot.

Flat Foot. With weight bearing, some children's feet appear flat because of a loss of the longitudinal arch. If the feet are otherwise normal, particularly the hind and foreparts of the foot, they need no treatment. In other children the feet collapse with weight bearing and display valgus on the hindfoot, or eversion, and pronation of the forefoot (Fig. 23–2). This collapse may be due to ligamentous laxity, muscular weakness, or a tight Achilles tendon. Valgus of less than 10° need not be treated. In more severe instances the bones of the foot will adapt to the abnormal position, with a "flat foot" configuration becoming permanent and sometimes with painful feet in adulthood.

The goal of treatment is to maintain the foot in as near normal shape as possible during growth so that the bones will develop normally. Because the underlying ligamentous laxity and muscular weakness remain unaltered, when maturity is reached, the feet may be flat but the bones relatively normal. Treatment may consist of exercises to strengthen the muscles or stretch the heel cord. Because these require active effort by the child, treatment is usually ineffective. If the condition is mild, the foot may be supported by an arch pad (usually 3/16–1/4 inch thick) glued into the shoe and a medial heel wedge (usually 1/8 inch thick). In the severe form a molded plastic insert ("UCB insert," University of California–Berkeley insert) designed to hold the foot in a neutral position can be worn inside the shoe. Occasionally, corrective surgery may be needed. The so-called Thomas Heel is ineffective.

In-toeing (Pigeon Toe, Ding Toe). There are three common reasons for in-toeing: (1) the forepart of the foot is turned medially (metatarsus varus or adductus); (2) the entire foot points inward while the knee points straight ahead (medial tibial torsion); and (3) the entire leg turns in so that both the knee and the foot are facing medially (medial femoral torsion or increased anteversion of the hips). The child should be observed standing and walking barefoot and with shoes on, and the position of the knees in relation to the line of gait should be noted. The simplest method of determining which of the three causes is responsible for the in-toed gait is to have the child lie prone with the knees bent to 90° (Fig. 23–3). This gives a good view of the sole of the foot to disclose metatarsus varus. A line drawn along the sole of the foot should line up with a similar line down the length of the thigh; any inward deviation of the foot is due to medial tibial torsion. The feet should be moved outward (Fig. 23–4) to demonstrate the degree of *medial* rotation of the femora in extension. Both feet should be moved simultaneously so that the pelvis stays in a neutral position. Similarly, the feet may be moved inward in order to measure the *lateral* rotation of

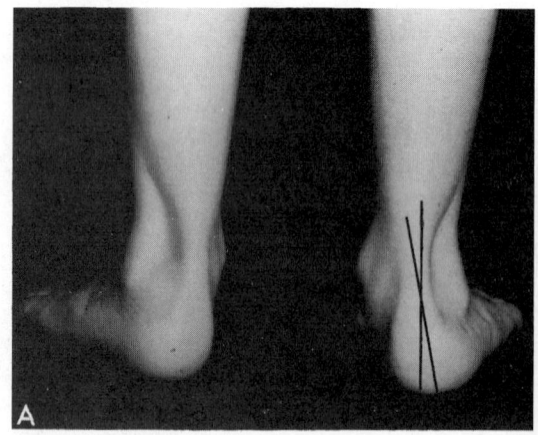
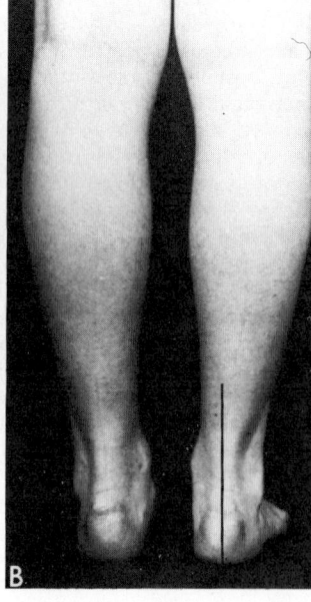

Figure 23–2. *A,* The heel in valgus. *B,* Normal heel.

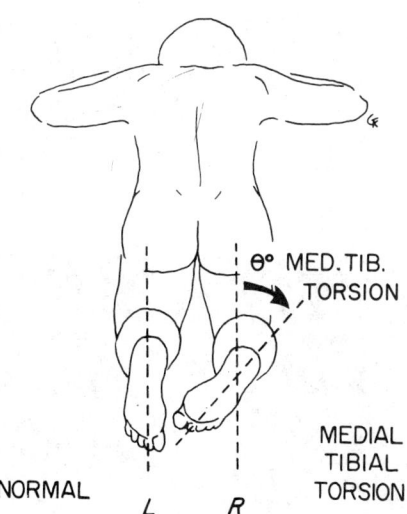

Figure 23–3. With the patient lying prone and the knees flexed 90°, the position of the foot is examined for medial tibial torsion. The left foot is normal; the right foot is in medial torsion.

the femora in extension. The femora normally rotate 45° in each direction; excessive medial rotation with a concomitant decrease in lateral rotation is called medial femoral torsion or increased anteversion.

Metatarsus varus of more than 10° that cannot be readily brought to the midline may cause problems with the proper fit of shoes and should be evaluated by an orthopedic surgeon. Otherwise, the condition can be ignored.

The problems of in-toeing from **medial tibial torsion** are more cosmetic than functional. In later childhood and adulthood, in-toeing from medial tibial torsion, even 20–30°, does not impair function and may even enhance it in athletics. Some children trip over their own feet, but this tendency vanishes by the age of 4 or 5 yr, even if there has been no change in rotation. Rarely, in later years, medial tibial torsion of greater than 20° may be a functional problem.

Medial femoral torsion (increased anteversion of the hips) usually becomes apparent to parents after the child reaches 2 yr of age. They frequently report that the children trip over their own feet, a problem that generally disappears spontaneously after the age of 4–5 yr. Only in extreme circumstances does this condition lead to any decrease in function; it is mainly a cosmetic concern. As the child passes the age of 10, parents usually learn to overlook the condition. Treatment is rarely required. The only realistic treatment for an axial deformity of a single long bone is surgical and requires division of the bone and realignment and fixation so that the bone heals in the new position. If needed, surgery can be performed as late as the age of 10. The longer the decision is delayed, the less likely it is that the parents or the child will want such treatment.

Out-toeing. When children start to walk, they often do so with their feet laterally rotated. Almost invariably this rotation corrects itself, and it deserves attention only if it persists beyond the age of 1–1.5 yr, with lateral rotation at the thighs.

Toewalking. A child who walks on tiptoes usually does so for one of three common reasons:

1. *Habit.* This may be treated by having the parents encourage the child to walk heel/toe and engage in exercises or game playing with the child walking on the heels.

2. *Cerebral palsy with mild spasticity.* Toewalking combined with limited abduction of the hips may provide the clue for the diagnosis of cerebral palsy in its milder form (Sec. 21.15).

3. *Congenital tight heelcords.* With the knees in extension the normal foot should be capable of dorsiflexion to 20° above a

right angle. If this cannot be attained, stretching exercises with assistance by the parents can help. Surgical lengthening of the tendon may be necessary if a 6 wk trial of immobilization in a plaster cast is unsuccessful.

Shoes. Shoes serve two purposes for the normal child: to protect the feet from sharp objects on the ground or floor and to keep the feet warm. They are not required to learn to walk. "Orthopedic shoes" (a term coined by the manufacturer) are of no benefit to a normal child and are potentially harmful by being too stiff. For the youngster learning to walk, shoes should be so soft so that the child can sense the contours of the ground. They should not have a heel which can catch on objects. High shoes are not needed for the support of a normal foot but may prevent a child from kicking them off. There is nothing inappropriate about the use of sneakers for a child with a normal foot. A new shoe should be long enough to allow for growth (a distance about the width of the child's thumb from the end of the big toe to the end of the shoe measured while the child stands). The shoe should be wide enough at the metatarsal heads so that when the child stands, a pinch of leather can be squeezed between the fingers.

The Older Child and Adolescent. *The Painful Foot.* A child or adolescent, especially if obese or undergoing a growth spurt, may complain of pain in the feet particularly after vigorous activity. If a general evaluation is unremarkable, the patient should be referred for orthopedic evaluation. If the pain is secondary to *pronated feet,* treatment by exercises and foot pads will often suffice. Occasionally, *flexible flat feet* that are painful may require surgical realignment of the tendons or bones.

Pain may also result from a *coalition between the tarsal bones.* Before the age of 10 yr coalition may be composed of cartilage of fibrous tissue not easily recognized on a roentgenogram, but the altered joint motion will lead to a painful subtalar joint with spasm of the peroneal muscles. Sharp medial motion of the hindfoot by the examiner will produce not only pain but a reactive spasm of the peroneal muscles. Prior to the age of 11 or 12 such a coalition may be excised. Older children usually require a triple arthrodesis to relieve the pain.

Pain may be caused by *osteochondritis dissecans of the talus,* a condition of unknown etiology. A small segment of the bone just under the articular cartilage becomes avascular. Occasionally, the fragment breaks free into the joint and requires surgical removal. Other causes of painful foot in the adolescent are *juvenile rheumatoid arthritis* (Sec. 10.58), which may present monarticular disease in the foot; *infection; Kohler disease,* avascular necrosis of the tarsal navicular; *Freiberg disease,* avascular necrosis of the head of the metatarsals, commonly the 2nd; and *stress fractures* of metatarsals.

Cavus Foot. The high arched foot is rarely brought to the pediatrician's attention by the parents, but should immedi-

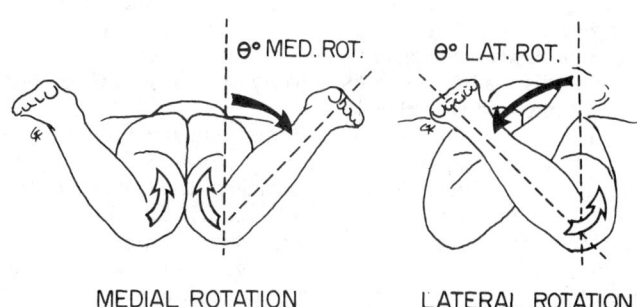

Figure 23–4. With the patient lying prone and the knees flexed 90°, the femurs are examined for their range of motion at the hips in extension.

ately suggest the possibility of a neurologic condition, such as spinal dysrhaphia or Charcot-Marie-Tooth disease.

Toe Conditions in the Adolescent. *Hallux valgus* may be seen in adolescents, especially in girls; commonly there is a family history of the deformity. Once the deformity begins, the forces created by growing bones generally make matters worse. Nonoperative treatments such as spacers between the 1st and 2nd toes and wider shoes are not usually successful in the adolescent; surgical correction may be necessary. This condition may reflect faulty development of the bones as in pseudohypoparathyroidism or pseudopseudohypoparathyroidism (Sec. 19.19).

Overlapping or Underlapping Fifth Toe. Such anomalies are very common. Underlapping of the 5th toe beneath the 4th is not a functional problem, but if wearing shoes causes pain, surgical correction may be necessary. In overlapping 5th toe, if the joint capsule and the extensor tendons become so tight that the fit of shoes is difficult, surgical correction is indicated.

Macrodactyly (Enlargement of One Toe). This may be associated with vascular anomalies or neurofibromatosis. Surgical fusion of the epiphyses at the appropriate age may ultimately result in normal length, but the diameter of the toe is not so easily controlled. When fitting of a shoe becomes a problem, amputation of all or part of the toe may be needed.

23.2 THE HIP

Congenital Dysplasia of the Hip. This lesion results from abnormal development of one or all of the components of the hip joint: the acetabulum, the femoral head, and the surrounding capsule and soft tissues. The head of the femur may be dislocated and may or may not be relocatable in the acetabulum. Alternatively, the hip joint may be so lax that the femoral head in the acetabulum is dislocatable and spontaneously relocates. In subluxation the capsule is lax enough that the femoral head may be partially displaced from its position within the acetabulum but cannot be dislocated. In acetabular dysplasia the femoral head is well seated and the capsule sufficiently tight that there is no subluxation, but the angle of the acetabulum faces laterally to such an extent that dislocation may occur later in childhood.

The etiology of congenital dysplasia of the hip is multifactorial. There are genetic factors, and girls are more commonly affected than boys. It also may be associated with other abnormalities such as clubfeet and arthrogryposis or with a breech delivery, in which case uterine position or the trauma of delivery may be important factors. Abnormal laxity of the surrounding capsule and the ligaments may reflect hormonal changes in the mother.

Diagnosis. The hips should be examined in every newborn child and re-examined at every routine follow-up visit during the first year of life. With the infant supine the examiner should inspect the contours of the lower extremities. While asymmetric folds may be seen in normal children, extra skin folds on the medial aspect of one thigh suggest that the femur has been dislocated proximally. *With the legs extended, the perineum should not be readily visible.* If it is, one should suspect bilateral dislocation, a condition likely to be missed when one hip is compared with the other.

The thighs should be flexed, then abducted fully. In the neonate each thigh should abduct to almost 90°; abduction less than 60–70° indicates an abnormality. The stability of the hip joint should also be evaluated to see whether the femoral head can be displaced from the acetabulum and then replaced. During this motion the examiner may get the sensation of the head "clunking" out of the acetabulum and over its posterior margin. Stability is determined in the following manner (Fig. 23–5A and B): both the tibia and the femur are held in the palm of the hand so that any clinking sensations in the knees

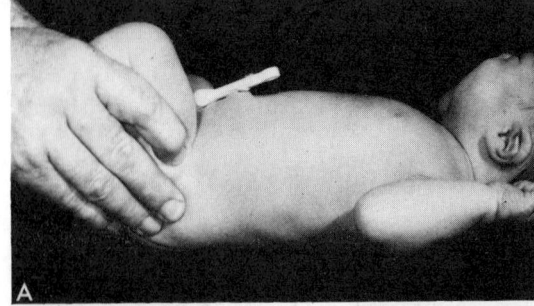
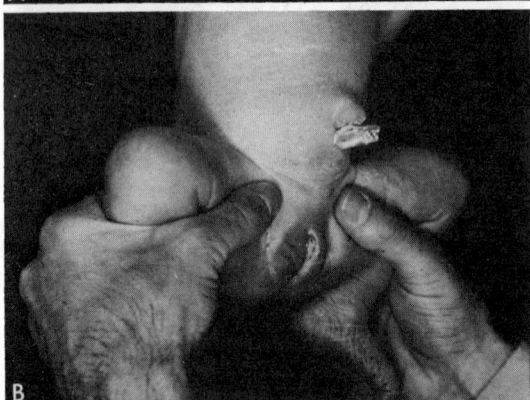
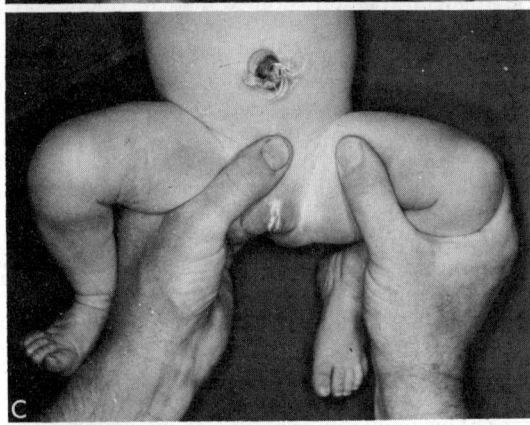
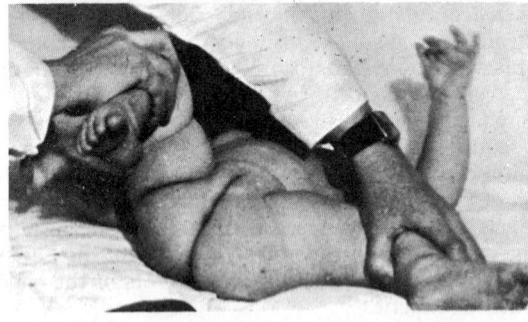

Figure 23–5. *A,* The newborn child is laid on its back with the hips and knees flexed, and the middle finger of each hand is placed over each greater trochanter. *B,* The thumb of each hand is applied to the inner side of the thigh opposite the lesser trochanter. *C,* In a doubtful case the pelvis may be steadied between a thumb over the pubis and fingers under the sacrum while the hip is tested with the other hand. *D,* Limitation of abduction is an early sign of congenital dislocation of the hip. Note restriction in abduction of right leg.

will not be confused with those in the hip. The long finger of the examiner is placed over the greater trochanter; the thumb is placed medially and just distal to the position of the long finger. The thighs are held in midabduction. The femoral head is then pulled out of the acetabulum by lateral pressure of the thumb and by rocking the knee medially with the knuckle of the index finger (Barlow test). If the femoral head can be displaced out of the acetabulum and over its posterior rim, the reverse maneuver is performed by pressing the long finger on the greater trochanter and rocking the knee laterally in order to replace the femoral head into the acetabulum (Ortolani maneuver).

If the femoral head can be felt to move laterally without coming out of the joint, the hip is classified as *subluxable*. If the head can be totally displaced out of the joint and replaced, it is classified as *dislocatable/relocatable*. The head may be found in the dislocated position and be relocatable but so unstable that dislocation immediately occurs again. This would be classified *dislocated/relocatable*. In the newborn period there are few dislocated hips that cannot be relocated, except in arthrogryposis. After the first weeks of life, however, an unstable hip may become fixed in the dislocated position. The adductor muscles and tendons will shorten so that limitation of abduction is even more obvious. At this point it is probable that the femoral head cannot be relocated by the Ortolani maneuver.

As the hip joint is moved through abduction, the examiner may feel the sensation of a high-pitched "click." This is not the same as the "clunk" that is felt as the femoral head is being displaced over the posterior acetabular margin and dropped either behind the acetabulum or back into it. The cause of the "click" is unknown. It usually disappears in the first weeks of life and is by itself of no significance.

Roentgenographic examination of the newborn's hips may be difficult to interpret because of the large ratio of cartilage to bone and absence of an ossified head. An anteroposterior roentgenogram will usually reveal lateral and superior displacement of the femoral head from the shadow acetabulum, which may be appreciated better after drawing certain lines in relation to the acetabula (Fig. 23–6) In the first few days of life dislocation may be seen on an anteroposterior roentgen-ogram of the pelvis and hips made with the femora abducted 45° and rotated medially (von Rosen maneuver).

Treatment. Therapy of the dysplastic hip depends on the age of the child at the time of diagnosis and the age of the abnormality on clinical examination. In a neonate with subluxation (i.e., femoral head and acetabulum are normal but the capsule is lax) the goal of treatment is to hold the legs in abduction until the capsule tightens, about 6 wk. This can be accomplished with a rigid device, such as a von Rosen splint or an Ilfeld brace, or one that allows some mobility, such as a Frejka pillow or Pavlik harness. The simple use of multiple diapers is not advised because adductor muscles of the thigh usually overpower soggy diapers and abduction is not maintained.

For the hip that is dislocatable and relocatable, a more reliable form of fixation is preferable, especially one which is not removed by the mother at each diaper change (e.g., Pavlik stirrups or von Rosen splint). Children under the age of 6–8 mo with a dislocated and unrelocatable hip should be treated with Pavlik stirrups directly. Over the succeeding 2–6 wk spontaneous reduction of the hip occurs in approximately 90% of children. The mechanism of this phenomenon is not understood, but after spontaneous reduction, the Pavlik stirrups should be maintained for several months until the hip is stable. If spontaneous reduction does not take place after 6 wk of treatment in Pavlik stirrups, or if the child is older than 6–8 months at the time of diagnosis, then the child should be treated by traction followed by closed reduction. An adductor tenotomy may be required to relocate the femoral head. Under no circumstances should be hips be forcefully relocated without preceding traction because of the increased risk of avascular necrosis of the femoral head. When traction has stretched the tissues sufficiently to allow the hip to be placed easily into the acetabulum, the dislocation is reduced under general anesthesia and held in a spica cast with the hips abducted about 45–60°. The cast is changed approximately every 6 wk to allow for the child's growth; immobilization is continued for a time equal to the age of the child at the time of diagnosis but not longer than 6 mo. Thereafter, a splinting device may be needed to maintain the hips in abduction until the acetabulum has developed satisfactorily. Occasionally, in spite of traction and an adductor tenotomy, the femoral head cannot be reduced. Under such circumstances open reduction should be performed.

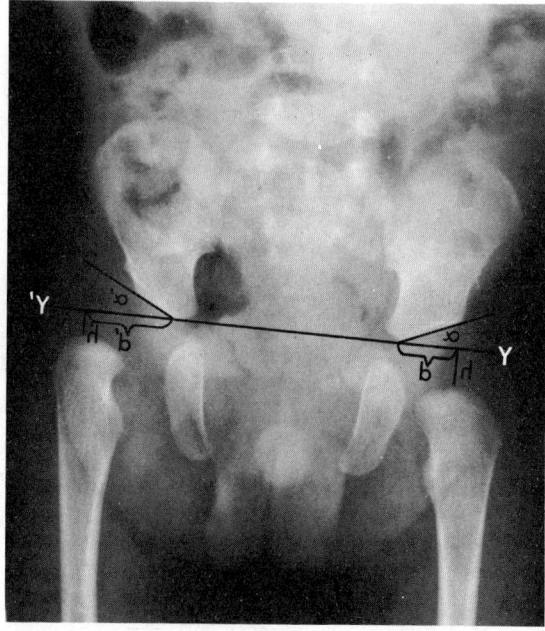

A

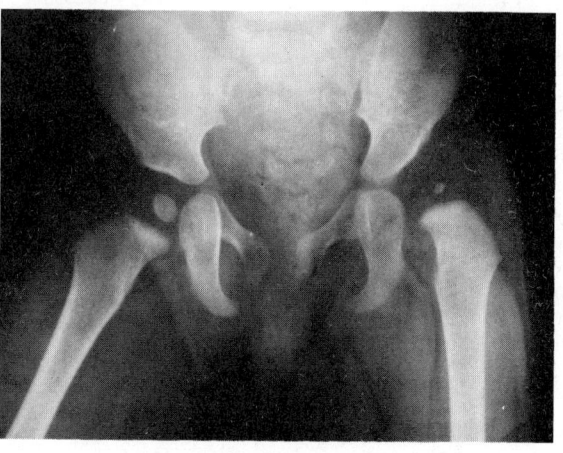

B

Figure 23–6. *A,* The Hilgenreiner method for identification of dysplasia of the hip prior to ossification of the capital femoral epiphysis: α' is greater than α, indicating greater obliquity of the acetabular roof. *d'* is greater than *d,* indicating lateral displacement of the femur. *h* is greater than *h',* indicating cephalic displacement of the femur. These relations indicate dysplasia of the patient's left hip. *B,* Congenital dislocation of left hip. The bony roof of the left acetabulum is quite oblique and there is the beginning of a false acetabulum above its most lateral aspect. The left femur is displaced laterally and superiorly. The left femoral capital epiphyseal center is smaller than the right.

In a child whose dislocation of the hip has not been discovered until after 18 mo of age, the most satisfactory form of therapy is usually open reduction with a simultaneous osteotomy of the pelvis to create a better roof over the femoral head (Salter innominate osteotomy). It may be necessary to combine this with shortening of the femur to achieve reduction in older children.

In **acetabular dysplasia** the acetabulum itself may be inadequately developed so that it faces more laterally than is normal; further maldevelopment may lead to a dislocation of the hip. The diagnosis of acetabular dysplasia is made on a roentgenogram taken because of limited hip abduction; the acetabular angle will be high, and the contour of the bony acetabulum will not be concave. The very young child may be treated by any device that holds the hip in abduction, usually for 3–6 mo. For a child over 18 mo of age, surgery may be required to provide better coverage for the femoral head and prevent dislocation.

In **congenital coxa vara** the neck of the femur makes less than the expected 135° angle with the shaft of the femur. It is not usually encountered under 2–3 yr of age, and the etiology is not known. The physical findings may simulate a dislocated hip because the shaft of the femur is located proximally relative to the normal side. On the other hand, the motion of the hip will be virtually normal, and there will be no laxity of the femoral head within the acetabulum. If this condition is left untreated, the varus deformity usually worsens. Treatment is osteotomy of the proximal femur to increase the femoral neck/shaft angle.

The Painful Hip. The causes of painful hip in a child and its evaluation vary considerably at different ages.

The Infant. The most likely cause of a painful hip joint in an infant is a **bacterial infection** (see Tuberculosis of the Hip, below). This infection may be caused by a bloodborne contamination of the hip joint or may be secondary to extension of osteomyelitis of the neck of the femur into the hip joint (Sec. 11.14–11.15). The capacity of the hip joint to hold an increased volume of fluid is maximal when the hip is held in about 20° of flexion, abduction, and lateral rotation (Fig. 23–7). Any attempt to move the thigh from this position will cause distress.

A roentgenogram of the infant's hip often reveals lateral displacement of the femoral head and of the fat adjacent to the capsule due to fluid accumulation. Aspiration of the hip will confirm the diagnosis and permit appropriate bacteriologic study. A needle of at least 18 gauge caliber is necessary for extraction of the thick pus. This procedure requires considerable expertise. General anesthesia is often helpful; fluoroscopic control should be used.

A septic hip joint should be treated immediately. The joint must be opened and the pus removed, with liberal irrigation and subsequent closed tube drainage. Antibiotics should be chosen initially with the knowledge that infecting agents commonly include *Haemophilus influenzae* and salmonella as well as *Staphylococcus aureus*.

The prognosis in an infant is poor. Not only is there destruction of the cartilage, but obstruction of the vascular supply to the femoral head, which passes across the joint space of the hip, may occur, causing avascular necrosis with lifelong crippling.

The Toddler. As with infants, infection is the most common cause of hip pain in the toddler, and the same discussion is applicable.

Children as young as 18 mo may suffer from **transient synovitis** ("toxic synovitis"). This is a disorder of unknown etiology which results in a painful hip and gives all the signs of mild inflammation. The episode may follow a viral upper respiratory tract infection by a few days to 2 wk. The major significance of the disorder is the possibility of overlooking a bacterial infection. Treatment is usually bed rest. Occasionally, the pain may be sufficiently severe to require in-hospital traction with the hip in flexion. The sedimentation rate can be elevated; however, the alpha$_2$-globulin is rarely greater than 1.0 mg/dL. The prognosis is excellent.

Other causes of painful hip in the toddler are *juvenile rheumatoid arthritis* and *leukemia* (in which monarticular pain is the first sign in 5% of cases).

The 2 to 10 Year Old. In the child of 4 yr and older, infection is much less common, but it results in severe damage to the joint if the diagnosis is delayed. It must always be suspected and excluded, but transient synovitis and Legg-Calvé-Perthes disease are more common causes of painful hip.

Legg-Calvé-Perthes disease is an avascular necrosis of the femoral head. Boys are affected more often than girls. The common age range is 5–9 yr, but children 2–11 may be affected.

At the onset of the avascular event the hip is painful and the symptoms indistinguishable from transient synovitis; a roentgenogram of the hips may show bulging of the capsule but will often be normal. If there has been disuse of the leg, the metaphysis may be more lucent than the epiphyseal center. A radioisotope bone scan (in anteroposterior and in frog leg lateral) may show decreased uptake in the femoral head (Fig. 23–8). Subsequently, in the repair process there is revascularization of the femoral head. As new bone is laid down upon the dead trabecular bone, resorption of the dead areas begins. At this point a roentgenogram will show increased density in the femoral head where new bone has been added. A subarticular fracture line may be seen anterolaterally, and there will be gradual distortion of the femoral head (Fig. 23–9). Healing occurs over 2–3 yr. While the repair proceeds, marked distortion of the femoral head and neck can lead to an imperfect joint.

The goal of *treatment* is to retain the normal spherical shape of the femoral head during the hip's natural repair process. In the past this was attempted by efforts to relieve the hip of weight bearing—by bed rest (up to several years) or by a variety of braces that kept the affected limb off the

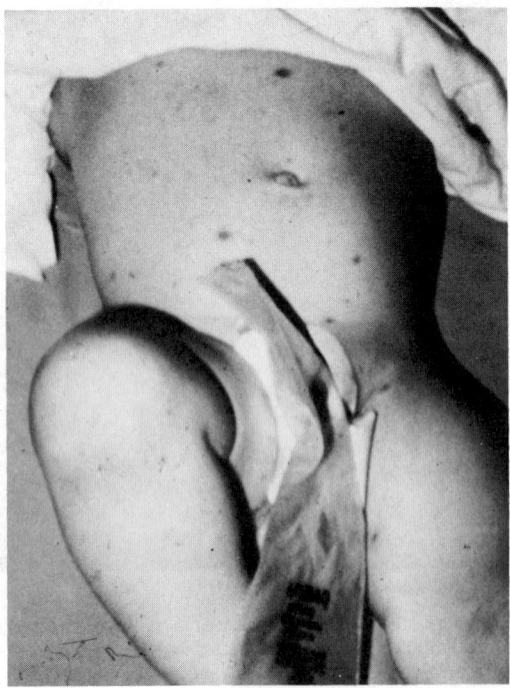

Figure 23–7. An infant with a bacterial infection of the hip holds the joint flexed, abducted, and laterally rotated.

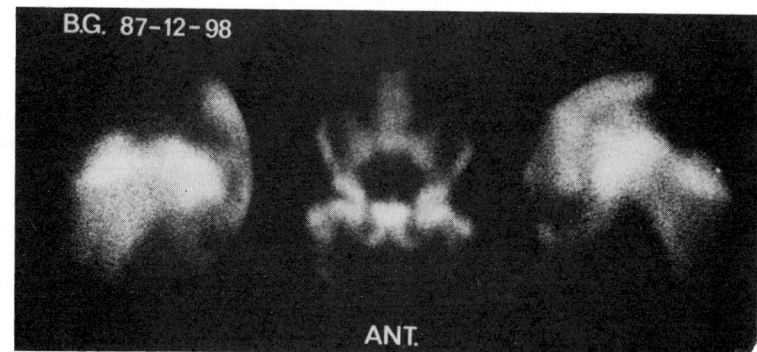

Figure 23–8. Legg-Calvé-Perthes disease. The radionuclide scan of the pelvis and hips reveals an area of decreased uptake in the head of the right femur. This is best seen in the isolated image on the right and can be compared with the normal left hip.

ground—but the proportion of patients who were left with distorted femoral heads was high. Current therapy allows the child to continue weight bearing but with the femur in an abducted position so that the head is well contained by the acetabulum. This decreases focal areas of increased load and minimizes distortion. Weight bearing in abduction may be accomplished by Petrie casts (long leg casts with the legs held in abduction and medial rotation by a bar between the two casts) or by braces which hold the legs in the same position. Surgical procedures have been developed to keep the femoral head abducted in relation to the acetabulum, either by varus osteotomy of the proximal femur or by Salter innominate osteotomy, which orients the acetabulum anterolaterally to cover the femoral head. Which of these methods of treatment is best has not been established.

TUBERCULOSIS OF THE HIP. The hip is the joint most often affected by tuberculosis. The disease may begin in the synovial membrane but usually starts as an infection in the femoral epiphysis or greater trochanteric apophysis with subsequent breakthrough into the joint. See also Sec. 11.46.

The first symptom is usually an intermittent slight limp, occurring when the patient first gets out of bed and after exercise. It may disappear for days or weeks at a time. Pain may be present at this stage or develop later and is usually referred to the knee or the medial aspect of the thigh. As destruction of the joint proceeds, the thigh is flexed and adducted, and rotation which initially was lateral becomes medial. Swelling about the hip increases and, if an abscess forms, pus may discharge anteriorly or be disseminated in other directions. Absorption of the head and neck of the femur may take place without evidence of suppuration.

Distinction must be made between Legg-Calvé-Perthes disease and tuberculous infections on the hip. In the former, roentgenographic changes do not extend beyond the femoral capital epiphysis and metaphysis, and the femoral capital epiphyseal center is relatively dense, not lucent. In the latter the acetabulum may also be affected. The two conditions may be indistinguishable in the early stage, and the clinical course and tuberculin reaction must be relied upon to differentiate them. The insidious onset of a tuberculous hip infection serves to distinguish it from rheumatic fever and acute arthritis.

Systemic isoniazid and ethambutol are indicated for 18 mo to treat tuberculosis of the hip and *tuberculous arthritis* of other joints. Intra-articular administration of drugs is not indicated. No controlled studies support bed rest immobilization, but it is recommended.

The Adolescent. Infection of the hip is rare in adolescents. More common causes of hip pain are slipped capital femoral epiphysis and traumatic avulsion of a muscle from its insertion.

In **slipped capital femoral epiphysis** the upper femoral epiphysis slips posteromedially off the metaphysis. This disorder occurs often in obese boys and can be bilateral. The slip may occur gradually or suddenly. Gradual slip may give

symptoms and signs like those of synovitis; often the diagnosis is delayed because the pain is referred to the medial aspect of the knee. Abduction and internal rotation are limited. Acute slip usually follows trauma, with pain, limited motion, and inability to walk.

The goal of *treatment* is to prevent further slipping. Threaded pins or screws may be inserted along the neck of the femur and across the epiphyseal cartilage. Occasionally, the slip may be so severe that there is marked limitation of medial rotation and flexion. In this situation the fixation of the epiphysis is accompanied by an osteotomy of the upper femur to regain the lost motions. Reduction of a slipped epiphysis may be successful but carries a very high risk of avascular necrosis.

Avulsion of muscles results when an adolescent does physical exertion more appropriate for an adult and pulls the origin or insertion of a muscle from its bony anchorage. The apophysis usually pulls free with the muscle. The sartorius can be pulled off the anterior superior iliac spine, the rectus femoris can be pulled off the anterior inferior spine, the iliopsoas from the lesser trochanter, or the hamstring muscles

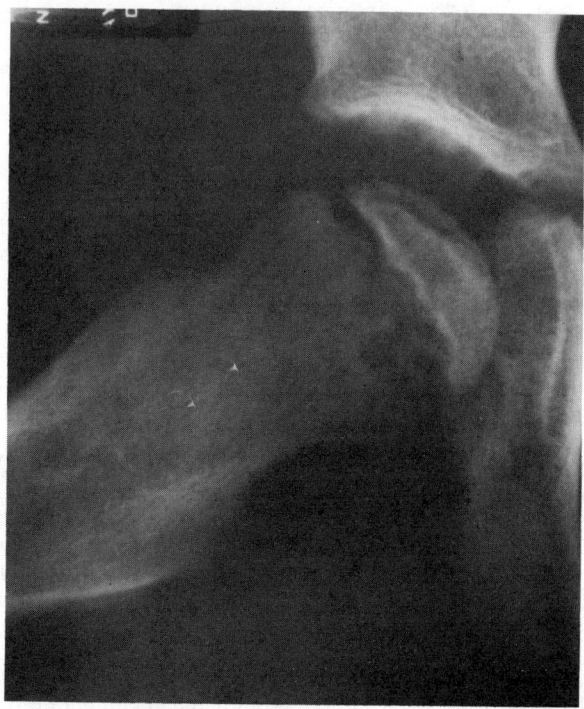

Figure 23–9. Legg-Calvé-Perthes disease. The lateral radiograph of the right hip reveals the epiphyseal line to be irregularly widened. The femoral capital epiphyseal center is flattened; there is a lucent defect in the anterior aspect of the center. Relative to the femoral neck, the secondary center is opaque.

from the ischial tuberosity. If the apophysis to which the muscle is attached is not ossified, the diagnosis by roentgenogram is more difficult. Suspicion of these possibilities and individually stressing these four muscles provide the clues for this diagnosis. The rectus femoris can be stressed by passive flexion of the knee with the hip extended, the psoas by medially rotating the thigh with the hip and knee fixed 90°, the hamstrings by flexing the hip with the knee extended, and the sartorius by placing the foot of the affected limb on top of the opposite knee and then resisting the patient's effort to flex the affected hip.

23.3   THE KNEE

Knee problems are not common in infants and young children, but the knee is a common site for disorders in the preadolescent and adolescent. Pain in the hip may be referred to the knee, and *an examination of the hip should be part of any examination of the knee joint.* The knee is also a common site of monarticular juvenile rheumatoid arthritis (Sec. 10.58); since this may be preceded by trauma, diagnostic confusion is common.

Popliteal Cysts. Characteristically, these are found posteriorly at the origin of the medial head of the gastrocnemius or the semitendinosus muscle. True Baker cysts (posterior herniations of the knee joint) are rare in childhood, but the term Baker cyst is commonly applied to popliteal cysts. These cysts most commonly resolve spontaneously and should not be treated. They may recur. Reasons to excise these benign lesions include persisting pain or limitation of motion, cosmetic concern, increasing size, or parental worry that cannot be alleviated.

Discoid Meniscus. This is a congenital disorder of the semilunar cartilage of the knee joint, almost invariably of the lateral side. Instead of being semilunar in configuration, the meniscus is disclike and may be cystic. Characteristically, it causes a popping sensation, and parents may notice a small mass that protrudes laterally at the knee joint. It is frequently bilateral. The treatment consists of excision of the meniscus to prevent later degenerative arthritis of the knee.

Osgood-Schlatter Disease. This is a disease of the anterior tibial tubercle. The apophysis is not well anchored on the infrapatellar ligament of the quadriceps, onto which it is attached, so that excessive activity involving the quadriceps results in pain and swelling in the region. The anterior tibial tubercle becomes prominent and is tender to direct pressure. Any activity that stresses the quadriceps reproduces this pain.

The goal of *treatment* is to decrease the stress at the tubercle. Often a period of 4–8 wk of restriction from strenuous physical activity, especially activities requiring deep knee bending, is sufficient. If the pain is not satisfactorily controlled in this manner, a cast may be required to rest the knee, a situation that is particularly difficult if the condition is bilateral. The problem ceases when the apophysis fuses to the metaphysis, but there may be several years of annoying pain. The bump at the anterior tubercle often alarms parents. Rarely, in the older adolescent excision of a residual ossicle deep to the ligament is needed to bring relief.

Osteochondritis Dissecans. In this condition of unknown etiology a small fragment of the bone underlying the articular cartilage of the knee becomes avascular. It characteristically occurs on the lateral aspect of the medial condyle of the femur but may occur anywhere over the distal femoral surface. Treatment is generally symptomatic. Application of a cast for as little as 6 wk may suffice, though the roentgenographic defect may persist for several years. Occasionally, the fragment and its adjacent articular cartilage break off and float freely in the knee joint. The fragment is either excised or repositioned and held in place with bone pegs or nails. The

prognosis for patients under 17 yr is good, for those over 17 only fair.

Dislocating Patella. The patella may dislocate laterally because of loose ligamentous structures (as seen in the child with Down syndrome) or a laterally inserted infrapatellar ligament. If the dislocation recurs, surgical reconstruction of the attachments of the patella may be needed. Sometimes a child's knee dislocates and then pops back prior to clinical examination. In such cases the knee should be examined in full extension and the patella pushed laterally as far as possible. The child who has a dislocating patella will have an involuntary contraction of the quadriceps to resist this maneuver, whereas the child with a normal knee will not.

Chondromalacia of the Patella. This condition of one or both patellae is characterized by pain within the knee whenever the leg is actively used with the knee flexed, as in going up or down stairs. There may be a sensation of buckling or giving way. Its cause is unknown, but it is often aggravated by poor mechanics of the patella sliding on the femur. It is most common in teenage girls. Examination of the knee in a child with chondromalacia rarely shows any effusion, which is common in adults. With the knee in full extension, downward pressure on the patella, impacting it against the femur, is very painful. This is exaggerated if the patient is asked to stress the quadriceps during the maneuver. Tenderness along the medial border of the articular margin of the patella is common.

Reassurance that the child is not suffering from juvenile rheumatoid arthritis or bone malignancy is often adequate treatment for the mild case. The next order of treatment, often with the administration of aspirin, is an exercise program aimed at strengthening the medial portion of the quadriceps muscle to realign the patella's motion on the femur. These exercises should be done with the knee in extension. Occasionally, surgery is required to realign the patella or to excise areas of softened cartilage and to drill the underlying cortical bone to allow the ingrowth of fibrocartilage.

23.4   THE LEG

Bowing of the Tibia. In the newborn, anterior or anterolateral bowing, as seen in neurofibromatosis, is often preliminary to fracture and ultimate nonunion (pseudoarthrosis), sometimes requiring amputation. It is important that affected infants have bone grafting procedures done early before the tibia breaks. Posterior bowing of the tibia is not associated with this sequence of events and may gradually remodel spontaneously.

Bowleg. Infants generally have bowing of the legs. By 12–18 mo of age the legs have straightened and progressed to mild knock knee; they will gradually assume their ultimate configuration by 6–7 yr of age (Fig. 23–10). If the bowing is outside the range shown in the graph, roentgenographic examination, with the child standing if possible, is required. In the absence of evidence for rickets of nutritional or of renal origin, the roentgenogram can be used to assess future change. Increasing bowing of the legs should be referred for evaluation.

Blount Disease (Tibia Vara). Of unknown etiology, this is a disorder of growth of the medial part of the proximal tibial epiphysis. Roentgenograms show irregularity of the medial aspect of the tibial metaphysis adjacent to the epiphysis, and distortion of the adjacent epiphyseal center (Fig. 23–11). The bowing begins as a sharp angulation at the metaphysis. Treatment is usually osteotomy of the proximal tibia and fibula, which may have to be repeated one or more times.

Knock Knees (Genu Valgum). This deformity can be assessed by measuring the distance between the medial malleoli of the ankles when the medial parts of the distal thighs are

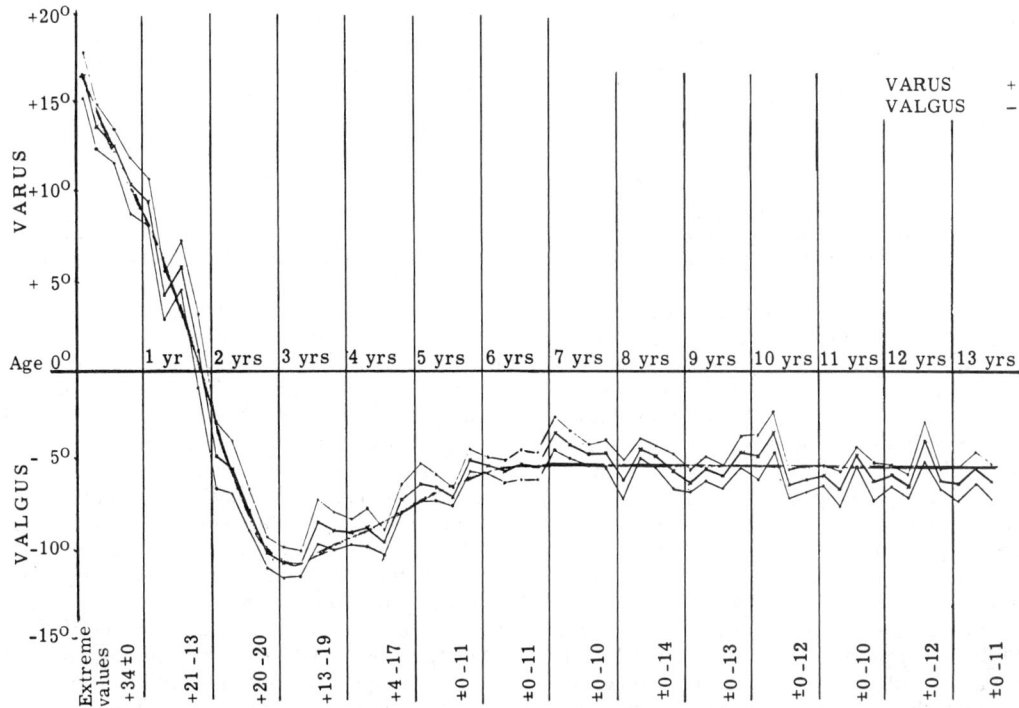

Figure 23–10. Development of the tibiofemoral angle during growth. (Salenius P, Vankka E: J Bone Joint Surg 57A:259, 1975.)

touching. Progressive knock knees after the age of 6 yr should be evaluated for an underlying abnormality and the need for surgical correction. There is no evidence that shoe wedges alter this abnormality or are needed to "protect" the feet from pronation.

"Growing Pains." Pain in the shins is common from the ages of 3–6 yr, especially at night after the child has gone to bed. The etiology is unknown but may involve edema of the muscle bodies within the tight fascial sheaths following a day of vigorous activity. Reassurance, the application of local heat, massage, and aspirin are usually adequate treatment. If the pain is severe and frequent, quinine sulfate given at supper-time can alleviate the problem.

Congenital Anomalies. Part or all of one of the bones of the lower extremity may be absent. Affected children should be cared for in centers where such deformities are frequently treated. Many of these children are best treated by appropriate removal of nonfunctional parts; rather than spending years in hospitals, they can then become fully active in prostheses. Small children readily accept prostheses for the lower extremity and should be fitted by the time they are ready to stand.

Congenital Short Femur. Children who are born with short femora can be divided into those who have a sound hip (or the elements from which a sound hip can be constructed) and those who do not. If the hip is sound and the knee and tibia appear to have the potential for normal development, lengthening the femur surgically may be possible, but most of these children require fusion of the shortened femur to the tibia. Removal of the foot then leaves a stump that will accept an appropriate prosthesis.

Inequality of Limb Length. Inequality of the lengths of the upper extremities is rarely of functional significance and seldom of cosmetic concern. Inequality of leg length, however, may require attention.

One side may be congenitally smaller (hemiatrophy) or larger (hemihypertrophy). *Congenital hemihypertrophy* is most likely due to faulty cell division of the zygote that results in two daughter cells of unequal size; it has been considered a form of incomplete twinning. Females are affected more often than males, the right side of the body more often than the left. The difference in the two sides is usually greatest in the extremities, the genitalia, and the trunk. Facial and palatal inequality may also be present. Paired internal organs are sometimes of unequal size. The bones of the larger size are longer and thicker than their counterparts and may differ in osseous maturation. Other malformations may be associated,

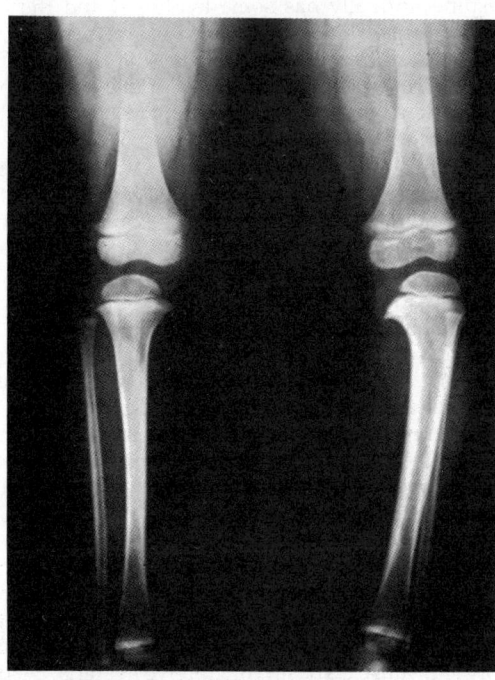

Figure 23–11. Blount disease. The medial aspect of the proximal end of the left tibia is irregular and "beaked." There is also minimal involvement of medial aspects of the proximal tibial epiphyseal center. As a consequence of the proximal tibial deformity, there was abnormal weight bearing, which in turn was responsible for the thickening shown in the medial cortex of the left tibia. The right tibia is normal.

such as aniridia, polydactyly, hypospadias, cryptorchidism, nevi, and hemangiomas. There is also an association with Wilms tumor and adrenal and hepatic neoplasms. Hemihypertrophy may be a feature of Beckwith-Wiedemann syndrome, in which the same neoplasms have been encountered.

Arteriovenous malformations, especially in the groin, may also result in significant overgrowth of a limb. Chronic inflammatory lesions about the knee, such as longstanding *juvenile rheumatoid arthritis*, may also stimulate growth, as may *fractures*, particularly those adjacent to epiphyseal cartilage plates.

A treatment plan begins with estimation of the ultimate limb length discrepancy at skeletal maturity through periodic (usually yearly) roentgenographic measurements of the extremities, together with an evaluation of the bone age in the left hand and wrist. Differences expected to be less than 2 cm at maturity usually do not need treatment. Anticipated greater differences can be treated by making the short leg longer or the long leg shorter. Usually the longer limb is shortened by surgically scraping away the epiphyseal cartilage at the appropriate end of the bone or by putting staples across it. The short leg continues growing and catches up with the long one. Shoe lifts are usually used until the child reaches the age for the definitive operation. Occasionally, the difference in leg length may be sufficiently large to warrant lengthening the short leg. While the surgical techniques are available, they require several stages and are fraught with complications. The procedure is best left in the hands of an experienced surgeon, and the parents need to be especially well informed about its limitations.

23.5 THE SPINE

The spinal problems most frequently encountered by the pediatrician often present as questions by parents about children's *poor posture*. The need is to determine whether the child's posture is merely habit or the result of an underlying skeletal deformity. Scoliosis is always abnormal, though it may not be a primary defect or always require treatment. The thoracic spine normally has some kyphosis, and the lumbar spine has lordosis. These are usually exaggerated in youngsters, gradually decreasing by the age of 8 or 9 yr. Only if these curves are excessive, either as primary or secondary problems, is there cause for concern. Scoliosis and kyphosis may be found together.

Posture. Many variations of standing posture are commensurate with health. The ramrod posture preferred by some patients is by no means ideal. Teenagers emulating their peers may slouch for no other reason than to irritate their parents. Shy teenage girls may prefer to slump, becoming round shouldered, in an attempt to hide their developing breasts.

Exercises aimed at strengthening the muscles of the upper trunk and developing "postural awareness" can combat slouching. An exercise program is only as useful as the child wants it to be, and insistent intervention by the pediatrician may only aggravate a conflict between parents and child. It is usually preferable and sufficient to reassure the parents that slouched posture does not lead to structural changes and that when the children are older and want to sit or stand differently, they will be able to do so.

Scoliosis. Side-to-side curves of the spine can be nonstructural or structural. Nonstructural curves have no axial rotation and show no residual deformity on bending as seen by roentgenograms. They are secondary to causes such as posture, short leg, muscle spasm, or, rarely, hysteria. Structural curves may be congenital in origin or secondary to metabolic problems, such as idiopathic juvenile osteoporosis or the Prader-Willi syndrome, or they may be secondary to a neuromuscular abnormality. Scoliosis is most commonly idiopathic. Idiopathic scoliosis is rarely seen within the 1st yr of

life ("infantile idiopathic") in North America, and uncommonly from 1–10 yr of age ("juvenile idiopathic"); it usually has its onset after 10 yr ("adolescent idiopathic").

Etiology. The etiology of idiopathic scoliosis is multifactorial, with an autosomal dominant genetic component and incomplete penetrance. Girls are much more commonly affected than boys. All members of the family should be carefully examined for scoliosis if one is found with the disorder. Patients with scoliosis should be warned to pay special attention to their offspring as they approach their teens.

Congenital scoliosis due to absence of a part of the spine or to a fusion of several segments of the spine is often associated with congenital anomalies of other organ systems within the same segmental level, particularly of the genitourinary tract and heart. One third of children with congenital scoliosis have abnormalities on intravenous urography.

Diagnosis. Structural curves can be separated from nonstructural curves on clinical examination by their associated spinal rotation. As the spine bends from side to side in scoliosis, there is an associated axial rotation. The bodies of the vertebral segments rotate toward the convexity and the spinous processes toward the concavity of the curve. Rotation of the spine is most readily appreciated if the patient is asked to bend forward with the arms hanging freely. In this position any prominence of one side of the rib cage is seen easily (more commonly on the right, as in Fig. 23–12). In the lumbar region only the short transverse processes protrude to push the paraspinous muscles posteriorly; therefore rotation is not as prominent. Patients who have rotational components to their curves should have a roentgenogram of the entire spine, anteroposterior, erect, preferably on a single film showing the full extent of the vertebral column from the chin to the anterior superior iliac spines.

The rotary component of scoliosis is its serious aspect. As the rotation of the thorax progresses, there is less room for the heart and lungs; pulmonary restriction may ultimately shorten the lifespan of the individual. In addition, curves of the lumbar region can be a source of significant pain in adult life.

Treatment. The goal of therapy is to keep the curve from increasing so that when growth ceases, the curve will be less than 40° (as measured by the Cobb method). This gives a reasonable expectation that progression thereafter will not present problems, whereas curves over 40° can increase after growth stops. For small curves (less than 10–15°) treatment is usually not required.

Curves from 20–40° in growing children can usually be managed with a brace worn 23 out of 24 hr a day throughout the period of growth. An alternative treatment consists of electrical stimulation. The usual technique is to apply two electrodes to the skin over the back or lateral aspect of the trunk. These electrodes are energized by a small portable power pack and are applied each night throughout the remaining years of spine maturation. This technique obviates the need to wear a spine brace throughout the day and is approximately as effective as brace treatment. However, some children cannot tolerate the discomfort of the electric current during their sleep. Treatment compliance is also harder to monitor, and the reliability of the apparatus has been variable. In most spine treatment centers the choice of brace or electrical stimulation is left up to the patient and parents.

Curves over 40° are generally managed by spinal fusion (most commonly posterior and the insertion of metal rod (Harrington rod) to obtain correction and to help hold the curve during the time required for the fusion to become solid. Some children must have their spines fused anteriorly. There has been concern that fusion before growth ceases will prevent that segment of the spine from growing. Fusion does prevent

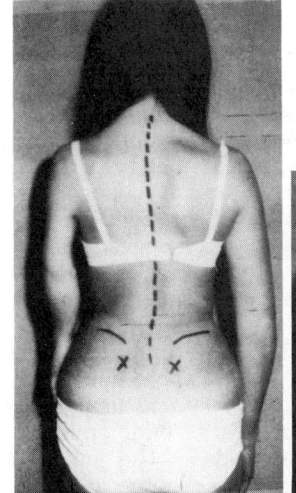
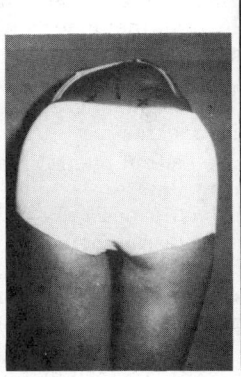
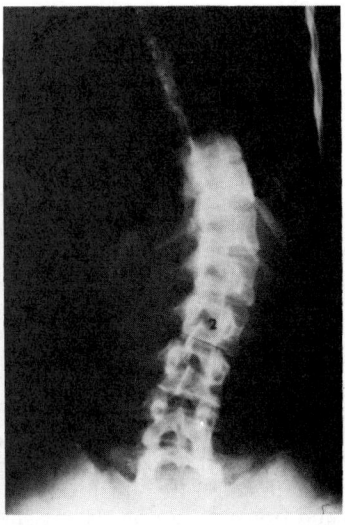

Figure 23–12. Scoliosis. The spine rotates as it curves, with the spinous processes moving toward the concavity. The severe curve of 46° seen by roentgenogram on the right is only partly recognizable when the patient stands upright. However, examination with the child's spine flexed shows the rotation on the right that indicates a structural scoliosis.

growth, but a spine with a marked curve is short anyway. A short straight spine is more desirable than a short crooked spine, particularly in congenital scoliosis in which lack of segmentation on one side of the spine will lead to an ever-progressing curve that must be fused as soon as it is recognized, even as early as a few months of age.

Kyphosis. Excessive thoracic kyphosis may be congenital or acquired. Congenital kyphosis is secondary to a lack of segmentation of the vertebral bodies anteriorly or to a lack of formation of one or more vertebral bodies. Generally, this requires surgical fusion; delay can lead to paraplegia.

Acquired kyphosis is a condition of unknown etiology. The child stands with an increased roundback in the thoracic region. There may be pain. Usually, there is a compensatory increase in lumbar lordosis.

The examiner should have the child bend forward as far as possible, allowing the arms to dangle freely. The spine is observed from the side. There should be a smooth curve going from the neck to the buttocks with no sharp angulation (Fig. 23–13). Normal lumbar lordosis should completely correct either to flat or to slight kyphosis. Any suspicion of abnormality is an indication for a standing lateral roentgenogram of the thoracolumbar spine. The thoracic kyphosis should not measure more than 40°; irregularity of the apophyseal growing areas of the vertebral bodies may be apparent (Scheuermann disease).

Excessive kyphosis may increase after the end of growth and become a major problem in later life if there is osteoporosis, a particular problem for females.

The goal of *treatment* is to reduce the thoracic kyphosis to less than 40°. Reduction can generally be achieved with brace treatment if the spine has not completed growth. If the curve is severe—for example, in excess of 60°—or if the spine has stopped growing, fusion may be required.

Spondylolysis and Spondylolisthesis. In these conditions of unknown etiology there is a discontinuity in the pars interarticularis of the posterior elements of the spine between the superior and inferior facet joints. The discontinuity (**spondylolysis**) may result in the forward slipping of one vertebral body on the one below, creating a lesion called spondylolisthesis. This occurs most frequently between L5 and the sacrum but may occur between L4 and L5, and even higher. A congenital variety of spondylolisthesis associated with an elongated pars interarticularis and defective facets allows forward slipping without a break in the pars. Trauma, especially stress in hyperextension, may cause a fracture in the pars interarticularis. Genetic factors are prominent.

Spondylolisthesis is usually associated with low back pain.

The propensity to slip forward is exaggerated during the growth spurt, and the forward slip can be so severe that the vertebral body can fall off the one below. Irritation of the L5 and S1 roots is common and results in limitation in straight leg raising with hamstringing spasm. The *diagnosis* of spondylolisthesis can be made from a standing lateral roentgenogram of the lumbosacral spine. Diagnosis of spondylolysis requires oblique roentgenograms of the lumbosacral spine to show the defective pars interarticularis. When roentgenograms are inconclusive, tomography or radionuclide bone scan may be helpful.

Treatment is directed at relieving pain and preventing further slipping. Excessive lumbar lordosis will increase the mechanical sheer forces leading to slipping; therefore exercises to reduce lumbar lordosis may relieve pain. Activities associated with hyperextension of the lumbar spine should be avoided. Braces may be helpful, or surgery may be required to relieve pain. Even if pain is under control, patients should be monitored for roentgenographic evidence of progressive slipping of the vertebrae. For progressive slipping, spinal fusion is necessary.

Tuberculous Spondylitis (see also Sec. 11.46). Tuberculous spondylitis originates in the body of one or more vertebrae, results in destruction of bone, and spreads to all of the tissues of the articulation. The spinous process and posterior arches are unaffected. Kyphosis is most common in midthoracic

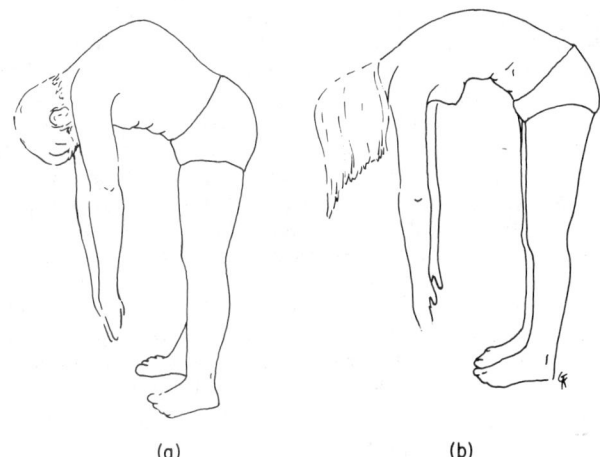

(a)   (b)

Figure 23–13. Note the sharp break in contour in the child with abnormal kyphosis (a) compared with the contour in the normal child (b).

lesions; scoliosis may accompany kyphosis if the lesion is disproportionately unilateral. The lower part of the thoracic spine is most likely to be involved, with the lumbar and the cervical segments next in order of frequency. Paraplegia may occur when the upper thoracic or cervical region is affected but is rarely associated with involvement below the midthoracic region. A *psoas abscess* results from the dissection of pus from an involved lumbar vertebra. A cold abscess in the cervical vertebrae may open into the pharynx (retropharyngeal abscess) or above the clavicle; one originating opposite the lower cervical or upper thoracic vertebrae may rupture into the pleura or penetrate into the scapula, but often it gravitates and points above Poupart ligament.

Clinical manifestations are insidious in onset. Persistent or intermittent pain may occur over the distribution of the spinal nerves arising adjacent to the affected vertebrae. This pain is increased by pressure on the head but not by pressure over the lesions. Muscular rigidity splints the back, and the child assumes a position that reduces weight on the diseased spine and prevents jarring. He or she may avoid bending to reach an object on the floor, may walk stiffly or carefully on the toes, or may prefer to lie on the abdomen and to rest frequently across a chair or over a parent's lap. With cervical involvement the child may hold the head stiffly or support it with a hand.

Acute nontuberculous osteomyelitis of the vertebrae can be distinguished by its greater toxicity, leukocytosis, and fever. Roentgenographic abnormalities are usually well established in a tuberculous lesion of the vertebrae when symptoms first become manifest, whereas they are not likely to be demonstrable during the first days of acute pyogenic osteomyelitis.

With *treatment* the reparative process may not begin for 1–3 yr, but recovery with ankylosis and little or no deformity can be expected in the majority of well-treated cases. Paraplegia may resolve completely. Traditional therapy consisted of holding the patient in continuous extension on a Bradford frame or in a plaster body jacket until there was no evidence of active infection. Immobilization has not been shown, however, to improve the results of antibiotic treatment of tuberculosis of the thoracic or lumbar vertebrae. In paraplegic patients or those with extensive bone destruction and necrosis, surgical debridement and bone grafting, with 18 mo of systemic administration of isoniazid and ethambutol, have produced the best results. A third drug may be indicated in areas of the world where resistant organisms are prevalent. When surgical facilities and skills are not available, ambulatory two-drug antibiotic treatment alone may be effective but is associated with increased morbidity (scoliosis or kyphosis).

Back Pain in Children. Back pain is frequently a sign of a significant underlying disorder. Roentgenographic examination should be made in order to identify Scheuermann disease, spondylolisthesis, evidence of infection in the vertebral bodies, or narrowing of the disc space that might indicate an adjacent bony infection ("discitis"). Lesions such as osteoid osteoma and infection may be the cause of considerable pain and yet be very difficult to locate by roentgenography; children with persistent back pain and no roentgenographic abnormalities should have a radionuclide bone scan.

Sacral Agenesis. This abnormality has a high incidence in infants of diabetic mothers (Sec. 8.58). There is an absence of one or more lumbar vertebral segments, the iliac wings are not anchored to any bone structure, and the femora and tibiae are usually short. There are marked flexion contractures and webbing of the skin between the leg and the thigh. The feet are usually abnormal. Renal anomalies are frequently associated.

For this devastating anomaly rehabilitation usually requires amputation of the lower extremities at the knees or hips, with prosthetic replacement. The absence of connection between the ilia and the lumbar vertebrae presents difficulties with spinal curvature.

23.6 THE NECK

Congenital Torticollis. It should be possible to turn the head of a newborn infant 90° in both directions, but limitation of motion of the neck may not become apparent until 1 wk of age. The inability to achieve this range of motion should suggest congenital torticollis, a condition in which the sternocleidomastoid muscle on one side is shortened. In early infancy the muscle may contain a firm mass in its midportion, but this is not evident after 2–3 mo. If this condition goes untreated, the muscle becomes fibrotic and shortened, the head and face become asymmetric, and there will be permanent limitation of motion in the neck. The etiology of this condition is unknown. (See also Sec. 22.6).

The initial treatment is exercise to stretch the involved sternocleidomastoid muscle. This requires turning the face toward the affected muscle but tilting it in the opposite direction and extending the neck. For example, if the right sternocleidomastoid muscle is affected, the chin should be turned to the right, the left ear brought down toward the left shoulder, and the neck extended. This position should be held for a count of 5 and repeated 10 times, twice daily. This exercise requires one person to hold the thorax and shoulders and another to hold the infant's head with a hand on each side. It is best done with the infant's head extended over the end of a table (Fig. 23–14). The exercise requires very explicit instruction to the parents. In addition, the crib should be placed so that the child who turns the head in the wrong direction sees less interesting objects. Similarly, the way in which the parents feed and play with the child can be used to encourage turning the head in the proper direction. If exercises do not give full correction, surgical release of the sternocleidomastoid muscle will be necessary.

Spastic Torticollis. After mild trauma or a tonsillar infection a child may complain of pain in the neck and hold the neck to one side in a fixed position. Such behavior immediately suggests a rotary subluxation of the atlantoaxial joint. If there is no roentgenographic evidence of subluxation, treatment with a soft collar (which can be readily made from a rolled towel pinned or taped in place), application of local heat, and the use of aspirin are usually sufficient. Occasionally, cervical traction is required. Mild or persistent cervical pain should

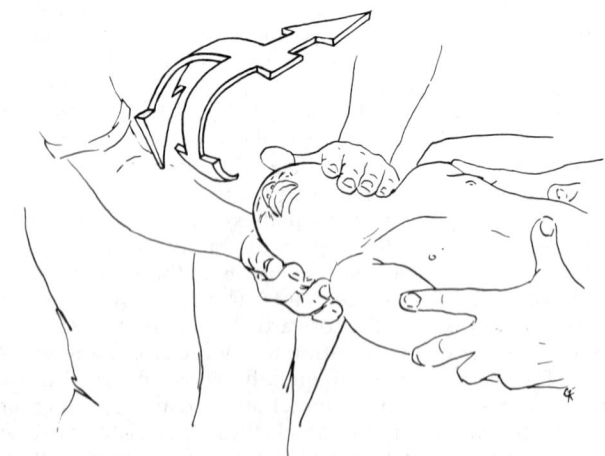

Figure 23–14. Exercises to stretch out a tight sternocleidomastoideus muscle in congenital torticollis. The motion is a combination of rotation toward the affected (right) side, tilting away from the affected side, and extension of the neck.

suggest the possibility of juvenile rheumatoid arthritis. Intraspinal tumors can also cause torticollis.

Klippel-Feil Disorder. This congenital dysgenesis consists of failure of segmentation of the cervical spine and is often associated with congenital anomalies of other skeletal parts of the same segment, such as Sprengel deformity (Sec. 23.8). Generally, no treatment is required for the cervical spine itself.

23.7 DEFORMITIES OF THE STERNUM

Fissure of the sternum is the term used when the halves of the sternum remain separated. *Pigeon breast* is prominence of the sternum and the cartilaginous parts of the ribs, with lateral depresssions of the thorax. A short sternum is a common manifestation of trisomy 18.

Pectus excavatum (Sec. 13.104), or indentation of the lower half of the sternum, may be rachitic in origin or the result of chronic obstruction to respiration. In most instances, however, the condition is congenital. The manubrium is at the normal level, but the inferior parts are depressed, the xiphoid approaching the vertebral bodies. The deformity can have adverse psychologic effects on the child. Surgical improvement may be attempted for cosmetic reasons if the deformity is severe or if compression adversely affects pulmonary function.

23.8 THE UPPER EXTREMITIES

Sprengel Deformity. In this congenital condition the scapula fails to descend completely from its embryonic position in the neck to its usual thoracic location. It may be unilateral or bilateral. There may be a fibrous, cartilaginous, or osseous connection between the scapula and the spine (an omovertebral connection). The scapula is smaller than usual, and abduction of the arm may be limited. There is webbing of the neck, which is often exaggerated by a short neck resulting from associated congenital anomalies of the cervical spine (Klippel-Feil disorder). There may be associated abnormalities of the kidneys and decreased hearing acuity. Treatment is directed at releasing the omovertebral connection to allow greater motion. Removal of the upper segment of the scapula and repositioning the scapula inferiorly improve the appearance.

Congenital Amputations of the Upper Extremity. Congenital amputations more commonly involve the upper extremity than the lower. They may involve only parts of fingers or may extend to the loss of an entire arm and represent intrauterine destruction of limbs that were originally normally formed. Children with congenital amputations of the upper extremities should be seen in specialized facilities as soon as possible. An appropriate prosthesis can be used after the child is able to sit. The first prosthesis is usually nothing more than a paddle to allow two-handed functions. When a child is 1.5–2 yr of age, an active terminal device can be fitted. If prosthetic management is not started early, children develop one-handed patterns that are virtually impossible to break. Cosmetic prostheses with actively operated hands are not available for children under about 5 yr of age and are very expensive. In the absence of sensory feedback children frequently abuse such structures (e.g., use a hand as a hammer); accordingly, most physicians are reluctant to prescribe expensive and delicate prosthetic devices.

Deformities of the Extremities. Severe deformities of the extremities are often associated with other malformations incompatible with life. Surviving children with extensive defects of the limbs were rare until the epidemic resulting from maternal ingestion of thalidomide. Limb defects due to primary inhibition of development or growth are called *reduc-*

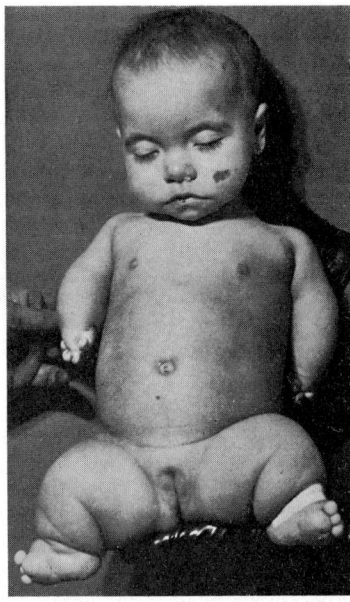

Figure 23–15. Partial phocomelia in an infant 11 mo of age, picture taken at autopsy.

tion malformations and frequently have terminal fingers or nails, indicating that no true amputation has occurred.

Amelia means absence of limbs. *Hemimelia* refers to defects of the distal parts of the extremities, such as absence of forearm and hand or lower leg and foot. *Phocomelia* signifies a great reduction in size of the proximal parts of the limb, resulting in an approach of distal parts toward the trunk (Fig. 23–15). In complete phocomelia the hand or foot seems to spring directly from the trunk. *Acheiria* and *apodia* are terms for absence of the hand or foot; *adactyly* for absence of digits (Fig. 23–16); and *aphalangia* for absence of phalanges.

Split hand and *split foot* are deep clefts in the anterior part of the hand or foot (Fig. 23–17), the foot appearing split where the 2nd or 3rd toe should be. Fingers and toes may have various degrees of syndactyly (Fig. 23–18). *Brachydactyly*, abnormal shortness of fingers or toes resulting from lack of or reduction in size of the phalanx or metacarpal bone, may be genetically determined. It may also be seen in pseudohypoparathyroidism, pseudopseudohypoparathyroidism, and Turner syndrome. *Clinodactyly*, incurving of the little finger, may be inherited as a dominant trait and is often seen in Down syndrome. *Camptodactyly*, permanently flexed fingers, can be transmitted as a dominant trait; it also occurs in trisomies D and E. *Macrodactyly* is a hypertrophy of one or several fingers and toes and may be a manifestation of neurofibromatosis.

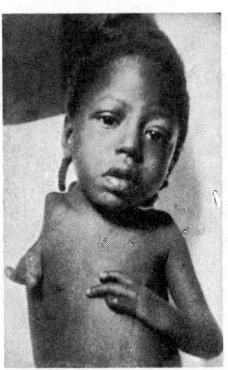

Figure 23–16. Phocomelia and partial adactyly in a girl 3.5 yr of age.

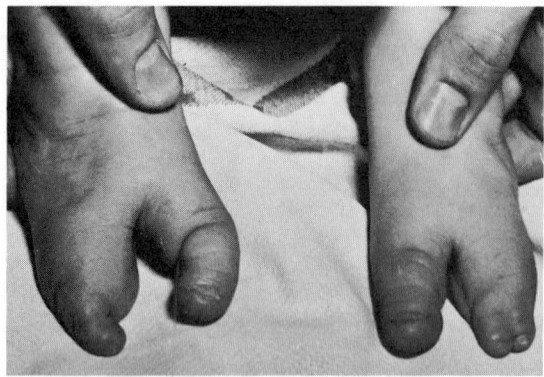

Figure 23–17. Split feet (lobster claws) in a child whose mother, maternal aunt, and maternal grandfather had similar malformations.

Congenitally Dislocated Radial Head. This dislocation of the proximal end of the radius is difficult to treat. Reduction is usually unsatisfactory, and removal of the head of the radius before the end of growth leads to shortening of the radius with radial deviation of the hand and consequent dysfunction of the wrist. After the child has attained full growth, the radial head may be removed if it is a cosmetic problem.

Congenital Radioulnar Synostosis. Fusion at birth of the proximal end of the radius and ulna results in an inability to pronate and supinate the forearm. Since attempts to divide this synostosis to allow motion have almost always failed, surgical treatment is directed at correcting extremes of position in order to leave the forearm in a useful neutral position.

Absence of the Radius or Ulna ("Club Hand"). Congenital absence of the radius or ulna is rare. In the former, which is more common, the soft tissues of the radial side of the arm act as a tension band, drawing the hand radially so that the wrist is pulled off the end of the ulna. Treatment is directed at stretching out the soft tissues during infancy, followed by surgical release and positioning the wrist on the ulna. Retention of this new position is a major problem; a number of operations may be required during the growing period to keep the hand appropriately placed. Radial anomalies of the hand, wrist, and forearm may be associated with congenital cardiac disease and certain blood dyscrasias (Sec. 15.4).

Pulled Elbow (Traumatic Subluxation of the Radial Head, Nursemaid's Elbow). This very common condition occurs in children from 1 to 4 yr of age. The child refuses to move the arm and holds it slightly flexed at the elbow and pronated at the forearm. The cause of this disorder is sudden forceful longitudinal traction upon the arm, which may happen when

a parent tries to drag a reluctant child by the arm or the child trips while being held by the arm. The sudden traction carries the head of the radius slightly distally and may partially tear the annular ligament at its attachment on the radius. When the traction is released, the annular ligament becomes impacted between the radius and the capitellum. Roentgenographic examination will not demonstrate the abnormality.

The condition is treated simply by supinating the arm fully, as may, on occasion unwittingly be done when positioning the forearm for a lateral roentgenogram. If a finger is held over the proximal radius as the arm is supinated, a click may be felt. Following reduction, the child may not move the arm immediately, but over the next 20–30 min spontaneous motion is usually noted. No postreduction fixation is needed unless the condition has recurred, in which case a collar-and-cuff sling is used. The parents should be alerted to the cause of the disorder to prevent recurrence.

Osteochondrosis of the Elbow. Children may suffer from osteochondrosis of the capitellum, the trochlea, or both. The etiology is unknown and is presumed to be analogous to that of osteochondritis dissecans of the knee. Trauma may play a role, especially in youngsters trying to emulate professional baseball pitchers. Treatment is usually supportive, but if fragments of the articular cartilage drop free into the joint, they must be surgically removed.

Polydactyly. Extra digits in the hand are most commonly seen at either the 5th finger or the thumb. These are frequently nothing more than skin tabs and can be readily removed. If they contain any bony element, it is preferable to delay their removal until the child is older than 9 mo, when there is more ossification of the cartilaginous anlage and a better assessment can be made of the amount of bone that must be removed.

Syndactyly. Syndactyly of the fingers (Fig. 23–18) generally requires surgical treatment. Because of the varied lengths of the metacarpals and phalanges in the different fingers, the joints of two adjacent and fused fingers do not line up side by side; their flexion and extension are therefore limited. If syndactyly is allowed to persist, there will be bony deformities at the joint with significant loss of function.

Tuberculous Dactylitis. This occurs most frequently in early childhood and involves one or more of the phalanges, the metacarpal bones, or the corresponding bones of the feet. The medullary canal of the involved bone becomes caseous; the cortex, thinned and expanded; and the periosteum, thickened. The entire digit develops a spindle-shaped, hard, red swelling as the soft tissues are affected. The process is comparatively painless, but it lasts many months and may leave a permanent deformity. The differential diagnosis involves chiefly the dactylitis of congenital syphilis (Sec. 11.49), which is more often multiple and symmetric. Dactylitis may also occur in sickle cell anemia (Sec. 15.18) and in coccidioidomycosis. The involved region should be put at rest with a splint or cast; surgical drainage is indicated if an abscess develops.

23.9 THE HEAD

Craniosynostosis. Premature closure of one or more sutures of the skull results in deformity of the head and, depending on which suture is involved, may cause damage to the brain and the eyes.

Etiology. Congenital craniosynostoses originate in embryonic life for unknown reasons and may be associated with other skeletal defects. In other instances craniostenoses may be postnatal and associated with rickets, hypophosphatasia, and idiopathic hypercalcemia and may follow shunt procedures for hydrocephalus.

In the normal newborn infant the bones of the cranium are

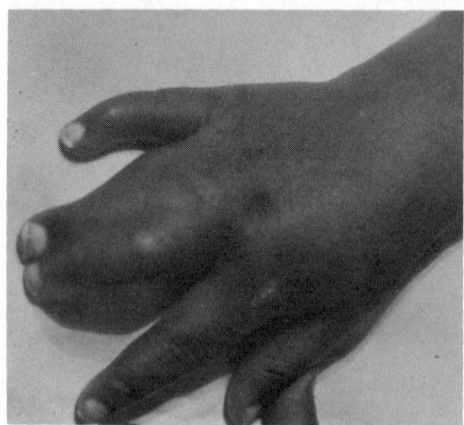

Figure 23–18. Syndactyly.

separated, but soon after birth the definitive sutures are established. The edges of the flat bones are separated by fibrous tissue in which growth takes place perpendicular to the line of the suture. Premature closure of a suture results in failure of growth of the vault at right angles to the involved suture and compensatory growth in regions where the sutures are patent.

Clinical Manifestations. When the *sagittal sutures* close prematurely, the head becomes long and narrow (scaphocephaly) and a bony ridge often marks the obliterated sutures. Males are affected more often than females. Ocular or neurologic abnormalities are rarely related to the abnormality of the suture.

Premature closure of the *coronal suture* results in severe deformity of the head (oxycephaly, acrocephaly) and in deformity of the face and orbits. The roof of the orbit is depressed, exophthalmos develops, and there may be strabismus, nystagmus, papilledema, optic atrophy, and loss of vision. The complications are more severe when both coronal sutures are obliterated or when other sutures are involved. Other malformations such as cardiac anomalies, choanal atresia, or defects of the elbow and knee joints may be associated. Syndactyly is the most commonly associated anomaly. A familial form of closure of the coronal sutures associated with hemolytic jaundice has been reported.

Acrocephalosyndactyly (Apert syndrome) consists of deformity of the skull secondary to closure of the coronal sutures and syndactyly of the hands and sometimes of the feet. It is thought to follow autosomal dominant transmission. **Acrocephalopolysyndactyly (Carpenter syndrome)** has certain similarities to the Apert syndrome and to the Laurence-Moon-Biedl syndrome. Besides acrocephaly, there is a peculiar facies, brachysyndactyly of the fingers, preaxial polydactyly and syndactyly of the toes, hypogenitalism, obesity, and mental retardation. Transmission is autosomal recessive. **Craniofacial dysostosis (Crouzon disease)** is characterized by acrocephaly, a beak-shaped nose, hypoplastic maxilla, short upper and protruding lower lips, hypertelorism, exophthalmos, and external strabismus. In **clover-leaf skull syndrome** (Kleeblattschädel) the severely deformed skull has a trilobed configuration as seen on a frontal roentgenogram. It is due to premature synostosis of some cranial sutures and is associated with marked hydrocephalus. The skull bulges toward the vertex and the temporal regions. It is often associated with skeletal dysplasias.

Oxycephaly or acrocephaly must be distinguished from a familial form of high skull in which premature closure of the sutures does not take place. In microcephaly the head is small, the vault is symmetric, and the sutures are patent; there is failure of the brain to grow. In craniosynostosis, roentgenograms of the skull reveal abnormality in shape depending on the suture or sutures involved. The involved suture may be obliterated or marked by a thin lucent line, but there is frequently thickening of bone along the suture and bony bridging.

Treatment. Closure of the sagittal suture is rarely associated with complications requiring therapy, except for the cosmetic problem of a long narrow head. In other congenital forms of craniosynostosis compression of the brain or cranial nerves may require surgery. When the lesion is one which may result in significant cerebral or visual damage, surgical intervention in early infancy may lessen or avoid such damage. Surgical treatment consists of linear craniectomy along the prematurely closed suture. Since there is rapid growth of the brain during the first 6 mo of life, surgery will be most effective when performed soon after birth. Secondary closure of one or more of the cranial sutures occurs months after birth and only rarely requires surgical treatment. In Crouzon and Apert syndromes, maxillary advancement, a complex surgical technique, may be of value.

Lacunar Skull. This cranial anomaly is characterized by defects in the vault in the form of shadow depressions or deep cavitations extending to the outer surface and occurring mainly in the frontal or parietal regions. The thinned areas of bone are lined by dura and bordered by regions of osseous tissue. The outer surface of the skull is smooth. The roentgenographic appearance is diagnostic and shows diminution in the thickness of the bones of the skull and variations in their density as irregular areas of rarefaction, or lacunae, separated by ridges of increased density (Fig. 23–19). Differentiation should be made from the generalized "hammered silver" or "digital impression" appearance of the bones of the skull, which is observed sometimes without apparent explanation or, in other instances, in associated with increased intracranial pressure, particularly in later childhood.

Lacunar skull is found roentgenographically in approximately half the infants with meningocele or myelomeningocele. When the latter is associated with the lacunar skull, progressive hydrocephalus is a frequent complication. As the cranium enlarges, the bony ridges become thin and the lacunae disappear.

Parietal Foramina. These are irregularly shaped congenital defects of varying size and well-defined margins symmetrically placed on each side of the posterior third of the sagittal suture. They are palpable but frequently discovered only roentgenographically. They may be transmitted through several generations or occur sporadically in otherwise normal persons. They must be distinguished from defects of the skull associated with meningoencephalocele or from defects caused by reticuloendotheliosis, infection, multiple myeloma, or metastases. Parietal foramina cause no discomfort, and no treatment is indicated.

Basilar Impression (Occipitalization of the Atlas; Platybasia). This condition may be primary or secondary. In primary basilar impression there is encroachment upon the cervical vertebral canal and posterior cranial fossa. The 1st and 2nd occipital segments and the 1st and 2nd cervical vertebrae may be fused into a bony mass. This anomaly is similar to the Klippel-Feil syndrome except that the latter involves the cervical segments below the 2nd. Secondary basilar impression occurs when the cranial bones are so softened by disease that they no longer support the weight of the head. It may occur in rickets (osteomalacia). The cranial vertex approaches the occiput, encroaching upon the posterior cranial fossa. Flattening of the base of the skull (platybasia or an increased basal angle) is at times associated with basilar impression.

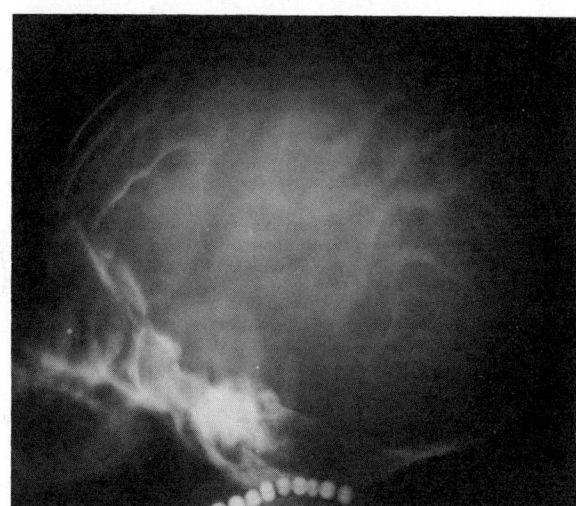

Figure 23–19. Lacunar skull. Multiple areas of decreased density in the frontal and parietal bones are delineated by thick bony ridges. The external surface of the cranial bones is smooth. The patient had a lumbar meningocele.

In either primary or secondary basilar impression, upward displacement of the odontoid process occurs which narrows the foramen magnum. Kinking of the medulla over the odontoid process may produce pressure upon the spinal cord. Localized thickening of the dura at the craniovertebral junction is frequently associated and contributes to constriction of the brain stem. This constriction may, in some instances, be relieved by surgery.

Ocular Hypertelorism. This condition consists of an abnormally large distance between the eyes and apparent broadening of the root of the nose; it is a nonspecific sign and not a disease entity. The diagnosis is made by determining the distance between the pupils rather than by inspection alone. It is often associated with mental deficiency or with other congenital defects. Mild forms occur in otherwise normal children. The lesser wings of the sphenoid bone are overdeveloped, the greater wings relatively small. Hypertelorism can be transmitted through several generations. Epicanthal folds may result in an appearance resembling hypertelorism, but with normal intrapupillary distance. Hypertelorism may be a sign of an ethmoid encephalocele.

23.10 TRAUMA

Epiphyseal Fractures. Fractures of an epiphysis can be innocuous or disastrous. In a growing bone the area of least resistance to stress is the junction between the metaphysis of the bone and the cartilaginous epiphyseal plate. If a bone breaks at this junction and is repositioned accurately, the rapid turnover of bone at this site allows for healing in 2–4 wk. Alternatively, a blow along the axis of a long bone that crushes the cartilaginous cells or injures the blood supply to them may destroy the epiphyseal cartilage plate, with subsequent loss of growth. If fractures at approximately right angles across the epiphyseal cartilage plate are not repositioned exactly, bone from the metaphysis will bridge to the epiphysis and there will be marked distortion of subsequent bony growth.

Salter-Harris type I fractures (Fig. 23–20) are not easily recognized on roentgenograms since there is no discontinuity in the outline of the bone. They are suspected only from the nature of the injury and from the swelling seen clinically or roentgenographically. "Ankle sprains" in young children are likely to involve Salter-Harris I epiphyseal fractures of the distal fibula.

Stress Fractures. Children, especially adolescents, engaging in intense physical activity after a period of decreased activity (such as football training after a summer's layoff) may develop pains in the region of the proximal tibia or at the junction of the distal three quarters of the femur and the metastases. These represent fractures through an area of remodeling where the body is trying to improve the structure of the bone (Sec. 23.12). Roentgenograms may show an area of reactive bone healing in the periosteum, often mistaken for a malignant tumor. Treatment is to refrain from such activity. Crutches may be needed.

Avulsion Injuries. Avulsions of the origins of muscles about the hip are common (Sec. 23.2). These may also be seen at the insertion of the peroneus brevis on the 5th metatarsal of the foot.

23.11 Sports Participation

The past decade has seen a marked increase in organized sports activities for adolescents and pre-adolescents and the inclusion of girls in many of them. This rapid growth has been accompanied by problems and controversies, including whether this age group's physical activities should be organized or spontaneous, individual or team-oriented. No consensus exists on these issues.

Advocates of organized sports believe that the availability of adult supervision reduces risks of bodily trauma. Trained coaches teach better techniques of play, which reduce injuries. Risk of injury is inherently less in children since the energy of collision (proportional to the mass and the square of the velocity) is smaller in children than in adults. Data show, for example, that football injuries in organized leagues of preadolescents are less frequent or serious than in college leagues.

Opponents argue, however, that poor leadership frequently leads growing children into physical activity more appropriate for adults. Injuries will increase in frequency as the number of participants and exposure time are increased, and recurrent minor trauma may ultimately exact a major toll upon the growing skeleton.

Advocates believe that children gain self-confidence and enjoyment from learning to play well under oganized coaching. They also find organized sports desirable as outlets for children's energies which might otherwise be spent in unwholesome activities. The substantial involvement of girls in organized sports can help eliminate some sex discrimination in expectation of gender roles. Opponents see the dangers of poor leadership, which can overemphasize and overvalue

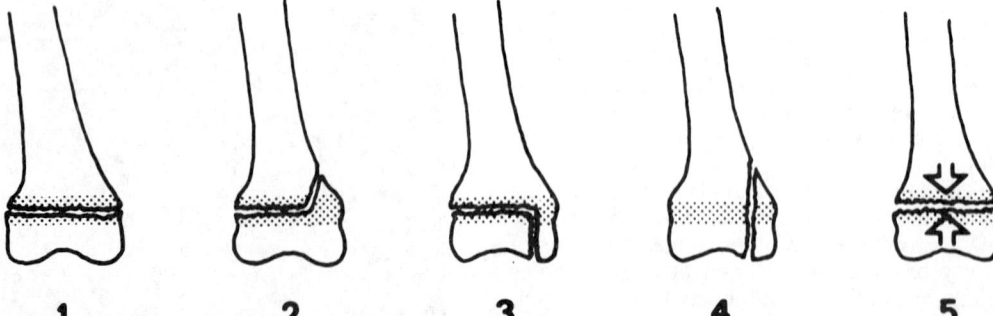

Figure 23–20. Salter-Harris classification of epiphyseal fractures. (1) The epiphysis separates from the metaphysis. The germinal cells remain with the epiphysis, usually uninjured. Healing is rapid and growth seldom arrested. (2) Similar to type 1, except that a small piece of metaphysis breaks free to remain with the epiphysis. Healing is rapid and growth is usually normal. Types 1 and 2 are the most common. (3) Separation passes a variable distance along the growth plate, then enters the joint. Accurate reduction of the intra-articular fracture is necessary to prevent later traumatic arthritis. Open reduction may be needed. Growth disturbances are not usually a problem. (4) The fracture extends from the joint, across the growth plate, and into the metaphysis. This usually requires open reduction to prevent unilateral growth arrest and traumatic arthritis from malposition. (5) This is a crushing injury which leads to death of the germinal cells of the epiphyseal cartilage and arrest of growth. This type is rare.

winning rather than sportsmanship, and undue emphasis on the trappings of the sport (in the form of uniforms and cheerleaders, for example) which can distort values and judgment as to what is good, desirable, and fair in play. "Not making the team" can represent serious emotional trauma for a child. The manner in which funds are allocated to the cost of equipment and transportation can easily be recognized in some communities as reflecting socially discriminatory decision making. Some of the organizations that promote certain sports have been blatantly sexist.

Advocates of team sports believe that they contribute to socialization in preparation for adult activities that involve "team efforts" and that teams may also provide good training for leadership, with players other than "stars" able to participate within the framework of the whole team. Critics of emphasis on teams point to the importance of individual sport to adult lives. They are concerned also that "team mentality" decreases self-reliance in thought and action.

23.12 Sports Injuries Peculiar to Children

The growing skeleton has special areas of susceptibility to injury not found in adults; these include the growth plate (physis), the epiphyses, and the apophyses.

Longitudinal growth occurs in the *physis*. Children can suffer ligamentous sprains, but ligaments are frequently not the points of greatest weakness under stress. When the energy of injury is transferred to the bone, it may break at its weakest point, the physeal cartilage. Such a break can lead to growth disturbances (Sec. 23.10). Chronic trauma to a growing shoulder caused by throwing can lead to the fracture of the proximal humerus through the physis ("Little League shoulder").

The *epiphysis*, in addition to the end of the bone and its articular cartilage, contains a layer of physeal cartilage (indistinguishable from the cells of the physis). The epiphysis is responsible for growth in diameter of the bone ends and for the sculpturing of the joint. The articular cartilage has beneath it a layer of physeal cells (like those of the growth plate) which are supported by the bony center in the epiphysis. Repeated excessive axial loading compresses these cells against the underlying bony support, causing not only temporary injury but also alteration of the joint configuration and lifelong arthritis, e.g., injury to the distal humerus (known as "Little League elbow") (Sec. 23.8). Osteochondritis dissecans, which characteristically afflicts the knee, may be secondary to trauma (Sec. 23.3).

Major tendons attach to bones at *apophyses* via an interfacing layer of physeal cartilage. Tendons that insert on the bones through apophyseal cartilaginous plates are prone to avulsion. This occurs most commonly around the hip, involving muscles that originate in the pelvis (Sec. 23.2). Osgood-Schlatter disease is a chronic partial avulsion of the infrapatellar ligament of the quadriceps from the anterior tibial tubercle (Sec. 23.3).

Stress Fractures. Stress fractures are not limited to children, but children's growing bones are especially susceptible. Cortical bone under unusual stress responds by seeking a structurally stronger form. Osteoclastic activity dissolves some bone, which is replaced with concentric lamellae. At the point where the bone substance has been weakened temporarily by osteoclasts (a process that may take several weeks) the bone may fracture under stress. Stress fractures are typically noted after a few weeks of vigorous physical activity that has followed a prolonged rest (for example, during the first weeks of spring training after a winter layoff). These are most commonly seen in tibia, distal fibula, and metatarsals (Sec. 23.10).

Excessive lumbar extension, such as back walk-overs in young gymnasts, may lead to stress fracture of the pars interarticularis of the lumbar spine (spondylolysis) (Sec. 23.5).

23.13 Prevention of Sports Injuries

Pre-participation Medical Evaluation. Physical examination prior to participation in organized sports is desirable, either to exclude children susceptible to injury or to counsel children and assign them to physically appropriate activities. Such pre-participation examinations provide a medical evaluation for many adolescents who never otherwise see a physician. On the other hand, there is serious question as to whether the goals of a general health evaluation can or should be attained in this way. The yield of abnormalities from such evaluations is low (about 1%), though the demand for medical examinations is enormous. It is estimated that there are 7 million high school children involved in interscholastic sports in the United States, as well as many involved in non–school related sport activities, and many pre-adolescents. Among the large number of examinations approximately 15% result in false-positive findings; these cause unnecessary anguish and considerable cost for the consultations required to determine that the affected children can participate. Some sports physicians have advised that children with lax ligaments should avoid contact sports or that they should be put on pre-participation training, but no substantial data indicate that these measures decrease the rate of injuries.

If pre-participation evaluation is done, the goals of the evaluation should be clear. If it is a yearly routine examination, then a complete physical examination can be done. If the goal is a matter of pre-sports evaluation, the aim is to find conditions that might interfere with the ability of the child to participate in a specific sport, be made worse by the sport, or indicate an increased susceptibility to injury.

The medical history is the primary source of significant findings, especially in respect to head injury, syncope with exercise, and recurrent sprains. Examination of the eyes, ears, nose, and throat, auscultation of the lungs, or eliciting deep tendon reflexes, for example, is usually of little value. Evaluation of tall athletes, such as basketball players, for ocular signs of Marfan syndrome (Sec. 23.43) may be an important exception. Blood pressure should be measured in all children. This is especially important for primarily isometric activities, such as weight-lifting, in which marked increases in pressure will occur. Assessment of sex maturity ratings (Tanner) has been advocated so that later-maturing children can be counseled to avoid collision sports; on the other hand, no data yet show that this advice decreases rates of injury. Estimation of joint laxity, either for individual joints or overall, is advocated by some, but awaits evaluation. Urine or blood analyses have not proved to be useful to these evaluations.

Education for Sports Participation. The child, parents, and coaches should understand the necessity for pre-season conditioning and for proper stretching and warming-up exercises prior to practice or competitive events. Such practices as achieving rapid weight loss to enter a lower wrestling weight category should be discouraged. Considerable effort may need to be expended in assessing the appropriateness of sport activities. An overenthusiastic coach may push children to excessively vigorous activity or to undue prolongation of an activity. In muscle-strengthening exercises children should be encouraged to work with less weight and increased frequency; the converse can be harmful. Some parents feel that certain practices, rule changes, or use of protective equipment designed to limit injuries are to protect "sissy kids." When this feeling leads to laxity on the part of officials (who may be the parents themselves), failure to enforce the rules may place the children in jeopardy. Education about these and other issues may require that the physician observe the sports program and talk with students, parents, and coaches.

Physicians may be in a strategic position to influence community attitudes toward sports. In an educational role the physician should be concerned with emotional as well as physical stress.

Protective Equipment. Advances have been made in protective equipment for children involved in violent sports; use of this protective equipment can sometimes be overdone, however, in the desire to emulate the adult model. Cleats on football shoes, for example, lead to a higher incidence of ankle injuries; the longer the cleats, the higher the accident rate. Playing in running shoes may appear less professional but can be safer. Equipment manufacturers have not always provided equipment of appropriate size for pre-adolescents. It is sometimes difficult to find the child inside the protective layer of padding; a child so equipped cannot move with good coordination.

Rule Changes. Organizations responsible for some sports have tried to alter the rules to make the games safer for children (for example, a rule limits pitching in Little League baseball to 6 innings/wk to minimize the likelihood of "Little League elbow"). Benefits of such rules can be undone by lack of awareness on the part of parents who allow the child to practice pitching at home considerably in excess of the rules. Prohibiting "spearing" and cross-body blocking in football and base-sliding in baseball has helped diminish injuries. Physicians who monitor such games should encourage vigorous enforcement of these rules.

Clinical. Injuries may be minimized by paying early attention to any child complaining of pain; minor microtrauma should be identified and/or stopped before disaster strikes.

INFECTIONS OF BONES AND JOINTS

See Sec. 11.14 and 11.15.

HUGH G. WATTS

Currarine G: Normal variants in congenital anomalies in the region of the obelion. Am J Roentgenol 127:487, 1976.

D'Angielis JA, Fisher RL, Ozonoff MB, et al: 99m Tc-polyphosphate bone imaging in Legg-Perthes disease. Radiology 115:407, 1975.

Dunn PM, Evans RE, Thearle MJ, et al: Congenital dislocation of the hip: Early and late diagnosis and management compared. Arch Dis Child 60:407, 1985.

Fraumani JF, Geiser GG, Manning MD: Wilms' tumor and congenital hemihypertrophy: Report of five new cases in review of literature. Pediatrics 40:886, 1967.

Garrick JG, Smith NJ: Preparticipation sports assessment. Pediatrics 66:803, 1980.

Hemple DJ, Harris LE, Svien HJ, et al: Craniosynostosis involving the sagittal suture only. Guilt by association? J Pediatr 58:342, 1961.

Ianaconne G, Guerlini G: So-called clover-leaf skull syndrome: Report of three cases with discussion of its relationships with thanatophoric dwarfism and the craniosynostosis. Pediatr Radiol 2:157, 1974.

Micheli LJ: Sports injuries in children and adolescents. In: Straus R (ed): Sports Medicine and Physiology. Philadelphia, WB Saunders, 1979, pp 288–303.

Moe JH, Winter RB, Bradford DS, et al: Scoliosis and Other Spinal Deformities. Philadelphia, WB Saunders, 1978.

Passarge E, Lenz W: Syndrome of caudal regression in infants of diabetic mothers. Pediatrics 37:672, 1966.

Rang M: Children's Fractures. Philadelphia, JB Lippincott, 1974.

Smith DW: Recognizable Patterns of Human Malformation. 3rd ed. Philadelphia, WB Saunders, 1982.

Tachdjian MO: Pediatric Orthopedics. Philadelphia, WB Saunders, 1972.

Warkany J: Congenital Malformations, Notes and Comments. Chicago, Year Book Medical Publishers, 1971.

23.14 GENETIC SKELETAL DYSPLASIAS

Developmental defects affecting the skeleton, while individually rare, contribute a major portion of the burden of short stature and skeletal deformity at all ages. They include dysplasias (disorders of growth), dysostoses (malformations of the bone), idiopathic osteolyses (pathologic resorption of bone), chromosomal aberrations with skeletal malformations, and metabolic disorders affecting the skeleton.

Nomenclature. The term "dwarfism" has been replaced by "dysplasia." The nomenclature of the skeletal dysplasias reflects clinical, genetic, and/or roentgenographic features. The name may describe the skeletal region involved or some characteristic feature of the disorder, or may be an eponym. Disorders with short stature are divided into short-trunk or short-limb conditions; the latter are divided into rhizomelic (shortening involving mainly the proximal segment of the limbs), mesomelic (shortening of the middle segments), and acromelic (shortening of the distal segments). In acromesomelic dysplasia both middle and distal segments are involved. Other names of skeletal dysplasias describe unique roentgenographic features (e.g., chondrodysplasia punctata) or the pattern of involvement of skeletal elements (e.g., epiphyseal, metaphyseal, or diaphyseal). With primary involvement of skull the prefix cranio- may be used; with significant involvement of the spine, spondylo- may be used.

Diagnosis and Assessment. The majority of skeletal dysplasias show disproportionate lengths of limbs and trunk. Usually, it is the limbs that are relatively short, even in conditions such as spondyloepiphyseal dysplasia congenita and metatropic dysplasia, in which, as the child grows, disproportion becomes manifestly greater in the shortened trunk than in the limbs. When the disproportion between limbs and trunk is not obvious, the disproportionately large head size may suggest dysplasia (e.g., with hypochondroplasia). Associated abnormalities aid in diagnosis. Cleft palate occurs with high frequency in Kniest dysplasia, in spondyloepiphyseal dysplasia (SED) congenita, and in Stickler arthroophthalmopathy; polydactyly is often associated with chondroectodermal dysplasia (Ellis–van Creveld), asphyxiating thoracic dysplasia, and other short rib–polydactyly syndromes.

In infants with the short rib–polydactyly syndromes, thanatophoric dysplasia, and lethal perinatal osteogenesis imperfecta, respiratory distress due to a short, small thorax is largely responsible for neonatal death.

Skeletal dysplasias vary in the ages at which they become apparent. When patients present beyond the newborn period, the most frequent reason for referral is disproportionate short stature, due either to relatively short limbs or to a short trunk, with kyphosis or scoliosis. Asymmetric growth of the limbs also occurs, as in chondrodysplasia punctata (Conradi-Hünermann), hemimelic epiphyseal dysplasia (Trevor), and multiple cartilaginous exostoses. Symptoms may arise from decreased density of the skeleton, as in osteogenesis imperfecta syndromes, or from increased density with hematologic or neurologic complications, as in osteopetrosis.

Whatever the presentation, the approach to these disorders of skeletal development is the same. Prenatal, perinatal, and postnatal growth history should be reviewed and the family history taken. Physical examination should assess the symmetry and proportions of the patient, with a search for associated skeletal or extraskeletal malformations. Measurements should include height, length of upper segment (US) and lower segment (LS), span, head circumference, and chest circumference; these measurements should be made periodically and plotted on appropriate growth charts. Specific growth charts exist for patients with achondroplasia, diastrophic dysplasia, and spondyloepiphyseal dysplasia. The upper segment/lower segment (US/LS) ratio and span/length ratio may aid in diagnosis. For example, a high US/LS ratio is characteristic of short-limb dysplasias (in which span is also usually less than height), whereas a decrease in US/LS ratio is found in short-trunk conditions, such as spondyloepiphyseal dysplasia.

Roentgenographic studies are required for the diagnostic

Table 23–1. Skeletal Dysplasias Associated with Immune Deficiency

	McKusick No.*
Metaphyseal chondrodysplasia, McKusick type	25025
Metaphyseal chondrodysplasia with thymolymphopenia	20090
Metaphyseal dysplasia with severe combined immunodeficiency (adenosine deaminase deficiency)	24275
Metaphyseal dysplasia with pancreatic insufficiency and neutropenia (Schwachman)	26040†
Metaphyseal dysplasia with short ribs, neutropenia, and pancreatic insufficiency	26040†

*McKusick VA: Mendelian Inheritance in Man. 6th ed. Baltimore, Johns Hopkins University Press, 1983.
†Probably two distinct syndromes.

Table 23–3. Skeletal Dysplasias Associated with Hearing Impairment

	McKusick No.*
Predominantly sensorineural	
Congenital	
Spondyloepiphyseal dysplasia congenita	18390
Kniest dysplasia	18655
Diastrophic dysplasia	22260
Otopalatodigital syndrome	31130
Stickler syndrome	10830
Due to progressive 8th nerve encroachment	
Osteopetrosis	16660
Craniodiaphyseal dysplasia	21830
Craniometaphyseal dysplasia	12300 and 21840
Endosteal hyperostosis (van Buchem)	23910
Sclerosteosis	26950
Hyperphosphatasia	23900
Frontometaphyseal dysplasia	13674
Predominantly conductive	
Achondroplasia†	10080
Hypochondroplasia‡	14600
Osteogenesis imperfecta (A.D.)	16620
Metaphyseal dysplasia and mental retardation	25042

*McKusick VA: Mendelian Inheritance in Man. 6th ed. Baltimore, Johns Hopkins University Press, 1983.
†Recurrent and chronic serous otitis media.
‡Infrequent.

differentiation of skeletal dysplasias; serial examinations are necessary for delineation of some conditions and for assessment of complications specific to each dysplasia.

At the first consultation a full series of skeletal views is usually required. These views include anteroposterior (AP), lateral, and Towne views of the skull, AP and lateral views of the spine, and AP views of the pelvis and extremities, with separate views of hands and feet. Lateral views of the foot are particularly helpful in identifying punctate calcification of the calcaneus and in detecting absence or hypoplasia of calcaneus and talus in the epiphyseal dysplasias.

In certain disorders radiologic features are diagnostic; others may require serial studies and consultation. Registries of skeletal dysplasias may be helpful.

Pathologic Studies. Specific histologic or ultrastructural changes are found in many dysplasias, especially in the lethal neonatal disorders. When affected infants die, autopsy should be obtained whenever possible, with specimens of costochondral junction and of growth plates of iliac crest and of long bones such as femur, tibia, or fibula preserved for study. During life a trephine biopsy of the iliac crest or a rib biopsy may be helpful. Appropriate studies may differentiate closely related conditions, but some dysplasias show only nonspecific histopathologic changes; in such cases pathologic examination is useful in excluding other diagnoses.

Biochemical Studies. Patients with severe congenital hypophosphatasia have a distinct pattern of abnormalities (Sec. 7.53 and 23.53), and patients with lysosomal storage disease have deficiencies of specific lysosomal enzymes (Sec. 7.24). On the other hand, the underlying biochemical defect in most cases of skeletal dysplasia is unknown.

Certain skeletal dysplasias, however, are characterized by disordered immune (Table 23–1), renal (Table 23–2), neurologic, cardiovascular, ophthalmologic, or hearing and speech functions (Table 23–3). These complications should be sought at the time of diagnosis and with periodic screening throughout life.

Table 23–2. Skeletal Dysplasias Frequently Associated with Renal Complications

	McKusick No.*
Lethal to newborn	
Short rib–polydactyly syndrome I (Saldino-Noonan)	26353
Short rib–polydactyly syndrome II (Majewski)	26352
Usually nonlethal	
Asphyxiating thoracic dysplasia	20850
Acrodysplasia with retinitis pigmentosa and nephropathy (Saldino-Mainzer)	26692

*McKusick VA: Mendelian Inheritance in Man. 6th ed. Baltimore, Johns Hopkins University Press, 1983.

Management. Effective management requires (1) precise diagnosis, (2) prompt recognition of specific skeletal and nonskeletal complications, (3) appropriate orthopedic and rehabilitative care, (4) emotional support and psychosocial counseling, and (5) genetic counseling. There is no specific cure for any of these conditions. Use of growth hormone is not presently indicated for short stature due to skeletal dysplasia. Use of androgenic hormones has limited value in most patients, but oxandrolone has been used in closely supervised situations for growth promotion in selected patients.

Orthopedic management aims at maximizing mobility and correcting deformity; if deformities in the lower limbs are left uncorrected beyond puberty, early onset of osteoarthritis may lead to mechanically unsound joints. Recognition of spinal deformity and its early treatment with bracing or minimal surgical intervention may reduce morbidity (from scoliosis, etc.) in adult life.

The need for educational and emotional support and counseling is often intense and chronic. Several lay organizations (see references) may help to provide emotional support and an environment in which short persons can learn together to adjust to a world of taller people.

23.15 DEFECTS OF THE GROWTH OF TUBULAR BONES AND/OR SPINE

23.16 ACHONDROPLASIA

Achondroplasia, the most common genetic skeletal dysplasia, is inherited as an autosomal dominant trait (Fig. 23–21). Achondroplasia occurs in about 1 in 25,000 births. About 80% of cases represent new mutations. The pathogenesis is unknown. Disordered growth mainly involves a reduced rate of qualitatively normal enchondral bone formation and a marked disturbance in craniofacial growth.

Clinical Manifestations. Rhizomelic shortening of the limbs can be recognized at birth, when most achondroplastic infants will already have large head size, frontal bossing, depression of the nasal bridge, and short stature. The limbs are covered with fatty folds of skin in infancy and early childhood. The

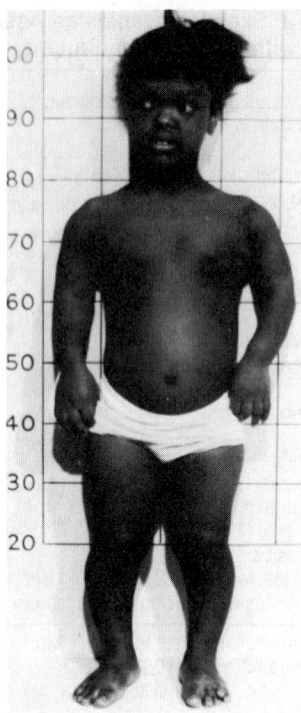

Figure 23–21. Achondroplasia demonstrating predominantly proximal (rhizomelic) limb shortening.

hands are short and broad, with an appearance resembling a trident consisting of the thumb, the 2nd and 3rd digits, and the 4th and 5th digits, a wedge-shaped gap separating the 3rd and 4th fingers. The trident appearance is usually lost in late childhood or adolescence, the hand remaining short and broad. The elbows may be limited in extension and pronation. A lumbar gibbus is common in infancy, but after the first year this almost always disappears, being replaced frequently by a straight back, invariably with a prominent lumbar lordosis.

Achondroplastic infants are often hypotonic with delayed motor development. Normal neuromuscular tone is usually gained by 2–3 yr of age. Joint laxity, particularly in the interphalangeal joints, may persist throughout childhood. In the absence of hydrocephalus, mental and motor development are usually normal.

The head is large throughout life, with prominent frontal bossing, hypoplasia of the maxilla, and relative mandibular prognathism. The mean head circumference in achondroplasia follows a growth curve above the 97th percentile for normal individuals. Specific growth curves for achondroplasia have been developed, which are particularly valuable in monitoring the rapid growth in head size in infancy since hydrocephalus may complicate achondroplasia.

Dental malocclusion with anterior open bite is common and should be managed by an orthodontist familiar with the problem of achondroplasia. High frequencies of recurrent otitis media and chronic serous otitis media are found in these children and lead to a high incidence of conductive hearing loss in adulthood if not recognized and treated in childhood.

Roentgenographic Manifestations. Roentgenograms show a short pelvis with broad iliac wings, horizontal acetabular roofs, and narrow, deep sacrosciatic notches. The vertebral interpedicular distance diminishes from L1 to L5, in contrast to the normal caudal widening; this is a distinctive feature of achondroplasia, though it may not be apparent in the newborn. The disc spaces are increased at the expense of the vertebral bodies, and the spinal canal is narrowed. There may

be anterior tonguing and wedging of a lower thoracic or upper lumbar vertebra. There is posterior scalloping of the lumbar vertebrae; the pedicles appear short on lateral view. The base of the skull is shortened, and the foramen magnum is small and irregular. The cranium is large relative to the face, with frontal prominence and maxillary hypoplasia. The long bones are decreased in length, particularly in proximal limb segments, and appear rather wide and squat. The metaphyses have some flaring and may appear V-shaped (circumflex sign). There is relative overgrowth of the fibulae. The short tubular bones of the hands and feet are shorter and wider than normal; the shortening is greatest in the phalanges. The chest has a decreased anteroposterior diameter, with anterior cupping of the ribs.

Management. Achondroplasia may be complicated by *hydrocephalus* (see above and Sec. 21.12), which results from obstruction of the foramen magnum, and by lumbar cord and nerve root compression syndromes, dental malocclusion, hearing impairment from repeated otitis media, and strabismus (resulting from craniofacial dysmorphism). *Bowing of the legs* and persistent *kyphosis* may also require attention. Besides the prompt recognition and appropriate treatment of these problems, management during childhood will mainly be concerned with the social and psychologic effects of severe short stature and unusual appearance and with genetic counseling. Prompt and appropriate therapy is particularly necessary for each episode of *acute otitis media*. Hydrocephalus is not common but must be recognized as early as possible. There is some evidence that physiotherapy and bracing during childhood can ameliorate the complications of prolonged infantile kyphosis or of the severe lordosis that may aggravate lumbar stenosis in adult life. Osteotomies may be indicated just prior to or during adolescence to correct severe progressive leg bowing.

Prognosis. Except for the rare patient with hydrocephalus or with severe complications of cervical or lumbar spinal cord compression, the life span in achondroplasia is normal. The mean adult height in achondroplasia is about 131.5 cm (51.8 in.) in men and 125 cm (49.2 in.) in women.

23.17 HYPOCHONDROPLASIA

This form of short-limbed (rhizomelic) short stature is usually recognized from 2–3 yr of age. It is distinct from achondroplasia, but there is wide variability in severity and much overlap in appearance with persons with achondroplasia. Morphologic studies of chondro-osseous tissue show qualitatively normal chondro-osseous transformation. Achondroplasia and hypochondroplasia appear to be allelic autosomal dominant disorders.

Clinical Manifestations. Hypochondroplasia is not usually recognized at birth. Head size commonly falls above the 50th percentile and may fall between the normal range and the range for achondroplasia. Usually, the nasal bridge is not depressed, nor is the mandible unusually prominent. Affected persons appear rather stocky and muscular. The hands and feet are short and broad but not trident, and the legs are usually straight, but mild genu varum may develop. There may be a mild lumbar lordosis, pelvic tilt, and mild limitation of extension at the elbows, features that are always prominent in achondroplasia.

Roentgenographic Manifestations. These resemble those in achondroplasia but may be very mild. Features include prominent deltoid tubercles, relatively short ulnae with prominent radial styloids, relatively long fibulae, and narrowing or constancy of the interpedicular distance between L1 and L5.

Complications. Hypochondroplasia causes little morbidity apart from short stature.

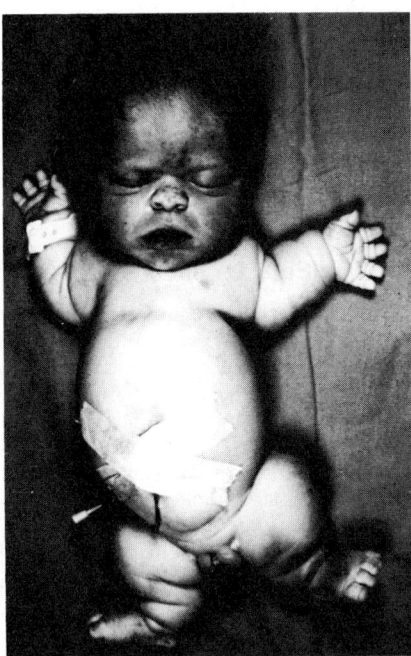

Figure 23–22. Thanatophoric dysplasia with short limbs, large head, prominent forehead, and depressed nasal bridge.

Management. The condition may require orthopedic management of problems such as leg bowing or lumbar spinal cord claudication.

23.18 THANATOPHORIC DYSPLASIA

Thanatophoric dysplasia is probably the most frequent lethal congenital skeletal dysplasia. Most cases have been sporadic. An instance of familial occurrence of thanatophoric dysplasia with clover-leaf skull deformity (Kleeblattschädel) has been reported.

Infants with thanatophoric dysplasia are shorter at birth than those with achondroplasia. They have a prominent forehead, depressed nasal bridge, and bulging eyes (Fig. 23–22). The limbs are extremely short and held extended from the body. The chest is small and pear-shaped. Affected infants are hypotonic and lack primitive reflexes. Roentgenograms show marked rhizomelic shortening of the long bones, bowing of the femora, metaphyseal flaring, marginal spicules, and cupping. The changes in lumbar vertebrae are characteristic: inverted-U-shaped appearance in the anteroposterior view and marked flattening of vertebrae with central narrowing in the lateral view. The pelvis resembles that of achondroplasia with short, flat acetabula and small sacrosciatic notches, but spicules of bone protrude from both acetabula and ischia. The cranium is large, with a constricted base and a small foramen magnum. Clover-leaf skull deformity is found in some babies with thanatophoric dysplasia, all of whom have had hydrocephalus at autopsy (Fig. 23–23).

23.19 ACHONDROGENESIS I (PARENTI-FRACCARO) AND ACHONDROGENESIS II (LANGER-SALDINO)

These rare lethal autosomal recessive conditions have clinical features in common and are distinguished by roentgenographic findings. Infants with achondrogenesis I have heads that appear large relative to the trunk, and the skull is extremely soft, with multiple small bone islands palpable in a membranous calvarium. The neck is very short, and the

arms are extremely short and stubby. The thorax is small and barrel-shaped rather than pear-shaped. Roentgenograms show no ossification in any vertebral body, although ossification of the pedicles and neural arches is present down to the mid-sacrum. The ribs are thin and may contain multiple fractures; there are usually no fractures of the long bones. The femora appear short and square with prominent bony projections at the border of the metaphyses.

Infants with achondrogenesis II (Fig. 23–24) have severe short limb stature, but the head is more proportionate to the body. The neck is short and hidden in skin folds; the trunk is short, with abdomen distended. The roentgenographic features differ from those of achondrogenesis I or of thanatophoric dysplasia. The skull is poorly mineralized but not so defective as in achondrogenesis I. The ribs are short but relatively normal in diameter. There is often lack of ossification of the vertebral bodies, but some infants show some ossification of the lower thoracic and upper lumbar vertebral centers. The ilia are small, with concave medial and inferior margins; ossification of the ischium and pubis is usually absent. The long bones are very short with metaphyseal flaring, spicules of ossification at both lateral and medial borders of the growth plate, and marked cupping.

23.20 SHORT RIB–POLYDACTYLY (SRP) SYNDROMES

SRP syndromes include lethal newborn skeletal dysplasias (Fig. 23–25), SRP I (Saldino-Noonan) and SRP II (Majewski), and the usually nonlethal disorders, asphyxiating thoracic dysplasia (ATD) and chondroectodermal dysplasia (Ellis–van Creveld). All are inherited as autosomal recessive conditions. They have in common respiratory distress due to pulmonary hypoplasia within a narrow dysplastic thorax with extremely short ribs. Polydactyly is almost always found in patients

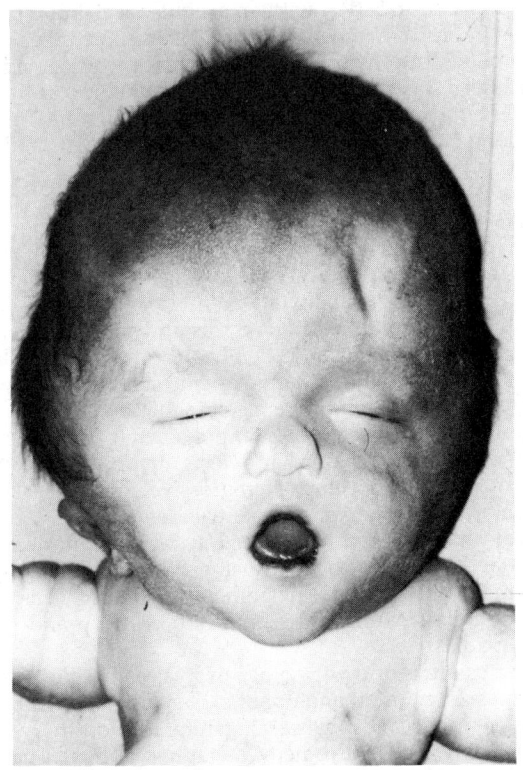

Figure 23–23. Cloverleaf skull deformity in association with thanatophoric dysplasia.

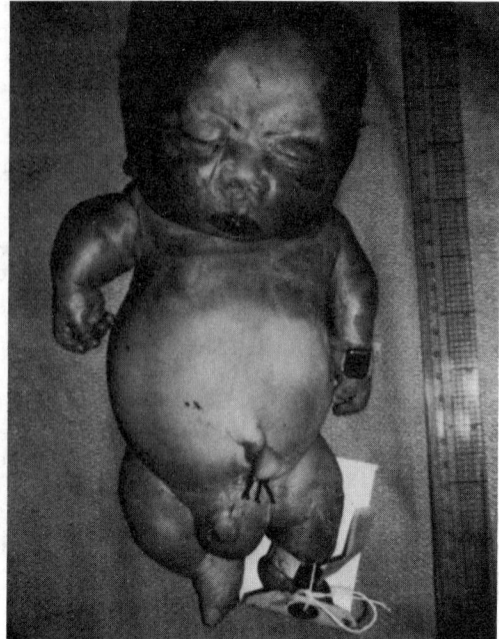

Figure 23–24. Achondrogenesis II (Langer-Saldino) showing extremely short limbs and globular body.

having SRP I, SRP II, and chondroectodermal dysplasia, but not as often in those having ATD.

SRP I is characterized by relatively high frequencies of cloacal abnormalities (anal atresia, urogenital sinus) and of postaxial polydactyly, whereas *SRP II* has high frequencies of associated cleft upper lip or palate, multiple internal anomalies including hypoplastic epiglottis, cardiovascular defects, and pre- as well as postaxial polydactyly. Roentgenographically, both show extremely short horizontal ribs. The pelvis is small and hypoplastic in SRP I, with an irregular acetabular margin, whereas in SRP II the pelvis is normal. In some cases of SRP I long bones are hypoplastic, with poor corticomedullary demarcation; other cases have longitudinal spurs at the margins of the metaphyses, with a convex central metaphysis. In SRP II long bones appear relatively normal apart from disproportionately short tibiae.

In the newborn it may be difficult to distinguish between *asphyxiating thoracic dysplasia* and *chondroectodermal dysplasia*. Both have short limbs and polydactyly and respiratory distress due to thoracic dysplasia. There is considerable clinical and roentgenographic variability in both. Roentgenograms may show short, horizontally oriented ribs and small pelvic bones with marked spur-like projections at the medial and lateral margins of the acetabula. Many patients survive the newborn period. Respiratory symptoms decrease with age.

In *asphyxiating thoracic dysplasia*, polydactyly may be absent or limited to the hands. Cardiac defects are uncommon. Many surviving patients develop a progressive renal disease that has glomerular, cystic, and interstitial elements.

Patients having *chondroectodermal dysplasia* often also have congenital cardiac anomalies (usually atrial septal defects) and ectodermal abnormalities including hypoplastic nails, natal teeth, multiple frenula of the upper lip, cleft lip and palate, and epispadias.

Short ribs are found with other dysplasias besides the SRP syndromes (e.g., in thanatophoric dysplasia, sometimes in spondyloepiphyseal dysplasia congenita, in chondrodysplasia punctata, and in a syndrome of metaphyseal dysplasia associated with neutropenia), but polydactyly is associated with none of these conditions.

The respiratory distress of infants with SRP I and SRP II is

not remediable. Some infants with asphyxiating thoracic dysplasia or severe chondroectodermal dysplasia who have severe respiratory distress will show spontaneous improvement in respiratory function. In asphyxiating thoracic dysplasia, surgical enlargement of the thoracic cage with prolonged respirator management has permitted survival beyond the newborn period. Survivors have a high incidence of chronic renal failure leading to death in infancy.

23.21 CAMPTOMELIC DYSPLASIAS

Camptomelic dysplasia is characterized by short-limbed short stature and bowing or bending of the long bones, particularly in the lower limbs; pretibial skin dimples at the site of the bowing; and associated anomalies. It is inherited as an autosomal recessive trait. The majority of reported cases are in phenotypic females, some of whom have 46,XY karyotypes; cases with intersex have been reported. The relationship between sex reversal and skeletal dysplasia is not understood.

The classic finding in camptomelic dysplasia is that the long bones are long and slender and usually bent at their midpoint. Cutaneous dimples may overlie the points of maximum curvature in tibia or fibula. Severe respiratory distress usually leads to early death, presumably due to small thoracic cage, narrow larynx, and hypoplasia of tracheal rings. Many other congenital abnormalities have been associated.

Roentgenograms show an enlarged dolichocephalic skull with narrow shallow orbits. The ribs usually number 11 and are often narrow. The cervical vertebral bodies may be hypoplastic and the lumbar interpedicular distance increased. The pelvis is usually tall, narrow, and hypoplastic.

Camptomelia (bent limbs) is observed in the camptomelic dysplasias, in osteogenesis imperfecta (at least four varieties), and in hypophosphatasia (dominant and recessive varieties).

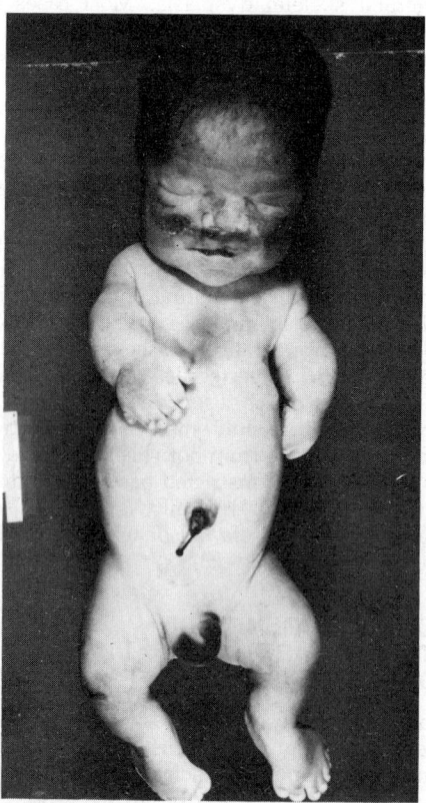

Figure 23–25. Short-rib polydactyly I (Saldino-Noonan) showing small thorax, postaxial hexadactyly in the fingers, and both pre- and postaxial heptadactyly of the feet.

Bowing or angulation of the limbs is found also with other skeletal dysplasias and malformations.

23.22 CHONDRODYSPLASIA PUNCTATA
(Punctate Epiphyseal Dysplasia)

Chondrodysplasia punctata comprises several dysplasias in which roentgenograms of the epiphyses, periarticular tissues, and growth plate zones show stippled calcification. At least three defined genetic skeletal dysplasias showing this finding have been referred to as Conradi disease, chondrodystrophia calcificans congenita, punctate epiphyseal dysplasia, stippled epiphyses, or other names. These defined syndromes include a severe autosomal recessive rhizomelic form, an autosomal dominant form (Conradi-Hünermann), and a milder X-linked form. Laryngomalacia with stippling of the laryngeal cartilages occurs in some patients, who may have significant respiratory distress from upper airway obstruction during inspiration. Asymmetry of the length of the lower limbs is characteristic of the Conradi-Hünermann form.

23.23 EPIPHYSEAL DYSPLASIAS

These are characterized by flattened, fragmented, or irregular epiphyses. The earliest feature may be delay in the development of certain epiphyses. The epiphyseal dysplasias can be broadly divided into those with spinal involvement (the spondyloepiphyseal dysplasias) and those without spinal involvement (the multiple epiphyseal or polyepiphyseal dysplasias). Many patients cannot be precisely classified.

Spondyloepiphyseal Dysplasias (SED). These are characterized by flattening and irregularity of the vertebrae and delay in ossification of the vertebral bodies. These changes are not pathognomonic of SED since vertebral irregularity, including an increased incidence of Schmorl nodes, also occurs in adults with multiple epiphyseal dysplasias. Accurate diagnosis can be made only from serial roentgenographic assessments of the vertebrae at various ages. In some spondyloepiphyseal dysplasias, skeletal dysplasia is evident at birth (SED congenita); in others, short stature develops during infancy or childhood (SED tarda). SED congenita has autosomal dominant inheritance with variable expressivity; SED tarda appears in both X-linked recessive and autosomal dominant forms.

Newborn infants wth **SED congenita** have rhizomelic shortening of the limbs, but these appear long relative to the trunk. Hands and feet are of normal size so that the fingers appear excessively long. Club feet are common. The head is also normal in size, but the neck is extremely short with limited flexion. Odontoid hypoplasia is common and may lead to atlanto-occipital dislocation with cervical cord and root compression. Exaggerated dorsal kyphosis contributes to a broad barrel chest, and scoliosis commonly develops during childhood or adolescence. Marked lumbar lordosis, often with genu valgum or varum, leads to a waddling gait. Cleft palate is common. Over 50% of patients have severe myopia predisposing to retinal detachment.

Roentgenographically, SED congenita is characterized by platyspondyly and epiphyseal dysplasia. In the newborn, ossification of the epiphyseal centers is retarded, especially at the ankles, knees, and hips. Epiphyseal ossification centers ultimately appear but are irregular, fragmented, and flattened. The proximal femoral epiphysis is severely affected; severe coxa vara results. The long bones appear shortened, especially the humerus and femur, but the hands are normal or show only minor abnormalities. In childhood the vertebrae are ovoid but later become flat and irregular with narrowed disc spaces. Odontoid hypoplasia may be found with subluxation of C1 on C2.

Some patients with SED congenita later show atypical features or have a relatively mild disorder, suggesting genetic heterogeneity.

Short stature in **SED tarda** (X-linked recessive type) is recognized from 5 to 10 yr of age, when spinal growth appears to be slowed and the shoulders assume a humped appearance. Mild to severe kyphoscoliosis may develop, and US/LS ratio is reduced. As adults, affected men have mild short stature, with short trunk, large chest capacity, and relatively normal limb length. The hands, head, and feet appear normal. During late childhood or adolescence vague back pain may occur; in early adulthood painful osteoarthritis with limited mobility of the back and hips is usually present. Symptoms may also affect the shoulders and, less commonly, the knees and ankles.

Roentgenograms in SED tarda reveal diagnostic changes in the lumbar vertebrae by childhood or adolescence. Vertebral bodies show generalized mild flattening, with a hump-shaped build-up of bones in the central and posterior portions of the superior and inferior plates. Ossification of the ring epiphyses is delayed. Disc spaces appear narrowed and may appear to be calcified, but the calcification is part of the vertebral body itself. Premature disc degeneration occurs, and osteospondylotic changes develop in early childhood. The acetabula are deep and the femoral neck short. Mild dysplastic changes are seen in all large joints, especially the hips.

Differential Diagnosis. A dominantly inherited form of SED tarda has variable onset of manifestations after infancy, with distinctive roentgenographic features. Several conditions having metaphyseal as well as epiphyseal changes are called spondyloepimetaphyseal dysplasia or spondylometepiphyseal dysplasia, depending on the relative severity of metaphyseal or epiphyseal lesions (Fig. 23–26). *Stickler syndrome* (hereditary arthro-ophthalmopathy) is charactaized by tall stature, myopia, and premature osteoarthritis. In the *Schwartz-Jampel* syndrome (myotonic chondrodysplasia) myotonia is associated with skeletal abnormalities. *Kniest dysplasia* is described below. Heterogeneity is marked among the spondyloepiphyseal dysplasias, many patients being unclassifiable.

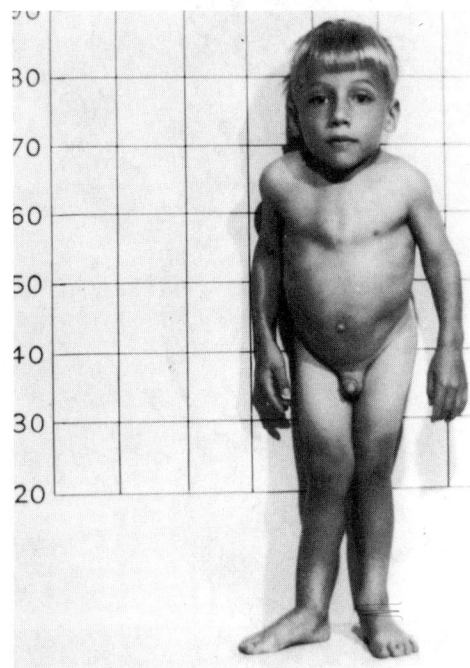

Figure 23–26. Spondylometepiphyseal dysplasia showing predominant shortening of the trunk characteristic of the spondylodysplasias.

Kniest Dysplasia. In this autosomal dominant condition there is a marked delay in epiphyseal ossification at the hips, short-trunk short stature, progressive kyphoscoliosis, and progressive joint limitation. The joint deformity and limitation are most marked at the knee and the small joints of the hands. The face is round and flat. Myopia and cleft palate are common. Roentgenographic features include coronal clefts in the vertebrae, hypoplastic iliac bones having wide and irregular acetabular margins, dysplastic femoral heads which are very delayed in appearance, and short, thin tubular bones having flared metaphyses. Epiphyseal ossification is irregular and punctate, and a peculiar stippling occurs at the epiphyses and adjacent metaphyses as the patient becomes older.

Kniest syndrome must be differentiated both from *Rolland-Desbuquois syndrome*, an autosomal recessive condition having many features in common with Kniest dysplasia but showing more severe vertebral segmentation defects, and from dyssegmental dysplasia, a lethal skeletal dysplasia of newborns that shows similar yet more severe vertebral malsegmentation and occipital encephalocele.

23.24 DIASTROPHIC DYSPLASIA

In this autosomal recessive disorder the dysplastic changes occur in auricular, tracheal, articular, and ligamentous tissues as well as in chondro-osseous tissues. Affected persons have short-limb (rhizomelic) short stature, severe club feet, joint contractures, and deformity of the hands with a proximally placed hypermobile (hitchhiker) thumb (Fig. 23–27). In about 85% of children the pinnae of the ears become acutely inflamed and swollen during the first 2–5 wk of life and remain thickened, firm, and irregular (cauliflower ear). With time, the ear lesions calcify and may ossify. The palate is broad and high arched; cleft palate occurs in about 25% of cases. Laryngomalacia may lead to respiratory distress. Midline frontal

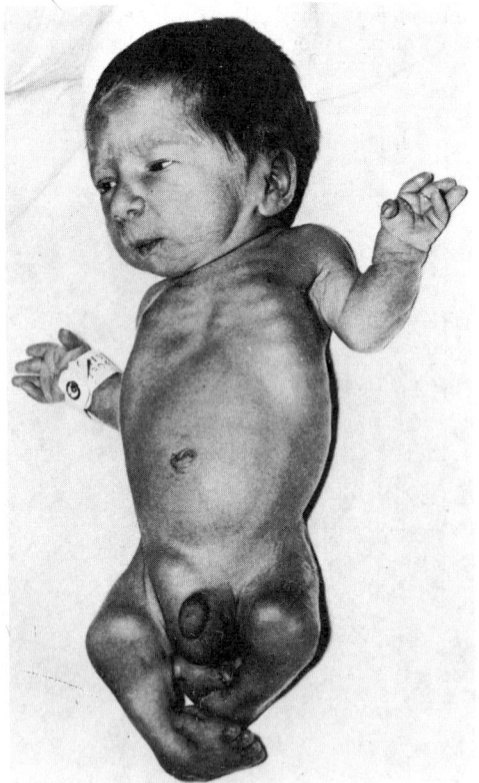

Figure 23–27. Diastrophic dysplasia showing fixed deformities of the knees and elbows, and hitch-hiker thumbs (and halluces).

hemangiomas are common. The hips are normal at birth, but hip and knee dislocations frequently develop on weight bearing. Both stiff joints and loose joints may occur in the same patient, with subluxations and dislocations as well as contractures. Progressive scoliosis may develop during the first year of life. Kyphosis may begin at adolescence and lead to respiratory difficulty in adults. The head and skull are normal. Some cases involving milder features of diastrophic dysplasia have been termed "diastrophic variant."

Roentgenographic manifestations include hypoplasia of the epiphyses and flaring of the metaphyses in long tubular bones, carpal bone irregularities (including extra carpal bones), and twisted or fused metatarsals with equinovarus deformity. Caudal narrowing of the spinal canal may be present, and the cervical spine may be kyphotic, with C2–C3 dislocation. Metacarpals and phalanges are short and wide, and the 1st metacarpal is oval or triangular in shape and set low on the carpus.

23.25 METATROPIC DYSPLASIA

Metatropic dysplasia is characterized by short extremities, bulbous enlargement of the joints, joint limitation, and progressive and ultimately severe kyphoscoliosis. It is probably genetically heterogeneous, having both dominant and recessive autosomal varieties. At birth, affected children have a short-limbed appearance, but kyphoscoliosis develops rapidly, and a short-trunk appearance supervenes. The kyphosis may produce neurologic complications due to acute angulation of the spinal cord. Some patients have a peculiar tail-like skin fold over the sacrum. Some patients die in infancy.

Roentgenographic findings at birth include extreme platyspondyly with tongue-like flattening of vertebrae and relatively large intervertebral spaces. The long bones are short and have irregularly expanded metaphyses resembling barbells. Epiphyses are deformed, flattened and irregular, and delayed in ossification. The tubular bones of the hands are short and broad with irregular epiphyses and metaphyses. Carpal ossification is delayed. The ribs are short and have flared and cupped costochondral junctions. Marked flaring of the iliac crests produces a "battle-axe" (halberd) appearance.

The kyphoscoliosis has generally been resistant to bracing or surgical treatment. Electrical stimulation to the sacrospinalis muscles with bracing has been reported to limit progression of the kyphoscoliosis.

23.26 MESOMELIC DYSPLASIAS

This heterogeneous group of skeletal dysplasias is characterized predominantly by shortening in the mesomelic segments of the limbs (Fig. 23–28). Modes of inheritance vary. Five syndromes manifest at birth are clearly delineated: the Nievergelt, Langer, Robinow, Rheinhardt, and Werner mesomelic dysplasias. The most common mesomelic dysplasia, dyschondrosteosis, is not manifest until late childhood. A number of other conditions with mesomelia, short stature, and other congenital abnormalities do not fit into these categories.

Dyschondrosteosis (Léri-Weill syndrome) results in mild mesomelic short stature with Madelung deformity at the wrist. Inheritance is autosomal dominant, with variable penetrance and expression. The bones of the forearm and leg are disproportionately shortened and widened. Hypoplasia and dorsal dislocation of the distal ends of the ulnae result in bilateral Madelung deformity. The carpal bones are wedged into a small triangular space between the deformed distal radius and ulna. The tibia and fibula appear widened. In some family members of normal stature the diagnosis is made solely on the basis of Madelung deformity.

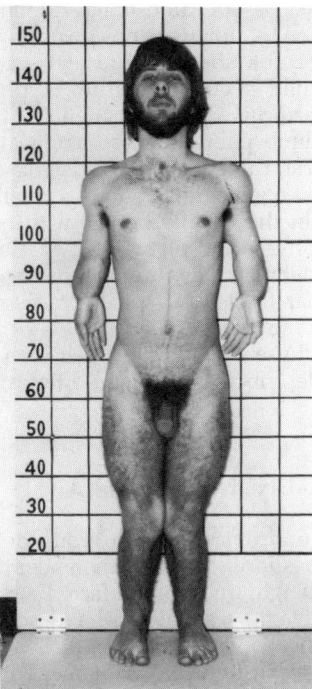

Figure 23–28. Mesomelic dysplasia with predominantly middle (mesomelic) limb shortening.

Robinow mesomelic dysplasia is an autosomal dominant condition recognizable by the flat facial profile, mesomelic shortening, and high frequency of genital hypoplasia. The distal ulna is hypoplastic; in some cases there is radial head dislocation. Prominent forehead, hypoplastic mandible and hypertelorism, down-slanting palpebral fissures, and a short, flat nose are characteristic. Genital hypoplasia may occur, with or without cryptorchidism. The nails are commonly hypoplastic.

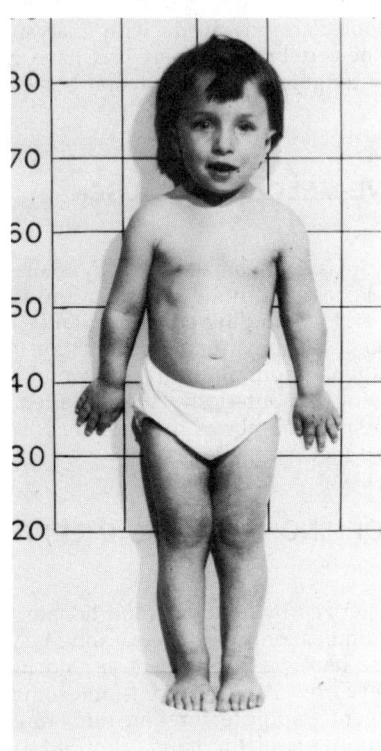

Figure 23–29. Peripheral dysostosis with disproportionate (acromelic) shortening of the fingers.

Acromesomelic dysplasias include several distinct skeletal dysplasias characterized by disproportionate shortening, predominantly affecting the forearms, hands, feet, and legs, which can be recognized at birth or within the first months of life (Fig. 23–29). In these the face and head are usually normal and the trunk only slightly shortened. The epiphyses and metaphyses of the long bones are unaffected.

23.27 CLEIDOCRANIAL DYSPLASIA

The disorder is characterized by varying degrees of hypoplasia of membranous bones. Inheritance is autosomal dominant, with variable expressivity. Hypoplasia of the anterior ends of the clavicles and sacral rami, delayed closure of the anterior fontanelle, and multiple wormian bones are characteristic. The hypoplasia of the clavicles leads to abnormally low positioning of the shoulders, which can commonly be apposed anteriorly. Frontal bossing, joint hyperlaxity leading to genu valgum, and dental anomalies are common. The primary dentition appears late and is frequently incomplete. The secondary dentition is similarly delayed and frequently malaligned, malformed, or hypoplastic. Proportionate short stature may occur.

Roentgenographically, there are variable degrees of hypoplasia of clavicles and scapulae, marked delay in ossification of the pubis and ischiopubic segments, and widening of the symphysis pubis.

23.28 LARSEN SYNDROME

This is a genetically heterogeneous group of disorders characterized by marked hyperlaxity and multiple dislocations, especially of the hips, knees, and elbows. Skin hyperlaxity and dermatorrhexis are not features. Autosomal dominant and, rarely, autosomal recessive transmissions occur. Affected patients characteristically have a prominent forehead, low nasal bridge, hypertelorism, a flattened face, disproportionate short stature, and, in about 50% of cases, cleft uvula and/or palate.

Roentgenographically, joint dislocations with secondary epiphyseal deformities are seen. Supernumerary carpal and tarsal ossification centers develop, and the 1st–4th metacarpals are short and broad. There may be premature fusion of the epiphysis and shaft of the 1st distal phalanx.

Larsen syndrome must be distinguished from Ehlers-Danlos syndrome, types III (benign hypermobility) and VII (arthrochalasis multiplex congenita), in which associated skeletal abnormalities and craniofacial disproportion are not present. Multiple joint dislocations occur also in the otopalatodigital syndrome.

23.29 OTOPALATODIGITAL SYNDROME

This disorder is characterized by a distinct facies, abnormalities of the hands and feet, proportionate short stature, and, sometimes, mental retardation. Inheritance is X-linked dominant, with complete expression in males and milder features in carrier females. The facies has prominent supraorbital ridges, a broad nasal root, flattening of the midface, and a small jaw. The thumbs and distal segments of the other fingers are short and broad. Dislocation of the radial heads and/or hips may be present. Midline cleft palate and conductive deafness are commonly associated.

23.30 METAPHYSEAL DYSPLASIAS

The metaphyseal dysplasias (formerly called *metaphyseal dysostoses*) are a heterogeneous group of disorders predominantly involving the metaphyses, with relatively normal epiphyses and spine. They should always be considered in the differential diagnosis of Vitamin D–resistant rickets. Four principal types are the Jansen type (autosomal dominant), the Schmid type (autosomal dominant), the Spahr type (autosomal recessive), and the McKusick type (autosomal recessive), which is also called cartilage-hair hypoplasia.

The *Jansen type* produces the most severe short stature (adult height about 125 cm) and can be recognized in the newborn period or early infancy by the predominantly rhizomelic short stature, severe bowing of the legs, and mandibular hypoplasia. Joints are large, with contractures, and since the legs are more severely affected than the arms, the arms appear to hang down around the knees. Roentgenographically, all metaphyses, including those of hands and feet, are severely involved, appearing markedly enlarged, wide, irregular, and cystic. Epiphyses and spine appear relatively normal. The long bones are broad and short, and bowing is evident. Deafness has been associated with hyperostosis of the calvarium. Serum calcium levels are elevated in some patients. Serum alkaline phosphatase activity is slightly elevated. New mutations account for most cases.

The *Schmid type* of metaphyseal dysplasia is characterized by mild to moderate short stature (adult height 130–160 cm), bowing of the legs, and a waddling gait. It is usually recognized when the infant commences walking. Enlarged wrists and flaring of the rib cage are usually present. Roentgenographically, the metaphyseal changes are much less severe than those of the Jansen type. The metaphyses are flared and irregular and may be fragmented, with radiolucent streaks. Changes are most prominent in the hips, shoulders, knees, ankles, and wrists. In contrast to the McKusick variety, involvement of the femoral neck may be quite severe and result in marked coxa vara. This disorder has been frequently confused with vitamin D–resistant rickets, but calcium and phosphorus metabolism appears to be normal.

The *Spahr type* is similar to the Schmid type but with autosomal recessive inheritance.

In the *McKusick type* of metaphyseal dysplasia (cartilage-hair hypoplasia) severe growth deficiency of postnatal onset, bowing deformities of the limbs, and particularly short, broad hands with loose joints are characteristic. Affected individuals also have an ectodermal dysplasia manifested by fine, light, sparse hair and a light complexion. Increased susceptibility to severe varicella infection in some patients reflects a deficiency in cellular immunity. Serum immunoglobulins may be abnormal in some families. Aganglionic megacolon may be associated.

Roentgenographically, cartilage-hair hypoplasia is characterized by multiple metaphyseal lesions in the long and short tubular bones, and a normal skull, spine, and epiphyses. Lesions especially involve the knees, and, in contrast to the Schmid type, the proximal femoral metaphyses are very mildly involved. The affected metaphyses are wide and irregular with sclerotic radiolucent cystic areas and linear streaks. The fibula is long relative to the tibia, producing an unstable ankle joint. Genu valgum is prominent. The ribs are short, with anterior cupping.

The *combination of metaphyseal abnormalities and immune deficiency* is found in at least three other autosomal recessive syndromes: (1) the Shwachman syndrome, in which skeletal lesions are associated with pancreatic exocrine insufficiency and chronic neutropenia; (2) metaphyseal chondrodysplasia–thymic alymphopenia syndrome; and (3) combined immunodeficiency due to adenosine deaminase deficiency, in which growth failure with metaphyseal irregularities and flaring of the ribs may occur.

23.31 SPONDYLOMETAPHYSEAL DYSPLASIAS (SMD)

In these conditions abnormalities primarily involve the vertebrae and metaphyses.

SMD Kozlowski is an autosomal dominant condition. Growth retardation is not usually apparent until 1–2 yr of age, when short-trunk short stature and waddling gait develop. There is mild pectus carinatum, kyphoscoliosis, and precocious osteoarthritis in some patients. Affected children frequently have limb pains that are aggravated by exercise and relieved by rest; these may be misdiagnosed as "growing pains." Skeletal roentgenograms show generalized metaphyseal irregularities in the tubular bones, with normal or small and irregular epiphyses and platyspondyly. On anteroposterior view the vertebral bodies appear flat and broad, with prominent articular facets and spinal processes contributing to an "open staircase" appearance.

Spondylometaphyseal dysplasias other than the Kozlowski type have been described, some with other modes of inheritance.

23.32 PSEUDOACHONDROPLASIA

The pseudoachondroplasias are a group of disorders producing short-limb short stature with moderately severe reduction of trunk height and normal face. Both dominant and autosomal recessive forms have been described, although recessive inheritance is very uncommon. Growth retardation is usually not apparent until 2–3 yr of age, with considerable variability in its severity. In some patients shortening is predominantly rhizomelic, in others predominantly mesomelic.

There is an exaggerated lumbar lordosis. Hypolaxity of the joint in the periphery may lead to valgus or varus deformities at the knees. Deformities of the legs lead to a waddling gait. The hands and feet are short and broad, ligamentous laxity permitting telescoping of the fingers similar to that seen in cartilage-hair hypoplasia. Dislocations may be troublesome, particularly at the knees. Contractures may also occur at the hips and knees, and there may be limitation of extension at the elbow. Ulnar deviation at the wrist is characteristic. The major complication is precocious osteoarthritis.

Roentgenographically, the epiphyses and metaphyses of the tubular bones are involved, with platyspondyly and irregularity of the vertebrae. The vertebrae have irregular endplates; anterior tonguing of the vertebral bodies is common in infancy.

23.33 DYGGVE-MELCHIOR-CLAUSEN SYNDROME

This rare dysplasia is characterized by short-trunk short stature, a barrel chest, accentuated lumbar lordosis, restricted joint mobility, and a waddling gait. Inheritance is autosomal recessive. In some sibships mental retardation has been associated. Roentgenographically, this is a spondyloepiphyseal dysplasia showing flat anteriorly beaked vertebral bodies, a fine lace-like ossification above the iliac crest, and irregular small carpal and metacarpal bones.

23.34 TRICHORHINOPHALANGEAL (TRP) SYNDROME

This is characterized by mild disproportionate short stature involving deformities of the fingers, and a typical facies including sparse hair, pear-shaped nose, and medial accentuation of the eyebrows. Inheritance is autosomal dominant. The main roentgenographic features are numerous phalangeal cone-shaped epiphyses of the hands (PhCSEH), often associated with brachymetacarpism and brachymetatarsism. Legg-Perthes–like changes may occasionally occur in the hips.

23.35 OSTEOCHONDRODYSPLASIAS WITH ANARCHIC DEVELOPMENT OF CARTILAGINOUS OR FIBROUS TISSUE

These form a group of disorders in which development of abnormally placed cartilage or fibrous elements leads to skeletal deformity during growth, with relative hyperplasia or hypoplasia of skeletal elements. Two subgroups can be distinguished according to whether the anarchic proliferation involves cartilage or fibrous tissue: those involving cartilage include dysplasia epiphysealis hemimelica, multiple cartilaginous exostoses, Langer-Giedion syndrome (multiple cartilaginous exostoses–peripheral dysplasia), multiple enchondromatosis (Ollier), enchondromatosis with hemangioma (Maffucci), and metachondromatosis. Those involving fibrous tissue include fibrous dysplasia (Jeffe-Lichtenstein), fibrous dysplasia with skin pigmentation and precocious puberty (McCune-Albright), cherubism and neurofibromatosis (Sec. 21.16 and 24.10).

Abnormally situated growths of osteocartilaginous tissue may be localized to the epiphyses, the metaphyses, or the diaphyses of the long bones. Dysplasia epiphysealis hemimelica or tarsomegaly affects the skeleton of only one portion of the lower extremity. Cartilage may develop within bone (i.e., as an enchondroma) or on the surface of bone, commonly at the edge of the metaphyses (i.e., as exostosis or enchondroma).

In **dysplasia epiphysealis hemimelica (Trevor disease)** there is asymmetric overgrowth of the epiphyses, tarsal centers, and, rarely, carpal centers. All cases have been sporadic, and there is a male predominance. Because there may be involvement of an entire epiphysis rather than half, the term "unilateral epiphyseal dysplasia" has been suggested as an alternative name.

This condition is usually recognized in the first years of life because of foot or knee deformity, a limp, or a painful gait. Usually, there is a medial or lateral firm swelling at the knee or tibiotarsal joint with minimal loss of length in the involved leg. Roentgenographically, fragmentation and excessive growth of the involved epiphysis are seen, which commonly involves only one part of the epiphysis. Simultaneous involvement of several epiphyses is common, especially of foot and knee. The talus, distal femoral, and distal tibial epiphyses are the most common sites of disease. Lesions of the upper extremities are rare.

Multiple cartilaginous exostoses (MCE) are bony projections found near the ends of the tubular bones and ribs, the vertebral bodies, the scapulae, and the iliac crest. Roentgenographically, these tumors appear to originate at the borders of metaphyses and sometimes along the shafts (diaphyses) of the long bones. They are distinct from enchondromata (chondromata), which arise within the metaphyses and sometimes the diaphyses and which appear to be expanding within the metaphyses into the epiphyses. Inheritance is autosomal dominant with high penetrance but widely variable expression. It is generally believed that the pathogenesis involves proliferation of normal cartilage at the borders of the metaphyses, along the diaphyses, or alongside the cartilaginous borders of the vertebrae and scapulae. Because regular endochondral ossification occurs within these cartilaginous tumors, the center of the tumor becomes ossified. The medullary cavity of this central ossified area may communicate with the marrow space of the shaft of the affected bone.

The tumors may undergo rapid growth during infancy but are rarely detected roentgenographically prior to 3 yr of age, when they appear as bony projections from the affected bones, which have a normal pattern of ossification. Exostoses at the ends of the long bones point away from the epiphyses. Involvement of metacarpals and phalanges frequently occurs,

but the exostoses are small and rarely deform the fingers. Exostoses of the shaft of the humerus characteristically occur at the junction of the upper and middle thirds on the medial surface. The exostoses are not only unsightly but disturbing to the growth of long bones, producing deformation and sometimes compression of nerves and blood vessels. Severe deformity of the distal ulna is often associated with an asymmetric growth disturbance, dislocation of the radial head, and ulnar deviation of the hand. Involvement of the lower limbs may lead to coxa valga, genu valgum, or obliquity of the distal tibial epiphyses and limb length discrepancy. Final adult height tends to be in the normal range, but mild skeletal disproportion may occur since limb involvement (often asymmetric) is much greater than spinal involvement. Malignant degeneration may occur, but rarely, if ever, in childhood.

Surgical treatment is indicated for cosmetically deforming lesions or those producing neurovascular complications. Wherever possible, surgery should be delayed until the end of growth because of the high chance of regression of the lesions.

Multiple cartilaginous exostoses–peripheral dysplasia (Langer-Giedion syndrome) is characterized by predominantly acromelic or acromesomelic short stature of postnatal onset, facial appearance similar to that in the trichorhinophalangeal syndrome (see above), mild microcephaly of postnatal onset, and multiple cartilaginous exostoses. All reported cases have been sporadic. The characteristic facies includes large, poorly developed, laterally protruding ears, sparse scalp hair with thick eyebrows, a large bulbous nose with a thick prominent septum, a simple prominent elongated philtrum, and a relatively recessed chin. Redundant or loose skin folds and hyperextensibility of skin and ligaments in infancy may lead to confusion with the Ehlers-Danlos syndrome.

Roentgenographically, two types of lesions are apparent: (1) multiple exostoses with all the possibilities for skeletal deformity produced by MCE alone, and (2) abnormalities in metacarpal and proximal phalanges consisting of cone-shaped epiphyses (see TRP syndrome), widening with lack of normal funnelization, and a hook-like, often asymmetric, projection of the metaphyses.

Enchondromata arise within bone, usually within areas of endochondral ossification. Single enchondromata of bone are not uncommon and may be incidentally detected. They may, on the other hand, produce local pain due to intramedullary expansion. *Multiple enchondromata* (Ollier disease) have widespread involvement of the skeleton, involving the hands; they are detected because of bone pain or deformity. Virtually all cases have been sporadic. Roentgenographically, the lesions may be detectable in early infancy as clear, homogeneous, oval lesions with axes parallel to the longitudinal axis of the bone.

Patients present because of growth disturbance, which may be asymmetric, leading to limp, or because of swelling of the fingers and toes in infancy. The tumors may produce visible or palpable swelling, particularly in the hands or the growing ends of the long bones; they are somewhat elastic and may limit mobility of neighboring joints. Phalangeal chondromas may lead to severe deformation of the fingers.

The effect of enchondromas on growth is usually much more serious than that of exostoses, and the prognosis is more serious than in MCE. Asymmetric growth disturbance is more severe. Involvement of distal ulna and radius may produce a severe deformation at the wrist leading to ulnar deviation of the hand. Malignant change is uncommon in childhood but has a higher frequency in adults. Pain and rapid growth in size and/or radiologic evidence of endosteal erosion may indicate malignant change.

Surgical intervention is indicated for lesions causing local symptoms for or growth plate deformation leading to marked limb asymmetry. Radionuclide scanning may be useful in investigating large enchondromata at risk of malignant change.

In **enchondromatosis with hemangiomatosis** (*Maffucci syndrome*) multiple enchondromata and hemangiomata of bone and overlying skin develop during childhood. The majority of affected persons are normal at birth; the lesions develop during infancy. All reported cases have been sporadic. The cutaneous lesions are usually cavernous or capillary hemangiomas, with or without lymphangiomas. Their distribution in skin appears to be independent of skeletal lesions; they may be found also in mucous membranes and intra-abdominal viscera. The skeletal lesions are typical enchondromata, involving metaphyses throughout the body; in some cases unilateral deformity predominates.

Maffucci syndrome produces a severe, cosmetically unsightly and often painful deformation of the skeleton. Neither the hemangiomata nor the enchondromata are amenable to surgical intervention except for palliation. The lesions lead to short stature or, if predominantly unilateral, to leg length discrepancy and scoliosis. The most serious complication is the development of malignancy, which has a higher incidence than malignant change in MCE. Chondrosarcomatous transformation of one or more enchondromata may occur; sarcomatous degeneration of hemangiomas and lymphangiomas has been reported.

Metachondromatosis is a condition in which typical multiple cartilaginous exostoses and multiple enchondromata are found in the same patient. Inheritance is autosomal dominant. Affected patients are normal at birth; in infancy they acquire lesions in digits and long bones. Short stature may occur, although the majority of patients have normal stature.

23.36 ABNORMALITIES OF DENSITY OR MODELING OF THE SKELETON AND COLLAGENOUS TISSUE

This group of genetic skeletal dysplasias includes heritable conditions associated with osteoporosis (diminished or fragile bone), osteopetrosis, and hyperostosis or hyperplasia of bone producing abnormal modeling of the skull, long bones, or axial skeleton.

23.37 INHERITED OSTEOPOROSES

Osteopenia (insufficiency of bone) is a roentgenographic feature of many inherited or acquired disorders of childhood; it results from reduced production or increased breakdown of bone, or both. Osteoporosis (the clinical syndrome resulting from osteopenia) is characterized by susceptibility to fractures and particularly to crush fractures of vertebrae. Osteogenesis imperfecta is the most prevalent of the osteoporosis syndromes in childhood and is characterized by fractures and skeletal deformities. Some of the affected die in the newborn period with extreme fragility of bone and numerous fractures (osteogenesis imperfecta congenita); others manifest bone fragility in life and live a normal life span (osteogenesis imperfecta tarda). At least four genetic syndromes account for variability in osteogenesis imperfecta. Serum alkaline phosphatase activity is normal or elevated in all forms.

OSTEOGENESIS IMPERFECTA TYPE I (OI Type I)

This is characterized by osteoporosis and excessive bone fragility, distinctly blue sclerae, and presenile conductive hearing loss in adolescents and adults. Inheritance is autoso-

mal dominant. This most common variety of osteogenesis imperfecta has an incidence of about 1:30,000 live births.

The sclerae are generally of a deep blue-black hue. Fractures result from minimal trauma, but not all accidental trauma produces fractures. About 10% of affected infants have a few fractures at birth. Occurrence of neonatal fractures does not predict more deformity, more handicap, or a greater number of fractures than in other patients who have their first fractures after 1 yr of age. Deformities of the limbs in OI type I are largely the result of fractures, but bowing, particularly of the lower limbs, is common. Other deformities such as genu valgum and flat feet with metatarsus varus are also common. About 20% of affected adults have progressive kyphoscoliosis which may be severe. Kyphosis alone is common in older adults but rarely seen in children. There is usually excessive hyperlaxity of ligaments, particularly at the small joints of the hands, feet, and knees, but this feature is less marked in adults. There is usually mild short stature; body proportions depend on the relative involvement of limbs or spine. During adolescence there is a marked spontaneous reduction in the frequency of fractures.

Hearing impairment affects 55% of patients; it is rare, however, before the end of the first decade.

Hereditary opalescent dentin (dentinogenesis imperfecta) is observed in some families with this trait. It produces distinctively yellow (or sometimes grayish-blue) transparent teeth, which are frequently prematurely eroded or broken. These teeth have short roots and constricted coronoradicular junctions. Opalescent dentin distinguishes a subgroup of patients with OI type I from a subgroup with normal teeth.

Roentgenographic studies in OI type I show generalized osteopenia, evidence of previous fractures, and normal callus formation at the site of recent fractures. Deformities are usually the result of angulation at the site of previous fractures, but bowing of the femora and tibia and fibula occurs as well as deformity in the bones of the feet, particularly metatarsus varus. Severe osteoporosis of the spine and codfish vertebrae are occasionally seen; kyphoscoliosis is not usually observed in childhood.

Osteogenesis Imperfecta Type II (OI Type II). This lethal syndrome is characterized by low birthweight and length and typical roentgenographic findings of crumpled long bones and beaded ribs. Autosomal recessive inheritance occurs in a proportion of cases, with some sporadic instances representing fresh autosomal dominant mutations. The condition affects about 1 infant in 60,000 live births.

Approximately 50% are stillborn, and the remainder die soon after birth of respiratory insufficiency due to a defective thoracic cage. The skull is soft and there are multiple palpable bone islands. The face may show beaking of the nose and apparent hypotelorism, and the limbs are extremely short, bent, and deformed. The thighs are broad and fixed at right angles to the trunk (Fig. 23–30). The skin is thin and fragile and may be torn during delivery.

Roentgenograms show multiple fractures of the ribs, which are often continuously beaded, and a crumpled (accordion-like) appearance of the long bones (especially the femora). There is diffuse osteopenia in the face and skull and multiple bone islands in the vault.

A number of distinct biochemical defects have been discovered in the α_1(I) and α_2(I) chains of type I collagen that have the common effect of a marked reduction in the synthesis of type I collagen, the principal collagen of bone.

Osteogenesis Imperfecta Type III (OI Type III). This syndrome is characteristically manifested in the newborn or young infant by severe bone fragility and multiple fractures, which lead to progressive skeletal deformity (Fig. 23–31). The sclerae may be blue at birth and become less blue with age. Inheritance is autosomal recessive; clinical variability suggests genetic heterogeneity.

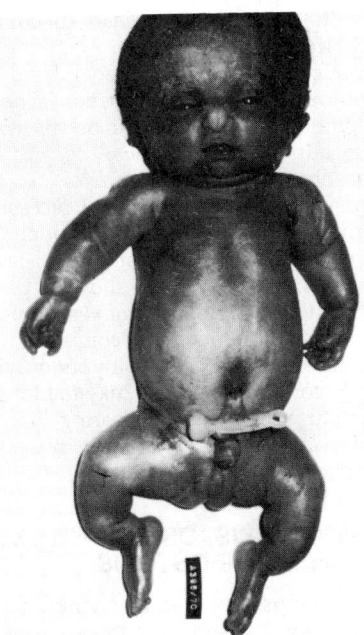

Figure 23–30. Osteogenesis imperfecta type II (lethal crumpled bone variety) with broad thighs and angulation deformities of the limbs.

Very few patients with OI type III reach adult life. Infants generally have normal birthweight and often normal birth length, but the latter may be reduced by deformities of the lower limbs. Fractures are present in the majority of cases at birth and occur frequently during childhood. Kyphoscoliosis develops during childhood and progresses into adolescence. Final stature is very short. Hearing impairment has not been reported. A considerable proportion of patients succumb to cardiorespiratory complications in infancy or childhood.

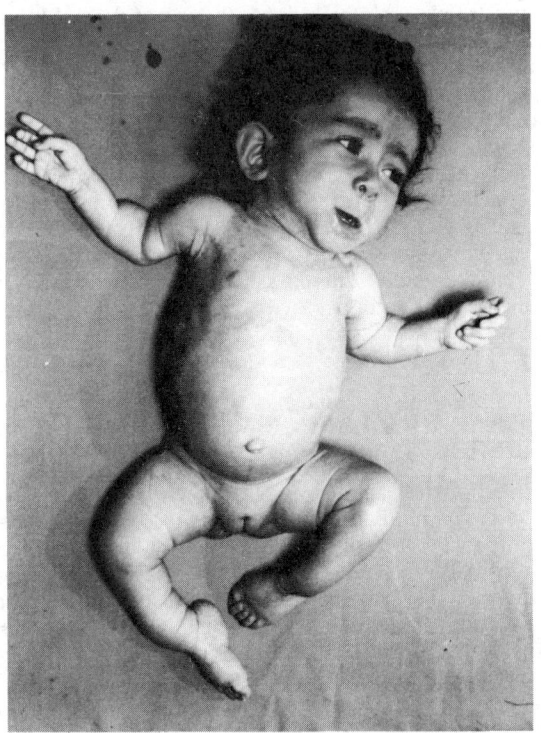

Figure 23–31. Osteogenesis imperfecta type III showing less shortening of limbs but angulation deformities of legs.

Skeletal roentgenograms in OI type III show generalized osteopenia and multiple fractures, without the beading of the ribs or crumpling of long bones seen in OI type II. Osteopenia appears to be progressive, with platyspondyly and codfish vertebrae. The skull shows osteopenia and multiple wormian bones.

Collagen gene and protein biochemical studies in one case showed absence of the $\alpha_2(I)$ chain of type I collagen.

Osteogenesis Imperfecta Type IV (OI Type IV). This syndrome is characterized by osteoporosis leading to bone fragility without other features of classic OI type I. Inheritance is autosomal dominant. The sclerae in OI type IV may be bluish at birth but become less blue as the patient matures. Hearing impairment is less common, but opalescent dentin has been observed in some families, suggesting heterogeneity within this group.

Patients with OI type IV have variable ages of onset of fractures, ranging from birth to adult life, and variable deformity of long bones and spine. Significant bowing of the lower limbs at birth may be the only feature of this syndrome, and progressive deformity of the long bones and spine has been reported without fractures. In several patients bowing has lessened with age. Like those with OI type I, patients with OI type IV show spontaneous improvement with puberty, few fractures showing up in adolescents and adults. Most patients, however, have short stature. Roentgenographically, there is generalized osteopenia. Multiple fractures may be observed at birth and occur throughout life, but these patients have less osteopenia and fewer fractures than infants with recessive varieties of osteogenesis imperfecta.

Management of Osteogenesis Imperfecta. For OI type II, no therapeutic intervention is effective. For other forms of OI careful nursing of the newborn on a firm mattress or pillows may prevent excessive fractures. Beyond the newborn period the mainstay of management is an aggressive orthopedic regimen aimed at prompt splinting of fractures and correction of deformities arising from fractures and from the progressive bowing or bending of the skeleton. Therapeutic regimens including supplements of calcium or fluoride, of vitamin C, or of magnesium oxide have shown no clear benefit. Calcitonin therapy has been reported to increase skeletal mass and decrease the frequency of fractures in some patients, but the use is still investigative. Genetic counseling for affected families should aim at primary prevention. Reliable antenatal diagnosis is not available for all types of osteogenesis imperfecta, but some severely affected fetuses with OI type II may be confidently recognized prenatally through a combination of ultrasound, roentgenographic, and biochemical studies.

Osteoporosis with Pseudogliomatous Blindness. This rare autosomal recessive syndrome is characterized by generalized osteoporosis leading to fractures and deformities of long bones and spine. Ocular pseudogliomas, which may be mistaken for retinoblastoma, develop in infancy. Mild mental retardation has been observed in several of those affected but may be unrelated.

23.38 OSTEOPETROSIS, PYKNODYSOSTOSIS, AND DYSOSTEOSCLEROSIS

These conditions are characterized by generalized increase in skeletal density. Individually, they are distinguished by their mode of inheritance, age of onset, and pattern of skeletal involvement. Several forms of **osteopetrosis** have been described with overlapping spectra of clinical and roentgenographic features. A form with manifestations in the newborn and a progressive course leading to death at an early age is called *osteopetrosis with precocious manifestations*. A usually milder disorder with delayed manifestations is known as *osteopetrosis tarda* or *Albers-Schönberg disease*.

Osteopetrosis with Precocious Manifestations. This form is most frequently discovered during the first months of life; it may appear as failure to thrive, malignant hypocalcemia, anemia with thrombocytopenia, or severe, perhaps overwhelming infection. Inheritance is generally autosomal recessive, but some cases may show autosomal dominant inheritance.

Rarely, fractures lead to medical attention. Hyperostosis may crowd the marrow cavity, with anemia and extramedullary hematopoiesis, hepatosplenomegaly, and thrombocytopenia. Anemia appears to result not from inadequate erythropoiesis but from excessive hemolysis. A defect in macrophage killing of bacteria may account for recurrent and sometimes overwhelming infection. Bony encroachment on the optic foramina may lead to optic atrophy and blindness, in some cases detectable at birth. Hypocalcemia is not uncommon, and serum phosphorus may be low. Serum alkaline phosphatase activity is elevated. Roentgenographically, the diagnostic findings are a generalized increase in bone density, with defective metaphyseal modeling and a "bone in bone" appearance most marked in the vertebral bodies. Diffuse hyperostosis leads to loss of demarcation between the cortex and the medullary cavity. Irregular condensation of bone at the metaphyses may produce the appearance of parallel plates of dense bone at the ends of the long bones. The base of the skull is dense, having normal to increased density of the vault and markedly increased density in the orbital margins.

Treatment is aimed at decreasing or arresting progressive hyperostosis, correcting anemia and thrombocytopenia, and treating infections promptly and vigorously; a regimen of oral cellulose phosphate, prednisone, and low calcium diet has been reported effective in some but not all patients. The prednisone arrests the progress of anemia. Neurosurgical unroofing of the optic foramina has been tried in some patients, but results are difficult to interpret. Bone marrow transplantation with appropriately HLA-matched donor marrow has been reported to be curative in several patients, but the long-term success of this treatment is unknown. Generally, the prognosis for survival is poor, and death in the first few months or years from anemia, bleeding, or overwhelming infection is not uncommon.

Osteopetrosis Tarda (Albers-Schönberg Disease). This condition presents in childhood, adolescence, or young adult life because of fractures (about 10% of patients), mild craniofacial disproportion, mild anemia, complications arising from neurologic involvement, or osteitis with osteonecrosis (usually of the mandible). Increased bone density may be discovered incidentally on a roentgenographic study made for some other problem. Most cases represent autosomal dominant inheritance, a few autosomal recessive.

Skeletal roentgenograms show generalized increase in density of cortical bone, with a club-shaped appearance of the long bones due to defective metaphyseal modeling. Over 50% of patients have longitudinal and transverse dense striations at the ends of the long bones. The vertebrae show alternating lucent and dense bands. The base of the skull is dense and thickened, but face and vault are less affected.

Management should be directed at recognition and treatment of complications, with frequent testing of visual fields and acuity and periodic roentgenograms of the optic foramina. Transfusion may be required for anemia, and splenectomy may be useful in some patients.

Pyknodysostosis. This autosomal recessive disorder is characterized by postnatal onset of short-limbed short stature and generalized hyperostosis. A disproportionately large skull, frontal and occipital bossing, and wide anterior fontanelle may bring the patient to the physician's attention. The hands and feet are short and broad, and the nails may be deformed and brittle. The sclerae are often blue; this evidence combined with a tendency to fractures may lead to confusion with osteogenesis imperfecta.

Roentgenographically, there is a generalized increase in bone density without metaphyseal striation. The distal phalanges are characteristically hypoplastic or aplastic. The skull has wide sutures and wormian bones; the face has a small mandible with an obtuse mandibular angle.

Dysosteosclerosis. This rare autosomal recessive disorder is characterized by generalized increase in bone density and short stature of postnatal onset. Dysosteosclerosis differs from osteopetrosis and pyknodysostosis in showing platyspondyly with superior and inferior irregularity of vertebral ossification. Developmental defects of the teeth are common, with delayed eruption of primary dentition, severe hypodontia, and early loss of the teeth. Secondary dentition may fail to erupt. Other complications (fractures, visual and hearing loss, and recurrent infections of mandible and paranasal sinuses) are similar to those of osteopetrosis.

23.39 OSTEOPOIKILOSIS, OSTEOPATHIA STRIATA, AND MELORHEOSTOSIS

These three conditions are usually asymptomatic and encountered incidentally through roentgenographic studies. Some patients have several types of lesions.

In *osteopoikilosis*, numerous small osteodense round or oval foci are seen in the skeleton, most commonly in the epiphyses and carpal and tarsal centers. Joint pain is associated in about 20% of cases, and skin lesions occur in some patients. The latter are slightly elevated whitish-yellow fibrocollagenous infiltrations (dermatofibrosis lenticularis disseminata). The incidence of keloid formation is increased. Inheritance is autosomal dominant.

In *osteopathia striata*, linear regular bands of increased density radiate from the metaphyses throughout the skeleton, with a fan-like array in the iliac wings. Inheritance is possibly autosomal dominant. The lesions should be differentiated from those of osteopetrosis, which are associated with modeling defects and transverse bands of osteodensity at the metaphyses. Osteopathia occurs with focal dermal hypoplasia (Goltz syndrome), in which linear lesions of dermal hypoplasia and herniation of the adipose tissue are associated with skeletal defects (hypoplasia or aplasia of limbs or syndactyly).

In *melorheostosis*, irregular linear osteodense lesions are seen along the axes of the tubular bones in single or multiple areas of the skeleton. No hereditary basis has been established. The osteodense lesions have been likened to wax flowing down the side of a candle. Since the pattern of lesions may follow the sensory sclerotomes, it has been suggested that melorheostosis may result from lesions of the sensory nerve supply to skeletal elements. The lesions may be associated with shortening of certain bones, with contractures of the joints or palmar and plantar fasciae, and with intermittently painful swelling of joints.

23.40 CRANIOTUBULAR REMODELING DISORDERS

A distinction has been drawn between craniotubular dysplasias, e.g., craniodiaphyseal dysplasia, in which modeling abnormalities are present, and craniotubular hyperostoses, e.g., endosteal hyperostosis (van Buchem), in which deformity is due to overgrowth of osseous tissue rather than to defective bone modeling. The distinction may be arbitrary since these disorders must be the result of bone resorption and bone deposition, albeit with different patterns of skeletal involvement. In all of them there is generally minimal involvement of the spine, as compared with osteopetrosis, pyknodysostosis, and dysosteoclerosis.

In diaphyseal dysplasia (Camurati-Engelmann), craniodiaphyseal dysplasia, the craniometaphyseal dysplasias, frontometaphyseal dysplasia, and pachydermoperiostosis, sclerosis in the region of optic foramina may lead to visual impairment, papilledema, and optic atrophy. Sclerosis of internal acoustic formina and the middle ear may also lead to conductive or sensorineural hearing loss. Encroachment on the facial nerve foramina may lead to facial paresis and encroachment on the foramen magnum to long tract signs, hyperreflexia, weakness, and even sudden death or paraplegia.

Diaphyseal Dysplasia (Camurati-Engelmann). This rare disorder, also known as progressive hereditary diaphyseal dysplasia, is associated with significant neuromuscular involvement. Inheritance is autosomal dominant, having variable penetrance and expression. Signs, symptoms, and severity vary among affected individuals within the same family. Symptoms usually begin at 4–10 yr of age but have occurred as early as 3 mo of age and as late as the 6th decade. Failure to thrive or gain weight, easy tiring, and abnormal gait are common presenting manifestations. Increasing leg pain may occur. The gait is waddling, with reduced muscle mass and poor muscle tone. Flexion contractures may develop at the elbows and knees. Bowleg or knock-knee may be seen; the feet may be flat and pronated. Deep tendon reflexes may be hypoactive or hyperactive, occasionally with ankle clonus. Lumbar lordosis, scoliosis, and back pain may occur. Symptoms and signs of encroachment on cranial nerves may be present. Exophthalmos is found in more than half of those affected.

The roentgenographic features include symmetric fusiform enlargement of the diaphyses of the long bones (especially the femur), with normal epiphyses and metaphyses. Diaphyseal cortex is enlarged by accretion of mottled endosteal and periosteal new bone. The lesions are often first noted in the centers of long bones, then gradual involvement of adjacent proximal and distal bone occurs. The skull may show sclerosis of frontal areas and base. Blood chemical findings are characteristically normal. There may be loss of individual muscle fibers and replacement by adipose tissue, atrophic muscle fibers, and slightly pyknotic sarcolemmal cell nuclei, with hyalinization and decreased prominence of cross-striations.

Management should aim for maximal mobility of the patient. Orthopedic correction of deformity of the lower limbs by appropriate osteotomy may help. A symptomatic response to low dose corticosteroid therapy has been reported.

Craniodiaphyseal Dysplasia. This rare disorder is characterized by massive hyperostosis and sclerosis of the skull and facial bones and by hyperostosis and defective modeling of the shafts of the tubular bones. Inheritance is autosomal recessive. The early respiratory symptoms may be due to narrowing of the nasal passages. Flattening of the nasal root may be noted at birth, and symptoms may occur as early as 3 mo of age. Progressive hyperostosis of the cranial and facial bones usually leads to prominence of nasal and adjacent maxillary bones by 1–2 yr of age. Symptoms and signs produced by encroachment on cranial foramina are marked. Affected patients are often of normal to tall stature. Serum alkaline phosphatase activity is markedly decreased.

Roentgenograms show massive hyperostosis of the cranial bones, which develops rapidly during infancy and completely obscures structural detail. The spine, ribs, clavicles, and scapulae appear hypermineralized but normal in shape. The metaphyses of the long bones show loss of normal funnelization and tubulation, which causes the long bones to appear broad and undermodeled.

No medical or surgical treatment can prevent progressive hyperostosis and sclerosis or their complications. Special attention should be given to amelioration of hearing and visual impairment and to psychosocial and genetic counseling.

Endosteal Hyperostosis and Sclerosteosis. These form a group of disorders characterized by marked accretion of osseous tissue at the endosteal (inner) surface of bone leading to narrowing of the medullary canal or obliteration of the medullary space.

A rare, dominantly inherited variety of *endosteal hyperostosis* (Worth type) is frequently associated with torus palatinus. A recessively inherited variety (*van Buchem disease*) is characterized by progressive mandibular enlargement from childhood; in adult life signs and symptoms result from sclerotic encroachment on optic and acoustic foramina. Serum alkaline phosphatase activity is markedly elevated. Roentgenographically, there is marked thickening of the skull, from base to vault, and increased density of the mandible after puberty. Cortices of tubular bones show increased density, with narrowing of the marrow cavity.

Sclerosteosis, an autosomal recessive trait, is clinically and roentgenographically almost indistinguishable from van Buchem disease, of which it may be a variant. It is differentiated by a high incidence of hyperostosis in nasal and facial bones, which produces a broad, flat nasal bridge and hypertelorism, and by minor hand malformations consisting of cutaneous syndactyly, radial deviation of the 2nd and 3rd fingers, and absent or hypoplastic nails.

Tubular Stenosis (Caffey-Kenny). This autosomal dominant syndrome is characterized by narrowing of the medullary canal. Features include delayed closure of the anterior fontanelle, tetanic seizures secondary to hypocalcemia, and myopia. Roentgenographically, the medullary cavity is reduced, often markedly, with normal or increased cortical thickness. The diploic space may be absent.

Frontometaphyseal Dysplasia. This X-linked dominant condition produces a clinically striking facial appearance: a pronounced supraorbital ridge resulting from a torus-like bony overgrowth of the supraorbital ridges of the frontal bones. Changes are more severe in males. Affected patients show hirsutism, conductive deafness, and wasting of the muscles of arms and legs and particularly of the hypothenar and interosseous muscles of the hands. The prominent supraorbital ridge extending across the entire frontal bone is associated with poor development of frontal and other paranasal sinuses and with mandibular hypoplasia. The metaphyses of all the long and short tubular bones are undermodeled.

Craniometaphyseal Dysplasias. These conditions manifest severe progressive cranial hyperostosis and undermodeling of the metaphyses. Both autosomal dominant and recessive transmissions are reported. The time of onset of symptoms and signs shows wide variability in families with dominant inheritance; some cases are recognized in infancy. Clinically, both dominant and recessively inherited forms show progressive facial dysmorphology, consisting of broad osseous prominence of the nasal root extending across the zygoma. Difficulty in breathing due to encroachment on the nasal passages may be recognized in early infancy. The severity of sclerotic encroachment on cranial foramina is variable.

The essential roentgenographic features are hyperostosis of the skull; of the nasal and maxillary bones, extending bilaterally across the zygoma, with failure of pneumatization of the paranasal sinuses and mastoids; and of the mandible. The long bones show flaring and decreased density of the metaphyses (Ehrlenmeyer flask deformity). Hyperostosis and sclerosis of the mandible are less severe than in craniodiaphyseal dysplasia.

23.41 OSTEODYSPLASTY
(Melnick-Needles)

This disorder or group of disorders is characterized by "abnormally shaped" bones. The majority of familial cases have shown autosomal dominant inheritance, but an autosomal recessive variant is reported. The age at diagnosis is variable, and affected children are usually first evaluated because of an abnormal gait and bowing of the extremities, occasionally because of dislocation of hips or delayed closure of the anterior fontanelle. On the whole, these patients do not have short stature, and psychomotor development and adult height are normal. Facial appearance is somewhat typical, consisting of slight exophthalmos, protruding cheeks, a high, narrow forehead, prominent orbital rims, micrognathia, and malaligned teeth. The lower thorax is narrow. Distal segments of the thumbs are incurved.

Roentgenographically, there is uneven thickening of the cortex of the long bones, in which irregular contours and multiple constrictions produce a wavy border. The diaphyses are slightly curved and show metaphyseal modeling defects.

Coxa valga and dislocation of the hips are common. The ribs are wavy in appearance. The supra-acetabular iliac wings appear narrowed.

HYPERPHOSPHATASIA WITH OSTEOECTASIA

See Sec. 23.56.

23.42 INFANTILE CORTICAL HYPEROSTOSIS
(Caffey Disease)

This condition of unknown cause must be differentiated from hyperphosphatasia with osteoectasia (Sec. 23.56). The disorder is usually recognized in the first 3 mo of life. The course is febrile, with marked swelling of soft tissues over the face and jaws and progressive cortical thickening of long bones and flat bones. Alkaline phosphatase activity is usually mildly increased. The condition has exacerbations and remissions with spontaneous regression after several years. Corticosteroids can relieve symptoms during exacerbations.

HYPOPHOSPHATASIA

See Sec. 23.53.

DAVID O. SILLENCE

General

Akeson WH, Bornstein P, Glimcher MJ: American Academy of Orthopaedic Surgeons Symposium on Heritable Disorders of Connective Tissue. St. Louis, CV Mosby, 1982.

Beighton P: Inherited Disorders of the Skeleton. Edinburgh, Churchill Livingstone, 1978.
Beighton P, Cremin B, Fauré C, et al: International nomenclature of constitutional diseases of bone. Ann Radiol 26:457, 1983.
Maroteaux P: Bone Disease of Children. Philadelphia, JB Lippincott, 1979.
McKusick VA: Heritable Disorders of Connective Tissues. St. Louis, CV Mosby, 1972.
McKusick VA: Mendelian Inheritance in Man. 6th ed. Baltimore, The Johns Hopkins Press, 1983.
Rimoin DL (ed): Skeletal dysplasias. Clin Orthop 114:2, 1976.
Rimoin DL, Horton WA: Short stature, Parts I and II. J Pediatr 92:523, 93:697, 1978.
Sillence DO, Lachman R, Rimoin DL: Neonatal dwarfism. Pediatr Clin North Am 25:453, 1978.
Temtamy SA, McKusick VA: The genetics of hand malformations. Birth Defects, Original Article Series 14(3), 1978.

Radiology

Lachman R: Radiology of pediatric syndromes. Curr Probl Pediatr 9(4):52, 1979.
Spranger JW, Langer LO, Wiedemann HR: Bone Dysplasias. An Atlas of Constitutional Disorders of Skeletal Development. Philadelphia, WB Saunders, 1974.

Chondro-osseous Morphology and Biochemical Investigation

Sillence DO, Horton WA, Rimoin DL: Morphologic studies in skeletal dysplasias. Am J Pathol 96:813, 1979.
Stanescu V, Stanescu R, Maroteaux P: Morphological and biochemical studies of epiphyseal cartilage in dyschondroplasias. Arch Franc Pediatr 34, Suppl 3:1, 1977.
Teitelbaum SL, Bullough PG: The pathophysiology of bone and joint disease. Am J Pathol 96:283, 1979.

Management

Amstutz HC, Sakai DN (eds): Equalization of leg length. Clin Orthop Rel Research 136:2, 1978.
Coccia PF, Krivit W, Cervenka J, et al: Successful bone-marrow transplantation for infantile malignant osteopetrosis. N Engl J Med 302:701, 1980.
Goldberg MJ: Orthopedic aspects of bone dysplasias. Orthop Clin North Am 7:445, 1976.
Horton WA, Rotter JI, Rimoin DL, et al: Standard growth curves for achondroplasia. J Pediatr 93:435, 1978.
Kopits SE: Orthopedic complications of dwarfism. Clin Orthop Rel Research 114:153, 1979.

Nonprofessional Organizations of and for Patients with Skeletal Short Stature

American Brittle Bone Society, National Headquarters, Suite LL-3, Cherry Hill Plaza, 1415 East Marlton Pike, Cherry Hill, N.J. 08034.
Human Growth Foundation, 11740 East 5th Street, Tulsa, Okla. 74128.
Little People of America, Inc., Box 126, Owatonna, Minn. 55060.
Osteogenesis Imperfecta Foundation, Inc., 632 Center Street, Van Wert, Ohio 45891.

23.43 MARFAN SYNDROME
(Arachnodactyly)

Marfan syndrome is an autosomal dominant disorder of connective tissue characterized by skeletal, ocular, and cardiovascular abnormalities. The basic nature of the metabolic defect is unknown, though abnormalities in elastin and collagen are present.

Clinical Manifestations. Patients with Marfan syndrome are tall and slender, lacking normal quantities of subcutaneous fat. The extremities are characteristically long, with the more distal bones demonstrating excessive length (Fig. 23–32). The lower segment measurement (pubis-to-sole) in these patients is greater than the upper segment measurement (pubis-to-vertex). The arm span is excessive and exceeds the height. The fingers are long and tapered (spider fingers). The thumb and fifth finger, when clasped around the wrist, overlap in patients with this disease (the wrist sign). The relatively long, narrow palm of the hand, together with a long thumb, forms the basis of the Steinberg thumb sign (the thumb opposed across the palm extends well beyond the ulnar border of the hand). The excessive longitudinal growth of the ribs in these children results in thoracic cage deformities, including pectus excavatum or pigeon-breast deformities. Weakness of joint capsules, ligaments, tendons, and fascia produces hyperextension of joints, flat feet, recurrent dislocations of hips, patella, and other joints, and femoral hernias. Underdeveloped muscle and cutaneous striae may also be present. Ocular abnormalities are common and include subluxation of the lens (ectopia lentis) which may be severe and is often bilateral, severe myopia, retinal detachment, strabismus, and nystagmus. The most common cardiovascular abnormalities (Sec. 14.68) are diffuse dilatation of the proximal segment of the

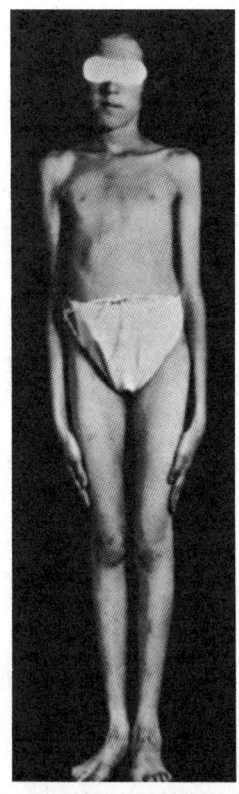

Figure 23–32. Arachnodactyly.

ascending aorta and aortic regurgitation secondary to dilatation and stretching of the aortic cusps. Mitral valve disease is common and presumably reflects stretching of the chordae tendineae; mitral valve prolapse also occurs. A variety of conduction abnormalities have been reported, and serious ventricular dysrhythmia may occur with or without valve disease and may progress with age. Congestive heart failure and rupture of the aorta secondary to a dissecting aneurysm are common causes of death. Spontaneous dissecting aneurysm of the ductus arteriosus has been reported in infancy.

Diagnosis. The clinical manifestations of Marfan syndrome are quite characteristic. However, significant variability occurs, and affected individuals may not have all the stigmata. The disease is most often confused with homocystinemia (Sec. 7.4), which may be differentiated by the character of the lens dislocation (upward dislodgment in Marfan syndrome), the presence of a malar flush, generalized osteoporosis, moderate mental retardation, a positive urinary nitroprusside test, and the identification of homocystine in the urine.

Treatment. No therapy is available for Marfan syndrome; orthopedic, cardiovascular, and ophthalmologic abnormalities should be identified and corrected.

Boucek RJ, Noble NL, Gunja-Smith Z, et al: The Marfan syndrome: A deficiency in chemically stable collagen cross-links. N Engl J Med 305:988, 1981.
Byers PH, Siegel RC, Peterson KE, et al: Marfan syndrome: Abnormal alpha-2 chain in type I collagen. Proc Natl Acad Sci USA 78:7745, 1981.
Gillan JE, Costigan DC, Keeley FW, et al: Spontaneous dissecting aneurysm of the ductus arteriosus in an infant with Marfan syndrome. J Pediatr 105:952, 1984.
Su-chiung C, Fagan LF, Soraya N, et al: Ventricular dysrhythmias in children with Marfan. Am J Dis Child 139:273, 1985.

23.44 ARTHROGRYPOSIS

Arthrogryposis multiplex congenita is a heterogeneous group of congenital disorders of unknown but probably multiple etiologies characterized by extreme stiffness and contracture of joints (usually flexion) and associated hypoplasia or absence of muscle development and soft tissues. Although it often occurs alone, arthrogryposis may be part of a complex of multisystemic congenital anomalies.

Epidemiology and Etiology. Most cases are sporadic, occurring in about 3 of 1000 live births, although rare instances of autosomal recessive inheritance are reported. Many of the etiologic theories postulate disorders of fetal joint mobility and include abnormalities of hormones, fetal blood supply, and mechanical restriction (e.g., bands) and in utero infection and neuropathy.

Pathology. Thick inelastic articular capsules and atrophic muscle fibers with fibrosis and fatty infiltration are noted at autopsy. Anterior horn cell degeneration in the spinal cord has also frequently been found.

Clinical Manifestations. Arthrogryposis multiplex congenita is occasionally associated with a prenatal history of reduced fetal movement, oligohydramnios, and breech presentation. It is present at birth, and, although the lesions are static, untreated deformities progress as the child grows.

The affected limbs appear cylindrical with loss of the normal contours and skin creases. The skin appears thickened, and there may be dimples near joints. Structural deformities are common, including flexion contractures of knees, elbows, wrists, and other joints, dislocation of the hips and other joints, clubfoot, and scoliosis. There may be webbing across affected joints. Similar deformities occur in association with mylomeningocele, myelodysplasia, and Potter syndrome. Defects of the palate or vertebrae and absence of the sacrum and fibula may also occur. The elbows and knees may also be ankylosed in extension. Some cases of arthrogryposis are associated with diastrophic dwarfism or with congenital muscular dystrophy. Mental retardation is relatively infrequent.

Treatment. This consists of massage, passive movements, gradual correction of deformities by splints and plaster casts, and orthopedic surgery.

RICHARD E. BEHRMAN

Beckerman RC, Buchino JJ: Arthrogryposis multiplex congenita as a part of an inherited symptom complex: Two case reports and a review of the literature. Pediatrics 61:417, 1978.
Wayne-Davies R, Lloyd-Roberts GC: Arthrogryposis multiplex congenita: Search for prenatal factors in 66 sporadic cases. Arch Dis Child 51:618, 1976.

23.45 METABOLIC BONE DISEASE

Bone is a dynamic organ capable of rapid turnover, weight-bearing, and withstanding the stresses of a variety of physical activities. It is constantly being formed (modeling) and re-formed (remodeling), and it is the major body reservoir for calcium, phosphorus, and magnesium. Disorders that affect this organ and the process of mineralization are designated "metabolic bone disease."

Since bone growth and turnover rates are high during childhood, many of the clinical features of metabolic bone disease are more marked in children than in adults. Recent advances in our knowledge of bone metabolism, the process of mineralization, interactions of the vitamin D–PTH–endocrine axis, and metabolism of vitamin D to active compounds have improved treatment of metabolic bone disease.

The human skeleton consists of a protein matrix, largely made up of a collagen-containing protein, osteoid, upon which is deposited a crystalline mineral phase. Although collagen-containing osteoid comprises 90% of bone protein, other proteins are present, including osteocalcin, which contains gamma-carboxyglutamic acid. Synthesis of osteocalcin is vitamin K–dependent and, in high bone turnover states, serum osteocalcin values are elevated.

The microfibrillar matrix of osteoid permits deposition of highly organized calcium phosphate crystals, including hydroxyapatite $[C_{10}(PO_4)_6 \cdot 6H_2O]$ and octacalcium phosphate $[Ca_8(H_2PO_4)_6 \cdot 5H_2O]$, plus less oganized amorphous calcium phosphate, calcium carbonate, sodium, magnesium, and citrate. Hydroxyapatite is deep within bone matrix, whereas amorphous calcium phosphate coats the surface of newly formed or remodeled bone.

In children bone growth occurs by the process of calcification of the cartilage cells present at the ends of bone. In accord with the prevailing extracellular fluid calcium and phosphate concentrations, mineral is deposited in those chondrocytes or cartilage cells set to undergo mineralization. The role of the vitamin D–PTH–endocrine axis is to maintain the extracellular fluid calcium and phosphate concentrations at appropriate levels to support mineralization.

Other hormones also appear to regulate the growth and mineralization of cartilalge, including growth hormone acting via somatomedins, thyroid hormones, insulin, and androgens and estrogens during the pubertal growth spurt. By contrast, supraphysiologic concentrations of glucocorticoids impair cartilage function and bone growth.

23.46 RICKETS

See also Sec. 3.29.

Rates of bone formation are coordinated with alterations in mineral metabolism at both the intestine and kidney. Inadequate dietary calcium intake or intestinal absorption causes a fall in serum calcium and its ionized fraction. This is the signal for PTH production and secretion, resulting in greater bone resorption to raise serum calcium, enhanced renal reabsorption of calcium, and higher rates of synthesis in the kidney of 1,25-dihydroxyvitamin D (1,25[OH]$_2$D or calcitriol), which is the most active metabolite of vitamin D (Fig. 23–33). Calcium homeostasis thus is controlled at the intestine, since the availability of 1,25(OH)$_2$D will determine the fraction of ingested calcium that is absorbed.

By contrast, phosphate homeostasis is regulated by the kidney, since intestinal phosphate absorption is nearly complete and renal excretion determines the serum level. Excessive intestinal phosphate absorption causes a fall in serum ionized calcium and a rise in PTH secretion, resulting in phosphaturia, which lowers serum phosphate and permits calcium to rise. Hypophosphatemia blocks PTH secretion and promotes renal 1,25(OH)$_2$D synthesis. This latter compound promotes greater intestinal phosphate absorption.

Understanding the metabolism of vitamin D is necessary to understand rickets (Fig. 23–33). The skin contains 7-dehydrocholesterol, which is converted to vitamin D$_3$ by ultraviolet radiation; other inactive vitamin D sterols are also produced. Reduced skin exposure to ultraviolet light (from smog or clothing) results in rickets (Sec. 3.29). Vitamin D$_3$ is then transported to the liver by a vitamin D–binding blood protein (DBP); DBP binds all forms of vitamin D. The plasma concentration of free or nonbound vitamin D is much lower than the level of DBP-bound vitamin D metabolites.

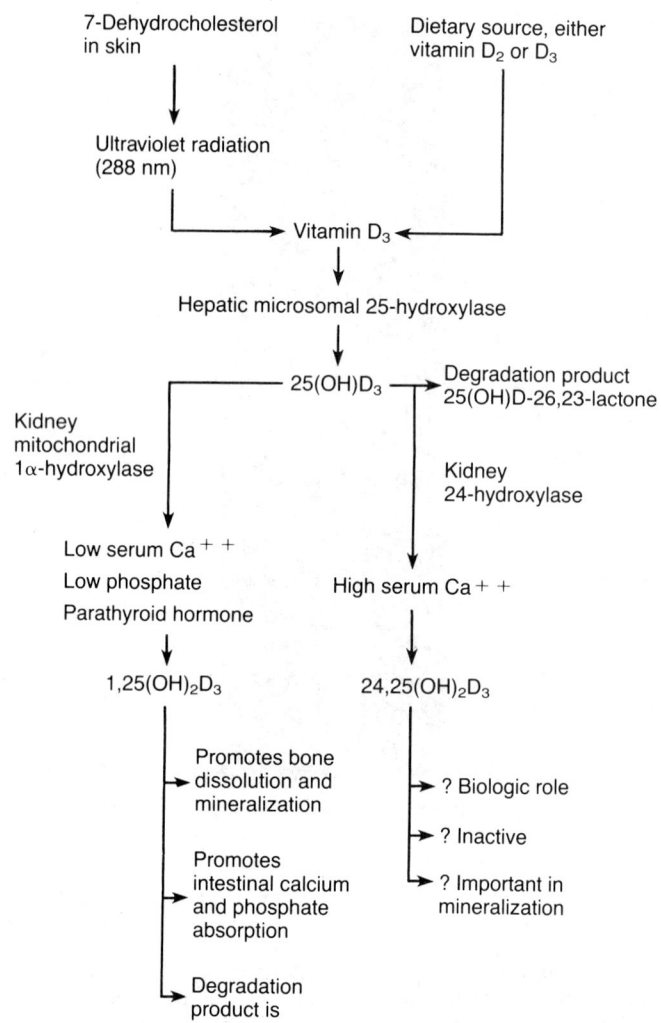

Figure 23–33. The metabolic pathway of vitamin D, indicating its conversion to the hormone 1,25(OH)$_2$D$_3$ and to 24,25(OH)$_2$D$_3$. Vitamin D$_2$ (ergosterol) of plant origin appears to undergo similar metabolic steps.

Vitamin D also can enter the metabolic pathway by ingestion of dietary vitamin D$_2$ (ergocalciferol) or vitamin D$_3$ (cholecalciferol), which are absorbed from the intestine along with other fat-soluble vitamins because of the action of bile salts. After absorption, ingested vitamin D is transported via chylomicrons to the liver where, along with skin-derived vitamin D$_3$, it is converted to 25-hydroxyvitamin D (25[OH]D) by the action of a hepatic microsomal enzyme requiring oxygen, NADPH, and magnesium to hydroxylate vitamin D at the 25th carbon atom. The 25(OH)D is next transported by DBP to the kidney, where it undergoes further metabolism. 25(OH)D is the main circulating vitamin D metabolite in man, at a concentration of 20–50 ng/mL (Table 23–4). Since its synthesis is weakly regulated by feedback, its plasma level rises in summer and falls in winter. High vitamin D intake raises the plasma level of 25(OH)D to many times above normal, but the parent vitamin D itself is absorbed by adipose tissue.

In the kidney, the 25(OH)D undergoes further hydroxylation, depending on the prevailing serum concentration of calcium, phosphate, and PTH. If calcium or phosphate is reduced or PTH is elevated, the enzyme 25(OH)D-1α-hydroxylase is activated and 1,25(OH)$_2$D is formed (Fig. 23–33). This metabolite circulates at a level that is only 0.1% of the level of 25(OH)D (Table 23–4). It also acts on the intestine to

Table 23–4. Vitamin D Metabolite Values in Plasma of Normal Healthy Subjects

Metabolite	Plasma Value	
Vitamin D$_2$	1–2	ng/mL
Vitamin D$_3$	1–2	ng/mL
25 (OH)D$_2$	4–10	ng/mL
25 (OH)D$_3$	12–40	ng/mL
Total 25 (OH)D	15–50	ng/mL
24, 25 (OH)$_2$D	1–4	ng/mL
1, 25 (OH)$_2$D		
—Infancy	70–100	pg/mL
—Childhood	30–50	pg/mL
—Adolescence	40–80	pg/mL
—Adulthood	20–35	pg/mL

increase the active transport of calcium and stimulate phosphate absorption. Since 1α-hydroxylase is a mitochondrial enzyme that is tightly regulated by feedback, the synthesis of 1,25(OH)$_2$D declines after serum calcium or phosphate returns to normal. Excessive 1,25(OH)$_2$D is converted to calcitroic acid, an inactive metabolite. In the presence of normal or elevated serum calcium and/or phosphate concentrations, the renal 25(OH)D-24-hydroxylase is activated, producing 24,25-dihydroxyvitamin D (24,25[OH]$_2$D), which may play a role in bone mineralization. The serum levels of 24,25(OH)$_2$D (1–5 ng/mL) become higher after ingestion of large amounts of vitamin D. Although hypervitaminosis D and production of inactive metabolites can occur after oral dosing (Sec. 3.31), extensive skin exposure to sunlight does not usually produce toxic levels of 25(OH)D$_3$, suggesting some natural regulation of the production of this metabolite.

Serum 1,25(OH)$_2$D levels are higher in children than in adults, are not subject to seasonal variability, and peak in the first year of life and again during the adolescent growth spurt. These values must be interpreted in light of the prevailing serum calcium, phosphate, and PTH values and with regard to the entire vitamin D metabolite profile.

Mineral deficiency prevents the normal process of bone mineral deposition. If mineral deficiency occurs at the growth plate, growth slows and bone age is retarded—a condition termed *rickets*. Poor mineralization of trabecular bone resulting in a greater proportion of unmineralized osteoid is the condition of *osteomalacia*. Rickets is found only in growing children prior to fusion of the epiphyses, whereas osteomalacia is present at all ages. All patients with rickets have osteomalacia, but not all patients with osteomalacia have rickets. These conditions should not be confused with *osteoporosis*, a condition of equal loss of bone volume and mineral, caused in childhood by glucocorticoid administration or found in Turner and Kleinfelter syndromes.

Rickets may be classified as calcium-deficient or phosphate-deficient rickets. Since both calcium and phosphate ions make up bone mineral, the insufficiency of either type in the extracellular fluid that bathes the mineralizing surface of bone results in rickets and osteomalacia. The two types of rickets are distinguishable by their clinical manifestations (Table 23–5).

23.47 FAMILIAL HYPOPHOSPHATEMIA
(Vitamin D–Resistant Rickets, X-Linked Hypophosphatemia)

The most commonly encountered form of rickets is familial hypophosphatemia. The usual mode of inheritance is X-linked dominant, indicating that some mothers of affected children exhibit clinical evidence of disease such as bowing or short stature, while others manifest only fasting hypophosphatemia. Autosomal recessive and sporadic cases have also been reported.

Pathogenesis. There are defects in the proximal tubular reabsorption of phosphate and the conversion of 25(OH)D to 1,25(OH)$_2$D. The latter defect is evidenced by low-normal serum 1,25(OH)$_2$D levels despite hypophosphatemia and by the finding that further phosphate depletion of subjects with familial hypophosphatemia does not stimulate 1,25(OH)$_2$D synthesis as it does in normal subjects. Both a renal tubular reabsorption defect and reduced 1,25(OH)$_2$D synthesis are found in an animal model of this disease (the X-linked hypophosphatemic mouse). In addition, oral phosphate supplementation alone cannot completely heal this bone disease, and the correction of osteomalacia requires 1,25(OH)$_2$D therapy.

Clinical Manifestations. Children with familial hypophosphatemia present with bowing of the lower extremities related to weight-bearing at the age of walking. Tetany is not present, and the profound myopathy, rachitic rosary, and Harrison's groove (pectus deformity) characteristic of calcium-deficient rickets are not evident. These children develop a waddling gait, smooth (rather than angular) bowing of the lower extremities, coxa vara, genu varus, genu valgum, and short stature. The adult height of untreated patients is 130–165 cm.

Pulp deformities and a lesion termed "intraglobular dentin" are characteristic tooth abnormalities, although enamel defects are found only occasionally. By contrast, calcium-deficient rickets usually results in enamel defects. Periapical infections are found in both forms of rickets.

Roentgenographic findings include metaphyseal widening and fraying and coarse-appearing trabecular bone. Cupping of the metaphysis occurs at the proximal and distal tibia and at the distal femur, radius, and ulna.

Laboratory Findings. There is a normal or slightly reduced serum calcium level (9.0–9.4 mg/dL), a moderately reduced serum phosphate level (1.5–3.0 mg/dL), elevated alkaline phosphatase activity, and no evidence of secondary hyperparathyroidism. Urinary phosphate excretion is large, despite hypophosphatemia, indicating a defect in renal tubular phosphate reabsorption. This disorder is typical of pure phosphate-deficient rickets; aminoaciduria, glucosuria, bicarbonaturia, and kaliuria are never found. In potential obligate heterozygotes, who later develop disease, serum phosphate levels may remain normal for several months, and the first laboratory abnormality is often a rise in serum alkaline phosphatase activity. The serum phosphate level probably remains normal for several months, since the glomerular filtration rate is quite low in neonates. Parathyroid hyperplasia with elevated serum PTH values is found occasionally, usually in sporadic cases.

Treatment. Oral phosphate supplements coupled with a vitamin D analog to offset the secondary hyperparathyroidism that may accompany an oral phosphate load is the preferred treatment. Oral phosphate is usually given every 4 hr at least 5 times a day, since urinary excretion is brisk and patients quickly become hypophosphatemic. Young children should receive 0.5–1.0 g/24 hr, while older children require 1.0–4.0 g daily. Phosphate can be given as Joulie solution (dibasic sodium phosphate, 136 g/L, and phosphoric acid, 58.8 g/L), which contains 30.4 mg of phosphate/mL. Thus, a 5.0 mL dose given every 4 hr, 5 times daily provides 760 mg of phosphate. Patient compliance is readily assessed, because nearly all of this dose is excreted in a 24 hr urine collection. The main side effect of oral phosphate therapy is diarrhea, which often improves spontaneously.

Providing a vitamin D analog is important for complete bone healing and for prevention of secondary hyperparathyroidism. Classically, vitamin D$_2$ was used at 2000 IU/kg/24 hr, but more recently dihydrotachysterol at a dose of 0.02 mg/kg/24 hr or 1,25(OH)$_2$D at 20–50 ng/kg/24 hr has been employed.

Familial hypophosphatemia was previously treated with 50,000–200,000 IU daily (1.25 to 10 mg) of vitamin D$_2$, but this

Table 23–5. **Clinical Variants of Rickets and Related Conditions**

Type	Serum Calcium Level	Serum Phosphorus Level	Alkaline Phosphatase Activity	Urine Concentration of Amino Acids	Genetics
I. Calcium deficiency with secondary hyperparathyroidism (Deficiency of vitamin D; low 25 (OH)D and no stimulation of higher 1,25(OH)₂D values)					
1. Lack of vitamin D					
a. Lack of exposure to sunlight	N or L	L	E	E	
b. Dietary deficiency of vitamin D	N or L	L	E	E	
c. Congenital	N or L	L	E	E	
2. Malabsorption of vitamin D	N or L	L	E	E	
3. Hepatic disease	N or L	L	E	E	
4. Anticonvulsive drugs	N or L	L	E	E	
5. Renal osteodystrophy	N or L	E	E	V	
6. Vitamin D–dependent type I	L	N or L	E	E	AR
II. Primary phosphate deficiency (no secondary hyperparathyroidism)					
1. Genetic primary hypophosphatemia	N	L	E	N	XD
2. Fanconi syndromes					
a. Cystinosis	N	L	E	E	AR
b. Tyrosinosis	N	L	E	E	AR
c. Lowe syndrome	N	L	E	E	XR
d. Acquired	N	L	E	E	
3. Renal tubular acidosis, type II proximal	N	L	E	N	
4. Oncogenic hypophosphatemia	N	L	E	N	
5. Phosphate deficiency or malabsorption					
a. Parenteral hyperalimentation	N	L	E	N	
b. Low phosphate intake	N	L	E	N	
III. End-organ resistance to 1,25(OH)₂D₃					
1. Vitamin D–dependent type II (several variants)	L	L or N	E	E	AR
IV. Related conditions resembling rickets					
1. Hypophosphatasia	N	N	L	Phosphoenthano-lamine elevated	AR
2. Metaphyseal dysostosis					
a. Jansen type	E	N	E	N	AD
b. Schmid type	N	N	N	N	AD

N, normal; L, low; E, elevated; V, variable; X, X-linked; A, autosomal; D, dominant; R, recessive.

caused hypervitaminosis D with nephrocalcinosis, hypercalcemia, and renal damage.

The term *vitamin D–resistant rickets* was used in the past to describe rickets in which patients failed to respond to a dose of vitamin D that would cure vitamin D deficiency. If appropriate doses of vitamin D or any of its metabolites fail to heal rickets, and if serum phosphate is not reduced, metaphyseal dysplasia should be considered (Sec. 23.54).

With early diagnosis and good compliance, the bowing deformities can be minimized, and an adult height above 170 cm is achievable. Corrective osteotomies always should be deferred until rickets appears healed roentgenographically and until the serum alkaline phosphatase level is in the normal range. Surgery prior to bone healing may be followed by redevelopment of deformity and bowing. In some patients, aggressive medical management may obviate the need for surgical intervention. Patients undergoing osteotomy should stop taking all vitamin D preparations before surgery and not restart them until they are again ambulating to avoid immobilization hypercalcemia. Since $1,25(OH)_2D$ has such a short half-life, it can be stopped just prior to surgery, while vitamin D_2 should be discontinued at least 1 mo before surgery. An additional advantage of $1,25(OH)_2D$ therapy is that it augments intestinal phosphate absorption and can improve phosphate balance. However, $1,25(OH)_2D$ should not be employed without concomitant oral phosphate.

Certain patients have hypophosphatemia and hyperphosphaturia but no roentgenographic evidence of rickets. This condition, inherited as an autosomal dominant disorder, has been termed *hypophosphatemic bone disease*. The serum concentration of $1,25(OH)_2D$ is normal, and the renal tubular phosphate excretion defect is not as marked as in familial hypophosphatemic rickets. Short stature also is not as marked. Oral phosphate and $1,25(OH)_2D$ have been used to treat this disorder.

23.48 VITAMIN D–DEPENDENT RICKETS
(Pseudovitamin D Deficiency, Hypocalcemic Vitamin D–Resistant Rickets)

Vitamin D–dependent rickets appears at age 3–6 mo in children who have been receiving doses of vitamin D (400–600 IU daily) that ordinarily prevent rickets. Serum calcium and phosphate levels are low, and alkaline phosphatase activity is elevated. This condition is a calcium-deficient form of rickets since patients have secondary hyperparathyroidism, aminoaciduria, glucosuria, renal tubular bicarbonate wasting, and renal tubular acidosis. These children also develop dental enamel hypoplasia. While the rickets and biochemical features of this autosomal recessive disorder can be treated with massive doses of vitamin D_2 (200,000 to 1 million IU daily), the use of relatively low dose $1,25(OH)_2D$ at 1–2 µg/24 hr will heal this disorder. The current hypothesis to account for these findings is that the enzyme activity of 25(OH)D-1α-hydroxylase is deficient or markedly reduced. As evidence of this hypothesis, the serum levels of $1,25(OH)_2D$ are low, despite hypocalcemia, hypophosphatemia, and elevated PTH levels.

Some patients with vitamin D–dependent rickets fail to reverse their rickets after treatment either with high-dose vitamin D_2 or $1,25(OH)_2D$ at 1–2 µ/day. Hypocalcemia, hypophosphatemia, aminoaciduria, and rickets persist in the presence of extremely high circulating levels of $1,25(OH)_2D$, usually above 180 pg/mL. A defect in the binding of $1,25(OH)_2D$ to either cytoplasmic or nuclear receptors in skin and bone cells is the pathophysiologic mechanism in this subset of patients; this form of the disease, which is particularly prevalent among children of first-cousin marriages, is termed *vitamin D dependency, type II*. Some patients have short

stature and alopecia totalis. Rickets can sometimes be reversed by administration of 15–30 µg/24 hr of $1,25(OH)_2D$, but lost hair does not return.

23.49 HEPATIC RICKETS

Rickets is not uncommon in children with hepatic disorders, particularly in extrahepatic biliary atresia, where failure of bile salt secretion prevents adequate absorption of vitamin D and other fat-soluble vitamins. Rickets also may occur in neonatal hepatitis and following hepatocellular damage induced by total parenteral nutrition. Although it was initially thought that hepatic disease would impair 25-hydroxylation and thereby reduce serum 25(OH)D levels, it is now believed that reduced absorption of vitamin D accounts for rickets. The usual findings of nutritional rickets are seen—reduced serum 25(OH)D values, hypocalcemia, roentgenographic evidence, and elevated serum alkaline phosphatase activity (bone and hepatic isoenzyme levels are raised). Since rickets mainly relates to vitamin D malabsorption, this form can be treated with high enough doses to overcome malabsorption. Thus, 4000–10,000 IU of vitamin D_2 (100–250 µg), 50µg of 25(OH)D or 0.2 µg/kg of $1,25(OH)_2D$ should be given daily, along with oral calcium. Calcium supplements are particularly indicated in infants having ascites who are receiving loop diuretics, such as furosemide, which result in hypercalciuria.

25.50 RICKETS ASSOCIATED WITH ANTICONVULSANT THERAPY

A small group of children receiving chronic anticonvulsant therapy will present with calcium-deficient rickets, despite apparently adequate vitamin D intake. This condition is far more common after the combination of phenobarbital and phenytoin, but it has been associated with nearly all anticonvulsant drugs. Affected patients have reduced serum levels of 25(OH)D and may have normal levels of $1,25(OH)_2D$. Because these anticonvulsants induce hepatic cytochrome P-450 hydroxylation enzyme activities, 25(OH)D is readily converted to more polar, inactive metabolites, thus accounting for lower serum 25(OH)D concentrations. However, this condition is far more complex, because many patients have a low intake of dairy products, which represent the major dietary source of calcium, and very poor exposure to sunlight. Thus, the relatively normal serum $1,25(OH)_2D$ values actually are subnormal in relation to the degree of hypocalcemia, hypophosphatemia, and secondary hyperparathyroidism.

In children receiving chronic anticonvulsant therapy, the serum values of calcium, phosphate, and alkaline phosphatase activity should be evaluated periodically. This form of rickets usually can be prevented by providing an extra 500 to 1000 IU of vitamin D_2 each day and by ensuring that the dietary intake of calcium is adequate.

23.51 ONCOGENOUS RICKETS
(Primary Hypophosphatemic Rickets Associated with Tumor)

Rickets associated with a tumor of mesenchymal origin that resolves upon removal of the tumor has been described in more than 30 cases. These tumors, which cause a phosphate-deficient form of rickets, are mostly benign, may become apparent only years after the development of rickets, and may be located in sites difficult to detect, such as the small bones of the hands and feet, abdominal sheath, nasal antrum, and pharynx. This syndrome also has been found in association with the epidermal nevus syndrome and neurofibromatosis (von Recklinghausen disease).

In addition to hypophosphatemia and hyperphosphaturia, glycinemia and glycinuria are sometimes found in this form of rickets. Evidence suggests that these tumors elaborate a still-unidentified substance which causes phosphaturia and impairs the conversion of 25(OH)D to 1,25(OH)$_2$D. Serum 25(OH)D levels are normal, and serum 1,25(OH)$_2$D levels are low but rapidly rise to normal after tumor excision. Such surgery also cures the bone pain and myopathy, which if untreated may confine the child to a wheelchair. Children with acquired or late-appearing hypophosphatemic rickets should undergo bone roentgenographic examination and/or bone scan to search for tumors. If a tumor cannot be removed or is metastatic, treatment with 1,25(OH)$_2$D and oral phosphate is often beneficial.

23.52 RICKETS ASSOCIATED WITH RENAL TUBULAR ACIDOSIS

Rickets may be present in primary renal tubular acidosis (RTA), particularly in type II or proximal RTA. Hypophosphatemia and phosphaturia are common in these syndromes, which are characterized by hyperchloremic metabolic acidosis, varying degrees of bicarbonaturia, and frequently hypercalciuria and hyperkaliuria (Sec. 17.29). Bone demineralization without overt rickets usually is detected in type I or distal RTA. In type I there is an inability to form an adequately acid urine at all levels of serum bicarbonate; in type II there is a lowered renal threshold for bicarbonate and impaired urinary acidification at normal levels of serum bicarbonate (Sec. 5.12). The metabolic bone disease that occurs in both types may also be characterized by bone pain, growth retardation, and osteopenia and occasionally by pathologic fractures. Although acute metabolic acidosis in vitamin D–deficient animals may impair the conversion of 25(OH)D to 1,25(OH)$_2$D, resulting in reduced levels of this active metabolite, the circulating levels of 1,25(OH)$_2$D in patients with either type of RTA are normal. If patients with RTA have azotemia and loss of renal mass, serum 1,25(OH)$_2$D levels may be reduced.

Bone demineralization in distal RTA probably relates to dissolution of bone, since the calcium carbonate in bone may serve as a buffer for the metabolic acidosis that is due to the hydrogen ions retained by patients with RTA.

Administration of sufficient bicarbonate to reverse acidosis will stop bone dissolution and the hypercalciuria that is common in distal RTA. Proximal RTA is treated with both bicarbonate and oral phosphate supplements to heal bone disease. Doses of phosphate similar to those used in familial hypophosphatemia should be employed (Sec. 23.47), and vitamin D is needed to offset the secondary hyperparathyroidism that complicates oral phosphate therapy.

23.53 HYPOPHOSPHATASIA

Hypophosphatasia is an autosomal recessive disorder that roentgenographically resembles rickets and is defined by low serum alkaline phosphatase activity. There is considerable heterogeneity in the severity of the disease. Some cases appear at birth, and diagnosis has even been made in utero by roentgenographic examination of the fetus. The disease may appear in a lethal neonatal form (*congenital lethal hypophosphatasia*), a severe infantile form, or a milder form occurring in childhood or late adolescence (*hypophosphatasia tarda*). The lethal form is characterized by a moth-eaten appearance at the ends of the long bones, by severe deficiency of ossification throughout the skeleton, and by marked shortening of the long bones. Patients with the mild disease may present with bowing of the legs and variable statural shortening. Since calcium accumulation by mature chondrocytes does not occur,

patients may appear to have rickets, and in the neonatal and infantile form, they may have hypercalcemia. In the childhood form, the only laboratory abnormality is a reduction in serum alkaline phosphatase activity.

Unusual clinical manifestations include wormian bones in the calvarium, poor calcification of the frontal, parietal, and occipital bones, and loss of deciduous and/or permanent teeth during childhood. Because of the hypercalcemia in the infantile form, nephrocalcinosis also is found. In the childhood form, bone pain, frequent fractures, and milder skeletal deformities are evident, as well as premature tooth loss. The metaphyseal defect consists of irregular ossification, punched-out areas, and metaphyseal cupping.

In hypophosphatasia, large quantities of phosphoethanolamine are found in the urine, because this compound cannot be degraded in the absence of adequate alkaline phosphatase activity. Although no satisfactory therapy has been found, infusion of plasma rich in alkaline phosphatase activity has been helpful in healing bone in short-term studies. The clinical course of this condition often improves spontaneously as the child matures, although early death from renal failure also may occur in the severe infantile form of the disorder. Rare patients presenting identical clinical and roentgenographic patterns have normal serum alkaline phosphatase activities. Their disease has been labeled pseudohypophosphatasia.

23.54 PRIMARY CHONDRODYSTROPHY
(Metaphyseal Dysplasia)

In this condition bowing of the legs, short stature, and a waddling gait appear in the absence of abnormalities of serum calcium or phosphate, alkaline phosphatase activity, or vitamin D metabolites. Metaphyseal chondrodysplasia (*Jansen type*) is typified by cupped and ragged metaphyses which develop mottled calcification at the distal ends of bone over time. Hypercalcemia, with serum values of 13–15 mg/dL may occur. The spine also may be deformed by the irregular growth of vertebrae. The *Schmidt type* of metaphyseal chondrodysplasia is less severe, although the roentgenographic appearance of the knees and extreme bowing of the lower limbs resemble signs seen in patients with familial hypophosphatemia. The hip abnormalities are more debilitating, however. Patients with both types of metaphyseal chondrodysplasia have lifelong short stature.

Metaphyseal dysostosis, or *Pyle disease*, results from defects in endochondral bone formation and metaphyseal modeling. The long ends of bones are splayed, resulting in an "Erlenmeyer flask" defect. Short stature is not present, and serum chemical levels are normal. Leonine features develop if the facial bones are involved.

No effective forms of treatment are available for the chondrodystrophies or the dysostosis.

23.55 IDIOPATHIC HYPERCALCEMIA

Medical attention was initially drawn to hypercalcemia shortly after World War II ended, when excessive quantities of vitamin D was used to enrich food for infants in England. Although many infants were exposed to high levels of vitamin D, only a few developed hypercalcemia, failure to thrive, and decline in renal function. These infants had roentgenographic evidence of osteosclerosis and dense bones at the metaphyses. This disorder disappeared with reduction in the vitamin D content of milk. Subsequently, at least three separate forms of hypercalcemia of unknown origin have been described.

Williams syndrome, or the elfin facies syndrome, consists of a constellation of manifestations, of which hypercalcemia is an infrequent finding. The characteristic facial features include a small mandible, prominent maxilla, and upturned nose. The upper lip has a Cupid's bow curve, and small peg-like teeth with numerous caries are common. Feeding problems and failure to thrive during the first year of life are usual. Mild mental retardation and an unusual "cocktail party patter" personality are typical. The types of cardiac lesions found separately or together include supravalvular aortic stenosis, peripheral pulmonic stenosis, hypoplasia of the aorta, and atrial or ventricular septal defects. In hypercalcemic patients, nephrocalcinosis and sclerotic long bones are sometimes evident.

Williams syndrome is sporadic, and some children have hypervitaminosis D without evidence of increased maternal or infantile vitamin D intake. Patients with this disorder slowly excrete an infused calcium load and have evidence for increased production of 25(OH)D from vitamin D. Treatment is directed at social and educational problems.

Children may also have mild *idiopathic hypercalcemia*, which is usually transient. None of the phenotypic features of Williams syndrome are found. These patients have hypercalciuria and sometimes nephrocalcinosis, possibly resembling the English infants who received excessive vitamin D after the war. However, no evidence for abnormalities in vitamin D metabolism has been found.

Familial hypocalciuric hypercalcemia is an autosomal dominant condition in which affected children have asymptomatic hypercalcemia without hypercalciuria. Pancreatitis may occur in some families and, in a few kindreds, neonates may present with life-threatening parathyroid hyperplasia. Instead of serum calcium levels of 12–15 mg/dL, typically found in the parent, these infants have levels exceeding 18 mg/dL. All these children have had mild parathyroid hyperplasia despite hypercalcemia, indicating that the parathyroid gland does not respond appropriately to the signal of hypercalcemia. Vitamin D metabolism is normal. Only the infants with serious hyperparathyroidism require treatment—an emergency parathyroidectomy. Serum magnesium also is elevated, but this is not a serious concern.

23.56 HYPERPHOSPHATASIA

Excessive elevation of the bone isozyme of alkaline phosphatase in serum and significant growth failure characterize hyperphosphatasia. Osteoid proliferation in the subperiosteal portion of bone results in separation of the periosteum from the bone cortex. Bowing and thickening of the diaphyses are common, along with osteopenia. The disease usually has its onset by age 2–3 yr, when painful deformity developing in the extremities leads to abnormal gait and sometimes fractures. Other common findings include pectus carinatum, kyphoscoliosis, and rib fraying. The skull is large and the cranium is thickened (widened diploë) and may be deformed. Roentgenographically the bony texture is variable; dense areas (showing a teased cotton-wool appearance) are interspersed with radiolucent areas and general demineralization. Long bones appear cylindrical, lose metaphyseal modeling, and contain pseudocysts showing a dense bony halo.

In this autosomal recessive disorder, serum levels of both calcium and phosphate are normal, while urinary leucine amino acid peptidase activity and serum acid phosphatase are increased. This disorder often is called *juvenile Paget disease* because, as in adult-onset Paget disease, calcitonin may re-

duce the rapid bone turnover found in this disorder; in children the disorder is more generalized and symmetric.

RUSSELL W. CHESNEY

Chesney RW: Metabolic bone diseases. Pediatr 5:227, 1984.
Chesney RW, Kaplan BS, Phelps M, et al: Renal tubular acidosis does not alter the circulating values of calcitriol (1,25(OH)₂-vitamin D). J Pediatr 104:51, 1984.
DeLuca HF: The vitamin D system in the regulation of calcium and phosphorus metabolism. W.O. Atwater Memorial Lecture. Nutr Rev 37:161, 1979.
Eil C, Lieberman UA, Rosen JF, et al: Cellular defect in hereditary vitamin D–dependent rickets type II: Defective nuclear uptake of 1,25-dihydroxyvitamin D in cultured skin fibroblasts. N Engl J Med 304:1588, 1981.
Finberg L: Metabolic bone disease. *In:* Gershwin ME, Robbins DL (eds): Musculoskeletal Diseases of Children. New York, Grune & Stratton, 1983, p 447.
Fraser DR: The physiological economy of vitamin D. Lancet 1:969, 1983.
Glorieux FH, Marie PJ, Pettifor JM, et al: Bone response to phosphate salts, ergocalciferol and calcitriol in hypophosphatemic vitamin D–resistant rickets. N Engl J Med 303:1023, 1980.
Harrison HE, Harrison HC: Disorders of Calcium and Phosphate Metabolism in Childhood and Adolescence. Philadelphia, WB Saunders, 1979.
Markowitz ME, Rosen JF, Smith C, et al: 1,25-Dihydroxyvitamin D₃–treated hypoparathyroidism: 35 patient years in 10 children. J Clin Endocrinol Metab 55:727, 1982.
Opshaug O, Maurseth K, Howlid H, et al: Vitamin D metabolism in hypophosphatasia: Case report. Acta Paediatr Scand 71:517, 1982.
Rosen JF, Chesney RW: Circulating calcitriol concentrations in health and disease of infancy and childhood. J Pediatr 103:1, 1983.
Scriver CR: Rickets and the pathogenesis of impaired tubular transport of phosphate and other solutes. Am J Med 57:43, 1974.
Scriver CR, Reade T, Halal F, et al: Autosomal hypophosphatemic bone disease responds to 1,25(OH)₂D₃. Arch Dis Child 56:203, 1981.

23.57 FANCONI SYNDROME
(Rickets Associated with Multiple Defects of the Proximal Renal Tubule; de Toni-Debré-Fanconi Syndrome)

Generalized aminoaciduria, renal glycosuria, and phosphaturia resulting in hypophosphatemia characterize Fanconi syndrome. Associated but inconstant renal tubular abnormalities include excessive bicarbonaturia leading to metabolic acidosis, hyperkaliuria leading to hypokalemia, sodium wasting, uricosuria, proteinuria, and hyposthenuria. Clinical hallmarks are linear growth failure and rickets resistant to doses of vitamin D that are ordinarily adequate for treatment of nutritional deficiency (Sec. 3.29).

Etiology. Fanconi syndrome occurs with genetically transmitted inborn errors of metabolism (cystinosis, fructose intolerance, galactosemia, glycogenosis, Lowe syndrome, tyrosinemia, and Wilson disease) and with some acquired diseases, including exposure to environmental toxins, e.g., heavy metals (Cd, Pb, Hg) or outdated tetracycline. Most commonly, it is idiopathic, and its occurrence in this form may be sporadic or inherited as a mendelian dominant or recessive trait, including X-linked recessive. The following description of the primary idiopathic form is representative of the syndrome in general.

Pathogenesis. Studies suggest an abnormality in some final common pathway for normal membrane transport in the proximal renal tubules. There may be deficient energy production, abnormalities in membrane structure, or both, leading to impaired tubular uptake or back-leak of solutes. Also, loss of bicarbonate in the urine leads to proximal renal tubular acidosis (Sec. 17.29 and 23.52). Renal potassium wasting results from excessive urinary losses of bicarbonate and glucose. Urinary sodium losses are obligatory because of the large excretion of urinary anions. Serum calcium level is normal to low; urinary calcium levels vary. A vasopressin-resistant urinary concentrating defect is often present but is unexplained. A syndrome similar to Fanconi syndrome occurs in the basenji breed of dogs in which excessive urinary losses of amino acids, sugar, and phosphate result from decreased proximal renal tubular reabsorption of the glomerular filtrate.

Rickets can result from the combined effects of metabolic acidosis and hypophosphatemia or from hypophosphatemia alone. Simple calcium deficiency does not appear to play a role in the bone disease. Vitamin D resistance may be due to impaired conversion of vitamin D to its biologically active metabolite, $1,25(OH)_2D_3$, by abnormal proximal tubular cells in the presence of metabolic acidosis.

Microscopic findings are nonspecific. Renal tubules may show dilatation, variation in size and shape, swelling of epithelial cells, and atrophy. Foci of interstitial fibrosis are common. Enlarged mitochondria may be seen on electron microscopy. Typically, glomerular architecture is preserved until late in the disease.

Clinical Manifestation. Primary Fanconi syndrome typically presents either in the first 6 mo of life or in the 3rd–4th decade. In infancy, vomiting, polydipsia, polyuria, and constipation occur. Episodes of weakness, fever with dehydration, and metabolic acidosis may also occur. Failure to thrive is often pronounced, especially in linear growth.

Roentgenographic signs of rickets or osteopenia may appear despite a history of adequate vitamin D intake and the absence of glomerular insufficiency, indicating a renal tubular cause.

Laboratory Data. Usually, a hyperchloremic metabolic acidosis is noted, with normal "anion gap" (Sec. 5.12), hypokalemia, hypophosphatemia, and hypouricemia. Fractional excretion of phosphate is elevated. Alkaline phosphatase activity is elevated if rickets is present. Glycosuria occurs at normal serum glucose concentrations. There is generalized nonspecific aminoaciduria. Urinary pH is inappropriately elevated, with low levels of urinary ammonia and titratable acid. When the glomerular filtration rate falls late in the course of the disease, there may be a "paradoxical" improvement in the levels of serum electrolytes and an amelioration of aminoaciduria, glycosuria, and phosphaturia.

Diagnosis. There is no definitive diagnostic test for idiopathic Fanconi syndrome. Aminoaciduria, diminished tubular reabsorption of phosphate, and elevated alkaline phosphatase activities accompany other forms of rickets. In a child with stunted growth and rickets refractory to ordinary doses of vitamin D the presence of renal glycosuria indicates multiple tubular dysfunction. Metabolic acidosis and hypokalemia are corroborative. Fluid deprivation to test urinary concentrating ability is risky in the face of obligatory hyposthenuria, and glucose loading may cause profound symptomatic hypokalemia by shifting potassium into cells.

Treatment. The clinical and biochemical expressions vary from patient to patient; accordingly, treatment is not uniform. For patients with secondary Fanconi syndrome, underlying causes should be sought. In those with primary Fanconi syndrome, symptomatic therapy can restore mineral and electrolyte balance, prolong survival, and often permit a normal life. Rickets can be corrected and skeletal deformities prevented, but fully normal growth rates are rarely achieved.

Rickets or osteopenia will respond to large doses of vitamin D. The usual starting dose is 5000 units/24 hr, which should be increased gradually to a maximal dose of 2000–4000 units/kg/24 hr. Most patients require at least 25,000 units to heal rickets. Dihydrotachysterol may be substituted for vitamin D at a starting dose of 0.05–0.1 mg/24 hr (1 mg is equivalent to 120,000 units of vitamin D) Several patients have been reported to have responded well to therapy with $1,25(OH)_2D_3$. Serum calcium levels must be followed closely (weekly at first, then monthly) to avoid hypercalcemia from vitamin D overdose. Hypophosphatemia can be treated by oral supplementation with 1–3 gm of neutral phosphate/24 hr given in 4–5 equally spaced doses through the waking hours. If abdominal pain or diarrhea ensues, therapy should be temporarily discontinued and then reinstituted at a lower dose. Phosphate should not be given without concomitant vitamin D to avoid causing or aggravating hypocalcemia.

Correcting metabolic acidosis due to excessive bicarbonaturia may require large amounts of alkali. From 2 to 15 mEq/kg/24 hr of alkali may be needed, as sodium bicarbonate solution (1 mEq of base = 1 mL). *Shohl* solution (140 g citric acid, 90 g sodium citrate qs to 1 L with water; 1 mEq of base = 1 mL), or *Polycitra* (5 mL = 550 mg potassium citrate, 500 mg sodium citrate, 334 mg citric acid; 2 mEq of base = 1 mL). Doses should be adjusted to raise serum bicarbonate only to near normal levels (18–20 mEq/L). Attempts to normalize serum bicarbonate may exaggerate urinary bicarbonate loss as a result of extracellular fluid volume expansion with excessive sodium loads. Alkali is administered 1–1½ hr after meals in 3–4 divided doses/day, and, if Polycitra is not used, extra potassium should be given at a starting dose of 2–3 mEq/kg/24 hr. Extra salt and water should be provided to counter excessive losses, especially in warm weather.

Chesney RW: Etiology and pathogenesis of the Fanconi syndrome. Miner Electrolyte Metab 4:303, 1980.
Cohn RM, Roth KS: Metabolic Disease: A Guide to Early Recognition. Philadelphia, WB Saunders, 1983, p 258.
Roth KS, Foreman JW, Segal S: The Fanconi syndrome and mechanisms of tubular transport dysfunction. Kidney Int 20:705, 1981.

23.58 CYSTINOSIS
(Lignac Syndrome; Fanconi Syndrome with Cystinosis)

Cystinosis presents the clinical and laboratory features of Fanconi syndrome with the additional distinctive finding of abnormal accumulation of cystine in various tissues (see also Sec. 7.5 and 23.57).

Pathogenesis. The cause is unknown. Cystine accumulates in lysosomes, where it cannot be maintained in reduced form. It is not clear whether there is failure in lysosomal release or in degradation of this amino acid. No specific enzyme defect has yet been identified. Tissue levels of cystine do not correlate with degree of renal tubular dysfunction; accordingly, a simple toxic effect of cystine on tubules is not the cause of Fanconi syndrome in cystinosis.

Cystine is deposited in the reticuloendothelial system, especially in spleen, liver, lymph nodes, and bone marrow. Deposits occur in renal tubular cells, cornea, and conjunctiva. Cystine also accumulates in peripheral blood leukocytes and fibroblasts. Early renal changes are similar to those of primary Fanconi syndrome; the characteristic "swan neck" lesion consists of atrophy and shortening of the proximal tubule just beneath the glomerulus. Birefringent cystine crystals may be seen in interstitial tissue and rarely in tubular cells; they are sometimes recognizable only on electron microscopy. With advancing renal failure, the kidneys become shrunken and contracted, with glomerular sclerosis and interstitial fibrosis.

Clinical Manifestations. Cystinosis is inherited as an autosomal recessive trait. There are three clinical patterns. Patients with the *infantile or nephropathic form* present with Fanconi syndrome at 3–6 mo of age. A generalized aminoaciduria is found without predominance of cystine. The glomerular filtration rate falls progressively, and chronic renal failure develops within the 1st decade. Severe growth failure and hypothyroidism accompany this state. Distinctive clinical features include blond hair and fair complexion, due to a defect in melanin synthesis, and photophobia secondary to deposit of cystine crystals on the conjunctivae. The *adolescent or intermediate form* is characterized by mild renal involvement, with onset in the 2nd decade and slow progression. Growth failure is not a feature of this form. The *adult type* of cystinosis (benign) causes no renal disease. Cystine crystals may be found in the cornea, bone marrow, and leukocytes.

Laboratory Data. Other than the deposition of cystine crystals, laboratory abnormalities are similar to those described for the Fanconi syndrome. Tubular proteinuria characterizes the early phase of nephropathic cystinosis, but glomerular proteinuria supervenes as renal failure ensues.

Diagnosis. In the asymptomatic newborn infant from an affected family the diagnosis of cystinosis can be made by measuring the cystine content of leukocytes or fibroblasts, which will be 80–100 times normal. Later, granular and circinate irregularities in the peripheral pigmentation of the retina may be noted. Cystine crystals may be detected in the bone marrow, lymph nodes, conjunctiva, and rectal mucosa. Slit lamp examination will show crystals in the cornea. Prenatal diagnosis can be made by finding an increased concentration of cystine in amniotic fluid cells. Cystinosis must not be confused with cystinuria, which is an inborn error of specific amino acid transport, with neither cystine deposition nor Fanconi syndrome.

Treatment. Early on, symptomatic therapy for tubular dysfunction is similar to that for primary Fanconi syndrome. In addition, cysteamine, a sulfhydryl binder, has been shown to lower intracellular cystine in vivo and to slow the rate of progression of renal (glomerular) failure in some children.

For patients with end-stage renal failure, hemodialysis and renal transplantation are recommended. Hemodialysis does not lower tissue cystine levels. Cystine will accumulate in the transplanted kidney, but the donor genome appears to be operative in that the Fanconi syndrome does not recur. Either cystine is stored in a different location or the cause of renal dysfunction is not cystine per se. Children with cystinosis appear to do as well after kidney transplantation as those with other forms of chronic kidney failure.

Broyer M, Guillot M, Gubler MC, et al: Infantile cystinosis: A reappraisal of early and late symptoms. Adv Nephrol 11:137, 1981.

Cohn RM, Roth KS: Metabolic Disease: A Guide to Early Recognition. Philadelphia, WB Saunders, 1983, p 237.

23.59 OCULOCEREBRORENAL DYSTROPHY
(Lowe Syndrome)

This rare disorder is transmitted as an X-linked recessive trait. In addition to Fanconi syndrome, organic aciduria, decreased production of urinary ammonia, and occasionally heavy proteinuria occur. Distinctive clinical features include congenital cataracts, glaucoma, and buphthalmos that lead to severe visual impairment. Severe hypotonia and hyporeflexia appear in the first year. Mental retardation is severe and often progressive. Rickets, marked osteopenia, and pathologic fracture may develop as a result of metabolic acidosis and phosphate depletion.

Pathogenesis. The pathogenesis is not known, but recent in vitro studies have suggested an abnormality in collagen metabolism. Pathologic studies have shown splitting of the glomerular basement membranes, with marked variation in their thickness. These changes may not be confined to the kidney.

Clinical Features. Early in life the eye findings and mental retardation predominate; the Fanconi syndrome becomes clinically apparent later. If the patient survives childhood, the Fanconi syndrome may resolve spontaneously, only to be supplanted by chronic renal failure. There is no specific therapy. Treatment is supportive, as in primary Fanconi syndrome.

Abbassi V, Lowe CU, Calcagno PL: Oculo-cerebro-renal syndrome. A review. Am J Dis Child 15:145, 1968.

For advice and support to families with Lowe syndrome, contact the Lowe's Syndrome Association, 607 Robinson Street, West Lafayette, IN 47906.

23.60 RENAL OSTEODYSTROPHY

The term renal osteodystrophy designates the alterations in skeletal growth and remodeling that occur in children with chronic renal disease because of abnormalities in mineral and bone metabolism. These abnormalities include malabsorption of calcium, hyperfunction of the parathyroid glands; cutaneous, vascular, and visceral calcifications; and impairment in the renal production of biologically active vitamin D. Renal osteodystrophy can ocur with tubular dysfunction while glomerular filtration remains intact (Sec. 17.28, 17.29, and 23.52) but more commonly follows progressive loss of nephrons, with glomerular insufficiency and uremia.

The condition was formerly called renal (uremic) rickets or renal dwarfism because severe linear growth failure was associated with rickets-like roentgenographic changes. These findings were first thought to be due primarily to a mineralization defect resulting from vitamin D deficiency, but secondary hyperparathyroidism is an equally important contributor to the clinical and roentgenographic findings. Since hemodialysis and kidney transplantation have become available to children, the major complication of chronic renal failure in childhood has become renal osteodystrophy (Sec. 17.36).

Pathogenesis. The bony abnormalities do not respond to physiologic doses of vitamin D adequate to treat simple vitamin D deficiency. This vitamin D resistance leads to a malabsorption of calcium and phosphate and, through unknown mechanisms, to defective mineralization of osteoid (osteomalacia). The fact that the kidney is the site of final synthesis of the major vitamin D metabolites may explain the vitamin D resistance.

Secondary hyperparathyroidism occurs as the glomerular filtration falls; serum phosphate levels rise and lead to hypocalcemia and release of parathyroid hormone (PTH). At some critical renal threshold, e.g., when glomerular filtration rate falls to approximately 25–30% of normal, the phosphaturic renal response to elevated PTH is lost, and compensatory hyperparathyroidism supervenes in an attempt to restore serum calcium to normal. The consequences are roentgenographic and histologic evidence of exaggerated osteoclast-mediated resorption of bone (osteitis fibrosa). Also, endosteal fibrosis, increased bone turnover, and replacement of regularly textured lamellar bone with disorganized and structurally deficient woven bone are seen. Chronic metabolic acidosis probably contributes to the bony changes by increasing calcium resorption from bone and increasing renal excretion before severe renal failure ensues.

The pathology varies. On biopsy, trabecular bone may show predominant osteomalacia, predominant osteitis fibrosa, or, most commonly, a mixed pattern. A subgroup of patients has been described in whom fracturing osteomalacia and low bone turnover have resulted from accumulation of aluminum at the mineralization front. The mineralization defect can be demonstrated by giving the patient tetracycline prior to biopsy; this fluorescent antibiotic is deposited at the mineralization front.

Roentgenographic abnormalities at the epiphyseal growth

plate may occasionally resemble those of nutritional rickets but are often quite distinct; histologically, they reflect osteitis fibrosa rather than rickets. The growth plate is not actually increased in longitudinal width but appears to be because of the formation of a bar of metaphyseal fibrosis with dysplastic trabeculae. The concomitant defect in mineralization leads to a failure in modeling, with persistence of cartilage, an expanded epiphyseal diameter, and frequent overriding of the lateral border of the metaphysis.

Clinical Manifestations. The younger the child at onset of chronic renal failure and the longer the duration of renal failure, the greater the incidence and severity of osteodystrophy. In children with congenital diseases of the kidney, which predominate under the age of 5 yr, the interval between onset of disease and end-stage renal failure is longer than it is in the glomerulonephritides, which occur later in childhood. However, in children with congenital nephropathies, bone disease is accelerated because it occurs at a time of maximal growth and bone modeling and remodeling.

The earliest sign of renal osteodystrophy is usually growth failure, to which metabolic acidosis, protein-calorie malnutrition, hormonal disorders, and trace mineral deficiencies associated with chronic renal failure may contribute. Growth failure may occur with no roentgenographic skeletal abnormalities. With advancing (untreated) disease, additional clinical manifestations appear, including muscle weakness, bone pain, bone deformities, slipped epiphyses, metaphyseal fractures, metastatic calcification, and pruritus. Genu varum, frontal bossing, and dental abnormalities are particularly evident in young children. Tetany is rare (despite hypocalcemia) because of the combined protective effects of metabolic acidosis and hyperparathyroidism.

Laboratory Data. There may be mild hypocalcemia, but the Ca × P product is usually elevated by increased levels of serum phosphorus. Elevated alkaline phosphatase activity reflects increased bone turnover but is not as reliable a sign in children as in adults.

In roentgenograms of the hands and wrists, subperiosteal erosions of the middle and distal phalanges may be sensitive early indicators of osteitis fibrosa. Erosions may also occur in the distal clavicle and on inner aspects of the distal femur and proximal tibia. Elevated serum levels of PTH will generally give the earliest indication of bone disease and may be found when glomerular filtration rates are reduced to as little as 40–50 mL/min/1.73 m². The degree of elevation of PTH correlates with roentgenographic and histologic evidence of osteitis fibrosa, but the degree of histologic osteomalacia does not correlate well with chemical abnormalities in serum or with roentgenographic evidence of rickets, osteopenia, or coarsening of trabeculae.

Treatment. Renal osteodystrophy can usually be successfully managed by (1) controlling hyperphosphatemia, (2) supplying adequate oral calcium intake, and (3) providing extra vitamin D. Treatment should begin early since growth failure in infancy can greatly influence the attainment of ultimate stature. An unresolved question is whether therapy should be initiated before definite roentgenographic or biochemical abnormalities appear.

Hyperphosphatemia should be controlled with oral administration of phosphate binders. Aluminum hydroxide or aluminum carbonate gel can be given at a starting dose of 20–30 mg/kg/24 hr in divided doses with meals and the dose adjusted to keep the serum phosphorus between 4 and 5 mg/dL.

The dose may have to be increased when vitamin D is given. However, prior to the beginning of dialysis, long-term treatment with high-dose aluminum-containing binders has been reported to cause osteomalacic osteodystrophy and a progressive, irreversible encephalopathy with dementia. Calcium supplementation in the form of calcium carbonate should be added to the diet to provide 1–1.5 g of elemental calcium per day. We prefer calcium carbonate because, of the available calcium preparations, it contains the highest percentage of elemental calcium and it affords some degree of phosphate binding. Strict control of acidosis should be achieved by administering sodium bicarbonate. Starting doses are usually 1–2 mEq/kg/24 hr, divided into thirds and given 1 hr after meals (see Sec. 23.57 for specific agents).

Some form of vitamin D appears necessary for successful treatment of uremic osteodystrophy. The preferred form is $1,25(OH)_2D_3$, although the long-term advantage of this form over dihydrotachysterol (DHT) has not been demonstrated. This therapy is indicated for symptomatic bone disease with hypocalcemia, secondary hypoparathyroidism, and evidence of osteitis fibrosa on roentgenography and/or bone biopsy. Starting doses are 15–40 ng/kg/24 hr and should be divided and given 8–12 hr apart to reduce the risk of hypercalcemia. Stepwise adjustments in the dose and indefinite biochemical monitoring are indicated, as with DHT treatment (below). When hypercalcemia ensues, it is usually very short-lived because of the extremely short half-life of $1,25(OH)_2D_3$.

DHT has been favored over vitamin D because it has a better ratio of therapeutic to toxic effects and because its shorter half-life will reduce complications if hypercalcemia occurs. Starting doses are 0.1–0.2 mg/24 hr, and the dosage is increased weekly or biweekly in stepwise fashion to normalize levels of serum calcium and to heal roentgenographic abnormalities. Doses can be lowered once these goals are achieved. Frequent measurements of serum calcium and phosphorus are required, weekly at first, then monthly.

Hemodialysis may either ameliorate or exacerbate bone disease; the effect cannot be predicted. Unrecognized or untreated hypercalcemia may accelerate renal insufficiency or foster metastatic calcification of the tympanic membranes, cornea, conjunctiva, skin, and vascular tree. When hypercalcemia is found, administration of vitamin D must be suspended until the serum calcium level is normal; therapy can then be reinstituted at a lower dose.

Parathyroidectomy is indicated in carefully selected patients with severe secondary hyperparathyroidism refractory to medical therapy. Indications include severe bone pain, mental aberrations, severe pruritus, fractures, chronic hypercalcemia, and, less commonly, metastatic calcification. In all cases marked elevation of serum PTH levels should be proved prior to surgery.

MICHAEL E. NORMAN

Alvioli LV, Teitelbaum SL: Renal osteodystrophy. In: Edelmann CM (ed): Pediatric Kidney Disease. Boston, Little, Brown, 1978.
Chesney RW, Moorthy AV, Jax DK, et al: Increased linear growth after long-term oral 1,25(OH)₂D therapy in childhood renal osteodystrophy. N Engl J Med 298:238, 1978.
Norman ME: Vitamin D in bone disease. Pediatr Clin North Am 29:947, 1982.
Norman ME, Mazur AT, Borden S, et al: Early diagnosis of juvenile renal osteodystrophy. J Pediatr 97:226, 1980.
Polinsky MS, Gruskin AB: Aluminum toxicity in children with chronic renal failure. J Pediatr 105:758, 1984.

24

THE SKIN

24.1 MORPHOLOGY OF THE SKIN

The Epidermis. The mature epidermis, a stratified epithelial tissue, is constantly renewed by mitotic division of the cells of the basal layer. In addition to the squamous cells or keratinocytes, the epidermis contains melanocytes (the pigment-forming cells) and Langerhans cells (dendritic cells of the mononuclear phagocyte system).

The continuous renewal of the surface cells of the epidermis normally proceeds in an orderly fashion as the cells of the basal cell layer move upward to the stratum corneum. The transit time of the epidermal cell is relatively fixed; the total life span is approximately 28 days. In hyperproliferative diseases the movement of the cells is more rapid, so that the newly arrived epidermal cells in the stratum corneum, being immature, form a defective barrier; this may alter permeability.

Epidermal melanocytes are derived from the neural crest and migrate to the skin during embryonic life. They reside in the interfollicular epidermis and in the hair follicles and multiply by mitosis to repopulate the epidermis. Melanocytes are responsible for skin color; melanosomes containing melanin are ingested by the keratinocytes, and the melanin is shed with the stratum corneum cells.

The Langerhans cells have a dendritic form like that of melanocytes, but rather than melanosomes, they contain a specific organelle, the Birbeck granule. These cells are derived from bone marrow and participate in immune reactions in the skin, playing an active role in antigen presentation and processing.

The Dermis. The dermis, or corium, forms a tough, pliable, fibrous supporting structure between the epidermis and the subcutaneous fat. It is composed of collagen and elastic and reticular fibers embedded in an amorphous ground substance; it contains blood vessels, lymphatics, neural structures, eccrine and apocrine sweat glands, hair follicles, sebaceous glands, and smooth muscle. Morphologically, the dermis can be divided into two layers, the superficial papillary layer that interdigitates with the rete ridges of the epidermis and the deeper reticular layer that lies beneath the papillary dermis. The papillary layer is less dense and more cellular, whereas the reticular layer appears more compact because of the coarse network of interlaced collagen and elastic fibers.

The predominant cell is a spindle-shaped fibroblast that is responsible for the synthesis of collagen, elastic fibers, and mucopolysaccharides. Phagocytic histiocytes, mast cells, and motile leukocytes are also present. The gelatinous ground substance serves as a supporting medium for the fibrillar and cellular components as well as a storage place for a substantial portion of body water. Nutrients are supplied to both epidermis and dermis via the dermal blood vessels.

The Subcutaneous Tissue. Panniculus, or subcutaneous tissue, is composed of fat cells, which form and store lipid, and of fibrous septa that divide it into lobules and anchor it to the underlying fascia and periosteum. Blood vessels and nerves are also present in this layer, which serves as a storage depot for lipid, an insulator to conserve body heat, and a protective cushion against trauma.

The appendageal structures are derived from aggregates of epidermal cells that become specialized during early embryonic development. Small buds (primary epithelial germs) appear during the 3rd fetal mo and give rise to hair follicles, sebaceous and apocrine glands, and the attachment bulges for the arrector pili muscles. Eccrine sweat glands are derived from separate epidermal downgrowths that arise during the 2nd fetal mo and are completely formed by the 5th mo. Formation of nails is initiated during the 3rd intrauterine mo.

The hair follicle is the most prominent structure in the pilary complex, which includes the sebaceous gland, the arrector pili muscle, and in areas such as the axillae, an apocrine gland. Hair follicles are distributed throughout the skin except in the palms, soles, lips, and glans penis; if destroyed, they cannot regenerate. Individual follicles extend from the surface of the epidermis to the deep dermis, where the matrix cells with the dermal papilla form a bulbous hair root. The growing hair consists of a bulb and a matrix from which the keratinized hair shaft is generated; the shaft is composed of an inner medulla, a cortex, and an outer cuticular layer.

Human hair growth is cyclical, with alternate periods of growth (anagen) and rest (telogen). The length of the anagen phase varies from months to years. At birth, all hairs are in the anagen phase. Subsequent generative activity lacks synchrony, so that an overall random pattern of growth and shedding prevails. Scalp hair usually grows about 0.35 mm/24 hr.

Sebaceous glands occur in all areas except the palms, soles, and dorsa of the feet, but are most numerous on the face, upper chest, and back. Their ducts open into the hair follicles except on the lips, prepuce, and labia minora, where they emerge directly onto the mucosal surface. These holocrine glands are saccular structures that are often branched and lobulated and consist of a proliferative basal layer of small flat cells peripheral to the central mass of lipidized cells. The latter cells disintegrate as they move toward the duct and form the lipid secretion known as sebum that is composed of cellular debris, triglycerides, phospholipids, and cholesterol esters.

Sebaceous glands are dependent upon hormonal stimulation and are activated by androgens at puberty. Fetal sebaceous glands are stimulated by maternal androgens, and their lipid secretion together with desquamated stratum corneum cells comprise the vernix caseosa.

The apocrine glands are located in the axillae, areolae, perianal and genital areas, and the periumbilical region. These large, coiled, tubular structures continuously secrete an odorless milky fluid which is discharged in response to adrenergic stimuli, usually the result of emotional stress. Bacterial decomposition of apocrine sweat accounts for the unpleasant odor associated with perspiration.

Apocrine glands remain dormant until puberty, when they enlarge and secretion begins in response to androgenic activity. The secretory coil of the gland consists of a single layer of cells enclosed by a layer of contractile myoepithelial cells. The duct is lined with a double layer of cuboidal cells and opens into the pilosebaceous complex. Although apocrine glands do not function in thermoregulation, they are involved in certain disease processes.

Eccrine sweat glands are distributed over the entire body surface including the palms and soles, where they are most abundant. Those on the hairy skin respond to thermal stimuli and serve to regulate the body temperature by delivering water to the skin surface for evaporation; in contrast, sweat glands on the palms and soles respond mainly to psychophysiologic stimuli.

Each eccrine gland is composed of a secretory coil located in the reticular dermis or subcutaneous fat, and a secretory duct that opens onto the skin surface. Sweat pores can be identified on the epidermal ridges of the palm and fingers with a magnifying lens but are not readily visualized elsewhere.

Two types of cells compose the single-layered secretory coil: small dark cells and large clear cells; these rest on a layer of contractile myoepithelial cells and a basement membrane. The glands are supplied by sympathetic nerve fibers, but the pharmacologic mediator of sweating is acetylcholine rather than epinephrine. The composition of sweat varies with the rate of sweating but is always hypotonic in normal children.

Nails are specialized epidermal structures that form convex, translucent plates on the distal dorsal surfaces of the fingers and toes. The nail plate, which is derived from a metabolically active matrix of multiplying cells situated beneath the posterior nail fold, grows forward at the rate of approximately 0.1 mm/24 hr. The nail plate is bounded by the lateral and posterior nail folds; a thin eponychium (the cuticle) protrudes from the posterior fold over a crescent-shaped white area called the lunula. The pink color above it reflects the underlying vascular bed.

24.2 EXAMINATION OF THE PATIENT

Though many skin disorders are easily recognized by simple inspection, a painstaking history and physical examination are often necessary for accurate assessment. In all instances the entire body surface, the mucous membranes, the hair, and nails should be thoroughly examined under adequate illumination. The color, turgor, texture, temperature, and moisture of the skin and the growth, texture, caliber, and luster of the hair and nails should be noted. Skin lesions should be palpated as well as inspected and should be classified on the bases of morphology, size, color, texture, firmness, configuration, location, and distribution. One must also decide whether the changes are those of the primary lesion itself or whether the clinical pattern has been altered by a secondary factor such as infection, trauma, or therapy.

Primary lesions are classified as macules, papules, nodules, tumors, vesicles, bullae, pustules, wheals, and cysts. A *macule* represents an alteration in skin color but cannot be felt. *Papules* are palpable solid lesions smaller than 1 cm, whereas *nodules* are larger in diameter. *Tumors* are usually larger than nodules and vary considerably in mobility and consistency. *Vesicles* are raised, fluid-filled lesions less than 0.5 cm in diameter; when larger, they are called *bullae*. *Pustules* contain purulent material. *Wheals* are flat-topped, palpable lesions of variable size and configuration that represent dermal collections of edema fluid. *Cysts* are circumscribed, thick-walled lesions that are located deep in the skin, are covered by a normal epidermis, and contain fluid or semisolid material. Aggregations of any of the primary lesions may be referred to as *plaques*.

Secondary lesions include scales, ulcers, excoriations, fissures, crusts, and scars. *Scales* are composed of compressed layers of stratum corneum cells that are retained on the skin surface. *Ulcers* are excavations of necrotic or traumatized tissue. Ulcerated lesions inflicted by scratching are often linear or angular in configuration and are called *excoriations*. *Fissures* are caused by splitting or cracking; they usually occur in diseased skin. *Crusts* consist of matted, retained accumulations of blood, serum, pus, and epithelial debris on the surface of a weeping lesion. *Scars* are end-stage lesions that can be

thin, depressed and atrophic, raised and hypertrophic, or flat and pliable; they are composed of fibrous connective tissue.

If the diagnosis is not clear after a thorough examination, one or more diagnostic procedures may be indicated. Besides those discussed below, others are identified in appropriate subsections (e.g., scrapings of scabies lesions and smears and cultures of vesicles and pustules for detection of bacteria).

Biopsy of skin by excision is rarely required for diagnosis in children. *Punch biopsy* is a simple and relatively painless procedure and usually provides adequate tissue for examination. A fresh but well-developed lesion should be selected for removal. Xylocaine, 1 or 2%, with or without epinephrine should be injected intradermally with a 27- or 30-gauge needle following cleansing of the site. A punch, 3 or 4 mm in diameter, is pressed firmly against the skin and rotated until it sinks to the proper depth. All three layers (epidermis, dermis, and subcutis) should be contained in the plug. The plug should be gently lifted with forceps or extracted with a needle and separated from the underlying tissue with an iris scissors. Bleeding abates with firm pressure; suturing is optional. The biopsy specimen should be placed in 10% formalin for appropriate processing.

The **Wood lamp** transmits ultraviolet light mainly in a wave length of 365 nm. The examination, which is performed in a darkened room, is useful mainly in certain superficial fungal infections of the scalp. Blue-green fluorescence is detectable at the base of each infected hair shaft in ectothrix and in some endothrix infections. Scales and crusts may appear pale yellow, but this is not evidence of a fungal infection. Dermatophyte lesions of the skin (tinea corporis) do not fluoresce; macules of tinea versicolor, however, have a golden fluorescence under the Wood lamp.

Discrete areas of altered pigment can often be visualized more clearly by use of a Wood lamp, particularly if the pigmentary change is epidermal. Hyperpigmented lesions appear darker and hypopigmented lesions lighter than the surrounding skin.

The **KOH preparation** provides a rapid and reliable method for the detection of fungal elements of both yeasts and dermatophytes. Scaly lesions should be scraped at the active border for optimal recovery of mycelia and spores. Vesicles should be unroofed, and the blister top should be clipped and placed on a slide for examination. In tinea capitis, infected hairs must be plucked from the follicle; scales from the scalp usually will not contain mycelia. A few drops of 10% potassium hydroxide are added to the specimen, which is then gently heated over an alcohol lamp until it begins to bubble. The preparation is examined under low-intensity light for fungal elements.

A **Tzanck smear** is useful in the diagnosis of some viral infections (herpes simplex, varicella, herpes zoster, and eczema herpeticum) as well as for detection of acantholytic cells in pemphigus. An intact, fresh blister should be ruptured and drained of fluid. The base of the blister is then vigorously scraped with a dull-edged instrument; the material is smeared on a clear glass slide and air-dried. Staining with Giemsa stain is preferable, but Wright stain is acceptable. Balloon cells and multinucleated giant cells are diagnostic of herpesvirus infection; acantholytic epidermal cells are characteristic of pemphigus.

Immunofluorescence studies of skin can be used to detect tissue-fixed antibodies to skin components; characteristic staining patterns are specific for certain skin disorders. Serum can be used for identification of circulating antibodies. Skin biopsies for direct immunofluorescence preparations should be obtained from involved sites except in those diseases for which paralesional skin or uninvolved skin is required. A punch biopsy is obtained, and the tissue is placed in a special transport medium or *immediately* frozen in liquid nitrogen for transport or storage. Thin cryostat sections of the specimen are incubated with fluorescein-conjugated goat or rabbit antihuman globulin or complement.

Serum of patients can be examined by indirect immunofluorescence techniques using sections of normal human skin, guinea pig lip, or monkey esophagus as substrate. A substrate is incubated with fresh or thawed frozen serum and then with fluorescein-conjugated antihuman globulin. If the serum contains antibody to epithelial components, its specific staining pattern can be seen on fluorescence microscopy. By serial dilutions, the titer of circulating antibody can be estimated.

DISEASES OF THE SKIN

24.3 TRANSIENT LESIONS OF THE NEONATE

Minor evanescent lesions of the newborn infant, particularly when florid, may cause undue concern. Most of the entities described in this section are relatively common, benign, and transient; they do not require therapy.

Sebaceous Hyperplasia. Minute profuse yellow-white papules are frequently found on the forehead, nose, upper lip, and cheeks of the term infant; they represent hyperplastic sebaceous glands. These tiny papules gradually diminish in size and disappear entirely within the first few weeks of life.

Milia. The milium is a superficial epidermal inclusion cyst that contains laminated keratinized material. The lesion is a firm papule, 1–2 mm in diameter and pearly, opalescent white in color. Milia may occur at any age but in the neonate are most frequently scattered over the face and gingivae and on the midline of the palate, where they are called *Epstein pearls.* Milia exfoliate spontaneously in most infants and may be ignored; those that appear in scars or sites of trauma in older children may be gently unroofed and "shelled out" with a fine-gauge needle.

Sucking Blisters. Solitary or scattered superficial bullae on the upper limbs and lips of infants at birth are presumed to be induced by vigorous sucking on the affected part in utero. Common sites are the radial aspect of the forearm, the thumb, the index finger, and the central portion of the upper lip. These bullae resolve rapidly without sequelae.

Cutis Marmorata. When the newborn infant is exposed to low environmental temperatures, an evanescent, lacy, reticulated red or blue cutaneous vascular pattern appears over most of the body surface. This vascular change represents an accentuated physiologic vasomotor response that disappears with increasing age, although it is sometimes discernible even in older children. Persistent and pronounced cutis marmorata occurs in the Cornelia de Lange, Down, and trisomy 18 syndromes. Cutis marmorata telangiectatica congenita (Sec. 24.7) is clinically similar, but the lesions are more intense and are persistent.

Harlequin Color Change. This rare but dramatic vascular event occurs in the immediate newborn period and is most common in infants of low birthweight. It probably reflects an imbalance in the autonomic vascular regulatory mechanism. When the infant is placed on his or her side, the body is bisected longitudinally into a pale upper half and a deep red dependent half. The color change lasts only a few minutes, and occasionally affects only a portion of the trunk or face. The pattern may be reversed by changing the infant's position. Muscular activity will cause generalized flushing and obliterate the color differential. Multiple episodes may occur but do not indicate permanent autonomic imbalance.

Salmon Patch (Macular Hemangioma, Nevus Simplex). Salmon patches are small, pale pink, ill-defined, flat vascular lesions that occur most commonly on the glabella, eyelids, upper lip, and nuchal area of 30–50% of normal newborn infants. These lesions, which represent localized plaques of vascular ectasia, persist for several months and may become more visible during crying or changes in environmental temperature. The lesions on the face eventually fade and disappear completely, but those on the posterior neck and occipital area often persist. When they become covered with hair, they are not noticeable. The facial lesions should not be confused with nevus flammeus, which is a permanent lesion.

Mongolian Spots. These blue or slate-gray macular lesions have variably defined margins; they occur most commonly in the presacral area but may be found over the posterior thighs, legs, backs, and shoulders. They may be solitary or multiple and often involve large areas. More than 80% of black, oriental, and East Indian infants have these lesions, whereas the incidence in white infants is less than 10%. The peculiar hue of these macules is due to the dermal location of melanin-containing melanocytes which are presumed to have been arrested in their migration from neural crest to epidermis. Mongolian spots usually fade during the first few years of life, but occasionally persist. Widespread multiple lesions, particularly those in unusual sites, are unlikely to disappear.

Erythema Toxicum. This benign, self-limited, evanescent eruption occurs in approximately 50% of fullterm infants; preterm infants are affected less commonly. The lesions are firm, yellow-white, 1–2 mm papules or pustules with a surrounding erythematous flare (Fig. 24–1, p. xxviii). At times, splotchy erythema is the only manifestation. Lesions may be sparse or numerous and clustered in several sites or widely dispersed over much of the body surface. Palms and soles are virtually always spared. Peak incidence occurs on the 2nd day of life, but new lesions may erupt during the 1st few days.

The pustules form below the stratum corneum or deeper in the epidermis and represent collections of eosinophils that also accumulate around the upper portion of the pilosebaceous follicle. The eosinophils can be demonstrated in Wright-stained smears of the intralesional contents. Cultures are sterile.

The cause of erythema toxicum is unknown. The lesions can mimic pyoderma, candidosis, herpes simplex, transient neonatal pustular melanosis, and miliaria but can be differentiated by the characteristic infiltrate of eosinophils and the absence of organisms on a stained smear. The course is brief, and no therapy is required.

Transient Neonatal Pustular Melanosis. Pustular melanosis, which is more common in black than in white infants, is a transient, benign, self-limited dermatosis of unknown cause that is characterized by three types of lesions: (1) evanescent superficial pustules; (2) ruptured pustules with a collarette of fine scale, at times with a central hyperpigmented macule; and (3) hyperpigmented macules (Fig. 24–2). The lesions are present at birth, and one or all types of lesions may be found in a profuse or sparse distribution. The pustules represent the early phase of the disorder, the macules, the late phase. Sites of predilection are the anterior neck, forehead, lower back, and shins, although the scalp, trunk, limbs, palms, and soles may be affected.

Biopsies of tissue during the active phase show an intracorneal or subcorneal pustule filled with polymorphonuclear leukocytes, debris, and an occasional eosinophil. The macules are characterized only by increased melanization of epidermal cells. Cultures and smears can be used to distinguish these pustules from those of erythema toxicum and pyoderma since

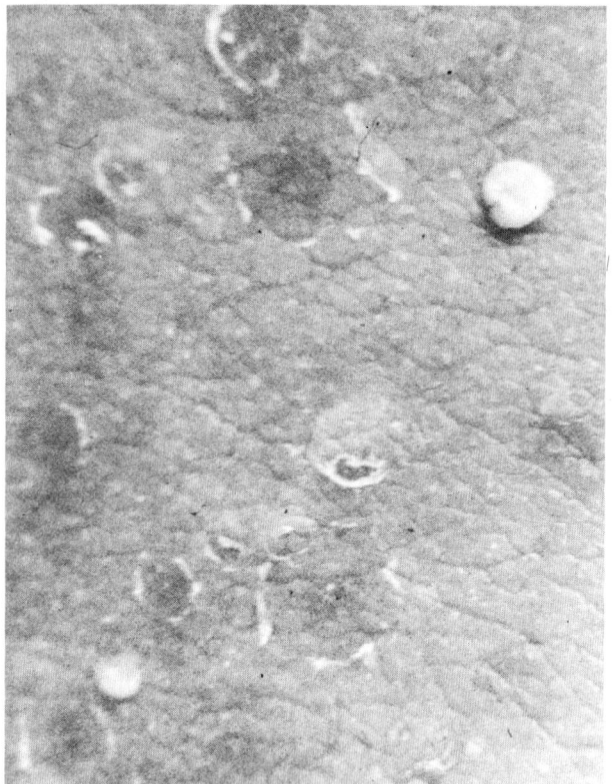

Figure 24–2. Transient neonatal pustular melanosis showing pustules, rings of scales, and hyperpigmented macules.

they do not contain bacteria or dense aggregates of eosinophils.

The pustular phase rarely lasts more than 2–3 days; hyperpigmented macules may persist for as long as 3 mo. No therapy is required.

24.4 DEVELOPMENTAL DEFECTS

24.5 CUTANEOUS DEFECTS

Skin Dimples. Deep dimpling over bony prominences and in the sacral area, at times associated with pits and creases, may occur in normal children as well as in association with some dysmorphologic syndromes, such as those of congenital rubella, deletion of the long arm of chromosome 18, Bloom, and the cerebrohepatorenal syndromes.

Redundant Skin. Loose folds of skin must be differentiated from cutis laxa, a congenital defect of elastic tissue. Redundant skin over the posterior neck is common in the Turner and Down syndromes; more generalized folds of the skin occur in infants with trisomy 18, with combined immunodeficiency disease, and with short-limbed dwarfism.

Amniotic Constriction Bands. Partial or complete constriction bands that produce defects in extremities and digits are found occasionally in otherwise normal infants. They are thought to result from intrauterine rupture of amnion with formation of fibrous strands which encircle the fetal parts and cause permanent depression of the underlying tissue. Rarely, amputation of 1 or more digits may result. Constriction bands on the limbs may be removed by plastic procedures.

Preauricular Sinuses and Pits. Pits and sinus tracts anterior to the pinna may be the result of imperfect fusion of the tubercles of the 1st and 2nd branchial arches, from which the tragus and pinna are derived. These anomalies may be unilateral or bilateral, at times associated with other anomalies

of the ears and face. When the tracts become chronically infected, retention cysts may form and drain intermittently; such lesions may require excision.

Accessory Tragi. Multiple or single, unilateral or bilateral, sessile or pedunculated skin tags may occur in the preauricular area or on the neck anterior to the sternocleidomastoid muscle. They may occur as isolated defects or in syndromes that include anomalies of the ears and face. Surgical excision is appropriate.

Branchial Cleft and Thyroglossal Cysts and Sinuses. Cysts and sinuses in the neck may be formed along the course of the 1st and 2nd branchial clefts as a result of improper closure during embryonic life. The lesions may be unilateral or bilateral and may open onto the cutaneous surface or drain into the pharynx. Secondary infection is an indication for systemic antibiotic therapy. These anomalies may be inherited as autosomal dominant traits.

Thyroglossal cysts and fistulas are similar defects located in or near the midline of the neck; they may extend to the base of the tongue. Occasionally these cysts contain aberrant thyroid tissue as well as the usual mucinous material. Surgical excision is the appropriate treatment, but care must be taken to preserve thyroid tissue (Sec. 19.10).

Supernumerary Nipples. Solitary or multiple accessory nipples may occur in a unilateral or bilateral distribution along a line from the midaxilla to the inguinal area. The accessory nipples may or may not have areolae and may be mistaken for congenital nevi. They may be excised for cosmetic reasons. Rarely, they undergo malignant change.

Aplasia Cutis Congenita (Congenital Absence of Skin). Developmental absence of skin is most frequently noted on the scalp as multiple or solitary, noninflammatory, well demarcated, oval or circular 1–2 cm ulcers. The majority occur at the vertex just lateral to the midline, but similar defects may also occur on the face, trunk, and limbs, where they are often symmetric. The depth of the ulcer is variable; it may involve only the epidermis and upper dermis, or it may extend to the deep dermis, subcutaneous tissue, and, rarely, to the periosteum, skull, and dura. Occasionally the defects are covered by a tough membrane and simulate a bulla. In some instances, multiple family members have been afflicted; both autosomal recessive and dominant patterns of inheritance have been observed. Defects of the limbs and trunk, usually symmetric, have been associated with intrauterine events such as placental infarcts and monozygotic twinning with fetus papyraceus.

The major complications are massive hemorrhage, secondary local infection, and meningitis. Associated developmental defects are rare; they include cleft lip and palate, hamartomas, vascular malformations, congenital heart disease, limb anomalies, and defects of the central nervous system. Aplasia cutis is also associated with malformation syndromes such as trisomy 13, 4p−, Johansson-Blizzard syndrome, and focal dermal hypoplasia. Congenital localized defects of skin, generalized recurrent blisters of skin and mucous membranes, and nail defects inherited as an autosomal dominant trait are known as Bart syndrome.

If the defect is small, recovery is uneventful with gradual epithelialization and formation of a hairless atrophic scar over a period of several weeks (Fig. 24–3). Small bony defects usually close spontaneously during the 1st yr of life. Large or multiple scalp defects may require excision and primary closure, if feasible, or rotation of a flap to fill the defect. Truncal and limb defects, despite large size, usually epithelialize and form atrophic scars, which can later be revised, if necessary.

Bitemporal aplasia cutis congenita, also called ectodermal dysplasia of the face, is a rare defect observed mostly in Puerto Rican children, who have a peculiar facies with widow's peak,

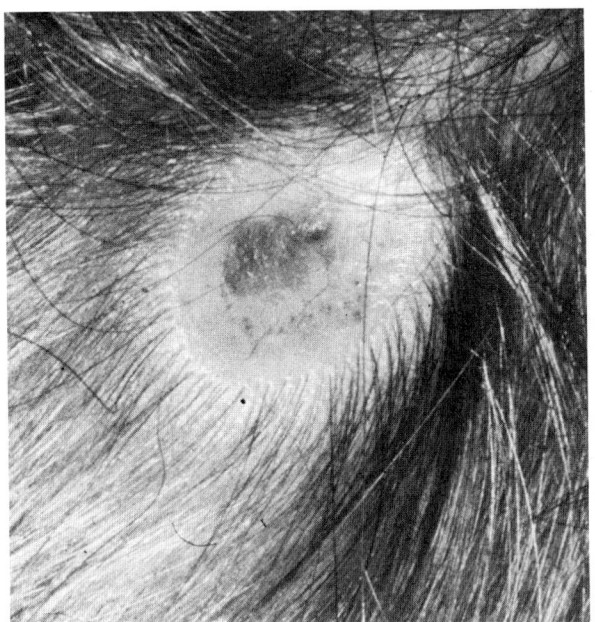

Figure 24–3. Healing solitary lesion of aplasia cutis.

frontal bossing, atrophic depressed defects of the temporal skin, upward slanting eyebrows, absence of or multiple rows of eyelashes, and a prominent chin with a median ridge. The pattern of inheritance is not established, but the defect may be an autosomal recessive trait in some instances.

Focal Dermal Hypoplasia (Goltz Syndrome). This rare congenital mesoectodermal disorder is characterized by herniations of fat through thinned, partially deficient dermis that are responsible for multiple soft, tan-colored papillomas. Other types of skin changes include linear cribriform atrophic lesions, reticulated hypopigmentation and hyperpigmentation, telangiectasia, congenital absence of skin, angiofibromas presenting as verrucous excrescences, and papillomas of the lips, tongue, circumoral region, vulva, anus, and the inguinal, axillary and periumbilical areas. Partial alopecia, sweating disorders, and dystrophic nails are additional less common ectodermal anomalies.

The most frequent skeletal defects include syndactyly, clinodactyly and polydactyly, and scoliosis and other spinal anomalies. Ocular abnormalities are legion, but the most common are colobomas, strabismus, nystagmus, and microphthalmia. Small stature, dental defects, soft tissue anomalies, and peculiar dermatoglyphic patterns are also common. Mental deficiency occurs occasionally.

This familial disorder occurs principally in girls. It has been postulated that an X-linked dominant gene, lethal in males, or an autosomal dominant sex-limited mode of inheritance may account for the sex distribution. This disorder is often confused with incontinentia pigmenti since it shares a sex predilection for females and has some similar skin manifestations and mesodermal anomalies. The cutaneous lesions may also superficially resemble epidermal nevi. Treatment should be directed at amelioration of specific anomalies; genetic counseling is advisable.

Congenital Dyskeratosis (Zinsser-Engman-Cole Syndrome). This rare familial syndrome usually affects males (rarely females) and is probably inherited in an X-linked fashion. The onset occurs during childhood; nail dystrophy is the usual initial manifestation. The nails become ridged and atrophic, and there is considerable loss of the nail plate. The skin changes resemble a poikiloderma with reticulated gray-brown pigmentation, atrophy, and telangiectasia, especially on the neck, face, and chest. Hyperhidrosis and hyperkeratosis of the palms and soles, acrocyanosis, and occasional bullae on the hands and feet are also characteristic. Blepharitis, ectropion, and excessive tearing due to atresia of the lacrimal ducts are occasional manifestations. Vesiculobullous lesions may occur on the oral mucous membranes and result in ulceration, formation of epithelial tags, atrophic changes of the tongue, and premalignant oral leukokeratosis. Similar changes have been noted in the urethral and anal mucosa. The scalp hair, eyebrows, and lashes may become sparse. Hypoplastic anemia, at times of the Fanconi variety, is a common complication; immune deficiency has been noted.

The differential diagnosis includes the ectodermal dysplasias, pachyonychia congenita, poikilodermas, epidermolysis bullosa, keratoderma of the palms and soles, and lichen sclerosus et atrophicus. The abnormalities noted in skin biopsies are those of poikiloderma. Congenital dyskeratosis is progressive and may be complicated by squamous cell carcinoma of the mouth and/or anus as well as by the potentially lethal hematologic abnormalities.

Cutis Verticis Gyrata. This bizarre alteration of the scalp, which is more common in males, may be present from birth or develop during adolescence. The scalp is characterized by convoluted elevated folds, 1–2 cm in thickness, usually in the fronto-occipital axis. Unlike the lax skin of other disorders, the convolutions cannot be flattened by traction.

Primary cutis gyrata is often associated with mental retardation, ocular defects, abnormal size and shape of the head, seizures, and spasticity. Secondary cutis gyrata may be due to chronic inflammatory diseases, tumors, nevi, acromegaly, and pachydermoperiostosis, a syndrome characterized by hypertrophy of the skin and bones.

24.6 ECTODERMAL DYSPLASIAS

The term ectodermal dysplasia has been used to designate a group of disorders characterized by a constellation of defects involving the teeth, skin, and appendageal structures, including hair, nails, and eccrine and sebaceous glands. Disturbances in tissue derived from embryologic layers other than ectoderm are not uncommon. Many of the syndromes have overlapping features and are distinguished by the presence or absence of a single defect.

Hypohidrotic (Anhidrotic) Ectodermal Dysplasia. This syndrome is manifested by a triad of defects: hypohidrosis, anomalous dentition, and hypotrichosis. It is usually inherited as an X-linked recessive trait, with full expression only in males; however, in some families an autosomal recessive mode of inheritance permits full expression in both sexes.

Affected children unable to sweat may experience episodes of high fever in warm environments and be mistakenly considered to have fever of unknown origin. The typical facies is characterized by frontal bossing, malar hypoplasia, a flattened nasal bridge and recessed columella, thick, everted lips, wrinkled, hyperpigmented periorbital skin, and prominent, low set ears (Fig. 24–4). The skin over the entire body is thin, dry, and hypopigmented, often with a prominent venous pattern. The hair is sparse, unruly, and lightly pigmented, and eyebrows and lashes are sparse or absent. Anodontia or hypodontia with widely spaced, peg-shaped teeth is a consistent feature (Fig. 24–4). Less commonly, stenotic lacrimal puncta, corneal dysplasia, cataracts, gonadal abnormalities, and conductive hearing loss have been observed. The incidence of atopic diseases in these children is relatively high.

The sweating deficit is a reflection of hypoplasia or absence of the eccrine glands; this may be confirmed by skin biopsy. The palmar skin is an appropriate site for biopsy. Reduction or absence of sweating can be documented by pilocarpine iontophoresis or by topical application of o-phthalaldehyde to the palmar skin. Sweat pores are not visible in the palmar

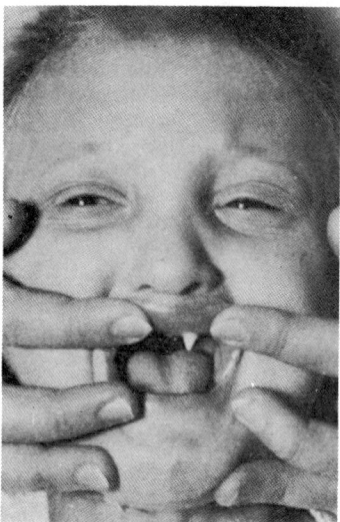

Figure 24–4. Hypohidrotic ectodermal dysplasia is characterized by pointed ears, wispy hair, periorbital hyperpigmentation, midfacial hypoplasia, and pegged teeth.

ridges in affected children and are decreased in number in carrier females. Diminished lacrimation and atrophic rhinitis are due to maldevelopment of the secretory glands. These glands are also deficient in the tracheobronchial mucosa, the esophagus, and the duodenum; recurrent pulmonary infections, hoarseness, and dysphonia are the clinical manifestations.

Children with hypohidrotic ectodermal dysplasia must be protected from exposure to high ambient temperatures. Early dental evaluation is necessary so that prostheses can be provided for cosmetic reasons and for adequate nutrition. The use of artificial tears will prevent damage to the cornea in patients with defective lacrimation. Alopecia may necessitate the wearing of a wig to improve the appearance.

Hidrotic Ectodermal Dysplasia (Clouston Type). Dystrophic, hypoplastic, or absent nails, sparse hair, and hyperkeratosis of the palms and soles are the salient features of this autosomal dominant disorder. The dentition is usually normal, although small teeth and rampant caries are occasionally associated. Sweating is always normal. Absence of eyebrows and lashes and hyperpigmentation over the knees, elbows, and knuckles have been noted in some affected individuals.

EEC Syndrome. Ectrodactyly, ectodermal dysplasia, and cleft lip and palate compose the EEC syndrome, which is probably inherited as an autosomal dominant trait of low penetrance and variable expressivity. The ectodermal dysplasia consists of a thin, dry, poorly pigmented integument, light-colored, wispy scalp hair and eyebrows, and absence of lashes. Decreased numbers of hair follicles and sebaceous glands have been demonstrated by biopsy.

Associated defects include anomalies of the hands and feet, nail hypoplasia, granulomatous perlèche frequently complicated by candidosis, defective dentition, ocular abnormalities such as blepharophimosis, atretic or absent lacrimal puncta, strabismus, and abnormalities of the urinary tract.

Rapp-Hodgkin ectodermal dysplasia is inherited as an autosomal dominant trait and consists of hypohidrosis with reduced numbers of sweat pores, sparse, fine hair, dysplastic nails, oral clefts, variable growth deficiency, and hypospadias.

Robinson-type ectodermal dysplasia, an autosomal dominant disorder, combines sensorineural deafness, nail dystrophy, and peg-shaped teeth with partial anodontia.

24.7 VASCULAR LESIONS

Developmental vascular anomalies may occur as isolated defects or as part of a syndrome. Hemangiomas (vascular nevi) are the most common vascular defects and, with rare exception, occur sporadically and without a genetic basis. Cutaneous hemangiomas are superficial in approximately 65% of instances, subcutaneous in 15%, and mixed in about 20%. The terms *capillary* and *cavernous* distinguish the histologic patterns. Capillary hemangiomas are composed of dilated capillaries with or without endothelial proliferation, whereas cavernous hemangiomas consist of large, blood-filled cavities that have a compressed single-layered endothelial lining.

Nevus Flammeus (Port Wine Nevus, Port Wine Stain). Port wine nevi are always present at birth; they consist of mature dilated capillaries and represent a permanent developmental defect. The lesions are macular, sharply circumscribed, pink to purple in color (or occasionally black in deeply pigmented infants), and tremendously varied in size, occasionally involving up to one half of the body surface (Fig. 24–5). The posterior surface of the neck is a common site (Unna nevus). The face is also a site of predilection; distribution is often unilateral, and the mucous membranes can be involved. With maturation, the port wine nevus may become slightly raised and pebbly in consistency; alternatively, the paler lesions may fade significantly.

True nevus flammeus should be distinguished from the common salmon patch of the neonate, which is, in contrast, a relatively transient lesion. When the nevus is localized to the trigeminal area of the face, the diagnosis of *Sturge-Weber syndrome* (leptomeningeal venous angioma, seizures, hemiparesis contralateral to the facial lesion, and intracranial calcification) must be considered. Associated glaucoma or other ocular defects may cause irreparable damage if not diagnosed and treated immediately. Rarely, Sturge-Weber syndrome is associated with a bilateral facial lesion or with a nevus flammeus elsewhere on the body surface. Nevus flammeus also occurs as a component of Klippel-Trenaunay-Weber syndrome and with moderate frequency in other syndromes, including the Rubinstein-Taybi, Cobb (spinal arteriovenous malformation and nevus flammeus), Wiedemann-Beckwith, and trisomy 13 syndromes.

Several types of therapy including cryosurgery, excision and grafting, and tattooing have been utilized in the management of this defect. Laser therapy is becoming the modality

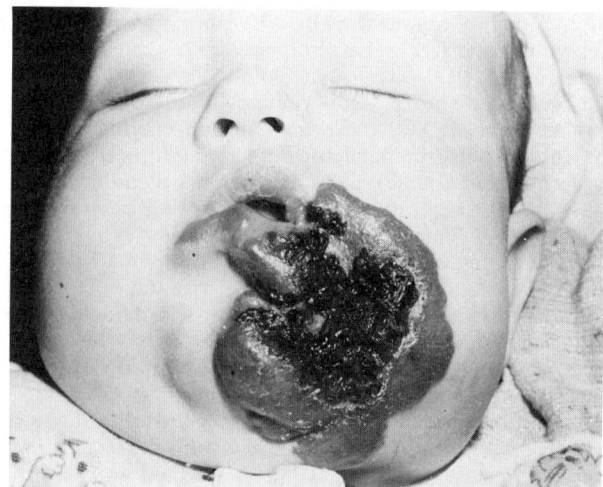

Figure 24–5. Large mixed capillary and cavernous hemangioma with central crusted ulcer.

of choice but has been most successful in adolescents and adults, particularly those with hemangiomas of darker hues. Makeup (e.g., Covermark) compounded to match the patient's normal facial skin provides a reasonable interim solution to the cosmetic problem.

Capillary Hemangioma (Strawberry Nevus). So-called strawberry hemangiomas are bright red, protuberant, compressible, sharply demarcated lesions that may occur on any area of the body. Although sometimes present at birth, more often they appear within the first 2 mo, heralded by an erythematous mark or by an area of pallor, which subsequently develops a fine telangiectatic pattern prior to the phase of expansion. Girls are affected more often than boys. Favored sites are the face, scalp, back, and anterior chest; lesions may be solitary or multiple.

Most strawberry hemangiomas undergo a phase of rapid expansion followed by a stationary period and finally by spontaneous involution. Regression may be anticipated when the lesion develops blanched or pale gray areas which are indicative of fibrosis. The course of a particular lesion is unpredictable, but approximately 60% of these lesions have involuted by the age of 5 yr, and 90–95% by the age of 9 yr. Spontaneous involution cannot be correlated with size or site of involvement, but lip lesions seem to persist most often. Complications include ulceration, secondary infection, and, rarely, hemorrhage.

In the usual patient who has no serious complications or extensive overgrowth that results in tissue destruction and severe disfigurement, a course of expectant observation should be followed. Since almost all of these lesions resolve spontaneously, interference is rarely indicated and may, in fact, cause further harm. Parents require repeated reassurance and support. After spontaneous resolution, approximately 10% of patients are left with small cosmetic defects such as puckering or discoloration of skin. These defects can be eliminated or minimized by judicious plastic repair if it is desired.

In the rare instance that intervention is required, excision may be advisable; the extent of scarring anticipated should influence the final decision. Radiation can be hazardous and should be considered only in life-threatening situations, such as the Kasabach-Merritt syndrome. Application of solid carbon dioxide is rarely effective and may produce scarring. Elastic bandages may reduce the amount of tissue distortion resulting from rapid growth, but they are appropriate only in selected patients with large hemangiomas. Systemic or intralesional administration of corticosteroids may be indicated for infants at risk for serious sequelae from exceptionally large or rapidly growing hemangiomas in vital areas (see below).

Cavernous Hemangiomas. These are more deeply situated than strawberry hemangiomas and, hence, appear more diffuse and ill-defined. The lesions are cystic, firm, or compressible, and the overlying skin may appear normal in color or have a bluish hue. Mixed hemangiomas consist of a cavernous component with a superimposed strawberry nevus (Fig. 24–5).

Cavernous hemangiomas progress from a growth phase to a stationary phase to a period of involution. These lesions are as likely to regress as strawberry hemangiomas, and the outcome cannot be predicted from size or site of involvement. A course of expectant observation should be followed in most instances. If involvement of underlying structures is suspected, appropriate radiologic studies should be performed for elucidation. Rarely, these lesions impinge on vital structures, interfere with functions such as vision or feeding, cause grotesque disfigurement because of rapid growth, or are associated with life-threatening complications such as thrombocytopenia and hemorrhage (see Kasabach-Merritt syndrome below). If it becomes necessary to intervene, a course of prednisone (2–4 mg/kg/24 hr) has proved effective in some infants. Termination of growth and sometimes regression may be evident after approximately 4 wk of therapy. When a response is obtained the dosage should be decreased gradually. Alternate day corticosteroid therapy has also been administered with success. Intralesional corticosteroid injection with the patient anesthetized can also induce rapid involution of a localized hemangioma. This technique has been particularly useful in patients with eyelid hemangiomas, which have a high incidence of complications including amblyopia, strabismus, and refractive errors.

Cavernous hemangiomas are associated with macrocephaly and pseudopapilledema in a rare autosomal dominant syndrome and occur with variable frequency in I cell disease and in Gorham disease (cavernous hemangiomas and disappearing bones).

Kasabach-Merritt syndrome is a combination of a rapidly enlarging hemangioma and thrombocytopenia; it is usually clinically evident during early infancy, but occasionally the onset is later. The hemangiomas are often present at birth and characteristically are solitary and large, although multiple and small hemangiomas have also been associated with thrombocytopenia. The vascular lesions are usually cutaneous and are only rarely located in viscera. The associated platelet defect may lead to precipitous hemorrhage accompanied by ecchymoses, petechiae, and a rapid increase in size of the hemangioma. Severe anemia may ensue. The platelet count is depressed, but the bone marrow contains increased numbers of normal or immature megakaryocytes. The thrombocytopenia has been attributed to sequestration or increased destruction of platelets within the hemangioma. Hypofibrinogenemia and decreased levels of consumable clotting factors are relatively common (Sec. 15.43–15.46).

Disseminated Hemangiomatosis. This is a serious condition in which multiple hemangiomas are widely distributed cutaneously and internally; on the skin there are usually numerous small, red or purple papular hemangiomas, but infrequently they may be sparse or absent. The internal hemangiomas may involve any of the viscera; the liver, gastrointestinal tract, central nervous system, and lung are the most common sites. The disorder is often fatal because of high-output cardiac failure, obstruction of the respiratory tract, and/or compression of central neural tissue. In a few instances systemic corticosteroid therapy alone or in combination with surgery and/or irradiation has apparently been lifesaving. Myriads of cutaneous hemangiomas may occur in the absence of visceral involvement; spontaneous regression of the lesions without complications is probable in such instances.

Multiple hemangiomas may also occur in several rare syndromes such as macrocephaly combined with pseudopapilledema or with lipomas.

Blue Rubber Bleb Nevus. This syndrome consists of multiple cavernous hemangiomas of the skin, mucous membranes, and gastrointestinal tract. Typical lesions are blue-purple in color and rubbery in consistency; they vary in size from a few mm to a few cm in diameter. At times they are painful or tender. Large disfiguring hemangiomas and irregular blue marks may also occur. The lesions, which can rarely be located in the liver, spleen, and central nervous system in addition to the skin, do not involute spontaneously. Recurrent gastrointestinal hemorrhage may lead to severe anemia. Palliation can be achieved by excision of involved bowel. Cutaneous angiomas have been removed successfully by laser therapy.

Maffucci Syndrome. The association of cavernous hemangiomas, phlebectasias, lymphangiomas, and lymphangiectasias with nodular echondromas in the metaphyseal or diaphyseal portion of long bones is known as the Maffucci syndrome. Onset occurs during childhood.

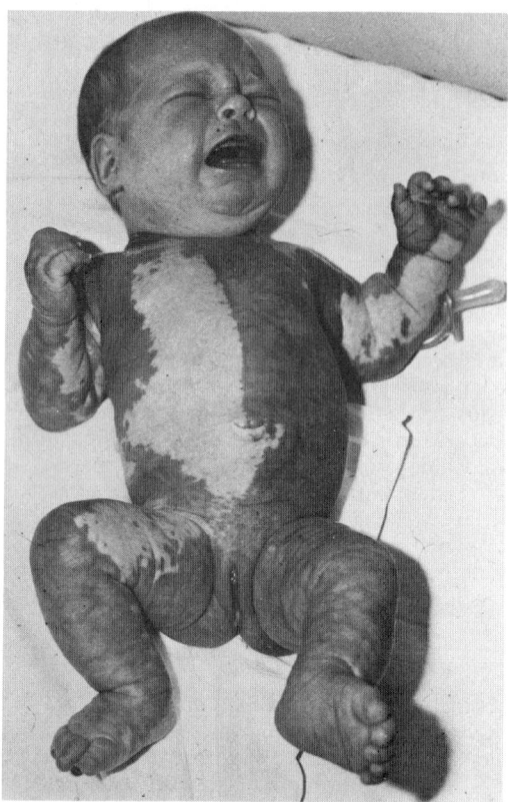

Figure 24–6. Widespread nevus flammeus in an infant with Klippel-Trenaunay-Weber syndrome.

Klippel-Trenaunay-Weber Syndrome. A macular vascular nevus (port-wine nevus) in combination with bony and soft tissue hypertrophy and venous varicosities constitutes the triad of defects of this nonheritable disorder. The anomaly may be confined to a single limb or involve more than one as well as portions of the trunk or face (Fig. 24–6). Enlargement of the soft tissues may be gradual and may involve the entire extremity, a portion of it, or selected digits. In addition to venous varicosities, arteriovenous fistulas can develop, and bruits are audible in the affected part. This disorder can be confused with Maffucci syndrome or, if the surface hemangioma is minimal, with Milroy disease. Thrombophlebitis, dislocations of joints, gangrene of the affected extremity, congestive heart failure, hematuria secondary to urinary tract hemangiomas, rectal bleeding from lesions of the gastrointestinal tract, pulmonary lesions, and malformations of the lymphatic vessels are infrequent complications. Arteriograms and venograms may delineate the extent of the anomaly, but surgical correction or palliation is often difficult. The indications for radiologic studies of viscera and bones are best determined by clinical evaluation.

Hereditary Hemorrhagic Telangiectasia (Osler-Weber-Rendu Disease). This disorder is inherited as an autosomal dominant trait. Affected children may experience recurrent epistaxis prior to detection of the characteristic skin and mucous membrane lesions. The mucocutaneous lesions, which usually develop at puberty, are 1–4 mm, sharply demarcated, red to purple macules, papules, or spider-like projections, each composed of a tightly woven mat of tortuous telangiectatic vessels. The nasal mucosa, lips, and tongue are usually involved; less commonly, cutaneous lesions occur on the face, ears, palms, and nail beds. Vascular ectasias may also arise in the conjunctivae, larynx, pharynx, gastrointestinal tract, bladder, vagina, bronchi, brain, and liver.

Massive hemorrhage is the most serious complication and may result in severe anemia. Bleeding may occur from the nose, mouth, gastrointestinal tract, genitourinary tract, and lungs. Persons with hereditary hemorrhagic telangiectasia have normal levels of clotting factors and an intact clotting mechanism. In the absence of serious complications, life span is normal. Local lesions may be temporarily ablated with chemical cautery or electrocoagulation. More drastic surgical measures may be required for lesions in critical sites such as the lung or gastrointestinal tract.

Spider Angiomas. The vascular spider (nevus araneus) consists of a central feeder artery with multiple dilated radiating vessels and a surrounding erythematous flush, varying from a few mm to several cm in diameter. Pressure over the central vessel will cause blanching; pulsations visible in larger nevi are evidence for the arterial source of the lesion. Spider angiomas are associated with conditions in which there are increased levels of circulating estrogens, such as cirrhosis and pregnancy, but they also occur in up to 15% of normal preschool-age children and 45% of school-age ones. Sites of predilection in children are the dorsum of the hand, forearm, face, and ears. Angiomas can be obliterated by application of liquid nitrogen or solid carbon dioxide or by electrocoagulation of the central vessel.

Generalized Essential Telangiectasia. A rare and presumably nevoid anomaly of unknown etiology, essential telangiectasia may have its onset in childhood or adulthood. Mild expression consists of patchy retiform telangiectases, particularly on the limbs, with occasional progression to involve large areas of the body surface. The condition must be distinguished from the secondary telangiectasia of connective tissue diseases, xeroderma pigmentosum, poikiloderma, and ataxia-telangiectasia. There is no treatment; however, patients can be reassured that their health will not be affected by the cutaneous disorder.

Unilateral Nevoid Telangiectasia. This unusual entity is characterized by the appearance of telangiectasia in a unilateral distribution, particularly in females at onset of menses or during pregnancy. The appearance of these lesions usually is coincident with elevated levels of circulating estrogens, whatever the cause. When initiated by pregnancy, the telangiectasia may fade or disappear postpartum.

Cutis Marmorata Telangiectatica Congenita (Congenital Generalized Phlebectasia). This benign vascular anomaly represents dilatation of superficial capillaries and veins and is apparent at birth. Involved areas of skin have a reticulated pattern of a red or purple hue which resembles physiologic cutis marmorata but is more pronounced and relatively unvarying (Fig. 24–7, p. xxviii). The lesions may be restricted to a single limb and a portion of the trunk or may be more widespread. The lesions become more pronounced during changes in environmental temperature, physical activity, or crying. In some instances, the underlying subcutaneous tissue is underdeveloped, and ulceration may occur within the reticulated bands. Nevus flammeus may also be associated. Rarely, defective growth of bone and soft tissue and other congenital abnormalities may be present. No specific therapy is indicated; the expected course is one of gradual steady improvement, with partial or complete resolution by adolescence.

Ataxia-Telangiectasia. (See also Sec. 21.20.) This disorder (*Louis-Bar syndrome*) is transmitted as an autosomal recessive trait. The characteristic telangiectasia develops at about 3 yr of age, first on the bulbar conjunctivae and later on the nasal bridge, malar areas, external ears, hard palate, upper anterior chest, and antecubital and popliteal fossae. Additional cutaneous stigmata include café-au-lait spots, premature graying of the hair, and sclerodermatous changes.

Angiokeratomas. Several forms of angiokeratomas have been described, but some of them do not occur during childhood or adolescence. *Angiokeratoma of Mibelli*, which is probably transmitted in an autosomal dominant pattern, is characterized by 1–8 mm red, purple, or black scaly, verrucous, occasionally crusted papules and nodules that appear on the dorsum of the fingers and toes and on the knees and the elbows. Less commonly, palms, soles, and ears may be affected. In many patients, onset has followed frostbite or chilblains. These nodules bleed freely following injury and may involute in response to trauma or may be effectively eradicated by cryotherapy or fulguration. *Angiokeratoma circumscriptum* is a rare solitary lesion that presents as a plaque of blue-red papules or nodules with a verrucous surface. These usually develop during infancy and early childhood, and they may increase in size at adolescence. The lower limb is the site of predilection. Excision is the treatment of choice.

Angiokeratoma corporis diffusum (Fabry disease) (Sec. 7.28), an inborn error of glycolipid metabolism, is an X-linked recessive disorder fully penetrant in males and of variable penetrance in carrier females. The skin lesions have their onset prior to puberty and occur in profusion over the genitalia, hips, buttocks, and thighs and in the umbilical and inguinal regions. They consist of 0.1–3.0 mm red to blue-black papules which may have a hyperkeratotic surface. Telangiectasias are seen in mucosa and in the conjunctivae. On light microscopy these angiokeratomas appear as blood-filled, dilated, endothelial-lined vascular spaces. Granular lipid deposits that stain with Sudan black and periodic acid–Schiff reagent are demonstrable in dermal macrophages, fibrocytes, and endothelial cells.

Additional clinical features include recurrent episodes of fever and agonizing limb pain, cyanosis and flushing of the acral areas, paresthesias of the hands and feet, corneal opacities detectable by slit-lamp examination, and hypohidrosis. Renal and cardiac involvement are the usual causes of death. The biochemical defect is a deficiency of the lysosomal enzyme α-galactosidase, with accumulation of ceramide trihexoside in tissues and its massive excretion in urine.

Similar cutaneous lesions have also been described in another lysosomal enzyme disorder, α-L-fucosidase deficiency, and in sialidosis, a storage disease with neuraminidase deficiency.

Nevus Anemicus. Although nevus anemicus is present at birth, it may not be detectable until early childhood. The nevus consists of solitary or multiple, sharply delineated, pale macules which are most often on the trunk but may also occur on the neck or limbs. These nevi may simulate plaques of vitiligo, leukoderma, or nevoid pigmentary defects, but they can be readily distinguished by their response to firm stroking. Stroking will evoke an erythematous line and flare in areas of pigment loss, but the skin of a nevus anemicus fails to redden. Although the cutaneous vasculature appears normal histologically, the blood vessels within the nevus do not respond to injection of vasodilators. It has been postulated that the persistent pallor may represent a sustained localized adrenergic vasoconstriction.

LYMPHANGIOMAS

See Sec. 16.27.

24.8 CUTANEOUS NEVI

The term *nevus* often causes semantic confusion because the precise definition of the word has been blurred by common usage. In this section it is used to designate skin lesions that histologically are characterized by collections of well-differentiated cell types normally found in the skin. Not all nevi, however, are discussed in this section; the most notable exceptions are vascular nevi (hemangiomas), which are described in the preceding section.

Acquired Pigmented Nevi. Common pigmented nevi or moles are also termed *nevocytic* or *nevocellular nevi* to distinguish them from the pigmented lesions arising from mature melanocytes. Nevus cells are closely related to melanocytes and may be derived from a common stem cell (*nevoblast*). An alternative theory is that nevus cells are of dual origin, with superficially located cells arising from melanocytes (*melanocytic nevus*) and cells in the deeper layers arising from Schwann cells (*neuroid nevus*).

Nevocellular nevi have a well-defined life history. Nevi are classified as junctional, compound, or dermal in accordance with the location of the nevus cells in the skin. Early lesions are usually junctional in type. Although some nevi remain junctional throughout life, most become compound or intradermal and change morphologically as well as histologically.

Junctional nevi may be present at birth but most often appear in early childhood or during adolescence. The lesions appear in varying shades of brown; they are relatively small, discrete, flat, and variable in shape. They may appear anywhere on the body; those on the palms, soles, and genitalia usually remain junctional throughout life. The melanized nevus cells are cuboidal or epithelioid in configuration and occur in nests on the epidermal side of the basement membrane.

With maturation *compound and intradermal nevi* may become raised, dome-shaped, verrucous, or pedunculated. Slightly elevated lesions are usually compound, i.e., the nevus cells inhabit both the epidermis and the dermis. Distinctly elevated lesions are usually intradermal. The amount of melanin in a lesion may vary greatly, or there may be none.

Acquired pigmented nevi are benign lesions and need be removed only to improve appearance or to avoid chronic irritation and infection if they are subject to repeated trauma. A very small percentage of nevi undergo malignant transformation; there is no way, however, to determine which are potentially dangerous, and random excision is neither feasible nor rational. Suspicious changes such as rapid increase in size, development of satellite lesions, induration, itching, or pain are indications for excision and histologic evaluation. Most of these changes will be due to irritation, infection, or maturation; color change and gradual increase in size and elevation normally occur during adolescence and should not be cause for concern. Nevertheless, if there is doubt about the benignity of a nevus, excision is a safe and simple outpatient procedure that may be justified to allay anxiety.

Congenital Pigmented Nevi. Nevocellular nevi are present in approximately 1% of newborn infants. They are viewed with more concern than are acquired nevocellular nevi because they pose an increased risk over a lifetime for development of malignant melanoma.

Sites of predilection are the lower trunk, upper back and shoulders, chest, and proximal limbs. The lesions may be flat, elevated, verrucous, or nodular; they may appear in various shades of brown, blue, or black, and may develop numerous coarse hairs or remain hairless and leathery in texture. The term giant congenital pigmented nevus is used for nevi measuring >20 cm (Fig. 24–8). Numerous smaller satellite nevi may be scattered elsewhere. The lesions, if significantly disfiguring, may cause severe emotional problems.

Some congenital nevi have the histologic features of ordinary junctional, compound, or intradermal nevi, but others are characterized by nevus cells dispersed between the collagen bundles of the lower 2/3 of the dermis with occasional extension into the underlying tissues. Less commonly, the histologic pattern is that of a neural nevus, blue nevus, or spindle and epithelioid cell nevus.

Giant congenital pigmented nevi are of special significance for 2 reasons: (1) the association of leptomeningeal melanocytosis and (2) the predisposition for development of malignant melanoma. Leptomeningeal involvement may cause hydrocephalus, seizures, retardation, and motor deficits and may result in melanoma. Malignancy can be identified by careful cytologic examination of the cerebrospinal fluid for

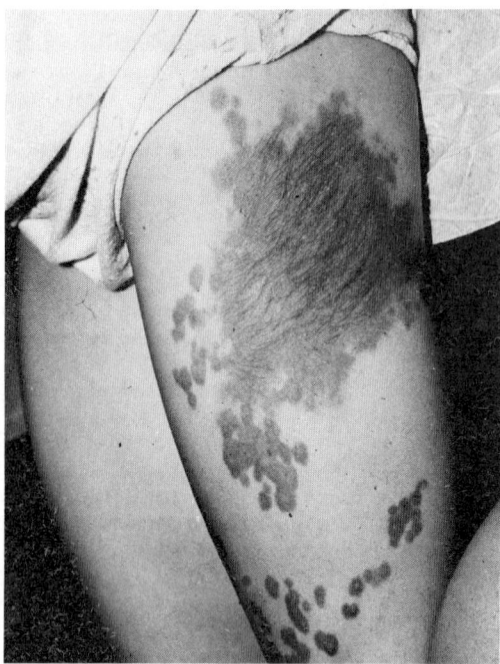

Figure 24–8. Congenital pigmented nevocytic nevus on the thigh.

melanin-containing cells. The incidence of malignant melanoma arising in giant congenital nevi is estimated to be approximately 6–10%. Affected patients usually succumb despite palliative measures. Early total excision and grafting is the treatment of choice. Extensive spotty involvement of peripheral skin with small nevi often limits the use of the patient's skin for grafting. If excision is delayed, frequent examinations and biopsy of enlarging nodules or suspicious areas are mandatory. Although there is agreement concerning the management of giant congenital nevi (larger than 20 cm), there is considerable controversy concerning the appropriate approach to medium-sized (1.5–20 cm) and small (smaller than 1.5 cm) congenital nevi. While there are no definitive data on the incidence of melanomas arising in these lesions, it is now the prevailing, but not universal, opinion that these nevi should be excised prior to adolescence. Benign-appearing macular lesions of uniform color may be observed expectantly until late childhood, when they can be removed under local anesthesia.

Halo Nevus (Leukoderma Acquisitum Centrifugum). Occasionally, the common pigmented nevus develops a peripheral zone of depigmentation up to 5 mm in width (Fig. 24–9). In tissue biopsy there is a dense inflammatory infiltrate of lymphocytes and histiocytes in addition to the nevus cells. The pale halo reflects disappearance of the melanocytes. This phenomenon has also been associated with blue nevi, neurofibromas, and primary and secondary malignant melanoma. Patients with certain organ-specific autoimmune disorders and vitiligo have an increased incidence of halo nevi.

These lesions occur primarily in children and young adults; development of the halo may coincide with puberty or pregnancy. Frequently, several pigmented nevi will develop halos simultaneously. Subsequent disappearance of the central nevus is the usual outcome, and the depigmented area may or may not be repigmented. Excision and histopathologic examination of the lesion is indicated only when the nature of the central lesion is in question.

Spindle and epithelioid cell nevus (Spitz nevus) is commonly referred to as a *juvenile melanoma;* however, since it is always benign, the anxiety-provoking term melanoma should be avoided. Spindle and epithelioid cell nevi are pink to red, smooth, dome-shaped, firm, hairless nodules, which appear

suddenly, grow rapidly, and are most often situated on the face, shoulder, or upper limb. They achieve a maximal size of about 1.5 cm. Rarely, they occur as multiple grouped lesions. Visually similar lesions include pyogenic granuloma, hemangioma, nevocellular nevus, juvenile xanthogranuloma, and basal cell carcinoma, but histologically these entities are distinguishable. The spindle and epithelioid cell nevus, a variant of the compound nevus, presents epidermal changes, vascular ectasias, and dermal and epidermal collections of pleomorphic, fusiform, and polygonal nevus cells, giant cells, and multinucleated giant cells. Although the histologic pattern may appear ominous to the inexperienced observer, the benign nature of the lesion permits conservative excision with little likelihood of reappearance or spread.

Zosteriform lentiginous nevus is a unilateral, linear, band-like lesion composed of multiple small brown or black macules on the face, trunk, or limbs. The lesions may be present at birth or develop during childhood; they represent collections of melanin-containing nevus cells at the tips of the dermal papillae.

Nevus spilus (speckled lentiginous nevus) is a flat, brown patch, within which are darker brown macules. These nevi vary considerably in size and can occur anywhere on the body. The darker macules usually develop gradually and represent nevus cells in a junctional or dermal location. These nevocellular nevi are benign and need not be excised.

Nevus of Ota is a permanent, blue-gray, macular, facial stain caused by aggregates of melanocytes in the dermis. The macular nevi resemble mongolian spots in color and occur unilaterally in the areas supplied by the 1st and 2nd divisions of the trigeminal nerve. They are sometimes present at birth, and in other cases may arise during the 1st or 2nd decade of life. Patchy involvement of the sclera and other ocular tissues and of the nasal and buccal mucosa occurs in some patients. Nevus of Ota is more common in females and in oriental and black patients.

Nevus of Ito is localized to the shoulder, supraclavicular area, lateral neck, and upper arm. It can also be regarded as a persistent mongolian spot. The only available treatment is masking with cosmetics.

Blue nevi are solitary lesions that may be present at birth or develop during childhood, most frequently on the face, neck, arms, buttocks, hands, and feet; they are more common in females. Typical lesions are smooth, dome-shaped, hairless, blue or black nodules that rarely exceed 1 cm in diameter. Microscopically, they are characterized by groups of intensely

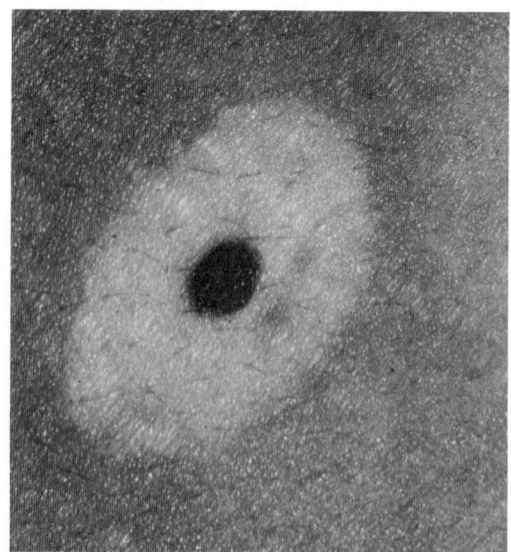

Figure 24–9. Well-developed halo nevus.

pigmented, spindle-shaped melanocytes in the dermis and around appendicular structures.

Cellular blue nevi, which differ somewhat histologically, are larger and occur most frequently on the buttocks and in the sacrococcygeal area. They have a low but definite incidence of malignant transformation, and hence excision is the treatment of choice.

Achromic nevi (nevus depigmentosus) are usually present at birth; they are localized macular hypopigmented patches or streaks, often with bizarre, irregular borders. They resemble hypomelanosis of Ito clinically except that they are smaller, more localized, and often unilateral. They appear to represent a focal defect in melanin production.

Epidermal nevi may be visible at birth or may develop within the first months or years of life. They affect both sexes equally and only very rarely occur in more than one family member. Initially the epidermal nevus may appear as a discolored, slightly scaly patch that, with maturation, becomes more thickened, verrucous, and hyperpigmented. Several morphologic types include: pigmented papillomas, often in a linear distribution; unilateral hyperkeratotic streaks (nevus unius lateris) involving a limb and perhaps a portion of the trunk; velvety hyperpigmented plaques; and feathered, whorled, or marbled hyperkeratotic lesions in localized plaques (Fig. 24–10) or over extensive areas of the body. An inflammatory linear verrucous variant that is markedly pruritic may become eczematized.

The histologic pattern evolves as the lesion matures; but epidermal hyperplasia of some degree is apparent in all stages of development. One or another dermal appendage may predominate in a particular lesion. The diagnosis can be confirmed by biopsy. These nevi must be distinguished from lichen striatus, lymphangioma circumscriptum, shagreen patch of tuberous sclerosis, congenital hairy nevi, and nevus sebaceus (Jadassohn). Keratolytic agents such as retinoic acid or salicylic acid may be moderately effective in reducing scaling and controlling pruritus, but definitive treatment requires full-thickness excision; recurrence is usual if more superficial removal is attempted. Alternatively, the nevus may be left intact.

With some frequency, epidermal nevi are associated with abnormalities of other organs; this combination has been designated as the *epidermal nevus syndrome*. The additional defects include localized soft tissue hypertrophy, hemangiomas, pigmentary changes, skeletal anomalies of various sorts, ocular defects, and neurologic abnormalities such as developmental delay, seizures, motor deficits, and cerebrovascular malformations. Associated malignancies such as Wilms tumor and astrocytoma, although rare, are being reported with increasing frequency.

Nevus sebaceus (Jadassohn) is a relatively small, sharply demarcated, oval or linear, yellow-orange, elevated plaque that is usually devoid of hair and occurs on the head and neck of infants. Although characterized histologically by an abundance of sebaceous glands, all elements of the skin are represented. With maturity, usually during adolescence, the lesions become verrucous and studded with large rubbery nodules. The changing clinical appearance reflects the histologic pattern, which is characterized by a variable degree of hyperkeratosis, hyperplasia of the epidermis, malformed hair follicles, and often a profusion of sebaceous and apocrine glands. During adulthood, these nevi are frequently complicated by secondary malignancies and benign adnexal tumors, most commonly basal cell carcinoma or syringocystadenoma papilliferum. The diagnosis can be established by biopsy; the treatment of choice is total excision prior to adolescence. Sebaceous nevi associated with central nervous system, skeletal, and ocular defects probably represent variants of the epidermal nevus syndrome.

Comedone nevi (nevus comedonicus) consist of linear plaques simulating comedones; they may be present at birth or appear during childhood. The horny plugs represent keratinous debris within dilated, malformed pilosebaceous follicles. The lesions are most often unilateral and may develop at any site. They appear to be a harmless developmental anomaly not associated with other congenital malformations. There is no effective treatment except full thickness excision; palliation of larger lesions may be achieved by regular applications of a retinoic acid preparation.

Connective tissue nevus may occur as a solitary defect or as a manifestation of an associated disorder. These nevi may occur at any site but are most common on the trunk. They are skin-colored, ivory, or yellow plaques, 2–15 cm in diameter, composed of multiple tiny papules or grouped nodules which are frequently difficult to appreciate visually because of the subtle color changes. The plaques have a rubbery or cobblestone consistency on palpation. Biopsy findings are variable and include increased amounts of dermal elastic tissue or a predominance of thickened collagen bundles. Similar lesions occurring with tuberous sclerosis are called shagreen patches. The association of multiple small papular connective tissue nevi with osteopoikilosis is called *dermatofibrosis lenticularis disseminata* (Buschke-Ollendorff syndrome).

24.9 DISORDERS OF PIGMENT

Alterations in skin color may be generalized or localized and may result from a variety of defects ranging from absence of melanocytes and defective melanization of melanosomes to overproduction of melanin and increased numbers of melanocytic cells. Some of these aberrations are induced by hormones (hyperpigmentation of Addison disease); others represent focal developmental defects (white spots of tuberous sclerosis); still others may be nonspecific and the result of cutaneous inflammation (postinflammatory hypopigmentation or hyperpigmentation).

24.10 HYPERPIGMENTED LESIONS

Ephelides or **freckles** are light or dark brown macules that occur in sun-exposed areas, such as the face, upper back, arms, and hands. They are induced by exposure to sun, particularly during the summer months, and may fade or disappear during the winter. They are more common in fair-haired individuals, appear first during the preschool years, and are probably genetically determined. Histologically, they are marked by increased melanin pigment in the epidermal

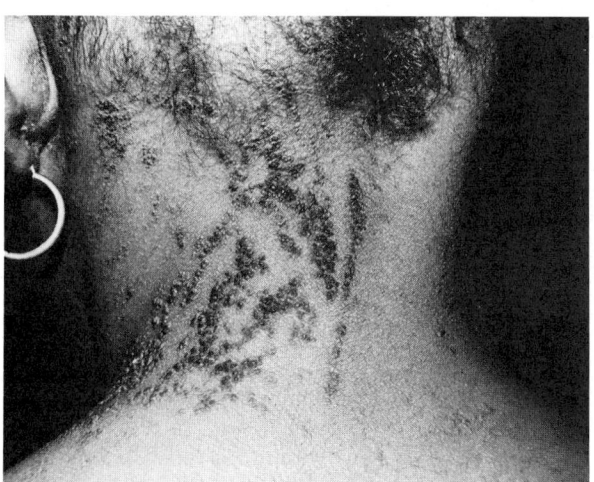

Figure 24–10. Verrucous streaky epidermal nevus on the neck.

basal layer with no increase in the number of melanocytes. Actually the freckle contains fewer but larger melanocytes than the surrounding paler skin.

Lentigines, often mistaken for freckles or pigmented nevi, are small (1–3 cm), round, dark brown macules that can appear anywhere on the body, are unrelated to sun exposure, and remain permanently. They differ from other hyperpigmented macules histologically in that they have elongated, club-shaped, epidermal rete ridges with increased numbers of melanocytes and dense epidermal deposits of melanin. The lesions are benign and, when few, may be viewed as a normal occurrence. Some juvenile lentigines may be precursors of nevocellular nevi (pigmented moles). The *multiple lentigines (leopard) syndrome* is an autosomal dominant entity consisting of a generalized distribution of lentigines in association with profound sensorineural deafness and other anomalies that include retarded growth, hypertelorism, cardiac defects such as pulmonic stenosis, and abnormalities of the genitalia.

The Peutz-Jeghers syndrome is characterized by melanotic macules on the lips and mucous membranes and by polyposis of the small intestine. It is inherited as an autosomal dominant trait. Onset is noted during early childhood when pigmented macules appear on the lips, buccal mucosa, and gingivae and occasionally on the nose, hands, and feet. Polyposis usually involves the small intestine but may also occur in the stomach and large intestine. Episodic abdominal pain, melena, and intussusception are frequent complications. Malignant degeneration has been reported, but the risk of malignancy is small, and a normal life span is usual in affected individuals. Peutz-Jeghers syndrome must be differentiated from other syndromes associated with multiple lentigines, from ordinary freckling, from Gardner syndrome, and from Cronkhite-Canada syndrome (a disorder characterized by gastrointestinal polyposis, alopecia, onychodystrophy, and skin pigmentation).

Café-au-lait spots are uniformly hyperpigmented, sharply demarcated, macular lesions, the hues of which vary with the normal depth of pigmentation of the individual: they are tan or light brown in white individuals and may be dark brown in black children. Café-au-lait spots vary tremendously in size and may be quite large, covering a significant portion of the trunk or limb. Generally, the borders are smooth, but some have an exceedingly irregular border. The lesions are characterized by increased numbers of melanocytes and melanin in the epidermis but lack the clubbed rete ridges that typify lentigines. One to 3 café-au-lait spots are common in normal children. They may be present at birth or develop during childhood.

Large, often unilateral café-au-lait spots with irregular borders are characteristic of patients with *McCune-Albright syndrome* (Sec. 19.7 and 23.14), a disorder that includes polyostotic bone dysplasia, precocious puberty, and multiple endocrine dysfunctions. The macular hyperpigmentation may be present at birth or develop late in childhood; if segmentally localized, it suggests an embryonic developmental defect.

Neurofibromatosis (von Recklinghausen disease). The café-au-lait spot is the most familiar cutaneous hallmark of this autosomal dominant neurocutaneous syndrome; it is present in up to 90% of affected children. Since these lesions occur in normal children and with certain other disorders, 6 lesions, each >1.5 cm in its largest diameter, are considered diagnostic of neurofibromatosis. The lesions may not be present at birth; accordingly, early definitive diagnosis may not be possible unless other evidence of the disease is present. Axillary freckling (Crowe sign) and speckled hyperpigmentation on the upper chest, groin, and perineal skin are also common manifestations of neurofibromatosis.

Neurofibromas are uncommon before late childhood or adolescence and may occur anywhere, including the oral

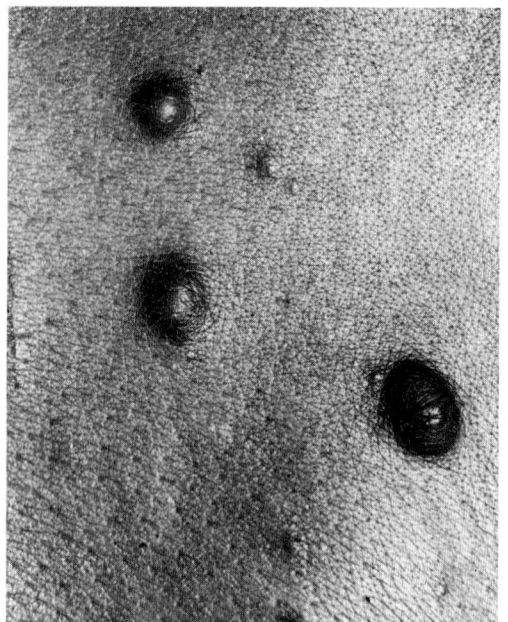

Figure 24–11. Multiple sessile neurofibromas.

mucous membranes and tongue. These lesions are soft, skin-colored, sessile or pedunculated nodules (Fig. 24–11) that may grow to considerable size and occasionally undergo sarcomatous change. Subcutaneous nodules may also occur along the course of nerve trunks. Deforming plexiform neuromas are another cutaneous feature. The histologic features of these lesions are diagnostic.

Neurofibromatosis also affects the musculoskeletal system, eye, gastrointestinal tract, vascular system, and central nervous system (Sec. 21.16). There is also an increased incidence of pheochromocytomas and central nervous system neoplasms in these patients.

Incontinentia pigmenti (Bloch-Sulzberger disease) is a rare, heritable, multisystem disorder that is thought to be transmitted as an X-linked dominant trait, lethal in males. The paucity of affected males and the high frequency of spontaneous abortions in carrier females lend credence to this supposition.

The cutaneous manifestations can be divided into three phases, which may not all be present in some patients:

1. The 1st phase is evident at birth or shortly thereafter and consists of erythematous, linear streaks and plaques of vesicles which are most pronounced on the limbs (Fig. 24–12A). The lesions may be confused with those of herpes simplex, bullous impetigo, or mastocytosis, but the linear configuration is unique, and smears of vesicle fluid prepared with Wright stain demonstrate masses of eosinophils. Blood eosinophilia up to 65% is common but disappears after 4–5 mo of age.

2. The vesicular phase is followed by an intermediate verrucous stage, which may persist up to approximately 6 mo of age. These lesions eventually involute, at times leaving atrophic or depigmented areas.

3. The final pigmentary stage is variable in time of onset; it may overlap the earlier phases and even be evident at birth or, more commonly, within the first few weeks of life; sites of involvement are not necessarily those of the preceding vesicular and warty lesions. The pigment is distributed in macular whorls, reticulated patches, flecks, splashes, and linear streaks and, once present, persists throughout childhood (Fig. 24–12B).

Histologically, an early vesicular lesion is characterized by epidermal edema and an intraepidermal vesicle filled with eosinophils. Epidermal hyperplasia, hyperkeratosis, and pap-

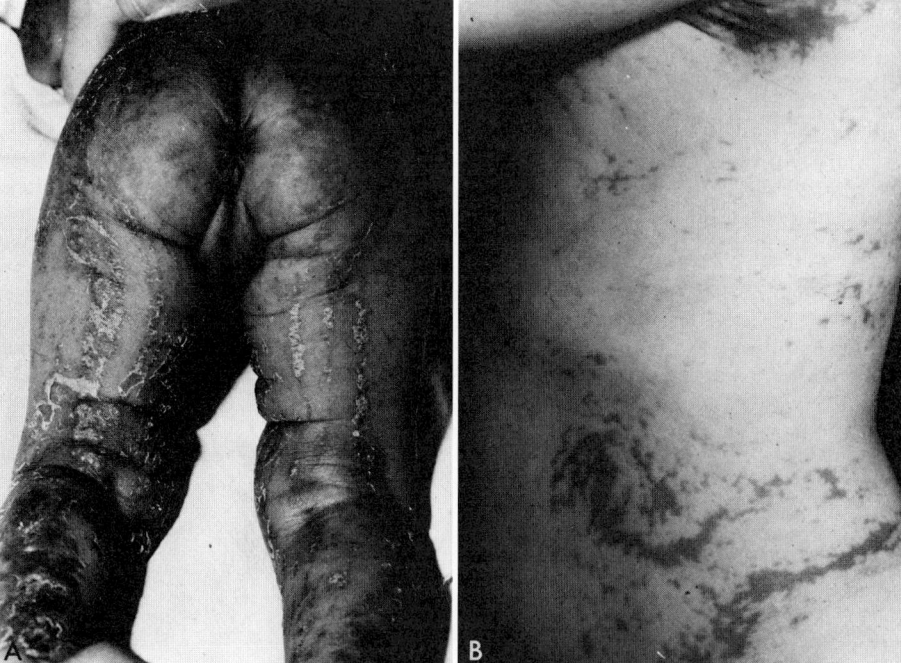

Figure 24–12. *A*, Vesicular and verrucous linear lesions on buttocks and legs of an infant girl with incontinentia pigmenti. *B*, Whorled macular hyperpigmentation of incontinentia pigmenti.

illomatosis are characteristic of the 2nd phase. The end-stage pigmentary lesion typically shows vacuolar degeneration of the epidermal basal cells and melanin in melanophages of the upper dermis. The name of the disease is derived from the latter histologic feature.

Although the skin lesions may constitute the only manifestation, approximately 80% of affected children have other defects. Alopecia, which may be scarring and patchy or diffuse, occurs in up to 40% of patients; dental anomalies, present in over half the children, consist of late dentition, conical teeth, and partial anodontia. Central nervous system manifestations, including developmental retardation, seizures, microcephaly, spasticity, and paralysis, are found in about a third of affected children; ocular anomalies resulting in severe impairment of vision or blindness occur in over 15% of children. Less common abnormalities include dystrophy of nails and skeletal defects. The choice of investigative studies and the plan of management depend on the occurrence of particular noncutaneous abnormalities since skin lesions are benign and often become less evident during adulthood. The high incidence of associated major anomalies warrants genetic counseling.

Postinflammatory Pigmentary Changes. Either hyperpigmentation or hypopigmentation can occur as a result of cutaneous inflammation. Alteration in pigmentation usually follows a severe inflammatory reaction but may result from mild dermatitis. Dark-skinned children are more likely to show these changes than fair-skinned ones. Although altered pigmentation may persist for weeks to months, patients can be reassured that these lesions are usually temporary. These changes must be distinguished from nevoid lesions and diseases manifested by pigmentary alterations such as vitiligo.

24.11 HYPOPIGMENTED LESIONS

Albinism. Several types of oculocutaneous albinism have been defined, each of which is inherited in an autosomal recessive fashion. The various forms of albinism may be distinguished by clinical manifestations, morphology of the melanosomes, and the hair bulb incubation test, which determines whether tyrosinase is present. The well-defined types of oculocutaneous albinism are as follows:

Tyrosinase-negative albinism is characterized by lack of visible pigment in hair, skin, and eyes that results in photophobia, nystagmus, defective visual acuity, white hair, and white skin. The irides are blue-gray in oblique light and pink in reflected light.

Tyrosinase-positive albinism may resemble the above pattern except that the hair may be straw colored or light brown. With aging, the irides may accumulate some brown pigment and hence some improvement in visual acuity. The skin color is cream or pink.

In *tyrosinase-variable albinism* (yellow mutant) the infant has white hair, pink skin, and gray eyes at birth but develops bright yellow hair, light tanning of skin on sun exposure, and some pigment in the iris. Photophobia and nystagmus are present but mild.

The *Hermansky-Pudlak syndrome* is tyrosinase-negative albinism with platelet defects and a hemorrhagic diathesis.

The *Cross-McKusick-Breen* syndrome consists of tyrosinase-positive albinism with microphthalmia, retardation, spasticity, and athetosis.

Because of the absence of normal protection by adequate amounts of epidermal melanin, persons with albinism are predisposed to develop actinic keratoses and cutaneous carcinoma secondary to skin damage by ultraviolet light. Protection with a broad-spectrum sunscreen preparation (Sec. 24.33) should be provided during exposure to sunlight.

Partial Albinism (Piebaldism). This autosomal dominant disorder is characterized by amelanotic plaques; they occur most frequently on the forehead, anterior scalp (producing a white forelock), thorax, elbows, and knees. Though sharply demarcated from normally pigmented skin, islands of normal pigmentation may be present within the amelanotic areas. The plaques are the result of localized absence or reduction in the number of melanocytes; the defect is permanent. Piebaldism must be differentiated from vitiligo, which is progressive and is not usually congenital; achromic nevus; and Waardenburg syndrome.

Waardenburg syndrome is characterized by a white forelock, heterochromic irides, broad nasal root, dystopia canthorum, congenital deafness, defects in fundus pigment, and cutaneous hypopigmentation; it is inherited as an autosomal dominant trait.

Chédiak-Higashi syndrome is an autosomal recessive disorder; the diffuse dilution in pigmentation results in a peculiar bluish hue of skin and hair, photophobia, decreased ocular pigmentation, and nystagmus. Hepatosplenomegaly and increased susceptibility to infections are also features (Sec. 10.32).

Tuberous sclerosis (Sec. 21.16), as is the case in many of the neurocutaneous syndromes, is a multisystemic disorder affecting primarily tissues derived from ectoderm but also involving organs of mesodermal and endodermal origin. It is inherited as an autosomal dominant trait of variable penetrance and expressivity. In addition to multiple cutaneous stigmata, it is characterized by mental retardation, epilepsy, cerebral calcification, tuberous nodules of the cortex and subependymal area, retinal phakomas, rhabdomyomas of the heart, renal cysts and tumors, and cysts of bone and lung.

The most reliable early cutaneous sign is the *white leaf macule*, which is present but not always easily detectable at birth. At least 80% of patients have these lesions, which may be identified by examination with the Wood lamp. They are sharply demarcated, pale, 0.5–3 cm lesions that often assume the shape of a mountain ash leaflet. Single or multiple lesions are most often found on the trunk (Fig. 24–13A) but also occur on the face and limbs. Small, confetti-like, hypopigmented macules are also present in some instances. Hypopigmentation reflects inadequate melanization of the melanosomes of the pigment-generating cells.

Adenoma sebaceum is the most commonly recognized cutaneous marker of tuberous sclerosis; the lesions appear on the face during mid to late childhood or adolescence in approximately 80% of patients. These pink or flesh-colored papulonodular growths may erupt in profusion on the cheeks, nose, forehead, and chin but often spare the upper lip (Fig. 24–13B). The term adenoma sebaceum is a misnomer since these growths are angiofibromas rather than tumors of the sebaceous glands. Similar fibromatous nodules may be scattered on the forehead, trunk, and limbs. Large, skin-colored, raised

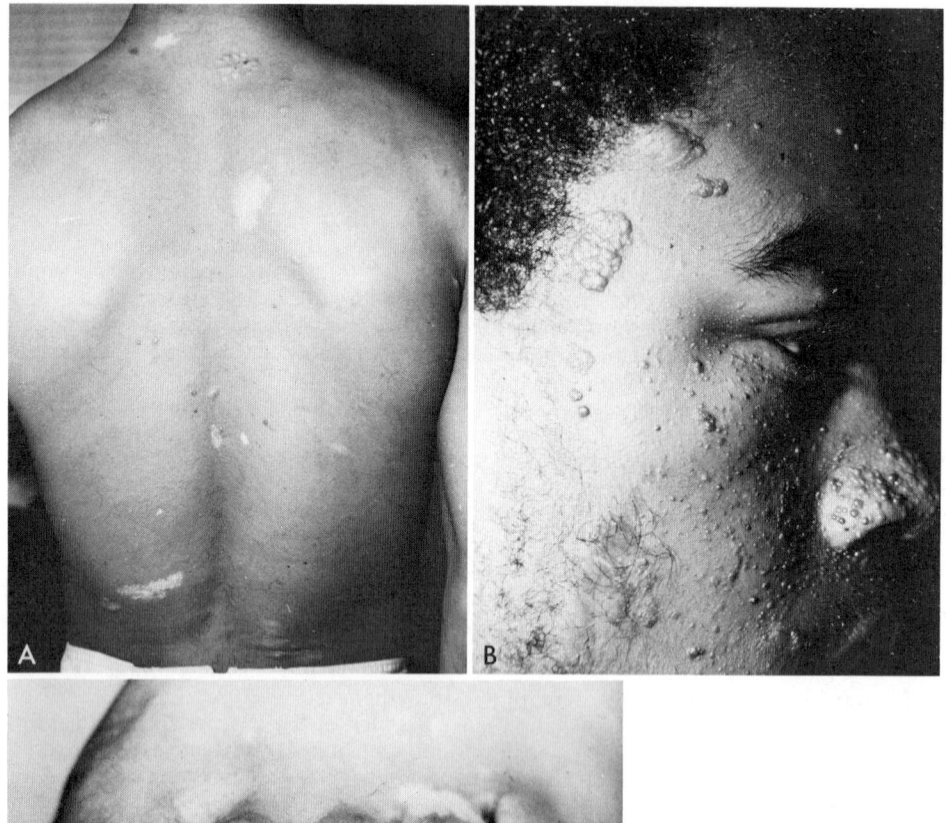

Figure 24–13. Tuberous sclerosis. A, Multiple white leaf macules, small papular fibromas, and shagreen patch on lower back. B, Adenoma sebaceum and angiofibromatous plaques on the temple. C, Periungual fibromas.

or flat collagenous plaques with an orange peel or cobblestone texture *(shagreen patches)* occur with some frequency in the lumbosacral area. At puberty, distinctive, clove-like, periungual fibromas (Fig. 24–13C) appear on the fingers and toes of some children; gingival fibromas may also occur, unassociated with the administration of anticonvulsant medications. Café-au-lait spots occur with increased frequency but are not as numerous as in neurofibromatosis.

The cutaneous markers of this disorder are incontrovertible evidence for tuberous sclerosis and should be sought in any child with suggestive central nervous system manifestations. Appreciation of the significance of white leaf macules with seizures and retardation can provide a focus for the diagnostic evaluation and permit effective genetic counseling.

Hypomelanosis of Ito (incontinentia pigmenti achromians) is a congenital skin disorder that affects children of both sexes, is frequently associated with defects in several organ systems, and should be regarded as a neurocutaneous syndrome. The role of genetic transmission has not been established. The skin lesions consist of bizarre, patterned, hypopigmented macules arranged in sharply demarcated whorls, streaks, and patches over the body surface (Fig. 24–14). The hypopigmentation remains unchanged throughout childhood but is said to fade during adulthood. Neither inflammatory nor vesicular lesions precede the development of the pigmentary changes as in Bloch-Sulzberger incontinentia pigmenti. Histologic changes in affected skin are nonspecific: decreased numbers of melanocytes are found on DOPA stains, and incomplete melanization of melanosomes is seen on electron microscopy. Commonly associated abnormalities include seizures, developmental retardation, scoliosis, limb asymmetry, and ophthalmologic defects.

Vitiligo is an acquired pigmentary defect that may occur at any age in persons of any skin color. The lesions are depigmented macules, sharply circumscribed, often with a hyperpigmented border; they vary in size and shape. Preferred sites are the face, particularly around the eyes or mouth (Fig. 24–15), the genitalia, hands and feet, elbows, knees, and upper chest. When the scalp or brow is affected, the hair may also lose its pigment.

Although no clear-cut pattern of genetic transmission has been established, vitiligo is known to occur with increased frequency in some families. It is also more prevalent in patients with hyperthyroidism, adrenal insufficiency, pernicious anemia, and diabetes mellitus; some patients have detectable circulating antibodies to thyroid, adrenal, and other tissues.

The cause is unknown, but trauma appears to play a role in induction of the lesions. An autoimmune mechanism has

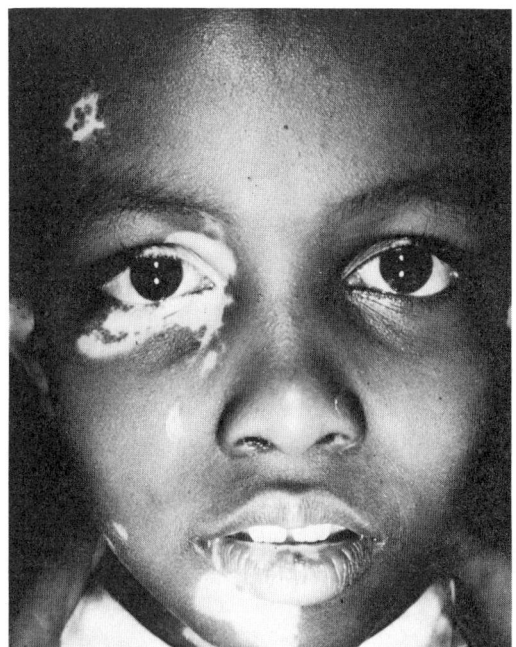

Figure 24–15. Multiple, sharply demarcated, depigmented areas of vitiligo.

been suggested; however, direct evidence to support it is lacking. Melanocytes are absent from involved sites and repopulate the epidermis from the hair follicle epithelium when repigmentation occurs. Although the diagnosis is usually made clinically, the disappearance of melanocytes can be confirmed by DOPA stains or electron microscopy of specimens obtained from depigmented skin. The course of vitiligo is variable; some lesions may remit spontaneously while others are developing, but relentlessly progressive depigmentation may occur. Treatment is difficult and usually involves administration of oral or topical psoralen compounds (8-methoxypsoralen or trioxsalen [Trisoralen]) in conjunction with exposure to sunlight or an ultraviolet light (UVA) source several times weekly. Repigmentation may be partial or complete, but many months of therapy may be required and should be carefully monitored by physicians experienced in the use of photosensitizing drugs. Small lesions may be camouflaged by application of a specially prepared makeup (Covermark). Because of the absence of melanin, vitiliginous skin will burn readily on sun exposure and should be protected at all times by the use of an appropriate sunscreen agent.

24.12 VESICOBULLOUS DISORDERS

Many diseases are characterized by vesicobullous lesions; they vary considerably in etiology, in age of occurrence, and in the pattern of the lesion. Some of them (e.g., varicella) are discussed in other chapters; some are described in other sections of this chapter since the vesicobullous lesions represent only a transient stage of the disease (e.g., incontinentia pigmenti and mastocytosis). The morphology of the blister often provides a visual clue to the location of the lesion within the skin. Blisters localized to the epidermal layers are thin-walled and relatively flaccid and tend to rupture easily. Subepidermal blisters are tense, thick-walled, and more durable. Biopsies of blisters can be diagnostic since the level of cleavage within the skin is constant and characteristic for a particular disorder. Blister cleavage sites are depicted schematically in Fig. 24–16.

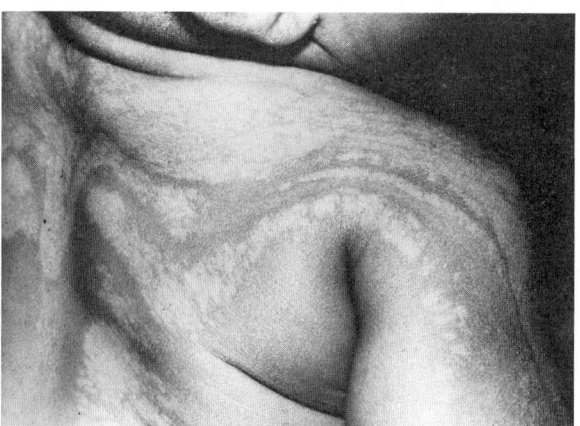

Figure 24–14. Marbled hypopigmented streaks of hypomelanosis of Ito (incontinentia pigmenti achromians).

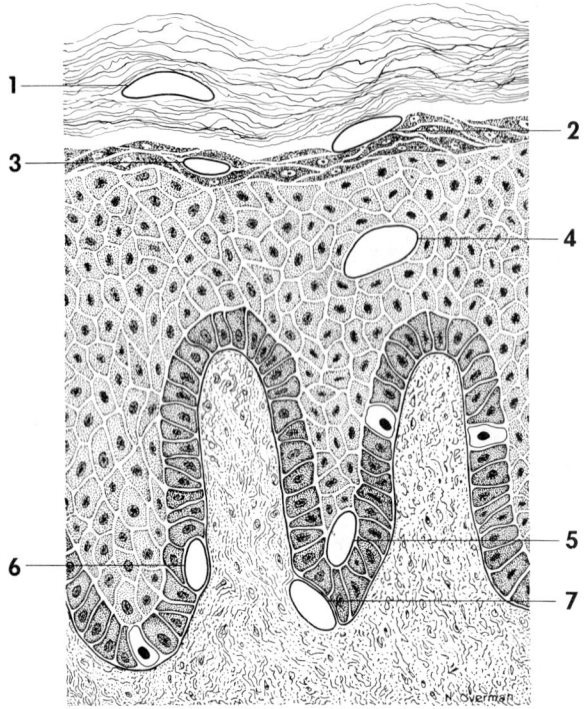

Figure 24–16. Blister cleavage sites in the skin: (1) intracorneal, (2) subcorneal, (3) granular layer, (4) intraepidermal, (5) suprabasal, (6) junctional (between basal cell membrane and basement membrane), and (7) subepidermal.

The freshest intact blister should be selected for biopsy since partial healing may obscure the true cleavage plane. The differential diagnosis of the disease process can often be narrowed by histologic examination in consideration with other diagnostic procedures (Table 24–1).

Erythema multiforme is an acute, sometimes recurrent, inflammatory disease of the skin and mucous membranes. It occurs at any age, but it is more common during childhood and more frequent in males than in females. The pathogenesis is unknown, but the disorder is generally regarded as a hypersensitivity reaction triggered by drugs, infections, and exposure to toxic substances. The causes of erythema multiforme are legion. Infectious agents include herpesvirus, *Mycoplasma pneumoniae*, coxsackievirus, echovirus, and influenza viruses, mumps virus, histoplasma, *Coccidioides immitis*, *S. typhi*, *M. tuberculosis*, *C. diphtheriae*, and hemolytic streptococci. Drugs include penicillins, tetracyclines, sulfonamides, hydantoins, barbiturates, phenylbutazone, phenolphthalein, chlorpropamide, and aspirin. Miscellaneous causes include collagen diseases, malignancies, vaccines (polio, BCG, vaccinia), radiation therapy, plant allergens, and 9-bromofluorine. There are several forms of the disease. In *erythema multiforme simplex*, the most common type, the diverse morphology of the skin lesions is the prominent manifestation. In *bullous erythema multiforme*, the mouth is often affected and the skin lesions are characteristically bullous. The *Stevens-Johnson syndrome* is a serious systemic disorder in which at least two mucous membranes as well as skin are involved (Sec. 10.78).

The cutaneous lesions of erythema multiforme are usually symmetrical, appear in crops, and show a predilection for the extensor surfaces of the hands, arms, feet, legs, palms, and soles. The eruption varies considerably in extent and severity and may involve the entire body except the scalp. Lesions may be macular, papular, nodular, or urticarial. Vesicobullous lesions arise centrally within pre-existent lesions; urticarial lesions may fuse to form annular polycyclic plaques of bizarre outline. Intradermal hemorrhage is common and may be florid

or may consist only of petechiae. Iris or target lesions, pathognomonic for erythema multiforme, are formed by urticarial lesions that have dusky centers and develop successively darker rings that may blister when the reaction is intense. Oral lesions occur in 25% of patients and consist of erythematous macules surmounted by vesicobullae that rapidly form painful necrotic ulcers, often with a pseudomembranous surface.

Skin lesions appear in crops for up to 3 wk and heal with hypo- or hyperpigmentation but without scarring. Pruritus is minimal to absent. The differential diagnosis includes bullous pemphigoid, pemphigus, urticaria, viral infections, Reiter disease, Behçet disease, allergic vasculitis, and periarteritis nodosa.

The diagnosis can usually be made from the clinical features, particularly when iris lesions are apparent. When the diagnosis is uncertain, a skin biopsy should be performed. The histologic changes vary with the severity of the lesions. There is intraepidermal edema with vesicular alteration in the epidermal basal layer and necrosis of individual epidermal cells. The dermis is edematous, with lymphocytic infiltration around the vessels and at the dermal-epidermal junction. When the changes are severe, red blood cells may be extravasated into the dermis, subepidermal bullae may form, and the epidermis may become necrotic. Eosinophils and neutrophils are sparse.

Treatment is local and symptomatic. Oral lesions should be cleaned with mouthwashes and glycerin swabs. Topical anesthetics (Benadryl, dyclonine, and viscous Xylocaine) may provide relief from pain, particularly when applied prior to eating. Denuded skin lesions can be cleansed with a Betadine-water solution. Patients with recurrent erythema multiforme may experience rapid relief following early systemic therapy with a corticosteroid or occasionally with a topical steroid preparation.

Toxic epidermal necrolysis (Lyell disease) appears to be a hypersensitivity phenomenon triggered by many of the same factors responsible for erythema multiforme: drugs, infections, vaccination, radiotherapy, and malignancies. It may represent the most devastating form of erythema multiforme; widespread epidermal necrosis rapidly follows blister formation at the dermal-epidermal junction.

The prodrome consists of fever, malaise, and localized skin tenderness and erythema. Flaccid bullae develop and full-thickness epidermis is lost in large sheets. Nikolsky sign (denudation of the skin with gentle pressure) is positive but only in the areas of blistering. Conjunctivitis and oral lesions are common and may mimic those of Stevens-Johnson syndrome. The course may be relentlessly progressive, complicated by severe dehydration, electrolyte imbalance, shock, and secondary localized infection and septicemia.

The differential diagnosis includes the staphylococcal scalded skin syndrome, in which the blister cleavage plane is intraepidermal; pemphigus; and the Stevens-Johnson syndrome. Appreciation of the specific etiologic factor is crucial, particularly when the disorder is drug-induced. Management is similar to that for severe burns: strict isolation, appropriately calculated fluid and electrolyte therapy, and daily cultures. Systemic antibiotic therapy is indicated when secondary infection is evident or suspected. Skin care consists of cleansing with isotonic saline or Betadine and applications of Silvadene. The case fatality rate is approximately 25%.

Epidermolysis Bullosa. The diseases categorized under this general term are a heterogeneous group of congenital, hereditary blistering disorders in which the lesions are induced by mechanical trauma and high environmental temperatures. They differ in severity and prognosis, clinical and histologic features, and inheritance patterns. The disorders can be categorized under three major headings: epidermolytic EB,

Table 24–1. **Sites of Blister Formation and Diagnostic Studies for the Vesicobullous Disorders**

Disorder	Blister Cleavage Site	Cutaneous Diagnostic Studies
Acrodermatitis enteropathica	IE	—
Bullous impetigo	GL	Smear, culture
Bullous pemphigoid	SE (junctional)	Direct and indirect immunofluorescence studies
Candidosis	SC	KOH preparation, culture
Chronic bullous dermatosis of childhood	SE	Direct immunofluorescence studies
Dermatitis herpetiformis	SE	Direct immunofluorescence studies
Dermatophytosis	IE	KOH preparation, culture
Dyshidrotic eczema	IE	—
Epidermolysis bullosa simplex	IE	—
hands and feet	IE	—
letalis	SE (junctional)	—
recessive dystrophic	SE	—
dominant dystrophic	SE	—
Epidermolytic hyperkeratosis	IE	—
Erythema multiforme	SE	—
Erythema toxicum	SC, IE	Smear for eosinophils
Incontinentia pigmenti	IE	Smear for eosinophils
Insect bites	IE	—
Mastocytosis	SE	Smear for mast cells
Miliaria crystallina	IC	—
Pachyonychia congenita	IC	—
Pemphigus foliaceus	GL	Direct and indirect immunofluorescence studies Tzanck smear
Pemphigus vulgaris	SB	Direct and indirect immunofluorescence studies Tzanck smear
Pseudomonas infection	IE, SE	Smear, culture
Scabies	IE	Scraping
Staphylococcal scalded skin syndrome	GL	Frozen section biopsy
Syphilis	SE	Darkfield preparation
Toxic epidermal necrolysis (Lyell)	SE	Frozen section biopsy
Transient neonatal pustular melanosis	SC, IE	Smear for cells
Viral blisters	IE	Tzanck smear for herpesvirus infections

GL, granular layer; IC, intracorneal; IE, intraepidermal; SB, suprabasal; SC, subcorneal; SE, subepidermal

junctional EB, and dermolytic EB. The pathogenesis is poorly understood in all types; some involve structural defects and others apparent enzymatic abnormalities. Since mechanical trauma and high environmental temperatures are provocative factors in all of the types, affected children should be protected to the extent warranted by the severity of their disease. Parents usually become quite knowledgeable about what their child will tolerate. Metal closures on clothing, tape of any kind, rough or tight clothing, and sharp-edged toys should be avoided. Hot baths may also initiate new lesions. Large blisters may be drained by puncturing, but the blister tops should be left intact to protect the underlying skin. Management must be individualized to permit maximum safe participation in childhood activities. Genetic counseling should be offered to families of affected children; therefore, early diagnosis of the type of the disease is critical.

Epidermolytic EB. Epidermolysis bullosa simplex is a nonscarring, autosomal dominant disorder. Blisters are usually present at birth or during the neonatal period. The bullae are intraepidermal and result from disintegration of the basal cells. These lesions may be mistaken for aplasia cutis. Sites of predilection are the hands, feet, elbows, knees, legs, and scalp; intraoral lesions are minimal, and nails may become dystrophic and may be shed but usually regrow. The infants are usually vigorous. Secondary infection is the only serious complication. The propensity to blister decreases with age, and the long-term prognosis is good.

Epidermolysis bullosa of hands and feet (Weber-Cockayne type) is also an autosomal dominant disorder. This nonscarring variant begins some time after the 1st yr of life. Bullae are usually restricted to the hands and feet, including the palms and soles; rarely, they occur elsewhere. The intraepidermal blisters involve the cells of the suprabasal and granular layers, which may be dyskeratotic with clumped tonofilaments. The disorder is only mildly incapacitating.

In a less common variant, *EB herpetiformis Dowling-Meara*, affected children are not heat-sensitive. Grouped blisters, intense inflammation and milia formation, later development of hyperkeratosis of palms and soles, and distinctive electron microscopic findings are characteristic.

Junctional EB. Epidermolysis bullosa letalis (Herlitz type), although basically a nonscarring condition, is life-threatening, and the complications are such that serious morbidity and disfigurement can be predicted. The infant is usually blistered at birth or develops lesions during the neonatal period, particularly on the perioral area, scalp, legs, diaper area, and thorax. Large, moist, erosive plaques may provide a portal of entry for bacteria, and septicemia is a frequent cause of death. Healing is delayed, and vegetating granulomas may persist for a long time. Mucous membrane lesions are mild. Defective dentition with early loss of teeth due to rampant caries is characteristic. In contrast to other variants of epidermolysis bullosa, sparing of the hands and feet is striking, with the exception of the distal digits and the nail plates; these are dystrophic or permanently lost. Growth retardation and recalcitrant anemia are almost invariable. A subepidermal blister is found on light microscopic examination, and electron microscopy demonstrates a cleavage plane between the plasma membranes of the basal cells and the basement membrane. Hypoplasia or absence of hemidesmosomes in the basal cell layer as seen on electron microscopy is diagnostic.

Therapy is supportive; an adequate caloric diet and iron

should be provided. Infections should be treated promptly with antibiotics. Transfusions of packed red blood cells may be required at times as supplementary therapy. In addition to infection, cachexia and circulatory failure are common causes of death. This disorder is an autosomal recessive disease; genetic counseling should be offered to the family.

Generalized atrophic benign EB, a milder autosomal recessive variant, is also nonscarring and is characterized by identical histologic changes. The course is compatible with normal growth and life span.

Dermolytic EB. *Dominant dystrophic epidermolysis bullosa* appears to occur sporadically in many instances, although an autosomal dominant mode of transmission has been documented in several generations of some families. Blisters may be present at birth and are often limited to the hands, feet, and sacrum. The lesions heal promptly with the formation of soft, wrinkled scars, milia, and alterations in pigmentation. The general health is unimpaired, and in many instances the blistering process is rather mild, causing little restriction of activity and unimpaired growth and development. Mucous membrane involvement tends to be minimal, but nail loss is common. The *Cockayne-Touraine* variant of dominant dystrophic EB is milder than the *Pasini* form, in which blistering is more widespread and flesh-colored papules called albopapuloid lesions develop on the trunk at adolescence. The blister is subepidermal in both variants, with separation beneath the basement membrane. On electron microscopy anchoring fibrils are abnormal and decreased in number over the entire skin in the Pasini type but only in areas of blister predilection in the Cockayne-Touraine variant.

Recessive dystrophic epidermolysis bullosa is probably the most incapacitating form of the disorder. Extensive erosions and blister formation may occur at birth and seriously impede the care and feeding of the infant. Mucous membrane lesions are common and may cause severe nutritional deprivation, even in older children, whose growth may be retarded. During

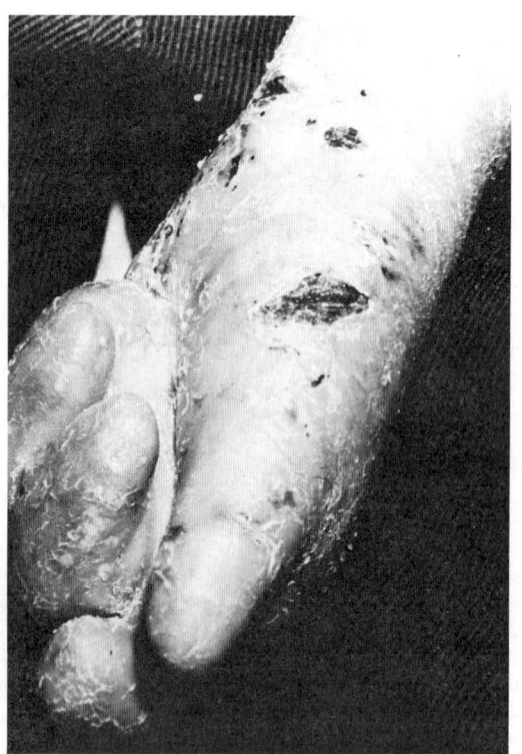

Figure 24–17. Mitten-hand deformity of recessive dystrophic epidermolysis bullosa.

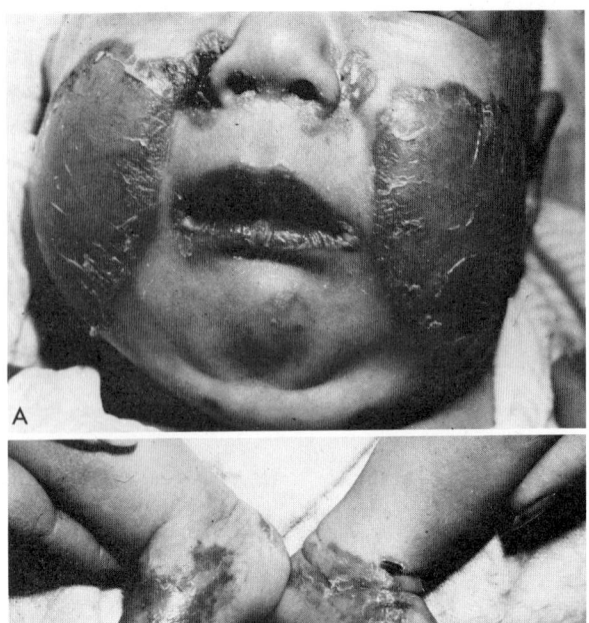

Figure 24–18. *A,* Psoriasiform facial lesions of acrodermatitis enteropathica. *B,* Similar lesions on the feet with secondary nail dystrophy.

childhood, esophageal erosions and strictures, scarring of the buccal mucosa, flexion contractures of joints secondary to scarring of the integument, and the development of the characteristic mitten deformity of the hands and feet due to digital fusion (Fig. 24–17) significantly limit the quality of life. The subepidermal bullae are located beneath the basement membrane, and absence of anchoring fibrils can be confirmed by electron microscopy. Excessive amounts of an aberrant collagenase are produced by dermal fibroblasts.

Although the skin becomes less sensitive to trauma with aging, the progressive and permanent deformities complicate management tremendously, and the overall prognosis is poor. If esophageal scarring develops, a semi-liquid diet and esophageal dilatations may be required. In infants, severe oropharyngeal involvement may necessitate the use of special feeding devices. Continuous iron therapy for anemia, intermittent antibiotic therapy for secondary infections, and periodic plastic procedures for release of digits may reduce morbidity.

Acrodermatitis enteropathica is a rare, autosomal recessive disorder of zinc deficiency that appears to be somewhat more common in girls. The onset is insidious, occurring usually during the 1st yr of life. Initial symptoms often are noted following weaning from breast milk to cow's milk. The cutaneous eruption consists of vesicobullous and eczematous skin lesions symmetrically distributed in the perioral, acral, and perineal areas as well as on the cheeks, knees, and elbows. Initially these lesions are intensely erythematous and erosive, but with chronicity they become dry, hyperkeratotic, and psoriasiform in appearance (Fig. 24–18A and B). The hair often has a peculiar reddish tint, and alopecia of some degree is characteristic. Ocular manifestations include photophobia, conjunctivitis, blepharitis, and corneal dystrophy, which is detectable by slit-lamp examination. Associated manifestations include chronic diarrhea, stomatitis, glossitis, paronychia, nail dystrophy, growth retardation, personality changes, intercurrent bacterial infections, and superinfection with *Can-*

dida albicans. The course without treatment is chronic and intermittent but often relentlessly progressive, terminating in severe marasmus and death. When the disease is less severe, only growth retardation and delayed development may be apparent.

The diagnosis is established by the constellation of clinical findings and low concentrations of plasma zinc and of alkaline phosphatase, a zinc-dependent enzyme. Histopathologic changes in the skin and gastrointestinal tract are nonspecific, except that a cytoplasmic inclusion body has been noted in the Paneth cells. The basic metabolic defect in the disease appears to relate to intestinal absorption of zinc. A possible deficiency in amount or function of a zinc-binding ligand has been suggested as a pathogenetic factor.

For many years, acrodermatitis enteropathica was treated empirically, but often successfully, with diiodohydroxyquin and breast milk; however, the possibility of serious untoward effects of the drug, particularly optic atrophy, was a hazard. Oral therapy with zinc compounds has replaced diiodohydroxyquin as the treatment of choice. Optimal doses range from 50 mg of zinc sulfate, acetate, or gluconate daily for infants up to 150 mg daily for children; plasma zinc levels should be monitored, however, to individualize the dosage. Zinc therapy rapidly abolishes the manifestations of the disease. A few patients with acrodermatitis enteropathica without hypozincemia have recovered when given pharmacologic doses of zinc. A syndrome resembling acrodermatitis enteropathica has been observed in patients of all ages receiving total parenteral nutrition without supplemental zinc.

Pemphigus occurs during childhood as pemphigus vulgaris or as pemphigus foliaceus.

Pemphigus vulgaris usually first appears as painful oral ulcers, which may be the only evidence of the disease for weeks or months. Subsequently, large, flaccid bullae emerge on nonerythematous skin, most commonly on the head and trunk. The lesions rupture and enlarge peripherally, producing painful, raw, denuded areas that have little tendency to heal. Malodorous verrucous and granulomatous lesions may develop at sites of ruptured bullae. Nikolsky sign (avulsion of epidermis on gentle pressure) is always present.

Histologically, the lesion is a suprabasal (intraepidermal) blister containing loose, acantholytic epidermal cells. IgG antibody to epidermal intercellular substance produces a characteristic pattern on direct immunofluorescent preparations. Serum antibody titers to the epidermal intercellular substance usually correlate with the clinical course; hence serial determinations may have predictive value.

The disease can be confused with erythema multiforme, bullous pemphigoid, Stevens-Johnson syndrome, and toxic epidermal necrolysis. Since the course may rapidly lead to debility, malnutrition, and death, prompt diagnosis is essential. The disease is best controlled initially with systemic corticosteroid therapy. Azathioprine, cyclophosphamide, and gold therapy have all been useful in maintenance regimens.

Pemphigus foliaceus is also characterized by intraepidermal blisters; the site of cleavage, however, is high in the epidermis rather than suprabasal. The blisters are very superficial, rupture quickly, and may be missed on examination. Crusting and scaling are typical manifestations. When generalized, the eruption may resemble exfoliative dermatitis or any of the chronic blistering disorders, but localized erythematous plaques simulate seborrheic dermatitis, psoriasis, impetigo, eczema, or lupus erythematosus. Focal lesions are usually localized to the scalp, face, neck, and upper trunk. Mucous membrane lesions are minimal or absent. Pruritus, pain, and a burning sensation are frequent complaints.

An intraepidermal acantholytic bulla high in the epidermis is diagnostic; it is imperative, however, to select an early lesion for biopsy. Tissue-bound and circulating intercellular

epidermal antibodies may be found. The course varies but is generally more benign than that of pemphigus vulgaris. Long-term remission is usual following suppression of the disease by systemic corticosteroid therapy. A topical corticosteroid preparation is occasionally sufficient.

Bullous pemphigoid rarely occurs in children, but it must be considered in the differential diagnosis of any chronic blistering disorder. Typically the blisters arise in crops on a normal, erythematous, or urticarial base. Individual lesions, varying greatly in size, are tense and filled with serous fluid, which may become hemorrhagic or turbid; oral lesions are common. Pruritus and a burning sensation may accompany the eruption, but constitutional symptoms are not prominent.

A subepidermal bulla can be identified by histologic examination. In sections of a blister or paralesional skin, a band of immunoglobulin (usually IgG) and C3 can be demonstrated in the basement membrane zone by means of immunofluorescent preparations. Indirect immunofluorescent studies of serum are usually positive for IgG antibodies to the basement membrane zone; the titers, however, do not correlate well with the clinical course.

The differential diagnosis includes bullous erythema multiforme, pemphigus, linear IgA dermatosis, bullous drug eruption, dermatitis herpetiformis, and bullous impetigo, which can be differentiated by histologic examination, immunofluorescent studies, and cultures. The cause of bullous pemphigoid is unknown, and the course is chronic and intermittent. Nevertheless, the disease can be successfully suppressed with systemic corticosteroid therapy alone or in combination with azathioprine, and ultimately it usually remits permanently. Local skin care consists of compresses and a drying lotion.

Dermatitis herpetiformis is characterized by grouped, small, tense, erythematous, pruritic papules and vesicles. The eruption tends to be symmetrically distributed; the sites of predilection are the knees, elbows, shoulders, buttocks, and scalp; mucous membranes are usually spared. When pruritus is severe, excoriations may be the only visible sign.

The cause is unknown; however, an association with gluten-sensitive enteropathy is found with some frequency (Sec. 12.49). Subepidermal blisters are found on skin biopsy, and IgA and C3 can be detected in the dermal papillae of paralesional skin by immunofluorescent studies. The frequent finding of immune complexes and autoimmune antibodies in serum, as well as the association with certain HLA types, suggests an immune mechanism.

Dermatitis herpetiformis may mimic other chronic blistering diseases and may also resemble scabies, papular urticaria, insect bites, contact dermatitis, and papular eczema. The most effective treatment is oral administration of sulfapyridine or dapsone. These drugs afford immediate relief from the intense pruritus, but must be used with caution because of possibly serious side effects. Local antipruritic measures may also be useful. The enteropathy will respond to a gluten-free diet more rapidly than the skin lesions will.

Linear IgA dermatosis (chronic bullous dermatosis of childhood) is more common in the 1st decade of life, with a peak incidence during the preschool years. The eruption consists of multiple large, tense bullae filled with clear or hemorrhagic fluid that emerge from a normal or erythematous base. Areas of predilection are the trunk, genitalia, and legs, as well as the face, scalp, and dorsum of the feet. In the smaller lesions sausage-shaped bullae may be arranged in an annular or rosette-like fashion around a central crust (Fig. 24-19). Erythematous plaques with gyrate margins bordered by intact bullae may develop over larger areas. Pruritus may be absent or very intense.

The cause of the eruption is unknown. Histologic examination discloses a subepidermal bulla infiltrated with a mix-

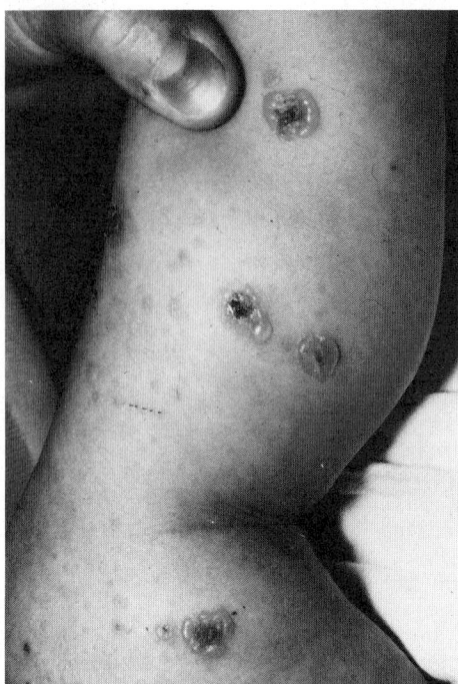

Figure 24–19. Rosette-like blisters around a central crust typical of linear IgA dermatosis (chronic bullous dermatosis of childhood).

ture of inflammatory cells. Direct immunofluorescent studies demonstrate linear deposition of IgA and sometimes C3 at the dermal-epidermal junction. Indirect immunofluorescent studies are sometimes positive for circulating antibodies. These studies serve to differentiate this eruption from pemphigus, bullous pemphigoid, dermatitis herpetiformis, and erythema multiforme, with which it may be confused. Gram stain and culture will exclude the diagnosis of bullous impetigo. The lack of bullous formation in response to trauma differentiates epidermolysis bullosa.

Many patients respond favorably to oral sulfapyridine or dapsone. During therapy with sulfapyridine, attention should be paid to urinary output and alkalinization of the urine to avoid crystal formation within the renal parenchyma. Hematologic and biochemical studies must be obtained at regular intervals during treatment with either drug to avoid serious side effects. Children who do not respond to either of these drugs may benefit from oral therapy with a corticosteroid or a combination of these drugs. The usual course is 2–4 yr; there are no long-term sequelae.

Infantile acropustulosis has its onset between 2 and 10 mo of age; occasionally lesions are noted at birth. Black males have a predisposition for this eruption, but infants of both sexes and all races may be affected. The cause is unknown.

The lesions are initially discrete, 1–2 mm erythematous papules that become vesiculopustular within 24 hr and subsequently crust prior to healing. They are intensely pruritic, and a fresh outbreak is usually accompanied by extreme fretfulness. Preferred sites are the palms and soles, where the lesions may develop in profusion. A less dense eruption may be found on the dorsum of the hands and feet, the ankles, and the wrists. Each episode lasts for 7–10 days, during which time pustules continue to appear in crops. After a 2–3 wk remission, a new outbreak follows. This cyclical pattern continues for about 2 yr; permanent resolution is often preceded by longer intervals of remission between periods of activity. Infants with acropustulosis are otherwise well, and there are no constitutional findings.

The white blood count and differential are normal. Wright-stained smears of intralesional contents show masses of neu-

trophils or, occasionally, a predominance of eosinophils. Cultures for all types of organisms are negative. Histologically the pustules are well circumscribed, subcorneal in location, and filled with polymorphonuclear leukocytes, with or without eosinophils.

The differential diagnosis in the neonate includes transient neonatal pustular melanosis, erythema toxicum, cutaneous candidosis and staphylococcal pustulosis. In the older infant and toddler additional diagnostic considerations include scabies, dyshidrotic eczema, pustular psoriasis, subcorneal pustular dermatosis, and hand, foot, and mouth disease.

Therapy is directed at minimizing discomfort; however, infantile acropustulosis is relatively unresponsive to topical corticosteroid preparations or oral antihistamines. Dapsone has been used effectively orally but has potentially serious side effects and should be used only with great caution.

24.13 ECZEMA

Eczema is a generic term used to designate a particular type of reaction pattern in the skin. Acute eczematous lesions are characterized by erythema, weeping, oozing, and the formation of microvesicles within the epidermis. Chronic lesions are generally thickened, dry, and scaly with coarse skin markings (lichenification) and altered pigmentation. Many types of eczema occur in children, of which the most common is atopic dermatitis (Sec. 10.49); however, seborrheic dermatitis, allergic and irritant contact dermatitis, nummular eczema, and dyshidrosis are also relatively common childhood eczemas. Pyoderma may become eczematized from scratching as may insect bites, papular urticaria, dermatophytosis, and a variety of dermatoses. Once the diagnosis of eczema has been established, it is important to classify the eruption more specifically for proper management. Pertinent historical data will often provide the clue. In some instances the subsequent course and character of the eruption permit classification. Histologic changes are relatively nonspecific, but all types of eczematous dermatitis are characterized by intraepidermal edema known as spongiosis.

Contact dermatitis can be subdivided into irritant dermatitis, resulting from nonspecific injury to the skin, and allergic contact dermatitis, in which the mechanism is a delayed hypersensitivity reaction. Of the two, irritant dermatitis is more frequent in children, particularly during the early years of life.

Irritant contact dermatitis can result from prolonged or repetitive contact with a variety of substances that include saliva, citrus juices, bubble bath, detergents, abrasive materials, strong soaps, and proprietary medications. Saliva is probably one of the most common offenders; it may cause dermatitis on the face and in the neck folds of the drooling infant or retarded child. The older child who habitually licks his lips because of dryness may develop a striking, sharply demarcated perioral rash (Fig. 24–20A). Among the exogenous irritants, citrus juices, proprietary medications, and bubble bath preparations are relatively common; bubble bath dermatitis is a cause of severe pruritus. Excessive accumulation of sweat and moisture as a result of wearing occlusive shoes may also be responsible for irritant dermatitis.

Clinically, irritant contact dermatitis may be indistinguishable from atopic dermatitis or allergic contact dermatitis. A detailed history and consideration of the sites of involvement, age of the child, and contactants will usually provide clues to the etiology. The propensity to develop irritant dermatitis varies considerably among children, and some may respond to minimal injury in this fashion. In general, all irritant contact dermatitis will clear after removal of the stimulus and temporary treatment with a topical corticosteroid preparation.

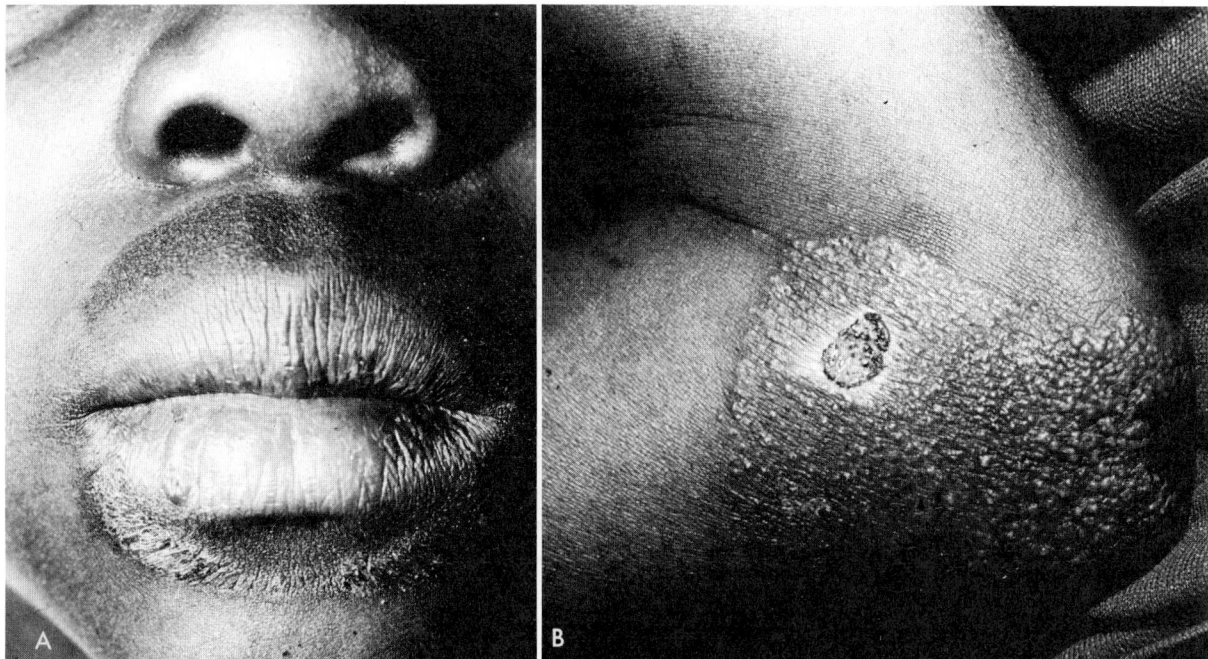

Figure 24–20. *A,* Perioral irritant contact dermatitis from lip-licking. *B,* Allergic contact dermatitis to Merthiolate spray. Note the sharp angular border of vesicular eruption.

Education of patient and parents as to the causes of contact dermatitis is crucial to successful therapy.

Diaper dermatitis can be regarded as the prototype of irritant contact dermatitis. As a reaction to friction, maceration, and prolonged contact with urine and feces, retained soaps, and topical preparations, the skin of the diaper area may become erythematous and scaly, often with papulovesicular or bullous lesions, fissures, and erosions. The eruption can be patchy or confluent, but the genitocrural folds are often spared. Chronic hypertrophic, flat-topped papules and infiltrative nodules may simulate syphilitic lesions. Secondary infection with bacteria and yeasts is common; discomfort may be marked because of intense inflammation. Such conditions as allergic contact dermatitis, seborrheic dermatitis, candidosis, atopic dermatitis, and rare disorders such as histiocytosis X and acrodermatitis enteropathica should be considered when the eruption is persistent or recalcitrant to simple therapeutic measures.

Diaper dermatitis will often respond to simple measures; however, some infants seem predisposed to diaper dermatitis, and management may prove difficult. The damaging effects of prolonged contact with feces and ammoniacal urine can be obviated by frequent changing of diapers and meticulous washing of the genitalia with warm water and mild soap. Occlusive plastic pants which accentuate maceration should not be used; disposable diapers are a practical substitute. Frequent applications of a bland protective topical agent (petrolatum or zinc oxide paste) following thorough gentle cleansing may suffice to prevent dermatitis.

When the above measures are not sufficient to promote healing, a light application of 0.5–1% topical hydrocortisone ointment after each diaper change for a limited time is often effective. Prior to initiation of such therapy the possibility of candidal infection should be excluded by a KOH preparation or culture. For infants requiring additional protection, zinc oxide paste can be applied after the steroid as a thick covering. Secondary complications can result from prolonged use of corticosteroids, especially fluorinated compounds.

Juvenile plantar dermatosis is a common form of irritant contact dermatitis occurring mainly in prepubertal children. The dermatitis characteristically involves the weight-bearing surfaces, is painful rather than pruritic, and causes a glazed appearance of the plantar skin. Fissuring may become extensive, producing considerable discomfort. The dermatitis results from alternating excessive hydration and rapid moisture loss, which causes chapping of the skin and cracking of the stratum corneum. Affected children often have hyperhidrosis, wear occlusive synthetic footwear, and subject their feet to rapid drying without moisturization. Immediate application of a thick emollient when socks and shoes are removed will usually prevent this condition.

Allergic contact dermatitis is a T cell–mediated hypersensitivity reaction that is provoked by application of an antigen to the skin surface. The antigen penetrates the skin, where it is conjugated with a cutaneous protein, and the hapten-protein complex is transported to the regional lymph nodes. A primary immunologic response occurs locally in the nodes and becomes generalized, presumably because of dissemination of sensitized T cells. Sensitization requires several days and, when followed by a fresh antigenic challenge, becomes manifest as allergic contact dermatitis. Generalized distribution may occur if enough antigen finds its way into the circulation. Once sensitization has occurred, each new antigenic challenge may provoke an inflammatory reaction within 8–12 hr; sensitization to a particular antigen usually persists for many years.

Acute allergic contact dermatitis is an erythematous, intensely pruritic, eczematous dermatitis, which, if severe, may be edematous and vesicobullous. Chronic contact dermatitis has the features of a longstanding eczema: lichenification, scaling, fissuring, and pigmentary change. The distribution of the eruption often provides a clue to the diagnosis. Volatile sensitizers usually affect exposed areas such as face and arms. Jewelry, topical agents, shoes, clothing, and plants cause dermatitis at points of contact.

Rhus dermatitis (poison ivy or poison oak) is often vesicobullous and may be distinguished by linear streaks of vesicles where the plant leaves have brushed against the skin. Contrary to popular opinion, fluid from ruptured vesicles does not spread the eruption; however, antigen retained on the skin, under the fingernails, and on clothing will initiate new plaques of dermatitis if not removed by washing. Antigen may also be carried by animals on their fur.

Nickel dermatitis usually develops from contact with jewelry or metal closures on clothing and is seen most frequently on the ear lobes, e.g., when nickel-containing posts rather than nonmetallic materials or stainless steel are used to keep a pierced tract open. Some children are exquisitely sensitive to nickel, with even the traces found in gold jewelry provoking eruptions.

Shoe dermatitis typically affects the dorsum of the feet and toes, sparing the interdigital spaces; it is usually symmetric. Allergic contact dermatitis, in contrast to irritant dermatitis, rarely involves the palms and soles. Common allergens are the antioxidants and accelerators in shoe rubber and the chromium salts in tanned leather or shoe dyes. These substances are often leached out by excessive sweating.

Wearing apparel contains a number of sensitizers, including dyes, mordants, fabric finishers, fibers, resins, and cleaning solutions. Dye may be poorly fixed to clothing and leached out with sweating, as are the partially cured formaldehyde resins. The elastic in garments is also a frequent cause of clothing dermatitis.

Topical medications and cosmetics may be unsuspected as allergens, particularly if the medication is being used for a pre-existing dermatitis. The most common offenders are neomycin, Merthiolate (Fig. 24–20B), topical antihistamines (e.g., Caladryl), anesthetics (e.g., Nupercaine and Surfacaine), preservatives (e.g., parabens), and ethylenediamine, a stabilizer present in many medications (e.g., Mycolog cream). All types of cosmetics can cause facial dermatitis; involvement of the eyelids is characteristic for nail polish sensitivity.

Contact dermatitis can be confused with other types of eczema, dermatophytosis, and vesicobullous diseases. Patch testing may clarify the situation but should be performed only by an experienced person. The essential principle in treatment is elimination of contact with the allergen. Acute dermatitis responds to cool compresses and a corticosteroid agent applied several times daily. Chronic dermatitis often requires a more potent fluorinated steroid ointment with protective covering at night. An antihistamine may be used orally for its sedative effect. Massive acute bullous reactions such as those of poison ivy are best treated by a short course of oral corticosteroid therapy. If secondary infection has occurred, appropriate systemic antibiotic therapy should be given. Desensitization therapy is rarely indicated.

Nummular eczema is unusual in children and unrelated to other types of eczema. The eczematous plaques are more or less coin-shaped. Common sites are the extensor surfaces of the extremities (Fig. 24–21), the buttocks, and the shoulders. The plaques are relatively discrete, boggy, vesicular, severely pruritic, and exudative; when chronic, they often become thickened and lichenified. The cause is unknown. Most frequently, these lesions are mistaken for tinea corporis, but plaques of nummular eczema are distinguished by the lack of a raised, sharply circumscribed border, and they often weep or bleed when scraped. A KOH study can be helpful in differentiation. Secondary infection is common. Control of pruritus is usually achieved with a fluorinated corticosteroid preparation with or without occlusion with a polyethylene wrap. Sedation with an antihistamine is helpful, particularly at night. Antibiotics are indicated for secondary infection.

Pityriasis alba occurs mainly in children; the lesions are hypopigmented, round or oval, macular or slightly elevated patches with fine adherent scales (Fig. 24–22, p. xxviii). They

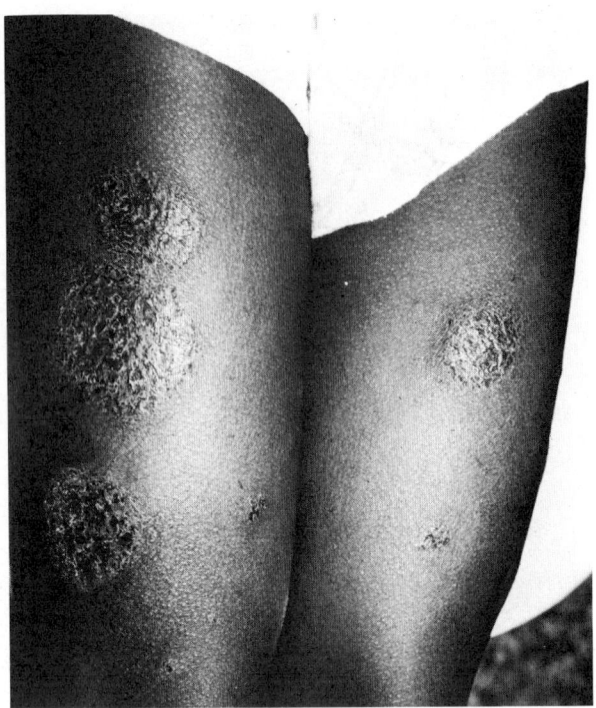

Figure 24–21. Multiple hyperpigmented scaly plaques of nummular eczema.

may be mildly erythematous and relatively well defined, but lack a sharply marginated border. Lesions occur on the face, neck, upper trunk, and proximal arms. Itching is minimal or absent.

The etiology is unknown, but the eruption appears to be exacerbated by dryness and is often regarded as a mild form of eczema. Pityriasis alba is frequently misdiagnosed as tinea versicolor or tinea corporis, each of which can be readily excluded by performing a KOH examination of surface scales. The lesions wax and wane but eventually disappear. Application of a lubricant may ameliorate the condition; if pruritus is troublesome, a topical 1% hydrocortisone preparation applied 3–4 times daily may be more effective. Normal pigmentation returns in weeks to months.

Lichen simplex chronicus is characterized by a chronic pruritic, eczematous, circumscribed, solitary plaque that is usually lichenified and hyperpigmented. The most common sites are the posterior neck, dorsum of the feet, wrists, and ankles. Trauma from rubbing and scratching accounts for persistence of the plaque, although the initiating event may be a transient lesion such as an insect bite. Pruritus must be controlled to permit healing. A topical fluorinated corticosteroid preparation is often helpful, but constant irritation to the skin must be avoided. A covering to prevent scratching may be necessary.

Dyshidrotic eczema (dyshidrosis, pompholyx) is a recurrent, sometimes seasonal, blistering disorder of the hands and feet; it occurs in all age groups but is uncommon in infancy. The pathogenesis is not known; there does not appear to be a genetic factor, although an increased incidence of atopy has been recorded in patients and their relatives.

The disease is characterized by recurrent crops of intensely pruritic, small vesicles on the hands and feet. Sites of predilection are the palms, soles, and lateral aspects of the fingers and toes. Primary lesions are noninflammatory and filled with clear fluid, which, unlike sweat, has a physiologic pH and contains protein. Larger vesicobullae may occur, and maceration and secondary infection are frequent because of scratching (Fig. 24–23). The chronic phase is characterized by

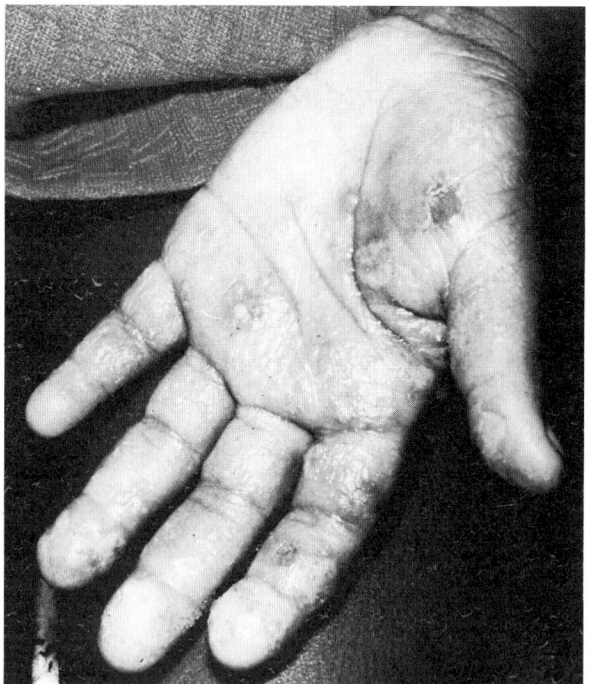

Figure 24–23. Vesicular palmar lesions of dyshidrotic eczema that have become secondarily infected.

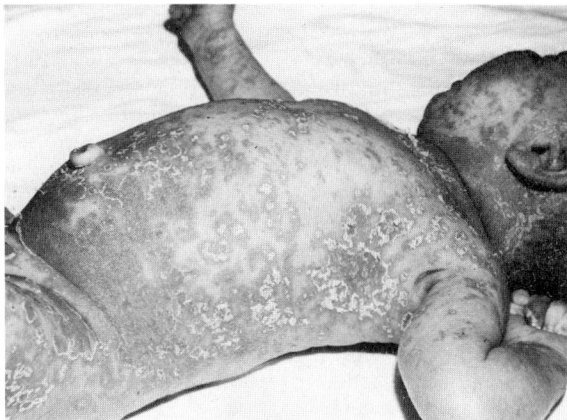

Figure 24–24. Widespread seborrheic dermatitis in an infant.

thickened, fissured plaques that may cause considerable discomfort. Hyperhidrosis is common in many patients, but the association may be fortuitous.

The diagnosis is made clinically. The disorder may be confused with allergic contact dermatitis, which usually affects the dorsal rather than the volar surfaces, and with dermatophytosis, which can be distinguished by a KOH preparation of the roof of a vesicle and by appropriate cultures.

Dyshidrotic eczema responds to wet dressings, followed by a topical corticosteroid preparation during the acute phase. Control of the chronic stage is difficult; lubricants containing mild keratolytic agents in conjunction with a potent topical fluorinated corticosteroid preparation and occlusion with a polyethylene wrap may be indicated. Secondary bacterial infection should be treated systemically with an appropriate antibiotic. Patients should be told to expect recurrence and should protect their hands and feet from the damaging effects of excessive sweating, chemicals, harsh soaps, and adverse weather.

Seborrheic dermatitis is a chronic inflammatory disease that occurs at all ages; in the pediatric age group it is most common during infancy and adolescence. The cause is unknown, as is the role of the sebaceous gland.

The disorder may begin within the 1st mo of life and be most troublesome during the 1st yr. Diffuse or focal scaling and crusting of the scalp, sometimes called *cradle cap,* may be the initial and at times the only manifestation. A dry, scaly, erythematous papular dermatitis, which is usually nonpruritic, may involve the face, neck, retroauricular areas, axillae, and diaper area. The dermatitis may be patchy and focal or may spread to involve almost the entire body (Fig. 24–24). Postinflammatory pigmentary changes are common, particularly in black infants. When the scaling becomes pronounced, the condition may resemble psoriasis and at times can be distinguished only with difficulty. The possibility of coexistent atopic dermatitis must be considered when there is an acute weeping dermatitis with pruritus. An intractable seborrhea-like dermatitis (*Leiner disease*) may reflect a functional disorder of complement. A seborrhea-like pattern may also result from cutaneous histiocytic infiltrates in infants with histiocytosis X.

During childhood and adolescence, seborrheic dermatitis is more localized and may be confined to the scalp and intertriginous areas. There may also be marginal blepharitis and involvement of the external auditory canal. Scalp changes may vary from diffuse, branny scaling to focal areas of thick, yellow crusts with underlying erythema. Loss of hair is not uncommon, and pruritus may be absent to marked. When the dermatitis is severe, erythema and scaling may occur at the frontal hairline, at the medial aspects of the eyebrows, and in the nasolabial and retroauricular folds. Red, scaly plaques may appear in the axillae, inguinal region, gluteal cleft, and umbilicus. On the extremities seborrheic plaques may be more eczematous and less erythematous and demarcated.

Seborrheic dermatitis is a condition that is reactivated in some patients by stressful situations, poor hygiene, and excessive perspiration. The differential diagnosis includes psoriasis, atopic dermatitis, dermatophytosis, and candidosis. Secondary bacterial infections and superimposed candidosis are not uncommon.

Scalp lesions should be controlled with an antiseborrheic shampoo, used daily if necessary. Inflamed lesions will usually respond promptly to topical corticosteroid therapy given 2–4 times daily. A 3% sulfur ointment in a washable base is an alternative means of therapy. Wet compresses should be applied to the moist or fissured lesions prior to application of the steroid ointment. Many patients require the continued use of an antiseborrheic shampoo for control. Response to therapy is usually rapid unless there are complicating factors or the diagnosis is in error.

24.14 PHOTOSENSITIVITY

Photosensitivity denotes a qualitatively or quantitatively abnormal cutaneous reaction to sunlight or, less commonly, to artificial light. The adverse effects of sunlight are due principally to wavelengths of light ranging from 250 to 800 nm, a range that includes both ultraviolet and visible light. Host factors play an important role, particularly natural skin pigmentation, since melanin serves to reflect, absorb, and scatter light.

Acute sunburn reaction is the most common light-induced effect seen in children; it is caused mainly by rays in the 290–320 nm band. Erythema appears 6–12 hr after initial exposure and reaches a peak in 24 hr when intense redness, exquisite tenderness, pain, edema, and blistering may occur. Additional effects of sun exposure include increase in thickness of the stratum corneum and increased formation and melanization of melanosomes, resulting in deepening of the skin color (tanning). Acute severe sunburn should be managed with cool tap water compresses and shake lotions and, if necessary, a mild oral analgesic. Topical corticosteroids, judiciously chosen, may diminish inflammation and pain. Proprietary preparations containing topical anesthetics are relatively ineffective and potentially hazardous because of their propensity to cause contact dermatitis. A bland emollient is effective in the desquamative phase.

Although the long-term sequelae of chronic and intense sun exposure are not often seen in children, pediatricians should advise patients regarding the harmful effects and irreversible skin damage that results from unduly prolonged sun exposure. Premature aging, senile elastosis, actinic keratoses, squamous and basal cell carcinomas, and probably melanomas all occur with greater frequency in sun-damaged skin. Adequate protection is readily provided by a wide variety of sunscreen agents.

Phototoxicity and Photoallergy. *Exogenous photosensitizers* in combination with a particular wavelength of light will cause dermatitis that can be classified as a phototoxic or a photoallergic reaction.

Phototoxic reactions occur in all individuals who accumulate adequate amounts of a photosensitizing drug or chemical within the skin. The eruption is confined to light-exposed areas and often resembles an exaggerated sunburn, but it may be urticarial or bullous, and it results in hyperpigmentation.

Photoallergic reactions, in contrast, occur only in a small percentage of persons exposed to photosensitizers and light and require a time interval for sensitization to take place. A photoallergic dermatitis is a T cell–mediated delayed hypersensitivity reaction in which the drug, acting as a hapten, combines with a skin protein to form the antigenic substance. Photoallergic reactions vary in morphology and may occur on partially covered as well as on light-exposed skin. Some of the important classes of drugs and chemicals responsible for photosensitivity reactions are listed in Table 24–2.

Although photodermatitis due to drugs or chemicals may be diagnosed by photopatch testing, facilities for this diagnostic procedure are not widely available. A high index of suspicion coupled with an appreciation of the distribution pattern of the eruption (sparing of eyelids, areas beneath the nose and chin, wrists, and antecubital fossae) and a history of application or ingestion of a known photosensitizing agent are all that is required to make a diagnosis. Discontinuation of the offending medication or avoidance of sun exposure, oral administration of an antihistamine, and application of a topical corticosteroid preparation to alleviate pruritus are appropriate therapeutic measures. Severe reactions may necessitate systemic corticosteroid therapy for a brief time.

The porphyrias are acquired or inborn abnormalities of specific enzymes in the heme biosynthetic pathway; they are quite diverse in their clinical manifestations (Sec. 7.55). Two in particular occur in children and have photosensitivity as a consistent feature. Signs and symptoms may be negligible during the winter, when sun exposure is minimal.

Congenital erythropoietic porphyria (Gunther) is a rare autosomal recessive disorder. Affected persons are exquisitely sensitive to light, which may induce repeated severe bullous eruptions that result in mutilating scars. Hyperpigmentation, hyperkeratosis, vesiculation, and fragility of skin in light-exposed areas are a consequence of permanent skin damage. Hirsutism, red urine, erythrodontia, hemolytic anemia, splenomegaly, and increased amounts of uroporphyrin I in urine, plasma, and erythrocytes and of coproporphyrin I in feces are additional characteristic manifestations.

Erythropoietic protoporphyria is inherited as an autosomal dominant trait; photosensitivity becomes apparent in early childhood and is manifested by pain, pruritus, and a sensation of burning within half an hour of sun exposure, followed by erythema, edema, urticaria, vesicles, and, rarely, bullae on

Table 24–2. Cutaneous Reactions to Sunlight

Sunburn
Photo-induced drug eruptions
   Systemic drugs include tetracyclines (Declomycin), psoralens, chlorothiazides, sulfonamides, barbiturates, griseofulvin, phenothiazines
   Topical agents include coal tar derivatives, furocoumarins (plants), psoralens, halogenated salicylanilides (soaps), perfume oils (e.g., oil of bergamot)
Genetic disorder with photosensitivity
   Xeroderma pigmentosum
   Bloom syndrome
   Cockayne syndrome
   Rothmund-Thomson syndrome
Disorders involving immune mechanisms
   Lupus erythematosus
   Dermatomyositis
   Scleroderma
   Solar urticaria
   Polymorphous light eruptions (?)
   Hydroa estivale and vacciniforme (?)
Inborn errors of metabolism
   Porphyrias
   Hartnup disease
   Pellagra
Infectious diseases associated with photosensitivity
   Recurrent herpes simplex infection
   Lymphogranuloma venereum
   Viral exanthems (accentuated photodistribution)
Skin disease exacerbated or precipitated by light
   Lichen planus
   Darier disease
   Granuloma annulare
   Psoriasis
   Erythema multiforme
   Sarcoid
   Atopic dermatitis
Deficient protection due to lack of pigment
   Vitiligo
   Oculocutaneous albinism
   Partial albinism
   Phenylketonuria
   Chediak-Higashi syndrome

light-exposed areas. Nail changes consist of opacification of the nail plate, onycholysis, pain, and tenderness. Mild systemic symptoms of malaise, chills, and fever may accompany the acute skin reaction. Recurrent sun exposure produces a chronic eczematous dermatitis with thickened, lichenified skin, especially over the finger joints, and persistent violaceous erythema, ulcers, and pitted or vermicular atrophic scars on the face and rims of the ears. Protoporphyrin is elevated in the red blood cells, plasma, and feces.

The *porphyrias* may be confused with other diseases characterized by photosensitivity. Biopsies of lesions from patients with porphyria have shown deposits of an amorphous material histochemically identifiable as a lipomucopolysaccharide-protein complex in perivascular areas and the papillary dermis.

The wavelengths of light mainly responsible for eliciting cutaneous reactions in porphyria are in the region of 400 nm. Window glass, which transmits wavelengths greater than 320 nm, is not protective. Patients must avoid direct sunlight, wear protective clothing, and use a sunscreen agent that effectively blocks wavelengths in the region of 400 nm. The administration of β-carotene (Solatene) quenches the fluorescence of the porphyrin molecule by imparting a yellow color to the skin; it effectively reduces the photosensitivity in patients with protoporphyria.

Colloid milium is a rare childhood disorder that occurs on the face and dorsum of the hands as a profuse eruption of ivory to yellow, firm, tiny, grouped papules. Although the translucent quality of the lesions suggests vesiculation, no fluid is obtained by puncture. The eruption is asymptomatic and usually remits spontaneously after puberty.

Polymorphous light eruption includes a wide spectrum of cutaneous lesions clearly attributable to photosensitivity that have not been accounted for by ingestion of drugs, use of topical medications, or known systemic diseases (see Table 24–2). The pathogenesis is obscure, but immune mechanisms have been implicated. The skin manifestations include erythematous plaques, urticaria, vesicles, bullae, papules, and eczematous dermatitis and are usually limited to sun-exposed areas. For some unknown reason, incidence peaks in spring and early summer, prior to the time when ultraviolet radiation is at a maximum. The greatest difficulty lies with light in the sunburn spectrum (290–320 nm), although patients with solar urticaria may have difficulty with the entire spectrum of ultraviolet light. Testing for light sensitivity with a monochromator is usually positive.

Patients must be instructed to avoid prolonged exposure during peak hours of sunlight. Appropriately selected sunscreens can afford excellent protection (Sec. 24.33). Pruritus may be alleviated by oral administration of an antihistamine and by applications of a mild corticosteroid preparation.

Children who have lesions clinically indistinguishable from other polymorphous light eruptions but who do not have a positive response to photo-testing with ultraviolet light are said to have *summer prurigo*. They must be protected from sunlight by an appropriate sunscreen agent.

Hydroa vacciniforme and **hydroa aestivale** are characterized by a vesicobullous eruption on portions of the body exposed to sunlight; the pathogenesis is unknown. Peak incidence occurs during the spring and summer months, a feature that is responsible for the designation of the milder form of the disease, hydroa aestivale, in which scarring does not result. It is possible that this disorder is a subtype of polymorphous light eruption. Itching and burning precede the eruption of lesions, which occur in crops in a symmetrical arrangement over the nose, cheeks, ears, lips, dorsum of the hands, and forearms. Severe lesions of hydroa vacciniforme resemble the vesicles of smallpox; they become ulcerated and crusted and heal as deep pitted scars. The disorder occurs with greater frequency in boys; it begins in early childhood and may remit at puberty. It must be distinguished from erythropoietic protoporphyria. Therapy with a topical corticosteroid preparation is effective in the inflammatory phase of the eruption. Protective sunscreens are mandatory for affected children.

Cockayne syndrome is inherited as an autosomal recessive trait and is characterized by photosensitivity, loss of adipose tissue, dwarfism, mental retardation, and thin, atrophic, hyperpigmented skin, particularly over the face. The ears are large and protuberant, the nose pinched, the teeth carious, the hands and feet cool and sometimes cyanotic. An unsteady gait with tremor, limitation of joint mobility, partial deafness, cataracts, retinal pigmentary abnormalities, optic atrophy, decreased sweating and tearing, and premature graying of the hair are additional features. The syndrome is distinguished from progeria (Sec. 26.4) by photosensitivity and the ocular abnormalities.

Rothmund-Thomson syndrome is also known as poikiloderma congenitale because of the striking skin changes; it is thought to be inherited as an autosomal recessive trait, although a preponderance of affected females has been reported. Skin changes are noted in infancy as early as the 3rd mo. Plaques of erythema and edema appear on the cheeks, buttocks, hands, and feet and are gradually replaced by reticulated, atrophic, hyperpigmented, telangiectatic plaques. Exposure to the sun may provoke formation of bullae. Short stature, small hands and feet, sparse eyebrows and eyelashes, sparse, prematurely gray hair or alopecia, dystrophic nails, defective dentition, bony defects, hypogenitalism, and mental retardation are common. Cataracts commonly become apparent at 2–7 yr of age.

Hartnup disease (Sec. 7.6) is a rare inborn error of metabolism with autosomal recessive inheritance; renal aminoaciduria is associated with a photo-induced, pellagra-like eruption. Approximately 20% of patients are mentally retarded and others evidence emotional instability and episodic cerebellar ataxia. The initial cutaneous manifestations are detectable during the early months of life when an eczematous, occasionally vesicobullous, eruption is noted on the face and on the extremities in a glove and stocking pattern. Hyperpigmentation and hyperkeratosis may supervene and are intensified by further exposure to sunlight. Episodic flares may be precipitated by febrile illness, sun exposure, emotional stress, and poor nutrition. Administration of nicotinamide and protection from sunlight result in improvement of both cutaneous and neurologic manifestations.

Bloom syndrome is characterized by erythema and telangiectasia in a butterfly distribution on the face, photosensitivity, and dwarfism of prenatal onset; inheritance is autosomal recessive. The facial erythema develops during infancy following exposure to sunlight. A bullous eruption may appear on the lips and telangiectatic erythema on the hands and forearms. Café-au-lait spots, ichthyosis, acanthosis nigricans, and hypertrichosis are less constant cutaneous manifestations. Defective dentition, prominent ears, pilonidal cysts, sacral dimples, syndactyly, polydactyly, clinodactyly of the 5th fingers, shortened lower extremities, and club feet are additional inconstant features. Mentation is normal. Chromosomal breaks and rearrangements are common, and affected children have an unusual tendency to develop lymphoreticular malignancies.

Xeroderma pigmentosum is a rare autosomal recessive genetic disorder in which skin changes are first noted during infancy or early childhood. Affected children, who are unable to repair DNA damaged by ultraviolet light, are sensitive to light in the wavelength range of 280–310 nm (UVB) and develop extensive solar changes in exposed skin. Sun-exposed areas such as the face, neck, hands, and arms are most severely involved, but lesions may occur at other sites including the scalp. The skin lesions consist of erythema, scaling, bullae, crusting, ephelides, telangiectasia, keratoses, basal and squamous cell carcinomas, and malignant melanomas. Ocular manifestations include photophobia, lacrimation, blepharitis, symblepharon, keratitis, corneal opacities, tumors of the lids, and possible eventual blindness. Neurologic abnormalities such as mental deterioration and sensorineural deafness may develop in some patients. The association of xeroderma pigmentosum with microcephaly, mental retardation, dwarfism, and hypogonadism is known as *De Sanctis–Cacchione syndrome*.

This disease is a serious, mutilating disorder, and the life span is often quite brief. Affected families should have genetic counseling. Amniocentesis and possible interruption of pregnancy can be offered inasmuch as the defect is detectable in cells cultured from amniotic fluid. Affected children should be protected from sun exposure; opaque broad-spectrum sunscreens should be employed even for mildly affected children. Early detection and removal of malignancies is mandatory. Grafting of skin from non–light-exposed areas may be helpful, as is the use of topical antimitotic agents such as 5-fluorouracil.

24.15 DISEASES OF THE EPIDERMIS

Psoriasis, a common, chronic skin disorder among adults, is first evident in approximately one third of affected individuals within the first 2 decades of life. When the onset occurs during childhood, about 50% have a positive family history of the disease, and girls are more frequently affected. The mode of transmission is unknown; a multifactorial type of inheritance has been proposed. The pathogenesis is also unknown; epidermal turnover time, however, is distinctly accelerated compared with that of normal epidermis.

The lesions consist of erythematous papules which coalesce to form plaques with sharply demarcated, irregular borders. If they are unaltered by treatment, a thick silvery or yellow-white scale develops; removal of it may result in pinpoint bleeding (Auspitz sign). The Koebner, or isomorphic, response in which new lesions appear at sites of trauma is a valuable diagnostic feature. Lesions may occur anywhere, but preferred sites are the scalp, knees (Fig. 24–25A), elbows, umbilicus, and genitalia. Scalp lesions may be confused with seborrheic dermatitis or tinea capitis. Small, raindrop-like lesions on the face are moderately common. Nail involvement,

a valuable diagnostic sign, is characterized by pitting of the nail plate (Fig. 24–25B), detachment of the plate (onycholysis), and accumulation of subungual debris.

Age is an important factor in determining the clinical pattern. Psoriasis is rare in the neonate but may be severe and recalcitrant and pose a diagnostic problem. The initial lesions may involve the diaper area and mimic seborrheic dermatitis, eczematous diaper dermatitis, or candidosis. Biopsy and/or prolonged observation may be required for definitive diagnosis. Other rare forms include psoriatic erythroderma, localized or generalized pustular psoriasis, and linear psoriasis. Hospitalization may be required for severe forms of the disease.

Guttate psoriasis, a variant that occurs predominantly in children, is characterized by an explosive eruption of profuse, small, oval or round lesions that morphologically are identical to the larger plaques of psoriasis (Fig. 24–25C). Sites of

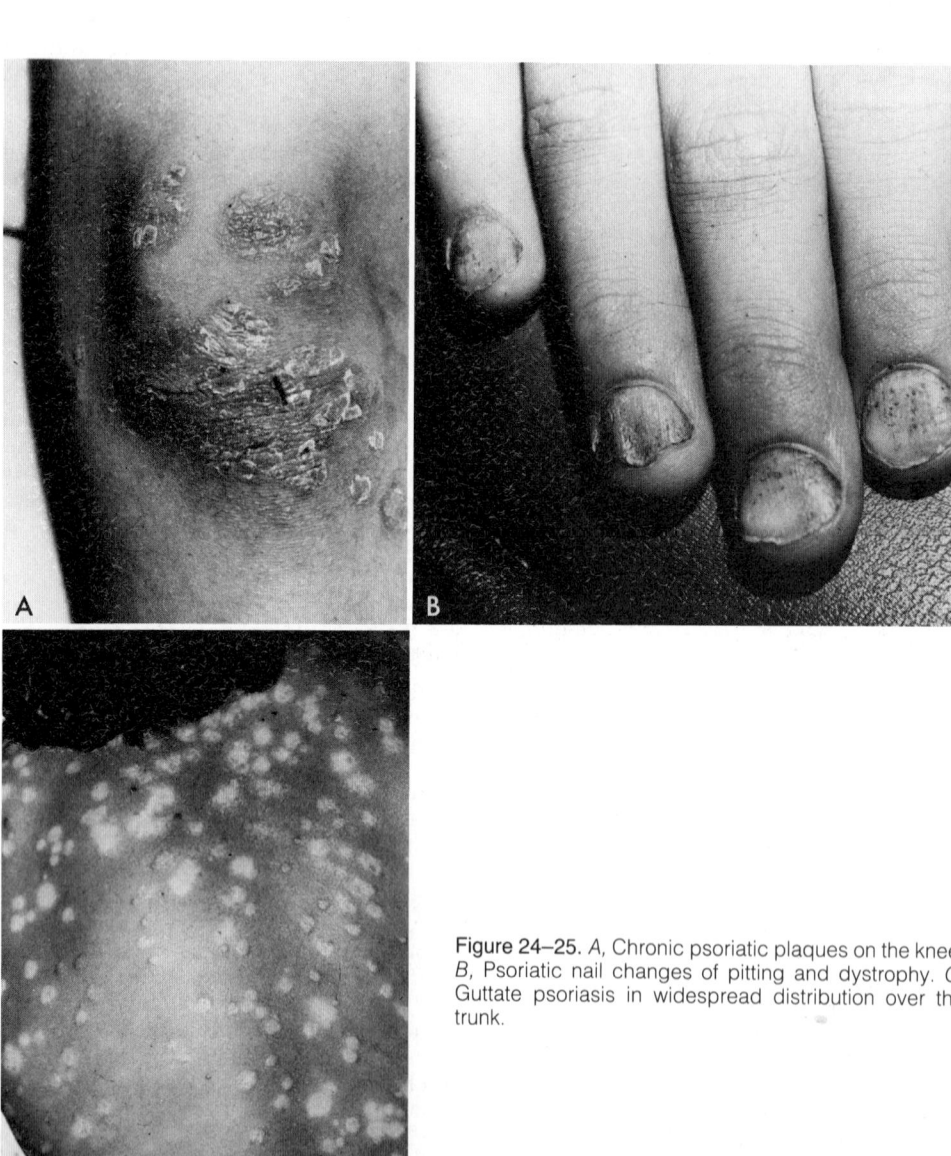

Figure 24–25. A, Chronic psoriatic plaques on the knee. B, Psoriatic nail changes of pitting and dystrophy. C, Guttate psoriasis in widespread distribution over the trunk.

predilection are the trunk, face, and proximal portions of the limbs. The onset frequently follows a recent streptococcal respiratory infection; a culture of the throat and serologic titers should be obtained. Guttate psoriasis has also been observed following viral infections, sunburn, and withdrawal of systemic corticosteroid therapy. The lesions may be confused with viral exanthems and guttate parapsoriasis (see below).

When the diagnosis is in question, a biopsy of skin may provide supportive evidence. In a typical psoriatic lesion, the stratum corneum is thickened and parakeratotic, and the epidermis is hyperplastic with irregular elongation of the rete ridges, thinning of the suprapapillary epidermis, and microabscesses. The dermis contains a proliferative vascular network and an infiltrate of inflammatory cells.

The therapeutic approach varies with the age of the child, type of psoriasis, sites of involvement, and extent of disease. Therapy is mainly palliative and should not be overly aggressive. Physical and chemical trauma to the skin should be avoided insofar as possible (see Koebner response, above).

Tar preparations may be used in the form of an emulsion added to the daily bath, gel preparations, or ointments such as crude coal tar (1–5%) and liquor carbonis detergens (5–15%) in petrolatum alone or in conjunction with ultraviolet light or natural sunlight (Sec. 24.14). Occasionally, sunlight has an adverse rather than a beneficial effect, and the use of tar preparations may have to be decreased during the summer to avoid phototoxic reactions. Salicylic acid ointment (1–3%) may provide an alternative for removal of scale, but extensive application may result in toxicity, particularly in small children. Topical corticosteroid preparations are extremely effective, but they must be used with caution; fluorinated compounds produce cutaneous atrophy if applied excessively or if occluded with polyethylene film for prolonged periods of time. The least potent effective preparation should be applied 1–2 times daily. For scalp lesions, applications of a phenol and saline solution (Baker P & S) followed by a tar shampoo are effective in the removal of scales. A corticosteroid in a lotion or gel base may be applied when the scaling is diminished. Rarely, the more severe forms of psoriasis may require systemic therapy; such management should be under the direction of an experienced physician. The use of psoralens and ultraviolet light (PUVA) is effective in severe psoriasis in adults, but the safety of PUVA has not been established for children. Psoriasis in infants and acute guttate psoriasis may flare with vigorous treatment and should be managed conservatively. Nail lesions are usually recalcitrant to therapy.

Guttate parapsoriasis (pityriasis lichenoides chronica), an uncommon chronic skin disorder, may occur at any age but most frequently affects older children. The etiology is not known. The eruption can be polymorphous, but typical lesions are small (1–5 mm), superficial, erythematous papules covered by a fine, white scale. Occasional lesions may become infiltrated, vesicular, hemorrhagic, and crusted. Prolonged postinflammatory pigmentary loss is usual and may be prominent in darker-skinned children. There is a predilection for involvement of the trunk, but all body sites may be affected except the nails and mucous membranes. An individual lesion may persist for 2–6 wk, but exacerbations and remissions persist for months to years.

Despite the prolonged course, guttate parapsoriasis is benign and unassociated with systemic manifestations. The lesions may be asymptomatic or cause minimal pruritus. The diagnosis is entirely clinical. Differential diagnosis includes guttate psoriasis, pityriasis rosea, drug eruptions, secondary syphilis, viral exanthems, lichen planus, and, occasionally, Mucha-Habermann disease. Since the pathologic changes are specific in some of these disorders, a skin biopsy may be indicated to exclude them. The chronicity of guttate para-

psoriasis helps to exclude pityriasis rosea, viral exanthems, and some drug eruptions.

No reliable treatment is known. Some patients show remarkable improvement following intense sun exposure. Topical corticosteroid-tar preparations and ultraviolet light have been employed with variable success. A lubricant to remove excessive scaling may be all that is necessary if the patient is asymptomatic. Parents may be reassured that the child will remain well.

Keratosis pilaris, a moderately common papular eruption, may vary in extent from sparse lesions over the extensor aspects of the limbs to involvement of most of the body surface. The lesions may resemble gooseflesh; they are noninflammatory, scaly, follicular papules that do not coalesce. Irritation of the follicular plugs occasionally causes folliculitis. Because the lesions are associated with and accentuated by dry skin, they are often more prominent during the winter months. They are more frequent in patients with atopic dermatitis and are most common during childhood and early adulthood, tending to subside during the 3rd decade of life. Mild or localized eruptions respond to lubrication with a bland emollient; more pronounced or widespread lesions require regular applications of a 10–25% urea cream, an α-hydroxy acid preparation such as lactic acid in an emollient, or topical retinoic acid.

Lichen spinulosus, an uncommon disorder, occurs principally in children and more frequently in boys. The cause is unknown. The lesions consist of sharply circumscribed irregular plaques of spiny, keratinous projections that protrude from the orifices of the pilosebaceous canals (Fig. 24–26). Plaques may occur anywhere on the body and are often distributed symmetrically on the trunk, elbows, knees, and extensor surfaces of the limbs. Although sometimes erythematous, the lesions are usually skin-colored. They are readily palpable and represent keratotic follicular plugs.

Lichen spinulosus is easily differentiated from keratosis pilaris since the latter lesions are never grouped to form plaques. More commonly, it is confused with papular eczema.

Treatment is usually unnecessary. For patients who regard the eruption as a cosmetic defect, keratolytic agents such as salicylic acid ointment (3–7%), urea-containing lubricants (10–25%), and retinoic acid preparations often are effective in

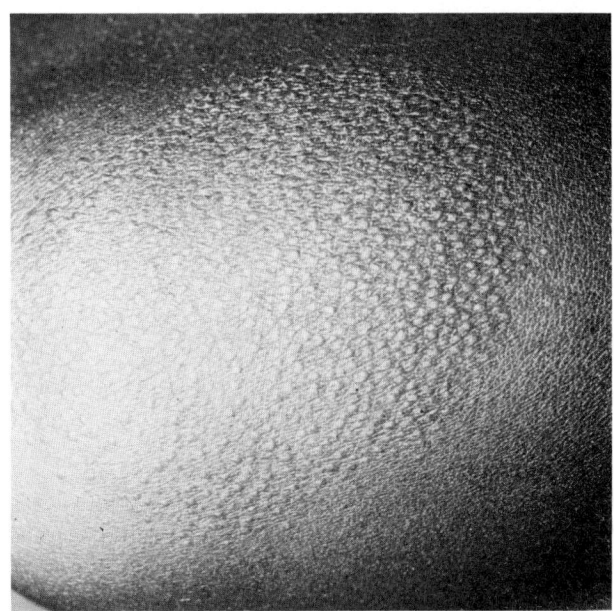

Figure 24–26. Sharply circumscribed plaque of follicular papules characteristic of lichen spinulosus.

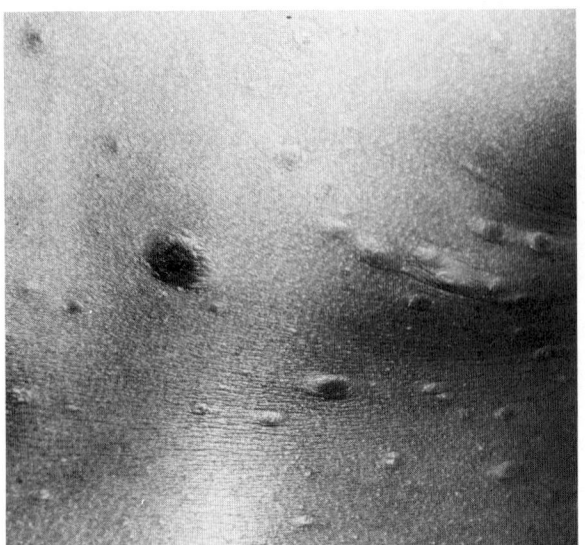

Figure 24–27. Ovoid, maculopapular lesions of pityriasis rosea. Note distribution along skin lines and herald patch on the chest.

flattening the projections. The plaques usually disappear spontaneously after several months or years.

Pityriasis rosea, a benign, common eruption, occurs most frequently in children and young adults. Although a prodrome of fever, malaise, arthralgia, and pharyngitis may precede the eruption, children rarely complain of such symptoms. A *herald patch,* a solitary, round or oval lesion that may occur anywhere on the body and is often but not always identifiable by its large size, usually precedes the generalized eruption. Herald patches vary from 1 to 10 cm in diameter, are annular in configuration, and have a raised border with fine, adherent scales. Approximately 5–10 days following appearance of the herald patch, a widespread, symmetrical eruption becomes evident involving mainly the trunk and proximal limbs (Fig. 24–27). When the disease is extensive, the face, scalp, and distal limbs may be involved, or, in the inverse form of pityriasis rosea, only those sites may be affected. Lesions may appear in crops over a period of several days. Typical lesions are oval or round, less than 1 cm in diameter, slightly raised, and pink to brown in color. The developed lesion is covered by a fine scale which gives the skin a crinkly appearance; some lesions clear centrally, producing a collarette of scale which is attached only at the periphery. Papular, vesicular, urticarial, hemorrhagic, and large, annular lesions are unusual variants. Usually the long axis of each lesion is aligned with the cutaneous cleavage lines, a feature that creates the so-called "Christmas tree" pattern on the back. Actually, conformation to skin lines is often more discernible in the anterior and posterior axillary folds and supraclavicular areas. Duration of the eruption varies from 2 to 12 wk. The lesions may be asymptomatic or mildly to severely pruritic. The cause of pityriasis rosea is unknown; a viral agent has been sought.

The diagnosis is entirely clinical. The herald patch may be mistaken for tinea corporis, a pitfall that can be avoided if a KOH preparation is obtained. The generalized eruption resembles a number of other diseases; of these, secondary syphilis is the most important. Drug eruptions, viral exanthems, guttate psoriasis, parapsoriasis, and eczema can also be confused with pityriasis rosea.

Treatment is unnecessary for the asymptomatic patient. If scaling is prominent, a bland emollient may suffice. Pruritus may be suppressed by a lubricating lotion containing menthol and phenol or by an oral antihistamine for sedation, particularly at night, when itching may be troublesome. Occasionally,

a nonfluorinated topical corticosteroid preparation may be necessary to alleviate pruritus. After the eruption has resolved, postinflammatory hypo- or hyperpigmentation may be pronounced, particularly in black patients; these changes disappear during subsequent weeks.

Pityriasis rubra pilaris, a rare chronic dermatosis, often has an insidious onset with diffuse scaling and erythema of the scalp, indistinguishable from seborrheic dermatitis, and with thick hyperkeratosis of the palms and soles. The characteristic primary lesion is a firm, dome-shaped, tiny, acuminate papule, which is pink to red in color and has a central keratotic plug pierced by a vellus hair. Masses of these papules coalesce to form large, erythematous, sharply demarcated plaques, within which islands of normal skin can be distinguished, creating a bizarre effect. Typical papules on the dorsum of the proximal phalanges are readily palpated and have been compared to the surface of a nutmeg grater. Gray plaques or papules resembling lichen planus may be found in the oral cavity. Dystrophic changes in the nails may occur and mimic those of psoriasis. In advanced stages, marked hyperkeratosis of scalp and face may cause alopecia and ectropion. Differential diagnosis includes ichthyosis, seborrheic dermatitis, keratoderma of the palms and soles, and psoriasis.

The etiology is unknown. A genetic form of pityriasis rubra pilaris with autosomal dominant transmission has been said to account for most of the cases in childhood, but most of the reported cases seem to be sporadic. Attempts to link the disease with a defect in vitamin A metabolism have not been definitive. Skin biopsy may help differentiate this condition from psoriasis and seborrheic dermatitis, which it resembles most closely.

Numerous therapeutic regimens have been recommended and are difficult to evaluate since the disease has a capricious course with exacerbations and remissions. Oral and topical retinoids as well as vitamin A have been used most frequently. When vitamin A or synthetic retinoids are administered orally, the child should be observed carefully for signs of toxicity. In childhood the prognosis for eventual resolution is relatively good.

Darier disease (keratosis follicularis) is a rare genetic disorder inherited as an autosomal dominant trait. Onset occurs usually during late childhood. Typical lesions are small, firm, skin-colored papules which are not always follicular in location. Eventually, the lesions acquire yellow, malodorous crusts; coalesce to form large, gray-brown, vegetative plaques; and usually involve the face, neck, shoulders, chest, back, and limb flexures in a symmetrical distribution. Papules, fissures, crusts, and ulcers may appear on the mucous membranes of the lips, tongue, buccal mucosa, pharynx, larynx, and vulva. Hyperkeratosis of the palms and soles and nail dystrophy with subungual hyperkeratosis are variable features. Severe pruritus, secondary infection, offensive odor, and aggravation of the dermatosis on exposure to sunlight are annoying features.

Darier disease is most likely to be confused with seborrheic dermatitis or juvenile flat warts. Histologic changes are diagnostic; hyperkeratosis, intraepidermal separation with formation of suprabasal clefts, and dyskeratotic epidermal cells are characteristic features.

Therapy is nonspecific. Some patients have responded to large oral doses of vitamin A or to topical retinoic acid, with or without occlusive dressings. Secondary infection may require local cleansing and systemically administered antibiotics. Affected individuals usually suffer more during the summer months.

Lichen nitidus is a chronic, benign, papular eruption characterized by minute (1–2 mm), flat-topped, shiny, firm papules of uniform size which are most often skin-colored but may be pink or red and, in black individuals, are usually

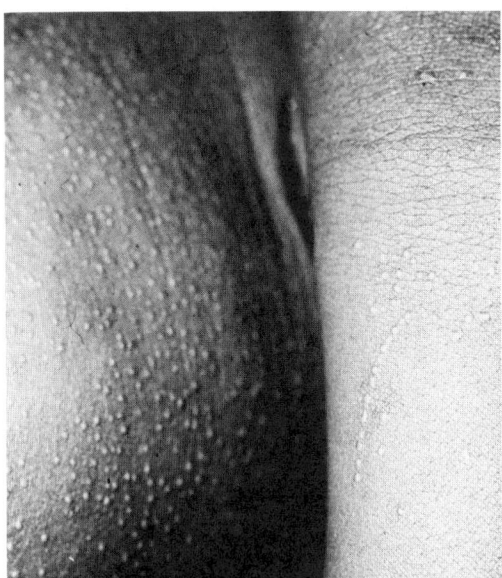

Figure 24–28. Tiny flat-topped papules of lichen nitidus on the arm and trunk. Note the Koebner response on the arm (papules in a line of scratch).

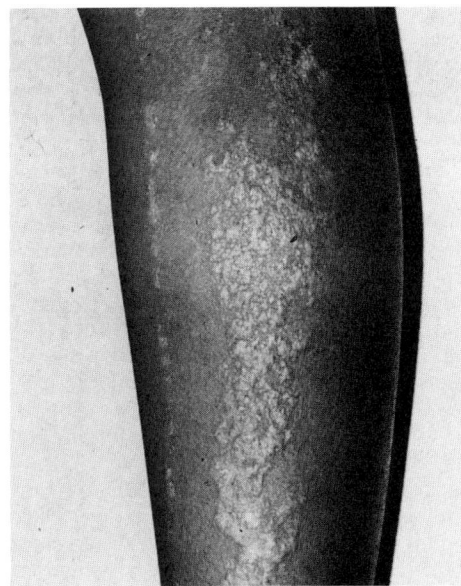

Figure 24–29. Multiple linear plaques and streaks of lichen striatus.

hypopigmented. Sites of predilection are the genitalia, abdomen, chest, forearms, wrists, and inner aspects of the thighs. The lesions may be sparse or numerous and form large plaques; careful examination will usually disclose linear papules in a line of scratch (Koebner phenomenon), a valuable clue to the diagnosis since it occurs in only a few diseases (Fig. 24–28).

Lichen nitidus occurs in all age groups. The cause is unknown. Patients are usually asymptomatic and constitutionally well. The lesions may be confused with and rarely coexist with those of lichen planus. Widespread keratosis pilaris also can be confused with lichen nitidus, but the follicular localization of the papules and the absence of the Koebner phenomenon in keratosis pilaris will distinguish them. Verruca plana (flat warts), if small and uniform in size, may occasionally resemble lichen nitidus. Although the diagnosis can be made clinically, a biopsy is occasionally indicated. Histopathologically, the lichen nitidus papule consists of sharply circumscribed nests of lymphocytes and histiocytes in the upper dermis enclosed by claw-like epidermal rete ridges. The course of lichen nitidus is months to years, but the lesions eventually involute completely. There is no effective therapy.

Lichen striatus, a benign, self-limited eruption, consists of a continuous or discontinuous linear band of papules in a zosteriform distribution. The primary lesion is a flat-topped red to violaceous papule covered with a fine scale. Aggregates of these papules form multiple bands or plaques (Fig. 24–29). In black patients the lesions may be hypopigmented.

The etiology and explanation for the linear distribution are unknown. The eruption evolves over a period of days or weeks in an otherwise healthy child, remains stationary for weeks to months, and finally remits without sequelae. Symptoms are usually absent; some children complain of itching. Nail dystrophy may occur if the eruption involves the posterior nail fold and matrix.

Lichen striatus is occasionally confused with other disorders. The initial plaque may resemble papular eczema or lichen nitidus until the linear configuration becomes apparent. Linear lichen planus and linear psoriasis are often associated with typical individual lesions elsewhere on the body. Linear epidermal nevi are permanent lesions that often become more hyperkeratotic and hyperpigmented than those of lichen stria-

tus. A lubricating lotion containing menthol and phenol or a mild corticosteroid preparation provides sufficient relief when pruritus is a problem.

Lichen planus is a rare disorder in the young child and uncommon in the older one. The primary lesion is a violaceous, sharply demarcated, polygonal papule with fine lines or thin white scales on the surface; papules may coalesce to form large plaques. The papules are intensely pruritic, and additional ones are often induced by scratching (Koebner phenomenon) so that lines of them are often detectable (Fig. 24–30). Sites of predilection are the flexor surfaces of the wrists, the forearms, and inner aspects of the thighs. Characteristic lesions of the mucous membrane consist of pinhead-sized, white papules that coalesce to form reticulated and lacy patterns on the oral mucosa and sometimes on the lips and tongue.

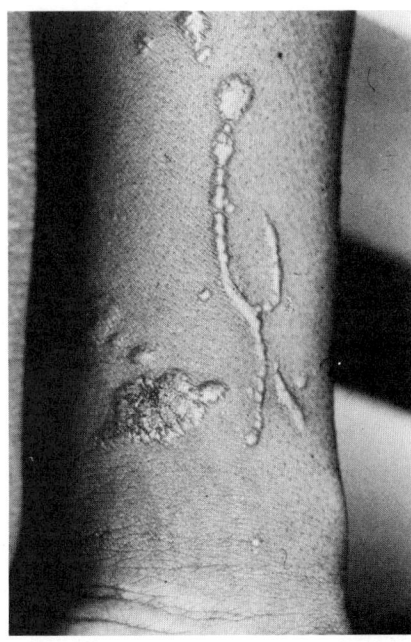

Figure 24–30. Violaceous polygonal papules of lichen planus. Note the striking Koebner response.

There are several subtypes of the disease. Acute eruptive lichen planus is probably the most common form in children. The lesions erupt in an explosive fashion, much like a viral exanthem, and spread to involve most of the body surface. Hypertrophic, linear, bullous, atrophic, annular, follicular, erosive, and ulcerative forms of lichen planus may also occur. Nail involvement may occur in the chronic forms but is rarely evident in children (twenty nail dystrophy, Sec. 24.22). The disorder may persist for months to years; the acute eruptive form is most likely to involute permanently. Frequently, intense hyperpigmentation persists for a long time following resolution of lesions. The pathology of lichen planus is quite specific, and a biopsy is indicated if the diagnosis is unclear.

Treatment is directed at alleviation of the intense pruritus as well as amelioration of the skin lesions. Oral antihistamines and/or tranquilizers are often helpful. The skin lesions respond best to regular applications of a topical corticosteroid preparation. Rarely, systemic corticosteroid therapy is necessary to gain control of widespread, intractable lesions.

Porokeratosis is a rare, chronic, progressive disease that is inherited as an autosomal dominant trait. Several forms have been delineated: solitary plaques, linear porokeratosis, hyperkeratotic lesions of the palms and soles, disseminated eruptive lesions, and superficial actinic porokeratosis. The last form, probably induced by excessive sun exposure, occurs more commonly in adult females. Other types of porokeratosis are more common in males and begin during childhood. Sites of predilection are the limbs, face, neck, and genitalia. The primary lesion is a small, keratotic papule that enlarges peripherally so that the center becomes depressed, the edge forming an elevated wall or collar. The configuration of the plaque may be round, oval, or gyrate; its elevated border is split by a thin groove from which minute cornified projections protrude. The enclosed central area is yellow, gray, or tan, sclerotic, smooth, and dry, whereas the hyperkeratotic border is a darker gray, brown, or black.

The differential diagnosis includes warts, epidermal nevi, lichen planus, granuloma annulare, and elastosis perforans serpiginosa. A skin biopsy will disclose the characteristic cornoid lamella (plug of stratum corneum cells with retained nuclei) which is responsible for the linear ridge of the lesion, an invariable clinical feature.

The disease is slowly progressive but relatively asymptomatic. Lesions are sometimes responsive to applications of liquid nitrogen or may be surgically excised, a procedure which may not be feasible.

Papular acrodermatitis of childhood (Gianotti-Crosti syndrome) is a distinctive eruption associated with malaise and low-grade fever but few other constitutional symptoms. The incidence peaks in early childhood. Occurrences are usually sporadic, but epidemics have been recorded.

The skin lesion is a monomorphous, usually nonpruritic, dusky or coppery red, flat-topped, firm papule ranging in size from 1 to 5 mm. The papules appear in crops and may become profuse but remain discrete forming a symmetrical eruption on the face, buttocks, and limbs including the palms and soles. At times the papules become hemorrhagic. Lines of papules (Koebner phenomenon) may be noted on the extremities. The trunk is relatively spared, as are the scalp and mucous membranes. Generalized lymphadenopathy and hepatomegaly constitute the only other abnormal physical findings. The eruption resolves spontaneously in about 3 wk. Lymphadenopathy and hepatomegaly may persist for several months.

This eruption is most often associated with primary infection with hepatitis B virus and is, therefore, associated with hepatitis B surface antigenemia. Subtyping of the HB$_s$Ag in most instances has demonstrated the determinant *ayw*. Elevation of serum transaminase and alkaline phosphatase values

without concomitant hyperbilirubinemia is usual, and histologic changes of viral hepatitis are demonstrable on liver biopsy. Skin biopsy is characterized by a perivascular mononuclear cell infiltrate and capillary endothelial swelling.

Generally the disease is benign and self-limited and does not recur. The hepatitis usually resolves in 2–3 mo but, occasionally, may progress to chronic hepatitis with persistent antigenemia and elevated transaminase activity. The surface antibody of the hepatitis B virus is not detected during the phase of dermatitis appearing approximately 6–12 mo later in patients who become HB$_s$Ag negative.

A similar cutaneous eruption has also been observed in patients infected with Epstein-Barr virus, coxsackievirus A16, and parainfluenza virus and undoubtedly accompanies other viral infections. Papular acrodermatitis can be confused with lichen planus, erythema multiforme, histiocytosis X, and Henoch-Schönlein purpura.

24.16 ICHTHYOSIS

The ichthyosiform dermatoses are a group of inherited keratinizing disorders characterized by visible scaling in distinctive patterns of distribution. They are usually distinguishable on the basis of inheritance patterns, clinical features, associated defects, and histologic changes. Since some of these conditions cause disfigurement and considerable mental anguish, early diagnosis is helpful in order to predict probable course and prognosis and to provide supportive management for the patient and family.

Harlequin fetus is a very rare keratinizing disorder that is inherited as an autosomal recessive trait. Affected infants are extremely grotesque. Markedly thickened, ridged, and cracked skin forms horny plates over the entire body, disfiguring the facial features and constricting the digits. Severe ectropion and chemosis obscure the orbits; the nose and ears are flattened, and the lips are everted and gaping. Nails and hair may be absent. Joint mobility is restricted, and the hands and feet appear fixed and ischemic. The infants have respiratory difficulty and suck poorly. Most succumb within the 1st wk of life; few live beyond 6 wk. The prognosis is hopeless. Prenatal diagnosis has been accomplished by fetoscopy and fetal skin biopsy.

The **collodion baby** is covered at birth by a thick, taut membrane resembling oiled parchment or collodion, which is subsequently shed. The condition is usually a primary manifestation of one of the ichthyoses, most often of the lamellar variety. Infrequently an affected infant has normal skin after the membrane is shed. There is ectropion, flattening of the ears and nose, and fixation of the lips in an O-shaped configuration (Fig. 24–31). Hair may be absent or may perforate the horny covering. The membrane cracks with initial respiratory efforts and, shortly after birth, begins to desquamate in large sheets. Complete shedding may take several weeks, and occasionally a new membrane may form in localized areas.

The nursery course may be complicated by cutaneous infection with yeasts and bacteria. The outcome is uncertain, and accurate prognosis is impossible with respect to the subsequent development of ichthyosis. Maintenance in a high-humidity environment and application of nonocclusive lubricants may facilitate shedding of the membrane.

Ichthyosis vulgaris, the most common type of ichthyosis, is transmitted as an autosomal dominant trait. Onset occurs sometime after the first year of life. Scaling is most prominent on the extensor aspects of the extremities and back. The flexures are spared, and the abdomen and face are relatively uninvolved. Accentuated markings and creases are apparent on palms and soles. Atopy is relatively common.

The histologic changes differ from those of other types of

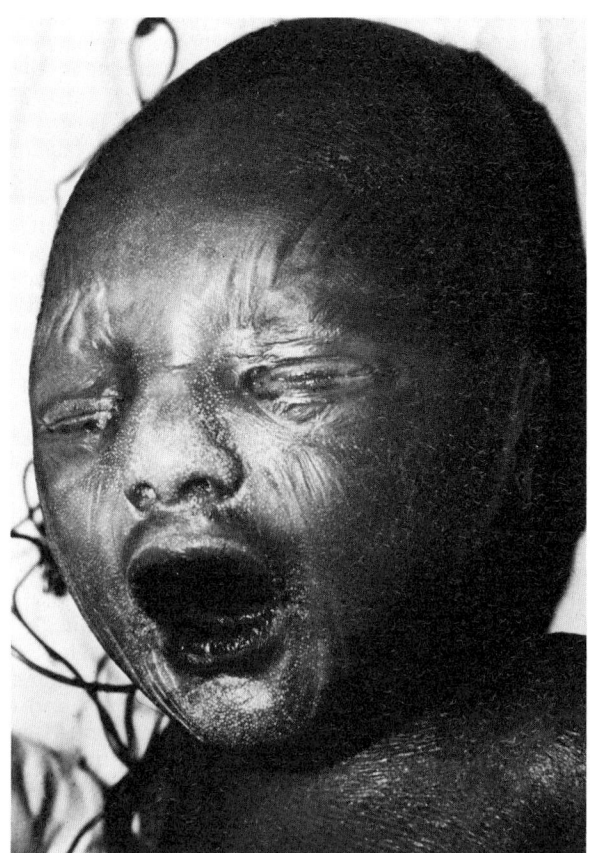

Figure 24–31. Typical facial appearance of a collodion baby.

ichthyosis in that the hyperkeratosis is associated with a decreased or absent granular layer. Abnormalities of kerato-hyalin structures and tonofilaments are found in epidermal cells on electron microscopy. Epidermal transit time is normal. Scaling is most pronounced during the winter months and may abate completely during warm weather. The condition may improve and even disappear with age. Scaling may be diminished by use of a bath oil and daily applications of an emollient or a urea-containing lubricant.

X-linked ichthyosis is limited to males and is often present at birth. Scaling is most pronounced on the scalp, neck, sides of the face, anterior trunk, and limbs. The face, palms, and soles are usually spared. The distribution pattern of scaling differs somewhat from that of ichthyosis vulgaris, but biopsy may be required to distinguish the two conditions. Histologic changes in X-linked ichthyosis include hyperkeratosis of the stratum corneum, a well-developed granular layer, a hyperplastic epidermis, and a mononuclear, perivascular dermal infiltrate. Epidermal transit time is normal.

The inherited biochemical defect in X-linked ichthyosis is a deficiency of the enzyme steroid sulfatase. This defect can be demonstrated in the fibroblasts and epidermal cells of affected males. Steroid sulfatase hydrolyzes cholesterol sulfate and other sulfate steroids; cholesterol sulfate accumulates in the stratum corneum and plasma in X-linked ichthyosis. The increase in plasma cholesterol sulfate can be detected by serum lipoprotein electrophoresis. Carrier mothers demonstrate a placental steroid sulfatase deficiency reflected by low urinary and serum estriol values, prolonged labors, and insensitivity of the uterus to oxytocin and prostaglandins. The role these enzymes play in the keratinization process is as yet unknown. The gene for steroid sulfatase is located on the short arm of the X chromosome, closely linked with the Xg^2 blood group locus.

Deep corneal opacities that do not interfere with vision develop during late childhood or adolescence and are a useful marker for the disease since they may also be present in carrier females. Although the disease does not represent a serious keratinizing defect, affected boys are usually embarrassed by the disfigurement and request treatment. Hydration by bathing with bath oil and daily application of emollients and a urea-containing lubricant are usually effective. Citric or lactic acid (5%) in an emollient base is an alternative form of topical therapy.

Lamellar ichthyosis, an autosomal recessive disorder, is always evident at birth; the neonate may have a "collodion membrane." Universal erythema is characteristic in infancy and may persist during childhood in some patients; in children so affected the disorder has been designated **congenital ichthyosiform erythroderma.** Scaling is often pronounced and involves the entire body surface including flexures and palms and soles (Fig. 24–32). Pruritus may be severe, and responds only minimally to antipruritic measures. Ectropion of variable degree is usually present. Some patients with this type of ichthyosis have relatively little erythema, large, dark, adherent scales, and a moderate degree of ectropion.

Skin biopsy shows hyperkeratosis, a well-developed granular layer, epidermal hyperplasia, and a mononuclear, perivascular dermal infiltrate. Epidermal transit time is decreased. Growth of hair may be curtailed, and patients may suffer in hot weather because of an inability to sweat freely through plugged sweat ducts. The unattractive appearance of the child and the malodor from bacterial colonization of macerated scales may create serious psychologic problems.

Effective measures include prolonged baths with bath oil to remove excessive scales. The restriction of bathing, on the erroneous premise that accentuation of dryness will occur, only promotes malodor and accumulation of keratinous debris and contributes to pruritus and discomfort. A high-humidity environment in winter and air conditioning in summer will lessen discomfort. Generous and frequent applications of emollients as well as keratolytic agents such as lactic or citric

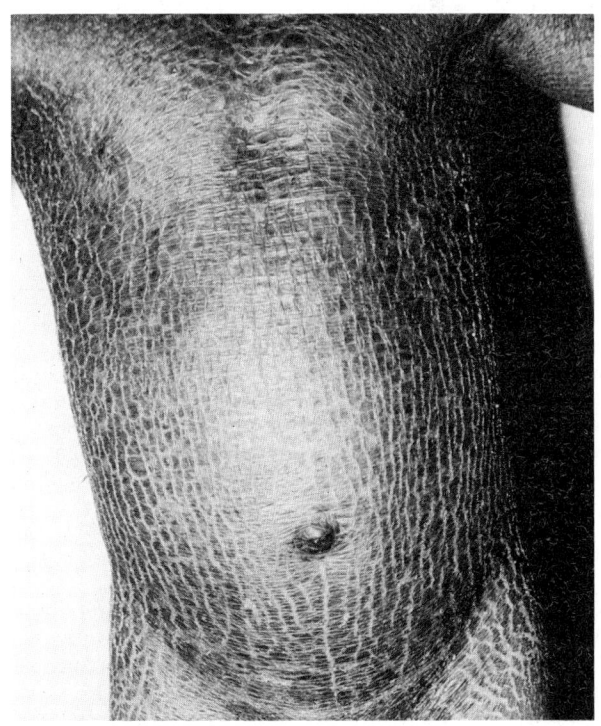

Figure 24–32. Generalized scaling of lamellar ichthyosis. Note involvement of axillary areas.

acid (5%), urea (10–25%), and retinoic acid (0.1% cream) may lessen the scaling to some extent. Ectropion requires ophthalmologic care and, at times, plastic procedures. Genetic counseling should be provided.

Epidermolytic hyperkeratosis (bullous congenital ichthyosiform erythroderma), an autosomal dominant keratinizing disorder, is characterized by onset at birth, generalized erythroderma, and severe hyperkeratosis with accentuation in the flexural areas. The scales are small, hard, and verrucous and in many areas assume a columnar configuration, thus differing from those of other forms of ichthyosis. Recurrent bullae, which are characteristic during childhood and are usually localized to the lower limbs, may be widespread in the neonate and cause diagnostic confusion with other blistering disorders. Secondary bacterial infection is common and requires appropriate antibiotic therapy.

The histologic pattern in this disorder is pathognomonic and consists of hyperkeratosis and vacuolization of the cells of the granular layer and mid-epidermis with abnormally large clumped keratohyaline granules. Epidermal transit time is decreased. Localized forms of the disease may resemble epidermal nevi (ichthyosis hystrix) or keratoderma of the palms and soles but share the distinctive histologic changes of epidermolytic hyperkeratosis.

Effective therapeutic agents are the same as those recommended for lamellar ichthyosis. Genetic counseling should be provided. Prenatal diagnosis has been accomplished by fetoscopy and fetal skin biopsy.

Ichthyosis linearis circumflexa, a rare autosomal recessive disorder, is characterized by migratory hyperkeratotic lesions, hyperkeratosis of the flexures, and hyperhidrosis of the palms and soles. The skin is diffusely red and scaly at birth. Superimposed serpiginous scaly plaques, bordered by a distinctive double-edged scale, appear at various sites on the trunk and limbs. This type of ichthyosis is characteristic of patients with the Netherton syndrome (see below).

Erythrokeratoderma variabilis is characterized by two types of lesions: sharply demarcated hyperkeratotic plaques with bizarre borders, and discrete areas of macular erythema which disappear or migrate but may eventually become hyperkeratotic and fixed. Sites of predilection are the face, buttocks, and extensor surfaces of the limbs. The palms and soles may be thickened, but hair, teeth, and nails are normal. The disorder is inherited as an autosomal dominant trait. Histologic changes include lamination of the stratum corneum, focal parakeratosis, papillomatosis, and irregular hyperplasia of the epidermis. The epidermal transit time is normal.

Ichthyosis Syndromes

Several syndromes that include ichthyosis as a constant feature have been established as distinct entities. Each of them is relatively rare.

Sjögren-Larssen syndrome, an autosomal recessive disorder, has three major and constant components: ichthyosis of the lamellar type, mental deficiency, and spastic diplegia. A degenerative defect of retinal pigment epithelium has been detected in 20–30% of affected individuals. Glistening dots in the foveal area, although easily overlooked, are believed to be a cardinal ophthalmologic sign (see also Table 25–1). Some patients may walk with the aid of braces, but most are confined to a wheelchair.

Rud syndrome, as described, consists of mental retardation, epilepsy, ichthyosis (type uncertain), and sexual infantilism. Associated defects of the skeleton, eyes, dentition, and hearing have also been reported.

Netherton syndrome is characterized by ichthyosis (usually ichthyosis linearis circumflexa but occasionally the lamellar type), trichorrhexis invaginata and other hair shaft anomalies,

and atopic diathesis. The ichthyosis is present at birth. Scalp hair is sparse and fractures easily; eyebrows, eyelashes, and body hair are also abnormal. The most frequent allergic manifestations are urticaria, angioedema, and asthma. Some patients are mentally retarded. Although the disease is believed to be inherited in an autosomal recessive fashion, a preponderance of females has been reported.

Refsum syndrome (see also Sec. 7.36), a multisystemic disorder, is inherited as an autosomal recessive trait and becomes symptomatic during the 1st or 2nd decade of life. The ichthyosis is relatively mild and not clinically distinctive. Chronic polyneuritis with progressive paralysis and ataxia, atypical retinitis pigmentosa, anosmia, deafness, bony abnormalities, and electrocardiographic changes are the most characteristic features. Affected patients have a deficiency of the enzyme alpha-decarboxylase and cannot degrade phytic acid (a constituent of chlorophyll), which accumulates in the serum and tissues. Dietary avoidance of chlorophyll-containing foods is all that is available therapeutically.

Chondrodysplasia punctata (see also Sec. 23.22) includes several genetically heterogeneous disorders. Three major types have been distinguished: *Conradi-Hunermann syndrome*, inherited as an autosomal dominant trait; *rhizomelic dwarfism*, transmitted as an autosomal recessive trait; and an *X-linked dominant* form affecting females only. Approximately 25% of patients with the recessive or dominant type have cutaneous lesions, ranging from severe, generalized erythema and scaling to mild hyperkeratosis. Patients with the X-linked dominant form have a distinctive ichthyosiform eruption at birth. Thick, yellow, tightly adherent keratinized plaques are distributed in a whorled pattern over the entire body, which may be intensely erythematous. The histologic changes include hyperkeratosis that penetrates to the depths of the hair follicles. The eruption disappears completely during the first few weeks of life and may be superseded by a follicular atrophoderma. Patchy alopecia may be associated. Additional features in all variants include cataracts with or without optic atrophy, an abnormal facies with saddle nose and hypertelorism, and cardiovascular and central nervous system abnormalities. The pathognomonic defect, which also disappears with age, is stippled epiphyses in the cartilaginous skeleton. Other bony abnormalities consist of shortened femora and humeri, flexion contractures of joints, dysplasia of the hips, and asymmetrical deformities of the limbs.

A number of other rare syndromes with ichthyosis as a consistent feature include the following: *ichthyosis with keratitis and deafness (KID syndrome); ichthyosis with defective hair having a banded pattern under polarized light and a low sulfur content, and mental and growth retardation (trichothiodystrophy); ichthyosis with atrophy, mental retardation, dwarfism, and generalized aminoaciduria;* and *ichthyosis with mental retardation, dwarfism, and renal impairment.*

Keratoderma of palms and soles (keratosis palmaris et plantaris) is due to excessive accumulation of stratum corneum and may occur as a manifestation of a focal or generalized congenital hereditary skin disorder or may result from such chronic skin diseases as psoriasis, eczema, or pityriasis rubra pilaris.

Although strict classification is difficult, the hereditary types of keratoderma may be categorized as follows:

Diffuse hyperkeratosis of palms and soles (tylosis) is an autosomal dominant disorder characterized by sharply demarcated areas of scaling. Striate and punctate forms have also been described.

Localized epidermolytic hyperkeratosis of palms and soles is an autosomal dominant defect with characteristic histologic changes.

Mal de Meleda is a rare, progressive autosomal recessive condition characterized by erythema and thick scales on palms, soles, and dorsal surfaces of the limbs, hyperhidrosis, EEG abnormalities, and mental retardation.

Keratoma hereditaria mutilans (progressive dystrophic hyperkeratosis) is a progressive autosomal dominant disease with honeycombed hyperkeratosis of palms and soles, starfish-like linear and annular keratoses on the dorsum of the hands and feet, and ainhum-like constriction of the digits that at times leads to autoamputation. This disorder may be associated with scarring, alopecia, and deafness.

Papillon-Lefèvre syndrome is an autosomal recessive erythematous hyperkeratosis of palms and soles characterized by periodontal inflammation and early shedding of teeth, nail dystrophy, and ectopic calcification of the dura.

Keratoderma of palms and soles also occurs in association with corneal dystrophy and with carcinoma of the esophagus as an autosomal dominant trait and as a feature of pachyonychia congenita, ichthyosis, ectodermal dysplasia, dyskeratosis congenita, and tyrosinemia as well as of several other conditions.

Patients with hyperhidrosis may develop macerated plaques that become secondarily infected and malodorous. Morbidity is lessened if the hyperkeratosis can be controlled; however, treatment is difficult, and only mild palliation is achieved with applications of lubricants, keratolytic agents (urea, salicylic acid, lactic acid), and retinoic acid. Excision and split-skin grafting have been successful in patients with extreme hyperkeratosis and painful fissuring that cause chronic disability.

Acanthosis nigricans is a symmetrical dermatosis characterized by papillary hypertrophy and hyperpigmentation, which give the skin a velvety appearance and texture. The neck, axillae, genitalia, groin, umbilicus, and inner aspects of the thighs, elbows, and knees are most often affected. Mucous membranes are occasionally involved as are the palms and soles. Four types of acanthosis nigricans have been delineated:

Benign acanthosis nigricans, usually inherited as an autosomal dominant trait, is present at birth or may develop during childhood. The lesions may resemble widespread epidermal nevi.

Pseudoacanthosis nigricans is common in obese, dark-complexioned individuals and may be related to exogenous factors such as friction or to various endocrine disorders. This type may be induced by administration of diethylstilbestrol and nicotinic acid. Pseudoacanthosis nigricans is often reversible.

Syndromal acanthosis nigricans occurs as a feature of a number of disorders including the Seip-Lawrence, Bloom, and Rud syndromes.

Malignant acanthosis nigricans is only rarely observed during childhood and occurs mainly in association with adenocarcinoma of the gastrointestinal tract, breast, and lung.

Pachyonychia congenita is a heritable disorder transmitted as an autosomal dominant trait with variable expressivity. The salient features include keratoderma of the palms and soles, follicular hyperkeratosis, hyperhidrosis, oral leukokeratosis, and nail dystrophy. Less common findings include epidermal cysts, corneal dystrophy, natal teeth, and abnormalities of the hair. The nail dystrophy is the most striking feature and may be present at birth or develop early in life. The nails are thickened and tubular, projecting upward at the free edge to form a conical roof over a mass of subungual keratotic debris. Repeated paronychial inflammation may result in shedding of the nails.

Treatment is relatively ineffective, although keratolytic agents may be of some benefit. The oral leukokeratosis should be evaluated periodically since malignant change may occur as early as the 2nd decade of life.

Essential fatty acid deficiency may be responsible for generalized, scaly dermatitis that resembles congenital ichthyosis. The eruption has also been observed in patients sustained on fat-free diets or fat-free parenteral alimentation and is caused by a deficiency of linoleic and arachidonic acids. Additional manifestations of essential fatty acid deficiency include alopecia, thrombocytopenia, increased susceptibility to bacterial infections, and failure to thrive. Daily application of sunflower seed oil, which contains linoleic acid, may ameliorate the clinical and biochemical manifestations, but it does not readily replenish tissue stores of linoleic acid. This condition should be distinguished from ichthyosis since it is amenable to therapy.

24.17 DISEASES OF THE DERMIS

Granuloma annulare is a common dermatosis that occurs predominantly in children; it can be polymorphous. Typical lesions begin as erythematous, firm, flat-topped papulonodules; they gradually enlarge to form ring-shaped plaques with a normal, slightly atrophic or discolored central area (Fig. 24–33) up to several cm in size. Lesions occur most frequently on the dorsum of the hands and feet and on the scalp, trunk, arms, and legs. *Annular lesions* are often mistaken for tinea corporis because of the elevated advancing border; they differ in that they are almost never scaly. *Papular lesions,* another variant, may simulate rheumatoid nodules, particularly when grouped on the fingers and elbows. The generalized papular form is rare in children. *Subcutaneous granuloma annulare,* a less common form, may appear on the palms, soles, scalp, and limbs, particularly in the pretibial area. These lesions are firm, usually nontender, skin-colored nodules. They may be confused with other nodular and cystic lesions; identification of typical annular lesions elsewhere on the body will resolve the diagnostic dilemma.

Occasionally a biopsy is required for identification. Histologic changes are sufficiently characteristic to confirm the diagnosis. The lesions consist of a granuloma with a central area of necrotic collagen, mucin deposition, and a peripheral palisading infiltrate of lymphocytes, histiocytes, and foreign body giant cells. The pattern resembles that of necrobiosis lipoidica and rheumatoid nodule, but subtle histologic differences usually permit differentiation. The cause of granuloma annulare is unknown. Affected children are usually healthy. The eruption persists for months to years, but spontaneous resolution without residual change is usual. Application of a potent topical corticosteroid preparation or intralesional injec-

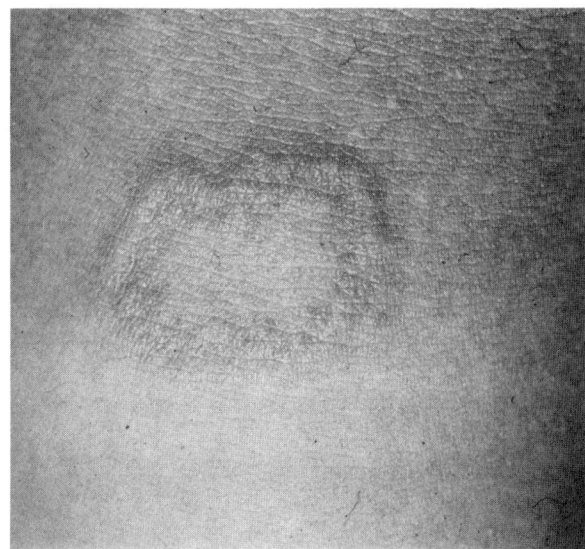

Figure 24–33. Annular lesion with a raised papular border and depressed center, characteristic of granuloma annulare.

tions of corticosteroid may hasten involution, but nonintervention is acceptable.

Lichen sclerosus et atrophicus, a dermatosis of unknown etiology, occurs rarely in children. Initial lesions consist of ivory-colored, shiny, indurated papules, often with violaceous halos that coalesce to form irregular atrophic plaques of variable size, in the margins of which hemorrhagic bullae may occur. Sites of predilection are the anogenital skin, buttocks, upper back, chest, forearms, and face. In boys, the prepuce and glans penis are involved most often. In girls, extensive involvement of the anogenital area may produce a sclerotic, atrophic plaque of hourglass configuration. Severe itching and burning are common.

Lichen sclerosus et atrophicus in children is most frequently confused with focal scleroderma (morphea). Biopsy is diagnostic, demonstrating hyperkeratosis, atrophy of the epidermis, edema and degeneration of the basal cell layer, homogenization of the collagen fibers, and edema of the upper dermis. The lesions may involute spontaneously and, in children, resolve without residua. Resolution has coincided with menarche. Corticosteroid creams have provided relief from pruritus. Topical estrogen and androgen preparations have been used for genital lesions. None has been invariably curative; the risks of side effects must be weighed against the benefits of therapy.

Macular atrophies (anetoderma) may occur in the absence of inflammation (primary macular atrophy) or as a sequel of an inflammatory process (secondary macular atrophy). Lesions vary from 0.5 to 1 cm in diameter and, if inflammatory, may initially be erythematous but subsequently become thinned, wrinkled, and blue-white in color or hypopigmented. Often the lesions protrude as small outpouchings that, on palpation, may be readily indented into the subcutaneous tissue because of the dermal atrophy. Secondary macular atrophy may follow cutaneous lesions of lupus erythematosus, sarcoidosis, and certain other dermatoses.

All types of macular atrophy show loss of elastic tissue on histopathologic examination, a change which is not recognizable unless special stains are used. These lesions occasionally resemble morphea, lichen sclerosus et atrophicus, or end-stage lesions of chronic bullous dermatoses.

Necrobiosis lipoidica is rare in children and is usually associated with diabetes mellitus. The lesions begin as erythematous papules and evolve into irregularly shaped, yellow, sclerotic plaques with central telangiectasia and a violaceous border. Scaling, crusting, and ulceration are frequent. Preferred sites are the pretibial areas, but plaques may occur on the arms, trunk, and scalp. Histologically, necrosis of collagen, a granulomatous infiltrate, deposition of lipid, and proliferation of the small dermal vessels are evident. Necrobiosis must be differentiated clinically from xanthomas, morphea, and pretibial myxedema. The lesions persist in spite of good control of the diabetes but may improve minimally after local injection of a corticosteroid.

Keloid is a sharply demarcated benign growth of connective tissue in the dermis; it is composed of whorled and interlaced hyalinized collagen fibers. The lesions are firm, raised, pink, and rubbery; they may be tender or extremely pruritic. Sites of predilection are the face, ears, sternum, and extremities. Keloids are usually induced by trauma and commonly follow ear piercing, burns and scalds, and surgical procedures. Certain individuals, especially blacks, seem predisposed to keloid formation. Keloids may enlarge to form grotesque excrescences with numerous claw-like projections, and, on the ear lobe, where they tend to be round, may hang in a pendulous fashion.

Keloids must be differentiated from hypertrophic scars, which differ histologically. Young keloids may diminish in size if injected intralesionally at 2 wk intervals with triamcin-

olone suspension (10 mg/mL). At times a more concentrated suspension is required. Large or old keloids may require surgical excision to be followed by intralesional injections of corticosteroid. The risk of recurrence at the same site argues against surgical excision alone.

Striae distensae are thinned, depressed, erythematous bands of atrophic skin that, with time, become silvery, opalescent, and smooth in consistency. They occur most frequently in areas that have been subject to distention, such as the lower back, buttocks, thighs, breasts, abdomen, and shoulders. The most frequent causes are rapid growth, pregnancy, obesity, Cushing disease, or prolonged corticosteroid therapy. The lesions result from rupture, retraction, and disintegration of the dermal elastic fibers.

Scleredema (scleredema adultorum, scleredema of Buschke) occurs in children as well as in adults. The onset is sudden with brawny edema of the face and neck that spreads rapidly to involve the thorax and arms but usually spares the abdomen, hands, and feet. The face acquires a waxy, mask-like appearance; the involved areas feel indurated and woody and are nonpitting. The overlying skin cannot be wrinkled, but it is normal in color and there are no atrophic changes. Systemic involvement, which is uncommon, is marked by thickening of the tongue, dysarthria, dysphagia, restriction of eye movements, and pleural, pericardial, and peritoneal effusions. Electrocardiographic changes may also be observed.

The disease often follows an infection such as tonsillitis, influenza, or scarlet fever after an interval of days or weeks, but its cause remains obscure. Onset may be heralded by a prodrome of fever, arthralgia, myalgia, and malaise. Laboratory data are not helpful. Skin biopsy demonstrates an increase in dermal thickness due to swelling and homogenization of the collagen bundles, which are separated by large interfibrous spaces. Increased amounts of mucopolysaccharides in the dermis can be identified by special stains.

The active phase of the disease persists for 2–8 wk; spontaneous and complete resolution usually occurs in 6 mo–2 yr. Recurrent attacks are unusual. The disorder must be differentiated from scleroderma, myxedema, trichinosis, dermatomyositis, and other conditions causing widespread edema. There is no specific therapy.

Lipoid proteinosis, an autosomal recessive disorder, may be initially noted in early infancy as hoarseness. Skin lesions appear during childhood and consist of yellowish papules and nodules which may coalesce to form plaques on the face, forearms, neck, genitalia, dorsum of the fingers, and scalp, where they result in patchy alopecia. Similar deposits are found on the lips, tongue, fauces, uvula, epiglottis, and vocal cords. Translucent nodules along the margins of the eyelids are the most characteristic clinical manifestation. Hypertrophic, hyperkeratotic nodules occur at sites of friction such as the elbows and knees; the palms may be diffusely thickened. The distinctive histologic pattern includes extreme dilatation of the dermal blood vessels and infiltration of the dermis with extracellular hyaline material, which is also deposited in the vessel walls. Calcification of the hippocampal gyri, identifiable roentgenographically, is pathognomonic but not always present. The biochemical defect is unknown; the infiltrates appear to contain both lipid and mucopolysaccharide substances. There is no specific treatment.

Cutis laxa (dermatomegaly, generalized elastolysis) is a congenital disorder inherited as an autosomal recessive or autosomal dominant trait. A newborn infant may appear prematurely aged. When onset appears to occur during childhood or adulthood, usually after a febrile illness or a course of drug therapy, the disorder is designated as acquired cutis laxa; such clinical expression may, however, represent the variable expressivity of the congenital types.

In all forms of cutis laxa, the skin hangs in pendulous folds.

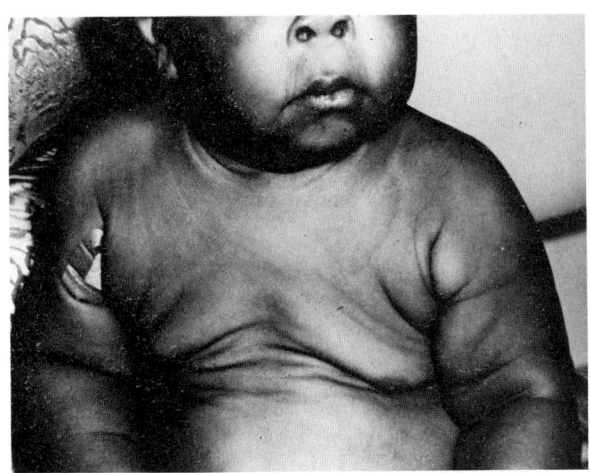

Figure 24-34. Pendulous folds of skin of an infant with cutis laxa. Note the long upper lip and upturned nose.

Characteristic facial features include an aged appearance with sagging jowls ("bloodhound" appearance), a hooked nose with everted nostrils, a short columella, a long upper lip, and everted lower eyelids. The skin is lax elsewhere on the body as well and may resemble an ill-fitting suit (Fig. 24-34). Hyperelasticity and hypermobility of the joints are not present as they are in the Ehlers-Danlos syndrome. Many infants have a hoarse cry, probably due to laxity of the vocal cords. Tensile strength of the skin is normal. Histologically, elastic tissue is reduced throughout the dermis, with fragmentation, distention, and clumping of the elastic fibers.

The dominant form of cutis laxa is generally benign and mainly of cosmetic significance; a few affected individuals have had mild cardiovascular or pulmonary manifestations. In contrast, the recessive form of the disease is prone to severe complications such as multiple hernias, diaphragmatic atony, diverticula of the gastrointestinal and genitourinary tracts, and cardiopulmonary disease with emphysema, peripheral pulmonary artery stenosis, and aortic dilatation. Patients often have a shortened life span. Skeletal anomalies, growth retardation, and developmental delay also occur. Plastic procedures may be helpful in ameliorating the cutaneous defect.

Ehlers-Danlos syndrome is a genetically heterogeneous connective tissue disorder whose severity varies because of mild or incomplete forms of the disease. Affected children appear normal at birth. The most striking feature is the hyperelasticity, fragility, and bruisability of the skin. It has been classified into 10 distinct clinical forms:

I. *Gravis type*—autosomal dominant. Skin hyperelasticity and fragility, easy bruising, generalized and severe joint hypermobility, preterm birth.

II. *Mitis type*—autosomal dominant. Mild skin and joint manifestations, the latter limited to hands and feet.

III. *Benign, hypermobile type*—autosomal dominant. Generalized severe joint hypermobility and minimal skin manifestations.

IV. *Ecchymotic (Sack) type*—autosomal dominant. Joint hypermobility limited to digits, skin hyperextensibility minimal, severe bruisability with prominent venous network, extensive ecchymoses from trauma, high incidence of keloids and contractures, rupture of bowel and great vessels common. Absence of type III collagen.

V. *X-linked type.* Limited joint hypermobility, extensive hyperelasticity, moderate bruising, fragility, and scarring. Lysyl oxidase deficiency.

VI. *Ocular type*—autosomal recessive. Ocular abnormalities (fragile cornea, sclera, deformed cornea), joint hyperextensi-

bility, skin hyperelasticity, fragile bones. Lysyl hydroxylase deficiency.

VII. *Arthrochalasis multiplex congenita*—autosomal recessive. Short stature, marked joint hyperextensibility and dislocation, moderate hyperelasticity and bruisability of skin. Procollagen peptidase deficiency.

VIII. *Periodontitis type*—autosomal dominant. Mild skin hyperelasticity, joint hypermobility and bruisability, moderate cutaneous fragility, and severe periodontitis leading to premature loss of teeth and alveolar bone.

IX. *X-linked skeletal type*—X-linked. Occipital exostoses, widening and bowing of long bones at tendinous and ligamentous insertion sites, deformed clavicles, mild skin hyperelasticity. Abnormal copper metabolism, lysyl oxidase deficiency.

X. *Dysfibronectinemic type*—autosomal recessive. Fibronectin-correctable failure of platelet aggregation, easy bruisability, joint hypermobility, skin hyperextensibility.

Ehlers-Danlos syndrome has been confused with cutis laxa, but the features of the two disorders differ considerably. The skin in Ehlers-Danlos syndrome is hyperextensible and snaps back into place when stretched. Because of its marked fragility, minor trauma results in ecchymoses, bleeding, and poor healing with atrophic cigarette-paper scars, which are most prominent on the forehead and lower legs and over pressure points. Surgical procedures are fraught with risk; dehiscence of wounds is common. Additional cutaneous manifestations include molluscoid pseudotumors over pressure points, small, subcutaneous, lipid-containing cysts that often calcify, and redundant skin on the palms and soles. Joint hypermobility with skeletal deformity, ocular defects, and ruptures of the bowel, great vessels, and lung are the major complications. Hernias and gastrointestinal diverticula may also occur.

All types of Ehlers-Danlos syndrome have been attributed to a defect of collagen; specific procollagen defects have been identified in types IV, VI, and VII disease.

There is no specific treatment for this group of disorders and, though death may occur secondary to the internal manifestations of the disease, life expectancy is usually normal. Orthopedic management with braces and physical therapy may improve musculoskeletal function; surgical intervention may be indicated to correct vascular or bleeding abnormalities.

Pseudoxanthoma elasticum is a rare, heritable, disorder of elastic tissue that involves the skin, eyes, cardiovascular system, and gastrointestinal tract. Of four distinct forms of the disease, two are transmitted in autosomal dominant fashion, two in autosomal recessive.

Onset of skin manifestations often occurs during childhood, but the changes produced by early lesions are subtle and may not be recognized. The characteristic cutaneous lesions are asymptomatic; 1–3 mm yellow papules are arranged in a linear or reticulated pattern or in confluent plaques. Preferred sites are the neck, axillary and inguinal folds, umbilicus, and antecubital and popliteal fossae. As the lesions become more pronounced, the skin acquires a velvety texture and droops in lax, inelastic folds. Mucous membrane lesions may involve lips, buccal cavity, rectum, and vagina. Additional manifestations include visual disturbances, angioid streaks and other chorioretinal changes, intermittent claudication, cerebral and coronary occlusion, hypertension, and hemorrhage from the gastrointestinal tract and uterus.

The four forms of the disorder can be distinguished by pedigree data and the clinical patterns. Most of the features described above occur in each of the two autosomal dominant forms of the disease; they differ principally in the incidence of vascular and ophthalmologic complications. Patients with the type 1 disorder tend to have extensive disease with numerous complications, whereas those with type 2 have a less prominent macular skin eruption and low incidences of vascular involvement and of debilitating ophthalmologic disease. Patients with the recessive type 1 form have the classic flexural skin changes, but vascular changes are minimal, and the degenerative retinopathy is localized. In the recessive type 2 form there is elastic tissue degeneration of the entire integument, in contrast to the flexural accentuation in the other forms of the disease, and systemic involvement does not occur.

The basic defect is unknown. Pathologic and clinical manifestations are related to deposition of calcium and to degenerative changes in the elastic fibers of the skin and blood vessels. Because of the serious nature of the systemic complications, even suggestive skin changes are an indication for skin biopsy. There is no effective therapy.

Elastosis perforans serpiginosa is an unusual skin disorder in which 1–3 mm, skin-colored, keratotic, firm papules tend to cluster in arcuate and annular patterns on the posterolateral neck and limbs and occasionally on the face and trunk. Onset usually occurs during childhood or adolescence. The etiology is unknown, but of particular interest is the frequent coexistence of this disorder with others such as osteogenesis imperfecta, Marfan syndrome, pseudoxanthoma elasticum, Ehlers-Danlos syndrome, Rothmund-Thomson syndrome, and Down syndrome.

Proliferation, thickening, and branching of dermal elastic fibers which perforate the epidermis and stimulate a reactive epidermal hyperplasia and inflammatory response are diagnostic. Differential diagnosis includes tinea corporis, granuloma annulare, lichen planus, creeping eruption, and porokeratosis of Mibelli. Treatment is ineffective; however, the lesions are asymptomatic and disappear spontaneously.

Xanthomas. (Sec. 7.39–7.46.)

Farber disease (lipogranulomatosis). (Sec. 7.33.)

The **mucopolysaccharidoses (MPS)** are distinguished by differences in clinical and genetic patterns and specific enzymatic defects (Sec. 7.24). In several of these disorders, thick, inelastic, rough skin, particularly on the extremities, and generalized hirsutism are characteristic but nonspecific features. Telangiectasias on the face, forearms, trunk, and legs have been observed in the Scheic and Morquio syndromes. In some patients with Hunter syndrome, distinctive lesions have been noted; they are skin- to ivory-colored papulonodules that aggregate to form plaques on the upper trunk, arms, and thighs. They are firm and have a corrugated surface texture. Onset of these unusual lesions occurs during the 1st decade, and spontaneous disappearance has been noted.

Biopsies of affected skin and nodular lesions demonstrate thickening of the dermis with swelling and separation of the collagen bundles and deposition of metachromatic material. The epidermal cells may be vacuolated, and large mononuclear "gargoyle" cells, which also contain metachromatic material, may be identified in the upper dermis.

Mastocytosis encompasses a spectrum of disorders that range from solitary cutaneous nodules to diffuse infiltration of skin associated with involvement of other organs. All the disorders are characterized by aggregates of tissue mast cells in the dermis; the local and systemic manifestations of the disease are due to release of histamine and heparin from mast cell granules. Biopsy of involved skin is diagnostic provided special stains such as Giemsa or toluidine blue are employed to identify the infiltrates of mast cells.

Affected children may have intense pruritus. Systemic signs of histamine release, such as episodic flushing, tachycardia, respiratory distress, headache, colic, diarrhea, hypotension, and syncope, occur most frequently in the more severe types of mastocytosis. Flushing can be precipitated by excessively hot baths, by vigorous rubbing of the skin, and by certain drugs such as codeine, aspirin, morphine, atropine, and polymyxin B. Avoidance of these triggering factors will reduce

discomfort considerably. For those patients who are symptomatic, oral antihistamines may be palliative.

The cause is unknown. Most cases are sporadic; rarely, other family members have been affected.

Mastocytomas are solitary lesions that constitute approximately 10% of childhood cases of mastocytosis. Lesions may be present at birth or arise during early infancy; they can occur at any site, although the wrist, neck, and trunk are sites of predilection. Initially the lesions may present as recurrent, evanescent wheals or bullae; however, in time, an infiltrated, rubbery, pink, yellow, or tan plaque develops at the site of whealing or blistering (Fig. 24–35A). The surface acquires a pebbly, orange-peel–like texture, and hyperpigmentation may become prominent. Stroking or trauma to the nodule may result in urtication (Darier sign); rarely, systemic signs of histamine release become apparent. The differential diagnosis includes recurrent bullous impetigo, nevi, and juvenile xanthogranuloma. Mastocytomas usually involute spontaneously during early childhood; troublesome lesions can be excised and do not recur. Only rarely do multiple cutaneous lesions develop.

Urticaria pigmentosa is the most common form of mastocytosis and occurs primarily in infants and children; onset occurs before the 2nd yr. Lesions may be present at birth but more often erupt in crops over a period of several months. In some cases, early lesions are bullous or urticarial and fade repeatedly only to recur at the same site until they become fixed and hyperpigmented; in others, the initial lesions are hyperpigmented. Vesiculation usually abates by age 2 yr. Individual lesions range in size from a few mm to several cm and may be macular, papular, or nodular; in color they range from yellow-tan to chocolate brown and often have ill-defined borders (Fig. 24–35B). Larger nodular lesions, like mastocytomas, may have a characteristic orange-peel texture (Fig. 24–35C).

Lesions may be sparse or numerous and are often symmetrically distributed. Palms, soles, and face are sometimes spared, as are the mucous membranes. The rapid appearance of erythema and whealing in response to vigorous stroking of a lesion (Darier sign) can usually be elicited; dermographism of intervening normal skin is also common. Urticaria pigmentosa can be confused with drug eruptions, postinflammatory pigmentary change, juvenile xanthogranuloma, pigmented nevi, ephelides, xanthomas, chronic urticaria, insect bites, and bullous impetigo.

The prognosis is good; spontaneous involution occurs in about 50% of patients by puberty; another 25% will have partial resolution by adulthood.

Diffuse mastocytosis is characterized by diffuse involvement of the skin rather than discrete hyperpigmented lesions. Rarely, there are no discernible skin changes, but usually the skin appears thickened and pink to yellow in color; it may also have a doughy feel and rough texture. Surface changes are accentuated in the flexural areas. Recurrent bullae, intractable pruritus, and flushing attacks are common, as is systemic involvement.

Systemic mastocytosis occurs in approximately 5–10% of patients with mastocytosis. Bone lesions may be silent but are detectable radiologically as osteoporotic or osteosclerotic areas, principally in the axial skeleton. Gastrointestinal tract involvement may produce diarrhea and steatorrhea. Mucosal infiltrates may be detectable by barium studies or by small bowel biopsy. Peptic ulcers also occur. Hepatosplenomegaly due to mast cell infiltrates and fibrosis has been described, as well as mast cell proliferation in lymph nodes, kidneys, periadrenal fat, bone marrow, and peripheral blood. The prognosis is guarded.

The need for laboratory studies is determined by the symptoms and physical findings. Urinary excretion of free hista-

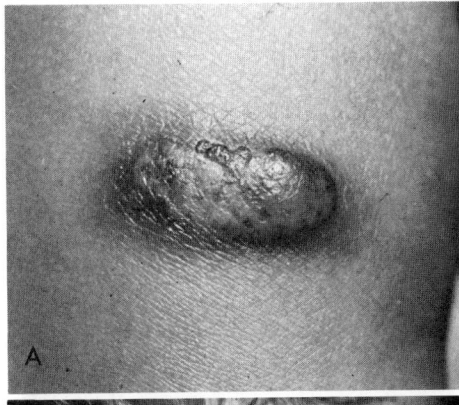
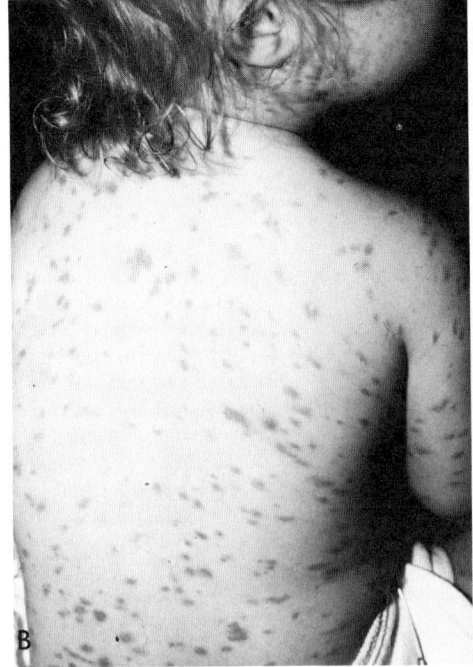
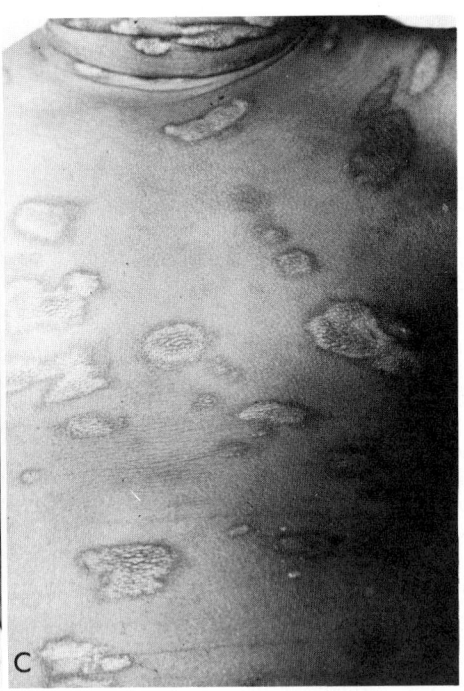

Figure 24–35. *A*, Solitary mastocytoma that is partially blistered. *B*, Hyperpigmented papular lesions of urticaria pigmentosa, some of which exhibit a surrounding flare. *C*, Infiltrated plaques of urticaria pigmentosa.

mine and its metabolites is increased. Coagulation abnormalities are rare.

Epidermal inclusion cysts are sharply circumscribed, firm, freely movable, skin-colored nodules, often with a central dimple or dilated pore. They form most frequently on the face, neck, or trunk and may periodically become inflamed and secondarily infected. The wall of the cyst is composed of stratified epithelium that surrounds a mass of layered keratinized material which may have a cheesy consistency. Epidermal cysts may be confused with dermatofibromas, branchial cleft cysts, and small lipomas. Excision of the cysts with removal of the entire sac and its contents is the appropriate procedure.

24.18 DISORDERS OF SUBCUTANEOUS TISSUE

Diseases involving the subcutis are usually characterized histologically by necrosis or inflammation; either may occur as a primary event or as a secondary response to a variety of stimuli or disease processes. Unfortunately, these disorders are not all separable on the basis of the histologic changes; the histologic pattern may merely reflect the stage of the lesion at biopsy. The principal diagnostic criteria the clinician must rely on are the appearance and distribution of the

lesions, the associated symptoms, and his or her appreciation of the exogenous provocative factors.

Lipogranulomatosis subcutanea (Rothmann-Makai syndrome) is a type of panniculitis that occurs mainly in children, most frequently on the legs but occasionally on the arms and trunk. Typically, nodules appear singly or a few at a time and are unaccompanied by fever or other constitutional symptoms. The nodules are 0.5–3 cm in diameter, tender, firm, and elastic; they may be skin-colored or hyperemic; and rarely they rupture and discharge liquefied material. Duration of an individual lesion is several weeks, but new ones appear over a period of 6–12 mo; the disease is usually self-limited.

Histologic findings vary with the stage of the lesion. In the acute stage, necrotic foci are surrounded by polymorphonuclear leukocytes. Subsequent granuloma formation with phagocytosis of fat by histiocytes is finally superseded by a fibrotic stage with homogenization of connective tissue fibers. Lipogranulomatosis subcutanea must be differentiated from Weber-Christian panniculitis, nodular vasculitis, erythema nodosum, and erythema induratum. There is no known effective treatment.

Weber-Christian panniculitis. (Sec. 10.81.)

Corticosteroid atrophy. The injection of a corticosteroid intradermally can produce deep atrophy accompanied by surface pigmentary changes and telangiectasia. These changes occur approximately 2 wk after injection and may last for months. The deltoid area is most susceptible to this complication; lesions also occur on the buttocks and thighs.

Postcorticosteroid panniculitis has been observed in children who have received corticosteroids orally for relatively short periods of time. Within 1–2 wk after discontinuation of the drug, multiple nodules appear on the face, trunk, and arms. Lesions range in size from 0.5 to 4.0 cm; they are erythematous or skin-colored and may be pruritic. The mechanism of the inflammatory reaction in the fat is unknown. Treatment is unnecessary, as the lesions remit spontaneously without scarring.

Cold panniculitis may result in localized lesions in infants after prolonged cold exposure, especially on the cheeks, or after prolonged application of a cold object such as an ice cube, ice bag, or Popsicle to any area of the skin. Erythematous, indurated lesions arise within hours of exposure, persist for 2–3 wk, and heal without residua. The pathogenic mechanism may be similar to that of subcutaneous fat necrosis (below and Sec. 14.85).

Lipodystrophy. Several rare conditions are associated with loss of fatty tissue in a partial or generalized distribution.

Partial lipodystrophy occurs more commonly in females, often with onset during the 1st decade. There is gradual symmetrical loss of subcutaneous tissue over the face, upper trunk, and arms, resulting in a cadaverous facies and marked disproportion between the upper and lower halves of the body. Loss of adipose tissue is not preceded by an inflammatory phase, and histologic examination reveals only absence of subcutaneous fat. Some patients have had associated renal disease, disordered glucose metabolism, or abnormal serum lipid profiles. The etiology of the disorder is not understood, and there is no effective treatment.

Congenital generalized lipodystrophy (Seip-Lawrence syndrome) is a progressive multisystem disorder inherited as an autosomal recessive trait. The earliest manifestation is generalized loss of subcutaneous and visceral fat; it may be evident at birth or occur during early infancy. Associated cutaneous changes include prominent superficial veins, hirsutism, and skin pigmentation with acanthosis nigricans. Accelerated skeletal and muscle growth and advanced bone age are seen. Abnormalities of carbohydrate homeostasis, insulin production, and growth hormone appear to be age-dependent. Hyperlipidemia, hyperinsulinism, and insulin-resistant nonketotic diabetes mellitus develop gradually and are reflected by increasing hepatomegaly due to fatty infiltration and cirrhosis. Serum levels of growth hormone may be normal, but its secretion in response to stimuli may be disturbed. Hypothalamic releasing factors not ordinarily found in plasma have been identified in affected patients and suggest a lack of hypothalamic regulation. There is no treatment.

Sclerema neonatorum is an uncommon disorder of adipose tissue that occurs primarily in preterm, sick, or debilitated infants. There is abrupt onset of a diffuse and generalized hardening of the skin, which becomes stony in consistency, cold, and nonpitting. Joint mobility may be compromised, and the face assumes a mask-like expression owing to inflexibility of the skin.

Sclerematous change is nonspecific and virtually always associated with serious illness such as sepsis, gastroenteritis, pneumonia, or multiple congenital anomalies. The appearance of sclerema in a sick infant should be regarded as an ominous prognostic sign. The outcome depends upon the response to treatment of the underlying disorder. When recovery is imminent, sclerema tends to disappear rapidly.

The histologic changes in sclerema consist only of edema and thickening of the connective tissue septa. Early and extensive subcutaneous fat necrosis may resemble sclerema, but the evolution of the process usually permits differentiation. Edema of the newborn is localized to dependent parts, pits easily with pressure, and should not be confused with sclerema.

Scleroderma. (Sec. 10.71.)

Subcutaneous fat necrosis is an inflammatory disorder of adipose tissue that occurs primarily in the newborn infant. Sites of predilection are the buttocks, thighs, back, upper arms, and face. Lesions may be focal or extensive and may be preceded by a brawny edema of the affected skin. Typical well-developed lesions are firm, irregular nodules that may be skin-colored or have a red or violaceous hue (Fig. 24–36, p. xxviii). They appear to be tender during the acute phase.

Uncomplicated lesions involute spontaneously within weeks to months, usually without scarring or atrophy. Occasionally, calcium deposition may occur within areas of fat necrosis and at times may result in rupture and drainage of liquid material. Rarely, constitutional symptoms such as hypotonia, poor feeding, vomiting, and fever are complications. Hypercalcemia and hyperlipemia have also been associated.

Fat necrosis in the infant has been attributed to birth trauma, asphyxia, overexposure to cold, and prolonged hypothermia, but in many of the affected infants no provocative factors are identified. Susceptibility has been attributed to differences in composition between the subcutaneous tissue of young infants and that of older infants and children. Clinical studies have demonstrated a high melting point and an altered ratio of saturated to unsaturated fatty acids. Nevertheless, the pathogenesis is poorly understood.

Subcutaneous fat necrosis can be confused with sclerema neonatorum, panniculitis, or hematoma. Histologic changes are diagnostic and consist of thickening of the fibrous septa, increased vascularity, crystal deposition within the fat cells, and a granulomatous cellular infiltrate composed of lymphocytes, histiocytes, foreign body giant cells, and fibroblasts. Lipid-stained frozen sections are required to demonstrate the crystals, which are dissolved by fixatives. Since the lesions are self-limited, therapy is not required. Careful needle aspiration of fluctuant lesions may prevent rupture and subsequent scarring; the possibility of introducing infection, however, must be considered.

24.19 DISEASES OF THE SWEAT GLANDS

Miliaria, or *prickly heat*, as it is known to the layman, results from retention of sweat in ducts and pores of the eccrine sweat glands when they are occluded by keratinous plugs. Retrograde pressure may result in rupture of the duct and leakage of sweat into the dermis, where an inflammatory response is evoked. The eruption is most often induced by hot, humid weather, but it may also be caused by high fever. Infants who are kept too warmly dressed indoors may develop this eruption even in wintertime.

In *miliaria crystallina* the lesions are very superficial and noninflammatory. The tiny clear vesicles rupture readily with gentle pressure. They can erupt suddenly and occur in profusion over large areas of the body surface (Fig. 24–37). The clarity of the fluid, the extreme superficiality of the vesicles, and the absence of inflammation permit differentiation from other blistering disorders. This type of miliaria occurs most frequently in newborn infants and in older patients with hyperpyrexia. *Miliaria rubra* is a less superficial eruption and is characterized by papulovesicles with intense erythema. The lesions are usually localized to sites of occlusion or to flexural areas where the skin may become macerated and eroded. This lesion may be confused with or superimposed on other diaper area eruptions including candidosis and folliculitis.

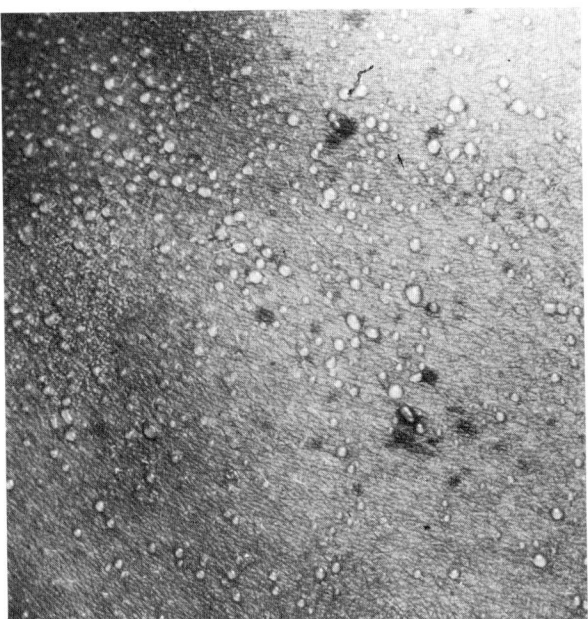

Figure 24–37. Superficial clear vesicles of miliaria crystallina in a patient with hyperpyrexia and lymphoma.

Pustular miliaria, unusual in children, is often a consequence of sweat retention associated with an underlying dermatitis.

All forms of miliaria respond dramatically to cooling the patient by regulation of environmental temperatures and removal of excessive clothing and, in patients with fever, to administration of antipyretics. Topical agents are usually ineffective and may exacerbate the eruption. A cool bath is often helpful in alleviating pruritus.

Hidradenitis suppurativa, an inflammatory suppurative disease of the apocrine glands, is a chronic, indolent disorder which involves the axillae and genitocrural area and, rarely, the scalp and mammary and umbilical skin. Onset usually occurs during puberty or early adulthood. The disease is probably initiated by plugging of apocrine gland ducts with keratinous debris. Progressive dilatation below the obstruction leads to rupture of the duct and inflammation and often to secondary bacterial infection. Healing is by fibrosis and scarring. Clinically, affected patients have solitary or multiple painful, erythematous nodules, deep abscesses, and contracted scars, sharply confined to areas of skin containing apocrine glands. When the disease is severe and chronic, sinus tracts, ulcers, and fistulas develop.

Early lesions are often mistaken for infected epidermal cysts or for furuncles (abscesses of the hair follicles), but the sharp localization to particular areas of the body should suggest hidradenitis.

Systemic antibiotics chosen on the basis of bacterial culture and sensitivity tests should be administered in the acute phase even though such therapy is not always effective. Warm compresses will encourage spontaneous rupture of abscesses; those which are "pointing" should be incised and drained. The addition of a limited course of prednisone (40–60 mg/24 hr) to the regimen of patients who respond poorly to antibiotics may decrease fibrosis and scarring. Axillary shaving and the use of deodorants should be avoided. Ultimately, surgical measures are required for control or cure. Solitary lesions can be excised and closed by primary intention, and sinus tracts and fistulas should be exteriorized and excised. Extensive involvement may require removal of all diseased tissue and placement of skin grafts. Surgical management should not be withheld in the mistaken belief that such an approach is radical.

Table 24–3. Causes of and Conditions Associated with Hypertrichosis

1. *Intrinsic factors*
   Racial and familial forms such as hairy ears, hairy elbows, intraphalangeal hair, or generalized hirsutism
2. *Extrinsic factors*
   Local trauma or casts
   Drugs
      Diazoxide, phenytoin, corticosteroids, corticotropin, androgens, anabolic agents, hexachlorobenzene, minoxidil
3. *Hamartomas or nevi*
   Congenital pigmented nevocytic nevus, nevus pilosus, Becker nevus, congenital smooth muscle hamartoma
4. *Endocrine disorders*
   Virilizing ovarian tumors, Cushing syndrome, acromegaly, congenital adrenal hyperplasia, adrenal tumors, gonadal dysgenesis, male pseudohermaphroditism, nonendocrine hormone–secreting tumors
5. *Congenital and genetic disorders*
   Hypertrichosis lanuginosa, mucopolysaccharidoses, leprechaunism, congenital generalized lipodystrophy, Cornelia de Lange syndrome, craniofacial dysostosis, trisomy 18, Rubinstein-Taybi syndrome, Bloom syndrome, congenital hemihypertrophy, gingival fibromatosis with hypertrichosis. Porphyrias

24.20 DISORDERS OF HAIR

Disorders of hair in infants and children may be due to intrinsic disturbances of hair growth; to structural anomalies of the hair shafts, or to underlying biochemical or metabolic defects. Excessive and abnormal hair growth is referred to as hypertrichosis or hirsutism. Deficient hair growth is known as hypotrichosis, and hair loss, partial or complete, is termed alopecia. Alopecia may be classified as nonscarring or scarring; the latter type is rare in children and, if present, is most often due to prolonged or untreated inflammatory conditions such as pyoderma or tinea capitis.

Hypertrichosis

Hypertrichosis is rare in children and may be localized or generalized, permanent or transient. Localized hypertrichosis is most often due to a heritable condition or to a nevoid defect. Generalized hypertrichosis has many causes; some are listed in Table 24–3.

Hypotrichosis and Alopecia

Some of the disorders associated with hypotrichosis and alopecia are listed in Table 24–4. True alopecia is only rarely congenital; it is more often related to infections, an inflammatory dermatosis, drug ingestion, or mechanical factors. Hair loss as well as alterations in texture and quality are

Table 24–4. Disorders Associated with Alopecia and Hypotrichosis

1. Congenital universal alopecia, atrichia with papular lesions
2. Localized congenital alopecia: aplasia cutis, alopecia triangularis
3. Ectodermal dysplasias
4. Heritable syndromes: Marie-Unna hypotrichosis, Cockayne, progeria, Rothmund-Thomson, dyskeratosis congenita, Seckel, cartilage-hair hypoplasia, Conradi, trichorhinophalangeal, pachyonychia congenita, Hallerman-Streiff, Treacher Collins, popliteal web, oculodentodigital, oral-facial-digital, incontinentia pigmenti, focal dermal hypoplasia, keratosis follicularis spirulosa decalvans
5. Metabolic defects: homocystinuria, acrodermatitis enteropathica
6. Hamartomas of the scalp and the hair follicles

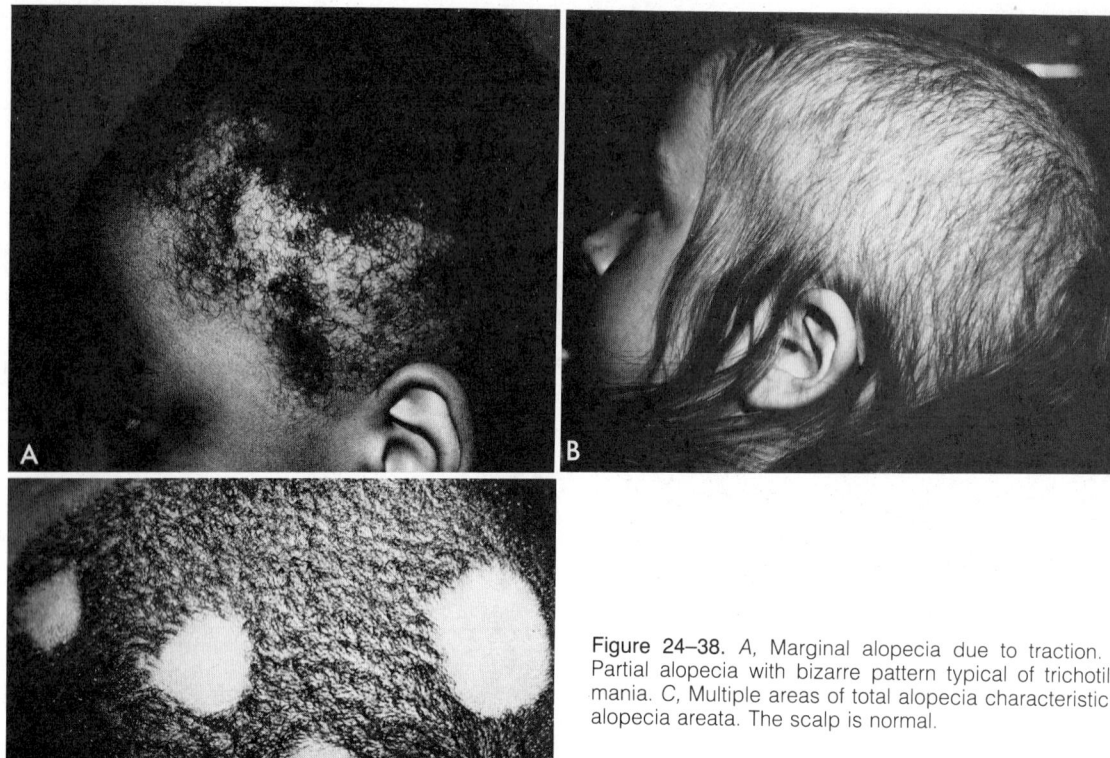

Figure 24–38. *A,* Marginal alopecia due to traction. *B,* Partial alopecia with bizarre pattern typical of trichotillomania. *C,* Multiple areas of total alopecia characteristic of alopecia areata. The scalp is normal.

associated with some of the endocrinopathies that involve the ovary, thyroid, parathyroid, adrenal, or pituitary glands. Bacterial, viral, and fungal infections of the scalp may also cause focal or diffuse hair loss. Metabolic disturbances, such as protein deprivation, celiac disease, hypervitaminosis A, and hypozincemia are additional causes. Any inflammatory condition of the scalp, such as atopic dermatitis or seborrheic dermatitis, if severe enough, may result in partial alopecia. In all these disorders, hair growth will return to normal if the underlying condition is treated successfully unless there has been permanent damage to the hair follicle.

Telogen effluvium, or loss of scalp hair because of premature conversion of growing hairs to the resting phase, accounts for the loss of hair by infants during the first few months of life, for postpartum loss, and for that lost 2–4 mo after an acute febrile illness. Telogen effluvium may also occur after discontinuation of oral contraceptives. There is no inflammatory reaction; the hair follicles remain intact, and telogen bulbs can be demonstrated microscopically on shed hairs. Since more than 50% of the scalp hair is rarely lost, alopecia is usually not severe; the sudden loss of large amounts of hair with brushing, combing, and washing of hair, however, can generate considerable anxiety. Parents should be reassured that normal hair growth will return shortly and alopecia will not be permanent.

Traction alopecia (marginal or traumatic alopecia) that results in follicular damage may be caused by tight braiding or "ponytails," headbands, rubber bands, curlers, and rollers (Fig. 24–38A). Associated folliculitis in the parietal areas, if severe, may cause scarring. The alopecia is usually reversible; children and parents must be encouraged to avoid these devices and, if necessary, alter the hair style. Otherwise, irreparable damage to hair follicles may occur.

Toxic alopecia is a side effect of radiation and certain drugs. Cancer chemotherapeutic agents, such as antimetabolites, alkylating agents, and mitotic inhibitors, inhibit synthesis of hair in growing (anagen) follicles. Hairs become dystrophic, and the hair shaft breaks at the narrowed segment. Loss is diffuse, rapid (1–3 wk after treatment), and temporary; regrowth occurs when administration of the drug(s) is discontinued. Thallium, heparin, and the coumarins induce shedding of the hair by converting it from the growing (anagen) to the resting (telogen) phase. Hair loss is diffuse and temporary.

Trichotillomania, or compulsive pulling, twisting, and breaking of hair, is responsible for irregular areas of incomplete hair loss. These are most often located on the crown and in the occipital and parietal areas of the scalp (Fig. 24–38B), but occasionally eyebrows, eyelashes, and body hair are traumatized. Some plaques of alopecia may have a linear outline. The hairs remaining within the areas of loss are of varying lengths and are typically blunt-tipped because of breakage. The scalp is normal in appearance.

The diagnosis of trichotillomania is often difficult and may require biopsy confirmation. Histologic changes include coexistent normal and damaged follicles, parafollicular hemorrhages, atrophy of some follicles, and catagen transformation of hair. Tinea capitis and alopecia areata must be considered in the differential diagnosis. Parents will often acknowledge that the child frequently plucks or twists the hair. Amelioration of the condition requires the patient's cooperation. Denial on the part of both patient and parents complicates management, and occasionally psychiatric counseling is required. Long-term repeated trauma may result in irreversible damage and permanent alopecia.

Alopecia areata is an idiopathic disorder characterized by rapid and complete loss of hair in round or oval patches on the scalp (Fig. 24–38C) as well as on other body sites. In *alopecia totalis* all the scalp hair is lost; in *alopecia universalis* body as well as scalp hair is nonexistent. Peripheral spread and confluence of plaques of alopecia areata often result in bizarre patterns. At the margin of active plaques, the hairs can often be extracted with gentle traction and, on examination, demonstrate an attenuated or catagen bulb at the termination of a tapered, poorly pigmented shaft. The skin within the plaques of hair loss is normal in appearance. In patients with severe alopecia, dystrophy of the nails is relatively common.

The cause of alopecia areata is unknown. A perifollicular infiltrate of inflammatory round cells is found in biopsy specimens from affected areas. Emotional factors and stress have been suggested as triggering factors, but supportive evidence is tenuous. About 20% of patients have a family history of alopecia areata. The infrequent but striking association with autoimmune diseases, such as Hashimoto thyroiditis, Addison disease, pernicious anemia, collagen diseases, and vitiligo, has suggested an autoimmune pathogenesis. Some patients have serum antibodies to thyroglobulin, parietal cells, and adrenal gland. An increased incidence of alopecia areata has been reported in patients with Down syndrome.

The differential diagnosis includes tinea capitis, seborrheic dermatitis, trichotillomania, traumatic alopecia, and lupus erythematosus. The course is unpredictable since spontaneous resolution is usual, but recurrences are common. In general, onset at a young age and extensive or prolonged hair loss are poor prognostic signs. Alopecia universalis and totalis as well as *ophiasis*, a type of alopecia areata in which hair loss is circumferential, are less likely to resolve permanently.

Treatment is difficult to evaluate since the course is erratic and unpredictable. The use of high-potency topical, fluorinated corticosteroids with occlusion at night is thought to be minimally effective in some patients. Intradermal injections of steroid may also stimulate hair growth locally, but this mode of treatment is impractical in young children or in those with extensive hair loss. Systemic corticosteroid therapy has, on occasion, been associated with good results; however, the permanence of cure is questionable, and the side effects are a serious deterrent. In general, parents and patients can be reassured that spontaneous remission will usually occur. New hair growth may initially be of finer caliber and lighter color, but replacement by normal terminal hair can be expected.

24.21 STRUCTURAL DEFECTS OF HAIR

Structural defects of the hair shaft can be congenital or acquired. Some reflect known biochemical aberrations; others are of unknown cause; and one, at least, appears to be related to damaging grooming practices. All the defects can be demonstrated by microscopic examination of affected hairs. Scanning and transmission electron microscopy has contributed greatly to an understanding of the structural abnormalities.

Trichorrhexis nodosa is the most common of the structural defects. Clinically, the defect appears as a node or swelling on the hair shaft. Microscopically, it has the appearance of two interlocking brushes. The defect is due to a fracture of the hair shaft with derangement of the cells in the cortex. Weakness at the nodal points accounts for the fragility of the shaft, resulting in broken stubs and partial alopecia. Trichorrhexis nodosa has been noted as a congenital defect in some families and has also been observed in some infants with argininosuccinic aciduria.

Acquired trichorrhexis nodosa, the most common cause of hair breakage, occurs in two forms. *Proximal defects* are found most frequently in black children, whose complaint is not of alopecia but of the failure of their hair to grow. The hair is short, often in brush-stroke patches; easy breakage is demonstrated by gentle traction on the hair shafts. A history of other affected family members may be obtained. The problem is thought to be caused by a combination of genetic predisposition and the cumulative mechanical trauma of rough combing and brushing, hair straightening procedures, and "permanents." The longitudinal splits, knots, and nodal defects can be demonstrated in hair mounts. The patient must be cautioned to avoid damaging grooming techniques. A soft, natural-bristle brush and a wide-toothed comb should be used. The condition is self-limited with resolution in 2–4 yr if the patient avoids damaging practices.

Distal trichorrhexis nodosa is seen more frequently in white and oriental children; it also is traumatic in origin. The distal portions of the hair shafts are thinned, ragged, and faded and may have white specks (sometimes mistaken for nits) along the shaft. Hair mounts reveal the paint-brush defect and the sites of excessive fragility and breakage. Avoidance of diverse insults, including saltwater soaking and traumatic grooming, as well as regular trimming of affected ends and the use of cream rinses to lessen tangling will ameliorate the condition.

Monilethrix, a rare defect of the hair shaft, is inherited as an autosomal dominant trait. The hair appears dry, lusterless, and brittle, and it fractures spontaneously or with mild trauma. Eyebrows, lashes, and body and sexual hair as well as scalp hair may be affected. Keratosis pilaris is always present, and, less commonly, there are other ectodermal defects. Microscopically, a distinctive, regular beading pattern of the hair shafts is evident; the narrowed internodal portions of the shaft lack a medulla and are the sites of fracture. The etiology is unknown; treatment is ineffective. Spontaneous improvement may occur at puberty.

Trichorrhexis invaginata (bamboo hair) is a distinguishing feature of the Netherton syndrome. Dry, fragile hair without apparent growth is characteristic. The nodal defects of the shaft have the appearance of a ball and socket joint in which the distal portion has been invaginated into the cup-like proximal portion. The abnormality is thought to result from a transient defect in keratinization. The defects may be identified in body hair as well as scalp hair and seem to decrease in frequency as the child matures. Hair growth may improve significantly at puberty.

Trichoschisis applies to a defect that has the appearance of a clean fracture perpendicular to the hair shaft. Under the light microscope, the hair resembles a flat ribbon and folds back on itself at intervals along the hair shaft. On scanning electron microscopy, near absence of the cuticular hair cells can be demonstrated along with ridging and fluting of the shaft. A zebra-striped pattern of alternating bright and dark bands is characteristic on polarizing microscopy.

Trichoschisis is associated with diminished hair sulfur content. Affected children have brittle hair as well as variable intellectual impairment, short stature, ichthyosis, and defects of the teeth, nails, and eyes. It has been suggested that this constellation of findings is inherited as an autosomal recessive trait, and the term trichothiodystrophy has been proposed for children with some or all of these features.

Pili torti is a structural defect in which the hair shaft is grooved and flattened at irregular intervals and twisted on its axis in varying degrees. Minor twists that occur in normal hair should not be misconstrued as pili torti. Pili torti is usually first recognized at about 2–3 yr of age, when the hair acquires a striking spangled appearance and increased fragility. The hair is often ash-blond in color.

Both autosomal dominant and recessive forms have been described; most cases, however, are sporadic. Pili torti has, on occasion, been associated with sensorineural hearing loss, mental retardation, and ectodermal defects of the hair and teeth. It has also been observed in patients with Menkes syndrome.

Pili annulati, ringed hair, is characterized by hair shafts banded with bright rings when viewed in reflected light. The bands are caused by reflection of light from focal aggregates of abnormal air-filled cavities within the hair shafts. The hair is not fragile. The defect may be familial or sporadic.

Pseudo–pili annulati is a variant of normal blond hair; an optical effect caused by the refraction and reflection of light from the flattened and twisted shaft creates the phenomenon of banding.

Wooly hair disease presents peculiarly tight, curly, abnormal hair at birth. Three types have been recognized: (1) an autosomal dominant form in which other ectodermal structures and hair color are normal; (2) an autosomal recessive type in which the scalp hair has a bleached appearance and body hair is short and pale; and (3) wooly hair nevus, a sporadic form in which only a portion of the scalp hair is involved.

24.22 DISEASES OF THE NAILS

Nail abnormalities in children may be manifestations of generalized skin disease or of systemic disease. They may also be due to trauma, localized bacterial and fungal infections, or skin diseases involving the nail fold. Nail changes occur in psoriasis, Reiter disease, Norwegian scabies, lichen planus, lichen striatus, Darier disease, alopecia areata, hypoparathyroidism, and acrodermatitis enteropathica. Nail anomalies are also common in certain congenital disorders (Table 24–5).

Anonychia is absence of the nail plate, usually the result of a congenital disorder or trauma. *Koilonychia* is flattening and concavity of the nail plate with loss of normal contour. *Macronychia* is an abnormally large nail, *micronychia* an unusually small one. *Leukonychia* is a white opacity of the nail plate that may involve the entire plate or may be punctate or striate; the nail plate, however, remains smooth and undamaged. Leukonychia can be traumatic or may be a benign hereditary defect. *Onychogryphosis* is an acquired defect characterized by a thickened, overgrown, distorted nail plate. *Onycholysis* indicates separation of the nail plate from the nail bed. Common causes are trauma, psoriasis, fungal infection (distal onycholysis), contact dermatitis, and drug-induced phototoxicity. *Beau lines* are transverse grooves in the nail plate that represent an inability of the nail matrix to produce a nail plate of normal thickness. Usually, Beau lines are indicative of periodic trauma or episodic shutdown of the nail matrix secondary to a systemic disease.

Pigmentation of an entire nail plate or linear bands of pigmentation are common in black individuals. The pigment is produced by melanocytes in the nail matrix and nail bed and is of no consequence. Pigmentation may also be due to nevus cells in the nail matrix (junctional nevus). Extension or

Table 24–5. Congenital Disease with Nail Defects

Large nails: Pachyonychia congenita, Rubinstein-Taybi syndrome, hemihypertrophy
Small or absent nails: Syndromes: the ectodermal dysplasias, nail-patella, dyskeratosis congenita, focal dermal hypoplasia, cartilage-hair hypoplasia, Ellis–van Creveld, Larsen, epidermolysis bullosa, incontinentia pigmenti, Rothmund-Thomson, Turner, popliteal web, trisomy 13, trisomy 18, Apert, Gorlin-Pindborg, long arm 21 deletion, otopalatodigital, fetal alcohol, and elfin facies

alteration in pigment in the latter lesion should be evaluated by biopsy because of the possibility of malignant change.

Paronychial inflammation is often responsible for dystrophies of the nail plate which are due to damage of the nail matrix; the lesions include bacterial infections, candidosis, eczema, psoriasis, and lichen striatus. Tumors in the paronychial area include pyogenic granulomas, mucous cysts, and junctional nevi. Periungual fibromas that appear during late childhood should suggest a diagnosis of tuberous sclerosis.

Twenty nail dystrophy is characterized by longitudinal ridging, fragility, distal notching, and opalescent discoloration of all the nails. The onset is insidious; there are no associated skin or systemic diseases and no other ectodermal defects. It has been suggested that nail dystrophy is due to lichen planus, but the typical skin lesions of lichen planus are never associated. The disorder must be differentiated from fungal infections, psoriasis, nail changes of alopecia areata, and nail dystrophy secondary to eczema. Eczema and fungal infections rarely produce changes of all the nails simultaneously. The disorder is self-limited and eventually remits; treatment is ineffective.

24.23 DISEASES OF THE MUCOUS MEMBRANES

The mucous membranes may be involved in developmental disorders, infections, acute and chronic skin diseases, genodermatoses, and benign and malignant tumors. A few of the more common diseases specific to mucous membranes are discussed below.

Fordyce disease is characterized by multiple, yellow-white papules which may be located on the mucosa of the lips and the buccal surface. They are aberrant sebaceous glands and may be found in otherwise normal individuals. They are asymptomatic and require no therapy.

Geographic tongue, or glossitis areata migrans, is seen most often in children and young adults. The lesions consist of sharply demarcated, irregular, smooth red plaques, often with elevated, gray margins. The erythematous areas are due to loss of the normal papillae other than the fungiform ones. The cause is unknown. Symptoms of mild burning or irritation are occasionally bothersome. Onset is rapid, and individual lesions may persist for months. These lesions should not be confused with mucous patches of secondary syphilis. No therapy other than reassurance is necessary.

Cheilitis, or inflammation of the lips and angles of the mouth (angular cheilitis), may be due to a variety of causes. In children it is commonly due to dryness, chapping, and constant lip-licking; excessive salivation and drooling, particularly in children with neurologic deficits, may also cause chronic irritation. The lesions of oral thrush may occasionally extend to the angles of the mouth. Protection can be provided by frequent applications of a bland ointment such as petrolatum. Candidosis should be treated with an appropriate antifungal agent and contact dermatitis of the perioral skin with a topical corticosteroid preparation and a lubricant for protection.

Lip pits and fistulas are usually located symmetrically in the vermilion of the lower lip; they represent the mucosa-lined sinus tracts from underlying minor salivary glands. They may occasionally exude a mucous secretion and should be excised for cosmetic reasons.

Mucoceles, or mucous retention cysts, usually form as a result of trauma to the lips or buccal mucosa. Severance of the duct of a mucous gland leads to retention of mucous secretion within the interrupted duct lumen and subsequent cystic dilatation. Lesions are common on the lips, tongue, palate, and buccal mucosa. Those on the floor of the mouth are known as *ranulas* when the submaxillary or sublingual salivary ducts are involved. Fluctuations in size are usual, and the lesions may disappear temporarily after traumatic rupture. Mucoceles must be excised to prevent recurrence.

Aphthous stomatitis (canker sores), recurrent painful ulceration of the oral mucous membranes, is a common condition in which several factors probably play a role. Solitary or multiple lesions occur on the labial, buccal, and lingual mucosa as well as on the sublingual, palatal, and gingival mucosa. Initial lesions are erythematous and indurated papules that erode rapidly to form sharply circumscribed, necrotic ulcers with a gray fibrinous exudate and an erythematous halo. The lesions heal spontaneously in 10–14 days. A more severe form of this disorder in which there are larger, more debilitating lesions is called *periadenitis aphthae.*

Aphthous stomatitis is often cyclical in occurrence. It has been attributed to a variety of causes that include food hypersensitivity, allergic or toxic drug reactions, infectious agents, endocrine factors, emotional stress, and trauma. Immunologic studies have demonstrated lymphocytotoxicity for oral epithelial cells, suggesting a cell-mediated pathogenesis. It is a common misconception that aphthous stomatitis is a manifestation of herpes simplex. Recurrent herpes infections remain localized to the lips and rarely cross the mucocutaneous junction; involvement of the oral mucosa occurs only in primary infections.

Treatment of aphthous stomatitis is extremely difficult and palliative at best. Relief of pain, particularly before eating, may be achieved by use of a topical anesthetic such as viscous Xylocaine or an oral rinse with 1 teaspoonful of elixir of Benadryl. A topical corticosteroid in a mucosal adhering agent (0.1% triamcinolone in Orabase) may be helpful if applied 2–3 times daily. Alternatively, Gelusil used as a rinse may provide some relief.

24.24 VASCULITIS

Cutaneous vasculitis can occur as a variable feature of a large number of disorders including connective tissue diseases, infections, and hypersensitivity reactions. Although the morphology of the skin lesions may vary considerably in these diseases, palpable purpura can be regarded as pathognomonic of vasculitis, reflecting the intense inflammatory process in the dermal vessels (Sec. 10.63).

Mucha-Habermann disease (pityriasis lichenoides et varioliformis acuta), which can occur at any age, is sometimes classified as a form of parapsoriasis but is, in fact, a type of vasculitis. The eruption is polymorphous; small, red-brown, scaly papules and varicelliform vesicles appear in crops and evolve as papulonecrotic, crusted, hemorrhagic lesions that heal as pitted scars. The anterior trunk and proximal limbs are preferred sites; the palms, soles, and mucous membranes are spared. There are no constitutional signs, and mild itching is often the only symptom.

The disease must be differentiated from varicella, other viral exanthems, papular urticaria, drug eruptions, and other vasculitides. The protracted episodic course of weeks to months (or even years) serves to exclude some of these disorders. The histologic changes are lymphocytic vasculitis, invasion of the epidermis by lymphocytes and erythrocytes, edema, necrosis, and vesicle formation. Cultures of intact lesions are always negative. The general health is unimpaired, and the process eventually resolves spontaneously. Oral administration of erythromycin can often control the eruption, but the response is slow. The medication must be given for several months, and the dose is reduced gradually when the disease appears to be quiescent.

24.25 CUTANEOUS BACTERIAL INFECTIONS

Impetigo contagiosa, a superficial form of pyoderma, occurs most commonly in children and is most prevalent during the hot, humid summer months. The infection is characterized by erythematous macules that very rapidly evolve into thin-walled vesicles and pustules (Fig. 24–39A). The vesicopustular stage is also brief, and, following rupture, sticky, heaped-up, honey-colored crusts are formed (Fig. 24–39B). Removal of crusts leaves a moist, red base over which a fresh exudate quickly accumulates. The lesions often spread peripherally and clear centrally to form circinate plaques and gyrate patterns. The infection may be spread to other parts of the body by the fingers, clothing, and towels. The sites usually involved are exposed areas such as the face, neck, and limbs, but lesions may develop anywhere on the body. Insect bites, scabies, cutaneous injuries, and preceding dermatitis serve as portals of entry for the organism, which does not penetrate intact skin. Regional lymphadenopathy is frequently associated.

Impetigo is usually initiated by infection with group A β-hemolytic streptococci, which are present on normal skin. Subsequently, superinfection with staphylococci, usually of nasal origin, can occur. Thus, streptococci alone or in combination with staphylococci can be isolated from impetiginous lesions. In later stages of the infection, staphylococci may be

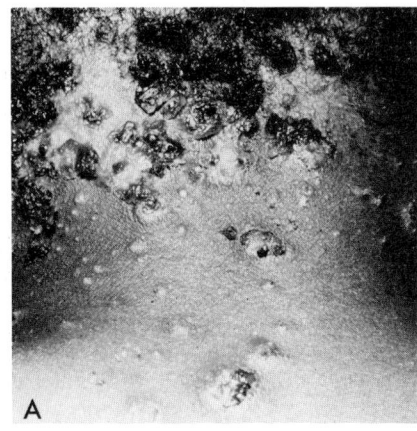
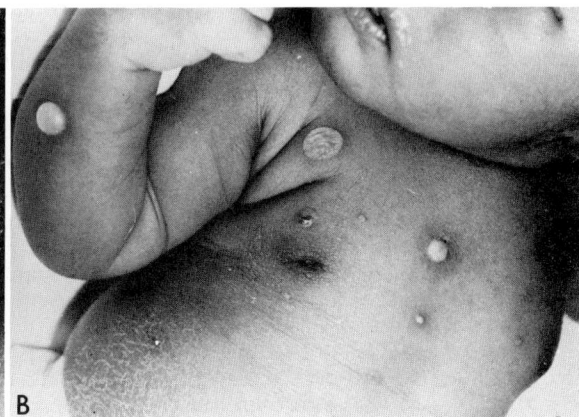

Figure 24–39. *A*, Multiple crusted and oozing lesions of streptococcal impetigo. *B*, Multiple tense and flaccid blisters of bullous impetigo on the trunk and arm of an infant.

the only agent isolated by usual means although streptococci are present. The belief that staphylococci were initiators of impetigo and could occur alone in this disease has been challenged by new data.

The strains of streptococci that colonize the skin and cause impetigo are different from the strains that are usually responsible for pharyngeal infection. Skin strains elaborate streptolysin, hyaluronidase, and DNase B, but ASO and antihyaluronidase titers are not consistently elevated; anti-DNase B titers are more frequently elevated. The white blood cell and differential counts and erythrocyte sedimentation rate are usually normal.

Type specificity and virulence of streptococci are associated with their M protein, and only certain types are associated with the development of poststreptococcal acute glomerulonephritis. The incidence of nephritis following streptococcal impetigo varies considerably in epidemiologic studies and is higher in areas where cutaneous infection is endemic (Sec. 17.5).

Impetigo is an indolent but self-limited disease. It should, however, be treated to decrease morbidity and prevent spread to other children. Local measures should include improvement of personal hygiene, compresses with Burow solution applied 4 times a day to remove crusts, and washing with an antibacterial soap. Systemic antibiotic therapy will result in more rapid recovery; penicillin is the drug of choice. Intramuscular benzathine penicillin is the most efficacious preparation when inadequate compliance with oral therapy can be expected. Oral erythromycin is a suitable alternative for penicillin-allergic patients. Topical antibiotics such as bacitracin or neosporin are less effective in eradicating the organisms. Associated staphylococci are often penicillin-resistant, but in most instances penicillin will eradicate the infection, a fact that further supports the thesis that the role of staphylococci in impetigo contagiosa is secondary. Early treatment of impetigo caused by nephritogenic strains of streptococci does not appear to lessen the occurrence of acute glomerulonephritis.

Ecthyma resembles impetigo in onset and appearance but gradually evolves into a deeper, more chronic infection. The initial lesion is a vesicle or vesicopustule with an erythematous base that erodes through the epidermis into the dermis to form an ulcer with elevated margins. The ulcer becomes obscured by a dry, heaped-up, tightly adherent crust that contributes to the persistence of the infection and to scar formation. Lesions vary in size and may be as large as 4 cm. Sites of predilection are the legs, where trauma probably plays a major role. Pruritic lesions such as insect bites, scabies, or pediculosis, which are subject to frequent scratching, act as a focus for the infection.

The causative agent is usually a β-hemolytic streptococcus; the lesions are infectious and may be spread by autoinoculation. Crusts should be softened by frequent warm compresses and then removed with an antibacterial soap or hydrogen peroxide. Systemic antibiotic therapy, as for impetigo, is indicated.

Blistering distal dactylitis is a β-hemolytic streptococcal infection of the fingertips. The superficial bullae are located over the volar fat pad on the distal portion of the fingers or thumb. If left untreated, they may continue to enlarge and extend to the paronychial area. Polymorphonuclear leukocytes and chains of gram-positive cocci are demonstrable in the purulent exudate obtained from the blister. The infection responds to incision and drainage and a 10 day course of systemic penicillin or erythromycin therapy.

Bullous impetigo is a localized skin infection that is sometimes regarded as a form of the staphylococcal scalded skin syndrome because it is also caused by group 2 phage types of *Staphylococcus aureus*. It is mainly an infection of infants and children. Typical bullae arise on normal skin or have a narrow, erythematous halo; they are filled with a clear, pale to dark yellow fluid which may become turbid if the bullae remain intact. The blisters are relatively superficial and rupture easily, leaving a moist denuded base that is rapidly covered with a thin crust. The skin adjacent to the blister is firmly attached to the underlying layers. The lesions occasionally become widespread, particularly in young infants, but they rarely have systemic manifestations.

The differential diagnosis in the neonate includes epidermolysis bullosa, bullous mastocytosis, herpetic infections, and early scalded skin syndrome. In older children, erythema multiforme, chronic bullous dermatosis of childhood, pemphigus, and pemphigoid must be considered, particularly if the lesions fail to respond to therapy. Examination of smears of blister fluid will disclose polymorphonuclear leukocytes and clusters of gram-positive cocci. Cultures of fluid from an intact blister should yield the causative agent; when the patient appears ill, blood cultures should be obtained. Bullae will rupture and dry rapidly with frequent application of wet compresses followed by gentle cleansing. Localized lesions can be treated topically with an antibiotic such as Polysporin, 3–4 times daily. Patients with widespread lesions and small infants should receive a 5–7 day course of oral therapy with a penicillinase-resistant penicillin, or with cephalexin or erythromycin in the case of the penicillin-allergic patient.

Staphylococcal scalded skin syndrome (Ritter disease) is, almost without exception, a disease of infants and children under 10 yr of age. In most instances it appears to be caused by a group 2 phage type *Staphylococcus aureus*; rarely, group 1 phage types have been isolated. The clinical manifestations are due to the elaboration of an exotoxin (exfoliatin) by the infecting strain of bacteria. This extracellular toxin is distinct from other staphylococcal toxins. The toxin has reproduced the disease in both animal models and human volunteers.

The onset of the rash may be preceded by a prodrome of malaise, fever, and irritability associated with exquisite tenderness of the skin, or the appearance of generalized erythema may be abrupt without preceding symptoms. Initially, the eruption is macular and involves the face, neck, axilla, and groin; rapid extension is usual, and the brightly erythematous skin may acquire a wrinkled appearance due to the formation of ill-defined flaccid bullae filled with clear fluid. At this stage, areas of epidermis may separate in response to gentle stroking (Nikolsky sign). Facial edema and perioral crusting are usual and result in a typically lugubrious facies. As large sheets of epidermis peel away, moist, glistening, denuded areas become apparent, initially in the flexures and subsequently over much of the body surface (Fig. 24–40, p. xxviii). These areas dry quickly and heal by postinflammatory desquamation, which begins within 2–3 days. Additional variable findings include pharyngitis, conjunctivitis, and superficial erosions of the oral mucous membranes. Although some patients appear desperately ill, many are reasonably comfortable except for the marked skin tenderness. Once the desquamative phase has started, healing proceeds at a rapid rate and is complete in 10–14 days.

A presumed abortive form of the disease (resembling *scarlet fever*) is less dramatic in presentation. The facial appearance is similar to that of the classic scalded skin syndrome, but the generalized scarlatiniform eruption, which may be accentuated in the flexural areas, does not progress to blister formation. In these patients the Nikolsky sign may be absent.

It is important to recognize that the portal of entry for the toxin-producing staphylococcus may be a preceding impetiginous skin eruption, conjunctivitis, gastroenteritis, or pharyngitis. Cultures, therefore, should be obtained from all suspected sites of infection and from the blood, although septicemia is a rare complication. Intact bullae are consistently sterile, unlike those of bullous impetigo; the organism, however, may be cultured from other cutaneous sites.

In staphylococcal scalded skin syndrome the site of blister cleavage is the granular layer, the feature that accounts for the rapid healing of denuded areas of skin. Scattered acantholytic cells are evident in the cleft-like bullae; mild edema and vascular ectasia are present in the dermis, but the absence of inflammatory infiltrate is striking. Ultrastructural studies have consistently demonstrated separation of the two halves of the desmosome without preceding cytolysis or demonstrable removal of the cellular surface.

The differential diagnosis varies with the presentation and age of the child. Incipient scalded skin syndrome in infants may be mistaken for bullous impetigo, epidermolysis bullosa, epidermolytic hyperkeratosis (a type of ichthyosis), or boric acid poisoning. Florid lesions of the scalded skin syndrome in older children may mimic erythema multiforme, toxic epidermal necrolysis of the drug-induced type (Lyell disease), pemphigus, and other blistering disorders. Toxic epidermal necrolysis can often be distinguished by a history of drug ingestion, absence of severe skin tenderness, presence of the Nikolsky sign only at the site of erythema, absence of perioral crusting, and a deeper blister cleavage plane. A frozen biopsy specimen of exfoliated epidermis provides a rapid means to distinguish the scalded skin syndrome from toxic epidermal necrolysis since the entire thickness of epidermis will be exfoliated only in the latter. The scarlatiniform variety of scalded skin syndrome is most frequently mistaken for streptococcal scarlet fever, but it lacks the palatal enanthem, strawberry tongue, and perioral pallor of scarlet fever. Drug eruptions and other hypersensitivity reactions must also be considered in the differential diagnosis.

Systemic therapy, either orally or parenterally, with a semisynthetic penicillinase-resistant penicillin should be prescribed since the staphylococci are usually penicillin-resistant. The skin should be gently moistened and cleansed with Burow solution, isotonic saline, or 0.25% silver nitrate compresses. During the desquamative phase, applications of a bland nonocclusive emollient will provide lubrication and decrease itching. Topical antibiotics are unnecessary. Recovery is usually rapid, but occasionally complicating factors such as excessive fluid loss, electrolyte imbalance, faulty temperature regulation, pneumonia, septicemia, and cellulitis cause increased morbidity. Uncomplicated skin lesions should heal without scarring.

Folliculitis is a superficial infection of the hair follicle which is most often caused by *Staphylococcus aureus*. The lesions are typically small, dome-shaped pustules with an erythematous base; they are located at the mouth of the pilosebaceous canals. Hair growth is unimpaired. Favored sites include the scalp, extremities, and perioral and paranasal areas. Poor hygiene, maceration, and drainage from wounds and abscesses can be provocative factors. Folliculitis can also occur as a result of tar therapy or occlusive wraps; the moist environment encourages bacterial proliferation.

The causative organism can be identified by Gram stain and culture of the pus. Treatment includes frequent cleansing; the use of an antibacterial soap may be helpful. Local antibiotic therapy is usually all that is required. In chronic recurrent folliculitis, daily application of a benzoyl peroxide lotion or gel may facilitate resolution.

Furuncles and **carbuncles** are follicular lesions that may originate from a preceding folliculitis or may arise initially as a deep-seated, tender, erythematous nodule. Although lesions are initially indurated, central necrosis and suppuration follow and lead to rupture and discharge of a central core of necrotic tissue. Pain may be intense if the lesion is situated in an area where the skin is relatively fixed such as in the external auditory canal or over the nasal cartilages. Sites of predilection are the face, neck, buttocks, and axillae. Con-

fluent furuncles with multiple drainage points are termed carbuncles. Furuncles may become chronic and recurrent, particularly in obese individuals and in those with poor hygiene and hyperhidrosis.

Patients with furuncles usually have no constitutional symptoms, whereas carbuncles may be accompanied by fever, leukocytosis, and bacteremia. The causative agent is almost always *Staphylococcus aureus*, but other bacteria or fungi may be responsible, and Gram stain and culture of the pus are indicated.

Initial treatment should consist of frequent applications of hot, moist compresses to encourage localization and drainage. Large lesions may be drained by a small incision or by repeated needle aspirations but should not be tampered with until fluctuant. Lesions in the paranasal area should not be incised because of the danger of extension to the cavernous sinus. Carbuncles and large or multiple furuncles should be treated with systemic antibiotics. Since penicillinase-producing staphylococci are frequently involved, a penicillinase-resistant penicillin (e.g., cloxacillin orally or oxacillin parenterally) should be used. The penicillin-allergic patient can be treated with a cephalosporin.

Treatment of chronic furunculosis is often difficult. Attention to personal hygiene, use of an antibacterial soap, and frequent hand washing may be beneficial.

Pitted keratolysis arises in chronically moist and macerated skin and is most often attributable to the wearing of occlusive footgear or to frequent swimming. The lesions consist of plaques of irregularly shaped, superficial erosions of the horny layer which produce crateriform defects on the soles. Occasionally they become secondarily infected. Although usually mild and asymptomatic, the lesions may be quite painful.

The etiologic agent is thought to be a species of keratinophilic diphtheroid. A KOH preparation of scrapings from the lesion demonstrates filamentous coccobacilli. Of the various therapeutic regimens that have been tried, 20% formalin solution in Aquaphor applied topically, with avoidance of maceration, has been the most effective.

Erythrasma is a benign chronic superficial infection of the skin in adolescents, particularly obese ones, and occurs more commonly in warmer climates. It is caused by the filamentous diphtheroid, *Corynebacterium minutissimum*. The most frequently affected sites are moist intertriginous areas such as the groin, axillae, and toe webs. Sharply demarcated, brownish-red, slightly scaly macular patches are characteristic of the disease. Mild pruritus is the only constant symptom.

The diagnosis is readily made with a Wood lamp; the lesions fluoresce to a brilliant coral-red color under ultraviolet light. The gram-positive pleomorphic coccobacilli can be cultured on routine laboratory media.

Erythrasma can be differentiated from dermatophyte infections and from tinea versicolor by the Wood lamp examination. A 10–14 day course of oral use of erythromycin therapy is usually curative. Recurrence may be inhibited by frequent use of an antibacterial soap.

Tuberculosis of the skin. See also Sec. 11.46. *Primary cutaneous tuberculosis* is rare in the United States but occurs with the greatest frequency in infants and children. Primary lesions result when *Mycobacterium tuberculosis* is inoculated at a site of injury on the skin or mucous membranes. Sites of predilection are the chin, lips, nose, limbs, and genitalia. The initial lesion, referred to as a *tuberculous chancre*, develops 2–3 wk after introduction of the organism into the damaged tissue. A red-brown papule gradually enlarges and ulcerates, forming an indolent, firm, sharply demarcated ulcer. Some lesions acquire a crust resembling impetigo, and others become heaped-up and verrucous at the margins. Regional adenopathy with or without lymphangitis appears at approximately 3–4 wk.

The primary lesion is a tuberculoid granuloma with caseation necrosis. *M. tuberculosis* is demonstrable in the skin lesion and local lymph nodes. Clinically, the lesions can resemble syphilitic chancres or deep fungal infections. Spontaneous healing coincides with acquisition of immunity, at which time the skin lesions and infected nodes may become calcified. Antituberculous therapy is indicated (Sec. 11.46).

Miliary tuberculosis may rarely be manifested cutaneously. The skin lesions result from bloodstream invasion by massive numbers of mycobacteria. The eruption consists of symmetrically distributed, erythematous papules that ulcerate and crust and may become purpuric. Subcutaneous gummatous nodules are often associated. Tubercle bacilli are readily identified in an active lesion. A fulminant course should be anticipated, and aggressive antituberculous therapy is indicated.

Lupus vulgaris is, fortunately, relatively rare today and represents reinfection tuberculosis in children with immunity induced by previous infection. Infection follows traumatic cutaneous inoculation of mycobacteria or the drainage of a tuberculous lymph node. Typical lesions consist of tiny red papules that evolve into small nodules. When examined by diascopy, these lesions are discerned as sharply marginated, yellow-brown macules. Relentless progression occurs by peripheral spread and coalescence of nodules to form irregular plaques of varying sizes, often with central spontaneous healing. These lesions usually ulcerate and cause extreme disfigurement with eventual formation of atrophic and hypertrophic scars.

Lupus vulgaris occurs most frequently on the head and neck, but no site is exempt. Lesions involving the nasal, buccal, and conjunctival mucosa may cause extensive facial deformity. Chronicity is characteristic, and persistence of plaques for many years is not uncommon. The histopathologic changes are those of a tuberculoid granuloma without caseation; organisms are extremely difficult to demonstrate. Small lesions can be excised; antituberculous drug therapy will usually halt further spread and induce involution.

Scrofuloderma is caused by infection of the skin from caseous tuberculous cervical lymph nodes. The infection is initiated in the larynx and is believed to be caused most often by the ingestion of milk containing *M. tuberculosis*. The lymph nodes become enlarged and fluctuant, stretching the overlying skin, which may slough, forming ulcerations and multiple draining sinuses. Healing results in cord-like cicatrices.

Caseous tubercles can be demonstrated in the deep dermis and subcutaneous tissue. Tubercle bacilli are readily identified.

Scrofuloderma may occasionally resemble actinomycosis, sporotrichosis, or pyogenic lymphadenitis. The course is predictably indolent, but constitutional symptoms are typically absent. Antituberculous therapy is usually effective.

Tuberculids represent a variety of noninfectious cutaneous lesions and have been ascribed to hypersensitivity to the tubercle bacillus. The most commonly observed reaction pattern is the *papulonecrotic tuberculid*; lesions appear in crops of symmetrically distributed, sterile papules that undergo central ulceration and eventually heal, leaving sharply delineated, circular, depressed scars. Preferred sites are the extensor aspects of the limbs and the dorsum of the hand and foot. Histologically, nonspecific inflammation, tubercles, and minimal caseation coexist with an obliterative vasculitis of the deep dermis. The duration of the eruption is variable, but disappearance usually follows eradication of the primary infection.

Lichen scrofulosorum, another form of tuberculid, is characterized by grouped, pinhead-sized, pink or red papules which form large plaques, mainly on the trunk. Clinically and histologically, the eruption can simulate sarcoidosis; in such instances hypersensitivity to tuberculin is supportive evidence of tuberculous disease. Healing occurs without scarring.

Atypical mycobacterial infection (swimming pool granuloma) may be responsible for cutaneous lesions in children; *M. marinum,* an organism found in saltwater fish and in swimming pools, is responsible for most of the infections. Swimming pool granulomas are usually initiated by traumatic abrasion of the skin, which serves as a portal of entry for the organism; the knees and elbows are most often affected. Approximately 3 wk after inoculation with the organism, single or multiple reddish papules develop and enlarge slowly to form violaceous nodules. Occasionally the lesions break down and become covered with adherent brown crusts. Systemic signs and symptoms, including regional lymphadenopathy, are absent.

M. marinum granulomas may mimic sporotrichosis or pyoderma. A biopsy specimen of a fully developed lesion will demonstrate a granulomatous infiltrate with tuberculoid architecture and caseation necrosis; intracellular organisms can be identified within the histiocytes with appropriate stains. Cultures of material obtained from the granuloma must be incubated at 30–33° C, since *M. marinum* does not grow at 37° C. This organism is a photochromogen; i.e., colonies will change color (white to yellow) on exposure to daylight.

There is no specific treatment, since these organisms are resistant to antituberculous drugs. Tetracycline, minocycline, and trimethoprim-sulfamethoxazole have been effective in some instances. Surgical excision may be curative for small lesions; however, recurrences are not uncommon. Spontaneous healing can be expected within a period of several years.

24.26 CUTANEOUS FUNGAL INFECTIONS

Tinea versicolor is a rather common, innocuous, chronic fungal infection caused by the dimorphic yeast *Pityrosporon orbiculare (Malassezia furfur).* The lesions vary widely in color; in whites they are typically reddish-brown, whereas in blacks they may be either hypo- or hyperpigmented. The characteristic macules are covered with a fine scale; they often begin in a perifollicular location, enlarge, and merge to form confluent patches, most commonly on the neck, upper chest, back, and upper arms (Fig. 24–41A). Facial lesions are not unusual in adolescents, and occasionally lesions appear on the forearms, the dorsum of the hands, and the pubis. There may be little or no pruritus. Involved areas do not tan following sun exposure.

P. orbiculare is part of the normal flora, predominantly in the yeast form, but proliferation of filamentous forms occurs in the disease state. Predisposing factors include excessive sweating, high plasma cortisol levels, debilitating diseases, and genetically determined susceptibility. The disease is most prevalent in adolescents and young adults.

Examination with a Wood lamp will disclose a deep gold fluorescence. A KOH preparation of scrapings is diagnostic, demonstrating groups of thick-walled spores and myriads of short, thick, angular hyphae (Fig. 24–41B).

Tinea versicolor must be distinguished from dermatophyte infections and scaling disorders such as seborrheic dermatitis and pityriasis alba. Nonscaling pigmentary disorders such as postinflammatory pigmentary change may be mimicked if the patient has removed the scales by scrubbing.

Many therapeutic agents can be used to treat this disease successfully; however, it must be appreciated that the causative agent is a normal human saprophyte, and the disorder will recur in predisposed individuals. Appropriate therapy may include one of the following: a selenium sulfide suspension applied for 4 consecutive evenings and repeated the following week; 25% sodium hyposulfite solution or 25% sodium thiosulfate lotion applied twice daily for 2–4 wk;

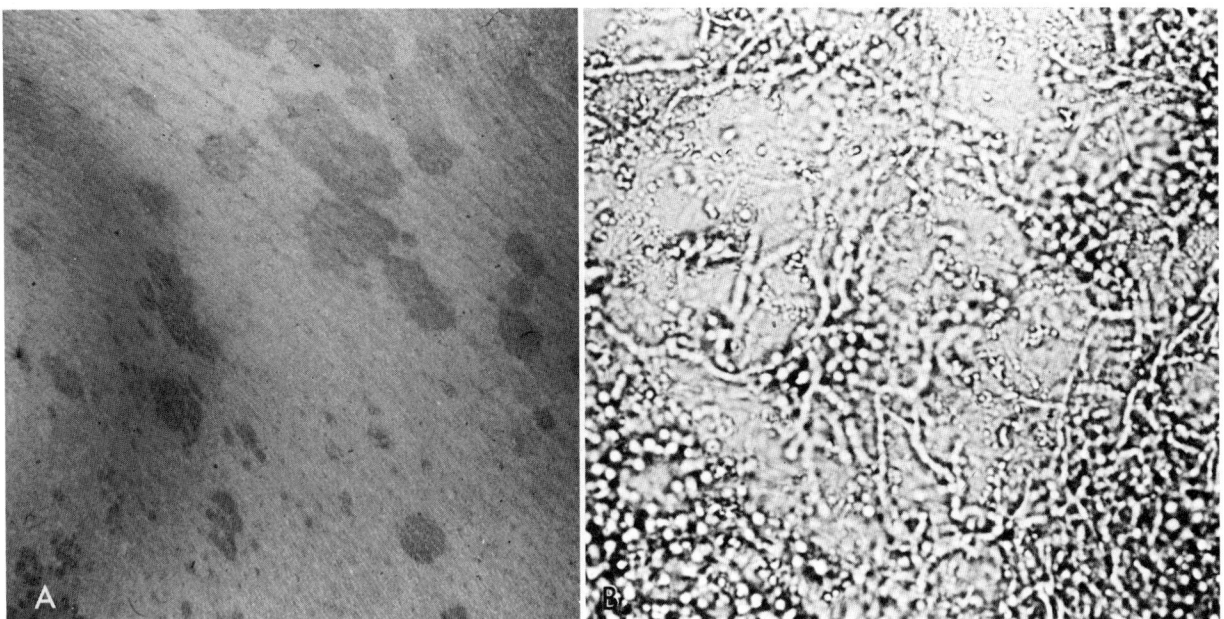

Figure 24–41. *A*, Hyperpigmented, sharply demarcated macules of varying sizes on the upper trunk characteristic of tinea versicolor. *B*, KOH preparation of *Pityrosporon orbiculare* demonstrating short, thick hyphae and clusters of spores.

lotions, ointments, or creams containing 3–6% salicylic acid twice daily for 2–4 wk; haloprogin, miconazole, clotrimazole or ketoconazole twice daily for 2–4 wk. The latter antifungal agents are relatively expensive. Recurrent episodes continue to respond promptly to the above agents.

24.27 THE DERMATOPHYTOSES

The dermatophytoses (ringworm) are caused by a group of closely related filamentous fungi with a propensity for invading the stratum corneum, hair, and nails. The three principal genera responsible for dermatophyte infections are *Trichophyton*, *Microsporum*, and *Epidermophyton*. The *Trichophyton* species cause lesions of all keratinized tissue, including skin, nails, and hair; the *Microsporum* species principally invade the hair, and the *Epidermophyton* species, the intertriginous skin. The dermatophytic infections are designated by the word tinea followed by the Latin word for the anatomic site of involvement. The dermatophytes are also classified according to source and natural habitat. Fungi acquired from the soil are called *geophilic*, those from animals, *zoophilic*; dermatophytes acquired from humans are referred to as *anthropophilic*. *Epidermophyton* infections are transmitted only by humans, but various species of *Trichophyton* and *Microsporum* can be acquired from both human and nonhuman sources.

Anthropophilic dermatophytes apparently elicit delayed-type hypersensitivity in the infected host; some dermatophytes, most notably the zoophilic species, tend to elicit a more severe, suppurative inflammation in humans. Some degree of resistance to reinfection apparently is acquired by most infected persons and may be associated with a positive delayed hypersensitivity response. Humoral immunity to dermatophytes can be detected by serologic techniques, but no relationship between antibody and resistance to infection has been demonstrated.

Occasionally a secondary skin eruption referred to as a dermatophytid or "id" reaction appears in sensitized individuals and has been attributed to circulating fungal antigens derived from the primary infection. The eruption occurs most frequently on the fingers, hands, and arms and is characterized by grouped papules, vesicles, and occasionally sterile pustules. Symmetric urticarial lesions and a more generalized maculopapular eruption can also occur. Id reactions are most often associated with tinea pedis but also occur with tinea capitis and, in the latter instance, most often appear as a generalized papulovesicular follicular eruption.

The important diagnostic procedures for the various dermatophyte diseases include examination with a Wood lamp of infected hairs, microscopic examination of potassium hydroxide (KOH) preparations of infected material, and cultural identification of the etiologic agent. Hairs infected with common *Microsporum* species fluoresce to a bright blue-green color; most *Trichophyton*-infected hairs do not fluoresce.

Tinea capitis is a dermatophyte infection of the scalp most often caused by the species *Microsporum audouini*, *M. canis*, or *Trichophyton tonsurans* and much less commonly by other microsporum and trichophyton species. In microsporum and some trichophyton infections, the spores are distributed in a sheath-like fashion around the hair shaft (ectothrix infection), whereas *T. tonsurans* produces an infection within the hair shaft. The clinical presentation of tinea capitis varies with the infecting organism. The pattern produced by *M. audouini* is characterized initially by a small papule at the base of a hair follicle. The infection spreads peripherally, forming an erythematous and scaly circular plaque within which the infected hairs become brittle and broken. Multiple, confluent patches of alopecia develop, and the patient may complain of severe pruritus. Although *M. audouini* infection was formerly the most common type of scalp ringworm, this organism is no longer ubiquitous. Endothrix infections such as those caused by *T. tonsurans* create a pattern known as "black-dot ringworm"; it is characterized initially by multiple, small, circular patches with only a few hairs involved; they are broken off close to the hair follicle and create a polka-dot appearance. This organism also may produce a chronic and more diffuse alopecia (Fig. 24–42*A*). A severe inflammatory response will produce elevated, boggy granulomatous masses (*kerions*), which are often studded with sterile pustules (Fig. 24–42*B*). Permanent scarring and alopecia may result. *Favus*, a form of tinea capitis that is rare in the United States, is caused by the fungus *T. schoenleini*; it is characterized by development of scaly, erythematous patches with yellow, honeycomb-like crust and a dull green fluorescence under the Wood lamp.

M. audouini and *T. tonsurans* are anthropophilic species

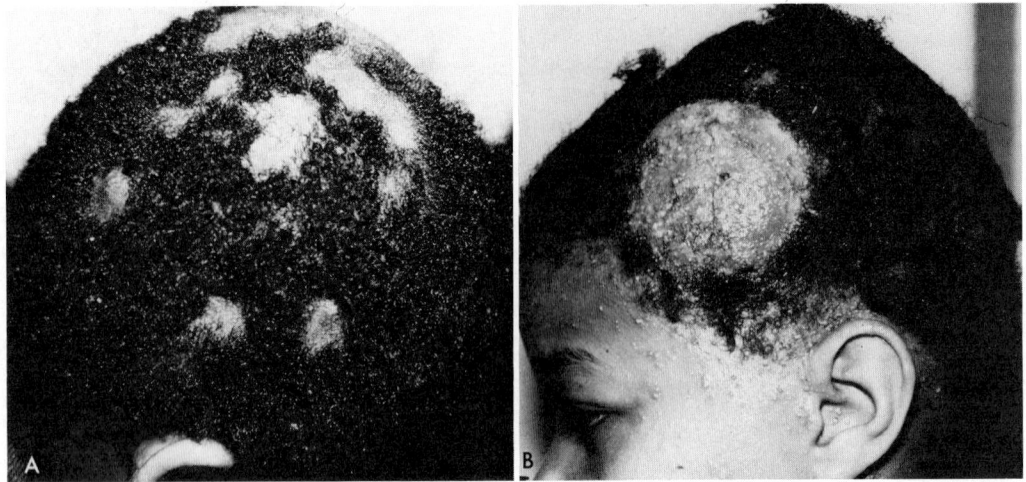

Figure 24–42. *A*, Patchy alopecia associated with tinea capitis. *B*, Elevated, boggy granuloma with multiple pustules (kerion) due to inflammatory tinea capitis.

acquired most often by contact with infected hairs and epithelial cells that are on such surfaces as theater seats, hats, and combs. Dermatophyte spores may also be airborne within the immediate environment, and high carriage rates have been demonstrated in noninfected schoolmates. *M. canis* is a zoophilic species whose preferred hosts are cats and dogs; children acquire it from them.

In microsporum-infected lesions a characteristic bright green fluorescence is seen at the base of each hair on examination with the Wood lamp, whereas lesions caused by *T. tonsurans* fail to fluoresce. Microscopic examination of a KOH preparation of infected hair from the active border of a lesion discloses tiny spores surrounding the hair shaft in microsporum infections and chains of spores within the hair shaft in *T. tonsurans* infections. Usually fungal elements are not seen in scales. A specific etiologic diagnosis of tinea capitis may be obtained by planting broken off infected hairs on Sabouraud medium or Mycosel agar; such identification may require 2 wk or more.

Tinea capitis can be confused with seborrheic dermatitis, psoriasis, alopecia areata, trichotillomania, and certain dystrophic hair disorders. When inflammation is pronounced, as in kerion, primary or secondary bacterial infection must also be considered. In adolescents, the patchy, motheaten type of alopecia associated with secondary syphilis may resemble tinea capitis.

Oral administration of griseofulvin microcrystalline (15 mg/kg/24 hr) is recommended for all forms of tinea capitis. Treatment may be necessary for 8–12 wk and should be terminated only after examination by the Wood lamp or KOH preparation is negative. Adverse reactions to griseofulvin are rare but include gastrointestinal disturbances, headache, blood dyscrasias, and hepatotoxicity. The possible carcinogenicity of this antibiotic is unconfirmed, but its use should be circumspect.

Topical therapy alone is ineffective; it may be an important adjunct since it may decrease the shedding of spores. For this purpose vigorous shampooing with a 2.5% selenium sulfide preparation is helpful. It is not necessary to shave the scalp.

Tinea corporis, or dermatophytic infection of the skin of the face, trunk, and extremities, can be caused by most of the dermatophyte species, although *T. rubrum* and *T. mentagrophytes* are the most prevalent etiologic organisms. In children, infections with *M. canis* are also frequent. The most typical clinical lesion begins as a dry, mildly erythematous, elevated, scaly papule or plaque and spreads centrifugally as it clears

centrally to form the characteristic annular lesion responsible for the designation "ringworm" (Fig. 24–43). At times plaques with advancing borders may spread over large areas. Grouped pustules are another variant. Most lesions clear spontaneously within several months, but some may become chronic. Central clearing does not always occur, and differences in host response may result in tremendous variability in the clinical appearance, e.g., granulomatous lesions and the kerion-like lesions referred to as tinea profunda.

Tinea corporis can be acquired by direct contact with infected persons or by contact with infected scales or hairs deposited on environmental surfaces. *M. canis* infections are usually acquired from infected pets. Not infrequently, a single dermatophyte lesion is responsible for dissemination.

Many skin lesions, both infectious and noninfectious, must be differentiated from the lesions of tinea corporis. Those most frequently confused are granuloma annulare, nummular eczema, pityriasis rosea, psoriasis, seborrheic dermatitis, and

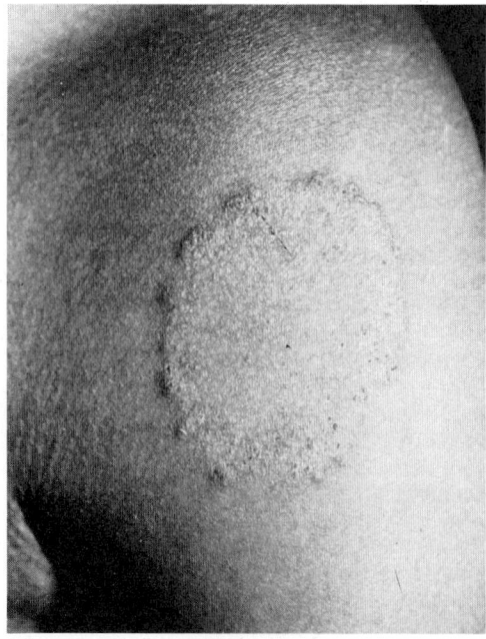

Figure 21–43. Circinate lesion of tinea corporis on the shoulder. Note the active papular border, scaling, and relative clearing centrally.

tinea versicolor. Microscopic examination of KOH wet mount preparations or cultures should always be obtained when fungal infection is considered.

Tinea corporis will usually respond to treatment with one of the topical antifungal agents (haloprogin, miconazole, clotrimazole, econazole) twice daily for 2–4 wk. In unusually severe or extensive disease, a course of therapy with oral griseofulvin microcrystalline may be required for several wk.

Tinea cruris, or dermatophyte infection of the groin, occurs most often in adolescent males and is usually caused by the anthropophilic species, *Epidermophyton floccosum* or *T. rubrum,* but occasionally by the zoophilic species *T. mentagrophytes.* The initial lesion is a small, raised, scaly, erythematous patch on the inner aspect of the thigh which spreads peripherally, often developing multiple tiny vesicles at the advancing margin. It eventually forms bilateral, irregular, sharply bordered patches with hyperpigmented, scaly centers. In some instances, particularly in infections of *T. mentagrophytes,* the inflammatory reaction is more intense, and the infection may spread beyond the crural region. Pruritus may be severe initially but abates as the inflammatory reaction subsides. Bacterial superinfection may alter the clinical appearance, and erythrasma or candidosis may coexist with the dermatophytosis. Tinea cruris is more prevalent in obese persons and in those who perspire excessively and wear tight-fitting clothing.

The diagnosis is confirmed by culture and by demonstrating septate hyphae on a KOH preparation of epidermal scrapings. Tinea cruris must be differentiated from intertrigo, allergic contact dermatitis, candidosis, and erythrasma. Bacterial superinfection must be excluded when there is a severe inflammatory reaction.

The patient should be advised to use a bland absorbent powder and to wear loose cotton underwear. Topical therapy with an imidazole is recommended for severe infection, especially since these agents are effective in mixed candidal-dermatophytic infections. Pure dermatophytic infection may also be treated with haloprogin or tolnaftate.

Tinea pedis (athlete's foot), a dermatophyte infection of the toe webs and soles of the feet, is uncommon in young children but occurs with some frequency in preadolescent and adolescent males. The usual etiologic agents are *T. rubrum, T. mentagrophytes,* and *E. floccosum.* Most commonly the toe webs in the 3rd and 4th interdigital spaces and the subdigital crevice are fissured with maceration and peeling of the surrounding skin. Severe tenderness, itching, and a persistent, foul odor are characteristic. These lesions may become chronic, but they can usually be treated effectively. Less commonly, a chronic, diffuse hyperkeratosis of the sole of the foot occurs with only mild erythema. This type of infection is more refractory to treatment and tends to recur.

An inflammatory, vesicular type of reaction may occur with *T. mentagrophytes* infection; this type is most common in young children. These lesions involve any area of the foot, including the dorsal surface, and are usually circumscribed. The initial papules progress to vesicles and bullae which may become pustular (Fig. 24–44). A number of factors, such as occlusive footwear and warm, humid weather, predispose to infection. The disease may be transmitted in shower facilities and swimming pool areas. Despite its severity, the infection tends to resolve spontaneously.

Tinea pedis must be differentiated from simple maceration and peeling of the interdigital spaces, which is common in children. Infection with *Candida albicans* and with a variety of bacterial organisms may cause confusion or may coexist with primary tinea pedis. Contact dermatitis, dyshidrotic eczema, and atopic dermatitis also simulate tinea pedis. Fungal mycelia can be seen on microscopic examination of a KOH preparation and/or by culture; the 4th toe web provides a high yield of infected scales; a blister top can also be used.

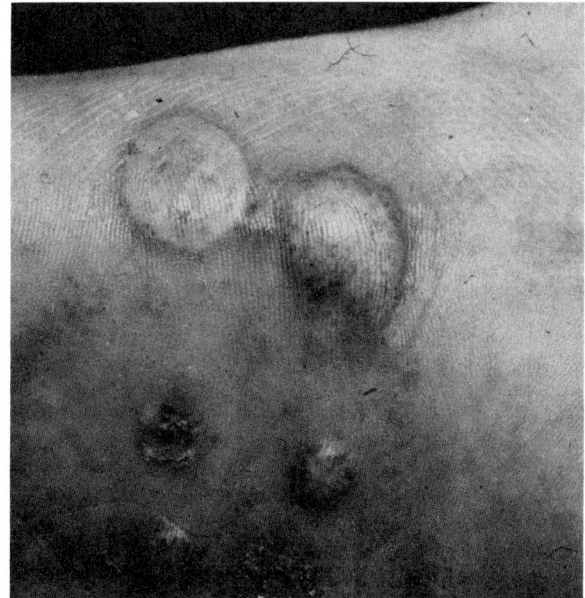

Figure 24–44. Multiple inflammatory bullae of tinea pedis.

Simple measures such as avoidance of occlusive footwear, careful drying between the toes after bathing, and the use of an absorbent antifungal powder such as zinc undecylenate may suffice for milder infections. Topical therapy with clotrimazole, miconazole, or econazole is curative in most instances; each of these agents is also effective against candidal infection. Haloprogin and tolnaftate can be used in uncomplicated dermatophyte infections. Several weeks of therapy may be necessary, and low-grade, chronic infections, particularly those caused by *T. rubrum,* may be refractory. In such patients, oral griseofulvin therapy may effect a cure, but recurrences are common.

Tinea unguium is a dermatophyte infection of the nail plate; it occurs most often in patients with tinea pedis, but it may occur as a primary infection. It can be caused by a number of dermatophytes, of which *T. rubrum* and *T. mentagrophytes* are the most common. The most superficial form of tinea unguium is often due to *T. mentagrophytes;* it is manifested by irregular, single, or multiple white patches on the surface of the nail unassociated with paronychial inflammation or deep infection. *T. rubrum* generally causes a more invasive, subungual infection that is initiated at the lateral distal margins of the nail and often preceded by mild paronychia. The middle and ventral layers of the nail plate, and perhaps the nail bed, are the sites of infection. The nail initially develops a yellowish discoloration and slowly becomes thickened, brittle, and loosened from the nail bed. In advanced infection the nail may turn dark brown to black and may crack or break off.

Tinea unguium must be differentiated from a variety of dystrophic nail disorders. Changes due to trauma, psoriasis, lichen planus, and eczema can all be confused with tinea unguium. Nails infected with *C. albicans* have several distinguishing features, most prominently the presence of pronounced paronychial swelling. Thin shavings taken from the infected nail, preferably from the deeper areas, should be examined microscopically with KOH and cultured. Repeated attempts may be required to demonstrate the fungus.

Therapy of tinea unguium is frequently disappointing. Prolonged therapy with griseofulvin and the application of topical fungistatic agents to the nail bed may be effective in some instances. Griseofulvin therapy may be required for more than 1 yr and should be reserved for especially severe disease in patients who are motivated to obtain a cure.

Tinea nigra palmaris is a rare but distinctive superficial fungal infection that occurs principally in children and adolescents. It is caused by the dimorphic fungus *Cladosporium wernecki*, which imparts a gray-black color to the affected palm. The characteristic lesion is a well-defined hyperpigmented macule; scaling and erythema are rare, and the lesions are asymptomatic. Tinea nigra is often mistaken for a junctional nevus, melanoma, or staining of the skin by contactants. A KOH preparation of scrapings will permit identification of the fungal hyphae; the organism can also be grown on Sabouraud agar. Treatment with Whitfield ointment, undecylenic acid ointment, or tincture of iodine is most successful.

24.28 CANDIDAL INFECTIONS
(Candidosis, Candidiasis, or Moniliasis)

The dimorphic yeasts of the genus *Candida* are ubiquitous in the environment, but *Candida albicans* is the one that usually causes candidosis in children. This yeast is not a member of the normal skin flora, but it is a frequent transient on skin and may colonize the human alimentary tract and the vagina as a saprophytic organism. Certain environmental conditions, notably elevated temperature and humidity, are associated with an increased frequency of isolation of *C. albicans* from the skin. Many bacterial species inhibit the growth of *C. albicans*, and alteration of normal flora by the use of antibiotics may promote overgrowth of the yeast.

Candidal infections in infants and children may be acute or chronic and localized or generalized; widespread lesions may occur in the newborn infant, in children with an immunodeficiency or with a serious disease of any etiology, and in patients with a multiple endocrinopathy syndrome (Sec. 10.20 and 20.4). In such instances, species other than *C. albicans* may also be important etiologic agents. In addition to the mucocutaneous lesions, candidosis may occur as a granulomatous process (candidal granuloma).

Oral candidosis (thrush). (Sec. 8.41 and 12.9.)

Vaginal candidosis. (Sec. 18.2.) *Candida albicans* is an inhabitant of the adult female vagina in at least 5% of women, and vaginal candidosis is not uncommon in adolescent girls. A number of factors can predispose to this infection, including antibiotic therapy, corticosteroid therapy, diabetes mellitus, pregnancy, and the use of oral contraceptives. The infection is manifested by cheesy white plaques on an erythematous vaginal mucosa and by a thick white-yellow discharge. The disease may be relatively mild or may produce pronounced inflammation and scaling of the external genitalia and surrounding skin with progression to vesiculation and ulceration. Patients often complain of severe itching and burning in the vaginal area. The infection may be eradicated by insertion of nystatin vaginal tablets or suppositories twice daily for 2 wk. If this regimen is ineffective, the addition of oral nystatin tablets, 1–2 tablets 3 times daily, may eliminate or decrease the candidal population in the gastrointestinal tract.

Congenital cutaneous candidosis is an infrequent intrauterine infection which may involve the umbilical cord and fetal adnexa. The infection is thought to occur from a cervical or vaginal focus. Premature rupture of the membranes is not usually associated. The skin lesions are often extensive and consist of erythematous macules, papules, and vesicopustules that are followed by a desquamative phase. The oral mucosa is usually spared, as is the diaper area. Palmar and plantar pustules are quite typical. Nail dystrophy may occur. Yellow-white, flat nodules, a few mm in diameter, may be discernible on the surface of the umbilical cord and fetal adnexa. The diagnosis can be made by culture or by KOH preparation of material obtained from an active lesion. Generalized application of an anticandidal agent (nystatin, amphotericin B, miconazole, or clotrimazole) 4 times daily will effect a cure

unless there is visceral involvement. Low birthweight infants are at increased risk for systemic infection. Early onset of severe respiratory symptoms portends an ominous prognosis. Infants with involvement of multiple organs require systemic anticandidal therapy but may not survive.

Candidal diaper dermatitis is a ubiquitous problem in infants and, although relatively benign, is often frustrating because of its tendency to recur. Predisposed infants usually carry *C. albicans* in their intestinal tract, and the warm, moist, occluded skin of the diaper area provides optimal environment for its growth. Usually a seborrheic, atopic, or primary irritant contact dermatitis provides a portal of entry for the yeast.

Candidal diaper dermatitis is an intensely erythematous, confluent plaque with a scalloped border and a sharply demarcated edge. It is formed by the confluence of numerous papules and vesicopustules; satellite pustules, those which stud the contiguous skin, are a hallmark of localized candidal infections. Usually the perianal skin, inguinal folds, perineum, and lower abdomen are involved (Fig. 24–45, p. xxviii). In males the entire scrotum and penis may be involved with an erosive balanitis of the perimeatal skin; in females the lesions may be found on the vaginal mucosa as well as on the labia. In some infants the process is generalized, with erythematous lesions distant from the diaper area; in some instances the generalized process may represent a fungal id (hypersensitivity) reaction.

The differential diagnosis includes other eruptions of the diaper area which may coexist with candidal infection. For this reason, it is important to establish a diagnosis by a KOH preparation or culture.

Treatment consists of applications of an anticandidal agent (nystatin, amphotericin B, miconazole, clotrimazole) with each diaper change or 4 times daily. Ointments are better tolerated than creams; lotions and creams may cause a burning sensation when applied to irritated skin, and powder may cake and cause erosion from friction during movement. The combination of a corticosteroid and antifungal agent is justified if inflammation is severe but may confuse the situation if the diagnosis is not firmly established. Protection of the diaper area by an application of thick zinc oxide paste overlying the anticandidal preparation may be helpful; the paste is more easily removed with mineral oil than with soap and water. Fungal id reactions will gradually abate with successful treatment of the diaper dermatitis or may be treated with a mild corticosteroid preparation. When recurrences of diaper candidosis are frequent, it may be helpful to prescribe a course of oral anticandidal therapy to decrease the yeast population in the gastrointestinal tract. Some infants seem to be receptive hosts for *C. albicans* and may reacquire the organism from a colonized adult.

Intertriginous candidosis occurs most often in the axillae and the groin, under the breasts, under pendulous abdominal fat folds, in the umbilicus, and in the gluteal cleft. Typical lesions are large, confluent areas of moist, denuded, erythematous skin with an irregular, macerated, scaly border. Satellite lesions are characteristic and consist of small vesicles or pustules on an erythematous base. With time, intertriginous candidal lesions may become lichenified, dry, scaly plaques. The lesions develop on skin subjected to irritation and maceration. Candidal superinfection is more prone to occur under conditions which lead to excessive perspiration, especially in obese children and in those with underlying disorders, such as diabetes mellitus.

A similar condition, *interdigital candidosis*, commonly occurs in individuals whose hands are constantly immersed in water; fissures occur between the fingers and have red, denuded centers, with an overhanging, white epithelial fringe. Similar lesions between the toes may be secondary to occlusive footgear. Treatment is the same as for other candidal infections.

Perianal candidosis. Perianal dermatitis is caused by irritation of the skin from occlusion, constant moisture, poor hygiene, anal fissures, and pruritus due to pinworm infestation. It may become superinfected with *C. albicans*, especially in children who are receiving oral antibiotic or corticosteroid medication. The involved skin becomes erythematous, macerated, and excoriated, and the lesions are identical to those of candidal intertrigo or candidal diaper rash. Application of a topical antifungal agent in conjunction with improved hygiene is usually effective. Underlying disorders such as pinworm infection must also be treated.

Candidal paronychia and onychia are characterized by tender, erythematous swellings at the base of the nails (posterior nail fold) that occasionally discharge purulent material. If the lesion becomes chronic, the nail is secondarily invaded and becomes brittle and thickened, initially in the proximal portion but subsequently over the entire nail plate. The nail may develop a brownish discoloration and prominent transverse ridges or grooves, or it may be completely destroyed. Associated infection with *Pseudomonas* imparts a green color to the nail plate, particularly at the lateral margins.

This type of onychia is more common on the fingers, particularly in thumb-sucking children and in those whose hands are frequently immersed in water. The candidal paronychia is often mistaken for a dermatophyte infection, which is rare in children and has different clinical characteristics. It may also be confused with bacterial paronychia. *C. albicans* can usually be cultured from the posterior nail fold and can often be identified on a KOH preparation of nail scrapings or a Gram stain of exudate. Effective management necessitates keeping the finger as dry as possible and applying nystatin, miconazole, or clotrimazole 3 times daily for weeks to months, until the nail plate grows in normally.

Candidal granuloma is a rare response to an invasive candidal infection of skin. Clinically the lesions appear as crusted, verrucous plaques and horn-like projections on the scalp, face, and distal limbs. Affected patients may have single or multiple defects in immune mechanisms and are often refractory to topical therapy. When antifungal agents prove ineffective, a systemic anticandidal agent may be required for palliation or eradication of the infection.

24.29 CUTANEOUS VIRAL INFECTIONS

Warts (Verrucae). All types of warts are caused by DNA viruses in the papova group; those which infect humans are not readily transmissible to animals. Warts can affect the skin and the mucous membranes, including the larynx (laryngeal papillomas). Histologically, the various types of verrucae differ in minor ways, but the basic changes consist of hyperplasia of the epidermal cells and vacuolization of the spinous keratinocytes, which may contain basophilic intranuclear inclusions (viral particles). Parakeratosis (retained stratum corneum cell nuclei), papillomatosis, and eosinophilic cytoplasmic inclusions thought to represent altered keratohyalin are additional variable histologic changes.

The incidence of all types of warts is highest in children and adolescents. The warts are probably transferred by direct contact, although transmission by contaminated fomites is possible. Incubation periods range from 1 to 8 mo. Once acquired, warts are spread by autoinoculation. Antibodies occur in response to infection but appear to have little protective effect.

Common warts (verruca vulgaris) occur most frequently on the fingers, dorsum of the hands, paronychial areas, face, knees, and elbows. They are well-circumscribed papules with a roughened, keratotic, irregular surface. When the surface is pared away, multiple black dots representing thrombosed dermal capillary loops are often visible. Periungual warts are less sharply circumscribed and often painful and may spread beneath the nail plate, separating it from the nail bed.

Filiform warts are frequently located on the face or neck; the lesion is a single projection of several mm which has a sharply circumscribed base. The digitate wart is a related morphologic type of verruca that is often found on the scalp and neck. It has multiple projections from a sessile base.

Plantar warts, although essentially similar to the common wart, are usually flush with the surface of the sole because of the constant pressure from weight bearing. Similar lesions (palmar) can also occur on the palms. They are sharply demarcated, often with a ring of thick callus. Sometimes the surface keratotic material must be removed before the boundaries of the wart can be appreciated; in contrast to calluses, warts obliterate normal skin markings. Several contiguous warts may fuse to form a large plaque, the so-called mosaic wart. Plantar warts may be exceedingly painful.

Juvenile flat warts (verruca plana) are slightly elevated, minimally hyperkeratotic papules that usually remain less than 3 mm in size and vary in color from pink to brown. They may occur in profusion on the face, arms, dorsum of the hands, and knees. The distribution of multiple lesions along a line of scratch is a helpful diagnostic feature. Lesions may be disseminated in the beard area by shaving and from the hairline onto the scalp by combing the hair.

Condylomata acuminata (mucous membrane warts) are moist, fleshy, papillomatous lesions that occur on the perianal mucosa (Fig. 24–46), the labia, vaginal introitus, and perineal raphe and on the shaft, corona, and glans penis. Occasionally, they may obstruct the urethral meatus or the vaginal introitus. Because they are located in intertriginous areas, they may become moist and friable. When untreated, condylomata proliferate and become confluent, at times forming large cauliflower-like masses. Condylomata acuminata can be transmitted by sexual contact and are often referred to as venereal warts. Lesions can also occur on the lips, gingivae, and tongue.

Differential Diagnosis. Common warts are most often confused with molluscum contagiosum. Plantar and palmar warts may be difficult to distinguish from punctate keratoses, corns, and calluses. Juvenile flat warts mimic lichen planus, lichen nitidus, adenoma sebaceum, syringomas, milia, and acne papules. Condylomata acuminata may resemble condylomata lata of secondary syphilis.

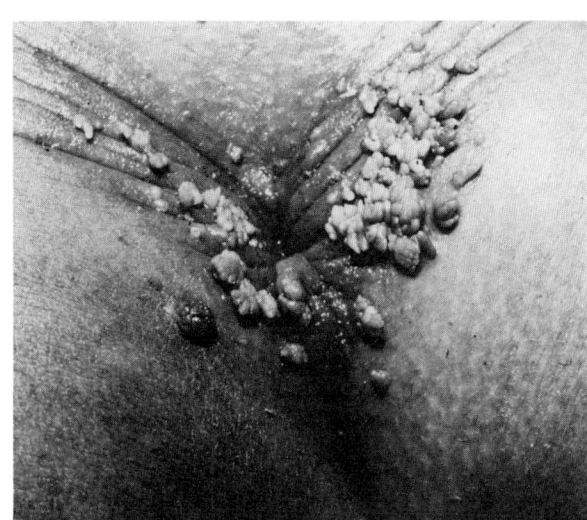

Figure 24–46. Condylomata acuminata in the perianal area of a toddler.

Treatment. A variety of therapeutic measures are effective in the treatment of warts. More than 50% of warts will disappear spontaneously within 2 yr, but failure to treat incurs the risk of spread to other sites. Warts are epidermal lesions and do not produce scarring unless they are managed surgically or treated in an overly aggressive fashion. Hyperkeratotic lesions (common, plantar, and palmar warts) are more responsive to therapy if the excess keratotic debris is gently pared with a scalpel only until thrombosed capillaries are apparent; further paring will induce bleeding.

Common warts can be destroyed by light electrodesiccation and curettage or by applications of liquid nitrogen or cantharidin. Daily applications of 10–17% lactic acid and 10–17% salicylic acid in flexible collodion is a slow but painless method of removal. Filiform, digitate, and periungual warts respond best to liquid nitrogen. Plantar and palmar warts may be treated with cantharidin, liquid nitrogen, salicylic and lactic acids in collodion, or 40% salicylic acid plasters. After prolonged soaking keratotic debris can be removed by an emery board or pumice stone. Condylomata respond best to weekly applications of 25% podophyllin in tincture of benzoin; the medication should be left on the warts for 4–6 hr and then removed by bathing. Condylomata localized to keratinized sites (e.g., buttocks) may not respond to podophyllin. Resistant lesions can usually be eradicated by weekly freezing with liquid nitrogen. With all types of therapy, extreme care should be taken to protect the surrounding normal skin from irritation.

Molluscum Contagiosum. This common cutaneous viral infection is caused by a DNA virus, the largest member of the poxvirus group and the largest true virus that infects man. The disease is acquired by direct contact with an infected person or from fomites and is spread by autoinoculation. The incubation period is estimated to be 2–8 wk.

The lesions are discrete, pearly, skin-colored, dome-shaped papules varying in size from 1 to 5 mm; typically they have central umbilication from which a plug of cheesy material can be expressed (Fig. 24–47). The papules may occur anywhere on the body, but the face, eyelids, neck, axillae, and thighs are sites of predilection. They may be found in clusters on the genitalia or in the groin of adolescents and may be associated with other venereal diseases in sexually active individuals. Mucosal lesions occur occasionally. An eczematous dermatitis may obscure the molluscum papules.

Although biopsy is not indicated, an appreciation of the histologic pattern of the lesions is helpful diagnostically. The molluscum papule consists of a lobulated adhesive mass of virus-infected epidermal cells which degenerate gradually as they move upward from basal layer to stratum corneum. The eosinophilic viral inclusions become more prominent as the cells reach the surface and pack the cytoplasm. The central plug of material that represents these virus-laden cells (molluscum bodies) may be shelled out from a lesion (see below) and examined under the microscope with 10% KOH or with Wright or Giemsa stain. The rounded, cup-shaped mass of homogeneous cells, often with identifiable lobules, is diagnostic.

Molluscum contagiosum is a self-limited disease, but lesions can persist for months to years, can be spread to distant sites, and may be transmitted to others. It is therefore advisable to eradicate the lesions in all infected children. It is mandatory to treat children who also have atopic dermatitis or an immunodeficiency since the infection may spread rapidly and produce hundreds of lesions. The papules can be destroyed by expressing the plug with a needle, a sharp curette, a comedo extractor, or a curved forceps; the base of the lesion can be touched with iodine. Brief application of liquid nitrogen is also very effective. Cantharidin 0.9% may be applied to each lesion without occlusion and frequently causes enough inflammation to facilitate spontaneous extrusion of the plug. Molluscum is an epidermal disease and should not be overtreated so that scarring results.

24.30 INSECT BITES AND PARASITIC INFESTATIONS

INSECT BITES

Insect bites are a common affliction of children and usually pose no problem in diagnosis. Occasionally, however, the patient is unaware of the source of the lesions or denies being bitten; in these instances, precise interpretation of the eruption may be difficult. Insect bites may occur as solitary, multiple, or profuse lesions but, when numerous, are usually grouped because of the tendency of a single insect to inflict several bites in a localized area.

The type of reaction that occurs depends on the species of insect and the age group and reactivity of the human host. Infants often display no reaction, young children manifest only a delayed hypersensitivity reaction, and older children experience both an immediate and a delayed reaction. By adolescence or adulthood, the delayed component of the insect bite reaction is lost, and the host responds only with an immediate reaction, which is characterized by an evanescent, erythematous wheal. Usually a central punctum is visible, but the punctum may disappear as the lesion ages, and, if edema is marked, the wheal may be surmounted by a tiny vesicle. Certain beetles produce bullous lesions through the action of cantharidin, and hemorrhagic lesions may be caused by a variety of insects including beetles and spiders. Delayed hypersensitivity reactions to insect bites are characterized by firm persistent papules which may become hyperpigmented and are often excoriated and crusted. Pruritus may be mild or severe, transient or persistent. The reaction is a response to introduction of insect toxins and antigens into the tissues. Severe hypersensitivity reactions that result from certain types of bites and stings are discussed in Chapters 10 and 28.

Acute local reactions may be ameliorated by cool water

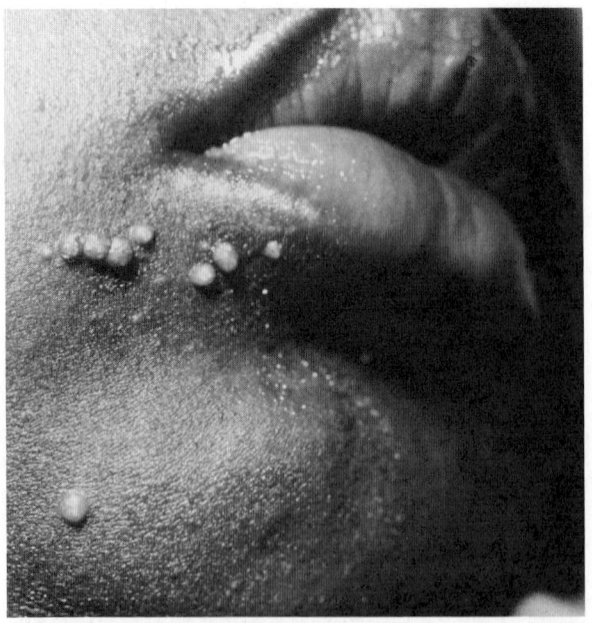

Figure 24–47. Grouped papules of molluscum contagiosum on the face.

compresses followed by application of a soothing shake lotion such as calamine, to which 0.25% menthol and 0.5% phenol can be added. Topical corticosteroids can also be helpful for control of pruritus. If lesions are extensive and extremely pruritic, an oral antihistamine may provide some relief. Topical antihistamines are potent sensitizers and have no role in the treatment of insect bite reactions or other skin diseases. Insect repellents containing diethyltoluamide or ethyl hexanediol may afford moderate protection against mosquitoes, fleas, flies, chiggers, and ticks but are relatively ineffective against wasps, bees, and spiders.

Papular urticaria is a persistent, annoying eruption that occurs principally in the 1st decade of life and appears to represent a delayed hypersensitivity reaction to the bites of insects, the most common of which are species of fleas and mites, bedbugs, gnats, mosquitoes, and animal lice. The disorder is most prevalent during the warmer months.

Typical lesions are firm, hyperpigmented, intensely pruritic, discrete papules which cluster mainly on the trunk and extensor surfaces of the extremities (Fig. 24–48). The initial and acute lesion may be an urticarial wheal that in turn is replaced by a papule. When new lesions are acquired, quiescent papules may flare and become erythematous and edematous. A central punctum is visible initially; however, when the lesions become severely excoriated, central crusting or a secondary pyoderma can obscure the typical morphologic aspects.

It is important to identify the etiologic agent. The nature of the eruption may not be suspected because older family members are usually not afflicted. When it is appreciated that papular urticaria represents a delayed hypersensitivity reaction to insect bites and that this phenomenon is age related, the sparing of others in the household becomes explicable.

Papular urticaria can be confused with papular exanthems, varicella, and scabies. The histologic changes are relatively nonspecific; they consist of dermal edema and a mixed inflammatory perivascular infiltrate. At times, however, the dermal cellular infiltrate is so dense that a lymphoma or foreign body reaction may be suspected.

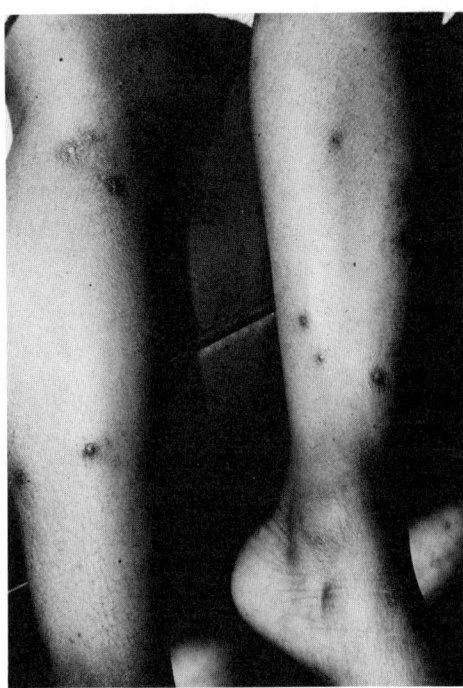

Figure 24–48. Hyperpigmented papulonodular lesions, some of which are grouped, characteristic of papular urticaria.

Treatment is directed at alleviation of pruritus by oral antihistamines, cool compresses, soothing lotions, and topical corticosteroid creams or lotions for the more annoying lesions. An effort should be made to identify the etiologic agent: pets should be carefully inspected; crawl spaces, eaves, and other sites of the house and/or outbuildings frequented by animals and birds should be decontaminated since insects such as fleas can survive for many months without feeding; baseboard crevices, mattresses, rugs, furniture, and animal sleeping quarters should also be sprayed with insecticide.

PARASITIC INFESTATIONS

Scabies is caused by the itch mite *Sarcoptes scabiei* var. *hominis*. A recent worldwide epidemic has resulted in an increased incidence of the disease in all age groups.

The intensely pruritic eruption consists of wheals, papules, vesicles, threadlike burrows, and a superimposed eczematous dermatitis. In older children and adolescents the clinical pattern is similar to that in adults; preferred sites are the interdigital spaces, wrists, elbows, ankles, buttocks, umbilicus, groin, genitalia, areolae, and axillae (Fig. 24–49A). The head, neck, palms and soles are generally spared. In infants, bullae and pustules are relatively common; burrows are absent, and the palms, soles (Fig. 24–49B), face, and scalp are often affected. Red-brown nodules, most often located in the axillae and groin and on the genitalia, are a less common variant. All lesions are extremely pruritic, particularly at night; scratching inevitably results in eczematization, excoriation, and secondary pyoderma, which may mask the true nature of the disorder.

Scabies is transmitted by direct contact with infected persons and only rarely by fomites since the isolated mite dies within 2–3 days. The adult female mite measures approximately 0.4 mm in length and has 4 sets of legs and a hemispherical body marked by transverse corrugations and brown spines and bristles on the dorsal surface. The male mite is approximately half her size and is similar in configuration. After fertilization on the skin surface, the gravid female burrows into the stratum corneum and gradually extends this tract as she deposits 1–3 oval eggs daily and numerous brown fecal pellets (scybala). When egg-laying is completed in 4–5 wk she dies within the burrow. The eggs hatch in 3 to 5 days, releasing larvae which grow and molt into nymphs on the skin surface. Maturity is achieved in about 2–3 wk. Mating occurs, and the gravid female invades the skin to complete the life cycle.

Diagnosis is made by microscopic identification of mites (Fig. 24–49C), ova, and scybala in epithelial debris. Scrapings are most often positive when obtained from burrows, eczematous lesions, or fresh papules. The most reliable method is application of a drop of mineral oil on the selected lesion, vigorous scraping of it with a dull-edged instrument, and transfer of the oil and scrapings to a glass slide. The mite can be detected microscopically by its movement.

The differential diagnosis depends on the types of lesions present. Burrows are virtually pathognomonic for human scabies. Papulovesicular lesions are confused with papular urticaria, canine scabies, chickenpox, viral exanthems, drug eruptions, dermatitis herpetiformis, and folliculitis. Eczematous lesions may mimic atopic dermatitis and seborrheic dermatitis, and the less common bullous disorders of childhood may be suspected in the infant with predominantly bullous lesions. Nodular scabies is frequently misdiagnosed as urticaria pigmentosa, histiocytosis X, and insect bite granuloma.

Treatment by application of 1% gamma benzene hexachloride cream or lotion to the entire body from the neck down, with particular attention to intensely involved areas, is effec-

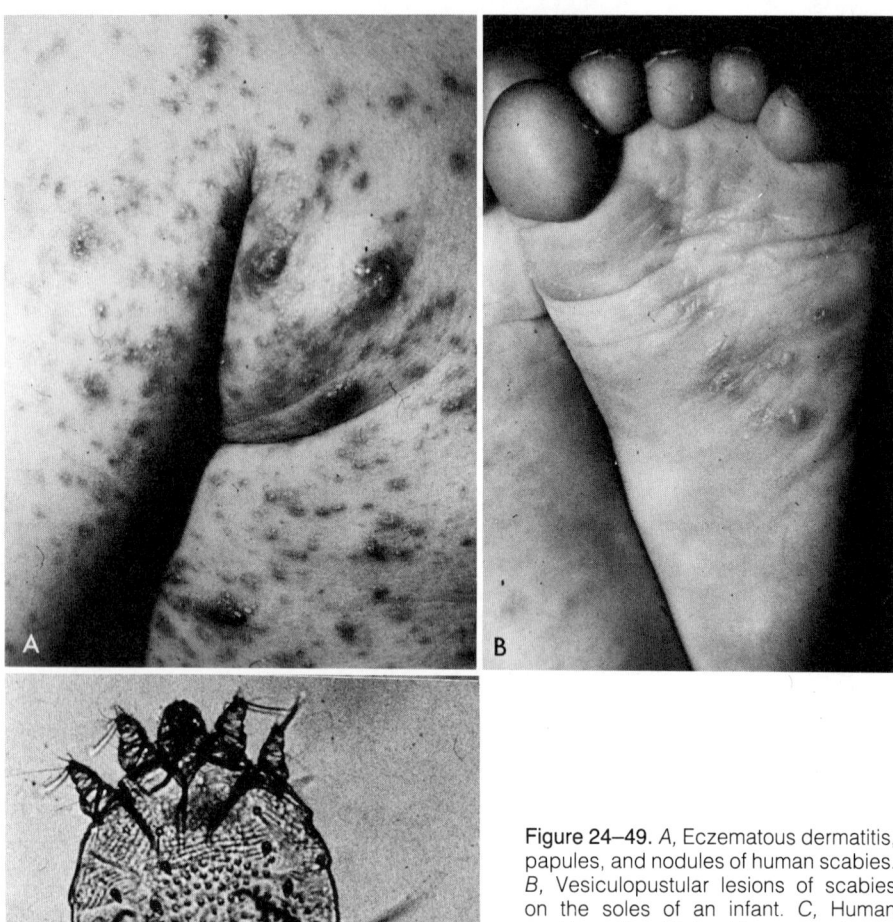

Figure 24–49. *A*, Eczematous dermatitis, papules, and nodules of human scabies. *B*, Vesiculopustular lesions of scabies on the soles of an infant. *C*, Human scabies mite obtained from scraping.

tive. The medication is left on the skin for 8–12 hr, and if necessary it may be reapplied in 1 wk for another 8–12 hr period. The vulnerability of small infants to percutaneous absorption of this potentially neurotoxic substance should dictate extreme caution in prescribing it for them. A shorter application time (6–8 hr) is less hazardous for infants under 1 yr of age. For infants less than 6 mo, as well as older individuals, alternative therapy includes 10% crotamiton cream or lotion applied twice during a 48 hr period or 6% sulfur in petrolatum applied for three consecutive 24 hr periods. Pruritus, which is due to hypersensitivity to mite antigens, may persist for a number of days and may be alleviated by a topical corticosteroid preparation. Nodules are extremely resistant to treatment and may not respond for several months. Persistent pruritus may not reflect inadequate treatment since the hypersensitivity reaction to the mite may outlast the presence of live parasites. The entire family should be carefully examined and all affected members treated appropriately. A latent period of approximately 1 mo follows infestation, so that itching may be absent and lesions relatively inapparent in family members who are asymptomatic carriers. Clothing, bed linens, and towels should be thoroughly laundered.

Norwegian scabies, a variant of human scabies, is highly contagious and occurs mainly in institutions among mentally and physically debilitated patients. Affected individuals are infested by myriads of mites which inhabit the crusts and exfoliating scales of the skin and scalp lesions. The nails may become thickened and dystrophic and are densely populated by mites. Management is extremely difficult; it requires scrupulous isolation measures and repeated but careful applications of antiscabetic preparations.

Canine scabies is caused by *Sarcoptes scabiei* var. *canis,* the dog mite that is associated with mange. The eruption in the human, which is most frequently acquired by cuddling an infested puppy, consists of tiny papules, vesicles, wheals, and excoriated eczematous plaques. Burrows are not present since the mite infrequently inhabits human stratum corneum. The rash is pruritic and has a predilection for the arms, chest, and abdomen, the usual sites of contact. Onset is sudden and usually follows exposure by 1–10 days, possibly resulting from development of a hypersensitivity reaction to mite antigens. Recovery of mites or ova from scrapings of human skin is rare. The disease is self-limited in humans, but removal and/or treatment of the infested animal is necessary. Symptomatic therapy for itching is helpful. In the rare instances that mites are demonstrated in scrapings from the affected child, they can be eradicated by the same measures applicable to human scabies.

Pediculosis. Three types of lice are obligate parasites of the human host: pubic or crab lice (*Phthirus pubis*), head lice (*Pediculus humanus capitis*), and body lice (*Pediculus humanus corporis*). Only the body louse is a vector for pathogens of human disease (typhus, trench fever, relapsing fever). Body and head lice are related and have similar physical characteristics; they are about 2–4 mm in length, whereas pubic lice have a striking crablike anatomy and are only 1–2 mm in length. Female lice live for approximately 1 mo and deposit up to 10 eggs daily on the human host. Ova hatch in 1 wk and require another wk to mature. Both nymphs and adult lice feed on human blood, injecting their salivary juices into the host and depositing their fecal matter on the skin.

Pediculosis pubis is usually encountered in adolescents, though small children may acquire pubic lice on the eyelashes by close contact with an infested individual. Patients experience moderate to severe pruritus and may develop a secondary pyoderma from scratching. Maculae caeruleae (blue spots) may appear in the pubic area and on the abdomen and thighs; they are thought to represent altered blood pigments or excretion from the salivary gland of the louse. Oval, translucent nits, which are firmly attached to the hair shafts, may be visible to the naked eye or may be readily identified by a hand lens or by microscopic examination (Fig. 24–50). Adult lice are occasionally detected.

Since the pubic louse may occasionally wander or be transferred to other sites on fomites, terminal hair on the trunk, thighs, axillary region, beard area, and eyelashes should be examined for nits. The patient also should be checked for manifestations of other venereal diseases. Infestation may be effectively treated by application of 1% gamma benzene hexachloride cream or lotion; it should be massaged into affected areas and permitted to remain for 12 hr. Alternatively, the shampoo is lathered for 4 min and removed by thorough rinsing. A 10 min application of a pyrethrin preparation has also proved to be curative. Retreatment may be required in 7–10 days. Nits can be removed with a fine-toothed comb.

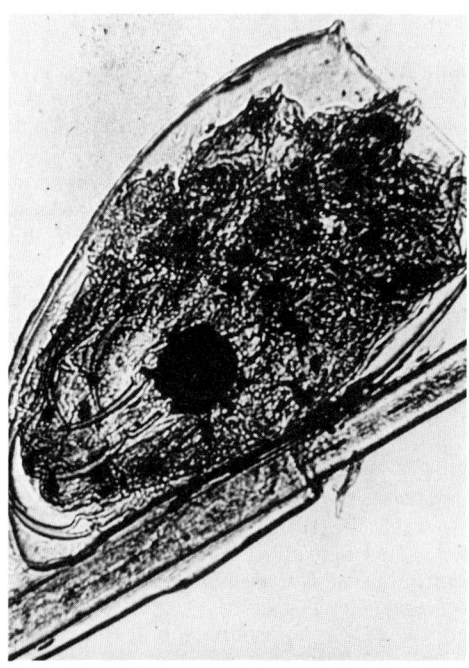

Figure 24–50. Intact nit on a human hair.

Infestation of eyelashes is eradicated by petrolatum or 0.25% physostigmine ophthalmic ointment applied twice daily for 8 days. Pubic lice survive for only a short time when separated from the host; nevertheless, clothing, towels, and bed linens may be contaminated with nit-bearing hairs and should be thoroughly laundered or dry-cleaned.

Pediculosis corporis is rare in children except under conditions of poor hygiene, since the parasite is transmitted mainly on contaminated clothing or bedding. The lesions consist of papules, wheals, excoriations, secondary eczematization, and pyoderma; itching is intense in all stages. Lice are found on the skin only when they are feeding; at other times they inhabit the seams of clothing, which are also a repository for nits. Therapy consists of improved hygiene and laundering or boiling all infested clothing and bedding. Gamma benzene hexachloride can be used to eradicate nits on body hair.

Pediculosis capitis is responsible for intense pruritus, and the infestation may be complicated by secondary pyoderma and lymphadenopathy. Pediculi are not always visible, but nits are detectable on the hairs, most commonly in the occipital region and above the ears. Dermatitis may also be noted on the neck and pinnae. Head lice can be transmitted on infested clothing, combs, brushes, and furniture or by direct human contact. Shampooing with 1% gamma benzene hexachloride for 4 min is effective; treatment may be repeated in 7–10 days. Alternative therapeutic agents include pyrethrin preparations, which are applied to the wet scalp for 10 min, and 0.5% malathion lotion, which is applied to dry hair and must remain in contact with the scalp for 8–12 hr in order to be effective. Nits can be removed with a fine-toothed comb or, if tenacious, by a 1:1 vinegar-water rinse followed by vigorous combing. Clothing and bed linens should be laundered in very hot water or dry-cleaned; brushes and combs should be discarded or thoroughly cleaned in boiling water.

Creeping eruption. (Sec. 11.116.)

24.31 ACNE

Acne Vulgaris. The appearance of this type of acne is often regarded as a physiologic event since it occurs almost universally during adolescence and frequently persists into adulthood. It is a self-limited inflammatory process of the pilosebaceous unit, and is somewhat more common in males. For girls the incidence peaks between 14 and 17 yr of age, for boys between 16 and 19 yr. Genetic factors probably play some role, but no clear-cut patterns of transmission are evident.

Pathology. The lesions of acne vulgaris develop in sebaceous follicles; these appendicular structures have a large, multilobular sebaceous gland and a wide follicular canal containing a rudimentary hair. The primary histologic alteration appears to be abnormal keratinization of the epithelium in the duct with impaction of the keratinized cells within the lumen. The initial lesions are comedones, which are impactions of lamellated keratinous material containing lipid and bacteria. Two types are recognized: open comedones, known as blackheads, and closed comedones, termed whiteheads. A patulous pilosebaceous orifice permits visualization of the plug (open comedo). Open comedones are presumed to be mature lesions since they less commonly become inflammatory. The closed comedo has only a pinpoint opening and represents a follicular sac filled with densely aggregated keratinous material, lipids, and bacteria.

Inflammatory papules and nodules develop from comedones in which the follicular epithelium has ruptured and extruded the follicular contents into the subjacent dermis, where a neutrophilic inflammatory response is induced. Suppuration and an occasional giant cell reaction to the keratin and hair are the cause of nodulocystic lesions; these are not true cysts but liquefied masses of inflammatory debris.

Etiology and Pathogenesis. The cause of acne vulgaris is not fully known, but certain aspects of the pathogenesis are understood. A functionally mature sebaceous gland is fundamental. At puberty, the sebaceous gland enlarges and sebum production increases in response to the increased activities of testicular, ovarian, and adrenal androgens. Adolescents with extensive acne usually have increased sebum production. Studies of testosterone metabolism in acne skin have implicated a local tissue abnormality as a possible mechanism in the pathogenesis.

Freshly formed sebum consists of a mixture of lipids with a predominance of triglycerides. Normal follicular bacteria convert sebum triglycerides to free fatty acids, and those of medium chain length (C8–C14) may be one of the minor provocative factors in initiating an inflammatory reaction. There is also evidence that free fatty acids may stimulate formation of comedones.

The sebaceous follicles are colonized by organisms of three types: an anaerobic diphtheroid, *Propionibacterium acnes;* coagulase-negative *Staphylococcus epidermidis;* and a dimorphic yeast, *Pityrosporon ovale.* Each of these organisms possesses lipolytic enzymes; however, *P. acnes* appears to be largely responsible for the formation of free fatty acids. It is probable that bacterial proteases, hyaluronidases, and chemotactic factors play significant roles in eliciting an inflammatory reaction.

Clinical Manifestations. Acne vulgaris is characterized by four basic types of lesions: open and closed comedones, papules, pustules, and nodulocystic lesions. The last may be firm and indolent, resembling true cysts, or fluctuant or draining, resembling furuncles. Pitted, atrophic or hypertrophic scars may be interspersed, depending on the severity and chronicity of the process. One or more types of lesions may predominate whether acne is mild or severe. Lesions may be confined to the face or also involve the chest, upper back, and deltoid areas. A predominance of lesions on the forehead, particularly closed comedones, is often attributable to prolonged use of greasy hair preparations (pomade acne). Marked involvement on the trunk is most often seen in males. The diagnosis is rarely difficult, although flat warts, folliculitis, and other types of acne may be confused with acne vulgaris.

Treatment. There is no evidence that early treatment will prevent the emergence of acne lesions; however, acne can be controlled and severe scarring prevented by judicious therapy maintained until the disease process has spontaneously abated.

It is important to establish rapport with the adolescent patient and to explain the basic pathogenetic events in clear language. Parents should be included in discussions since their misconceptions about acne may lead to needless harassment of the afflicted adolescent.

GENERAL MEASURES. Diet plays *no* significant role in the pathogenesis of the usual case of acne. There is little evidence that ingestion of particular foods can trigger acne flares. When a patient is convinced that certain dietary items exacerbate acne, it is permissible to omit those foods; it is unnecessary, however, to impose unwarranted restrictions on most teenagers. A balanced diet should be encouraged for reasons of general health.

Climate appears to influence acne in that improvement frequently occurs during the summer months, and flares are more common during the wintertime. Remission during summer may relate, in part, to the relative absence of stress. Emotional tension and fatigue seem to exacerbate acne in many individuals.

Additional factors that should be discussed are cleansing, cosmetics, hair preparations, and facial manipulation. Cleansing with soap and water removes surface lipid and renders the skin less oily in appearance, but there is no evidence that surface lipid is harmful in acne. Only minimal drying and peeling are achieved by cleansing; repetitive cleansing can be harmful since it irritates and chaps the skin. Greasy cosmetic and hair preparations must be discontinued as they will exacerbate pre-existing acne and cause further plugging of follicular pores. Manipulation and squeezing of facial lesions will serve only to rupture intact lesions and provoke localized inflammatory reactions.

TOPICAL THERAPY. Cleansing agents that contain keratolytic agents, such as sulfur, salicylic acid, and benzoyl peroxide, may exert a mild drying and peeling effect and are acceptable if tolerated. Cleansers containing abrasives probably provide little additional help and may be excessively drying and irritating. There is no evidence that preparations containing alcohol or hexachlorophene decrease acne, since surface bacteria are not involved in the pathogenesis.

Topical lotions, creams, and gels containing sulfur, salicylic acid, and resorcinol may be added for additional mild keratolytic effect. Tinted preparations intended to replace cosmetics often mismatch normal skin color and highlight rather than mask the lesions.

The most effective topical preparations, particularly for comedones and papulopustular acne, include the benzoyl peroxide gels and retinoic acid. Benzoyl peroxide is an organic peroxide and oxidizing agent that dries and peels the skin and suppresses growth of *P. acnes.* Preparations are available in concentration of 2½%, 5% and 10% (e.g., Desquam-X, Benzagel, PanOxyl) and may be applied as a thin film once or twice daily as tolerated. Water-based gels are less irritating than alcohol-based gels for patients with sensitive skin. Retinoic acid (Retin-A) affects keratinization in the sebaceous follicle by increasing turnover of epidermal cells and by decreasing the cohesiveness of the squamous cells; it thus aids in elimination of the keratinous plug. Some erythema and peeling may be expected, and pustular flares due to rupture of microcomedones are common. Retinoic acid may be applied once daily, a half hour after washing, in the form best tolerated (0.025% gel; 0.01% gel; 0.1% cream; 0.05% cream, in decreasing order of potency). Increased sensitivity to sunlight may occur, and a sunscreen should be provided until partial tanning has occurred.

Topical antibiotics in a vehicle appropriate for use in patients with acne are now commercially available. These products contain either clindamycin (Cleocin-T) or erythromycin (T-Stat) and may be applied once or twice daily. While not as effective as orally administered antibiotics, they serve as a useful therapeutic adjunct.

All topical preparations require several weeks for a demonstrable positive effect. They may be used alone or together in selected patients, e.g., benzoyl peroxide gel in the morning and retinoic acid at night.

SYSTEMIC THERAPY. Certain antibiotics, especially tetracycline and erythromycin, have been used in the treatment of papulopustular and nodulocystic acne. These drugs appear to act by suppressing the normal follicular flora, mainly *P. acnes,* and by decreasing the inflammatory reaction. For most patients, initiation of therapy with 1 g daily for 4 wk and gradual decrease in dosage to a maintenance dose of 250–500 mg daily will be effective. The drugs should always be administered in combination with topical therapy. Patients should be instructed to take the drug between meals and should be forewarned of such side effects as secondary candidal vaginitis and transient nausea. Tetracycline is contraindicated in pregnant adolescents.

Estrogen therapy is appropriate only for young women with premenstrual flares of acne; it is sometimes effective in such circumstances. The hazards of side effects must be considered. Diuretics, oral vitamin A, and staphylococcal vaccines are ineffective.

PHYSICAL THERAPY. Ultraviolet light, cryotherapy, and radiation therapy may be included under this heading. Ultraviolet light appears to be beneficial in some patients who tan easily, possibly because of the peeling effect of tanning. It is best provided by natural sunlight. Periodic applications of CO_2 snow or slush for a peeling effect may be therapeutic for some patients. Radiation therapy is contraindicated.

SURGICAL THERAPY. Extraction of open and closed comedones, needle aspiration of nodulocystic lesions, and injection of corticosteroid into acne cysts are additional helpful measures in selected patients. Planing of the skin by dermabrasion to minimize scarring is indicated only after the active process is quiescent. Not all patients, however, will be improved by dermabrasion, and some risks accompany it.

Steroid Acne. Pubertal and postpubertal patients who are receiving systemic corticosteroid therapy or potent topical steroids are predisposed to steroid-induced acne, a monomorphous folliculitis that occurs on the face, neck, chest (Fig. 24–51A), shoulders, upper back, arms, and, rarely, the scalp. Onset follows the initiation of steroid therapy by 2 wk. The lesions are small, erythematous papules or pustules that may erupt in profusion and are all in the same stage of development. Comedones may occur subsequently, but nodulocystic lesions and scarring are rare. Pruritus is occasional. The steroid appears to induce focal degeneration of the follicular epithelium with a localized neutrophilic inflammatory response. Although steroid acne is relatively refractory if there is continued use of the drug, the eruption may respond to use of retinoic acid and a benzoyl peroxide gel.

Endogenous steroid (androgen) production may produce acne in children with congenital adrenal hyperplasia, of which severe acne in adolescence may be the only clinical manifestation. Studies of adrenal function are indicated in appropriate patients (Sec. 19.23).

Halogen Acne. Administration of medications containing iodides or bromides or, rarely, ingestion of massive amounts of vitamin-mineral preparations or iodine-containing "health foods" such as kelp may induce halogen acne. The lesions are often very inflammatory. Discontinuation of the provoc-ative agent and appropriate topical preparations will usually achieve reasonable therapeutic results.

Infantile Acne. Acne vulgaris may occur in infants, principally in males; it has been attributed to a hypersensitive end-organ response to hormones, but the etiology is unknown. Onset may occur within the 1st mo of life, and lesions are confined to the face (Fig. 24–51B). Papules, pustules, and open and closed comedones are usual, but only occasionally do nodulocystic lesions develop; pitted scarring is rare. The course may be relatively brief, or the lesions may persist for many months. Rarely, an unusual exposure to an occlusive ointment, a halogenated compound, or a topical fluorinated corticosteroid may cause the acneiform eruption, and appropriate history should be sought. The use of a mild acne lotion or a benzoyl peroxide gel will usually clear the eruption within a few weeks. Often there is a history of severe acne in one or both parents, and the child may be predisposed to more severe acne in adolescence.

Tropical Acne. A severe form of acne occurs in tropical climates and is believed to be due to the intense heat and humidity. Lesions occur mainly on the back, chest, and buttocks, with a predominance of suppurating nodulocystic lesions. Secondary infection with *S. aureus* may be a complication. The eruption is refractory to acne therapy if the environmental factors are not eliminated.

Acne Conglobata. This rare disorder is a chronic, progressive inflammatory disease that occurs mainly in adult males but may begin during adolescence. Papules, pustules, nodules, cysts, abscesses, sinus tracts, and severe scarring are characteristic. The face is relatively spared, but, in addition to the back and chest, the buttocks, abdomen, arms, and thighs may be involved. Constitutional symptoms and anemia may accompany the inflammatory process. Acne conglobata has been related to hidradenitis suppurativa and may occur coincidentally. Routine acne therapy is generally ineffective. Systemic therapy with a corticosteroid or sulfones may be required to suppress the intense inflammatory activity. Isotretinoin (Accutane) appears to be the most effective form of therapy for most of these patients. It is mandatory that physicians prescribing this drug be familiar with its side effects, including teratogenicity in pregnancy.

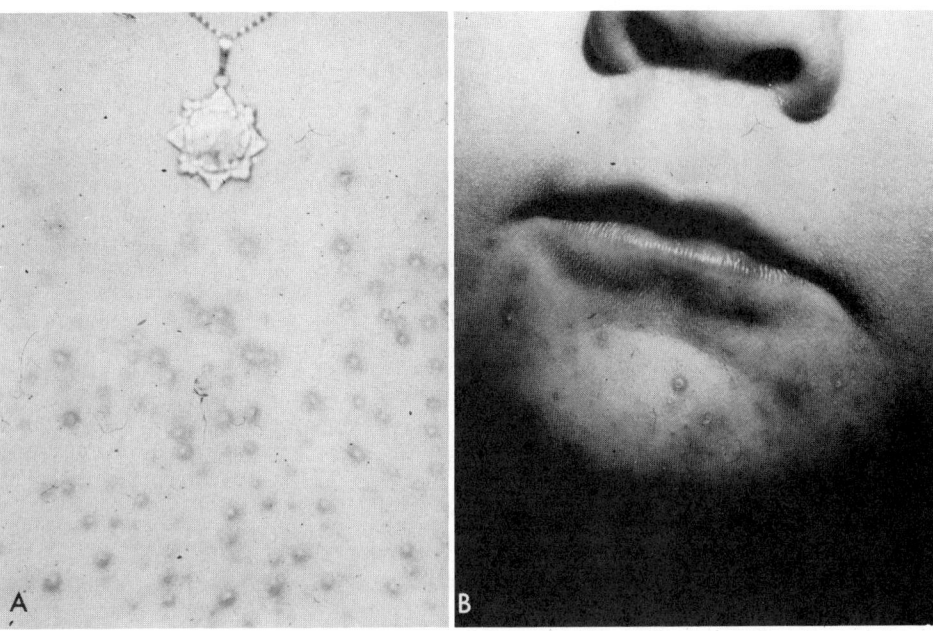

Figure 24–51 A, Monomorphous papular eruption of steroid acne. B, Acne in a male infant.

24.32 TUMORS OF THE SKIN

See also Sec. 16.24.

Pyogenic granuloma (telangiectatic granuloma) is a small, red, moist, sessile or pedunculated growth that often has a discernible epithelial collarette (Fig. 24–52). The surface may be weeping and crusted, or completely epithelialized. Pyogenic granulomas initially grow rapidly and bleed easily when traumatized since they are composed of exuberant granulation tissue. They are relatively common in children, particularly on the face, arms, and hands. Generally they arise at sites of injury, but often a history of trauma cannot be elicited. Clinically, they resemble and often are indistinguishable from small hemangiomas.

Microscopically, the lesions consist of a dense proliferation of capillaries and fibroblastic stroma. Masses of polymorphonuclear leukocytes that infiltrate the stroma account for the name pyogenic granuloma. These lesions are benign but a nuisance, since they bleed easily with trauma and may recur if incompletely removed. Small lesions may regress after cauterization with silver nitrate; larger lesions require excision and electrodesiccation of the base of the granuloma.

Infantile digital fibromatoses are benign but destructive tumors identifiable as firm, smooth, erythematous or skin-colored nodules on the dorsal or lateral surfaces of the distal phalanges of the fingers and toes. More than 80% of reported tumors have been in infants less than 1 yr of age. Lesions may be solitary or multiple. Generally, they are asymptomatic, but flexion deformity of the digits may occur.

Clinically, the lesions resemble fibromas, leiomyomas, angiofibromas, and mucous cysts. The diagnosis is confirmed by finding characteristic pyroninophilic intracellular inclusion bodies within the proliferating fibroblasts on biopsy. A viral etiology has been postulated. Local recurrence following simple excision of this tumor has been reported in 60% of patients. Since the tumor does not metastasize and occasionally may regress spontaneously, a course of expectant observation is advised. If functional impairment or flexion deformity of the digit becomes apparent, prompt full excision of the tumor is indicated.

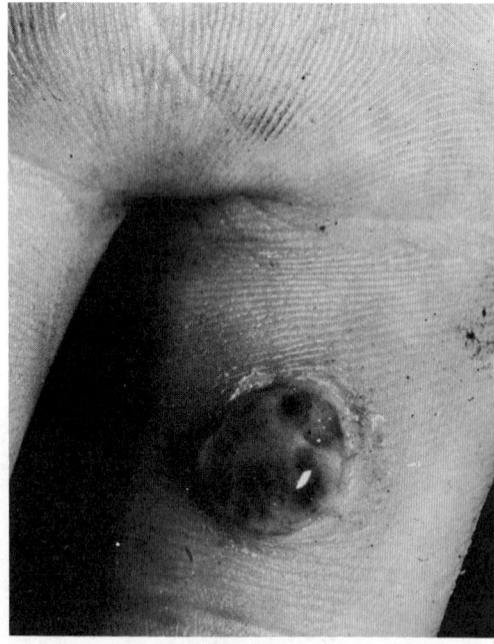

Figure 24–52. Pyogenic granuloma with a moist surface and epithelial collarette at the base.

Dermatofibromas (histiocytomas) are benign dermal tumors which rarely exceed 1 cm and arise most frequently on the limbs. They may be nodular, flat, or pedunculated and are usually firm and well circumscribed but occasionally feel soft on palpation. The overlying skin is usually hyperpigmented. The differential diagnosis includes sclerosing hemangioma, epidermal inclusion cyst, juvenile xanthogranuloma, hypertrophic scar, and neurofibroma. Dermatofibromas may be excised or left intact according to the patient's preference. They represent collections of histiocytes, fibroblasts, and small capillaries in the dermis.

Basal cell epithelioma (basal cell carcinoma) is rare in children in the absence of a predisposing condition such as nevoid basal cell carcinoma syndrome, xeroderma pigmentosum, nevus sebaceus of Jadassohn, or prior exposure to irradiation. Isolated lesions have been reported in children as young as 7 yr of age. Sites of predilection are the face, scalp, and upper back; the lesions are yellow to pink, smooth, crusted or verrucous papulonodules which enlarge slowly and may bleed occasionally or become chronically irritated. The differential diagnosis includes pyogenic granuloma, nevocellular nevus, epidermal inclusion cyst, closed comedo, dermatofibroma, and the various adnexal tumors. Simple excision is usually curative; occasional recurrences have been reported.

Nevoid basal cell carcinoma syndrome includes a wide spectrum of defects involving the skin, eyes, central nervous system, bones, and endocrine system. The typical facies of this autosomal dominant syndrome is characterized by temporoparietal bossing, prominent supraorbital ridges, a broad nasal root, ocular hypertelorism or dystopia canthorum, and prognathism. Appearing in early childhood, basal cell carcinomas erupt in crops and vary in size, color, and number, mimicking numerous other types of skin lesions. Sites of predilection are the periorbital skin, nose, malar areas, and upper lip, but the lesions can develop on the trunk and limbs and are not restricted to sun-exposed areas. Ulceration, bleeding, and crusting can occur, with considerable destruction of surrounding tissue if the lesions are not removed. Small milia, epidermal cysts, pigmented lesions, hirsutism, and palmar and plantar pits are additional cutaneous findings.

Cysts in the maxilla and mandible occur in 65–75% of these patients; they may result in maldevelopment of the teeth and cause pain, fever, swelling of the jaw, facial deformity, bone erosion, pathologic fractures, and suppurating sinus tracts. Osseous defects such as anomalous rib development, spina bifida, kyphoscoliosis, and brachymetacarpalism occur in two thirds of patients, and ocular abnormalities including cataracts, coloboma, strabismus, and blindness in approximately one third. Neurologic manifestations include calcification of the falx, seizures, mental retardation, partial agenesis of the corpus callosum, hydrocephalus, and nerve deafness. There is increased incidence of medulloblastoma and ovarian fibroma.

The management of these patients requires participation of various specialists according to individual clinical problems. Genetic counseling is also indicated.

Syringomas are benign adnexal tumors which are inherited in an autosomal dominant fashion but are more frequent in females. They develop during childhood or adolescence. The tumors are soft, small, skin-colored, red, or brown papules which erupt in profusion on the face, particularly in the periorbital regions, and on the neck, upper chest, lower abdomen, and pubic area. Syringomas are derived from the sweat gland ducts and are readily distinguishable from other adnexal tumors by their histologic pattern. They are of cosmetic significance only. Sparse lesions may be excised, but they are often too numerous to remove.

Trichoepitheliomas (epithelioma adenoides cysticum) are benign nevoid tumors derived from the hair follicles; inheritance is autosomal dominant. Trichoepitheliomas occur on the face in a symmetrical distribution but may also appear on the scalp, ears, neck, upper trunk, arms, and thighs. They arise during childhood and adolescence as firm, pink, yellow, or skin-colored papules which enlarge gradually, reaching a final size of 0.5–2 cm. They may be distinguished from other adnexal tumors, basal cell epitheliomas, syringomas, and adenoma sebaceum by biopsy. Surgical excision is the only available therapy.

Lipomas are benign collections of fatty tissue that appear on the trunk, neck, and proximal limbs. They are soft, compressible, lobulated growths which form skin-colored masses that are usually subcutaneous. They reach their maximal size and thereafter persist indefinitely. Occasionally, multiple lesions may occur, particularly in association with neurofibromatosis. At times atrophy, calcification, liquefaction, or xanthomatous change may complicate their course. They represent a cosmetic defect and may be surgically excised, or subjected to biopsy if diagnosis is in doubt.

Juvenile xanthogranulomas (nevoxanthoendothelioma) may be present at birth or develop within the first several months of life. The lesions are firm, dome-shaped, yellow, pink, or orange papules or nodules, varying in size from a few mm to approximately 4 cm in diameter. Rarely, they are macular, annular, or reticulated. Sites of predilection are the scalp (Fig. 24–53), face, and upper trunk, where they may erupt in profusion or remain as solitary lesions. Affected infants are otherwise normal, and blood lipid values are never elevated, as they are with xanthomas of hyperlipoproteinemic disorders.

The lesions may resemble papulonodular urticaria pigmentosa, dermatofibromas, or xanthomas of hyperlipoproteinemia. Biopsy is helpful diagnostically; mature lesions are characterized by a dermal infiltrate of lipid-laden histiocytes, admixed inflammatory cells, and Touton giant cells (multinucleated vacuolated cells with a wreath of nuclei and a peripheral rim of foamy cytoplasm) that are pathognomonic. Lipid deposits may be demonstrated by special stains. There is no need to remove these lesions since virtually all of them regress spontaneously during the first few years.

Rare instances of similar lesions in the lung, testes, and pericardium have been reported. More commonly, juvenile

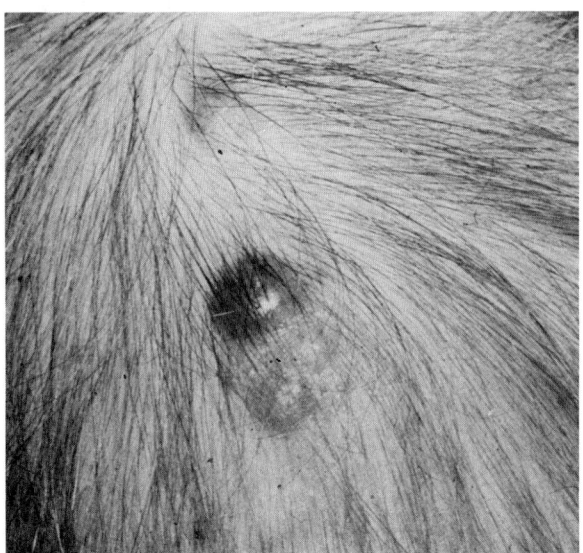

Figure 24–53. Multiple papulonodular juvenile xanthogranulomas on the scalp.

xanthogranulomas occur in the ocular tissues, presenting as infiltrates in the orbit, iris, episclera, or ciliary body or as glaucoma, hyphema, uveitis, heterochromia iridum, iritis, or sudden proptosis (see Chapter 25). There appears to be an association among juvenile xanthogranuloma, neurofibromatosis, and childhood leukemia, most frequently juvenile chronic myelogenous leukemia.

Mucosal neuroma syndrome (Sipple syndrome) is inherited as an autosomal dominant trait and is easily recognized during the first few weeks of life by characteristic physical features. An asthenic or marfanoid habitus is accompanied by scoliosis, pectus excavatum, pes cavus, and muscular hypotonia. There are thick, patulous lips and soft tissue prognathism simulating acromegaly. Multiple mucosal neuromas or neurofibromas appear as pink, pedunculated, or sessile nodules on the the anterior third of the tongue, at the commissures of the lips, and on the buccal mucosa and palpebral conjunctiva. A variety of ophthalmologic defects and intestinal ganglioneuromatosis with recurrent diarrhea are additional common findings.

Of major concern in these patients is the high incidence of medullary thyroid carcinoma associated with high calcitonin levels, pheochromocytoma, and hyperparathyroidism, probably a compensatory response to the high levels of circulating calcitonin. Rarely, these patients are mistakenly diagnosed as having neurofibromatosis. Periodic screening tests for the associated malignant tumors are mandatory.

24.33 PRINCIPLES OF THERAPY

Dermatologic therapy is a mixture of art and science in which the nuances often determine the success of management. Competent skin care requires a specific diagnosis and knowledge of the natural course of the disease as well as an appreciation of primary versus secondary lesions. If the diagnosis is uncertain, it is better to err on the side of less rather than more aggressive treatment. Even when the diagnosis is clear, an acute dermatitis may require gentle and bland therapy initially.

In the use of topical medication, consideration of vehicle is as important as the specific therapeutic agent. Acute weeping lesions respond best to wet compresses, followed by lotions, aerosols, or creams. For dry, thickened, and scaly skin, an ointment base is more effective. Gels and solutions are most useful for the scalp and other hairy areas. The site of involvement is of considerable importance since the most desirable vehicle may not be cosmetically or functionally appropriate, e.g., ointment on the face or hands. The patient's preference should also play a role in choice of vehicle, since compliance is poor if the medication is not acceptable to the patient.

Therapy should be kept as simple as possible, and specific written instructions as to frequency and duration of application should be provided. Drug combinations in a single vehicle may exacerbate a dermatitis and cause diagnostic confusion. The physician should become familiar with one or two preparations in each category and learn to use them appropriately. The careless prescribing of nonspecific proprietary medications that often contain sensitizing agents is not to be condoned. Certain preparations such as topical antihistamines and anesthetics are never indicated in good dermatologic practice.

Wet dressings will alleviate pruritus, burning, and stinging sensations; they are indicated for any acutely inflamed moist or oozing dermatitis. Although a variety of astringent and antiseptic substances may be added to the solution, tap water compresses are just as effective.

Open wet dressings cool and dry the skin by evaporation and cleanse by removal of crusts and exudates that cause further irritation if permitted to remain. The solution should be cool or tepid and consist of tap water, isotonic saline, or aluminum acetate (Burow solution) in a 1:20 or 1:40 dilution. Potassium permanganate is messy and offers no advantage. Boric acid can be toxic if absorbed and should *never* be used for compresses. Dressings of multiple layers of Kerlix, gauze, or soft cotton material should be saturated with the solution and remoistened as often as necessary. Compresses should be applied for 10–20 min at least every 4 hr and continued usually for 24–48 hr.

Closed wet dressings are indicated for abscesses and cellulitis. The solution should be warm, and the dressings should be covered with plastic to prevent evaporation. Closed wet dressings, if prolonged, cause maceration, as they prevent evaporation and heat loss.

Bath oils, colloids, soaps. *Bath oil* may be added to the bath or to compressing solutions when the skin is dry. Bath oils, which are highly dispersible and have surfactant activity, may be obtained scented or unscented for the allergic patient. These preparations leave a fine film of oil on the skin for lubrication; parents should be cautioned that the child and tub will be slippery. Alpha Keri oil, Lubath, and Domol are examples of commercial preparations. Bath oils containing tar (Balnetar, Zetar) can be prescribed for psoriasis and atopic dermatitis.

Colloids such as starch powder or Aveeno are soothing and antipruritic for some patients when added to the bath water. Oilated Aveeno contains mineral oil and lanolin derivatives for lubrication if the skin is dry.

Ordinary toilet *soaps* may be irritating and drying if patients have dry skin or dermatitis. Examples of soaps that are usually not harmful to skin are Dove, Lowila, Aveeno, Neutrogena, Basis, Alpha Keri, Lubriderm, and Oilatum. When skin is acutely inflamed, avoidance of soap is advised.

Lubricants, such as lotions, creams, and ointments, can be used as emollients for dry skin and as vehicles for topical agents such as corticosteroids and keratolytics. In general, ointments are the most effective emollients. Numerous commercial preparations are available in addition to standard U.S.P. items, such as petrolatum, cold cream, stearin-lanolin cream, and hydrophilic ointment. Some patients do not tolerate ointments, and some may be sensitized to a component of the lubricant; some preservatives of creams (most commonly parabens) are sensitizers.

Useful lubricating lotions include Lubriderm, Shepard's lotion, Nutraderm, and Nivea. Creams include Eucerin, Neutrogena, Nutraderm, Lubriderm, and Complex 15. Aquaphor is a cosmetically acceptable alternative to petrolatum. These preparations can be applied several times a day if necessary. Maximal effect is achieved when they are applied *immediately* following a bath or shower. Sarna lotion contains menthol and phenol in an emollient vehicle for control of pruritus as well as dryness.

Shampoos. Special shampoos containing sulfur, salicylic acid, antiseptics, and selenium sulfide (Selsun, Exsel) are useful for conditions in which there is scaling of the scalp. Most shampoos also contain surfactants and detergents. Shampoos with sulfur and/or salicylic acid include Ionil, Sebulex, Fostex, and Vanseb. Those with only antiseptic agents include DHS-zinc, Danex, and Head and Shoulders. Tar-containing shampoos such as T-gel, Ionil-T, Sebutone, and Polytar are useful for psoriasis and severe seborrheic dermatitis. In general, they can be used as frequently as necessary to control scaling, but use must be limited to avoid irritation. Patients should be instructed to leave the lathered shampoo in contact with the scalp for 5–10 min.

Shake lotions are useful antipruritic agents; they consist of a suspension of powder in a liquid vehicle. A water-dispersible oil may be added for lubrication. Calamine lotion is acceptable but tends to cake on the skin. A prototype lotion is zinc oxide 20 g, talc 20 g, glycerine 20 g, Alpha Keri 5 g, and water to make 120 g. These preparations can be used effectively in combination with wet dressings for exudative dermatitis. Cooling occurs as the lotion evaporates and moisture is absorbed by the powder deposited on the skin.

Powders are hygroscopic and serve as effective absorptive agents in areas of excessive moisture. They are most useful in the intertriginous areas and between the toes, where maceration and abrasion may result from friction on movement. Coarse powders may cake; therefore they should be of fine particle size and inert unless medication has been incorporated in the formulation. Zeasorb is a bland, finely milled, general purpose powder that can be applied to any area of the body.

Pastes contain a fine powder in an ointment vehicle and are not often prescribed in current dermatologic therapy; in certain situations, however, they can be used effectively to protect vulnerable or damaged skin. For example, a stiff zinc oxide paste is bland and inert and can be applied to the diaper area to avert irritant diaper dermatitis. Zinc paste should be applied in a thick layer completely obscuring the skin and is more easily removed with mineral oil than with soap and water.

Keratolytic agents. *Urea*-containing agents are hydrophilic; they hydrate the stratum corneum and make the skin more pliable. In addition, because urea dissolves hydrogen bonds and epidermal keratin, it is effective in treatment of scaling disorders. Concentrations of 10–25% are available in several commercial lotions and creams (Carmol 20, Carmol 10, Nutraplus, Ultra Mide, Aquacare HP), which can be applied once or twice daily as tolerated.

Salicylic acid is an effective keratolytic agent and can be incorporated into a variety of vehicles in concentrations up to 6% to be applied 2–3 times daily. Salicylic acid preparations should not be used in the treatment of small infants or on large surface areas or denuded skin; percutaneous absorption may result in salicylism.

The α-hydroxy acids, particularly *lactic acid* and *citric acid*, can be incorporated in an ointment vehicle such as petrolatum or Aquaphor in concentrations up to 5%. These preparations are useful for the treatment of keratinizing disorders and may be applied once or twice daily. Some patients complain of burning; in this event, the frequency of application should be decreased.

Tar compounds. Tars are obtained from bituminous coal, shales, and petrolatum (coal tars), and from wood. They are antipruritic and astringent and appear to promote normal keratinization. They are particularly useful for chronic eczema and psoriasis, and their efficacy may be increased if the affected area is exposed to ultraviolet light. (The tar should be removed prior to exposure to light; otherwise a phototoxic dermatitis may ensue.) Tars *should not be used* in acute inflammatory lesions.

Tars may be incorporated into shampoos, bath oils, lotions, and ointments. A useful preparation for pediatric patients is liquor carbonis detergens (LCD) 2–5% in a cream or ointment vehicle. Tar gels (Psorigel and Estargel) and tar in a light body oil (T-Derm) are relatively pleasant cosmetic preparations which cause minimum staining of skin and fabrics. Tars can also be incorporated into a vehicle with a topical corticosteroid. The frequency of application varies from 1 to 3 times daily according to tolerance.

Antifungal agents are now available as powders, lotions, creams, and ointments for the treatment of dermatophyte and yeast infections. Nystatin and amphotericin B (Fungizone) are specific for *Candida* and are ineffective in other fungal disorders. Tolnaftate (Tinactin) is effective against the dermatophytes and somewhat effective in the treatment of tinea versicolor. The spectrum for haloprogin (Halotex) includes the dermatophytes, *Pityrosporon orbiculare* and *Candida albicans*. The newest agents, miconazole (Monistat-Derm), clotrimazole (Lotrimin), and econazole (Spectazole) have a spectrum similar to haloprogin. They should be applied 2–3 times a day for most fungal infections. All these agents have low sensitizing potential; however, additives such as preservatives and stabilizers in the vehicles may cause allergic contact dermatitis. Whitfield ointment (6% benzoic acid and 3% salicylic acid) is a potent keratolytic agent that has also been used for the treatment of dermatophyte infections. Irritant reactions are common.

Topical antibiotics have been used to treat local cutaneous infections for many years; recently their efficacy has been questioned. Ointments are the preferable vehicle, and combinations with other topical agents, such as corticosteroids, are in general inadvisable. Whenever possible, the etiologic agent should be identified and treated specifically. Antibiotics in wide use as systemic preparations should be avoided because of the risk of sensitization. The sensitizing potential of certain other antibiotics (e.g., neomycin, Furacin) should be kept in mind. Polysporin and bacitracin are probably the two most useful preparations for pyoderma; Silvadene cream is effective in the treatment of patients with denuded areas of skin.

Topical corticosteroids are potent antiinflammatory agents and effective antipruritic agents. Successful therapeutic results have been achieved in a wide variety of skin conditions. In general, corticosteroids fall into two classes: nonfluorinated preparations such as hydrocortisone (Hytone) and desonide (Tridesilon); and fluorinated compounds including triamcinolone (Kenalog, Aristocort), flurandrenolone (Cordran), fluocinolone (Synalar), betamethasone (Valisone, Benisone, Flurobate), and flumethasone (Locorten). The nonfluorinated steroids are of lesser potency but also cause fewer local and systemic side effects, whereas fluorinated steroids are potentially more harmful, particularly with long-term use. Other fluorinated compounds, e.g., fluocinonide (Lidex), halcinonide (Halog), betamethasone dipropionate (DiProlene), and clobetasol propionate (Temovate), are extremely potent and should be prescribed with care. Some of these compounds are formulated in several strengths.

Virtually all of the corticosteroids can be obtained in a variety of vehicles, including creams, ointments, solutions, gels, and aerosols. Absorption is enhanced by an ointment or gel vehicle, but the selection of the vehicle should be based on the type of disorder and site of involvement. Frequency of application should be determined by the potency of the preparation and the severity of the eruption. In general, the application of a *thin film* 2 times daily will suffice. Adverse local effects include cutaneous atrophy, striae, telangiectasia, hypopigmentation, and increased hair growth.

Percutaneous absorption of corticosteroids can be enhanced up to 100-fold by the use of occlusive pliable plastic wraps (Handi-Wrap, Saran Wrap). The steroid is applied in a thin film and tightly covered with a strip of plastic which is taped to the skin. Baggies may be used for the feet and disposable plastic gloves for the hands. Occlusion should be carried out for no more than 8–10 hr, since prolonged occlusion may produce undesirable side effects such as pyoderma, folliculitis, miliaria, and malodor from maceration and bacterial overgrowth. This procedure is appropriate in chronic recalcitrant disorders such as lichen simplex chronicus, dyshidrotic eczema, and psoriasis. The possibility of systemic absorption and adrenal suppression must be considered if large areas are occluded. Fluorinated corticosteroids with or without occlusion are seldom indicated in infancy.

In selected circumstances, corticosteroids may be administered by intralesional injection (for acne cysts, keloids, psoriatic plaques, alopecia areata, and persistent insect bite re-

actions). This method of administration should be used only by physicians experienced in techniques of dermatologic therapy.

Sunscreens are of two general types: those which reflect all wavelengths of the ultraviolet and visible spectrums, such as zinc oxide and titanium dioxide; and a heterogeneous group of chemicals that selectively absorb energy of various wavelengths within the ultraviolet spectrum. Some sunscreens permit tanning without burning; others prevent both. In addition to the spectrum of light that is blocked, other factors to be considered include cosmetic acceptance, sensitizing potential, retention on skin while swimming or sweating, required frequency of application, and cost. Effective opaque total barrier agents are A-Fil, zinc oxide ointment, and RVPaque. Para-aminobenzoic acid–ethanol (Pabanol, PreSun) and cinnamate-benzophenone combinations (Maxafil, Solbar, Uval) effectively prevent transmission of UVB and at least some UVA wavelengths. PABA-esters (Eclipse, Pabafilm, Sundown) afford partial protection. Lip protectants that absorb in the UVB range (Sunstick, RVPaba lipstick, Uval Sun 'N Wind Stick) are also available for patients with photoinduced lip disorders such as recurrent herpesvirus infections. Sunscreens are now designated by sun protection factor (SPF) values ranging from 2 (minimal protection) to 15 (maximal protection) and are so labeled on the container. Examples of sunscreens offering maximal protection are Supershade 15 and Total Eclipse. The efficacy of these agents depends on careful attention to instructions for use. PABA-containing sunscreens should be applied at least 1/2 hr prior to sun exposure to permit penetration of the epidermis. Most patients with photosensitivity eruptions will require protection by agents that absorb UVB wavelengths; patients with porphyria, phototoxic eruptions, and some types of solar urticaria require agents with a broader spectrum of prevention.

NANCY B. ESTERLY

General

Arndt KA: Manual of Dermatologic Therapeutics. 3rd ed. Boston, Little, Brown, 1983.
Cunliffe WJ, Cotterill JA: The Acnes. London, WB Saunders, 1975.
Hurwitz S: Clinical Pediatric Dermatology. Philadelphia, WB Saunders, 1981.
Moschella SL, Hurley HM: Dermatology. 2nd ed. Vols I and II. Philadelphia, WB Saunders, 1985.
Rasmussen JE (ed): Pediatric dermatology. Pediatr Clin North Am 30(3) and 30(4), 1983.
Solomon LM, Esterly NB, Loeffel ED: Adolescent Dermatology. Philadelphia, WB Saunders, 1978.
Weston WL: Practical Pediatric Dermatology. Boston, Little, Brown, 1979.

Specific Diseases

Altman J, Perry HO: The variations of course of lichen planus. Arch Dermatol 84:179, 1961.
Arons MS, Hurwitz S: Congenital nevocellular nevus: A review of the treatment controversy and a report of 46 cases. Plast Reconstr Surg 72:355, 1983.
Beckett IH, Jacobs AH: Recurring digital fibrous tumors of childhood. Pediatrics 59:401, 1977.
Beighton P: The dominant and recessive forms of cutis laxa. J Med Genet 9:216, 1972.
Brown SH Jr, Neerhout RC, Fonkalsrud FW: Prednisone therapy in the management of large hemangiomas in infants and children. Surgery 71:168, 1972.
Carney RG Jr: Incontinentia pigmenti. A world statistical analysis. Arch Dermatol 112:535, 1976.
Chalhub EG: Neurocutaneous syndromes in children. Pediatr Clin North Am 23:499, 1976.
Cooper PH, Frierson HF, Kayne AL, et al: Association of juvenile xanthogranuloma with juvenile myeloid leukemia. Arch Dermatol 120:371, 1984.
Cooper TW, Bauer EA: Epidermolysis bullosa: A review. Pediatr Dermatol 1:181, 1984.
Dajani AS, Ferrieri P, Wannamaker LW: Natural history of impetigo. II. Etiologic agents and bacterial interactions. J Clin Invest 51:2863, 1972.
Dicken CH: Retinoids: A review. J Am Acad Dermatol 11:541, 1984.
Elias PM, Fritsch P, Epstein J: Staphylococcal scalded skin syndrome. Arch Dermatol 113:207, 1977.
Epstein EH Jr, Oren ME: Popsicle panniculitis. N Engl J Med 282:966, 1970.

Ferrieri P, Dajani AS, Wannamaker LW, et al: Natural history of impetigo. I. Site sequence of acquisition and familial patterns of spread of cutaneous streptococci. J Clin Invest 51:2851, 1972.

Fost NC, Esterly NB: Successful treatment of juvenile hemangiomas with prednisone. J Pediatr 72:351, 1968.

Friedman Z, Schochat SJ, Maisela MJ, et al: Correction of essential fatty acid deficiency in newborn infants by cutaneous application of sunflower seed oil. Pediatrics 58:650, 1976.

Gianotti F: Papular acrodermatitis of childhood and other papulo-vesicular acrolocated syndromes. Br J Dermatol 100:49, 1979.

Golitz LE, Weston WL, Lane AT: Bullous mastocytosis: Diffuse cutaneous mastocytosis with extensive blisters mimicking scalded skin syndrome or erythema multiforme. Pediatr Dermatol 1:288, 1984.

Greaves WL, Juranek DD, Washington AE: Treatment of scabies and pediculosis pubis. Rev Infect Dis 4:S857, 1982.

Hazelrigg DE, Duncan C, Jarrett M: Twenty-nail dystrophy of childhood. Arch Dermatol 113:73, 1977.

Holder KR, Pilchard WA: Diffuse neonatal hemangiomatosis. Pediatrics 46:411, 1971.

Jacobs AH, Walton RG: The incidence of birthmarks in the neonate. Pediatrics 58:281, 1976.

Kaplan EN: The risk of malignancy in large congenital nevi. Plast Reconstr Surg 53:421, 1974.

King LE Jr: Darier's disease: Genetic and isolated forms. Arch Dermatol 110:657, 1974.

Kopf AN, Bart RS, Hennessey P: Congenital nevocytic nevi and malignant melanomas. J Am Acad Dermatol 1:123, 1979.

Kraemer KH: Xeroderma pigmentosum. Arch Dermatol 116:541, 1980.

Krieger I, Evans GW: Acrodermatitis enteropathica without hypozincemia: Therapeutic effect of a pancreatic enzyme preparation due to a zinc-binding ligand. J Pediatr 96:32, 1980.

Krowchuk DP, Lucky AW, Primmer SI, et al: Current status of the identification and management of tinea capitis. Pediatrics 72:625, 1983.

Laymon CW, Peterson WC: Lipogranulomatosis subcutanea (Rothmann-Makai). Arch Dermatol 90:288, 1954.

Lees MH, Stroud CE: Bone lesions of urticaria pigmentosa in childhood. Arch Dis Child 34:205, 1959.

Mabry CC, Hollingsworth DR, Upton GV, et al: Pituitary-hypothalamic dysfunction in generalized lipodystrophy. J Pediatr 82:625, 1973.

Mannino FL, Jones KL, Benirschke K: Congenital skin defects and fetus papyraceus. J Pediatr 91:559, 1977.

Marsden RA, McKee PH, Bhogal B, et al: A study of benign chronic bullous dermatosis of childhood and comparison with dermatitis herpetiformis and bullous pemphigoid in childhood. Clin Exp Dermatol 5:159, 1980.

Mikat DM, Ackerman HR Jr, Mikat KW: Balanitis xerotica obliterans: Report of a case in an 11-year-old and review of the literature. Pediatrics 52:25, 1973.

Milstone EG, Helwig EB: Basal carcinoma in children. Arch Dermatol 108:523, 1973.

Mulbauer JE: Granuloma annulare. J Am Acad Derm 3:217, 1980.

Neldner KH, Hambidge KM: Zinc deficiency of acrodermatitis enteropathica. N Eng J Med 292:879, 1975.

Nelson LB, Melick JE, Harley RD: Intralesional corticosteroid injections for infantile hemangiomas of the eyelids. Pediatrics 74:241, 1984.

Nyfors A, Lemholt K: Psoriasis in childhood. Br J Dermatol 92:437, 1975.

Ortega JA, Swanson VL, Landing BH, et al: Congenital dyskeratosis. Am J Dis Child 124:701, 1972.

Papa CM, Mills OH Jr, Hanshaw W: Seasonal trichorrhexis nodosa. Arch Dermatol 106:888, 1972.

Pope FM: Two types of autosomal recessive pseudoxanthoma elasticum. Arch Dermatol 110:209, 1974.

Prockop DJ: Genetic defects of collagen. Hosp Pract, Feb 15, 1986, pp 125–140.

Prockop DJ, Kivirikko KI: Heritable diseases of collagen. N Engl J Med 311:376, 1984.

Prystowsky SD, Maumenee IH, Freeman RG, et al: A cutaneous marker in the Hunter syndrome. Arch Dermatol 113:602, 1977.

Rand RE, Baden HP: The ichthyoses: A review. J Am Acad Dermatol 8:285, 1983.

Rasmussen J: Erythema multiforme: Responses to treatment with systemic corticosteroid. Br J Dermatol 95:181, 1976.

Rhodes AR, Melski JW: Small congenital nevocellular nevi and the risk of cutaneous melanoma. J Pediatr 100:219, 1982.

Roenigk HH, Haserick JR, Arundell FD: Poststeroid panniculitis. Arch Dermatol 90:387, 1964.

Rook A: Papular urticaria. Pediatr Clin N Am 8:817, 1961.

Rosenmann A, Shapira T, Cohen MM: Ectrodactyly, ectodermal dysplasia and cleft palate (EEC syndrome). Clin Genet 9:347, 1976.

Schachner L, Young D: Pseudoxanthoma elasticum with severe cardiovascular disease in a child. Am J Dis Child 127:571, 1974.

Schmidt H, Knitker G, Thomson K, et al: Erythropoietic protoporphyria. A clinical study based on 29 cases in 14 families. Arch Dermatol 110:58, 1974.

Schwartz MF Jr, Esterly NB, Fretzin DF, et al: Hypomelanosis of Ito (incontinentia pigmenti achromians): A neurocutaneous syndrome. J Pediatr 90:236, 1977.

Solomon LM, Esterly NB: Epidermal and other congenital organoid nevi. Curr Probl Pediatr 6:1, 1975.

Solomon LM, Keuer EJ: The ectodermal dysplasias. Arch Dermatol 116:1295, 1980.

Spear KL, Winkelmann RK: Gianotti-Crosti syndrome: A review of 10 cases not associated with hepatitis B. Arch Dermatol 120:891, 1984.

Wanzl JE, Bugert EO Jr: The spider nevus in infancy and childhood. Pediatrics 33:227, 1964.

Watson W, Farber EM: Psoriasis in childhood. Pediatr Clin North Am 18:875, 1971.

Wilkin JK: Unilateral nevoid telangiectasia. Three new cases and the role of estrogen. Arch Dermatol 113:486, 1977.

25

PEDIATRIC OPHTHALMOLOGY

THE EYE IN INFANCY AND CHILDHOOD

25.1 GROWTH AND DEVELOPMENT

At birth the eye of the normal full-term infant is approximately three quarters of adult size. Postnatal growth is maximal during the 1st yr, proceeds at a rapid but decelerating rate until the 3rd yr, and continues at a slower rate thereafter until puberty, after which little change occurs. In general, the anterior structures of the eye are relatively large at birth and thereafter grow proportionately less than the posterior structures. This growth pattern results in a progressive change in the shape of the globe; it becomes more nearly spherical.

In the infant the *sclera* is thin and translucent, with a bluish tinge. The *cornea* is relatively large in the newborn (averaging 10 mm) and attains adult size (nearly 12 mm) by the age of 2 yr or earlier. Its curvature tends to flatten with age, with progressive change in the refractive properties of the eye. The normal cornea is perfectly clear. In infants born prematurely there may be a transient opalescent haze. The anterior chamber in the newborn appears shallow, and the angle structures, so important to the maintenance of normal intraocular pressure, must undergo further differentiation after birth. The *iris*, typically light blue at birth in Caucasians, undergoes progressive change of color as the pigmentation of the stroma increases in the early months and years. The pupils of the newborn infant tend to be small and are often difficult to dilate. Often remnants of the pupillary membrane (anterior vascular capsule) are evident on ophthalmoscopic examination as cobweb-like lines crossing the pupillary aperture, especially in preterm infants; these developmental remnants tend to disappear but sometimes persist in sufficient density to warrant surgical intervention.

The *lens* of the newborn infant is more nearly spherical than that of the adult; its greater refractive power helps to compensate for the relative shortness of the young eye. The lens continues to grow throughout life; new fibers added to the periphery continually push older fibers toward the center of the lens. With age, the lens becomes progressively more dense and more resistant to change of shape during accommodation.

The *fundus* of the newborn eye is less pigmented than that of the adult; the choroidal vascular pattern is highly visible, and the retinal pigmentary pattern often has a fine "peppery" or mottled appearance. In addition, the macular landmarks, particularly the foveal light reflex, are less well defined and not readily apparent to ophthalmoscopic examination. The peripheral retina appears pale or grayish, and the peripheral retinal vasculature is immature, especially in the premature infant. The optic nervehead color varies from pink to slightly pale, sometimes grayish. Within 4–6 mo the appearance of the fundus more nearly approximates that of the mature eye.

Superficial retinal hemorrhages may be observed in many newborn infants. These are usually absorbed promptly and rarely leave any permanent effect. Conjunctival hemorrhages also may occur at birth and are resorbed spontaneously without consequence.

Remnants of the primitive hyaloid vascular system may also be seen as small tufts or worm-like structures projecting from the disc (Bergmeister papilla) or as a fine strand traversing the vitreous; in some cases only a small dot (Mittendorf dot) remains on the posterior aspect of the lens capsule.

As a rule, the infant eye is somewhat hyperopic (farsighted), but the refractive state at any time in life depends on the net effect of many factors, the principal ones being the size of the eye, the state of the lens, and the curvature of the cornea.

Newborn infants tend to keep their eyes closed much of the time, but the normal newborn can see, will respond to changes in illumination, and can fixate points of contrast. The visual acuity in the newborn is estimated to be in the range of 20/600. One of the earliest responses to a formed visual stimulus is the infant's regard for the mother's face, evident especially during feeding. By 2 wk of age the infant shows more sustained interest in large objects, and by 8–10 wk of age the normal infant can follow an object through an arc of 180°. The acuity improves rapidly and may reach 20/30–20/20 by the age of 3 yr or earlier.

In many normal infants there may be imperfect coordination of the *eye movements* and *alignment* during the early days and weeks, but proper coordination should be achieved by age 4–6 mo, usually sooner. Persistent deviation of an eye in an infant requires evaluation.

Catford GV, Oliver A: Development of visual acuity. Arch Dis Child 48:47, 1973.

Gordon RA, Donzis PB: Refractive development of the human eye. Arch Ophthalmol 103:785, 1985.

Hendrickson AE, Youdelis C: The morphological development of the human fovea. Ophthalmology 91:603, 1984.

Khodadoust AA, Ziai M, Biggs SL: Optic disc in normal newborns. Am J Ophthalmol 66:502, 1968.

Krishnamohan VK, Wheeler MB, Testa MA, et al: Correlation of postnatal regression of the anterior vascular capsule of the lens to gestational age. J Pediatr Ophthalmol Strab 19:28, 1982.

Robb RM: Increase in retinal surface area during infancy and childhood. J Pediatr Ophthalmol Strab 19:16, 1982.

Roth AM: Retinal vascular development in premature infants. Am J Ophthalmol 84:636, 1977.

Wilmer HA, Scammon RE: Growth of the components of the human eyeball: Diagrams, calculations, computation and reference tables. Arch Ophthalmol 43:599, 1950.

25.2 EXAMINATION OF THE EYE

Examination of the eye should be a routine part of the periodic pediatric assessment. Screening in schools and community programs can also be effective in detecting problems early. The child should be examined by an ophthalmologist whenever a significant ocular abnormality or vision defect is noted. Ideally, every child should have a thorough ophthalmologic examination sometime in early childhood, preferably by the age of 3–4 yr; these are the crucial years for the detection and treatment of amblyopia, strabismus, high refractive errors, and certain tumors of childhood.

Basic examination, whether done by the pediatrician or ophthalmologist, must include evaluation of visual acuity and the visual fields, assessment of the pupils, ocular motility and alignment, a general external examination, and an ophthalmoscopic examination of the media and fundi. When indicated, biomicroscopy (slit lamp examination), cycloplegic refraction, and tonometry are performed by the ophthalmologist. In some cases special diagnostic procedures, such as ultrasonic examination, fluorescein angiography, electroretinography (ERG), or visual evoked response (VER) testing, are also indicated.

Visual acuity is best measured by the standard Snellen chart (Fig. 25–1), and this method should be used as early as the child's ability to name, copy, or match letters or numbers will allow. The "E" chart, consisting of rows of the letter E in various sizes and directions, can also be used; children are asked to indicate the direction of the selected E by pointing their hand or fingers (or a matching cardboard E) up, down, right, or left. For the very young child or the retarded, shy, or frightened child, a calibrated picture test can be used. In infants and toddlers, in the very retarded, and in the psychiatrically disturbed youngster, vision can be estimated by the response to balls and familiar objects of various sizes, recording the distance at which the response is elicited. Optokinetic nystagmus (the response to a sequence of moving targets; "railroad" nystagmus), can also be used to assess vision; this can be calibrated by various sized targets (stripes or dots) or a rotating drum at specified distances. The VER, an electrophysiologic method of evaluating the response to light and special visual stimuli, such as a changing checkerboard pattern, can also be used to study visual function in selected cases. Preferential looking tests are also coming into use for evaluation of vision in infants and children who cannot respond to standard acuity tests. This is a behavioral technique based on the observation that, given a choice, an infant prefers to look at patterned rather than unpatterned stimuli.

Subnormal vision in one or both eyes warrants further evaluation.

Visual field assessment, like visual acuity testing, must be geared to the child's age and abilities. Formal visual field examination (perimetry and scotometry) can often be accomplished in the school age child. Often, however, the examiner must rely on confrontation techniques and finger counting in quadrants of the visual field. In many children only testing by attraction can be accomplished; the examiner observes the child's response to familiar objects brought into each of the four quadrants of the visual field of each eye in turn. The child's bottle, a favorite toy, and lollipops are particularly effective attention-getting items. Even such gross methods can often detect diagnostically significant field changes such as the bitemporal hemiopsia of a chiasmal lesion or the homonymous hemianopsia of a cerebral lesion.

Color vision testing can be accomplished whenever the child is able to name or trace the test symbols; these may be either numbers or Xs, Os, and triangles. Color vision testing is not frequently necessary in young children, but parents will sometimes request it, particularly if the child seems to be slow in learning colors. Defective color vision is not uncommon in males but rare in females. Occasionally, there is achromatopsia, a total color vision defect with subnormal visual acuity, nystagmus, and photophobia. A change in color discrimination can be a sign of optic nerve or retinal disease.

The pupillary examination includes evaluation of both the direct and consensual reactions to light, the reaction on near gaze, and the response to reduced illumination, noting the size and symmetry of the pupils under all conditions. Special care must be taken to differentiate the reaction to light from the reaction to near gaze; the natural tendency of a child is to look directly at the approaching light, inducing the near gaze reflex when one is attempting to test only the reaction to light; accordingly, every effort must be made to control fixation. The swinging flashlight test is especially useful for detecting unilateral or asymmetric prechiasmatic afferent defects in children (see Marcus Gunn pupil, Sec. 25.5).

Ocular motility is tested by having the child follow an object into the various positions of gaze. Movements of each eye individually (ductions) and of the two eyes together (versions, conjugate movements, and convergence) are assessed. Alignment is judged by the symmetry of the corneal light reflexes and by the response to alternate occlusion of each eye (see *cover tests for strabismus*, Sec. 25.6).

External examination begins with general inspection in good illumination, noting size, shape, and symmetry of the orbits; position and movement of the lids; and the position and symmetry of the globes. Viewing the eyes and lids from above will aid in detection of orbital asymmetry, lid masses, proptosis (exophthalmos), and abnormal pulsations. Palpation too is important in detection of orbital and lid masses.

The lacrimal apparatus is assessed by looking for evidence of tear deficiency, overflow of tears (epiphora), and erythema and swelling in the region of the tear sac or gland. The sac is massaged to check for reflux when obstruction is suspected. The presence and position of the puncta are also checked.

The lids and conjunctiva are specifically examined for focal lesions, foreign bodies, and inflammatory signs; loss and maldirection of lashes are also to be noted. When necessary, the lids can be everted in the following manner: (1) instruct the patient to look down; (2) grasp the lashes of the patient's upper lid between the thumb and index finger of one hand; (3) place a probe, a cotton-tipped applicator, or the thumb of

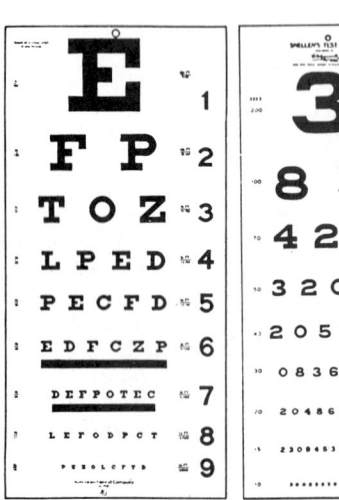
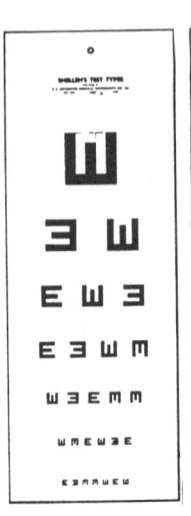
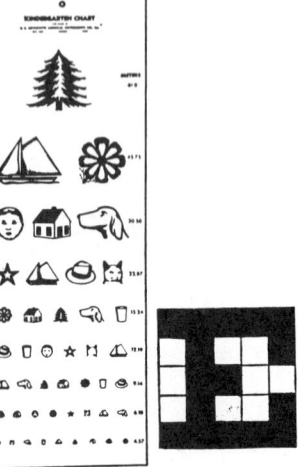

Figure 25–1. Various types of visual acuity charts. As illustrated by the Snellen E, each optotype is designed to subtend 5 min of arc, each component 1 min of arc.

the other hand at the upper margin of the tarsal plate; and (4) pulling the lid down and outward, evert it over the probe, using the instrument as a fulcrum. Skill at eversion of the lid should be acquired. Foreign bodies commonly lodge in the concavity just above the lid margin and are exposed only by fully everting the lid.

The anterior segment of the eye is then evaluated with oblique focal illumination, noting luster and clarity of the cornea, depth and clarity of the anterior chamber, and features of the iris. Transillumination of the anterior segment will aid in detecting opacities and in demonstrating atrophy or hypopigmentation of the iris; these latter signs are important when ocular albinism is suspected. Fluorescein dye will also aid in the diagnosis of abrasions, ulcerations, and foreign bodies.

Biomicroscopy (slit lamp examination) provides a highly magnified view of the various structures of the eye and an optical section through the media of the eye—that is, the cornea, aqueous humor, lens, and vitreous. Lesions can be not only identified but also localized as to their depth within the eye, and the resolution is sufficient to allow detection even of individual inflammatory cells in the aqueous and vitreous. With addition of special lenses and prisms, the angle of the anterior chamber and regions of the fundus also can be examined with the slit lamp. Biomicroscopy is often crucial in trauma and in examination for iritis. It is also helpful in the diagnosis of many metabolic diseases of childhood.

Fundus examination is best done with the pupil dilated unless there are neurologic or other contraindications. Tropicamide (Mydriacyl), 0.5–1% and phenylephrine (Neo-Synephrine), 2.5%, are recommended as mydriatics of short duration. These are safe for most children, but the possibility of adverse systemic effects must be recognized. For very small infants more dilute preparations may be advisable. Beginning with posterior landmarks, the disc and the macula, the four quadrants are systematically examined by following each of the major vessel groups to the periphery. More of the fundus can be seen if the child is directed to look up, down, right, and left. Even with care, only a limited amount of the fundus can be seen with the direct or handheld ophthalmoscope. For examination of the far periphery the indirect ophthalmoscope is used, and full dilation of the pupil is essential.

It should be noted that before an examination of the retina is made, the ophthalmoscope is used to examine the clarity of the media; with a high plus lens ($+8$ or $+10$) in place, the ophthalmoscope can also be used for examination of external lesions and foreign bodies as it provides magnification and good illumination.

Refraction determines the refractive state of the eye; that is, the degree of nearsightedness, farsightedness, or astigmatism. Retinoscopy gives an objective determination of the amount of correction needed and can be done at any age. In young children it is best done with cycloplegia. Subjective refinement of refraction involves asking the patient for preferences in the strength and axis of corrective lenses; it can be accomplished in many school age children. Refraction and determination of visual acuity with appropriate corrective lenses in place are essential steps in deciding whether or not the patient has a visual defect or amblyopia.

Tonometry measures intraocular pressure; it is usually done by the indentation method with the Schiøtz gauge or by the applanation method with the slit lamp. Alternative methods are pneumatic and electronic tonometry. When accurate measurement of the pressure is necessary in a child who cannot cooperate, it may be done with sedation or general anesthesia. A gross estimate of pressure can be made by palpating the globe with the index fingers placed side by side on the upper lid above the tarsal plate.

Examination of the Eye

Hoyt CS: The clinical usefulness of the visual evoked response. J Pediatr Ophthalmol Strab 21:231, 1984.

Isenberg S, Everett S, Parelhoff E: A comparison of mydriatic eyedrops in low-weight infants. Ophthalmology 91:278, 1984.

Linksz A: Color vision tests in clinical practice. Trans Am Acad Ophthalmol Otolaryngol 75:1078, 1971.

Marsh WR, Rawlings SC, Mumma JV: Evaluation of clinical stereoacuity tests. Ophthalmology 87:1265, 1980.

Sokol S, Hansen VC, Moskowitz A, et al: Evoked potentials and preferential looking estimates of visual acuity in pediatric patients. Ophthalmology 90:552, 1983.

Sturner RA, Green JA, Funk S, et al: A developmental approach to preschool vision screening. J Pediatr Ophthalmol Strab 18:61, 1981.

25.3 ABNORMALITIES OF REFRACTION AND ACCOMMODATION

If parallel rays of light come to focus on the retina with the eye in a state of rest (nonaccommodating), emmetropia exists. Such an ideal optical state is not uncommon, but more often the opposite condition, ametropia, exists. Three principal types occur: hyperopia (farsightedness), myopia (nearsightedness), and astigmatism. The majority of children are physiologically hyperopic at birth, but a significant number, especially those born prematurely, are myopic, and there is often some degree of astigmatism. With growth, the refractive state tends to change and should be evaluated periodically.

The refractive state of the eye in children is most accurately measured by cycloplegic refraction, with the use of such drugs as tropicamide (Mydriacyl), cyclopentolate hydrochloride (Cyclogyl), homatropine hydrobromide, or atropine sulfate to relax accommodation.

Hyperopia. If parallel rays of light come to focus posterior to the retina with the eye in a state of rest (nonaccommodating), hyperopia or farsightedness exists. This may result because the anteroposterior diameter of the eye is too short, because the refractive power of the cornea or lens is less than normal, or because the lens is dislocated posteriorly.

In hyperopia, accommodation is used to bring objects into focus for both far and near gaze. If the accommodative effort required is not too great, the child will have clear vision and will be comfortable for both distant and close work. In high degrees of hyperopia requiring greater accommodative effort, vision may be blurred, and the child may complain of "eye strain," headaches, or fatigue. Squinting, eye rubbing, lid inflammation, and lack of interest in reading are also frequent manifestations. There may be associated esotropia (convergent strabismus, accommodative esotropia, Sec. 25.6). Convex lenses (spectacles) of sufficient strength to provide clear vision and comfort are prescribed when indicated.

Myopia. In myopia parallel rays of light come to focus anterior to the retina, possibly because the anteroposterior diameter of the eye is too long, because the refractive power of the cornea or lens is greater than normal, or because the lens is dislocated forward. The principal symptom is blurred vision for distant objects. The far point of clear vision varies inversely with the degree of myopia; as the myopia increases, the far point of clear vision comes closer. With myopia of 1 diopter, for example, the far point of clear focus is 1 meter from the eye; with myopia of 3 diopters, the far point of clear vision is only one third of a meter from the eye. Thus myopic children tend to hold objects and reading matter close, prefer to be close to the blackboard, and may be uninterested in distant activities. Frowning and squinting are common since the visual acuity is improved when the lid aperture is reduced; the effect is similar to that achieved by closing or "stopping down" the aperture of the diaphragm of a camera.

Concave lenses (spectacles or contact lenses) of appropriate strength to provide clear vision and comfort are prescribed. Yearly re-evaluation is advised; simple myopia tends to increase through adolescence. There is a hereditary tendency to myopia, and children of myopic parents should be examined at an early age. In some cases of myopia there are associated degenerative changes of the retina.

Some practitioners advocate the use of cycloplegic agents and bifocals in an effort to retard progression of myopia, but the value of such treatment is controversial.

Astigmatism. In astigmatism there is a difference in the refractive power of the various meridians of the eye. Most cases are due to irregularity in the curvature of the cornea; some astigmatism is due to changes in the lens. Mild degrees of astigmatism are very common and may produce no symptoms. With greater degrees there may be distortion of vision. In an effort to achieve a clearer image, the person with astigmatism will use accommodation or frown or squint to obtain a pinhole effect, as in myopia. Symptoms include "eye strain," headache, and fatigue. Eye rubbing and lid hyperemia, indifference to schoolwork, and holding reading matter close are common manifestations in childhood. Cylindric or spherocylindric lenses are used to provide optical correction when indicated. Glasses may be needed constantly or only part-time, depending on the degree of astigmatism and the severity of the attendant symptoms.

Anisometropia. When the refractive state of one eye is significantly different from the refractive state of the fellow eye, anisometropia exists. Uncorrected, this may lead to sensory deprivation amblyopia or "lazy eye." Early detection and correction are essential if normal visual development in both eyes is to be achieved.

Paralysis of Accommodation. The most frequent cause of paralysis of accommodation in children is the intentional or inadvertent use of cycloplegic substances, topically or systemically; included are all the anticholinergic drugs and poisons as well as plants and plant substances containing naturally occurring alkaloids. Neurogenic causes of accommodative paralysis include lesions affecting the oculomotor nerve (3rd cranial nerve) in any part of its course. Differential diagnosis includes tumors, degenerative diseases, vascular lesions, and trauma. Infectious diseases also may affect accommodation; diphtheria, for example, may cause paralysis of the ciliary muscle. Rarely, inability to accommodate is due to a congenital defect of the ciliary muscle. An apparent defect in accommodation may be psychogenic in origin; it is not uncommon for a child to feign inability to read when it can be demonstrated that visual acuity and ability to focus are normal.

Brodstein RS, Brodstein DE, Olson RJ, et al: The treatment of myopia with atropine and bifocals: A long-term prospective study. Ophthalmology 91:1373, 1984.

Curtin BJ: Physiologic vs pathologic myopia: Genetics vs environment. Ophthalmology 86:681, 1979.

Fulton AB, Dobson V, Salem D, et al: Cycloplegic refractions in infants and young children. Am J Ophthalmol 90:239, 1980.

Mäntyjärvi MI: Changes in refraction in schoolchildren. Arch Ophthalmol 103:790, 1985.

25.4 DISORDERS OF VISION

Amblyopia. Amblyopia is subnormal visual acuity in one or both eyes despite correction of any significant refractive error. The term may embrace a variety of vision defects of organic or nonorganic origin (for example, organic amblyopia designates vision loss directly attributable to trauma or to an organic lesion or disease of the eye or visual pathways), but the term is preferentially used to denote a specific developmental disorder of visual function arising from (1) sensory stimulation deprivation or (2) abnormal binocular interaction

(i.e., malalignment or strabismus). In the latter sense amblyopia is familiarly known as "lazy eye."

Under normal conditions the development of visual acuity proceeds rapidly in infancy and early childhood. Anything that interferes with the formation of a clear retinal image during this early developmental period can produce *sensory deprivation amblyopia.* For example, during a critical developmental period in early life a cataract can interfere with retinal stimulation to such a degree that even after the cataract is successfully removed and the aphakic refractive error is corrected with glasses or a contact lens that provides a clear retinal image, vision will be relatively poor. Similarly, uncorrected anisometropia in the young child can lead to amblyopia; in this condition the eye with the more normal refractive state and clearer retinal image is used for definitive seeing and the eye with the greater refractive error and blurred retinal image becomes amblyopic from sensory deprivation or disuse.

In children with strabismus there is a tendency to suppress or "tune out" the image of the deviating eye as a sensory adaptation to avoid diplopia. If allowed to persist untreated in the young child, such suppression can result in amblyopia.

Susceptibility to amblyopia is greatest within the first 2–3 yr of life and especially in the first months of life, but risk of amblyopia lasts until full visual potential and stability have been achieved, generally by the age of 5–6 yr.

Amblyopia can be treated; the key to success is early detection and prompt intervention. In an infant amblyopia can often be reversed in a matter of days or weeks. In an older child with longstanding amblyopia, months or years of treatment may be required.

Treatment of amblyopia involves (1) providing the clearest possible retinal image (for example, by correction of refractive error, removal of cataract), and (2) stimulation or forced use of the amblyopic eye. The latter is accomplished by occlusion therapy, often referred to as "patching"; the better eye is simply covered to force use of the amblyopic eye. In many cases best results are achieved with complete and constant occlusion throughout the waking hours by the use of adhesive eye pads or "patches"; in some cases part-time occlusion is sufficient or preferred. Occluders placed on spectacles allow peeking, and the adjustable head band type of cloth or plastic occluder is too easily removed by the child. In selected cases an opaque contact lens or a contact lens of sufficiently high power to blur the vision in the better eye is used. In certain cases cycloplegic drops are used to blur the image in the better eye. Most children and their families tolerate occlusion therapy well. In some cases the child resists therapy because of the severity of the vision defect, the cosmetic blemish of the patching, or related psychologic disturbances. The goals of treatment must be thoroughly understood and the treatment carefully supervised. Close monitoring of occlusion therapy is essential, especially in the very young, to avoid deprivation amblyopia in the occluded eye.

Amaurosis. The term amaurosis refers to partial or total loss of vision; it is usually reserved for profound impairment, blindness or near blindness. When amaurosis exists from birth, primary consideration in differential diagnosis must be given to developmental malformations, damage consequent to gestational or perinatal infection, anoxia or hypoxia, perinatal trauma, and the genetically determined diseases that can affect the eye itself or the visual pathways. In certain cases the reason for the amaurosis can be readily determined by objective ophthalmic examination; examples are severe microphthalmia, corneal opacification, dense cataracts, atrophic chorioretinal scars, macular colobomata, retinal dysplasia, and severe optic nerve hypoplasia. In some cases there is intrinsic retinal disease that may not be apparent on initial ophthalmoscopic examination; an example is Leber congenital retinal amaurosis. In this retinal dystrophy the fundus may appear normal or near normal for some time before ophthalmoscopically appreciable signs of retinal degeneration (pigmentary deposits, arteriolar attenuation, optic pallor, etc.) develop; in such cases electroretinography is highly important in diagnosis, as the electroretinographic response in this condition will be markedly reduced or absent. In many cases of amaurosis the defect lies not in the eye or optic nerve but in the brain, requiring neurologic and neuroradiologic evaluation, including computed tomography or magnetic resonance imaging.

Amaurosis that develops in a child who once had useful vision has somewhat different implications. In the absence of obvious ocular disease (cataract, chorioretinitis, retinoblastoma, retinitis pigmentosa, etc.) consideration must be given to many neurologic and systemic disorders that can affect the visual pathways. Amaurosis of rather rapid onset may indicate an encephalopathy (such as might occur with hypertension), infectious or parainfectious processes, vasculitis, leukemia, toxins, or trauma. It may be due to acute demyelinating disease affecting the optic nerves, chiasm, or cerebrum. In some cases precipitous loss of vision is the result of increased intracranial pressure, a rapidly progressive hydrocephalus, or dysfunction of a shunt. More slowly progressive visual loss suggests tumor or neurodegenerative disease. Gliomas of the optic nerve and chiasm and craniopharyngiomas are primary diagnostic considerations in children who show progressive loss of vision.

Manifestations of impairment of vision vary with the age and abilities of the child, the mode of onset, and the laterality and severity of the deficit. The first clue to amaurosis in an infant may be nystagmus or strabismus, the vision defect itself passing undetected for some time. Timidity, clumsiness, or behavioral change may be the initial clues in the very young. Deterioration in school progress and indifference to school activities are common signs in the older child. School age children will often try to hide their disability and, in the case of very slowly progressive disorders, may not themselves realize the severity of the problem; some will detect and promptly report small changes in their vision.

Any evidence of loss of vision requires prompt and thorough ophthalmic evaluation. More often than not, the complete delineation of childhood amaurosis and its etiology will require extensive investigation involving neurologic evaluation, electrophysiologic tests, neuroradiologic procedures, and sometimes metabolic and genetic studies. Management will require that special educational, social and emotional needs be met.

Nyctalopia. Nyctalopia or "night blindness" refers to vision that is defective in reduced illumination. It generally implies impairment in function of the rods, particularly in dark adaptation time and perceptual threshold. *Stationary congenital night blindness* may occur as an autosomal dominant, autosomal recessive, or X-linked recessive condition. It may be associated with myopia and disc anomaly. *Progressive night blindness* usually indicates primary or secondary retinal, choroidal, or vitrioretinal degeneration (Sec. 25.13); it occurs also in vitamin A deficiency or as the result of retinotoxic drugs such as quinine.

Diplopia. Diplopia or "double vision" is most frequently due to malalignment of the visual axes—that is, displacement or deviation of the eye. It is common in heterophoria, in heterotropia of recent onset (particularly when due to acquired nerve palsy), and in proptosis. Because in such cases occluding one eye relieves the diplopia, affected children commonly squint, cover one eye with a hand, or assume abnormal head postures (a face turn or head tilt) to alleviate the bothersome sensation. These mannerisms, especially in preverbal children, are important clues to diplopia. The onset of diplopia in any child warrants prompt evaluation; it may signal the onset of a serious problem such as increased intracranial

pressure, a brain tumor, an orbital mass, or myasthenia gravis.

Monocular diplopia results from dislocation of the lens or some defect in the media or macula.

Psychogenic Disturbances of Vision. Vision problems of psychogenic origin are not uncommon in school age children. Both conversion reactions and willful feigning are encountered. The usual manifestation is a report of reduced visual acuity in one or both eyes. Another common manifestation is constriction of the visual field. In some cases the symptom is diplopia or polyopia.

Important clues to the diagnosis are inappropriate affect, excessive grimacing, inconsistency in performance, and suggestibility. Thorough ophthalmologic examination is essential to differentiate organic from functional visual disorders.

As a rule, affected children do well with reassurance and positive suggestion. In some cases psychiatric care is indicated. In all cases the approach must be supportive and nonpunitive.

Dyslexia. The term dyslexia is used to describe a specific reading disability that is attributable to a primary or developmental defect in the higher cortical processing of graphic symbols. It is to be differentiated from (1) reading retardation that may be secondary to other causes such as intellectual impairment, maturational delay, cultural or educational deprivation, emotional disturbances, organic brain disease, or sensory defects, and from (2) acquired word blindness (alexia) occurring as the result of a lesion in the dominant cerebral hemisphere.

Neither dyslexia nor the often associated symptoms such as letter or word reversal and so-called mirror writing are due to any defect in the eye or visual acuity per se, nor are they attributable to a defect in ocular motility or binocular alignment, but ophthalmologic evaluation of the child with a reading problem is recommended because (1) such assessment is of value in differential diagnosis, (2) correction of any concurrent ocular problems such as a refractive error, amblyopia, or strabismus will ensure the best possible visual function for the child's education, and (3) the ophthalmologist can be of help in counseling patient and family.

The approach to treatment is remedial instruction. Treatment directed to the eyes themselves cannot be expected to correct developmental dyslexia.

Barnet AB, Manson JI, Wilmer E: Acute cerebral blindness in childhood. Six cases studied clinically and electrophysiologically. Neurology 30:1147, 1970.
Duffy FH, Burchfield JL, Snodgrass SR: The pharmacology of amblyopia. Ophthalmology 86:489, 1978.
Francois J: Diagnosis of blindness in the infant. Ann Ophthalmol (Sept):533, 1970.
Flynn JT, Cassady JC: Current trends in amblyopia therapy. Ophthalmology 85:428, 1978.
Hittner HM, Borda RP, Justice J Jr: X-linked recessive congenital stationary night blindness, myopia, and tilted discs. J Pediatr Ophthalmol 18:15, 1981.
Jastrzebski GR, Hoyt CS, Marg E: Stimulus deprivation amblyopia in children: Sensitivity, plasticity, and elasticity (SPE). Arch Ophthalmol 102:1030, 1984.
Kushner BJ: Functional amblyopia associated with organic ocular lesions. Am J Ophthalmol 91:39, 1981.
Mäntyjärvi MI: The amblyopic schoolgirl syndrome. J Pediatr Ophthalmol Strab 18:30, 1981.
Mellor DH, Fields AR: Dissociated visual development: Electrodiagnostic studies in infants who are "slow to see." Dev Med Child Neurol 22:327, 1980.
Stager DR: Amblyopia and the pediatrician. Pediatr Ann (Feb):91, 1977.
Tongue AC: Low vision examination in children with visual impairment. J Pediatr Ophthalmol Strab 17:175, 1980.
von Noorden GK, Milane JB: Penalization in the treatment of amblyopia. Am J Ophthalmol 88:511, 1979.

25.5 ABNORMALITIES OF PUPIL AND IRIS

Aniridia. With this developmental anomaly there is almost complete absence of iris. The defect is usually accompanied by photophobia, nystagmus, and defective vision. There may be associated glaucoma, progressive corneal degenerative changes, cataracts, macular hypoplasia, and optic nerve hypoplasia. The condition may be familial (the transmission being dominant) or sporadic. Sporadic aniridia is associated with an increased incidence of Wilms tumor; periodic abdominal examination, supplemented by ultrasound examination or intravenous pyelography, is advised in children with sporadic aniridia. (See also Sec. 16.13.)

Coloboma of the Iris. Coloboma is a developmental defect that may take the form of a defect in a sector of the iris, a hole in the substance of the iris, or a notch in the pupillary margin. Simple colobomata are frequently transmitted as an autosomal dominant characteristic, and may occur alone or be associated with other anomalies. An iris coloboma may be part of an extensive coloboma involving the fundus and optic nerve as a result of malclosure of the embryonic fissure (Sec. 25.13). Such defects may be associated with chromosomal abnormalities, particularly trisomies 13 and 18.

Heterochromia. In heterochromia the two irides are of different color, or a portion of an iris differs in color from the remainder. Simple heterochromia may occur as an autosomal dominant characteristic. Congenital heterochromia is also a feature of Waardenburg syndrome, an autosomal dominant condition characterized principally by lateral displacement of the inner canthi and puncta, pigmentary disturbances (usually a median white forelock and patches of depigmentation of the skin), and defective hearing. Change in the color of the iris (acquired heterochromia) may occur as the result of trauma, hemorrhage, intraocular inflammation (iridocyclitis, uveitis), intraocular tumor (especially retinoblastoma), intraocular foreign body, glaucoma, iris atrophy, or oculosympathetic palsy (Horner syndrome).

Other Iris Lesions. Discrete nodules of the iris may be seen in patients with neurofibromatosis. The lesions vary from slightly elevated pigmented areas to distinct ball-like excrescences. Slit lamp examination may aid in diagnosis of neurofibromatosis.

In leukemia there may be infiltration of the iris, sometimes with hypopyon, an accumulation of white cells in the anterior chamber which may herald relapse or involvement of the central nervous system.

The lesion of juvenile xanthogranuloma (nevoxanthoendothelioma) may occur in the eye as a yellowish fleshy mass or plaque of the iris. Spontaneous hyphema (blood in the anterior chamber), glaucoma, or a red eye with signs of uveitis may be associated. A search for the skin lesions of xanthogranuloma (see also Sec. 24.32) should be made in any infant or young child with spontaneous hyphema. In many cases the ocular lesion will respond to topical corticosteroid therapy.

Dyscoria and Corectopia. Dyscoria is abnormal shape of the pupil, and corectopia is abnormal pupillary position. They may occur together or independently as congenital anomalies. Corectopia may be associated with dislocation of the lens. Distortion and displacement of the pupil are frequently the result of trauma and are important signs of prolapse of the iris in perforating injuries of the eye; they may also be seen with tears of the iris, with segmental iridoplegia, and with synechiae (adhesions of iris to lens or cornea).

Leukocoria. This term describes any white pupillary reflex or so-called cat's eye reflex. Primary diagnostic considerations in any child with leukocoria are cataract, persistent hyperplastic primary vitreous, cicatricial retinopathy of prematurity, retinal detachment and retinoschisis, larval granulomatosis, and retinoblastoma (Fig. 25–2). Also to be considered are endophthalmitis, organized vitreous hemorrhage, leukemic ophthalmopathy, exudative retinopathy (as in Coats disease), and a few rare conditions such as medulloepithelioma, massive retinal gliosis, the retinal pseudotumor of Norrie disease, the so-called pseudoglioma of the Bloch-Sulzberger syndrome,

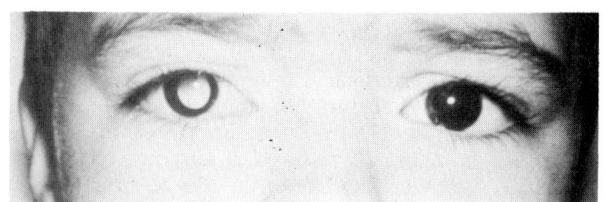

Figure 25–2. Leukocoria. White pupillary reflex in a child with retinoblastoma.

and the retinal lesions of the phakomatoses, to name just a few. A white reflex may also be seen with fundus coloboma, large atrophic chorioretinal scars, and ectopic medullation of retinal nerve fibers.

Often the diagnosis can readily be made by direct examination of the eye by ophthalmoscopy and biomicroscopy. Ultrasonographic and radiologic examinations are helpful. In some cases the final diagnosis rests with the pathologist.

Anisocoria. This is inequality of the pupils. As a general rule, if the inequality is more pronounced in the presence of bright focal illumination or on near gaze, the larger pupil is abnormal, whereas if the anisocoria is worse in reduced illumination, the smaller pupil is abnormal. Neurologic causes of anisocoria (parasympathetic or sympathetic lesions) must be differentiated from local causes such as synechiae (adhesions), congenital iris defects (colobomata, aniridia), and pharmacologic effects. Simple, central anisocoria may occur in otherwise healthy individuals.

The Dilated Fixed Pupil. Differential diagnosis of the dilated unreactive pupil includes internal ophthalmoplegia due to a central or peripheral lesion, the Hutchinson pupil of transentorial herniation, tonic pupil, pharmacologic blockade, and iridoplegia secondary to ocular trauma.

The most common cause of a dilated unreactive pupil is the purposeful or accidental instillation of a cycloplegic agent, particularly atropine and related substances. Internal ophthalmoplegia may occur with central lesions, and in children the possibility of pinealoma must be considered. The "blown pupil" of transentorial herniation, as occurs with subdural hematoma and increasing intracranial pressure, is usually unilateral, and usually the patient is obviously ill. The pilocarpine test can help to differentiate neurologic iridoplegia from pharmacologic blockade. In the case of neurologic iridoplegia the dilated pupil will constrict within minutes after the instillation of 1 or 2 drops of 0.5–1.0% pilocarpine; if the pupil has been dilated with atropine, the pilocarpine will have no effect. Because pilocarpine is a long-acting drug, this test is not to be used in acute situations in which pupillary signs must be carefully monitored.

Tonic Pupil. This is typically a large pupil that reacts poorly to light (the reaction may be very slow or essentially nil), reacts poorly and slowly to accommodation, and redilates in a slow, tonic manner. A distinctive feature of the tonic pupil is its sensitivity to dilute cholinergic agents, such as 0.125% pilocarpine. The condition is usually unilateral. Its occurrence in association with decreased deep tendon reflexes in young women is referred to as *Adie syndrome*. It may also occur in familial dysautonomia. Tonic pupil is usually attributed to a lesion affecting the ciliary ganglion in the orbit, and sometimes referred to as ciliary ganglionitis. It is usually benign.

Marcus Gunn Pupil. The Marcus Gunn pupil sign indicates an asymmetric, prechiasmatic, afferent conduction defect. It is best demonstrated by the swinging flashlight test; this allows comparison of the direct and consensual pupillary responses in both eyes. With the patient fixing on a distant target (to control accommodation) a bright focal light is directed alternately into each eye in turn. In the presence of an afferent lesion, both the direct response to light in the affected eye and the consensual response in the fellow eye will be defective. Swinging the light to the better or normal eye causes both pupils to react (constrict) normally. Swinging the light back to the affected eye causes both pupils to redilate to some degree, reflecting the defective conduction. This is a very sensitive and useful test for detecting and confirming optic nerve and retinal disease. A relative afferent defect may be found in some children with amblyopia.

Horner Syndrome. The principal signs of oculosympathetic paresis (Horner syndrome) are homolateral miosis, mild ptosis, and apparent enophthalmos with slight elevation of the lower lid. There may also be decrease in facial sweating, increased amplitude of accommodation, and transient decrease in intraocular pressure. If paralysis of the ocular sympathetic fibers occurs before the age of 2 yr, there may be heterochromia iridis with hypopigmentation of the iris on the affected side.

Oculosympathetic paralysis may be due to a lesion in the midbrain, brain stem, upper spinal cord, neck, middle fossa, or orbit. Congenital oculosympathetic paresis due to birth trauma is common, though the ocular signs, particularly the anisocoria, may pass undetected for years. Acquired oculosympathetic paresis may be due to mediastinal disease, including neuroblastoma.

The cocaine test is useful in the diagnosis of oculosympathetic paralysis; a normal pupil will dilate within 20–45 min after instillation of 1 or 2 drops of 4% cocaine while the miotic pupil of an oculosympathetic paresis will dilate poorly if at all to cocaine. In some cases there is denervation supersensitivity to dilute phenylephrine; 1 or 2 drops of a 1% solution will dilate the affected but not the normal pupil. Furthermore, the instillation of 1% hydroxyamphetamine hydrobromide will dilate the pupil only if the postganglionic sympathetic neuron is intact.

Francois J: Differential diagnosis of leukokoria in children. Ann Ophthalmol 10:1375, 1978.
Grant WM, Walton DS: Progressive changes in the angle in congenital aniridia with development of glaucoma. Am J Ophthalmol 78:842, 1974.
Greenwald MJ, Folk ER: Afferent pupillary defects in amblyopia. J Pediatr Ophthalmol Strab 20:63, 1983.
Hittner HM, Riccardi VM, Ferrell RE, et al: Variable expressivity in autosomal dominant aniridia by clinical, electrophysiologic, and angiographic criteria. Am J Ophthalmol 89:531, 1980.
Jaffe N, Cassady JR, Filler RM, et al: Heterochromia and Horner syndrome associated with cervical and mediastinal neuroblastoma. J Pediatr 87:75, 1975.
Lewis RA, Riccardi VM: Von Recklinghausen neurofibromatosis: Incidence of iris hamartomata. Ophthalmology 88:348, 1981.
Loewenfeld IE: "Simple, central" anisocoria: A common condition seldom recognized. Trans Am Acad Ophthalmol Otolaryngol 83:832, 1977.
Mackman G, Brightbill FS, Opitz JM: Corneal changes in aniridia. Am J Ophthalmol 87:497, 1979.
Maloney WF, Younge BR, Moyer NJ: Evaluation of the causes and accuracy of pharmacologic localization in Horner's syndrome. Am J Ophthalmol 90:394, 1980.
McCrary JA: Light reflex anatomy and the afferent pupil defect. Trans Am Acad Ophthalmol Otolaryngol 83:820, 1977.
Thompson HS: Segmental palsy of the iris sphincter in Adie's syndrome. Arch Ophthalmol 96:1615, 1978.
Thompson HS, Newsome DA, Loewenfeld IE: The fixed dilated pupil: Sudden iridoplegia or mydriatic drops? A simple diagnostic test. Arch Ophthalmol 86:21, 1971.
Weinstein JM, Zweifel TJ, Thompson HS: Congenital Horner's syndrome. Arch Ophthalmol 98:1074, 1980.
Zimmerman L: Ocular lesions of juvenile xanthogranuloma (nevoxanthoendothelioma). Trans Am Acad Ophthalmol Otolaryngol 69:412, 1965.

25.6 DISORDERS OF EYE MOVEMENT AND ALIGNMENT

STRABISMUS
(Squint, Cast; Tropia, Phoria; Cross-Eye, Wall-Eye)

The development of normal vision in each eye, the maintenance of proper alignment of the visual axes (orthophoria), and the ability to integrate the images from the two eyes into a single visual perception are essential to normal depth perception, or stereopsis. Any variation from normal sensorimotor development in early life may result in lifelong patterns of defective vision or abnormal ocular alignment. Early detection and treatment of strabismus in children is of primary importance; and proper assessment and management require knowledge of the various types of strabismus, the methods of detection, and the principles of treatment.

Clinical Types of Strabismus; Classification and Terminology. The two principal types of deviation or malalignment of the eyes are heterophoria and heterotropia. *Heterophoria* is a latent tendency to malalignment; the eye deviates only under certain conditions (such as fatigue, illness, stress, or dissociative testing) that interfere with maintenance of normal fusion. Phorias are common and may or may not give rise to bothersome symptoms such as transient diplopia, asthenopia ("eye strain"), or headaches. When the deviation exceeds the amplitude of fusion and becomes manifest, the malalignment is termed *heterotropia* or simply tropia. The condition may be monocular or alternating, depending on the vision and fixation pattern. In *alternating strabismus* the patient uses either eye for fixation or definitive seeing while the fellow eye deviates; since each eye is being used in turn, vision develops more or less equally in both. The patient in effect learns to suppress the image in the deviating (nonfixating) eye. When only one eye is used (or preferred) for fixation and the fellow eye consistently deviates, the deviation may be referred to as monocular or as right or left strabismus; in this situation the child is prone to amblyopia or defective central vision in the deviating eye as the result of disuse or misuse.

Strabismus is further described according to the direction of the deviation. Convergent deviation, a crossing or turning in of the eyes, is designated by the prefix *eso-* (hence esotropia, esophoria), while a divergent deviation or turning outward of the eyes (commonly referred to as wall-eye) is designated by the prefix *exo-*. Vertical deviations are indicated by the prefixes *hyper-* and *hypo-*. These may occur singly or in various combinations; in addition, torsional or cyclovertical deviations may occur.

The etiologic classification of strabismus is complex and knowledge of the causative factors and mechanisms incomplete. Certain major types must be distinguished; these are paralytic (noncomitant), nonparalytic (comitant), accommodative, and nonaccommodative.

Paralytic strabismus is due to weakness or paralysis of one or more of the extraocular muscles. The deviation characteristically worsens on gaze into the field of action of the affected muscle. Hence, in the case of a right abducent paresis the eyes appear crossed on looking to the right but appear straight (orthophoric) on looking to the left. The subjective manifestation is diplopia; to avoid this bothersome sensation, the child may turn the head to compensate for the paretic muscle or may close or cover one eye to eliminate the double image. Such mannerisms are important clues to the presence of an extraocular muscle palsy. With few exceptions, acquired extraocular muscle palsies are ominous signs of a serious pathologic process; the development of a noncomitant strabismus may be the first sign of an intracranial tumor, an infectious or parainfectious process (meningitis, encephalitis, neuritis), a demyelinizing or neurodegenerative disease, myasthenia gravis, or a progressive myopathy. A notable exception is benign 6th nerve palsy (see below). Congenital paralytic strabismus is more commonly due to developmental defects of the cranial nerve nuclei or fibers, to muscle anomalies, to congenital infection syndromes, or to birth trauma.

Nonparalytic strabismus is the more common type. There is no defect in the action of the individual extraocular muscles, and the amount of deviation is constant or relatively constant in all directions of gaze. The majority of the congenital or infantile esotropias are of the nonparalytic or comitant type; this type is best treated surgically, but successful treatment must also involve treatment of any concurrent amblyopia.

Some cases of nonparalytic strabismus are due to underlying ocular or visual defects, such as may occur with cataracts, lesions of the optic nerve or macula, high refractive errors, or asymmetric refractive errors (anisometropia). When possible, the underlying ocular condition is corrected first; in selected cases surgery may then be offered to "straighten" the eyes.

A special type of nonparalytic strabismus is *accommodative esotropia* (Fig. 25–3). This type depends on the relationship between the accommodation and convergence reflexes. In certain individuals activation of accommodation results in overconvergence or crossing of the eyes; in some cases also the amount of crossing with near gaze is greater than that with gaze into the distance. This type of deviation most commonly appears at 2–3 yr of age, with a range of onset from approximately 6 mo–7 or 8 yr. The majority of affected children have some degree of hyperopia (farsightedness). In most cases the crossing can be controlled with glasses that correct the hyperopia; some children require the use of bifocal lenses to control fully the excessive convergence for near gaze. Some respond to topical miotics such as phospholine iodide, but these must be used with great care as they are long-acting cholinesterase inhibitors. With early treatment of accommodative esotropia good vision should be maintained in both eyes; when amblyopia occurs, it is necessary to use occlusion therapy as well as glasses. A few children with accommodative esotropia require surgery for a residual amount of crossing that cannot be controlled with glasses alone.

True strabismus must be differentiated from the false impression of deviation created by certain anatomic variations. Children with prominent epicanthal folds and broad, flat nasal bridges will often appear cross-eyed when they are in fact orthophoric; this is *pseudoesotropia*. Similarly, an orthophoric child may appear to have a divergent strabismus because of an increased interpupillary distance or a slight disparity between the position of the corneal light reflex and the pupillary axis; this is *pseudoexotropia*. Various types of facial asymmetry can also contribute to the false impression of vertical malalignment of the eyes.

Methods of Testing for Strabismus. Two relatively simple and reliable techniques for assessing the alignment of the eyes in children are the Hirschberg or corneal light reflex test and the cover, uncover, and cross-cover tests. The *Hirschberg test* involves simply observing the position of the corneal reflexes (reflections) when a small focal light is directed toward the patient's face. If the light reflex is well centered in each eye or falls symmetrically on corresponding points of both eyes simultaneously, the eyes are properly aligned. If the light reflex in one eye is well centered while the light reflex in the fellow eye falls nasally or temporally, superiorly or inferiorly, a deviation exists. The amount of prism needed to recenter the light reflex in the deviating eye gives an accurate measurement of the degree of deviation.

In the *cover, uncover, and cross-cover tests* the eyes are observed for compensatory or adjustive refixation movements. With the patient fixating a distant target, the examiner alternately covers each eye in turn with an occluder. If no movement of either eye occurs as the occluder is moved back and forth from one eye to the other, alignment is normal (orthophoria). If there is esotropia, the deviating eye will be seen to move outward as the fixating eye is occluded; if there is exotropia, the deviating eye will move inward as the fixating eye is occluded. In the case of a phoria or latent deviation it is the occluded eye that tends to deviate because of the temporary disruption of binocular fusion; the adjustive or refixation movement will be seen at the moment of uncovering. The tests should be performed both for distance and for near gaze to assure detection of any accommodative component or any abnormality of the distance-near relationship; the tests should also be done in the cardinal positions of gaze to assure detection of any incomitancy. In addition, the extraocular muscle functions of each eye should be tested individually. Simple toys, particularly those that create a gentle noise, are especially useful in attracting the attention of young children for these tests, but detailed targets such as letters, numbers, and pictures are needed to elicit accommodative deviations.

Before proceeding with the light reflex and cover testing it is advisable to take time simply to observe the child at a nonthreatening distance in quiet, pleasant surroundings while the child plays or sits comfortably with a parent, particularly when the child is very young, shy, fearful, or retarded.

Principles of Treatment. The first goal of treatment is to develop the best possible vision in each eye, and, if possible, equal or nearly equal vision in both eyes. Any correctable underlying defect such as a cataract must be dealt with, contributing refractive errors must be corrected with lenses, and any amblyopia must be vigorously treated with occlusion therapy.

The second goal is to achieve the best possible ocular alignment, especially for the primary or forward gaze position and for the reading or eyes-down position. In many cases surgery is required. Surgical treatment is particularly important in congenital strabismus, and it should be accomplished at the earliest possible time to give the child the best possible opportunity to develop normal sensorimotor patterns. The longer the deviation persists untreated, the less chance there is for development of good or reasonably good function. Surgery is also required in some children with accommodative or partially accommodative esotropia when there is some degree of residual crossing that cannot be controlled with glasses and/or miotics. Surgical correction of a deviation is also offered in selected cases for cosmetic reasons, particularly when there is an underlying ocular defect such as an optic nerve or macular lesion or a dense amblyopia that cannot be altered. In some cases multiple surgical procedures are required for strabismus, but the majority of uncomplicated cases can be corrected with only one or two procedures.

The ultimate goal of treatment is to develop fusion and

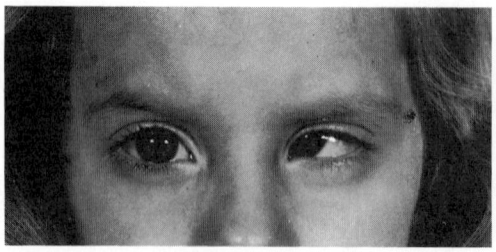 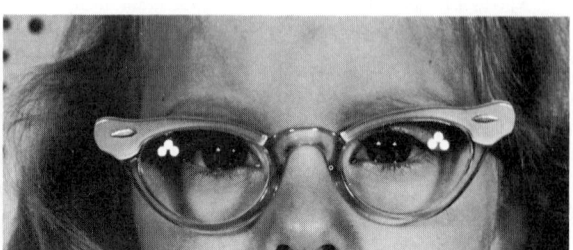

Figure 25–3. Accommodative esotropia; control of deviation with corrective lenses.

depth perception. In some cases the ophthalmologist and the patient must be satisfied with less than the ideal functional result.

OTHER DISORDERS

Duane Syndrome. This is a congenital ocular motor disorder in which there is a defect in abduction with an associated retraction of the globe on adduction. The retraction is typically accompanied by narrowing of the palpebral fissure. There may also be a defect in adduction of the affected eye, with vertical or oblique movement of the eye on attempted adduction. The condition may be unilateral or bilateral, may occur as an isolated defect or with other anomalies, and in some instances is familial. Associated defects have included fibrosis or abnormal insertion of the lateral rectus, hypoplasia of cranial nerve VI, aberrant innervation of the lateral rectus by cranial nerve III, and dual innervation of the lateral rectus muscle by cranial nerves VI and III. Electrophysiologic evidence has been found for a co-contraction phenomenon or supranuclear disorder.

Moebius Syndrome. This consists of congenital facial palsy and inability to abduct the eye. The etiology is unknown. The facial palsy is commonly bilateral, frequently asymmetric, and often incomplete, tending to spare the lower face and platysma. Ectropion, epiphora, and exposure keratopathy may develop. The abduction defect may be unilateral or bilateral. It is usually complete, and esotropia is common. Associated developmental defects may include ptosis, palatal and lingual palsy, hearing loss, pectoral and lingual muscle defects, micrognathia, syndactyly, supernumerary digits, or absence of hands, feet, fingers, or toes. Surgical correction of the esotropia can be done in selected cases.

Gradenigo Syndrome. This is an acquired abducens palsy with pain in the distribution of the homolateral trigeminal nerve, indicating involvement of the petrous portion of the 6th cranial nerve and the adjacent gasserian ganglion. The usual causes are otitis media or mastoiditis with inflammation extending into the petrous bone, its meninges, and the inferior petrosal sinus. Tumor is rarely the cause. Principal signs and symptoms are weakness of the lateral rectus, diplopia, ocular and facial pain, photophobia, lacrimation, and sometimes corneal hypesthesia. There may also be involvement of the 7th nerve, with facial palsy.

Benign Sixth Nerve Palsy. This is a painless acquired abducens palsy that resolves spontaneously, usually without residua. The palsy typically develops 1–3 wk after a nonspecific febrile illness or upper respiratory infection; in some cases the palsy precedes other symptoms of infection or occurs during the prodrome of an exanthem. Improvement usually begins within 3–6 wk after onset, and recovery is usually complete within 10–12 wk. Episodes may be recurrent. The paresis is thought to be a neurotropic effect of a viral infection. Except for benign 6th nerve palsy the development of a cranial nerve palsy in a child is usually a sign of a serious pathologic process, such as intracranial tumor, increased intracranial pressure, meningitis, or demyelinating disease.

Brown Syndrome. In this syndrome elevation of the eye in the adducted position is restricted or absent. Often, there is an associated downward deviation of the affected eye in adduction. There may be a compensatory tilt of the head. Various causes have been described. In some cases there is congenital shortening of the anterior sheath of the superior oblique tendon; in others there are fine adhesions between the sheath and the tendon. In many cases no anatomic abnormality is found. Acquired and intermittent cases have been related to inflammation or injury in the region of the trochlea of the superior oblique. Surgery is helpful in selected cases.

Parinaud Syndrome. This eponym designates a palsy of vertical gaze, isolated or associated with pupillary or nuclear oculomotor (cranial nerve III) paresis. It indicates a lesion affecting the mesencephalic tegmentum. The ophthalmic signs of midbrain disease include vertical gaze palsy, dissociation of the pupillary responses to light and to near focus, general pupillomotor paralysis, corectopia, dyscoria, accommodative disturbances, pathologic lid retraction, ptosis, extraocular muscle paresis, and convergence paralysis. In some cases there are spasms of convergence, convergent retraction nystagmus, and vertical nystagmus, particularly on attempted vertical gaze. Combinations of these signs are referred to as the Koerber-Salus-Elschnig or sylvian aqueduct syndrome.

A principal cause of vertical gaze palsy and associated mesencephalic signs in children is tumor of the pineal gland or 3rd ventricle. Differential diagnosis includes trauma and demyelinating disease. In children with hydrocephalus, impairment of vertical gaze and pathologic lid retraction are referred to as the *setting sun sign*. A transient supranuclear disorder of gaze is sometimes seen in healthy infants.

Congenital Ocular Motor Apraxia. This congenital disorder of conjugate gaze is characterized by (1) a defect in voluntary horizontal gaze, (2) compensatory jerking movement of the head, and (3) retention of slow pursuit and reflexive eye movements. Additional features are absence of the fast (refixation) phase of optokinetic nystagmus and obligate contraversive deviation of the eyes on rotation of the body. Typically, the affected child is unable to look quickly to either side voluntarily in response to command or in response to an eccentrically presented object but may, however, be able to follow a slowly moving target to either side. To compensate for the defect in purposive lateral eye movements, the child jerks the head to bring the eyes into the desired position and may also blink repetitively in an attempt to change fixation.

The pathogenesis of congenital ocular motor apraxia is unknown; it may be due to delayed myelination of the ocular motor pathways. The condition tends to become less conspicuous with age. It may be associated with some clumsiness and with slowness in reading.

A disorder of eye movement resembling congenital ocular motor apraxia may occur in patients with certain metabolic neurodegenerative diseases (particularly Gaucher disease) or with ataxia-telangiectasia, or as a sign of brain tumor.

Nystagmus. Nystagmus (rhythmic oscillations of one or both eyes) may be due to abnormality in any one of the three basic mechanisms that regulate position and movement of the eyes: the fixation, conjugate gaze, or vestibular mechanisms. In addition, physiologic nystagmus may be elicited by appropriate stimuli.

Congenital pendular nystagmus is commonly associated with ocular and visual defects; it typically occurs with albinism, aniridia, achromatopsia, congenital cataracts, congenital macular lesions, congenital optic atrophy, and high refractive errors. In some instances pendular nystagmus occurs as a dominant or X-linked characteristic without obvious ocular abnormalities. There may be associated rhythmic movements of the head.

Congenital jerky nystagmus is characterized by horizontal jerky oscillations with gaze preponderance; the nystagmus is coarser in one direction of gaze than in the other, with the jerk toward the direction of gaze. There is usually a point of reversal or null point in which the nystagmus lessens and in which position vision is best; compensatory posturing, turning of the head to bring the eyes into the position of least nystagmus, is characteristic. The cause of congenital jerky nystagmus is unknown; in some instances it is familial.

Acquired nystagmus requires prompt and thorough evaluation. Worrisome pathologic types are the gaze-paretic or gaze-evoked oscillations of cerebellar, brain stem, or cerebral disease.

Nystagmus retractorius or *convergent nystagmus* is repetitive jerking of the eyes into the orbit or toward each other. It is usually seen with vertical gaze palsy as a feature of the Parinaud or Koerber-Salus-Elschnig (sylvian aqueduct) syndrome. The causal condition may be neoplastic, vascular, or inflammatory. In children nystagmus retractorius suggests particularly the presence of pinealoma or hydrocephalus.

Spasmus nutans is a special type of acquired nystagmus in childhood (see also Sec. 21.13). In its complete form it is characterized by the triad of pendular nystagmus, head nodding, and torticollis. The nystagmus is characteristically very fine, very rapid, horizontal, and pendular; it is often asymmetric, sometimes unilateral. Signs usually develop within the first year or two of life. Components of the triad may develop at varying times. The cause is unknown, but poor illumination and deprivation have been implicated. The condition is benign and self-limited, usually lasting a few months though sometimes years. Certain insidious lesions such as optic glioma may produce a fine rapid nystagmus (asymmetric or monocular) that initially mimics spasmus nutans. The differential diagnosis also includes congenital nystagmus, midbrain glioma (Sec. 21.22), and encephalopathy (Sec. 21.24). Children with nystagmus warrant close follow-up.

To be differentiated from true nystagmus are certain special types of abnormal eye movements, particularly opsoclonus, ocular dysmetria, and flutter.

Opsoclonus. Opsoclonus and ataxic conjugate movements are terms which describe spontaneous, nonrhythmic, multidirectional, chaotic movements of the eyes. The eyes appear to be in agitation, with bursts of conjugate movement of varying amplitude in varying directions. Opsoclonus is most often associated with encephalitis. It may be the first sign of neuroblastoma.

Ocular Motor Dysmetria. This is analogous to dysmetria of the limbs. There is lack of precision in performing movements of refixation, characterized by an overshoot (or undershoot) of the eyes with several corrective to and fro oscillations on looking from one point to another. Ocular motor dysmetria is a sign of cerebellar or cerebellar pathway disease.

Flutter-Like Oscillations. These intermittent to and fro horizontal oscillations of the eyes may occur spontaneously or on change of fixation. They are characteristic of cerebellar disease.

Anthony JH, Ouvrier RA, Wise G: Spasmus nutans: A mistaken identity. Arch Neurol 37:373, 1980.

Apt L, Beckwitt MC, Isenberg S: Emotional aspects of hospitalization of children for strabismus surgery. Ann Ophthalmol (Jan):11, 1974.

Baker JD, Parks MM: Early-onset accommodative esotropia. Am J Ophthalmol 90:11, 1980.

Bixenman WW, von Noorden GK: Benign recurrent VI nerve palsy in childhood. J Pediatr Ophthalmol Strab 18:29, 1981.

Chan CC, Sogg RL, Steinman L: Isolated oculomotor palsy after measles immunization. Am J Ophthalmol 89:446, 1980.

Cogan DG: Ocular dysmetria: flutter-like oscillations of the eyes, and opsoclonus. Arch Ophthalmol 51:318, 1954.

Cogan DG: Congenital ocular motor apraxia. Can J Ophthalmol 1:253, 1966.

Cogan DG: Heredity of congenital ocular motor apraxia. Trans Am Acad Ophthalmol Otolaryngol 76:60, 1972.

Grover WD, Naiman JL: Progressive paresis of vertical gaze in lipid storage disease. Neurology 21:896, 1971.

Grunt JA, Destro RL, Hamtil LW, et al: Ocular palsies in children with diabetes mellitus. Diabetes 25:459, 1976.

Harley RD: Paralytic strabismus in children: Etiologic incidence and management of the third, fourth and sixth nerve palsies. Ophthalmology 87:24, 1980.

Harley RD, Rodrigues MM, Crawford JS: Congenital fibrosis of the extraocular muscles. J Pediatr Ophthalmol Strab 15:346, 1978.

Hiatt RL: Medical management of accommodative esotropia. J Pediatr Ophthalmol Strab 20:199, 1983.

Hoyt CS, Mousel DK, Weber AA: Transient supranuclear disturbance of gaze in healthy neonates. Am J Ophthalmol 89:708, 1980.

Ing M: Early surgical alignment for congenital esotropia. Ophthalmology 90:132, 1983.

Katz NNK, Whitmore PV, Beauchamp GR: Brown's syndrome in twins. J Pediatr Ophthalmol Strab 18:32, 1981.

Kornder LD, Nursey JN, Pratt-Johnson JA, et al: Detection of manifest strabismus in young children: 1. A prospective study. Am J Ophthalmol 77:209, 1974.

Kornder LD, Nursey JN, Pratt-Johnson JA, et al: Detection of manifest strabismus in young children. 2. A retrospective study. Am J Ophthalmol 77:211, 1974.

Kushner BJ: Ocular causes of abnormal head postures. Ophthalmology 86:2115, 1979.

Magoon EH: Botulinum toxin chemo-denervation for strabismus in infants and children. J Pediatr Ophthalmol Strab 21:110, 1984.

Miller NR: Solitary oculomotor nerve palsy in children. Am J Ophthalmol 83:106, 1977.

Mohindra I, Zwann J, Held R, et al: Development of acuity and stereopsis in infants with esotropia. Ophthalmology 92:691, 1985.

Norton EWD, Cogan DG: Spasmus nutans: A clinical study of twenty cases followed two years or more since onset. Arch Ophthalmol 52:442, 1954.

O'Malley ER, Helveston EM, Ellis FD: Duane's retraction syndrome—plus. J Pediatr Ophthalmol Strab 19:161, 1982.

O'Neill JF: Strabismus in childhood. Pediatr Ann 6:10, 1977.

Pfaffenbach DD, Cross HE, Kearns TP: Congenital anomalies in Duane's retraction syndrome. Arch Ophthalmol 88:635, 1972.

Richard JM, Parks M: Intermittent exotropia: Surgical results in different age groups. Ophthalmology 90:1172, 1983.

Scott WE, Kraft SP: Surgical treatment of compensatory head position in congenital nystagmus. J Pediatr Ophthalmol Strab 21:85, 1984.

Sevel D: Brown's syndrome—a possible etiology explained embryologically. J Pediatr Ophthalmol Strab 18:26, 1981.

Shetty T, Rosman NP: Opsoclonus in hydrocephalus. Arch Ophthalmol 88:585, 1972.

Smith JL, Walsh FB: Opsoclonus—ataxic conjugate movements of the eye. Arch Ophthalmol 64:244, 1960.

Smith JL, Ziepes I, Gay AJ, et al: Nystagmus retractorius. Arch Ophthalmol 62:864, 1959.

Solomon GE, Chutorian AM: Opsoclonus and occult neuroblastoma. N Engl J Med 279:475, 1968.

Utrata J: Gradenigo's syndrome—bilateral occurrence. The Eye, Ear, Nose and Throat Monthly 52:54, 1973.

Van Allen MW, Blodi FC: Neurologic aspects of the Möbius syndrome. A case study with electromyography of the extraocular and facial muscles. Neurology 10:249, 1960.

van Pelt W, Andermann F: On the early onset of ophthalmoplegic migraine. Am J Dis Child 107:228, 1964.

Wang FM, Wertenbaker C, Behrens MM, et al: Acquired Brown's syndrome in children with juvenile rheumatoid arthritis. Ophthalmology 91:23, 1984.

Wybar K: Disorders of ocular motility in brain stem lesions in children. Ann Ophthalmol 3:645, 1971.

Zaret CR, Behrens MM, Eggers HM: Congenital ocular motor apraxia and brainstem tumor. Arch Ophthalmol 98:328, 1980.

25.7 ABNORMALITIES OF THE LIDS

Ptosis. Blepharoptosis exists when the upper eyelid droops below its normal level. Congenital ptosis is usually due to faulty development of the levator muscle or its innervating branch of the 3rd nerve. There may be associated involvement of the superior rectus muscle and attendant impairment in elevation of the eye. The condition may be familial, transmitted as a dominant trait. Congenital ptosis can be corrected surgically; the age at which surgery is done depends on its degree, its cosmetic and functional severity, the presence or absence of compensatory posturing, the wishes of the parents, and the discretion of the surgeon; unless the ptosis is of marked degree, surgery is generally deferred until the child is 3–4 yr old. In some cases associated anisometropia and amblyopia will require early treatment.

Congenital ptosis occurs with a large number of syndromes. In the Marcus Gunn jaw winking syndrome of aberrant innervation, there is abnormal synkinesis of lid and jaw movements; paradoxical elevation of the ptotic lid occurs as the child sucks, chews, or cries. In the congenital fibrosis syndrome, a hereditary condition, ptosis is associated with paralysis or "fibrosis" of other extraocular muscles. Minimal ptosis occurs in the Horner syndrome (oculosympathetic palsy). In the Sturge-Weber syndrome ptosis is often secondary to hemangiomatous involvement of the upper lid, and in von Recklinghausen syndrome there may be ptosis due to plexiform neuroma of the upper lid.

Differential diagnosis of acquired ptosis in childhood includes myasthenia gravis, progressive external ophthalmoplegia, progressive intracranial lesions affecting the 3rd nerve, and inflammation or tumors affecting the levator, the orbit, or lid. Ptosis may also result from trauma. Aberrant regeneration of injured 3rd nerve fibers may produce paradoxic lid and eye movements.

Epicanthal Folds. These vertical or oblique folds of skin extend on either side of the bridge of the nose from the brow or lid area, covering the inner canthal region. They are present to some degree in most young children and become less apparent with age. The folds may be sufficiently broad to cover the medial aspect of the eye, making the eyes appear crossed (pseudoesotropia).

Epicanthal folds are a common feature of many syndromes, including chromosomal aberrations (particularly the trisomies) or disorders of single genes.

Lagophthalmos. This exists when complete closure of the lids over the globe is difficult or impossible. It may be paralytic, owing to a facial palsy involving the orbicularis muscle, or spastic, as in thyrotoxicosis. It may be structural when retraction or shortening of the lids results from scarring or atrophy consequent to injury (e.g., burns) or disease. Infants with collodion membrane may have temporary lagophthalmos due to the restrictive effect of the membrane on the lids. Lagophthalmos may accompany proptosis or buphthalmos when the lids, although normal, cannot effectively cover the enlarged or protuberant eye. A degree of physiologic lagophthalmos may occur normally during sleep, but functional lagophthalmos in the unconscious or debilitated can be a problem.

When lagophthalmos exists, exposure of the eye may lead to drying, infection, corneal ulceration, or perforation; the result may be loss of vision, even loss of the eye. In lagophthalmos protection of the eye by means of artificial tear preparations, ophthalmic ointment, or moisture chambers is essential. Gauze pads are to be avoided as the gauze may abrade the cornea. In some cases surgical closure of the lids (tarsorrhaphy) may be necessary for long term protection of the eye.

Lid Retraction. Pathologic retraction of the lid may be myogenic or neurogenic. Myogenic retraction of the upper lid occurs in thyrotoxicosis, in which it is associated with three classic signs: a staring appearance (Dalrymple sign), infrequent blinking (Stellwag sign), and lag of the upper lid on downward gaze (von Graefe sign).

Neurogenic retraction of the lids may occur in conditions affecting the anterior mesencephalon. Lid retraction is a feature of the syndrome of the sylvian aqueduct. In children it is commonly a sign of hydrocephalus. It may occur with meningitis.

Paradoxical retraction of the lid is a feature of the Marcus Gunn jaw winking syndrome. Paradoxical lid retraction may also occur during recovery from a 3rd nerve palsy as a result of aberrant regeneration or misdirection of oculomotor fibers.

To be differentiated from pathologic lid retractions are simple staring and the physiologic or reflexive lid retraction ("eye popping") that occurs in infants in response to sudden reduction in illumination or as a startle reaction.

Entropion. Entropion is inversion of the lid margin, which may cause discomfort and corneal damage due to the inward turning of the lashes (trichiasis). A principal cause is scarring secondary to inflammation such as occurs in trachoma. There is also a rare congenital form. Surgical correction is effective.

Ectropion. Ectropion is eversion of the lid margin; it may lead to overflow of tears (epiphora) and subsequent maceration of the skin of the lid, to inflammation of exposed conjunctiva, or to superficial exposure keratopathy. Common causes are scarring consequent to inflammation, burns, or

trauma, or weakness of the orbicularis muscle due to facial palsy; these forms may be corrected surgically. Protection of the cornea is essential. Eversion of the lids may occur during delivery; this can resolve with conservative management.

Ectropion is also seen in certain children who have faulty development of the lateral canthal ligament; this may occur in Down syndrome.

Blepharospasm. This is spastic or repetitive closure of the lids. It may be due to irritative disease of the cornea, conjunctiva, or facial nerve, to fatigue or uncorrected refractive error, or to common tic, but thorough ophthalmic examination for pathologic causes such as trichiasis, keratitis, conjunctivitis, or foreign body is indicated.

Blepharitis. This inflammation of the lid margins is characterized by erythema and crusting or scaling; the usual symptoms are irritation, burning, and itching. The condition is commonly bilateral and chronic or recurrent. There are two main types: staphylococcal and seborrheic. In *staphylococcal blepharitis* ulceration of the lid margin is common, the lashes tend to fall out, and there is often associated conjunctivitis and superficial keratitis. In *seborrheic blepharitis* the scales tend to be greasy, the lid margins are less red, and ulceration does not occur. The blepharitis is often of mixed type.

Thorough daily cleansing of the lid margins with a cloth or moistened cotton applicator to remove scales and crusts is important in the treatment of both forms of blepharitis. Staphylococcal blepharitis is treated with antistaphylococcal antibiotic or sulfonamide ophthalmic ointment applied directly to the lid margins daily at bedtime. When seborrhea exists, concurrent treatment of the scalp is important.

Pediculosis of the eyelashes may produce the clinical picture of blepharitis. The lice can be smothered with ophthalmic grade petrolatum ointment applied to the lid margin and lashes. Nits should be mechanically removed from the lashes.

Hordeolum. Infection of the glands of the lid may be acute or subacute; there is tender focal swelling and redness. The usual agent is *Staphylococcus aureus.*

When the meibomian glands are involved, the lesion is referred to as an *internal hordeolum;* the abscess tends to be large and may point through either the skin or conjunctival surface. When the infection involves the glands of Zeis or Moll, the abscess tends to be smaller and more superficial and points at the lid margin; it is then referred to as an *external hordeolum* or *stye.*

As with abscesses elsewhere, treatment is frequent warm compresses and, if necessary, surgical incision and drainage. In addition, topical antibiotic or sulfonamide preparations are often used. Untreated, the infection may progress to cellulitis of the lid or orbit, requiring use of systemic antibiotics. Recurrence is common, possibly by reinfection through contaminated hands. Itching due to an underlying allergy is a common contributory factor. Recurrent styes in children may also signal an immunologic defect.

Chalazion. Chalazion is granulomatous inflammation of a meibomian gland characterized by a firm, nontender nodule in the upper or lower lid. This lesion tends to be chronic and differs from internal hordeolum in the absence of acute inflammatory signs. When a chalazion is large enough to distort vision (it may cause astigmatism by exerting pressure on the globe) or to be a cosmetic blemish, excision is advised. In some cases chalazion will subside spontaneously.

Vaccinia. Vaccinia of the lids or conjunctiva has followed accidental inoculation. Corneal involvement may produce dense scarring and visual loss.

Coloboma of the Eyelid. This cleft-like deformity may vary from a small indentation or notch of the free margin of the lid to a large defect involving almost the entire lid. If the gap is extensive, xerosis, ulceration, and corneal opacities may result from exposure. Early surgical correction of the lid defect is recommended. Other deformities frequently associated with lid colobomata include dermoid cysts or dermolipomata on the globe; often, they occur in a position corresponding to the site of the lid defect. Lid colobomata may also be associated with extensive facial malformation, as in mandibulofacial dysostosis (Franceschetti or Treacher Collins syndrome).

Tumors of the Lid. A number of lid tumors arise from surface structures (the epithelium and sebaceous glands). Nevi may appear in early childhood; most are junctional. Compound nevi tend to develop in the prepubertal years, dermal nevi at puberty. Malignant epithelial tumors (basal cell carcinoma and squamous cell carcinoma) are rare in children, but the basal cell nevus syndrome, and the malignant lesions of xeroderma pigmentosum and of the Rothmund-Thomson syndrome may develop in childhood. Adenoma sebaceum (vascular fibroma) may also occur in the lid, sometimes forming extensive masses. The small yellowish papules of juvenile xanthogranuloma may occur on the lids, with or without cutaneous lesions elsewhere; these usually appear in infancy and regress spontaneously by the age of 1–2 yr.

Other lid tumors arise from deeper structures (the neural, vascular, and connective tissues). Hemangiomas are especially common. The majority tend to regress spontaneously, though they may show alarmingly rapid growth in infancy. In many cases, the best management of such hemangiomas is patient observation, allowing spontaneous regression to occur (Sec. 24.32). In the case of a rapidly expanding lesion that threatens to obstruct vision and produce sensory deprivation amblyopia, corticosteroid treatment should be considered.

Nevus flammeus (port wine stain), a noninvoluting hemangioma, occurs as isolated lesions or in association with other signs of Sturge-Weber syndrome. Affected patients should be examined for glaucoma.

Lymphangiomas of the lid appear as firm masses at or soon after birth and tend to enlarge slowly during the growing years. Associated conjunctival involvement, appearing as a clear, cystic, sinuous conjunctival mass, may provide a clue to the diagnosis. In some cases there is also orbital involvement. The treatment is surgical excision.

Plexiform neuromas of the lids occur in children with neurofibromatosis, often with ptosis as the first sign.

The lids may also be involved by other tumors such as retinoblastoma, neuroblastoma, and rhabdomyosarcoma of the orbit; these conditions are discussed elsewhere.

Crawford JS: Congenital eyelid anomalies in children. J Pediatr Ophthalmol Strab 21:140, 1984.

Crawford JS, Iliff CE, Stasier OG: Symposium on congenital ptosis. J Pediatr Ophthalmol Strab 19:245, 1982.

Johnson CC: Epicanthus and epiblepharon. Arch Ophthalmol 96:1030, 1978.

Kushner BJ: Intralesional corticosteroid injection for infantile adnexal hemangioma. Am J Ophthalmol 93:496, 1982.

Masaki S: Congenital bilateral facial paralysis. Arch Otolaryngol 94:260, 1971.

McCully JP, Dougherty JM, Deneau DG: Classification of chronic blepharitis. Ophthalmology 89:1173, 1982.

Merriam WW, Ellis FD, Helveston EM: Congenital blepharoptosis, anisometropia, and amblyopia. Am J Ophthalmol 89:401, 1980.

Moainie R, Kopelowitz N, Rosenfeld W, et al: Congenital eversion of the eyelids: A report of two cases treated with conservative management. J Pediatr Ophthalmol Strab 19:326, 1982.

Paine RS: Facial paralysis in children: Review of the differential diagnosis and report of ten cases treated with cortisone. Pediatrics 19:303, 1957.

Picó G: Congenital ectropion and distichiasis. Etiologic and hereditary factors. A report of cases and review of the literature. Am J Ophthalmol 47:363, 1959.

Pratt SG, Beyer CK, Johnson CC: The Marcus Gunn phenomenon: A review of 71 cases. Ophthalmology 91:27, 1984.

Ruben FL, Lane JM: Ocular vaccinia: An epidemiologic analysis of 348 cases. Arch Ophthalmol 84:45, 1970.

Stigmar G, Crawford JS, Ward CM, et al: Ophthalmic sequelae of infantile hemangiomas of the eyelid and orbit. Am J Ophthalmol 85:806, 1978.

Zak TA: Congenital primary upper eyelid entropion. J Pediatr Ophthalmol Strab 21:69, 1984.

25.8 DISORDERS OF THE LACRIMAL SYSTEM

Dacryostenosis and Dacryocystitis. Normally, tears produced by the lacrimal gland and the secretions produced by the accessory glands of the lid and conjunctiva drain medially into the punctal openings of the lid margins and flow through the canaliculi into the lacrimal sac, and then through the nasolacrimal duct into the nose. When partial or complete obstruction to the drainage system occurs, the condition is commonly referred to as dacryostenosis; in many cases more specific terms are applicable.

In infants and children the problem most often is congenital, due to maldevelopment or incomplete canalization of some portion of the drainage system. In most cases there is a congenital narrowing, a membranous or valve-like obstruction of the nasolacrimal duct, more often involving the distal or nasal segment than the proximal portion. In some cases there is involvement of the puncta, the canaliculi, the opening into the sac, or the sac itself. Rarely there may be a more complex anomaly or atresia of some portion of the system.

Signs may appear days or weeks after birth, and are often aggravated by upper respiratory infection or by exposure to cold or wind. The usual manifestations of nasolacrimal obstruction are "tearing," ranging in degree from a "wetness" of the eye (an increase in the tear lake, "pooling," or "puddling") to frank overflow of tears (epiphora), accumulation of mucoid or mucopurulent discharge (often described by the parents as "matter"), and crusting. There may be erythema or maceration of the skin owing to irritation and rubbing produced by dripping of tears and discharge. In many cases, reflux of clear fluid or mucopurulent discharge can be elicited by massaging the nasolacrimal sac, proving obstruction to outflow.

Infants with obstruction may have acute infection and inflammation of the nasolacrimal sac (dacryocystitis), inflammation of the surrounding tissues (pericystitis), or even periorbital cellulitis. With dacryocystitis, the sac area is swollen, red, and tender, and there may be systemic signs of infection such as fever and irritability.

Rarely, nasolacrymal obstruction will lead to distention of the nasolacrimal sac, producing a tense bluish mass (nasolacrimal mucocele, amniotocele or amniocele) that in some cases will transilluminate.

The primary treatment of uncomplicated nasolacrimal obstruction is a regimen of nasolacrimal massage, usually two to three times a day, often accompanied by cleansing of the lids with warm water and instillation of an antibacterial drop. In most cases, the problem will resolve with conservative management by the age of 1 yr, if not earlier. In persistent or severe cases, dilatation, probing, and irrigation of the nasolacrimal system may be indicated. In more complicated cases, placement of tubes or more extensive reconstructive surgery (such as dacryocystorhinostomy) may be required to provide adequate drainage.

Acute dacryocystitis or cellulitis requires prompt treatment with antibiotics. In such cases some form of definitive surgical intervention is usually indicated.

Nasolacrimal obstruction in children is most often congenital. Lacrimal problems may develop later in life as the result of acquired infection, inflammation, or trauma.

It should be noted that not all tearing in infants and children is due to nasolacrimal obstruction. Tearing may be a sign also of glaucoma, of intraocular inflammation, or of external irritation such as that from a corneal abrasion or foreign body.

Dacryoadenitis. Dacryoadenitis, or inflammation of the lacrimal gland, is uncommon in childhood. It may occur with mumps (in which case it is usually acute and bilateral, subsiding in a few days or weeks), or with infectious mononucleosis. Chronic dacryoadenitis is associated with certain systemic diseases, particularly sarcoidosis, tuberculosis, and syphilis. Some systemic diseases may produce enlargement of the lacrimal and salivary glands (Mikulicz syndrome).

Alacrima and "Dry Eye." Marked deficiency of tears may occur as an isolated unilateral or bilateral congenital defect or in association with other nervous system anomalies, such as aplasia of cranial nerve nuclei. It occurs congenitally in familial dysautonomia (Riley-Day syndrome) and in the anhidrotic type of ectodermal dysplasia; it may occur with glucocorticoid deficiency, sometimes in association with swallowing dysfunction. Tear deficiency may be a sign of Sjögren syndrome, in which it is sometimes associated with salivary gland enlargement and with arthritis. Deficiency of tears may also follow inflammation; it is not uncommon after Stevens-Johnson syndrome. Drying of the eye, corneal ulceration, and scarring may result. Preventive care includes the frequent instillation of an artificial tear preparation. In some cases occlusion of the lacrimal puncta is helpful. In severe cases tarsorrhaphy may be necessary to protect the cornea.

Caccamise WC, Townes PL: Congenital absence of the lacrymal puncta associated with alacrima and aptyalism. Am J Ophthalmol 89:62, 1980.

Geffner ME, Lippe BM, Kaplan SA, et al: Selective ACTH insensitivity, achalasia, and alacrima: A multisystem disorder presenting in childhood. Pediatr Res 17:532, 1983.

Goldberg MF, Payne JW, Brunt PW: Ophthalmologic studies of familial dysautonomia. Arch Ophthalmol 80:732, 1966.

Kushner BJ: Congenital nasolacrymal system obstruction. Arch Ophthalmol 100:597, 1982.

Mondino BJ, Brown SI: Hereditary congenital alacrima. Arch Ophthalmol 94:1478, 1976.

Paul TO: Medical management of congenital nasolacrymal duct obstruction. J Pediatr Ophthalmol Strab 22:68, 1985.

Pinsky L, DiGeorge AM: Congenital familial sensory neuropathy with anhidrosis. J Pediatr 68:1, 1966.

Sevel D: Developmental and congenital abnormalities of the nasolacrymal apparatus. J Pediatr Ophthalmol Strab 18:13, 1981.

Weinstein GS, Biglan AW, Patterson JH: Congenital lacrimal sac mucoceles. Am J Ophthalmol 94:106, 1982.

Welham RAN, Hughes SM: Lacrimal surgery in children. Am J Ophthalmol 99:27, 1985.

25.9 DISORDERS OF THE CONJUNCTIVA

CONJUNCTIVITIS

The conjunctiva reacts to a wide range of bacterial and viral agents, allergens, irritants, toxins, and systemic diseases. Conjunctivitis is common in childhood and may be infectious or noninfectious.

Acute purulent conjunctivitis is characterized by more or less generalized conjunctival hyperemia, edema, mucopurulent exudate, and various degrees of ocular discomfort. It is usually due to bacterial infection. The most frequent causes are staphylococci, pneumococci, *Haemophilus influenzae*, and streptococci. Conjunctival smear and culture are helpful in differentiating specific types. These common forms of acute purulent conjunctivitis usually respond well to warm compresses and frequent topical instillation of antibiotic drops.

Ophthalmia neonatorum is acute conjunctivitis in the newborn infant. Any of the common bacterial conjunctivitides can occur in the newborn period, but emphasis in differential diagnosis must be given to recognition of gonococcal and chlamydial infections.

Ophthalmia neonatorum due to *Neisseria gonorrhoeae* usually appears from 1 to 4 days after birth; there is generally profuse discharge with marked edema and hyperemia of the eyelids and conjunctiva. Gonococcal infection can lead to corneal perforation and blindness. Prompt diagnosis is aided by identification of gram-negative diplococci in smears of conjunctival scrapings. Culture and fermentation tests must differentiate the gonococcus from other members of the *Neisseria* group. Systemic treatment with penicillin with or without the frequent topical instillation of antibiotic drops is usually effective, but the emergence of penicillinase-producing *Neisseria gonorrhoeae* in the United States makes it necessary to determine the antibiotic susceptibility in individual cases. Great care must be taken in handling infected infants to avoid spread to others.

Ophthalmia neonatorum due to *Chlamydia trachomatis* (also known as inclusion conjunctivitis) is common. The infant is infected during birth by organisms in the maternal genital tract. The incubation period is usually 1 wk or more. The clinical picture is commonly that of an acute purulent conjunctivitis. The diagnosis can be made on demonstration of intracytoplasmic inclusion bodies, by fluorescent antibody tests, or by tissue culture of the organism. Systemic administration of erythromycin is recommended (Sec. 11.57). There is risk of associated systemic infection and of late conjunctival scarring or corneal complications.

To be differentiated from the infectious types of ophthalmia neonatorum is the chemical conjunctivitis due to prophylactic use of silver nitrate. This usually develops 12–24 hr after instillation and lasts only 24–48 hr; no pathogen is grown on culture.

Viral conjunctivitis is generally characterized by a watery discharge. Often, there are follicular changes (small aggregates of lymphocytes) in the palpebral conjunctiva. Conjunctivitis due to adenovirus infection is relatively common, sometimes with corneal involvement (below). Topical sulfonamides are often used in treatment.

Conjunctivitides are commonly associated with such systemic viral infections as the childhood exanthems, particularly measles. These are self-limited.

Epidemic keratoconjunctivitis is caused by adenovirus type 8 and is transmitted by direct contact. Initially, there is a sensation of a foreign body beneath the lids with itching and burning. Edema and photophobia develop rapidly, and large oval follicles appear within the conjunctiva. Preauricular adenopathy and a pseudomembrane on the conjunctival surface occur frequently. Blurring of vision results from subepithelial corneal infiltrates; these usually disappear but may reduce visual acuity permanently. Corneal complications are less common in children than in adults. Children may have associated upper respiratory infection.

Membranous and pseudomembranous conjunctivitis can be seen in a number of diseases. The classic membranous conjunctivitis is that of diphtheria, accompanied by a fibrin-rich exudate that forms on the conjunctival surface and permeates the epithelium; the membrane is removed with difficulty and leaves raw bleeding areas. In pseudomembranous conjunctivitis the layer of fibrin-rich exudate is superficial and can often be stripped with ease, leaving the surface smooth. This type occurs with many bacterial and viral infections, including staphylococcal, pneumococcal, streptococcal, or chlamydial conjunctivitis, and in epidemic keratoconjunctivitis. It is seen also in vernal conjunctivitis and in Stevens-Johnson disease.

Allergic conjunctivitis is usually accompanied by intense itching, tearing, and conjunctival edema. It is commonly seasonal. Cold compresses and decongestant drops give symptomatic relief. Topical corticosteroids are used only under ophthalmic supervision.

Vernal conjunctivitis usually begins in the prepubertal years and may recur for many years. Atopy appears to play a role in its origin, but the pathogenesis is uncertain. Extreme itching and tearing are the usual complaints. Large flattened cobble-stone-like papillary lesions of the palpebral conjunctivae are characteristic. A stringy exudate and a milky conjunctival pseudomembrane are frequently present. There may be small elevated lesions of the bulbar conjunctiva adjacent to the limbus (limbal form). Smear of the conjunctival exudate will show many eosinophils. Topical corticosteroid therapy and cold compresses afford some relief. Cromolyn sodium may help.

Chemical conjunctivitis can result when an irritating substance enters the conjunctival sac (as in the acute but benign conjunctivitis due to silver nitrate in the newborn). Other common offenders are household cleaning substances, sprays, smoke, smog, and industrial pollutants.

Alkalis tend to linger in the conjunctival tissues and continue to inflict damage over a period of hours or days. Acids precipitate the proteins in tissues and so produce their effect immediately. In either case, prompt, thorough, and copious irrigation is crucial. Extensive tissue damage, even loss of the eye, can result, especially if the offending agent is an alkali.

OTHER CONJUNCTIVAL DISORDERS

Subconjunctival hemorrhage is manifested by bright or dark red patches in the bulbar conjunctiva and may result from injury or inflammation. It may occasionally result from severe sneezing or coughing or be a manifestation of a blood dyscrasia.

Pingueculum is a yellowish-white, slightly elevated mass on the bulbar conjunctiva, usually in the interpalpebral region. It represents elastic and hyaline degenerative change of the conjunctiva. No treatment is required except for cosmetic reasons, in which case simple excision suffices.

Pterygium is a fleshy triangular conjunctival lesion that may encroach on the cornea. It typically occurs in the nasal interpalpebral region. The pathologic findings are similar to those of a pingueculum. Irritation such as exposure to dust and wind is thought to aggravate the lesion. Removal is suggested when the lesion encroaches far onto the cornea.

Phlyctenular keratoconjunctivitis is discussed in Sec. 25.10.

Dermoid cyst and dermolipoma are benign lesions, clinically similar in appearance. They are smooth, elevated, round to oval lesions of various sizes. The color varies from yellowish-white to a fleshy pink. The most frequent site is the upper outer quadrant of the globe; they commonly also occur near or straddle the limbus. The dermolipoma is composed of adipose and connective tissue. Dermoid cysts may also contain glandular tissue, hair follicles, and hair shafts. Excision for cosmetic reasons is feasible.

Conjunctival nevus is a small, slightly elevated lesion that may vary in pigmentation from pale salmon to dark brown. It is usually benign, but careful observation for progressive growth or changes suggestive of malignancy is advised.

Symblepharon is a cicatricial adhesion between the conjunctiva of the lid and the globe; the lower lid is usually affected. It follows operation or injuries, especially burns from lye, acids, or molten metals. It may interfere with motion of the eyeball and cause diplopia. The band should be separated and the raw surfaces kept from uniting during healing. Grafts of oral mucous membrane may be necessary.

American Academy of Pediatrics Committee on Drugs, Committee on Fetus and Newborn, Committee on Infectious Diseases: Prophylaxis and treatment of neonatal gonococcal infections. Pediatrics 65:1047, 1980.

Brook I: Anaerobic and aerobic bacterial flora of acute conjunctivitis in children. Arch Ophthalmol 98:833, 1980.

Clark SW, Culbertson WW, Forster RK: Clinical findings and results of treatment in an outbreak of acute hemorrhagic conjunctivitis in southern Florida. Am J Ophthalmol 99:45, 1983.

Cohen KL, McCarthy LR: *Haemophilus influenzae* ophthalmia neonatorum. Arch Ophthalmol 98:1214, 1980.

Doraiswamy B, Hammerschlag MR, Pringle GF, et al: Ophthalmia neonatorum caused by β-lactamase-producing *Neisseria gonorrhoeae*. JAMA 12:790, 1983.

Forster RK, Dawson CR, Schachter J: Late followup of patients with neonatal inclusion conjunctivitis. Am J Ophthalmol 69:467, 1970.

Gigliotti F, Williams WT, Hayden FG, et al: Etiology of acute conjunctivitis in children. J Pediatr 98:531, 1981.

Knopf HLS, Hierholzer JC: Clinical and immunologic responses in patients with viral keratoconjunctivitis. Am J Ophthalmol 80:661, 1975.

Raucher HS, Newton MJ, Stern RH: Ophthalmia neonatorum caused by penicillinase-producing *Neisseria gonorrhoeae*. J Pediatr 100:925, 1982.

Rowe DS, Aicardi EZ, Dawson CR, et al: Purulent ocular discharge in neonates: Significance of *Chlamydia trachomatis*. Pediatrics 63:628, 1979.

Stenson S, Newman R, Fedukowicz H: Conjunctivitis in the newborn: Observations on incidence, cause and prophylaxis. Ann Ophthalmol 13:329, 1981.

25.10 ABNORMALITIES OF THE CORNEA

Megalocornea denotes a developmental anomaly in which the diameter of the cornea is greater than 13 mm. The condition is nonprogressive and produces no ill effects, although there is often a high refractive error. Megalocornea is often familial and may be associated with other developmental abnormalities.

Pathologic corneal enlargement due to glaucoma is to be differentiated from this anomaly. Any progressive increase in the size of the cornea, especially when accompanied by photophobia, lacrimation, or haziness of the cornea, requires prompt ophthalmologic evaluation.

Microcornea, or anterior microphthalmia, describes an abnormally small cornea in an otherwise relatively normal eye. It may be familial, transmission being dominant more often than recessive. More commonly, a small cornea is just one feature of an otherwise developmentally abnormal or microphthalmic eye; associated defects include colobomata, microphakia, congenital cataract, and glaucoma.

Keratoconus or conical cornea is characterized by ectasia and increased curvature of the central or axial portion of the cornea. It commonly appears in adolescence and with increased frequency in Down syndrome. It may occur as a late complication of congenital rubella. The etiology is obscure. There is usually considerable impairment of vision due to a high degree of astigmatism, though vision can often be improved with contact lenses. In some cases acute ectasia and corneal edema (hydrops) develop. In selected cases perforating keratoplasty (corneal transplant) is done.

Keratoconus is to be differentiated from keratoglobus, a globular configuration of the cornea present at or soon after birth. Both anomalies can be associated with other developmental abnormalities, including blue sclera, hearing impairment, abnormal teeth, and hyperextensible joints.

Sclerocornea (also known as scleralization of the cornea) is a congenital malformation in which part or all of the cornea is opaque, having the appearance of sclera. This anomaly may be sporadic or familial, and it may be associated with other developmental defects of the eye, with defects of other systems, or with chromosomal abnormalities. In generalized sclerocornea, early keratoplasty should be considered in an effort to provide vision.

In **dendritic keratitis,** infection of the eye with the virus of herpes simplex produces a characteristic lesion of the corneal epithelium, referred to as a dendrite; it has a branching tree-like pattern that can be demonstrated by fluorescein staining. The acute episode is accompanied by pain, photophobia, tearing, blepharospasm, and conjunctival injection. Specific treatment is 5-iodo-2'-deoxyuridine (IDU) in the form of drops or ointment, or topical vidarabine. In addition, a cycloplegic agent is used, preferably atropine. Recurrent infection and deep stromal involvement can lead to corneal scarring.

It has been clearly demonstrated that topical use of corticosteroids causes exacerbation of superficial herpetic disease of the eye; eyedrops combining steroids and antibiotics, are, therefore, to be avoided in treatment of "red eye" unless there are clear-cut indications for their use and close supervision during therapy.

Infants born to mothers infected with herpes simplex should be examined carefully for signs of ocular involvement.

In **corneal ulcers,** the usual signs and symptoms are focal or diffuse corneal haze, hyperemia, lid edema, pain, photophobia, tearing, and blepharospasm. Often, there is hypopyon (pus in the anterior chamber).

Corneal ulcers require prompt treatment. They result most frequently from traumatic lesions that become secondarily infected. Many organisms are capable of infecting the cornea. One of the most troublesome is *Pseudomonas aeruginosa;* it can rapidly destroy stromal tissue and lead to corneal perforation. *Neisseria gonorrhoeae* also is particularly damaging to the cornea. Indolent ulcers are often found to be due to fungi. In each case scrapings of the cornea must be studied in an effort to identify the infectious agent and to determine the best therapy. Generally, both systemic and local treatment are needed to save the eye. Perforation or scarring due to corneal ulceration is an important cause of blindness throughout the world and is estimated to be responsible for 10% of blindness in the United States.

Unexplained corneal ulcers in infants and young children should raise the question of a sensory defect, as in Riley-Day or Goldenhar-Gorlin syndrome, or of a metabolic disorder such as tyrosinemia.

Phlyctenules are small, yellowish, slightly elevated lesions usually located at the corneal limbus; they may encroach on the cornea and extend centrally. Often, there is a small corneal ulcer at the head of the advancing lesion, with a fascicle of blood vessels behind the head of the lesion. Phlyctenular keratoconjunctivitis was earlier thought most commonly to represent hypersensitivity to tuberculin proteins, but the cause is not really known. Staphylococcal infections may be associated with phlyctenular changes. There is strong evidence for an immunologic factor. The condition usually responds to topical corticosteroid therapy, sometimes leaving superficial stromal pannus and scarring.

Interstitial keratitis denotes inflammation of the corneal stroma. The most common cause is syphilis, interstitial keratitis being one of the characteristic late manifestations of congenital syphilis. The deep inflammation produces pain, photophobia, tearing, circumcorneal injection, and corneal haze. Corneal vascularization and opacities develop and generally remain as permanent stigmata of the disease.

Cogan syndrome is a nonluetic interstitial keratitis associated with hearing loss and vestibular symptoms. Both the corneal changes and the auditory involvement may respond to corticosteroids.

Less frequently, interstitial keratitis is due to other infectious diseases, such as tuberculosis or leprosy.

Peters anomaly is a condition in which maldevelopment of the anterior segment of the eye may affect the cornea, anterior chamber angle, and iris. The terms "mesodermal dysgenesis," "anterior cleavage syndrome," and a number of eponyms describe these defects and various combinations thereof.

Peters anomaly consists of a congenital corneal opacity (leukoma) with corresponding defects in the posterior corneal stroma and Descemet membrane and endothelium, often with associated iridocorneal or lenticulocorneal adhesions. The condition is usually bilateral. It is generally sporadic, but recessive and dominant inheritances have been suggested.

Other anomalies within the spectrum of anterior chamber cleavage syndrome are abnormalities of the peripheral cornea and angle including a prominent anteriorly displaced ring of Schwalbe, Axenfeld anomaly (fine iris strands that cross the chamber to the displaced ring of Schwalbe), or Rieger anomaly. There may be associated glaucoma or lens abnormalities.

Corneal Manifestations of Systemic Disease. Several metabolic diseases produce distinctive corneal changes in childhood. Refractile polychromatic crystals are deposited throughout the cornea in cystinosis. Corneal deposits producing various degrees of corneal haze also occur in certain of the mucopolysaccharidoses, particularly MPS IH (Hurler), MPS IS (Scheie), MPS I H/S (Hurler-Scheie compound), MPS IV (Morquio), MPS VI (Maroteaux-Lamy), and sometimes MPS VII (Sly). Corneal deposits may develop in patients with GM_1 (generalized) gangliosidosis. In Fabry disease fine opacities radiating in a whorl or fan-like pattern occur, and corneal changes can be important in identifying the carrier state. A spray-like pattern of corneal opacities may also be seen in the Bloch-Sulzberger syndrome. In Wilson disease the distinctive corneal sign is the Kayser-Fleischer ring, a golden brown ring in the peripheral cornea due to changes in Descemet membrane. Corneal changes may occur in autoimmune hypoparathyroidism, and band keratopathy in patients with hypercalcemia. Transient keratitis may occur with rubeola, sometimes with rubella.

Beauchamp GR, Gillette TE, Friendly DS: Phlyctenular keratoconjunctivitis. J Pediatr Ophthalmol Strab 18:22, 1981.

Biglan AW, Brown SI, Johnson BL: Keratoglobus and blue sclera. Am J Ophthalmol 83:225, 1977.

Boger WP III, Peterson RA, Robb RM: Keratoconus and acute hydrops in mentally retarded patients with congenital rubella syndrome. Am J Ophthalmol 91:231, 1981.

Burns RB: Soluble tyrosine aminotransferase deficiency: An unusual cause of corneal ulcers. Am J Ophthalmol 73:400, 1972.

Cobo LM, Haynes BF: Early corneal findings in Cogan's syndrome. Ophthalmology 91:903, 1984.

Deckard PS, Bergstrom TJ: Rubeola keratitis. Ophthalmology 88:810, 1981.

Elliott JH, Feman SS, O'Day DM, et al: Hereditary sclerocornea. Arch Ophthalmol 103:676, 1985.

Goldberg MF: A review of selected inherited corneal dystrophies associated with systemic disease. Birth Defects: Original Article Series VII:13, 1971.

Goldberg MF, Payne JW, Brunt PW: Ophthalmologic studies of familial dysautonomia. Arch Ophthalmol 80:732, 1966.

Hutchison DS, Smith RE, Haughton PB: Congenital herpetic keratitis. Arch Ophthalmol 93:70, 1975.

Kraft SP, Judisch GF, Grayson DM: Megalocornea: A clinical and echographic study of an autosomal dominant pedigree. J Pediatr Ophthalmol Strab 21:190, 1984.

Mohandessan MM, Romano PE: Neuroparalytic keratitis in Goldenhar-Gorlin syndrome. Am J Ophthalmol 85:111, 1978.

Schanzlin DJ, Goldberg DB, Brown SI: Transplantation of congenitally opaque corneas. Ophthalmology 87:1253, 1980.

Stieglitz LM, Kind HP, Kazden JJ, et al: Keratitis with hypoparathyroidism. Am J Ophthalmol 84:467, 1972.

Stone DL, Kenyon KR, Green WR, et al: Congenital central corneal leukoma (Peters' anomaly). Am J Ophthalmol 81:173, 1976.

Tso MOM, Fine BS, Thorpe HE: Kayser-Fleischer ring and associated cataract in Wilson's disease. Am J Ophthalmol 79:479, 1975.

25.11 ABNORMALITIES OF THE LENS

Cataracts may be defined simply as any opacity of the lens. Cataracts vary, however, in their etiology, morphology, and effects on vision.

Early developmental processes in the lens may lead to a number of different types of congenital cataract. Not uncommon are discrete dots or small white plaque-like opacities of the lens capsule, sometimes with involvement of the contiguous subcapsular region. Such opacities of the posterior capsule may be associated with persistent remnants of the hyaloid system, while those of the anterior capsule may be associated with persistent strands of the pupillary membrane or vascular sheath of the lens. Congenital opacities of this type are usually stationary and rarely interfere with vision; in some cases significant progression occurs.

To be differentiated from capsular and capsulolenticular opacities are congenital cataracts involving the central nucleus of the lens or the developing lamellae laid down immediately around the fetal nucleus. Some are hereditary, dominant transmission being more common than recessive or sex-linked, and examination of other family members is important in the differential diagnosis of congenital cataracts. Some are the result of intrauterine infection, rubella being a more frequent cause than syphilis or toxoplasmosis. In congenital rubella the cataract tends to be a dense, pearly, nuclear opacity surrounded by clearer cortex, often with associated ocular abnormalities such as microphthalmos, iris hypoplasia, inflammatory iris adhesions (synechiae), glaucoma, pigmentary retinopathy, and optic atrophy. In many cases congenital cataract is just one facet of a complex syndrome; in Lowe syndrome, for example, congenital cataract and glaucoma are associated with mental retardation, hypotonia, renal tubular dysfunction, and aminoaciduria. In this sex-linked disorder affected males tend to have a dense nuclear or total cataract readily visible at birth, whereas fine punctate cortical opacities can be detected in many carrier females.

As lens growth continues throughout life, opacities of various layers may occur as the result of disease at particular ages. Metabolic diseases are major considerations in the differential diagnosis of cataracts. In infants with galactosemia, cataracts may form in the 1st weeks of life; opacities in the cortex create a refractive ring and an "oil droplet" appearance on ophthalmoscopic examination, best seen with the pupil well dilated. Infants and children with hypocalcemic tetany may develop cataracts; these opacities are zonular, affected lamellae often being separated by clear layers. Young persons with diabetes mellitus may develop cataracts that progress rapidly, with the formation of fine vacuoles and punctate "snowflake" opacities in the subcapsular layers occurring in a matter of hours, days, or weeks. Development of the cataract may be heralded by rapid changes in the refractive state. This may occur in adolescence, rarely earlier. In Wilson disease a brilliant array of anterior capsular and subcapsular opacities arranged in a radiating pattern ("sunflower cataract") may develop.

Certain drugs and toxins may produce cataract at various ages. Cataract not rarely is an effect of prolonged corticosteroid therapy, and all children being treated long term with steroids should have periodic eye examinations. As a rule, steroid-induced lens opacities develop in the posterior subcapsular region. The effect on vision depends on the extent and density of the opacity. In many cases, the acuity is only minimally or moderately impaired.

Trauma at any age can produce cataracts. Opacities may result either from contusion or from penetrating injury. Other physical agents such as radiation can also damage the lens and result in cataract.

Cataract may also develop secondary to such intraocular processes as retrolental fibroplasia, retinal detachment, retinitis pigmentosa, and uveitis.

A special type of lens change seen in some newborns is the so-called cataract of prematurity. The opacities appear as clusters of tiny vacuoles in the distribution of the "Y" sutures of the lens; they can be visualized with the ophthalmoscope and are best seen with the pupil well dilated. The etiology is unclear; in most cases the opacities disappear spontaneously, often within a few weeks.

The treatment of cataracts that significantly interfere with vision involves (1) surgical removal of lens material to provide an optically clear visual axis; (2) correction of the resultant aphakic refractive error with spectacles, contact lenses, intraocular lens implantation, or possibly refractive corneal surgery; and (3) treatment of any associated sensory deprivation amblyopia. The last may be the most demanding and difficult step in the visual rehabilitation of a child with cataract.

The prognosis depends on numerous factors, including the nature of associated ocular abnormalities (such as microphthalmia, retinal lesions, optic atrophy, nystagmus, strabismus, etc.). In addition, affected children may have cardiac, renal, skeletal, or central nervous system disorders. There is often amblyopia requiring intensive treatment. The ultimate management decisions must rest jointly with the ophthalmologist, the pediatrician, and the family.

Dislocation of the Lens (Ectopia Lentis). Dislocation or subluxation of the lens in children is usually associated with trauma, Marfan syndrome, Marchesani syndrome, or homocystinuria; displacement of the lens is also seen in aniridia, sulfite oxidase deficiency, hyperlysinemia, and Ehlers-Danlos syndrome. Simple ectopia of the lens may occur as a dominant condition, or in association with ectopia of the pupil as an autosomal recessive condition. Abnormal position of the lens produces refractive changes with various degrees of impairment of vision. In many instances vision can be improved with corrective lenses. In selected cases surgery is performed. Complications associated with subluxation of the lens are glaucoma and retinal detachment. The external sign of dislocation is iridodonesis, a shimmering movement of the iris due to its loss of support by the lens.

Chrousos GA, Parks MM, O'Neill JF: Incidence of chronic glaucoma, retinal detachment and secondary membrane surgery in pediatric aphakic patients. Ophthalmology 91:1238, 1984.
Cotlier E: Congenital varicella cataract. Am J Ophthalmol 86:627, 1978.
Cross HE, Jensen AD: Ocular manifestations in the Marfan syndrome and homocystinuria. Am J Ophthalmol 75:405, 1973.
Forman AR, Loreto JA, Tina LU: Reversibility of corticosteroid-associated cataracts in children with the nephrotic syndrome. Am J Ophthalmol 84:75, 1977.
Francois J: Late results of congenital cataract surgery. Ophthalmology 86:1586, 1979.
Hiles DA: Intraocular lens implantation in children with monocular cataracts, 1974–1983. Ophthalmology 91:1231, 1984.
Jaafar MS, Robb RM: Congenital anterior polar cataract: A review of 63 cases. Ophthalmology 91:249, 1984.
Jensen AD, Cross HE, Paton D: Ocular complications in the Weill-Marchesani syndrome. Am J Ophthalmol 77:261, 1975.
Kirkam TH: Mandibulofacial dysostosis with ectopia lentis. Am J Ophthalmol 70:947, 1979.
Kohn BA: The differential diagnosis of cataracts in infancy and childhood. Am J Dis Child 130:184, 1976.
Maumenee IH: Classification of hereditary cataracts in children by linkage analysis. Ophthalmology 86:1554, 1979.
Morgan KS, Stephenson GS, McDonald MB, et al: Epikeratophakia in children. Ophthalmology 91:780, 1984.
Parks MM: Visual results in aphakic children. Am J Ophthalmol 94:441, 1982.
Seetner AA, Crawford JS: Surgical correction of lens dislocation in children. Am J Ophthalmol 91:106, 1981.
Townes PL: Ectopia lentis et pupillae. Arch Ophthalmol 94:1126, 1976.
Wets B, Milot JA, Polomeno RC, et al: Cataracts and ketotic hypoglycemia. Ophthalmology 89:999, 1982.

25.12 DISORDERS OF THE UVEAL TRACT

Uveitis (Iritis, Cyclitis, Chorioretinitis). The uveal tract (the inner vascular coat of the eye consisting of iris, ciliary body, and choroid) is subject to inflammatory involvement in a number of systemic diseases, both infectious and noninfectious, and in response to exogenous factors, including trauma and toxic agents. Inflammation may affect any one portion of the uveal tract preferentially or all parts together.

Iritis may occur alone or in conjunction with inflammation of the ciliary body as iridocyclitis or in association with pars planitis. Pain, photophobia, and lacrimation are the characteristic symptoms of acute anterior uveitis, but the inflammation may develop insidiously without disturbing symptoms. Signs of anterior uveitis include conjunctival hyperemia, particularly in the perilimbal region (ciliary flush), cells and protein ("flare") in the aqueous humor, inflammatory deposits on the posterior surface of the cornea (keratic precipitates, or "KP"), congestion of the iris, and sometimes neovascarization of the iris. In more chronic cases there may be degenerative changes of the cornea (band keratopathy), lenticular opacities (cataract), and impairment of vision. The etiology of anterior uveitis is often obscure; primary considerations in children are rheumatoid disease, particularly pauciarticular rheumatoid arthritis, and sarcoidosis. Iritis may be secondary to corneal disease, such as herpetic keratitis or a bacterial or fungal corneal ulcer, or to a corneal abrasion or foreign body. Traumatic iritis and iridocyclitis are especially common in children.

Choroiditis, inflammation of the posterior portion of the uveal tract, invariably also involves the retina; when both are obviously affected, the term chorioretinitis is used (Fig. 25–4). The causes of posterior uveitis are protean; the more common are toxoplasmosis, histoplasmosis, cytomegalic inclusion disease, sarcoidosis, syphilis, tuberculosis, and toxocariasis. Depending on the etiology, the inflammatory signs may be diffuse or focal. Often there is vitreous reaction as well. With many types the result is atrophic chorioretinal scarring demarcated by pigmentation, often with visual impairment. Secondary complications include retinal detachment, glaucoma, or phthisis.

Panophthalmitis is inflammation involving all parts of the eye. It is frequently suppurative, most often as a result of a perforating injury or of septicemia. It produces severe pain, marked congestion of the eye, inflammation of the adjacent orbital tissues and eyelids, and loss of vision. In many cases the eye is lost despite intensive treatment of the infection and inflammation. Enucleation of the eye or evisceration of the orbit may be necessary.

Sympathetic ophthalmia is a rare type of inflammatory response that affects both eyes following perforating injury of one eye. It may occur weeks or even months after the injury. A hypersensitivity phenomenon is the most probable cause. Loss of vision may result.

Treatment of the various forms of intraocular inflammation varies with the etiologic factors. In a few cases an identified process can be treated specifically. A primary goal of treatment is prevention or reduction of the inflammatory sequelae, often with topical or systemic use of corticosteroids. Cycloplegic agents, particularly atropine, are also used to reduce inflammation and to prevent adhesion of the iris to the lens, especially in anterior uveitis.

Burke MJ, Rennebohm RM: Eye involvement in Kawasaki disease. J Pediatr Ophthalmol Strab 18:7, 1981.
Contreras F, Pereda J: Congenital syphilis of the eye with lens involvement. Arch Ophthalmol 96:1052, 1978.
Hart WM, Reed AB, Freedman HL, et al: Cytomegalovirus in juvenile iridocyclitis. Am J Ophthalmol 86:329, 1978.
Kanski JJ: Anterior uveitis in juvenile rheumatoid arthritis. Arch Ophthalmol 96:1794, 1977.
Lonn LL: Neonatal cytomegalic inclusion disease chorioretinitis. Arch Ophthalmol 88:434, 1972.
Lou P, Kazdan J, Basu PK: Ocular toxoplasmosis in three consecutive siblings. Arch Ophthalmol 96:613, 1978.
Makley TA, Azar A: Sympathetic ophthalmia: A long-term follow-up. Arch Ophthalmol 96:257, 1978.
Molk R: Ocular toxocariasis: A review of the literature. Ann Ophthalmol 15:216, 1983.
Ryan SJ, Hardy PH, Hardy JM, et al: Persistence of virulent *Treponema pallidum* despite penicillin therapy in congenital syphilis. Am J Ophthalmol 73:258, 1972.
Smith ME, Zimmerman LE, Harley RD: Ocular involvement in congenital cytomegalic inclusion disease. Arch Ophthalmol 76:696, 1966.
Stern GA, Romano PE: Congenital ocular toxoplasmosis: Possible occurrence in siblings. Arch Ophthalmol 96:615, 1978.
Wilkinson CP, Welch RB: Intraocular toxocara. Am J Ophthalmol 71:921, 1971.

25.13 DISORDERS OF THE RETINA AND VITREOUS

Retinopathy of Prematurity (Retrolental Fibroplasia). This disorder is due to immaturity of the developing retinal vasculature and pathologic alteration of vasoformative elements. It occurs predominantly in preterm infants, low birthweight infants, and in infants who have required supplemental oxygen in the newborn period to sustain life and neurologic function (see also Sec. 8.17). Clinical manifestations range from mild or transient changes of the peripheral retina to severe progressive vasoproliferation, cicatrization, and potentially blinding retinal detachment. The term *retinopathy of prematurity* (ROP) applies to all stages of the disease; it is often used, however, to designate specifically the early active phases, whereas the older term *retrolental fibroplasia* (RLF) is now reserved for the cicatricial stages of the disease.

Pathogenesis. Retinal angiogenesis normally proceeds from the disc to the periphery. Two zones are recognized in the developing vasculature. The first (the vanguard) consists principally of meridionally aligned spindle-shaped cells of mesenchymal origin. The vanguard appears around the papilla at 16 wk gestation and advances as a wave in the inner retina to the periphery, reaching the ora serrata nasally by 36 wk and temporally by approximately 40 wk. In newborn infants, and particularly in preterm infants, the peripheral retina (especially the temporal region) may be incompletely vascularized and susceptible to insults and pathologic changes that can lead to retinopathy.

The initial pathologic event in the development of ROP appears to be activation of the spindle cells of the vanguard, with an increase in gap junctions between adjacent cells. Studies indicate that oxygen tension greater than that of the relatively hypoxic intrauterine environment can induce a pathologic increase in gap junctions. Those conditions that require the therapeutic use of supplemental oxygen and that alter the amount of oxygen carried in the blood and delivered to tissues increase the risk for development of ROP in susceptible infants.

The gap junction linkage interferes with further normal retinal vascular development. This may lead to ischemia of the unvascularized retinal areas and in some cases to extraretinal neovascularization and intravitreal fibrovascular proliferation. It is postulated that retinal ischemia provides the stimulus for release of a vasoactive factor that directly causes neovascularization.

Clinical Manifestations. The early or active phases of ROP comprise four clinical stages (International Classification

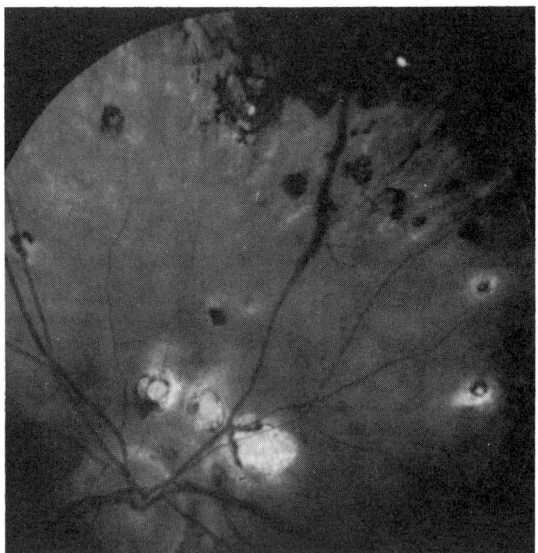

Figure 25–4. Focal atrophic and pigmented scars of chorioretinitis.

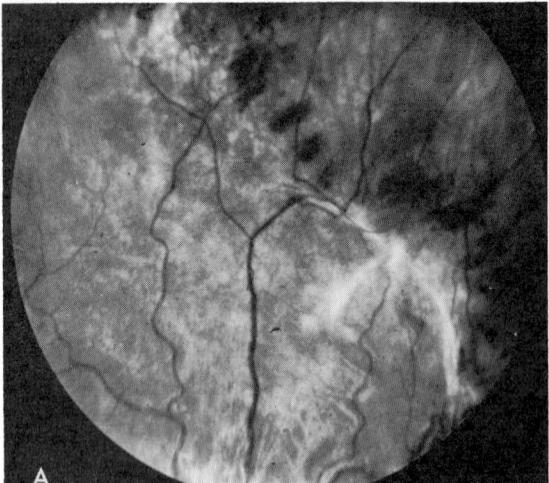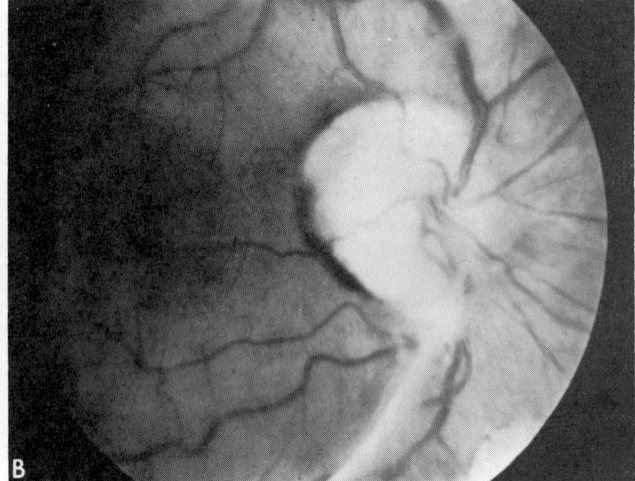

Figure 25–5. A, Developing retinopathy of prematurity in the temporal periphery. B, "Dragged disc" phenomenon in cicatricial retinopathy of prematurity.

1984). Stage 1 ROP is characterized by a distinct demarcation line that separates the avascular retina peripherally from the vascularized retina proximally (Fig. 25–5A). The demarcation line appears white and relatively flat; it lies within the plane of the retina. There is abnormal branching or arcading of vessels leading up to the line. Stage 2 is characterized by a ridge. In this stage, the line of stage 1 has grown, increasing in height, width, and volume, and it now extends up and out of the plane of the retina. It may change from white to pink. Vessels may leave the plane of the retina to enter the ridge. Stage 3 is characterized by the finding of extraretinal fibrovascular proliferative tissue, in addition to the ridge of stage 2. In stage 4, detachment of the retina is added to the aforementioned changes. The detachment may be due to exudative effusion of fluid, to traction, or to both. During the active stages progressive dilatation and tortuosity of the retinal vessels, iris vascular engorgement, pupillary rigidity, and vitreous haze also may develop.

The course is variable. In most cases the progress arrests and the signs regress, leaving little or no residua or visual disability. In other cases progression leads to cicatrization and sequelae of varying severity. Many of the characteristic signs of cicatricial RLF are due to foreshortening of the retina. These include so-called dragging of the disc and retinal vessels (Fig. 25–5B), displacement of the macula, retinal folds, detachment of the retina, and retinal pigmentary changes. In advanced cases, a "V" or funnel-shaped detachment of the retina is common. Subsequently, the "V" or funnel may be altered by closure anteriorly and/or posteriorly. The final clinical picture is that of a retrolental membrane, producing leukocoria (a white or cat's eye reflex in the pupil). Some patients also develop cataracts, glaucoma, and signs of inflammation. The end stage is often a painful blind eye or a degenerated phthisic eye. The spectrum of ROP-RLF also includes myopia; this is often progressive and of significant degree in infancy. There may also be an increased incidence of anisometropia, strabismus, amblyopia, and nystagmus in affected children.

In order to detect ROP, systematic examination of infants at risk is recommended. Guidelines generally include infants born at less than 36 wk gestation, those weighing less than 2000 g, and those requiring supplemental oxygen in the newborn period. Some data suggest that the optimal time for an initial screening ophthalmic examination is from age 7–9 wk. Follow-up is planned on the basis of the initial findings and risk factors.

Treatment. Therapy for ROP-RLF remains controversial.

The value of retinal photocoagulation, cryotherapy, and scleral buckling in active ROP and the possible benefits of retinal and vitreous surgery in cicatricial RLF are being evaluated.

Prevention of ROP ultimately rests with the prevention of premature birth and attendant risks. Failing this, efforts must be directed at controlling factors that induce the pathologic changes of ROP. Data suggest that for preterm infants at high risk continuous supplementation with vitamin E to physiologic levels from the first hours of life until retinal vascularization is complete may suppress the development of severe ROP, although treatment with this antioxidant does not appear to alter the overall incidence of the disease. The untoward effects of vitamin E are discussed in Sec. 8.17.

Persistent Hyperplastic Primary Vitreous (PHPV). This entity comprises a spectrum of manifestations due to persistence of various portions of the fetal hyaloid vascular system and associated fibrovascular tissue.

During development of the eye, the hyaloid artery extends from the optic disc to the posterior aspect of the lens; it sends branches into the vitreous (vasa hyaloidea propria) and ramifies to form the posterior portion of the vascular capsule of the lens (tunica vasculosa lentis). The posterior portion of the hyaloid system normally regresses by the 7th fetal mo, the anterior portion by the 8th fetal mo. Small remnants of the system, such as a tuft of tissue at the disc (Bergmeister papilla) or a tag of tissue on the posterior capsule of the lens (Mittendorf dot) are common findings in healthy persons. More extensive remnants and associated complications constitute PHPV. Two major forms are described: anterior PHPV and posterior PHPV. Variability is great, and mixed or intermediate forms occur.

The usual manifestation of anterior PHPV is the presence of a vascularized plaque of tissue on the back surface of the lens, in an eye that is microphthalmic or slightly smaller than normal. The condition is usually unilateral and may occur in persons with no other abnormalities and with no history of prematurity. The fibrovascular tissue tends to undergo gradual contracture. The ciliary processes characteristically become elongated, and the anterior chamber may become shallow. The lens usually is smaller than normal. The lens may be clear, but it often becomes cataractous and may swell or absorb fluid. Large or anomalous vessels of the iris may be present. There may be abnormalities of the anterior chamber angle. In time, the cornea may become cloudy.

Anterior PHPV is usually noted in the first weeks or months

of life. The most frequent presenting signs are leukocoria (white or cat's eye reflex), strabismus, or nystagmus. The course is usually progressive and ill fated. Major complications are spontaneous intraocular hemorrhage, swelling of the lens owing to rupture of the posterior capsule, and glaucoma. The eye may eventually deteriorate. In selected cases, surgery can be done in an effort to prevent complications, to preserve the eye and a reasonably good cosmetic appearance, and, in some cases, to salvage vision. Surgical treatment usually involves aspirating the lens and excising the abnormal tissue. If useful vision is to be attained, refractive correction and aggressive amblyopia therapy are required, but the visual results tend to be disappointing.

In some cases, the affected eye is enucleated, as the differential diagnosis between this white mass and that of retinoblastoma can be difficult. Ultrasonography and computed tomography are valuable aids in differential diagnosis.

The spectrum of posterior PHPV includes fibroglial veils around the disc and macula, vitreous membranes and stalks containing hyaloid artery remnants projecting from the disc, and meridional retinal folds. Traction detachment of the retina may occur. Vision may be impaired, but the eye is usually retained.

Retinoblastoma (Fig. 25–6). Retinoblastoma is the most common primary malignant intraocular tumor of childhood. It usually appears before the age of 5 yr, most commonly in the earlier years. The most frequent first sign is leukocoria, a white or cat's eye reflex in the pupil. Another frequent sign is strabismus, secondary to impairment of vision. Some children present ocular inflammation, intraocular hemorrhage, glaucoma, or heterochromia iridis.

On examination, the tumor appears as a white mass, sometimes small and relatively flat, sometimes large and protuberant. It may appear nodular. Vitreous haze or tumor seeding may be evident.

Differential diagnosis includes lesions such as retrolental fibroplasia, nematode endophthalmitis, persistent hyperplastic primary vitreous, and retinal dysplasia. As calcification occurs in the majority of retinoblastomas, standard orbital roentgenograms, computed tomography of the eye and orbit, and ultrasonography can be helpful in the diagnosis.

The goals of treatment are to destroy the tumor and to retain useful vision whenever possible without endangering life. The primary treatment of unilateral retinoblastoma is usually enucleation, though in selected cases alternative treatment such as cryotherapy, photocoagulation, or irradiation can be considered. In the treatment of bilateral retinoblastoma much depends on the number, size, location, and symmetry of the lesions in the two eyes. In some cases adjunctive chemotherapy is used.

Central nervous system involvement may occur by extension along the optic nerve; or hematogenous metastasis may occur to other organs, particularly bone, liver, kidney, and the adrenal glands. Patients with germinal mutation (hereditary) retinoblastoma are at increased risk also for other malignancies; the most common is osteogenic sarcoma; others include rhabdomyosarcoma, leukemia, melanoma, thyroid adenosarcoma, fibrosarcoma, malignant mesenchymoma, chondrosarcoma, angiosarcoma, and midline neuroblastic brain tumors, particularly pinealoma.

Other features of retinoblastoma and its management are discussed in Sec. 16.20.

Retinitis Pigmentosa. This is a progressive retinal degeneration characterized by pigmentary changes, arteriolar attenuation, usually some degree of optic atrophy, and progressive impairment of visual function. Dispersion and aggregation of the retinal pigment produce a variety of ophthalmoscopically visible changes, ranging from granularity or mottling of the retinal pigment pattern to distinctive focal pigment aggregates with the configuration of bone spicules (Fig. 25–7).

Impairment of night vision or dark adaptation is often the first symptom. Progressive loss of peripheral vision, often in the form of an expanding ring scotoma or concentric contraction of the field, is usual. There may or may not be loss of central vision. Retinal function as measured by electroretinography (ERG) is characteristically reduced. Manifestations commonly begin in childhood. The disorder may be autosomal recessive, autosomal dominant, or sex-linked.

In *Leber congenital retinal amaurosis* pigmentary retinal degenerative changes are pleomorphic, with varying degrees of pigment disorder, anteriolar attenuation, and optic atrophy. Vision impairment is usually evident soon after birth, and the ERG is abnormal early.

To be differentiated from retinitis pigmentosa are clinically similar, secondary, pigmentary retinal degenerations that occur in a wide variety of metabolic diseases, neurodegenerative processes, and multifaceted syndromes. Examples include the progressive retinal changes of the mucopolysaccharidoses

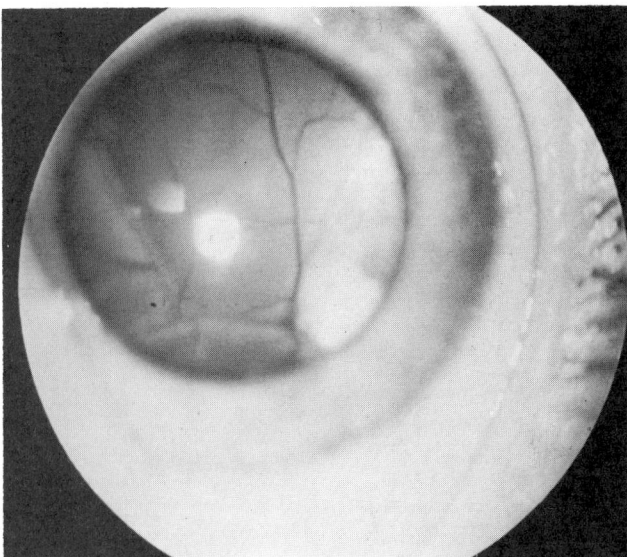
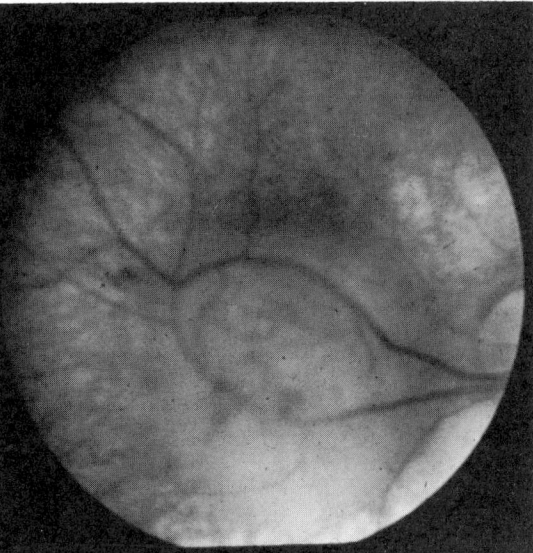

Figure 25–6. Retinoblastoma.

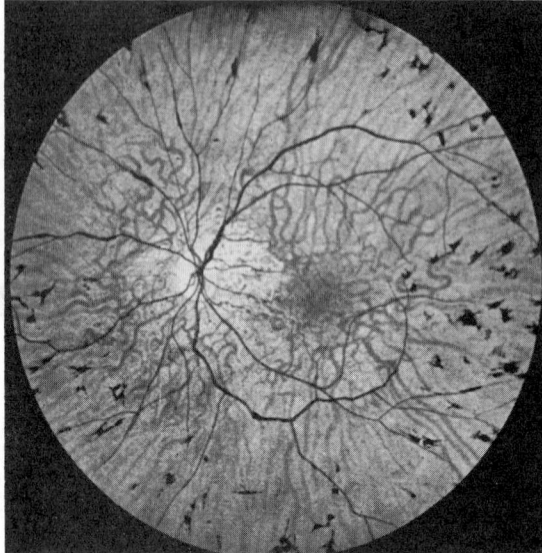

Figure 25–7. Retinitis pigmentosa.

macula surrounded and accentuated by a grayish-white or yellowish halo. The halo is the result of loss of transparency of the multilayered ganglion cell ring due to edema or lipid accumulation or to both. The sign occurs typically in certain sphingolipidoses, principally in Tay-Sachs disease (GM$_2$ type 1), in the Sandhoff variant (GM$_2$ type 2), and in generalized gangliosidosis (GM$_1$ type 1). Similar but less distinctive macular changes occur in some cases of metachromatic leukodystrophy (sulfatide lipidosis), in some forms of neuronopathic Niemann-Pick disease, and in certain mucolipidoses. To be differentiated from the cherry red spot of neurodegenerative disease is the cherry red spot that characteristically occurs as the result of retinal ischemia secondary to vasospasm, ocular contusion, or occlusion of the central retinal artery.

Phakomata. These are the herald lesions of the hamartomatous disorders. In Bourneville disease (tuberous sclerosis) the distinctive ocular lesion is a refractile, yellowish, multinodular cystic lesion arising from the disc or retina; the appearance of this typical lesion is often likened to that of an unripe mulberry (Fig. 25–8). Equally characteristic and more common in tuberous sclerosis are flatter, yellow to whitish retinal lesions, varying in size from minute dots to large lesions approaching the size of the disc. These lesions are benign astrocytic proliferations. Similar retinal phakomata occur in von Recklinghausen disease (neurofibromatosis). In von Hippel-Lindau disease (angiomatosis of the retina and cerebellum) the distinctive fundus lesion is a hemangioblastoma; this vascular lesion usually appears as a reddish globular mass with large paired arteries and veins passing to and from the lesion. In Sturge-Weber syndrome (encephalofacial angiomatosis) the fundus abnormality is a choroidal hemangioma; the hemangioma may impart a dark color to the affected area of the fundus, but the lesion is best seen with fluorescein angiography.

Retinoschisis. Congenital retinoschisis is a splitting of the retina into an inner and outer layer. This hereditary disorder is transmitted as a sex-linked recessive or autosomal dominant condition. It may be stationary or progressive. Often good vision is retained.

The most characteristic ophthalmoscopic sign is an elevation of the inner layer of the retina, most commonly in the inferotemporal quadrant of the fundus, often with round or oval holes visible in the inner layer. There are often associated cystoid macular changes. In some cases frank retinal detachment or vitreous hemorrhage occurs.

(particularly the syndromes of Hurler, Hunter, Scheie, and Sanfilippo) and certain of the late-onset gangliosidoses (the syndromes of Batten-Mayou, Spielmeyer-Vogt, and Jansky-Bielschowsky), the retinal manifestations of abetalipoproteinemia (Bassen-Kornzweig syndrome), the progressive retinal degeneration that is associated with progressive external ophthalmoplegia (as in Kearns-Sayre syndrome), and the retinitis pigmentosa–like changes in the Laurence-Moon-Biedl syndrome, to name just a few. There is also a high association of retinitis pigmentosa and hearing loss, as in Usher syndrome.

Stargardt Disease. This autosomal recessive retinal disorder is characterized by slowly progressive bilateral macular degeneration and vision impairment. It usually appears from 8–14 yr of age. The foveal reflex becomes obtunded or appears grayish; pigment spots develop in the macular area; and eventually macular depigmentation and chorioretinal atrophy occur. Macular hemorrhages also may develop. Central visual acuity is reduced, often to 20/200, but total loss of vision does not occur. ERG findings vary.

In some patients, there are also white or yellow spots beyond the macula or pigmentary changes in the periphery; in such cases, the term "fundus flavimaculatus" is applied. The condition is not associated with CNS abnormalities and is to be differentiated from the macular changes of many progressive metabolic neurodegenerative diseases.

Best Vitelliform Degeneration. This macular dystrophy is characterized by a distinctive yellow or orange discoid subretinal lesion in the macula, resembling the intact yolk of a fried egg. Diagnosis is usually made from 5–15 yr of age; usually, vision is normal at this stage. The condition may be progressive; the yolk-like lesion may eventually degenerate ("scramble") and result in pigmentation, chorioretinal atrophy, and vision impairment. There is no association with systemic abnormalities. Inheritance is usually autosomal dominant.

In vitelliform macular degeneration the electroretinographic response is normal. The electro-oculogram, however, is abnormal in affected patients and in carriers and is therefore a useful test in diagnosis and in genetic counseling.

Cherry Red Spot. Because of the special histologic features of the macula, certain pathologic processes affecting the retina produce an ophthalmoscopically visible sign referred to as a cherry red spot, a bright to dull red spot at the center of the

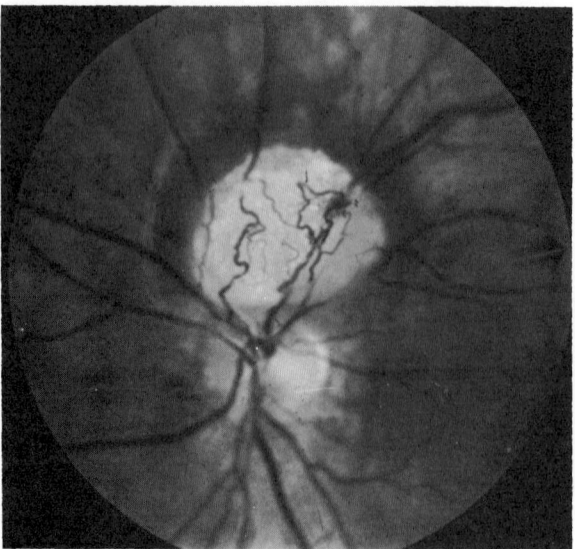

Figure 25–8. Retinal phakoma of tuberous sclerosis.

Retinal Detachment. In retinal detachment the neuroretina separates from the underlying layers. The most common cause of retinal detachment in children is trauma; there is usually a tear of the retina, with accumulation of subretinal fluid. Retinal detachment may also be associated with retinopathy of prematurity (cicatricial retrolental fibroplasia), myopia, aphakia (following cataract surgery), lattice degeneration, or congenital retinoschisis; may occur secondary to inflammatory or exudative processes, such as uveitis, hypertensive renal disease, or leukemia; or may be associated with a variety of congenital anomalies.

The principal effect is blurring or loss of vision in the corresponding field of vision, although in some cases retinal detachment can be asymptomatic. Some patients experience a shower of floaters or flashes of light.

In most cases treatment is surgical. Prompt care is important if vision is to be salvaged.

Coats Disease. This is an exudative retinopathy of obscure etiology, characterized by telangiectasis of retinal vessels with leakage of plasma to form intraretinal and subretinal exudates, and with retinal hemorrhages and detachment. The condition is usually unilateral. It affects predominantly boys, usually appearing in the 1st decade. The condition is nonfamilial and for the most part occurs in otherwise healthy children. The most frequent presenting signs are blurring of vision, leukocoria, and strabismus. Rubeosis of the iris, glaucoma, and cataract may develop. Treatment with photocoagulation or cryotherapy may be helpful.

Familial Exudative Vitreoretinopathy (FEV). This progressive retinovascular disorder is of unknown etiology, but clinical and angiographic findings suggest an aberration of vascular development. A significant finding in most cases is avascularity of the peripheral temporal retina, with abrupt cessation of the retinal capillary network in the region of the equator. The avascular zone often has a wedge- or V-shaped pattern in the temporal meridian. There may be glial proliferation or well-marked retinochoroidal atrophy in the avascular zone. Excessive branching of retinal arteries and veins, dilatation of the capillaries, arteriovenous shunt formation, neovascularization, and leakage from retinal vessels of the farthest vascularized retina occur. Vitreoretinal adhesions are usually present at the peripheral margin of the vascularized retina. Traction, retinal dragging and temporal displacement of the macula, falciform retinal folds, and retinal detachment are common. Intraretinal or subretinal exudation, retinal hemorrhage, and recurrent vitreous hemorrhages may develop. Patients may also develop cataracts and glaucoma. Vision impairment of varying severity occurs. The condition is usually bilateral. FEV is an autosomal dominant condition; sporadic cases have been reported.

The findings in FEV may resemble those of retinopathy of prematurity in the cicatricial stages (RLF); but unlike RLF, the neovascularization of FEV seems to develop years after birth and in most patients with FEV there is no history of prematurity, of oxygen therapy, of prenatal or postnatal injury or infection, or developmental abnormalities.

FEV is also to be differentiated from Coats disease, angiomatosis of retina, peripheral uveitis, and other disorders of the posterior segment.

Hypertensive Retinopathy. In the early stages of hypertension there may be no observable retinal changes. Generalized constriction and irregular narrowing of the arterioles are usually the first signs in the fundus. Other alterations include retinal edema, flame-shaped hemorrhages, "cotton-wool patches," and papilledema (Fig. 25–9). These changes are reversible if the disease can be controlled in the early stages, but in hypertension of long standing, irreversible changes may occur. Thickening of the vessel wall may produce a silver- or copper-wire appearance.

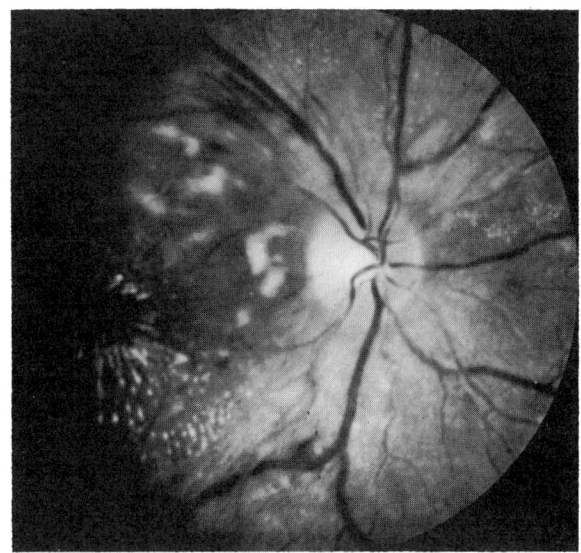
Figure 25–9. Hypertensive retinopathy.

Hypertensive retinal changes in the child should alert the physician to renal disease, pheochromocytoma, collagen disease, and cardiovascular disorders, particularly coarctation of the aorta.

The Retina in Subacute Bacterial Endocarditis. At some time during the course of the disease, retinopathy is present in approximately 40% of cases of subacute bacterial endocarditis; the lesions include hemorrhages, hemorrhages with white centers (Roth spots), papilledema, and, rarely, embolic occlusion of the central retinal artery.

The Retina in Blood Disorders. In primary and secondary anemias retinopathy in the form of hemorrhages and "cotton-wool patches" may occur. Vision can be affected if hemorrhage occurs in the macular area. The hemorrhages may be light and feathery or dense and preretinal. In polycythemia vera, the retinal veins are dark, dilated, and tortuous. Retinal hemorrhages, retinal edema, and papilledema may be observed. In leukemia the veins are characteristically dilated, with sausage-shaped constrictions; and hemorrhages, particularly white-centered hemorrhages and exudates, are common during the acute stage. In the sickling disorders fundus changes include vascular tortuosity, arterial and venous occlusions, "salmon patches," refractile deposits, pigmented lesions, arteriolar-venous anastomoses, and neovascularization (with "sea-fan" formations), sometimes leading to vitreous hemorrhage and retinal detachment.

Diabetic Retinopathy. The retinal changes of diabetes mellitus are classified as simple or nonproliferative (early) or proliferative (more advanced).

Nonproliferative diabetic retinopathy is characterized by retinal microaneurysms, venous dilatation, and retinal hemorrhages and exudates. The microaneurysms appear as tiny red dots. The hemorrhages may be of both the dot and blot type representing deep intraretinal bleeding and the splinter or flame-shaped type involving the superficial nerve fiber layer. The exudates tend to be deep and to appear waxy. There may also be superficial nerve fiber infarcts called cytoid bodies or "cotton wool spots," and retinal edema. These signs may wax and wane. They are seen primarily in the posterior pole, around the disc and macula, well within the range of direct ophthalmoscopy.

Proliferative retinopathy, the more serious form, is characterized by neovascularization and proliferation of connective tissue on the retina, extending into the vitreous. The vision-threatening complications of proliferative diabetic retinopathy are retinal and vitreous hemorrhages, cicatrization, traction, and retinal detachment. Rubeosis of the iris and secondary glaucoma may develop.

Diabetic retinopathy involves alteration and nonperfusion of retinal capillaries, retinal ischemia, and neovascularization, but its pathogenesis is not yet completely understood, either as to location of the primary pathogenetic mechanism (retinal vessels versus surrounding neuronal or glial tissue) or as to the specific biochemical factors involved. The relationship between control of blood glucose and the genesis or progression of retinopathy remains controversial, but data suggest that the better the degree of long-term metabolic control, the lower the risk of diabetic retinopathy.

Clinically, the prevalence and course of retinopathy relate to patient's age and to duration of disease. Detectable microvascular changes are rare in prepubertal children, the prevalence of retinopathy increasing significantly after puberty, and especially after the age of 15 yr. The incidence of retinopathy is low during the first 5 yr of disease and increases progressively thereafter, the incidence of proliferative retinopathy becoming substantial after 10 yr, with increased risk of visual impairment after 15 yr or more. Periodic ophthalmologic evaluation is recommended for all patients with diabetes mellitus.

In addition to retinopathy, patients with juvenile-onset diabetes may develop optic neuropathy, characterized by swelling of the disc and blurring of vision. Patients with diabetes may also develop cataracts, even at an early age, sometimes with rapid progression.

Recent advances in ocular therapy, such as retinal photocoagulation and vitrectomy, offer hope in reducing the visual morbidity in some patients with diabetes. Whether technologic advances such as insulin infusion pumps and pancreatic transplantation will be of value in the prevention of the ocular complications has yet to be determined.

Medullated Nerve Fibers. Myelination of the optic nerve fibers normally terminates at the level of the disc, but in some individuals ectopic medullation extends to nerve fibers of the retina. The condition is most commonly seen adjacent to the disc, although more peripheral areas of the retina may be involved. The characteristic ophthalmoscopic picture is a focal white patch with a feathered edge or brush-stroke appearance. In many cases, vision is not affected, but there may be relative or absolute visual field defects corresponding to areas of ectopic medullation. The eye is usually otherwise normal, but various abnormalities have been associated with ectopic medullation, including coloboma, cranial anomalies, anisometropic myopia, strabismus, and amblyopia, which may respond to treatment.

Coloboma of the Fundus. The term "coloboma" describes a defect such as a gap, notch, fissure, or hole. The typical fundus coloboma is due to malclosure of the embryonic fissure, which leaves a gap in the retina, retinal pigment epithelium, and choroid, thus baring the underlying sclera. The defect may be extensive, involving the ciliary body, iris, and even lens, or it may be localized to one or more portions of the fissure. The usual appearance is of a well-circumscribed, wedge-shaped white area extending inferonasally below the disc, sometimes involving or engulfing the disc. In some cases there is ectasia or cyst formation in the area of the defect. Less extensive colobomatous defects may appear as only single or multiple focal "punched-out" chorioretinal defects or anomalous pigmentation of the fundus in the line of the embryonic fissure. Colobomata may occur in one or both eyes. Usually a visual field defect corresponds to the chorioretinal defect. Visual acuity may be impaired, particularly if the defect involves the disc or macula.

Fundus colobomata may occur in isolation as sporadic defects or inherited as a dominant or recessive condition, or

may be associated with such abnormalities as microphthalmia, cyclopia, or anencephaly. They occur frequently in patients with trisomy 13 or trisomy 18. They may be associated with congenital heart disease, choanal atresia, and other abnormalities in the CHARGE* syndrome, or with cerebellar vermis agenesis in Joubert syndrome.

Aaby AA, Kushner BJ: Acquired and progressive myelinated nerve fibers. Arch Ophthalmol 103:542, 1985.

Abramson DH, Ellsworth RM, Kitchin FD, et al: Second nonocular tumors in retinoblastoma survivors: Are they radiation-induced? Ophthalmology 91:1351, 1984.

Barr CC, Glaser JS, Blankenship G: Acute disc swelling in juvenile diabetes: Clinical profile and natural history of 12 cases. Arch Ophthalmol 98:2185, 1980.

Bateman JB, Riedner E, Levin LS, et al: Heterogeneity of retinal degeneration and hearing impairment syndromes. Am J Ophthalmol 90:755, 1980.

Berson EL, Rosner B, Siminoff E: Risk factors for genetic typing and detection in retinitis pigmentosa. Am J Ophthalmol 89:763, 1980.

Biglan AW, Brown DR, Reynolds JD, et al: Risk factors associated with retrolental fibroplasia. Ophthalmology 91:1504, 1984.

Burns RP, Lourien EW, Cibis AB: Juvenile sex-linked retinoschisis: Clinical and genetic studies. Trans Am Acad Ophthalmol Otolaryngol 75:1011, 1971.

Chang M, McLean IW, Merritt JC: Coats' disease: A study of 62 histologically confirmed cases. J Pediatr Ophthalmol Strab 21:163, 1984.

Cogan DG, Kuwabara T: The sphingolipidoses and the eye. Arch Ophthalmol 79:437, 1968.

Cotlier E: Café-au-lait spots of the fundus in neurofibromatosis. Arch Ophthalmol 95:1990, 1977.

Doft BH, Kingsley LA, Orchard TJ, et al: The association between long-term diabetic control and early retinopathy. Ophthalmology 91:763, 1984.

Dryja TP, Cavena W, White R, et al: Homozygosity of chromosome 13 in retinoblastoma. N Engl J Med 319:550, 1984.

Duane TD, Osher RH, Green WR: White centered hemorrhages: Their significance. Ophthalmology 87:66, 1980.

Eagle RC, Lucier AC, Bernardino VB Jr, et al: Retinal pigment epithelial abnormalities in fundus flavimaculatus. Ophthalmology 87:1189, 1980.

Fishman GA: Retinitis pigmentosa: Genetic percentages. Arch Ophthalmol 96:822, 1978.

Flynn JT, O'Grady GE, Herrera J, et al: Retrolental fibroplasia: I. Clinical observations. Arch Ophthalmol 95:217, 1977.

Foos RY: Chronic retinopathy of prematurity. Ophthalmology 92:563, 1985.

Frank RN: On the pathogenesis of diabetic retinopathy. Ophthalmology 91:626, 1984.

Frank RN, Hoffman WH, Podgor MJ, et al: Retinopathy in juvenile-onset diabetes of short duration. Ophthalmology 87:1, 1980.

Gallie BL, Phillips RA: Retinoblastoma: A model of oncogenesis. Ophthalmology 91:666, 1984.

Goldberg MF, Cotlier E, Fichenscher LG, et al: Macular cherry-red spot, corneal clouding, and β-galactosidase deficiency. Arch Intern Med 128:387, 1971.

Goldberg MF, Mafee M: Computed tomography for diagnosis of persistent hyperplastic primary vitreous (PHPV). Ophthalmology 90:442, 1983.

Hanada S, Ellsworth RM: Congenital retinal detachment and the optic disc anomaly. Am J Ophthalmol 71:460, 1971.

Hardwig P, Robertson DM: Von Hippel-Lindau disease: A familial, often lethal, multi-system phakomatosis. Ophthalmology 91:263, 1984.

Hittner HM, Rudolph AJ, Kretzer FL: Suppression of severe retinopathy of prematurity with vitamin E supplementation: Ultrastructural mechanism of clinical efficacy. Ophthalmology 91:1512, 1984.

Holt JM, Gordon-Smith EC: Retinal abnormalities in diseases of the blood. Br J Ophthalmol 53:145, 1969.

Jackson RL, Ide CH, Guthrie RA, et al: Retinopathy in adolescents and young adults with onset of insulin-dependent diabetes in childhood. Ophthalmology 89:7, 1982.

JuanVerdaguer T: Juvenile retinal detachment. Am J Ophthalmol 93:145, 1982.

Kline R, Klein BEK, Moss SE, et al: The Wisconsin epidemiologic study of diabetic retinopathy: II. Prevalence and risk of diabetic retinopathy when age at diagnosis is less than 30 years. Arch Ophthalmol 102:520, 1984.

Knobloch WH, Layer JM: Clefting syndromes associated with retinal detachment. Am J Ophthalmol 73:517, 1972.

Kushner BJ: Strabismus and amblyopia associated with regressed retinopathy of prematurity. Arch Ophthalmol 100:256, 1982.

Kushner BJ, Essner D, Cohen IJ, et al: Retrolental fibroplasia: II. Pathologic correlation. Arch Ophthalmol 95:29, 1977.

Kushner BJ, Sondheimer S: Medical treatment of glaucoma associated with cicatricial retinopathy of prematurity. Am J Ophthalmol 94:313, 1982.

Laverda AM, Saia OS, Drigo P, et al: Chorioretinal coloboma and Joubert syndrome: A nonrandom association. J Pediatr 105:282, 1984.

Mann E, Kut LJ, Lee CB: Rheumatogenous retinal detachment in infancy. Arch Ophthalmol 95:1774, 1971.

Margo C, Hidayat A, Kopelman J, et al: Retinocytoma: A benign variant of retinoblastoma. Arch Ophthalmol 101:1519, 1983.

*C, coloboma; H, heart disease; A, atresia choanae; R, retarded growth and development and/or CNS anomalies; G, genetic anomalies and/or hypogonadism; E, ear anomalies and/or deafness.

Miller SJH: Ophthalmic aspects of the Sturge-Weber syndrome. Proc Roy Soc Med 56:419, 1963.

Miyakulo H, Hashimoto K, Miyakulo S: Retinal vascular pattern in familial exudative vitreoretinopathy. Ophthalmology 91:1524, 1984.

Mohler CW, Fine SL: Long-term evaluation of patients with Best's vitelliform dystrophy. Ophthalmology 88:688, 1981.

Noble KG, Carr RE: Leber's congenital amaurosis: A retrospective study of 33 cases and a histopathological study of one case. Arch Ophthalmol 96:818, 1978.

Noble KG, Carr RE: Stargardt's disease and fundus flavimaculatus. Arch Ophthalmol 97:1281, 1979.

Nyboer JH, Robertson DM, Gomez MR: Retinal lesions in tuberous sclerosis. Arch Ophthalmol 94:1277, 1976.

Pagon RA: Ocular coloboma. Survey Ophthalmol 25:223, 1981.

Pagon RA, Graham JM, Zonana J, et al: Coloboma, congenital heart disease, and choanal atresia with multiple anomalies: CHARGE association. J Pediatr 99:223, 1981.

Palmer EA: Optimal timing of examination for acute retrolental fibroplasia. Ophthalmology 88:662, 1981.

Pruett RC, Schepens CI: Posterior hyperplastic primary vitreous. Am J Ophthalmol 69:535, 1970.

Ridgeway EW, Jaffe N, Walton DS: Leukemic ophthalmopathy in children. Cancer 38:1744, 1976.

Ridley ME, Shields JA, Brown GC, et al: Coats' disease: Evaluation of management. Ophthalmology 89:1381, 1982.

Riley FC, Campbell RJ: Double phakomatosis. Arch Ophthalmology 97:518, 1979.

Romayananda N, Goldberg MF, Green WR: Histopathology of sickle cell retinopathy. Ophthalmology 77:652, 1973.

Rosenthal AR: Ocular manifestations of leukemia. Ophthalmology 90:899, 1983.

Salazar FG, Lamiell JM: Early identification of retinal angiomas in a large kindred with von Hippel-Lindau disease. Am J Ophthalmol 89:540, 1980.

Shields JA, Augsburger JJ: Current approaches to the diagnosis and management of retinoblastoma. Surv Ophthalmol 25:347, 1981.

Stark WJ, Lindsey PS, Fagadau WR, et al: Persistent hyperplastic primary vitreous: Surgical treatment. Ophthalmology 90:452, 1983.

Stein MR, Gay AJ: Acute chorioretinal infarction in sickle cell trait. Arch Ophthalmol 84:485, 1970.

Straatsma BR, Foos RY, Heckenlively JR, et al: Myelinated retinal nerve fibers. Am J Ophthalmol 91:25, 1981.

Tasman W: Late complications of retrolental fibroplasia. Ophthalmology 86:1724, 1979.

The Committee for the Classification of Retinopathy of Prematurity: An international classification of retinopathy of prematurity. Arch Ophthalmol 102:1130, 1984.

Topilow HW, Ackerman AL, Wang FM: The treatment of advanced retinopathy of prematurity by cryotherapy and scleral buckling surgery. Ophthalmology 92:379, 1985.

Trese MT: Surgical results of stage V retrolental fibroplasia and timing of surgical repair. Ophthalmology 91:461, 1984.

Tso MOM, Jampol LM: Pathophysiology of hypertensive retinopathy. Ophthalmology 89:1132, 1982.

Walsh JB: Hypertensive retinopathy: Description, classification and prognosis. Ophthalmology 89:1127, 1982.

Yassur Y, Nissenkorn I, Ben-Sira I, et al: Autosomal dominant inheritance of retinoschisis. Am J Ophthalmol 94:338, 1982.

Zimmerman LE, Buras RP, Wankum G, et al: Trilateral retinoblastoma: Ectopic intracranial retinoblastoma associated with bilateral retinoblastoma. J Pediatr Ophthalmol Strab 19:320, 1982.

25.14 ABNORMALITIES OF THE OPTIC NERVE

Optic nerve hypoplasia is a developmental deficiency of optic nerve fibers. It has been attributed to primary failure in the differentiation of retinal ganglion cells or their axons. Alternatively, it may result from prenatal degeneration of the ganglion cell axons. In typical cases the nervehead is small and pale, with a pale or pigmented peripapillary halo or "double ring sign." This anomaly is associated with defects of vision and of visual fields of varying severity, ranging from blindness to normal or near-normal vision in the affected eye. Hypoplasia may be unilateral or bilateral, clinical findings varying with severity and laterality of the condition. Unilateral or asymmetric hypoplasia commonly presents as deviation (heterotropia, strabismus) of the more severely affected eye; the deviation usually develops early in life, but often the underlying visual defect is not suspected or detected until a later age. When there is bilateral hypoplasia of relatively severe degree, the defect in vision is usually appreciated early, and there is often obvious strabismus or secondary nystagmus. Mild hypoplasia may be unrecognized for years.

Optic nerve hypoplasia may occur alone or with other developmental abnormalities, including microphthalmia, anencephaly, hydrocephalus, and encephalocele. Optic nerve hypoplasia is a principal feature of septo-optic dysplasia of de Morsier, a developmental disorder characterized by association of anomalies of the midline structures of the brain with hypoplasia of the optic nerves, optic chiasm, and optic tracts; typically, there is agenesis of the septum pellucidum and malformation of the fornix, with a large chiasmatic cistern. There may be hypothalamic abnormalities and endocrine defects, ranging from panhypopituitarism to isolated deficiency of growth hormone, hypothyroidism, diabetes insipidus, or diabetes mellitus. The condition does not appear to be familial, although it has occurred in siblings. There is no regularly associated chromosomal defect. It may occur with somewhat increased frequency in infants of diabetic mothers.

Morning Glory Syndrome. This term describes a congenital anomaly of the optic nerve characterized by an enlarged, excavated, funnel-shaped disc with an elevated rim, resembling the flower for which it is named. There often is whitish tissue in the funnel; the abnormal vessel pattern involves multiple branches emerging radially; and there is usually pigmentary mottling of the peripapillary region. One or both eyes may be affected. There may be other developmental defects of the affected or fellow eye. Vision is usually impaired, and strabismus may be the first sign. Detachment of the retina occurs. The anomaly may rarely be associated with developmental midline defects, including cleft lip and palate, agenesis of the corpus callosum, and encephalocele.

Papilledema. The term papilledema ("choked disc") can be applied to swelling of the nervehead of diverse etiologies, but it preferentially denotes the disc changes of increased intracranial pressure, including edematous blurring of the disc margins, fullness or elevation of the nervehead, partial or complete obliteration of the disc cup, capillary congestion and hyperemia of the disc, generalized engorgement of the veins, loss of spontaneous venous pulsation, nerve fiber layer hemorrhages around the disc, and peripapillary exudates. In some cases there may be edema extending into the macula, producing a fan- or star-shaped figure. In addition, there may be concentric peripapillary retinal wrinkling. Typically, the blind spot enlarges, and there may be transient obscuration of vision, lasting seconds. Visual acuity is generally preserved. Normally, when the intracranial pressure is relieved, the papilledema will resolve and the disc return to a normal or nearly normal appearance within 6–8 wk. Sustained chronic papilledema or longstanding unrelieved increased intracranial pressure may, however, lead to permanent nerve fiber damage, atrophic changes of the disc, and impairment of vision.

The sequence of events as increased intracranial pressure leads to papilledema is probably as follows: elevation of intracranial subarachnoid cerebrospinal fluid pressure, elevation of cerebrospinal fluid pressure in the sheath of the optic nerve, elevation of tissue pressure in the optic nerve, stasis of axoplasmic flow and swelling of the nerve fibers in the optic nervehead, and secondary vascular changes and the characteristic ophthalmoscopic signs of venous stasis.

The common causes of increased intracranial pressure and choked disc in childhood are intracranial tumors and obstructive hydrocephalus, intracranial hemorrhage, the cerebral edema of trauma, meningoencephalitis and toxic encephalopathy, and certain metabolic diseases. Whatever the etiology, the disc signs of increased intracranial pressure in early childhood may be modified by the distensibility of the young skull.

To be differentiated from true papilledema are certain

structural changes of the disc ("pseudopapilledema," "pseudoneuritis," drusen, and medullated fibers), with which it may be confused, and the disc swelling of hypertension and diabetes mellitus.

Optic Neuritis. This term is used to describe any inflammation, demyelinization, or degeneration of the optic nerve with attendant impairment of function. The process is usually acute, with rapidly progressive loss of vision. It may be unilateral or bilateral. Pain on movement of the globe or pain on palpation of the globe may precede or accompany the onset of visual symptoms.

When the retrobulbar portion of the nerve is affected without ophthalmoscopically visible signs of inflammation at the disc, the term retrobulbar neuritis is applied. When there is ophthalmoscopically visible evidence of inflammation of the nervehead, the term papillitis or intraocular optic neuritis is used. When there is involvement of both the retina and papilla, the term optic neuroretinitis is used.

In childhood, optic neuritis rarely occurs as an isolated condition but is usually a manifestation of a neurologic or systemic disease. It may occur with bacterial meningitis or with viral infection (often accompanying encephalomyelitis following an exanthem). It may signify one of the many demyelinizing diseases of childhood. It may be the first manifestation of disseminated sclerosis. Alternatively, the cause may be an exogenous toxin or drug; optic neuritis may develop, for example, with lead poisoning or as a complication of long term, high dose treatment with chloramphenicol.

In most cases of acute optic neuritis there is some improvement in vision beginning within 1–4 wk after the onset, and vision may improve to normal or near normal within weeks or months. In some cases there is permanent impairment of vision. The course varies with etiology.

Optic Atrophy. This denotes degeneration of optic nerve axons with attendant loss of function. The ophthalmoscopic signs of optic atrophy are pallor of the disc and loss of substance of the nervehead, sometimes with enlargement of the disc cup. The associated vision defect varies with the nature and site of the primary disease or lesion.

Optic atrophy is the common expression of a wide variety of congenital or acquired pathologic processes. The cause may be traumatic, inflammatory, degenerative, neoplastic, or vascular; intracranial tumors and hydrocephalus are principal causes of optic atrophy in children. Progressive optic atrophy occurs with many metabolic neurodegenerative diseases, and with several developmental anomalies of the skull, particularly the craniosynostoses. In some instances optic atrophy is hereditary. Dominantly inherited infantile optic atrophy is a relatively mild heredodegenerative type that tends to progress through childhood and adolescence. Autosomal recessively inherited congenital optic atrophy is a rare condition that is evident at birth or develops at a very early age; the visual defect is usually profound. Behr optic atrophy is a hereditary type associated with hypertonia of the extremities, increased deep tendon reflexes, mild cerebellar ataxia, some degree of mental deficiency, and possibly external ophthalmoplegia; this disorder afflicts principally males from 3–11 yr of age. Leber hereditary optic atrophy, now defined as an optic neuropathy, occurs predominantly in males and usually appears from 18–23 yr of age; in the early stages inflammatory changes at the disc may be evident. Some forms of heredodegenerative optic atrophy are associated with sensorineural hearing loss, as may occur in some children with juvenile onset (insulin-dependent) diabetes mellitus.

Optic Glioma. The most frequent tumor of the optic nerve in childhood is optic glioma. This neuroglial tumor may develop in the intraorbital, intracanalicular, or intracranial portion of the nerve; often the chiasm is involved.

Histologically, optic glioma is a benign lesion; its deleterious effects vary with its location and growth pattern. The principal manifestations of intraorbital optic glioma are unilateral loss of vision, proptosis, and deviation of the eye; there may be optic atrophy or congestion of the optic nervehead. With chiasmal gliomas there may be defects of vision and visual fields (often bitemporal hemianopsia), increased intracranial pressure, papilledema or optic atrophy, hypothalamic dysfunction, pituitary dysfunction, and even evidence of brain stem effects such as nystagmus.

Optic glioma occurs with increased frequency in patients with neurofibromatosis.

The natural clinical course of optic glioma often involves relatively slow, often self-limited progression; there may, however, be relentless progression to death.

Management of optic glioma is controversial. When the tumor is confined to the intraorbital, intracanalicular, or prechiasmal portion of the nerve, resection is often done, especially when there is unsightly proptosis with complete or nearly complete loss of vision of the affected eye. When the chiasm is involved, surgery is not advised, though surgical intervention to control secondary hydrocephalus may be necessary. Radiation may or may not alter growth of the tumor. Chemotherapy is under trial.

Barr CC, Glaser JS, Blankenship G: Acute disc swelling in juvenile diabetes: Clinical profile and natural history of 12 cases. Arch Ophthalmol 98:2185, 1980.

Blodi FC: Developmental anomalies of the skull affecting the eye. Arch Ophthalmol 57:593, 1957.

Danoff BF, Kramer S, Thompson N: The radiotherapeutic management of optic nerve gliomas in children. J Radiation Oncol Biol Phys 6:45, 1980.

Haik BG, Greenstein SH, Smith ME, et al: Retinal detachment in the morning glory anomaly. Ophthalmology 91:1638, 1984.

Harley RD, Huang NN, Macri CH, et al: Optic neuritis and optic atrophy following chloramphenicol in cystic fibrosis patients. Trans Am Acad Ophthalmol Otolaryngol 74:1011, 1970.

Hayreh SS: Optic disc edema in raised intracranial pressure: V. Pathogenesis. Arch Ophthalmol 95:1553, 1977.

Hayreh SS: Optic disc edema in raised intracranial pressure: VI. Associated visual disturbances and their pathogenesis. Arch Ophthalmol 95:1566, 1977.

Kazarian EL, Gager WE: Optic neuritis complicating measles, mumps and rubella vaccination. Am J Ophthalmol 86:544, 1978.

Kennedy C, Carter S: Relation of optic neuritis to multiple sclerosis in children. Pediatrics 28:377, 1961.

Kennedy C, Carroll FD: Optic neuritis in children. Arch Ophthalmol 63:747, 1960.

Kindler P: Morning glory syndrome: Unusual congenital optic disc anomaly. Am J Ophthalmol 69:376, 1970.

Kline LB, Glaser JS: Dominant optic atrophy: The clinical profile. Arch Ophthalmol 97:1680, 1979.

Koenig SB, Naidich TP, Lissner G: The morning glory syndrome associated with sphenoidal encephalocele. Ophthalmology 89:1368, 1982.

Layman PR, Anderson DR, Flynn JT: Frequent occurrence of hypoplastic optic discs in patients with aniridia. Am J Ophthalmol 77:513, 1974.

Lessell S, Rosman P: Juvenile diabetes mellitus and optic atrophy. Arch Neurol 34:759, 1977.

Lewis RA, Gerson LP, Axelson KA, et al: von Recklinghausen neurofibromatosis: II. Incidence of optic gliomata. Ophthalmology 91:929, 1984.

Lloyd LA: Gliomas of the optic nerve and chiasm in childhood. Trans Am Ophthalmol Soc LXXI:488, 1978.

McLeod AR: Acute blindness in childhood optic glioma caused by hematoma. J Pediatr Ophthalmol Strab 20:31, 1983.

Meadows SP: Retrobulbar and optic neuritis in childhood and adolescence. Trans Ophthalmol Soc UK 89:603, 1970.

Nikoskelainen E: New aspects of the genetic, etiologic, and clinical puzzle of Leber's disease. Neurology 34:1482, 1984.

O'Dwyer JA, Newton TH, Hoyt WF: Radiologic features of septo-optic dysplasia: deMorsier syndrome. AJNR 1:443, 1980.

Petersen RA, Walton DS: Optic nerve hypoplasia with good visual acuity and visual field defects: A study of children of diabetic mothers. Arch Ophthalmol 95:254, 1977.

Rosenberg MA, Savino PJ, Glaser JS: A clinical analysis of pseudopapilledema: I. Population, laterality, acuity, refractive error, ophthalmoscopic characteristics, and coincident disease. Arch Ophthalmol 97:65, 1979.

Rush JA, Younge BR, Campbell RJ, et al: Optic glioma: Long-term follow-up of 85 histopathologically verified cases. Ophthalmology 89:1213, 1982.

Schwartz JF, Chutorian AM, Evans RA, et al: Optic atrophy in childhood. Pediatrics 34:670, 1964.

Selbst RG, Selhorst JB, Harbison JW, et al: Parainfectious optic neuritis: Report and review following varicella. Arch Neurol 40:347, 1983.

Skarf B, Hoyt CS: Optic nerve hypoplasia in children: Association with anomalies of the endocrine and CNS. Arch Ophthalmol 102:62, 1984.

Walton DS, Robb RM: Optic nerve hypoplasia: A report of 20 cases. Arch Ophthalmol 84:572, 1970.

25.15 DISORDERS OF OCULAR PRESSURE

Glaucoma. This term refers to conditions in which there is abnormal elevation of intraocular pressure of a degree sufficient to cause ocular damage and changes in vision. In infants and young children the principal signs are tearing, photophobia, blepharospasm, corneal clouding (edema), and progressive enlargement of the eye ("buphthalmos"). Optic nerve-head cupping, optic atrophy, and visual loss may result.

Childhood glaucoma is usually due to a developmental abnormality of the angle of the anterior chamber; commonly there is residual mesodermal tissue blocking drainage through the trabecular meshwork. Primary or simple congenital glaucoma is inherited as a recessive condition, although glaucoma associated with dominantly inherited goniodysgenesis has been described. Glaucoma may also be associated with other ocular anomalies such as aniridia, mesodermal dysgenesis of the anterior segments, and spherophakia, with certain of the hamartomatoses (neurofibromatosis, Sturge-Weber syndrome), and with a variety of syndromes such as those of Lowe and Marfan. Glaucoma in infants and children may also be secondary to trauma, intraocular hemorrhage, inflammatory processes (uveitis), and intraocular tumor.

Treatment of congenital and infantile glaucoma is primarily surgical; surgery should be performed as early as the child's general medical condition will allow. Procedures currently used to reduce and control ocular tension are goniotomy, goniopuncture, trabeculotomy, trabeculectomy, and, in some cases, cyclocryotherapy. Frequently, multiple surgical procedures are required. In many cases, even after surgery, long-term medical therapy also is required. The prognosis for vision depends on normalization of intraocular pressure and prevention of optic nerve damage. Even following early normalization of tension, further therapy must be directed toward the correction of amblyopia and refractive errors. In some children there are also such complicating factors as cataracts, corneal opacities, retinal disease, and abnormalities of the optic nerve.

Hypotony. Abnormally low intraocular pressure may result from perforating ocular injury, or from ocular inflammation (cyclitis/uveitis) that impairs aqueous secretion. Acute hypotony occurs in infants or children with moderate to severe dehydration.

Boyer WP III, Walton DS: Timolol in uncontrolled childhood glaucomas. Ophthalmology 88:253, 1981.

Cibis GW, Tripathi RC, Tripathi BJ: Glaucoma in Sturge-Weber syndrome. Ophthalmology 91:1061, 1984.

Jerndal T: Dominant goniodysgenesis with late congenital glaucoma. Am J Ophthalmol 74:28, 1972.

McPherson SD Jr, Berry DP: Goniotomy vs external trabeculotomy for developmental glaucoma. Am J Ophthalmol 95:427, 1983.

Robin AL, Quigley HA, Pollack IP, et al: An analysis of visual acuity, visual fields, and disc cupping in childhood glaucoma. Am J Ophthalmol 88:847, 1979.

25.16 ORBITAL ABNORMALITIES

Hypertelorism. This term denotes wide separation of the eyes or an increased interorbital distance, which may occur as a morphogenetic variant, a primary deformity, or a secondary phenomenon in association with developmental abnormalities, such as frontal meningocele or encephalocele or the persistence of a facial cleft. There is often associated strabismus, generally exotropia, and sometimes optic atrophy.

Hypotelorism. This term denotes narrowness of the interorbital distance, which may occur as a morphogenetic variant alone or in association with other anomalies, such as epicanthus, or secondary to a cranial dystrophy, such as scaphocephaly.

Exophthalmos. Protrusion of the eye is referred to as exophthalmos or proptosis. It may be due to shallowness of the orbits as seen in many craniofacial malformations or to increased tissue mass within the orbit as occurs with neoplastic, vascular, and inflammatory disorders. Ocular complications include exposure keratopathy, ocular motor disturbances, and optic atrophy with loss of vision.

Enophthalmos. Posterior displacement or sinking of the eye back into the orbit is referred to as enophthalmos. This may occur with orbital fracture or with atrophy of orbital tissue. It is a feature of Horner syndrome.

Orbital Cellulitis. This describes a condition involving inflammation of the tissues of the orbit, with proptosis, limitation of movement of the eye, edema of the conjunctiva (chemosis), and inflammation and swelling of the eyelids. There is often some discomfort, usually with general symptoms of toxicity, fever, and leukocytosis.

In general, orbital cellulitis may follow (1) direct infection of the orbit from a wound, (2) metastatic deposition of organisms during bacteremia, or (3) direct extension or venous spread of infection from contiguous sites such as the lids, the conjunctiva, the globe, the lacrimal gland, the nasolacrimal sac, or the paranasal sinuses. In some cases primary or metastatic tumor in the orbit can produce the clinical picture of orbital cellulitis.

By far the most common cause of orbital cellulitis in children is paranasal sinusitis, the most frequent pathogenic organisms being *Haemophilus influenzae*, *Staphylococcus aureus*, group A beta-hemolytic streptococci, and *Streptococcus pneumoniae*.

The orbital inflammatory manifestations of paranasal sinusitis vary with the location and extent of involvement. Stage 1 is swelling of the lids—the edema of impaired venous drainage or the reactive inflammation of underlying periostitis; in this stage the infection is still confined to the sinus. The 2nd stage is subperiosteal abscess, a collection of pus between the periosteum and the wall of the orbit, often with localized tenderness, displacement of the globe, and some limitation of eye movement. The 3rd stage is true orbital cellulitis, diffuse inflammation of the tissues within the orbit, with proptosis and impairment of ocular motility. The 4th stage is orbital abscess, resulting from localization of infection in the orbit or from extension of a subperiosteal abscess through the periosteum.

The potential for complications is great. Involvement of the optic nerve may result in loss of vision. Extension of infection from the orbit into the cranial cavity may lead to cavernous sinus thrombosis or meningitis or to epidural, subdural, or brain abscess.

Orbital cellulitis must be recognized promptly and treated aggressively. In most cases hospitalization and systemic antibiotic therapy are indicated. In some cases surgical intervention is necessary to drain infected sinuses or a subperiosteal or orbital abscess.

Periorbital Cellulitis. Inflammation of the lids and periorbital tissues without signs of true orbital involvement (such as proptosis or limitation of eye movement) is generally referred to as periorbital or preseptal cellulitis. This is common in young children and may be due to trauma, or to an infected wound or abscess of the lid or periorbital region (such as pyoderma, hordeolum, conjunctivitis, or dacryocystitis); it may be associated with respiratory infection or bacteremia, often with *H. influenzae*, streptococcus, or *Staph. aureus*. What initially appears to be periorbital or preseptal cellulitis may be the first sign of sinusitis that may progress to true orbital cellulitis. Prompt antibiotic therapy and careful monitoring for signs of progression are essential.

Tumors of the Orbit. A variety of tumors occur in and about the orbit in childhood. Among benign tumors, the most common are vascular lesions (principally hemangiomas) and dermoids. Among malignant neoplasms rhabdomyosarcoma, lymphosarcoma, and metastatic neuroblastoma are the most frequent. Optic gliomata and retinoblastomas that extend into the orbit also occur.

The effects of orbital tumors vary with their locations and growth patterns. The principal signs are proptosis, resistance to retroplacement of the eye, and impairment of eye movement. There may be a palpable mass. Other significant signs are ptosis, optic nervehead congestion, optic atrophy, and loss of vision. Bruit and visible pulsation of the globe are important clues to vascular lesions.

The differential diagnosis of orbital tumors is difficult; ultrasonography and computed tomography may be particularly helpful. Pseudotumor of the orbit also must be considered in children with signs of a mass lesion.

Haik BG, Jakobiec FA, Ellsworth RM, et al: Capillary hemangioma of the lids and orbit: An analysis of the clinical features and therapeutic results in 101 cases. Ophthalmology 86:760, 1979.
Hawkins DB, Clark RW: Orbital involvement in acute sinusitis: Lessons from 24 childhood patients. Clin Pediatr 16:464, 1977.
Mottow LS, Jakobiec FA: Idiopathic inflammatory orbital pseudotumor in childhood. Arch Ophthalmol 96:1410, 1978.
Pollard ZF, Calhoun J: Deep orbital dermoid with draining sinus. Am J Ophthalmol 79:310, 1975.
Porterfield JF: Orbital tumors in children: A report of 214 cases. Int Ophthalmol Clin 2:319, 1962.
Shields JA, Bakewell B, Augsberger JJ, et al: Classification and incidence of space-occupying lesions of the orbit: A survey of 645 biopsies. Arch Ophthalmol 102:1606, 1984.
Smith TF, O'Day D, Wright PF: Clinical implications of preseptal (periorbital) cellulitis in childhood. Pediatrics 62:1006, 1978.
Weiss A, Friendly D, Eglin K, et al: Bacterial periorbital cellulitis in childhood. Ophthalmology 90:195, 1983.

25.17 INJURIES TO THE EYE

About one third of all blindness in children results from trauma, usually avoidable. Injuries are caused by air rifles, arrows, darts, stones and missile-throwing toys, sticks, sharp tools, explosives, and strong chemicals. Many injuries cause acute pain, photophobia, tearing, blepharospasm, redness, or bleeding, prompting immediate consultation with a physician; unfortunately, some injuries do not produce such signs and symptoms and are often ignored.

Ecchymoses and swelling of the eyelids are common after blunt trauma. Hemorrhage into the lids and periorbital region (the "black eye" or "shiner") is usually of no consequence and will absorb spontaneously, but it should prompt careful examination of the eye for deeper, more serious injury, such as intraocular hemorrhage or rupture of the globe.

Lacerations of the eyelids require careful management. Horizontal laceration of the upper lid may involve the levator, the tarsal plate, or the orbital septum. Faulty repair can result in ptosis, distortion of the lid, or herniation of orbital fat. Lacerations involving the lid margins require meticulous surgical apposition to prevent notching, eversion, or inversion of the margin or misdirection of the lashes that might lead to epiphora (tear overflow) and chronic irritation. Lacerations situated near the medial canthus may involve the punctum, canaliculi, or nasolacrimal duct and may require the attention of an experienced ophthalmic surgeon. In all cases of lid laceration, examination of the globe for perforating injury is mandatory.

Superficial abrasions of the cornea usually produce pain or a foreign body sensation, sensitivity to light, tearing, redness, blepharospasm, and sometimes blurring of vision. The diagnosis is facilitated by fluorescein staining. Sterile paper strips impregnated with fluorescein dye are available. When the strip is moistened and applied to the conjunctiva, the yellow dye diffuses in the tear film and will "stain" any epithelial defect; the stain is best seen with the aid of a blue light.

Most superficial corneal abrasions heal promptly without complication. The injury is best treated initially by instillation of an antibiotic eye drop or ophthalmic ointment to prevent infection and application of a firm bandage (eye pad) to reduce eyelid movement and promote healing. The eye should then be examined within a day, preferably by an ophthalmologist, to determine the progress of healing and the need for further treatment (such as removal of a foreign body). In some cases attendant iritis will require the topical use of a cycloplegic agent and/or corticosteroid.

A foreign body on or in the cornea or conjunctiva usually produces acute discomfort, lacrimation, and inflammation. Most foreign bodies can be detected by examination in good light with the aid of magnification; the direct ophthalmoscope set on a high plus lens (+10 or +12) is helpful. In many cases slit lamp examination will be necessary, especially if the particle is deep or metallic. Some conjunctival foreign bodies tend to lodge under the upper eyelid, producing the sensation of corneal foreign body as they come into contact with the globe on eyelid movement; eversion of the lid may be necessary to detect such foreign particles (Sec. 25.2). If a foreign body is suspected but not found, further examination is indicated. If the history suggests injury with a high velocity particle, roentgenographic examination of the eye may be needed to explore the possibility of intraocular foreign body.

Removal of a foreign body can be facilitated by the instillation of a drop of topical anesthetic. Many foreign bodies can be removed by irrigating or by gently wiping them away with a moistened cotton-tipped applicator. Embedded foreign bodies should be handled by an ophthalmologist. Removal of corneal foreign bodies may leave epithelial defects; these are treated as corneal abrasions. Metallic foreign bodies may cause rust to form in the corneal tissues; examination by an ophthalmologist a day or two after removal of a foreign body is recommended since a rust ring would require further treatment (curettage).

Lacerations and perforating wounds of the cornea or sclera require immediate referral to an ophthalmologist and prompt surgical repair if the eye and vision are to be saved. Important clues to perforating injury of the eye are collapse of the anterior chamber, distortion and displacement of the pupil, and protrusion of dark tissue (uvea) into the wound. Emergency treatment consists of protecting the injured eye from further damage by applying a sterile bandage and a rigid eye shield. If these medical supplies are not on hand, an adequate eye shield can be fashioned from a plastic or styrofoam cup or from a piece of cardboard bent into a box or cone shape. Manipulation must be kept to a minimum, and no medication should be instilled except under the direction of an ophthalmologist.

Hyphema is the presence of blood in the anterior chamber of the eye. It may occur with either blunt or perforating injury. Hyphema appears as a bright or dark red fluid level between the cornea and iris or as a diffuse murkiness of the aqueous humor. The treatment of hyphema is bed rest, with the head elevated 30–45 degrees to promote settling and resorption of the blood. In some cases secondary bleeding occurs 3–5 days after the initial hemorrhage, increasing the risk of sequelae. The blood in the anterior chamber may produce elevation of intraocular pressure and blood staining of the cornea. These complications may affect vision. In such

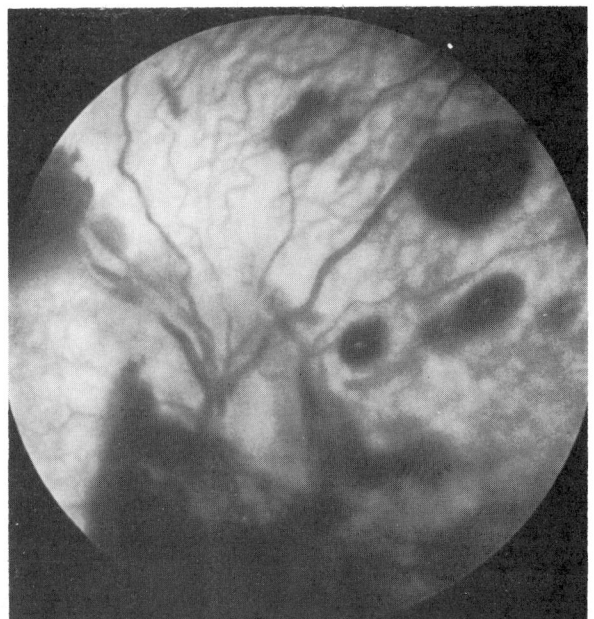

Figure 25–10. Retinal hemorrhages in abused child with subdural hematoma.

(resulting in restriction of movement of the eye and diplopia) and (2) herniation of orbital fat or of the eye itself (resulting in enophthalmos); such cases require surgical repair.

Penetrating wounds of the orbit demand careful evaluation for possible damage to the eye, the optic nerve, or the brain. Examination should include investigation for retained foreign body. Orbital hemorrhage and infection are common with penetrating wounds of the orbit; such injuries must be treated as emergencies.

Child abuse is a major cause of injuries to the eye and orbital region. The manifestations are numerous and may play a prominent role in the recognition of this syndrome. The possibility of nonaccidental trauma must be considered in any child with ecchymosis or laceration of the lids, hemorrhage in or about the eye, cataract or dislocated lens, retinal detachment, or fracture of the orbit (Fig. 25–10).

LOIS J. MARTYN

Emery JM, von Noorden GK, Schlernitzauer DA: Orbital floor fractures: Long-term follow-up of cases with and without surgical repair. Trans Am Acad Ophthalmol Otolaryngol 75:802, 1971.

Friendly DS: Ocular manifestations of physical child abuse. Trans Am Acad Ophthalmol Otolaryngol 75:318, 1971.

Hofman RF, Paul TO, Pentelei-Molner J: The management of corneal birth trauma. J Pediatr Ophthalmol Strab 18:45, 1981.

Pfister RR: Chemical injuries of the eye. Ophthalmology 90:1246, 1983.

Vinger PF: Sports eye injuries: A preventable disease. Ophthalmology 88:108, 1981.

Wilson FM: Traumatic hyphema: Pathogenesis and management. Ophthalmology 87:910, 1980.

General References

Duke-Elder S (ed): System of Ophthalmology. Vol III. Part 2: Congenital Deformities. St Louis, CV Mosby, 1963.

Francois J: Heredity in Ophthalmology. St Louis, CV Mosby, 1961.

Harley RD (ed): Pediatric Ophthalmology. 2nd ed. Philadelphia, WB Saunders, 1983.

McKusick VA: Mendelian Inheritance in Man. Catalogue of Autosomal Dominant, Autosomal Recessive, and X-linked Phenotypes. 5th ed. Baltimore, The Johns Hopkins University Press, 1978.

Salmon MA: Developmental Defects and Syndromes. Aylesbury, England, HM&M Publishers, Ltd, 1978.

Stanbury JB, Wyngaarden JB, Fredrickson DS, et al (eds): The Metabolic Basis of Inherited Disease. 5th ed. New York, McGraw-Hill Book Co, 1983.

Walsh FB, Hoyt WF: Clinical Neuro-Ophthalmology. Baltimore, Williams & Wilkins, 1969.

cases surgical evacuation of the clot and irrigation of the anterior chamber may be necessary.

Chemical injuries require immediate, thorough, and copious irrigation. Whereas acids do their damage on contact, caustic alkalis may continue to penetrate and damage the tissue long after the initial contact and require long term ophthalmic care. In some cases reparative surgery is necessary for resultant corneal and conjunctival scarring.

Fracture of the orbit is a common result of blunt trauma. Routine roentgenograms may fail to show the fracture; tomography is frequently necessary. Any portion of the orbital rim or any wall may be involved, but fracture of the floor of the orbit ("blow-out" fracture) is of special concern. Possible complications are (1) entrapment of the extraocular muscles

Table 25–1. Ocular Changes in Developmental Pediatric Syndromes

1. CNS Anomalies	10. Demyelinating Scleroses
2. Craniostenosis Syndromes	11. Hamartomatoses/Phakomatoses
3. Miscellaneous Craniofacial Defects and Syndromes	12. Neurocutaneous Syndromes
4. Chromosomal Abnormalities	13. Special Neurobiotrophies
5. Disorders of Amino Acid Metabolism	14. Disorders of Connective Tissues, Bones, and Joints
6. The Mucopolysaccharidoses (MPS)	15. Dermatologic Disorders
7. Sphingolipidoses	16. Syndromes of Multiple Developmental Abnormalities
8. Ceroid Lipofuscinoses	17. Miscellaneous Multisystem Disorders
9. Leukodystrophies	18. Congenital Infection Syndrome

Clinical Features

1. CNS ANOMALIES

Anencephaly
  See Sec. 21.10; Optic nerve aplasia or hypoplasia

Holoprosencephaly
  See Sec. 21.11; Hypotelorism; in extreme form, cyclopia; in some cases, iris coloboma

Cyclopia
  A single eye of variable complexity, usually accompanied by proboscis-like structure on forehead; often associated with holoprosencephaly; sometimes fusion of both eyes with duplication of lenses, corneas, and other structures; rosette formation in retina; optic nerve rudimentary or absent; orbit diamond shaped

Arnold-Chiari malformation
  See Sec. 21.12; Nystagmus, usually vertical, often downbeat; ocular motor palsies with diplopia; sometimes skew deviation

Dandy-Walker syndrome
  See Sec. 21.12; Ophthalmic manifestations of increased intracranial pressure

Septo-optic dysplasia (deMorsier syndrome)
  Malformation of anterior midline structures (agenesis of septum pellucidum, primitive optic ventricle, with hypoplasia of optic nerves, chiasm, and infundibulum); sometimes associated endocrine abnormalities; vision defects, strabismus, nystagmus; in some cases, other anomalies of eyes.

Table continued on following page

Table 25–1. **Ocular Changes in Developmental Pediatric Syndromes** (*Continued*)

2. CRANIOSTENOSIS SYNDROMES

Apert syndrome (acrocephalosyndactyly)
See Sec. 23.9; Orbits shallow, eyes protuberant (proptosis) and widely spaced; antimongoloid slant of palpebral fissures; ocular motor abnormalities (strabismus, partial ophthalmoplegia, nystagmus); papilledema; optic atrophy; cataracts; sometimes dislocated lenses; occasionally iris and fundus colobomata

Carpenter syndrome (acrocephalopolysyndactyly)
See Sec. 23.9; Orbits shallow; lateral displacement of medial canthi; epicanthus; antimongoloid slant of palpebral fissures; optic atrophy; microcornea and corneal opacities in some cases

Crouzon syndrome (dysostosis craniofacialis)
See Sec. 23.9; Eyes protuberant (proptosis) and widely spaced; luxation of globe may occur; antimongoloid slant of palpebral fissures; strabismus; papilledema; optic atrophy; vision loss; cataracts in some patients

Kleeblattschädel syndrome (cloverleaf skull)
See Sec. 23.9; Shallow orbits with proptosis; high risk of corneal ulceration

3. MISCELLANEOUS CRANIOFACIAL DEFECTS AND SYNDROMES

Frontonasal dysplasia (median cleft-face syndrome)
Hypertelorism (radiographic interorbital distance 2 SD above normal for age); in some cases, anophthalmia, microphthalmia, epibulbar dermoids, lid colobomata, congenital cataracts

Opitz syndrome
Hypertelorism, particularly associated with hypospadias; antimongoloid slant of palpebral fissures; epicanthus; strabismus

Waardenburg syndrome
Lateral displacement of medial canthi and inferior puncta; heterochromia iridis, total or partial; in some cases both irides completely blue (isochromia)

Oculodentodigital dysplasia (Meyer-Schwickerath syndrome)
Hypotelorism, microphthalmos, microcornea, dental anomalies and enamel hypoplasia, camptodactyly, syndactyly, and other skeletal defects; persistent pupillary membrane; glaucoma

Hallermann-Streiff syndrome (dyscephalia oculomandibulofacialis)
Microphthalmos, cataract, sparse eyebrows and lashes, blue sclerae, nystagmus

Pierre Robin syndrome
Congenital glaucoma; retinal detachment; strabismus

Treacher Collins syndrome (mandibulofacial dysostosis; Franceschetti-Klein syndrome)
Antimongoloid slant of palpebral fissures; underdevelopment of supraorbital ridges; coloboma of lower eyelids and in some cases of iris or choroid

Goldenhar syndrome (oculo-auriculo-vertebral dysplasia)
Antimongoloid slant of palpebral fissures; colobomata of eyelid, upper lid more commonly involved than lower; hypoplasia or coloboma of iris; hypertelorism; sometimes microphthalmos

4. CHROMOSOMAL ABNORMALITIES

Trisomy 21 (Down syndrome)
See Sec. 6.11; monogoloid slant of palpebral fissures; epicanthus; dacryostenosis; blepharitis; Brushfield spots of iris; peripheral thinning of iris stroma; keratoconus and corneal hydrops; cataracts; high refractive errors; strabismus; nystagmus

Trisomy 18 (Edwards syndrome)
See Sec. 6.12; ptosis; short palpebral fissures; epicanthus; hypoplastic supraorbital ridges; microphthalmia; corneal opacities; anisocoria; cataracts; fundus and disc colobomata; retinal hypopigmentation

Trisomy 13 (Patau syndrome)
See Sec. 6.13; microphthalmos; anophthalmos; cyclopia in some cases; dysgenesis of anterior segment (iris hypoplasia, iris adhesions, chamber angle abnormalities); corneal opacities; congenital glaucoma; cataracts; persistent hyperplastic primary vitreous; retinal dysplasia; colobomata of iris, ciliary body, fundus; intraocular cartilage; optic nerve hypoplasia

Trisomy 9
Antimongoloid slant of palpebral fissures; deeply set eyes; corectopia; strabismus

Trisomy 8
Dysmorphic skull; strabismus

Syndrome 45X (Turner) (and mosaic variants)
See Sec. 6.22 and 19.29; ptosis; epicanthus; blue sclerae; defective color vision; cataracts; strabismus; nystagmus

47,XXY; 48,XXXY; 49,XXXXY (Klinefelter) syndromes
See Sec. 6.23 and 19.30; hypertelorism; epicanthus; Brushfield spots of iris; myopia; strabismus

Partial deletion short arm chromosome 4 (4p−)
See Sec. 6.18; ptosis; hypertelorism; epicanthus; colobomata

Partial deletion short arm chromosome 5 (5p−) (cri-du-chat syndrome)
See Sec. 6.18; antimongoloid slant of palpebral fissures; hypertelorism; epicanthus; strabismus

Partial deletion short arm chromosome 9 (9p−)
See Sec. 6.18; mongoloid slant of palpebral fissures; epicanthus; arched brows

Partial deletion long arm chromosome 13 (13q−)
Ptosis; epicanthus; hypertelorism; microphthalmos; colobomata; retinoblastoma

Partial deletion long arm chromosome 18 (18q−)
See Sec. 6.18; horizontal palpebral fissures; epicanthus; deeply set eyes; optic disc pallor; tapetoretinal degeneration; nystagmus

Partial deletion long arm chromosome 21 (21q−)
Downward slanting palpebral fissures

Partial deletion long arm chromosome 22 (22q−)
Ptosis; epicanthus

Extrachromosomal material (cat eye syndrome)
Antimongoloid slant of palpebral fissures; epicanthus; hypertelorism; microphthalmos; colobomata of iris, fundus, optic nerve; macular defects; pale discs; cataracts; strabismus; nystagmus

Table continued on opposite page

Table 25–1. Ocular Changes in Developmental Pediatric Syndromes (*Continued*)

5. DISORDERS OF AMINO ACID METABOLISM

Albinism*

Defect in the formation of melanin; several forms include:

(1) *Oculocutaneous albinism, tyrosine negative;* generalized hypopigmentation

Iris blue or gray; generalized hypopigmentation of eye; typical pink or orange reflex; fundus bright, with increased choroidal vascular pattern; macula/fovea poorly defined (hypoplastic); photophobia; nystagmus; subnormal vision; often high refractive error

(2) *Oculocutaneous albinism, tyrosinase positive;* pigmentation may increase with age

Iris color blue, yellow, or brownish; color increasing with age; photophobia; nystagmus; subnormal vision, which may improve with age

(3) *Amish* or *yellow* mutant; generalized albinism in which a yellowish pigment is produced instead of melanin, providing some skin and hair color

(4) *Hermansky-Pudlak syndrome;* tyrosine negative albinism associated with a hemorrhagic diathesis; iris blue-gray to brown; photophobia; nystagmus; slight to moderate vision defect

(5) *Cross syndrome,* tyrosine positive; a syndrome of hypopigmentation, gingival fibromatosis, spasticity, athetoid movements, and microphthalmos; iris blue-gray; microphthalmos; cataracts; severe vision defect; nystagmus

(6) *Ocular albinism*; pigment deficiency limited to the eye; generalized ocular hypopigmentation; macular hypoplasia; nystagmus (in Blacks, fundus tessellated)

Alcaptonuria

See Sec. 7.3; black discoloration of sclera, most noticeable at insertion of extraocular muscles

Tyrosinemia (Richner-Hanhart syndrome)

See Sec. 7.3; corneal ulceration, "herpetiform"

Cystinosis

See Sec. 7.5; accumulation of refractile crystals in cornea (best seen with slit lamp, but corneal haze may be detected grossly); photophobia; pigmentary retinopathy; fundi generally hypopigmented, with fine to coarse spotty pigmentation, most marked peripherally; vision usually normal to nearly normal

Homocystinemia, type I

See Sec. 7.4; ectopia lentis; cataract; secondary glaucoma; peripheral cystic degeneration of retina

Sulfite oxidase deficiency

See Sec. 7.5; subluxation of lens; spherophakia; strabismus

Hartnup disease

See Sec. 7.6; photophobia; nystagmus; strabismus

Maple syrup urine disease

See Sec. 7.7; strabismus, varying with condition of child

6. THE MUCOPOLYSACCHARIDOSES (MPS)

Hurler syndrome (MPS IH; α-L-iduronidase deficiency)

See Sec. 7.24; hypertelorism, prominent eyes; puffy lids; heavy brows; deposition of MPS and attendant cellular changes throughout most regions of eye, particularly the conjunctiva, cornea, sclera, iris, ciliary body, retina, and optic nerve; characteristic corneal clouding, clinically evident early in life, and progressing to dense milky "ground-glass" haze, often with associated photophobia; progressive retinal degeneration with pigmentary dispersion and clumping, arteriolar attenuation and disc pallor, and reduced ERG; optic atrophy; vision loss, owing principally to corneal, retinal, and optic nerve changes; hydrocephalus and cerebral changes; glaucoma in some cases

Scheie syndrome (MPS IS; α-L-iduronidase deficiency)

See Sec. 7.24; progressive corneal clouding, diffuse but sometimes more dense peripherally than centrally; progressive retinal degeneration; visual symptoms, field loss and night blindness often commencing in 2nd or 3rd decade; glaucoma in some cases

Hurler-Scheie Compound (MPS IH/S; α-L-iduronidase deficiency)

See Sec. 7.24; corneal clouding, diffuse and progressive; glaucoma in some cases; vision loss owing to corneal clouding or to optic nerve effects of arachnoid cysts

Hunter syndrome (MPS II; iduronosulfate sulfatase deficiency)

Phenotypically similar to MPS IH; both mild and severe forms occur; progressive retinal degeneration with pigmentary changes, arteriolar attenuation, optic atrophy, vision, loss, reduced ERG; corneas macroscopically (clinically) clear, but microscopic corneal changes documented; papilledema secondary to hydrocephalus in some cases

Sanfilippo syndrome (MPS III; types A [heparan sulfate sulfatase deficiency], B [*N*-acetyl α-D-glucosaminidase deficiency], and C [acetyl-Co A:α-glucosaminide *N*-acetyl transferase deficiency])

Retinal changes in some patients—arteriolar narrowing; reduced ERG; corneas clinically clear but some microscopic changes reported

Morquio syndrome (MPS IV; galactosamine-6-sulfate sulfatase deficiency in classic form; β-galactosidase deficiency reported in variants)

See Sec. 7.24; fine corneal clouding in many patients; slowly progressive; often not clinically apparent for several years

Maroteaux-Lamy syndrome (MPS VI; arylsulfatase-B deficiency)

See Sec. 7.24; diffuse corneal clouding, usually evident within 1st few yr of life; tortuosity of retinal vessels in some patients; papilledema and 6th nerve paresis in some patients with hydrocephalus

Sly syndrome (MPS VII; β-D-glucuronidase deficiency)

Some diversity of phenotype; corneas clear or cloudy; corneal haze of either fine or coarse type

Di Ferreni syndrome (MPS VIII: *N*-acetylglucosamine-6-sulfate sulfatase deficiency)

Short stature; mild dysostosis multiplex; odontoid hypoplasia; hepatosplenomegaly; mental retardation; ophthalmologic abnormalities not yet described

7. SPHINGOLIPIDOSES

Generalized gangliosidosis (GM$_1$ gangliosidosis type 1; β-galactosidase deficiency)

See Sec. 7.25; diffuse corneal clouding (MPS accumulation); macular cherry red spot of retinal ganglioside accumulation; retinal vascular tortuosity and retinal hemorrhages; optic atrophy; vision loss, nystagmus, strabismus

---

*To be differentiated from these forms of albinism is the **Chédiak-Higashi syndrome**, in which the defect is in morphology of the melanosomes, not in formation of melanin. Ocular signs include hypopigmentation of iris and fundus, photophobia, nystagmus, and papilledema with lymphocytic infiltration of optic nerve.

Table continued on following page

Table 25-1. **Ocular Changes in Developmental Pediatric Syndromes** (*Continued*)

Juvenile GM₁ gangliosidosis (GM₁ gangliosidosis type 2; β-galactosidase deficiency)
    See Sec. 7.32; corneas clinically clear; histologic changes of retinal ganglioside storage without clinically obvious signs; optic atrophy and vision loss; nystagmus and strabismus

Tay-Sachs disease (GM₂ gangliosidosis type 1; hexosaminidase A deficiency)
    See Sec. 7.26; macular cherry red spot; optic atrophy (demyelination and degeneration of optic nerves, chiasm, and tracts); progressive loss of vision, owing both to ocular and to cerebral abnormalities; sequential deterioration of eye movements

Sandhoff variant (GM₂ gangliosidosis type 2; hexosaminidase A and B deficiency)
    See Sec. 7.26; macular cherry red spot; optic atrophy and progressive loss of vision; corneas clinically clear or slightly opalescent; histologic evidence of storage cytosomes in cornea

Juvenile GM₂ gangliosidosis (GM₂ gangliosidosis type 3; partial deficiency of hexosaminidase A)
    See Sec. 7.26; retinal pigmentary degeneration; macular changes (cherry-red spot type) in some cases; optic atrophy; blindness later in course of disease

Krabbe globoid cell leukodystrophy (galactosyl ceramide lipidosis; galactosylceramide β-galactosidase deficiency)
    See Sec. 7.32; cortical blindness and optic atrophy, owing to degenerative changes in brain and visual pathways; nystagmus; strabismus

Gaucher disease (glycosyl ceramide lipidosis; glucosyl ceramide β-glucosidase deficiency)
    See Sec. 7.29; paralytic strabismus due to brain stem and cranial nerve involvement in neuronopathic forms; nystagmus; macular changes (grayness) in some cases; retinal hemorrhages secondary to anemia, thrombocytopenia; discrete white spots in or on retina reported in juvenile form; pingueculae (wedgeshaped conjunctival lesions) in chronic non-neuronopathic form; possibly corneal clouding

Niemann-Pick disease (sphingomyelin lipidoses; sphingomyelinase deficiency)
    See Sec. 7.30; macular cherry red–like spot or grayish macular haze in classic infantile neuronopathic form (type A), and in subacute neurovisceral or juvenile form (type C); corneal clouding, lens opacities in some cases (Type A); vertical gaze palsy in some patients

Fabry disease (glycosphingolipid lipidosis; α-galactosidase A deficiency)
    See Sec. 7.28; corneal dystrophy related to epithelial lipid deposits (radiating lines/whorls in affected males and in carrier females); aneurysmal dilatation and tortuosity of conjunctival and retinal vessels; renovascular signs of renal hypertension; papilledema; orbital and lid edema; cataracts (spoke-like posterior cortical lens opacities—anterior lens opacities in some cases)

Farber disease (ceramide lipidosis; ceramidase deficiency)
    See Sec. 7.33; cherry red–like spot; grayish posterior pole; retinal pigmentary mottling; granulomata in and around eye

8. CEROID LIPOFUSCINOSES (See also Sec. 7.37, 21.17, and 21.18)
    Infantile (Finnish variant; unsaturated fatty acid lipidosis)
        Microcephaly; marked atrophy of brain; loss of vision; granular inclusions; ataxia, myoclonus; profound dementia, decorticate state; onset 1–2 yr; death by 10 yr
    Late infantile (Jansky-Bielschowsky)
        Intellectual deterioration, seizures, ataxia; pigmentary retinal degeneration, in some cases, predominantly macular; ERG abnormal; optic atrophy; inclusions of curvilinear type; onset 2–4 yr; death by 10 yr
    Juvenile (Batten-Mayou-Spielmeyer-Vogt)
        Intellectual deterioration, seizures, ataxia, progressive loss of motor function; pigmentary retinal degeneration, resembling retinitis pigmentosa, with progressive loss of vision; in some cases predominantly macular degeneration; ERG abnormal; optic atrophy as a late manifestation; mixed inclusion bodies including curvilinear and fingerprint types, and lipofuscin in brain; onset 5–8 yr, sometimes later; death in teens or 20's
    Late juvenile or adult (Kufs)
        Behavior disturbances and intellectual impairment; ataxia, spasticity, myoclonic seizures; vision and fundi usually normal; macular degeneration in some cases; mostly lipofuscin in brain; onset in childhood, adolescence, or early adult life
    Cherry red spot myoclonus syndrome
        Macular cherry red spot; vision loss; intention myoclonus; variable inclusions in brain; light inclusions in hepatocytes and Kupffer cells; onset in childhood; survival to adulthood

9. LEUKODYSTROPHIES (See also Sec. 7.35 and 21.19)
    Metachromatic leukodystrophy (arylsulfatase A deficiency)
        Retinal degeneration resembling retinitis pigmentosa; in some cases, early macular involvement (macular grayness with accentuation of central red spot); optic atrophy; vision loss; strabismus and nystagmus
    Pelizaeus-Merzbacher syndrome
        "Eye-rolling" (rhythmic eye movements) noted soon after birth, sometimes with rotary movements of the head; optic atrophy as a late manifestation
    Canavan disease
        Vacuolization of ganglion cell layer of retina reportedly detectable with slit lamp; retinal pigmentary changes; optic atrophy; blindness early in course; ERG normal; VER reduced; strabismus, roving eye movements, and nystagmus

10. DEMYELINATING SCLEROSES (See Sec. 21.19)
    Schilder disease (encephalitis periaxialis diffusa)
        Involvement of visual pathways, producing retrobulbar neuritis, optic atrophy, central scotomas, chiasmal syndromes, homonymous field defects; disorders of cortical gaze functions; nystagmus
    Multiple sclerosis
        Retrobulbar neuritis (episodic loss of vision, typically a central scotoma, unilateral more often than bilateral, often with retrobulbar pain); other visual pathway lesions (variety of field defects); internuclear ophthalmoplegia; supranuclear gaze palsies; nystagmus; sheathing of peripheral retinal vessels in some cases
    Neuromyelitis optica (Devic disease)
        Optic neuritis (usually papillitis with visible disc edema), with resultant optic atrophy; other visual pathway lesions (variety of visual field defects); in some cases extraocular muscle palsies, conjugate gaze palsies, nystagmus, pupil abnormalities

11. HAMARTOMATOSES/PHAKOMATOSES
    Tuberous sclerosis (Bourneville disease)
        See Sec. 21.16 and 24.11; retinal phakomata (glial hamartomas, ranging from small flat or slightly elevated white or yellowish lesions to large elevated refractile yellowish multinodular or cystic masses often likened to an unripe mulberry); fibroangioma of the lids; in some, papilledema or optic atrophy, vision defects, pupil or ocular motor signs related to CNS changes (tumors, hydrocephalus)

Table continued on opposite page

Table 25–1. **Ocular Changes in Developmental Pediatric Syndromes** (*Continued*)

Neurofibromatosis (von Recklinghausen syndrome)
　　See Sec. 21.16 and 24.10; plexiform neuromas of eyelids, often producing ptosis; episcleral and conjunctival neurofibromas; prominent
　　corneal nerves; iris nodules; uveal hypercellularity; glaucoma (related to angle anomalies, uveal hypercellularity, neovascularization,
　　or synechiae); hamartomas (phakomata) of disc and retina; fundus pigmentary changes likened to café-au-lait spots; optic gliomas
　　and vision loss (presenting with proptosis, strabismus, nystagmus if intraorbital—with signs of increased intracranial pressure,
　　hydrocephalus, or diencephalic syndrome when intracranial); orbital asymmetry; orbital wall defects; pulsatile exophthalmos,
　　intraorbital neurofibromas, with proptosis
Angiomatosis of the retina and cerebellum (von Hippel–Lindau disease)
　　See Sec. 21.16; retinal hemangioblastoma (reddish or yellowish globular mass with paired vessels coursing to and from the lesion,
　　sometimes likened to a toy balloon in the fundus); may lead to hemorrhage, exudates, retinal detachment
Encephalofacial angiomatosis (Sturge-Weber syndrome)
　　See Sec. 21.16; lid and conjunctival involvement of facial nevus flammeus; choroidal hemangioma; dilated and tortuous retinal vessels;
　　glaucoma, congenital or later in infancy or childlhood (related to possible angle anomalies, vascular lesion, or hypersecretion); visual
　　field defects associated with CNS lesions; hemianopsia in some cases
Angiomatosis of mid-brain and retina (Wyburn-Mason syndrome)
　　Extensive vascular malformations involving principally the midbrain and eye; angiomatosis of the retina; vessels dilated and tortuous;
　　angiomatosis affecting optic nerve and orbit

12. NEUROCUTANEOUS SYNDROMES
Ataxia-telangiectasia (Louis-Bar syndrome)
　　See Sec. 21.20; telangiectasias of bulbar conjunctivae, usually by the age of 4–6 yr; apraxic disorder of conjugate eye movements;
　　horizontal and vertical gaze performed in halting dyssynergic fashion; difficulty in maintaining eccentric gaze; sometimes
　　convergence defect; nystagmus
Sjögren-Larsson syndrome
　　See also Sec. 24.16; chorioretinal lesions; discrete defects in retinal pigment epithelium of unknown etiology; circumscribed
　　symmetrical lesions of varying size in and about the macula in approximately 25% of cases
Incontinentia pigmenti (Bloch-Sulzberger Syndrome)
　　See Sec. 24.10; intraocular retrolental masses ("pseudogliomas") and membranes, apparently secondary to an underlying retinal
　　vascular disorder characterized by aneurysmal dilatation, abnormal arteriovenous connections, and vasoproliferative changes;
　　sometimes intraocular hemorrhage and inflammation; microphthalmos; corneal opacities; cataracts; optic atrophy
Linear nevus sebaceus of Jadassohn
　　See also Sec. 24.8; coloboma of the eyelids, iris, and fundus; corectopia; epibulbar lipodermoids; orbital teratomas; proptosis; aberrant
　　lacrimal gland; corneal vascularization; ocular motor palsies; nystagmus; defective vision
Xerodermic idiocy of de Sanctis and Cacchione
　　See Sec. 24.14; atrophy of eyelids; loss of cilia, ectropion, entropion, symblepharon, ankyloblepharon; drying and infection of
　　conjunctiva; ulceration of cornea; iritis; photophobia
Klippel-Trenaunay-Weber syndrome
　　See Sec. 24.7; conjunctival telangiectasia; choroidal hemangioma; iris coloboma; heterochromia; glaucoma; strabismus

13. SPECIAL NEUROBIOTROPHIES
Subacute sclerosing panencephalitis (Dawson disease; Van Bogaert disease)
　　See Sec. 11.79; focal retinitis (edema, hemorrhage, pigmentary changes), with chorioretinal scarring (usually macular or paramacular,
　　usually bilateral)—may precede other neurologic manifestations; papilledema; optic atrophy; visual symptoms of retinal and optic
　　nerve involvement; field defects of cerebral involvement; nystagmus; extraocular muscle palsies; ptosis
Subacute necrotizing encephalomyopathy (Leigh disease)
　　See Sec. 7.20 and 21.18; abnormal eye movements (bizarre rolling eye movements, disconjugate eye movements, horizontal and
　　vertical nystagmus, saccadic ocular movements); extraocular muscle palsies (sometimes complete external ophthalmoplegia);
　　blepharoptosis; progressive optic atrophy and vision loss; sometimes retinal changes (diminished macular reflex); afferent and
　　efferent pupil defects
Hepatolenticular degeneration (Wilson disease)
　　See Sec. 12.77 and 21.21; Kayser-Fleischer ring of cornea (copper deposition in periphery of Descemet membrane, particularly in
　　deepest zone adjacent to endothelium, seen as granules of golden, greenish, grayish, or brown hue); Sonnenblumenkatarakt
　　("sunflower" cataract); occasionally ocular motor abnormalities (jerky oscillations of eyes, involuntary upward deviation of eyes, or
　　paresis of upward gaze); accommodation sometimes affected; in some cases, optic neuritis secondary to penicillamine therapy
Trichopoliodystrophy (Menkes disease; kinky hair disease)
　　See Sec. 7.54 and 21.18; decrease in retinal ganglion cells, thinning of retinal nerve fiber layer, and partial atrophy of optic nerve;
　　progressive vision loss; abnormal ERG; microcysts of pigment epithelium of iris
Abetalipoproteinemia (acanthocytosis; Bassen-Kornzweig disease)
　　See Sec. 7.48 and 21.20; pigmentary retinal degeneration with progressive impairment of visual function (pigment dispersion, arteriolar
　　attenuation, disc pallor, impaired dark adaptation); cataracts, ptosis, and ocular motor abnormalities; in some cases, progressive
　　exotropia, paresis of medial recti, and dissociated nystagmus on lateral gaze
Heredopathia atactica polyneuritiformis (Refsum syndrome; phytanic acid α-hydrolase deficiency)
　　See Sec. 7.36, 21.20, and 24.16; pigmentary retinal degeneration (pigmentary clumping, arteriolar attenuation, optic atrophy,
　　progressive impairment of night vision and visual field); ERG abnormal; sometimes vitreous opacities; cataracts, cornea guttata,
　　miosis; ophthalmoparesis; nystagmus
Familial dysautonomia (Riley-Day syndrome)
　　See Sec. 21.29; depressed or absent corneal sensation, with corneal ulceration and scarring common; defective lacrimation; tortuosity
　　of retinal vessels; tonic pupil in some cases; myopia and exotropia common
Congenital familial sensory neuropathy with anhidrosis (Pinsky-DiGeorge syndrome)
　　See Sec. 22.3; defective corneal sensation, with defective lacrimation; corneal ulceration and scarring may result

14. DISORDERS OF CONNECTIVE TISSUES, BONES, AND JOINTS
Arachnodactyly (Marfan syndrome)
　　See Sec. 23.43; ectopia lentis (lens dislocation, usually upward) and iridodonesis (tremulous iris); microphakia, spherophakia; cataract;
　　myopia; glaucoma; retinal changes: degeneration, detachment

Table continued on following page

Table 25–1. Ocular Changes in Developmental Pediatric Syndromes (*Continued*)

Cutis hyperelastica (Ehlers-Danlos syndrome)
  See Sec. 7.54 and 24.17; epicanthus; blue sclera; keratoconus; subluxation of lens; retinal detachment
Pseudoxanthoma elasticum
  See Sec. 24.17; angioid streaks (breaks in Bruch membrane appearing as dark lines in the fundus radiating from the disc); tendency to retinal hemorrhage
Osteogenesis imperfecta
  See Sec. 23.37; blue sclera; prominent eyes; in some cases, megalocornea, keratoconus, corneal opacities
Polyostotic fibrous dysplasia (McCune-Albright syndrome)
  See Sec. 19.7 and 24.10; thickening of bones of orbit
Osteopetrosis (Albers-Schönberg disease; "marble bones")
  See Sec. 23.38; vision loss and extraocular muscle palsies, due to bony overgrowth of cranial foramina; in some cases, retinal degeneration, optic atrophy
Chondrodystrophia calcificans congenita (Conradi syndrome)
  See Sec. 23.22; cataract; optic atrophy; hypertelorism
Spondyloepiphyseal dysplasia congenita
  See Sec. 23.23; myopia; retinal detachment; cataract; buphthalmos
Spondyloepiphyseal dysplasia variants
  See Sec. 23.23; punctate corneal dystrophy without impairment of vision
Hereditary onchyo-osteodysplasia (nail-patella syndrome)
  Dark "cloverleaf" pigmentation of iris; cataract; microphakia; microcornea; keratoconus; ptosis
Progressive arthro-ophthalmopathy (Stickler syndrome)
  Pain and stiffness of joints with bony enlargement; kyphosis; cleft palate; Pierre Robin anomaly; deafness; progressive myopia; retinal detachment; glaucoma

15. DERMATOLOGIC DISORDERS
Focal dermal hypoplasia (Goltz syndrome)
  See Sec. 24.5; nystagmus; strabismus; microphthalmos; coloboma
Hypohidrotic (anhidrotic) ectodermal dysplasia
  See Sec. 24.6; deficiency of tears, leading to keratopathy, photophobia; stenosis of the lacrimal puncta; cataracts; lashes and brows sparse
Dyskeratosis congenita
  See Sec. 24.5; bullous conjunctivitis, with minimal scarring of cornea; chronic blepharitis, loss of lashes and ectropion; keratinization of lacrimal puncta
Ichthyosis
  See Sec. 24.16; conjunctivitis, ectropion, and corneal erosions in lamellar and sex-linked forms; cataracts in congenital and vulgaris forms
Basal cell nevus syndrome
  See Sec. 24.32; prominent supraorbital ridges; hypertelorism or dystopia canthorum; cataracts; coloboma; vision defects; strabismus
Juvenile xanthogranuloma (nevoxanthoendothelioma)
  See Sec. 24.32; xanthogranuloma in ocular tissues, as infiltrates in orbit, iris, episclera, ciliary body; presenting signs may be proptosis, heterochromia, spontaneous hyphema, uveitis, glaucoma
Poikiloderma congenitale (Rothmund-Thomson syndrome)
  See Sec. 24.14; sparse eyebrows and eyelashes; cataracts (onset 2–7 yr); corneal dystrophy
Bloom syndrome
  See Sec. 24.14; conjunctivitis; conjunctival telangiectasias; drusen at posterior pole of fundus

16. SYNDROMES OF MULTIPLE DEVELOPMENTAL ABNORMALITIES
Cornelia de Lange syndrome
  Microbrachycephaly, short neck, low hair line, anteverted nares, micrognathism, and low set ears; physical and mental retardation; limb defects including micromelia, phocomelia, oligodactyly, polydactyly; cardiac and urogenital anomalies; synophrys (confluent eyebrows) and long curly eyelashes; ptosis; epicanthus; microphthalmos with eccentric pupils; corneal opacities; optic atrophy; strabismus
Fraser syndrome
  Facial, genitourinary, skeletal anomalies (including lateral cleft of nostril, ear deformity, renal agenesis, hydronephrosis, hypospadias, cryptorchidism, syndactyly); cerebral defects, meningoencephalocele; cryptophthalmos (eye hidden, fused lids—absence of palpebral fissure), sometimes with symblepharon (adhesion of lid to globe); microphthalmos in some cases; flat supraorbital ridge
Rieger syndrome
  Various dental and limb anomalies; occasionally intellectual retardation, muscular dystrophy, and myotonic dystrophy; dysplasia of anterior segment of the eye; posterior embryotoxon (prominence and anterior displacement of Schwalbe line), often with bands of iris tissue attached (Axenfeld syndrome); iris hypoplasia; glaucoma; cataracts; ectopia lentis; colobomata; micro- or megalocornea; strabismus; ptosis; optic atrophy
Peter syndrome
  Skeletal anomalies; developmental defects of the gastrointestinal tract and central nervous system; hydrocephalus and mental retardation; central defect of Descemet membrane, with central corneal leukoma, shallow anterior chamber, peripheral anterior synechia; cataracts
Lenz syndrome
  Microcephaly, mental retardation; short stature, digital anomalies, and dental defects; colobomatous microphthalmos; blepharoptosis; nystagmus; strabismus
Meckel syndrome (Meckel-Gruber syndrome)
  Microcephaly, occipital encephalocele, or anencephaly; polycystic kidneys; polydactyly; congenital heart disease; genital abnormalities; microphthalmos, anophthalmos, cryptophthalmos; sclerocornea; partial aniridia; cataract; retinal dysplasia; optic nerve hypoplasia
Otopalatodigital syndrome (Rubinstein-Taybi syndrome)
  Intellectual and growth retardation; abnormally broad thumbs and broad great toes; characteristic facies with hypoplasia of maxilla and mandible, beaked nose, posterior rotation of ears; hypertrichosis; cryptorchidism; cardiac and renal anomalies; hypertelorism, with epicanthus, ptosis, and antimongoloid slant of palpebral fissures; cataract; colobomata; strabismus

Table continued on opposite page

Table 25–1. **Ocular Changes in Developmental Pediatric Syndromes** (*Continued*)

Seckel syndrome
  Growth retardation, with small head circumference and characteristic face, narrow with beak-like nose ("bird head"); micrognathism and apparent prominence of maxilla; sometimes musculoskeletal and genitourinary anomalies; hypertelorism, with antimongoloid slant of palpebral fissures, prominent eyes; strabismus
Freeman-Sheldon syndrome
  Syndrome characterized by mask-like face with small pursed mouth, "whistling-face"; ulnar deviation of the hand and fingers; talipes equinovarus; deep-set eyes; epicanthus, blepharophimosis, ptosis; strabismus
Aicardi syndrome
  Agenesis of the corpus callosum, with cortical heterotopia; seizures; mental retardation; costovertebral anomalies; multiple discrete chorioretinal defects of varying size; sometimes microphthalmos
Wildervanck syndrome
  Association of the Klippel-Feil malformation with congenital deafness and *Duane syndrome*, unilateral or bilateral (congenital defect in abduction with retraction of the globe or attempted adduction of the affected eye); epibulbar dermoid cysts
Falls-Kertesz syndrome
  Pterygium colli; later onset of lymphedema of lower extremities; distichiasis of all 4 lids; partial ectropion of lower lids
Kartagener syndrome
  See Sec. 14.31; pigmentary retinal disorder; cataracts

17. MISCELLANEOUS MULTISYSTEM DISORDERS
Oculocerebrorenal syndrome (Lowe syndrome)
  See Sec. 23.59; congenital cataracts in affected males; fine lens opacities in carrier females; glaucoma; rarely microphthalmos
Cerebrohepatorenal syndrome (Zellweger syndrome)
  Profound hypotonia, growth retardation, and failure to thrive; hepatomegaly, jaundice, hypoprothrombinemia; renal cortical cysts; characteristic facies, flat profile; accumulation of iron in various organs; mild hypertelorism, flat supraorbital ridges, and epicanthal folds; cataracts; glaucoma (also, nonglaucomatous corneal haze); vitreous opacities; optic nerve hypoplasia; retinal pigmentary disorder (fundi generally hypopigmented, with fine to coarse spotty pigmentation, most marked peripherally)
Laurence-Moon-Biedl syndrome
  See Sec. 19.31; pleomorphic pigmentary retinal degeneration (retinitis pigmentosa type, with prominent macular involvement in some cases), with progressive vision impairment
Prader-Willi syndrome
  A syndrome of hypotonia, hypomentia, hypogonadism, and obesity, with tendency to diabetes mellitus; strabismus
Cockayne syndrome
  See Sec. 24.14; pigmentary retinal degeneration; optic atrophy; cataracts; photophobia
Werner syndrome
  A syndrome of premature aging; in the 2nd decade, with cessation of growth, graying of the hair, alopecia, scleroderma-like changes of the skin, atherosclerosis, and diabetes mellitus; hypogonadism; increased risk of neoplasia; cataracts, juvenile onset; pigmentary retinal degeneration ("retinitis pigmentosa"); macular degeneration; glaucoma
Asphyxiating thoracic dysplasia (Jeune syndrome)
  See Sec. 13.105; pigmentary retinal degeneration, with progressive vision impairment in some cases
Alstrom disease
  Nerve deafness, diabetes mellitus, and obesity in childhood; pigmentary retinal degeneration; cataracts
Renal-retinal dystrophy
  Interstitial nephritis; progressive pigmentary retinal degeneration, with attenuation of arterioles, reduced ERG, optic atrophy, and loss of vision
Usher syndrome
  Nerve deafness; mental retardation; epilepsy; pigmentary retinal degeneration ("retinitis pigmentosa"); cataracts
Norrie disease
  A syndrome of retinal malformation, mental retardation, and deafness; congenital retinal pseudoglioma; persistent hyperplastic primary vitreous, with vision loss; degenerative changes with phthisis bulbi; corneal opacities; cataracts

18. CONGENITAL INFECTION SYNDROMES
Congenital rubella
  See Sec. 8.69; ophthalmic sequelae both teratogenic and inflammatory; bilateral or unilateral effects; persistence of virus in the eye for months or years; microphthalmia; cataract (usually a dense pearly nuclear opacity with relatively clearer cortical rim); iris hypoplasia, atrophy synechiae (pupils often difficult to dilate); congenital glaucoma; transient nonglaucomatous corneal clouding in the newborn; retinopathy (pigmentary mottling "salt and pepper," focal or generalized, without loss of function); acute maculopathy (submacular neovascularization) as a delayed complication later in childhood in some cases, with attendant vision impairment; optic atrophy; vision defects and ocular motor abnormalities (nystagmus, strabismus) related not only to ocular involvement but also to effects of encephalomyelitis
Congenital cytomegalovirus infection
  See Sec. 6.68 and 11.68; chorioretinitis (single or multifocal atrophic and pigmented fundus lesions, more often peripheral than macular—sometimes perivascular retinal exudates and hemorrhages); anterior uveitis, conjunctivitis, and corneal clouding; optic atrophy; optic nerve hypoplasia; coloboma; microphthalmos; vision defects with strabismus, nystagmus
Congenital toxoplasmosis
  See Sec. 11.107; retinochoroiditis (retinitis, with secondary choroiditis, often with exudate into vitreous in early stages, resulting in single or multifocal atrophic and pigmented scars); often large macular lesions; satellite lesions and recurrent inflammation common in later years due to persistence of organism in eye; vision loss, optic atrophy, retinal detachment, cataract, and glaucoma common; attendant oculomotor abnormalities (strabismus, nystagmus) attributed to ocular and/or CNS involvement; congenital anomalies of eye (e.g., microphthalmos)
Congenital syphilis
  See Sec. 11.49; perivascular infiltration by *T. pallidum*, with inflammation in the cornea, uvea, retina, and optic nerve; persistence of the organism in the eye for years; interstitial keratitis, usually appearing after age 5 or 6 yr (iridocyclitis and intense photophobia in acute phase, vascularization and corneal opacification later, with decreased vision); retinopathy ("salt and pepper" pigmentary changes, frequently with arteriolar attenuation and disc pallor); retinal periphlebitis, sometimes with vascular occlusion; exudative uveitis in some cases; phthisis may result; disc edema; optic atrophy

26

UNCLASSIFIED DISEASES

26.1 SUDDEN INFANT DEATH SYNDROME (SIDS)

Definition. The sudden and unexpected death of an infant, for reasons that are unclear even after an autopsy, is the most common manner of death in the first year of life following the neonatal period. In the typical case this *sudden infant death syndrome (SIDS)* occurs in an apparently healthy infant of 2–3 mo of age who has been put to bed without suspicion that anything is out of the ordinary. Some time later the infant is found dead, and a conventional autopsy fails to reveal a cause of death. Although these infants appear healthy before death, detailed perinatal histories and more intensive studies of cardiorespiratory and neurologic function have produced evidence that some affected children have not been normal earlier. The needs to separate this tragic condition from child abuse and to supply stricken families with psychologic support have been highlighted in recent years largely through the efforts of families who have had infants die in this way.

Epidemiology. SIDS is a worldwide phenomenon; incidence rates vary from 0.2 to 3.0/1000 live births. Part of this variability may reflect the thoroughness with which other diagnoses are sought and the accuracy of reporting. In the United States the average incidence ranges from 1.6 to 2.3/1000 live births, with considerable ethnic variation. The rates per 1000 live births are 0.5 among Asians; 1.3 among whites; 1.7 among Hispanics; 2.9 among blacks; and 5.9 among American Indians. Incidence peaks at 2–3 mo of age; few cases occur before 2 wk or after 6 mo of age. Males are at higher risk than females. The incidence of SIDS is higher during the colder months of the year.

Since the greatest number of deaths occur between midnight and 9 AM, SIDS has been presumed to take place during sleep, but it is difficult to prove that SIDS actually occurs during sleep; the association with sleep may only reflect the larger proportion of time that infants in the susceptible age group spend sleeping. However, there may be additional vulnerability to cardiorespiratory collapse during sleep (see below).

A variety of genetic, environmental, and social factors have been associated with increased risk of SIDS, including premature births, especially with history of apnea or bronchopulmonary dysplasia; low birthweight for gestational age; cold weather; young unmarried mother; poor socioeconomic conditions, including crowding; maternal history of smoking, anemia, or narcotic ingestion; history of a sibling with SIDS; and history of a "near miss" or aborted episode of SIDS (i.e., an episode in which an infant ceases to breathe, develops cyanosis or pallor, and becomes unresponsive, but is successfully resuscitated). The risk of SIDS varies inversely with maternal age and directly with parity. The Apgar scores of infants with SIDS average lower than those of their surviving peers. Breast feeding is not associated with a decreased risk. The peak incidence of SIDS (2–3 mo) coincides with normally low levels of circulating immunoglobulins, but no specific pathogens have been found.

In a family having an infant with SIDS the risk for the next or a subsequent child varies from 5/1000 to 10/1000 or about 5 times the usual risk. Although the data are conflicting, twins or triplets are probably not at higher risk for SIDS than subsequent siblings, nor is the risk higher for monozygotic than for dizygotic twins. Evidence suggests that environmental factors (prenatal or postnatal) are important rather than genetic factors, with no evidence for mendelian inheritance of susceptibility.

Pathology. Although their significance is controversial, a wide variety of findings have been reported in infants dying of SIDS: retarded postnatal growth, increased pulmonary arterial smooth muscle, increased right ventricular muscle mass, increased extramedullary hematopoiesis, retention of brown fat, hyperplastic adrenal chromaffin tissue, brain stem gliosis, and intrathoracic petechiae. Attention has been particularly focused on the increase in smooth muscle in the larger pulmonary arteries extending to smaller blood vessels close to the alveoli. This suggests that infants with SIDS had been subjected to chronic hypoxia. However, there is no direct evidence of this hypoxia, and the failure to find hyperplasia of the carotid bodies postmortem weighs against the presence of chronic hypoxia.

Pathogenesis. It seems likely that SIDS may have several etiologies. In addition, several rare conditions may masquerade as SIDS. For example, prolonged sleep apnea in infancy has been associated with a space-occupying lesion (left temporal lobe astrocytoma), with a congenital CNS anomaly (absence of the corpus callosum), and with the neuromuscular dysfunction accompanying infantile botulism. Sudden death has also been caused by vascular rings, usually with antecedent evidence of upper airway obstruction. Infants with familial prolongation of the Q-T interval on electrocardiogram (*Romano-Ward* and *Jervell and Lange-Nielsen* syndromes) may die suddenly; on the other hand, infants with near-miss or aborted SIDS have been found to have shorter than normal Q-T intervals. When such conditions as the above are excluded, a majority of patients with SIDS may share a common etiology involving an abnormality in cardiorespiratory control in which state of consciousness or central nervous system activity plays a modulating role. Since there is no satisfactory animal model, much of the research in this field has focused on respiratory and cardiovascular controls in groups of infants believed to be at increased risk for SIDS, including siblings of infants with SIDS and infants with near-SIDS (aborted SIDS). Recently prospective studies have become available on large populations of infants who died of SIDS.

Respiratory Pauses. The precise role of apneic episodes or respiratory pauses in the pathogenesis of SIDS remains unclear. Prolonged apnea and cyanosis during sleep have been observed in infants who subsequently died of what was presumed to be SIDS, and upper airway obstruction, with prolonged pauses in respiration and bradycardia, has been noted in infants with aborted SIDS. It is uncertain, however, whether apnea of central or of obstructive origin is more important in the genesis of SIDS. Difficulties in reconciling much of the reported data stem from arbitrary definitions of apnea and from absence of standards for the normal frequency and duration of respiration pauses. In studies of a group of normal fullterm infants during the first 4 mo of life, the mean

1480

duration of respiratory pauses (defined as durations of expiratory phase greater than average by 2 standard deviations or more) was 5–7 sec, with some lasting as long as 13 sec. Pauses were longer and less frequent in quiet than in REM sleep in these infants. In infants with aborted SIDS or near-SIDS the pauses were not abnormal with respect either to frequency or to duration. None of the normal or high-risk infants studied had any apneic episode longer than 13 sec during the first 4 mo of life. In a prospective study of more than 9000 infants, Southall did not observe respiratory pauses in those who subsequently died of SIDS that were longer than those seen in the survivors. In contrast, others have noted prolonged apneic periods (15 sec or longer) in study populations that have included prematurely born infants with apnea. In addition, transient decreases of the instantaneously recorded heart rate during sleep to approximately 70/min have been noted in both normal infants and those with near-SIDS without cyanosis or other evidence of cardiorespiratory embarrassment.

Brain Stem Defect. Some evidence suggests that infants with SIDS have an abnormality in the central nervous system, presumably at the level of the brain stem: abnormalities in evoked auditory brain stem potentials have been observed in some infants with aborted SIDS; a higher than normal resting $PaCO_2$ and a blunted ventilatory response to CO_2 have been found in a group of infants with aborted SIDS. However, the data with respect to ventilatory responsiveness are conflicting, other studies showing that responsiveness to CO_2 in infants with aborted SIDS is normal or increased. Infants with markedly decreased responses to CO_2, especially during sleep, may have other disorders, such as failure of automatic control of ventilation or Ondine's curse, that should not be confused with SIDS.

Abnormal Upper Airway Function. UPPER AIRWAY OBSTRUCTION. The young infant may be vulnerable to upper airway obstruction for anatomic and developmental reasons, including posterior displacement of the tongue and decreased airway diameter following flexion of the neck. Immature or abnormal neuromuscular control of the oropharyngeal muscle may also lead to airway obstruction. Patency of the upper airway may be maintained by muscles such as the genioglossus, the activation of which is coordinated with excitation of respiratory muscles; phase shifts in the contraction of these muscles could lead to upper airway obstruction, but it is not known whether this occurs in SIDS.

HYPERREACTIVE AIRWAY REFLEXES. The laryngeal chemoreflex system, mediated through the superior laryngeal nerve, is capable of overriding central and peripheral respiratory drive mechanisms, and a number of studies are focusing on the maturation of this system in early life. Because the introduction of some fluids into the larynx can stimulate this reflex, presumably leading to apnea, gastroesophageal reflux with aspiration might be an underlying mechanism for SIDS in some infants. With massive reflux there are clear-cut episodes of apnea and severe bradycardia. Moreover, such episodes cease when feedings are thickened and the infants are kept continuously upright. On the other hand, the normal infant demonstrates gastroesophageal reflux at least up to 2 mo of age, and it is difficult, therefore, to know to what extent apneic episodes can be attributed to mild or moderate reflux.

Cardiac Abnormalities. Although electrical instability may be present in the young heart, there is no convincing evidence to indicate that cardiac arrhythmias play a role in SIDS. Southall's prospective study did not detect a difference between the infants who died of SIDS and the normal infants with respect to cardiac rhythm.

Findings in Infants Who Later Died of SIDS. Several infants who subsequently died of SIDS have been studied before death. Shannon found that such infants have abnormal heart rate variability, and Southall observed that some of the infants

who subsequently died of SIDS had a greater number of episodes of tachycardia than age-matched normal fullterm infants. In response to auditory stimuli one infant has shown greater than normal lability and poorer stabilization of cardiac rate.

Findings in Infants at High Risk for SIDS. SIBLINGS OF INFANTS WITH SIDS. Although one group of infant siblings of infants with SIDS was found to have an increased incidence and longer duration of periodic breathing in sleep than a control group, another group of siblings of SIDS victims had an increased respiratory rate and decreased incidence of breathing pauses in sleep; these latter siblings could not be differentiated from normal infants in terms of the frequency of long pauses (more than 10 sec). Siblings of SIDS victims also have had a faster heart rate in early infancy than control infants, with a delay in the normal decrease in heart rate with age. Finally, siblings of infants with SIDS have had longer sleep cycles during both quiet and active or REM sleep before 12 wk of age compared with normal controls, raising the possibility of a higher arousal threshold.

INFANTS WITH NEAR-SIDS OR ABORTED SIDS. In one group of infants with near-SIDS, detailed neurologic examination has revealed consistent abnormalities of muscle tone, particularly shoulder hypotonia in infants under 3 mo of age. Another group of 21 infants with near-SIDS (found to be unresponsive, cyanotic, and apneic, and having had mouth-to-mouth resuscitation) studied during the first 4 mo of life had, in comparison with normal infants, faster heart rates, less heart rate variability (both beat-to-beat and overall variability), shorter Q-T intervals even when corrected for the increased heart rate, and normal or increased ventilatory responses to elevated concentrations of inspired CO_2. Similar groups of infants with near-SIDS have been noted to have an increase in the frequency and duration of respiratory pauses on exposure to gases with low oxygen tension. Although the ventilatory or arousal responses to increased CO_2 or decreased O_2 have been proposed as potentially important mechanisms in SIDS, neither discriminates between the normal and the high risk for SIDS group.

Two studies of the respiratory control mechanisms of parents of SIDS victims have given conflicting results; in one there was no abnormal finding in the ventilatory response to hypoxia or to hypercapnia during wakefulness in either parent; in the other a significantly lower ventilatory response to CO_2 was found, with or without the imposition of added resistance to breathing.

Differences in results among investigations of infants at risk for SIDS may be due to differences in the techniques used to measure cardiorespiratory function, in the criteria used for patient selection and the populations studied, in the methods used to stage sleep, and in the sleep states of the infants who are studied.

Abnormal Autonomic Nervous System and Chemical Mediators. The increased heart rate and decreased heart rate variability, the smaller Q-T index, and the greater variability response to CO_2 found in infants at high risk for SIDS suggests that these infants have an abnormality in the autonomic nervous system, possibly an increase in sympathetic nervous activity. Consistent with this is the finding of increased levels of dopamine in the carotid bodies of infants who have died of SIDS; dopamine could inhibit carotid discharge, especially during hypoxia. Whether the hypothetical increase in sympathoadrenal activity is likely to be secondary to hypoxia or to some other stimulus is unknown. The possible roles of such chemical mediators as catecholamines, endorphins, and serotonin in cardiorespiratory function, in the response to such stresses as hypoxia and hypercapnia, and in the maturation of these responses during sleep represent important areas of research.

Diagnosis. Some infants at risk for SIDS may have physiologic handicaps before birth. In the neonatal period they may demonstrate low Apgar scores and abnormalities in control of respiration, heart rate, and temperature, and they may have postnatal growth retardation. Near-SIDS or aborted SIDS remains a diagnosis that can be made only by exclusion of such conditions as seizure disorders, other neurologic abnormalities, metabolic abnormalities (including hypoglycemia), cardiac anomalies and arrhythmias, vascular anomalies (especially vascular ring), massive gastroesophageal reflux, infantile botulism, and fulminant infection.

In suspected cases investigation should include (1) blood chemistries (serum glucose, Na, K, Cl, Ca, P, Mg, and BUN); (2) pH and blood gas analysis; (3) chest roentgenogram (including magnification films of the upper airways) and upper gastrointestinal study with barium swallow; (4) a 12-lead electrocardiogram (ECG) and 12–24 hr ECG monitoring for rhythm analysis; (5) an electroencephalogram; and (6) esophageal pH studies made concomitantly with measurements of respiration.

Home Monitoring of High-Risk Infants. As technology has improved and more parents have become informed about SIDS, their desire to monitor ventilation or heart rate has increased. This monitoring requires knowledge of the normal ranges during sleep of heart rate, of heart rate variability, of respiratory rate, and of frequency and duration of respiratory pauses so that infants most likely to benefit from monitoring can be identified.

Apnea monitors based on impedance may not detect complete airway obstruction as infants continue to make respiratory movements. Since serious apnea may be missed if only thoracoabdominal movements are monitored, monitoring of heart rate should also be included. It is unknown whether measuring heart rate and heart rate variability with a high degree of precision will increase the ability to detect the infant at high risk for SIDS.

There is little objective information available on which to base a decision about whether home monitoring is necessary or desirable or how long it should go on. The abilities of members of the household to handle monitors and to make the appropriate responses to true or false alarms are critical factors in the decision. When monitoring is used for infants thought to be at special risk after a thorough evaluation, parents should receive appropriate training in cardiopulmonary resuscitation and the proper use of the monitoring equipment. There should also be documentation of the monitoring, timely re-evaluation of the patient at least by 6 mo of age, supportive counseling, and planned termination of monitoring. Some think that home monitoring programs should not be independent from research evaluating the program and its effects.

Even if, in all infants at high risk, it were possible to prevent SIDS, some cases would occur among those not recognized as being at risk. For this reason, and because, by definition, death comes swiftly and without forewarning, psychologic and emotional support should be provided to all members of the family in cases of SIDS and confusion with child abuse should be avoided.

ROBERT B. MELLINS
GABRIEL G. HADDAD

Haddad GG, Bazzy AR, Chang SL, et al: Heart rate pattern during respiratory pauses in normal infants during sleep. J Develop Physiol 6:329, 1984.
Haddad GG, Leistner HL, Lai TL, et al: Ventilation and ventilatory pattern during sleep in aborted sudden infant death syndrome. Pediatr Res 15:879, 1981.
Harper RM, Leake B, Hoffman H, et al: Periodicity of sleep states is altered in infants at risk for the sudden infant death syndrome. Science 213:1030, 1981.
Harper RM, Leake B, Hoppenbrouwers T, et al: Polygraphic studies of normal infants and infants at risk for the sudden infant death syndrome: Heart rate and heart rate variability as a function of state. Pediatr Res 12:778, 1978.
Leistner HL, Haddad GG, Epstein RA, et al: Heart rate and heart rate variability during sleep in aborted sudden infant death syndrome. J Pediatr 97:51, 1980.
Naeye RL: Pulmonary arterial abnormalities in the sudden infant death syndrome. N Engl J Med 289:1167, 1973.
Naeye RL, Ladis B, Drage JS: Sudden infant death syndrome: A prospective study. Am J Dis Child 130:1207, 1976.
Perrin DG, Becher LE, Madapallimatum A, et al: Sudden infant death syndrome: Increased carotid-body dopamine and noradrenalin content. Lancet 2:535, 1984.
Peterson DR: Evolution of the epidemiology of sudden infant death syndrome. Epidemiol Rev 2:97, 1980.
Shannon DC, Kelly DH: SIDS and near-SIDS. N Engl J Med 306:959, 1022, 1982.
Southall DP, Richards JM, de Swiet D, et al: Identification of infants destined to die during infancy; evaluation of predictive importance of prolonged apnea and disorders of cardiac rhythm or conduction: First report of a multicentered prospective study into the sudden infant death syndrome. Br Med J 286:1092, 1983.
Steinschneider A: Prolonged apnea and the sudden infant death syndrome: Clinical and laboratory observations. Pediatrics 50:646, 1972.
Valdes-Dapena MA: Sudden infant death syndrome: A review of the medical literature 1974–1979. Pediatrics 66:597, 1980.
Williams A, Vawter G, Reid L: Increased muscularity of the pulmonary circulation in victims of sudden infant death. Pediatrics 63:18, 1979.

26.2 THE AMYLOID DISEASES

Definition and Classification. The amyloid diseases include a number of entities of diverse etiology having in common the extracellular deposition of a proteinaceous material which displays a green birefringence when stained with Congo red and viewed under a polarizing microscope. The amyloid deposits appear homogeneous by light microscopy, but reveal 10–15 nm wide fibrils on electron microscopy. On x-ray crystallography the fibrils show a β-pleated sheet structure. Amyloid deposits compress and destroy involved tissues.

Based on the clinical features of the amyloid diseases and the nature of the major protein component of the fibrils, the classification shown in Table 26–1 has been proposed.

Etiology and Pathogenesis. Significant insight into the complexity of these diseases has come with recognition of their heterogeneity and the elucidation of the nature of some of the amyloid fibrils. Each type of amyloid deposit in man and in all experimental animals consists of two components. One of these, the P component, is common to all types of amyloid though it constitutes only about 5% of the deposits. It is derived from a 220,000 dalton serum component, a globulin which is composed of 10 identical subunits. It is closely related in structure and perhaps also in function to C-reactive protein. It is present in all types of amyloid, but its role in pathogenesis is unknown, though it seems possible that it may serve as a scaffold for the fibril deposition. The major component of all amyloid deposits, which constitutes 70–90% of the mass, is the 10–15 nm fibril. The different protein subunits of the fibrils of the several types of amyloid confer distinctive properties upon each of them. In spite of their biochemical differences, reflected slightly by the staining

Table 26–1. **Classification of the Amyloid Disease**

Proposed Designation	Clinical Features	Protein Subunit*
Light chain (AL)	Primary and myeloma-associated	AL
AA protein (AA)	Secondary	AA
Familial (AF)	Familial (many types)	AF
Endocrine (AE)	Endocrine	AE
Dermal (AD)	Localized (dermal, cutaneous)	AD
Senile (AS)	Senile	AS

*The 1st A stands for amyloid; among the 2nd letters, L = immunoglobulin light chain, A = A protein, F = familial, E = endocrine, D = dermatologic, S = senile. When the nature of the protein is known, a subscript is added (e.g., p for prealbumin, c for cardiac, t for thyrocalcitonin, etc.).

properties, the ultrastructural appearance of the various types of fibrils is identical.

Because the nature of the associated disorders varies with the amyloid protein subunits, it is necessary to consider the pathogenesis of the major types of amyloid individually. Some researchers suggest disordered functioning of the immune system in the pathogenesis of amyloidosis; others view all types of amyloidosis as the result primarily of the overproduction of normal or, perhaps in some instances, an unusual "amyloidogenic" protein. Overproduction, however, is not a sufficient explanation, since only a fraction of the patients overproducing such proteins develop amyloid. Other factors related to the nature of the host's response and to the processing of the precursor of the fibril may also play a role. However, current data support the fibril precursor processing concept only for the types of amyloid related to the L chain and AA protein.

In the AA type of amyloid, the 8000 dalton AA protein appears to be derived by proteolysis from a 12,000 dalton precursor known as SAA. SAA, a molecule of unknown function, exists in plasma complexed to other proteins, predominantly the high density lipoproteins. Subtle structural polymorphisms have been observed in the SAA and AA proteins, but these seem insufficient to account for differences in susceptibility to amyloidosis noted among different individuals. Consequently, differences in processing of the precursor or the fibril have been suggested as responsible for predisposing certain individuals to amyloidosis. Serum SAA levels are of little value in the diagnosis of amyloidosis since SAA behaves as an acute phase reactant.

AL fibrils consist of fragments of L chains or sometimes of an entire light chain. Since amyloid fibrils can be created in vitro by the proteolysis of certain L chains, it seems likely that in vivo degradation of L chains is responsible for the formation of AL amyloid deposits. Some light chains appear to be more "amyloidogenic" than others. It seems likely that proteolysis of a soluble precursor may also affect proteins such as prealbumin in some of the familial forms of amyloidosis, peptide hormones in the endocrine types, and the proteins with β-pleated sheet structure in some of the other variants.

Even though proteolysis of the amyloid precursors seems to play a role in the deposition of the fibrils, when once formed they resist phagocytosis and proteolytic degradation. The body has few mechanisms to remove these deposits, a factor which may well account for the generally relentless progression of the diseases.

Incidence. Amyloidosis is a rare disease. The most common type of amyloidosis in adults is the AL (primary) type, which is seen in association with myeloma and related plasma cell dyscrasias; these disorders are exceedingly rare among children. Among the diseases giving rise to AA (secondary) amyloidosis in children are rheumatoid arthritis, regional ileitis, cystic fibrosis, and, on rare occasions, chronic suppurative disorders. Among children in the United States with juvenile rheumatoid arthritis the frequency of amyloidosis is low; for unknown reasons it is more common in certain European countries. Regional ileitis is more frequently complicated by amyloidosis than ulcerative colitis. Amyloidosis in children is rarely associated with Hodgkin disease, renal carcinoma, or chronic suppurative conditions. In young adults amyloidosis is beginning to be seen with some frequency as a consequence of the suppurative and infectious complications of drug addiction. In developing countries such endemic infectious diseases as leprosy and malaria often give rise to secondary amyloidosis.

Some of the rare familial forms of amyloidosis, especially those associated with familial Mediterranean fever (most common among Sephardic Jews) as well as the Portuguese type,

can affect children. The localized forms of amyloidosis, such as those involving the skin, are rare in children.

Clinical Manifestations. The clinical features of all types of amyloidosis stem from the infiltration of tissues by amyloid deposits, with the ultimate destruction of the affected organs. Symptoms depend upon the tissues involved; particularly when the liver, kidney, or heart is affected, functional impairment may lead to death. In certain localized forms of amyloidosis, for example, the cutaneous ones, the disease remains limited; otherwise it tends to be progressive, and even with control or treatment of the underlying disease significant regression is rare. An exception is familial Mediterranean fever, the amyloidosis of which often improves with the administration of colchicine.

Secondary (AA) amyloidosis occurs with underlying disorders that are usually severe and protracted; sometimes, however, amyloid deposits appear rapidly or with mild disease. In secondary amyloidosis, deposits occur predominantly in the kidneys, spleen, liver, and adrenals and rarely involve the heart, musculoskeletal, or gastrointestinal systems. Since amyloid in the kidney is deposited primarily in the glomeruli, the major manifestations are proteinuria, hyposthenuria, and hematuria; as the disease progresses, the nephrotic syndrome and ultimately renal failure make their appearance and, if left untreated, lead to death. Renal vein thrombosis is a common complication; hypertension is rare.

Hepatic and splenic enlargement may be massive but are generally asymptomatic or give rise only to abdominal discomfort, since liver function usually is not significantly impaired. Tests of liver function may be only minimally altered, with increased hepatic alkaline phosphatase activity and Bromsulphalein retention, with or without increased transaminase activities.

AL amyloid is rarely seen in children, whether idiopathic (primary) or associated with myeloma, macroglobulinemia, or other plasmacytic or lymphocytic neoplasms. In addition to producing the hepatic, splenic, and renal infiltrates seen in secondary amyloidosis, L chain amyloid also infiltrates the tongue, heart, skeletal muscles, subcutaneous tissues, ligaments, skin, and gastrointestinal tract. Accordingly, macroglossia, carpal tunnel syndrome, peripheral neuropathy, arrhythmias and congestive heart failure, purpura, subcutaneous infiltrates, and gastrointestinal bleeding and malabsorption may be early signs of this type of amyloidosis.

There are many familial forms of amyloidosis, each with characteristic clinical features and often with unique geographic distribution. Because of their variety and rarity, the review by Andrade et al should be consulted for a complete clinical description. Table 26–2 summarizes the salient features of four of the most common hereditary types. It is noteworthy that the Portuguese and Japanese forms have prominent neuropathic components in addition to marked visceral involvement.

Probably the most common and widespread of the familial forms of amyloidosis is associated with **familial Mediterranean fever** (FMF) in Sephardic Jews and certain other ethnic groups of the Middle East. It is manifested as recurrent bouts of fever at irregular intervals, accompanied by abdominal, chest, or joint pains. In most patients the symptoms begin at 5–15 yr. The appearance of amyloidosis, which resembles the AA form clinically, is not related to the frequency or severity of attacks. In some patients a deficiency of C5a inhibitor occurs, which may play a role in the pathogenesis of the inflammatory attacks.

Independent inheritance of FMF and amyloidosis is suggested by the appearance in certain individuals and families of amyloidosis as the first or sole clinical manifestation of the syndrome and by the absence in Armenians of amyloidosis in the FMF syndrome. FMF is inherited as an autosomal

Table 26–2. **Comparison of the Hereditary Amyloidoses**

Types	Portuguese-Japanese Families	Indiana-Maryland Families	Iowa Family	Familial Mediterranean Fever
Genetic mode of transmission	Autosomal dominant	Autosomal dominant	Autosomal dominant	Autosomal recessive
Ethnicity	Portuguese and Japanese	Swiss and German	Scotch-English-Irish	Mediterranean Jews
Age of onset (decades)	3rd–4th	4th–5th	3rd–5th	1st–2nd
Time from clinical onset to death (yr)	10–12	16–35	1–26	2–10
Neuropathy	+ + + + in lower extremities	+ + + + in upper extremities	+ + + + in lower extremities; + + in upper extremities	—
Nephropathy	—	—	+ + + +	+ + + +
Vitreous opacities	—	+ +	—	—

Adapted from Andrade et al., 1970.

recessive trait, although most of the familial forms of amyloidosis are inherited in an autosomal dominant fashion.

The diagnosis of FMF is based on the typical clinical features in the proper familial setting. The amyloidosis of FMF is unique in that its appearance can be delayed or prevented and the deposits made to regress by the administration of colchicine, 0.6 mg 2–3 times/day, a regimen which also aborts the febrile attacks. Since colchicine can produce chromosomal alterations and azoospermia, it should be used with caution in children and in adults in their reproductive period. To date, however, no fetal abnormalities have been attributed to the drug.

Diagnosis. Amyloidosis can be suspected clinically, but histologic studies with proper staining of the tissues are needed to establish the diagnosis. Ideally, biopsy is made of a clinically involved organ, but if biopsy of an affected organ is not advisable, rectal or gingival biopsy will yield positive results in over 90% of cases even when the rectum or gums are not obviously clinically involved. However, a positive rectal biopsy does not necessarily prove that renal or hepatic dysfunction is due to amyloidosis; the patients may have another associated disease.

In the differential diagnosis other causes of nephrotic syndrome must be ruled out when renal involvement is prominent or other causes of hepatosplenomegaly must be ruled out when liver involvement prevails.

Treatment. With the exception of the amyloidosis associated with FMF, there is no effective treatment for amyloidosis because the material resists resorption. However, treatment of the underlying disease may halt progression, and perhaps may also achieve some spontaneous resorption. In the AA protein type, eradication of a septic focus may be of help. Administration of colchicine may prevent, arrest, or at times even cause regression of the amyloid deposits in FMF but has been disappointing in the treatment of the other types. Use of dimethyl sulfoxide is currently under investigation. Amyloidosis associated with myeloma and primary amyloidosis are treated with chemotherapy, most often using melphalan or cyclophosphamide, in regimens similar to those used in myeloma. The renal manifestations can be managed by dialysis and, if necessary, transplantation, which has been about as effective as in other types of renal failure. Amyloid has been found to involve transplanted kidneys after periods of 5–10 yr.

Prognosis. In the absence of effective therapy the systemic forms of amyloidosis tend to be progressive and result in death in 1–5 yr, most often from renal failure or sepsis. The course can be slowed by dialysis or transplantation.

RICHARD E. BEHRMAN*

---

*Modified from original by E. C. Franklin.

Andrade C, Araki S, Block WD, et al: Hereditary amyloidosis. Arthritis Rheum 13:902, 1970.
Benson MD, Skinner M, Cohen S: Amyloid deposition in a renal transplant in familial Mediterranean fever. Ann Intern Med 87:31, 1977.
Castile R, Shwachman H, Travis W, et al: Amyloidosis as a complication of cystic fibrosis. Am J Dis Child 139:728, 1985.
Filipowicz-Sosnowski AM, Roztropowicz-Densiewicz K, Rosenthal CJ, et al: The amyloidosis of juvenile rheumatoid arthritis—comparative studies in Polish and American children. Arthritis Rheum 21:699, 1978.
Glenner GG: Amyloid deposits and amyloidosis. The β-fibrilloses. N Engl J Med 302:1283, 1333, 1980.
Glenner GG, Costa PP, Freitas F (eds): Amyloid and Amyloidosis. Amsterdam, Excerpta Medica, 1980.
Kuhlbäck B, Falck H, Törnroth T, et al: Renal transplantation in amyloidosis. Acta Med Scand 205:169, 1979.
Kyle RA, Bayrd ED: Amyloidosis: Review of 236 cases. Medicine 54:271, 1975.
Levy M, Eliakim M: Long-term colchicine prophylaxis in familial Mediterranean fever. Br Med J 2:808, 1977.
Matzner Y, Brzezinski A: C5a inhibitor deficiency in peritoneal fluids from patients with familial Mediterranean fever. N Engl J Med 311:287, 1984.
Rosenthal CJ, Franklin EC: Variation with age and disease of an amyloid A protein-related serum component. J Clin Invest 55:746, 1975.
Wolff SM: Familial Mediterranean fever: A status report. Hosp Pract, Nov, 1978, p 113.

26.3 SARCOIDOSIS

Sarcoidosis, a chronic, multisystemic disease of obscure origin and variable pattern, occurs in children but is uncommon under the age of 10 yr. Weight loss, cough, fatigue, bone and joint pain, and anemia are the most frequent clinical manifestations.

The pathologic lesion is a noncaseating granuloma, and the basic abnormalities simulate those of chronic granulomatous diseases, especially tuberculosis. *Mycobacterium tuberculosis* has not been demonstrated in the lesions, and most patients with sarcoidosis do not have dermal reactions to tuberculin. Perturbations in immune reactions in the lungs have been described in adults but have not been studied in children.

The epidemiology is far from clear, but sarcoidosis is diagnosed most commonly in blacks, in young adults, and in rural areas of the southeastern United States.

The lung is the most frequently affected organ; pulmonary involvement is variable in its extent and characteristics. Parenchymal infiltrates, miliary nodules, and hilar and paratracheal lymphadenopathy (Fig. 26–1) occur. Pulmonary function tests primarily show restrictive changes. Peripheral lymphadenopathy, eye changes consisting of uveitis or iritis, skin lesions, and hepatic involvement occur frequently. The clinical manifestations of sarcoidosis in the older child are different from those of the very young, which consist of a maculopapular erythematous rash, uveitis, and arthritis; pulmonary changes are minimal. The arthritis, which can be confused with rheumatoid arthritis, produces large, painless, boggy synovial effusions of the tendon sheaths; there is little limitation of motion.

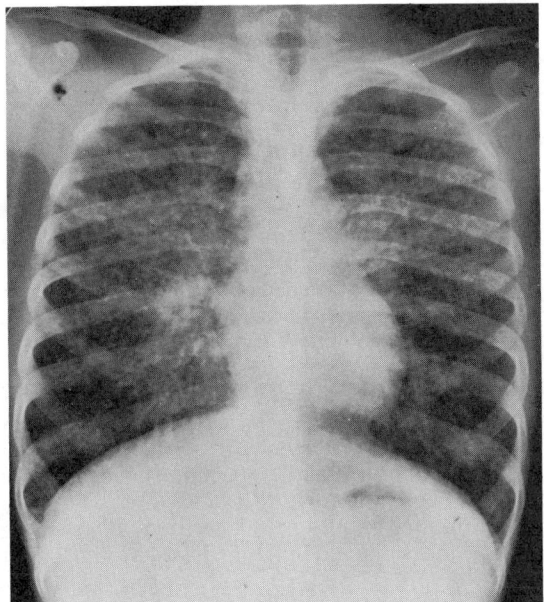

Figure 26–1. Sarcoidosis in a white 10 yr old girl. There are widely disseminated peribronchial infiltrations, multiple small nodular densities, overaeration of the lungs, and hilar adenopathy.

There are no specific diagnostic tests. An elevated erythrocyte sedimentation rate, hyperproteinemia, hypercalcemia, hypercalciuria, eosinophilia, and an elevated angiotensin-converting enzyme level are common. The Kveim test, consisting of intradermal injection of material from a sarcoid lesion and observation for the formation of a granuloma several weeks later, is used infrequently for diagnosis because of difficulty in obtaining a standardized test material and reports of varying sensitivity and specificity of the test. Biopsy of tissue from affected areas is the most valuable diagnostic measure.

Because of its protean manifestations, the differential diagnosis of sarcoidosis is extremely broad; it includes tuberculosis, the various pulmonary mycoses, lymphoma, and inflammatory ocular lesions such as phlyctenular conjunctivitis.

Treatment is symptomatic and supportive. Adrenal corticosteroids may suppress the acute manifestations, especially the inflammatory ocular lesions, progressive pulmonary disease, and the hypercalcemia/hypercalciuria. Pulmonary function tests are useful in following the progress of lung involvement, and angiotensin-converting enzyme levels have been shown to correlate with disease activity.

The prognosis and natural history of sarcoidosis in children are uncertain. Spontaneous recovery may occur after a prolonged illness of several months to several years, or the condition may be very chronic, involving progressive lung disease. Eye involvement may lead to blindness.

FLOYD W. DENNY

Bresnitz EA, Strom BL: Epidemiology of sarcoidosis. Epidemiol Rev 5:124, 1983.
Hetherington S: Sarcoidosis in young children. Am J Dis Child 136:13, 1982.
Jasper PL, Denny FW: Sarcoidosis in children: With special emphasis on the natural history and treatment. J Pediatr 73:499, 1968.
Kendig EL Jr, Brummer DL: The prognosis of sarcoidosis in children. Chest 70:351, 1976.
Mitchell DN, Scadding JG: Sarcoidosis. Am Rev Respir Dis 110:774, 1974.
Pattishall EN, Strope GL, Spinola SM, et al: Childhood sarcoidosis. J Pediatr, 108:169, 1986.
Rodriguez GE, Shin BC, Abernathy RS, et al: Serum angiotensin-converting enzyme activity in normal children and in those with sarcoidosis. J Pediatr 99:68, 1981.

26.4 PROGERIA

The Hutchinson-Gilford progeria syndrome has been reported in 86 patients in the medical literature. The author is also personally aware of 16 patients who have not been reported. This condition may be an autosomal dominant trait. It has occurred in one of a twin pair and in two sets of identical twins. Paternal age is also significantly increased.

Children with progeria are usually considered to be normal in early infancy, but manifestations such as "scleroderma," midfacial cyanosis, and "sculptured nose" may suggest the existence of the syndrome at birth. Profound growth failure occurs during the first year of life. The characteristic facies, alopecia, loss of subcutaneous fat, abnormal posture, stiffness of joints, and bone and skin changes become apparent during the second year (Fig. 26–2). Motor and mental development are normal.

Features almost *always* present when the condition has become apparent are short stature; weight distinctly low for height; failure to complete sexual maturation; diminished subcutaneous fat; head disproportionately large for face; micrognathia; prominent scalp veins; generalized alopecia; prominent eyes; "plucked-bird appearance"; delayed and abnormal dentition; pyriform thorax; short, dystrophic clavicles; "horse-riding" stance; widebased shuffling gait; and coxa valga, thin limbs, and prominent, stiff joints.

Features *frequently* present are skin that is thin, taut, dry, wrinkled, brown-spotted in various areas, or "sclerodermatous" over lower abdomen, proximal thighs, and buttocks; prominent superficial veins; loss of eyebrows and eyelashes; persistently patent anterior fontanel; "sculptured," beaked nasal tip; faint nasolabial cyanosis; thin lips; protruding ears; absence of ear lobes; thin, high-pitched voice; dystrophic nails; and progressive radiolucency of terminal phalanges.

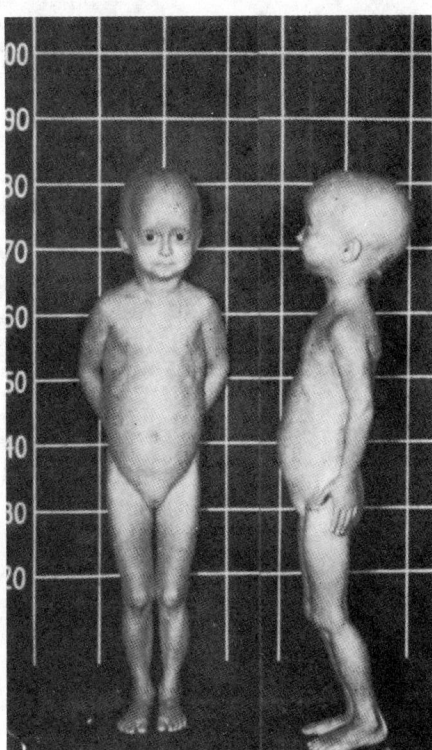

Figure 26–2. A, 4.5 yr old girl with height age of 1.75 yr and bone age of 4 yr. (From Wilkins, L.: Diagnosis and Treatment of Endocrine Disorders in Childhood and Adolescence. 3rd ed. Springfield, IL, Charles C Thomas, 1965.)

Insulin resistance, abnormal collagen, increased metabolic rate, and variable abnormalities of serum lipids are found, but there are no demonstrable abnormalities of thyroid, parathyroid, pituitary, or adrenal function. Growth hormone responses are normal. Studies of cultured skin fibroblasts show reduced replicative life spans, increased fractions of heat-labile cellular enzymes, and increased tissue procoagulant activity. Increased hyaluronic acid is noted in the urine of some patients.

Progeric patients ordinarily develop atherosclerosis and die of cardiac or cerebral vascular disease between 7 and 27 yr of age, with a median age of 13.4 yr at death. Many features associated with normal aging such as cataracts, presbycusis, presbyopia, arcus senilis, osteoarthritis, or senile personality changes are not found.

No effective treatment for this condition exists, but physiotherapy has been effective in preventing contractures. There are now support groups for the families of children with progeria, and a Progeria Registry now exists which may help to better define the incidence and genetic basis of the disorder.

FRANKLIN L. DeBUSK

Brown TW: Personal communications.
DeBusk FL: The Hutchinson-Gilford progeria syndrome. J Pediatr 80:697, 1972.
Goldstein S: Studies on age-related diseases in cultured skin fibroblasts. J Invest Dermatol 73:19, 1979.

26.5 HISTIOCYTOSIS X

Three clinical conditions have been described that share the common histologic feature of an infiltrating histiocytosis but have widely varied clinical manifestations (Fig. 26–3). *Eosinophilic granuloma* of bone usually presents as a solitary lesion in an older child. The *Hand-Schüller-Christian syndrome* characteristically seen in younger children is also associated with bony lesions but to a variable degree affects soft tissues as well; exophthalmos and diabetes insipidus form part of the classic triad of this syndrome. *Letterer-Siwe syndrome*, as originally described, is a disseminated histiocytosis occurring in younger children and primarily affecting soft tissues, particularly the skin, bone marrow, liver, and lungs.

These syndromes represent a spectrum of severity and prognosis of the same underlying disorder. Most patients

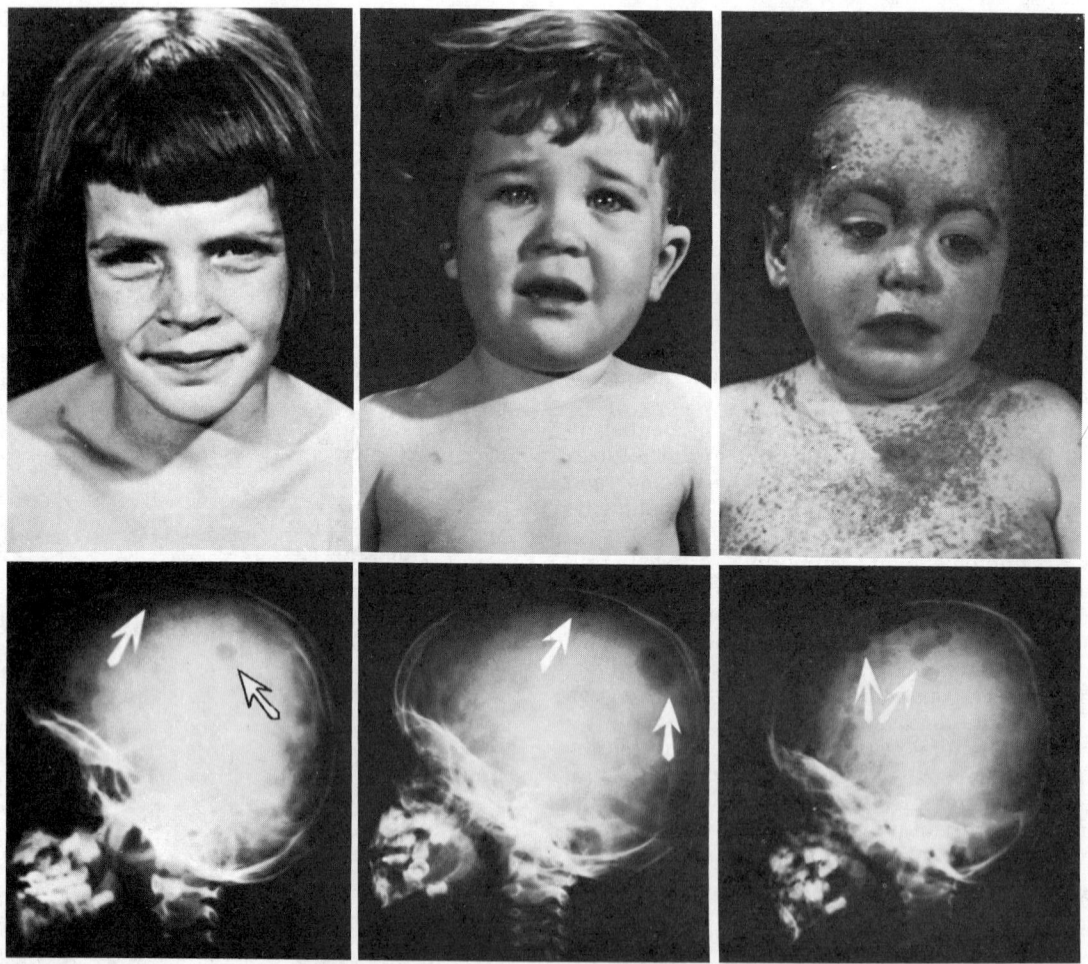

Figure 26–3. Common clinical patterns. Girl on left did not progress beyond brief involvement and isolated bone lesions that could be categorized as eosinophilic granuloma, and had good recovery. Girl in middle had several dozen bone lesions, a papular skin eruption, scalp "seborrhea," stomatitis, vaginitis, pulmonary infiltration, and diabetes insipidus. The diagnostic term Hand-Schüller-Christian syndrome is applicable here. Her disease responded well to chlorambucil therapy. Girl on right had extensive bone disease, plus a febrile course, anemia, severe skin eruption, generalized adenopathy, hepatosplenomegaly, pulmonary infiltration, and a fatal outcome in spite of antitumor chemotherapy. This patient fits the category of Letterer-Siwe syndrome.
Early biopsies of bone lesions from all 3 patients showed a similar type of histiocytic granuloma.

who present with a solitary bone lesion do well with minimal or no therapy, while the prognosis of those with the disseminated form of the disease is relatively poor but may be significantly improved by systemic chemotherapy or local radiation.

Etiology. Although the syndrome is usually sporadic, it has occurred in monozygotic twins and also in a familial pattern consistent with autosomal recessive inheritance. Abnormalities in immune function are present in many of these patients. It is not clear whether this disease represents an underlying abnormality in immune function or is a true malignancy. The fatal outcomes, especially in infants, and the responsiveness of some patients to anticancer drugs suggest the latter, although there are frequent regressions without therapy, particularly in children with disease limited to bone. Alternatively, the heterogeneous nature of the cellular infiltrate is consistent with the clonal proliferation of a single cell within the immune system, which is capable of releasing lymphokines or other chemotactic factors to attract a varied cell population to the lesions.

Pathology. The characteristic histiocytic cells have a deeply indented nucleus and cytoplasmic structures known as Langerhans granules. These cells closely resemble the normal Langerhans cells, which are widely distributed in normal skin and some reticuloendothelial organs. There are also variable numbers of other inflammatory and reactive cells such as eosinophils, neutrophils, and, less commonly, lymphocytes and plasma cells. The younger the patient and the more disseminated and rapidly progressive the disease, the more likely the lesions will contain a greater proportion of histiocytosis X cells. With healing, the lesions are gradually replaced by fibrosis. This infiltrative process can affect tissues in any region of the body, but marrow, skin, lymph nodes, lung, liver, and meninges are the more common sites. Variable degrees of histologic and functional abnormalities of the involved normal tissue are found.

Clinical Manifestations. The three classic presentations have been described above. This disease has an acute phase in which patients may quickly recover, e.g., with healing of a single bone lesion, or quickly succumb, e.g., owing to disseminated pulmonary disease, but there may also be a chronic phase with recurrent or persistent disease that may lead to significant impairment of growth and function. The skeleton is the most commonly involved tissue and in the child over 5 yr of age may be the only site of involvement. The lesions may be single or multiple and are most commonly found in the skull, long bones, spine, and pelvis. They may be asymptomatic or associated with pain and local swelling. Involvement of the spine may result in collapse of the vertebral body, which can be seen radiographically and may result in secondary compression of the spinal cord. In flat and long bones, osteolytic lesions with sharp borders occur and there is no evidence of reactive new bone formation (Fig. 26–3). Lesions involving weight-bearing long bones may result in pathologic fractures. Chronically draining infected ears are commonly associated with destruction in the mastoid area. Bony destruction of the mandible and maxilla may result in teeth that appear on roentgenograms to be floating free. With response to therapy there may be complete healing and reformation of normal bony support.

Skin involvement occurs in about one third of the patients at some time during their course, usually a seborrheic dermatitis of the scalp. The lesions may spread to involve the trunk and the palms and soles. The exanthem may be petechial or hemorrhagic even in the absence of thrombocytopenia. Localized or disseminated lymphadenopathy is present in about 50% of patients. Hepatosplenomegaly occurs in about 20%. Varying degrees of hepatic malfunction may occur, including jaundice and ascites.

Exophthalmos, when present, is often bilateral and is caused by retro-orbital accumulation of granulomatous tissue. Gingival mucous membranes may be involved with infiltrative lesions that appear superficially like candidosis.

In 10–15% of patients, pulmonary infiltrates are found on roentgenograms. The lesions may vary from diffuse fibrosis and disseminated nodular infiltrates to diffuse cystic changes. Rarely, pneumothorax may be a complication. If the lungs are severely involved, tachypnea and progressive respiratory failure may result.

Pituitary dysfunction or hypothalamic involvement may result in growth retardation. In addition there may be diabetes insipidus and, rarely, panhypopituitarism. Other symptomatic involvement of the central nervous system is uncommon but may be serious; histiocytosis X cells can be demonstrated in the cerebrospinal fluid when neurologic disease is present.

More severely affected patients may have systemic manifestations including fever, weight loss, malaise, irritability, and failure to thrive. Bone marrow involvement may cause anemia and thrombocytopenia with resulting pallor and bleeding.

Laboratory Findings. Tissue biopsy is diagnostic. Any involved area may be helpful, but the skin lesions, when present, are the easiest site from which to obtain the diagnosis. The infiltrating abnormal histiocytes can also be demonstrated on bone marrow examination. Blood counts may be normal, even in patients with disseminated disease; anemia, thrombocytopenia, or pancytopenia may occur secondary to marrow infiltration. Roentgenographic examinations should be performed to assess the degree of bony and pulmonary involvement. Hepatic infiltration may result in intrahepatic bile duct obstruction with superimposed parenchymal damage. Pituitary function should be assessed, including evaluation for the presence of diabetes insipidus.

Treatment. The design of appropriate therapy has been hampered by the uncertainty surrounding the nature of this condition. For patients with localized bony disease curettage may be curative, but full evaluation of the extent of the disease should be performed. For patients with disseminated and progressive disease, treatment programs incorporate a variety of cancer chemotherapeutic agents including cyclophosphamide, vinca alkaloids, prednisone, methotrexate, 6-mercaptopurine, and chlorambucil. Single agents appear to be as useful as combination chemotherapy and carry less risk of toxic side effects, although prednisone is often combined with another agent to reduce systemic manifestations such as fever. About 50% of patients will respond to chemotherapy.

Prognosis. Impaired organ function is the single most important prognostic factor. About 40% of patients will show organ dysfunction: hematopoietic function (36%), hepatic function (10%), and pulmonary function (5%). Patients who are over 2 yr of age and have no evidence of organ dysfunction have a good prognosis; about 90% of these children survive 5 yr. Those who are less than 2 yr of age at diagnosis and have no organ dysfunction have an intermediate prognosis; about 65% of these survive 5 yr. Patients who have organ involvement regardless of age have the worst prognosis; about 45% of these survive 5 yr. In an evaluation of patients who had survived 5 yr, it was found that at least half had active disease for the 5 yr period, while the other half had apparently cleared their disease. It should be emphasized that this is a disease that may come and go even without therapy. Of these long-term survivors, about half had significant functional impairment either from disease or from treatment. Diabetes insipidus, growth failure, intellectual impairment, or other neurologic deficits were the most common, although chronic lung disease was the most severe complication, resulting in pulmonary failure and death.

BRIGID G. LEVENTHAL

Berry DH, Gresik MV, Humphrey GB, et al: Natural history of histiocytosis X. A POG study. Med Pediatr Oncol 14:1, 1986.
Falletta JM, Fernbach DJ, Singer DB, et al: A fatal X linked recessive reticuloendothelial syndrome with hyperglobulinemia and X linked recessive reticuloendotheliosis. J Pediatr 83:549, 1973.
Lahey ME: Histiocytosis X: An analysis of prognostic factors. J Pediatr 87:184, 1975.
Lichtenstein L: Histiocytosis X. Integration of eosinophilic granuloma of bone, Letterer-Siwe disease and Schüller-Christian disease as related manifestations of a single nosologic entity. Arch Pathol 56:84, 1953.
Komp DM, El Mahdi A, Starling KA, et al: Quality of survival in histiocytosis X: A Southwest Oncology Group study. Med Pediatr Oncol 8:35, 1980.
Komp DM, Herson J, Starling KA, et al: Staging system for histiocytosis X: A Southwest Oncology Group study. Cancer 47:798, 1981.

27

RADIATION INJURY

The possibility of untoward biologic effects of radiation is of special interest in pediatrics since these effects may be most serious in growing tissues. By judicious limitation of roentgen procedures during childhood a margin of safety for unavoidable radiation exposure later in life can be preserved (Sec. 5.55).

Ionizing radiation produces injury in the same manner regardless of the type of particle or ray emitted. The variation is quantitative rather than qualitative. Absorption of energy may cause molecules in the path of the radiations to become ionized. In attaining stability these molecules may form substances that alter, temporarily or perhaps permanently, biochemical processes within the cell or its environment. These effects upon cellular structures result in the deaths of persons exposed to ionizing radiations, the death of certain cancer cells treated with roentgen rays, genetic mutations, and the production of cancer as a late effect of exposures to radiations.

Susceptibility of tissues to roentgen rays is generally greater in the more rapidly mitosing and in the more undifferentiated cells. Because of an abundance of this type of tissue in the abdomen, a patient is more likely to have radiation sickness from roentgen therapy to this region than from comparable exposure elsewhere.

Dosage Factors. Radiation absorption increases with the volume of the child's body exposed, with prolongation of exposure, or with an increase in amperage or voltage. Absorption decreases in relation to the effectiveness of filters used and with an increase in distance between the patient and the roentgen tube.

Adverse acute effects of roentgen rays are diminished when the total dose is administered in several exposures separated by sufficient time for recovery from the subclinical effects of each. Repeated exposures may produce pathologic effects not manifested until years later. Some of the chemical changes produced in cells by roentgen rays are irreversible and may lie dormant until aging, infection, hormonal alterations, or further exposure to toxic agents activates them.

The infant may be more susceptible to the effects of roentgen rays than the adult. Moreover, even if there are no essential differences in susceptibility, the infant's longer life span provides more time for such changes to develop.

Early Effects of Irradiation. Exposure of the entire body to 100 roentgens usually produces illness in humans. A dose of about 450 roentgens will cause death in 50% of exposed persons. Higher doses can be tolerated if only a part of the body is exposed. Death results within hours to days when the entire body is exposed to the overwhelming dosage of an atomic bomb.

Symptoms of radiation sickness, which vary with the exposure, are malaise, fever, nausea, vomiting, and diarrhea. Leukopenia develops rapidly, and in more severe instances thrombocytopenia may appear within 1 wk. When the initial symptoms are not severe, they are followed by a temporary period of well-being. Epilation begins about 2 wk after the exposure. The leukopenia increases susceptibility to infection, and the low platelet count predisposes to hemorrhage. When autopsy does not reveal the cause of death, one can only assume that the radiation injury was responsible for lethal "cytochemical changes." If the patient survives for 6 wk, death is not likely from these effects of radiation.

Only a small percentage of deaths caused by an atomic explosion can be attributed to radiation effects alone; thermal and blast injuries account for most of them. Traumatic injuries do not heal effectively in persons with radiation sickness.

Clinical observation of the effects of radiation on children with genetic disease has led to a new understanding of molecular biology. Children with *ataxia-telangiectasia* are markedly predisposed to lymphoma and when treated for it with the usual doses of radiotherapy, sometimes suffer severe reactions. These patients have defective repair of DNA after damage by γ radiation, analogous to defective repair of DNA damage by ultraviolet light (UV) in *xeroderma pigmentosum*. The defects in repair after γ or UV damage are enzyme-mediated and nonoverlapping. Another interaction involving genetics, neoplasia, and radiosensitivity may occur in the heritable (usually bilateral) form of retinoblastoma. For example, radiogenic tumors of the orbit occur more frequently and after a shorter latent period than in patients with nonheritable cancers given similar doses of radiotherapy.

Late Effects of Irradiation. Within the decade following the detonations of the atomic bombs in Japan there was a significant rise in the incidence of leukemia in proportion to exposure to the explosions. An increase in leukemia rates has been observed at doses as low as 20–49 rads among Hiroshima survivors of all ages. Children 10 yr of age at the time of the bombing were more susceptible to leukemogenesis than were older persons.

When girls (under 10 yr of age) exposed to 50 rad or more reached the usual age for breast cancer (i.e., 35–45 yr), the frequency of breast cancer was increased; in the future, this frequency may exceed that for females who were older when exposed.

In Britain and in the United States, in utero exposures to diagnostic radiation have been reported to increase the relative risk of death from cancer before 10 yr of age by about 50%. No such effect was found among children exposed in utero to the atomic bomb.

Among persons exposed in utero to radiation from the Hiroshima atomic bomb (beginning at 10–19 rads) before the 18th wk of gestation, small head circumference occurred with excessive frequency. The effect increased in frequency and severity with increasing dose. Mental retardation occurred in those exposed to doses of 50 rads and above and affected the majority exposed before the 18th wk of gestation to 150 rads or more. There was a dose-response effect for the group exposed in utero suggesting that 1 rad absorbed by the fetus at 8–15 wk of gestation doubled the frequency of severe mental retardation. Because of the catastrophic effects of the bomb, the observations at low doses may not apply directly to medical radiology. This question might be clarified by studying the head size of Soviet children exposed under 18 wk of gestational age to radiation from the nuclear reactor accident at Chernobyl.

Complex chromosomal abnormalities are still found in the

peripheral lymphocytes of atomic bomb survivors more than 35 yr after exposure, including those who were in utero—even in the 1st trimester—but not among persons conceived after the explosion. On the basis of animal experimentation, there is no doubt that point mutations occurred, but no effect could be demonstrated among the 75,000 first generation offspring examined.

Small opacities of the posterior capsule of the lens have developed in 85% of those who epilated soon after the bomb explosion; the lesions are asymptomatic. Only 10 of the thousands of survivors have grade III or IV radiation-induced cataracts.

Radiation-induced premature aging has been described in animals, characterized by early senescence and death in middle age from diseases that ordinarily beset the elderly members of the species. This has not been demonstrated in humans.

Therapeutic doses of partial-body radiation may predispose to cancer. This is indicated by reports of a greater incidence of leukemia among adults treated for ankylosing spondylitis and of thyroid tumors among persons treated in early infancy for thymic enlargement. That repeated small doses of radiation to the entire body may predispose to leukemia is indicated by the increased occurrence of this disease among radiologists in the past.

Effects of exposure of parts of the body include temporary sterility, dermatitis, bone and skin tumors, and developmental defects of teeth. Arrest in bone growth may occur in children who received cancericidal doses of roentgen rays.

Low-Level Radiation. Claims that low levels of radiation can induce cancer are based on data from persons in the area of fallout from nuclear weapons tests in Nevada in the 1950's. Increased mortality from leukemia has been reported in children in southwestern Utah and in military participants on maneuvers at the test site. The exposures were presumably low. Worries about low-dose exposures were amplified by the near meltdown at a nuclear power plant at Three Mile Island. In addition, controversial claims have been made that atomic energy workers in decades past now have increased cancer rates. The findings are not in accord with expectation based on a linear or quadratic extrapolation from effects at high or intermediate levels, as among Japanese atomic-bomb survi-

vors. The question about low-level effects is unlikely to be solved by further epidemiologic studies because the number of exposed persons needed for study far exceeds the number available. However, the Chernobyl accident, if appropriately studied, could provide important insights into this issue. Judgments will probably eventually be based on a knowledge of the fundamental biology of radiation carcinogenesis.

Preventive Measures. Exposures to ionizing radiation should be limited to situations in which commensurate benefits are expected. The average *whole-body* exposure of the general population, based on the genetically significant dose, should not exceed 100 mrem/yr, according to the National Council on Radiation Protection and Measurements.

It is thought that radiation changes within somatic cells are *incompletely* additive throughout life. The child of today is likely to have repeated exposures to ionizing radiations, and there is a possibility that tolerance may be dissipated. The pediatrician should limit as much as possible the exposure of patients (and self) to the emanations of roentgen ray machines and radioisotopes, but should not refrain from using them for essential diagnostic and therapeutic procedures (Sec. 5.55). The patient's gonads should be shielded whenever possible.

Roentgen therapy should never be used except when the indications are unmistakable or the risk justified, as, for example, in the treatment of malignant tumors. Great care must be exercised to avoid unnecessary damage to osseous growth centers and tooth buds.

ROBERT W. MILLER

Boice JD Jr, Fraumeni JF Jr; (eds): Radiation Carcinogenesis. Epidemiology and Biological Significance. New York, Raven Press, 1984, p 489.

Land CE, McKay FW, Machado SG: Childhood leukemia and fallout from the Nevada nuclear tests. Science 223:139, 1984.

Lyon JL, Klauber MR, Gardner JW, et al: Childhood leukemias associated with fallout from nuclear testing. N Engl J Med 300:397, 1979.

Miller RW, Boice JD Jr: Radiogenic cancer after prenatal or childhood exposure. *In* Upton AC, Albert RE, Burns F, et al (eds): Radiation Carcinogenesis. New York, Elsevier-North Holland, 1986, p 379.

Miller RW, Mulvihill JJ: Small head size after atomic irradiation. Teratology 14:355, 1976.

Otake M, Schull WJ: In utero exposure to A-bomb radiation and mental retardation: A reassessment. Br J Radiol 57:409, 1984.

United Nations Scientific Committee on Effects of Atomic Radiation 1982 Report to the General Assembly, with annexes: Ionizing Radiation: Sources and Biological Effects. New York, United Nations Publ. E. 82 IX. 8, 1982.

28

POISONINGS FROM FOOD, DRUGS, CHEMICALS, POLLUTANTS, AND VENOMOUS BITES; MAMMALIAN BITES

FOOD POISONING

The inadvertent consumption of poisonous foodstuffs is a significant cause of illness worldwide. In 1982, more than 12,000 instances of salmonella food poisoning were reported in the United Kingdom, a 19% increase over the previous year. In the United States, the incidence of mushroom poisoning has increased dramatically over the past 5 yr. With the availability of rapid transportation of foodstuffs, poisoning by *Vibrio parahaemolyticus*, once limited to Japan, now occurs worldwide. Not only is the incidence of foodborne illness increasing, but also the types of poisoning have increased.

Food poisoning occurs by two mechanisms. First, contamination of usually innocuous foodstuffs by toxins or bacteria is the most common cause of poisoning; foods may either intrinsically contain toxins that manifest themselves under certain conditions (e.g., solanine poisoning and fish poisoning) or foods may become contaminated by bacterial or chemical toxins. Second, ingestion of intrinsically poisonous foodstuffs may occur; mushroom poisoning is the major example.

28.1 BACTERIAL FOOD POISONING

Salmonella Food Poisoning

Species of salmonella (Sec. 11.26) account for most cases of food poisoning in the United States and the United Kingdom. In 1982, 612 of 702 outbreaks of food poisoning in the United Kingdom were attributed to salmonella; *S. typhimurium* accounted for 44% of the cases.

Epidemiology. Poultry is the most frequently implicated identifiable contaminated food source. Meat products, particularly pork, are also associated with outbreaks. In rural epidemics of salmonella food poisoning, unpasteurized milk is often the cause. Sporadically, contaminated chocolate bars, roast beef, and marijuana have been linked to epidemics of salmonellosis; in the latter cases, unusual strains are often involved. In 1982, there were 26 outbreaks of salmonella food poisoning in hospitals.

Because the organism is readily killed at normal cooking temperatures and by pasteurization, improper storage of precooked food and consumption of raw milk are the most common causes of salmonella poisoning. Cream-filling of pastries that have been baked and are subsequently stored above 7° C may also lead to contamination.

Pathophysiology. Large inocula of the organism are required to produce illness in humans. As a result, the attack rate of salmonella poisoning following ingestion of contaminated food ranges from 25–65%. Salmonella species produce disease by invasion and infection of the gastrointestinal mucosa.

Clinical Manifestations. The incubation period after ingestion of contaminated food ranges from 12–48 hr. The most common manifestation is diarrhea, which is often bloody. Vomiting and abdominal pain are less prominent clinical features. Headache, chills, and fever may also occur. These symptoms usually resolve within 48 hr. Gastrointestinal infection may disseminate in newborns, in persons with immunoincompetence, and in patients with chronic diseases. Bacteremia and meningitis may occur, and the mortality rate is about 3/1000.

Treatment. Oral or parenteral replacement of fluid and electrolytes is suggested for patients with gastroenteritis. The routine use of antimicrobial therapy is not indicated, as prolongation of carriage occurs in adults and relapses occur in children.

Many isolates are resistant to ampicillin, particularly salmonella acquired from animals fed tetracycline or other antimicrobial agents. Chloramphenicol, trimethoprim-sulfamethoxazole, or a third-generation cephalosporin such as cefotaxime or ceftriaxone should be included in the initial therapy of patients with bacteremia or meningitis. Uncomplicated salmonella gastroenteritis should be treated in the neonate, in patients undergoing immunosuppressive therapy, and in the chronically ill.

Staphylococcal Food Poisoning

Ingestion of foodstuffs contaminated by enterotoxigenic strains of *Staphylococcus aureus* or, less commonly, coagulase-negative staphylococci is one of the major causes of epidemic food poisoning in the United States (Sec. 11.17). Between 1977 and 1981, 131 outbreaks involving 7126 persons in 42 states were reported to the Centers for Disease Control.

Epidemiology. Contamination of food by *S. aureus* results from improper storage of previously cooked, proteinaceous food or from poor hygiene by food handlers. Whereas milk and milk products are the most frequently identified sources of staphylococcal poisoning, ham, salads containing potatoes or eggs, and cream-filled baked goods account for 50% of the outbreaks. Food that has been cooked but stored above 7° C for more than 4 hr is responsible for two thirds of the outbreaks. The remainder have been attributed to food handlers who were either staphylococcal carriers or who were actively infected.

Most epidemics occur wherever large numbers of people are fed from a common source. Fifty percent of the 131 outbreaks between 1977 and 1981 occurred in restaurants or schools, and 30% occurred at home.

From a public health standpoint, it is imperative to diagnose and confirm an outbreak of staphylococcal food poisoning.

1491

The acute onset of gastrointestinal illness in two or more individuals with exposure to a common food source should raise suspicion, which may be confirmed if one of the following are documented: (1) demonstration of staphylococcal enterotoxin in food; (2) identical staphylococcal phage types isolated from food, food handler, and patient; (3) identical phage types recovered from six or more persons; or (4) presence of more than 10^5 colony-forming units of *S. aureus* per gram of food.

Pathogenesis. Staphylococcal gastroenteritis is caused by the ingestion of one of five immunologically distinct enterotoxins: A, B, C, D, and E. Enterotoxin A is the most frequently encountered; enterotoxins C and D are often associated with milk outbreaks whose incidence has decreased in recent years. All of the staphylococcal enterotoxins produce an identical clinical syndrome, but the mechanisms by which they produce disease are unknown. Staphylococcal enterotoxins do not directly affect the gut or mucosal lining. Recent evidence suggests that the effector site for the toxin is within the autonomic nervous system.

Clinical Manifestations. The incubation period between ingestion and the onset of clinical symptoms is about 4 hr (range 1–8 hr). Usually, nausea and abdominal pain precede vomiting and diarrhea. The illness is generally self-limited, resolving within 48 hr.

Treatment. Hospitalization for the correction of fluid and electrolyte abnormalities is rarely required. Parenteral rehydration may be required in severe cases. There is no antitoxin available, and the mortality rate is 0.03%, with most fatalities occurring in the severely debilitated.

Clostridium Botulinum Food Poisoning (Botulism)

Clostridium botulinum is an unusual cause of foodborne illness in the United States. Over the last decade, approximately 40 cases per year have been reported; most have occurred in infants. (See Sec. 11.39 for clinical manifestations and treatment.)

The ingestion of preformed toxin is responsible for the clinical manifestations of botulism in adults, whereas gastrointestinal colonization with toxin-producing strains causes the illness in infants. Eight antigenically distinct but physiologically similar neurotoxins have been identified: A, B, C_1, C_2, D, E, F, and G. Botulinum toxin affects the peripheral nervous system by blocking the presynaptic release of acetylcholine. Although the exact mechanism of inhibition of release of acetylcholine is unclear, in vitro studies have shown that the toxin negatively influences Ca^{++}-dependent acetylcholine release. Higher than physiologic concentrations of Ca^{++} are required to counter the action of the neurotoxin.

Because the spores of *Clostridium botulinum* are ubiquitous, contamination of foodstuffs occurs frequently. Anaerobic conditions, temperatures below 121° C, and pH above 4.5 are required for bacterial growth and toxin production. Most outbreaks of botulism are associated with improperly canned foods, particularly with foods that have been canned at home. The incidence of botulism is particularly high in Alaska, where local dishes such as fermented fish heads and seal flippers have been linked to outbreaks. In infants, honey is frequently identified as a source of poisoning.

Botulinum toxin serotypes causing infantile botulism have a distinct geographic distribution in the United States; west of the Mississippi River, most sporadic cases are caused by *C. botulinum* type A, whereas eastern cases tend to involve type B. Type F has also been identified from infants with botulism.

Other Bacterial Food Poisonings

Clostridium perfringens. In the United Kingdom, the incidence of food poisoning caused by *C. perfringens* is second only to salmonella in frequency; in the United States it is comparable to that of shigella. Meat products other than poultry are the typical sources of outbreaks. Following ingestion of contaminated foodstuffs, the organism replicates in the small intestine, producing a heat-labile enterotoxin. The toxin acts throughout the small intestine, where it impairs glucose absorption and promotes secretion of fluid. (See Sec. 11.38 for clinical manifestations and treatment.)

Bacillus cereus. This is an unusual cause of food poisoning in the United States. Outbreaks have resulted from the ingestion of contaminated Chinese food, lamb, and vegetables. Illness results either from the ingestion of preformed toxin or from gastrointestinal colonization and subsequent in vivo toxin production. The toxin activates intestinal adenyl cyclase, resulting in hyperperistalsis and secretory diarrhea. Ingestion of the preformed toxin gives rise to a clinical syndrome indistinguishable from that of staphylococcal food poisoning. Gastrointestinal colonization produces a syndrome with a longer incubation period. In both instances, the illness is self-limited and does not typically require specific therapy.

Vibrio parahaemolyticus. This also is an unusual cause of food poisoning in the United States. Because this is a marine organism, ingestion of raw or improperly prepared seafood is the most common source of outbreaks. The organism produces a hemolysin, which causes gastrointestinal hypersecretion in vitro. The organism is also capable of invading the intestinal mucosa. Abdominal pain, diarrhea, vomiting, and nausea occur 4–96 hr after consumption of contaminated food. The illness is self-limited, usually resolving within 72 hr without specific therapy.

28.2 NONBACTERIAL FOOD POISONING

Mushroom Poisoning

The consumption of wild mushrooms, a favorite pastime in Europe, is becoming increasingly popular in the United States, with concomitant increases in fatal cases of mushroom poisoning.

There are 4 clinical syndromes and 7 classes of toxins associated with wild mushroom poisoning. The clinical syndromes are divided according to the predominant system involved and the rapidity of onset of symptoms. The toxins produced by wild mushrooms are categorized as follows: cyclopeptides, monomethylhydrazine, muscarine, coprine, ibotenic acid, psilocybin, and unknown.

Gastrointestinal–Delayed Onset. *Amanita Poisoning.* Poisoning from species of *Amanita* and *Galerina* account for 95% of the fatalities from mushroom intoxication, although the mortality rate for this group is 5–10%. Most species produce 2 classes of cyclopeptide toxins: (1) phalloidins, which are heptapeptides believed to be responsible for the early symptoms of *Amanita* poisoning; and (2) amanitotoxin, which is an octapeptide that inhibits RNA polymerase and subsequent production of messenger RNA. Cells with high turnover rates, such as those in the gastrointestinal mucosa, kidney, and liver, are the most severely affected.

Histopathologically, *Amanita* poisoning causes cellular necrosis which may occur throughout the gastrointestinal tract, the most heavily exposed site. Acute yellow atrophy of the liver and necrosis of the proximal renal tubules are found in lethal cases.

The clinical course produced by poisoning with *Amanita* or *Galerina* species is biphasic, after an initial 6–12 hr latent period. Six to 24 hr following ingestion, patients develop nausea, vomiting, and severe abdominal pain. Profuse, watery diarrhea follows shortly thereafter and may last for 12–24 hr. During this time, as much as 9 liters of fluid may be lost. Twenty-four to 48 hr after poisoning, jaundice, hypertransaminasemia (peaking at 72–96 hr), renal failure, and coma are noted. Death occurs 4–7 days after the ingestion.

The treatment of *Amanita* poisoning is both supportive and specific. Fluid loss during the early course of the illness is profound, requiring aggressive replacement therapy in patients with severe diarrhea. In the late phase of the disease, management of renal and hepatic failure is also necessary.

Specific therapy for *Amanita* poisoning is designed to remove the toxin rapidly and to block binding at its target site. Because amanitotoxin may be recovered from the duodenum up to 36 hr after ingestion, aspiration of duodenal contents will significantly decrease toxin load. Charcoal hemoperfusion is recommended in severe poisonings (two or more mushrooms). Forced diuresis should be avoided, as this increases renal exposure.

Although cytochrome C protects mice from lethal doses of amanitotoxin, clinical trials with this agent have been inconclusive. Intravenous penicillin G (250 mg/kg/24 hr) administered as a continuous infusion may offer some protection. Thioctic acid has been shown to be effective in several studies; it is administered intravenously, often in combination with penicillin, in a dosage of 100–200 mg every 6 hr. Although corticosteroids and vitamin B complexes have also been used in the treatment of *Amanita* poisoning, their therapeutic efficacy has not been demonstrated.

Monomethylhydrazine Intoxication. Species of *Gyromitra* contain monomethylhydrazine (CH_3NHNH_2), which inhibits central nervous system (CNS) enzymatic production of gamma-aminobutyric acid (GABA). Monomethylhydrazine also oxidizes iron in hemoglobin, resulting in methemoglobinemia. Patients with *Gyromitra* poisoning develop vomiting, diarrhea, hematochezia, and abdominal pain within 6–24 hr of ingestion of the toxin. Symptoms of CNS depression and seizures develop later in the clinical course. Hemolysis and methemoglobinemia are potential life-threatening complications of monomethylhydrazine poisoning. Severe methemoglobinemia may require dialysis.

Hypovolemia from gastrointestinal fluid losses and seizures require supportive intervention. Pyridoxal phosphate, the coenzyme that catalyzes the production of GABA, can reverse the effects of monomethylhydrazine when administered in high dosages. Pyridoxine hydrochloride (25 mg/kg) is administered intravenously at a frequency dependent on clinical improvement. Parenteral administration of methylene blue is indicated if the methemoglobin concentration exceeds 30%. Blood transfusions may be required for significant hemolysis.

Autonomic Nervous System–Rapid Onset. *Muscarine Poisoning.* Mushrooms of the genera *Inocybe* and, to a lesser degree, *Clitocybe* contain muscarine or muscarine-related compounds. These quaternary ammonium derivatives bind to postsynaptic receptors, producing an exaggerated cholinergic response.

The clinical syndrome is characterized by the following hypercholinergic response: the onset of symptoms is rapid (30 min–2 hr after consumption) and consists of diaphoresis, excessive lacrimation, salivation, miosis, urinary and fecal incontinence, and vomiting. Respiratory distress caused by bronchospasm and increased bronchopulmonary secretions is the most serious complication. The symptoms subside spontaneously within 6–24 hr.

Atropine sulfate, the specific antidote, is administered intravenously (0.1 mg/kg). This is repeated until the pulmonary symptoms resolve or the patient becomes overtly tachycardic.

Coprine Ingestion. *Coprinus atramentarius* and *Clitocybe clavipes* contain coprine. Like disulfiram (Antabuse), coprine inhibits the metabolism of acetaldehyde following ethanol ingestion. The clinical symptomatology results from accumulation of acetaldehyde.

Coprine intoxication becomes apparent after ethanol ingestion and may occur up to 5 days after consuming the mushroom. Hyperemia of the face and trunk, tingling of the hands, metallic taste, tachycardia, and vomiting occur acutely. Hypotension may result from intense peripheral vasodilatation.

The syndrome is typically self-limited and lasts only several hours. No specific antidote is available. If hypotension is severe, vascular reexpansion with isotonic parenteral solutions may be required. Small doses of oral propranolol have also been suggested.

Central Nervous System–Rapid Onset. *Ibotenic Acid and Muscimol Intoxication.* Although *Amanita muscaria* and *Amanita pantherina* may contain muscarine (see above), the toxins responsible for the central nervous system symptoms following ingestion of these mushrooms are muscimol and ibotenic acid. Muscimol, a hallucinogen, and ibotenic acid, an insecticide, have an anticholinergic effect. One half to 2 hr following ingestion, ataxia, hallucinations, and euphoria occur. Nausea and vomiting may be associated. With large ingestions, coma and seizures may also develop. If large amounts of muscarine are contained in the mushroom, symptoms of cholinergic crisis may also occur.

Specific therapy must be carefully selected. If an exaggerated cholinergic response is observed, atropine should be administered. Because ingestions of *A. muscaria* are frequently associated with anticholinergic findings, the acetylcholinesterase inhibitor physostigmine is used to reverse the delirium and coma.

Indole Intoxication. Mushrooms belonging to the genus *Psilocybe* ("magic mushrooms") contain psilocybin and psilocin, two psychotropic compounds. Within half an hour after ingestion, patients develop euphoria and hallucinations, often accompanied by tachycardia and mydriasis. Fever and seizures have also been observed in children with psilocybin poisoning. These symptoms are short-lived, usually lasting 6 hr after consumption of the mushroom. Severely agitated patients may respond to diazepam.

Gastrointestinal–Rapid Onset. Many mushrooms from a variety of genera produce local gastrointestinal symptoms. The causative toxins are diverse and largely unknown.

Within an hour of ingestion, patients develop acute abdominal pain, nausea, vomiting, and diarrhea. Symptoms may last from hours to days, depending on the species.

Treatment is mainly supportive. Patients with large fluid losses may require parenteral fluid therapy. It is imperative to differentiate ingestion of mushrooms of this class from ingestions of *Amanita* and *Galerina* species containing cyclopeptide toxins (see above).

Solanine Poisoning

Solanine is a mixture of several related toxins found in "greened" and sprouted potatoes. Potatoes exposed to light and allowed to sprout produce a number of alkaloidal glycosides containing the cholesterol derivative, solanidine. Two of these glycosides, alpha-solanine and alpha-chaconine, are found in highest concentration in the peels of greened potatoes and in the sprouts. The solanine alkaloids bind to serum cholinesterase, suggesting a possible pathophysiological mechanism.

Clinical manifestations of solanine intoxication occur within 7–19 hr after ingestion. The most common symptoms are vomiting and diarrhea; in more severe instances of poisoning, fever, generalized abdominal pain, coma, and hypovolemic shock occur.

Treatment of solanine poisoning is largely supportive. In the most severe cases, symptoms resolve within 11 days. Atropine treatment has not been evaluated.

Seafood Poisoning

Ciguatera Fish Poisoning. Major outbreaks of ciguatera fish poisoning have been reported in Florida, Hawaii, and the

Virgin Islands; however, with modern methods of transportation, the illness now occurs worldwide. Grouper is the most frequently identified source of the toxin, followed by snapper, kingfish, amberjack, dolphin, and barracuda.

The source of this poisoning is the dinoflagellate *Gambierdiscus toxicus*, a microscopic organism found in the food chain along coral reefs, which contains high concentrations of ciguatoxin and maitotoxin. After ingestion of the organism by small fish, the toxin is absorbed and concentrated in fish flesh and musculature. Larger fish consume the smaller fish, and again the toxin is absorbed from the gastrointestinal tract and concentrated in the musculature.

Ciguatoxin, a lipid with a molecular weight of approximately 1100 daltons, increases the sodium permeability of excitable membranes. This action is inhibited by calcium and tetrodotoxin.

The onset of symptoms following ingestion of fish containing ciguatoxin is rapid, usually occurring within 2–30 hr. The illness is often biphasic. The earliest symptoms are diarrhea, vomiting, and abdominal pain; the second phase includes myalgias and circumoral or extremity dysesthesias. The dysesthesia is characterized by reversal of hot and cold sensation. Tachycardia, bradycardia, and hypertension occur infrequently.

Treatment of ciguatera fish poisoning is supportive. Gastric lavage is recommended to remove any remaining toxin. Intravenous fluids may be required for severe diarrhea, and parenteral administration of calcium can be used to treat hypotension. Most cases are self-limited; symptoms may last up to 3 wk.

Scombroid (Pseudoallergic) Fish Poisoning. Epidemics have been associated with the ingestion of members of the *Scombresocidae* or *Scombridae* families, notably albacore, mackerel, tuna, bonita, and kingfish. Nonscombroid fish and marine mammals, such as mahi-mahi (dolphin) and bluefish, have also been linked to outbreaks of poisoning.

Although the identity of "scombrotoxin" remains unknown, the product of the action of the toxin on fish flesh, histamine, appears to be responsible for the clinical syndrome. Histidine is found in high concentrations in the flesh of scombroid fish; the action of bacterial decarboxylases during putrification converts the histidine to histamine. Fish containing greater than 20 mg of histamine per 100 g of flesh are toxic. In patients receiving isoniazid, a potent histaminase-blocker, ingestion of fish flesh containing lower concentrations of histamine may be toxic.

The onset of clinical illness is acute and occurs within 10 min–2 hr following ingestion. The most common symptoms include diarrhea, flushing, diaphoresis, urticaria, nausea, and headache. Abdominal pain, tachycardia, oral burning, dizziness, respiratory distress, and facial swelling also occur. The illness is usually self-limited, terminating within 8–10 hr.

Treatment is mainly supportive. Gastric lavage decreases continued absorption of histamine. With severe diarrhea, fluid replacement may be necessary. Antihistamines have been variably successful. Four patients with severe toxicity treated with cimetidine (a histamine blocker) responded rapidly. Since data are limited, cimetidine or ranitidine should be reserved for severe cases.

Paralytic Shellfish Poisoning. Filter-feeding mollusks, such as the black mussel and sea scallop, may become contaminated during dinoflagellate blooms, or "red tides." The dinoflagellates *Gonyaulax catenella, G. tamerensis,* and *G. grindleyi* are often responsible for these "red tides" and contain several potent neurotoxins. Saxitoxin is the most important of the neurotoxins responsible for paralytic shellfish poisoning. This toxin prevents nerve conduction by inhibiting the sodium-potassium pump. Although 6 other toxins have been isolated from contaminated scallops, these toxins may be bioconverted to less toxic structures.

The onset of clinical symptoms of paralytic shellfish poisoning occurs rapidly, 30 min–2 hr after ingestion. Paresthesias are the most common complaints and occur circumorally or in a stocking-glove distribution, or both. Vertigo, ataxia, and the sensation of floating occur less commonly. In severe cases, respiratory failure due to diaphragmatic paralysis may result.

There is no known antidote for paralytic shellfish poisoning. Supportive care, including mechanical ventilation, may be needed. Although the symptoms are usually self-limited and short-lived, weakness and malaise may persist for weeks following ingestion.

STEPHEN C. ARONOFF

Salmonella

Holmberg SD, Osterholm MT, Senger KA, et al: Drug-resistant salmonella from animals fed antimicrobials. N Engl J Med 311:617, 1984.
Public Health Laboratory Service: Food poisoning and Salmonella surveillance in England and Wales: 1982. Br Med J 288:306, 1984.

Staphylococcal Food Poisoning

Breckinridge JC, Bergdoll MS: Outbreak of food-borne gastroenteritis due to a coagulase-negative enterotoxin-producing staphylococcus. N Engl J Med 284:541, 1972.
Carpenter CCJ: Mechanisms of bacterial diarrheas. Am J Med 68:313, 1980.
Holmberg SD, Blake PA: Staphylococcal food poisoning in the United States: New facts and old misconceptions. JAMA 251:457, 1984.

Botulism

CDC. Botulism in the United States, 1979. J Infect Dis 142:302, 1980.

Vibro Parahaemolyticus

Rodrick GE, Hood MA, Blake NJ: Human *Vibrio* gastroenteritis. Med Clin North Am 66:665, 1982.

Mushroom Poisoning

Editorial: Mushroom poisoning. Lancet 2:351, 1980.
Hanrahan JP, Gordon MA: Mushroom poisoning. Case reports and a review of therapy. JAMA 251:1057, 1984.
Litten W: The most poisonous mushrooms. Sci Am 232:90, 1975.
McCormick DJ, Avbel AJ, Biggons RB: Nonlethal mushroom poisoning. Ann Intern Med 90:332, 1979.
McDonald A: Mushrooms and madness. Hallucinogenic mushrooms and some psychopharmacological implications. Canad J Psychiatr 25:586, 1980.
Mitchell DH: Amanita mushroom poisoning. Ann Rev Med 31:51, 1980.
Rumack BH (ed): POISINDEX®, A Computerized Poison Information System. 44th ed. Micromedex, Inc., Englewood, CO, 1985.

Solanine Poisoning

Editorial: Potatoe poisoning. Lancet 2:681, 1979.
McMillan M, Thompson JC: An outbreak of suspected solanine poisoning in school boys: Examination of criteria of solanine poisoning. Q J Med 48:227, 1979.

Scombroid Fish Poisoning

Blakesley ML: Scombroid poisoning: Prompt resolution of symptoms with cimetidine. Ann Emerg Med 12:104, 1983.
Gilbert RJ, Hobbs G, Murray CK, et al: Scombrotoxic fish poisoning: Features of the first 50 incidents to be reported in Britain (1976–9). Br Med J 281:71, 1980.
Uragoda CG: Histamine poisoning in tuberculous patients after ingestion of tuna fish. Am Rev Respir Dis 121:157, 1980.

Ciguatera Fish Poisoning

Lawrence DN, Enriquez MB, Lumish RM, et al: Ciguatera fish poisoning in Miami. JAMA 244:254, 1980.
Morris JG, Lewin P, Hargrett NT, et al: Clinical features of ciguatera fish poisoning. Arch Intern Med 142:1090, 1982.
Withers NW: Ciguatera fish poisoning. Ann Rev Med 33:97, 1982.

Paralytic Shellfish Poisoning

Hughes JM, Merson MH: Fish and shellfish poisoning. N Engl J Med 295:1117, 1976.
Popkiss MEE, Horstman DA, Harpur D: Paralytic shellfish poisoning: A report of 17 cases in Cape Town. South Afr Med J 55:1017, 1979.
Shimizu Y, Yoshioka M: Transformation of paralytic shellfish toxins as demonstrated in scallop homogenates. Science 212:547, 1981.

CHEMICAL AND DRUG POISONING

28.3 PRINCIPLES OF MANAGEMENT

In 1984, 251,012 poisoning cases were reported by the 16 centers that participated in the National Data Collection System of the American Association of Poison Control Centers (AAPCC). More than 90% of the cases occurred in the home. Children age 5 yr and under accounted for 64.1% of all cases. Accidental cases composed 87.1%, while 5.4% were reported as suicidal. More than 90% of instances involved a single substance. Only 95 fatalities were reported: 10 in those 5 yr of age or less; 0 in those 6–12 yr; 3 in those 13–17 yr; and 82 in those greater than 17 yr old. Extrapolation of these data would indicate more than 2.3 million total exposures to poisons throughout the United States for all reasons.

The AAPCC data likely represent some skewing of cases away from reports of suicide with heavier emphasis on accidental cases, owing to the kinds of questions referred to a poison center. Many suicidal patients are taken directly to an emergency facility, which may or may not report to or request consultation from a poison information center. The peak age of suicide attempts for children is 13–17 yr (Sec. 2.44 and 9.3). Thus, pediatricians have to contend with two major groups of children in regard to poisoning: (1) those age 5 and under exposed to plants, household products, medications, and so on; and (2) the adolescent exposed most frequently to medications. Once the diagnosis of poisoning or potential poisoning is entertained, the pediatrician should follow a specific management plan to ensure optimum care.

Management Plan for Poisoning and Overdose

Initial contact with a poisoned patient will usually be over the telephone. The following data should be obtained at the time of initial contact.

Phone Number. Getting the caller's telephone number is necessary in case the phone contact is accidentally broken and to permit follow-up calls.

Address. This may be crucial if emergency equipment needs to be dispatched or if the person on the phone becomes hysterical or develops lethargy, convulsions, etc.

Evaluation of Severity. Although many callers may begin with a description of symptoms or signs such as a convulsion, it is vital to evaluate the current status of the patient in terms of immediate danger, potential danger, and no danger. Further history may be necessary to evaluate an asymptomatic patient.

Weight and Age. This permits estimation of potential toxicity.

Time of Ingestion. This permits interpretation of onset of symptoms or signs as well as evaluation of laboratory data and other prognostic information.

Past Medical History. Brief information should be elicited to determine the usual health status of the patient as a basis for interpreting signs. It will also suggest interactions of chronic medications or allergies with the current ingestion.

Type of Exposure. Product names and ingredients should be obtained from labels or, if unavailable, from the POISIN-DEX.

Amount of Exposure. How many tablets or how much fluid has been consumed should be estimated. Pills or fluid remaining in the container should be counted or measured.

Route of Exposure. It should be determined if the exposure was by ingestion, inhalation, local application to the eyes or skin, or parenteral route.

Such basic information should be a standard procedure in every office or clinic where such cases may be reported. Written records should be kept of each event. It may be acceptable practice either to see the patient or to treat and observe the patient at home, depending on the exposure and patient's condition. If treatment is at home, then follow-up calls *must* be made at approximately 1/2, 1, and 4 hr after exposure. Any change in the patient's condition may warrant a change in the decision to treat at home. Since as many as half the histories obtained from poisoned patients will have an error of some magnitude, the physician must be ready to change treatment or disposition decisions in light of changes in onset of symptoms or new history. Lomotil is an example of a drug for which even careful follow-up may be inadequate. Owing to the idiosyncratic nature of its ingestion, *all* children consuming this drug under age 6 yr *must* be hospitalized and monitored for 24 hr; delayed onset of coma for 8–12 hr requires that these patients receive intensive medical observation.

Initial Medical Care

If after telephone consultation or direct primary evaluation the decision is made to have the patient seen by others, transportation appropriate to the patient's condition should be arranged. The site of initial medical contact should also be considered in relation to the exposure history. For example, if it is expected that respiratory support will be required, then paramedic transport to a well-equipped emergency facility is mandatory. Once the decision is made, then the receiving personnel should be notified so that proper preparation can be made, including notification of the poison center if that has not yet been done. Prior to transport, all product containers thought likely to be related to the exposure should be gathered up and brought with the patient. If the patient has vomited spontaneously or by induction with syrup of ipecac, this emesis should be saved and brought with the patient.

Once the patient has arrived in the appropriate medical care setting, initial attention should focus on life support with primary emphasis on cardiorespiratory care. Shock, arrhythmias, and convulsions must be dealt with as in the case of any other critically ill patient (Sec. 5.38–5.40). There are few poisons for which there is an antidote. Except for the few poisons listed below, specific treatment directed at the poison can be delayed until the physician is satisfied that the patient's condition is stable. The following poisons require simultaneous use of an antagonist with life support measures:

Carbon Monoxide. Oxygen (100%) should be administered as early as possible to reduce the concentration of carbon monoxide in the blood and increase oxygen transport to tissues. Symptomatic patients or those with high levels may be candidates for hyperbaric oxygen therapy.

Cyanide. Oxygen should be supplied immediately, followed by specific antidotal treatment. Although the antidote currently available in the United States is not ideal, appropriate doses should be administered to a symptomatic patient with cyanide poisoning. The antidote kit contains (1) amyl nitrite inhalers that may be broken under the patient's nose for 30 sec of each minute, while the sodium nitrite solution is being readied; (2) sodium nitrite 3% solution should be administered at a dose of 0.33 mL/kg (10 mg/kg) to a maximum dose of 10 mL/patient with normal hemoglobin; (3) sodium thiosulfate 25% solution should be administered next at a dose of 1.65 mL/kg to a maximum dose of the entire ampoule. These agents produce methemoglobin, which may help remove cyanide by competition for the cytochrome. An alternative antidote, a hydroxocobalamin-thiosulfate mixture, is available outside the United States; it should be given in doses of 4–10 g. Hydroxocobalamin alone cannot be given in sufficient quantity to be effective.

Opiates and Related Poisons. Naloxone in sufficient doses is very effective in treating these poisonings. A minimum dose of 0.4 mg can be given to any patient, regardless of age or weight. If there is failure of response, up to 2.0 mg should be administered rapidly intravenously to larger children and adolescents. Newborns to infants 6 mo of age should be given a second dose of 0.8 mg.

Substances Producing Methemoglobinemia. Although relatively uncommon, exposure to aniline dyes, nitrobenzene, azo compounds, and nitrites may produce methemoglobinemia that is unresponsive to oxygen administration. The diagnosis is suggested by comparing a drop of the patient's blood with that of the physician. If there is at least 15% methemoglobinemia, the patient's blood will be relatively brown when dried on a sheet of filter paper; the color would be red at a lower percentage of methemoglobin. Methylene blue at a dose of 0.1–0.2 mL/kg (1–2 mg/kg) of a 1% solution is therapeutic. If two doses are unsuccessful, exchange transfusion may be required.

Cholinergic Agents. Children exposed to organophosphate insecticides and carbamates may develop salivation, lacrimation, urination, defecation, and fasciculations. Atropine at a dose of 0.05 mg/kg to a maximum initial dose of 1–2 mg should be administered while the patient is being decontaminated with soap and water. Repeated doses of atropine may be necessary if the patient is unresponsive. In severe cases or when the cholinesterase level falls to 25% of normal or lower, pralidoxime, a cholinesterase regenerator, may be indicated. The dosage is 250 mg/dose slowly intravenously every 8–12 hr in young children, to a maximum of 1 g/dose in older children.

Other "Antidotes." These are not generally required immediately and may be administered after the diagnosis is confirmed, e.g., ethanol for ethylene glycol or methanol poisoning, or N-acetyl-L-cysteine for acetaminophen overdose.

Preventing Absorption

The goal of these procedures is to reduce the amount of the poison taken up by the body. In some cases, this may be preventative (e.g., a child who ingested something just prior to calling the physician may have absorbed very little). In other cases, it may be desirable to reduce further absorption (e.g., oral activated charcoal following oral or intravenous theophylline overdosage). Before using any of these techniques, their safety should be evaluated for the particular child.

Emesis. Administration of syrup of ipecac, 15–30 mL, followed by a clear liquid such as water results in vomiting in over 95% of children under the age of 5 yr. The airway may be protected by positioning the patient on the left side with the head down (spanking position). Emesis should not be induced if the patient is comatose, convulsing, or has ingested strong acids or bases. Treatment of hydrocarbon ingestions with emesis is controversial (Sec. 28.6). Emesis should be avoided when there is a significant risk of aspiration. Data in adolescents and adults have brought into question whether emesis affects outcome; it produces only an average of 8–30% recovery of ingested material. The initial emesis should be saved for diagnostic analysis. Apomorphine is contraindicated in children and adolescents.

Lavage. Gastric washout is relatively fast and about as effective as emesis. Complications in adults have included esophageal perforation. It is probably unsafe in young children in whom there may be airway obstruction and in whom cuffed endotracheal tubes cannot be used. Only in rare instances does lavage change the outcome of poisoning. If the procedure is done, warm saline should be used in young children and warm tap water in older children; a large bore tube, 32–36 French, should be employed in order to remove fragments of tablets and capsules.

Charcoal. The administration of a good grade of activated charcoal (*not* burned toast or universal antidote) may be the most effective and safest procedure to prevent absorption. Charcoal is capable of adsorbing almost all drugs and many other chemicals. It should be given as a water slurry with a minimum dose of 30–50 g in a child and 50–100 g in an adolescent. Repeat doses of 20 g should be administered every 2 hr until the charcoal appears in the stool. Super activated carbon is three to five times as adsorptive as regular charcoal and comes premixed in a liquid.

Cathartic. Sorbitol (maximum 1 g/kg), magnesium sulfate (maximum 250 mg/kg), sodium citrate (maximum 250 mg/kg), or phosphosoda (maximum 250 mg/kg) can be used to hasten emptying of the gastrointestinal tract once the ingested material has passed through the stomach. These agents should be used cautiously in young children. They may be useful in older children following administration of activated charcoal, especially for hydrocarbons and agents that delay bowel motility.

Enhancing Excretion

Forced diuresis is an overused technique for treating poisoned children. It has little general use, and its administration is even questionable in phenobarbital and salicylate ingestion, since alkalinization without diuresis may be just as effective. Acid diuresis is contraindicated for agents such as amphetamines, phencyclidine, and so on, owing to aggravation of renal problems with myoglobinuria and methoglobinemia.

Hemodialysis, once heralded as the answer to many poisonings, is now used rarely and selectively. Many drugs have very large volumes of distribution so that even if there is good clearance by dialysis, total body removal may be extremely small. For example, after a digoxin or tricyclic antidepressant overdose, only a small percentage of the drug can be removed by dialysis. The major indications for hemodialysis are severe salicylate intoxication unresponsive to standard care, poisoning with methanol and ethylene glycol with blood levels above 20 mg/dL and acidosis, and symptomatic theophylline overdoses with blood levels at 60–100 μg/dL or higher.

Hemoperfusion over activated charcoal or resin may be helpful in some situations when there is a small volume of distribution and the agent is well adsorbed. It may be valuable in theophylline, salicylate, and paraquat poisoning of patients who have not responded well to other forms of therapy. It is not recommended for poisonings with tricyclics, acetaminophen, digoxin, etc., as it does not remove substantial amounts of total body load or change the clinical outcome.

Laboratory Evaluation

In some cases (e.g., salicylates, acetaminophen, iron, methanol, and ethylene glycol), the laboratory provides data sufficient to change the treatment plan. In other instances (e.g., opiates, in which there is definitive treatment unrelated to levels, and cyanide, in which it would be too late if the physician waited for laboratory assistance), the laboratory data may be helpful but will not likely change treatment. "Drug screens" are generally not helpful. The best way to use the laboratory is to discuss the case with the technologist and provide appropriate samples and clinical data so that specific analysis can be interpreted. There is little use in doing certain portions of the screen if it is already known what the patient has consumed and that symptoms are consistent with its toxicity. If a "toxic screen" is obtained, it is important to know the specific drugs that are included in the test.

Bayer MJ, Rumack BH, Wanke LA: Toxicologic Emergencies. Bowie, MD, Brady-Prentice Hall, 1984.

Blumer JL, Reed MD (eds): Pediatric Toxicology. Pediatr Clin North Am 33(2), 1986.

Dine MS, McGoven ME: Intentional poisoning of children: An overlooked category of child abuse. Pediatrics 70:32, 1982.

Goldfrank LR: Toxicologic Emergencies: A Comprehensive Handbook of Problem Solving. New York, Appleton-Century-Crofts, 1982.
Matthew H, Lawson AAH: Treatment of Common Acute Poisonings. 4th ed. New York, Churchill-Livingstone, 1979.
Rumack BH: POISINDEX®, A Computerized Poison Information System. 47th ed. Englewood, CO, Micromedex Inc, 1986.
Rumack BH: Poisoning. In: Kempe CH, Silver HR, O'Brien D (eds): Current Pediatrics Therapy. Los Altos, CA, Lange Medical Publications, 1984.
Rumack BH, Rosen P: Emesis: Safe and Effective? Ann Emerg Med 10:551, 1981.
Veltri JC, Litovitz TL: 1983 Annual Report of the American Association of Poison Control Centers National Data Collection System. Am J Emerg Med 2:420, 1984.

28.4 ACETAMINOPHEN

Acetaminophen has become the most widely used analgesic antipyretic, owing, in part, to the finding of a relationship between Reye syndrome and salicylates (Sec. 12.82). Consequently, acetaminophen is more available for accidental or intentional use by young children and adolescents in the home. There are significant differences in the degree of toxicity that may occur in children under age 6 yr and in the older child.

Pathophysiology. Acetaminophen is primarily metabolized to the sulfate or glucuronide (94%), and the shift from sulfate to glucuronide predominance between ages 9–12 yr parallels the change in degree of toxicity at these ages. A small amount of acetaminophen is excreted unchanged, and the remaining approximately 4% is metabolized via cytochrome P450 and glutathione to the mercapturic acid conjugate. This latter pathway produces the toxicity of acetaminophen; when hepatic stores of glutathione are depleted to less than 70% of normal, the highly reactive intermediate metabolites combine with hepatic macromolecules and produce cellular damage.

Although therapeutic peak plasma levels of acetaminophen usually occur at 1–2 hr when hepatic function is normal, measurement prior to 4 hr cannot be used to determine the severity of an overdose. If there is pre-existing hepatic disease, or if the therapeutic half-life ($t_{1/2}$) is measured after the onset of hepatotoxicity, then the $t_{1/2}$ may be extended to 4 or more hours. Because the $t_{1/2}$ primarily reflects the sulfate and glucuronide pathways and not the toxic metabolite, it does not relate to the degree of toxicity. The volume of distribution is approximately 1 L/kg and does not vary with the quantity of absorbed drug as does salicylate.

Clinical and Laboratory Manifestations. Untreated overdose patients pass through four stages of toxicity (Table 28–1). Without a history of ingestion or high index of suspicion the pediatrician may not diagnose the ingestion. If there is a history of acetaminophen ingestion, plasma level should be assessed at 4 or more hours after ingestion. Interpretation of this level should be plotted on the nomogram (Fig. 28–1) to determine whether antidotal treatment is indicated. SGOT, SGPT, bilirubin, and prothrombin time should be followed

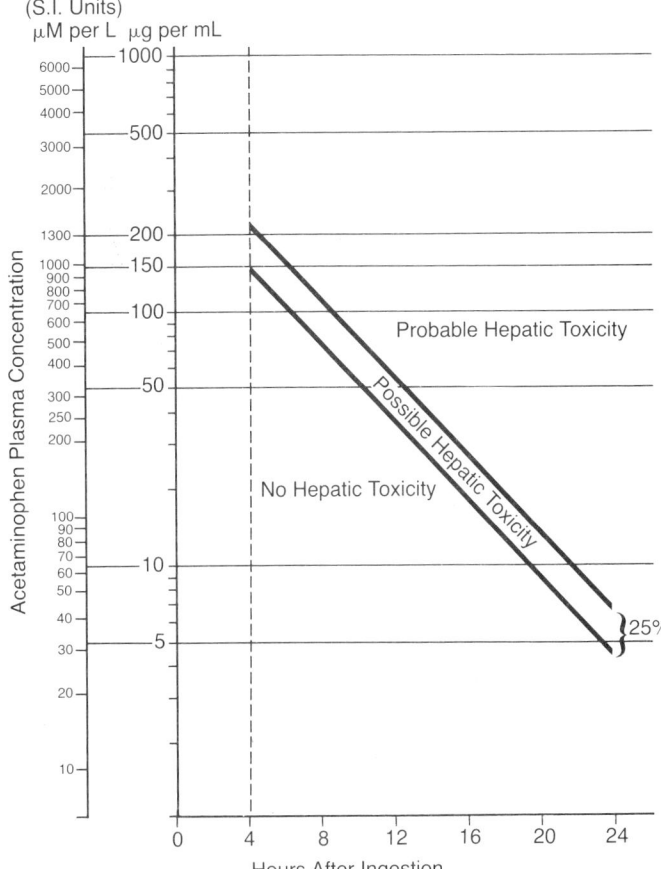

Figure 28–1. Rumack-Matthew nomogram for acetaminophen poisoning. Semi-logarithmic plot of plasma acetaminophen levels versus time. *Cautions for the use of this chart:* (1) the time coordinates refer to time after *ingestion.* (2) Serum levels drawn before 4 hr may not represent peak levels. (3) The graph should be used only in relation to a single acute ingestion. (4) The lower solid line 25% below the standard nomogram is included to allow for possible errors in acetaminophen plasma assays and estimated time from ingestion of an overdose. (From Rumack BH: POISINDEX: A COMPUTERIZED POISON INFORMATION SYSTEM. Ed 47. Copyright © Micromedex, Inc., Denver, CO, 1986. Adapted from Rumack BH, Matthew H: Acetaminophen poisoning and toxicity. Pediatrics 55:871–876, 1975.)

daily in all patients with levels in the toxic range on the nomogram.

Treatment. Therapy of patients with potentially toxic plasma levels of acetaminophen as determined from the nomogram is most effective if oral N-acetyl-L-cysteine (Mucomyst) is administered prior to 16 hr postingestion. It should be administered until up to 24 hr after ingestion, and the mode of administration should be as an initial loading dose of 140 mg/kg. Follow-up doses of 70 mg/kg should be given at 4 hr intervals for 17 additional doses (3 days). The drug should be diluted to a 5% concentration, which may be swallowed by the patient or instilled into the stomach or duodenum by gastric tube.

Intravenous use of this agent is not possible in the United States since there is no approved nonpyrogenic form. Additionally, the incidence of hepatotoxicity is significantly higher with intravenous N-acetyl-L-cysteine (58%) than with the oral form (29%). Cysteamine and methionine have been abandoned as therapies for this ingestion.

Prognosis. Children less than age 6 yr are unlikely to develop significant toxicity following ingestion of even relatively large doses of acetaminophen. In a large series, 55 of 417 developed potentially toxic plasma levels following inges-

Table 28–1. **Stages in the Clinical Course of Acetaminophen Toxicity**

Stage	Time Following Ingestion	Characteristics
I	½–24 hr	Anorexia, nausea, vomiting, malaise, pallor, diaphoresis
II	24–48 hr	Resolution of above; upper quadrant abdominal pain and tenderness; elevated bilirubin, prothrombin time, hepatic enzymes; oliguria
III	72–96 hr	Peak liver function abnormalities; anorexia, nausea, vomiting, malaise may reappear
IV	4 days–2 wk	Resolution of hepatic dysfunction

tion, but only 3 of the 417 developed SGOT peaks of greater than 1000 IU/L, which is considered a toxic response. In two other series totaling 2787 cases, there were none with toxic plasma levels, and only 35 hospitalized. Nevertheless, at this time children with a significant ingestion should have plasma level measured and receive treatment with the antidote if the level falls within the toxic range on the nomogram. Adolescents have a higher incidence (23.2%) of toxic plasma levels following ingestion than children, and 29% of those with toxic levels are likely to develop SGOT of greater than 1000 IU/L. Even after a serious case of hepatotoxicity, the mortality rate is well under 0.5%. Patients who recover have no sequelae when followed at 3–12 mo after the acute toxicity.

Lauterburg BH, Vaishnav Y, Stillwell WG, et al: The effects of age and glutathione depletion on hepatic glutathione turnover in vivo determined by acetaminophen probe analysis. J Pharmacol Exp Ther 213:54, 1980.

Linden CH, Rumack BH: Acetaminophen overdose. Emerg Clin North Am 2:103, 1984.

Mancini RE, Sonaware BR, Yaffe SJ: Developmental susceptibility to acetaminophen toxicity. Res Commun Chem Pathol Pharmacol 27:603, 1980.

Miller RP, Roberts RJ, Fisher LJ: Acetaminophen elimination kinetics in neonates, children, and adults. Clin Pharmacol Ther 19:284, 1976.

Mitchell JR, Jollow DJ, Potter WZ, et al: Acetaminophen-induced hepatic necrosis: I. Role of drug metabolism. J Pharmacol Exp Ther 187:185, 1973.

Peterson RG, Rumack BH: Age as a variable in acetaminophen overdose. Arch Intern Med 141:390, 1981.

Rumack BH: Acetaminophen overdose in young children. AJDC 138:428, 1984.

Rumack BH, Matthew H: Acetaminophen poisoning and toxicity. Pediatrics 55:871, 1975.

Rumack BH, Peterson RG: Acetaminophen overdose: Incidence, diagnosis and management in 416 patients. Pediatrics 62:898, 1978.

Rumack BH, Peterson RG, Koch GC, et al: Acetaminophen overdose: 662 cases with evaluation of oral acetylcysteine treatment. Arch Intern Med 141:380, 1981.

28.5 SALICYLATES

Incidence of ingestion of this drug has gradually dropped as the use of acetaminophen has increased. Toxicity related to salicylates must be considered in therapeutic situations as well as when there has been an overdose.

Pathopharmacology. Understanding the pharmocokinetics of salicylates permits a clearer evaluation of the plasma levels of salicylate and other laboratory data. The usual $t_{1/2}$ of salicylate is 1–2 hr. This may be extended to 25–30 hr once the urine becomes acidic and ion excretion becomes limited. The normal volume of distribution of salicylate is 0.15 L/kg, but with significant toxicity this may increase to 0.3–0.4 L/kg as protein binding is saturated and central nervous system and other distribution occurs. In cases of chronic toxicity, the metabolism of salicylates plays an insignificant role, urine excretion becomes minimal, and further doses add to the accumulated pool of drug in the patient.

Ionization of salicylate is related to the absorption and excretion of salicylate. In an alkaline state (e.g., urine of pH 7), this weak acid (pK approximately 3.0) is mostly ionized. Thus, it does not cross cell membranes very well and stays in the glomerular filtrate, permitting the drug to be excreted. As the urine pH becomes acid, less and less of the drug is ionized, reabsorption from glomerular filtrate occurs, and excretion decreases. Therapy directed at changing urine pH, therefore, affects urine excretion. In some circumstances, patients with various illnesses (e.g., juvenile rheumatoid arthritis) who are doing well on aspirin will suddenly develop problems after dietary changes. A large increase in use of orange juice, for example, will enhance excretion and reduce the plasma salicylate level, perhaps exacerbating the basic disease. Conversely, large ingestions of cranberry juice may acidify the urine, decrease excretion of salicylate, and raise plasma levels to toxic ranges.

Clinical Manifestations. Young infants may have few signs other than dehydration or hyperpnea. Temperature elevation

Table 28–2. Salicylate Intoxication

	Plasma pH*	Urine pH†
Phase 1	Alkaline	Alkaline
Phase 2	Alkaline	Acid
Phase 3	Acid	Acid

*Plasma pH is defined as alkaline or acid when it is above or below the normal range.

†Urine pH is defined as relatively alkaline above pH 6 and relatively acid when pH 6 or less.

may occur, leading to increased dosages of salicylates in a patient with salicylate toxicity. Older children demonstrate hyperpnea, vomiting, and progressive lethargy as the drug is distributed throughout the central nervous system. Tinnitus and sudden deafness may occur early in patients with salicylate toxicity. In adolescents, salicylate level measurement is required to distinguish hyperpnea from the "hyperventilation syndrome" (Sec. 5.34).

Although a large number of complex metabolic phenomena are involved following a salicylate ingestion, the clinically important relationships can be easily summarized. Table 28–2 lists the pH to be expected in each phase of salicylate intoxication in both plasma and urine. Understanding the progression permits a clear approach to diagnosis and treatment.

Phase 1. Salicylates directly stimulate the respiratory center following absorption. The increased respiratory rate results in respiratory alkalosis and obligate alkaluria as a compensatory mechanism. Both K^+ and Na^+ are lost along with bicarbonate in the urine. This phase may last for as long as 12 hr after ingestion in an adolescent and may be totally missed in a young infant.

Phase 2. When sufficient K^+ has been lost to deplete the kidney of this ion, an exchange of K^+ for H^+ occurs and the urine becomes relatively acid. The hypokalemia is initially limited to renal tissue and is not reflected either in serum K^+ or on the electrocardiogram. This "paradoxical aciduria" occurs in the presence of a continued respiratory alkalosis. As this phase progresses, hypokalemia is reflected throughout the rest of the body. This phase may begin within hours after ingestion in a young child and may last as long as 12–24 hr in an adolescent.

Phase 3. Eventually dehydration, hypokalemia, and progressive accumulation of lactic acid and other metabolic acids predominate over the respiratory alkalosis. The patient's rapid breathing is in response to the acidosis rather than to primary respiratory center drive. The plasma level of salicylate is generally higher than in phase 1 or 2 because of inability to excrete salicylate in an acid urine and because of continued absorption from the intestine. Uncoupling of oxidative phosphorylation and other metabolic activity contribute a small amount to this phenomenon. The patient is acidotic, with an even more acid urine. This phase may begin 4 to 6 hr after ingestion in a young infant, or 24 or more hr after ingestion in an adolescent. This is also the presentation of chronic salicylate poisoning following repeated therapeutic dosing in the face of dehydration.

The more severe cases may develop pulmonary edema or hemorrhage, although both of these complications are rare. Hyperglycemia or hypoglycemia has also been observed. Virtually all seriously poisoned patients will be more than 5% dehydrated, usually 10% or more.

Laboratory Data. Following a single acute ingestion of salicylate, plasma level should be measured 6 hr or more after ingestion and plotted on the nomogram (Fig. 28–2). Levels observed before 6 hr may not reflect peak levels. The nomogram cannot be used when the drug has accumulated over several ingestions, because patients with chronic salicylate

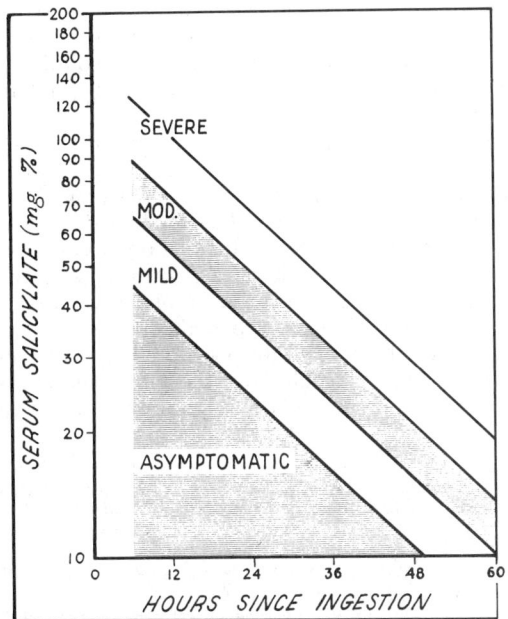

Figure 28–2. The Done nomogram for salicylate poisoning. *This nomogram should be used with the following cautions taken:* (1) The patient has taken a single acute ingestion and is not suffering from chronic toxicity. (2) The blood level to be plotted on the nomogram was drawn 6 hr after *ingestion*. (3) Levels in the toxic range drawn before 6 hr should be treated. (4) If levels measured before 6 hr are in the nontoxic range, further measurements should be taken to see if the level is increasing. (From Done AK: Salicylate intoxication. Significance of measurements of salicylate in blood in cases of acute ingestion. Pediatrics 26:800–807, 1960. Copyright 1960. Reproduced by permission of Pediatrics.)

toxicity may have very low levels in relation to the severity of their illness, owing to a 3- to 4-fold increase in the volume of distribution. Levels in chronic toxicity may be in the therapeutic range of 10–20 mL/dL.

In all patients with salicylate poisoning serious enough to be hospitalized, the plasma levels should be plotted on semilog paper against time. Although the concept of t½ is not precisely correct in salicylate overdoses, calculation of this value from these plots is important. By seeing whether the apparent t½ decreases with therapy, the success of that therapy can be monitored. As long as the relative t½ is greater than 10–15 hr, treatment is not optional.

Urine pH and volume should be measured hourly in all seriously poisoned children. Plasma pH should be done at regular intervals. K$^+$ and other electrolytes are critical to calculating replacement fluid therapy; serum K$^+$ will lag behind the K$^+$ status of the kidney. Prothrombin time should also be measured in all severely poisoned patients. Arterial blood gas measurements, as well as other ancillary laboratory measures required for the general support of the patient, should be performed. Hepatotoxicity from salicylate in severe, chronic cases will be demonstrated by SGOT, SGPT, bilirubin, and prothrombin abnormalities. Ferric chloride or Phenistix only indicate presence of the drug and should not be substituted for salicylate measurements. Neither of these tests will detect unhydrolized aspirin (acetylsalicylic acid) in tablets or vomitus.

Treatment. Dehydration and electrolyte abnormalities should be corrected after initiating activated charcoal, emesis, and other general acute measures (Sec. 5.29 and 28.3).

Phase 1. If this has been going on for several hours, the patient may have a relative depletion of body bicarbonate, which requires treatment. Failure to administer sufficient bicarbonate, *even in the face of an alkaline plasma,* may result in progression to phase 2. Plasma pH should be carefully monitored throughout bicarbonate infusion. Potassium should be carefully administered, even if the serum potassium is normal; urine potassium may be measured to document quantitative excretion.

Phase 2. It is critical to replace bicarbonate and potassium in patients in this phase. Insufficient potassium results in further depletion of body stores and continued failure to alkalinize the urine. At least 20–40 mEq/L of potassium is required.

Phase 3. Following correction of the usual severe dehydration, therapy is directed toward replacing potassium and administering bicarbonate. Usually at least 40 mEq/L of potassium is required.

In all of these phases, alkalinization of the urine assists in excretion of salicylate.

Forced diuresis of 3–6 mL/kg/hr is not as important as alkalinization. Minimum fluid maintenance should result in at least 2 mL/kg/hr of urine flow. However, forced diuresis may aggravate pulmonary edema and adds little therapeutically once good alkalinization of the urine has been achieved. Acetazolamide and tris(hydroxymethyl)aminomethane are not recommended, because of associated complications. Glucose should be administered and carefully monitored throughout the course of treatment.

Hemodialysis may be useful in severe toxicity when alkalinization has not been successful. No specific plasma levels should be used as an indication for this modality, as even very high levels of salicylate, above 100 mL/dL, have responded to alkalinization. *Peritoneal dialysis* is almost totally useless, even with addition of albumin. *Charcoal hemoperfusion* may be a useful adjunct; however, it is easier to correct fluid and electrolyte problems with hemodialysis.

Anderson RJ, Potts DE, Gabow PA, et al: Unrecognized adult salicylate intoxication. Ann Intern Med 85:745, 1976.
Done AK: Salicylate intoxication: Significance of measurements of salicylates in blood in cases of acute ingestion. Pediatrics 26:800, 1960.
Garrettson LK, Procknal JA, Levy G: Fetal acquisition and neonatal elimination of a large amount of salicylate. Study of a neonate whose mother regularly took therapeutic doses of aspirin during pregnancy. Clin Pharmacol Ther 17:98, 1975.
Gaudreault P, Temple AR, Lovejoy FH: The relative severity of acute versus chronic salicylate poisoning in children: A clinical comparison. Pediatrics 70:566, 1982.
Hill JB: Experimental salicylate poisoning: Observations on the effects of altering blood pH on tissue and plasma salicylate concentrations. Pediatrics 47:658, 1971.
Levy G: Clinical pharmacokinetics of aspirin. Pediatrics 62 (Suppl 5):867, 1978.
Levy G, Yaffe SJ: Relationship between dose and apparent volume of distribution of salicylate in children. Pediatrics 54:713, 1974.
Prescott LF, Balali-Mood M, Critchley JA, et al: Diuresis or urinary alkalinization for salicylate poisoning? Br Med J 285:1381, 1982.
Rumack CM, Guggenheim MA, Rumack BH, et al: Neonatal intracranial hemorrhage and maternal use of aspirin. Obstet Gynecol 58 (Suppl):52, 1981.
Snodgrass W, Rumack BH, Peterson RG: Salicylate toxicity following therapeutic doses in young children. Clin Toxicol 18:247, 1981.
Temple AR: Pathophysiology of aspirin overdosage toxicity with implications for management. Pediatrics 62 (Suppl):873, 1978.

28.6 HYDROCARBONS

Accidental ingestion of products containing hydrocarbons involves an extremely wide array of chemical substances, and many factors are involved in determining whether a particular exposure will produce systemic or local toxicity. The following general classification of hydrocarbons relates to acute exposure and lists only representative examples.
1. High likelihood of systemic toxicity following ingestion.
   Halogenated and aliphatic hydrocarbons
   Trichloroethane
   Trichlorethylene
   Carbon tetrachloride
   Methylene chloride

Aromatic
   Benzene
Hydrocarbons with additives
   Heavy metals
   Insecticides
   Herbicides
   Nitrobenzene
   Aniline
2. Systemic and local toxicity unlikely.
   Toluene
   Xylene
   Petroleum ether (benzine)
   Petroleum naphtha ("lighter fluid")
   VM & P naphtha ("paint thinner")
   Mineral spirits (stoddard solvent, white spirit, mineral turpentine, petroleum spirits)
   Turpentine
3. Local toxicity (e.g. aspiration) highly likely after ingestion. Systemic toxicity unlikely.
   Mineral seal oil
   Signal oil
   Furniture polish mixtures
   Gasoline
   Kerosene
   Charcoal lighter fluid
4. Generally non-toxic after ingestion in over 95% of cases.
   Asphalt or tar
   Lubricants (motor oil, transmission oil, cutting oil, household oil and heavy grease)
   Mineral or liquid petrolatum

Pathophysiology. Once absorbed through ingestion, inhalation, or dermal routes, hydrocarbons can produce many kinds of *systemic toxicity.* The most common is central nervous system depression related to the anesthetic properties of certain hydrocarbons. Because most commercial products are mixtures or impure distillates, it is not possible to be precise about each product. In most cases, even following ingestion of hazardous hydrocarbons, the blood concentration may remain low enough to avoid central nervous system depression. Myocardial sensitization may follow ingestion of halogenated or nonhalogenated hydrocarbons. Hepatic toxicity, while usually related to carbon tetrachloride, is associated with many substances. Primary respiratory irritation with chemical pneumonitis, as well as irritation of the gastrointestinal tract, may occur. Renal and hematologic toxicity is usually related to long-term exposure. In some instances when there is high concentration of a hydrocarbon in the atmosphere, inhaling oxygen-poor air may produce anoxia or other findings not related to the toxicity of the actual hydrocarbon. Methylene chloride, found in most paint strippers, is an example of a substance that is metabolized after absorption to another substance, carbon monoxide, which produces systemic toxicity. Nitrobenzene or aniline-related compounds produce methemoglobinemia.

Local toxicity includes defatting of skin, irritation of mucous membranes, and most importantly, **aspiration pneumonitis** (see Sec. 13.69). Furniture polishes are the most common products containing mineral seal oil, the most notorious of the substances producing aspiration pneumonitis. During the act of swallowing, the very small amount of this substance that passes into the pulmonary tree is all that is required to produce significant pneumonitis. The chemical has very low viscosity and consequently is capable of spreading to involve large surface areas of the lung after only 0.1–0.2 mL are inhaled. Interstitial inflammation, hyperemia (sometimes with hemorrhage), and alveolar necrosis result.

Clinical Manifestations. Aspiration pneumonia is characterized by coughing, which usually is the first clinical finding. Chest roentgenograms may be unremarkable for as long as 8–12 hr after aspiration. Most commonly, however, infiltrates will be seen by 2–3 hr postingestion. Fever occurs later and may persist for as long as 10 days after ingestion. Accompa-

nying leukocytosis may be misleading, since in most cases of aspiration pneumonitis, no bacteria are present in the lung. Later in the course of this illness, after resolution of most clinical findings and 2–3 wk after exposure, pneumatoceles may appear on the chest roentgenogram.

Treatment. Emesis may be useful in patients who have no other contraindication to vomiting and have consumed a hydrocarbon whose primary toxicity is systemic. When aspiration pneumonitis is likely and systemic toxicity is unlikely, emesis should not be induced. Instillation of vegetable oils or mineral oil into the stomach in an attempt to prevent absorption is contraindicated. Similarly, steroids should be avoided, as they do not provide any benefit and may be harmful. Antibiotics should not be given prophylactically. Fever and leukocytosis usually result from the pyrogenic effect of the agent; bacterial pneumonia occurs in only a small percentage of cases.

Anas N, Nanasonthi V, Ginsburg CM: Criteria for hospitalizing children who have ingested products containing hydrocarbons. JAMA 246:840, 1981.
Banner W, Walson PD: Systems toxicity following gasoline aspiration. Am J Emerg Med 3:292, 1983.
Bergson PS, Hales SW, Lustganter MP: Pneumatoceles following hydrocarbon ingestion. AJDC 129:49, 1975.
Brown J, Burke B, Dajani AS: Experimental kerosene pneumonia: Evaluation of some therapeutic regimens. J Pediatr 84:396, 1984.
Dice WH, Ward G, Kelley J: Pulmonary toxicity following gastrointestinal ingestion of kerosene. Ann Emerg Med 11:138, 1982.
Kulig K, Rumack BH: Hydrocarbon ingestion. Curr Topics Emerg Med 3:1, 1981.
Marsh WW: Butane firebreathing in adolescents: A potentially dangerous practice. J Adolesc Health Care 5:59, 1984.
Rumack BH: Hydrocarbon ingestions in perspective. JACEP 6:4, 1977.

28.7 IRON

Iron poisoning occurs frequently in childhood, related partially to the prevalence of iron-containing tablets in many homes and to the resemblance of many iron tablets to candy. Although iron poisoning rarely results in death, prompt action may be lifesaving. The severity of iron poisoning is related to the amount of elemental iron absorbed. Death has been reported after ingestion of as little as 650 mg of elemental iron, an amount contained in only ten iron sulfate tablets. Absorption of 60 mg/kg is probably necessary for development of significant iron poisoning.

Clinical Manifestations. The diagnosis of iron poisoning is usually made by history. Roentgenographic confirmation is often possible, because undisintegrated iron tablets are radiopaque.

Five phases may be observed with serious iron poisoning:
1. The local irritative effects of iron on the gastrointestinal mucosa have their onset 30 min–2 hr postingestion and usually subside after 6–12 hr. They are the result of local necrosis and hemorrhage at the sites of iron contact. Nausea, vomiting, diarrhea, abdominal pain, hematemesis, and bloody diarrhea result. Severe hypotension may also occur.
2. The next phase of 2–6 hr is seen as a period of apparent recovery. The patient appears better, which may lead the physician to a false sense of security. During this time iron accumulates in mitochondria and various organs.
3. About 12 hr after ingestion the cellular damage produced by the iron produces manifestations. Hypoglycemia and a metabolic acidosis may occur, attributable to an impairment of electron transport by the damaged mitochondrial membranes. Lactic and citric acids accumulate owing to development of anaerobic metabolism and interference with the Krebs cycle.
4. Following apparent recovery, 2–4 days after ingestion, severe hepatic necrosis with elevation of SGOT, SGPT, and abnormalities of bilirubin and prothrombin may occur.
5. There may be scarring and stenosis of the pyloric area

2–4 wk after ingestion as a result of the local irritative action during the first phase. This stenosis may be symptomatic and occasionally requires surgical intervention.

Not all patients demonstrate the phases in easily discernible increments. Most children with a history of ingestion develop few, if any, signs or symptoms, but they should be followed for 4–6 hr before being considered free of toxicity.

Laboratory Findings. The measurement of free iron in the serum is the best way to determine the potential for toxicity. This should be done by assessing levels of total serum iron and of total serum iron-binding capacity; if the total iron exceeds the iron-binding capacity, then free iron exists. Toxicity is unlikely unless there is at least 50 mg/kg or more of free iron. Total iron levels in excess of 350 mg/kg, regardless of iron-binding capacity, may also be toxic. In many instances, it is not possible to obtain a rapid assay. Usually, levels of serum iron greater than 300 mg/kg will be seen in patients who have diarrhea, vomiting, leukocytosis, hyperglycemia, and positive abdominal roentgenograms. Vomiting has some correlation with high toxicity, and its absence with low toxicity.

Treatment. If the patient has not vomited, emesis should be induced. Lavage with a large bore tube may be useful. Whereas 250 mg/kg oral dose of a saline cathartic may be helpful, activated charcoal is of little value. Emergency gastrotomy to remove tablets may be considered if large numbers remain in the stomach after lavage in a symptomatic patient.

Oral bicarbonate (2%) or dilute phosphosoda (1:4) forms a less soluble complex, but clinical benefits are questionable. Oral deferoxamine is expensive, may increase absorption, and is generally not used by this route in treating an acute overdose.

Supportive care for hypotension and the other severe problems associated with phases 1 and 3 should be instituted as for any other life-threatening illness (Sec. 5.41 and 28.3). If there is free serum iron of greater than 50 mg/dL, if the total iron level is greater than 350 mg/dL, or if the patient is symptomatic, then *parenteral deferoxamine* should be given. In severe cases, 10–15 mg/kg/hr for up to 24 hr may be given intravenously. For less severe cases, 90 mg/kg up to a 1 g/dose may be given intramuscularly every 8 hr for 3 doses. The total dose should not exceed 6.0 g intravenously or intramuscularly. Once the deferoxamine iron chelate is achieved, the complex will be excreted, imparting a reddish (vin rosé) color to the urine. Although some believe that administering deferoxamine in this way can be used to predict serum free iron by evaluating urine color, at best this gives an indication of presence but not severity. The use of chelation in renal failure requires hemodialysis to remove the complex.

Bayer MJ, Rumack BH: Poisoning and Overdose. Rockville, MD, Aspen Systems Corp, 1983.

Czajka PA, Conrad JD, Duffy JP: Iron poisoning: An in vitro comparison of bicarbonate and phosphate lavage solutions. J Pediatr 98(3):491, 1981.

Fischer DS, Parkman R, Finch SC: Acute iron poisoning in children. JAMA 218:1179, 1971.

Gleason WA Jr, deMello DE, deCastro FJ, et al: Acute hepatic failure in severe iron poisoning. J Pediatr 38:140, 1979.

Helfer RE, Rodgerson DO: The effect of deferoxamine on the determination of serum iron and iron-binding capacity. J Pediatr 68:804, 1966.

Lacouture PG, Wason S, Temple AR, et al: Radiopacity of drugs and plants in vitro—limited usefulness. Vet Hum Toxicol 23:2, 1981.

Lovejoy FH: Chelation therapy in iron poisoning. J Toxicol Clin Toxicol 19(8):871, 1982–83.

28.8 CYCLIC ANTIDEPRESSANTS

This group of drugs includes the tricyclics and a variety of associated agents primarily used as antidepressants. Table 28–3 lists these agents by structural classification as well as by relative toxicity. The mortality rate from all of these agents is estimated to be 7–12%. If exposures involving only acciden-

Table 28–3. Cyclic Antidepressants

Generic	Trade Name	Structural Classification	CNS Toxicity	CV Toxicity
Amitriptyline	Elavil Amitid Endep Amitril	Tricyclic	+ + +	+ + + +
Amoxapine*	Ascendin	Tricyclic	+ + + +	+
Clomipramine	INV	Tricyclic	+ + + +	+ + + +
Desipramine	Norpramin Pertofrane	Tricyclic	+ + +	+ + + +
Doxepin	Adapin Sinequan	Tricyclic	+ + +	+ + + +
Imipramine	Tofranil Presamine SK-Pramine Janimine	Tricyclic	+ + +	+ + + +
Loxapine	Loxatane	Tricyclic	+ + +	+
Maprotiline†	Ludiomil	Tetracyclic	+ + +	+ + +
Mianserin	INV‡	Tetracyclic	?	?
Nortriptyline	Aventyl Pamelor	Tricyclic	+ + +	+ + + +
Protriptyline	Vivactyl	Tricyclic	+ + +	+ + + +
Trazodone	Desyrel	Miscellaneous¶	+	+
Trimipramine	Surmontil	Tricyclic	+ + +	+ + + +
Viloxazine	INV§	Bicyclic	?	?
Zimelidine	INV§	Bicyclic	?	?

*Amoxapine is structurally similar to loxapine, an antipsychotic agent, and appears to have similar toxicity. Amoxapine is an active metabolite of loxapine.

†Available evidence suggests that maprotiline may have less cardiovascular toxicity when compared with the tricyclic antidepressants.

‡Investigational or newly released drug; tetracyclic antidepressant toxicity to be determined.

§Investigational or newly released drug; bicyclic antidepressant toxicity to be determined.

¶This agent has a unique dual bicyclic structure.

Combination products: Combination products containing tricyclic antidepressants include Limbitrol (amitriptyline and chlordiazepoxide); Etrafon, Perphenyline, Triavil, and Triptazine (amitriptyline and perphenazine).

From Rumack BH (ed): POISINDEX®. 47th ed. Englewood, CO, Micromedex Inc, 1986, with permission of author and publisher.

tal ingestion reported to poison centers in children less than 5 yr old are considered, then the mortality rate is lower.

Pathophysiology. Cyclic antidepressants, notably the tricyclics, are structurally similar to the phenothiazines and have similar anticholinergic, adrenergic, and alpha-blocking properties. Following absorption, these agents are extensively bound to plasma proteins and also bind to tissue and cellular sites, including the mitochondria. The blood:tissue ratio varies from 1:10 to 1:30, which explains the ineffectiveness of forced diuresis and dialysis techniques in removal of the drug. They block the neuronal reuptake of norepinephrine, 5-hydroxytryptamine, serotonin, or dopamine. Therapeutic doses, initially, may cause drowsiness and difficulty concentrating and thinking; dulling of depressive ideation may explain the efficacy of these agents in depressive disorders. Hallucinations, excitement, and confusion have occurred in a small percentage of patients during antidepressant therapy. These agents also have a slight alpha-adrenergic blocking effect. Trazodone inhibits the neuronal uptake of serotonin and has antiserotonin and alpha-adrenergic blocking properties.

Clinical Manifestations. The initial presentation is the onset of the anticholinergic syndrome including tachycardia, pupillary dilatation, dryness of mucus membranes, urinary retention, hallucinations, and flushing. Although hypertension also may initially occur, hypotension rapidly develops and is a serious sign. Convulsions, coma, and major arrhythmias

1502 28 • POISONINGS FROM FOOD, DRUGS, CHEMICALS, POLLUTANTS, AND VENOMOUS BITES; MAMMALIAN BITES

ensue as tissue saturation occurs. Cardiac findings include quinidine-like effects such as slowing of myocardial conduction, multifocal premature ventricular contractions, ventricular tachycardia, flutter, and fibrillation. In addition to widening of the QRS complex, Q-T prolongation occurs with T-wave flattening or inversion, S-T segment depression, right bundle branch block, and complete heart block.

Central nervous system (CNS) toxicity includes manifestations of depression, lethargy, and hallucinations. Choreoathetosis and myoclonus have been reported and must be differentiated from generalized seizures. Coma, when it occurs, has a mean duration of 6.4 hr but may last for longer than 24 hr.

A withdrawal syndrome in neonates delivered of patients who have been taking tricyclics has occurred, with tachypnea, irritability, and restlessness lasting the 1st mo of life. Amoxapine differs from other tricyclics; there is significantly greater incidence of seizures and coma. Cardiovascular toxicity is less prominent, and seizures and coma may be associated with normal QRS complexes.

Loxapine is similar to its metabolite amoxapine in having a greater incidence of CNS toxicity and a lesser incidence of cardiovascular toxicity.

Exposure to the tetracyclics appears to be associated with a higher incidence of cardiovascular effects than does exposure to the tricyclics. Bicyclics are similar to tetracyclics but additionally appear to cause less anticholinergic toxicity. Trazodone, which has a uniquely different structure, appears to result in little CNS or cardiovascular toxicity.

Children should be observed and their electrocardiogram monitored for at least 6 hr. If any tissue manifestations (such as a QRS interval longer than 0.12 or an altered mental status) are present, then patients should be monitored for 24 hr. Catastrophic deterioration has been observed in patients who at first appear mildly, if at all, poisoned and whose condition then rapidly becomes seriously toxic. Only completely asymptomatic children should be discharged after 6 hr. Others should be admitted to intensive care and monitored for at least 24 hr.

Laboratory Findings. These may be helpful in establishing the type of agent ingested. However, because these agents have extremely high volumes of distribution, blood level measurements may not be helpful in establishing severity. The observation of signs and symptoms is extremely helpful and should be relied on in the face of negative laboratory data.

Treatment. Following general life support measures, efforts should be made to *prevent absorption*. Emesis should be avoided in children showing clinical manifestations, because of the danger of aspiration from vomiting following onset of coma. Activated charcoal should be administered at a dose of 50–100 g in adolescents and 15–30 g in younger children. Repeated doses of activated charcoal should be given to all symptomatic children at a dose of 10–20 g every 2–6 hr. Obtunded patients may have this agent administered through a small bore nasogastric tube. Multiple-dose charcoal will remove drug being re-excreted in the gastrointestinal tract. *Cathartics* such as sorbitol, magnesium, or sodium sulfate should be administered.

Although there is controversy as to which *antiarrhythmic drugs* should be given and in what order, the following is generally accepted. Sodium bicarbonate should be administered in doses sufficient to achieve a pH of 7.4–7.5. Phenytoin is indicated, if conduction defects occur, such as QRS increased beyond 0.12 or prolonged QT. The dose of phenytoin is 15 mg/kg, up to 1.0 g intravenously, not to exceed a rate of 0.5 mg/kg/min. Some experts prefer prophylactic loading of phenytoin. Children with ventricular arrhythmias should have their acidosis corrected immediately with bicarbonate or mechanical hyperventilation. Phenytoin should be the first

agent administered, followed by lidocaine at a loading dose of 1 mg/kg/dose and by appropriate maintenance doses thereafter. Bretylium tosylate should not be used in hypotensive patients or in those with fixed cardiac output. In adolescents, propranolol may be used at a dose of 1.0 mg intravenously every 2–5 min, until a response occurs. In younger children, the dose is 0.1 mg intravenously, until a maximum of 1.0 mg has been given. Physostigmine should be used only rarely. It is an exceptionally dangerous agent, especially if given rapidly. It is most useful in supraventricular arrhythmias. In children, 0.5 mg IV should be given over 2–3 min; it may be repeated two to three times.

Patients with *seizures* should be primarily treated with diazepam at a dose of up to 10 mg intravenously in an adolescent or 0.1–0.3 mg/kg, up to 10 mg, in a child. Phenytoin should then be given. Physostigmine may be used for myoclonic seizures or choreoathetosis but is not very effective for generalized seizures.

Hypotension may respond to norepinephrine but usually does not respond to dopamine. Severe hypotension is very serious and may require fluids and an intra-aortic balloon. *Hypertension* usually responds to physostigmine. Patients who have a seriously deteriorating course may have such a significant degree of tissue loading that they cannot be saved. Although hemodialysis and charcoal hemoperfusion have been attempted, these procedures are rarely helpful in such overdoses.

Bader TF, Newman K: Amitriptyline in human breast milk and the nursing infant's serum. Am J Psychol 137(7):855, 1980.
Burks JS, Walker JE, Rumack BH, et al: Tricyclic antidepressant poisoning—reversal of coma, choreoathetosis, and myoclonus by physostigmine. JAMA 230(10):1405, 1974.
Callaham M, Kassel D: Epidemiology of fatal tricyclic antidepressant ingestion: Implications for management. Ann Emerg Med 14:1, 1985.
Kulig K, Rumack BH, Sullivan JB, et al: Amoxapine overdose: Coma and seizures without cardiotoxic effects. JAMA 248:1092, 1982.
Molloy DW, Penner SB, Rabson J, et al: Use of sodium bicarbonate to treat tricyclic antidepressant-induced arrhythmias in a patient with alkalosis. Canad Med Assoc J 130:1457, 1984.
Rumack BH: Anticholinergic poisoning: Treatment with physostigmine. Pediatrics 52:449, 1973.
Rumack BH: POISINDEX® A Computerized Poison Information System. 37th ed. Englewood, CO, Micromedex Inc, 1985.
Sjöqvist F, Bergfors PG, Borga O, et al: Plasma disappearance of nortriptyline in a newborn infant following placental transfer from an intoxicated mother: Evidence of drug metabolism. J Pediatr 80:1046, 1972.
Swartz CM, Sherman A: The treatment of tricyclic antidepressant overdose with repeated charcoal. J Clin Psychopharmacol 4:336, 1984.

28.9 ALKALIS AND ACIDS

The incidence of severe injury from this variety of ingestion has dropped dramatically following the removal from the market of liquid corrosive drain cleaners. These agents had the tenacious capacity to coat the esophagus and produce major tissue destruction.

Pathophysiology. *Alkaline agents* tend to produce liquefaction necrosis (e.g., when the strong base binds to the fats and oils in the tissue and produces a soap [saponification]). Tablets such as Clinitest tend to lodge at about the level of the aortic arch in the esophagus and produce circumferential burns. Crystalline drain cleaners may produce a small streak-like burn; they result in circumferential burns in only 15% of all cases. Solutions of greater than 4% NaOH may produce very widespread circumferential burns. Linear streak burns usually do not constrict and form obstructions, but circumferential burns are likely to develop esophageal strictures, which may become totally occlusive. Alkaline agents in the crystal form may spare the mouth and hypopharynx as they travel across these areas on the saliva. Once in the esophagus, they may then produce damage. Common household bleach (5.4% or less), while producing hyperemia, is unlikely to produce burns.

Strong acid agents, such as sulfuric, nitric, or hydrochloric acid, are frequently concentrated at the pyloric end of the stomach, resulting in scarification and eventually stricture formation. They may also seriously damage the esophagus and other areas of the stomach, leading to necrosis and perforation.

Clinical Manifestations. When burns of the esophagus or hypopharynx have occurred, swallowing is likely to be impeded, and consequently the child may drool excessively. Burns on lips and tongue may be seen. No correlation exists between oral and esophageal burns; either can exist without the other. Pain and difficulty swallowing may be encountered. Occasionally, when the diagnosis has been missed, the patient will present with esophageal strictures and vomiting.

Treatment. If the patient can swallow safely, milk or water should be administered, 1–2 cups in the first few minutes after ingestion. Following this, the child should be kept from having anything orally. Steroids such as decadron at a dose of 1 mg every 4–6 hr may be given. Esophagoscopy should be performed between 12–24 hr after ingestion, to determine whether or not a circumferential burn exists. Performing this procedure earlier may be of less value, as the full extent of the burns may not be apparent. If there are significant burns, the patient should remain on clear liquids and steroids to avoid possible esophageal perforation. At approximately 2–3 wk postinjury, patients may develop strictures, necessitating a feeding gastrostomy. A colonic interposition or a gastric tube may then be necessary as a more definitive procedure.

Administering acids (such as fruit juice) to children who have consumed bases and bases to children after acid ingestion are contraindicated, as an exothermic reaction may occur and aggravate the injury. Surgical evaluation in significant cases is mandatory.

French RJ, Tabb HG, Rutledge LJ: Esophageal stenosis produced by ingestion of bleach. South Med J 63:1140, 1970.

Gaudreault P, Parent M, McGuigan MA: Predictability of esophageal injury from signs and symptoms: A study of 378 children. Pediatrics 71:761, 1983.

Haller JA, Andrews HG, White JJ, et al: Pathophysiology and management of acute corrosive burns of the esophagus. J Pediatr Surg 6:578, 1971.

Leape LL, Ashcraft KW, Scarpelli DG, et al: Hazard to health—liquid lye. N Engl J Med 284:578, 1971.

Linden CH, Buner JM, Kulig K, et al: Acid ingestion: Toxicity following systemic absorption. Vet Human Toxicol 25:282, 1983.

O'Konek S, Bierbach H, Atzpodien W: Unexpected metabolic acidosis in severe lye poisoning. Clin Toxicol 18(2):225, 1981.

Penner GE: Acid ingestion: Toxicology and treatment. Ann Emerg Med 9:374, 1980.

Rumack BH: Soap solution contraindicated in acid ingestion (letter). J Am Coll Emerg Phys 8:124, 1979.

Rumack BH, Burrington JD: Caustic ingestions: A rational look at diluents. Clin Toxicol 11:27, 1977.

Scher LA, Maull KI: Emergency management and sequelae of acid ingestion. J Am Coll Emerg Phys 7:206, 1978.

28.10 IBUPROFEN

This anti-inflammatory agent, which recently became available as an over-the-counter drug, is likely to be involved in progressively more accidental and intentional overdoses because of its wider distribution.

Pathophysiology. Peak plasma levels occur after 1–1½ hr. The volume of distribution is 0.11–0.13 L/kg, which is similar to that seen with salicylates. Only about 1% of the drug is excreted unchanged; the rest is metabolized in the liver. About 99% of a therapeutic dose of ibuprofen is bound to protein, and its half-life is about 2 hr.

Laboratory Findings. The drug can be measured in plasma; levels of 20–30 µg/mL at 2 hr are therapeutic. Levels in the 70–100 µg/mL range 2 hr after ingestion are not associated with symptoms, but mild symptoms of gastrointestinal upset and lethargy occur at 3 hr in the range of 80–200 µg/mL (Fig. 28–3). Seriously toxic findings have been seen at a 2 hr level of 360 µg/mL, but levels as high as 704 µg/mL have been seen without toxicity.

Clinical Manifestations. Gastrointestinal disorders including nausea, epigastric pain, and upper gastrointestinal bleeding have been seen. Renal failure and toxicity have been reported in adults and children with marked increase in serum potassium and creatinine and blood urea nitrogen. Hypotension has occurred but is rare. Nystagmus, diplopia, headache, tinnitus, and transient deafness have all been observed.

The most serious problems with this drug are lethargy, coma, and transient apnea. While not reported in adults or adolescents, children 1–1½ yr of age have developed apnea following ingestion of 2.8–7.6 g. Lethargy and drowsiness are common and occur in pediatric patients following ingestion of 120–230 mg/kg. Acid base disturbances are not common. Acidosis is seen especially in younger children. Anaphylactoid reactions have been reported with circulatory collapse, angioedema, and pruritus.

Treatment. Respiratory and cardiovascular support should be given immediately. Emesis, unless contraindicated by the patient's condition, may be useful. Ingested amounts of less than 100 mg/kg are not likely to produce toxicity (Fig. 28–3); however, as with any ingestion, the history should be cautiously interpreted. Hypotension should be treated with dopamine or norepinephrine. Although the manufacturer recommends alkaline diuresis, this is unlikely to be beneficial because of 99% protein binding. Hemodialysis and charcoal hemoperfusion may be of benefit because of the small volume of distribution.

In general, good supportive care of coma or apnea until the drug is metabolized should permit resolution of the overdose in 24 hr. Children with a history of ingestion should be observed at least 6 hr to be certain that apnea and central nervous system depression do not occur.

Barry WS, Meinzinger MM, Howse CR: Ibuprofen overdose and exposure in utero: Results from a postmarketing voluntary reporting system. Am J Med 77:35, 1984.

Court H, Streete P, Volans GN: Acute poisoning with ibuprofen. Hum Toxicol 2:381, 1983.

Court H, Street RJ, Volans GN: Overdose with ibuprofen causing unconsciousness and hypotension. Br Med J 282:1073, 1981.

Hall AH, Smolinske SC, Conrad FL, et al: Ibuprofen overdose: 126 cases. Ann Emerg Med 15:1308, 1986.

Hunt DP, Leigh RJ: Overdose with ibuprofen causing unconsciousness and hypotension. Br Med J 281:1458, 1980.

Joubert DW: Zomepirac overdose and review of literature on acute toxicity of nonsteroidal antiinflammatory agents. Drug Intell Clin Pharmacol 16:328, 1982.

Poirier TI: Reversible renal failure associated with ibuprofen: Case report and review of the literature. Drug Intell Clin Pharmacol 18:27, 1984.

Rumack BH: POISINDEX®, A Computerized Poison Information System. 37th ed. Englewood, CO, Micromedex Inc, 1985.

28.11 PLANTS

Ingestion or exposure to plants both inside the home and outside in backyards and fields is one of the most common accidental poisoning problems. Table 28–4 lists the 20 most frequent exposures in young children. Fortunately, most plant ingestions result in little or no toxicity, and those children developing clinical manifestations usually can be dealt with symptomatically. The following are some of the common groups, their major findings, and treatment.

Arum Family

Examples are dieffenbachia, caladium, and philodendron. In this family, the entire plant contains various concentrations of calcium oxalate crystals. The most common problems occur in the oropharynx and include irritation of the lips, tongue, and mucous membrane. Intense pain and swelling may be seen. Washing of the affected area may be helpful, along with

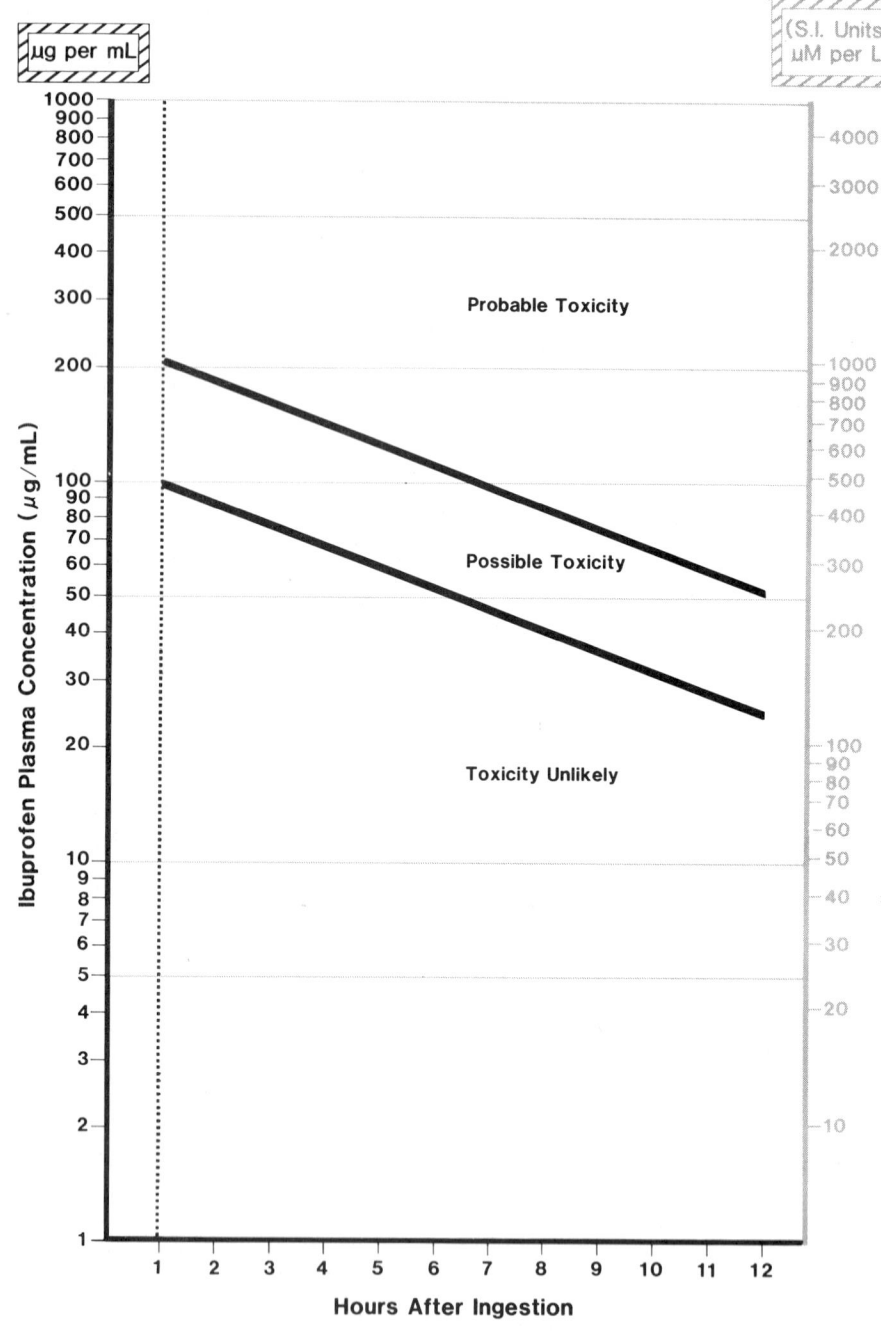

Figure 28–3. Nomogram for ibuprofen poisoning. *Cautions for use of this chart*: (1) The time coordinates refer to time after *ingestion*. (2) Plasma levels obtained sooner than 1 hr or later than 12 hr after ingestion cannot be interpreted. (3) The nomogram may aid in predicting which initially asymptomatic or mildly symptomatic patients have the potential to develop symptoms or more severe symptomatology later. (From Hall AH, et al: Ibuprofen overdose: 126 cases. Ann Emerg Med 15:1308, 1986.)

Nomogram Prediction of Toxicity Development

	Portion of Nomogram		
	Probable Toxicity	Possible Toxicity	Toxicity Unlikely
Severe Symptoms	24%	17%	0%
Symptoms	65%	33%	24%
Asymptomatic	35%	67%	76%

Table 28–4. Plants Most Frequently Involved in Human Exposure Cases Reported to Poison Centers

Table 28–4. Plants Most Frequently Involved in Human Exposure Cases Reported to Poison Centers

Plant	No. of Yearly Exposures
Philodendron spp. (Philodendron)	2010
Dieffenbachia spp. (Dumbcane)	1009
Euphorbia pulcherrima (Poinsettia)	714
Crassula argentea (Jade plant)	630
Pyracantha spp. (Firethorn)	586
Ilex spp. (Holly)	533
Brassaia actinophylla (Schefflera)	478
Phytolacca americana or rigida (Pokeweed)	347
Anthericum and Chlorophytum (Spiderplant)	242
Lonicera spp. (Honeysuckle)	213
Ficus elastica (Rubber plant)	211
Nephthytis spp. (Arrowhead vine)	203
Capsicum annuum conides ("Fiesta" pepper)	200
Episcia reptans (Flame violet)	199
Scindapsus aureus or pictus Pothos	199
Aloe spp. (Medicine aloe)	179
Asparagus officinalis (Asparagus fern)	169
Ficus benjamina (Weeping fig tree)	151
Solanum dulcamara (Climbing nightshade)	149
Toxicodendron radicans (Poison ivy)	144
Rhododendron spp. (Rhododendron, azalea)	141
Pittosporum tobira (Pittosporum)	141
Mohonia spp. (Oregon grape)	138
Quercus spp. (Oak)	125
Nerium oleander (Oleander)	125
Chrysanthemum spp. (Chrysanthemum)	122
Solanum pseudocapsicum (Jerusalem cherry)	121
Phorandendron flavescens (Mistletoe)	121
Begonia spp. (Begonia)	119
Sorbus spp. (Mountain-ash)	111

ice chips to chew and relieve pain. Steroids may be helpful in very serious cases. Systemic toxicity is extremely rare.

Anticholinergic (Solanum and Related) Family

Examples are jimson weed, nightshade, and potato (see also Sec. 28.2). All parts of these plants, especially the green portions, contain solanaceous (atropinic) alkaloids. Findings include tachycardia, dryness, flushing, hypertension, delirium, hallucinations, thirst, and in some cases coma and convulsions. If the syndrome is very severe, physostigmine may be used in doses similar to that with the cyclic antidepressants. If the findings are mild, then the patient should receive no treatment but be carefully observed.

Castor Bean and Jequirity Bean

These contain toxalbumins: ricin in castor bean, and abrin in jequirity bean. Severe, crampy diarrhea along with nausea, vomiting, central nervous system depression, shock, and convulsions may occur. Hemolytic anemia may occur with ricin, whereas renal failure is more common with abrin. There is no specific treatment. Children should be managed symptomatically, and urine flow should be monitored. Activated charcoal should be administered.

Foxglove

These plants contain the classic cardiac glycoside, digitalis. Substantial similarity to overdose with any of the digitalis glycosides exists. Bradycardia with nausea and vomiting are seen as heart block gradually progresses. FAB fragments are effective in treatment. Potassium levels should be monitored.

Treatment by phenytoin loading should be considered, as well as activated charcoal to prevent further absorption.

Oleander

Oleander contains cardiac glycosides somewhat different from those of foxglove. In addition to local irritation, patients exhibit nausea, vomiting, diarrhea, and in severe cases, AV block, with S-T segment depression and severe bradycardia. It is unknown whether FAB fragments will help. Potassium levels should be carefully followed. Phenytoin or atropine may be useful, as well as oral activated charcoal.

Hemlock

Poison hemlock contains the alkaloid coniine, which initially produces hyperactivity followed by central nervous system depression and respiratory failure. There is no specific treatment. Activated charcoal should be administered soon after ingestion, and respirations should be monitored. The intoxication is similar to that of nicotine.

Water hemlock contains the agent cicutoxin, which is likely to cause the rapid onset of hyperactivity, leading to convulsions within 1/2 hr. Abdominal pain, emesis, and salivation are usually seen. Dilatation of the pupils is usual after onset of major signs. There is no specific treatment. Control of seizures with diazepam and administration of activated charcoal, if the patient can swallow, may be helpful. Supportive care should be provided.

BARRY H. RUMACK

Hardin JW, Arena JM: Human Poisoning from Native and Cultivated Plants. Durham, NC, Duke University Press, 1974.

Kingsbury JM: Poisonous Plants of the United States and Canada. Englewood Cliffs, NJ, Prentice-Hall, 1964.

Rumack BH (ed): POISINDEX®, A Computerized Poison Information System. 44th ed. Englewood, CO, Micromedex, Inc, 1985.

Veltri JC, Litovitz TL: 1983 Annual Report of the American Association of Poison Control Centers, National Data Collection System. Am J Emerg Med 2:420, 1984.

MERCURY

Mercury, both inorganic and organic, causes acute and chronic poisoning. However, it is still widely used today in the household, in medicine, in agriculture, and in industry. Its effects may be either reversible or irreversible, depending on the compound and quantity of exposure. In acute poisoning, the effects of mercury exposure appear predominantly in the gastrointestinal tract and kidney, and in chronic poisoning in the central nervous system and skin. Incidents of mercury poisoning of human communities have occurred in many areas of the world. Therefore, understanding the implications and mechanisms of environmental pollution by mercurial compounds has become essential for preventing and remedying contamination.

28.12 Acute and Chronic Mercury Poisoning

Etiology. Mercury vapor is highly toxic. Mercurous chloride, or calomel, is still used as an antiseptic in some skin creams. Aqueous thimerosal (Merthiolate) has been serving for years as a topical antiseptic. The mercurial diuretic chlormerodrin has been employed in the roentgenographic scanning of kidney and brain. Phenylmercuric salts are used in paints and as a fungicide for seeds. Methylmercury compounds have been used extensively as fungicides and have been the reported cause of poisonings resulting from the ingestion of bread made from wheat treated with these compounds. Mercuric salts have wide application in industries whose pollution has led to problems of environmental contamination, notably of methylmercury poisoning, which results from the ingestion of contaminated fish.

Clinical Manifestations. Exposure to high concentrations of mercury vapor may cause pulmonary irritation or pneumonitis, nausea, vomiting, diarrhea, abdominal pain, and headache.

Oral intake of mercury may cause stomatitis; gingivitis; esophagitis; gastroenteritis with excessive salivation; nausea, vomiting, and abdominal pain; and severe, bloody diarrhea. Patients with kidney damage develop anuria, albuminuria, and uremia and frequently die. Central nervous system symptoms include ataxia, slurring of speech, numbness of the hands and feet, visual and hearing impairment, and delirium.

Treatment. Emergency treatment of acute mercury poisoning consists of (1) intravenous replacement of fluid and electrolytes to prevent peripheral vascular collapse, and (2) gastric lavage to remove the mercury in the stomach. Lavage is done first with milk and then repeated with 2–5% sodium bicarbonate.

The most effective antidote for acute mercury poisoning is BAL, British antilewisite, or dimercaprol. The drug is administered intramuscularly in a 10% solution with a recommended dosage of 5 mg/kg for the first injection and 3 mg/kg every 4 hr for 2 days; this dose is then tapered to every 6 hr for 1 day, followed by administration every 12 hr for 7 days. BAL may protect against kidney damage from acute poisoning when given within 3 hr after ingestion of mercury. It may produce unpleasant side effects, such as nausea, vomiting, and fever, as the dose is increased. Penicillamine (N-acetyl-D,L-penicillamine) is used in patients who have side reactions to BAL. One method of administration is to give 100 mg/kg orally in four divided doses, to a maximum of 1000 mg/day.

Symptomatic treatment is also important. Hydroxyzine and chlorpromazine may be useful for restlessness and tolazoline hydrochloride for tachycardia.

Peritoneal dialysis or hemodialysis may be indicated for acute renal failure.

Chronic mercury poisoning generally results from occupational exposure in adults and is rare in children. However, both acrodynia and Minamata disease are important clinical conditions in children in which the central nervous system and skin are most frequently involved. The symptoms are diverse and variable, and in severe cases are irreversible.

28.13 Acrodynia
(Pink Disease, Swift Disease; Feer Disease;
Erythredema; Dermatopolyneuritis)

Acrodynia (Greek, "painful extremities"), principally a syndrome of chronic mercury poisoning in infants and young children, consists of many unusual symptoms that in the well-established cases are so distinctive that there is practically no differential diagnosis. In few other conditions does extreme and persistent misery play such a prominent part of the clinical picture.

Etiology. Most cases of acrodynia represent the clinical response to repeated contact with or ingestion of mercury in products such as house paints, wallpapers, teething powders, vermifuges, and diaper rinses. The interval between mercury exposure and onset of symptoms may vary from 1 wk to several months. The condition is probably the manifestation of a sensitization to mercury in the hypersensitive child.

Pathology. Pathologic findings are mainly present in the central nervous system. Degeneration and chromatolysis of the cerebral and cerebellar cortex are prominent.

Clinical Manifestations. The natural course of acrodynia is prolonged, extending from several months to a year. There are all grades of severity. The child becomes listless, no longer interested in play, restless, and irritable. Generalized inconstant rashes, which are protean, recur from time to time. Early, the tips of the fingers, toes, and nose acquire a pinkish color, and later the hands and feet become a dusky pink, with patchy areas of ischemia and cyanotic congestion. The coloring shades off at the wrists and ankles. These changes in the extremities are the most distinctive features of the syndrome and are responsible for the term "pink disease." Frequently the cheeks and the tip of the nose acquire a scarlet color.

As the disease becomes established, the sweat glands are enormously dilated and enlarged, and perspiration is profuse. Secondary infection may lead to a severe pyoderma. There is desquamation of the soles and palms, which, though usually superficial, may be severe and recur during the course of the disease. The fingers and toes appear edematous; the swelling is due to hyperplasia and hyperkeratosis of the skin. An outstanding symptom is constant pruritus with excruciating pain in the hands and feet. Children will rub their hands together for hours, and older children will complain of a severe burning sensation.

The nails become dark and frequently drop off. Occasionally, gangrene of the toes and fingers develops, and trophic ulcers may result from the constant rubbing of the hands and feet. The hair tends to fall out and is often pulled out by the child.

There is photophobia without evidence of local inflammation of the eyes. The children shield their eyes or bury their faces in their pillows. The lax ligaments and hypotonia permit the children to assume unusual positions (Fig. 28–4).

In extreme cases the teeth may be lost; necrosis of the jaw bones frequently follows. Initially, the gums appear normal except for a slightly deeper red color; later they become inflamed and swollen. Salivation then becomes pronounced,

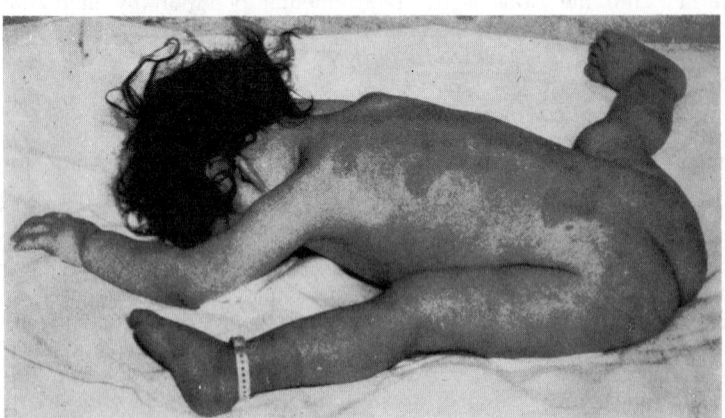

Figure 28–4. Extreme hypotonia and photophobia in an infant with acrodynia. This bizarre position may be maintained for hours.

and the saliva often flows from the mouth in a constant stream. Anorexia is prominent, but because of the excessive perspiration large quantities of water are consumed. There may be diarrhea, and prolapse of the rectum is a frequent complication. The blood pressure and pulse rate may be increased significantly. Fever is usually not present unless there is some complication such as a urinary tract infection or bronchopneumonia.

Neurologic symptoms are an important part of the syndrome and include neuritis, mental apathy, and irritability. Early in the disease the tendon reflexes may be normal or increased, but later disappear. There is not a true motor paralysis, but because of the soft, flabby musculature the child has no desire to walk and remains hypotonic, listless, and hypomotile. Severe pain prevents normal sleep. A child with acrodynia never appears happy or comfortable; the child does not play or smile but appears dejected and melancholic, a picture of abject misery.

Laboratory Data. There are no characteristic changes in the blood or cerebrospinal fluid. Proteinuria may occur, and a nephrotic syndrome may develop. Slit lamp examination may show a lenticular gray or red brown reflex.

Prevention. The withdrawal of mercury from various household products has led to a marked decrease in the incidence of acrodynia. However, mercurial drugs should be avoided in pediatric practice whenever possible, and the physician should be alert to other sources of mercury, especially food contaminated by agricultural processes and industrial waste.

Treatment. The treatment of acrodynia includes (1) the removal of mercury, (2) the administration of antidotes, and (3) careful initiation of supportive measures.

BAL is an effective antidote, especially when given early in the disease. The dose and possible side effects are the same as for acute poisonings (Sec. 28.12). L-Penicillamine (*N*-acetyl-D,L-penicillamine) has been used to successfully treat acrodynia and has an advantage over BAL in that it can be given orally. The effective dose is 30 mg/kg daily in 2–3 divided doses for 4 wk or until symptoms improve. Side effects include fever, rashes, proteinuria, leukopenia, and thrombocytopenia.

Barbiturates, paraldehyde, hydroxyzine, or chlorpromazine may be used for irritability and pain. Nourishing foods containing proteins, minerals, and vitamins should be given. Frequently, nasogastric tube feeding is necessary for severe anorexia. Intravenous replacement of fluid and electrolytes may be required for dehydration. Appropriate antibiotics should be given for secondary pyogenic infections of the skin and urinary system.

28.14 Minamata Disease

Minamata disease is a form of mercury poisoning that occurred among adults and children living in towns facing Minamata Bay, Kumamoto prefecture, Japan, from 1953–1966. The disease has become symbolic of the catastrophic health risks of industrial pollution (Sec. 28.16).

Etiology. The causative agent of this disease is methylmercury, released as industrial waste during the manufacture of acetaldehyde and vinyl chloride and absorbed into the body by the ingestion of contaminated fish and shellfish. Congenital Minamata disease was produced by placental transfer of methylmercury to the fetus from the pregnant mother who had eaten contaminated fish. The fetus is more sensitive than the mother or the postnatal infant to toxic effects of methylmercury.

Pathology. Various degrees of regressive changes in the brain have been observed. Degeneration and loss of granular cells in the cortex of the cerebellum and central convolutions are prominent. In the congenital type more severe and widespread damage of the nerve cells in the cerebral and cerebellar cortices has been demonstrated.

Clinical Manifestations. The principal symptoms in the infantile form of Minamata disease include disturbance in hand coordination, in gait, and in speech. Difficulty in masticating and swallowing and visual blurring also occur. Some patients complain of numbness and pain in the extremities, and in severe cases there are involuntary movements. Tremor, clouded consciousness, convulsions, and rigidity of the extremities are observed. Some patients have impaired hearing and constriction of the visual field. More generalized damage to the nervous system results from fetal poisoning, the principal clinical features of which include: physical retardation, severe mental disturbance, delay in development, abnormal movement, or lack of smoothness in movement.

Laboratory Data. Mercury content in the hair of most Minamata disease patients is high, more than 20 ppm. Some patients have abnormal electroencephalograms and constricted visual fields. In the congenital form most patients have an abnormal pneumoencephalogram, cortical atrophy, and microcephalus. Chromosomal aberrations are not found.

Prevention. The environment should be kept free of mercury hazards. Pregnant women should be especially careful because of the high sensitivity of fetuses to mercury. The maximum safe concentration of mercury in food is 0.3 ppm of methylmercury. A level of over 40–50 ppm of mercury in the hair is considered dangerous.

Treatment. In the early stages elimination of organic mercury exposure may be sufficient. Foods suspected of contamination should not be eaten. Since mercury is transmitted to infants in human milk, breast feeding should be discontinued. BAL is effective in eliminating systemic mercury, and the dosage regimen is identical to that prescribed in acrodynia and acute poisonings. The diet should contain nourishing food rich in proteins, minerals, and vitamins. In severe cases tube feeding is necessary. Symptomatic treatment is increasingly important as time goes on. Anticonvulsive drugs are indicated for seizures. Damage is irreversible, and survivors require extensive rehabilitation, re-education, and long-term care.

TARO AKABANE

Amin-Zaki L, Elhassani S, Majeed MA, et al: Studies of infants postnatally exposed to methylmercury. J Pediatr 85:81, 1974.
Harada Y, Moriyama H: Congenital Minamata disease. Bull Inst Constitut Med Kumamoto Univ 26:1, 1976.
Jaffe KM, Shurtleff DB, Robertson WO: Survival after acute mercury vapor poisoning. Am J Dis Child 137:749, 1983.
Rohyans J, Walson PD, Wood GA, et al: Mercury toxicity following merthiolate ear irrigations. J Pediatr 104:311, 1984.
Rumack BH: Acute poisoning. In: Gellis SS, Kagan BM (eds): Current Pediatric Therapy. 11th ed. Philadelphia, WB Saunders, 1984.
Takeuchi T: Study group of Minamata disease. In: Katsuma M (ed): Minamata Disease, Japan. Kumamoto University, 1966.
Warkany J, Hubbard DM: Acrodynia and mercury. J Pediatr 42:365, 1953.

28.15 INCREASED LEAD ABSORPTION AND LEAD POISONING

Among children in the United States, 3.9% have increased lead (Pb) absorption. Plumbism is most prevalent in children 1–6 yr of age who live in old, deteriorated dwellings, and most affected children are being identified through screening programs. Most patients are asymptomatic, although biochemical evidence of disturbed heme synthesis is generally present, and such children are at increased risk for future neurobehavioral and cognitive deficits, which can impede progress in school. Acute lead colic and lead encephalopathy, the most severe forms of this chronic disorder, are now rare. Chelation therapy substantially reduces mortality, but 50% or more of the survivors of encephalopathy treated *after* the onset of symptoms have sustained, severe, permanent brain damage. This emphasizes the importance of treating cases in the early asymptomatic phase, if the degree of residual injury is to be reduced. In many areas of the United States, lead poisoning is a reportable disease.

Exposure. Food, water, and air contain small amounts of lead: the amount ingested daily in food and beverages is less than 120 µg Pb; in drinking water, less than 50 µg Pb/liter; in air, less than 1 µg Pb/m³. Such usual exposures are associated with average blood lead level (PbB) of 9.6 µg (range, 5–25 µg) and are without evident adverse effects on health. (See Table 28–5 for abbreviations used in this section.)

Children may have multiple nondietary sources of exposure to lead. The powdering of paint from the surfaces of old buildings and the lead in automotive exhausts are major contributors to the lead content of surface soil and dust. Although average daily diets may contain less than 120 µg Pb, house dust in old housing may average from 750–11,000 µg Pb/g, and multilayered chips of old lead pigment paints may contain 20,000–100,000 µg Pb/cm². Increased absorption of lead occurs among children living near lead processing smelters and among children of workers who bring leaded dust into their homes on their work clothes. Sporadic cases of clinical plumbism have been traced to other sources with very high concentrations of lead, including (1) lead shot, fishing or curtain weights, and leaded jewelry, swallowed and retained in the stomach, where the lead is dissolved and absorbed; (2) juices conveyed or stored in improperly lead-glazed earthenware; (3) lead type or toys; (4) Asiatic and Mexican folk medicines and cosmetics (azarcon, greta, pay-looah, surma, al kohl); (5) "soft" drinking water conveyed in lead pipes or stored in lead-lined cisterns; (6) lead-soldered vessels used in cooking; (7) fumes from burning painted wood or casings of storage batteries; and (8) dust from sanding and burning of paint containing lead. The above exposures cause *inorganic* lead poisoning. Sniffing of leaded gasoline by older children and adolescents causes *organic* lead poisoning characterized by toxic encephalopathy.

Epidemiology. The 2nd National Health and Nutrition Examination Survey (NHANES II) (1976–1980) revealed that 3.9% of children ages 6 mo–5 yr, an estimated 675,000 children (of whom 325,000 were black), had PbB of at least 30 µg. The percentage was lowest in rural white children (1.2%) and highest in poor, inner-city black children (18.6%). The reduction in the use of leaded gasoline has left pre-1960 housing as the major environmental source of lead for children in the United States. At least 75% of the more than 50,000,000 dwelling units built before 1960 have lead paint on surfaces exposed to children. As these dwellings fall into disrepair, they present an immediate hazard; household dust is often rich in lead, and the adjacent exterior surface soil generally has a high lead content. In young children, PbB is most closely correlated with Pb on the surface of their hands and the Pb content of household dust. The usual hand-to-mouth activity of preschool children can, if they are exposed to dust containing greater than 1000 µg Pb/g of dust, produce PbB values in groups II and III (Table 28–5). The more severe degrees of poisoning (group IV, Table 28–5) are generally associated with repetitive ingestion (pica) of lead paint flakes or some uncommon source (see under Exposure). PbB fluctuates seasonally, being highest in summer, when most symptomatic episodes occur.

Metabolism. Lead absorption from the gastrointestinal tract is affected by age, diet, and nutritional deficiencies. Although adults absorb 5–10% of dietary lead and retain little of it, young children absorb 40–50% and retain 20–25%. Spontaneous urinary excretion of lead is less than 50 µg/24 hr; it may increase in acute poisoning. Animal studies show that diets high in fat, and especially those low in calcium, magnesium, iron, zinc, or copper, increase the absorption of lead. Diets suboptimal in calcium and iron are prevalent among children in low income groups. The total body lead burden is divided into two major components: bone, in which the amount increases with age and has a half-life of about 20 yr; and soft tissues, in which the half-life is 20–30 days. Lead sequestered in bone is removed from the active metabolic pool. The toxicity of lead is related to its concentration in the small, mobile, soft tissue pool.

Pathophysiology. The principal toxic effects occur in the

Table 28–5. Laboratory Test Results Usually Associated with Various Levels of Lead Absorption

Blood Lead (PbB) Groups*	Normal	Increased Lead Absorption		
	I	II	III	IV
Indicators of internal dose (soft tissue concentrations)				
PbB (µg/dL w.b.)	5–24	25–49	50–69	≥70
PbU-EDTA†	0.20 ± 0.08		>0.75	>2.2
Indicators of disturbed heme synthesis				
PBGS‡			<10–15%	<10–15%
ALAU§	1.1 ± 0.37		>3	>6
EP (µg/dL w.b.)¶	≤35	35–109	110–249	≥250
FEP (µg/dL rbc)**	50 ± 20	92–288	289–655	≥658

*Adapted from Statement by Centers for Disease Control, 1985.

†Results expressed as µg Pb excreted/mg CaEDTA administered during 24 hr following a single intramuscular injection of CaEDTA in a dosage of 500 mg/m². Mean normal value for PbB is 10 µg.

‡Results vary according to method; however, for most methods when PbB≥50–60 µg, then PBGS ≤10–15% of normal for each method, PbU-EDTA ≥ 0.75 and ALA-U begins to increase exponentially from 3 mg/m²/24 hr.

§ALAU results expressed as mg/m²/24 hr. Less specific screening methods give values for ALAU (1) 0.5–1.0 mg/M²/24 hr higher than values shown above. See Nordberg GF: Effects and Dose-Response Relationships of Toxic Metals. New York, Elsevier, 1976, Chapter B16.

¶Note results expressed as µg erythrocyte protoporphyrin (EP)/dL whole blood as used in many screening programs.

**Normal values based on several reports. FEP values for groups II, III, and IV calculated from EP values on basis of 38% hematocrit. EP and FEP values are for microfluorometric extraction methods.

Abbreviations:

PBGS = porphobilinogen synthase (formerly δ-aminolevulinate de-hydratase) in erythrocytes.
ALAU = δ-aminolevulinic acid in urine.
CaEDTA = edathamil calcium disodium.
EP = erythrocyte protoporphyrin (as µg/dL whole blood).
FEP = "free" erythrocyte protoporphyrin (as µg/dL erythrocytes).

Pb = lead.
PbB = µg Pb/dL whole blood.
PbU = µg Pb/24 hr in urine.
PbU-EDTA = chelatable lead (µg Pb excreted in urine after standard dose of CaEDTA).

erythroid cells of the bone marrow, the central and peripheral nervous systems, and the kidney. Abnormal cardiac conduction and thyroid function have also been reported in severe cases. Lead causes partial inhibition in the synthesis of heme at several enzymatic steps (see Fig. 7–34). Ferrochelatase and porphobilinogen synthase (PBGS) are the enzymes most sensitive to inhibition by lead. The following combination is pathognomonic for lead poisoning: increased activity of δ-aminolevulinate synthase and decreased activity of porphobilinogen synthase in erythrocytes, increased δ-aminolevulinic acid in plasma and urine, normal or slightly increased urinary porphobilinogen and uroporphyrin, increased urinary coproporphyrin, and increased "free" erythrocyte protoporphyrin (FEP). Although the porphyrin found in the circulating erythrocytes in lead poisoning and in iron deficiency is zinc protoporphyrin, this metabolite is generally measured as FEP. Compensatory erythroid hyperplasia and reticulocytosis result. Basophilic stippling is best seen in bone marrow normoblasts. There is a dose-dependent decrease in 5-pyrimidine nucleotidase activity, which underlies the basophilic stippling of erythrocytes. As the concentration of lead in blood increases above 50–60 μg/dL, hemoglobin decreases. The microcytic, hypochromic anemia of plumbism is usually morphologically indistinguishable from that of iron deficiency. The dose-dependent decrease in plasma 1,25-dihydroxy vitamin D has been linked to impaired heme production in the kidney.

Severe acute lead poisoning may be responsible for the Fanconi syndrome (generalized renal aminoaciduria, melituria, hyperphosphaturia, and hypophosphatemia) because of acute proximal renal tubular injury; the lesion is reversible. Lead nephropathy, characterized by hyperuricemia with or without gout, has been reported as a sequel of chronic plumbism in Australian children. Acute lead encephalopathy in the very young is characterized by massive cerebral edema due primarily to a generalized increase in vascular permeability. Neuronal destruction also occurs. In suckling animals, but not in mature animals, slowness in learning and behavioral changes can be induced by doses of lead insufficient to produce histopathologic changes.

Clinical Manifestations. The chronic course of unrecognized lead poisoning is characterized by recurrent symptomatic episodes, which may abate spontaneously. The earliest symptoms are hyperirritability, anorexia, and decreased play activity. Sporadic vomiting, intermittent abdominal pain, and constipation are manifestations of lead colic. Colic may occur at blood levels of lead as low as 60 μg/dL, but children with levels of up to 250 μg/dL may appear clinically well. Loss of recently acquired developmental skills may occur. Anemia may be present.

The above symptoms usually, but not always, appear 4–6 wk prior to the start of acute encephalopathy, which is heralded by the sudden onset of persistent vomiting, ataxia, impairment of consciousness, coma, and seizures. In younger children massive cerebral edema is almost always present, although the classic signs of increased intracranial pressure may not be found. In older children and adolescents a toxic encephalopathy without massive cerebral edema is more likely. Subtle premonitory behavioral changes may not be appreciated.

Acute encephalopathy, in which blood lead concentration almost always exceeds 100 μg/dL and usually exceeds 150 μg/dL, is most common during the summer months. The diagnosis can usually be made without lumbar puncture, which is very dangerous. If examination of the cerebrospinal fluid is considered essential for differential diagnosis, the least amount of fluid required should be obtained (several drops). In lead encephalopathy, the fluid changes consist of mild pleocytosis, mild to moderate increase in protein, and increased pressure. Observation for inappropriate secretion of

antidiuretic hormone, partial heart block, and profoundly impaired renal function must be maintained in the seriously ill child. Peripheral neuropathy, manifested in adults principally by motor weakness in the distal muscles of the arms and legs, is rare in children.

Clinical Diagnosis. Symptoms are subtle and nonspecific, and physical examination generally reveals little or nothing abnormal unless there is acute encephalopathy. Plumbism should be included in the differential diagnosis of anemia, seizure disorders, mental retardation, severe behavioral disorders, colicky abdominal pain, and the cerebral and abdominal crises of sickle cell disease. Isolated seizures and self-limited episodes of vomiting during the recent past may represent episodes of clinical plumbism, particularly if the child lives in or visits an old house, if a parent is unavailable for much of the time, and if a history of pica for any substance is obtained. Recent changes of address, recent renovations in the home, and especially, time spent unsupervised or with babysitters and relatives should be ascertained, as persistent pica is particularly associated with such histories. This information is essential in planning the appropriate management for each patient. Emphasis must be placed on environmental sampling for sources of lead and laboratory data. Whenever an index case is found, all housemates should be examined. The possibility of uncommon sources should be ascertained (see under Exposure).

Laboratory Diagnosis. Because clinical diagnosis is exceedingly difficult in children prior to the occurrence of severe injury to the nervous system, early diagnosis depends on laboratory determinations. At least two tests are required: (1) an indicator of the internal accumulation of lead and (2) an indicator of adverse metabolic effect (Table 28–5). Blood lead and FEP can be determined in micro blood samples, as well as in venous blood obtained in hematology Vacutainers containing EDTA as anticoagulant. Special precautions are needed to prevent contamination of blood and urine samples by exogenous lead. Serial tests are needed to determine trends. Iron deficiency may cause FEP to be as high as 500 μg/dL of packed red blood cells when the blood lead level is normal; higher values generally indicate lead toxicity (blood lead groups III and IV, Table 28–5) with or without iron deficiency. In groups III and IV, toxic effects increase exponentially. In emergencies, when these tests are not immediately available and acute lead encephalopathy is a diagnostic possibility, a strongly positive qualitative urinary coproporphyrin test result, many stippled erythroblasts in bone marrow, glycosuria, and hypophosphatemia constitute presumptive evidence of plumbism. The diagnostic edathamil calcium disodium (CaEDTA) mobilization test for chelatable lead in urine *should not be used in patients with symptoms compatible with plumbism.* Radiopaque flecks in the intestinal tract indicate recent ingestion of foreign matter containing lead. Broad bands of increased density at the metaphyses of the long bones usually represent increased storage of lead in bone, but roentgenograms of long bones may be normal or equivocal in severe acute plumbism.

Short-term responses to treatment may be monitored by changes in PbB and ALAU. FEP, which tends to change slowly, is not predictive of chelatable lead (PbU-EDTA, Table 28–5); however, serial FEP tests are useful to monitor long-term responses to therapy and trends in lead absorption. Blood lead values should be obtained, since laws requiring the abatement of housing hazards are directly correlated to the measurement of lead in the child.

Treatment. The cornerstone of therapy is prompt separation of the child from the source(s) of lead, followed by timely reduction of lead hazards in the home environment. Removal of hazards is usually the local health agency's responsibility. Children and pregnant women should remain out of the home *day and night* until the burning and sanding to remove old leaded paint have been completed, the premises have been thoroughly scrubbed with high phosphate detergents 2–3 times to remove the fine particulate lead generated by the deleading process, and the deleaded areas have been re-painted. Thereafter, regular wet cleaning with high phosphate detergents for dust control should be continued, particularly in old housing areas. Play in dirt areas adjacent to such housing should also be avoided. Pre–school aged children should be tested periodically according to Centers for Disease Control (CDC) and Early Periodic Screening, Diagnosis and Treatment (EPSDT) guidelines, to determine trends in lead absorption.

Most children detected in current screening programs are asymptomatic and fit the requirements for groups II and III (Table 28–5). For those in group II, the above measures and improved diet should suffice, and chelation therapy is probably not advisable.

Chelation therapy is advised for children in groups III and IV, including the asymptomatic ones. Intramuscular therapy with CaEDTA should be limited to 5 days at a daily dose of 1000 mg/m² in two divided portions, when venous PbB is greater than 50 but less than 90–100 μg/dL whole blood. Chelation therapy prior to the onset of symptoms may lessen the risk of cerebral injury. Treatment with oral CaEDTA is contraindicated. Oral D-penicillamine is effective only if current exposure to lead is definitely excluded. In the United States, D-penicillamine is at present classed by the FDA as an investigational drug when it is used for lead poisoning. Side effects of this drug include allergic reactions, nephrotic syndrome, and bone marrow suppression—especially neutropenia.

Patients who have symptomatic plumbism (colic, seizures, acute encephalopathy) should be treated promptly with chelating agents if presumptive laboratory test results are positive. Because the onset and clinical course of encephalopathy are unpredictable, the risk of delay outweighs the risk of a few days of chelation therapy. If subsequent tests do not indicate an increased absorption of lead, treatment should be discontinued and the presumptive diagnosis reconsidered.

When acute encephalopathy is present or when PbB is greater than 90–100 μg/dL whole blood, a regimen of BAL and CaEDTA is recommended; the dose for BAL is 500 mg/m²/24 hr and for CaEDTA, 1500 mg/m²/24 hr. The drugs are injected simultaneously at separate intramuscular sites in six divided doses each day for 5 days, after an initial priming dose of BAL only. In moderately ill children who show immediate clinical improvement after initiation of this regimen, BAL may be stopped after 3 days, and the total daily dose of CaEDTA should be reduced by one third after 72 hr. If repeated 5 day courses are needed, a daily dose of 1000 mg/m²/24 hr of CaEDTA is safer and adequate. If the patient becomes anuric, administration of CaEDTA, but not BAL, should be temporarily withheld. CaEDTA is a nonmetabolizable drug that is excreted solely by the kidney; side effects include hypercalcemia, elevation of blood urea nitrogen, and renal injury. Side effects of BAL include vomiting, hypertension, and tachycardia. The side effects of each drug require careful evaluation, because some of them are also features of acute lead encephalopathy. BAL may occasionally evoke intravascular hemolysis in patients with severe glucose-6-phosphate dehydrogenase deficiency.

Fluid and electrolyte management is critical in lead encephalopathy. After an initial infusion of 10% dextrose in water (and of mannitol, if necessary to decrease intracranial pressure) to establish urine flow, continuous intravenous infusion should be restricted to basal requirements and a minimal estimate of the amounts required for replacement of losses due to vomiting, dehydration, and activity associated with

seizures. It is prudent to administer parenteral fluids initially in the same manner in mildly symptomatic patients and in asymptomatic ones who have very high tissue levels of lead, until the trend of the clinical course becomes clear. The use of enemas to remove lead from the lower bowel should never be permitted to delay treatment of symptomatic patients.

Seizures can be controlled initially with diazepam and thereafter with repeated doses of paraldehyde until the patient's state of consciousness is significantly improved. As the dose of paraldehyde is lowered, long-term anticonvulsant therapy with diphenylhydantoin or phenobarbital is started (see Table 29–1 B and Sec. 21.7–21.8). When lead poisoning results from ingestion of lead paint, effective long-term management requires the cooperative efforts of local health department personnel, the medical social worker, the psychologist or psychiatrist, and the pediatrician. Control of hand-to-mouth activity and pica are very difficult to accomplish, although behavioral modification may help.

Prognosis. Sequelae are related to the degree and duration of excessive lead ingestion. Recurrence of clinical manifestations increases the chance of permanent injury. Residual brain damage may not be evident until the child reaches school age. Some survivors of encephalopathy may require residential care; sequelae include seizure disorders, impaired mentation, and attentional deficit. Seizures and altered behavior tend to abate during adolescence, but intellectual deficits persist. Blindness and hemiparesis are restricted to the most severe cases of encephalopathy.

There is general agreement that PbB, if sustained during early childhood in the range of groups III and IV, presents an unacceptable risk for long-lasting but subtle injury to the nervous system, even if no symptoms are ever detected. An increased frequency of learning difficulties in school has been reported among groups of children with a previous record of PbB values in groups III and IV, who had no symptoms and were never treated. There is some evidence that chelation therapy to reduce body lead burden and prompt steps to reduce further excess Pb intake may improve prognosis in asymptomatic children in groups III and IV. Recently, in a study of over 2000 children, a dose-response relationship was shown between the frequency of behavioral and attentional problems in school and the dentin Pb content of shed deciduous teeth. Some of these children had earlier PbB values in the range of group II (Table 28–5).

Prevention. Various agencies in the United States have taken steps during the past decade to reduce air Pb levels, enforce the drinking water standard for Pb, and reduce the Pb content of foods—particularly canned foods; lead additives in automotive fuels will be eliminated in 1988. The use of lead additives in residential paints was banned by the United States Consumer Product Safety Commission in 1977. However, until the large stock of older residential housing is renovated or replaced, screening programs will be needed for early detection of lead toxicity in young children.

J. JULIAN CHISOLM, JR.

Baker EL Jr, Folland DS, Taylor TA, et al: Lead poisoning in children of lead workers. Home contamination with industrial dust. N Engl J Med 296:260, 1977.

Boeckx RL, Posti B, Coodin FJ: Gasoline sniffing and tetraethyl lead poisoning in children. Pediatrics 60:140, 1977.

Centers for Disease Control: Lead Poisoning: Associated Death from Asian Indian Folk Remedies—Florida. Morbidity Mortality Weekly Report 33:638, 1984.

Centers for Disease Control: Preventing lead poisoning in young children, 1985 Statement.

Charney E, Kessler B, Farfel M, et al: Childhood lead poisoning: A controlled trial of the effect of dust control measures on blood lead levels. N Engl J Med 309:1089, 1983.

Chisolm JJ Jr: The use of chelating agents in the treatment of acute and chronic lead intoxication in childhood. J Pediatr 73:1, 1968.

Chisolm JJ Jr, Barltrop D: Recognition and management of children with increased lead absorption. Arch Dis Child 54:249, 1979.

Emmerson BT: The clinical differentiation of lead gout from primary gout. Arthritis Rheum 11:623, 1968.

Lourie RS, Layman EM, Millican FK: Why children eat things that are not food. Children 10:143, 1963.

Mahaffey KR: Nutritional factors in lead poisoning. Nutr Rev 39:353, 1981.

Mahaffey KR, Annest JL, Roberts J, et al: National estimates of blood lead levels: United States, 1976–1980: Association with selected demographic and socioeconomic factors. N Engl J Med 307:573, 1982.

Needleman HL, Gunnoe C, Leviton A, et al: Deficits in psychologic and classroom performance of children with elevated dentine lead levels. N Engl J Med 300:689, 1979.

Nriagu JO: Lead and Lead Poisoning In Antiquity. New York, John Wiley & Sons, 1983, pp 1–437.

Perlstein MA, Attala R: Neurologic sequelae of plumbism in children. Clin Pediatr 5:292, 1966.

Piomelli S, Rosen JF, Chisolm JJ Jr, et al: Management of childhood lead poisoning. J Pediatr 105:523, 1984.

Rabinowitz MB, Wetherill GW, Kopple JD: Kinetic analysis of lead metabolism in healthy humans. J Clin Invest 58:260, 1976.

Rutter M: Low level lead exposure: Sources, effects and implications. In: Rutter M, Jones RR (eds): Lead versus Health: Sources and Effects of Low Level Lead Exposure. New York, John Wiley & Sons, 1982, p 333.

28.16 CHEMICAL POLLUTANTS

As chemicals increasingly permeate our environment, there is a need to consider the special exposures and vulnerability of the fetus and child. Each pediatrician should be alert for evidence of new environmental effects on child health. Virtually all known human teratogens and carcinogens have been discovered by alert clinicians.

Intrauterine Effects

Methylmercury. In the mid 1950's methylmercury caused the first epidemic of congenital cerebral palsy attributable to intrauterine exposures to a chemical pollutant (Sec. 28.14). It was associated with severe, sometimes fatal, neurologic disorders in the population at large and was traced to contamination of fish by waste dumped into Minamata Bay, Japan, by a factory that made vinyl plastics. Similar episodes have occurred in Alamogordo, New Mexico and Iraq due to grain treated prior to planting with a methylmercury-containing fungicide, which was mistakenly used for animal feed or baking.

Polychlorinated Biphenyls (PCB's). In 1968, in Kyushu, Japan, there was an epidemic of chloracne, and women who were pregnant at the time gave birth to infants who were small for gestational age and had, among other findings, dark skin that cleared with time. The outbreak was traced to contamination of cooking oil by PCB's, a heat-transfer agent, through pinhole erosions in pipes during the manufacture of the oil. PCB's from factory waste have now been found in major waterways of the United States and other countries. In Taiwan an episode virtually identical to that in Kyushu has occurred. Compounds similar to PCB's, polybrominated biphenyls (PBB's), were accidentally mixed with animal feed in Michigan and widely distributed within the state. Animals became ill and died, but no fetal effects or overt illnesses have been found in human beings.

Dioxin. In 1976 a runaway reaction in a factory in Seveso, Italy, spewed a chemical cloud downwind over farms and homes. Many animals died, and 2 wk later about 40 exposed children developed chloracne. The chemical in the cloud was dioxin, a potent teratogen in laboratory animals. No human teratogenesis has been found among the abortuses or liveborn children of Seveso women exposed early in pregnancy. In Missouri, horse arenas and roads were sprayed with waste oil to which dioxin had been added; about 60 horses died, and foals were malformed. Transient illness, but not chloracne, occurred in one arena owner and her two children. Further contamination from the same source was subse-

quently recognized in Times Beach, Missouri, and the inhabitants had to be relocated.

Cigarette Smoke. On the average, the birthweight of infants whose mothers smoke heavily during pregnancy is 200 g less than normal, and perinatal morbidity is increased when medical care is inadequate (Sec. 8.17).

Transplacental Carcinogenesis. The discovery that cancer of the cervix or vagina occurs in women after intrauterine exposure to diethylstilbestrol raises the possibility that other chemicals, including pollutants, may also be transplacental carcinogens. Four children have now been reported with fetal hydantoin syndrome and neuroblastoma, suggesting that diphenylhydantoin is a transplacental carcinogen. Among other possible carcinogens is benzene, which causes leukemia after heavy occupational exposures.

Asbestos. Although asbestos is a naturally occurring chemical, its capacity to induce cancer is related to its physical properties. Long, thin fibers are carcinogens, whereas short, thick ones are not. The latent period from exposure until the development of mesothelioma is usually more than 30 yr. Exposure in childhood may thus induce cancer in adulthood. Asbestos dust brought home on a father's workclothes has been implicated as the cause of mesothelioma in his daughter (onset at 34 yr), as well as in his wife.

Bronchogenic carcinoma is induced by exposure to asbestos, especially among cigarette smokers; the risk is about five times greater than it is in cigarette smokers not exposed to asbestos and 54 times greater than in people exposed to neither. From 1947–1973, asbestos fibers were sprayed on new schoolroom ceilings in the United States; about 10,000 schools were treated. With time and abuse, the asbestos frayed and fibers floated through the schoolrooms. In theory the exposure could increase the frequencies of mesothelioma and bronchogenic carcinoma. As yet, no increases have been observed in young adults, but sufficient time may not yet have passed to allow for both deterioration of asbestos and the latent period. Asbestos in schools is being removed, sealed with plastic, or contained by dropped ceilings. The interaction between asbestos exposure and the use of cigarettes in causing lung cancer adds to the reasons for urging young people not to smoke.

Lactational Effects

Because of chemical pollution, new questions are being raised about the safety of breast feeding. PCB's, PBB's, dioxin, and certain pesticides are stored in fat and are not readily cleared from the body except in the fat of breast milk. Japanese infants whose mothers were exposed postpartum to PCB-contaminated cooking oil were exposed to high levels in their mothers' milk while nursing. Elsewhere, samples of breast milk to date have rarely shown high levels of these chemicals. When unusual exposures occur, however, before advice on breast feeding is given, the milk should be tested, e.g., for dioxin in Seveso, for PBB's in Michigan, or for PCB's in upper New York State. No general recommendation against breast feeding should be made because of its many benefits. Cow's milk may also contain these chemicals, but tests are routinely made to determine that the milk sold commercially does not exceed limits set by federal regulation. Game fish have also been contaminated from PCB-polluted waters.

Effects of Other Exposures

Water. About 200 chemicals have been found in small amounts in various water supplies. Some are known to cause human cancer after heavy occupational exposure, but the claim that regional increases in cancer mortality rates are attributable to chemicals in the water supply is not generally accepted. Fluoride, added to water or naturally occurring, is not associated with human cancer.

Air. Major air pollutants generated by fossil fuel consumption are sulfur oxides, carbon monoxide, photochemical oxidants (especially ozone), and nitrogen oxides. The most common respiratory diseases associated with these pollutants are asthma, chronic bronchitis, and emphysema. Automotive exhausts add lead to the atmosphere and, in enclosed spaces, can cause intense pollution with carbon monoxide to which children have been especially susceptible, as in underground garages or at skating rinks where gasoline-powered vehicles were used to scrape the ice. Some industries have caused specific diseases in neighboring residential areas through air pollution with asbestos, beryllium, lead, methylmercury, or dioxin. There is an increased mortality from lung cancer among persons living in counties with arsenic-emitting smelters or petrochemical industries.

Workclothes. Illnesses in the child are at times traceable to a parent's workclothes; toxicity from lead, beryllium, and asbestos has occurred. Pediatricians, in considering the origins of noninfectious diseases, should ask about parental occupation, unusual household exposures, and neighborhood factories.

Food. In addition to the foregoing chemical pollutants that may enter the food chain, many other chemicals are intentionally added to food to improve appearance, taste, texture, or preservation. Evaluation of the safety of these chemicals is difficult because of problems in measuring exposures and in separating them from the effects of the myriad of variables which may confound interpretation of the alleged untoward effects.

Interactions

Little is known about the interactions of chemicals with one another, with physical or viral agents, or with susceptibilities. Furthermore, chemicals may be activated or inactivated by metabolic processes, thus altering their disease potential. One would expect children with heritable methemoglobin reductase deficiency to be especially susceptible to the effects of nitrates or aniline dyes. Other children from the general population may be exceptionally resistant. Some chemicals photosensitize the skin as a consequence of an interaction with a physical agent, ultraviolet light. Asbestos greatly potentiates the capacity of cigarette smoke to induce lung cancer. An interaction between old viruses and new chemicals may explain the increased frequency of diseases such as the mucocutaneous lymph node syndrome.

Susceptibility to chemical pollutants varies markedly from conception through adolescence. Exposures also vary as the environment changes from that within the uterus to the nursery, home, school, neighborhood, recreational area, and, occasionally, the hospital. Greater attention must be given by pediatricians to the effects of chemical pollutants, and environmental experts must become more aware of the special biology and surroundings of the fetus and child.

ROBERT W. MILLER

Chisolm JJ Jr: Fouling one's own nest. Pediatrics 62:614, 1978.
D'Itri PA, D'Itri FM: Mercury Contamination. A Human Tragedy. New York, John Wiley & Sons, 1977.
Finberg L (ed): Eighty-fourth Ross Conference on Pediatric Research: Chemical and Radiation Hazards. Columbus, OH, Ross Laboratories, 1982.
IARC Monographs on the Evaluation of Carcinogenic Risk of Chemicals to Man. Asbestos. Lyon, France, International Agency for Research on Cancer, v14,1977.
Miller RW: Environmental causes of cancer in childhood. Adv Pediatr 25:97, 1978.
Miller RW: Areawide chemical contamination: Lessons from case histories. JAMA 245:1548, 1981.
Miller RW: Congenital PCB poisoning: A reevaluation. Environ Health Perspect 60:211, 1985.
Rogan WJ: The sources and routes of childhood chemical exposures. J Pediatr 97:861, 1980.
Spooner CM: Asbestos in schools—a public health problem. N Engl J Med 301:782, 1979.

28.17 VENOM DISEASES; POISONING BY VENOMOUS SNAKES, LIZARDS, AND MARINE ANIMALS

The fear of venomous animals dates from antiquity, but the knowledge of venomous disease remains limited. As modern transportation makes remote areas of the world more accessible and interest in outdoor recreational activities expands, contact with venomous animals is likely to increase.

SNAKE BITE

Of the more than 3500 known species of snakes, only 200 that belong to the following four families are poisonous to humans. They have in common a modified salivary gland that secretes and stores venom and maxillary fangs for conducting the venom to the victim.

The Colubridae family includes most of the world's snakes, but only the African boomslang (*Disholidus typus*) and the vine, twig, or bird snake (*Thelotornis kirtlandi*) have been associated with human fatalities.

The Elapidae family includes many of the world's deadliest snakes. The Afro-Asian cobras, the African mambas, the Indo-Malayan kraits, and the New World coral snakes are poisonous members of this family. The elapids are particularly numerous and diverse in Australia, where all dangerous land snakes are elapids (black tiger snake, brown snake, death adder, taipan, and copperheads).

The Hydrophidae family includes 52 different species of poisonous sea snakes that inhabit tropical waters throughout the world.

The Viperidae (true vipers) are all poisonous and inhabit Europe, Africa, and Asia; the subfamily Crotalidae (pit vipers) are common in the Americas and Southeast Asia. Many species have adapted to relatively cool climates, spending the winter in hibernation and, therefore, showing seasonal variations in growth and reproduction. Species common to North America include rattlesnakes, water moccasins, and copperheads.

Epidemiology. It has been estimated that 300,000 poisonous snake bites responsible for 30,000 to 40,000 deaths occur throughout the world each year. The largest number of fatalities occurs in Southeast Asia; most are due to cobra bites. In the Western Hemisphere most fatalities from snake bites occur in Brazil. About 45,000 people are bitten by snakes every year in the United States, and about 20% of these are bitten by poisonous snakes; the fatalities number fewer than 20 and are usually due to bites by rattlesnakes, water moccasins, or coral snakes.

Clinical Manifestations. The most important clinical sign of envenomation is hypotension or shock secondary to hypovolemia due to extravasation of blood or to a direct effect of venom on blood vessels and/or the myocardium.

Local Effects. Bites by members of the Viperidae (true vipers) and Crotalidae (pit vipers) are characterized by localized pain and swelling. Necrosis of the skin with formation of bullae, ecchymoses, and discoloration soon follows. There is extensive local edema with oozing of serosanguineous fluid into the bullae and subcutaneous tissue.

The bites by members of the Elapidae family vary among species. The Eastern coral snake bite causes minimal pain and tissue destruction; cobra bites are characterized by severe pain with extensive necrosis and sloughing. Bites by the Hydrophidae are painless, fang marks are often inconspicuous, and no local reaction is observed.

Systemic Effects. A bite by a member of the Viperidae family or the subfamily Crotalidae produces predominantly hemorrhagic symptoms. Disseminated intravascular coagulation develops rapidly and leads to ecchymoses, epistaxis, hematuria, hemoptysis, and hematemesis. Acute renal insufficiency may develop. Neurologic abnormalities are then manifest as delirium, disorientation, coma, and seizures. Death is usually secondary to intracranial hemorrhage.

The venoms of other species of poisonous snakes are neurotoxic, and death is secondary to respiratory paralysis. Cobra bites often produce drowsiness within 15 min, followed by progressive involvement of cranial nerves, including ptosis and ophthalmoplegia. Palatal and pharyngeal involvement leads to slurred speech and difficulty in handling oral secretions. Varying degrees of motor paralysis ensue as do seizures and coma. The reaction to the bite of the sea snake differs from that of the cobra bite in that the above sequence is heralded by diffuse myalgia and progressive muscular weakness. The bite of the Eastern coral snake initially produces paresthesia in the involved extremity followed rapidly by involvement of the cranial nerves, respiratory insufficiency, and death.

Treatment. Initially, one should determine whether the attacking snake is poisonous; knowledge of the species indigenous to the geographic area is helpful. Examination of the wound may be informative, as bites by nonpoisonous species lack distinct fang punctures and do not cause local pain or swelling. There is also a lack of progressive symptomatology from nonpoisonous snake bites. Bites on the extremities and into adipose tissue are less dangerous than bites into highly vascularized areas such as the face.

When the victim has been bitten on an extremity, a tourniquet should be placed above the bite area, tightly enough to occlude venous and lymphatic return but loosely enough to preserve a distal pulse. The involved extremity should be immobilized, and, if possible, the patient should avoid exercise, including walking, thus lessening the spread of the venom. Applying ice directly to the wound or cooling the involved extremity may be harmful and should be avoided. Incision and suction soon after the bite can remove substantial amounts of venom from the wound, and should be performed when transportation to a medical facility cannot be accomplished within a period of hours. The skin should be cleaned and a single linear incision 1 cm in length and 0.5 cm in depth made through each fang mark. Suction with cups provided in commercial snake bite kits or oral suction should be continued for at least 1 hr before the tourniquet is released. The risks of this procedure are considerable and include infection, particularly when nonsterile equipment or mouth suction is used, and persistent bleeding in patients with incoagulable blood. Amputation of the involved digit or extremity is not indicated, and every effort should be made to remove the patient as quickly and as comfortably as possible to a medical facility.

The wound should be cultured, irrigated with saline, and treated with a topical antiseptic preparation. Extensive swelling that compromises the peripheral circulation is an indication for immediate fasciotomy. The administration of aspirin and/or intramuscular injections are contraindicated in patients with hypocoagulable blood. Surgical debridement of vesicles and necrotic skin can often be delayed for 1 wk.

Systemic Measures. Specific therapy with antivenom (see below) should be followed by appropriate supportive therapy, which often consists of blood transfusions for bites by snakes with a strongly hematotoxic venom. Adjustment of fluid and electrolyte balance is indicated in the presence of vomiting, renal insufficiency, and shock. Systemic complications include paralysis, respiratory insufficiency, disseminated intravascular coagulation, and cardiac arrhythmias. Tetanus prophylaxis with toxoid or antitoxin is indicated if the child has not been adequately immunized, and parenteral therapy with penicillin is indicated to prevent secondary bacterial infection. Pain is often severe and may require narcotic administration.

Nonpoisonous snake bites generally require no treatment.

Serum Therapy. Snake venom antisera or antivenoms are prepared by hyperimmunization of horses against one or more venoms. Though the chemical composition of snake venom varies from species to species, there is enough antigenic similarity between venoms of related species to produce clinically useful polyvalent antisera. Two antivenin preparations are commercially available in the United States.* Antivenom for the treatment of bites by exotic species can usually be obtained through local zoological societies. These products can cause anaphylaxis and will cause serum sickness in 30–75% of patients, depending on the amount administered. Administration, therefore, is best performed in a hospital setting following skin testing with the normal horse serum present in the commercial antivenin kits. Severe allergic reactions have occurred after a negative test, and some patients have been safely treated even after a positive test. Some clinicians routinely give epinephrine subcutaneously or antihistamines intravenously before infusing antivenom. After bites by unidentified snakes or snakes known not to be highly poisonous, antivenom treatment should be withheld until the development of local symptoms.

GILA MONSTER

This is the only lizard poisonous to humans. The two species inhabit the Sahuaro desert regions of Arizona and New Mexico as well as the desert regions of Mexico. Most bites occur during attempted capture or in handling captive animals. After a bite it is often difficult to remove the lizard. There is considerable injury locally, severe pain, erythema, and edema. The venom contains a potent neurotoxin. Initial systemic symptoms include nausea and vomiting and are followed rapidly by generalized weakness, cranial nerve paralysis, and respiratory insufficiency. Fatalities are uncommon. No antivenom is available. Treatment consists of local care of the wound and supportive therapy as described for snake bites.

VENOMOUS MARINE ANIMALS

Venomous fish include certain sharks, scorpion fish, weeverfish, toadfish, catfish, and stingrays. Among the venomous bony fish of the world, the family Scorpaenidae is considered the most dangerous in both the number and severity of injuries produced. These fish inhabit tropical waters and are especially plentiful around coral reefs; well camouflaged with their environment, they pose a risk for scuba divers, snorkelers, swimmers, and surfers. In addition, many species including the lionfish are imported into this country each year by private and commercial collectors. Accordingly, aquarists are also at risk for envenomation.

The clinical manifestations of poisoning are remarkably similar in all cases. There is immediate pain at the puncture sight that spreads to involve the entire extremity. The venom produces local ischemia and circumscribed cyanosis, followed by edema and erythema that may spread to involve the entire extremity. Tissue necrosis may be locally extensive and con-

---

*Wyeth Antivenin (Crotalidae) polyvalent: venom effective against rattlesnakes, water moccasins, and copperheads. Wyeth Antivenin (*Micrurus fulvius*): effective against North American coral snake venom.

tributes to secondary bacterial infection. The wound produced by stingrays is unique in that the laceration is several cm deep and often contains bony and epithelial fragments of the venom apparatus. Systemic manifestations include pallor, nausea, vomiting, diaphoresis, and loss of consciousness. Convulsions, paralysis, and death have been reported.

Treatment consists of the appropriate application of a tourniquet and copious irrigation of the wound to remove fragments of the venom apparatus. The only available antivenom is one for stonefish venom. Although effective for most types of Scorpaenidae, this product is only indicated for stonefish envenomations.* Many venoms are heat labile; for this reason immersion of the involved extremity in water as hot as can be tolerated is recommended. Tetanus toxoid or antitoxin should be administered except when the immune status of the patient is adequate. Broad spectrum antibiotic therapy should be prescribed to prevent superinfection. Narcotics may be required to control pain.

COELENTERATE STINGS

The venomous coelenterates include hydroids, jellyfish, sea anemones, and coral. They are equipped with tentacles that have a venom apparatus consisting of nematocysts or nettle cells. The stings vary from a mild stinging sensation produced by the smaller jellyfish to an extremely painful, almost shock-like sensation produced by the most dangerous member of the phylum (Portuguese man-of-war). The local signs include erythema and urticaria. Systemic involvement may be manifested by weakness, chills, fever, nausea, and vomiting. In extreme situations there may be respiratory failure and death.

The intensity of symptoms depends upon the length of time the tentacles remain in contact with the skin; the tentacles should therefore be removed as promptly as possible. Caution must be observed since some species of jellyfish have powerful nematocysts which may penetrate gloves and other clothing. Topical treatment consists of warm soaks with normal saline. Antihistamines and corticosteroids are indicated in the presence of extensive swelling and urticaria.

Prevention of stings is best accomplished by caution when swimming in tropical waters. Damaged tentacles, which often float in water following a storm, are capable of inflicting stings, as are jellyfish washed up on beaches and often presumed to be dead.

WILLIAM T. SPECK

Bücherl W: Venomous Animals and Their Venoms, Vols I and II. New York, Academic Press, 1968.
Halstead BW: Poisonous and Venomous Marine Animals of the World, Vols I and II. Washington DC, US Government Printing Office, 1965 and 1967.
Kizer KW, McKinney HE, and Auerbach PS: Scorpaenidae envenomation: a five year poison center experience. JAMA 253:307, 1985.
Watt CH: Poisonous snakebite: Treatment in the United States. JAMA 240:654, 1978.

28.18 MAMMALIAN BITES: DOG, HUMAN, CAT, AND RAT

Mammalian bites are a common cause of morbidity and a rare cause of mortality among children. Bite wounds account for 1% of all emergency room visits; the incidence varies from 300 to over 1000 bites/100,000. A large proportion of the bite victims are children. However, there are probably fewer than 50 bite-related deaths/yr.

Epidemiology. Dog bites account for 50–95% of bite injuries; children are commonly victims, and males sustain almost 60% of the bites. More than 70% of dog bites to the face occur in children under 15 yr old. Most dog bites occur in summer months and in the afternoon. Fewer than 25% of bites involve stray dogs. Large breed dogs account for 50% of bite injuries.

Human bite injuries consist of self-inflicted wounds of the lips, tongue, or of other soft tissues, and injuries to hands when they strike the tooth of another person. Rat bites are uncommon; most occur in the summer, on the extremities, and to children less than 6 yr old, usually while the child is asleep.

Clinical Manifestations. Animal and human bites consist of scratches, lacerations, punctures, and abrasions. Dogs and humans have the strength also to produce crush injuries. Because cats have long, thin, sharp teeth, their puncture wounds are often deep. Hand wounds resulting from striking the teeth of another person are usually seen on the dorsal surface near the metacarpophalangeal joint. Such wounds may involve only the joint or spread to other parts of the hand; when the hand is unclenched, folds of skin may partially cover the wound and prevent adequate drainage.

Infectious Complications. Animal and human bite wounds should be presumed to be contaminated with bacteria, which may result in a variety of immediate and/or long-term infections. *Tetanus* is discussed in Sec. 11.36 and *rabies* in Sec. 11.78; other infectious etiologies are presented here.

A history of a bite, and the time of the bite referable to the time the physician sees the patient and to the time the lesions appear are the most important factors in evaluating infection. Animal bite infections vary with the species, but *tetanus* is always a serious risk. *Pasteurella multocida* is commonly associated with the bites of cats and, somewhat less frequently, of dogs and other animals. *P. pneumotropica* has been implicated as the cause of infection from dog and cat bites. *Staphylococcus epidermidis, Streptococcus viridans,* and diphtheroids have also been cultured from cat bite wounds. Although most rat bites heal without sequelae, rare local and systemic complications are caused by *Streptobacillus moniliformis* or *Spirillum minus* (Sec. 11.54). Alligator bites may be contaminated by *Aeromonas hydrophila,* a facultative anaerobic asporogenous gram-negative rod. *Human bites* are usually infected with anaerobic bacteria found in the oropharynx or with *Staphylococcus aureus,* streptococci, or *Eikenella corrodens.* Hepatitis B can also be transferred by human bite.

When there is swelling, erythema, and a purulent discharge, a Gram stain of the exudate is indicated to facilitate initial selection of a potentially appropriate antibiotic prior to the availability of culture and sensitivity reports. If the purulent material has no foul odor and if clumps of gram-positive cocci are seen, staphylococcal infection may be suspected. If the purulent discharge has no foul odor and gram-negative rods are present, infection with enteric or soil organisms or with *Pasteurella multocida* or *P. pneumotropica* should be suspected.

If there is a foul odor or crepitation in the wound, or both, anaerobic infection should be considered: gram-negative rods suggest *Bacterioides* infection; whereas gram-positive rods with spores suggest *Clostridium sp.,* and gram-positive cocci in chains suggest infection with anaerobic streptococci. Gram-negative anaerobes may be present in purulent material even in the absence of foul-smelling discharge.

Noninfectious Complications. Depending on the location and severity of the bite, cosmetic and/or functional problems may also arise. Psychologic sequelae are probably rare if the child receives adequate support from the family in the postinjury period. However, vivid memories of the bite episode may persist, and serious personality changes have been known to occur.

---

*Health Services Department, Sea World in San Diego (619-222-6363), Steinbart Aquarium, San Francisco (415-221-8014), and Sea World of Ohio in Aurora (216-562-8101).

Prevention. Children should be kept away from animals or people who might bite them, and they and their parents should be educated about safe interaction with animals. All dogs should be leashed or confined in a fenced yard. All strays should be removed from streets by the animal warden. Rat bites can be prevented only by appropriate public health measures to clean up breeding grounds and upgrade homes to prevent infestation.

Treatment. The management of bite injuries should include scrupulous cleansing, debridement of devitalized tissue, and care to ensure that neural and vascular structures are not injured or are repaired. Osteomyelitis must be considered in deep or crush wounds. Tetanus prophylaxis should be administered if indicated (Sec. 11.36).

Cleansing should be performed by high pressure irrigation with large volumes of isotonic saline using a syringe connected to a large bore needle. In some medical centers, povidone-iodine is used for cleansing. Quaternary ammonia compounds, such as 1:100 benzalkonium chloride (Zephiran), may be used when exposure to rabies is considered a possibility.

Bite lacerations, except for those of the hand, seen within several hours of injury can be closed primarily after adequate irrigation and debridement. Lacerations of the face may be closed primarily up to 6–8 hr after the injury. Lacerations presenting after these time limits should be cultured and allowed to close by secondary intention. Scar revision can be done at a later date. Puncture wounds, except those of the hand, should be excised and irrigated prior to closure. Dirty wounds, deep puncture wounds, or crush injuries that cannot be cleansed adequately and debrided should be left unsutured. Some surgeons suggest that all bites inflicted by humans be left unsutured, because of the high probability of local infection. If the wound is potentially disabling or disfiguring, the child should be referred to a plastic surgeon, hand surgeon, or other qualified individual for appropriate management.

Culture of fresh wounds and the use of prophylactic antibiotics are not indicated for most bites. However, such therapy is justified after obtaining a culture if the wound appears infected or there is more than a superficial injury. Generally, for dog and cat bites penicillin G should be given in doses of 125–250 mg orally, four times a day, for 7–10 days; this is effective against *P. multocida, P. pneumotropica, Spirillum minus, Streptobacillus moniliformis, E. corrodens,* and a number of other pathogens. For human bites, which are infected with *Staphylococcus aureus* more commonly than are animal bites, a penicillinase-resistant drug such as dicloxacillin (50 mg/kg/24 hr in four divided doses) may be indicated. A foul-smelling discharge suggesting anaerobic infection should be treated with high doses of penicillin (75,000 units/kg/24 hr) or with clindamycin (30 mg/kg/24 hr in three divided doses) if *Bacillus fragilis* is a consideration.

Patients allergic to penicillin may be given clindamycin, tetracycline, or erythromycin. If the allergic reaction has not included anaphylaxis, exfoliative dermatitis, or an urticarial response, these patients may be treated with a cephalosporin such as cephalexin (40 mg/kg/24 hr in four divided doses).

If there is purulent drainage and if gram-negative rods are seen, ampicillin or amoxicillin plus an aminoglycoside such as gentamicin should be prescribed.

A patient presenting with an uninfected or only superficially infected hand wound may be managed as an outpatient. The wound should be well irrigated, left open, and elevated. The hand should be soaked frequently and checked daily. Some authorities recommend the prophylactic use of antibiotics, with coverage including penicillinase-producing staphylococci. A patient presenting with an infected hand wound—swollen, stiff, tender finger, involvement of other structures—should be admitted. The wound should be cleaned, debrided,

and left open. After cultures are taken, the patient should be started on a semisynthetic penicillin or similar antibiotic and the hand kept elevated. *E. corrodens* is sensitive to penicillin but not to the semisynthetic penicillins.

Patients who have high fever and such complications as septic arthritis, osteomyelitis, septicemia, visceral abscesses, or endocarditis should be hospitalized and appropriately treated.

Berzon DR: The animal bite epidemic in Baltimore, Maryland: Review and update. Am J Pub Health 63:593, 1978.

Berzon DR, DeHoff JB: Medical costs and other aspects of dog bites in Baltimore. Pub Health Reports 89:377, 1979.

Callahan ML: Treatment of common dog bites: Infection risk factors. JACEP 7:83, 1978.

Callahan ML: Prophylactic antibiotics in common dog bite wounds: A controlled study. Ann Emerg Med 9:410, 1980.

Gislason IL, Call JD: Dog bite in infancy. Trauma and personality development. J Am Acad Child Psychol 21:203, 1982.

Goldstein EJC, Citron DM, Finegold SM: Dog bite wounds and infections: A prospective clinical study. Ann Emerg Med 9:508, 1980.

Goldstein EJC, Citron DM, Wield B, et al: Bacteriology of human and animal bite wounds. J Clin Microbiol 8:667, 1970.

Harris D, Imperato PJ, Oken B: Dog bites—an unrecognized epidemic. Bull NY Acad Med 50:981, 1979.

Jaffe AC: Animal bites. Pediatr Clin North Am 30:405, 1983.

Kizer KW: Epidemiologic and clinical aspects of animal bite injuries. JACEP 8:134, 1979.

Malinowski RW, Strate RG, Perry JF, et al: The management of human bite injuries of the hand. J Trauma 19:655, 1979.

Marr JS, Beck AM, Lugo JA: An epidemiologic study of the human bite. Pub Health Reports 94:514, 1979.

28.19 SPIDER, SCORPION, AND ANT BITES

Spiders (Order Araneae, which includes tarantulas) and scorpions (Order Scorpionida) are feared, although the incidence of morbidity and mortality is very low.

In the United States the spiders that may cause problems include members of the *Latrodectus* genus, especially the *L. mactans mactans* or black widow, and members of the *Loxosceles* genus, especially the *L. reclusa* or brown recluse. Tarantulas in the United States have a venom that is not toxic to humans, and the two scorpions that can cause severe systemic reactions are *Centruroides sculpturatus* and *Centruroides gertschi. Hadrurus arizonensis* is a scorpion whose venom causes only local reactions.

Latrodectus Bites. Patients usually contact these spiders outdoors in trash piles, outhouses, and stacks of old lumber. The black widow is found in the eastern United States, although there are members of the *Latrodectus* in other parts of the country.

The bite initially produces a local, mild to moderate pain. After a brief period of time, systemic symptoms occur, including sweating, nausea, headache, apprehension, hyperesthesias and paresthesias, muscular cramps with a rigid abdomen, and fever. The blood pressure is elevated, and there may be ECG changes. Coma may occur. The symptoms resolve over a period of hours or days.

Latrodectus antivenom is made in horses and may be given intravenously after appropriate skin tests. Cramps, headache, and nausea may be treated with intravenous calcium gluconate. Muscle relaxants such as methocarbamol have been used but are ineffective. Morphine or meperidine can be used for analgesia. Tetanus prophylaxis and antibiotics may be indicated.

Loxosceles Bites. Patients usually contact these spiders in abandoned houses, cellars, wood piles, and trash piles. The recluse spider is found predominantly in the central and southern United States, but other *Loxosceles* spiders are found throughout the south and west.

The venom of *Loxosceles* spiders contains enzymes that cause endothelial damage, which is followed by thrombocytopenia, decreased fibrinogen, and a prolonged partial thromboplastin time. Small vessel thrombosis accounts for skin necrosis.

The *Loxosceles* bite has local and systemic manifestations. The bite is initially painless. Two–4 hr later itching, swelling, pain, and redness occur locally. A blister, which may be hemorrhagic, may form. Over several days the area becomes necrotic. It then becomes mummified over the next 1–2 wk, and eventually an ulcer develops which, if larger than 1 cm, may last for weeks to months. The ulcer may become secondarily infected. Systemic reactions, while rare, are more common in children. These include fever, chills, malaise, weakness, nausea, vomiting, chest pain, petechiae, seizures, and intravascular hemolysis.

There is no antivenom for *Loxosceles* bites. It is unclear whether treatment other than supportive therapy is beneficial. Some authorities recommend excision of the bite to limit the size of the resultant ulcer; others recommend the use of steroids for treatment of the systemic reactions. Tetanus prophylaxis and antibiotics may be indicated.

Scorpion Bites. *C. sculpturatus* and *C. gertschi* are nocturnal and usually encountered in the desert Southwestern United States. Bites are most common in May through August.

The venom contains neurotoxins, enzymes, and other substances. The bite causes local pain followed by paresthesias. Systemic reactions, which are rare, consist of difficulty in speaking and swallowing, salivation, sweating, nausea, vomiting, restlessness, and hyperreflexia. Seizures may occur in children.

Local application of ice as soon as possible is the first treatment. Antivenom is available for severe cases. Barbiturates will control seizures; paraldehyde is contraindicated. Nerve blocks should be used for pain control; morphine, meperidine, and other morphine derivatives are contraindicated.

Solenopsis Bites. Bites of the fire ant are a problem in the Southeastern United States; *S. invicta* is the dangerous species. These ants live in large hills housing tens of thousands of the arthropods. They swarm when disturbed, and the patient usually sustains multiple bites. The venom is an insoluble alkaloid.

The bite causes a papule that progresses into a sterile pustule within 24 hr. There may be localized tissue necrosis and subsequent scar formation. Secondary infection is common.

Some individuals develop hypersensitivity reactions to solenopsis stings. Desensitization, as with hymenoptera, is possible.

No antivenom is available. Treatment is primarily supportive and directed at the secondary infection, if present.

JEROME A. PAULSON

Arnold RE: What to do about bites and stings of venomous animals. New York, Macmillan, 1973.

Auer AI, Hershey FB: Surgery for neurotic bites of the brown spider. Arch Surg 108:612, 1979.

Hunt GR: Bites and stings of uncommon arthropods. 1. Spiders. 2. Reduvids, fire ants, pus caterpillars, and scorpions. Postgrad Med 70:91–102, 107-110, 1982.

Minton SA: Venomous arthropods. *In:* Hubbert WT, McCulloch WF, Schnurenberger PR (eds): Diseases Transmitted from Animals to Man. 6th ed. Springfield, Ill, Charles C Thomas, 1975.

Wasserman GS, Siegel C: Loxoscelism (brown recluse spider bites): A review of the literature. Clin Tox 19:353, 1979.

29

APPENDIX

TABLES 29–1*A* AND *B*: DRUGS*

Table 29–1*A*. Selected Drugs for Systemic Therapy Grouped Alphabetically by Category of Indication for Their Use
Individual drugs with their dosages are listed alphabetically by generic names in Table 29–1*B*, p. 1520.

ACTIVATED CHARCOAL
ANALGESIC AGENTS
1. Narcotic analgesics
    codeine phosphate, codeine sulfate
    meperidine hydrochloride, DEMEROL hydrochloride
    morphine sulfate
    pentazocine hydrochloride, TALWIN hydrochloride
    propoxyphene hydrochloride, DARVON, ‡
2. Non-narcotic analgesics
    acetaminophen, LIQUIPRIN, TYLENOL, ‡
    acetylsalicylic acid, ASPIRIN, BUFFERIN, ‡
    sodium salicylate
ANTACID
aluminum hydroxide, AMPHOGEL
aluminum hydroxide + magnesium hydroxide, MAALOX
ANTHELMINTIC AGENTS
1. Against *Giardia lamblia (Lamblia intestinalis)*
    quinacrine, ATABRINE
2. Against pinworms (*Enterobius vermicularis*), roundworms (*Ascaris lumbricoides*), and hookworms (*Necator americanus, Ancylostoma duodenale*)
    mebendazole, VERMOX
    pyrantel pamoate, ANTIMINTH
3. Against tapeworms (*Diphyllobothrium latum, Taenia saginata, Taenia solium, Hymenolepis nana*)
    niclosamide, YOMESAN
4. Against whipworms (*Trichuris trichiura*)
    mebendazole, VERMOX
ANTIALLERGIC AGENTS
1. Antihistamines
    brompheniramine maleate, DIMETANE
    carbinoxamine maleate, CLISTIN
    chlorpheniramine maleate, CHLOR-TRIMETON
    dimenhydrinate, DRAMAMINE
    diphenhydramine hydrochloride, BENADRYL
    tripelennamine hydrochloride, PYRIBENZAMINE
2. Antihistamine and antiserotonin
    cyproheptadine, PERIACTIN
3. Inhibition of immunologic reaction
    corticosteroid
ANTIASTHMA MEDICATION
1. Bronchodilators
    β-adrenergic stimulants
        bronchodilator inhalation

epinephrine
metaproterenol sulfate, ALUPENT, METAPREL
terbutaline sulfate, BRETHINE, BRICANYL
Phosphodiesterase inhibitors
    theophylline, ELIXOPHYLLIN, LUFYLLIN, SLO-PHYLLIN, ‡ and many combinations
    aminophylline, SOMOPHYLLIN ‡
2. In status asthmaticus resistant to other treatment modalities
    corticosteroid, in addition to other supportive measures
3. Inhibition of mastocyte degranulation (only for prevention)
    cromolyn sodium inhalation, AARANE, INTAL Spinhaler
4. Topical corticosteroid treatment (in steroid-dependent cases)
    beclomethasone aerosol, VANCERIL Inhaler
ANTICHOLINERGIC AGENTS
atropine sulfate
propantheline, PRO-BANTHINE
scopolamine methylbromide, PAMINE
ANTICONVULSANT DRUGS
1. Treatment of partial cortical seizures with elementary symptomatology (focal motor epilepsy, focal somatosensory epilepsy, or autonomic or compound forms thereof), and generalized tonic-clonic seizures (grand mal epilepsy)
    carbamazepine,† TEGRETOL
    phenobarbital,† LUMINAL
    phenytoin,† DILANTIN
    primidone, MYSOLINE
2. Treatment of partial seizures with complex symptomatology (temporal lobe or psychomotor epilepsy)
    carbamazepine,† TEGRETOL
    phenytoin,† DILANTIN
    primidone, MYSOLINE
3. Treatment of petit mal (with 3/sec spike and wave pattern)
    clonazepam, CLONOPIN
    ethosuximide,† ZARONTIN
    phenobarbital† (to prevent secondary generalization to tonic-clonic seizures)
    trimethadione, TRIDIONE
    valproate sodium, DEPAKENE
4. Treatment of mixed seizure patterns (akinetic seizures, myoclonic seizures, petit mal variant, and combinations thereof with tonic-clonic seizures): use rational combination of drugs listed above, including, in particular, valproate sodium, DEPAKENE. At times, addition of acetazolamide, DIAMOX.

Table continued on following page

---

*To be used in conjunction with Sec. 5.50, p. 231. Consult also the following:

1517

Table 29–1A. Selected Drugs for Systemic Therapy Grouped Alphabetically by Category of Indication for Their Use (Continued)

5. Treatment of status epilepticus (by parenteral route)
    diazepam,† VALIUM
    paraldehyde
    phenobarbital, LUMINAL
    phenytoin sodium, DILANTIN
6. Treatment of infantile spasms (by parenteral route) adrenocorticotropic hormone (ACTH), ACTHAR, CORTROSYN

ANTICROUP MEDICATION
epinephrine racemic, VAPONEFRINE

ANTIDIURETIC HORMONE REPLACEMENT (by nasal route) desmopressin acetate, DDAVP

ANTIEMETIC MEDICATION
chlorpromazine, THORAZINE
dimenhydrinate, DRAMAMINE
promethazine, PHENERGAN

ANTIFUNGAL AGENTS
amphotericin B, FUNGIZONE
griseofulvin, FULVICIN, GRISACTIN,‡
miconazole, MONISTAT
nystatin, MYCOSTATIN, NILSTAT

ANTIHYPERTENSIVE AGENTS (See Table 14–15)
1. Diuretics: see chlorothiazide, hydrochlorothiazide
2. Agents with antiadrenergic effect
    methyldopa, ALDOMET
    propranolol, INDERAL
    reserpine, SANDRIL, SERPASIL, ‡
3. Vasodilators
    hydralazine, APRESOLINE
    in hypertensive emergency: diazoxide, HYPERSTAT; nitroprusside, NIPRIDE
    minoxidil, LONITEN
4. Against hypertension associated with catecholamine-secreting tumors
    phenoxybenzamine (α-adrenergic blockade), DIBENZYLINE
    phentolamine (α-adrenergic blockade), REGITINE
    See Sec. 19.27 on catecholamine-secreting tumors.
5. Against hypertension associated with adrenocortical hyperfunction
    See Sec. 14.88, 17.35, and 19.25.
6. Angiotensin I–converting enzyme inhibitor captopril, CAPOTEN

ANTIMALARIAL AGENTS
1. For prevention of clinical manifestations of disease
    chloroquine diphosphate, ARALEN, RESOCHIN
    pyrimethamine, DARAPRIM
2. For treatment of malarial attack
    chloroquine diphosphate, ARALEN, RESOCHIN
    quinine sulfate or dihydrochloride, with either tetracycline or pyrimethamine and sulfadiazine
3. For "radical" cure
    primaquine diphosphate

ANTIMICROBIAL AGENTS (mechanism of action)
1. Aminoglycosides (interfere with function of ribosomes in sensitive bacteria)
    amikacin sulfate, AMIKIN
    gentamicin sulfate, GARAMYCIN
    kanamycin sulfate, KANTREX
    neomycin sulfate, MYCIFRADIN, NEOBIOTIC
    streptomycin sulfate
    tobramycin, NEBCIN
2. Cephalosporins (interfere with cell wall synthesis in sensitive bacteria)
    cefaclor, CECLOR
    cefadroxil, DURICEF
    cefamandole, MANDOL
    cefoperazone, CEFOBID
    cefotaxime, CLAFORAN
    cefoxitin, MEFOXIN
    ceftizoxime, CEFIZOX
    cefuroxime, ZINACEF
    cephalexin, KEFLEX
    cephazolin, ANCEF, KEFZOL
    cephalothin sodium, KEFLIN
    cephapirin, CEFADYL
    cephradine, ANSPOR, VELOSEF
    moxalactam, MOXAM
3. Chloramphenicol (impairs peptide bond formation by ribosomes in sensitive bacteria)
    chloramphenicol, CHLOROMYCETIN
4. Macrolides (impair peptide bond formation by ribosomes in sensitive bacteria)
    clindamycin hydrochloride, clindamycin palmitate hydrochloride, clindamycin phosphate, CLEOCIN
    erythromycin, ILOTYCIN, ‡
    erythromycin estolate, ILOSONE
    erythromycin ethylsuccinate, ERYTHROCIN ethylsuccinate, PEDIAMYCIN
    erythromycin stearate, ERYTHROCIN stearate, ETHRIL, ‡
    lincomycin, LINCOCIN
5. Penicillins (interfere with cell wall synthesis in sensitive bacteria)
    amoxicillin, AMOXIL, LAROTID, ‡
    amoxicillin + clavulanic acid, AUGMENTIN
    ampicillin sodium, OMNIPEN-N, PENBRITIN-S, ‡
    ampicillin trihydrate, OMNIPEN, PENBRITIN, ‡
    benzathine penicillin G, BICILLIN
    benzylpenicillin, penicillin G, PENTIDS, PFIZERPEN G, ‡
    carbenicillin disodium, GEOPEN
    cloxacillin sodium, TEGOPEN
    dicloxacillin sodium, DYNAPEN, PATHOCIL
    methicillin sodium, CELBENIN, STAPHCILLIN
    nafcillin sodium, NAFCIL, UNIPEN
    oxacillin sodium, BACTOCILL, PROSTAPHLIN
    phenoxymethylpenicillin, penicillin V, PEN-VEE K, VEETIDS, ‡
    piperacillin, PIPERACIL
    procaine penicillin G, DURACILLIN, WYCILLIN
    ticarcillin disodium, TICAR
6. Polypeptide antimicrobials (increase permeability of cytoplasmic membrane in sensitive bacteria)
    colistimethate sodium, COLY-MYCIN M
    colistin sulfate, COLY-MYCIN S
7. Complex glycopeptide (inhibits cell wall synthesis in gram positive organisms)
    vancomycin, VANCOCIN
8. Sulfonamides (inhibit tetrahydrofolic acid synthesis in sensitive bacteria)
    sulfadiazine
    sulfamethoxazole, GANTANOL
    sulfisoxazole, GANTRISIN, ‡
    trimethoprim-sulfamethoxazole, BACTRIM, SEPTRA
    trisulfapyrimidines
9. Tetracyclines (interfere with function of ribosomes in sensitive microorganisms)
    chlortetracycline, AUREOMYCIN
    demeclocycline, DECLOMYCIN
    doxycycline, VIBRAMYCIN
    methacycline, RONDOMYCIN
    minocycline, MINOCIN, VECTRIN
    oxytetracycline, TERRAMYCIN, UROBIOTIC
    tetracycline, ACHROMYCIN, TETRACYN, ‡
10. Additional antimicrobial agents used in urinary tract infections
    methenamine mandelate, MANDELAMINE, ‡
    nalidixic acid, NEGGRAM
    nitrofurantoin, FURADANTIN, MACRODANTIN, ‡

ANTIPYRETIC AGENTS
acetaminophen, LIQUIPRIN, TEMPRA, TYLENOL, ‡
acetylsalicylic acid, ASPIRIN, BUFFERIN, ‡
sodium salicylate

ANTIRHEUMATIC AGENTS
acetylsalicylic acid, ASPIRIN, BUFFERIN, ‡
sodium salicylate
Other nonsteroidal anti-inflammatory agents have not been conclusively evaluated in the pediatric age group. See Sec. 10.58.

Table continued on opposite page

Table 29–1A. Selected Drugs for Systemic Therapy Grouped Alphabetically by Category of Indication for Their Use (Continued)

ANTITUBERCULOUS AGENTS
aminosalicylate sodium, PAS, PARASAL-sodium, ‡
ethambutol, MYAMBUTOL
isoniazid, INH, NYDRAZID, ‡
rifampin, RIFADIN, RIMACTANE
streptomycin

ANTITUSSIVE AGENTS
codeine phosphate or sulfate (addictive on long-term use)
dextromethorphan hydrobromide, ROMILAR, component in many combinations

ANTIVIRAL AGENTS
acyclovir, ZOVIRAX

CALCIUM PREPARATIONS
calcium gluconate
calcium lactate

CARDIOACTIVE AGENTS
1. Agents with inotropic effect
   digitoxin, CRYSTODIGIN, PURODIGIN
   digoxin,† LANOXIN
   dobutamine, DOBUTREX
   dopamine, INTROPIN
   isoproterenol, ISUPREL
2. Antiarrhythmic agents
   a. against sinus node disturbances
      sinus bradycardia
         atropine sulfate (anticholinergic effect)
      sinus tachycardia
         associated with congestive heart failure
            digoxin (inotropic effect), LANOXIN
         associated with increased sympathetic tone or induced by excess of catecholamines
            propranolol (β-adrenergic blockade), INDERAL
   b. against paroxysmal atrial tachycardia, supraventricular tachycardia, atrial flutter, or atrial fibrillation
      measures to increase vagal tone (cholinergic stimulation) (carotid massage)
         cholinesterase-inhibiting agents
            edrophonium, TENSILON
            neostigmine methylsulfate, PROSTIGMIN
         triggering of reflex vagal discharge
            phenylephrine hydrochloride, NEO-SYNEPHRINE (α-adrenergic agent, peripheral vasoconstrictor)
      digoxin,† LANOXIN
      β-adrenergic blockade
         propranolol hydrochloride, INDERAL (in association with digoxin, if digoxin not effective alone)
         After reversal of arrhythmia, for protection from recurrence: digoxin,† quinidine,† procainamide, propranolol
   c. in atrioventricular conduction block
      isoproterenol IV† (β-adrenergic agonist), ISUPREL (ventricular pacing)
   d. against paroxysmal ventricular tachycardia or tachyarrhythmia
      lidocaine hydrochloride IV,† XYLOCAINE
      procainamide hydrochloride, PRONESTYL
      quinidine gluconate, QUINAGLUTE prn associated with propranolol hydrochloride, INDERAL
      phenytoin, DILANTIN (cardioconversion)
      After reversal of arrhythmias, for protection from recurrence: quinidine,† procainamide, propranolol†
   e. against digitalis-induced arrhythmia
      (correct hypokalemia, if present)
      lidocaine hydrochloride IV, XYLOCAINE
      phenytoin, DILANTIN
      propranolol,† INDERAL
   f. calcium channel blocker
      verapamil, CALAN, ISOPTIN

CENTRAL STIMULANTS
caffeine
dextroamphetamine sulfate, DEXEDRINE, ‡
methylphenidate hydrochloride, RITALIN
pemoline, CYLERT

CHELATING AGENT FOR IRON INTOXICATION
deferoxamine, DESFERAL

CHOLINERGIC AGENTS (cholinesterase inhibitors)
edrophonium chloride, TENSILON
pyridostigmine bromide, MESTINON

CORTICOSTEROIDS
for physiologic replacement
for pharmacologic effects

DIURETICS
1. osmotic diuretic
   mannitol, OSMITROL
2. saluretic agents
   with moderate effect
      chlorothiazide, DIURIL
      chlorthalidone, HYGROTON
      hydrochlorothiazide, ESIDRIX, HYDRODIURIL, ‡
      triamterene, DYRENIUM
   with rapid and accentuated effect
      ethacrynic acid, EDECRIN
      furosemide, LASIX
3. aldosterone antagonist
   spironolactone, ALDACTONE

DUCTUS ARTERIOSUS CLOSURE
indomethacin, INDOCIN

ENURESIS (adjunct medication used in enuresis)
imipramine, TOFRANIL, W.D.D., ‡

GASTRIC ACID SECRETION INHIBITION
cimetidine, TAGAMET

HYPNOTIC AND SEDATIVE AGENTS
amobarbital, amobarbital sodium, AMYTAL
chloral hydrate, NOCTEC
pentobarbital, pentobarbital sodium, NEMBUTAL
phenobarbital, phenobarbital sodium, LUMINAL
secobarbital, secobarbital sodium, SECONAL
For selected uses, see diazepam, diphenhydramine, and "lytic cocktail" (Table 29–1B).

ION EXCHANGE RESIN
cholestyramine, QUESTRAN

IRON PREPARATIONS
ferrous sulfate
iron-dextran complex, IMFERON

LAXATIVES, CATHARTICS, DEMULCENTS
bisacodyl, DULCOLAX
cascara sagrada (extract containing anthraquinones), component of PERI-COLACE
dioctyl sodium sulfosuccinate, COLACE, ‡
magnesium hydroxide, magnesium sulfate, milk of magnesia, components of HALEY'S M-O
mineral oil, component of AGORAL, HALEY'S M-O
phenolphthalein, PRULET, component of AGORAL
senna (extract of senna fruit), SENOKOT, X-PREP
sodium sulfate

MAGNESIUM
magnesium sulfate

MOTION SICKNESS MEDICATION (in ascending order of effectiveness)
cyclizine, MAREZINE
dimenhydrinate, DRAMAMINE
promethazine, PHENERGAN

MUCOLYTIC AGENT
acetylcysteine, MUCOMYST

NASAL DECONGESTANTS
phenylephrine, NEO-SYNEPHRINE, component of many combinations
pseudoephedrine hydrochloride, D-FEDA, SUDAFED, component of many combinations

Table continued on following page

DRUGS

Table 29–1A. Selected Drugs for Systemic Therapy Grouped Alphabetically by Category of Indication for Their Use *(Continued)*

NEUROLEPTIC AGENTS
chlorpromazine hydrochloride, THORAZINE
hydroxyzine hydrochloride, or pamoate, ATARAX, VISTARIL
"lytic cocktail"
methotrimeprazine, LEVOPROME
prochlorperazine, COMPAZINE
promethazine hydrochloride, PHENERGAN
thioridazine, MELLARIL

OPIATE ANTAGONIST
naloxone hydrochloride, NARCAN

PRESSOR AGENTS
epinephrine
phenylephrine hydrochloride, NEO-SYNEPHRINE

RENAL TUBULAR SECRETION (inhibition of renal tubular secretion)
probenecid, BENEMID

URIC ACID LOWERING AGENT (inhibition of synthesis)
allopurinol, ZYLOPRIM

VASCULAR HEADACHE
1. in acute attack
   acetylsalicylic acid, ASPIRIN, BUFFERIN, ‡
   atropine sulfate
   caffeine, component in many combinations
   ergotamine tartrate, GYNERGEN, component in many combinations
   sedative (amobarbital, pentobarbital, secobarbital, phenobarbital)
2. for prevention of attacks
   cyproheptadine hydrochloride, PERIACTIN
   phenytoin, DILANTIN
   propranolol hydrochloride, INDERAL

†First-line drug; drug of choice.
‡Available also under other brand name(s).
The drug tables in several recent editions were prepared by Harry C. Shirkey, M.D.

D R U G S

Table 29–1B. Drug Doses* (Drugs Listed Alphabetically by Generic Name)

KEY:

NB	newborn (birth to end of 1st mo)		†	available as generic preparation
IN	infant (1–12 mo)		‡	available also under other brand name(s)
CH	child (1–12 yr)			
AD	adult			

caps	capsules		g	gram
div	divided		mg	milligram = 10^{-3} g
D/W	dextrose in water		μg	microgram = 10^{-6} g
IM	intramuscular			(sometimes abbreviated "mcg")
inj	injection		ng	nanogram = 10^{-9} g
IV	intravenous		kg	kilogram = 10^{3} g
LO	linguo-occlusal		mL	milliliter = 10^{-3} liter ≃
ointm	ointment			cm^3 = cc
PO	per os, oral			(cubic centimeter)
PR	per rectum		℞	Prescription
SC	subcutaneous			
SL	sublingual			
sol	solution			
susp	suspension			
tabl	tablets			

Acetaminophen, paracetamol, APAP, NAPAP
℞ antipyretic, analgesic: IN, CH = PO: 30–40 mg/kg/24 hr, div, every 4–6 hr, prn
†, LIQUIPRIN, TYLENOL, ‡; tabl, liquid preparations
Caution: Massive overdose may cause hepatic necrosis through formation of a toxic metabolite. Lesser overdoses frequently cause reversible jaundice (Sec. 28.4).

Acetazolamide, carbonic anhydrase inhibitor
℞ as adjunct in the treatment of convulsive disorders (ketotic effect): CH = PO: 8–30 mg/kg/24 hr, div, every 6–8 hr
†, DIAMOX; tabl

Acetylcysteine, mucolytic agent; detoxifying agent in acetaminophen overdose
℞ to loosen tenacious bronchial secretions by local application to the bronchial tree with nebulizer: 3–5 mL 20% sol diluted with equal volume of sterile water or saline, or 6–10 mL of 10% sol, every 6-8 hr; or by direct instillation: 1–2 mL of 10% or 20% sol every 1–4 hr
℞ in acetaminophen overdose: CH, AD = PO: 140 mg/kg/1st dose, followed by 70 mg/kg/dose every 4 hr for a total of 72 hr
MUCOMYST; vials 10% (100 mg/mL) or 20% (200 mg/mL)

Acetylsalicylic acid, ASA
℞ antipyretic, analgesic, anti-inflammatory: IN, CH = PO: 30–65 mg/kg/24 hr, div, every 4–6 hr, prn. This dosage corresponds to 27–58 mg salicylate sodium/kg/24 hr, or 20–50 mg salicylic acid/kg/24 hr.
℞ antirheumatic: CH = PO: 65–130 mg/kg/24 hr, div, every 4–6 hr
†, ASPIRIN, BUFFERIN, ‡: tabl; also contained in many combination products
Caution: Acute or chronic overdose may cause life-threatening poisoning syndrome (Sec. 5.29 and 28.5).

ACTH, adrenocorticotropic hormone
℞ of infantile spasms: IM: 24–40 units q 12 hr, or 2.5–4.0 units/kg q 12 hr. Observe for hypertension, use with caution in presence of congestive heart failure, acute psychosis, ocular herpes
10 units/mL, 20 units/mL, 40 units/mL vials
CORTICOTROPIN, CORTROSYN, ACTHAR; inj

Activated Charcoal, adsorbent for treatment of oral drug overdose
PO: 10 times (by weight) estimated quantity of drug ingested or 1 g/kg orally; may repeat every 4 hr when necessary

Table continued on opposite page

See KEY to abbreviations, above; for further information about drugs, see package insert.

Table 29–1B. Drug Doses *(Continued)*

Commercial ready-to-use suspensions may contain sorbitol, which induces osmotic diarrhea in some patients
Multiple products

Acyclovir, antiviral agent against herpes simplex and varicella-zoster virus by selective inhibition of viral DNA synthesis
  ℞ in clinical herpes simplex infection in neonates: NB = IV (over 60 min): 10 mg/kg/dose every 8 hr, for 10 days.
    Dosing interval should be increased to 24 hr if renal function is less than 25% of normal
  ℞ in immunocompromised individuals with herpes simplex or varicella-zoster virus infection: CH = IV (over 60 min): 250 mg/m²/dose every 8 hr; AD = IV (over 60 min): 5 mg/kg/dose every 8 hr
  ℞ in severe first episode of herpes genitalis: CH, AD = LO: 5% ointm
ZOVIRAX; inj, ointm

Allopurinol, analogue of hypoxanthine; inhibitor of xanthine oxidase and thereby of the terminal steps of uric acid biosynthesis
  ℞ against hyperuricemia and urate deposition in tissues and kidneys, especially in patients receiving antineoplastic chemotherapy: CH = PO: 10 mg/kg/24 hr, div or in single daily dose. Note that allopurinol and its metabolite alloxanthine (oxypurinol) inhibit xanthine oxidase, and that reduced glomerular filtration requires lowering the dose to compensate for delayed excretion. A high urine output should be established—with a neutral or slightly alkaline urine pH—to allow for excretion of uric acid precursors.
  Caution: If azathioprine or mercaptopurine, which are metabolized by xanthine oxidase, are to be given concomitantly with allopurinol, the dosage of azathioprine or mercaptopurine should be reduced substantially (to ¼–⅓ of usual dosage).
ZYLOPRIM; tabl

*No attempt has been made to reproduce a comprehensive list of adverse side effects or of formulations available for the drugs listed. For these, the reader is again referred to standard textbooks of pharmacology, to the package inserts accompanying the commercial preparations of each drug, and to *Physicians' Desk Reference,* distributed annually in the United States by Physicians' Desk Reference, Box 210, Westwood, N.J. 07675.

Dosages listed in the Table are not specifically intended for premature and newborn infants unless so indicated.

All doses are average doses and are approximate. Variability of individual response may require alteration of dosage upward or downward. Doses based on different criteria (e.g., body weight, surface area) frequently do not correspond. Surface area may be calculated from Figures 29–1 and 29–2.

Doses are generally expressed as grams or milligrams per kilogram of body weight per 24 hours (g or mg/kg/24 hr), even for drugs ordinarily administered on a prn (as needed or indicated) basis.

For teratogenic effects of drugs, see Sec 6.31, package inserts, and Physicians' Desk Reference.

Because of the multiplicity of proprietary names and formulations of the drugs listed, only a few representative examples have been given of the many proprietary preparations available in most instances. We have intended no bias in selecting the proprietary names used, and make due apology to any manufacturers and distributors whose products may appear to have been slighted.

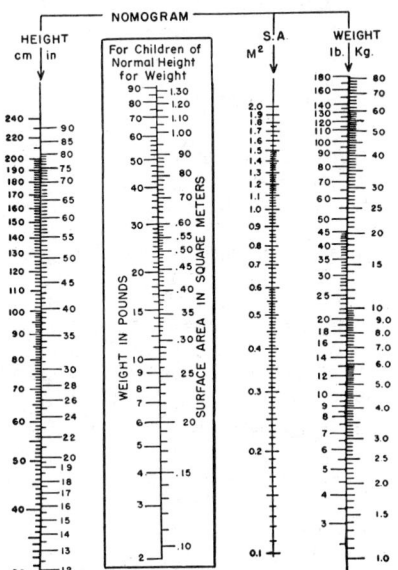

Figure 29–1. Nomogram for estimation of surface area. The surface area is indicated where a straight line which connects the height and weight levels intersects the surface area column; or the patient is roughly of average size, from the weight alone (enclosed area). (Nomogram modified from data of E. Boyd by C.D. West.)

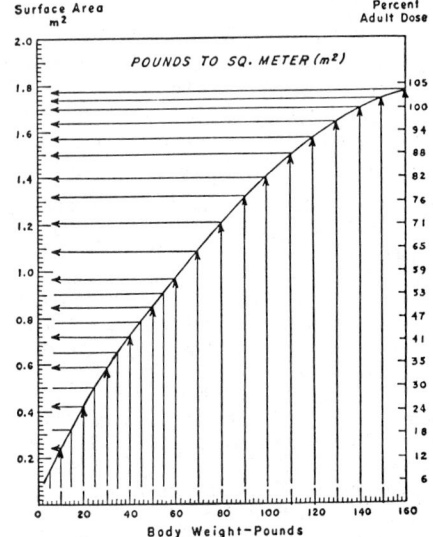

Figure 29–2. Relations between body weight in pounds, body surface area, and adult dosage. The surface area values correspond to those set forth by Crawford et al (1950). Note that the 100% adult dose is for a patient weighing about 140 lb and having a surface area of about 1.7 m². (From Talbot NB, et al: Metabolic Homeostasis—A Syllabus for Those Concerned with the Care of Patients. Cambridge, Harvard University Press, 1959.)

See KEY to abbreviations, p. 1520; for further information about drugs, see package insert.

Table 29–1B. Drug Doses (Continued)

Aluminum hydroxide, antacid
  ℞ for treatment of peptic ulcer: CH = PO: 5–15 mL/dose every 3–6 hr, or 1 and 3 hr after meals and at bedtime
  ℞ for prophylaxis of gastrointestinal bleeding:
    IN = PO(by nasogastric tube): 2–5 mL every 1–2 hr
    CH = PO(by nasogastric tube): 5–15 mL every 1–2 hr
  ℞ against hyperphosphatemia: IN, CH = PO: 50–150 mg/kg/24 hr, div, every 4–6 hr
  Note: May cause constipation, phosphorus depletion. Inhibits gastric emptying. Interferes with absorption of tetracyclines
  †, AMPHOJEL; susp (320 mg/5 mL), tabl (300 mg, 600 mg), gel liquid (600 mg/5 mL)

Aluminum hydroxide and magnesium hydroxide, antacid
  Note: Magnesium-containing antacids are laxative. In renal failure, magnesium and aluminum may be retained. Interferes with absorption of tetracyclines
  ℞ for treatment of peptic ulcer: same as for aluminum hydroxide alone.
  †, MAALOX, ‡; susp, tabl

Amikacin, antimicrobial aminoglycoside
  NB (≤2000 g and/or ≤7 days old) = IM, IV (over 20–30 min): 15 mg/kg/24 hr, div, every 12 hr
  NB (>2000 g and >7 days old), IN, CH = IM, IV (over 20–30 min): 15–22.5 mg/kg/24 hr, div, every 8 hr
  Usual duration of treatment: 7–10 days.
  AMIKIN; inj

Aminosalicylate sodium, para-aminosalicylate sodium, PAS sodium; structural analogue of para-aminobenzoic acid with weak bacteriostatic activity against *Mycobacterium tuberculosis,* used only in combination with other antituberculous agents
  ℞ as adjunct to isoniazid therapy: CH = PO: 200–300 mg/kg/24 hr, div, every 4–6 hr
  †, PAMISYL-Sodium, PARASAL-Sodium, ‡; tabl, caps
  Note: Frequent nausea, vomiting, diarrhea, abdominal pain, and poor acceptance by patients restrict the usefulness of this substance. 1 g of aminosalicylate sodium contains 4.7 mEq Na⁺

Amobarbital, central nervous system depressant with intermediate duration of action. Tolerance to its hypnotic effect may develop on continued use. Initially, hypnotic effect lasts 3–8 hr.
  ℞ for sedation: IN, CH = PO, IM: 1–2 mg/kg/24 hr, div, every 6 hr
  ℞ for sleep: IN, CH = PO, IM: 2–3 mg/kg/dose, repeat prn after 12–24 hr
  †, AMYTAL; tabl, elixir • amobarbital sodium, †, AMYTAL sodium; inj, caps

Amoxicillin, acid-resistant ampicillin congener
  IN, CH = PO: 20–40 mg/kg/24 hr, div, every 8 hr
  †, AMOXIL, LAROTID; ‡, caps, oral susp, pediatric drops

Amoxicillin + clavulanic acid; combination of a β-lactam antibiotic with a β-lactamase (penicillinase) inhibitor. The addition of clavulanic acid extends the activity of amoxicillin from Group A and other streptococci, *Streptococcus pneumoniae,* many strains of *E. coli* and *Proteus mirabilis,* non–β-lactamase-producing strains of staphylococci, *Neisseria gonorrhoeae,* and *Haemophilus influenzae* to include β-lactamase-producing strains of *H. influenzae, E. coli, P. mirabilis* as well as *Klebsiella pneumoniae, Staphylococcus aureus* (but not methicillin-resistant strains), *Branhamella catarrhalis, Bacteroides fragilis,* and *Legionella pneumophila. Pseudomonas aeruginosa,* many strains of *Serratia,* and *Enterobacter* are resistant.
  ℞ for otitis media, sinusitis, lower respiratory tract, skin, soft tissue, and urinary tract infections: CH = PO: amoxicillin 20–40 mg/kg/24 hr + clavulanic acid 5–10 mg/kg/24 hr, div, every 8 hr
  Note: May cause diarrhea, abdominal pain, urticaria and other rashes, due possibly to clavulanic acid alone. Amoxicillin is available as single component.
  AUGMENTIN; tabl of 2 strengths: 250 mg amoxicillin + 125 mg clavulanic acid, and 500 mg amoxicillin + 125 mg clavulanic acid; oral susp with amoxicillin 125 mg + clavulanic acid 31.25 mg/5 mL, or amoxicillin 250 mg + clavulanic acid 62.5 mg/5 mL

Amphotericin B; antifungal agent of the "polyene" type (nystatin, another example); insoluble in water, unstable below pH 4, must be given IV. Effective through binding to sterol components of the membrane of sensitive fungi, thereby altering its permeability; interference with renal function of patients seems an extension of the mode of action of this drug, demanding caution and continued monitoring during amphotericin B therapy.
  Owing to potential toxicity for a variety of biologic functions, amphotericin B should be used only in progressive and potentially fatal infections with fungi sensitive to it. Guidelines not available at this time for dosage in children as compared with adults.
  Use as solution of amphotericin B at concentration of 0.1 mg/mL in 5% dextrose (all other drugs, including antimicrobial agents, and electrolytes must be kept away from the colloidal suspension of amphotericin B).
  See Sec. 11.98 for dose and administration. Optimal dose and duration of therapy not clearly determined.
  Available as lyophilized powder containing sodium deoxycholate as emulsifier. Colloidal suspension prepared by adding required volume of sterile water and shaking appropriately, subsequently diluted in 5% sterile dextrose in water to a final concentration of amphotericin B of 0.1 mg/mL, for slow IV administration; FUNGIZONE intravenous; inj

Ampicillin; acid-resistant penicillin congener
  NB (≤7 days old) = IV (over 15–30 min), IM: 50 mg/kg/24 hr, div, every 12 hr
    ℞ for meningitis: IV: 100 mg/kg/24 hr, div, every 4 hr
  NB (>7 days old) = IV (over 15–30 min), IM: 75 mg/kg/24 hr, div, every 8 hr
    ℞ for meningitis: IV: 200 mg/kg/24 hr, div, every 4 hr
  IN, CH = PO: 50–100 mg/kg/24 hr, div, every 6 hr
    ℞ for septicemia: IV (over 15–30 min), IM: 100–200 mg/kg/24 hr, div, every 4 hr (IV) or every 6 hr (IM)
    ℞ for meningitis: IV (over 15–30 min): 400 mg/kg/24 hr, div, every 4 hr
  ampicillin sodium, for injection, OMNIPEN-N, PENBRITIN-S, ‡; inj • ampicillin trihydrate, †, OMNIPEN, PENBRITIN, ‡; caps, oral susp, pediatric drops

Atropine sulfate, *dl*-hyoscyamine; anticholinergic agent used mainly in premedication for anesthesia, as antiarrhythmic agent and as antispasmodic. Dosage varies according to indications and sensitivity of patients. On the average for IN, CH = SC, PO (IV): 0.01 mg/kg/dose, to be repeated prn after 2 hr until desired effect is obtained or adverse effects preclude further increase; for continued ℞: PO: 0.04 mg/kg/24 hr, div, every 6 hr, preferably with meals
  †; inj, tabl
  Caution: As for belladonna, below.

Beclomethasone dipropionate, chlorinated synthetic corticosteroid
  ℞ topical treatment to the bronchial tissues in long-term, steroid-dependent asthma. Delivered from metered-dose aerosol unit, releasing approximately 50 µg beclomethasone by activation of the dispenser unit: CH (6–12 yr): 1–2 inhalations every 6–8 hr. Effect usually apparent within 1–4 wk after beginning of steroid inhalations
  Caution: On transfer from systemic steroid therapy for asthma to inhalation therapy, adrenocortical competency of the patient must be watched and supported, if indicated, since inhalation therapy does not contribute to systemic corticosteroid supply.
  VANCERIL inhaler

Belladonna tincture, aqueous-alcoholic extract of belladonna leaves; anticholinergic preparation; used chiefly as antispasmodic
  Contains the equivalent of approximately 0.3 mg atropine sulfate per mL. Usual dose: 1 drop/4.5 kg (10 lbs) body weight 15–30 min before meals, 3 times per day
  Caution: Erythematous skin, persistently dilated pupils, or tachycardia are indications for discontinuing, then lowering dose. Extreme hypersensitivity may exist in patients with Down syndrome.

Bisacodyl, cathartic, structurally related to phenolphthalein
  ℞ laxative: PO: 0.3 mg/kg/dose, 6–8 hr before desired large bowel action. *Note:* tablets are enteric-coated and should be swallowed whole, with the added precaution of avoiding oral antacids or milk within at least 1 hr of ingestion.
  DULCOLAX; tabl, suppos

Table continued on opposite page

Table 29–1*B*. **Drug Doses** (*Continued*)

Brompheniramine maleate; alkylamine; antihistamine with mild anticholinergic and mild sedative effects

℞ antiallergic effect: CH = PO: 0.5 mg/kg/24 hr, div, every 6 hr

†, DIMETANE; elixir, tabl, inj

Bronchodilator aerosols

℞ in acute asthmatic attack, provided effective inhalation is possible, e.g., in early stage of attack, or with assisted ventilation (IPPB). Effectiveness of a delivered dose depends on the microdispersion in the aerosol generated from different types of nebulizers. Onset of effect 2–5 min after inhalation of aerosol. Risk of overuse or overdosage in children is high with aerosol treatment, particularly in emergency situations. These limitations apply to all bronchodilator aerosols (epinephrine, racemic epinephrine, isoproterenol, metaproterenol, isoetharine), some of which can be dispensed from "metered" nebulization nozzles in products for use in adults.

Caffeine, CNS stimulant and vasoconstrictor of cerebral vessels

℞ against vascular headache and as an analeptic: CH = PO: 10 mg/kg/24 hr, div, prn every 4–6 hr; single dose usually 2–3 mg/kg/dose.

Note: In newborn, caffeine elimination markedly diminished compared with adult (including parturient woman) so that transplacentally acquired blood concentrations of caffeine are maintained within possibly effective range for several days after delivery. Danger of toxic manifestations by cumulation if additional caffeine administered without adjustment for this particular situation.

Calcium gluconate $[CH_2OH(CHOH)_4COO]_2Ca \cdot H_2O$

1 g equivalent to 89 mg elemental calcium or to 4.46 mEq Ca^{++}. Solution "10%" contains 100 mg/mL of calcium gluconate. This concentration equivalent to elemental calcium, 8.9 mg/mL or Ca^{++} 0.45 mEq/mL.

℞ to compensate for manifestations of hypocalcemia (tetany, seizures, myocardial insufficiency, hypoparathyroidism). Urgency and severity of clinical situation dictate dose and route of administration: IN, CH = IV (infused slowly, with monitoring of heart for bradycardia, arrest): "10%" calcium gluconate solution: 1–2 mL/kg/dose, equivalent to Ca^{++} 0.45–0.90 mEq/kg/dose, repeat prn after 6 hr. Daily dose needed might be as high as Ca^{++} 2.7 mEq/kg/24 hr.

Caution: Do not use any calcium preparation for intramuscular injection because of risk of sterile abscess formation. Extravascular leakage may cause local necrosis.

IN, CH = PO: calcium gluconate 500 mg/kg/24 hr, equivalent to elemental calcium 45 mg/kg/24 hr or Ca^{++} 2.3 mEq/kg/24 hr, div, every 4–8 hr

Note: Concomitant oral intake of phosphate exerts a major influence on the amount of calcium made available for absorption in the intestine;

†, powder, tabl

Calcium lactate $[CH_3CHOHCOO]_2Ca \cdot 5H_2O$

1 g of Ca lactate equivalent to 130 mg elemental calcium or to 6.49 mEq Ca^{++}.

IN, CH = PO: 500 mg/kg/24 hr, equivalent to elemental calcium 65 mg/kg/24 hr or Ca^{++} 3.2 mEq/kg/24 hr, div, every 4–8 hr

Note: Concomitant oral intake of phosphate exerts major influence on amount of calcium available for absorption in intestine. To ensure appropriate absorption in neonatal transient hypoparathyroidism, a calcium:phosphorus ratio of 4:1 (by weight, corresponding to 3:1 on molar basis) should be achieved in the feeding. This would require 10 g calcium lactate powder added to a daily formula containing 500 mL of whole cow milk.

†; powder, tabl

Captopril, competitive inhibitor of angiotensin I–converting enzyme, antihypertensive agent

℞ in hypertension: CH(> 12 yr old) = PO: initially 75 mg/24 hr, div, every 8 hr, followed, if necessary, by increments of 25 mg/dose up to a maximum of 450 mg/24 hr

Note: May cause renal impairment, neutropenia, immunodeficiency, rashes, and disturbances of taste. Adjust dose with renal failure. There is only limited experience in children.

CAPOTEN; tabl

Carbamazepine, anticonvulsant agent; structurally related to tricyclic antidepressants

CH = PO: initially 10 mg/kg/24 hr, div, every 8–12 hr; to be increased progressively, if needed, to 20 mg/kg/24 hr, div, every 12 hr or as a single daily dose, if tolerated. On the basis of presently available information 25 mg/kg/24 hr should not be exceeded.

TEGRETOL; tabl

Carbenicillin disodium; semisynthetic penicillin susceptible to destruction by penicillinase

℞ for systemic use: NB = IV (over 15–30 min), IM: initial dose 100 mg/kg, followed by maintenance therapy according to the following criteria:

≤2000 g + ≤7 days old: 225 mg/kg/24 hr, div, every 8 hr
≤2000 g + >7 days old: 400 mg/kg/24 hr, div, every 6 hr
>2000 g + ≤7 days old: 300 mg/kg/24 hr, div, every 6 hr
>2000 g + >7 days old: 400 mg/kg/24 hr, div, every 6 hr

IN, CH = IV (over 15–30 min), IM: 400–600 mg/kg/24 hr, div, every 4 hr (IV) or every 6 hr (IM)

GEOPEN; inj; 1 g carbenicillin disodium contains 6.5 mEq Na^+

℞ for treatment of urinary tract infection only: CH = PO: 10–30 mg/kg/24 hr, div, every 6 hr carbenicillin indanyl sodium, GEOCILLIN; tabl

Carbinoxamine maleate, ethanolamine; antihistamine with mild anticholinergic effect and low incidence of sedation and drowsiness

℞ antiallergic effect: IN, CH = PO: 0.6 mg/kg/24 hr, div, every 6 hr

CLISTIN; elixir, tabl; component of many combination products

Cascara sagrada aromatic fluid extract; contains anthraquinones as active ingredients

℞ laxative: IN = PO: 1–2 mL/dose; CH = PO: 2–8 mL/dose

Cephalosporins, semisynthetic derivatives of 7-aminocephalosporanic acid, structurally related to penicillins

a. **First generation cephalosporins:** active against most gram-positive cocci (excluding enterococci and methicillin-resistant *Staphylococcus aureus*), some strains of *Escherichia coli, Klebsiella pneumoniae,* and *Proteus mirabilis*

Cefadroxil; relatively resistant against β-lactamases; absorption appears unaffected by food intake; minimal inhibitory concentrations for *E. coli, P. mirabilis, Klebsiella* species may be maintained in urine for about 20 hr after single dose

℞ for treatment of urinary tract infections: CH = PO: 30 mg/kg/24 hr, div, every 12 hr

DURICEF; caps, powder for oral susp

Cephazolin sodium: NB = IV (over 15–30 min), IM: 40 mg/kg/24 hr, div, every 12 hr; IN, CH = IV (over 15–30 min), IM: 50–100 mg/kg/24 hr, div, every 6 hr

ANCEF, KEFZOL; inj

Cephalexin: IN, CH = PO: 25–50 mg/kg/24 hr, div, every 6 hr

KEFLEX; inj

Cephalothin: NB = IV (over 15–30 min), IM: ≤ 7 days old: 40 mg/kg/24 hr, div, every 12 hr; >7 days old: 60 mg/kg/24 hr, div, every 8 hr; IN, CH = IV: 80–160 mg/kg/24 hr, div, every 4 hr

KEFLIN; inj

Cephapirin sodium: CH = IV, IM: 40–80 mg/kg/24 hr, div, every 6 hr

CEFADYL; inj

Cephradine: CH = PO: 50–100 mg/kg/24 hr, div, every 6 hr; IV, IM: 50–100–300 mg/kg/24 hr, div, every 6 hr

ANSPOR, VELOSEF; caps, oral susp, inj

b. **Second generation cephalosporins:** more active against gram-negative bacteria such as *Haemophilus influenzae* type b, *Neisseria gonorrhoeae,* and enteric gram-negative bacilli

Cefaclor: effective against some β-lactamase–producing ampicillin-resistant strains of *H. influenzae;* absorption not affected by food intake.

℞ for treatment of otitis media and infections of the upper and lower respiratory tracts, urinary tract, skin, and soft tissues with susceptible organisms: IN, CH = PO: 20–40 mg/kg/24 hr, div, every 8 hr

See KEY to abbreviations, p. 1520; for further information about drugs, see package insert.

Table continued on following page

DRUGS

Table 29–1B. Drug Doses (Continued)

CECLOR: powder for oral susp, caps
  Cefamandole: IN, CH = IV, IM: 50–150 mg/kg/24 hr, div, every 4–6 hr
Note: May cause renal and hepatic impairment, rash, neutropenia, and cross-reaction with penicillin. Adjust dose with renal failure.
MANDOL; vials, plastic bags, inj
  Cefoxitin: IN(>3 month old), CH = IV, IM: 80–160 mg/kg/24 hr, div, every 4–6 hr
Note: May cause renal impairment and cross-reaction with penicillin.
MEFOXIN; vials, infusion bottles, inj
  Cefuroxime: IN (>3 month old), CH: IV, IM: 50–100 mg/kg/24 hr, div, every 6–8 hr
  ℞ in bacterial meningitis: IN, CH = IV: 200–240 mg/kg/24 hr, div, every 6–8 hr
Note: May cause renal impairment and cross-reaction with penicillin. Interacts with aminoglycosides or furosemide to cause nephrotoxicity.
ZINACEF; vials, infusion bottles, inj
  c. **Third generation cephalosporins:** less active against gram-positive cocci than older cephalosporins but more active against most strains of enteric gram-negative bacilli (except *Clostridium difficile*), moderately active against *Pseudomonas aeruginosa*, highly active against *H. influenzae* and *N. gonorrhoeae.*
  Ceftriaxone sodium; biliary and renal excretion.
  ℞ misc. infection 50–75 mg/kg/24 hr (not to exceed 2 g) divided q 12 hr; meningitis 100 mg/kg/24 hr (not to exceed 4 g) divided q 12 hr.
  Cefotaxime: IN, CH = IV, IM: 50–150 mg/kg/24 hr, div, every 4–6 hr
  ℞ in neonatal meningitis: NB = IV 150–200 mg/kg/24 hr, div, every 4–6 hr
Note: May cause hypersensitivity reactions in penicillin-sensitive patients. Adjust dose with renal failure. Nephrotoxicity may develop with combined use of a cephalosporin and an aminoglycoside.
CLAFORAN; vials, inj
  Ceftizoxime: not metabolized, excreted unchanged by the kidneys. Safety and effectiveness in children have not been established.
CEFIZOX; vials, inj
  Moxalactam (lamoxactam): not metabolized, almost entirely excreted by kidneys; effective against *H. influenzae*
  IN, CH = IV, IM: 150 mg/kg/24 hr, div, every 6–8 hr
  ℞ in neonatal meningitis: NB = IV: initial dose of 100 mg/kg, followed by 100 mg/kg/24 hr in NB 1–7 days old, div, every 12 hr; and 150 mg/kg/24 hr in NB 8–28 days old, div, every 8 hr
Note: Can interfere with hemostasis through three different mechanisms: hypoprothrombinemia, platelet dysfunction, or immune-mediated thrombocytopenia, resulting in bleeding. Local irritation after IM injection and phlebitis from IV administration are common.
MOXAM; vials, inj

Chloral hydrate; trichloro derivative of acetaldehyde; tolerance to its hypnotic effect may develop
  ℞ for sedation: IN, CH = PO: 25 mg/kg/24 hr, div, every 6–8 hr
  ℞ for sleep: IN, CH = PO, (PR): 20 mg/kg/dose, to be repeated prn after 12–24 hr (maximum total daily dose: 50 mg/kg/24 hr)
†, NOCTEC, SOMNOS, ‡; elixir, syrup, suppos

Chloramphenicol; derivative of dichloracetic acid combined to a structure containing a nitrobenzene ring
  NB = IV (over 15–30 min), (PO):
    ≤ 14 days old, irrespective of weight: 25 mg/kg/24 hr, div, every 4 hr
    15–30 days old and ≤2000 g: 25 mg/kg/24 hr, div, every 4 hr
    15–30 days old and >2000 g: 50 mg/kg/24 hr, div, every 4 hr
  IN, CH = PO: 50–100 mg/kg/24 hr, div, every 6 hr; IV (over 15–30 min): 100 mg/kg/24 hr, div, every 4 hr
Caution: Newborn infants susceptible to development of high blood levels and gray-baby syndrome on usual doses; therefore, careful monitoring (of blood levels, if available) mandatory. Dose-duration–related suppression of erythrocyte production universal; weekly hematocrit or hemoglobin and reticulocyte count mandatory. Idiosyncratic aplastic anemia occasionally occurs without warning and may be lethal. **Use only when specifically indicated.**
CHLOROMYCETIN; caps ● chloramphenicol palmitate, CHLOROMYCETIN palmitate; oral susp ● chloramphenicol sodium succinate, CHLOROMYCETIN sodium succinate; inj

Chloroquine, a 4-aminoquinoline antimalarial agent; drug of choice for the treatment of attacks of malaria caused by *Plasmodium vivax, P. ovale, P. malariae,* and susceptible strains of *P. falciparum.* Not advised for use in treatment of juvenile rheumatoid arthritis.
  ℞ oral treatment of uncomplicated attacks (excluding those caused by chloroquine-resistant *P. falciparum*):
    Chloroquine diphosphate: CH = PO:
    first day: 25 mg/kg/first 24 hr (equivalent to base: 15 mg/kg/first 24 hr), div in initial dose of 16.5 mg/kg (equivalent to base 10 mg/kg) and subsequent dose of 8.5 mg/kg (equivalent to base 5 mg/kg) 6 hr later;
    second and third day: 8.5 mg/kg/24 hr (equivalent to base 5 mg/kg/24 hr), as single daily dose
  ℞ intramuscular treatment of severe illness (excluding malaria caused by chloroquine-resistant *P. falciparum*):
    Chloroquine dihydrochloride: CH = IM: 6 mg/kg/dose (equivalent to base 5 mg/kg/dose), every 12 hr, until clinical response is obtained and treatment can be completed by the oral route
  ℞ clinical prophylaxis of malaria (prevention of clinical manifestations from infection with any of the *Plasmodium* species):
    Chloroquine diphosphate: CH = PO: 8.5 mg/kg/dose (equivalent to base 5 mg/kg/dose) once every 7 days, beginning 2 wk before entering the malarious area and continuing for 8 wk after return. For eradication of *P. vivax* and *P. ovale,* treatment for 14 days with primaquine should be considered on leaving malarious area.
chloroquine diphosphate, ARALEN diphosphate, (RESOCHIN) diphosphate, tabl; chloroquine dihydrochloride, ARALEN dihydrochloride, inj; (1 mg chloroquine base is equivalent to 1.65 mg chloroquine diphosphate or 1.2 mg chloroquine dihydrochloride)
Caution: Irreversible retinal damage may occur with prolonged use; frequent ophthalmologic examination necessary to detect early changes. *Note:* Chloroquine does *not* cause hemolysis in individuals with G-6-PD deficiency

Chlorothiazide; saluretic, inhibiting sodium reabsorption and interfering with dilution of urine
  IN, CH = PO: 20 mg/kg/24 hr, div, every 12 hr
†, DIURIL; tabl, oral susp

Chlorpheniramine maleate; alkylamine; antihistamine with anticholinergic and mild sedative effects
  ℞ antiallergic effect: CH = PO: 0.35 mg/kg/24 hr, div, every 6 hr
†, CHLORTRIMETON, ‡; tabl, syrup, inj

Chlorpromazine; phenothiazine with aliphatic side chain
  ℞ for sedation: CH = PO: 2 mg/kg/24 hr, div, every 4–6 hr, prn; IM: 1.6 mg/kg/24 hr, div, every 6–8 hr, prn
THORAZINE; suppos; chlorpromazine hydrochloride, THORAZINE hydrochloride; tabl, syrup, inj
Caution: Overdose may produce parkinsonian syndrome. Diphenhydramine may be antidotal.

Chlortetracycline; see Tetracyclines

Chlorthalidone; nonthiazide saluretic with protracted duration of action
  CH = PO: 2 mg/kg/dose, as single dose; to be repeated with adjusted single dose 3 times/wk
HYGROTON; tabl

Cholestyramine, ion-exchange resin for treatment of cholestatic jaundice and hyperlipidemia
  Toxicity includes constipation, vitamin A, D, and K deficiencies, and altered medication absorption.
  PO: 120 mg/kg q 8–12 hr with meals
QUESTRAN; 4 g packets, 378 g tins, 4 g cholestyramine per 9 g Questran

Table 29-1B. Drug Doses (Continued)

Cimetidine; H$_2$-receptor antagonist inhibiting gastric acid secretion
R for treatment of duodenal and gastric ulcers and for relief of symptoms caused by gastroesophageal reflux; compatible with concomitant treatment with oral antacids (which should be given at frequent intervals and in adequate dosage) and/or anticholinergic antispasmodics. Clinical experience in children is extremely limited, and the benefit/risk ratio should be carefully considered: PO: 20–40 mg/kg/24 hr, div and given with every meal, have been used, as well as same dosage, IV, div, every 4 hr.
TAGAMET; tabl, inj

Clindamycin; semisynthetic derivative of lincomycin
IN, CH = PO: 10–25 mg/kg/24 hr, div, every 6–8 hr (expressed in terms of the base); IV (infusion over 30–60 min), IM: 25–40 mg/kg/24 hr, div, every 6–8 hr (expressed in terms of the base)
clindamycin hydrochloride, CLEOCIN hydrochloride; caps ● clindamycin palmitate hydrochloride, CLEOCIN pediatric; oral susp ● clindamycin phosphate, CLEOCIN phosphate; inj

Clonazepam; benzodiazepine with selective anticonvulsant effect
CH = PO: start with 0.01–0.03 mg/kg/24 hr, div, every 8 hr, and progressively increase up to 0.3 mg/kg/24 hr, div, every 8 hr, if needed.
Caution: Concomitant use of clonazepam and valproate sodium may lead to petit mal status.
CLONOPIN; tabl

Cloxacillin sodium monohydrate; penicillinase-resistant penicillin
IN, CH = PO: 50–100 mg/kg/24 hr, div, every 6 hr (expressed in terms of the base)
TEGOPEN; caps, oral susp

Codeine phosphate or sulfate; narcotic analgesic
R as antitussive: CH = 1–1.5 mg/kg/24 hr, div, every 4 hr, prn
R against moderately severe pain: CH = PO: 4 mg/kg/24 hr, div, every 4–6 hr, prn; SC: 3 mg/kg/24 hr, div, every 4–6 hr, prn
†; tabl, oral susp, inj; mostly in combination with other drugs

Colistin sodium methanesulfonate, colistimethate sodium, and **colistin** sulfate, polymyxin E; polypeptide antimicrobial agent with cationic detergent activity
R inhibition of gastrointestinal flora, justified only in selected cases (gastroenteritis with susceptible organism): IN, CH = PO (colistin sulfate): 5–15 mg/kg/24 hr, div, every 8 hr; IM, IV (by slow infusion): 3–5 mg/kg/24 hr, div, every 8 hr
Caution against overgrowth of abnormal organisms
colistimethate sodium, COLY-MYCIN N; inj ● colistin sulfate, COLY-MYCIN S; oral susp

Corticosteroids
R physiologic replacement: *cortisone:* PO: 1 mg/kg/24 hr, div, every 8 hr; IM: 0.5 mg/kg/24 hr, every 24 hr. (*Note:* "Increased demand" under stressful situation; e.g., in children with congenital adrenogenital syndrome, receiving replacement therapy, for stressful situation in which 2 mg/kg/24 hr of cortisol may be safer)
R use in pharmacologic doses (leukemia, lymphoma, nephrosis, rheumatic carditis, certain types of tuberculosis, immunologic reactions, and other types of autoimmune disease): adjust dosage to the specific situation.
cortisone: PO: 10 mg/kg/24 hr, div, every 6–8 hr; IM: 3–6 mg/kg/24 hr, div, every 12 hr
prednisone: PO: 2 mg/kg/24 hr, div, every 6–8 hr (or analogue in equally effective dosage; see Table)
(For continued treatment after initial response, adjust dosage, frequency of administration, and duration of treatment according to type of disease and side effects to be avoided.)
R in status asthmaticus refractory to other types of treatment: hydrocortisone sodium phosphate or succinate: IV: 10–20 mg/kg/24 hr, div, every 6 hr *or* 4 mg/kg/dose every 4 hr until response is obtained
R in endotoxic shock: hydrocortisone sodium phosphate or succinate: IV: 50 mg/kg/initial dose, followed by 50–75 mg/kg/24 hr, div, every 6 hr

Relative Potencies of Corticosteroids:

	Anti-inflammatory Effect, Gluconeogenesis	Sodium-Retaining Effect
hydrocortisone (cortisol)	1	1
cortisone	0.8	0.8
prednisolone	4	0.8
prednisone	4	0.8
methylprednisolone	5	0.5
triamcinolone	4	0
dexamethasone	25	0
desoxycorticosterone	0	100
aldosterone	0.3	3000

dexamethasone, DECADRON, GAMMACORTEN, ‡; tabl, elixir ● dexamethasone sodium phosphate, DECADRON phosphate; inj
hydrocortisone, †, CORTEF, HYDROCORTONE, ‡; tabl, oral susp ● hydrocortisone sodium phosphate, †, HYDROCORTONE phosphate; inj ● hydrocortisone sodium succinate, †, SOLU-CORTEF; inj
methylprednisolone, MEDROL; tabl ● methylprednisolone sodium succinate, SOLU-MEDROL; inj
prednisone, †, DELTASONE, METICORTEN, ‡; tabl ● prednisolone, †, DELTA-CORTEF, METICORTELONE, ‡; tabl
triamcinolone, ARISTOCORT, KENACORT; tabl, syrup
Caution: May inhibit clinical signs of infection.

Cortisone; see Corticosteroids

Cromolyn sodium
R topical prophylaxis of bronchial asthma; not useful in the treatment of acute asthmatic attack since it is not a bronchodilator. CH (5 yr and older) = inhalation of the content of 1 capsule every 6 hr through the specially devised turbo-inhaler; 1 capsule contains 20 μg cromolyn sodium
AARANE, INTAL; inhalation with Spinhaler

Cyclizine hydrochloride; antihistamine, antiemetic, and anticholinergic agent
R for prevention and relief of symptoms of motion sickness: CH (6–10 yr) = PO: 3 mg/kg/24 hr, div, every 8 hr. The 1st dose should be taken about 20 min before departure.
MAREZINE; tabl; cyclizine lactate for IM inj

Cyproheptadine hydrochloride; piperidine; serotonin and histamine antagonist with mild anticholinergic and mild sedative effects
R antiallergic effect: CH = PO: 0.25 mg/kg/24 hr, div, every 6 hr
PERIACTIN; tabl, syrup

Deferoxamine, chelating agent for treatment of iron intoxication. May cause hypotension; contraindicated in renal failure or acute anuria unless concomitant hemodialysis is used.
IV: 10–15 mg/kg/hr infusion
DESFERAL; 500 mg/vial inj

Demeclocycline; see Tetracyclines

Desmopressin acetate, synthetic analogue of vasopressin indicated as replacement therapy in the management of central diabetes insipidus. Toxicities include headache, abdominal cramping, and excessive water retention. Nasal insufflation: 0.03–0.05 mL/day divided BID or TID, dose determined by patient response, DDAVP, 0.1 mg/mL for nasal insufflation

Dexamethasone; see Corticosteroids

Dextroamphetamine sulfate; noncatecholamine sympathomimetic agent
R in minimal brain dysfunction: drug treatment not recommended below age of 3 yr or in nonstructural therapeutic situation. CH (above 3 yr) = PO: initiate treatment with 2.5 mg/dose given at onset of daytime activities and again 4–6 hr later. If needed, increase at weekly intervals by increments of 2.5 mg/dose and adjust respective size of separate doses according to response. Daily dose should not exceed 1 mg/kg/24 hr.

Table continued on following page

Table 29–1B. **Drug Doses** (Continued)

℞ in narcolepsy: PO: proceed for dosage as in minimal brain dysfunction. End points: control of symptoms, maximal dose. To avoid insomnia do not administer closer than 6 hr before bedtime. **Caution** against diversion of CNS stimulants from legitimate use in patient to misuse in adults.
†, DEXEDRINE; tabl
Caution: Severe mental depression may follow withdrawal. Overdose may produce extreme restlessness and psychotic behavior.

Dextromethorphan hydrobromide; D-isomer of a codeine analogue, and probably free of addictive effects
℞ antitussive agent: IN, CH = PO: 1 mg/kg/24 hr, div, every 6–8 hr
†, ROMILAR; syrup; contained in many combination products

Diazepam; benzodiazepine with anxiolytic and muscle-relaxant effects
℞ in status epilepticus: NB, IN, CH = IV (slowly, as controlled "push" injection): 0.3 mg/kg/dose; may be repeated 2 times after intervals of 5 min; give IM if impossible to give it IV (efficacy diminished)
℞ for symptomatic relief of anxiety: CH = PO: 0.2–0.3 mg/kg/24 hr, div, every 6 hr; adjust dosage according to response
VALIUM; tabl and VALIUM injectable
Caution: Confusion and prolonged extreme drowsiness may follow overdose or concurrent ingestion of alcohol in any form.

Diazoxide, nondiuretic benzothiadiazine derivative with several prominent actions: (1) relaxation of smooth muscles in the peripheral arterioles after IV injection only; (2) hyperglycemic effect (beginning 1 hr after administration and lasting for approximately 8 hr) through inhibition of release of insulin; (3) retention of sodium and concomitantly of water; (4) hyperuricemic effect
℞ for emergency reduction of hypertension: CH = IV (injection within 30 sec of calculated amount of undiluted diazoxide solution into a peripheral vein): 5 mg/kg/dose. If 1st injection fails to elicit adequate response within 30 min, administer a 2nd complementary dose. Hypotensive effect usually lasts 2–12 hr. Successive injections frequently give a better response than the initial dose. As soon as possible, switch to oral regimen with alternative antihypertensive medication (Table 14–15).
Note: Diazoxide is ineffective against hypertension due to pheochromocytoma. A concurrently administered thiazide diuretic (which characteristically exerts a diuretic response) may potentiate the antihypertensive, hyperglycemic, and hyperuricemic effects of diazoxide.
Caution: hypotensive circulatory failure (responding to catecholamine such as norepinephrine), congestive heart failure (responding to plasma volume depletion by saluretic), and hyperosmolar coma in patients with diabetes mellitus (responding to insulin) may occur.
HYPERSTAT; inj

Dicloxacillin sodium monohydrate; penicillinase-resistant penicillin
IN, CH = PO: 12.5–25 mg/kg/24 hr, div, every 6 hr
DYNAPEN; caps, oral susp

Digitoxin; cardiac glycoside with long half-life (5–9 days); main glycoside in digitalis leaf
℞ for digitalization: 0.5 × digitalizing dose initially, 0.25 × digitalizing dose 8 and 16 hr later. (Digitalizing dose: NB = IV, IM: 0.035 mg/kg, div in fractions, or PO: 0.050 mg/kg, div in fractions.
IN = IV, IM 0.050 mg/kg, div in fractions, or PO: 0.070 mg/kg, div in fractions
CH = IM, PO: 0.030 mg/kg, divided into fractions as indicated above)
℞ for maintenance: begin maintenance dosage 24 hr after 1st fraction of digitalizing dose. NB, IN, CH = 0.1 × digitalizing dose, every 24 hr
Note: Digitalizing and maintenance doses must be adjusted to condition of patient.
†, CRYSTODIGIN, PURODIGIN; tabl, inj
Caution: Fatal arrhythmia may follow overdose.

Digoxin; cardiac glycoside with rapid onset of action and half-life of approximately 48 hr
℞ for digitalization: 0.5 × digitalizing dose initially, 0.25 × digitalizing dose 8 and 16 hr later.
(Digitalizing dose: NB = IV, IM: 0.010–0.030 mg/kg div in fractions, or PO: 0.040 mg/kg, div in fractions.
IN = IV, IM 0.030–0.040 mg/kg div in fractions, or PO: 0.050 mg/kg, in fractions
CH = IV, IM, PO: same doses as indicated for NB)
℞ for maintenance: begin maintenance dosage 24 hr after 1st fraction of digitalizing dose. NB = PO: 0.010 mg/kg/24 hr, div, every 12 hr. IN, CH = PO: 0.015 mg/kg/24 hr, div, every 12 hr
Note: Digitalizing and maintenance doses must be adjusted to the condition of the patient.
†, LANOXIN; tabl, elixir, inj
Caution: Fatal arrhythmia may follow overdose.

Dimenhydrinate, chlorotheophylline salt of diphenhydramine
℞ for the prevention and treatment of motion sickness: CH = PO: 5 mg/kg/24 hr, div, every 6 hr
DRAMAMINE; tabl, oral susp, suppos

Dioctyl sodium sulfosuccinate; wetting agent, emulsifier, demulcent
℞ as stool softener: IN, CH = PO: 5 mg/kg/24 hr, div, with meals
†, COLACE, DOXINATE, ‡; caps, oral sol, syrup

Diphenhydramine hydrochloride; ethanolamine; antihistamine with mild anticholinergic, sedative, antiemetic and antitussive effects
℞ antiallergic effect; sometimes used as sedative. IN, CH = PO, IM, IV: 5 mg/kg/24 hr, div, every 6–8 hr
†, BENADRYL; caps, elixir, inj

Dobutamine, β-adrenergic inotropic agent used for short-term treatment of cardiac failure due to depressed cardiac contractility. Heart rate, blood pressure, and cardiac electrical activity should be monitored during infusion. Do not mix with sodium bicarbonate. IV: 0.0025–0.010 mg/kg/min constant infusion, depending on patient response.
DOBUTREX; 250 mg vials for injection

Dopamine, α- and β-adrenergic as well as dopaminergic agent (positive inotropic effect on heart)
℞ to increase cardiac output and improve organ perfusion: IV infusion (into large vein): Example: to prepare a solution containing 0.400 mg/mL, mix 100 mg dopamine HCl in 250 mL 5% D/W or appropriate electrolyte solution with pH below 7.0 (do not include bicarbonate!), and infuse at rate adjusted to response in patient, beginning with 0.002–0.005 mg/kg/min and increasing by increments of 0.005 mg/kg/min if needed up to 0.050 mg/kg/min. In case of extravasation causing peripheral ischemia, use phentolamine (REGITINE) for local infiltration.
INTROPIN; inj

Doxycycline; see Tetracyclines

Edrophonium chloride; cholinesterase inhibitor with short duration of action
℞ for myasthenia in NB of myasthenic mother = IV (slowly) or IM: 0.2 mg/kg/dose. Symptoms should be relieved almost immediately. Continue cholinesterase-inhibiting treatment, if indicated, with pyridostigmine.
℞ for differential diagnosis of myasthenic crisis, or as adjunct treatment to carotid massage in supraventricular tachycardia: NB, IN, CH = IV: 0.05 mg/kg/dose, and watch for effect after 15–30 sec, *or* IM: 0.1 mg/kg/dose, and expect effect after 2–10 min
If edrophonium test is given during "cholinergic crisis," weakness of affected muscles, including respiratory muscles, will worsen or not improve. Ventilation should be assisted, if needed, and bradycardia can be influenced by atropine. If recovery from weakness occurs, continuation of cholinesterase inhibition is indicated using inhibitors with longer duration of action, such as pyridostigmine, neostigmine, ambenonium. Their dosage must be individually titrated and adjusted.
Manifestations of overdosage with cholinesterase-inhibiting medication: increase in muscle weakness and worsening of respiratory difficulty and dysphagia after each dose of drug; fascicula-

Table continued on opposite page

tions of muscles; excessive salivation, increase in bronchial secretion; vomiting, diarrhea, pallor, sweating, bradycardia.
TENSILON; inj
Caution: Administration during cholinergic crisis may cause paralysis of respiratory muscles. Use only when ventilatory assistance is available.

Ephedrine, phenylethylamine (direct and indirect sympathomimetic)
℞ for treatment of asthma in subacute stage; tolerance develops. CH = PO: 3 mg/kg/24 hr, div, every 4–6 hr. Contained in many antiasthma preparations; should be replaced with more selectively active drug
ephedrine hydrochloride; ephedrine sulfate; caps, tabl, syrup
Caution: Acute overdose may produce seizures and coma.

Epinephrine, catecholamine (α- and β-adrenergic agonist)
℞ bronchodilator (β$_2$ stimulatory effect), in acute asthma attack: IN, CH = SC: 0.01 mg/kg/dose, repeat prn every 20 min, 2 times
Note: With epinephrine solution 1:1000 this corresponds to 0.01 mL/kg/dose.
Caution: Cardiac arrhythmia and/or acute hypertension may follow overdose.

Epinephrine racemic, Inhalation treatment of acute spasmodic croup. Inhalation: 0.25–0.5 mL of 2.25% solution diluted in 3 mL of saline given via nebulizer.
VAPONEPHRINE; Inhalation 2.25% solution

Ergotamine, adrenergic blocking agent as well as direct vasoconstrictor of vessels to the brain, and serotonin antagonist
℞ against acute attack of vascular headache (migraine): older child and adolescent = IM, SC (in acute attack): 0.25–0.50 mg/dose, in single application. Minimal effective dose should be established for each patient by titration of the amount required to control headaches in that patient. Older child and adolescent = SL, PO (at 1st symptoms of attack): 1 mg/dose; if no improvement within following 30 min, repeat same dose once.
Note: Signs of therapeutic overdosage: nausea, vomiting, diarrhea, tingling of hands and feet, weakness, muscle pain.
ergotamine tartrate: CYNERGEN; inj, tabl ● ergotamine tartrate + caffeine: CAFERGOT, tabl, suppos ● dihydroergotamine mesylate: D.H.E.45, inj

Erythromycin; macrolide antimicrobial agent
IN, CH = PO: 30–50 mg/kg/24 hr, div, every 6 hr; IV: 15–20 mg/kg/24 hr, div, every 6 hr
erythromycin, †, ILOTYCIN, ‡; tabl ● erythromycin estolate, ILOSONE; tabl, oral susp ● erythromycin ethylsuccinate, PEDIAMYCIN, ‡; tabl, oral susp, drops ● erythromycin glucepate, ILOTYCIN glucepate IV; inj ● erythromycin lactobionate, ERYTHROCIN lactobionate IV; inj ● erythromycin stearate, ERYTHROCIN stearate, ‡; tabl

Ethacrynic acid; saluretic, inhibiting chloride and sodium reabsorption and interfering mainly with concentration of urine
CH = PO: approximately 1 mg/kg/dose, as single daily dose. Adjust according to effect, and repeat prn on alternate days; dosage in infants and children not firmly established (PO, IV)
EDECRIN; tabl ● ethacrynate sodium, IV, sodium EDECRIN; inj (IV only)

Ethambutol hydrochloride; antituberculous agent used concomitantly with isoniazid
℞ in the treatment of tuberculosis as part of multiple drug regimen. Conditions for safe use in children not firmly established. In adults: 15–25 mg/kg/24 hr, as single daily dose, for course of treatment or retreatment. *Because of rare side effects of optic neuritis and decreased visual acuity,* eye examinations are indicated before inception of treatment and at monthly intervals thereafter.
MYAMBUTOL; tabl

Ethosuximide; anticonvulsant agent of the succinimide type
CH = PO: 20 mg/kg/24 hr, div, every 12 hr
ZARONTIN; caps, syrup

Furosemide; saluretic with a duration of action of about 2 hr when given IV; inhibits chloride and sodium reabsorption and interferes with concentration of urine
IN, CH = PO: start with 2 mg/kg/dose; if needed, increase progressively to 3–6 mg/kg/dose, at intervals of 6–8 hr. IV: start with 1 mg/kg/dose; if needed, increase progressively to 6 mg/kg/dose, with an interval of at least 2 hr between doses
LASIX; tabl, oral sol, inj

Gentamicin sulfate; antimicrobial aminoglycoside
NB = IM, IV (over 1–2 hr). ≤ 7 days old: 5 mg/kg/24 hr, div, every 12 hr; > 7 days old: 7.5 mg/kg/24 hr, div, every 8 hr. CH = IM, IV (over 0.5–2 hr): 6–7.5 mg/kg/24 hr, div, every 8 hr
Usual duration of treatment: 7–10 days.
GARAMYCIN; inj
Caution: Ototoxic; nephrotoxic, perhaps especially with concomitant administration of cephalosporins

Griseofulvin; antifungal agent
℞ against deep-seated mycotic infections (skin, hair, nails) with organisms of the species *Microsporum, Trichophyton, Epidermophyton:* CH = PO (microcrystalline): 10 mg/kg/24 hr for 4–6 wk (4–6 mo for fingernails, 6–12 mo for toenails)
Note: "Ultramicrosize" form is an ultramicrocrystalline suspension for which 125 mg is biologically equivalent to 250 mg of a "microsize" preparation. The daily dose of an ultramicrosize preparation is reduced to 5 mg/kg/24 hr and offers comparable efficacy without additional advantages.
griseofulvin, microcrystalline, †, FULVICIN-U/F, GRIFULVIN V, ‡; tabl, oral susp ● griseofulvin, ultramicrocrystalline GRIS-PEG; tabl

Hydralazine hydrochloride; phthalazine derivative; causes relaxation of vascular smooth muscles, especially of arterioles
℞ as antihypertensive in long-term treatment: CH = PO: initially 0.75 mg/kg/24 hr, div, every 6 hr; increase progressively until desired response or daily maximum dose of 3.5 mg/kg/24 hr is reached
℞ for emergency reduction of hypertension: IV (immediate onset of action), IM (onset of action after 15–20 min): 0.15 mg/kg/dose; repeat prn every 30–90 min up to daily dose of 1.7–3.6 mg/kg/24 hr; switch to oral administration if conditions permit
Note: Hydralazine may produce sodium retention and usually increases plasma renin activity.
Caution: May induce lupus erythematosus–like syndrome; frequency related to dosage.
†, APRESOLINE, ‡; tabl, inj

Hydrochlorothiazide; saluretic, inhibiting sodium reabsorption and interfering with dilution of urine
IN, CH = PO: 2 mg/kg/24 hr, div, every 12 hr
†, ESIDRIX, HYDRODIURIL, ‡; tabl

Hydroxyzine hydrochloride; neuroleptic agent of the piperazine type, with sedative and antihistamine effects
℞ for sedation and/or antihistamine effect: CH = PO: 2 mg/kg/24 hr, div, every 6–8 hr, prn
ATARAX: tabl, syrup; VISTARIL I.M.: inj (IM) ● hydroxyzine pamoate, VISTARIL; caps, oral susp

Imipramine hydrochloride; tricyclic antidepressant
℞ against enuresis, as adjunct therapy to proper medical and educational approach, after age 4 yr: CH (after age 4 yr) = PO: 25 mg/24 hr, to be given in single dose 1 hr before bedtime; if response unsatisfactory, dose may be increased to 50 mg in children between 25–40 kg, and to 75 mg in adolescents
After a 1 mo trial without result, the drug should be discontinued as ineffective under existing circumstances. After a favorable response for a continued treatment period of 3 mo, drug should be skipped on alternate days and finally discontinued.
†, TOFRANIL; tabl

Indomethacin, pharmacologic management of patent ductus arteriosus in premature infants.
Note: May cause GI irritation and bleeding and decreased GFR.
IN = IV: <48 hr, 0.2 mg/kg for 1 dose, then 0.1 mg/kg q 12–24 hr for 2 doses; >48 hr, 0.2 mg/kg q 12–24 hr up to a total of 3 doses.
INDOCIN; PO, inj

Table continued on following page

Iron preparations

℞ Daily maintenance iron requirement: elemental iron: PO: 0.5–1 mg/kg/24 hr, in single dose or divided

℞ In iron deficiency anemia, as elemental iron: PO: 6 mg/kg/24 hr, div, with meals

Note: Iron supply at this dosage level ought to be continued for 2–3 mo to compensate for the deficits in erythrocytes and iron stores. Only iron in the ferrous form (Fe^{++}) is absorbed from the gastrointestinal tract. The content of elemental iron in different preparations varies. The percentage of dry weight as elemental iron of ferrous choline citrate is 20; ferrous fumarate, 33; ferrous gluconate, 12; ferrous lactate, 19; ferrous sulfate, 20; and iron-dextran complex (ferric hydroxide), 2.

℞ Dose calculation for parenteral iron administration: elemental Fe deficit = 2.5 mg/kg × deficit of hemoglobin concentration (in g/dL) in blood. (The deficit of the hemoglobin concentration is obtained as the difference between the measured and the desirable value, expressed in g/dL.) When iron has to be supplied by the parenteral route, deep IM injection is preferable to IV administration. In either case, a test dose of approximately 25 mg elemental Fe in the form of the dextran complex should precede the administration of the total dose. If the total dose is large, it should be divided in separate daily doses of which none should exceed 5 mg/kg/24 hr of elemental iron.

Note: An additional 20–30% of the calculated deficit is needed to restore the tissue iron reserves.

Caution: Acute overdose may lead to shock, CNS depression, death (Sec 28.7).

Isoniazid, INH, isonicotinic acid hydrazide; tuberculostatic agent

℞ in the treatment of active tuberculosis, in combination with other antituberculous drugs: IN, CH = PO, IM: 10–20 mg/kg/24 hr, div, every 8–12 hr; maximum daily dose: 500 mg/24 hr. AD = PO, IM: 5–10 mg/kg/24 hr, div, every 8–12 hr; maximum daily dose: 300 mg/24 hr

℞ for prophylaxis of complications in recent conversion to positive tuberculin reaction (primary tuberculosis), or after suspected exposure: IN, CH = PO: 5–10 mg/kg/24 hr, as single dose, or div, every 12 hr; maximum daily dose: 300 mg/24 hr

Note: "Slow" acetylators (homozygous) need only about 0.20–0.50 of this dose to reach therapeutically effective plasma concentrations achieved by "rapid" acetylators (homozygous and heterozygous). Higher than necessary plasma concentrations of unmetabolized isoniazid seem not to be associated with risk of isoniazid hepatotoxicity.

†, INH; tabl, syrup, inj

Caution: Formation of toxic metabolite in some patients may lead to hepatic necrosis with usual doses (rare under 20 yr of age).

Isoproterenol hydrochloride; β-adrenergic agent

℞ to overcome atrioventricular block: IV infusion: Example: to prepare a solution containing 0.004 mg/mL, mix 1 mg isoproterenol in 250 mL 5% D/W or appropriate electrolyte solution and infuse at rate adjusted to response in patient (beginning with approximately 0.0001–0.0002 mg/kg/min)

†, ISUPREL; inj

Kanamycin sulfate; antimicrobial aminoglycoside

NB = IM, IV (over 20–30 min):

≤ 2000 g and ≤ 7 days old: 15 mg/kg/24 hr, div, every 12 hr
≤ 2000 g and > 7 days old: 20 mg/kg/24 hr, div, every 12 hr
> 2000 g and ≤ 7 days old: 20 mg/kg/24 hr, div, every 12 hr
> 2000 g and > 7 days old: 30 mg/kg/24 hr, div, every 8 hr
IN, CH = IM, IV (over 20–30 min): 6–15 mg/kg/24 hr, div, every 8–12 hr. Usual duration of therapy: 7–10 days; not indicated in long-term therapy because of ototoxic hazard. **Caution:** Ototoxic, nephrotoxic.
KANTREX; inj

Lidocaine hydrochloride; anesthetic agent used systemically for its antiarrhythmic effects; delayed slow diastolic depolarization, diminished automaticity. Does not affect normal conduction but seemingly improves conduction velocity in damaged areas of myocardium. In therapeutic doses does not depress myocardial contractility or atrioventricular conduction.

℞ against ventricular tachyarrhythmia: IN, CH = IV (slowly, as 20 mg/mL sol): 1 mg/kg/dose, to be repeated prn after 20 min, or continuous IV infusion as 1 mg/mL sol: 0.020–0.050 mg/kg/min, to a maximum total dose of 5 mg/kg/24 hr
XYLOCAINE hydrochloride IV; inj

Caution: Excessive depression of cardiac conductivity may occur; ECG monitoring indicated during treatment.

Lincomycin hydrochloride; antimicrobial macrolide

CH = PO: 30–60 mg/kg/24 hr, div, every 8 hr. IM, IV (over 1–4 hr, as 10 mg/mL sol): 10–20 mg/kg/24 hr, div, every 8–12 hr
LINCOCIN; caps, syrup, inj

"Lytic cocktail," mixture of narcotic analgesic, antihistamine, and phenothiazine

℞ for temporary heavy sedation: IM (deep, after mixing the 3 components in 1 syringe): meperidine (DEMEROL), 2 mg/kg/dose, plus promethazine (PHENERGAN), 1 mg/kg/dose, plus chlorpromazine (THORAZINE), 1 mg/kg/dose (maximum single dose not to exceed meperidine, 50 mg, promethazine, 25 mg, and chlorpromazine, 25 mg)

Magnesium hydroxide, Mg(OH)$_2$

℞ as cathartic: PO: 40 mg/kg/dose
milk of magnesia, susp, "8%" containing Mg(OH)$_2$ 80 mg/mL

Magnesium sulfate, MgSO$_4$·7H$_2$O, Epsom salt; 1 g of the salt is equivalent to 98.6 mg elemental Mg or to 8.11 mEq Mg^{++}

℞ as cathartic: PO: (MgSO$_4$·7H$_2$O): 250 mg/kg/dose

℞ in hypomagnesemia: IM (in solution containing MgSO$_4$·7H$_2$O 500 mg/mL, equivalent to Mg^{++} 4 mEq/mL, also labeled "50%"): MgSO$_4$·7H$_2$O 100 mg/kg/dose, equivalent to Mg^{++} 0.8 mEq/kg/dose, repeat every 4–6 hr
IV (in solution containing MgSO$_4$·7H$_2$O 100 mg/mL, equivalent to Mg^{++} 0.08 mEq/mL, also labeled "10%"): Infuse slowly MgSO$_4$·7H$_2$O up to 100 mg/kg/dose, equivalent to Mg^{++} 0.08 mEq/kg/dose

†; crystalline salt, sterile sol for inj available as 50%, 25%, and 10%

Mannitol; osmotic diuretic

℞ test dose for oliguria: CH = IV: 0.2 g/kg/dose, injected within 3–5 min

℞ in cerebral edema: CH = IV: 1–2.5 g/kg/dose, injected as 15–25% sol over 30–60 min

†, OSMITROL, ‡; IV inj

Mebendazole; anthelmintic agent which blocks glucose uptake by the susceptible parasites and interferes with their survival

℞ against pinworms (Enterobius vermicularis; cure rate 90–100%): CH = PO: 100 mg/dose; as single dose; against whipworms (Trichuris trichiura; cure rate 61–75%), roundworms (Ascaris lumbricoides; cure rate 91–100%) and hookworms (Ancylostoma duodenale, Necator americanus; cure rate 96%): alternative method = PO: 200 mg/24 hr, div, every 12 hr, for 3 consecutive days. If patient is not free of parasites 3 wk after treatment a 2nd course is indicated

Note: Not extensively studied in children under 2 yr of age.
VERMOX; chewable tabl

Meperidine hydrochloride; synthetic narcotic analgesic agent; addictive

℞ against severe pain: CH = PO, SC, IM: 6 mg/kg/24 hr, div, prn every 4–6 hr (maximum single dose: 100 mg)

†, DEMEROL hydrochloride, ‡; tabl, elixir, inj

Caution: May produce respiratory depression, seizures, coma in some sensitive patients. Test dose advisable. Naloxone is antidote.

Mercaptomerin sodium; mercurial diuretic

Outmoded regimen for reducing edema in congestive heart failure, in patients with normal kidney function: CH = SC, IM: 0.035 mL "mercaptomerin sol"/kg/dose, equivalent to approximately 1.4 mg mercury/kg/dose. Dose and frequency of administration to be adjusted to the situation of the patient (once daily to once/wk). 125 mg mercaptomerin sodium is equivalent to 40 mg mercury
THIOMERIN; inj

Table 29–1B. **Drug Doses** (Continued)

Metaproterenol sulfate; analogue of catecholamine; selective β₂ adrenergic agent
℞ bronchodilator: dosage in children not yet firmly established. PO: 1–1.5 mg/kg/24 hr, div, every 6 hr
ALUPENT, METAPREL; syrup, tabl, inhalation

Methacycline; see Tetracyclines

Methenamine mandelate; urinary antibacterial agent effective in a nonspecific manner against microorganisms by liberating formaldehyde on decomposing in urine at pH below 5.5
℞ for prevention of bacterial growth in urine, provided pH is sufficiently low: CH = PO: initially 100 mg/kg/24 hr, div, every 6 hr, followed by 50 mg/kg/24 hr, div, every 6 hr
Note: Should not be used (and is useless) when urine acidification is contraindicated or not attainable (as in infections with urea-splitting bacteria). If situation permits, acidification of urine below pH 5.5 might be implemented by adjusting acid load of intake.
†, MANDELAMINE, tabl, oral susp ● methenamine hippurate, HIPREX; tabl

Methicillin sodium; semisynthetic penicillinase-resistant penicillin
NB = IM, IV (over 15–30 min): according to the following criteria:
≤ 2000 g and ≤ 14 days old: 50 mg/kg/24 hr, div, every 12 hr
≤ 2000 g and 15–30 days old: 75 mg/kg/24 hr, div, every 8 hr
> 2000 g and ≤ 14 days old: 75 mg/kg/24 hr, div, every 8 hr
> 2000 g and 15–30 days old: 100 mg/kg/24 hr, div, every 6 hr
IN, CH = IV (over 15–30 min), IM: 200–400 mg/kg/24 hr, div, every 4 hr (IV) or every 6 hr (IM)
CELBENIN, STAPHCILLIN; inj

Methyldopa; antihypertensive agent, inhibitor of aromatic amino acid decarboxylase, and precursor of α-methylnorepinephrine. Probably lowers arterial blood pressure by stimulation of central inhibitory α-adrenergic receptors, false neurotransmission, and/or reduction of plasma renin activity
℞ as antihypertensive in long-term treatment: CH = PO: initially 10 mg/kg/24 hr, div, every 6–12 hr; decrease or increase the dose progressively at intervals of 2 days until adequate response achieved; maximum daily dosage: 65 mg/kg/24 hr
Caution: Positive direct Coombs test develops in 10–20% of patients on prolonged treatment, usually between 6–12 mo of continued administration. Positive indirect Coombs test, fever, and liver dysfunction occur less frequently. If evidence of hemolysis or liver dysfunction present, methyldopa should be discontinued and not reinstituted.
ALDOMET; tabl

Methylphenidate hydrochloride; piperidine derivative structurally related to amphetamine; CNS stimulant with more prominent effects on mental than on motor activities
℞ in minimal brain dysfunction (MBD): drug treatment of MBD not recommended below the age of 3 yr or in nonstructured therapeutic situation. CH (over 3 yr) = PO: initiate treatment with 5 mg dose given at the onset of daytime activities and again 4–6 hr later; if needed, increase the dose at weekly intervals by increments of 5 mg/dose and adjust the size of the respective doses (early morning and mid-day) according to the response in the patient; daily dose usually should not exceed 2 mg/kg/24 hr. To avoid insomnia do not administer closer than 6 hr before bedtime. (For MBD, see Sec. 2.46, 2.63, 2.66.)
Caution: Reduction of growth rate and weight gain might accompany prolonged use. Chronic abuse can lead to tolerance.
℞ in narcolepsy: PO: proceed for dosage adjustment as in MBD, with correction of the abnormal symptomatology as the end point.
RITALIN; tabl

Miconazole; synthetic antifungal imidazole derivative effective against systemic infections with *Coccidioides immitis, Candida albicans, Cryptococcus neoformans, Paracoccidioides brasiliensis.* IV infusion alone is inadequate in the treatment of fungal meningitis and urinary bladder infection; intrathecal administration and bladder instillation must also be carried out.
℞ for treatment of proven coccidioidomycosis, candidosis, cryptococcosis, or paracoccidioidomycosis: CH = IV (after dilution with isotonic saline or 5% D/W and over 30–60 min): 20–40 mg/kg/24 hr, div, every 8 hr, until clinical and laboratory tests no longer indicate activity of fungal infection. Dose may vary with type of fungus involved.
MONISTAT IV; ampoules for IV inj

Mineral oil; indigestible liquid hydrocarbon with limited absorbability; lubricant
℞ mild laxative: PO: 0.5 mL/kg/dose
†, liquid petrolatum; plain liquid or emulsion

Minocycline; see Tetracyclines

Minoxidil; direct-acting peripheral vasodilator
℞ in severely hypertensive patients who do not adequately respond to maximum therapeutic doses of a diuretic and 2 other antihypertensive agents. Usually a beta-adrenergic blocking agent has to be given concomitantly to prevent tachycardia and increased myocardial workload, as well as a diuretic such as hydrochlorothiazide, chlorthalidone, or furosemide to prevent serious fluid retention. CH = PO: initial dosage 0.2 mg/kg/24 hr as single dose; thereafter dosage may be increased stepwise to 0.25–1.0 mg/kg/24 hr under careful titration of the size and frequency of administration of the doses according to the individual needs of the patient.
LONITEN; tabl

Morphine sulfate; narcotic analgesic agent; addictive
℞ against severe pain: CH = SC: 0.6–1.2 mg/kg/24 hr, div, prn every 4 hr, equivalent to 0.1–0.2 mg/kg/dose, to be repeated prn every 4 hr
†; inj
Caution: Overdose produces severe respiratory depression, hypothermia, coma. Naloxone antidotal.

Nafcillin sodium; semisynthetic penicillinase-resistant penicillin
NB = IM, IV (over 15–30 min): ≤ 7 days old: 40 mg/kg/24 hr, div, every 12 hr; > 7 days old: 60 mg/kg/24 hr, div, every 8 hr. IN, CH = PO: 50–100 mg/kg/24 hr, div, every 6 hr; IM, IV (over 15–30 min): 100–200 mg/kg/24 hr, div, every 6 hr (IM) or every 4 hr (IV)
UNIPEN; caps, tabl, oral susp, inj

Nalidixic acid, antimicrobial agent effective against a selected group of gram-negative bacteria, apparently by inhibiting DNA synthesis
℞ for treatment of selected cases of urinary tract infection, when infective organisms can be shown to be sensitive: IN (>3 mo), CH = PO: 55 mg/kg/24 hr, div, every 6 hr, for 10–14 days
Note: If prolonged treatment is indicated, daily dose should be reduced to 33 mg/kg/24 hr, div, every 6 hr, and periodic evaluation for adverse side effects should be made. Resistance of initially sensitive microorganisms develops in about 25% of infections, and can occur within 48 hr. If resistance suspected, a therapeutic alternative must be chosen. Action of nalidixic acid is antagonized by nitrofurantoin.
NEGGRAM; oral susp, caplets
Caution: Even therapeutic doses may cause increased intracranial pressure, toxic psychosis, seizures in some patients.

Naloxone hydrochloride; opioid antagonist; nonaddictive
℞ in respiratory depression due to opioids: NB, IN, CH = IV, IM, SC: 0.01 mg/kg/dose, to be repeated prn after 2–3 min up to 3 times. After satisfactory response the dose must be repeated every 1–2 hr, as long as opioid depression persists
NARCAN, NARCAN neonatal; inj

Neomycin sulfate; antimicrobial aminoglycoside
℞ inhibition of gastrointestinal flora; justified only in selected cases (danger of hyperammonemia, enterocolitis with pathogenic *E. coli*): IN, CH = PO: 50–100 mg/kg/24 hr, div, every 6–8 hr
Caution: Possible overgrowth of abnormal organisms.
†, MYCIFRADIN sulfate, ‡; oral susp, tabl

Niclosamide; anthelmintic agent useful particularly against cestodes, which under the effect of the drug become susceptible to the proteolytic action of intestinal secretions

Table continued on following page

℞ against *Diphyllobothrium latum* (fish tapeworm) and *Taenia saginata* (beef tapeworm): CH = PO: 1000 mg, as single dose; Adult = PO: 1500 mg, as single dose

℞ against *Taenia solium* (pork tapeworm): same dose as for fish and beef tapeworms. Since viability of ova contained in the segments is not affected by the drug and there is risk of cysticercosis with *Taenia solium* if ova spill out of digested segments, it is **mandatory** to give an adequate purge 1 hr after niclosamide, to clear the bowel of all dead segments before they can be digested

℞ against *Hymenolepis nana* (dwarf tapeworm): CH = PO: 1000 mg/24 hr, as single daily dose, for 5 consecutive days. Adult = PO: 1500 mg/24 hr, as single daily dose, for 5 consecutive days

Note: Niclosamide tablets must be thoroughly chewed before swallowing or finely ground and mixed with some liquid before ingested to be fully effective. Niclosamide is available in the U.S.A. from the Parasitic Disease Drug Service, Bureau of Epidemiology, Centers for Disease Control, Atlanta, GA 30333. YOMESAN; tabl

Nitrofurantoin; nitrofuran-substituted hydantoin; antimicrobial agent effective against selected organisms, by interfering with enzyme systems of the microorganisms

℞ in the treatment of urinary tract infections, when infecting organisms are shown to be sensitive or likely to respond by clinical experience: IN (>3 mo), CH = PO: 5–7 mg/kg/24 hr, div, every 6 hr (with meals to minimize gastric upset), for 10–14 days. Repeated treatment courses with nitrofurantoin should be separated by "rest" periods. For long-term suppressive therapy dosage should be reduced, possibly to as low as 2 mg/kg/24 hr, div, every 6 hr.

Note: Because of rapid elimination by the kidneys, bacteriostatic concentrations are achieved only in urine. Better antibacterial activity is obtained in acid urine.

Caution: hemolysis occurs in G-6-PD–deficient individuals and in newborns because of insufficient detoxification capabilities. Nitrofurantoin should not be given to pregnant women at term or to women who breast feed.

†, FURADANTIN, MICRODANTIN, ‡; oral susp, tabl, caps

Nitroprusside; sodium nitrosylpentacyanoferrate, $Na_2Fe(CN)_5 \cdot NO \cdot 2H_2O$; vasodilator by direct action on smooth muscles of blood vessels; effect appears almost immediately and ends promptly, 1–10 min after stopping of administration of nitroprusside

℞ for emergency reduction of hypertension: IV infusion: Example: to prepare a solution of nitroprusside containing 0.1 mg/mL, dissolve 50 mg nitroprusside first in 2–3 mL 5% dextrose in water, and transfer this amount to 500 mL 5% dextrose water,* and start continuous infusion using a microdrip regulator or an infusion pump that allows precise measurement of flow; begin with infusion rate of 0.003 mg/kg/min (equivalent to 0.03 mL/kg/min of solution containing 0.1 mg/mL nitroprusside), and decrease or increase dosage according to response, for which there exists a wide dosage range (0.0005–0.008 mg/kg/min)

*Only 5% dextrose in water solution should be used to prepare nitroprusside solution, and no other drug should be added. To prevent decomposition of nitroprusside by exposure to light, protect infusion bottle and possibly tubing from light; for instance, by wrapping in aluminum foil.

Caution: Fall in arterial blood pressure is dose-dependent, with risk of hypotensive circulatory failure on overdosage if careful monitoring of blood pressure does not lead to prompt adjustment of infusion rate.

Note: In patients receiving concomitant antihypertensive medications, a smaller dosage of nitroprusside is required for comparable reduction of hypertension.

NIPRIDE; powder for preparation of solution prior to inj

Nystatin; antifungal agent; 1 mg = 2000 units; seems to be active by altering permeability of cell membrane of yeasts

℞ for topical treatment of candidosis of the buccal cavity (thrush) and the gastrointestinal tract. Very poorly absorbed. In oral candidosis, spread nystatin suspension into recesses of mouth: NB (<2000 g) = PO: 200,000–400,000 units/24 hr, div, every 4–6 hr. NB (>2000 g), IN = PO: 400,000–800,000 units/24 hr, div, every 4–6 hr. CH = PO: 800,000–2,000,000 units/24 hr, div, every 4–6 hr

†, MYCOSTATIN, NILSTAT; oral susp, tabl

Oxacillin sodium; semisynthetic penicillinase-resistant penicillin NB = IV (over 15–30 min), IM: for dosage same criteria apply as for methicillin in newborns; see Methicillin sodium. IN, CH = PO: 50–100 mg/kg/24 hr, div, every 6 hr; IV (over 15–30 min), IM: 100–200 mg/kg/24 hr, div, every 4 hr (IV) or every 6 hr (IM) BACTOCILL, PROSTAPHLIN; caps, oral susp, inj

Paraldehyde; cyclic ether compound which decomposes to acetaldehyde on exposure to light and air; rapidly acting hypnotic agent

℞ in status epilepticus: CH = IM (injection remote from nerves because of risk of damage): 0.15 g/kg/dose, corresponding to 0.15 mL/kg/dose of paraldehyde solution containing 1 g/mL; occasionally 1 additional dose may be given after 30 min, prn

Note: Use glass syringe, since paraldehyde reacts with plastic equipment. When given IV, injection should be slow and paraldehyde solution should be diluted with isotonic sodium chloride solution to lessen risk of thrombophlebitis. IV use is not recommended.

℞ to calm agitation: CH = PO, IM (PR, diluted in equal amount of olive oil): 0.15 mL/kg/dose, to be repeated prn after 4–6 hr

Caution: Before use, make sure that drug is not decomposed (acetaldehyde, acetic acid).

†, PARAL; liquid for inj, oral use (risk of gastric irritation), and rectal use

Pemoline, an oxazolidone; structurally different from amphetamine and methylphenidate; CNS stimulant with minimal sympathomimetic effects

℞ in minimal brain dysfunction: drug treatment of MBD not recommended below the age of 3 yr or in nonstructured therapeutic situation: CH (so far insufficient data have been accumulated in children below the age of 6 yr to assess efficacy and safety in this age group) = PO: initiate treatment with approximately 1 mg/kg/24 hr, as single dose each morning. If needed, increase dosage at weekly intervals by increments of 0.5 mg/kg/24 hr. On this schedule of titration of dose therapeutic response may not become evident until 4th wk of continued administration. Daily dose should not exceed 3 mg/kg/24 hr

Note: Insomnia, anorexia, and weight loss have been observed. The degree of reduced growth pattern on continued treatment is not yet established. Drug treatment of MBD should be discontinued at appropriate intervals to observe behavior of the patient and assess indication for further treatment. (See Sec. 7.46.) CYLERT; tabl

Penicillin G, benzylpenicillin; potassium penicillin G (1 mg = 1595 units); sodium penicillin G (1 mg = 1667 units). One million units of these salts of penicillin contains either 1.68 mEq K^+ or Na^+; in other terms, 1 g contains either 2.7 mEq K^+ or 2.8 mEq Na^+

NB = IV (over 15–30 min), IM:

≤ 7 days old: 50,000 units/kg/24 hr, equivalent to 31 mg/kg/24 hr, div, every 12 hr

   ℞ for meningitis: 100,000–150,000 units/kg/24 hr, div, every 4 hr

> 7 days old: 75,000 units/kg/24 hr, equivalent to 47 mg/kg/24 hr, div, every 8 hr

   ℞ for meningitis: 150,000–250,000 units/kg/24 hr, div, every 4 hr

(The higher doses should be chosen for meningitis caused by group B streptococci)

IN, CH = PO, IM, IV (over 15–30 min): 25,000–50,000 units/kg/24 hr, equivalent to 15.5–31 mg/kg/24 hr, div, every 4–6 hr; if given PO, administer penicillin G 0.5 hr before or 2 hr after the meal.

   ℞ in severe infections: IV: 200,000–400,000 units/kg/24 hr, equivalent to 125–250 mg/kg/24 hr, as continuous drip infusion or div, every 2–4 hr

   ℞ for prophylaxis of rheumatic fever: PO: 200,000 units/dose, equivalent to 125 mg/dose, twice daily, spaced from meals (see Sec 9.81)

Table continued on opposite page

DRUGS

Table 29–1B. Drug Doses (Continued)

Penicillin G benzathine, for injection: combination of 1 mole of diben-zylethylenediamine with 2 moles of penicillin G; 1 mg = 1211 units

℞ for prophylaxis of rheumatic fever: CH = IM: 600,000–1,200,000 units, equivalent to 500–1000 mg penicillin G, once a month

†, BICILLIN L-A, PERMAPEN, ‡; susp for inj

†, PENTIDS, PFIZERPEN G, ‡; tabl, caps, oral susp, inj (IV)

Penicillin G procaine, for injection; combination of penicillin G with procaine, mole for mole (1 mg = 1009 units)

NB = IM: 50,000 units/kg/24 hr, equivalent to 50 mg/kg/24 hr, in single daily dose. IN, CH = IM: 25,000–50,000 units/kg/24 hr, equivalent to 25–50 mg/kg/24 hr, in single daily dose

†, CRYSTICILLIN, DURACILLIN A.S., ‡; susp for IM inj

Penicillin V, phenoxymethyl penicillin; acid-resistant penicillin; 1 mg = 1695 units

IN, CH = PO: 25,000–50,000 units/kg/24 hr, equivalent to 15–30 mg/kg/24 hr, div, every 6–8 hr. *Note:* 400,000 units = 250 mg (approx).

†, PEN-VEE K, VEETIDS, ‡; tabl, oral susp, drops

Pentazocine hydrochloride; narcotic analgesic of the benzomorphan type; addictive

℞ against severe pain: Clinical experience in children under 12 yr of age is limited. Adult = PO: 50 mg/dose, to be repeated prn after 3–4 hr; IM, SC (pentazocine lactate); 30 mg/dose, to be repeated prn after 4 hr

FORTRAL, TALWIN; tabl (hydrochloride); inj (lactate)

Caution: As for *morphine,* above.

Pentobarbital, central nervous system depressant with short duration of action; tolerance to hypnotic effect may develop on continued use; initially, hypnotic effect of 3–5 hr

℞ for sedation: IN, CH = PO, IM: 1–2 mg/kg/24 hr, div, every 6 hr

℞ for sleep: IN, CH = PO, IM: 2–3 mg/kg/dose, repeat prn after 12–24 hr

†, NEMBUTAL elixir ● pentobarbital sodium, †, NEMBUTAL sodium; inj, caps, suppos

Phenobarbital, central nervous system depressant with long duration of action; initially, hypnotic effect of 8–12 hr; tolerance to hypnotic effect may develop on continued use

℞ for sedation: IN, CH = PO, IM: 2–3 mg/kg/24 hr, div, every 8–12 hr

℞ for sleep: IN, CH = PO, IM: 2–3 mg/kg/dose, repeat prn after 12–24 hr

℞ as anticonvulsant for long-term therapy: IN, CH = PO: start with 1.5 mg/kg/24 hr, div, every 12 hr; increase according to tolerance and therapeutic effect to 4–6 mg/kg/24 hr, div, every 12 hr, or as single daily dose, preferably at bedtime in order to minimize daytime drowsiness from hypnotic effect (see also Table 21–6)

℞ as adjunct in treatment of status epilepticus: CH = IV: 5–7.5 mg/kg/1st dose, by slow IV injection; followed prn after interval of 5 min by 2.5–3 mg/kg/dose, to be repeated once prn. If status epilepticus has been interrupted by drugs not including a barbiturate, phenobarbital can be given IM: 5–10 mg/kg/dose, followed by PO anticonvulsant regimen

†, LUMINAL; elixir, tabl ● phenobarbital sodium, †, LUMINAL sodium; inj

Phenolphthalein; laxative acting primarily on the colon

CH = PO: 1 mg/kg/dose

†, tabl, oral susp; component of several preparations

Phenylephrine hydrochloride; catecholamine with exclusively α-adrenergic action; peripheral vasoconstrictor

℞ to increase blood pressure in orthostatic hypotension, or

℞ to trigger vagal reflex in response to blood pressure increase, in the treatment of atrial tachyarrhythmia: PO: 1 mg/kg/24 hr, div, every 4 hr; SC, IM: 0.1 mg/kg/dose, repeat prn by monitoring response

Caution: With regard to hypertensive state and peripheral ischemia.

†, NEO-SYNEPHRINE hydrochloride; inj, elixir; also available as nose drops for local decongestant effect

Phenytoin, diphenylhydantoin; anticonvulsant agent; effective also in certain types of cardiac arrhythmias; antiarrhythmic effects similar to those of lidocaine: delayed slow diastolic depolarization, diminished automaticity; may facilitate conduction in damaged myocardial areas; does not depress myocardial activity

℞ as anticonvulsant for long-term therapy: IN, CH = PO: 3–8 mg/kg/24 hr, div, every 12 hr

℞ as adjunct in the treatment of status epilepticus: CH = IV (slow infusion under monitoring of heart rate): 10–15 mg/kg/dose (see also Table 21–6)

℞ as adjunct in the treatment of ventricular tachyarrhythmia: CH = IV (over 5 min): 2–3 mg/kg/dose, to be repeated prn after 20 min

†, DILANTIN; oral susp ● phenytoin sodium, †, DILANTIN sodium; caps, inj

Piperacillin, semisynthetic penicillin with predominant gram-negative spectrum.

CH (>2 mo) = IV: 200–300 mg/kg/day, div, q 4–6 hr

PIPERACIL; 1, 3, 6 g/vial; inj

Primaquine, 8-aminoquinoline antimalarial agent, used for prophylaxis against *Plasmodium vivax, P. ovale,* and *P. malariae* and for "radical" cure for *P. vivax* and *P. ovale*

IN, CH = PO: 0.55 mg/kg/24 hr (equivalent to 0.3 mg/kg/24 hr of base), as single daily dose, for 14 days

Note: Degree of intravascular hemolysis in individuals with G-6-PD deficiency is related to dosage and particular variant of the deficiency.

Primaquine diphosphate; tabl

Primidone; a deoxybarbiturate which is partially metabolized to phenobarbital; anticonvulsant agent

℞ for long-term therapy of selected types of convulsive disorder: CH = PO: 10 mg/kg/24 hr, div, every 8–12 hr (see also Table 21–6)

MYSOLINE; oral susp, tabl

Probenecid, competitive inhibitor of tubular secretion and reabsorption of organic acids

℞ for uricosuric action (acetylsalicylic acid antagonizes this effect), or

℞ in conjunction with penicillin G or V, or ampicillin, methicillin, oxacillin, cloxacillin, nafcillin to achieve longer persistence of therapeutic blood and tissue concentrations of the antimicrobial agent. CH = PO: initial dose of 25 mg/kg, followed by 40 mg/kg/24 hr, div, every 6 hr

BENEMID; tabl

Procainamide hydrochloride; antiarrhythmic agent with general cardiodepressant effects; diminished myocardial excitability (decreased threshold potential, prolonged refractory period), reduced conduction velocity, diminished automaticity; decreases myocardial contractility; effects similar to those of quinidine

℞ against ventricular tachyarrhythmia: IN, CH = IV (infused slowly, diluted in 5% dextrose in water): 2–5 mg/kg/dose; to be repeated at intervals of 20 min up to a total of 30 mg/kg in a 24 hr period. IM: 20–30 mg/kg/24 hr, div, every 6 hr; PO: 40–60 mg/kg/24 hr, div, every 4–6 hr

†, PRONESTYL; tabl, caps, inj

Prochlorperazine; piperazine-type phenothiazine with pronounced antiemetic effect

℞ for sedation: CH (over 2 yr old) = PO: 0.4 mg/kg/24 hr, div, every 6–8 hr, prn. IM: 0.2 mg/kg/24 hr, div, every 8–12 hr, prn

COMPAZINE; suppos ● prochlorperazine edisylate, COMPAZINE edisylate; oral liquid, syrup, inj

Caution: May produce parkinsonian syndrome. Diphenhydramine may be antidotal.

Promethazine hydrochloride; phenothiazine with aliphatic side chain

℞ for sedation, prevention or treatment of motion sickness, and as antihistamine; CH = PO: 1 mg/kg/24 hr, divided into half dose at bedtime and quarter doses every 6 hr of the remaining daytime

†, PHENERGAN; syrup, tabl, suppos

See KEY to abbreviations, p. 1520; for further information about drugs, see package insert.

Table continued on following page

DRUGS

Table 29–1B. Drug Doses (Continued)

Propantheline bromide, antispasmodic synthetic antimuscarinic agent as well as partial ganglionic blocking drug
℞ as adjunctive therapy against spasms in the gastrointestinal tract: CH = PO: 1.5 mg/kg/24 hr, div, every 6 hr, with meals, if applicable. IM: 0.8 mg/kg/24 hr, div, every 6 hr
PRO-BANTHINE; tabl, inj

Propoxyphene hydrochloride, and propoxyphene napsylate; opioid analgesic with less dependence liability than seen with codeine
℞ against mild to moderately severe pain: CH = PO: 2–3 mg/kg/24 hr, div, every 6 hr
propoxyphene hydrochloride, †, DARVON, ‡; caps • propoxyphene napsylate, DARVON-N; oral susp, tabl

Propranolol hydrochloride; β-adrenergic blocking agent (β₁ and β₂); racemic mixture of D- and L-propranolol, of which only L form has adrenergic blocking activity
℞ against selected forms of supraventricular and ventricular tachycardia: IN, CH = IV: 0.02–0.03 mg/kg/dose, given slowly; repeat prn every 20 min. PO: 0.3–1.2 mg/kg/24 hr, div, every 6 hr
℞ as antihypertensive in long-term therapy: CH = PO: initially 1 mg/kg/24 hr, div, every 6 hr, and progressive increase of dosage, if needed to achieve adequate response, up to 5 mg/kg/24 hr, div, every 6 hr. Combination with diuretic and/or hydralazine indicated, since propranolol blocks physiologic compensatory mechanisms such as adrenergic inotropic and chronotropic responses, as well as renin activity. See also Table 14–15.
℞ for prevention of migraine attack in severe cases and to combat the manifestations of thyrotoxicosis: Propranolol requirements vary widely from patient to patient because of individual differences in severity of underlying disease, endogenous sympathetic neuronal activity, sensitivity of β-adrenergic receptors to blockade, degree of protein binding, hepatic blood flow. For comparable effect, oral dose 6–10 times higher than intravenous dose in spite of good absorption from the gut because of inactivation of important fraction of propranolol in liver after entrance through portal vein.
Measures in case of exaggerated response: against bradycardia, atropine; if no response, isoproterenol, cautiously; against cardiac failure, digitalization and diuretics; against hypotension, epinephrine; against bronchospasm, isoproterenol, theophylline (aminophylline)
INDERAL; tabl, inj

Pseudoephedrine hydrochloride; indirectly acting sympathomimetic
℞ as nasal decongestant by systemic route: CH = PO: 4 mg/kg/24 hr, div, every 6 hr
†, SUDAFED, ‡; syrup, caps; contained in many combination products

Pyrantel pamoate, anthelmintic agent effective by means of neuromuscular paralysis of the parasite
℞ against pinworms (Enterobius vermicularis), Ascaris lumbricoides, and hookworms (Necator americanus, Ancylostoma duodenale): pyrantel pamoate has not been extensively studied in infants and children below 2 yr of age, hence particular attention should be given to children of this age group during treatment of parasitic infestation with pyrantel. CH = PO: 11 mg/kg/dose, as single dose and without regard to food intake or time of day; purging not necessary prior to, during, or after therapy
Note: In pinworm infestation, in which possibility of reinfection with eggs from the host exists, a 2nd treatment 2–3 wk after the 1st might be indicated.
ANTIMINTH; oral susp

Pyridostigmine bromide, cholinesterase inhibitor
℞ for diagnosis of myasthenia gravis: see Edrophonium chloride
℞ in myasthenia gravis: NB, IN, CH = IM: 0.1 mg/kg/dose, and continue with PO medication. PO: frequency of dosage and size of dose must be adjusted individually to provide optimum compensation during cycle of daily activities; average effective dose: 7 mg/kg/24 hr, div, every 4–5 hr
℞ for reversal of nondepolarizing muscle relaxants (tubocurarine, gallamine, pancuronium): IV (preceded by IV injection of atropine to prevent excessive secretions and bradycardia): 0.15 mg/kg/dose, and watch for recovery that ought to occur after 15–30 min; assure appropriate ventilation until complete recovery
MESTINON; tabl, syrup, inj
Caution: As for Edrophonium chloride.

Pyrimethamine, inhibitor of dihydrofolate reductase, antimalarial agent; for use in treatment of toxoplasmosis (see Sec 11.107)
℞ for clinical prophylaxis of malaria, especially effective against Plasmodium falciparum: IN, CH = PO: 0.5–0.75 mg/kg/dose, once every 7 days. Begin prophylaxis 2 wk before entering malarious area and continue for 8 wk after leaving. To eradicate P. vivax and P. ovale infections, treatment for 14 days with primaquine should be considered immediately on leaving malarious area while pyrimethamine prophylaxis is still in effect; see also Sec 11.104
Note: Hematologic abnormalities (anemia, thrombocytopenia, leukopenia) secondary to folic and folinic acid depletion can be prevented or reversed by IM administration of folinic acid (leucovorin) without affecting the efficacy of pyrimethamine.
DARAPRIM; tabl

Quinacrine hydrochloride, mepacrine hydrochloride; acridine derivative formerly used as antimalarial agent and against infestation with tapeworms, presently regarded as drug of choice against giardiasis
℞ against Giardia lamblia (Lamblia intestinalis): CH = PO: 6 mg/kg/24 hr, div, every 8 hr, for 5 consecutive days; maximum daily dose: 300 mg/24 hr
ATABRINE; tabl

Quinidine gluconate, quinidine sulfate, and quinidine polygalacturonate; alkaloid with general cardiodepressant effects: diminished myocardial excitability (decrease in threshold potential), reduced conduction velocity (widening of QRS complex, possibility of A-V block), increased refractory period, diminished automaticity, especially in ectopic sites; depresses myocardial contractility with risk of congestive heart failure if myocardial damage present
℞ against atrial tachycardia (usually after digitalization), and/or ventricular tachyarrhythmia: IN, CH = 2 mg/kg test dose PO, IM, (IV) to exclude idiosyncrasy. For treatment: PO (quinidine sulfate): 30 mg/kg/24 hr, div, every 4–5 hr. IV, IM (quinidine gluconate): 2–10 mg/kg/dose, prn every 3–6 hr
quinidine gluconate, QUINAGLUTE; tabl, inj • quinidine sulfate, †, QUINIDEX, ‡; tabl quinidine polygalacturonate. CARDIOQUIN; tabl
Caution: Overdose may lead to cardiac arrest.

Quinine sulfate and quinine dihydrochloride; alkaloid with effects on such a variety of biologic systems that it has been called "general protoplasmic poison."
℞ for treatment of chloroquine-resistant strains of Plasmodium falciparum, quinine used either with tetracycline or with a combination of pyrimethamine and a sulfonamide (see Table 11–38)
Oral treatment: quinine sulfate: CH = PO: 25 mg/kg/24 hr, div, every 8 hr, for 10–14 days, and either tetracycline: CH = PO: 40 mg/kg/24 hr, div, every 6 hr, for 10 days or pyrimethamine: CH = PO: 0.75 mg/kg/24 hr, div, every 12 hr, for 3 days, and sulfadiazine: CH = PO: 150 mg/kg/24 hr, div, every 6 hr, for 6 days
Intravenous treatment (severe cases when PO treatment not indicated): quinine dihydrochloride: IN, CH = IV (use dilute solution containing 200 mg in 200 mL half-isotonic sodium chloride solution): give 10 mg/kg/dose, by slow infusion over 1–2 hr; repeat at intervals of 12 hr until clinical response is obtained. Complete course of treatment (14 days) by oral route.
In addition: either tetracycline: IN, CH = IV: 20 mg/kg/24 hr, div, every 12 hr, until oral administration of oral dosage (see above) becomes possible, for a course of treatment of 10 days; or pyrimethamine: IN, CH = PO: 0.75 mg/kg/24 hr, div, every 12 hr, for 3 days, and sulfadiazine: IN, CH = IV: 100 mg/kg/24 hr, div, every 6 hr, until oral administration of oral dosage (see above) becomes possible, for a total of 6 days

See KEY to abbreviations, p. 1520; for further information about drugs, see package insert.   Table continued on opposite page

Note: In case quinine dihydrochloride for injection (powder to be dissolved) not available, quinidine, the D-isomer of quinine, can be substituted until quinine becomes available. Quinidine for injection comes as the gluconate. Also see *note* under Tetracyclines.

Quinine sulfate, tabl; quinine dihydrochloride, inj, available in U.S.A. from Parasitic Disease Drug Service, Bureau of Epidemiology, Centers for Disease Control, Atlanta, GA 30333

Reserpine, alkaloid which depletes stores of catecholamines and serotonin in many organs, including the brain

℞ as antihypertensive in long-term treatment: CH = PO: initially 0.02 mg/kg/24 hr, as single daily dose or div, every 12 hr; for maintenance, dose usually reduced to 0.005–0.01 mg/kg/24 hr

Note: See Table 14–15. Reserpine may induce mental depression, nasal congestion.

†, SANDRIL, SERPASIL; tabl, elixir

Rifampin; macrocytic antimicrobial and antimycobacterial agent, interfering with RNA-polymerase of infecting organisms

℞ in treatment of tuberculosis, in conjunction with at least 1 other antituberculous agent (isoniazid), and

℞ in carriers of *Neisseria meningitidis* resistant to penicillin and sulfonamide; treatment course of 4 consecutive days (possibility of rapid emergence of resistance): IN, CH = PO: 10–20 mg/kg/24 hr, in single daily dose (1 hr before or 2 hr after meal); maximum daily dose: 600 mg (= adult dose)

RIFADIN, RIMACTANE; caps

Salicylate sodium

℞ antipyretic, analgesic, anti-inflammatory: CH, Adolescents = PO: 25–50 mg/kg/24 hr, div, every 4–6 hr, prn

℞ antirheumatic: CH, Adolescents = PO: 50–100 mg/kg/24 hr, div, every 6 hr

†, tabl

Caution: See Sec 28.5.

Scopolamine methylbromide; also methscopolamine bromide, an antimuscarinic agent and quaternary ammonium compound that essentially lacks the central nervous system actions (sedation or excitement, amnesia, euphoria, hallucinations, unexpected behavior) of scopolamine

℞ as adjunctive therapy in the treatment of spasms in the gastrointestinal and urinary tracts: CH = PO: 0.15 mg/kg/24 hr, div, every 6 hr; SC, IM: 0.01 mg/kg/dose, repeat prn every 6–8 hr

PAMINE; tabl, inj

Caution: As for Belladonna.

Secobarbital, central nervous system depressant with short duration of action; tolerance to the hypnotic effect may develop on continued use; initially, hypnotic effect of 3–5 hr

℞ for sedation: IN, CH = PO, IM: 1–2 mg/kg/24 hr, div, every 6 hr

℞ for sleep: IN, CH = PO, IM: 2–3 mg/kg/dose, repeat prn after 12–24 hr

†, SECONAL elixir ● secobarbital sodium, †, SECONAL sodium; inj, caps, suppos

Senna syrup; contains anthraquinones, sennosides A and B, which stimulate the intramural nerve plexuses of the colon

℞ as laxative: CH = PO: 0.15 mL/kg/dose; to be repeated only once per wk, if indicated, so as not to interfere with normal bowel motility and not to induce laxative dependence

†; syrup

Sodium sulfate, $Na_2SO_4 \cdot 10H_2O$, Glauber salt; 1 g of salt traps about 30 mL of water to make the solution isosmotic

℞ as salinic cathartic: CH = PO: 300 mg/kg/dose

†; crystalline substance to be dissolved in a liquid for PO administration

Spironolactone; aldosterone antagonist and potassium-sparing diuretic, which interferes with sodium reabsorption

℞ as diuretic in selected cases (with normal renal function), most effective in combination with a potassium-wasting diuretic: CH = PO: 1.5–3 mg/kg/24 hr, div, every 4–8 hr

Note: Monitoring of serum concentration of potassium, of potassium intake, and of renal function is indicated during treatment with spironolactone.

ALDACTONE; tabl

Streptomycin sulfate; antimicrobial aminoglycoside

Caution: Because this drug when administered in large doses and/or for long periods can damage the 8th cranial nerve in adults, children, and transplacentally in fetuses, its indications are stringently selective today.

℞ in tuberculous meningitis and progressive tuberculosis, in association with isoniazid and other anti-tuberculous medication: CH = IM: 20–40 mg/kg/24 hr, div, every 12 hr, for 2–3 mo; maximum daily dose irrespective of weight: 1 g/24 hr. See Sec. 11.46 and Table 11–22.

†; susp, inj

Sulfonamides; analogues of para-aminobenzoic acid, interfering with the synthesis of tetrahydrofolic acid in sensitive bacteria

Sulfadiazine, sulfisoxazole, and *trisulfapyrimidines:* IN, CH = PO: initial dose 75 mg/kg/1st dose, followed by 120–150 mg/kg/24 hr, div, every 4–6 hr. IV (over 30 min), SC: 100–110 mg/kg/24 hr, div, every 4–6 hr

Sulfadiazine, †; tabl ● sulfadiazine sodium, †; inj ● sulfisoxazole, †, GANTRISIN; tabl sulfisoxazole acetyl, GANTRISIN acetyl; oral susp, syrup ● sulfisoxazole diolamine, GANTRISIN diolamine; inj ● trisulfapyrimidines (equal parts of sulfadiazine, sulfamerazine, and sulfamethazine), †, ‡; tabl, oral susp

Sulfamethoxazole: IN, CH = PO: initial dose 50–60 mg/kg/1st dose, followed by 50–60 mg/kg/24 hr, div, every 12 hr

GANTANOL; oral susp, tabl

Trimethoprim-sulfamethoxazole (combination of TMP + SMX): IN (>2 mo old), CH = PO: 6–12 mg TMP + 30–60 mg SMX/kg/24 hr, div, every 12 hr

℞ in severe urinary tract or *Shigella* infection: CH = PO, IV: 8–10 mg TMP + 40–60 mg SMX/kg/24 hr, div, every 6–8 hr

℞ against *Pneumocystis carinii:* CH = PO, IV: 15–20 mg TMP + 75–100 mg SMX/kg/24 hr, div, every 6–8 hr

Caution: Do not use in infants less than 2 mo old. Reduce dose in severe renal insufficiency. May cause bone marrow depression.

BACTRIM, SEPTRA; susp: 40 mg TMP + 200 mg SMX/5 mL; tabl: 80 mg TMP + 400 mg SMX/tabl or 160 mg TMP + 800 mg SMX/tabl; ampule: 80 mg TMP + 400 mg SMX/5 mL

Terbutaline sulfate, catecholamine; β-adrenergic receptor agonist with preferential effect on $β_2$-adrenergic receptors

℞ bronchodilator: Dosage in pediatric age group not firmly established. PO: 0.10–0.15 mg/kg/24 hr, div, every 8 hr. $β_2$-selectivity is reduced with increasing dosage or on parenteral administration. SC: 0.005 mg/kg/dose, to be repeated prn after 20 min, once only

BRETHINE, BRICANYL; tabl, inj

Tetracyclines; a group of derivatives of polycyclic naphthacenecarboxamide

Chlortetracycline hydrochloride: CH = PO: 25–50 mg/kg/24 hr, div, every 6 hr

AUREOMYCIN; caps, inj (IV)

Demeclocycline and *demeclocycline hydrochloride:* CH = PO: 7–13 mg/kg/24 hr, div, every 6–12 hr

DECLOMYCIN; pediatric drops, syrup ● DECLOMYCIN hydrochloride; caps, tabl

Doxycycline monohydrate and *doxycycline hyclate:* CH = PO: 5 mg/kg/24 hr, div, every 12 hr

†, VIBRAMYCIN monohydrate; oral susp ● †, VIBRAMYCIN hyclate; caps, inj (IV)

Methacycline hydrochloride: CH = PO: 7–13 mg/kg/24 hr, div, every 6–12 hr

RONDOMYCIN; caps, syrup

Minocycline hydrochloride: CH = PO, IV: initial dose 4 mg/kg, followed by 4 mg/kg/24 hr, div, every 12 hr

MINOCIN, VECTRIN; caps, syrup, inj (IV)

Table continued on following page

DRUGS

Table 29–1B. Drug Doses (Continued)

Oxytetracycline, oxytetracycline hydrochloride, oxytetracycline calcium: same dosage as tetracycline hydrochloride, below TERRAMYCIN; tabl, inj (IM) • TERRAMYCIN hydrochloride; †, caps, inj (IV, IM) • TERRAMYCIN calcium; pediatric drops, syrup

Tetracycline hydrochloride: CH = PO: 25–50 mg/kg/24 hr, div, every 8 hr; IM (often very painful): 15–25 mg/kg/24 hr, div, every 8–12 hr; IV: 10–20 mg/kg/24 hr, div, every 12 hr
    †, ACHROMYCIN V, PANMYCIN, ‡; caps, inj (IV, IM); sol for IM inj contains local anesthetic. Pediatric drops, oral susp, and syrup prepared with tetracycline base

Note: Tetracyclines have limited indications in infancy and childhood because of their accumulation in bone and teeth and their potential to interfere with growth. Their use should be avoided insofar as possible until formation of dental enamel is complete in most permanent teeth (at about 8 yr), to avoid unsightly discolored, pitted teeth. Tetracyclines may cause increased intracranial pressure in infants (pseudotumor cerebri).

Theophylline, inhibitor of phosphodiesterase, analeptic, cardiotonic, diuretic
    ℞ in status asthmaticus: initial loading dose IV: 7 mg/kg/dose, infused after dilution in equal volume of intravenous fluid over 20–30 min, followed by maintenance IV: 20 mg/kg/24 hr, div, every 4–6 hr, or by continuous IV drip; switch to PO maintenance as soon as possible
    ℞ oral maintenance: PO: 20 mg/kg/24 hr, div, every 6 hr; as conditions permit, taper to lowest effective dosage, usually around 10 mg/kg/24 hr, div, every 6 hr

Note the content of theophylline in the following formulations: theophylline (anhydrous), 100%; aminophylline, 85%; theophylline monoethanolamine, 75%; dihydroxypropyltheophylline, 70%; oxtriphylline, choline salt, 64%; theophylline sodium glycinate, 50%; theophylline calcium salicylate, 48%.

theophylline, †, ELIXOPHYLLIN elixir, ELIXICON oral susp, SLO-PHYLLIN caps, oral susp, SOMOPHYLLIN caps, ‡: component of many combination products • aminophylline, †, SOMOPHYLLIN oral liquid, ‡; inj, oral preparations

Caution: Circulatory collapse, seizures, coma may result from acute or chronic overdose.

Thioridazine hydrochloride; phenothiazine of the piperidine type
    ℞ for sedation and neuroleptic effect: CH = PO: 1 mg/kg/24 hr, div, every 8 hr
MELLARIL; oral liquid, tabl

Caution: Overdose may produce parkinsonian syndrome. Diphenhydramine may be antidotal.

Ticarcillin disodium; semisynthetic penicillin which is not resistant to penicillinase; low degree of toxicity permits high serum and tissue concentrations in selected severe infections; 1 g contains 5.3 mEq Na⁺

Note: Experience with ticarcillin disodium in the pediatric age group is limited at this time and recommendations are not firmly established.
NB = IV (over 20–30 min), IM: ≤ 2000 g and ≤ 7 days old: 225 mg/kg/24 hr, div, every 8 hr; > 2000 g and ≤ 7 days old: 300 mg/kg/24 hr, div, every 6 hr; > 7 days old: 600 mg/kg/24 hr, div, every 4 hr
IN, CH = IV (over 20–30 min): 200–300 mg/kg/24 hr, div, every 4 hr
TICAR; IV and IM inj

Tobramycin, aminoglycoside antibiotic. Serum concentration and renal function should be monitored during therapy. Excessive doses may cause 8th nerve toxicity.
NB = IM, IV: 4–5 mg/kg/24 hr, div, q 12 hr
IN = IM, IV: 7.5 mg/kg/24 hr, div, q 8 hr
CH = IM, IV: 2.5 mg/kg q 8 hr
Patients with cystic fibrosis may require doses up to 12 mg/kg/day, div, q 4 hr. Peak serum concentrations should be maintained below 12 µg/mL and trough below 2 µg/mL.
NEBCIN; IM, IV; 10, 40 mg/mL, 2 mL vials

Triamterene; potassium-sparing diuretic; inhibits the reabsorption of Na⁺ in exchange for K⁺ and H⁺; its effect is potentiated by concomitant use of diuretics which act more proximally
CH = PO: initially 4 mg/kg/24 hr, div, every 12 hr (after meals).
Note: For maintenance, dosage must be adjusted to needs of individual patient; in conjunction with other diuretics dosage usually can be decreased.

Caution: Because of the risk of hyperkalemia, serum potassium concentrations and potassium intake should be watched.
DYRENIUM; caps

Trimethadione; oxazolidinedione; anticonvulsant agent
    ℞ as an adjunct in the treatment of convulsive disorders: CH = PO: 20 mg/kg/24 hr, div, every 8 hr; if needed, dosage can be progressively adjusted to 40 mg/kg/24 hr, div, every 8 hr
Note: The methylated metabolite of trimethadione accumulates progressively in the body and is partially responsible for anticonvulsant effect.
TRIDIONE; tabl, caps, oral susp

Trimethoprim; see Sulfonamides

Tripelennamine hydrochloride: an ethylenediamine with antihistamine, mild cholinergic, and slight sedative effects
    ℞ antiallergic effect: CH = PO: 5 mg/kg/24 hr, div, every 6 hr
    †, PYRIBENZAMINE hydrochloride; tabl • tripelennamine citrate, PYRIBENZAMINE citrate; elixir

Valproate sodium, dipropylacetate sodium; anticonvulsant agent with singular mode of action (effective probably by increasing γ-aminobutyric acid in brain tissues)
    ℞ in the treatment of simple petit mal, and of complex absence seizures, either alone or in combination with other drugs (see reservation below) according to the results: CH = PO: start with 15 mg/kg/24 hr, div, every 8–12 hr; if needed, dosage increased by weekly increments of 5–10 mg/kg/24 hr up to a maximum recommended dose of 30 mg/kg/24 hr, div, every 8 hr

Caution: Concomitant use of valproate sodium and clonazepam might result in petit mal status. Blood concentrations of phenobarbital and phenytoin may be affected by addition of valproate sodium to the regimen.
DEPAKENE; caps (valproic acid), syrup (valproate sodium)

Vancomycin, complex glycopeptide that inhibits synthesis of cell wall in gram-positive bacteria and is effective against methicillin-resistant staphylococci; in oral application effective in pseudomembranous colitis caused by toxin-producing bacteria such as *Clostridium difficile* and *Staphylococcus aureus;* excreted mainly by kidneys
NB = IV: 30 mg/kg/24 hr, div, every 12 hr if ≤1 wk old, every 8 hr if >1 wk old
CH = IV (<500 mg/30 min): 40 mg/kg/24 hr, div, every 6 hr (maximum 2 g/24 hr)
Note: Reduce dosage in renal insufficiency. May cause ototoxicity and renal impairment, skin rashes, peripheral neuropathy
VANCOCIN; vials

Verapamil; calcium channel blocker. Toxic effects include allergic reactions, urticaria, bronchospasm, hypotension, decreased cardiac output, and asystole. Cardiac monitoring should be used during administration.
IN = IV: 0.1–0.2 mg/kg infused over 2 min
CH = IV: 0.1–0.3 mg/kg infused over 2 min
Maintenance dose = 1–2 mg/kg q 8 hr
CALAN, ISOPTIN; IV 2.5 mg/mL vial inj; PO Tabs: 80, 120 mg

Vidarabine, antiviral agent used for treatment of neonatal herpes simplex infections.
IN = IV: 15–30 mg/kg infused over 12 hr q 24 hr for 10 days.
Note: May rarely cause hepatic and hematologic toxicity.
VIRA-A; 200 mg/mL vial inj

SANFORD N. COHEN
RALPH E. KAUFFMAN
LEON STREBEL

TABLE 29–2: REFERENCE RANGES FOR LABORATORY TESTS

Reference ranges are guides for judging health and disease. For many years, the method of defining the normal range was to make a series of measurements in healthy individuals and then calculate the mean and standard deviation of those measurements. By convention the normal range was defined as the mean $\pm$ 2 SD. This system does not work in most medical situations because the distribution of measurements does not fit a gaussian distribution. Most biologic measurements are skewed. A more appropriate normal distribution or reference range can be defined as the central 90% (5th–95th percentiles) of a group of measurements in normal individuals. This listing of reference ranges uses the measured or reasonable estimate of the central 90% of a normal distribution of values. These ranges have proved to be clinically useful in our pediatric wards and clinics. More complete catalogues are referenced. The pertinent prefixes denoting the decimal factors are listed below.

Prefixes Denoting Decimal Factors

Prefix	Symbol	Factor
mega	M	10^6
kilo	k	10^3
hecto	h	10^2
deka	da	10^1
deci	d	10^{-1}
centi	c	10^{-2}
milli	m	10^{-3}
micro	μ	10^{-6}
nano	n	10^{-9}
pico	p	10^{-12}
femto	f	10^{-15}

To preserve space, the following common abbreviations are used.

Abbreviations

ΔA	change in absorbance
ACD	acid-citrate-dextrose
AI	angiotensin I
ALL	acute lymphocytic leukemia
AML	acute myeloid leukemia
AMML	acute myelomonocytic leukemia
AU	arbitrary unit
BMD	Boehringer Mannheim Diagnostics
cAMP	adenosine 3',5'-cyclic phosphate
cap.	capillary
CH_{50}	dilution required to lyse 50% of indicator RBC
CHF	congestive heart failure
CNS	central nervous system
conc.	concentration
CSF	cerebrospinal fluid
d	diem, day, days
EDTA	ethylenediaminetetraacetate; edetic acid
F	female
g	gram
G-D	General Diagnostics
hr	hour, hours
Hb	hemoglobin
HbCO	carboxyhemoglobin
hpf	high power field
HPLC	high performance liquid chromatography
IRP-2-hMG	2nd International Reference Preparation of Human Menopausal Gonadotropin
IU	International Unit of hormone activity
L	liter
L→P	lactate to pyruvate reaction
M	male
MB	heart CK isoenzyme
MCV	mean corpuscular value
mEq/L	milliequivalents per liter
min	minute, minutes
mm^3	cubic millimeter; equivalent to microliter (μL)
mmHg	millimeters of mercury
mo	month, months
mol	mole
mOsmol	milliosmoles
M.W.	relative molecular weight
P→L	pyruvate to lactate reaction
Pa	pascals
RBC	red blood cell(s); erythrocyte(s)
RIA	radioimmunoassay
RID	radial immunodiffusion
RT	room temperature
s	second, seconds
SD	standard deviation
std.	standard
therap.	therapeutic
U	International Unit of enzyme activity
V	volume
WBC	white blood cell
WHO	World Health Organization
wk	week, weeks
yr	year, years

Symbols

$>$	greater than
$\geq$	greater than or equal to
$<$	less than
$\leq$	less than or equal to
$\pm$	plus/minus
$\simeq$	approximately equal to

C. CHARLTON MABRY

Hicks JM, Boeckx RL (ed): Pediatric Clinical Chemistry. Philadelphia, WB Saunders, 1984.

Hung W, August GP, Glasgow AM: Pediatric Endocrinology. New Hyde Park, NY, Medical Examination Publ Co, 1983.

Meites S (ed): Pediatric Clinical Chemistry. 2nd ed. Washington, DC, Am Assoc Clin Chem, 1981.

Tietz NW (ed): Clinical Guide to Laboratory Tests. Philadelphia, WB Saunders, 1983.

Wallach J: Interpretation of Pediatric Tests. Boston, Little, Brown, 1983.

Table 29–2. **Reference Ranges**

Test	Specimen	Reference Range	Factor	Reference Range International Units
Acetaminophen	Serum, plasma (heparin, EDTA)	Therap. conc.: 10–30 µg/mL Toxic conc.: >200	×6.62	66–200 µmol/L >1300
Acetone *Semiquantitative*	Serum or plasma (oxalate)	Negative (<3 mg/dL)	×0.1722	Negative (<0.5 mmol/L)
Quantitative		0.3–2.0 mg/dL		0.05–0.34 mmol/L
Semiquantitative	Urine	Negative		Negative
Activated Partial Thromboplastin Time (APTT) *Microtechnique (Miale)*	Whole blood (Na citrate) Remove plasma immediately Capillary blood (siliconized micropipets; Na citrate)	25–35 s (Differs with method) Infants: <90 s Reaches adult levels by 2–6 mo		25–35 s <90 s
Adrenocorticotropic Hormone (ACTH)	Plasma (heparin)	*pg/mL* Cord: 130–160 1–7 d postnatal: 100–140 Adult, 0800 hr: 25–100 1800 hr: <50	×1	*ng/L* 130–160 100–140 25–100 <50
Alanine Aminotransferase (ALT, GPT)	Serum	Newborn/Infant: 5–25 U/L Thereafter: 8–20		5–25 U/L 8–20
Albumin	Serum	*g/dL* Premature: 3.0–4.2 Newborn: 3.6–5.4 Infant: 4.0–5.0 Thereafter: 3.5–5.0	×10	*g/L* 30–42 36–54 40–50 35–50
	CSF	10–30 mg/dL		100–300 mg/L
Qualitative	Urine	<20 mg/dL		<200 mg/L
Quantitative		<80 mg/d	×1	<80 mg/d
Aldolase	Serum	1.0–7.5 U/L (30 °C) 0.3–3.0 U/L at bed rest 1.5–12.0 U/L (37 °C) Children: 2× adults Newborn: 4× adults		1.0–7.5 U/L (30 °C) 0.3–3.0 U/L at bed rest 1.5–12.0 U/L (37 °C) Children: 2× adults Newborn: 4× adults
Aldosterone	Plasma (heparin, EDTA) or serum	*ng/dL* Newborn: 5–60 1 wk–1 yr: 1–160 1–3 yr: 5–60 3–5 yr: <5–80 5–7 yr: <5–50 7–11 yr: 5–70 11–15 yr: <5–50 Adult, *Average sodium diet* Supine: 3–10 Upright, F: 5–30 M: 6–22 2–3× higher during pregnancy Adrenal vein: 200–800 ng/dL *Low sodium diet:* increases 2- to 5-fold: Florinef suppression: <4 ng/dL ACTH or angiotensin stimulation, 1 hr: 2- to 5-fold	×0.0277	*nmol/L* 0.14–1.7 0.03–4.4 0.14–1.7 <0.14–2.2 <0.14–1.4 0.14–1.9 <0.14–1.4 0.08–0.3 0.14–0.8 0.17–0.61 5.5–22 nmol/L <0.1 nmol/L

Aldosterone (continued), Urine, 24 hr:

Total Urinary Na *mmol/d*	Plasma Renin Activity *ng AI/mL/hr*	Urinary Aldosterone *µg/d*	Factor	Urinary Aldosterone *nmol/d*
<20	5–24	>35–80	×2.77	>97–220
50	2–7	13–33		36–91
100	1–5	5–24		14–66
150	0.5–4	3–19		8–53
200		1–16		3–44
250		1–13		3–36

(assuming normal serum Na, K, and extracellular volume)

Test	Specimen	Reference Range	Factor	Reference Range International Units
Alkaline Phosphatase, Leukocyte, see *Neutrophil Alkaline Phosphatase*				
Alkaline Phosphatase, Serum, see *Phosphatase, Alkaline*				
δ-Aminolevulinic Acid (δ-ALA)	Serum Urine, 24 hr	15–23 µg/dL; lower in children 1.3–7.0 mg/d	×0.076 ×7.626	1.1–1.8 µmol/L 9.9–53.4 µmol/d

Table continued on opposite page

Table 29–2. **Reference Ranges** *(Continued)*

Test	Specimen	Reference Range		Factor	Reference Range International Units
Ammonia Nitrogen *Resin or enzymatic*	Serum or plasma (Na-heparin)		*μg N/dL*		*μmol/L*
		Newborn:	90–150	× 0.714	64–107
		0–2 wk:	79–129		56–92
		>1 mo:	29–70		21–50
		Thereafter:	15–45		11–32
	Urine, 24 hr	500–1200 mg/d		× 0.0714	36–86 mmol/d
Amniotic Fluid Analysis, ΔA_{450nm}	Amniotic fluid	28 wk: 0–0.048 *A*			0–0.048 *A*
		40 wk: 0–0.02 *A*			0–0.02 *A*
Amphetamine	Serum, plasma (heparin, EDTA)	Therap. conc.: 20–30 ng/mL		× 7.396	150–220 nmol/L
		Toxic conc.: >200			>1500
Amylase *(Beckman; BMD)*	Serum	Newborn: 5–65 U/L			5–65 U/L
		>1 yr: 25–125			25–125
	Urine, timed specimen	1–17 U/hr			1–17 U/hr
Androstenedione	Serum		*ng/dL*		*nmol/L*
		Child:	8–50	× 0.0349	3–18
		Adult, M:	75–205		26–72
		F:	85–275		30–96
Anion Gap [Na − (Cl + CO_2)]	Plasma (heparin)	7–16 mmol/L			7–16 mmol/L
Anti-Deoxyribonuclease B Titer (Anti-DNAse Titer)	Serum	≤170 units			≤170 units
Antidiuretic Hormone (hADH, Vasopressin)	Plasma (EDTA)	*Plasma mOsmol/kg*	*Plasma ADH pg/mL*		*Plasma ADH ng/L*
		270–280:	<1.5	× 1	<1.5
		280–285:	<2.5		<2.5
		285–290:	1–5		1–5
		290–295:	2–7		2–7
		295–300:	4–12		4–12
Anti-Streptolysin-O Titer (ASO Titer)	Serum	≤166 Todd Units 170–330 Todd Units in school-aged children			
α_1-Antitrypsin	Serum	Newborn: 145–270 mg/dL		× 0.222	32.2–60.0 μmol/L
		Thereafter: 105–200			23.3–44.4
Ascorbic Acid, see *Vitamin C*					
Aspartate Aminotransferase (AST, SGOT, 30 °C)	Serum	Newborn/Infant: 15–60 U/L			15–60 U/L
		Thereafter: 8–20			8–20
Base Excess	Whole blood (heparin)		*mmol/L*		*mmol/L*
		Newborn:	(−10)–(−2)		(−10)–(−2)
		Infant:	(−7)–(−1)		(−7)–(−1)
		Child:	(−4)–(+2)		(−4)–(+2)
		Thereafter:	(−3)–(+3)		(−3)–(+3)
Bicarbonate	Serum	Arterial: 21–28 mmol/L			Arterial: 21–28 mmol/L
		Venous: 22–29			Venous: 22–29
Bile Acids, Total	Serum, fasting	0.3–2.3 μg/mL		× 1	0.3–2.3 mg/L
	Serum, 2 hr postprandial	1.8–3.2 μg/mL			1.8–3.2 mg/L
	Feces	120–225 mg/d		× 1	120–225 mg/d
Bilirubin			*Premature mg/dL*	*Full Term mg/dL*	
Total	Serum				*μmol/L*
		Cord:	<2.0	<2.0	× 17.10	<34 <34
		0–1 d:	<8.0	<6.0		<137 <103
		1–2 d:	<12.0	<8.0		<205 <137
		2–5 d:	<16.0	<12.0		<274 <205
		Thereafter:	<2.0	0.2–1.0		<34 3.4–17.1
	Urine	Negative			Negative
	Amniotic fluid	28 wk: <0.075 mg/dL (or ΔA_{450} <0.048)		× 17.10	<1.3 μmol/L (or ΔA_{450} <0.048)
		40 wk: <0.025 mg/dL (or ΔA_{450} <0.02)			<0.43 μmol/L (or ΔA_{450} <0.02)
Conjugated (Direct)	Serum	0–0.2 mg/dL		× 17.10	0–3.4 μmol/L
Bleeding Time (BT) *Ivy*	Blood from skin puncture	Normal: 2–7 min			2–7 min
		Borderline: 7–11 min			7–11 min
Simplate (G-D)		2.75–8 min			2.75–8 min

Table continued on following page

Table 29–2. **Reference Ranges** *(Continued)*

Test	Specimen	Reference Range	Factor	Reference Range International Units
Blood Volume	Whole blood (heparin)	M: 52–83 mL/kg F: 50–75 mL/kg	× 0.001	M: 0.052–0.083 L/kg F: 0.050–0.075 L/kg
Brucellosis, Agglutinins	Serum	≤1:8	× 1	≤1:8
C-Peptide	Serum	≤4.0 ng/mL	× 1	≤4.0 µg/L
C-Reactive Protein	Serum	Cord: 10–350 ng/mL Adult: 68–8200	× 1	10–350 µg/L 68–8200
CSF, see *Cerebrospinal Fluid*				
Calcitonin (hCT)	Serum or plasma (heparin or EDTA)	*pg/mL* Newborn, Term, cord: 30–240 48 hr: 91–580 7 d: 77–293 Premature, cord: 30–265 48 hr: 108–670 7 d: 79–570 Adult, M: <100 F: 4 times lower (increases in pregnancy) Concentrations decrease with age	× 1	*ng/L* 30–240 91–580 77–293 30–265 108–670 79–570 <100
Calcium, Ionized (iCa)	Serum, plasma, or whole blood (heparin)	*mg/dL* Cord: 5.0–6.0 Newborn, 3–24 hr: 4.3–5.1 24–48 hr: 4.0–4.7 Thereafter: 4.48–4.92 or 2.24–2.46 mEq/L	× 0.25 × 0.5	*mmol/L* 1.25–1.50 1.07–1.27 1.00–1.17 1.12–1.23 1.12–1.23
Calcium, Total	Serum	*mg/dL* Cord: 9.0–11.5 Newborn, 3–24 hr: 9.0–10.6 24–48 hr: 7.0–12.0 4–7 d: 9.0–10.9 Child: 8.8–10.8 Thereafter: 8.4–10.2	× 0.25	*mmol/L* 2.25–2.88 2.3–2.65 1.75–3.0 2.25–2.73 2.2–2.70 2.1–2.55
	Urine, 24 hr	*Ca in Diet mg/d* Ca Free: 5–40 Low to average: 50–150 Average (20 mmol/d): 100–300	× 0.025	*mmol/d* 0.13–1.0 1.25–3.8 2.5–7.5
	CSF	2.1–2.7 mEq/L or 4.2–5.4 mg/dL	× 0.50 × 0.25	1.05–1.35 mmol/L 1.05–1.35 mmol/L
	Feces	Avg.: 0.64 g/d	× 25	16 mmol/d
Carbamazepine	Serum, plasma (heparin, EDTA); collect at trough conc.	Therap. conc.: 8–12 µg/mL Toxic conc.: >15	× 4.233	34–51 µmol/L >63
Carbon Dioxide, Partial Pressure (*p*CO₂)	Whole blood (heparin)	*mmHg* Newborn: 27–40 Infant: 27–41 Thereafter, M: 35–48 F: 32–45	× 0.1333	*kPa* 3.6–5.3 3.6–5.5 4.7–6.4 4.3–6.0
Carbon Dioxide, Total (tCO₂)	Serum or plasma (heparin)	*mmol/L* Cord: 14–22 Premature: 14–27 Newborn: 13–22 Infant: 20–28 Child: 20–28 Thereafter: 23–30		*mmol/L* 14–22 14–27 13–22 20–28 20–28 23–30
Carbon Monoxide	Whole blood (EDTA)	Nonsmokers: <2% HbCO Smokers: <10% Lethal: >50%	× 0.01	HbCO fraction: <0.02 <0.10 >0.5
Carboxyhemoglobin, see *Carbon Monoxide*				
β-Carotene	Serum	*µg/dL* Infant: 20–70 Child: 40–130 Thereafter: 60–200	× 0.0186	*µmol/L* 0.37–1.30 0.74–2.42 1.12–3.72

Table continued on opposite page

Table 29–2. **Reference Ranges** *(Continued)*

Test	Specimen	Reference Range		Factor	Reference Range International Units
Catecholamines, Fractionated	Plasma (EDTA-sodium metabisulfite)	Norepinephrine,			
		Supine:	100–400 pg/mL	×5.911	591–2364 pmol/L
		Standing:	300–900		1773–5320
		Epinephrine,			
		Supine:	<70 pg/mL	×5.458	<382 pmol/L
		Standing:	<100		<546
		Dopamine:	<30 pg/mL	×6.528	<196 pmol/L
		(no postural change)			(no postural change)
	Urine, 24 hr	Norepinephrine,	μg/d		nmol/d
		0–1 yr:	0–10	×5.911	0–59
		1–2 yr:	0–17		0–100
		2–4 yr:	4–29		24–171
		4–7 yr:	8–45		47–266
		7–10 yr:	13–65		77–384
		Thereafter:	15–80		87–473
		Epinephrine,	μg/d		nmol/d
		0–1 yr:	0–2.5	×5.458	0–13.6
		1–2 yr:	0–3.5		0–19.1
		2–4 yr:	0–6.0		0–32.7
		4–7 yr:	0.2–10		1.1–55
		7–10 yr:	0.5–14		2.7–76
		Thereafter:	0.5–20		2.7–109
		Dopamine,	μg/d		nmol/d
		0–1 yr:	0–85	×6.528	0–555
		1–2 yr:	10–140		65–914
		2–4 yr:	40–260		261–1697
		Thereafter:	65–400		424–2611
Catecholamines, Total Free	Urine, 24 h		μg/d		μg/d
		0–1 yr:	10–15	×1	10–15
		1–5 yr:	15–40		15–40
		6–15 yr:	20–80		20–80
		Thereafter:	30–100		30–100
Cerebrospinal Fluid Pressure	CSF	70–180 mm water			70–188 mm water
Cerebrospinal Fluid Volume	CSF	Child: 60–100 mL		×0.001	0.006–0.10 L
		Adult: 100–160			0.1–0.16
Ceruloplasmin	Serum		mg/dL		μmol/L
		Newborn:	1–30	×0.0662	0.06–1.99
		6 mo–1 yr:	15–50		0.99–3.31
		1–12 yr:	30–65		1.99–4.30
		Thereafter:	14–40		0.93–2.65
Chloral Hydrate	Serum	As Trichloroethanol:			
		Therap. conc.: 2–12 μg/mL		×6.694	13–80 μmol/L
		Toxic conc.: >20			>134
Chloride	Serum or plasma (heparin)		mmol/L		mmol/L
		Cord:	96–104		96–104
		Newborn:	97–110		97–110
		Thereafter:	98–106		98–106
	CSF	118–132 mmol/L			118–132 mmol/L
	Urine, 24 h		mmol/d		mmol/d
		Infant:	2–10		2–10
		Child:	15–40		15–40
		Thereafter:	110–250		110–250
		(varies greatly with Cl intake)			
	Sweat		mmol/L		mmol/L
		Normal			
		(homozygote):	0–35		0–35
		Marginal:	30–60		30–60
		Cystic fibrosis:	60–200		60–200
		Increases by 10 mmol/L during lifetime			Increases by 10 mmol/L during lifetime
Cholesterol, Total	Serum or plasma (EDTA or heparin)		mg/dL		mmol/L
		Cord:	45–100	×0.0259	1.17–2.59
		Newborn:	53–135		1.37–3.50
		Infant:	70–175		1.81–4.53
		Child:	120–200		3.11–5.18
		Adolescent:	120–210		3.11–5.44
		Adult:	140–310		3.63–8.03
		Recommended (desirable) range for adults:			
			140–250		3.63–6.48

Table continued on following page

Table 29–2. **Reference Ranges** (Continued)

Test	Specimen	Reference Range		Factor	Reference Range International Units
Chorionic Gonadotropin, β-Subunit (β-hCG)	Serum or plasma (EDTA)	Child and M: nondetectable			
		F, post-conception	*mIU/mL*		*IU/L*
		7–10 d:	>5.0	× 1.0	>5.0
		30 d:	>100		>100
		40 d:	>2000		>2000
		10 wk:	50,000–100,000		50,000–100,000
		14 wk:	10,000–20,000		10,000–20,000
		Trophoblastic disease:	>100,000		>100,000
Clotting Time *Lee-White, 37 °C*	Whole blood (no anticoagulant)	Glass tubes: 5–8 min (5–15 min at RT) Silicone tubes: about 30 min prolonged			Glass tubes: 5–8 min (5–15 min at RT) Silicone tubes: about 30 min prolonged
Coagulation Factor Assays *Factor I, see Fibrinogen* *Factor II*	Plasma (citrate)	0.5–1.5 U/mL or 60–150% of normal		× 1	0.5–1.5 kU/L 60–150 AU
Factor IV, see Calcium *Factor V*		0.5–2.0 U/mL or 60–150% of normal		× 1	0.5–2.0 kU/L 60–150 AU
Factor VII		65–135% of normal		× 1	65–135 AU
Factor VIII		60–145% of normal		× 1	60–145 AU
Factor VIII antigen		50–200% of normal		× 1	50–200 AU
Factor IX		60–140% of normal		× 1	60–140 AU
Factor X		60–130% of normal		× 1	60–130 AU
Factor XI		65–135% of normal		× 1	65–135 AU
Factor XII		65–150% of normal		× 1	65–150 AU
Factor XIII (Fibrin Stabilizing Factor, FSF)	Whole blood (citrate or oxalate)	Minimal hemostatic level: 0.02–0.05 U/mL or 1–2% of normal		× 1000 × 1	20–50 U/L or 1–2 AU
Complement Components *Total hemolytic complement activity*	Plasma (EDTA)	75–160 U/mL or >33% of plasma CH_{50}		× 1	75–160 kU/mL >0.33 of plasma CH_{50}
Total complement decay rate (functional)	Plasma (EDTA)	~10–20% Deficiency: >50%		× 0.01	~0.10–0.20 (fraction of decay rate) 0.50 (fraction of decay rate)
Classic pathway components *C1q*	Serum		*mg/dL*		*mg/L*
		Cord:	1.0–14.9	× 10	10–149
		1 mo:	2.2–6.2		22–62
		6 mo:	1.2–7.6		12–76
		Adult:	5.1–7.9		51–79
C1r	Serum	2.5–3.8 mg/dL		× 10	25–38 mg/L
C1s (C1 esterase)	Serum	2.5–3.8 mg/dL		× 10	25–38 mg/L
C2	Serum		*mg/dL*		*mg/L*
		Cord:	1.6–2.8	× 10	16–28
		1 mo:	1.9–3.9		19–39
		6 mo:	2.4–3.6		24–36
		Adult:	1.6–4.0		16–40
C3			*mg/dL*		*g/L*
RID	Serum	Cord:	65–112	× 0.01	0.65–1.12
		1 mo:	61–130		0.61–1.30
		Adult:	111–171		1.11–1.71
		Maternal:	161–175		1.61–1.75
		At birth, conc. is 50–75% of adult values			At birth, conc. is 50–75% of adult values
Nephelometry	Serum	Newborn:	58–120 mg/dL	× 0.01	0.58–1.20 g/L
C4					
RID	Serum	Newborn:	16–39 mg/dL	× 10	160–390 mg/L
		Adult:	15–45		150–450
Nephelometry	Serum	Newborn:	10–26 mg/dL	× 10	100–260 mg/L
		Adult:	13–37		130–370
C5	Serum		*mg/dL*		*mg/L*
		Cord:	3.4–6.2	× 10	34–62
		1 mo:	2.3–6.3		23–63
		6 mo:	2.4–6.4		24–64
		Adult:	3.8–9.0		38–90

Table continued on opposite page

Table 29–2. **Reference Ranges** (Continued)

Test	Specimen	Reference Range		Factor	Reference Range International Units
C6	Serum		*mg/dL*	× 10	*mg/L*
		Cord:	1.0–4.2		10–42
		1 mo:	2.2–5.2		22–52
		6 mo:	3.7–7.1		37–71
		Adult:	4.0–7.2		40–72
C7	Serum	4.9–7.0 mg/dL		× 10	49–70 mg/L
C8	Serum	4.3–6.3 mg/dL		× 10	43–63 mg/L
C9	Serum	4.7–6.9 mg/dL		× 10	47–69 mg/L
Alternative pathway components					
C4 binding protein	Serum	18.0–32.0 mg/dL		× 10	180–320 mg/L
Factor B (C3 proactivator)					
RID	Plasma (EDTA)		*mg/dL*	× 10	*mg/L*
		Cord:	7.8–15.8		78–158
		1 mo:	6.2–28.6		62–286
		6 mo:	16.9–29.3		169–293
		Adult:	14.7–33.5		147–335
Nephelometry	Serum	Newborn:	14–33 mg/dL	× 10	140–330 mg/L
		Adult:	20–45		200–450
Properdin	Serum		*mg/dL*	× 10	*mg/L*
		Cord:	1.3–1.7		13–17
		1 mo:	0.6–2.2		6–22
		6 mo:	1.3–2.5		13–25
		Adult:	2.0–3.6		20–36
Regulatory proteins					
β1H-globulin (C3b inactivator accelerator)	Serum		*mg/dL*	× 10	*mg/L*
		Cord:	26–42		260–420
		1 mo:	24–56		240–560
		6 mo:	33–61		330–610
		Adult:	40–72		400–720
C1 inhibitor (Esterase inhibitor)					
RID	Plasma (EDTA)	17.4–24.0 mg/dL		× 10	174–240 mg/L
Complement decay rate (functional)	Serum	<20% decay		× 0.01	<0.20 (fraction of decay rate)
		Deficiency: >50% decay			>0.50 (fraction of decay rate)
C3b inactivator (KAF)	Serum		*mg/dL*	× 10	*mg/L*
		Cord:	1.8–2.6		18–26
		1 mo:	1.5–3.9		15–39
		6 mo:	2.3–4.3		23–43
		Adult:	2.6–5.4		26–54
S protein	Serum	41.8–60.0 mg/dL		× 10	418–600 mg/L
Copper	Serum		*µg/dL*		*µmol/L*
		Birth-6 mo:	20–70	× 0.157	3.14–10.99
		6 yr:	90–190		14.13–29.83
		12 yr:	80–160		12.56–25.12
		Adult, M:	70–140		10.99–21.98
		F:	80–155		12.56–24.34
	Erythrocytes (heparin)	90–150 µg/dL		× 0.157	14.13–23.55 µmol/L
	Urine, 24 h	15–30 µg/d		× 0.0157	0.24–0.47 µmol/d
Coproporphyrin	Urine, 24 hr	34–234 µg/d		× 1.5	51–351 nmol/d
	Feces, 24 hr	<30 µg/g dry wt		× 1.5	<45 nmol/g dry wt
		400–1200 µg/d			600–1800 nmol/d
Corticobinding Globulin (CBG), see *Transcortin*					
Cortisol	Serum or plasma (heparin)		*µg/dL*		*nmol/L*
		Newborn:	1–24	× 27.59	28–662
		Adults, 0800 hr:	5–23		138–635
		1600 hr:	3–15		82–413
		2000 hr:	≤50% of 0800 h	× 0.01	Fraction of 0800 hr: ≤0.50
Cortisol, Free	Urine, 24 hr		*µg/d*		*nmol/d*
		Child:	2–27	× 2.759	5.5–74
		Adolescent:	5–55		14–152
		Adult:	10–100		27–276

Table continued on following page

Table 29–2. **Reference Ranges** (*Continued*)

Test	Specimen	Reference Range		Factor	Reference Range International Units
Creatine Kinase (CK, CPK; 30 °C)					
Total	Serum		*U/L*		*U/L*
		Newborn:	68–580		68–580
		Adult, M:	12–70		12–70
		F:	10–55		10–55
		Ambulatory,			
		M:	25–90		25–90
		F:	10–70		10–70
		Higher after exercise			Higher after exercise
Isoenzymes	Serum	Fraction 2 (MB) <5% of total			Fraction of total: <0.05
Creatinine					
Jaffe, kinetic or enzymatic	Serum or plasma		*mg/dL*		*μmol/L*
		Cord:	0.6–1.2	×88.4	53–106
		Newborn:	0.3–1.0		27–88
		Infant:	0.2–0.4		18–35
		Child:	0.3–0.7		27–62
		Adolescent:	0.5–1.0		44–88
		Adult, M:	0.6–1.2		53–106
		F:	0.5–1.1		44–97
Jaffe, manual	Serum or plasma	0.8–1.5 mg/dL		×88.4	70–133 μmol/L
	Amniotic fluid	After 37 wk gestation: >2.0 mg/dL		×88.4	After 37 wk gestation: >180 μmol/L
	Urine, 24 hr		*mg/kg/d*		*μmol/kg/d*
		Infant:	8–20	×8.84	71–180
		Child:	8–22		71–195
		Adolescent:	8–30		71–265
		Adult:	14–26		124–230
		or:	*mg/d*		*mmol/d*
		M:	800–2000	×0.00884	7–18
		F:	600–1800		5.3–16
Creatinine Clearance (Endogenous)	Serum or plasma and urine	Newborn: 40–65 mL/min/1.73 m² <40 yr, M: 97–137 F: 88–128 Decreases ~6.5 mL/min/decade			
Cyclic AMP	Plasma (EDTA)	*ng/mL* M: 5.6–10.9 F: 3.6–8.9		×3.03	*nmol/L* M: 17–33 F: 11–27
	Urine, 24 hr	<3.3 mg/d or <1.64 mg/g creatinine			1000–11,500 nmol/d <6000 nmoles cAMP/g creatinine
Dehydroepiandrosterone (DHEA)	Serum		*ng/mL*		*nmol/L*
		Cord:	5.6–20.0	×3.467	19.4–69.3
		Child:	1.0–3.0		3.5–10.4
		Adult, M:	1.7–4.2		5.9–14.6
		F:	2.0–5.2		6.9–18.0
		Pregnancy:	0.5–12.5		1.7–43.3
	Urine, 24 hr		*mg/d*		*μmol/d*
		Child,			
		0–1 yr:	<0.1	×3.467	<0.35
		10–15 yr:	<0.4		<1.4
		Adult, M:	0–2.3		0–8.0
		F:	0–1.2		0–4.2
Dehydroepiandrosterone Sulfate (DHEA-SO₄)	Serum or plasma (heparin or EDTA)		*μg/mL*		*μmol/L*
		Newborn:	<300	×2.608	<780
		1–4 d:	<20		<52
		Child:	0.60–2.54		1.6–6.6
		Adult, M:	1.99–3.34		5.2–8.7
		F:			
		Premenopausal:	0.82–3.38		2.1–8.8
		Pregnancy, term:	0.23–1.17		0.6–3.0
Diazepam	Serum, plasma (heparin, EDTA); collect at trough conc.	Therap. conc.: 100–1000 ng/mL Toxic conc.: >5000		×3.512	350–3500 nmol/L >17,500
Differential Count, see *Leukocyte Differential Count*					
Digitoxin	Serum, plasma (heparin, EDTA); collect at least 6 hr after dose	Therap. conc.: 20–35 ng/mL Toxic conc.: >45		×1.307	26–46 nmol/L >59
Digoxin	Serum, plasma (heparin, EDTA); collect at least 12 hr after dose		*ng/mL*		*nmol/L*
		Therap. conc.,			
		CHF:	0.8–1.5	×1.281	1–1.9
		Arrhythmias:	1.5–2.0		1.9–2.6
		Toxic conc.,			
		Child:	>2.5		>3.2
		Adult:	>3.0		>3.8

Table continued on opposite page

Table 29–2. **Reference Ranges** (Continued)

Test	Specimen	Reference Range	Factor	Reference Range International Units
Dihydrotestosterone (DHT)	Serum	*ng/dL*	× 0.03443	*nmol/L*
		Prepubertal: <3.5		<0.12
		Pubertal M F		M F
		stage I: <10 <10		<0.34 <0.34
		II: <20 <15		<0.7 <0.5
		III: <35 <25		<1.2 <0.86
		IV–V: <75 <25		<2.6 <0.86
		Adult: 30–85 4–22		1.03–2.92 0.14–0.76
Diphenylhydantoin, see *Phenytoin*				
Disaccharide Absorption Test	Serum	*mg/dL*	× 0.055	*mmol/L*
		Change in glucose from fasting		Change in glucose from fasting value:
		value: Normal: >30		>1.67
		Inconclusive: 20–30		1.11–1.67
		Abnormal: <20		<1.11
Dithionite Tube Test, see *Sickle Cell Tests*				
Electrophoresis, Hemoglobin, see *Hemoglobin Electrophoresis*				
Eosinophil Count	Whole blood (EDTA or heparin); capillary blood	50–350 cells/mm³ (µL)	× 10⁶	50–350 × 10⁶ cells/L
Epinephrine, see *Catecholamines, Fractionated*				
Erythrocyte Count (RBC Count)	Whole blood (EDTA)	*millions of cells/mm³ (µL)*	× 1	*× 10¹² cells/L*
		Cord blood: 3.9–5.5		3.9–5.5
		1–3 d (cap.): 4.0–6.6		4.0–6.6
		1 wk: 3.9–6.3		3.9–6.3
		2 wk: 3.6–6.2		3.6–6.2
		1 mo: 3.0–5.4		3.0–5.4
		2 mo: 2.7–4.9		2.7–4.9
		3–6 mo: 3.1–4.5		3.1–4.5
		0.5–2 yr: 3.7–5.3		3.7–5.3
		2–6 yr: 3.9–5.3		3.9–5.3
		6–12 yr: 4.0–5.2		4.0–5.2
		12–18 yr, M: 4.5–5.3		4.5–5.3
		F: 4.1–5.1		4.1–5.1
		18–49 yr, M: 4.5–5.9		4.5–5.9
		F: 4.0–5.2		4.0–5.2
Erythrocyte Sedimentation Rate (ESR)				
Westergren, modified	Whole blood (EDTA)	*mm/hr*		*mm/hr*
		Child: 0–10		0–10
		Adult: M, <50 yr: 0–15		0–15
		F, <50 yr: 0–20		0–20
Wintrobe		Child: 0–13		0–13
		Adult: M, 0–9		0–9
		F, 0–20		0–20
ZETA		41–54%		41–54 AU
Erythropoietin				
RIA	Serum	<5–20 mU/mL	× 1	<5–20 U/L
Hemagglutination		25–125		25–125
Bioassay		5–18		5–18
Estradiol	Serum or plasma (heparin or EDTA)	*pg/mL*	× 3.671	*pmol/L*
		M, pubertal		
		stage I: 2–8		7–29
		II: 11		40
		III: >20		>73
		Adult, M: 8–36		29–132
		F, pubertal		
		stage I: 0–23		0–84
		II: 0–66		0–242
		III: 0–105		0–385
		IV: 20–300		73–1101
		Follicular: 10–90		37–330
		Midcycle: 100–500		367–1835
		Luteal: 50–240		184–881

Table continued on following page

Table 29–2. **Reference Ranges** *(Continued)*

Test	Specimen	Reference Range		Factor	Reference Range International Units
Estradiol *(Continued)*	Urine, 24 hr		*µg/d*		*nmol/d*
		Adult, M:	0–6	×3.671	0–22
		F:			
		Follicular:	0–3		0–11
		Ovulatory peak:	4–14		15–51
		Luteal:	4–10		15–37
Estriol (E$_3$), Free	Serum	*Weeks of gestation*			*nmol/L*
			µg/L		
		25:	3.5–10.0	×3.47	12.1–34.7
		28:	4.0–12.5		13.9–43.4
		30:	4.5–14.0		15.6–48.6
		32:	5.0–16.0		17.4–55.5
		34:	5.5–18.5		19.1–64.2
		36:	7.0–25.0		24.3–86.8
		37:	8.0–28.0		27.8–97.2
		38:	9.0–32.0		31.2–111.0
		39:	10.0–34.0		34.7–118.0
		40–41:	10.5–25.0		36.4–86.8
	Amniotic fluid	*Weeks*	*ng/mL (95% range)*		*nmol/L (95% range)*
		16–20:	1.0–3.2	×3.47	3.5–11.1
		20–24:	2.1–7.8		7.3–27.1
		24–28:	2.1–7.8		7.3–27.1
		28–32:	4.0–13.6		13.9–47.2
		32–36:	3.6–15.5		12.5–53.8
		36–38:	4.6–18.0		16.0–62.5
		38–40:	5.4–19.8		18.7–68.7
Estriol (E$_3$), Total	Serum		*ng/mL*		*nmol/L*
		Pregnancy (wk),			
		24–28:	30–170	×3.468	104–590
		28–32:	40–220		140–760
		32–36:	60–280		208–970
		36–40:	80–350		280–1210
		Adult, M and nonpregnant F:	<2		<7
	Urine, 24 hr		*mg/d*		*µmol/d*
		Pregnancy (wk),			
		30:	6–18	×3.468	21–62
		35:	9–28		31–97
		40:	13–42		45–146
		Decrease of >40% of previous value suggests fetus at risk			Fraction of previous value of <0.60 suggests fetus at risk
Estrogens, Total	Serum		*pg/mL*		*ng/L*
		Child:	<30	×1	<30
		M:	40–115		40–115
		F, cycle—days			
		1–10 d:	61–394		61–394
		11–20 d:	122–437		122–437
		21–30 d:	156–350		156–350
		Prepubertal:	≤40		≤40
	Urine, 24 hr		*µg/d*		*µg/d*
		Child:	<10	×1	<10
		Adult, M:	5–25		5–25
		F, Preovulation:	5–25		5–25
		Ovulation:	28–100		28–100
		Luteal peak:	22–80		22–80
		Pregnancy:	<45,000		<45,000
		Postmenopausal:	<10		<10
Ethanol	Whole blood (oxalate), serum	Toxic conc.: 50–100 mg/dL		×0.2171	11–22 mmol/L
		Depression of CNS: >100			>22
Ethosuximide	Serum, plasma (heparin, EDTA); collect at trough conc.	Therap. conc.: 40–100 µg/mL		×7.084	280–700 µmol/L
		Toxic conc.: >150			>1060
Fat, Fecal	Feces, 72 hr		*g/d*		*g/d*
		Infant, breast-fed:	<1	×1	<1
		0–6 yr:	<2		<2
		Adult:	<7		<7
		Adult (fat-free diet):	<4		<4
		Coefficient of fat absorption (%)			*Absorbed fraction*
		Infant, breast-fed:	>93	×0.01	>0.93
		Infant, formula-fed:	>83		>0.83
		>1 y:	≥95		≥0.95

Table continued on opposite page

Table 29–2. **Reference Ranges** (Continued)

Text	Specimen	Reference Range		Factor	Reference Range International Units
Fatty Acids, Nonesterified (Free)	Serum or plasma (heparin)	Adults: 8–25 mg/dL Children and obese adults: <31		× 0.0354	0.30–0.90 mmol/L <1.10
Ferric Chloride Test	Urine, fresh random	Negative			Negative
Ferritin	Serum		*ng/mL*	× 1	*μg/L*
		Newborn:	25–200		25–200
		1 mo:	200–600		200–600
		2–5 mo:	50–200		50–200
		6 mo–15 yr:	7–140		7–140
		Adult, M:	15–200		15–200
		F:	12–150		12–150
α_1-Fetoprotein	Serum	Adult: <40 ng/mL		× 1	<40 μg/L
		Fetal: peak of 200–400 mg/dL in first trimester		× 0.01	peak of 2–4 g/L in first trimester
		1 yr: <30 ng/mL		× 1	<30 μg/L
	Amniotic fluid	*weeks*	*mg/dL*	× 10	*mg/L*
		10–12	0.5–3.3		5–33
		13–14	0.3–3.7		3–37
		15–16	0.4–2.7		4–27
		17–18	0.1–2.6		1–26
		19–20	<0.1–1.4		<1–14
		21–22	<0.1–1.1		<1–11
		23–24	<0.1–0.7		<1–7
Fibrin Degradation Products *Agglutination (Thrombo-Wellco test[R])*	Whole blood; special tube containing thrombin and proteolytic inhibitor	<10 μg/mL		× 1	<10 mg/L
	Urine: 2 mL in special tube (see above)	<0.25 μg/mL		× 1	<0.25 mg/L
Fibrinogen	Whole blood (Na citrate)	Newborn: 125–300 mg/dL Adult: 200–400		× 0.01	1.25–3.00 g/L 2.00–4.00
Folate	Serum	Newborn: 7.0–32 ng/mL Thereafter: 1.8–9		× 2.265	15.9–72.4 nmol/L 4.1–20.4
	Erythrocytes (EDTA)	150–450 ng/mL cells			340–1020 nmol/L cells
Follicle Stimulating Hormone (hFSH)	Serum or plasma (heparin)		*mU/mL* *(IRP-2-hMG)*	× 1	*IU/L*
		Birth–1 yr, M:	<1–12		<1–12
		F:	<1–20		<1–20
		1–8 yr, M:	<1–6		<1–6
		F:	<1–4		<1–4
		9–10 yr, M:	<1–10		<1–10
		F:	2–8		2–8
		11–12 yr, M:	2–12		2–12
		F:	3–11		3–11
		13–14 yr, M:	3–15		3–15
		F:	3–15		3–15
			mU/mL		*IU/L*
		Adult, M:	4–25		4–25
		F,			
		Premenopause:	4–30		4–30
		Midcycle peak:	10–90		10–90
		Pregnancy: Low to undetectable			Low to undetectable
Galactose	Serum	Newborn: 0–20 mg/dL Thereafter: <5		× 0.0555	0–1.11 mmol/L <0.28
	Urine	Newborn: ≤60 mg/dL Thereafter: <14 mg/d		× 0.0555 × 0.00555	≤3.33 mmol/L <0.08 mmol/d
Gastrin	Serum	<100 pg/mL		× 1	<100 ng/L
Glucose	Serum		*mg/dL*		*mmol/L*
		Cord:	45–96	× 0.0555	2.5–5.3
		Premature:	20–60		1.1–3.3
		Neonate:	30–60		1.7–3.3
		Newborn,			
		1 d:	40–60		2.2–3.3
		>1 d:	50–90		2.8–5.0
		Child:	60–100		3.3–5.5
		Adult:	70–105		3.9–5.8
	Whole blood (heparin)	Adult:	65–95		3.6–5.3
	CSF	Adult:	40–70		2.2–3.9
Quantitative, enzymatic	Urine	<0.5 g/d		× 5.55	<2.8 mmol/d
Qualitative	Urine	Negative			Negative

Table continued on following page

Table 29–2. **Reference Ranges** (Continued)

Text	Specimen	Reference Range	Factor	Reference Range International Units
Glucose, 2 hr Postprandial	Serum	<120 mg/dL Diabetes: see *Glucose Tolerance Test, Oral*	× 0.0555	<6.7 mmol/L
Glucose-6-phosphate Dehydrogenase (G-6-PD) in Erythrocytes	Whole blood (ACD, EDTA, or heparin)			
Bishop, modified		Adult: 3.4–8.0 U/g Hb 98.6–232 U/10^{12} RBC 1.16–2.72 U/mL RBC Newborn: 50% higher	× 0.0645 × 10^{-3} × 1	Adult: 0.22–0.52 MU/mol Hb 0.10–0.23 nU/RBC 1.16–2.72 kU/L RBC Newborn: 50% higher

Glucose Tolerance Test (GTT), Oral — Serum

Dose, Adult: 75 g
Child: 1.75 g/kg
of ideal weight up to
maximum of 75 g

	mg/dL		× 0.0555	mmol/L	
	Normal	Diabetic		Normal	Diabetic
Fasting:	70–105	>115		3.9–5.8	>6.4
60 min:	120–170	≥200		6.7–9.4	≥11
90 min:	100–140	≥200		5.6–7.8	≥11
120 min;	70–120	≥140		3.9–6.7	≥7.8

Text	Specimen	Reference Range	Factor	Reference Range International Units
γ-Glutamyltransferase (GGT), 37 °C	Serum	M: 9–50 U/L F: 8–40	× 1	M: 9–50 U/L F: 8–40

Growth Hormone (hGH, Somatotropin) — Serum or plasma (EDTA, heparin); Fasting, at rest

	ng/mL	× 1	μg/L
Cord:	10–50		10–50
Newborn:	10–40		10–40
Child:	<5		<5
Adult, M:	<5		<5
F:	<8		<8

Ham's Test, see *Acidified Serum Test*

Text	Specimen	Reference Range	Factor	Reference Range International Units
Haptoglobin (Hp)	Serum; avoid hemolysis			
RID		30–175 mg/dL	× 0.155*	6.20–27.90 μmol Hb bound/L of serum = 300–1750 mg/L
Sephadex		40–180 mg Hb bound/dL of serum		
Nephelometry		Newborn: 5–48 mg/dL Thereafter: 25–175 mg/dL	× 10	50–480 mg/L 250–1750 mg/L

HDL-Cholesterol (HDLC) — Serum or plasma (EDTA)

	mg/dL		× 0.0259	mmol/L	
	M	F		M	F
Mean:	45	55		1.17	1.42
Range,					
Cord blood:	5–50	5–50		0.13–1.30	0.13–1.30
0–14 yr:	30–65	30–65		0.78–1.68	0.78–1.68
15–19 yr:	30–65	30–70		0.78–1.68	0.78–1.81
20–29 yr:	30–70	30–75		0.78–1.81	0.78–1.94
30–39 yr:	30–70	30–80		0.78–1.81	0.78–2.07
40 + yr:	30–70	30–85		0.78–1.81	0.78–2.20
Values for blacks ~10 mg/dL higher					

Hematocrit (HCT, Hct) — Whole blood (EDTA)

Calculated from MCV and RBC (electronic displacement or laser)

	% of packed red cells (V red cells/V whole blood × 100)	× 0.01	Volume fraction (V red cells/V whole blood)
1 d (cap):	48–69		0.48–0.69
2 d:	48–75		0.48–0.75
3 d:	44–72		0.44–0.72
2 mo:	28–42		0.28–0.42
6–12 yr:	35–45		0.35–0.45
12–18 yr, M:	37–49		0.37–0.49
F:	36–46		0.36–0.46
18–49 yr, M:	41–53		0.41–0.53
F:	36–46		0.36–0.46

Hemoglobin (Hb) — Whole blood (EDTA)

	g/dL	× 0.155*	mmol/L
1–3 d (cap):	14.5–22.5		2.25–3.49
2 mo:	9.0–14.0		1.40–2.17
6–12 yr:	11.5–15.5		1.78–2.40
12–18 yr, M:	13.0–16.0		2.02–2.48
F:	12.0–16.0		1.86–2.48
18–49 yr, M:	13.5–17.5		2.09–2.71
F:	12.0–16.0		1.86–2.48

Text	Specimen	Reference Range	Factor	Reference Range International Units
	Serum or plasma (heparin, ACD, EDTA)	<10 mg/dL <3 mg/dL with butterfly set-up and 18 g needle	× 0.1551*	<1.55 μmol/L <0.47 μmol/L with butterfly set-up and 18 g needle
	Urine, fresh random	Negative		Negative

*Based on hemoglobin MW 64,500.

Table continued on opposite page

Table 29–2. **Reference Ranges** (Continued)

Test	Specimen	Reference Range	Factor	Reference Range International Units
Hemoglobin, glycosylated	Whole blood (heparin, EDTA, or oxalate)			*Fraction of Hb*
Electrophoresis		5.6–7.5% of total Hb	×0.01	0.056–0.075
Column		6–9% of total Hb		0.06–0.09
HPLC		HbA_{1a} 1.6% total Hb		0.016
		HbA_{1b} 0.8		0.008
		HbA_{1c} 3–6		0.03–0.06
Hemoglobin A	Whole blood (EDTA, citrate, or heparin)	>95%	×0.01	Fraction of Hb: >0.95
Hemoglobin A_2 (HbA$_2$)	Whole blood (EDTA, oxalate)	Adult: 1.5–3.5% (2 SD) Lower in infants <1 yr		*Mass fraction* 0.015–0.035 (2 SD)
Hemoglobin (Hb) Electrophoresis	Whole blood (EDTA, citrate, or heparin)	HbA >95% HbA$_2$ 1.5–3.5% HbF <2%	×0.01	*Mass fraction* HbA >0.95 HbA$_2$ 0.015–0.035 HbF <0.02
Hemoglobin F	Whole blood (EDTA)	*% HbF*	×0.01	*Mass fraction HbF*
Alkali denaturation (White)		1 d: 63–92		0.62–0.92
		5 d: 65–88		0.65–0.88
		3 wk: 55–85		0.55–0.85
		6–9 wk: 31–75		0.31–0.75
		3–4 mo: <2–59		<0.02–0.59
		6 mo: <2– 9		<0.02–0.09
		Adult: <2		<0.02
Hemoglobin H (HbH) *Isopropanol precipitation*	Whole blood (ACD, EDTA, or heparin)	No precipitation at 40 min		No precipitation at 40 min
Homovanillic Acid (HVA)	Urine, 24 hr	Child: 3–16 µg/mg creatinine Thereafter: <15 mg/d	×0.621 ×5.489	1.9–10 mmol/mol creatinine <82 µmol/d
17-Hydroxycorticosteroids (17-OHCS)	Urine, 24 hr	*mg/d*	×2.76	*µmol/d*
		0–1 yr: 0.5–1.0		1.4–2.8 (Conversion
		Child: 1.0–5.6		2.8–15.5 based on
		Adult, M: 3.0–10.0		8.2–27.6 hydrocortisone,
		F: 2.0–8.0		5.5–22 M.W. 362)
		or: 3–7 mg/g creatinine	×0.312	or: 0.9–2.5 mmol/mol creatinine
5-Hydroxyindoleacetic Acid (5-HIAA)				
Qualitative	Fresh random urine	Negative		Negative
Quantitative	Urine, 24 hr	2–8 mg/d	×5.230	10.5–42 µmol/d
17-Hydroxyprogesterone (17-OHP)	Serum	*ng/mL*		*nmol/L*
		M,		
		Pubertal stage I: 0.1–0.3	×3.026	0.3–0.9
		Adult: 0.2–1.8		0.6–5.4
		F,		
		Pubertal stage I: 0.2–0.5		0.6–1.5
		Follicular: 0.2–0.8		0.6–2.4
		Luteal: 0.8–3.0		2.4–9.0
		Postmenopausal: 0.04–0.5		0.12–1.5
Immunoglobulin A (IgA)	Serum	*mg/dL*		*mg/L*
		Cord: 0–5	×10	0–50
		Newborn: 0–2.2		0–22
		1/2–6 mo: 3–82		30–820
		6 mo–2 yr: 14–108		140–1080
		2–6 yr: 23–190		230–1900
		6–12 yr: 29–270		290–2700
		12–16 yr: 81–232		810–2320
		Thereafter: 60–380		600–3800
Immunoglobulin D (IgD)	Serum	Newborn: None detected Thereafter: 0–8 mg/dL	×0.055	None detected 0–0.44 µmol/L
Immunoglobulin E (IgE)	Serum	M: 0–230 IU/mL F: 0–170	×1	0–230 kIU/L 0–170
Immunoglobulin G (IgG)	Serum	*mg/dL*		*g/L*
		Cord: 760–1700	×0.01	7.6–17
		Newborn: 700–1480		7–14.8
		1/2–6 mo: 300–1000		3–10
		6 mo–2 yr: 500–1200		5–12
		2–6 yr: 500–1300		5–13

Table continued on following page

Table 29–2. **Reference Ranges** (*Continued*)

Test	Specimen	Reference Range	Factor	Reference Range International Units
Immunoglobulin G (IgG) (*Continued*)		6–12 yr: 700–1650 12–16 yr: 700–1550 Adults: 600–1600 (higher in blacks)		7–16.5 7–15.5 6–16 (higher in blacks)
Immunoglobulin M (IgM)	Serum	*mg/dL* Cord: 4–24 Newborn: 5–30 1/2–6 mo: 15–109 6 mo–2 yr: 43–239 2–6 yr: 50–199 6–12 yr: 50–260 12–16 yr: 45–240 Thereafter: 40–345 Results vary with std. preparation	× 10	*mg/L* 40–240 50–300 150–1090 430–2390 500–1990 500–2600 450–2400 400–3450
Insulin (12 hr Fasting)	Serum or plasma (no anticoagulant)	Newborn: 3–20 µU/mL Thereafter: 7–24	× 1.0	3–20 mU/L 7–24
Insulin with Oral Glucose Tolerance Test	Serum	*Min* *Insulin, µU/mL* 0: 7–24 30: 25–231 60: 18–276 120: 16–166 180: 4–38	× 1	*mU/L* 7–24 25–231 18–276 16–166 4–38
Iron	Serum	*µg/dL* Newborn: 100–250 Infant: 40–100 Child: 50–120 Thereafter, M: 50–160 F: 40–150 Intoxicated child: 280–2550 Fatally poisoned child: >1800	× 0.179	*µmol/L* 17.90–44.75 7.16–17.90 8.95–21.48 8.95–28.64 7.16–26.85 50.12–456.5 >322.2
Iron-Binding Capacity, Total (TIBC)	Serum	Infant: 100–400 µg/dL Thereafter: 250–400	× 0.179	17.90–71.60 µmol/L 44.75–71.60
17-Ketogenic Steroids (17-KGS)	Urine, 24 hr	*mg/d* 0–1 yr: <1.0 1–10 yr: <5 11–14 yr: <12 Thereafter, M: 5–23 F: 3–15	× 3.467	*µmol/d* <3.5 (Conversion based <17 on dehydroepi- <42 androsterone, 17–80 M.W. 288) 10–52
Ketone Bodies				
Qualitative	Serum Urine, random	Negative Negative		Negative Negative
Quantitative	Serum	0.5–3.0 mg/dL	× 10	5–30 mg/L
17-Ketosteroids (17-KS), Total *Zimmerman rection*	Urine, 24 hr	*mg/d* 14 d–2 yr: <1 2–6 yr: <2 6–10 yr: 1–4 10–12 yr: 1–6 12–14 yr: 3–10 14–16 yr: 5–12 Thereafter, M, 18–30 yr: 9–22 M, >30 yr: 8–20 F: 6–15 Decreases with age	× 3.467	*µmol/d* <3.5 (Conversion based <7 on dehydroepi- 3.5–14 androsterone, 3.5–21 M.W. 288) 10–35 17–42 31–76 28–70 21–52 Decreases with age
Chromatography	Urine, 24 hr	Adult, M: 5.0–12.0 F: 3.0–10.0	× 3.467	Adult, M: 17–42 F: 10–35
LDL-Cholesterol (LDLC)	Serum or plasma (EDTA)	*mg/dL* M F Cord blood: 10–50 10–50 0–19 yr: 60–140 60–150 20–29 yr: 60–175 60–160 30–39 yr: 80–190 70–170 40–49 yr: 90–205 80–190 *Recommended* (desirable) range for adults: 65–175 mg/dL	× 0.0259	*mmol/L* M F 0.26–1.30 0.26–1.30 1.55–3.63 1.55–3.89 1.55–4.53 1.55–4.14 2.07–4.92 1.81–4.40 2.33–5.31 2.07–4.92 1.68–4.53
Lactate	Whole blood (heparin)	*mmol/L* Venous: 0.5–2.2 Arterial: 0.5–1.6 Inpatients, Venous: 0.9–1.7 Arterial: <1.25		*mmol/L* 0.5–2.2 0.5–1.6 0.9–1.7 <1.25

Table continued on opposite page

Table 29–2. Reference Ranges (Continued)

Test	Specimen	Reference Range	Factor	Reference Range International Units
Lactate Dehydrogenase (LDH), 30 °C	Serum	*U/L*		*U/L*
Total (L→P)		Newborn: 160–450		160–450
		Infant: 100–250		100–250
		Child: 60–170		60–170
		Thereafter: 45–90		45–90
Total (P→L)				
30 °C		Adult: 150–320 U/L		150–320 U/L
37 °C		Adult: 210–420		210–420
	CSF	~10% of serum value	×0.01	~0.10 fraction of serum value
Isoenzymes	Serum		×0.01	*Fraction of total*
		Fraction 1: 15–29%		0.15–0.29
		Fraction 2: 28–45%		0.28–0.45
		Fraction 3: 16–27%		0.16–0.27
		Fraction 4: 5–15%		0.05–0.15
		Fraction 5: 3–12%		0.03–0.12
Lead	Whole blood (heparin)	*μg/dL*		*μmol/L*
		Child: <30	×0.0483	<1.45
		Adult: <40		<1.93
		Acceptable for industrial exposure: <60		<2.90
		Toxic: ≥100		≥4.83
	Urine, 24 hr	<80 μg/L	×0.00483	<0.39 μmol/L
Lecithin/Sphingomyelin (L/S) Ratio	Amniotic fluid	2.0–5.0 indicates probable fetal lung maturity (>3.0 in diabetics)		2.0–5.0 indicates probable fetal lung maturity
Lecithin Phosphorus	Amniotic fluid	>0.10 mg/dL indicates probable adequate fetal lung maturity	×0.3229	>0.33 mmol/L indicates probable adequate fetal lung maturity
Leukocyte Count (WBC Count)	Whole blood (EDTA)	*×1000 cells/mm³ (μL)*		*×10⁹ cells/L*
		Birth: 9.0–30.0	×10⁶	9.0–30.0
		24 hr: 9.4–34.0		9.4–34.0
		1 mo: 5.0–19.5		5.0–19.5
		1–3 yr: 6.0–17.5		6.0–17.5
		4–7 yr: 5.5–15.5		5.5–15.5
		8–13 yr: 4.5–13.5		4.5–13.5
		Adult: 4.5–11.0		4.5–11.0
	CSF	*cells/μL*		*×10⁶ cells/L*
		Premature: 0–25 mononuclear		0–25
		0–100 polymorphonuclear		0–100
		0–1000 RBC		0–1000
		Newborn: 0–20 mononuclear		0–20
		0–70 polymorphonuclear		0–70
		0–800 RBC		0–800
		Neonate: 0–5 mononuclear		0–5
		0–25 polymorphonuclear		0–25
		0–50 RBC		0–50
		Thereafter: 0–5 mononuclear		0–5
		(Numbers of cells in very young infants are greater than those in older individuals' CSF, without substantial implications for growth and development in most instances.)		
Leukocyte Differential Count	Whole blood (EDTA)	*%*		*Number fraction*
Myelocytes		0	×0.01	0
Neutrophils—"bands"		3–5		0.03–0.05
Neutrophils—"segs"		54–62		0.54–0.62
Lymphocytes		25–33		0.25–0.33
Monocytes		3–7		0.03–0.07
Eosinophils		1–3		0.01–0.03
Basophils		0–0.75		0–0.0075
		Cells/mm³ (μL)		*×10⁶ cells/L*
		0	×1	0
		150–400		150–400
		3000–5800		3000–5800
		1500–3000		1500–3000
		285–500		285–500
		50–250		50–250
		15–50		15–50
Leukocyte Differential Count	CSF	*%*		*Number fraction*
		Lymphocytes 62 ± 34	×0.01	0.62 ± 0.34
		Monocytes* 36 ± 20		0.36 ± 0.20
		Neutrophils 2 ± 5		0.02 ± 0.05
		Histiocytes 0–rare		0–rare
		Ependymal cells 0–rare		0–rare
		Eosinophils 0–rare		0–rare
		*Includes pia-arachnoid mesothelial cells.		

Table continued on following page

Table 29–2. **Reference Ranges** (Continued)

Text	Specimen	Reference Range	Factor	Reference Range International Units
Leukocyte Peroxidase Stain	Whole blood	+ + + in AML – in ALL ± in AMML		
Lipase *Tietz method (37 °C)* *BMD (30 °C)*	Serum	 0.1–1.0 U/mL <140 U/L	 ×280 ×1	 28–280 U/L <140 U/L
Lipoprotein Electrophoresis	Serum	Distinct beta band; negligible chylomicron and pre-beta bands		
Lithium	Serum, plasma (heparin, EDTA); at least 12 hr after last dose	Therap. conc.: 0.6–1.2 mmol/L Toxic conc.: >2		0.6–1.2 mmol/L >2
Long Acting Thyroid Stimulating Hormone (LATS)	Serum	Undetectable		Undetectable

Luteinizing Hormone (hLH) — Serum or plasma (heparin)

	mIU/mL	Factor	*IU/L*
Child:	1–6	×1	1–6
M, 10–13 yr:	4–12		4–12
12–14 yr:	6–12		6–12
12–17 yr:	6–16		6–16
15–18 yr:	7–19		7–19
F, 8–12 yr:	2–12		2–12
9–14 yr:	2–14		2–14
12–18 yr:	3–29		3–29
Adult, M:			6–23
F, Follicular phase:			5–30
Midcycle:	6–23		75–150
Luteal:	5–30		3–40
Postmenopausal:	75–150		30–200
	3–40		
	30–200		

Text	Specimen	Reference Range	Factor	Reference Range International Units
Lysergic Acid Diethylamide	Plasma (EDTA) Urine	After hallucinogenic dose: 0.005–0.009 µg/mL 0.001–0.050 µg/mL	 ×3089	After hallucinogenic dose: 15.5–27.8 nmol/L 3.1–155 nmol/L

Mean Corpuscular Hemoglobin (MCH) — Whole blood (EDTA)

	pg/cell	Factor	*fmol/cell*
Birth:	31–37	×0.0155	0.48–0.57
1–3 d (cap.):	31–37		0.48–0.57
1 wk–1 mo:	28–40		0.43–0.62
2 mo:	26–34		0.40–0.53
3–6 mo:	25–35		0.39–0.54
0.5–2 yr:	23–31		0.36–0.48
2–6 yr:	24–30		0.37–0.47
6–12 yr:	25–33		0.39–0.51
12–18 yr:	25–35		0.39–0.54
18–49 yr:	26–34		0.40–0.53

Mean Corpuscular Hemoglobin Concentration (MCHC) — Whole blood (EDTA)

	%Hb/cell or g Hb/dL RBC	Factor	*mmol Hb/L RBC*
Birth:	30–36	×0.155	4.65–5.58
1–3 d (cap.):	29–37		4.50–5.74
1–2 wk:	28–38		4.34–5.89
1–2 mo:	29–37		4.50–5.74
3 mo–2 yr:	30–36		4.65–5.58
2–18 yr:	31–37		4.81–5.74
>18 yr:	31–37		4.81–5.74

Mean Corpuscular Volume (MCV) — Whole blood (EDTA)

	µm³	Factor	*fL*
1–3 d (cap):	95–121	×1	95–121
0.5–2 yr:	70–86		70–86
6–12 yr:	77–95		77–95
12–18 yr, M:	78–98		78–98
F:	78–102		78–102
18–49 yr, M:	80–100		80–100
F:	80–100		80–100

Table continued on opposite page

Table 29–2. **Reference Ranges** (*Continued*)

Test	Specimen	Reference Range		Factor	Reference Range International Units
Metanephrine, Total	Urine, 24 hr	*µg/mg creatinine*		× 0.5735	*mmol/mol creatinine*
		<1 yr:	0.001–4.60		0.0006–2.64
		1–2 yr:	0.27–5.38		0.15–3.08
		2–5 yr:	0.35–2.99		0.20–1.71
		5–10 yr:	0.43–2.70		0.25–1.55
		10–15 yr:	0.001–1.87		0.0006–1.07
		15–18 yr:	0.001–0.67		0.0006–0.38
		Thereafter:	0.05–1.20		0.03–0.69
Methemoglobin (MetHb)	Whole blood (EDTA, heparin, or ACD)	0.06–0.24 g/dL or		× 155	9.3–37.2 µmol/L
		0.78 ± 0.37% of total Hb		× 0.01	0.0078 ± 0.0037 (mass fraction)
Microsomal Antibodies, Thyroid see *Thyroid Microsomal Antibodies*					
Myoglobin	Serum	6–85 ng/mL		× 1	6–85 pg/L
	Urine, random	Negative			Negative
Neutrophil Alkaline Phosphatase (Leukocyte Alkaline Phosphatase)	Finger-stick blood	Score: 13–130			
Niacin (Nicotinic Acid)	Urine, 24 hr	0.3–1.5 mg/d		× 8.113	2.43–12.17 µmol/d
Occult Blood	Feces, random	Negative (<2 mL blood/d in ~100–200 g stool)			Negative
	Urine, random	Negative			Negative
Osmolality	Serum	Child, Adult: 275–295 mOsmol/kg H_2O			
	Urine, random	50–1400 mOsmol/kg H_2O, depending on fluid intake. After 12 hr fluid restriction: >850 mOsmol/kg H_2O			
	Urine, 24 hr	≈300–900 mOsmol/kg H_2O			

Osmotic Fragility Test (RBC Fragility) *pH 7.4, 20 °C*	Whole blood (heparin)	*% NaCl (g/dl)*	*% Hemolysis*		*NaCl (g/L)*	*Hemolyzed fraction*
		0.30	97–100	× 10 = g/L NaCl	3.0	0.97–1.00
		0.35	90–99	× 0.01 = Hem. frac.	3.5	0.90–0.99
		0.40	50–95		4.0	0.50–0.95
		0.45	5–45		4.5	0.05–0.45
		0.50	0–6		5.0	0.00–0.06
		0.55	0		5.5	0.00
Sterile incubation at 37 °C		*% NaCl (g/dL)*	*% Hemolysis*		*NaCl (g/L)*	*Hemolyzed fraction*
		0.20	95–100	× 10 = g/L NaCl	2.0	0.95–1.00
		0.30	85–100	× 0.01 = Hem. frac.	3.0	0.85–1.00
		0.35	75–100		3.5	0.75–1.00
		0.40	65–100		4.0	0.65–1.00
		0.45	55–95		4.5	0.55–0.95
		0.50	40–85		5.0	0.40–0.85
		0.55	15–70		5.5	0.15–0.70
		0.60	0–40		6.0	0.00–0.40
		0.65	0–10		6.5	0.00–0.10
		0.70	0–5		7.0	0.00–0.05
		0.85	0		8.5	0.00

Oxygen, Partial Pressure (*p*O$_2$)	Whole blood (heparin), arterial	*mmHg*			*kPa*
		Birth:	8–24	× 0.133	1.1–3.2
		5–10 min:	33–75		4.4–10.0
		30 min:	31–85		4.1–11.3
		>1 hr:	55–80		7.3–10.6
		1 d:	54–95		7.2–12.6
		Thereafter:	83–108		11–14.4
		(Decreases with age)			
Oxygen Saturation	Whole blood (heparin), arterial				Fraction saturated:
		Newborn: 40–90%		× 0.01	0.40–0.90
		Thereafter: 95–99%			0.95–0.99
*p*O$_2$, see *Oxygen, Partial Pressure*					
*p*O$_2$ at half saturation (*p*O$_2$(0.5) or P$_{50}$)	Whole blood (heparin), arterial	25–29 mmHg		× 0.133	3.3–3.9 kPa

Table continued on following page

Table 29–2. **Reference Ranges** (Continued)

Test	Specimen	Reference Range		Factor	Reference Range International Units
Paraldehyde	Serum, plasma (heparin, EDTA)	*µg/mL*			*µmol/L*
		Therap. conc.,			
		Sedation:	10–100	× 7.567	75–750
		Anesthesia:	>200		>1500
		Toxic conc.:	20–40		150–300
		Lethal conc.:	>50		>375
Parathyroid Hormone (hPTH)	Serum	Vary with laboratory, e.g., Mayo Clinic, Bioscience:			
		N-terminal 230–630 pg/mL		× 1	230–630 ng/L
		C-terminal 410–1760 pg/mL			410–1760 ng/L
		Nichols Institute:			
		C-terminal 40–100 µLEq/mL			40–100 mLEq/L
Partial Thromboplastin Time (PTT)	Whole blood (Na citrate)				
Nonactivated		60–85 s (Platelin)			60–85 s
Activated		25–35 s (differs with method)			25–35 s
pH	Whole blood (heparin), arterial				*H⁺ concentration:*
		Premature (48 hr):	7.35–7.50		31–44 nmol/L
		Birth, full term:	7.11–7.36		43–77
		5–10 min:	7.09–7.30		50–81
		30 min:	7.21–7.38		41–61
		>1 hr:	7.26–7.49		32–54
		1 d:	7.29–7.45		35–51
		Thereafter:	7.35–7.45		35–44
		Must be corrected for body temperature			
	Urine, random	Newborn/neonate:	5–7		0.1–10 µmol/L
		Thereafter:	4.5–8		0.01–32 µmol/L
		(average ≈6)			(average ≈1.0 µmol/L)
	Stool		7.0–7.5		31–100 nmol/L
Phenacetin	Plasma (EDTA)	Therap. conc.: 1–20 µg/mL		× 5.580	5.6–110 µmol/L
		Toxic conc.: 50–250			280–1400
Phenobarbital	Serum, plasma (heparin, EDTA); collect at trough conc.	*µg/mL*			*µmol/L*
		Therap. conc.:	15–40	× 4.306	65–170
		Toxic conc., Slowness, ataxia,			
		nystagmus:	35–80		150–345
		Coma with reflexes:	65–117		280–504
		Coma without reflexes:	>100		>430
Phensuximide (both parent and N-desmethyl metabolite)	Serum, plasma (heparin, EDTA)	Therap. conc.: 40–60 µg/mL		× 5.71	228–343 µmol/L
Phenylalanine	Serum	*mg/dL*			*mmol/L*
		Premature:	2.0–7.5	× 0.06054	0.12–0.45
		Newborn:	1.2–3.4		0.07–0.21
		Thereafter:	0.8–1.8		0.05–0.11
	Urine, 24 hr	*mg/d*		× 6.054	*µmol/d*
		10 d–2 wk:	1–2		6–12
		3–12 yr:	4–18		24–110
		Thereafter:	trace–17		trace–103
Phenylpyruvic Acid, Qualitative	Urine, fresh random	Negative by FeCl₃ test			Negative by FeCl₃ test
Phenytoin	Serum, plasma (heparin, EDTA); collect at steady-state trough conc.	Therap. conc.: 10–20 µg/mL		× 3.964	40–80 µmol/L
		Toxic conc.: >20			>80
Phosphatase, Acid	Serum	<3.0 ng/mL		× 1	<3.0 µg/L
Prostatic (RIA)					
Roy, Brower, and Hayden, 37 °C		0.11–0.60 U/L			0.11–0.60 U/L
Phosphatase, Alkaline (*p*-nitrophenyl phosphate)	Serum				
SKI method; 30 °C		*U/L*			*U/L*
		Infant:	50–155		50–155
		Child:	20–150		20–150
		Adult:	20–70		20–70
Bowers and McComb, 30 °C		25–90 U/L			25–90 U/L

Table continued on opposite page

Table 29–2. **Reference Ranges** (Continued)

Text	Specimen	Reference Range	Factor	Reference Range International Units
Phospholipids, Total	Serum or plasma (EDTA)	*mg/dL* Newborn: 75–170 Infant: 100–275 Child: 180–295 Adult: 125–275	×0.01	*g/L* 0.75–1.70 1.00–2.75 1.80–2.95 1.25–2.75
Phosphorus, Inorganic	Serum	*mg/dL* Cord: 3.7–8.1 Premature (1 wk): 5.4–10.9 Newborn: 4.3–9.3 Child: 4.5–6.5 Thereafter: 3.0–4.5	×0.3229	*mmol/L* 1.2–2.6 1.7–3.5 1.4–3.0 1.45–2.1 0.97–1.45
Plasma Volume	Plasma (heparin)	M: 25–43 mL/kg F: 28–45	×0.001	M: 0.025–0.043 L/kg F: 0.028–0.045
Platelet Count (Thrombocyte Count)	Whole blood (EDTA)	$\times 10^3/mm^3$ (µL) Newborn: 84–478 (After 1 wk, same as adult) Adult: 150–400	$\times 10^6$	$\times 10^9/L$ 84–478 150–400
Porphobilinogen (PBG) *Quantitative* *Qualitative*	Urine, 24 hr Urine, fresh random	0–2.0 mg/d Negative	×4.42	0–8.8 µmol/d Negative
Potassium	Serum	*mmol/L* Newborn: 3.9–5.9 Infant: 4.1–5.3 Child: 3.4–4.7 Thereafter: 3.5–5.1		*mmol/L* 3.9–5.9 4.1–5.3 3.4–4.7 3.5–5.1
	Plasma (heparin)	3.5–4.5 mmol/L		3.5–4.5 mmol/L
	Urine, 24 hr	2.5–125 mmol/d varies with diet		2.5–125 mmol/d varies with diet
Prealbumin (PA, Tryptophan-Rich, Thyroxine-Binding, TBPA) *RID*	Serum	*mg/dL* Cord: 13 1yr: 10 Maternal: 23 Adult: 10–40	×10	*mg/L* 130 100 230 100–400
Pregnanetriol	Urine, 24 hr	*mg/d* 2 wk–2 yr: 0.02–0.2 2–5 yr: <0.5 5–15 yr: <1.5 >15 yr: <2.0	×2.972	µmol/d 0.06–0.6 <1.5 <4.5 <5.9
Primidone	Serum, plasma (heparin, EDTA); collect at trough conc.	Therap. conc.: 5–12 µg/mL Toxic conc.: >15	×4.582	23–55 µmol/L >69
Progesterone	Serum	*ng/mL* M, Pubertal stage I: 0.11–0.26 Adult: 0.12–0.3 F, Pubertal stage I: 0–0.3 II: 0–0.46 III: 0–0.6 IV: 0.05–13.0 Follicular: 0.02–0.9 Luteal: 6.0–30.0	×3.18	*nmol/L* 0.35–0.83 0.38–1 0–1 0–1.5 0–2 0.16–41 0.06–2.9 19–95
Prolactin (hPRL)	Serum	*ng/mL* Adults, M: <20 F, Follicular phase: <23 Luteal phase: 5–40 Pregnancy, 1st trimester: <80 2nd trimester: <160 3rd trimester: <400 Newborn: >10-fold adult levels	×1	*µg/L* <20 <23 5–40 <80 <160 <400 >10-fold adult levels
Propranolol	Serum, plasma (heparin, EDTA); collect at trough conc.	Therap. conc.: 50–100 ng/mL	×3.856	190–380 nmol/L
Protein *Total*	Serum	*g/dL* Premature: 4.3–7.6 Newborn: 4.6–7.4 Child: 6.2–8.0 Adult, Recumbent: 6.0–7.8 ~0.5 g higher in ambulatory patients	×10	*g/L* 43.0–76.0 46.0–74.0 62.0–80.0 60.0–78.0 ~5 g higher in ambulatory patients

Table continued on following page

1553

Table 29–2. **Reference Ranges** (Continued)

Text	Specimen	Reference Range	Factor	Reference Range International Units
Electrophoresis		*g/dL*		*g/L*
		Albumin,		
		Premature: 3.0–4.2		30–42
		Newborn: 3.6–5.4		36–54
		Infant: 4.0–5.0		40–50
		Thereafter: 3.5–5.0		35–50
		α_1-Globulin,		
		Premature: 0.1–0.5		1–5
		Newborn: 0.1–0.3		1–3
		Infant: 0.2–0.4		2–4
		Thereafter: 0.2–0.3		2–3
		α_2-Globulin,		
		Premature: 0.3–0.7		3–7
		Newborn: 0.3–0.5		3–5
		Infant: 0.5–0.8		5–8
		Thereafter: 0.4–1.0		4–10
		β-Globulin,		
		Premature: 0.3–1.2		3–12
		Newborn: 0.2–0.6		2–6
		Infant: 0.5–0.8		5–8
		Thereafter: 0.5–1.1		5–11
		γ-Globulin,		
		Premature: 0.3–1.4		3–14
		Newborn: 0.2–1.0		2–10
		Infant: 0.3–1.2		3–12
		Thereafter: 0.7–1.2		7–12
		Higher in blacks		Higher in blacks
Total	Urine, 24 hr	1–14 mg/dL		10–140 mg/L
		50–80 mg/d (at rest)		50–80 mg/d
		<250 mg/d after intense exercise		<250 mg/d after intense exercise
Electrophoresis		*Average % of Total Protein*		*Fraction of Total*
		Albumin 37.9	×0.01	0.379
		Globulin, α_1 27.3		0.273
		α_2 19.5		0.195
		β 8.8		0.088
		γ 3.3		0.033
Total	CSF			
Column		Lumbar: 8–32 mg/dL	×10	80–320 mg/L
Turbidimetry		*mg/dL*		*mg/L*
		Lumbar,		
		Premature: 40–300		400–3000
		Newborn: 45–120		450–1200
		Child: 10–20		100–200
		Adolescent: 15–20		150–200
		Thereafter: 15–45		150–450
Electrophoresis		*% of Total*		*Fraction of Total*
		Prealbumin: 2–7	×0.01	0.02–0.07
		Albumin: 56–76		0.56–0.76
		α_1-Globulin: 2–7		0.02–0.07
		α_2-Globulin: 4–12		0.04–0.12
		β-Globulin: 8–18		0.08–0.18
		γ-Globulin: 3–12		0.03–0.12
Prothrombin Time (PT)				
One-stage (Quick)	Whole blood (Na citrate)	In general: 11–15 s (varies with type of thromboplastin)		11–15 s
		Newborn: prolonged by 2–3 s		Prolonged by 2–3 s
Two-stage modified (Ware and Seegers)	Whole blood (Na citrate)	18–22 s		18–22 s
Quinidine	Serum, plasma (heparin, EDTA); collect at trough conc.	Therap. conc.: 2–5 μg/mL	×3.083	6.2–15.5 μmol/L
		Toxic conc.: >6		>18.5
RBC Count, see *Erythrocyte Count*				
RBC Fragility, see *Osmotic Fragility*				
Red Cell Volume	Whole blood (heparin)	M: 20–36 mL/kg	×0.001	M: 0.020–0.036 L/kg
		F: 19–31		F: 0.019–0.031
Renin (Renin Activity, Plasma; PRA)	Plasma (EDTA)	*ng/mL/hr*		*μg/L/hr*
		0–3 yr: <16.6	×1	<16.6
		3–6 yr: < 6.7		< 6.7
		6–9 yr: < 4.4		< 4.4
		9–12 yr: < 5.9		< 5.9
		12–15 yr: < 4.2		< 4.2
		15–18 yr: < 4.3		< 4.3

Table continued on opposite page

Table 29–2. **Reference Ranges** (Continued)

Text	Specimen	Reference Range	Factor	Reference Range International Units
Renin (Renin Activity, Plasma; PRA) (Continued)	Plasma (EDTA) (Continued)	Normal sodium diet:		
		Supine: 0.2–2.5		0.2–2.5
		Upright: 0.3–4.3		0.3–4.3
		Low sodium diet:		
		Upright 2.9–24		2.9–24
Reticulocyte Count	Whole blood (EDTA, heparin, or oxalate)	Adults: 0.5–1.5% of erythrocytes or	×0.01	0.005–0.015 (number fraction)
		25,000–75,000/mm³ (μL)	×10⁶	25,000–75,000 × 10⁶/L
	Capillary	%		Number fraction
		1 d: 0.4–6.0	×0.01	0.004–0.060
		7 d: <0.1–1.3		<0.001–0.013
		1–4 wk: <0.1–1.2		<0.001–0.012
		5–6 wk: <0.1–2.4		<0.001–0.024
		7–8 wk: 0.1–2.9		0.001–0.029
		9–10 wk: <0.1–2.6		<0.001–0.026
		11–12 wk: 0.1–1.3		0.001–0.013
Retinol-Binding Protein (RBP) *RID*	Serum, plasma	mg/dL		mg/L
		2–10 yr: 2.2–4.5	×10	22–45
		16 yr and older, M: 4.5–9.0		45–90
		F: 2.5–9.0		25–90
Reverse Triiodothyronine (rT₃)	Serum	ng/dL		nmol/L
		1–5 yr: 15–71	×0.0154	0.23–1.1
		5–10 yr: 17–79		0.26–1.2
		10–15 yr: 19–88		0.29–1.36
		Adults: 30–80		0.46–1.23
Riboflavin (Vitamin B₂)	Urine, random, fasting	μg/g creatinine		μmol/mol creatinine
		1–3 yr: 500–900	×0.3	150–270
		4–6 yr: 300–600		90–180
		7–9 yr: 270–500		81–150
		10–15 yr: 200–400		60–120
		Adult: 80–269		24–81
Salicylates	Serum, plasma (heparin, EDTA); collect at trough conc.	Therap. conc.: 15–30 mg/dL	×0.0724	1.1–2.2 mmol/L
		Toxic conc.: >30		>2.2
Sediment *Casts*	Urine, fresh random	Hyaline: occasional (0–1) casts/hpf		Hyaline: occasional (0–1) casts/hpf
		RBC: not seen		RBC: not seen
		WBC: not seen		WBC: not seen
		Tubular epithelial: not seen		Tubular epithelial: not seen
		Transitional and squamous epithelial: not seen		Transitional and squamous epithelial: not seen
Cells		RBC: 0–2/hpf		RBC: 0–2/hpf
		WBC,		WBC,
		Males: 0–3/hpf		Males: 0–3/hpf
		Females and children: 0–5/hpf		Females and children: 0–5/hpf
		Epithelial: few; more frequent in newborn		Epithelial: few; more frequent in newborn
		Bacteria, unspun: no organisms/oil immersion field		Bacteria, unspun: no organisms/oil immersion field
		spun: <20 organisms/hpf		spun: <20 organisms/hpf
Sedimentation Rate, see *Erythrocyte Sedimentation Rate*				
Sickle Cell Tests *Sodium Metabisulfite*	Whole blood (EDTA, heparin, or oxalate)	Negative		
Dithionite Test	Whole blood (EDTA, heparin, or oxalate)	Negative		
Sodium	Serum or plasma (heparin)	mmol/L		mmol/L
		Newborn: 134–146	×1	134–146
		Infant: 139–146		139–146
		Child: 138–145		138–145
		Thereafter: 136–146		136–146
	Urine, 24 hr	40–220 (diet dependent)		40–220
	Sweat	10–40		10–40
		Cystic fibrosis >70		>70

Table continued on following page

Table 29–2. **Reference Ranges** (Continued)

Text	Specimen	Reference Range	Factor	Reference Range International Units
Somatomedin C	Plasma (EDTA)	Vary with laboratory, e.g., Nichols Institute		

Nichols Institute

		U/mL		U/L
		M	F		M	F
0–2 yr:		0.10–0.72	0.10–1.7	×1000	100–720	100–1700
3–5 yr:		0.12–1.5	0.15–2.3		120–1500	150–2300
6–10 yr:		0.19–2.2	0.44–3.6		190–2200	440–3600
11–12 yr:		0.22–3.6	1.50–6.9		220–3600	150–6900
13–14 yr:		0.79–5.5	0.81–7.4		790–5500	810–7400
15–17 yr:		0.76–3.3	0.59–3.1		760–3300	590–3100
18–64 yr:		0.34–1.9	0.45–2.2		340–1900	450–2200

Endocrine Sciences

	Reference Range		International Units
Cord:	0.25–0.66		250–660
0–1 yr:	0.17–0.62		170–620
1–5 yr:	0.14–0.94		140–940
6–12 yr:	0.87–2.06		870–2060
13–17 yr:	1.35–3.00		1350–3000
18–25 yr:	0.92–2.06		920–2060
Thereafter:	0.70–2.04		700–2040

Text	Specimen	Reference Range	Factor	Reference Range International Units
Specific Gravity	Urine, random	Adult: 1.002–1.030 After 12 hr fluid restriction: >1.025		Adult: 1.002–1.030 After 12 hr fluid restriction: >1.025
	Urine, 24 hr	1.015–1.025		
Sucrose Hemolysis and Sugar-Water Tests for Paroxysmal Nocturnal Hemoglobinuria (PNH)	Whole blood (citrate or oxalate)	≤5% lysis Questionable: 6–10% lysis	×0.01	Lysed fraction: ≤0.05 0.06–0.10
T₃, see *Triiodothyronine*				
T₄, see *Thyroxine*				

Testosterone, Total — Serum

	ng/dL	Factor	nmol/L
Prepubertal,			
M:	1.6–11.6	×0.03467	0.06–0.40
F:	1.6–11.6		0.06–0.40
Adult,			
M:	302–842		10.47–29.19
F:	17–57		0.59–1.98

Theophylline — Serum, plasma (heparin, EDTA)

	µg/mL	Factor	µmol/L
Therap. conc.,			
Bronchodilator:	8–20	×5.550	44–110
Prem. apnea:	6–13		33–72
Toxic conc.:	>20		>110

Text	Specimen	Reference Range	Factor	Reference Range International Units
Thiamine (Vitamin B₁)	Serum	0–2.0 µg/dL	×37.68	0.0–75.4 nmol/L
	Urine, acidify with HCl			

	µg/g creatinine	Factor	µmol/mol
1–3 yr:	176–200	×0.426	75–85
4–6 yr:	121–400		52–170
7–9 yr:	181–350		77–149
10–12 yr:	181–300		77–128
13–15 yr:	151–250		64–107
Thereafter:	66–129		28–55

Text	Specimen	Reference Range	Factor	Reference Range International Units
Thrombin Time	Whole blood (Na citrate)	Control time ± 2 s when control is 9–13 s		Control time ± 2 s when control is 9–13 s
Thromboplastin Time, Activated, see *Activated Partial Thromboplastin Time (APTT)*				
Thyroglobulin (Tg)	Serum	<50 ng/mL	×1	<50 µg/L
Thyroid Microsomal Antibodies	Serum	Nondetectable (hemagglutination) or <1:10 (IFA)		Nondetectable (hemagglutination) or <1:10 (IFA)
Thyroid Thyroglobulin Antibodies	Serum			
Tanned RBC agglutination test		Children: ≤1:4 dilution Thereafter: ≤1:10		≤1:4 dilution ≤1:10

Thyroid Stimulating Hormone (hTSH) — Serum or plasma (heparin)

	µU/L	Factor	mU/L
Cord:	3–12	×1	3–12
Newborn:	3–18		3–18
Thereafter:	2–10		2–10

Text	Specimen	Reference Range	Factor	Reference Range International Units
Thyroid Uptake of Radioactive Iodine	Activity over thyroid gland	2 hr: <6% 6 hr: 3–20% 24 hr: 8–30%	×0.01	2 hr: <0.06 6 hr: 0.03–0.20 24 hr: 0.08–0.30

Table continued on opposite page

Table 29–2. **Reference Ranges** (Continued)

Test	Specimen	Reference Range	Factor	Reference Range International Units
Thyroid Uptake of $^{99m}TcO_4^-$	Activity over thyroid gland	After 24 hr: 0.4–3.0%	×0.01	Fractional uptake: 0.004–0.03
Thyrotropin Releasing Hormone (hTRH)	Plasma	5–60 pg/mL	×2.759	14–165 pmol/L
Thyroxine Binding Globulin (TBG)	Serum		×10	

mg/dL (Range) / mg/L (Range)

	mg/dL (Range)	mg/L (Range)
Cord:	1.4–9.4	14–94
1–4 wk:	1.0–9.0	10–90
1–12 mo:	2.0–7.6	20–76
1–5 yr:	2.9–5.4	29–54
5–10 yr:	2.5–5.0	25–50
10–15 yr:	2.1–4.6	21–46
Adult:	1.5–3.4	15–34

Test	Specimen	Reference Range	Factor	Reference Range International Units
Thyroxine, Free (FT₄)	Serum	0.8–2.4 ng/dL	×12.87	10–31 pmol/L
Thyroxine, Total (T₄)	Serum		×12.87	

	µg/dL	nmol/L
Cord:	8–13	103–168
Newborn:	11.5–24	148–310
(lower in low birth weight infants)		
Neonate:	9–18	116–232
Infant:	7–15	90–194
1–5 yr:	7.3–15	94–194
5–10 yr:	6.4–13.3	83–172
Thereafter:	5–12	65–155
Newborn screen (filter paper):	6.2–22	80–284

Test	Specimen	Reference Range	Factor	Reference Range International Units
Tourniquet Test (Capillary Fragility)		<5–10 petechiae in 2.5 cm circle on forearm (halfway between systolic and diastolic pressure for 5 min); 0–8 petechiae in 6 cm circle (50 torr for 15 min); 10–20 petechiae in 5 cm circle (80 mm Hg)		<5–10 petechiae in 2.5 cm circle on forearm (halfway between systolic and diastolic pressure for 5 min); 0–8 petechiae in 6 cm circle (50 torr for 15 min); 10–20 petechiae in 5 cm circle (80 mm Hg)
Transcortin	Serum		×10	

	mg/dL	mg/L
M:	1.5–2.0	15–20
F, Follicular:	1.7–2.0	17–20
Luteal:	1.6–2.1	16–21
Postmenopausal:	1.7–2.5	17–25
Pregnancy,		
21–28 wk:	4.7–5.4	47–54
33–40 wk:	5.5–7.0	55–70

Test	Specimen	Reference Range	Factor	Reference Range International Units
Transferrin	Serum	Newborn: 130–275 mg/dL Adult: 200–400	×0.01	1.3–2.7 g/L 2.0–4.0
Triglycerides (TG)	Serum, after ≥12 hr fast		×0.01	

	mg/dL M	mg/dL F	g/L M	g/L F
Cord blood:	10–98	10–98	0.10–0.98	0.10–0.98
0–5 yr:	30–86	32–99	0.30–0.86	0.32–0.99
6–11 yr:	31–108	35–114	0.31–1.08	0.35–1.14
12–15 yr:	36–138	41–138	0.36–1.38	0.41–1.38
16–19 yr:	40–163	40–128	0.40–1.63	0.40–1.28
20–29 yr:	44–185	40–128	0.44–1.85	0.40–1.28

Recommended (desirable) levels for adults:
Male: 40–160 mg/dL
Female: 35–135

Recommended (desirable) levels for adults:
Male: 0.40–1.60 g/L
Female: 0.35–1.35

Test	Specimen	Reference Range	Factor	Reference Range International Units
Triiodothyronine, Free	Serum		×0.01536	

	pg/dL	pmol/L
Cord:	20–240	0.3–3.7
1–3 d:	200–610	3.1–9.4
6 wk:	240–560	3.7–8.6
Adult (20–50 yr):	230–660	3.5–10.0

Test	Specimen	Reference Range	Factor	Reference Range International Units
Triiodothyronine Resin Uptake Test (T₃RU)	Serum	Newborn: 26–36% Thereafter: 26–35%	×0.01	Fractional uptake: 0.26–0.36 0.26–0.35
Triiodothyronine, Total (T₃-RIA)	Serum		×0.0154	

	ng/dL	nmol/L
Cord:	30–70	0.46–1.08
Newborn:	75–260	1.16–4.00
1–5 yr:	100–260	1.54–4.00
5–10 yr:	90–240	1.39–3.70
10–15 yr:	80–210	1.23–3.23
Thereafter:	115–190	1.77–2.93

Table continued on following page

Table 29–2. **Reference Ranges** (Continued)

Test	Specimen	Reference Range		Factor	Reference Range International Units
Tyrosine	Serum		*mg/dL*	×0.0552	*mmol/L*
		Premature:	7.0–24.0		0.39–1.32
		Newborn:	1.6–3.7		0.088–0.20
		Adult:	0.8–1.3		0.044–0.07
Urea Nitrogen	Serum or plasma		*mg/dL*	×0.357	*mmol urea/L*
		Cord:	21–40		7.5–14.3
		Premature (1 wk):	3–25		1.1–9
		Newborn:	3–12		1.1–4.3
		Infant/Child:	5–18		1.8–6.4
		Thereafter:	7–18		2.5–6.4
Uric Acid	Serum		*mg/dL*	×59.48	*μmol/L*
Phosphotungstate		Newborn:	2.0–6.2		119–369
		Adult, M:	4.5–8.2		268–488
		F:	3.0–6.5		178–387
Uricase		Child:	2.0–5.5		119–327
		Adults, M:	3.5–7.2		208–428
		F:	2.6–6.0		155–357
Urinary Sediment, see *Sediment*					
Urine Volume	Urine, 24 hr		*mL/d*	×0.001	*L/d*
		Newborn:	50–300		0.050–0.300
		Infant:	350–550		0.350–0.500
		Child:	500–1000		0.500–1.000
		Adolescent:	700–1400		0.700–1.400
		Thereafter, M:	800–1800		0.800–1.800
		F:	600–1600		0.600–1.600
		(varies with intake and other factors)			
Valproic Acid	Serum, plasma (heparin, EDTA); collect at trough conc.	Therap. conc.: 50–100 μg/mL Toxic conc.: >100		×6.934	350–700 μmol/L >700
Vanillylmandelic Acid (Vanilmandelic Acid)	Urine, 24 hr		*mg/d*	×5.046	*μmol/d*
		Newborn:	<1.0		<5.0
		Infant:	<2.0		<10.1
		Child:	1–3		5–15
		Adolescent:	1–5		5–25
		Thereafter:	2–7		10–35
		or: 1.5–7 μg/mg creatinine		×0.571	or: 0.86–4 mmol/mol creatinine
Vitamin A	Serum		*μg/dL*	×0.0349	*μmol/L*
		Newborn:	35–75		1.22–2.62
		Child:	30–80		1.05–2.79
		Thereafter:	30–65		1.05–2.27
Vitamin B$_1$, see *Thiamine*					
Vitamin B$_2$, see *Riboflavin*					
Vitamin B$_6$	Plasma (EDTA)	3.6–18 ng/mL		×4.046	14.6–72.8 nmol/L
Vitamin B$_{12}$	Serum	Newborn: 175–800 pg/ml Thereafter: 140–700		×0.738	129–590 pmol/L 103–517
Vitamin C	Plasma (oxalate, heparin, or EDTA)	0.6–2.0 mg/dL		×56.78	34–113 μmol/L
Vitamin D$_2$, 25-Hydroxy	Plasma (heparin)	Summer: 15–80 ng/mL Winter: 14–42		×2.496	37–200 nmol/L 35–105
Vitamin D$_3$, 1,25-Dihydroxy (Calcitriol)	Serum	25–45 pg/mL		×2.4	60–108 nmol/L
Vitamin E	Serum	5.0–20 μg/mL		×2.32	11.6–46.4 μmol/L
WBC, see *Leukocyte*					
Xylose Absorption Test	Whole blood (Na-fluoride) 0.5 g/kg in H$_2$O:		*mg/dL*	×0.0667	*mmol/L*
	25 g:	Child, 1 hr:	>20		>1.33
		Adult, 2 hr:	>25		>1.67
	Urine, 5 hr	Child: 16–33% of ingested dose		×0.01	Fraction ingested dose: 0.16–0.33
		Adult,	*g/5 hr*	×6.66	*mmol/5 hr*
		5 g dose:	>1.2		>8.00
		25 g dose:	>4.0		>26.64
Zinc	Serum	70–150 μg/dL		×0.153	10.7–22.9 μmol/L

MILLIOSMOLAL AND MILLIOSMOLAR SOLUTIONS

The total osmotic pressure of a solution is dependent on the number of particles in the solution, regardless of their charge, size, or shape. In principle, 1 mole of an ideal substance (assumed to be a nonelectrolyte) dissolved in a kilogram of water will lower the freezing point of the solvent (water) by 1.8557° C. Such a solution would have 1 osmol *per kilogram of water*. One milliosmol is equal to one thousandth of an osmol. The osmometer used in the clinical laboratory measures the osmolality of serum, urine, or other biologic fluids by comparing their freezing points with that of a carefully prepared sodium chloride solution of known osmotic pressure. The lowering of the freezing point is proportional to the mole fraction (gram-mole of solute *per kg of solvent*), and gives the millios*molal* concentration, which is slightly different from the millios*molar* concentration; the latter represents milliosmoles of solute *per liter of solution*. For dilute solutions these two values approach each other and are often used without distinction. Osmo*lality* is the preferred term, because that is what is measured by the osmometer.

In studying osmotic pressure relations in solutions containing electrolytes it is useful to express the osmotic activity in terms of ionic concentrations. The term "milliosmolar" supplements the term "millimolar" in appreciation of the additive osmotic effect of the particles formed by ionization.

For example: A millimolar solution of glucose (180 mg/L) is also a milliosmolar solution (1 milliosmol/L), because the number of osmotically active particles is not increased in solution through ionization. On the other hand, owing to the nearly complete ionization of sodium chloride in solution, a millimolar solution of sodium chloride (58.5 mg/L) contains 1 milliequivalent of sodium ions and 1 milliequivalent of chloride ions. The milliosmolar concentration is 2 milliosmols per liter, because 1 chemical milliequivalent of sodium or of chloride ions is equal to 1 milliosmol of sodium or of chloride ions, respectively.

A milliequivalent equals a milliosmol for all univalent ions. The chemical milliequivalence of a divalent ion is twice the milliosmolar value. In a millimolar solution of calcium chloride ($CaCl_2$), for example, there are 2 chemical milliequivalents of calcium ions, but only 1 milliosmol of calcium ions.* The millimolar solution of calcium chloride contains 2 chemical milliequivalents of chloride ions or 2 milliosmols of chloride ions per liter. Accordingly, a millimolar solution of calcium chloride contains 3 milliosmols per liter, because this salt ionizes into 1 calcium ion and 2 chloride ions. In blood serum containing 10 mg of calcium per dL (100 mL), there are 5 chemical milliequivalents of calcium* per liter, but only 2.5 milliosmols of calcium per liter.

The average normal total ionic concentration of blood serum is 290 milliosmols per *kg* H_2O, to which cations contribute 151 milliosmols and anions 139. In blood plasma the milliosmols accounted for by glucose or urea (3–6 mOsm/kg H_2O) or by protein (1.2–1.4 mOsm/kg H_2O) are small compared to the osmotic effect of the electrolytes. One milliosmol generates an osmotic pressure of about 19.3 mm Hg. The osmotic pressure of the blood serum of infants and children is comparable to that of adults.

VICTOR C. VAUGHAN III

*Calcium has an atomic weight of 40; a millimolar solution has 40 mg/L (4 mg/dL). (See also Table 29–3.)

Table 29–3 to 29–7: CONVERSION TABLES

Table 29–3. Method for Conversion of Milligrams to Milliequivalents per Liter (or to Millimoles per Liter)

mg = milligrams
g = grams
mL = milliliter
1 mL = 1.000027 cc
dL = deciliter = 100 mL

$$mEq/l \text{ (milliequivalents per liter)} = \frac{mg \text{ per liter}}{equivalent\ weight}$$

$$Equivalent\ weight = \frac{atomic\ weight}{valence\ of\ element}$$

For example: A sample of blood serum contains 10 mg of Ca in 1 dL (100 mL). The valence of Ca is 2, and the atomic weight is 40. The equivalent weight of Ca is therefore 40 ÷ 2, or 20. The milliequivalents of Ca per liter are 10 (mg/dL) × 10 (dL/L) ÷ 20, or 5 milliequivalents per liter.

$$mM/L \text{ (millimoles per liter)} = \frac{mg/liter}{molecular\ weight}$$

Vol. % (volumes per cent) = mM/liter × 2.24 for a gas whose properties approach that of an ideal gas, such as oxygen or nitrogen. For carbon dioxide the factor is 2.226.

Table 29–4. Factors for Conversion of Concentration Expressed in Milliequivalents per Liter to Milligrams per Deciliter (100 mL), and Vice Versa, for Common Ions That Occur in Physiologic Solutions

Element or Radical	mEq/L	to	mg/dL	mg/dL	to	mEq/L
Sodium	1		2.30	1		0.4348
Potassium	1		3.91	1		0.2558
Calcium	1		2.005	1		0.4988
Magnesium	1		1.215	1		0.8230
Chloride	1		3.55	1		0.2817
Bicarbonate (HCO_3)	1		6.1	1		0.1639
Phosphorus valence 1	1		3.10	1		0.3226
Phosphorus valence 1.8	1		1.72	1		0.5814
Sulfur valence 2	1		1.60	1		0.625

Example: To convert milliequivalents of magnesium per liter to milligrams per deciliter (100 mL), multiply by the factor 1.215.

To convert milligrams of potassium per deciliter (100 mL) to milliequivalents per liter, multiply by the factor 0.2558.

Table 29–5. Milliequivalents and Milligrams of Cations and Anions Present in a Millimole of Salts Commonly Used in Physiologic Solutions

Salt	mM/L	mg/L	Cation	Anion	mEq/L	mg/L	mEq/L	mg/L
Sodium chloride (NaCl)	1	58.5	Na^+	Cl^-	1	23.0	1	35.5
Potassium chloride (KCl)	1	74.6	K^+	Cl^-	1	39.1	1	35.5
Sodium bicarbonate ($NaHCO_3$)	1	84.0	Na^+	HCO_3^-	1	23.0	1	61.0
Sodium lactate ($CH_3CHOHCOONa$)	1	112.0	Na^+	Lactate$^-$	1	23.0	1	89.0
Potassium phosphate (K_2HPO_4) dibasic	1	174.2	K^+	HPO_4^{--}	2	78.2	1	96.0
Potassium phosphate (KH_2PO_4) monobasic	1	136.1	K^+	$H_2PO_4^-$	1	39.1	1	97.0
Calcium chloride anhydrous ($CaCl_2$)		111.0	Ca^{++}	Cl^-	2	40.0	2	71.0
Calcium chloride dihydrate ($CaCl_2 \cdot 2H_2O$)	1	147.0	Ca^{++}	Cl^-	2	40.0	2	71.0
Magnesium chloride anhydrous ($MgCl_2$)	1	95.2	Mg^{++}	Cl^-	2	24.3	2	71.0
Magnesium chloride hexahydrate ($MgCl_2 \cdot 6H_2O$)	1	203.3	Mg^{++}	Cl^-	2	24.3	2	71.0
Ammonium chloride (NH_4Cl)	1	53.5	NH_4^+	Cl^-	1	18.0	1	35.5

Table 29–6. Conversion of Apothecary's Measures to Metric Equivalents

1 grain = 64 mg
60 minims = 1 fl dram = 3.7 mL
1 mL = 16.23 minims

Table 29–7. Equivalent Temperature Readings (Celsius and Fahrenheit)*

C	F	C	F	C	F	C	F
0	32.0	37.2	99	39.2	102.6	41.2	106.2
20	68.0	37.4	99.3	39.4	102.9	41.4	106.5
30	86.0	37.6	99.7	39.6	103.3	41.6	106.9
31	87.8	37.8	100.1	39.8	103.7	41.8	107.2
32	89.6	38.0	100.4	40.0	104	42	107.6
33	91.4	38.2	100.8	40.2	104.4	43	109.4
34	93.2	38.4	101.2	40.4	104.7	44	111.2
35	95.0	38.6	101.5	40.6	105.1	100	212
36	96.8	38.8	101.8	40.8	105.4		
37	98.6	39.0	102.2	41.0	105.8		

*To convert Celsius (centigrade) readings to Fahrenheit, multiply by 1.8 and add 32. To convert Fahrenheit readings to Celsius, subtract 32 and divide by 1.8.

TABLES 29–8 TO 29–10: NUTRITIONAL VALUES

Table 29–8. Composition of Commonly Used Oral and Parenteral Solutions

Fluid	CHO g/dL	Prot*	Calories per L	Na mEq/L	K mEq/L	Cl mEq/L	HCO_3† mEq/L	Ca mEq/L	P‡ mEq/L	Mg mEq/L	Osm§ mOsm/kgH_2O
					Oral						
Apple juice¶	11.9	0.1	480	0.4	26			3	4.5		700
Coca-Cola¶	10.9		435	4.3	0.1		13.4				656
Gatorade	5.9		250	21	2.5	17			6.8		377
Ginger ale¶	9.0		360	3.5	0.1		3.6				565
Grape juice¶	16.6	0.2	672	0.4	30		32				1027
Grapefruit juice¶ (canned, sugar added)	17.8	0.6	736	0.2	35			6.5			591
Hydra-lyte	2.5		100	84	10	59	15	<1	<1		300
Lytren	7.0		280	30	25	25	36	4	5	4	267**
Milk	4.9	3.5	670	22	36	28	30	60	54		260**
Orange juice¶	10.4	0.7	444	0.2	49		50				654
Pedialyte	5.0		200	30	20	30	28	4		4	387
Pepsi-Cola	12.0		480	6.5	0.8		7.3				—
Pineapple juice (canned)¶	13.5	0.4	556	0.2	38			7.5	9		783
Prune juice¶	19	0.4	776	0.9	60			7	20		—
Root beer¶				3.5	3.9						588
Seven-Up¶	8.0		320	7.5	0.2			0.3			564
Tomato juice (canned, salted)¶	4.3		172	100	59	150	10	3	18		592

Table continued on opposite page

Table 29–8. Composition of Commonly Used Oral and Parenteral Solutions (Continued)

Fluid	CHO g/dL	Prot*	Calories per L	Na mEq/L	K mEq/L	Cl mEq/L	HCO₃† mEq/L	Ca mEq/L	P‡ mEq/L	Mg mEq/L	Osm§ mOsm/kgH₂O
						Parenteral					
CHO†† in H₂O	5–10		200–400								266–532
Isotonic saline	0–5		0–200	154		154					292–558
½ Isotonic saline	2.5–5		100–200	77		77					280–415
3% (M/2) saline				513		513					969
5% Saline				855		855					1616
2.14% Ammonium chloride						400					
M/6 Sodium lactate				167			167				
5% Sodium bicarbonate				595			595				
Lactated Ringer solution	0–5–10		0–200–400	130	4	109	28	3			261–531–801
Modified Butler 1 (a)	5		200	25	20	22	23		3	3	360
Modified Butler 2 (b)	5–10		200–400	56	25	49	26		12	5	423–719**
Talbot (c)	5		200	40	35	40	20		15		409
Ordway (d)	3.5		140	26	27	53					281**
Gastric replacement (e)	5–10		200–400	63	17	150	(contains 71 mEq/L NH₄⁺)				555–812**
Intestinal replacement (f)	10		390	80	36	64	60	5		3	800**
Protein hydrolysate 5% (g)		5	850	35	19	20		5	30	2	430**
Protein hydrolysate 10% (h)		10	1700	60	31	44		10	60	4	860**
Amino-acid preparation (i)		8.5		10					20		850**
Human plasma protein fraction (j)		5		110	2	50	50				
Blood††		3		95	4	50	40		2	1–2	
Dextran 10% (low mol. wt.) (k)	5		200								
Dextran 10% in saline (l)				154		154					
Dextran 6% (high mol. wt.) (m)	5–10		200–400								
Dextran 6% in saline (n)				154		154					
Mannitol 20%§§											

AVAILABLE ADDITIVES

Glucose 50%	0.5 g per mL
Sodium chloride	0.5, 1, 2.5 and 5 mEq per mL
Sodium lactate	4 and 5 mEq per mL
Sodium bicarbonate	5 (4.2%) and 9 (7.5%) mEq per mL
Potassium chloride	1, 2 and 3 mEq per mL
Potassium phosphate	3 mEq per mL
Potassium acetate	2 and 2.5 mEq per mL
Calcium gluconate 10%	9.0 mg (0.45 mEq) calcium per mL
Calcium chloride 10%	27.2 mg (1.36 mEq) calcium per mL
Ammonium chloride	4 mEq per mL
Magnesium sulfate (Mg SO₄ · 7 H₂O) 50% (also 10%, 12.5% and 25% available)	4 mEq per mL

SELECTED U.S. COMMERCIAL PREPARATIONS
(possible slight variations in composition from values in Table)

(A, Abbott; C, Cutter; M, McGaw; P, Pharmacia; T, Travenol)

(a)	Ionosol MB in D5W (A); Isolyte P with 5% Dextrose (M)
(b)	Ionosol B in D5W (A); Electrolyte #2 with 10% invert sugar (C,M); 10% Travert in Electrolyte #2 (T)
(c)	Ionosol T in D5W (A); Isolyte M (M)
(d)	Ordway solution with 3.5% Dextrose (C)
(e)	Ionosol G in D10W (A); Isolyte G with 5% Dextrose (M)
(f)	Ionosol D with 10% Invert Sugar (A); 10% Travert with Electrolyte #1 (T)
(g)	Amigen 5% (T)
(h)	Amigen 10% (T)
(i)	Free Amine 2 (M)
(j)	Plasmatein (A); Plasmanate (C)
(k)(l)	LMD 10% (A); Dextran 40 (C,M); Rheomacrodex (P); Gentran 40 (T)
(m)(n)	Dextran 75 (A); Macrodex (P); Gentran 75 in 10% Travert (T)

*Protein or amino acid equivalent.
†Actual or potential bicarbonate, such as acetate, lactate, citrate.
‡Calculated according to valence of 1.8.
§Osmolality except for values shown ** which are osmolarity (in mOsm/L).
¶Composition varies slightly depending on source.
**See § above.
††Glucose (dextrose, fructose or invert sugar).
‡‡Red cell contents not included in calculations.
§§Also available: mannitol 5%, 10%, 15%, and 20%.
(Sources: Church CF, Church HN: Food Values of Portions Commonly Used (Bowes and Church). 11th ed. Philadelphia, JB Lippincott, 1970; Kastrup EK, Boyd JR: Facts and Comparisons. 1978. St. Louis, Facts and Comparisons, Inc., 1978; Murray BN, Peterson LJ: Unpublished observations. Additional values in Wendland BE, Arbus GS: Can Med Assoc J 121:564, 1979.)

Table 29–9. Food Composition Table For Short Method of Dietary Analysis

Food and Approximate Measure	Weight g	Food Energy kcal	Protein g	Fat g	Carbohydrate g	Calcium mg	Iron mg	Vitamin A Value IU	Thiamine mg	Riboflavin mg	Niacin mg	Ascorbic Acid mg
Milk, cheese, cream; related products												
Cheese: blue, cheddar (1 cu in, 17 g), cheddar process (1 oz). Swiss (1 oz)	30	105	6	9	1	165	0.2	345	0.01	0.12	Trace	0
cottage (from skim) creamed (½ c)	115	120	16	5	3	105	0.4	190	0.04	0.28	0.1	0
Cream: half-and-half (cream and milk) (2 tbsp)	30	40	1	4	2	30	Trace	145	0.01	0.04	Trace	Trace
For light whipping add 1 pat butter												
Milk: whole (3.5% fat) (1 c)	245	160	9	9	12	285	0.1	350	0.08	0.42	0.1	2
fluid, nonfat (skim) and buttermilk (from skim)	245	90	9	Trace	13	300	Trace	—	0.10	0.44	0.2	2
milk beverage (1 c): cocoa, chocolate drink made with skim milk. For malted milk add 4 tbsp half-and-half (270 g)	245	210	8	8	26	280	0.6	300	0.09	0.43	0.3	Trace
milk desserts, custard (1 c) 248 g, ice cream (8 fl oz) 142 g		290	8	17	29	210	0.4	785	0.07	0.34	0.1	1
cornstarch pudding (248 g), ice milk (1 c) 187 g		280	9	10	40	290	0.1	390	0.08	0.41	0.3	2
White sauce, med (½ c)	130	215	5	16	12	150	0.2	610	0.06	0.22	0.3	Trace
Egg: 1 large	50	80	6	6	Trace	25	1.2	590	0.06	0.15	Trace	0
Meat, poultry, fish, shellfish, related products												
Beef, lamb, veal: lean and fat, cooked, inc. corned beef (3 oz) (all cuts)	85	245	22	16	0	10	2.9	25	0.06	0.19	4.2	0
lean only, cooked; dried beef (2 + oz) (all cuts)	65	140	20	5	0	10	2.4	10	0.05	0.16	3.4	0
Beef, relatively fat, such as steak and rib, cooked (3 oz)	85	350	18	30	0	10	2.4	60	0.05	0.14	3.5	0
Liver: beef, fried (2 oz)	55	130	15	6	3	5	5.0	30,280	0.15	2.37	9.4	15
Pork, lean and fat, cooked (3 oz) (all cuts)	85	325	20	24	0	10	2.6	0	0.62	0.20	4.2	0
lean only, cooked (2 + oz) (all cuts)	60	150	18	8	0	5	2.2	0	0.57	0.19	3.2	0
ham, light cure, lean and fat, roasted (3 oz)	85	245	18	19	0	10	2.2	0	0.40	0.16	3.1	0
Luncheon meats: bologna (2 sl), pork sausage, cooked (2 oz), frankfurter (1), bacon, broiled or fried crisp (3 sl)		185	9	16	—	5	1.3	—	0.21	0.12	1.7	0
Poultry chicken: flesh only, broiled (3 oz)	85	115	20	3	0	10	1.4	80	0.05	0.16	7.4	0
fried (2 + oz)	75	170	24	6	1	10	1.6	85	0.05	0.23	8.3	0
turkey, light and dark, roasted (3 oz)	85	160	27	5	0	—	1.5	—	0.03	0.15	6.5	0
Fish and shellfish salmon (3 oz) (canned)	85	130	17	5	0	165	0.7	60	0.03	0.16	6.8	0
fish sticks, breaded, cooked (3-4)	75	130	13	7	5	10	0.3	—	0.03	0.05	1.2	0
mackerel, halibut, cooked	85	175	19	10	0	10	0.8	515	0.08	0.15	6.8	0
bluefish, haddock, herring, perch, shad, cooked (tuna canned in oil, 20 g)	85	160	19	8	2	20	1.0	60	0.06	0.11	4.4	0
clams, canned: crab meat, canned; lobster; oyster, raw; scallop; shrimp, canned	85	75	14	1	2	65	2.5	65	0.10	0.08	1.5	0
Mature dry beans and peas, nuts, peanuts, related products												
Beans: white with pork and tomato, canned (1 c)	260	320	16	7	50	140	4.7	340	0.20	0.08	1.5	5
red (128 g). Lima (96 g), cowpeas (125 g), cooked (½ c)		125	8	—	25	35	2.5	5	0.13	0.06	0.7	—
Nuts: almonds (12), cashews (8), peanuts (1 tbsp), peanut butter (1 tbsp), pecans (12), English walnuts (2 tbsp), coconut (¼ c)	15	95	3	8	4	15	0.5	5	0.05	0.04	0.9	—
Vegetables and vegetable products												
Asparagus, cooked, cut spears (⅔ c)	115	25	3	Trace	4	25	0.7	1055	0.19	0.20	1.6	30
Beans: green (½ c) cooked 60 g; canned 120 g		15	1	Trace	3	30	0.4	340	0.04	0.06	0.3	8
Lima, immature, cooked (½ c)	80	90	6	1	16	40	2.0	225	0.14	0.08	1.0	14
Broccoli spears, cooked (⅔ c)	100	25	3	Trace	4	90	0.8	2500	0.09	0.20	0.8	90
Brussels sprouts, cooked (⅔ c)	85	30	3	Trace	5	30	1.0	450	0.07	0.12	0.7	75
Cabbage (110 g); cauliflower, cooked (80 g); and sauerkraut, canned (150 mg) (reduced ascorbic acid value by one third for kraut) (⅔ c)		20	1	Trace	4	35	0.5	80	0.05	0.05	0.3	37
Carrots, cooked (⅔ c)	95	30	1	Trace	7	30	0.6	10,145	0.05	0.05	0.5	6
Corn, 1 ear, cooked (140 g); canned (130 g) (½ c)		75	2	Trace	18	5	0.4	315	0.06	0.06	1.1	6
Leafy greens: collards (125 g), dandelions (120 g), kale (75 g), mustard (95 g), spinach (120 g), turnip (100 g cooked, 150 g canned) (⅔ c cooked and canned) (reduce ascorbic acid one half for canned)		30	3	Trace	5	175	1.8	8570	0.11	0.18	0.8	45

Table continued on opposite page

Table 29–9. **Food Composition Table for Short Method of Dietary Analysis** (*Continued*)

Food and Approximate Measure	Weight g	Food Energy kcal	Pro-tein g	Fat g	Carbo-hy-drate g	Cal-cium mg	Iron mg	Vitamin A Value IU	Thia-mine mg	Ribo-flavin mg	Niacin mg	Ascor-bic Acid mg
Peas, green (½ c)	80	60	4	1	10	20	1.4	430	0.22	0.09	1.8	16
Potatoes, baked, boiled (100 g), 10 pc. French fried (55 g) (for fried, add 1 tbsp cooking oil)	85	85	3	Trace	30	10	0.7	Trace	0.08	0.04	1.5	16
Pumpkin, canned (½ c)	115	40	1	1	9	30	0.5	7295	0.03	0.06	0.6	6
Squash, winter, canned (½ c)	100	65	2	1	16	30	0.8	4305	0.05	0.14	0.7	14
Sweet potato, canned (½ c)	110	120	2	—	27	25	0.8	8500	0.05	0.05	0.7	15
Tomato, 1 raw, ⅔ c canned, ⅔ c juice	150	35	2	Trace	7	14	0.8	1350	0.10	0.06	1.0	29
Tomato catsup (2 tbsp)	35	30	1	Trace	8	10	0.2	480	0.04	0.02	0.6	6
Other, cooked (beets, mushrooms, onions, turnips) (½ c)	95	25	1	—	5	20	0.5	15	0.02	0.10	0.7	7
Other commonly served raw, cabbage (½ c, 50 g), celery (3 sm stalks, 40 g), cucumber (¼ med, 50 g), green pepper (½, 30 g), radishes (5, 40 g)		10	Trace	Trace	2	15	0.3	100	0.03	0.03	0.2	20
carrots, raw (½ carrot)	25	10	Trace	Trace	2	10	0.2	2750	0.02	0.02	0.2	2
lettuce leaves (2 lg)	50	10	1	Trace	2	34	0.7	950	0.03	0.04	0.2	9
Fruits and fruit products												
Cantaloupe (½ med)	385	60	1	Trace	14	25	0.8	6540	0.08	0.06	1.2	63
Citrus and strawberries: orange (1), grapefruit (½), juice (½ c), strawberries (½ c), lemon (1), tangerine (1)		50	1	—	13	25	0.4	165	0.08	0.03	0.3	55
Yellow, fresh: apricots (3), peach (2 med); canned fruit and juice (½ c) or dried, cooked, unsweetened: apricot, peaches (½ c)		85	—	—	22	10	1.1	1005	0.01	0.05	1.0	5
Other, dried: dates, pitted (4), figs (2), raisins (¼ c)	40	120	1	—	31	35	1.4	20	0.04	0.04	0.5	—
Other, fresh: apple (1), banana (1), figs (3), pear (1)		80	—	—	21	15	0.5	140	0.04	0.03	0.2	6
Fruit pie: to 1 serving fruit add 1 tbsp flour, 2 tbsp sugar, 1 tbsp fat												
Grain products												
Enriched and whole grain: bread (1 sl, 23 g), biscuit (½), cooked cereals (½ c), prepared cereals (1 oz) Graham crackers (2 lg), macaroni, noodles, spaghetti (½ c, cooked), pancake (1, 27 g), roll (½), waffle (½, 38 g)		65	2	1	16	20	0.6	10	0.09	0.05	0.7	—
Unenriched: bread (1 sl, 23 g), cooked cereal (½ c), macaroni, noodles, spaghetti (½ c), popcorn (½ c), pretzel sticks, small (15), roll (½)		65	2	1	16	10	0.3	5	0.02	0.02	0.3	—
Desserts												
Cake, plain (1 pc), doughnut (1). For iced cake or doughnut add value for sugar (1 tbsp). For chocolate cake add chocolate (30 g)	45	145	2	5	24	30	0.4	65	0.02	0.05	0.2	—
Cookies, plain (1)	25	120	1	5	18	10	0.2	20	0.01	0.01	0.1	—
Pie crust, single crust (⅐ shell)	20	95	1	6	8	3	0.3	0	0.04	0.03	0.3	—
Flour, white, enriched (1 tbsp)	7	25	1	Trace	5	1	0.2	0	0.03	0.02	0.2	0
Fats and oils												
Butter, margarine (1 pat, ½ tbsp)	7	50	Trace	6	Trace	1	0	230	—	—	—	—
Fats and oils, cooking (1 tbsp). French dressing (2 tbsp)	14	125	0	14	0	0	0	0	0	0	0	0
Salad dressings, mayonnaise type (1 tbsp)	15	80	Trace	9	1	2	0.1	45	Trace	Trace	Trace	0
Sugars, sweets												
Candy, plain (½ oz), jam and jelly (1 tbsp), syrup (1 tbsp), gelatin dessert, plain (½ c), beverages, carbonated (1 c)		60	0	0	14	3	0.1	Trace	Trace	Trace	Trace	Trace
Chocolate fudge (1 oz), chocolate syrup (3 tbsp)		125	1	2	30	15	0.6	10	Trace	0.02	0.1	Trace
Molasses (1 tbsp), caramel (½ oz)		40	Trace	Trace	8	20	0.3	Trace	Trace	Trace	Trace	Trace
Sugar (1 tbsp)	12	45	0	0	12	0	Trace	0	0	0	0	0
Miscellaneous												
Chocolate, bitter (1 oz)	30	145	3	15	8	20	1.9	20	0.01	0.07	0.4	0
Sherbet (½ c)	96	130	1	1	30	15	Trace	55	0.01	0.03	Trace	2
Soups: bean, pea (green) (1 c)		150	7	4	22	50	1.6	495	0.09	0.06	1.0	4
noodle, beef, chicken (1 c)		65	4	2	7	10	0.7	50	0.03	0.04	0.9	Trace
clam chowder, minestrone, tomato, vegetable (1 c)		90	3	2	14	25	0.9	1880	0.05	0.04	1.1	3

From Wilson ED, Fisher KH, Fuqua ME: Principles of Nutrition. 2nd ed. New York, John Wiley & Sons, 1965, pp 528–33.

Table 29–10. **Nutritive Value of Baby Foods (Per Serving)**

Food	Serving g	Energy kcal	Pro-Tein g	Fat g	Carbo-hydrate g	Sodium mg	Calcium mg	Iron mg	Vitamin A Value IU	Thiamin mg	Ribo-flavin mg	Niacin mg	Ascorbic Acid mg
Cereals, precooked, dry and other products													
Barley, added nutrients	15	50	1	0	10	5	95	7	(0)	0.2	0.3	2	0
High protein, added nutrients	15	50	5	1	6	3	95	7	—	0.2	0.3	24.0	0
Mixed, added nutrients	15	40	2	0	9	4	95	7	—	0.2	0.3	22.3	0
Oatmeal, added nutrients	15	50	2	1	9	5	95	7	(0)	0.2	0.3	21.3	0
Rice, added nutrients	15	40	1	0	9	4	95	7	(0)	0.2	0.3	19.7	0
Dinners, canned: cereal, vegetable, meat mixtures (approx. 2–4% protein)													
Beef with vegetables	128	110	7	5	9	40	10	0.7	600	0.04	0.05	2	2
Chicken with vegetables	128	130	8	7	8	35	95	0.8	2200	0.03	0.05	1.5	3
Cottage cheese with pineapple	135	150	8	2	26	200	96	0.3	0	0.05	6	0.4	2
Ham with vegetables	128	110	8	4	10	30	8	0.8	400	0.15	6	1.5	3
Turkey with vegetables	128	120	8	6	9	40	50	0.9	350	0.03	6	2	4
Veal with vegetables	128	90	8	3	9	35	8	1.0	100	0.04	7	2.5	3
Fruits and fruit products with or without thickening, canned													
Applesauce	128	50	0	0	14	2	5	0.1	40	0.01	0.02	0.1	15
Applesauce and apricots	128	80	0	1	18	5.5	5.7	0.1	288	0.01	0.04	0.2	1.5
Bananas (with tapioca or cornstarch added ascorbic acid), strained	128	80	1	0	16		13	0.1	50	0.02	0.02	0.2	15
Bananas and pineapple (with tapioca or cornstarch)	128	70	0	1	16	8.0	20	0.1	45	0.01	0.01	0.1	15
Peaches	128	70	1	1	14	5	6	0.1	300	0.01	0.02	0.7	15
Pears	128	70	1	1	15	3	7	0.1	50	0.02	0.02	0.2	15
Pears and pineapple	128	80	1	1	16	2	7	0.1	45	0.03	0.02	0.2	15
Plums with tapioca, strained	128	90	1	1	19	5	5	0.1	150	0.01	0.02	0.2	1
Prunes with tapioca	135	110	1	1	25	15	7	0.3	300	0.02	0.06	0.4	7
Meats, poultry, and eggs; canned													
Beef:													
Strained	99	90	13	4	0	59	7	1	91	0.01	0.16	3.5	2
Junior	99	100	14	4	1	61	6	1.6	74	0.02	0.20	3.6	2
Chicken junior, strained	99	140	14	9	0	41	8	1	52	0.02	0.16	3.5	2
Egg yolks, strained	94	180	9	16	1	57	79	3.0	542	0.12	0.22	Trace	2
Ham junior	99	120	15	6	1	43	6	1	32	0.01	0.16	2.8	2
Lamb:													
Strained	99	100	14	4	1	51	4	1	99	0.02	0.17	3.3	1
Junior	99	100	15	4	1	54	5	1.6	19	0.01	0.16	3.0	1
Liver, strained	99	90	14.1	3	2	53	4	5.6	25,000	0.05	2.00	7.6	19
Veal:													
Strained	99	0	13	4	1	55	4	1	61	0.03	0.20	4.3	3
Junior	99	100	15	4	0	55	5	1	28	0.01	0.15	4	2
Vegetables, canned													
Beans, green	128	40	2	0	7	1	40	0.7	400	0.02	0.06	0.3	6
Beets, strained	128	40	1	0	10	90	13	0.3	20	0.02	0.03	0.1	3
Carrots	128	40	1	0	8	50	25	0.5	17,000	0.02	0.03	0.4	10
Mixed vegetables, including vegetable soup	128	60	2	1	10	15	14	0.9	7000	0.05	0.04	0.6	3
Peas, strained	128	60	4	1	10	5	14	1.2	600	0.08	0.09	1.2	10
Spinach, creamed	128	70	4	2	9	65	130	1.5	7000	0.02	0.13	0.3	6
Squash	128	40	1	0	8	3	24	0.4	2000	0.02	0.04	0.3	11
Sweet potatoes	135	80	1	0	19	25	16	0.4	6500	0.04	0.03	0.4	11

From various manufacturers.

INDEX

Note: Page numbers in *italics* refer to illustrations. Page numbers followed by t refer to tables. Pages xxv to xxviii are in color plate section.

Bonding (*Continued*)
  in mental retardation, 104
  optimal timing of, 10
  parent-infant, 364–365
  with premature infant, 10, 379
Bone, benign tumors in, 1107–1108
  eosinophilic granuloma of, 1486, *1486*
  fibrous cortical defect of, 1108
  formation of, 150
  neoplasms of, 1100–1103
Bone age, determination of, 30–31
Bone infection, arthritis in, 536
  atypical mycobacterial, 639
Bone marrow, aplasia of, 1057
  aspiration of, 1033
  biopsy of, 1033
  differential cell counts in, 1033t
  hypertrophy of, in hemolytic anemia, 1044
  red, 1033
  replacement of, pancytopenia due to, 1059
  suppression of, chemotherapeutic, correction of, 1084
  yellow, 1033
Bone marrow transplantation, 1083–1084
  autologous, 1084
  chemotherapy vs, 1084
  graft-vs-host disease in, 1084
  HLA-matched siblings in, 1084
  in combined immunodeficiency, 465
  liver disease in, 840
  oropharyngeal candidosis prophylaxis in, 765
  psychological considerations in, 75
Bone scan, 239
Bone survey, roentgenographic, in physical abuse, 81
Bone trauma, 1358, *1358*
  in physical abuse, 81
  rare bone disease resembling, 81
Bordetella pertussis infection, 596–598. See also *Pertussis.*
Bornholm disease, 692–694
Bottle feeding. See *Formula feeding.*
Bottle propping, 128
Botulism, 622–623, 1492
  clinical manifestations of, 622
  diagnosis and differential diagnosis of, 622
  epidemiology of, 622
  etiology of, 622
  food-borne, 622–623
  infant, 622–623
  pathogenesis of, 622
  prevention of, 622
  prognosis in, 623
  treatment of, 622–623
  wound, 622–623
Bourneville disease, 1309, *1309*
Bowleg, 1350, *1351*
Bowman capsule, anatomy of, 1111
Boxing, accident prevention and, 156
Brachial cleft cysts, 1388
Brachial palsy, in birth trauma, 388, *388*
Brachydactyly, 1355
Bradyarrhythmia, 1008–1009, *1008–1009*
Bradycardia, fetal, 368
  sinus, 1004
    in premature infant, 361
Bradycardia-tachycardia syndrome, 1009
Bradykinin, in hypersensitivity reactions, 485
Brain, computed tomography of, 1283
  degenerative disease of, 1311–1319
  developmental changes in, 1301, *1302*
  growth of, in second year of life, 14

Brain (*Continued*)
  magnetic resonance imaging of, 1283
  progressive degenerative disease of, 103
  tentorial herniation of, 1283, *1284*
Brain abscess, *1322*, 1322–1323
  anaerobic, 623–624
  cerebrospinal fluid findings in, 548t
  in otitis media, 883
  in tetralogy of Fallot, 966
Brain death, 1284
Brain injury, prenatal factors in, 55
  psychiatric problems in, 55
Brain scan, radionuclide, 1283
Brain stem, developmental defects in, 1306–1307
  glioma of, 1320
  in sudden infant death syndrome, 1481
Brain stem auditory evoked potentials (BAEP), 1282
Brain tumors, 1319–1322
  cerebral hemisphere, 1321–1322
  clinical manifestations of, 1319
  incidence of, 1319
  infratentorial, 1320
  intracranial pressure in, 1319
  supratentorial, 1320–1321
Branched chain amino acid defects, hypoglycemia in, 1268
Brazelton Neonatal Behavioral Assessment Scale, 9
  in learning disability prediction, 94–95
Breast, asymmetry of, 450
  carcinoma of, 1107
  cysts of, 450–451
  disorders of, in adolescence, 450–451
  examination of, in adolescence, 453
  infection of, in newborn, 415
  mass of, 450
  newborn, maternal hormonal effects on, 8, 362
  nipple discharge from, 451
  pubertal development of, 21
  sex maturity ratings of, 20t, *21*
Breast feeding, 124–128
  advantages of, 124–125
  beriberi in, 145
  breast emptying time in, 127
  breast hygiene in, 126
  burping after, 127
  cessation of, stopping milk production in, 128
  contraindications to, 125
    acute maternal infection, 125
    hemolytic disease of newborn, 125
    maternal, 125
    menstruation and pregnancy, 125
    premature or low birth weight infant, 125
  diet in, 126
  drug therapy and, 126, 364t, 365
  fibroadenoma of, 1107
  galactogenic substances in, 126
  gastrointestinal flora in, 125
  hospital practices and, 364–365
  hypocalcemic tetany due to, 209
  immune advantages of, 458
  in developing world, 165
  in maternal hepatitis B infection, 685
  insufficient milk in, 127
  jaundice and, 407
  manual expression of milk in, 127–128
  maternal nutritional requirements in, 114t
  milk supply for, 125–126, 127
  newborn reflexes and, 127
  nipple care in, 126
  one or both breasts in, 127

Breast feeding (*Continued*)
  parenteral vitamin K for infant in, 125
  PCB contaminated fish consumption and, 126
  pollution effects on, 1511
  position for, 126
  preparation of mother for, 125
  psychologic advantages of, 125, 126
  schedule for, 126
  stool in, 8, 12, 136
  supplemental feeding in, 126, 128
  supplemental iron in, 125
  technique of, 126–128
  vitamin C and, 148
  vs formula feeding, 128
  weaning from, 128
Breath, first, 393
Breath-holding, 1297
  in early childhood, 63
Breath hydrogen analysis, 801
Breathing. See also *Respiration.*
  disruption of, in language disorders, 99
  fetal, 6
  in newborn, 361, 393
  periodic, 393, 861
  primary failure of, 391, 942
  work of, 859
Breech deformation sequence, 275, *275*
Breech presentation, in dysmorphology, 274
Broca aphasia, 1274–1275
Bronchial challenge testing, in allergy, 487–488
  inhalational, 497
Bronchiectasis, 920
  clinical manifestations in, 920
  congenital, 920
  etiology of, 920
  in cystic fibrosis, 927
  middle lobe syndrome in, 920
  pathology in, 920
  therapy in, 921
Bronchiectatic cysts, in cystic fibrosis, 927
Bronchiolectasia, in cystic fibrosis, 927
Bronchioles, postnatal development of, 854
Bronchiolitis, acute, 897–898
  asthma vs, 498, 897
  clinical manifestations of, 897
  course and prognosis in, 897–898
  differential diagnosis of, 897
  etiology and epidemiology of, 897
  pathophysiology of, 897
  ribavirin in, 898
  treatment in, 898
  in cystic fibrosis, 927
  respiratory syncytial viral, 680–682
    apnea in, 681
    clinical manifestations of, 681
    diagnosis of, 681
    epidemiology of, 680
    immunologic injury in, 680–681
    pathology and pathogenesis of, 680–681
    prevention of, 681–682
    prognosis in, 681
    treatment of, 681
Bronchiolitis obliterans, 895, 898
Bronchitis, acute, 895
  air pollution and, 895–896
  arachidic, 892
  asthmatic, 895
  chronic, 895–896
  cigarette smoking and, 895–896
  vegetal, 892
Bronchobiliary fistula, 887
Bronchodilator therapy, in cystic fibrosis, 932–933

Complement (*Continued*)
immune complexes and, 474
in host defense, 472
in hypersensitivity reactions, 485
in rheumatic disease, 514
nomenclature for, 470
secondary deficiencies of, 474–475
total hemolytic activity of, assay for, 475
Complement receptor 1 deficiency, 474
Compliance, in drug therapy, 237
parental, 53
Computed tomography, 240
in pulmonary diagnosis, 861
of brain, 1283
ultrasonography vs, 239t
Concrescence, of teeth, 756
Concussion, 1325
dental, 764
Condom, 445
Conduct disorder, attention deficit disorder and, 64
in early childhood, 63–64
Condylomata acuminata, 1172t, 1435
in adolescence, 447–448
Condylomata lata, syphilitic, 645
Confidence limits, statistical, 162
Confounding bias, 162
Congenital heart disease, 962–1002. See also individual types.
Congenital malformations, 268–269
association of, 268
clinical evaluation in, 268–269
etiology of, 268
in low birthweight and premature infants, 378
major, 268
minor, 268, 268t
morphogenic complex or anomalad as, 268
normal variations vs, 268, 268t
parental reactions to, 386
syndromes of, 268
teratogens in, 268
underlying mechanisms in, 268
Congenital stigmata, in mental retardation, 103, 105t
Congestive heart failure, 1018–1022
after open heart surgery, 1002
afterload reducing agents in, 1021–1022
arterial blood gases and electrolytes in, 1020
captopril in, 1022
chest roentgenogram in, 1020
chlorothiazide in, 1021
clinical manifestations of, 1019
diet in, 1021
digitalis in, 1020–1021
intravenous, 1020–1021
maintenance therapy in, 1021
serum level measurement of, 1021
toxicity in, 1021
diuretics in, 1021
dobutamine in, 1022
dopamine in, 1022
drugs and dosages in, 1020t
echocardiography in, 1020
electrocardiography in, 1020
feeding problems in, 1019
Frank-Starling curve in, 1019, *1019*
furosemide in, 1021
general therapy measures in, 1020
high output failure in, 1019
hydralazine in, 1022
in children, 1019
in infants, 1019
in tetralogy of Fallot, 966
isoproterenol in, 1022

Congestive heart failure (*Continued*)
laboratory data in, 1020
liver disease in, 839
nitroprusside in, 1022
parenteral fluid therapy in, 193
pathophysiology of, 1019, *1019*
prazosin in, 1022
sodium intake in, 1021
treatment of, 1020–1022
Congo-Crimean hemorrhagic fever, 707–710
Conjunctiva, disorders of, 1459–1460
foreign body in, 1472
in vitamin A deficiency, 143
nevus of, 1460
Conjunctivitis, 1459–1460
acute hemorrhagic, enteroviral, 694
adenoviral, 682
allergic, 511
chlamydial, 652–653
clinical manifestations of, 652
diagnosis and differential diagnosis of, 652–653
follicular, adenoviral, 682
treatment of, 653
herpesvirus infection and, 664
in newborn, 429–430
vernal, 511
Connective tissue disorders, eye in, 1477t–1478t
inflammatory, 513–543
Conradi disease, 1365
Conradi-Hunermann disease, 1365
Consanguineous matings, 244
Conscience, cognitive development of, 41–42
formation of, 35, 41–42
Kohlberg's theory of, 41–42
psychoanalytic theory of, 41
socialization in, 41
Consensual light reflex, 1278
Constipation, causes of, 768
gastroenterologic disorders causing, 770t
in first year, 136
in newborn, 403
non–digestive tract causes of, 769t
treatment of, 136
Constitutional growth delay, 1180–1181
Consumption coagulopathy, 1073–1074
Contact dermatitis, 1404–1405
allergic, 1405
in external otitis, 879
irritant, 1405
Continuing education, for physicians, 4–5
Continuous ambulatory peritoneal dialysis, 1146, 1146t
Continuous negative chest pressure, in hyaline membrane disease, 396
Continuous positive airway pressure, in drowning, 222
in hyaline membrane disease, 396
Contraception, barrier, 445
combination, 445
hormonal, 445–446, 1029
in adolescence, 47, 157, 445–446
intrauterine device, 446
postcoital, 446
spermicidal, 445
Contractures, of fingers, in heroin abuse, 439
Contusion, athletic, 213
Conversion reactions, 55–56, 59
neurologic evaluation in, 1281
Conversion tables, 1559t–1560t
Convoluted tubule, in sodium excretion, 177, *177*

Convulsion, 1285–1295. See also *Epilepsy; Seizure.*
febrile, 1287–1288
Cooley anemia, *1052*, 1052–1053
Coombs test, in hemolytic anemia, 1055
Copper, deficiency or excess of, 118t
dietary sources of, 118t¯
function and metabolism of, 118t
Coprine intoxication, 1493
Coproporphyria, hereditary, 351, 356
Copying skills, delay in, 85
Corectopia, 1452
Cornea, abnormalities of, 1460–1461
abrasion of, 1472
foreign body in, 1472
growth and development of, 1447
in herpesvirus infection, 664
in newborn, 361
in systemic disease, 1461
in vitamin A deficiency, 143
lacerations and perforations of, 1472
ulcer of, 1461
Corneal dystrophy, macular, protein defect in, 348
Cornelia de Lange syndrome, 276
Coronary arteries, anomalous origin of, *999*, 999–1000
calcinosis of, myocarditis in, 1016
fistula of, 990
Coronavirus, 869–870
Corpus callosum, agenesis of, 1301
Corpuscular volume, mean, 1043t
Cortical hyperostosis, infantile, 1374
Cortical nephron, in sodium regulation, 177
Corticosteroids, adrenal production of, 1214
atrophy of subcutaneous tissue due to, 1421–1422
dietary changes with, 122
guidelines for systemic use of, 492
in allergic rhinitis, 495
in allergy, 491–492
in asthma, 501
in shock, 219
in ulcerative colitis, 796
myopathy due to, 1338
topical, 1445
Corticotropin (ACTH), 1177
deficiency of, 1215–1216
Corticotropin-releasing factor, 1177, 1215
Cortisol, 1214
normal and defective synthesis of, *1218*
Cortisone, 1214
Corynebacterium diphtheriae infection, 593–596. See also *Diphtheria.*
Cosmetics, allergens in, 1406
Costochondral junction, in rickets, *150*, 152
rickets vs scurvy and, 152
Costochondritis, arthritis in, 536
Costs of health care, 4
Cot death, 1480–1482. See also *Sudden infant death syndrome.*
Cough, chronic, etiologic significance of, 923t
laboratory tests in, 923
differential diagnosis of, 923t
in airway obstruction, 855
in cystic fibrosis, 927
in particle clearance, 856
physical examination in evaluation of, 923
recurrent or persistent, 922–923, 923t
sputum examination in evaluation of, 923
Cough syncope, 942

Dyshidrosis, 1406–1407, *1407*
Dyshidrotic eczema, 1406–1407, *1407*
Dyskeratosis, 1389
Dyskeratosis congenita, 1058
Dyskinetic cilia syndrome, 896
Dyslexia, 1275, 1451
  developmental, as low-severity handicap, 84
Dysmenorrhea, in adolescence, 450
Dysmetria, ocular motor, 1456
Dysmorphology, 273–276
  multifactorial inheritance in, 274
  multiple malformation syndromes in, 274, 275–276
    associations in, 276
    intrauterine infection in, 276
    single mutant genes in, 276
    teratogens in, 276
  single primary defects in, 273, 274–275
    deformations as, 274
    disruptions as, 274–275
    malformations as, 274
    sequences as, 275, *275*
Dysnomia, 91
Dysorthographia, 91
Dysosteosclerosis, 1372
Dysostosis multiplex, 323
Dysphagia, due to neuromuscular disease, 773, 773t
  gastroenterologic disorders causing, 770t
  transfer, 767
Dysplasia epiphysealis hemimelica, 1369
Dysplastic nevus syndrome, melanoma in, 1107
Dyspraxia, fine motor, 89
Dysthymic disorder, 60
Dystonia, 1276
Dystonia musculorum deformans, 1318–1319

Eagle-Barrett syndrome, 1157, *1157*
Ear, 877–884
  cauliflower, 883
  congenital malformations of, 878
  cyst or fistulous tract of, 878
  examination of, 877–878
  external, flora of, 878
  foreign bodies in, 883
  frostbite of, 883
  hematoma of, 883
  inflammatory disease of, 878–883. See also *Otitis media.*
  inner, infection of, 883
  lop, 878
  middle, abnormal pressure in, 878
    aspiration of, 878
    eosinophilic granuloma of, 884
    in newborn, 7
    perilymphatic fistula of, 878, 883
    rhabdomyosarcoma of, 884
    static compliance measure of muscles of, 97
  of newborn, 361
  signs and symptoms of disease of, 877
  skin tags of, 878
  swimmer's, 878–879
  traumatic injury of, 883–884
  tumors of, 884
Early Language Milestone Scale, 99
Early school years, growth and development in, 17
  physical development in, 17
  psychosocial development in, 17
Eating habits, poor, 140–141

Eating problems, mother and, 122
Ebola hemorrhagic fever, 708–710
Ebstein disease, 976
Ecchymoses, 1070
  in forceps delivery, 386
  subcutaneous, in newborn, 414
Eccrine sweat glands, 1385–1386
Echinococcosis, 751–752
Echinococcus granulosus, 751–752
Echinococcus multilocularis, 752
Echocardiography, 240, 951–953
  contrast, 953, *954*
  Doppler, 952–953, *954*
  in cardiovascular performance measurement, 952t
  normal, 952, *952*
  two-dimensional, 952
Echovirus infection, asymptomatic, 692
  clinical manifestations of, 693t
  gastrointestinal manifestations of, 694
  in aseptic meningitis, 695
  in encephalitis, 695
  in myositis and arthritis, 694–695
  in newborn infant, 695–696
  in pericarditis and myocarditis, 694
  nonspecific febrile, 692
  pathology in, 690
  respiratory manifestations of, 692–694
Echovirus 9 infection, 695
Ecthyma, 1428
Ecthyma gangrenosum, in *Pseudomonas* infection, 609
Ectodermal dysplasia, 1389–1390, *1390*
  anhidrotic, 1389–1390, *1390*
  hidrotic, 1390
  hypohidrotic, 1389–1390, *1390*
  Rapp-Hodgkin, 1390
  Robinson-type, 1390
  teeth in, 757
Ectomorph, 29
Ectopia cordis, 980–981
Ectopia lentis, 1462
  in homocystinemia, 286
Ectropion, 1457
Eczema, 1404–1407
  atopic, 501–504. See also *Dermatitis, atopic.*
  dyshidrotic, 1406–1407, *1407*
  nummular, 1406, *1406*
Eczema herpeticum, *663*, 663–664
Eczematoid dermatitis, in external otitis, 879
Edema, angioneurotic, fluid distribution in, 175
  cerebral, in intracranial hemorrhage, 388
    in Reye syndrome, 841–842
    pharmacologic prevention of, 560
  generalized, in newborn, 360
  in nephrotic syndrome, 1130, 1131
  in septic shock, 218
  localized, in newborn, 360
  neonatal, 416–417
  pulmonary, 918–919
    in burns, 226
    in drowning, 222
    in heroin abuse, 440
EEC syndrome, 1390
Education, continuing, for physicians, 4–5
  for handicapped children, 109
  in hearing loss, 97–98
  in mental retardation, 104
  sex, materials for, 69
Effectance, as intrinsic motivation, 42
Effeminacy, in boys, 72
Eggs, in child's diet, 135
Ego ideal, 41

Ehlers-Danlos syndrome, collagen metabolism in, 268, 349
  cutaneous manifestations of, 1419
  hydroxylysine-deficient collagen in, 305
Eighth nerve deafness, syphilitic, 645
Eisenmenger syndrome, 978, *978*
Ejaculation, in early puberty, 22
Ejection clicks, 945
Elastase, function of, 818
Elastolysis, generalized, 1418–1419, *1419*
Elastosis perforans serpiginosa, 1420
Elbow, Little League, 1359
  nursemaid's, 1356
  osteochondrosis of, 1356
  pulled, 1356
Electrocardiography, 947–950
  after open heart surgery, 1002
  in adult, 948, *949*
  in newborn infant, 947–948, *948*
  in older child, 948, *948*
  in potassium depletion or increase, 180, 1142
  in ventricular hypertrophy, 948, *949*
  P wave in, 948–949, *949*
  Q-T interval in, 950, *950–951*
  S-T segment and T wave in, 950, *951*
Electroencephalography, 1282
  in epilepsy, 1288–1289, *1289*
Electrolytes. See *Fluid and electrolytes;* individual types.
Electromyography, 1282–1283
Elliptocytes, *1046*
Elliptocytosis, hereditary, 1045–1047, *1046*
Ellis–van Creveld syndrome, 1363–1364
Emancipated minor, 452
Embden-Meyerhof pathway, 1264, *1265*
Embolism, 1027
  pulmonary, 919, 1027
    vascular collapse in, 217
Embryo, hematopoietic system in, 1033
  hemoglobin of, 1034
  physical development of, 6
Embryonic period, 6
  mortality in, 7
Embryonic testicular regression syndrome, 1242
Emergencies, delivery room, 391–392
Emergency services, patient needs vs wants in, 74
  patterns of use of, 74
Emesis, in poisoning, 1496
Emotional abuse, 80
  hypopituitarism vs, 1181
  in failure to thrive, 210
Emotional disorder(s), 58–63
  depression as, 59–61
  neuroses as, 58–59
  suicidal behavior in, 61–63
Emotional factors, in growth and development, 6
Emotional state, of mother, fetal and newborn activity and, 7
Emotional support, of cancer patients and families, 1084–1085
Emphysema, 916–918
  alpha₁-antitrypsin deficiency and, 918
  bullous, 917
  interstitial, 917
  lobar, congenital obstructive, 916, *916*
  obstructive, *892*, 892–893
  pulmonary interstitial, in newborn, 400–401, *401*
  subcutaneous, 917–918
Empty-sella syndrome, hypopituitarism in, 1178
Empyema, 937–938
  clinical manifestations in, 937

SolidWorks 2015
Part I - Basic Tools

Introductory Level Tutorials
Parts, Assemblies and Drawings

Written by: Sr. Certified SolidWorks Instructor
Paul Tran, CSWE, CSWI

SDC Publications
P.O. Box 1334
Mission, KS 66222
913-262-2664
www.SDCpublications.com
Publisher: Stephen Schroff

ISBN-13: 978-1-58503-943-2
ISBN-10: 1-58503-943-8

Printed and bound in the United States of America.

Acknowledgments

Thanks as always to my wife Vivian and my daughter Vylan for always being there and providing support and honest feedback on all the chapters in the textbook.

I would like to give a special thanks to Karla Werner and Rachel Schroff for their editing and corrections. Additionally thanks to Kevin Douglas, Dave Worcester and Peter Douglas for writing the forewords.

I also have to thank SDC Publications and the staff for its continuing encouragement and support for this edition of **SolidWorks 2015 Part I – Basic Tools**. Thanks also to Zach Werner for putting together such a beautiful cover design.

Finally, I would like to thank you, our readers, for your continued support. It is with your consistent feedback that we were able to create the lessons and exercises in this book with more detailed and useful information.

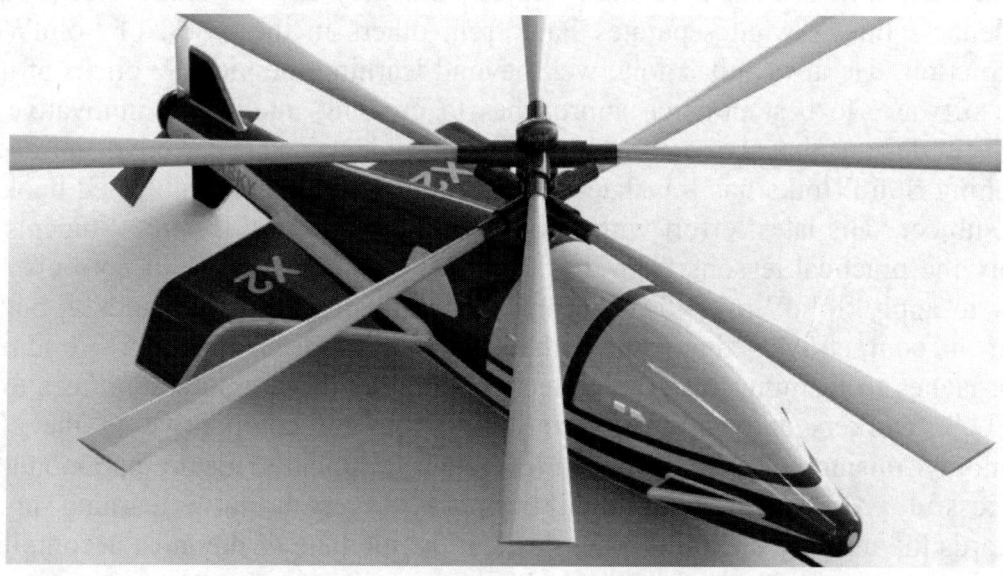

Foreword

For more than two decades, I have been fortunate to have worked in the fast-paced, highly dynamic world of mechanical product development providing computer-aided design and manufacturing solutions to thousands of designers, engineers and manufacturing experts in the western US. The organization where I began this career was US CAD in Orange County CA, one of the most successful SolidWorks Resellers in the world. My first several years were spent in the sales organization prior to moving into middle management and ultimately President of the firm. In the mid 1990's is when I met Paul Tran, a young, enthusiastic Instructor who had just joined our team.

Paul began teaching SolidWorks to engineers and designers of medical devices, automotive and aerospace products, high tech electronics, consumer goods, complex machinery and more. After a few months of watching him teach and interacting with students during and after class, it was becoming pretty clear – Paul not only loved to teach, but his students were the most excited with their learning experience than I could ever recall from previous years in the business. As the years began to pass and thousands of students had cycled through Paul's courses, what was eye opening was Paul's continued passion to educate as if it were his first class and students in every class, without exception, loved the course.

Great teachers not only love their subject, but they love to share that joy with students – this is what separates Paul from others in the world of SolidWorks Instruction. He always has gone well beyond learning the picks & clicks of using the software, to best practice approaches to creating intelligent, innovative and efficient designs that are easily grasped by his students. This effective approach to teaching SolidWorks has translated directly into Paul's many published books on the subject. His latest effort with SolidWorks 2015 is no different. Students that apply the practical lessons from basics to advanced concepts will not only learn how to apply SolidWorks to real world design challenges more quickly, but will gain a competitive edge over others that have followed more traditional approaches to learning this type of technology. As the pressure continues to rise on U.S. workers and their organizations to remain competitive in the global economy, raising not only education levels but technical skills are paramount to a successful professional career and business. Investing in a learning process towards the mastery of SolidWorks through the tutelage of the most accomplished and decorated educator and author in Paul Tran will provide a crucial competitive edge in this dynamic market space.

Kevin Douglas
Vice President Sales/Board of Advisors, GoEngineer

Foreword

I first met Paul Tran when I was busy creating another challenge in my life. I needed to take a vision from one man's mind, understand what the vision looked like, how it was going to work and comprehend the scale of his idea. My challenge was I was missing one very important ingredient, a tool that would create a picture with all the moving parts.

Research led me to discover a great tool, SolidWorks. It claimed to allow one to make 3D components, in picture quality, on a computer, add in all moving parts, assemble it and make it run, all before money was spent on bending steel and buying parts that may not fit together. I needed to design and build a product with thousands of parts, make them all fit and work in harmony with tight tolerances. The possible cost implications of failed experimentation were daunting.

To my good fortune, one company's marketing strategy of selling a product without an instruction manual and requiring one to attend an instructional class to get it, led me to meet a communicator who made it all seem so simple.

Paul Tran has worked with and taught SolidWorks as his profession for 30 years. Paul knows the SolidWorks product and manipulates it like a fine musical instrument. I watched Paul explain the unexplainable to baffled students with great skill and clarity. He taught me how to navigate the intricacies of the product so that I could use it as a communication tool with skilled engineers. *He teaches the teachers*.

I hired Paul as a design engineering consultant to create the thousands of parts for my company's product. Paul Tran's knowledge and teaching skill has added immeasurable value to my company. When I read through the pages of these manuals, I now have an "instant replay" of his communication skill with the clarity of having him looking over my shoulder - *continuously*. We can now design, prove and build our product and know it will always work and not fail. Most important of all, Paul Tran helped me turn a blind man's vision into reality and a monument to his dream.

Thanks Paul.

These books will make dreams come true and help visionaries change the world.

Peter J. Douglas

CEO, Cake Energy, LLC

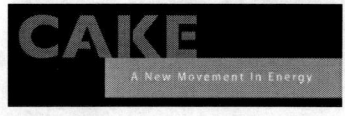

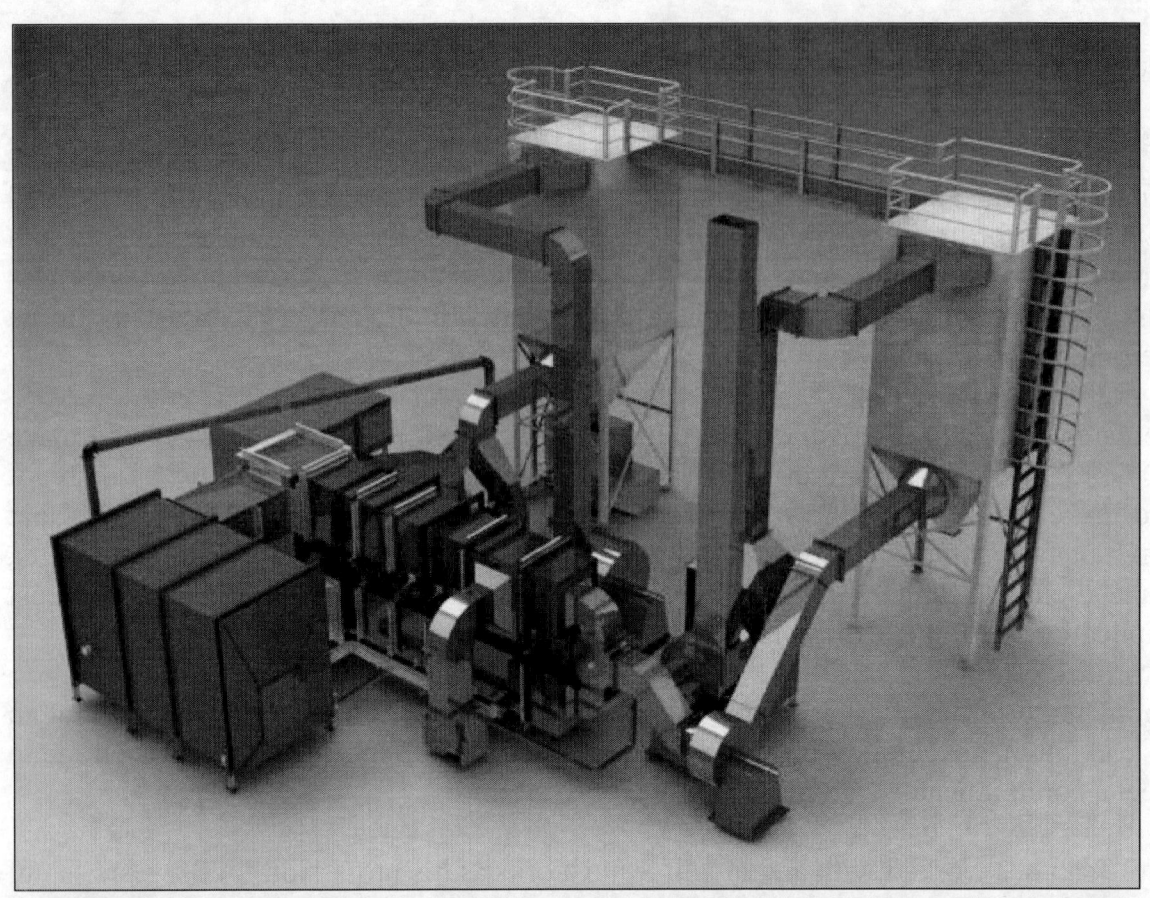

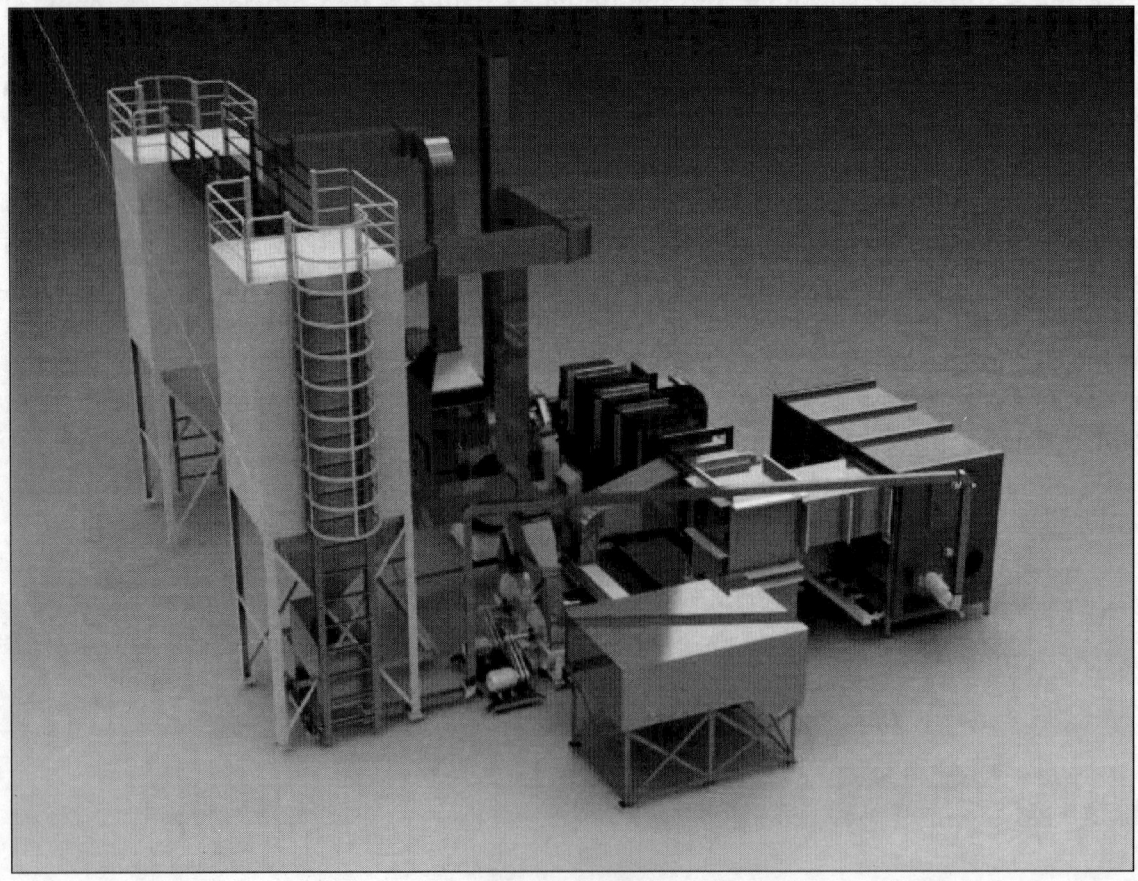

Images courtesy of C.A.K.E. Energy Corp., designed by Paul Tran

Preface

The modern world of engineering design and analysis requires an intense knowledge of Computer Aided Design (CAD) tools. To gain this deep understanding of unique CAD requirements one must commit the time, energy, and use of study guides. Paul Tran has invested countless hours and the wealth of his career to provide a path of easy to understand and follow instructional books. Each chapter is designed to build on the next and supplies users with the building blocks required to easily navigate SolidWorks 2015. I challenge you to find a finer educational tool whether you are new to this industry or a seasoned SolidWorks veteran.

I have been a part of the CAD industry for over twenty five years and read my share of instructional manuals. I can tell you Paul Tran's SolidWorks books do what most promise; however what others don't deliver. This book surpasses any CAD instructional tool I have used during my career. Paul's education and vast experience provides a finely tuned combination, producing instructional material that supports industry standards and most importantly, industry requirements.

Anyone interested in gaining the basics of SolidWorks to an in-depth approach should continue to engage the following chapters. All users at every level of SolidWorks knowledge will gain tremendous benefit from within these pages.

Dave Worcester
System Administer
Advanced Sterilization Products - A Johnson & Johnson Company

Author's Note

SolidWorks 2015 Basic Tools and Advanced Techniques are comprised of lessons and exercises based on the author's extensive knowledge on this software. Paul has 30 years of experience in the fields of mechanical and manufacturing engineering; 19 years were in teaching and supporting the SolidWorks software and its add-ins. As an active Sr. SolidWorks instructor and design engineer, Paul has worked and consulted with hundreds of reputable companies including; IBM, Intel, NASA, US- Navy, Boeing, Disneyland, Medtronic, Guidant, Terumo, Kingston and many more. Today, he has trained nearly 8,000 engineering professionals, and given guidance to nearly ½ of the number of Certified SolidWorks Professionals and Certified SolidWorks Expert (CSWP & CSWE) in the state of California.

Every lesson and exercise in this book was created based on real world projects. Each of these projects have been broken down and developed into easy and comprehendible steps for the reader. Learn the fundamentals of SolidWorks at your own pace, as you progress form simple to more complex design challenges. Furthermore, at the end of every chapter, there are self test questionnaires to ensure that the reader has gained sufficient knowledge from each section before moving on to more advanced lessons.

Paul believes that the most effective way to learn the "world's most sophisticated software" is to learn it inside and out, create everything from the beginning, and take it step by step. This is what the **SolidWorks 2015 Basic Tools & Advanced Techniques** manuals are all about.

About the Training Files

The files for this textbook are available for download on the publisher's website at **www.SDCpublications.com/downloads/978-1-58503-943-2**. They are organized by the chapter numbers and the file names that are normally mentioned at the beginning of each chapter or exercise. In the Built Parts folder you will also find copies of the parts, assemblies and drawings that were created for cross references or reviewing purposes.

It would be best to make a copy of the content to your local hard drive and work from these documents; you can always go back to the original training files location at anytime in the future, if needed.

Who this book is for

This book is for the mid-level user, who is already familiar with the SolidWorks program. It is also a great resource for the more CAD literate individuals who want to expand their knowledge of the different features that SolidWorks 2015 has to offer.

The organization of the book

The chapters in this book are organized in the logical order in which you would learn the SolidWorks 2015 program. Each chapter will guide you through some different tasks, from navigating through the user interface, to exploring the toolbars, from some simple 3D modeling and move on to more complex tasks that are common to all SolidWorks releases. There is also a self-test questionnaire at the end of each chapter to ensure that you have gained sufficient knowledge before moving on to the next chapter.

The conventions in this book

This book uses the following conventions to describe the actions you perform when using the keyboard and mouse to work in SolidWorks 2015:

Click: means to press and release the mouse button. A click of a mouse button is used to select a command or an item on the screen.

Double Click: means to quickly press and release the left mouse button twice. A double mouse click is used to open a program, or show the dimensions of a feature.

Right Click: means to press and release the right mouse button. A right mouse click is used to display a list of commands, a list of shortcuts that is related to the selected item.

Click and Drag: means to position the mouse cursor over an item on the screen and then press and hold down the left mouse button; still holding down the left button, move the mouse to the new destination and release the mouse button. Drag and drop makes it easy to move things around within a SolidWorks document.

Bolded words: indicated the action items that you need to perform.

Italic words: Side notes and tips that give you additional information, or to explain special conditions that may occur during the course of the task.

Numbered Steps: indicates that you should follow these steps in order to successfully perform the task.

Icons: indicates the buttons or commands that you need to press.

SolidWorks 2015

SolidWorks 2015 is program suite, or a collection of engineering programs that can help you design better products faster. SolidWorks 2015 contains different combinations of programs; some of the programs used in this book may not be available in your suites.

Start and exit SolidWorks

SolidWorks allows you to start its program in several ways. You can either double click on its shortcut icon on the desktop, or go to the Start menu and select the following: All Programs / SolidWorks 2015 / SolidWorks, or drag a SolidWorks document and drop it on the SolidWorks shortcut icon.

Before exiting SolidWorks, be sure to save any open documents, and then click File / Exit; you can also click the X button on the top right of your screen to exit the program.

Using the Toolbars

You can use toolbars to select commands in SolidWorks rather than using the drop down menus. Using the toolbars is normally faster. The toolbars come with commonly used commands in SolidWorks, but they can be customized to help you work more efficiently.

To access the toolbars, either right click in an empty spot on the top right of your screen or select View / Toolbars.

To customize the toolbars, select Tools / Customize. When the dialog pops up, click on the Commands tab, select a Category, and then drag an icon out of the dialog box and drop it on a toolbar that you want to customize. To remove an icon from a toolbar, drag an icon out of the toolbar and drop it into the dialog box.

Using the task pane

The task pane is normally kept on the right side of your screen. It display various options like SolidWorks resources, Design library, File explorer, Search, View palette, Appearances and Scenes, Custom properties, Built-in libraries, Technical alerts and news, etc,.

The task pane provides quick access to any of the mentioned items by offering the drag and drop function to all of its contents. You can see a large preview of a SolidWorks document before opening it. New documents can be saved in the task pane at anytime, and existing documents can also be edited and re-saved. The task pane can be resized, close or move to different location on your screen if needed.

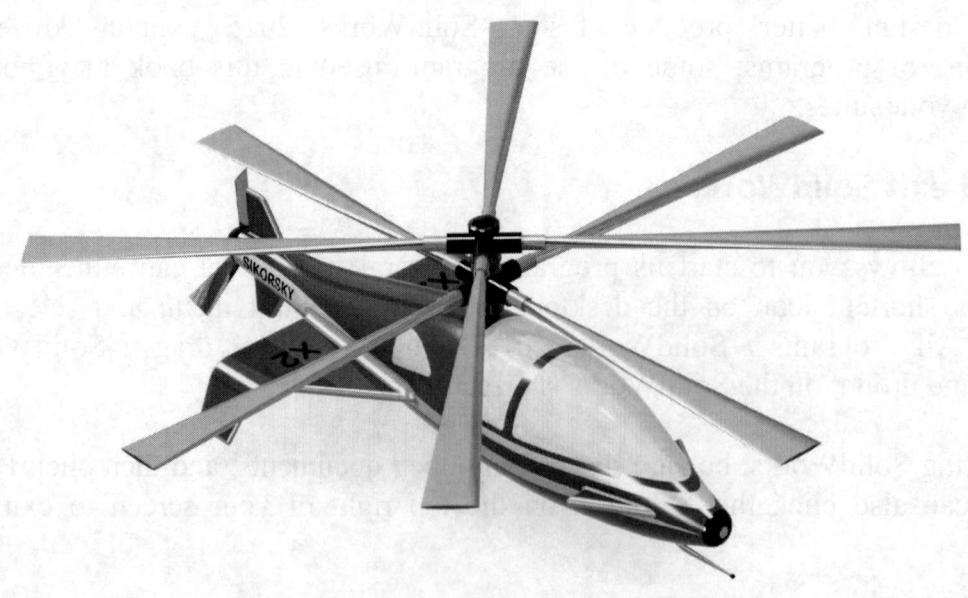

Table of Contents

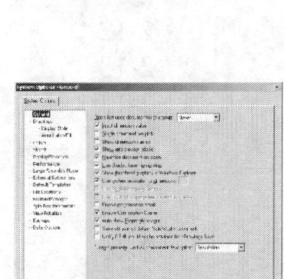

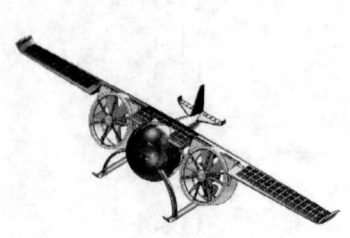

Drawing Topics

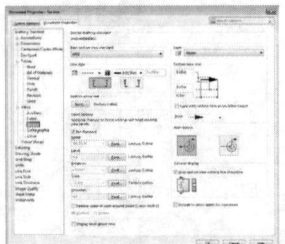

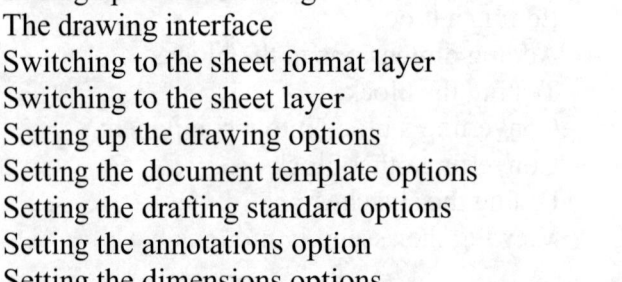

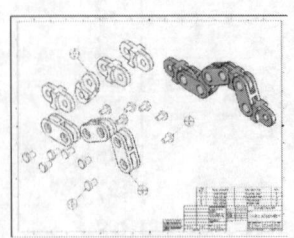

Glossary

Index

SolidWorks 2015 Quick-Guides:

Quick Reference Guide to SolidWorks 2015 Command Icons and Toolbars.

Introduction

SolidWorks User Interface

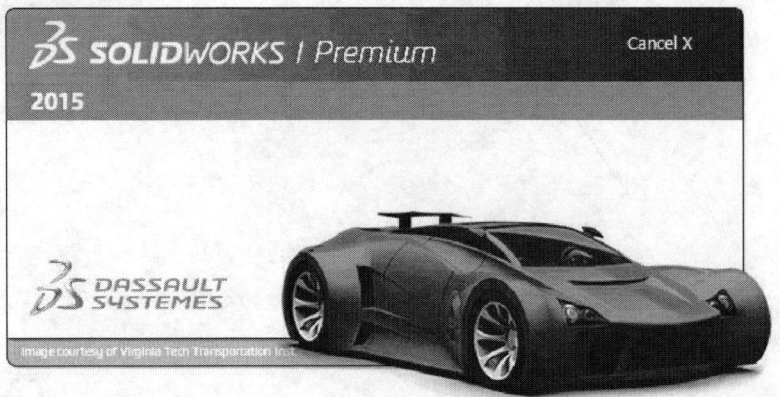

The SolidWorks 2015 User Interface

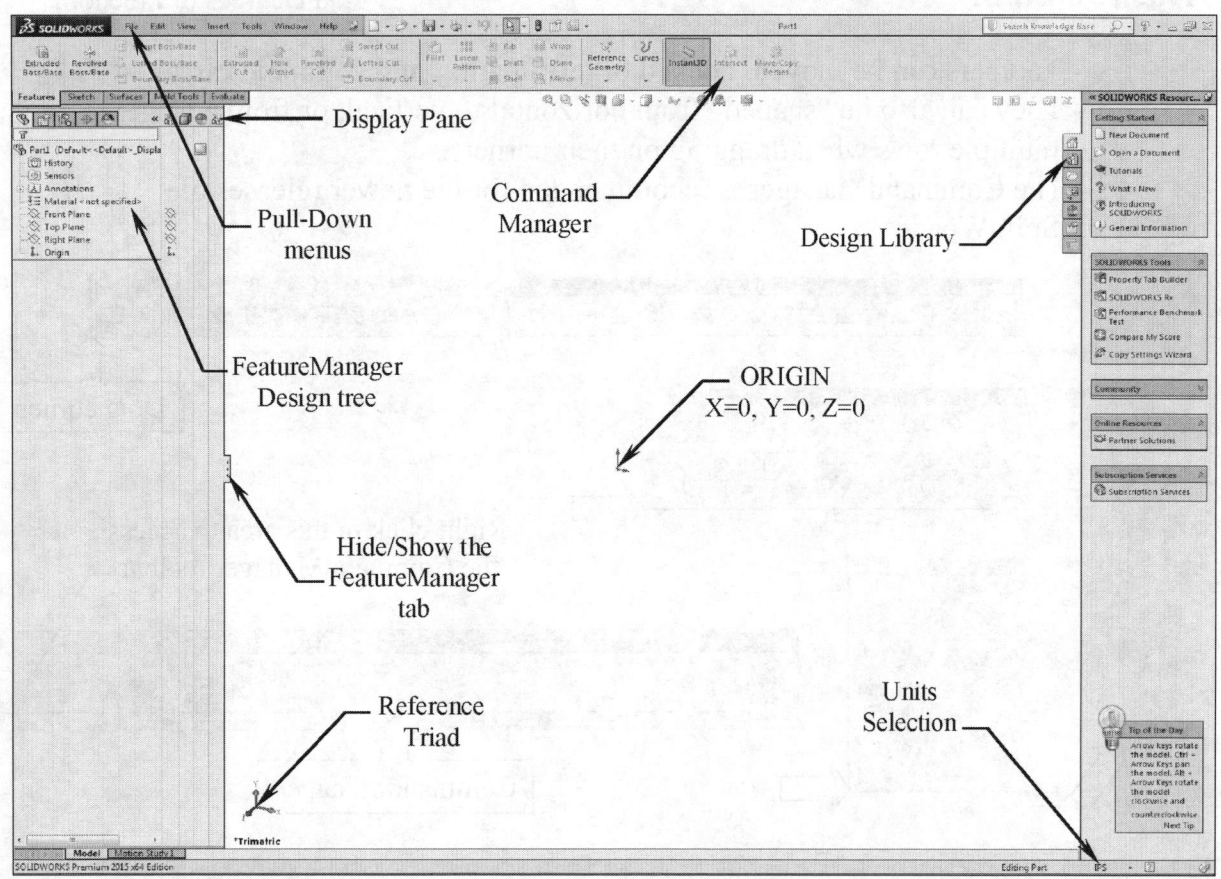

Display Pane

Command Manager

Design Library

Pull-Down menus

FeatureManager Design tree

ORIGIN
X=0, Y=0, Z=0

Hide/Show the FeatureManager tab

Reference Triad

Units Selection

The 3 reference planes:

- The Front, Top and the Right plane are 90° apart. They share the same center point called the Origin.

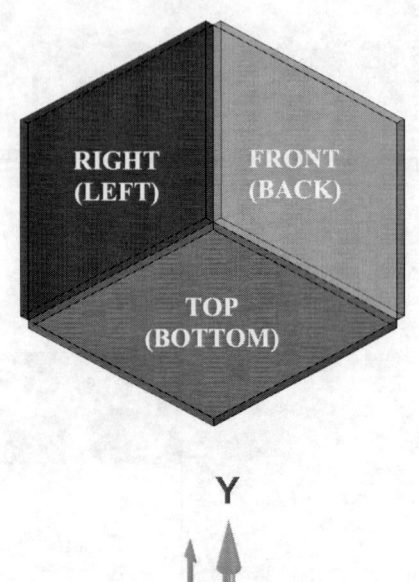

RIGHT (LEFT) FRONT (BACK)

TOP (BOTTOM)

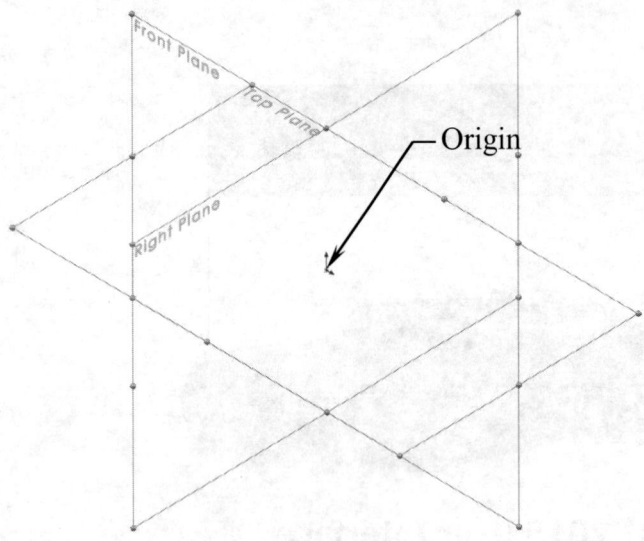

Front Plane

Top Plane

Right Plane

— Origin

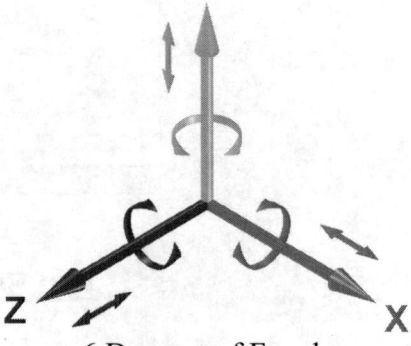

Y

Z   X

6 Degrees of Freedom

The Toolbars:

- Toolbars can be moved, docked or left floating in the graphics area.
- They can also be "shaped" from horizontal to vertical, or from a single to multiple rows when dragging on their corners.
- The CommandManager is recommended for the newer releases of SolidWorks.

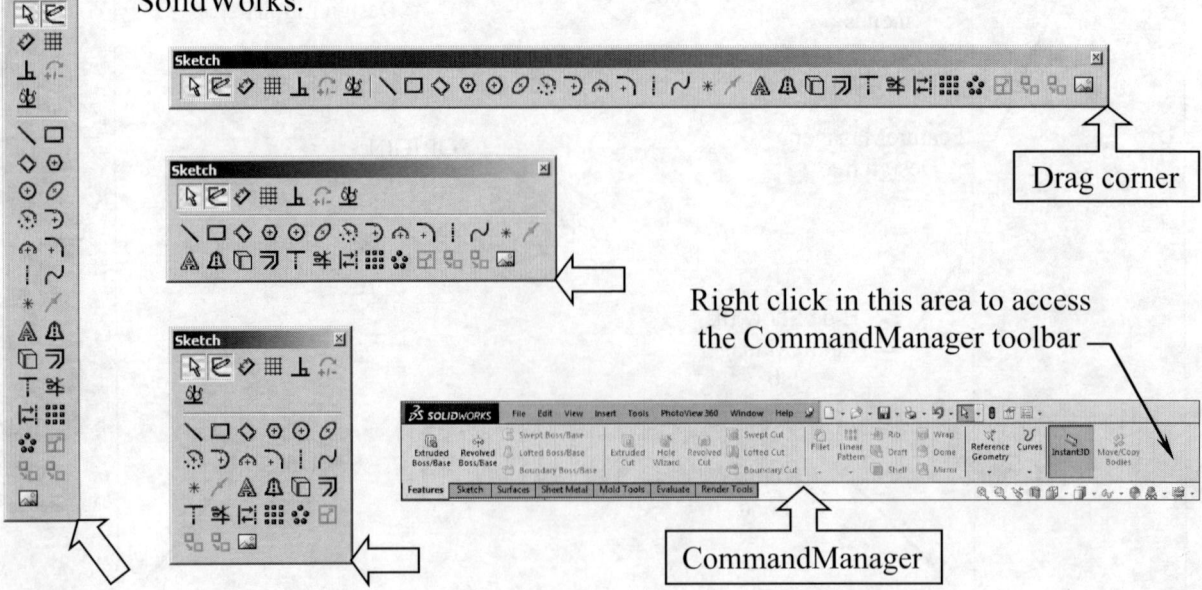

Drag corner

Right click in this area to access the CommandManager toolbar

CommandManager

- If the CommandManager is not used, toolbars can be docked or left floating.

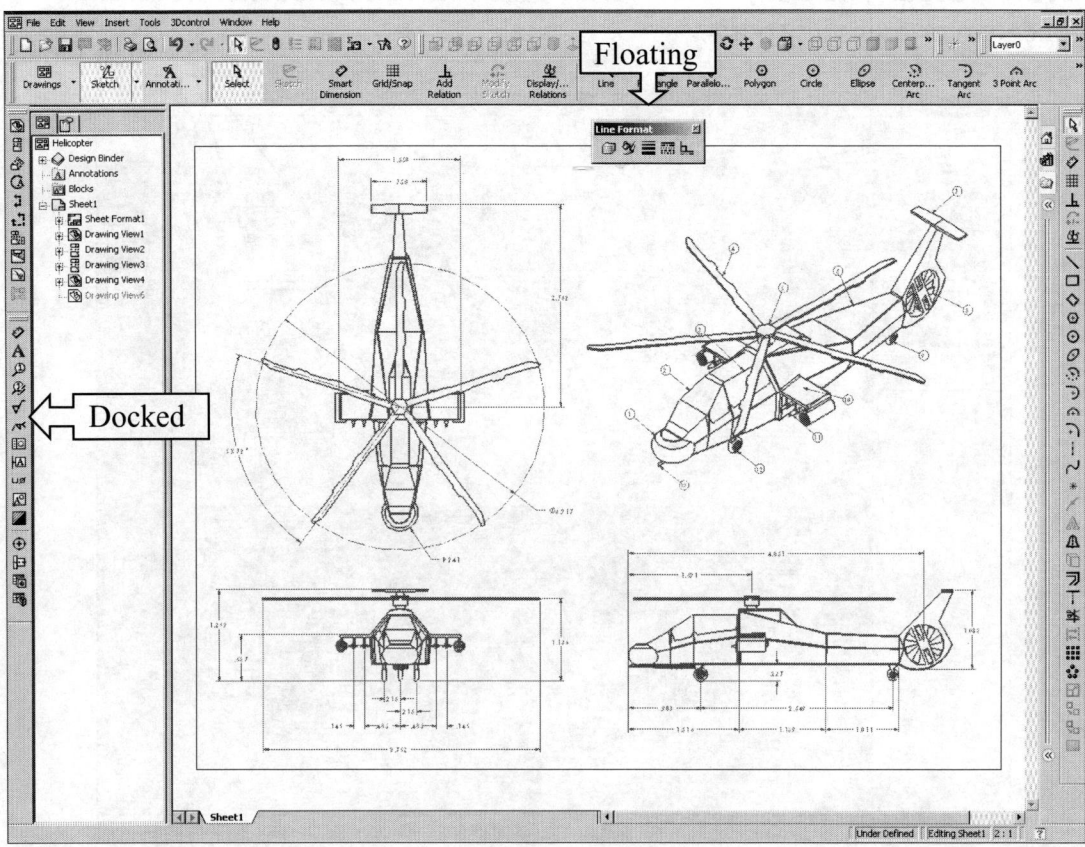

- Toolbars can be toggled off or on by activating or de-activating their check boxes:

- Select **Tools / Customize / Toolbars** tab.

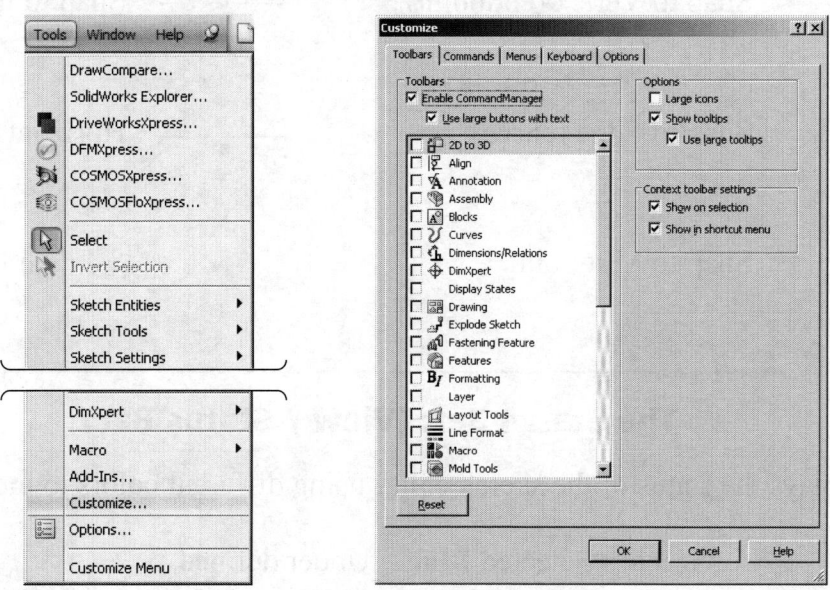

- The icons in the toolbars can be enlarged when its check box is selected

The View ports: You can view or work with SolidWorks model or an assembly using one, two or four view ports.

View Orientation

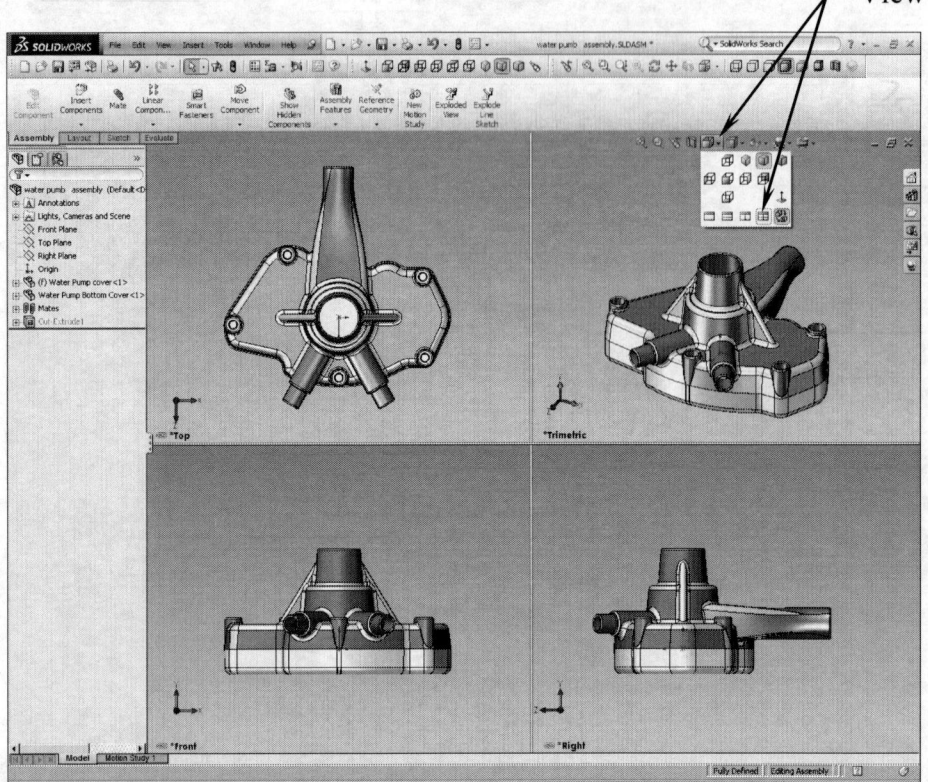

- Some of the **System Feedback symbols** (Inference pointers):

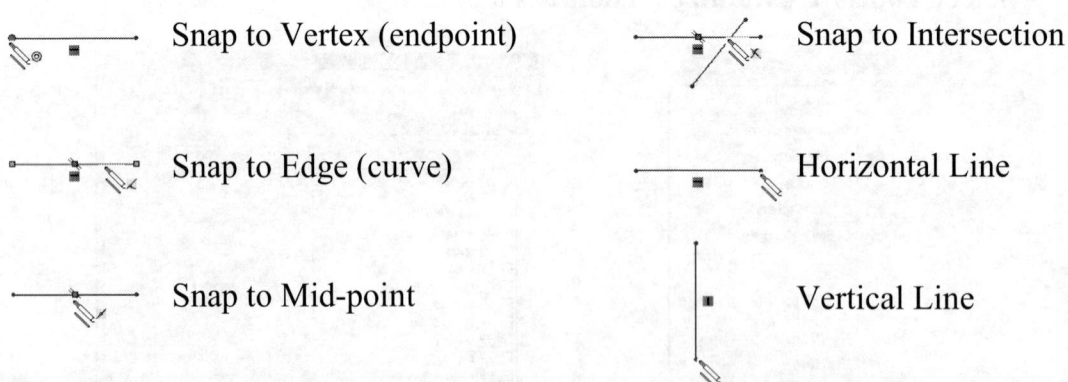

Snap to Vertex (endpoint)   Snap to Intersection

Snap to Edge (curve)   Horizontal Line

Snap to Mid-point   Vertical Line

The Status Bar: (View / Status Bar)

Displays the status of the sketch entity using different colors to indicate:

Green = Selected **Blue** = Under defined

Black = Fully defined **Red** = Over defined

2D Sketch examples:

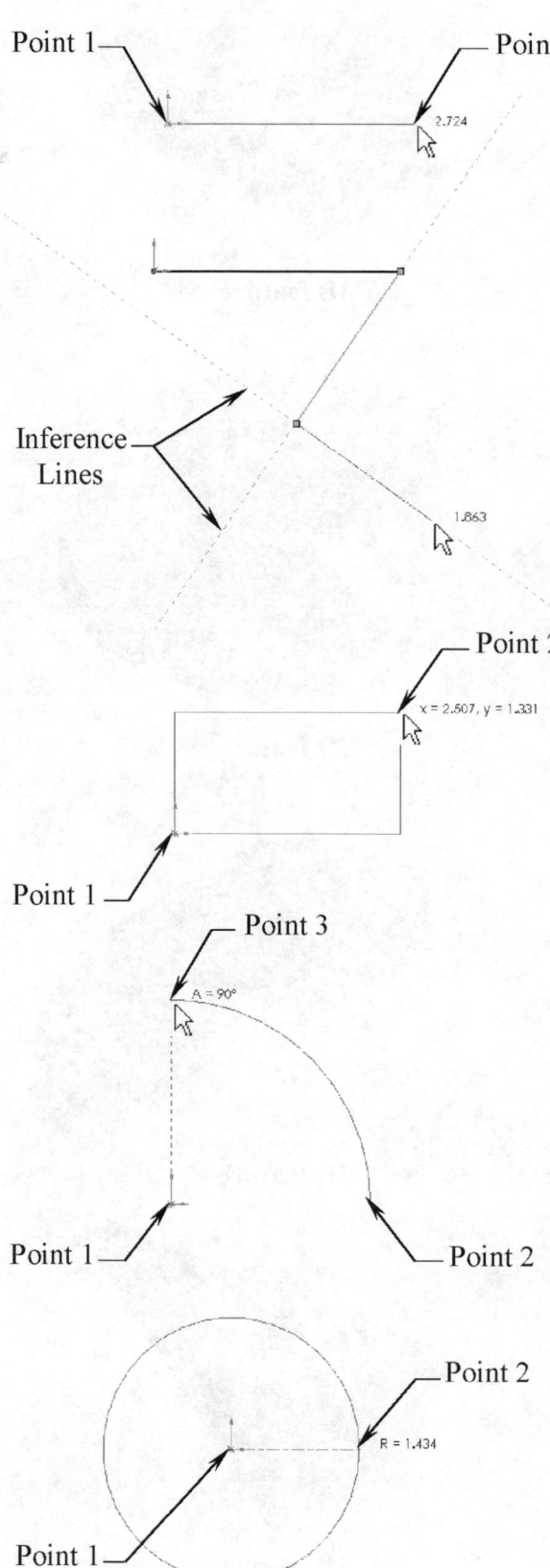

Click-Drag-Release: Single entity.

(Click Point 1, hold the mouse button, drag to point 2 and release).

Click-Release: Continuous multiple entities.

(The Inference Lines appear when the sketch entities are Parallel, Perpendicular or Tangent with each other).

Click-Drag-Release: Single Rectangle

(Click point 1, hold the mouse button, drag to Point 2 and release).

Click-Drag-Release: Single Centerpoint Arc

(Click point 1, hold the mouse button and drag to Point 2, release; then drag to Point 3 and release).

Click-Drag-Release: Single Circle

(Click point 1 [center of circle], hold the mouse button, drag to Point 2 [Radius] and release).

3D Feature examples:

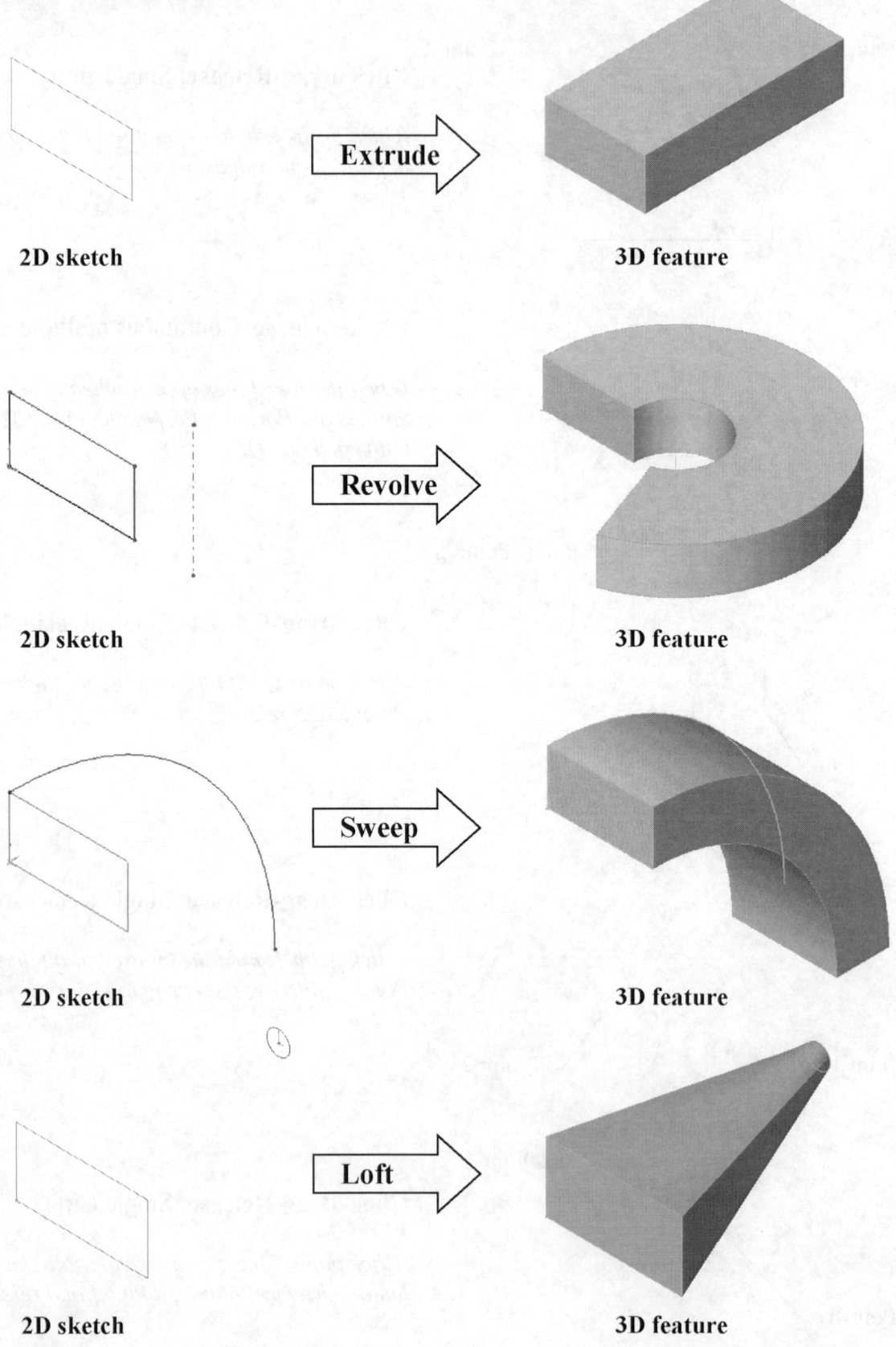

2D sketch   **Extrude**   3D feature

2D sketch   **Revolve**   3D feature

2D sketch   **Sweep**   3D feature

2D sketch   **Loft**   3D feature

Box-Select: Use the Select Pointer [cursor] to drag a selection box around items.

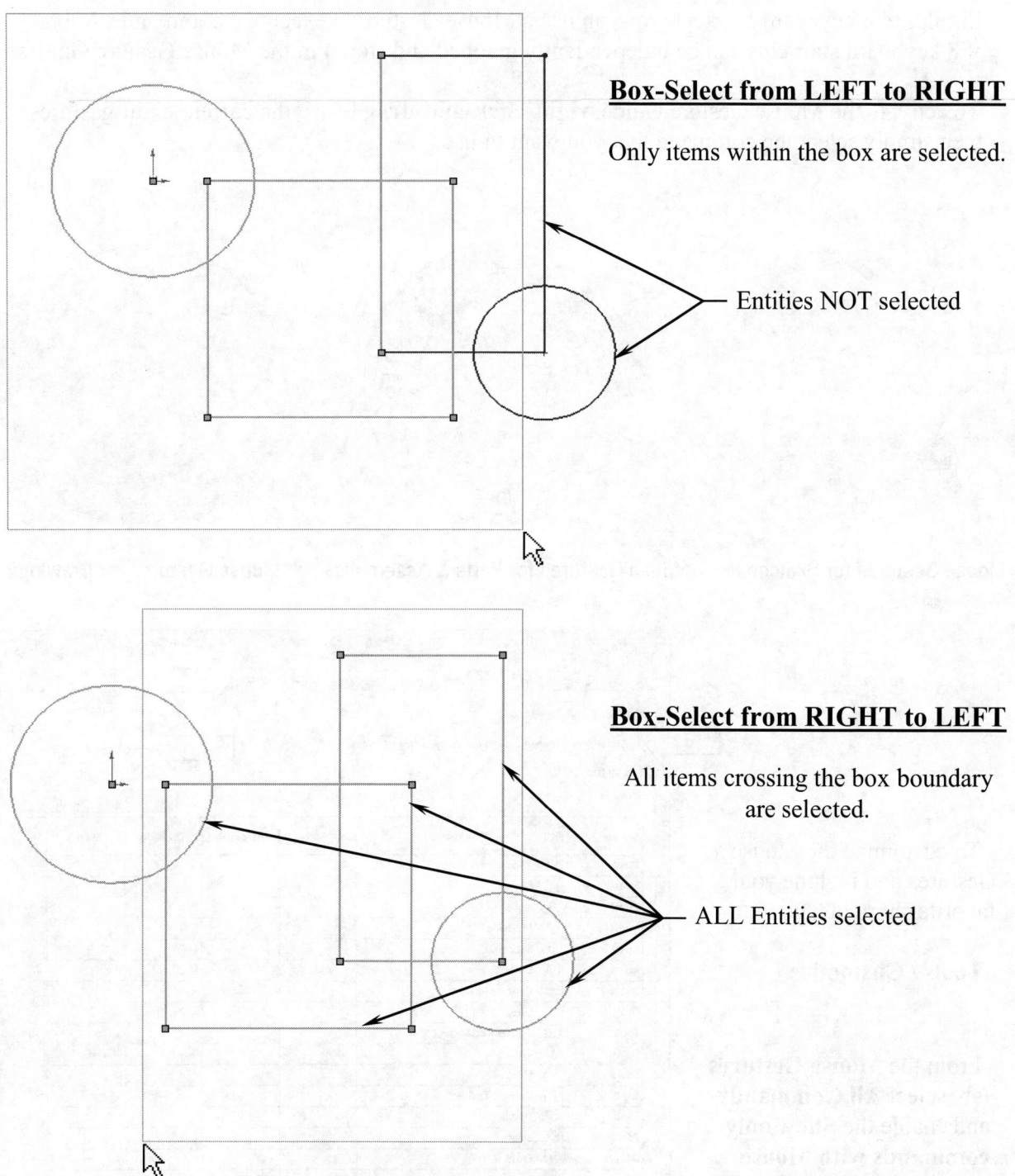

Box-Select from LEFT to RIGHT

Only items within the box are selected.

Entities NOT selected

Box-Select from RIGHT to LEFT

All items crossing the box boundary
are selected.

ALL Entities selected

The default geometry type selected is as follows:

* Part documents – edges * Assembly documents – components * Drawing documents - sketch entities,
dims & annotations. * To select multiple entities, hold down **Ctrl** while selecting after the first selection.

The <u>Mouse Gestures</u> for Sketches, Drawings and Parts

- Similar to a keyboard shortcut, you can use a Mouse Gesture to execute a command. A total of 8 keyboard shortcuts can be independently mapped and stored in the Mouse Gesture Guides.

- To activate the Mouse Gesture Guide, **right-click-and-drag** to see the current eight-gestures, then simply select the command that you want to use.

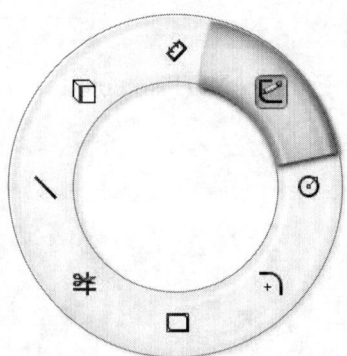
Mouse Gestures for Sketches

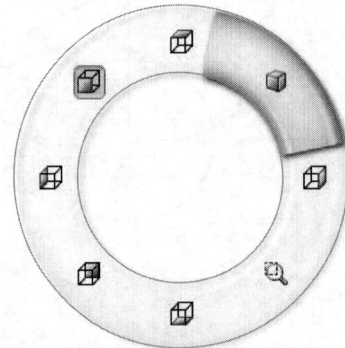
Mouse Gestures for Parts & Assemblies

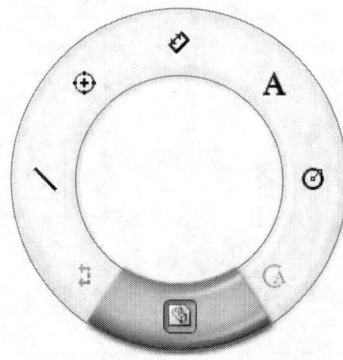
Mouse Gestures for Drawings

- To customize the Mouse Gestures and include your favorite shortcuts, go to:

   Tools / Customize.

- From the **Mouse Gestures** tab, select **All Commands** and enable the **Show only commands with Mouse Gestures assigned** checkbox.

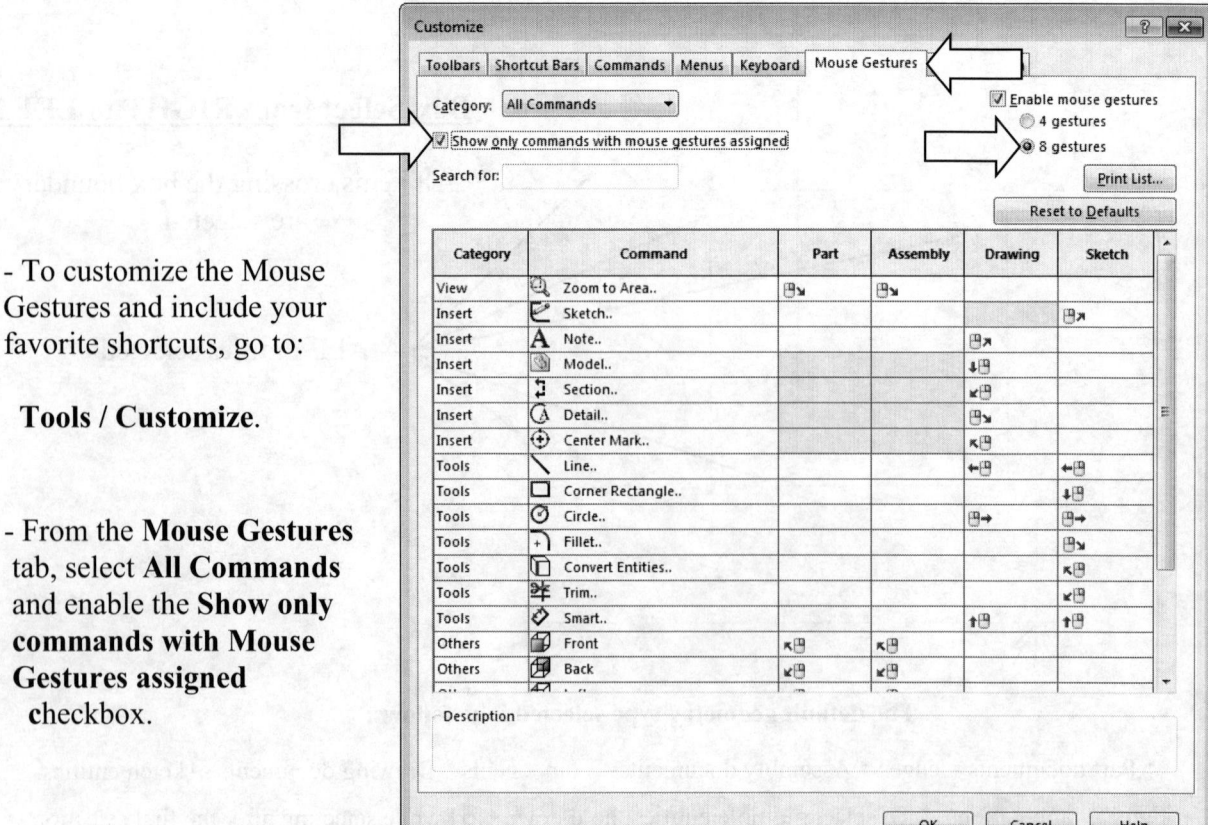

Fit to Left display ———   ——— Fit to Right display

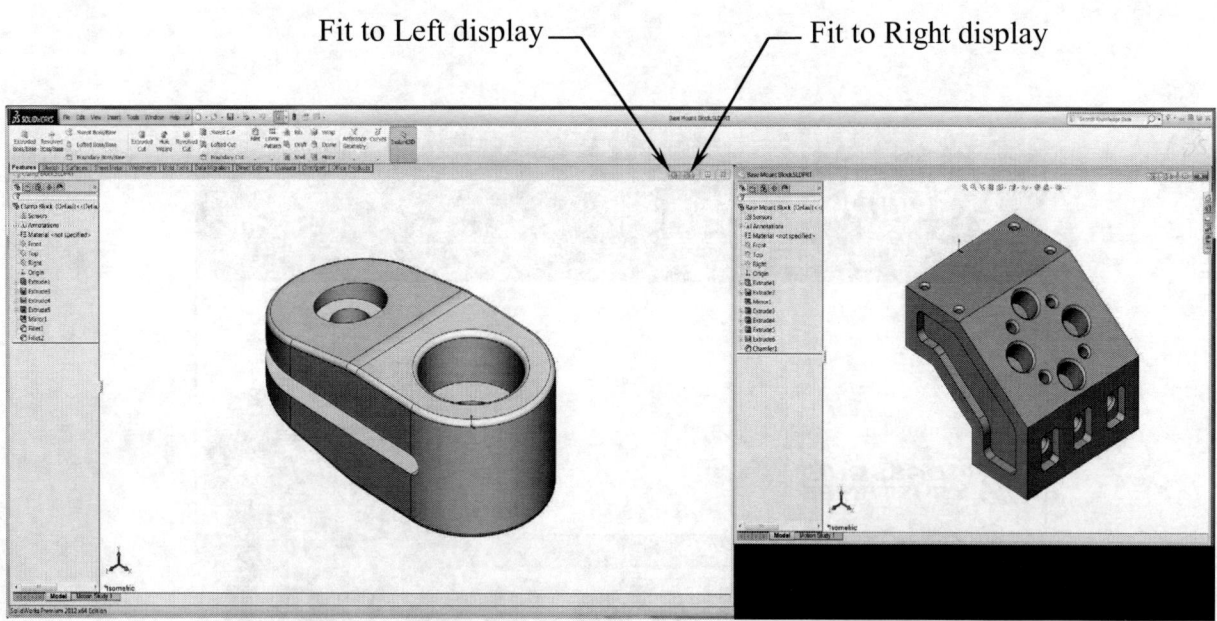

Dual monitors display

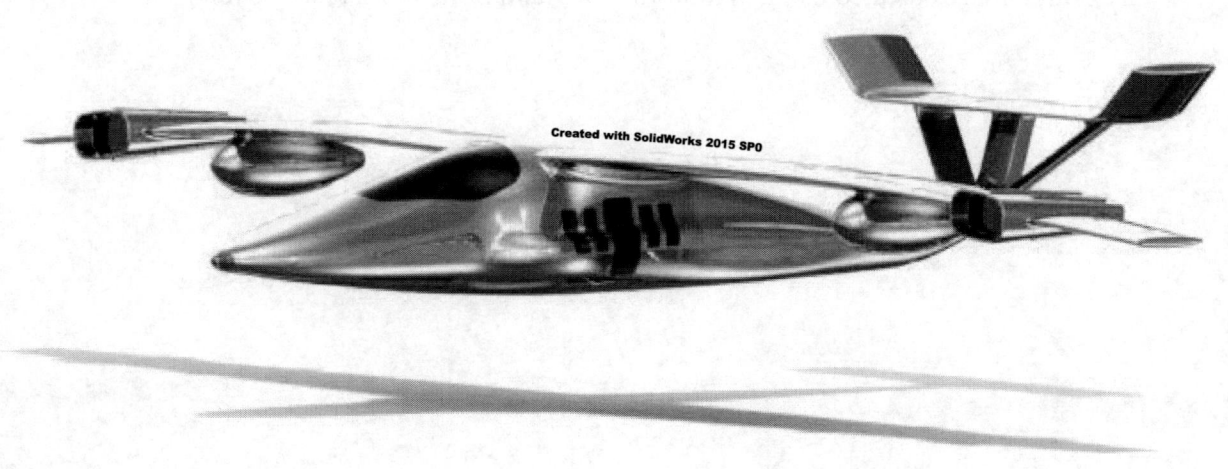

Created with SolidWorks 2015 SP0

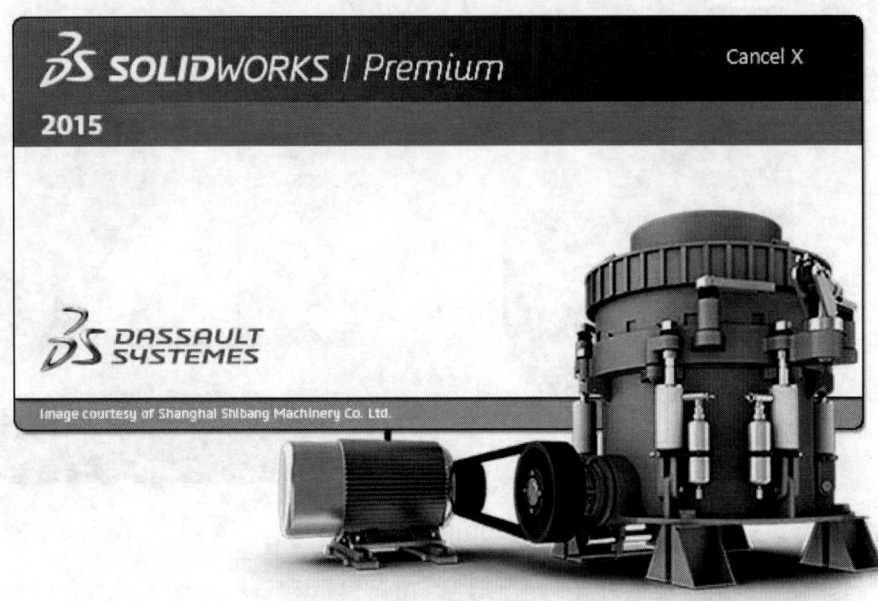

Text and images created using Windows 7 SP1 and SolidWorks 2015 64bit SP0

CHAPTER 1

System Options

Setting Up The System Options

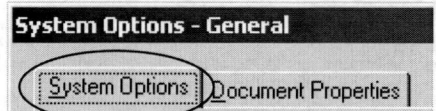

One of the first things to do after installing the SolidWorks software is to setup the system options to use as the default settings for all documents.

System Options such as:

- Input dimension value, Face highlighting…

- Drawing views controls, edge and hatch display.

- System colors, errors, sketch, text, grid, etc.

- Sketch display, Automatic relation.

- Edges display and selection controls.

- Performance and Large assembly mode.

- Area hatch/fill and hatch patterns.

- Feature Manager and Spin Box increment controls.

- View rotation and animation.

- Backup files and locations, etc.

The settings are all set and saved in the **system registry**. While not part of the document itself, these settings affect all documents, including current and future documents.

This chapter will guide you through some of the options settings for use with this textbook; you may need to modify them to ensure full compatibility with your applications or company's standards.

System Options

The **General** Options

- To start setting up the system options, go to: **Tools / Options.**

- Select the **General** options.

- Select only the check boxes as shown in the General Options dialog box.

- Go down the list and select the **Drawings** Options.

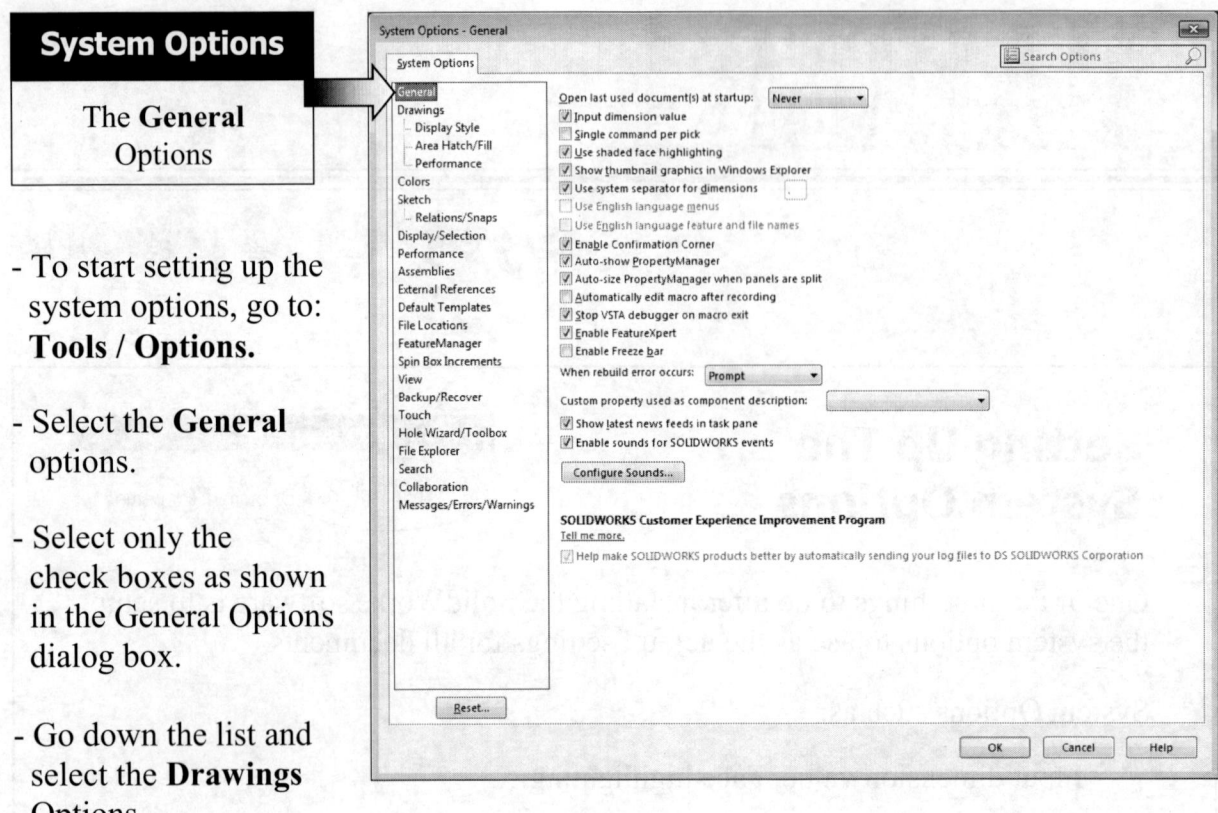

System Options

The **Drawings** Options

- Enable only the check boxes as indicated in this dialog box.

(These settings are intended for use with this training manual only, you may need to change them to meet your company's requirements).

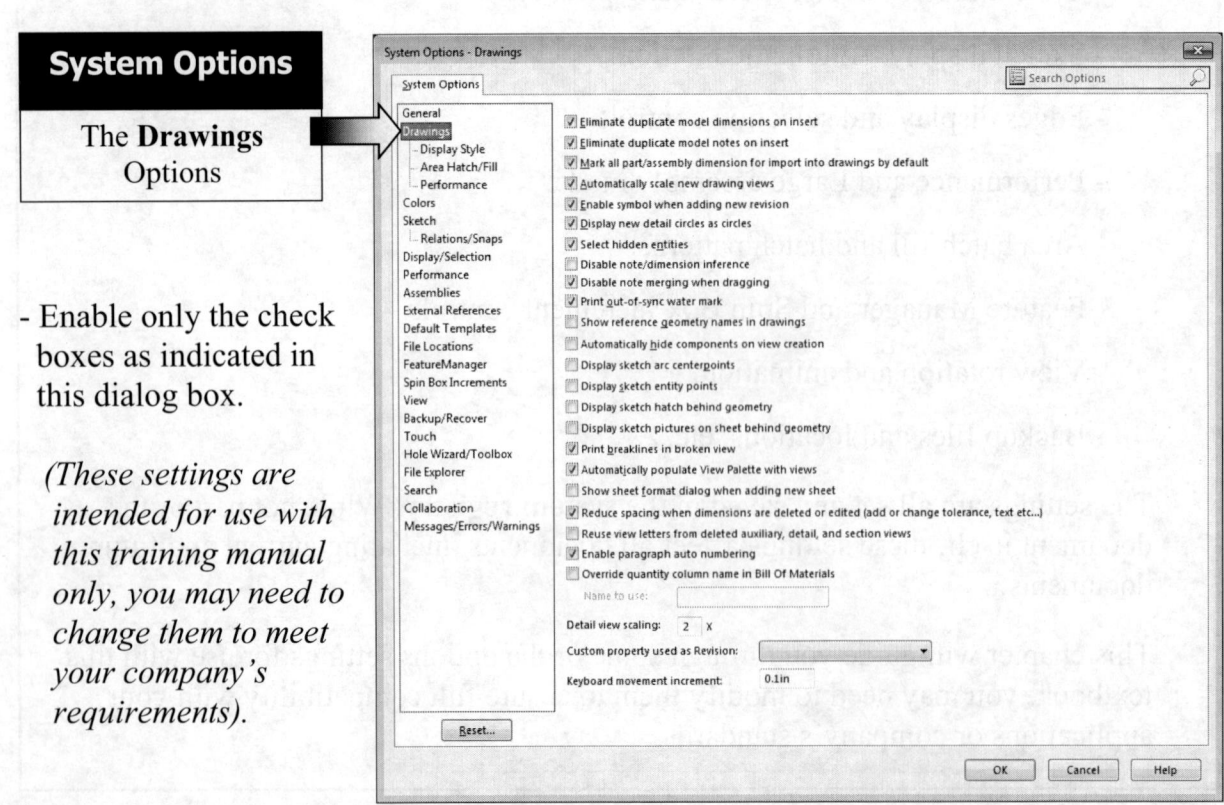

System Options

The **Display Style** Options

- Continue going down the list and follow the sample settings shown in the dialog boxes to setup your System Options.

- For more information on these settings click the Help button at the lower right corner of the dialog box (arrow).

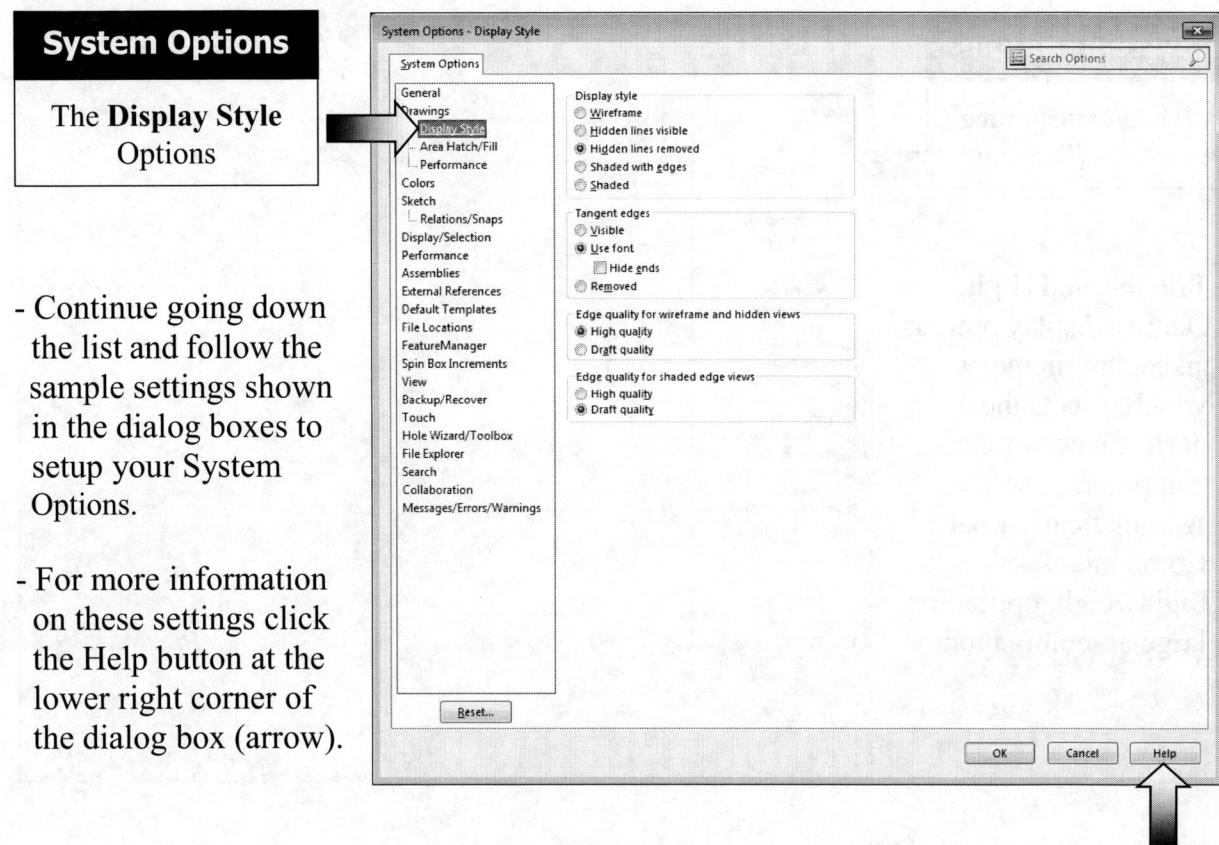

System Options

The **Area Hatch/Fill** Options

- The Area Hatch/Fills option sets the hatch pattern and Spacing (Scale).

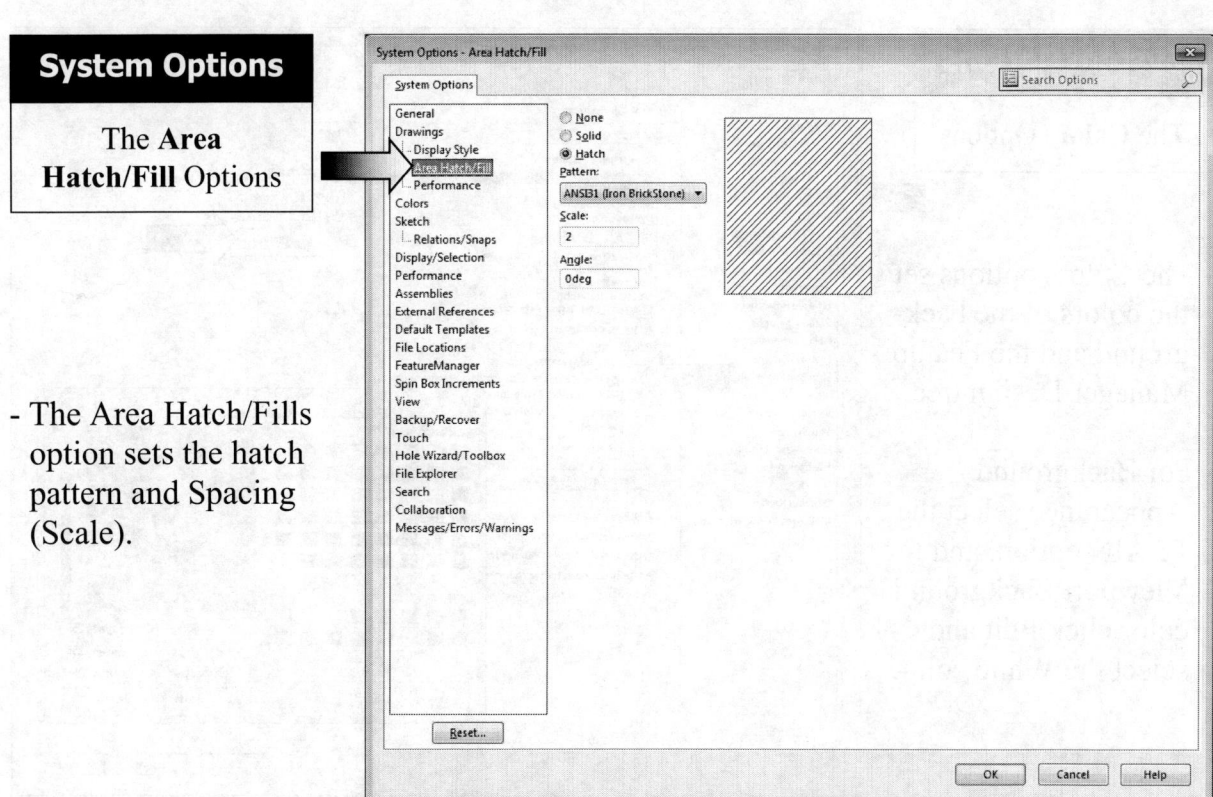

System Options

The **Performance** Options (Drawing)

- Preview and High Quality display options take extra memory, which effects the performance of the computer. (Use the Automatically Load Components Lightweight option in large assembly mode).

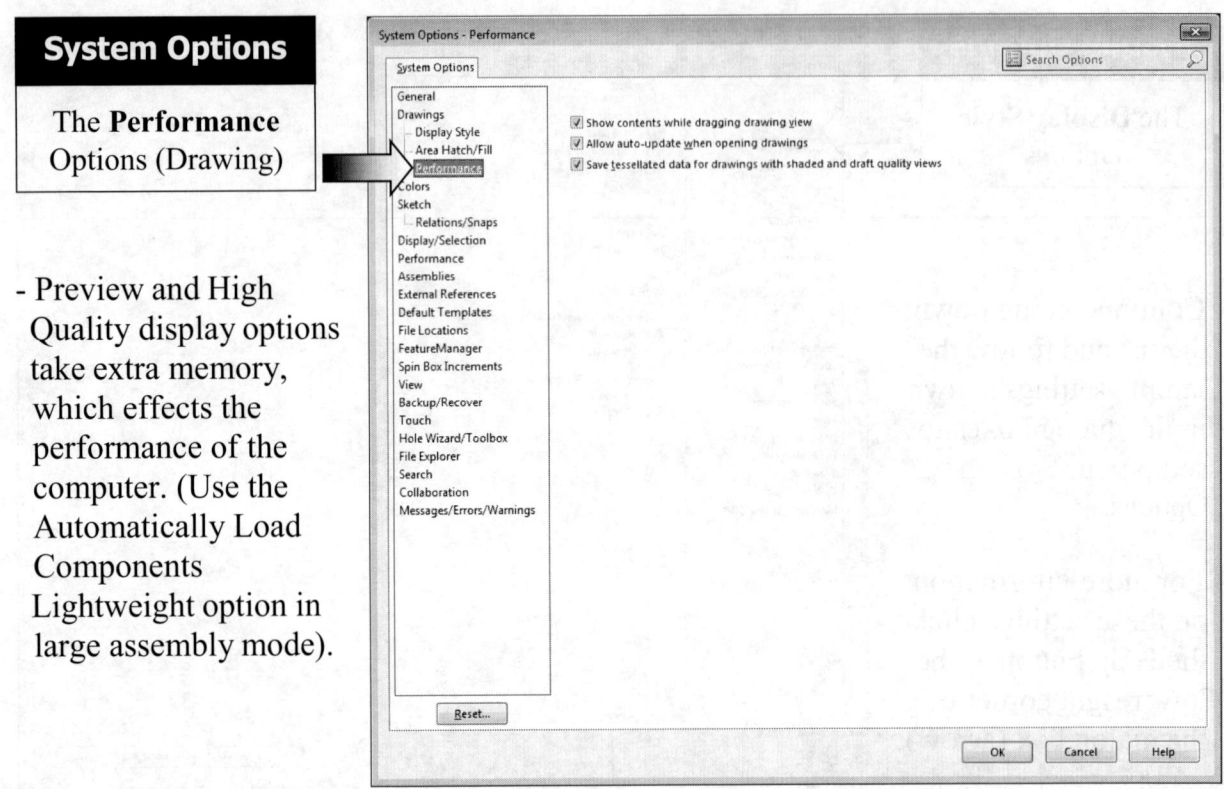

System Options

The **Colors** Options

- The Colors options set the colors of the background and the Feature-Manager Design tree.

- For Background-Appearance select the PLAIN option, and for Viewport Background color click Edit and select the White color.

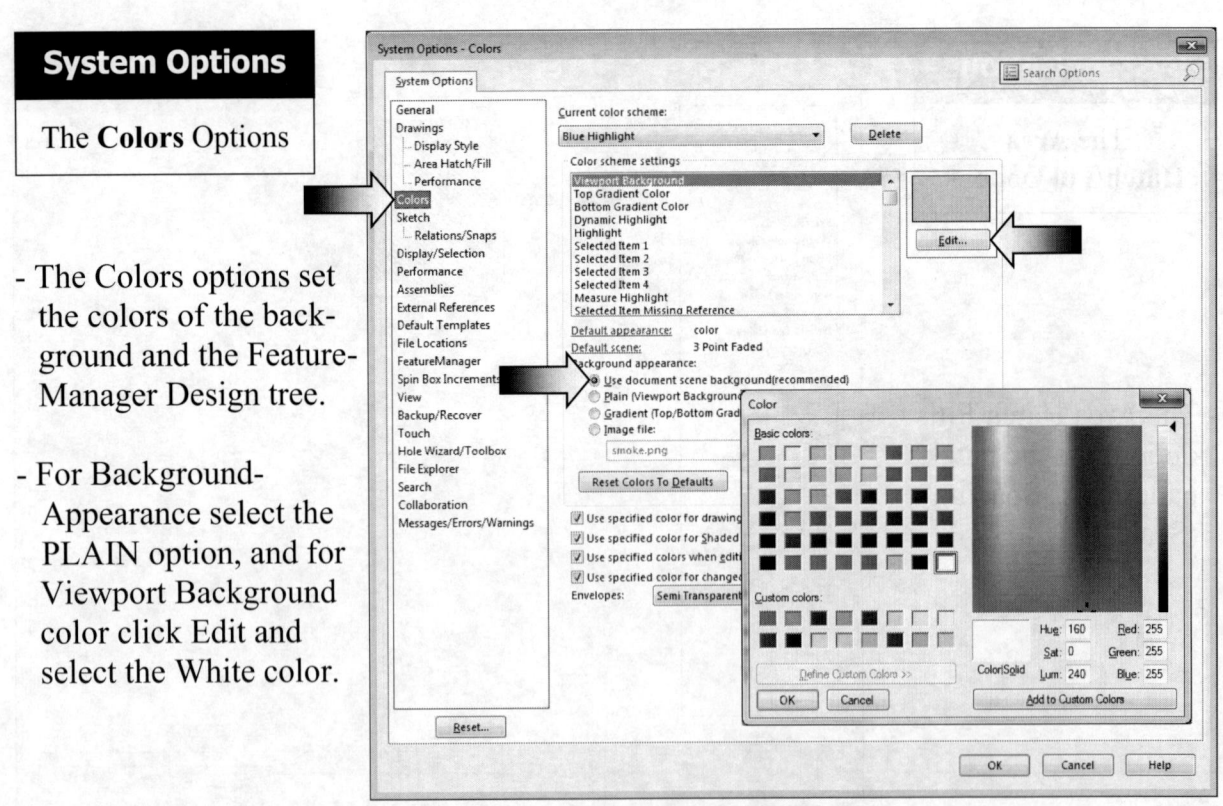

System Options

The **Sketch** Options

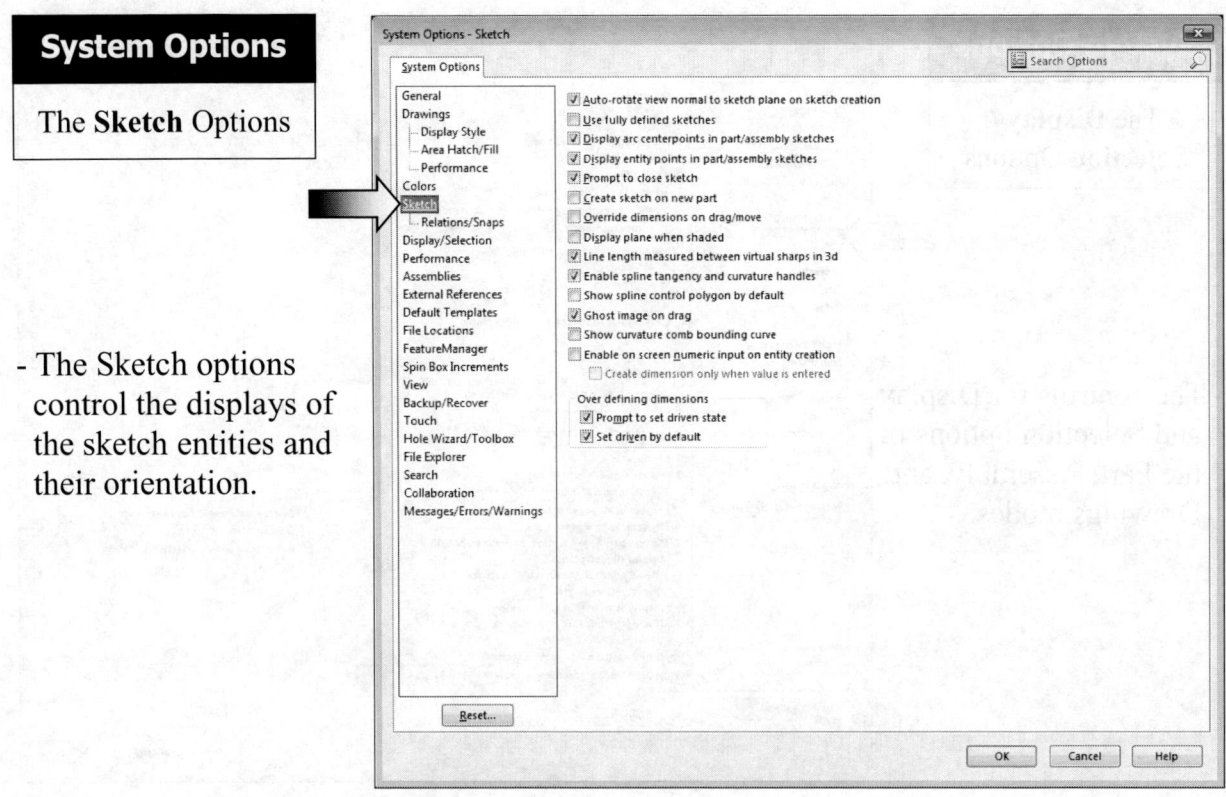

- The Sketch options
control the displays of
the sketch entities and
their orientation.

System Options

The **Relations /
Snaps** Options

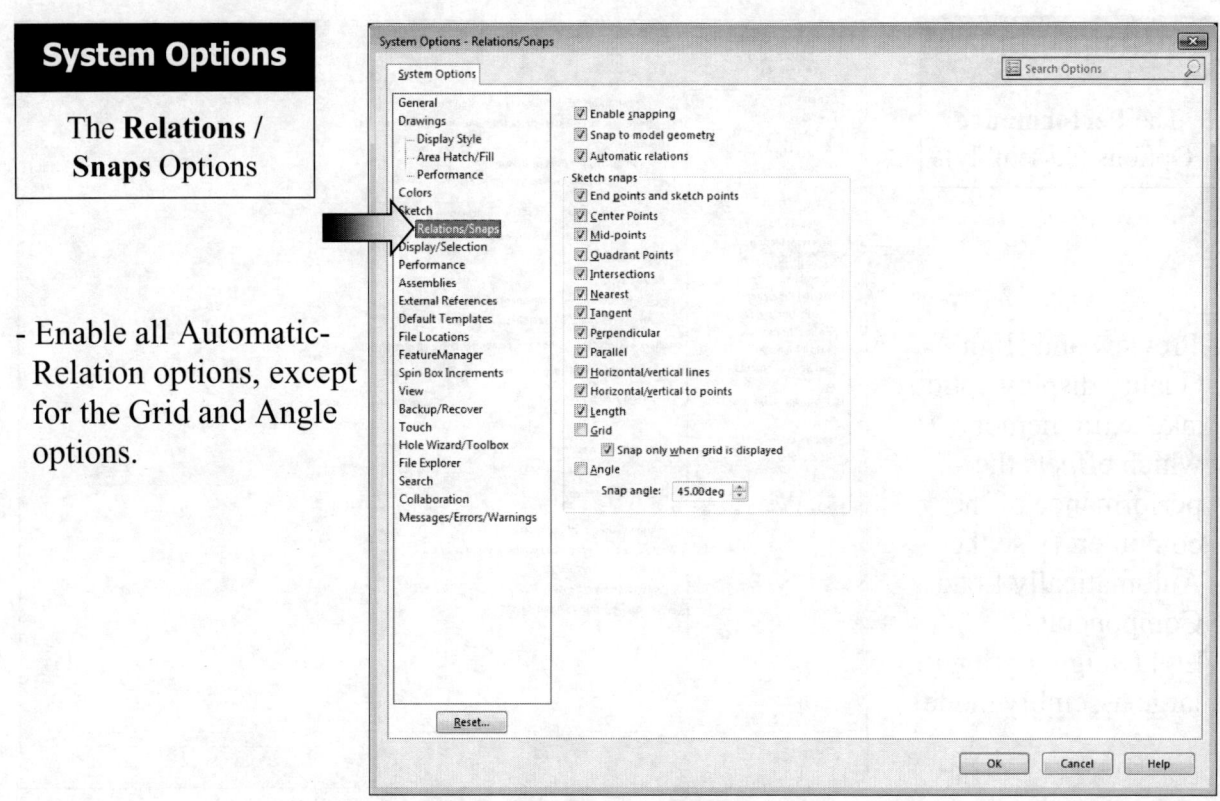

- Enable all Automatic-
Relation options, except
for the Grid and Angle
options.

System Options

The **Display /
Selection** Options

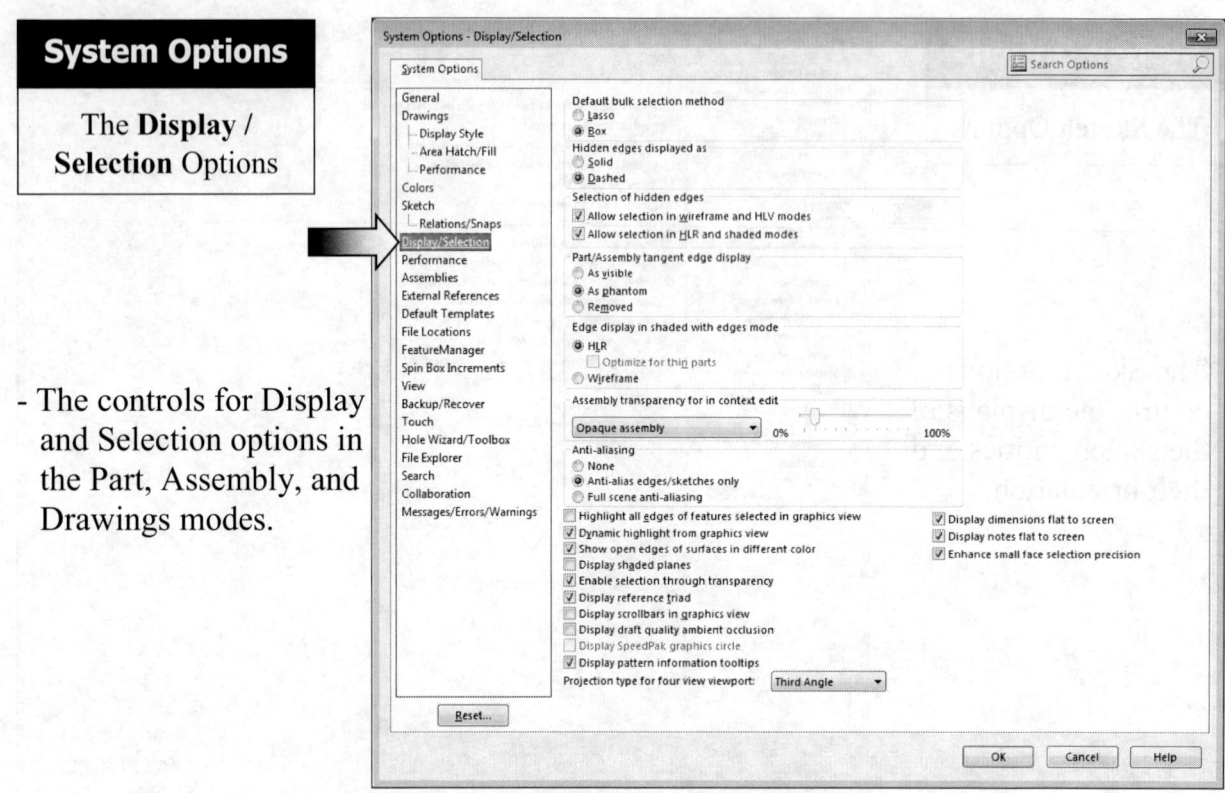

- The controls for Display
and Selection options in
the Part, Assembly, and
Drawings modes.

System Options

The **Performance**
Options (Assembly)

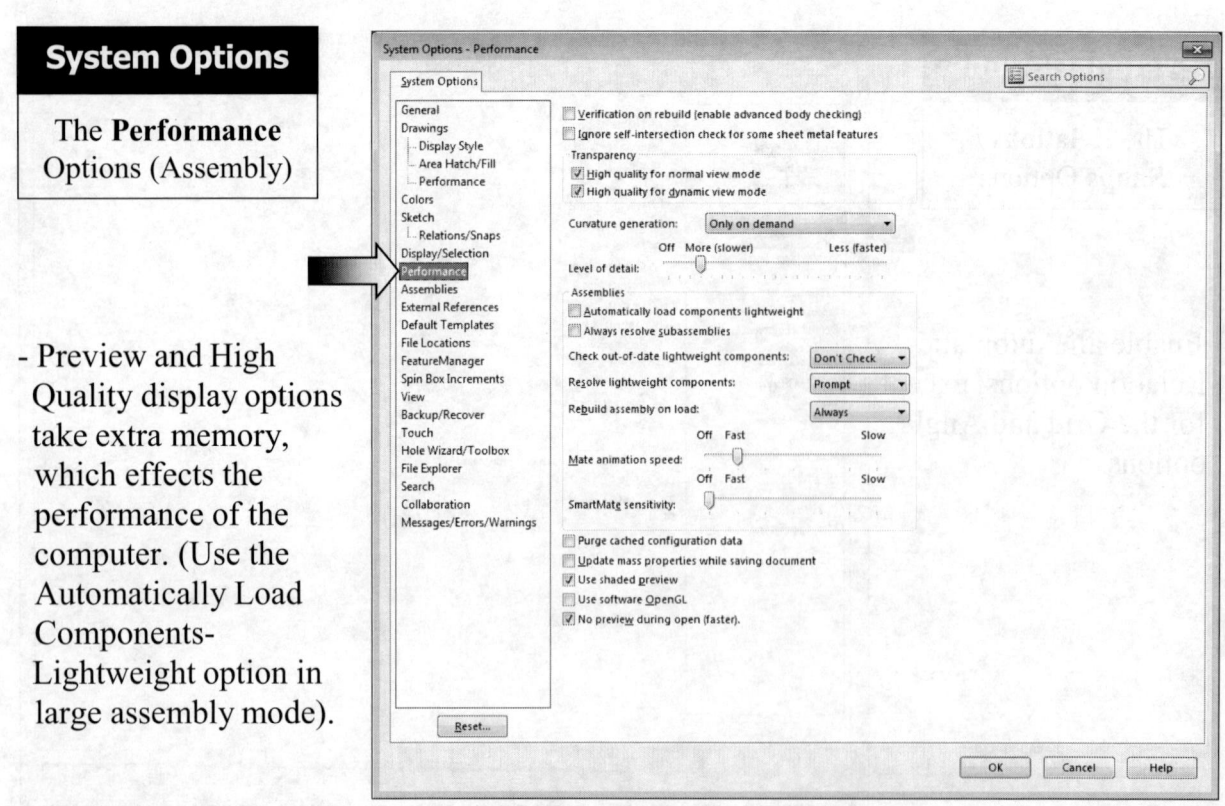

- Preview and High
Quality display options
take extra memory,
which effects the
performance of the
computer. (Use the
Automatically Load
Components-
Lightweight option in
large assembly mode).

System Options

The **Assemblies**
Options

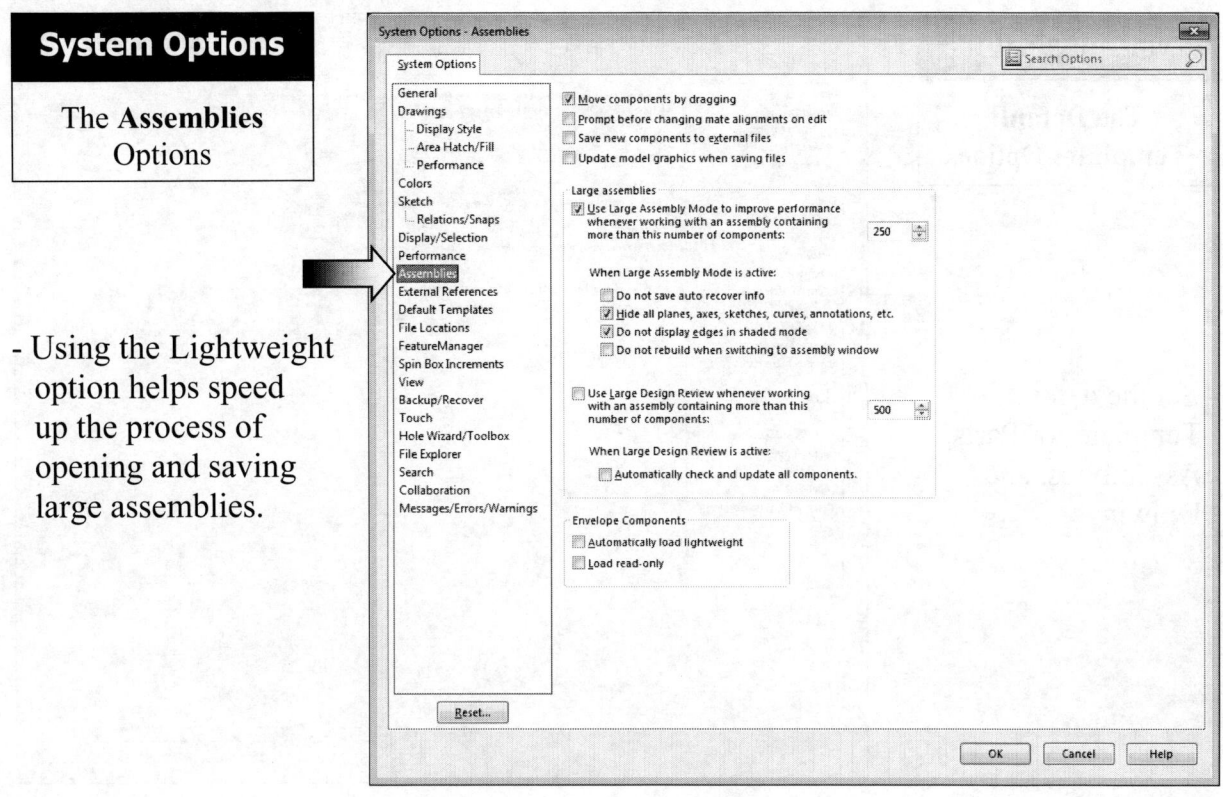

- Using the Lightweight
option helps speed
up the process of
opening and saving
large assemblies.

System Options

The **External
References** Options

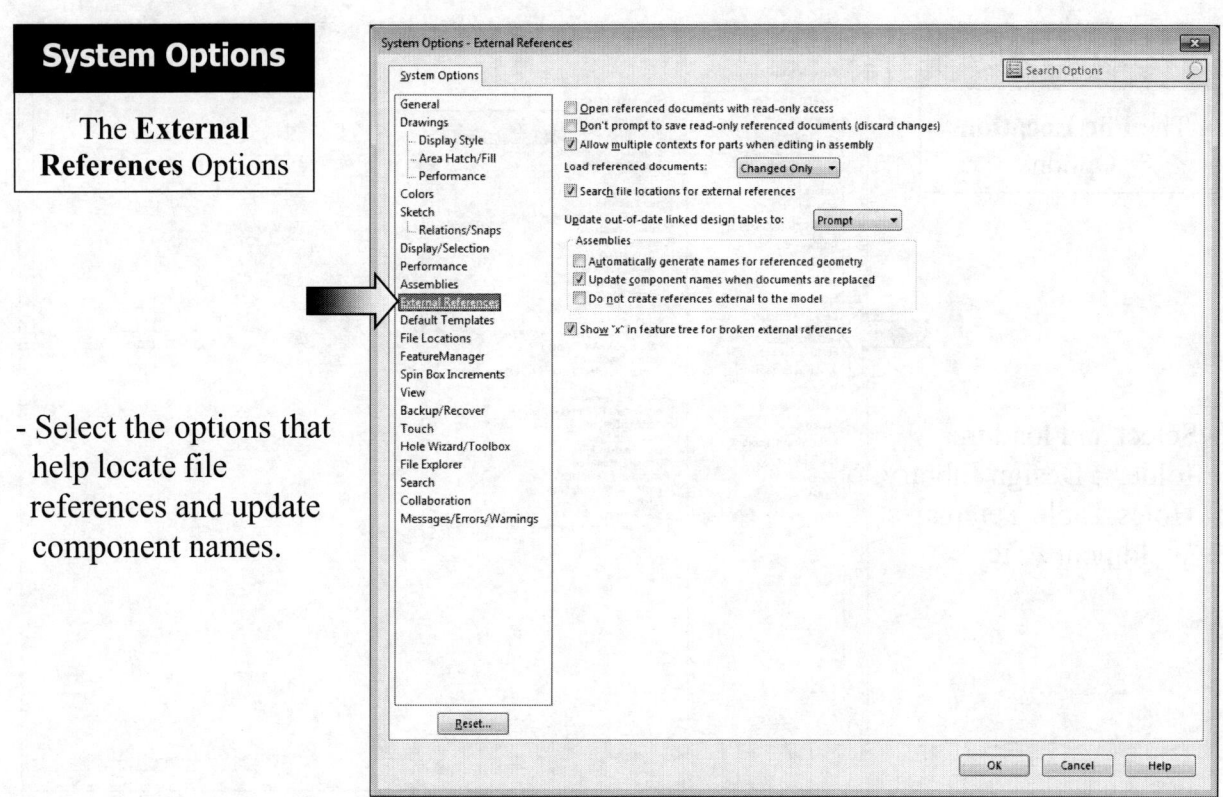

- Select the options that
help locate file
references and update
component names.

System Options

The **Default Templates** Options

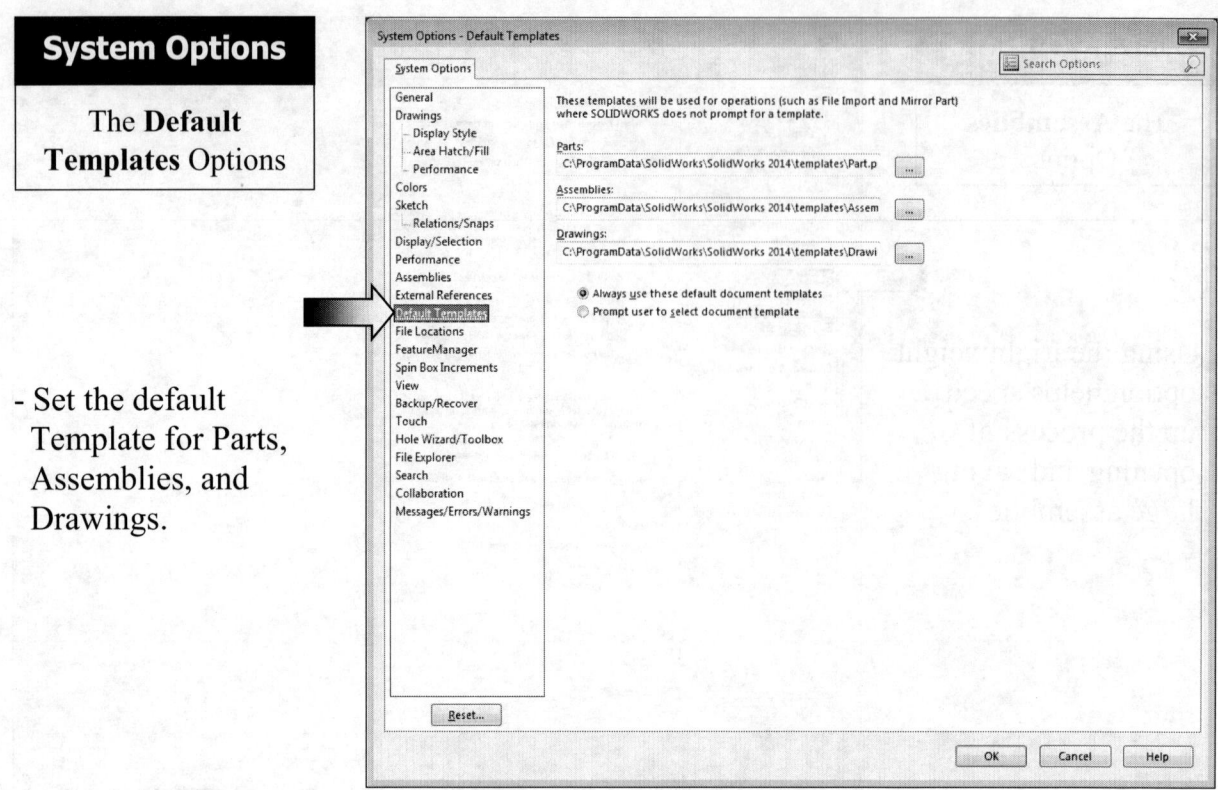

- Set the default Template for Parts, Assemblies, and Drawings.

System Options

The **File Locations** Options

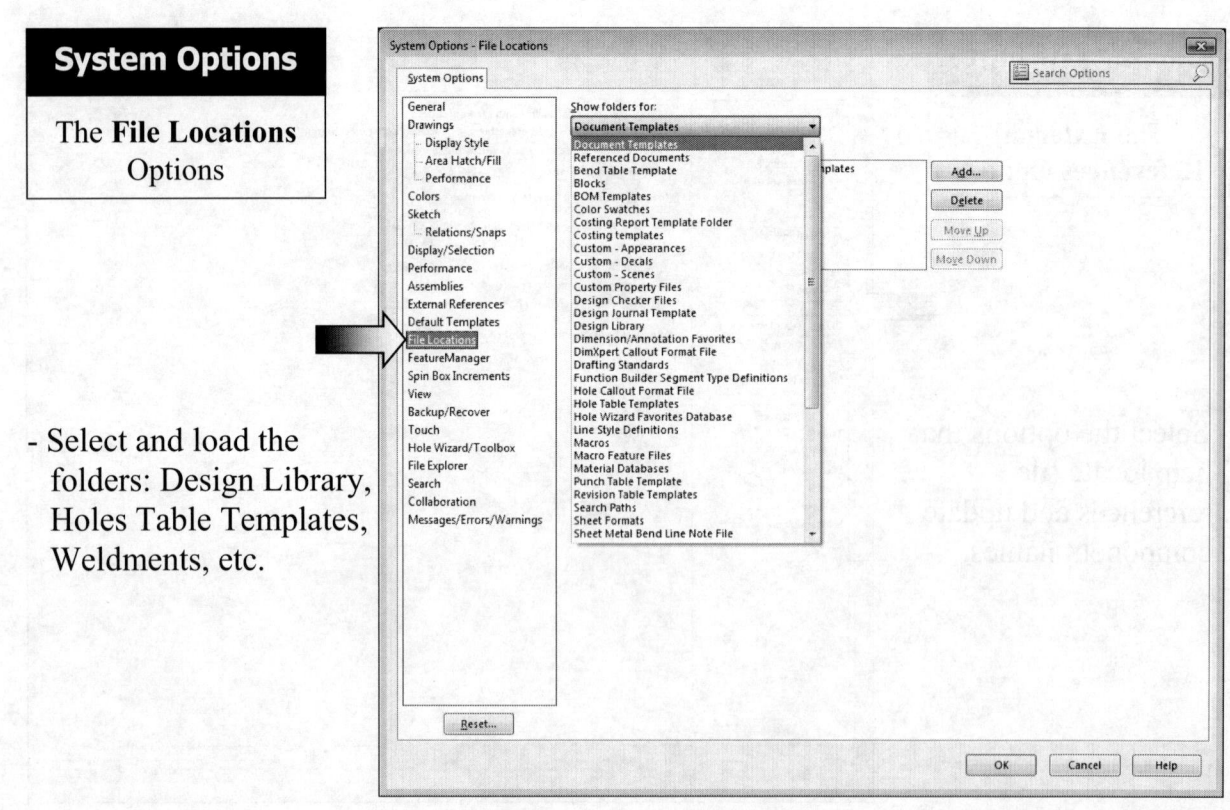

- Select and load the folders: Design Library, Holes Table Templates, Weldments, etc.

System Options

The **Feature-Manager** Options

- Select the Folders that you want to show on the FeatureManager Design tree.

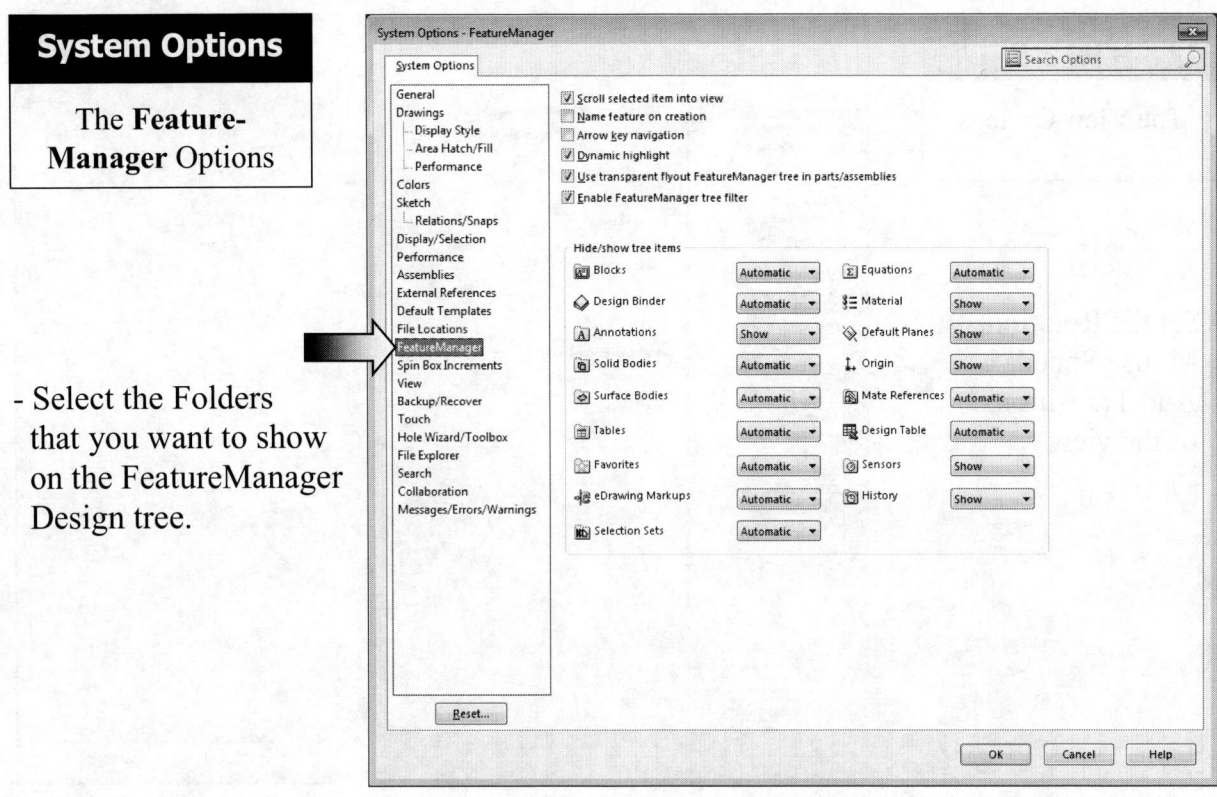

System Options

The **Spin Box Increments** Options

- Set the default increments for the Modify Spin Box (when creating or Editing dimensions).

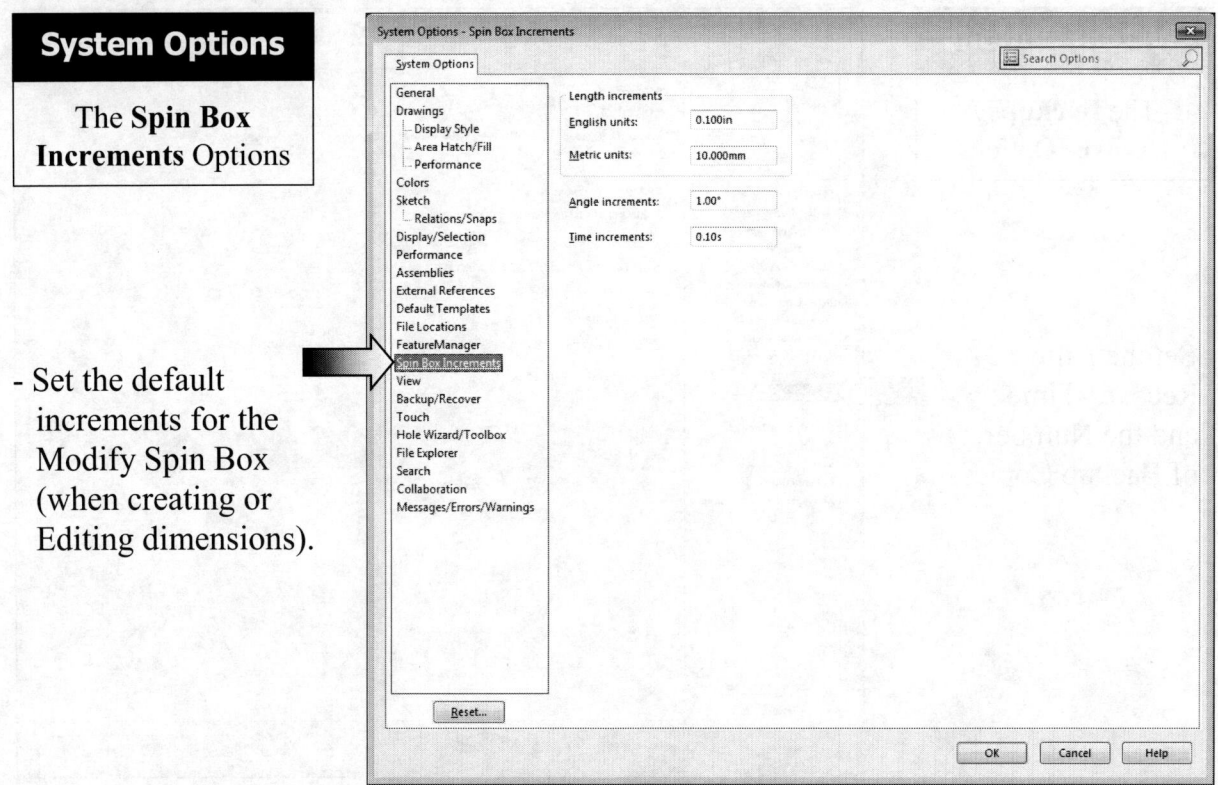

System Options

The **View** Options

- Set the Rotation,
Mouse Speed,
And Transitions
of the view.

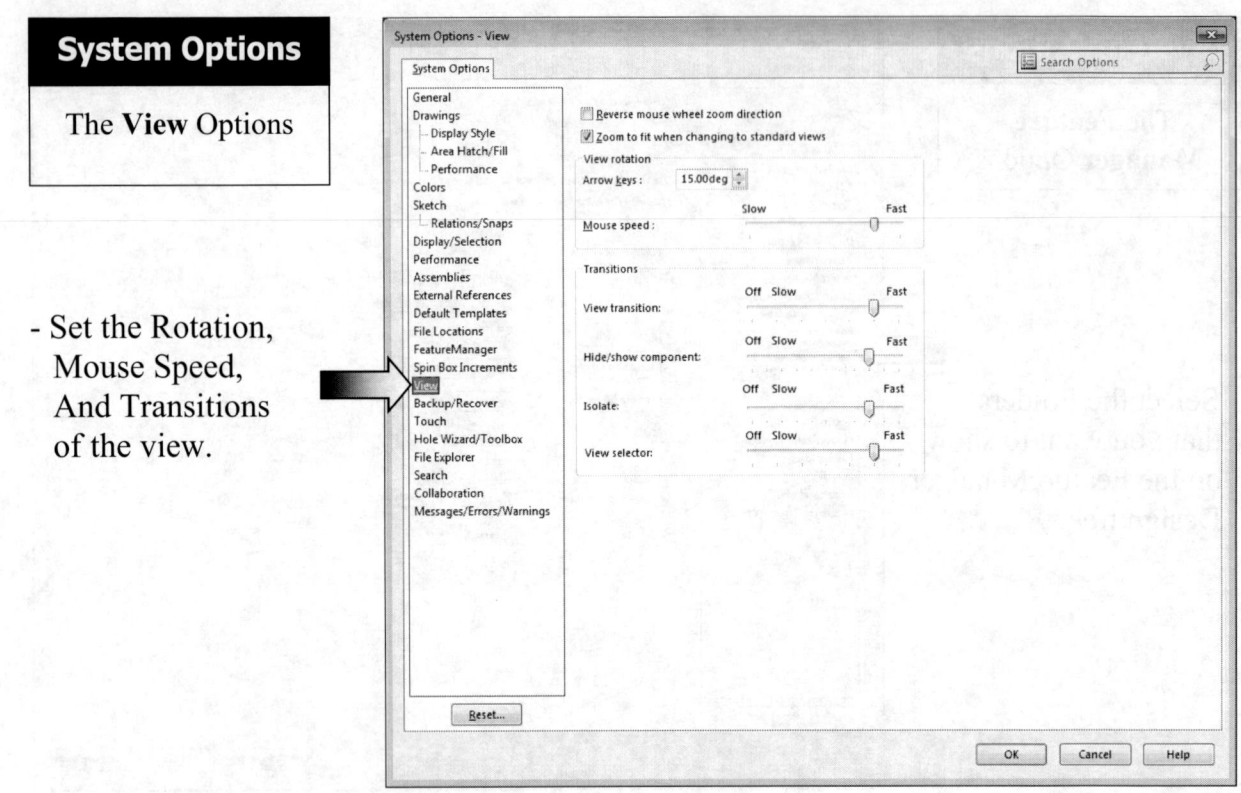

System Options

The **Backups /
Recover** Options

- Set the Auto-
Recover-Time
and the Number
of Backup Copies.

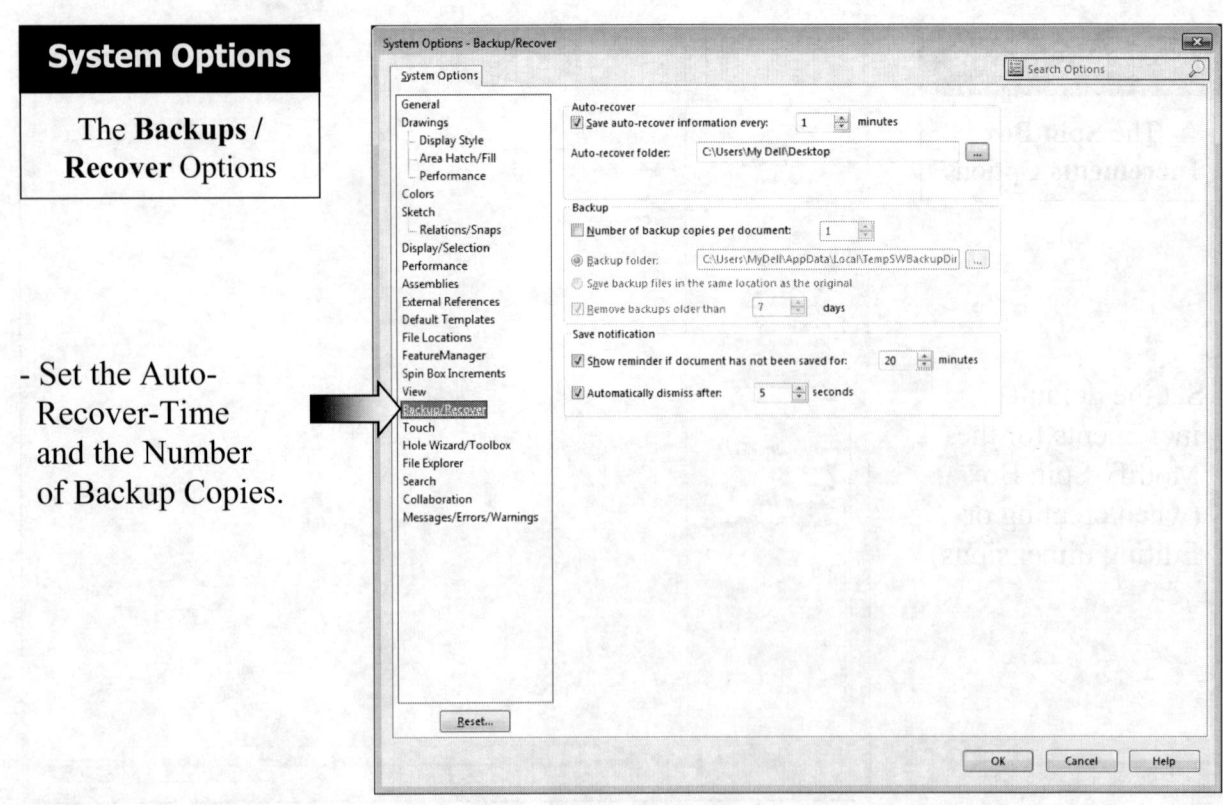

System Options

The **Touch**
Options

- With a Touch-enabled
computer, you
can use flick
touch and multi-
touch gestures in
SolidWorks 2015.

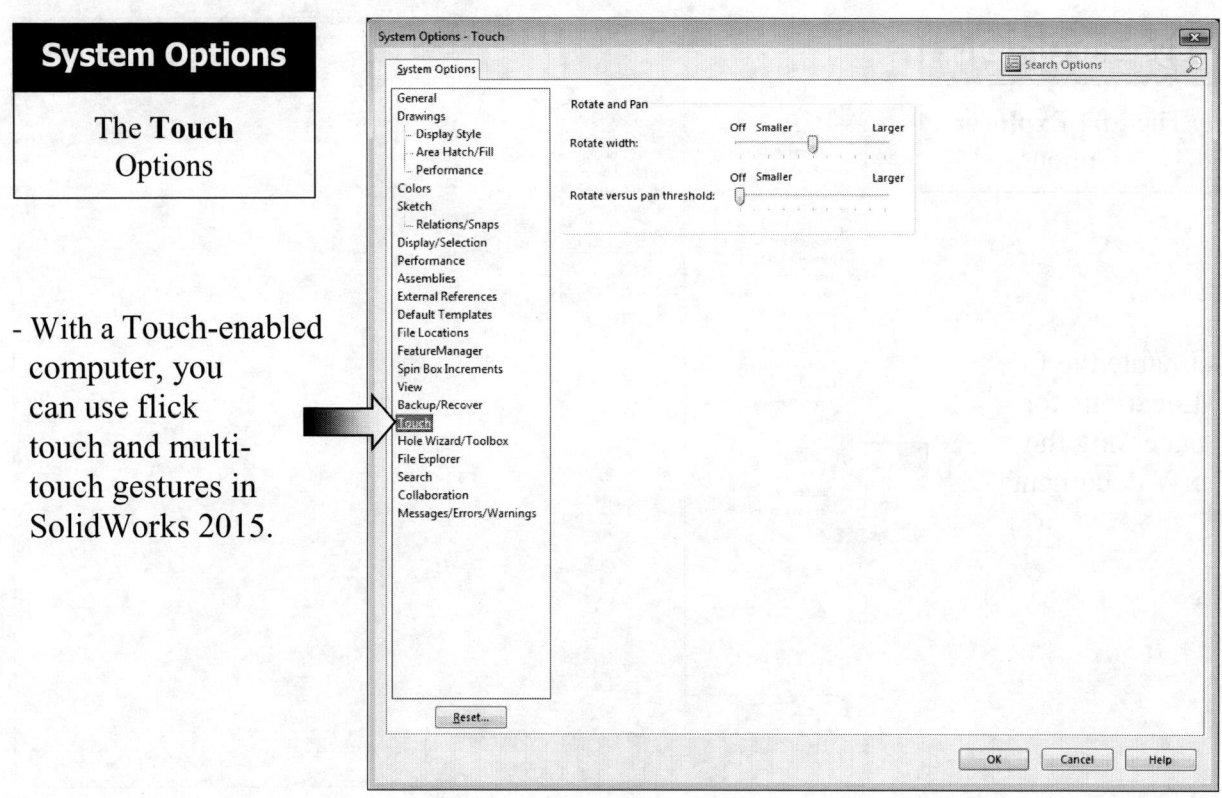

System Options

The **Hole-
Wizard/Toolbox**
Options

- Locate the Hole
Wizard and
Toolbox folder.

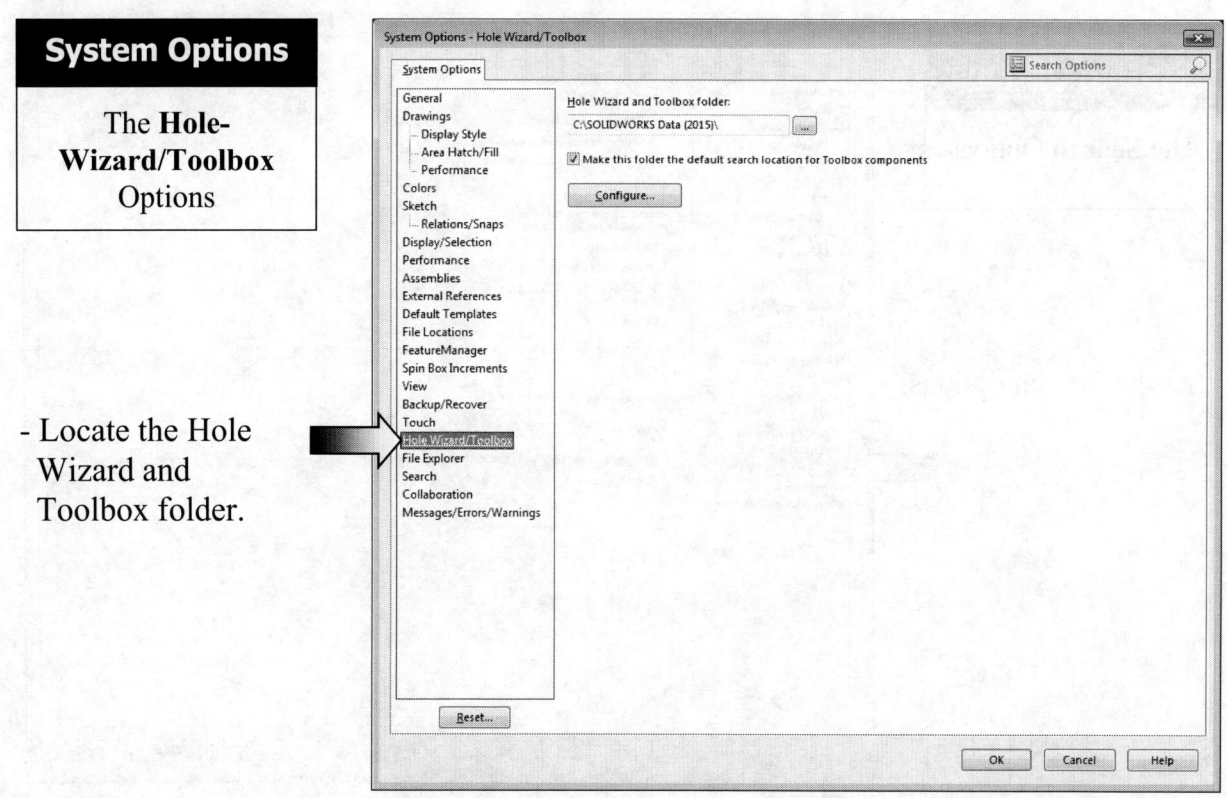

System Options

The **File Explorer**
Options

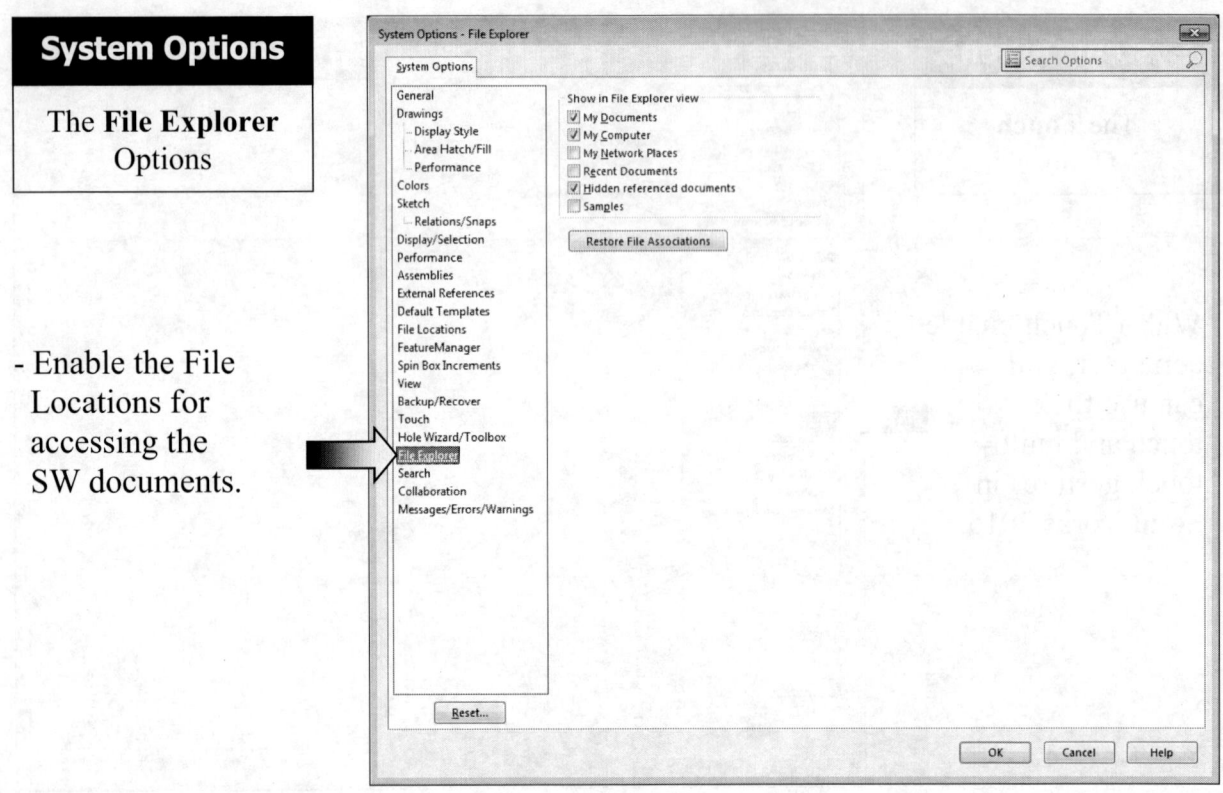

- Enable the File
Locations for
accessing the
SW documents.

System Options

The **Search** Options

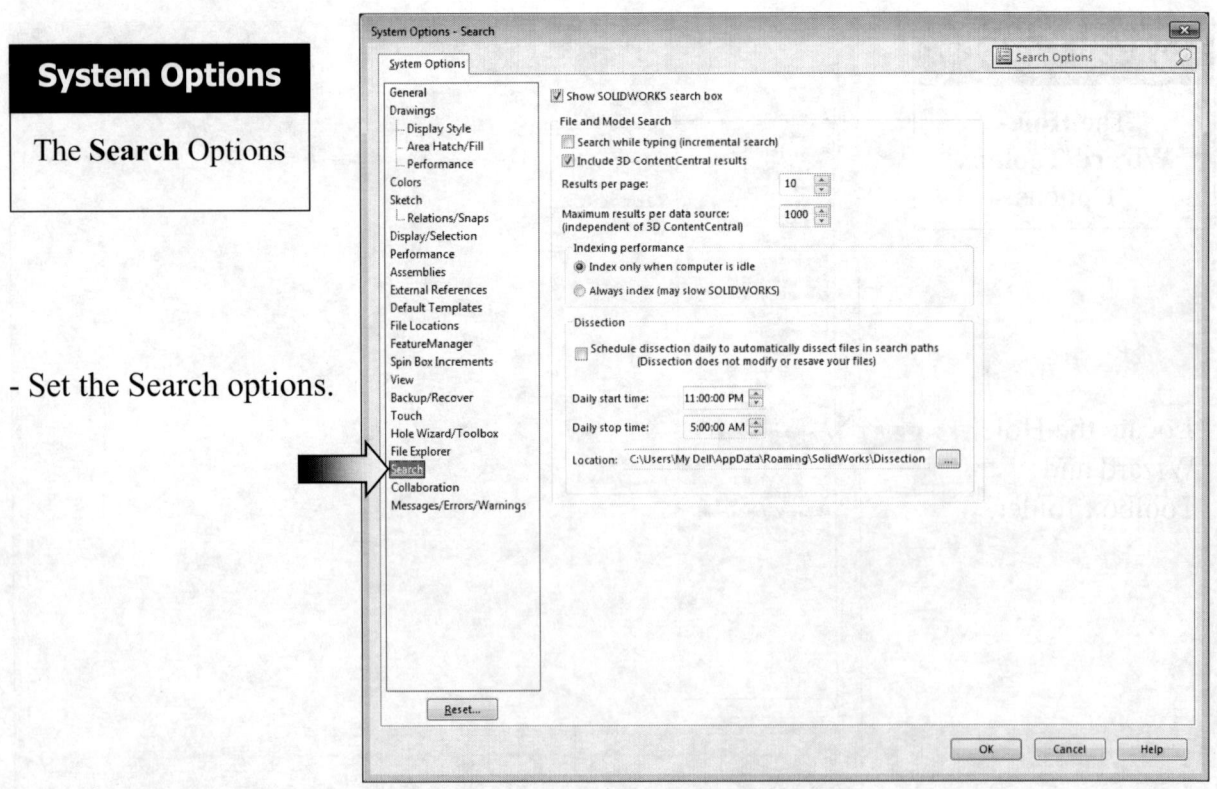

- Set the Search options.

System Options

The **Collaboration**
Options

- Enable / Disable
the Multi-User
Environment.

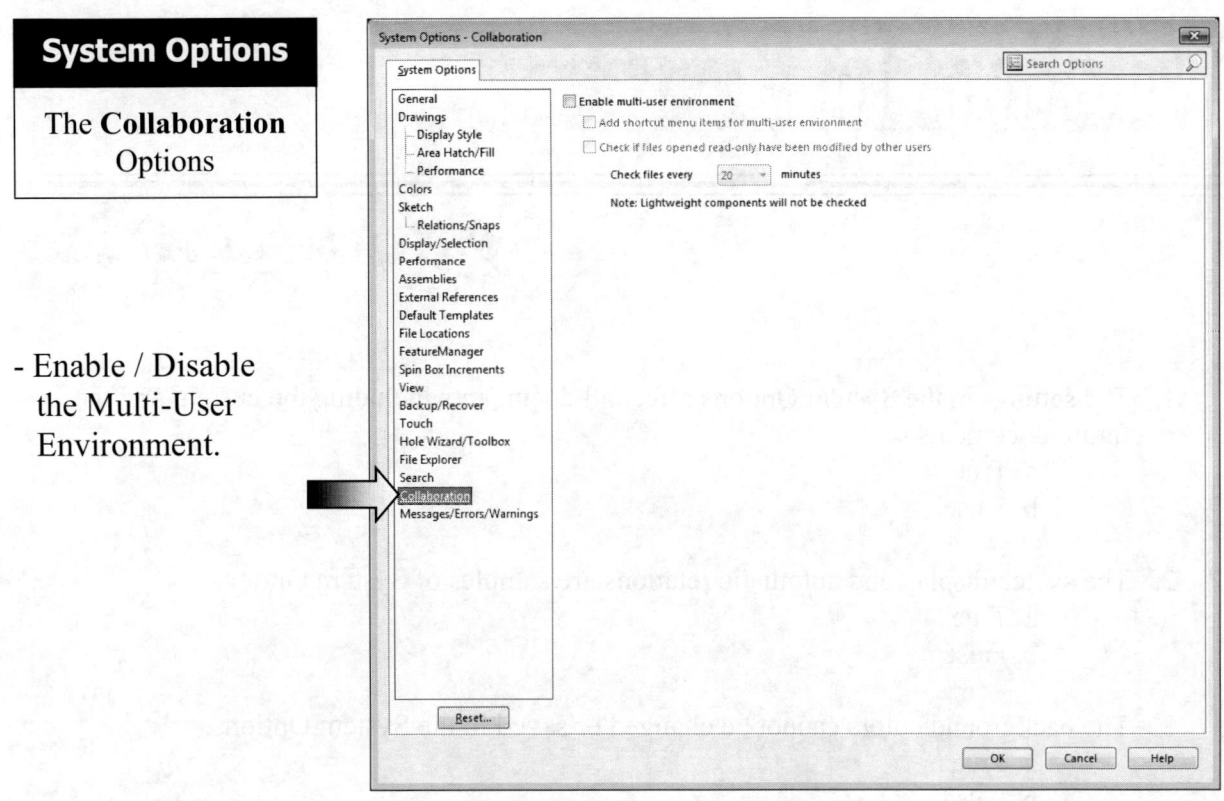

System Options

The **Advanced**
Options

- Set the Error and
Warning messages.

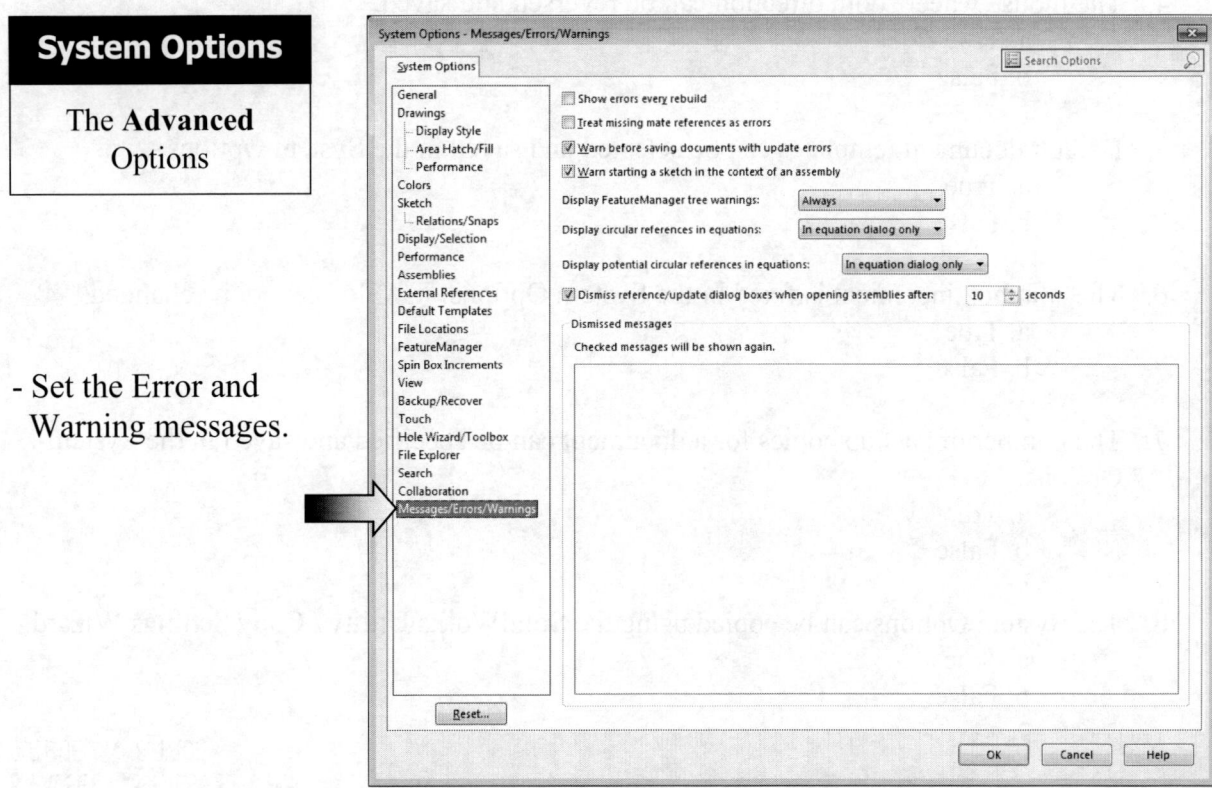

- Continue to setup the Document Properties in Chapter 2…

Questions for Review

System Options

1. The settings in the System Options affect all documents including the current and the future documents.
   - a. True
   - b. False

2. The sketch display and automatic relations are samples of System Options.
   - a. True
   - b. False

3. The background colors cannot be changed or saved in the System Options.
   - a. True
   - b. False

4. The mouse wheel zoom direction can be reversed and saved.
   - a. True
   - b. False

5. Default document templates can be selected and saved in the System Options.
   - a. True
   - b. False

6. The spin box increment is fixed in the System Options; its value cannot be changed.
   - a. True
   - b. False

7. The number of backup copies for a document can be specified and saved in the System Options.
   - a. True
   - b. False

8. The System Options can be copied using the SolidWorks Utility / Copy Settings Wizard.
   - a. True
   - b. False

7. TRUE   8. TRUE
5. FALSE   6. FALSE
3. FALSE   4. TRUE
1. TRUE   2. TRUE

CHAPTER 2

Document Templates

Setting Up The Document Properties

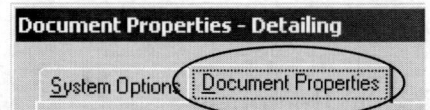

After setting up the System Options, the next task is to setup a document template, where drafting standards and other settings can be set, saved and used over and over again as a template. The Document Properties such as:

- Drafting Standard (ANSI, ISO, DIN, JIS, etc.).

- Dimension, Note, Balloon, and Fonts Sizes.

- Arrowhead sizes.

- Annotation display.

- Grid spacing and grid display.

- Units (Inches, Millimeters, etc.) and Decimal places.

- Feature Colors, Wireframe, and Shading colors.

- Material Properties.

- Image quality controls.

- Plane display controls.

These settings are all set and saved in the templates, all settings affect only the **current document** (C:\Program Files\SolidWorks Corp\SolidWorks Data\ Templates) OR (C:\Program Files\SolidWorks Corp\SolidWorks\Lang\English\ Tutorial).

The following are examples of various document settings which are intended for use with this textbook only; you may need to modify them to ensure full compatibility with your applications.

Document Properties

The **Drafting Standard** options

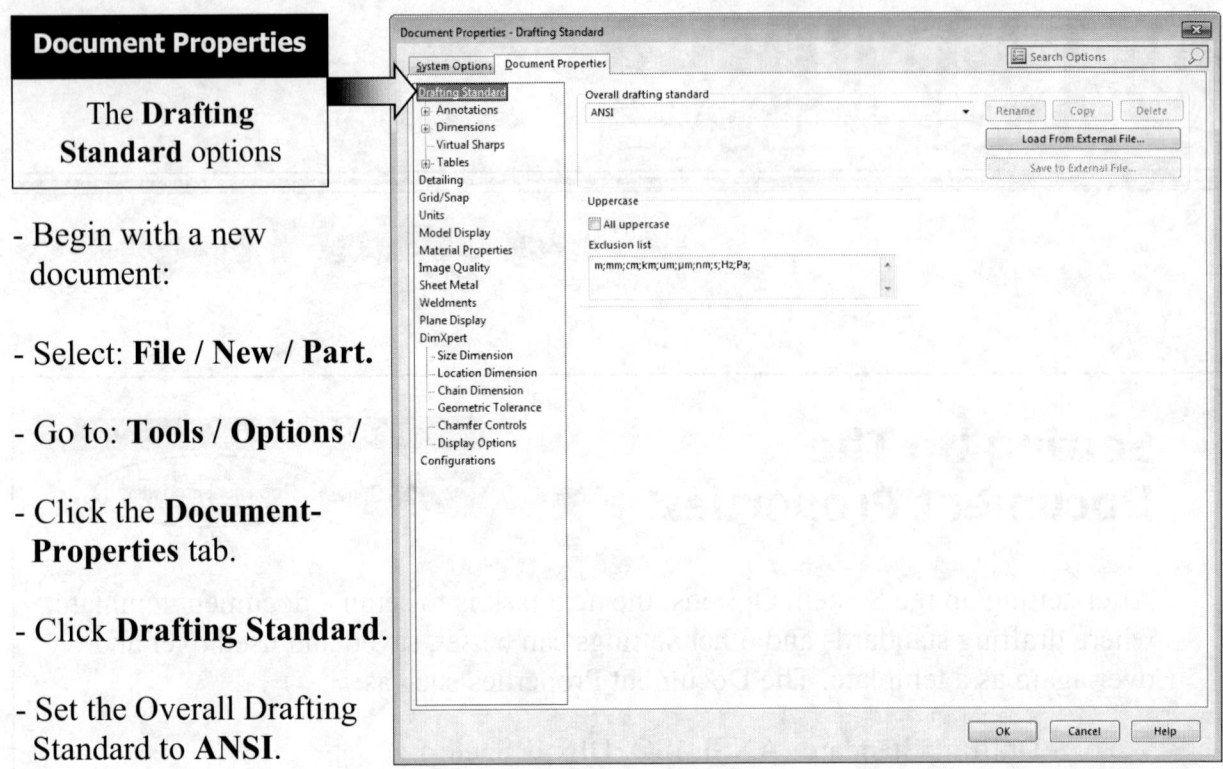

- Begin with a new document:

- Select: **File / New / Part.**

- Go to: **Tools / Options /**

- Click the **Document-Properties** tab.

- Click **Drafting Standard**.

- Set the Overall Drafting Standard to **ANSI**.

Note: If your Units are in Millimeters, skip to the Units options on page 2-13 and set your units to IPS, then return to where you left off and continue with your template settings.

Document Properties

The **Annotations** options

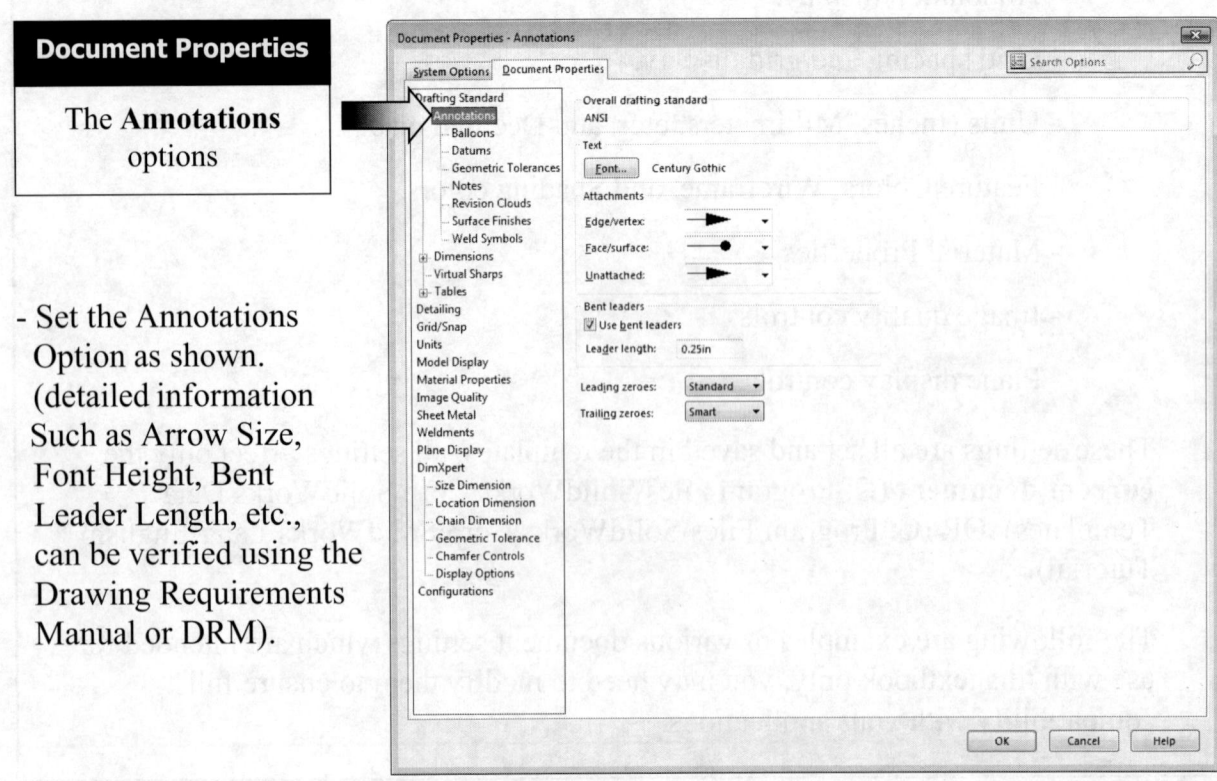

- Set the Annotations Option as shown. (detailed information Such as Arrow Size, Font Height, Bent Leader Length, etc., can be verified using the Drawing Requirements Manual or DRM).

Document Properties

The **Annotations / Balloons** options

- Set the Balloons standard to ANSI and the other options as shown.

- Click on the Help button at any time to access the information on these topics.

Document Properties

The **Annotations / Datums** options

- Set the Datums standard to ANSI and other options as shown.

Note:

1982 Datum symbol – A –

1994 Datum symbol A

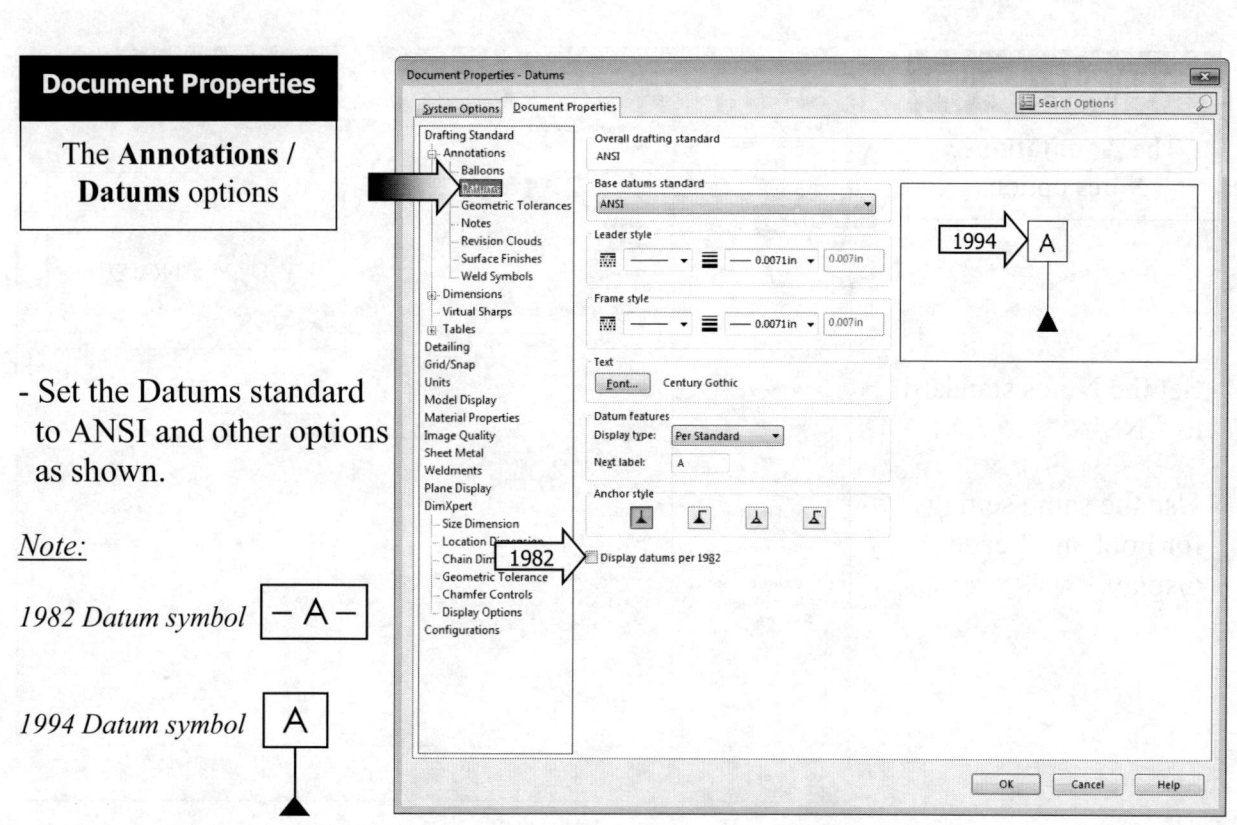

Document Properties

The **Annotations /
Geo. Tol.** options

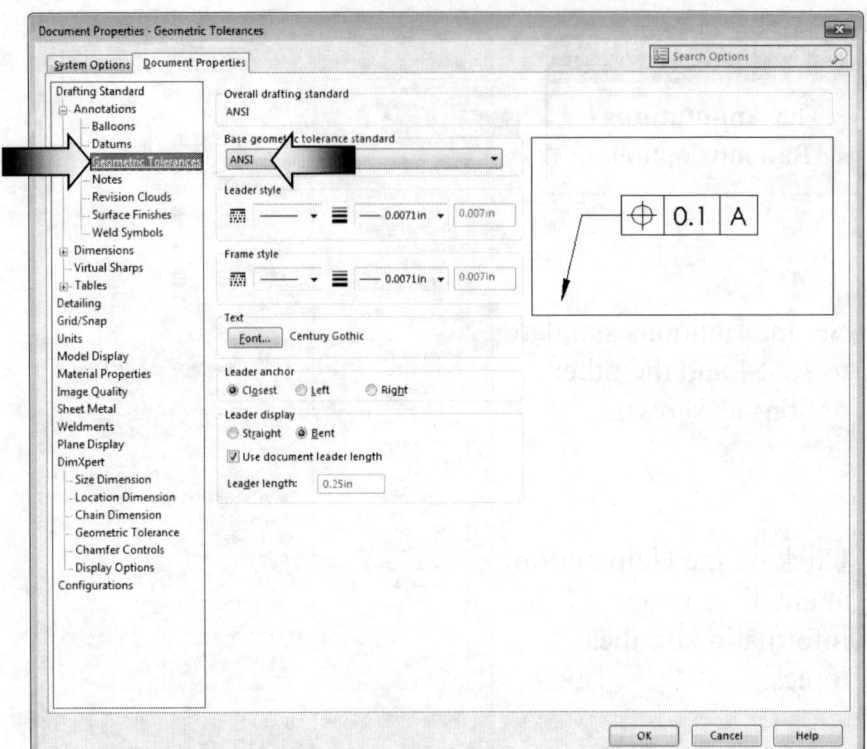

- Set the Geometric-
Tolerance standard to
ANSI.

- The Font selection
should match the other
options for all
annotations.

Document Properties

The **Annotations /
Notes** options

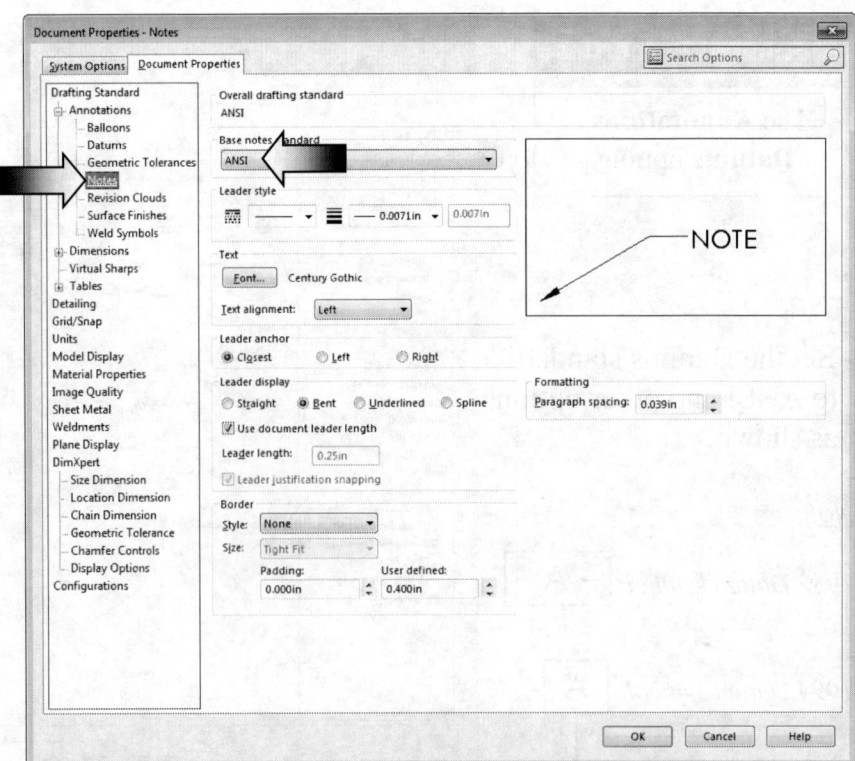

- Set the Notes standard
to ANSI.

- Use the same settings
for Font and Leader
display.

Document Properties

The **Revision Clouds** options

- Use Revision Clouds to call attention to geometry changes in a drawing.

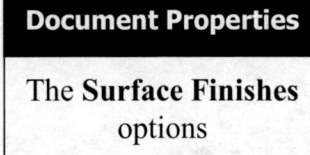

Document Properties

The **Surface Finishes** options

- Set the Surface Finish standard to ANSI and set the Leader Display to match the ones in the previous options.

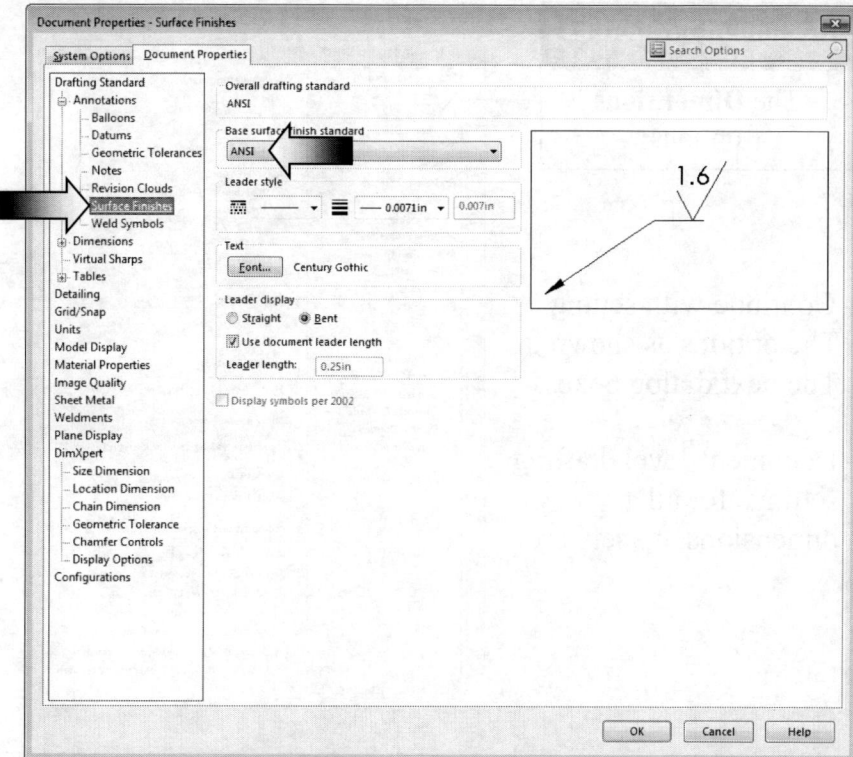

Document Properties

The **Annotations / Weld Symbols** options

- Set the Weld Symbols standard to ANSI.

- Clear the Fixed Size Weld Symbols checkbox to scale the size of the symbol to the symbol font size.

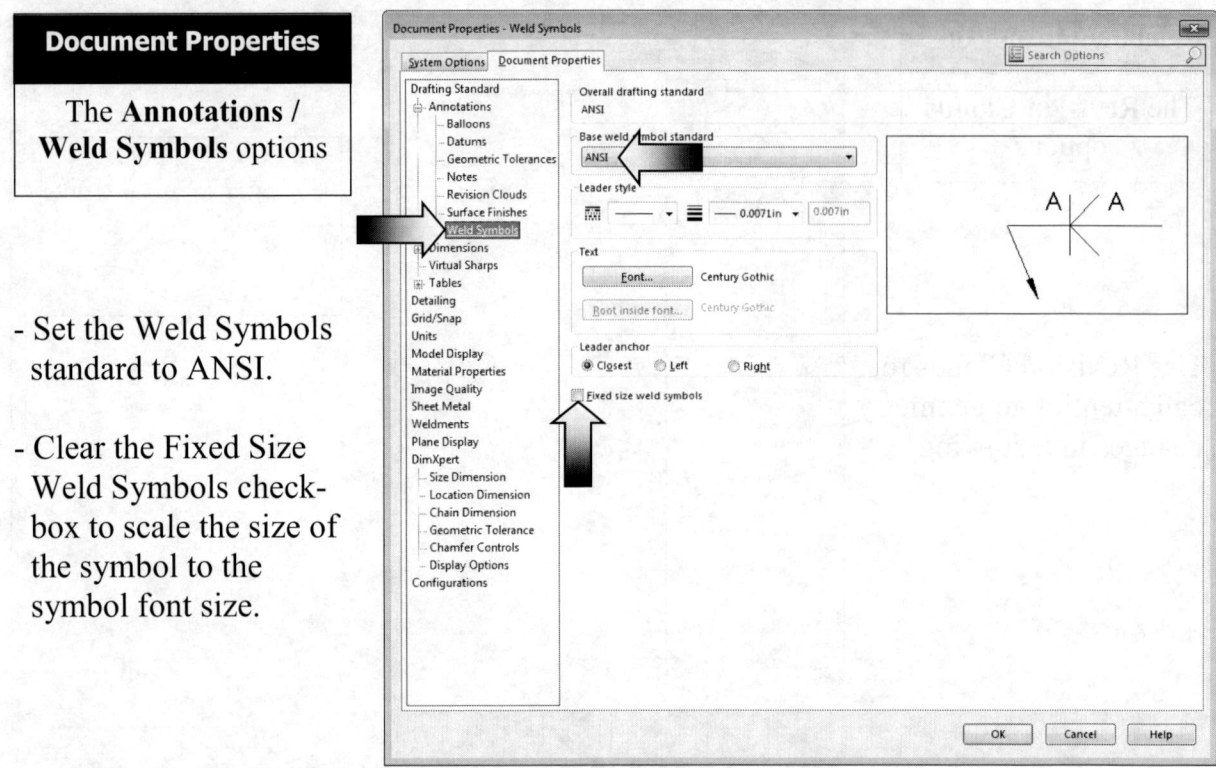

Document Properties

The **Dimensions** options

- Continue with setting The options as shown in The next dialog boxes.

- Document-level drafting settings for all dimensions are set here.

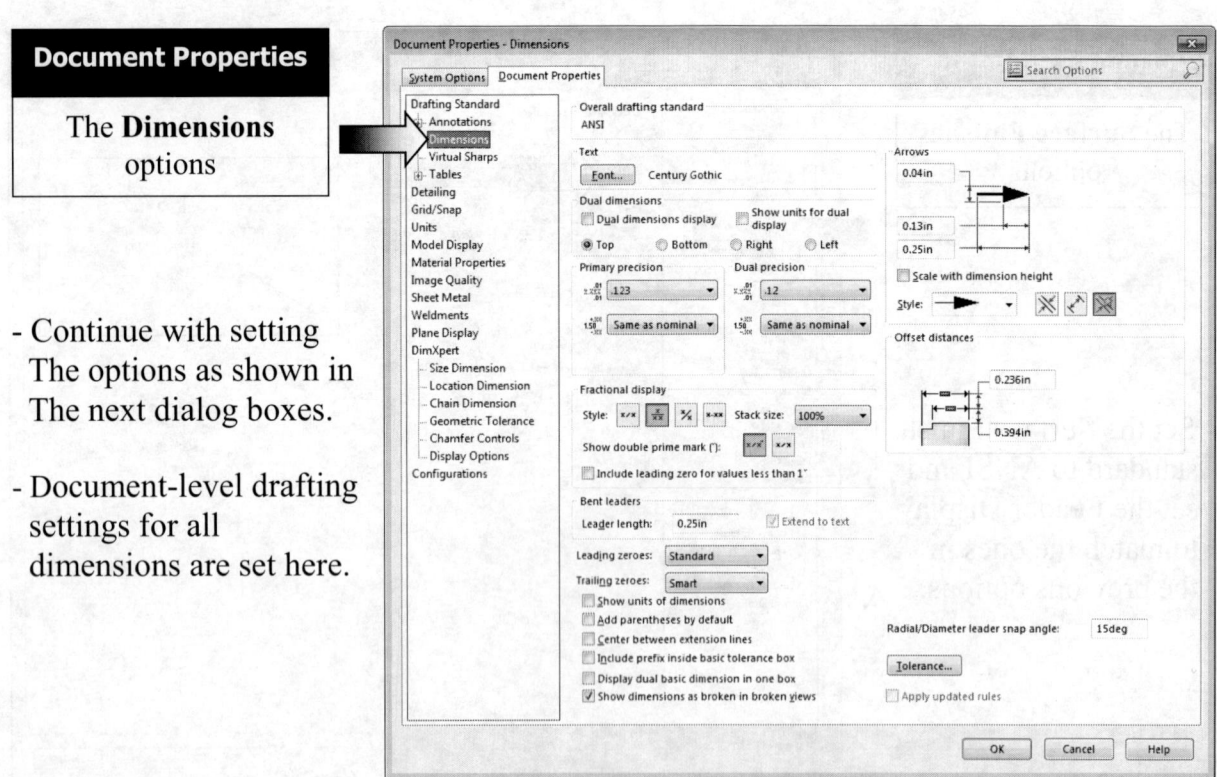

Document Properties

The **Dimensions /
Angle** options

- Set the Angle Dimension
standard to ANSI and set
the other options shown.

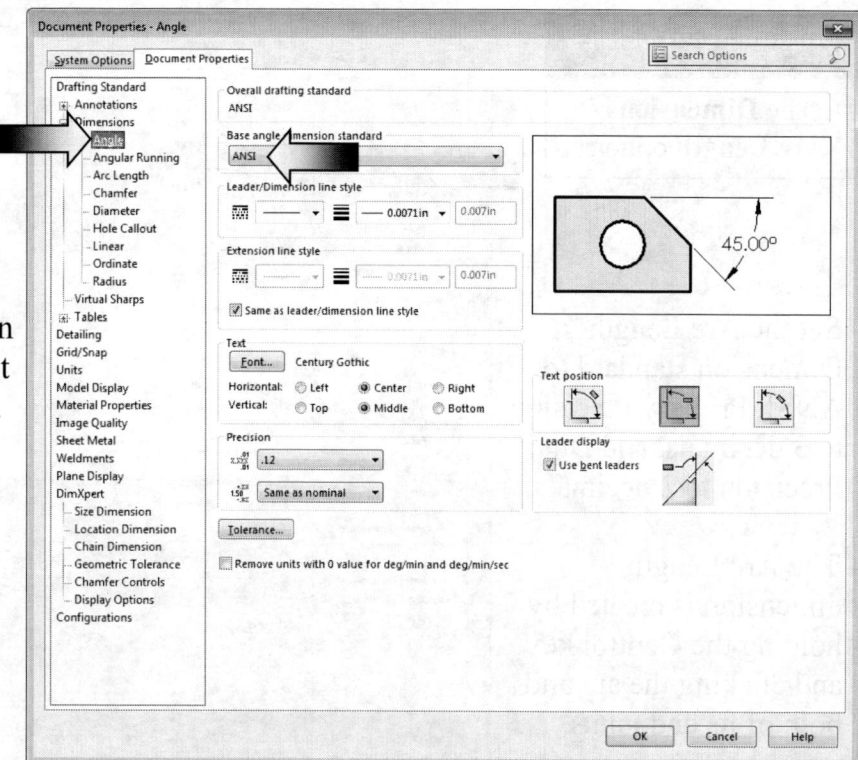

Document Properties

The **Angular
Running** options

- A set of dimensions
measured from a zero-
degree dimension in a
sketch or drawing.

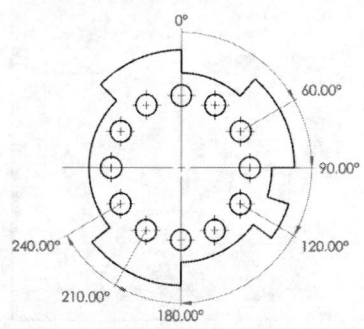

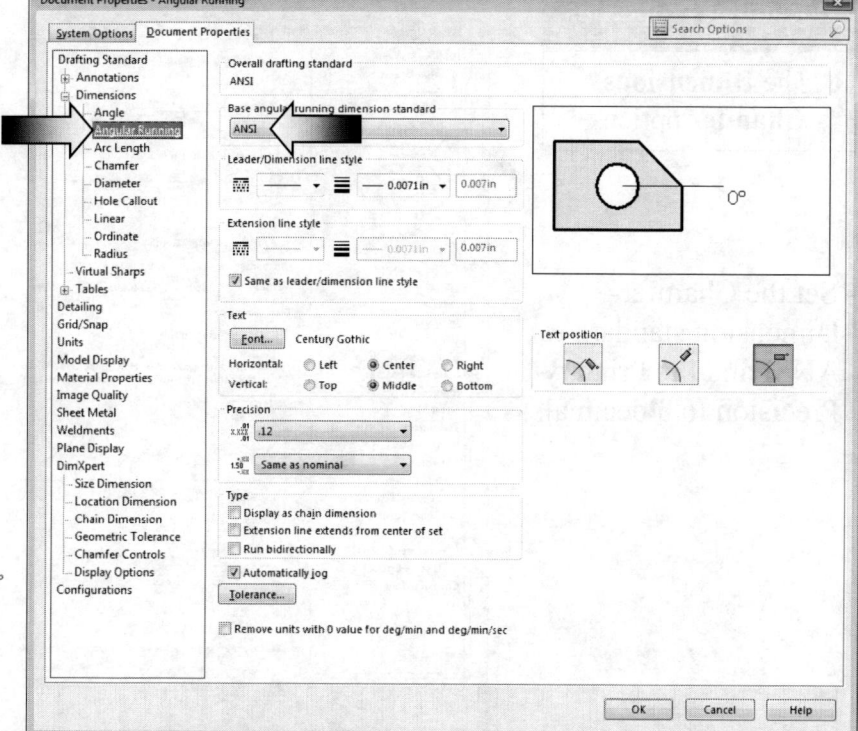

Document Properties

The **Dimensions** / **Arc Length** options

- Set the Arc Length Dimension standard to ANSI, Primary Precision to 3 decimals, and Dual Precision to 2 decimals.

- The Arc Length dimension is created by holding the Control key and clicking the arc and both of its endpoints.

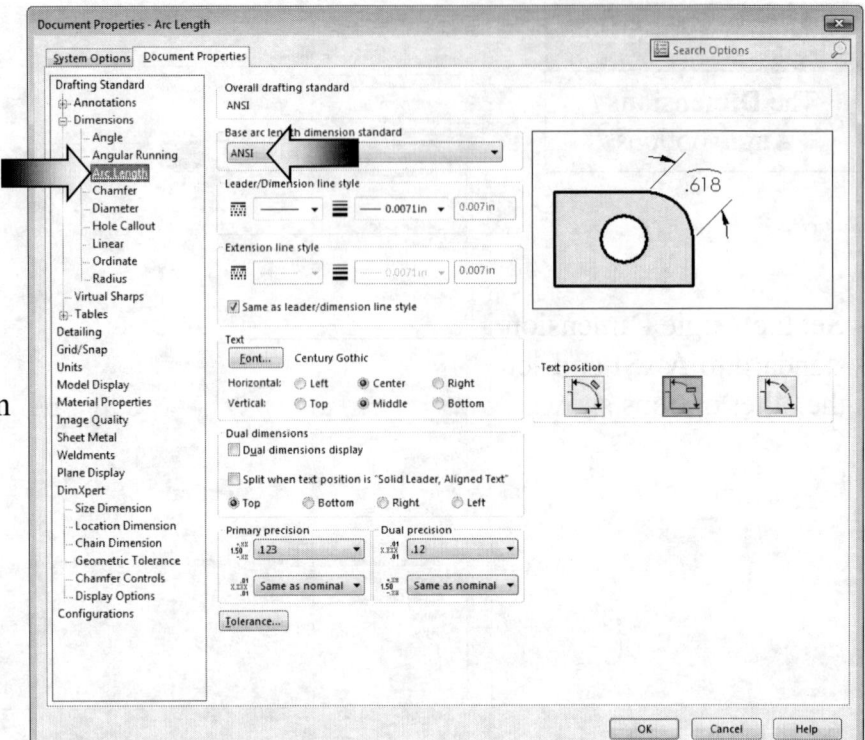

Document Properties

The **Dimensions** / **Chamfer** options

- Set the Chamfer-Dimension standard to ANSI and the Primary-Precision to 3 decimals.

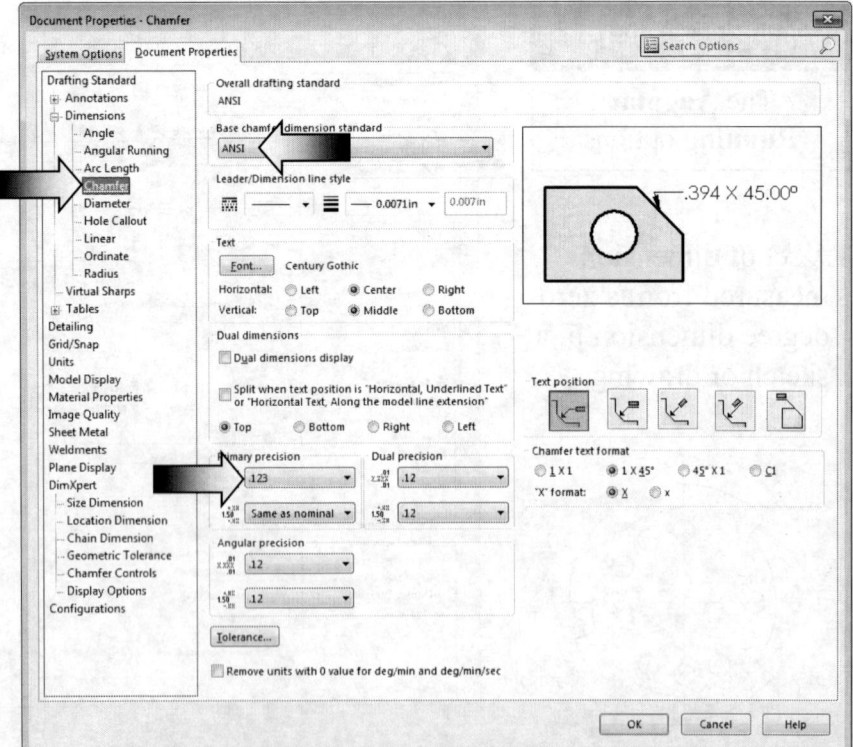

Document Properties

The **Dimensions /
Diameter** options

- Set the Diameter-
Dimension standard to
ANSI.

- Set the Leader Style and
thickness here.

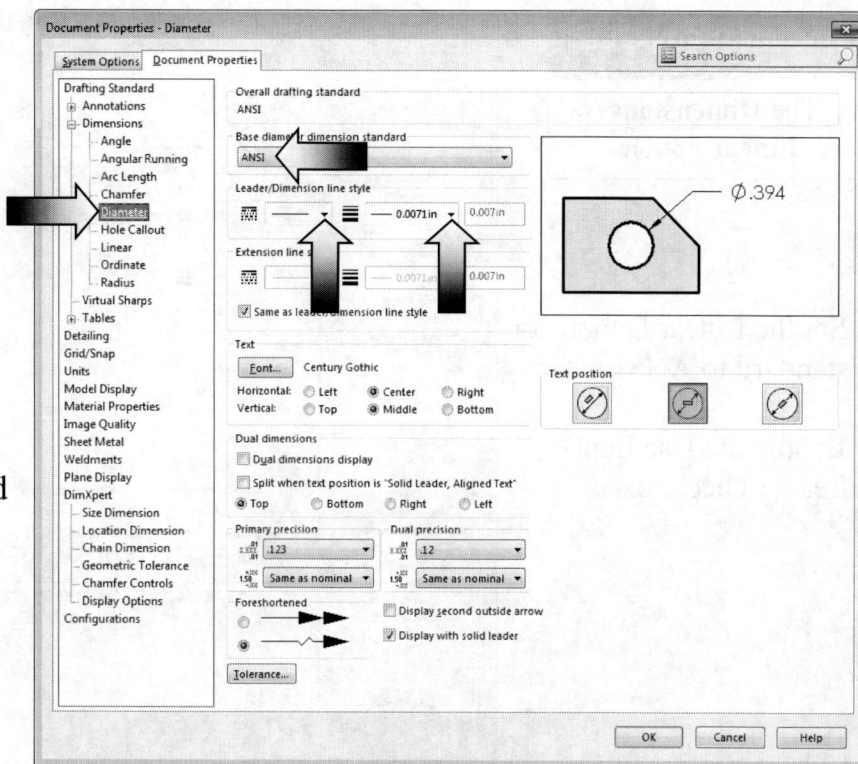

Document Properties

The **Dimensions /
Hole Callout** options

- Set the Hole Callout
Dimension standard
to ANSI.

- Set the Text justification
positions to Center and
Middle.

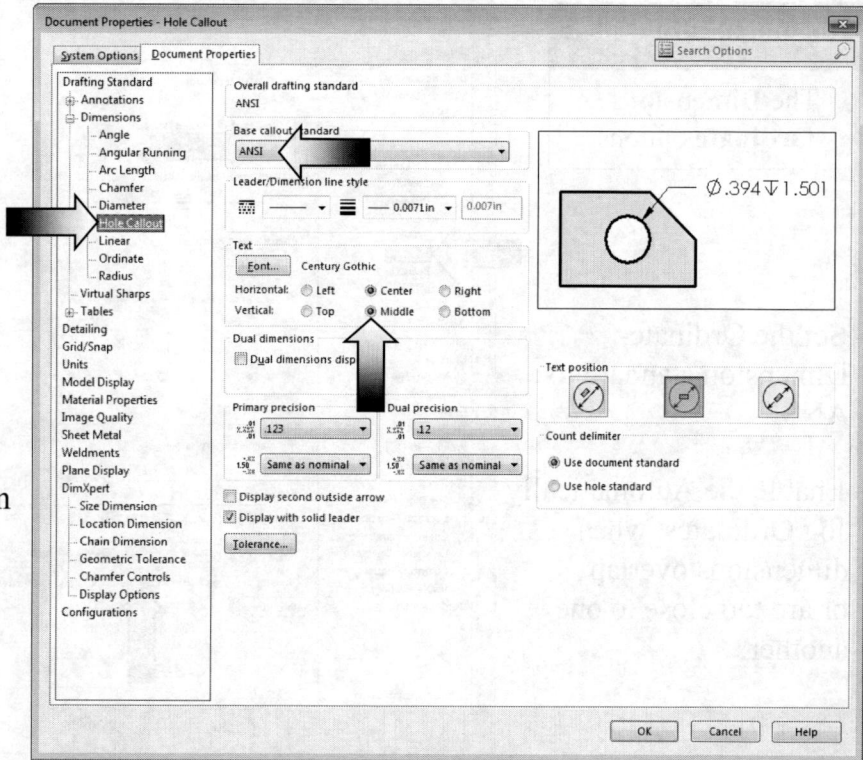

Document Properties

The **Dimensions** /
Linear options

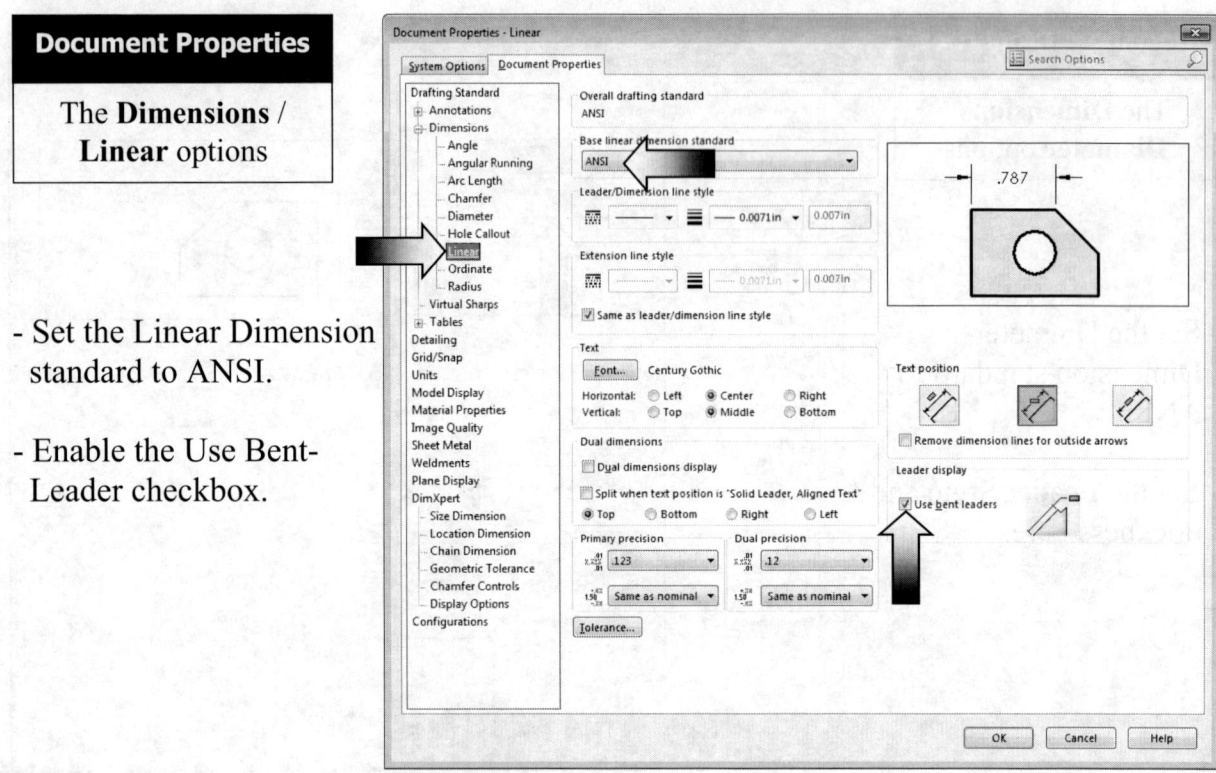

- Set the Linear Dimension
standard to ANSI.

- Enable the Use Bent-
Leader checkbox.

Document Properties

The **Dimensions** /
Ordinate options

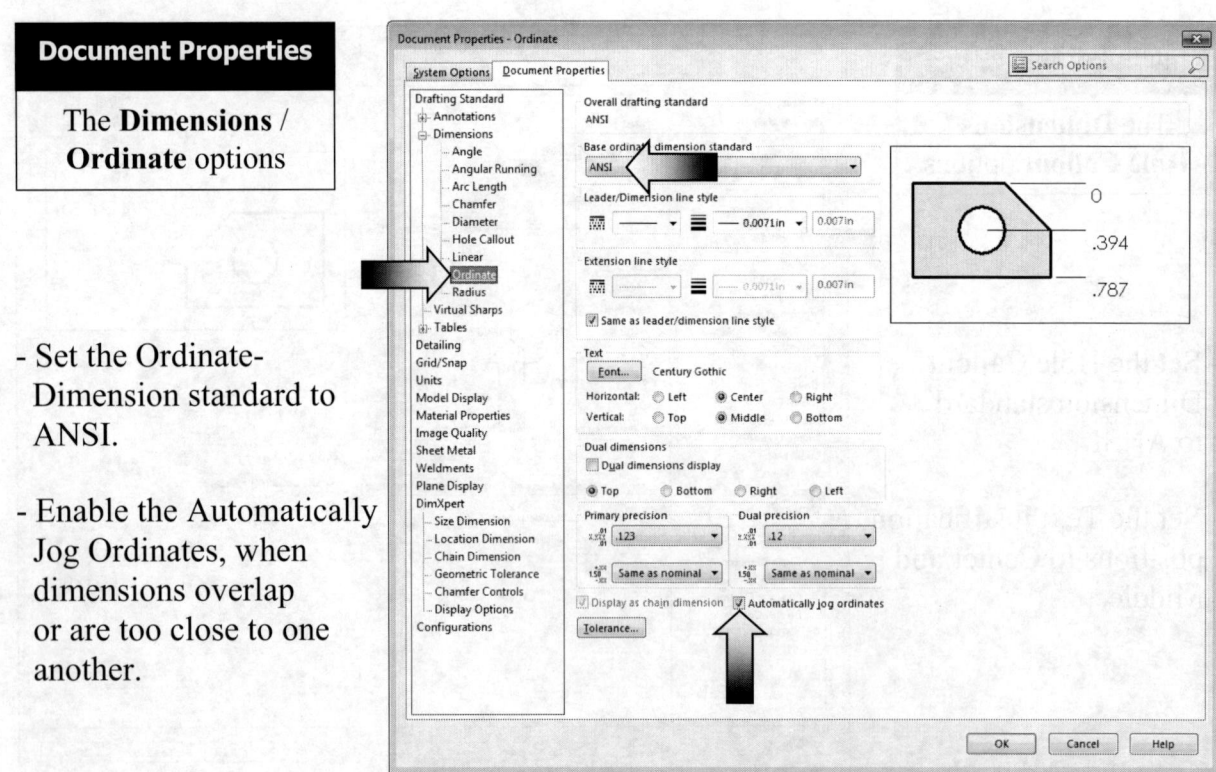

- Set the Ordinate-
Dimension standard to
ANSI.

- Enable the Automatically
Jog Ordinates, when
dimensions overlap
or are too close to one
another.

Document Properties

The **Dimensions /
Radius** options

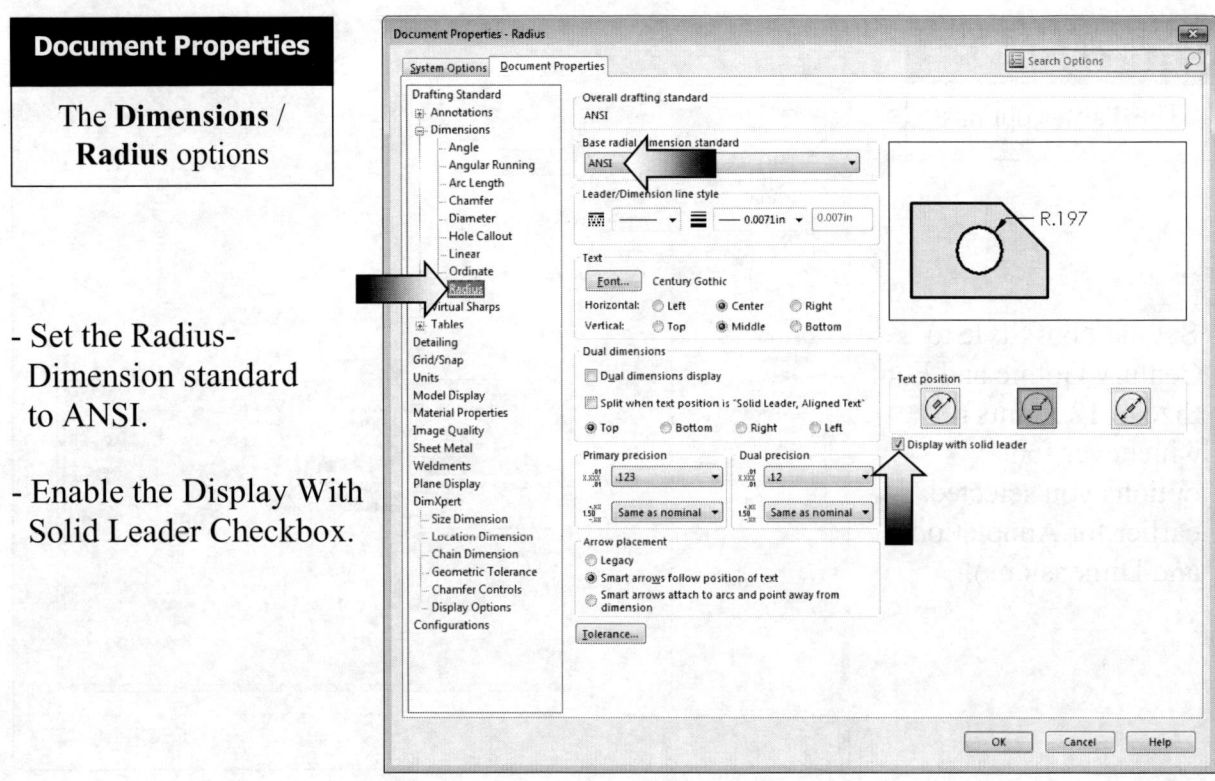

- Set the Radius-
Dimension standard
to ANSI.

- Enable the Display With
Solid Leader Checkbox.

Document Properties

The **Virtual Sharps**
options

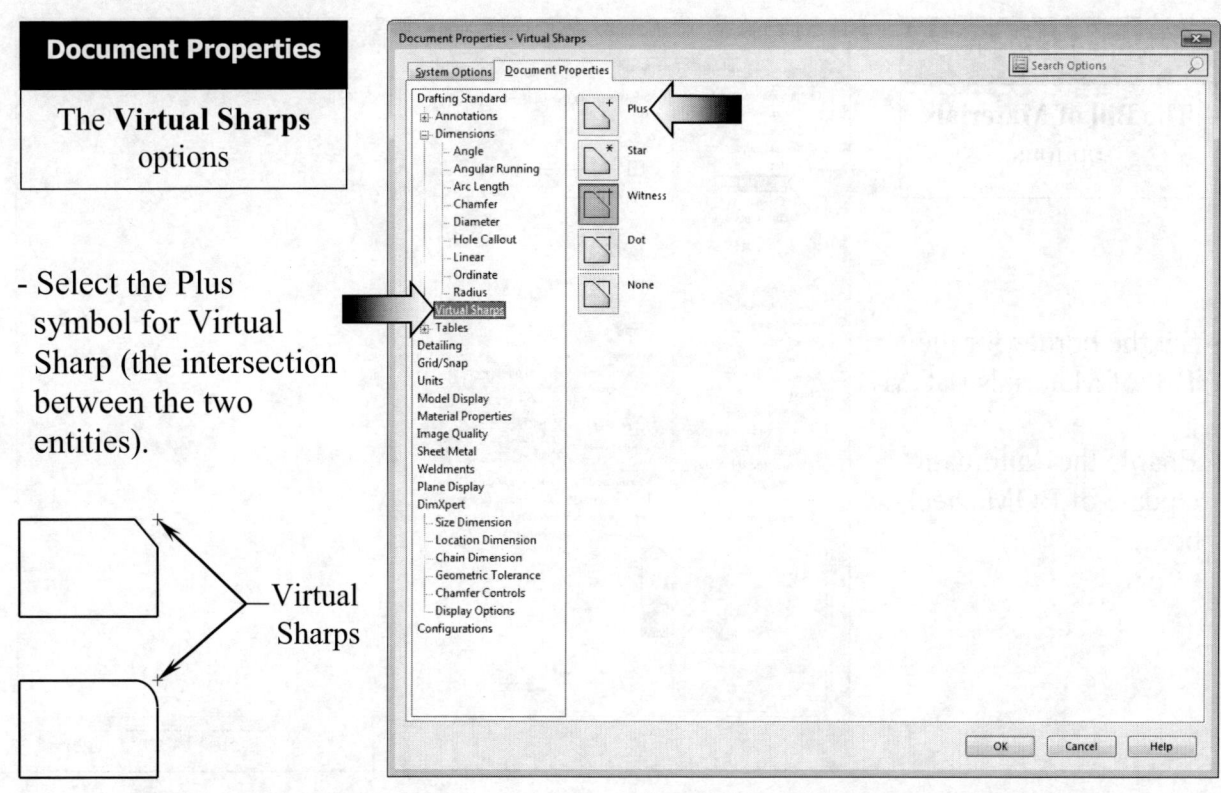

- Select the Plus
symbol for Virtual
Sharp (the intersection
between the two
entities).

Virtual
Sharps

Document Properties

The **Tables** options

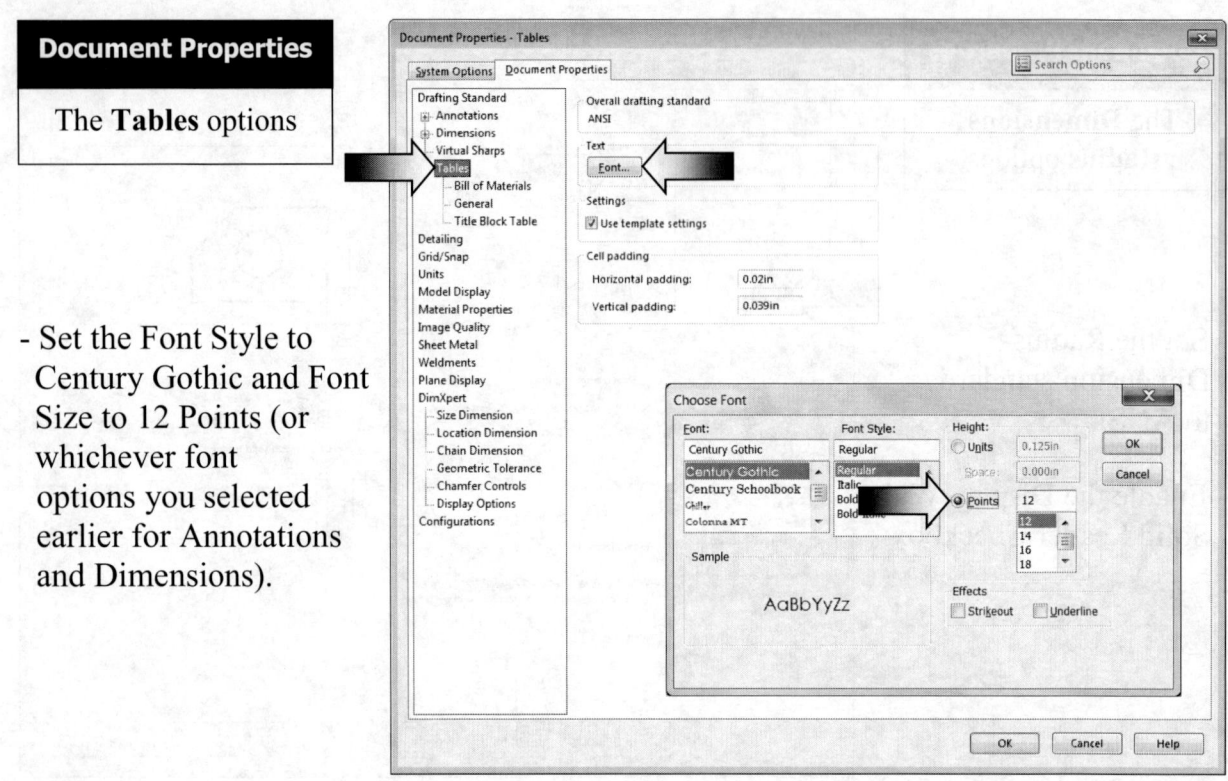

- Set the Font Style to
Century Gothic and Font
Size to 12 Points (or
whichever font
options you selected
earlier for Annotations
and Dimensions).

Document Properties

The **Bill of Materials**
options

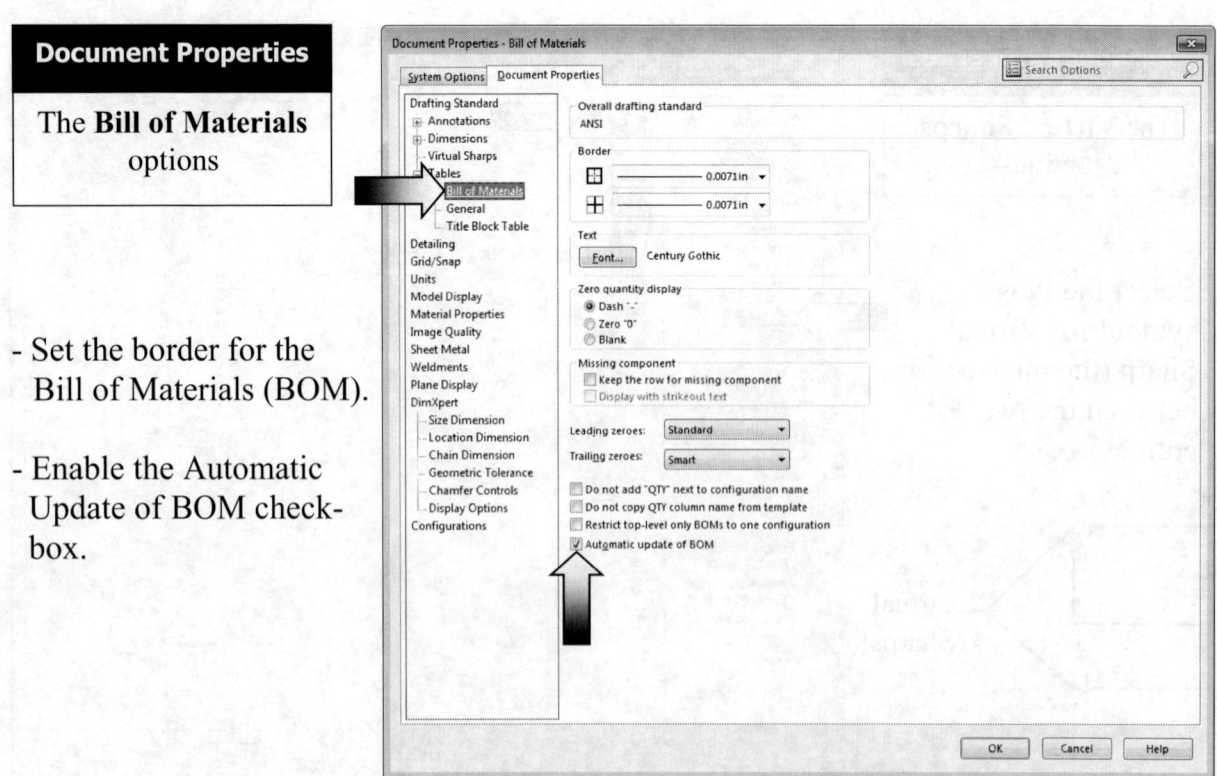

- Set the border for the
Bill of Materials (BOM).

- Enable the Automatic
Update of BOM check-
box.

Document Properties

The **General** options

- Create a General Table to use in a drawing. The user inputs data in the cell manually.

- Set the line thickness for the border of the table here.

Document Properties

The **Title Block Table** options

- Set the border for the Title Block Table.

- Set the thickness and the Font for the Title Block Table to match the BOM border.

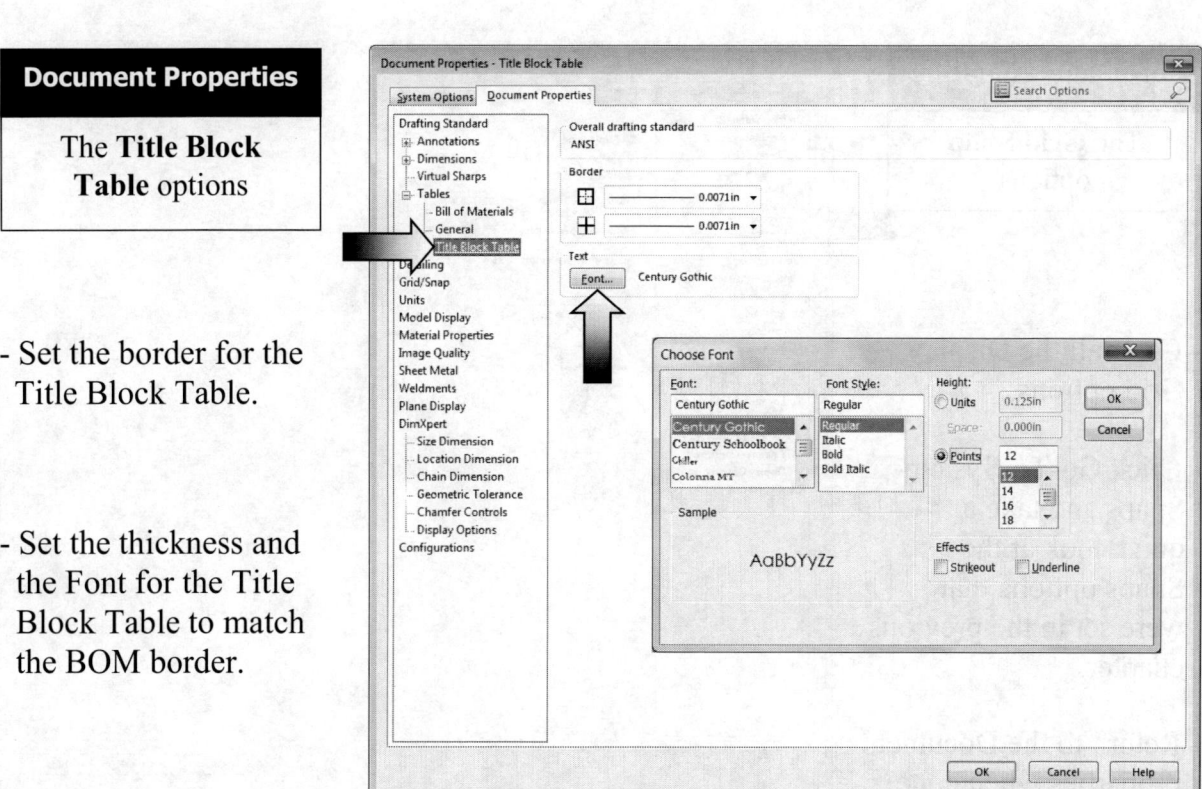

Document Properties

The **Detailing** options

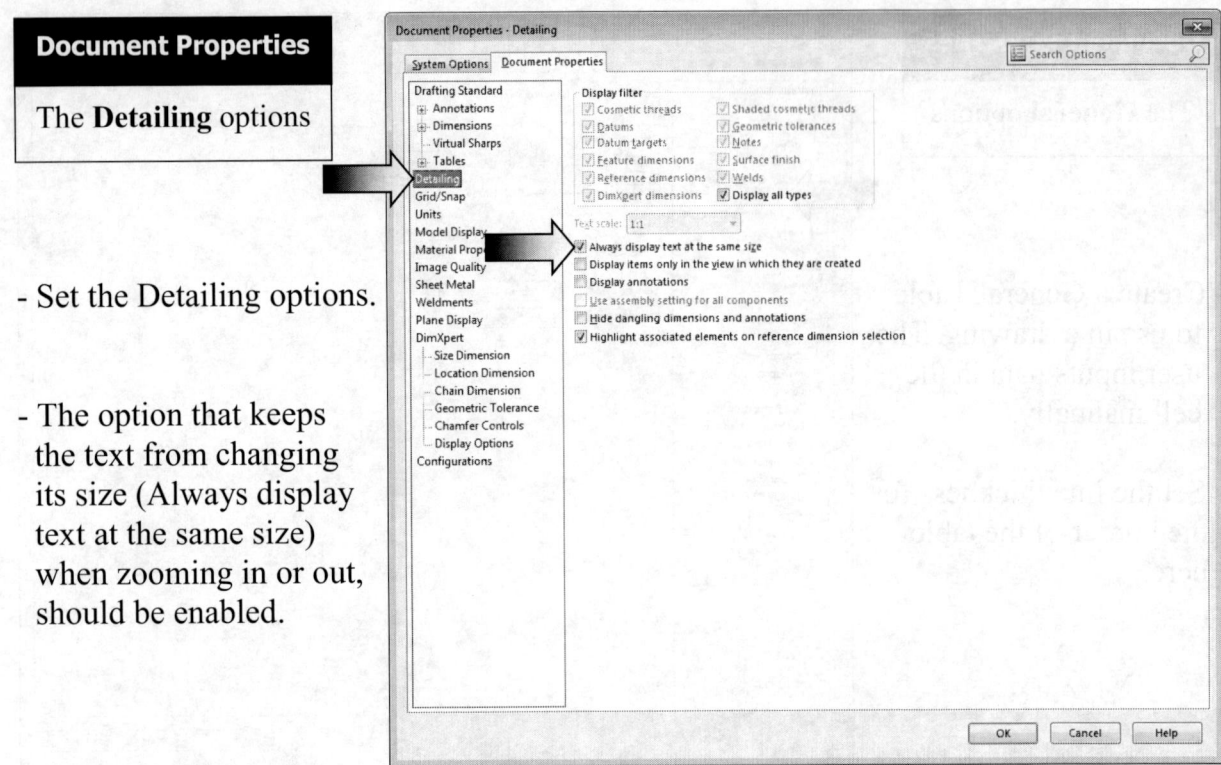

- Set the Detailing options.

- The option that keeps the text from changing its size (Always display text at the same size) when zooming in or out, should be enabled.

Document Properties

The **Grid/Snap** options

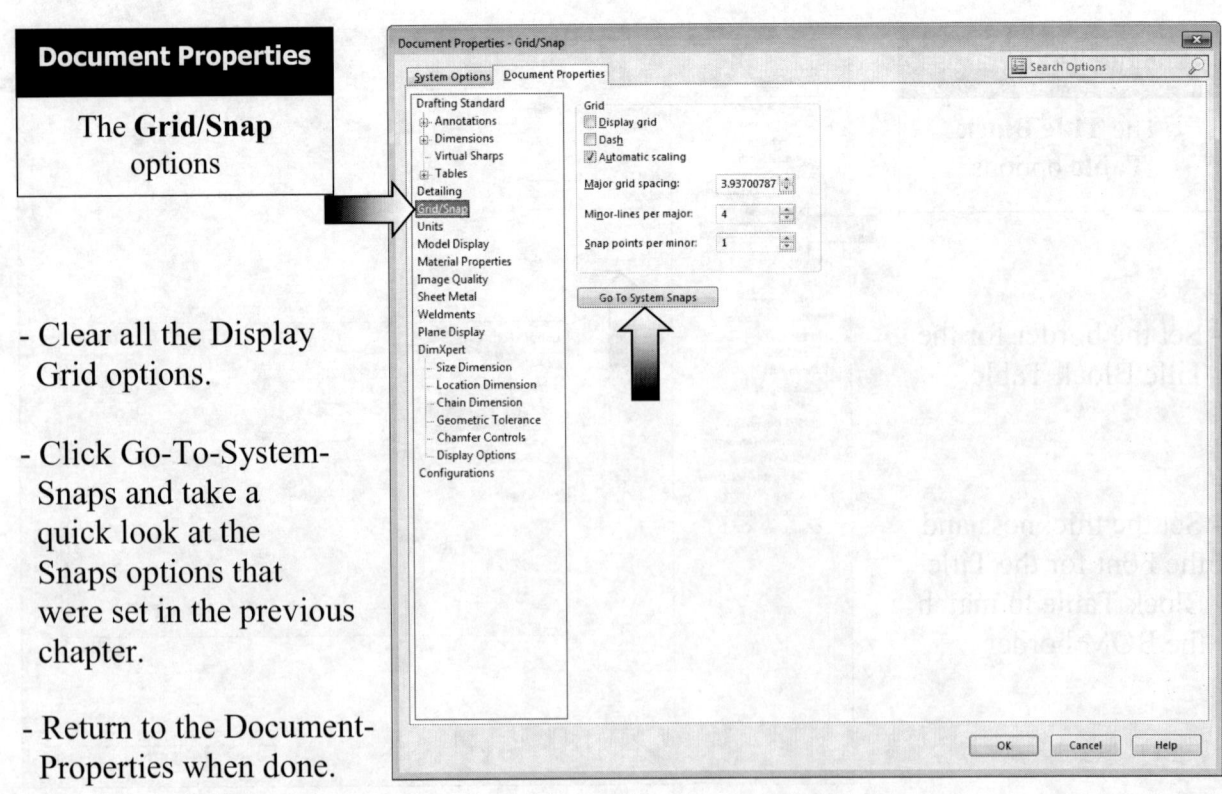

- Clear all the Display Grid options.

- Click Go-To-System-Snaps and take a quick look at the Snaps options that were set in the previous chapter.

- Return to the Document-Properties when done.

Document Properties

The **Units** options

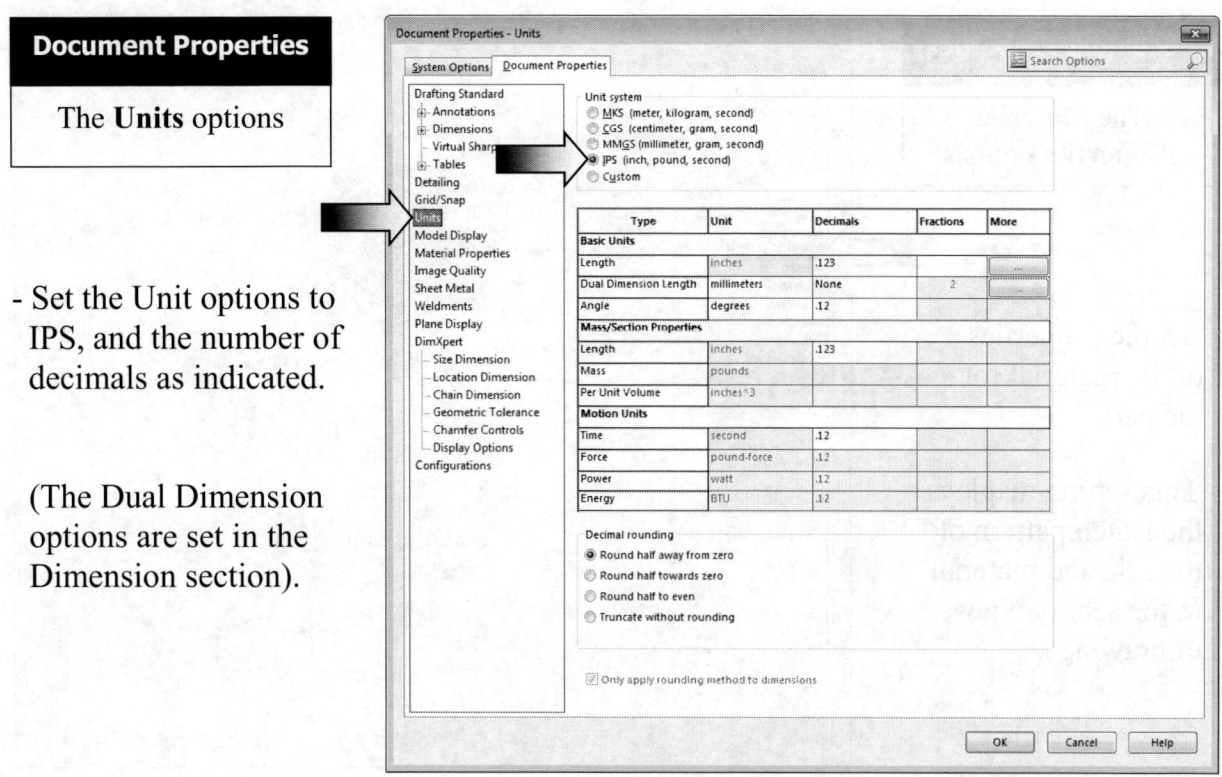

- Set the Unit options to IPS, and the number of decimals as indicated.

(The Dual Dimension options are set in the Dimension section).

Document Properties

The **Model Display** options

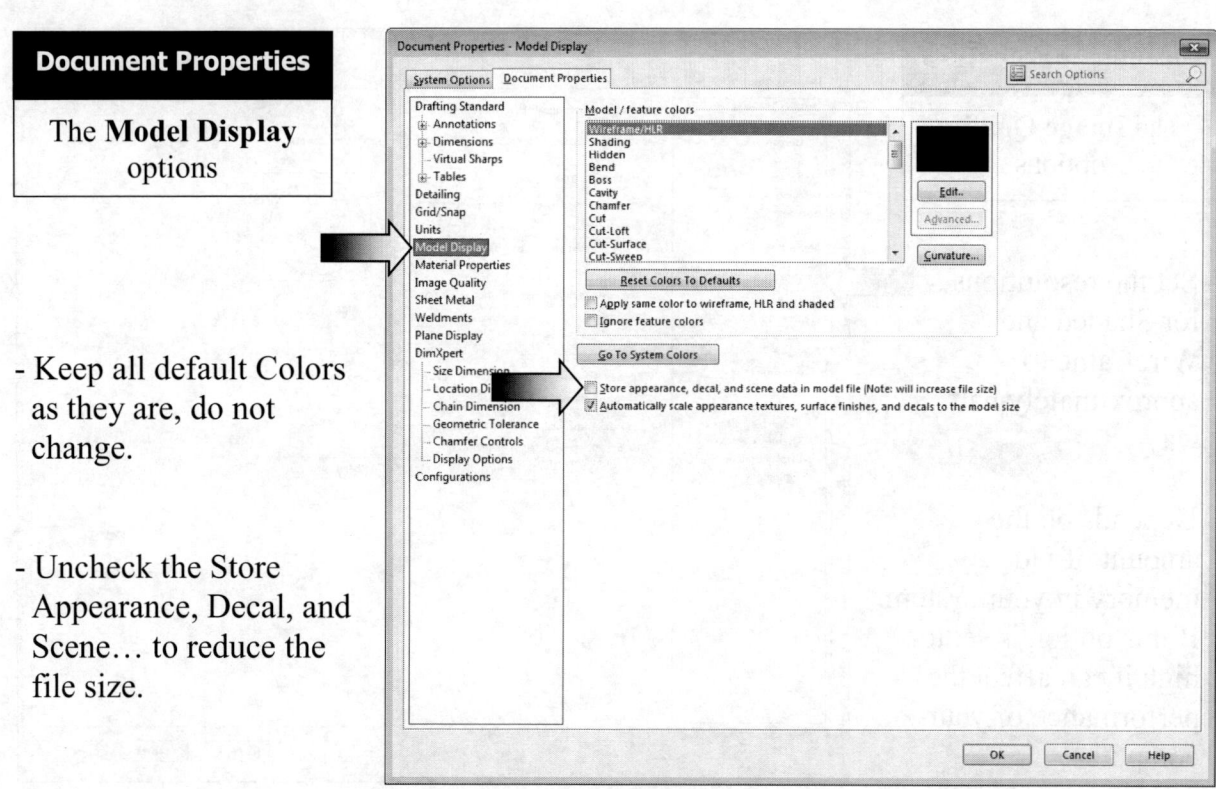

- Keep all default Colors as they are, do not change.

- Uncheck the Store Appearance, Decal, and Scene… to reduce the file size.

Document Properties

The **Material Properties** options

- Set the properties of the material for the part.

- This setting displays the Hatch pattern of the selected material in the section views of drawings.

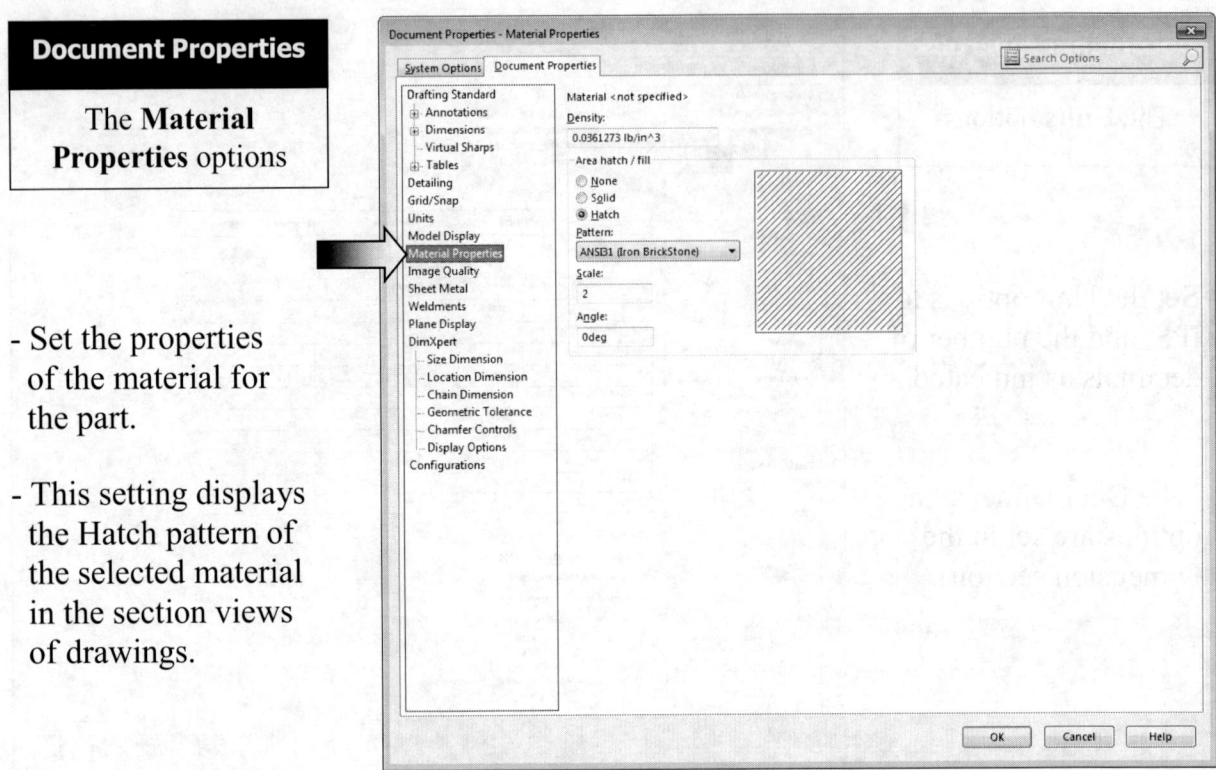

Document Properties

The **Image Quality** options

- Set the resolutions for Shaded and Wireframe to approximately half way...

- Depends on the amount of video memory in your system. If this option is set too high it can affect the performance of your computer.

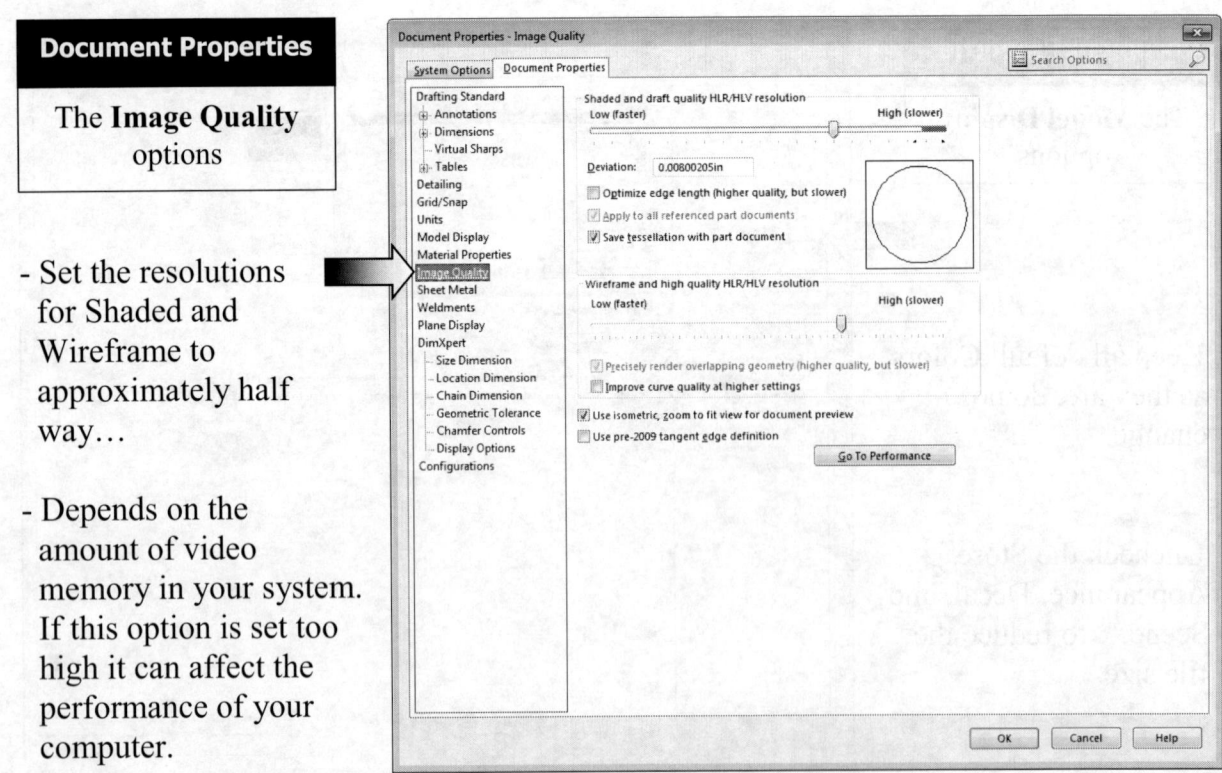

Document Properties

The **Sheet Metal**
options

- Set the Sheet Metal
options as shown.

- These options vary
depending on
whether you are
working with a part,
assembly, or drawing.
Click the Help button
for more information
about these settings.

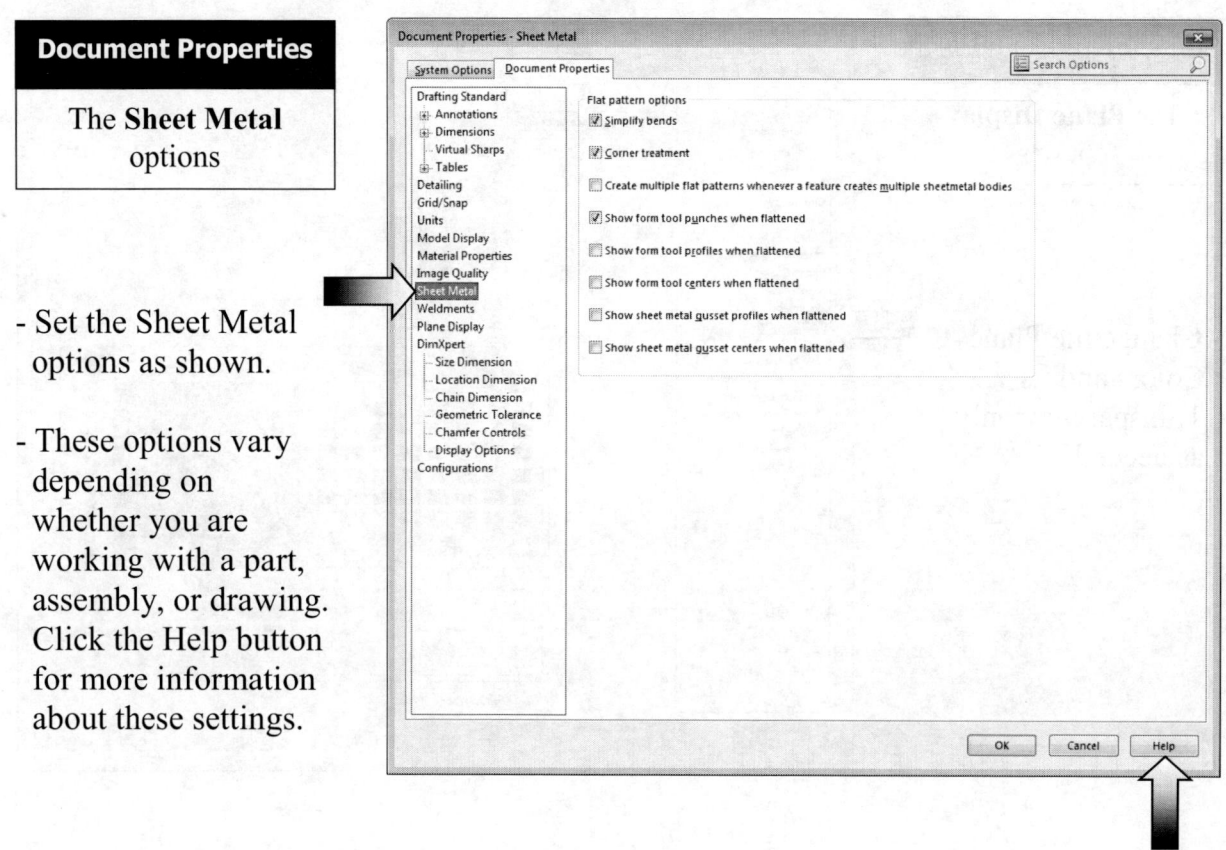

Document Properties

The **Weldments**
options

- Sets the weldments
behaviors per document
basis.

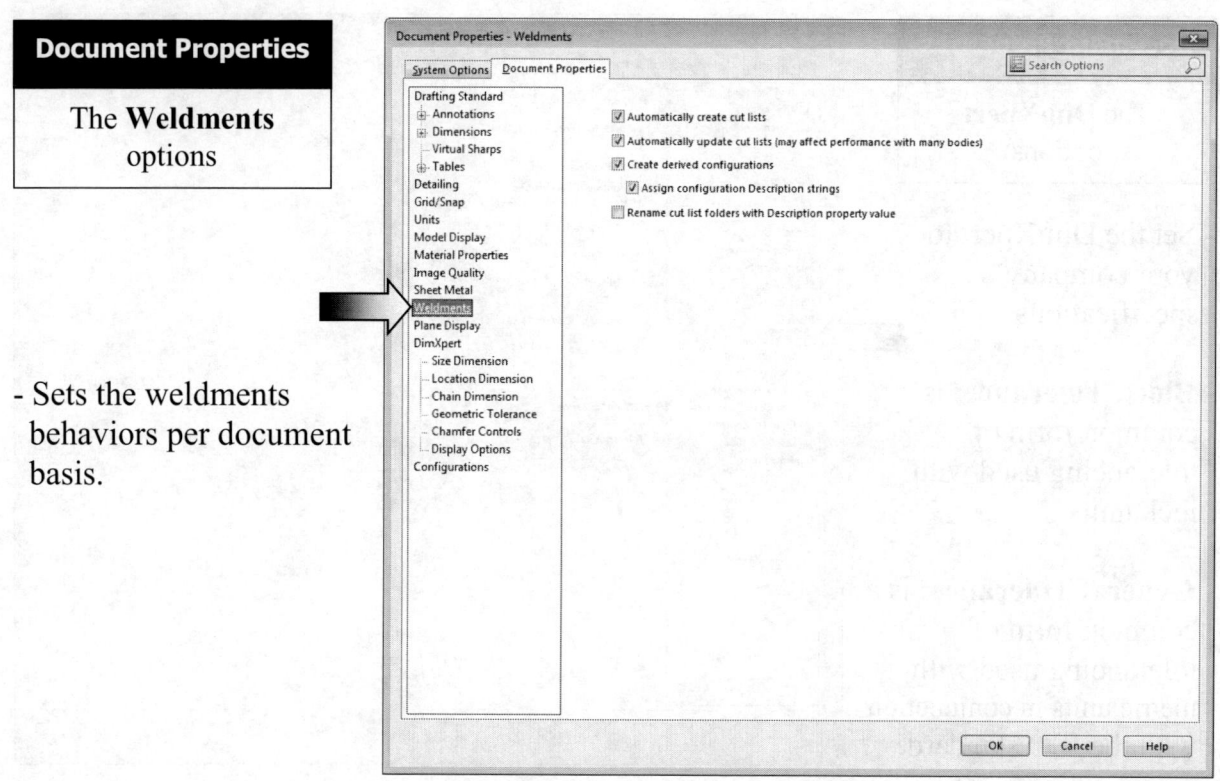

Document Properties

The **Plane Display** options

- Change the Plane Colors and its Transparency only as needed.

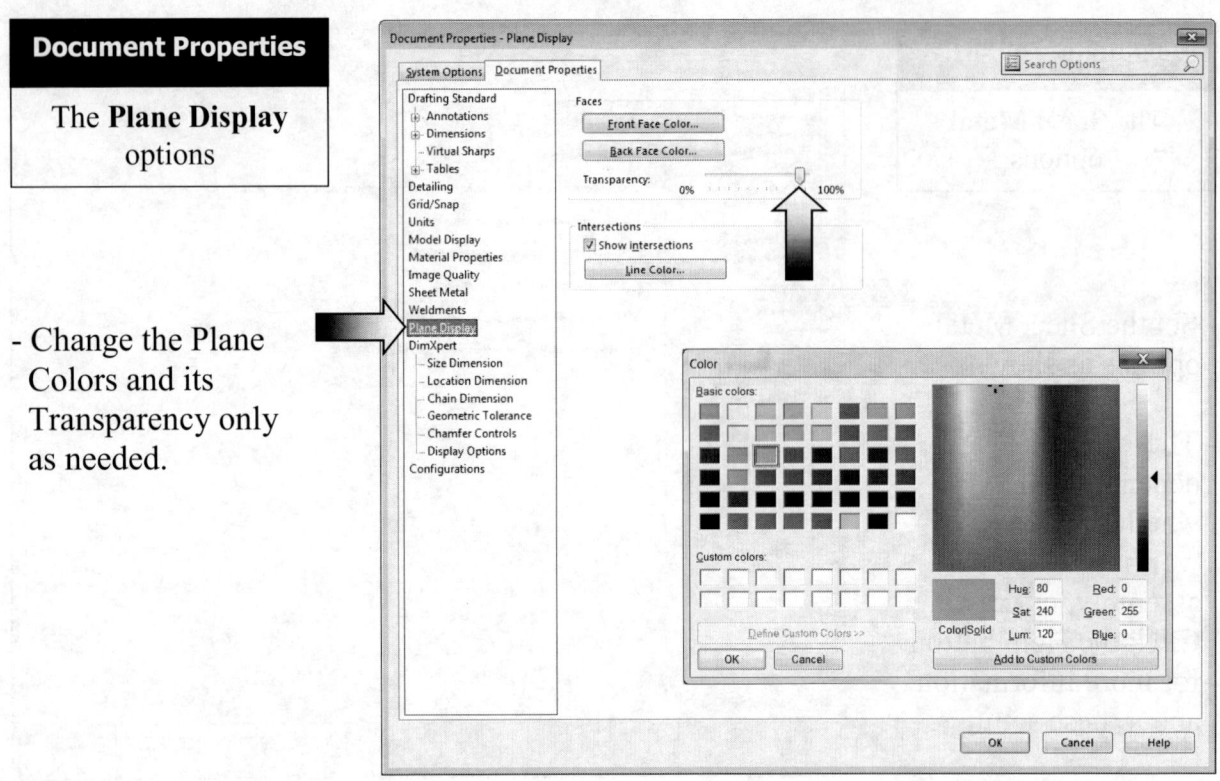

Document Properties

The **DimXpert** options

- Set the DimXpert to your company's specifications.

- **Block Tolerance:** is a common form of tolerancing used with inch units.

- **General Tolerance:** is a common form of tolerancing used with metric units in conjunction with the ISO standard.

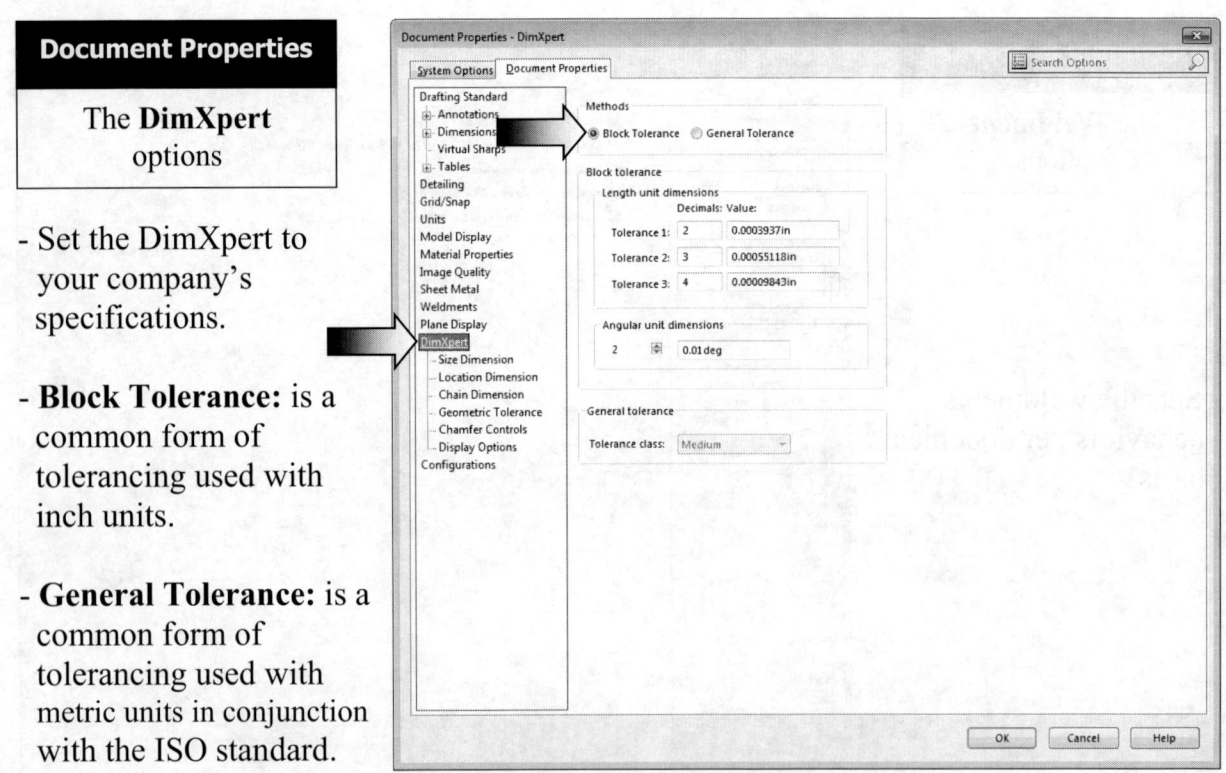

Document Properties

The **Size Dimension** options

- Set per company Std.

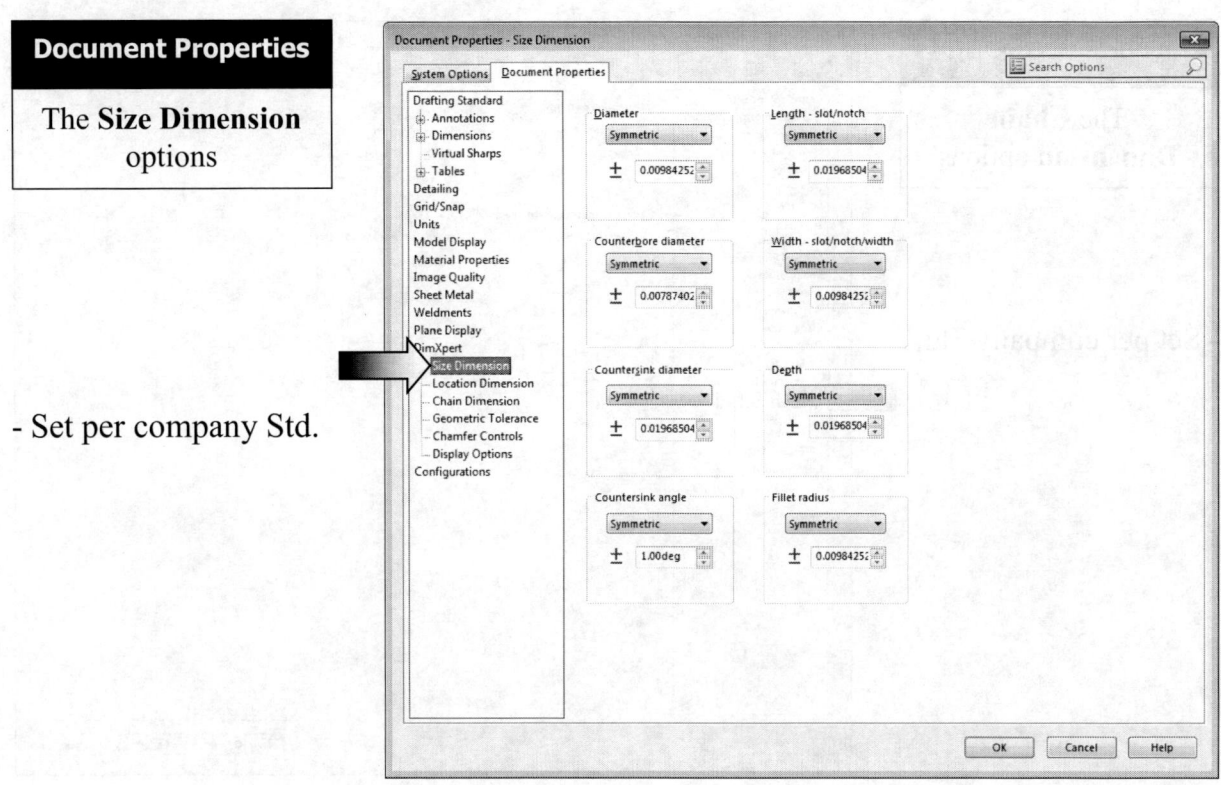

Document Properties

The **Location-Dimension** options

- Set per company Std.

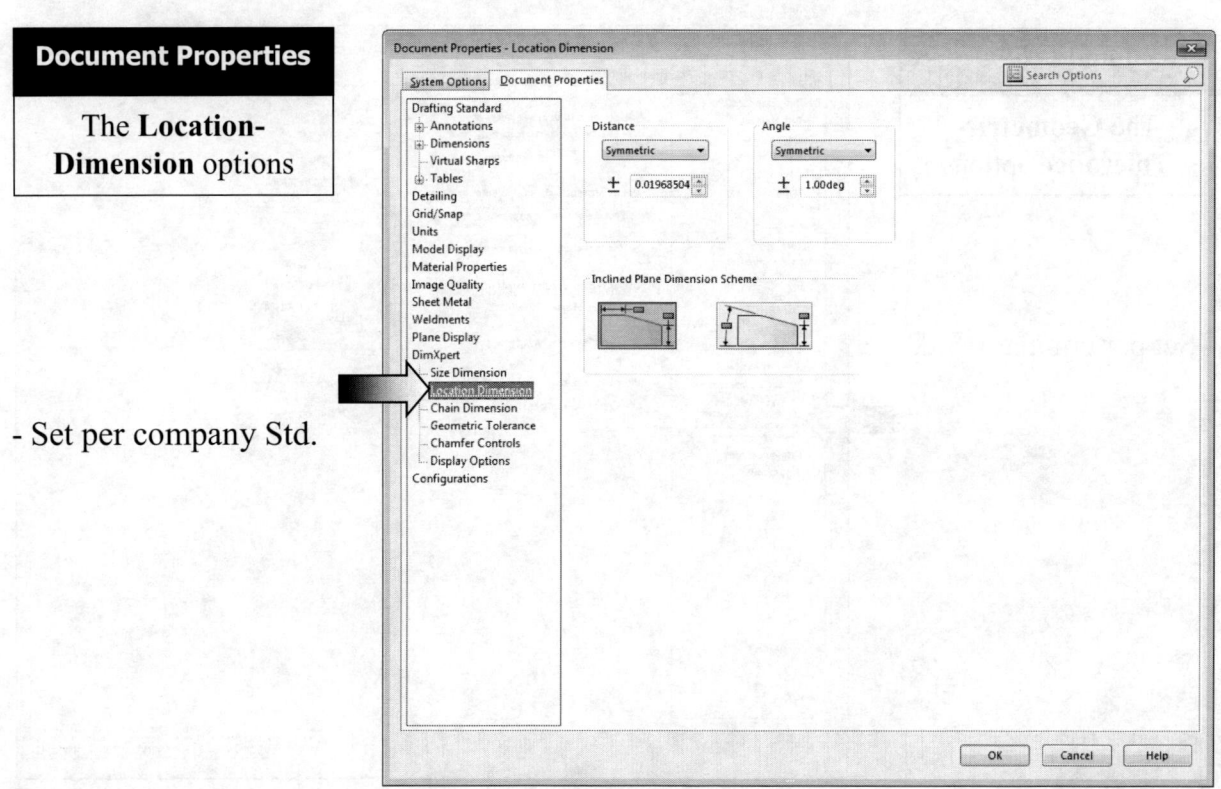

Document Properties

The **Chain Dimension** options

- Set per company Std.

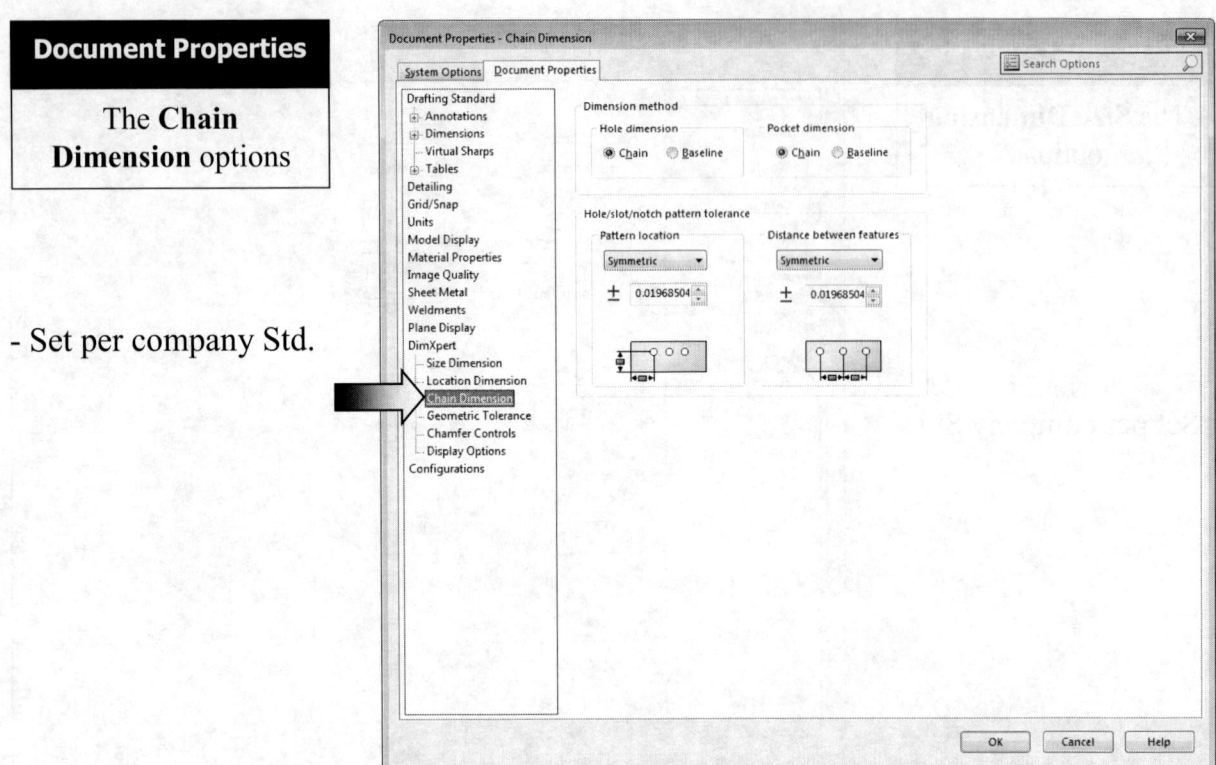

Document Properties

The **Geometric-Tolerance** options

- Set per company Std.

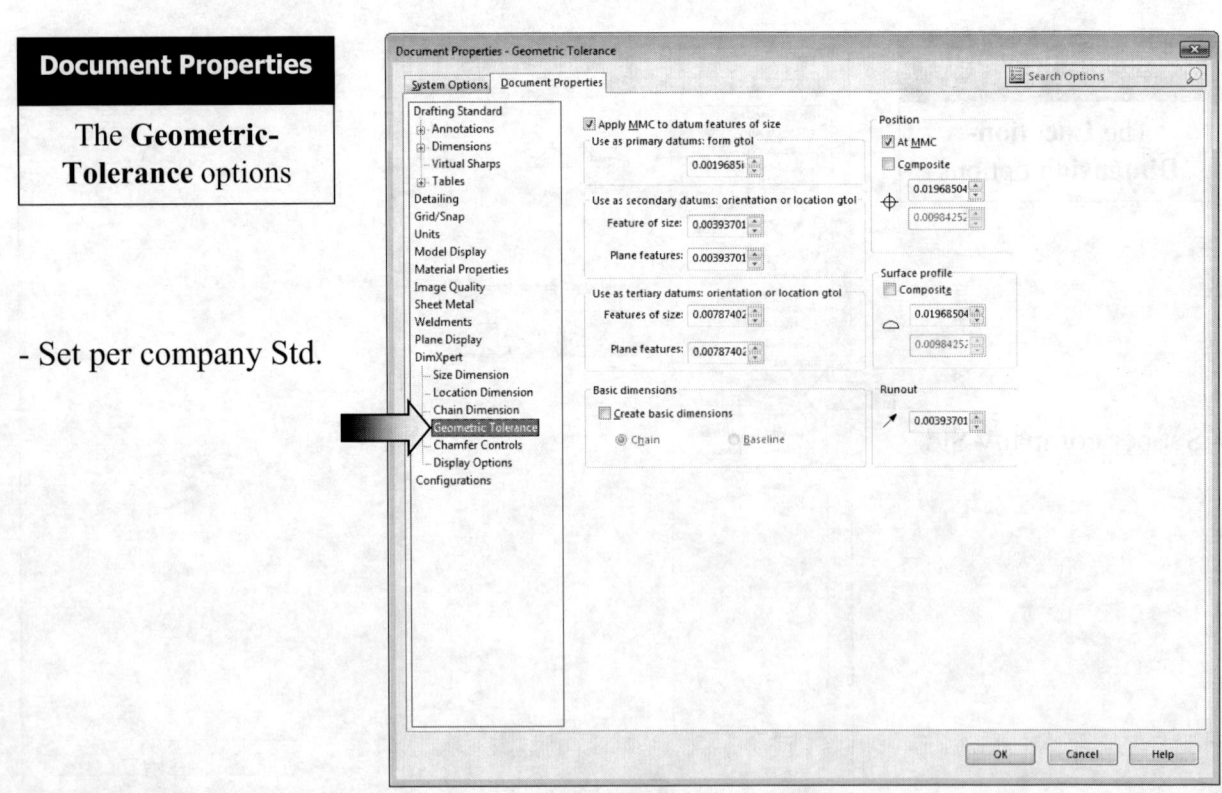

Document Properties

The **Chamfer-Controls** options

- Set per company Std.

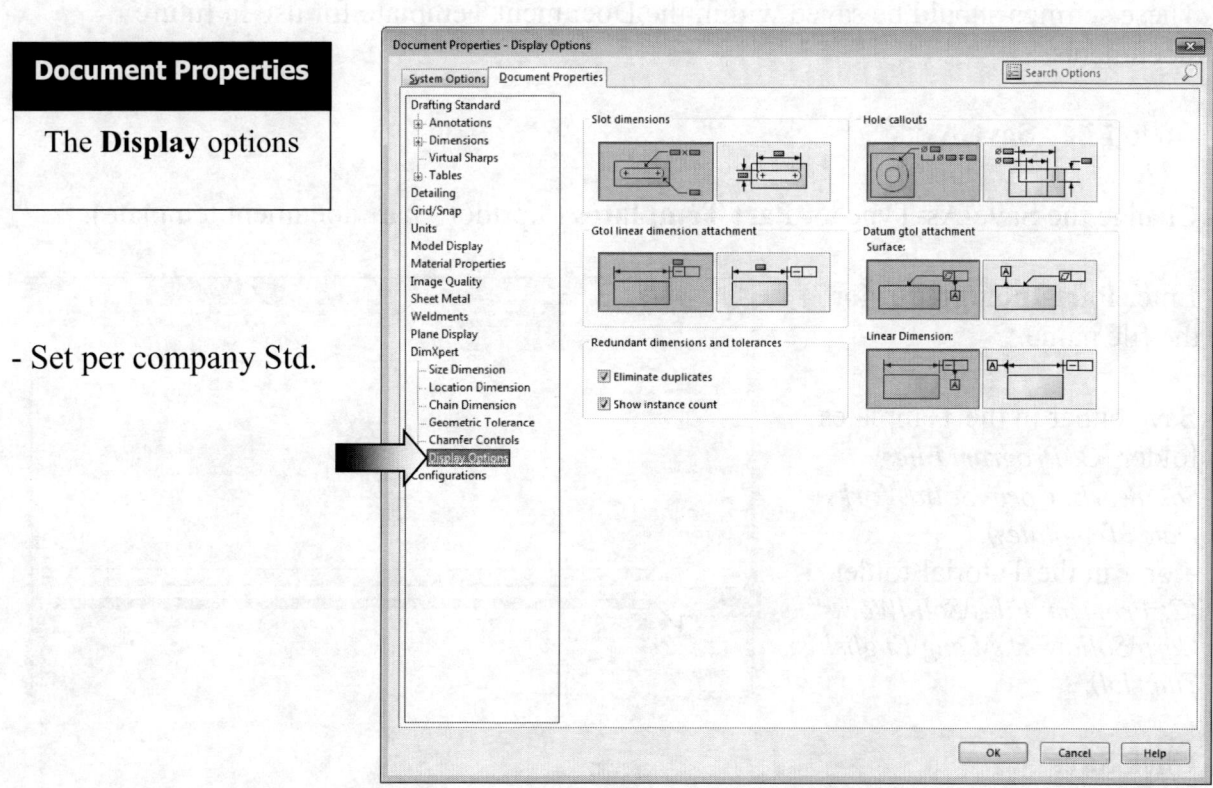

Document Properties

The **Display** options

- Set per company Std.

Document Properties

The **Configurations** option

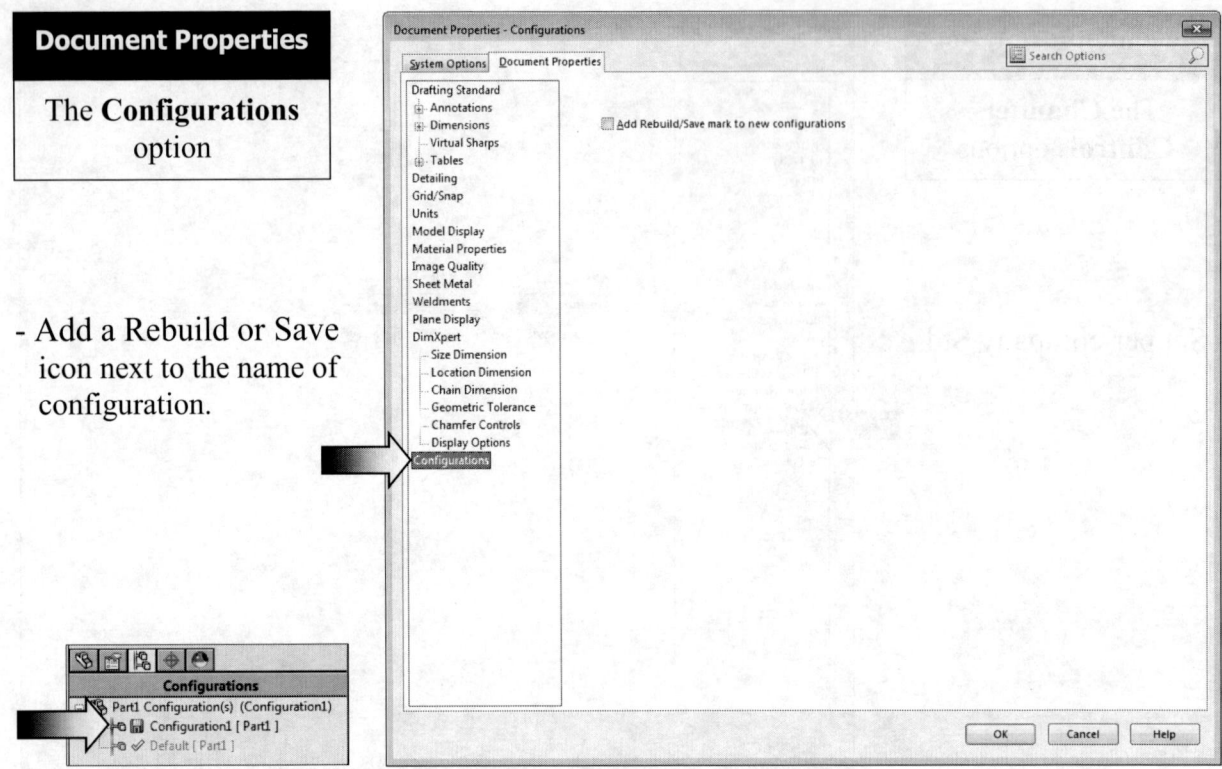

- Add a Rebuild or Save icon next to the name of configuration.

Saving the settings as a Part Template:

- These settings should be saved within the Document Template for use in future documents.

- Go to **File / Save As.**

- Change the Save-As-Type to: **Part Templates** (*.prtdot - part document template).

- Enter **Part-Inch.prtdot** for the file name.

- Save either in the Templates folder *(C:\Program Files\ Solidworks Corp\ SolidWorks\ Data\ Templates).*
  – or – in the Tutorial folder *(C:\Program Files\SolidWorks Corp\Solidworks\Lang\English\ Tutorial).*

- Click **Save**.

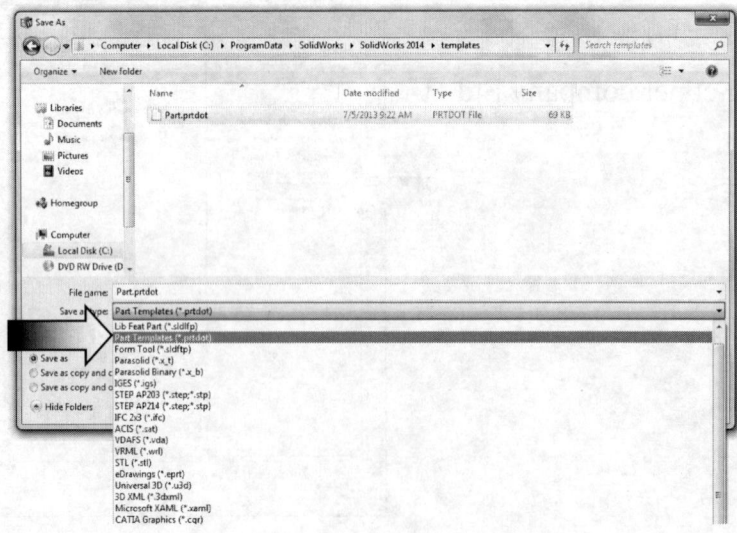

Questions for Review

Document Templates

1. The ANSI dimensioning standard (American National Standards Institute) can be set and saved in the System Options.
   - a. True
   - b. False

2. The size of dimension arrows can be controlled globally from the Document Templates.
   - a. True
   - b. False

3. The balloon's size and shape can be set and saved in the Document Templates.
   - a. True
   - b. False

4. Dimension and note fonts can be changed and edited both locally and globally.
   - a. True
   - b. False

5. The Grid option is only available in the drawing environment, not in the part or assembly.
   - a. True
   - b. False

6. The number of decimal places can be set up to 10 digits.
   - a. True
   - b. False

7. The feature colors can be pre-set and saved in the Document Templates.
   - a. True
   - b. False

8. The display quality of the model can be adjusted using the settings in the Image Quality option.
   - a. True
   - b. False

9. The plane colors and transparency can be set and saved in the Document Templates.
   - a. True
   - b. False

	9. TRUE
8. TRUE	7. TRUE
6. FALSE	5. FALSE
4. TRUE	3. TRUE
2. TRUE	1. FALSE

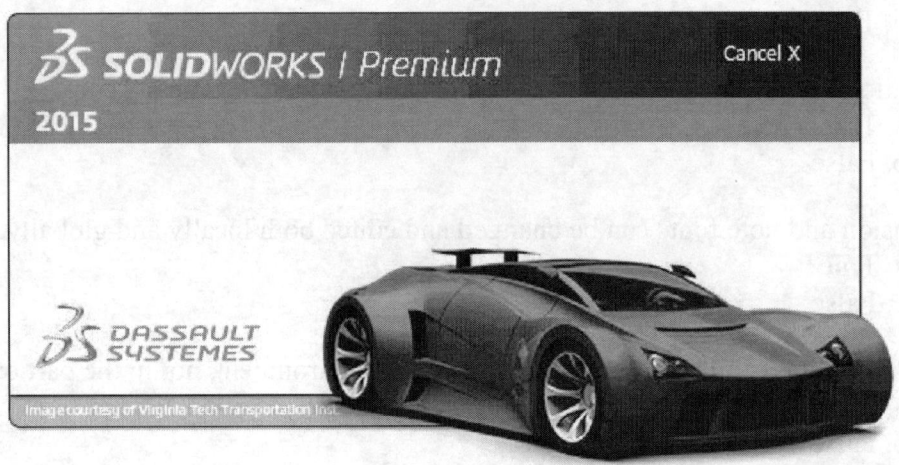

CHAPTER 3

Basic Solid Modeling

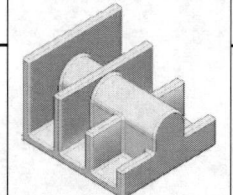

Basic Solid Modeling
Extrude Options

- Upon successful completion of this lesson, you will be able to:

   * Sketch on planes and/or planar surfaces.

   * Use the sketch tools to construct geometry.

   * Add the geometric relations or constraints.

   * Add/modify dimensions.

   * Explore the different extrude options.

- The following 5 basic steps will be demonstrated throughout this exercise:

   * Select the sketch plane.

   * Activate Sketch pencil ✏.

   * Sketch the profile using the sketch tools ╲ ⊙ ⌐ .

   * Define the profile with dimensions ◇ or relations ⊥ .

   * Extrude the profile ▣ .

- Be sure to review the self-test questionnaires at the end of the lesson, prior to moving to the next chapter.

Basic Solid Modeling
Extrude Options

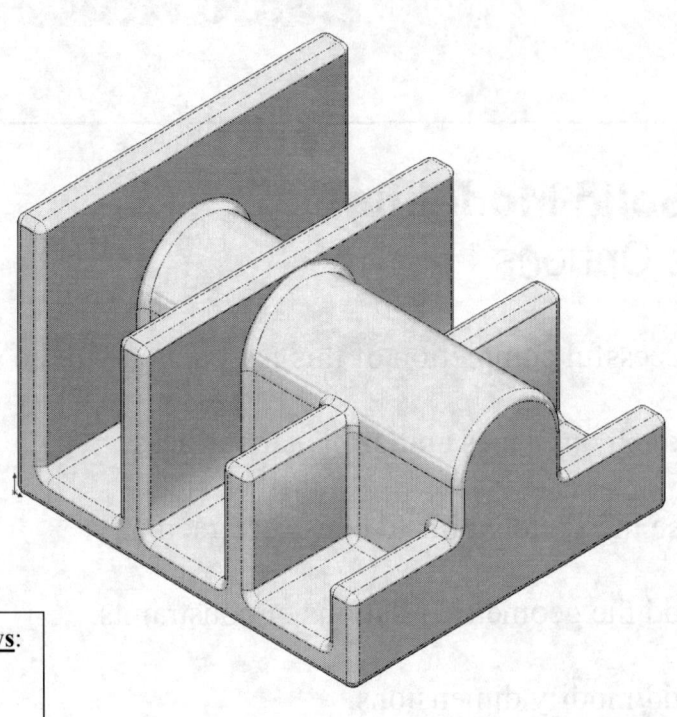

Dimensioning Standards: **ANSI**

Units: **INCHES** – 3 Decimals

Tools Needed:

 Insert Sketch

Line

 Circle

 Add Geometric Relations

Dimension

 Sketch Fillet

 Trim Entities

 Boss / Base Extrude

1. Starting a new Part:

- From the **File** menu, select **New / Part**, or click the **New** icon.

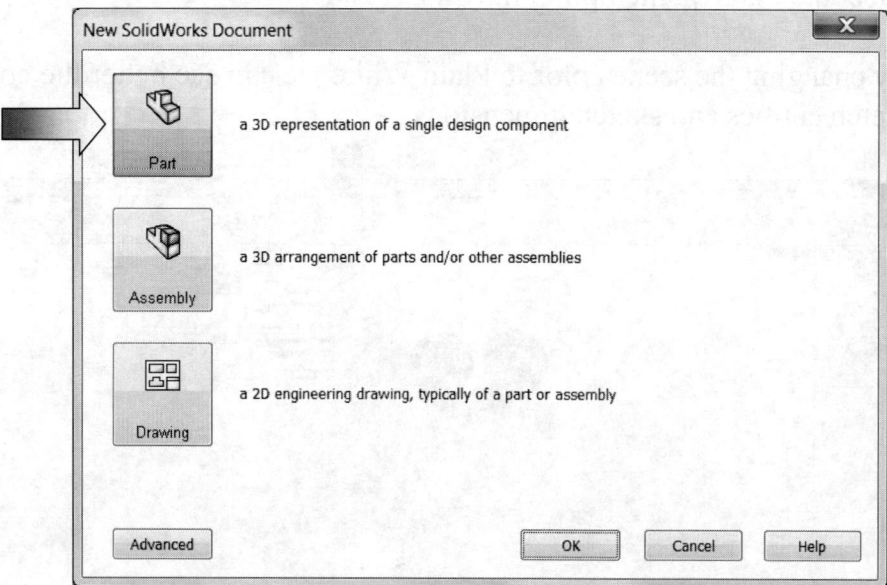

- Select the **Part** template from either the Templates or Tutorial folders.

- Click **OK** [OK]; a new part template is opened.

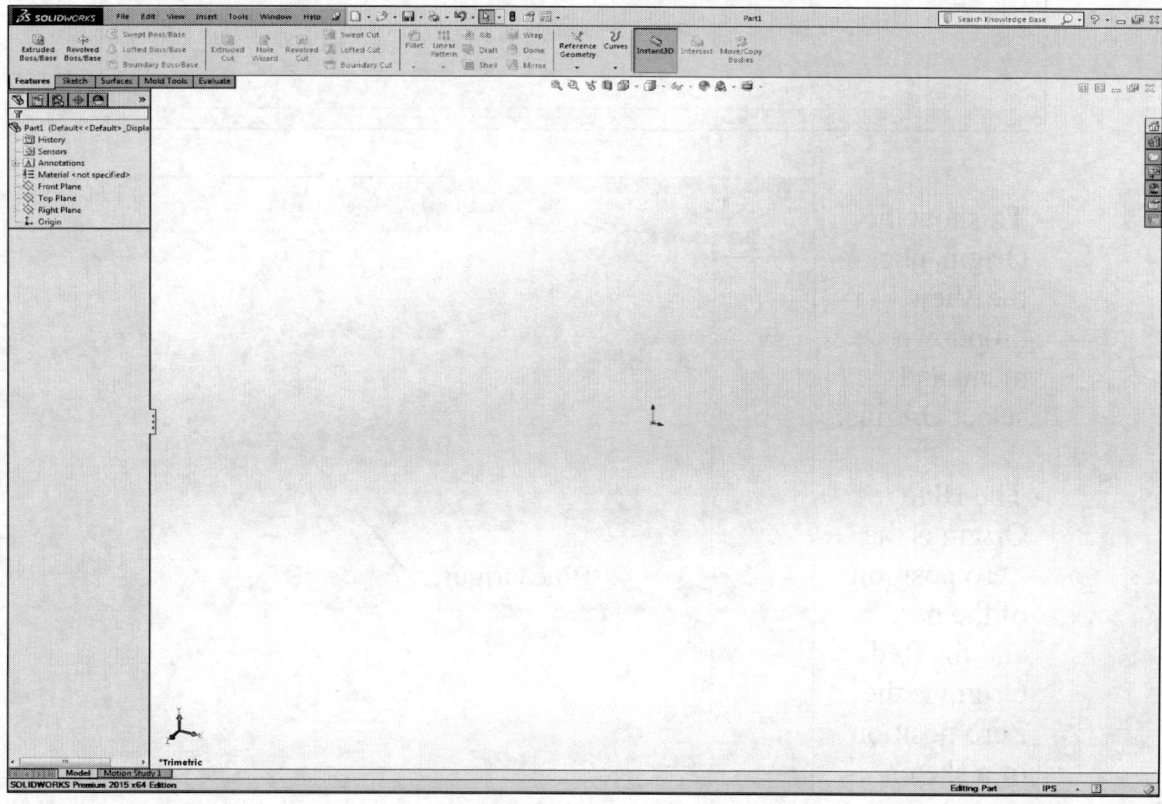

2. Changing the Scene:

- From the View (Heads-up) toolbar, click the Apply Scene button (arrow) and select the Plain White option (arrow).

- By changing the scene color to Plain White we can see better the colors of the sketch entities and sketch dimensions.

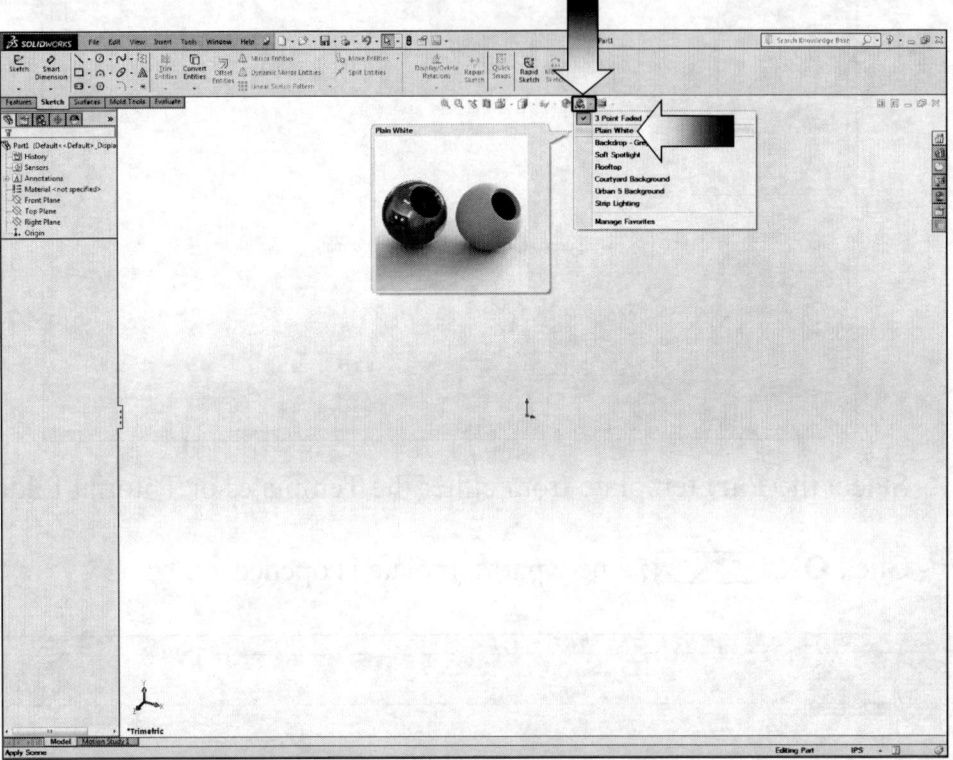

- To show the Origin, click the **View** dropdown menu and select Origins.

- The Blue Origin is the Zero position of the part and the Red Origin is the Zero position of a sketch.

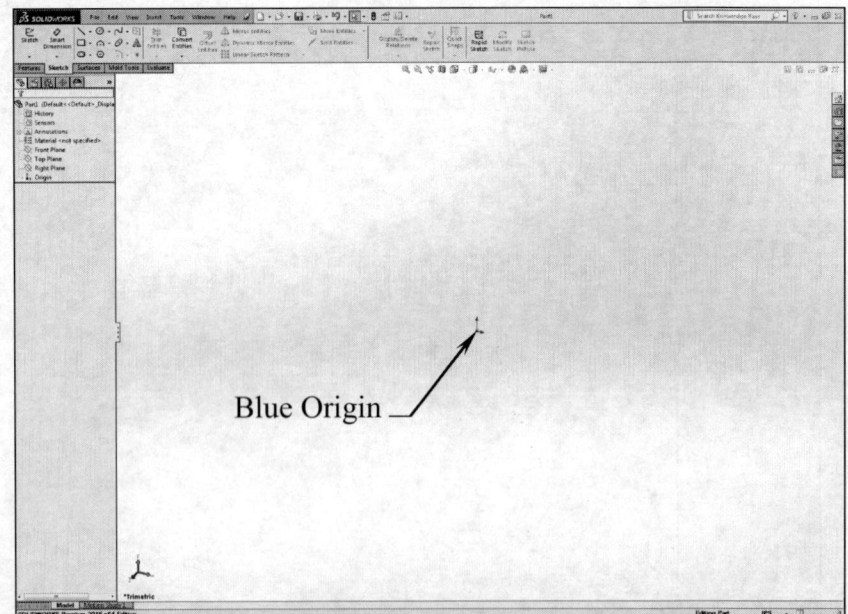

3. Starting a new Sketch:

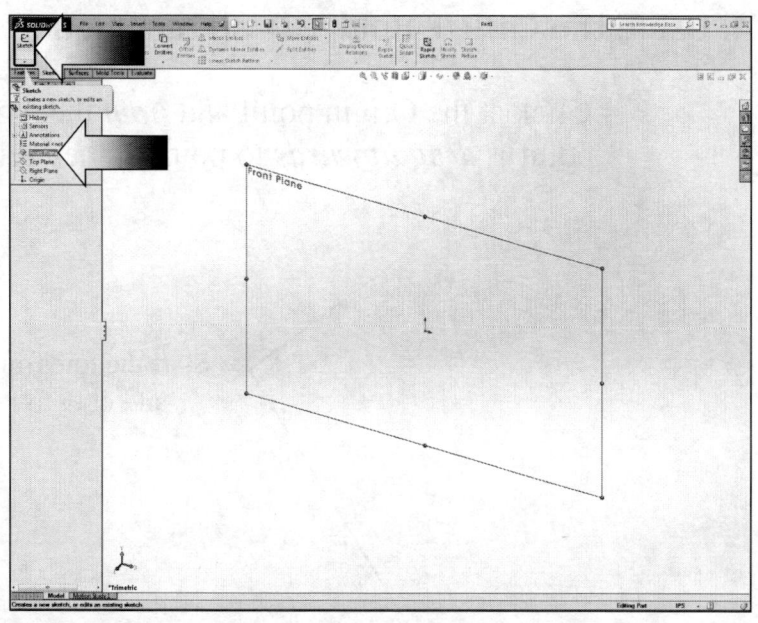

- Select the Front plane from the Feature-Manager tree and click the Pencil icon 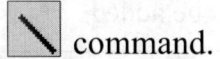 to start a new sketch.

- A sketch is normally created first, relations and dimensions are added after, and then it gets extruded into a 3D feature.

- From the Command-Manager toolbar, select the **Line** command.

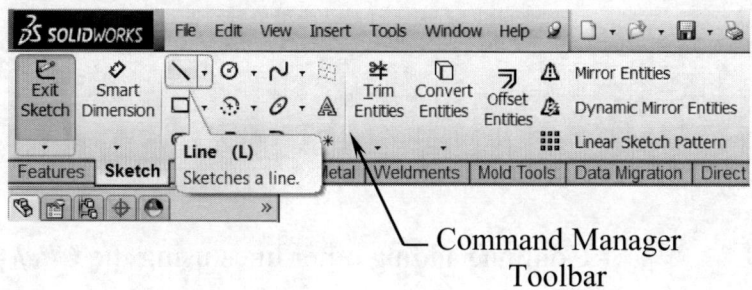

Command Manager Toolbar

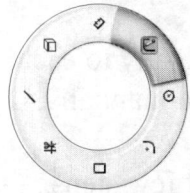

Mouse Gesture

OPTION:
Right-Drag to display the Mouse Gesture guide and select the Line command from it. (See the Introduction section, page XVIII for details on customizing the Mouse Gesture).

- Position the mouse cursor at the Red Origin point, a yellow feedback symbol appears to indicate a relation (Coincident) is going to be added automatically to the 1st endpoint of the line. This endpoint will be locked at the zero position.

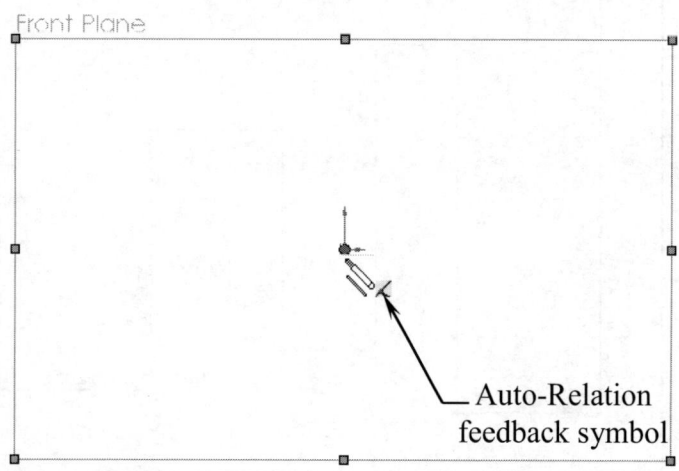

Auto-Relation feedback symbol

4. Using the Click + Hold + Drag technique:

- Click at the Origin point and *hold* the mouse button to start the line at point 1, *drag upwards* to point 2, then release the mouse button.

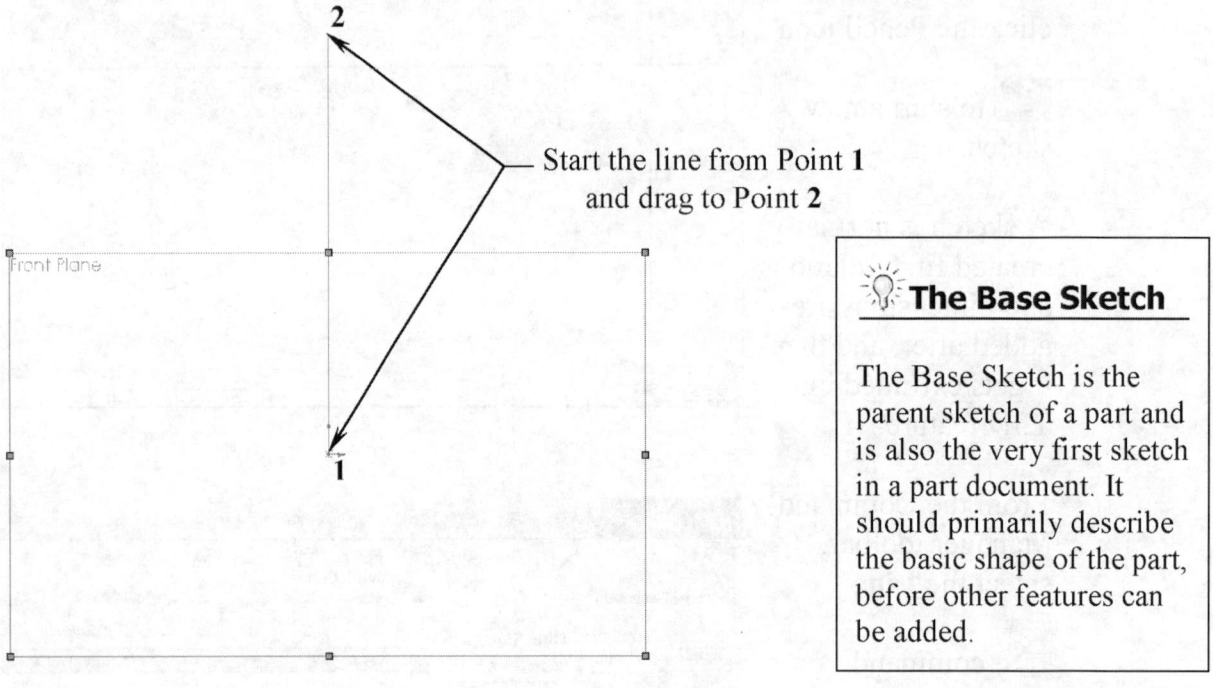

Start the line from Point **1**
and drag to Point **2**

Front Plane

💡 The Base Sketch

The Base Sketch is the parent sketch of a part and is also the very first sketch in a part document. It should primarily describe the basic shape of the part, before other features can be added.

- Continue adding other lines using the *Click-Hold-Drag* technique.

- The relations like Horizontal and Vertical are added automatically to each sketch line. Other relations like Collinear and Equal are added manually.

- The size and shape of the profile will be corrected in the next few steps.

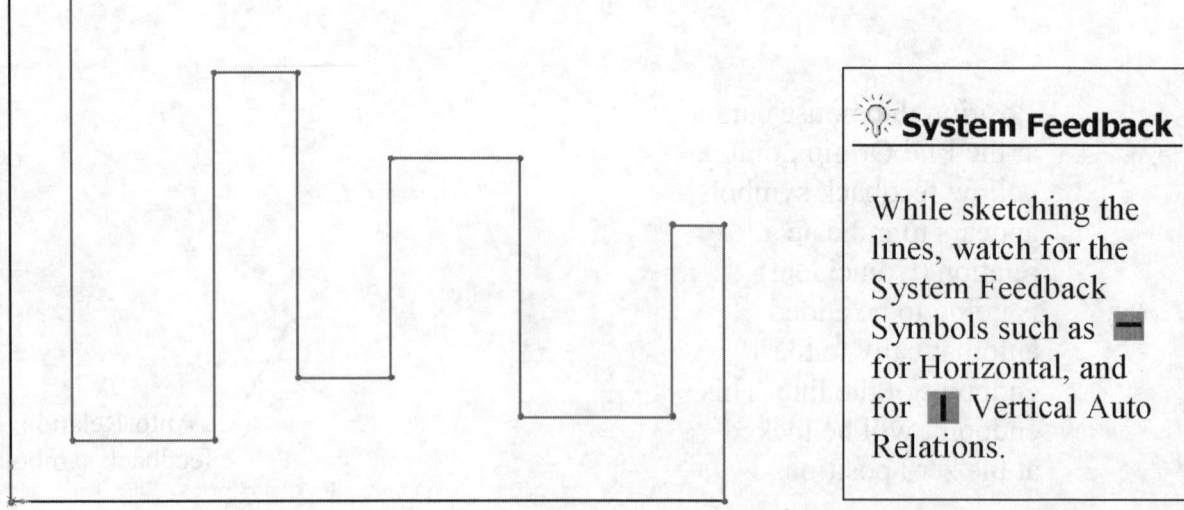

💡 System Feedback

While sketching the lines, watch for the System Feedback Symbols such as ▬ for Horizontal, and for ▮ Vertical Auto Relations.

5. Adding Geometric Relations*:

- Click **Add Relation** ⊥ under Display/Delete Relations - OR - select **Tools / Relations / Add**.

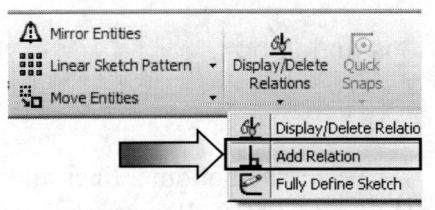

- Select the 4 lines shown below.

- Click **Equal** from the Add Geometric Relation dialog box. This relation makes the length of the two selected lines equal.

* Geometric relations are one of the most powerful features in SolidWorks. They are used in the sketch level to control the behaviors of the sketch entities when they are moved or rotated and to keep the associations between one another.

When applying geometric relations between entities, one of them should be a 2D entity and the other can either be a 2D sketch entity or a model edge, a plane, an axis, or a curve, etc.

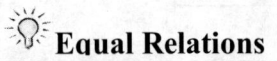 **Equal Relations**

Adding the EQUAL relations to these lines eliminates the need to dimension each line.

Geometric relations can be created manually or automatically. The next few steps in this chapter will demonstrate how geometric relations are added manually.

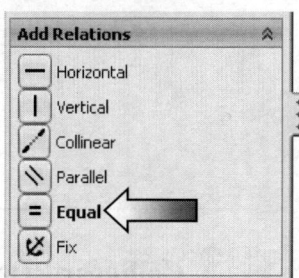

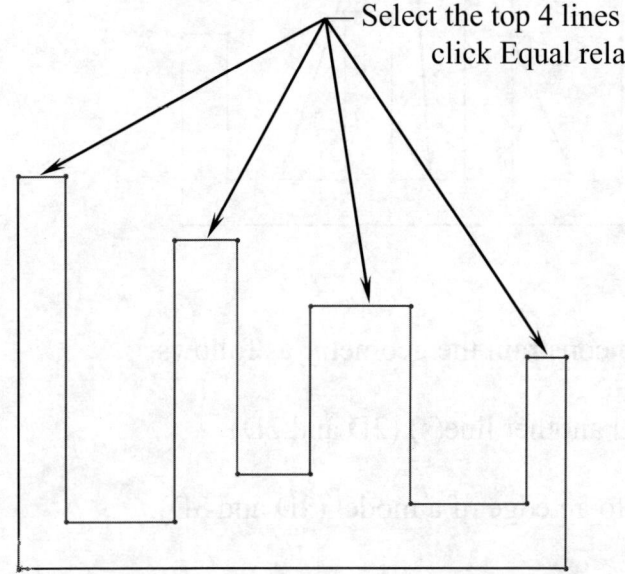

Select the top 4 lines and click Equal relation

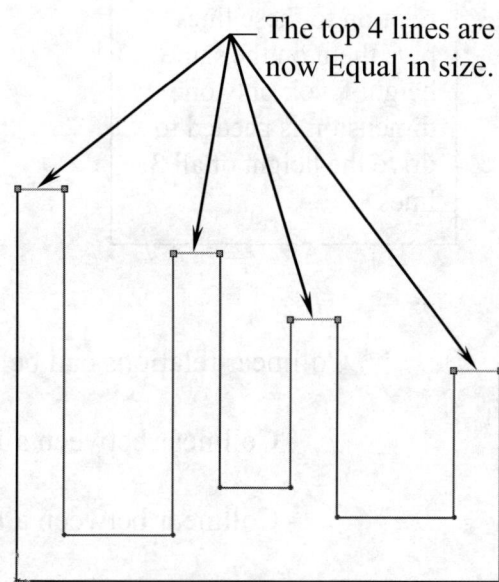

The top 4 lines are now Equal in size.

6. Adding a Collinear relation**:

- Select the **Add Relation** 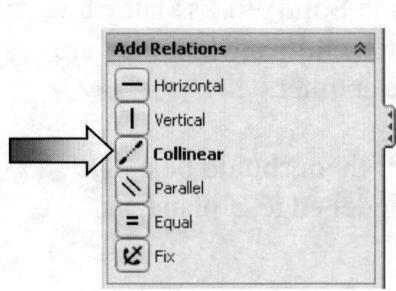 command again.

- Select the 3 lines as shown below.

- Click **Collinear** from the Add Geometric Relations dialog box.

- Click **OK** ⊘.

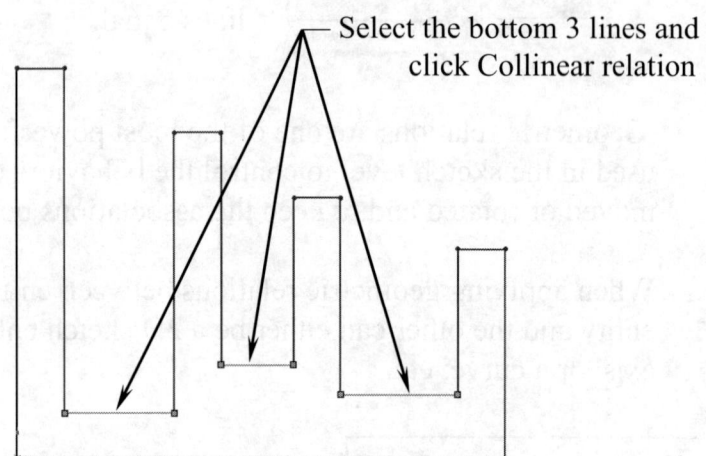

Select the bottom 3 lines and click Collinear relation

Collinear Relations

Adding a Collinear relation to these lines puts them on the same height level; only one dimension is needed to drive the height of all 3 lines.

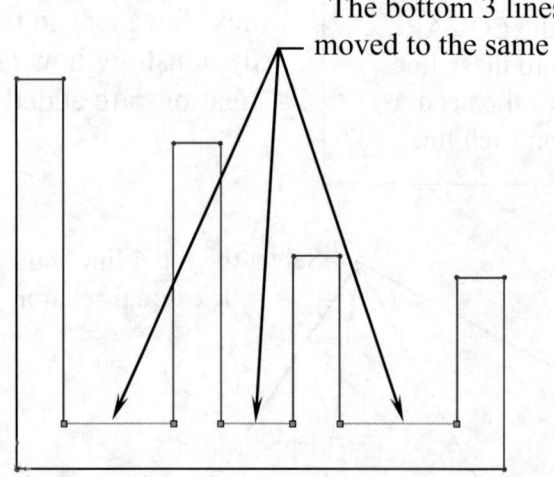

The bottom 3 lines are moved to the same level.

** Collinear relations can be used to constrain the geometry as follows:

- Collinear between a line and another line(s) (2D and 2D).

- Collinear between a line(s) to an edge of a model (2D and 3D).

Geometric Relations Examples

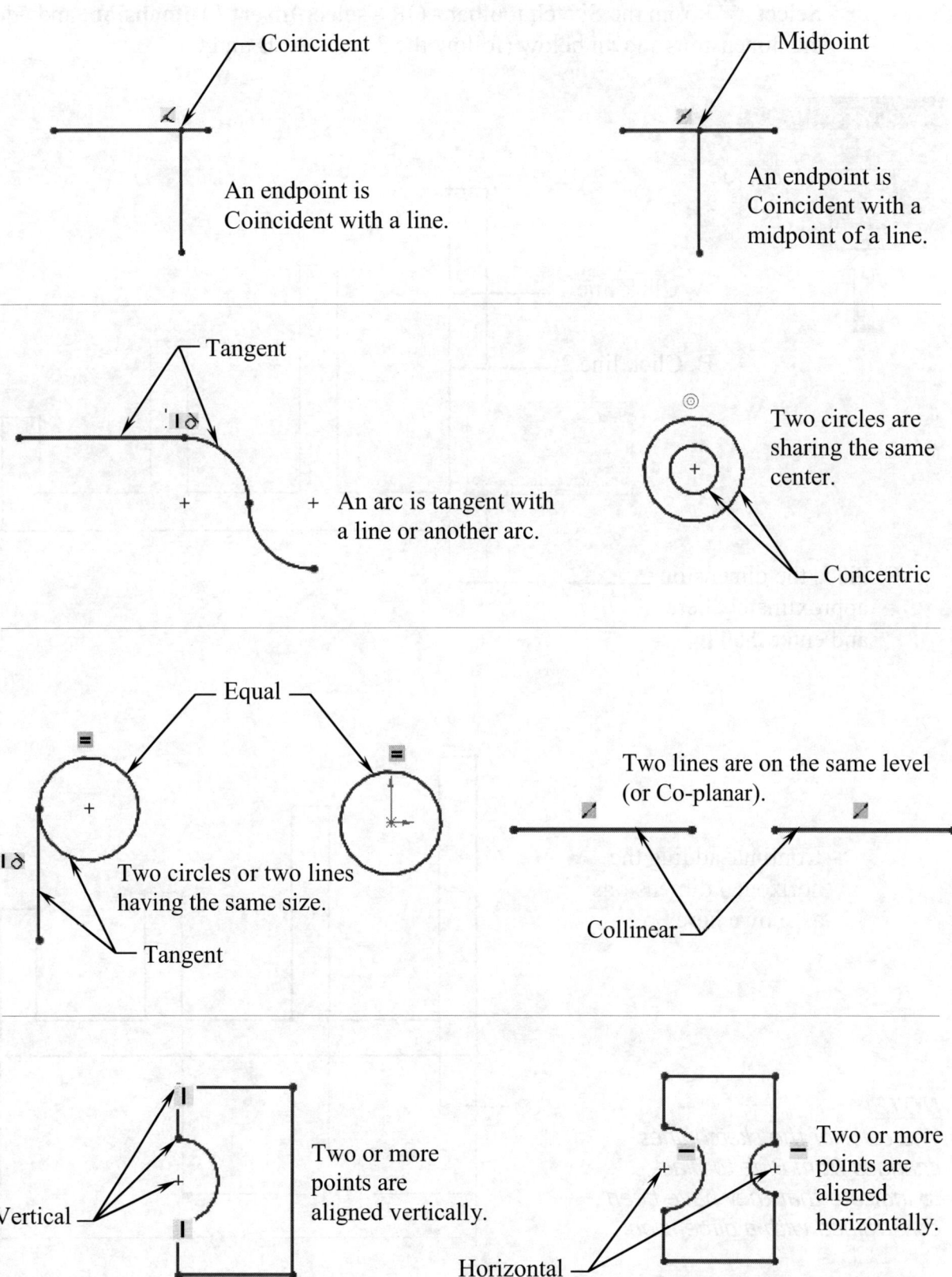

Coincident

An endpoint is Coincident with a line.

Midpoint

An endpoint is Coincident with a midpoint of a line.

Tangent

An arc is tangent with a line or another arc.

Two circles are sharing the same center.

Concentric

Equal

Two circles or two lines having the same size.

Tangent

Two lines are on the same level (or Co-planar).

Collinear

Vertical

Two or more points are aligned vertically.

Two or more points are aligned horizontally.

Horizontal

7. Adding the horizontal dimensions:

- Select 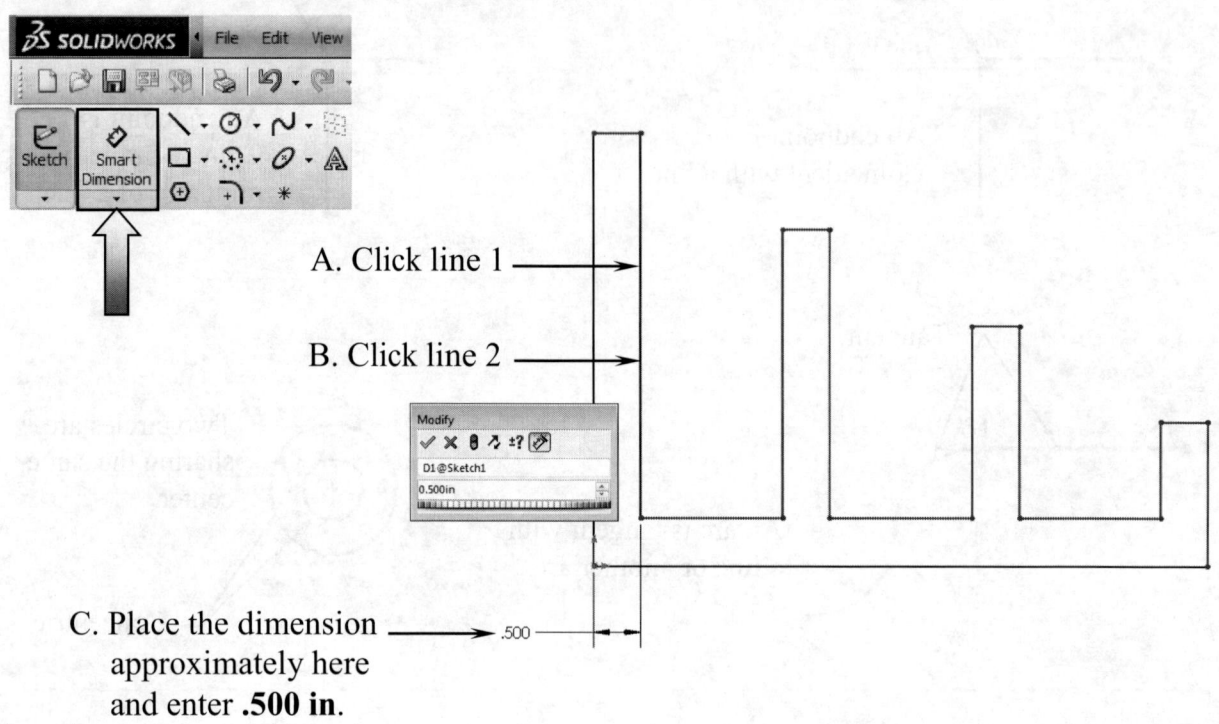 from the Sketch toolbar - OR - select **Insert / Dimension**, and add the dimensions shown below (follow the 3 steps A, B and C).

A. Click line 1

B. Click line 2

C. Place the dimension approximately here and enter **.500 in**.

- Continue adding the horizontal dimensions as shown here.

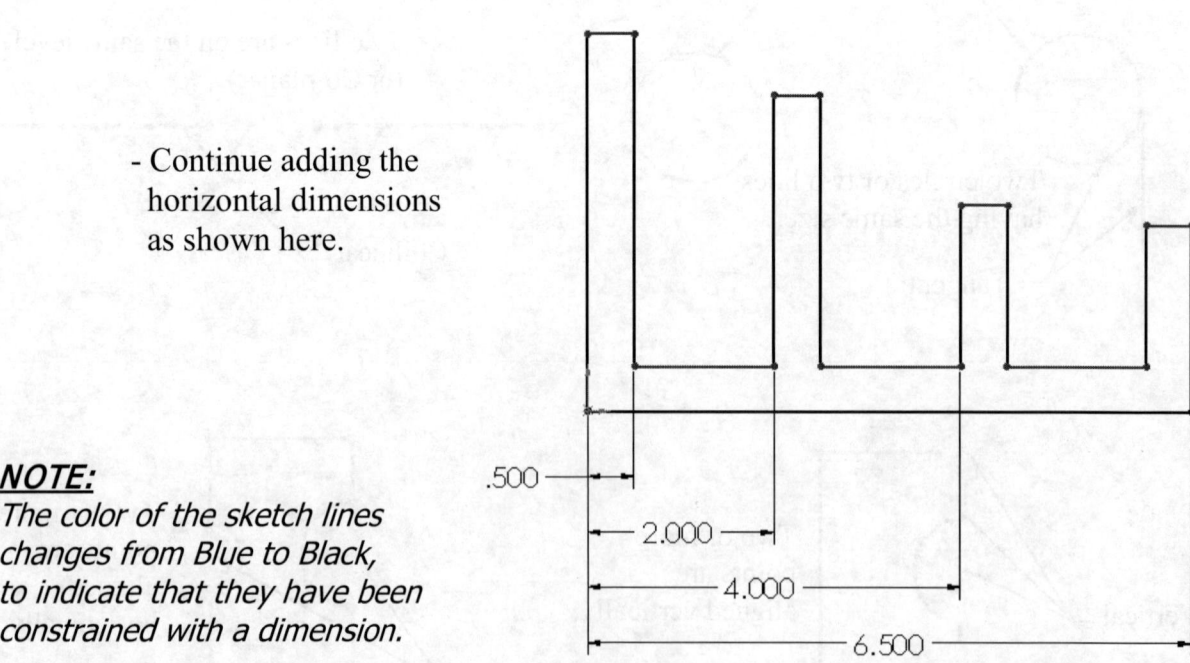

<u>**NOTE:**</u>
The color of the sketch lines changes from Blue to Black, to indicate that they have been constrained with a dimension.

8. Adding the Vertical dimensions:

- With the Smart-
 Dimension tool
 still selected, click
 on line 1 and line 2;
 place the dimension
 approximately as
 shown, and change
 the value to **.500 in**.

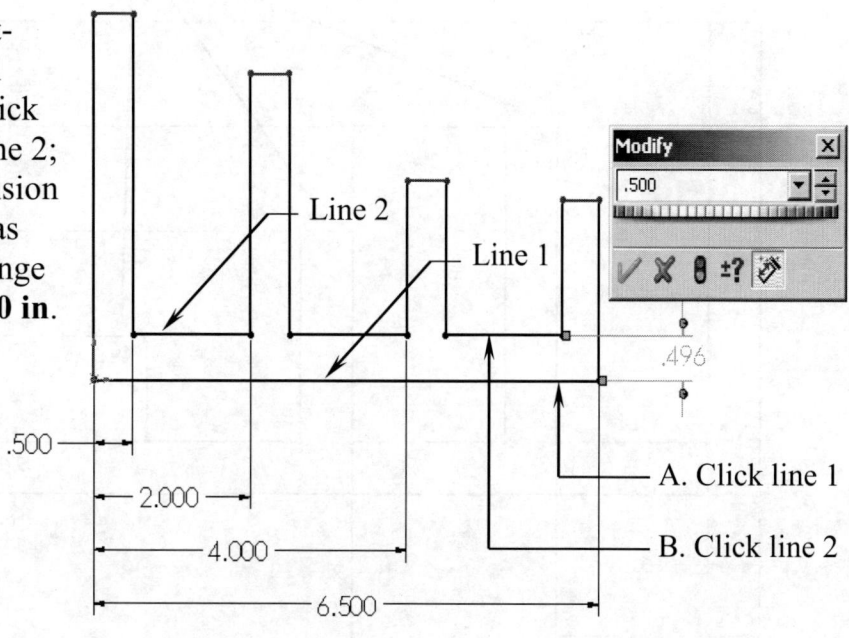

Line 2

Line 1

A. Click line 1

B. Click line 2

- Continue adding
 other dimensions
 until the entire
 sketch turns into
 the Black color.

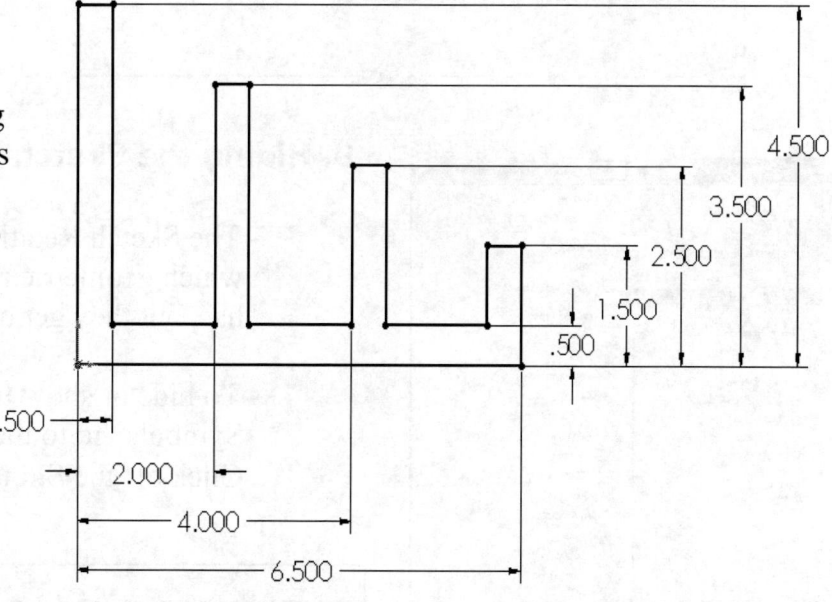

The Status of a Sketch:

The current status of a sketch is displayed in the lower right corner of the screen.

Fully Defined	=	**Black**	Fully Defined
Under Defined	=	**Blue**	Under Defined
Over Defined	=	**Red**	Over Defined

Sketch Relation Symbols

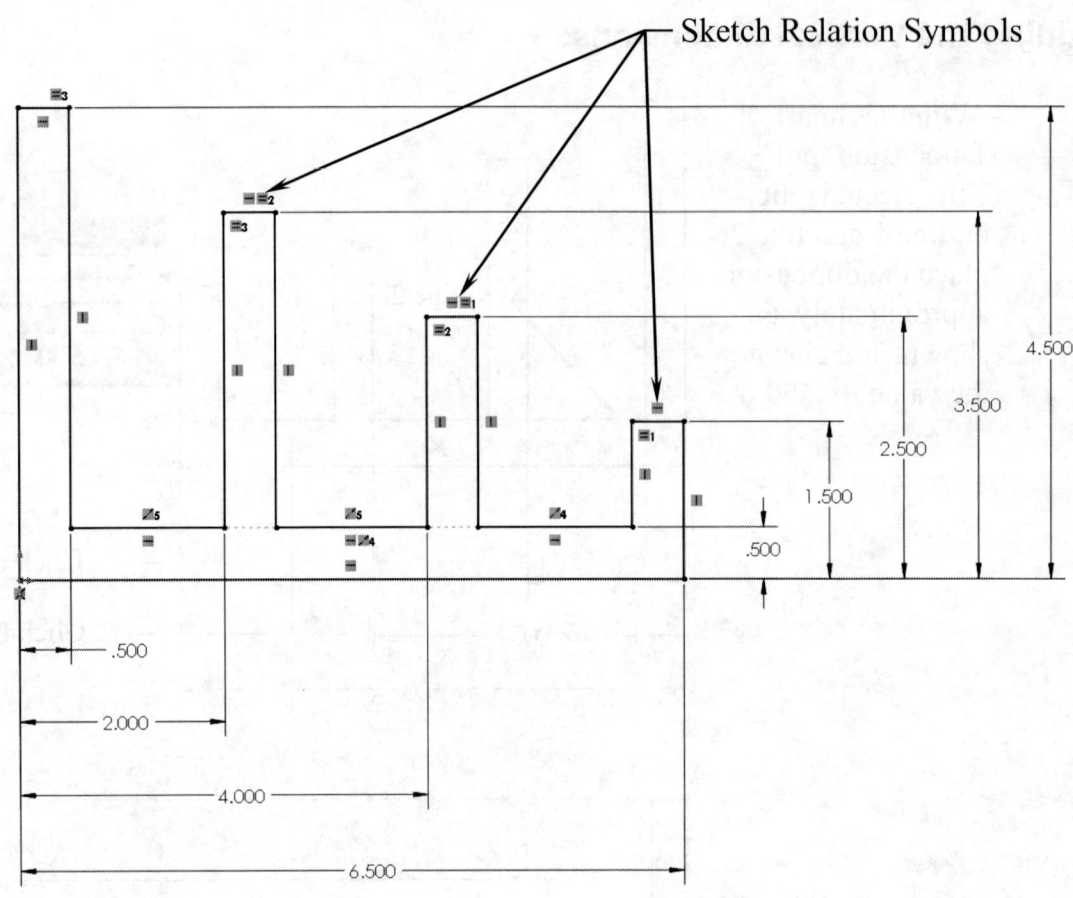

4.500

3.500

2.500

1.500

.500

.500

2.000

4.000

6.500

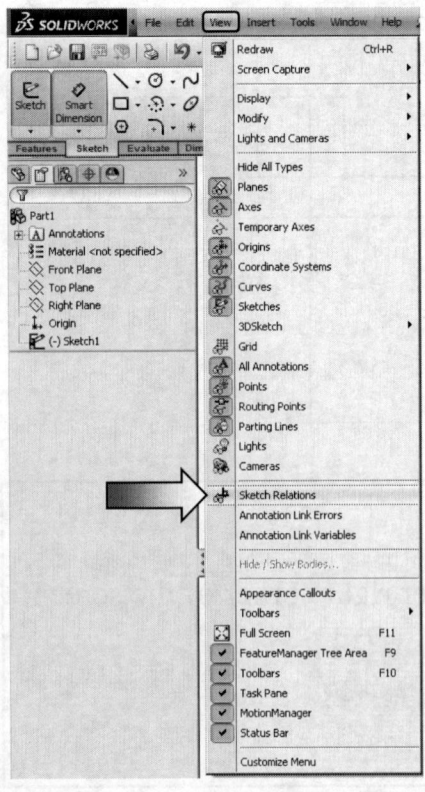

9. Hiding the Sketch Relation Symbols:

- The Sketch Relation Symbols indicate which geometric relation a sketch entity has, but they get quite busy as shown.

- To hide or show the Sketch Relation Symbols, go to the **View** menu and Click off the **Sketch Relations** option.

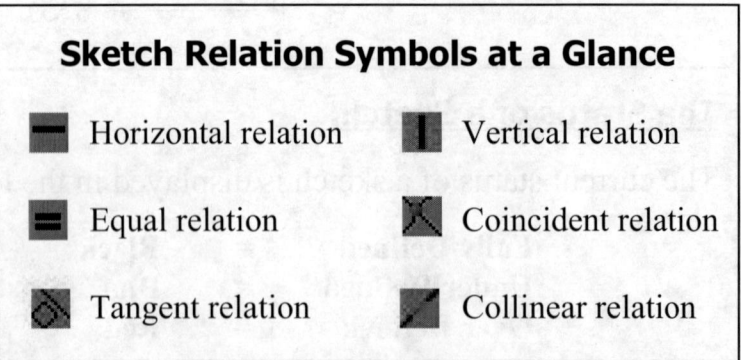

Sketch Relation Symbols at a Glance

▬	Horizontal relation	▌	Vertical relation
▬	Equal relation	✕	Coincident relation
◎	Tangent relation	╱	Collinear relation

10. Extruding the Base:

- The **Extrude Boss/Base** command is used to define the characteristic of a 3D linear feature.

- Click 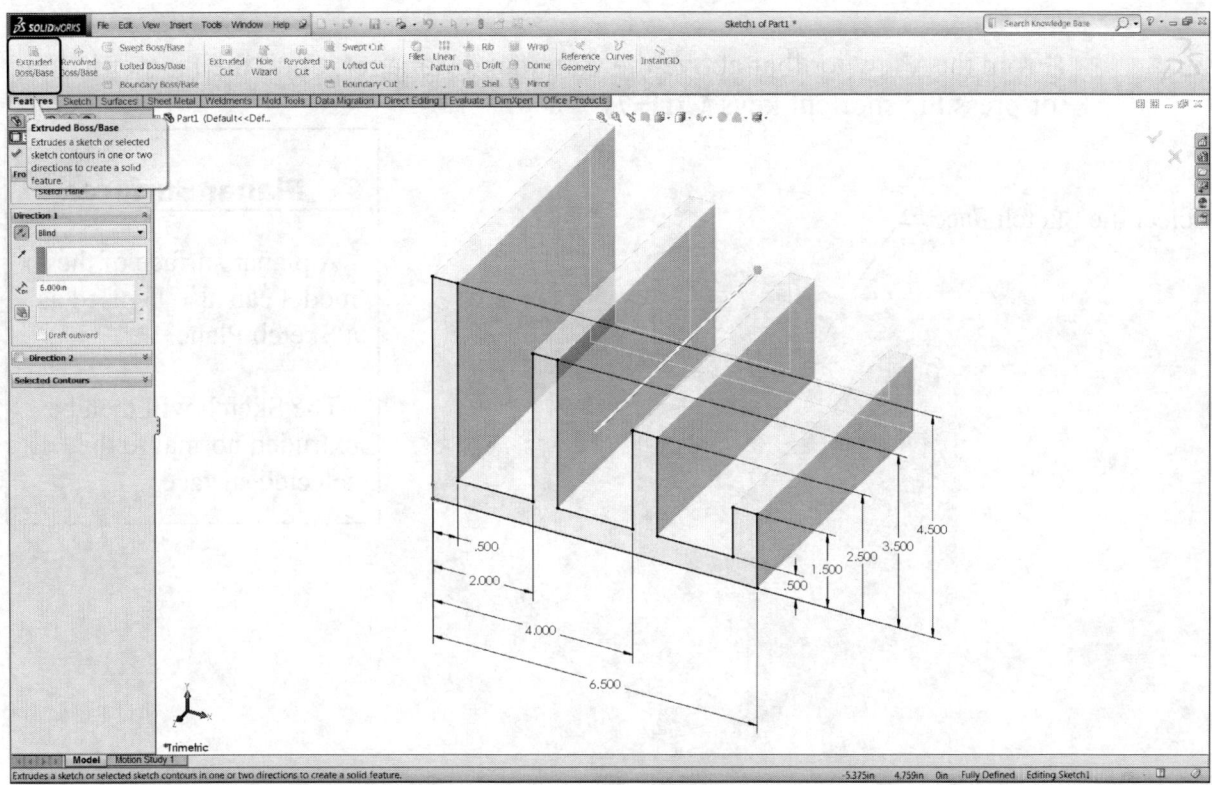 from the Features toolbar - OR- select **Insert / Boss Base / Extrude**.

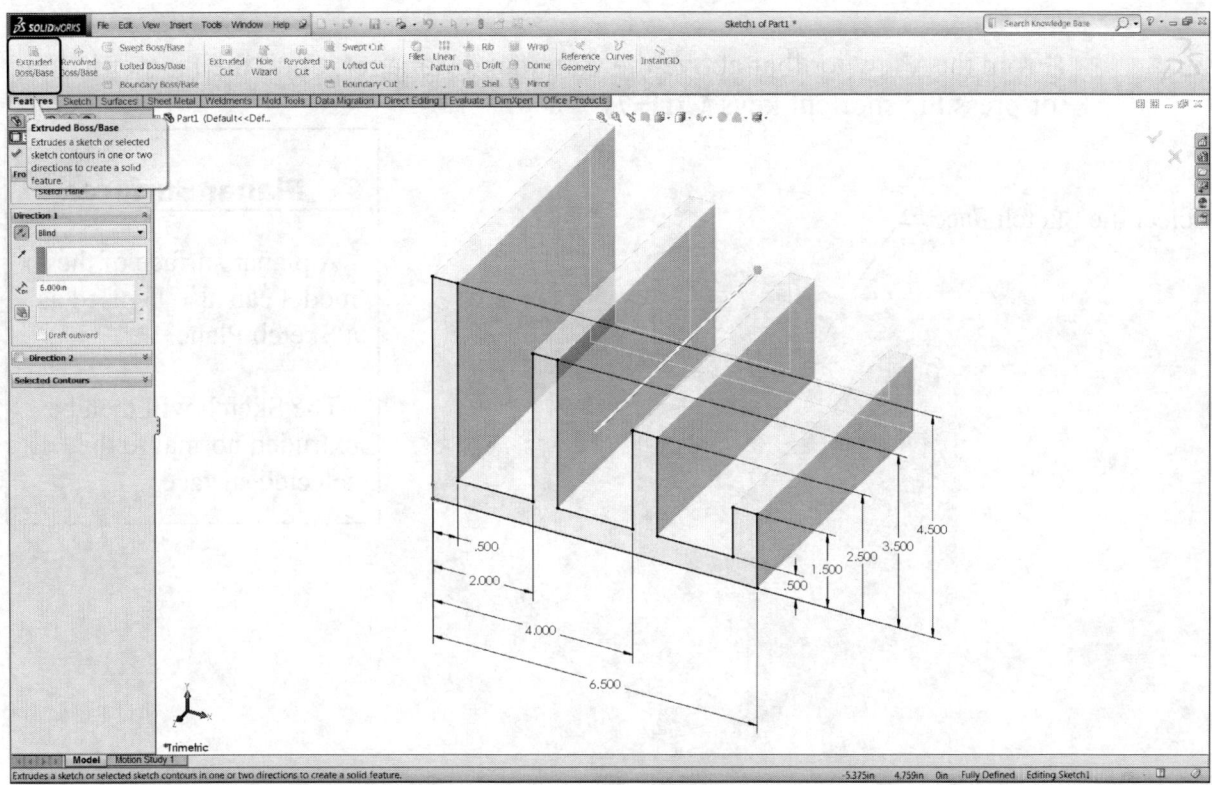

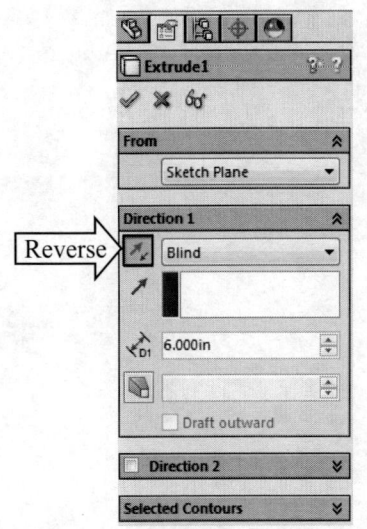

- Set the following:

- Direction: **Blind**.

- Depth: **6.00 in**.

- Enabled **Reverse** direction.

- Click **OK** ✓.

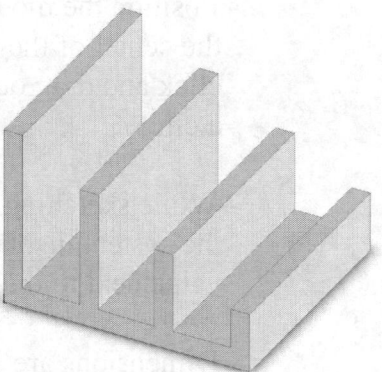

11. Sketching on a Planar Face:

- Select the face as indicated.

- Click [icon] or select **Insert/Sketch**.

- Click [icon] from the Sketch Tools toolbar
  Or select **Tools / Sketch Entity / Circle**.

(From the View toolbar above the CommandManager, click the Isometric icon or press the shortcut keys **Ctrl+7**).

Select the Sketch Face ——

> **Planar Surfaces**
>
> - A planar surface of the model can also be used as a Sketch Plane.
>
> - The Sketch will then be extruded normal to the selected surface.

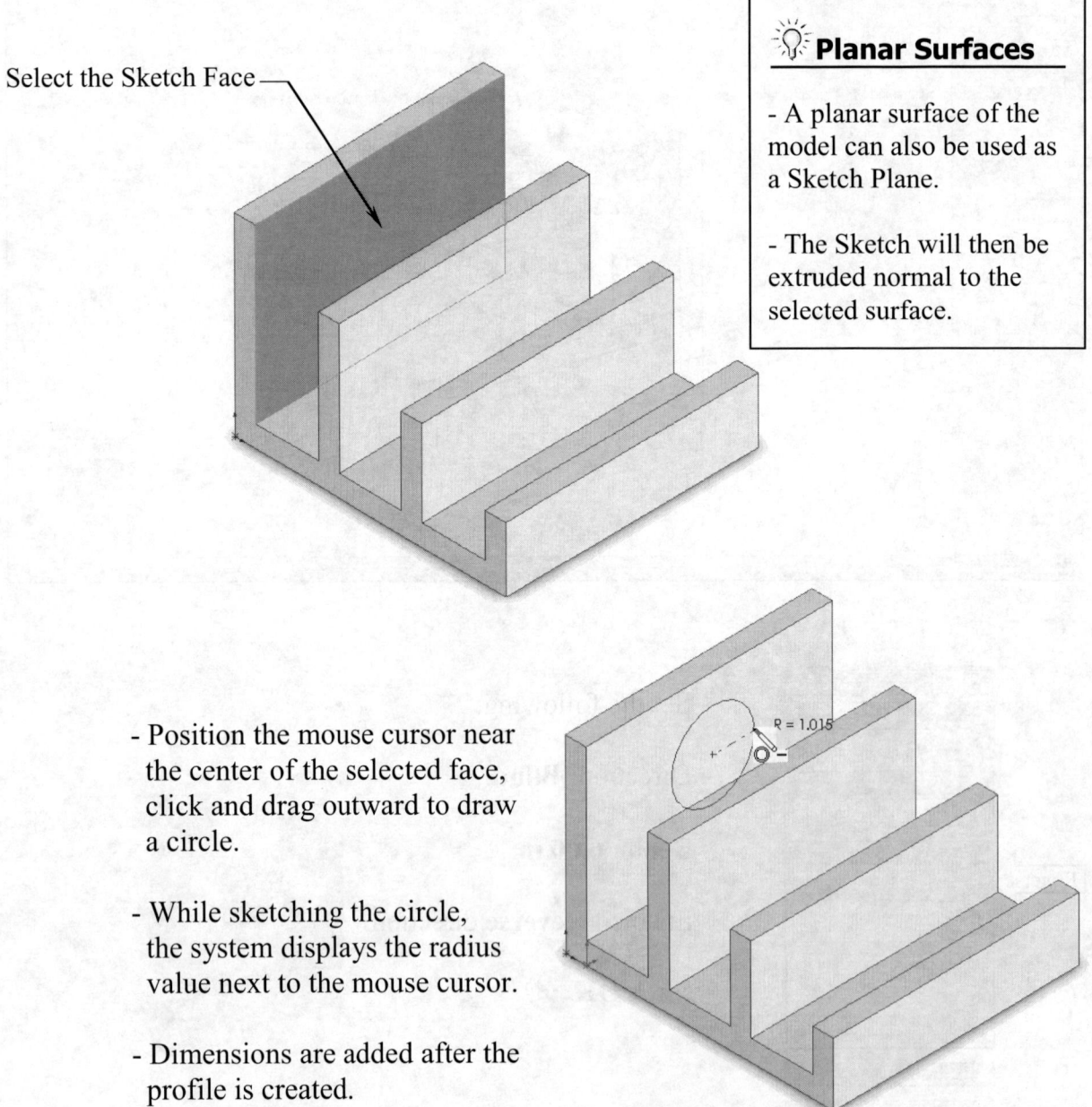

- Position the mouse cursor near the center of the selected face, click and drag outward to draw a circle.

- While sketching the circle, the system displays the radius value next to the mouse cursor.

- Dimensions are added after the profile is created.

- Select the **Smart Dimension**

command 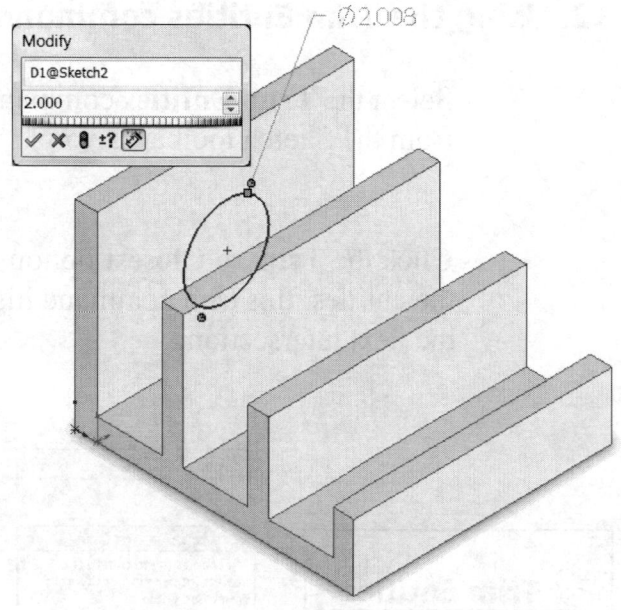 and add a
diameter dimension to the
circle.

(Click on the circle and move
the mouse cursor outward, at
approximately 45 degrees and
place it).

- To add the location dimensions
click the edge of the circle and
the edge of the model, place
the dimension, then correct
the value.

- Continue adding the
location dimensions
as shown, to fully
define the sketch.

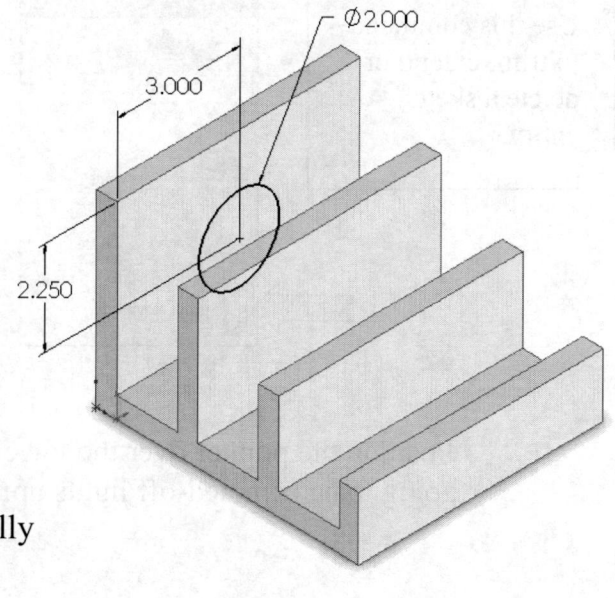

- Select the Line command
and sketch the 3 lines as shown
below. Snap to the hidden edge
of the model when it lights up.

- The color of the sketch should
change to black at this point (Fully
Defined).

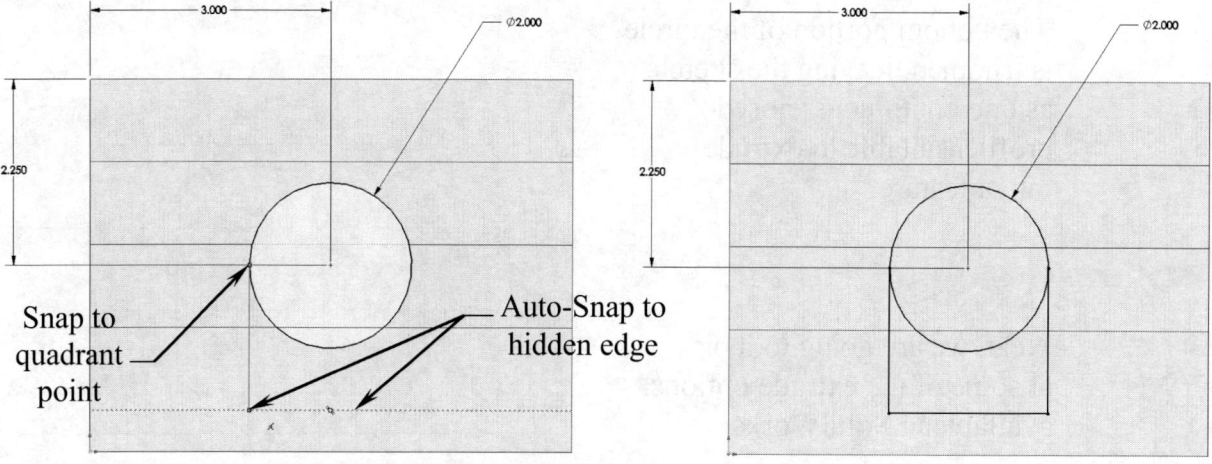

12. Using the Trim Entities command:

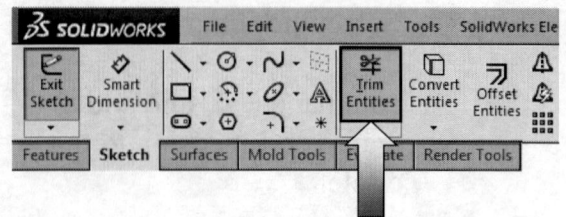

- Select the **Trim Entities** command from the Sketch toolbar (arrow).

- Click the **Trim to Closest** option (arrow). When the pointer is hovered over the entities, this trim command highlights the entities prior to trimming to the next intersection.

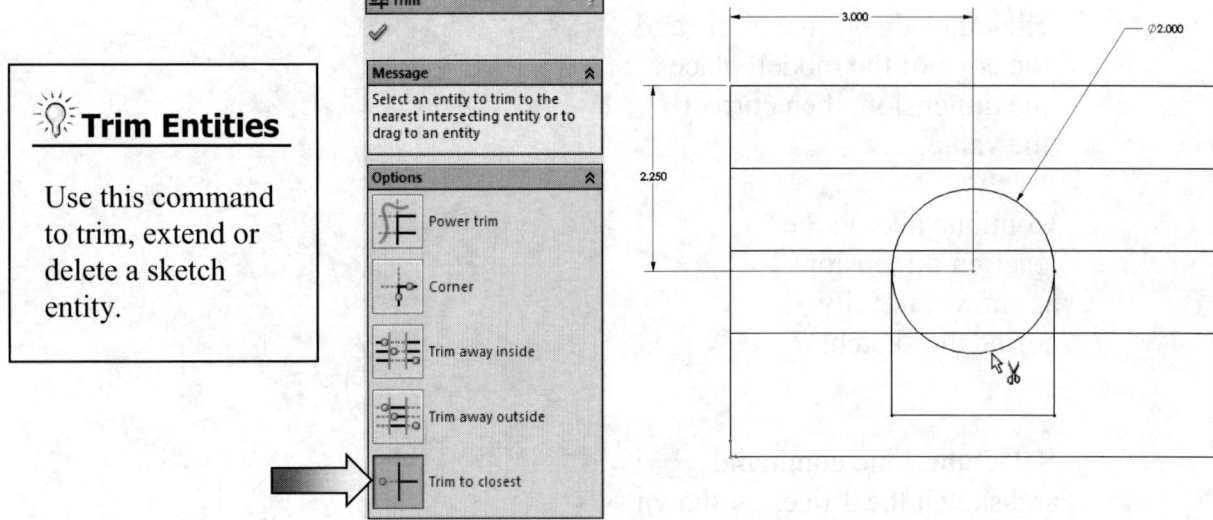

Trim Entities

Use this command to trim, extend or delete a sketch entity.

- Position the pointer over the lower portion of the circle, the portion that is going to be trimmed-off lights up. Click the mouse to trim.

- The bottom portion of the circle is trimmed, leaving the sketch as one-continuous-closed-profile, suitable to extrude into a feature.

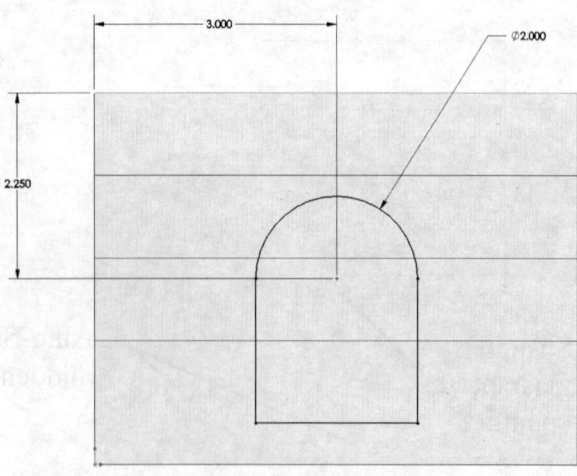

- Next, we are going to look at some of the extrude options available in SolidWorks.

13. Extruding a Boss:

- Switch to the Feature toolbar and click 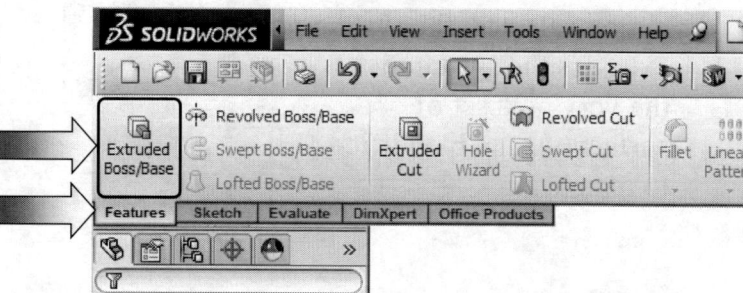 or select:
  Insert / Boss-Base / Extrude.

Extrude Options...

Explore each extrude option to see the different results.
Press Undo to go back to the original state after each one.

(A) Using the Blind option:

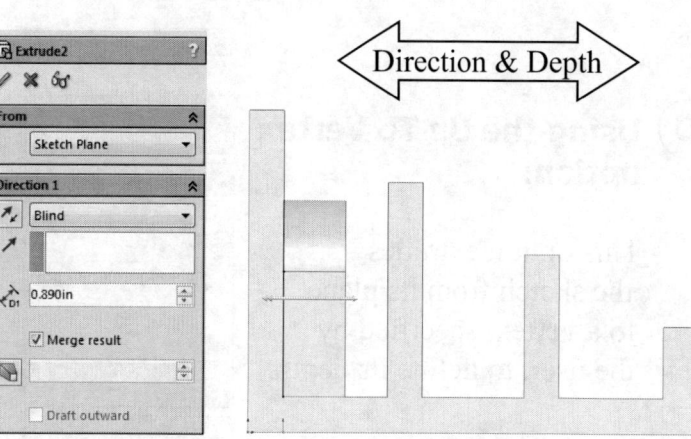

- When extruding with the Blind option, the following conditions are required:

  * Direction

  * Depth dimension

- Drag the direction arrow on the preview graphics to define the direction, then enter a dimension for the depth.

Blind
Condition

(B) Using the Through All option:

- When the Through All option is selected, the system automatically extrudes the sketch to the length of the part, normal to the sketch plane.

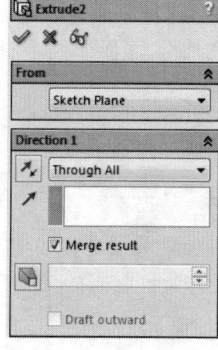

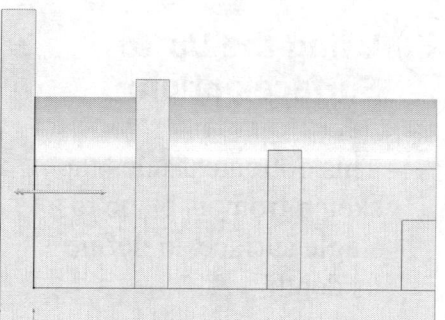

Through All
Condition

C **Using the Up To Next option:**

- With the Up To Next option selected, the system extrudes the sketch to the very next set of surface(s), and blends it to match.

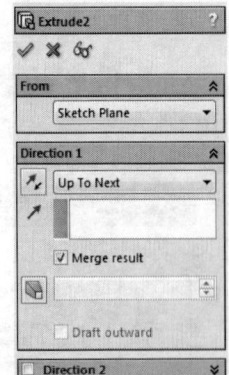

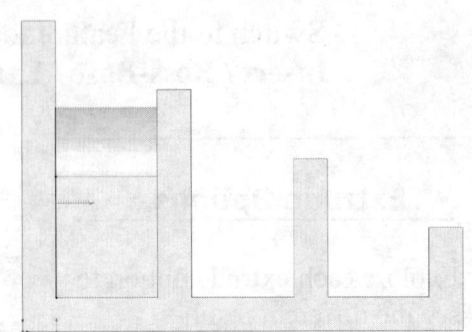

Up To Next
Condition

D **Using the Up To Vertex option:**

- This option extrudes the sketch from its plane to a vertex, specified by the user, to define its depth.

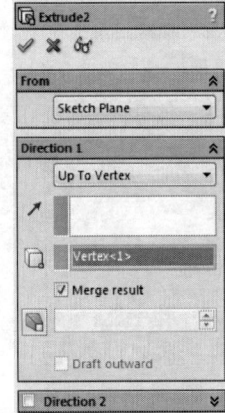

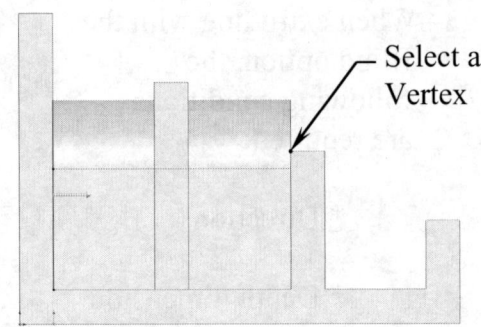

Select a Vertex

Up To Vertex
Condition

E **Using the Up To Surface option:**

- This option extrudes the sketch from its plane to a single surface, to define its depth.

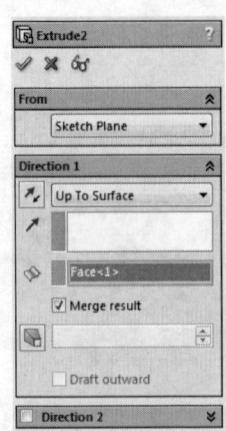

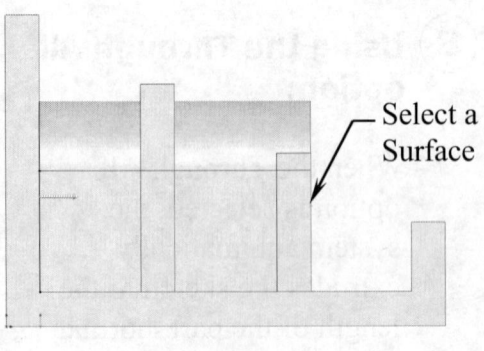

Select a Surface

Up To Surface
Condition

(F) Using the Offset From Surface option:

- This option extrudes the sketch from its plane to a selected face, then offsets at a specified distance.

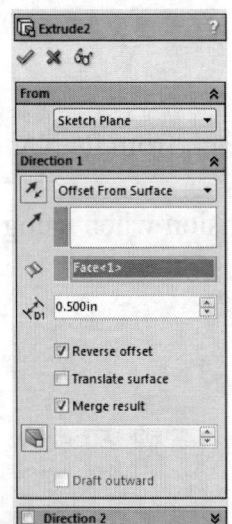

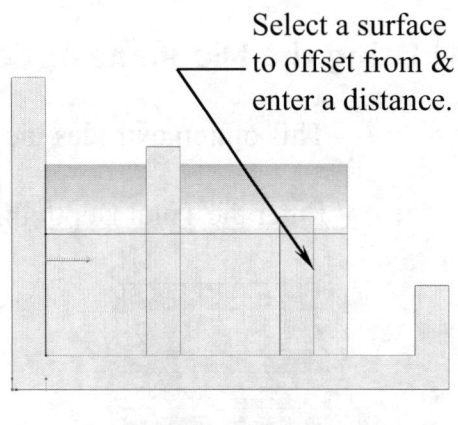

Select a surface to offset from & enter a distance.

Offset From Surface
Condition

(G) Using the Up To Body option:

- This option extrudes the sketch from its sketch plane to a specified body.

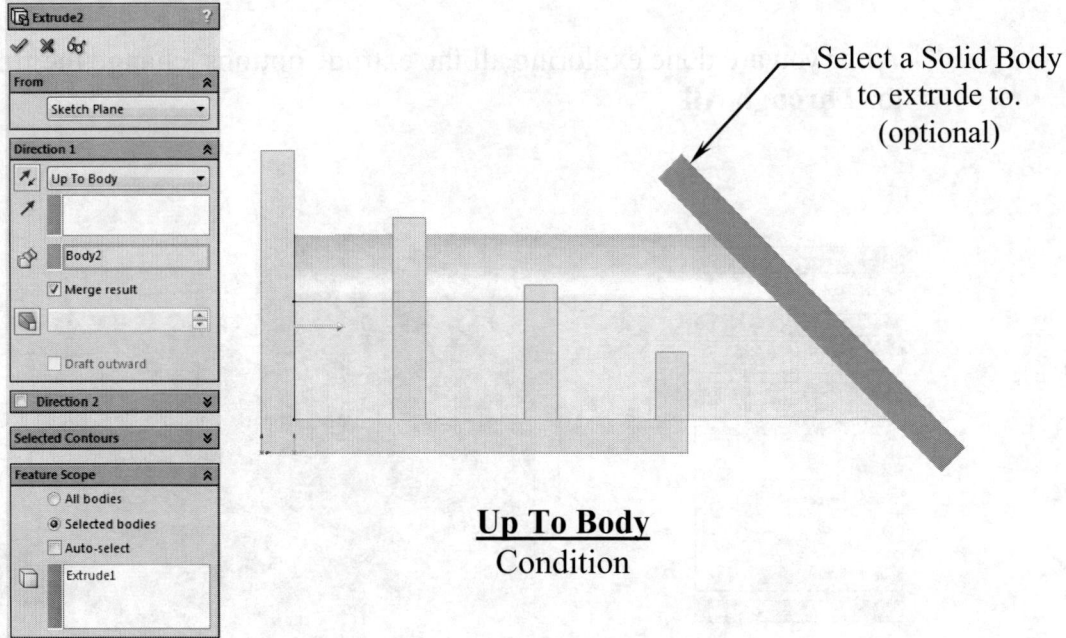

Select a Solid Body to extrude to. (optional)

Up To Body
Condition

- The Up To Body option can also be used in assemblies or multi-body parts.

- The Up To Body option works with either a solid body or a surface body. It is also useful when making extrusions in an assembly to extend a sketch to an uneven surface.

(H) Using the Mid Plane option:

- This option extrudes the sketch from its plane equally in both directions.

- Enter the Total Depth dimension when using the Mid-Plane option.

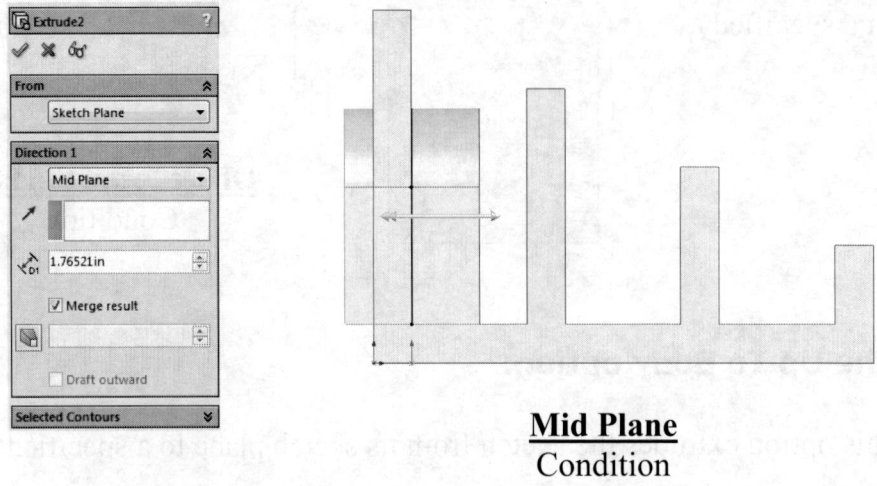

Mid Plane
Condition

- After you are done exploring all the extrude options, change the final condition to: **Through All**

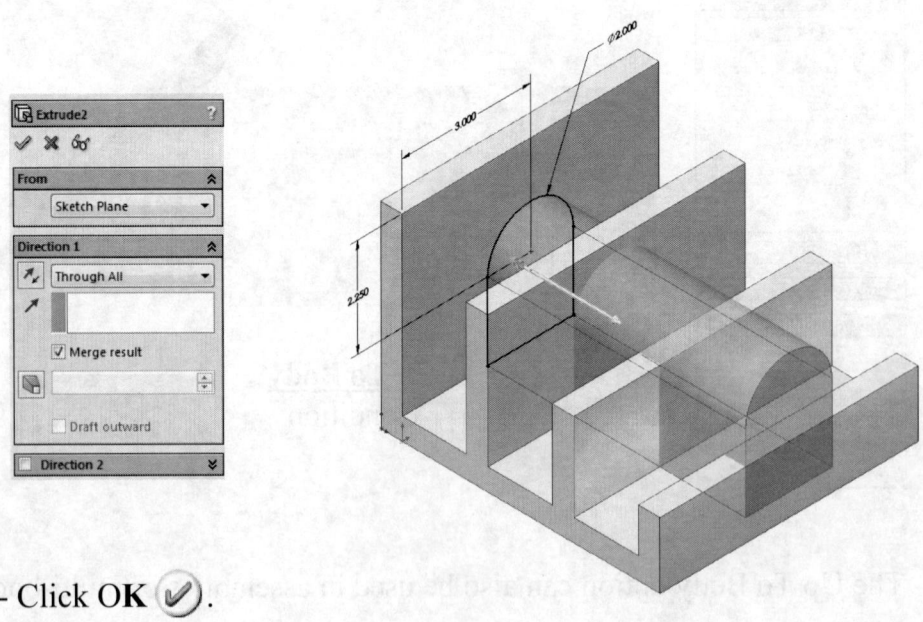

- Click **OK** ✓.

- The system extrudes the circle to the outer most surface as the result of the Through All end condition.

- The extra material between the first and the second extruded features
is removed automatically.

- Unless the Merge Result checkbox is cleared, all interferences will be
detected and removed.

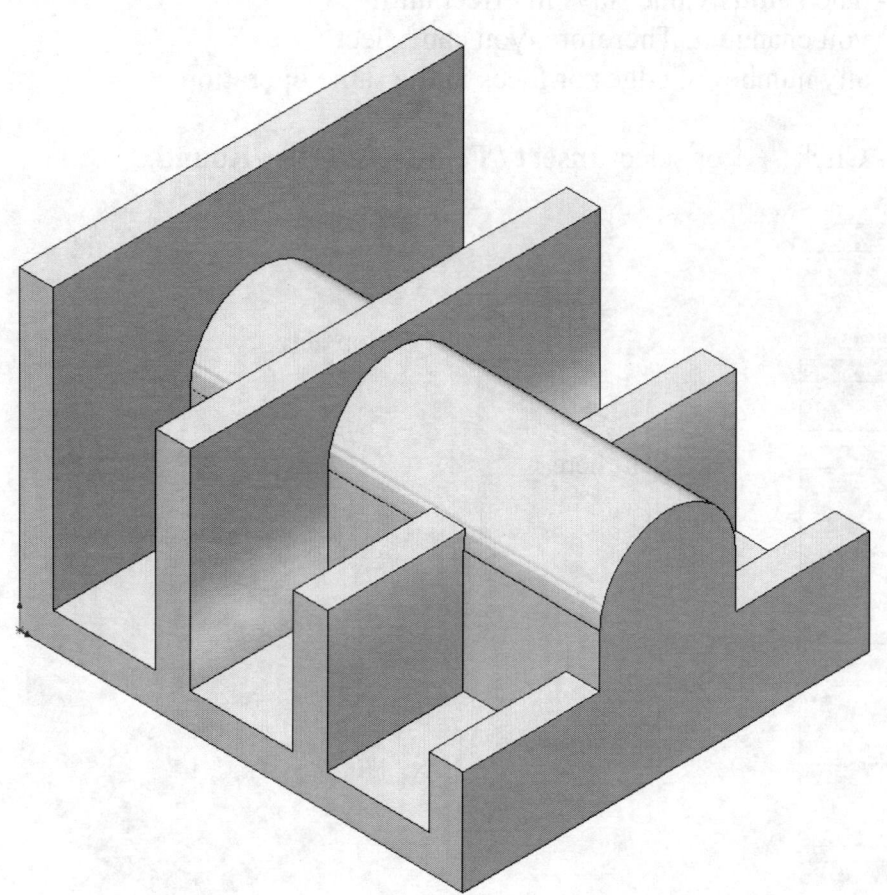

Extrude summary:

* The Extrude Boss/Base command is used to add thickness to a sketch and to
define the characteristic of a 3D feature.

* A sketch can be extruded in both directions at the same time, from its sketch
plane.

* A sketch can also be extruded as a solid or a thin feature.

14. Adding the model fillets by Lasso*:

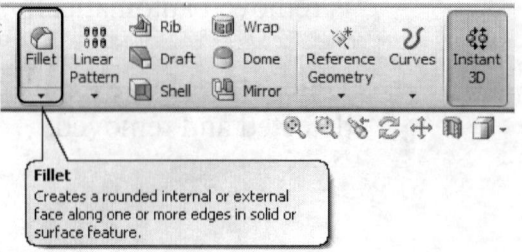

- Fillet/Round creates a rounded internal or external face on the part. You can fillet all edges of a face, select sets of faces, edges, or edge loops.

Fillet
Creates a rounded internal or external face along one or more edges in solid or surface feature.

- The **radius** value stays in effect until you change it. Therefore, you can select any number of edges or faces in the same operation.

- Click 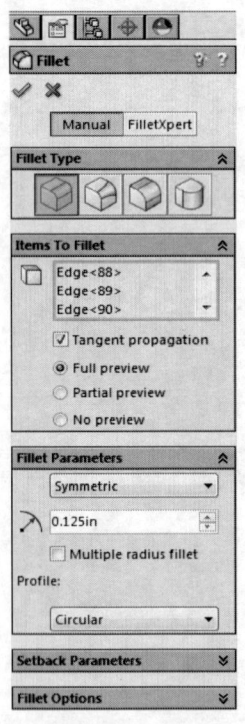 or select **Insert / Features / Fillet/Round**.

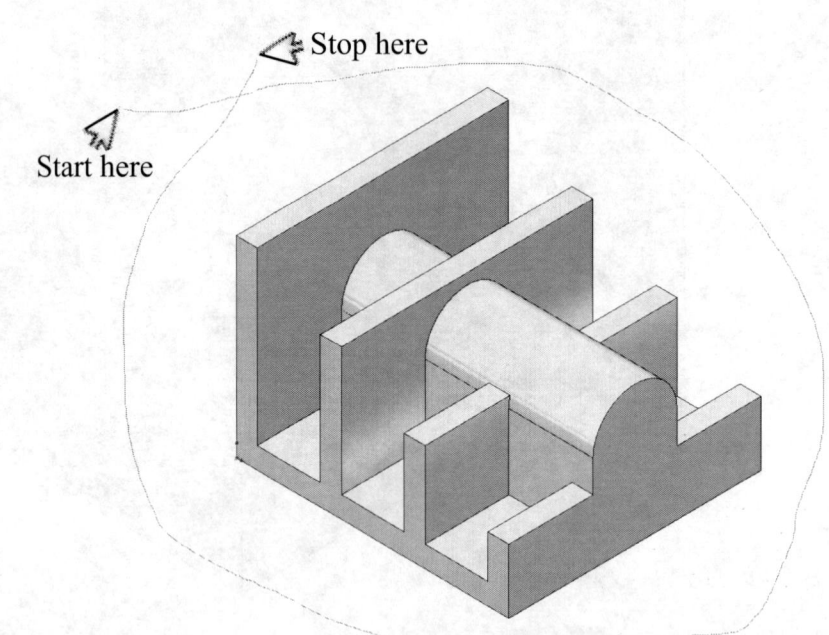

Stop here

Start here

- Enter **.125 in**. for radius value.

- Click-Hold the mouse approximately at the "Start here" position and drag the pointer around the entire model to select all of its edges.

- Click **OK** ✓.

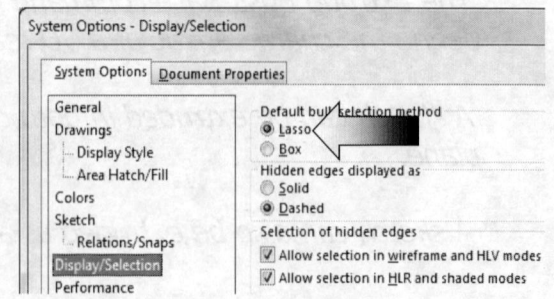

* To set the Lasso Selection as the default, go to: **Tools / Options / Display Selection / Default Bulk Selection Method / Lasso** (arrow).

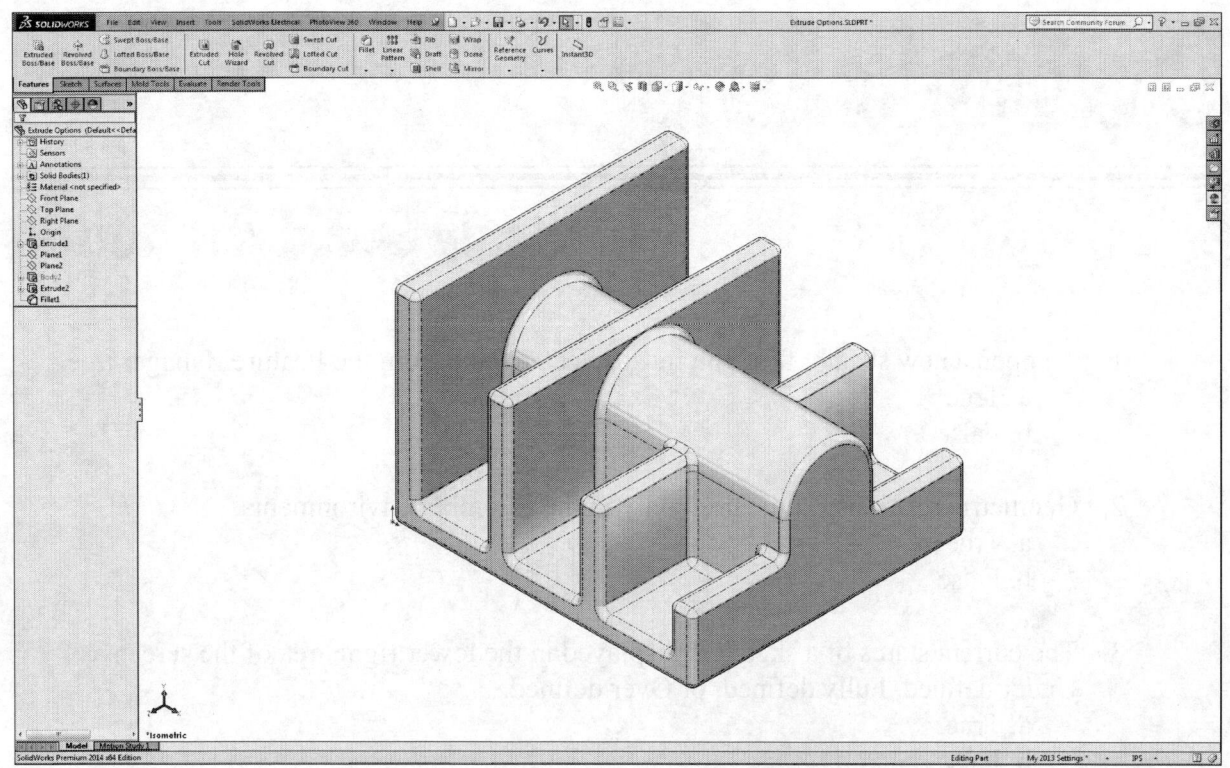

* *In the Training Files folder, in the <u>Built Parts folder</u> you will also find copies of the parts, assemblies, and drawings that were created for cross referencing or reviewing purposes.*

Fillet
(adds material)

* *Fillets and Rounds:*

Using the same Fillet command, SolidWorks "knows" whether to add material (Fillet) or remove material (Round) to the faces adjacent to the selected edge.

Round
(removes material)

15. Saving your work:

- Select **File / Save As**.

- Change the file type to **Part** file (.sldprt).

- Enter **Extrude Options** for the name of the file.

- Click **Save**.

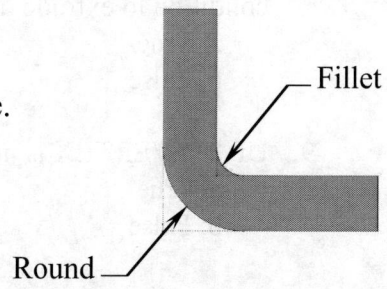

Fillet

Round

Questions for Review

Basic Solid Modeling

1. To open a new sketch, first you must select a plane from the FeatureManager tree.
   a. True
   b. False

2. Geometric relations can be used only in the assembly environments.
   a. True
   b. False

3. The current status of a sketch is displayed in the lower right area of the screen as: Under defined, Fully defined, or Over defined.
   a. True
   b. False

4. Once a feature is extruded, its extrude direction cannot be changed.
   a. True
   b. False

5. A planar face can also be used as a sketch plane.
   a. True
   b. False

6. The Equal relation only works for Lines, not Circles or Arcs.
   a. True
   b. False

7. After a dimension is created, its value cannot be changed.
   a. True
   b. False

8. When the UP TO SURFACE option is selected, you have to choose a surface as an end-condition to extrude up to.
   a. True
   b. False

9. UP TO VERTEX is not a valid Extrude option.
   a. True
   b. False

9. FALSE
8. TRUE   7. FALSE
6. FALSE   5. TRUE
4. FALSE   3. TRUE
2. FALSE   1. TRUE

Exercise: Extrude Boss & Extrude Cut

NOTE: *In an exercise, there will be less step-by-step instruction than those in the lessons, which will give you a chance to apply what you have learned in the previous lesson to build the model on your own.*

1. Dimensions are in inches, 3 decimal places.
2. Use Mid-Plane end condition for the Base feature.
3. The part is symmetrical about the Front plane.
4. Use the instructions on the following pages if needed.

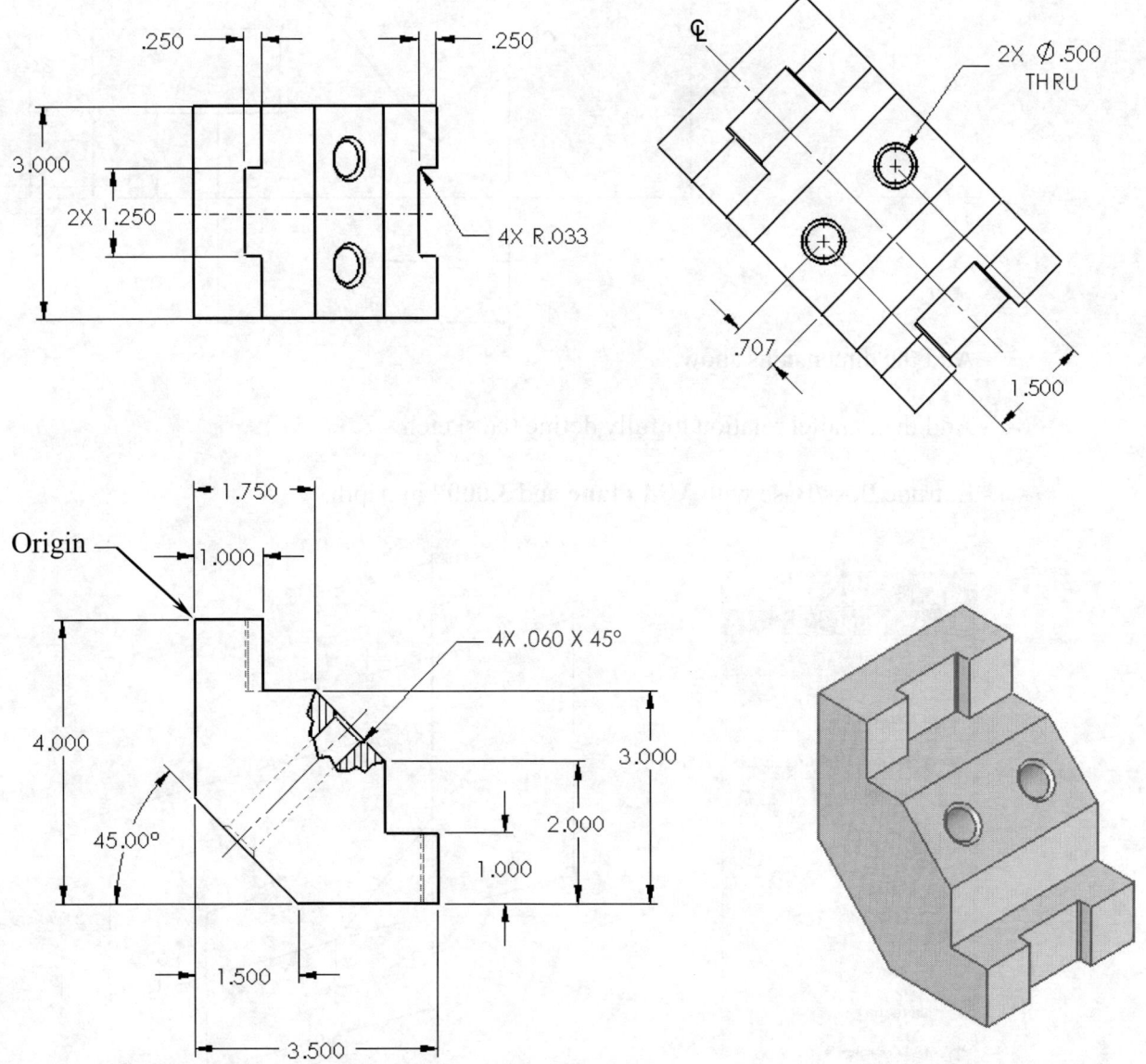

1. Starting with the base sketch:

- Select the <u>Front</u> plane and open a new sketch.

- Starting at the top left corner, using the line command, sketch the profile below.

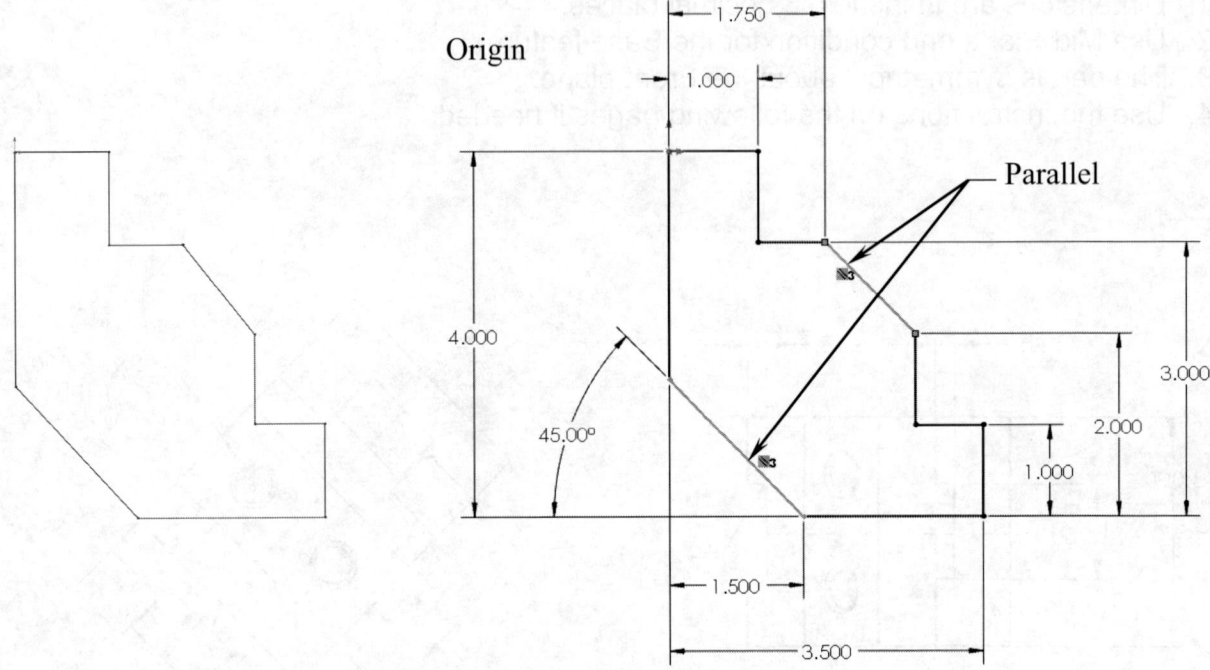

- Add the dimensions shown.

- Add the Parallel relation to fully define the sketch.

- Extrude Boss/Base with **Mid Plane** and **3.000"** in depth.

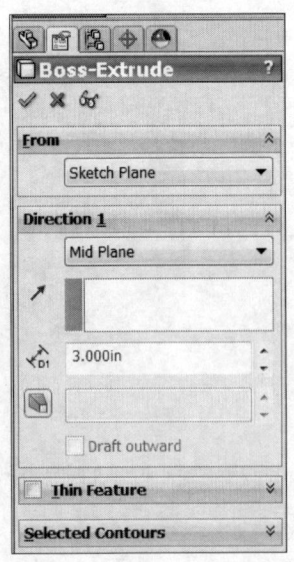

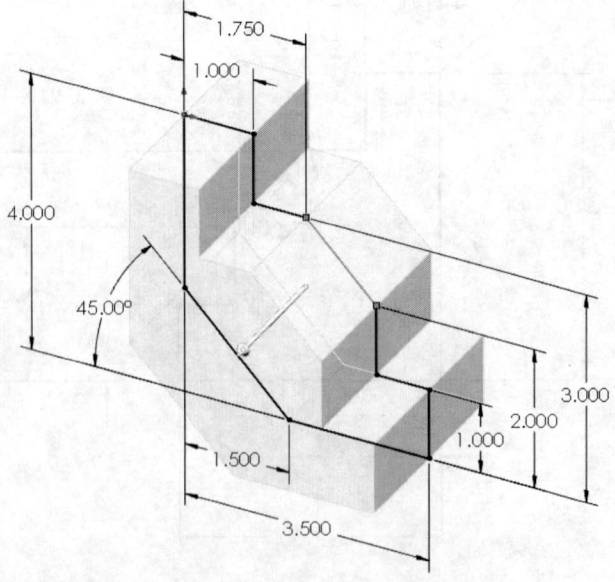

2. Adding the through holes:

- Select the <u>face</u> as indicated and click the Normal-To button.

- This command rotates the part normal to the screen.

- The hot-key for this command is **Ctrl + 8**.

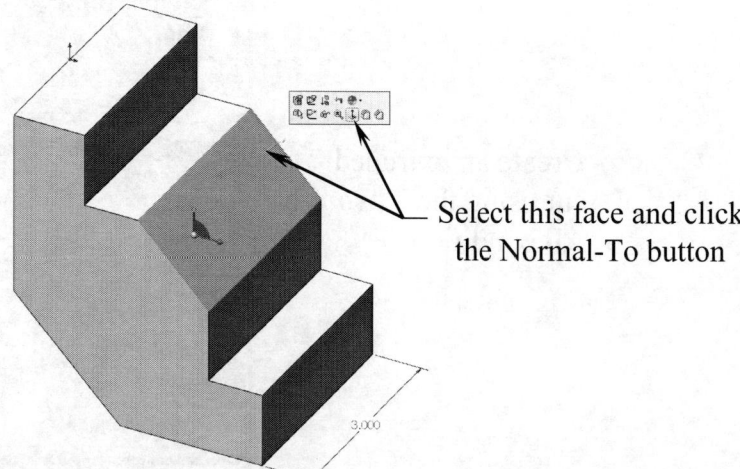

Select this face and click the Normal-To button

- Open a new sketch and draw a centerline that starts from the origin point.

- Sketch 2 circles on either side of the centerline.

- Add the diameter and location dimensions shown. Push Escape when done.

Both circles are Symmetric about the Centerline

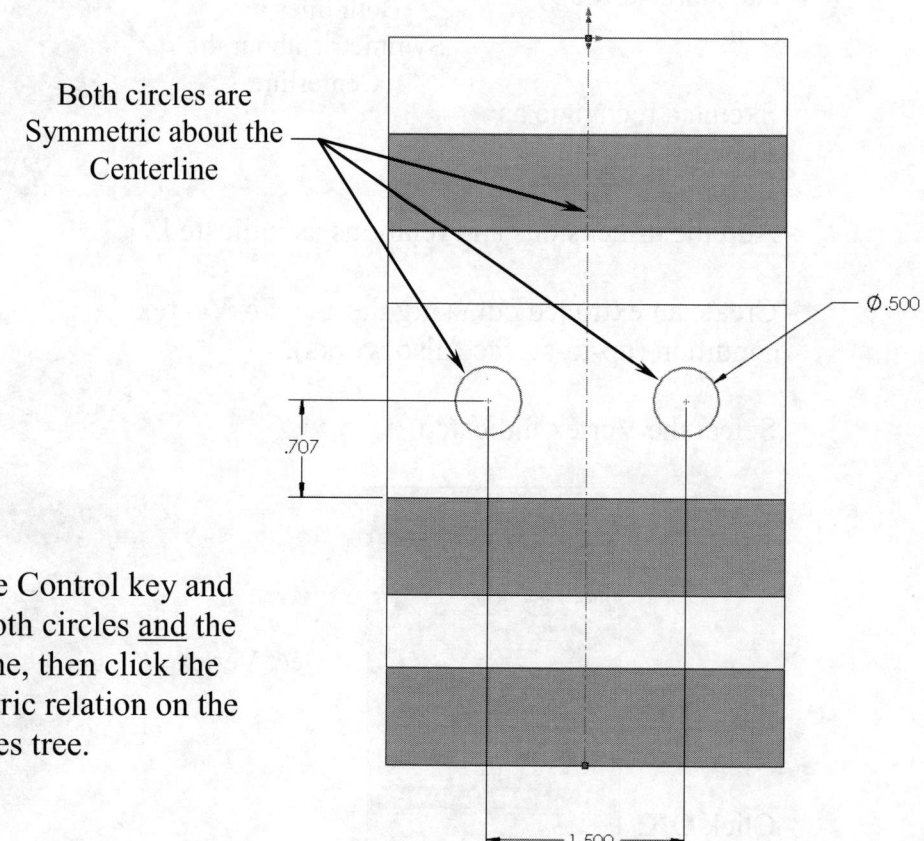

Ø.500

.707

1.500

- Hold the Control key and select both circles <u>and</u> the centerline, then click the Symmetric relation on the properties tree.

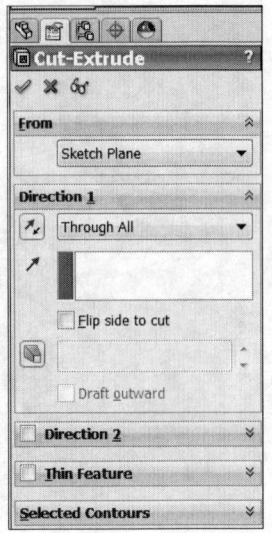

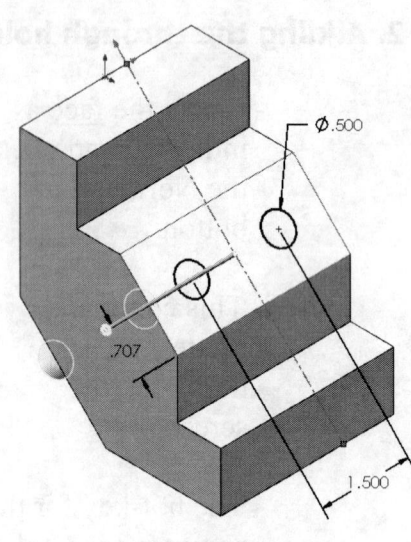

- Create an extruded cut using the **Through-All** condition.

3. Adding the upper cut:

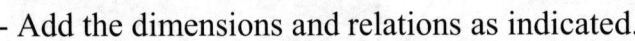

- Select the <u>upper face</u> and click the Sketch pencil to open a new sketch.

- Sketch a centerline that starts at the Origin.

Both lines are Symmetric about the Centerline

- Sketch a rectangle as shown.

- Add the dimensions and relations as indicated.

- Create an extruded cut using the **Up-To-Vertex** condition (up-to-surface also works).

- Select the Vertex indicated.

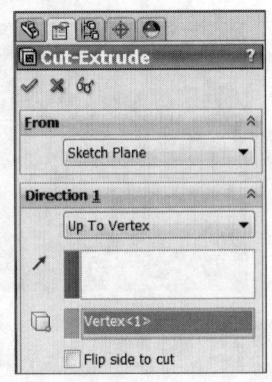

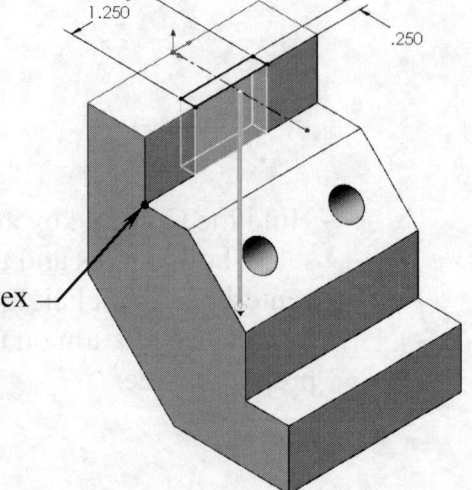

Select Vertex

- Click **OK**.

4. Adding the lower cut:

- Select the <u>lower face</u> of the part and open a new sketch.

- Sketch a rectangle on this face.

- Add a Collinear <u>and</u> an Equal relations to the lines and the edges as noted.

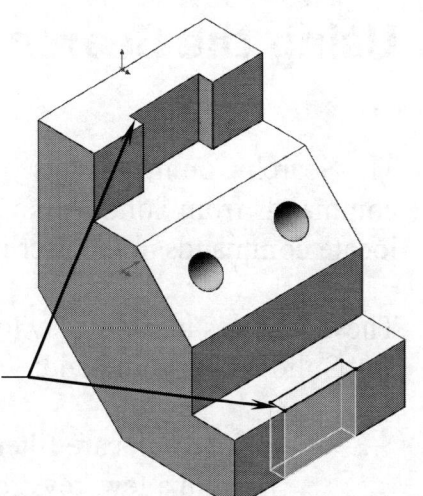

The line is Collinear <u>and</u> Equal with the edge on both sides.

- Extrude a cut using the Through All condition.

5. Adding a chamfer:

- Click **Chamfer** under the Fillet button.

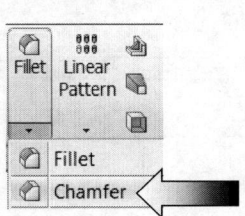

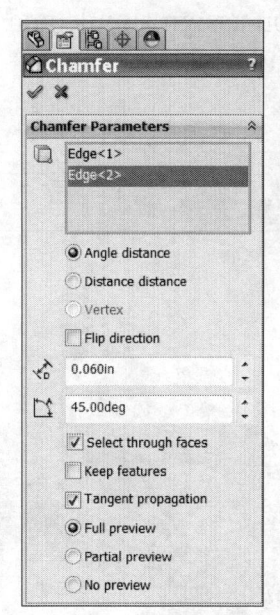

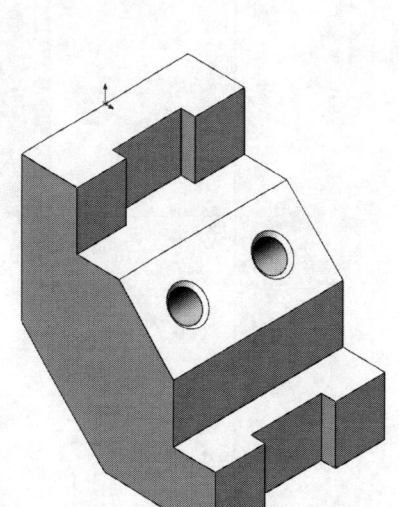

Select 4 edges

- Enter **.060** for depth.

- Select the 4 circular edges of the 2 holes.

- Click **OK**.

6. Saving your work:

- Click **File / Save As**.

- Enter **Extrudes_Exe1** for the file name.

- Select a location to save the file.

- Click **Save**.

Using the Search Commands:

The Search Commands lets you find and run commands from SolidWorks Search or locate commands in the user interface.

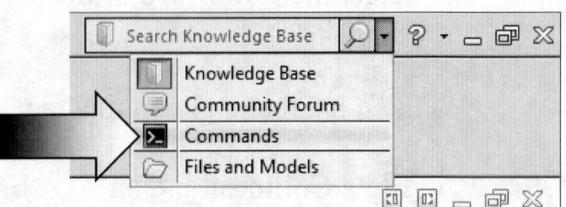

These features make it easy to find and run any SolidWorks command:

- The results are filtered as you type and typically find the command you need within a few keystrokes.

- When you run a command from the results list for a query, Search Commands remembers that command and places it at the top of the results list when you type the same query again.

- Search shortcuts lets you assign simple and familiar keystroke sequences to Commands you use regularly.

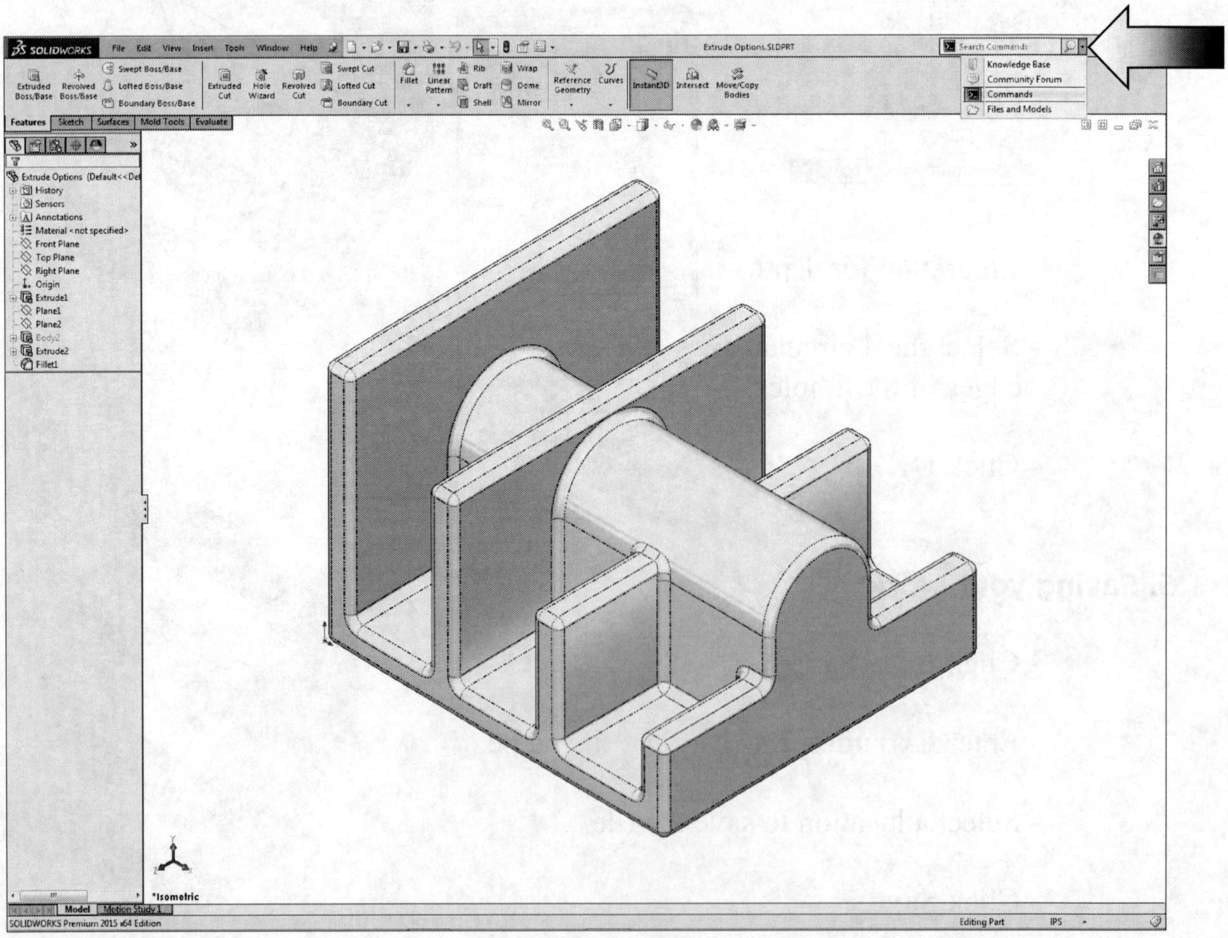

1. Search Commands in Feature Mode:

- The example below shows how you might use Search Commands to find and run the **Lasso Selection** command in the <u>Feature Mode</u>.

- With the part still open, start typing the command **Lasso Selection** in Search Commands. As soon as you type the first few letters of the word Lasso, the results list displays only those commands that include the character sequence **"lasso"**, and **Lasso Selection** appears near the top of the results list.

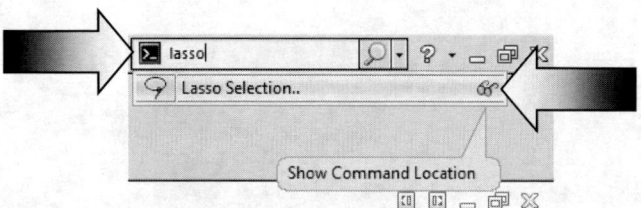

- Click **Show Command Location** 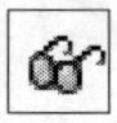 🔍, a red arrow indicates the command in the user interface.

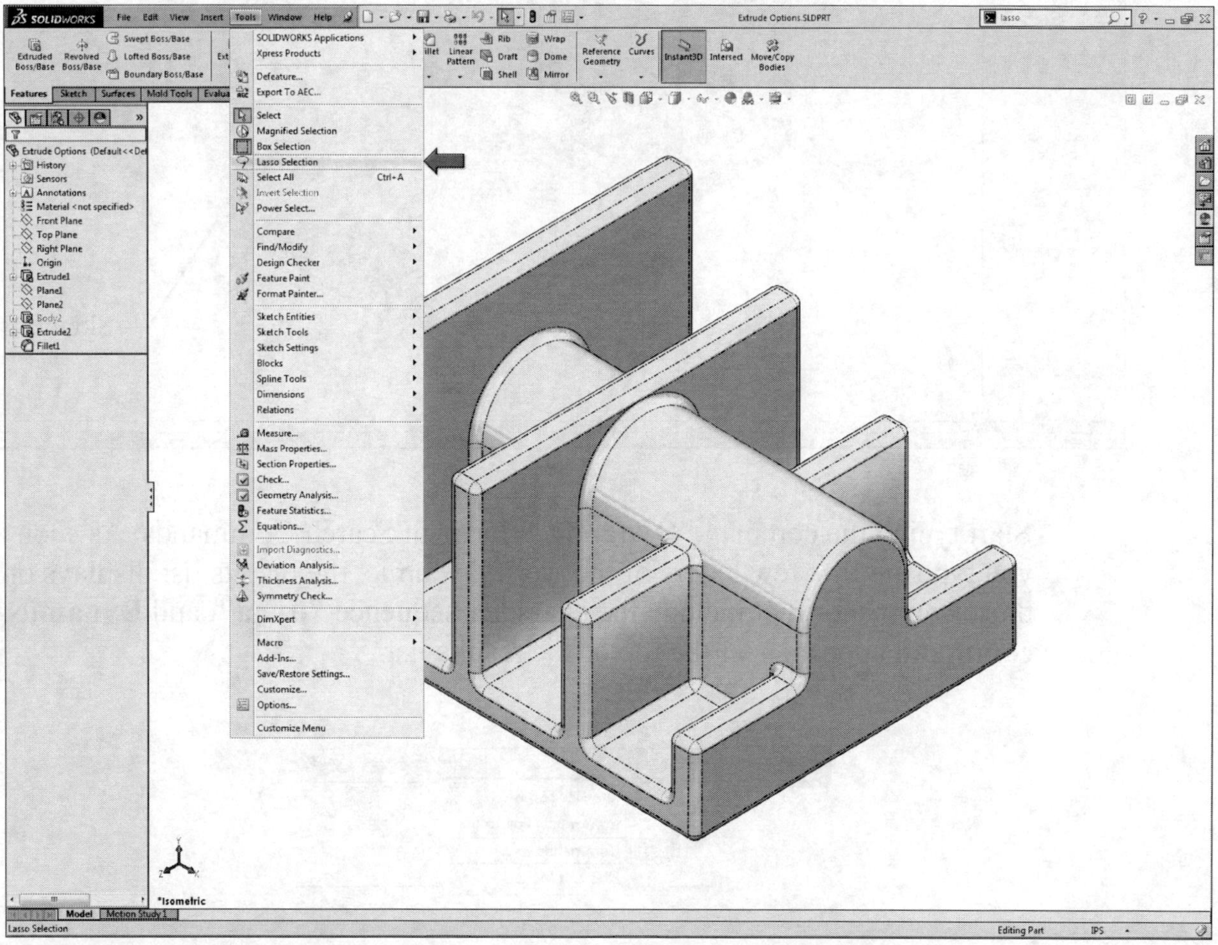

2. Search Commands in Sketch Mode:

- The example below shows how you might use Search Commands to find and run the **Dynamic Mirror** command in the <u>Sketch Mode</u>.

- Using the same part, open a **new sketch** on the <u>side face</u> of the model as noted.

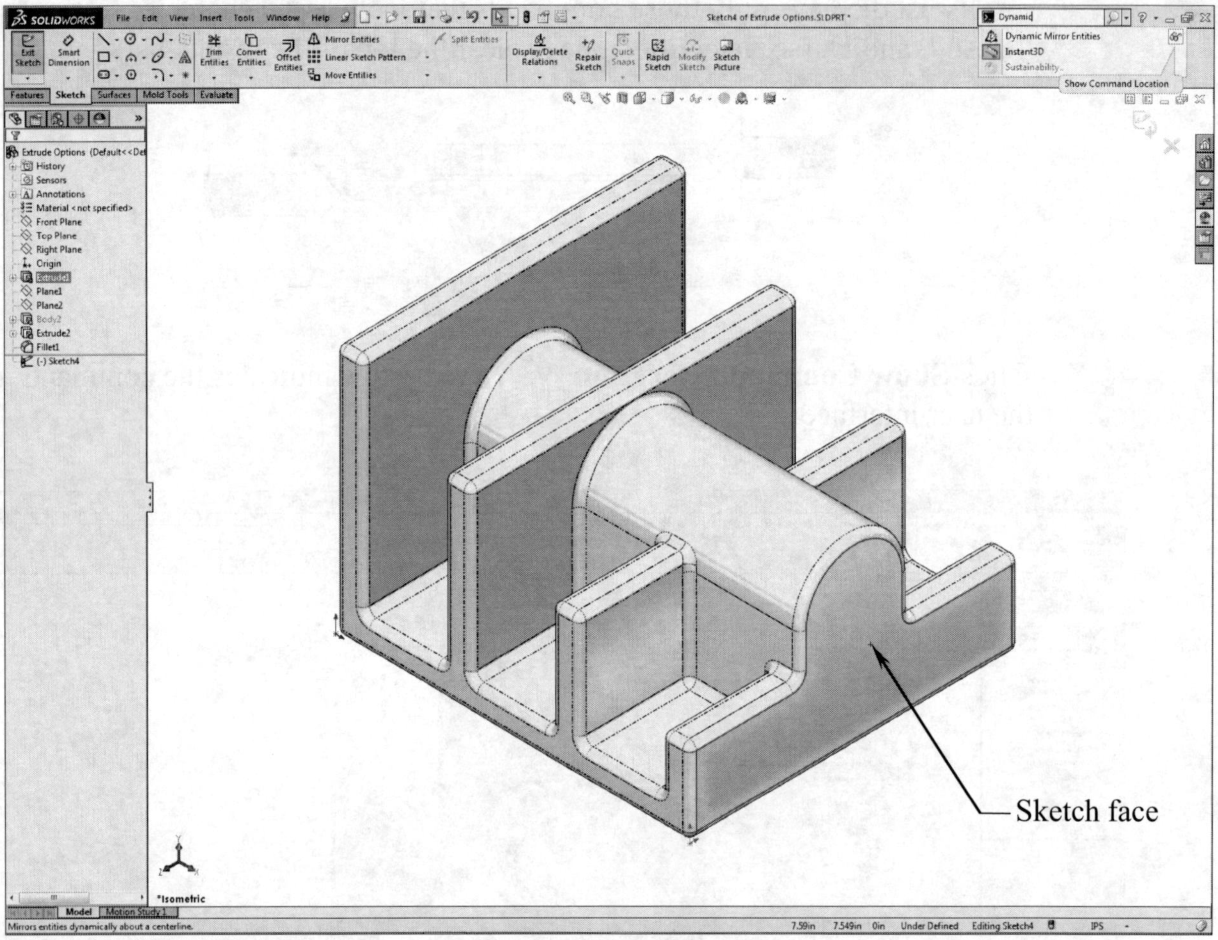

Sketch face

- Start typing the command **Dynamic Mirror** in Search Commands. As soon as you type the first few letters of the word Dynamic, the results list displays only those commands that include the character sequence **"dyna"**, and **Dynamic command** appears near the top of the results list.

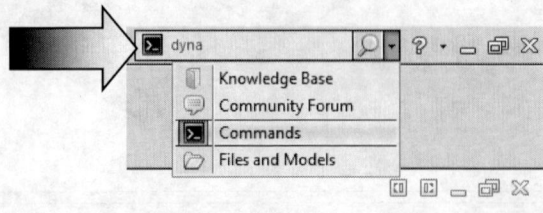

- Click **Show Command Location** 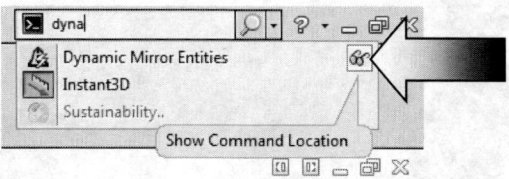, a red arrow indicates the command in the user interface.

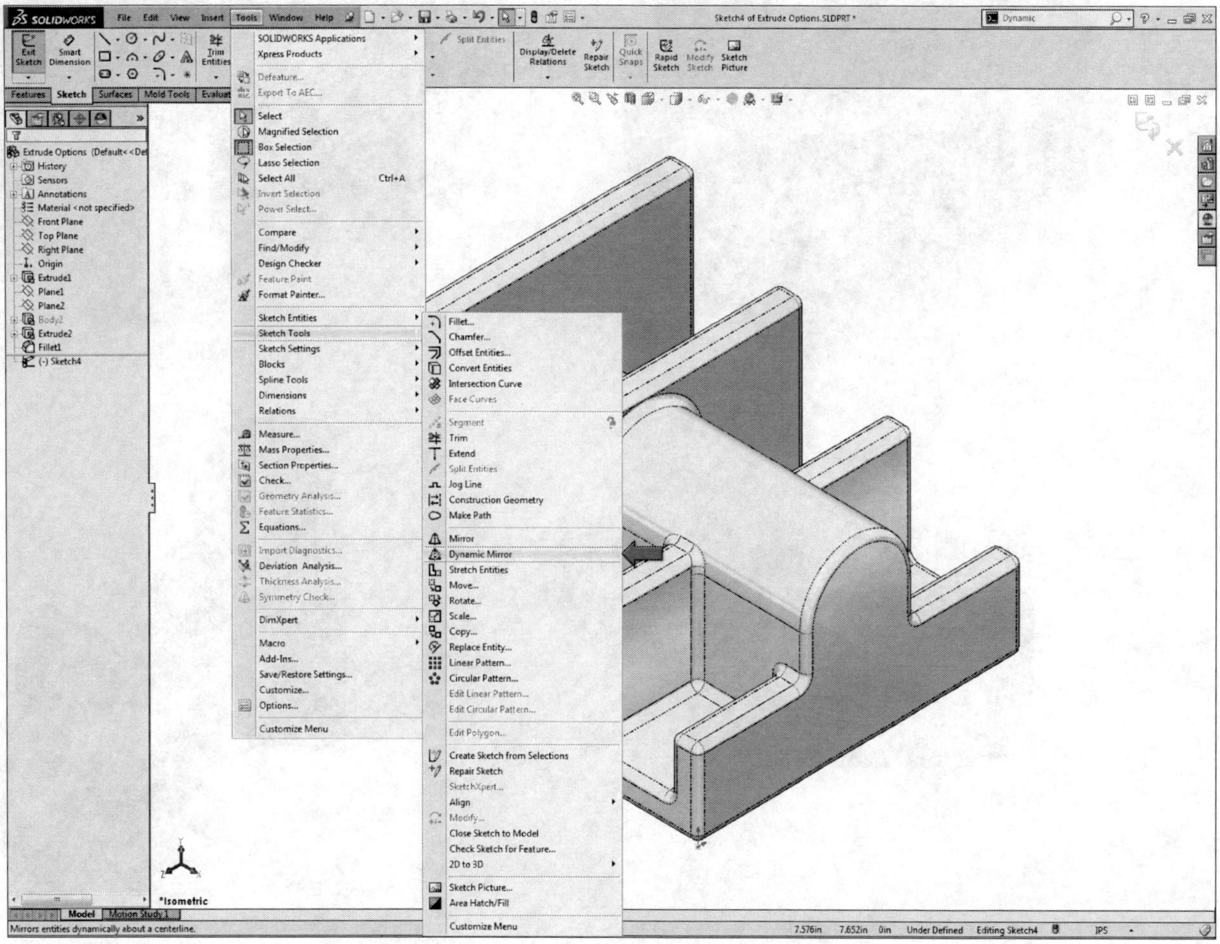

- Additionally, a Search Shortcut can be assigned to any command to help find it more quickly (see Customize Keyboard in the SolidWorks Help for more info):

1. Click **Tools / Customize**, and select the **Keyboard** tab.
2. Navigate to the command to which you want to assign a search shortcut.
3. In the Search Shortcut column for the command, type the shortcut letter you want to use, then click OK.

- Save and close all documents.

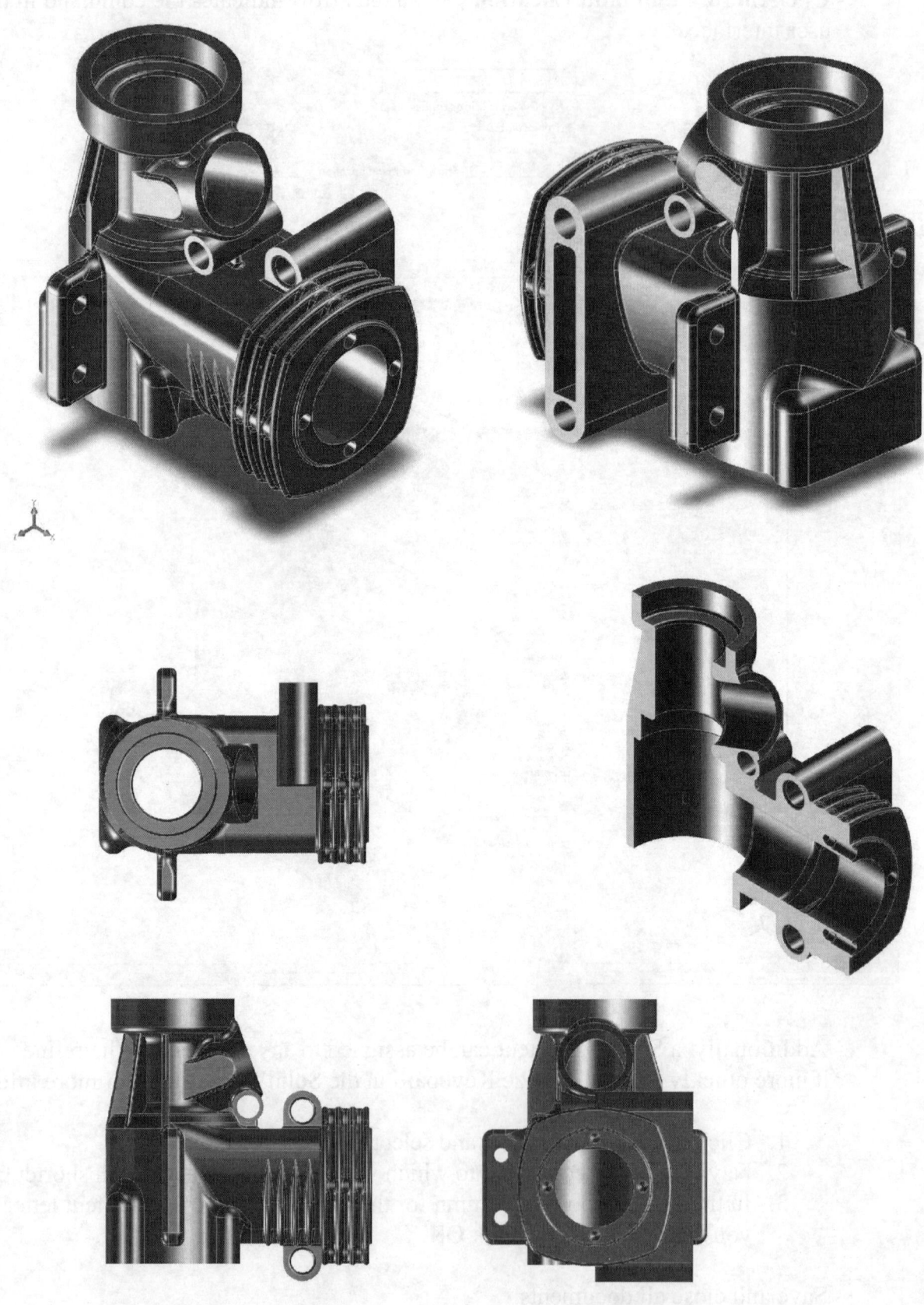

CHAPTER 4

Basic Solid Modeling

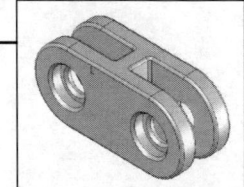

Basic Solid Modeling
Extrude & Revolve

- Upon successful completion of this lesson, you will be able to:

    * Perform basic modeling techniques.

    * Sketch on planar surfaces .

    * Add dimensions .

    * Add geometric relations or constraints .

    * Use extrude with Boss / Base .

    * Use Extruded Cut .

    * Create revolved features .

    * Create Fillets and Chamfers .

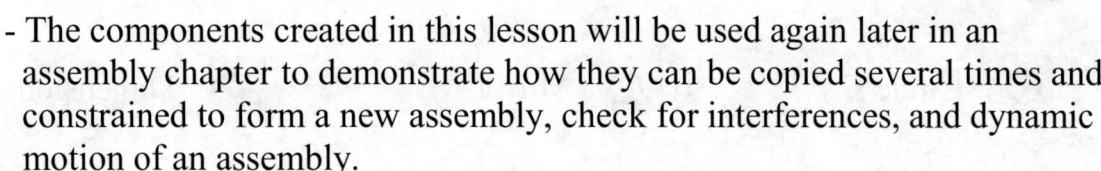

- The components created in this lesson will be used again later in an assembly chapter to demonstrate how they can be copied several times and constrained to form a new assembly, check for interferences, and dynamic motion of an assembly.

- Be sure to review self-test questionnaires at the end of the lesson, prior to going to the next chapter. They will help to see if you have gained enough knowledge required in the following chapters.

Link Components
Basic Solid Modeling

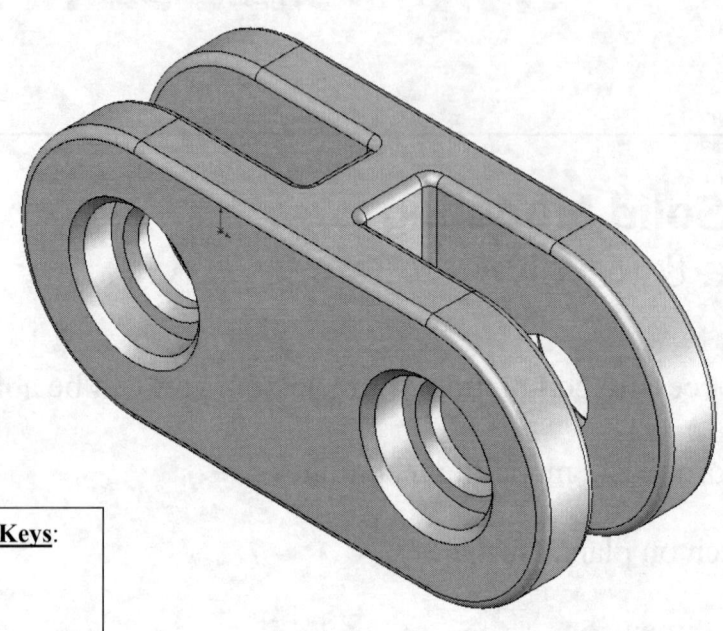

View Orientation Hot Keys:

Ctrl + 1 = Front View
Ctrl + 2 = Back View
Ctrl + 3 = Left View
Ctrl + 4 = Right View
Ctrl + 5 = Top View
Ctrl + 6 = Bottom View
Ctrl + 7 = Isometric View
Ctrl + 8 = Normal To
      Selection

Dimensioning Standards: **ANSI**

Units: **INCHES** – 3 Decimals

Tools Needed:

Insert Sketch	Line	Centerline
 Circle	Mirror	Dimension
Add Geometric Relations	Fillet	Chamfer
Extruded Boss/Base	Extruded Cut	Boss/Base Revolve

1. Sketching the first profile:

- Select the <u>Front</u> plane from the FeatureManager tree.

- Click ![icon] (Insert Sketch) and select the **Straight Slot** command ![icon] .

- First start at the origin, sketch a straight line and then move downward (or upward) to complete the slot (arrows).

- Add 2 circles on the same centers of the arcs.

- Add Dimensions ![icon] and Relations ![icon] as shown.

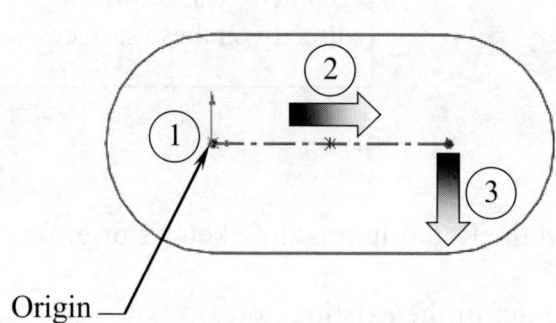

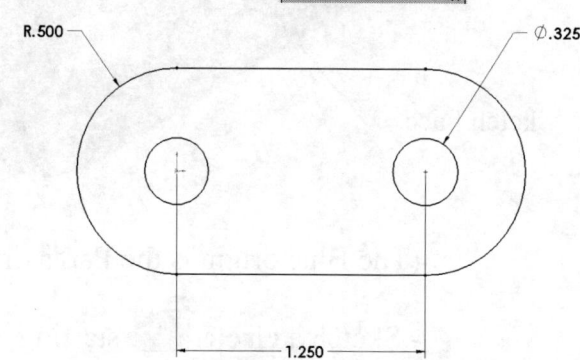

Origin

2. Extruding the first solid:

- Click ![icon] on the Features toolbar or select **Insert / Boss-Base / Extrude**.

- End condition: **Mid Plane**

- Extrude depth: **.750 in**.

- Click **OK** ![icon] .

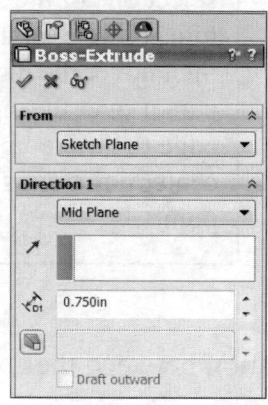

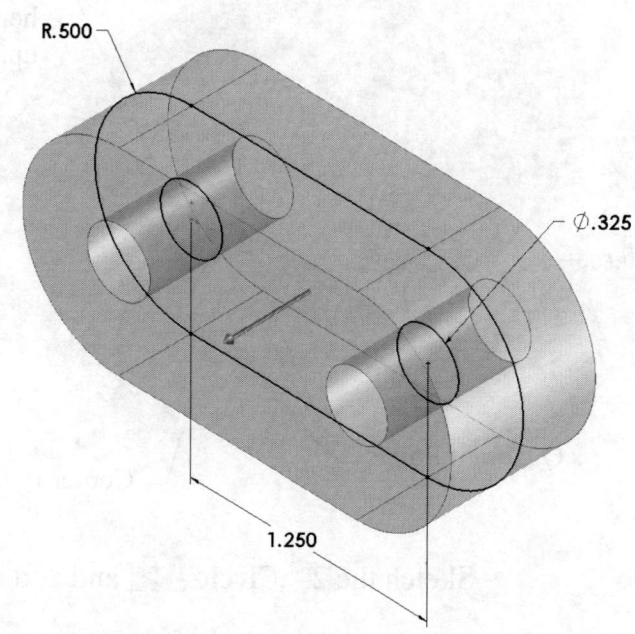

3. Creating the Bore holes:

- Select the front <u>face</u> as indicated and click 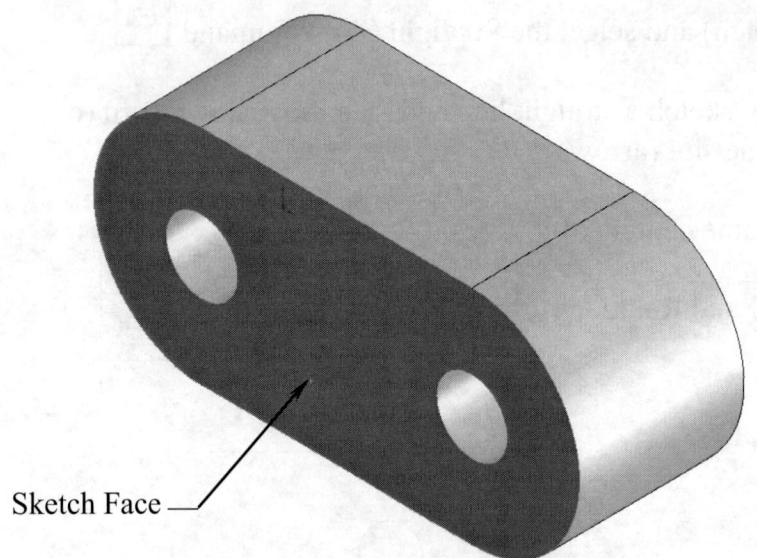 (Insert / Sketch).

Sketch Face —

> ### ☼ Planar Surfaces
>
> The planar surfaces of the model can also be used as sketch planes; sketch geometry can be drawn directly on these surfaces.

(The Blue origin is the Part's origin and the Red origin is the Sketch's origin).

- Sketch a **circle** ⊕ starting at the center of the existing hole.

- Add **Ø.500** dimension ✎ as shown.

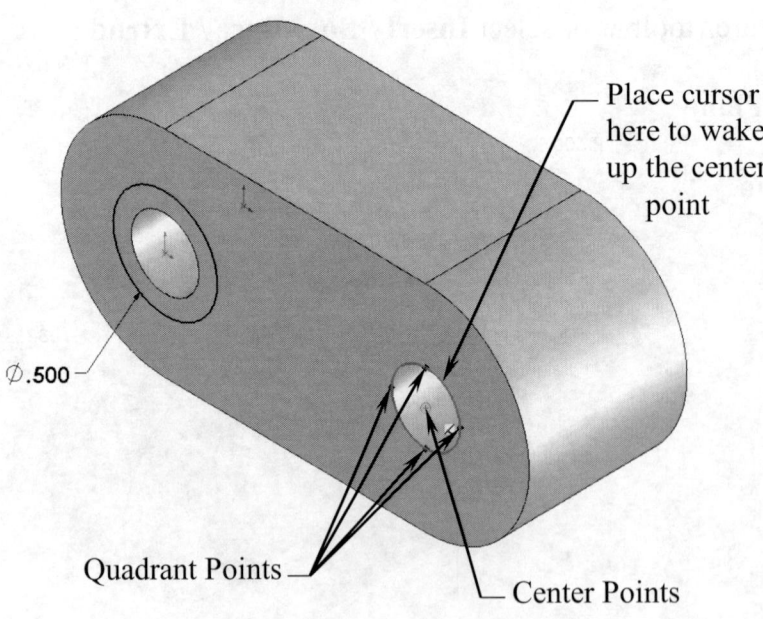

— Place cursor here to wake up the center point

Ø.500 —

Quadrant Points —

— Center Points

> ### ☼ Wake-Up Entities*
>
> To find the center (or the quadrant points) of a hole or a circle:
>
> * In the Sketch mode, select one of the sketch tools (Circle, in this case), then hover the mouse cursor over the circular edge to "wake-up" the center point & its quadrant points.

- Sketch the 2ⁿᵈ **Circle** ⊕ and add an **Equal** relation between the 2 circles.

- Click off the Circle command. Hold the **Control** key, select the 2 Circles and click the **Equal** relation (arrow).

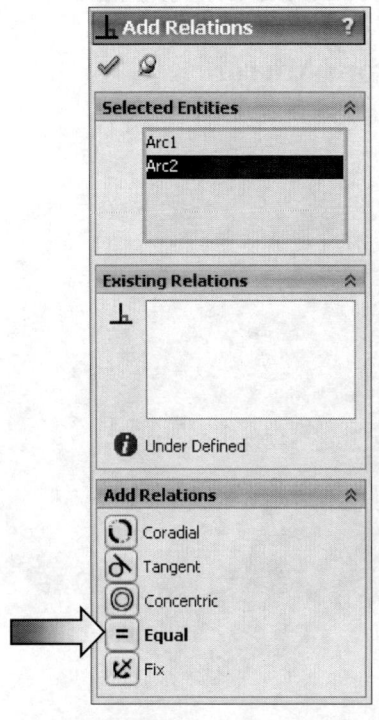

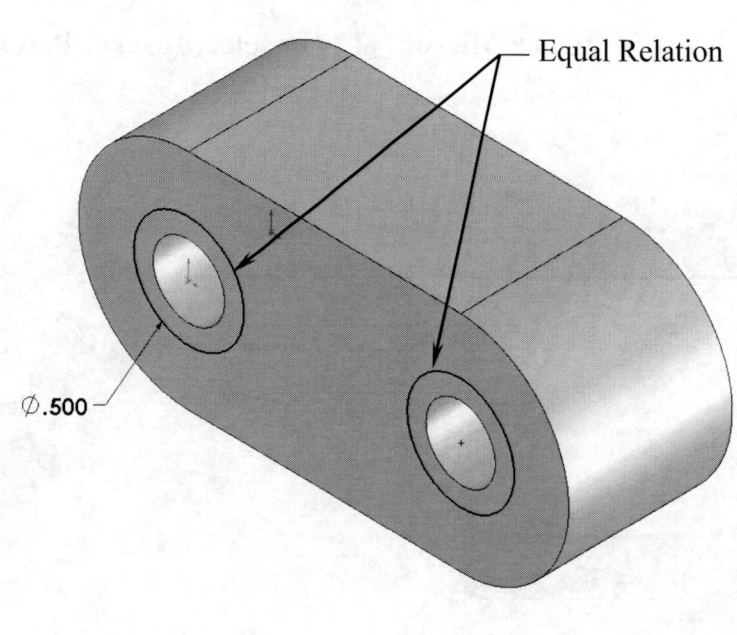

Equal Relation

⌀.500

4. Cutting the Bore holes:

- Click **Extruded Cut** or select **Insert / Cut / Extrude**.

- End Condition: **Blind**

- Extrude Depth: **.150 in**.

- Click **OK**.

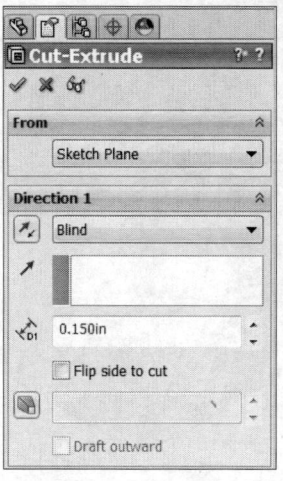

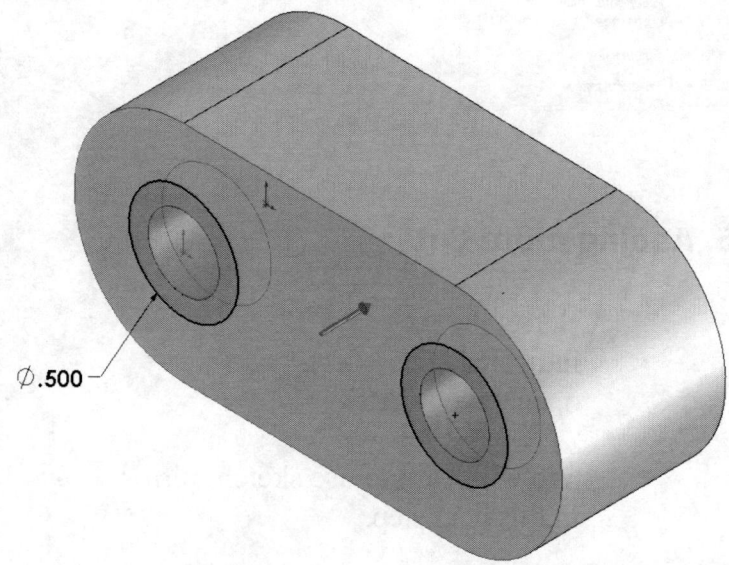

⌀.500

5. Mirroring the Bore holes:

- Select the <u>Front</u> plane from the FeatureManager Tree as the Mirror Plane.

- Click **Mirror** or select **Insert / Patent Mirror / Mirror**.

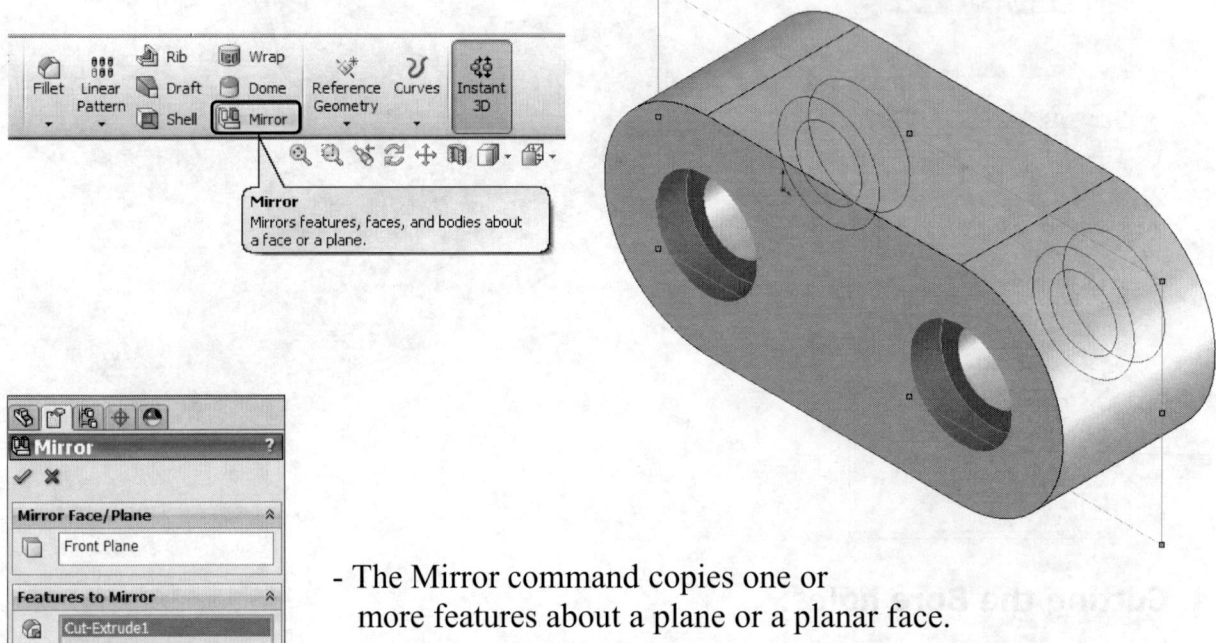

- The Mirror command copies one or more features about a plane or a planar face.

- Select the **Cut-Extrude1** from the FeatureManager Tree, or click one of the Bore holes from the graphics area.

- Click **OK** .

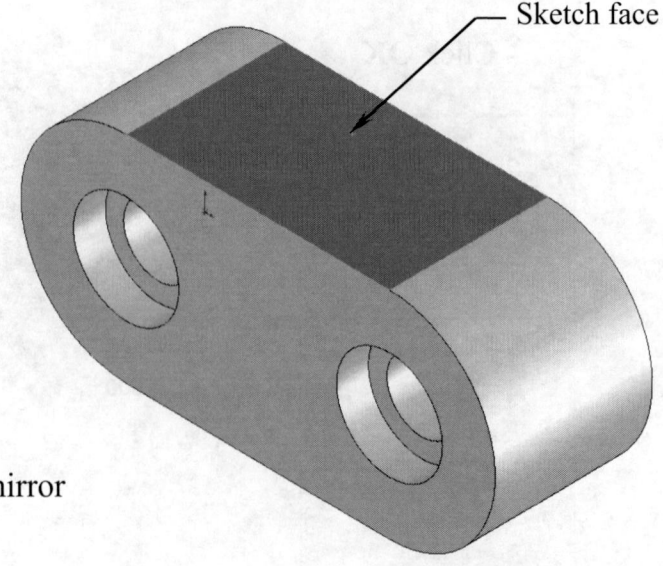

Sketch face

6. Adding more Cuts:

- Select the <u>face</u> as indicated and open a new sketch .

- We will learn to use sketch mirror in this next step.

- Sketch 2 Centerlines ⦙ one vertical and one horizontal as shown.

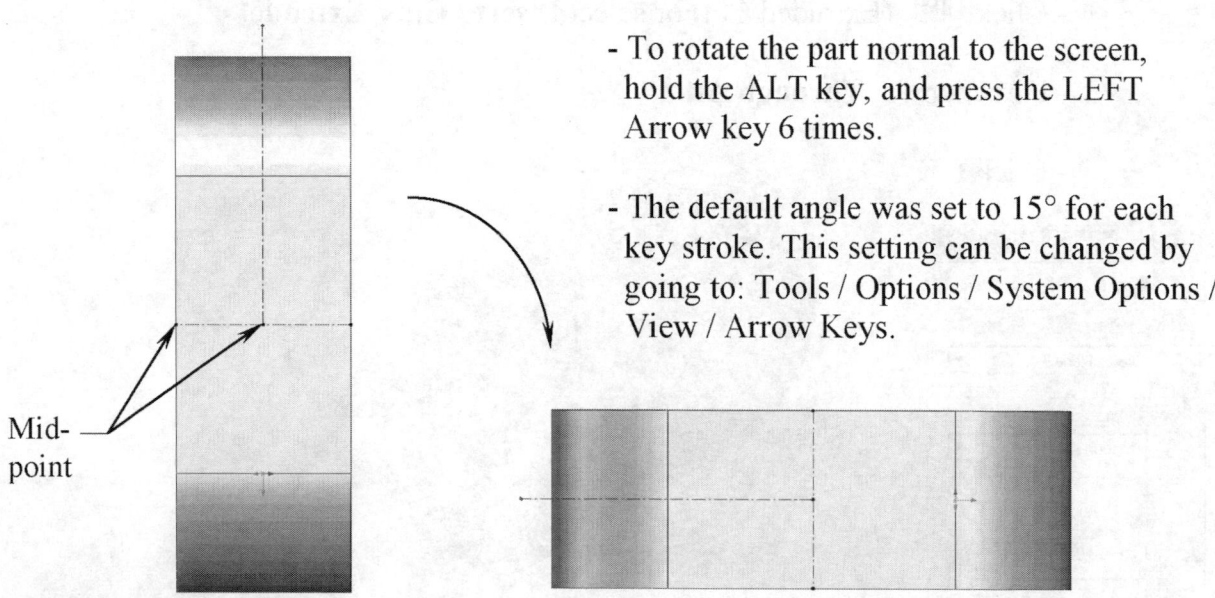

- To rotate the part normal to the screen, hold the ALT key, and press the LEFT Arrow key 6 times.

- The default angle was set to 15° for each key stroke. This setting can be changed by going to: Tools / Options / System Options / View / Arrow Keys.

Mid-point

- Select the vertical centerline and click the **Dynamic Mirror** command 🔲 or click: **Tools, Sketch Tools, Dynamic Mirror**.

- Sketch a Rectangle 🔲 on one side of the centerline; it will get mirrored to the other side automatically.

- Click off the Dynamic mirror button. Add a Symmetric relation to the 3 lines as noted .

- Add dimensions 🔷 to fully define the sketch.

- Click **OK** ✅ .

.230

Mid-Point

.300

Coincident

Symmetric

7. Extruding a Through All cut:

- Click 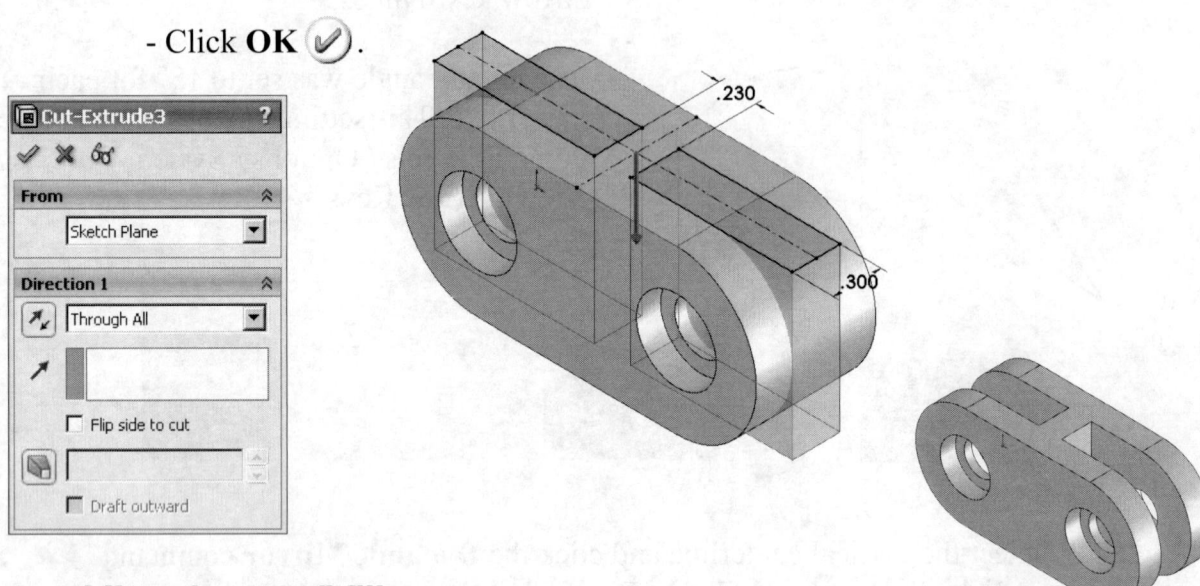 (Extruded Cut) or select **Insert / Cut / Extrude**.

- Direction 1: **Through All**

- Click **OK** ✓.

.230

.300

Cut-Extrude3

From

Sketch Plane

Direction 1

Through All

☐ Flip side to cut

☐ Draft outward

8. Adding the .032" fillets:

- Click **Fillet** or select **Insert / Features / Fillet/Round**.

- Enter **.032 in.** for Radius.

- Select the edges as indicated below.

- Click **OK** ✓.

Radius 0.032in

Fillet Type

Items To Fillet

Edge<8>
Edge<9>
Edge<10>

☑ Tangent propagation

⦿ Full preview
○ Partial preview
○ No preview

Fillet Parameters

Symmetric

0.032in

☐ Multiple radius fillet

Profile:

Circular

Select ALL edges (except for the holes)

9. Adding the .032" chamfers:

- Click **Chamfer** 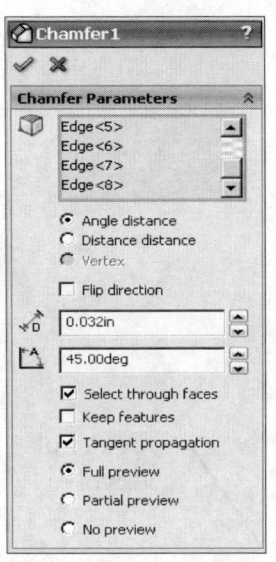 or select **Insert / Features / Chamfer.**

- Enter **.032 in.** for the depth of the chamfer and select the <u>edges</u> of the 4 holes.

- Click **OK** ✓.

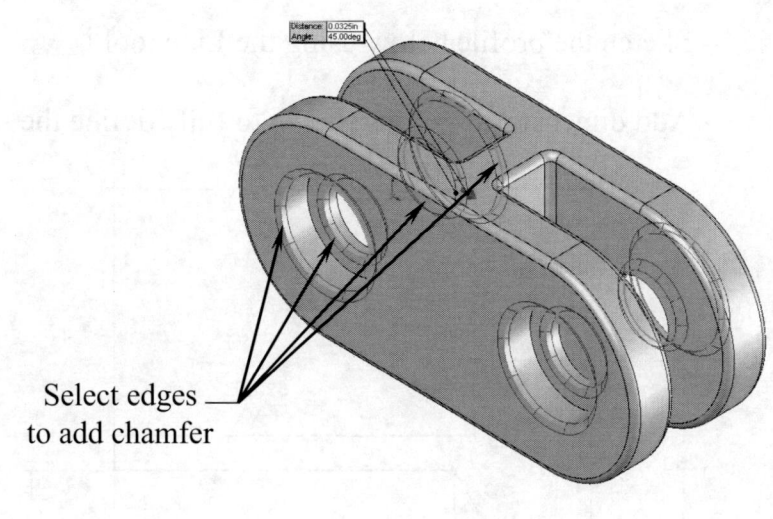

Select edges
to add chamfer

10. Saving your work:

- Select **File / Save As / Double Link / Save.**

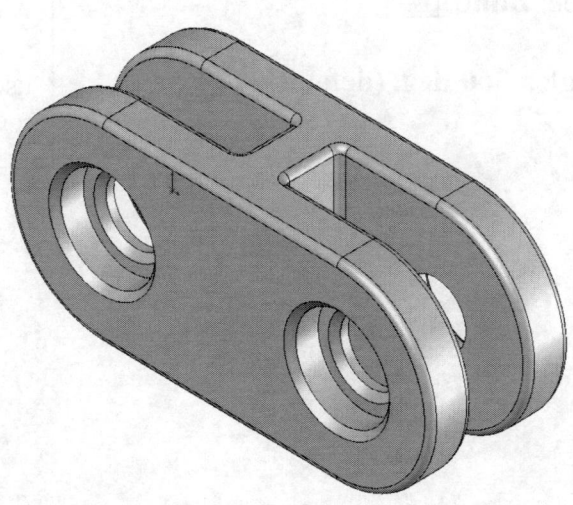

11. Creating the Sub-Components:

- The 1st sub-component is the **Alignment Pin**.

- Select the <u>Right</u> plane from the FeatureManager Tree.

- Click ✎ or select **Insert / Sketch**.

- Sketch the profile below using the Line tool ╲ .

- Add dimensions ◇ as shown to fully define the sketch.

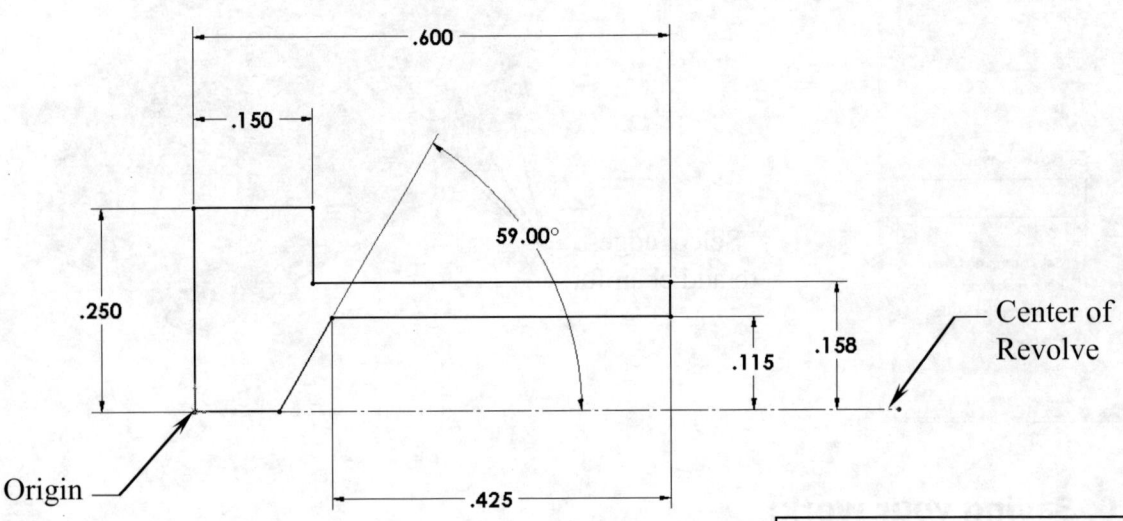

.600
.150
59.00°
.250
.115 .158
— Center of Revolve
Origin —
.425

12. Revolving the base feature:

- Click ⊕ or select **Insert / Boss-Base / Revolve**.

- Revolve Type: **Blind** 🔄 .

- Revolve Angle: **360 deg**. (default) 📐 .

- Click **OK** ✔ .

> ### 💡 Center of Revolve
>
> A centerline is used when revolving a sketch profile.
>
> A model edge, an axis, or a sketch line can also be used as the center of the revolve.

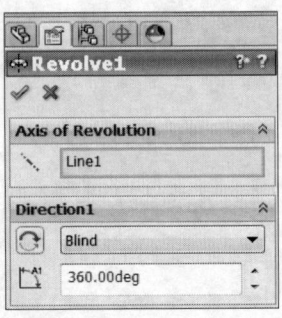

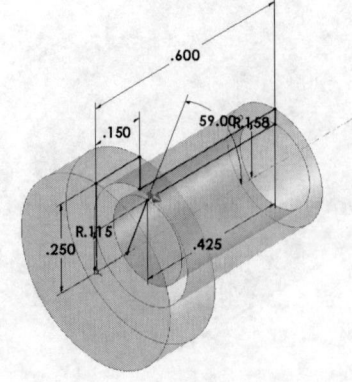

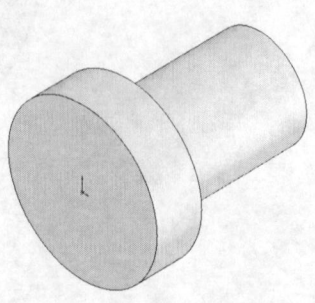

13. Adding chamfers:

- Click **Chamfer** 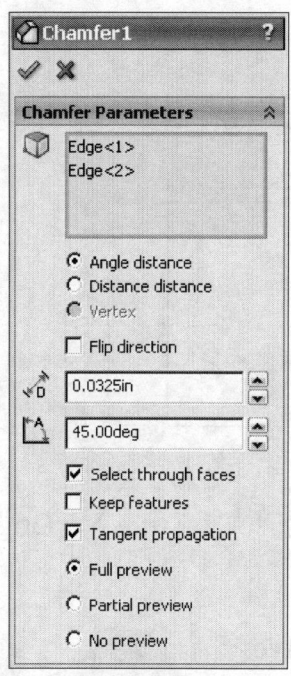 or select **Insert / Features / Chamfer**.

- Enter **.0325** for Distance .

- Enter **45 deg**. for Angle .

- Select the <u>2 Edges</u> as indicated.

- Click **OK** .

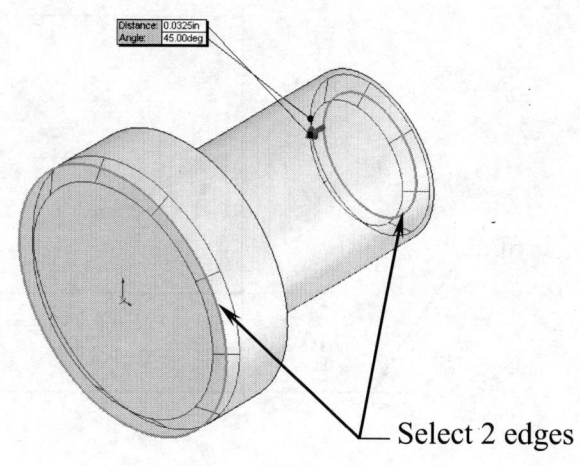

Select 2 edges

14. Saving your work:

- Select **File / Save As / Alignment Pin / Save**.

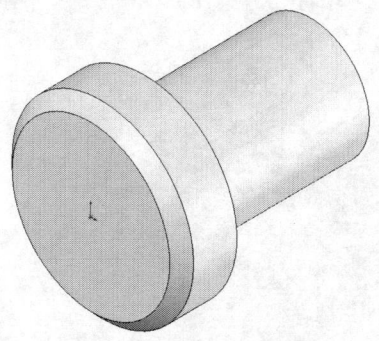

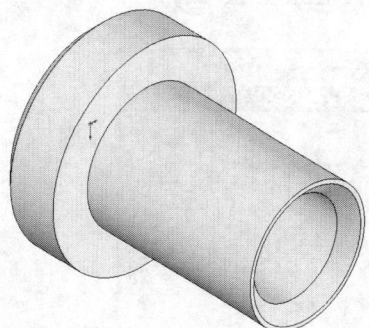

15. The 2ⁿᵈ Sub-Components:

- The 2ⁿᵈ sub-component is the **Pin Head**:

- Select the <u>Front</u> plane from the FeatureManager Tree.

- Click 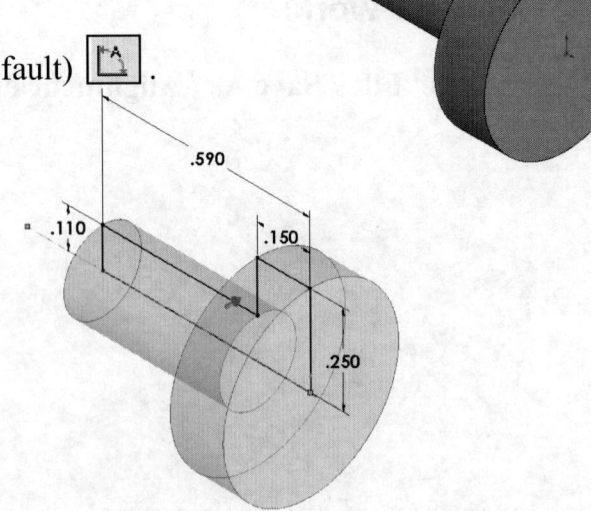 or select **Insert / Sketch**.

- Sketch the profile below using the Centerline and the Line tools .

- Add dimensions as shown to fully define the sketch.

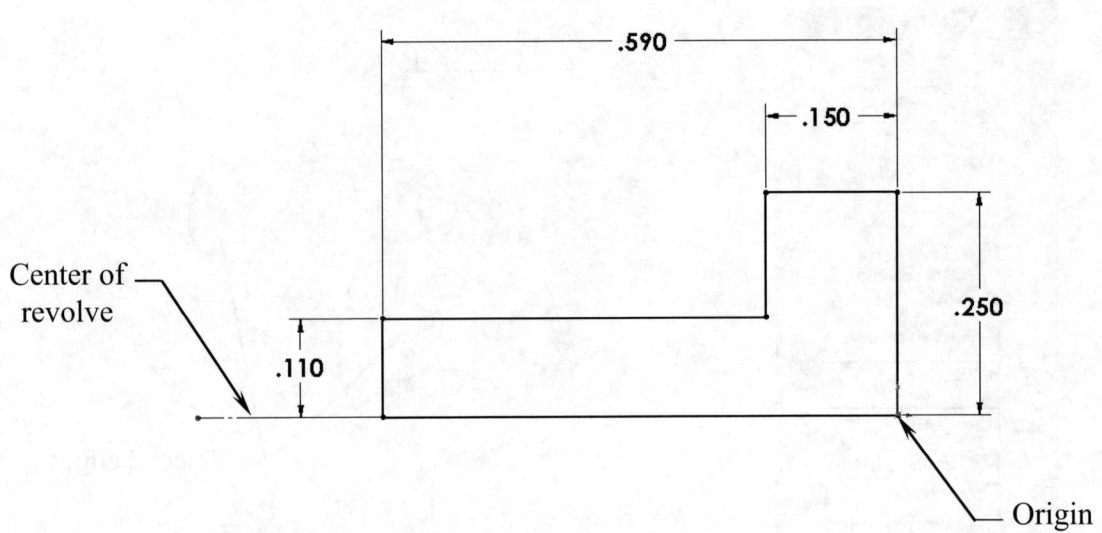

Center of revolve

.590

.150

.250

.110

Origin

16. Revolving the base feature:

- Click or select **Insert / Boss-Base / Revolve**.

- Revolve Type: **Blind** .

- Revolve Angle: **360 deg**. (default) .

- Click **OK** .

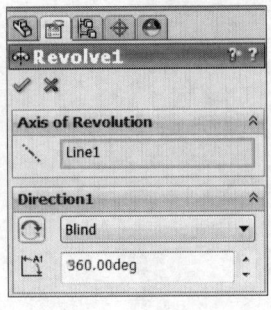

Revolve1

Axis of Revolution

Line1

Direction1

Blind

360.00deg

.590

.110

.150

.250

17. Adding a chamfer:

- Click **Chamfer** 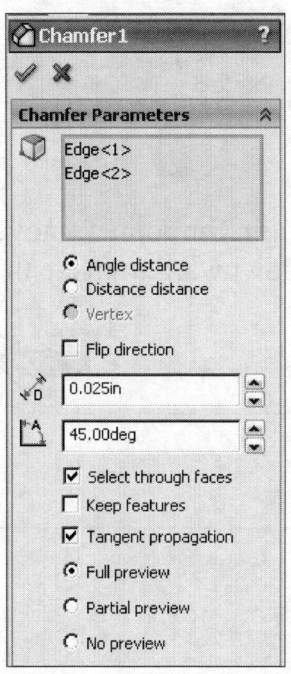 or select **Insert / Features / Chamfer**.

- Enter **.025** for Distance 🔑.

- Enter **45 deg**. for Angle 📐.

- Select the <u>Edge</u> as indicated.

- Click **OK** ✅.

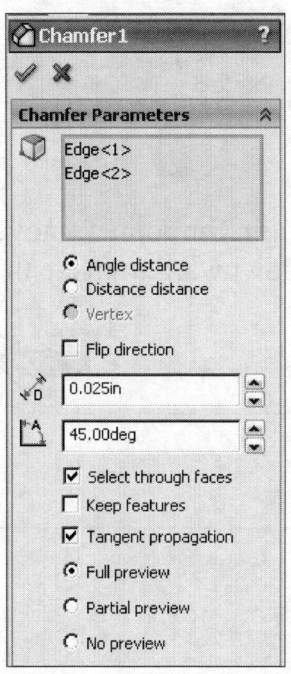

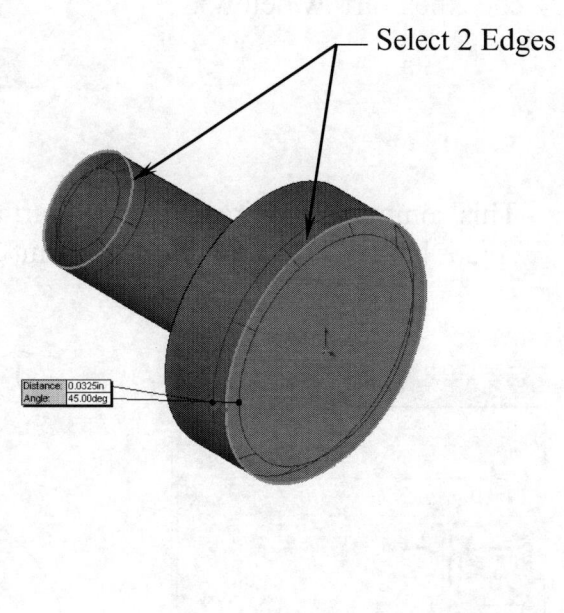

Select 2 Edges

18. Saving your work:

- Select **File / Save As / Pin Head / Save**.

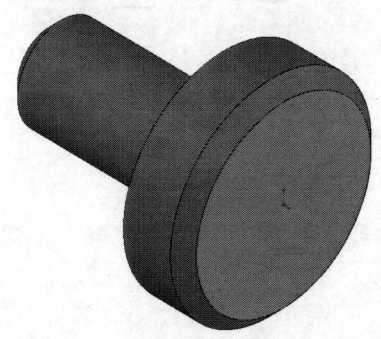

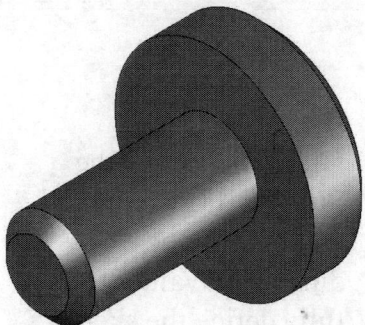

19. Creating the 3ʳᵈ Sub-Components:

- The 3ʳᵈ sub-component is the **Single Link**:

- Select <u>Front</u> plane from FeatureManager Tree.

- Click 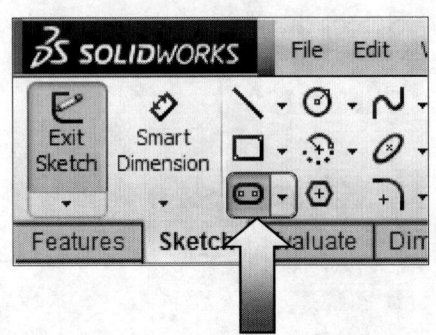 Insert Sketch and select the **Straight Slot** command.

- Enable the **Add Dimensions** checkbox (arrow below).

- This command requires 3 clicks. Start at the origin for point 1, move the cursor horizontally and click the point 2, then downward to make the point 3.

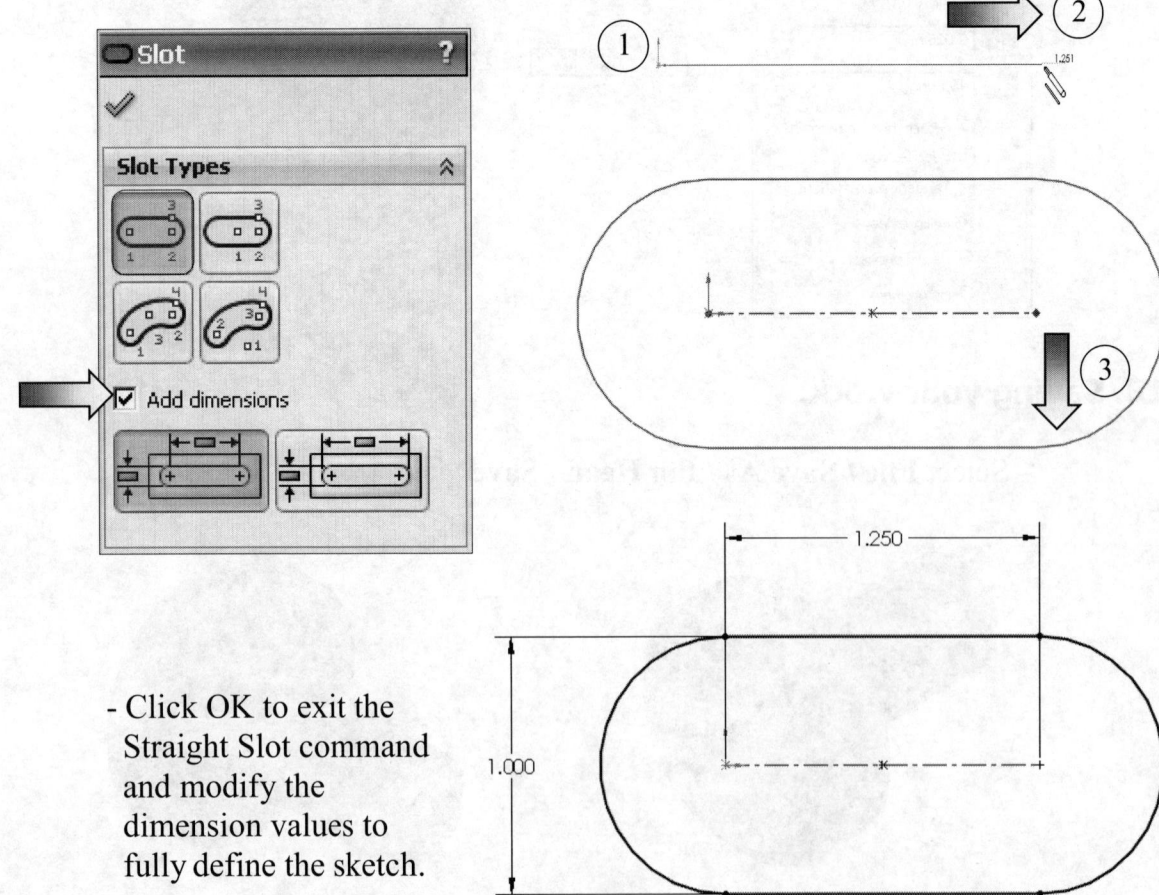

- Click OK to exit the Straight Slot command and modify the dimension values to fully define the sketch.

20. Extruding the base:

- Click **Extruded Boss-Base** 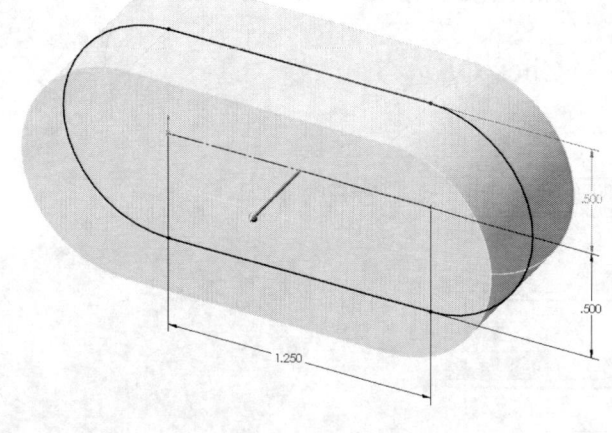 or select **Insert / Boss-Base / Extrude**.

- End condition: **Mid Plane**

- Extrude depth: **.750 in**.

- Click **OK** ✓.

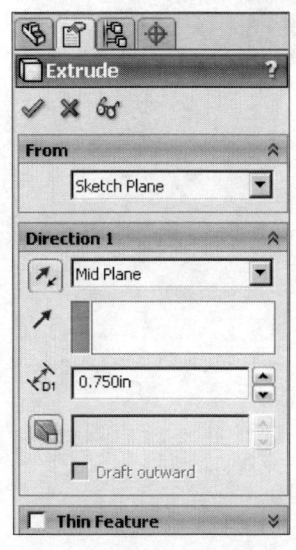

21. Sketching the Recess Profiles:

- Select the <u>face</u> indicated and open a new sketch 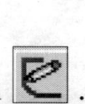 .

Sketch Face

- Sketch 2 Circles 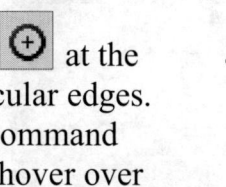 at the centers of the circular edges. (with the Circle command already selected, hover over the circular edge to see its center)

- Add a **Ø1.020 in.** dimension 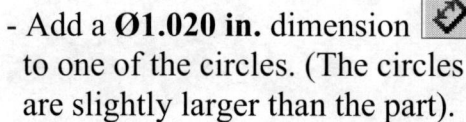 to one of the circles. (The circles are slightly larger than the part).

- Add an Equal relation 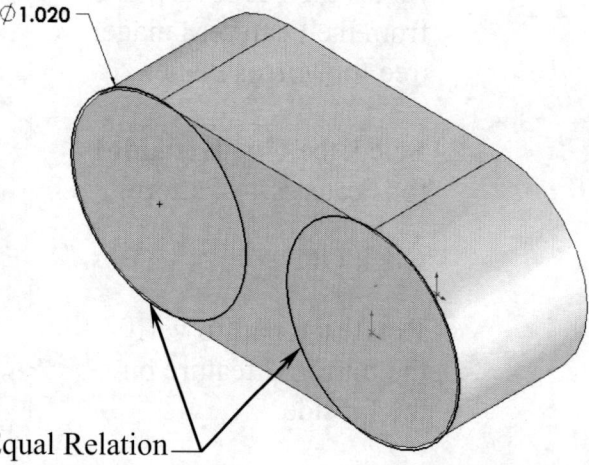 between the 2 circles.

Ø1.020

Equal Relation

22. Extruding a blind cut:

- Click **Extruded Cut** 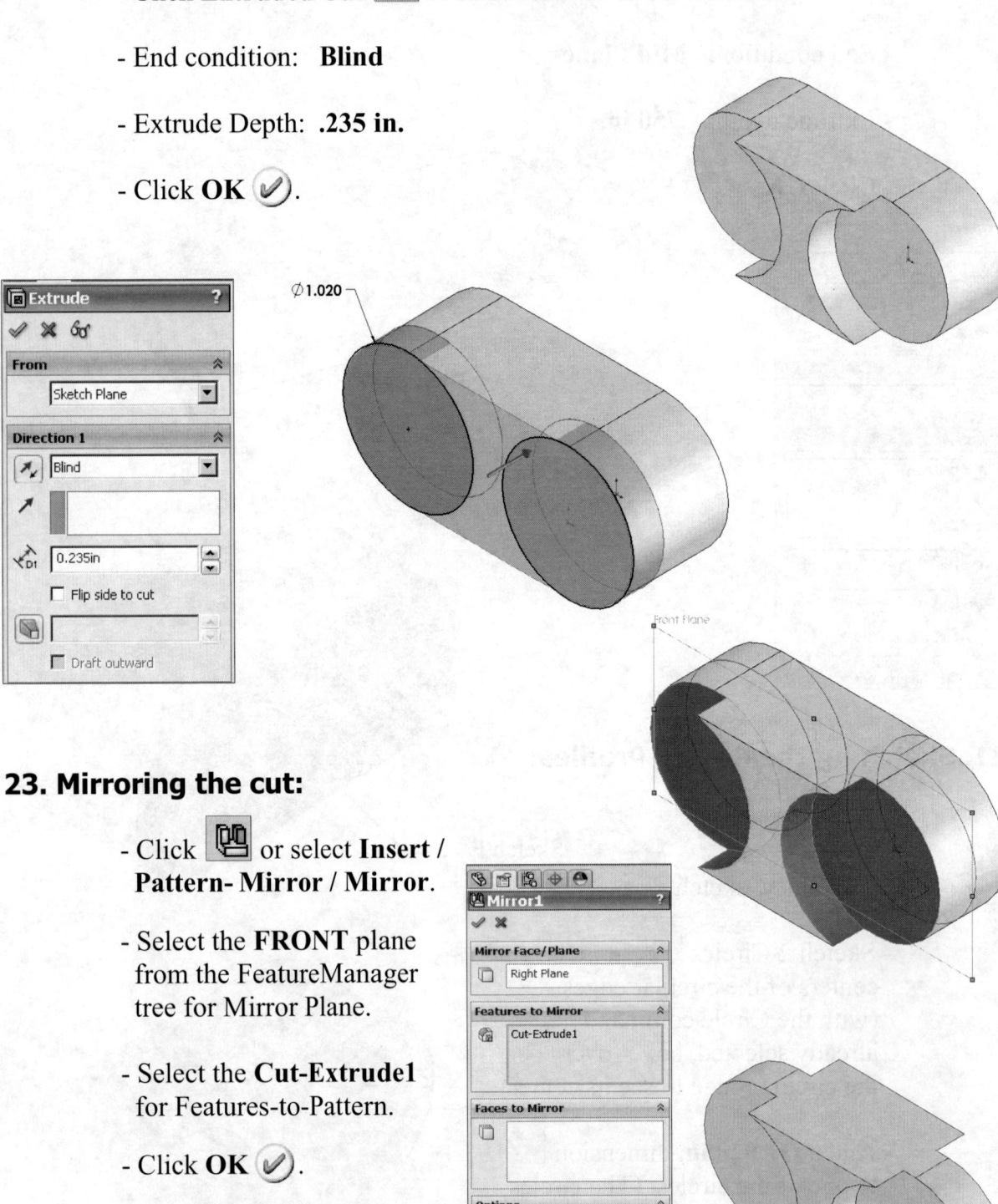 or select **Insert / Cut / Extrude**.

- End condition: **Blind**

- Extrude Depth: **.235 in.**

- Click **OK** ✓.

23. Mirroring the cut:

- Click 🔲 or select **Insert / Pattern- Mirror / Mirror**.

- Select the **FRONT** plane from the FeatureManager tree for Mirror Plane.

- Select the **Cut-Extrude1** for Features-to-Pattern.

- Click **OK** ✓.

- Rotate the part to verify the mirrored feature on the far side.

24. Adding the Holes:

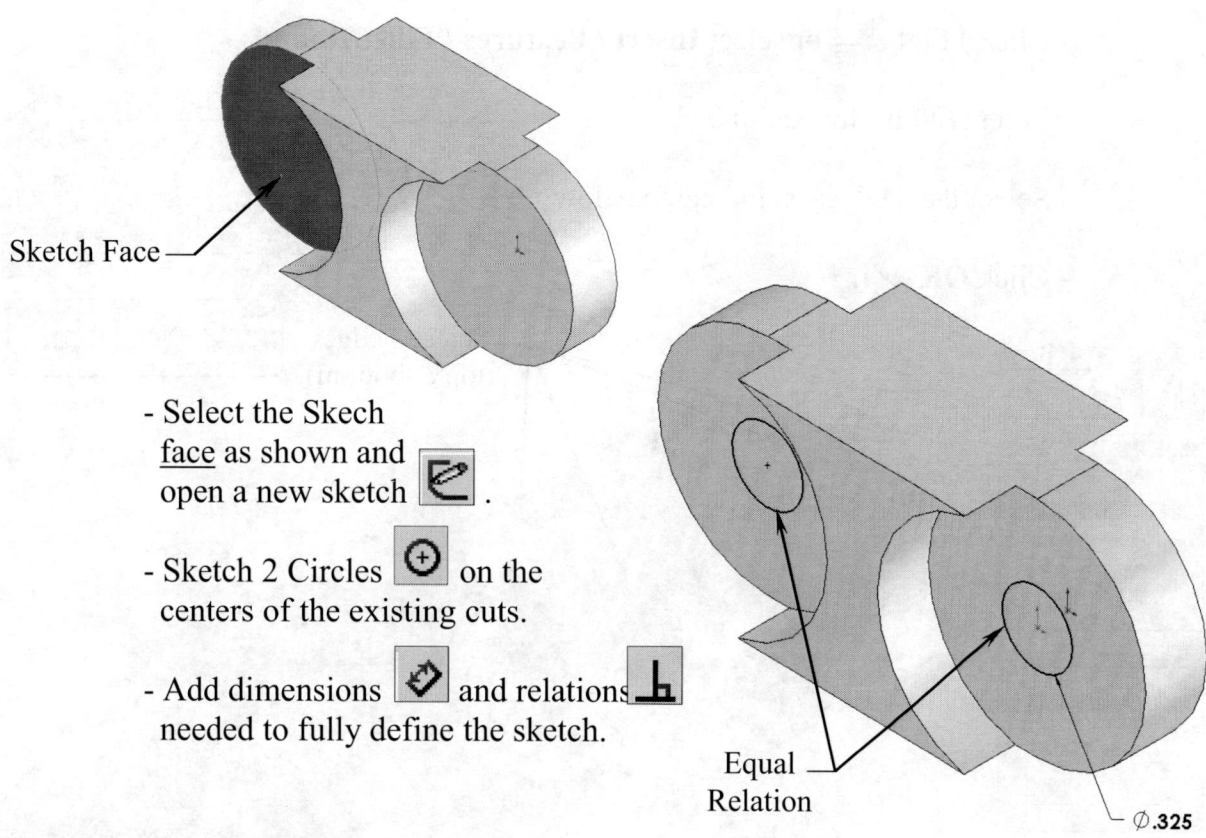

Sketch Face

- Select the Skech <u>face</u> as shown and open a new sketch 🖉 .

- Sketch 2 Circles ⊙ on the centers of the existing cuts.

- Add dimensions 🔷 and relations 🔳 needed to fully define the sketch.

Equal Relation

⌀.325

25. Cutting the holes:

- Click **Extruded Cut** 🔲 or select **Insert / Cut / Extrude**.

- End condition: **Through All**

- Click **OK** ✅.

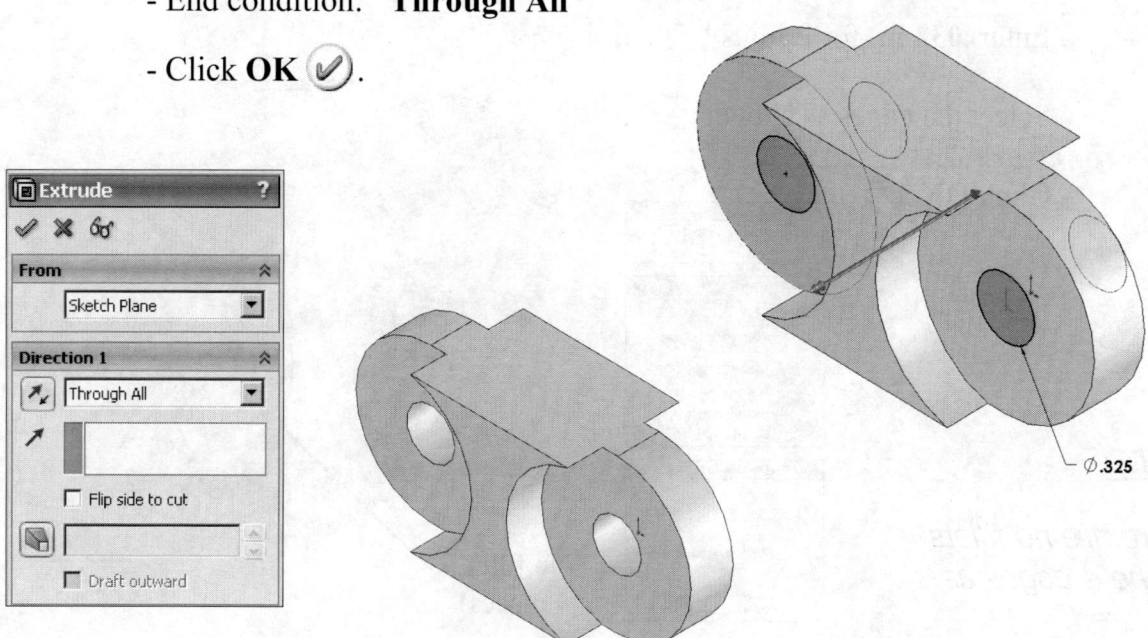

⌀.325

26. Adding the .100" fillets:

- Click **Fillet** 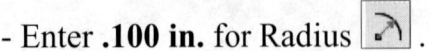 or select **Insert / Features / Fillet/Round**.

- Enter **.100 in.** for Radius.

- Select the 8 edges as indicated below.

- Click **OK**.

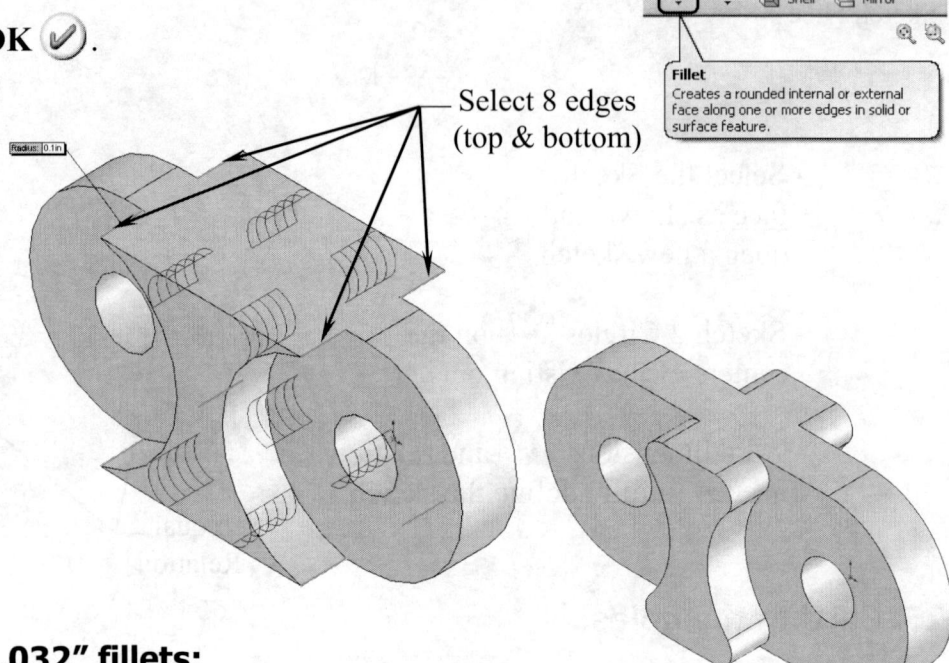

Select 8 edges
(top & bottom)

Fillet
Creates a rounded internal or external face along one or more edges in solid or surface feature.

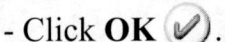

27. Adding the .032" fillets:

- Click **Fillet** 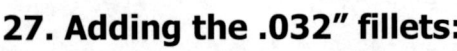 or select **Insert / Features / Fillet/Round**.

- Enter **.032 in.** for Radius.

- Select the edges as shown.

- Click **OK**.

<u>*NOTE:*</u>

There are no fillets on the 4 edges as indicated.

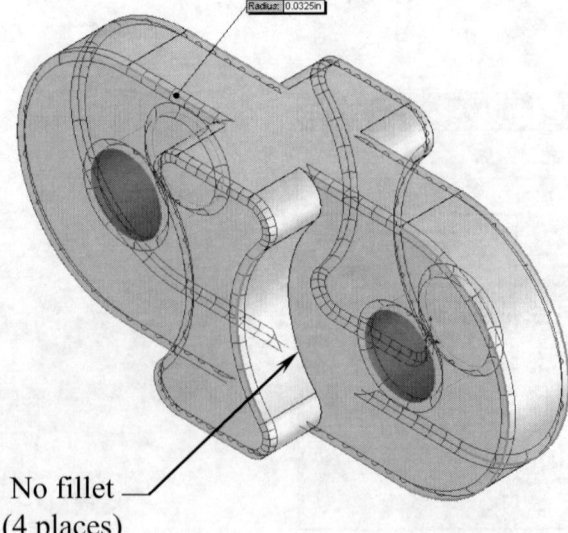

No fillet
(4 places)

28. Saving your work:

- Click **File / Save As / Single Link / Save.**

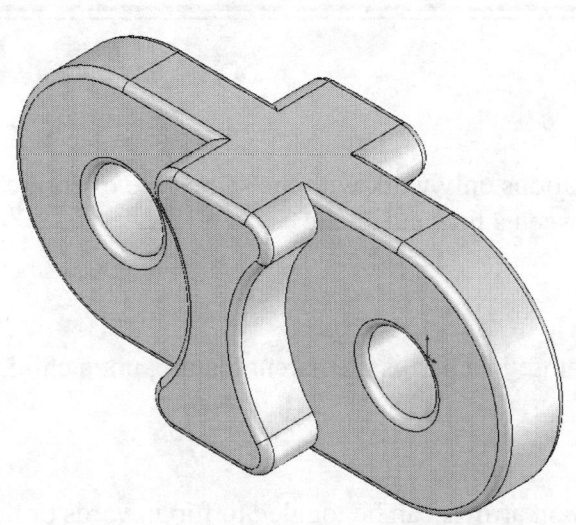

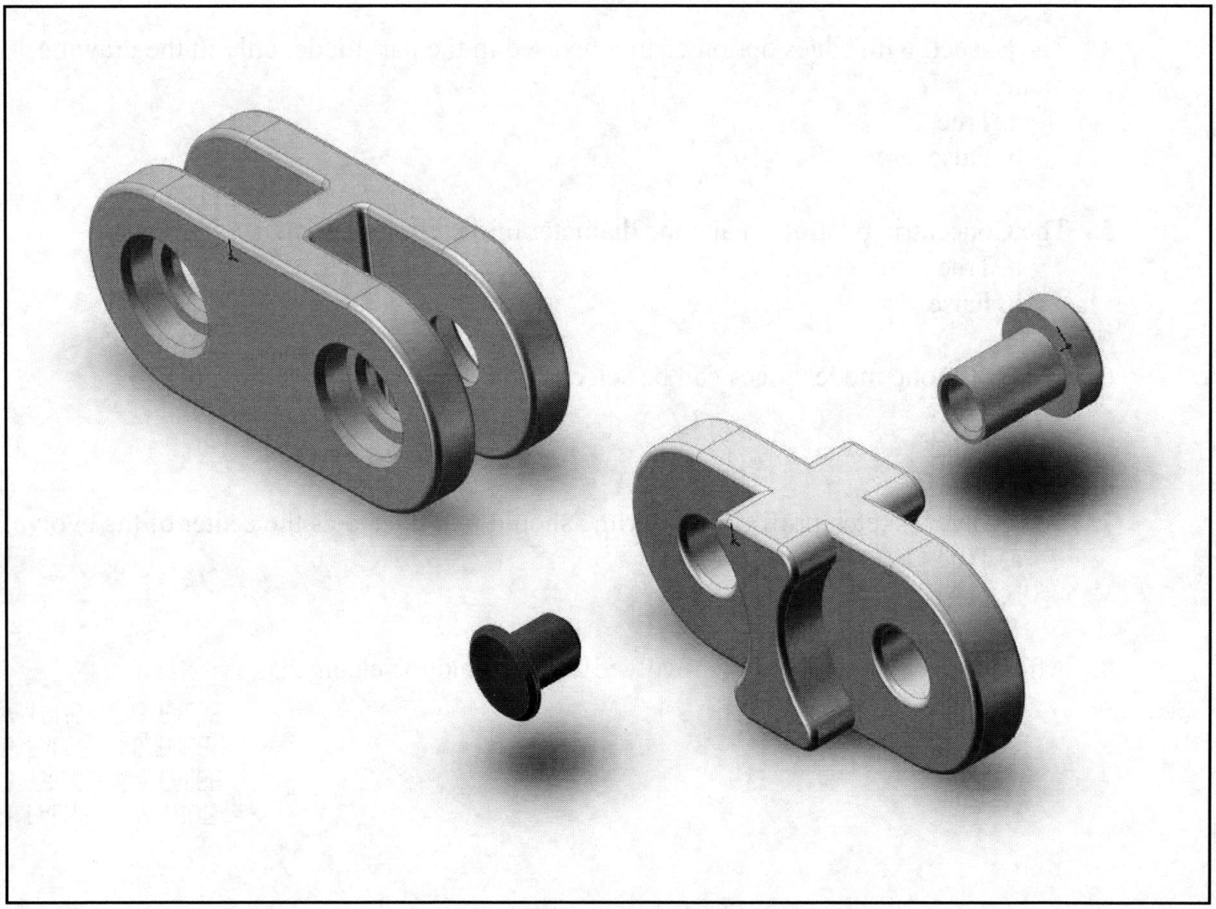

Questions for Review

Basic Solid Modeling

1. Tangent relations only work with the same type of entities such as an arc to another arc, not between a line and an arc.
   a. True
   b. False

2. The first feature in a part is the parent feature, not a child.
   a. True
   b. False

3. The dimension arrows can be toggled to flip inwards or outwards when clicking on its handle points.
   a. True
   b. False

4. The Shaded with edges option cannot be used in the part mode, only in the drawing mode.
   a. True
   b. False

5. The Concentric relations make the diameter of the circles equal.
   a. True
   b. False

6. More than one model edges can be selected and filleted at the same time.
   a. True
   b. False

7. To revolve a sketch profile, a centerline should be selected as the center of the evolve.
   a. True
   b. False

8. After a sketch is revolved, its revolved angle cannot be changed.
   a. True
   b. False

7. TRUE   8. FALSE
5. FALSE   6. TRUE
3. TRUE   4. FALSE
1. FALSE   2. TRUE

Exercise: Extrude Boss & Extrude Cut

1. Create the solid model using the drawing provided below.
2. Dimensions are in Inches, 3 decimal places.
3. Tangent relations between the transitions of the Arcs should be used.
4. The Ø.472 holes are Concentric with R.710 Arcs.
5. Use the instructions on the following pages, if needed.

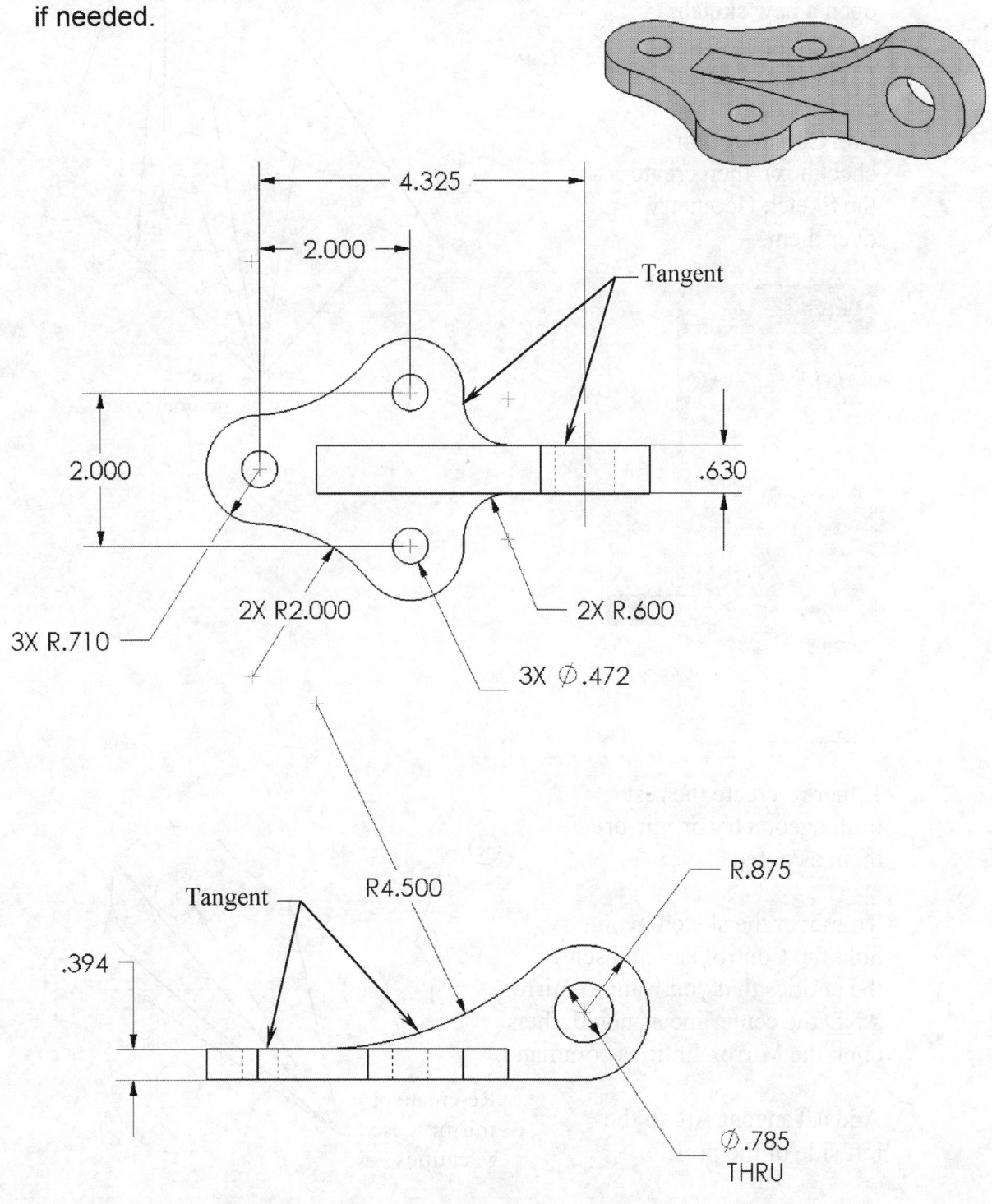

1. Creating the Base sketch:

- There are many ways to create this part but let's try this basic method first.

- Select the <u>Top</u> plane and open a new sketch.

- Create the construction circles (toggle the **For Construction** checkbox), then create the Sketch Geometry over them.

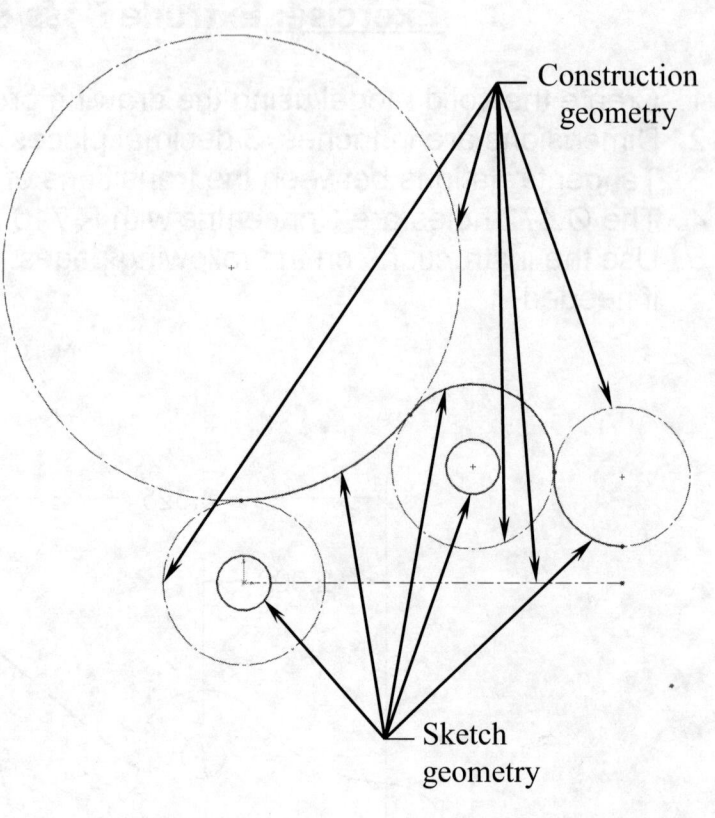

Construction geometry

Sketch geometry

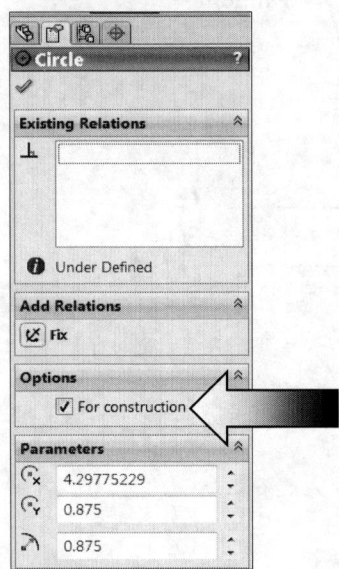

- Either re-create the rest of the geometry or mirror them as noted.

- To mirror the sketch geometry, hold the Control key and select the entities that you want to mirror <u>AND</u> the centerline as noted, then click the Mirror-Entities command.

(*) Add a Tangent Arc to the left side of the profile.

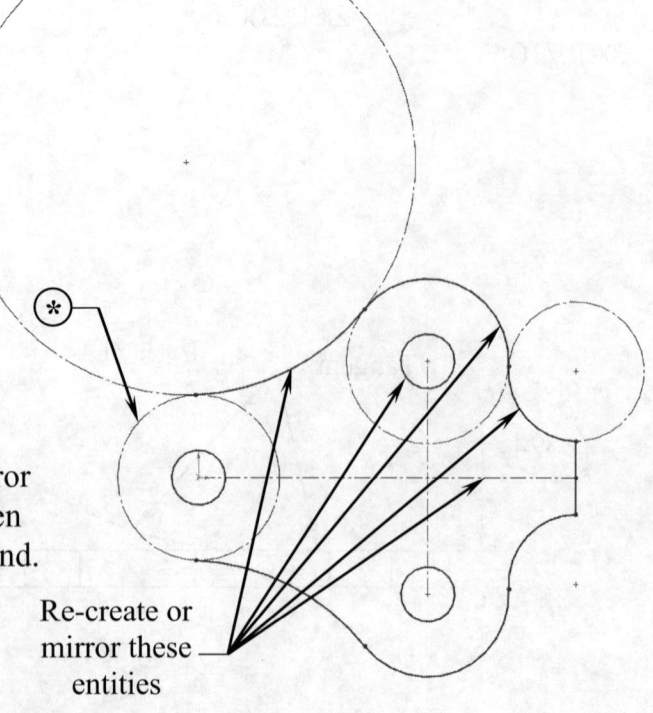

Re-create or mirror these entities

- Add the geometric relations as indicated. Remember to add the Equal relations to the circles and the arcs.

- Add the Smart-Dimensions to fully define the sketch.

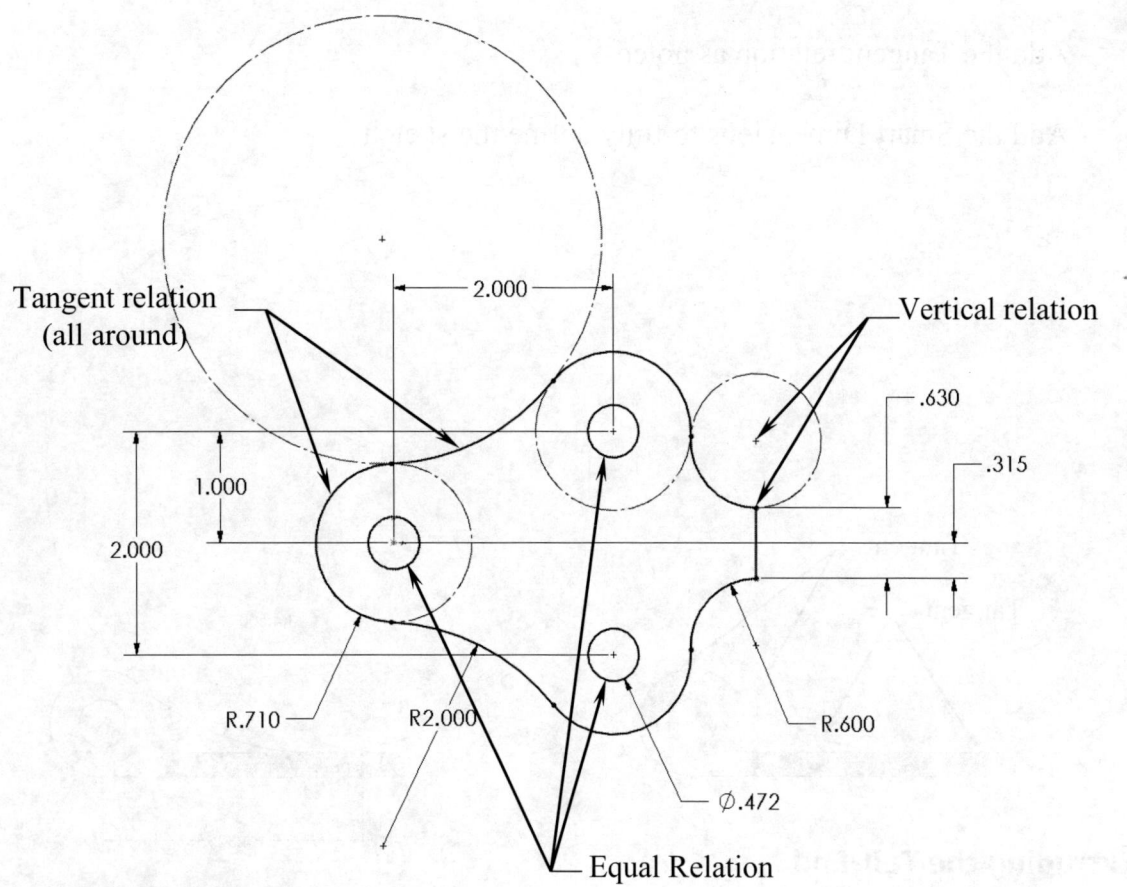

Tangent relation (all around)

Vertical relation

2.000

.630

.315

1.000

2.000

R.710

R2.000

R.600

⌀.472

Equal Relation

2. Extruding the Base:

- Click **Extruded Boss-Base**.

- Use the **Blind** type for Diretion1.

- Enter **.394"** for extrude Depth.

- Click **OK**.

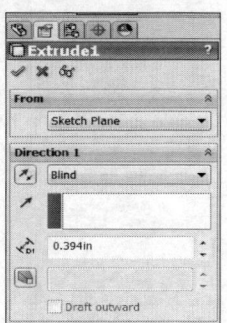

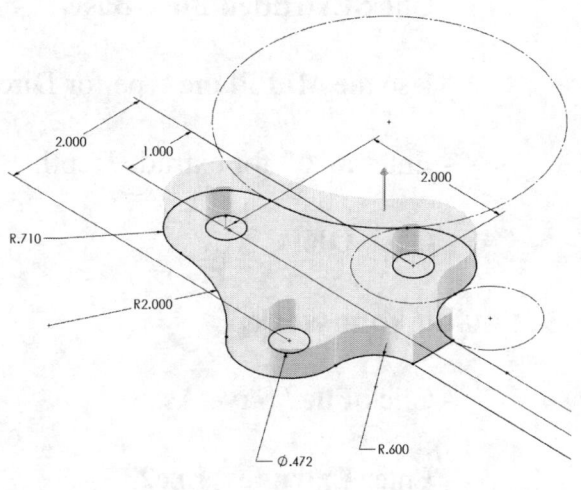

3. Creating the Tail-End sketch:

- Select the <u>Front</u> reference plane from the Feature tree and open another sketch.

- Sketch the construction circles and add the sketch geometry right over them.

- Add the Tangent relation as noted.

- Add the Smart Dimensions to fully define the sketch.

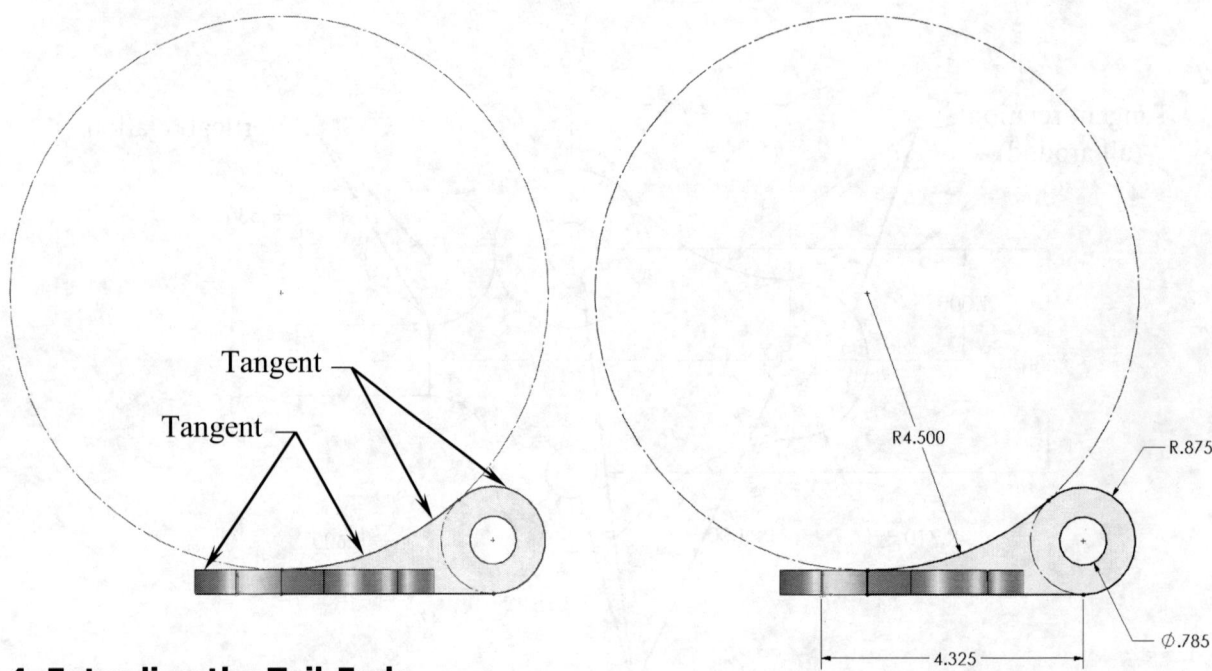

Tangent

Tangent

R4.500

R.875

4.325

∅.785

4. Extruding the Tail-End:

- Click **Extruded Boss-Base**.

- Use the **Mid Plane** type for Diretion1.

- Enter **.630"** for extrude Depth.

- Click **OK**.

5. Saving your work:

- Click **File / Save As**.

- Enter **Extrudes_Exe2**.

- Click **Save**.

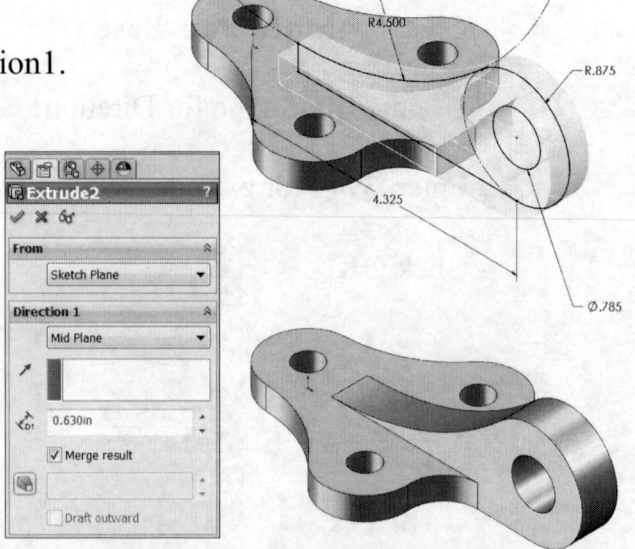

CHAPTER 5

Revolved Parts

Revolved Parts
Ball Joint Arm

- The Revolve command rotates one or more sketch profiles around a centerline, up to 360° to create a <u>thin</u> or a <u>solid</u> feature.

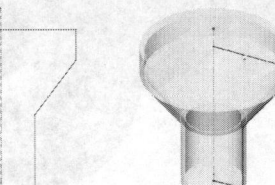 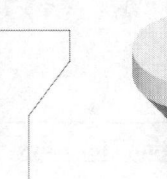 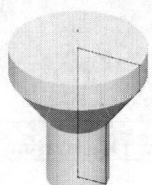

Open profile
= Thin Feature

Closed profile
= Solid Feature

- The revolved sketch should have a continuous closed contour and it can either be a polygon, a circle, an ellipse, or a closed spline.

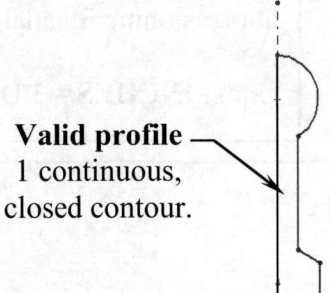 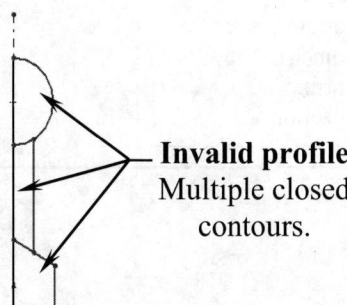

Valid profile
1 continuous,
closed contour.

Invalid profile
Multiple closed
contours.

- If there is more than one centerline in the same sketch, the center of rotation must be selected when creating the revolve.

- In the newer releases of SolidWorks, the center of the revolve (centerline) can be replaced with a line, an axis, or a linear model edge.

- The revolve feature can be a cut feature (which removes material) or a revolve boss feature (which adds material).

- This chapter will guide you through the basics of creating the revolved parts.

Ball Joint Arm
Revolved Parts

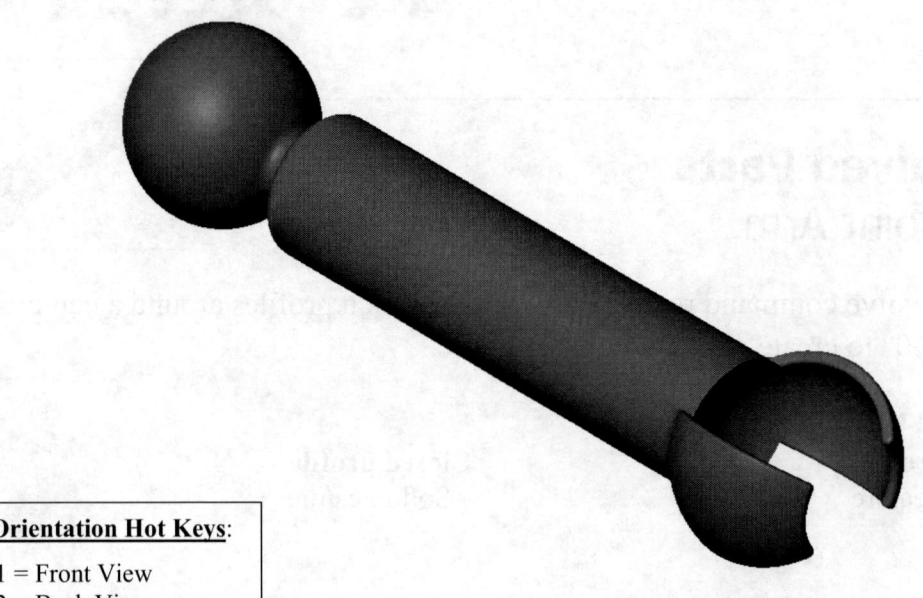

View Orientation Hot Keys:

Ctrl + 1 = Front View
Ctrl + 2 = Back View
Ctrl + 3 = Left View
Ctrl + 4 = Right View
Ctrl + 5 = Top View
Ctrl + 6 = Bottom View
Ctrl + 7 = Isometric View
Ctrl + 8 = Normal To
       Selection

Dimensioning Standards: **ANSI**

Units: **INCHES** – 3 Decimals

Tools Needed:

Insert Sketch	Line	Circle
Rectangle	Sketch Fillet	Trim
Add Geometric Relations	Dimension	Centerline
Base/Boss Revolve	Fillet/Round	Mirror Features

1. Creating the Base Profile:

- Select the <u>Front</u> plane from the FeatureManager tree.

- Click 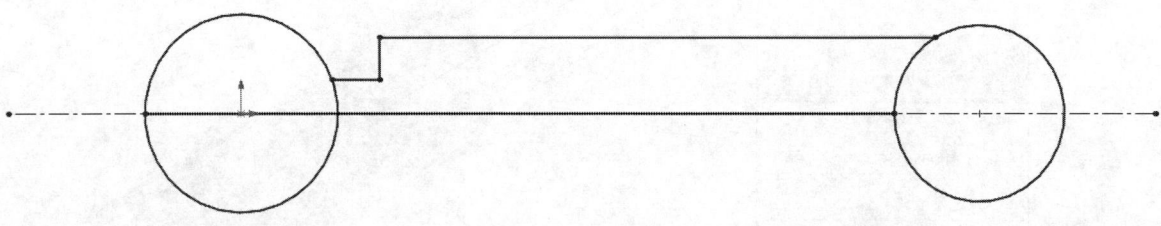 or select **Insert / Sketch**.

- Sketch the profile using the Line ＼ and Circle ⊕ commands.

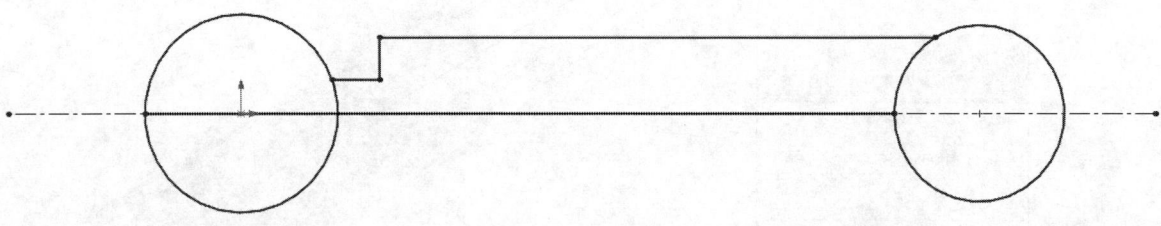

- Trim ⅀ the circles as shown.

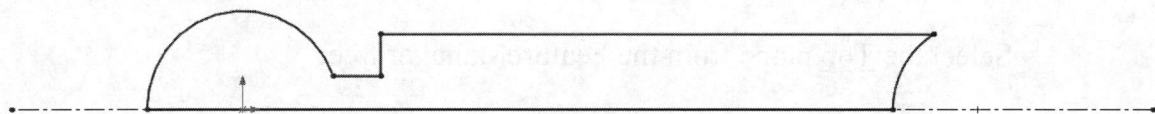

- Add Dimensions ◇ and Relations ┺ needed to fully define the sketch.
  (It is easier to add the R.050" fillets after the sketch is fully defined).

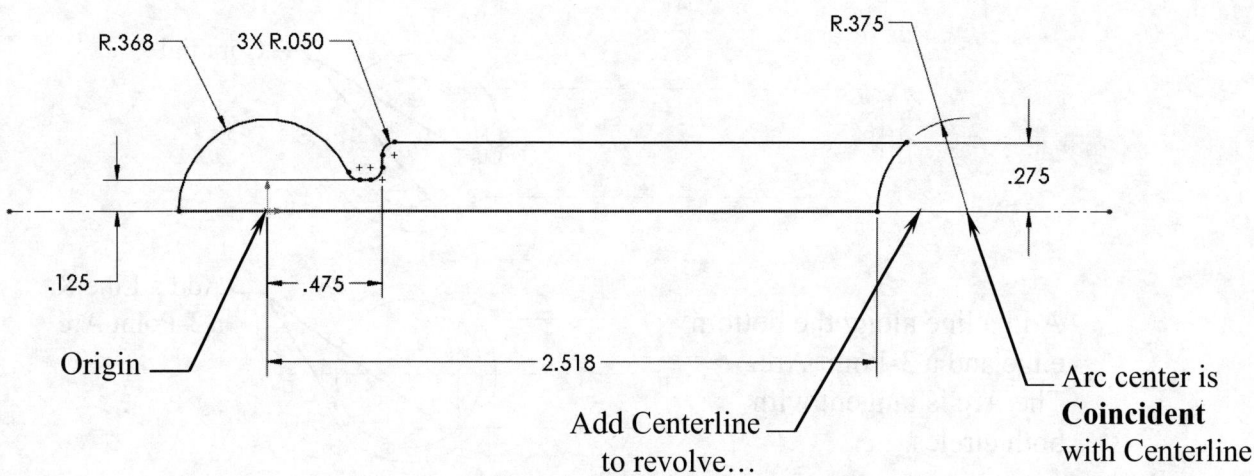

R.368   3X R.050   R.375

.275

.125   .475

Origin   2.518

Add Centerline to revolve…

Arc center is **Coincident** with Centerline

2. Revolving the Base Feature:

- Click **Revolve** or select **Insert / Boss-Base / Revolve**.

- Revolve Type: **Blind** .

- Revolve Angle: **360 deg.** .

- Click **OK** .

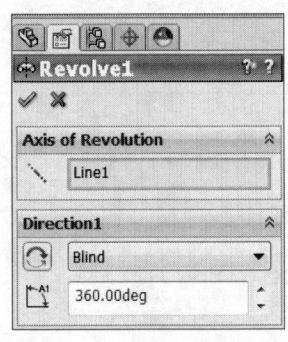

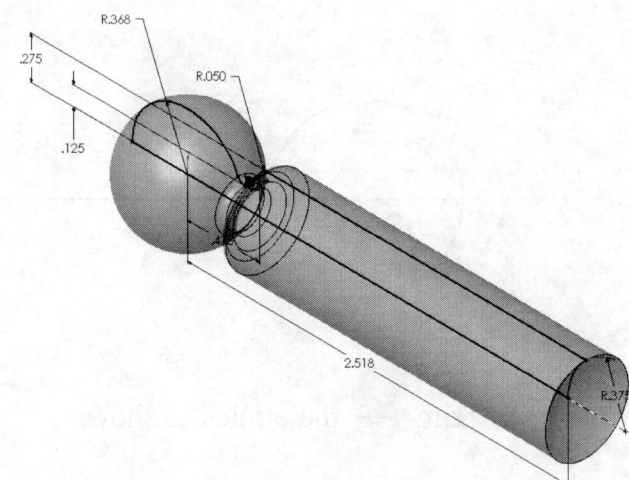

3. Sketching the Opened-End Profile:

- Select the <u>Top</u> plane from the FeatureManager tree.

- Click or select **Insert / Sketch**.

- Switch to Hidden Lines Visible mode: click on the VIEW toolbar.

- Sketch 2 circles as shown.

- Add a **Coradial** relation between the small circle and the hidden edge.

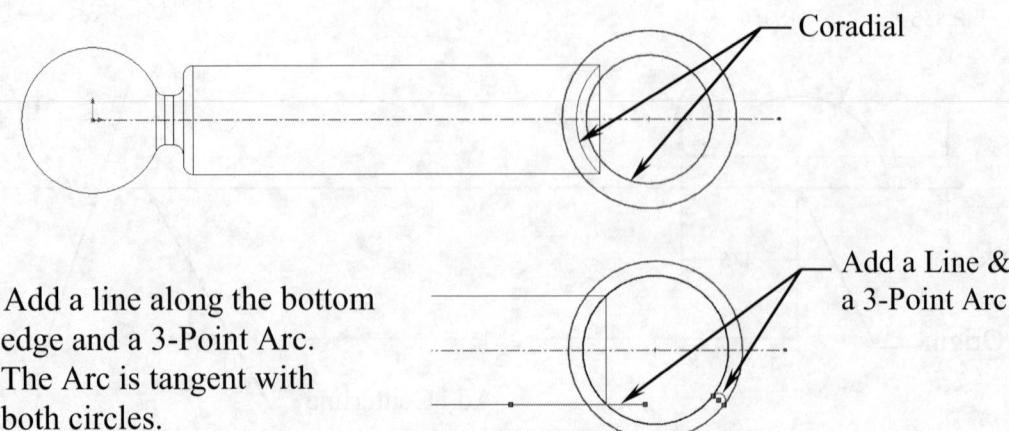

Coradial

- Add a line along the bottom
  edge and a 3-Point Arc.
  The Arc is tangent with
  both circles.

Add a Line &
a 3-Point Arc

- Trim 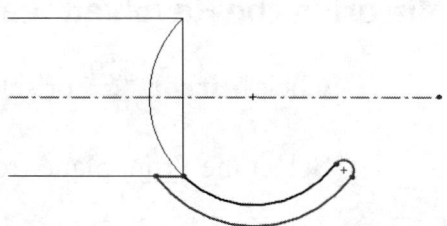 the line and the 2 circles.

- Add a Collinear relation ⊥ between
  the line and the bottom edge of the part.

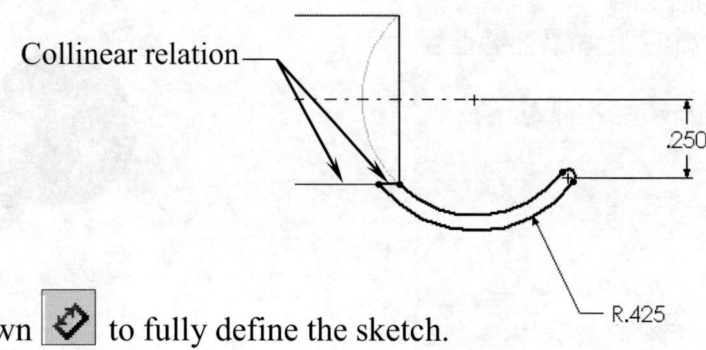

Collinear relation

.250

R.425

- Add the dimensions shown ✎ to fully define the sketch.

4. Revolving the Opened-End Feature:

- Click **Revolve** ⚙ or select **Insert / Boss-Base / Revolve**.

- Revolve Type: **Mid Plane** ⚙ .

- Revolve Angle: **75 deg.** ⚙ .

- Click **OK** ✓ .

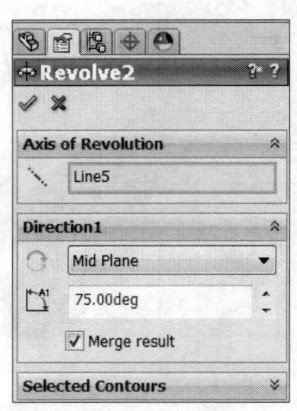

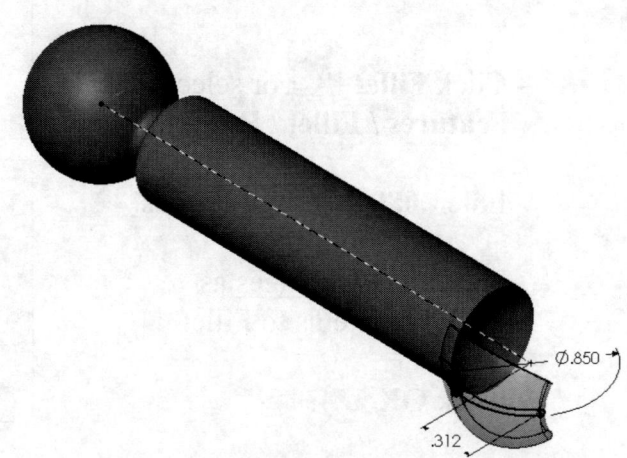

Ø.850

.312

5. Mirroring the Revolved feature:

- Click **Mirror** 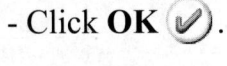 or select **Insert / Pattern Mirror / Mirror**.

- Select the <u>Front</u> plane from the FeatureManager tree as mirror plane 🔲 .

- Select the Revolve2 feature either from the graphics area or from the Feature-Manager tree, as Features to Mirror 🔳 .

- Click **OK** ✅ .

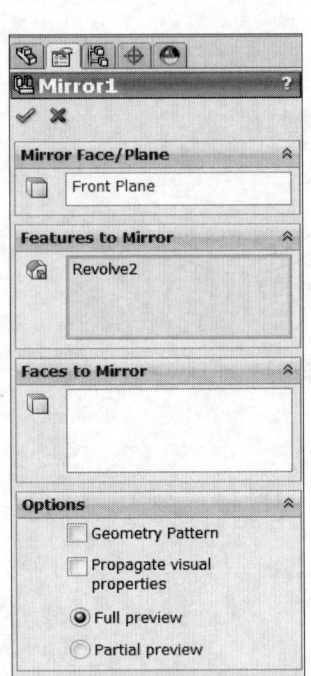

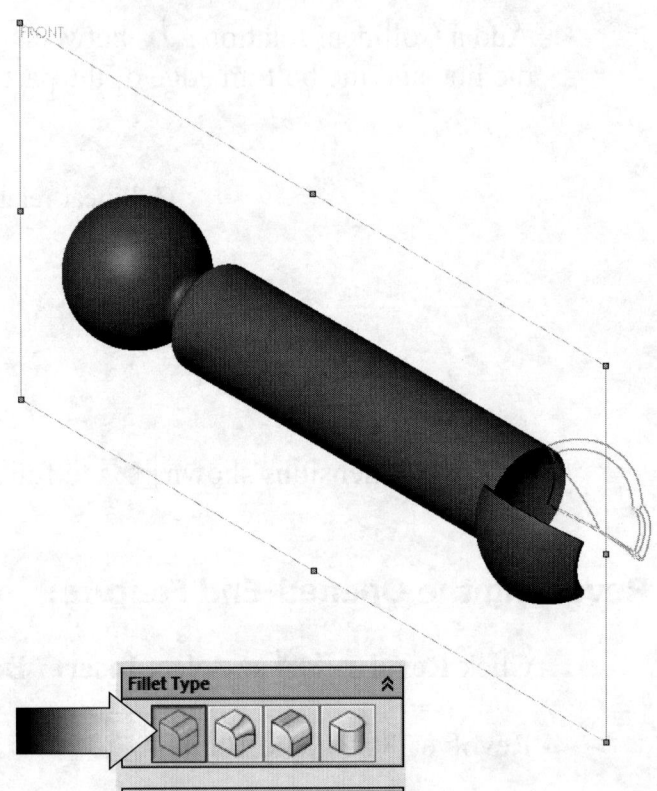

6. Adding the .080" Fillets:

- Click **Fillet** 🔘 or select **Insert / Features / Fillet / Round**.

- Enter **.080** in. as the Radius 🔘 .

- Select the <u>two edges</u> as shown for Items to Fillet 🔲 .

- Click **OK** ✅ .

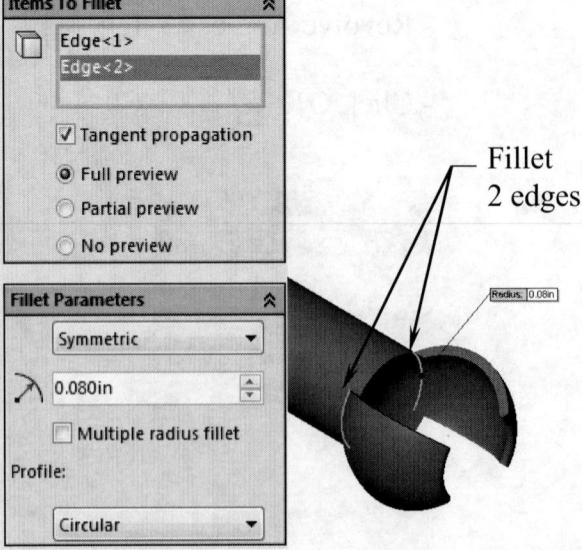

Fillet
2 edges

7. Adding the .015" Fillets:

- Click **Fillet** 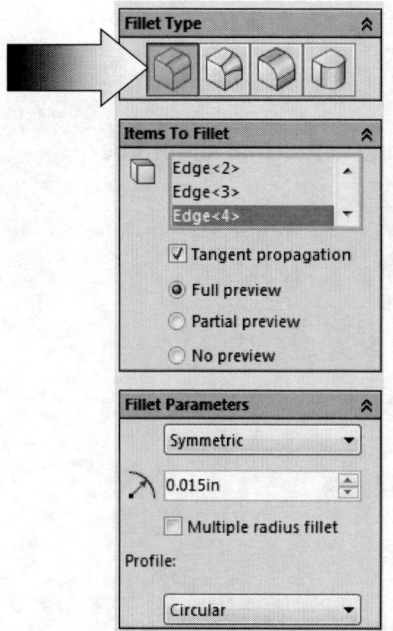 or select **Insert / Features / Fillet / Round**.

- Enter **.015** in. as the Radius .

- Select the <u>edges</u> of the 2 revolved features as shown.

- Click **OK** .

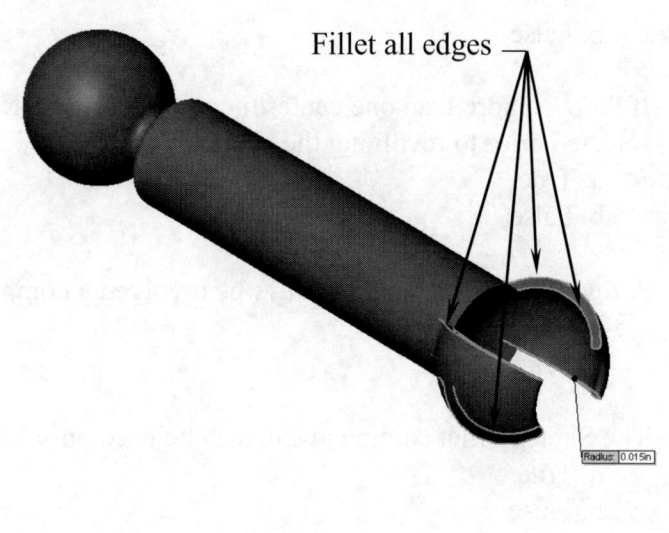

Fillet all edges

8. Saving Your Work:

- Select **File / Save As / Ball-Joint-Arm / Save**.

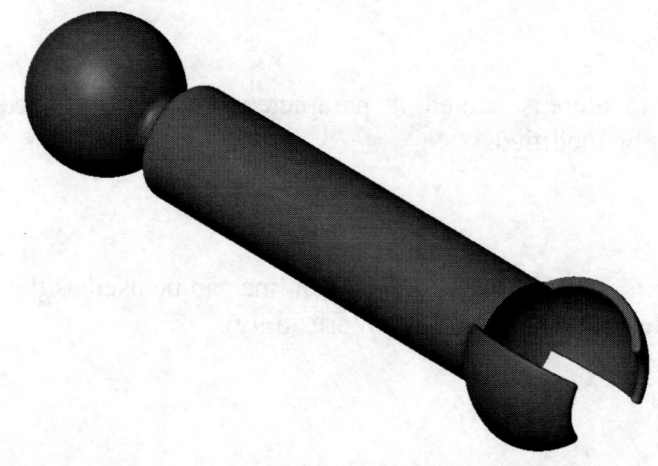

Questions for Review

Revolved Parts

1. A proper profile for use in a revolved feature is a single closed contour, created on one side of the revolved centerline.
   a. True
   b. False

2. If there is more than one centerline in the same sketch, one centerline should be selected prior to revolving the sketch.
   a. True
   b. False

3. A revolve feature should *always* be revolved a complete 360°.
   a. True
   b. False

4. The Sketch Fillet command can also be used on solid features.
   a. True
   b. False

5. To mirror a 3D feature, a plane, or a planar surface should be used as a mirror plane.
   a. True
   b. False

6. To mirror a series of features, a centerline can be used as a mirror plane.
   a. True
   b. False

7. After a fillet feature is created, its parameters (selected faces, edges, fillet values, etc.) cannot be modified.
   a. True
   b. False

8. Either an axis, a model edge, or a sketch line can be used as the center of the revolve. (Newer releases of SolidWorks only).
   a. True
   b. False

7. FALSE   8. TRUE
5. TRUE   6. FALSE
3. FALSE   4. FALSE
1. TRUE   2. TRUE

<u>Exercise</u>: Flat Head Screw Driver

1. Create the part using the drawing provided below.
2. Dimensions are in inches, 3 decimal places.
3. The part is symmetrical about the Top plane.
4. Unspecified radii to be R.050 max.
5. Use the instructions on the following pages, if needed.

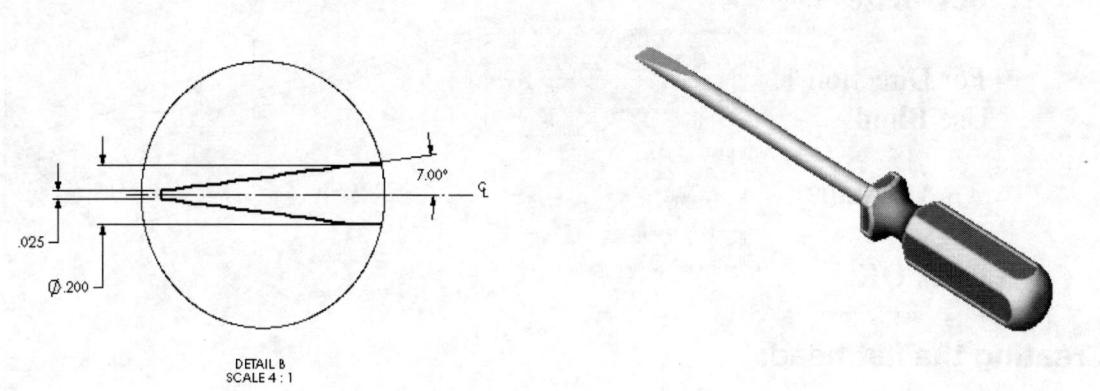

DETAIL B
SCALE 4 : 1

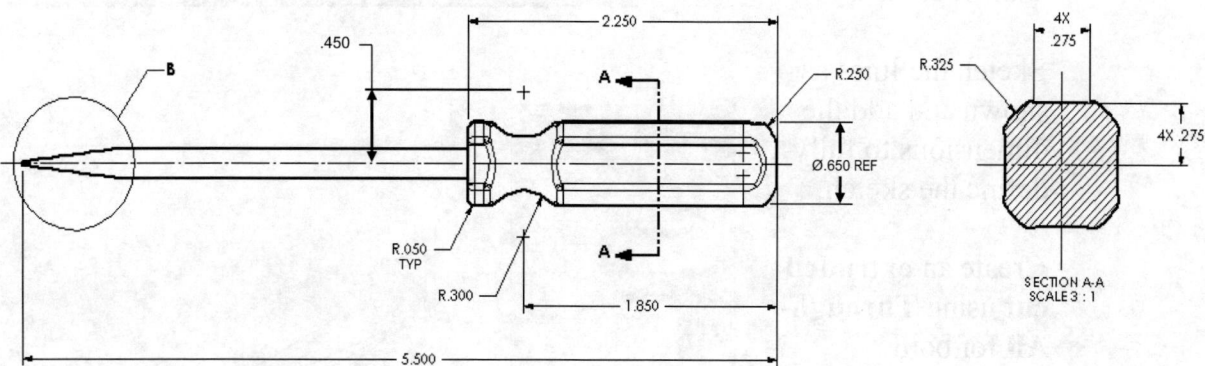

6. Save your work as: **Flat Head Screw Driver**.

1. Creating the base sketch:

- Select the <u>Front</u> plane and open a new sketch.

- Sketch the profile shown and add the dimensions noted.

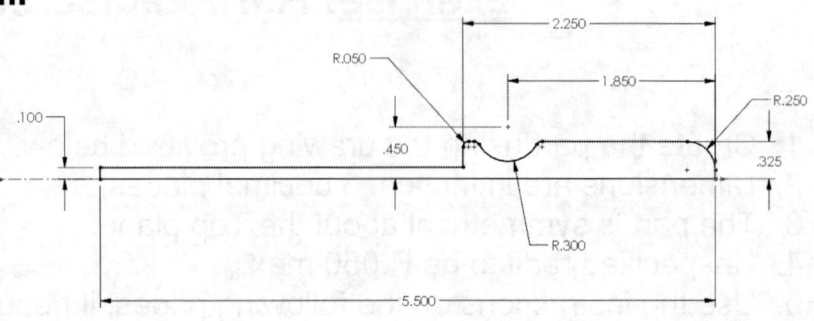

2. Revolving the base:

- Click **Revolve / Boss-Base**.

- For Direction 1: Use **Blind**.

- Angle = **360°**

- Click **OK**.

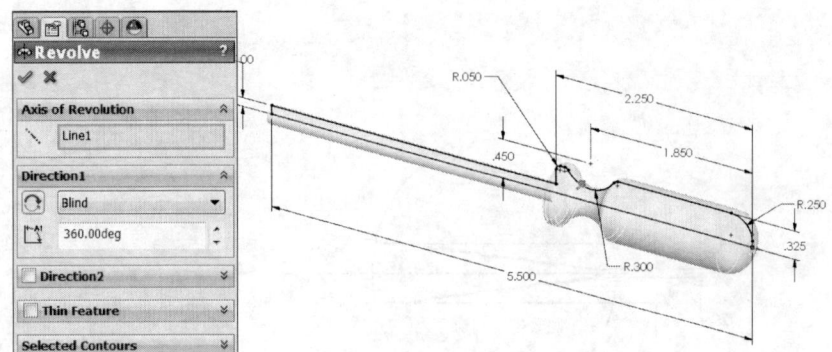

3. Creating the flat head:

- Select the <u>Front</u> plane and open another sketch.

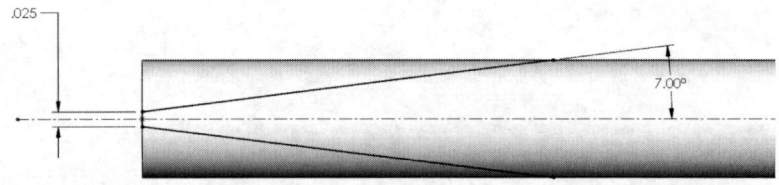

- Sketch the lines as shown and add the dimensions to fully define the sketch.

- Create an **extruded cut** using **Through-All** for both directions.

- Since the sketch was open, Through All is the only extrude option in this case.

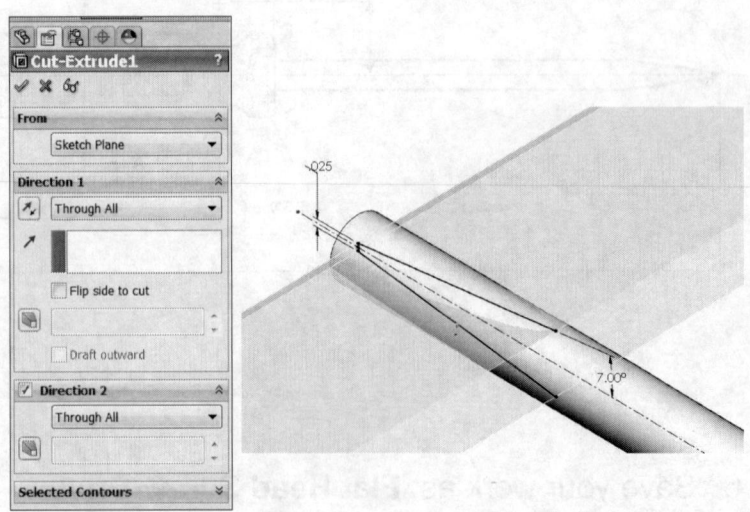

4. Creating the flat handle:

- Select the <u>flat surface</u> on the right end of the handle and open a new sketch.

- Sketch a rectangle and mirror it using the vertical and horizontal centerline (the sketch can be left under defined for this example).

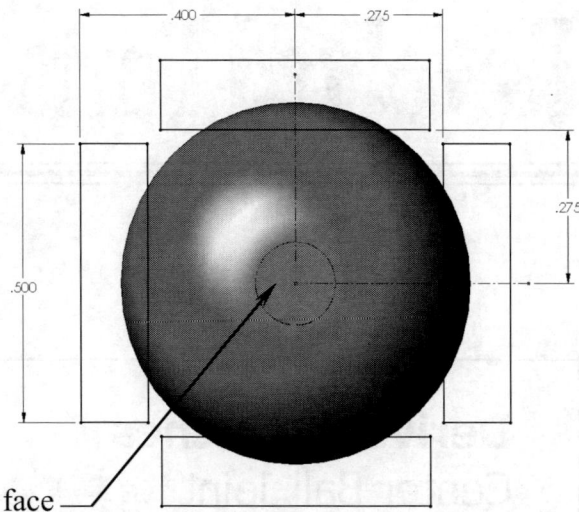

Sketch face ⟵

- Create an extruded cut using the opposite end of the handle as the end condition for the Up-To-Surface option. (Through-All can also be used to achieve the same result).

⟵ Up to Surface

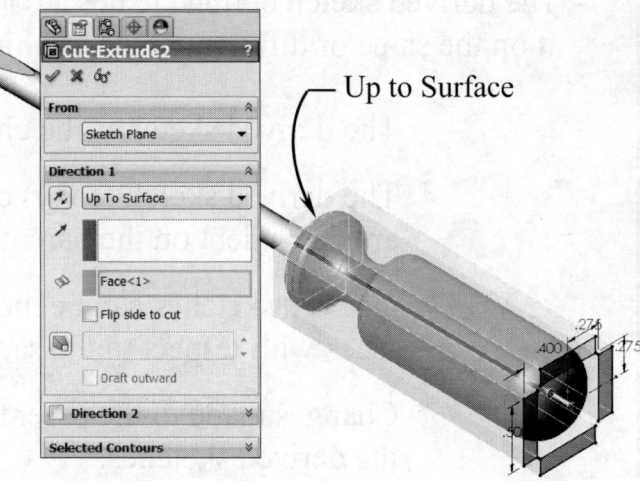

5. Adding the .050" fillets:

- Apply a **.050"** fillet to the 2 faces as indicated.

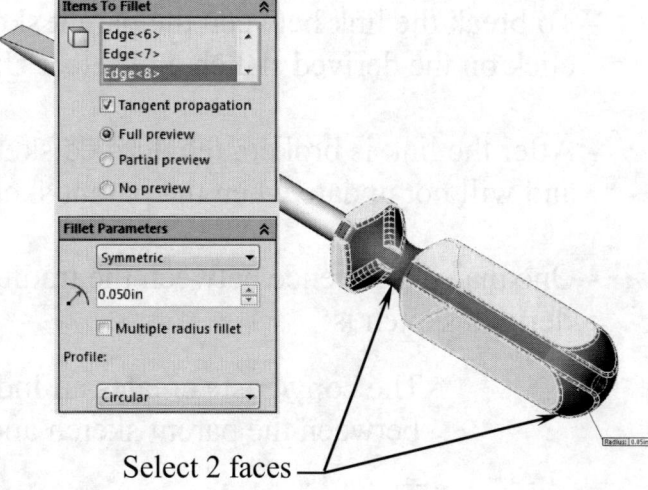

Select 2 faces ⟵

6. Saving your work:

- Save your work as **Flat Head Screw Driver**.

Revolved Parts (cont.)

Derived Sketches

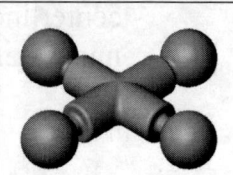

Derived Sketches
Center Ball Joint

- The derived sketch option creates a copy of the original sketch and places it on the same or different plane, within the same part document.

  * The derived sketch is the child feature of the original.

  * The derived sketch (copy) cannot be edited. Its size and shape are dependent on the parent sketch.

  * Derived sketches can be moved and related to different planes or faces with respect to the same model.

  * Changes made to the parent sketch are automatically reflected in the derived sketches.

- To break the link between the parent sketch and the derived copies, right click on the derived sketch and select **Underived**.

- After the link is broken, the derived sketches can be modified independently and will not update when the parent sketch is changed.

- One major difference between the traditional copy / paste option and the derived sketch is:

  * The copy/paste creates an Independent copy. There is no link between the parent sketch and the derived sketch.

  * The derived sketch creates a dependent copy. The parent sketch and the derived sketch are fully linked.

Center Ball Joint
Derived Sketches

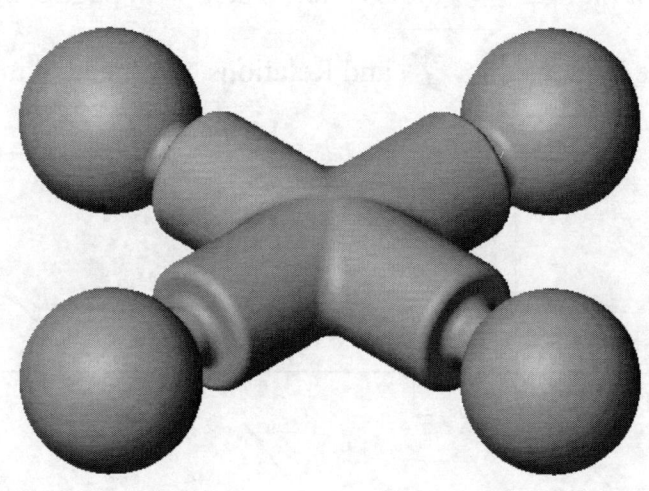

Dimensioning Standards: **ANSI**

Units: **INCHES** – 3 Decimals

Tools Needed:

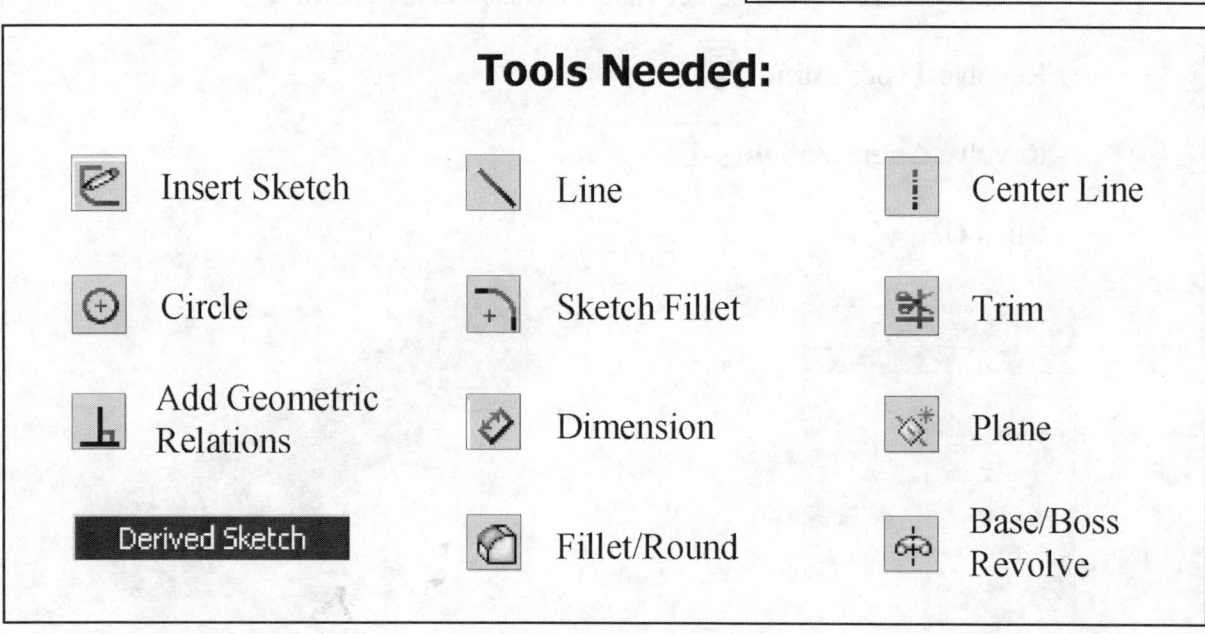

Insert Sketch	Line	Center Line
Circle	Sketch Fillet	Trim
Add Geometric Relations	Dimension	Plane
Derived Sketch	Fillet/Round	Base/Boss Revolve

1. Creating the Base Profile:

- Select the <u>Front</u> plane from the Feature Manager tree.

- Click 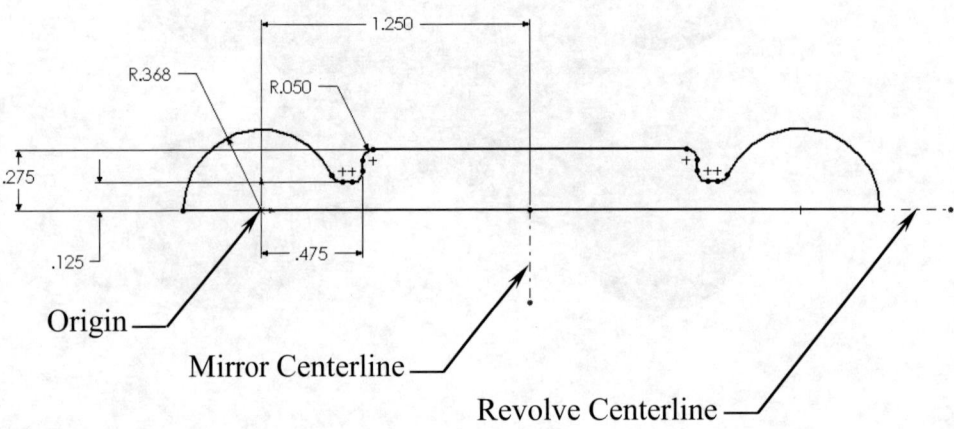 or select **Insert / Sketch**.

- Sketch the profile using Lines , Circles , Sketch Fillets and

the Trim Entities tools (refer to step 1 on page 5-3 for reference).

- Add the Dimensions and Relations needed to fully define the sketch.

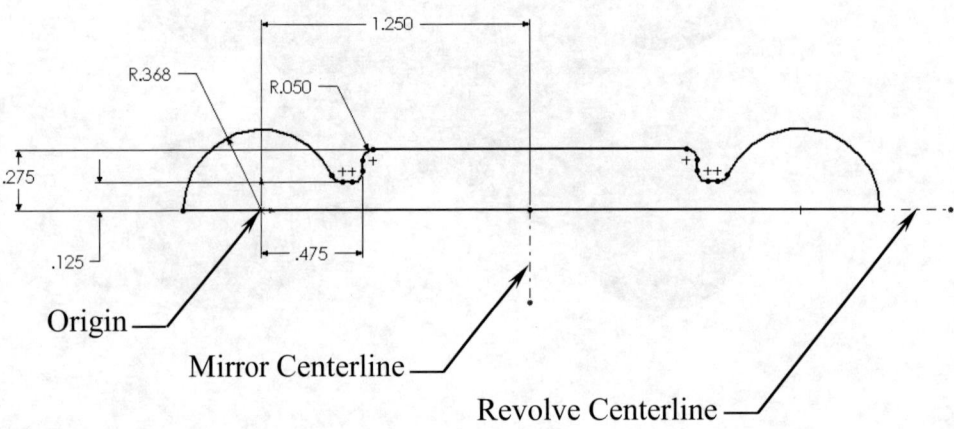

R.368

R.050

1.250

.275

.125

.475

Origin

Mirror Centerline

Revolve Centerline

2. Revolving the Base Feature:

- Click **Revolve** or select **Insert / Boss-Base / Revolve**.

- Revolve Type: **Blind** .

- Revolve Angle: **360 deg**. .

- Click **OK** .

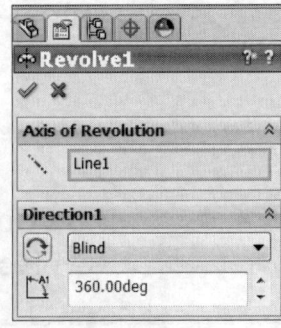

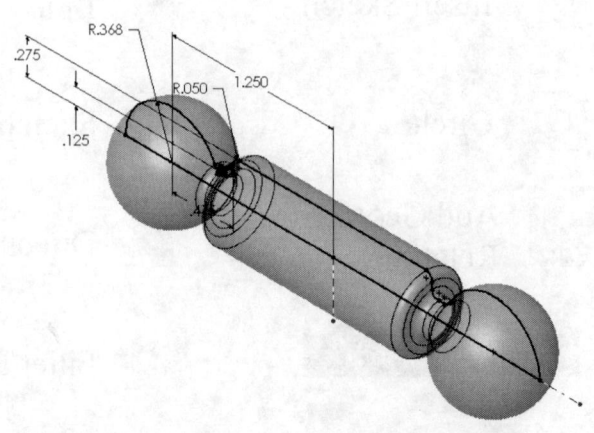

3. Creating a new work plane*:

- Click **Plane** 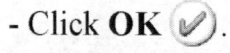 or select **Insert / Reference Geometry / Plane**.

- Select the <u>Right</u> plane from the FeatureManager tree 🔲.

- Choose the **Offset Distance** option.

- Enter **1.250** in. (place the new plane on the right side).

- Click **OK** ✓.

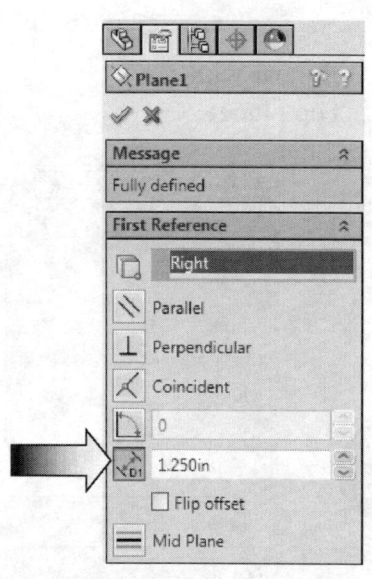

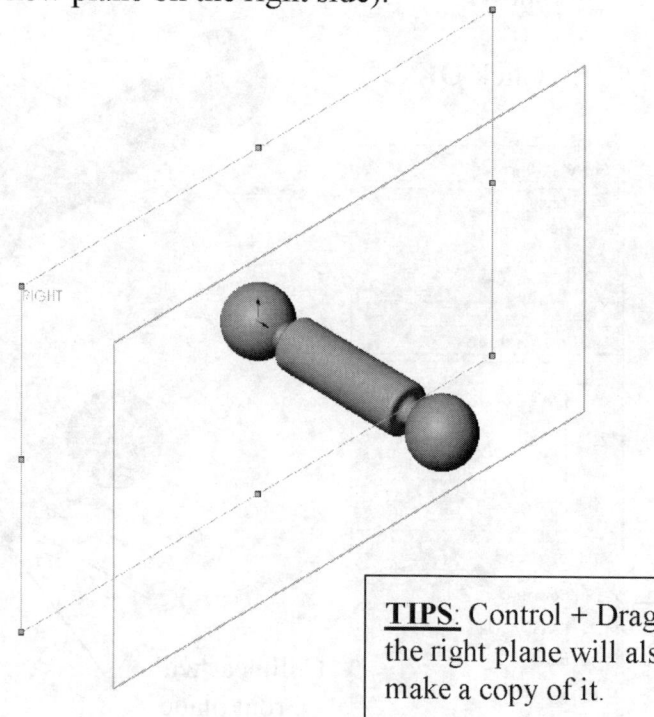

TIPS: Control + Drag the right plane will also make a copy of it.

4. Creating a Derived Sketch:

- Hold the **Control** key, select the new plane (**Plane1**) and the **Sketch1** (under Base-Revolved1) from the FeatureManager tree.

- Select **Derived Sketch** under the **Insert** menu.

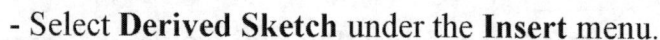

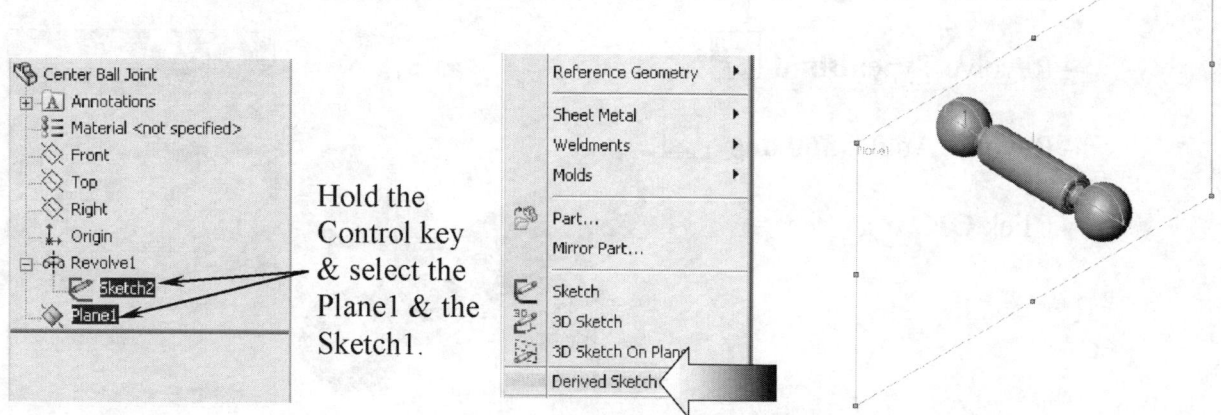

Hold the Control key & select the Plane1 & the Sketch1.

- A copy of Sketch1 is created and placed on Plane1, and is automatically activated for positioning.

5. Positioning the Derived Sketch:

- Add a **Collinear** relation between the Top plane and the Line as indicated.

- Add a **Collinear** relation between the Front plane and the Centerline as shown.

- Click **OK** ✓.

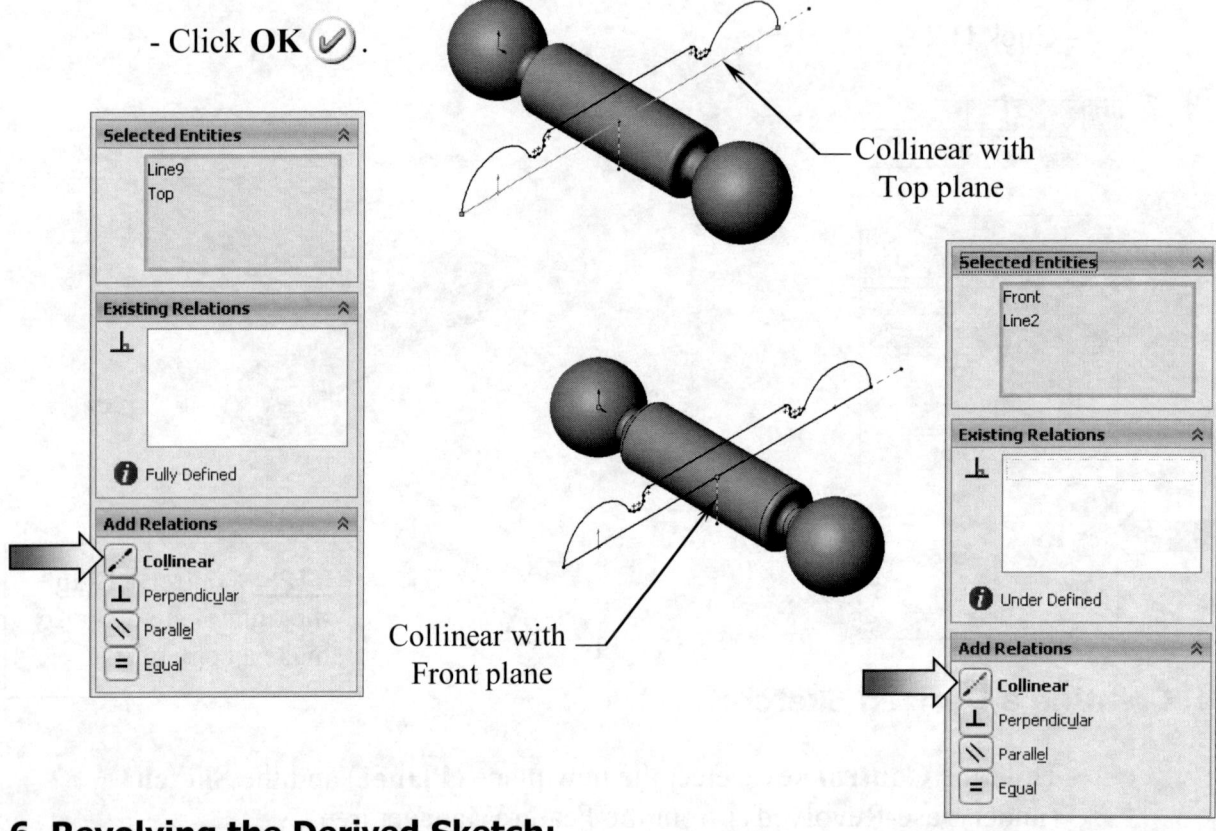

Collinear with
Top plane

Collinear with
Front plane

6. Revolving the Derived Sketch:

- Click **Revolve** or select **Insert / Boss-Base / Revolve**.

- Revolve Type: **Blind** .

- Revolve Angle: **360 deg**. .

- Click **OK** ✓.

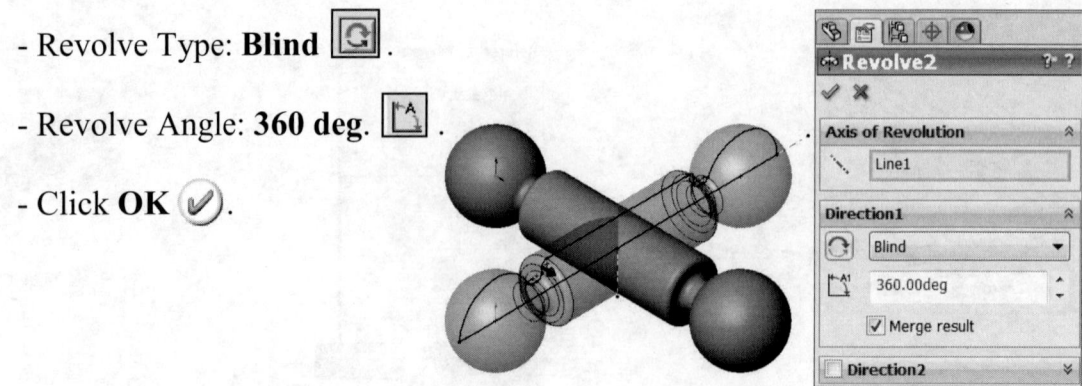

7. Adding Fillets:

- Click **Fillet** 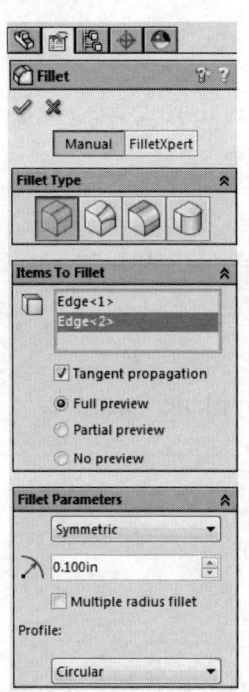 or select **Insert / Features / Fillet / Round**.

- Enter **.100 in.** for Radius size ⬚.

- Select the <u>edges</u> shown as the Edges-To-Fillet ⬚.

- Click **OK** ✓.

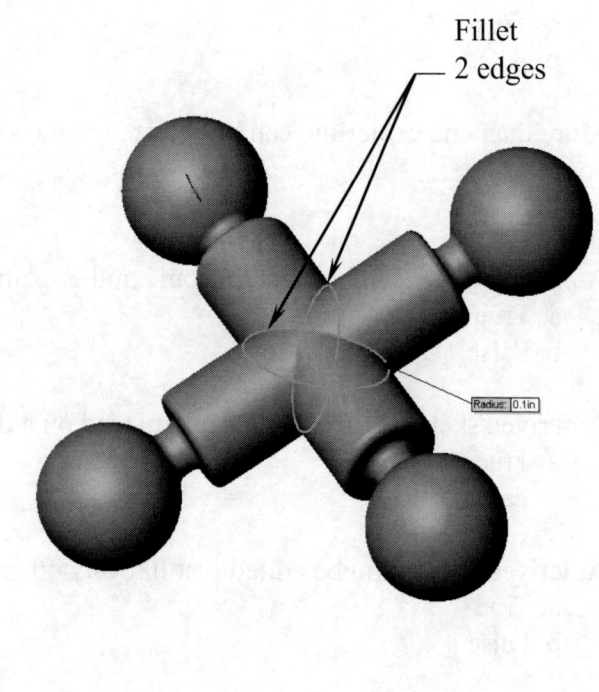

Fillet
2 edges

8. Saving Your Work:

- Select **File / Save As / Center Ball Joint / Save**.

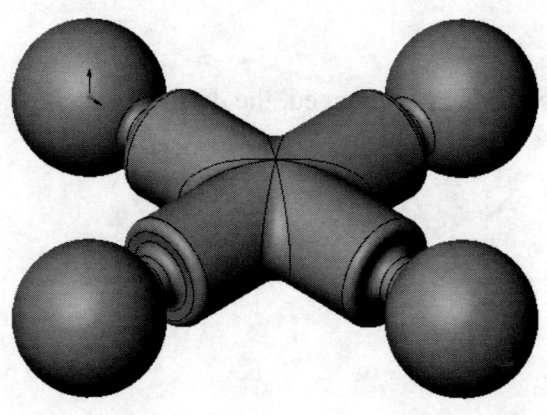

Questions for Review

Derived Sketches

1. The first feature in a part is the parent feature.
   a. True
   b. False

2. More than one centerline can be selected at the same time to revolve a sketch profile.
   a. True
   b. False

3. A parallel plane can be created from another plane or a planar surface.
   a. True
   b. False

4. A derived sketch can be copied and placed on a different plane / surface.
   a. True
   b. False

5. A derived sketch can be edited just like any other sketch.
   a. True
   b. False

6. A derived sketch is an independent sketch. There is no link between the derived sketch and the parent sketch.
   a. True
   b. False

7. A derived sketch can only be positioned and related to other sketches / features.
   a. True
   b. False

8. When the parent sketch is changed, the derived sketches will be updated automatically.
   a. True
   b. False

7. TRUE   8. TRUE
5. FALSE   6. FALSE
3. TRUE   4. TRUE
1. TRUE   2. FALSE

Exercise: Revolved Parts - Wheel

1. Create the 3D model using the drawing provided below.
2. Dimensions are in inches, 3 decimal places.
3. The part is Symmetrical about the horizontal axis.
4. The 5 mounting holes should be created as a Circular Pattern.
5. Use the instructions on the following pages if needed.

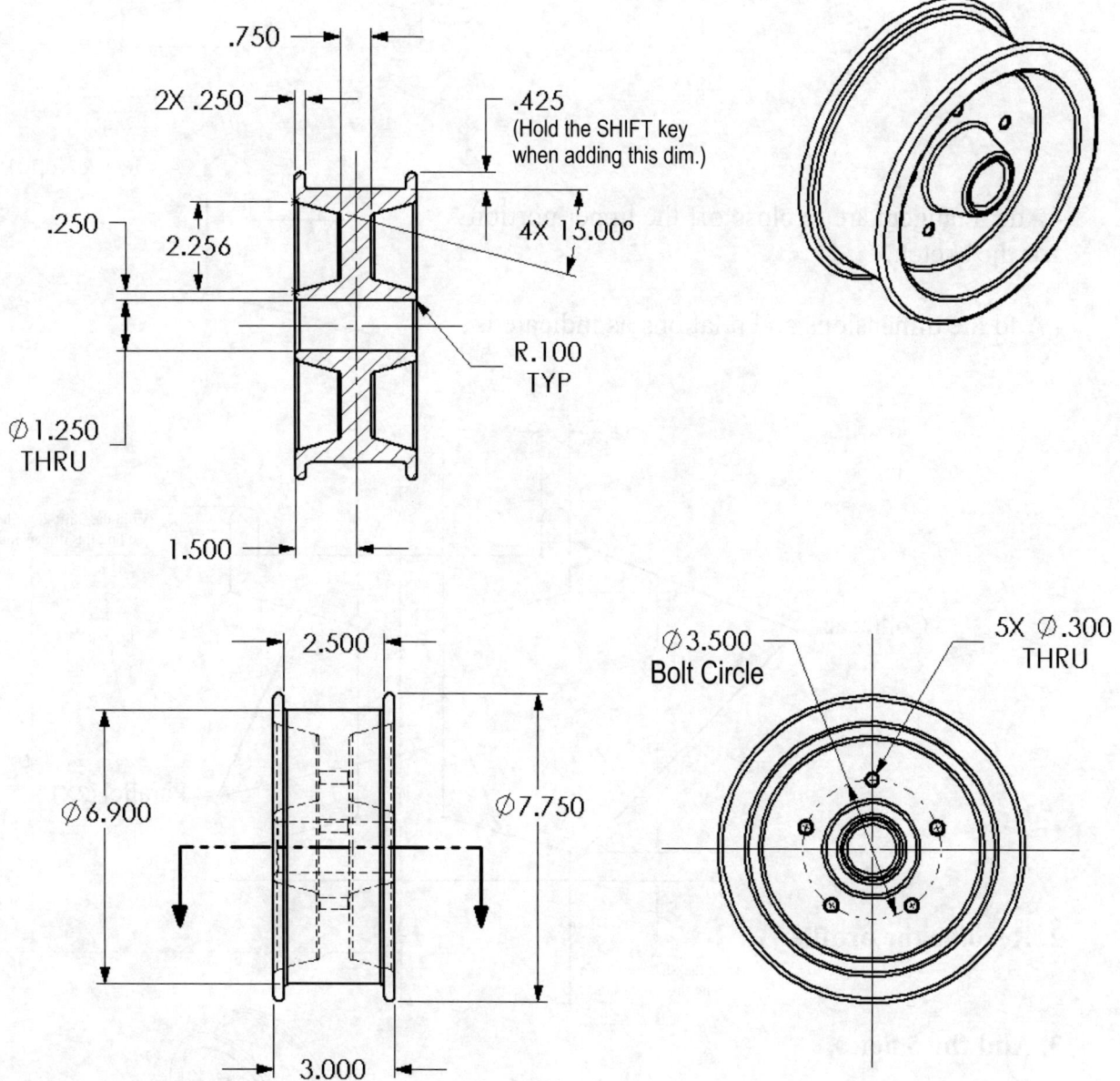

6. Save your work as: **Wheel_Exe**.

1. Start with the Front plane.

- Sketch 2 centerlines
  and use the vertical
  centerline for Dynamic
  Mirror.

- Sketch the profile
  as shown.

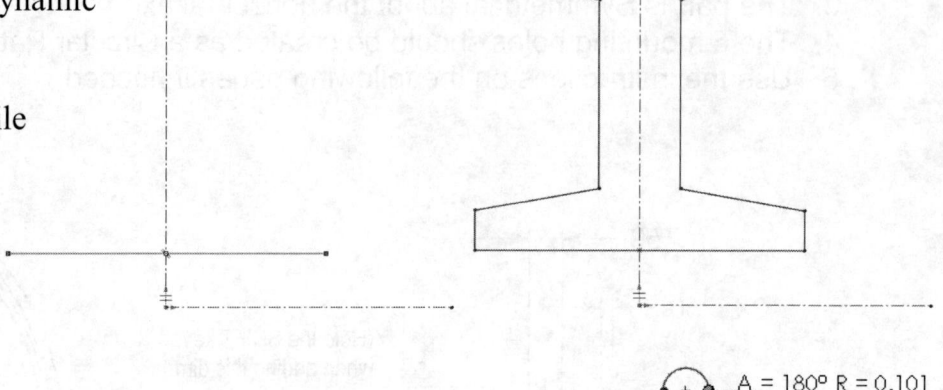

- Add a tangent arc to close off the upper portion
  of the sketch.

- Add the dimensions and relations as indicated.

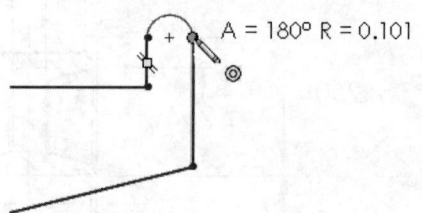

A = 180° R = 0.101

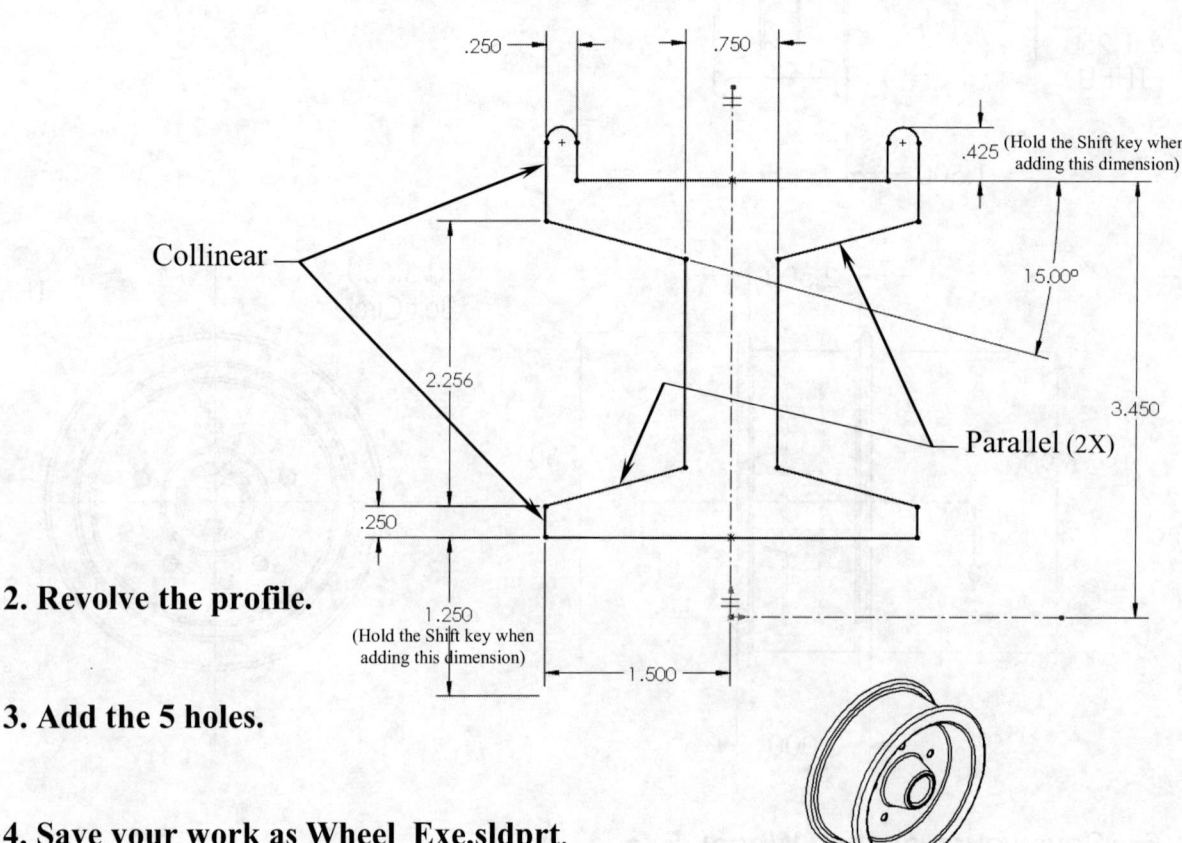

.250 — .750

Collinear

.425 (Hold the Shift key when adding this dimension)

15.00°

2.256

Parallel (2X)

3.450

.250

2. Revolve the profile.

1.250
(Hold the Shift key when
adding this dimension)

1.500

3. Add the 5 holes.

4. Save your work as Wheel_Exe.sldprt.

Exercise: Revolved Parts - Bottle
Extrude / Revolve / Sweep and Circular Pattern

1. Copying the document:

Go to:
Training Files folder, browse to
the file named:
Basic Solid Modeling_Bottle

Make a Copy of this file
and **Open the copy**.

(To review how this part
was made, open the sample
part from the Training Files
folder, in the Built-Parts
folder).

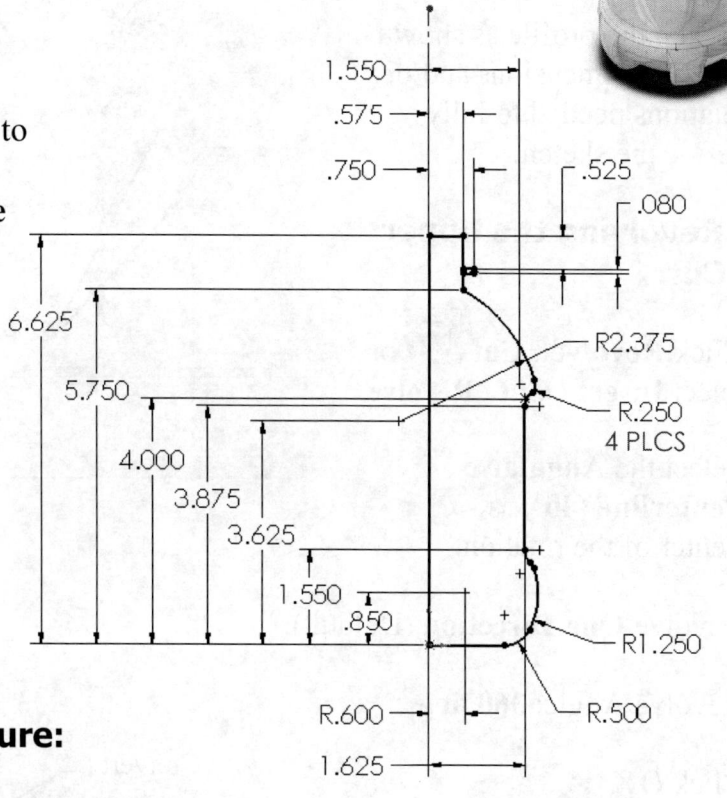

2. Revolving the Base feature:

- Click **Revolve** or select **Insert /
Boss-Base / Revolve**

- Select the **Vertical Centerline** as the
Center of the rotation.

- Direction: **Blind** (Default).

- Revolve Angle: **360 deg**.

- Click **OK**.

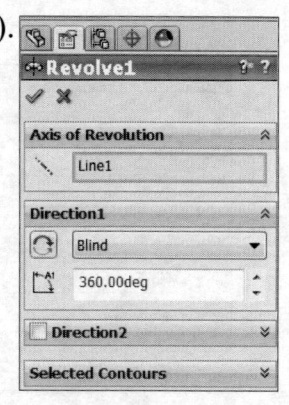

Revolve line

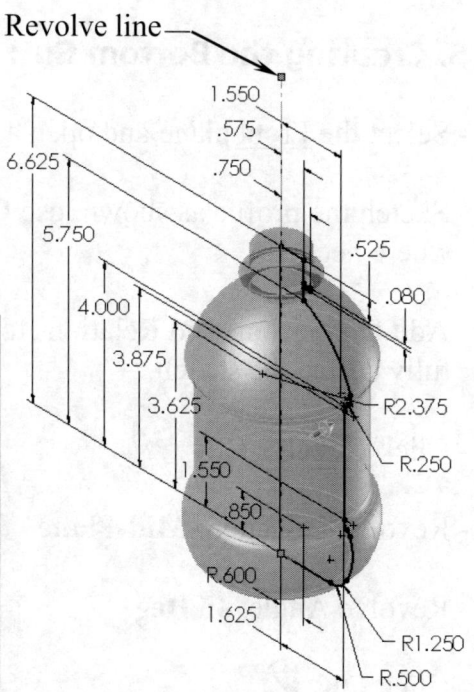

3. Creating the Upper Sketch:

- Select the <u>Front</u> plane and open a new sketch.

- Sketch the profile as shown **and** add dimensions and/or relations needed to fully define the sketch.

4. Revolving the Upper Cut:

- Click **Revolved Cut** 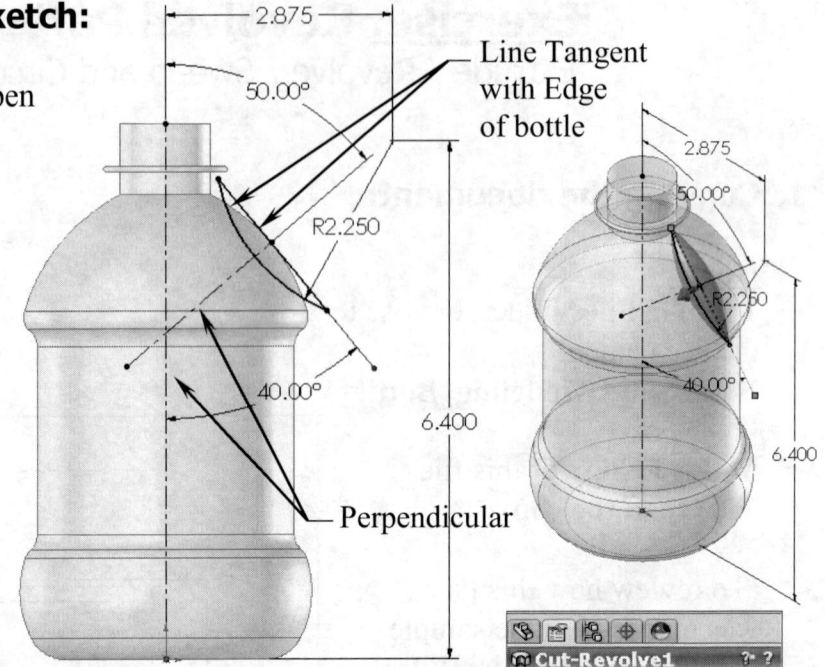 or select **Insert / Cut / Revolve**.

- Select the **Angular Centerline (40°)** as Center of the rotation.

- Revolve **One-Direction** (Default).

- Revolve Angle: **360 deg**.

- Click **OK** ✅.

5. Creating the Bottom Cut:

- Select the <u>Front</u> plane and open a new sketch.

- Sketch the profile as shown, use **Convert-Entities** where needed.

- Add Dimensions and Relations to fully define the sketch.

- Click **Revolve Cut** 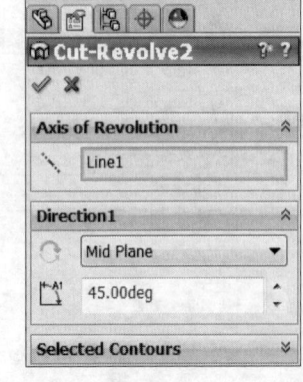.

- Revolve Direction: **Mid-Plane**

- Revolve Angle: **45 Deg**.

- Click **OK** ✅.

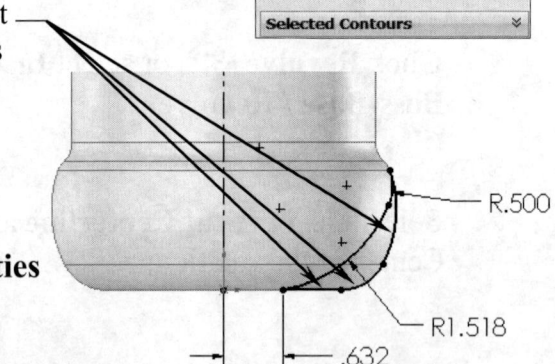

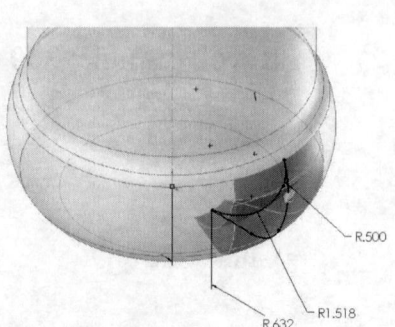

6. Adding .075" Fillets:

- Click **Fillet** 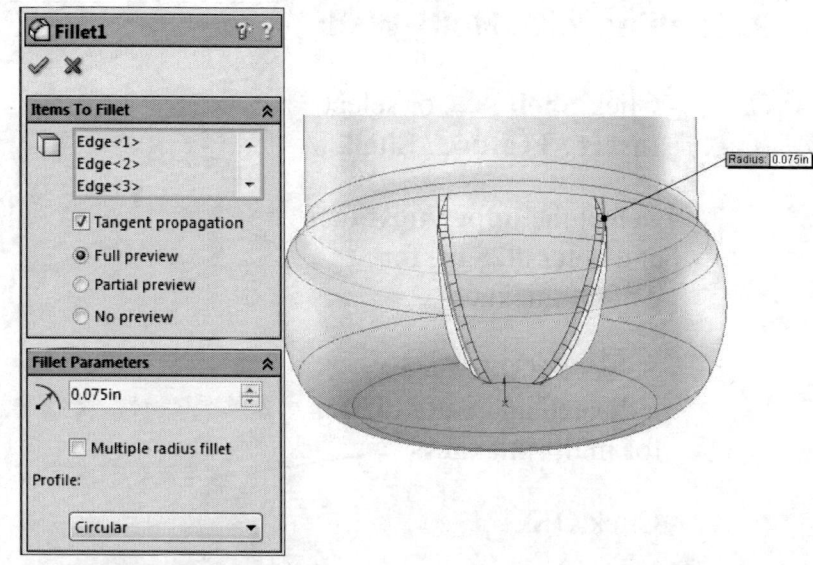 or select: **Insert / Feature / Fillet-Round**

- Enter **.075 in**. for Radius.

- Select the **2 inner edges**.

- Click **OK** ✅.

7. Adding .125" Fillets:

- Click Fillet 🔲 or select: **Insert / Feature / Fillet-Round**

- Enter **.125 in**. for Radius.

- Select the **2 outer edges**.

- Click **OK** ✅.

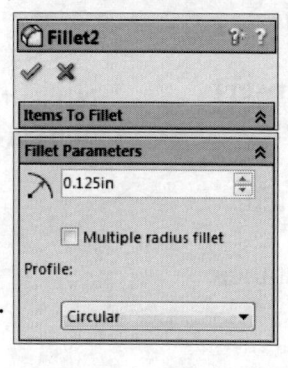
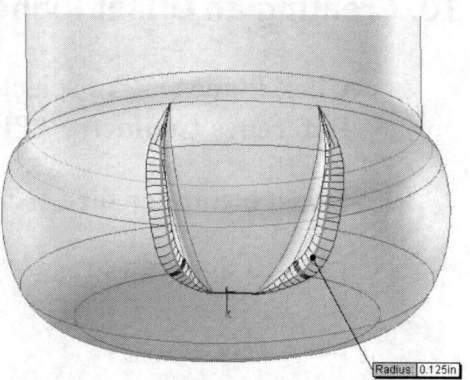

8. Circular Pattern the Cutouts:

- Click **Circular Pattern** 🔷 or select **Insert / Pattern-Mirror /Circular Pattern**.

- Select the **Center Axis** for use as the Pattern-Axis.

- Pattern Angle: **360deg**.

- **Equal Spacing** enabled.

- Number of Copies: **5**

- Select the **Upper Cut,** the **Lower Cut,** the **Fillet 1,** and **Fillet 2**.

- Click **OK** ✅.

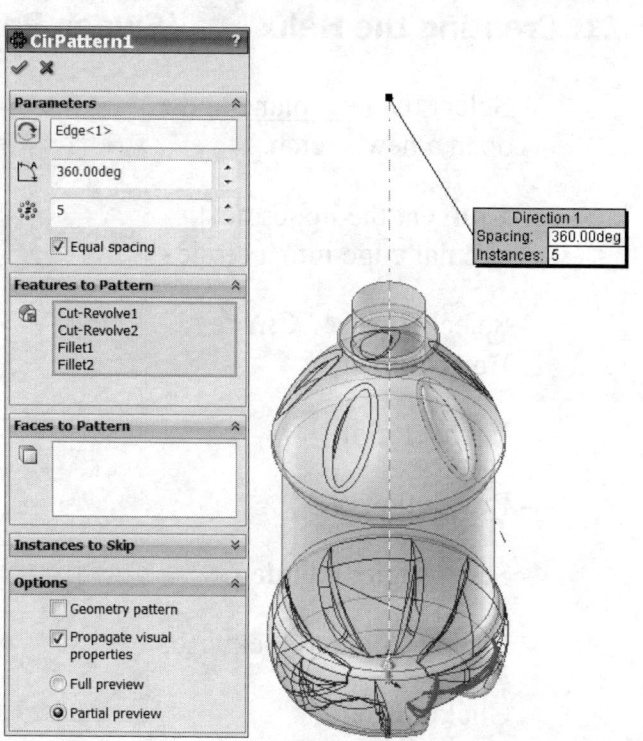

9. Shelling with Multi-Wall:

- Click **Shell** or select: **Insert / Feature / Shell.**

- Select the **uppermost face** and enter **.025 in**. for default thickness

- Select the **side face** as indicated and enter **.050 in**. for multi-thickness

- Click **OK**.

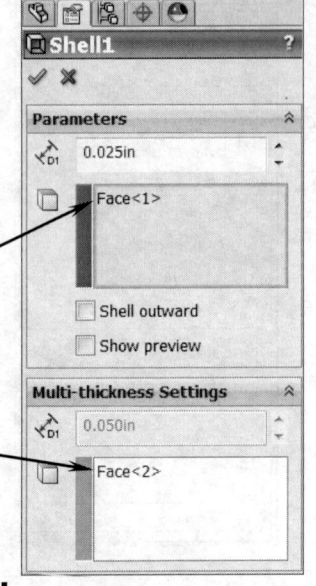

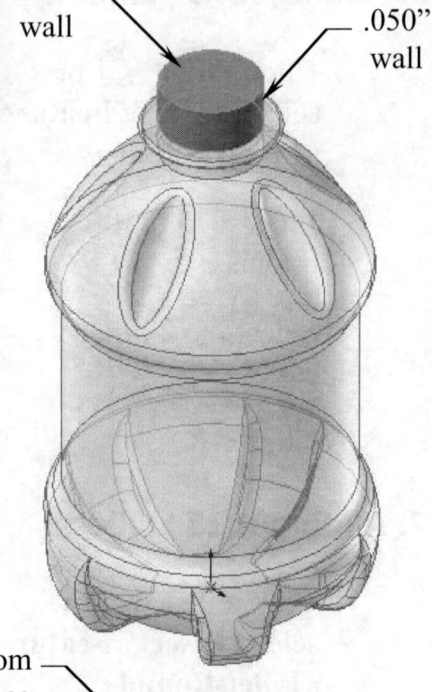

.025" wall

.050" wall

10. Creating an Offset Plane:

- Click **Plane** or select **Insert / Reference Geometry / Plane.**

- Select the **upper face** as noted.

- Enter **.450 in**. for offset Distance.

- Click **OK**.

Offset from top surface

11. Creating the Helix (Sweep Path):

- Select the new plane and open a new sketch.

- **Convert** the uppermost circular edge into a circle.

- Select: **Insert / Curve / Helix-Spiral.**

- Pitch: **.115 in**.

- Revolution: **3.5**

- Start Angle: **0.00deg**.

- Enable Counterclockwise.

- Click **OK**.

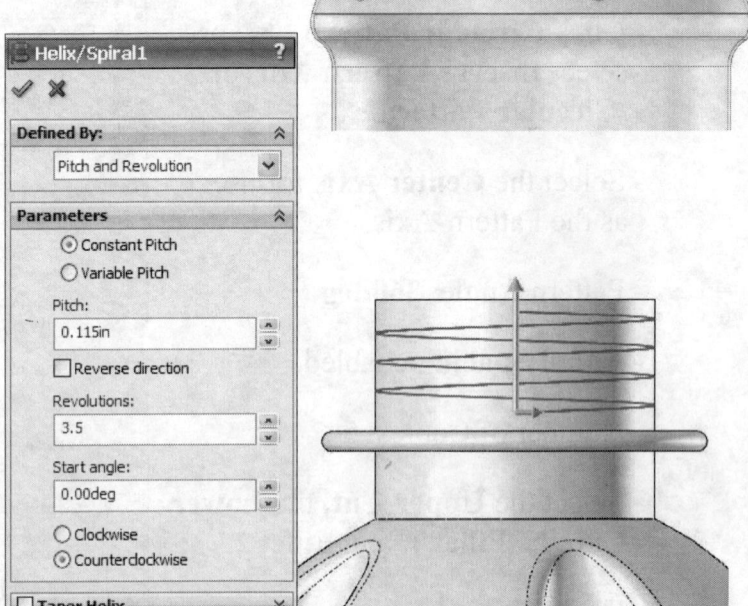

12. Sketching the Thread Profile:

- Select the <u>Right</u> plane and open a new sketch.

- Sketch the profile (Triangle), add the dimensions and relations needed to fully define the sketch.

- Use Dynamic Mirror 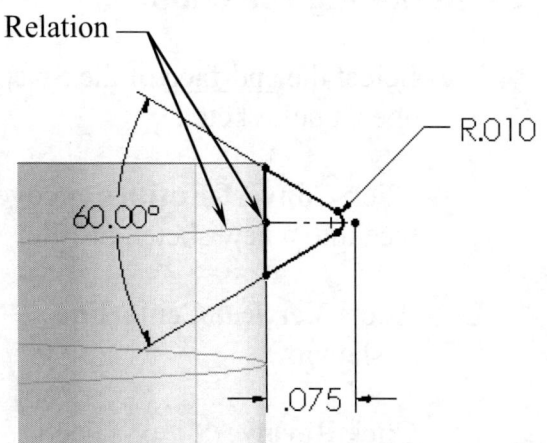 to keep all sketch entities symmetrical.

- Add a **Pierce** relation (between the the endpoint of the centerline and the helix) to properly snap the sweep profile on the Helix.

- **Exit** the Sketch .

13. Adding the Threads:

- Click **Swept Boss Base** or select: **Insert / Boss-Base / Sweep**.

- Select the Sketch Profile (the triangle) for use as the Sweep Profile.

- Select the Helix for use as the Sweep Path.

- Click **OK** .

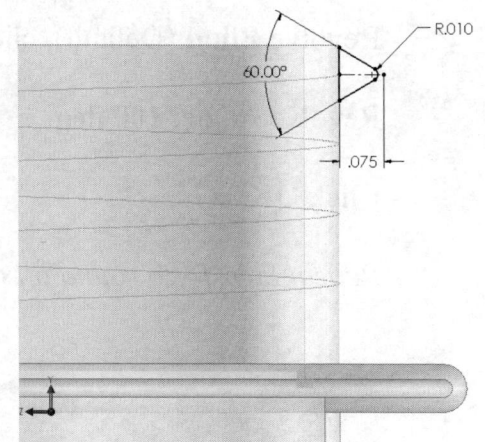

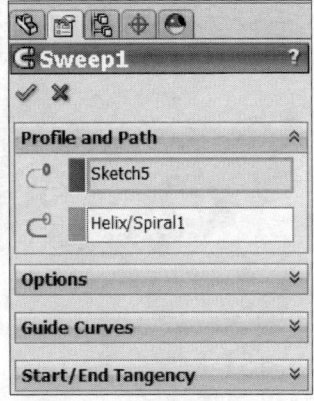

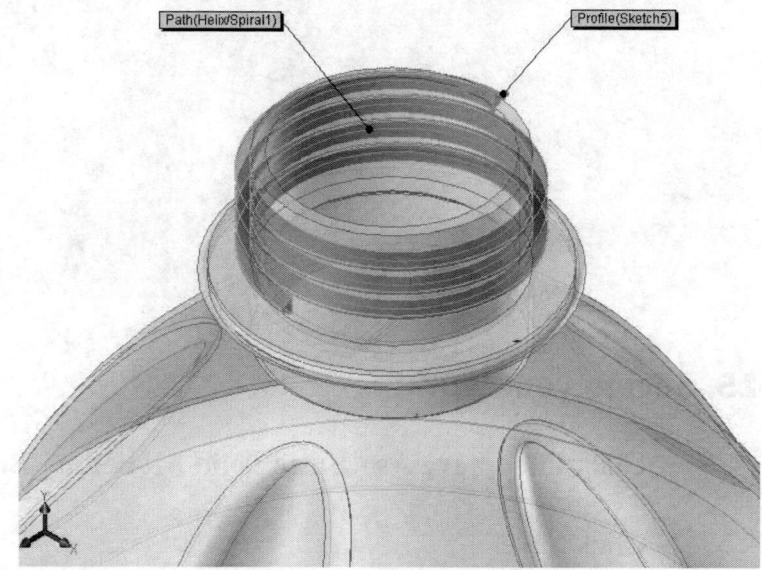

14. Rounding the ends:

- Select the <u>end-face</u> of the Swept feature and open a new sketch.

- Click **Convert-Entities** to covert the selected face into a new sketch profile.

- Add a **Vertical Centerline** as shown.

- Click **Revolve** 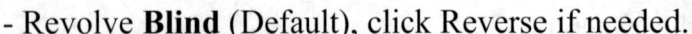 or select:
Insert / Boss-Base / Revolve.

- Revolve **Blind** (Default), click Reverse if needed.

- Revolve Angle: **100 deg**.

- Click **OK** ✅.

- Repeat Step 14 to round off the other end of the threads.

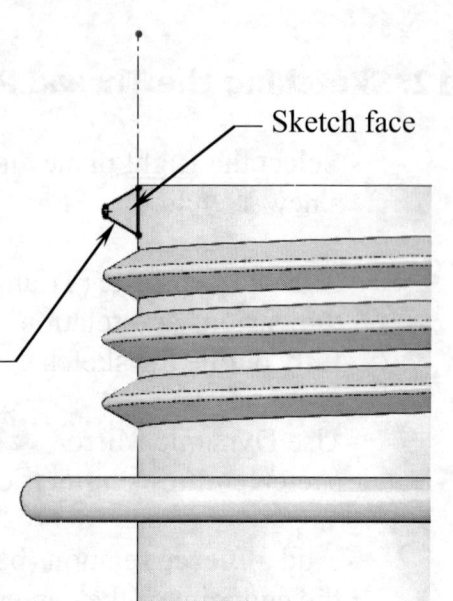

Sketch face

Convert Entities

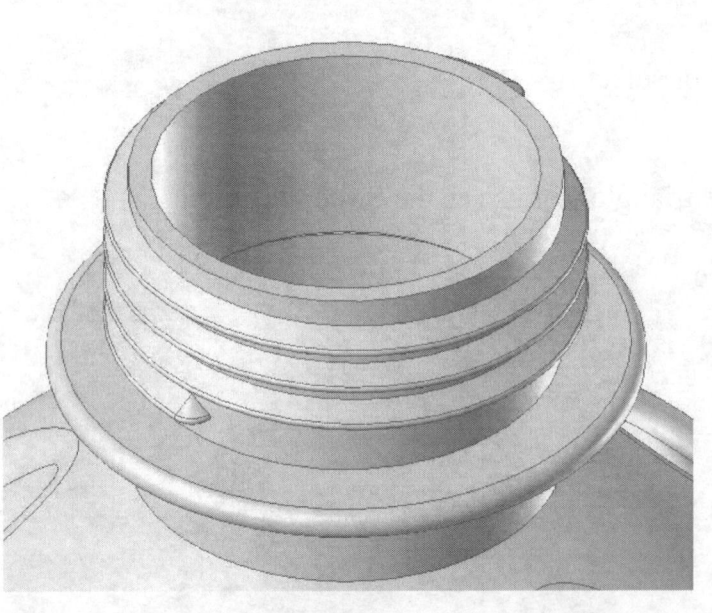

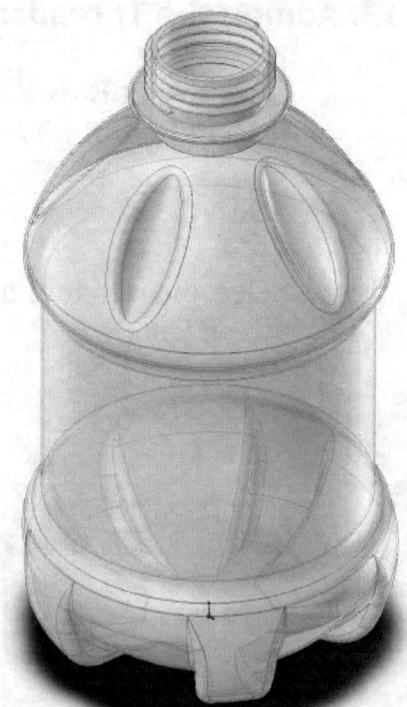

15. Saving your work:

- Click **File / Save As / Basic Solid Modeling_Bottle**.

- Click **Save**.

CHAPTER 6

Rib & Shell Features

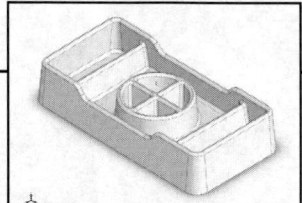

The Rib and Shell Features
Formed Tray

- A **Rib** is a special type of extruded feature created from open or closed sketched contours. It adds material of a specified thickness in a specified direction between the contour and an existing part. A rib can be created using single or multiple sketches.

- Rib features can have draft angles applied to them either inward, or outward.

- The **Detailed Preview** Property Manager can be used with multi-body parts to enhance detail and select entities to display.

- The **Shell** tool hollows out a part, leaves selected faces open, and creates thin walled features on the remaining faces. If nothing (no face) is selected on the model, a solid part can be shelled, creating a closed hollow model.

- Multiple thicknesses are also supported when shelling a solid model.

- In most cases, the model fillets should be applied before shelling a part.

- One of the most common problems when the shell fails is when the wall thickness of the shell is smaller than one of the fillets in the model.

- If errors appear when shelling a model, you can run the **Error Diagnostics**. The shell feature displays error messages and includes tools to help you identify why the shell feature failed. The diagnostic tool **Error Diagnostics** is available in the **Shell** Property Manager.

Formed Tray
Rib & Shell Features

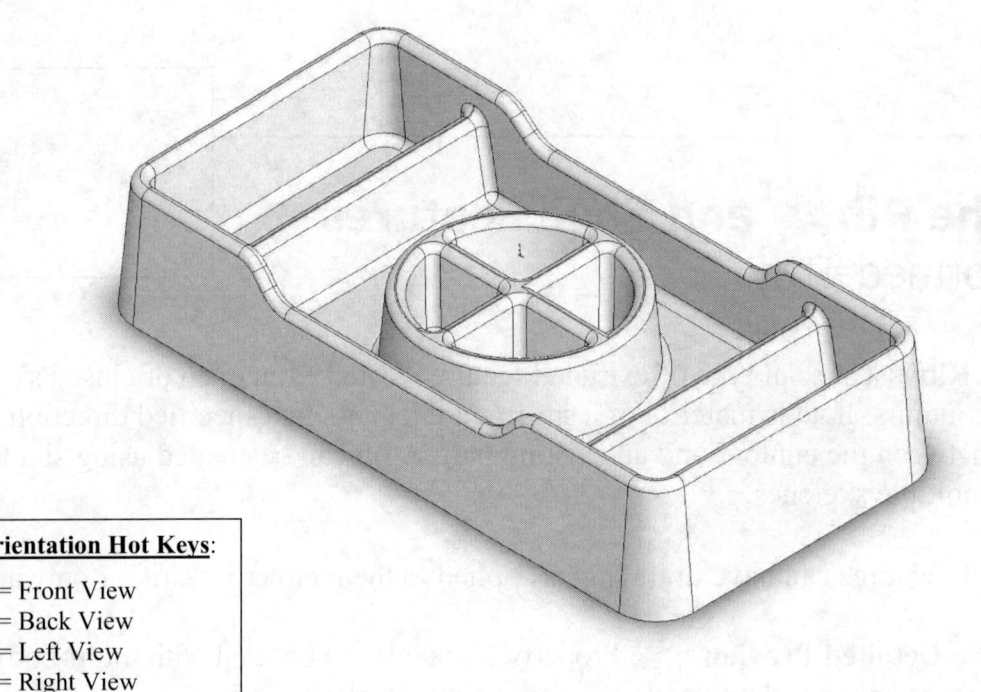

View Orientation Hot Keys:

Ctrl + 1 = Front View
Ctrl + 2 = Back View
Ctrl + 3 = Left View
Ctrl + 4 = Right View
Ctrl + 5 = Top View
Ctrl + 6 = Bottom View
Ctrl + 7 = Isometric View
Ctrl + 8 = Normal To
            Selection

Dimensioning Standards: **ANSI**

Units: **INCHES** – 3 Decimals

Tools Needed:

Insert Sketch	Line	Circle
Add Geometric Relations	Dimension	Fillet
Boss/Base Extrude	Rib	Shell

1. Sketching the Base Profile:

- Select the <u>Top</u> plane from the FeatureManager tree.

- Click Sketch 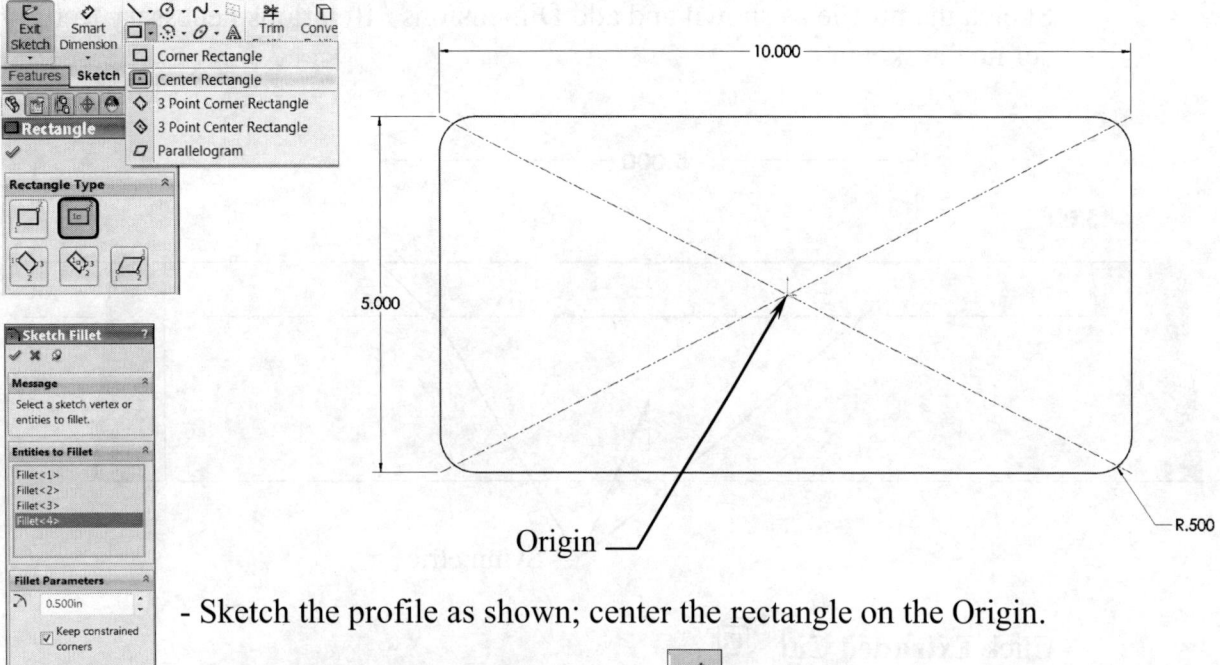 or select **Insert / Sketch**.

- Sketch the profile as shown; center the rectangle on the Origin.

- Add sketch fillets and dimensions as shown to fully define the sketch.

2. Extruding the Base feature:

- Click **Extruded Boss-Base** or select **Insert / Boss-Base / Extrude**.

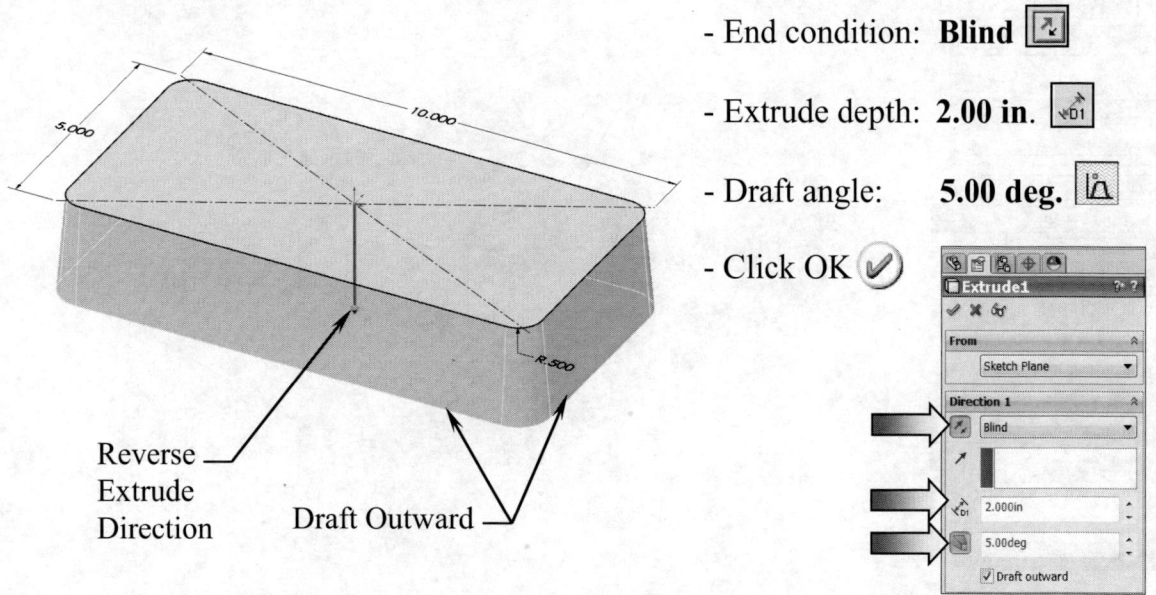

- End condition: **Blind**

- Extrude depth: **2.00 in**.

- Draft angle: **5.00 deg.**

- Click OK

Reverse Extrude Direction

Draft Outward

3. Adding the Side Cutouts:

- Select the <u>Front</u> plane from the FeatureManager tree.

- Click Sketch 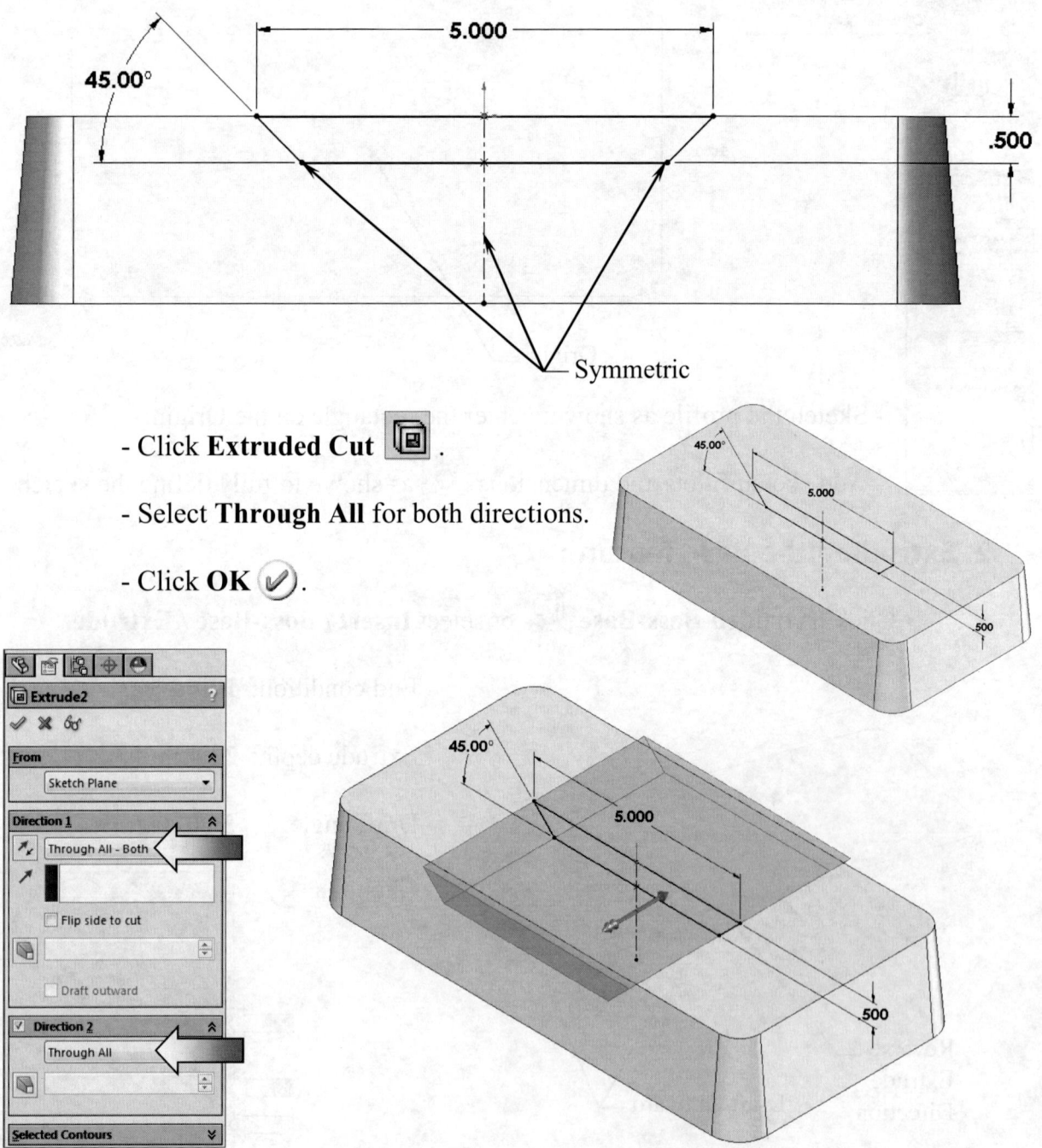 or select **Insert / Sketch.**

- Sketch the profile as shown and add Dimensions / Relations necessary to fully define the sketch.

- Click **Extruded Cut** .

- Select **Through All** for both directions.

- Click **OK** .

4. Removing more material:

- Select the top surface and open a new sketch.

- Select the outer edges and create an **offset** of **.250"** as indicated.

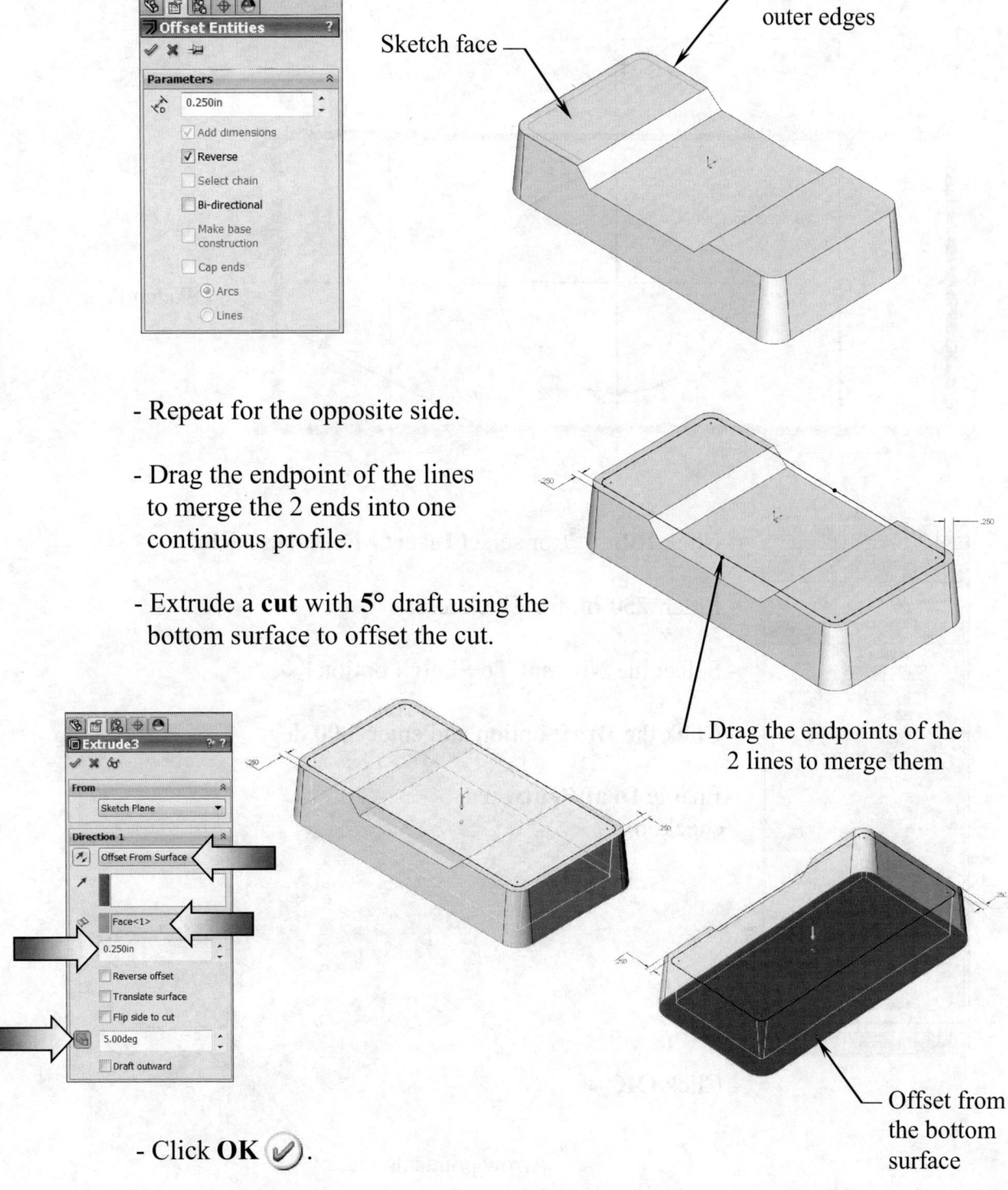

- Repeat for the opposite side.

- Drag the endpoint of the lines to merge the 2 ends into one continuous profile.

- Extrude a **cut** with **5°** draft using the bottom surface to offset the cut.

- Click **OK** ✓.

5. Creating the Rib Profiles:

- Select the <u>face</u> as indicated and open a new sketch .

- Sketch the profile and add dimensions / relations needed to fully define the sketch.

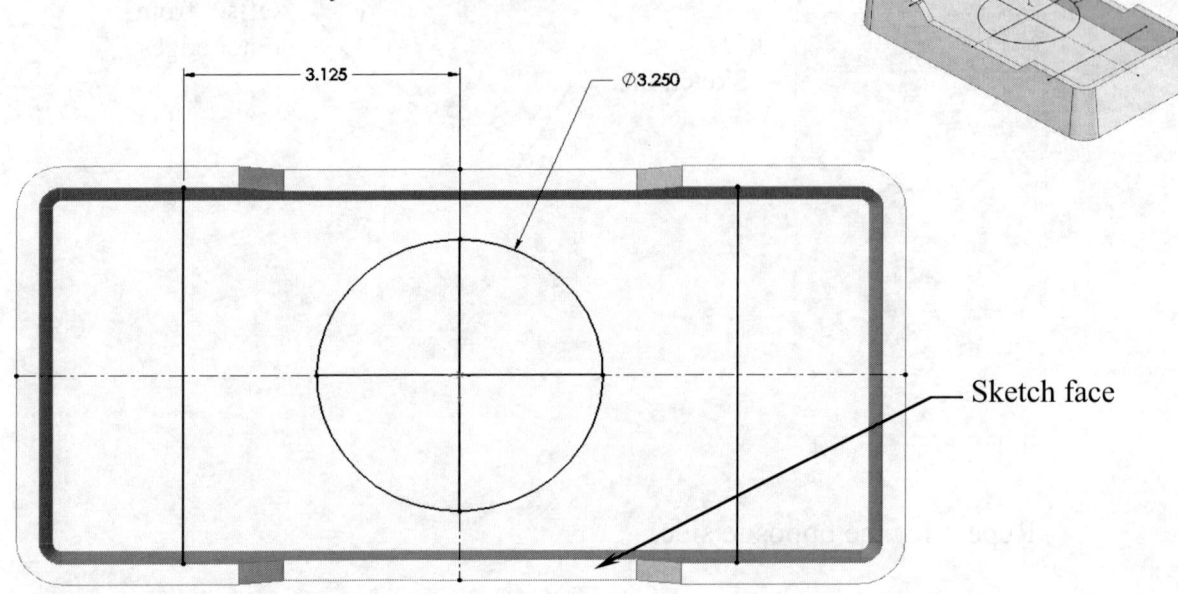

Sketch face

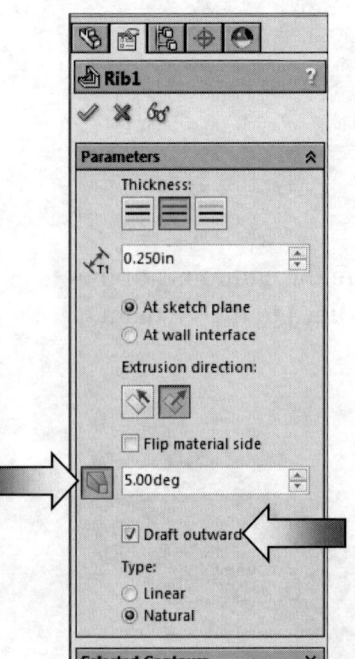

- Click **Rib** 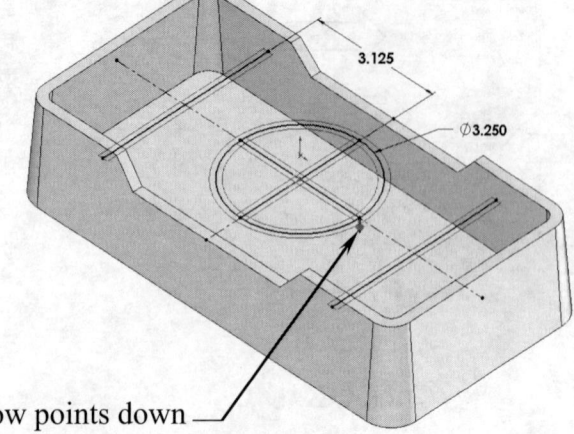 or select **Insert / Features / Rib**.

- Enter **.250 in.** for Thickness.

- Select the **Normal To Sketch** option.

- Click the **Draft** option and enter **5.00** deg.

- Enable **Draft Outward** checkbox.

- Click **OK**.

Arrow points down

6. Adding the .500" Fillets:

- Click **Fillet** 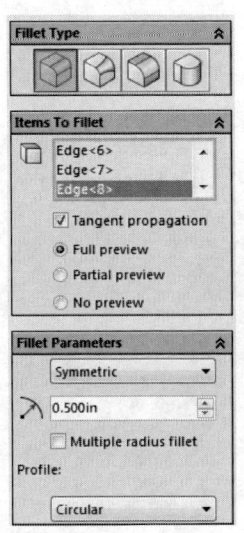 or select **Insert / Features / Fillet-Round**.

- Enter **.500 in.** as the Radius and select the 8 Edges as shown.

- Click **OK** ⊘.

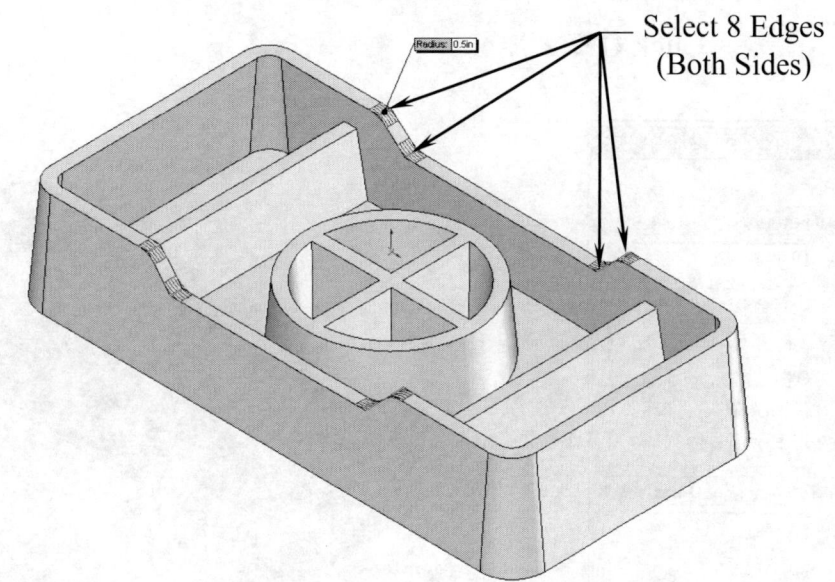

Select 8 Edges
(Both Sides)

7. Adding the .125" Fillets:

- Click **Fillet** 🔲 or select **Insert / Features / Fillet-Round**.

- Enter **.125 in.** for radius size
  and select all edges **except**
  for the bottom edges.

- Click **OK** ⊘.

Box select

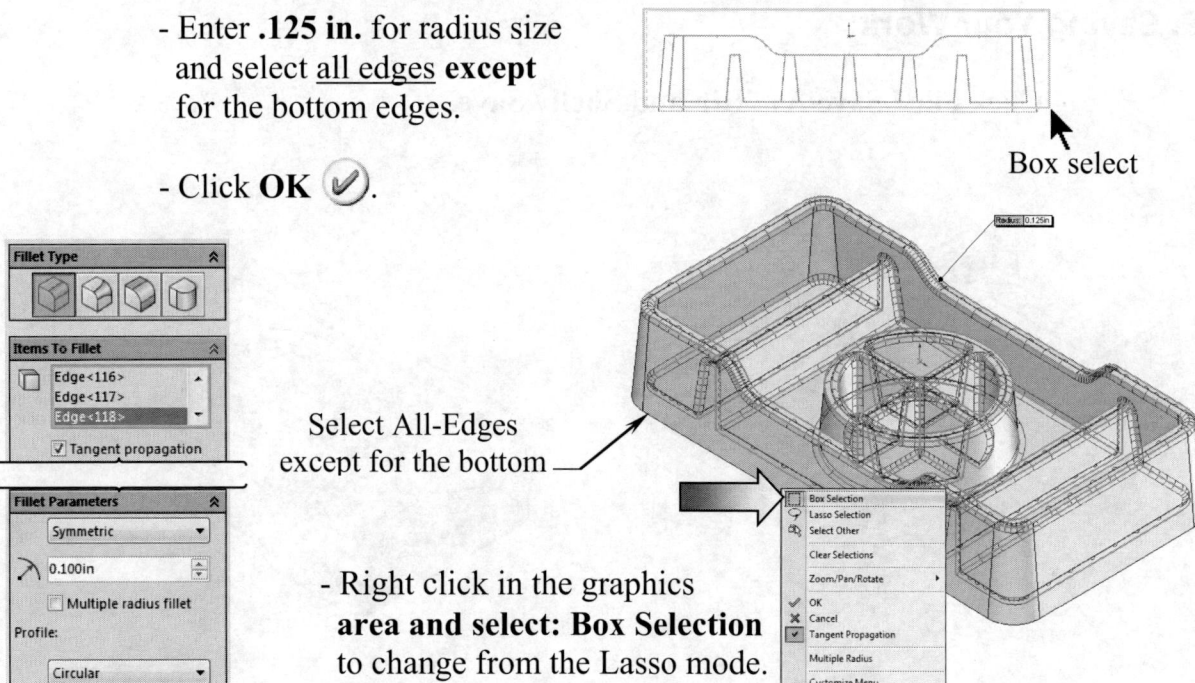

Select All-Edges
except for the bottom

- Right click in the graphics
  area and select: Box Selection
  to change from the Lasso mode.

8. Shelling the lower portion:

- The Shell command hollows out a part, leaves open the faces that you select.

- Click **Shell** 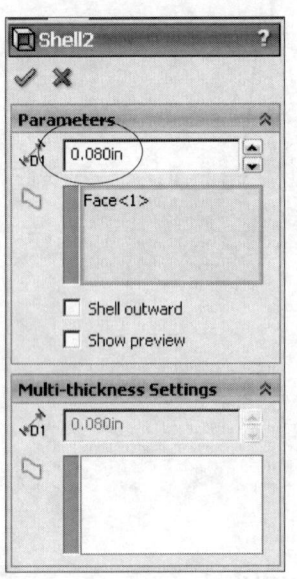 or select **Insert / Features / Shell**.

- Select the <u>bottom face</u> and enter **.080** in. for Thickness.

- Click **OK**.

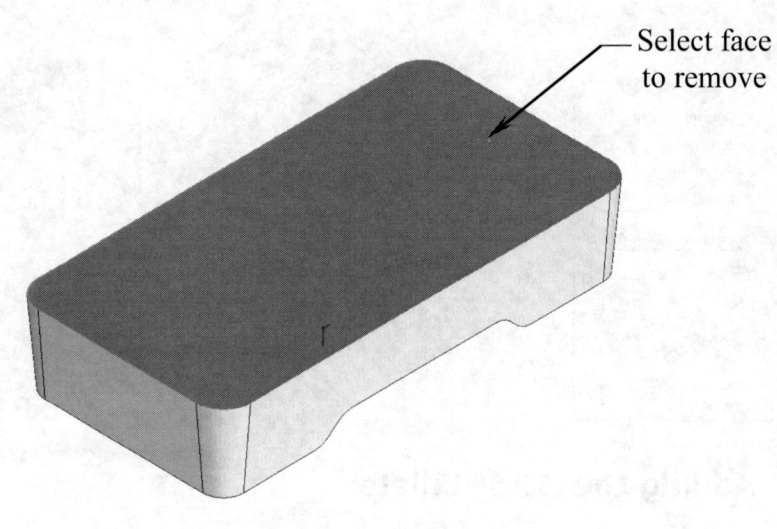

Select face
to remove

9. Saving Your Work:

- Click **File / Save As / Rib and Shell / Save**.

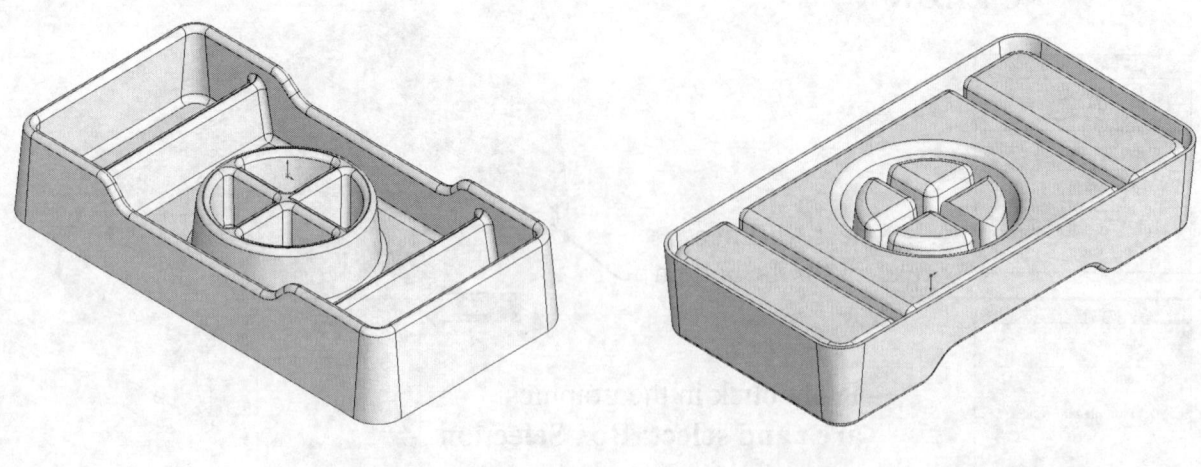

Questions for Review

Rib & Shell Features

1. A fully defined sketch can be re-positioned after its relations/dimensions to the origin have been removed.
   - a. True
   - b. False

2. The Mid-Plane extrude option extrudes the profile in both directions and at equal depths.
   - a. True
   - b. False

3. Draft Outward is the only option available; the Draft Inward option is not available.
   - a. True
   - b. False

4. The Shell feature hollows out the part starting with the selected face.
   - a. True
   - b. False

5. If nothing (no face) is selected, a solid model cannot be shelled.
   - a. True
   - b. False

6. A Rib is a special type of extruded feature; no drafts may be added to it.
   - a. True
   - b. False

7. 7. A Rib can only be created with a closed-sketch profile; opened-sketch profiles may not be used.
   - a. True
   - b. False

8. The Rib features can be fully edited, just like any other feature in SolidWorks.
   - a. True
   - b. False

7. FALSE	8. TRUE
5. FALSE	6. FALSE
3. FALSE	4. TRUE
1. TRUE	2. TRUE

CHAPTER 6 (cont.)

Using Shell & Mirror

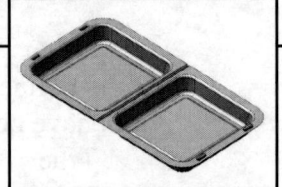

Using Shell & Mirror
Styrofoam Box

- In most cases, creating a model as a solid and then shell it out towards the end of the process would probably be easier than creating the model as a thin walled from the beginning.

- Although the model can be made as a thin walled part in the newer releases of SolidWorks, but this lesson will guide us through the process of creating the solid model, and the shell feature will be added in the end.

- The shell command hollows out a model, it deletes the faces that you select and creates thin walled feature on the remaining faces. But if you do not select any faces of the model, it will still get shelled, and the model will become a closed hollow part. Multi-thickness can be created at the same time.

- Mirror, on the other hand, offers a quick way to make a copy of one or more features, where a plane or a planar surface is used to mirror about.

- The options that are available for mirror are:

  * Mirror Features: is used to mirror solid features such as Extruded Boss, Cuts, Fillets and Chamfers.

  * Mirror Faces: is used when the model, or an imported part, has faces that make up the features, but not the solid features themselves.

  * Mirror Bodies: is used to mirror solid bodies, surface bodies, or multibodies.

- If Mirror bodies option is selected, the Merge Solids and the Knit Surfaces options appear, requiring you to select the appropriate checkboxes, prior to completing the mirror function.

Using Shell & Mirror
Styrofoam Box

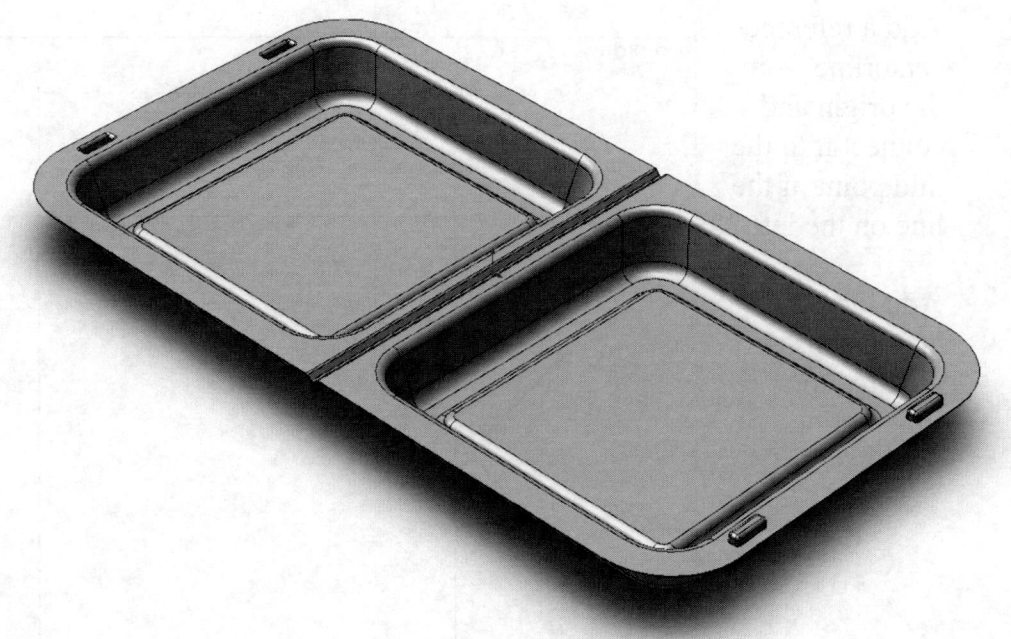

Dimensioning Standards: **ANSI**

Units: **INCHES** – 3 Decimals

Tools Needed:

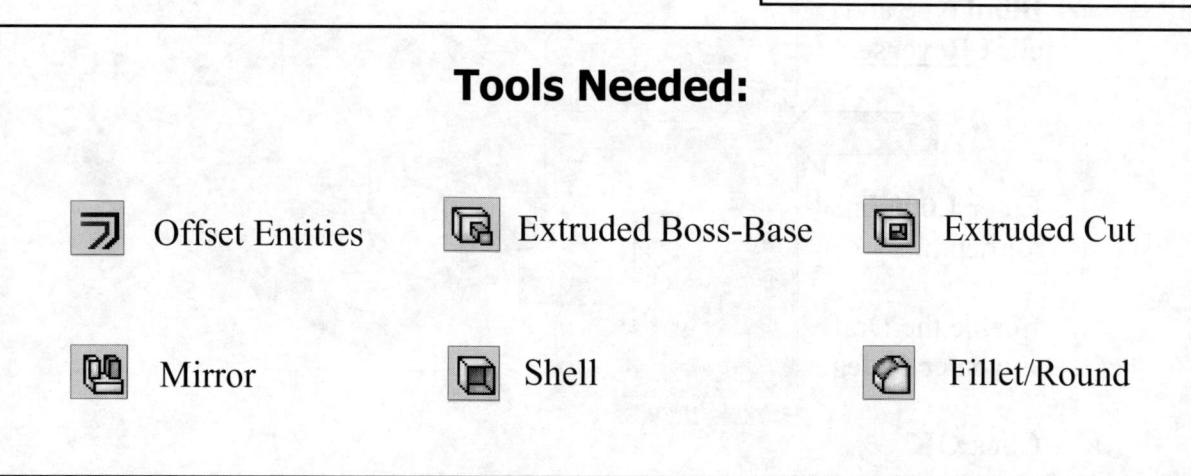

Offset Entities

Extruded Boss-Base

Extruded Cut

Mirror

Shell

Fillet/Round

1. Starting a new part:

- Click **File / New / Part**. Set the Units to Inches and number of Decimal to 3.

- Select the Top plane and open a new sketch 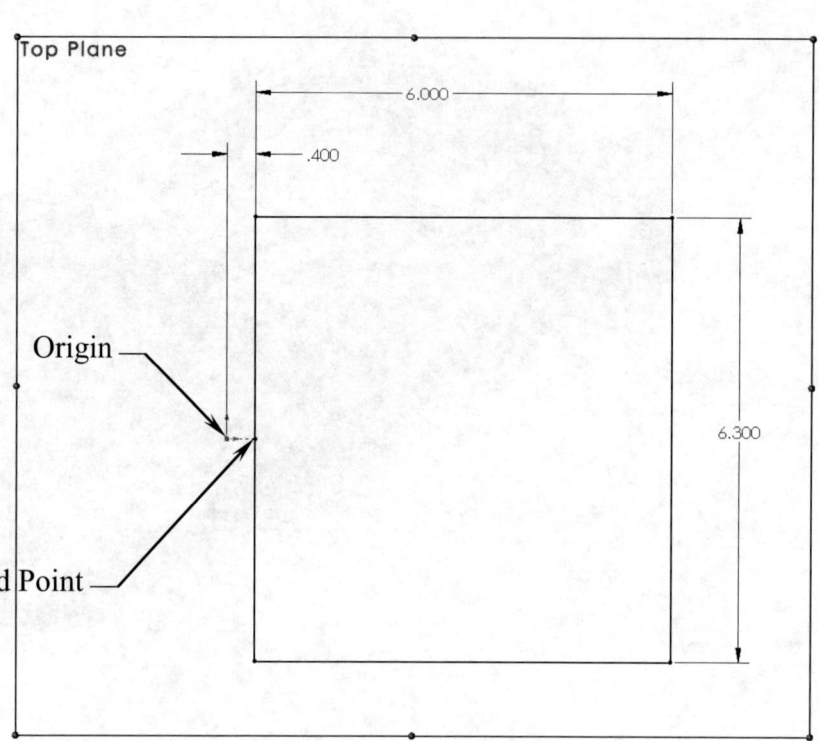.

- Sketch a **rectangle** a little bit to the right of the Origin as shown below.

- Add a reference centerline from the origin and connect it to the mid point of the line on the left.

- Add the dimensions as pictured to fully define this sketch.

2. Extruding the base:

- Click **Extruded Boss-Base** .

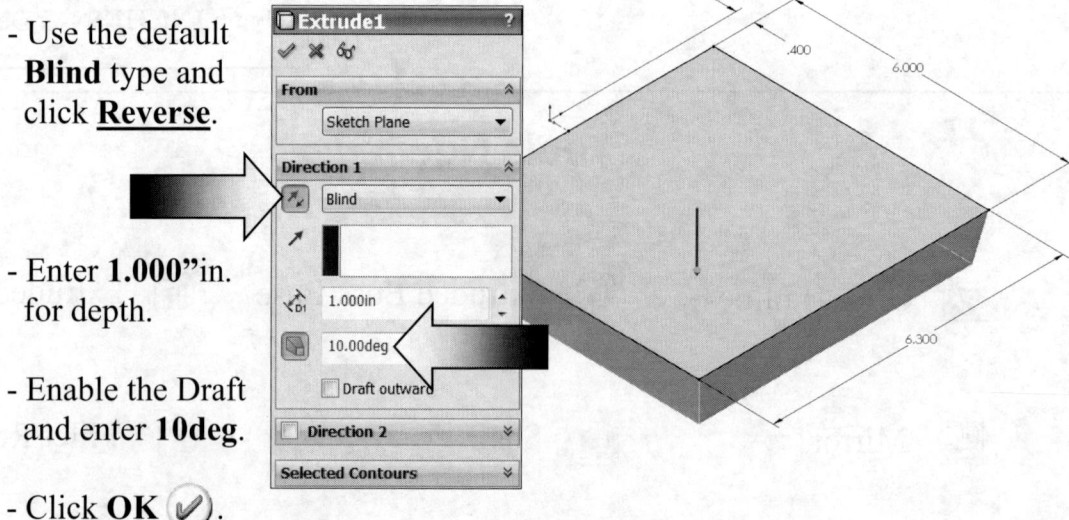

- Use the default **Blind** type and click **Reverse**.

- Enter **1.000"**in. for depth.

- Enable the Draft and enter **10deg**.

- Click **OK** .

3. Adding the .750" fillets:

- Click the **Fillet** 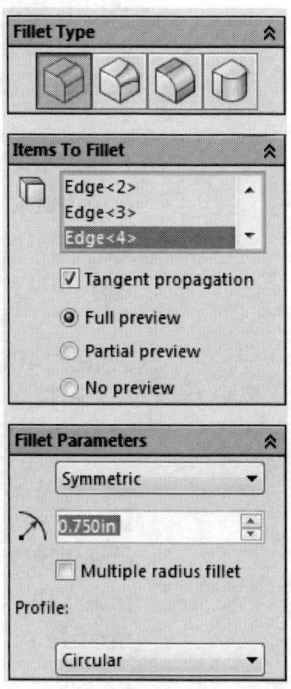 command from the Features toolbar.

- Enter **.750in** for radius.

- Select the **4 edges** as noted.

- Click **OK** ✓.

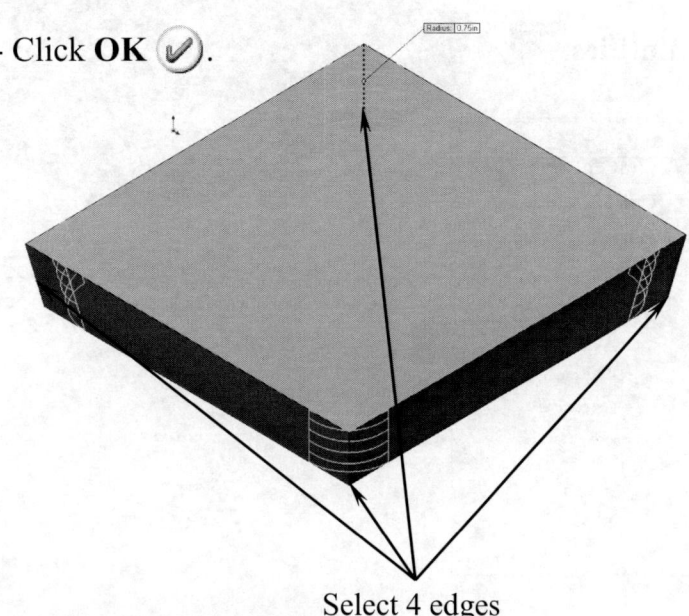

Select 4 edges

4. Adding the .250" fillets:

- Press **Enter** to <u>repeat</u> the previous command or click the Fillet command again.

- Enter **.250in** for radius.

- Select one of the edges at the <u>bottom</u> of the part. The fillet should propagate automatically because the Tangent Propagation checkbox was enabled by default.

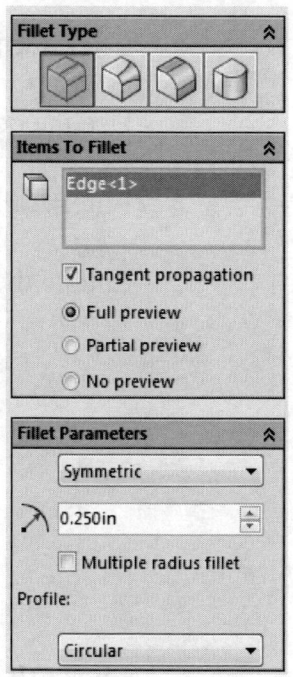

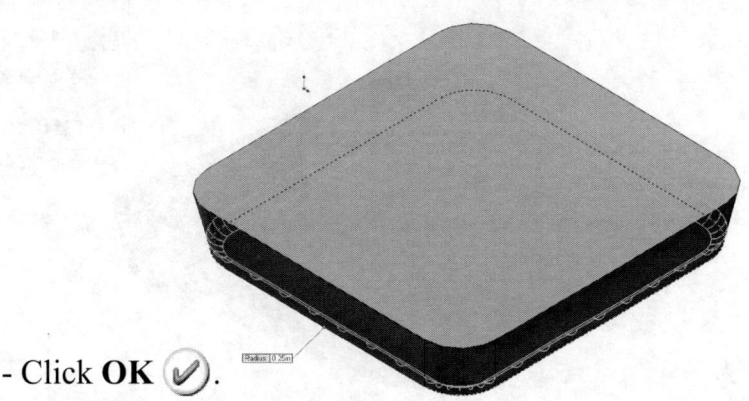

- Click **OK** ✓.

5. Creating an offset sketch:

- Open a new sketch 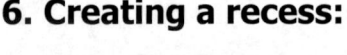 on the <u>bottom face</u> as indicated.

- Right click on one of the edges as noted and pick: **Select Tangency**.

- Click the **Offset Entities** command on the Sketch toolbar.

- Enter **.400in** for offset dimension and click the **Reverse** checkbox to place the new profile on the <u>inside</u>.

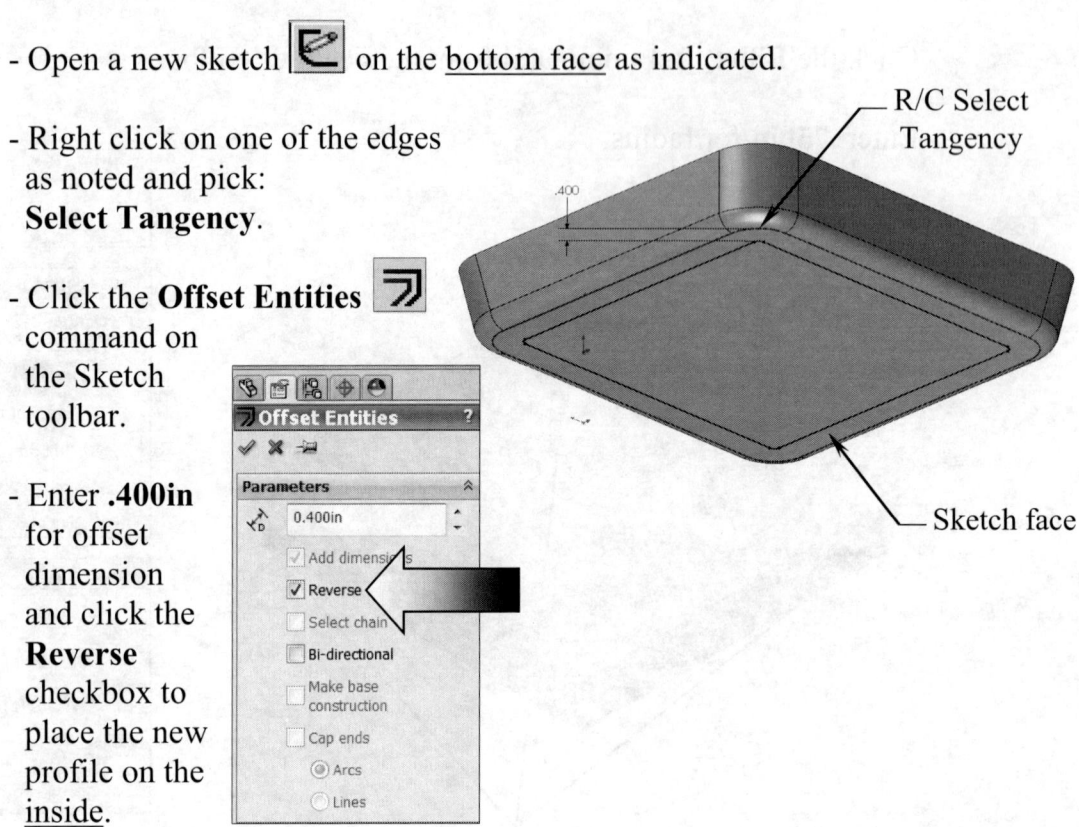

R/C Select Tangency

Sketch face

6. Creating a recess:

- Click **Extruded Cut** .

- Use the default **Blind** type.

- Enter **.200in** for extrude depth.

- Enable the Draft button and enter **10.00deg**. for angle.

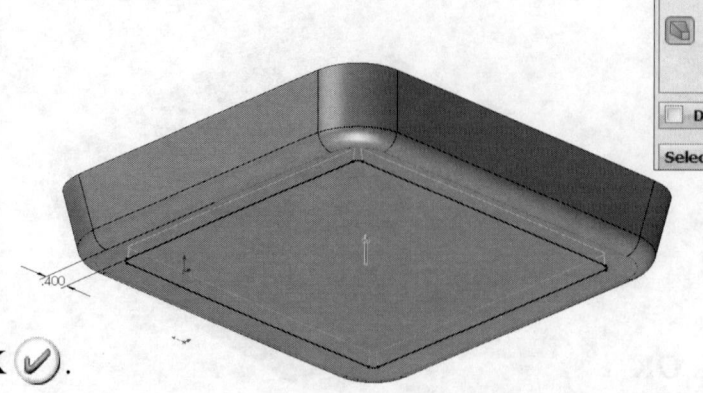

- Click **OK** ✅.

7. Adding the .125" fillets:

- From the Features toolbar, click the **Fillet** command .

- Enter **.125in** for radius value.

- Select the rectangular <u>face</u> of the recess instead. The fillet propagates along all edges of the selected face.

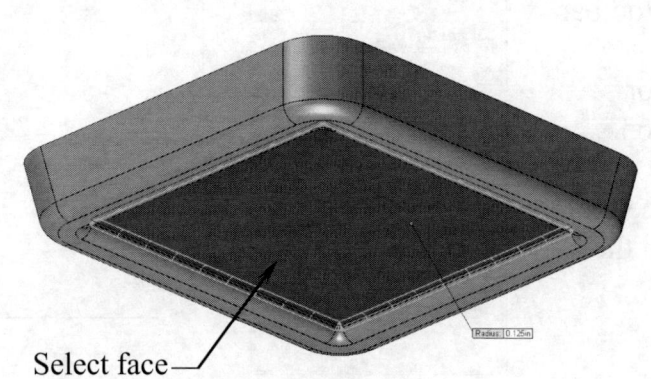

Select face

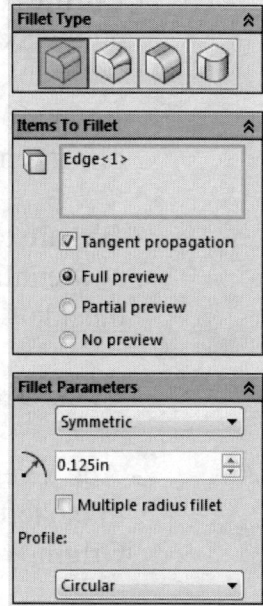

- Click **OK** ✅.

8. Adding the .200" fillets:

- Press **Enter** to repeat the last command (or click the Fillet command again).

- Enter **.200in** for radius value.

- Select one of the <u>upper</u> edges of the recess. The fillet propagates around the recess feature.

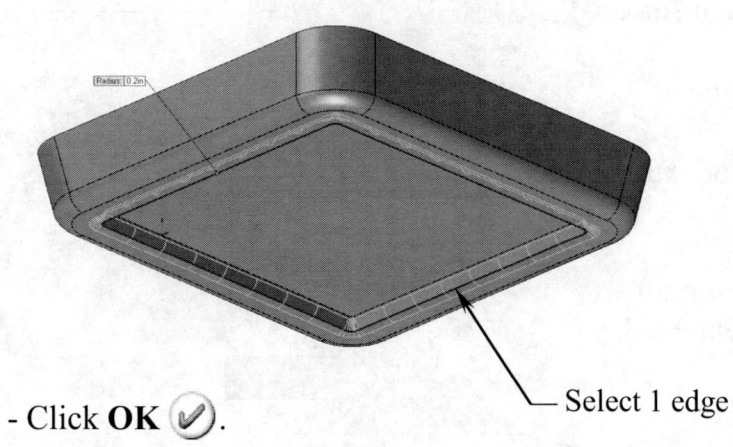

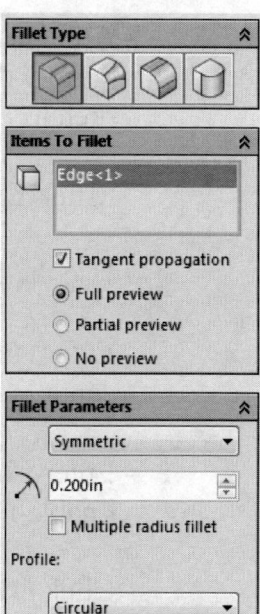

Select 1 edge

- Click **OK** ✅.

9. Creating the rim:

- Select the <u>upper face</u> of the part and open a new sketch .

- Hold the Control key and select the <u>5 edges</u> as noted.

- Click the **Offset Entities** command on the Sketch toolbar.

- Enter **.600in** for offset dimension.

- Be sure to place the new entities on the <u>outside</u>.

- Click **OK** ✓.

- Add a vertical line to the left of the Origin.

- Extend the line to close off both ends of the profile.

- Add the **.600"** spacing dimension to fully define the sketch.

- Click **Extruded Boss**.

- Use the **Blind** type.

- Enter **.400in** for extrude depth.

- Enter **10deg** for draft. Enable Draft Outward.

- Click **OK** ✓.

Sketch face

Select 5 edges

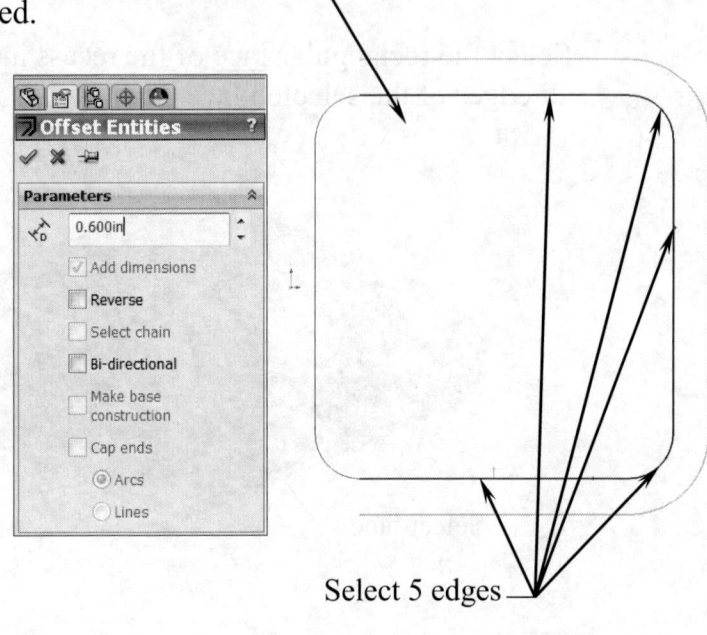

Trim / Extend to close off both ends

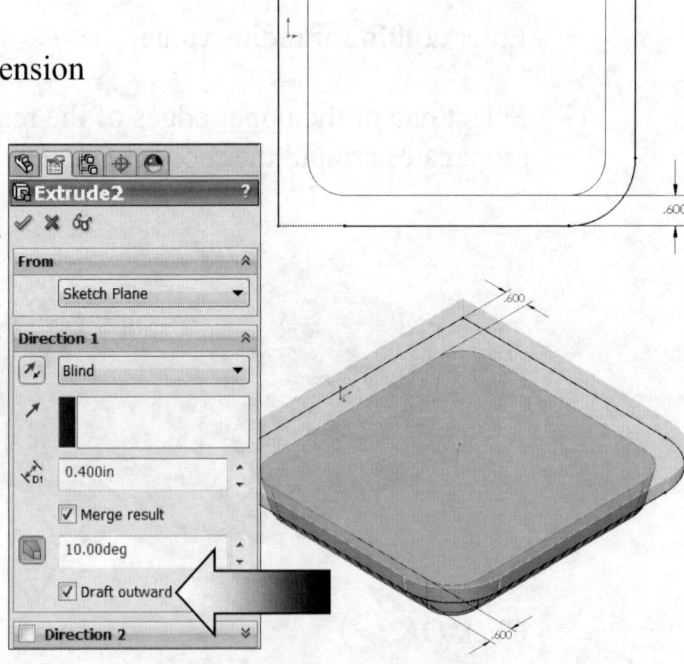

10. Adding another .125" fillet:

- Click the **Fillet** command 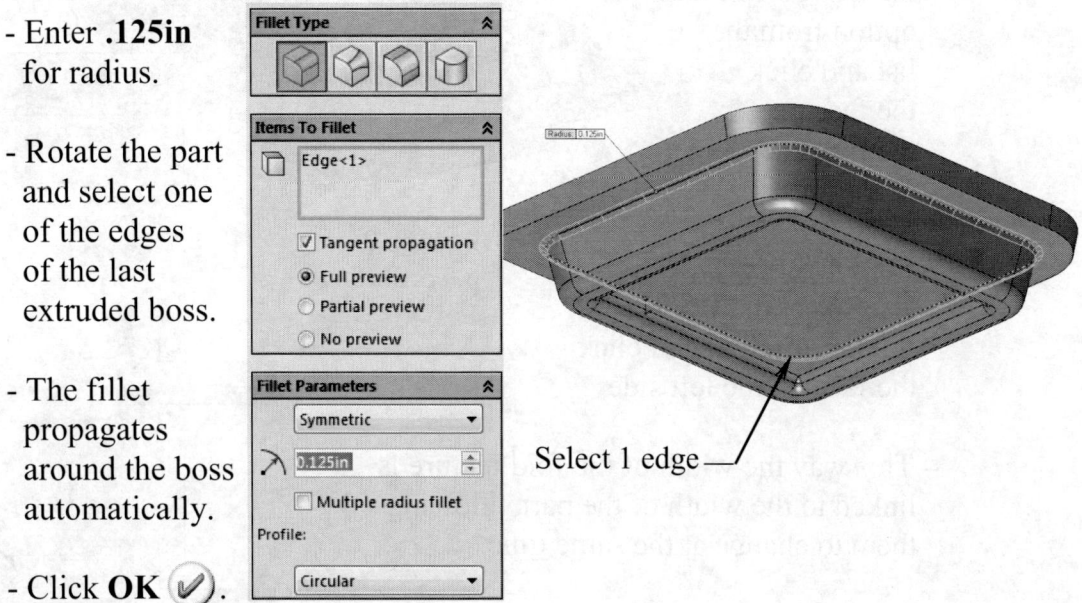 from the Feature toolbar.

- Enter **.125in** for radius.

- Rotate the part and select one of the edges of the last extruded boss.

- The fillet propagates around the boss automatically.

- Click **OK** ✅.

Fillet Type

Items To Fillet

Edge<1>

☑ Tangent propagation
◉ Full preview
○ Partial preview
○ No preview

Fillet Parameters

Symmetric ▾

0.125in

☐ Multiple radius fillet

Profile:

Circular ▾

Radius: 0.125in

Select 1 edge

11. Creating the fold feature:

- Select the <u>Front</u> plane and open a new sketch 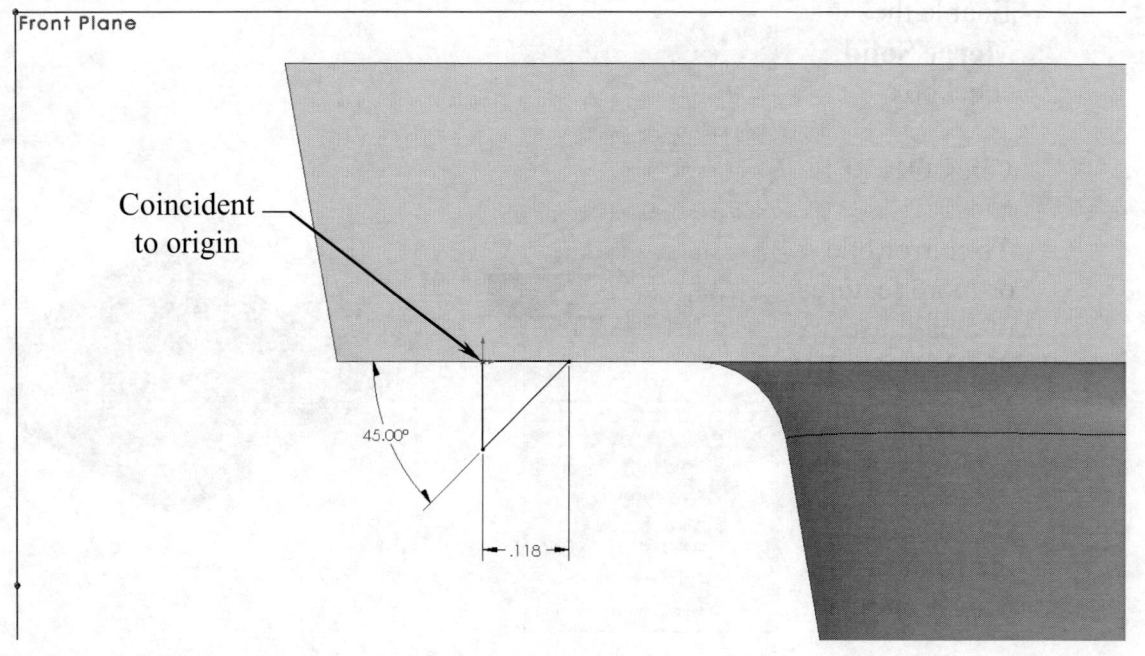. Press **Ctrl + 8** to rotate the view normal to the sketch.

- Sketch a triangle using the line tool. Add the dimensions shown.

Front Plane

Coincident to origin

45.00°

.118

- Click **Extruded Boss-Base**.

- For **Direction 1**, select the **Up-To-Surface** option from the list and click the face on the right side of the part.

- For Direction 2, also select the **Up-To-Surface** option, and click the face on the left side.

- This way the width of the fold feature is linked to the width of the part, allowing them to change at the same time.

- Click **OK** ✓.

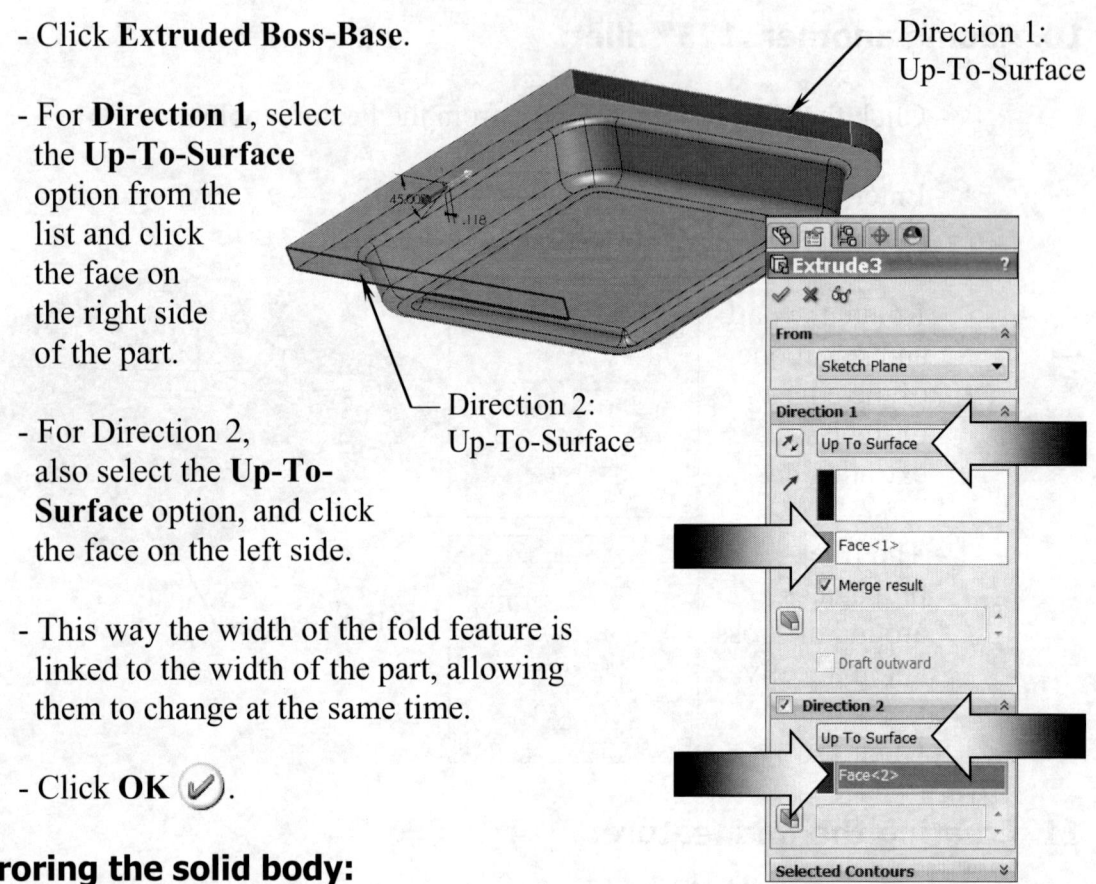

Direction 1: Up-To-Surface

Direction 2: Up-To-Surface

12. Mirroring the solid body:

- Select the <u>Right</u> plane from the Feature tree and click the **Mirror** button.

- Expand the **Bodies to Mirror** section and click the part in the graphics area.

- Enable the **Merge Solid** checkbox

- Click **OK** ✓.

- To mirror one or more features of a part, use the Features-To-Mirror option.

- To mirror the entire part, use the Bodies-to-Mirror option.

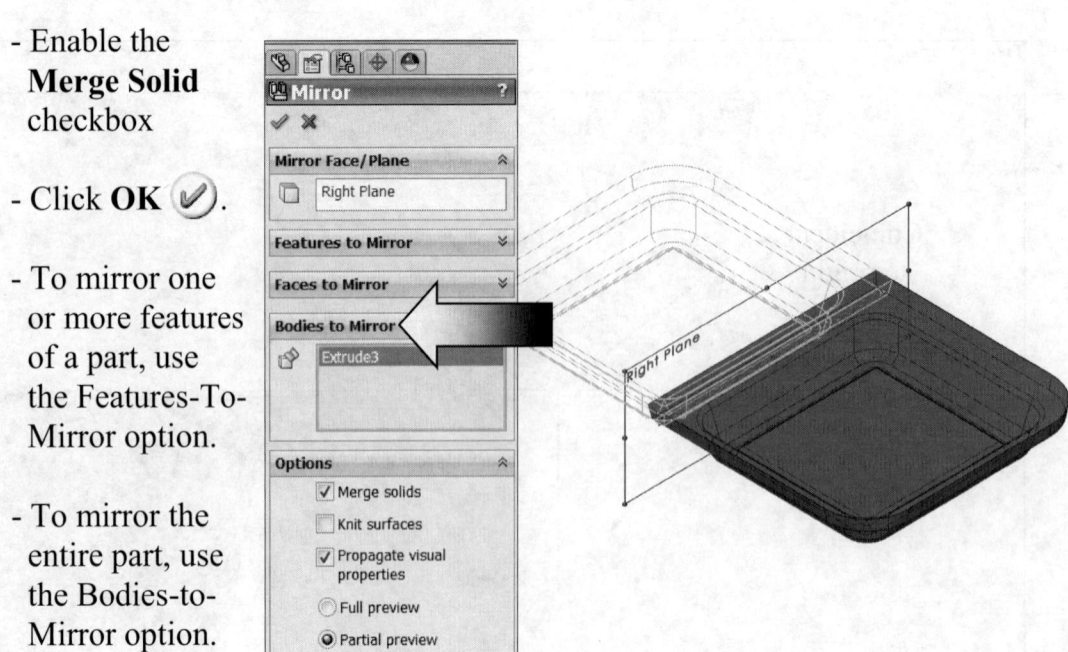

13. Creating the lock feature:

Sketch face

- Rotate the part, select the <u>bottom face</u> of the rim and open a new sketch 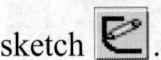.

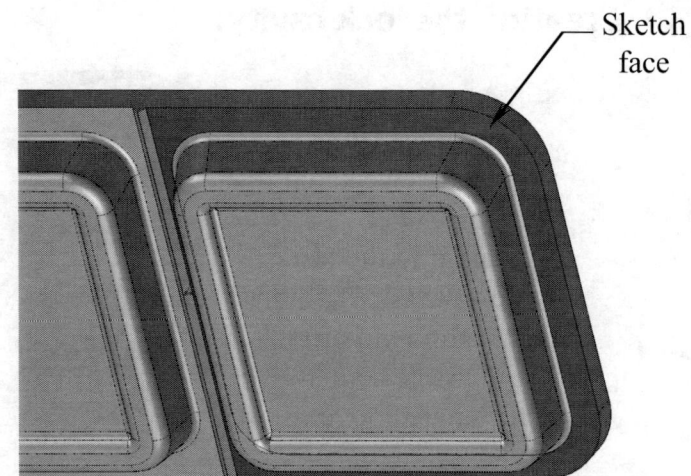

- Sketch a centerline from the origin and use it as the mirror line.

- Sketch a small rectangle above the centerline.

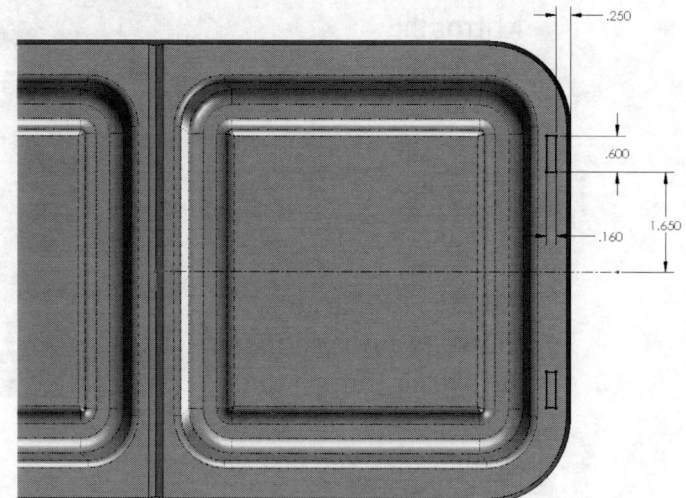

- Use one of the mirror options to mirror the rectangle below the centerline.

- Add the dimensions shown to fully define the sketch.

- Click **Extruded Cut** .

- Use the default **Blind** type.

- Enter **.150in** for depth.

- Enable the Draft checkbox and enter **3deg** for taper angle.

- Click **OK** .

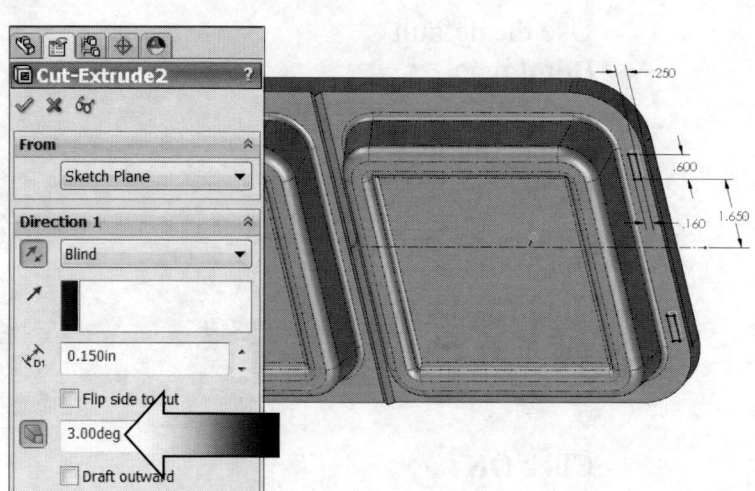

14. Creating the lock cavity:

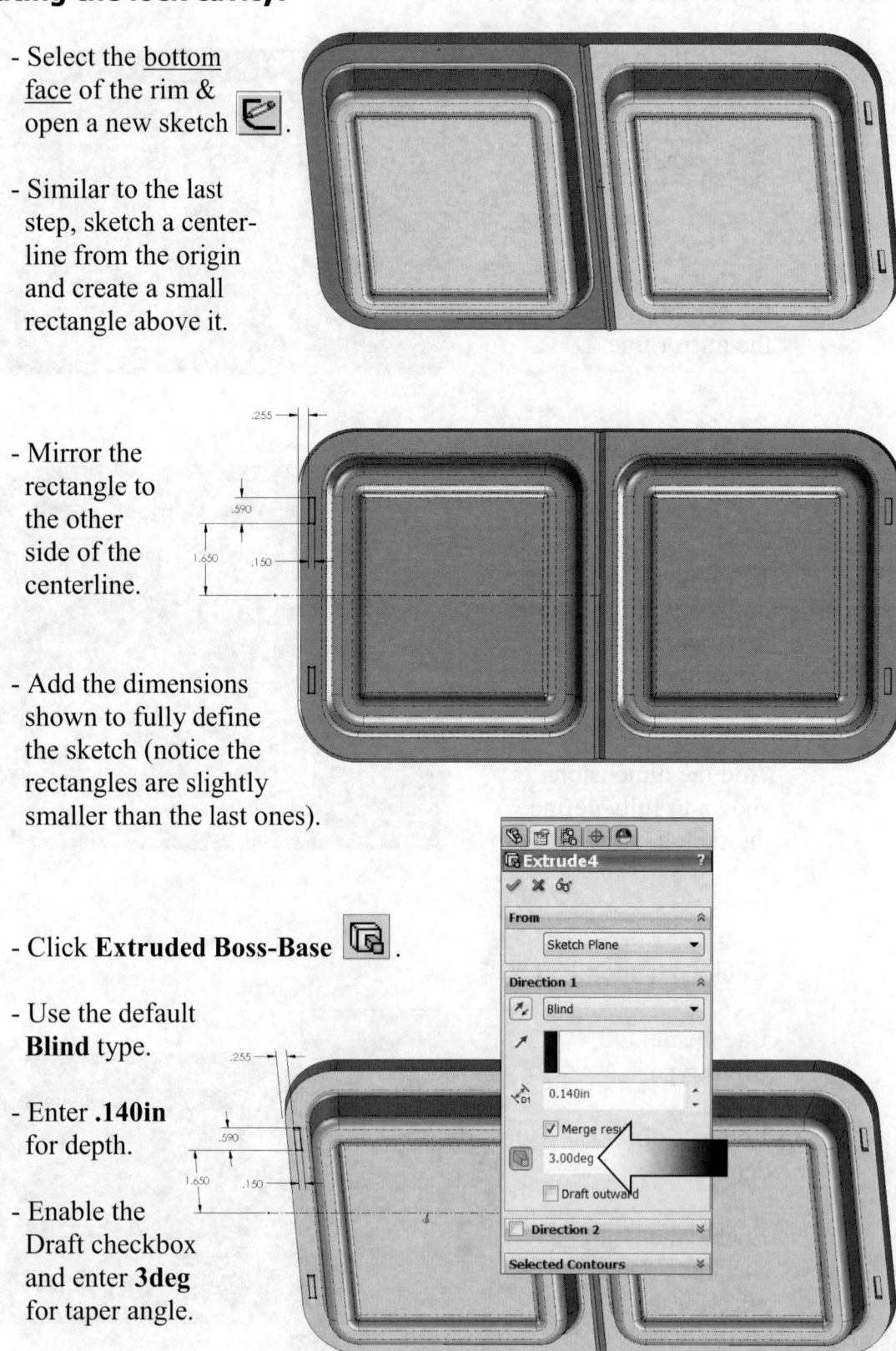

- Select the <u>bottom face</u> of the rim & open a new sketch.

- Similar to the last step, sketch a center-line from the origin and create a small rectangle above it.

- Mirror the rectangle to the other side of the centerline.

- Add the dimensions shown to fully define the sketch (notice the rectangles are slightly smaller than the last ones).

- Click **Extruded Boss-Base**.

- Use the default **Blind** type.

- Enter **.140in** for depth.

- Enable the Draft checkbox and enter **3deg** for taper angle.

- Click **OK**.

15. Adding the .032" fillets:

- Click the **Fillet** command 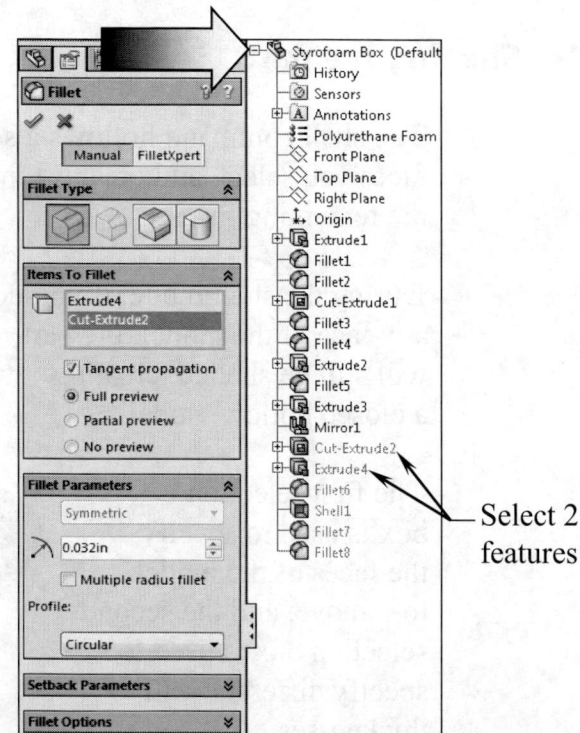 from the Features toolbar.

- Enter **.032in** for radius.

- Expand the FeatureManager tree (push the + symbol) and select the last 2 features, the **Cut-Extrude2** and the **Extrude4**.

- This method is a little bit quicker than selecting the edges individually.

- All edges of the selected features are filleted using the same radius value. Create the fillets separately if you want the features to have different radiuses.

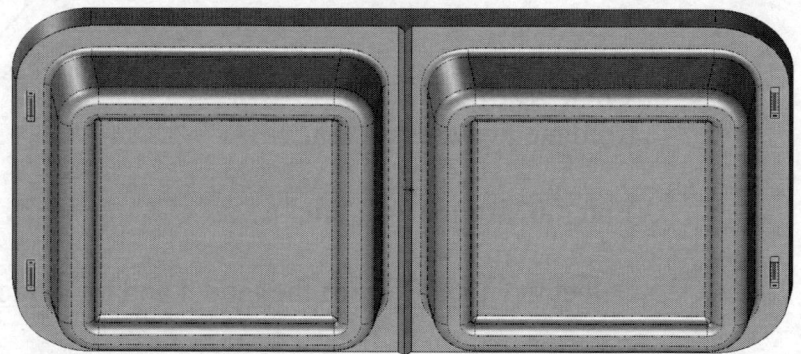

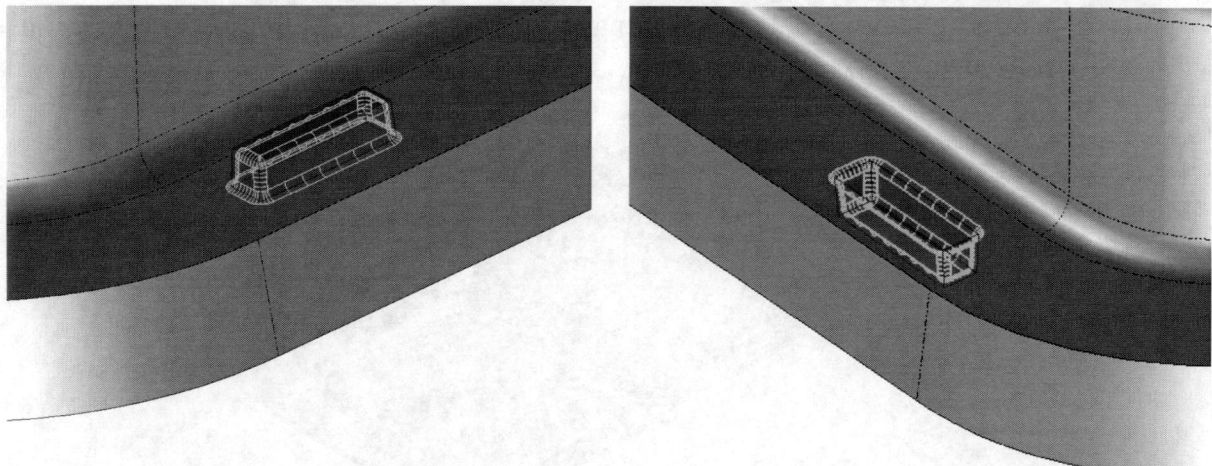

- Rotate and zoom a little closer to verify the fillets on both features.

16. Shelling the part:

- The shell command hollows a solid model, deletes the faces you select, and creates thin walled features on the remaining faces.

- During the shell mode, if you do not select any face of the model, the part will still be shelled, creating a closed hollow model.

- The first selection box is used to specify the faces of the model to remove, and the second selection box is used to specify different wall thicknesses.

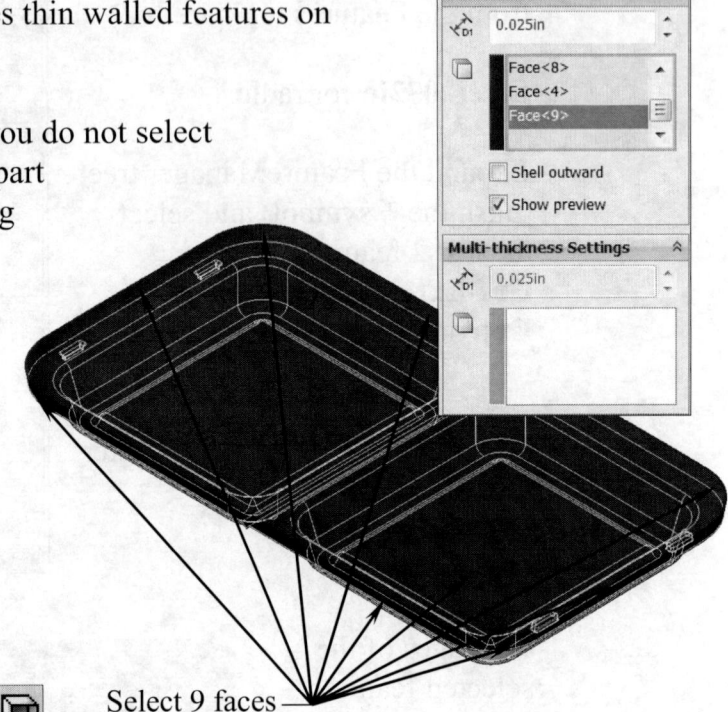

Select 9 faces

- Click the **Shell** command ⬚. from the Features toolbar.

- Enter **.025in** for wall thickness.

- Select the <u>upper face</u> of the model and the <u>8 faces</u> of the rim to remove.

- Click **OK** ✅.

- Compare your model with the image shown below. Edit the shell to correct it if needed.

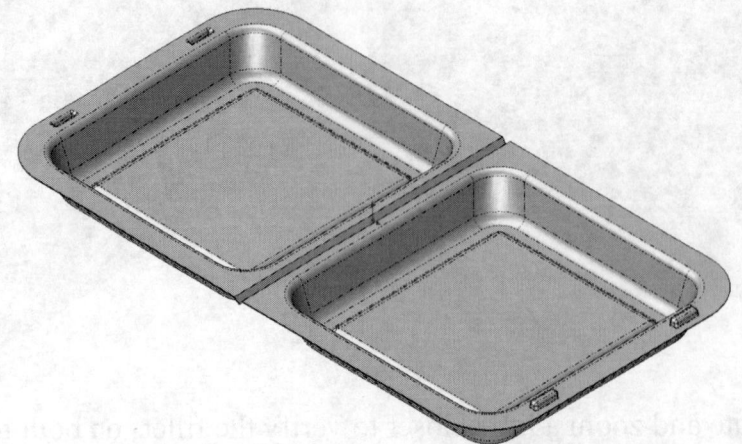

17. Adding the .050" fillets:

- Zoom in on the fold section in the middle of the part.

- Click **Fillet**

- Enter **.050in** for radius.

- Select the <u>3 edges</u> as noted, (2 on the top and 1 on the bottom).

- Click **OK**.

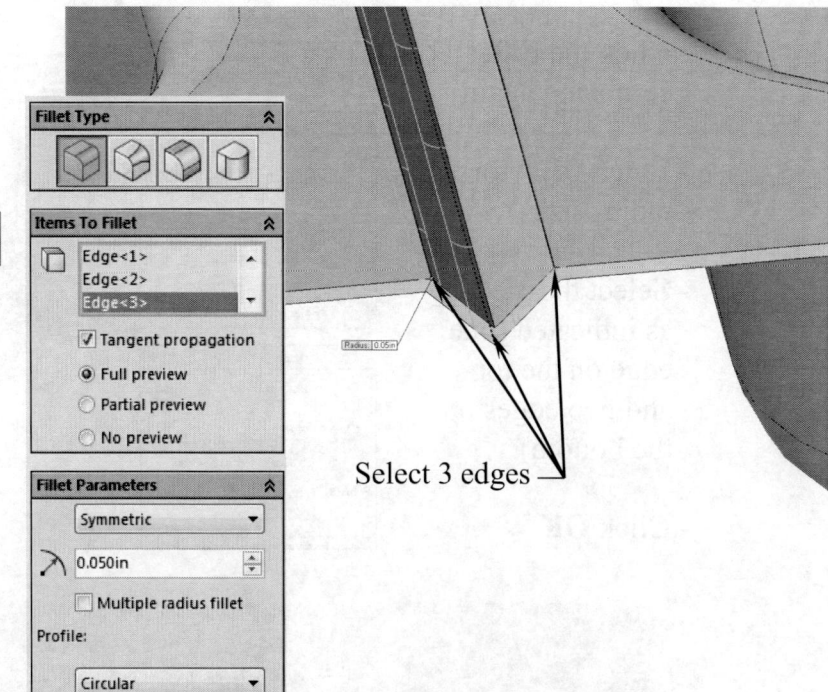

Select 3 edges

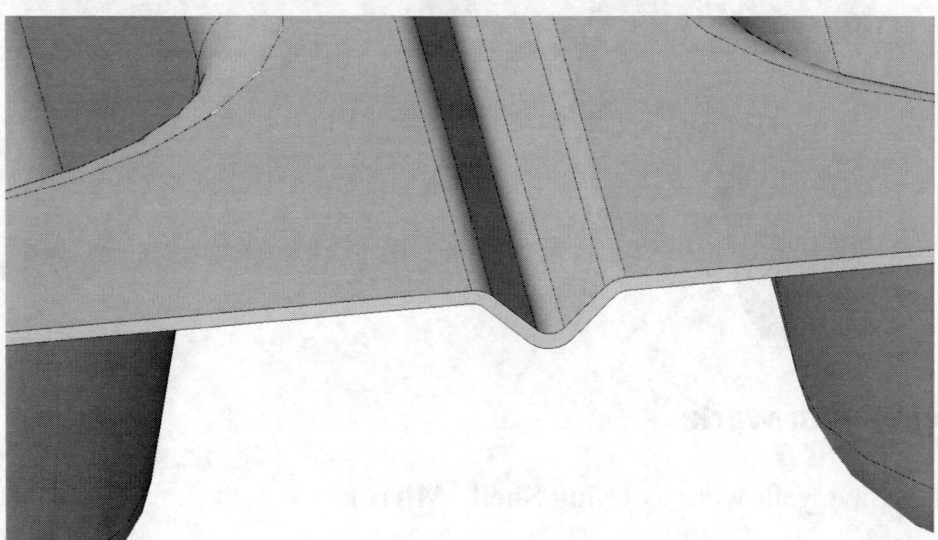

- Verify the resulting fillets.

- We could have used the Multiple Radius option to create both fillets, the .050" and the .032" (in the next step), but the screen will get very busy, hard to see which edge is which to apply the correct fillets.

- Instead, we are going to create the two fillets separately, that will also give you a chance to practice using the fillet command once again.

18. Adding the .032" fillets:

- Click the **Fillet** command again.

- Enter .032" for radius size.

- Select the 3 edges as indicated (one edge on the top and two edges on the bottom).

- Click **OK**.

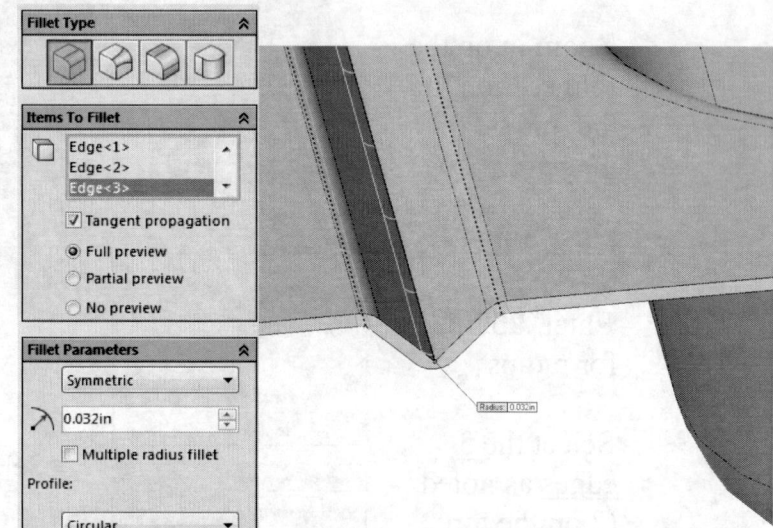

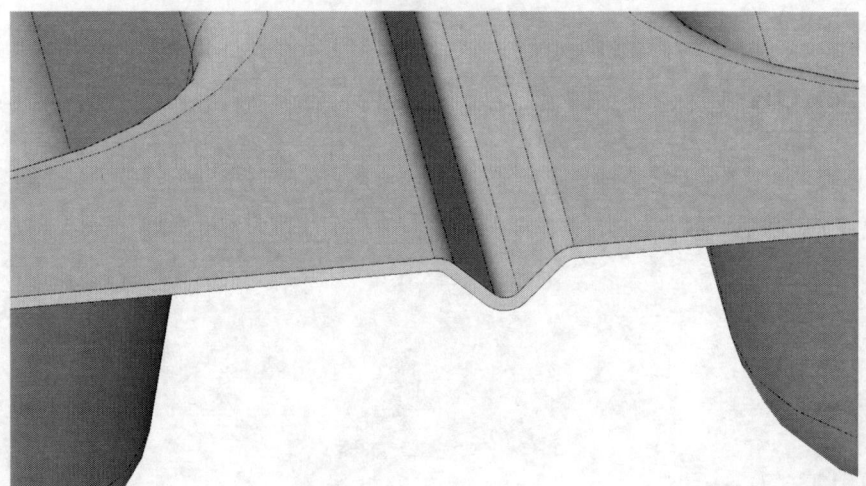

19. Saving your work:

- Save your work as **Using Shell_ Mirror**.

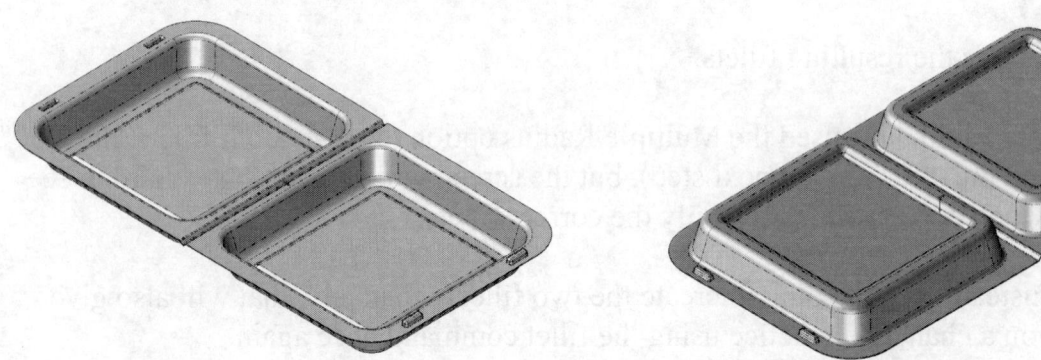

Questions for Review

Using Shell & Mirror

1. It is easier to create a thin walled part by making it out of solid and then shell it out in the end.
    - a. True
    - b. False

2. The shell commands hollows out a solid model and removes the faces that you select.
    - a. True
    - b. False

3. If you do not select any faces of the model the part will still be shelled into a closed volume.
    - a. True
    - b. False

4. Only one wall thickness can be created with the shell command.
    - a. True
    - b. False

5. To mirror a feature, you must use a centerline to mirror about.
    - a. True
    - b. False

6. To mirror one or more features, a planar face or a plane is used as the center of the mirror.
    - a. True
    - b. False

7. To mirror the entire part you must use mirror-features and select all features from the tree.
    - a. True
    - b. False

8. To mirror the entire part you must use mirror-body and select the part from the graphics area.
    - a. True
    - b. False

7. FALSE   8. TRUE
5. FALSE   6. TRUE
3. TRUE   4. FALSE
1. TRUE   2. TRUE

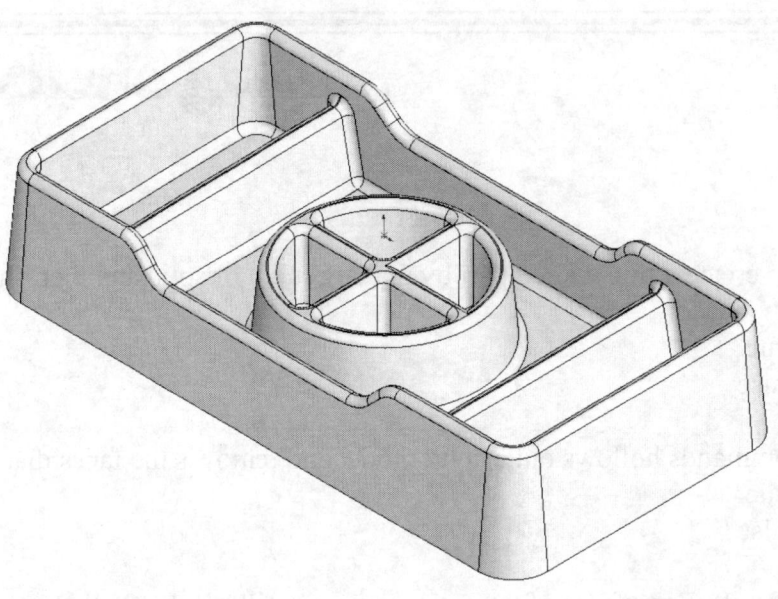

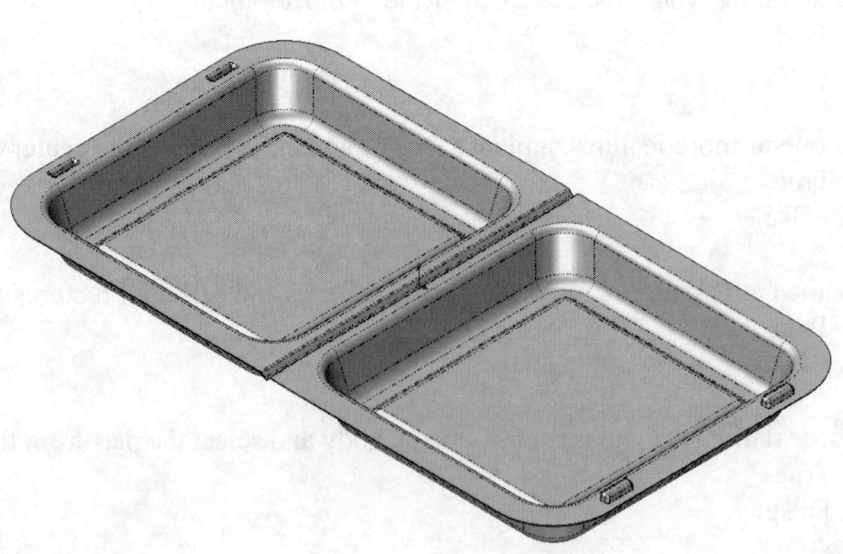

CHAPTER 7

Linear Patterns

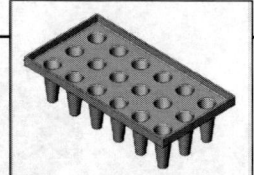

Linear Patterns
Test Tray

- The Linear Pattern is used to arrange multiple instances of selected features along one or two linear paths.

- The following 4 elements are needed to create a linear pattern:

    * Direction of the pattern (linear edge of the model or an axis) .

    * Distance between the pattern instances .

    * Number of pattern instances in each direction .

    * Feature(s) to the pattern .

- If the features used to create the pattern are changed, all instances within the pattern will be updated automatically.

- The options available in Linear Patterns:

    * Pattern instances to skip. This option is used to hide / skip some of the instances in a pattern.

    * Pattern seed only. This option is used when only the original feature gets repeated, not its instances.

- This chapter will guide you through the use of the pattern commands such as: Linear, Circular, and Curve Driven Patterns.

Test Tray
Linear Patterns

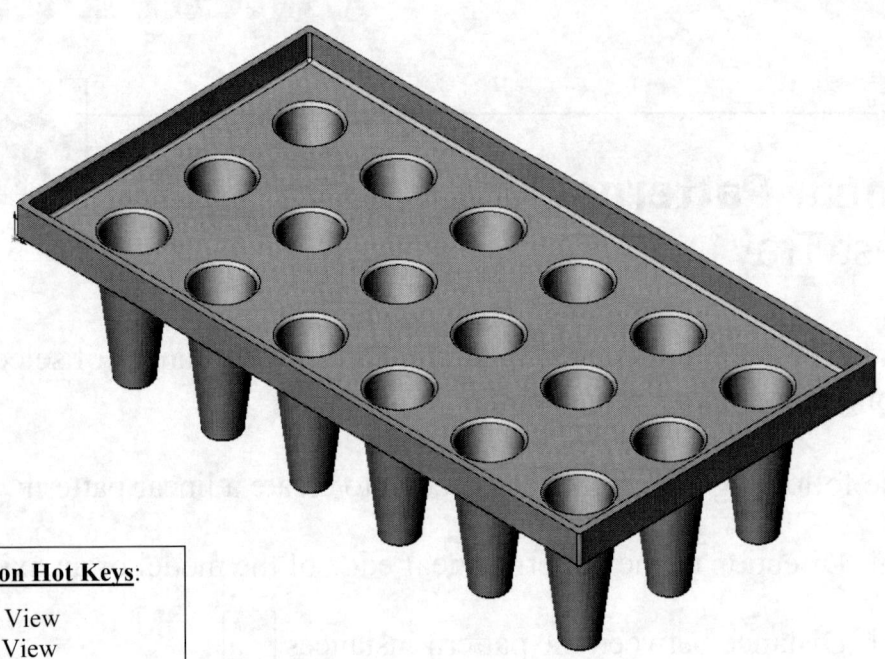

View Orientation Hot Keys:

Ctrl + 1 = Front View
Ctrl + 2 = Back View
Ctrl + 3 = Left View
Ctrl + 4 = Right View
Ctrl + 5 = Top View
Ctrl + 6 = Bottom View
Ctrl + 7 = Isometric View
Ctrl + 8 = Normal To
        Selection

Dimensioning Standards: **ANSI**

Units: **INCHES** – 3 Decimals

Tools Needed:

Insert Sketch	Rectangle	Circle
Dimension	Add Geometric Relations	Base/Boss Extrude
Shell	Linear Pattern	Fillet/Round

1. Sketching the Base Profile:

- Select the <u>Top</u> plane from the FeatureManager tree.

- Click 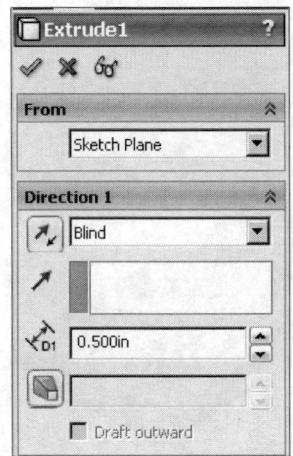 or select **Insert /Sketch**.

- Sketch a **Corner Rectangle** ▢ starting at the Origin.

- Add the dimensions ◇ shown.

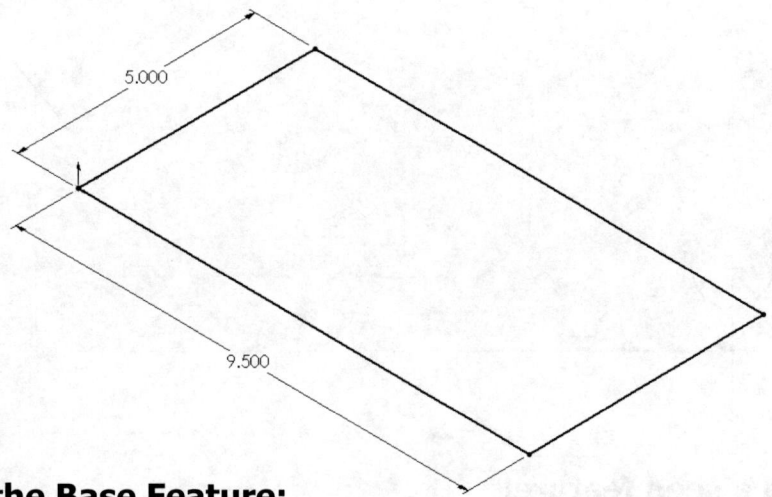

2. Extruding the Base Feature:

- Click 🗔 or select **Insert / Boss-Base / Extrude**.

- End Condition: **Blind.**

- Extrude Depth: **.500 in**.

- Click **OK** ✓.

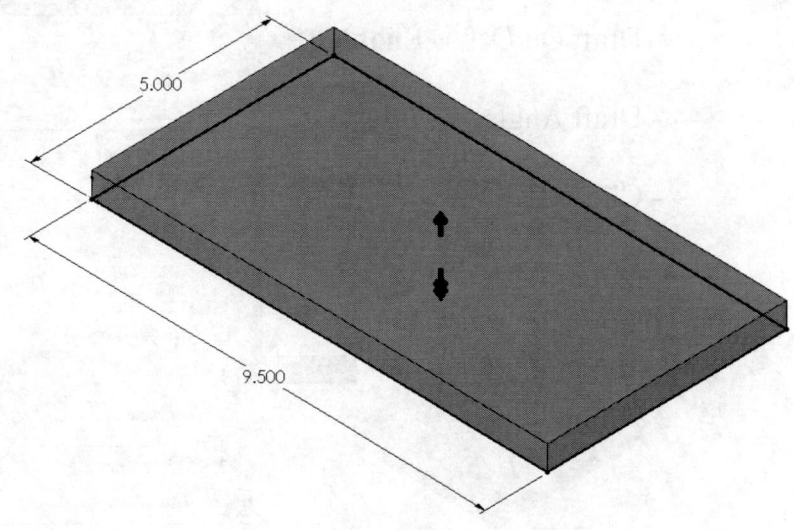

3. Sketching the seed feature:

- Select the <u>face</u> indicated as the sketch plane.

- Click 🗒 or select **Insert / Sketch**.

- Sketch a **circle** ⊕ and add dimensions ◇ as shown.

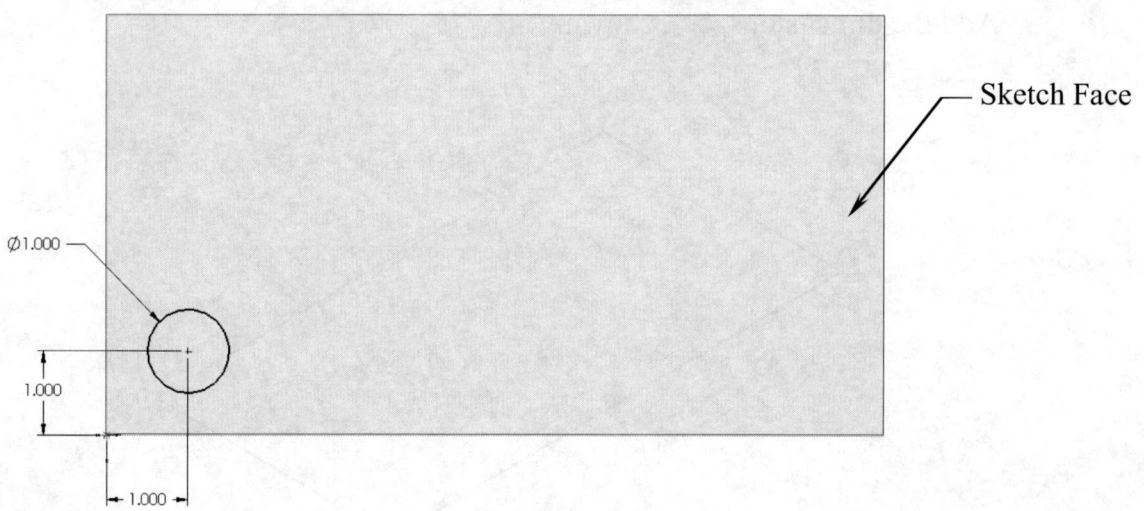

Sketch Face

Ø1.000

1.000

1.000

4. Extruding a seed feature:

- Click 🗔 or select **Insert / Boss-Base / Extrude**.

- End Condition: **Blind.**

- Extrude Depth: **2.00 in**.

- Draft On/Off: **Enabled.**

- Draft Angle: **7 deg**.

- Click **OK** ✓.

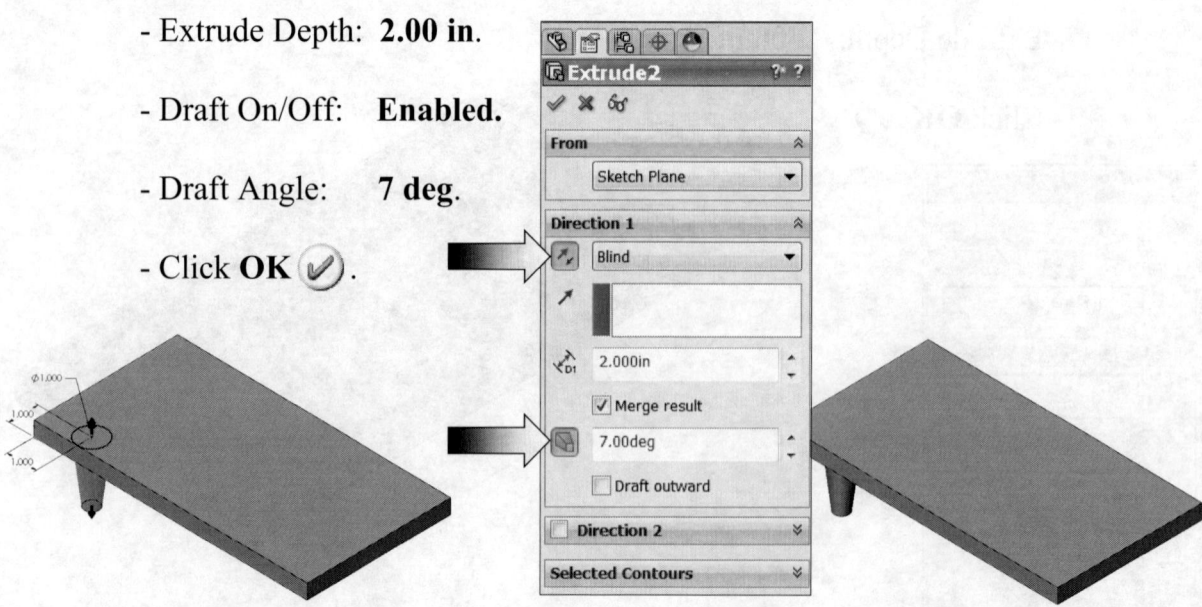

5. Creating a Linear Pattern:

- Click 🔢 or select **Insert / Pattern Mirror / Linear Pattern**.

For <u>Direction 1</u>:

- Select the bottom **horizontal edge** as Pattern Direction1 ↗.

- Enter **1.500** in. as the Spacing.

- Enter **6** as the Number Of Instances.

For <u>Direction 2</u>:

- Select the **vertical edge** as Pattern Direction2 ↗.

- Enter **1.500** in. as the Spacing.

- Enter **3** as the Number of Instances.

- Click Extrude2 as the Features to Pattern.

- Click **OK** ✓.

> 💡 **Linear Patterns**
>
> The Linear Pattern option creates multiple instances of one or more features uniformly along one or two directions.

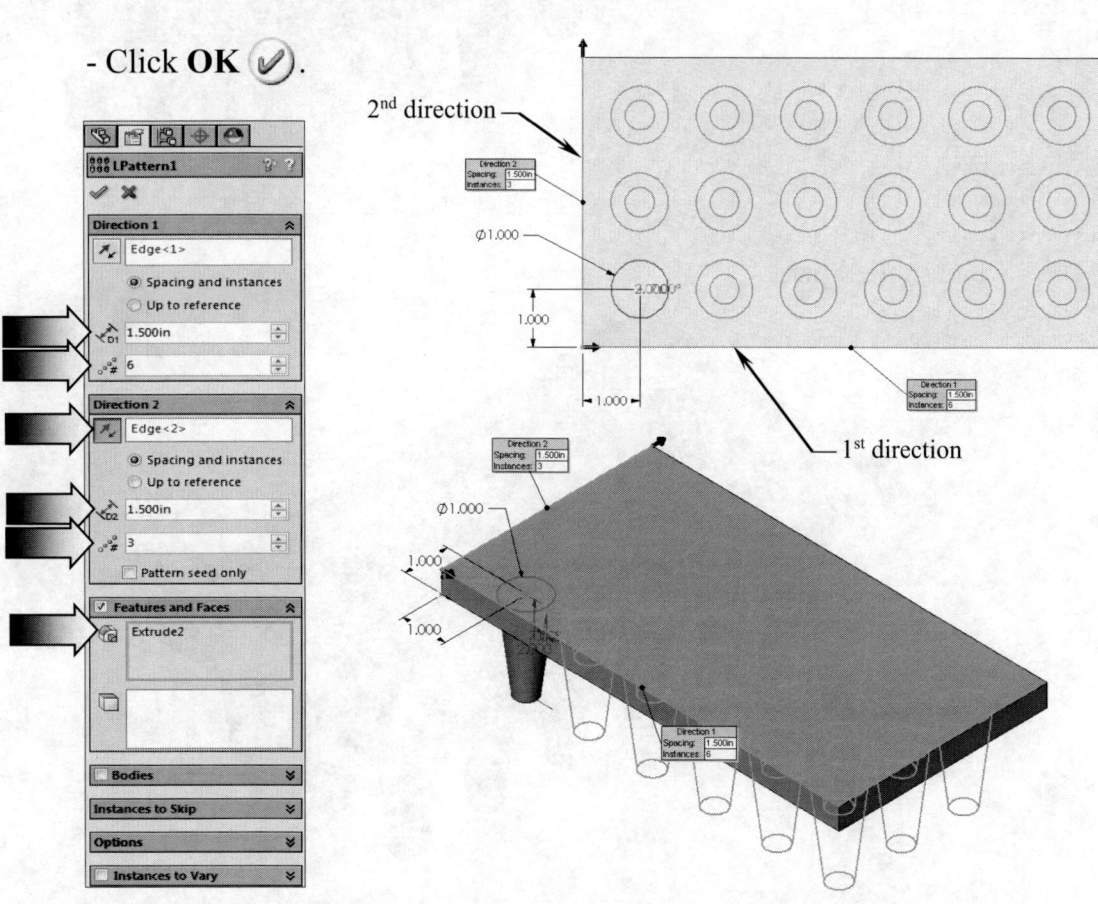

6. Shelling the Base feature:

- Select the <u>upper face</u> as shown.

- Click 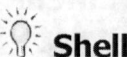 or select **Insert / Features / Shell**.

- Type **.100** in. for the Thickness.

- Click **OK** ✓ .

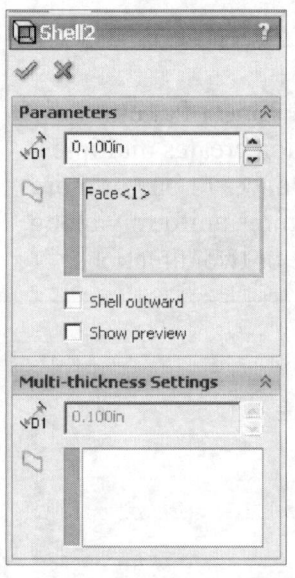

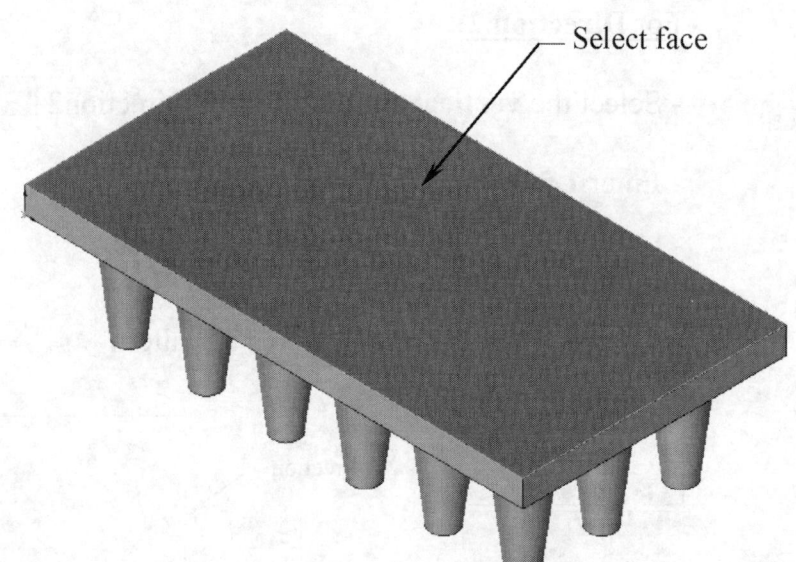

Select face

> ### 💡 Shell
>
> The Shell command
> hollows out the part,
> starting with the selected
> face.
> Constant or multi-wall
> thickness can be done in
> the same operation.

- The shelled part.

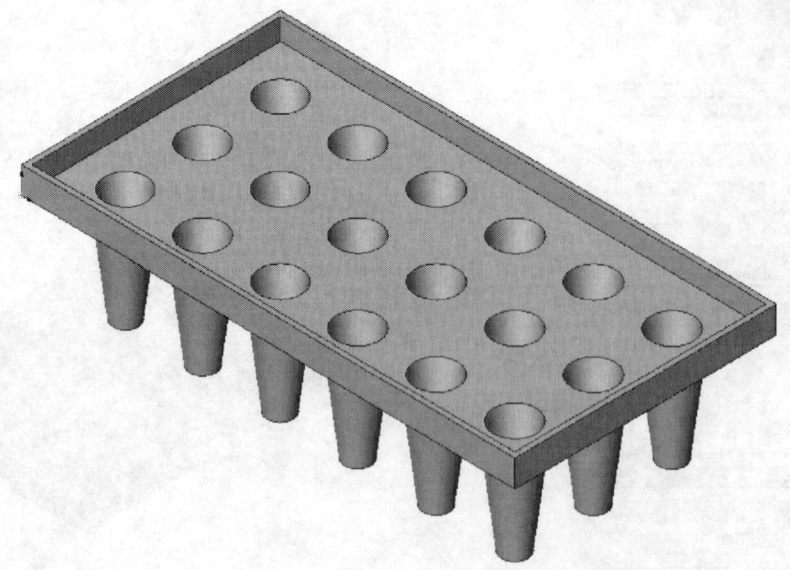

7. Adding Fillets:

- Click **Fillet** 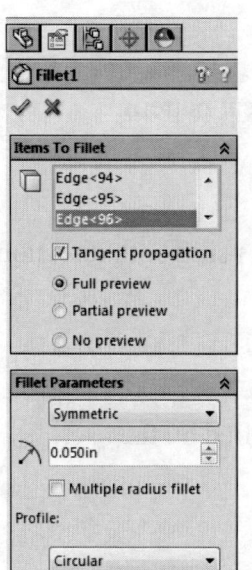 or select **Insert / Features / Fillet / Round.**

- Enter **.050** in. for Radius size ⟋ .

- Select the <u>all edges</u> ⬚ .
  (To use Box-Select method right click in the
  graphics area and select: Box-Selection).

- Click **OK** ✓ .

> 💡 **Fillets**
>
> A combination of faces
> and edges can be selected
> within the same fillet
> operation.
> (Box-select the entire part
> to select all edges).

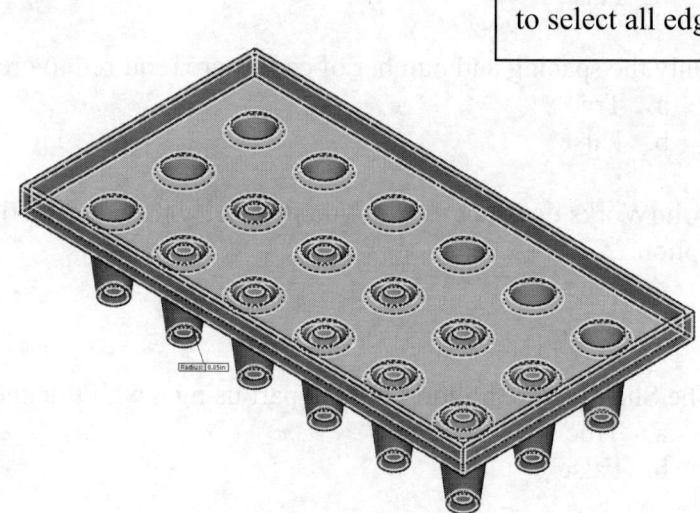

8. Saving your work:

- Select **File / Save As / Test Tray / Save.**

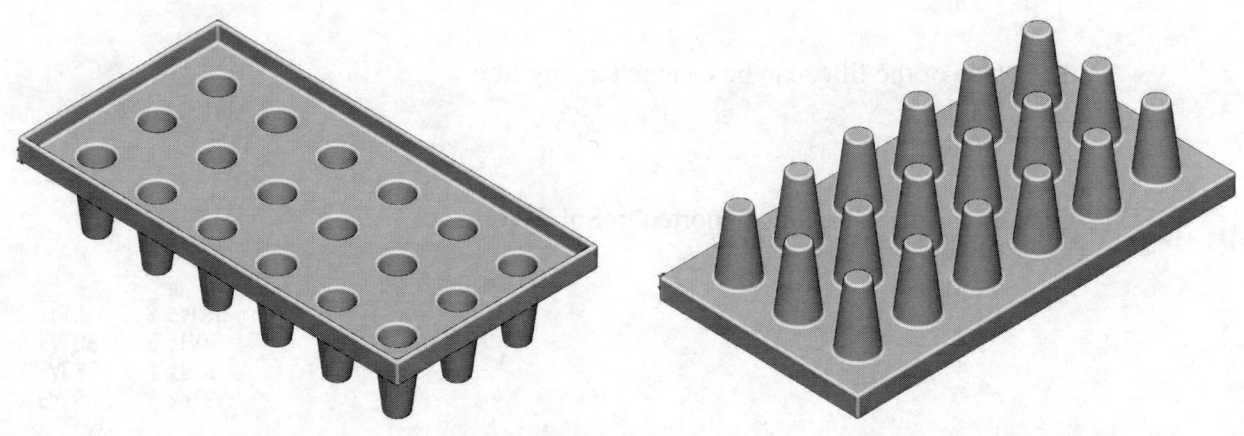

Questions for Review

Linear Patterns

1. SolidWorks only allows you to pattern one feature at a time. Patterning multiple features is not supported.
   a. True
   b. False

2. Only the spacing and number of copies are required to create a linear pattern.
   a. True
   b. False

3. SolidWorks does not require you to specify the 2nd direction when using both directions option.
   a. True
   b. False

4. The Shell feature hollows out the part using a wall thickness specified by the user.
   a. True
   b. False

5. After the Shell feature is created, its wall thickness cannot be changed.
   a. True
   b. False

6. A combination of faces and edges of a model can be selected in the same fillet operation.
   a. True
   b. False

7. The value of the fillet can be changed at anytime.
   a. True
   b. False

8. "Pattern a pattern" is not supported in SolidWorks.
   a. True
   b. False

7. TRUE	8. FALSE
5. FALSE	6. TRUE
3. FALSE	4. TRUE
1. FALSE	2. FALSE

CHAPTER 7 (cont.)

Circular Patterns

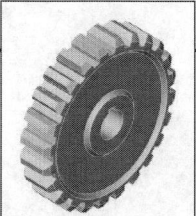

Circular Patterns
Spur Gear

- One or more instances can be copied in a circular fashion or around an Axis.

- The center of the pattern can be defined by a circular edge, an axis, a temporary axis, or an angular dimension.

- In the newer releases of SolidWorks, a circular edge can be used as the center of the pattern, instead of an axis.

- The information required to create a circular pattern is:

    * Center of rotation.

    * Spacing between the instances.

    * Number of copies.

    * Feature(s) to copy.

- Only the original feature can be edited; changes made to the original are automatically updated within the pattern.

- The features to the pattern can be selected directly from the graphics area or from the Feature Manager tree.

- The instances in a pattern can be skipped. The skipped instances can be edited during or after the pattern is made.

Spur-Gear
Circular Patterns

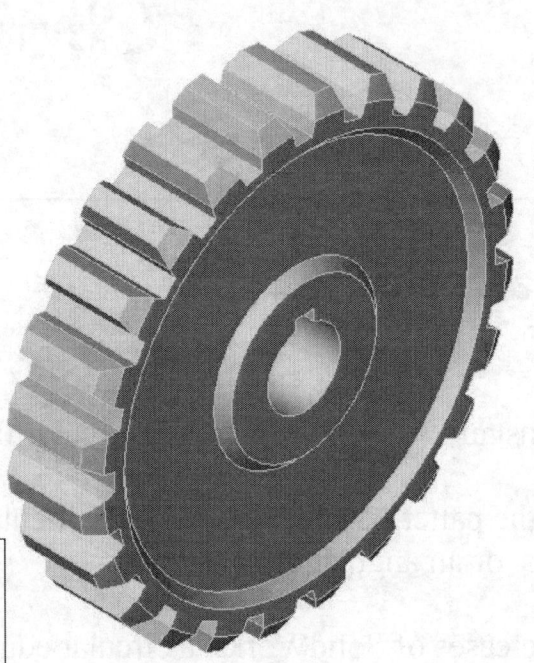

View Orientation Hot Keys:

Ctrl + 1 = Front View
Ctrl + 2 = Back View
Ctrl + 3 = Left View
Ctrl + 4 = Right View
Ctrl + 5 = Top View
Ctrl + 6 = Bottom View
Ctrl + 7 = Isometric View
Ctrl + 8 = Normal To
      Selection

Dimensioning Standards: **ANSI**

Units: **INCHES** – 3 Decimals

Tools Needed:

 Insert Sketch   Line    Center Line

 Dynamic Mirror   Add Geometric Relations   Dimension

 Convert Entities   Trim Entities   Base/Boss Revolve

 Circular Pattern   Base/Boss Extrude   Extruded Cut

1. Sketching the Body profile:

- Select the <u>Front</u> plane from the FeatureManager Tree.

- Click or select **Insert / Sketch**.

- Sketch a **Centerline** starting at the Origin.

- Select the **Mirror** tool and click the centerline to active the Dynamic-Mirror mode (or select: **Tools / Sketch Tools / Dynamic Mirror**).

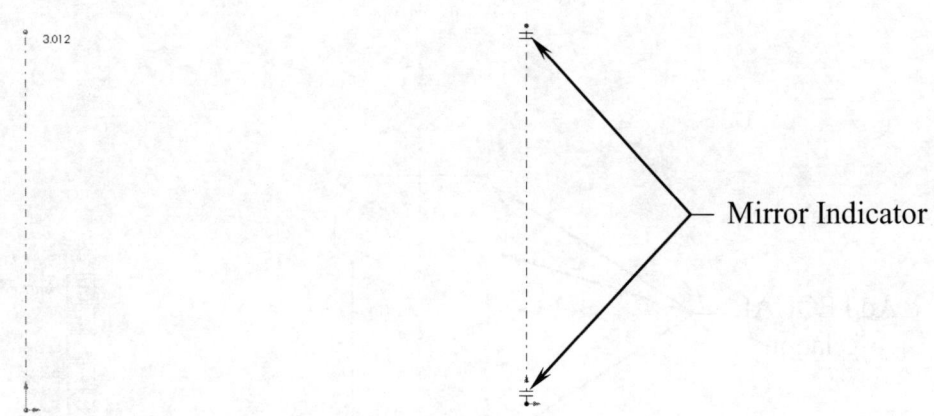

Mirror Indicator

- Sketch the profile below using the Line tool .

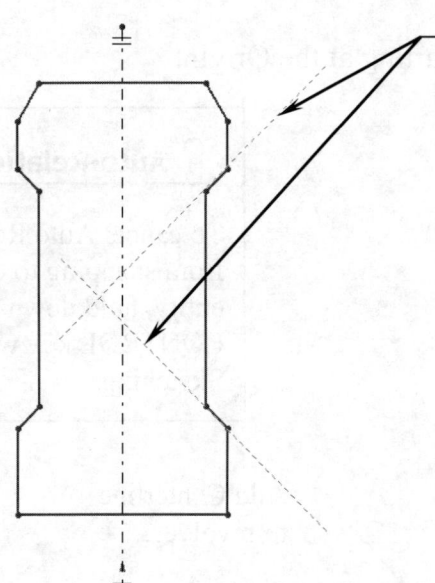

To cancel Auto-Relations (dotted inference lines), either hold down the Control key while sketching the lines – OR – just simply avoid sketching over the dotted lines.

Using the Dynamic Mirror:

- Sketch on one side of the centerline only.

- The sketch should not cross the centerline.

- The system creates **Symmetric** relations between all mirrored sketch entities.

- Add the following Geometric Relations 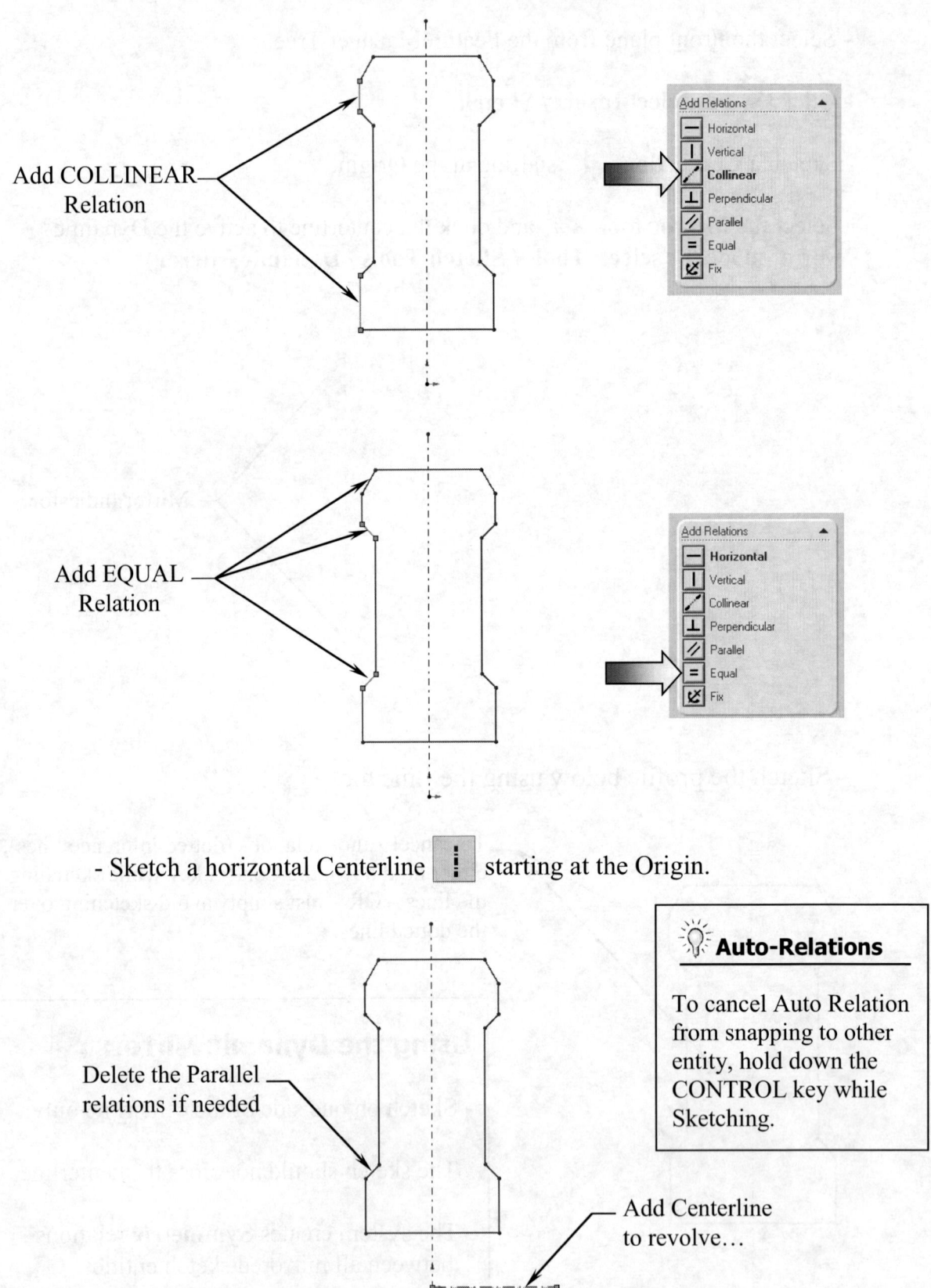 to the entities indicated below:

Add COLLINEAR Relation

Add EQUAL Relation

- Sketch a horizontal Centerline ⋮ starting at the Origin.

Delete the Parallel relations if needed

💡 **Auto-Relations**

To cancel Auto Relation from snapping to other entity, hold down the CONTROL key while Sketching.

Add Centerline to revolve…

- Add the **dimensions** 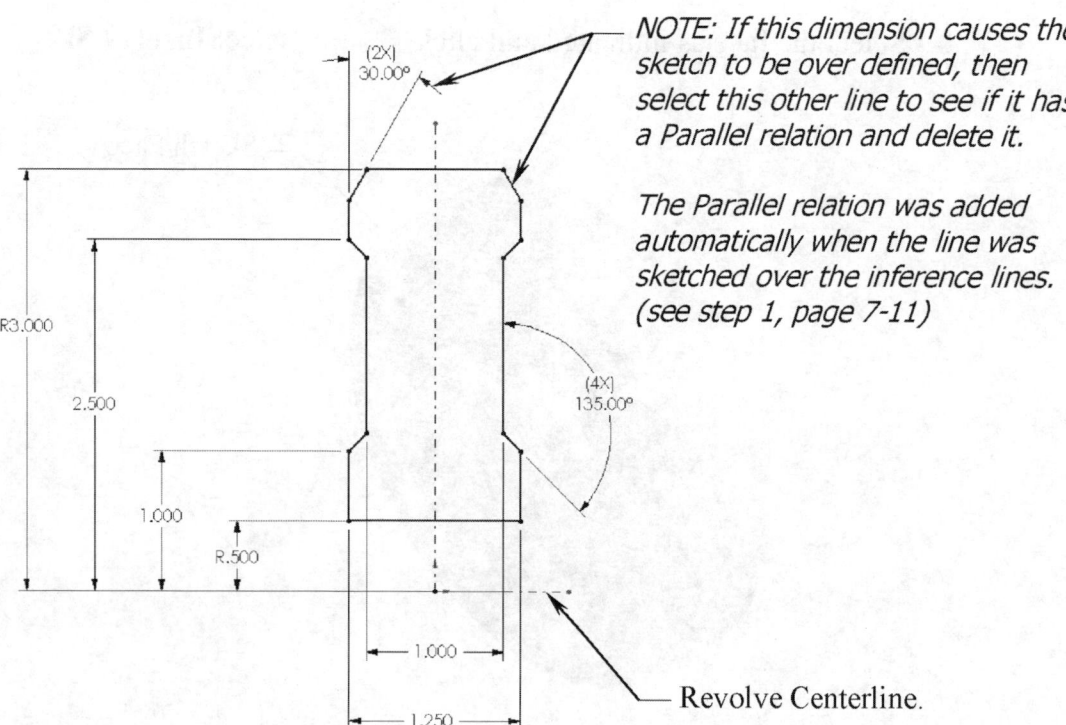 as shown below:

NOTE: If this dimension causes the sketch to be over defined, then select this other line to see if it has a Parallel relation and delete it.

The Parallel relation was added automatically when the line was sketched over the inference lines. (see step 1, page 7-11)

Revolve Centerline.

2. Revolving the Base Body:

- Select the horizontal centerline as indicated above.

- Click 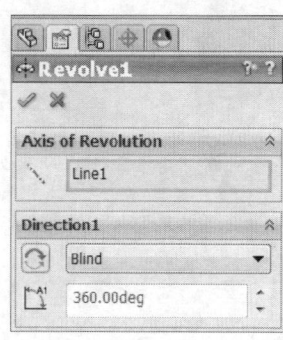 or select **Insert / Boss-Base / Revolve**.

- Revolve direction: **One Direction**

- Revolve Angle: **360°**

- Click **OK** ✓.

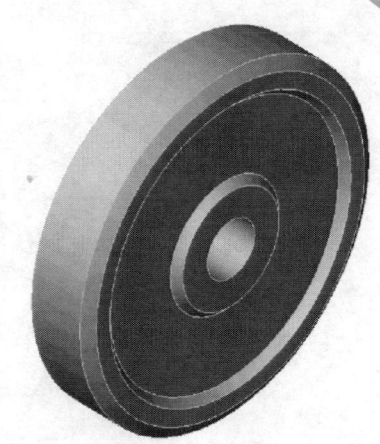

3. Sketching the Thread Profile:

- Select the <u>face</u> as indicated and click 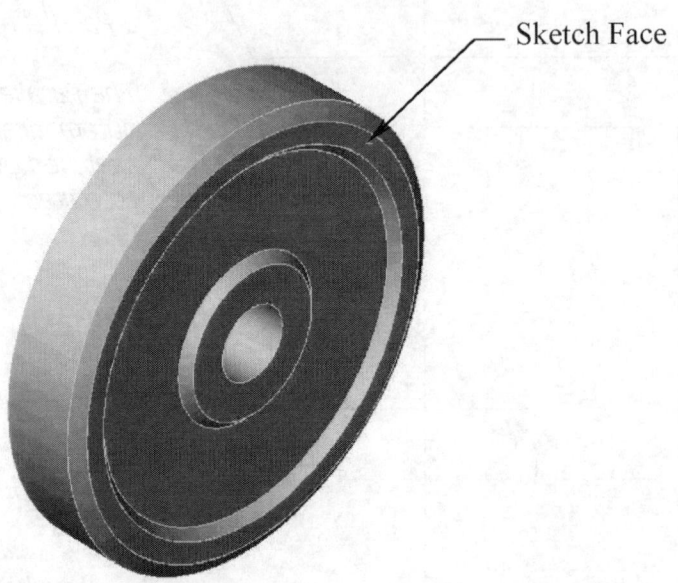 or select **Insert / Sketch**.

— Sketch Face

- Click **Normal To** from the Standard View Toolbar.

- Sketch a vertical **Centerline** starting at the origin.

- Select the **Mirror** tool and click the centerline to active the Dynamic-Mirror mode.

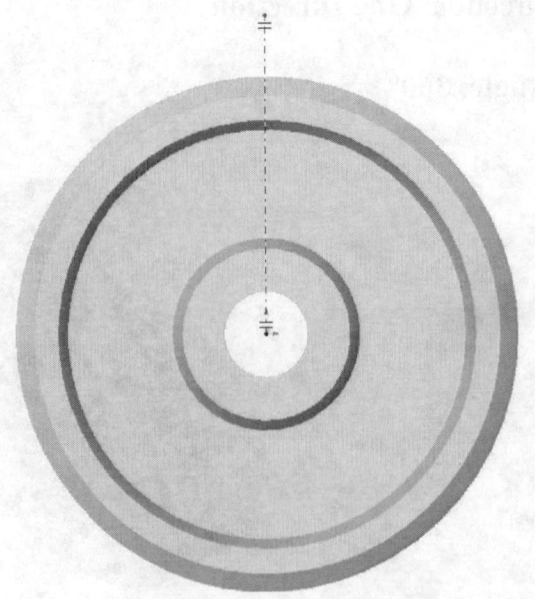

- Sketch the profile using the Line 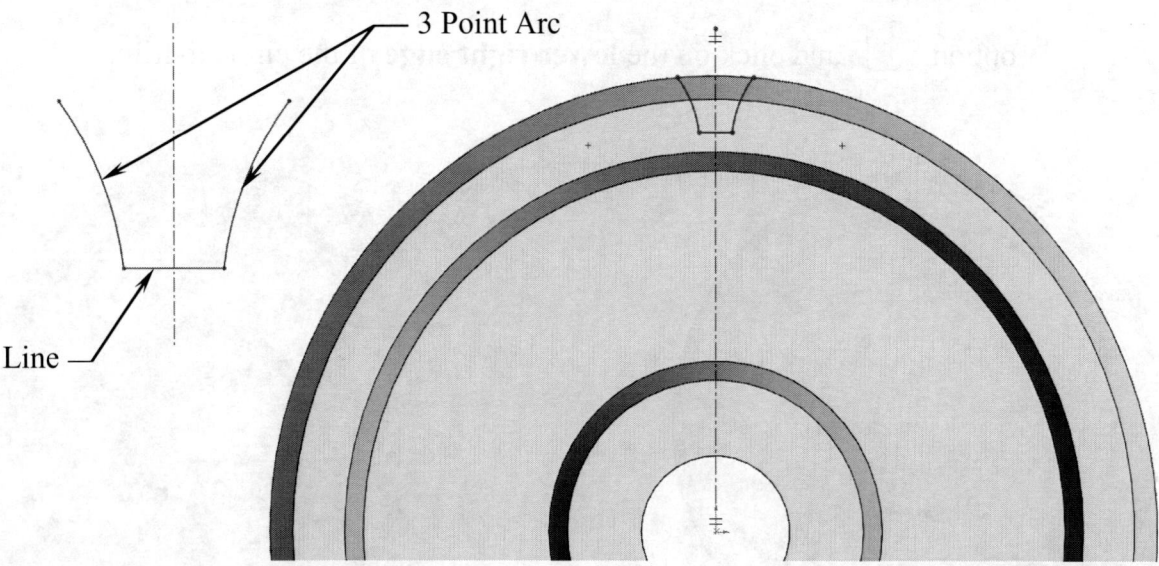 and the 3-Point-Arc tools.

3 Point Arc

Line

4. Converting the entities:

- Select the **outer edge** of the part and click **Convert Entities** from the Sketch toolbar.

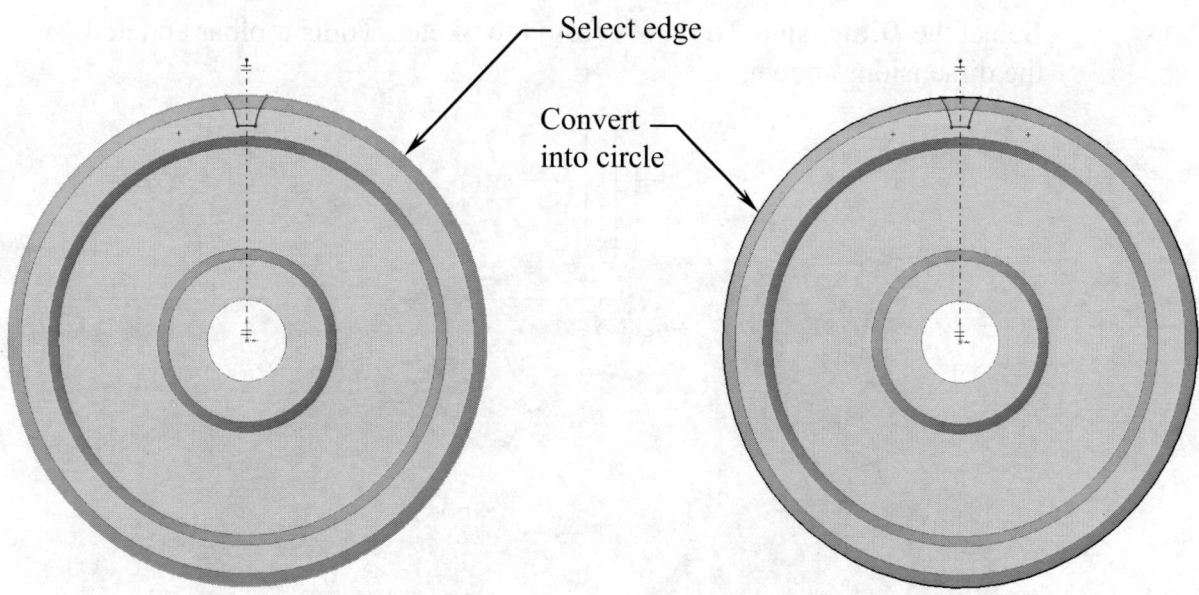

Select edge

Convert into circle

- The selected edge is converted into a circle.

5. Trimming the Sketch Entities:

- Select the **Trim** tool ![icon] from the Sketch toolbar; select the **Trim-to-Closest** option ![icon] , and click on the **lower right edge** of the circle to trim.

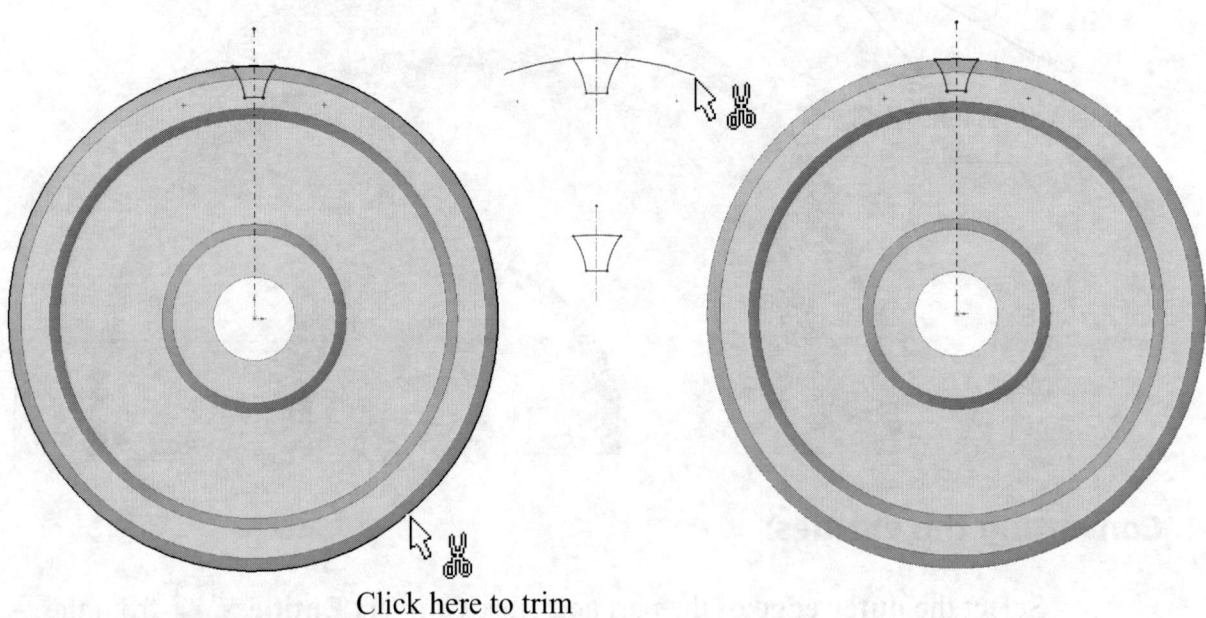

Click here to trim

6. Adding Dimensions:

- Select the **Dimension** Tool ![icon] from the Sketch-Tools toolbar and add the dimensions shown.

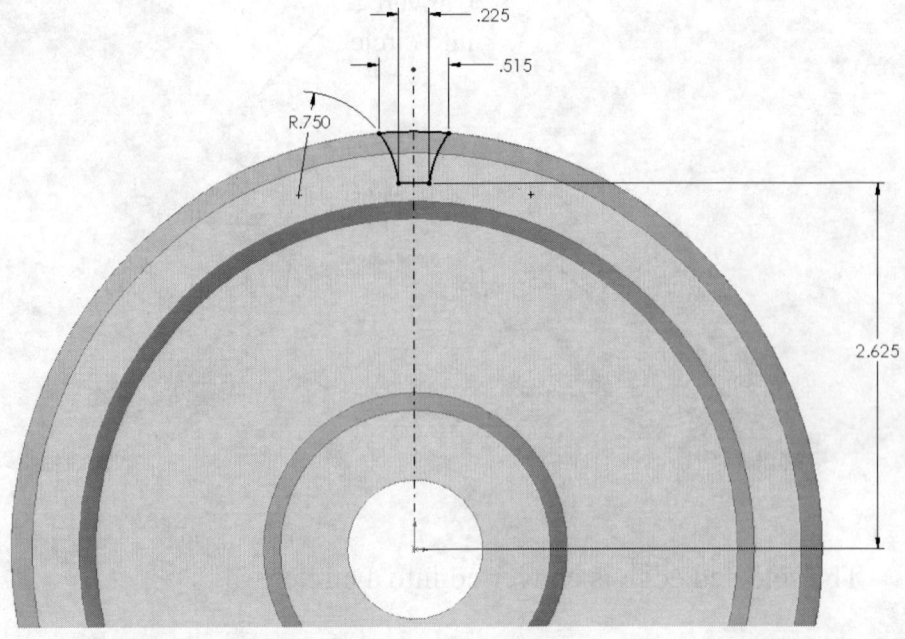

- Switch to the Isometric View 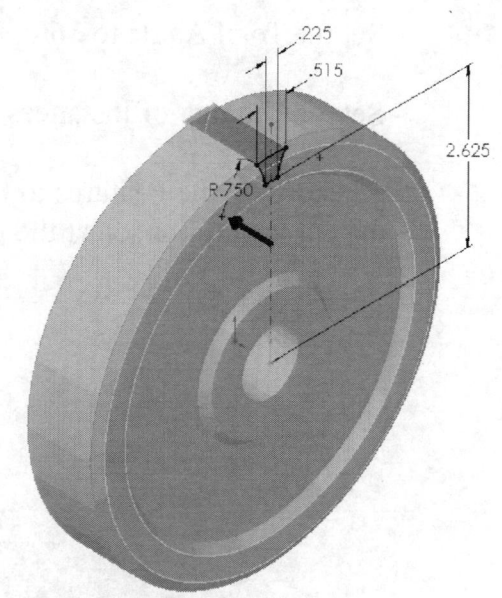 or press **Ctrl + 7**.

7. Cutting the First Tooth:

- Click **Extruded Cut** ⬚ from the Features toolbar.

- End Condition: **Through All**.

- Click **OK** ✓.

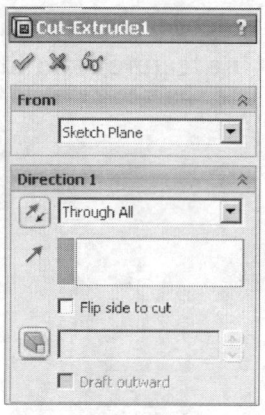

8. Circular Patterning the Tooth:

- Select **Temporary Axis** from the **View** pull-down menu. An axis in the center of the hole is created automatically; this axis will be used as the center of the pattern.

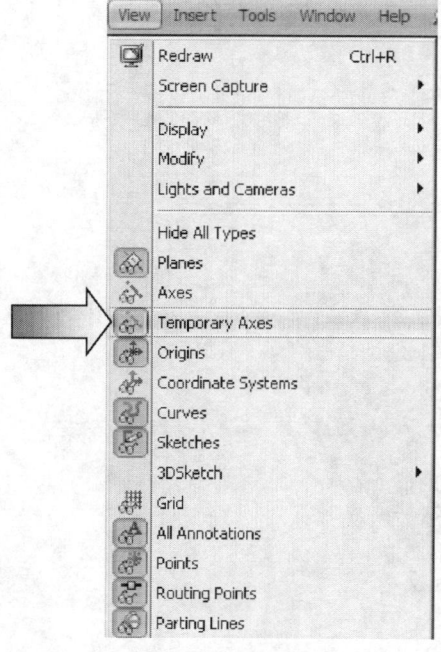

For pattern direction
select the Axis
– or –
the Circular Edge

- Click **Circular Pattern** from the Features toolbar.

- Click on the center **axis** as Direction 1 .

- Click the **Equal Spacing** check box.

- Set the Total Angle to **360°** .

- Set the Number of Instances to **24** .

- Click inside the Features to Pattern box and select one of the faces of the cut feature (or select the previous **Extruded-Cut** feature from the tree).

- Click **OK** .

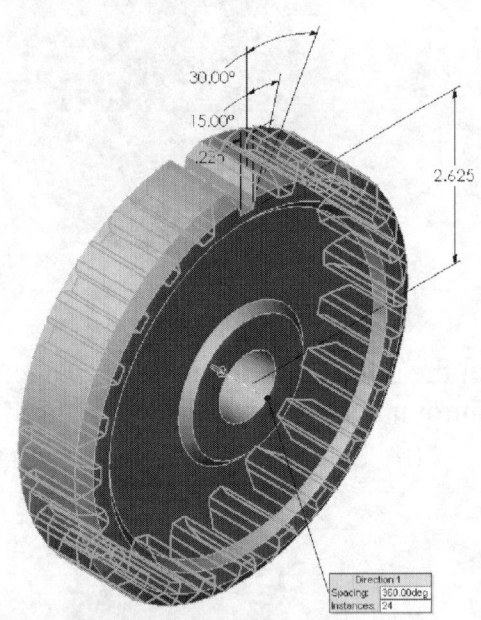

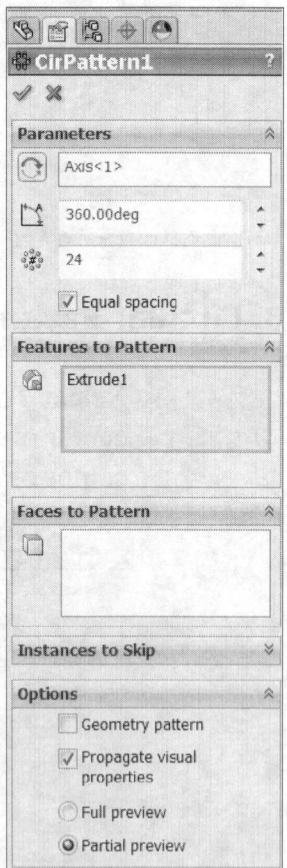

- The resulting circular Pattern.

9. Adding the Keyway:

- Select the <u>face</u> as indicated and click 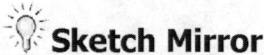 or select **Insert / Sketch**.

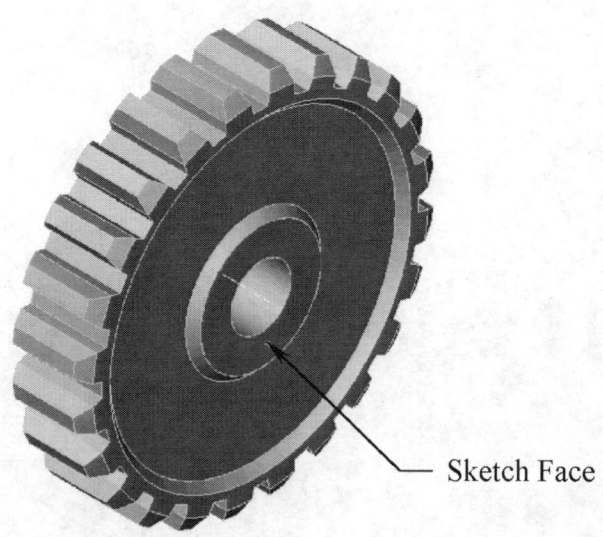

Sketch Face

- Click **Normal To** from the Standard Views toolbar (Ctrl + 8).

- Sketch a vertical **Centerline** starting at the Origin.

- Select the **Mirror** tool and click the centerline to activate the Dynamic-Mirror mode.

> ### ᯼ Sketch Mirror
>
> Use the Mirror option in a sketch to make a symmetrical profile.
>
> When a sketch entity is changed, the mirrored image will also change.

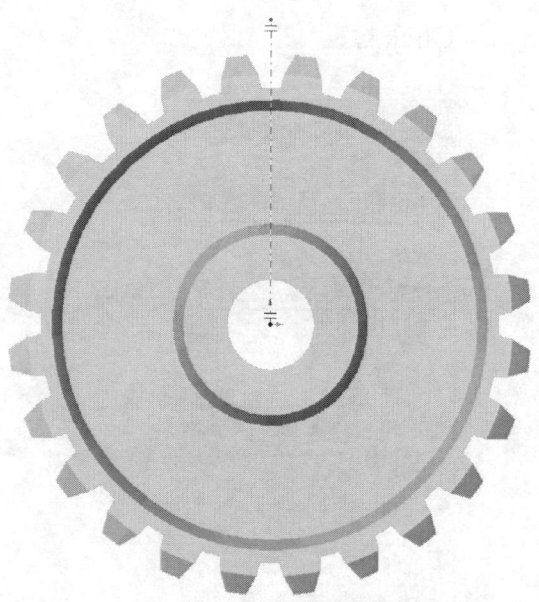

- Sketch the profile of the keyway and add dimension 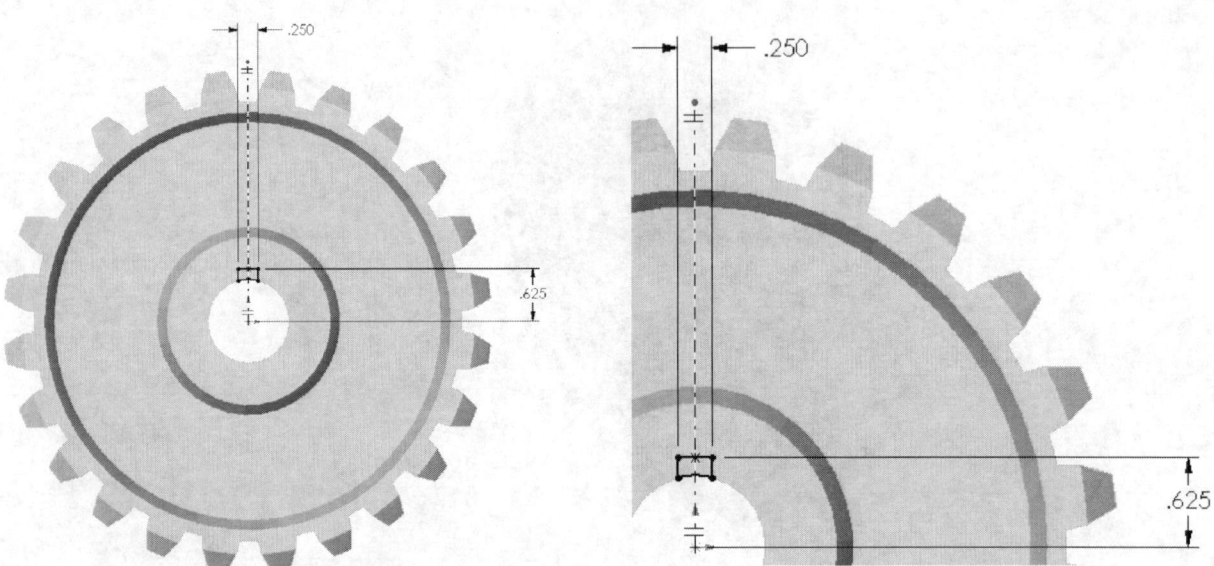 as shown:

10. Extruding a Cut:

- Click on **Extruded Cut** 🔲 from the Features toolbar.

- End Condition: **Through All**

- Click **OK** ✓.

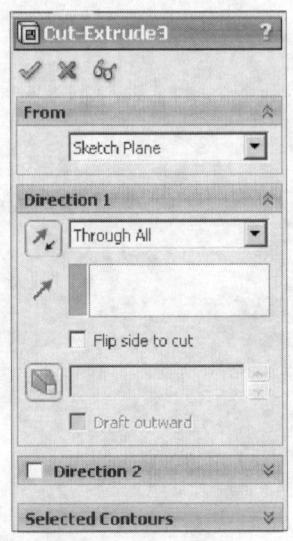

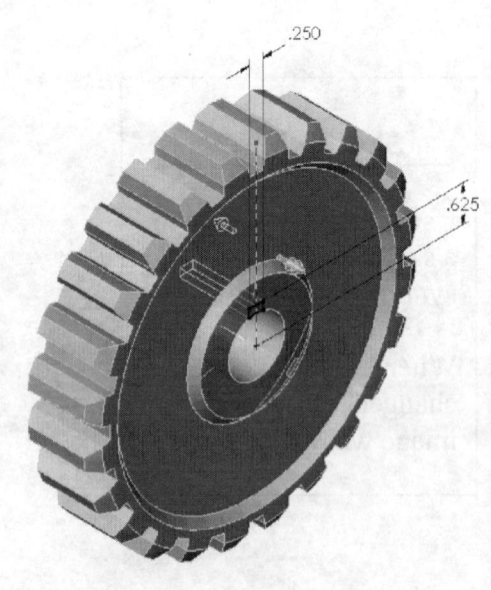

11. Saving Your Work:

- Select **File / Save As**.

- Enter **Spur Gear** for the file name.

- Click **Save**.

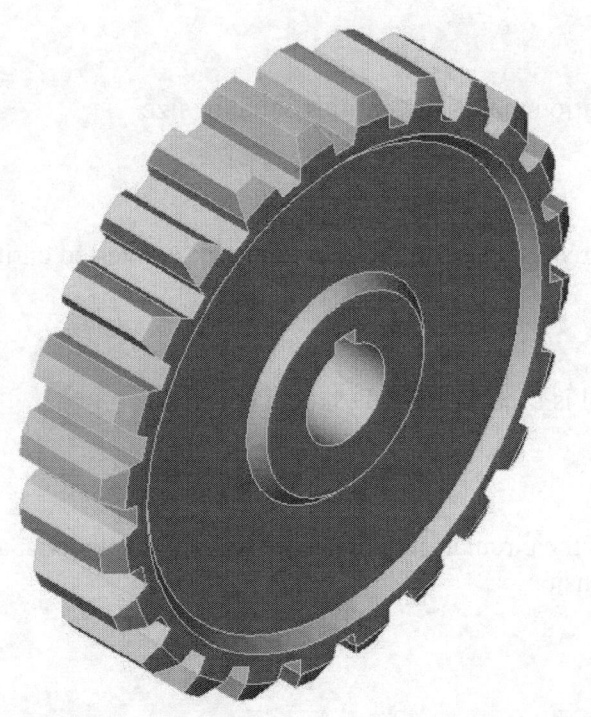

Questions for Review

Circular Patterns

1. The Revolve sketch entities should not cross the Revolve centerline.
   a. True
   b. False

2. The system creates **symmetric** relations to all mirrored sketch entities.
   a. True
   b. False

3. An Equal relation makes the entities equal in size.
   a. True
   b. False

4. The system creates an On-Edge relation to all converted entities.
   a. True
   b. False

5. The Trim tool is used to trim 2D sketch entities.
   a. True
   b. False

6. The center of the circular pattern can be defined by an axis, a linear edge, or an angular dimension.
   a. True
   b. False

7. The center of rotation, spacing, number of copies, and features to copy are required when creating a circular pattern.
   a. True
   b. False

8. When the original feature is changed, all instances in the pattern will also change.
   a. True
   b. False

7. TRUE	8. TRUE
5. TRUE	6. TRUE
3. TRUE	4. TRUE
1. TRUE	2. TRUE

CHAPTER 7 (cont.)

Circular Patterns

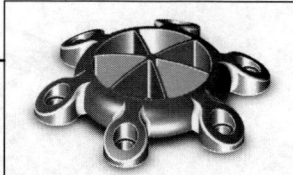

Circular Patterns

Circular Base Mount

- As mentioned in the 1st half of this chapter, the Circular Pattern command creates an array of feature(s) around an axis.

- The elements required to create circular patterns are:

    * Center axis (Temporary Axis, Axis, an Edge, etc.)

    * Spacing between each instance

    * Number of instances in the pattern

    * Feature(s) to the pattern

- Only the original feature may be edited and changes made to the original feature will automatically be passed onto the instances within the pattern.

- The features to the pattern can be selected directly from the graphics area or from the Feature Manager tree.

- Instances in a pattern can be skipped. The skipped instances can be edited during or after the pattern is complete.

- The Temporary axis can be toggled on or off (View/Temporary Axis).

- This 2nd half of the chapter will guide you through the use of the Circular Pattern command, as well as the Curve Driven Pattern command.

Circular Base Mount
Circular Patterns

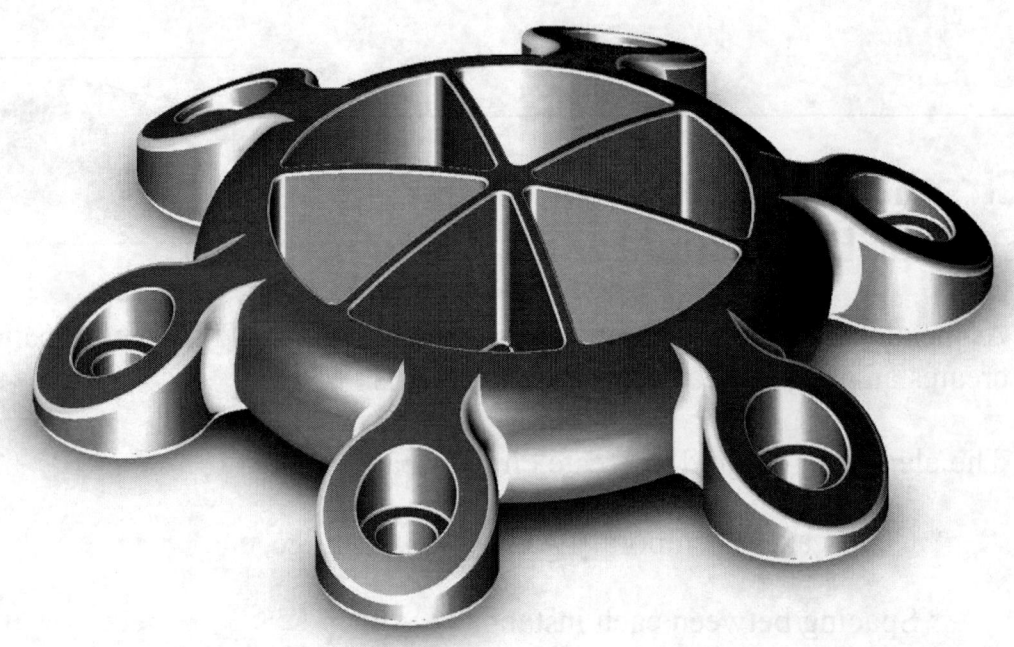

Dimensioning Standards: **ANSI**
Units: **INCHES** – 3 Decimals

Tools Needed:

Insert Sketch	Line	Mirror Dynamic
Add Geometric Relations	Dimension	Base/Boss Revolve
Revolve Cut	Circular Pattern	Fillet/Round

1. Creating the Base Sketch:

- From the <u>Front</u> plane, start a new Sketch 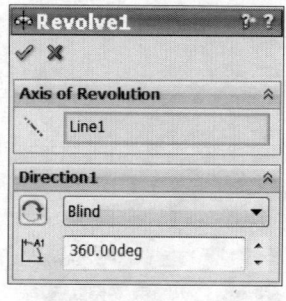.

- Sketch the profile on the right side of the revolve centerline as shown.

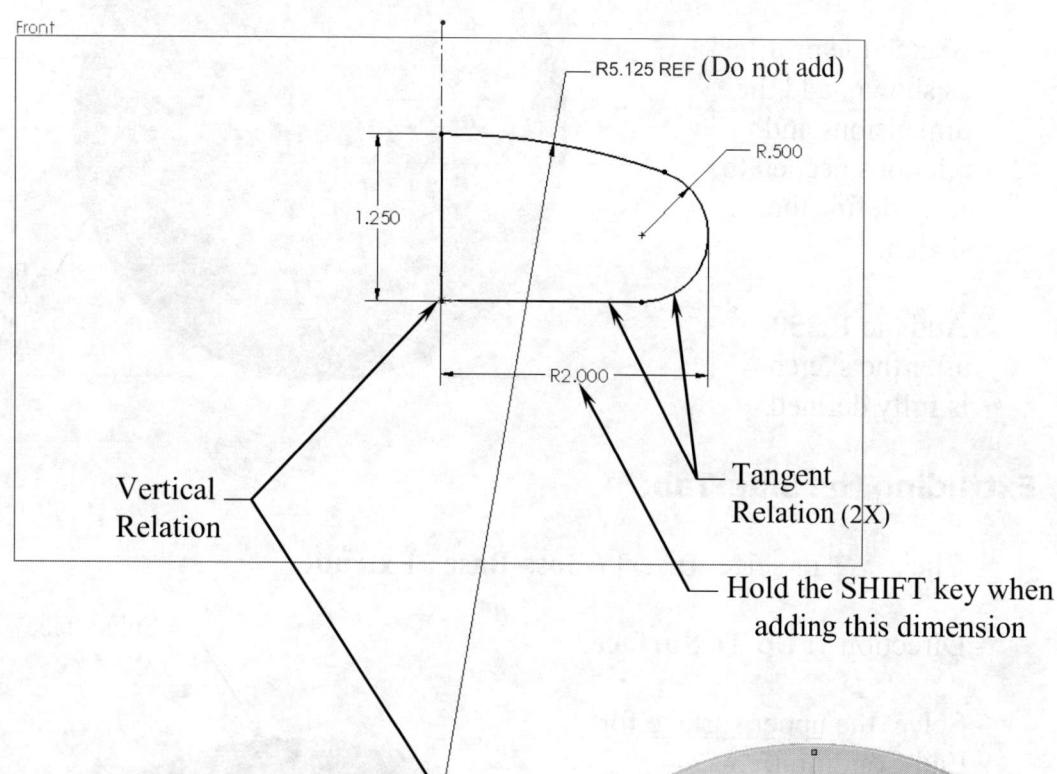

Front

R5.125 REF (Do not add)

R.500

1.250

Vertical Relation

R2.000

Tangent Relation (2X)

Hold the SHIFT key when adding this dimension

2. Revolving the Base Feature:

- Click 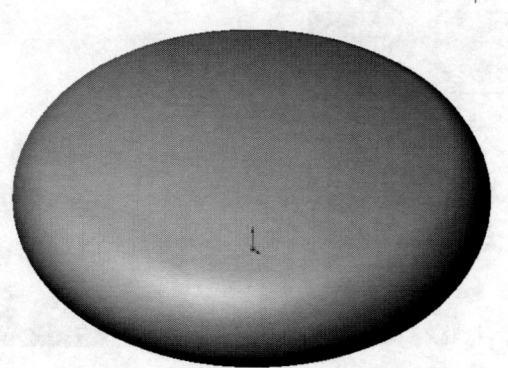 or select: **Insert / Boss Base / Revolve**.

- Revolve Direction: **Blind**.

- Revolve Angle: **360 deg**.

Revolve1

Axis of Revolution

Line1

Direction1

Blind

360.00deg

- Click **OK** ✔.

3. Creating the first Side-Tab sketch:

- Select the <u>Top</u>
  plane and open
  a new Sketch.

- Sketch the profile
  as shown; add the
  dimensions and
  relations needed to
  fully define the
  sketch.

- Add the **R.250**
  after the sketch
  is fully defined.

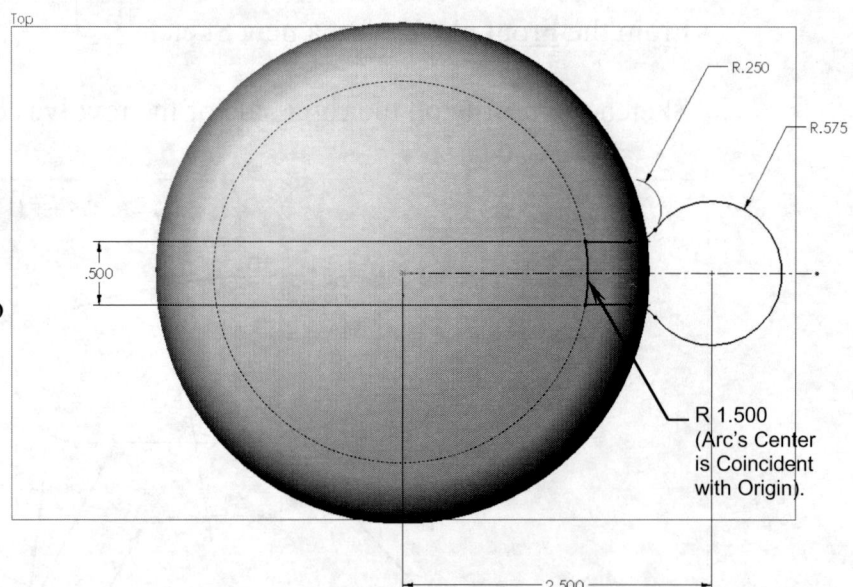

4. Extruding the Side-Tab:

- Click 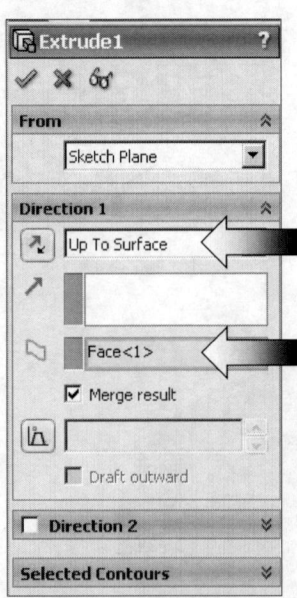 or select **Insert / Boss-Base / Extrude**.

- Direction 1: **Up To Surface**.

- Select the <u>upper surface</u> for
  End Condition.

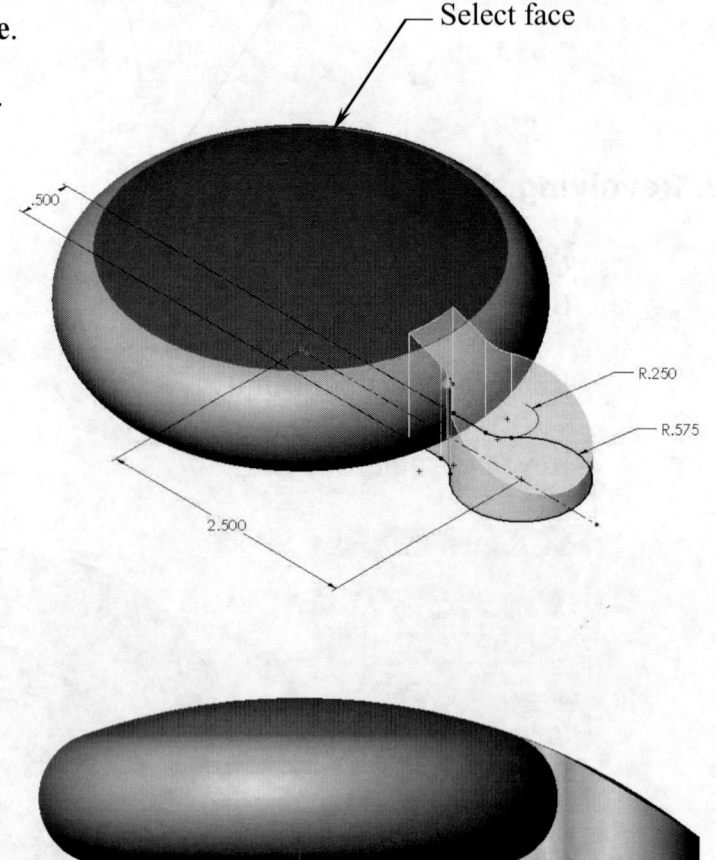

- Click **OK** ✅.

5. Adding a CounterBore Hole:

- Using the "traditional method" sketch the profile of the Counter-Bore on the <u>Front</u> plane.

(To create the "Virtual Diameter" dimensions 1st click the centerline then any other entity and place the dimension on the other side of the centerline).

- Add the 2 Diameter and the 2 Depth dimensions.

- Add the relations needed to fully define the sketch.

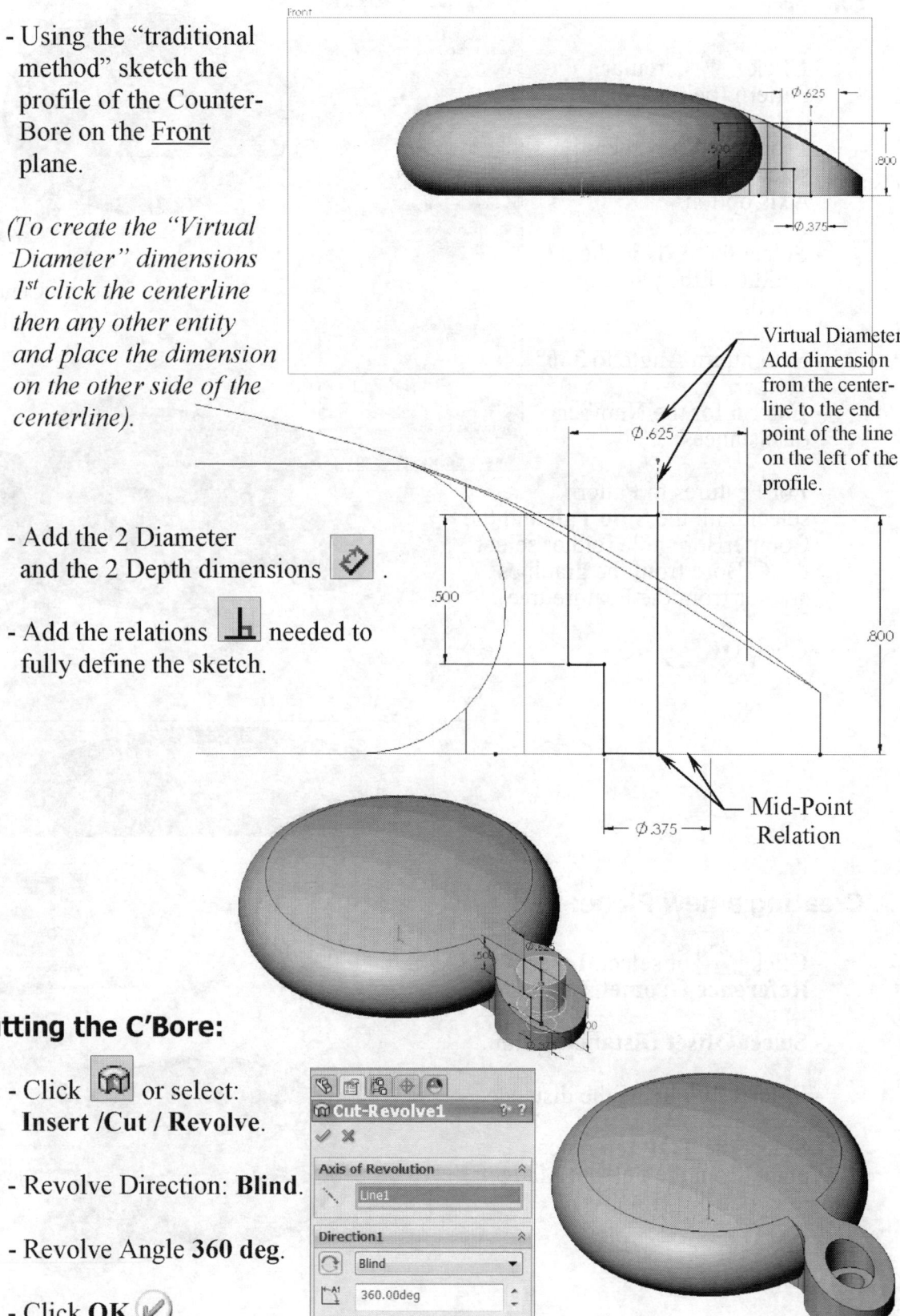

Virtual Diameter: Add dimension from the center-line to the end point of the line on the left of the profile.

Mid-Point Relation

6. Cutting the C'Bore:

- Click or select: **Insert /Cut / Revolve**.

- Revolve Direction: **Blind**.

- Revolve Angle **360 deg**.

- Click **OK**.

7. Creating the circular pattern:

- Click 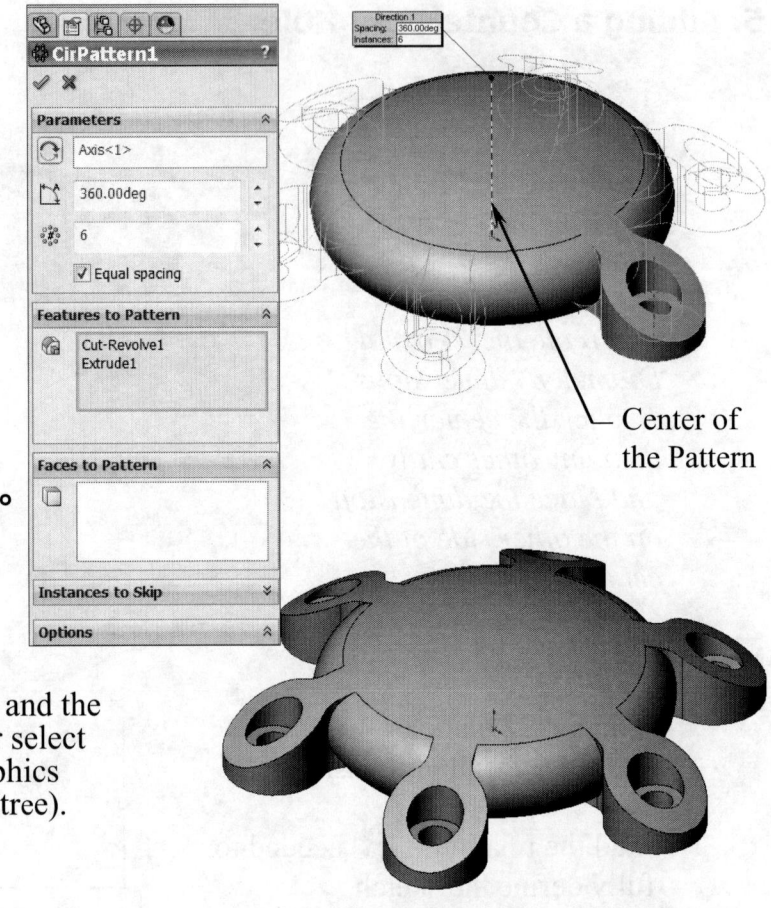 Circular Pattern (below Linear).

- From the **View** menu, select the **Temporary-Axis** option.

- Select the **Axis** in the middle of the part as noted.

- Set Pattern Angle to **360°**

- Enter **6** for the Number of Instances.

- For Features to Pattern, select both the **Side Tab** and the CounterBore hole (either select the C'Bore from the graphics area or from the Feature tree).

- Click **OK** ⊘.

Center of the Pattern

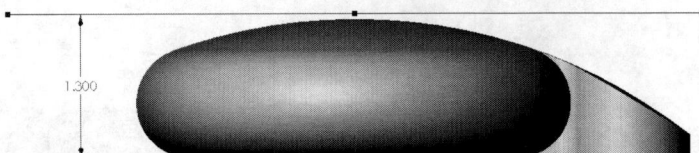

8. Creating a new Plane:

- Click 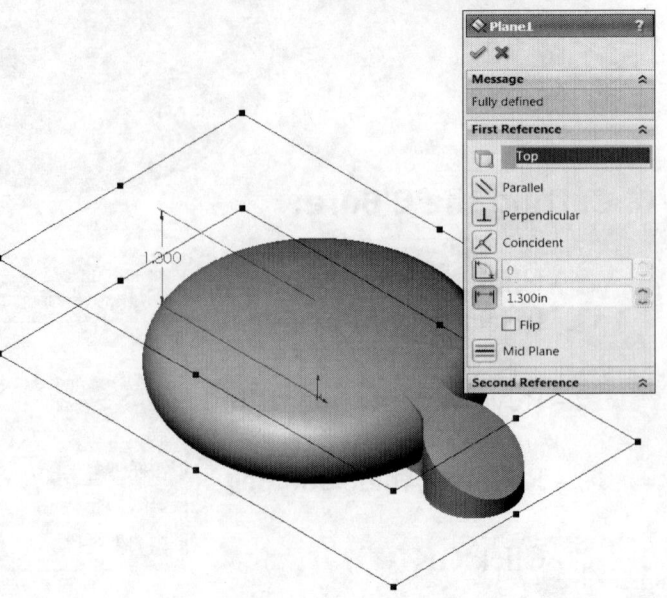 or select: **Insert / Reference Geometry / Plane**.

- Select **Offset Distance** option.

- Enter **1.300 in.** as the distance.

- Select the **TOP** reference plane from the Feature Manger tree to offset from.

- Click **OK** ⊘.

9. Creating the Pockets Sketch:

- Select the <u>new plane</u> (Plane1) and open a new sketch.

- Use the **Dynamic Mirror** 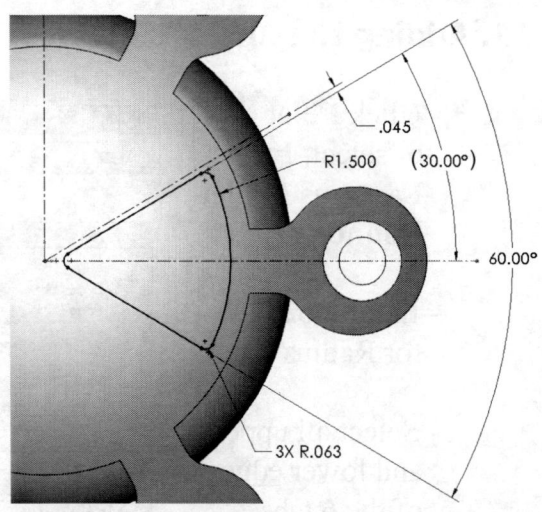 and sketch the profile as shown.

- Add the dimensions and relations as needed to fully define the sketch.

- Use **Circular Sketch Pattern** to make a total of 6 instances of the pocket.

10. Cutting the Pockets:

- Click or select:
Insert / Cut / Extrude.

- For direction 1: use
Offset From Surface.

- Select the **bottom surface** to offset from.

- Enter **.125 in**. for Depth.

- Click **OK** ✅.

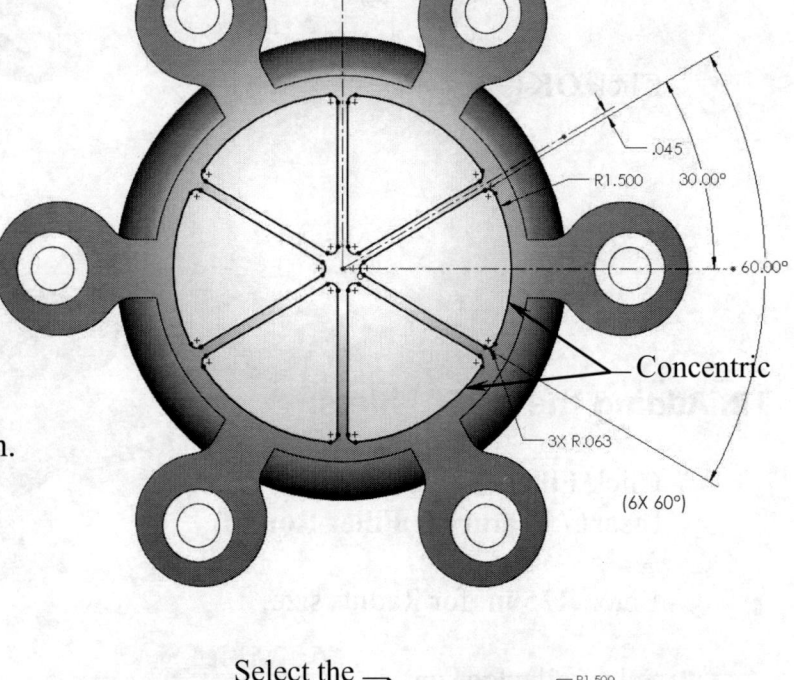

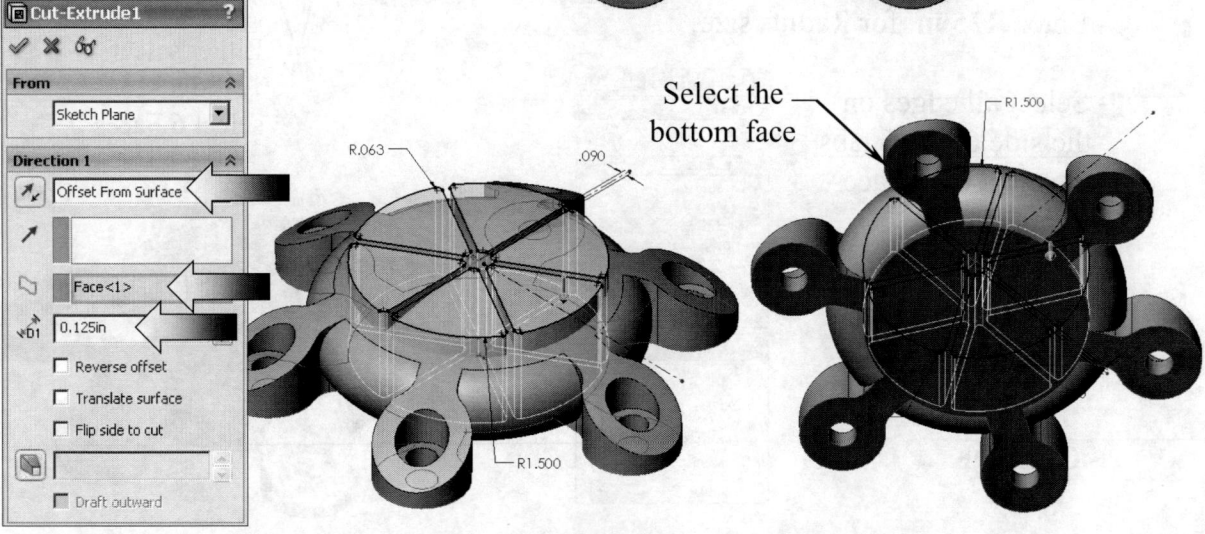

Select the bottom face

11. Adding the .0625" Fillets:

- Click **Fillet** 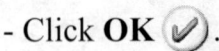 or select: **Insert / Features / Fillet-Round**.

- Enter **.0625 in**. for Radius size.

- Select all upper and lower <u>edges of the 6 tabs</u>.

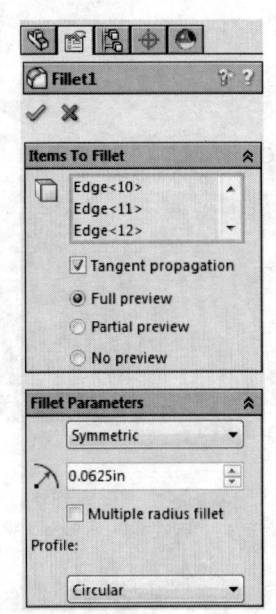

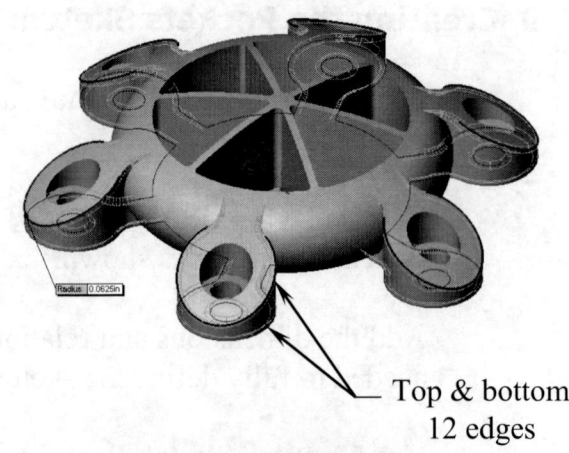

Top & bottom 12 edges

- Click **OK** .

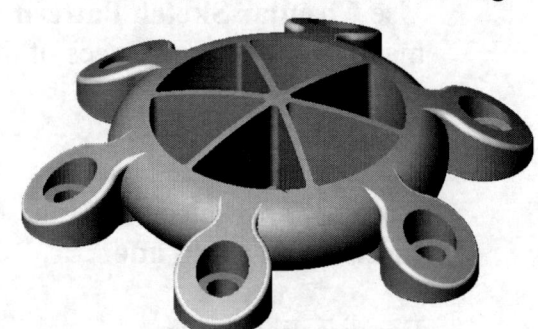

12. Adding the .125" Fillets:

- Click **Fillet** 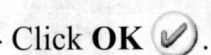 or select: **Insert / Features / Fillet-Round.**

- Enter **.125 in**. for Radius size.

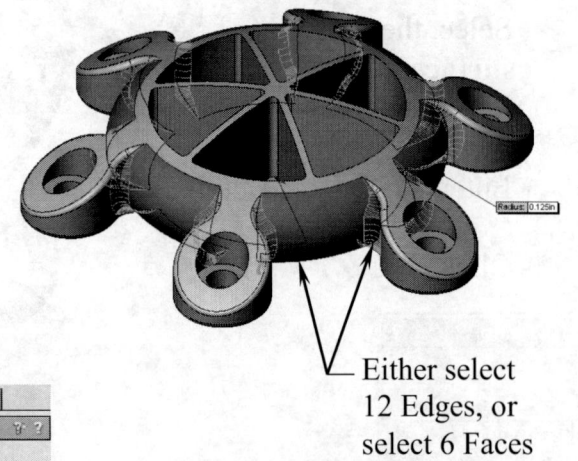

Either select 12 Edges, or select 6 Faces

- Select all edges on <u>the side of the 6 tabs</u> or select the 6 faces as noted.

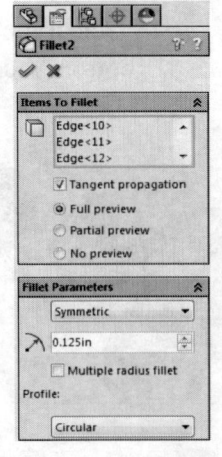

- Click **OK** .

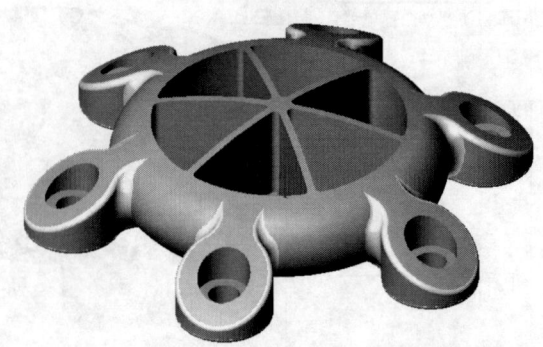

13. Adding the .015" Fillets:

- Click **Fillet** 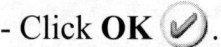 or select
Insert / Features / Fillet-Round.

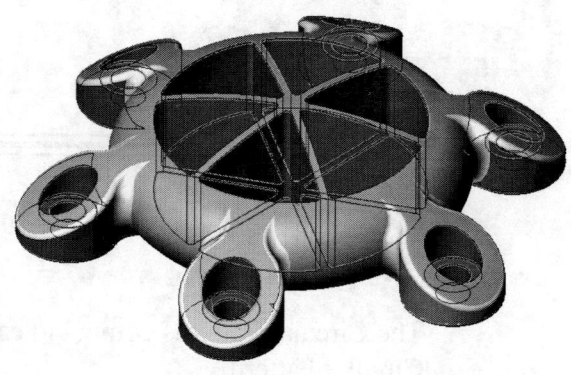

- Enter **.015 in**. for radius size.

- Select <u>all edges</u> of the 6 Pockets and the 6 Counterbores.

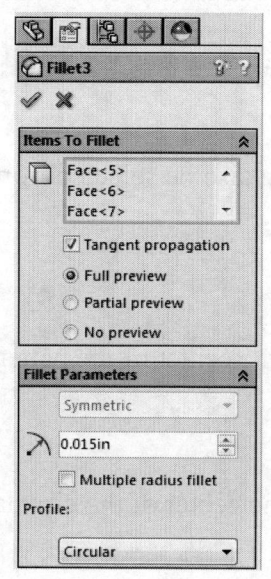

- Click **OK** ✅.

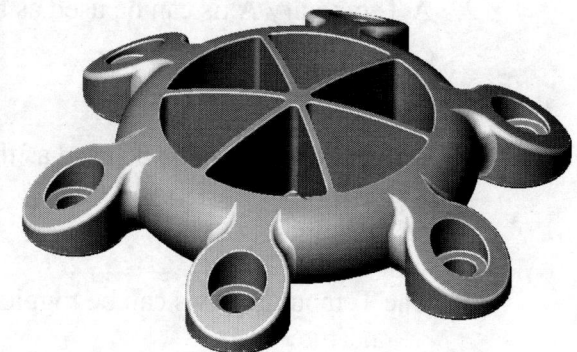

14. Saving your work:

- Click **File / Save As**.

- Enter **Circular Base Mount** for file name.

- Click **Save**.

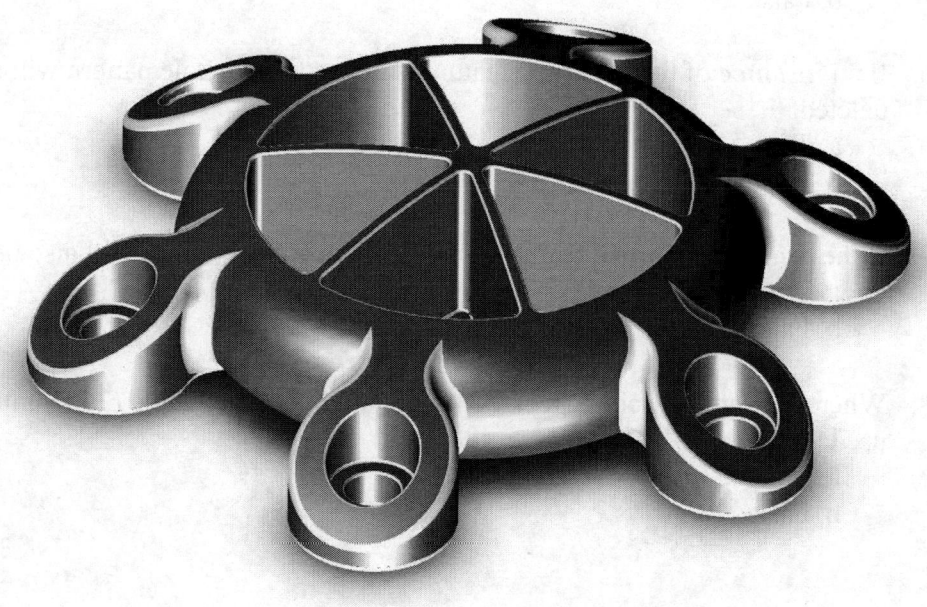

Questions for Review

Circular Patterns

1. The Circular Patterns command can also be selected from Insert / Pattern Mirror / Circular Pattern.
   - a. True
   - b. False

2. A Temporary Axis can be used as the center of the pattern.
   - a. True
   - b. False

3. A linear edge can also be used as the center of the circular pattern.
   - a. True
   - b. False

4. The Temporary Axis can be toggled ON / OFF under View / Temporary Axis.
   - a. True
   - b. False

5. The instances in the circular pattern can be skipped during and after the pattern is created.
   - a. True
   - b. False

6. If an *instance* of the patterned feature is deleted, the whole pattern will also be deleted.
   - a. True
   - b. False

7. If the *original* patterned feature is deleted, the whole pattern will also be deleted.
   - a. True
   - b. False

8. When the Equal spacing check box is enabled, the total angle (360°) must be used.
   - a. True
   - b. False

7. TRUE   8. FALSE
5. TRUE   6. FALSE
3. TRUE   4. TRUE
1. TRUE   2. TRUE

CHAPTER 7 (cont.)

Curve Driven Patterns

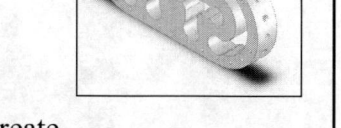

Curve Driven Patterns
Universal Bracket

- The **Curve Drive Pattern** PropertyManager appears when you create
a new curve driven pattern feature or when you edit an existing curve driven pattern feature.

- The PropertyManager controls the following properties:

   Pattern Direction: Select a curve, edge, sketch entity, or select a sketch from the FeatureManager to use as the path for the pattern. If necessary, click Reverse Direction to change the direction of the pattern.

   Number of Instances: Set a value for the number of instances of the seed feature in the pattern.

   Equal spacing: Sets equal spacing between each pattern instance. The separation between instances depends on the curve selected for Pattern Direction and on the Curve method.

   Spacing: (Available if you do not select Equal spacing) Set a value for the distance between pattern instances along the curve. The distance between the curve and the Features to Pattern is measured normal to the curve.

Curve method: Defines the direction of the pattern by transforming how you use the curve selected for Pattern Direction. Select one of the following:

   * Transform curve. The delta X and delta Y distances from the origin of the selected curve to the seed feature are maintained for each instance.

   * Offset curve: The normal distance from the origin of the selected curve to the seed feature is maintained for each instance.

Alignment method: Select one of the following:

   * Tangent to curve: Aligns each instance tangent to the curve selected for Pattern direction

   * Align to seed: Aligns each instance to match the original alignment of the seed feature of **Curve method** and **Alignment method** selections.

   * Face normal: (For 3D curves only) Select the face on which the 3D curve lies to create the curve driven pattern.

Curve Driven Pattern and Hole Wizard
Universal Bracket

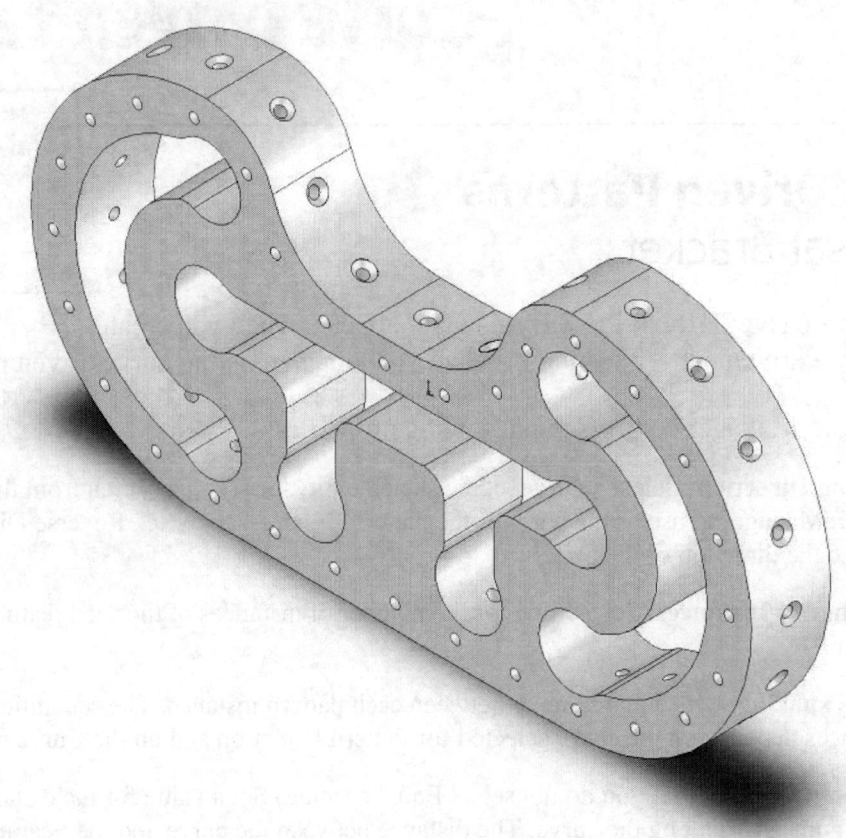

Dimensioning Standards: **ANSI**
Units: **INCHES** – 3 Decimals

Tools Needed:

Insert Sketch	Convert Entities	Offset Entities
Boss Base Extrude	Hole Wizard	Curve Driven Pattern

1. Opening the existing file:

- Go to: The Training Files folder
          Open a copy of the file named:
          Curve Driven Pattern.sldprt

- **Edit** the **Sketch1.**

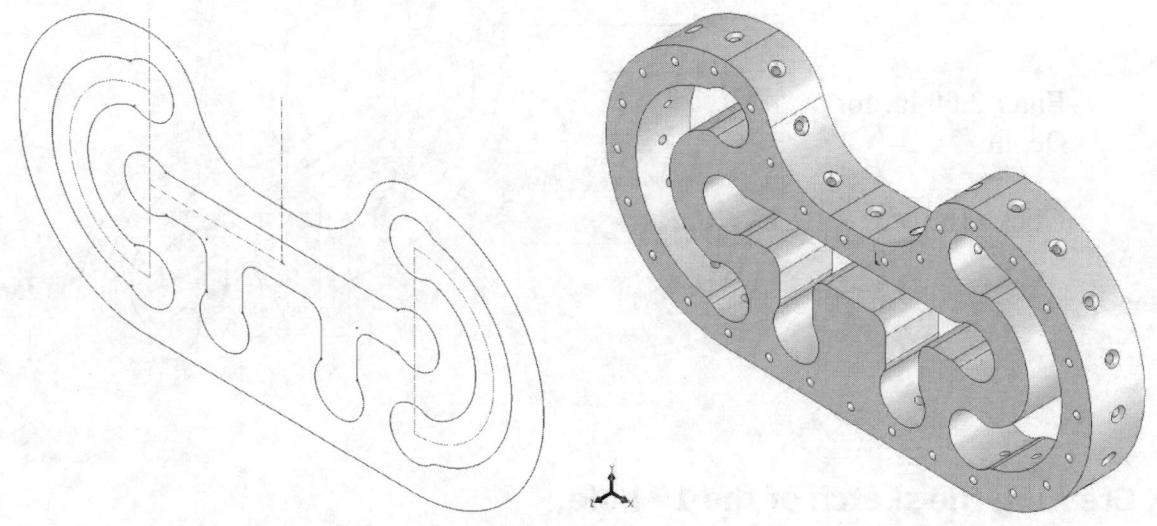

- Make sure the sketch1 is fully defined before extruding.

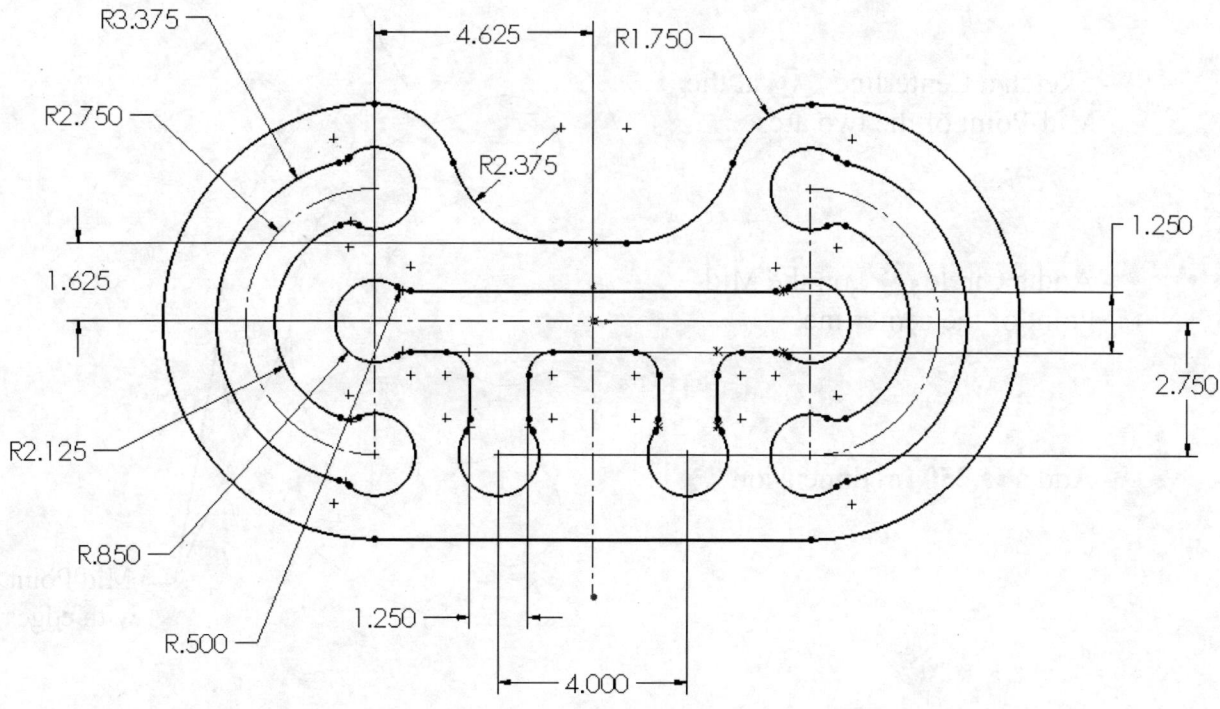

2. Extruding the Base:

- Click 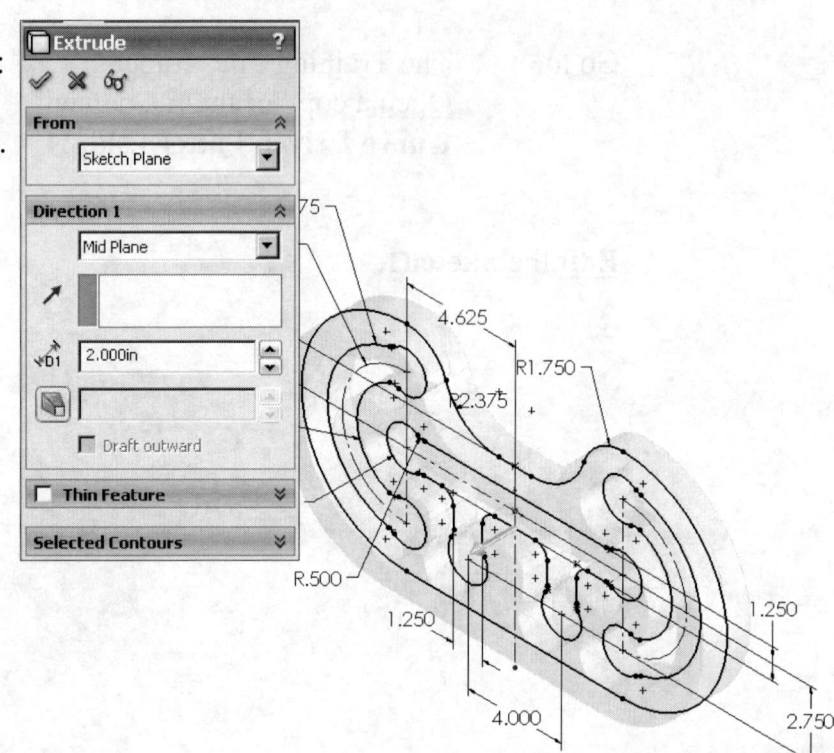 or select:
**Insert / Features /
Boss Base Extrude**.

- Use **Mid Plane**
for Direction1.

- Enter **2.00 in**. for
Depth.

- Click **OK**.

3. Creating the sketch of the 1ˢᵗ hole:

- Select the <u>face</u> as indicated and open a new sketch .

- Sketch a Centerline at the
Mid-Point of the two arcs.

- Add a Circle on the Mid-
Point of the centerline.

- Add a **Ø.250 in**. dimension .

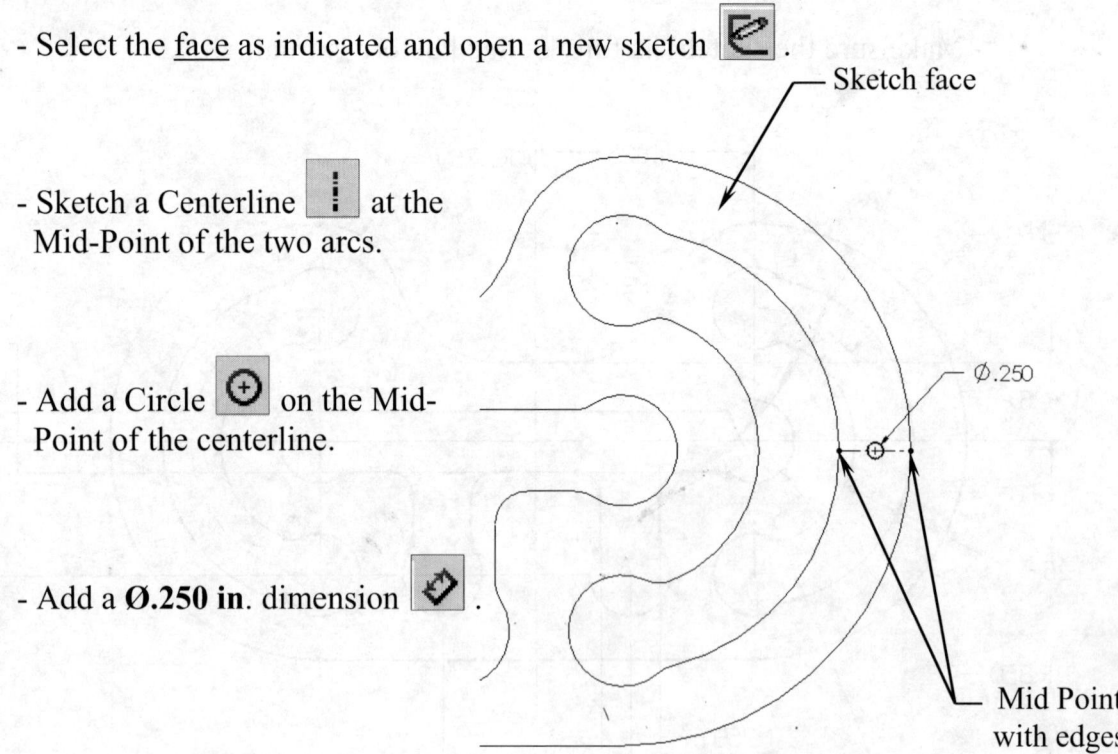

Sketch face

Ø.250

Mid Point
with edges

4. Cutting the hole:

- Click 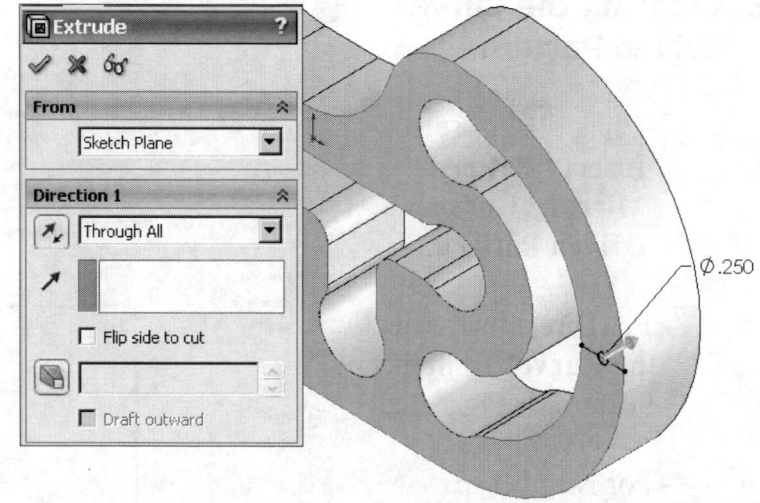 or select:
Insert / Cut / Extrude.

- Select **Through All**
for Direction1.

- Click **OK** ✅ .

5. Constructing the Curve-Sketch to drive the Pattern:

- Select the <u>face</u> as noted* and open a new sketch ✏️ .

- Select all Outer-Edges of the part (Right mouse click on an edge & Select-Tangency).

- Click ↗ or select **Tools / Sketch Entities / Offset Entities**.

- Enter **.563 in**. for Offset Distance.

- Click Reverse if necessary to place the new profile on the **INSIDE**.

- **Exit** the sketch mode and change the name of the sketch to **CURVE1**.

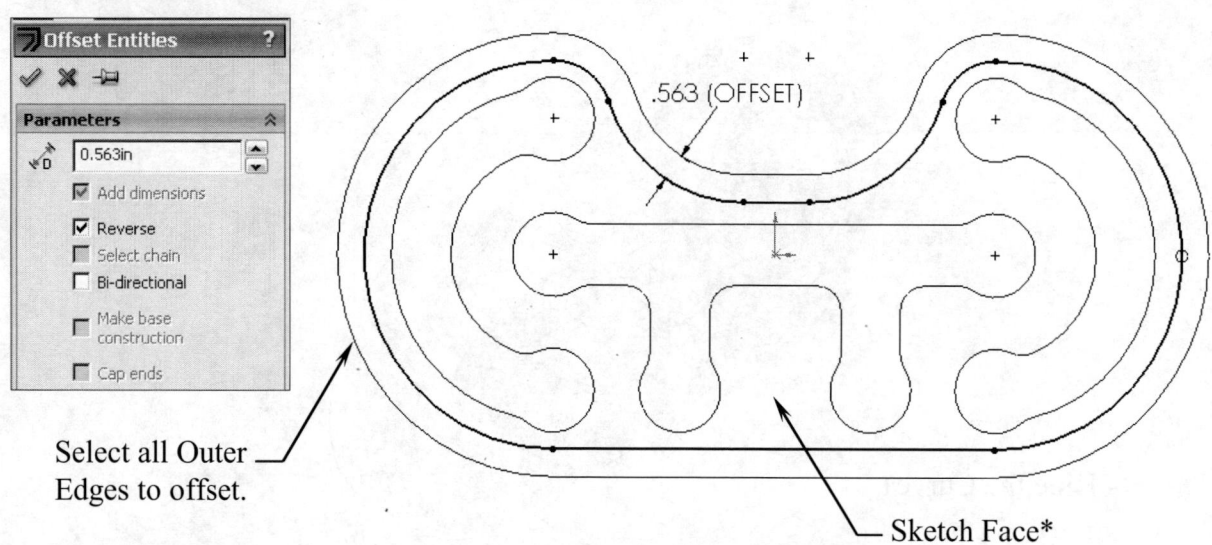

Select all Outer Edges to offset.

Sketch Face*

6. Creating the Curve-Driven Pattern:

- Click 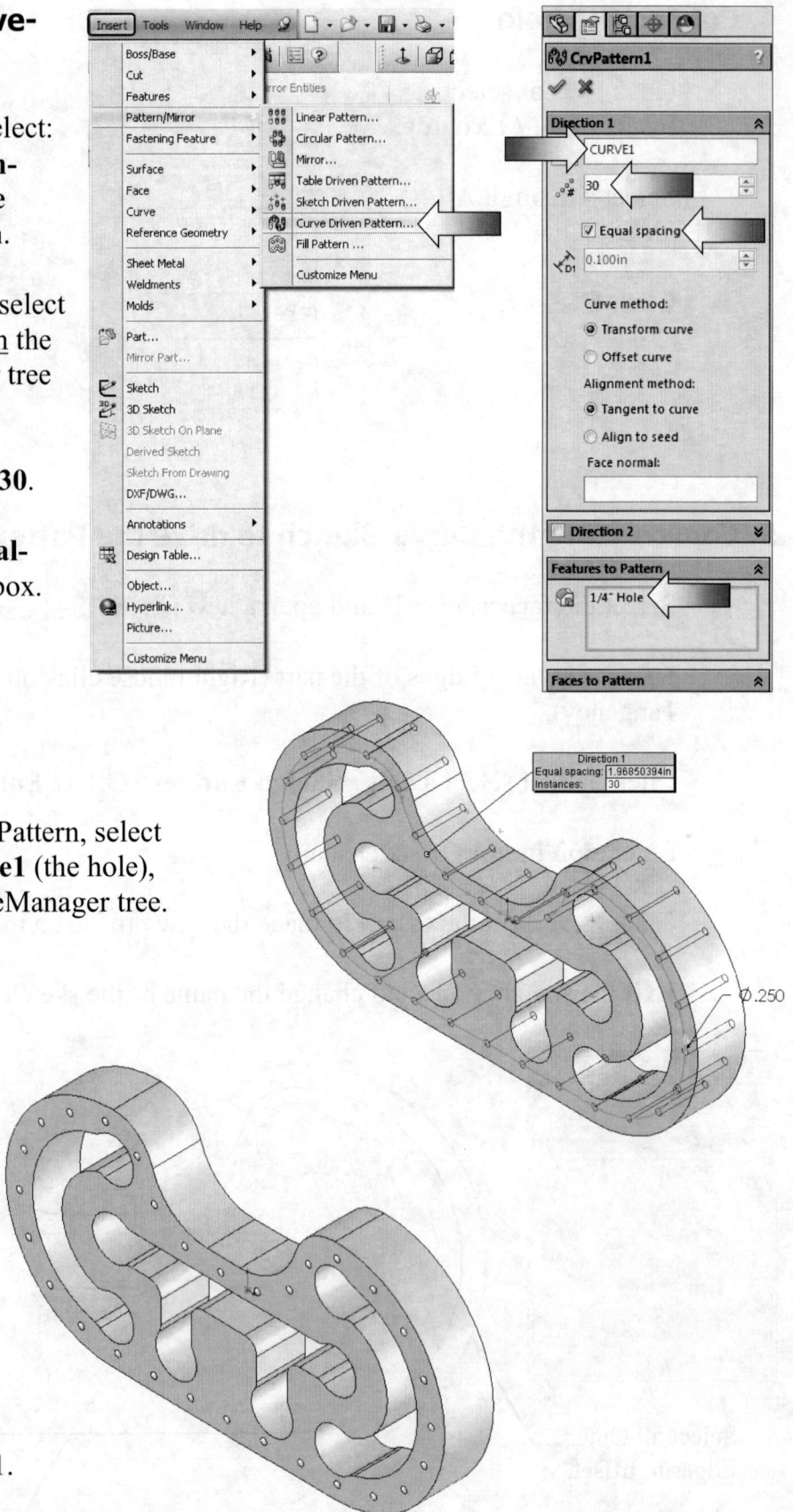 or select:
Insert / Pattern-Mirror / Curve Driven Pattern.

- For Direction1, select the **Curve1** from the FeatureManager tree

- For Number of Instances, enter **30**.

- Enable the **Equal-Spacing** check box.

- For Features to Pattern, select the **Cut-Extrude1** (the hole), from the FeatureManager tree.

- Click **OK** ✅.

- Hide the Curve1.

7. Constructing the 2nd Curve:

- Select the <u>Front</u> plane and open a new sketch.

- Select all **Outer-Edges** of the

part and click 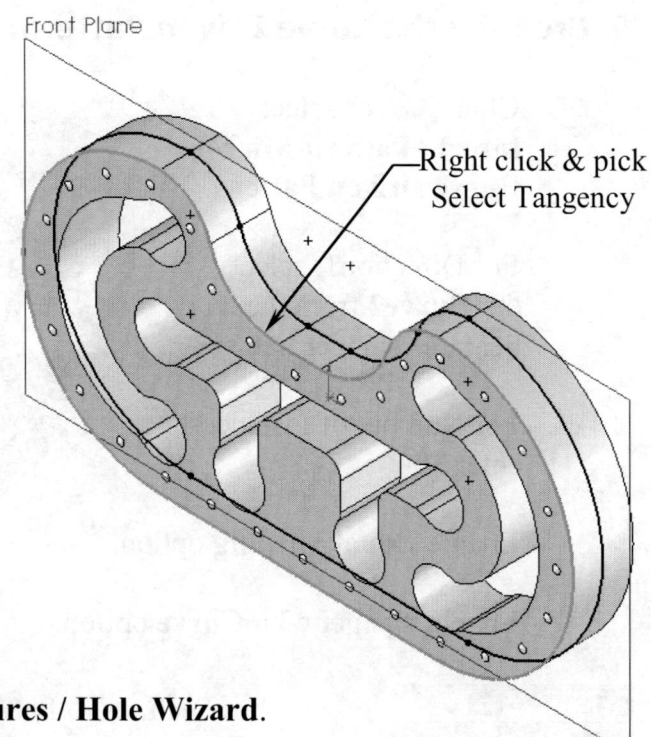 or select: **Tools / Sketch Entities / Convert Entities**.

- **Exit the Sketch** and change the sketch name to: **CURVE2**.

Front Plane

—Right click & pick Select Tangency

8. Adding the Hole Wizard:

- Click or select **Insert / Features / Hole Wizard**.

- Select the Counter-Sink button and set the following:

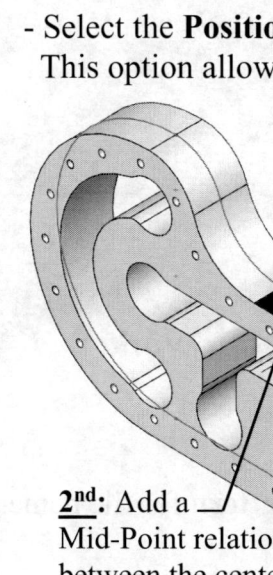

* Standard: **Ansi Inch**
* Type: **Flat Head Screw** (100)
* Size: **1/4**
* Fit: **Normal**
* End Condition: **Blind**
* Depth: **1.250 in**.

- Select the **Position** tab (arrow) and click the **3D Sketch** button 3D Sketch
This option allows the holes to be placed on non-planar surfaces as well.

1st: Place the center of hole approx. here, on the flat surface...

- Click **OK** .

2nd: Add a Mid-Point relation between the center point and the line.

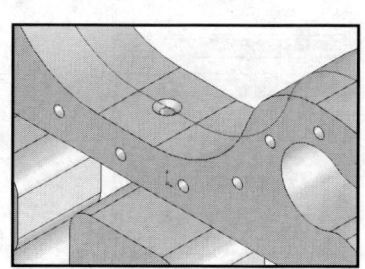

9. Creating the Curve Driven Pattern:

- Click 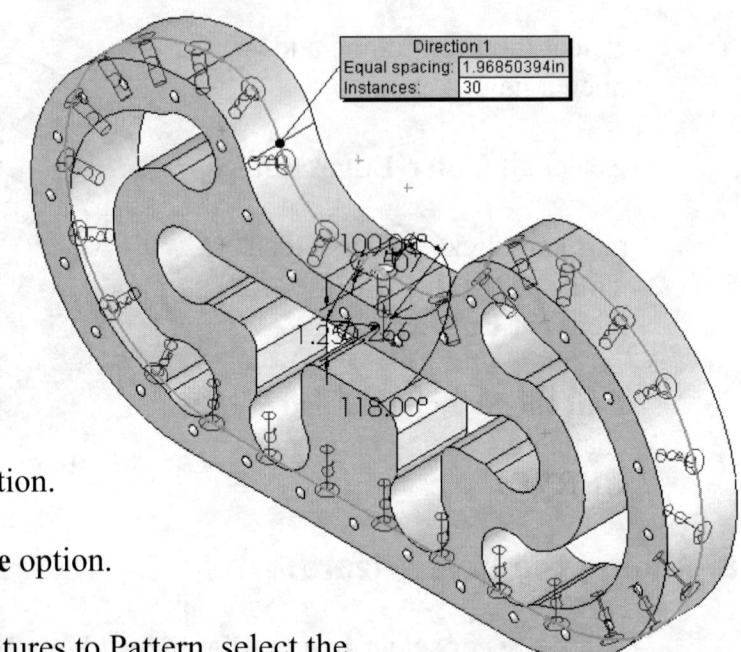 or select:
**Insert / Pattern-Mirror
Curve Driven Pattern**.

- For Direction1, select
the **Curve2** from the
FeatureManager tree.

- For Number of Instances,
enter **30**.

- Enable **Equal Spacing** option.

- Enable **Tangent To Curve** option.

- For Features to Pattern, select the
CSK-Hole from the FeatureManager tree.

- Click **OK** ✅.

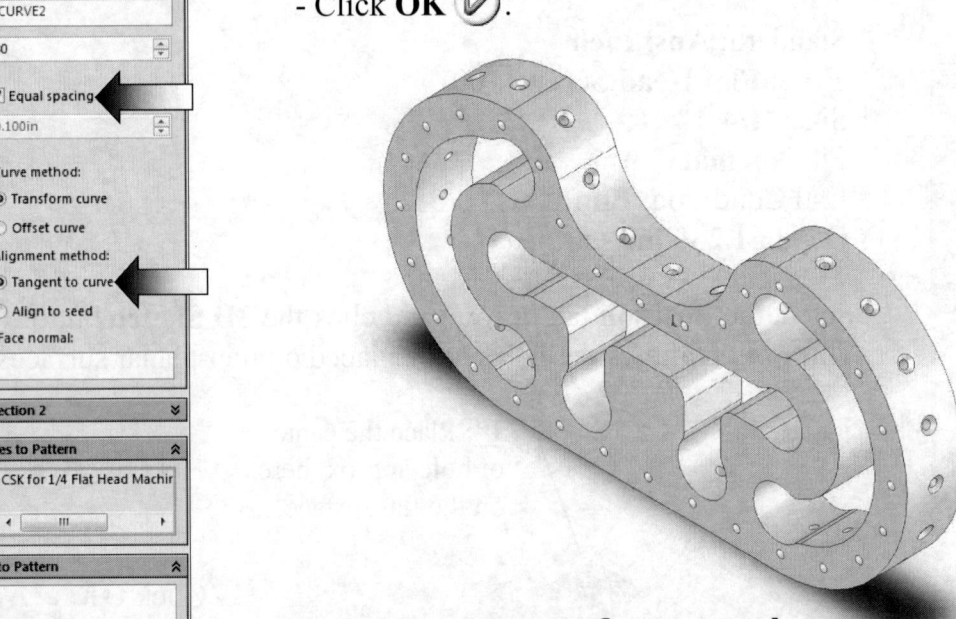

10. Saving a copy of your work:

- Click **File / Save As**.

- Enter **Curve Driven Pattern** for file name.

- Click **Save**.

CHAPTER 8

Part Configurations

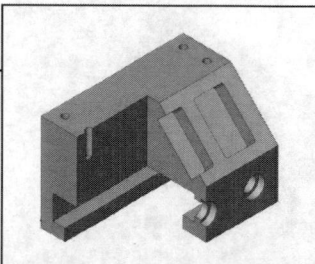

Part Configurations
Machined Block

- This chapter reviews most of the commands that were covered in the previous chapters. Upon successful completion of this lesson, you will have a better understanding of how and when to:

        * Sketch on planes and planar surfaces.

        * Sketch fillets and model fillets.

        * Dimensions and Geometric Relations.

        * Extruded Cuts and Bosses.

        * Linear Patterns.

        * Using the Hole-Wizard option.

        * Create new Planes.

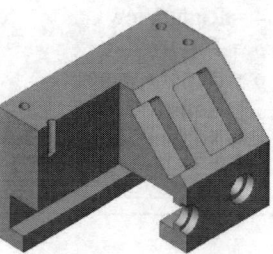

        * Mirror features.

        * Create new Part Configurations; an option that allows the user to develop and manage families of parts and assemblies.

- Configuration options are available in Part and Assembly environments.

- After the model is completed, it will be used again in a drawing chapter to further discuss the details of creating an Engineering drawing.

Machined Block
Part Configurations

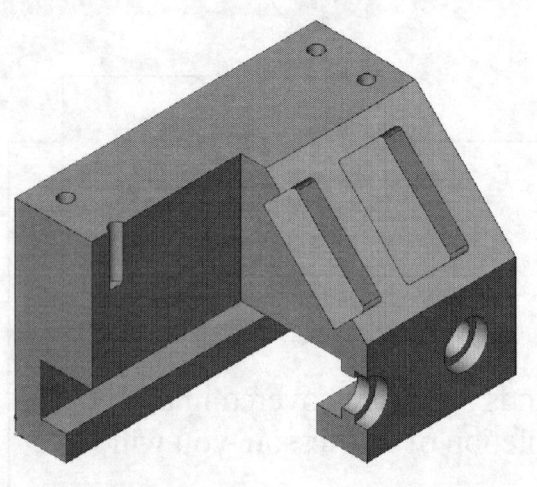
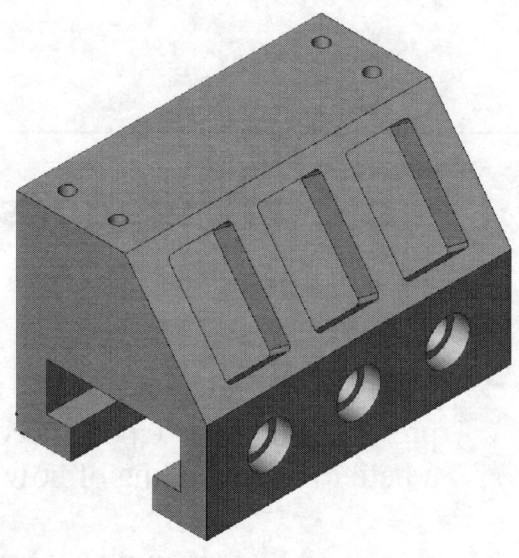

Dimensioning Standards: **ANSI**
Units: **INCHES** – 3 Decimals

Tools Needed:

Insert Sketch	Line	Rectangle
Circle	Sketch Fillet	Dimension
Add Geometric Relations	Extruded Boss/Base	Extruded Cut
Hole Wizard	Fillet	Linear Pattern

1. Sketching the base profile:

- Select the <u>Front</u> plane from the FeatureManager tree.

- Click 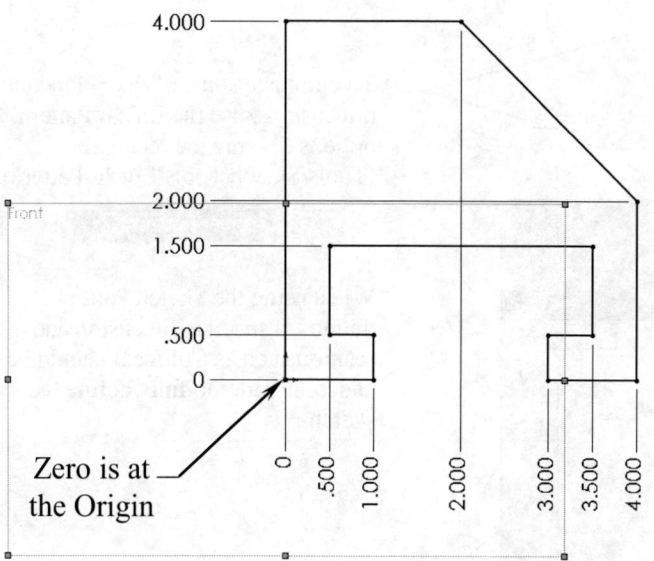 or select **Insert / Sketch**.

- Sketch the profile below using the Line tool .

- Add the dimensions shown.

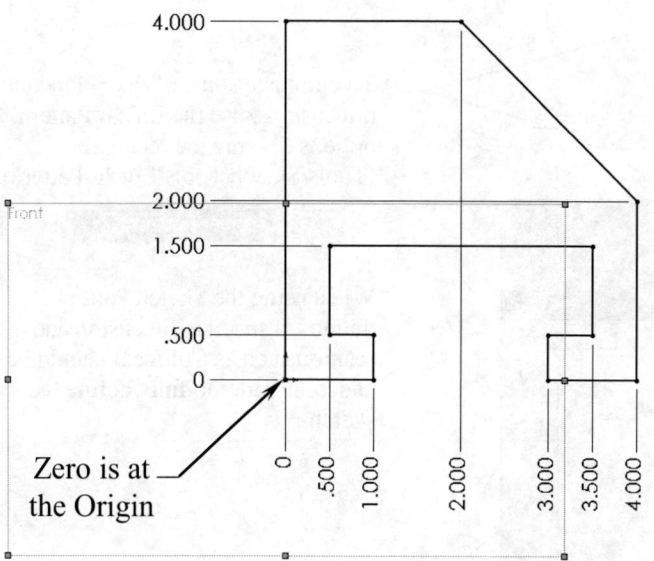

Zero is at
the Origin

> ### Ordinate Dimensions
>
> To create Ordinate dimensions:
>
> 1. Click the small drop down arrow below the Smart-Dimension command and select either Vertical or Horizontal Ordinate option.
>
> 2. First click at a vertex to determine the Zero dimension, then click the next entity to create the next dimension.
>
> 3. Repeat step 2 for the other entities / dimensions.

2. Extruding the base feature:

- Click or select **Insert / Boss-Base / Extrude**.

- End Condition: **Blind** .

- Extrude Depth: **6.00 in**. .

- Click **OK** .

Reverse Direction

Extrude1

From
Sketch Plane

Direction 1
Blind

6.000in

Draft outward

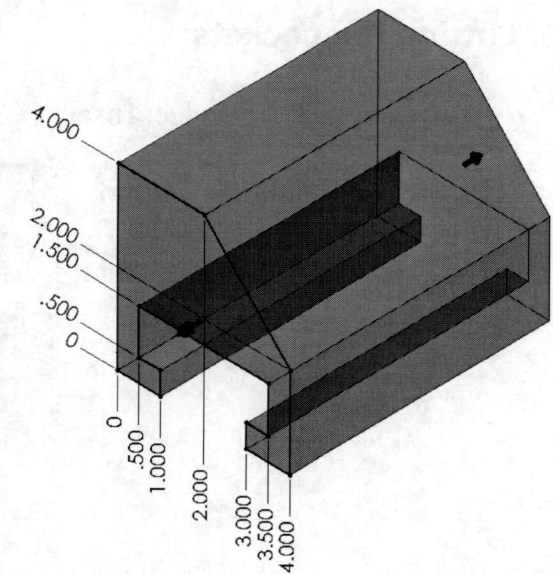

3. Creating the pocket profiles:

- Select the <u>face</u> as indicated below for sketch plane.

- Click 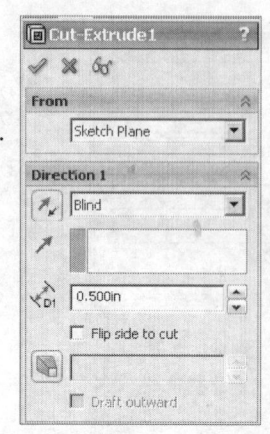 or select **Insert / Sketch**.

- Sketch the profile below using Rectangle and Sketch Fillet tools.

- Add dimensions* or Relations needed to fully define the sketch.

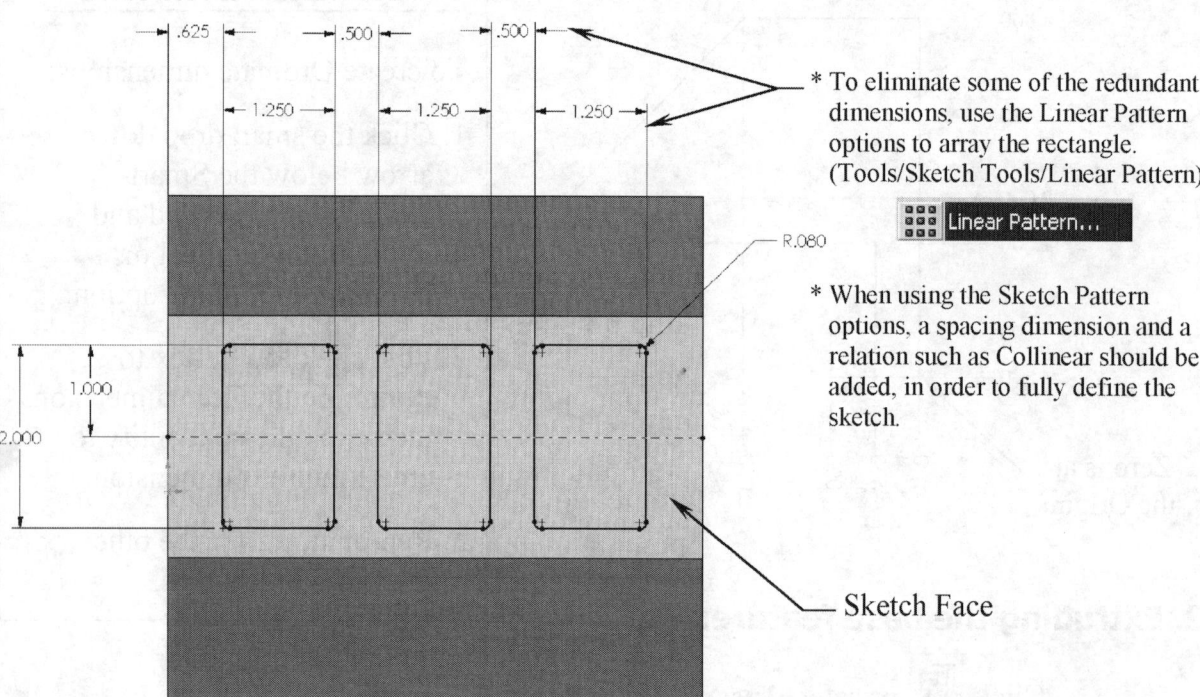

* To eliminate some of the redundant dimensions, use the Linear Pattern options to array the rectangle. (Tools/Sketch Tools/Linear Pattern).

Linear Pattern...

* When using the Sketch Pattern options, a spacing dimension and a relation such as Collinear should be added, in order to fully define the sketch.

Sketch Face

4. Cutting the pockets:

- Click or select **Insert / Cut / Extrude**.

- End Condition: **Blind**.

- Extrude Depth: **.500 in**.

- Click **OK** .

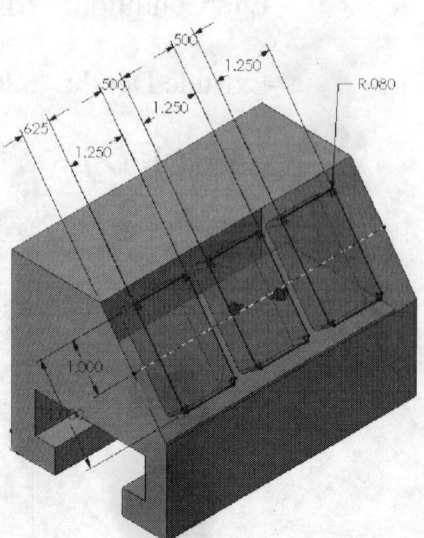

5. Adding a CounterBore from the Hole Wizard:

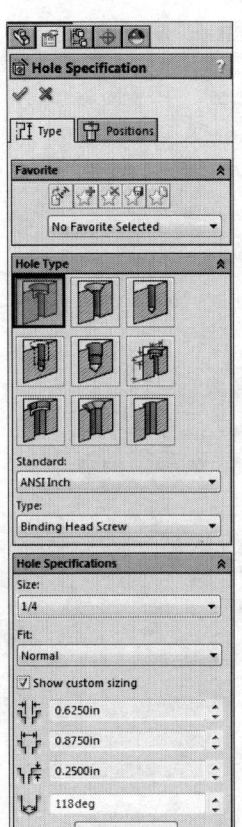

- Select the <u>face</u>* as shown for sketch plane.

- Click 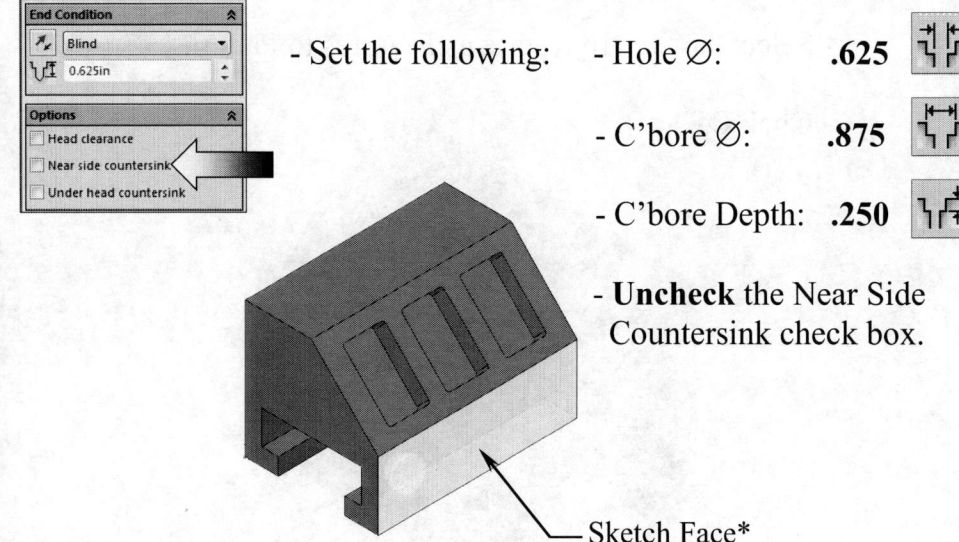 or select **Insert / Features / Hole / Wizard**.

- Click the **Counterbore** button (Circled).

 - Use CBORE for ¼ Binding Head Machine Screw.

- Set the following: - Hole ∅:   **.625**

  - C'bore ∅:   **.875**

  - C'bore Depth: **.250**

- **Uncheck** the Near Side Countersink check box.

Sketch Face*

- Select the **Positions Tab** (arrow). (Note: We need to review the pattern and mirror commands, so only one hole will be created and then pattern and mirror it to create the others).

- Add Dimensions 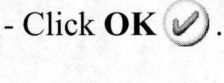 as shown to position the C'bore.

- Click **OK** 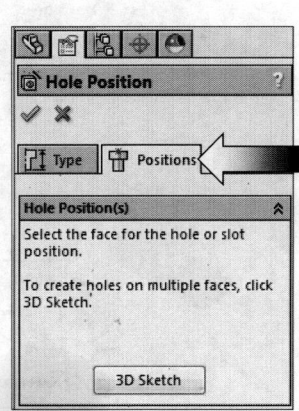.

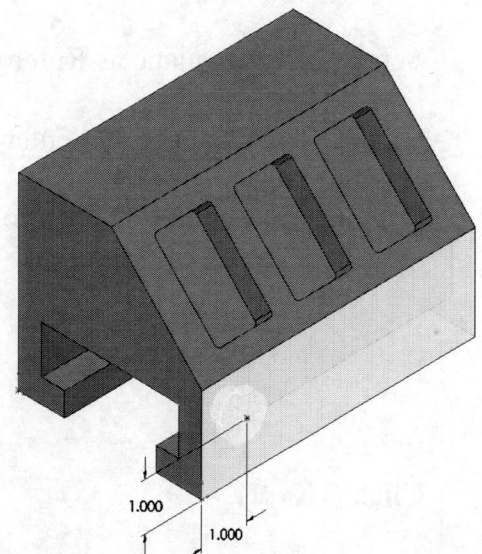

1.000

1.000

6. Patterning the Counterforce:

- Click 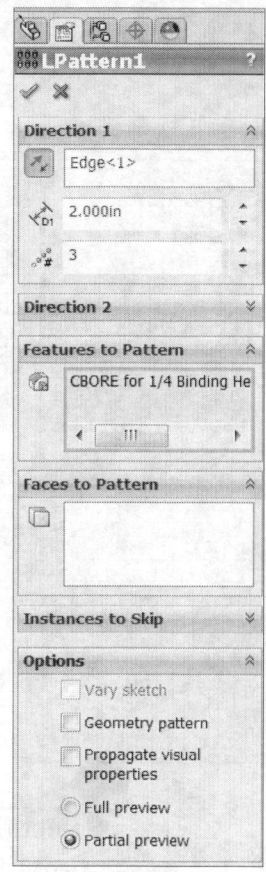 or select **Insert / Pattern Mirror / Linear Pattern**.

- Select the **bottom edge** as direction .

- Enter **2.00 in**. for Spacing .

- Type **3** for Number of Instances .

- Select the C'bore feature as Features to Pattern .

- Click **OK** .

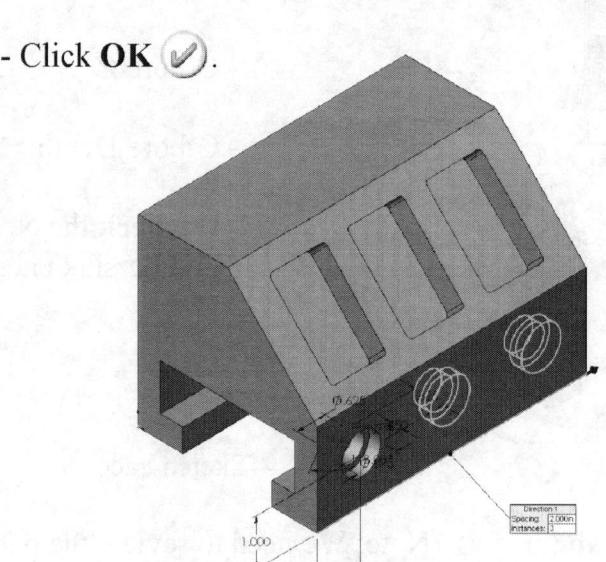

7. Creating the Mirror-Plane:

- Click or select **Insert / Reference Geometry / Plane.**

- Select the <u>Right</u> plane as Reference Entities .

- Click Offset Distance and enter **2.00 in**. .

- Use the Flip option if needed to place
  the new plane on the **right side**.

- Click **OK** .

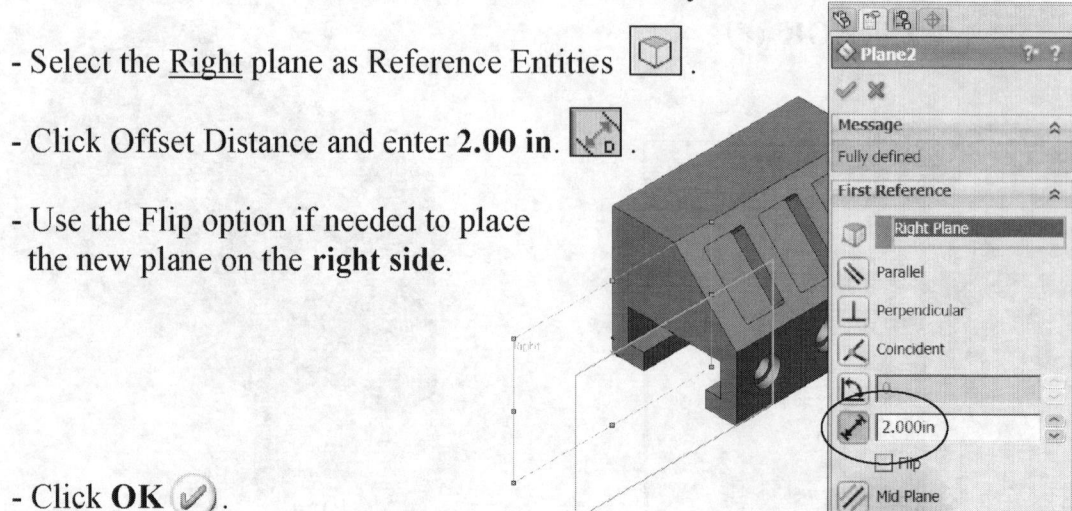

8. Mirroring the C'bores:

- Click 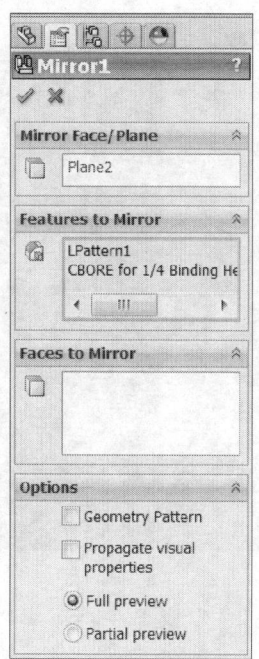 or select **Mirror** under **Insert / Pattern Mirror menu**.

- Select the <u>new plane</u> (Plane1) as Mirror Face/Plane ☐ .

- Choose the C'bore and its Pattern as Features to Pattern ☐ .

- Click **OK** ✓ .

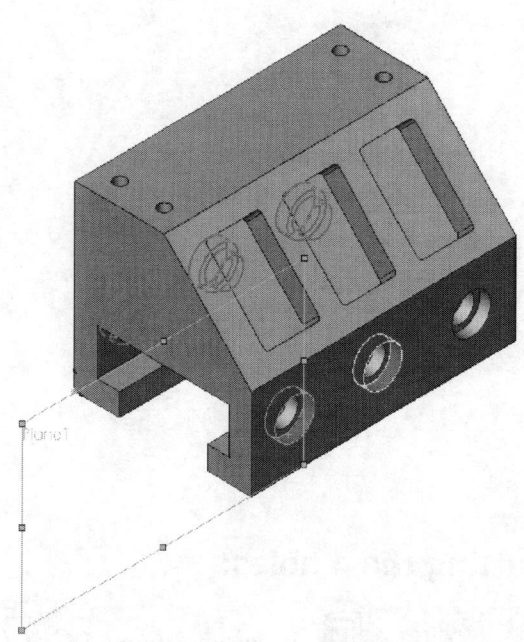

- Rotate ⟳ the model around to verify the results of the mirror.

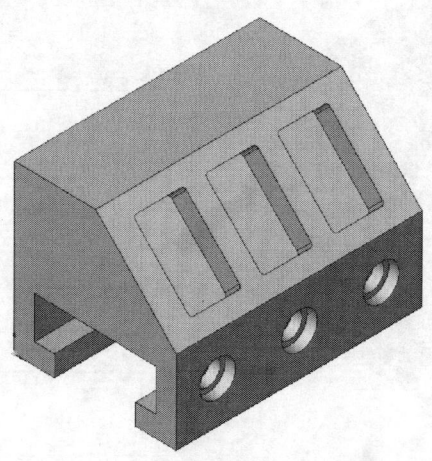

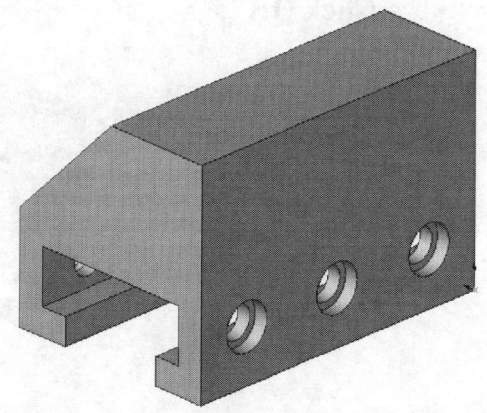

9. Creating the blind holes on the top surface:

- Select the <u>top face</u>* as the new sketch plane.

- Click 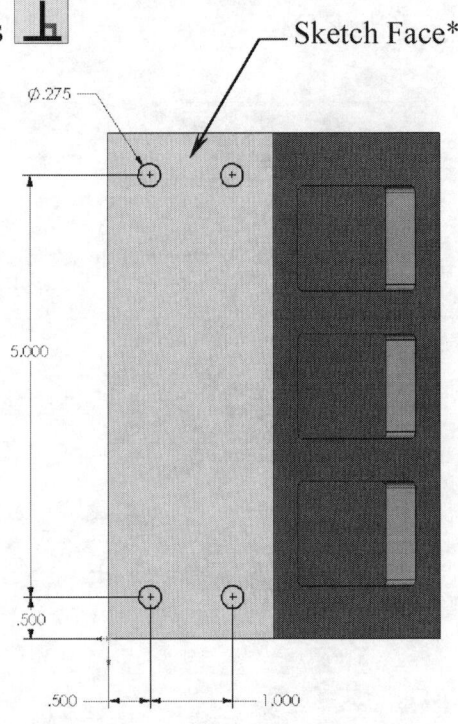 or select **Insert / Sketch**.

- Sketch 4 Circles as shown.

- Add Dimensions and Relations needed to fully define the sketch.

Sketch Face*

10. Cutting the 4 holes:

- Click or select **Insert / Cut / Extrude**.

- End Condition: **Blind.**

- Extrude Depth: **1.00 in**.

- Click **OK**.

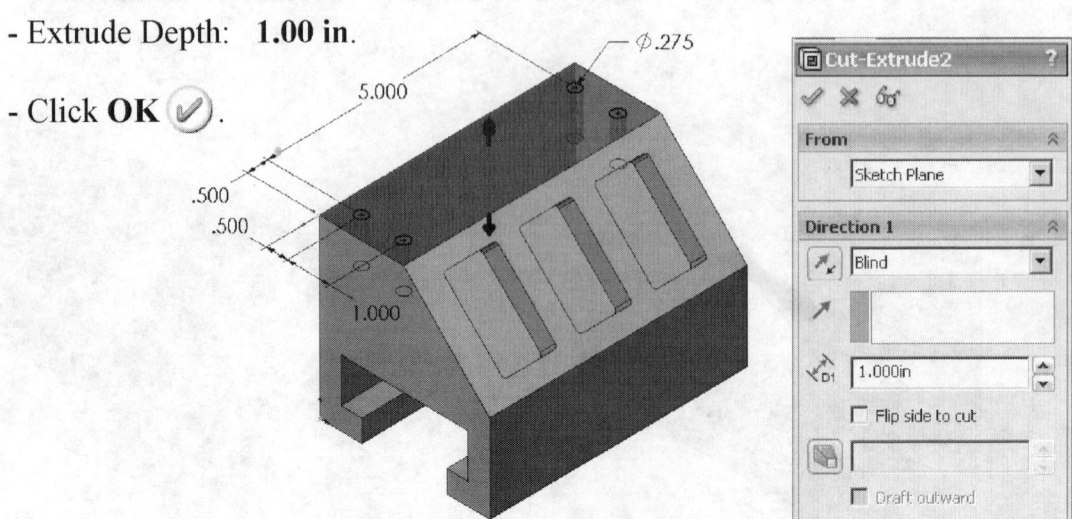

11. Creating a Cutaway section: (in a separate configuration).

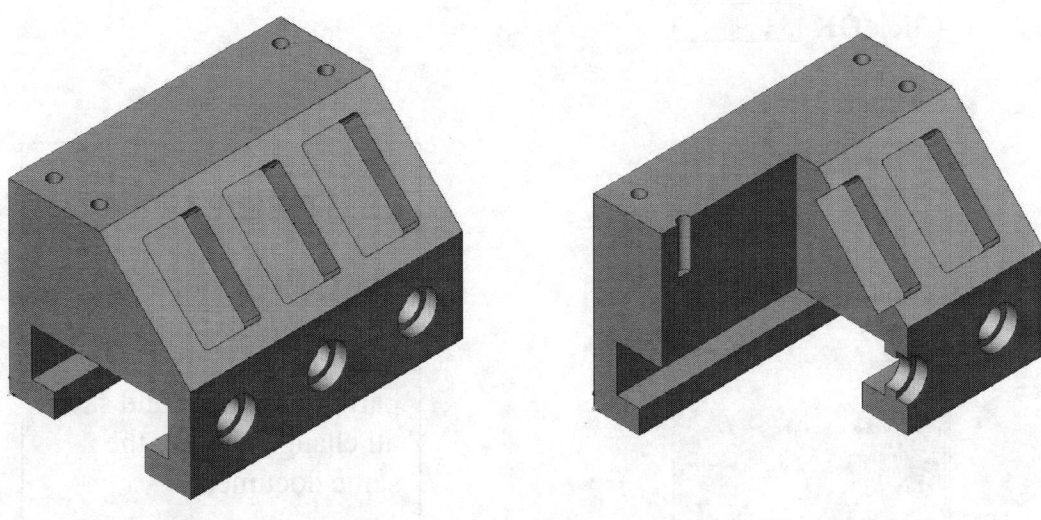

Default Configuration   **New Cutaway Configuration**

- At the top of the FeatureManager tree, select the Configuration tab.

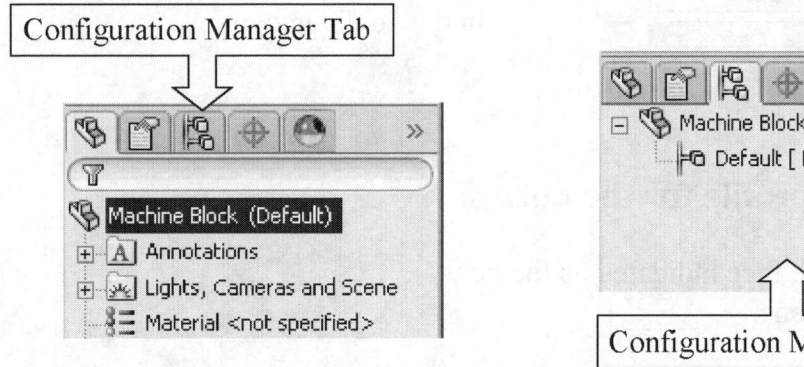

- Right click on the name of the part and select **Add Configuration**.

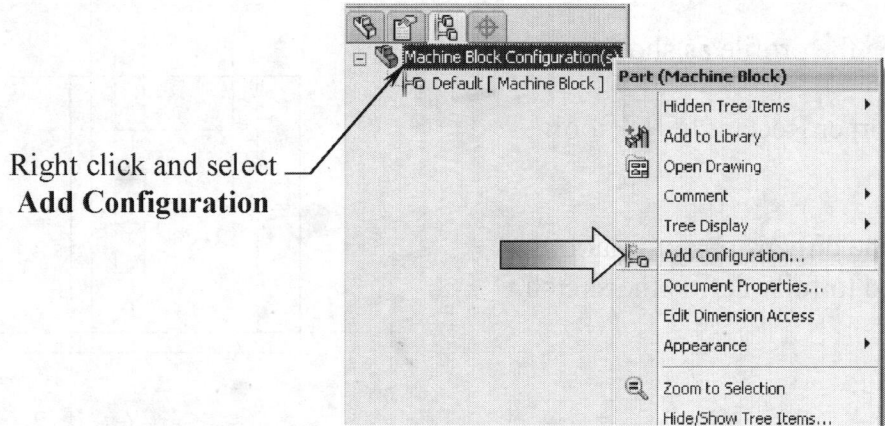

Right click and select
Add Configuration

- Under Configuration Name, enter: **Cutaway View.**

- Click **OK**   OK

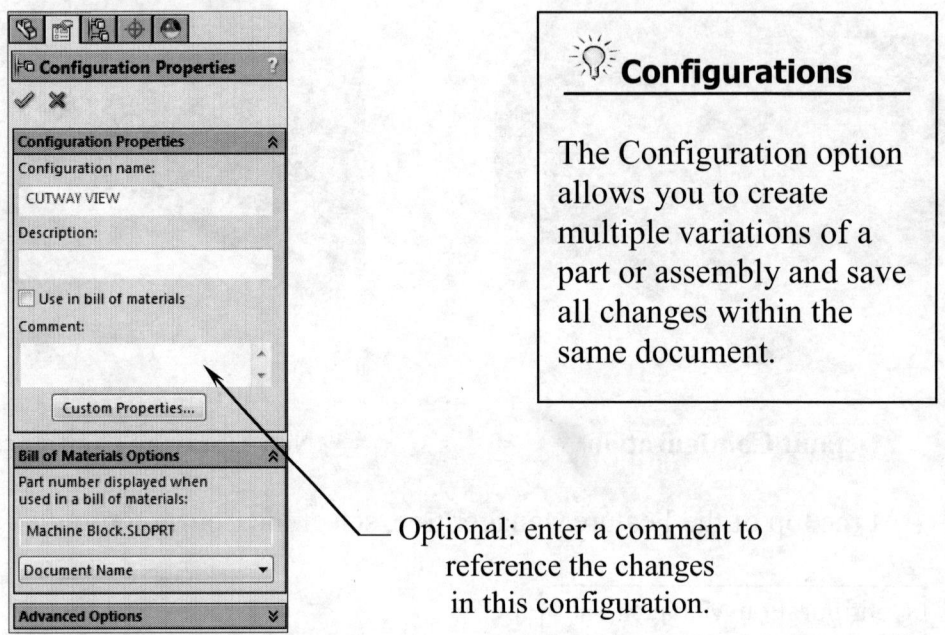

Configurations

The Configuration option allows you to create multiple variations of a part or assembly and save all changes within the same document.

Optional: enter a comment to
reference the changes
in this configuration.

12. Sketching a profile for the cut:

- Select the face indicated as the new sketch plane.

- Click or select **Insert / Sketch**.

- Sketch the profile as shown using the Corner Rectangle tool.

- Add the dimensions or relations needed to fully define the sketch.

Sketch face

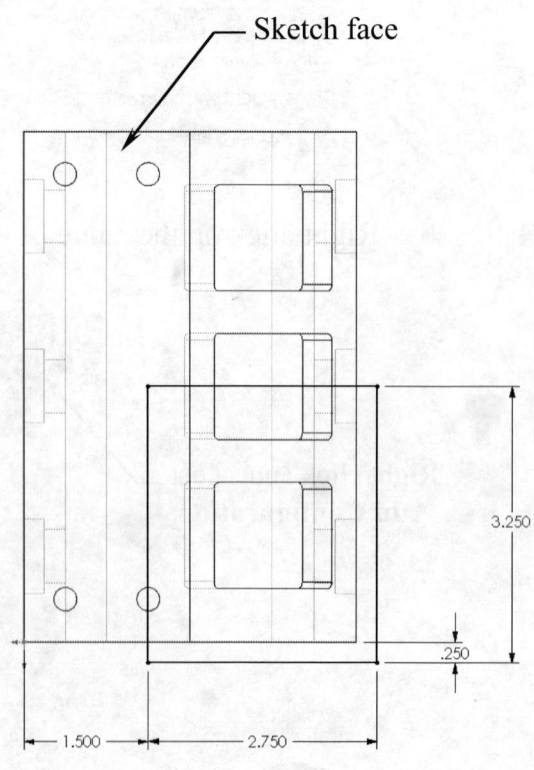

3.250

.250

1.500   2.750

13. Making the section cut:

- Click 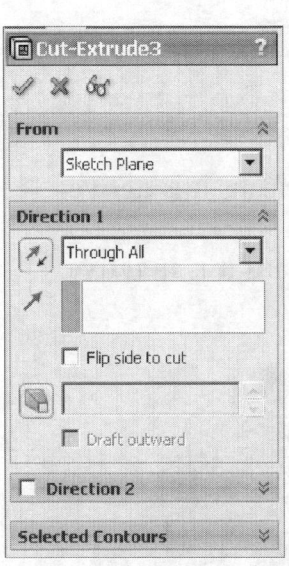 or select **Insert / Cut / Extrude**.

- End Condition: **Through All.**

- Click **OK** ✅.

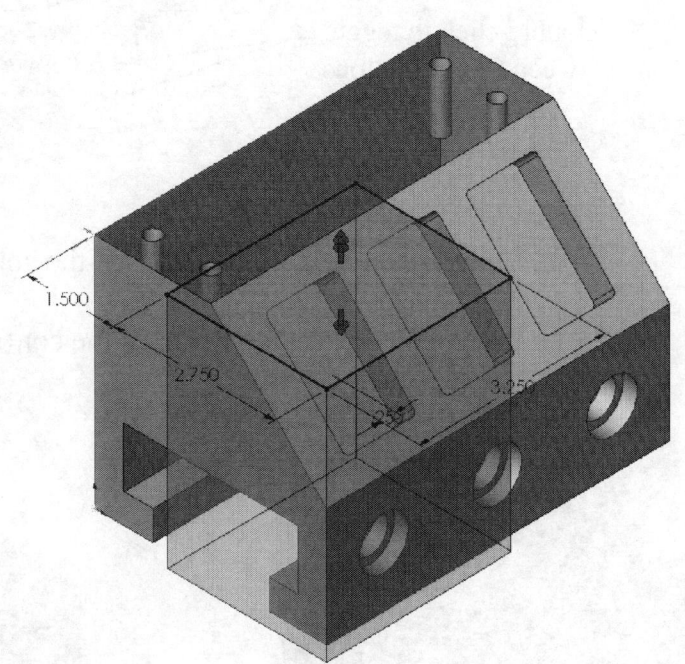

- The Cutaway section view.

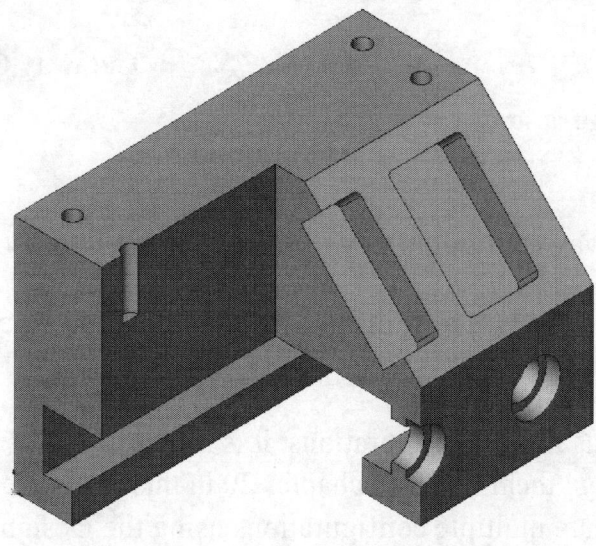

14. Switching between the Configurations:

- Double-click on Default configuration to see the original part.

- Double-click on Cutaway View configuration to see the cut feature.

Double-click to toggle between Configurations*

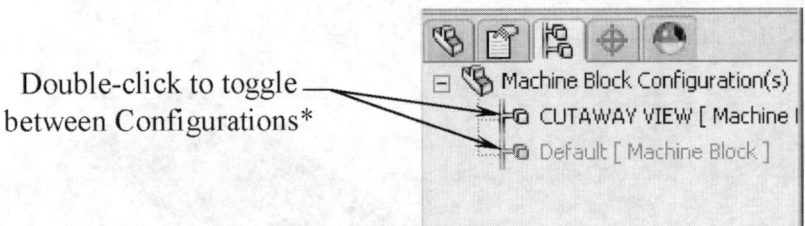

* The **Yellow** icon next to the name of the configuration means it is **active**.

* The **Grey** icon next to the name of the configuration means it is **inactive**.

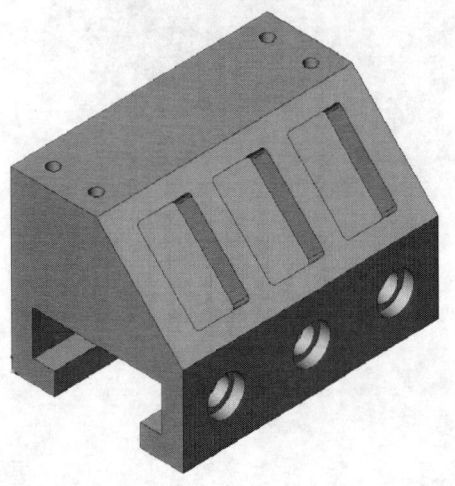

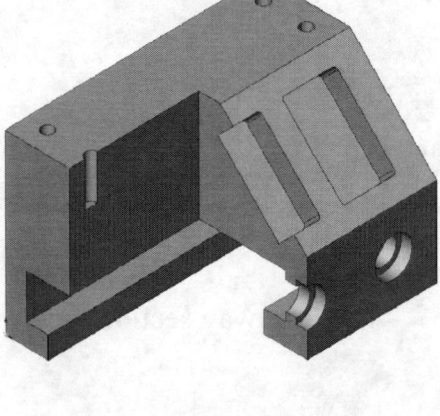

Cutaway Configuration

Default Configuration

- The Cutaway configuration will be used again in one of the drawing chapters.

- There is no limit on how many configurations can be created and saved in a part document.

- If a part has many configurations, it is might be better to use a design table to help manage them (refer to chapter 20 in this textbook for more infomation on how to create multiple configurations using the Design Table option).

15. Splitting the FeatureManager pane:

- Locate the Split Handle on top of the FeatureManager tree and drag it down about half way.

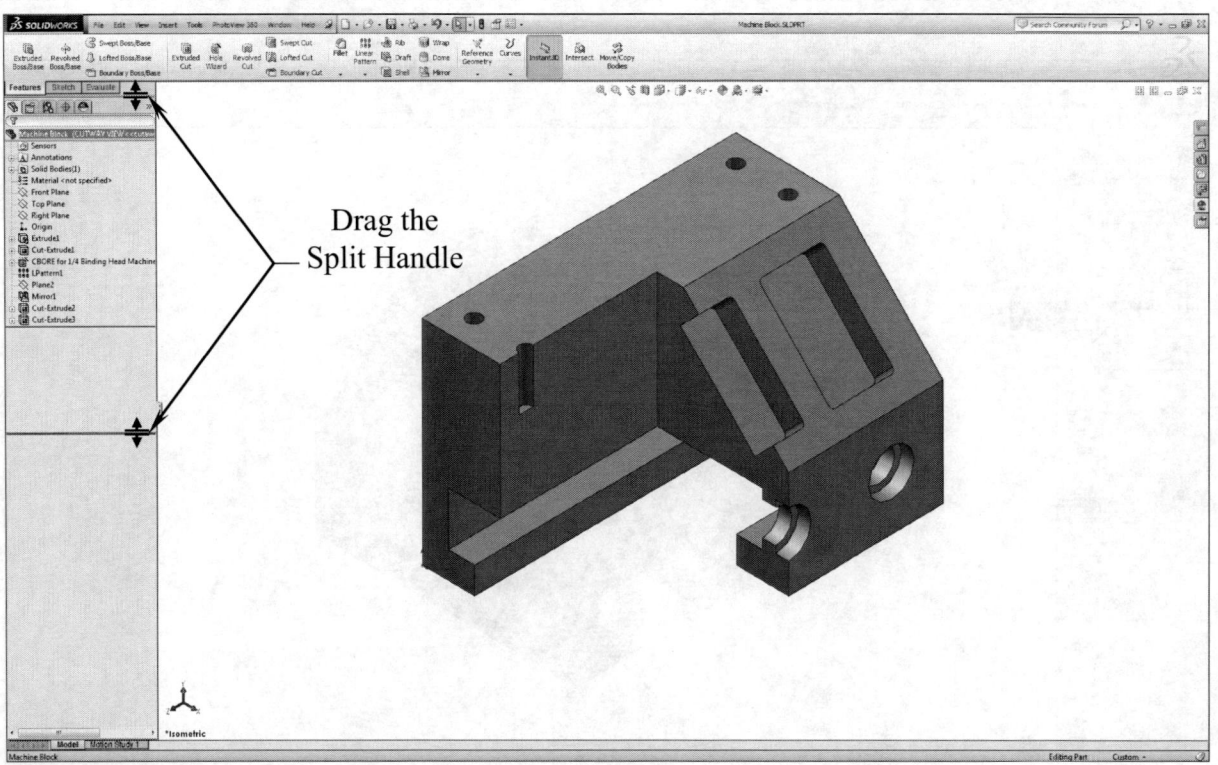

Drag the
Split Handle

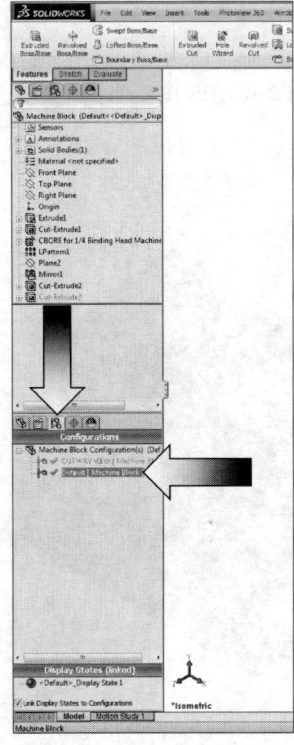

- Click the ConfigurationManager tab (arrow) to change the lower half to ConfigurationManager.

- Double click on the **Default** configuration to activate it.

16. Creating a new configuration:

- Right click the name of the part (arrow) and select: **Add Configuration** (arrow).

- For the name of the new configuration, enter: **Machine Features Suppressed**.

- Click **OK** to close the config. dialog (see next page)

- Hold the Control key and select the following cut features from the tree: **Cut-Extrude1, C'Bore for 1/4 Binding Head, LPattern1, Mirror1,** and **Cut-Extrude2**.

- Release the Control key and click the **Suppress** button from the popup window.

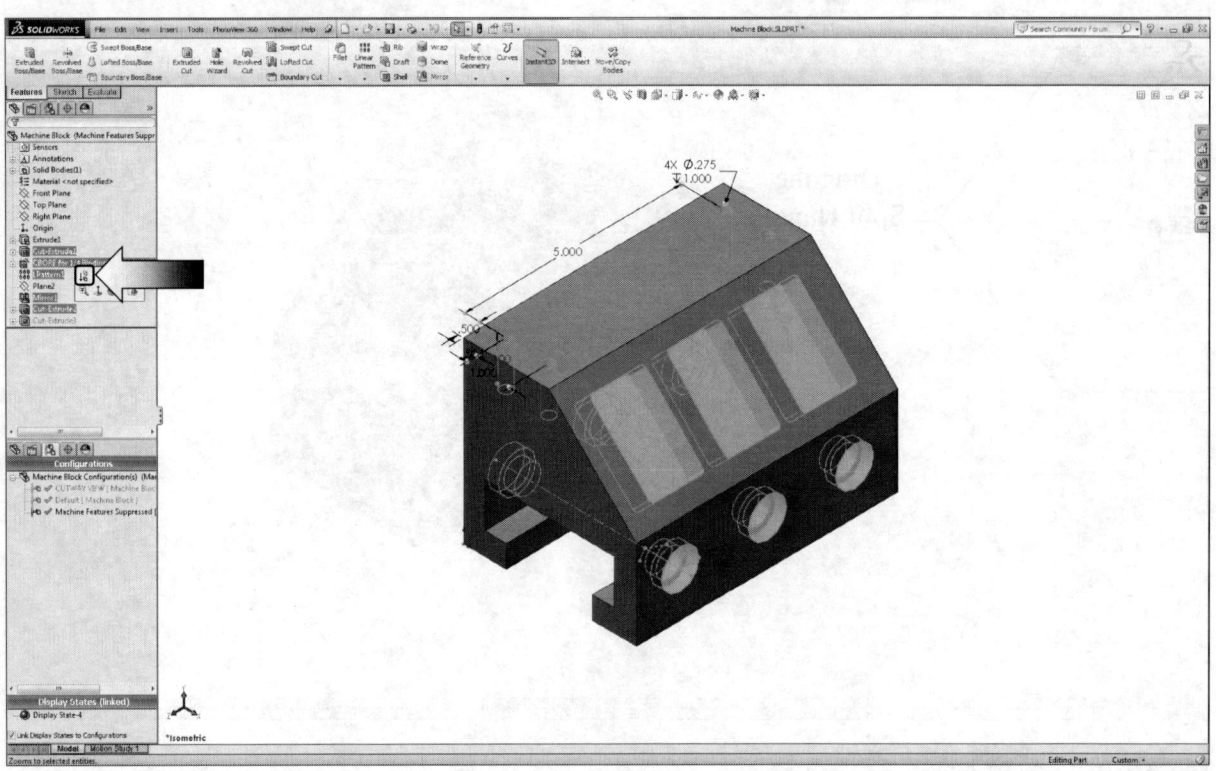

- The machine features are now suppressed and their feature icons are diplayed in grey color on the feature tree.

The machine features are now suppressed

- Double click on each configuration to see the changes between each one.

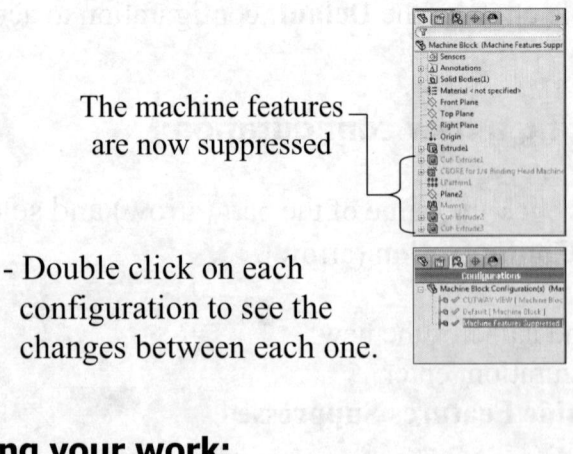

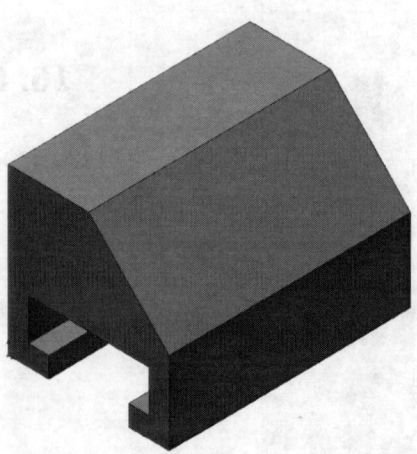

17. Saving your work:

- Select **File / Save As / Machined Block / Save**.

Questions for Review

Part Configurations

1. The five basic steps to create an extruded feature are:
   - Select a sketch Plane OR a planar surface
   - Activate Sketch Pencil (Insert / Sketch)
   - Sketch the profile
   - Define the profile (Dimensions / Relations)
   - Extrude the profile
   a. True
   b. False

2. When the extrude type is set to Blind, a depth dimension has to be specified as the End-Condition.
   a. True
   b. False

3. More than one closed sketch profiles on the same surface can be extruded at the same time to the same depth.
   a. True
   b. False

4. In the Hole Wizard definition, the Counter bore's parameters such as bore diameter, hole depth, etc. cannot be changed.
   a. True
   b. False

5. Holes created using the Hole Wizard cannot be patterned.
   a. True
   b. False

6. Configurations in a part can be toggled ON / OFF by double clicking on their icons.
   a. True
   b. False

7. Every part document can only have *one* configuration in it.
   a. True
   b. False

Exercise: Using Vary-Sketch.

1. The Vary Sketch allows the pattern instances to change dimensions as they repeat.
2. Create the part as shown, focusing on the Linear Pattern & Vary-Sketch option.

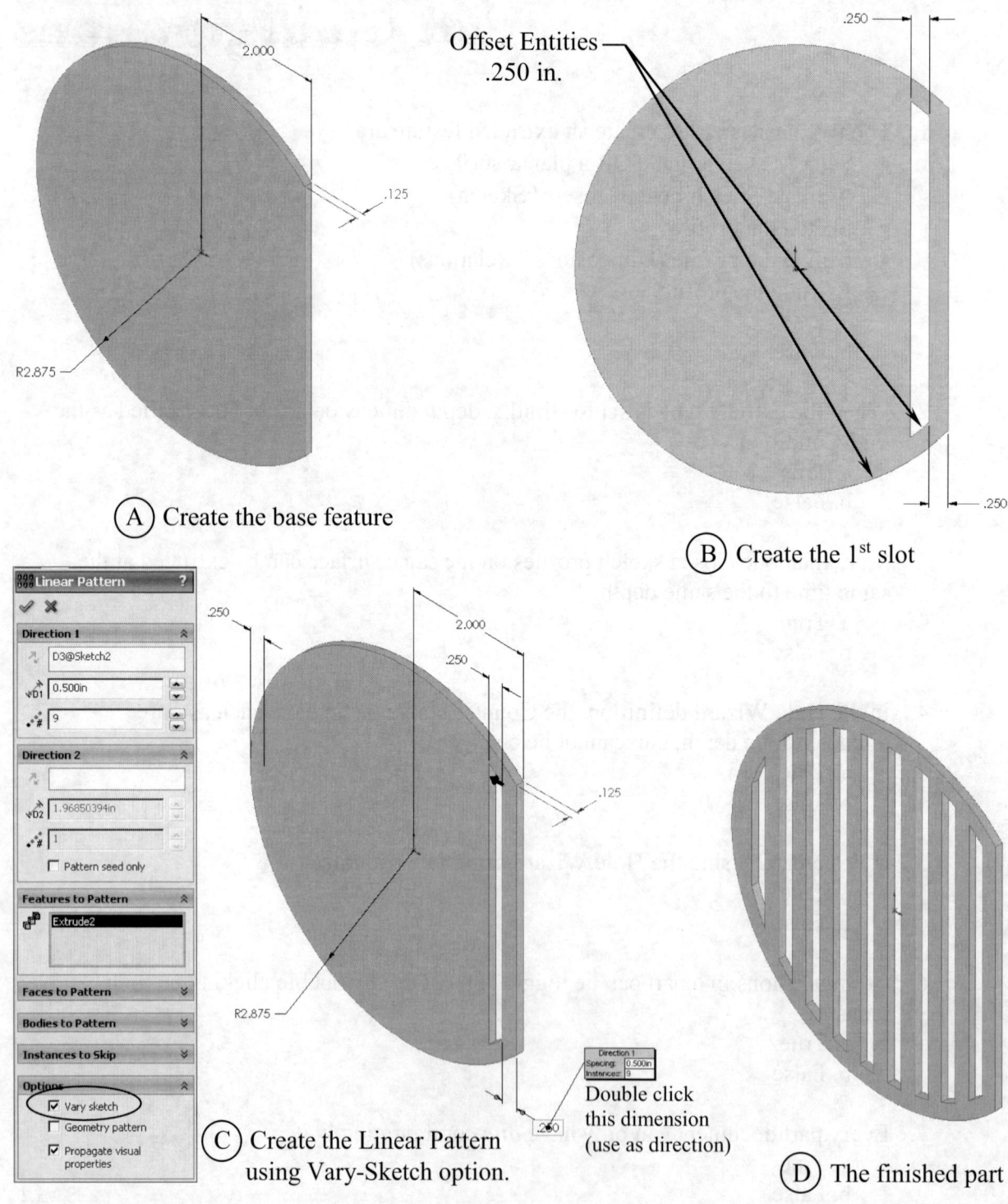

Ⓐ Create the base feature

Offset Entities .250 in.

Ⓑ Create the 1st slot

Ⓒ Create the Linear Pattern using Vary-Sketch option.

Double click this dimension (use as direction)

Ⓓ The finished part

3. Save your work as: **Vary Sketch_Exe**.

CHAPTER 8 (cont.)

Contour Selection

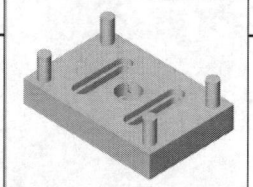

Contour Selection
Fixture

- The **Contour Selection** tool allows the SolidWorks user to select one or more closed contours in a sketch for use in a feature.

- Any sketches created in SolidWorks or imported from another CAD program, can be <u>reused</u> by using the Contour Select tool. This useful command allows the user to use a partial sketch to create features.

- The examples below show many possible contours available for extruding solid features within a single sketch.

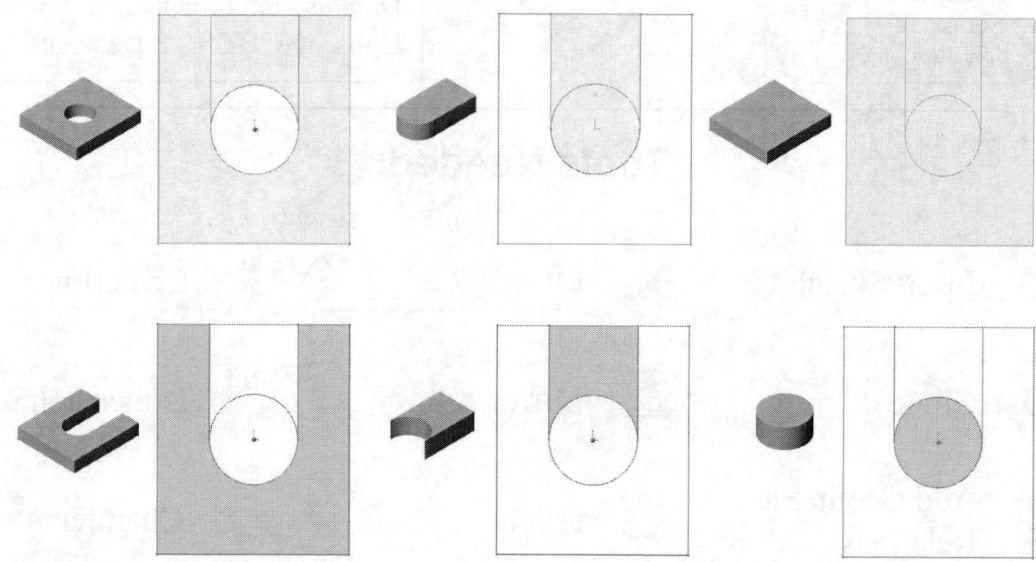

- This chapter and its exercise will guide you through the use of the Contour-Selection tool to convert 2D sketches into 3D models.

Fixture
Using Contour Selection

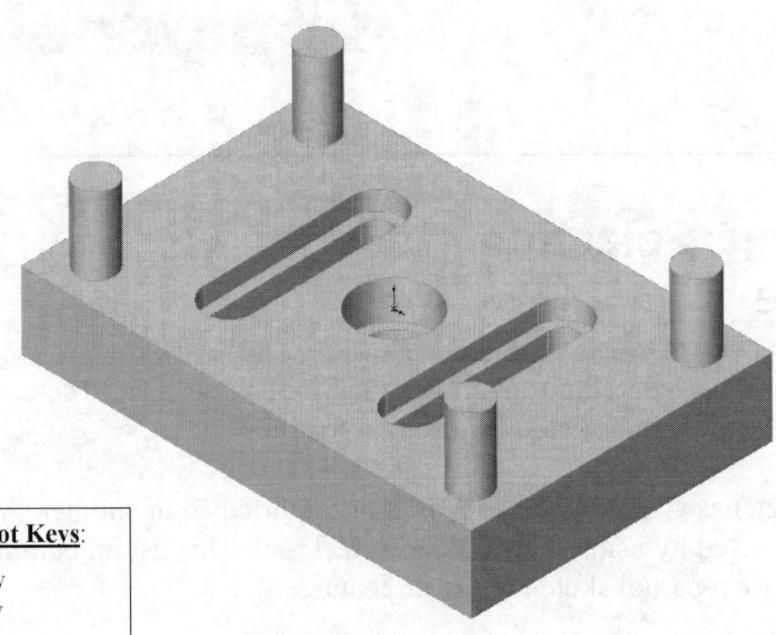

View Orientation Hot Keys:

Ctrl + 1 = Front View
Ctrl + 2 = Back View
Ctrl + 3 = Left View
Ctrl + 4 = Right View
Ctrl + 5 = Top View
Ctrl + 6 = Bottom View
Ctrl + 7 = Isometric View
Ctrl + 8 = Normal To
          Selection

Dimensioning Standards: **ANSI**
Units: **INCHES** – 3 Decimals

Tools Needed:

Insert Sketch		Line		Centerline	
Circle		Mirror		Dimension	
Add Geometric Relations		Fillet		Chamfer	
Extruded Boss/Base		Extruded Cut		Contour Select Tool	

1. Opening the main sketch:

- From the Training Files folder, open the SolidWorks document named:
  Contour Selection.sldprt

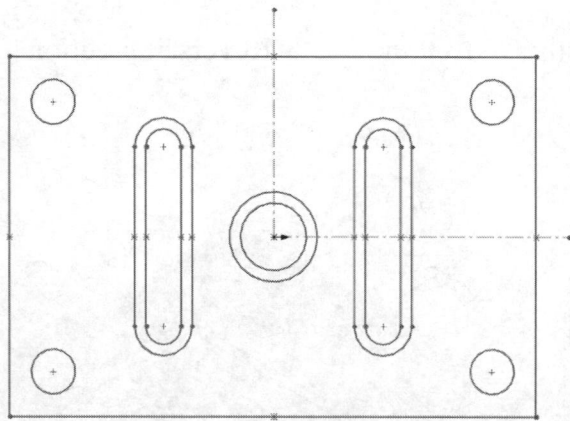

- **Edit** the sketch. Verify that the sketch is fully defined.

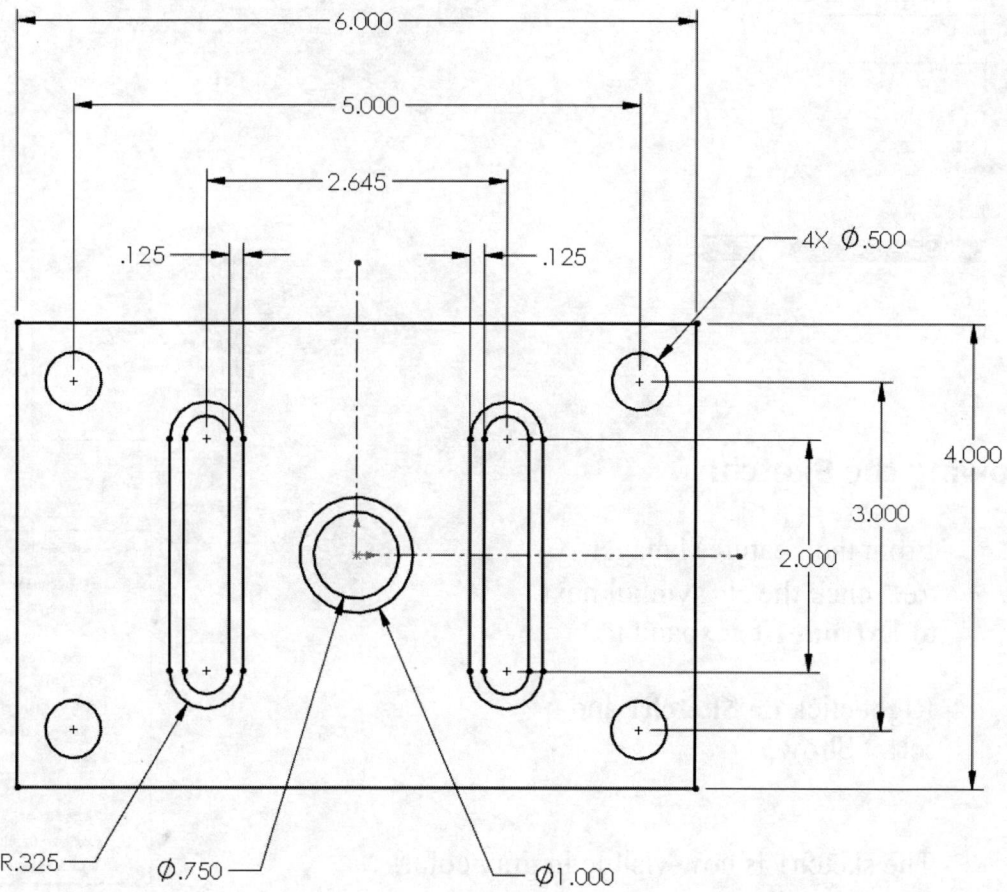

2. Extruding the Base:

- Click 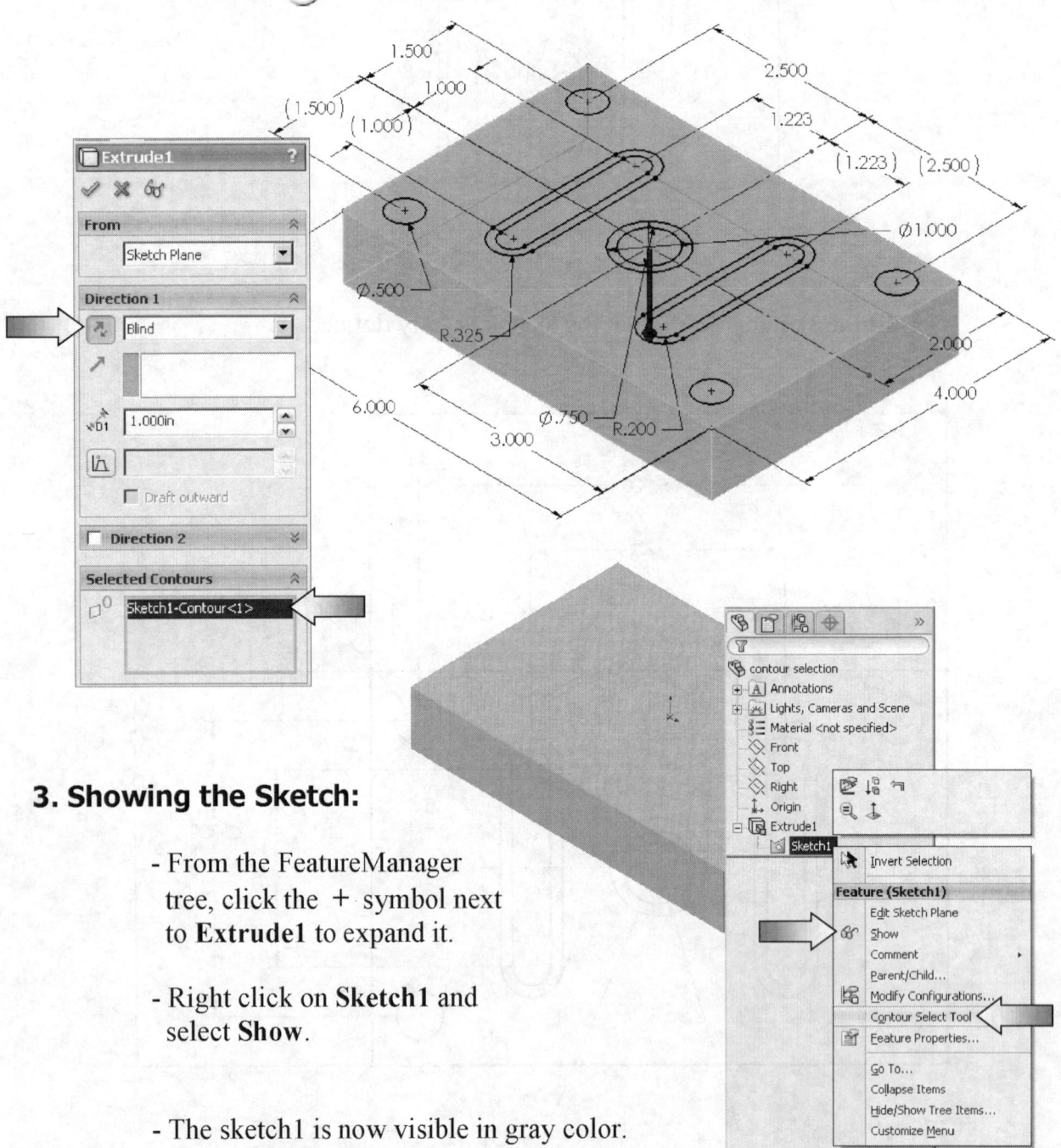 or select **Insert / Boss-Base / Extrude**.

- End Condition: **Blind**.

- Extrude Depth: **1.00 in**.   - Reverse Direction   **Enabled**

- Click **OK** .

3. Showing the Sketch:

- From the FeatureManager
  tree, click the **+** symbol next
  to **Extrude1** to expand it.

- Right click on **Sketch1** and
  select **Show**.

- The sketch1 is now visible in gray color.

4. Using the Contour Selection Tool:

- Right click on the line as indicated and select **Contour Selection Tool** .

Right click on
one of the lines…

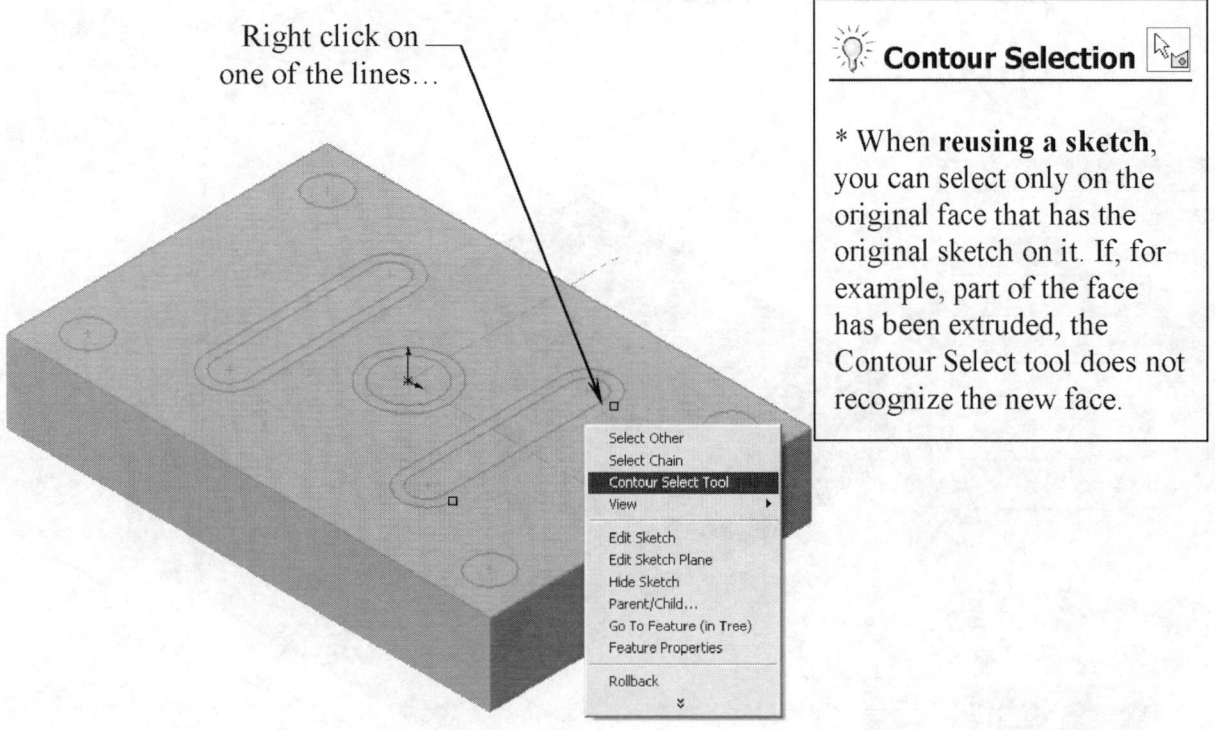

Select Other
Select Chain
Contour Select Tool
View ▶

Edit Sketch
Edit Sketch Plane
Hide Sketch
Parent/Child...
Go To Feature (in Tree)
Feature Properties

Rollback
⌄

💡 **Contour Selection** 🔲

* When **reusing a sketch**,
you can select only on the
original face that has the
original sketch on it. If, for
example, part of the face
has been extruded, the
Contour Select tool does not
recognize the new face.

- Hold down the CONTROL key and select the areas as indicated.

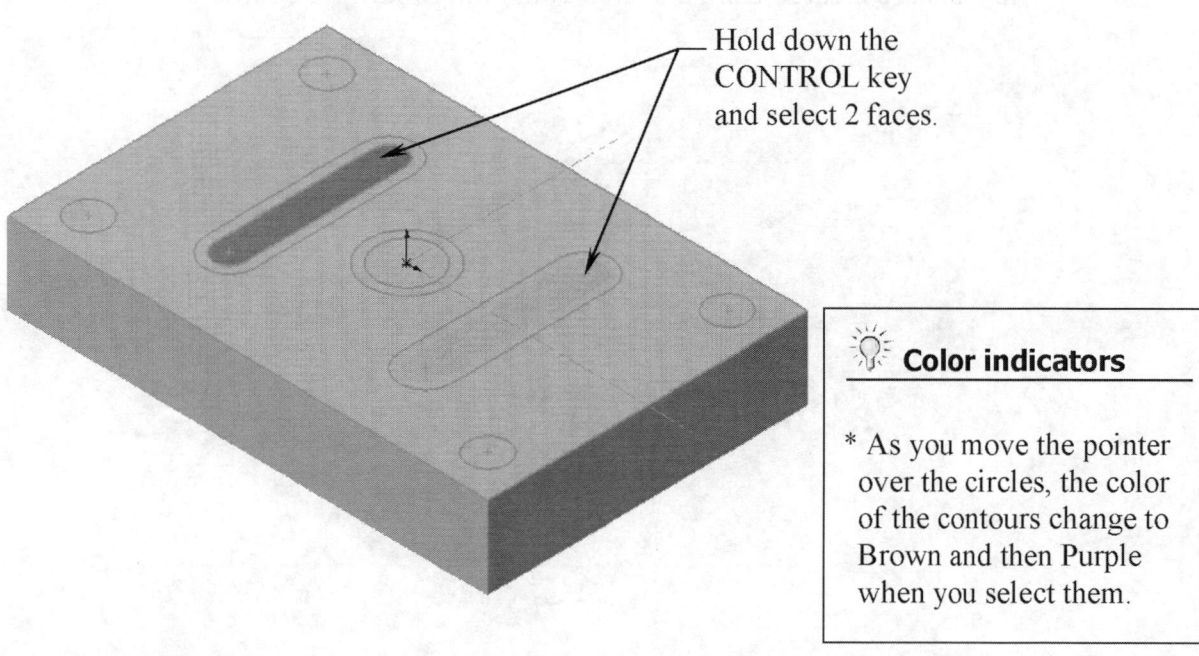

Hold down the
CONTROL key
and select 2 faces.

💡 **Color indicators**

* As you move the pointer
over the circles, the color
of the contours change to
Brown and then Purple
when you select them.

5. Extruding the selected contours as cut features:

- Click 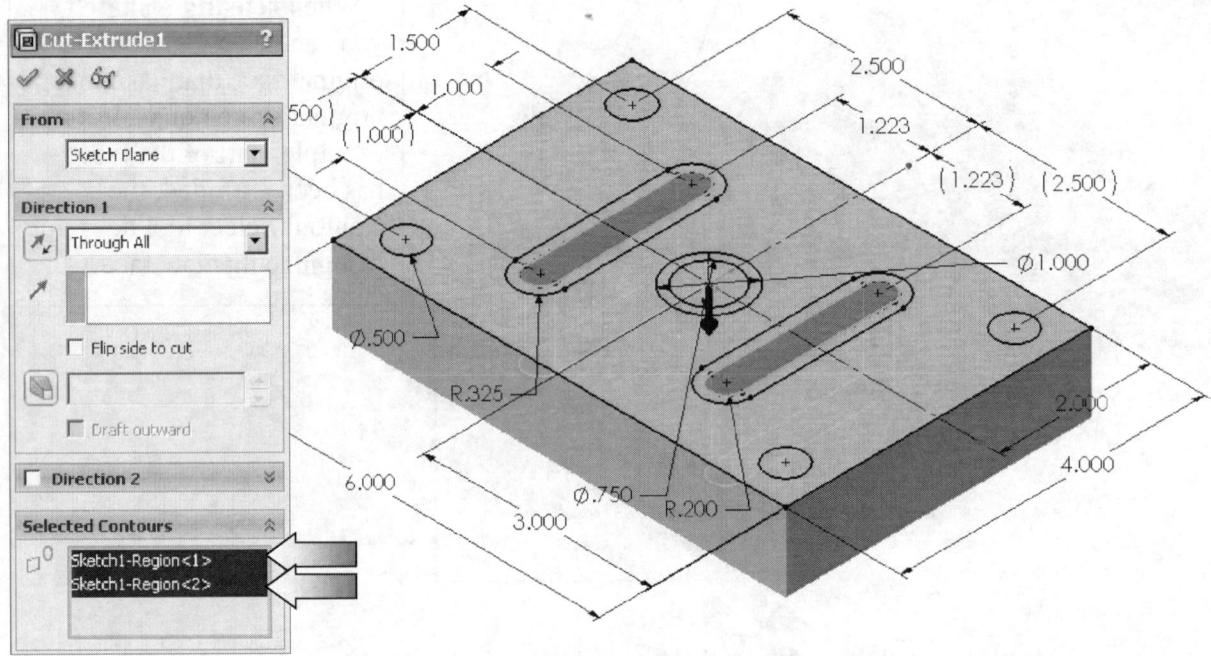 or select **Insert / Cut / Extrude**.

- End Condition: **Though All**

- Click **OK** ✓.

- The slots are created from a sketch containing multiple contours.

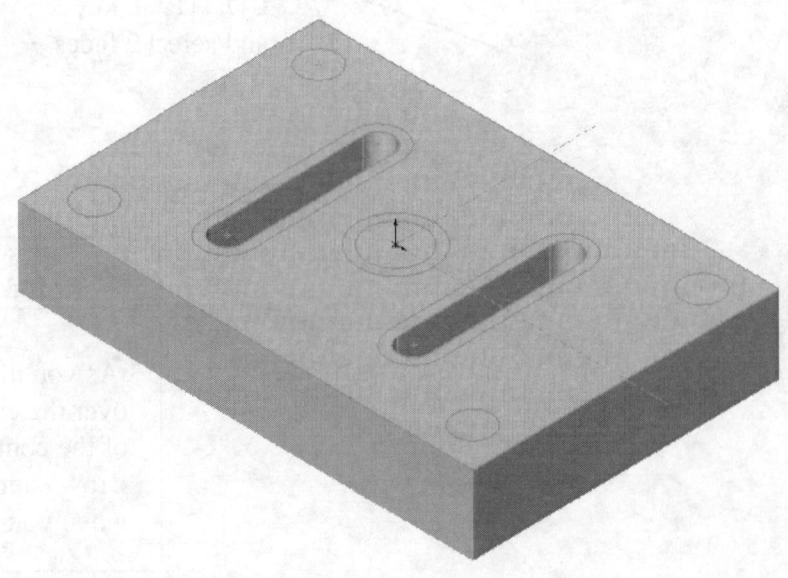

6. Re-using the same sketch:

- Right click on the line indicated and select **Contour Selection Tool** .

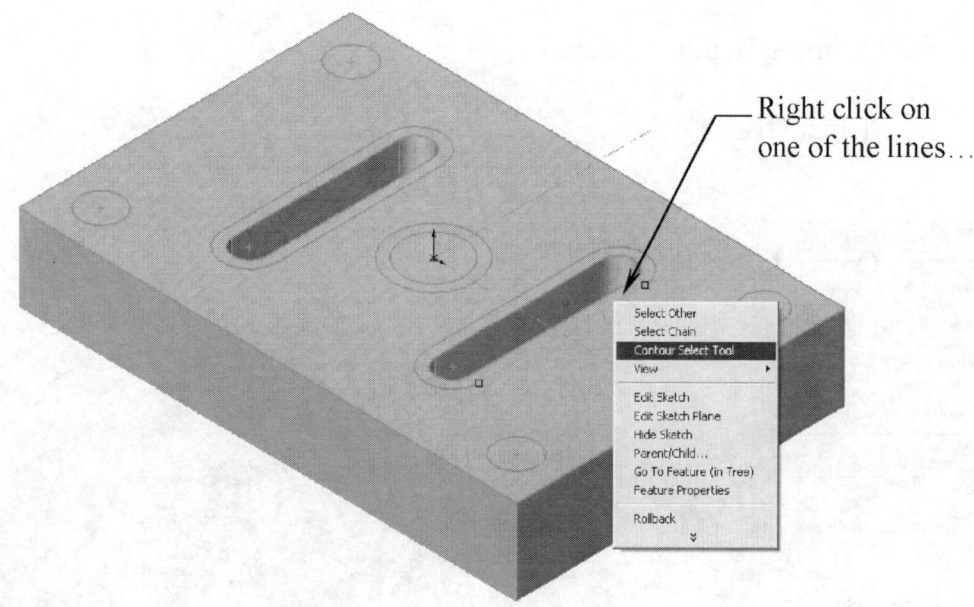

Right click on
one of the lines...

- Hold down the *CONTROL* key and select inside the faces as indicated.

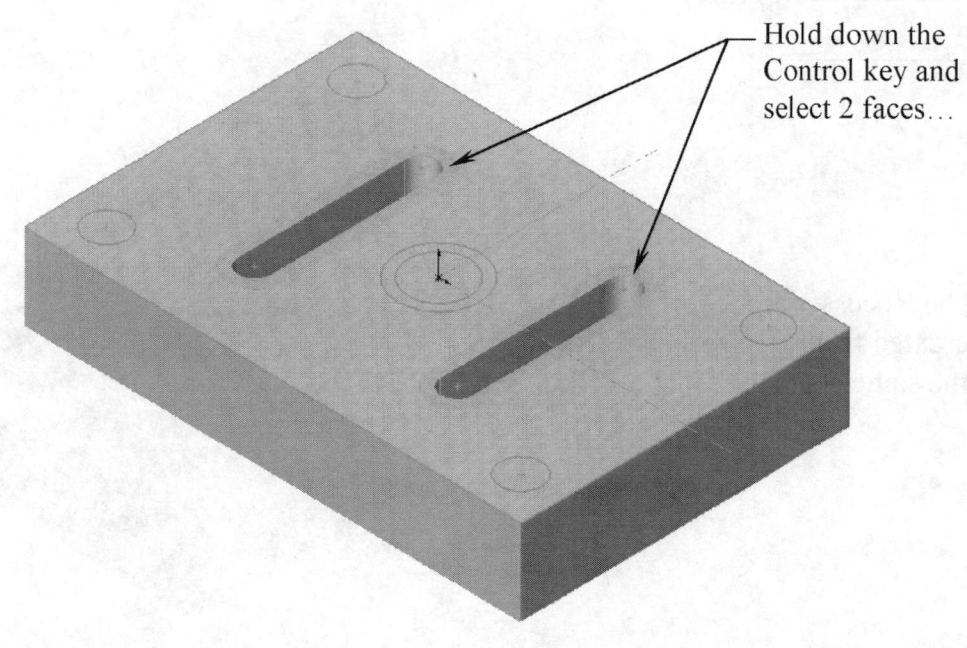

Hold down the
Control key and
select 2 faces...

7. Cutting the selected contours:

- Click 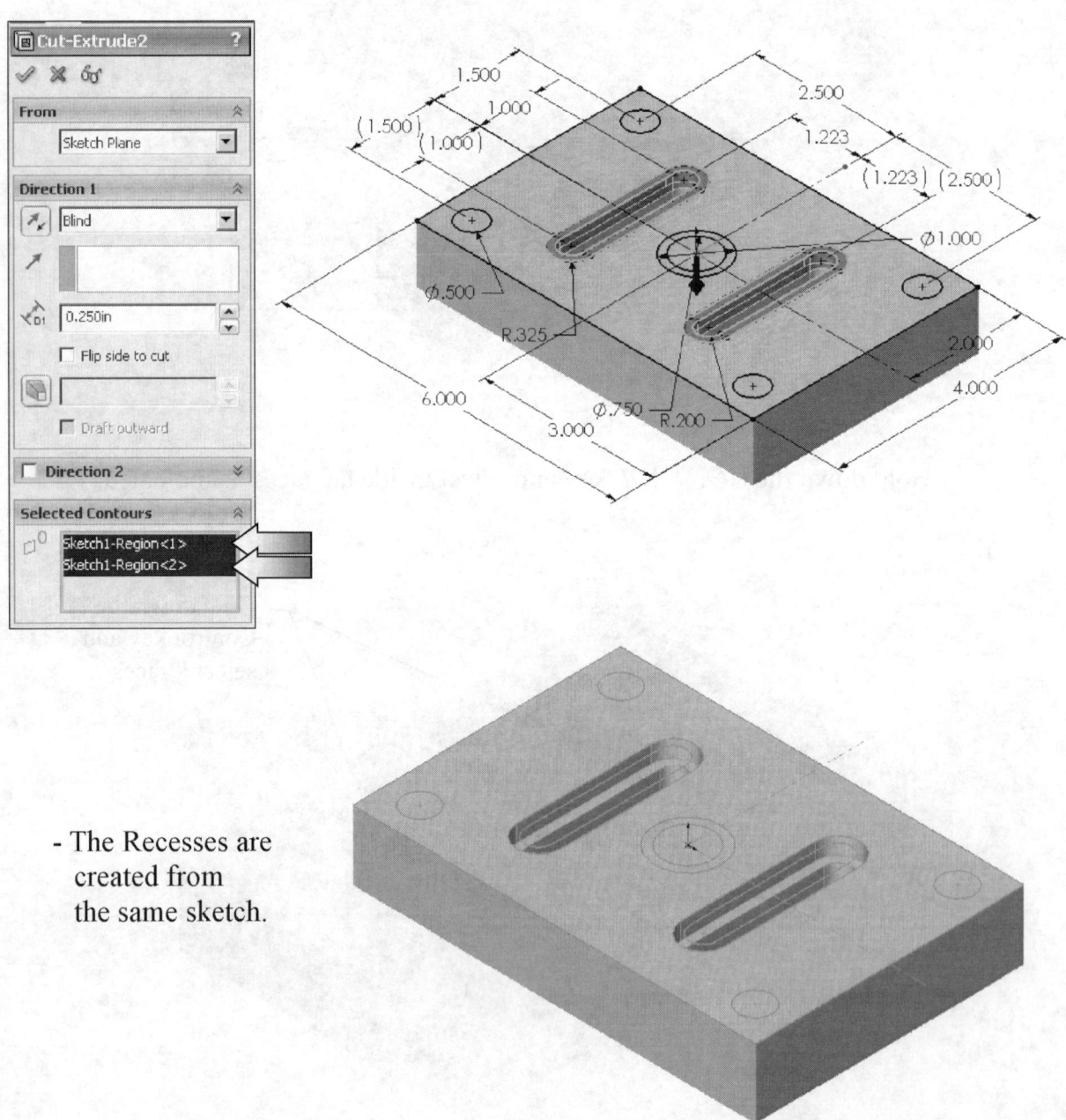 or select **Insert / Cut / Extrude**.

- End Condition: **Blind.**

- Extrude Depth: **.250 in**.

- Click **OK** ✅.

- The Recesses are
  created from
  the same sketch.

8. Continuing with other contours:

- Right click on the circle indicated and select: **Contour Selection Tool** .

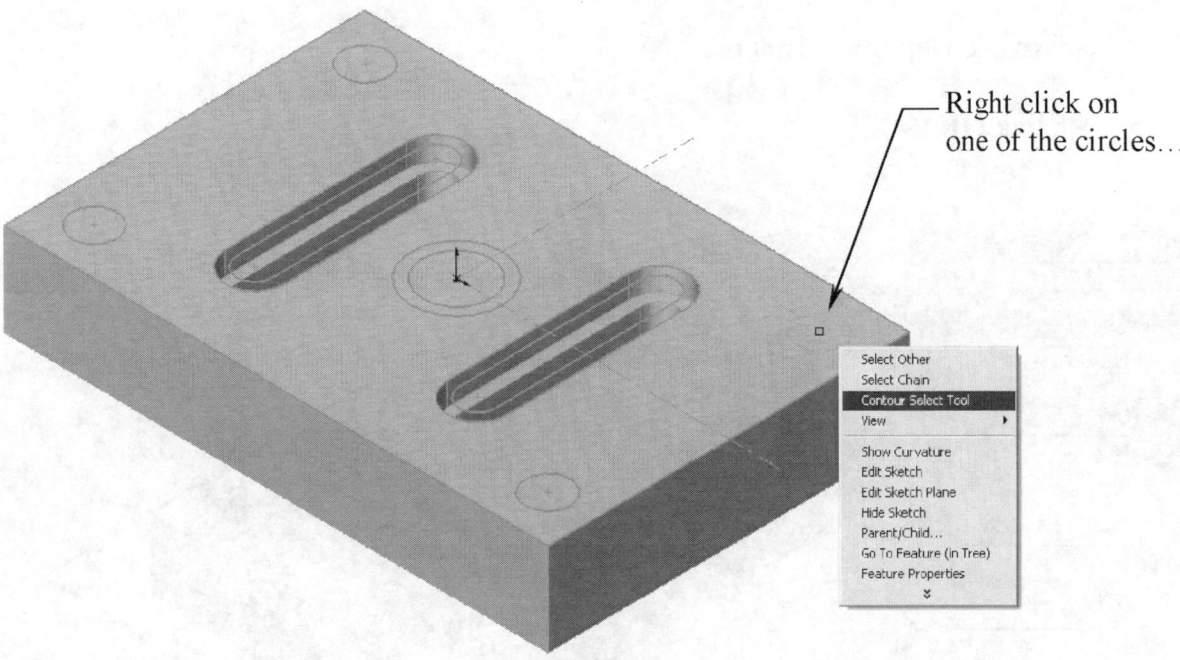

Right click on
one of the circles...

- Hold down the CONTROL key and select the faces as shown below.

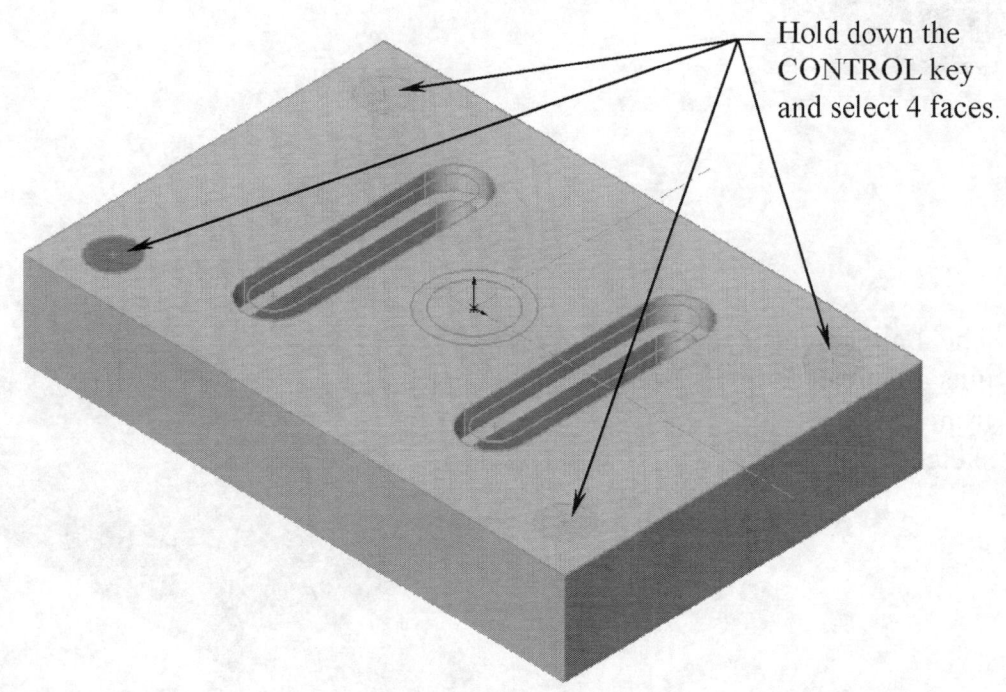

Hold down the
CONTROL key
and select 4 faces.

9. Extruding the selected contours:

- Click 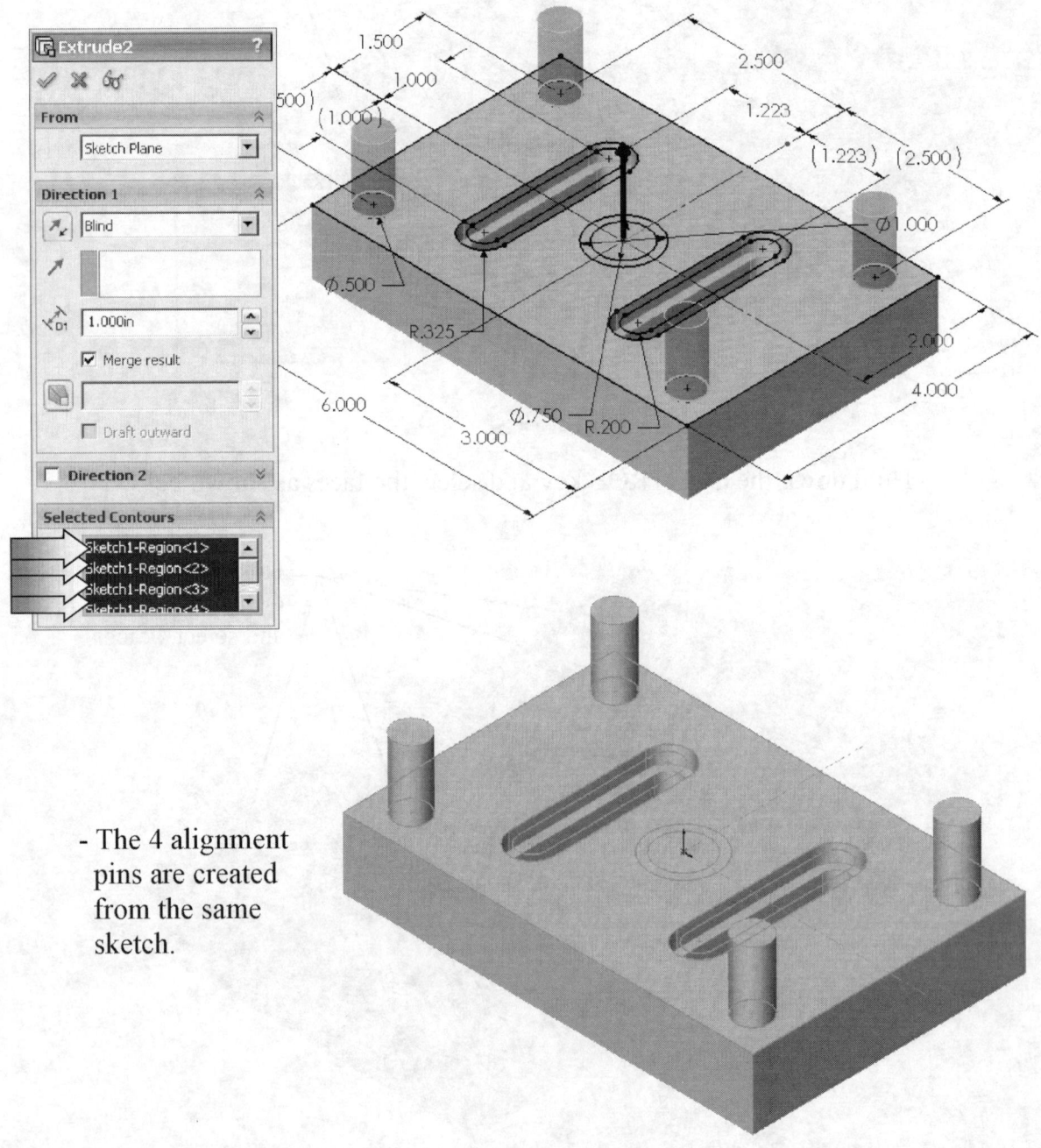 or select **Insert / Boss-Base / Extrude**.

- End Condition: **Blind.**

- Extrude Depth: **1.00 in**.

- Click **OK** .

- The 4 alignment pins are created from the same sketch.

10. Selecting the center contours:

- Right click on the circle indicated and select: **Contour Selection Tool** .

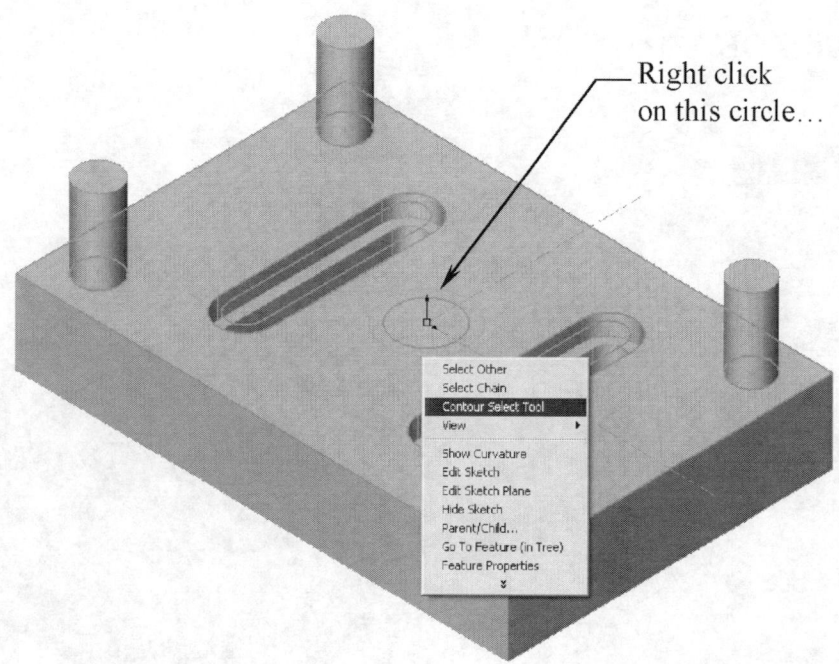

Right click
on this circle...

Select Other
Select Chain
Contour Select Tool
View
Show Curvature
Edit Sketch
Edit Sketch Plane
Hide Sketch
Parent/Child...
Go To Feature (in Tree)
Feature Properties

- Hover the mouse cursor over the circle in the center, select the contour when the color changes to Brown.

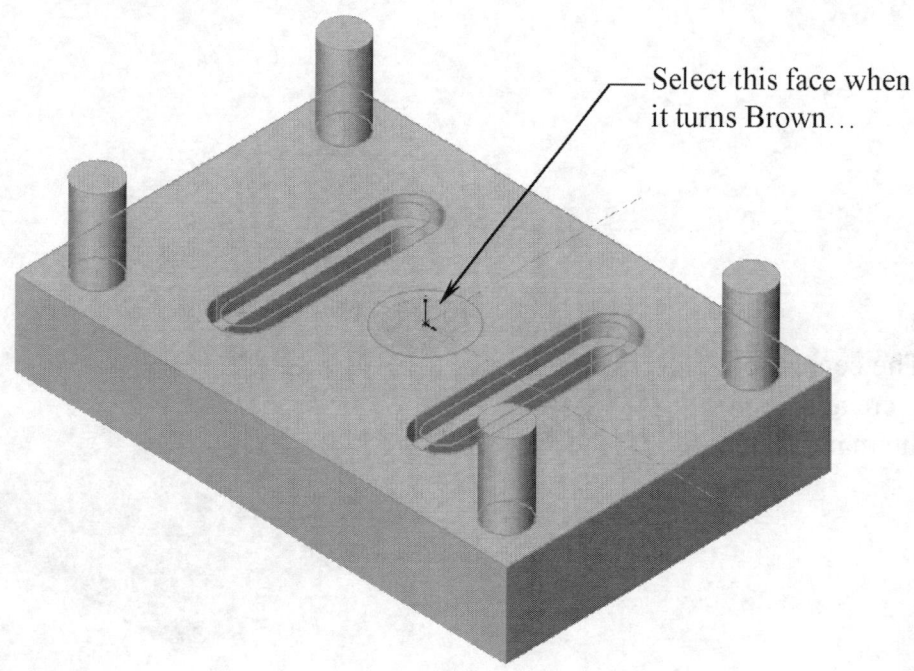

Select this face when
it turns Brown...

11. Extruding the selected contours as cut features:

- Click ⬚ or select **Insert / Cut / Extrude**.

- End Condition: **Though All.**

- Click **OK** ✓.

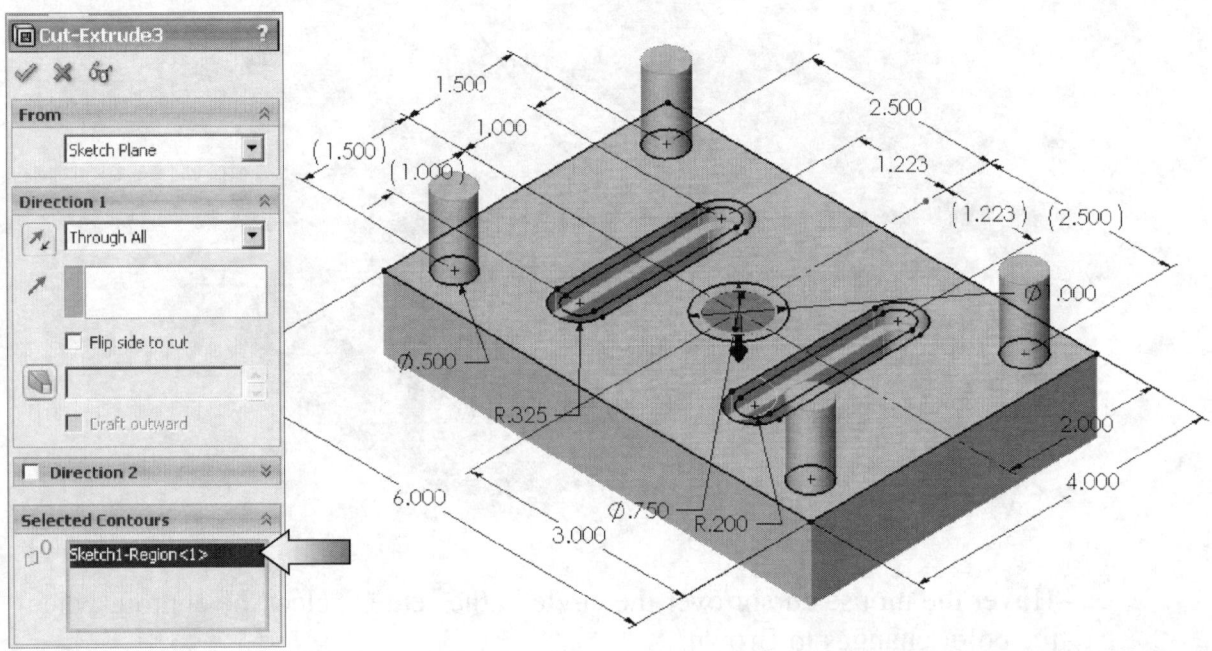

- The center hole
  is created from
  the main sketch.

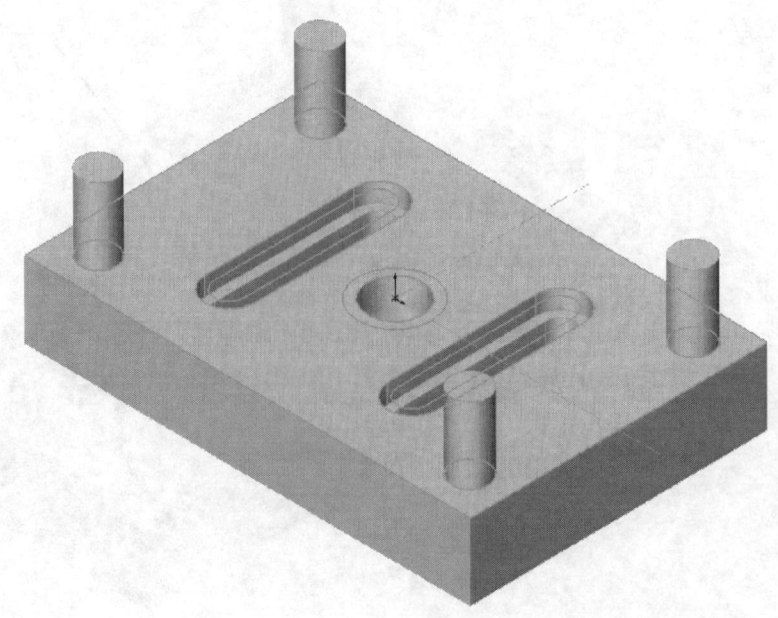

12. Selecting the next contour:

- Right click on the circle indicated and select: **Contour Selection Tool** .

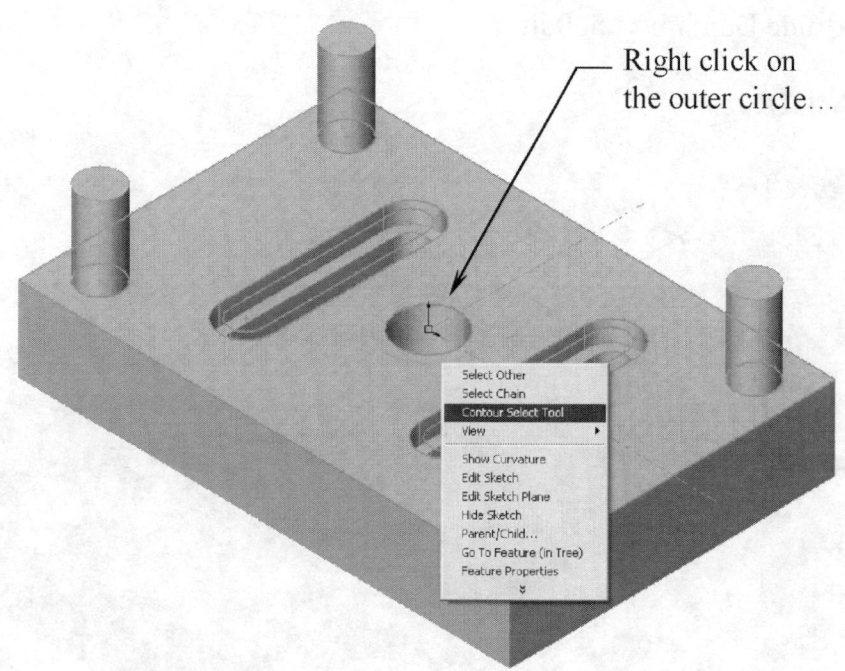

Right click on
the outer circle...

- Select the face as indicated when its color changes to Brown.

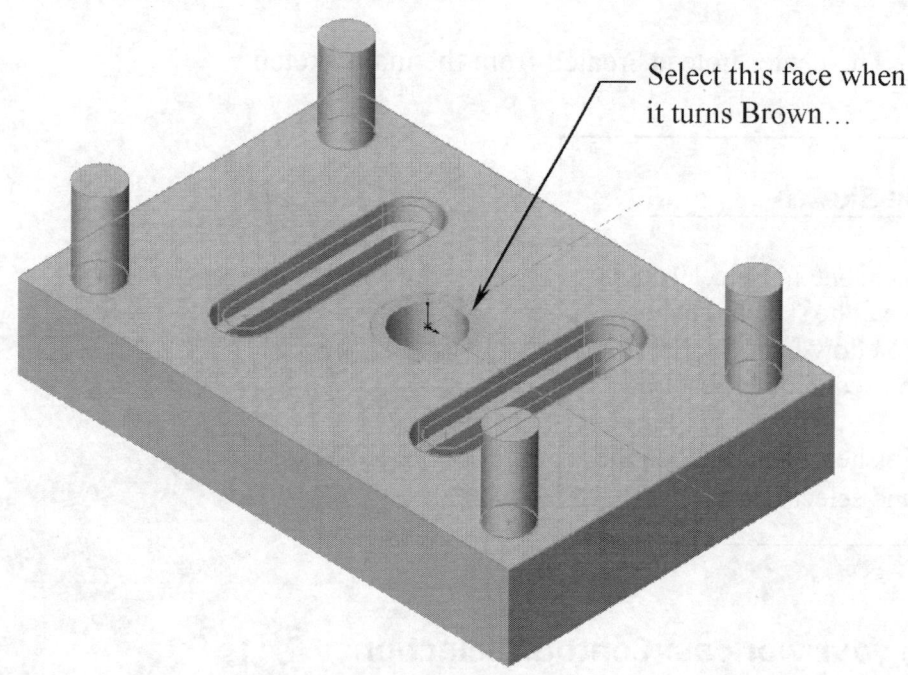

Select this face when
it turns Brown...

13. Cutting the center hole:

- Click 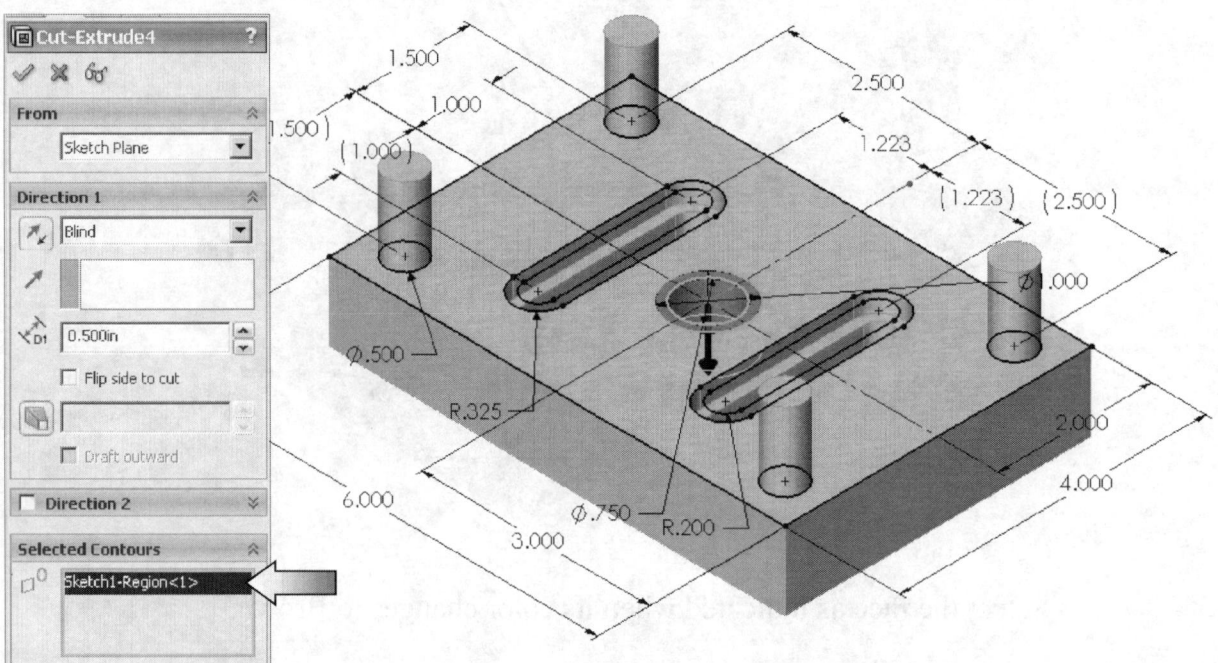 or select **Insert / Cut / Extrude**.

- End Condition: **Blind.**

- Extrude Depth: **.500 in**.

- Click **OK** ✓.

- The center hole is created from the main sketch.

☼ Hide Sketch

* When the Contour Select Tool is being used, the sketch remains visible (Yellow Icon) so that it can be reused in other features.

* When finished, right-click on the sketch and select **Hide**.

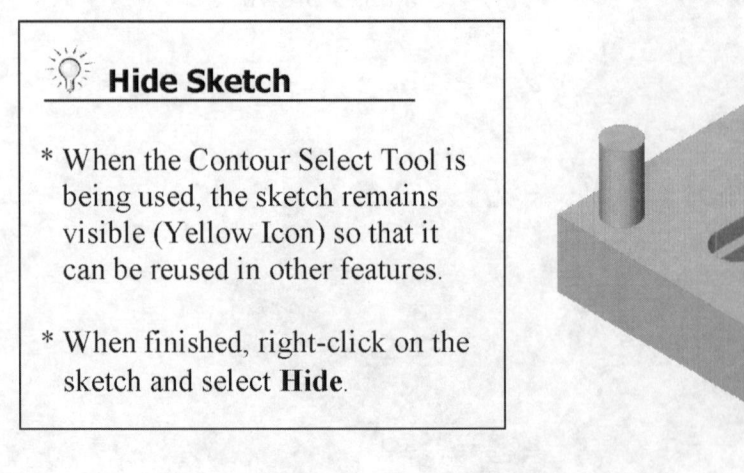

14. Save your work as: Contour Selection.

Questions for Review

Contour Selection

1. The Contour Select Tool allows you to select one or more closed contours in a sketch to convert into a feature.
   a. True
   b. False

2. When extruding several contours at the same time, they can have different depths.
   a. True
   b. False

3. Opened contours can be selected and extruded.
   a. True
   b. False

4. If several contours are selected, they will have to be extruded to the same depth.
   a. True
   b. False

5. As you drag the pointer over the contours, their colors change from Brown to Purple when selected.
   a. True
   b. False

6. The sketches cannot be reused; a new sketch has to be made each time.
   a. True
   b. False

7. The selected contours can be edited at any time.
   a. True
   b. False

8. To select multiple contours, hold down the key:
   a. Shift
   b. Control
   c. Alt

1. True   2. False
3. False   4. True
5. True   6. False
7. True   8. B

Exercise: Contour Selection

1. From the Training Files folder, open the document named:
   Contour Selection_Exe.
2. Use the Contour Selection tool to extrude all features.
3. The 4 holes are thru holes.
4. The upper boss is centered of the thickness.
5. Use the instructions on the next page, if needed.

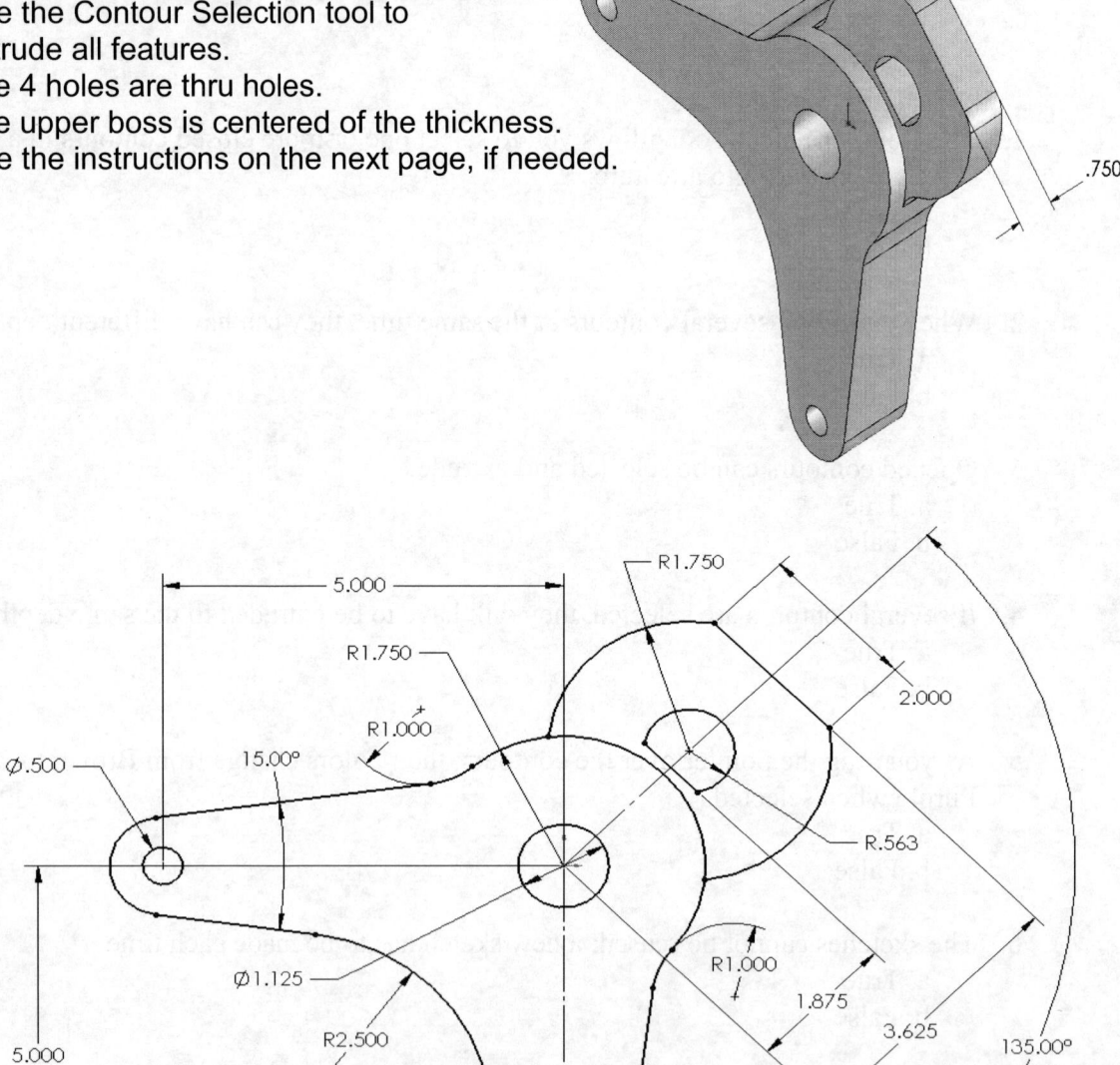

6. Save a copy of your work as: **Contour Selection_Exe**.

1. Activating the Contour Select tool:

- Right click on one of the lines and pick: **Contour-Select Tool**.

- Hove the mouse in the area as noted and select it when the color changes to magenta.

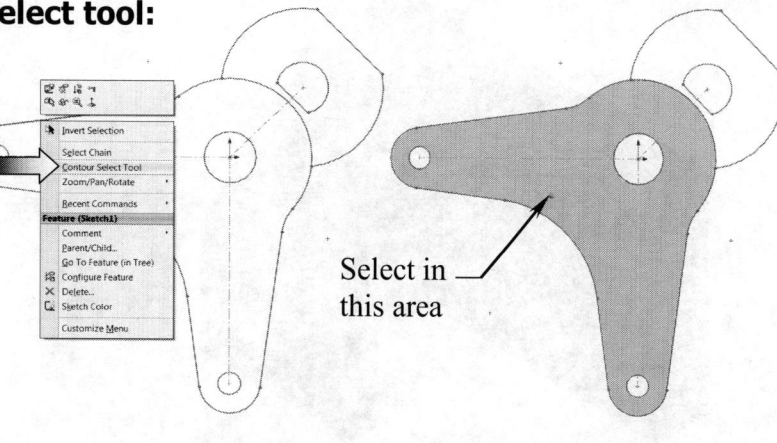

Select in this area

2. Extruding the base:

- Create an **Extruded Boss-Base** using **Mid Plane** at **1.500"** thick.

3. Selecting another contour:

- Expand the Boss-Extrude1 feature and <u>show</u> the **Sketch1**.

- Right click on one of the lines and pick: **Contour Select Tool**.

- Select the upper contour when the color changes to magenta.

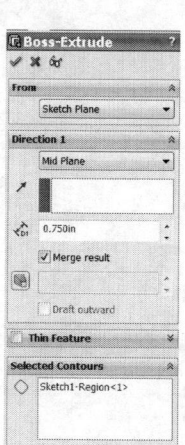

Select this contour

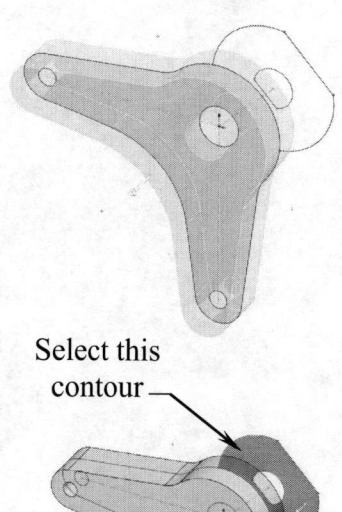

4. Extruding the upper boss:

- Extrude the selected contour using **Mid Plane** at **.750"** thick.

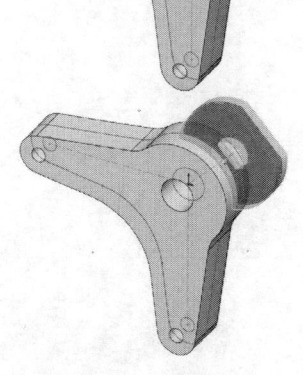

5. Adding fillets:

- Add a **.500"** fillet to the 4 edges as indicated.

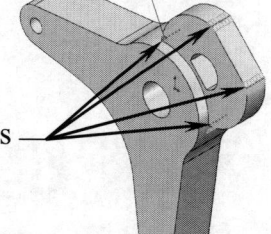

Fillet 4 edges

6. Saving your work:

- Save a copy of your work as: **Contour_Selection_Exe**.

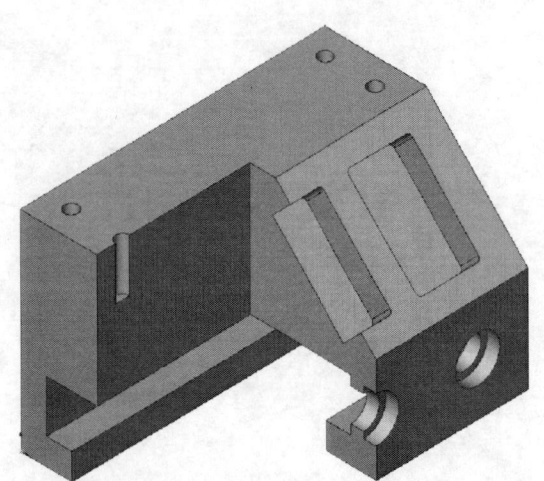

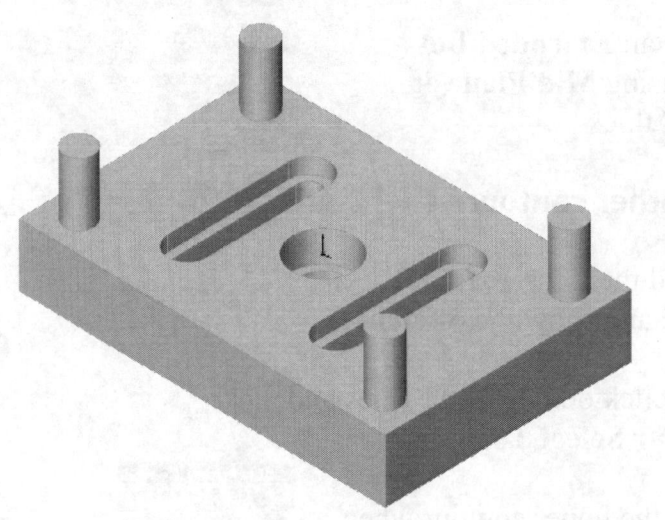

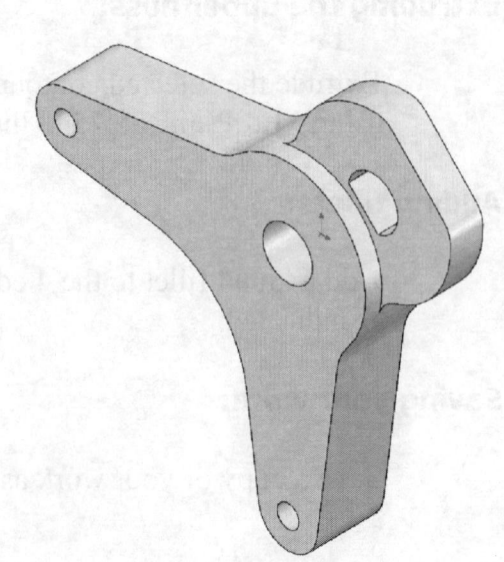

CHAPTER 9

Modeling Threads

Modeling Threads (external)
Threaded Insert

- Most of the time threads are not modeled in the part, instead they are represented with dashed lines and callouts in the drawings. But for non-standard threads they should be modeled in the part for use in some applications such as Stereo Lithography, Finite Element Analysis, etc.

- Two sketches are involved in making the threads:

  * A sweep path (a helix that controls the pitch, revolutions, starting angle, and left or right hand threads).

  * A sweep profile (shape and size of the threads).

- The sweep profile should be related to the sweep path with a **pierce** relation, which will move the sketch profile to the end of the path.

- The profile is swept along the path with the command swept cut and the interfered material is removed as the result of the cut.

- Most of the time the sweep cut command is used when creating threads but in some cases, the sweep boss command can also be used to add material to the sweep path when making the external threads.

- This chapter and its exercises will guide you through some special techniques on how internal and external threads can be modeled in SolidWorks.

Modeling Threads – External
Threaded Insert

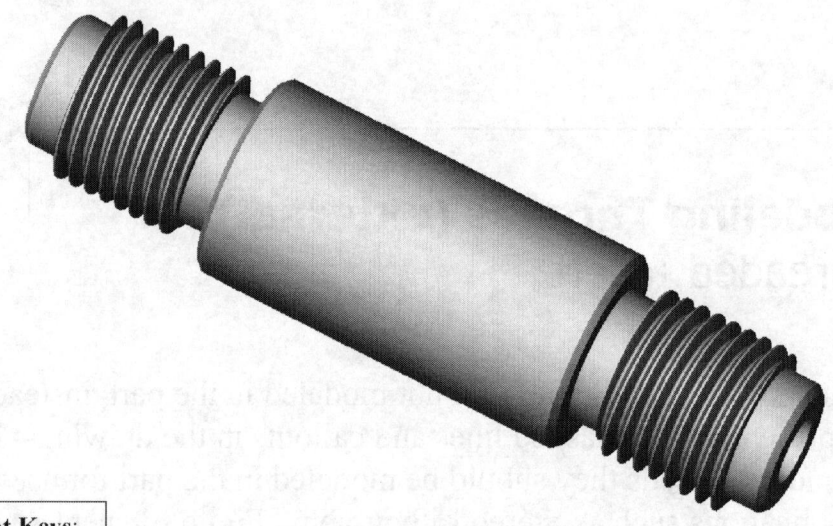

View Orientation Hot Keys:

Ctrl + 1 = Front View
Ctrl + 2 = Back View
Ctrl + 3 = Left View
Ctrl + 4 = Right View
Ctrl + 5 = Top View
Ctrl + 6 = Bottom View
Ctrl + 7 = Isometric View
Ctrl + 8 = Normal To
      Selection

Dimensioning Standards: **ANSI**

Units: **INCHES** – 3 Decimals

Tools Needed:

Insert Sketch	Line	Convert Entities
Dimension	Add Geometric Relations	Helix/Spiral
Extruded Base / Revolve	Cut Sweep	Mirror

1. Sketching the base profile:

- Select the <u>Front</u> plane from the FeatureManager Tree.

- Click Sketch 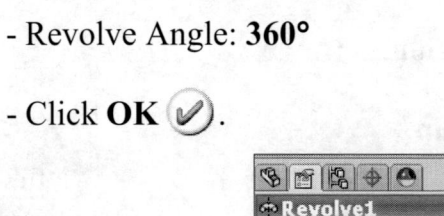 or select: **Insert / Sketch**.

- Sketch the profile as shown below using the Line tool .

- Add dimensions to fully define the sketch.

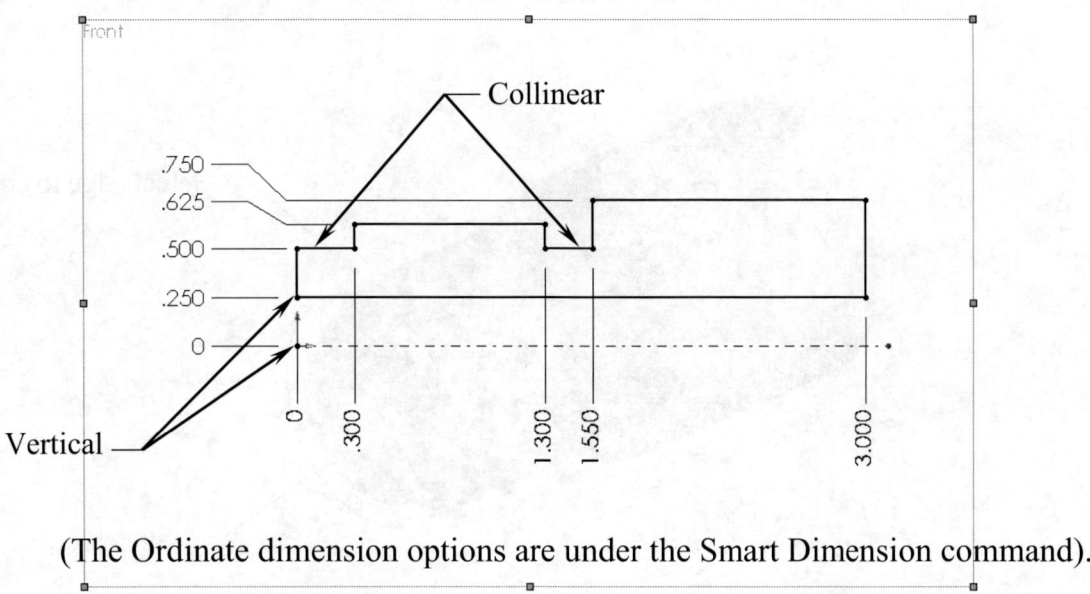

(The Ordinate dimension options are under the Smart Dimension command).

2. Revolving the base feature:

- Click **Revolve** or select **Insert / Base / Revolve**.

- Revolve Direction: **Blind**.

- Revolve Angle: **360°**

- Click **OK** .

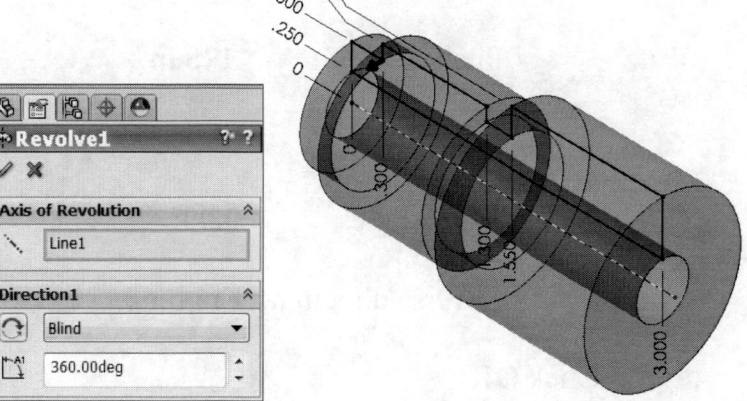

3. Creating the Sweep path:

- Select the <u>face</u> indicated as sketch face.

- Click Sketch 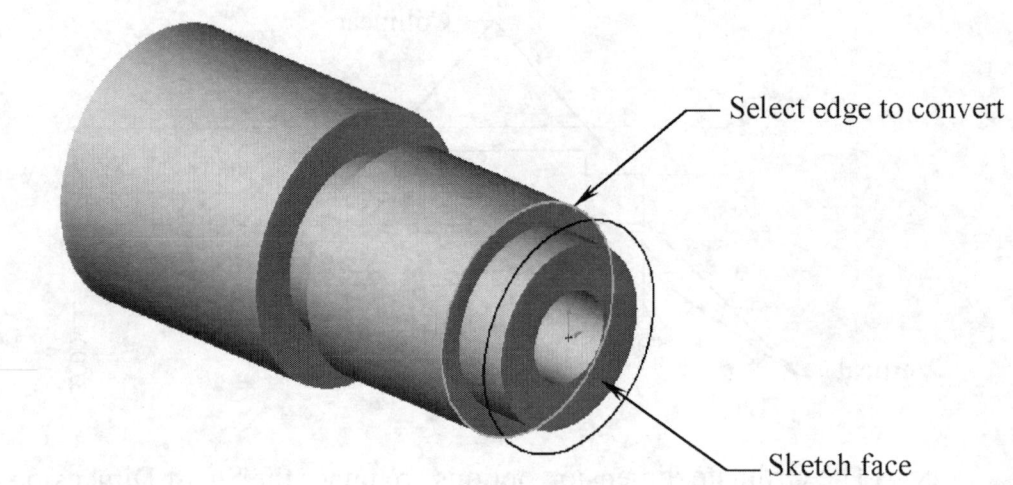 or select: **Insert / Sketch**.

- Select the **circular edge** as indicated.

- Click **Convert Entities** , the select edge is converted to a circle and brought to the sketch face.

Select edge to convert

Sketch face

4. Creating the Helix:

- Switch to the Features tool tab and select the helix command under the Curves button or select: **Insert / Curve / Helix Spiral**.

- Defined by: **Pitch and Revolution.**

       * Pitch: **.125 in**.

       * Revolution: **11.00**

       * Start Angle: **0.00°**

       * Reverse direction: **Enabled.**

- Click **OK** .

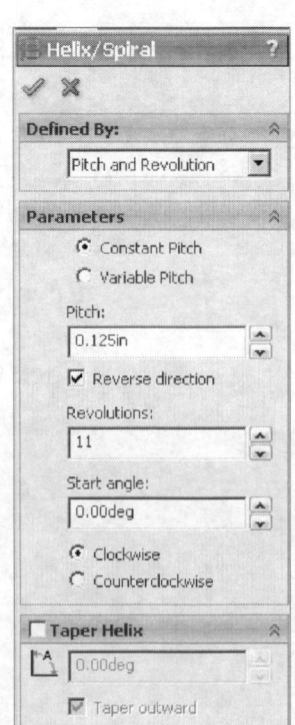

- The resulting Helix (the sweep path).

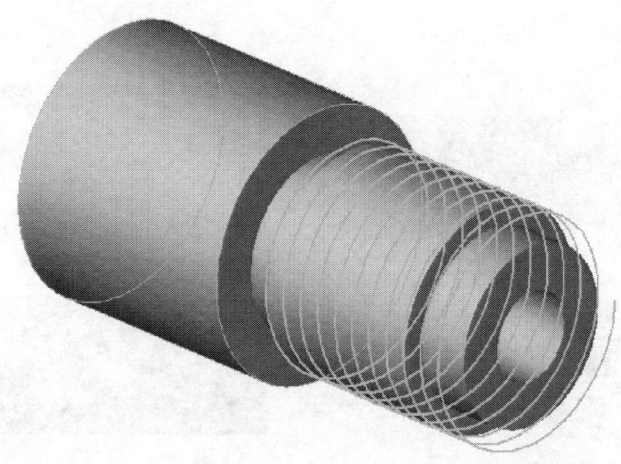

5. Sketching the Sweep profile:

- Select the <u>Top</u> plane from the FeatureManager Tree.

- Click 🖋 or **Insert / Sketch**.

- Sketch a Triangle ◣ and dimension ◈ as shown.

- Add a Pierce relation between the upper endpoint of the centerline and the Helix.

(Either use the Mirror option to create this sketch, or add a Symmetric relation between the two angled lines and the centerline).

Virtual Sharp

R.010

.100

60.00°

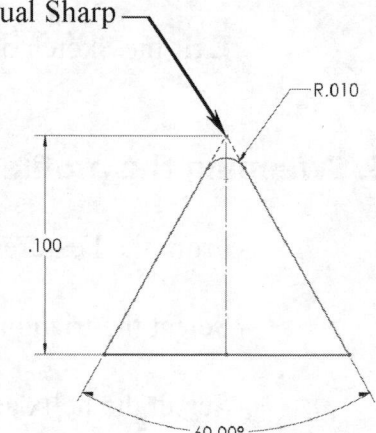

Pierce relation between the Helix & Endpoint (Click on the helix, near the end of the last revolution and the end-point of the centerline).

R.010

.100

60.00°

- The sketch should be fully defined at this point.

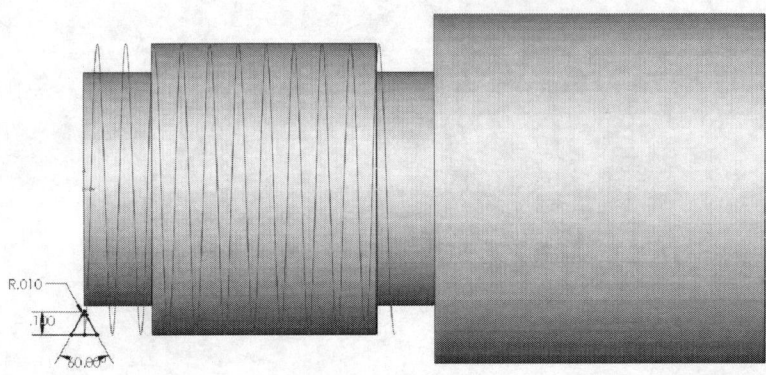

- **Exit** the Sketch or click [ ] .

6. Sweeping the profile along the path.

- From the Features tool tab click [ ] or Select **Insert / Cut / Sweep**.

- Select the triangular profile as sweep profile [ ] .

- Select the helix as sweep path [ ] .

- Click **OK** [ ] .

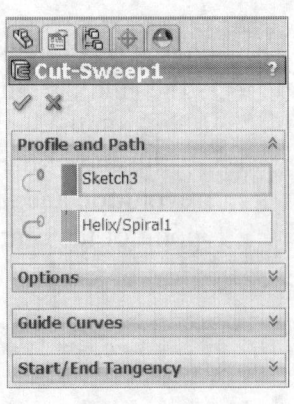

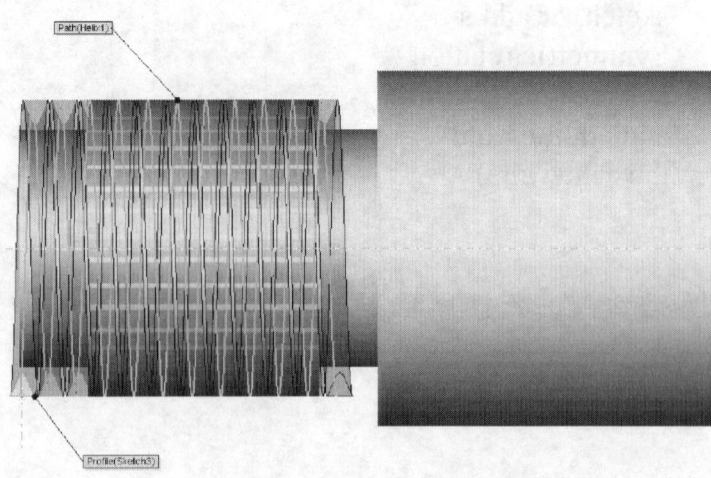

- The 1st half of the threads, clockwise direction (right hand).

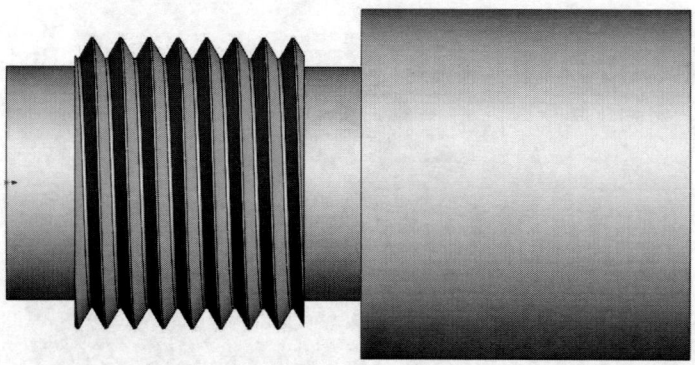

7. Using the Mirror Bodies option:

- Select **Mirror** 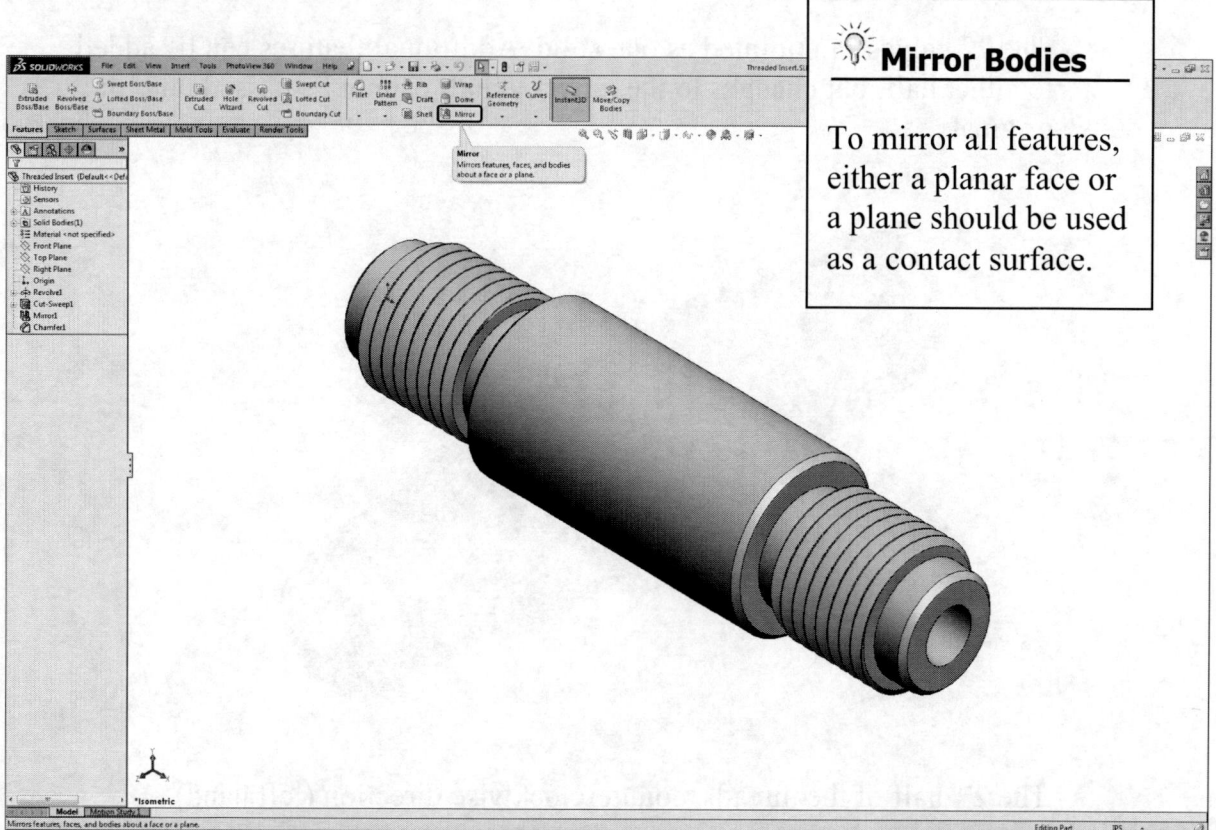 from the Features tool tab or click: **Insert / Pattern-Mirror/Mirror**.

> ### Mirror Bodies
>
> To mirror all features, either a planar face or a plane should be used as a contact surface.

- Select the mirror face as indicated.

- Expand the Bodies-To-Mirror section and select the part from the graphics area as noted.

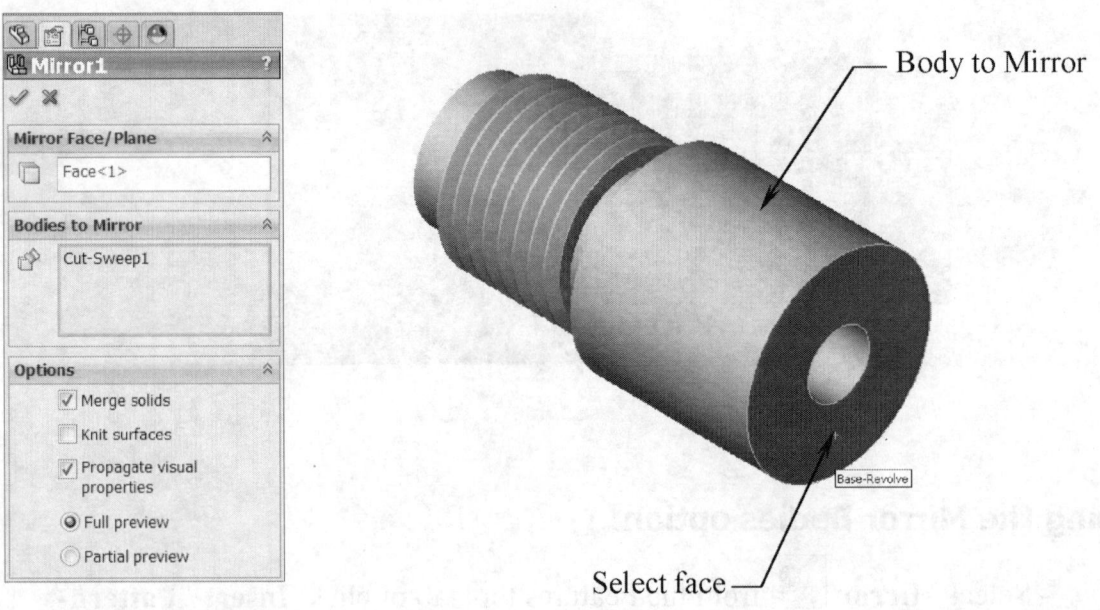

Body to Mirror

Base-Revolve

Select face

- Click **OK** ✅.

- The "2 halves" are jointed as one solid. Additional features can be added to either half, but changes to the mirrored half cannot be passed onto the original.

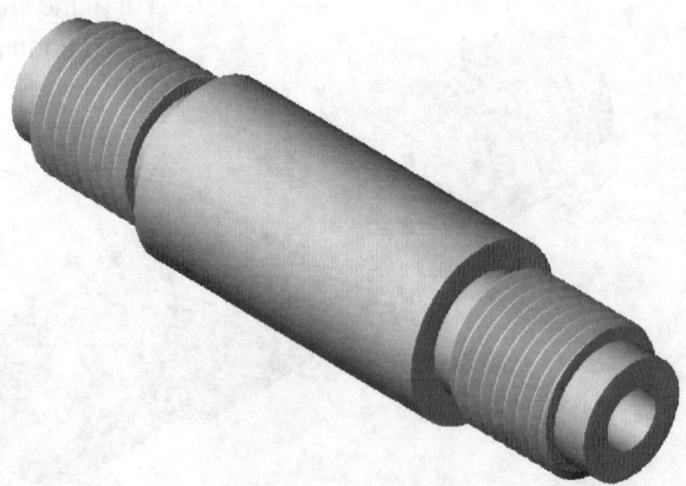

- The 2nd half of the threads, counterclockwise direction (left hand).

8. Adding chamfers:

- Click **Chamfer** 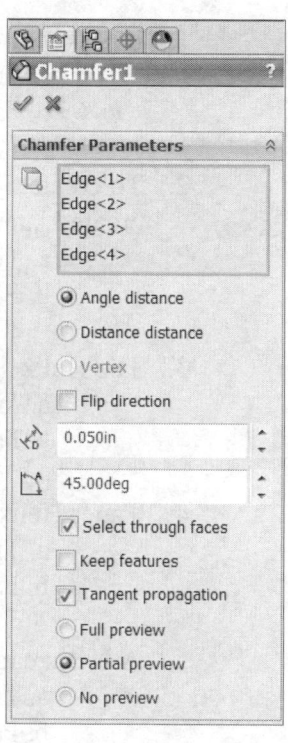 or **Insert / Features / Chamfers**.

- Select the **4 edges** as indicated.

- Enter **.050 in**. for Depth.

- Enter **45°** for Angle.

- Click **OK**.

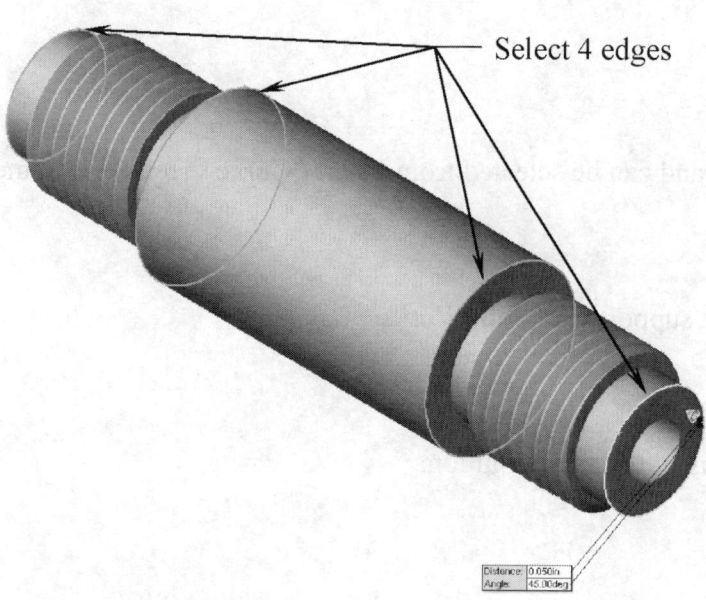

Select 4 edges

9. Saving the finished part.

- Select **File / Save as / Threaded Insert / Save**.

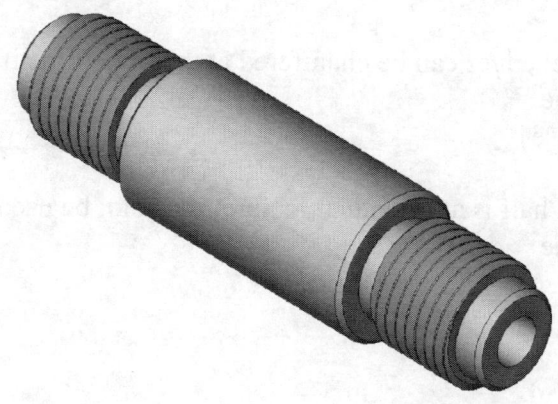

Questions for Review

Modeling Threads

1. It is proper to select the sketch plane first before activating the sketch pencil.
   - a. True
   - b. False

2. To create a sweep feature, the sweep path should be created first and the sweep profile created later.
   - a. True
   - b. False

3. The Helix / Spiral command can be selected from Insert / Curve / Helix-Spiral menus.
   - a. True
   - b. False

4. Taper Helix option is not supported in SolidWorks.
   - a. True
   - b. False

5. A Helix can be defined by pitch and revolution.
   - a. True
   - b. False

6. The Sweep profile should not have any relations with the sweep path.
   - a. True
   - b. False

7. Either a planar surface or a plane can be used to perform a Mirror-Bodies (All) feature.
   - a. True
   - b. False

8. Several model edges can be chamfered at the same time if their values are the same.
   - a. True
   - b. False

9. The mirrored half is a dependent feature; it cannot be used to change the original half.
   - a. True
   - b. False

	9. TRUE
7. TRUE	8. TRUE
5. TRUE	6. FALSE
3. TRUE	4. FALSE
1. TRUE	2. TRUE

Exercise: Modeling Threads - Internal

1. Dimensions provided are for solid modeling practice purposes.
2. Dimensions are in Inches, 3 decimal places.
3. Use the instructions on the following pages, if needed.
4. Save your work as **Nut – Internal Threads**.

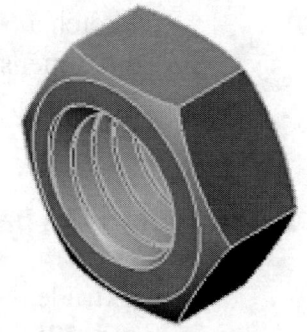

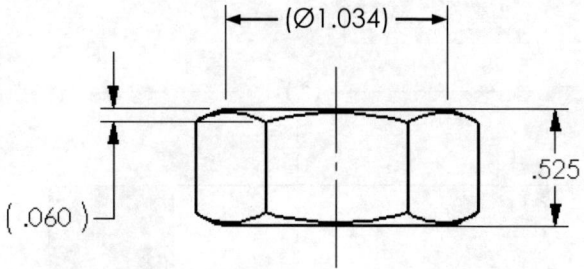

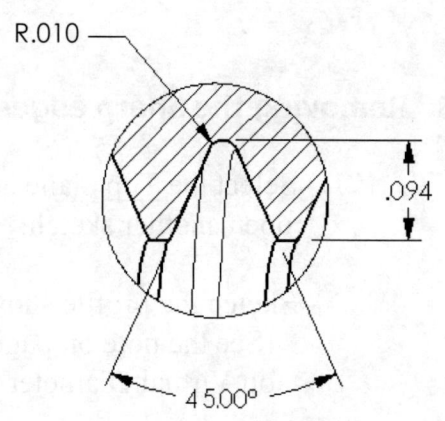

DETAIL B

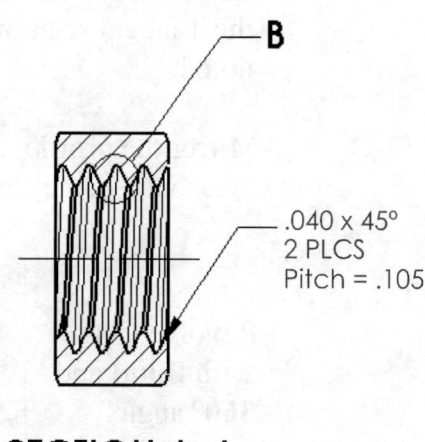

SECTION A-A

1. Starting with the base sketch:

- Select the <u>Front</u> plane and open a new sketch.

- Sketch a 6 sided Polygon and add the dimensions and relation shown.

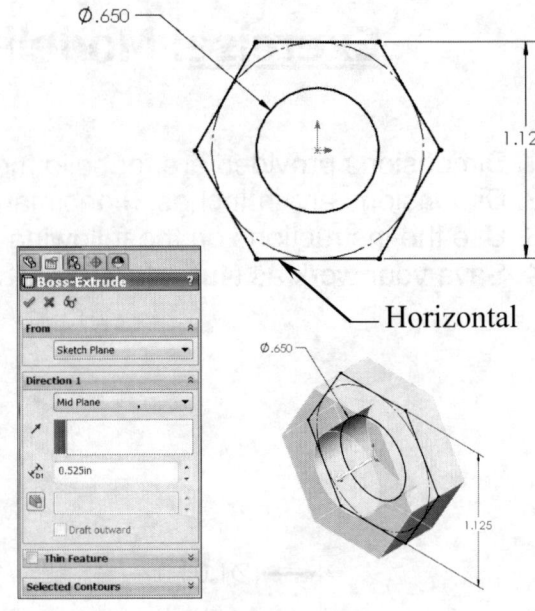

2. Extruding the base:

- Extrude the sketch using **Mid Plane** and **.525"** thick.

3. Removing the Sharp edges:

- Select the <u>Top</u> plane and open another sketch.

- Sketch the profile shown.
  * (See the note on page 9-15 on Virtual Diameter dim).

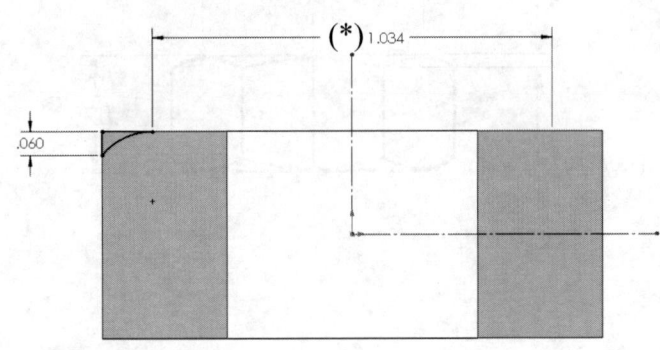

- Add the dimensions and the Tangent relation as noted.

- Mirror the profile using the horizontal centerline.

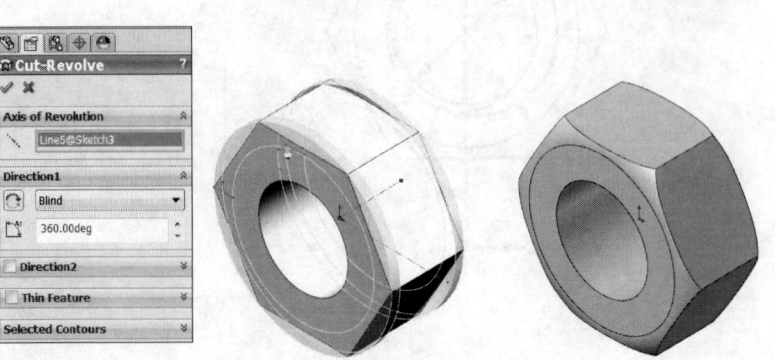

- Revolve Cut with **Blind** and **360°** angle.

- Click **OK**.

4. Creating a new plane:

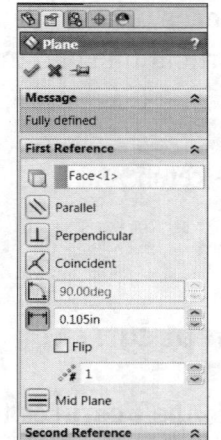

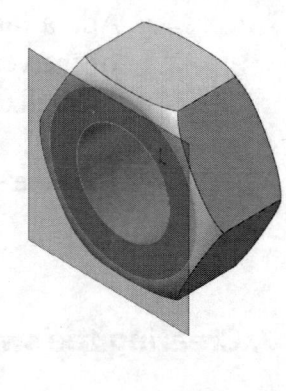

- Select the <u>front face</u> of the part and click **Insert / Reference Geometry / Plane**.

- The **Offset Distance** should be selected automatically; enter **.105"** for distance.

- Click **OK**.

5. Creating the sweep path:

- Select the <u>new plane</u> and open a new sketch. (Starting from this offset location will prevent an undercut from happening where the thread starts).

Convert this edge

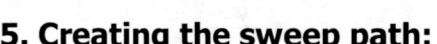

-Select the circular edge as indicated and click: **Convert Entities**.

- The selected edge turns into a sketch circle.

- Click the **Helix** command or select: **Insert / Curve / Helix-Spiral**.

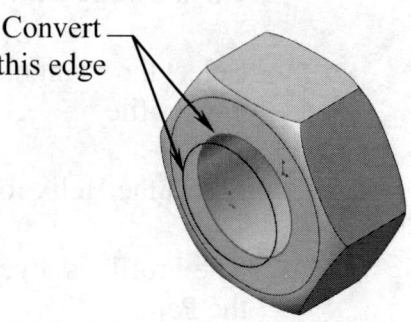

- Enter the following:
  * Pitch = **.105"**
  * Reverse Direction: **Enabled**.
  * Revolutions: **7**
  * Start Angle: **0.00 deg**.
  * **Clockwise**

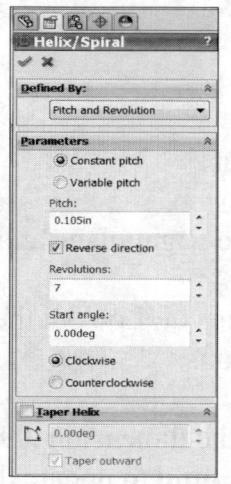

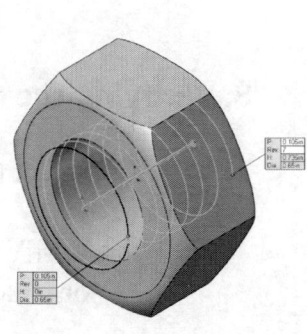

- Click **OK**.

6. Creating the sweep profile:

- Select the <u>Top</u> plane, open a new sketch and sketch the profile using Dynamic Mirror.

- Add the dimensions as shown to fully define the sketch.

- Add a **.010"** sketch fillet to the tip.

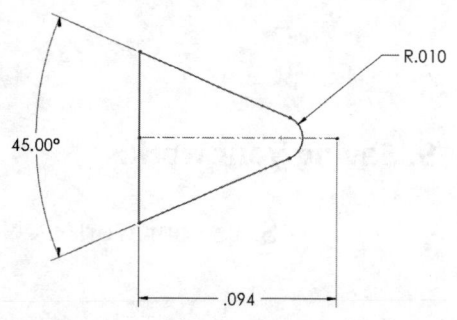

R.010

45.00°

.094

- Add a **Pierce** relation between the midpoint
  of the vertical line and the 1st revolution of
  the helix.

- **Exit** the sketch.

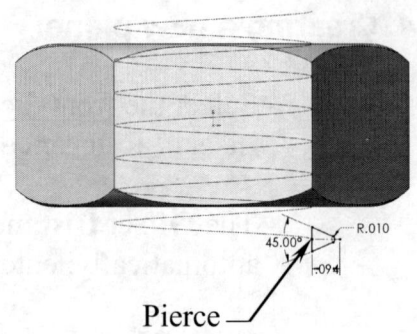

7. Creating the swept cut:

- Change to the **Features** toolbar.

- Click **Swept Cut**.

- Select the triangular sketch
  for Profile.

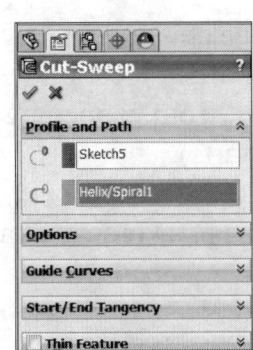

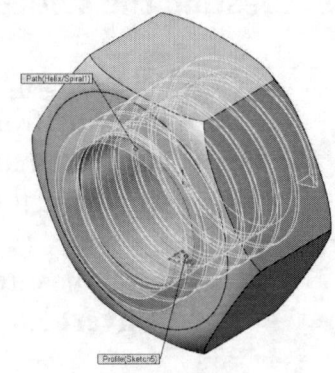

- Select the Helix for Path.

- The Profile is Swept along
  the Path.

- Click **OK**.

8. Verifying the cut:

- Select the <u>Right</u> plane and click **Section View**.

- Verify the cut. Look at the section view from different
  orientations.

- Change the dimension **.094"** in the profile sketch to **.100"**.
  Click **Rebuild** to update the change.

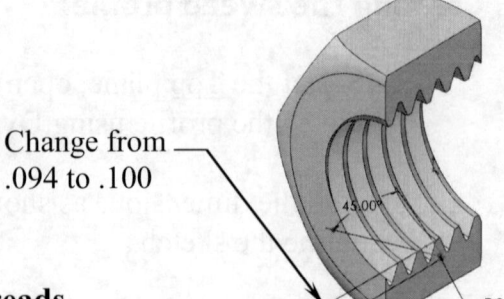

Change from
.094 to .100

9. Saving your work:

- Save your work as **Nut – Internal Threads**.

Exercise: Internal & External Thread

A. Internal Threads:

1. Creating the Revolve Sketch:

- Select the <u>Front</u> plane and open a new sketch plane as shown.

- Sketch the profile and add relations & dimensions as shown.

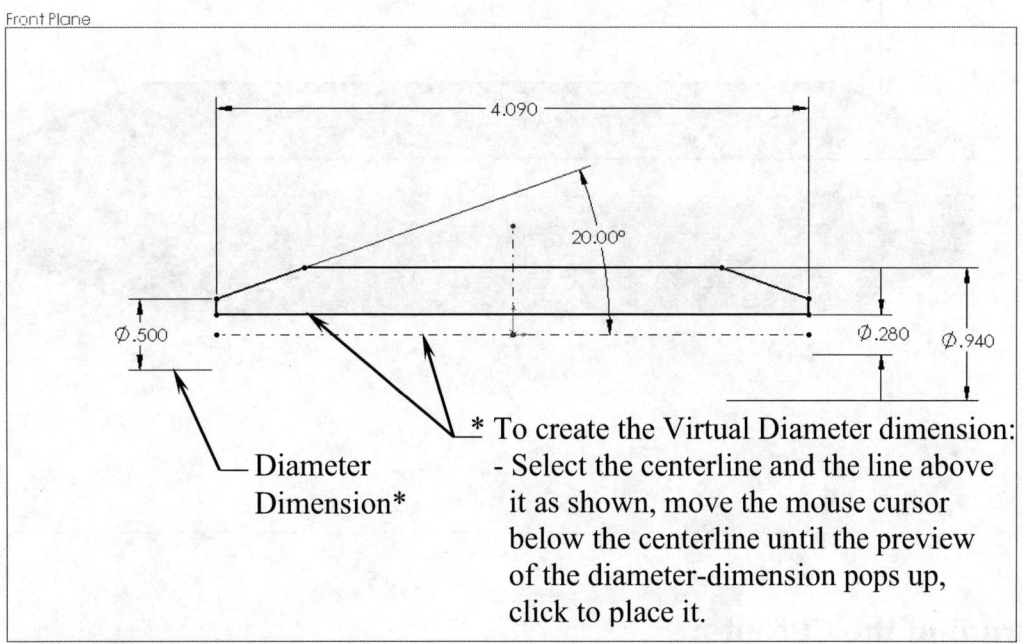

Front Plane

4.090

20.00°

Ø.500   Ø.280   Ø.940

Diameter Dimension*

* To create the Virtual Diameter dimension:
- Select the centerline and the line above
  it as shown, move the mouse cursor
  below the centerline until the preview
  of the diameter-dimension pops up,
  click to place it.

2. Revolving the Body:

- Revolve the sketch a full 360 deg. and click **OK** ✓.

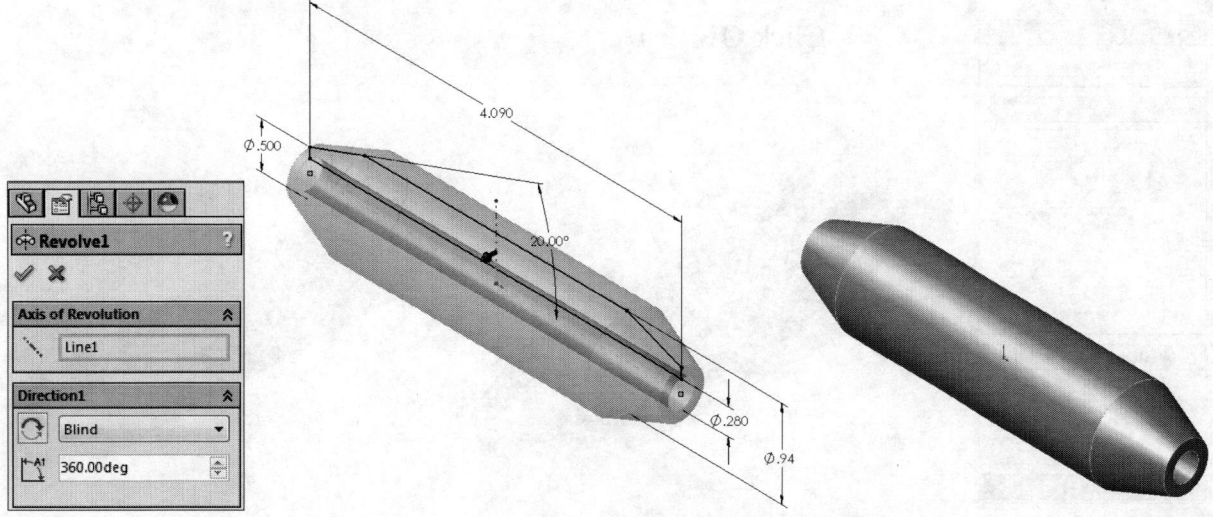

Revolve1

Axis of Revolution
Line1

Direction1
Blind
360.00deg

4.090
Ø.500
20.00°
Ø.280
Ø.94

3. Creating the cutout features:

- From the <u>Front</u> plane, sketch the profiles of the cutouts.

- Use the Mirror function where applicable. Add Relations & Dimensions to fully define the sketch.

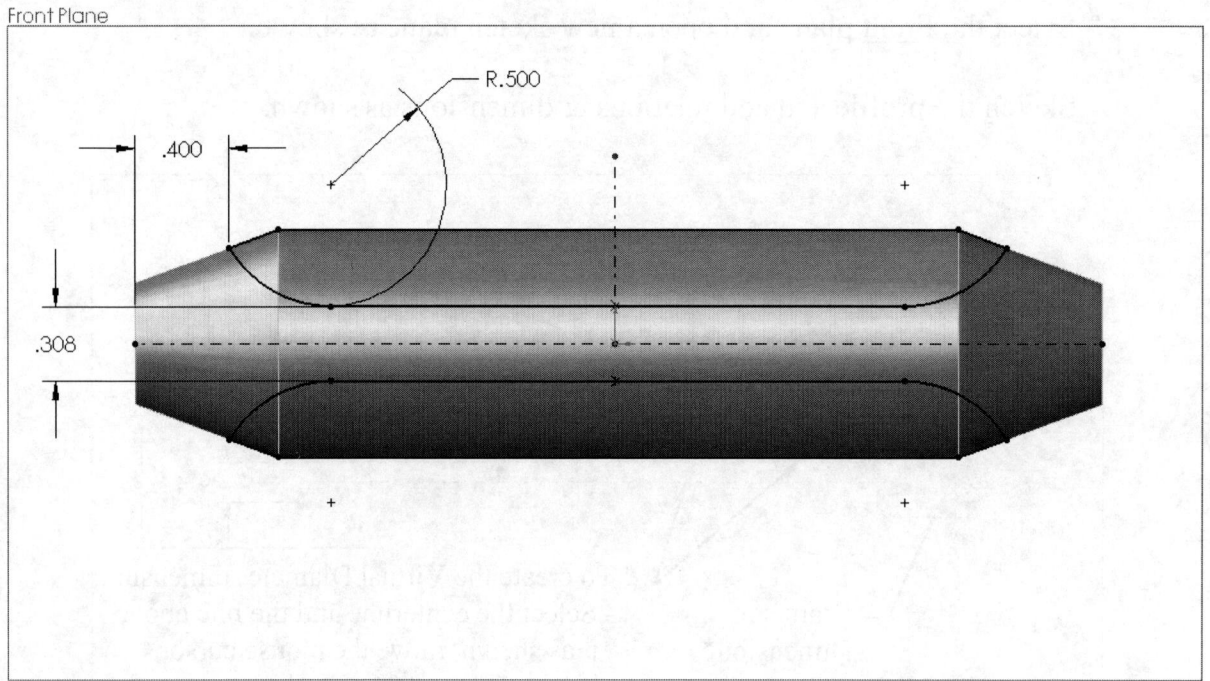

4. Extruding the Cutouts:

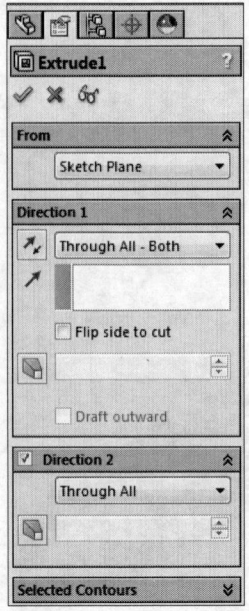

- Click **Extruded Cut** and select **Through All** for **Both-Directions**.

- Click **OK** ✅.

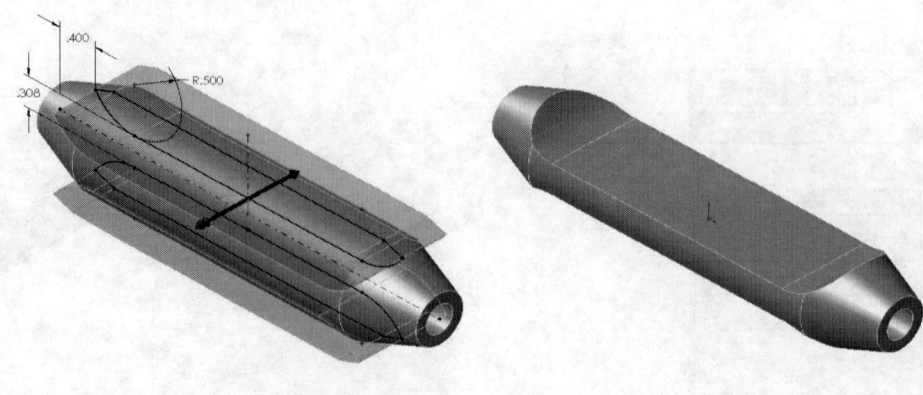

5. Sketching the Slot Profile:

- From the <u>Top</u> plane, sketch the profile of the slot (use the Straight Slot options).

- Add Relations & Dimensions to fully define the sketch.

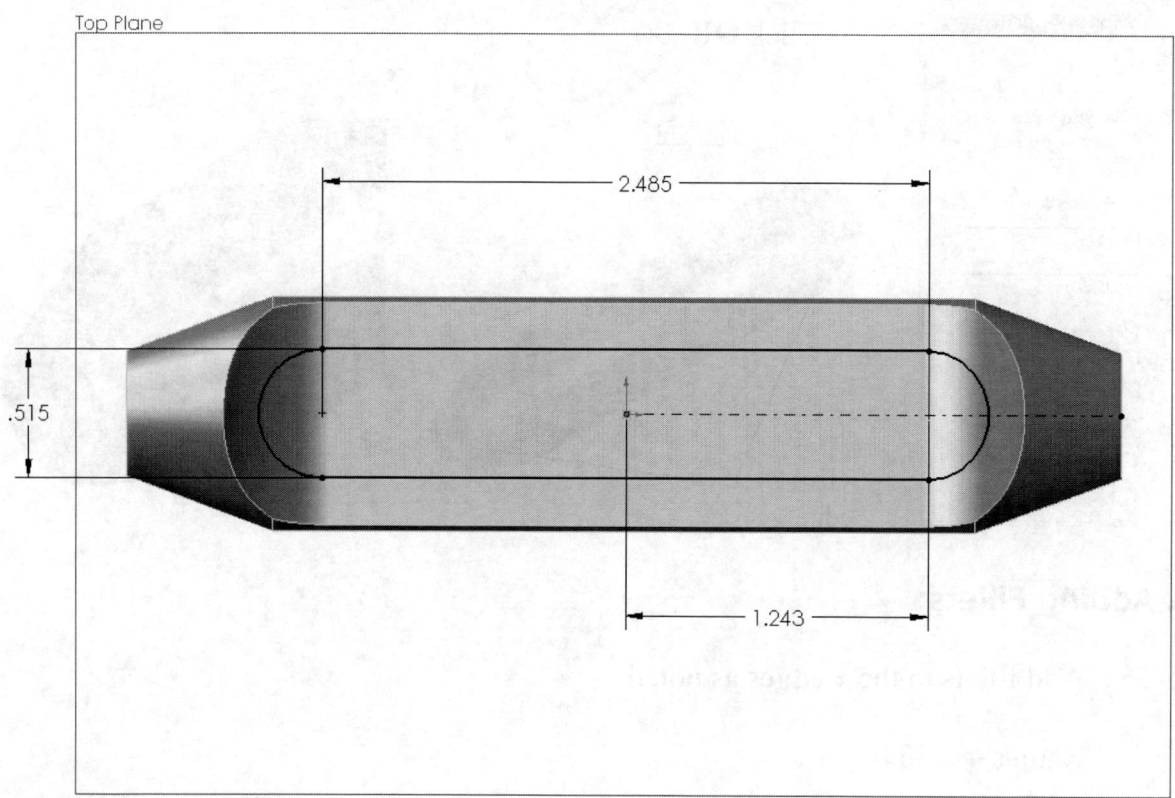

6. Cutting the Slot:

- Click **Extruded Cut** and select **Through All** for Both-Directions.

- Click **OK** .

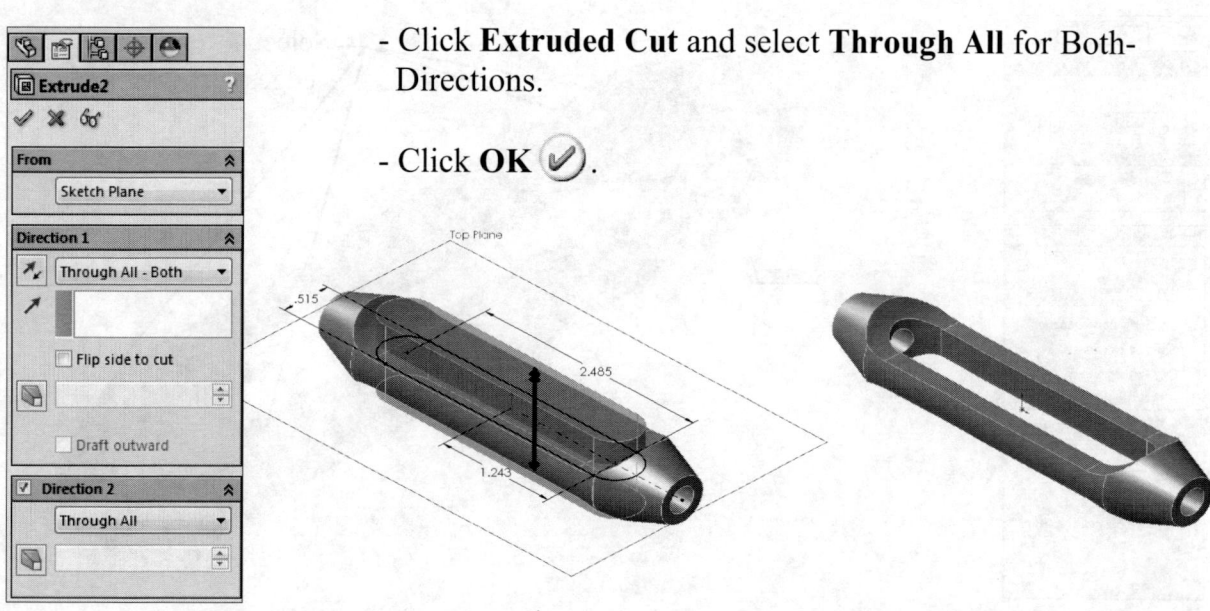

7. Adding Chamfers:

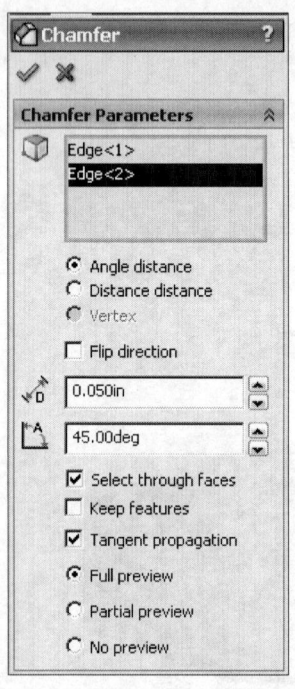

- Add a **chamfer** to both ends of the holes.

- Chamfer Depth = **.050 in**.   - Chamfer Angle = **45 deg**.

- Click **OK** ✓.

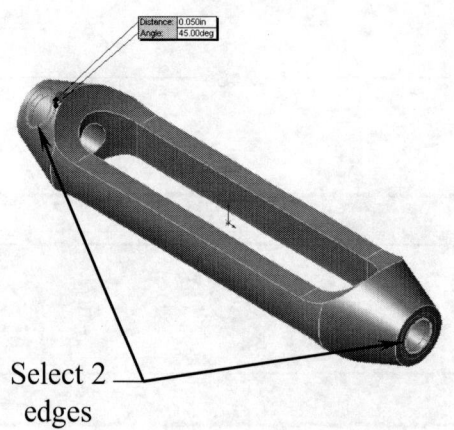

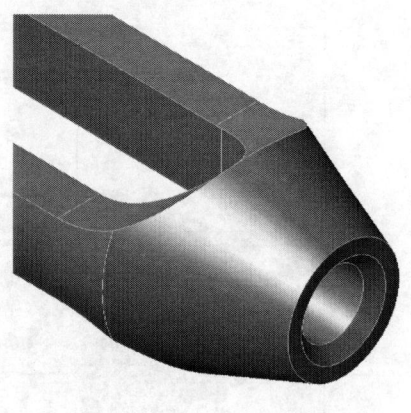

Select 2 edges

8. Adding Fillets:

- Add **fillets** to the **4 edges** as noted.

- Radius = **.250 in**.

- Click **OK** ✓.

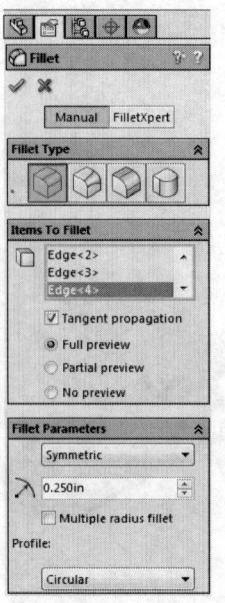

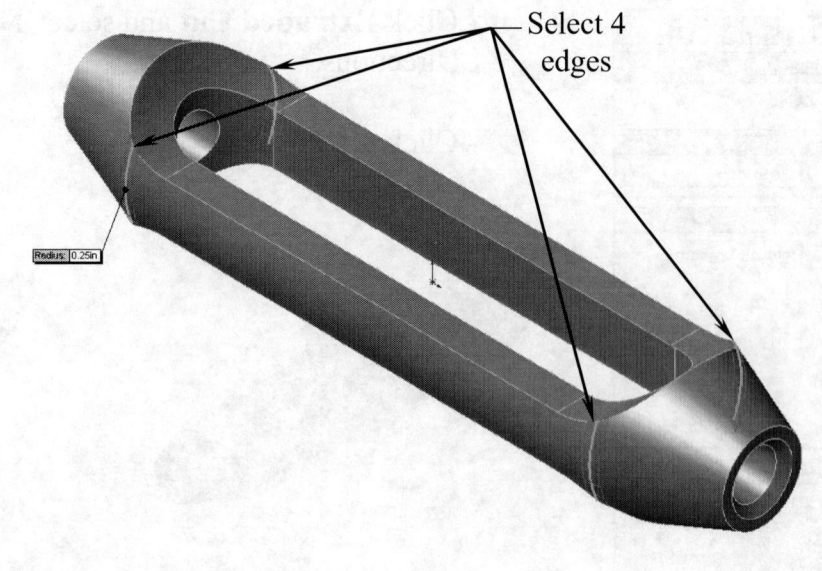

Select 4 edges

9. Filleting all edges:

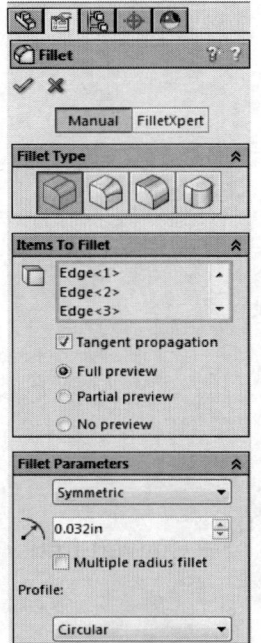

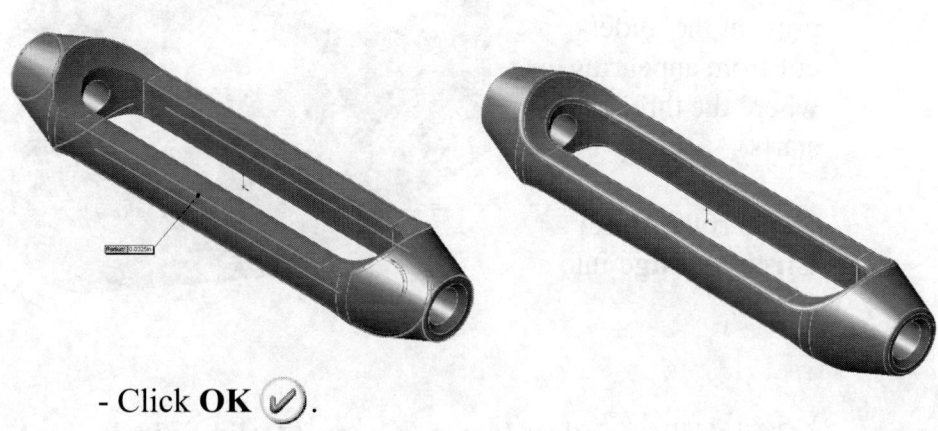

- Box-Select the entire part and add a fillet of **.032 in**. to all edges. (If Lasso-Selection was the default, right click in the graphics area and choose: **Box Selection**).

- Click **OK** .

10. Creating an Offset-Distance Plane:

- Click **Plane** or select **Insert / Reference Geometry / Plane**.

- Click **Offset-Distance** option and enter **2.063 in**.

- Select the <u>Right</u> plane to copy from; place the new plane on the right hand side.

- Click **OK** .

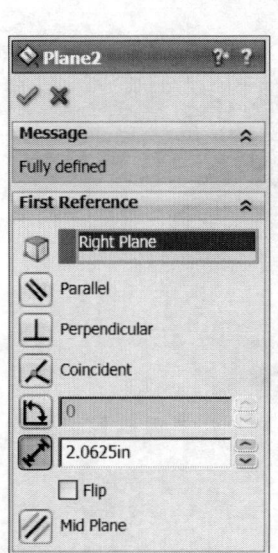

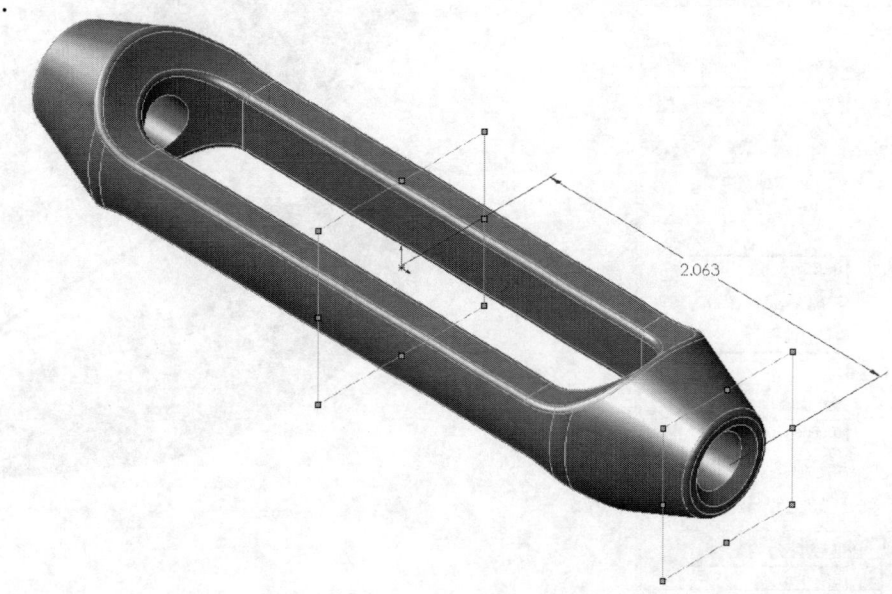

11. Creating the Helix (the sweep path):

- Select the <u>new plane</u> and open a new sketch.

(Using an offset of "1-pitch" can help prevent the under-cut from appearing where the thread starts).

- Convert the **Inner Circular Edge** into a Circle.

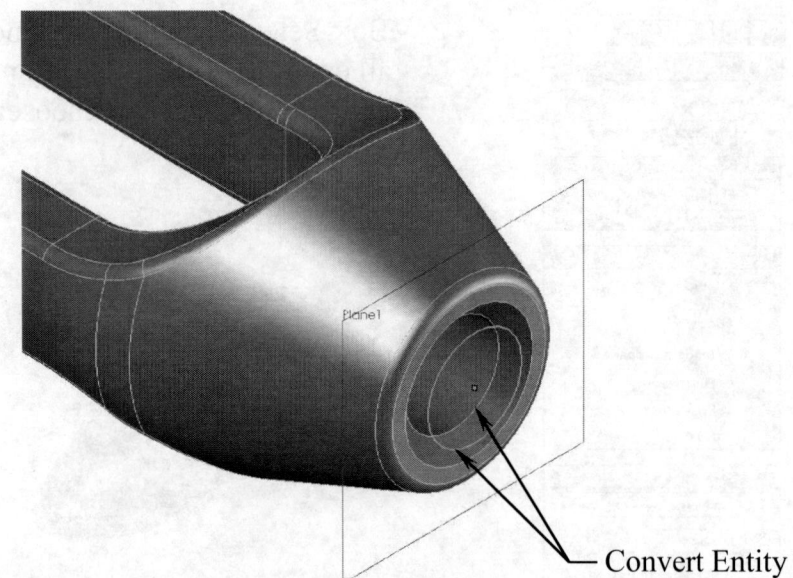

Convert Entity

- Click **Helix** or select **Insert / Curve / Helix-Spiral**.

- Pitch: **.055 in**.

- Revolutions: **11**

- Start Angle: **0 deg**.

- Clockwise   - Click **OK** ✅.

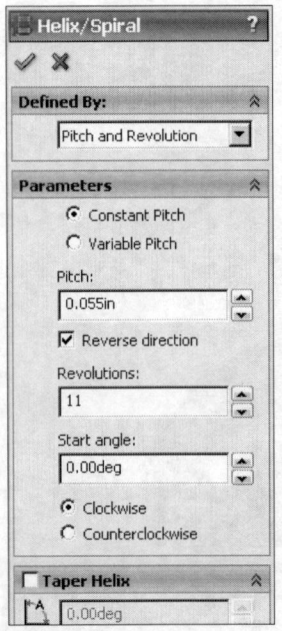

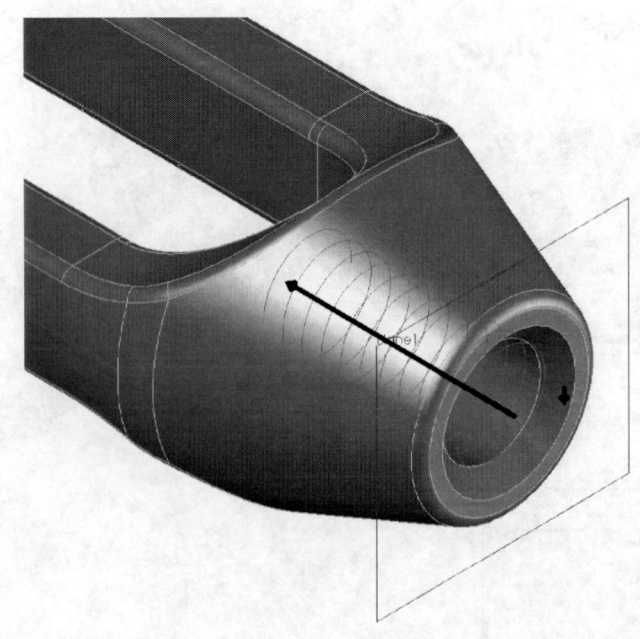

12. Sketching the Thread Profile:

- Select the Top reference plane and open a new sketch.

- Sketch the thread profile as shown. Add the relation and dimensions needed to define the profile.

- **Exit** the Sketch.

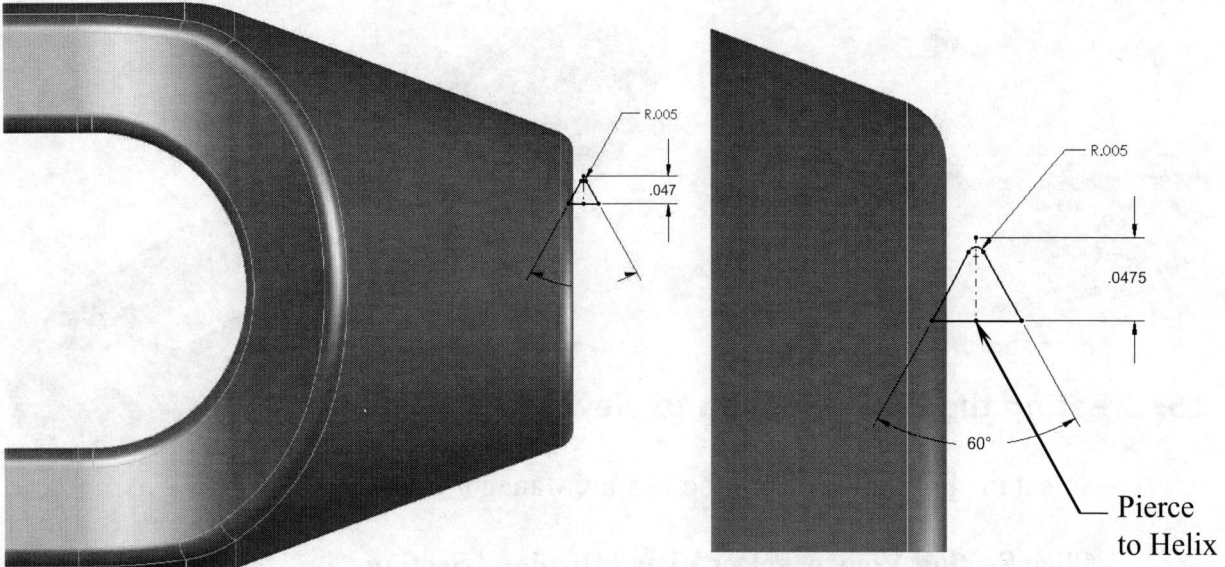

13. Sweeping the Cut:

- Click **Cut-Sweep** or select **Insert / Cut / Sweep**.

- Select the triangular sketch as Profile and select the helix as Sweep Path.

- Click **OK** ✅.

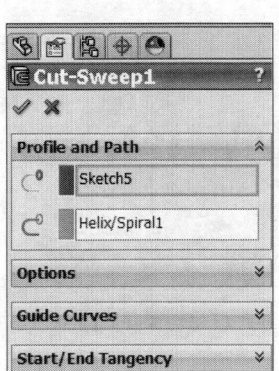

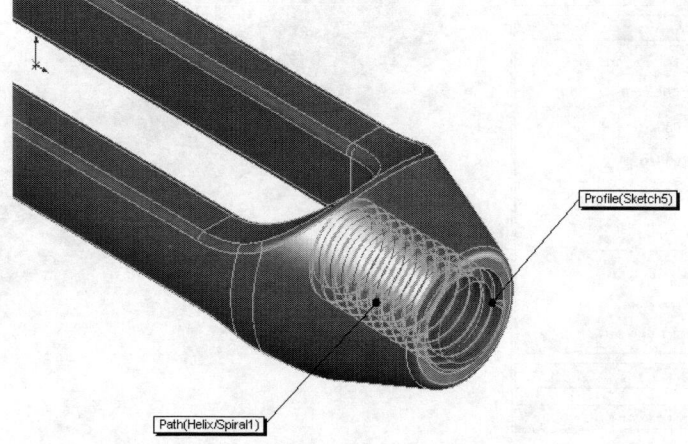

14. Mirroring the Threads:

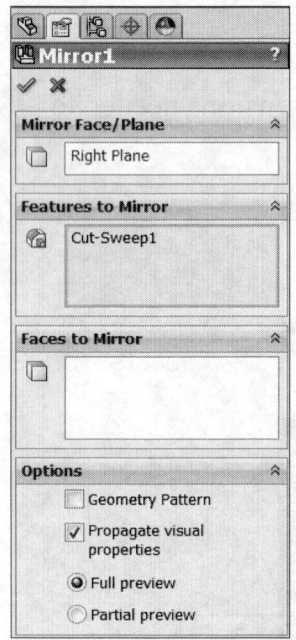

- Click **Mirror** or select **Insert / Pattern Mirror / Mirror**.

- Select the **Right** plane as the Mirror Plane.

- For Features to Mirror select the **Cut-Sweep1** feature.

- Click **OK** ✅.

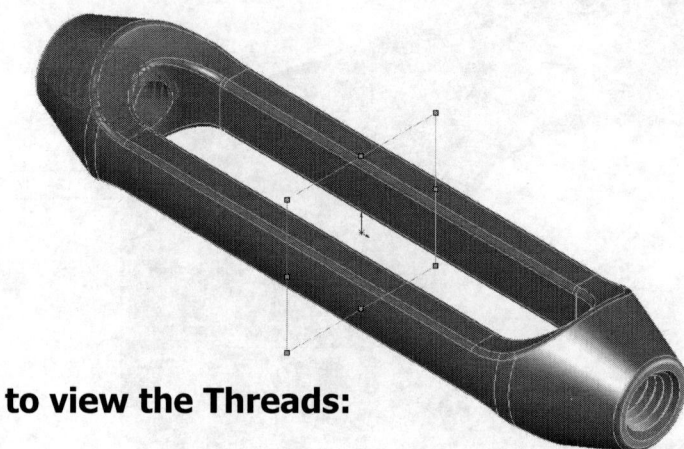

15. Creating the Cross-Section to view the Threads:

- Select the <u>Front</u> plane from the FeatureManager tree.

- Click **Section View** or select **View / Display / Section**.

- Zoom in on the threaded areas and examine the thread details.

- Click **Cancel** when you are done viewing.

- Save the part as **Internal Threads**.

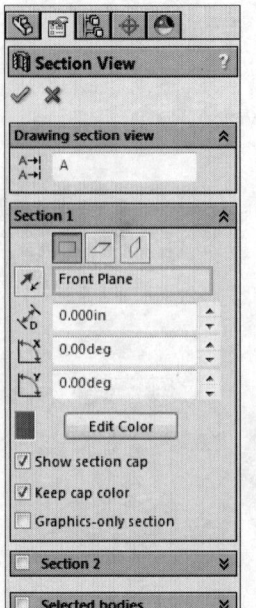

B. External Threads:

1. Sketching the Sweep Path:

- Select the <u>Front</u> plane and open a new sketch.

- Sketch the profile shown; add Relations & Dimensions needed to fully define.

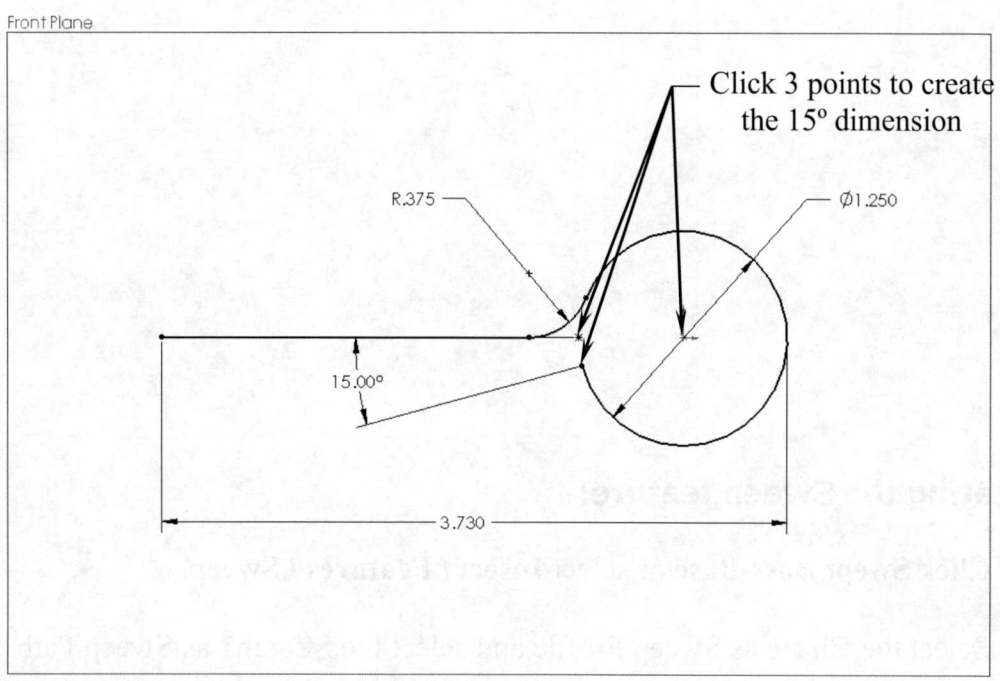

Front Plane

R.375

Ø1.250

Click 3 points to create the 15° dimension

15.00°

3.730

2. Creating a plane Perpendicular to the line:

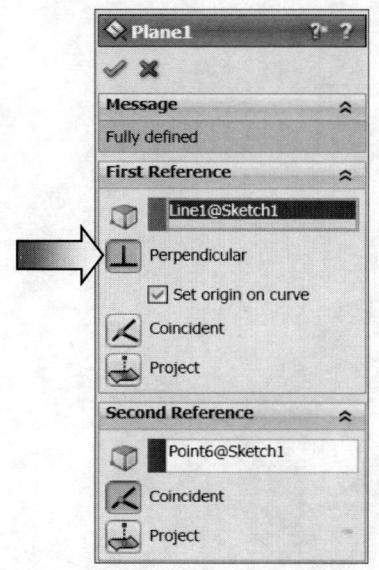

- Click **Plane** or select **Insert / Reference Geometry/ Plane**.

- Select the Horizontal line and the Endpoint on the left side.

- A new plane is created normal to the line

- Click **OK** 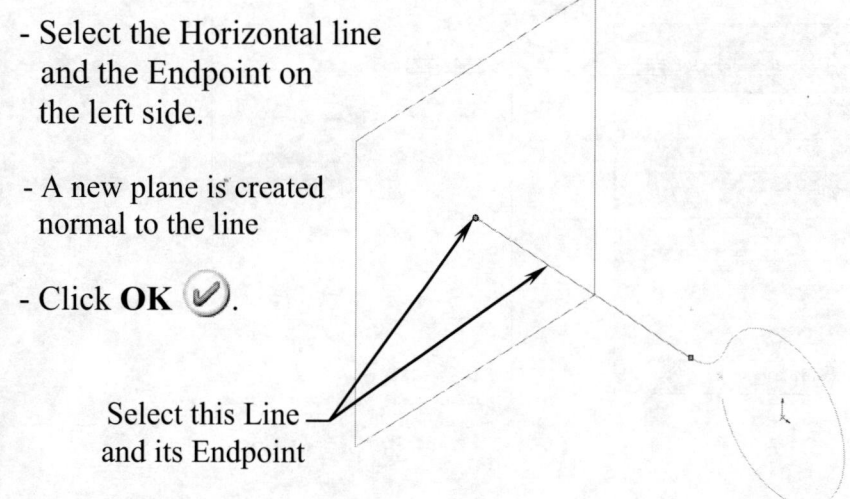.

Select this Line and its Endpoint

3. Sketching the Sweep Profile:

- Select the <u>new plane</u> and open a new sketch.

- Sketch a **Circle** as shown and add
  a diameter dimension.

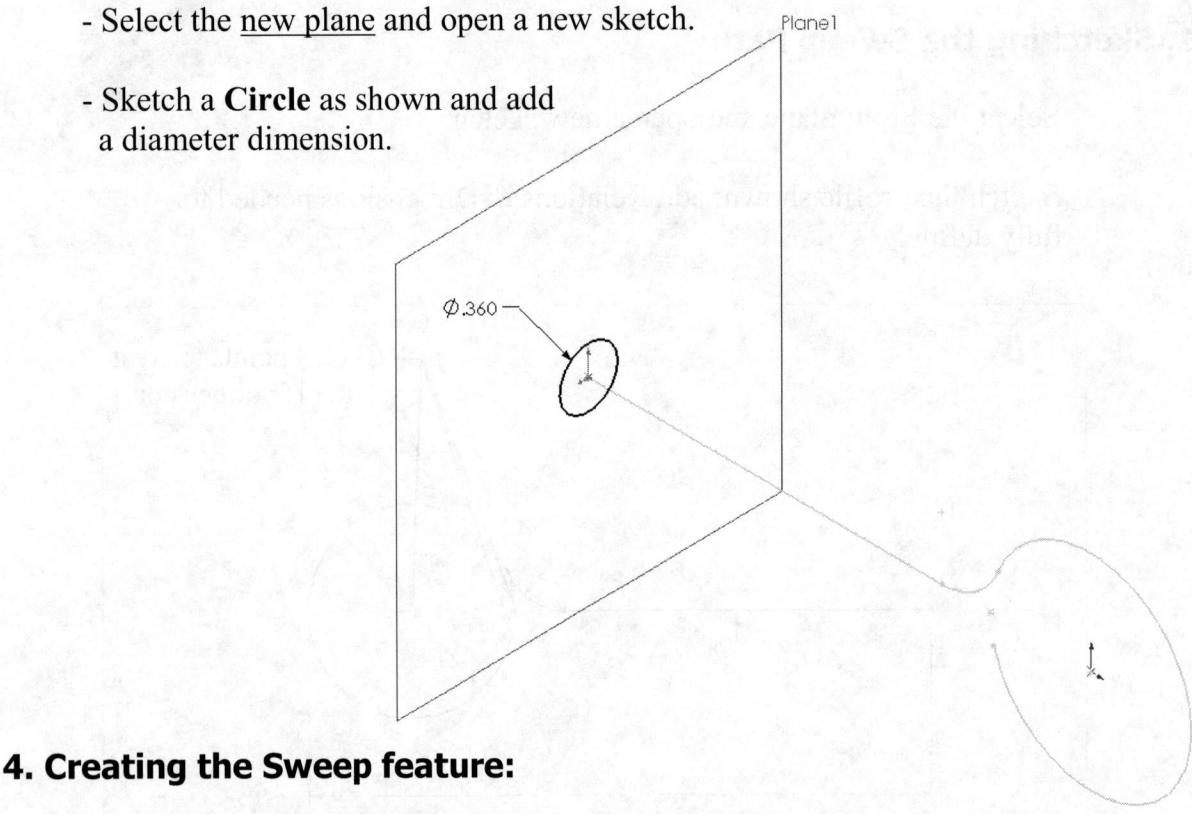

4. Creating the Sweep feature:

- Click **Swept Boss-Base** or select **Insert / Features / Sweep**.

- Select the **Circle** as Sweep Profile and select the **Sketch1** as Sweep Path.

- Click **OK** ✓ .

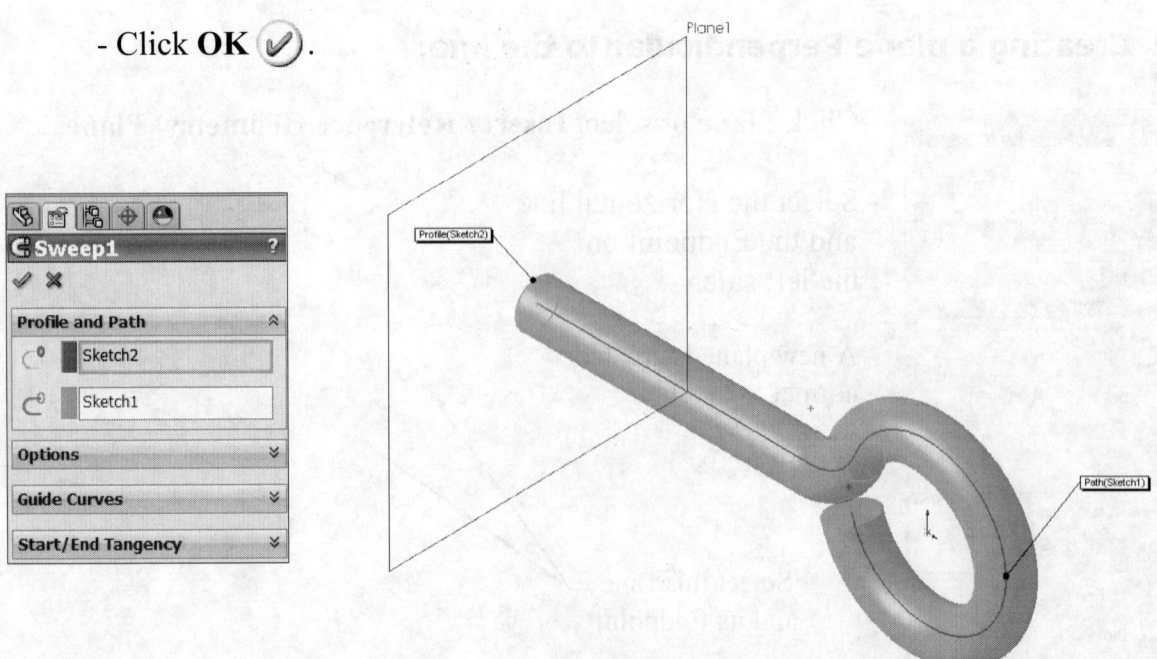

5. Adding Chamfers:

- Click **Chamfer** or select **Insert / Features / Chamfer**.

- Select the **2 Circular Edges** at the 2 ends.

- Enter **.050 in**. for Depth.

- Enter **45 deg**. for Angle.

- Click **OK** 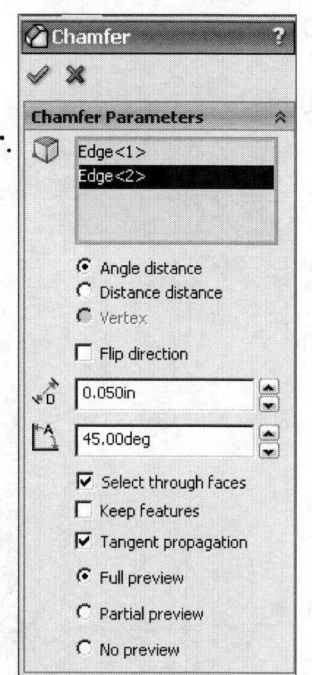.

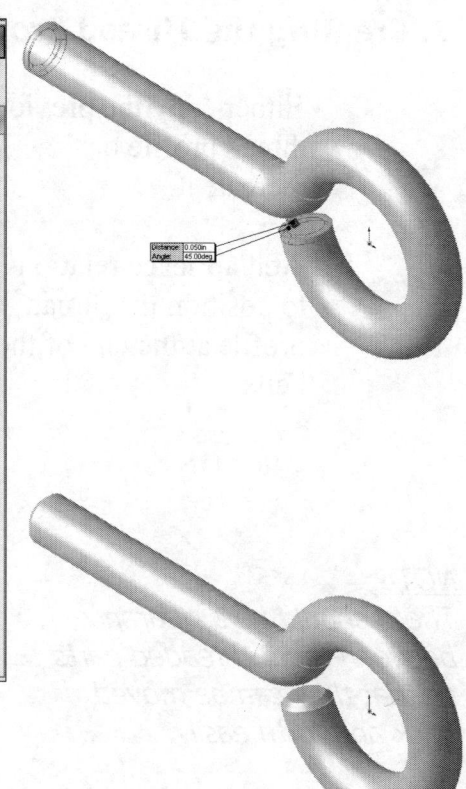

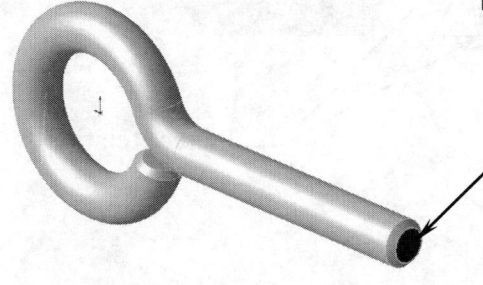

— Sketch face

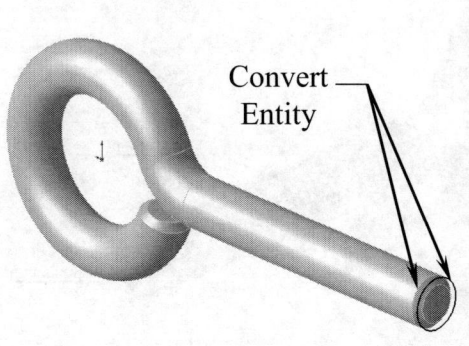

Convert Entity

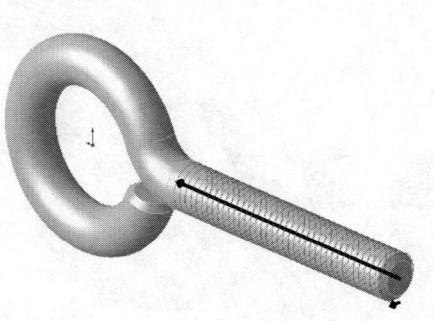

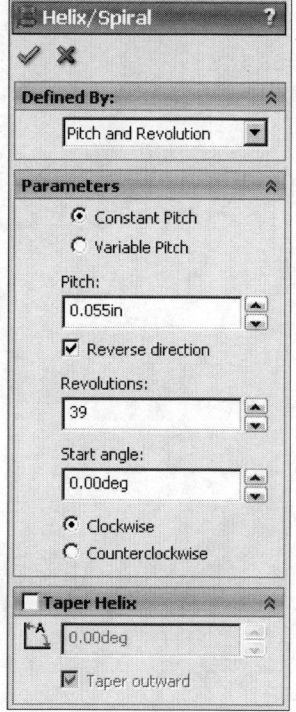

6. Creating the Helix:

- Select the face as indicated and open a new sketch.

- Select the **circular edge** at the end as shown and click Convert Entities or select: **Tools/Sketch Tools/Convert Entities**.

- Click **Helix** or select **Insert/ Curve/Helix-Spiral**.

- Enter **.055** in. for Pitch.

- Enter **39** for Revolutions.

- Enter **0 deg**. for Start Angle.

- Click **OK** 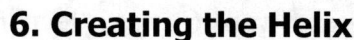.

7. Creating the Thread Profile:

- Either copy the previous thread profile or recreate it.

- Add a **Pierce** relation to position the thread profile at the end of the helix.

- Click **OK** ✅.

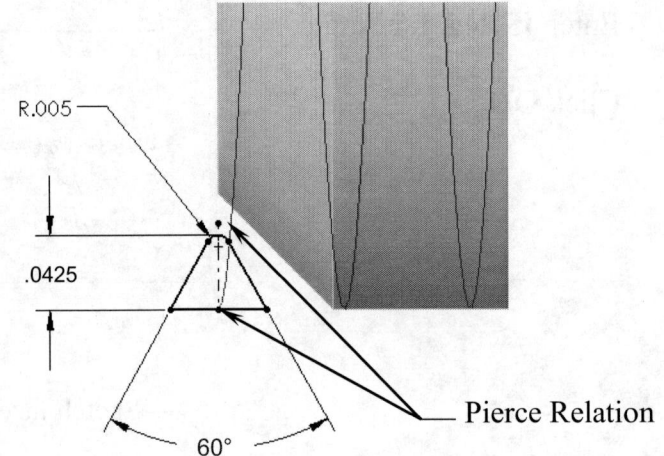

NOTE:
There should be a clearance between the 2 threaded parts so that they can be moved back and forth easily.

R.005

.0425

60°

Pierce Relation

8. Sweeping Cut the Threads:

- Click **Swept Cut** or select **Insert / Cut / Sweep.**

- Select the **triangular sketch** as the Sweep Profile.

- Select the **Helix** as the Sweep path.

- Click **OK** ✅.

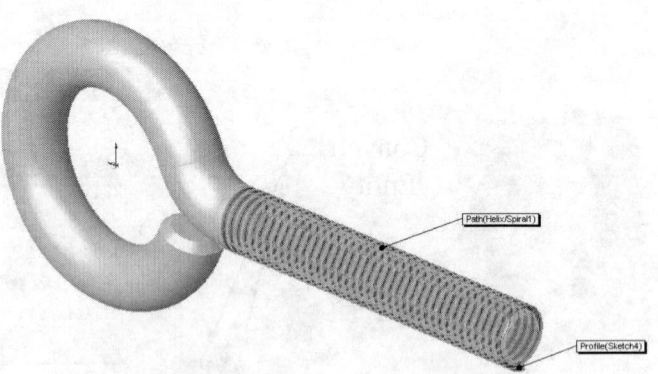

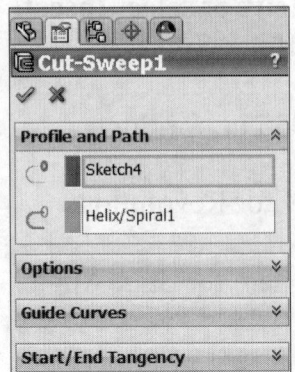

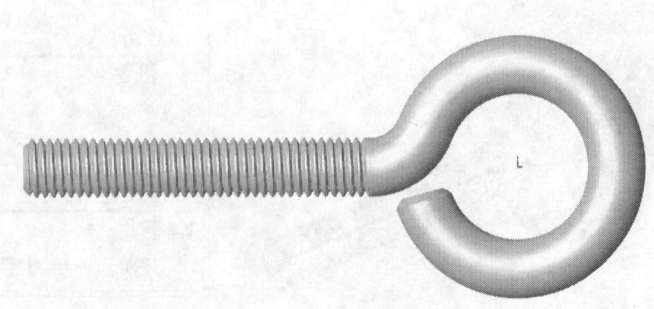

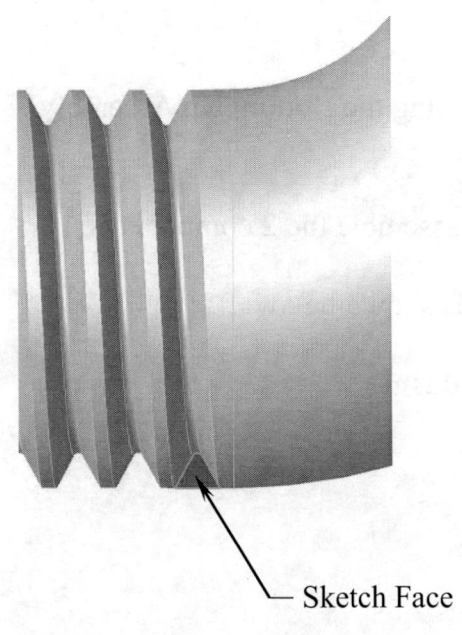

— Sketch Face

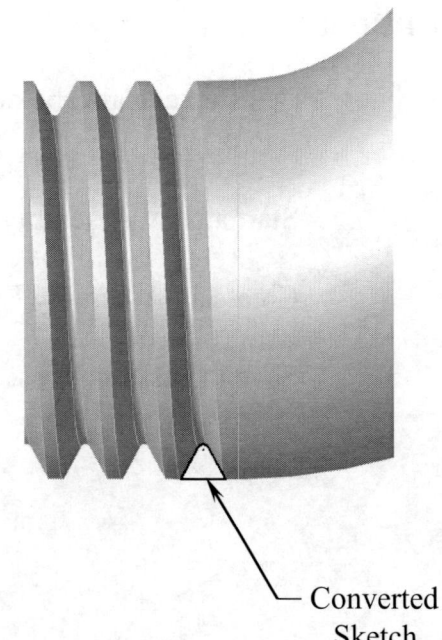

— Converted
Sketch

9. Removing the Undercut:

- Select the <u>face</u> as noted and open a new sketch.

- **Convert** the selected **face** into a new triangular sketch.

- Click Extruded-Cut or select **Insert / Cut / Extrude**.

- Select **Through All** for End Condition.

- Click **OK** ✓.

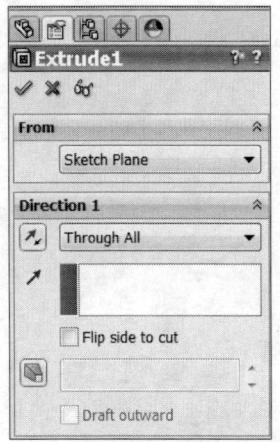

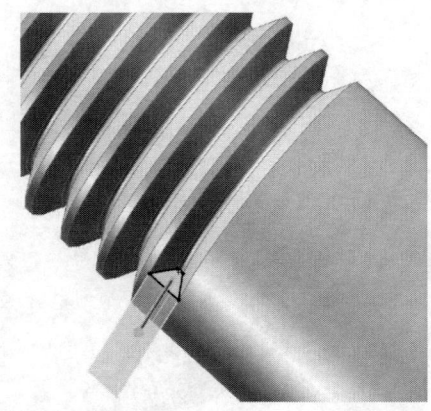

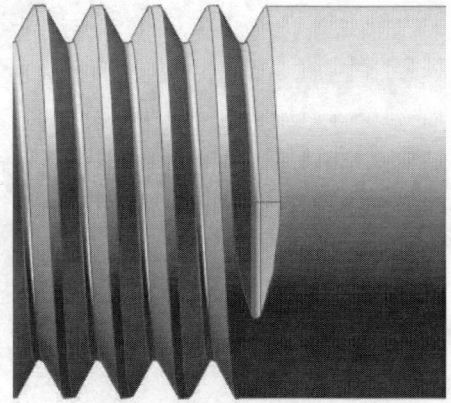

10. Saving your work:

- Save a copy of your work as **External Threads**.

11. Optional:

(This step can also be done after completing the Bottom Up Assembly chapter).

- Start a New Assembly document and assemble the 2 components.

- Create an Assembly Exploded View as shown below.

- Save the assembly as: **TurnBuckle.sldasm**

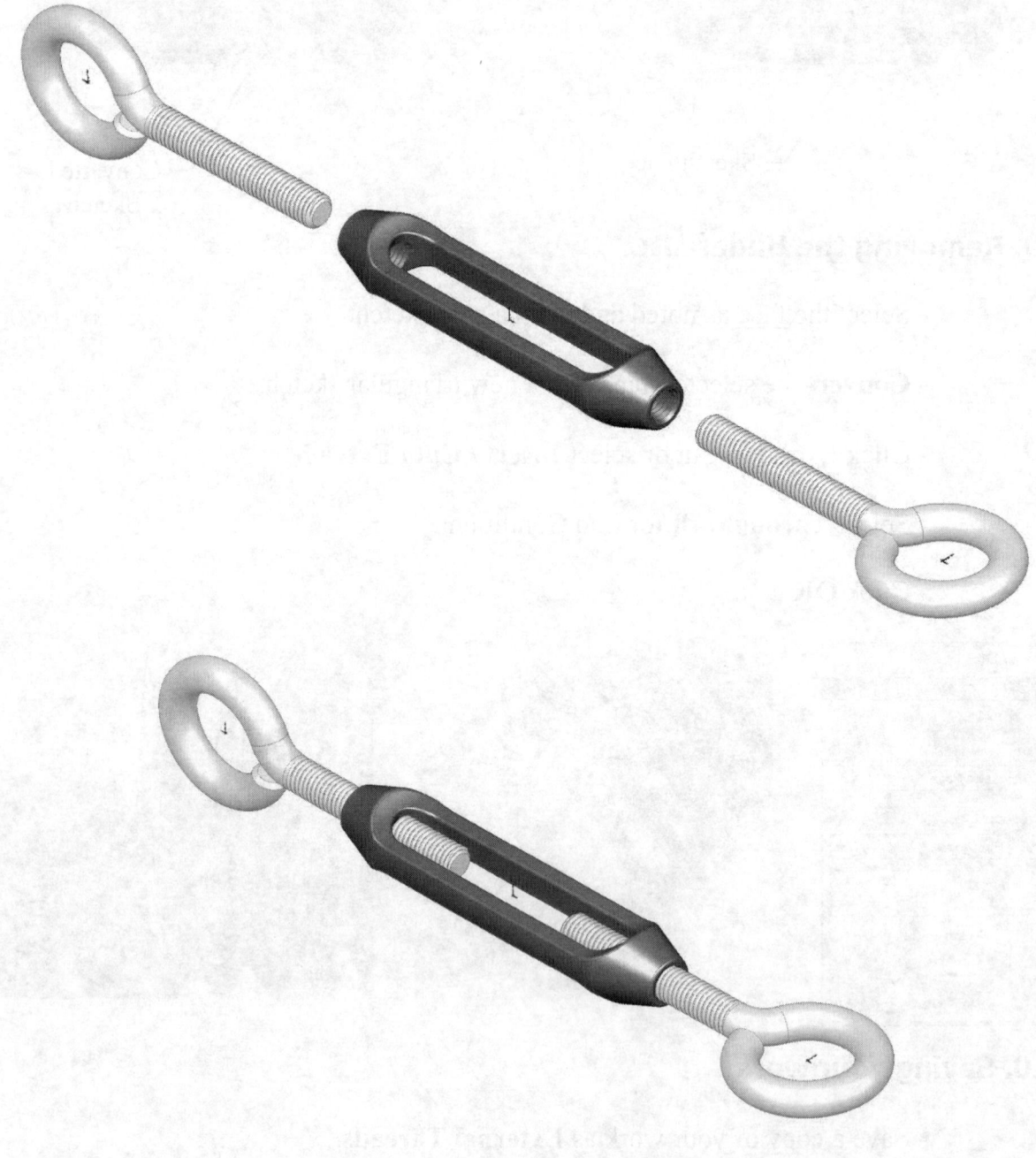

CHAPTER 9 (cont.)

Working with MultiBody Parts

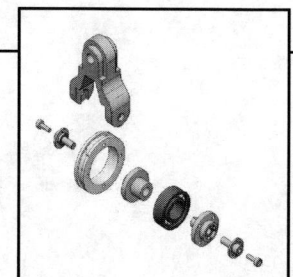

MultiBody Parts
Creating Mates & Exploded Views

- Use the **Insert Part** command 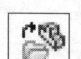 to insert a base part into another part document.

- When you insert a part into another part, it becomes a MultiBody Part, and the part you insert becomes a Solid Body.

- If the inserted part contains mate references, you can use them to position the inserted part.

- There are 3 options available to help locate a solid body: Constraints, Translate, and Rotate. You can move or rotate the body after it is placed in the graphics area. A feature Body-Move/Copy is then added to the FeatureManager design tree.

- The inserted body can also be constrained with the mate options. Some of the standard mates are available in the part mode to help position the solid bodies.

- An exploded view is created after all solid bodies are positioned. Exploded views are stored in the ConfigurationManager. They can be edited, deleted, or more than one exploded views can be created, if needed.

- This chapter will guide you through the use of multibodies parts, where an existing part document with a number of solid bodies is used. Other parts will then get inserted into the same document and constrained with some mates. After all solid bodies are positioned, an exploded view will be created in the same part mode, and the Solid Bodies folder is used to help keep track of the number of solid bodies exist in the part document.

MultiBody Parts
Creating Mates and Exploded Views

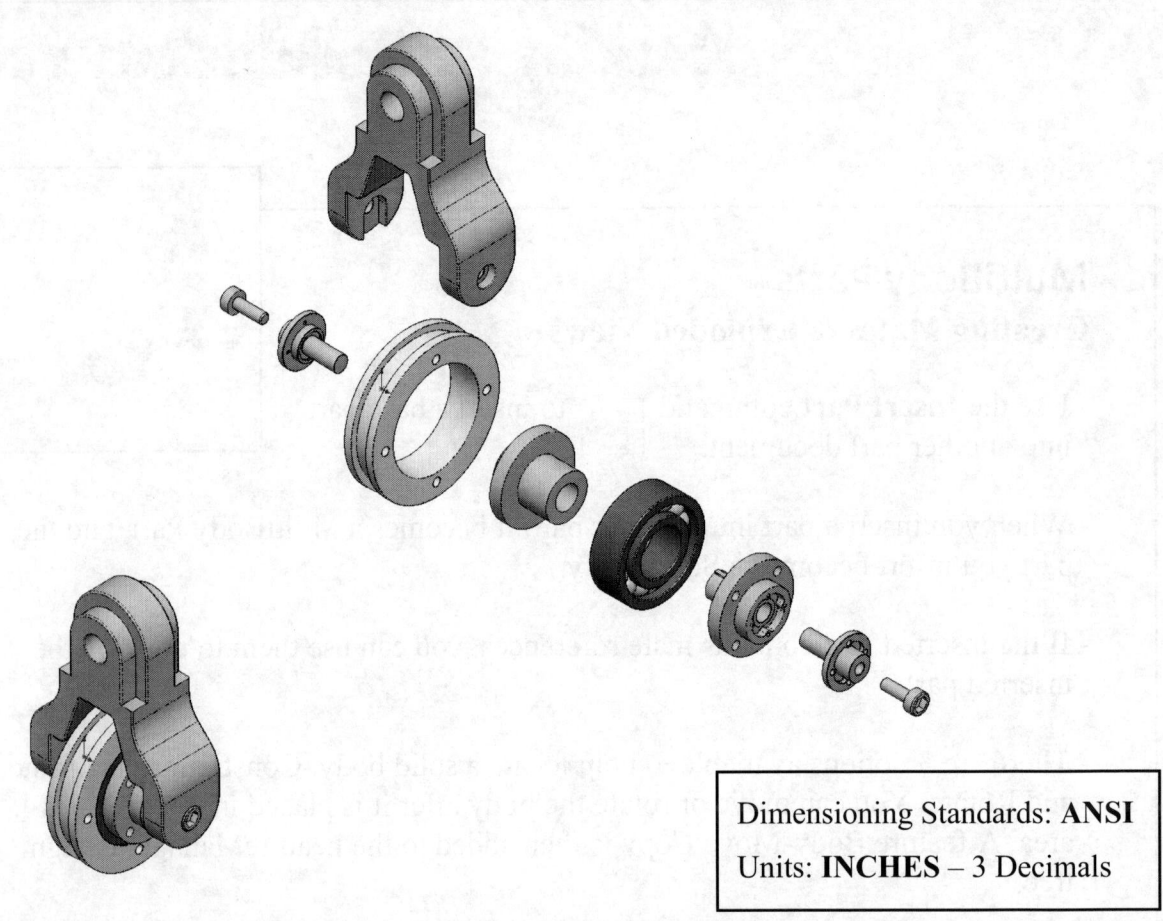

Dimensioning Standards: **ANSI**

Units: **INCHES** – 3 Decimals

Tools Needed:

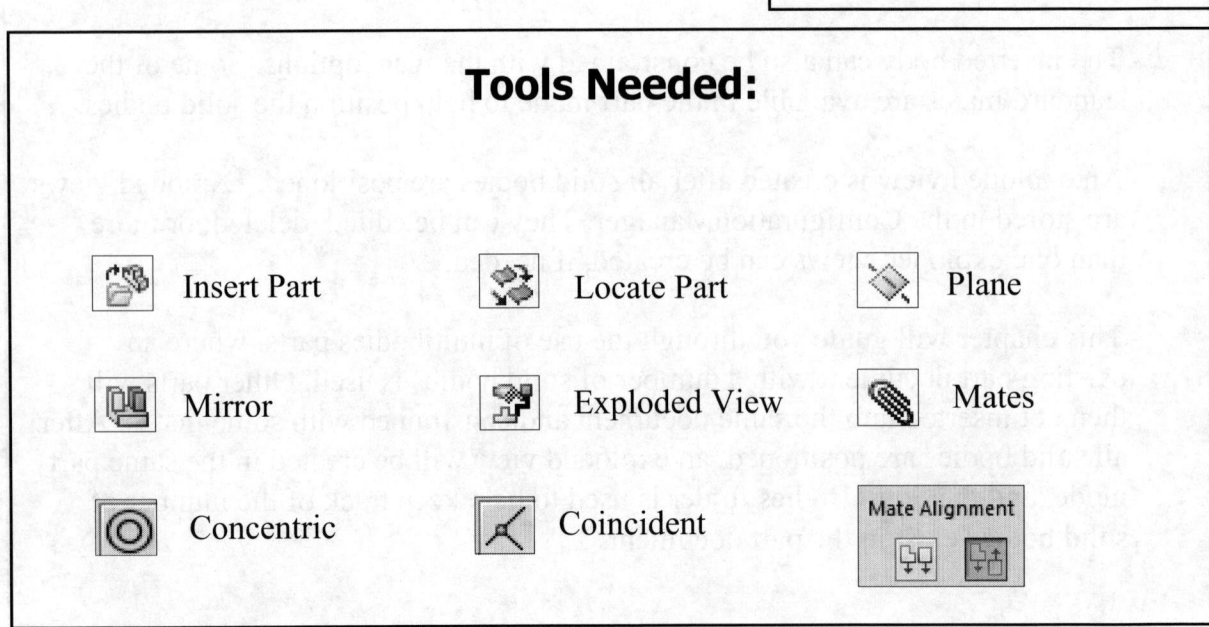

Insert Part

Locate Part

Plane

Mirror

Exploded View

Mates

Concentric

Coincident

Mate Alignment

1. Opening a part document:

- Go to **File / Open**.

- Browse to the Training Files folder. Locate the part document named: **MultiBodies Parts** and open it.

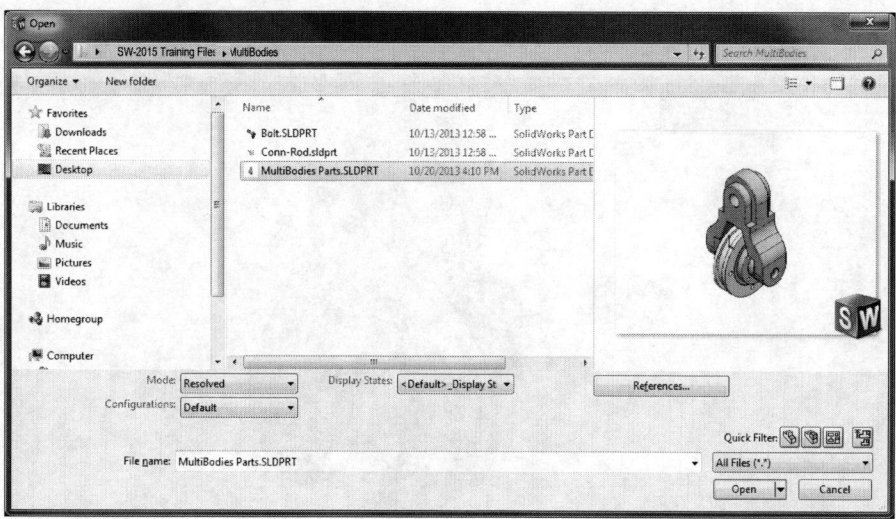

- When opening a non-SolidWorks native document, the program will prompt you with a couple of options such as Import Diagnostics or Feature-Recognition. We will not discuss these options in this chapter but focus on the use of MultiBodies instead.

- If prompted, click **No** to cancel the Import Diagnostics option.

- Click **No** once again to cancel the Feature Recognition options

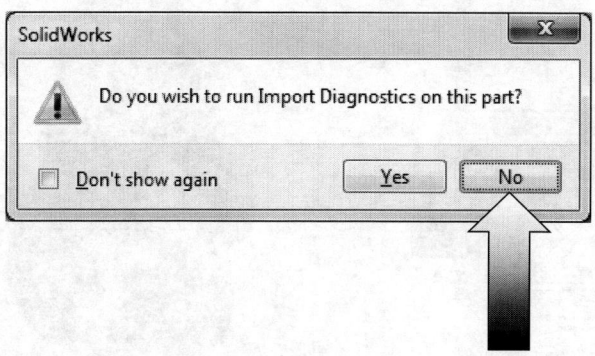

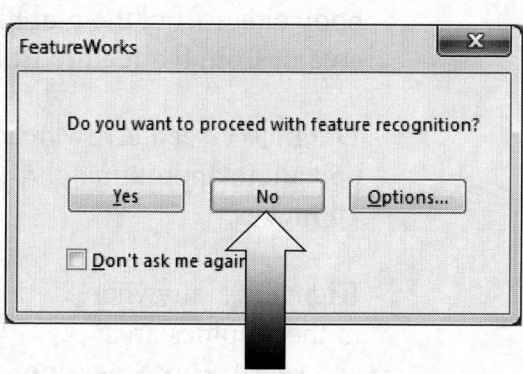

2. Creating an exploded view:

- An exploded view is going to be created so that the collapse / explode stages can be toggled back and forth in the future.

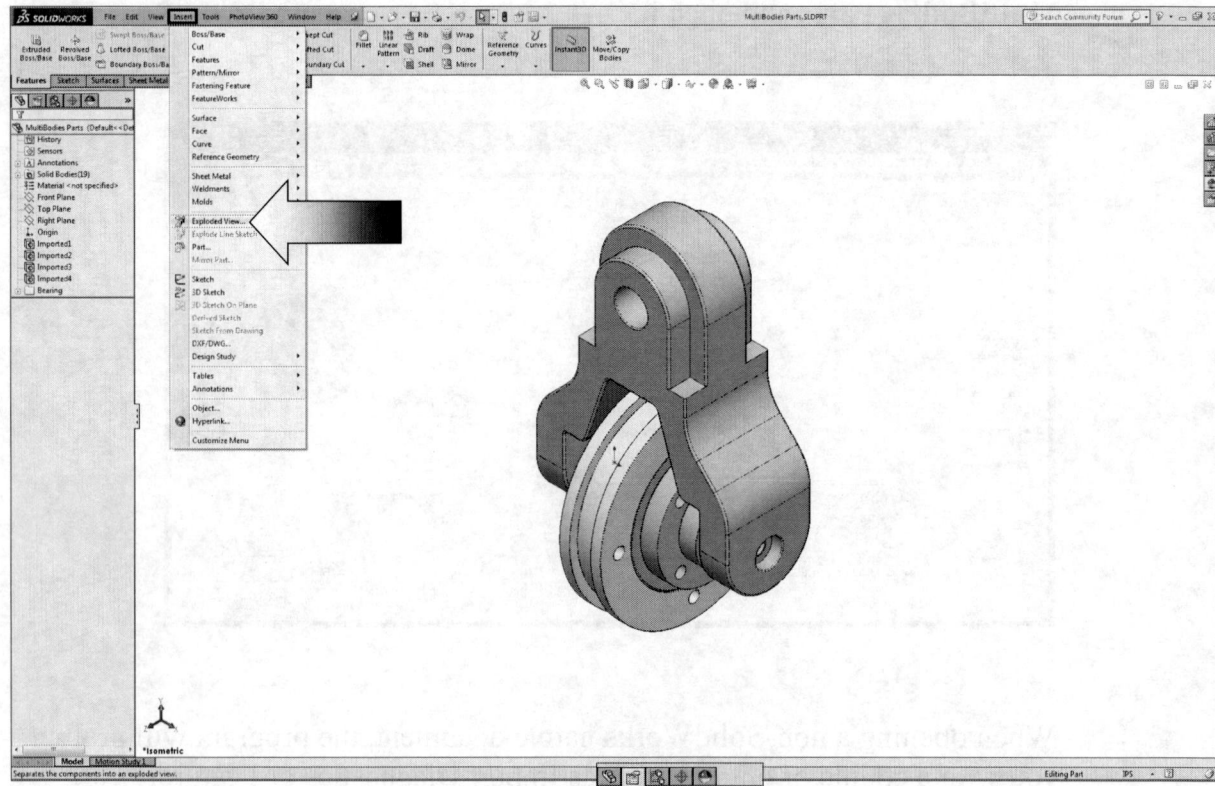

- Select **Insert/ Exploded View**.

- The Exploded dialog appears similar to the one seen in the assembly mode.

- Select the **Imported2** solid body either from the graphics area or from the feature tree.

- Drag the **Green** arrow head upward to approximately **10 inches**.

- Right click anywhere in the graphics area and select: **Box Selection**.

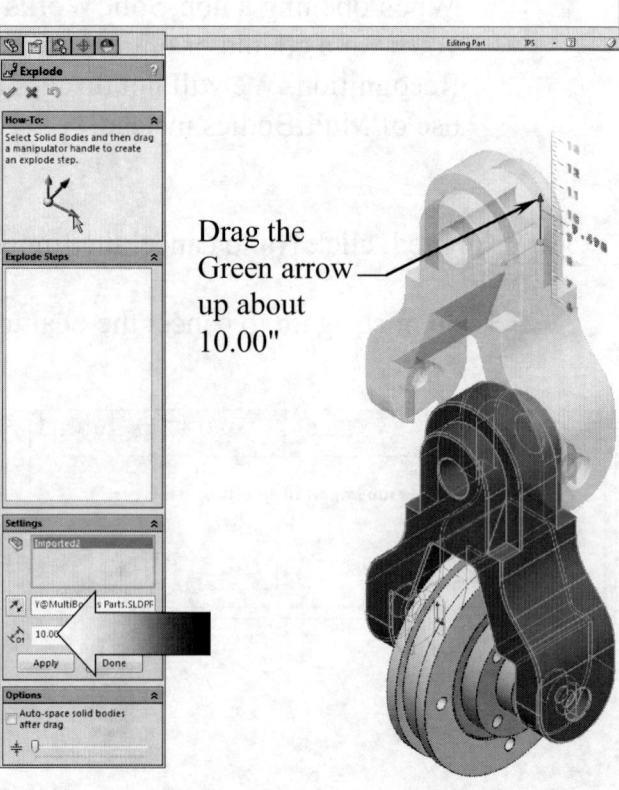

Drag the Green arrow up about 10.00"

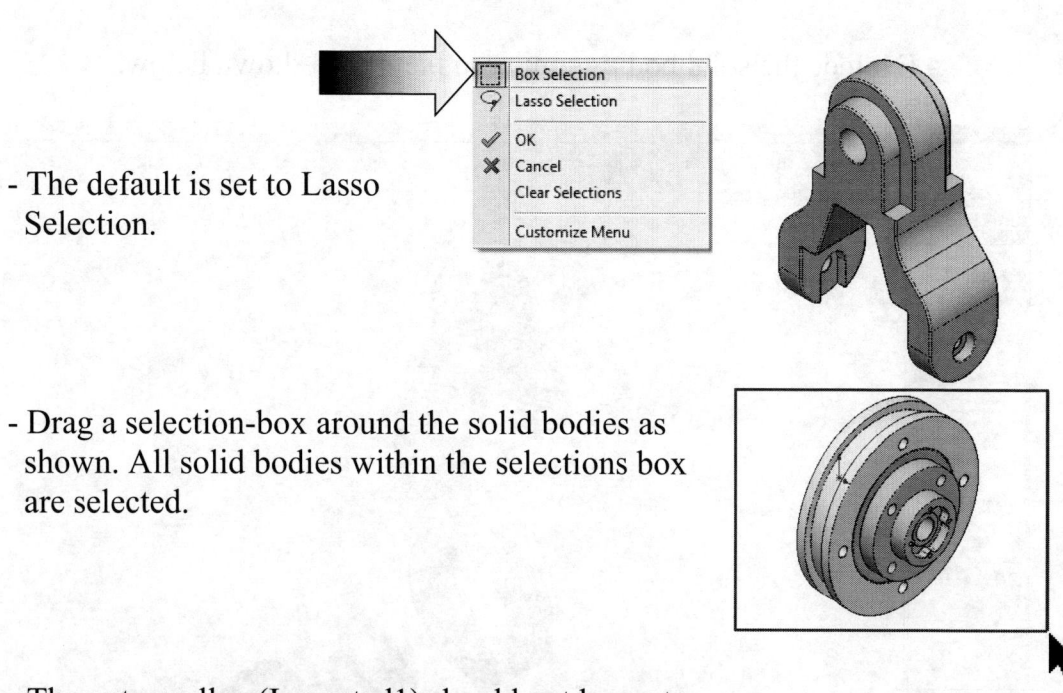

- The default is set to Lasso Selection.

- Drag a selection-box around the solid bodies as shown. All solid bodies within the selections box are selected.

- The outer pulley (Imported1) should not be part of this group, so we are going to unselect it before exploding this group of solid bodies.

- Either hold the Control key and click the Imported1 body to exclude it from the group, or delete it from the list under the Settings section.

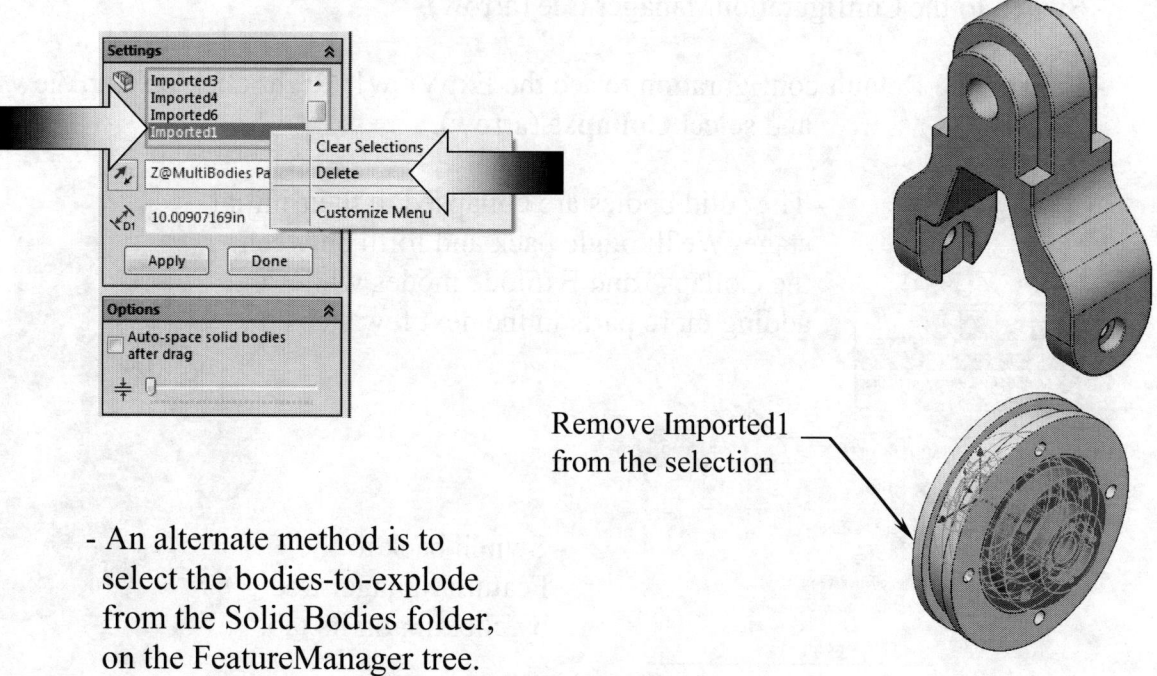

Remove Imported1
from the selection

- An alternate method is to select the bodies-to-explode from the Solid Bodies folder, on the FeatureManager tree.

- Explode the solid bodies similar to the image shown below.

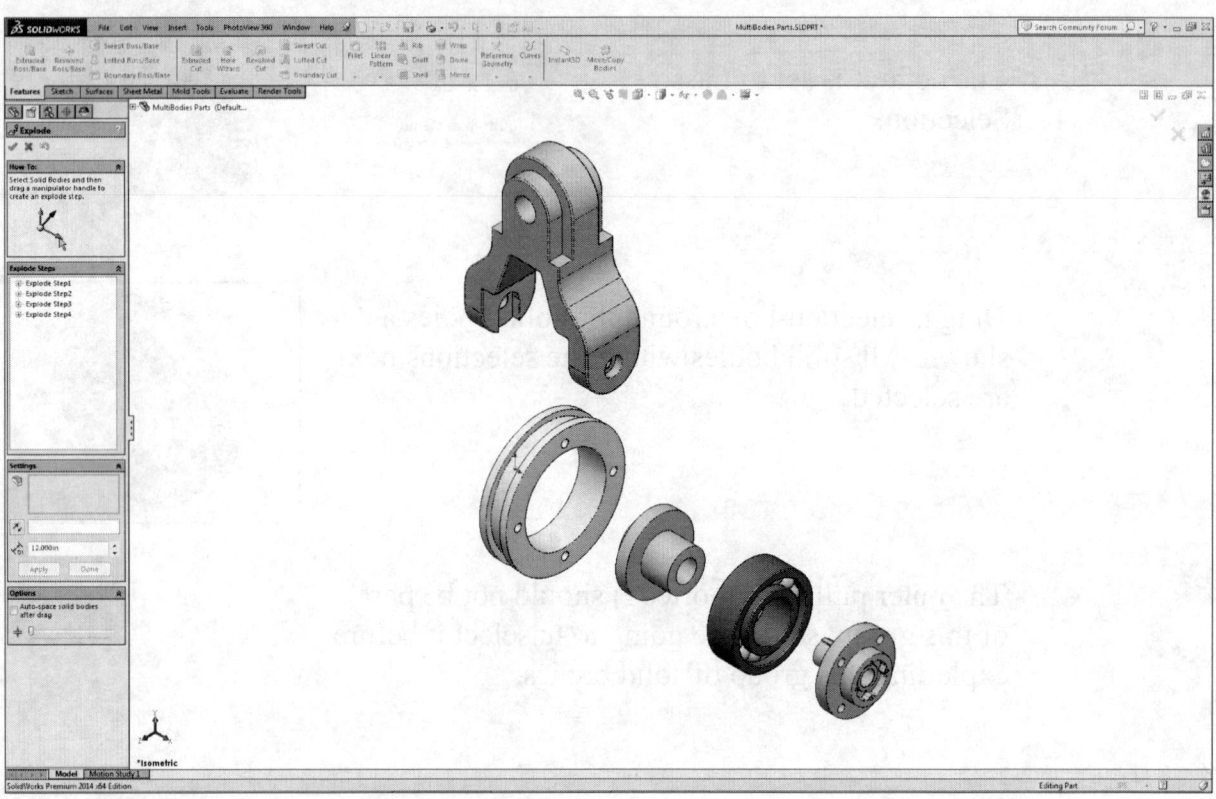

3. Collapsing the solid bodies:

- Switch to the ConfigurationManager tree (arrow).

- Expand the Default configuration to see the ExpView1. Right click on ExpView1 and select **Collapse** (arrow).

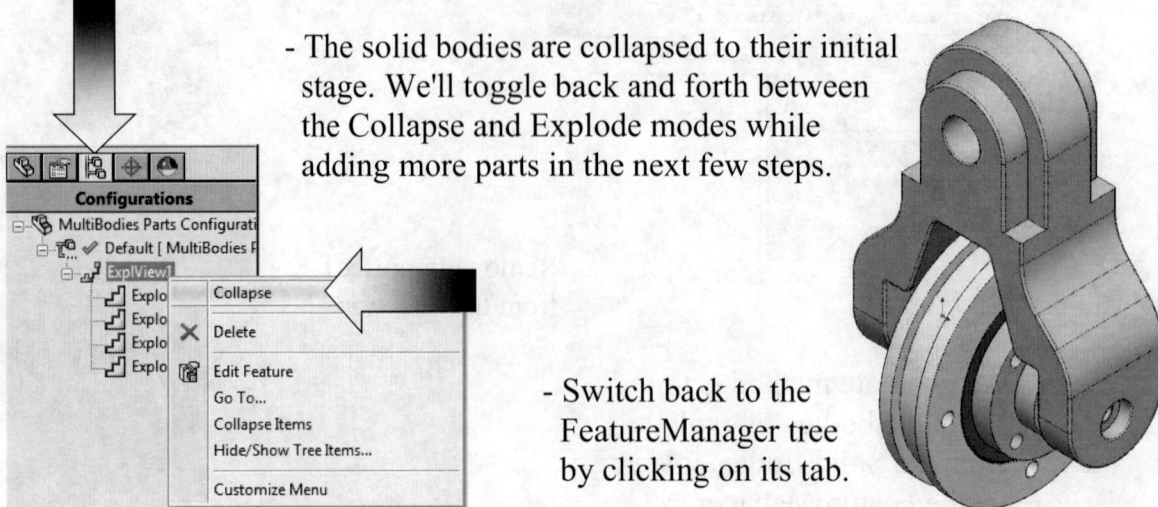

- The solid bodies are collapsed to their initial stage. We'll toggle back and forth between the Collapse and Explode modes while adding more parts in the next few steps.

- Switch back to the FeatureManager tree by clicking on its tab.

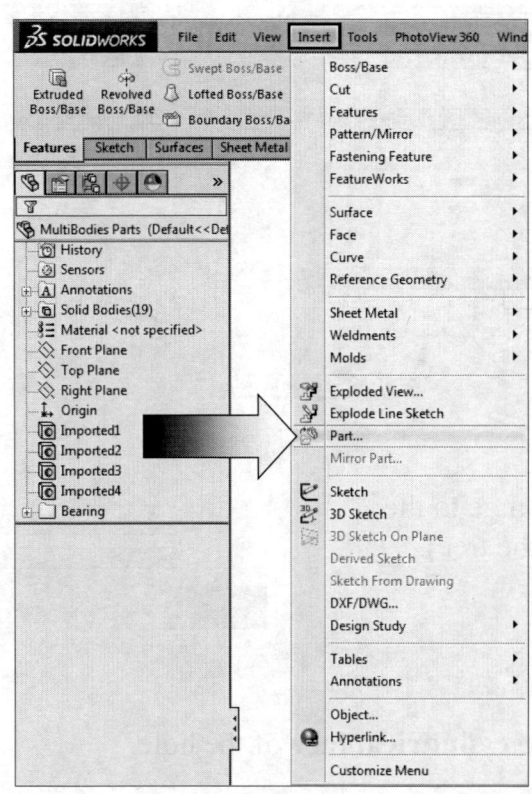

4. Inserting another part:

- Other parts can be inserted into an existing part document. Once inserted they will become Solid Bodies, and the original part becomes a Multibody Part.

- Click **Insert / Part**.

- Select the part document named: **Conn-Rod.sldprt** from the same training files directory and open it.

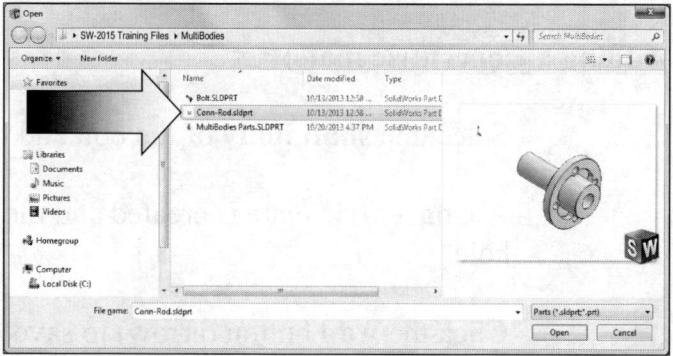

- Place the new part on the right side of the others, approx. as shown below.

- The **Insert Part** dialog box appears.

- Select the following options:

    * **Solid Bodies**

    * **Planes**

    * **Locate Part with Move/ Copy feature**

- Uncheck all other checkboxes.

- Click **OK**.

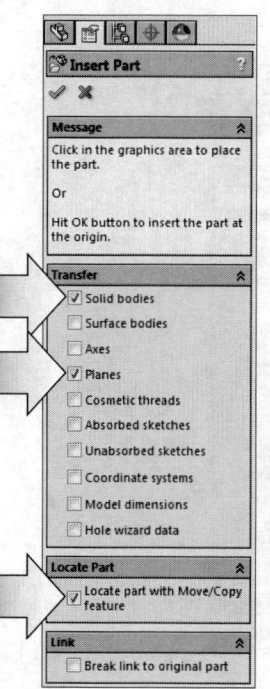

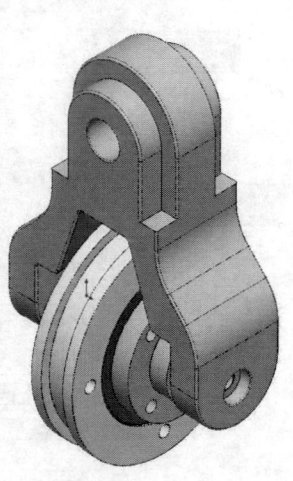

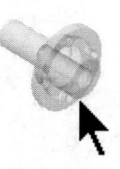

5. Constraining the solid bodies:

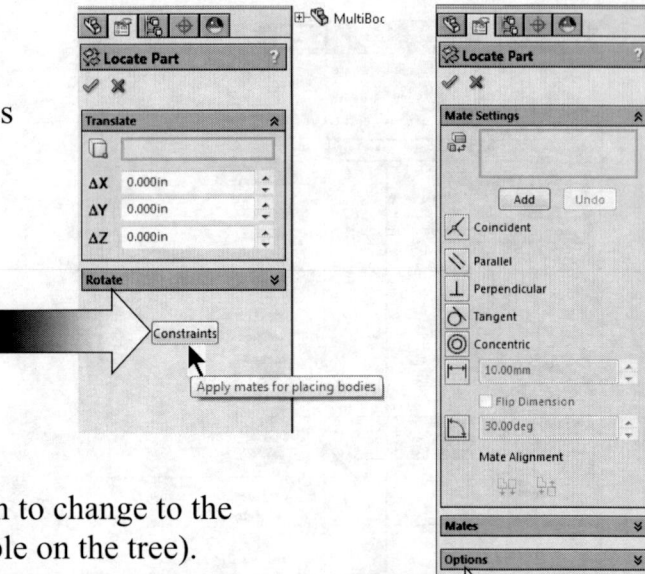

- By clicking OK from the previous step the **Locate Part** section is activated.

- Click the **Constraints** button to switch to the Mate Settings mode (arrow).

(Click the Translate / Rotate button to change to the Constraints section if it is not visible on the tree).

Adding a Concentric mate:

- Select the **shaft body** of the bolt and the **cylindrical face** of the hole.

- A **Concentric** mate is created and the bolt moves to the same center with the hole.

- Click the **Add** button (arrow) to save the mate in its mate group below.

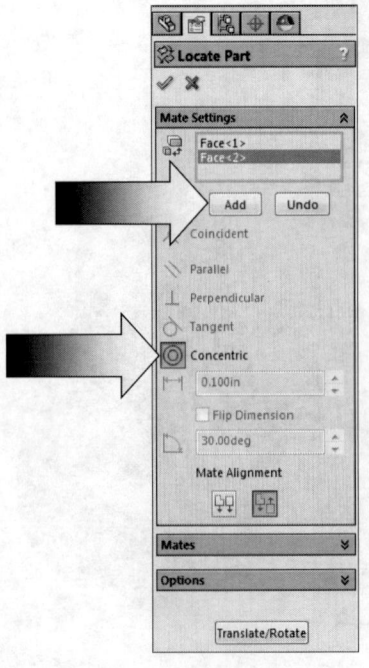

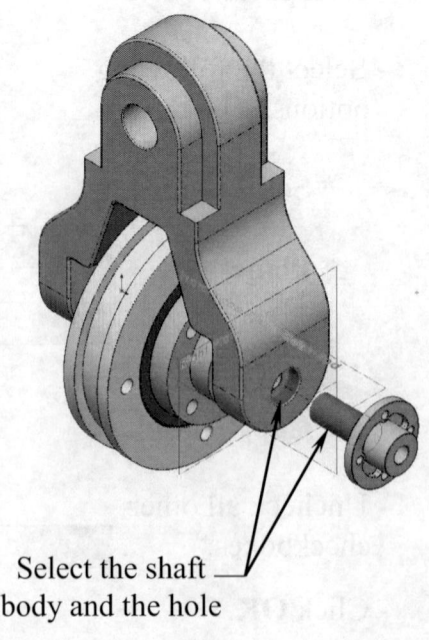

Select the shaft body and the hole

Adding a Coincident mate:

- Select the 1st **planar face** (face1) as indicated.

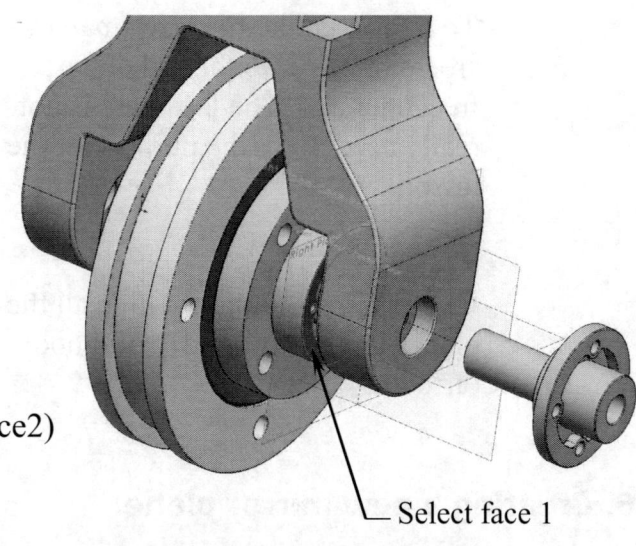

- Select the 2nd **planar face** (face2) as noted.

Select face 1

- A **Coincident** mate is created and the 2 selected faces are now coincide or occupying the same place.

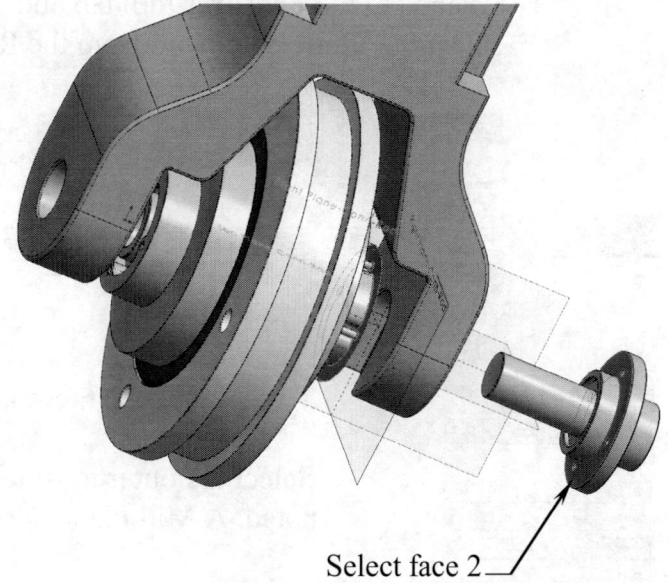

Select face 2

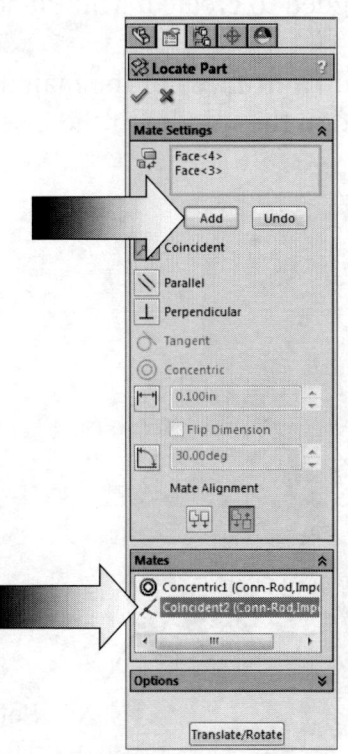

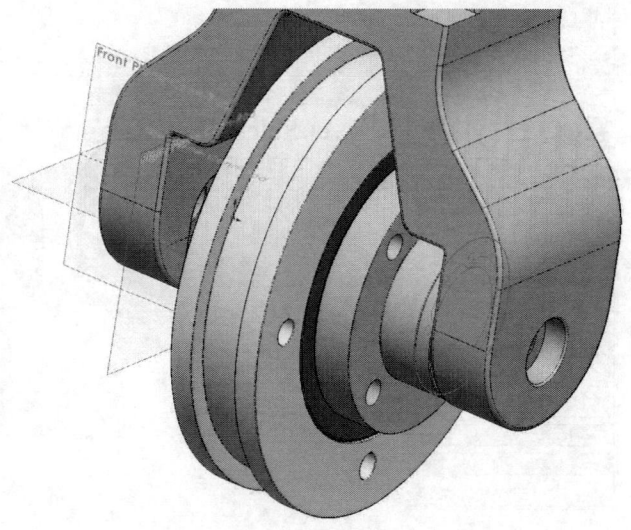

- To help keep the file size smaller, we are going to leave the 3rd degree of freedom open. The last mate is not really needed for the purpose of the lesson.

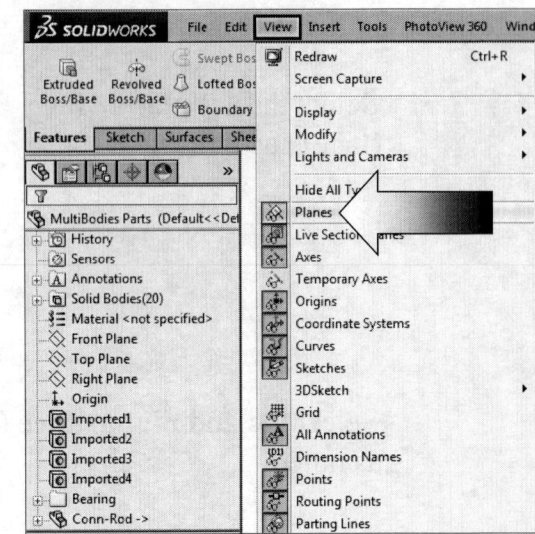

- Click: **View / Planes** to hide all the planes in the Imported1 solid body (arrow).

6. Creating a new mirror plane:

- Change to the **Features** tool tab and select the **Plane** command from the Reference Geometry drop down arrow.

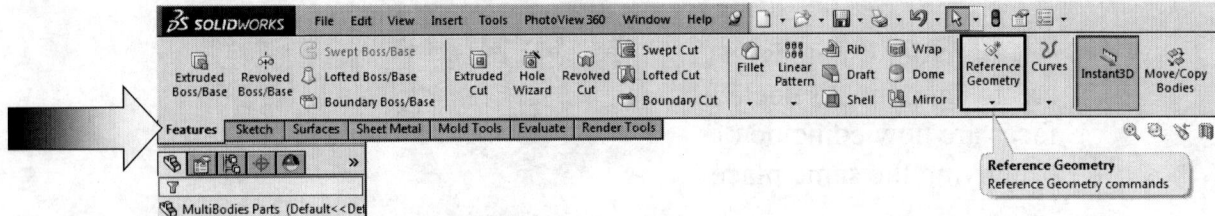

- Two **planar surfaces** are needed to create a Mid Plane.

- Select the outer most **left** and **right** faces of the main housing as noted. A Mid Plane is created in the middle of the 2 selected faces.

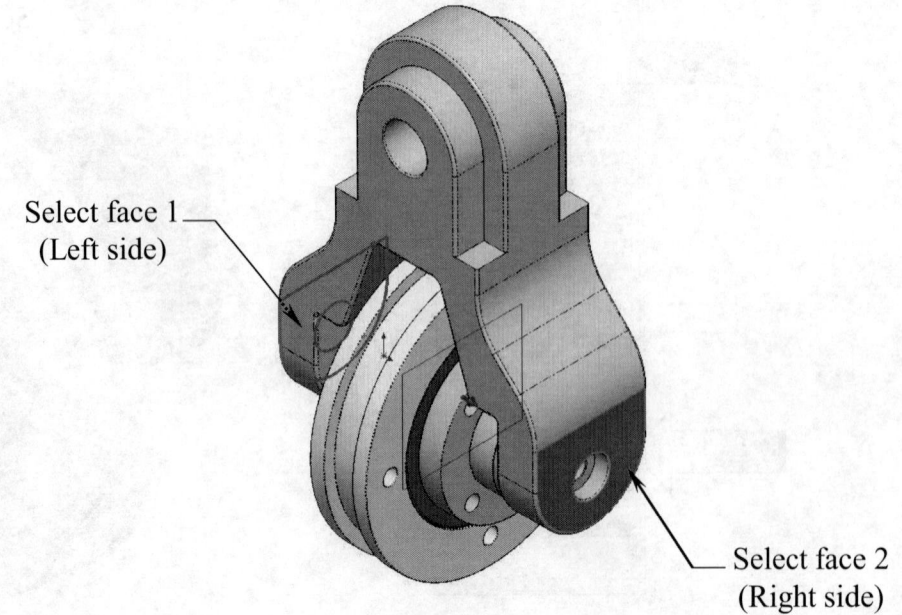

Select face 1
(Left side)

Select face 2
(Right side)

7. Creating a mirror body:

- Click the **Mirror** command from the Features tool tab.

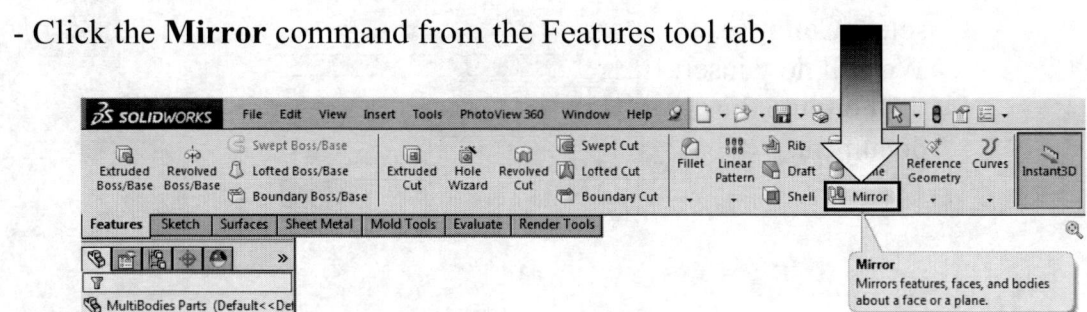

- Select the **new plane** for **Mirror Face / Plane** (arrow).

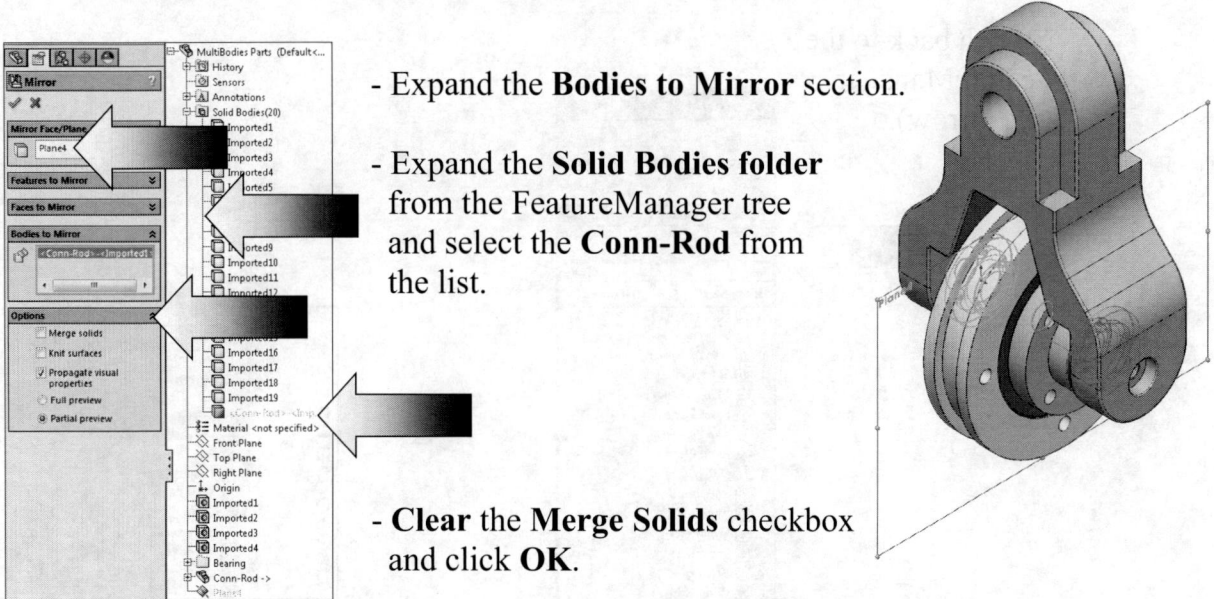

- Expand the **Bodies to Mirror** section.

- Expand the **Solid Bodies folder** from the FeatureManager tree and select the **Conn-Rod** from the list.

- **Clear** the **Merge Solids** checkbox and click **OK**.

- **Edit** the Exploded view and move the solid bodies to the positions approx. as shown.

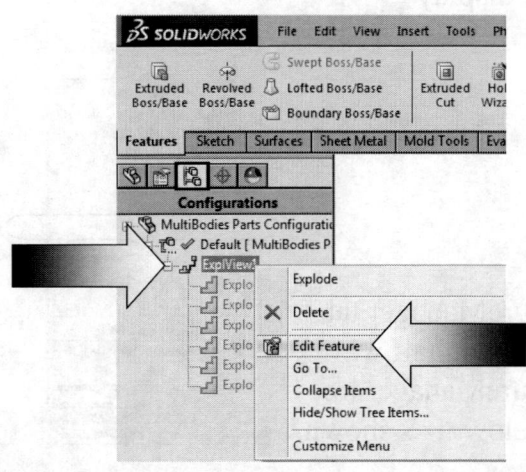

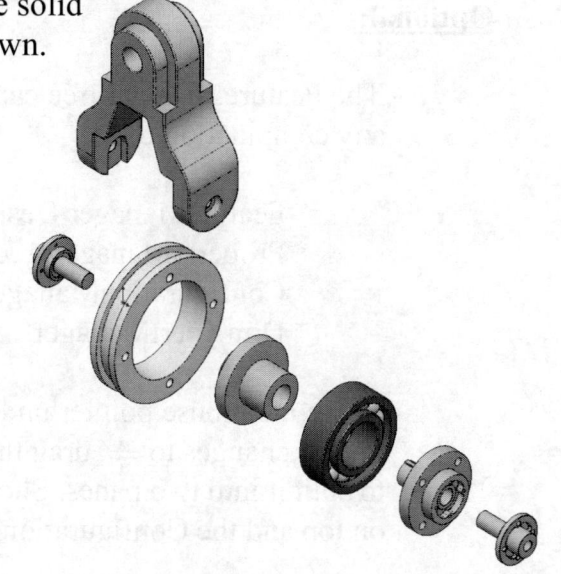

- Right click on ExplView1 and select **Collapse**. We will now insert the bolt into this document.

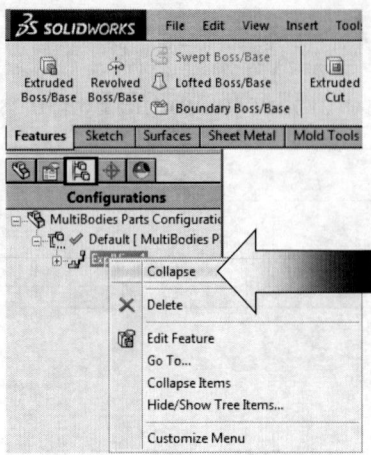

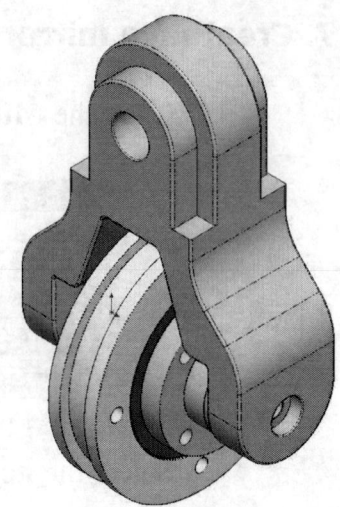

- Switch back to the FeatureManager tree (arrow).

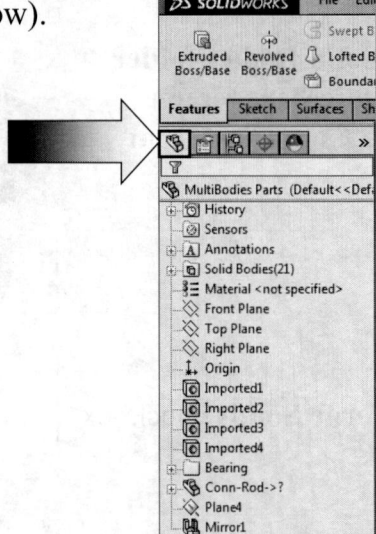

Optional:

- The FeatureManager tree can be split to display any combination of:

    * FeatureManager Design tree
    * PropertyManager tree
    * ConfigurationManager
    * DimXpertManager

- Move the mouse pointer under the FeatureManager tab until it changes to ⇕, drag the split bar down half way to split it into two panes. Show the FeatureManager tree on top and the ConfigurationManager below it as shown.

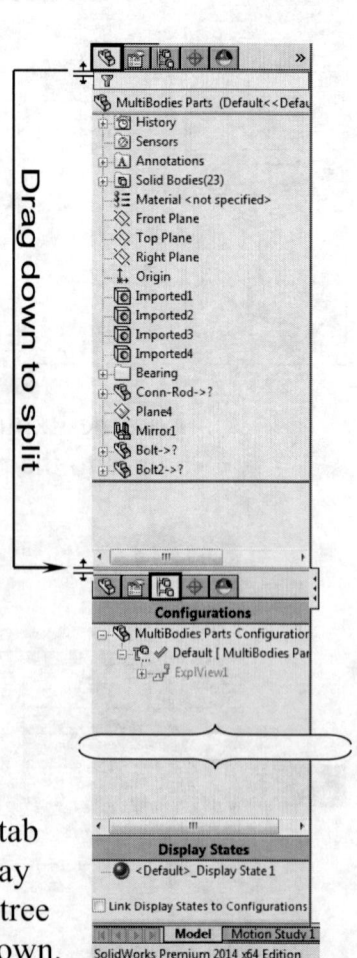

8. Inserting another part:

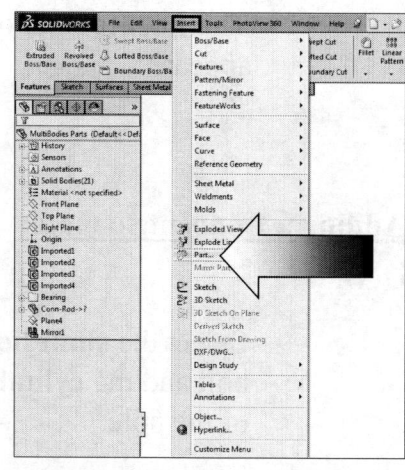

- The Bolt is going to be inserted into the same part document, it will become another solid body, and the part document is called Multi-Body Part.

- Click **Insert / Part**.

- Select the part **Bolt.sldprt** from the previous training files folder.

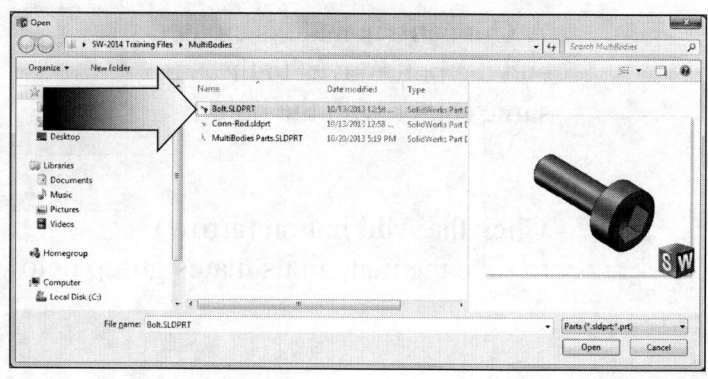

- Place the new part on the right side of the main housing.

- Click **YES** to change the units of the new part to match the units of the MultiBody part.

- Select the **3 checkboxes** as noted and click **OK**.

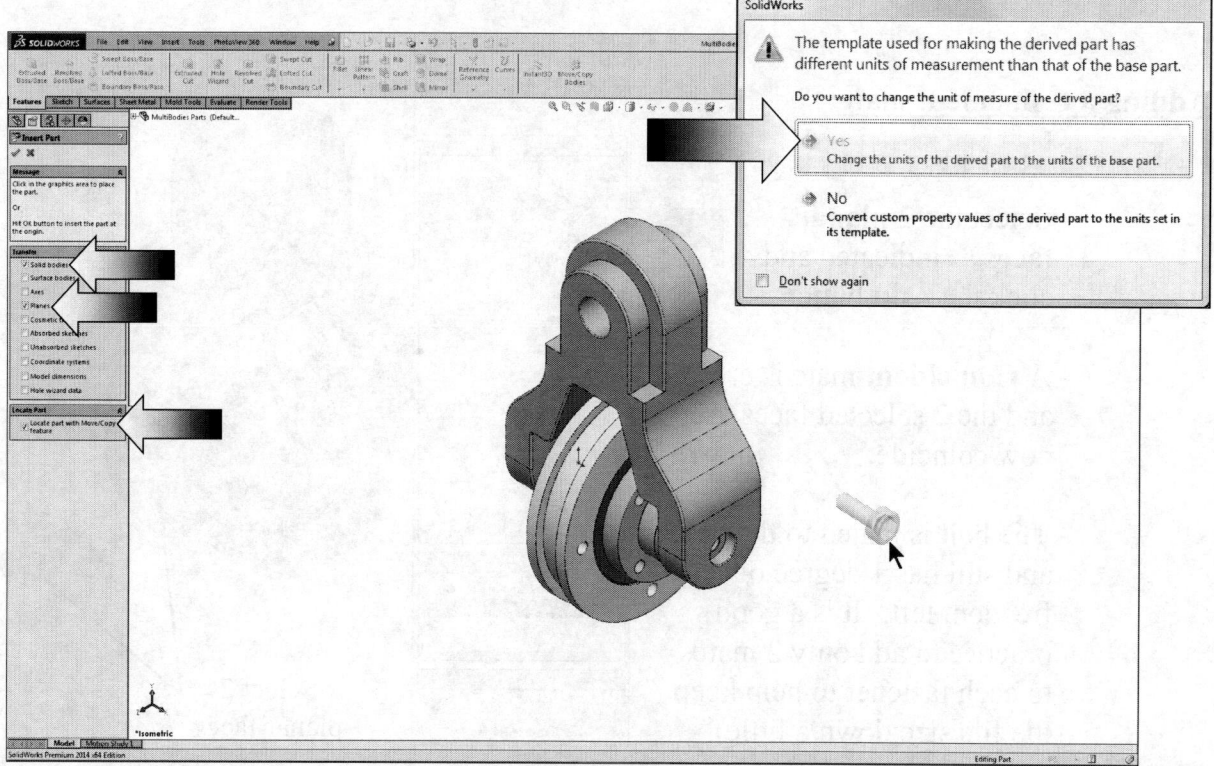

- The **Locate Part** options appear.

Adding a Concentric mate:

- Select the **shaft body** of the bolt and the **cylindrical face** of the hole.

- A **Concentric** mate is created and the bolt moves to the same center with the hole.

- Click the **Add** button (arrow) to save the mate in its mates group below.

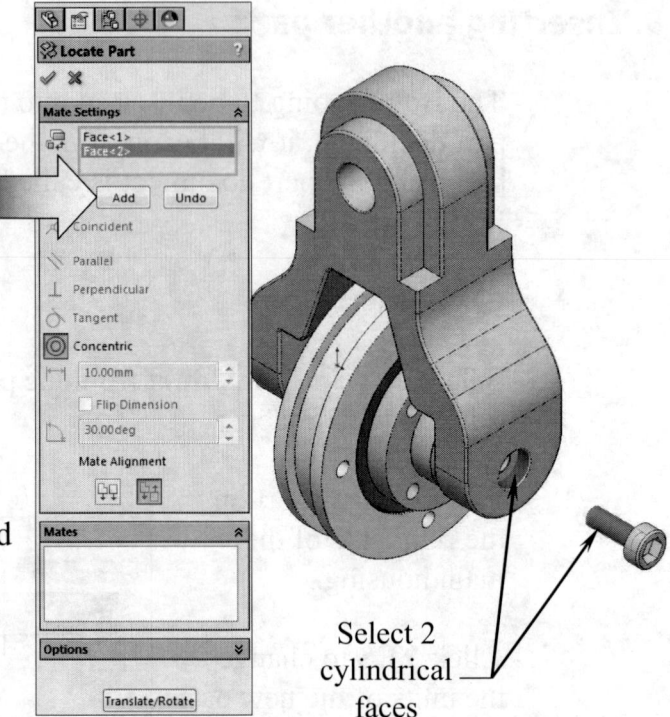

Select 2 cylindrical faces

Adding a Coincident mate:

- Select the 2 **planar-faces** as indicated and click the **Add** button.

- A **Coincident** mate is created and the 2 selected faces are now coincide.

- The bolt is mated to the hole and still has 1 degree of freedom left. (It is a good practice to add only 2 mates to each fastener to help keep the file size down a little).

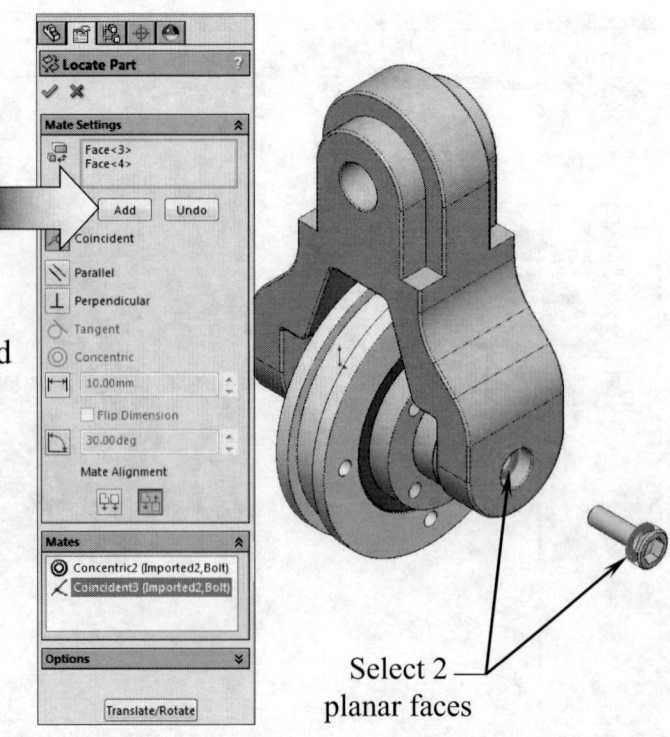

Select 2 planar faces

9. Adding another instance of the bolt:

- A second instance of the bolt is needed on the opposite side of the main housing.

- Click **Insert / Part**.

- Select the part **Bolt.sldprt** once again from the previous directory.

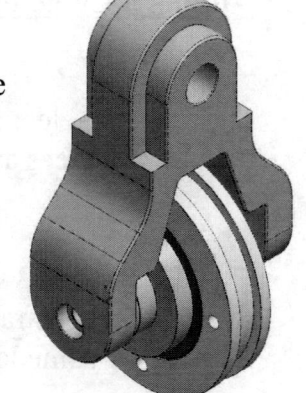

- Rotate the view and place the new part on the left side on the of the main housing.

Adding a Concentric mate:

- Select the body of the bolt and the side hole of the main housing to add a **Concentric** mate.

- Click the **Anti-Aligned** button to flip the bolt 180 degrees (arrow), and then click the **Add** button to save the new mate in its Mates group.

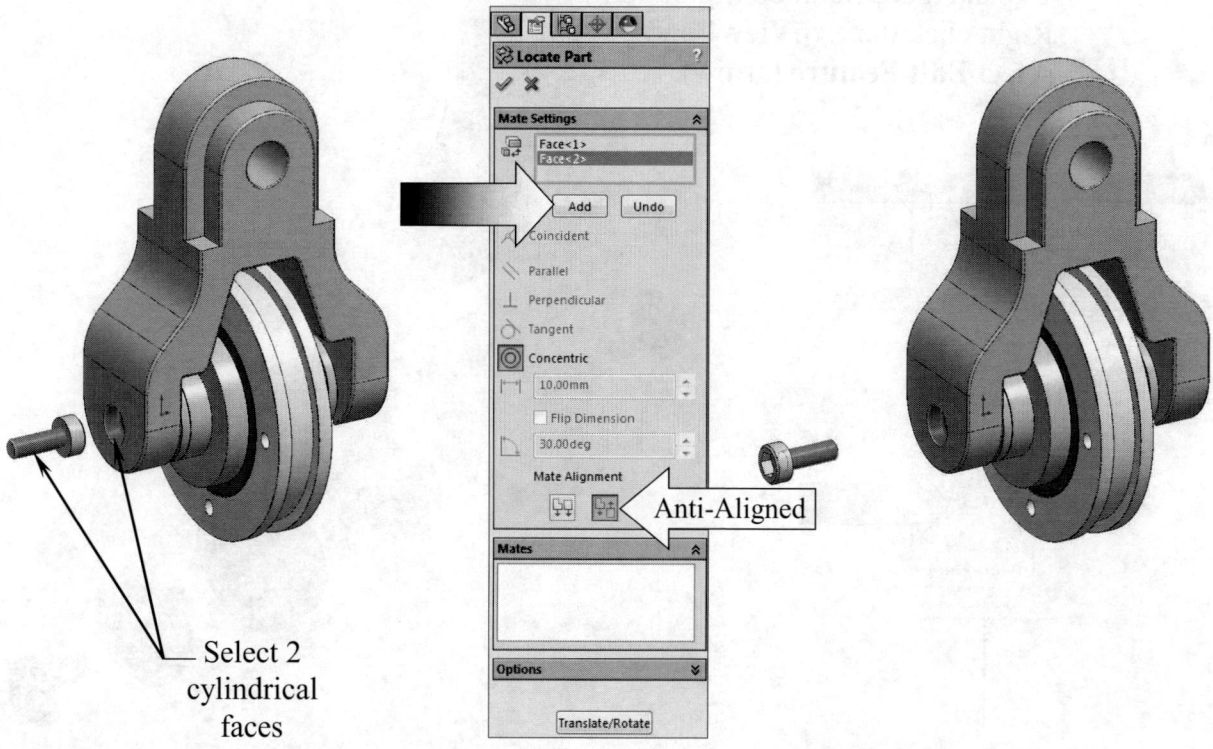

Select 2 cylindrical faces

Anti-Aligned

Adding a Coincident mate:

- Select the 2 **planar-faces** as indicated.

- The 2 selected faces are constrained to share the same location.

- Click the **Add** button to save the new mate.

- Click **OK** to exit the Locate Part mode.

Select 2 planar faces

10. Editing the exploded view:

- Switch to the ConfigurationManager.

- Expand the Default configuration. Right click the **ExpView1** and select **Edit Feature** (arrow).

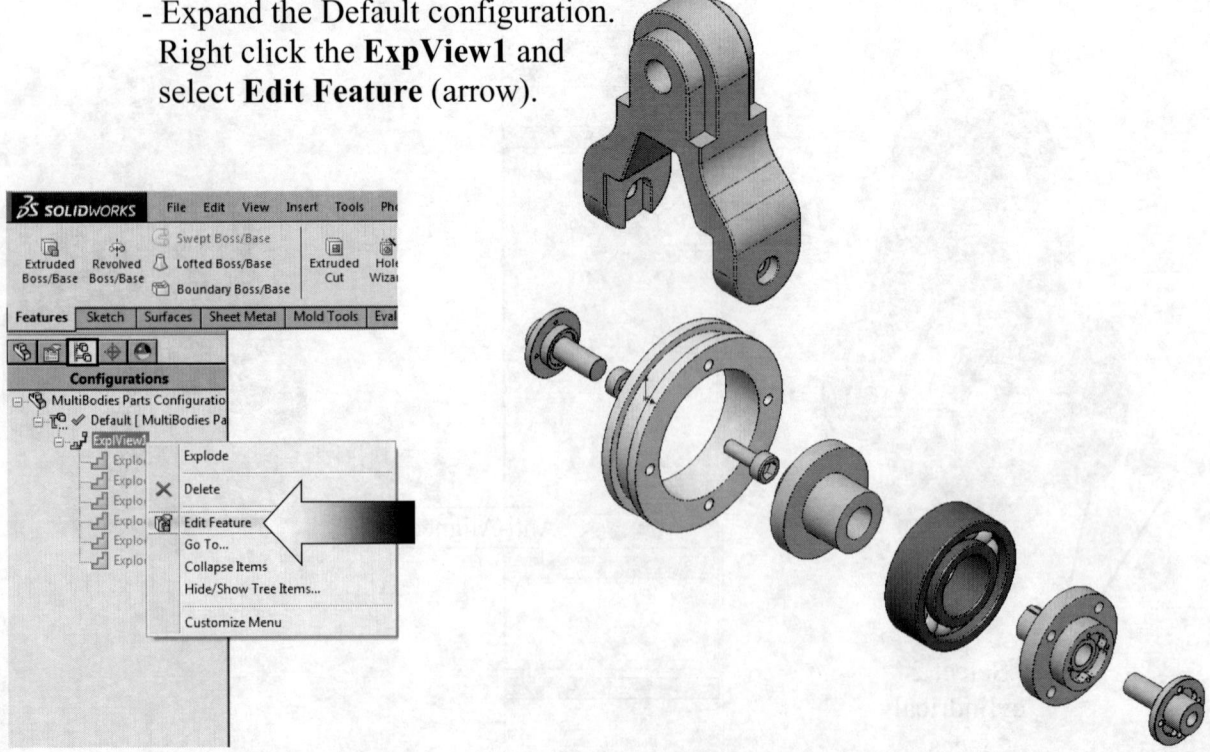

- Select the bolt on the right.

- Drag the head of the **Red arrow** to move the bolt along the X direction.

NOTE: _Enter a dimension* if a precise distance is preferred._

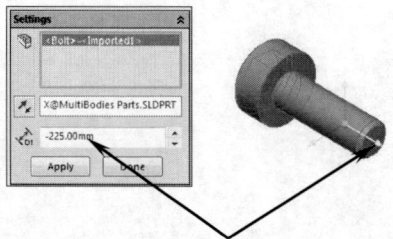

* If distance is used: Select a direction arrow (red), enter a dimension then click Apply and Done.

- Select the bolt on the left.

- Drag the head of the **Red arrow** to the left to move the bolt along the -X direction.

- Click **OK** to exit the exploded View mode.

11. Saving your work:

- Click **File / Save As**.

- Enter: **MultiBodies Parts** for the name of the file.

- Click **Save**.

- Close all documents.

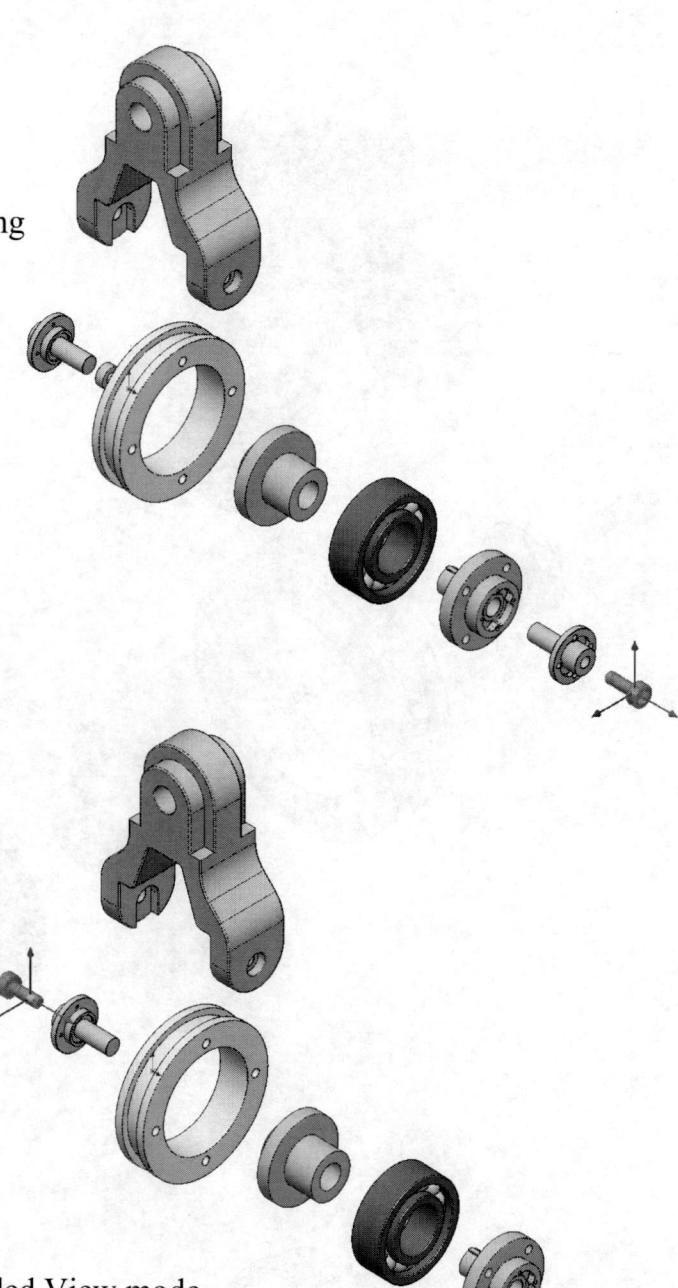

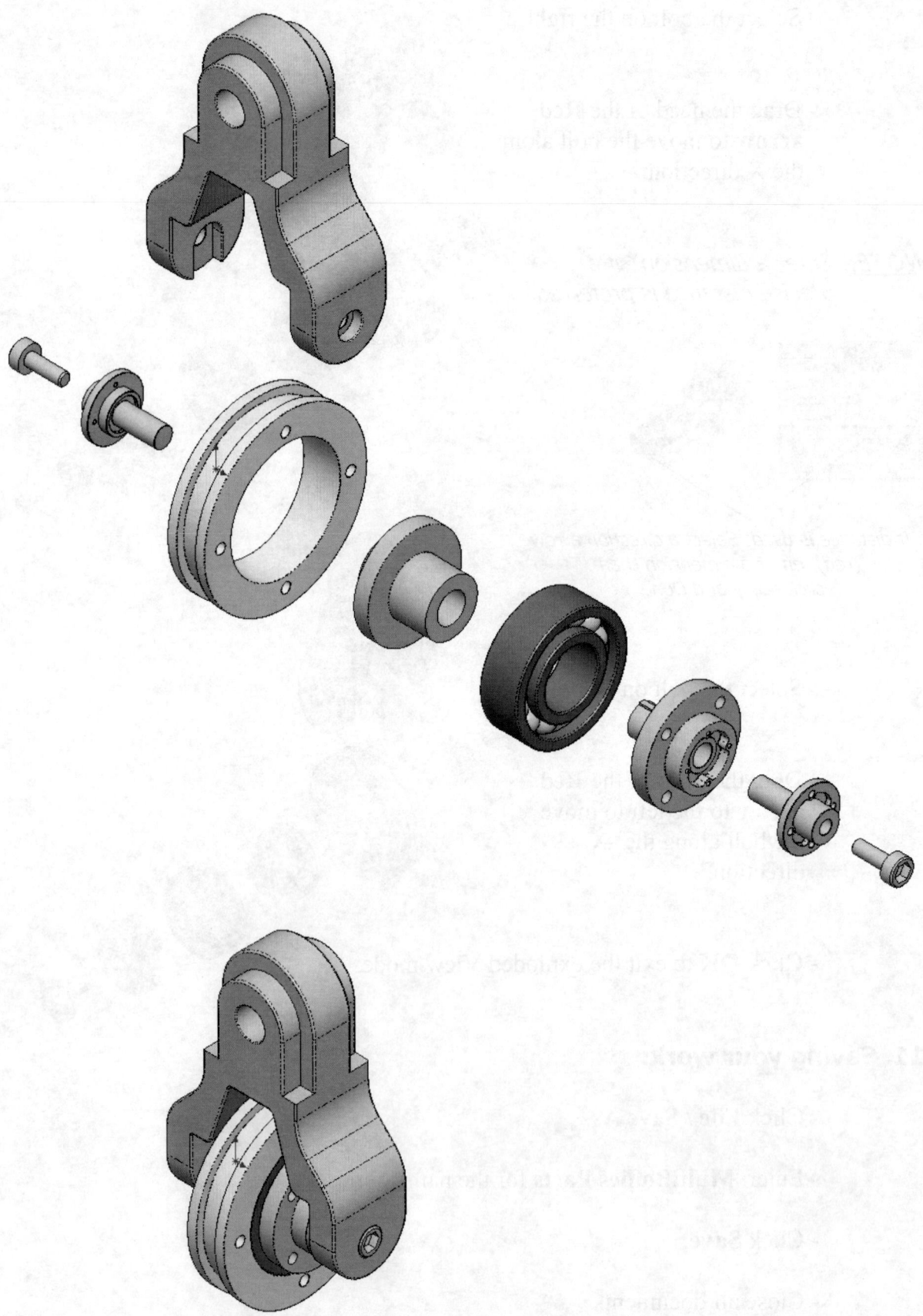

CHAPTER 10

Bottom Up Assembly

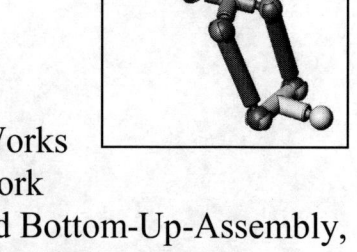

Bottom Up Assembly
Ball Joint Assembly

- When your design involves multiple parts, SolidWorks offers 4 different assembly methods to help you work faster and more efficient. The first method is called Bottom-Up-Assembly, the second method is called Layout-Assembly, the third Top-Down-Assembly, and the fourth, Master-Modeling.

- We will explore the first two methods, the Bottom-Up and the Lay-Out Assemblies in this Part-1 textbook.

- When individual components get inserted into an assembly document and mated (constrained) together, is called Bottom Up Assembly.

- The first component inserted into the assembly will be fixed by the system automatically. If it is placed on the Origin, then the Front, Top, and the Right planes of the first component will automatically be aligned with the assembly's planes.

- Only the first part will be fixed by default, all other components are free to move or be re-oriented.

- Each component has a total of 6 degrees of freedom; depending on the mate type, once a mate is assigned to a component one or more of its degrees of freedom are removed, causing the component to move or rotate only in the desired directions.

- All Mates (constraints) are stored in the FeatureManager tree under the Mates group. They can be edited, suppressed, or deleted.

Ball Joint Assembly
Bottom-Up Assembly

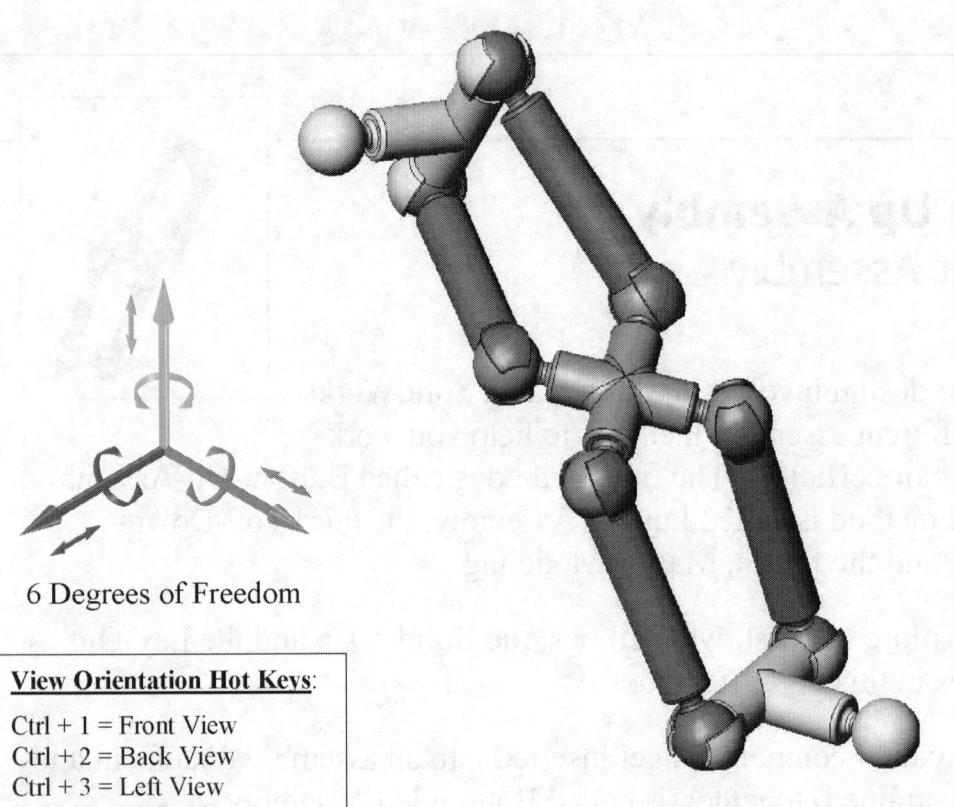

6 Degrees of Freedom

View Orientation Hot Keys:

Ctrl + 1 = Front View
Ctrl + 2 = Back View
Ctrl + 3 = Left View
Ctrl + 4 = Right View
Ctrl + 5 = Top View
Ctrl + 6 = Bottom View
Ctrl + 7 = Isometric View
Ctrl + 8 = Normal To
Selection

Dimensioning Standards: **ANSI**

Units: **INCHES** – 3 Decimals

Tools Needed:

 Mates

 Move Component

 Rotate Component

 Concentric Mate

 Inference Origins

 Placing New Component

1. Starting a new Assembly template:

- Select **File / New / Assembly / OK**.

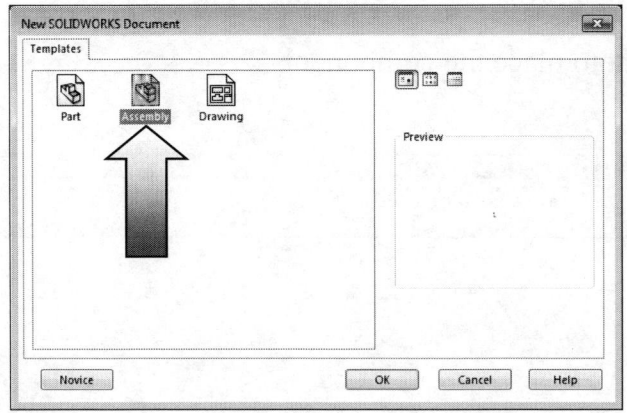

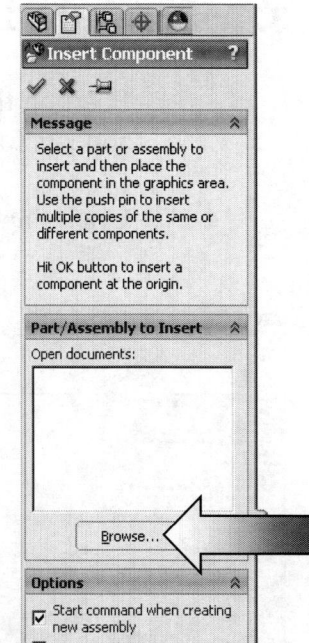

- In the Insert Component dialog, click Browse | Browse... | .

- Select the **Center Ball Joint** document from the Training folder and click **Open**.

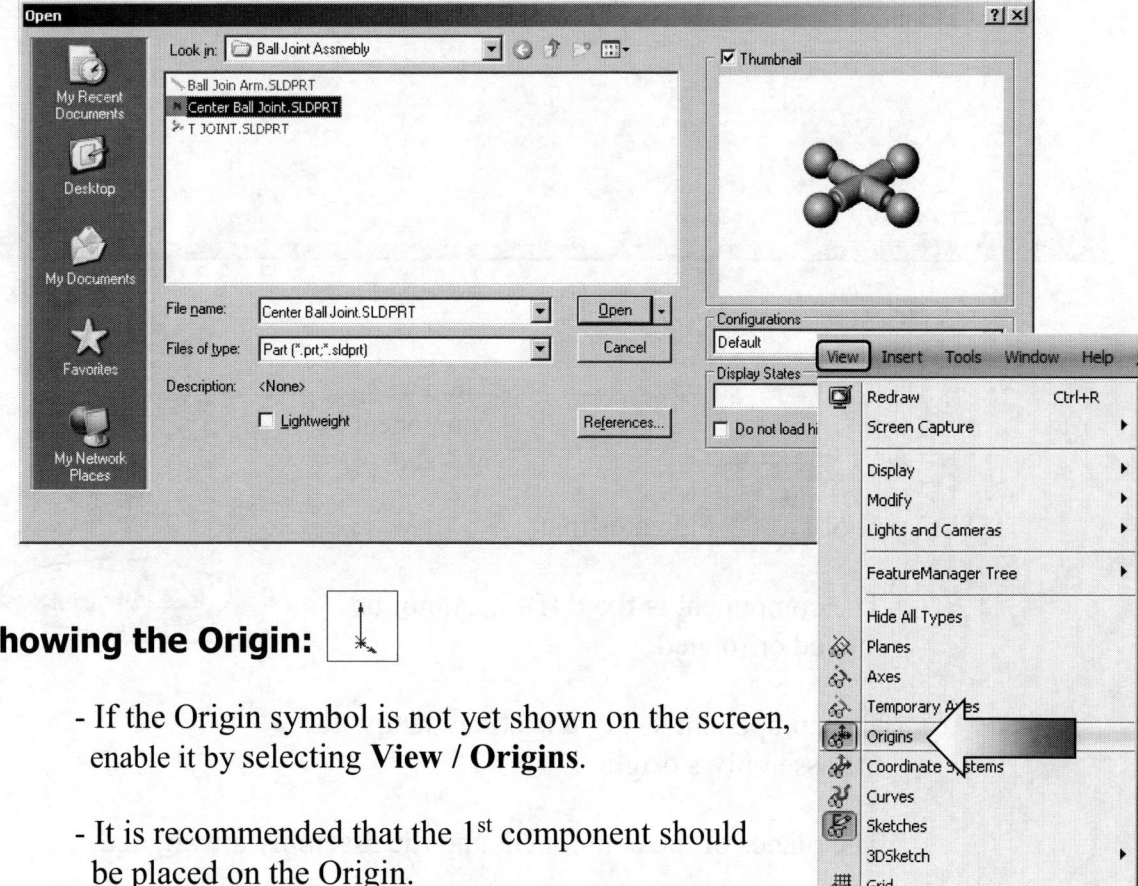

2. Showing the Origin:

- If the Origin symbol is not yet shown on the screen, enable it by selecting **View / Origins**.

- It is recommended that the 1st component should be placed on the Origin.

3. Inserting the 1st component (the Parent) on the Origin:

- Position the mouse cursor on the origin, an Origin-Inference symbol appears to confirm the location of the 1st component.

- Click the Origin point to place the component.

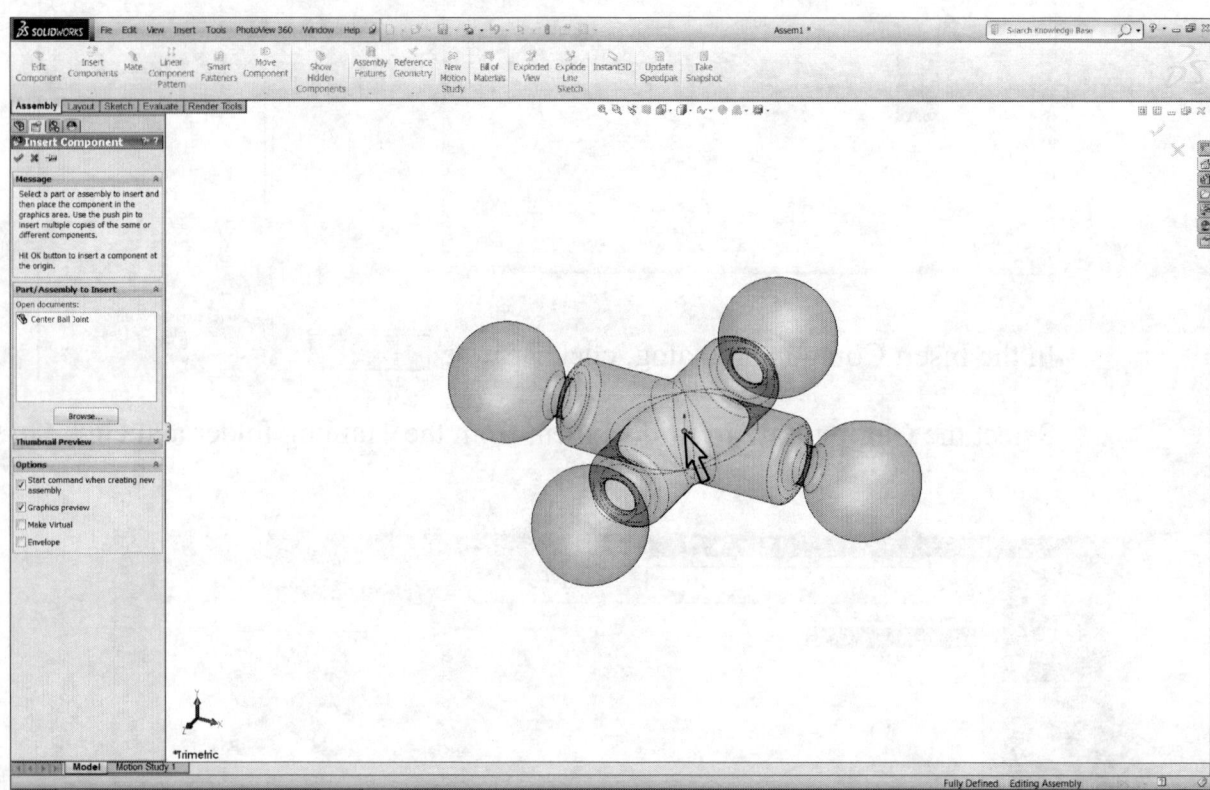

The 1st component is Fixed.

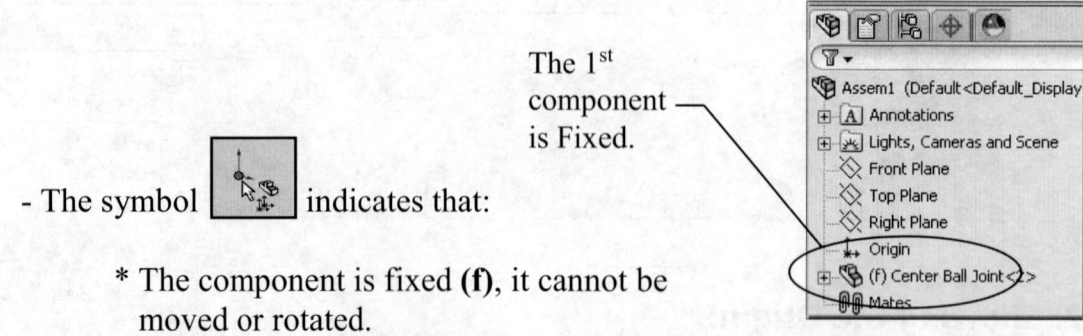

- The symbol indicates that:

* The component is fixed (**f**), it cannot be moved or rotated.

* The component's origin is coincident with the assembly's origin.

* The planes of the component and the assembly are aligned.

4. Inserting the second component (a child) into the assembly:

- Click [Insert Compon...] or Select **Insert / Component / Existing Part/Assembly**.

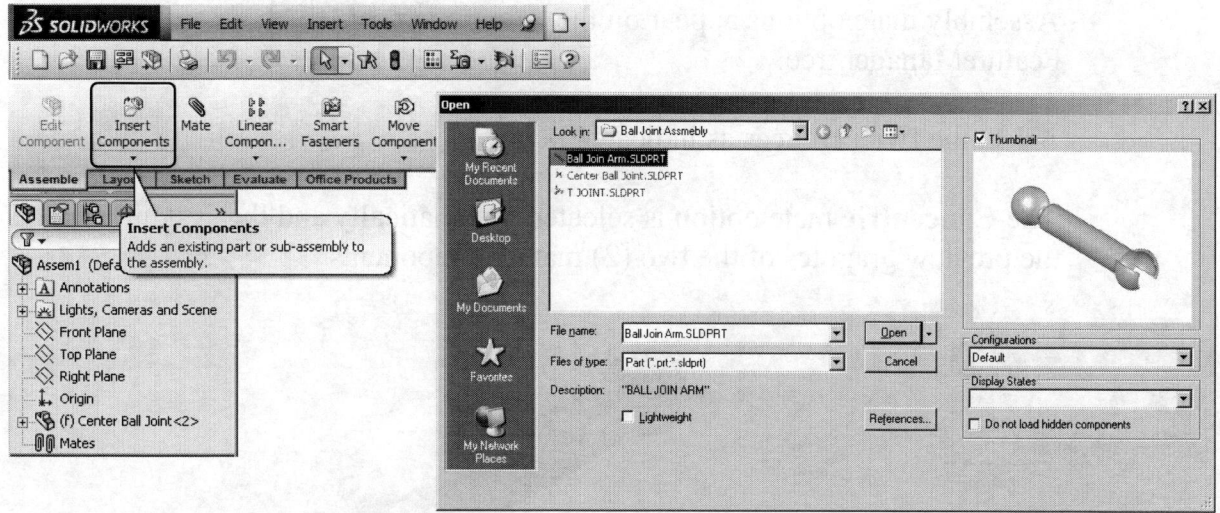

- Click **Browse** [Browse...].

- Select **Ball Joint Arm.sldprt** from the Training Files folder and click **Open**.

- The preview graphic of the component is attached to the mouse cursor.

- Place the new Child component above the Parent component as shown below.

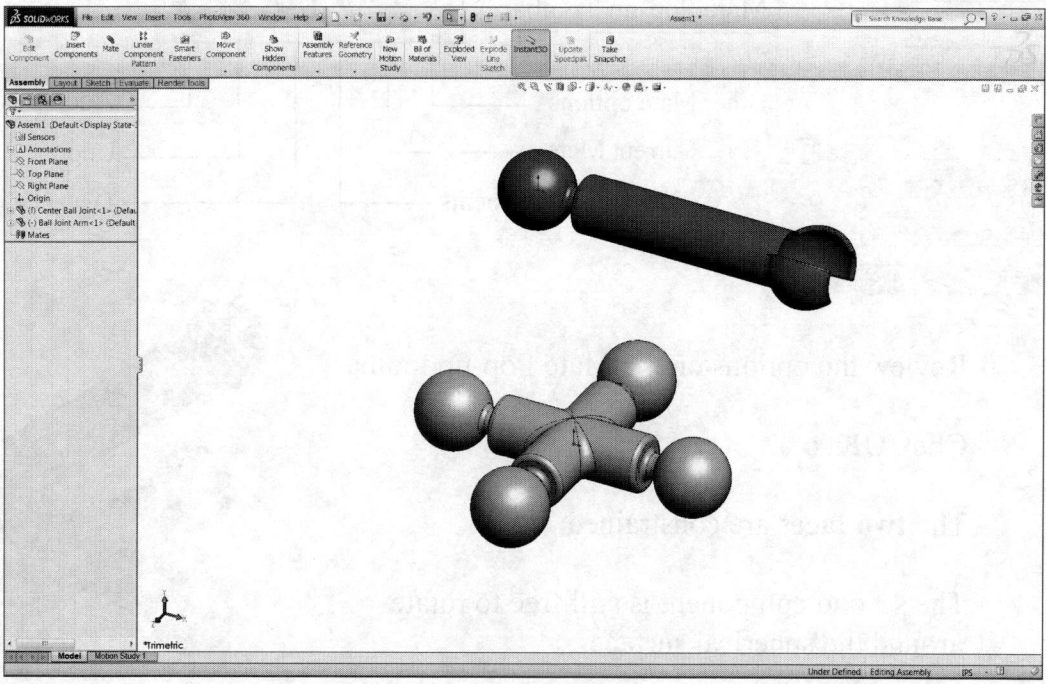

5. Mating the components:

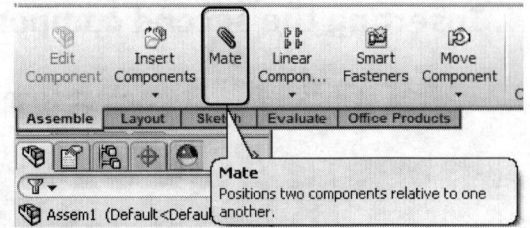

- Click or select **Insert / Mate**.

- Assembly mate options appear on the FeatureManager tree.

- Select the **two (2) faces** as indicated below.

- The **Concentric** mate option is selected automatically and the system displays the preview graphics of the two (2) mated components.

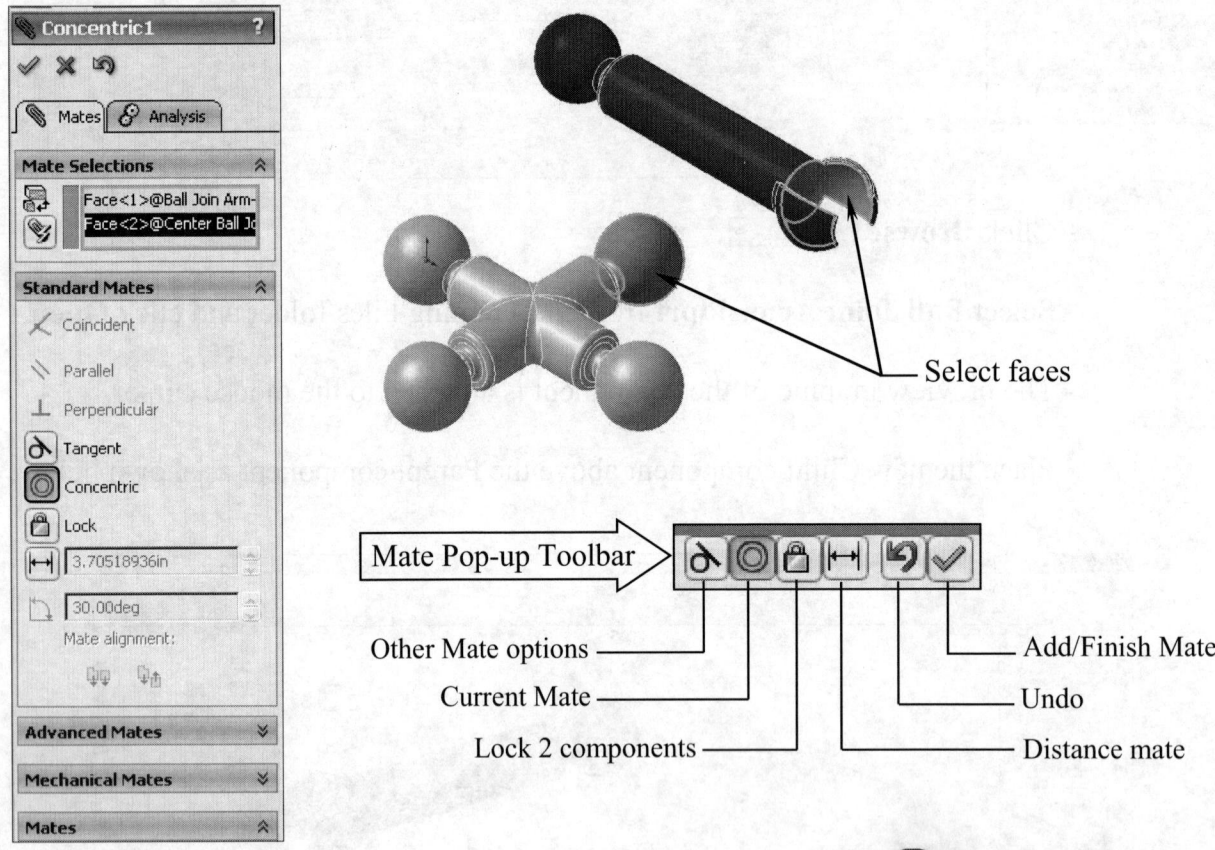

Select faces

Mate Pop-up Toolbar

Other Mate options ———— Add/Finish Mate

Current Mate ———— Undo

Lock 2 components ———— Distance mate

- Review the options on the Mate Pop-up toolbar.

- Click **OK** ✅.

- The **two faces** are constrained.

- The second component is still free to rotate around the spherical surface.

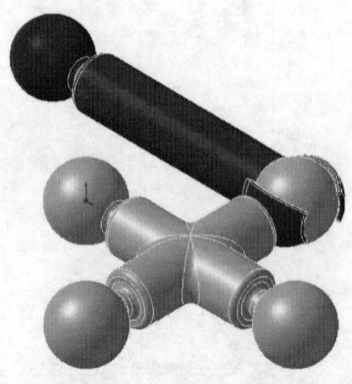

6. Moving the component:

- Click 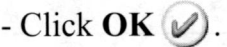 **Move Component**.

- Click and drag the **face** as noted.

- Move the component to the approximate shown position.

- Click **OK** ✅.

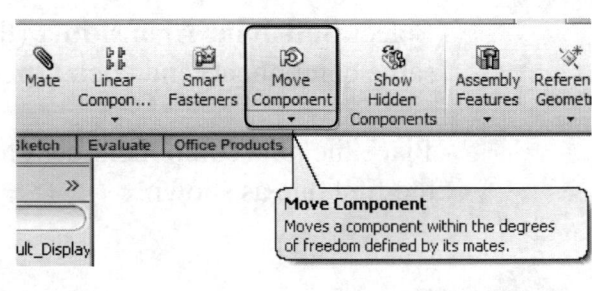

Drag here ——

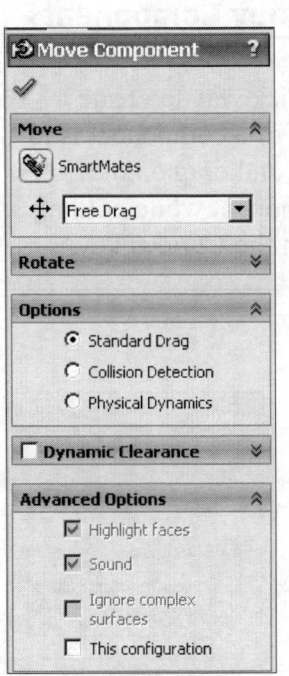

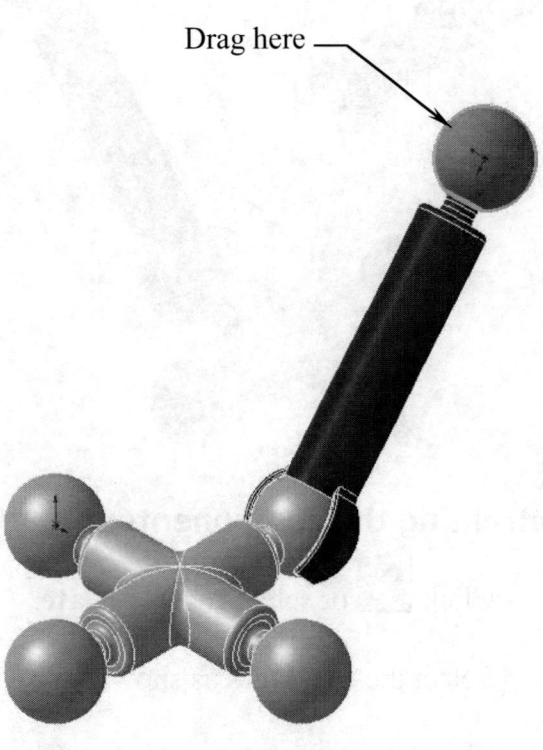

7. Inserting another instance into the assembly:

- Click [Insert Compon...] Select **Insert / Component / Existing Part/ Assembly**.

- Click [Browse...].

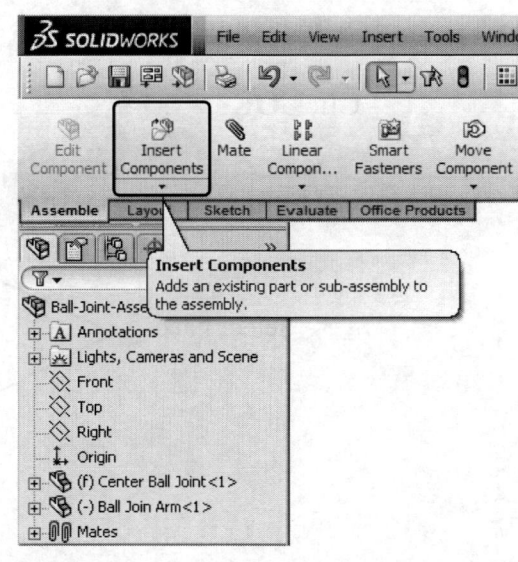

NOTE: Not all assemblies are fully constrained. In an assembly with moving parts, leave at least one degree of freedom open so that the component can still be moved or rotated.

- Select **Ball Joint Arm.sldprt** (the same component) and click **Open**.

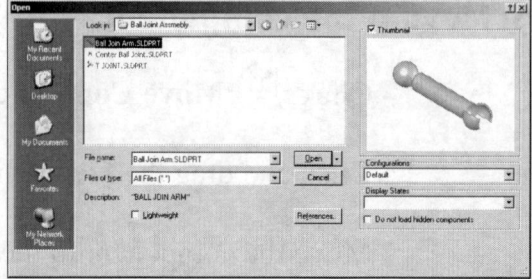

- Place the new component next to the first one as shown.

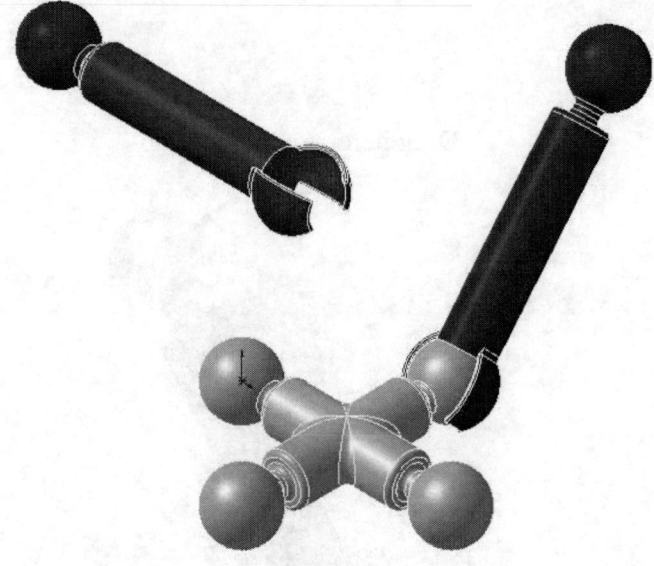

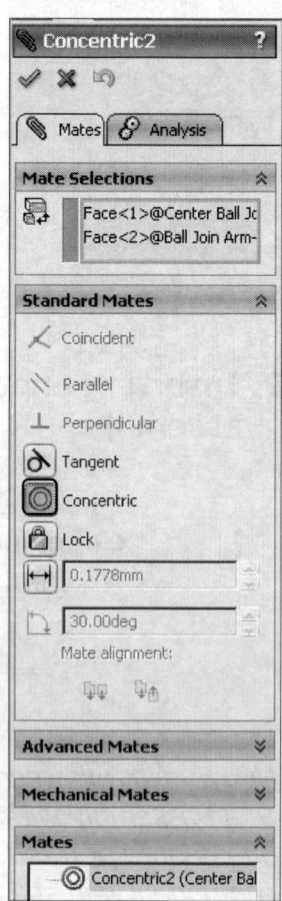

☼ Copy Components

A quick way to create a copy of a component is to click and drag on the component while holding down the *Control* key.

8. Constraining the components:

- Click ✎ or select **Insert / Mate**.

- Select the **two faces** as shown.

- The **Concentric** mate option is selected automatically and the system displays the preview graphics of the two mated components.

- Click **OK** ✅.

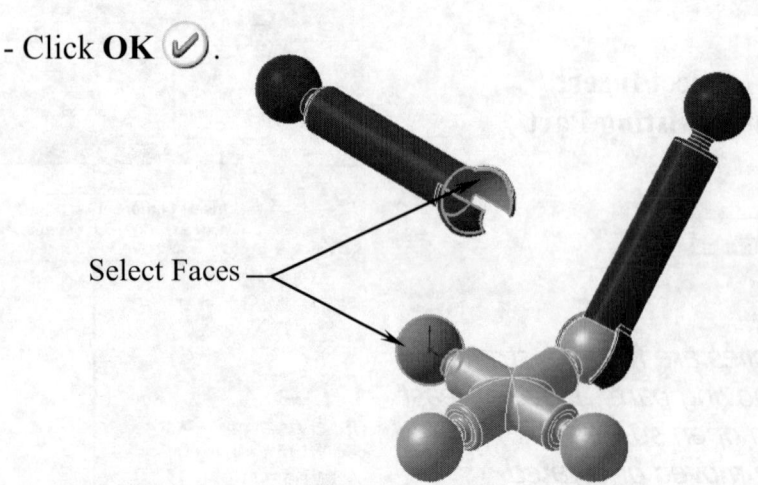

Select Faces

- The two selected faces are mated together with a Concentric mate.

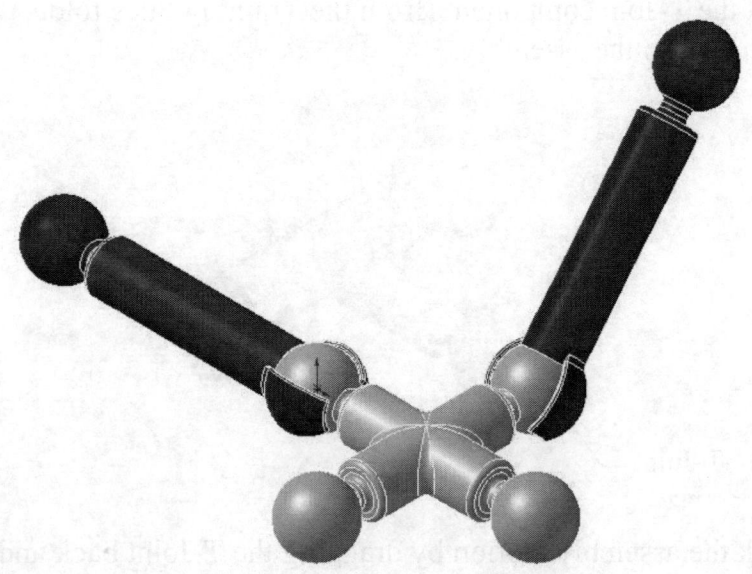

9. Repeating the step 5:

- Insert (or copy) two more instances of the **Ball Joint Arm** and add the mates to assemble them as shown.

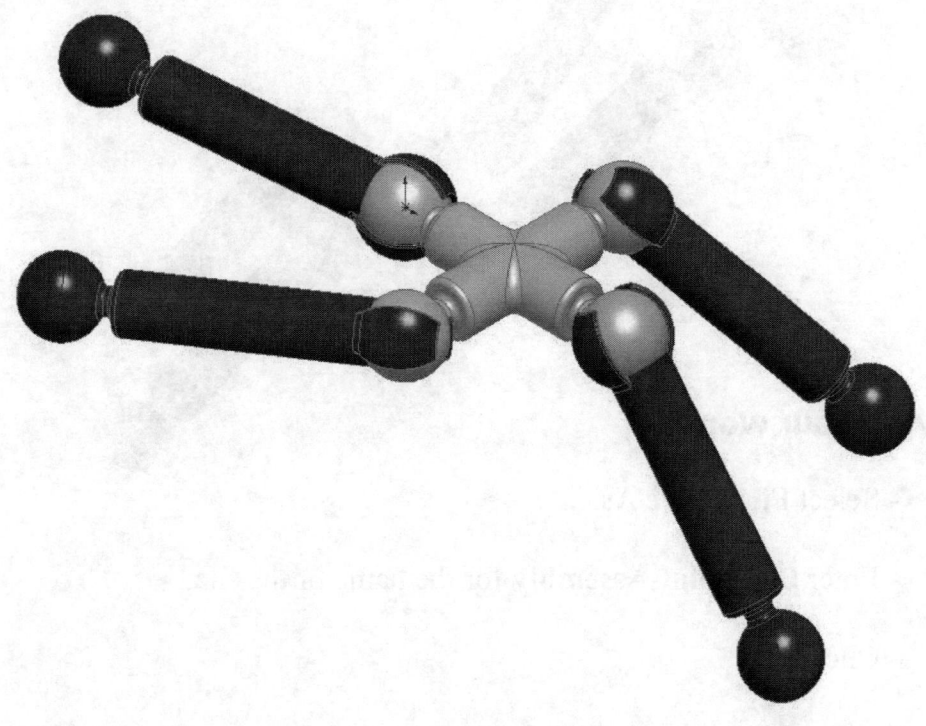

<u>**Optional**</u>:

- Insert the T-Join component (from the Training Files folder) as pictured below and mate it to the assembly.

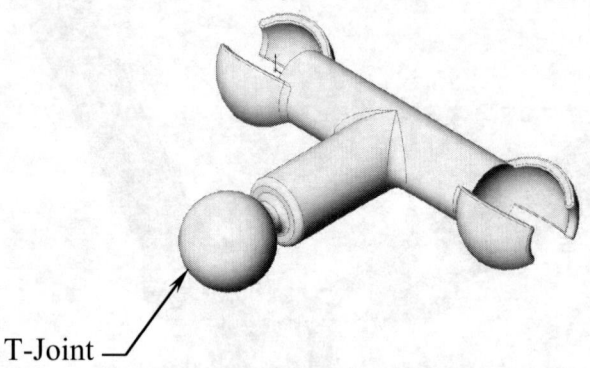

T-Joint —

- Check the assembly motion by dragging the T-Joint back and forth.

- Each component has only one mate applied, they are still free to move or rotate around their constrained geometry.

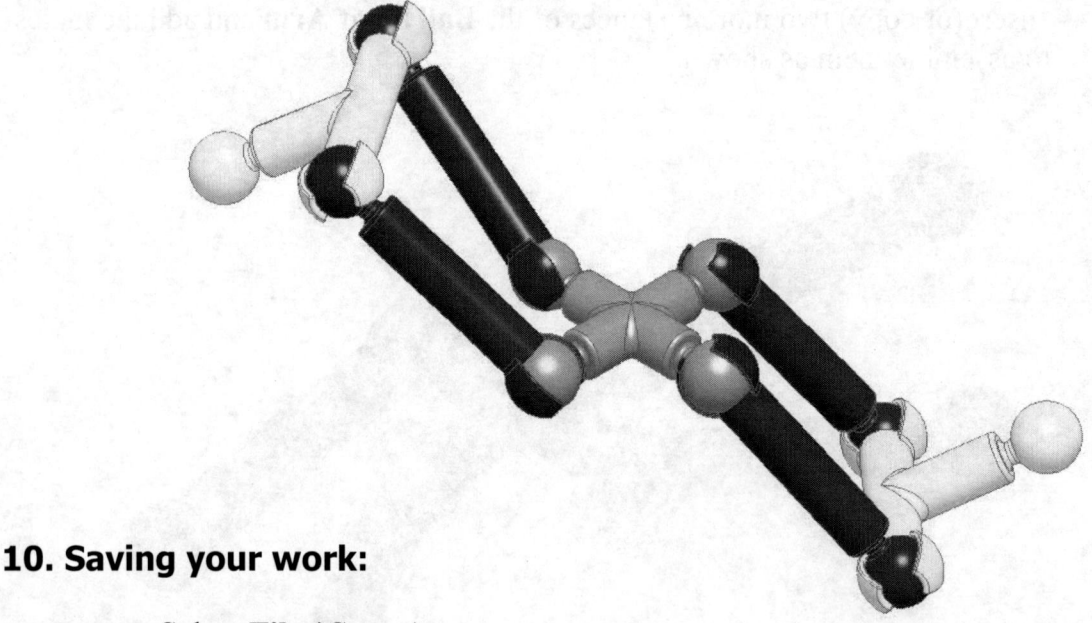

10. Saving your work:

- Select **File / Save As**.

- Enter **Ball-Joint-Assembly** for the name of the file.

- Click **Save**.

(Open the completed assembly in the Training Files folder, to check your work against it, if needed).

Questions for Review

Bottom Up Assembly

1. The 1st component should be fixed on the Origin.
   a. True
   b. False

2. The symbol (f) next to a file name means:
   a. Fully defined
   b. Failed
   c. Fixed

3. After the first component is inserted into an assembly, it is still free to be moved or re-oriented.
   a. True
   b. False

4. Beside the first component, if other components are not yet constrained they cannot be moved or rotated.
   a. True
   b. False

5. You cannot copy multiple components in an assembly document.
   a. True
   b. False

6. To make a copy of a component, click and drag that component while holding the key:
   a. Shift
   b. Control
   c. Alt
   d. Tab

7. Once a mate is created, its definitions (mate alignment, mate type, etc.) cannot be edited.
   a. True
   b. False

8. Mates can be suppressed, deleted, or changed.
   a. True
   b. False

1. TRUE   2. C
3. FALSE   4. FALSE
5. FALSE   6. B
7. FALSE   8. TRUE

CHAPTER 10 (cont.)

Bottom Up Assembly

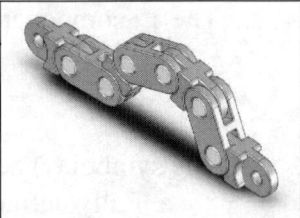

Bottom Up Assembly
Links Assembly

- After the parts are inserted into an assembly document, they are now called components. These components will get re-positioned and mated together. This method is called Bottom Up Assembly.

- The first component inserted into the assembly will be fixed by the system automatically. If it is placed on the Origin, then the Front, Top, and Right planes of the first component will also be aligned with the assembly's planes.

- Only the first part will be fixed by default, all other components are free to be moved or re-oriented. Depending on the mate type, once a mate is assigned to a component, one or more of its degrees of freedom are removed, causing the component to move or rotate only in the desired directions.

- Standard mates [icon] are created one by one to constraint components.

- Multi-Mates [icon] can be used to constrain more than one component, where a common entity is used to mate with several other entities.

- This second half of the chapter will guide you through the use of the Bottom Up assembly method once again. Some of the components are exactly identical. We will learn how to create several copies of them and then add 2 mates to each one, leaving one degree of freedom open, so that they can be moved or rotated when dragged. There will be an instance number <1> <2> <3> etc., placed next to the name of each copy, to indicate how many times the components are used in an assembly.

Links Assembly
Bottom-Up Assembly

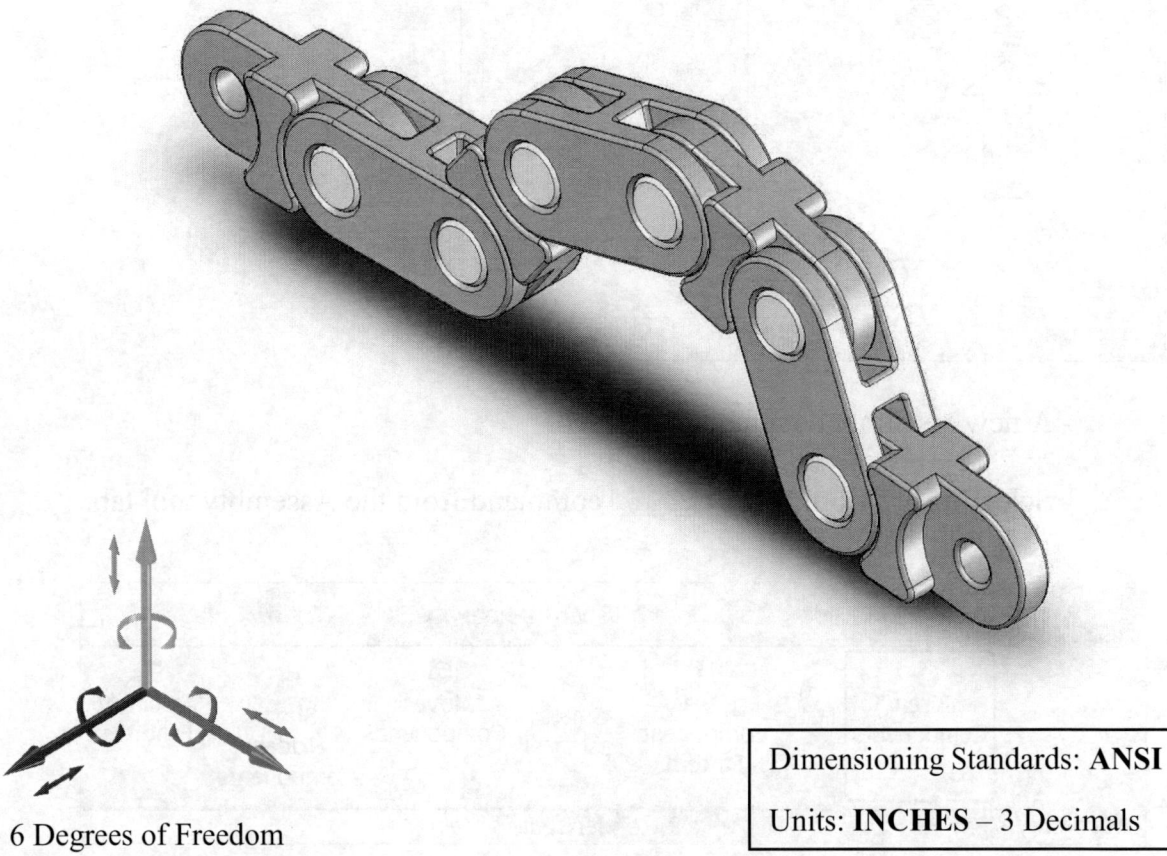

6 Degrees of Freedom

Dimensioning Standards: **ANSI**

Units: **INCHES** – 3 Decimals

Tools Needed:

	Mates		Insert New Component		Rotate Component
	Move Component		Inference Origins		Place/Position Component
	Align & Anti-Align		Concentric Mate		Coincident Mate

1. Starting a new Assembly Template:

- Select **File / New / Assembly / OK**.

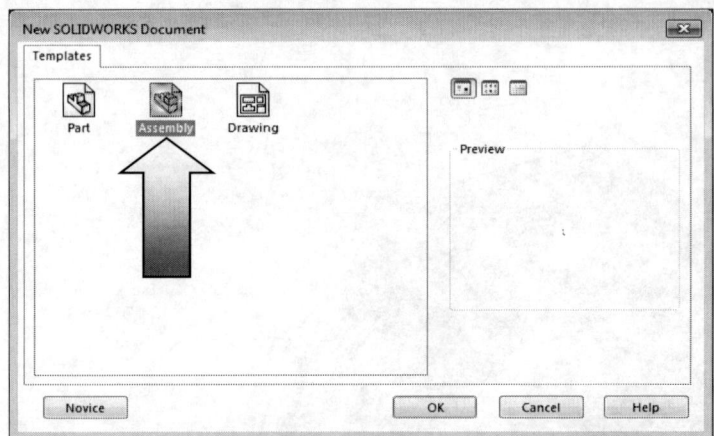

- A new assembly document is opened.

- Select **Insert Component** command from the Assembly tool tab.

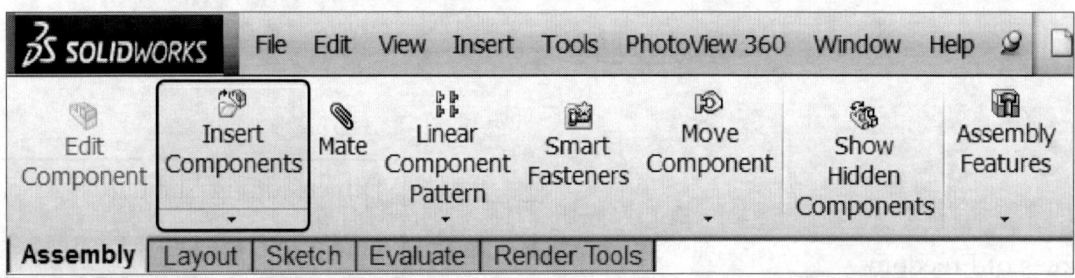

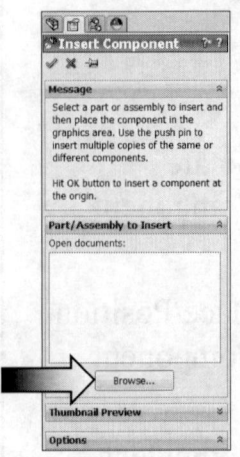 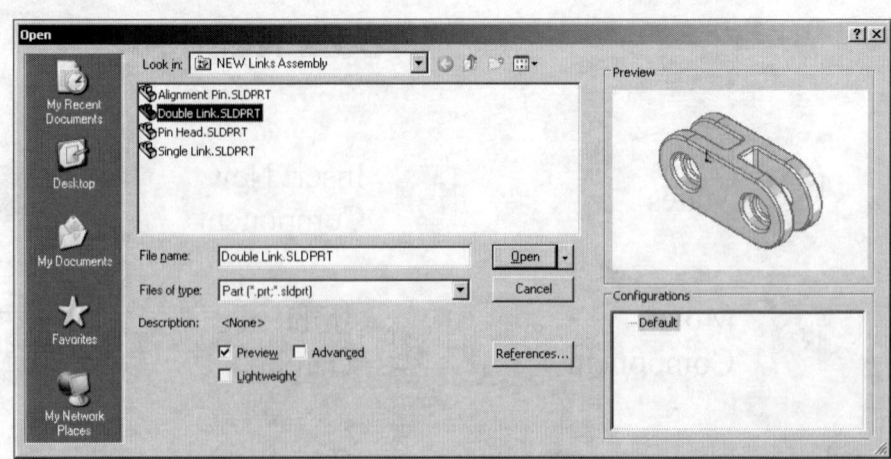

- Click the **Browse** button (arrow).

2. Inserting the 1ˢᵗ Component:

- Go to: The Training Files folder and open the part **Double Link.sldprt**.

- Place the part Double Link on the assembly Origin.

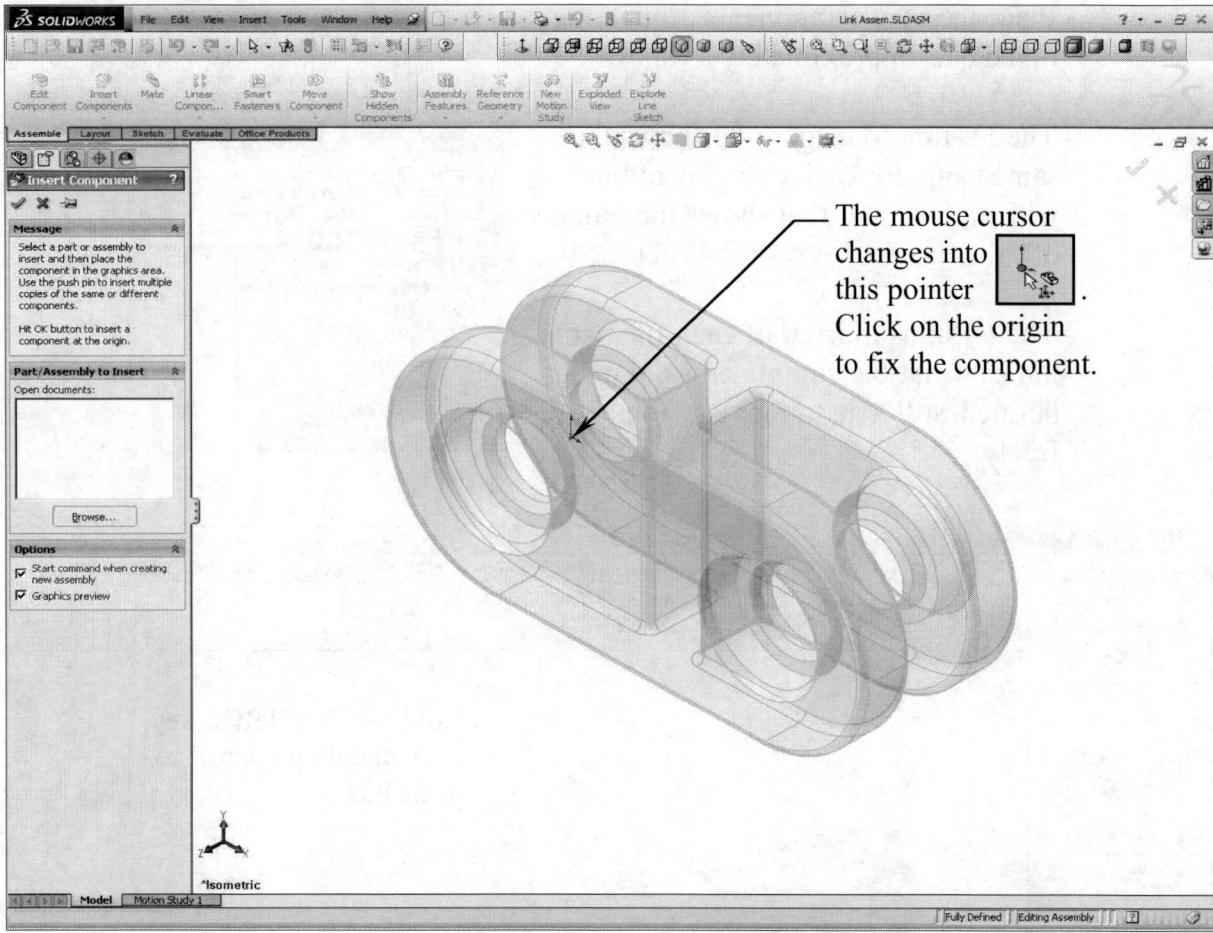

The mouse cursor changes into this pointer. Click on the origin to fix the component.

💡 **"Fixing" the 1ˢᵗ component**

- The first component inserted into the assembly will be fixed automatically by the system, the symbol (f) next to the document's name means the part cannot be moved or rotated.

- Other components can be added and mated to the first one using one of the three options:

       1. Drag & Drop from an opened window
       2. Use the Windows Explorer to drag the component into the assembly.
       3. Use the Insert Component command.

3. Adding other components:

- Select **Insert / Component / Existing Part/Assembly** (or click 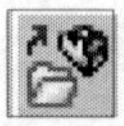 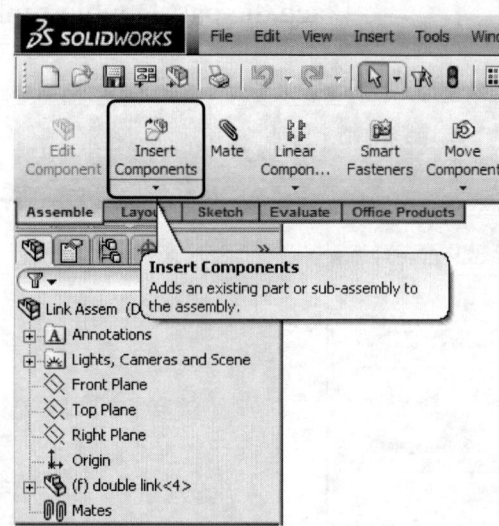) and add five (**5**) more copies of the first component into the Assembly document.

- Place the new components around the Fixed one, approximately as shown.

- The Feature Manager tree shows the same name for each component but with an indicator that shows the number of times used **<2>**, **<3>**, **<4>**, etc...

- The **(-)** signs in front of each file name indicate that the components are under defined, still able to move or rotate freely.

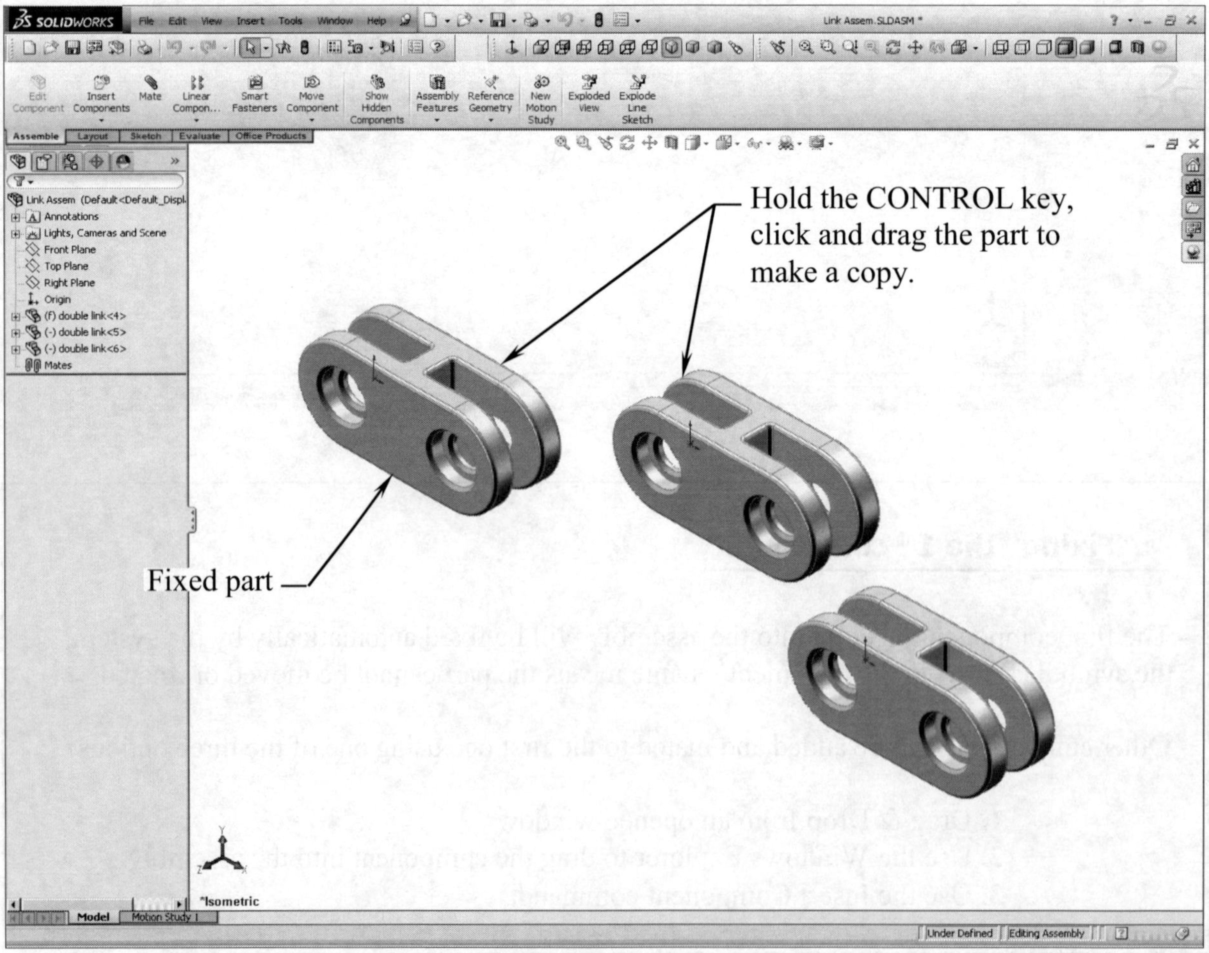

Hold the CONTROL key, click and drag the part to make a copy.

Fixed part

4. Changing colors:

- For Clarity, change the color of the 1st component to a different color, this way we can differentiate the parent component from the copies.

- Click the 1st component and select the **Appearances** button (the beach ball) and click the **Edit Part Color** option (arrow).

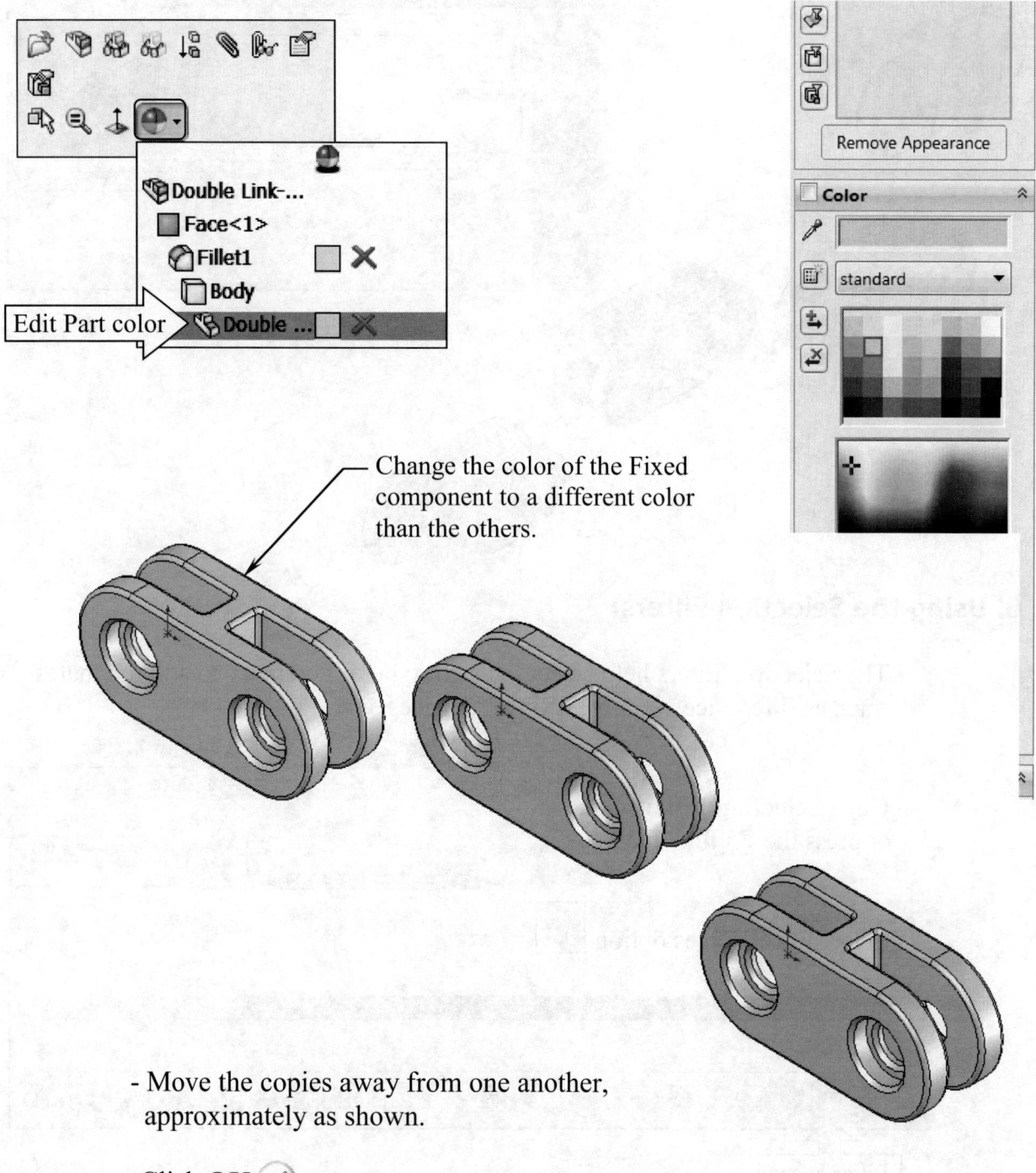

Change the color of the Fixed component to a different color than the others.

- Move the copies away from one another, approximately as shown.

- Click **OK**.

5. Inserting the Single Link into the assembly:

- Click **Insert Component** 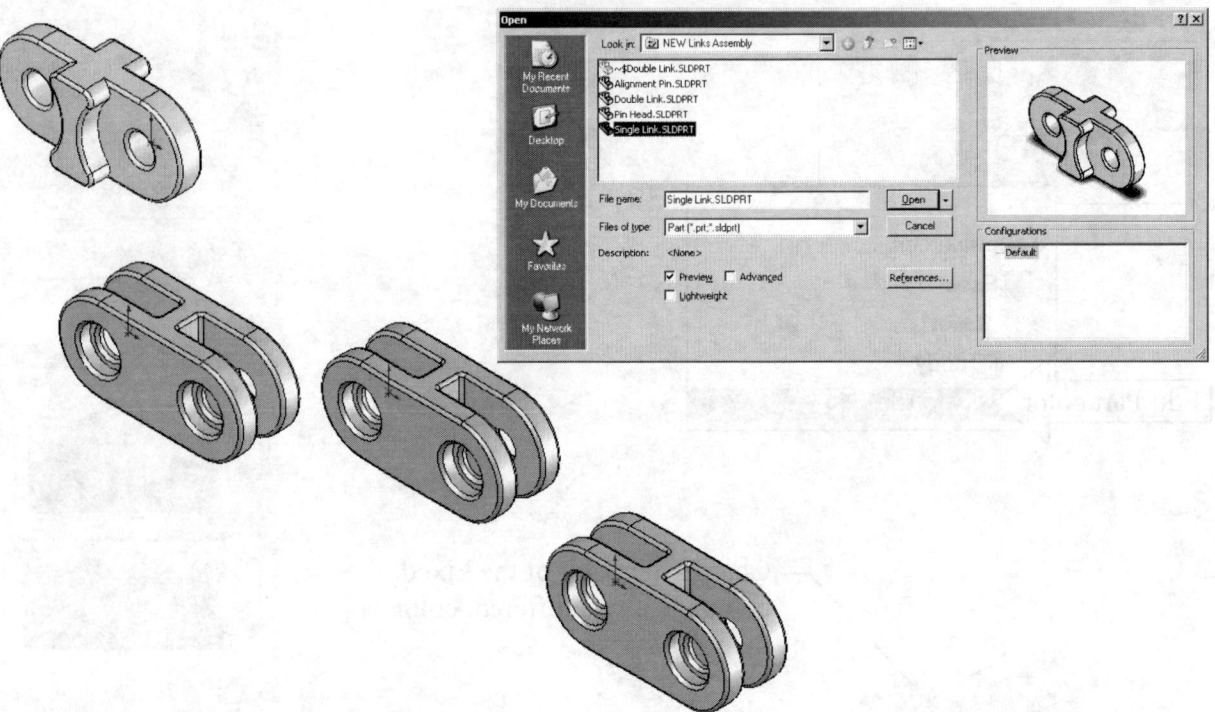 on the Assembly toolbar and select the part **Single Link**, from the previous folder.

- Place the Single Link approximately as shown.

6. Using the Selection Filters:

- The Selection Filters help select the right type of geometry to add the mates such as filter Faces, Edges, Axis or Vertices, etc…

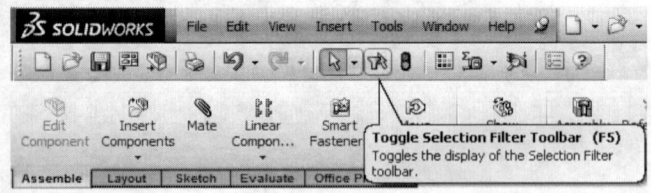

- Click **Selection Filter** icon, or press the **F5** function key.

- Select **Filter Faces** option 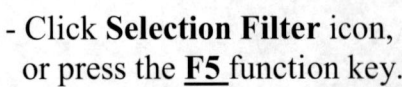.

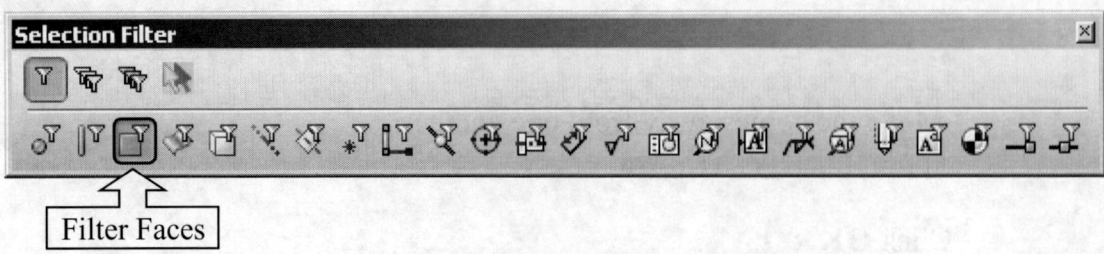

Filter Faces

7. Adding Mates:

- Click **Mate** 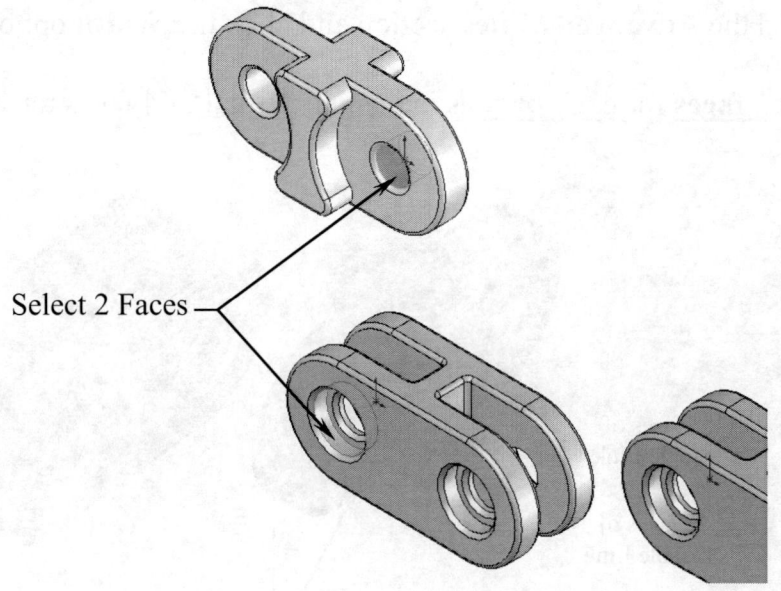 on the Assembly toolbar or select **Insert / Mate**.

- Select the faces of the **two holes** as indicated.

Select 2 Faces

- The **Concentric** mate option is selected automatically and the system displays the preview graphics for the two mated components.

- Click **OK** to accept the concentric mate.

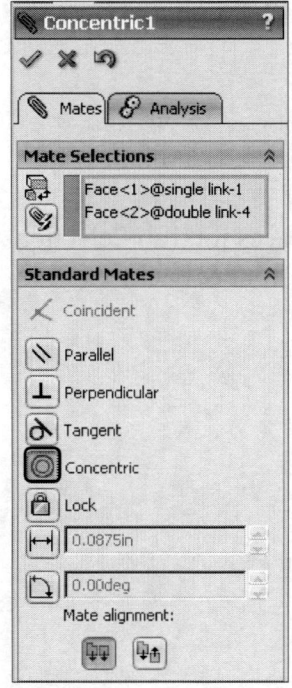

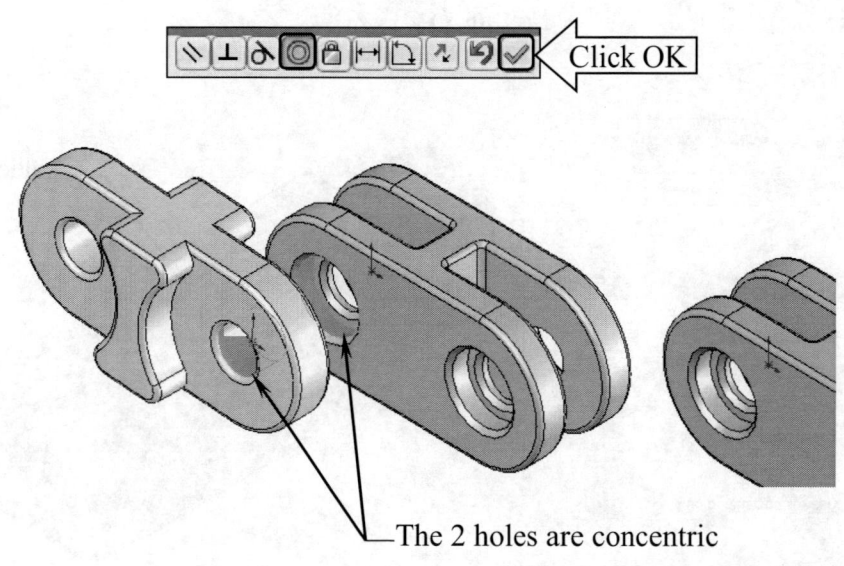

Click OK

The 2 holes are concentric

8. Adding a Width mate:

- The Width mate centers the 2 parts (width of part 1 and groove/tab of part 2).

- Click **Mate** on the Assembly toolbar or select **Insert / Mate**.

- Expand the **Advanced Mates** section and click the **Width** option.

- Select **2 faces** for **each part** as indicated. A total of 4 faces must be selected.

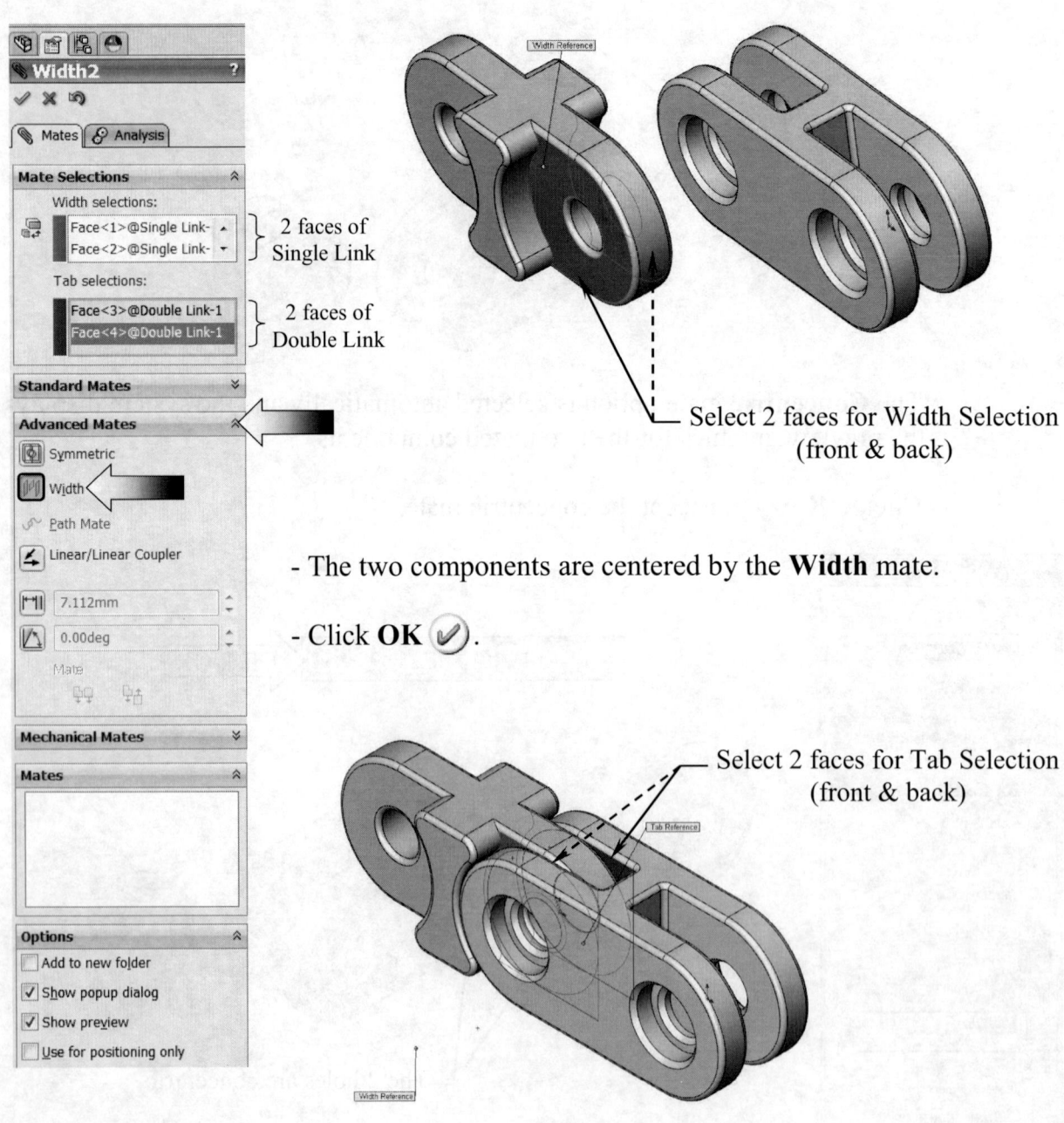

2 faces of Single Link

2 faces of Double Link

Select 2 faces for Width Selection (front & back)

- The two components are centered by the **Width** mate.

- Click **OK**.

Select 2 faces for Tab Selection (front & back)

9. Making copies of the component:

- Select the part Single-Link and click **Edit / Copy**, then click anywhere in the graphics area and select **Edit / Paste** – OR – Hold down the CONTROL key, click/hold and drag the part Single Link to make a copy.

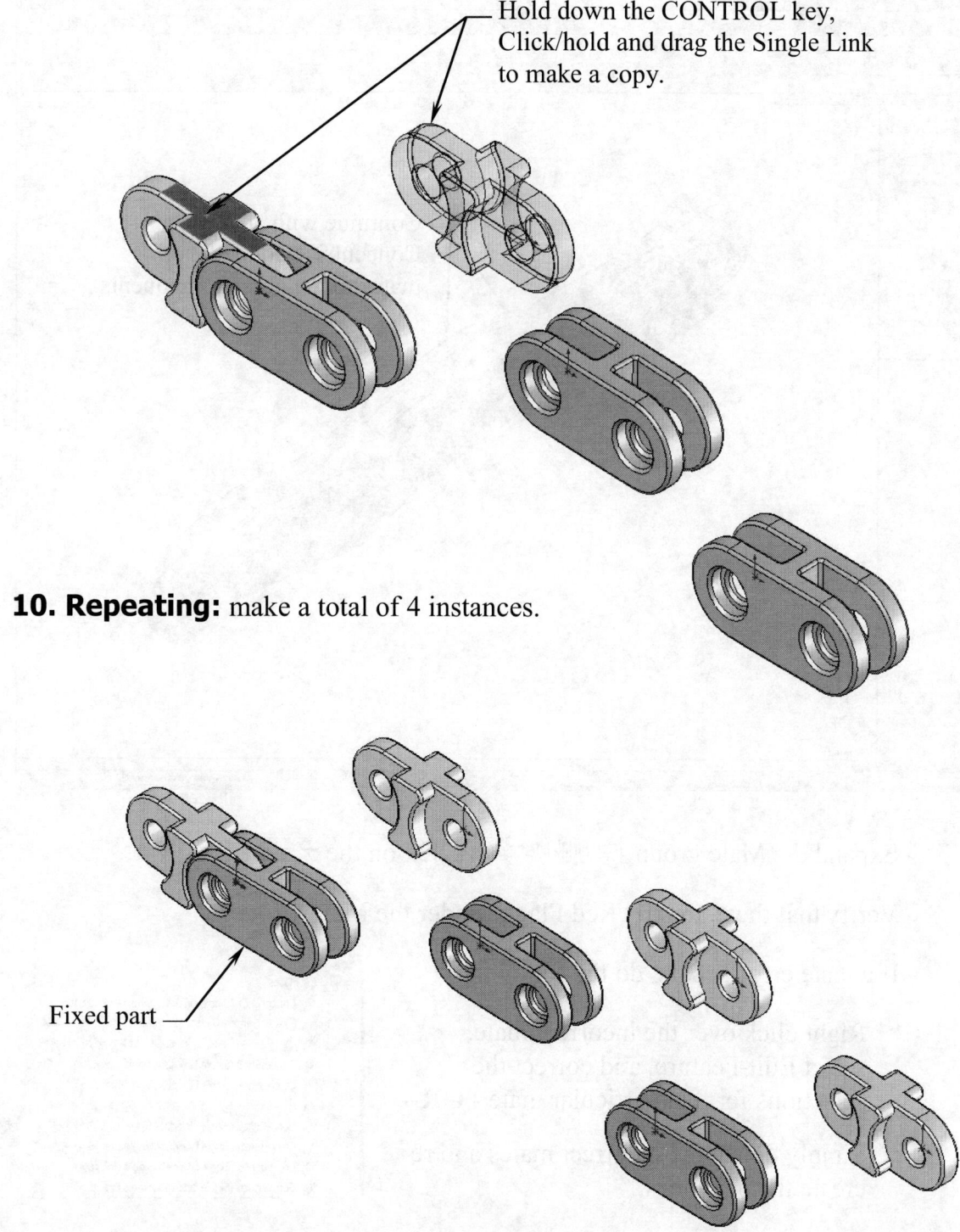

Hold down the CONTROL key,
Click/hold and drag the Single Link
to make a copy.

10. Repeating: make a total of 4 instances.

Fixed part

Notes:

- *The correct mates are displayed in Black color* 🔗 *on the FeatureManager tree.*

- *The Incorrect mates are displayed with a red X* 🔗 ⊗ (+) *or a yellow*

exclamation mark 🔗 ⚠ (+) *next to them.*

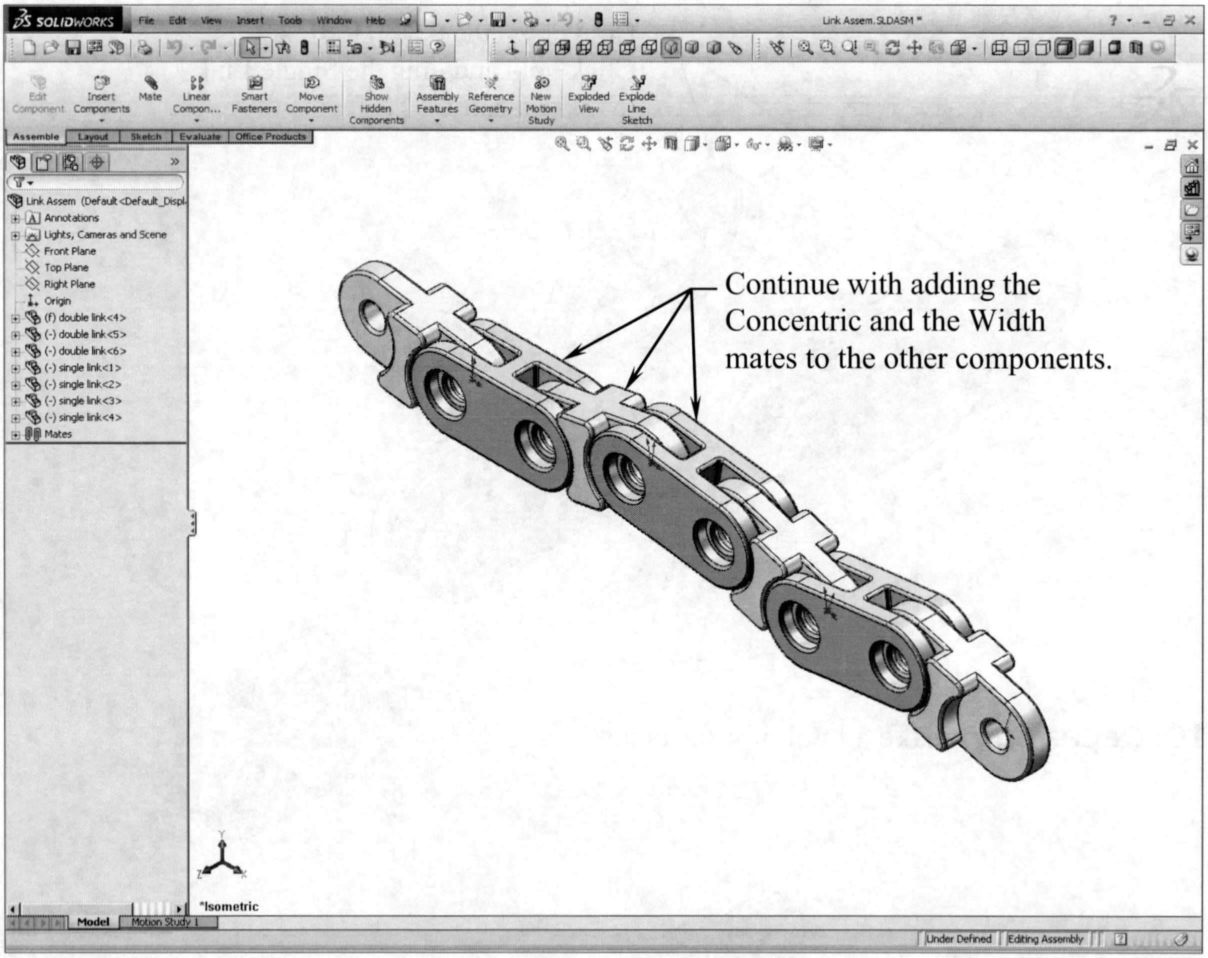

Continue with adding the
Concentric and the Width
mates to the other components.

- Expand the Mate group ⊟ 🔗 Mates (Click on the + sign).

- Verify that there are no "Red Flags" under the Mate Group.

- If a mate error occurs, do the following:

** Right click over the incorrect mate,
select Edit-Feature, and correct the
selections for that particular mate - **OR** -

** Simply delete the incorrect mates and recreate the new ones.

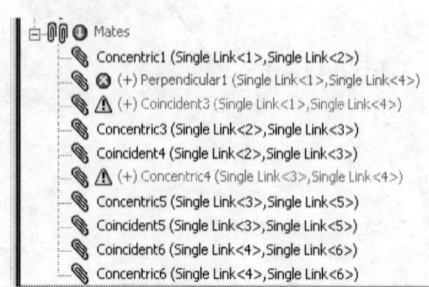

11. Inserting other components into the Assembly:

- Click 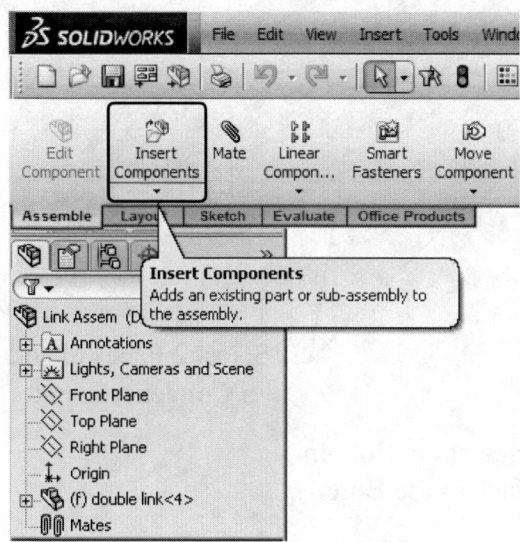 or select **Insert / Component / Existing Part/Assembly.**

- Click **Browse**, select **Alignment Pin** and click **Open**.

- Place the component on the left side of the assembly as shown.

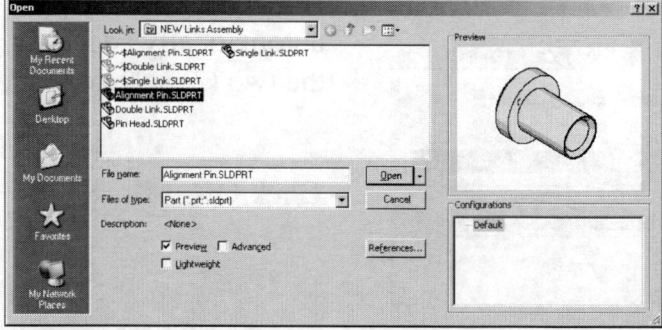

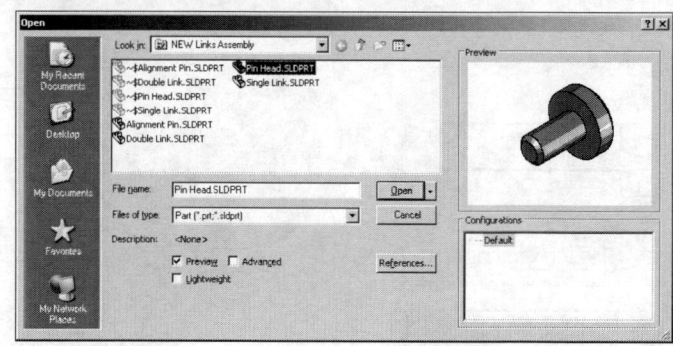

- Insert the **Pin Head** and place it on the right side.

12. Rotating the Pin Head:

- Select the Rotate Component command and rotate the Pin-Head to the correct orientation.

Make 5 more copies of both, the Pin-Head and the Alignment Pin.

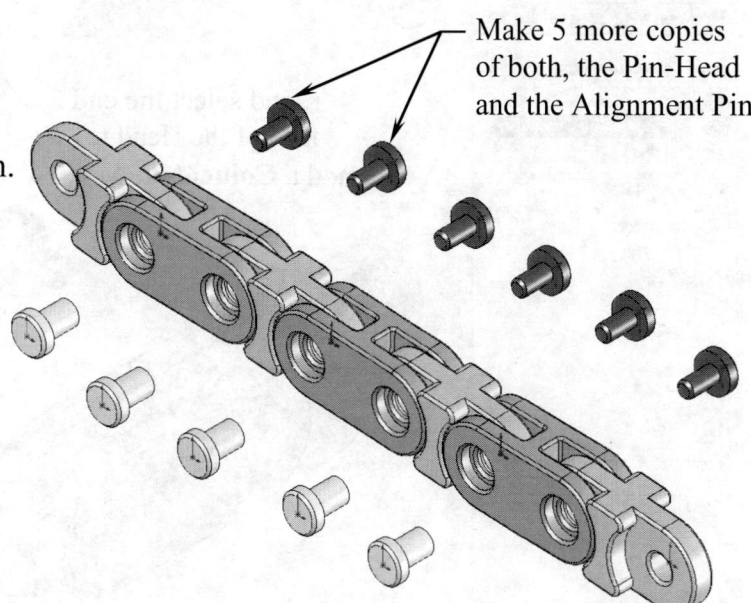

13. Constraining the Alignment Pin:

- Click 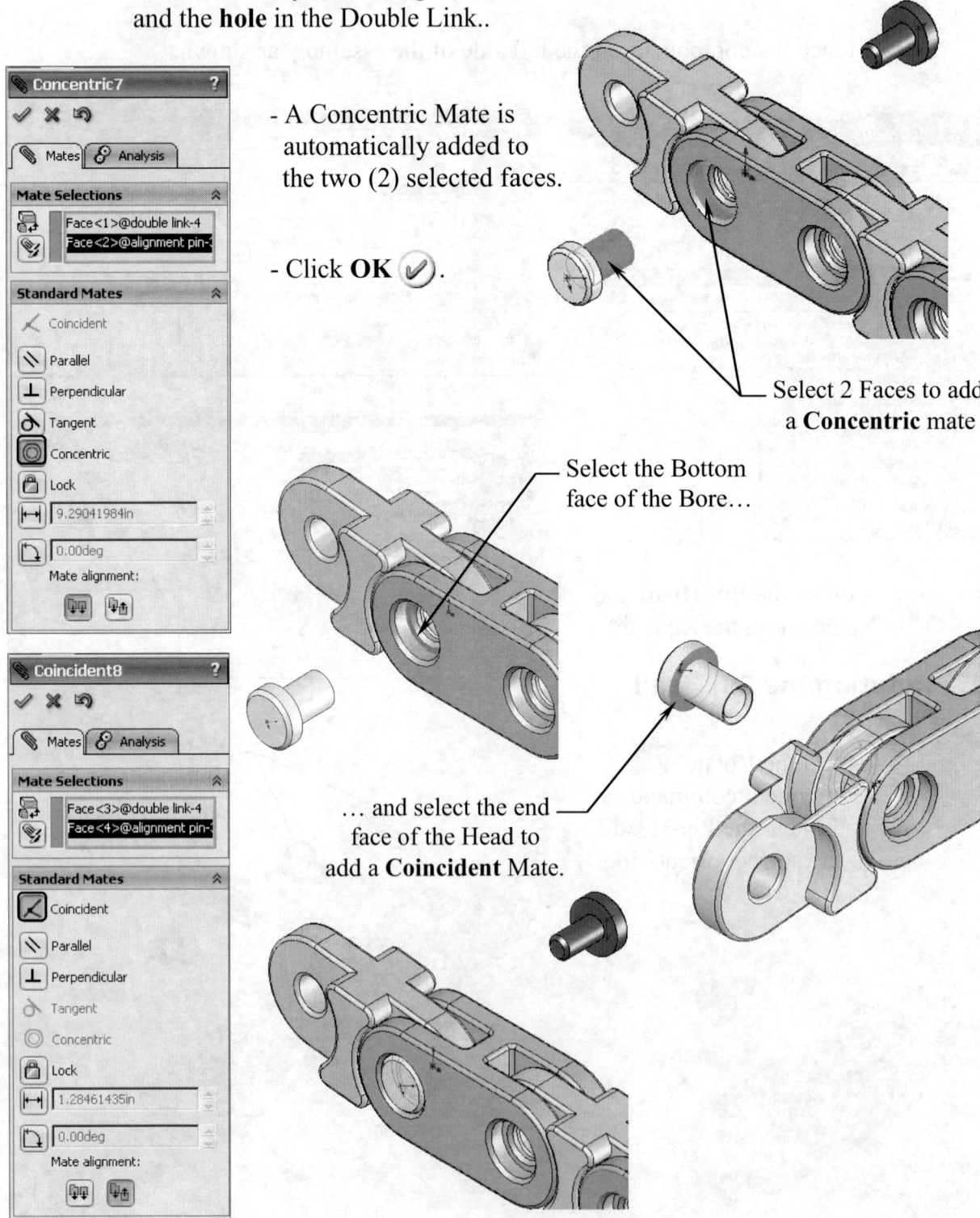 **Mate** on the Assembly toolbar.

- Select the **body** of the Alignment Pin and the **hole** in the Double Link..

- A Concentric Mate is automatically added to the two (2) selected faces.

- Click **OK**.

Select 2 Faces to add a **Concentric** mate

Select the Bottom face of the Bore…

… and select the end face of the Head to add a **Coincident** Mate.

14. Constraining the Pin-Head:

- Align the Pin-Head with its mating hole, using a **Concentric Mate**.

Select the cylindrical
body of the Pin-Head...

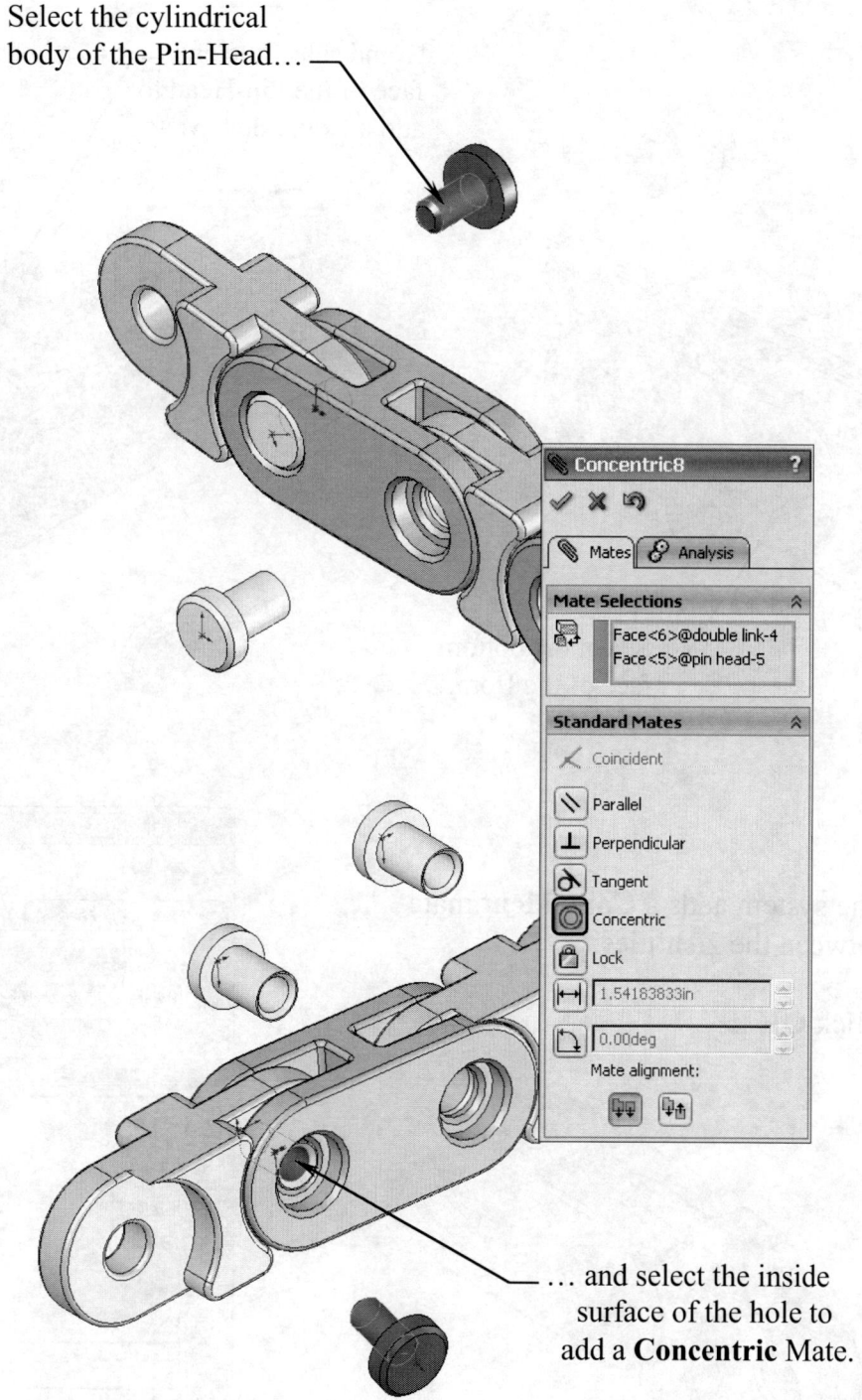

... and select the inside
surface of the hole to
add a **Concentric** Mate.

- Click **OK** ✅.

- Click 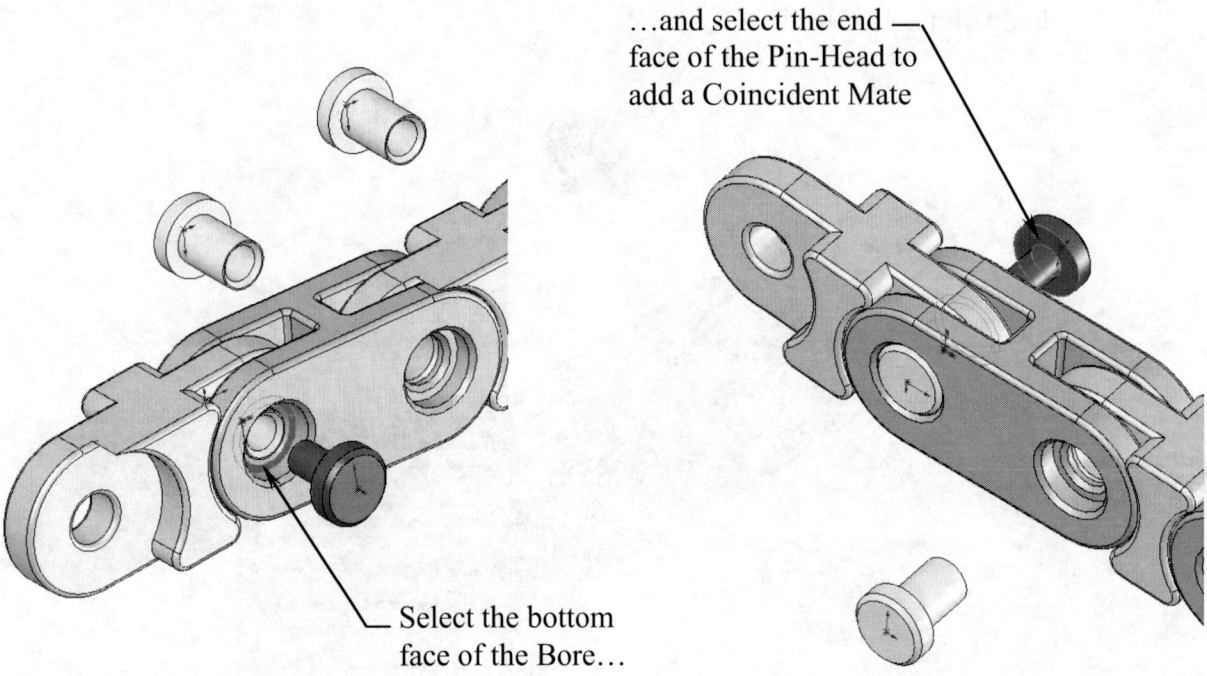 **Mate** again, if you have already closed out of it from the last step.

- Select the **two faces** as indicated to add a Coincident Mate.

…and select the end
face of the Pin-Head to
add a Coincident Mate

Select the bottom
face of the Bore…

- The system adds a **Coincident** mate
  between the 2 entities.

- Click **OK** 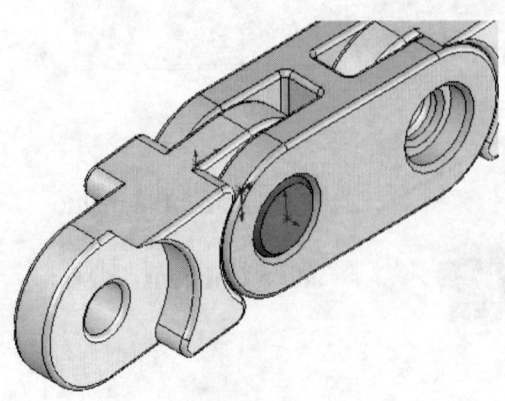.

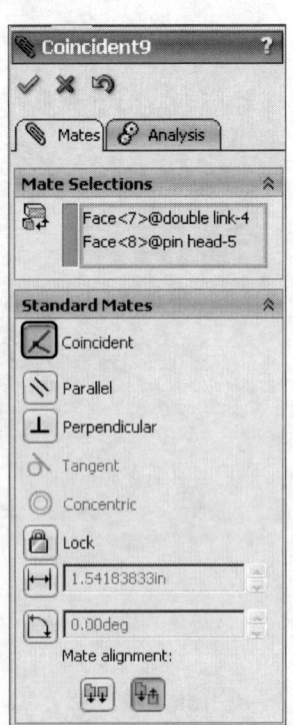

15. Using the Align & Anti-Align Options:

- When the Mate command is active, the options **Align** and **Anti-Align** are also available in the Mate dialog box.

- Use the alignment options to flip the mating component 180º 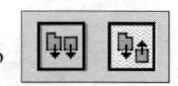 .

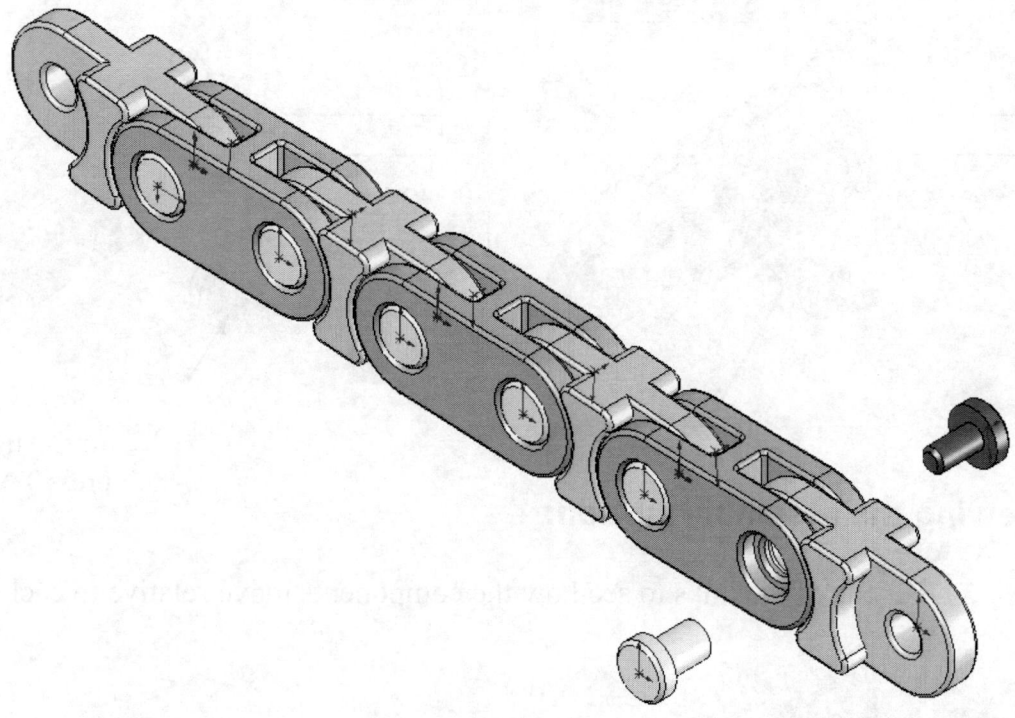

- The last two (2) pins will be used to demonstrate the use of Align 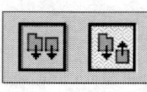 and Anti-Align (see step 16).

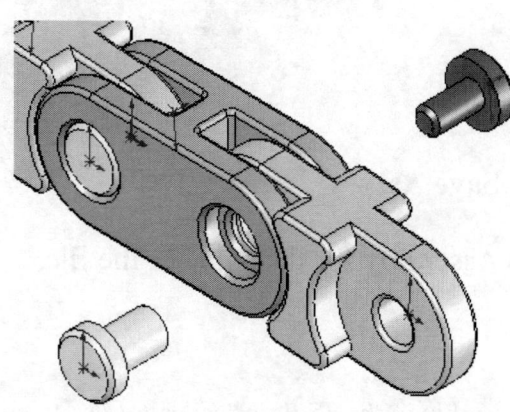

16. Using Align and Anti-Align:

- When mating the components using the **Concentric** option, the **TAB** key can be used to flip the component 180° or from Align into Anti-Align.

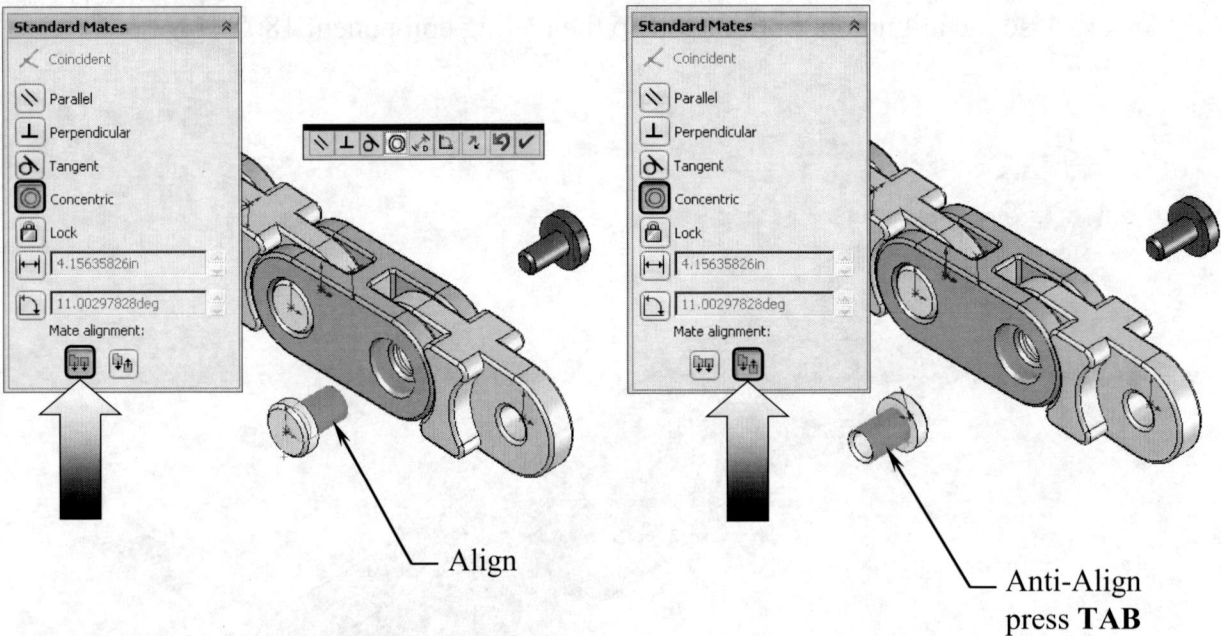

Align

Anti-Align
press **TAB**

17. Viewing the assembly motion:

- Drag one of the links to see how the components move relative to each other.

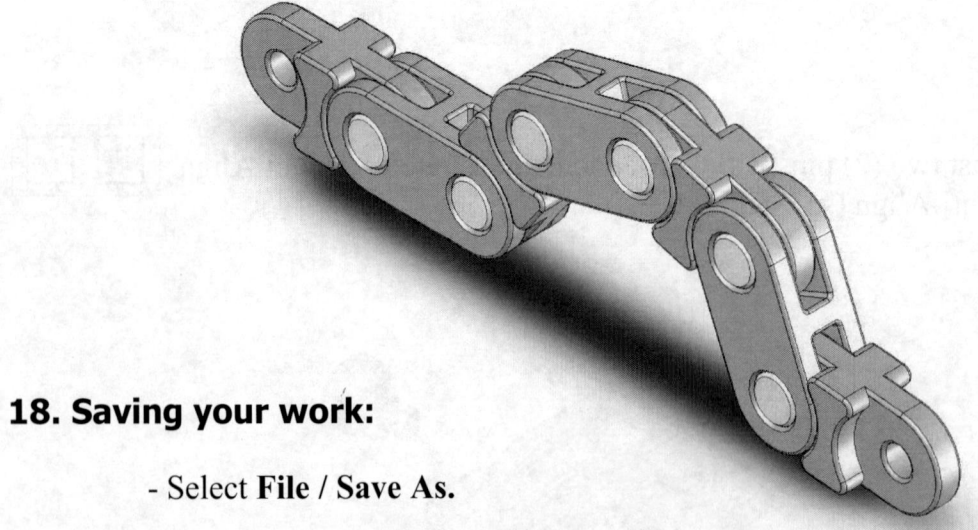

18. Saving your work:

- Select **File / Save As.**

- Enter **Links Assembly** for the name of the file.

- Click **Save**.

(Open the pre-built assembly in the Training Files folder, to compare your work).

Questions for Review

Bottom Up Assembly

1. Parts inserted into an assembly document are called documents.
   a. True
   b. False

2. Each component in an assembly document has six degrees of freedom.
   a. True
   b. False

3. Once a mate is applied to a component, depends on the mate type, one or more of its degrees of freedom is removed.
   a. True
   b. False

4. Standard mates are created one by one to constrain the components.
   a. True
   b. False

5. A combination of a Face and an Edge can be used to constraint with a Coincident mate.
   a. True
   b. False

6. Align and Anti-Align while in the Mating mode can toggle by pressing:
   a. Control
   b. Back space
   c. Tab
   d. Esc.

7. Mates can be deferred so that several mates can be done and solved at the same time.
   a. True
   b. False

8. Mates can be:
   a. Suppressed
   b. Deleted
   c. Edited
   d. All of the above

1. FALSE 2. TRUE
3. TRUE   4. TRUE
5. TRUE   6. C
7. TRUE   8. D

Exercise: Gate Assembly

Go to: The Training Files folder
      Gate Assembly Folder.

1. Create an Assembly document from
   the components provided.
2. Create a Mirror plane at **26.125 in**.
   offset from the RIGHT plane.

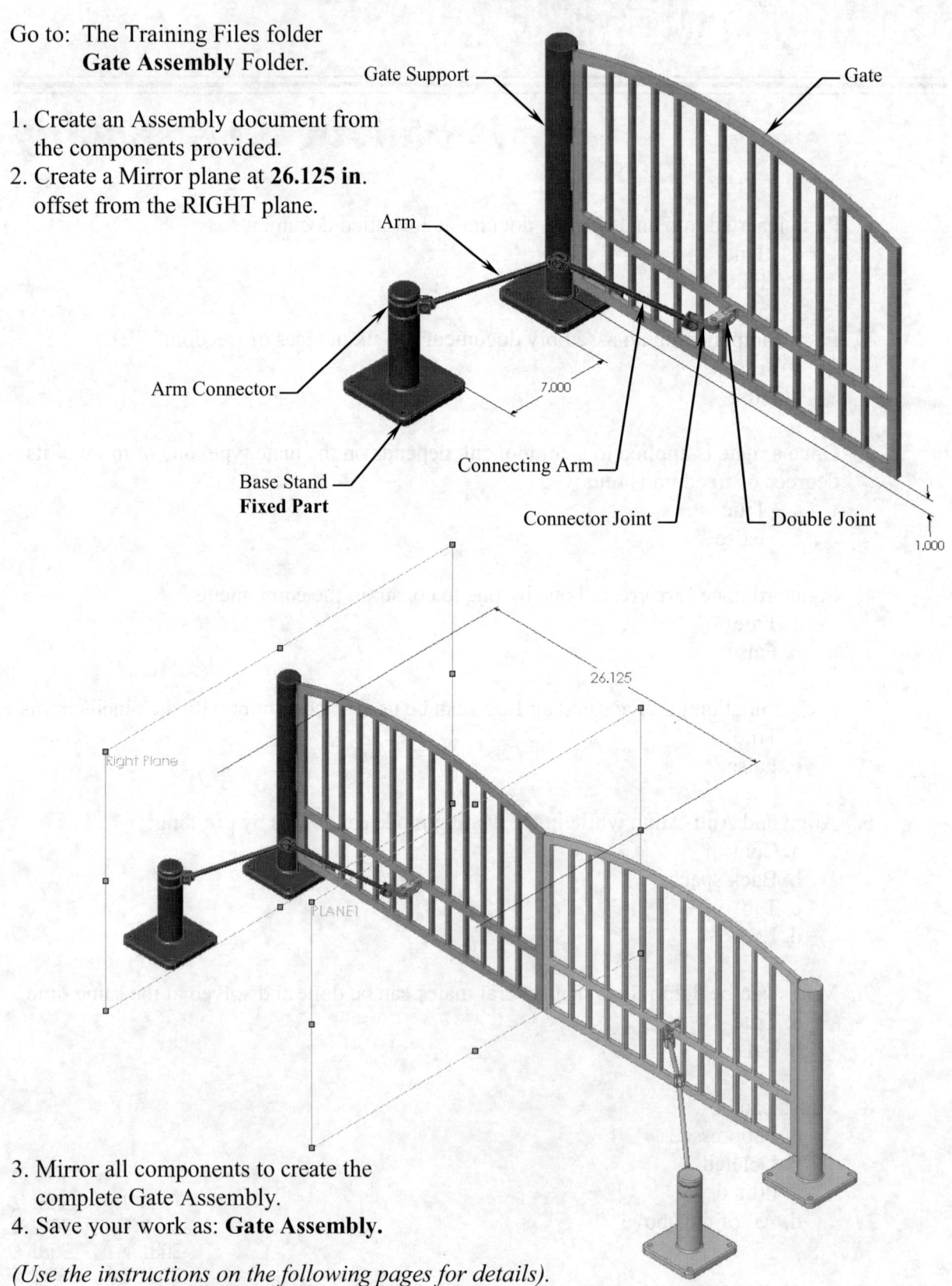

Gate Support

Gate

Arm

Arm Connector

Base Stand
Fixed Part

7.000

Connecting Arm

Connector Joint

Double Joint

1.000

Right Plane

26.125

PLANE1

3. Mirror all components to create the
   complete Gate Assembly.
4. Save your work as: **Gate Assembly.**

(Use the instructions on the following pages for details).

1. Starting a new assembly:

- Click **File / New / Assembly**.

- From the Assembly tool-bar, select **Insert / Components**.

- Browse to the part **Base Stand** and place it on the assembly's origin.

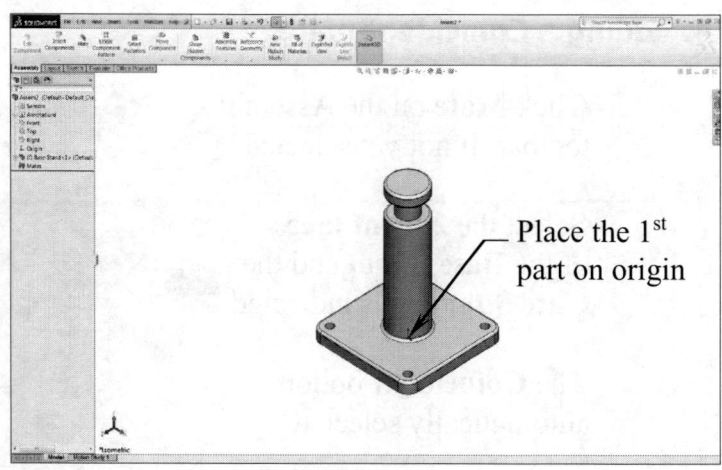

Place the 1st part on origin

2. Inserting other components:

- Insert all components (total of 8) into the assembly.

- **Rotate** the **Gate** <u>and</u> the **Gate-Support** approximately **180 degrees**.

- Move the Gate and the Gate-Support to the positions shown.

- By rotating and positioning the components before mating them, it helps seeing the mating entities a little easier.

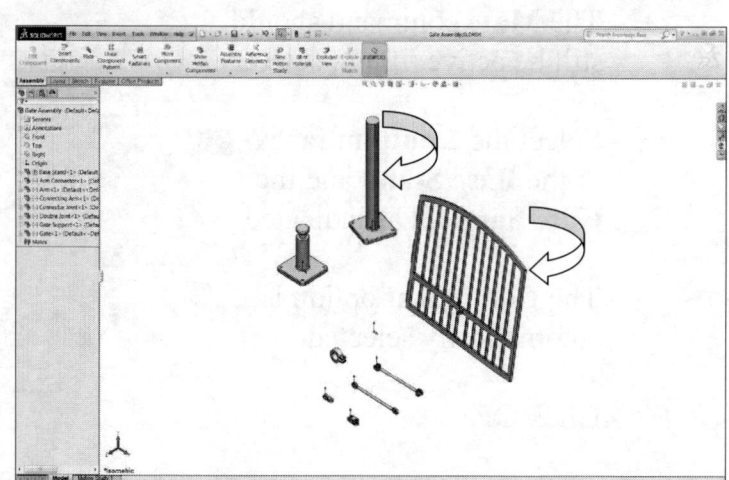

3. Adding a Distance mate:

- Click **Mate** on the Assembly toolbar.

- Select the **2 side faces** of the **Base Stand** and the **Gate-Support** as indicated.

- Click the **Distance** button and enter **7.00"**.

- Click **OK**.

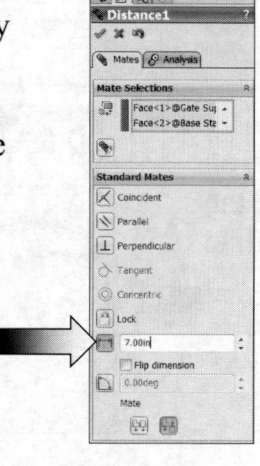

Select 2 side faces

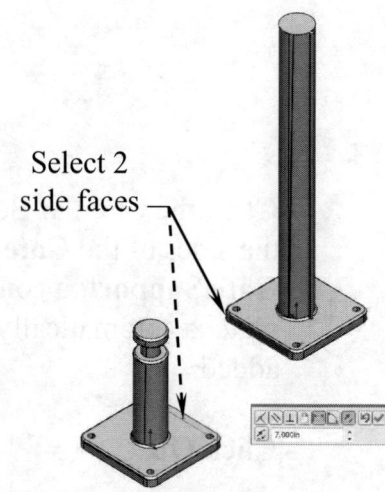

4. Adding a Coincident mate:

- Click **Mate** on the Assembly toolbar, if not yet selected.

- Select the **2 front faces** of the **Base Stand** and the **Gate Support** as indicated.

- The **Coincident** option is automatically selected.

- Click **OK**.

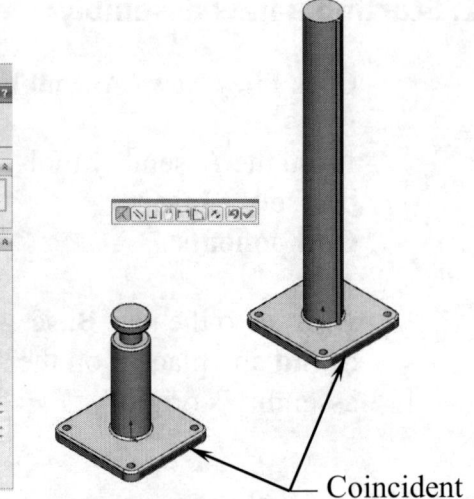

Coincident

5. Adding other mates:

- The **Mate** command should still be active, if not, select it.

- Select the **2 bottom faces** of the **Base Stand** and the **Gate Support** as indicated.

- The **Coincident** option is automatically selected.

- Click **OK**.

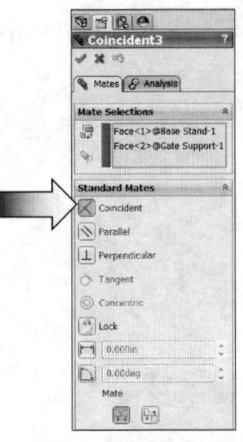
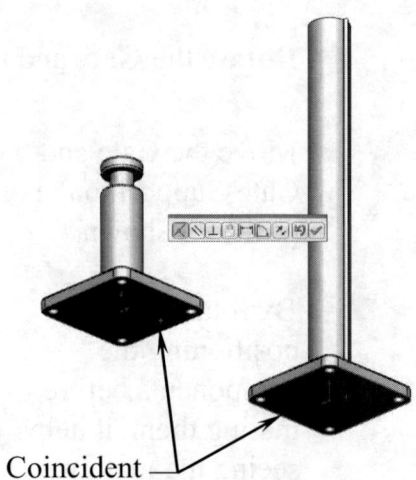

Coincident

Concentric

- Click the Circular Bosses on the sides of the **Gate** and the **Gate Support**; a **concentric** mate is automatically added.

- Click **OK**.

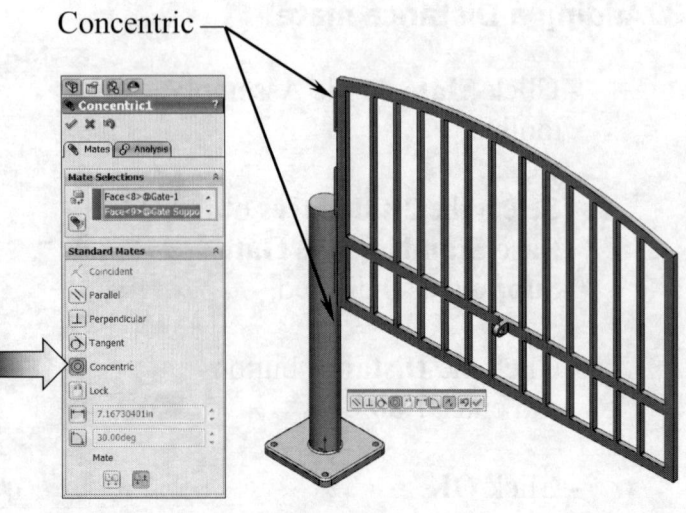

- Add a **Distance** mate of **1.000"** between the **upper face** of the Gate Support and the **bottom face** of the Gate, as noted.

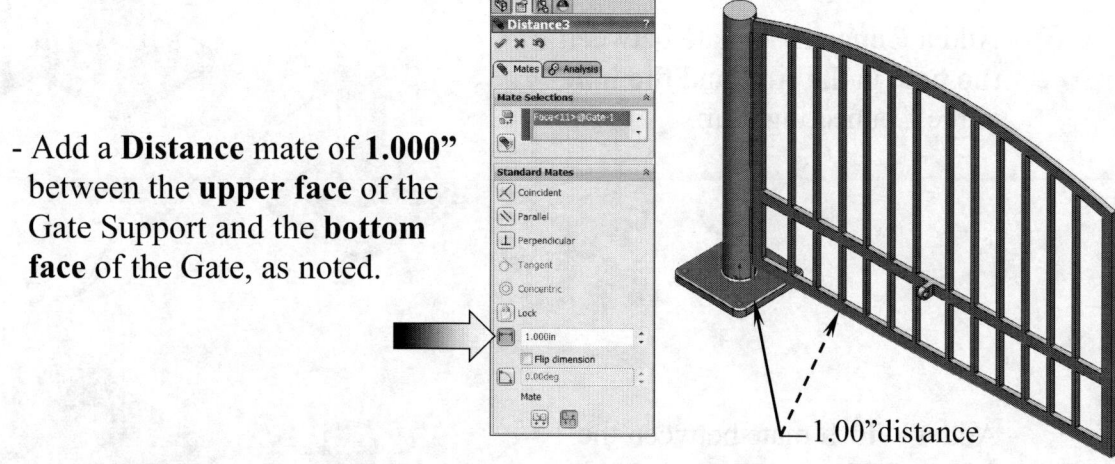

1.00"distance

- Add a **Concentric** mate between the **circular face** of the Base-Stand and the **center hole** of the Arm-Connector.

- Add a **Width** mate between the **4 faces** of the same components.

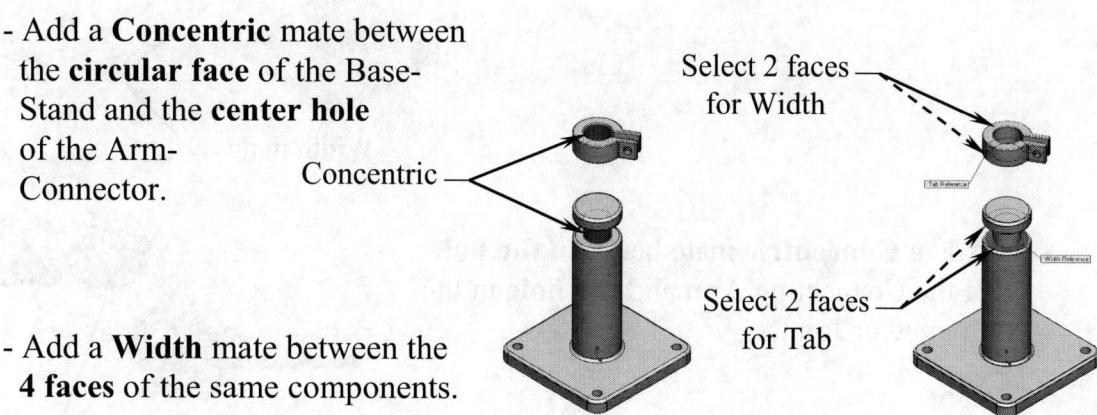

Concentric

Select 2 faces for Width

Select 2 faces for Tab

- Add a **Concentric** mate between the side Hole of the Arm Connector and **the hole** in the Arm.

Concentric mate

- Add another **Width** mate between the **4 faces** of these two components.

Width mate

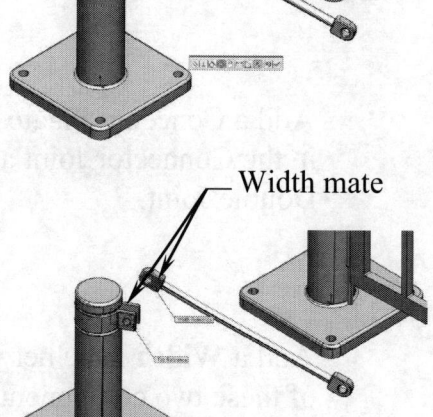

- Add a **Concentric** mate between
  the hole in the Arm and **the hole**
  in the Connecting Arm.

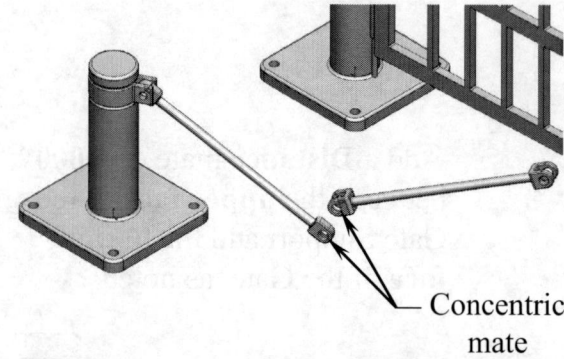

Concentric
mate

- Add a **Width** mate between the
  4 faces of the same components.

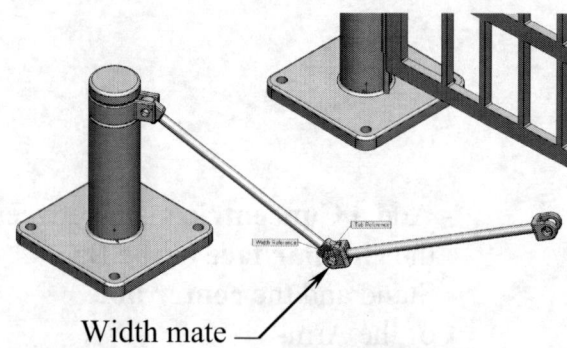

Width mate

- Add a **Concentric** mate between **the hole**
  of the Connecting Arm and **the hole** in the
  Connector Joint.

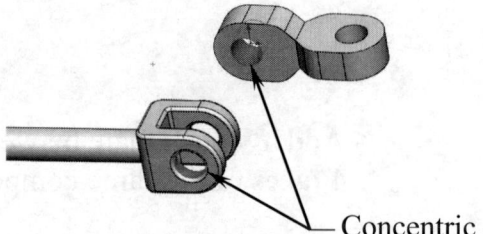

Concentric

- Add another **Width** mate between the **4 faces**
  of these two components.

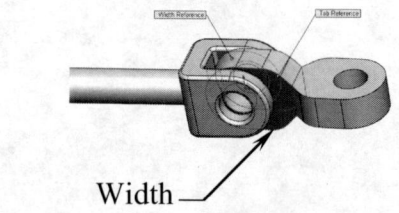

Width

- Add a Concentric mate between **the hole**
  in the Connector Joint and **the hole** in the
  Double Joint.

Concentric

- Add a **Width** mate between the **4 faces**
  of these two components.

Width

- Click **OK**.

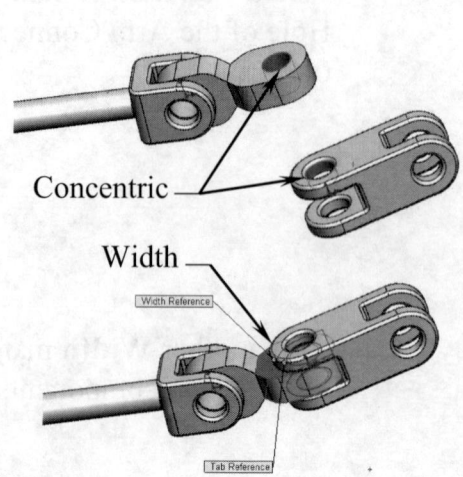

- Move the components to the position shown.

- Since the Double Joint has several components connected to its left side, this time it might be a little easier if we create the Width mate before the Concentric mate.

6. Adding more mates:

- Click the **Mate** command again, if not yet selected.

Move the components to approx. here

- Select the **Advanced** tab.

- Click the **Width** option.

- Select the **2 faces** of the **Double Joint** for Width selection.

- Select the other **2 faces** of the tab on the **Gate** for Tab selection.

- Click **OK**.

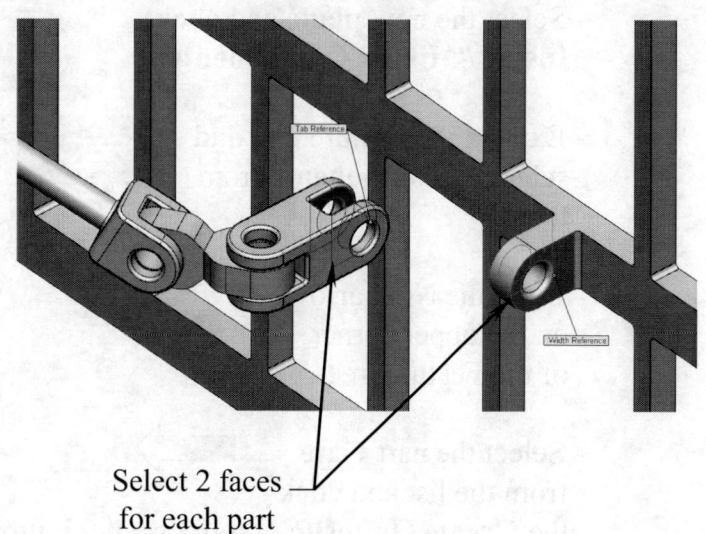

Select 2 faces for each part

- Change to the **Standard Mates** tab.

Concentric mate

- Select **the hole** in the Double-Joint and **the hole** on the tab of the Gate.

- A **Concentric** mate is added automatically to the selected holes.

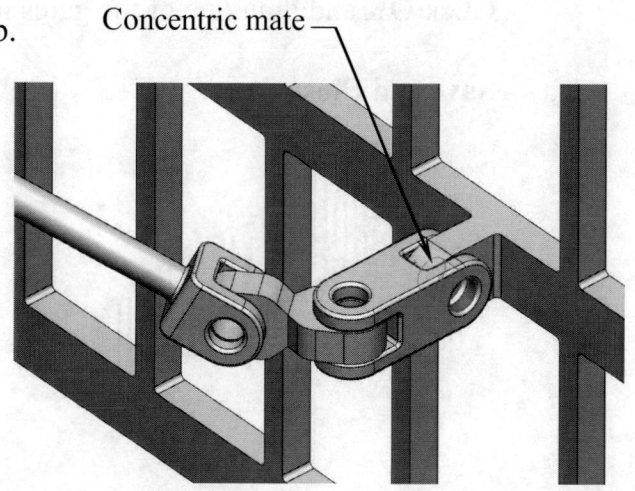

- Click **OK** twice to close out of the mate mode.

7. Creating an Offset Distance plane:

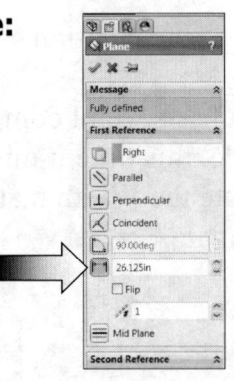

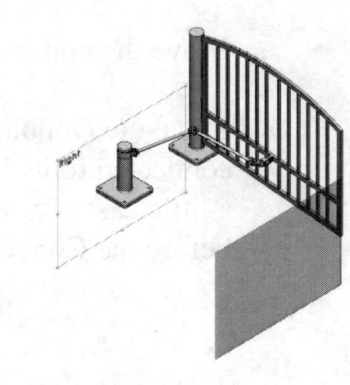

- Select the **Right** plane of the assembly and click the **Plane** command, or **select Insert / Reference Geometry / Plane**.

- The **Offset Distance** button is selected by default.

- Enter **26.125"** for distance.

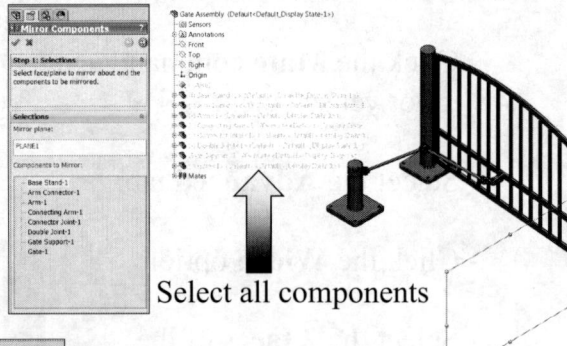

- Click **OK**.

8. Mirroring the components:

- Select the **new plane** and click: **Insert / Mirror Components**.

Select all components

- Expand the Feature tree and **select all components** from there.

NEXT

- Click the **Next** arrow on the upper corner of the Feature tree.

- Select the part **Gate** from the list and click the **Create Opposite Hand Version** button.

- Click **OK** and drag one of the gates to test out your assembly.

- **Save** and **Close**.

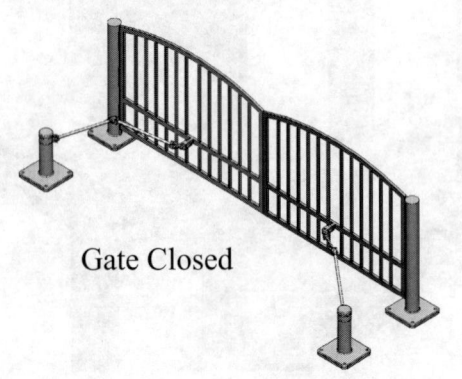

Gate Closed

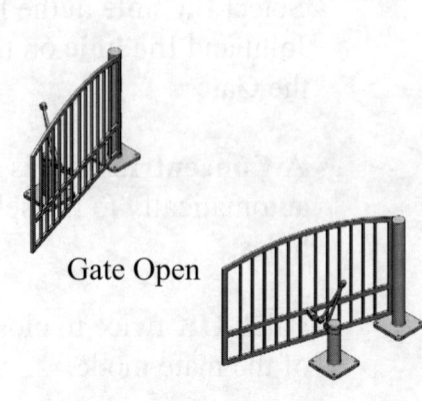

Gate Open

Assembly Motions exercise

1. Opening an existing assembly document:

- Browse to the Training Files location and open the assembly document named:
HeliDrone Assembly.sldasm

- This assembly contains 1 component and 2 sub-assemblies.

- The sub-assemblies are set to **Rigid** by default; they will need to be changed to **Flexible** so that the blades inside the fan housings can be rotated when needed.

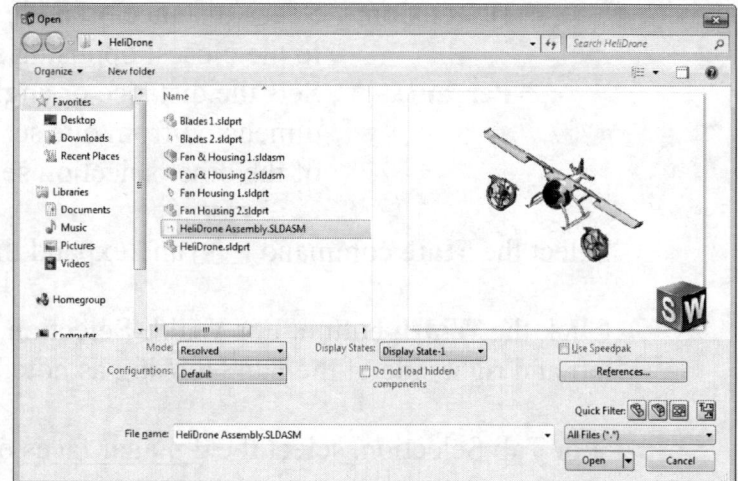

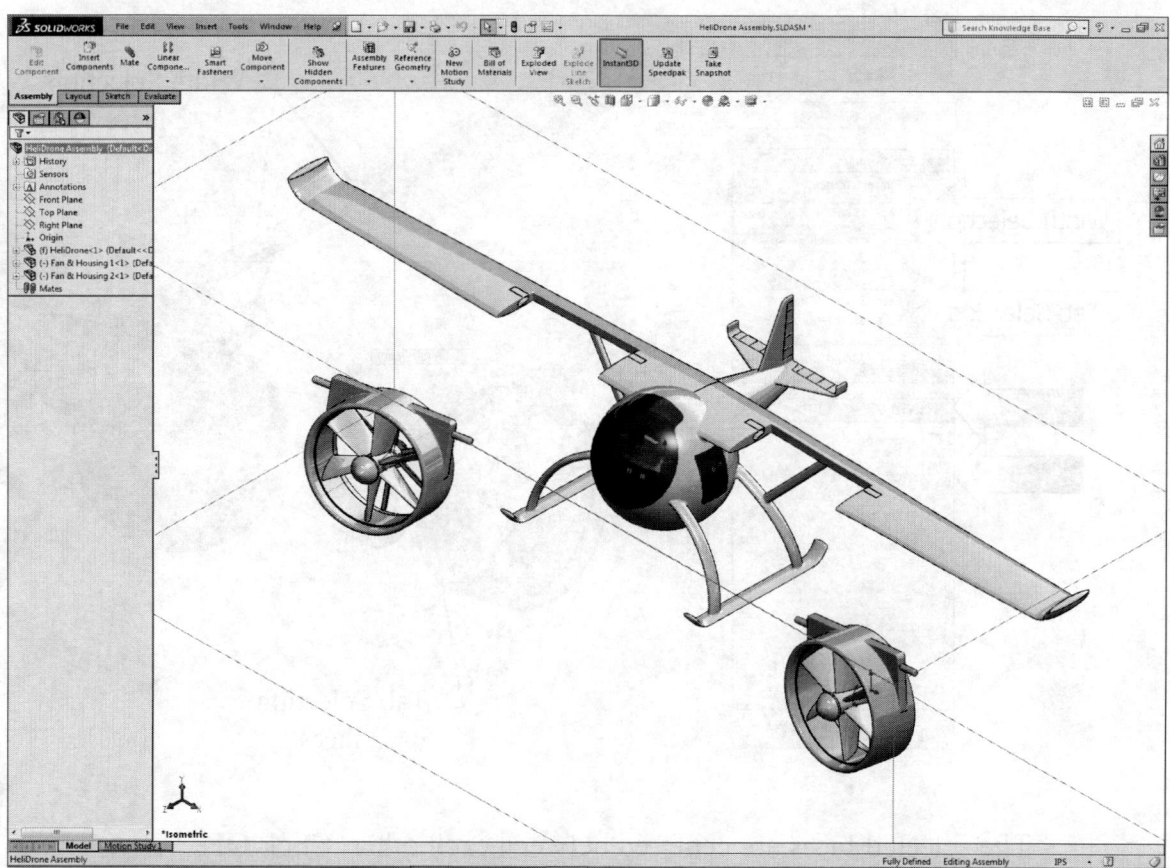

2. Using the Width mate:

- Use the following options to define the limits of the mate: (Note: A width mate must be created prior to selecting one of the options below).

* **Centered:**   Centers a tab within the width of a groove.
* **Free:**   Lets the components move freely within the limits of the selected or planes with respect to the components.
* **Dimension:**   Sets a distance or angle dimension from one selection set to the closest opposing selection set of faces or planes.
* **Percent:**   Sets the distance or angle based on a percentage value dimension from one set of the selection set to the center of the other selection set.

- Select the **Mate** command 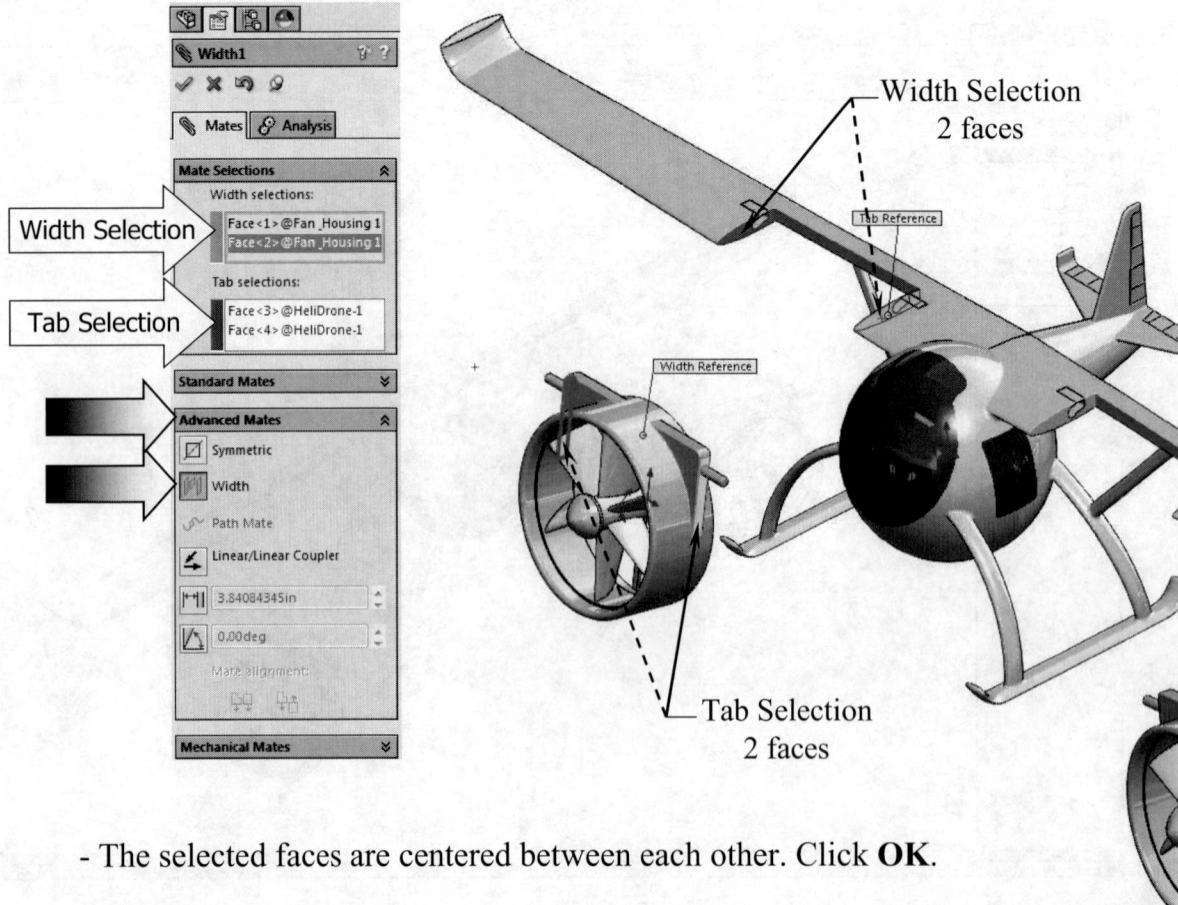 and expand the **Advanced Mate** section.

- Click the **Width** button. For Width-Selection, select the 2 planar faces on the left and right side of the Fan Housing as noted.

- For Tab-Selection, select the 2 planar faces on the left and right side of the wing.

- The selected faces are centered between each other. Click **OK**.

3. Adding a Concentric mate:

- Concentric mate can be added between a circular edge, a cone or a cylinder, a line, a point, or a sphere.

- Switch back to the **Standard Mates** section (arrow).

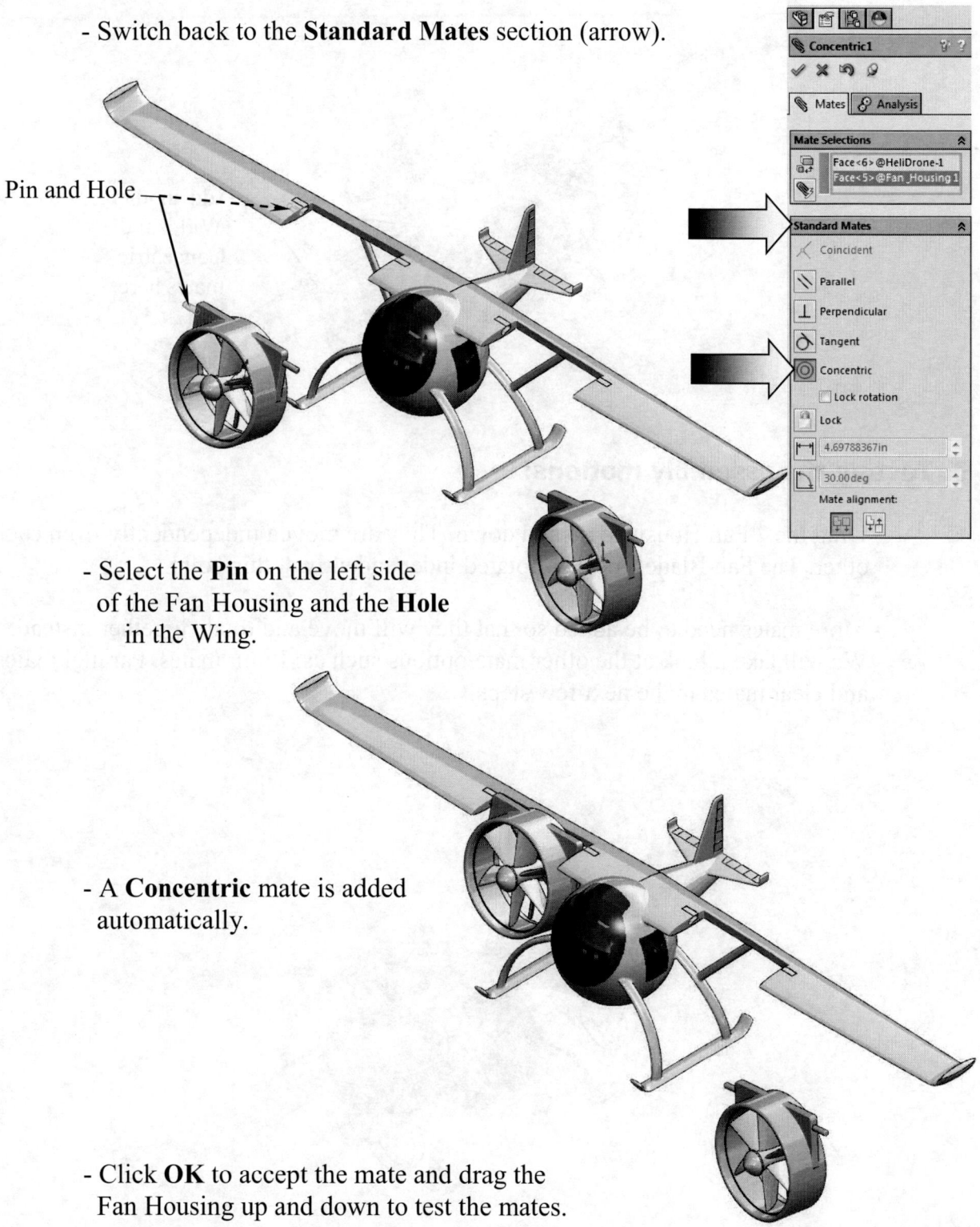

Pin and Hole

- Select the **Pin** on the left side of the Fan Housing and the **Hole** in the Wing.

- A **Concentric** mate is added automatically.

- Click **OK** to accept the mate and drag the Fan Housing up and down to test the mates.

4. Adding another Concentric mate:

- Repeat the last step and mate the second Fan Housing to the opposite wing.

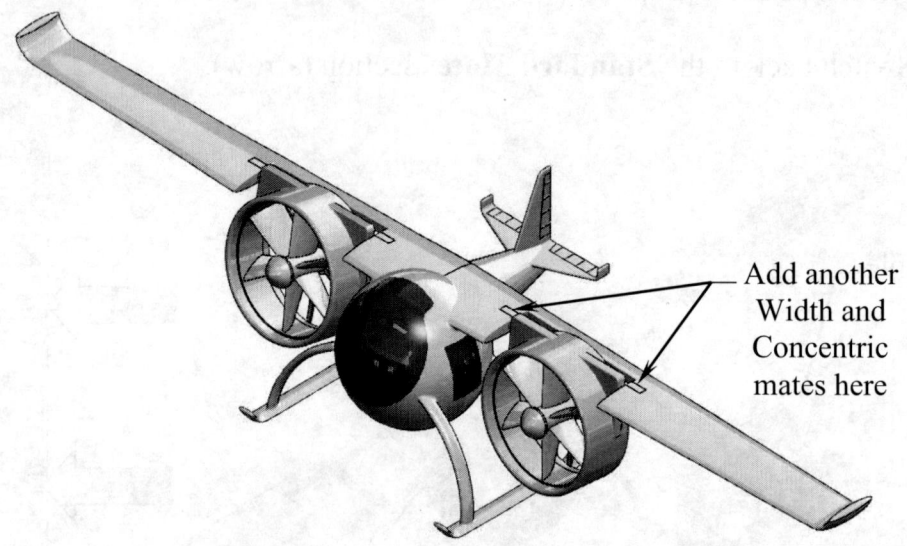

Add another
Width and
Concentric
mates here

5. Testing the assembly motions:

- Drag the 2 Fan Housings up and down. They are moved independently from each other. The Fan Blades are also rotated independently at this point.

- More mates need to be added so that they will move and rotate together instead. We will take a look at the other mate options such as: Limit mates, Parallel mates, and Gear mates in the next few steps.

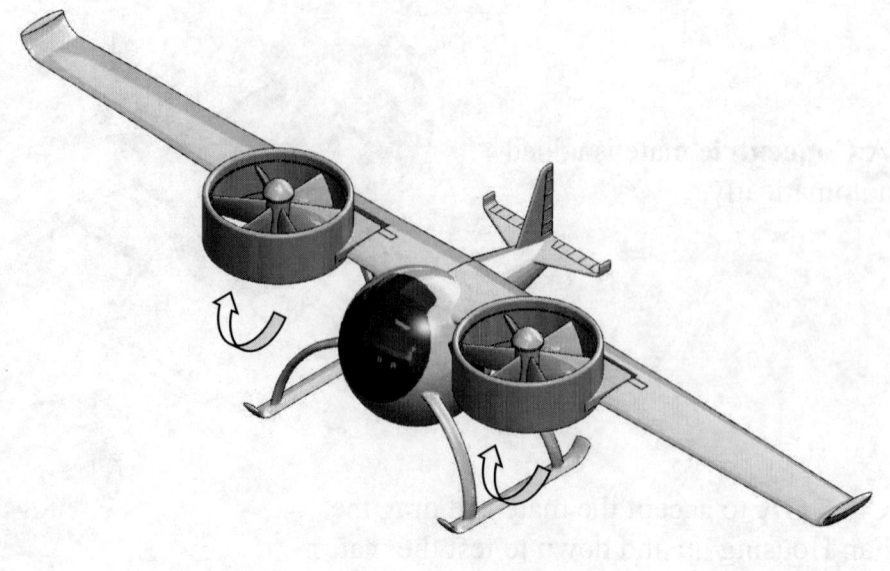

6. Adding a Limit-Angle mate:

- Limit Angle mate allows components to move within a range of specified angles.

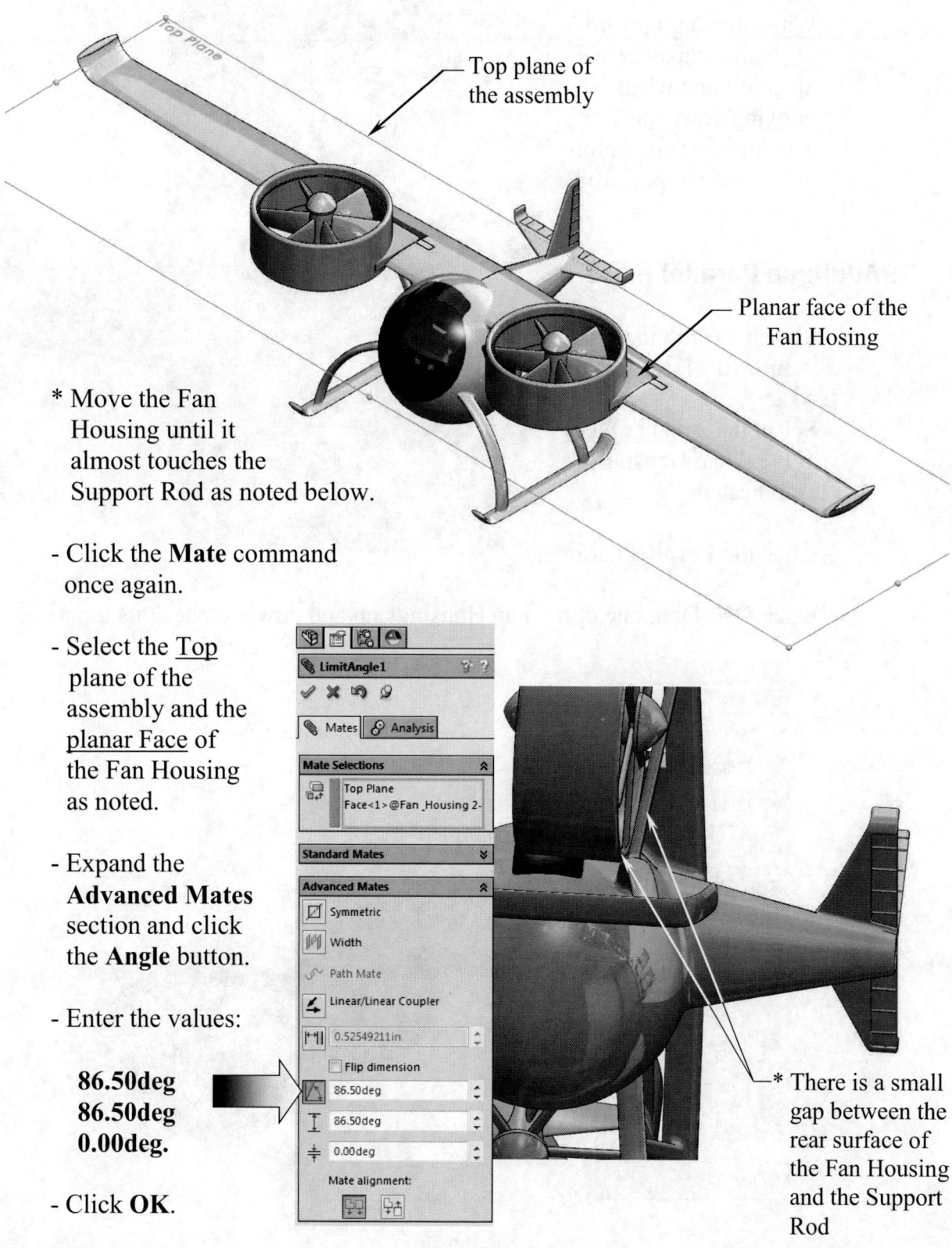

Top plane of the assembly

Planar face of the Fan Hosing

* Move the Fan Housing until it almost touches the Support Rod as noted below.

- Click the **Mate** command once again.

- Select the Top plane of the assembly and the planar Face of the Fan Housing as noted.

- Expand the **Advanced Mates** section and click the **Angle** button.

- Enter the values:

86.50deg
86.50deg
0.00deg.

- Click **OK**.

* There is a small gap between the rear surface of the Fan Housing and the Support Rod

- Drag the Fan Housing up and down to test its limits.

- When moving upward it should stop at zero degrees; and when moving downward it should stop right before it hits the Support Rod.

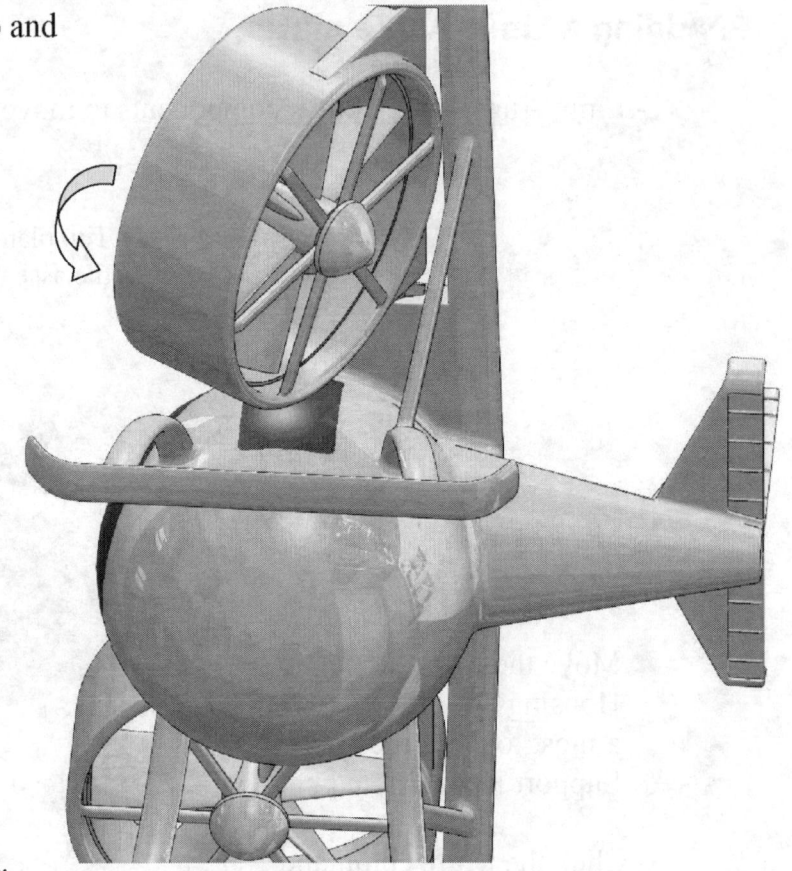

7. Adding a Parallel mate:

- Switch back to the **Standard Mates** section.

- Select the <u>2 planar faces</u> of the 2 Fan Housings as indicated.

- Click the **Parallel** button.

- Click **OK**. Drag one of the Fan Housings up and down to check its motions.

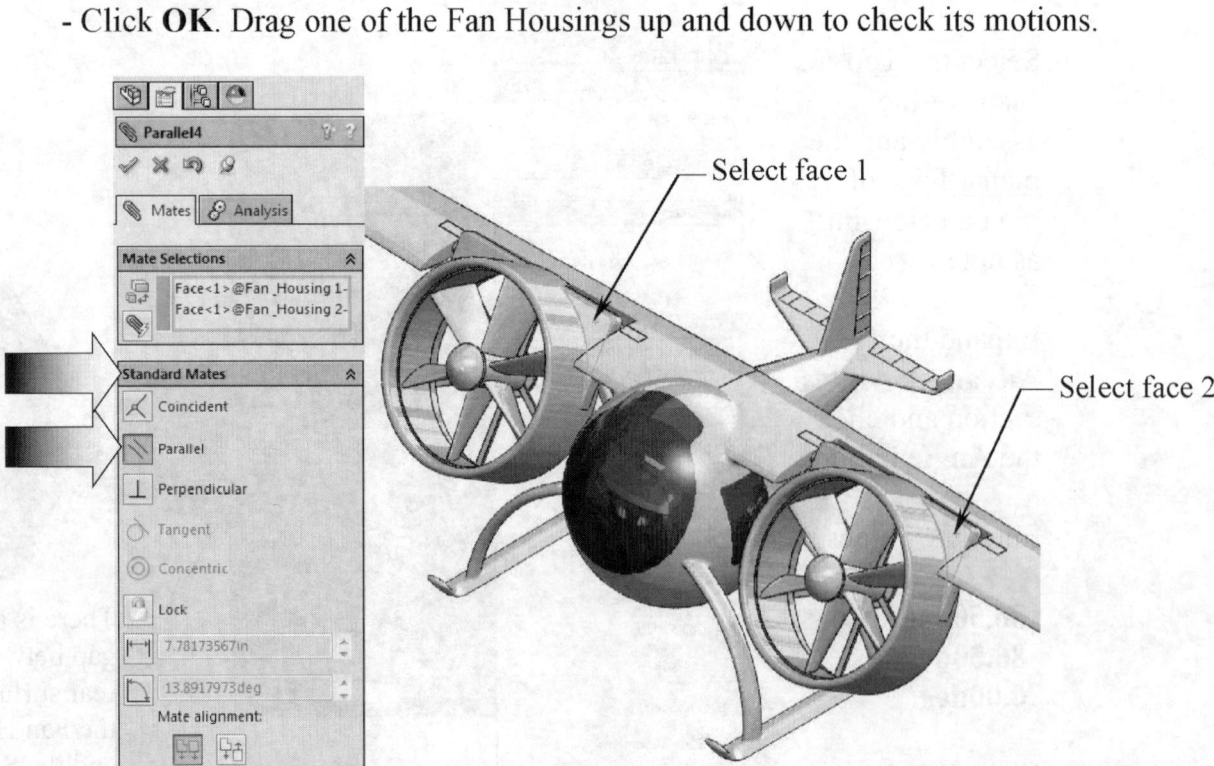

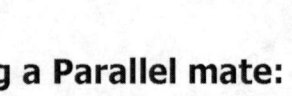

Select face 1

Select face 2

8. Adding a Gear mate:

- A Gear mate forces two components to rotate relative to one another about selected axes.

- Switch to the **Mechanical Mates** section (arrow).

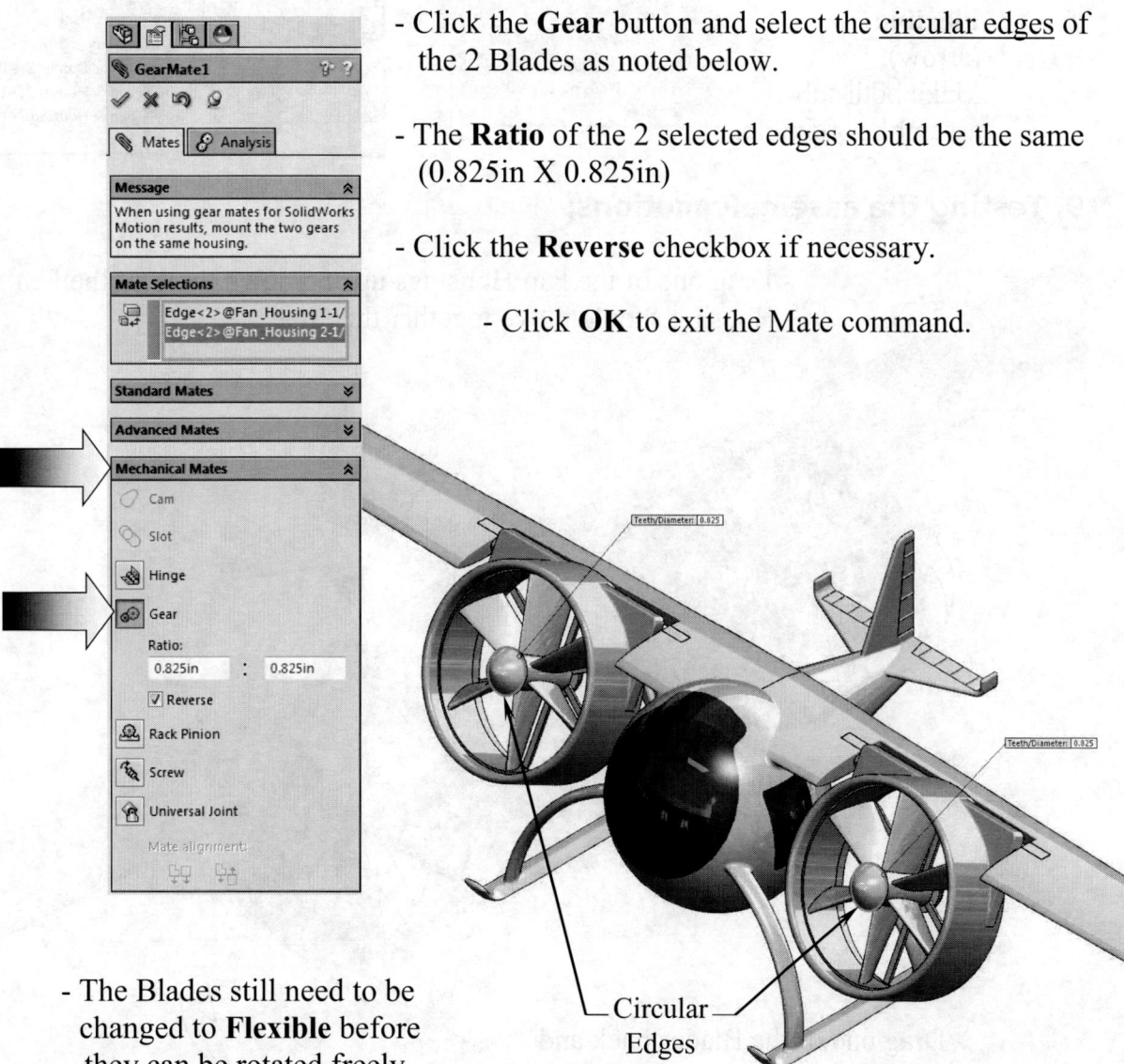

- Click the **Gear** button and select the circular edges of the 2 Blades as noted below.

- The **Ratio** of the 2 selected edges should be the same (0.825in X 0.825in)

- Click the **Reverse** checkbox if necessary.

- Click **OK** to exit the Mate command.

Circular Edges

- The Blades still need to be changed to **Flexible** before they can be rotated freely.

- Click on the
Sub-Assembly
icon and select
the option:
**Make Sub-
Assembly
Flexible**
(arrow).
Make both sub-
assemblies flexible.

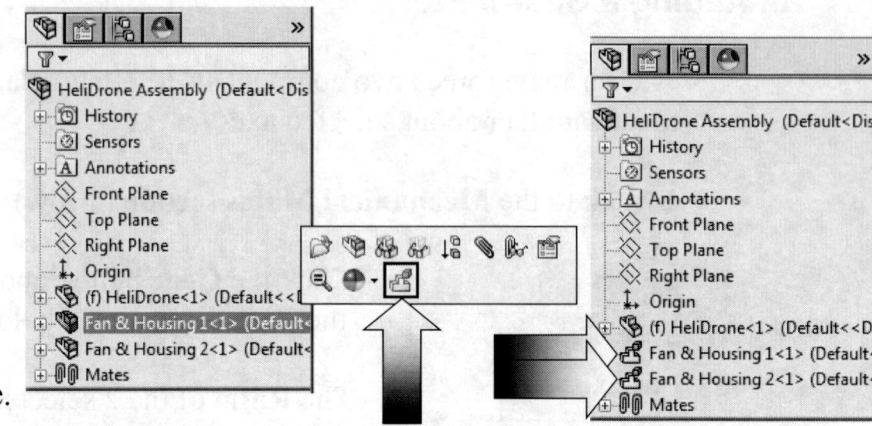

9. Testing the assembly motions:

- Drag one of the Fan Housings up and down, both of the Fan
Housing should move together this time.

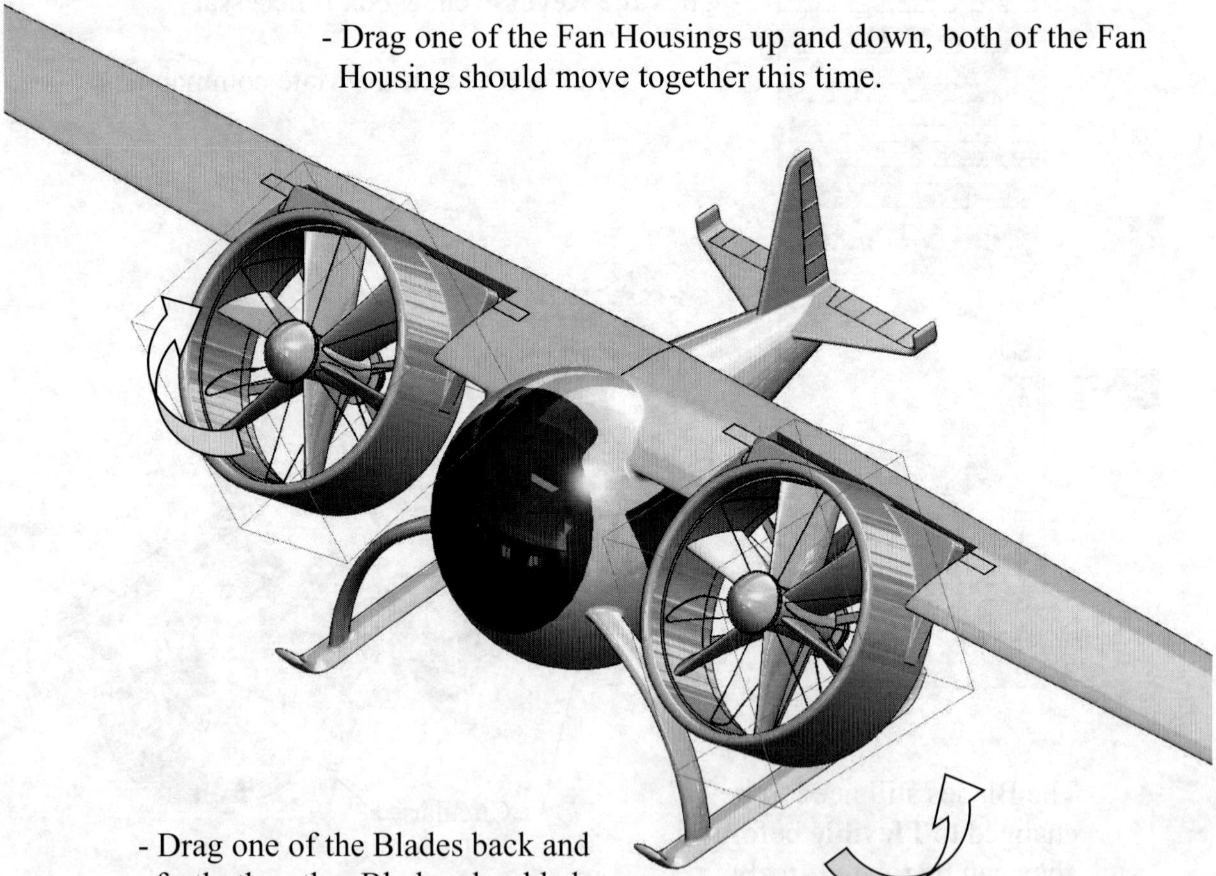

- Drag one of the Blades back and
forth, the other Blades should also
rotate at the same time.

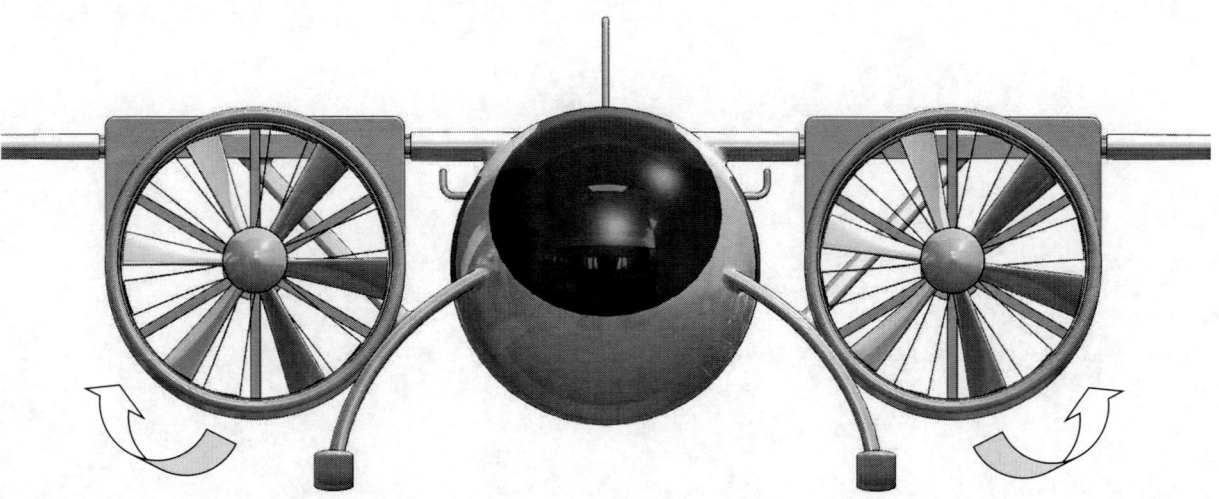

10. Saving your work:

- Press **Save** (or Control + S) and click **Yes** to overwrite the existing assembly document with your completed one.

CHAPTER 11

Using Advanced Mates

Rack and Pinion
Using Advanced-Mates

- Beside the standard mates such as Concentric, Coincident, Tangent, Angle, etc., which must be done one by one, SolidWorks offers an alternative option that is much more robust called: Smart-Mates.

- There are many advantages for using Smart-mates. It can create several mates at the same time, depending on the type of entity selected. For example: If you drag a circular edge of a hole and drop it on a circular edge of another hole, SolidWorks will automatically create 2 mates, a concentric mate between the two cylindrical faces of the holes and a coincident mate between the two planar faces.

- Using Smart-mates, you do not have to select the Mate command every time. Simply hold the ALT key and drag an entity of a component to its destination, a smart-mate symbol will appear to confirm the types of mates it is going to add. At the same time, a mate toolbar will also pop up offering some additional options such as Flip Mate Alignment, change to a different mate type, or simply undo the selection.

- Using the Alt + Drag option, the Tab key is used to flip the mate alignments. This is done by releasing the Alt key and pressing the Tab key, while the mouse button is still pressed. This option works well even if your assembly is set to lightweight.

- In addition to the Alt + Drag, if you hold the Control key and Drag a component, SolidWorks will create an instance of the selected component and apply the smart-mates to it at the same time. Using this option you will have to click the Flip Mate Alignment button on the pop-up toolbar to reverse the direction of the mate, the Tab key does not work.

- This lesson will guide you through the use of the Smart-mate options, and for some of the steps, use the standards mate options as well.

Rack & Pinion
Using Advanced-Mates

Rack & Pinion Mates

The Rack and Pinion mate option allows linear translation of the Rack to cause circular rotation in the Pinion, and vice versa.

For each full rotation of the Pinion, the Rack translates a distance equal to π multiplied by the Pinion diameter. You can specify either the diameter or the distance by selecting either the Pinion Pitch Diameter or the Rack Travel / Revolution options.

1. Open an assembly document:

- From the Training Files folder, browse to the Rack & Pinion folder and open the assembly named **Rack & Pinion mates**.

- The assembly has two components, the Rack and Gear1. Some of the mates have been created to define the distances between the centers of the two components.

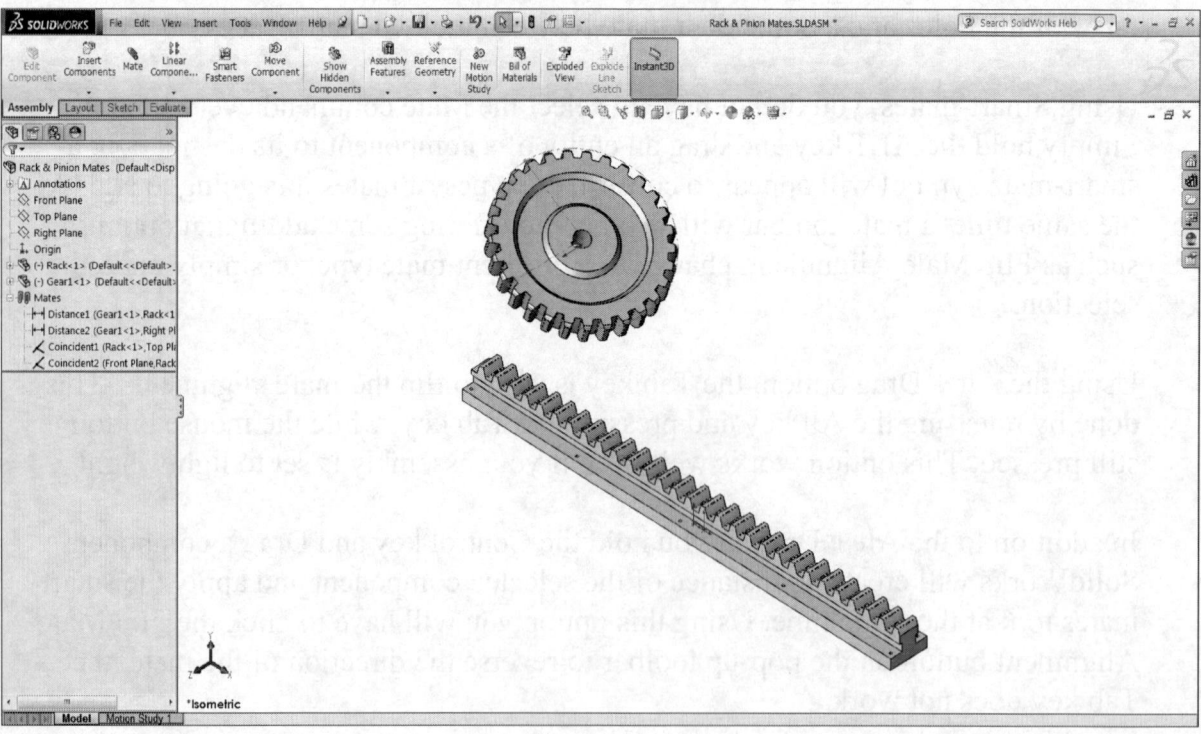

2. Adding standard mates:

- Click the **Mate** command [Mate] from the assembly toolbar, or select **Insert / Mate**.

- Expand the FeatureManager tree and select the **Front planes** for both components. A coincident mate is automatically created for the two selected planes.

- Click **OK** ✓.

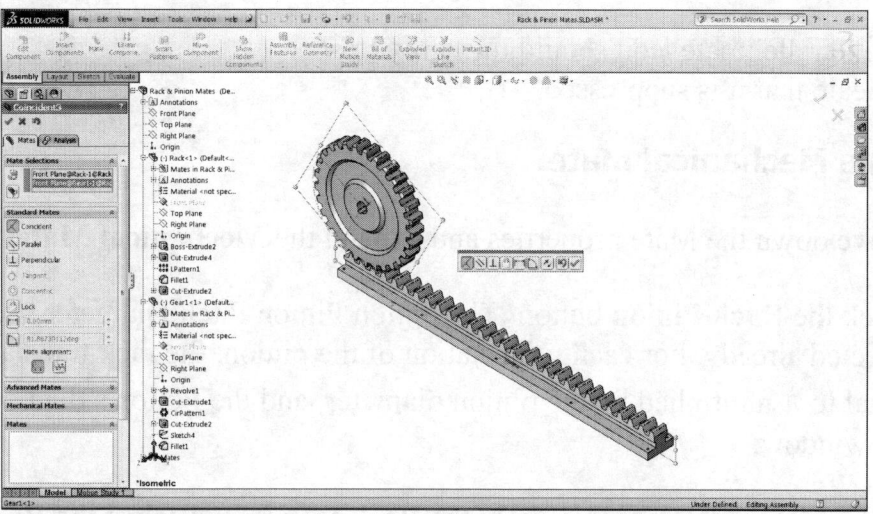

- Click the **Mate** command if not already selected.

- Select the **Right planes** for both components and click the **Parallel** mate option.

- Click **OK** ✓.

- This mate is used to position the starting position of the Gear1, but it needs to be suppressed prior to adding the Rack & Pinion mate.

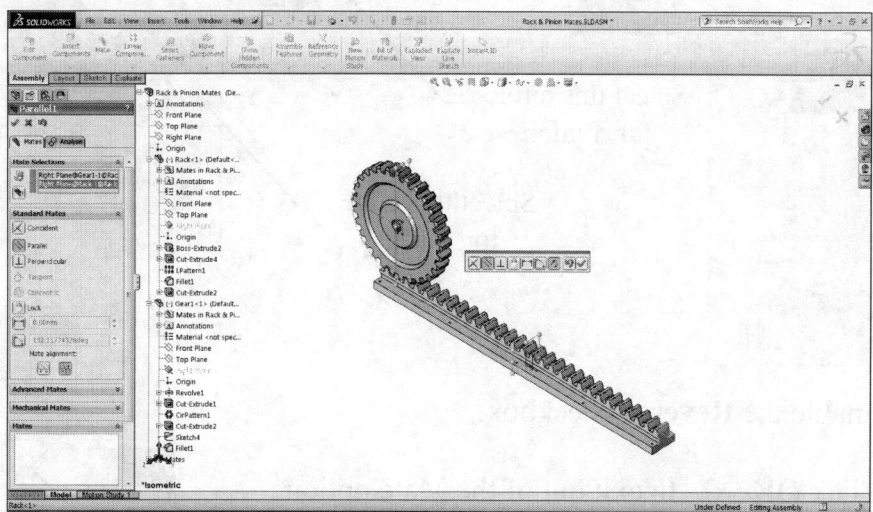

3. Suppressing a mate:

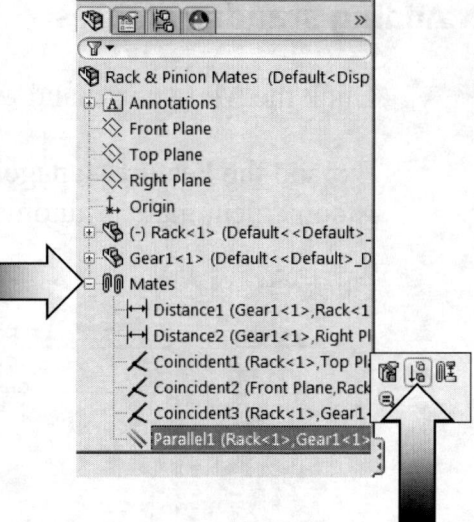

- Expand the **Mate Group** (click the + sign) at the bottom of the FeatureManager tree.

- Right click the Parallel mate and select the **Suppress** button from the pop-up window (arrow).

- The Parallel mate icon should turn grey to indicate that it is suppressed.

4. Adding a Mechanical mate:

- Move down the Mate properties and expand the **Mechanical Mates** section (arrow).

- Click the **Rack Pinion** button. The option Pinion Pitch Diameter should be selected already. For each full rotation of the pinion, the rack translates a distance equal to π multiplied by the pinion diameter, and the Pinion's diameter appears in the window.

- In the Mate Selections, highlight the Rack section and select the **Bottom-Edge** of one of the teeth on the Rack as indicated.

- Click in the Pinion section and select the **Construction-Circle** on the gear as noted.

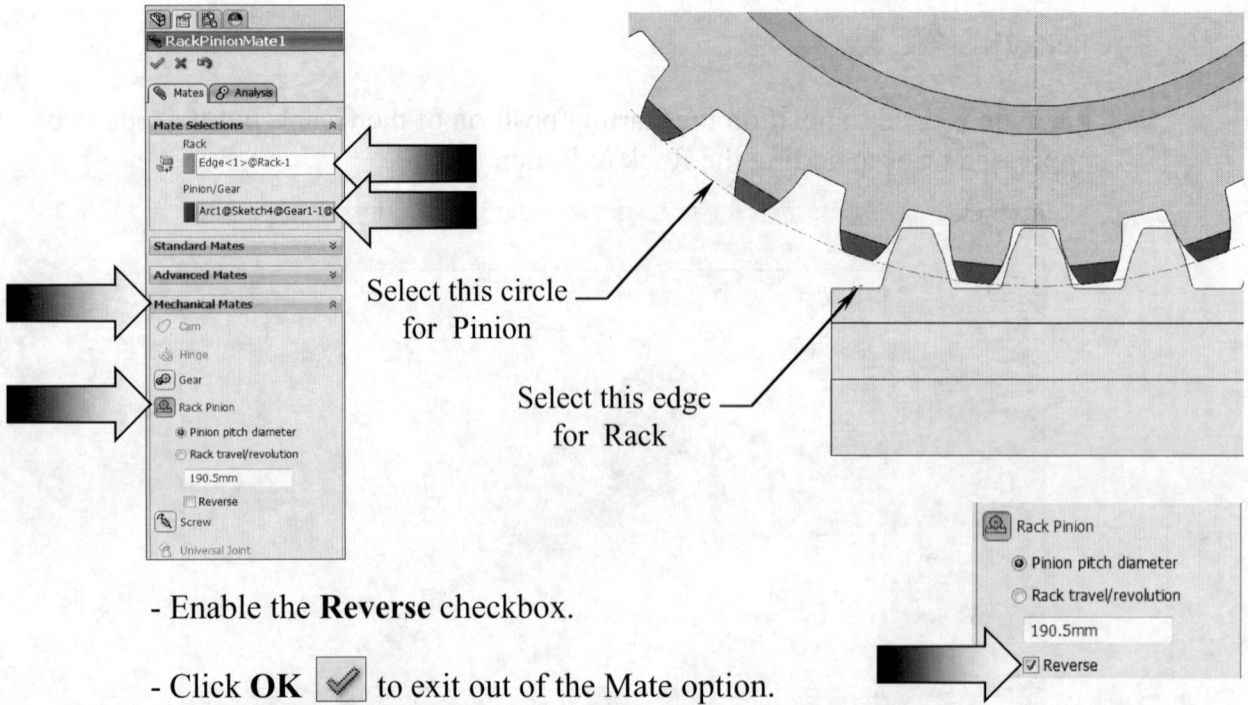

Select this circle for Pinion

Select this edge for Rack

- Enable the **Reverse** checkbox.

- Click **OK** to exit out of the Mate option.

5. Testing the mates:

- Change to the Isometric orientation (Control + 7).

- Drag either the Rack or the Gear1 back and forth and see how the two components will move relative to each other.

- Hide the construction circle. Next we will create an animation using a linear motor to drive the motions.

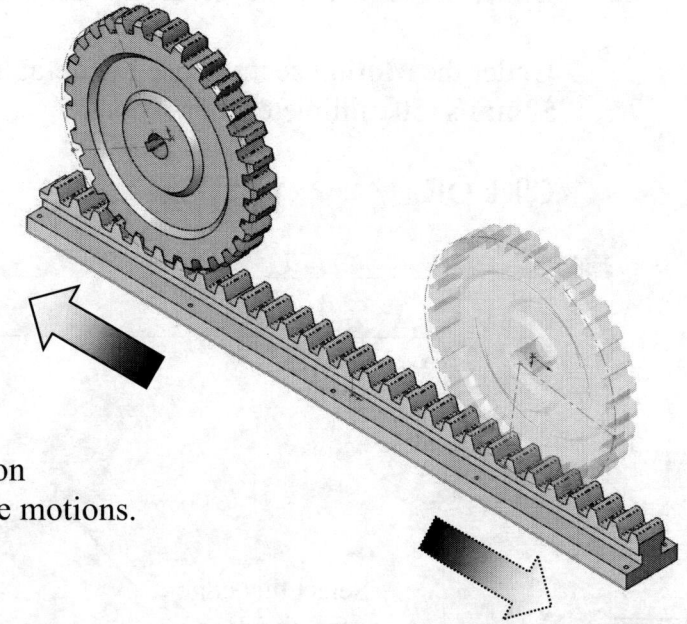

6. Creating a Linear Motion:

- Remain in the Isometric view, click the **Motion Study1** tab on the lower left corner of the screen.

- The screen is split into 2 viewports showing the Animation program on the bottom.

- Click the **Motor** button (arrow) on the Motion Study toolbar.

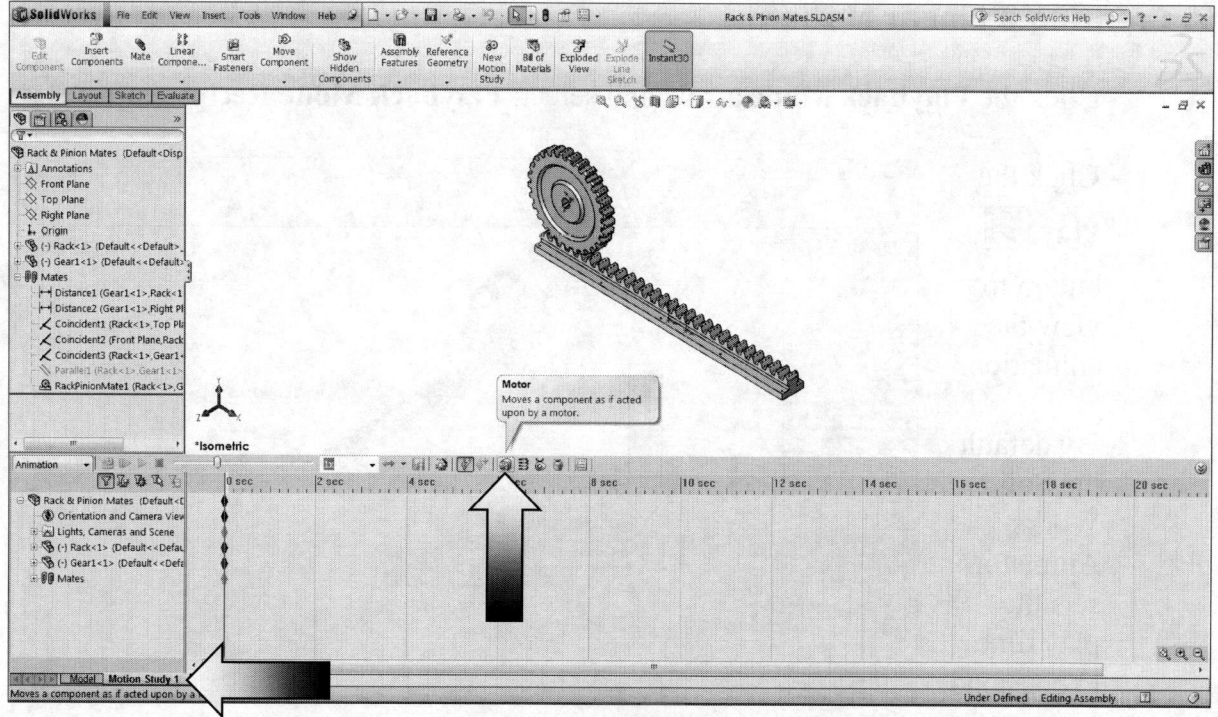

- Under the **Motor Type**, select the **Linear Motor (Actuator)** option.

- Under the **Motion** section, use the default **Constant Speed** and set the speed to **50mm/s** (50 millimeters per second).

- Click **OK** .

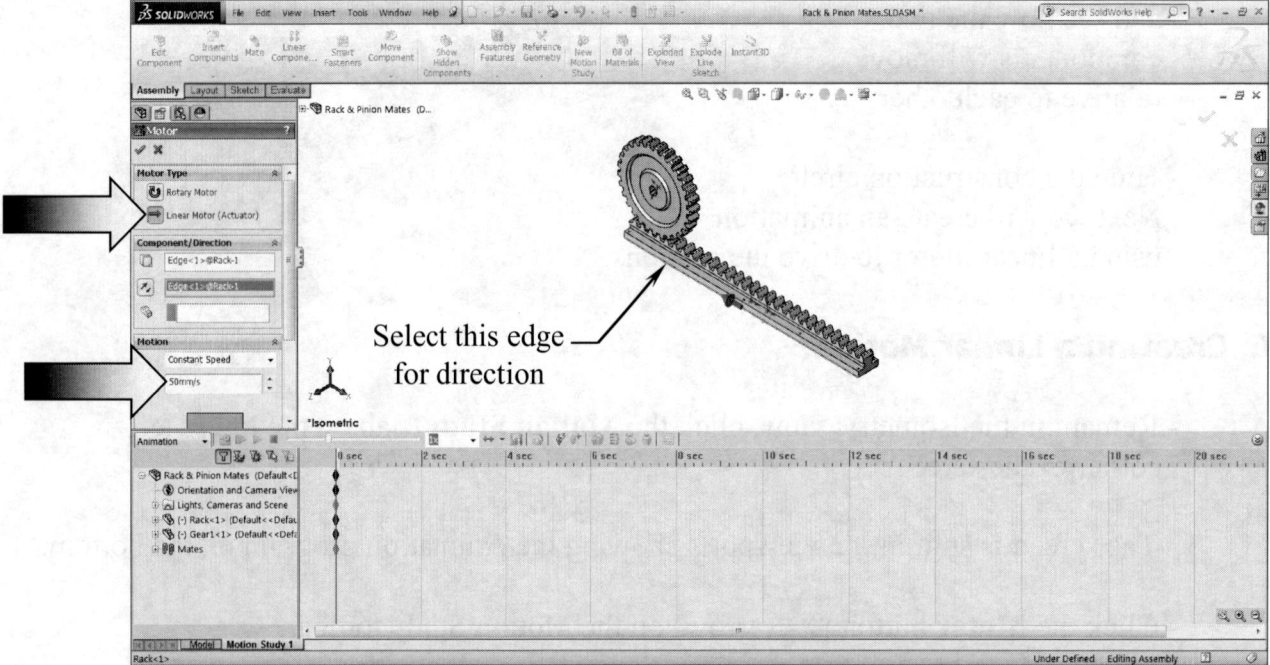

Select this edge for direction

7. Creating a Linear Motion:

- Click the **Playback Mode** arrow and select: **Playback Mode Reciprocate**.

- Click the **Play** button to view the animation.

- By default the Solid-Works-Animator sets the play time to 5 seconds.

- To change the **Playback Time**, drag the diamond key to **10 second** spot (arrow).

- To change the **Playback Speed**, click the drop down arrow and select **5X** (arrow).

- Click the **Play** ▷ button again to re-run the animation.

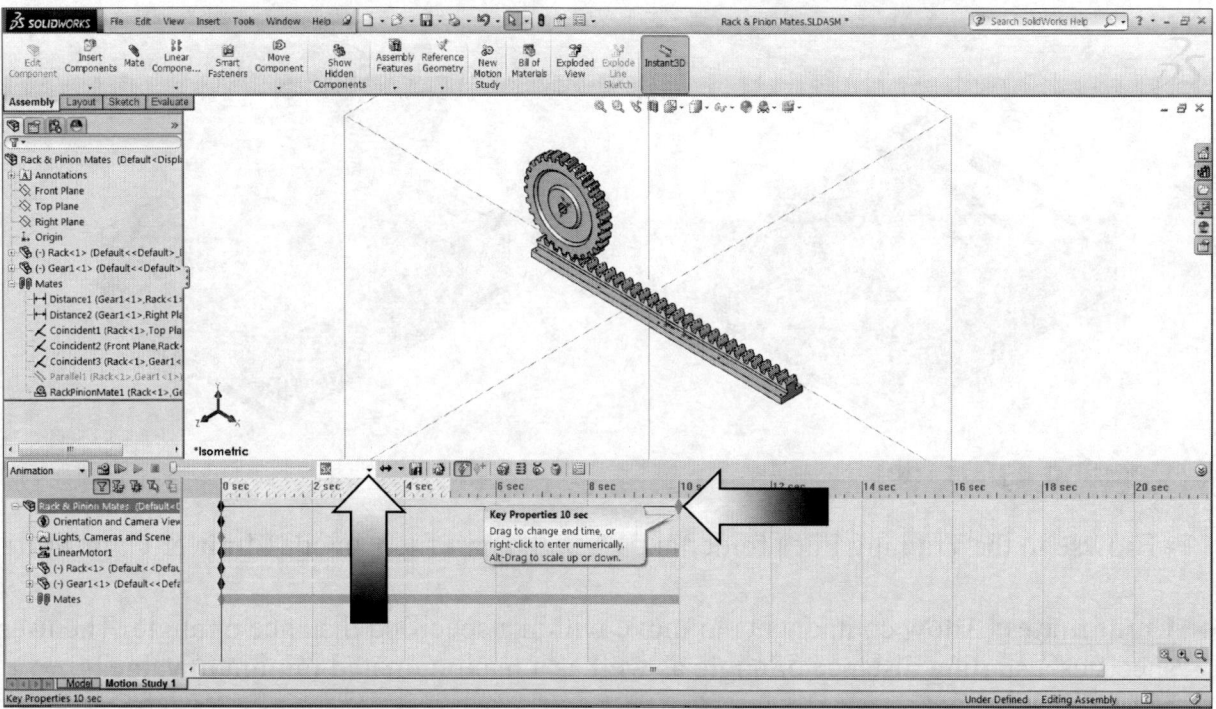

8. Saving your work:

- Click **File / Save As**.

- Enter **Rack & Pinion Mates** for the name of the file.

- Overwrite the old file when prompted.

- Click **Save**.

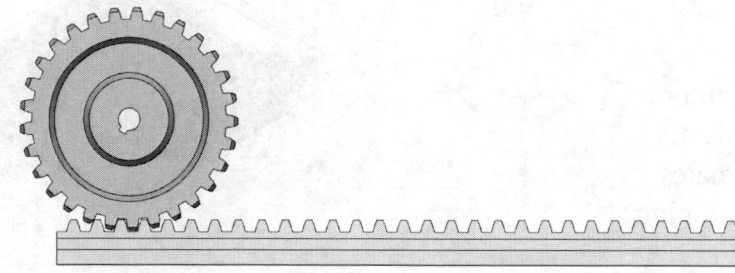

CHAPTER 11 (cont.)

Limit & Cam Mates

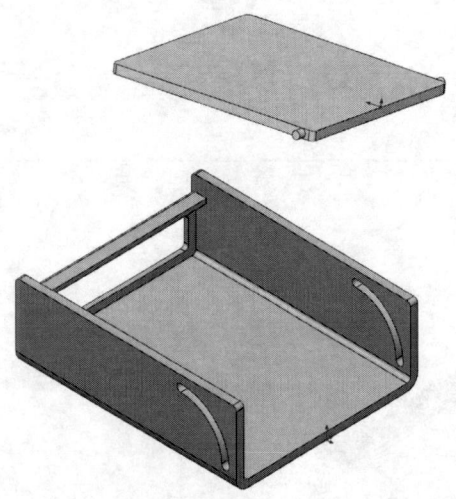
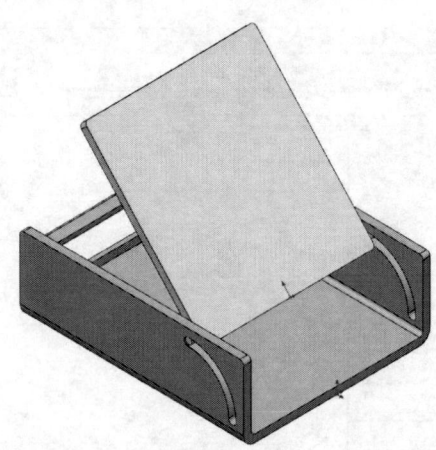

1. Opening a part file:

- Browse to the Training Files folder and open the part file named: **Limit & Cam Mates**.

Limit mates: Allow components to move within a specified distance or angle. The user specifies a starting distance or angle as well as a maximum and minimum value.

Cam Mate: is a type of coincident or tangent mate. Where a cylinder, a plane, or a point can be mated to a series of tangent extruded faces.

- This assembly document has 2 components. The Part1 has been fixed by the Inplace1 and the Part2 still has 6 degrees of freedom.

- We will explore the use of Limit and Cam mates when positioning the Part2.

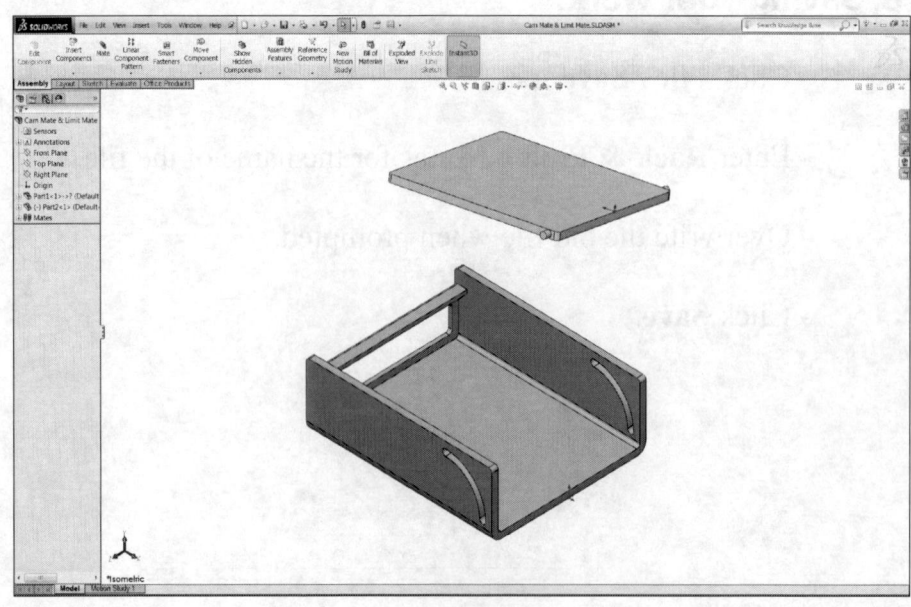

2. Adding a Width mate:

- Click the **Mate** command from the Assembly tab.

- Click the **Advanced Mates** tab and select the **Width** option.

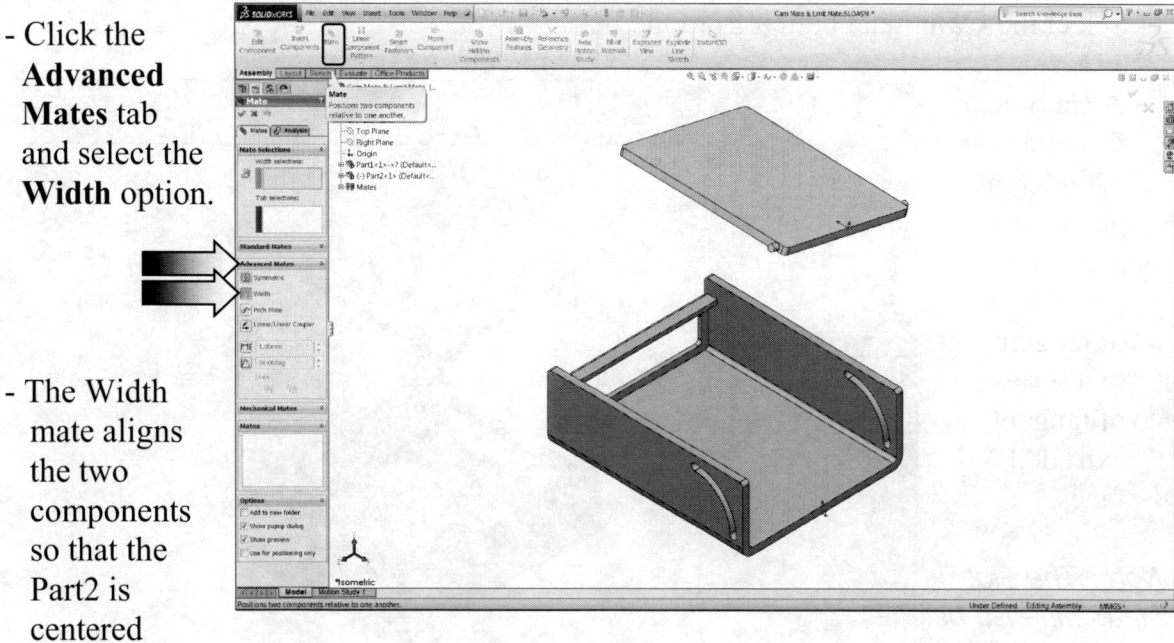

- The Width mate aligns the two components so that the Part2 is centered between the faces of the Part1 (Housing). The Part2 can translate along the center plane of the Housing and rotate about the axis that is normal to the center plane. The width mate prevents the Part2 from translating or rotating side to side.

- For the **Width Selection**, select the **2 side faces** of the **Part2** (arrow).

- For the **Tab Selection**, select the **2 side faces** of the **Part1** (Housing).

- It does not matter which component you select first or second, just be sure to select both faces of the same part before selecting the next set.

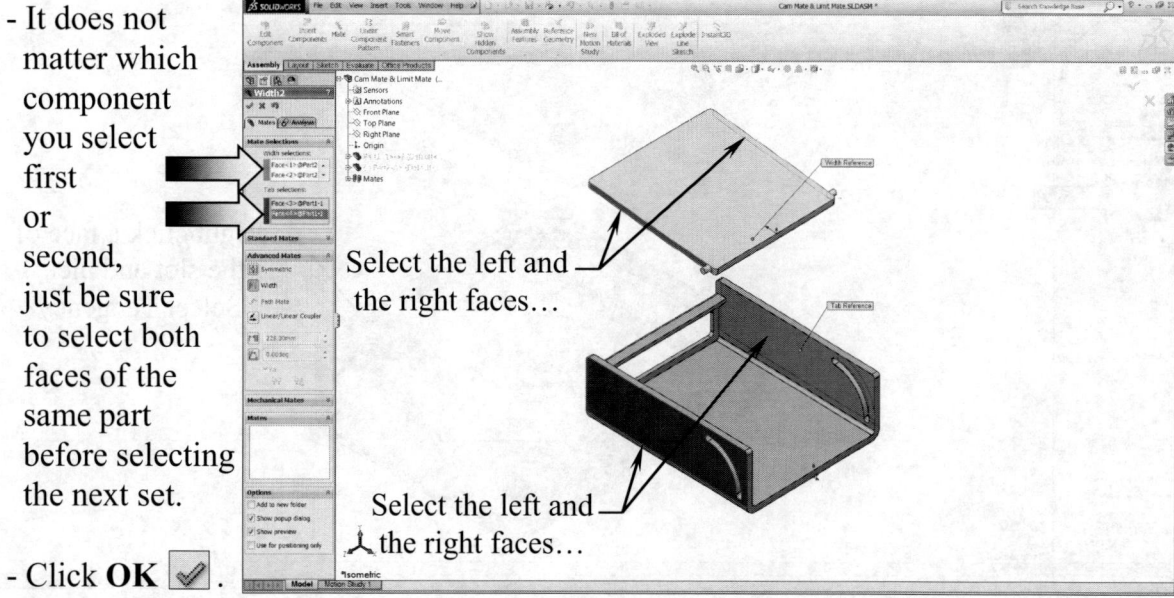

Select the left and the right faces…

Select the left and the right faces…

- Click **OK** ✓ .

3. Adding a Cam mate:

- Click the **Mechanical Mates** tab below the Standard and Advanced tabs (Arrow).

- Select the **Cam** mate button from the list.

- A Cam mate forces a cylinder, a plane, or a point to be coincident or tangent to a series of tangent extruded faces.

Note: The Slot-Mate can also be used to achieve the same result.

- For the **Cam Selection**, right click a face of the slot and pick: **Select Tangency**.

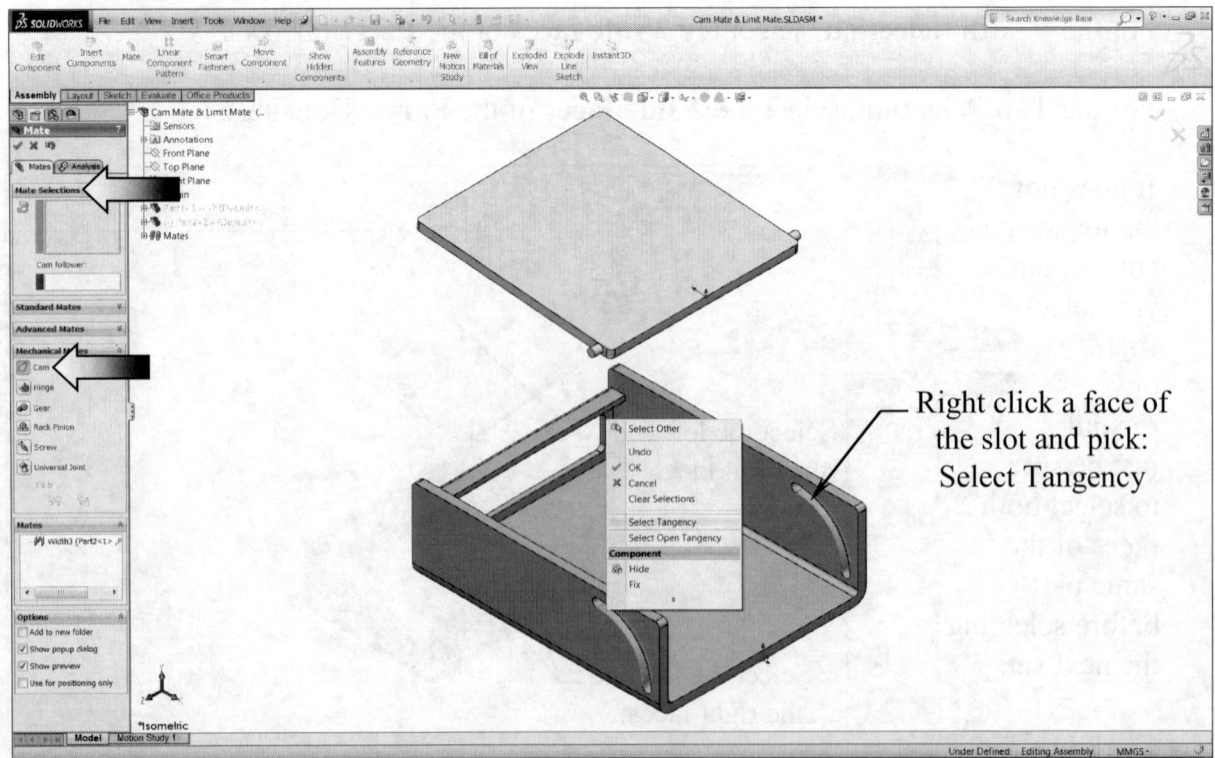

Right click a face of the slot and pick: Select Tangency

- For the **Cam Follower**, select the <u>cylindrical face</u> of one of the pins.

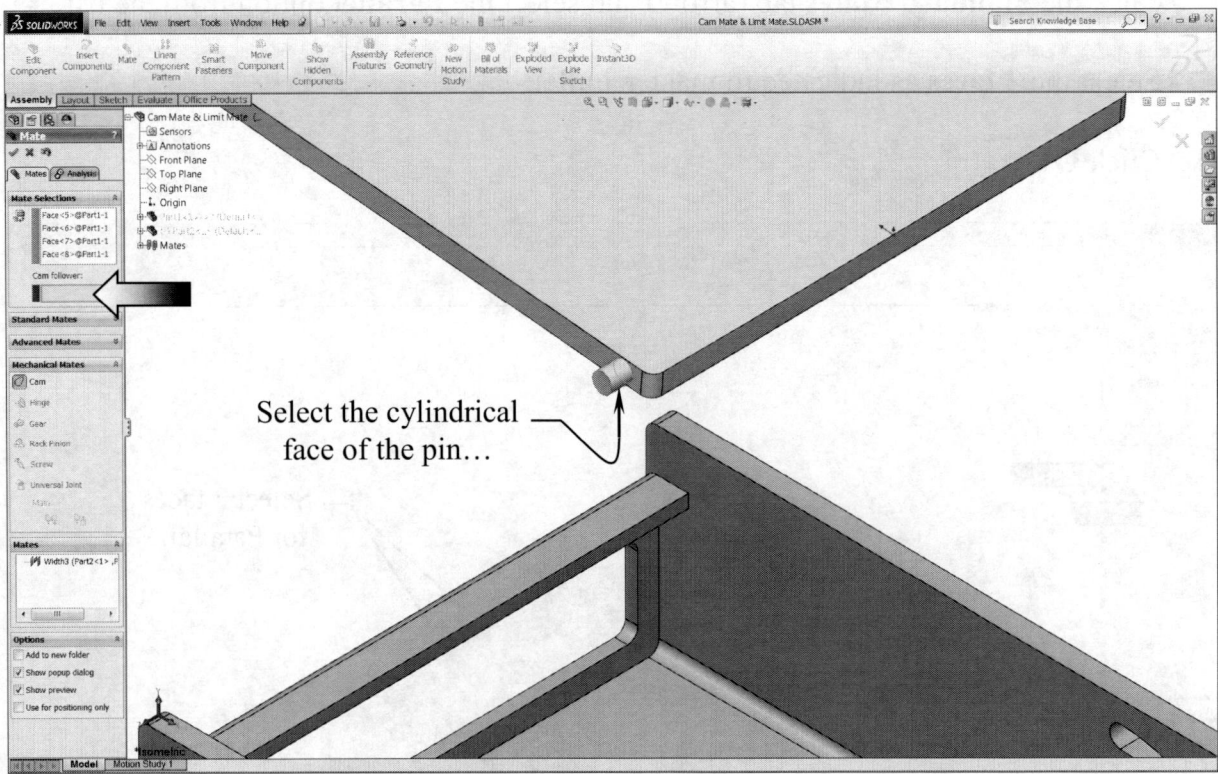

Select the cylindrical
face of the pin…

- Zoom in and check the alignment between the pin and the slot.

- Toggle between
the 2 mate
alignment
buttons (arrow)
to make sure
the two
components
are properly
oriented.

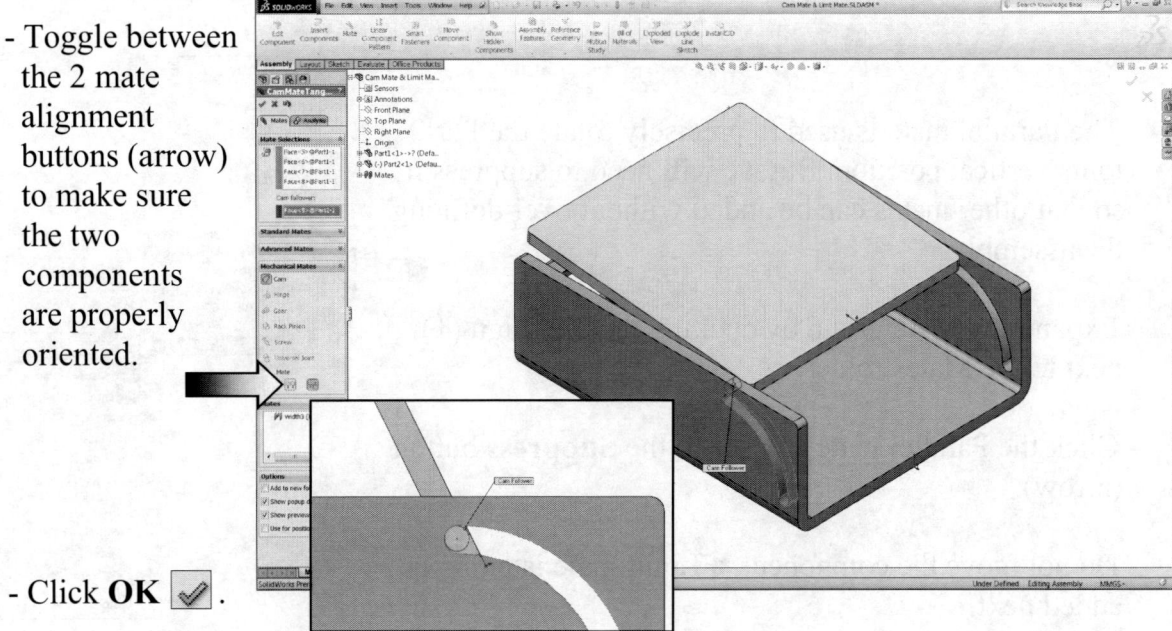

- Click **OK** .

4. Adding a Parallel mate:

- Click the **Standard Mates** tab (arrow) and select the **Parallel** option from the list.

- Select the **2 faces** as indicated to make parallel.

- Click **OK** .

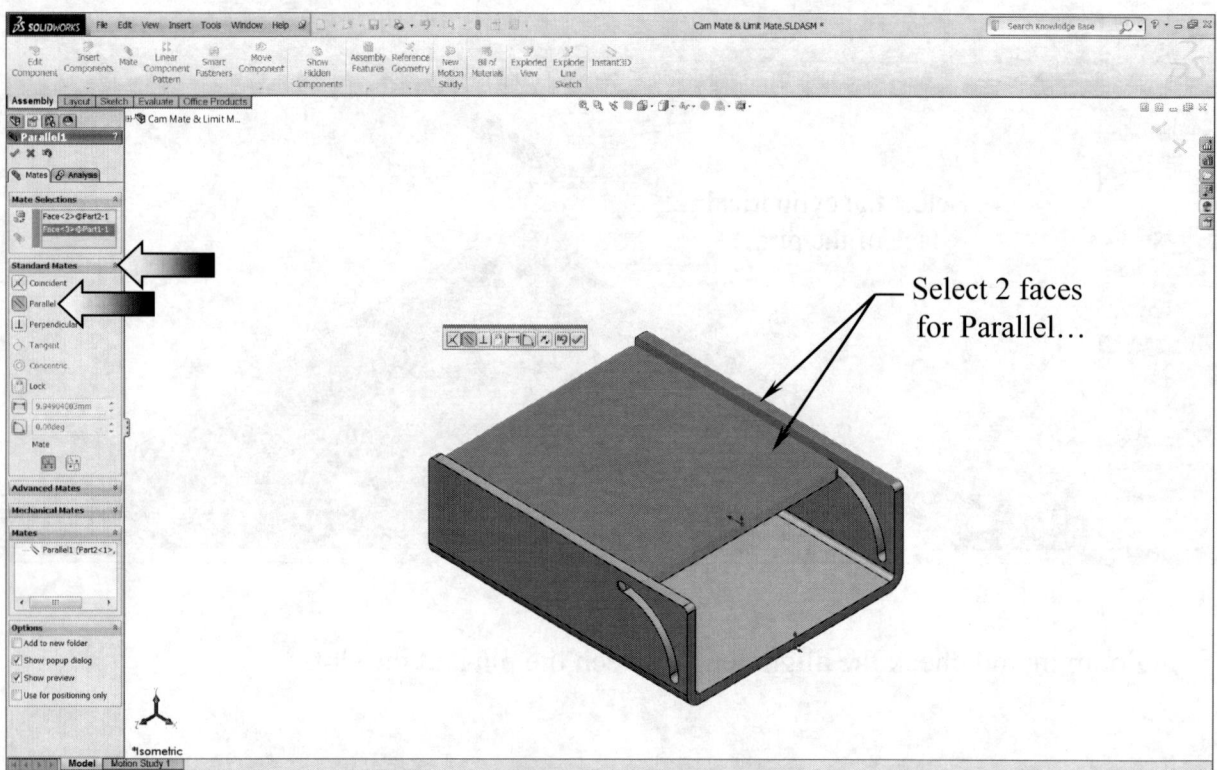

Select 2 faces
for Parallel...

- The Parallel mate is used to precisely rotate the Part2 to its vertical position. But we will need to suppress it so that other mates can be added without over defining the assembly.

- Expand the Mate group by clicking the plus sign (+) next to the Mates folder.

- Click the Parallel mate and select the **Suppress** button (arrow).

- Do not move the component, a Limit mate is going to be added next.

5. Adding a Limit mate:

- Click the **Advanced Mates** tab (arrow) and select the **Angle** option from the list.

- Select the **2 faces** of the 2 components as indicated.

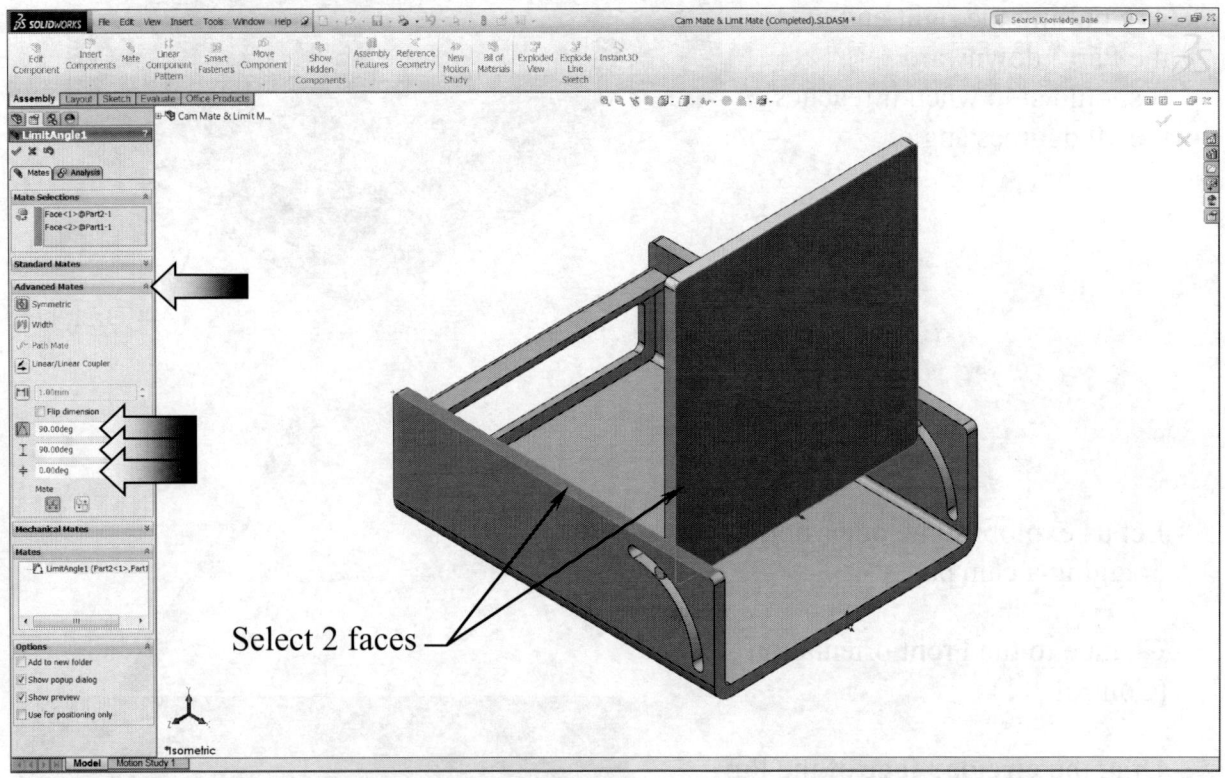

Select 2 faces

- Enter the following:

    90.00 deg for "starting" Angle.
    0.00 deg for **Maximum** value.
    0.00 deg for **Minimum** value.

- Click **OK**

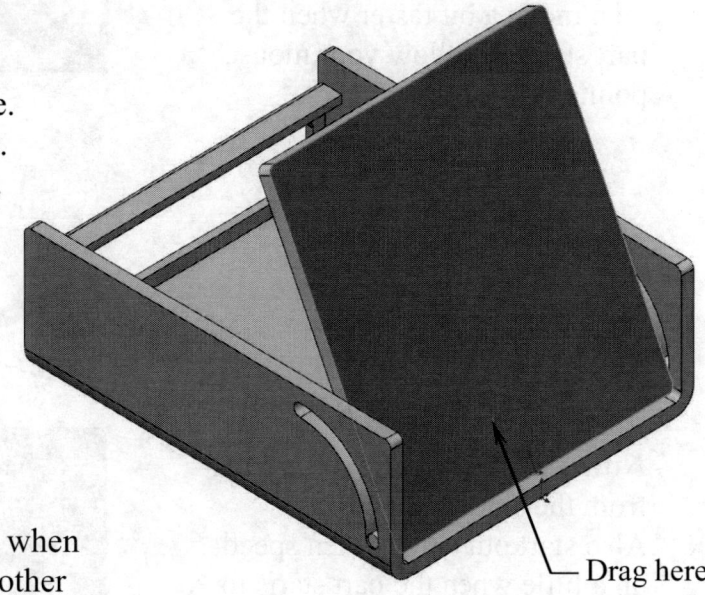

Drag here

- Test the mates by dragging the Part2 up and down.

- It may take a little getting used to when moving a cam part. (Changing to other orientations may make it easier).

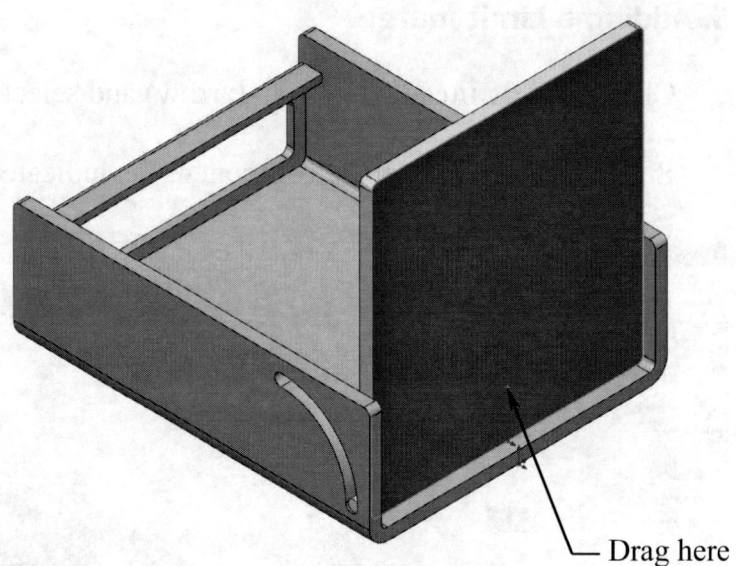

- Try pulling the right end of
  the Part2 downward.
  It should stop when it reaches
  the 90 degrees angle.

Drag here

- Let us explore some other options of
  dragging a cam part.

- Change to the Front orientation
  (Control + 1).

- Drag the **circular face** of the Pin
  upward. Start out slowly at first,
  then move a bit faster when the
  part starts to follow your mouse
  pointer.

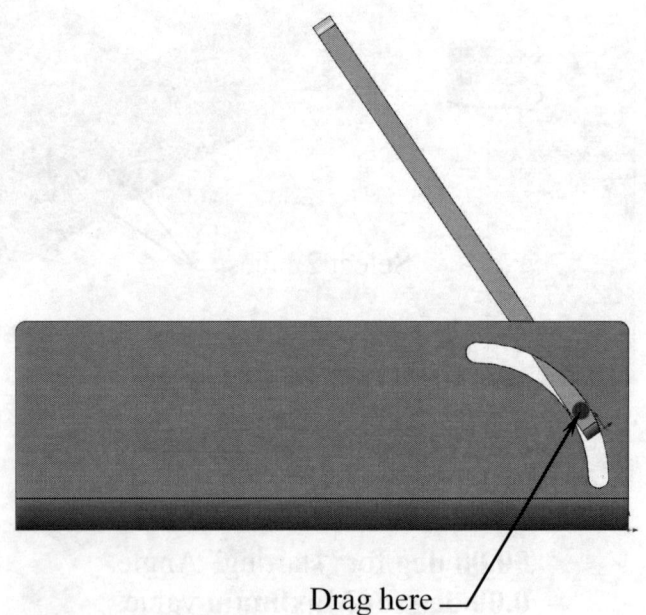

Drag here

Drag here

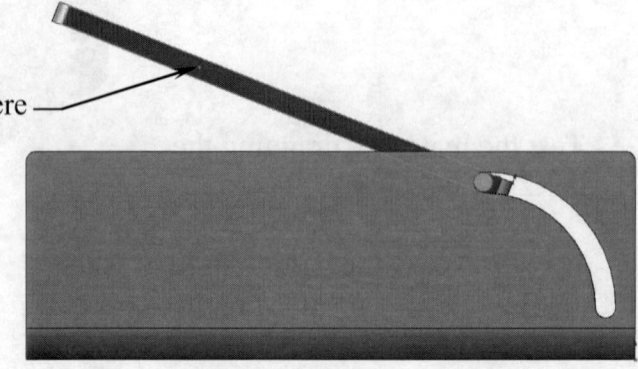

- Now try dragging the same part
  from the side as shown here.
  Also start out slowly then speed
  up a little when the part starts to
  catch on.

6. Saving your work:

- Click **File / Save As**.

- Enter **Limit & Cam Mates** for file name.

- Click **Save**.

- Overwrite the document if prompted.

(In the Training Files folder, locate the Built-Parts folder; open the pre-built assembly and check your work against it).

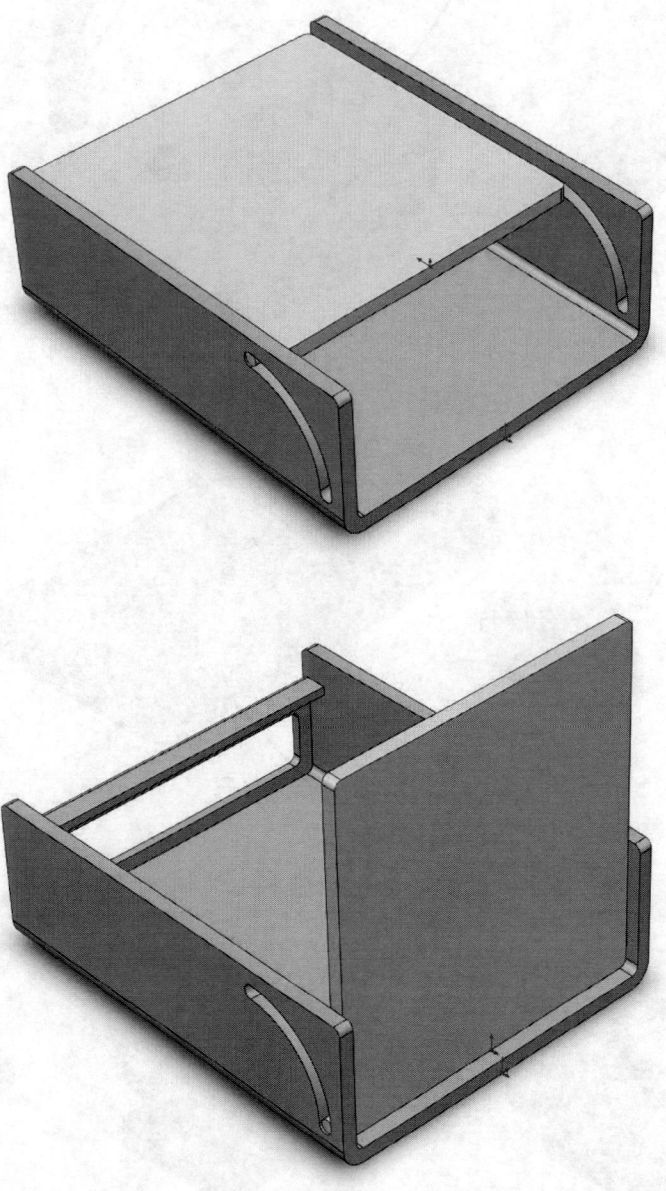

Exercise: Using Cam Followers*

1. Copying the Cam Followers Assembly folder:

- Go to: The Training Files folder.
- Copy the entire folder named **Cam Followers** to your desktop.

A Cam-Follower mate is a type of tangent or coincident mate. It allows you to mate a cylinder, a plane, or a point to a series of tangent extruded faces, such as you would find on a cam. You can make the profile of the cam from lines, arcs, and splines, as long as they are tangent and form a closed loop.

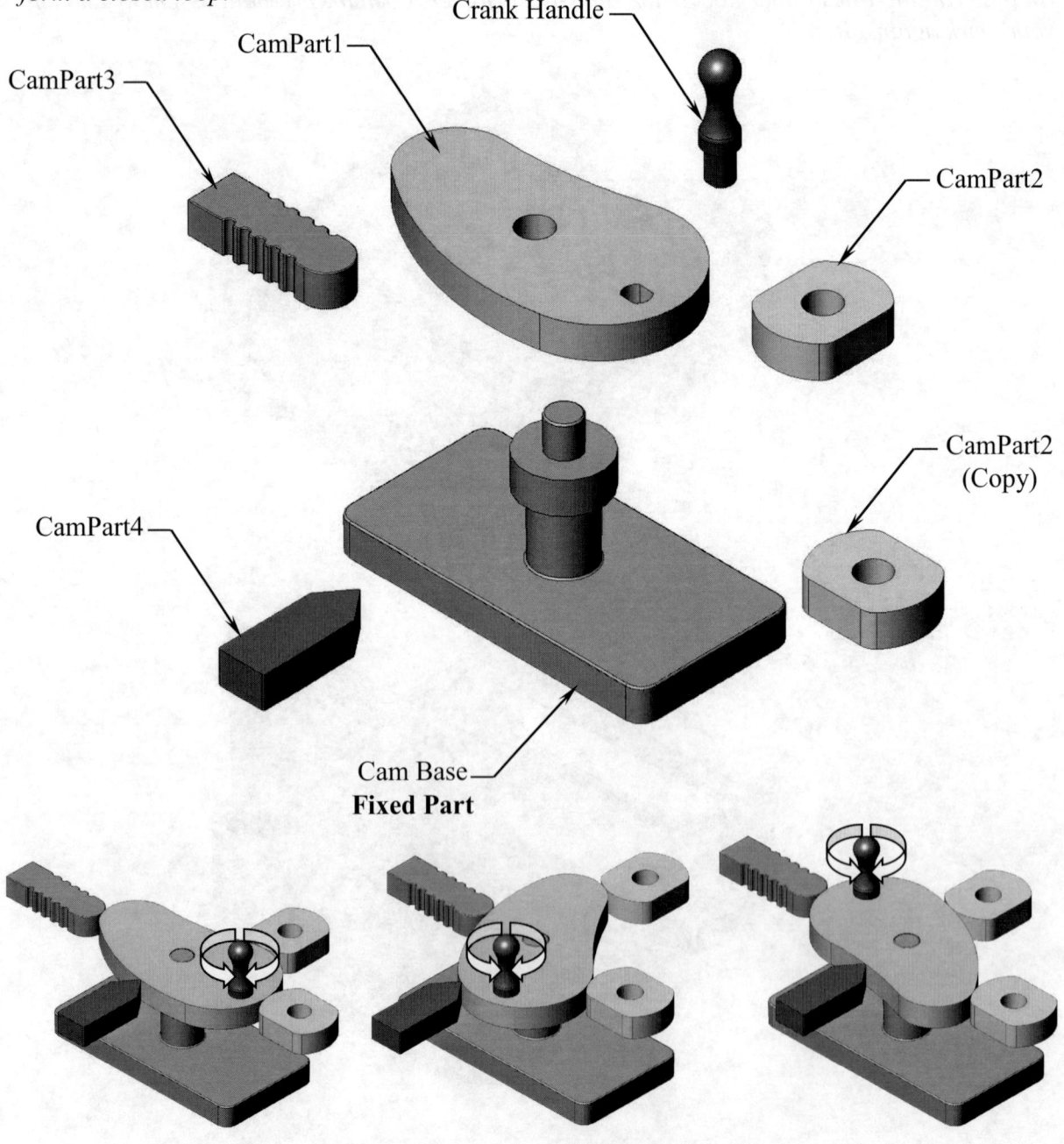

Crank Handle

CamPart1

CamPart3

CamPart2

CamPart2 (Copy)

CamPart4

Cam Base
Fixed Part

2. Assembling the components using the Standard Mates:

- Create a **Concentric** mate between the **shaft** and the **hole** as shown below.

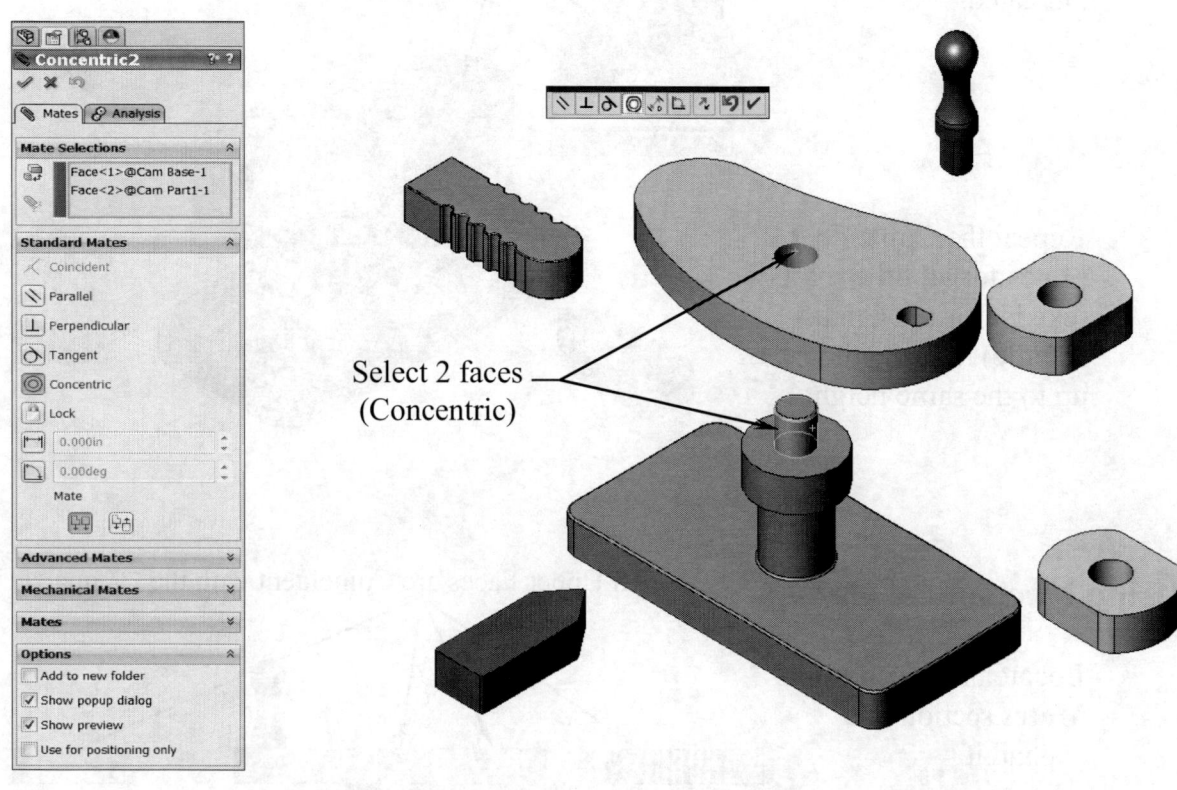

Select 2 faces
(Concentric)

- Create a **Coincident** mate between the **two faces** as shown below.

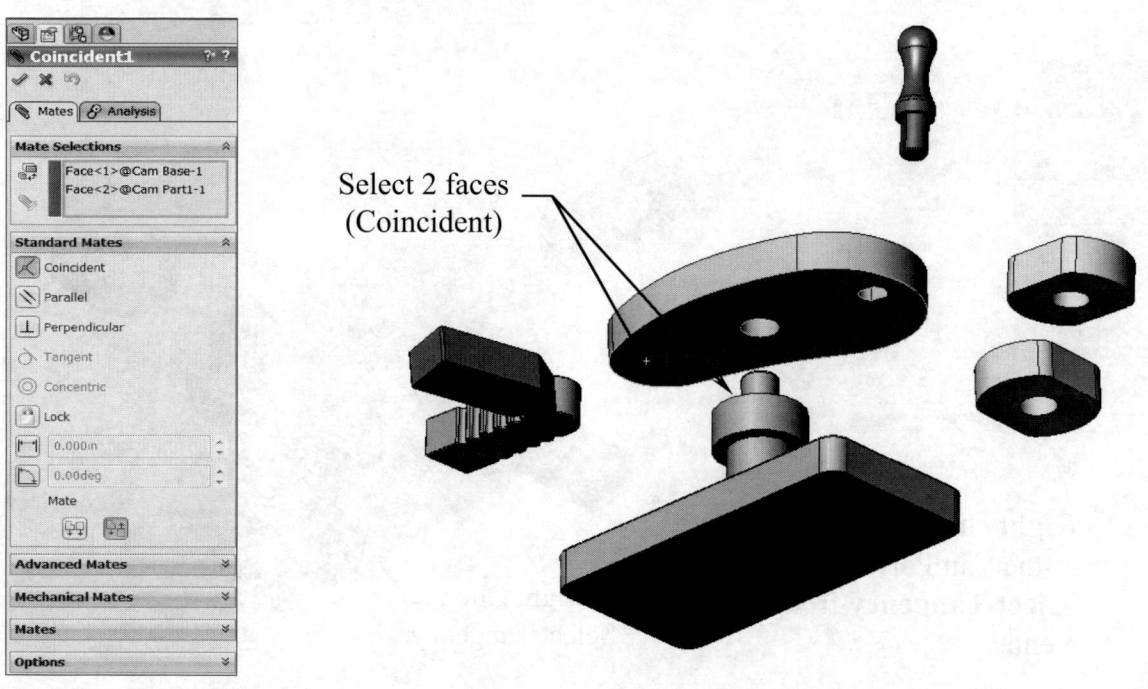

Select 2 faces
(Coincident)

- Create a **Coincident** Mate between the **2 upper surfaces** of the 2 components as indicated.

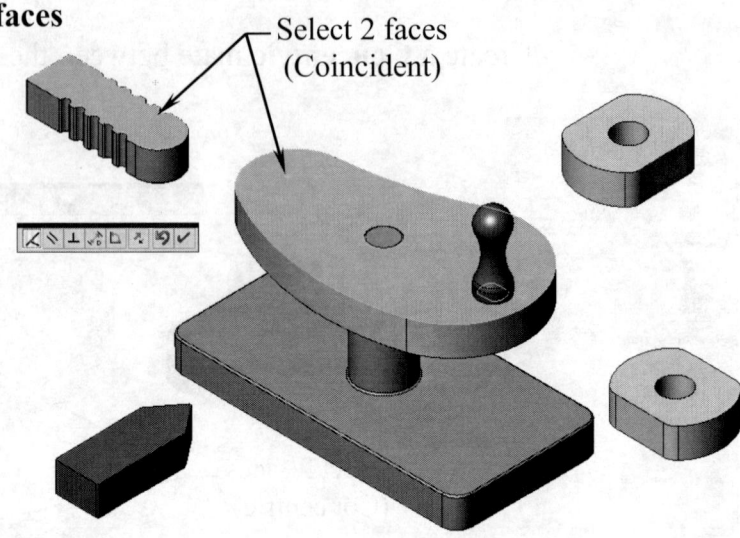

Select 2 faces
(Coincident)

- Repeat the Coincident Mates for all other parts (except for the Crank-Handle) to bring them up to the same height.

3. Using Mechanical Mates:

All Upper Faces are Coincident with the Campart1.

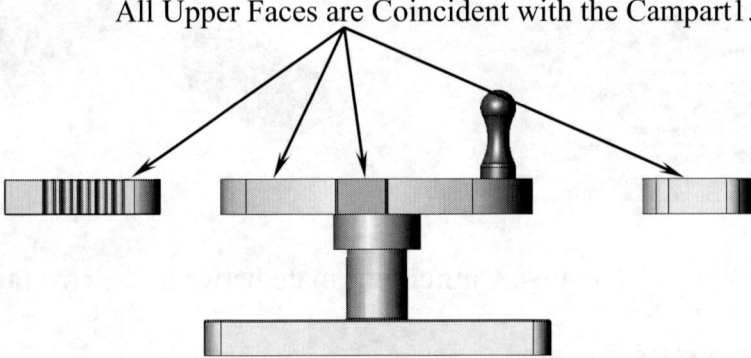

- Locate the **Mechanical Mates** section and expand it.

- Select the **Cam** option (arrow).

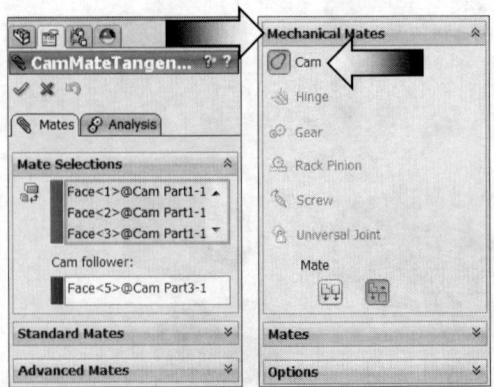

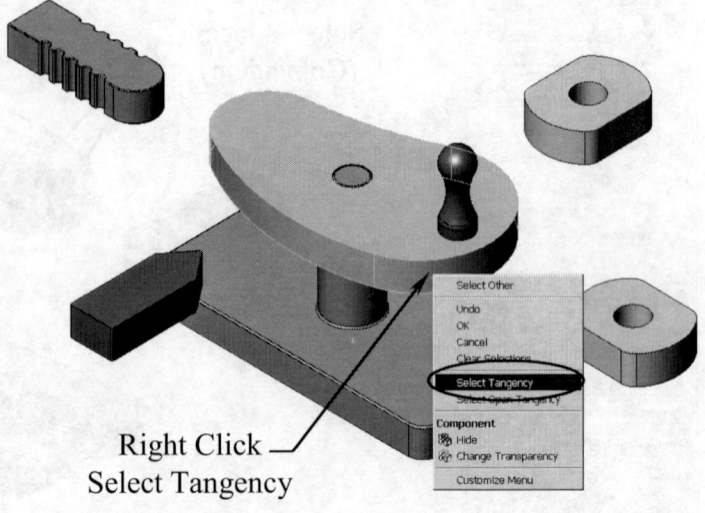

- **Right click** on the side of the CamPart1 and pick **Select-Tangency** from the menu.

Right Click
Select Tangency

- Click in the **Cam-Follower** section (circled) and select the **left face** of the part CamPart2,

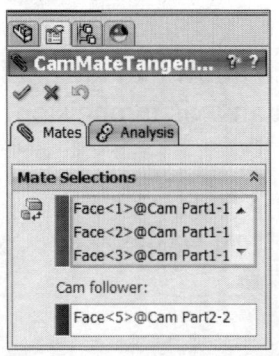

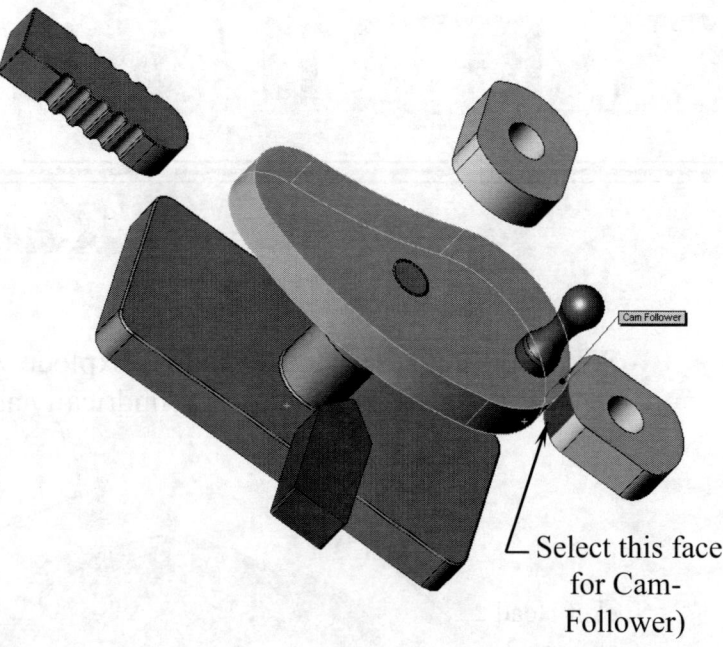

Select this face for Cam-Follower)

NOTES:

- In order for the components to "behave" properly when they're being rotated, their center-planes should also be constrained.

- Create a Coincident Mate between the FRONT plane of the CamPart1 and the FRONT plane of the CamPart3, then repeat the same step for the others.

4. Viewing the Cam Motions

Move the Crank Handle to test the Cam Motions

- Drag the Crank Handle clockwise or counter-clockwise to view the Cam-Motion of your assembly.

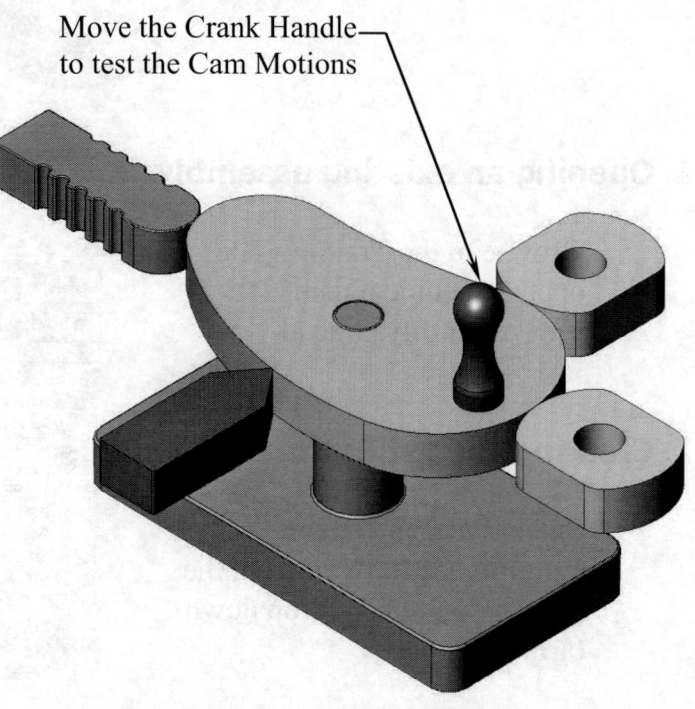

5. Saving your Work:

- Click **File / Save As**.

- Enter **Cam Follower** for the name of the file.

- Click **Save**.

CHAPTER 11 (cont.)

Radial Explode

- SolidWorks 2015 introduces Radial Explode which allows you to explode components aligned radially or cylindrically about an axis in one step.

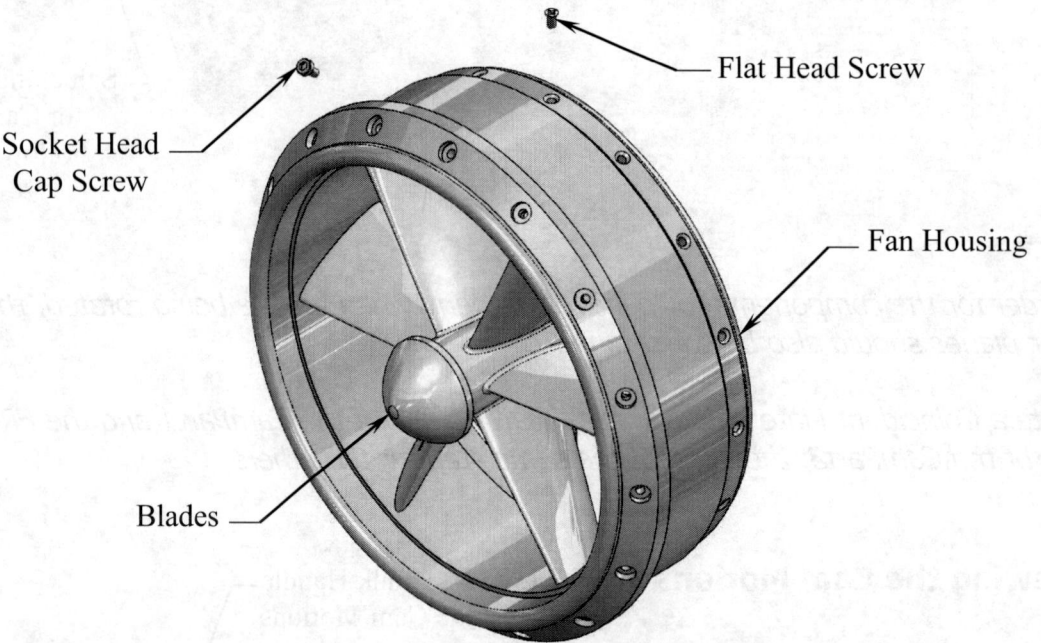

Flat Head Screw

Socket Head Cap Screw

Fan Housing

Blades

1. Opening an existing assembly:

- Browse to the Training Files and open a document named:
Fan Assembly.sldasm

2. Creating the 1st Pattern Driven:

- Select **Pattern Driven Component Pattern** from the Linear Component drop down (arrow).

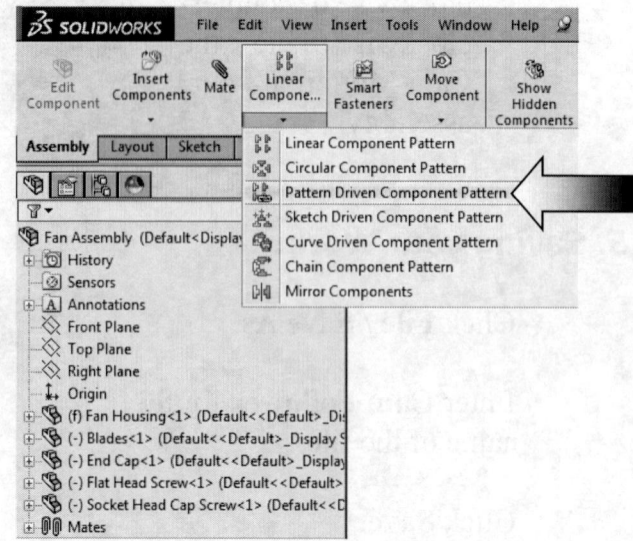

- Expand the FeatureManager tree and select the **Flat Head Screw** to use as the Component-To-Pattern.

- For Driving Feature or Component, select **one of the holes** in the existing pattern as noted.

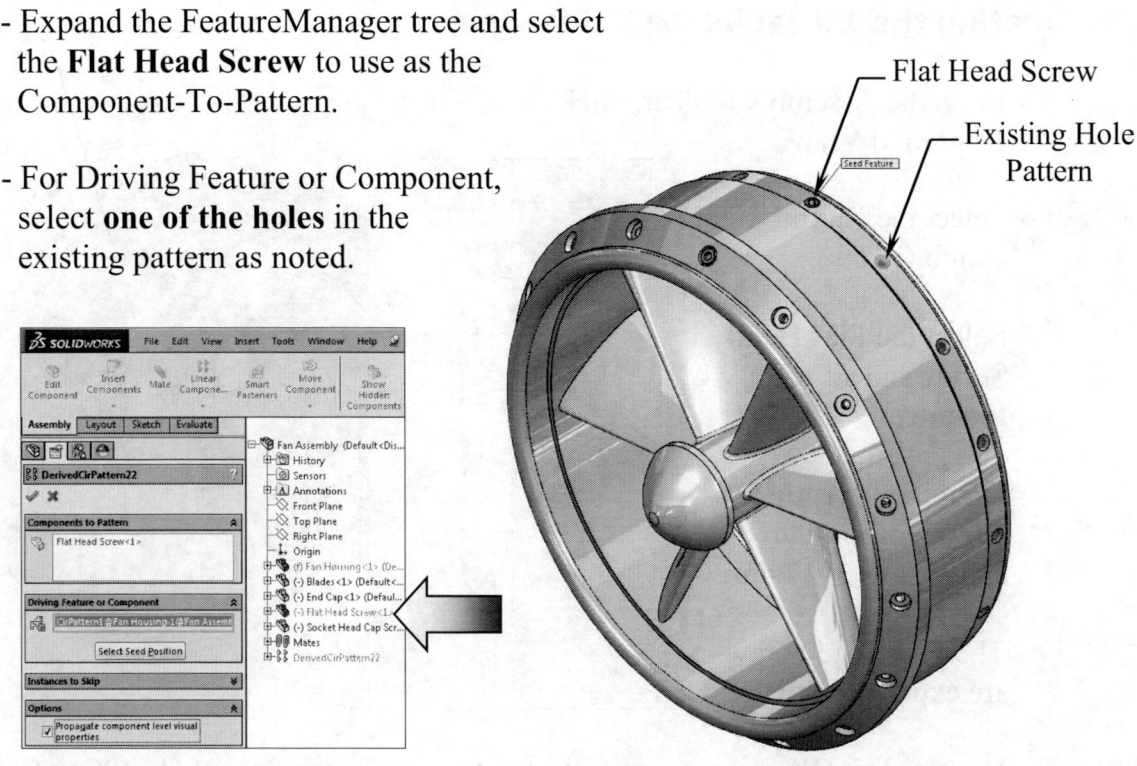

Flat Head Screw

Existing Hole Pattern

- Click **OK**.

3. Creating the 2nd Pattern Driven:

- Select the **Driven Component Pattern** option once again.

- Select the **Socket Head Cap Screw** for Component to Pattern.

- Select **one of the holes** in the existing pattern as indicated for Driving Feature.

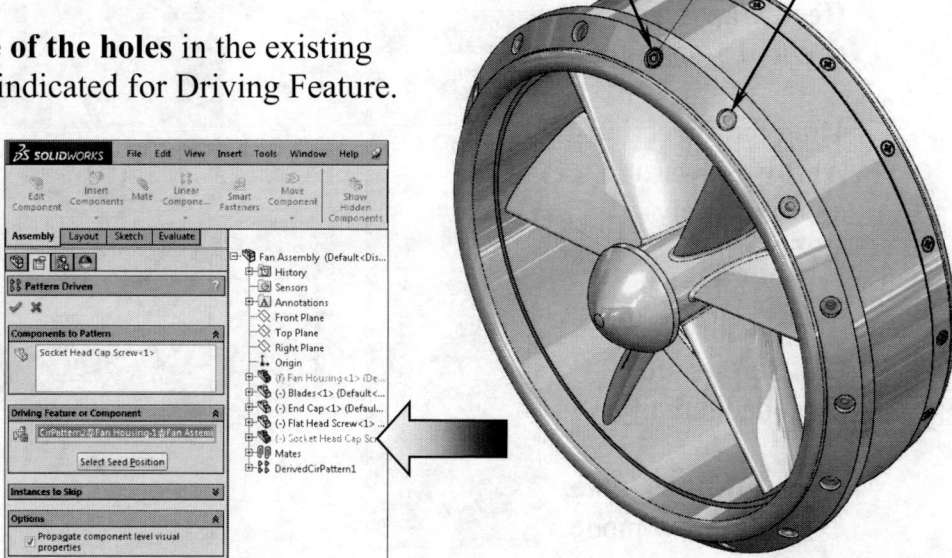

Socket Head Cap Screw

Existing Hole Pattern

- Click **OK**.

4. Creating the 1st radial exploded view:

- From the Assembly toolbar, click:
  Exploded View.

- Select the **Radial Step**
  option (arrow).

- Select the **Flat Head
  Screw** and all **15
  Instances**.

- Drag the **Direction-
  Arrow** outward to
  approximately **.700in**.

- The Flat Head Screws
  are exploded radially.

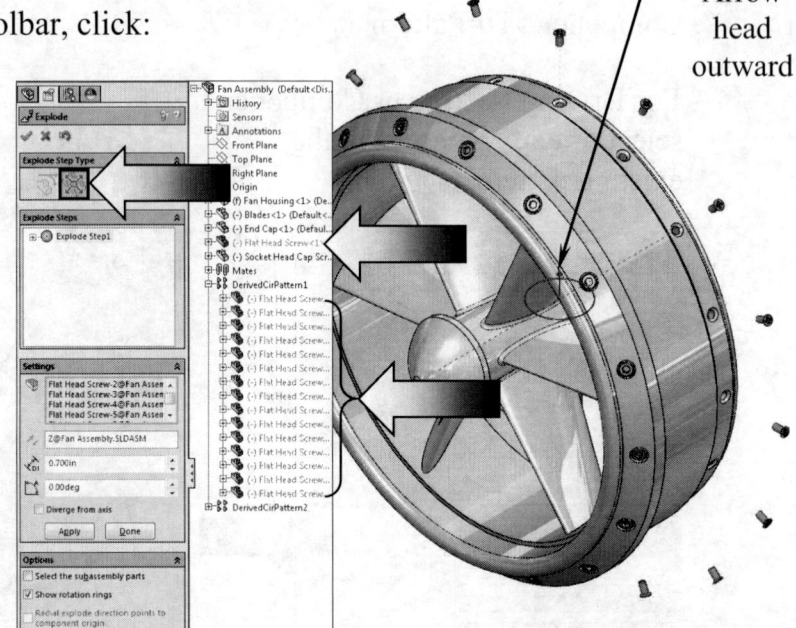

Drag the
Arrow
head
outward

- Do not click OK just yet, we will need to explode the Socket Head Cap Screws
  as the next explode step.

5. Creating the 2nd radial exploded view:

- The Radial Step option should
  be selected already.

- Select the **Socket
  Head Cap Screw**
  and its **15 Instances**.

- Drag the **Direction-
  Arrow** outward to
  approximately
  1.250in.

- The Socket Head
  Cap Screws are
  exploded radially.

- Click **OK** to exit the
  exploded view mode.

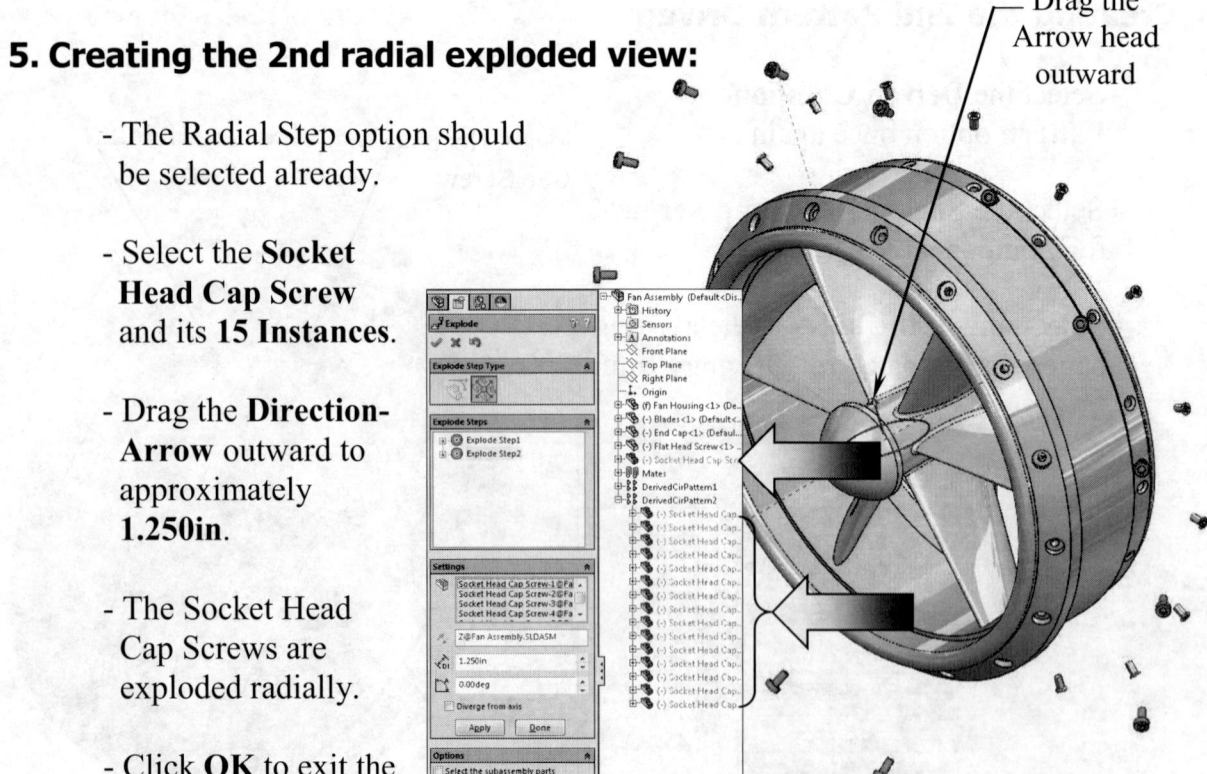

Drag the
Arrow head
outward

6. Verifying the exploded view:

- Change to the **Front** orientation (Control + 1).

- Your exploded view should look similar to the image shown on the right.

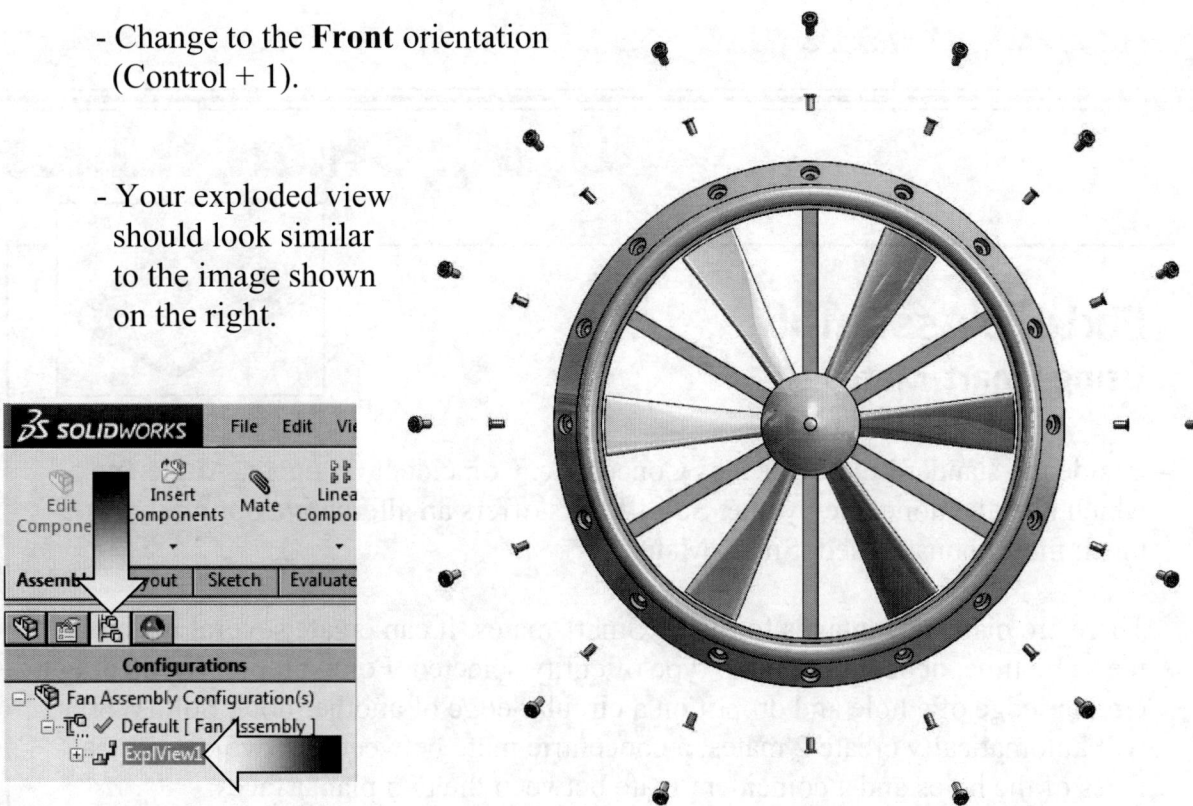

- Switch to the **Configuration Manager** tree (arrow) and expand the **Default** configuration to see or to edit the Exploded View (arrow).

- Double click on the **ExplView1** to Collapse or to Explode the assembly.

7. Saving your work:

- Click **File / Save As**.

- Enter **Radial Explode** for the name of the document.

- Select the option: **Save As Copy and Continue**, and click **Save**.

CHAPTER 11 (cont.)

Using Smart-Mates

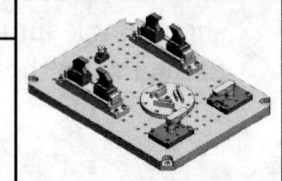

Fixture Assembly
Using Smart-Mates

- Beside the standard mates such as Concentric, Coincident, Tangent, Angle, etc., which must be done one by one, SolidWorks offers an alternative option that is much more robust called: Smart-Mates.

- There are many advantages for using Smart-mates. It can create several mates at the same time, depending on the type of entity selected. For example: If you drag a circular edge of a hole and drop it on a circular edge of another hole, SolidWorks will automatically create 2 mates, a concentric mate between the two cylindrical faces of the holes and a coincident mate between the two planar faces.

- Using Smart-mates, you do not have to select the Mate command every time. Simply hold the ALT key and drag an entity of a component to its destination, a smart-mate symbol will appear to confirm the types of mates it is going to add. At the same time, a mate toolbar will also pop up offering some additional options such as Flip Mate Alignment, change to a different mate type, or simply undo the selection.

- Using the Alt + Drag option, the Tab key is used to flip the mate alignments, this is done by releasing the Alt key and pressing the Tab key, while the mouse button is still pressed. This option works well even if your assembly is set to lightweight.

- In addition to the Alt + Drag, if you hold the Control key and Drag a component, SolidWorks will create an instance of the selected component and apply the smart-mates to it at the same time. Using this option you will have to click the Flip Mate Alignment button on the pop-up toolbar to reverse the direction of the mate, the Tab key does not work.

- This lesson will guide you through the use of the Smart-mate options, and for some of the steps, use the standards mate options as well.

Fixture Assembly
Using Smart-Mates

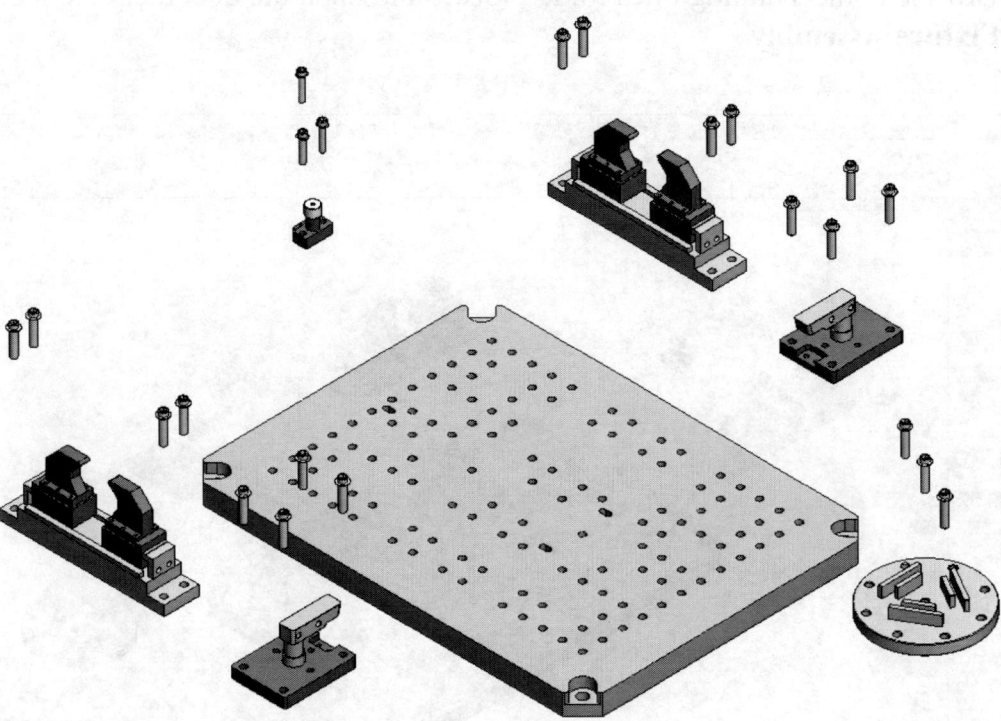

View Orientation Hot Keys:

Ctrl + 1 = Front View
Ctrl + 2 = Back View
Ctrl + 3 = Left View
Ctrl + 4 = Right View
Ctrl + 5 = Top View
Ctrl + 6 = Bottom View
Ctrl + 7 = Isometric View
Ctrl + 8 = Normal To Selection

Dimensioning Standards: **ANSI**

Units: **INCHES** – 3 Decimals

Tools Needed:

 Concentric &
Coincident

 Concentric two
cylindrical faces

 Coincident
two edges

 Coincident
two planar faces

 Coincident
two vertices

 Coincident
two origins

1. Opening an existing assembly document:

- Select **File / Open**.

- Browse to the Training Files folder, locate and open the document named:
  Fixture Assembly.

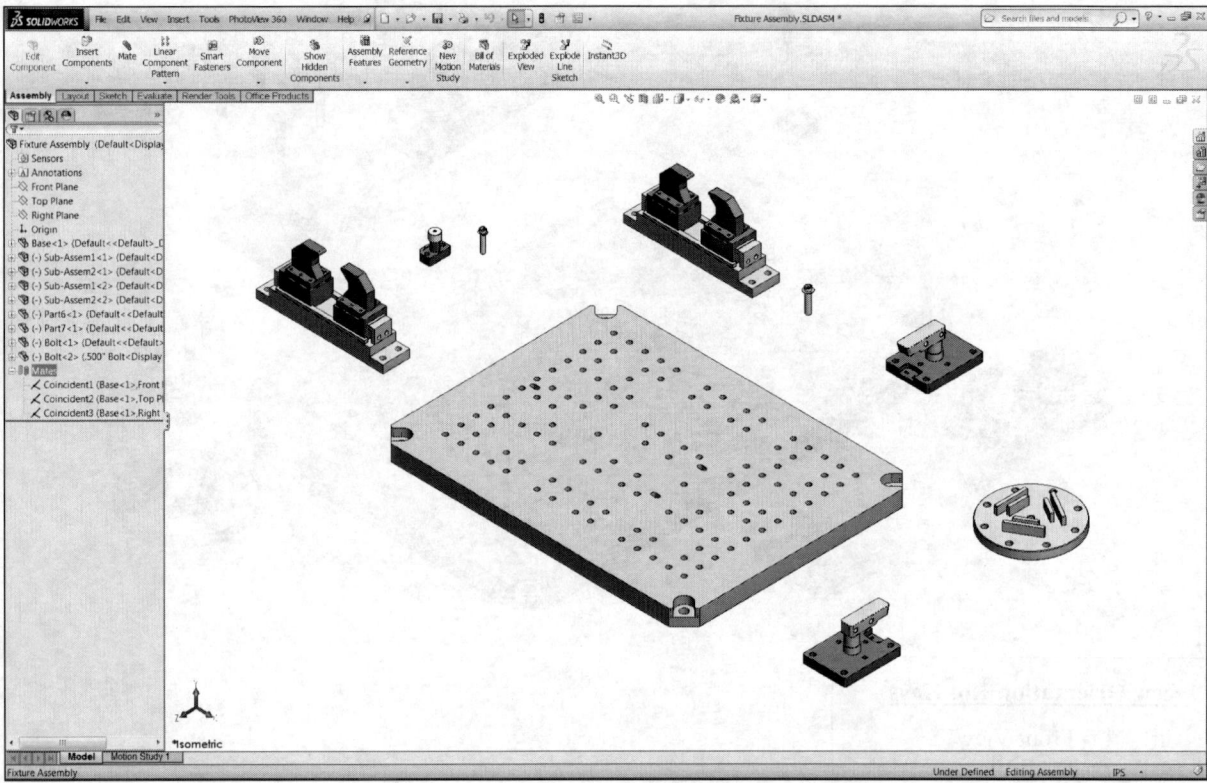

2. Enabling the Selection options:

- Go to **Tools / Options / Display / Selection** and enable the two checkboxes:
  * Allow Selection in Wireframe...
  * Allow selection in HLR and...

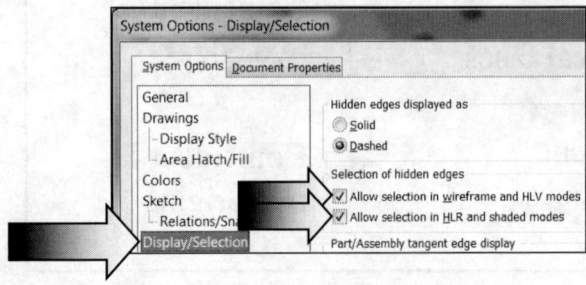

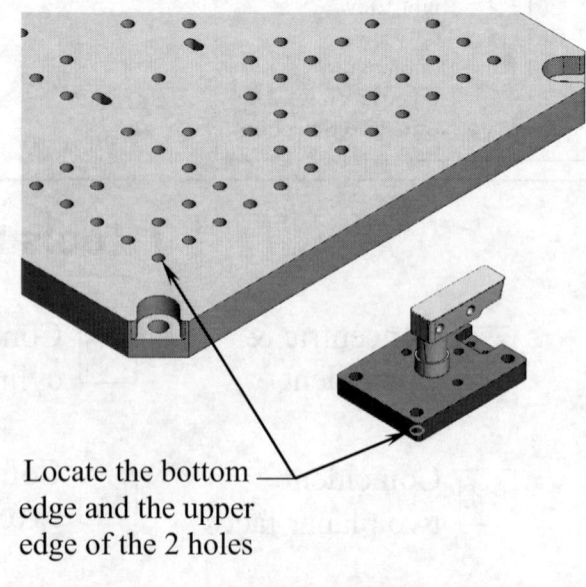

Locate the bottom edge and the upper edge of the 2 holes

3. Exploring the Smart-Mate options:

- Some types of Smart-Mates can be created in an assembly by dragging and dropping one entity to another.

- Depending on the entity that you drag. You will get different mate result. Use either a linear or circular edge of the model, a planar or cylindrical face, or a vertex to drag with Smart-Mates.

	Concentric & Coincident 2 circular edges
	Concentric 2 cylindrical faces
	Coincident 2 linear edges
	Coincident 2 planar faces
	Coincident 2 vertices
	Coincident 2 origins or coordinate systems

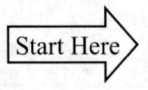 Start Here - <u>Hold</u> the **ALT** key, drag the <u>hidden edge</u> of the hole to the <u>upper edge</u> of the mating hole but <u>do not</u> release the mouse. Hover the cursor over the edge of the hole until the Smart-Mate symbol appears, then release the mouse button.

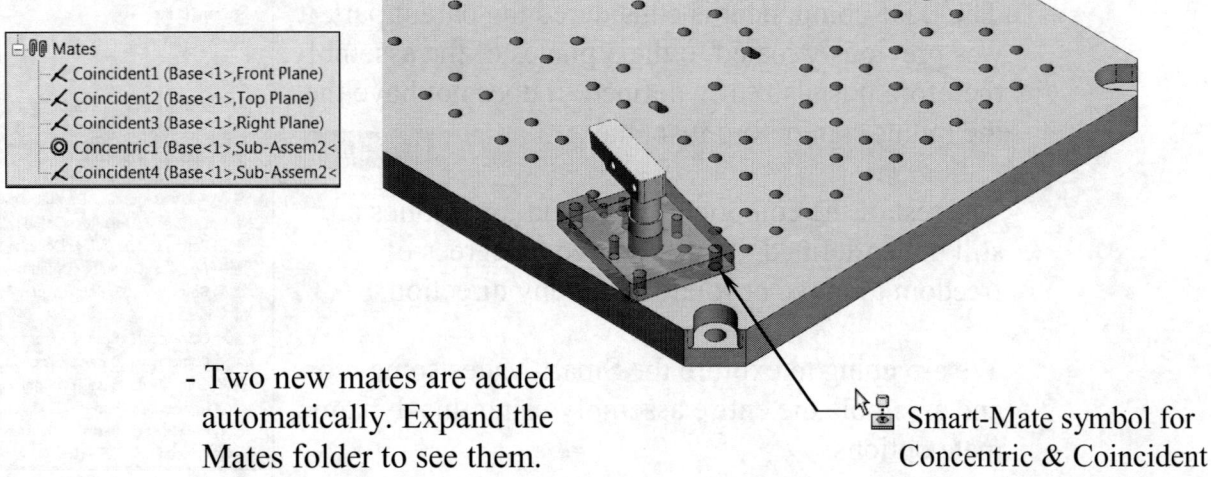

Mates
- Coincident1 (Base<1>,Front Plane)
- Coincident2 (Base<1>,Top Plane)
- Coincident3 (Base<1>,Right Plane)
- Concentric1 (Base<1>,Sub-Assem2<
- Coincident4 (Base<1>,Sub-Assem2<

- Two new mates are added automatically. Expand the Mates folder to see them.

Smart-Mate symbol for Concentric & Coincident

4. Using Smart-Mate Concentric:

- The concentric mate is created when two cylindrical surfaces are dragged and dropped onto one another.

- <u>Hold</u> the **ALT** key, drag the <u>cylindrical face</u> of the 1st hole and drop on the <u>cylindrical face</u> of the 2nd hole. The mouse cursor must be stopped on an entity and must not be moving, in order for the Smart-Mate symbol to appear.

- Release the mouse cursor when the concentric symbol pops up, click the **OK** on the pop-up toolbar to accept the concentric mate.

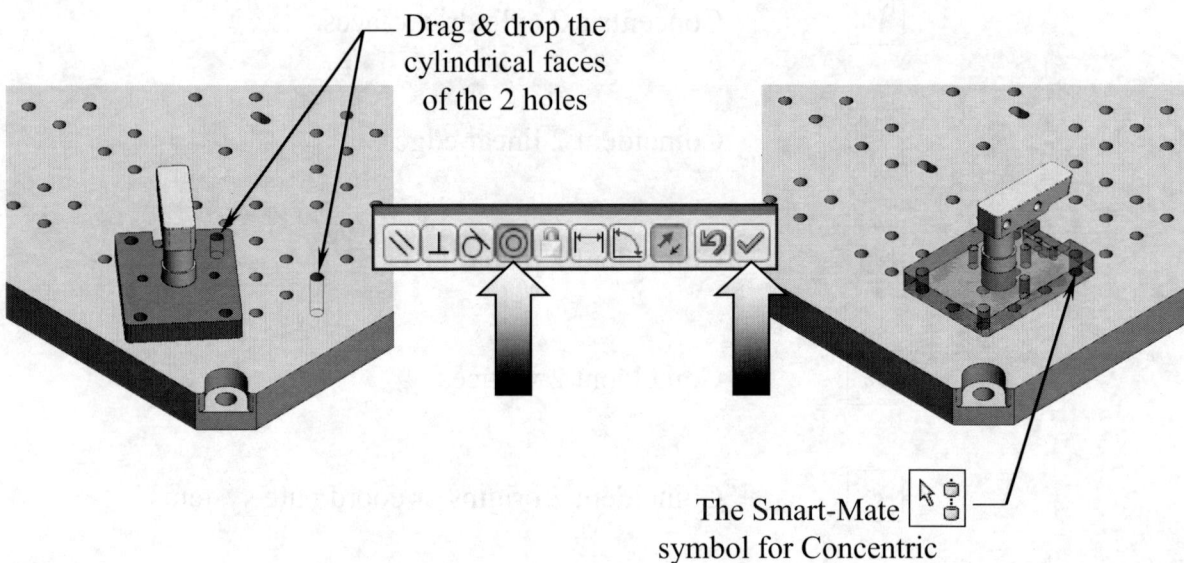

Drag & drop the cylindrical faces of the 2 holes

The Smart-Mate symbol for Concentric

- The sub assembly becomes fully defined. There is no minus sign (-) before the name Sub-Assem2.

- The Base component is considered the parent part, it was previously mated to the 3 planes of the assembly, therefore it is also fully defined. It does not have the the minus sign before its name.

- The rest of the components and sub-assemblies are still under defined, they still have 6 degrees of freedom to move or rotate about any direction.

- We are going to explore the Smart-Mates some more and assemble the entire assembly using this dynamic mate options.

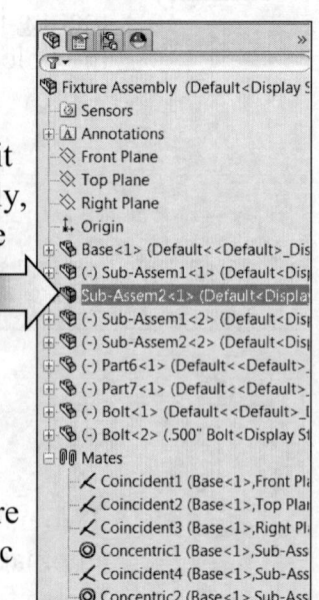

5. Creating a Smart-Mate Concentric & Coincident:

- Zoom in closer between the two components that will get mated next.

- <u>Hold</u> the **ALT** key, drag and drop the <u>hidden edge</u> of the hole1 onto the <u>upper edge</u> of the hole2 as noted.

- Keep the mouse cursor steady until the Smart mates symbol appears, and then release the mouse button.

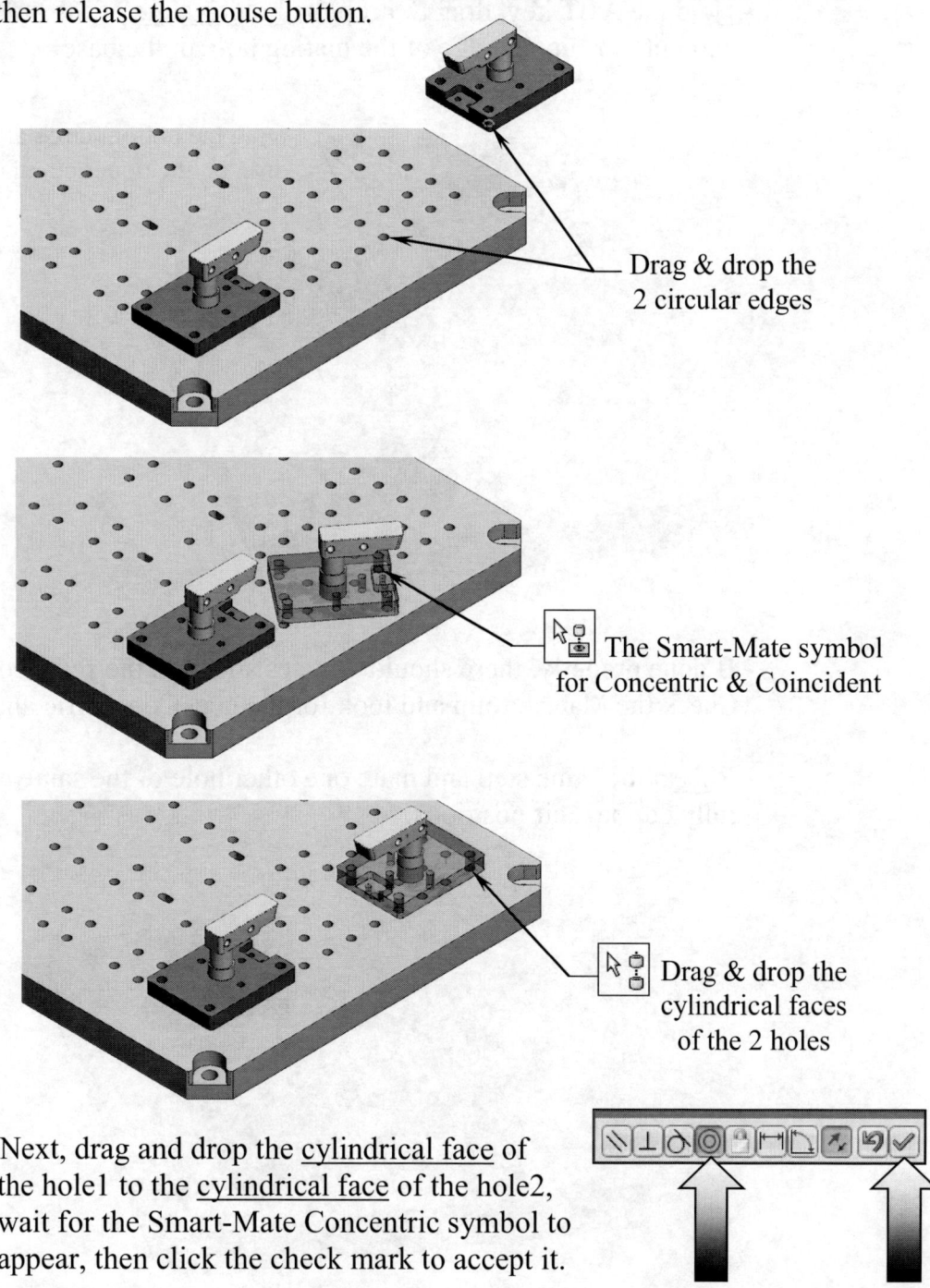

Drag & drop the 2 circular edges

The Smart-Mate symbol for Concentric & Coincident

Drag & drop the cylindrical faces of the 2 holes

- Next, drag and drop the <u>cylindrical face</u> of the hole1 to the <u>cylindrical face</u> of the hole2, wait for the Smart-Mate Concentric symbol to appear, then click the check mark to accept it.

6. Repeating the previous Mate:

- Move the cylindrical part above the base as shown.

- We are going to use the same mate techniques to assemble this part.

- The Explode Lines are added for clarity only, you do not have to add them.

- Hold the **ALT** key, drag & drop the hidden edge of the hole in the cylindrical part onto the upper edge of the mating hole in the base.

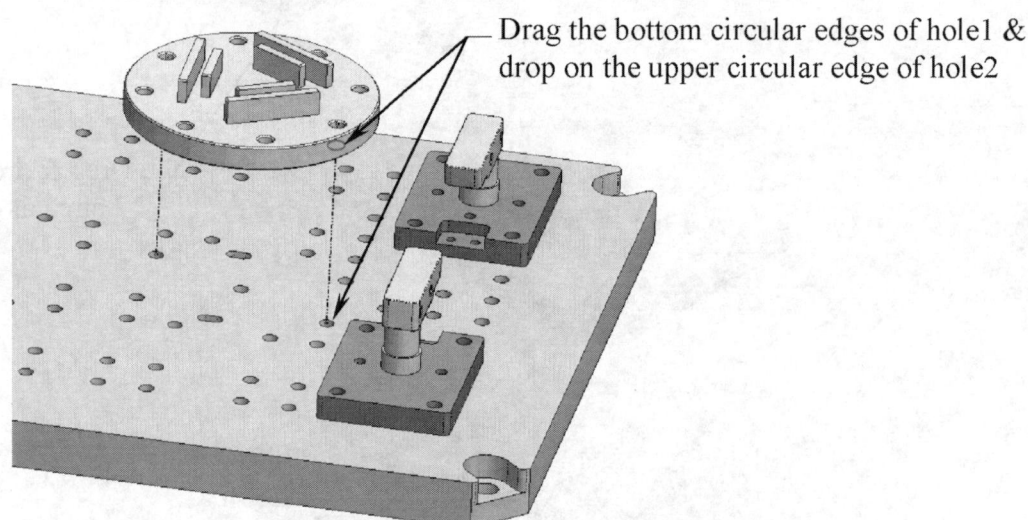

Drag the bottom circular edges of hole1 & drop on the upper circular edge of hole2

- If done properly, there should 2 mates added to the selected entities already. Check the Mates group and look for the new Concentric and Coincident mates.

- Repeat the same step and mate one other hole of the same components, to fully define their positions.

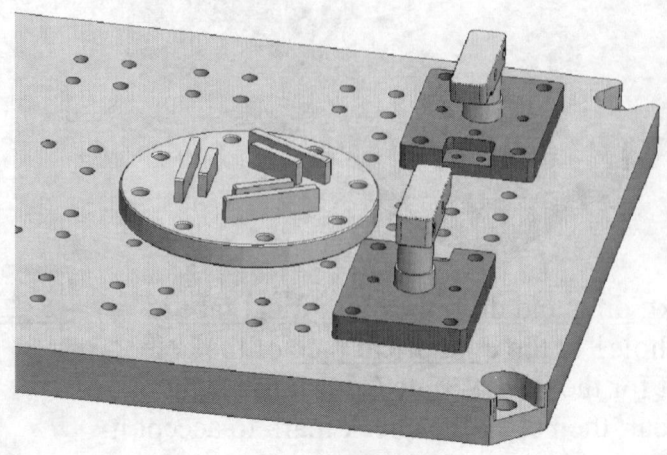

7. Mating other components:

- Since the holes in the components were patterned and have the exact same diameters, two mates per component would be enough to fully define them.

- The Explode Lines are added for clarity again, you do not need to add them.

- Use the same techniques and add the Smart-Mates to the other components, use the explode lines for reference locations, and only create two mates for each component.

- Do not mate the bolts just yet, we are going to take a look at the configurations that come with the bolts, and switch them to different sizes and use in them different locations.

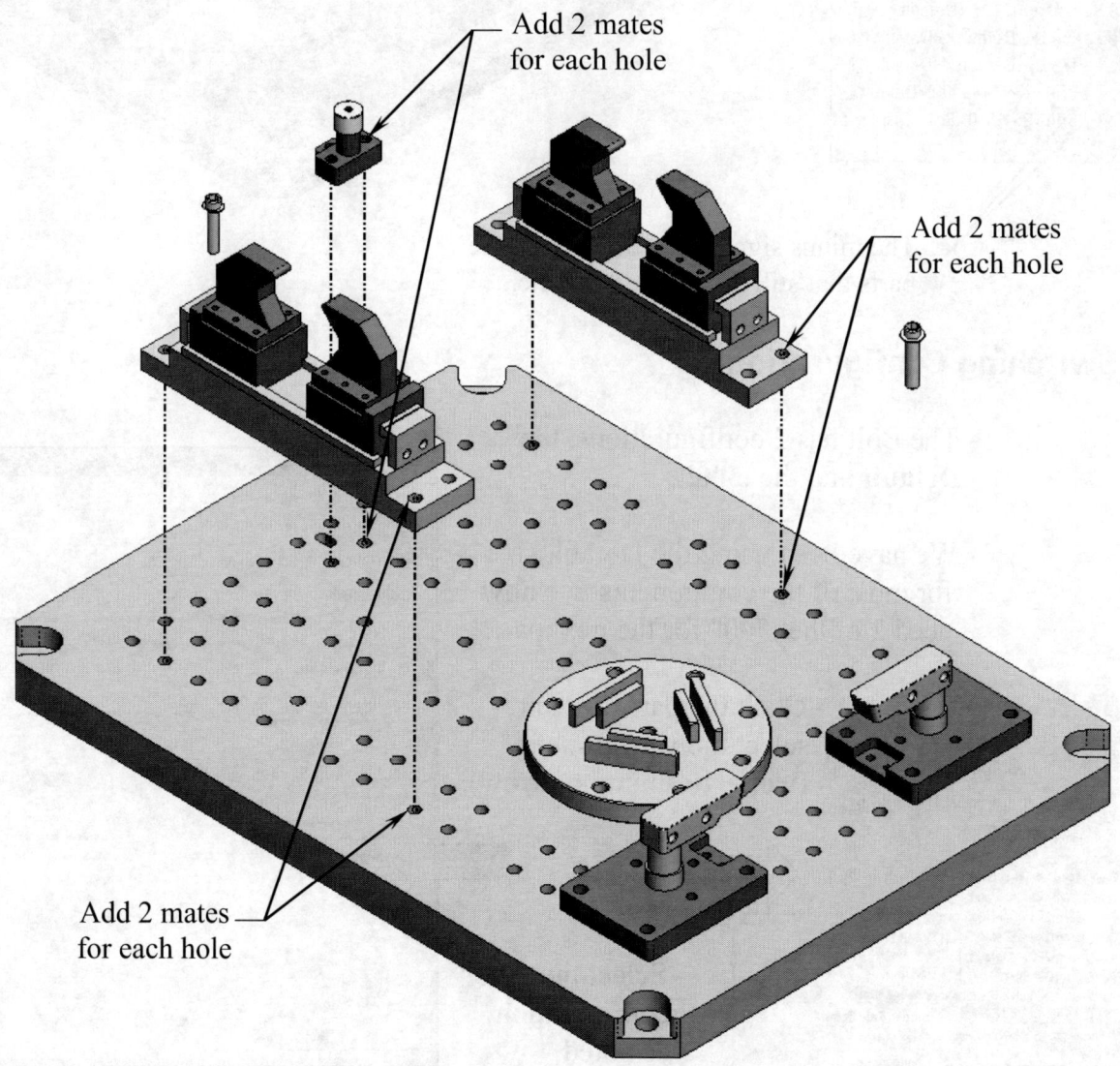

Add 2 mates for each hole

Add 2 mates for each hole

Add 2 mates for each hole

8. Checking the status of the components:

- After adding two mates to each component, the FeatureManager updates and shows only the minus signs (-) before the bolts.

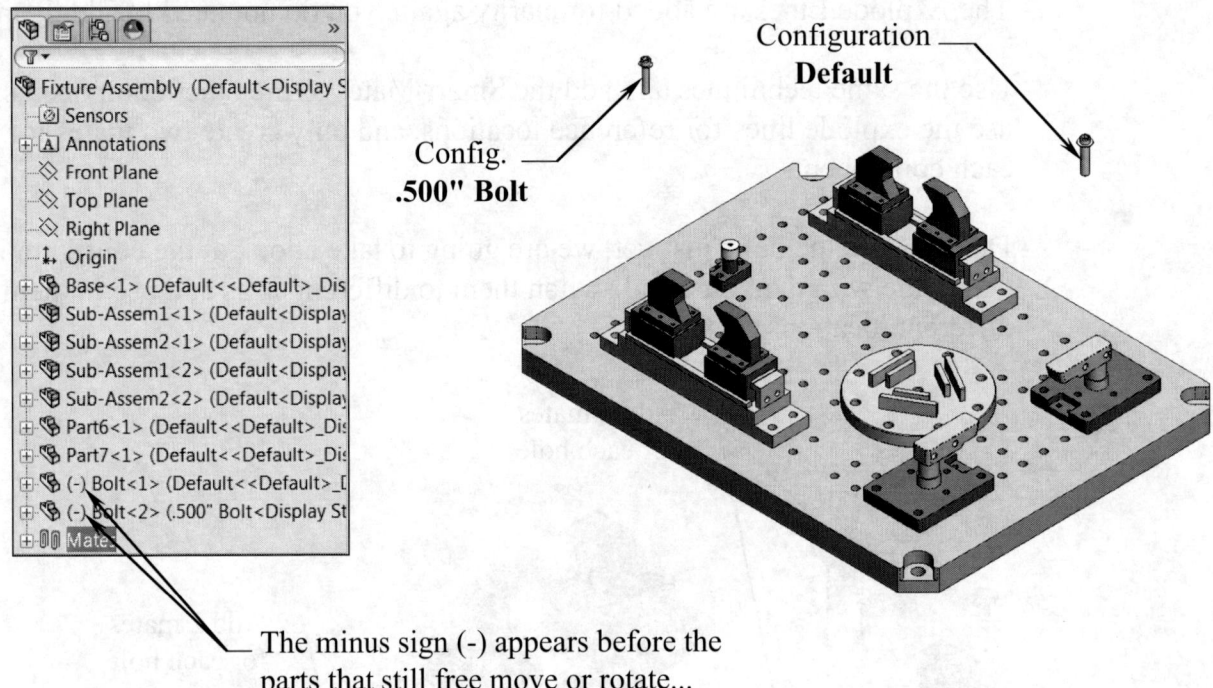

Configuration
Default

Config.
.500" Bolt

The minus sign (-) appears before the parts that still free move or rotate...

9. Switching Configuration:

- The Bolt has 2 configurations, the **Default** and the **.500"**.

- We have been using the Default size for most of the components, we now need 2 of the .500" for the next part.

- Click the part Bolt and select the **Component-Properties** button (arrow).

- Select the **.500"** configuration as noted.

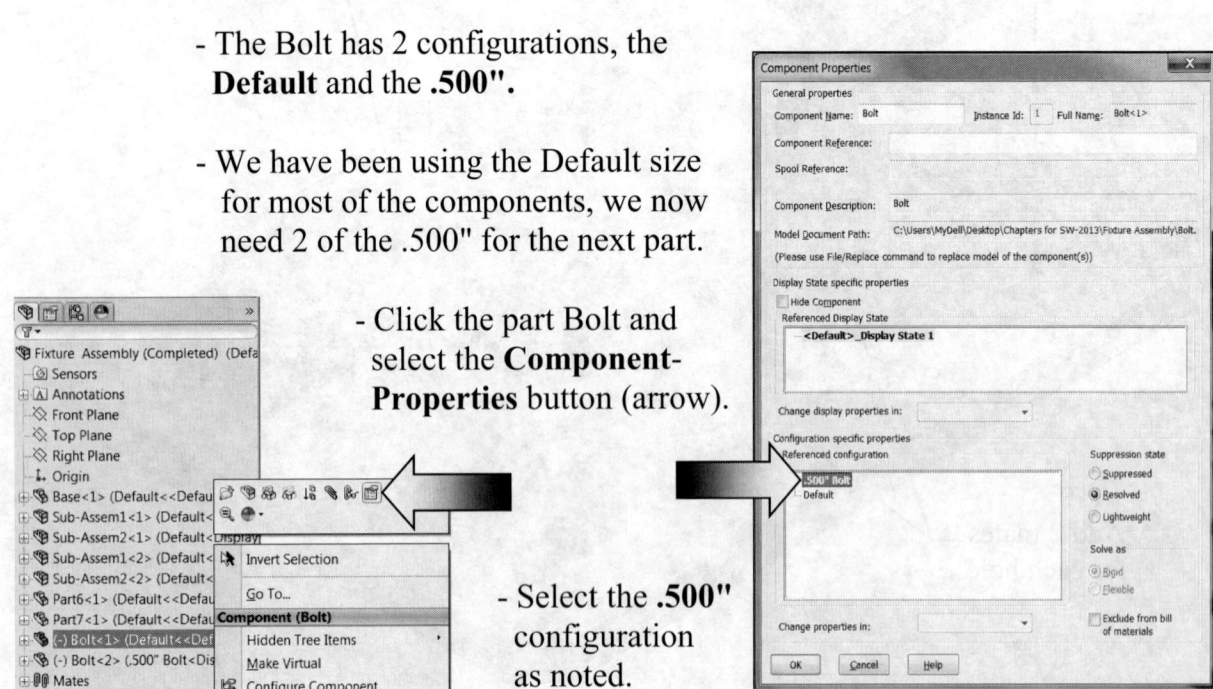

10. Creating an instance of the .500" bolt:

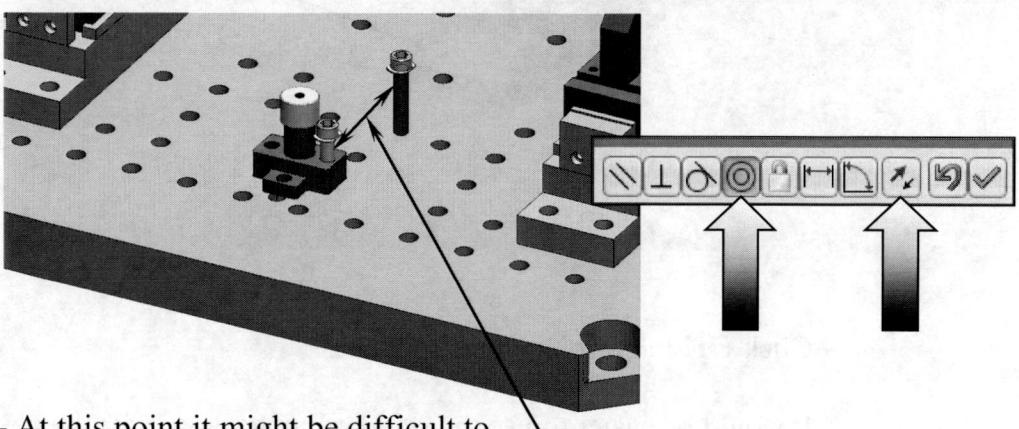

An instance of the bolt is mated to the hole

- When holding the Alt key and dragging a component the smart-mate is activated for mating the 2 components.

- But if you hold the Control key and drag a component, SolidWorks makes a copy of the component and smart-mates it to the other component at the same time.

- <u>Hold</u> the **Control** key, drag and drop (the shaft body) <u>an instance</u> of the bolt to the mating hole as pictured below. Release the mouse button when the smart-mate symbol appears. Click the Flip Alignment button if needed (arrow).

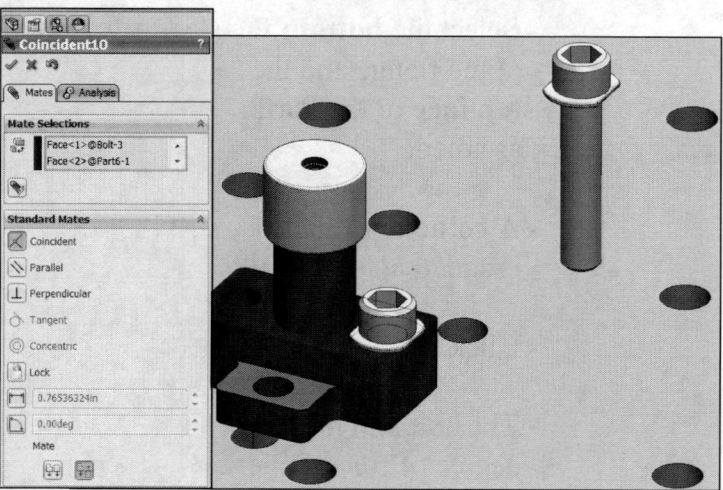

Hold the Control key drag & drop a copy of the bolt to the hole

- At this point it might be difficult to see the 2 faces to apply the next mate. Let's use the standard mates instead.

- Click the **Mate** command from the Assembly toolbar.

- Select the **bottom face** of the flange and the **top face** of the Part6.

- A coincident mate is added. Click **OK** to exit the mate.

11. Creating another instance of the bolt:

- Move the Default-Bolt closer to the Sub-Assembly1 on the right as noted.

- Hold the **Control** key, drag and drop an instance of the (default) bolt to the mating hole as noted. Look for the smart-mate symbol before releasing the mouse button.

- Click the Flip Mate Alignment button if needed (arrow).

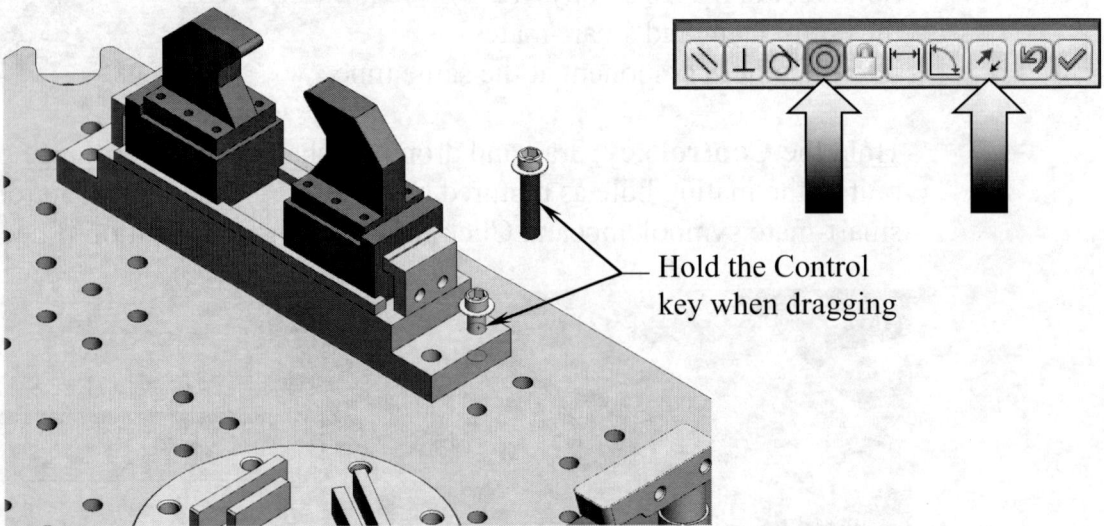

— Hold the Control key when dragging

- Click **OK** to close the mate toolbar.

- It would be easier to use the standard mates again for the next mate.

- Click the **Mate** command [icon] from the assembly toolbar.

- Select the **bottom face** of the flange and the **top face** of the Part2 as noted.

- A **coincident** mate is added automatically.

- Click **OK**.

- The bolt still has one degree of freedom left.

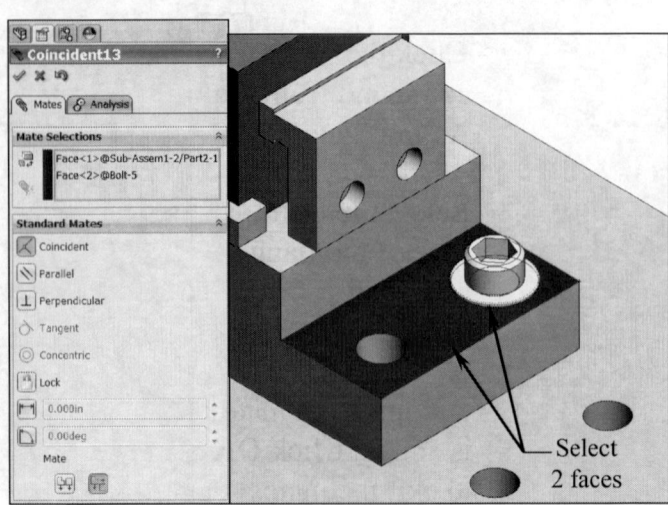

Select 2 faces

12. Adding more bolts:

- Rotate around to the other side of the sub-assembly1.

- Hold the CONTROL key and drag the default-bolt to make a copy and place it on the right of the Part2.

- Hold the Control key again, drag the copy of the default bolt to the mating hole as indicated. Look for the smart-mate symbol before releasing the mouse button. Click the Flip Mate Alignment if needed (arrow).

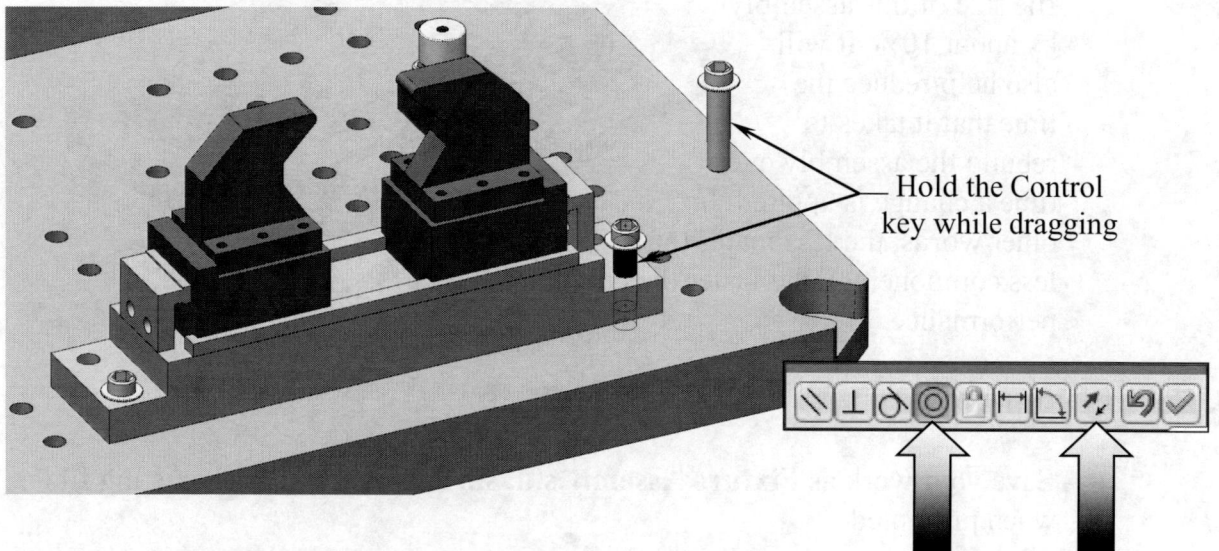

Hold the Control key while dragging

- Once again, it would be easier to use the standard mates for the next step, since we cannot really see the 2 two mating faces very well.

- Click **Mate** 📎 .

- Select the **bottom face** of the flange and the **top face** of the Part2.

- Another **coincident** mate is added.

- Click **OK** to exit the mate mode.

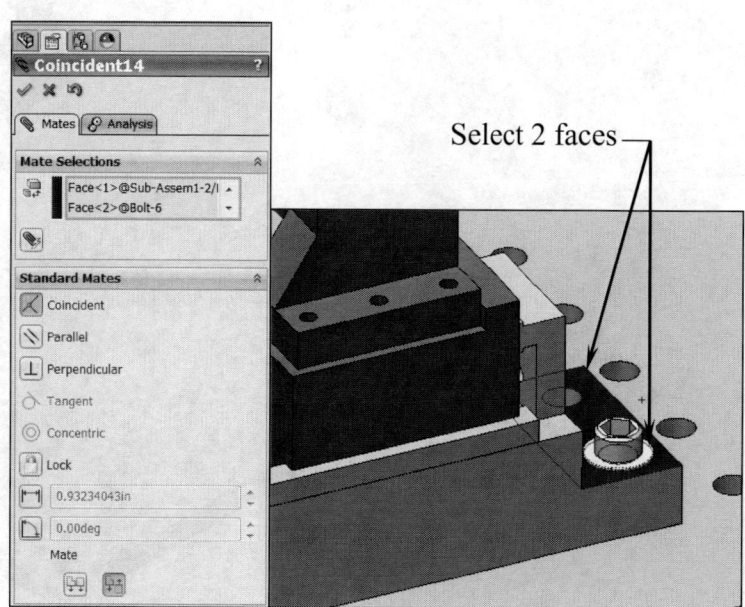

Select 2 faces

13. Repeating:

- For practice purposes, we are going to add more instances of the bolts to the other components.

- Keep in mind that fasteners do not have to be fully defined. Each bolt only needs two mates, and even though they still rotate the assembly will not be affected.

- By using one less mate for each component you can reduce the file size of this assembly by about 10%. It will also help reduce the time that it takes to rebuild the assembly every time a change is applied. In other words, the less mates (and less components), the faster the computer performance.

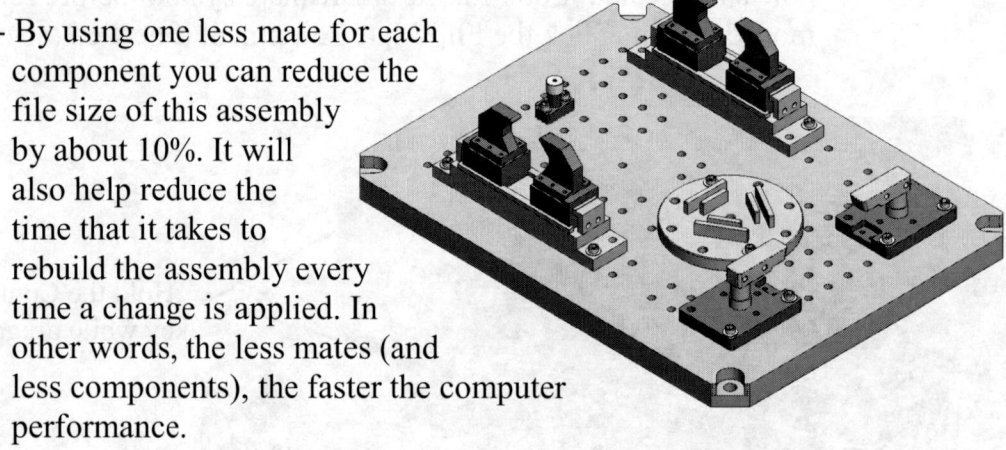

14. Saving your work:

- Save your work as **Fixture Assemly.sldasm** and overwrite the existing file when prompted.

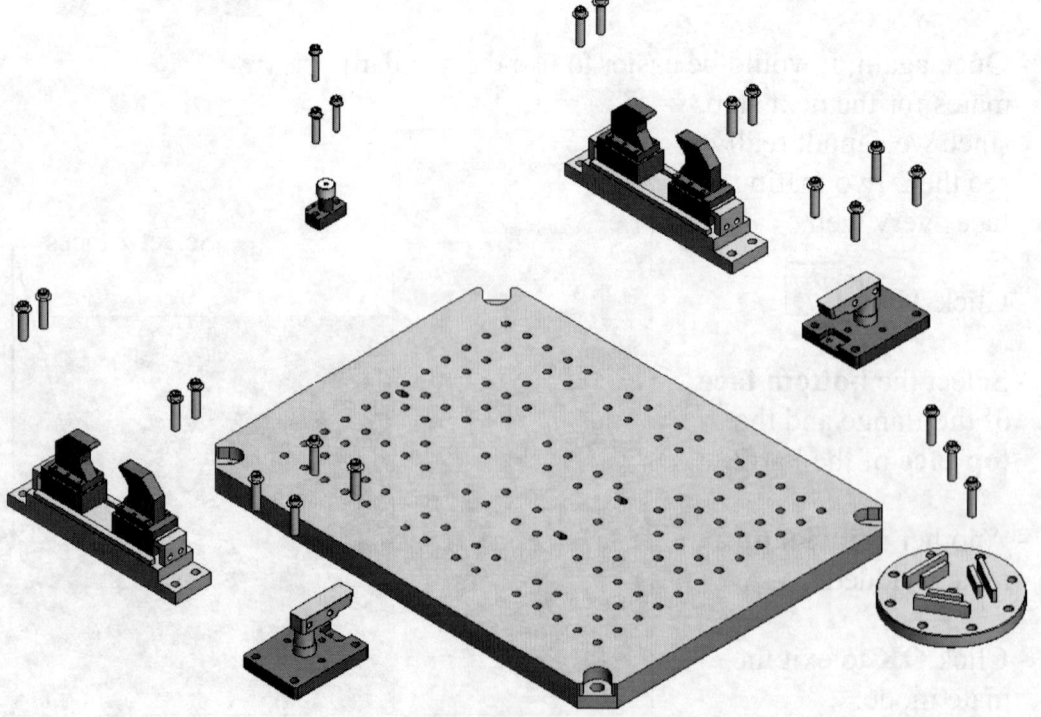

Questions for Review

Using Smart-Mates

1. When using the smart-mate options, you will need to select the Mate command first.
   a. True
   b. False

2. To activate the smart-mates, hold the Alt key while dragging the component.
   a. True
   b. False

3. To make a copy of a component and apply smart-mates to it at the same time, hold both the Control & Alt keys, and then drag the component to its destination.
   a. True
   b. False

4. Smart-mates will work with either a set of model edges, faces, or vertices, as mating entities.
   a. True
   b. False

5. Smart-mates also work with reference geometry such as planes and axis, as mating entities.
   a. True
   b. False

6. To flip the component direction during the smart-mate mode, push the "esc" key.
   a. True
   b. False

7. Using the Alt + Drag option, the tab key is used to flip the mate alignment (still holding the mouse button, release the Alt key and push Tab).
   a. True
   b. False

8. Hold the Control key while dragging a component to make a copy and smart-mate it at the same time.
   a. True
   b. False

7. TRUE   8. TRUE
5. TRUE   6. FALSE
3. FALSE   4. TRUE
1. FALSE   2. TRUE

Exercise: Bottom Up Assembly

<u>Files location</u>: Training Files folder.
Bottom Up Assembly Folder.
Copy the entire folder to your
Desktop.

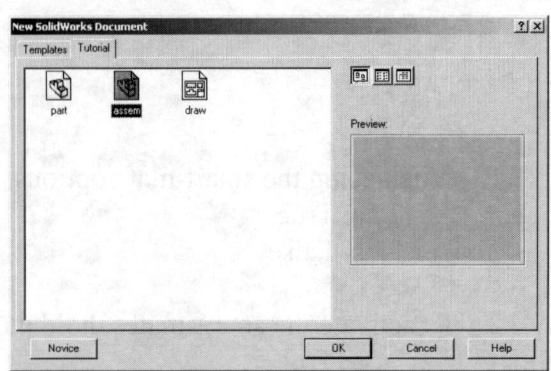

1. Starting a new Assembly document:

- Select **File / New / Assem**. (Assembly)
from either the Template or the
Tutorial folder.

2. Inserting the Fixed component:

- Click the **Insert Component** command from the Assembly toolbar.

- Locate the **Molded Housing** and place it on the assembly's origin.

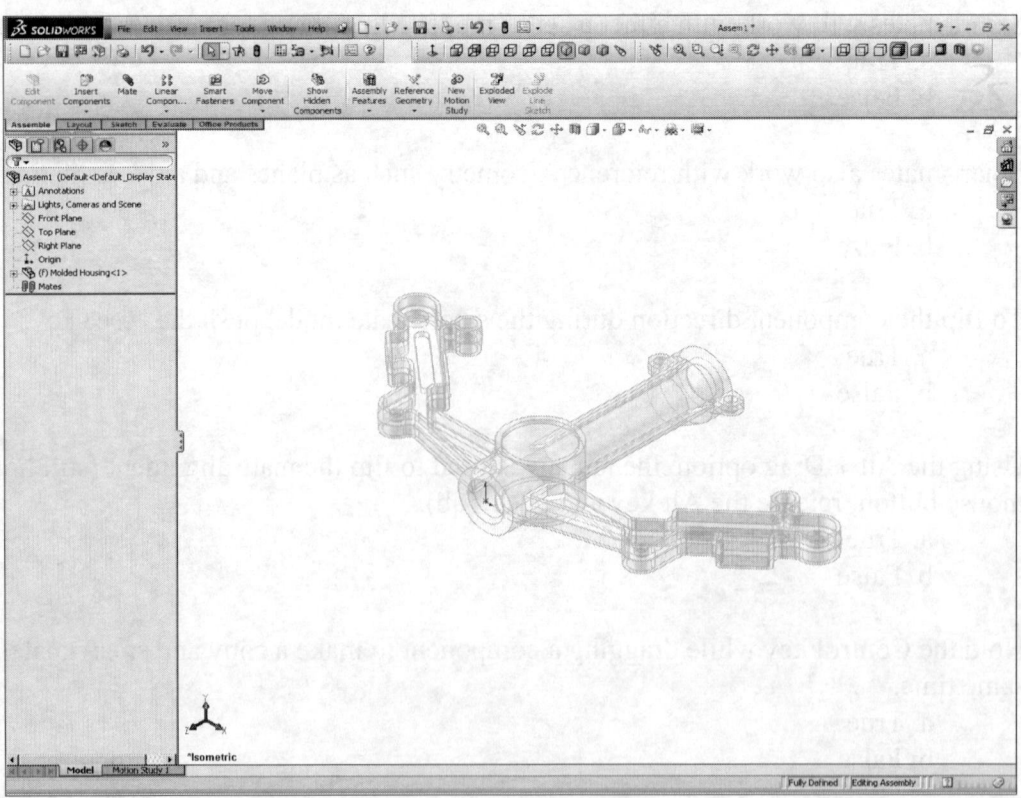

Note: *To show the Origin symbol, click **View / Origins.***

3. Inserting the other components:

- Insert the rest of the components as labeled, from the Bottom Up Assembly folder into the assembly.

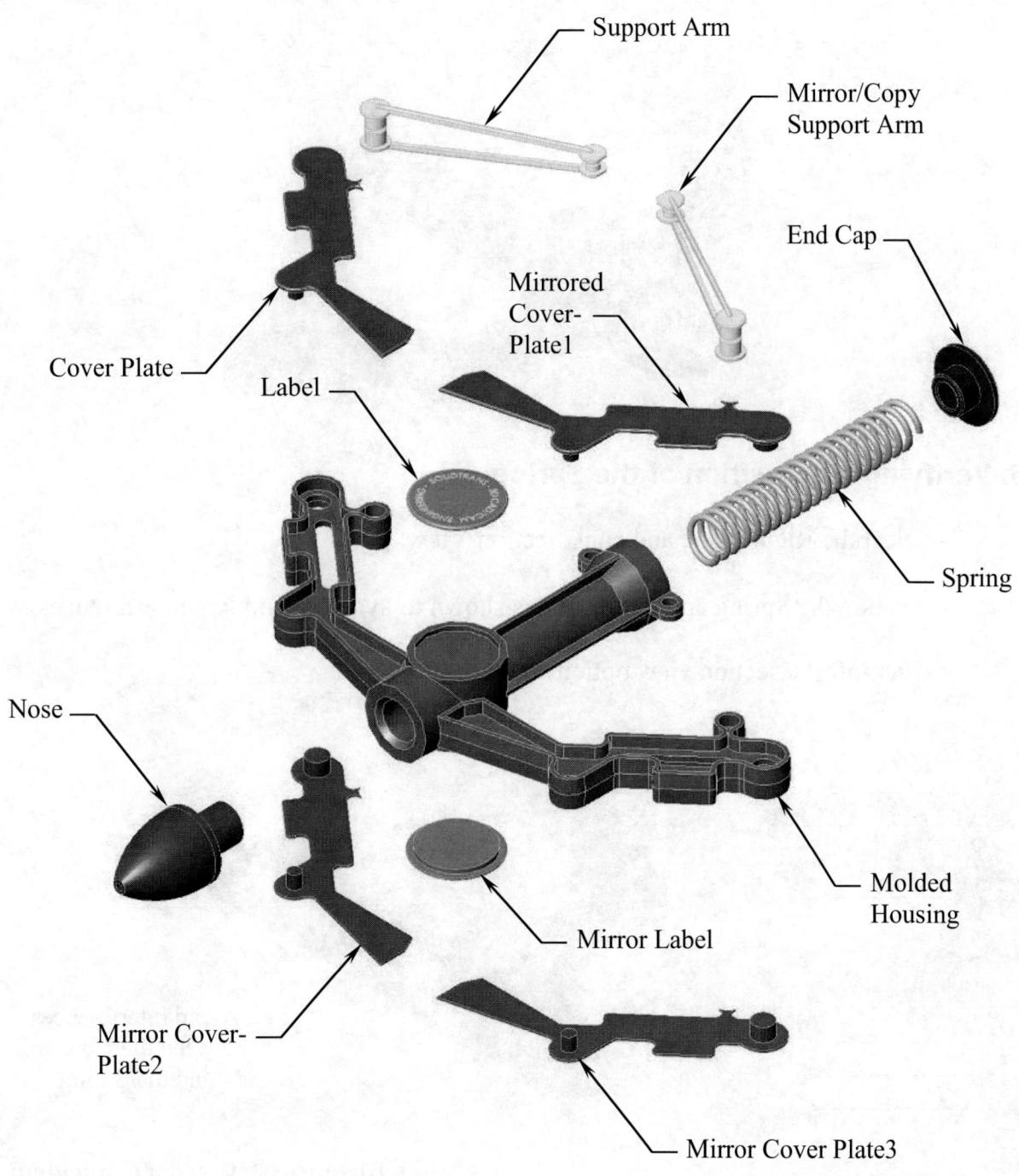

4. Mating the components:

- Assign the Mate conditions such as Concentric, Coincident, etc., to assemble the components.

- The finished assembly should look like the one pictured below.

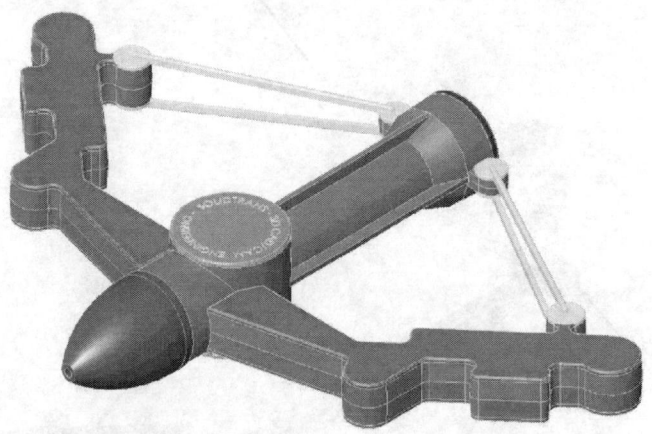

5. Verifying the position of the Spring:

- Select the Right Plane and click Section View.

- Position the Spring approximately as shown to avoid assembly's interferences.

- Click-off the section view option when finished.

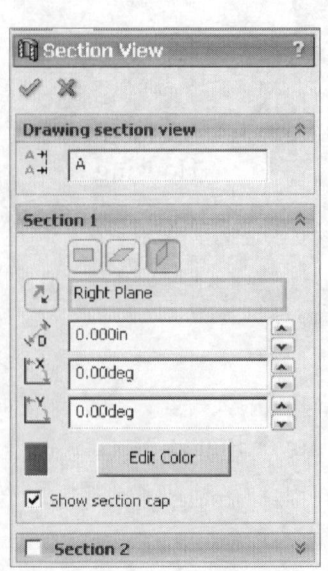

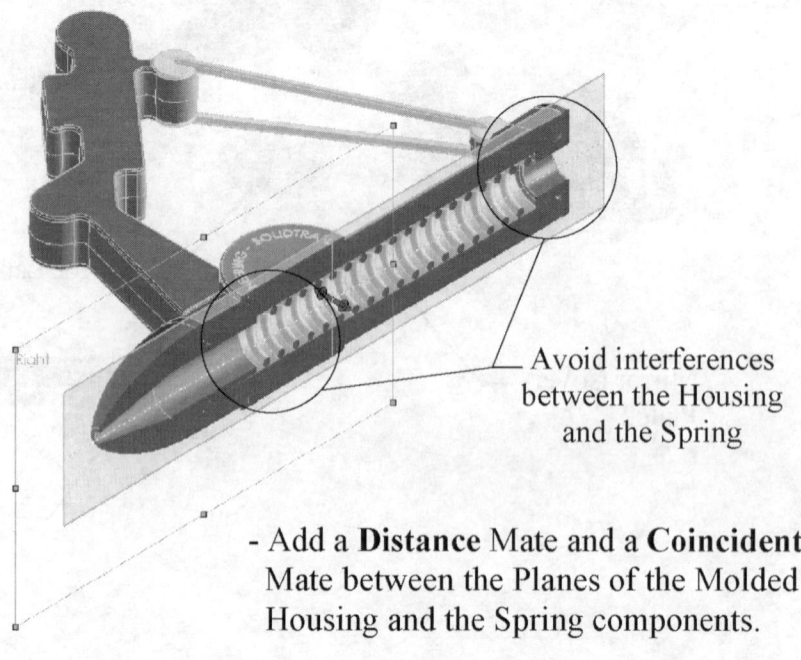

— Avoid interferences
between the Housing
and the Spring

- Add a **Distance** Mate and a **Coincident** Mate between the Planes of the Molded Housing and the Spring components.

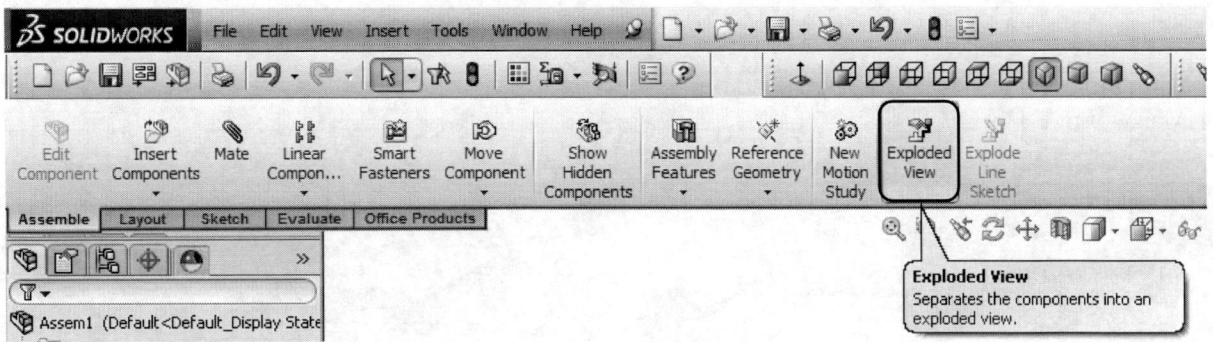

6. Creating the Assembly Exploded View:

- Click 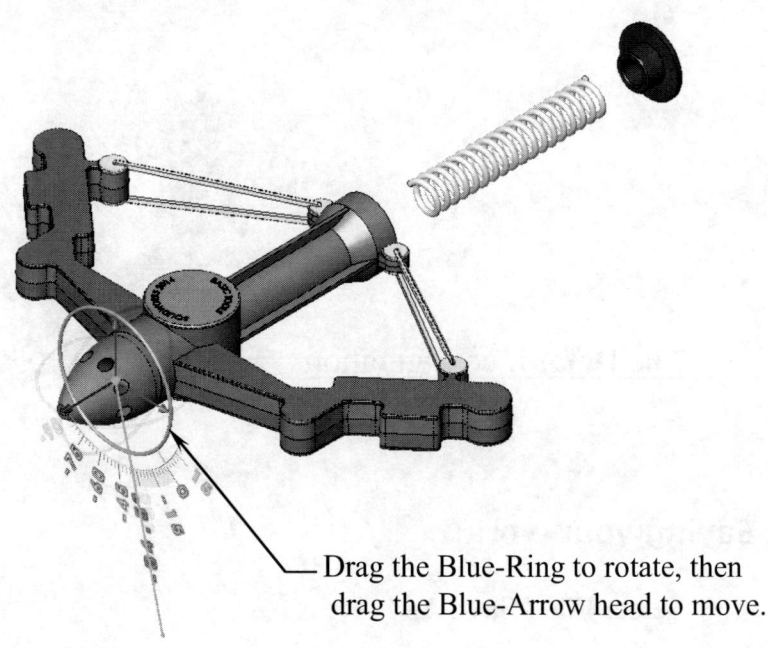 or Select **Insert / Exploded View**.

- Select a component either from the Feature tree or directly from the Graphics area.

- Drag one of the three Drag-Handles to move the component along the direction you wish to move.

- Repeat the same step to explode all components.

- For editing, right click on any of the steps on one of the Explode-Steps and select Edit-Step.

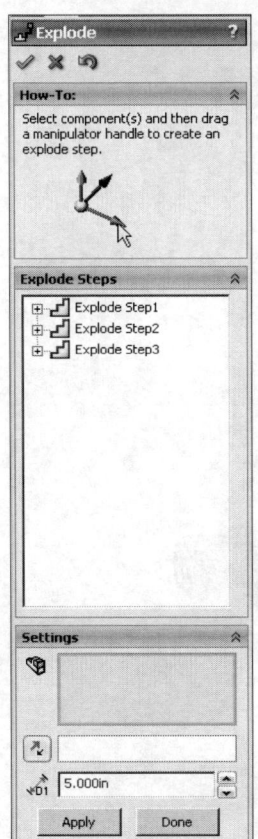

Drag the Blue-Ring to rotate, then drag the Blue-Arrow head to move.

**Note:** _The finished exploded view can be edited by accessing the ConfigurationManager under the Default Configuration._

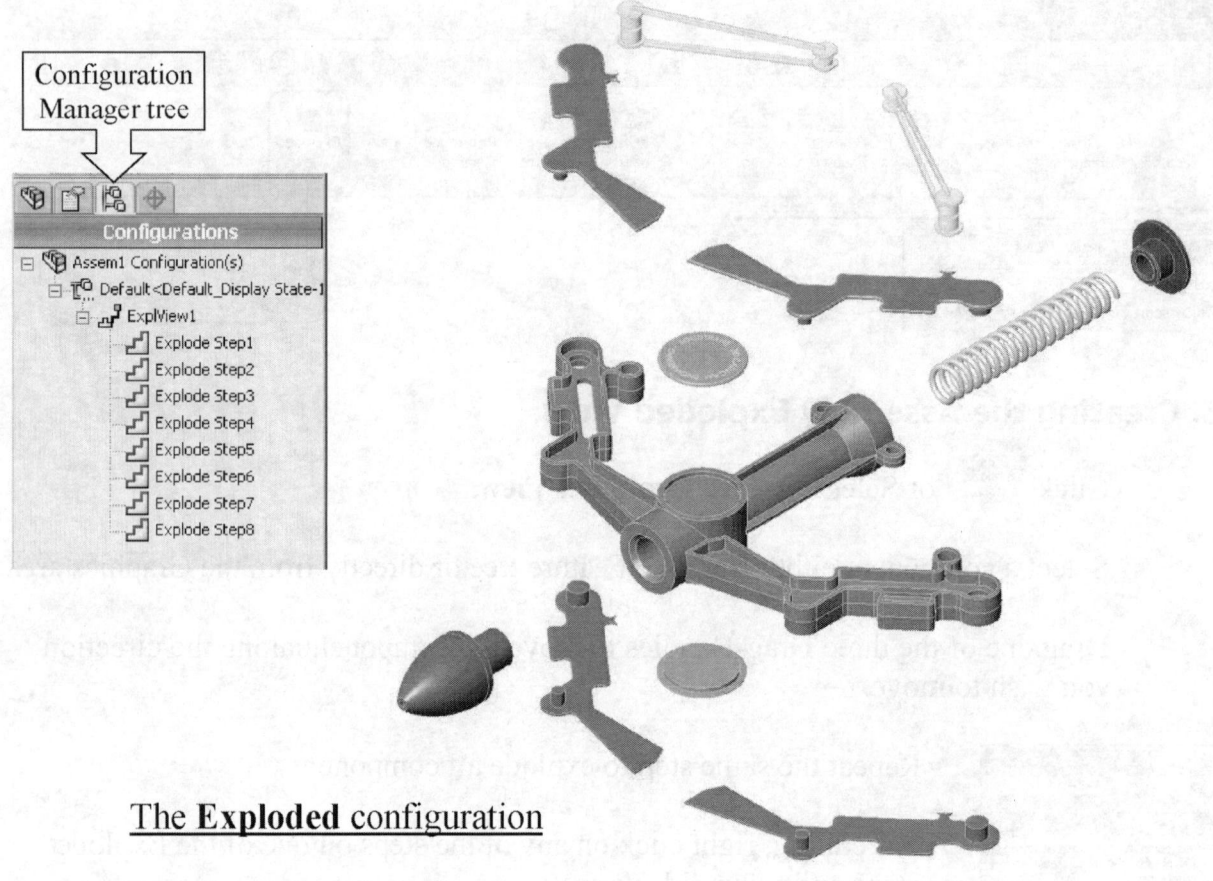

Configuration
Manager tree

The **Exploded** configuration

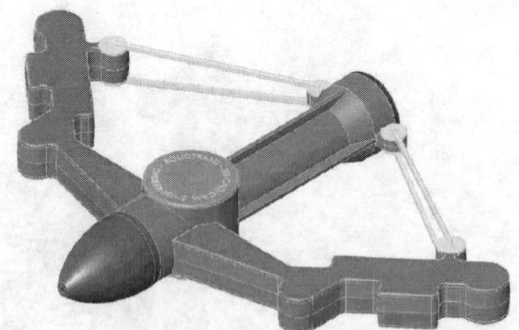

The **Default** configuration

7. Saving your work:

- Select **File / Save As**.

- Enter **Bottom Up Assembly Exe** for the name of the file.

- Click **Save**.

(From the Training Files folder, locate the Built-Parts folder; open the pre-built assembly to check your work against it).

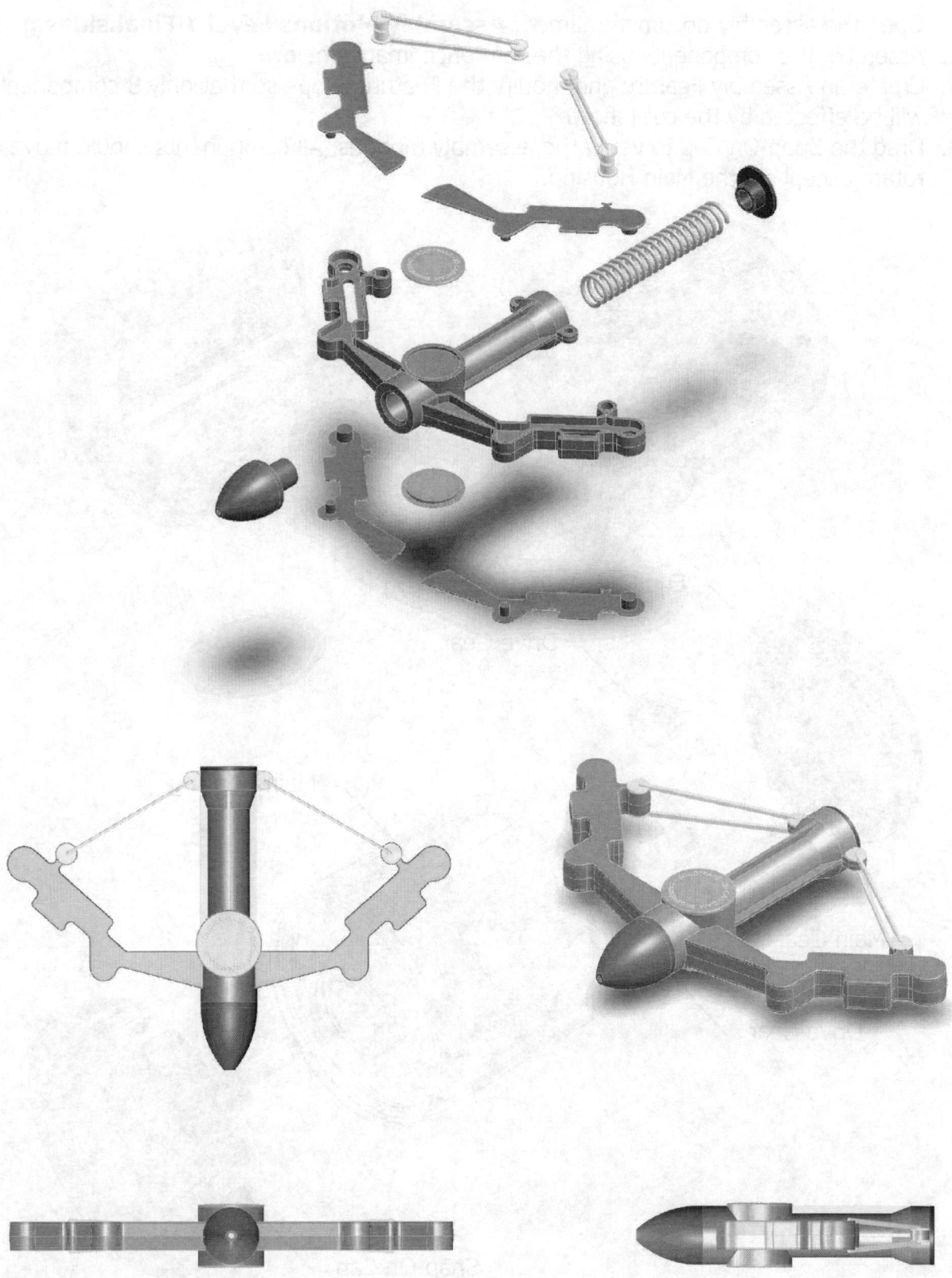

Level 1 Final Exam: Assembly Motions

1. Open the assembly document named: **Assembly Motions Level 1 Final.sldasm**
2. Assemble the components using the reference images below.
3. Create an Assembly Feature and modify the Feature Scope so that only 3 components will be effected by the cut (shown).
4. Drag the Snap-On Cap to verify the assembly motions. All components should move or rotate except for the Main Housing.

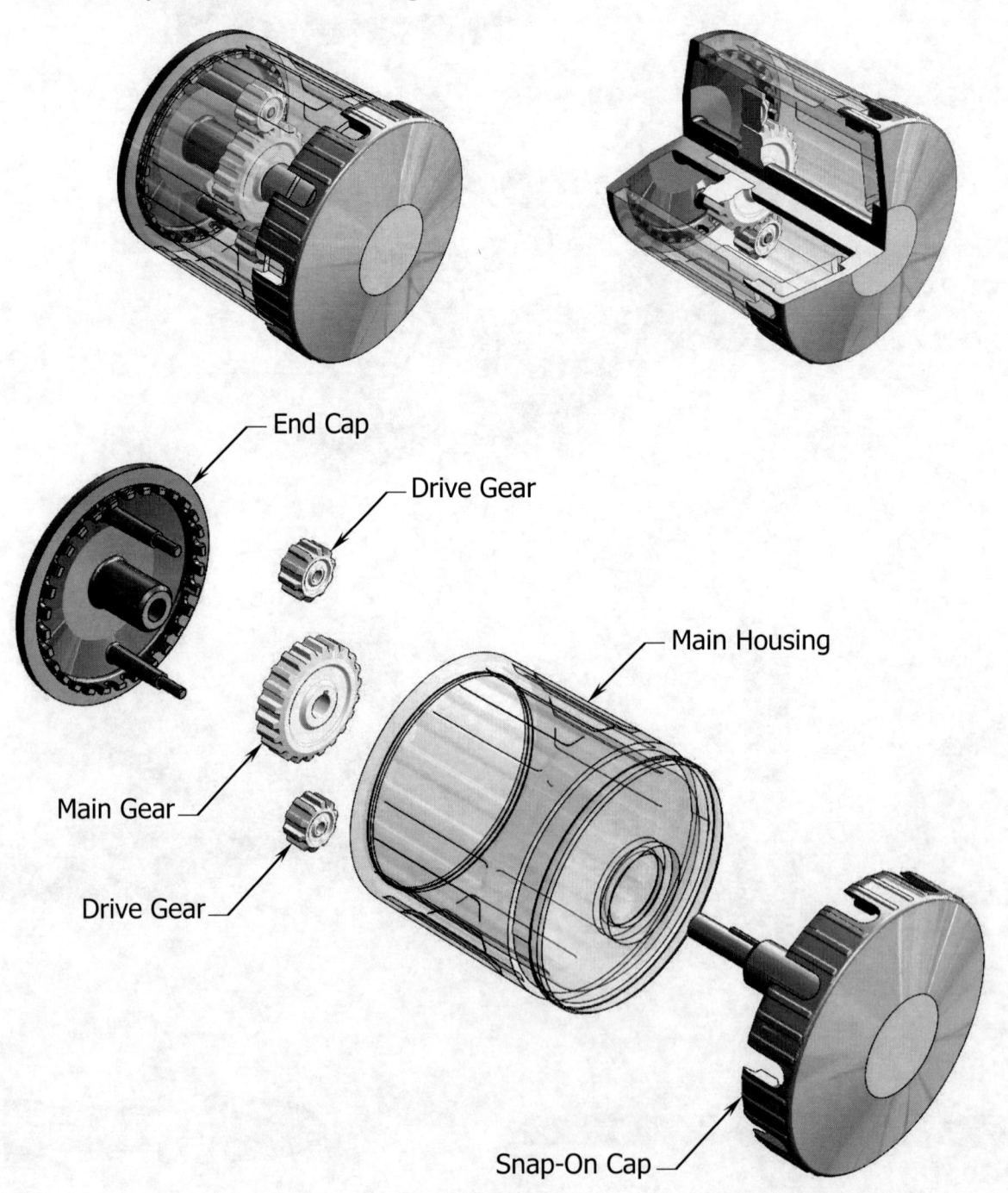

End Cap

Drive Gear

Main Housing

Main Gear

Drive Gear

Snap-On Cap

Testing the Assembly Motions:

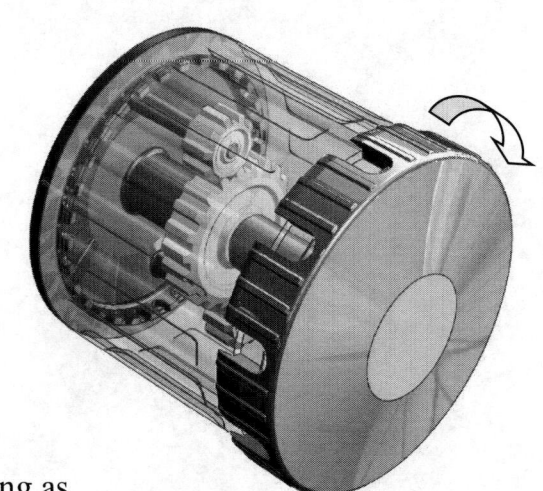

- Drag the Snap-On Cap in either direction to verify the motions of the assembly.

- The Main Gears, the two Drive Gears, and the Snap-On Cap should rotate at the same time.

- If the mentioned components are not rotating as expected, check your mates and recreate them if needed.

Creating a Section View:

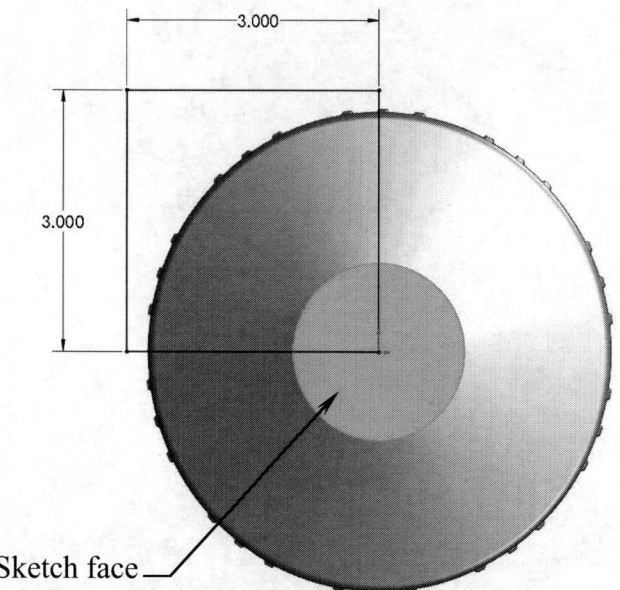

- Open a new sketch on the <u>face</u> as indicated.

- Sketch a rectangle and add the dimensions shown.

- Create an Extruded Cut Through All components.

Sketch face

- Verify that the Keyway on the Snap-On Cap is properly mated to the Main Gear, and there is no interference between them.

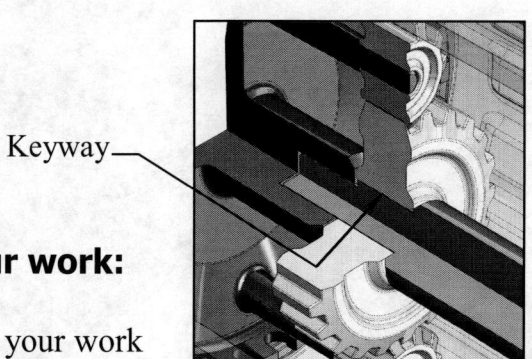

Keyway

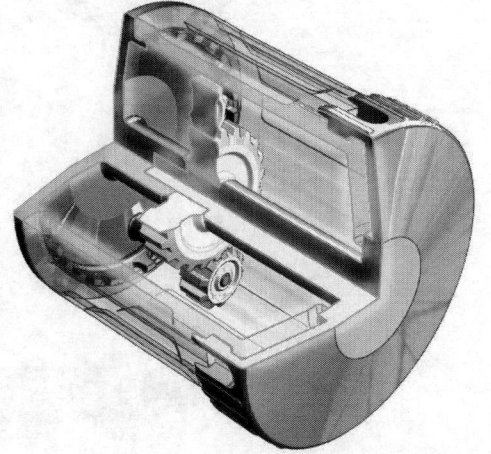

Saving your work:

- Save your work as: **Level 1 Final**.

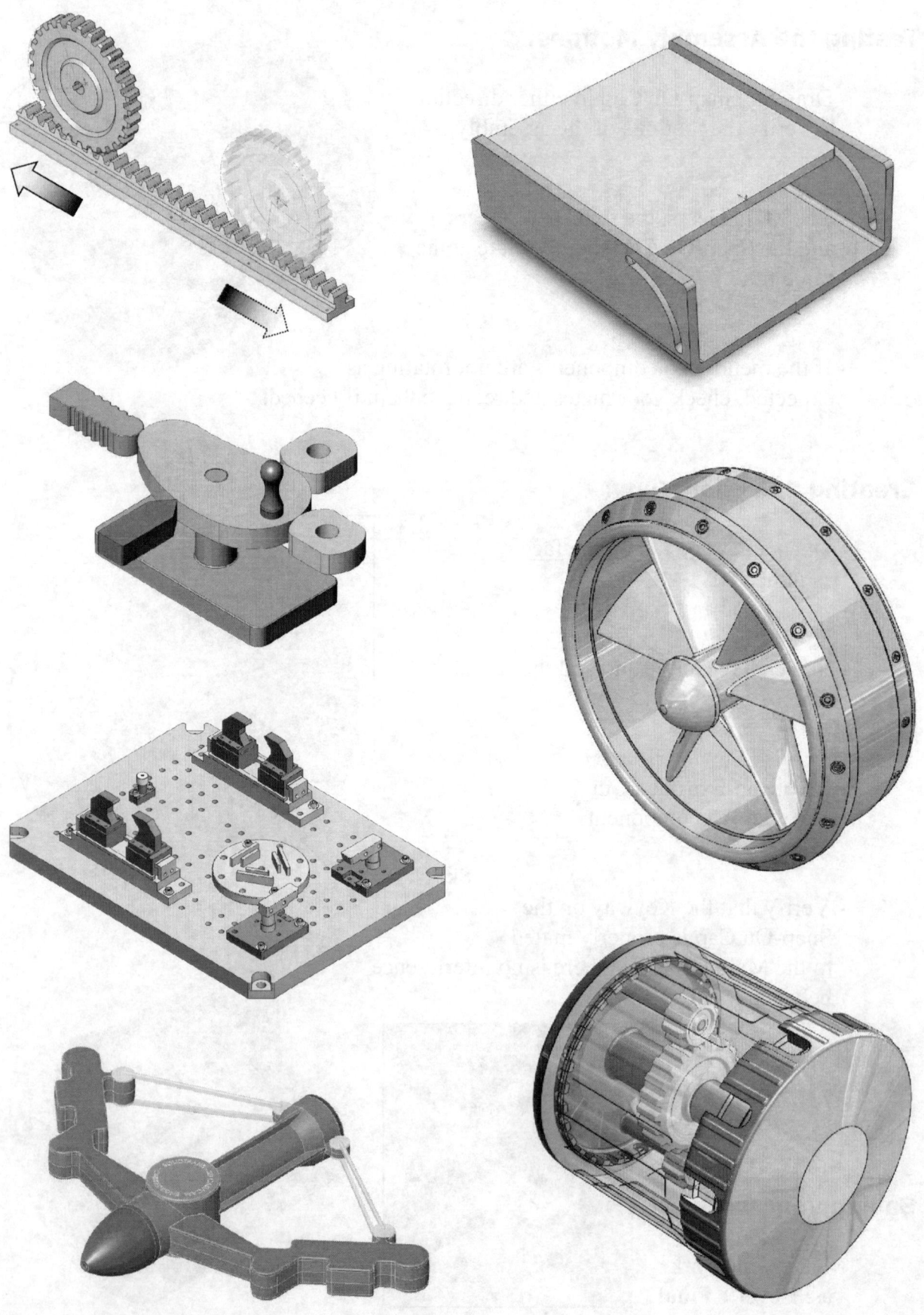

CHAPTER 12

Layout Assembly

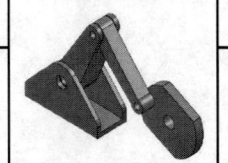

Layout Assembly

- You can design an assembly from the top-down using layout sketches. You can construct one or more sketches showing where each assembly component belongs. Then, you can create and modify the design before you create any parts. In addition, you can see the assembly motions ahead of time and how the components are going to behave when they are being moved around.

- The major advantage of designing an assembly using a layout sketch is that if you change the layout sketch, the assembly and its parts are automatically updated. You can make changes quickly, and in just one place.

- In a Layout Assembly, blocks are created from each sketch to help handle them more efficiently. A block is created by grouping the sketch entities, dimensions, callouts, etc., into one unit and then saving them as a Block. A block can easily be moved, positioned, or re-used in other assembly documents.

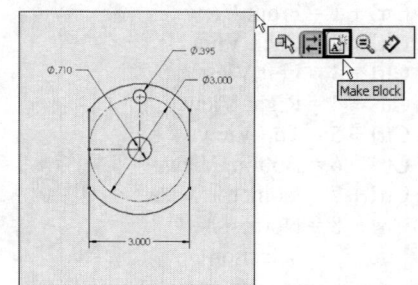

- In layout-based assembly design, you can switch back and forth between top-down and bottom-up design methods. You can create, edit, and delete parts and blocks at any point in the design cycle without any history-based restrictions. This is particularly useful during the conceptual design process, when you frequently experiment with and make changes to the assembly structure and components.

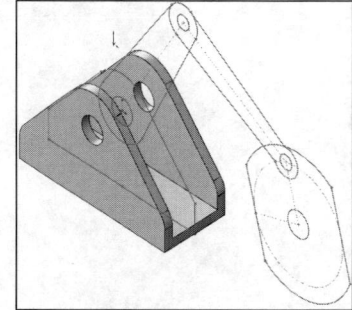

- This chapter will guide you through the use of Layout Assembly, as well as making new blocks and converting them to 3D models.

Assembly Motions
Layout Assembly

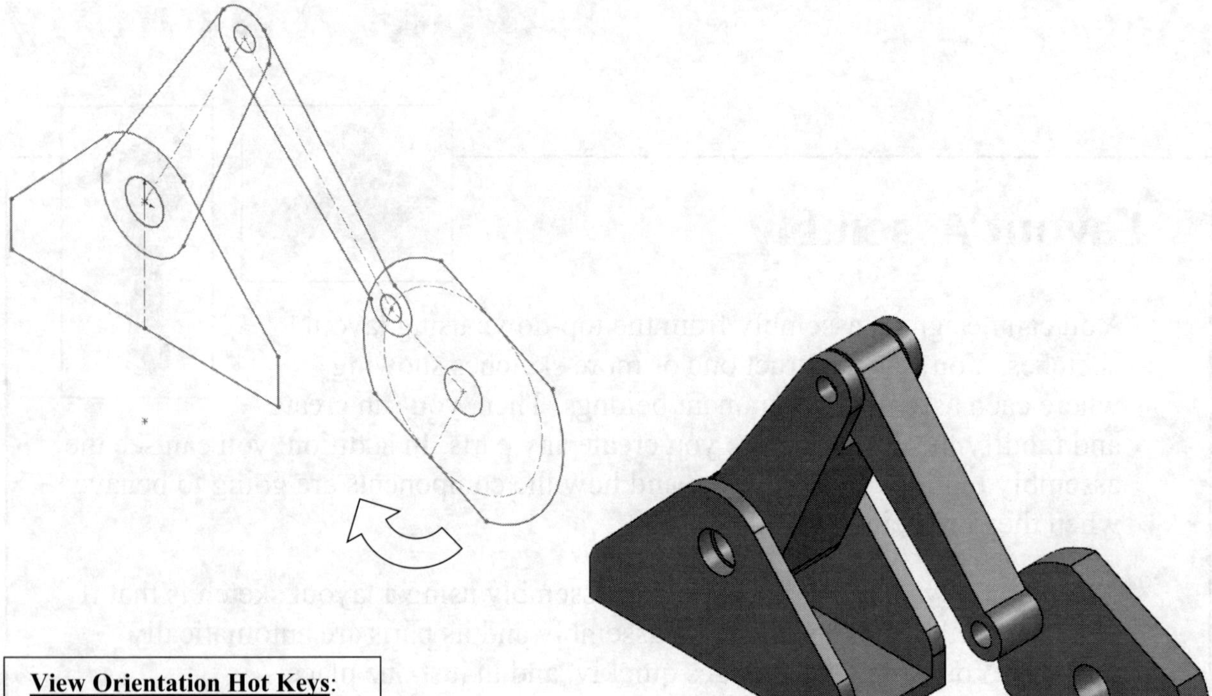

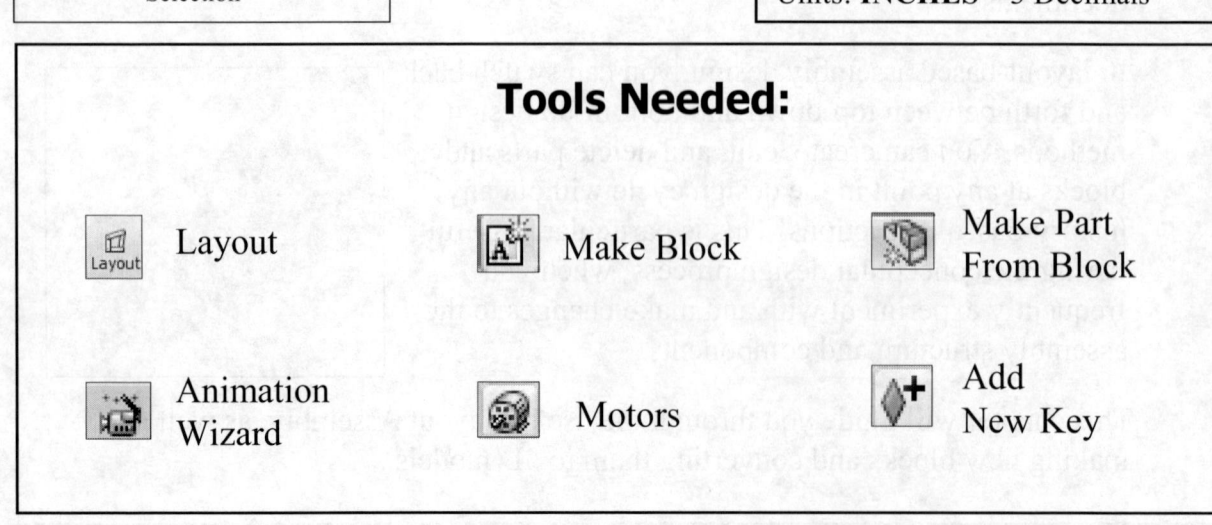

Dimensioning Standards: **ANSI**

Units: **INCHES** – 3 Decimals

Tools Needed:

Layout

Make Block

Make Part
From Block

Animation
Wizard

Motors

Add
New Key

1. Opening an assembly document:

- Browse to the Training Files folder and open the document named: **Layout Assembly.sldasm**.

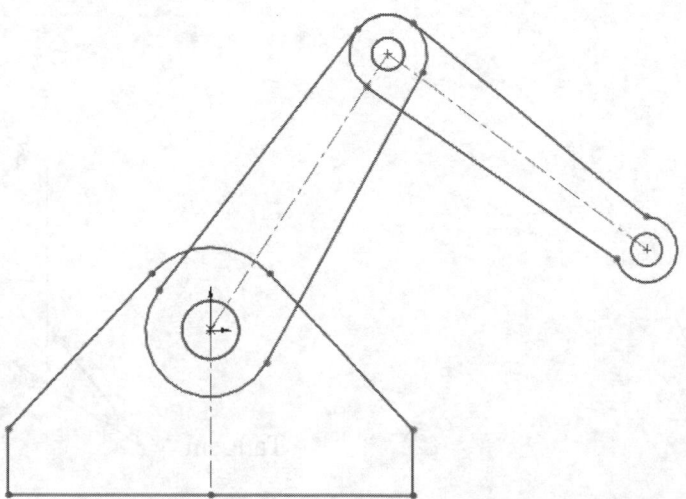

2. Activating the layout mode:

- In order to see the motions in the Layout mode, each sketch must be converted into a Block.

- In a block, a set of sketch entities and Dimensions are grouped into one unit or one block so that they can be moved, positioned easily, or re-used in other assembly documents.

- Click the **Layout** button on the Layout tab, next to the Assembly toolbar (arrow).

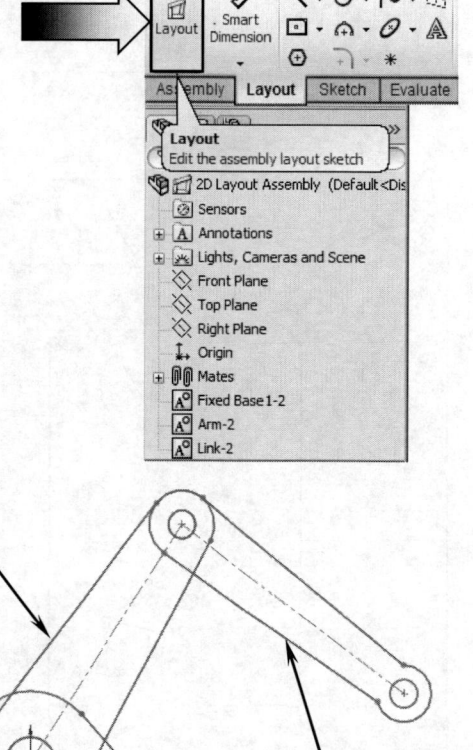

Block 2

Block 1

Block 3

NOTE: _Recreate the mates if needed._

3. Creating a new sketch:

- Sketch the profile below and add the dimensions as shown.

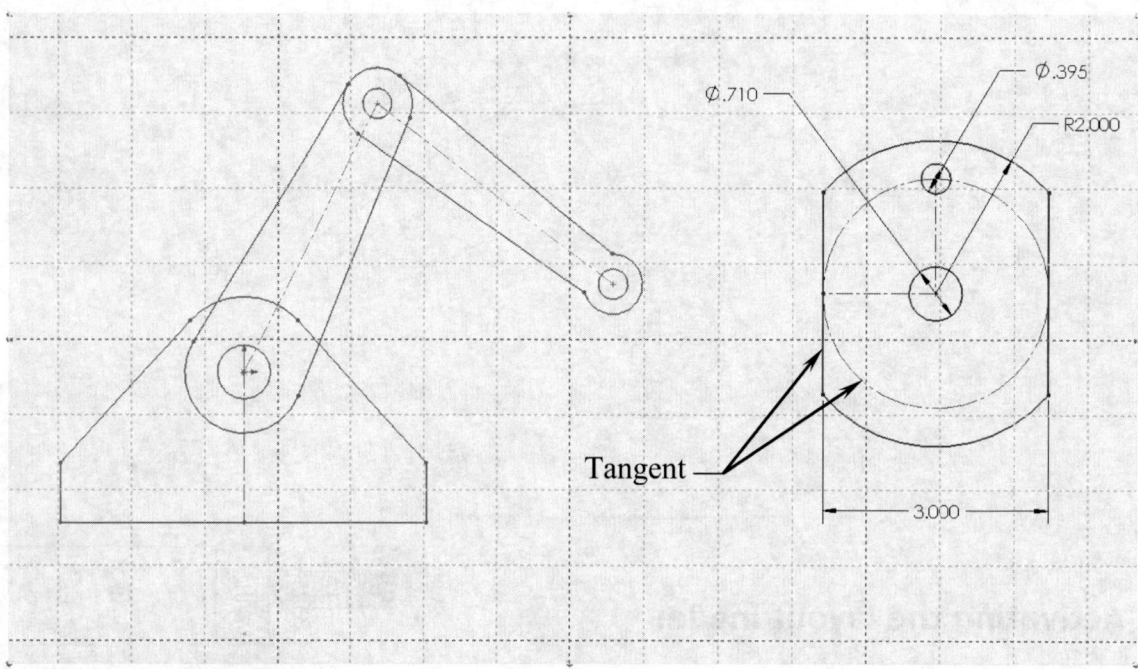

Tangent

4. Making a Block:

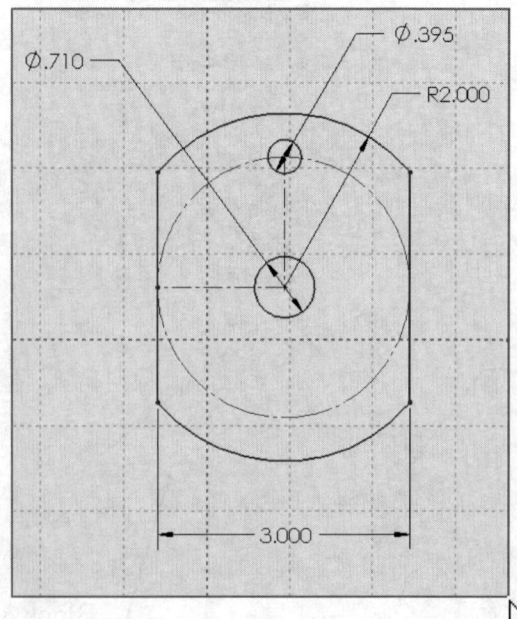

- A block is created by grouping the Sketch entities, dimensions, callouts, etc., into one unit and then saving them as a Block.

- Box-select the entire profile, click the **Make Block** button 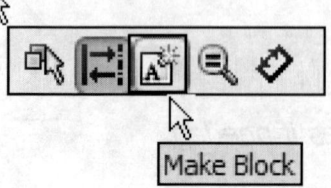 from the pop up toolbar – OR – select **Tools / Block / Make** from the pull down menus.

Make Block

5. Setting the Insertion Point:

- Each block should have an Insertion Point (or Handle Point), which will allow
the block to move and position more easily.

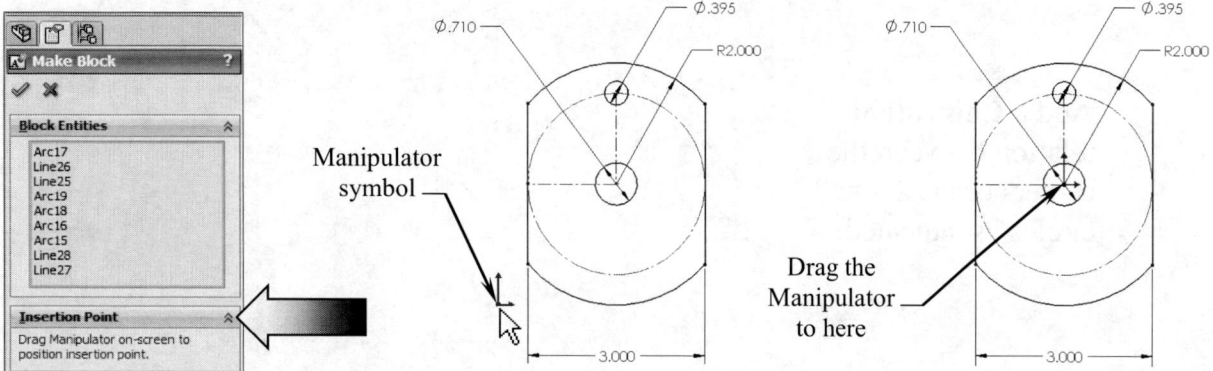

- Expand the **Insertion Point** option (arrow) and drag the Blue Manipulator symbol
and place it on the center of the middle circle.

- Click **OK** .

6. Editing a block:

- To edit a block simply double click on one of its sketch entities - or - Right click
one of the lines and select: **Edit Block** (arrow).

- Click-Off the Edit Block button on the Layout tool bar when finished (arrow).

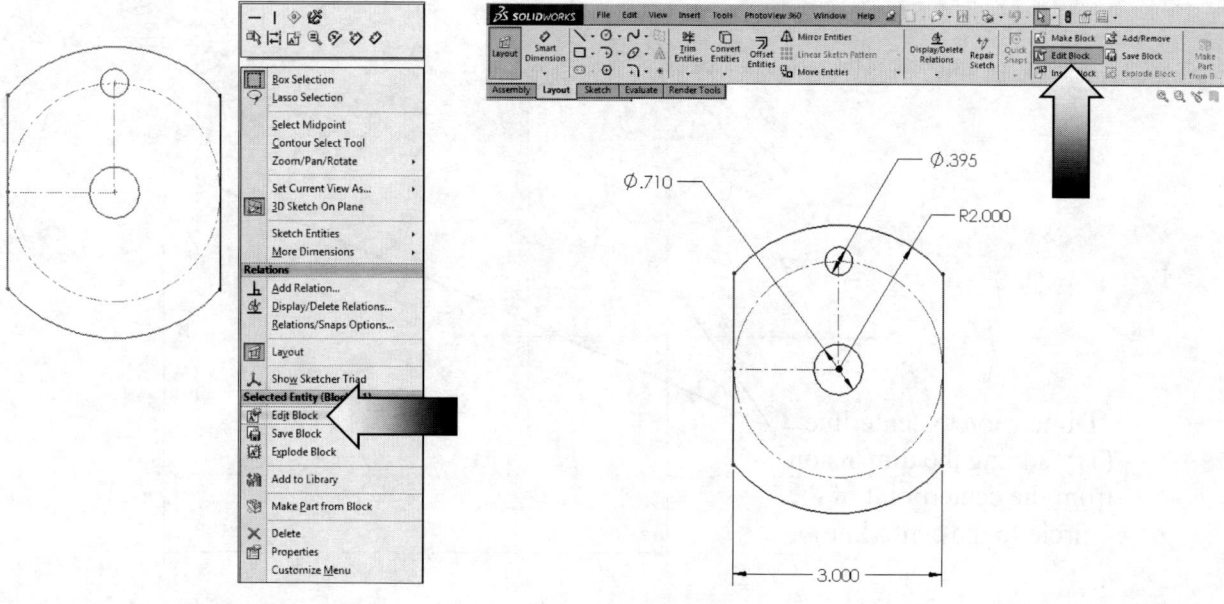

- Ensure that the Edit Block mode is off.

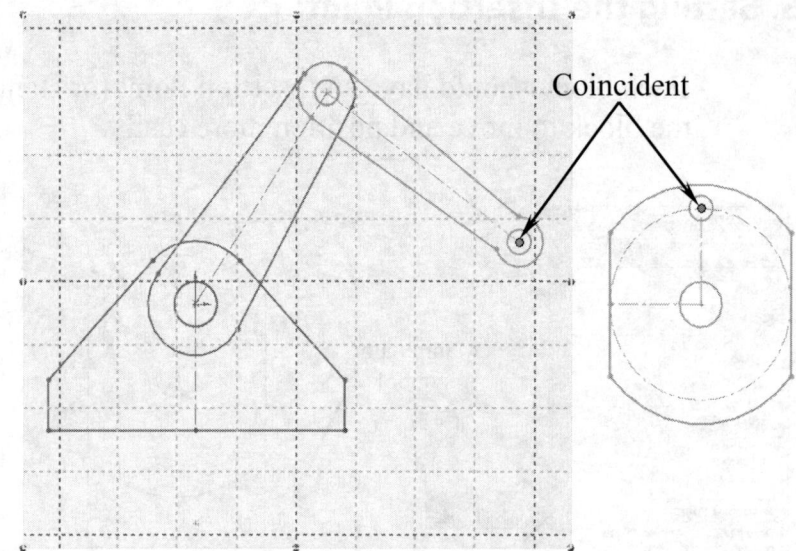

Coincident

- Add a **Coincident** relation between the centers of the 2 small circles as indicated.

7. Adding dimensions:

- Add a **6.000 in** dimension to define the spacing between the 2 blocks.

**Note:** _Dimension from the vertical centerline of the 1st block to the center of the 4th block as noted below._

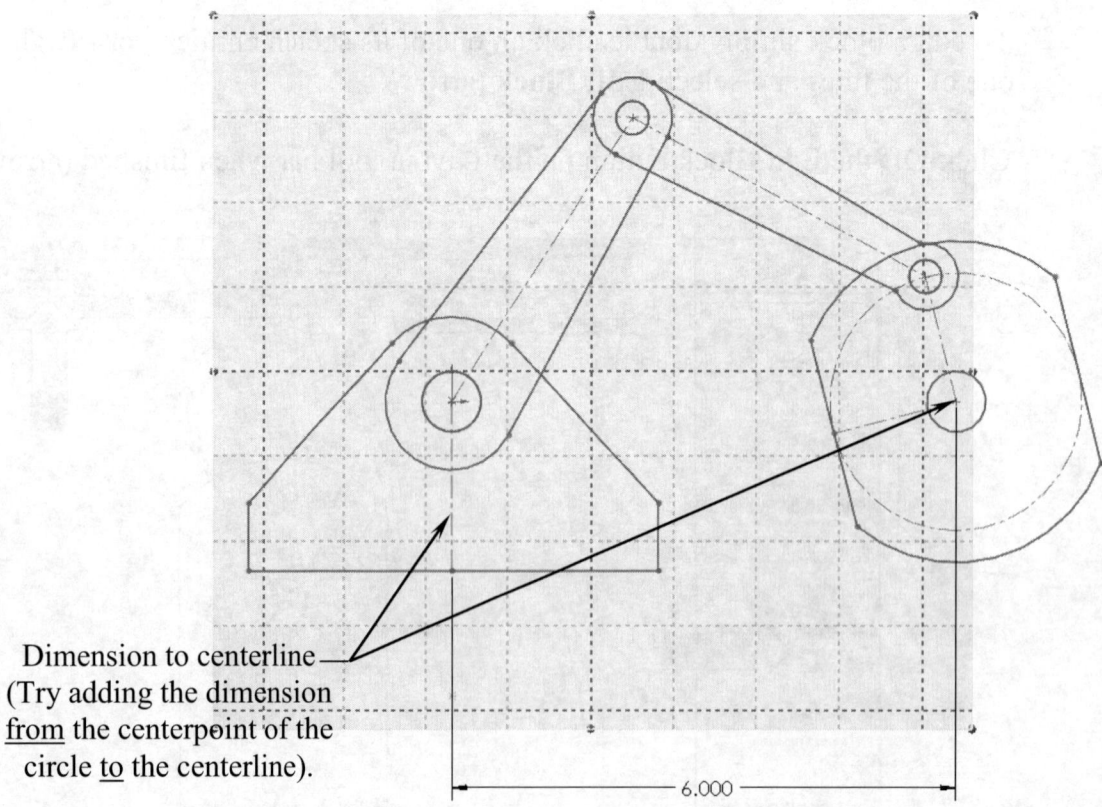

Dimension to centerline
(Try adding the dimension
from the centerpoint of the
circle to the centerline).

6.000

8. Testing the relations between the blocks:

- Drag one of the vertices of the new part to see how the blocks respond.

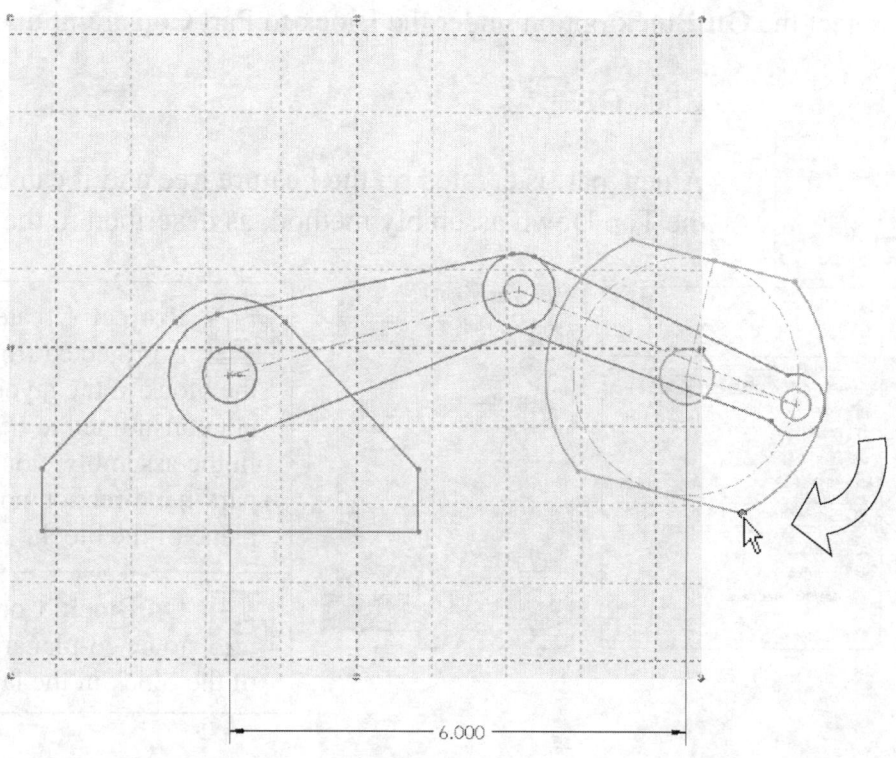

6.000

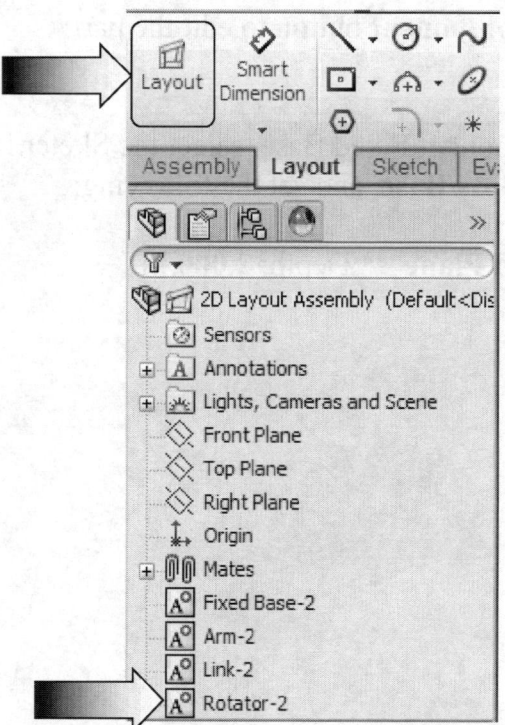

- **Click-off** the Layout command (arrow).

- Rename the new block to: **Rotator** (arrow).

- So far we have 4 different blocks, created as 2D-sketches in the assembly environment. The next step is to convert these blocks into 3D solid parts.

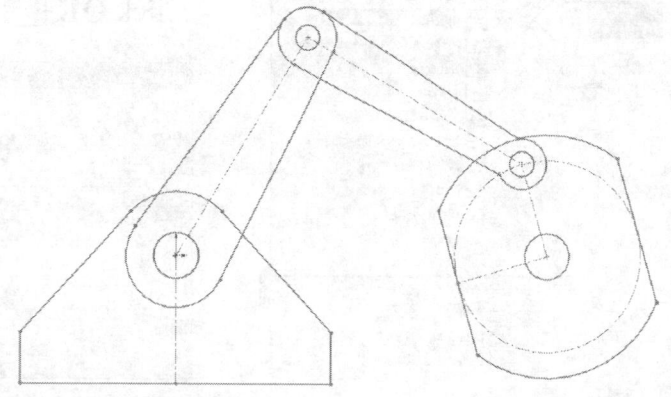

9. Converting a Block into a Component:

- Right click the name of the 1ˢᵗ block (Fixed Base) select **Make Part from Block**.

- Select the **On Block** option under the Block to Part Constraint dialog.

- Click **OK** ☑.

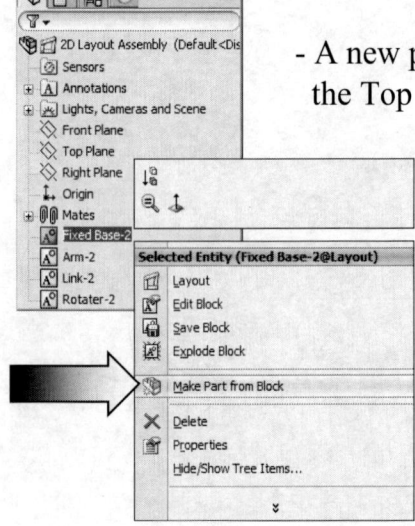

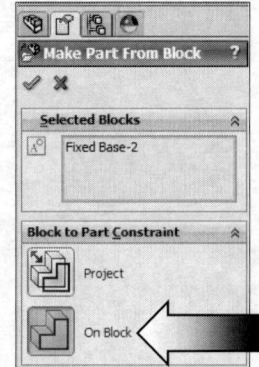

- A new part is created on the Feature tree and it can be edited using the Top Down assembly method, as described in the next few steps.

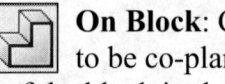
Project: Creates a part that is projected from the plane of the block in the layout sketch, but not constrained to be co-planar with. In the assembly, you can drag the part in a direction normal to the plane of the block.

On Block: Constrains the part to be co-planar with the plane of the block in the layout sketch.

10. Extruding the Fixed Base:

- Click the **Edit Component** button to edit the part Fixed Base.

- **Expand** the component Fixed Base, select the Sketch1, click **Extruded Boss/Base**, and set the following:

     * Type: **Mid Plane**   * Depth: **2.000 in**

- Click **OK** ☑.

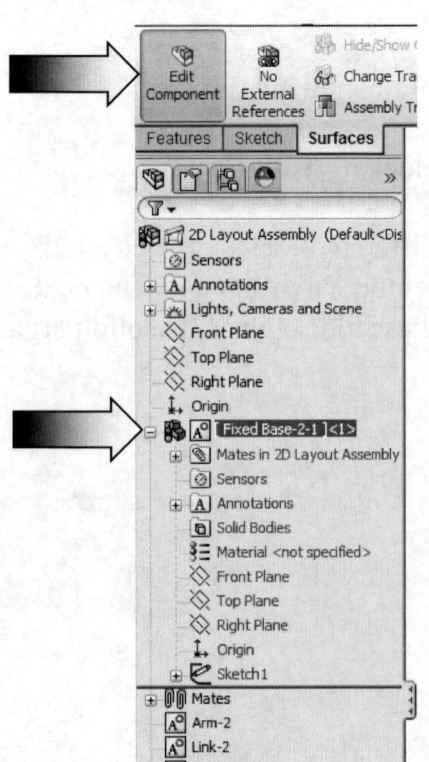

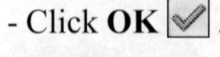

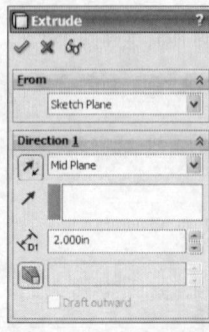

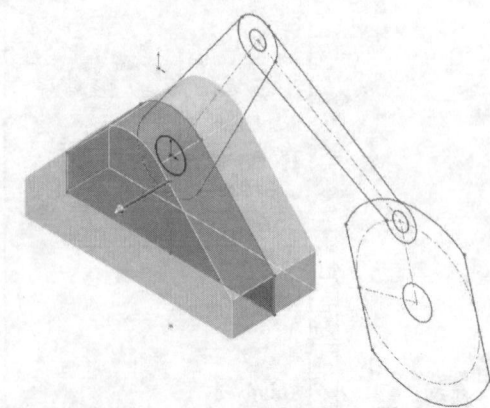

11. Adding fillets:

- Click the **Fillet/ Round** command.

- Enter **.500 in** for radius.

- Select the **2 edges** as indicated.

- Click **OK** ✓.

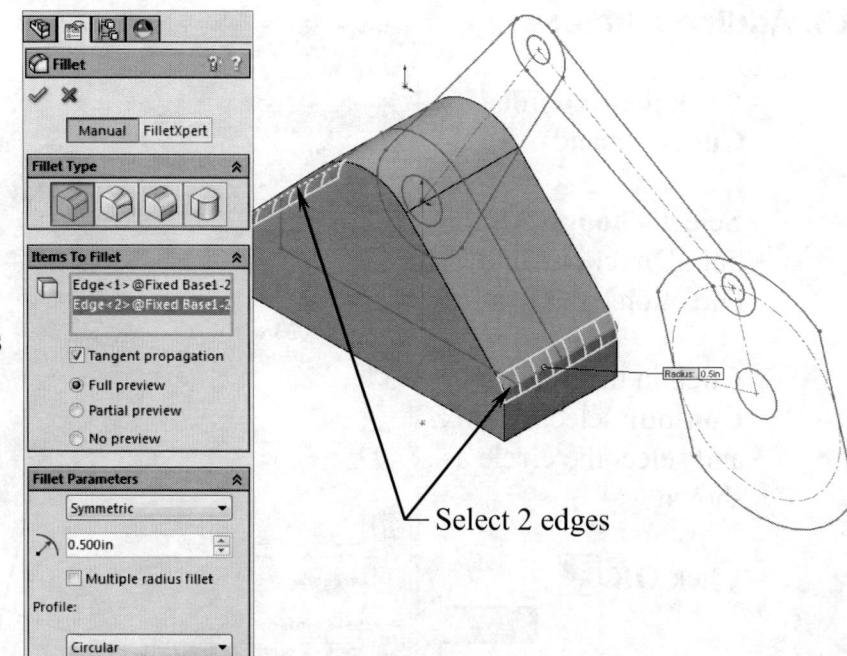

Select 2 edges

12. Shelling the part:

- Click the **Shell** command from the Features toolbar.

- Enter **.250 in** for wall thickness.

- Select the **7 faces** as noted.

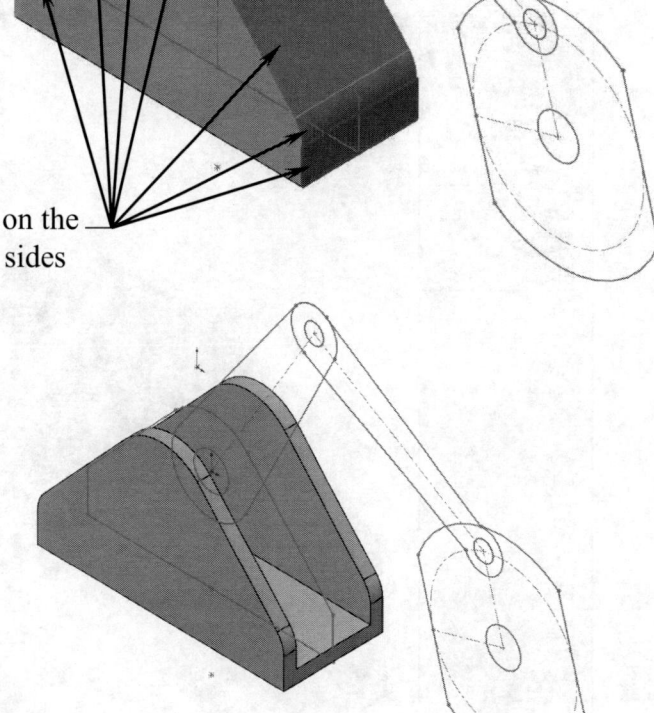

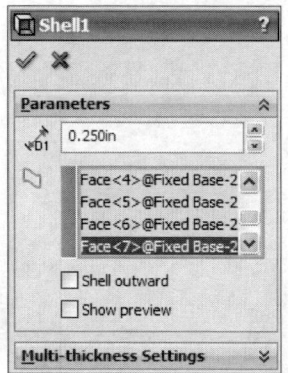

Select 7 faces on the left and right sides

- Click **OK** ✓.

13. Adding a hole:

- Click the **Extruded Cut** command.

- Select **Though All** for both Direction1 and Direction2.

- Click in the **Selected-Contour** selection box and select the **circle** as shown.

- Click **OK** ✓.

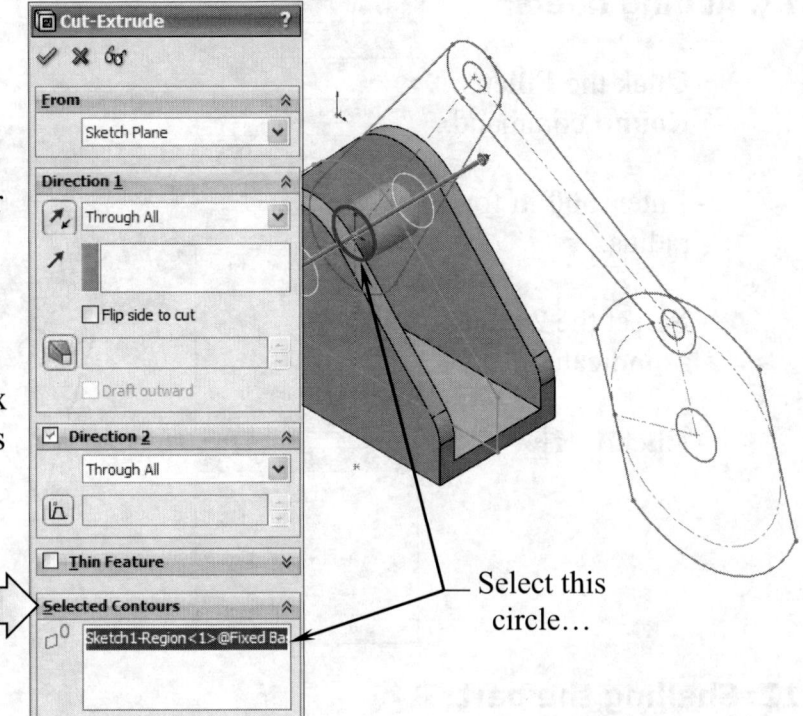

Select this circle…

- Click off the **Edit Component** command 🔲, the first part is completed.

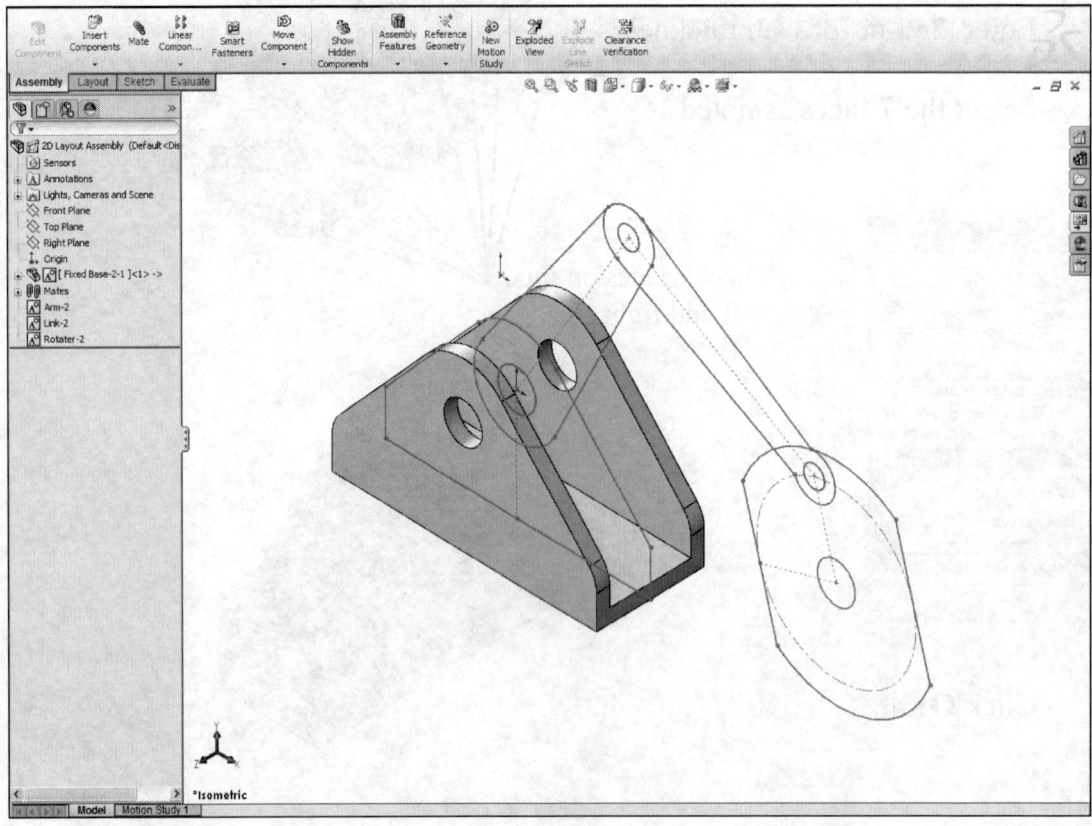

14. Converting the next block: (Repeating from step no. 8)

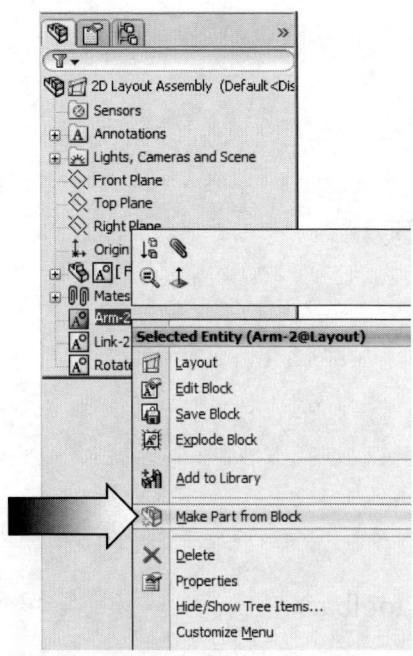

- Right click on the block named **Arm** and select **Make Part from Block**.

- Select the **On Block** option once again, from the **Block to Part Constraint** section.

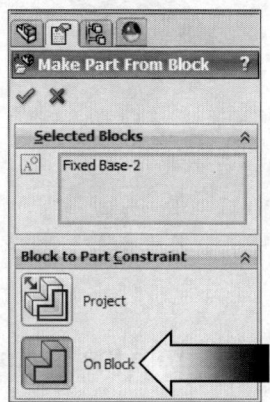

- A new part is created on the Feature Tree and it can be edited using the same method as the last one.

- Click **OK** .

15. Extruding the Arm:

- Select the part **Arm** from the Feature tree and click the **Edit Component** button.

- **Expand** the part **Arm**, select its sketch and click **Extruded Boss/Base**.

- Set the following:

  * Type: **Mid Plane**

  * Depth: **1.400 in**

- Click **OK** .

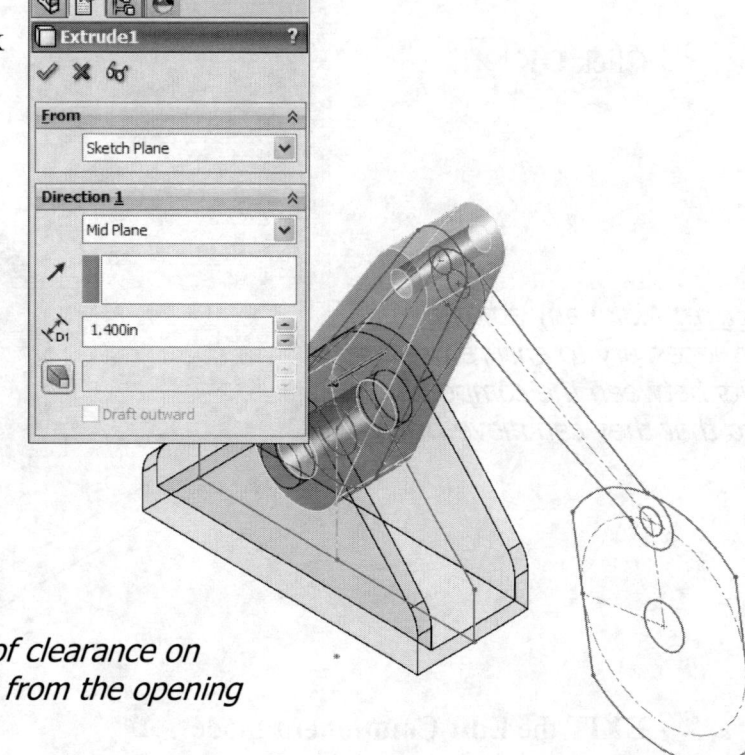

**Note:** There should be a .050" of clearance on each side of this part, measured from the opening of the Fixed Base.

16. Adding a cut:

- Select the **Front** plane of the Part Arm and sketch the profile as shown.

- Use **Convert Entities** if needed and add the relations/dimensions to fully define the sketch.

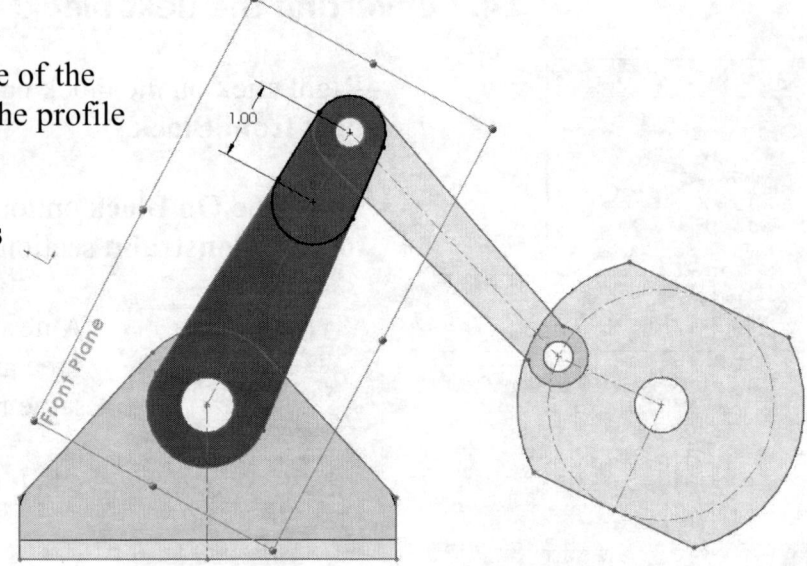

- Select the **Extruded Cut** command from the Features toolbar.

- Set the following:

  * Type: **Mid Plane**

  * Depth: **.900 in**

- Click **OK** ✓ .

Note: Make any adjustments if necessary to ensure proper fits between the components so that they can move freely.

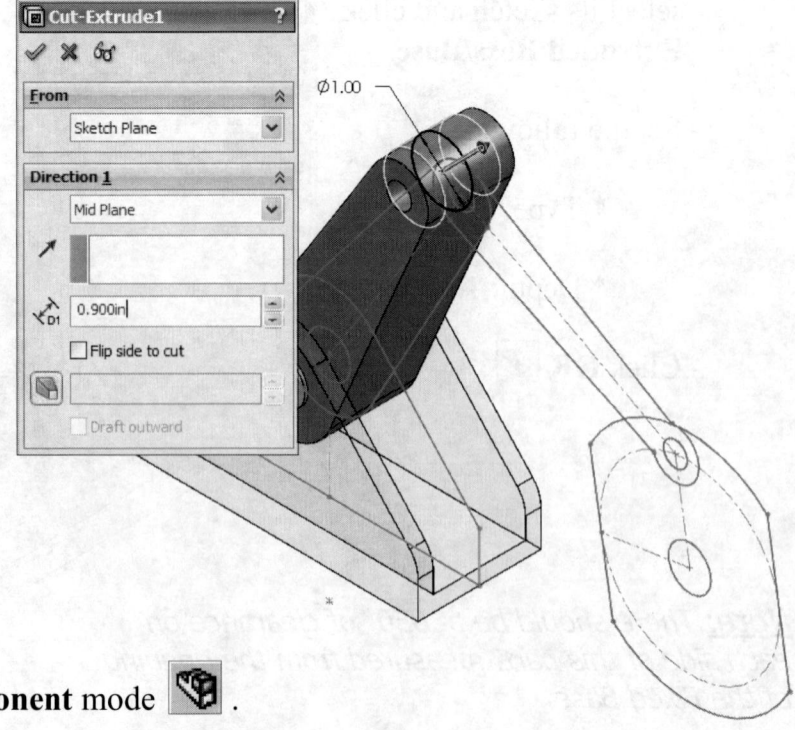

- **EXIT** the **Edit Component** mode 🗗 .

17. Repeating:

- Repeat either **step 8** or **step 13** and convert the next two blocks the same way.

- Make the part **Link .800 in** thick as shown.

- Extrude with the **Mid Plane** type to keep the Link on the center of the Arm.

- **EXIT** the **Edit Component** mode 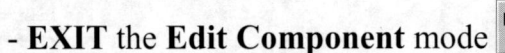.

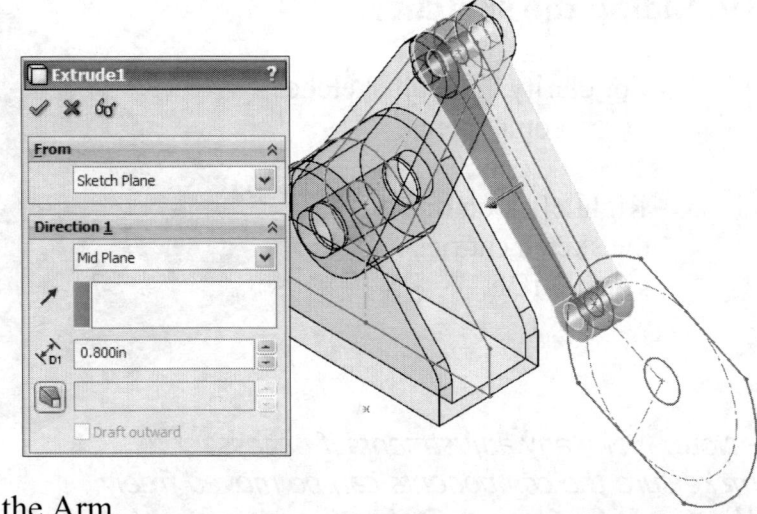

18. Using the Extrude-From option:

- The Extrude-From option allows a sketch to be extruded from a different location rather than from its own sketch plane. This new "location" can be either a plane, a surface of a part, or an offset distance which the user can control.

- Select the part **Rotator** and click **Edit Component** 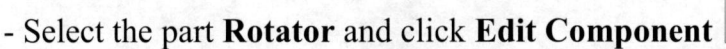.

- Set the following:

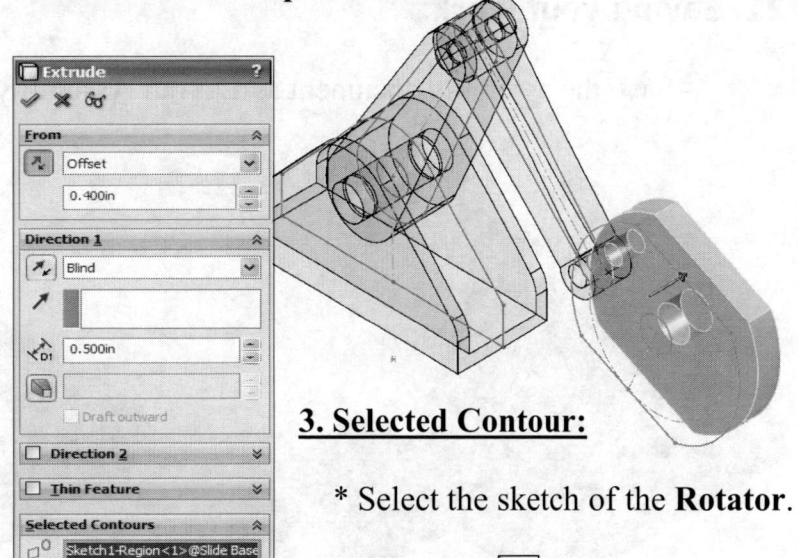

1. Extrude From:

    * **Offset**

    * **.400 in**

    * **Reverse Direction**

2. Direction 1:

    * **Blind**

    * **.500 in**

    * **Reverse Direction**

3. Selected Contour:

    * Select the sketch of the **Rotator**.

    * Click **OK** ✓.

    * **EXIT** the **Edit Component** 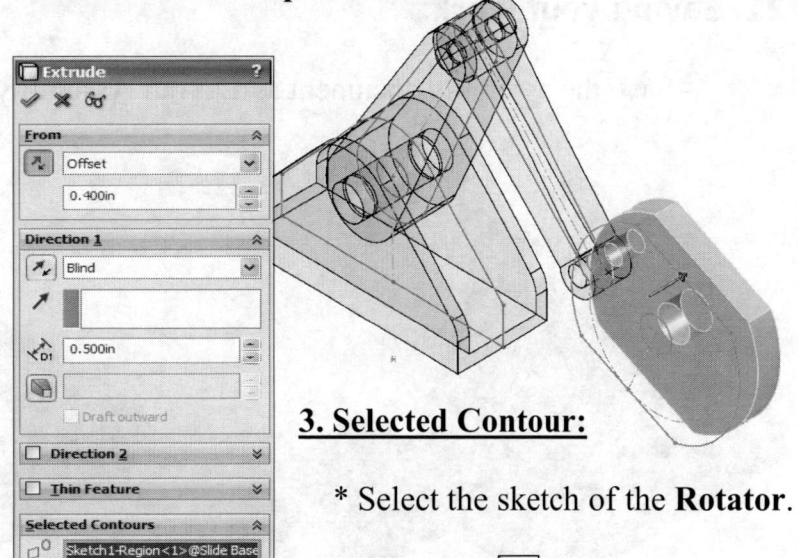.

19. Hiding the sketches:

- For clarity, hide all sketches of the components.

- Right click on one of the sketch entities and select HIDE.

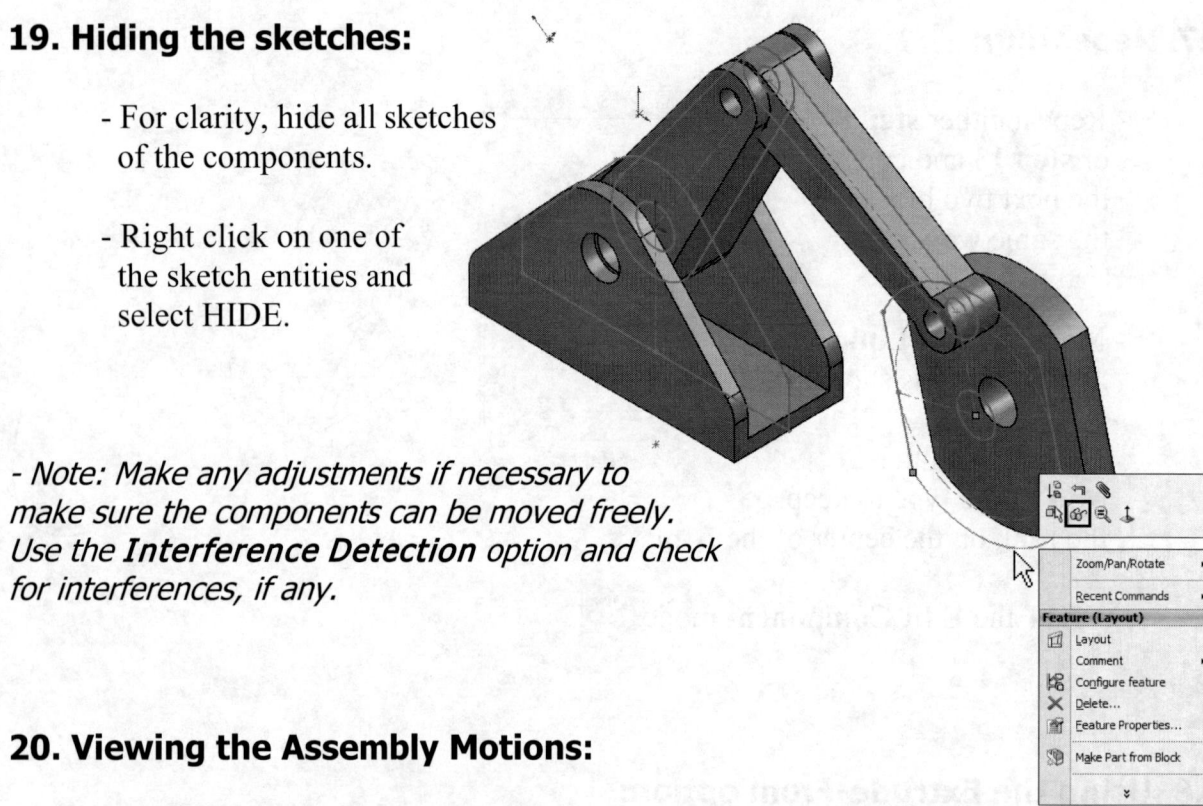

*- Note: Make any adjustments if necessary to make sure the components can be moved freely. Use the **Interference Detection** option and check for interferences, if any.*

20. Viewing the Assembly Motions:

- Drag the part **Rotator** back and forth to see how the components will move.

- Keep the part Fixed Base fixed and recreate any mates if necessary.

21. Saving your work:

- Save the assembly document as **Layout Assembly.sldasm**

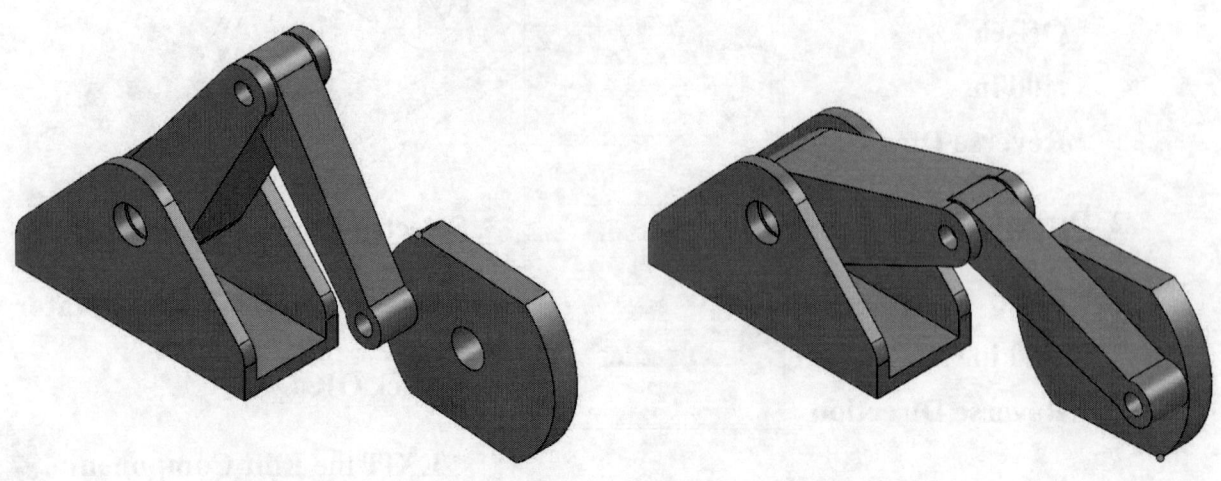

SolidWorks Animator – The Basics

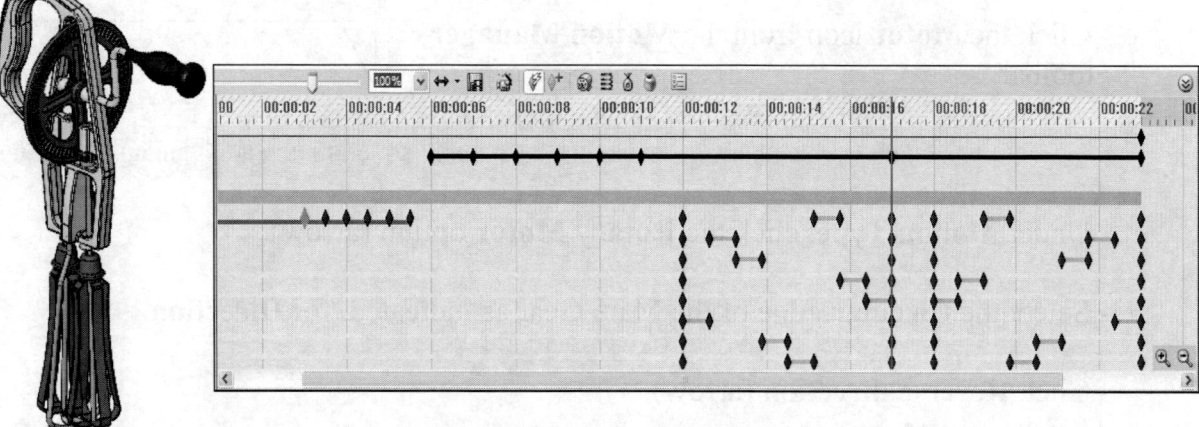

- You can use animation motion studies to simulate the motion of assemblies.

- The following techniques can be used to create animated motion studies:

  * Create a basic animation by dragging the timeline and moving components.
  * Use the Animation Wizard to create animations or to add rotation, explodes, or collapses to existing motion studies.
  * Create camera-based animations and use motors or other simulation elements to drive the motion.

- This exercise discusses the use of all techniques mentioned above.

1. Opening an existing Assembly document:

- Open the file named: **Egg-Beater.sldasm** from the Training Files folder.

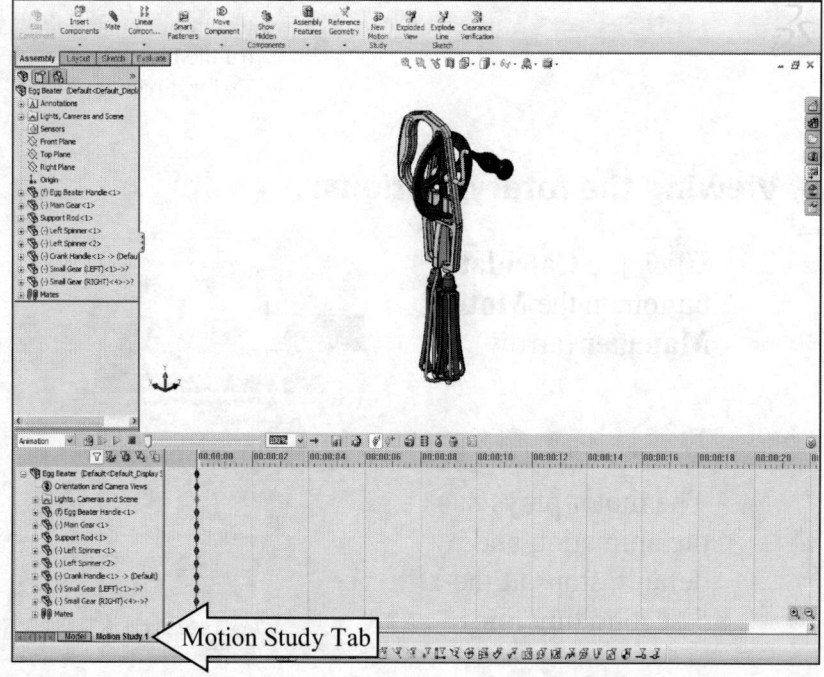

- Click the **Motion Study** tab to switch to the SolidWorks-Animation program (Motion Study1).

2. Adding a Rotary Motor:

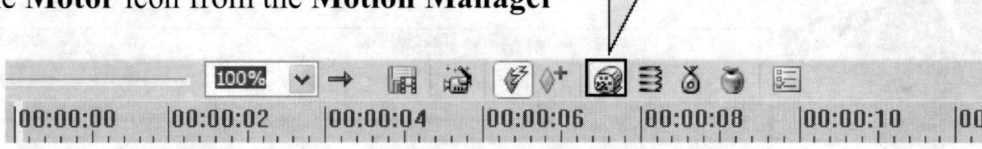

- Click the **Motor** icon from the **Motion Manager** toolbar.

- Under **Motion Type**, click the **Rotary Motor** option (arrow).

- Select the **Circular edge** of the Main Gear as indicated, for **Direction**.

- Click **Reverse direction** (arrow).

- Under **Motion**, select **Constant Speed**.

- Set the speed to: **30 RPM** (arrow).

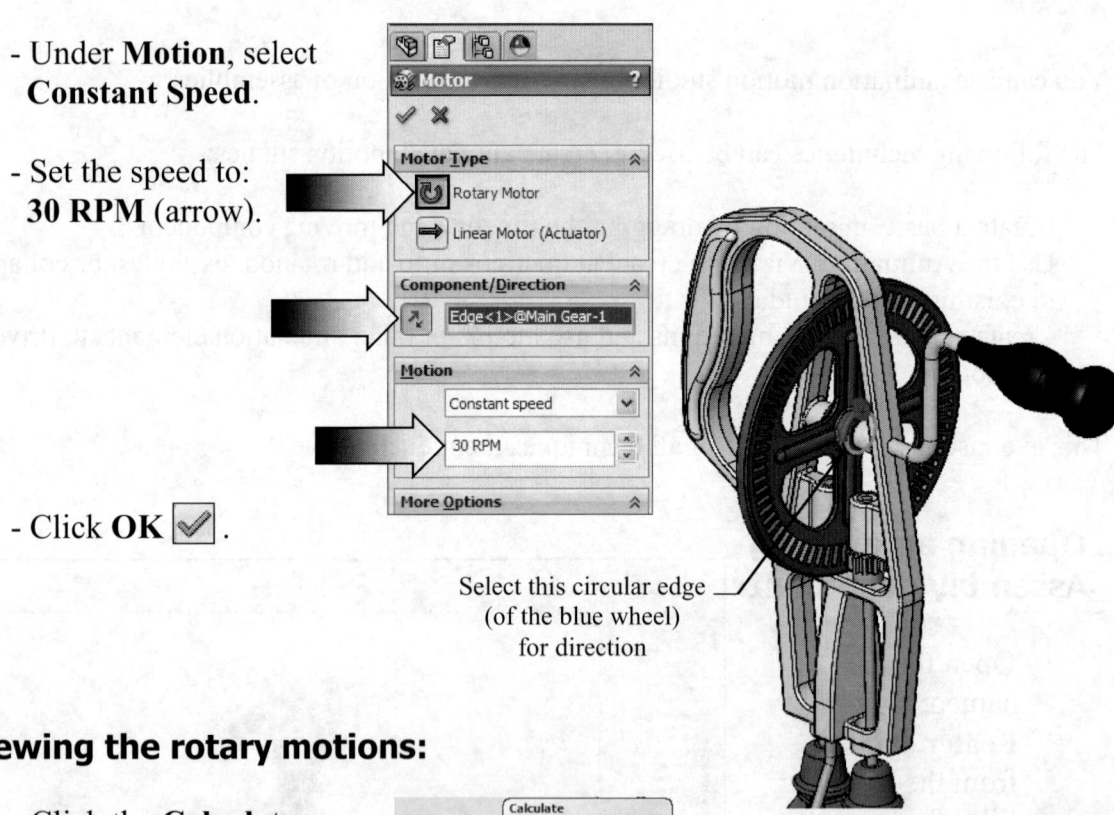

- Click **OK** .

Select this circular edge (of the blue wheel) for direction

3. Viewing the rotary motions:

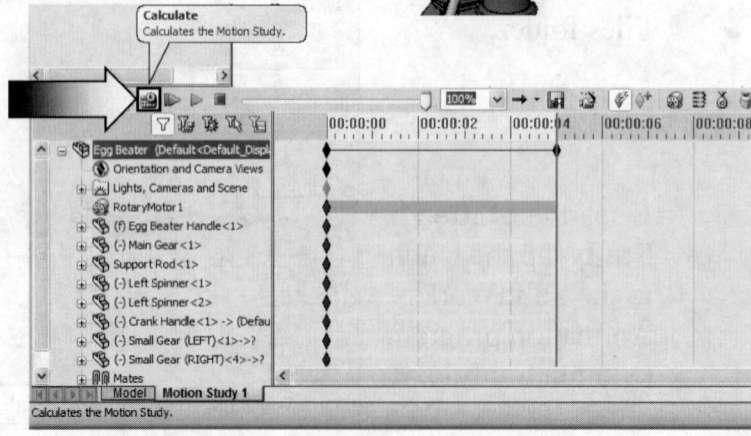

- Click the **Calculate** button on the **Motion Manager** (arrow).

- The motor plays back the animation and by default, stops at the 5-second timeline.

4. Using the Animation Wizard:

- Click the **Animation Wizard** button on the **Motion Manager** toolbar.

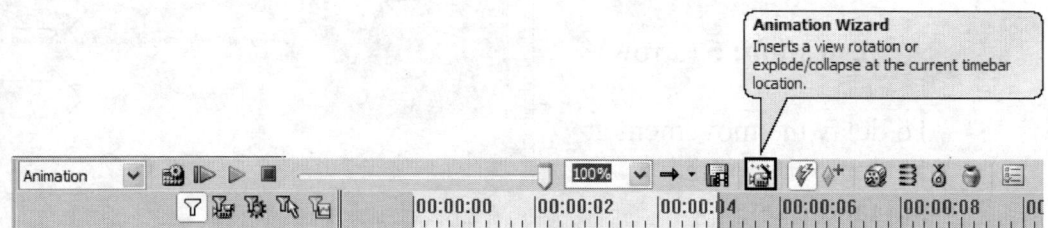

- Select the **Rotate Model** Option from the **Animate Type** dialog.

- As noted in this dialog box, in order to animate the Explode or Collapse of an assembly, an exploded view must be created prior to making the animation.

- Click **Next** Next > .

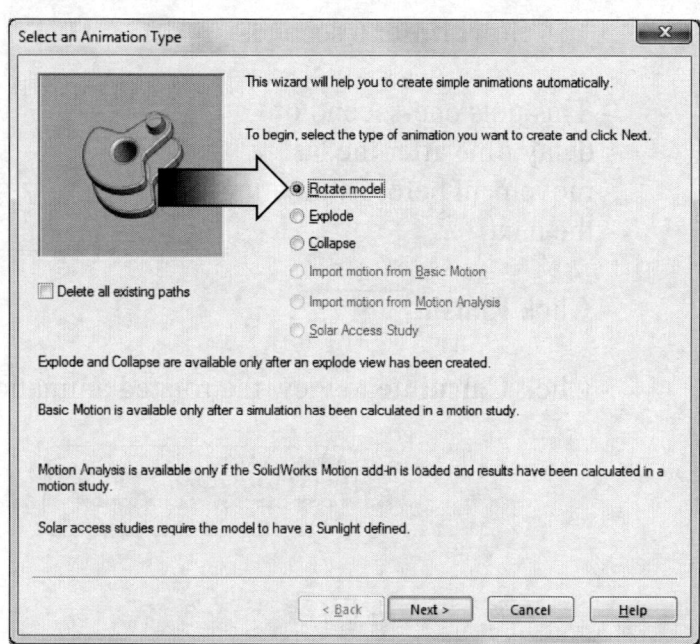

- For **Axis of Rotation**, select the **Y-axis**.

- For **Number of Rotation**, enter **1**.

- Select the **Clockwise** option.

- Click **Next** Next > .

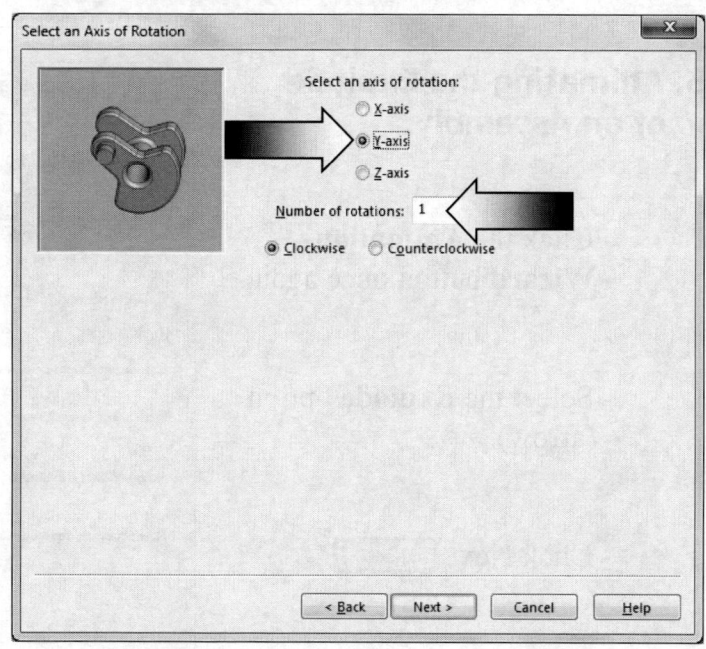

- To control the speed of the animation, the duration should be set (in seconds).

    * **Duration: 5** (arrow)

- To delay the movement at the beginning of the animation, set:

    * **Start time: 6** seconds

- This puts one-second of delay time after the last movement before animating the next.

- Click **Finish** Finish .

- Click **Calculate** to view the rotated animation.

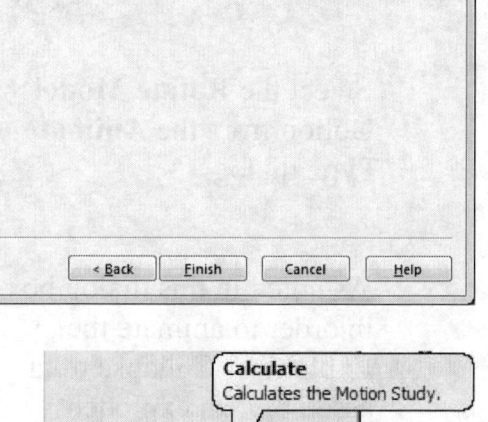

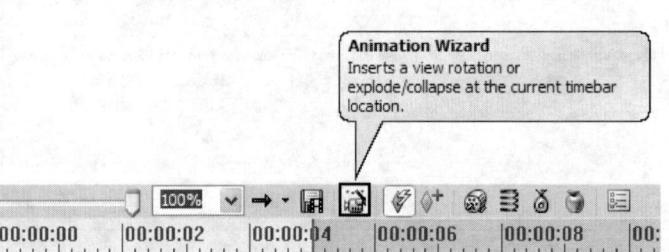

5. Animating the Explode of an Assembly:

- Click the **Animation-Wizard** button once again.

- Select the **Explode** option (arrow).

- Click **Next** Next > .

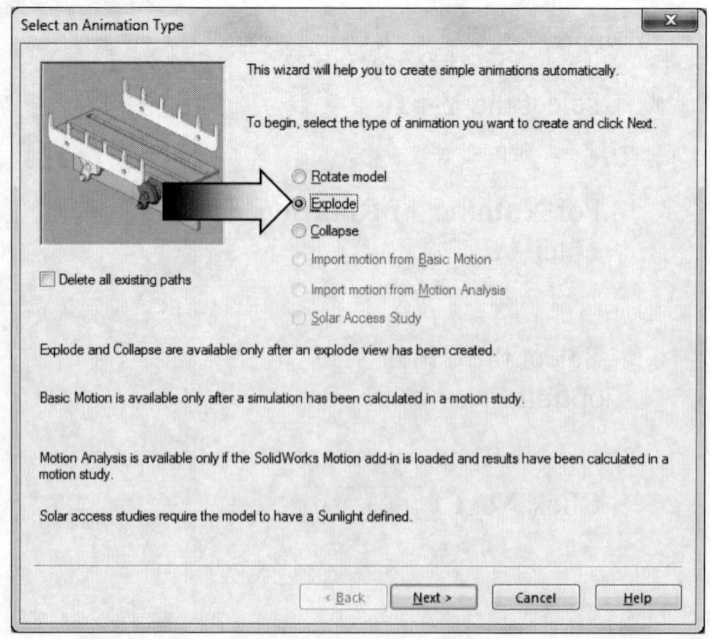

- Use the same speed as the last time

> * **Duration: 5 seconds** (arrow).

- Also put one-second of delay time at the end of the last movement.

> * **Start Time: 12 seconds** (arrow).

- Click **Finish** [Finish] .

- Click **Calculate** to view the new animated movements.

- To view the entire animation, click:

Play from Start.

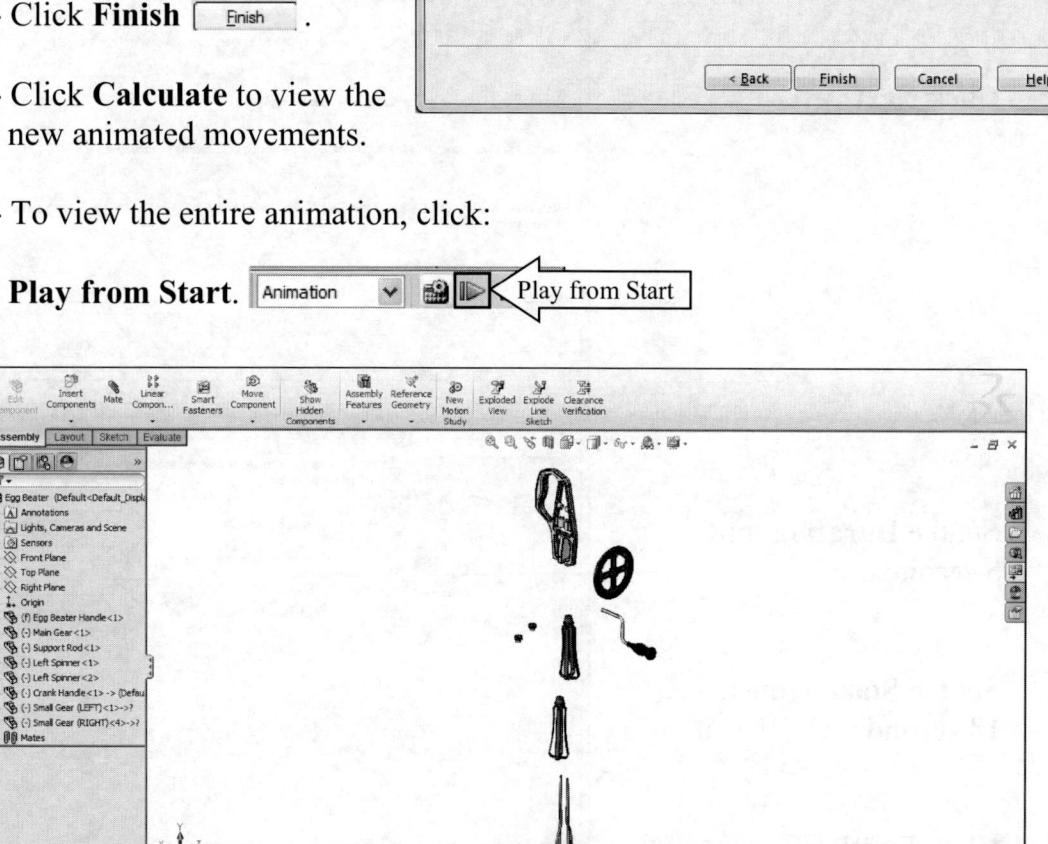

6. Animating the Collapse of the Assembly:

- Click the **Animation Wizard** button on the **Motion-Manager** toolbar.

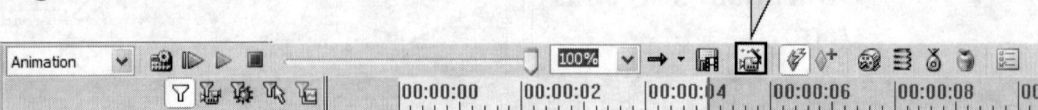

- Select the **Collapse** option from the **Animate Type** dialog.

- Click **Next** Next > .

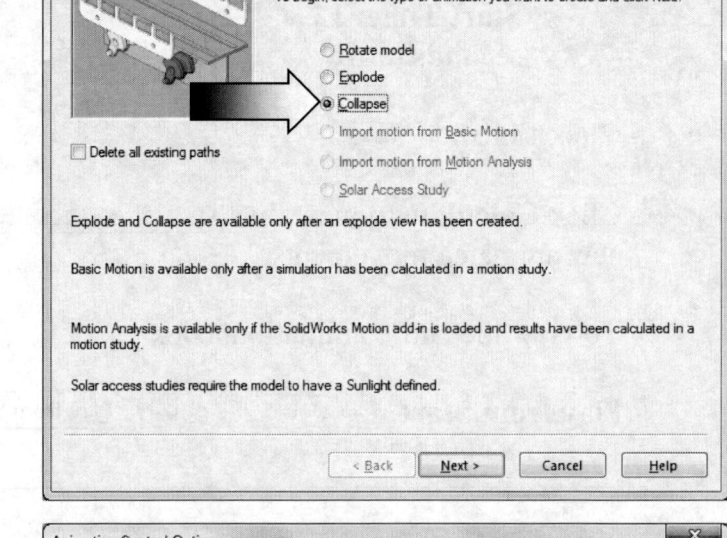

- Set the **Duration** to: **5 seconds**.

- Set the **Start Time** to: **18 seconds**.

- Click **Finish** Finish .

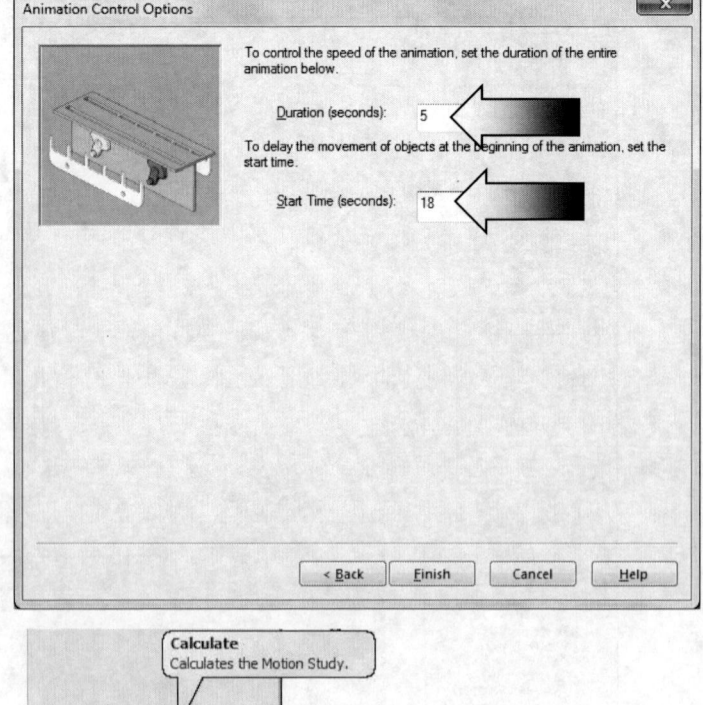

- Click **Calculate** to view the new animated movements.

- Click the **Play from Start** button
to view the entire animation.

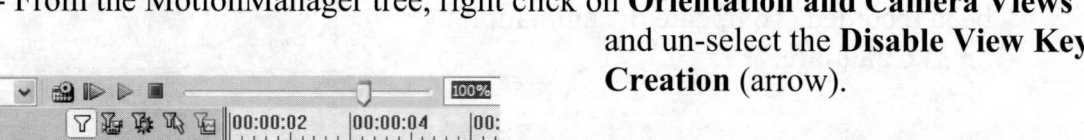

Notice the change in the view? We now need to change the view orientation.

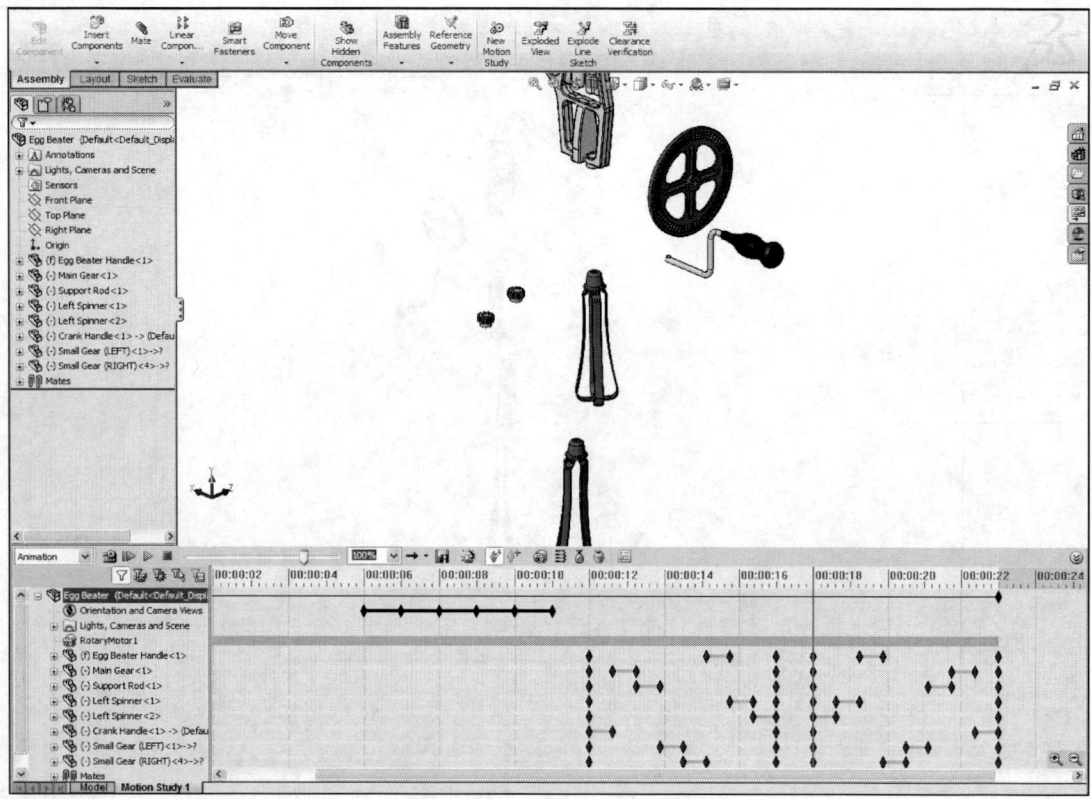

7. Changing the View Orientation of the assembly at 17-second:

- Drag the timeline to the **17-second position**.

- From the MotionManager tree, right click on **Orientation and Camera Views** and un-select the **Disable View Key Creation** (arrow).

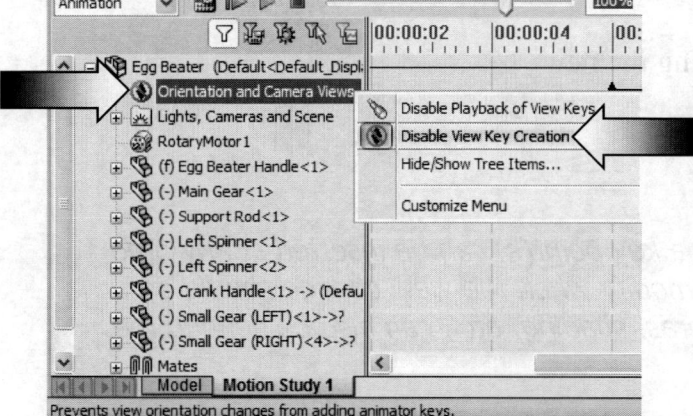

- Click the **Add/Update Key** (below).

- This key will allow modifications to the steps recorded earlier.

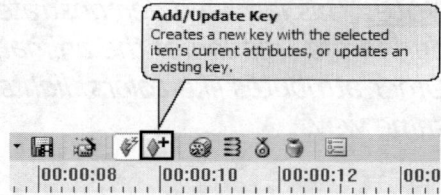

Add/Update Key
Creates a new key with the selected item's current attributes, or updates an existing key.

- Press the **F** key on the keyboard to change to the full screen – or – click Zoom to fit.

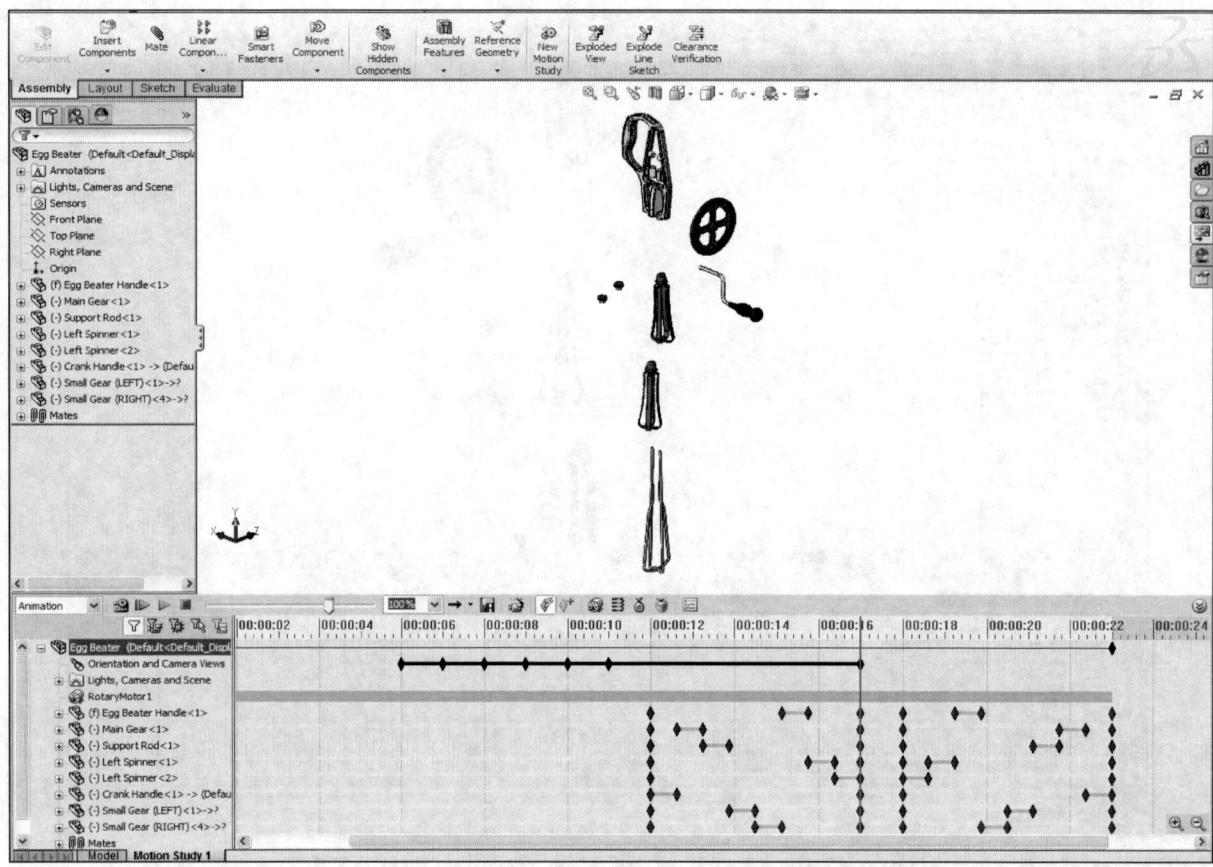

- The change in the view orientation from a zoomed-in position to a full-screen has just been recorded. To update the animation, press **Calculate.**

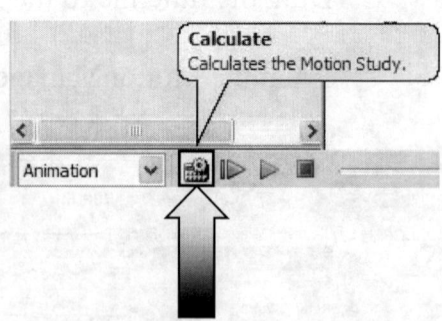

- The animation plays back showing the new Zoomed position.

<u>Note:</u> *This last step demonstrated that a key point(s) can be inserted at any time during the creation of the animation to modify when the view change should occur. Other attributes like colors, lights, cameras, shading, etc., can also be defined the same way.*

- When the animation reaches the 23 second timeline, the assembly is shown as collapsed. We'll need to add another key and change the view orientation to full screen once again.

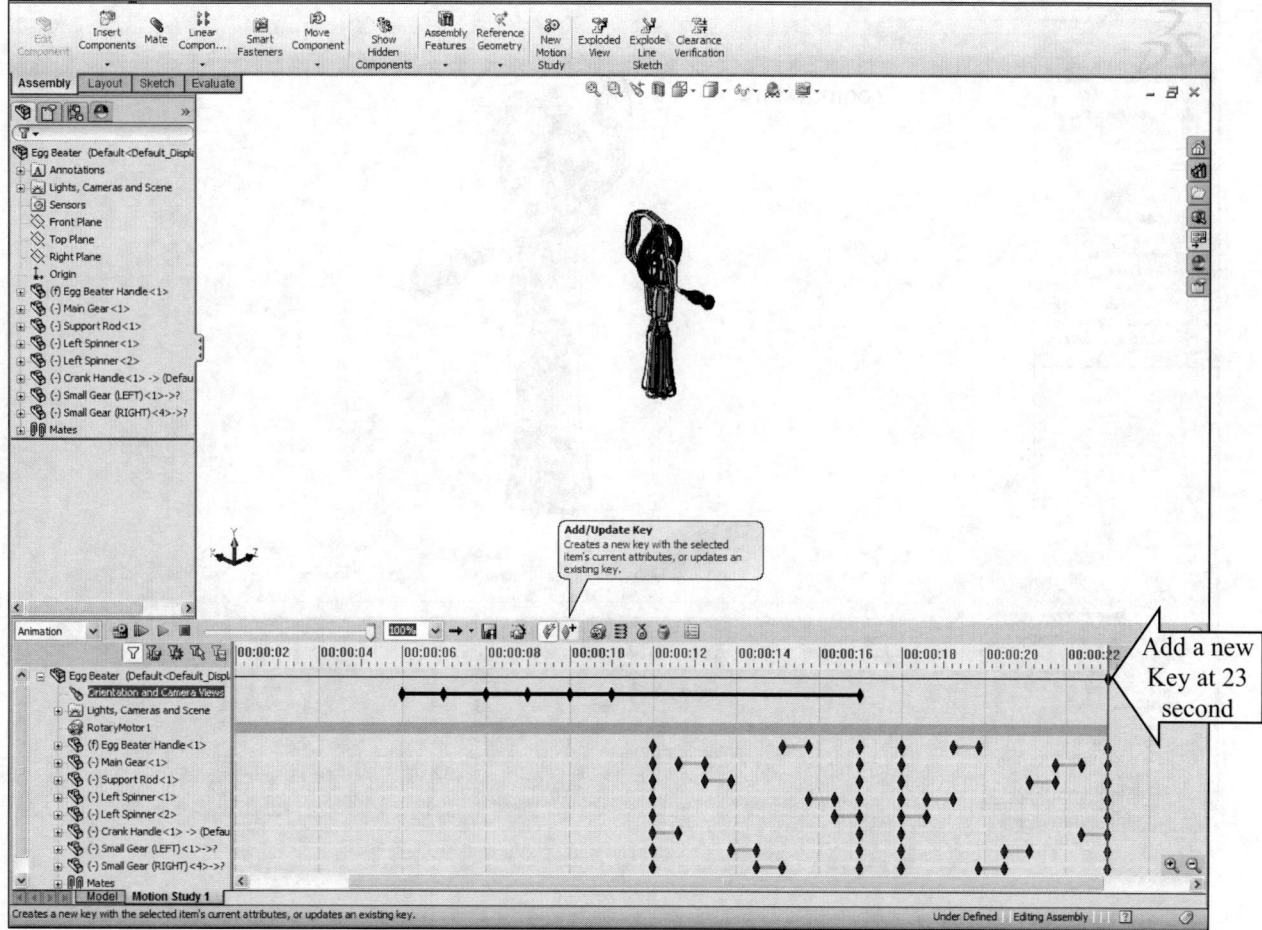

8. Changing the View Orientation of the Assembly at 23 second:

- Make sure the timeline is moved to the **23 second position**.

- Click the **Add/Update Key** button on the MotionManager toolbar.

Note:

In order to capture the changes in different positions, a new key should be added each time. We will need to go back to the full screen so that more details can be viewed.

- Press the **F** key on the keyboard to change to the full screen – or – click Zoom to fit.

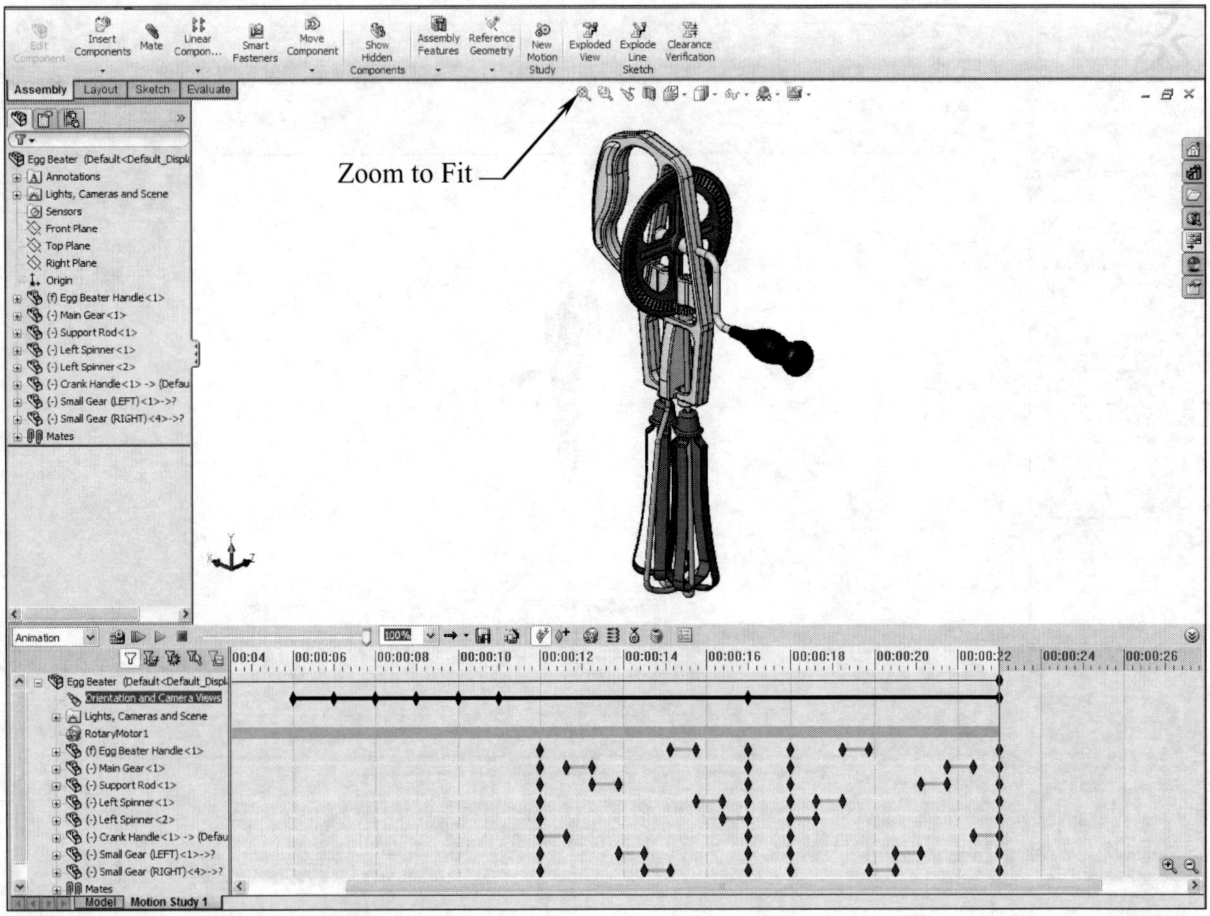

Zoom to Fit

- Similar to the previous step, the change in the view orientation has just been captured.

- To update the animation, press **Calculate.**

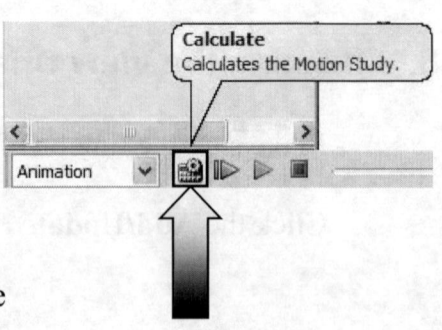

Calculate
Calculates the Motion Study.

Animation

- The system plays back the animation showing the new zoom to fit position.

- Save your work before going to the next steps.

9. Creating the Flashing effects:

- Move the timeline to the **3-second position**.

- Click the **Add/Update Key** button.

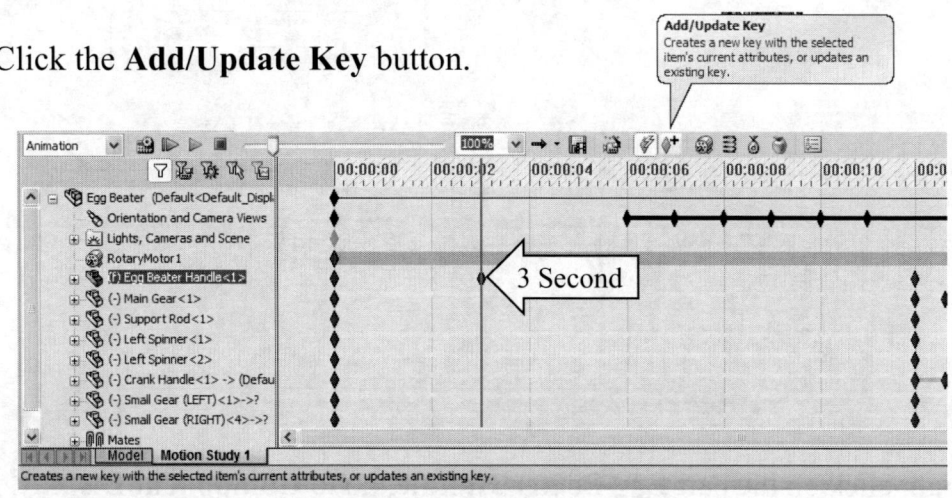

- We are going to make the Handle flash 3 times.

- Right click the part **Egg-Beater-Handle** from the Animation tree, go to **Component Display** and select **Wireframe**.

- Click **Calculate** .

- At this point, the Handle turns into Wireframe when the animation reaches the 3 second timeline and stays that way until the end.

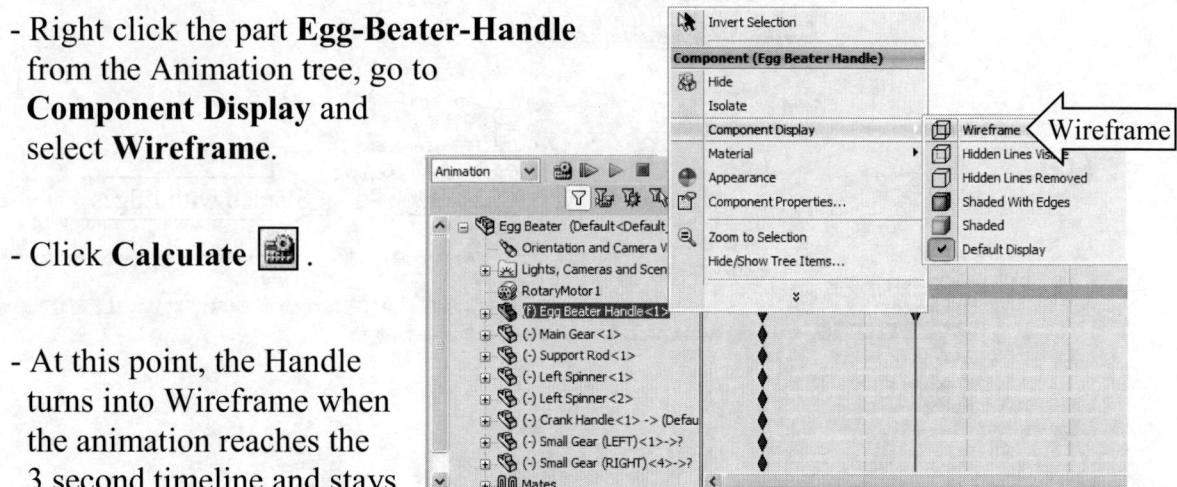

- Hover the cursor over the key point to display its key properties.

Place the mouse cursor over this key

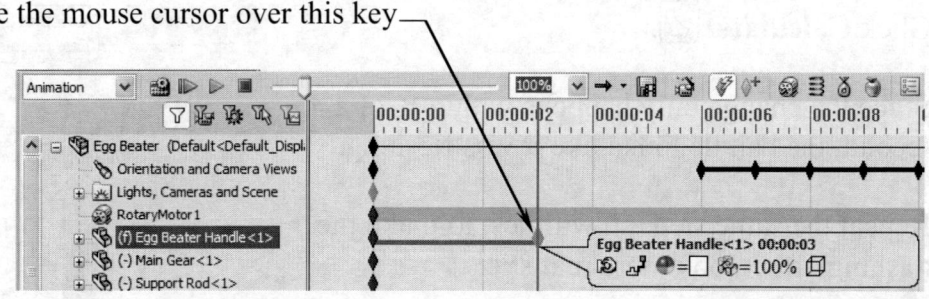

- Next, move the timeline to the **3.5 second position**.

- This time we are going to change the Handle back to shaded mode.

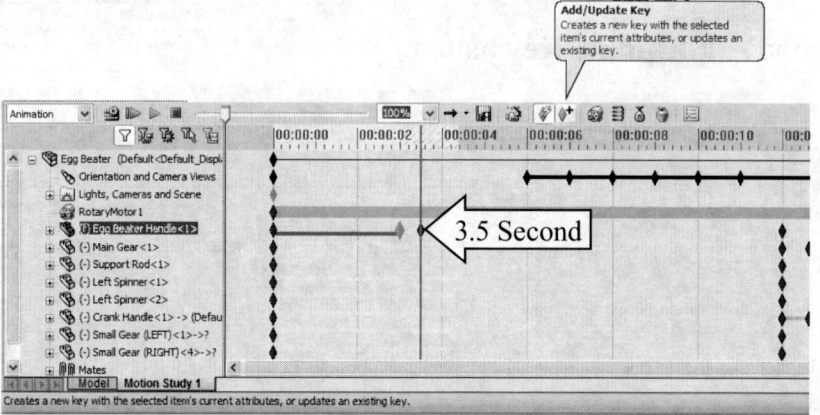

- Right click on the part **Egg Beater Handle**, go to **Component Display**, and select **Shaded with Edges**.

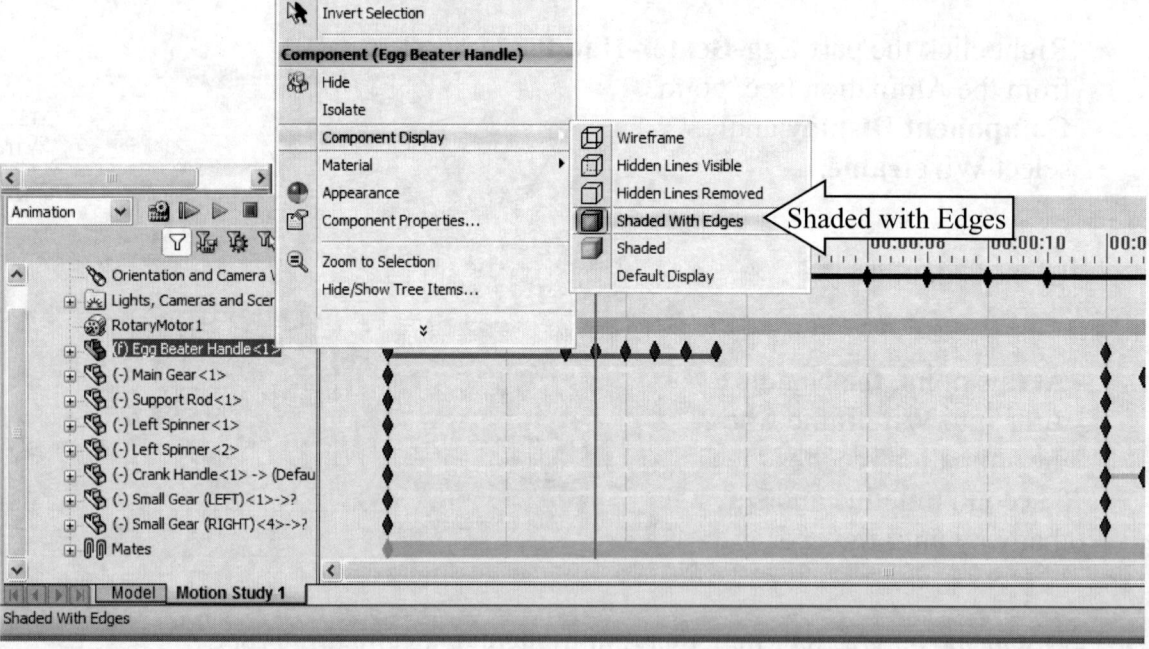

- Click **Calculate** .

- Since the change only happens within ½ of a second, the handle looks like it was flashing.

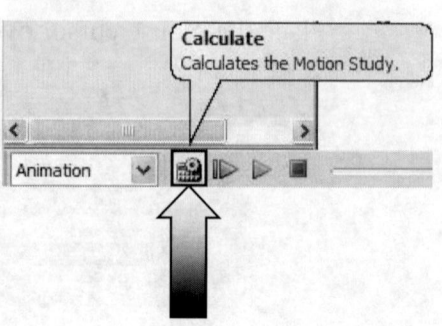

- Repeat the same step a few times, to make the flashing effect look more realistic.

4-second = Wireframe

3.5-second = Shaded with Edges

3-second = Wireframe

4.5-second = Wireframe

5-second = Shaded with Edges

5.5-second = Wireframe

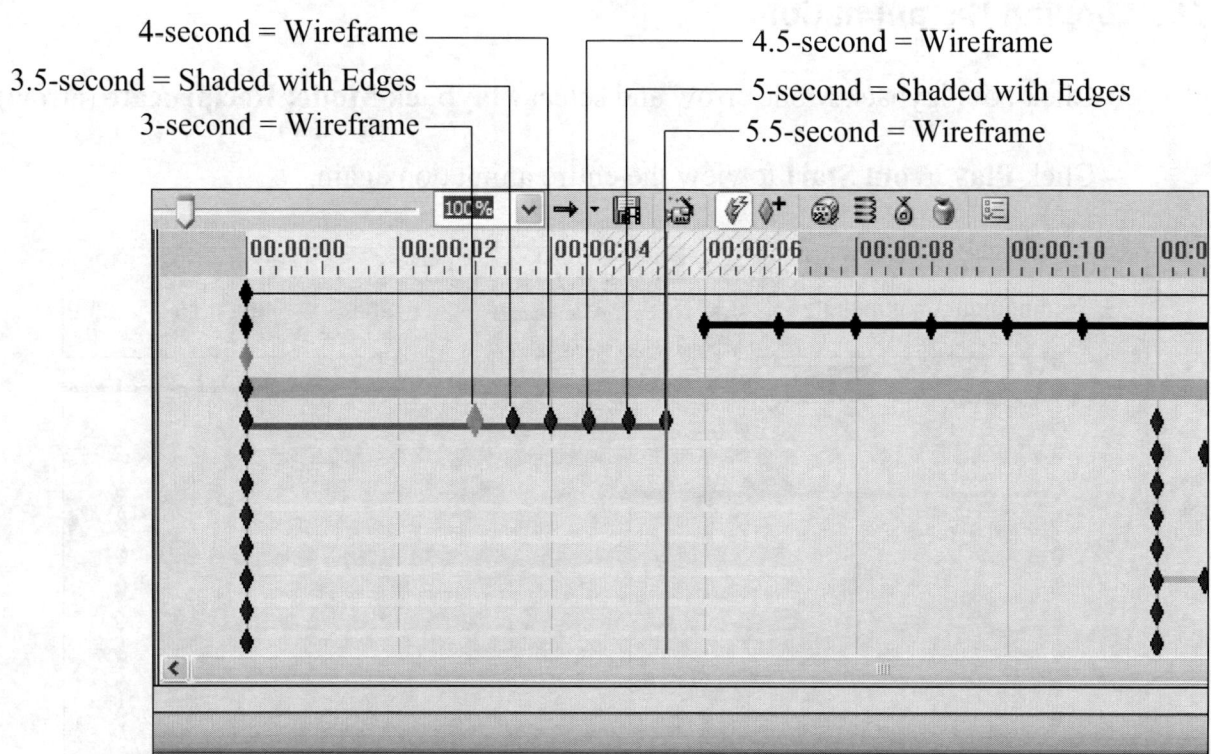

- Use the times chart listed above and repeat step number 9 at least 3 more times.

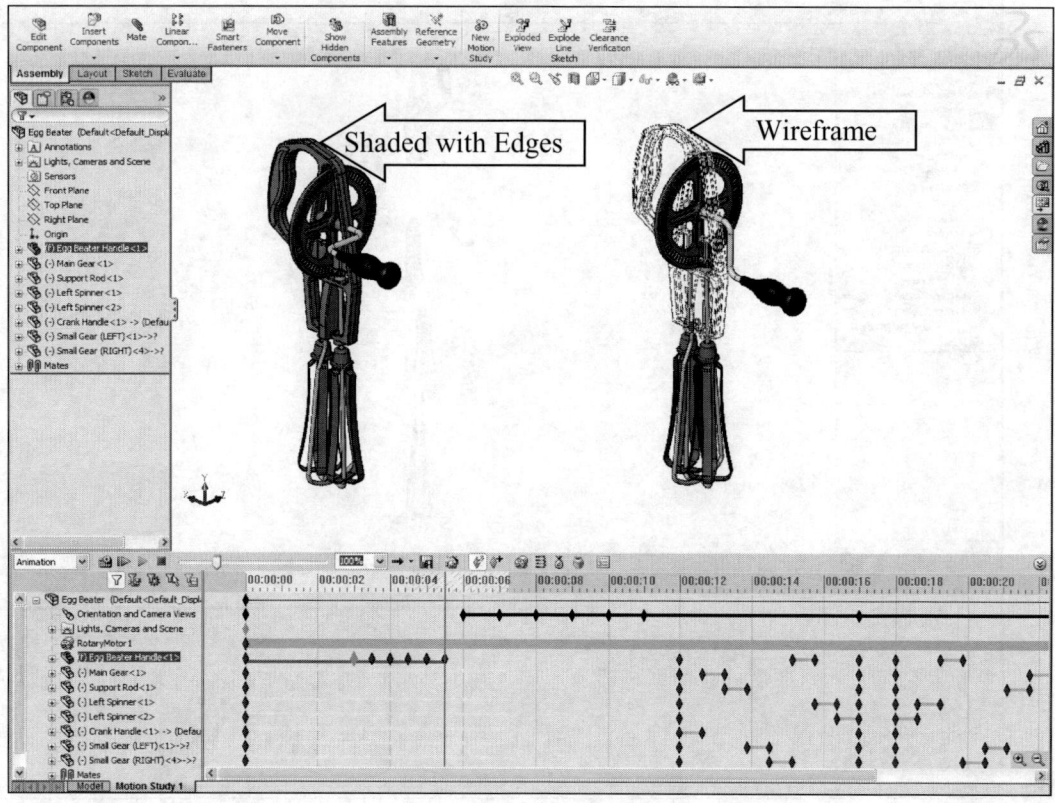

Shaded with Edges

Wireframe

10. Looping the animation:

- Click the Playback Mode arrow and select **Playback Mode: Reciprocate** (arrow).

- Click **Play From Start** to view the entire animation again.

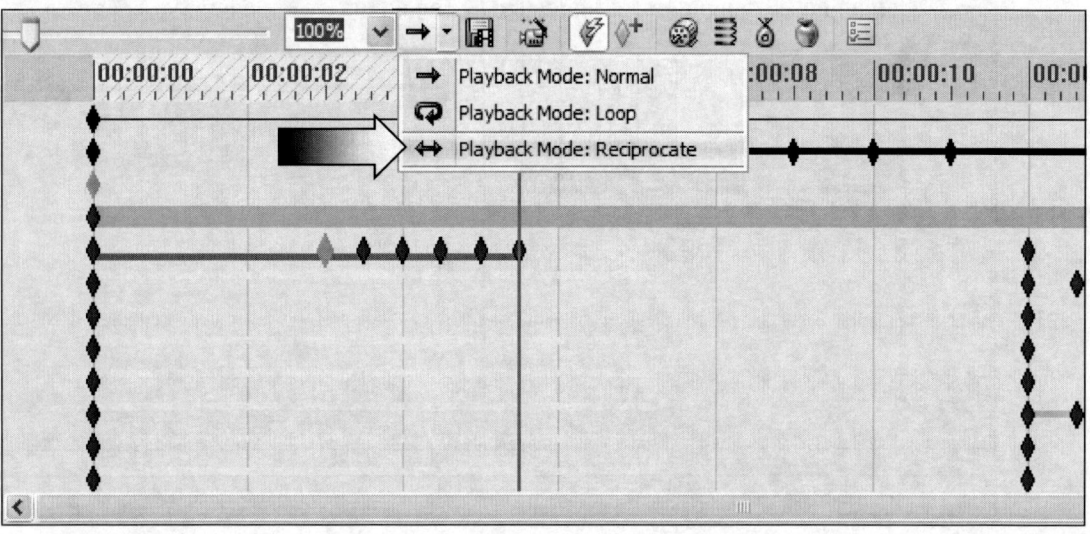

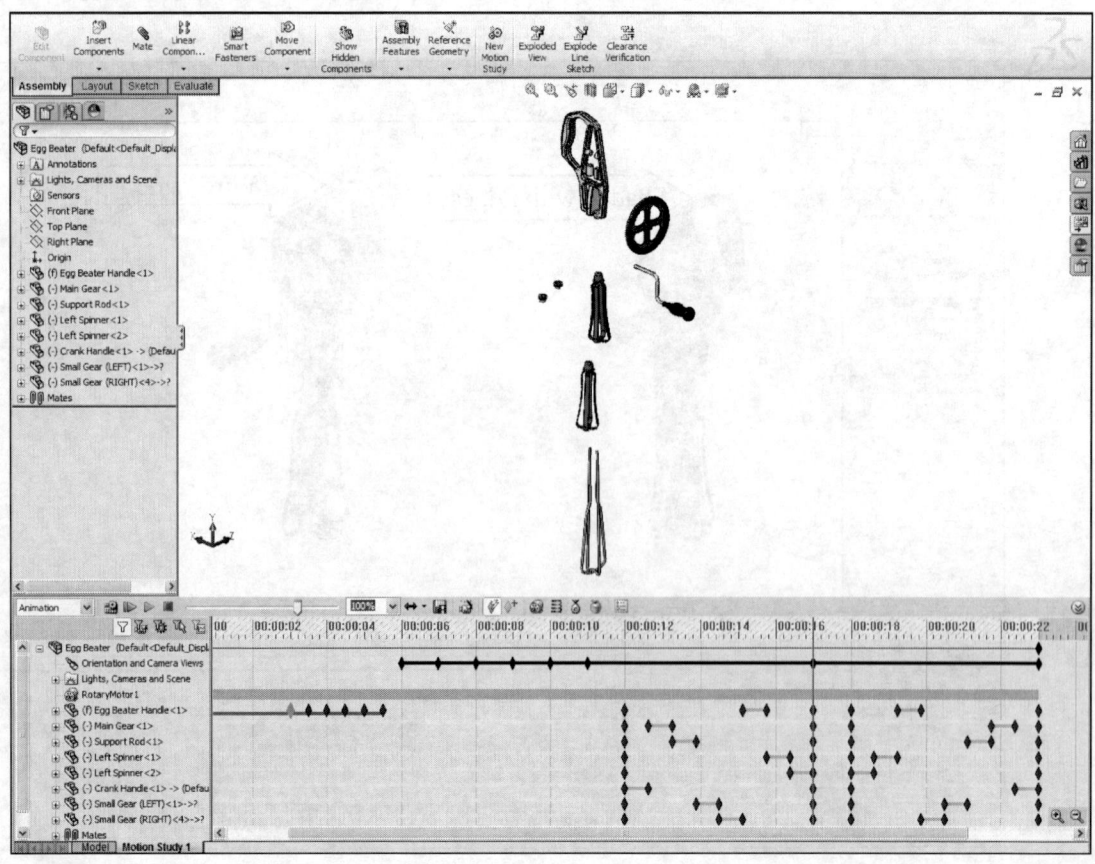

11. **Saving the animation as AVI:** (Audio Visual Interleaving):

- Click the **Save Animation** icon on the Motion Manager toolbar.

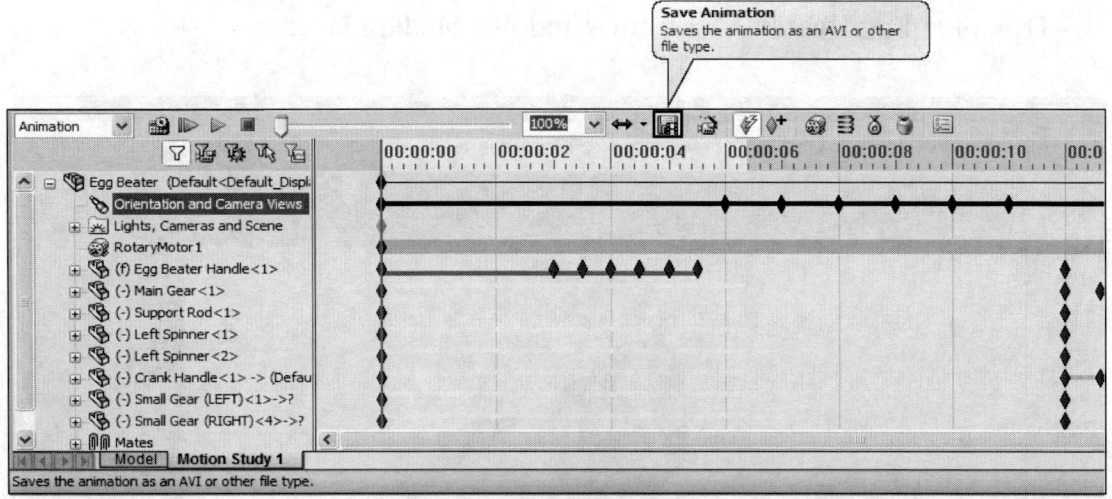

- Use the default name (Egg Beater) and other default settings.

- Click **Save**.

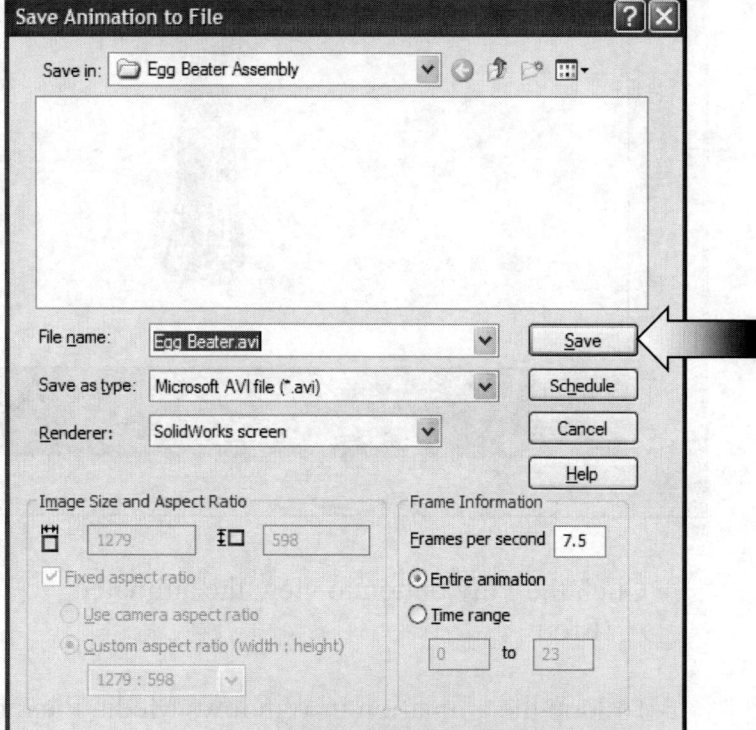

- The **Image Size** and **Aspect Ratio** (grayed-out) adjusts size and shape of the display. It becomes available when the renderer is PhotoWorks buffer.

- **Compression** ratios impact image quality. Use lower compression ratios to produce smaller file sizes of lesser image quality.

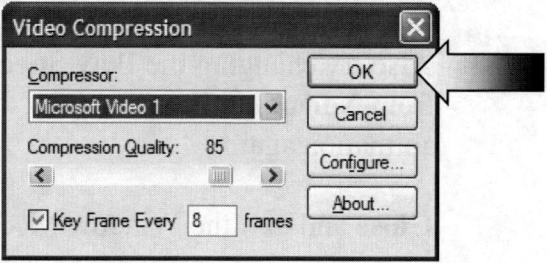

12. Viewing the Egg Beater AVI with Windows Media Player:

- **Exit** the SolidWorks program, locate and launch your **Windows Media Player**.

- **Open** the **Egg Beater.AVI** from Windows Media Player.

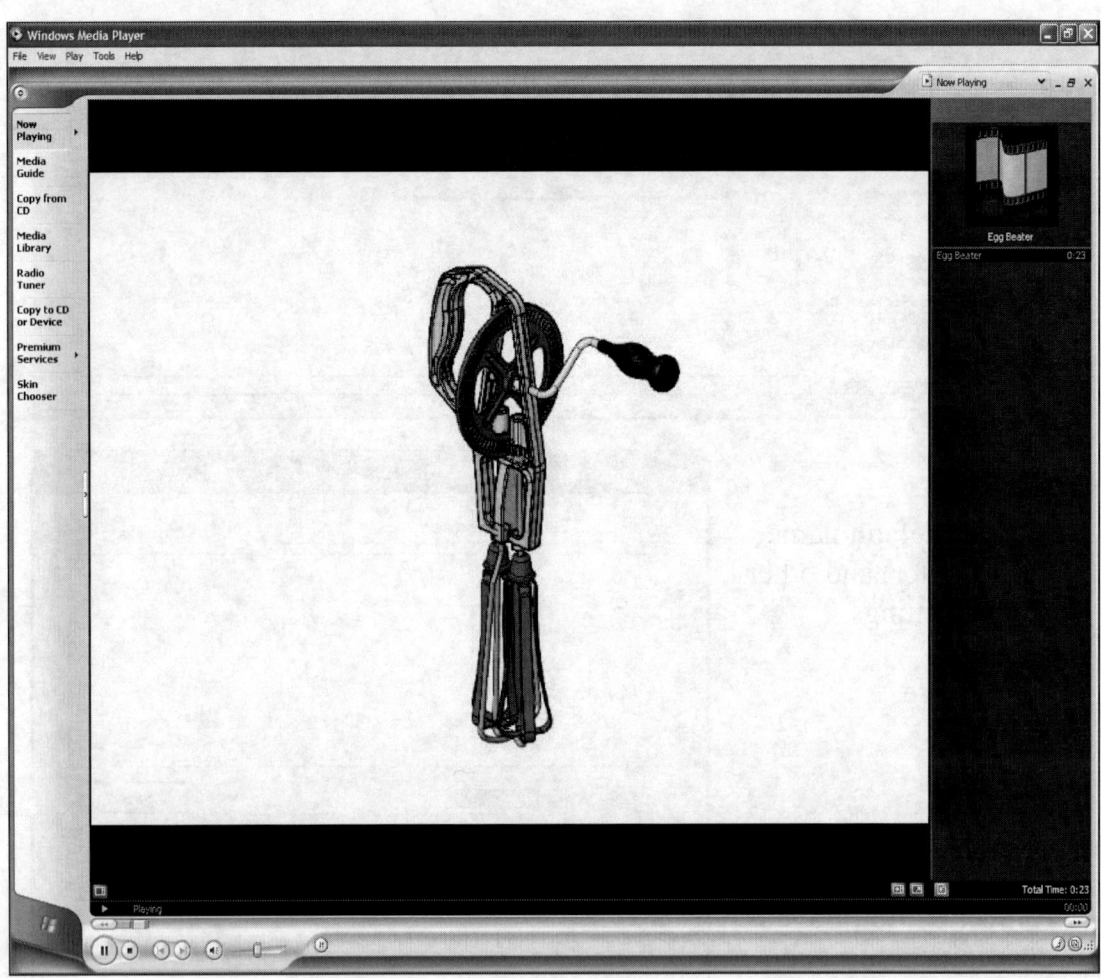

- Click the **Play** button to view the animated AVI file.

- To loop the animation in Windows Media Player, select **Repeat** from the Play dropdown menu.

- Also try changing the **Play Speed** from **Normal** to **Fast** and Play the animation again.

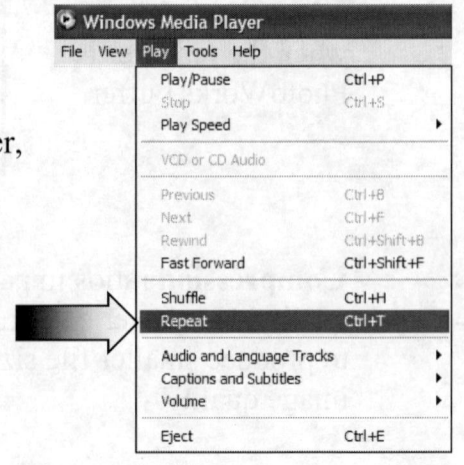

- **Close** and **exit** the Window Media Player.

CHAPTER 13

Working with Sketch Pictures

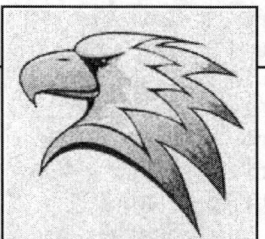

Working with Sketch Pictures
Using the Spline tool

- A digital image can be used as a reference to model a part. Each image can be placed on its own planes, so several images can be inserted to help define the shape of the model from different orientations.

- The formats such as jpg, tif, bmp, gif, png, etc., are supported in SolidWorks. They can be inserted and converted into a sketch, so that a feature can be made from it.

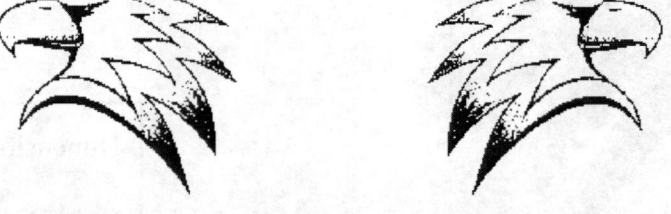

- When scanning or saving the digital images, it is best to use fine resolution and high contrast pictures. Sketching over the sharp edges would be so much easier than the blurry edges.

- Splines are often used to do the tracing of the images due to its flexibilities in manipulating the shapes, and splines offer a set of control tools to assist you with creating and maintaining the smoothness of the curves.

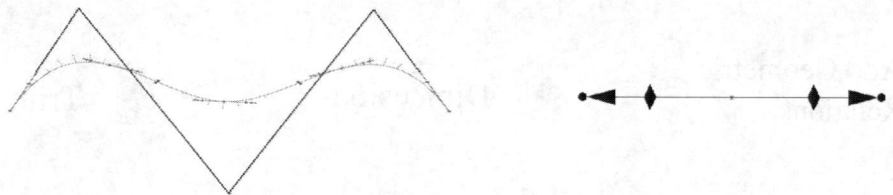

- The digital or scanned image can be scaled to size and repositioned with reference to the origin so that dimensions can be added for accuracy.

Working with Sketch Pictures
Using Splines

View Orientation Hot Keys:

Ctrl + 1 = Front View
Ctrl + 2 = Back View
Ctrl + 3 = Left View
Ctrl + 4 = Right View
Ctrl + 5 = Top View
Ctrl + 6 = Bottom View
Ctrl + 7 = Isometric View
Ctrl + 8 = Normal To
          Selection

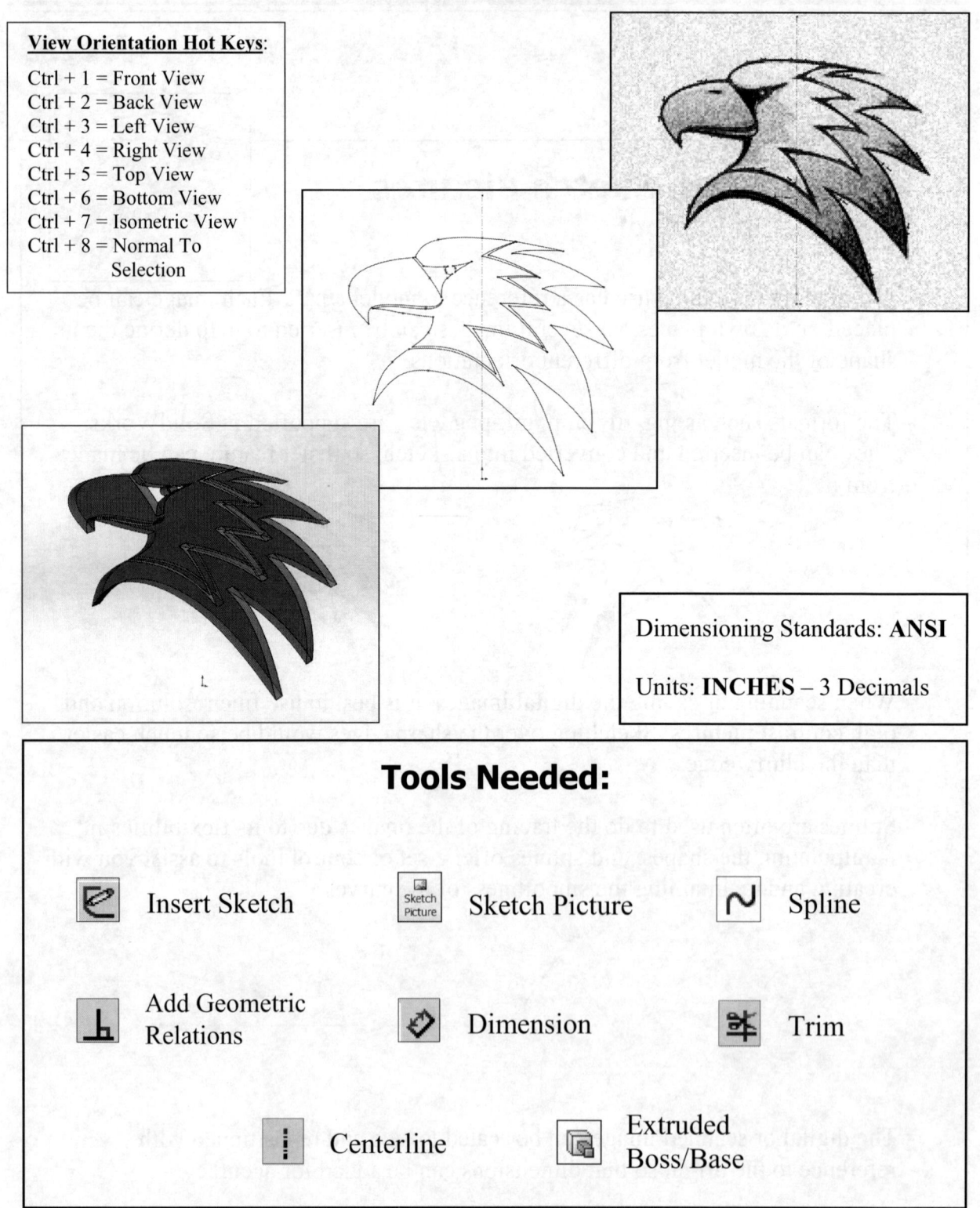

Dimensioning Standards: **ANSI**

Units: **INCHES** – 3 Decimals

Tools Needed:

Insert Sketch	Sketch Picture	Spline
Add Geometric Relations	Dimension	Trim
Centerline	Extruded Boss/Base	

1. Inserting the scanned image:

     - The scanned image must be inserted into an active sketch.

     - Select the <u>Front</u> plane and open a new sketch.

     - From the **Tools** menu, click **Sketch Tools / Sketch Picture**.

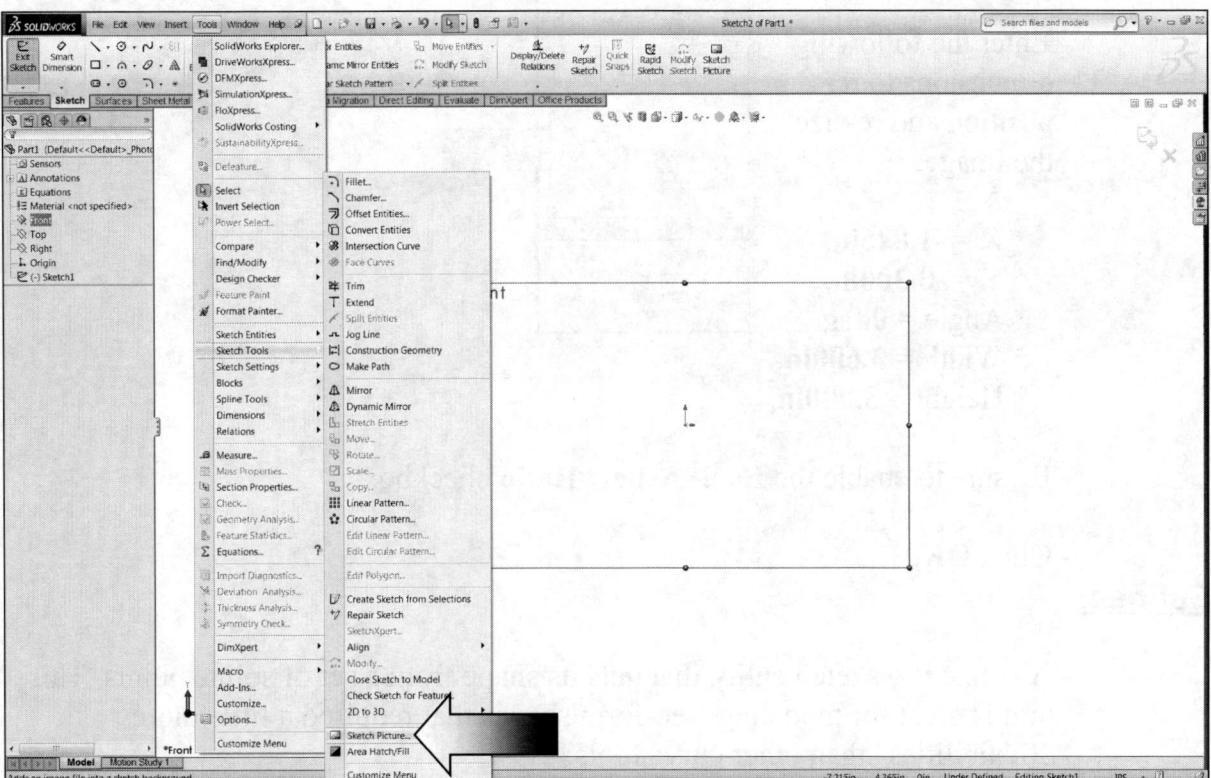

     - Browse to the Training Files folder and select the file named: **Eagle Head.jpg** and open it.

     - The lower left corner of the image is placed on the origin.

     - The image size and locations appear on the properties tree; we will modify those dimensions in the next step.

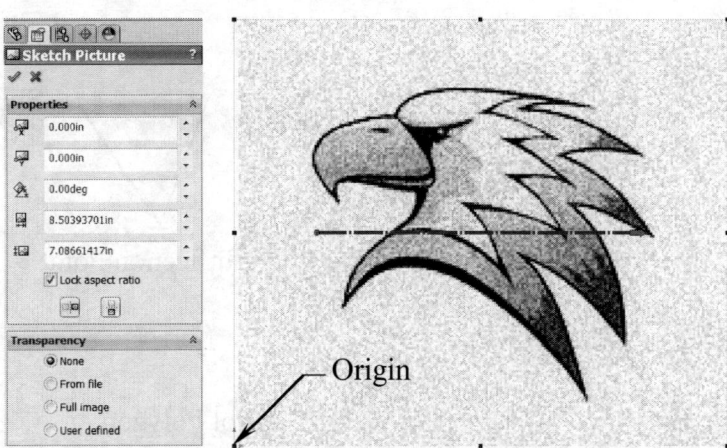

2. Positioning and sizing the scanned image:

- Sketch a **vertical centerline** to help center the image

- Double click the image to activate it.

- Enter the following dimensions to re-position and re-size the image:

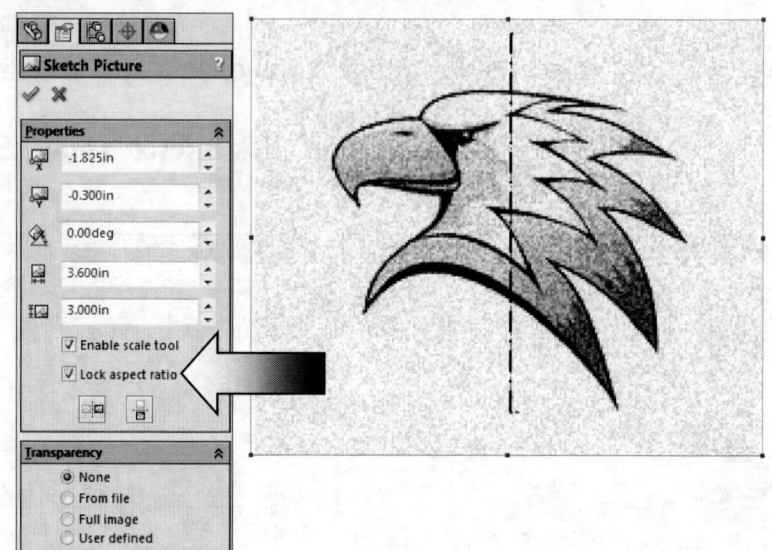

    * X = **-1.825in**.
    * Y = **-0.300in**.
    * Angle = **0deg**.
    * Width = **3.600in**.
    * Height = **3.000in**.

- Be sure to enable the **Lock Aspect Ratio** checkbox.

- Click **OK**.

Splines:

- A spline is a sketch entity that gets its shape from a set of spline points. This tool is great for modeling free-form shapes that required a little more "flexibilities" than other curve tools.

- During the creation of a spline, each click creates a spline point and these points can be added or deleted when needed.

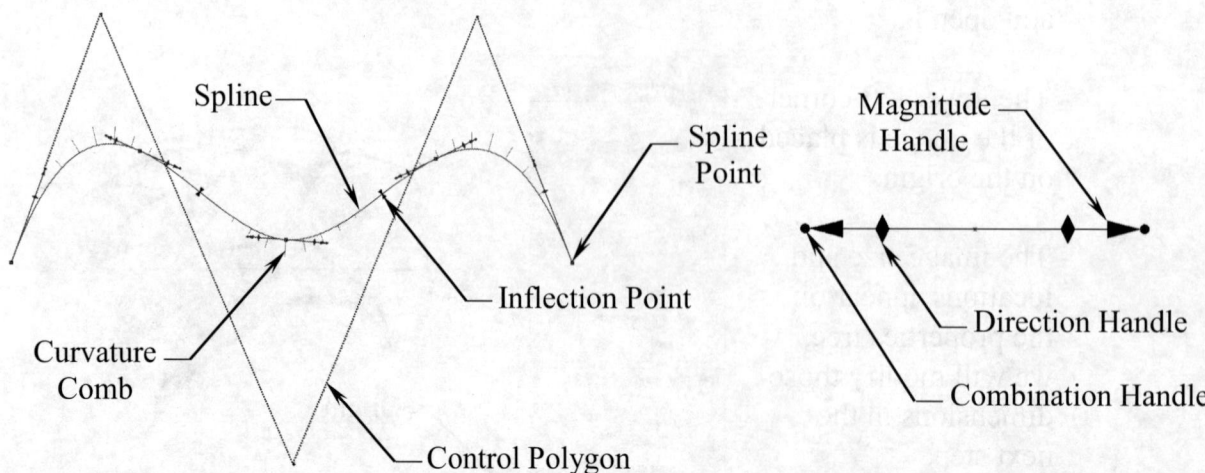

- Try to use as few spline points as possible in the general, long curving areas. Only use more spline points on tighter, smaller radiuses.

- Use the spline handles to drag freely, or hold the ALT key to drag symmetrically. The spline handles are used to change the direction and magnitude of the tangency at a spine point.

- Use the Control Polygons in place of the spline handles. Drag its control points to manipulate the spline.

- The Curvature Combs displays the curvature of the spline in a form of a series of lines called a comb. The length of the lines represents the curvature. The longer the line, the larger the curvature, and smaller the radius.

- Inflection Points or Markers are used to show where the inflection changes in a spline, whether it is convex or concave.

3. Tracing the image with the spline tool:

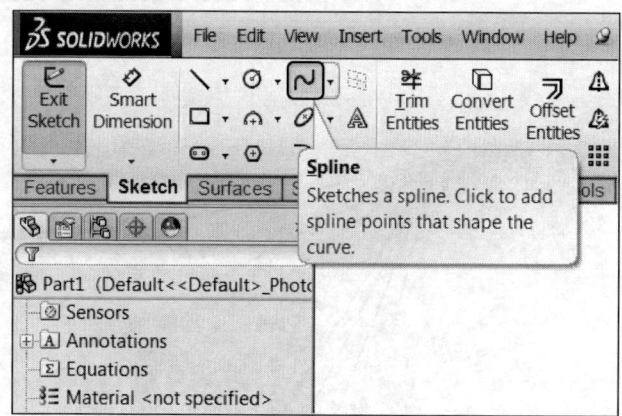

- The sketch should still be active at this time, select the Spline command from the Sketch toolbar.

- Keep in mind that the simpler the spline, the easier to manipulate it. So we are going to create one spline with two or three spline points each time, and then adjust it to match the outline of the image as closely as possible. (Zoom in a little closer).

- Start at "point 1", and "point 2", then "point 3" as indicated.

- Push the **Escape** key when done.

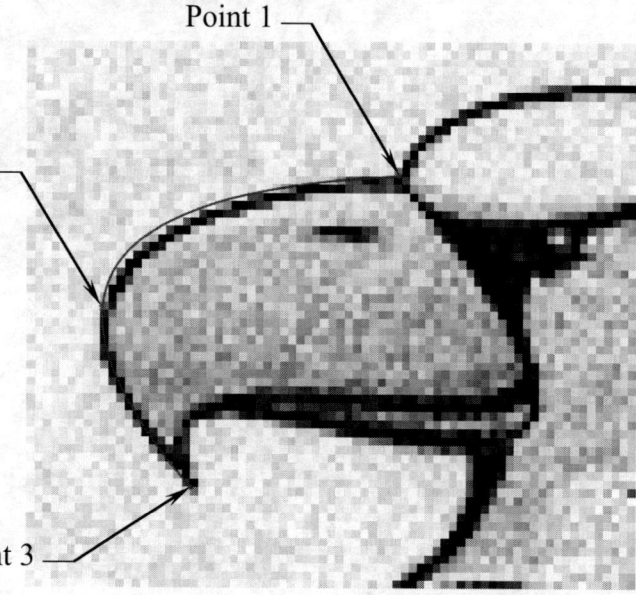

- Zoom in even closer so that You can adjust the spline a little easier.

Drag the Spline-Handles to adjust the curvature

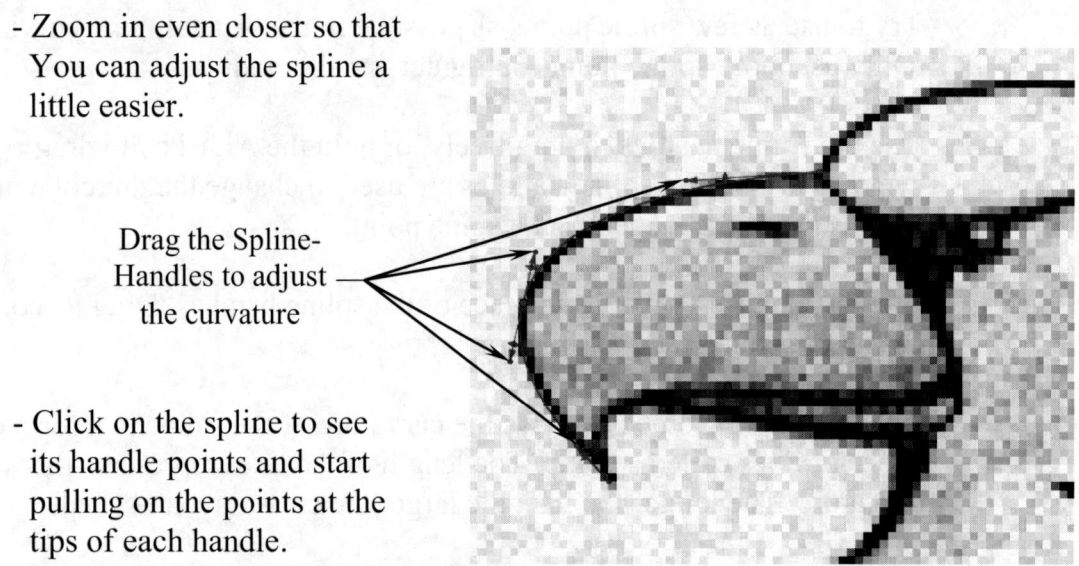

- Click on the spline to see its handle points and start pulling on the points at the tips of each handle.

- It may take some getting used to, so work on a small area each time. Create only one spline each time, and each spline should have two or three points only.

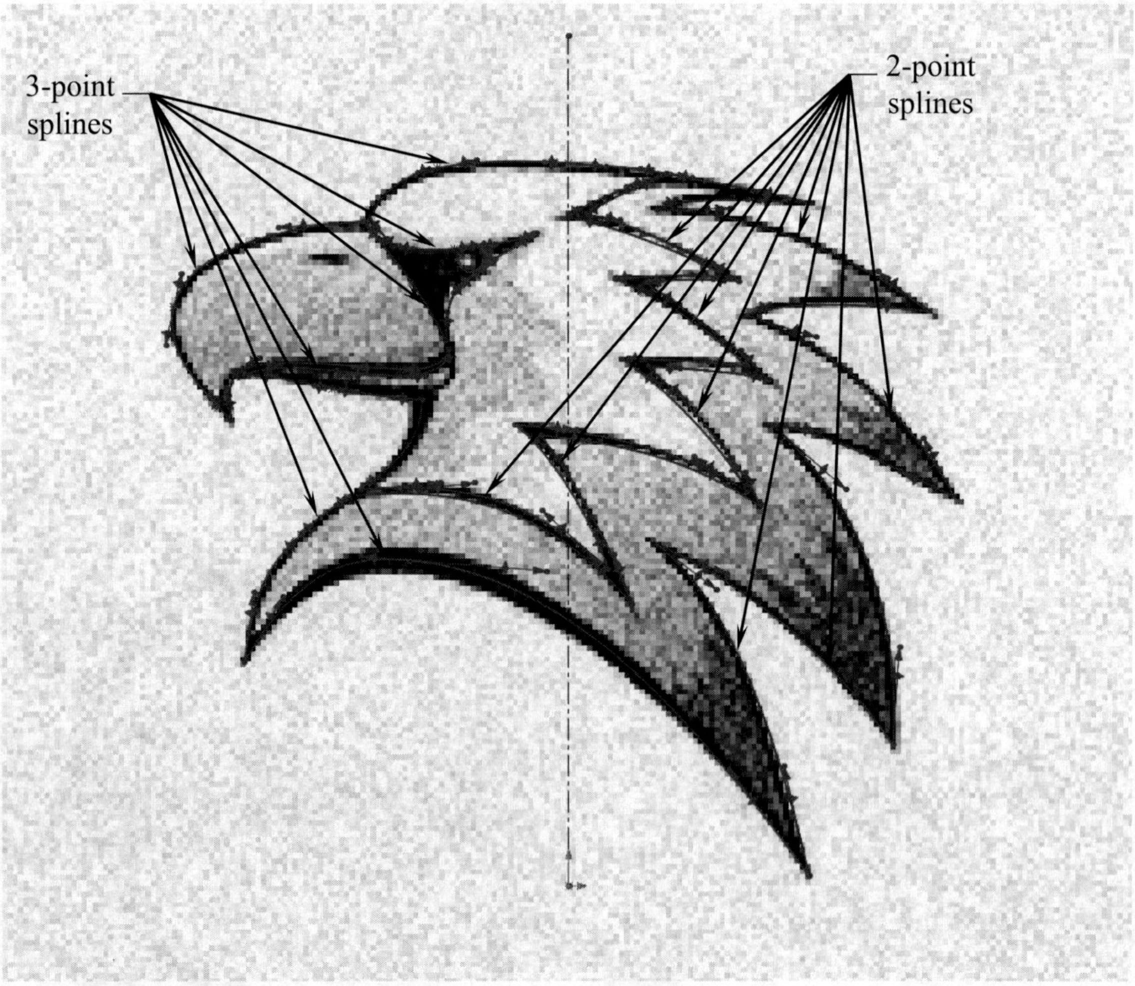

3-point splines

2-point splines

- There should be a small gap
  around the sketch (as noted),
  so that a single sketch
  can be extruded
  into a feature.

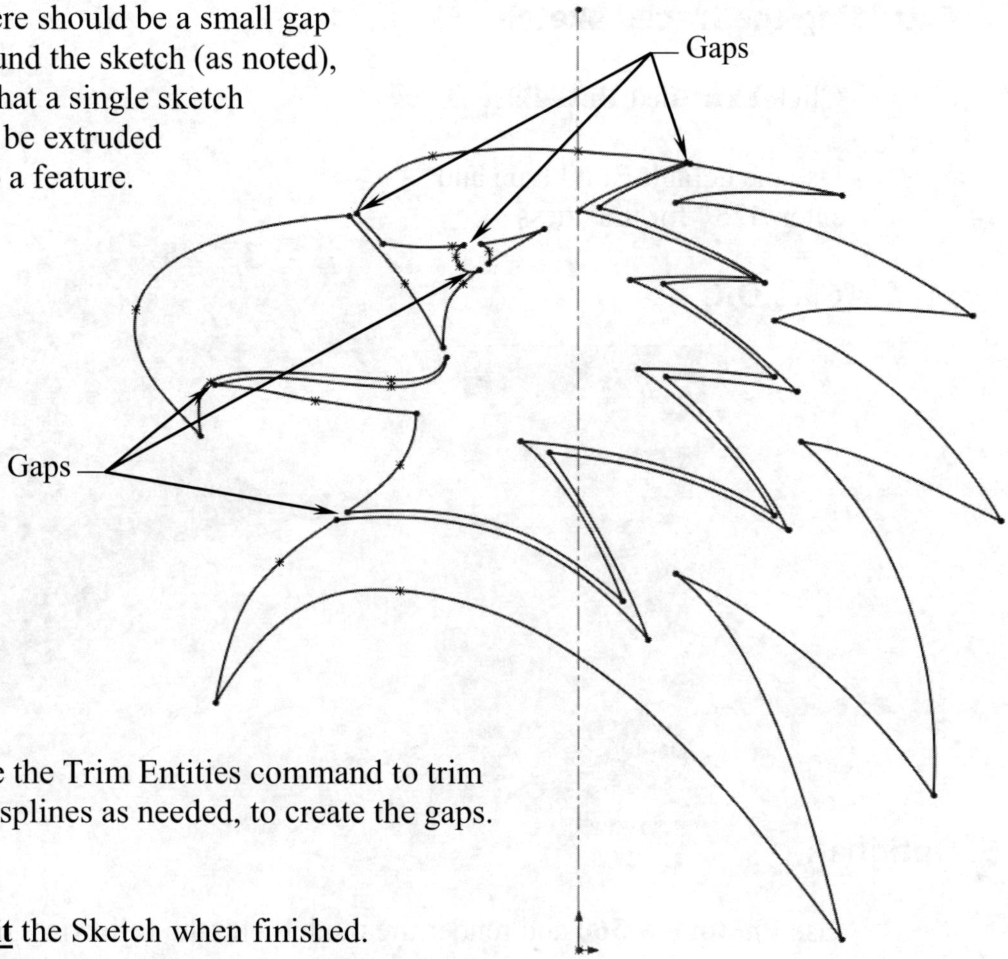

Gaps

Gaps

- Use the Trim Entities command to trim
  the splines as needed, to create the gaps.

- **Exit** the Sketch when finished.

- Expand the Sketch1 from the tree and
  Suppress the Sketch Picture.

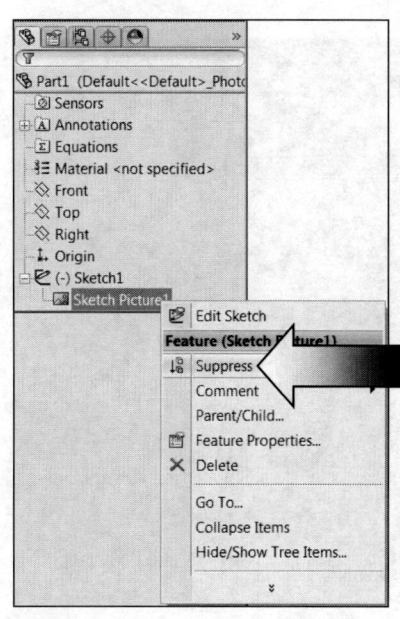

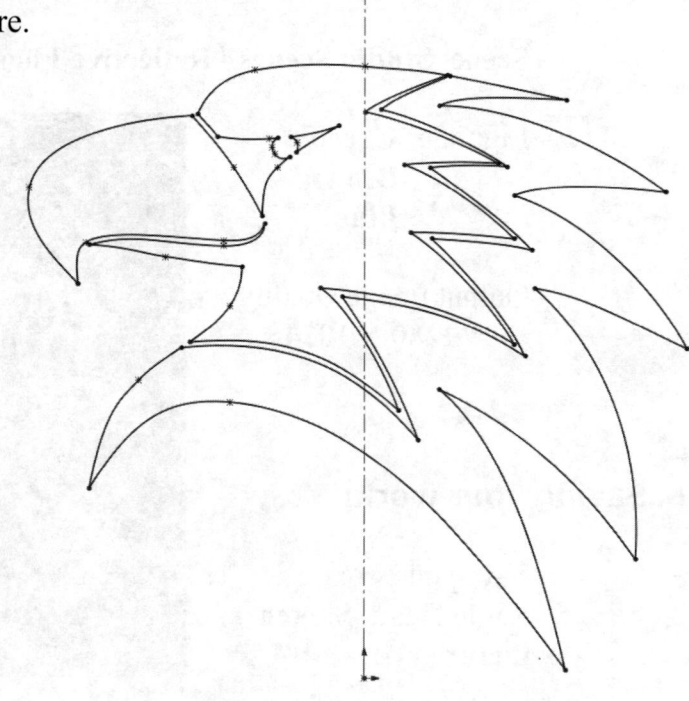

4. Extruding the traced sketch:

- Click **Extruded Boss-Base**.

- Use the default Blind type and enter **.125"** for thickness

- Click **OK**.

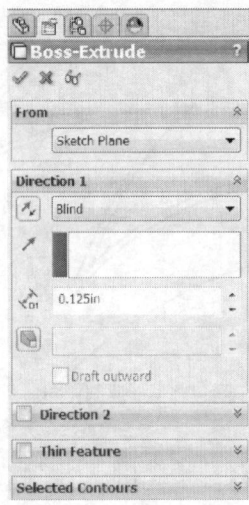

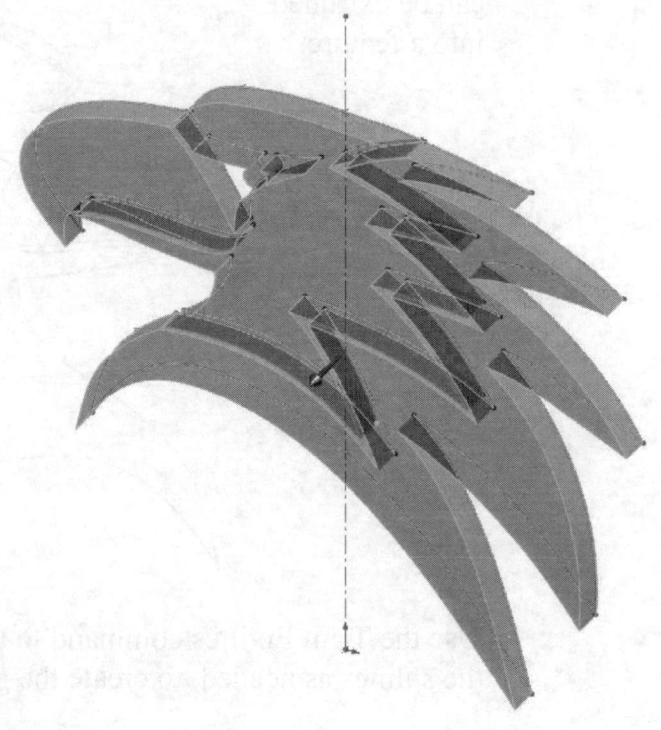

5. Optional:

- Use **Photoview 360** and render the model with the following settings:

- Appearances: **Glass / Clear Thick Gloss / Clear Thick Glass**

- Scene: **Studio Scenes / Reflective Floor Black**.

- Lighting: **Green**
  Brown
  Blue

- Output Image Quality:
  1280 X 1024

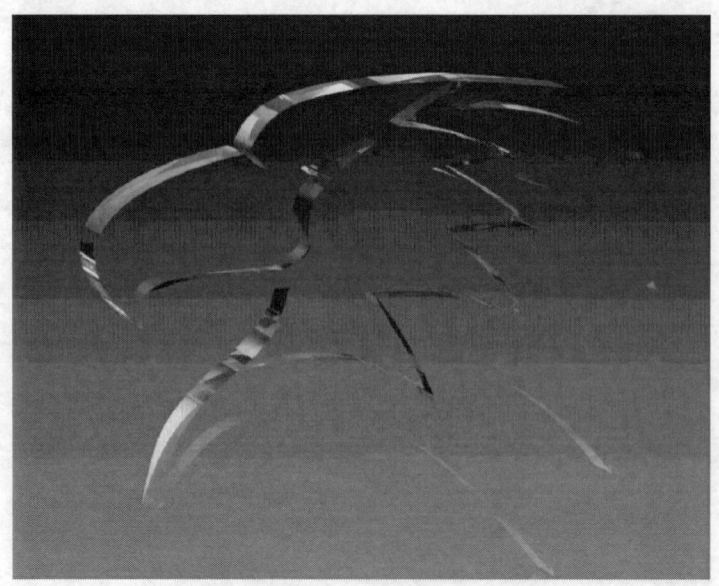

6. Saving your work:

- Save your work as:
  Eagle Head_Sketch Picture.

Questions for Review

Working with Sketch Pictures

1. A digital image can be inserted into a sketch to reference a model.
   a. True
   b. False

2. Most picture formats are supported such as: bmp, jpg, gif, tif, png.
   a. True
   b. False

3. A digital image can be copied and pasted into a sketch plane, and used as a background for tracing.
   a. True
   b. False

4. A scanned picture should be scanned as low-resolution and has multi-colors is best for tracing.
   a. True
   b. False

5. To open a digital image, you should use the command Sketch Picture to insert it into a plane.
   a. True
   b. False

6. A digital image can be opened in SolidWorks like any part or assembly file.
   a. True
   b. False

7. The spline command creates curves that are fixed and cannot be changed or manipulated.
   a. True
   b. False

8. To see the spline handles, simply click on the spline.
   a. True
   b. False

7. FALSE   8. TRUE
5. TRUE   6. FALSE
3. FALSE   4. FALSE
1. TRUE   2. TRUE

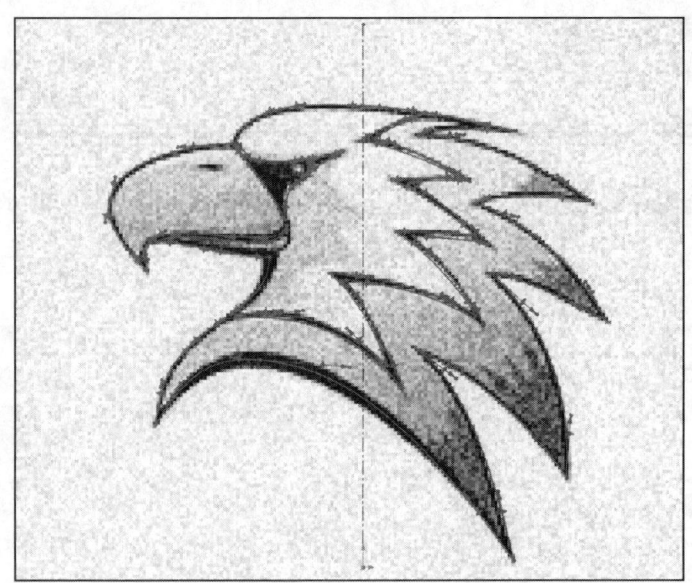

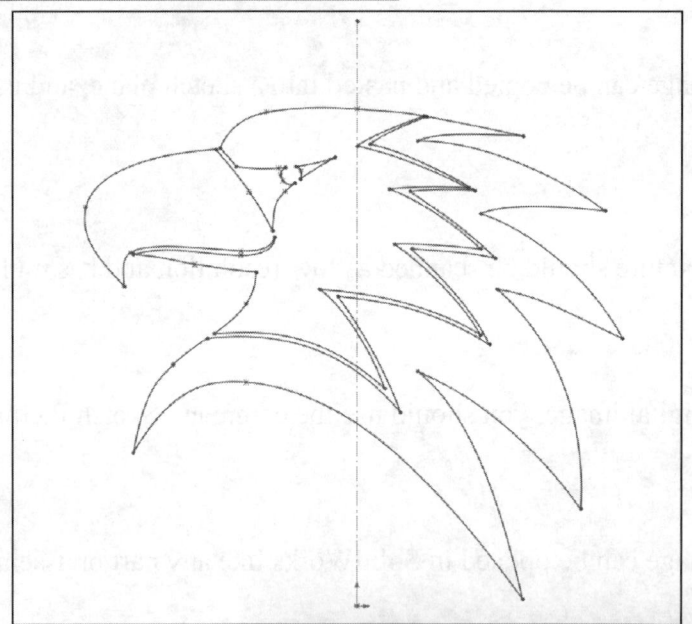

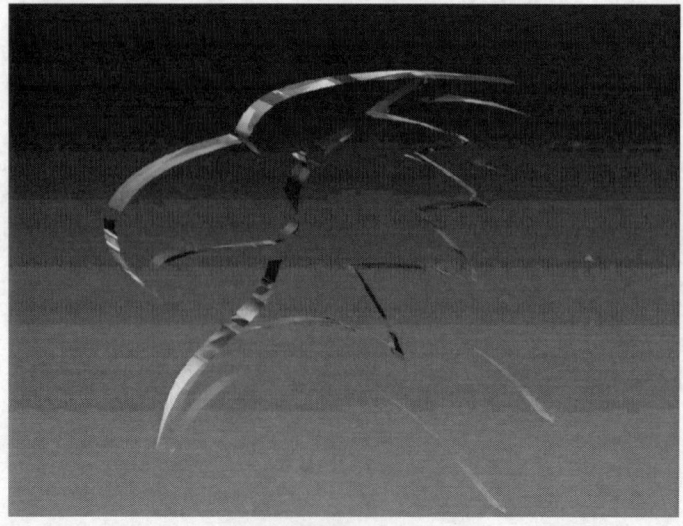

CHAPTER 13 (Cont.)

PhotoView 360 Basics

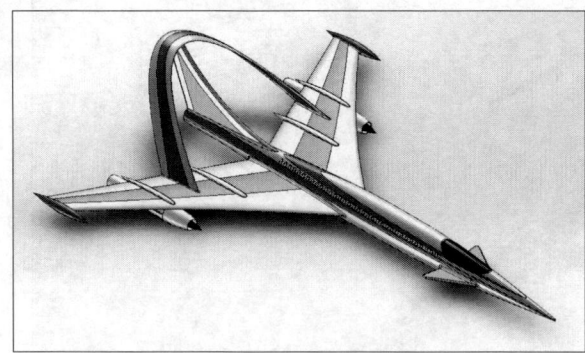
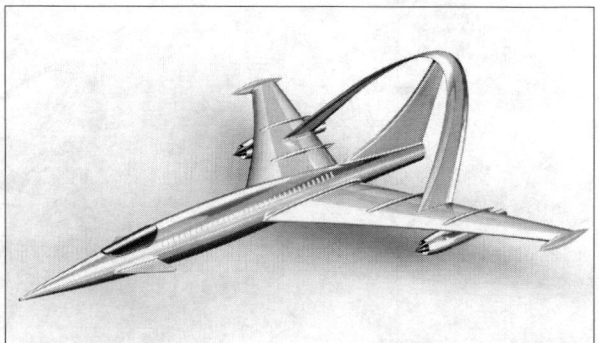

PhotoView 360 enables the user to create photo-realistic renderings of the SolidWorks models. The rendered image incorporates the appearances, lighting, scene, and decals included with the model. PhotoView 360 is available with SolidWorks Pro or SolidWorks Premium only.

- Open the document named **Supersonic Green Aircraft** from the Training Files folder.

1. Activating the PhotoView 360 Add-In:

- Click **Tools / Add-Ins**...

- Select the **PhotoView 360** checkbox.

- Click **OK**.

<u>NOTE:</u>

Enable the checkbox on the right of the PhotoView 360 add-in if you wish to have it available at startup. Otherwise only activate it for each use.

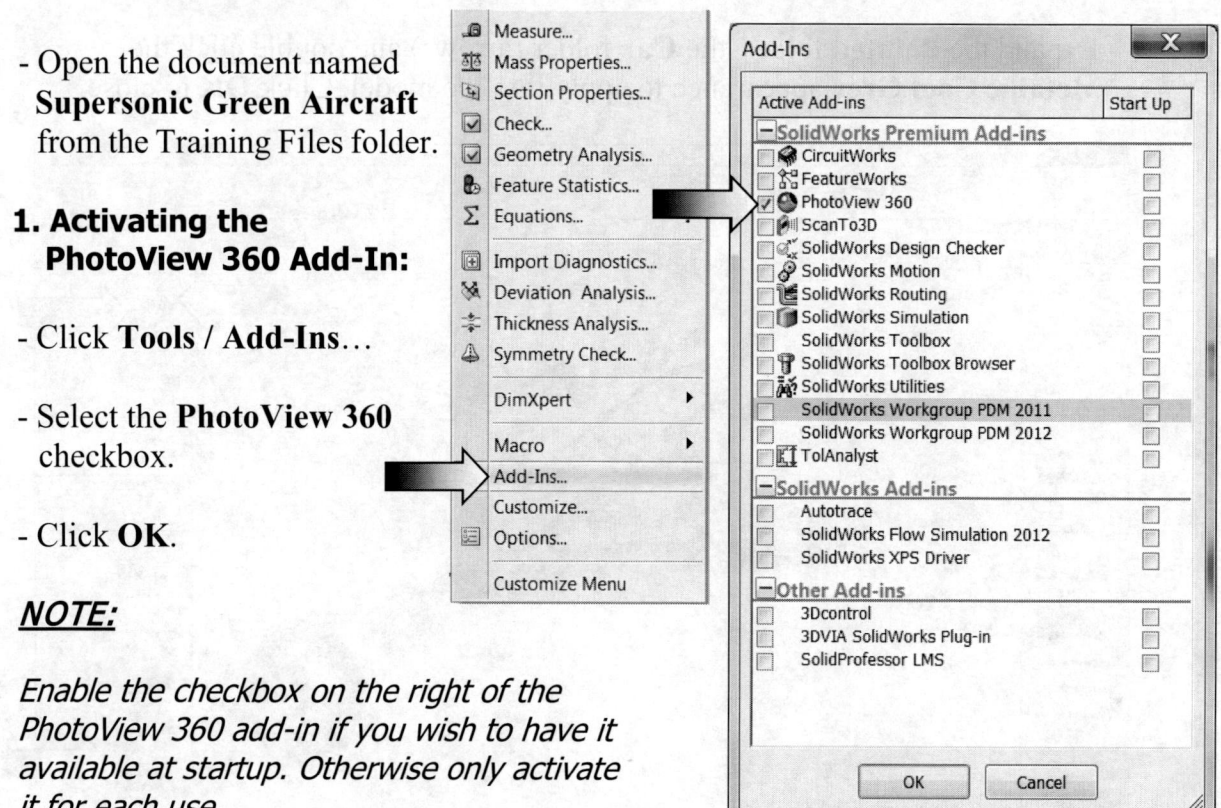

2. Setting the Appearance: (right click the Sketch tab and enable the Render tools).

- Click the **Edit Appearance** button from the Render tool tab (arrow).

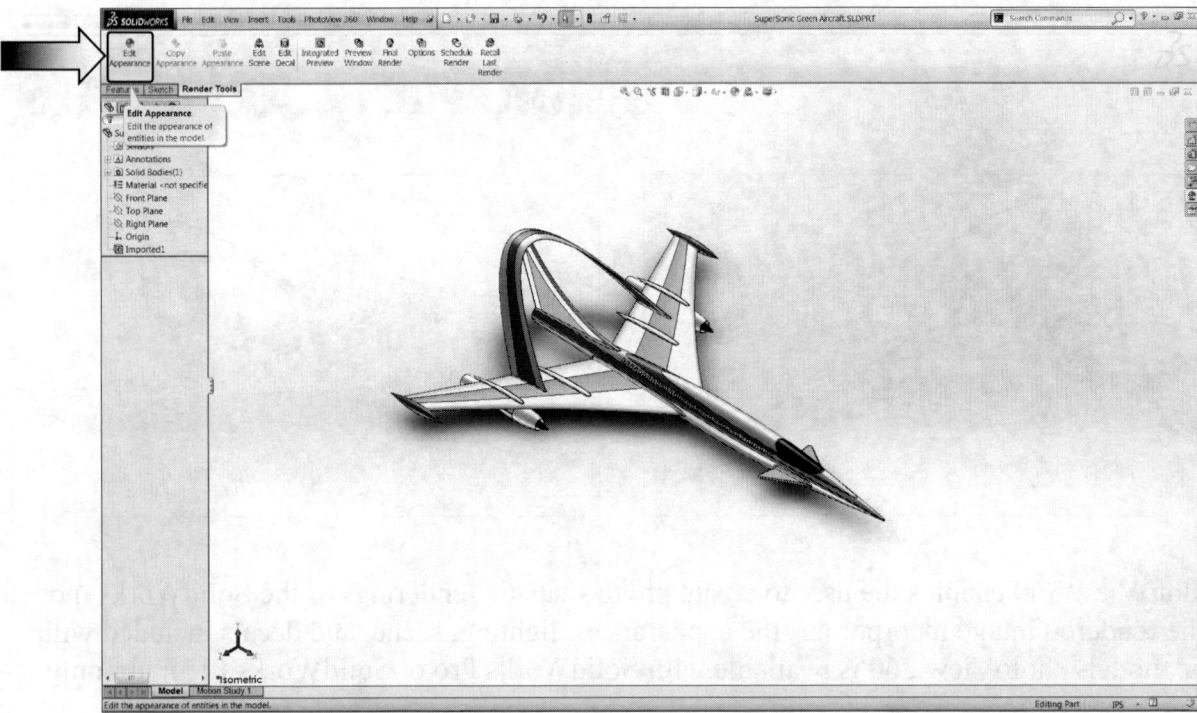

- Expand the **Painted** folder, the **Car** folder (arrows) and <u>double click</u> the **Metallic Cool Grey** appearance to apply it to the model. Click **OK** to close.

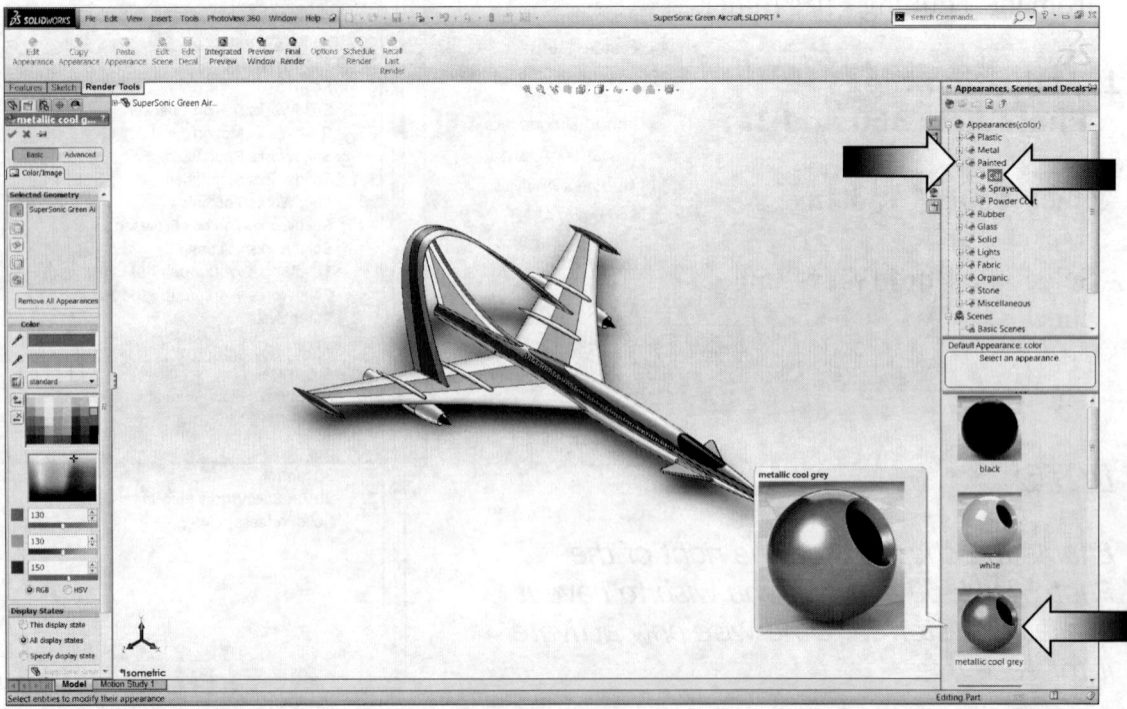

3. Setting the Scene:

- Click the **Edit Scene** button from the Render tool tab (arrow).

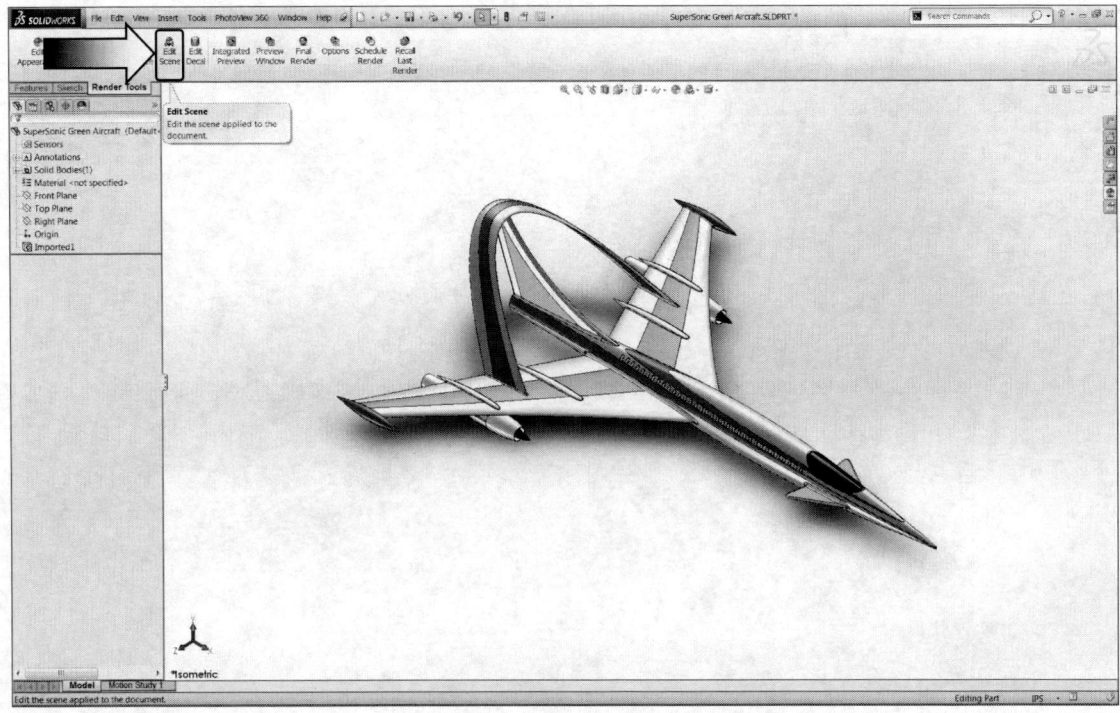

- Expand the **Scenes** folder, the **Basic Scenes** folder (arrows) and <u>double click</u> the **Backdrop - Studio Room** scene to apply it. Set the other settings as noted.

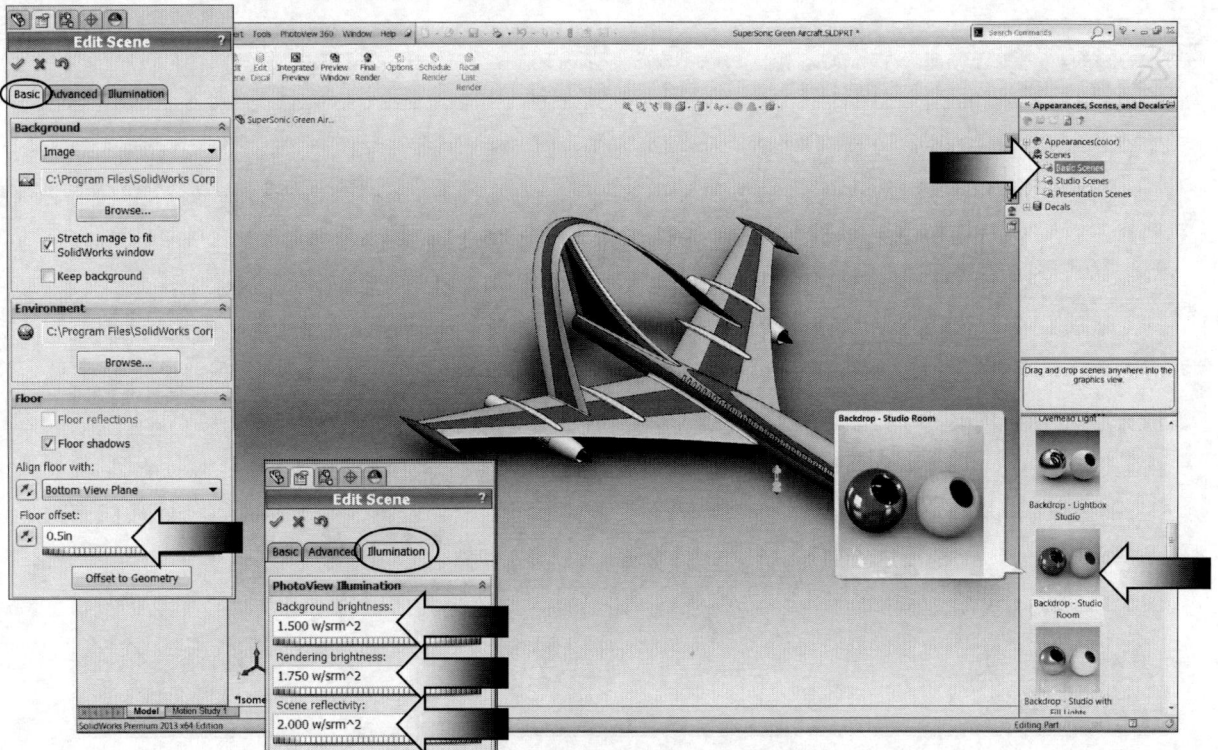

4. Setting the Image Quality options:

- Click the **Options** button from the Render tool tab (arrow).

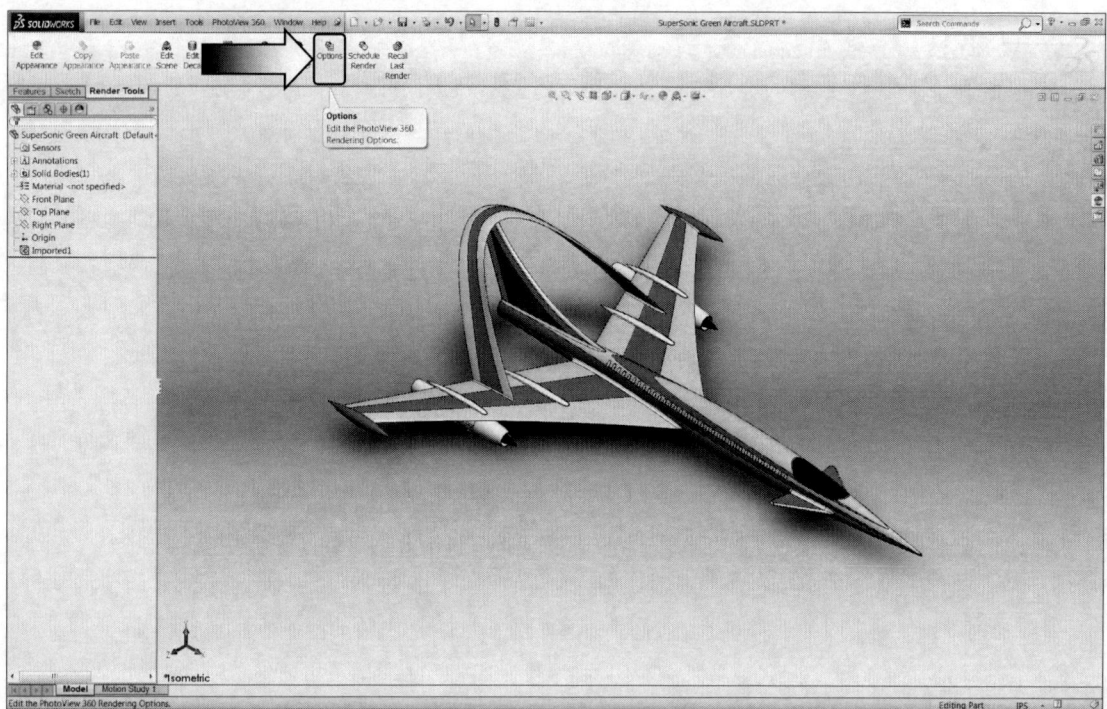

- Set the **Output Image** to **1920x1080** from the drop down list.
- Set the other options as indicated with the arrows. Click **OK** to close.

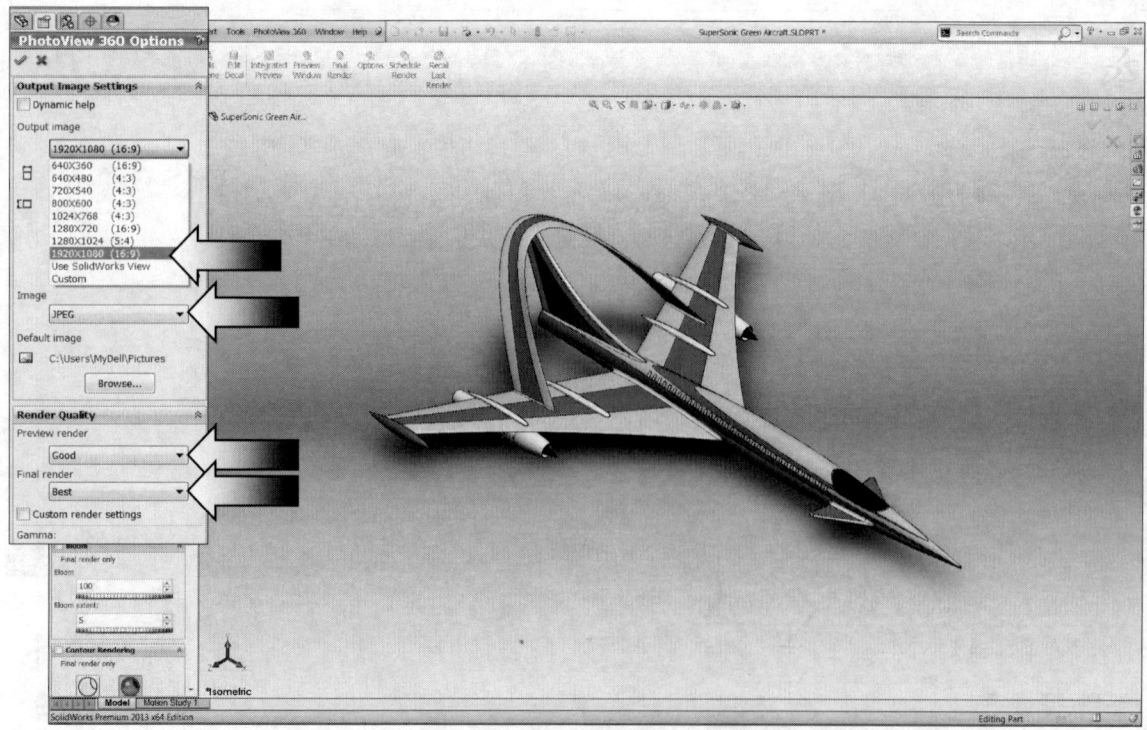

5. Rendering the image:

- Click the **Final Render** button from the Render tool tab (arrow).

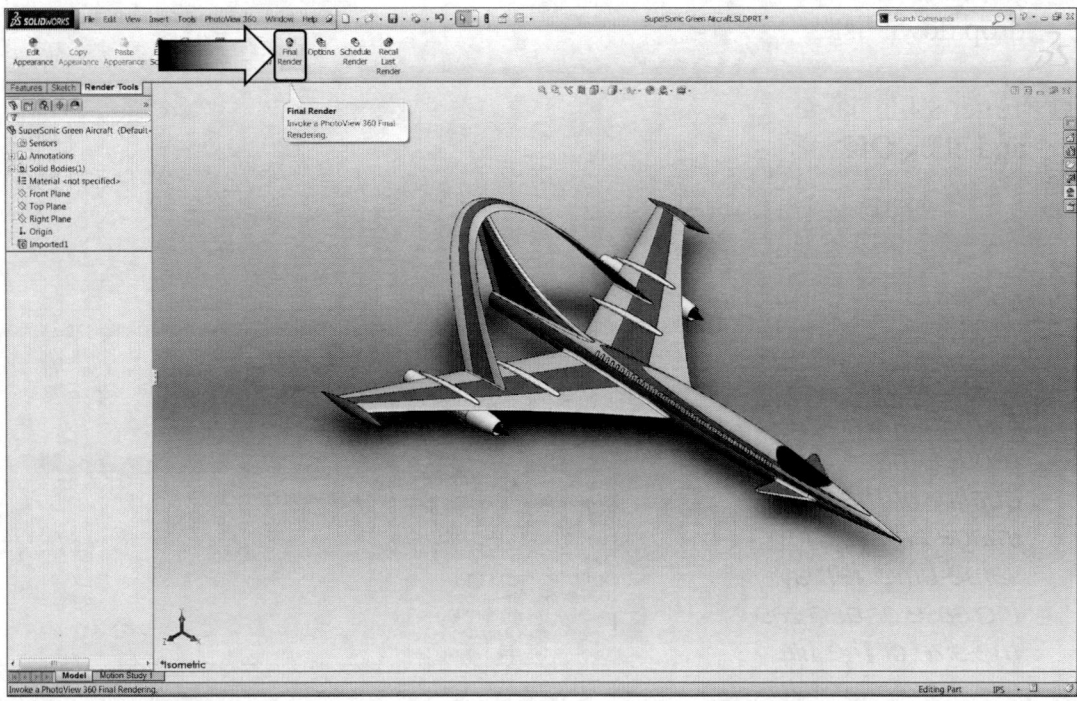

6. Saving the image:

- Select the **Best Fit** option from the drop down list and click **Save Image** (arrows).

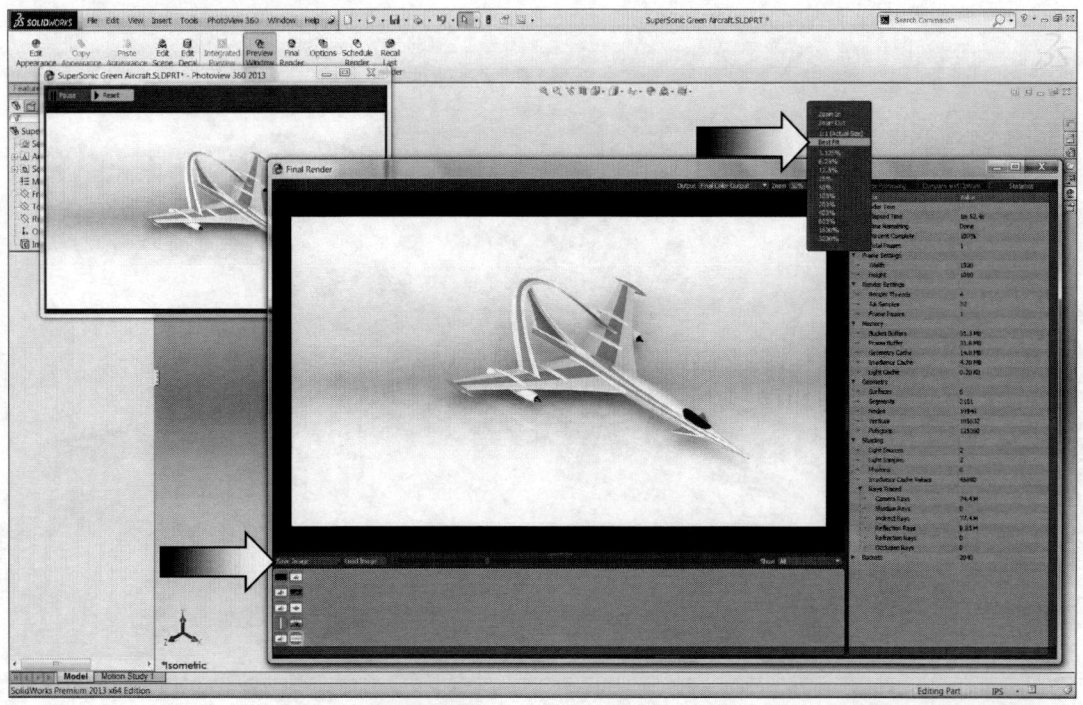

- Select the **JPEG** format from the Save-as-Type drop down list.

- Enter a file name and click **OK**.

NOTE:

- *Different file formats may reduce the quality of the image and at the same time, it may increase or decrease the size of the file.*

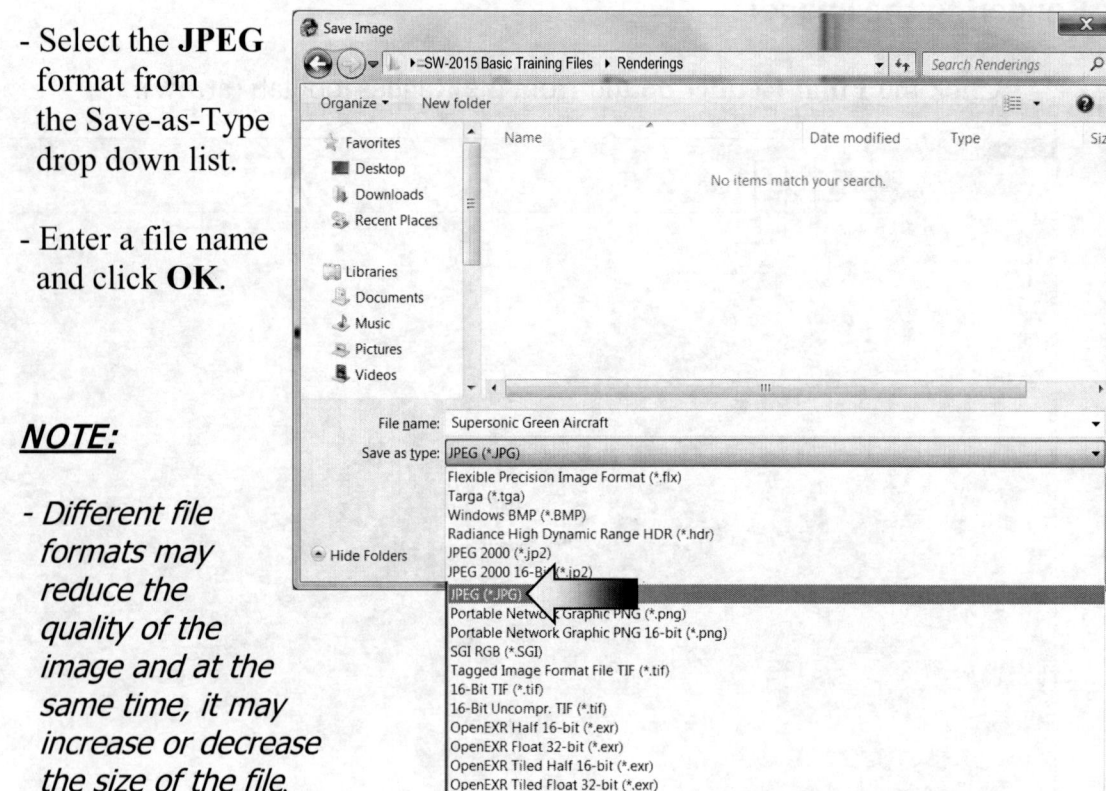

- Close all documents when finished.

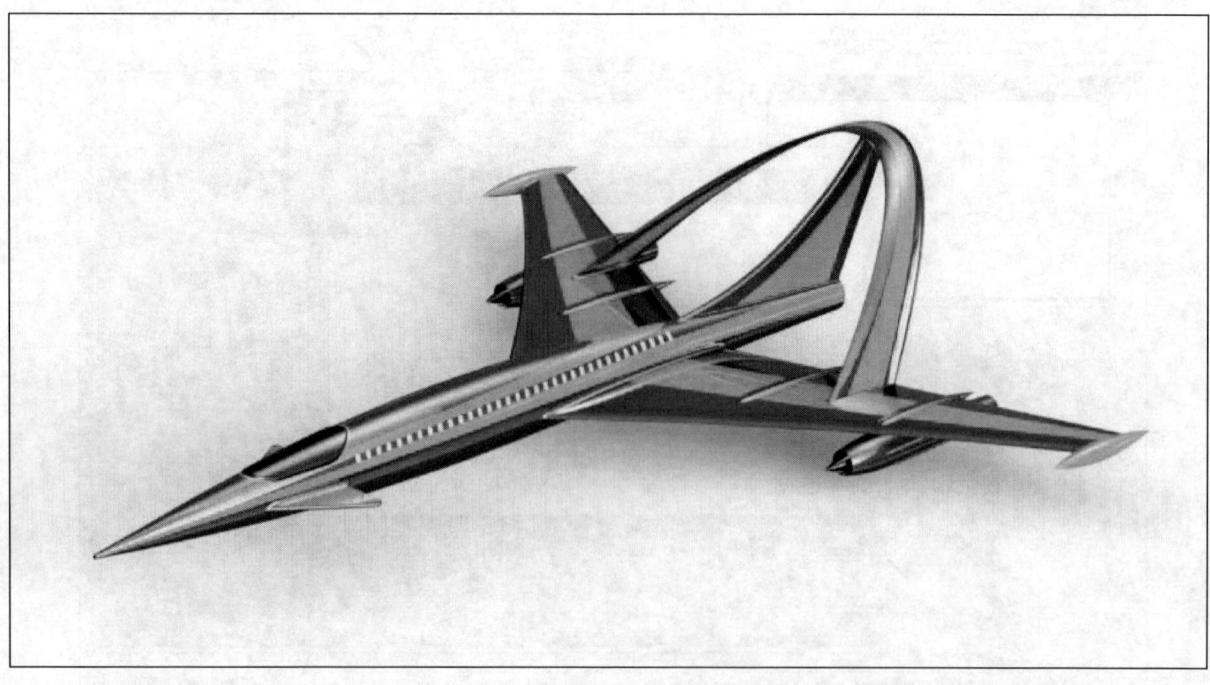

PhotoView 360 Exercise

PhotoView 360 is a SolidWorks add-in that produces photo-realistic renderings of SolidWorks models.

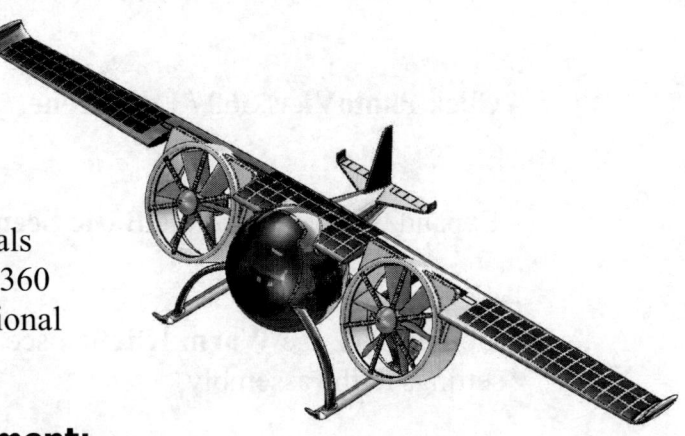

The rendered image incorporates the appearances, lighting, scene, and decals included with the model. PhotoView 360 is available with SolidWorks Professional or SolidWorks Premium.

1. Opening an assembly document:

- Open an assembly document named: **Helidrone.sldasm**.

- Drag/drop the **Polished Platinum** appearance to the drone's body (arrows).

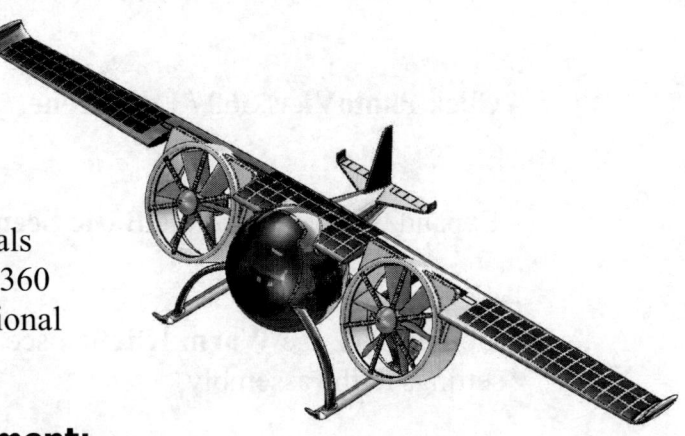

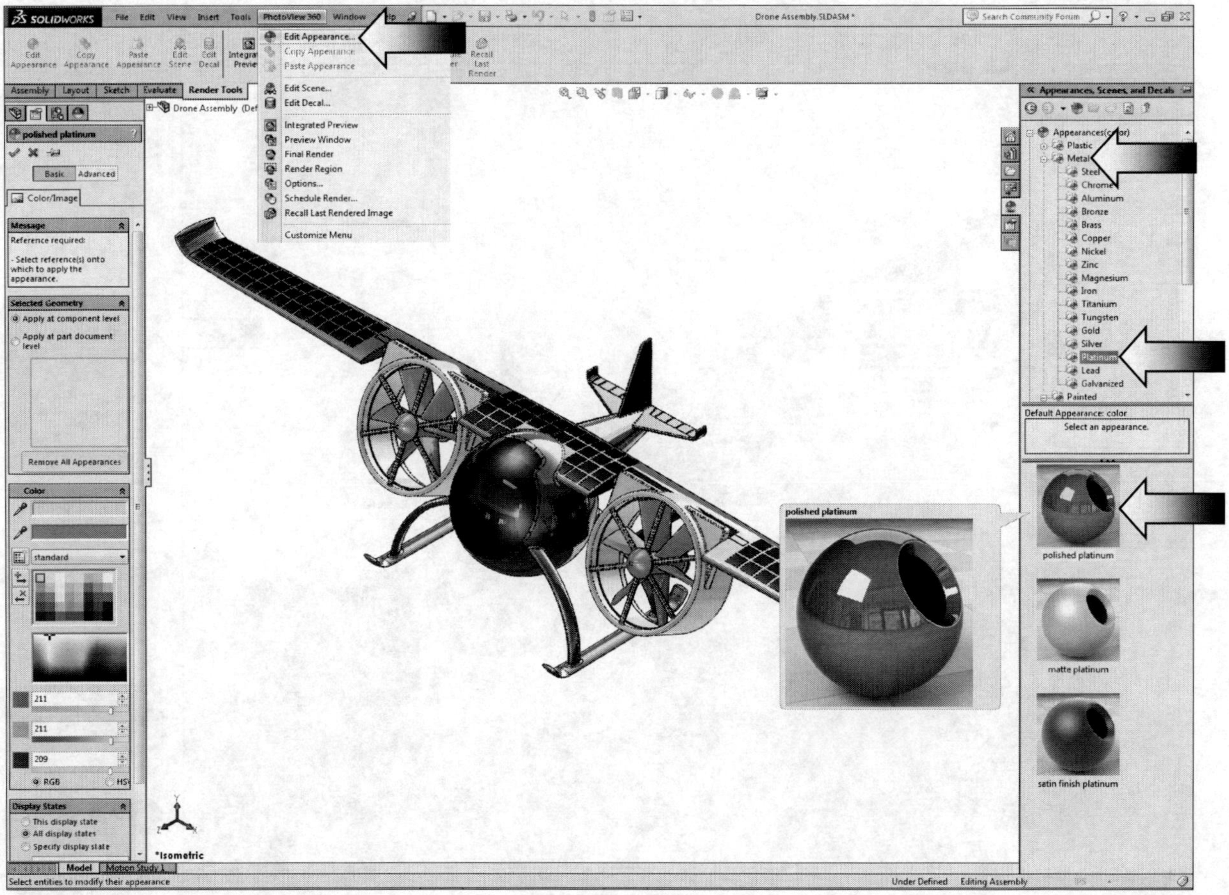

2. Applying the Scene:

- Apply the scene after the appearance is set.

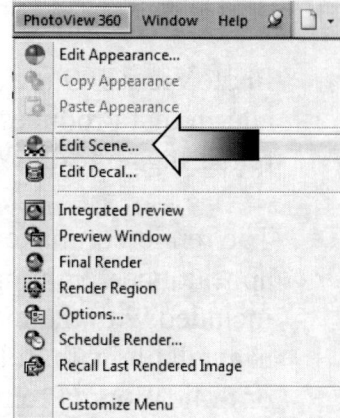

- Click **PhotoView 360 / Edit Scene**.

- Expand the **Scene** and the **Basic Scene** folders.

- Double click the **Warm Kitchen** scene to apply its settings to the assembly.

- Use the options in the **Edit Scene** sections, on the left side of the screen, to modify the lightings, floor reflections, and environment rotation.

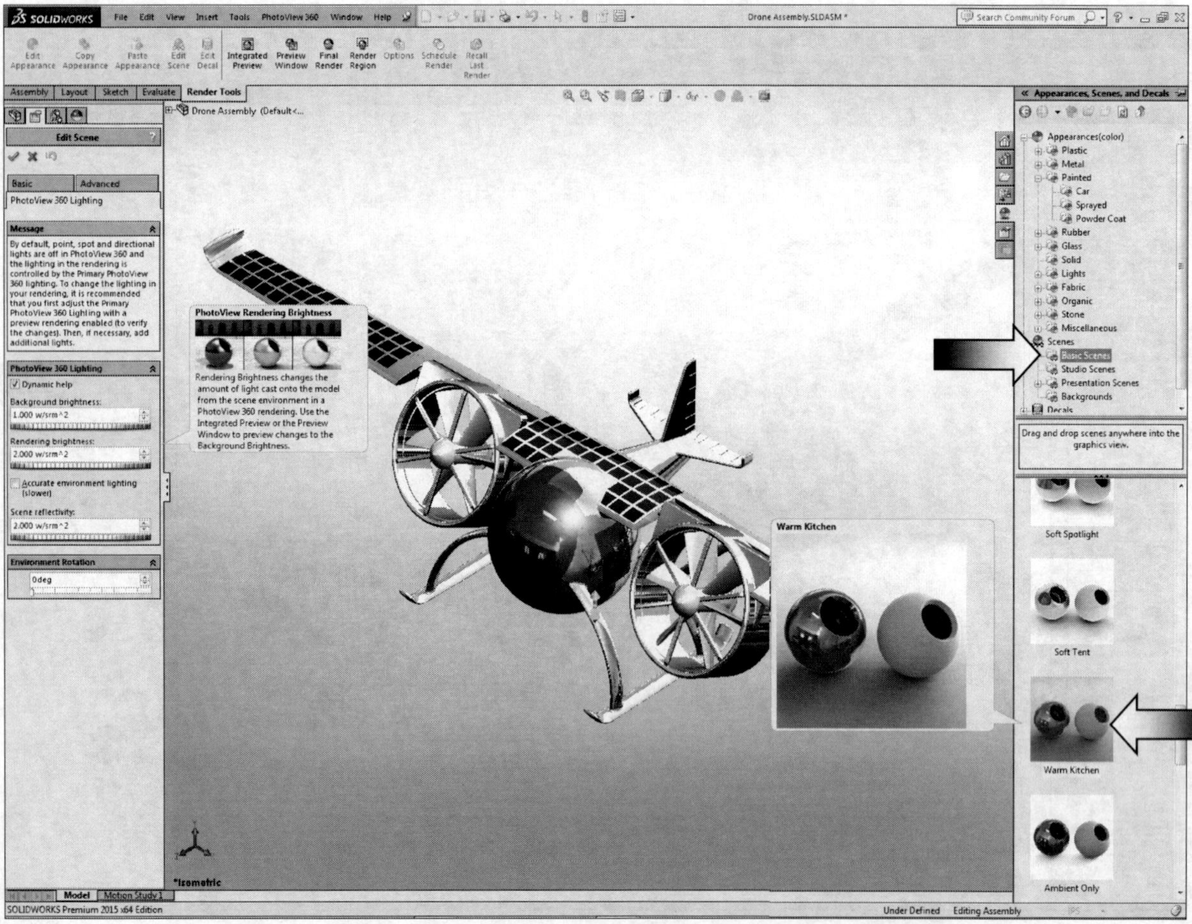

3. Setting the Render Region:

- The render region provides an accelerator that lets you render a subsection of the current scene without having to zoom in or out, or change the window size.

- Select the **Render Region** option from the PhotoView 360 pull down menu.

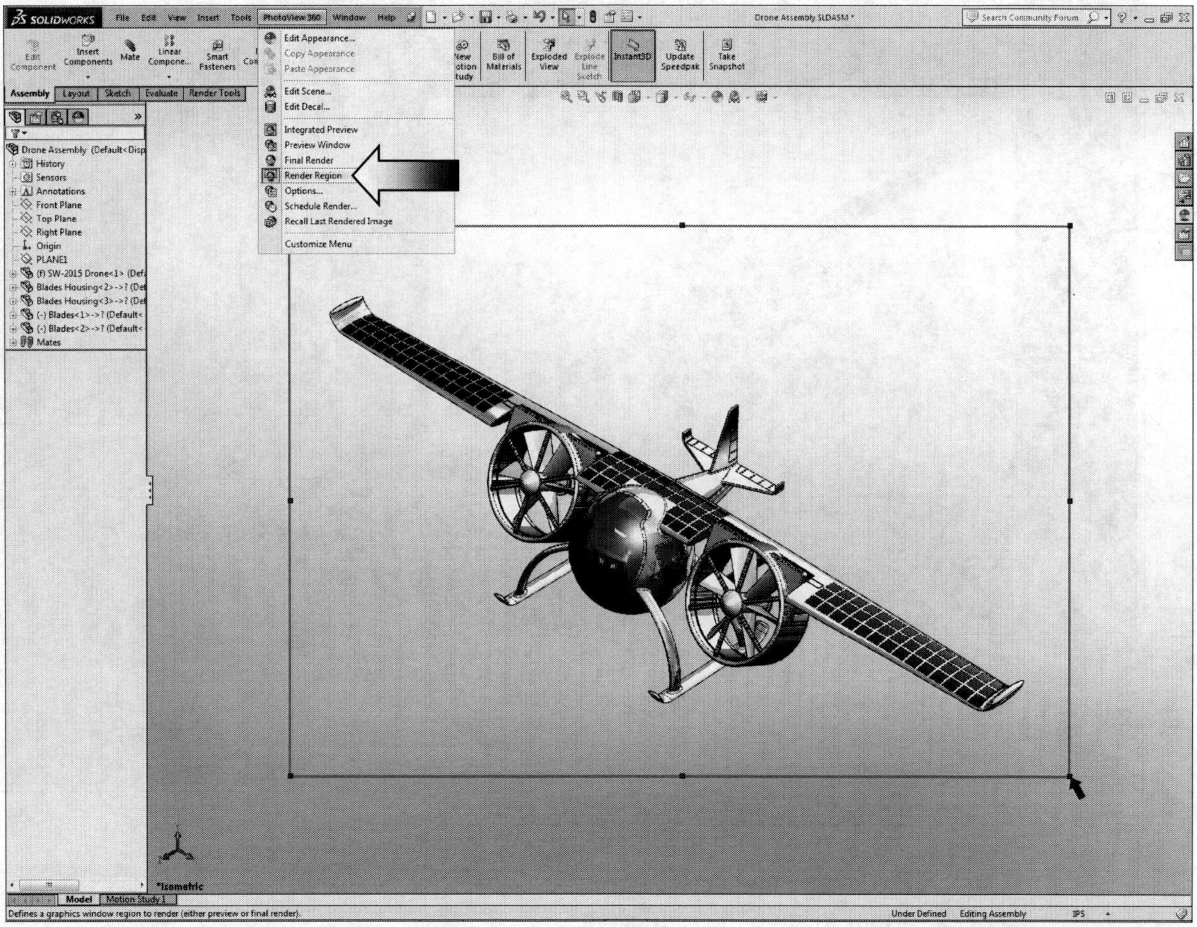

- Drag one of the handle points to define the region to render.

4. Setting the Image Size:

- Select **Options** under the PhotoView 360 pull down.

- The height and width of the render image can be selected from some of the pre-set image sizes.

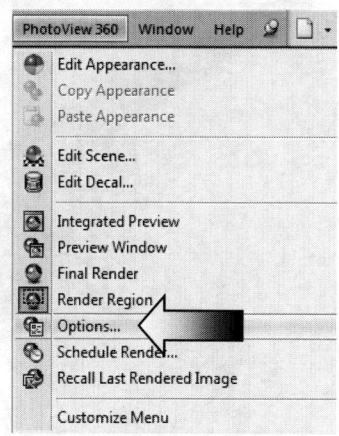

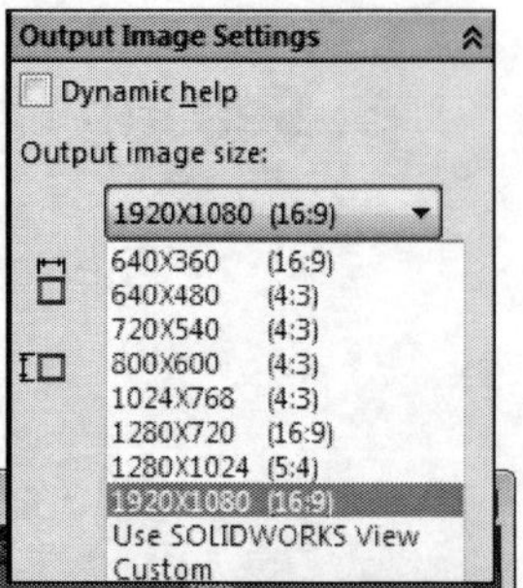

- Select the **1920x1080** (16:9) from the Image Size pull
  down options (The larger the image size the more time required)

- Select **Final Render** from the PhotoView 360.

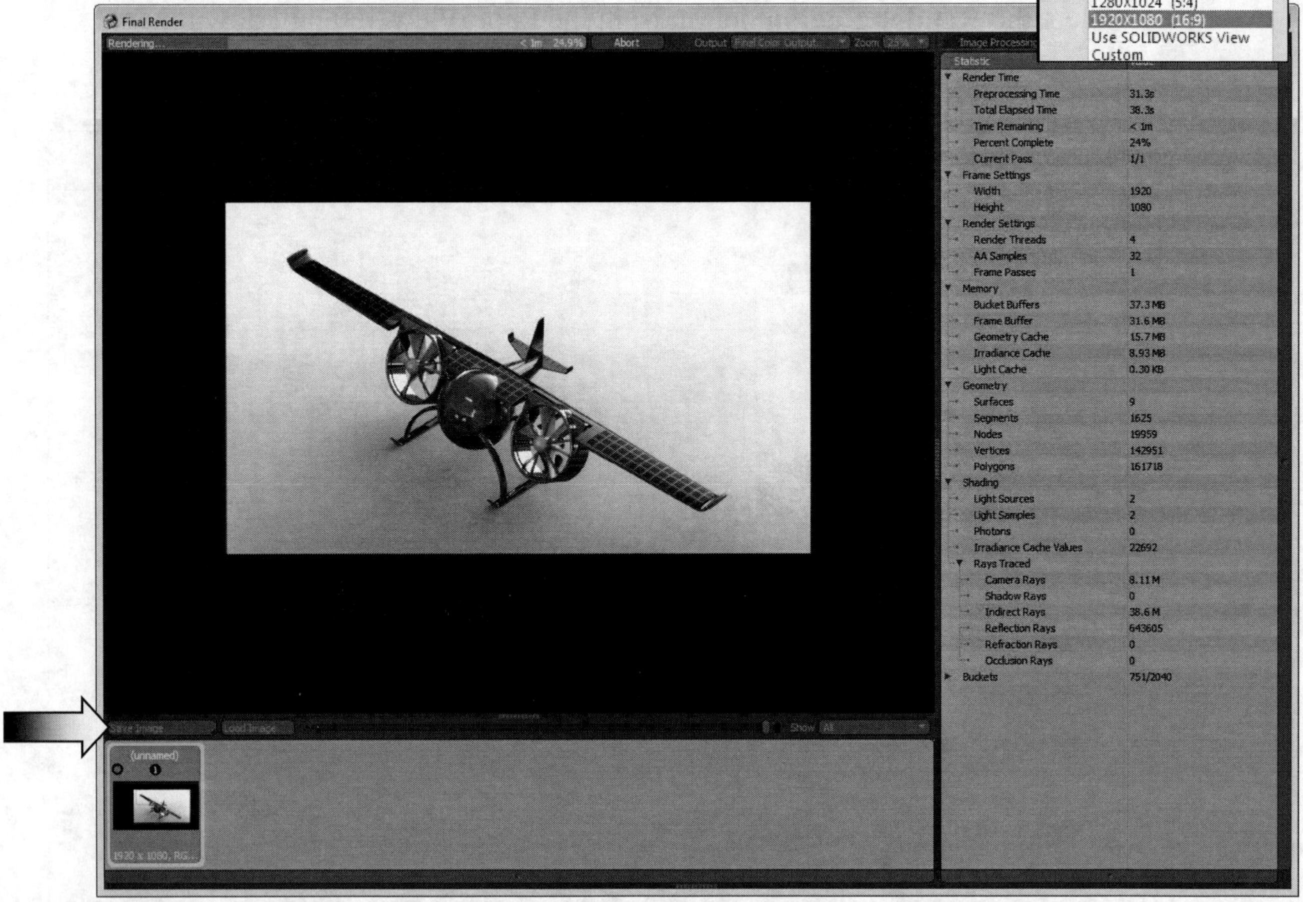

Output Image Settings

☐ Dynamic help

Output image size:

| 1920X1080 (16:9) | ▼ |

640X360	(16:9)
640X480	(4:3)
720X540	(4:3)
800X600	(4:3)
1024X768	(4:3)
1280X720	(16:9)
1280X1024	(5:4)
1920X1080	(16:9)
Use SOLIDWORKS View
Custom

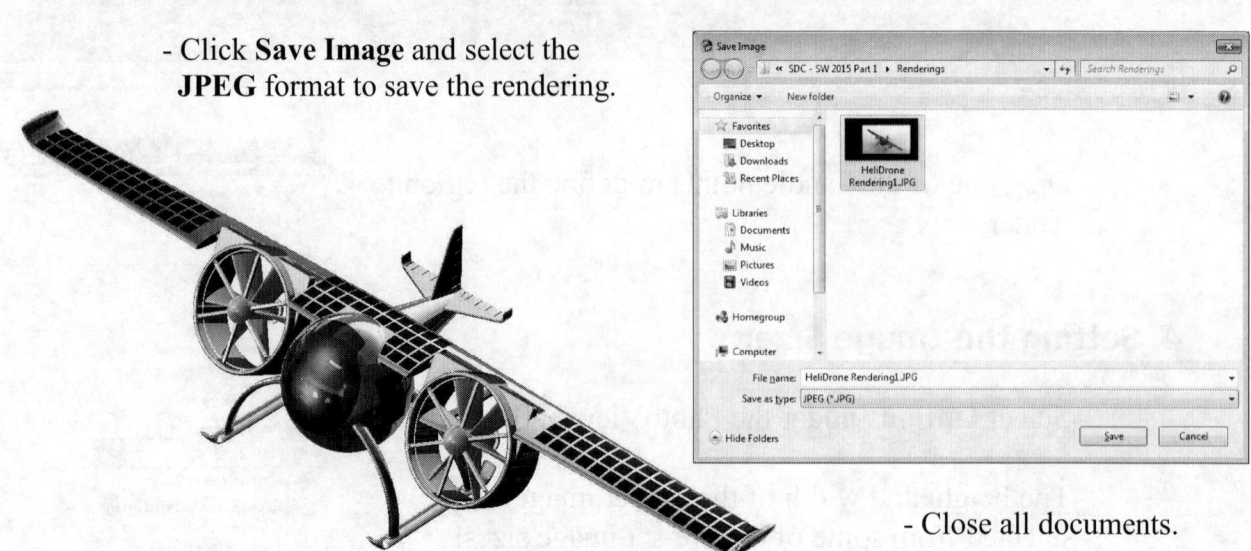

Final Render

Rendering...   < 1m 24.9%   Abort   Output Final Color Output ▼ Zoom 25% ▼   Image Processing

Statistic	
▼ Render Time	
Preprocessing Time	31.3s
Total Elapsed Time	38.3s
Time Remaining	< 1m
Percent Complete	24%
Current Pass	1/1
▼ Frame Settings	
Width	1920
Height	1080
▼ Render Settings	
Render Threads	4
AA Samples	32
Frame Passes	1
▼ Memory	
Bucket Buffers	37.3 MB
Frame Buffer	31.6 MB
Geometry Cache	15.7 MB
Irradiance Cache	8.93 MB
Light Cache	0.30 KB
▼ Geometry	
Surfaces	9
Segments	1625
Nodes	19959
Vertices	142951
Polygons	161718
▼ Shading	
Light Sources	2
Light Samples	2
Photons	0
Irradiance Cache Values	22692
▼ Rays Traced	
Camera Rays	8.11 M
Shadow Rays	0
Indirect Rays	38.6 M
Reflection Rays	643605
Refraction Rays	0
Occlusion Rays	0
▶ Buckets	751/2040

Save Image   Load Image   Show All ▼

(unnamed)

1920 x 1080, RG...

- Click **Save Image** and select the
  JPEG format to save the rendering.

Save Image

SDC - SW 2015 Part 1 ▶ Renderings   ▼ ↻ Search Renderings

Organize ▼   New folder

☆ Favorites
  🖥 Desktop
  📥 Downloads
  📍 Recent Places

📚 Libraries
  📄 Documents
  🎵 Music
  🖼 Pictures
  🎬 Videos

🖧 Homegroup

💻 Computer

HeliDrone
Rendering1.JPG

File name: HeliDrone Rendering1.JPG
Save as type: JPEG (*.JPG)

▲ Hide Folders   Save   Cancel

- Close all documents.

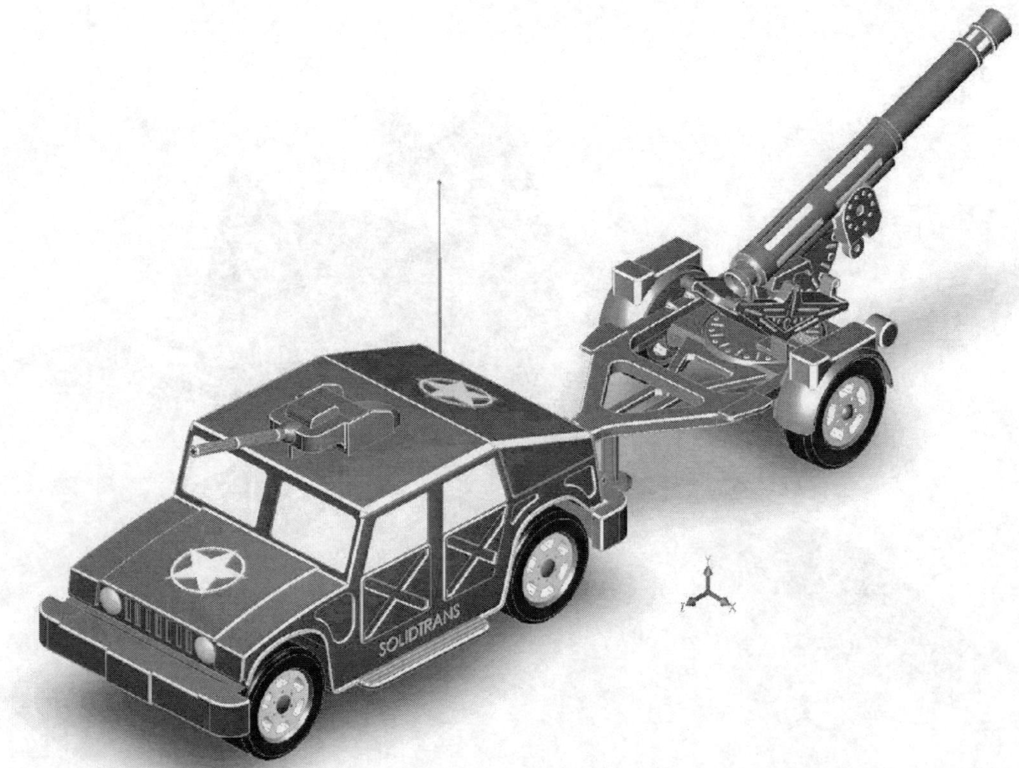

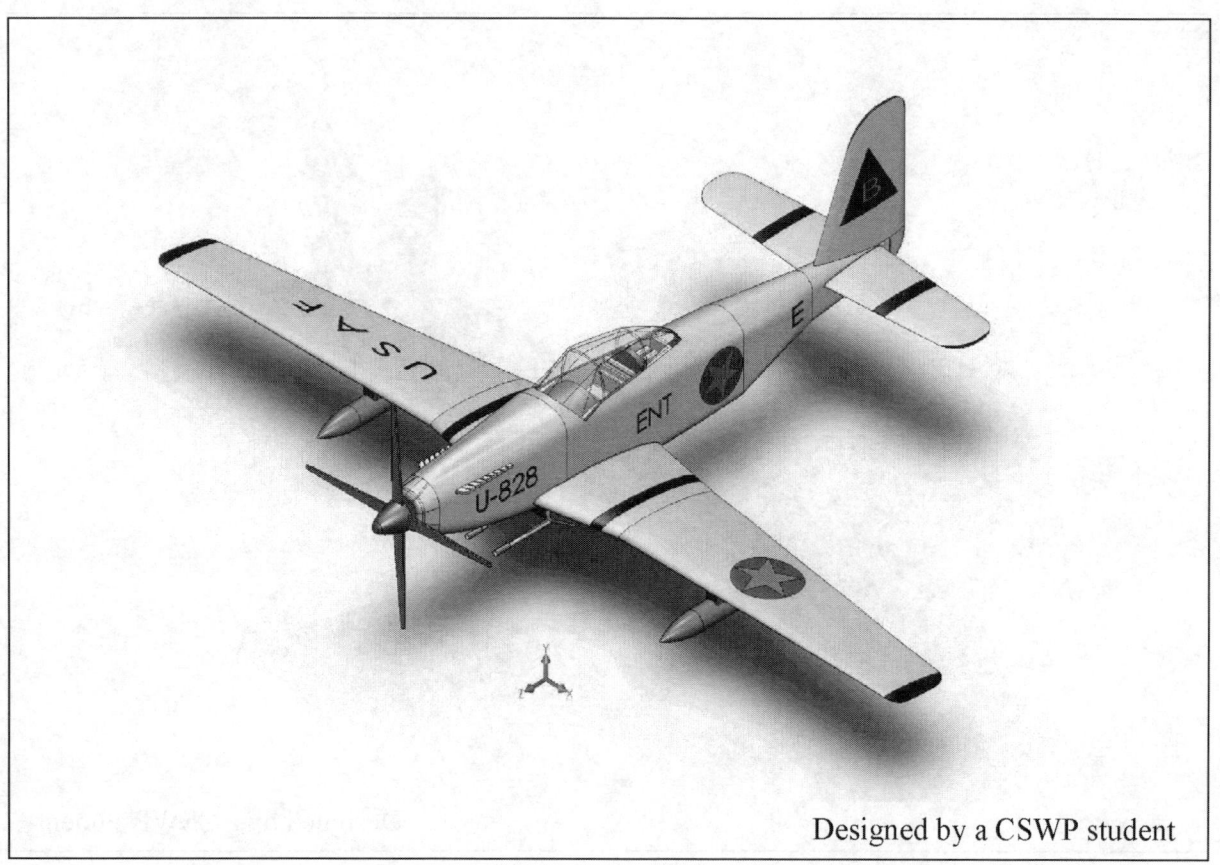

Designed by a CSWP student

Designed by a CSWP student

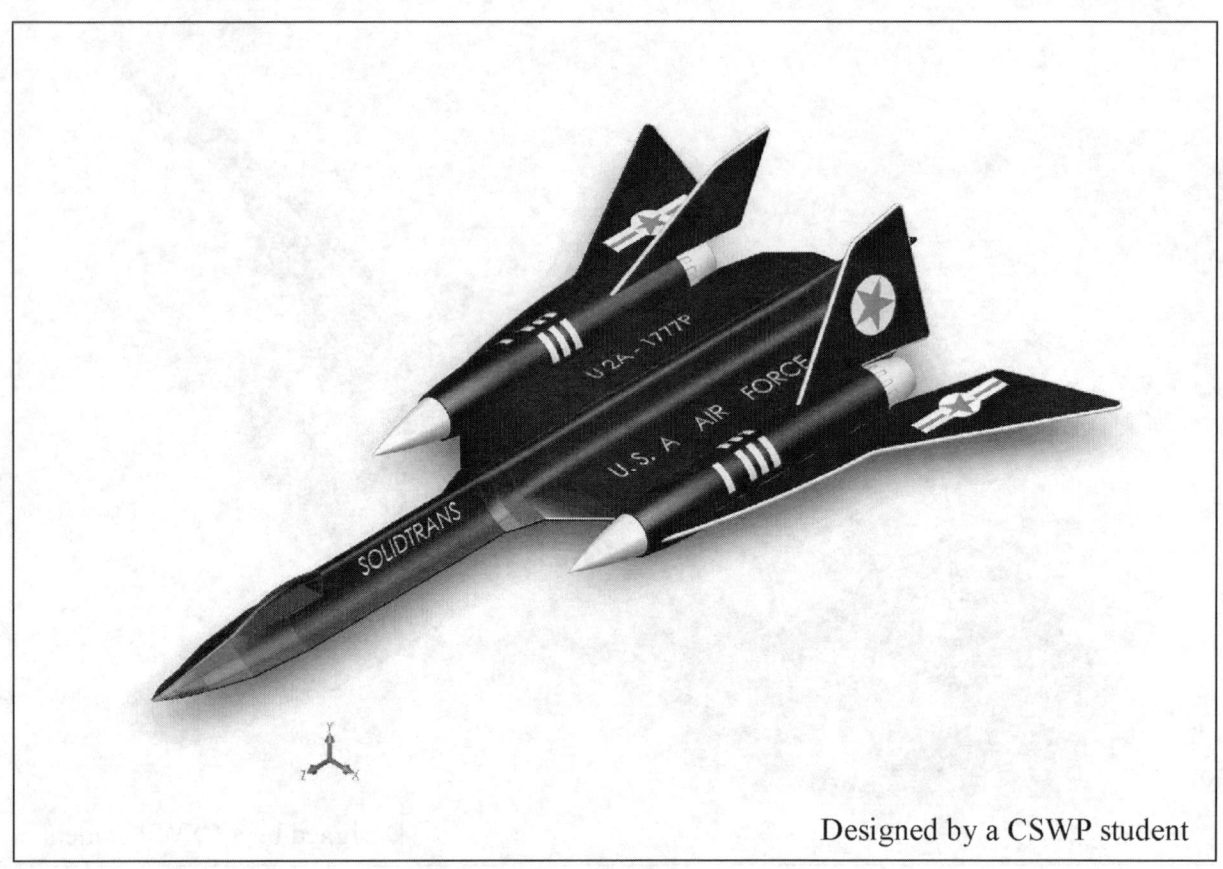

Designed by a CSWP student

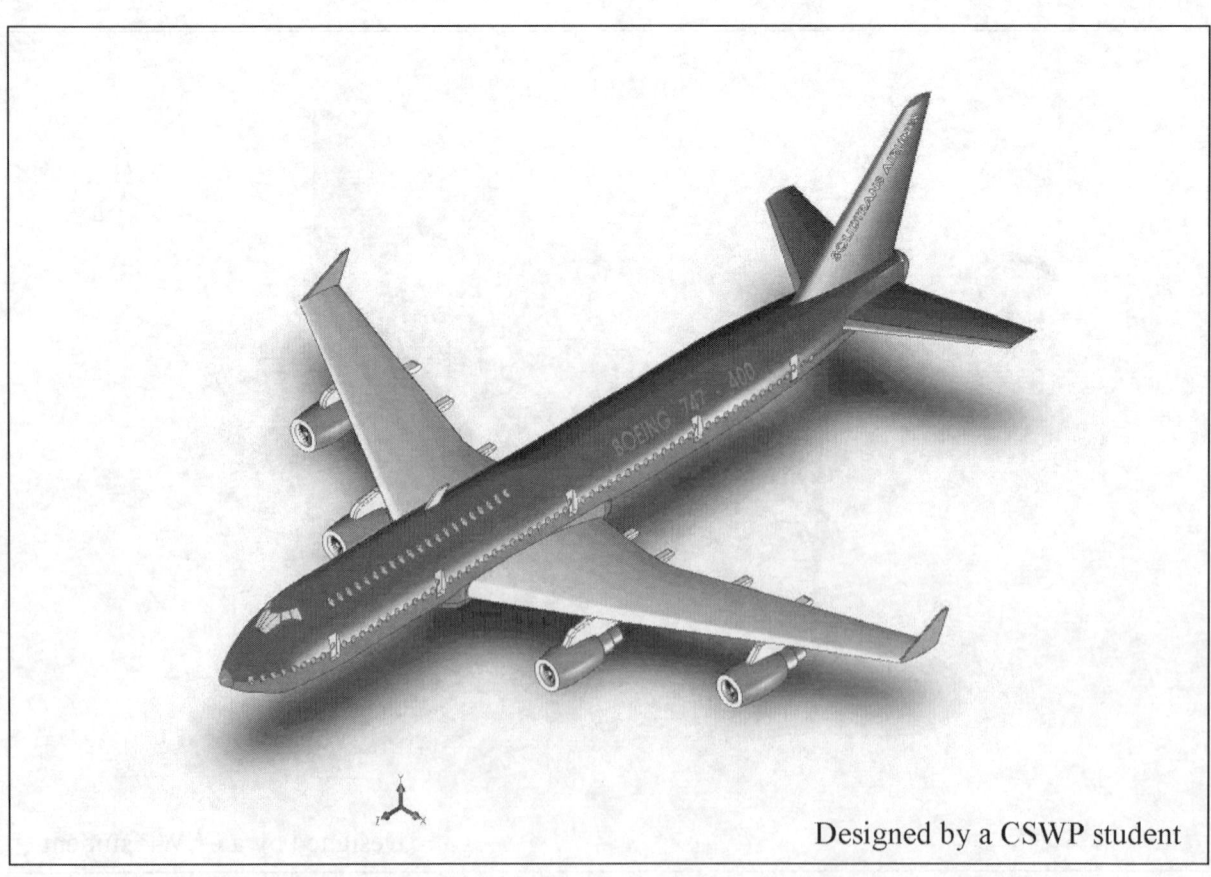

Designed by a CSWP student

CHAPTER 14

Drawing Preparations

Customizing the Document Template

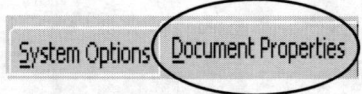

- Custom settings and parameters such as: ANSI standards, units, number of decimal places, dimensions and note fonts, arrow styles and sizes, line styles and line weights, image quality, etc., can be set and saved in the document template for use with the current drawing or at any time in the future.

- All Document Templates are normally stored either in the templates folder or in the Tutorial folder:

    * (C:\Program Files\SolidWorks Corp\ SolidWorks\Data\Templates)
    * (C:\Program Files\SolidWorks Corp\ SolidWorks\Lang\English\Tutorial)

- By default, there are 2 "layers" in every new drawing. The "top layer" is called the **Sheet**, and the "bottom layer" is called the **Sheet Format**.

- The **Sheet** layer is used to create the drawing views and annotations. The **Sheet-Format** layer contains the title block information, revision changes, BOM-anchor, etc.

- The 2 layers can be toggled back and forth by using the FeatureManager tree, or by right clicking anywhere in the drawing and selecting: Edit Sheet Format / Edit Sheet.

- When the settings are done they will get saved in the Document Template with the extension: **.drwdot** (Drawing Document Template).

- This chapter will guide us through the settings and the preparations needed prior to creating a drawing.

Drawing Preparations

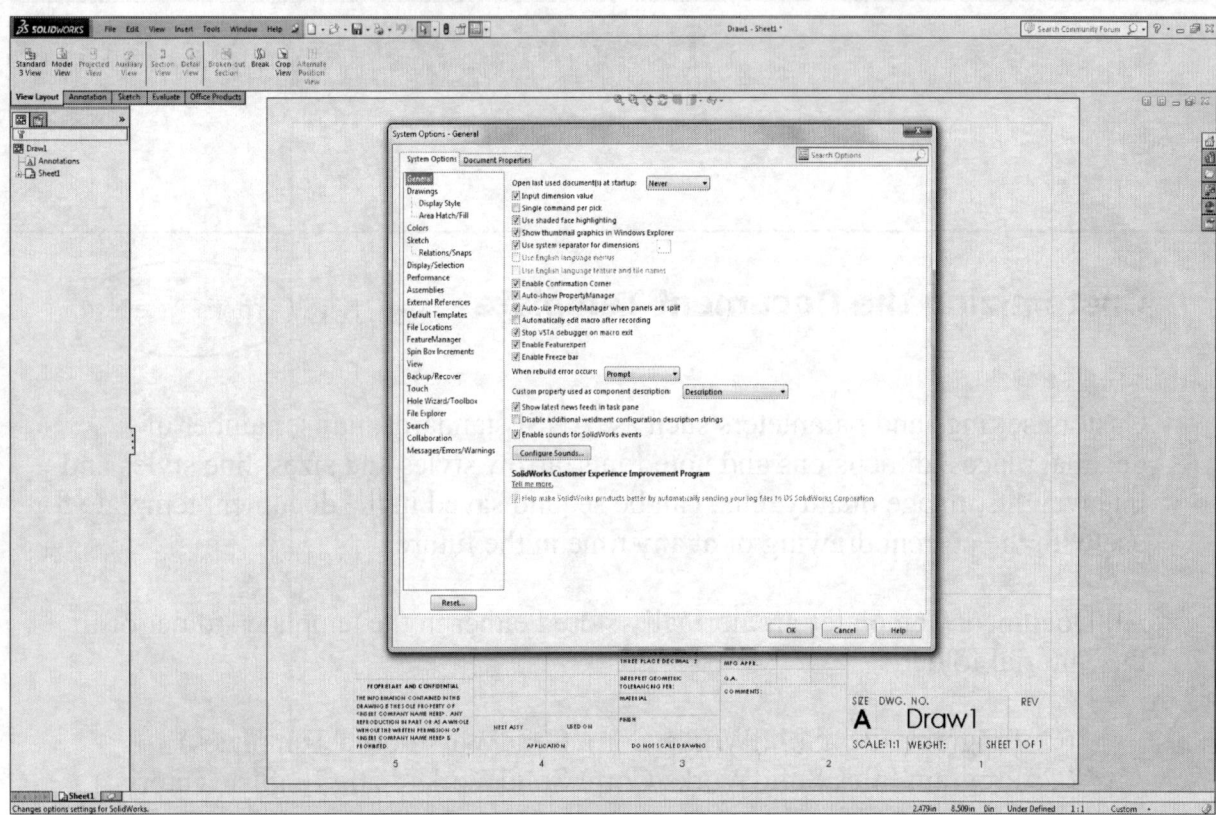

Dimensioning Standards: **ANSI**	Third Angle Projection
Units: **INCHES** – 3 Decimals	

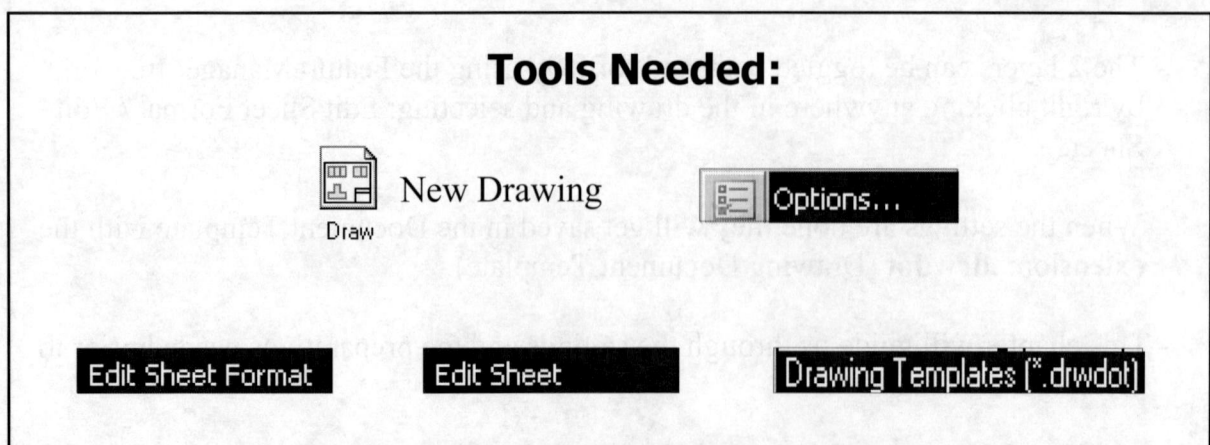

Tools Needed:

New Drawing
Draw

Options...

Edit Sheet Format   Edit Sheet   Drawing Templates (*.drwdot)

1. Setting up a new drawing:

- Select **File / New / Draw** (or Drawing) / **OK** `OK` .

- Change the option Novice to **Advanced** as noted.

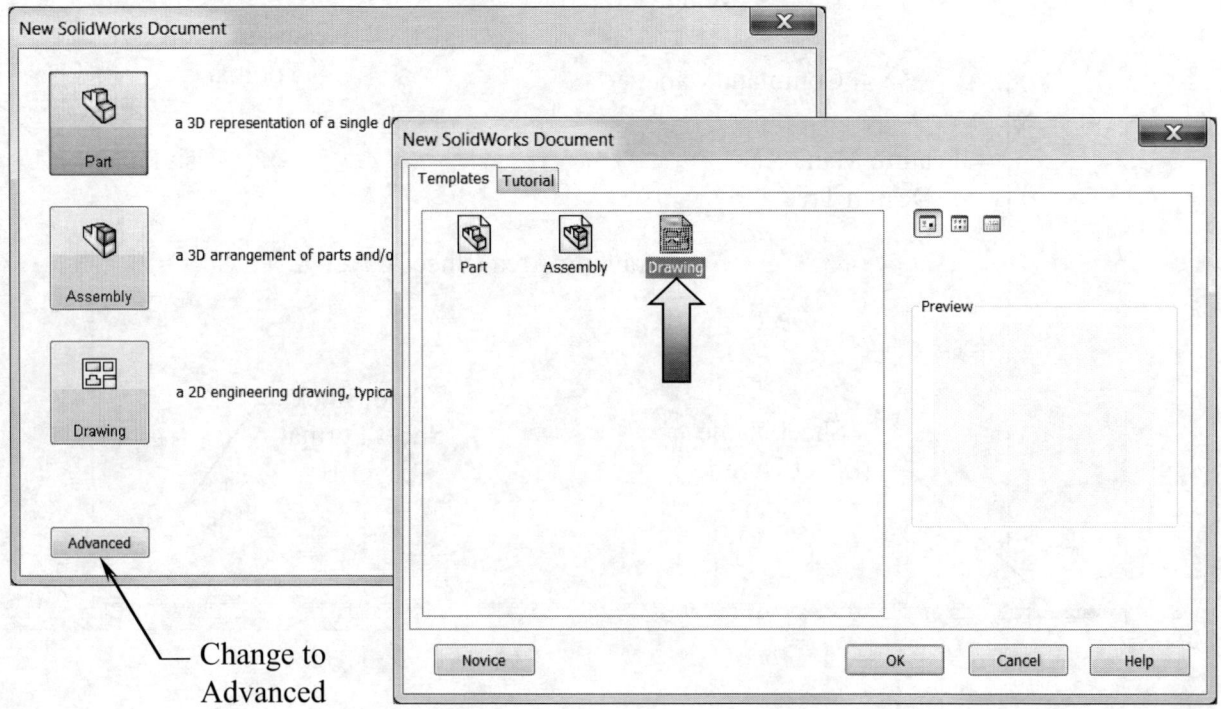

Change to
Advanced

- By clicking on either **Advanced** or **Novice** (Circled), you can switch to the appropriate dialog box.

- Set the following options:

  * **Scale: 1:2**

  * **Third Angle Projection**

  * View Label and Datum Label set them both to A.

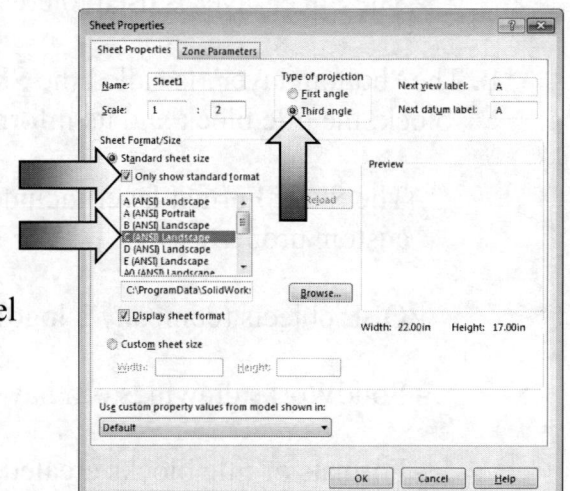

- Under Standard Sheet Size, choose: **C-Landscape**.

- Uncheck the **Only Show Standard Format** checkbox (arrow).

- Click **OK** `OK`

- The SolidWorks Drawing User Interface

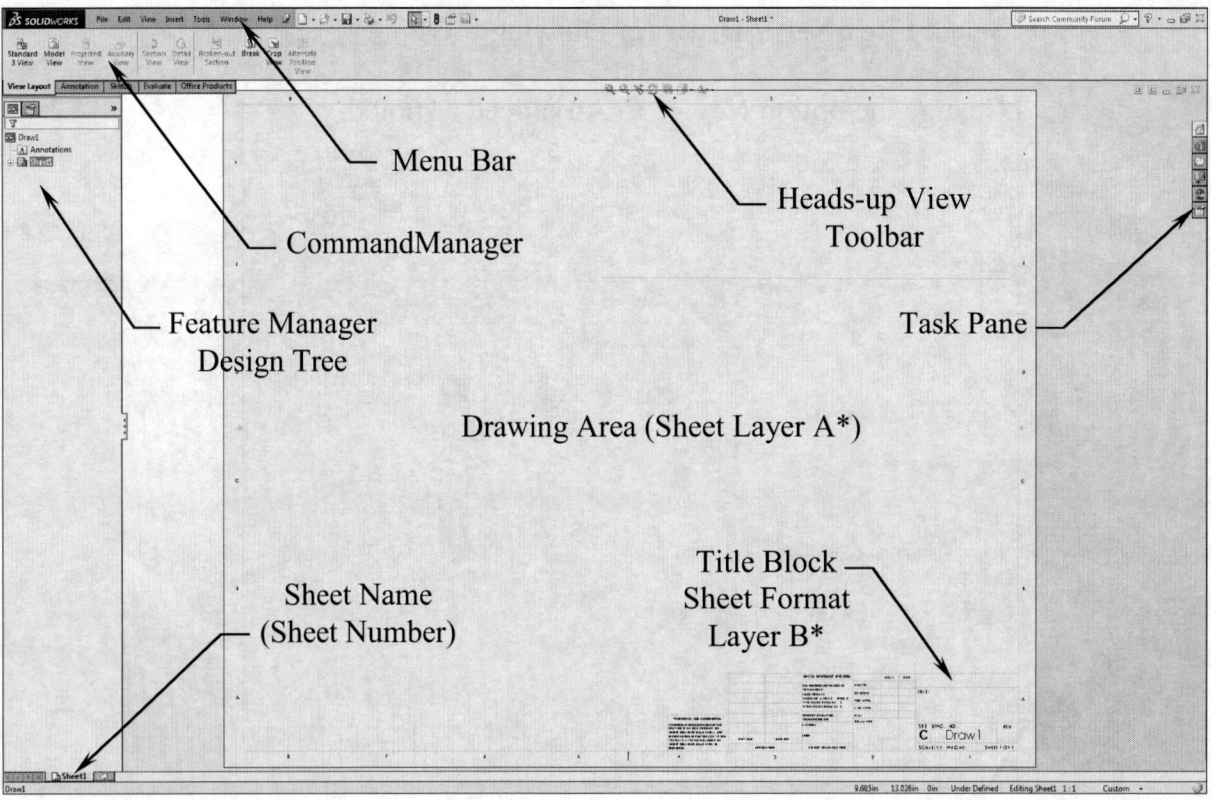

Menu Bar

CommandManager

Heads-up View Toolbar

Feature Manager Design Tree

Task Pane

Drawing Area (Sheet Layer A*)

Sheet Name (Sheet Number)

Title Block
Sheet Format
Layer B*

*A. By default, the **Sheet** layer is active and placed over the **Sheet Format** layer.

- The **Sheet** layer is used to create drawing views, dimensions, and annotations.

*B. The "bottom layer" is called the **Sheet Format** layer, which is where the revision block, the title block and its information are stored.

- The Sheet Format layer includes some links to the system properties and the custom properties.

- OLE objects (company's logo) such as .Bmp or .Tif can be embedded here.

- SolidWorks drawings can have different Sheet Formats or none at all.

- Formats or title blocks created from other CAD programs can be opened in SolidWorks using either DXF or DWG file types, and saved as SolidWorks' Sheet Format.

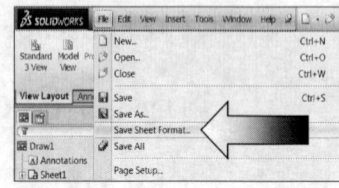

2. Switching to the Sheet Format layer:

- Right click in the drawing and select **Edit Sheet Format**.

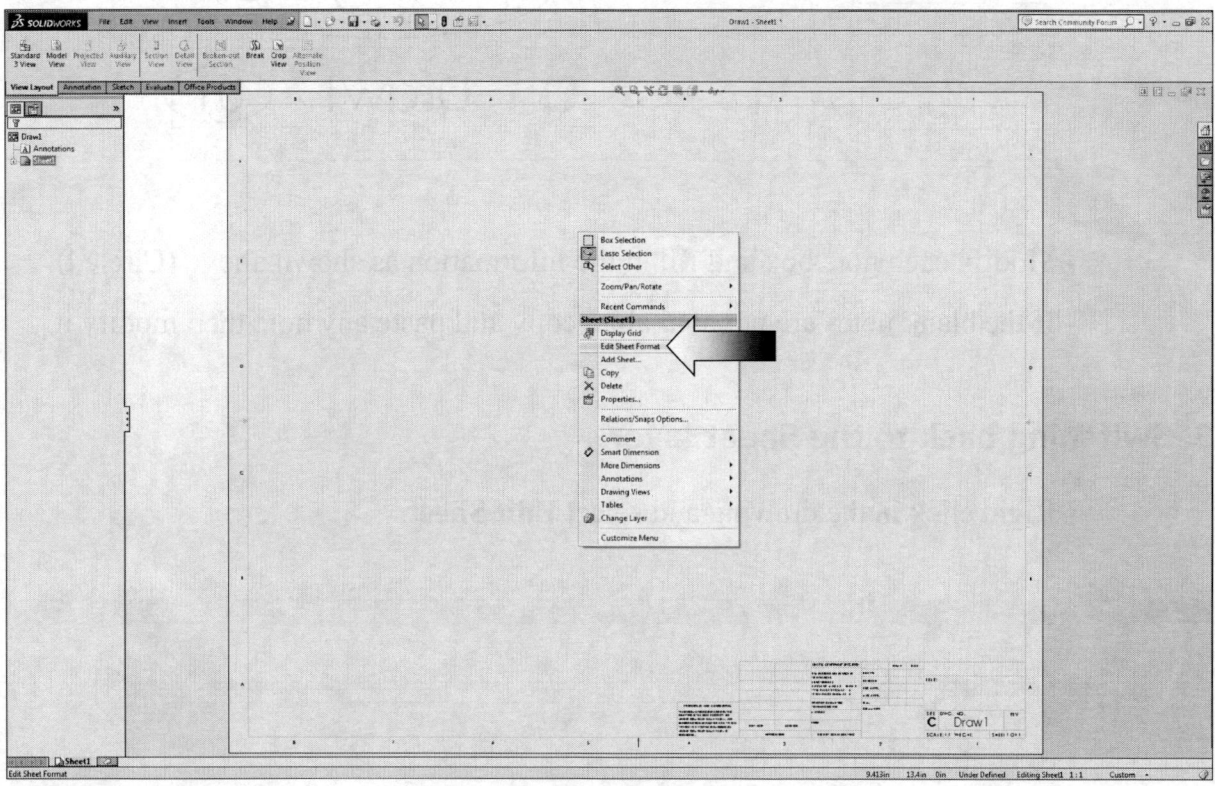

- Using the SolidWorks drawing templates, there are "blank notes" already created for each field within the title block.

- Double click the blank note in the Company-Name field and enter: **SolidWorks.**

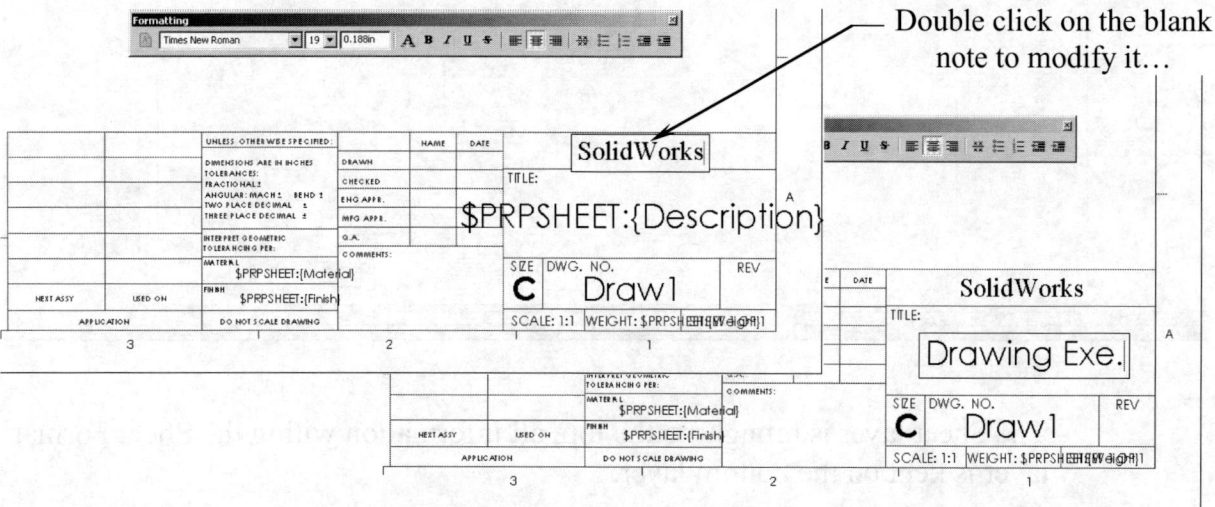

Double click on the blank note to modify it...

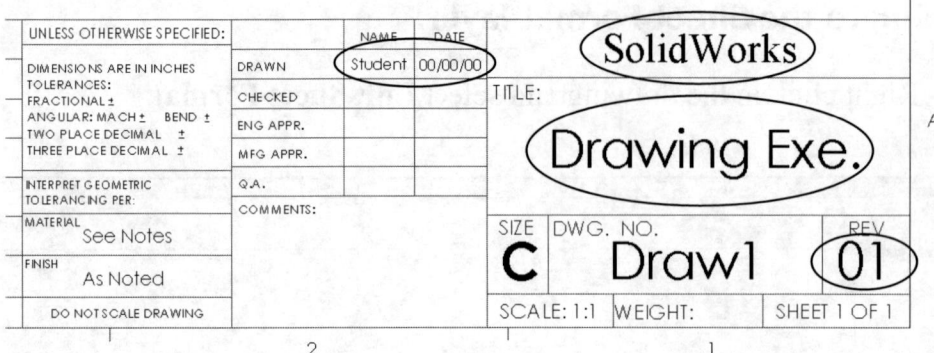

- Modify each note box and fill in the information as shown above (Circled).

- If the blank notes are not available, copy and paste any note then modify it.

3. Switching back to the Sheet layer:

- Right click in the drawing and select **Edit Sheet**.

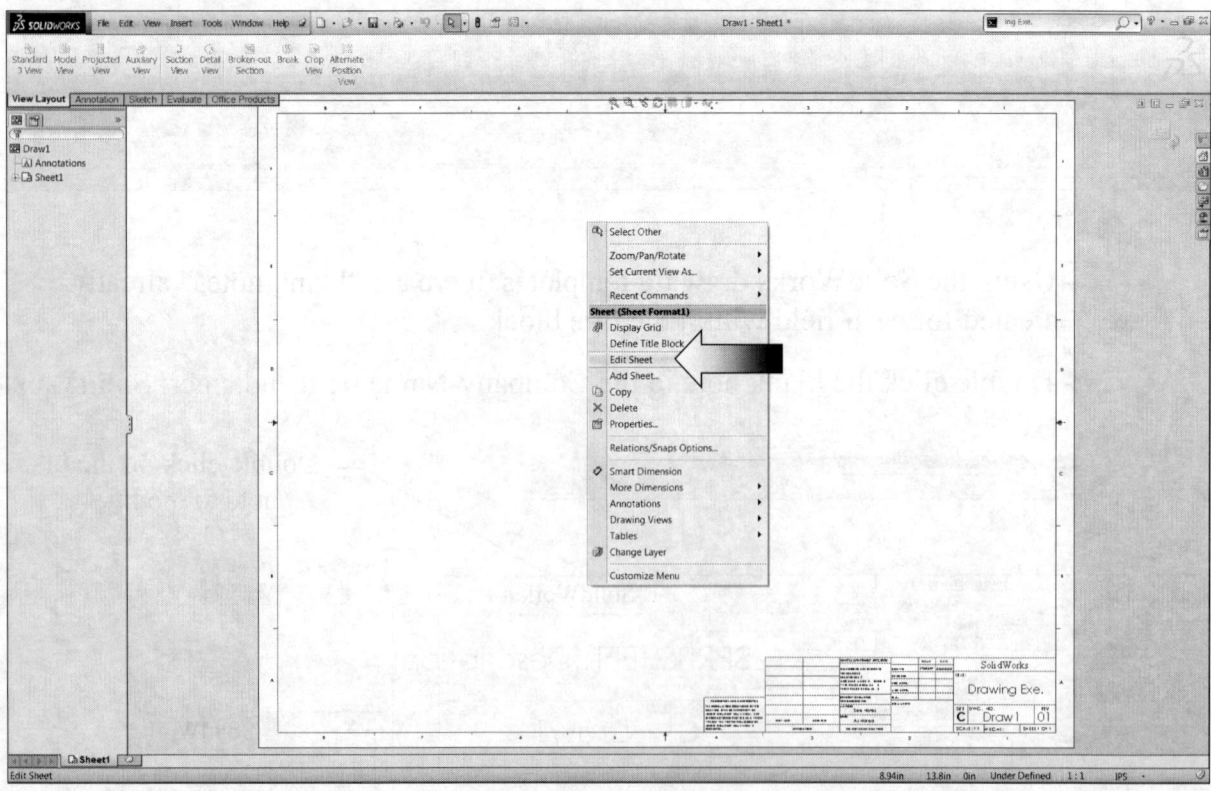

- The Sheet layer is brought to the top, all information within the Sheet Format layer is kept on the bottom layer.

4. Setting up the Drawing Options:

- Go to **Tools / Options**

- Select the **Drawings** options from the list.

- Enable and/or disable the drawing options by clicking on the check boxes as shown below.

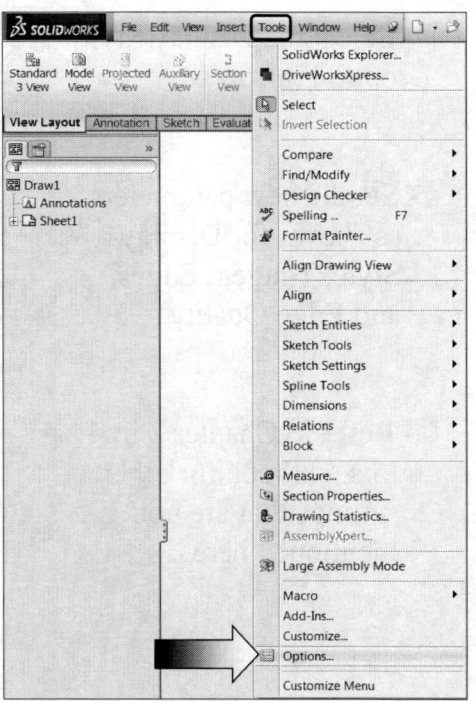

<u>NOTE:</u>
For further information about these options, please refer to Chapter 2 in the: SolidWorks 2015 Part I - Basic Tools textbook (Essential Parts, Assemblies and Drawings).

- These parameters are examples for use with this textbook only; you may have to modify them to work with your application or company's standards.

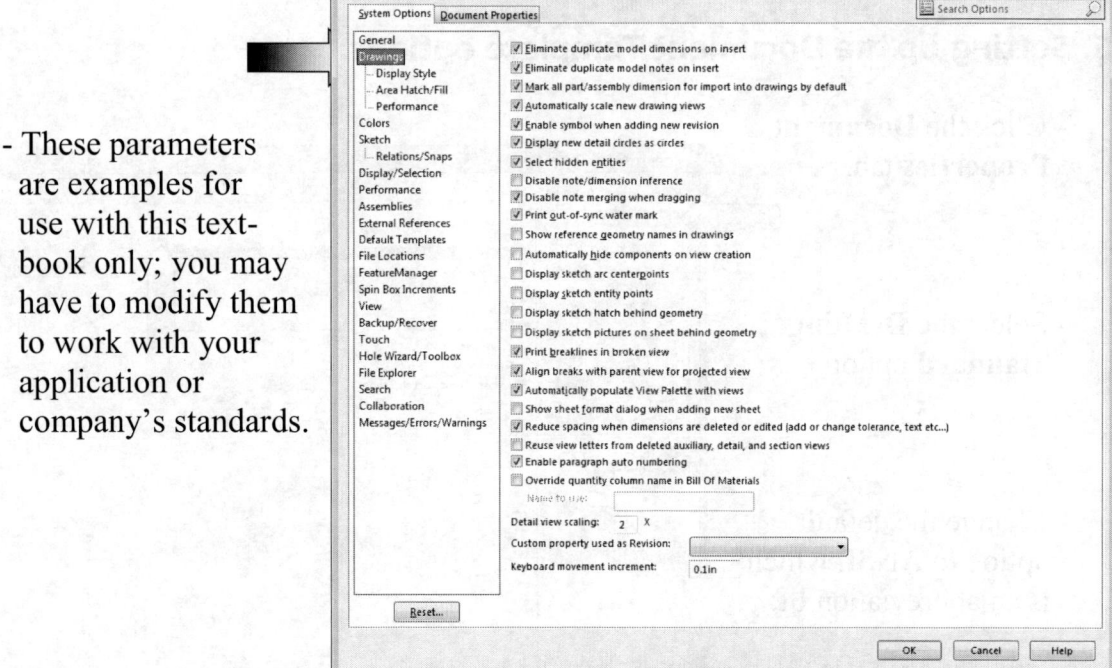

- The parameters that you are setting here will be saved as the default system options, and they will affect the current as well as all future documents.

- Once again, enable only the check boxes as shown in the dialog above.

- Select the Display Style option (arrow).

- Set the new parameters as shown for Display-Style, Tangent Edges, and Edge Quality.

- Refer to Chapter 2 in this textbook for other settings that are not mentioned here.

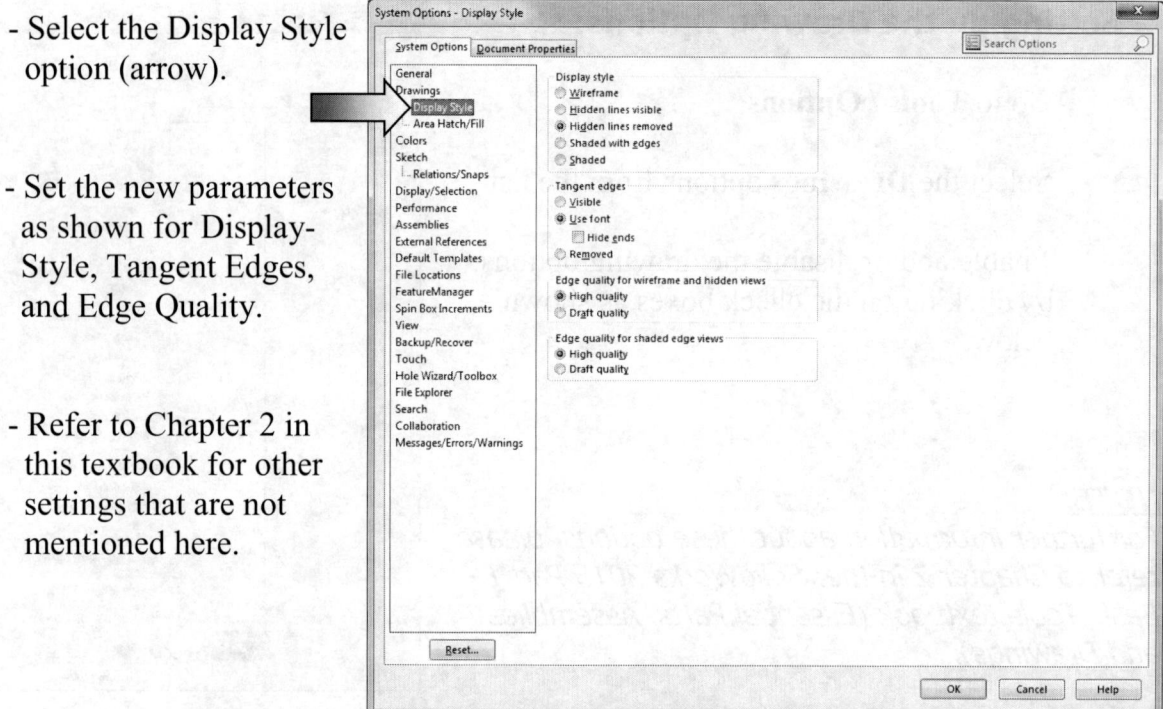

5. Setting up the Document Template options:

- Click the **Document Properties** tab.

- Select the **Drafting Standard** option.

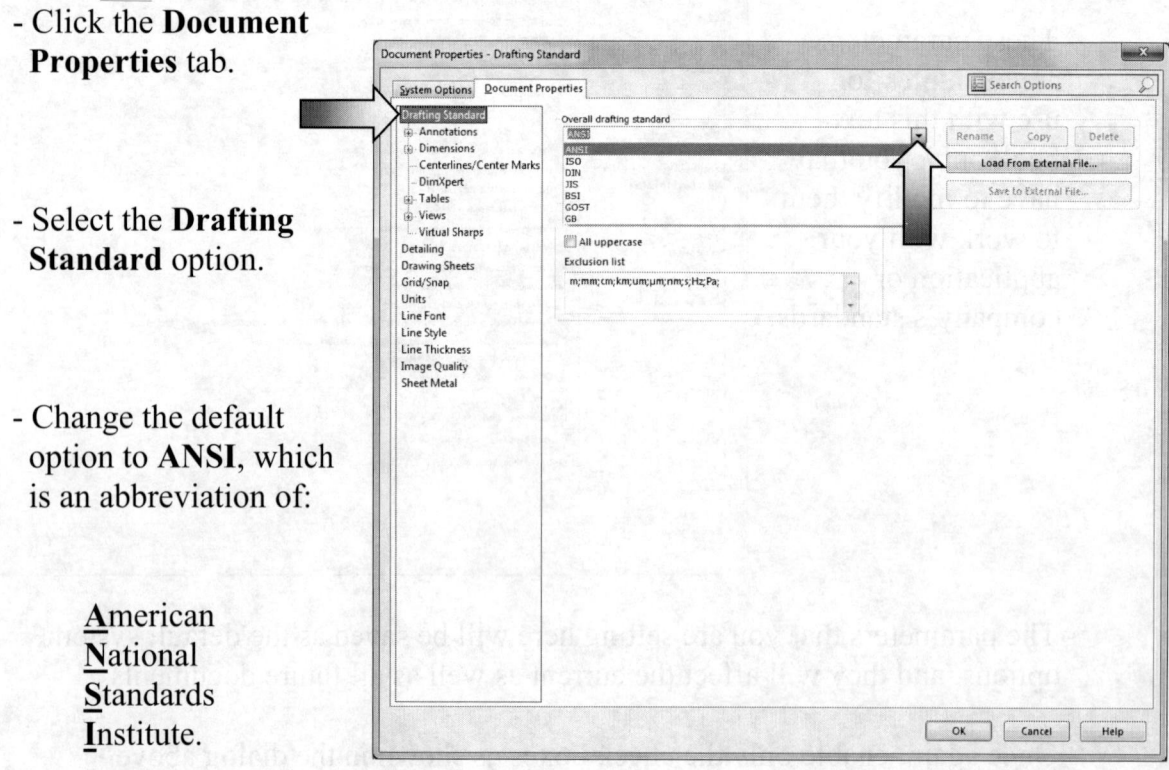

- Change the default option to **ANSI**, which is an abbreviation of:

 American
 National
 Standards
 Institute.

- Select the **Annotations** option (arrow).

- Set the new parameters as shown.

- Click the **Font** button and select the following:

  Century Gothic
  Regular
  13 points

- Set the Note, Dimension, Surface Finish, Weld-Symbol, Tables, and Balloon to match the settings for Annotations.

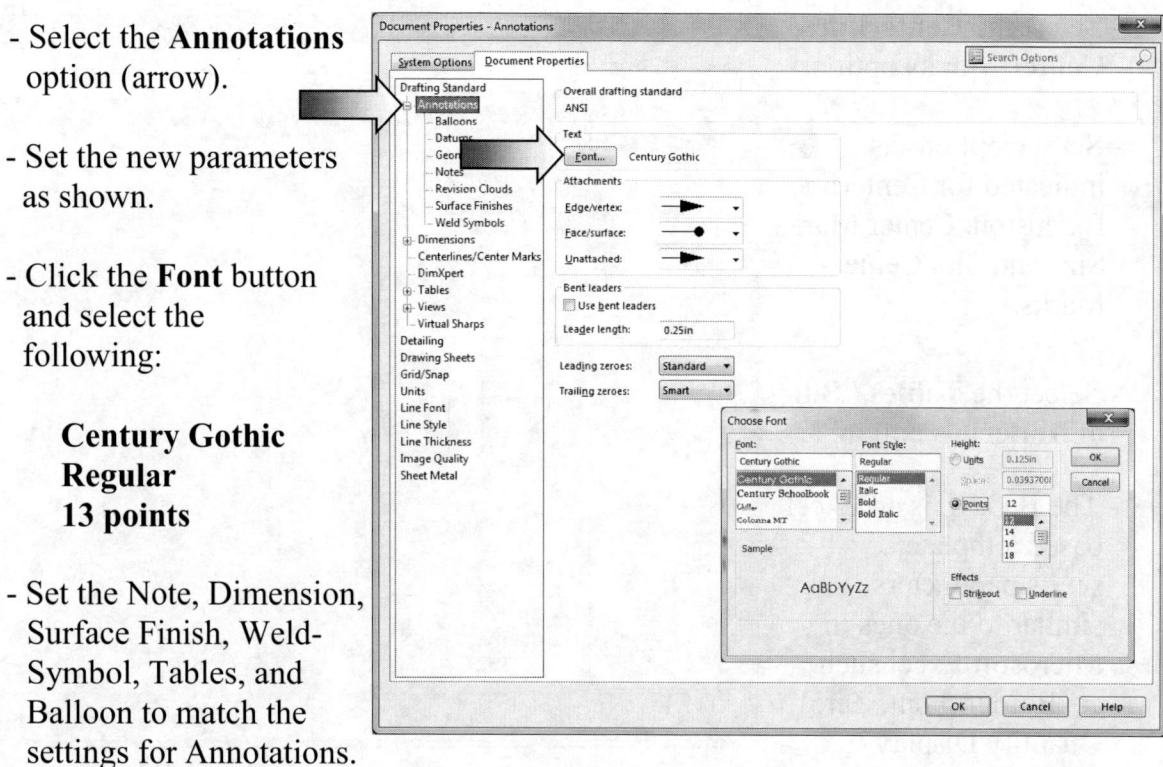

- Select the **Dimensions** option (arrow).

- Set the parameter in this section to match the ones shown in this dialog box.

- If the Dual Dimension Display is selected, be sure to set the number of decimal places for both of your Primary and Secondary dimensions.

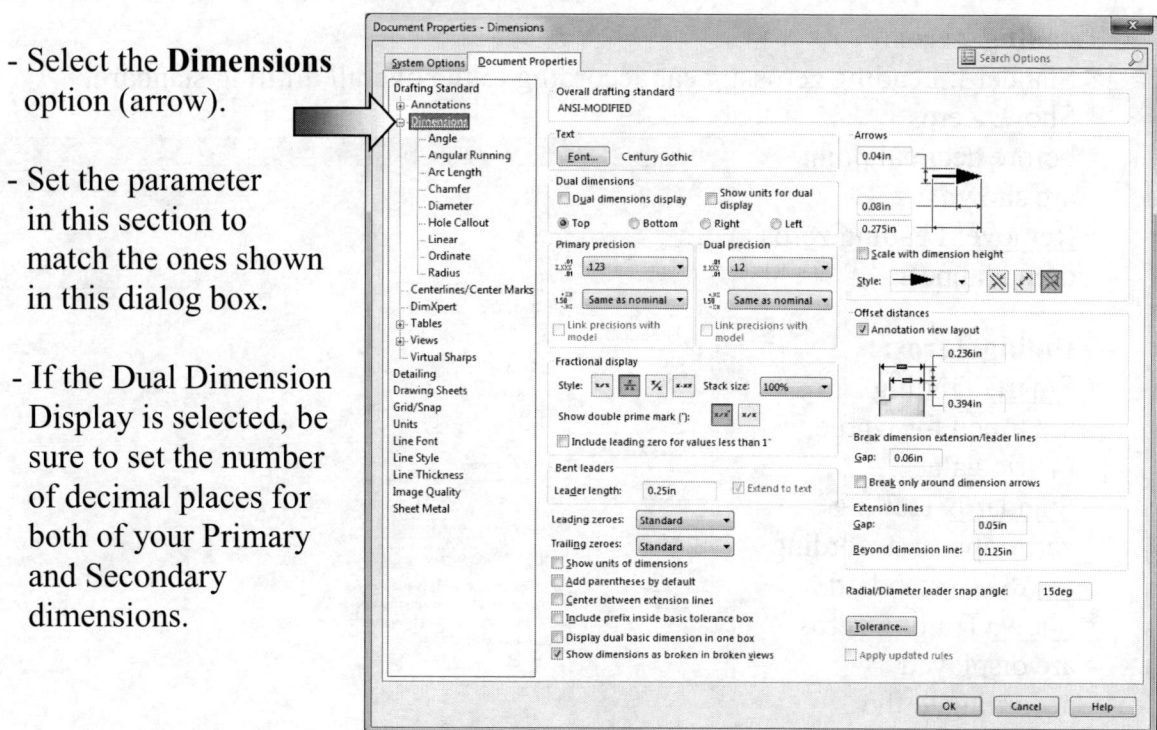

NOTE: *Skip to the Units option below, if you need to change your Primary unit from Millimeter to Inches, or vice versa.*

- Select the **Centerlines/ Center Marks** option.

- Set the options as indicated for Centerline Extension, Center Marks Size and Slot Center-Marks.

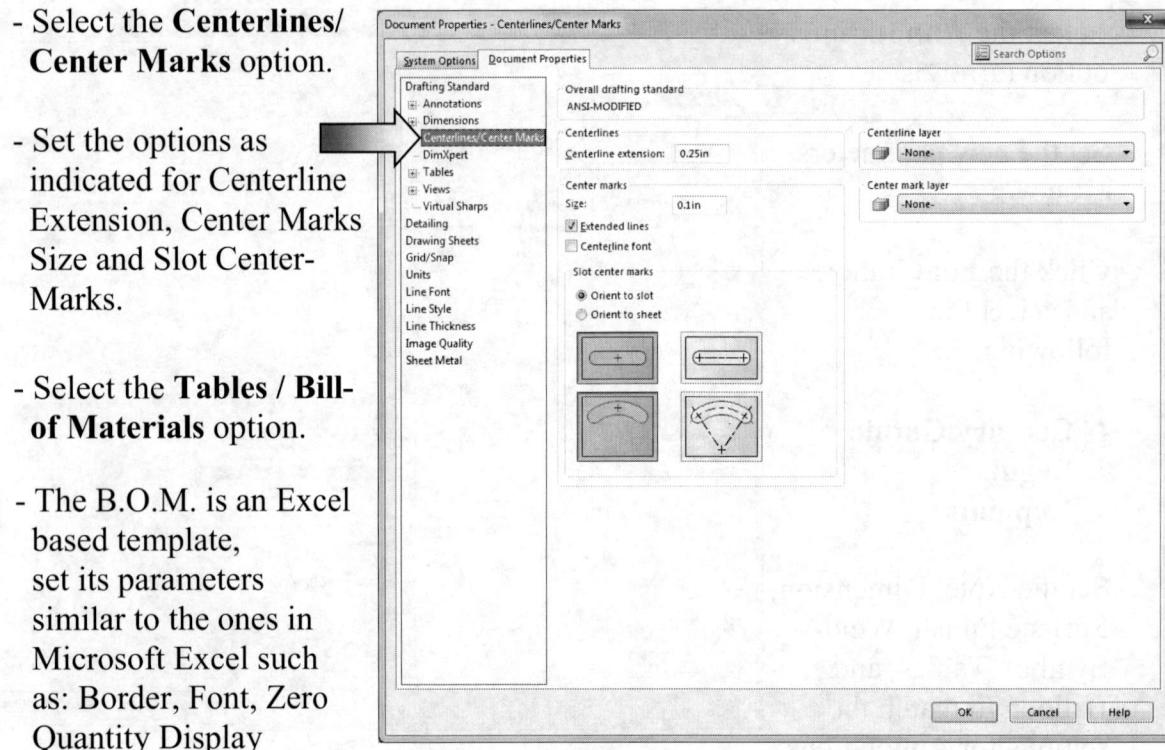

- Select the **Tables / Bill-of Materials** option.

- The B.O.M. is an Excel based template, set its parameters similar to the ones in Microsoft Excel such as: Border, Font, Zero Quantity Display Missing Component, Leading and Trailing Zeros, etc.

- **Leading Zeros:**
  * Standard: Leading zeros appear according to the overall drafting standard.
  * <u>Show:</u> Zeros before decimal point are shown.
  * <u>Remove:</u> Leading zeros do not appear.

- **Trailing Zeros:**
  * <u>Smart:</u> Trailing zeros are timed for whole metric values.
  * <u>Standard:</u> Trailing zeros appear according to ASME standard.
  * <u>Show:</u> Trailing zeros are displayed according to the decimal places specified in Units.
  * <u>Remove:</u> Trailing zeros do not appear.

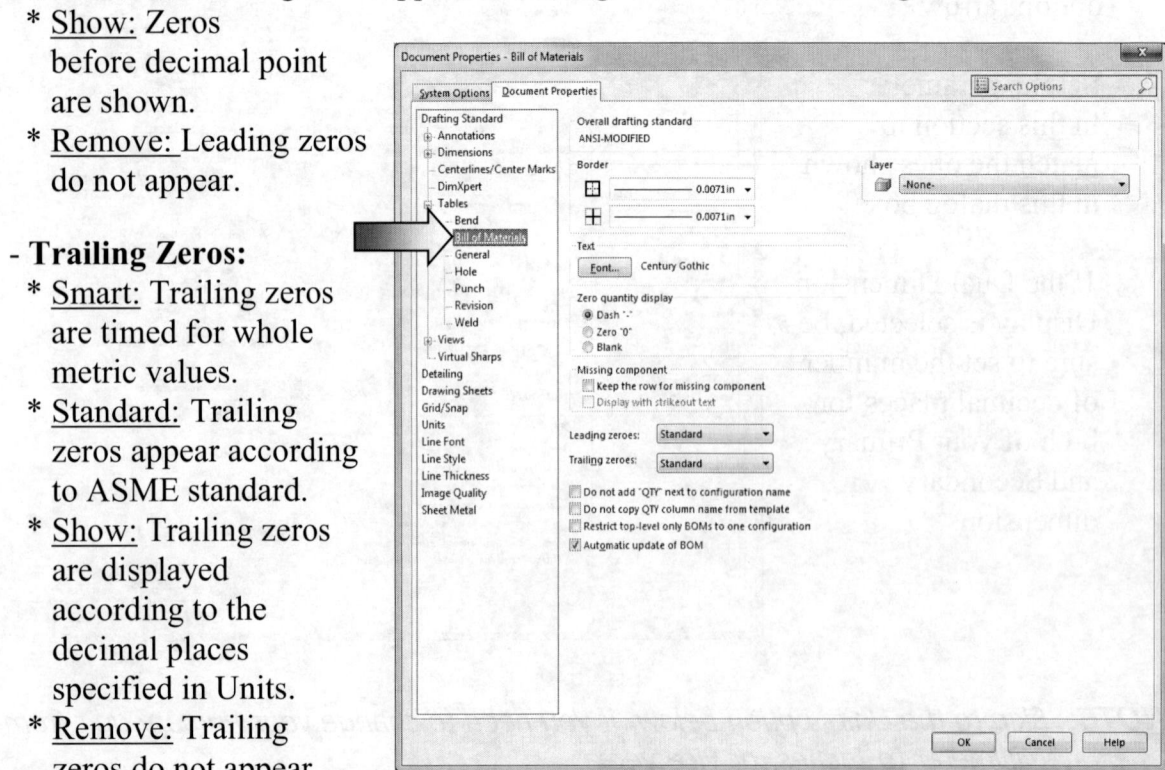

- Select the **Tables / Revision** option.

- Set the document-level drafting settings for revision table like: Border, Font, Alphabet Numerical Control, Multiple Sheet Style and Layer.

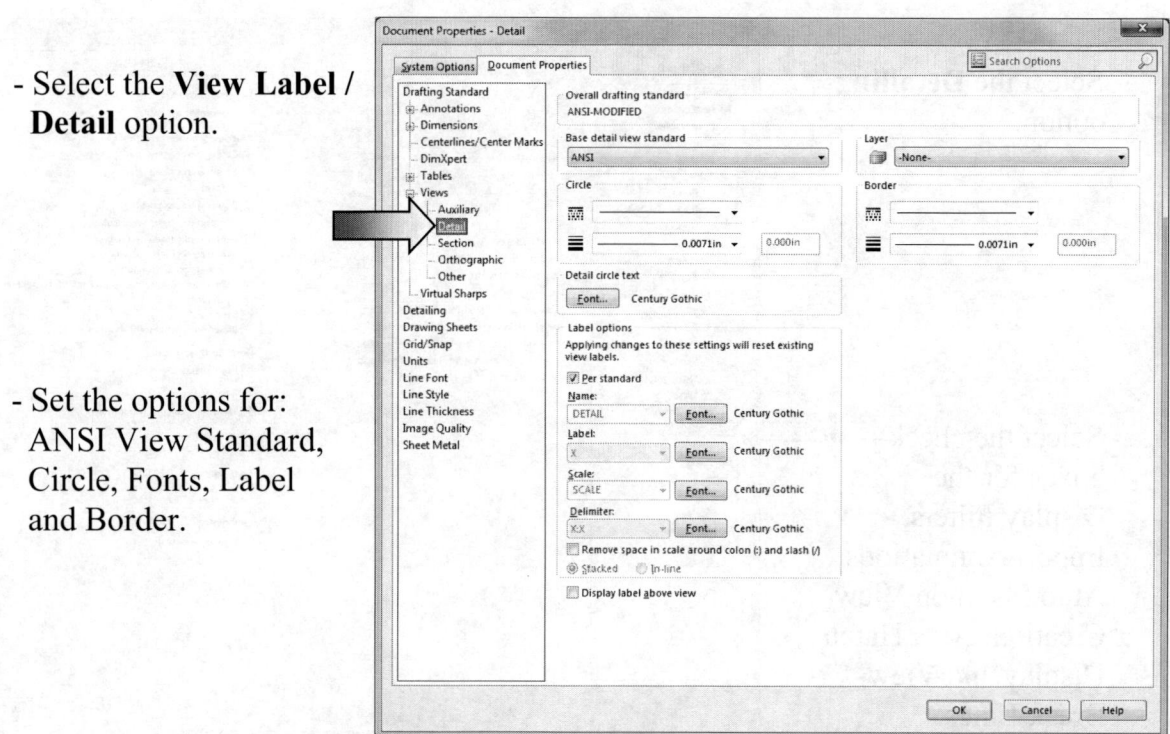

- Select the **View Label / Detail** option.

- Set the options for: ANSI View Standard, Circle, Fonts, Label and Border.

- Select the **View Label /
Section** option.

- Set the Line Style, Line
Thickness, Fonts, Label,
Scale, Layer, and
Section Arrow
Size.

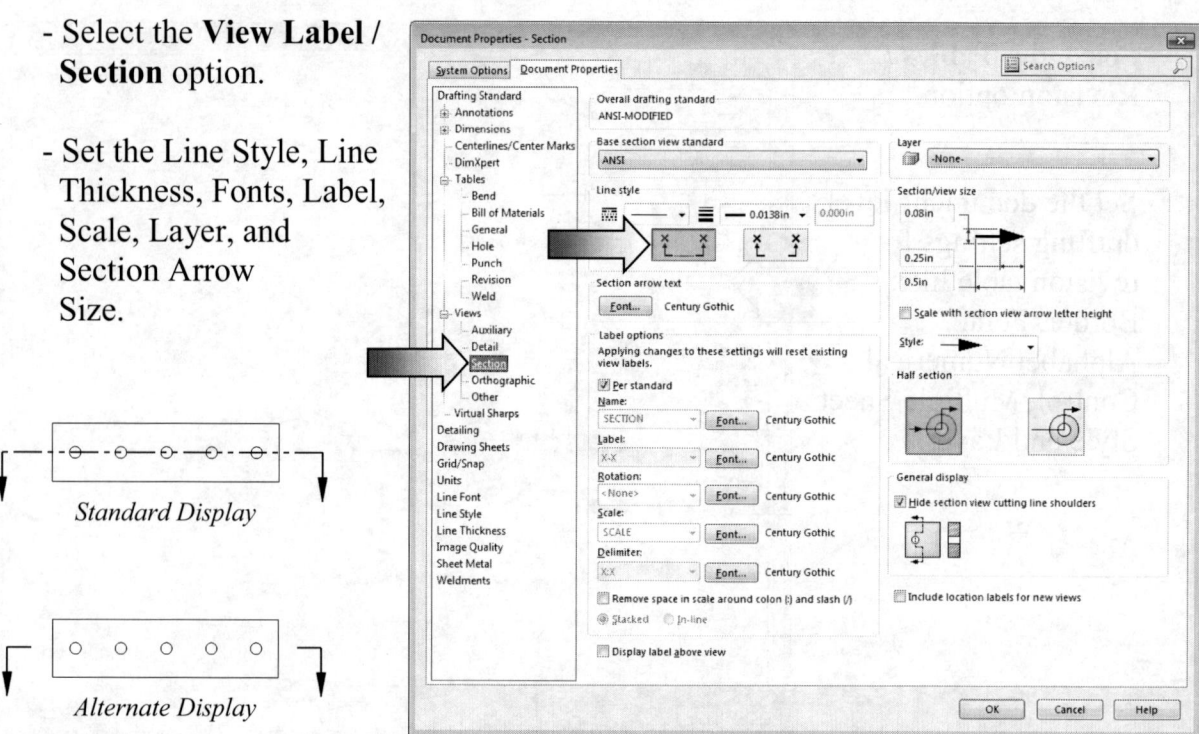

Standard Display

Alternate Display

- Select the **Detailing**
option.

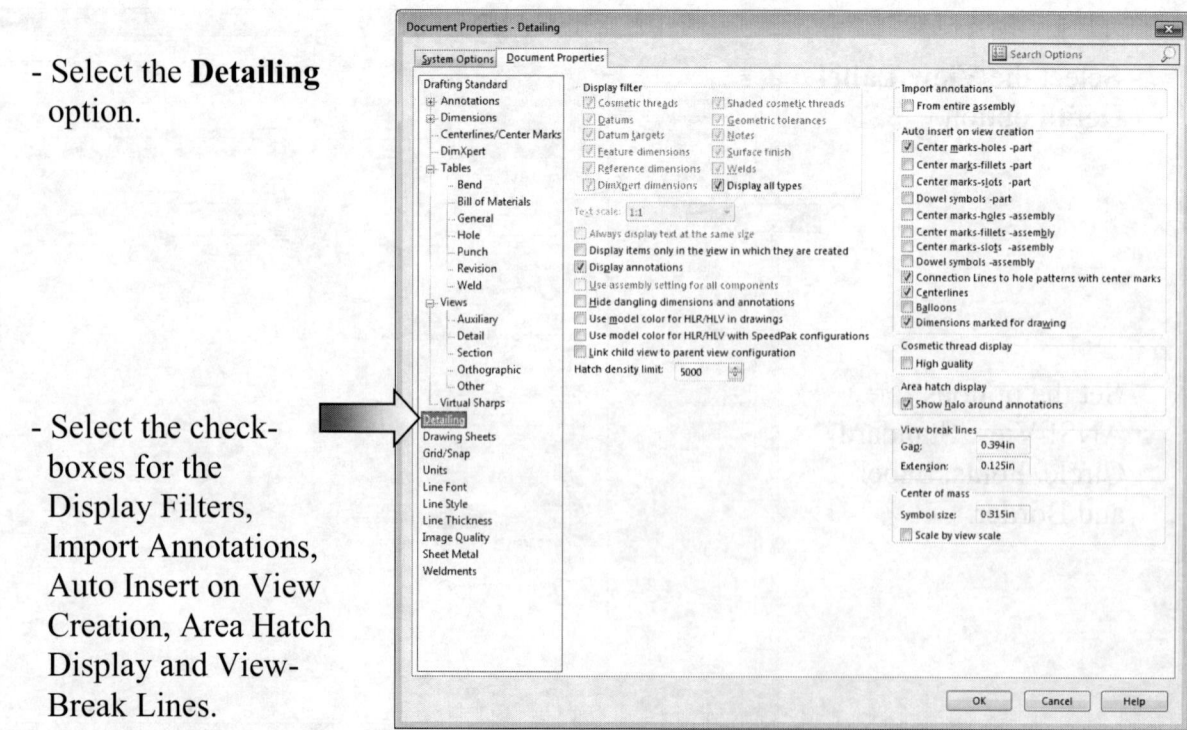

- Select the check-
boxes for the
Display Filters,
Import Annotations,
Auto Insert on View
Creation, Area Hatch
Display and View-
Break Lines.

- Select the **Drawing-Sheet** option.

- Enable the checkbox: **Use Different Sheet Format** if sheet 2 uses a different (or partial) title block.

- This property lets you automatically have one sheet format for the first sheet and a separate sheet format for all additional sheet.

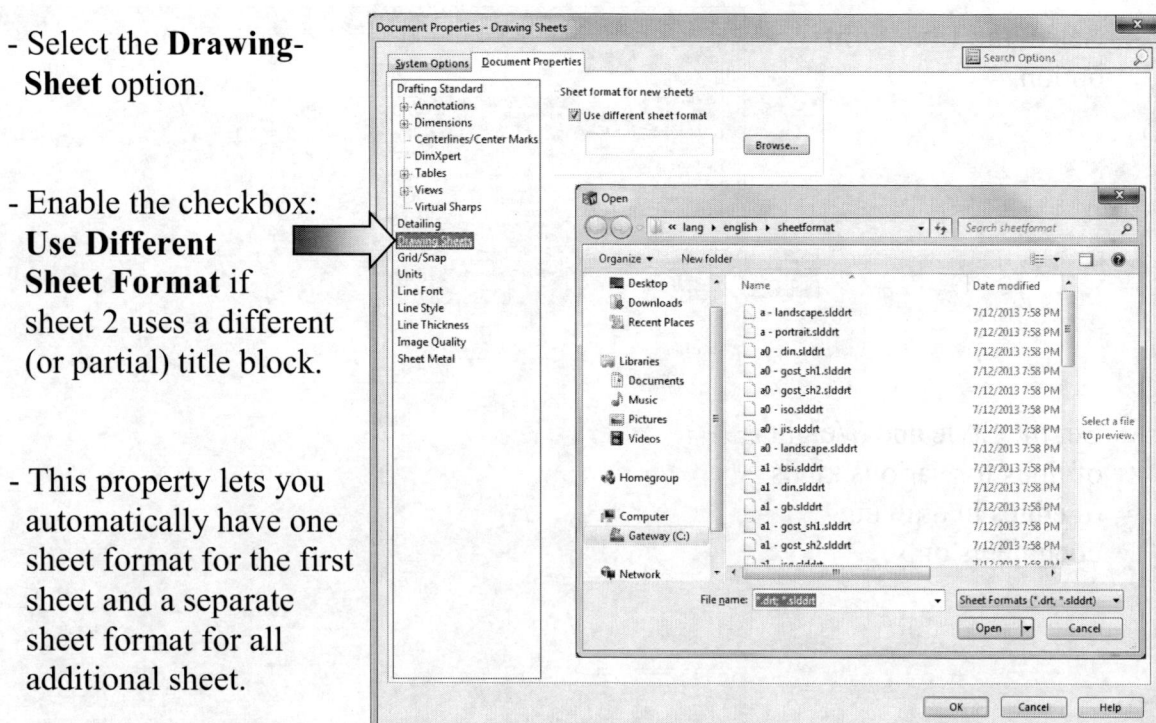

- Select the **Units** option.

- Click the **IPS (Inch, Pound, Second)** system.

- Set the Length Units to: **3 Decimal Places (.123)**

- Other options can be set to meet your company's standards.

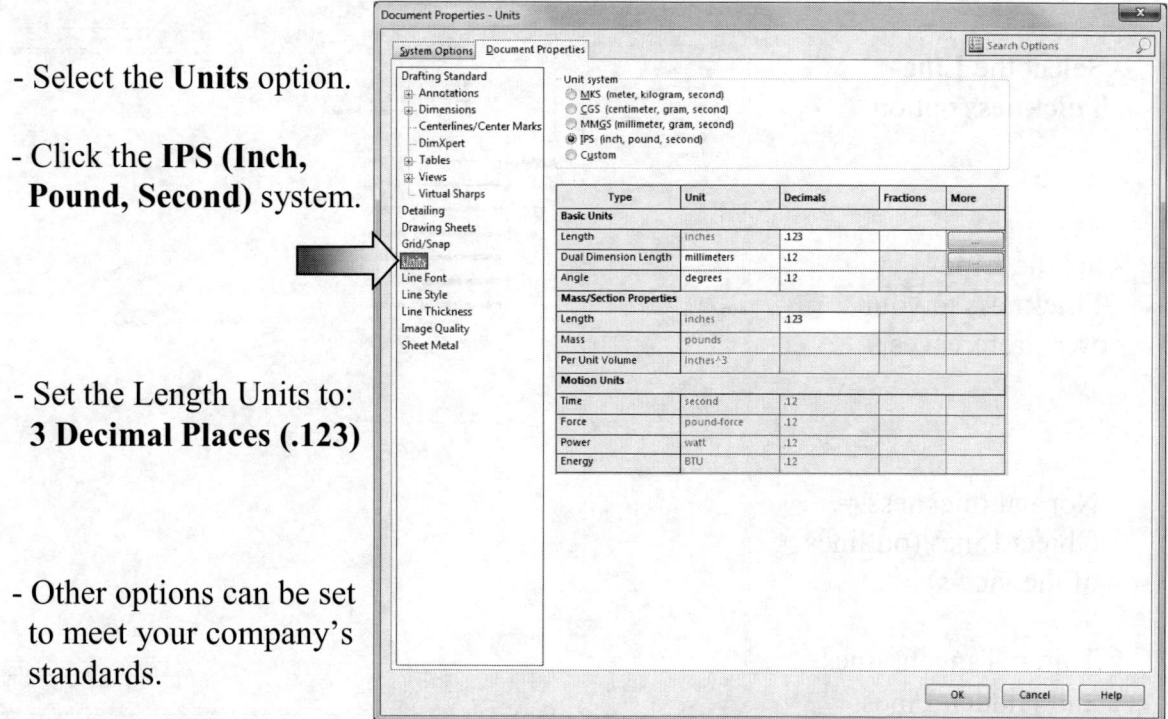

- Select the **Line Font** option.

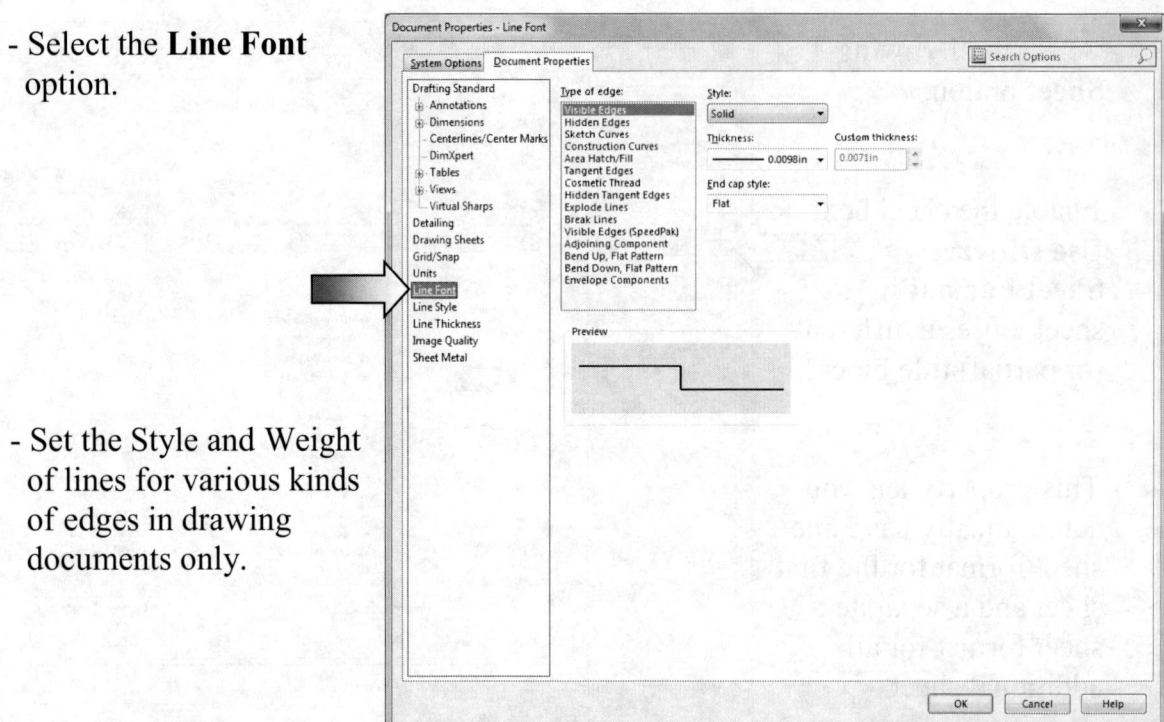

- Set the Style and Weight of lines for various kinds of edges in drawing documents only.

- Select the **Line-Thickness** option.

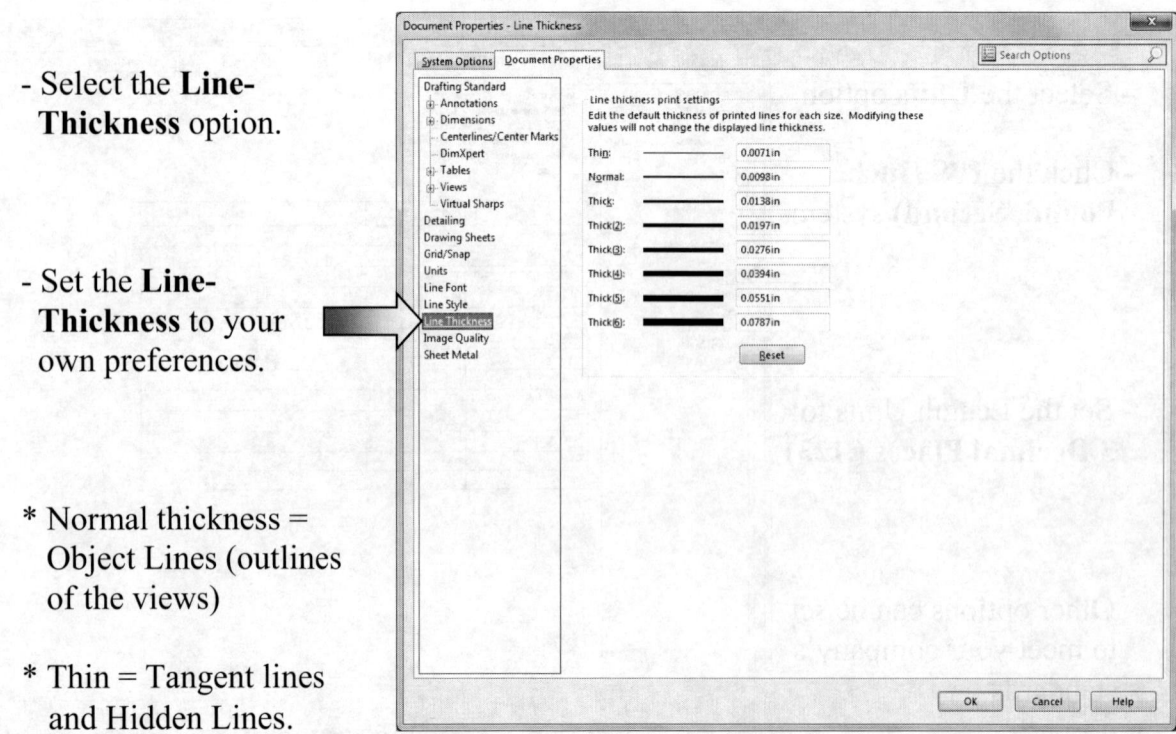

- Set the **Line-Thickness** to your own preferences.

* Normal thickness = Object Lines (outlines of the views)

* Thin = Tangent lines and Hidden Lines.

- Select the **Image-Quality** option.

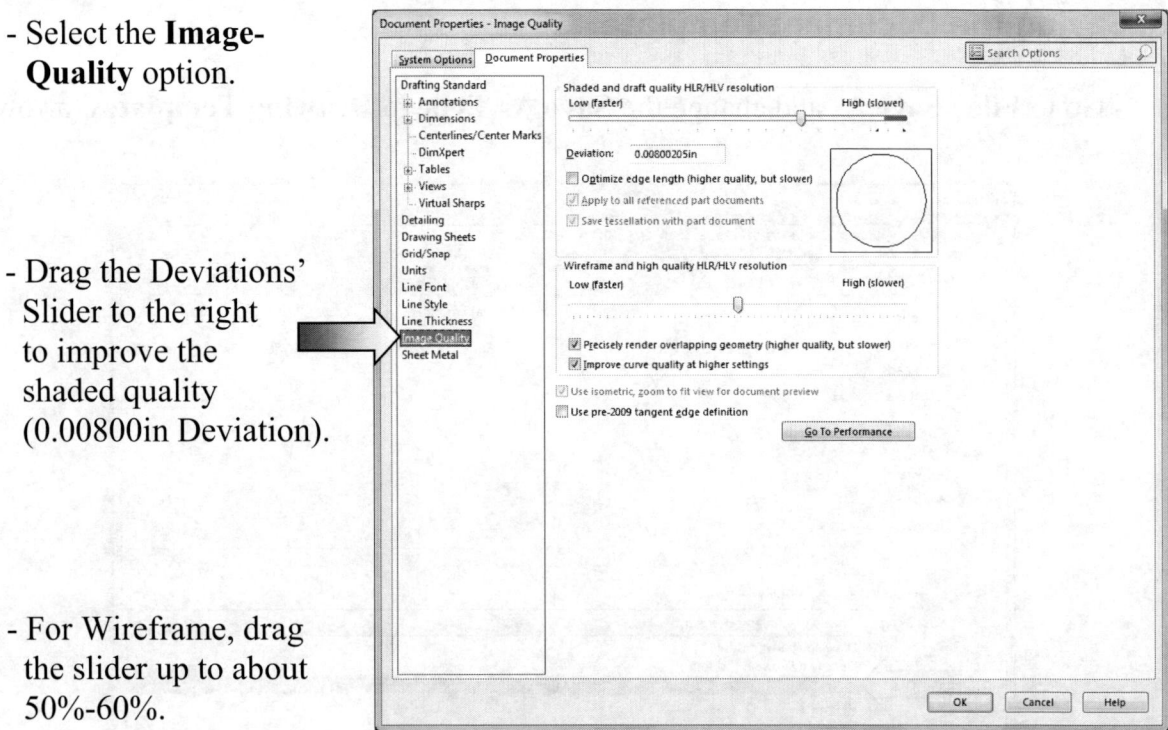

- Drag the Deviations' Slider to the right to improve the shaded quality (0.00800in Deviation).

- For Wireframe, drag the slider up to about 50%-60%.

- Select the **Sheet Metal** option.

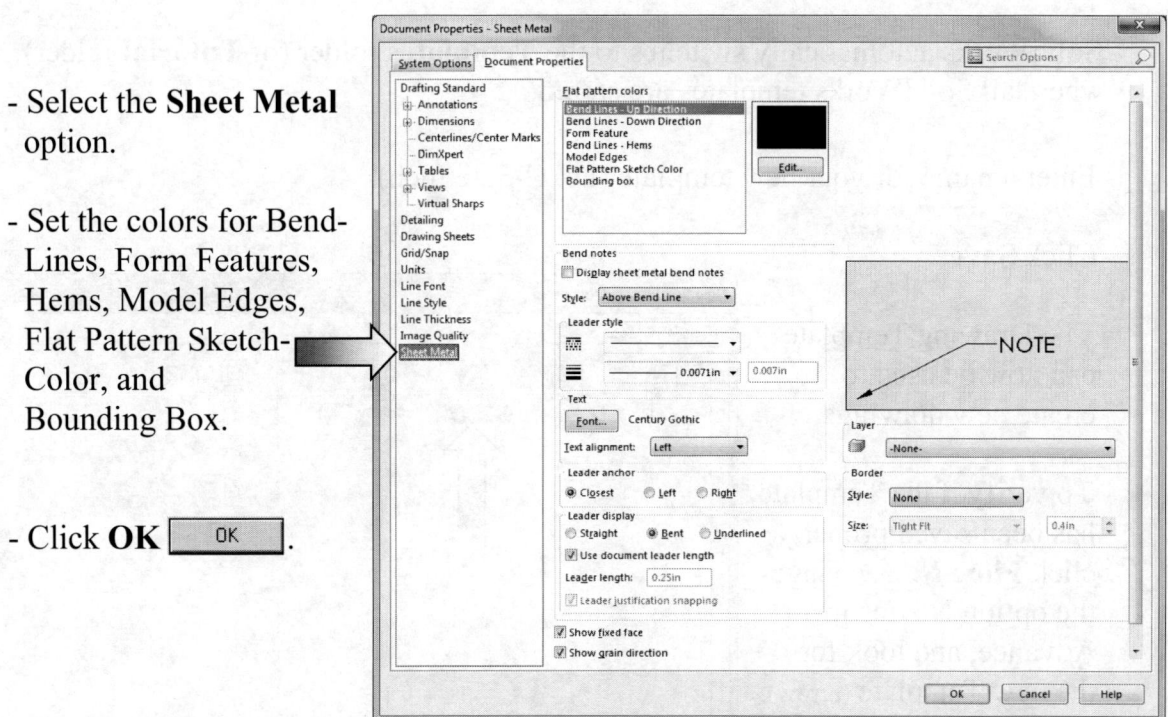

- Set the colors for Bend-Lines, Form Features, Hems, Model Edges, Flat Pattern Sketch-Color, and Bounding Box.

- Click **OK** [OK].

- These settings control the tessellation of curved surfaces for shaded rendering output. A higher resolution setting results in slower model rebuilding but more accurate curves.

6. Saving the Document Template:

- Go to **File / Save As** and change the **Save As Type** to **Drawing Templates** (arrow).

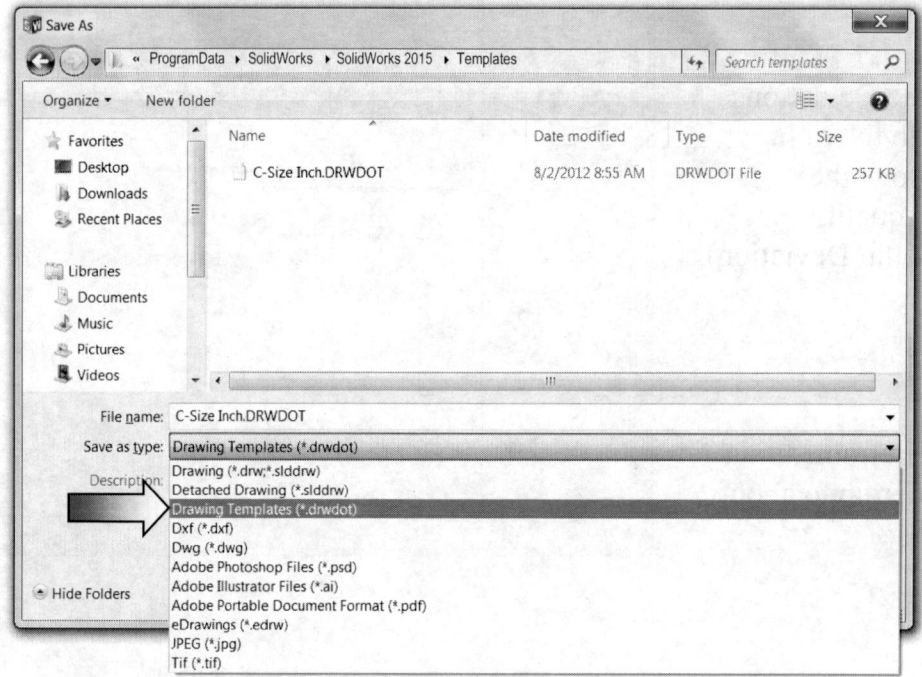

- SolidWorks automatically switches to the **Templates** folder (or **Tutorial** folder), where all SolidWorks templates are stored.

- Enter a name for your new template (i.e. C-Size Inch).

- Click **Save**.

- The Drawing Template can now be used to create new drawings.

- To verify if the Template has been saved properly, click **File / New**, change the option Novice to Advance, and look for the new Template (arrow).

- **Close** the document template.

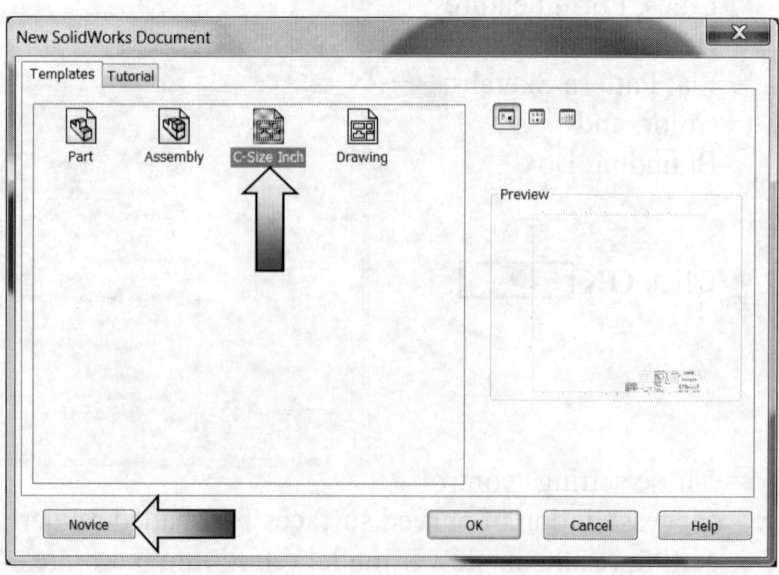

Questions for Review

Drawing Preperations

1. Custom settings and parameters can be set and saved in the Document Template.
   a. True
   b. False

2. Document Templates are normally stored either in: (C:\Program Files\SolidWorks Corp\SolidWorks\Data\Templates) OR (C:\Program Files\SolidWorks Corp\Lang\English\Tutorial).
   a. True
   b. False

3. To access the sheet format and edit the information in the title block:
   a. Right click in the drawing and select Edit Sheet Format.
   b. Right click the Sheet Format icon from the Feature Tree and select Edit Sheet-Format.
   c. All of the above.

4. The **Sheet** layer is where the Title Block information and Revisions changes are stored.
   a. True
   b. False

5. The **Sheet Format** layer is used to create the drawing views, dimensions, and annotations.
   a. True
   b. False

6. Information in the Title Block and Revision Block are Fixed, they cannot be modified.
   a. True
   b. False

7. The Document Template is saved with the file Extension:
   a. DWG
   b. DXF
   c. SLDPRT
   d. DRWDOT
   e. SLDDRW

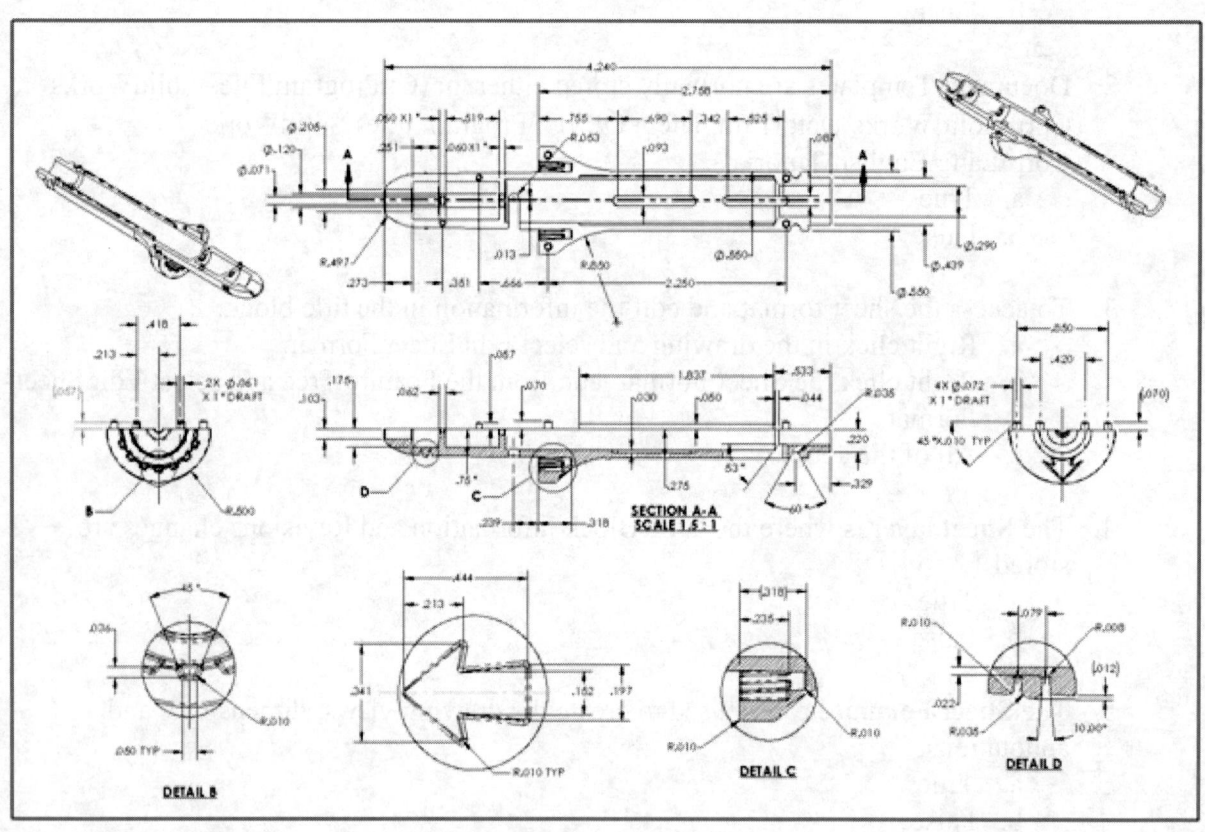

CHAPTER 15

Assembly Drawings

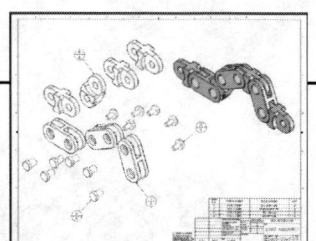

Assembly Drawings
Links Assembly

- Assembly drawings are created in the same way as part drawings, the same drawing tools and commands are used to create the drawing views and annotations. In an assembly drawing all components are shown together as assembled or as exploded.

- The standard drawing views like the Front, Top, Right, and Isometric views can be created with the same drawing tools, or they can be dragged and dropped from the View Pallet.

- When a cross section view is created, it will be cross hatched automatically and the hatch patterns that represent the material of the part can be added and easily edited as well.

- A parts list or a Bill of Materials (B.O.M.) is created to report the details of the components such as:

       * Materials.

       * Vendors.

       * Quantities.

       * Part numbers, etc.

4	004-12345	Single Link	4
3	003-12345	Pin Head	6
2	002-12345	Alignment Pin	6
1	001-12345	Double Link	3
ITEM NO.	PART NUMBER	DESCRIPTION	QTY.

- The components will then be labeled with Balloons (or Dash Numbers) for verification against the Bill of Materials.

- This chapter discusses the basics of creating an assembly drawing using SolidWorks 2015.

Links Assembly
Assembly Drawings

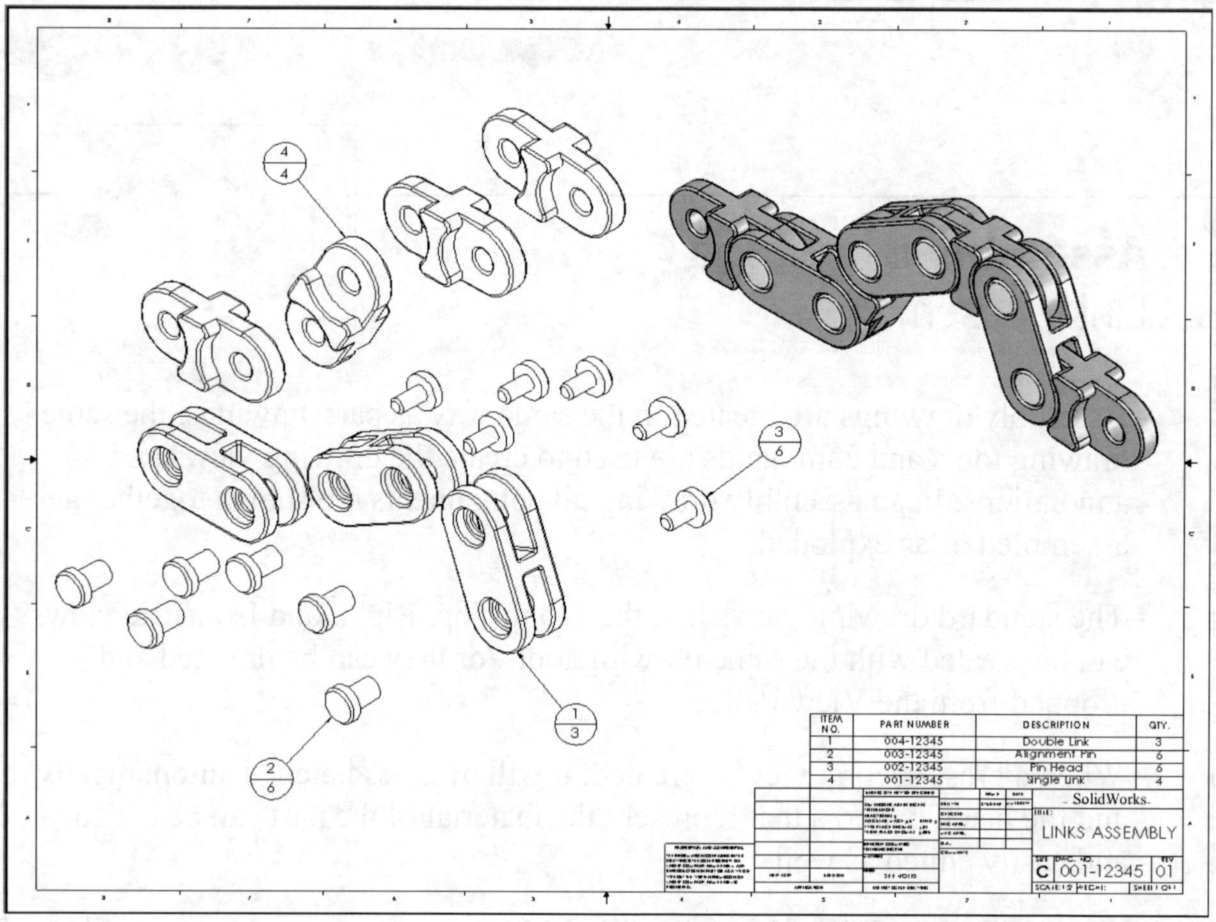

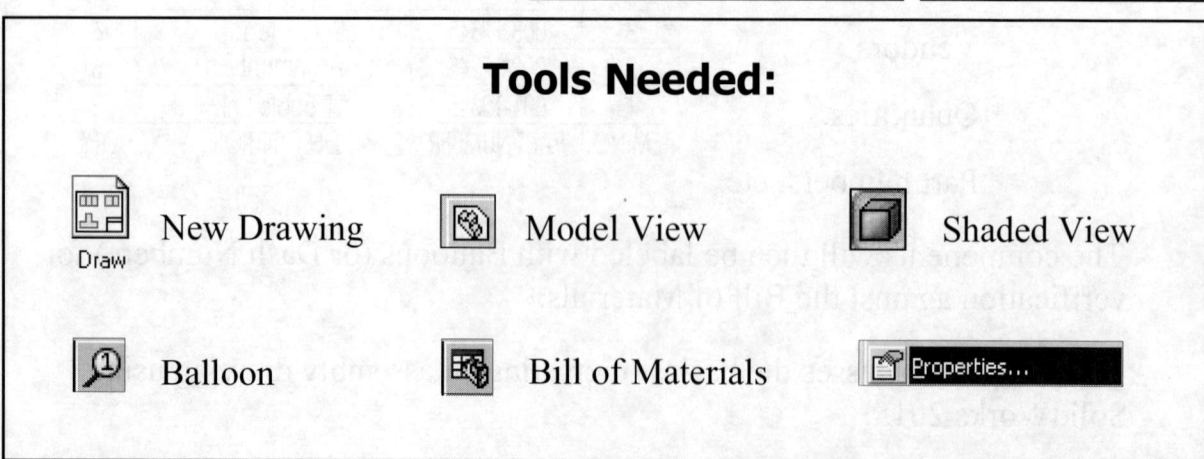

ITEM NO.	PART NUMBER	DESCRIPTION	QTY.
1	004-12345	Double Link	3
2	003-12345	Alignment Pin	6
3	002-12345	Pin Head	6
4	001-12345	Single Link	4

SolidWorks.

TITLE: LINKS ASSEMBLY

C | 001-12345 | REV 01

SCALE:2 | WEIGHT: | SHEET 1 OF 1

Dimensioning Standards: **ANSI**	Third Angle Projection
Units: **INCHES** – 3 Decimals	

Tools Needed:

New Drawing
Draw

Model View

Shaded View

Balloon

Bill of Materials

Properties...

1. Creating a new drawing:

- Select **File / New / Draw** (or Drawing) / **OK**.

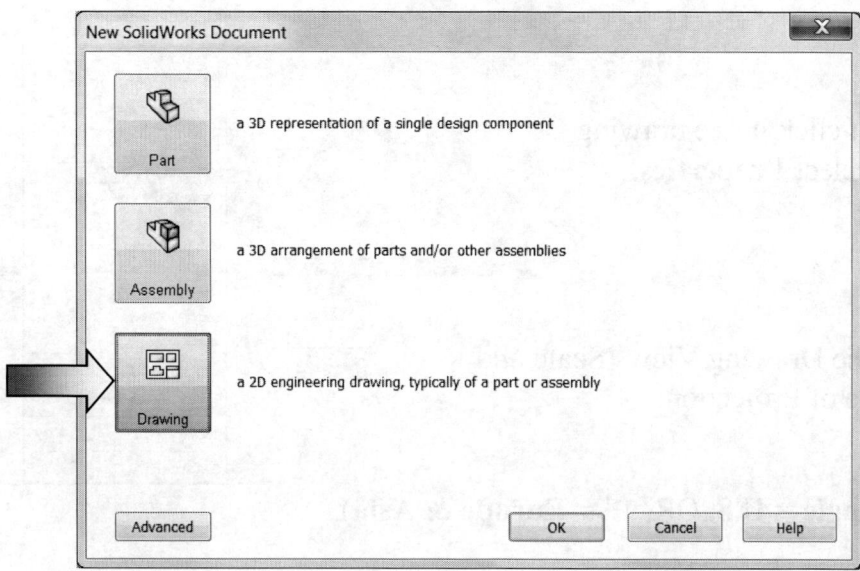

- Under Standard Sheet Size, select **C-Landscape** for paper size.

A = 8.5"   x   11.00"   (Landscape)
B = 17.00"   x   11.00"   (Landscape)
C = 22.00"   x   17.00"   (Landscape)
D = 34.00"   x   22.00"   (Landscape)
E = 44.00"   x   34.00"   (Landscape)

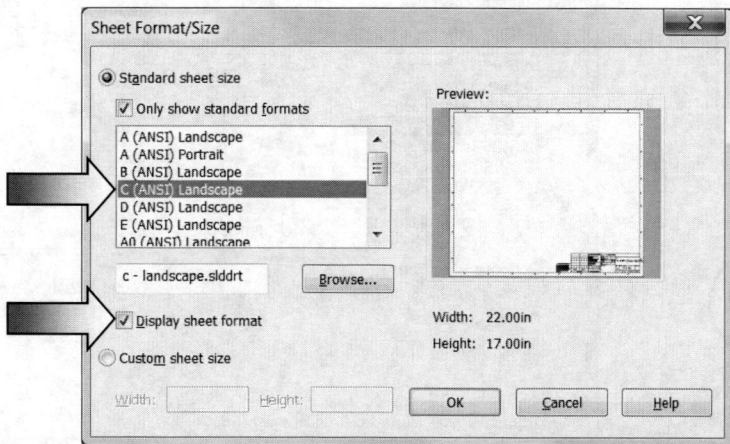

- Enable **Display Sheet Format** checkbox to display the revision and title blocks.

- Click **OK** ☐ OK .

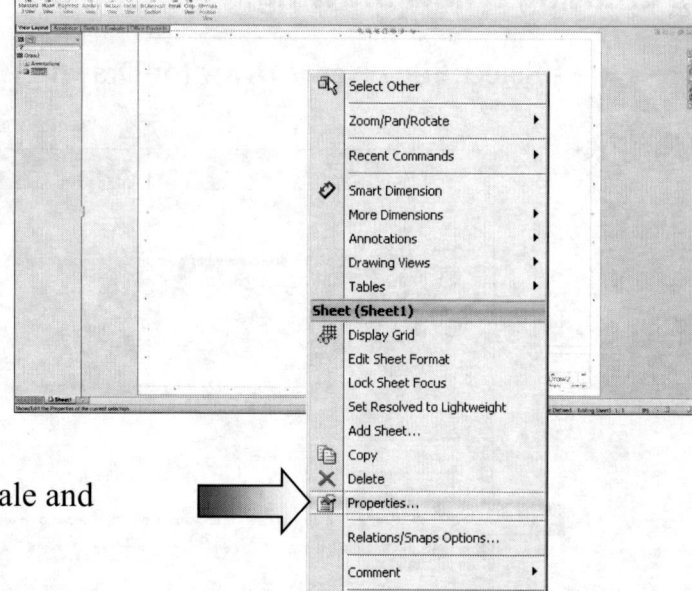

- The Drawing template appears in the graphics area.

- Right click in the drawing and select **Properties**.

- Set the Drawing Views Scale and Angle of Projection:

(**3rd Angle = U.S. <u>OR</u> 1st = Europe & Asia**).

- Set **Scale** to **1:1** (full scale)

- Set **Type of Projection** to: **Third Angle**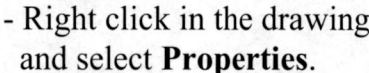

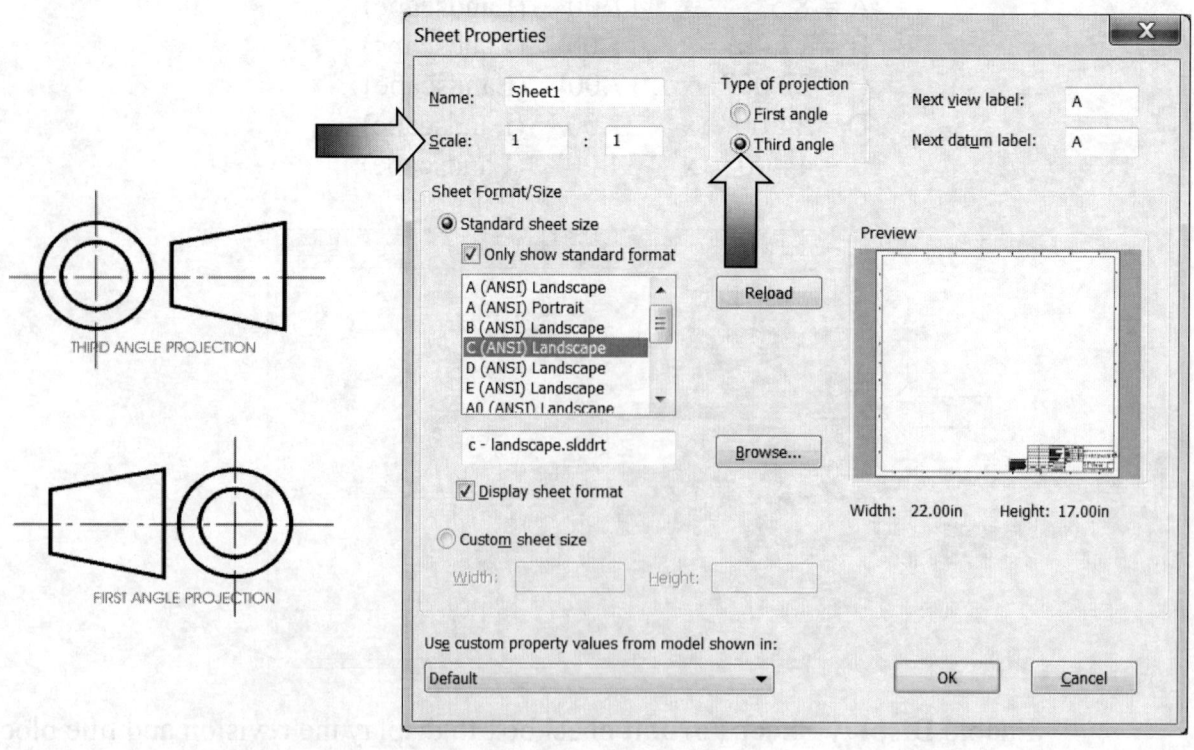

- Click **OK** [OK] .

2. Editing the Sheet Format:

- Right click inside the drawing and select **Edit-Sheet-Format**.

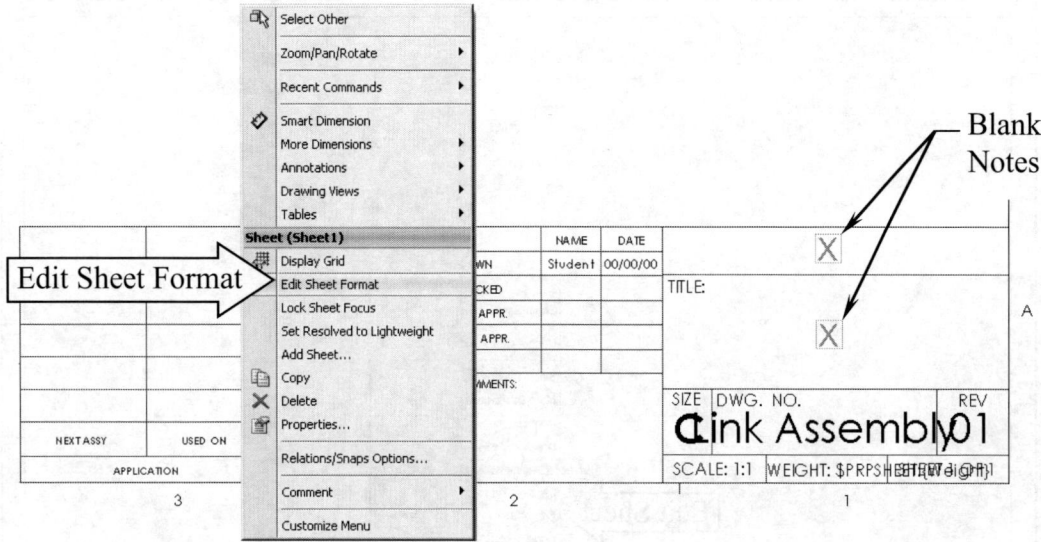

- The **Format** layer is brought up to the top.

3. Setting up the anchor point to attach the B.O.M.:

- Zoom in on the lower right side of the title block.

- Right click on the end point of the line (as shown) and select **Set-As-Anchor / Bill Of Materials.**

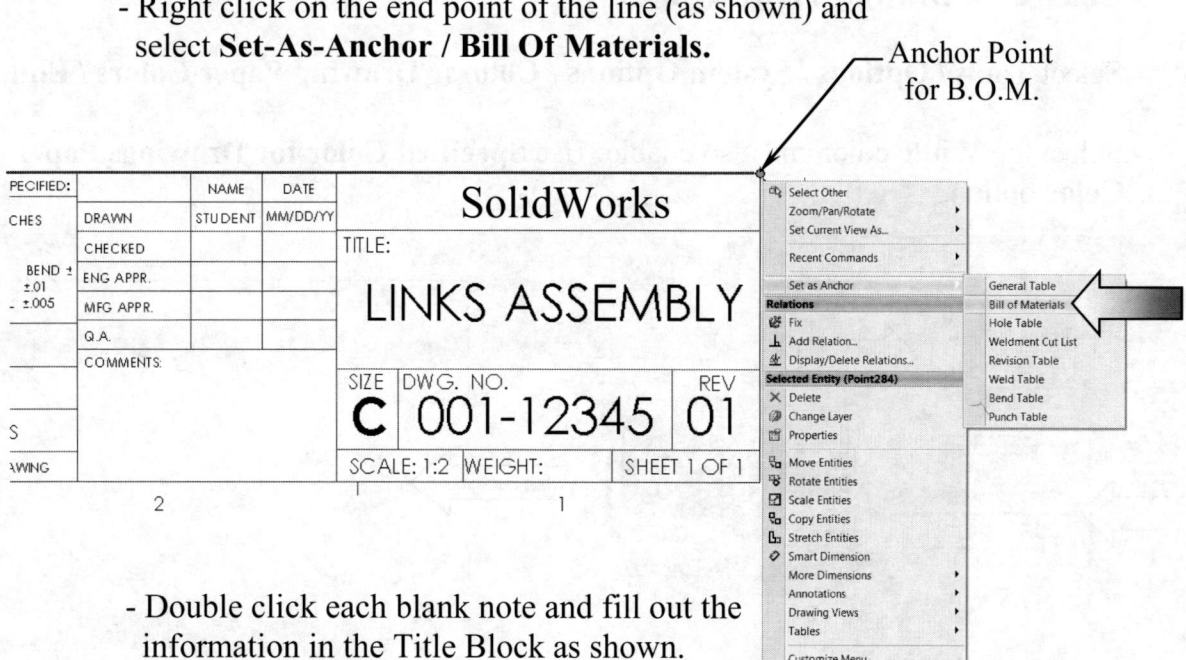

- Double click each blank note and fill out the information in the Title Block as shown.

4. Switching back to the Sheet layer:

- Right click inside the drawing and select **Edit-Sheet.**

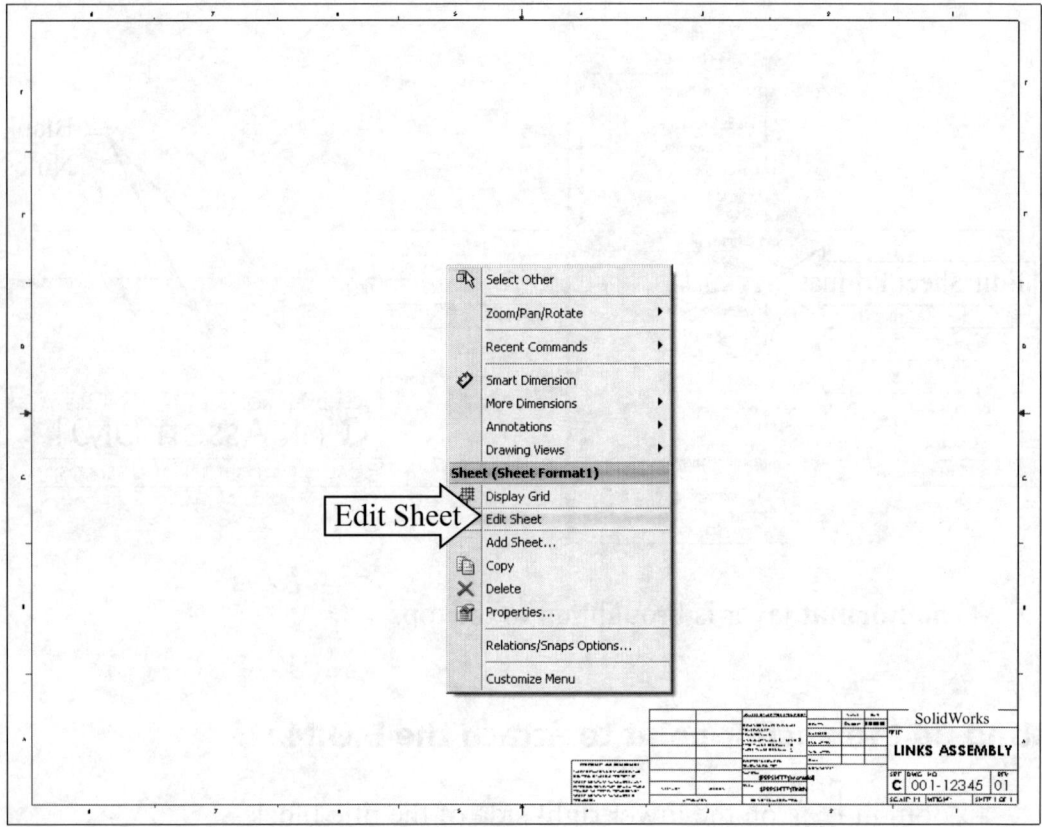

- **Change the Drawing Paper's color:**

- Select **Tools / Options / System Options / Colors / Drawing Paper Colors / Edit**.

- Select the **White** color and also enable: **Use Specified Color for Drawings Paper-Color** option.

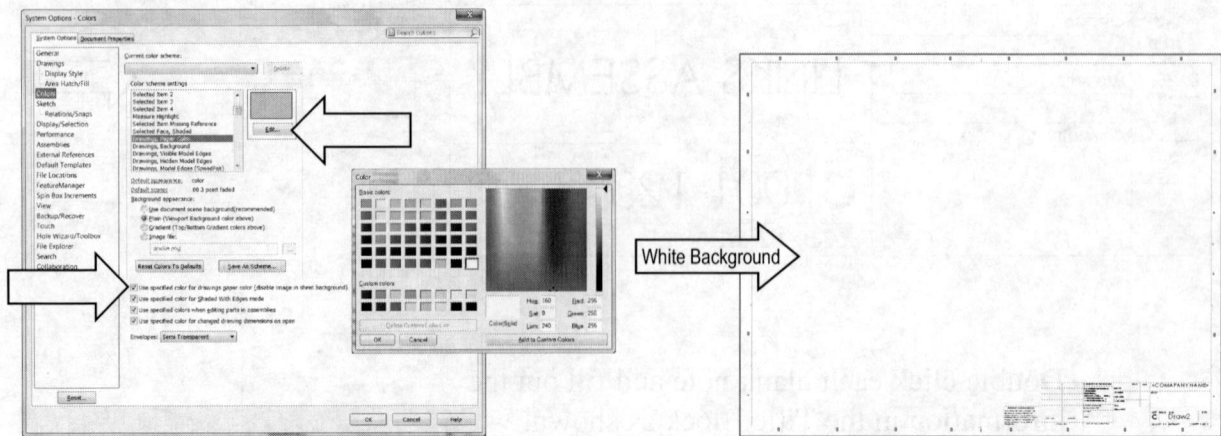

5. Opening an existing assembly document:

- Click the **Model View** command from the View Layout toolbar.

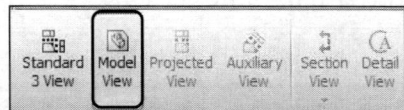

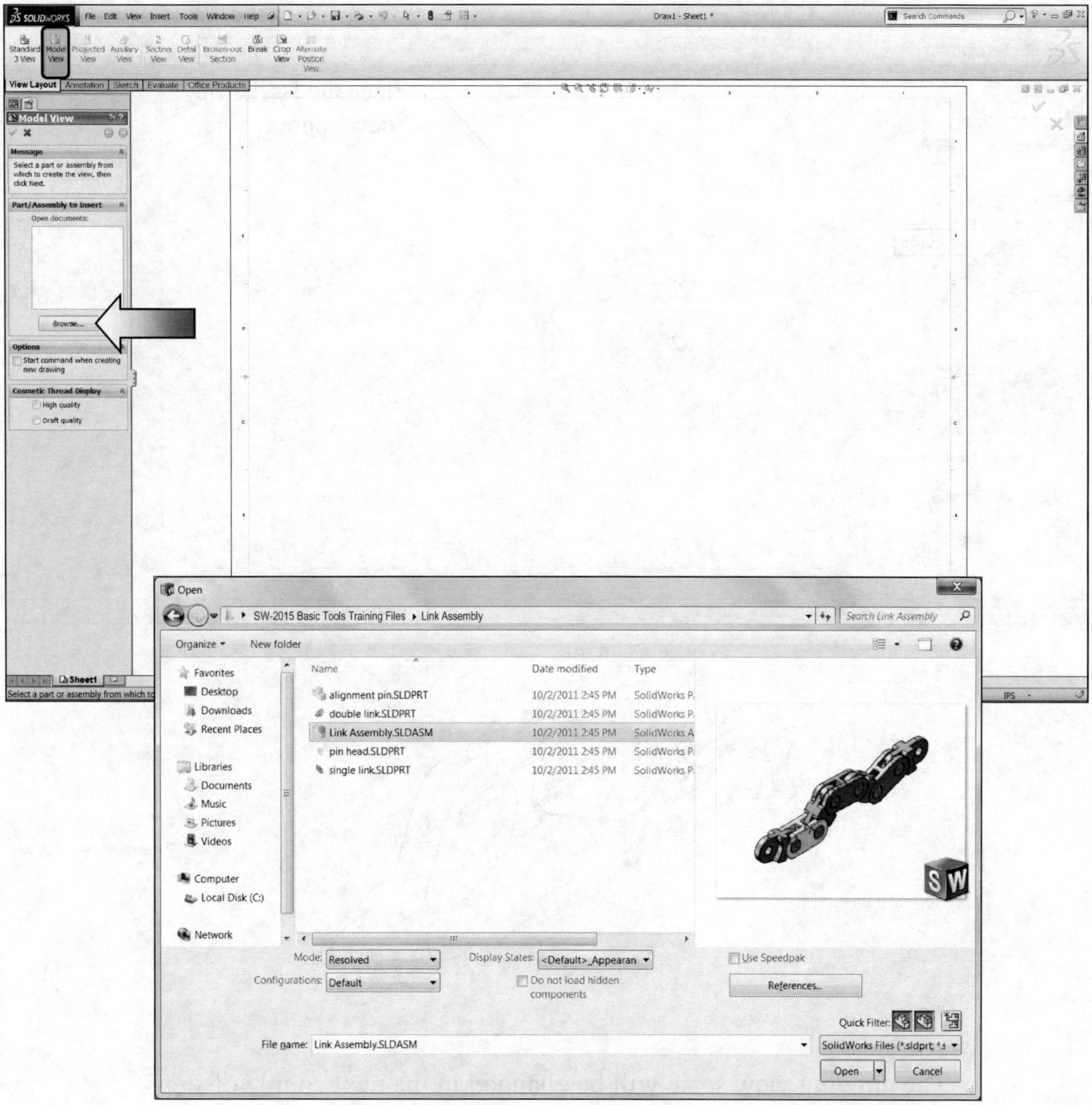

- Click the **Browse** button, from the Training Files folder, locate and open the **Links Assembly** document.

- There are several different methods to create the drawing views; in this lesson, we will discuss the use of the **Model-View** command first.

- Select the **Isometric** view button (arrow) and place the drawing view approximately as shown.

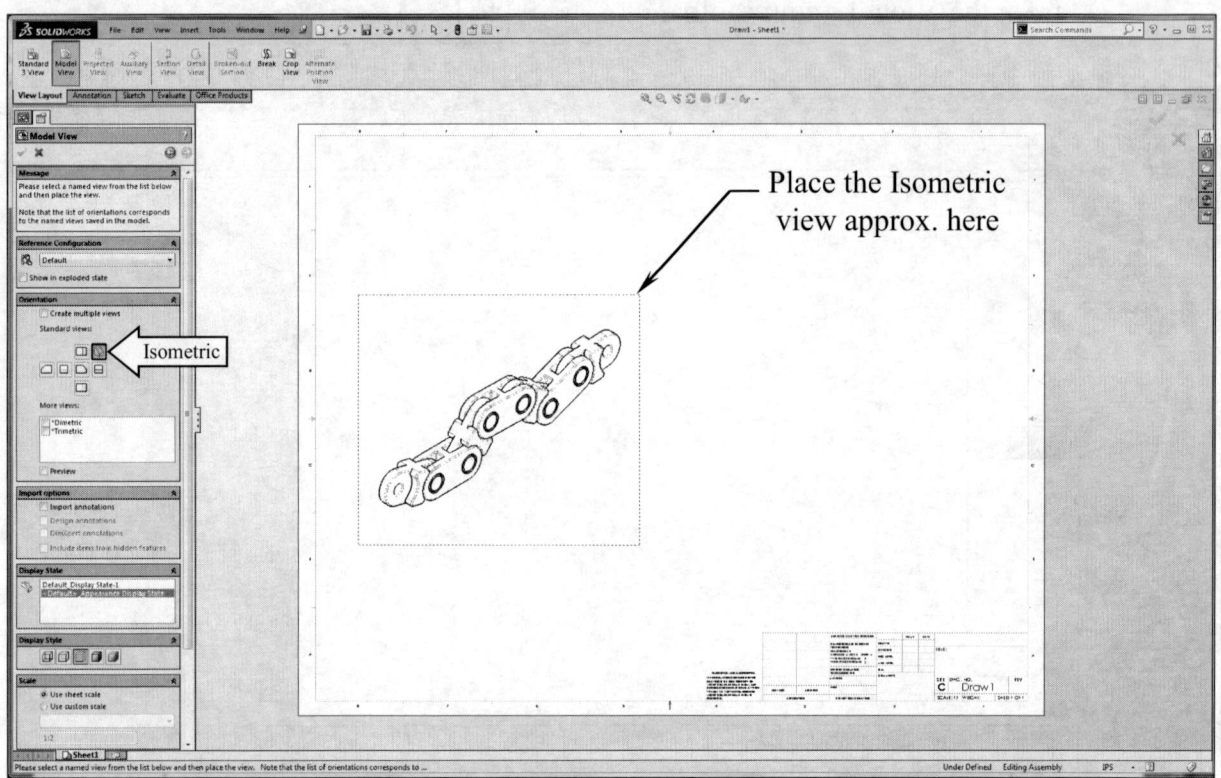

Place the Isometric view approx. here

Isometric

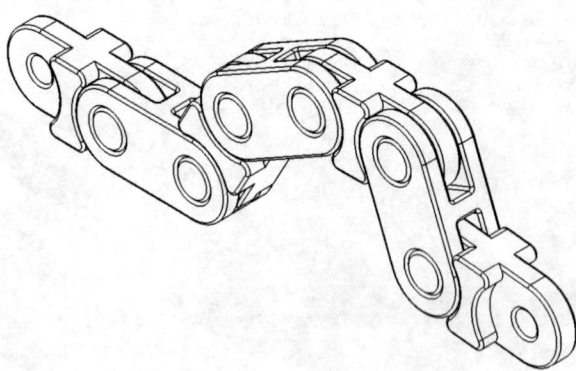

- The drawing view scale will be changed in the next couple of steps.

- The isometric view is created based on the default orientations of the last saved assembly document.

NOTE: If the Assembly document is already opened, press **Ctrl + Tab** to toggle back and forth between the Drawing and the Assembly documents.

6. Switching to the Exploded View state:

- Right click on the drawing view's border and select **Properties**.

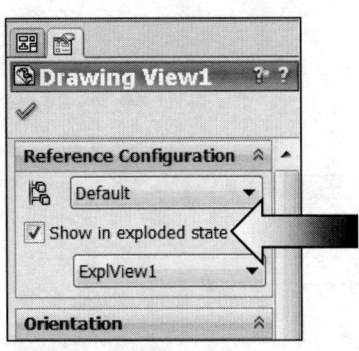

(In the newer releases of SolidWorks, the Explode option is also available on the top left of the properties tree).

Right click on the drawing view border and select Properties...

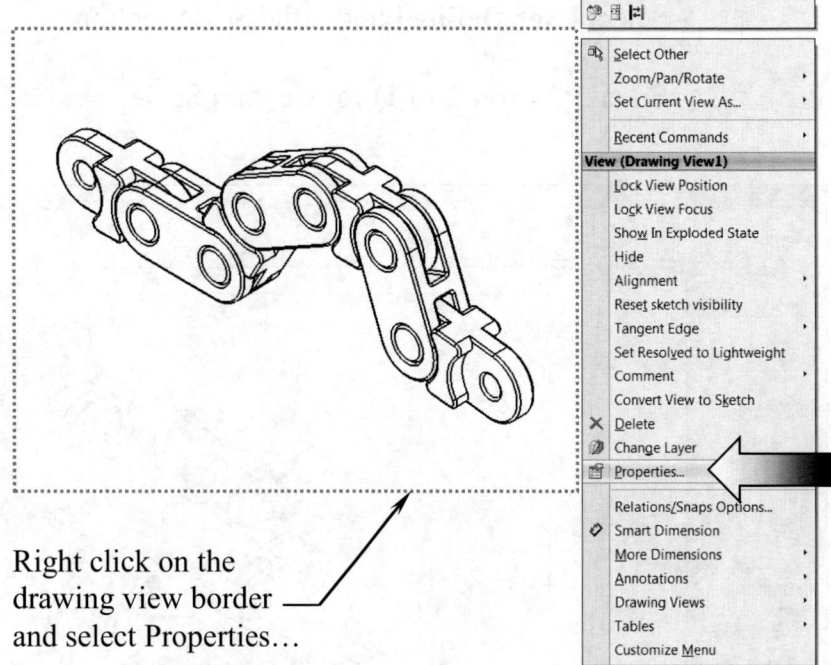

- Enable the **Show In - Exploded State** check box.

- The exploded checkbox is only available if an exploded view has been created earlier in the assembly level.

- Click **OK** [OK].

7. Changing the Scale of the Isometric Exploded view:

- Click the drawing view border to access the Properties tree.

- Select **User Defined** under the Scale section.

- Enter **3:2 (or 1.5 to 1)** for Custom Scale.

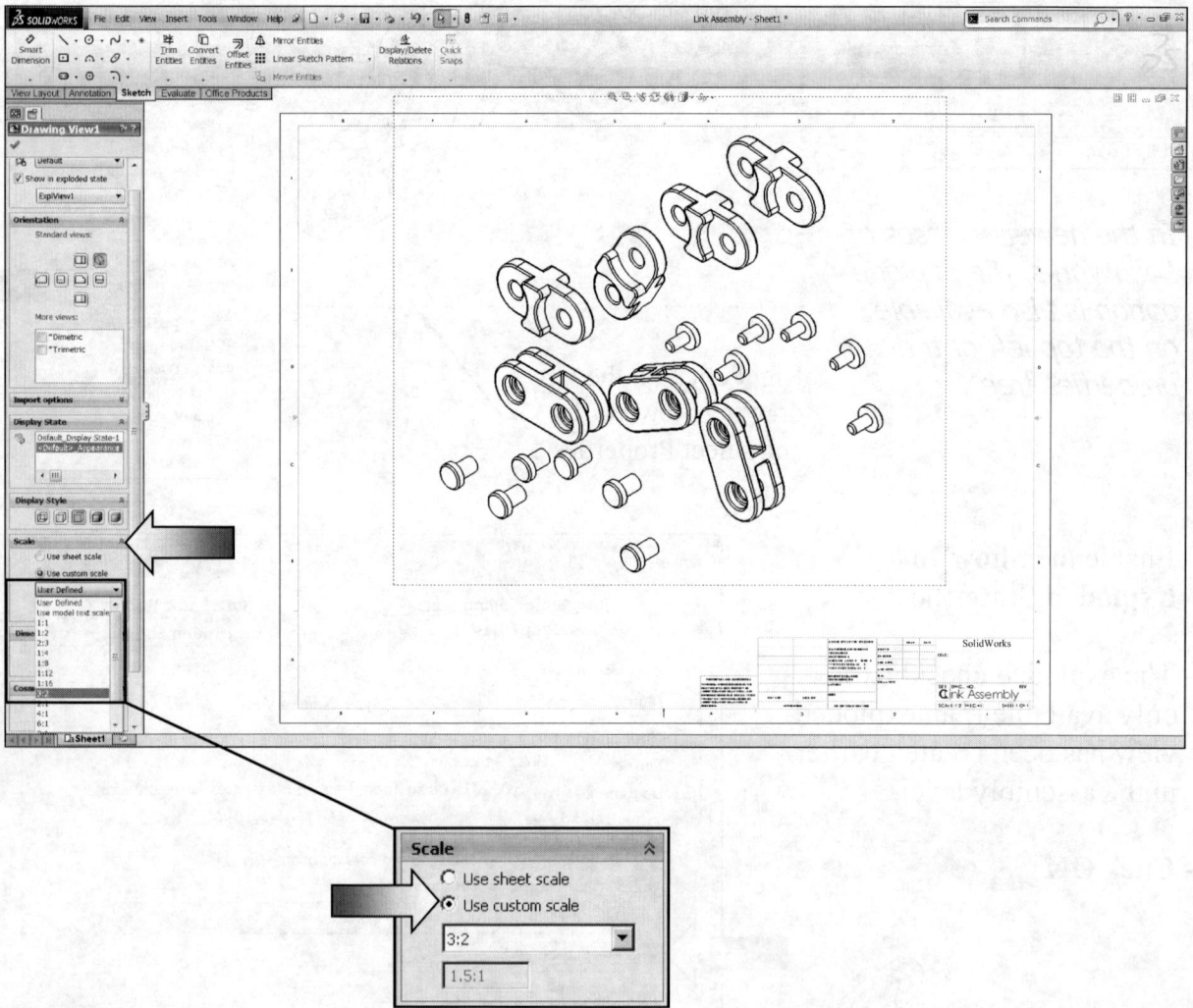

Notes:

- *When changing the Scale from the Properties tree, only the selected drawing view(s) will be affected.*

- *To change the scale of all drawing views on the same sheet, right click on the drawing, select Properties, and change the scale from there.*

- *The Scale can be pre-set and saved in the Drawing Template.*

8. Creating the 2nd Isometric View:

- Click the **Model View** command.

- Click **Next** , select the ISOMETRIC view button (arrow) under the Orientation Section.

- Place the drawing view approximately as shown.

- Click **OK** .

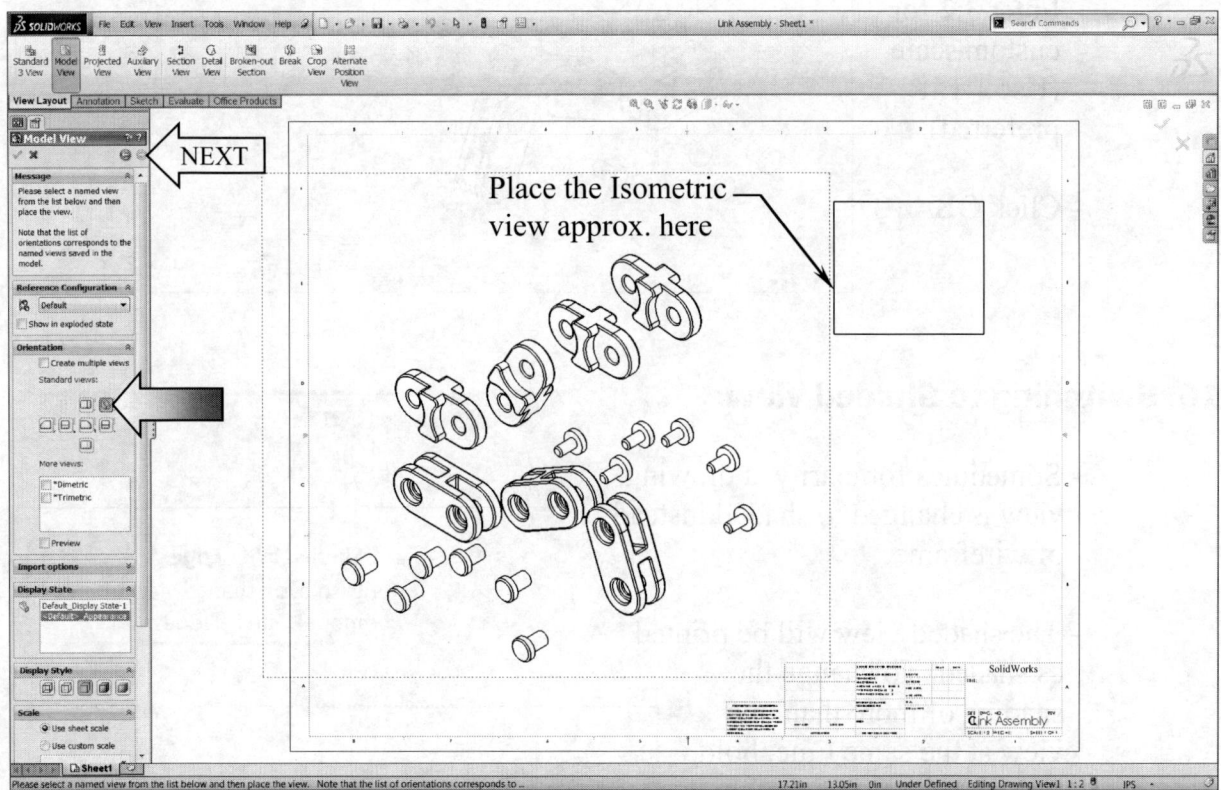

Place the Isometric view approx. here

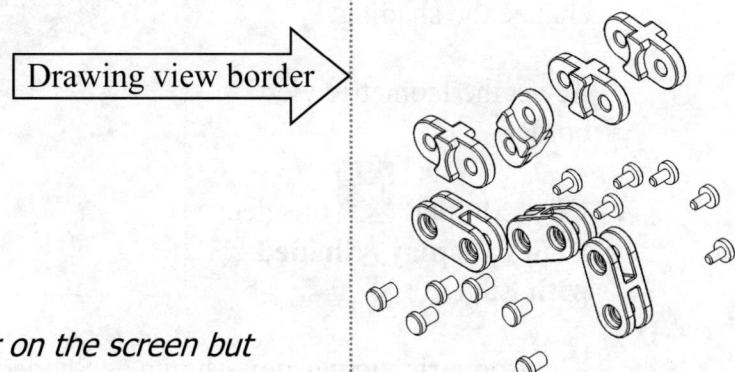

Drawing view border

Note:

The drawing view borders appear on the screen but not on the printouts.

9. Changing Scale:

- Set the Scale option to: **Use Custom Scale**.

- Select from the list: **User Define**.

- Enter **3:2** for custom scale. (Use 1:1 if preferred).

- Click **OK** .

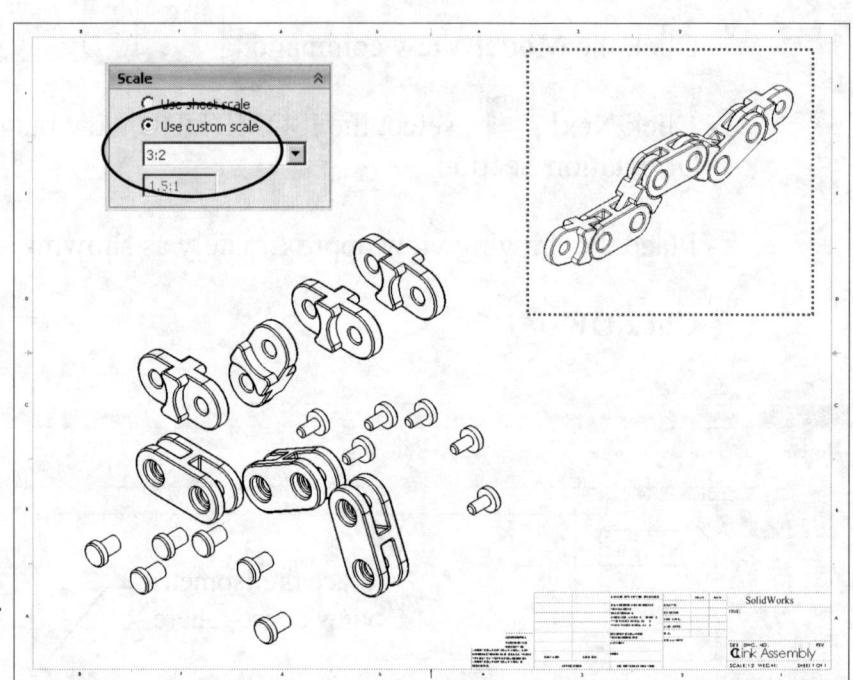

10. Switching to Shaded view:

- Sometimes for clarity, a drawing view is changed to shaded instead of wireframe.

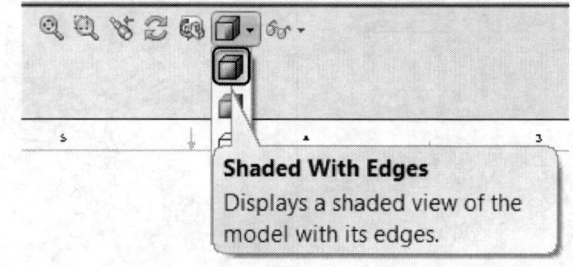

- The shaded view will be printed as shaded. To change the shading of more than one view at the same time, hold the control key, select the borders of the views then change the shading.

- Select the Isometric view border.

- Click **Shaded** or select **View / Display / Shaded with Edges**.

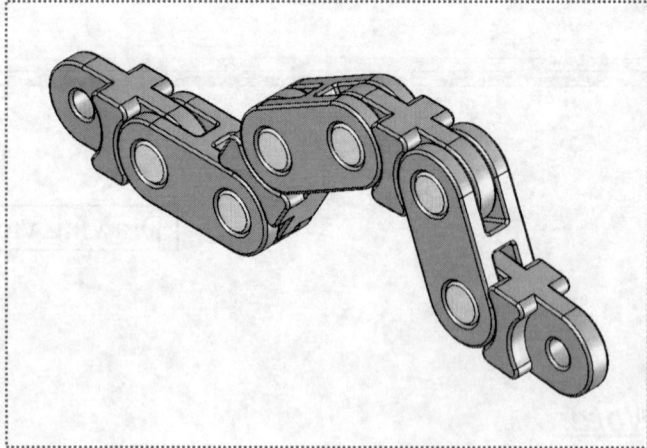

- The Isometric view is now shown as Shaded with Edges.

11. Creating a Bill of Materials (B.O.M.):

- Click the Isometric view's border.

- Select **Insert / Tables / Bill of Materials** – OR – Click the B.O.M. command from the **Tables** button.

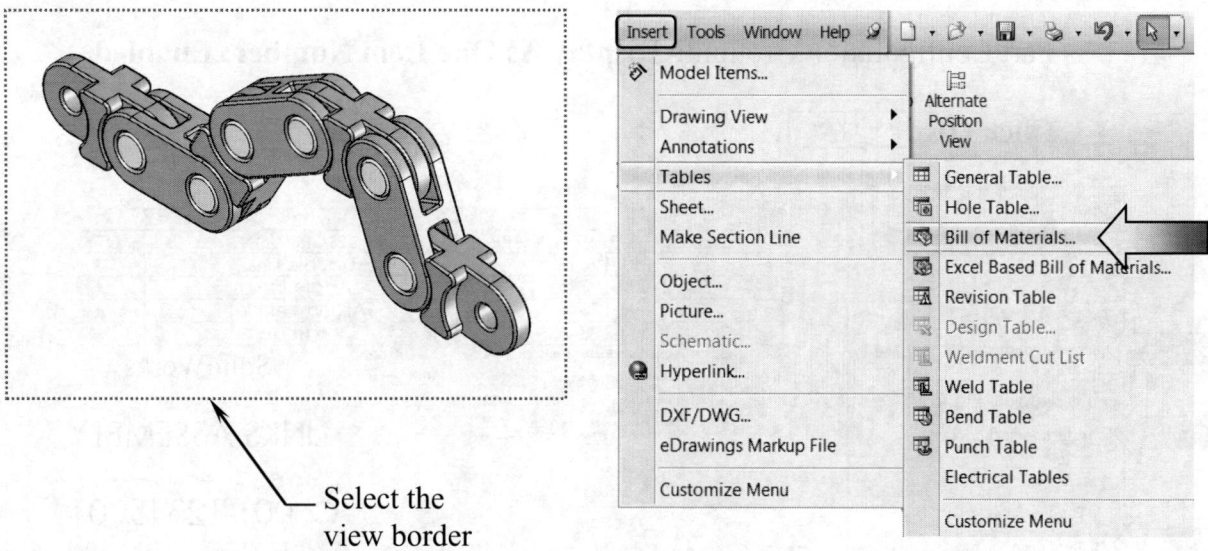

Select the view border

- A BOM is created automatically and the information in the assembly document is populated with item numbers, description, quantities and part numbers.

- When the Bill of Materials properties tree appears, select **Bom-Standard** (Circled) from the Table Template list (Circled) and Click **Open** .

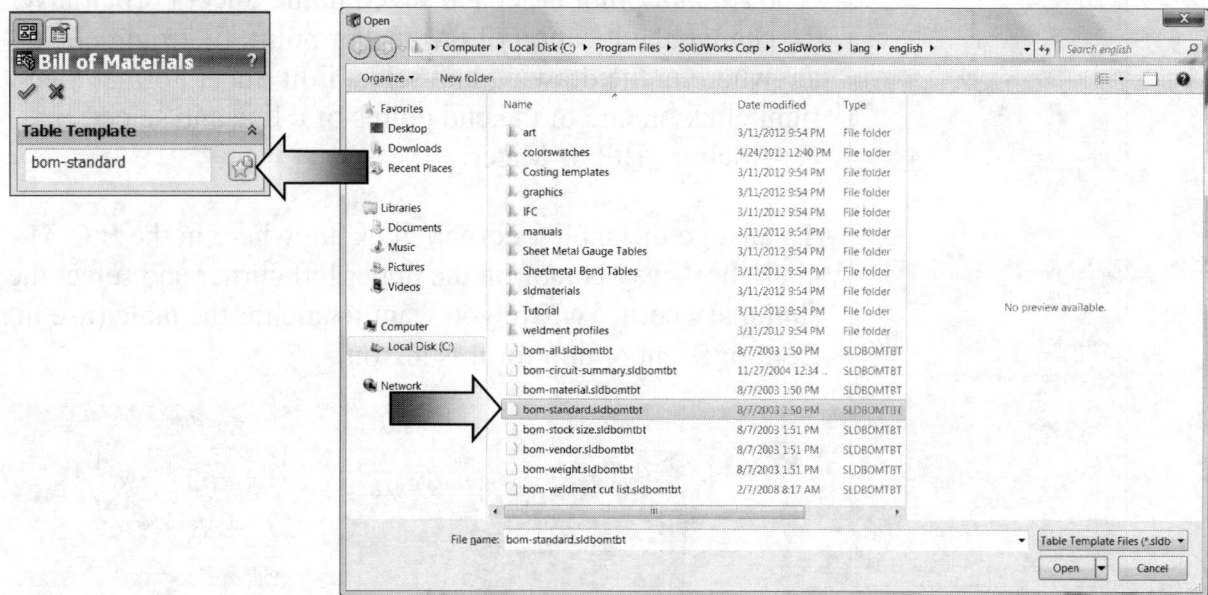

12. Selecting the B.O.M. options:

- Table Template: **BOM Standard.**

- Attach to Anchor Point*: **Enabled**.

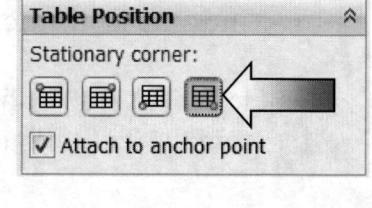

- BOM Type: **Parts only**.

- Part Configuration Grouping **Display As One Item Number: Enabled**.

- Click **OK** 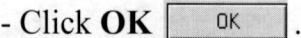.

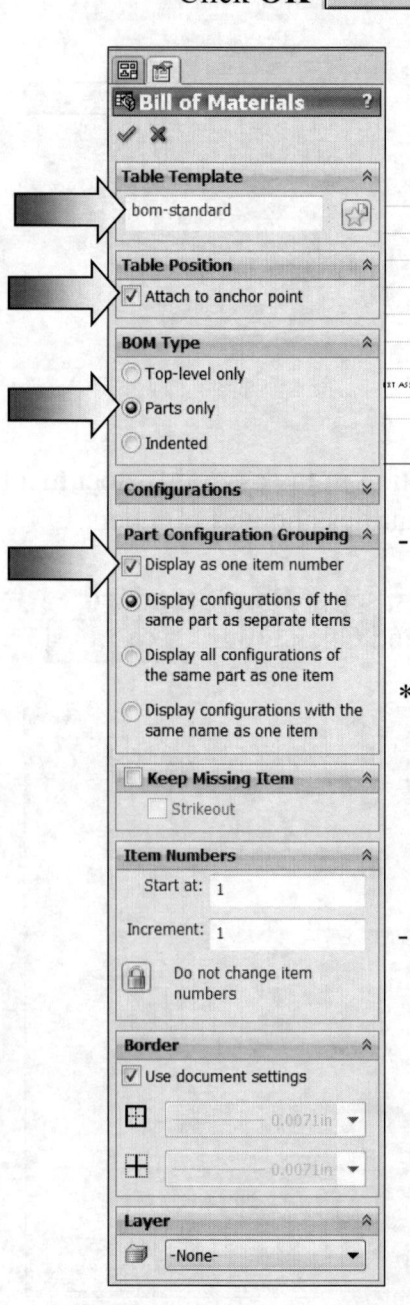

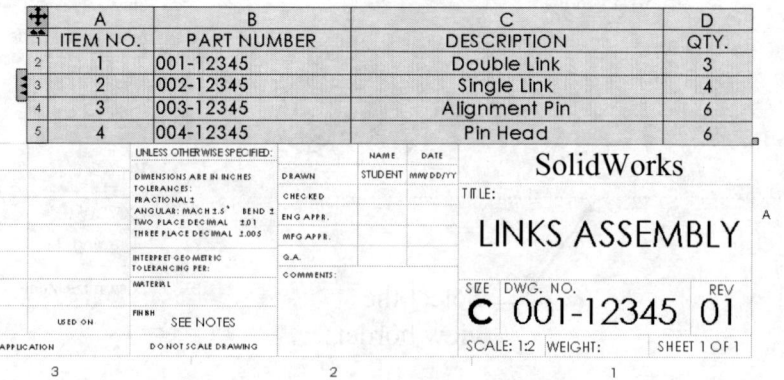

- The Bill of Materials is created and anchored to the lower right corner of the title block, where the anchor point was set earlier.

* The Anchor point is set and saved in the Sheet Format layer. To change the location of the anchor point, first right click anywhere in the drawing and select Edit Sheet Format then right click on one of the end points of a line and select: Set-As-Anchor / Bill of Material.

- To change the anchor corner, click anywhere in the B.O.M, click the 4-way cursor on the upper left corner and select the stationary corner where you want to anchor the table (use the Bottom Right option for this lesson).

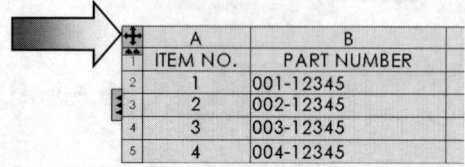

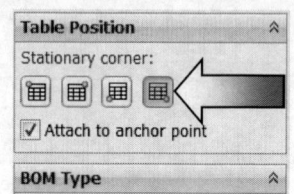

13. Modifying the B.O.M.:

- Double-click on the B.O.M. table to edit its content.

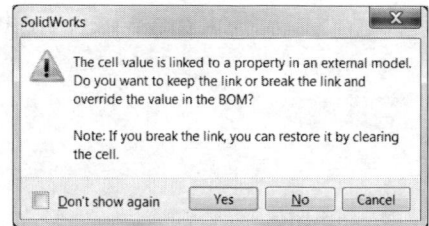

- Transfer the Part Number column over to the Description column.

- **To transfer Cell-By-Cell:**

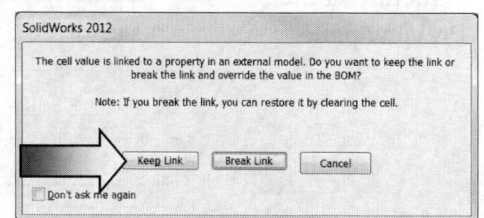

In the Part Number column, double-click in a cell and select **Keep Link**.

Press **Control + X** (Cut).

Enter a New Part Number.

Double-click a cell in the Description column and press **Control + V** (Paste) or simply re-enter the part name.

	A	B	C	D
1	ITEM NO.	PART NUMBER	DESCRIPTION	QTY.
2	1	Double Link	← Double Click	3
3	2	Alignment Pin		6
4	3	Pin Head		6
5	4	Single Link		4

- Click OK or click anywhere in the drawing when finished with editing. The BOM is updated accordingly.

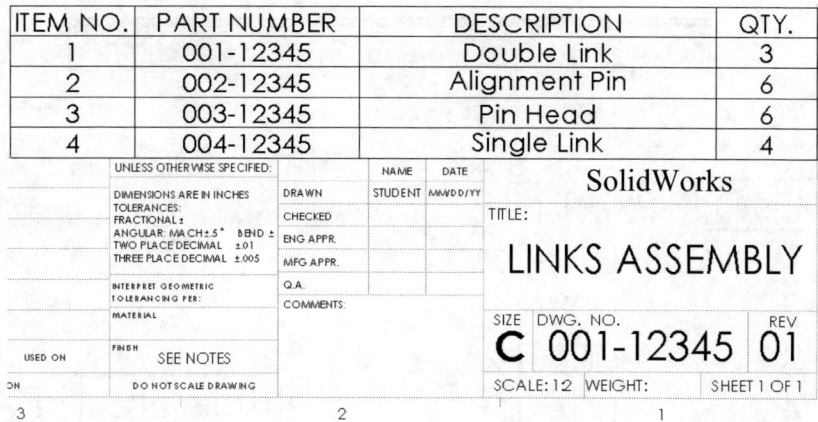

ITEM NO.	PART NUMBER	DESCRIPTION	QTY.
1	001-12345	Double Link	3
2	002-12345	Alignment Pin	6
3	003-12345	Pin Head	6
4	004-12345	Single Link	4

Note: Refer to SolidWorks Online Help to learn more about customizing the B.O.M and how to create Custom Properties such as Part Numbers, Materials, etc.

14. Reversing the column headers:

- Click anywhere in the B.O.M. table to access its **Properties**.

Click anywhere in
the BOM to access
its Properties...

Assembly
Structure and
Preview pane

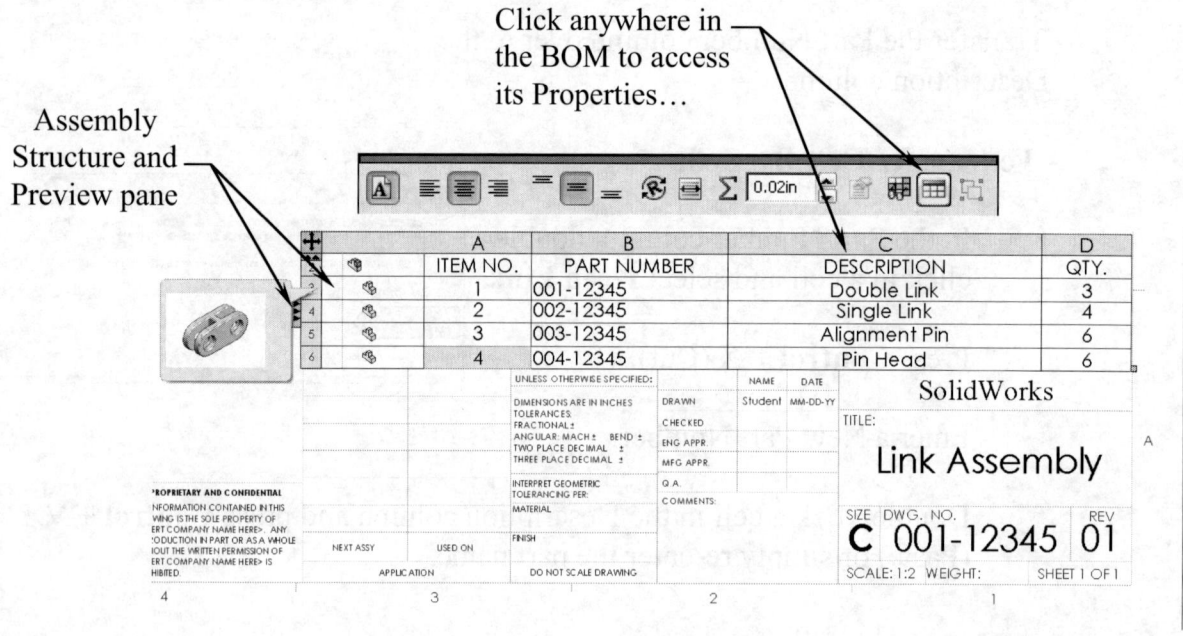

	A	B	C	D
	ITEM NO.	PART NUMBER	DESCRIPTION	QTY.
1	1	001-12345	Double Link	3
2	2	002-12345	Single Link	4
3	3	003-12345	Alignment Pin	6
4	4	004-12345	Pin Head	6

- Click the Assembly Structure arrow-tab to see the preview of the components.

- The Formatting toolbar pops up on top of the BOM.

- Click the **Table Header** button.

- Click **OK** ✓.

Table Header
Top/Bottom

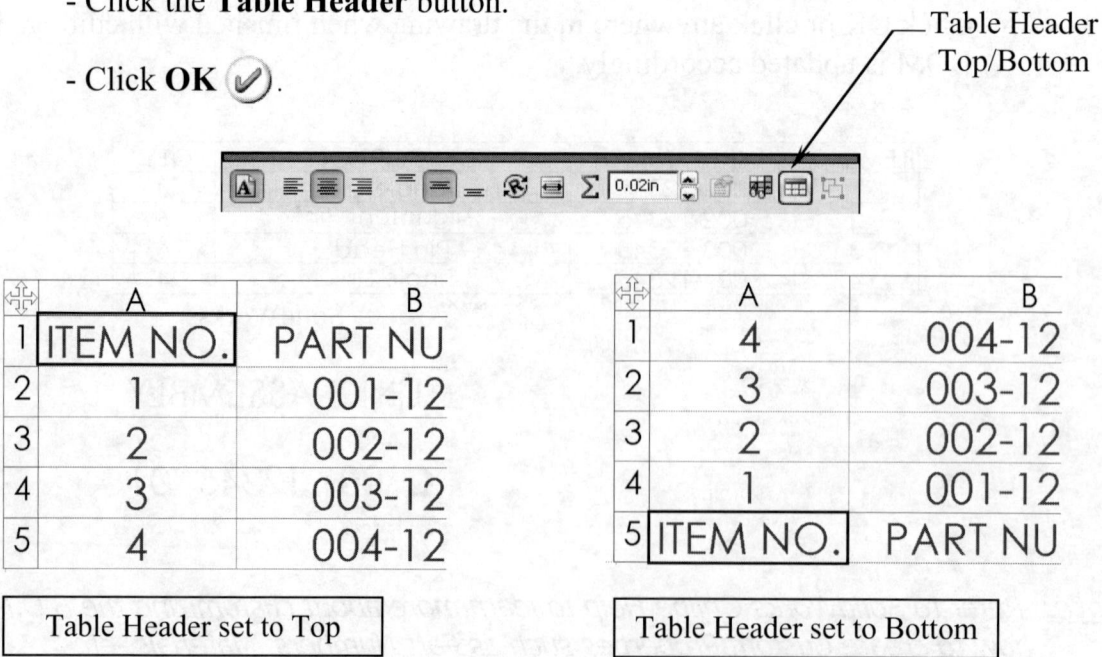

	A	B
1	ITEM NO.	PART NU
2	1	001-12
3	2	002-12
4	3	003-12
5	4	004-12

Table Header set to Top

	A	B
1	4	004-12
2	3	003-12
3	2	002-12
4	1	001-12
5	ITEM NO.	PART NU

Table Header set to Bottom

15. Adding Balloon callouts:

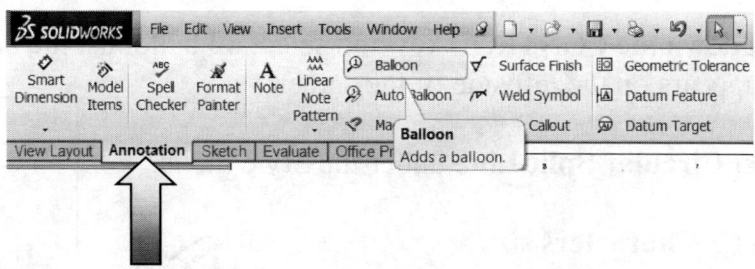

- Click 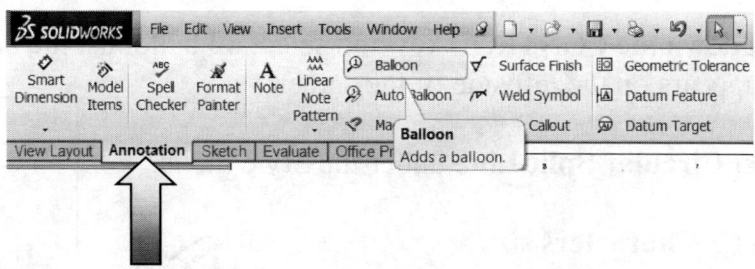 or select **Insert / Annotations / Balloon**.

- Click on the **edge** of the Single-Link. The system places a balloon on the part.

- The Item Number matches the one in the B.O.M. automatically.

- Click on the Double Link, the Alignment Pins, and Pin Heads to assign balloons to them.

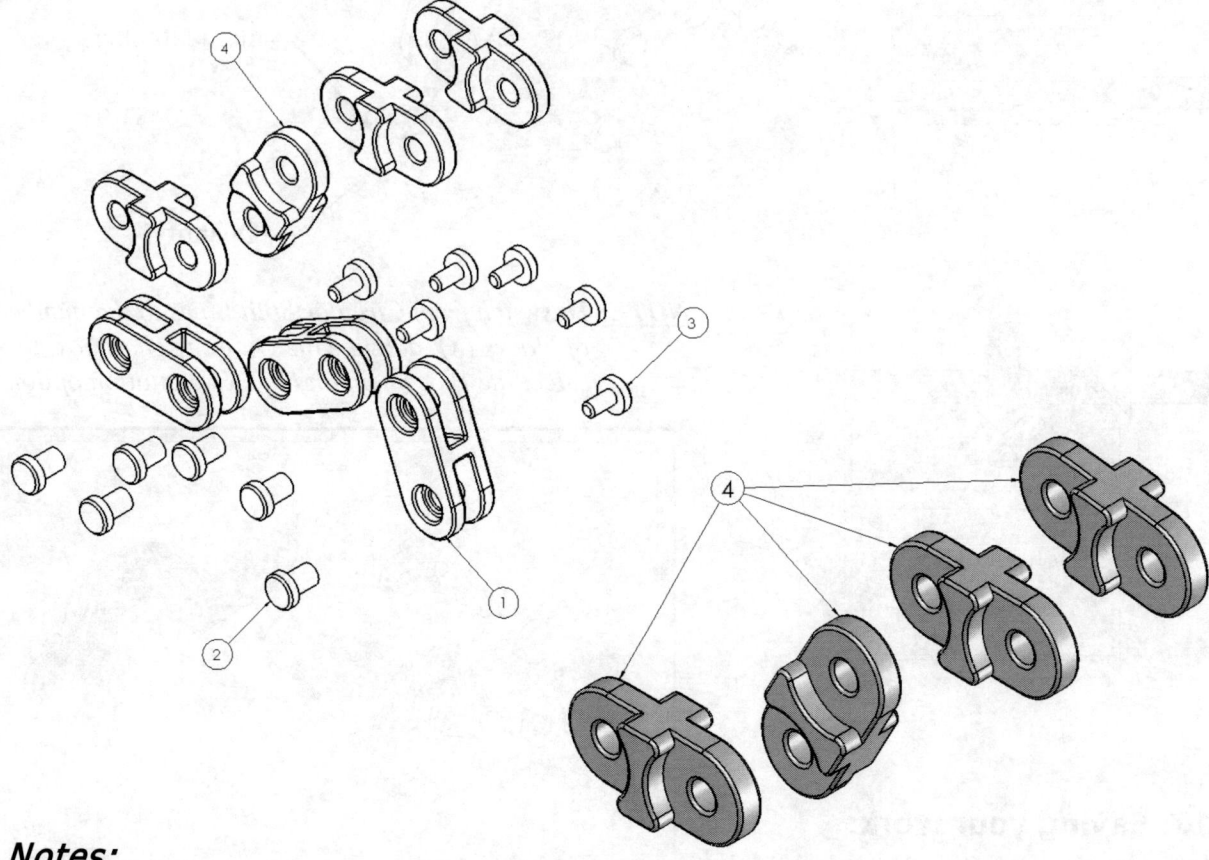

Notes:

Balloons are similar to notes; they can have multiple leaders or attachment points. To copy the leader line, hold down the CONTROL key and drag the tip of one of the arrows.

16. Changing the balloon style:

- Hold down the CONTROL key and select all balloons, the balloon Properties tree appears on the left side of the screen.

- Select **Circular Split Line** under the Style menu.

- Select **2 Characters** size.

- Click **OK** ✓.

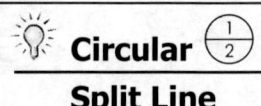

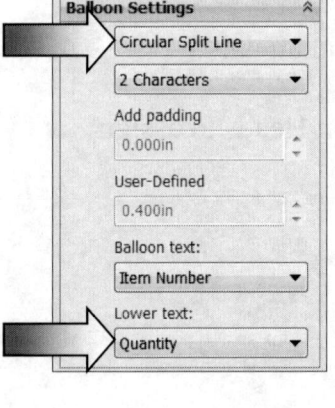

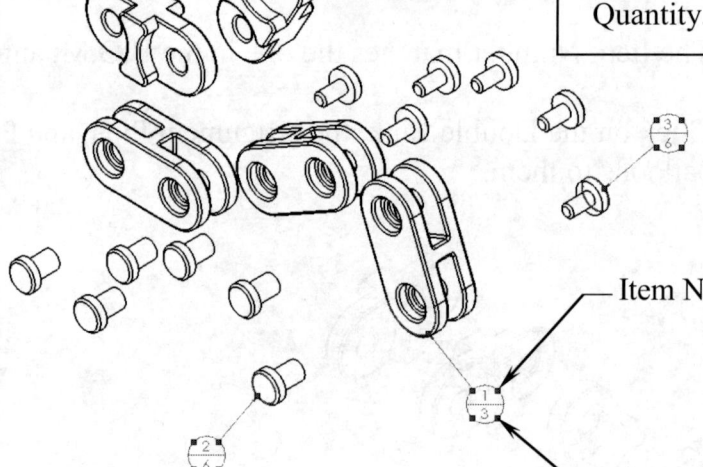

> ⚡ **Circular** ①/②
> ___
> **Split Line**
>
> - The Upper Number represents the Item-Number.
> - The Lower Number represents the Quantity.

Item Number

Quantity

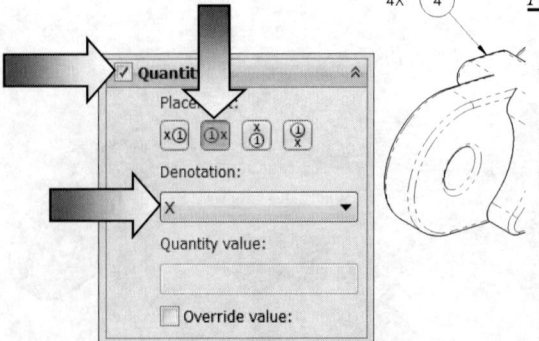

NOTE: *To switch from Circular Split Lines to the number of places (X), activate the Quantity checkbox, then select the Placement and the X denotation options.*

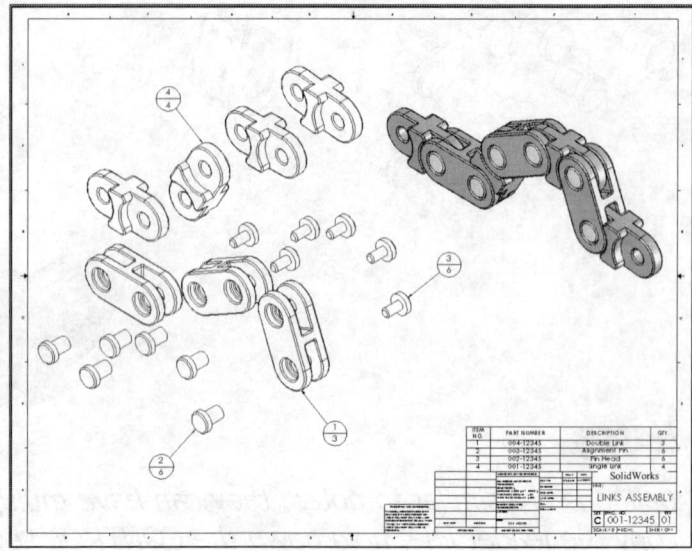

17. Saving your work:

- Select **File / Save As / Links-Assembly / Save**.

Questions for Review

Assembly Drawings

1. The drawing's paper size can be selected or changed at any time.
    a. True
    b. False

2. The First or Third angle projection can be selected in the sheet setup.
    a. True
    b. False

3. To access the sheet format and edit the information in the title block:
    a. Right click in the drawing and select Edit Sheet Format
    b. Right click the Sheet Format icon from the Feature Tree and select: Edit Sheet Format.
    c. All of the above.

4. The BOM anchor point should be set on the Sheet Format not on the drawing sheet.
    a. True
    b. False

5. A Model View command is used to create Isometric views.
    a. True
    b. False

6. The Drawing views scale can be changed individually or all at the same time.
    a. True
    b. False

7. A Bill of Materials (BOM) can automatically be generated using Excel embedded features.
    a. True
    b. False

8. The Balloon callouts are linked to the Bill of Materials and driven by the order of the Feature Manager Tree.
    a. True
    b. False

1. TRUE   2. TRUE
3. C   4. TRUE
5. TRUE   7. TRUE
8. TRUE   9. TRUE

Exercise: Assembly Drawings

Go to: Training Files folder.
Mini Vise folder.

1. Create an Assembly Drawing
   from the components provided.

2. Create a Bill of Materials and
   modify the Part Number and the
   Description columns as shown.

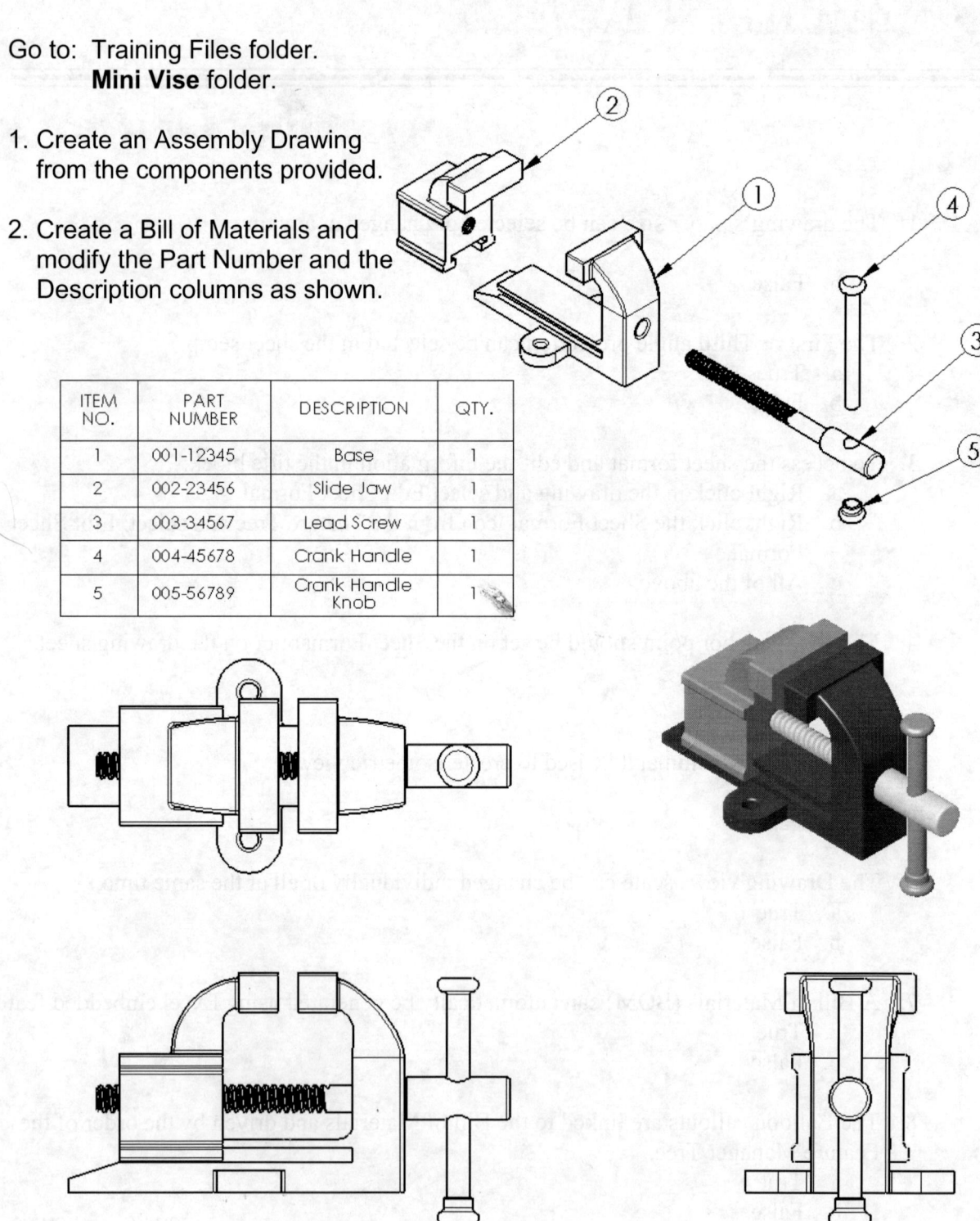

ITEM NO.	PART NUMBER	DESCRIPTION	QTY.
1	001-12345	Base	1
2	002-23456	Slide Jaw	1
3	003-34567	Lead Screw	1
4	004-45678	Crank Handle	1
5	005-56789	Crank Handle Knob	1

3. Save your work as: **Mini Vise Assembly.slddrw**

Exercise: Assembly Drawings

File Location:
Training Files folder
Egg Beater.sldasm

ITEM NO.	PART NUMBER	DESCRIPTION	QTY.
1	010-8980	Egg Beater Handle	1
2	010-8981	Main Gear	1
3	010-8982	Support Rod	1
4	010-8983	Right Spinner	1
5	010-8984	Left Spinner	1
6	010-8985	Crank Handle	1
7	010-8986	Small Gear (RIGHT)	1
8	010-8987	Small Gear (LEFT)	1

1. Create an Assembly Drawing with 5 views.

2. Add Balloons and a Bill Of Materials.

3. Save your work as: **Egg Beater Assembly**.

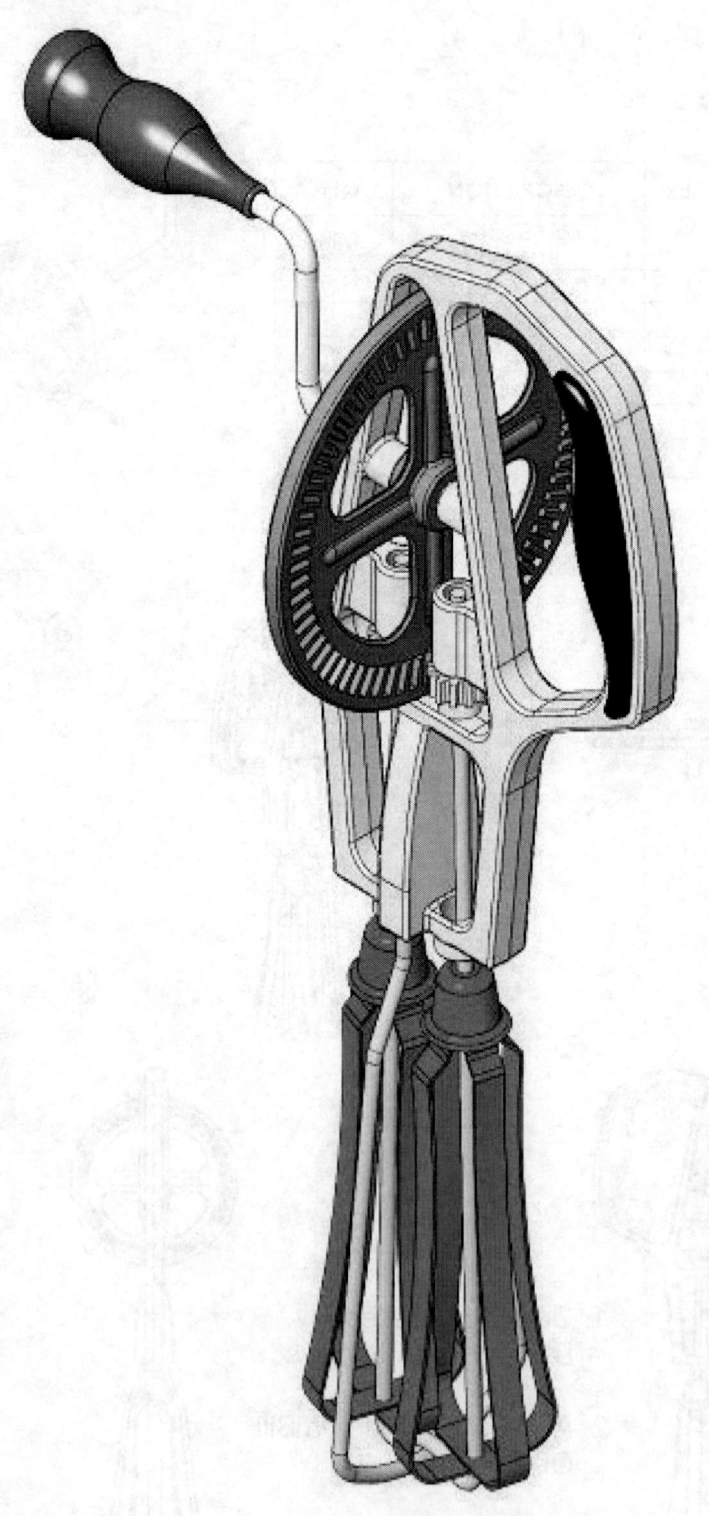

CHAPTER 15 (cont.)

Alternate Position Views

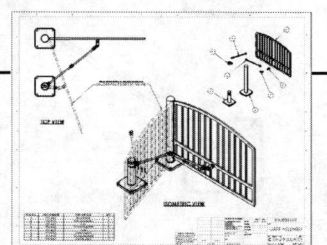

Assembly Drawings
Alternate Position Views

- Assembly drawings are created in the same way as part drawings, except for all components that are shown together as assembled or exploded.

- A Bill of Materials is created to specify the details of the components, such as: Part Number, Material, Weight, Vendor, etc.

- The BOM template can be modified to have more columns, rows, or different headers.

- Balloons are also created on the same drawing to help identify the parts from its list (B.O.M). These balloons are linked to the Bill of Materials parametrically, and the order of the balloon numbers is driven by the Assembly's Feature tree.

Alternate Position Views

- The Alternate Position View allows users to superimpose one drawing view precisely on another (open/close position as an example).

- The alternate position(s) is shown with phantom lines.

- Dimension between the primary view and the Alternate Position View can be added to the same drawing view.

- More than one Alternate Position View can be created in a drawing.

- Section, Detail, Broken, and Crop views are currently not supported.

Alternate Position Views
Assembly Drawings

ITEM NO.	PART NUMBER	DESCRIPTION	QTY.
1	011-4321	Base Stand	1
2	012-4321	Arm Connector	1
3	013-4321	Arm	1
4	014-4321	Connecting Arm	1
5	015-4321	Gate	1
6	016-4321	Gate Support	1
7	017-4321	Connector Joint	1
8	018-4321	Double Joint	1

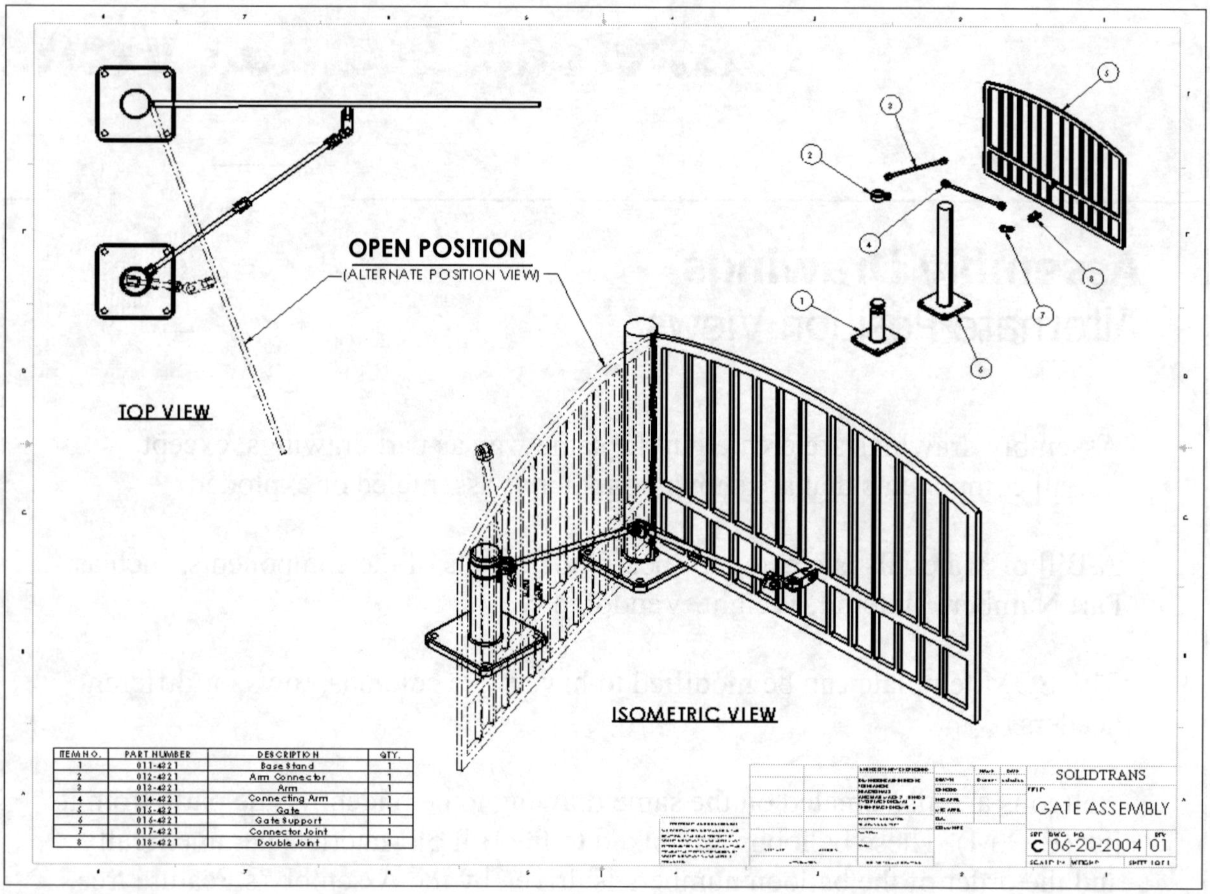

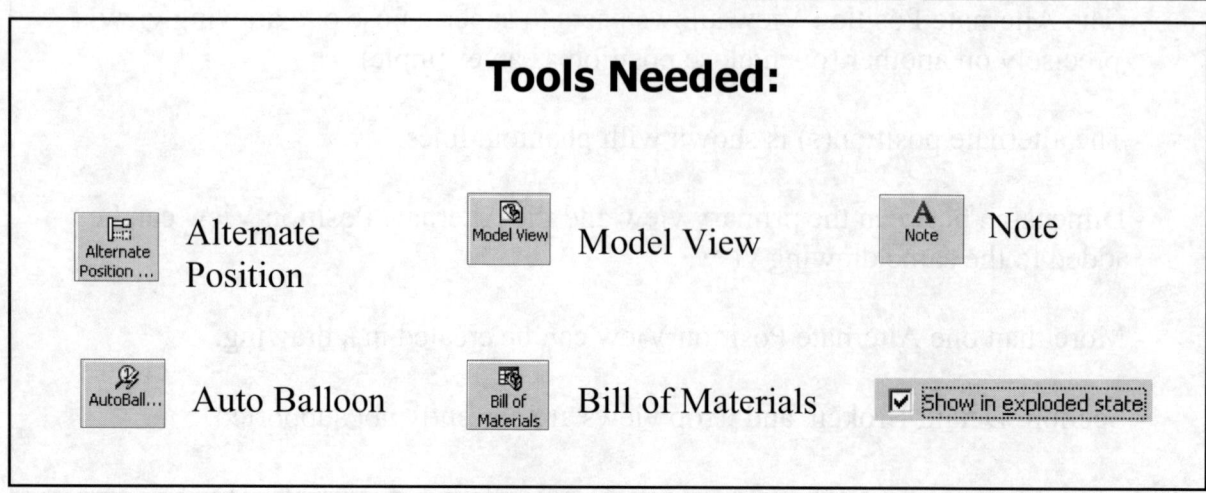

Dimensioning Standards: **ANSI**
Units: **INCHES** – 3 Decimals

Third Angle Projection

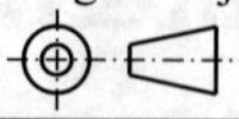

Tools Needed:

Alternate Position

Model View

Note

Auto Balloon

Bill of Materials

Show in exploded state

1. Creating a new drawing:

- Select **File / New / Draw** (or Drawing) / **OK**.

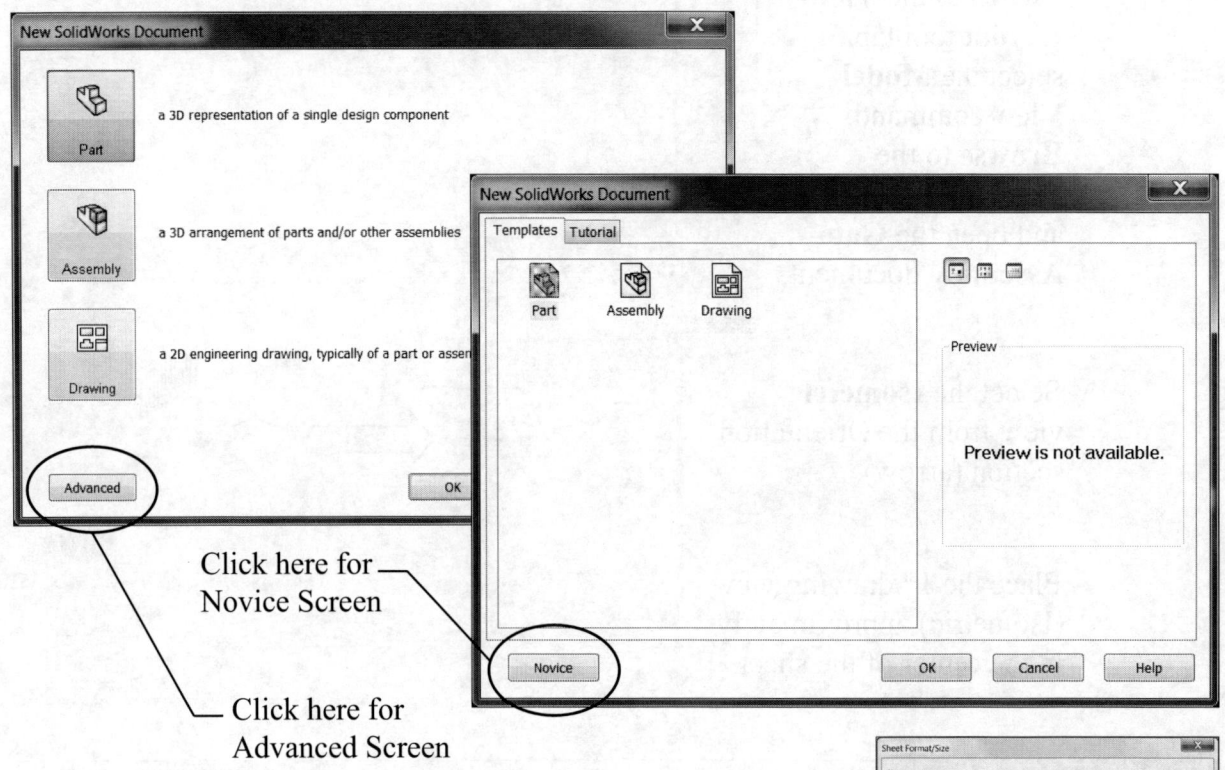

Click here for
Novice Screen

Click here for
Advanced Screen

- Under Standard Sheet Size, choose **C-Landscape**.

- Enable the **Display Sheet Format** check box.

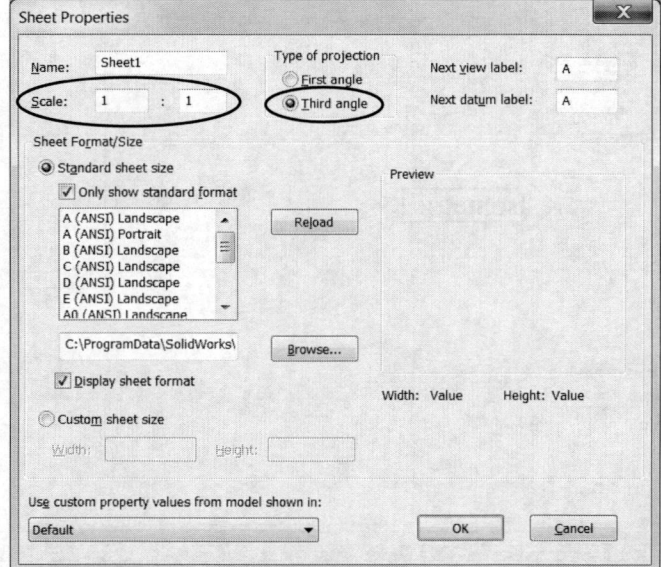

- Click **OK** [OK].

- Right click in the drawing
  and select **Properties.**

- Set **Scale** to **1:1**
  (full scale)

- Set **Type of Projection** to:
  Third Angle [⦿ Third angle].

- Click **OK** [OK].

2. Creating the Isometric Drawing View:

- Switch to the **View-Layout** tool tab, select the **Model-View** command, **Browse** to the Training Files folder and open the **Gate-Assembly** document.

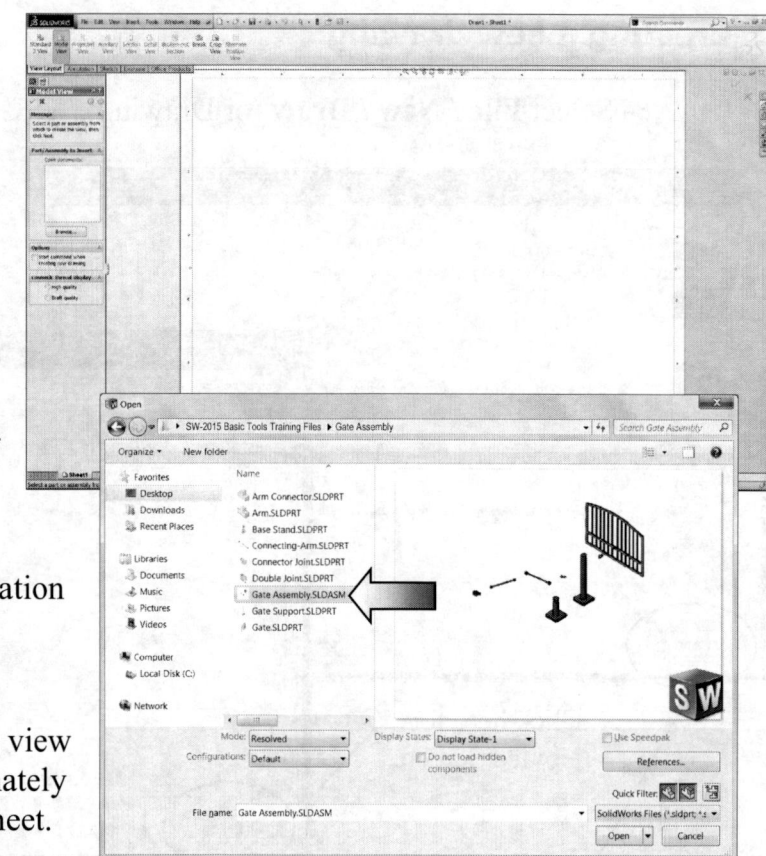

- Select the **Isometric** view from the Orientation section (arrow).

- Place the 1st drawing view (Isometric) approximately in the center of the sheet.

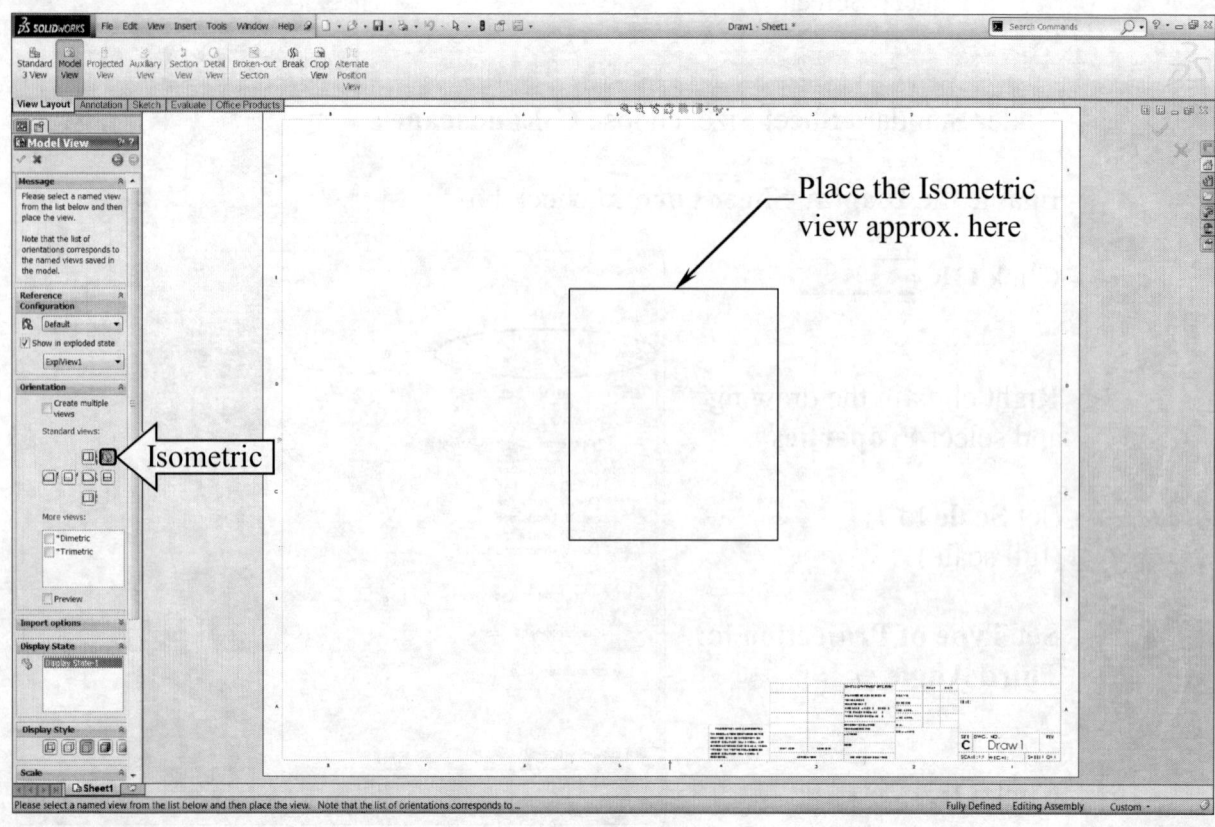

Place the Isometric view approx. here

Isometric

3. Changing the Drawing View Scale:

- Click on the drawing view border and change the Scale to:

* Use Custom Scale.

* User Defined.

* Scale 1:3

- Click **OK** ✅.

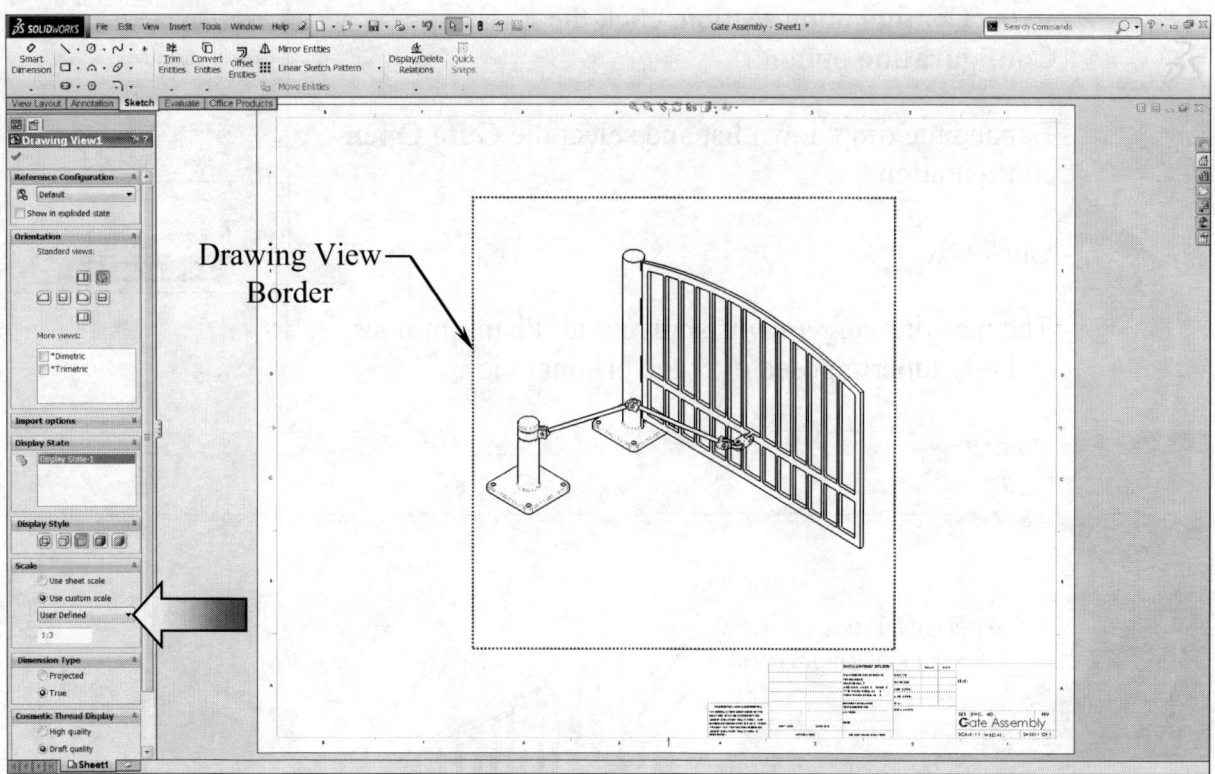

Drawing View Border

- The Isometric View is scaled to (1:3) or 1/3 time the actual size.

- When selecting the User Defined option you can enter your own scale, if the scale option that you want is not on the list.

- The scale in the Sheet properties is linked to the scale callout in the title block (page 14-25). Changing the scale in the Properties will automatically update the one in the title block.

4. Creating an Alternate Position drawing view:

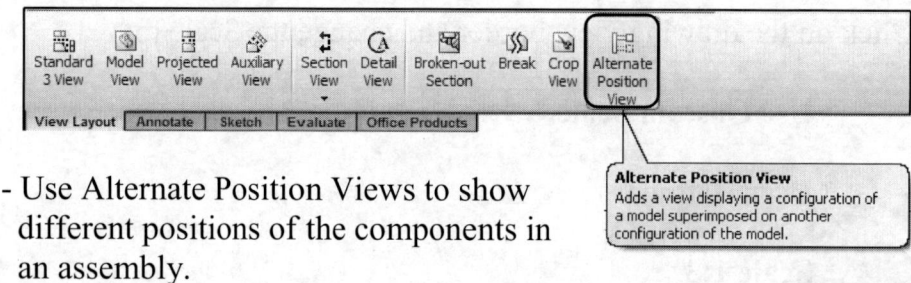

- Use Alternate Position Views to show different positions of the components in an assembly.

- From the Drawing Toolbar, click Alternate Position... or select **Insert / Drawing View / Alternate Position View**.

- In the Configuration section, click the **Existing-Configuration** option.

- Expand the drop down list and select the **Gate Open** configuration.

- Click **OK** ✓.

- The new drawing view is shown with Phantom lines and it is superimposed over the original view.

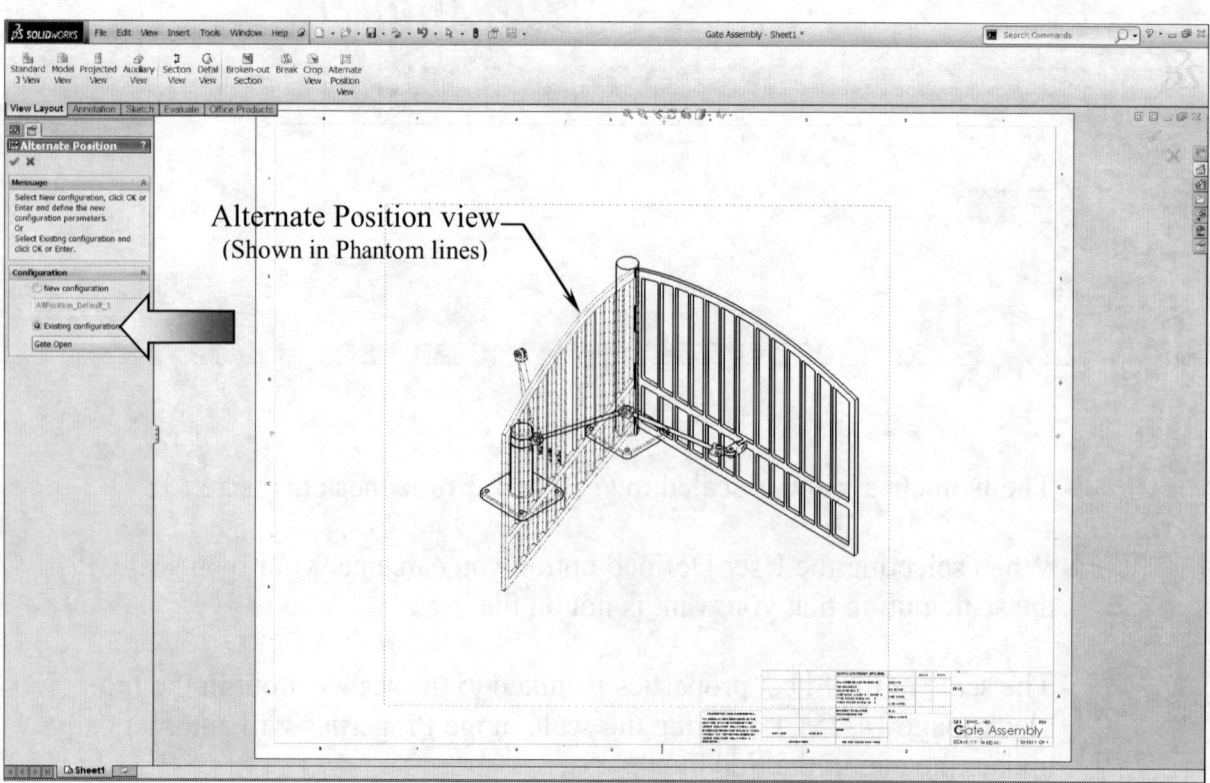

Alternate Position view
(Shown in Phantom lines)

5. Adding the Top Drawing view:

- From the Drawing Toolbar, click **Model View** 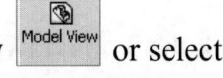 or select: **Insert / Drawing View / Model**.

- Click the **NEXT** arrow.

- Select the **TOP** view from the Orientation dialog.

- Place the Top drawing view approximately as shown.

- Click **OK** ✔.

- For clarity, change the view line style to Tangent Edges With Font. (Right click on the view's border, select Tangent Edge, and then click Tangent Edges with Font).

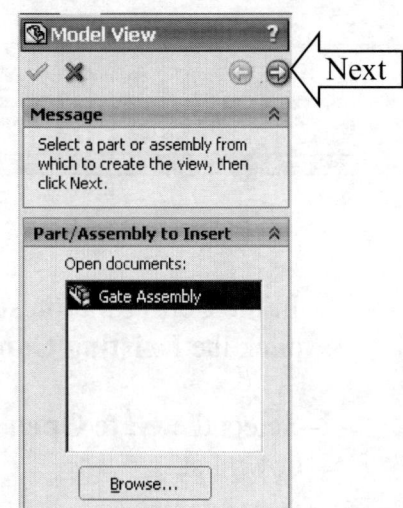

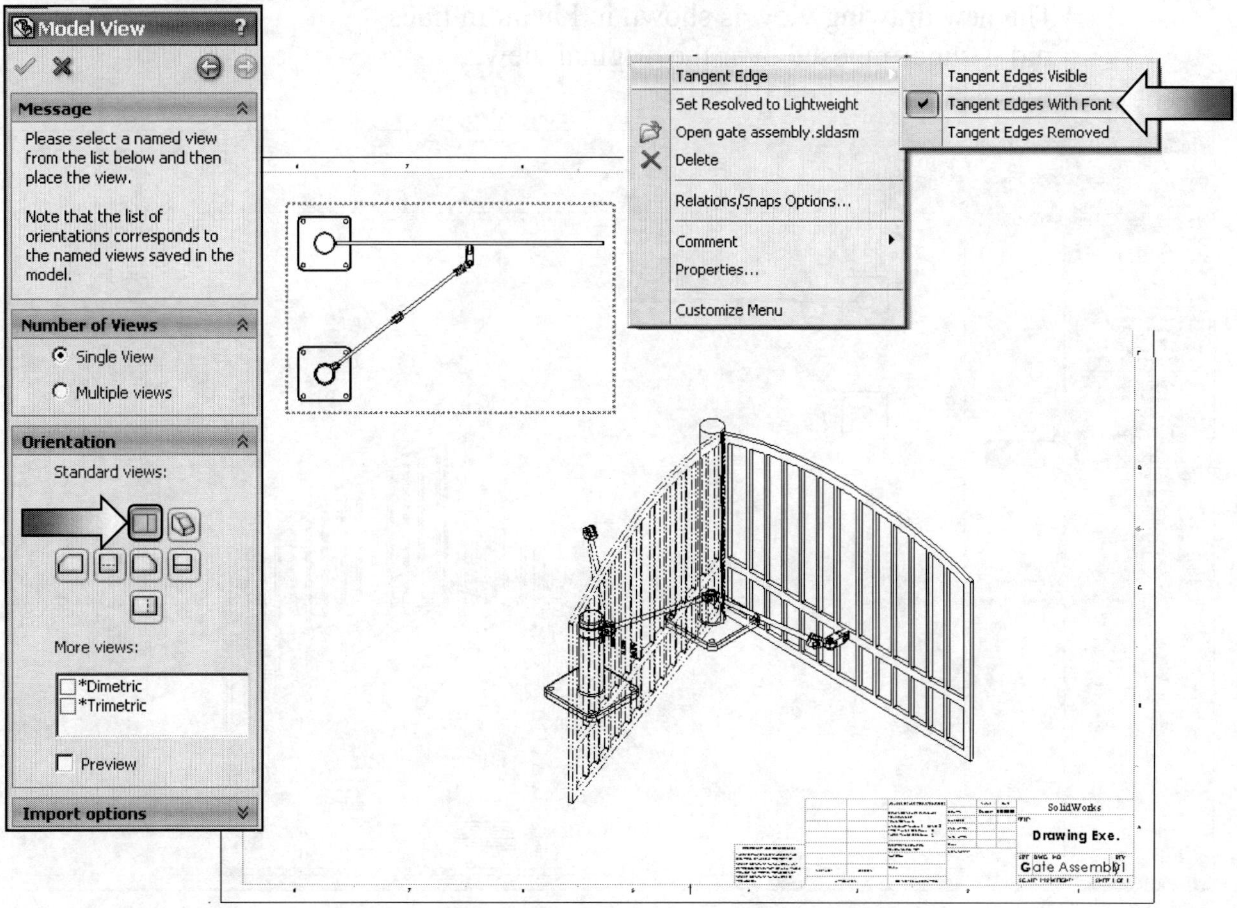

6. Creating the 2nd Alternate Position View:

- Click the Top Drawing View's Border to activate.

- Click **Alternate Position ...** or select **Insert / Drawing View / Alternate Position**.

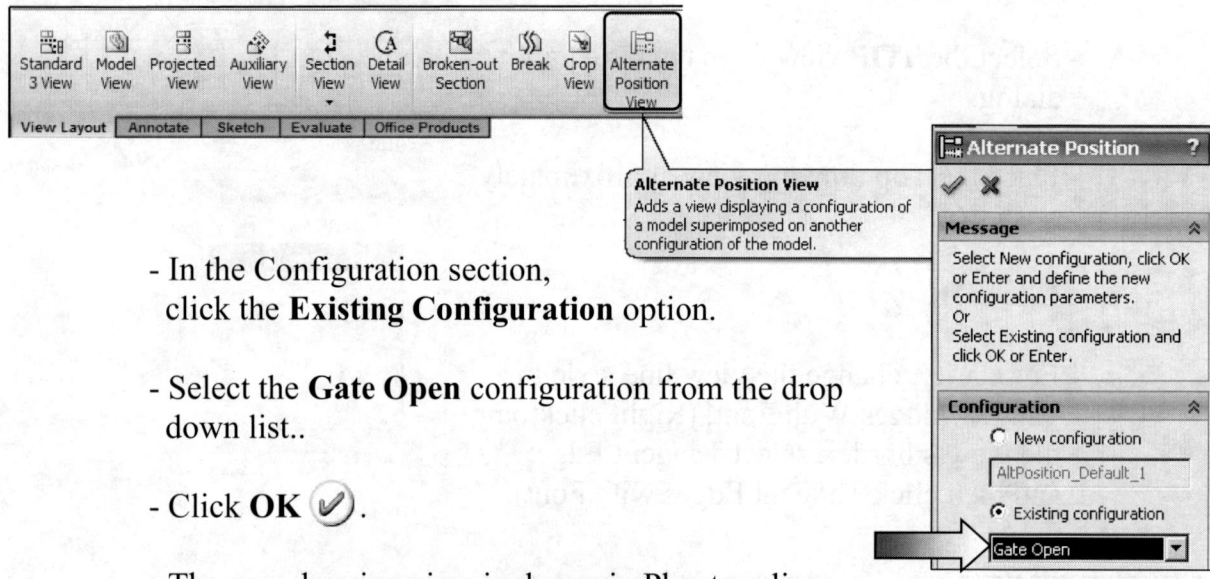

- In the Configuration section,
click the **Existing Configuration** option.

- Select the **Gate Open** configuration from the drop
down list..

- Click **OK**.

- The new drawing view is shown in Phantom lines
and is superimposed over the original view.

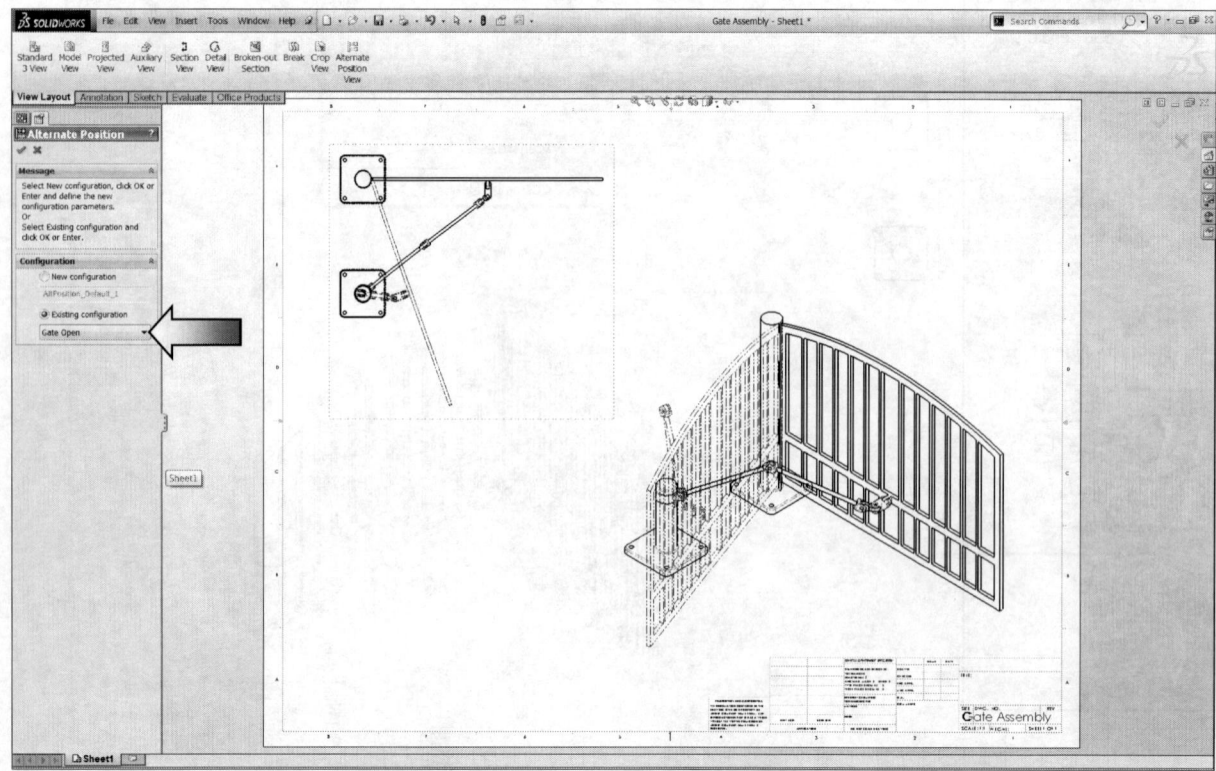

7. Adding Text / Annotations:

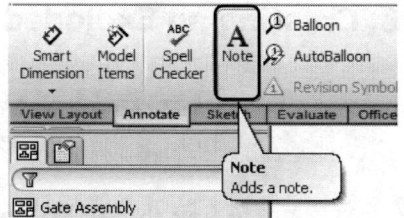

- Select the Top drawing view's Border to activate the view and then click **Note** [A Note] .

- Add the notes: **Top View** and **Isometric View** as shown.

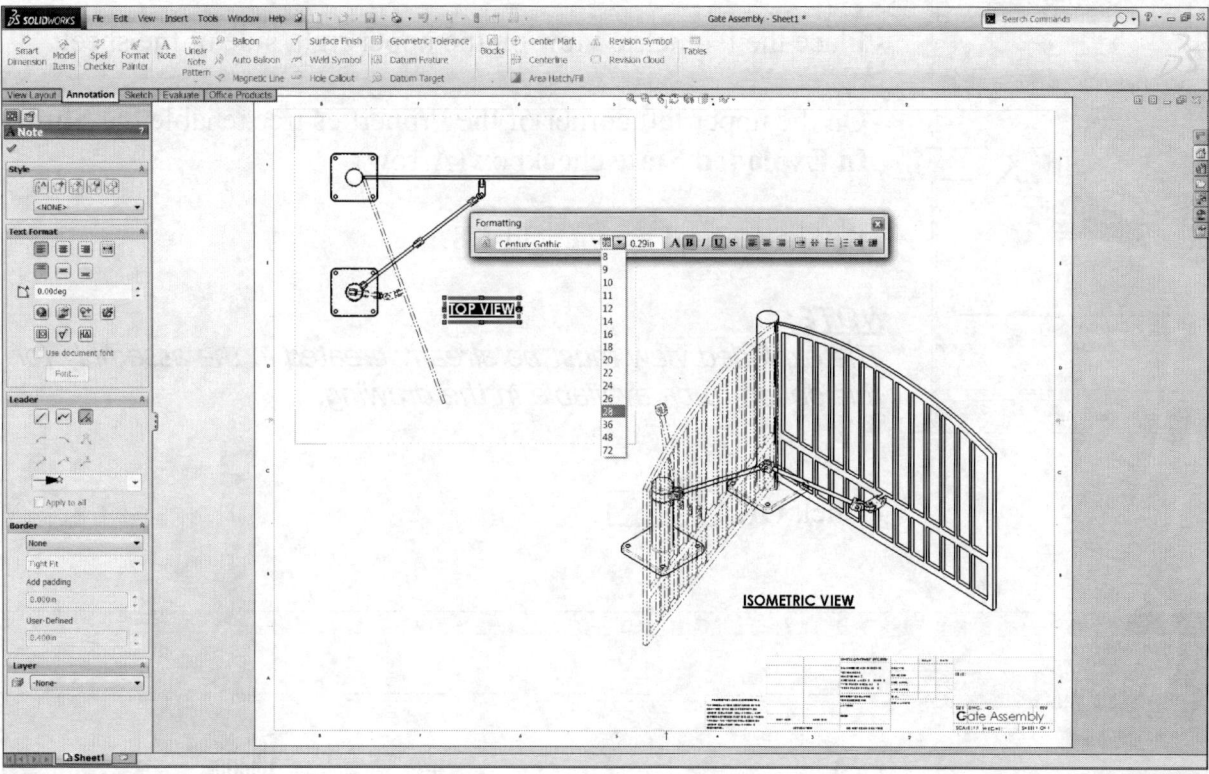

- Use the options in the Formatting toolbar to modify the text.

- Highlight the text and change it to match the settings below:

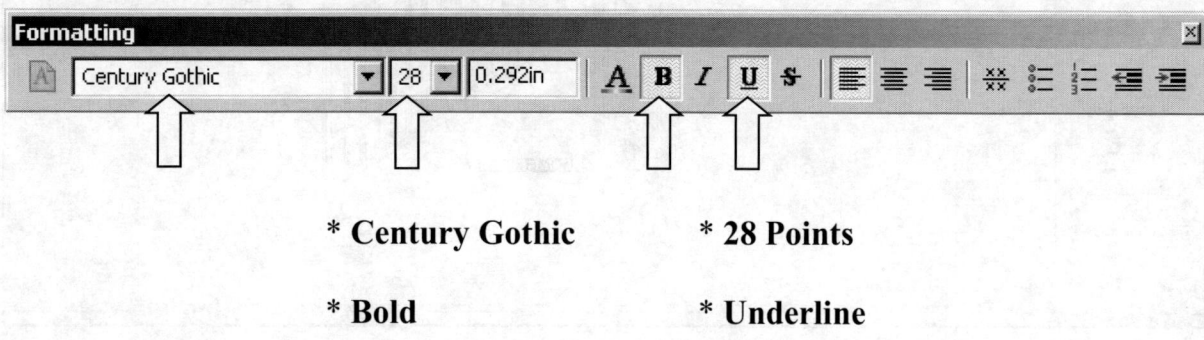

           * **Century Gothic**   * **28 Points**

           * **Bold**   * **Underline**

8. Creating an Exploded Isometric view:

- Click 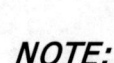 or select **Insert / Drawing View / Model**.

- Click the **NEXT** arrow 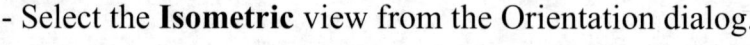 .

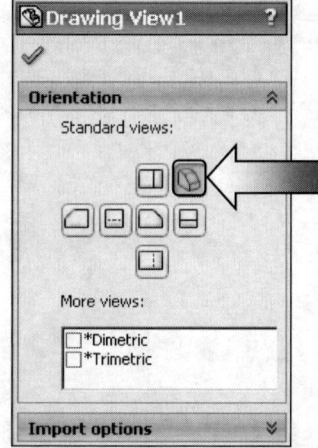

- Select the **Isometric** view from the Orientation dialog.

- Place the Isometric view on the upper right side of the sheet.

- On the upper left corner of the Properties tree, enable the **Show-In Exploded State** checkbox (Arrow).

- Set the scale of the view to **1:8**.

<u>NOTE:</u>
The exploded view must be already created in the assembly for this option to be available in the drawing.

- Click **OK**   OK   .

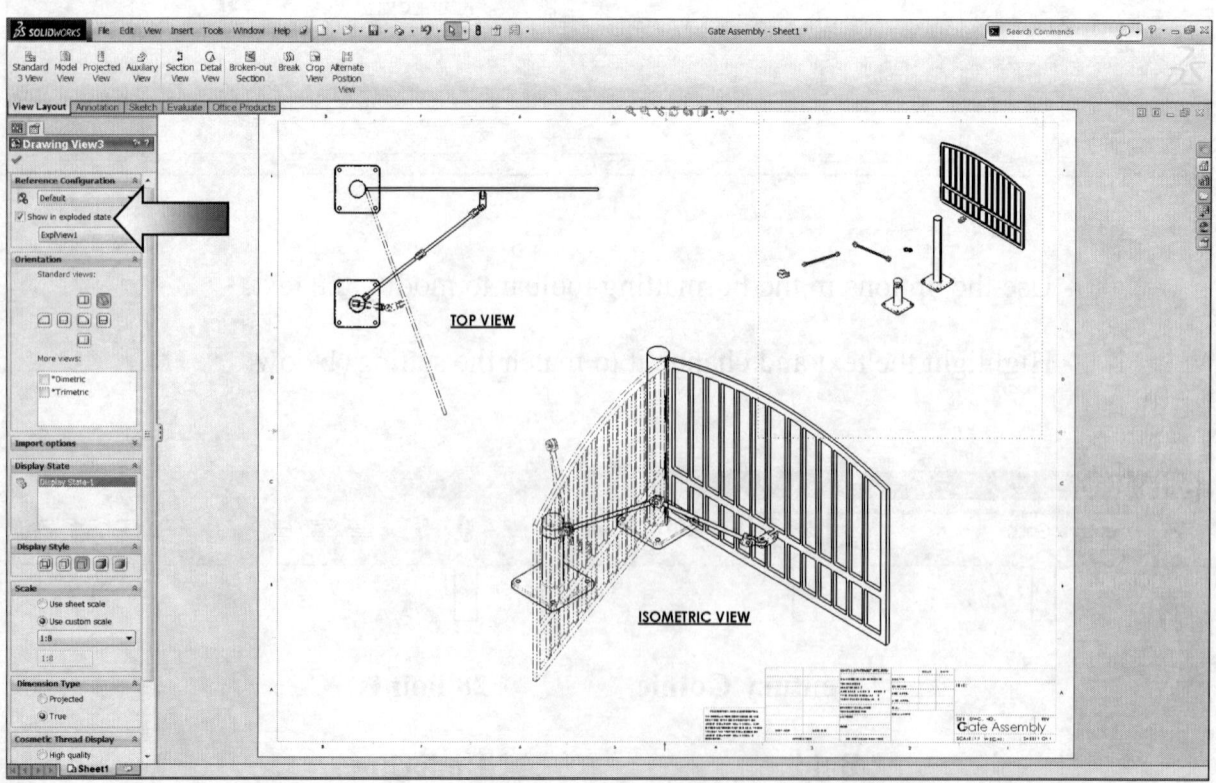

9. Adding Auto-Balloons to the Exploded view:

- Switch to the **Annotation** tool tab.

- Select the Isometric drawing view's border.

- Click AutoBall... or select **Insert / Annotations / AutoBalloon**.

- In the Auto Balloon properties tree, set the following:

    * Balloon Layout: **Square**

    * Ignore Multiple Instances: **Enable**

    * Style: **Circular**

    * Size: **2 Character**

    * Balloon Text: **Item Number**

- Click **OK** [OK] .

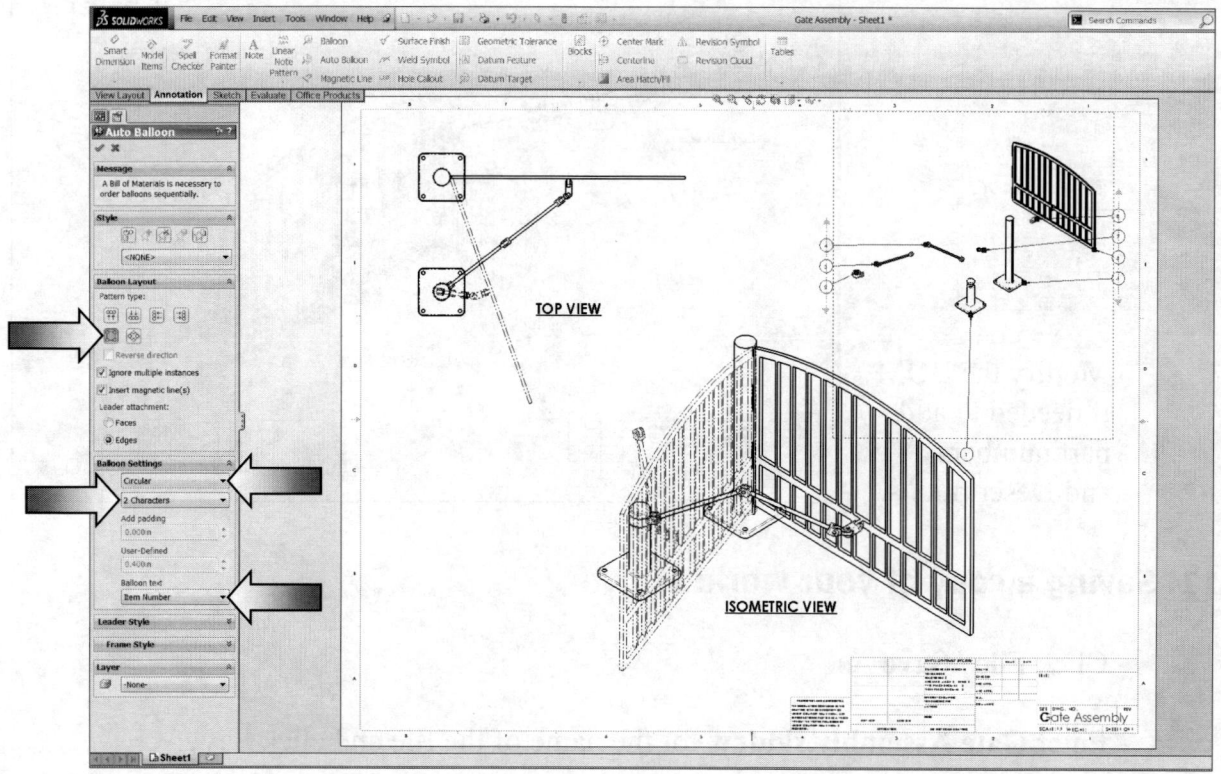

10. Adding a Bill of Materials to the Drawing:

- Click 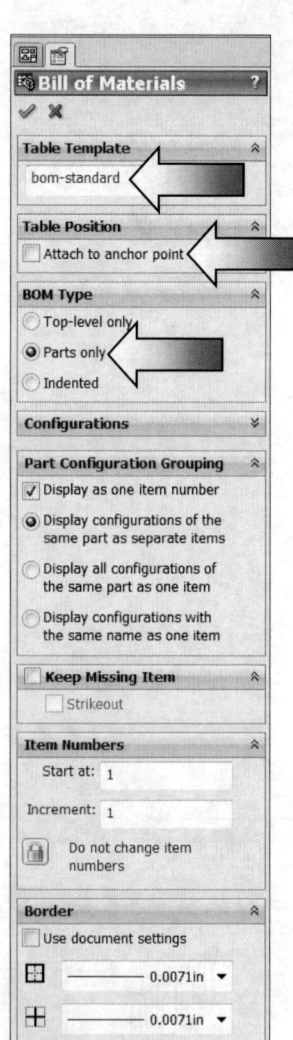 or select **Insert / Tables / Bill of Materials**.

- Select **Bom-Standard** under Table Templates.

- **Disable** Attached To Anchor.

- Select **Parts Only** for BOM Type.

- Click **OK** [OK] .

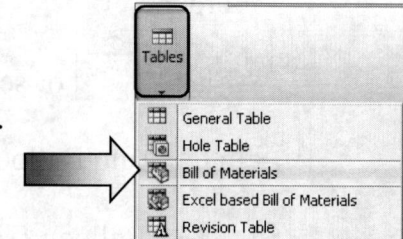

	A	B	C	D
1	ITEM NO.	PART NUMBER	DESCRIPTION	QTY.
2	1	011-4321	Base Stand	1
3	2	012-4321	Arm Connector	1
4	3	013-4321	Arm	1
5	4	014-4321	Connecting-Arm	1
6	5	015-4321	Gate	1
7	6	016-4321	Gate Support	1
8	7	017-4321	Connector Joint	1
9	8	018-4321	Double Joint	1

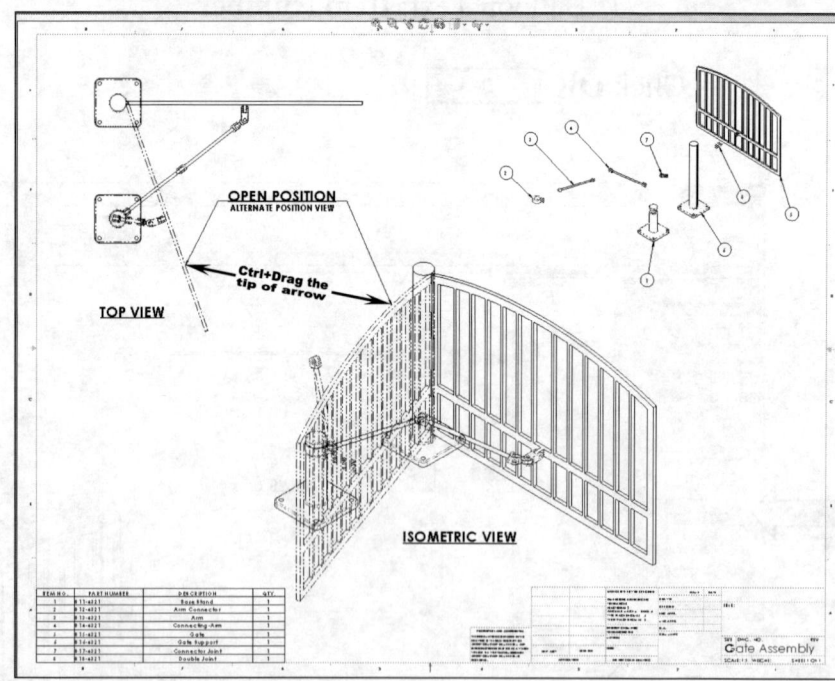

- Modify the BOM if needed to add part numbers and Descriptions.

11. Saving a copy of your work:

- Click **File / Save As**.

- Enter **Gate Assembly.slddrw** for the name of the file and click **Save**.

Questions for Review

Assembly Drawings

1. The Alternate Position command can also be selected from Insert / Drawing View / Alternate Position.
   a. True
   b. False

2. The Alternate Position command precisely places a drawing view on top of another view.
   a. True
   b. False

3. The types of views that are not currently supported to work with Alternate Position are:
   a. Broken and Crop Views
   b. Detail View
   c. Section View
   d. All of the above.

4. Dimensions or annotations cannot be added to the superimposed view.
   a. True
   b. False

5. The Line Style for use in the Alternate Position view is:
   a. Solid line
   b. Dashed line
   c. Phantom line
   d. Centerline

6. In order to show the assembly exploded view on a drawing, an exploded view configuration must be created first in the main assembly.
   a. True
   b. False

7. Balloons and Auto Balloons can also be selected from: Insert / Annotations / (Auto) Balloon.
   a. True
   b. False

8. The Bill of Materials contents can be modified to include the Material Column.
   a. True
   b. False

7. TRUE   8. TRUE
5. C   6. TRUE
3. D   4. FALSE
1. TRUE   2. TRUE

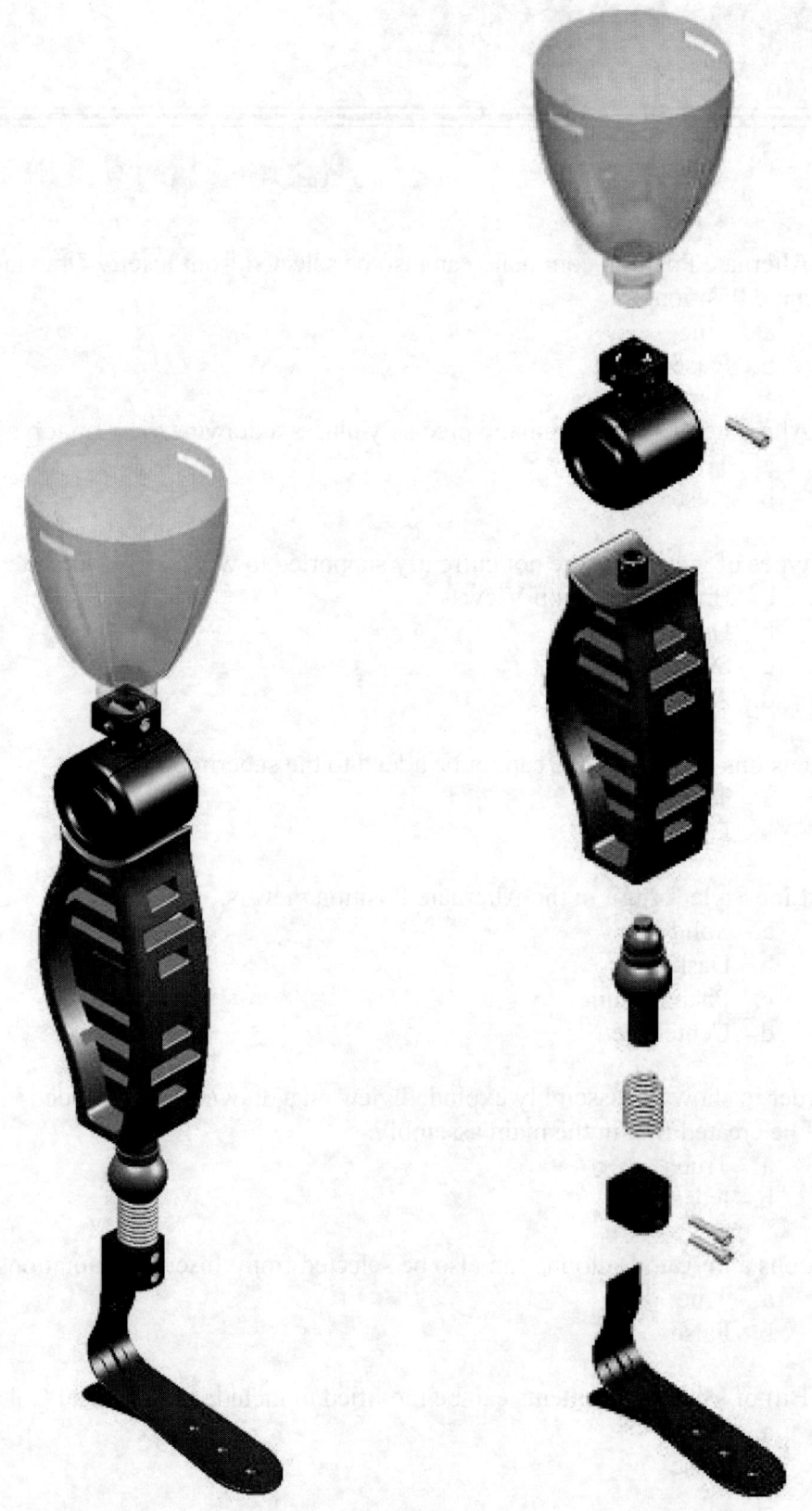

CHAPTER 16

Drawing Views

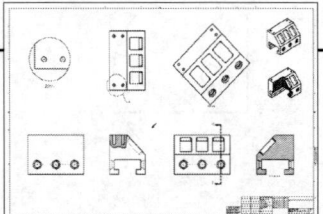

Drawing Views
Machined Block

- When creating an engineering drawing, one of the first things to do is to layout the drawing views such as:

  * The standard Front, Top, Right, and Isometric views.

  * Other views like Detail, Cross section, Auxiliary views, etc., can be created or projected from the 4 standard views.

- Most of the drawing views in SolidWorks are automatically aligned with one another (default alignments); each one can only be moved along the direction that was defined for that particular view (vertical, horizontal, or at projected angle).

- Dimensions and annotations will then be added to the drawing views.

- The dimensions created in the part will be inserted into the drawing views, so that their association between the model and the drawing views can be maintained. Changes done to these dimensions will update all drawing views and the solid model as well;

- Configurations are also used in this lesson to create some specific views.

- This chapter will guide you through the creation of some of the most commonly used drawing views in an engineering drawing like: 3 Standard views, Section views, Detail views, Projected views, Auxiliary views, Broken Out Section views, and Cross Hatch patterns.

Machined Block
Drawing Views Creation

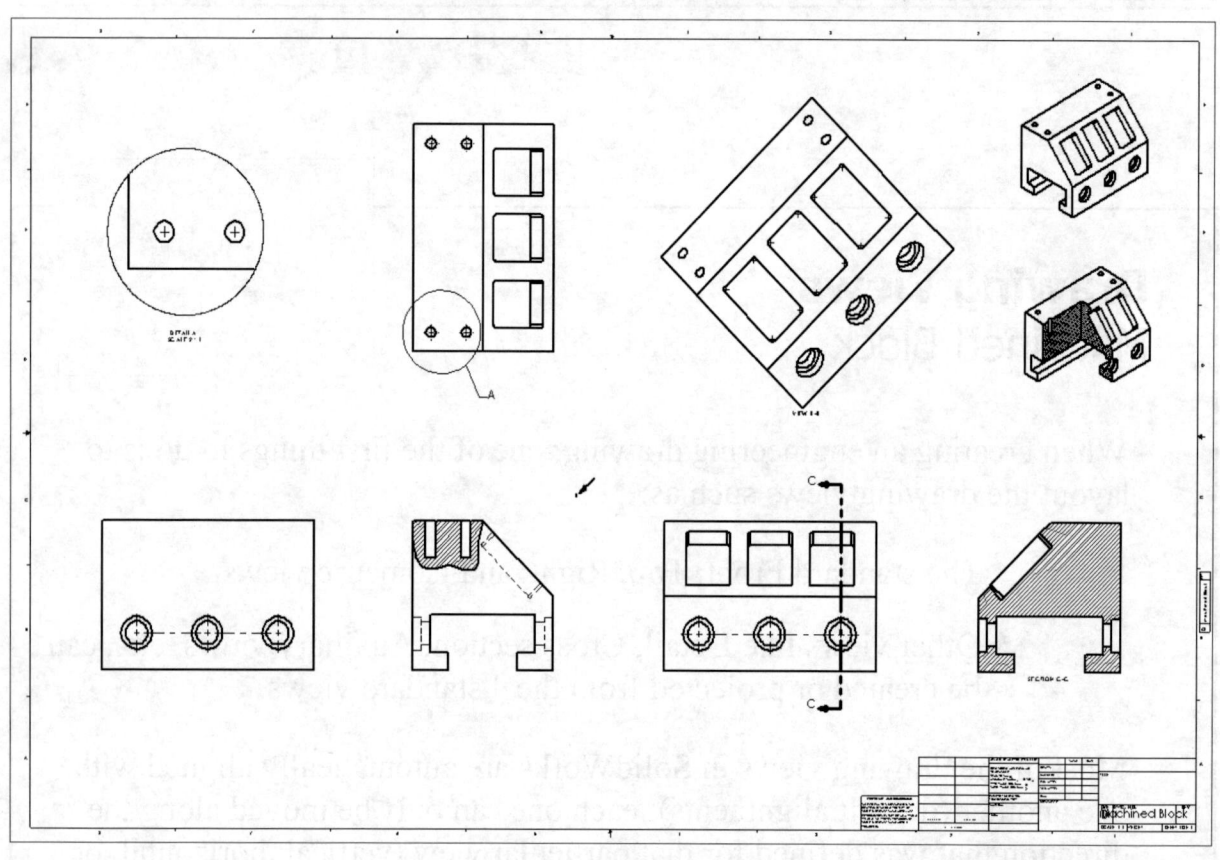

| Dimensioning Standards: **ANSI** | Third Angle Projection |
| Units: **INCHES** – 3 Decimals | |

Tools Needed:

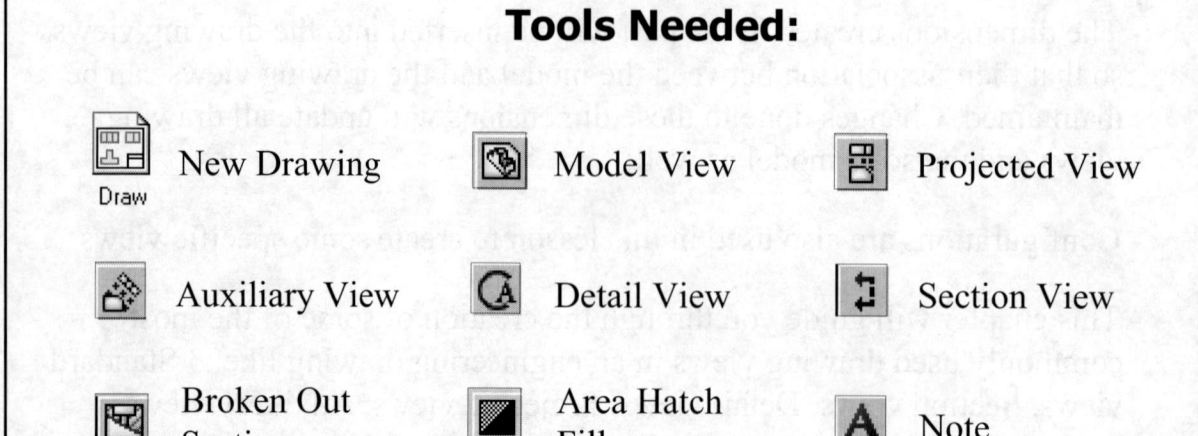

	New Drawing		Model View		Projected View
	Auxiliary View		Detail View		Section View
	Broken Out Section		Area Hatch Fill		Note

1. Creating a new drawing:

- Select **File / New / Drawing** template.

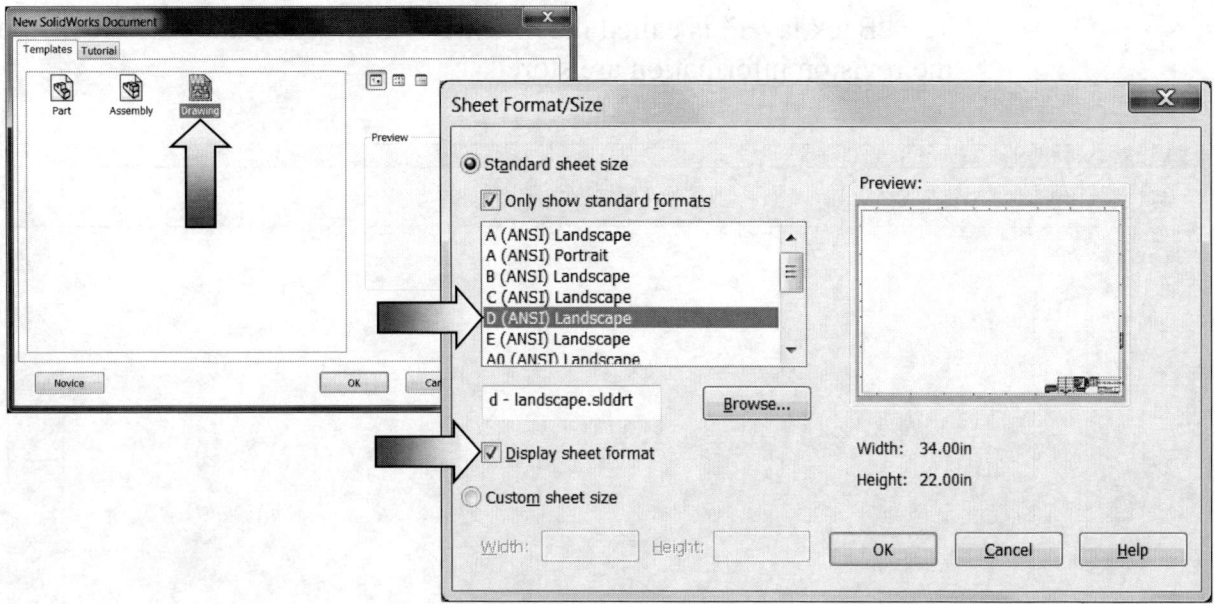

- Choose **D-Landscape*** under Standard Sheet Size. (34.00 in. X 22.00 in.)

- Enable the **Display Sheet Format** check box to include the title block.

- Click **OK**.

* If the options above are not available, **right click** inside the drawing and select **Properties**.

- Select the **Third Angle** option under Type of Projection.

- Set the default view scale to **1:2**.

- The Units can be changed later on.

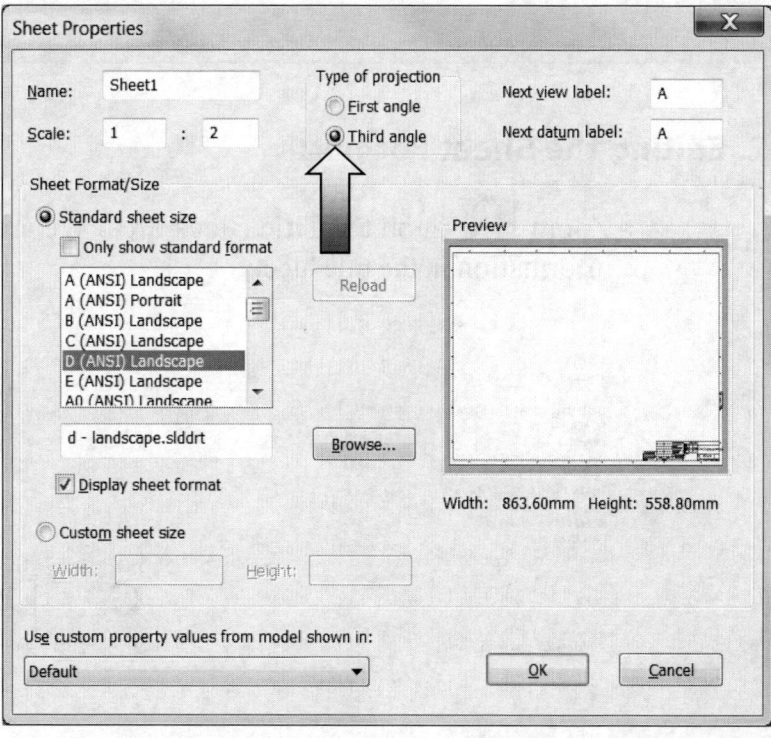

- The drawing template comes with 2 default "layers":

    * The "Front layer" is called the **Sheet** layer, where drawings are created.

    * The "Back layer" is called the **Sheet Format**, where the title block and the revision information are stored.

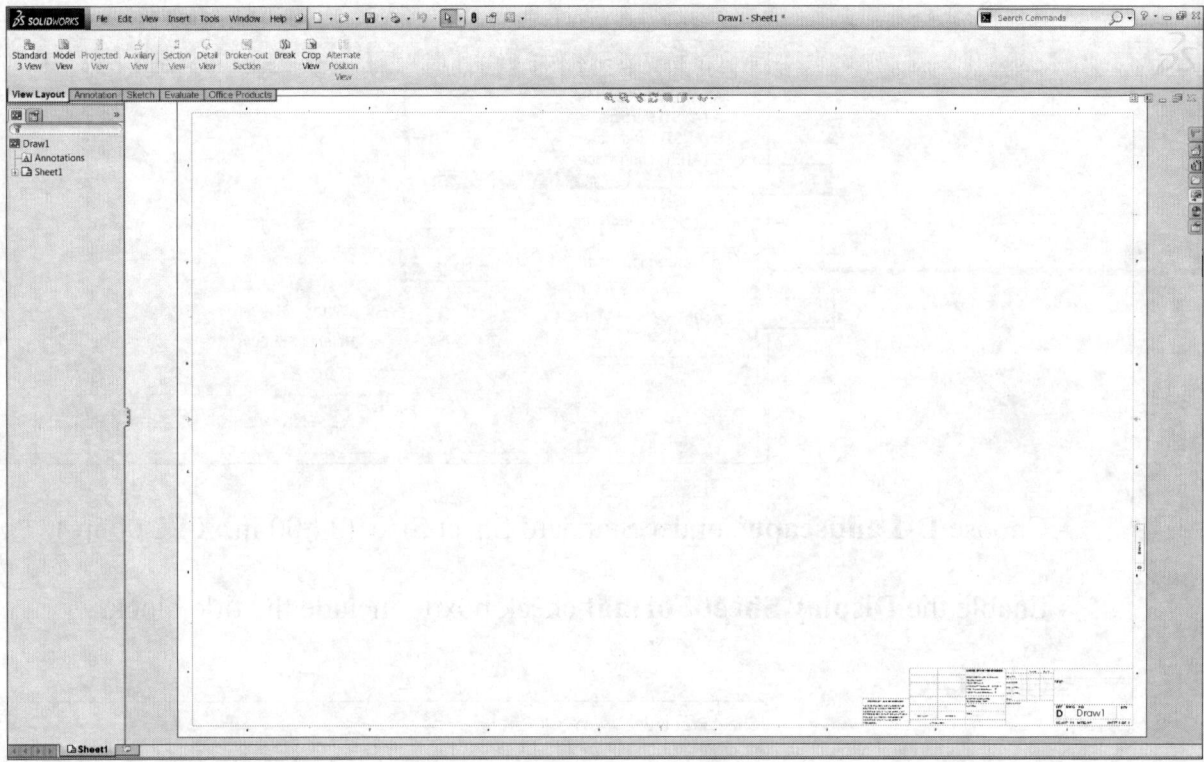

2. Editing the Sheet Format:

- Zoom 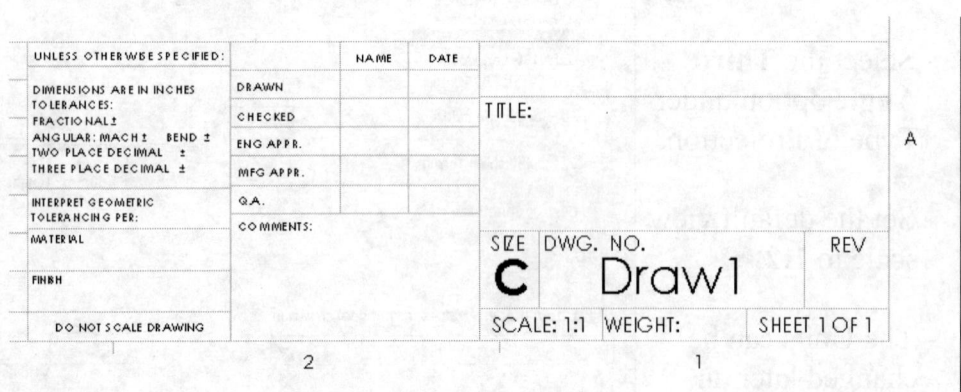 in on the Title Block area. We are going to first fill out the information in the title block.

UNLESS OTHERWISE SPECIFIED:		NAME	DATE		
DIMENSIONS ARE IN INCHES TOLERANCES: FRACTIONAL±	DRAWN			TITLE:	A
ANGULAR: MACH± BEND ± TWO PLACE DECIMAL ± THREE PLACE DECIMAL ±	CHECKED				
	ENG APPR.				
	MFG APPR.				
INTERPRET GEOMETRIC TOLERANCING PER:	Q.A.				
MATERIAL	COMMENTS:			SIZE **C** DWG. NO. Draw1 REV	
FINISH					
DO NOT SCALE DRAWING				SCALE: 1:1 WEIGHT: SHEET 1 OF 1	

- Right click in the drawing area and select **Edit Sheet Format.**

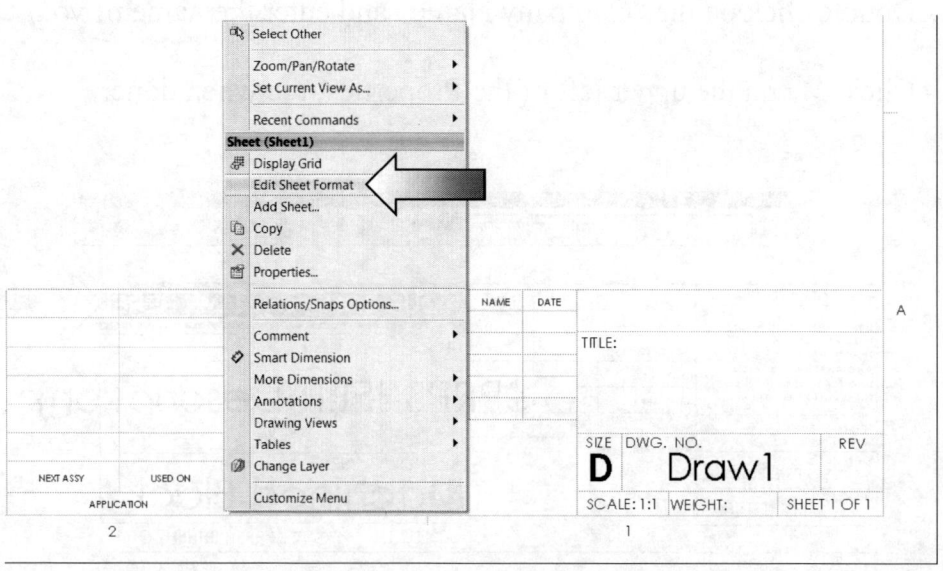

- The Sheet Format is brought up on top.

- New annotation and sketch lines can now be added.

- Any existing text or lines can now be modified.

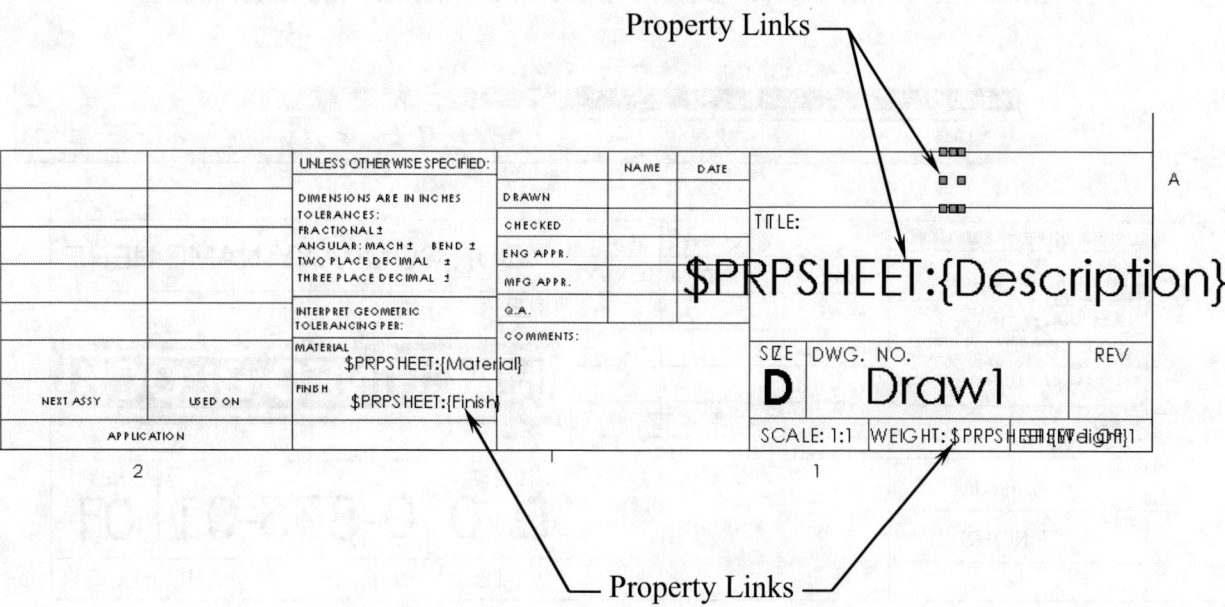

- Notice the link to properties text strings: "$PRPS". Some of the annotations have already been linked to the part's properties.

3. Modifying the existing text:

- Double click on the "Company Name" and enter the name of your company.

- Click ✅ on the upper left of the Properties tree when done.

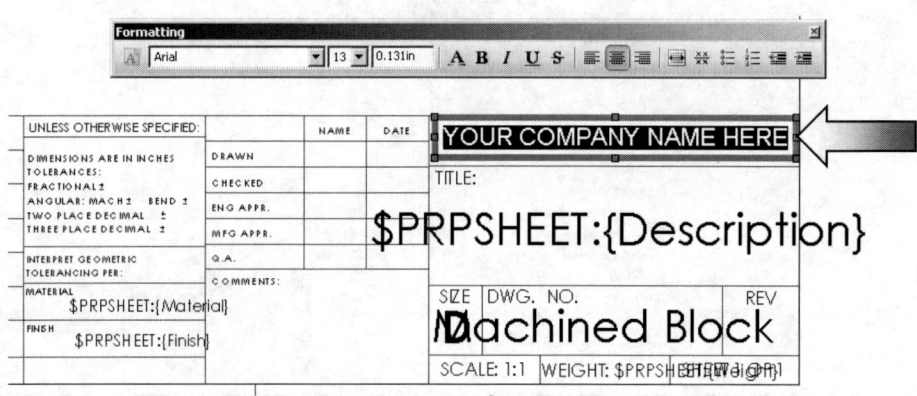

4. Adding the Title of the drawing:

- Double click on the Property-Link in the Title area ($PRPSHEET:{Description})

- Type **Machined Block** for the title of the drawing.

- Enter the information as shown in the title block for the other areas.

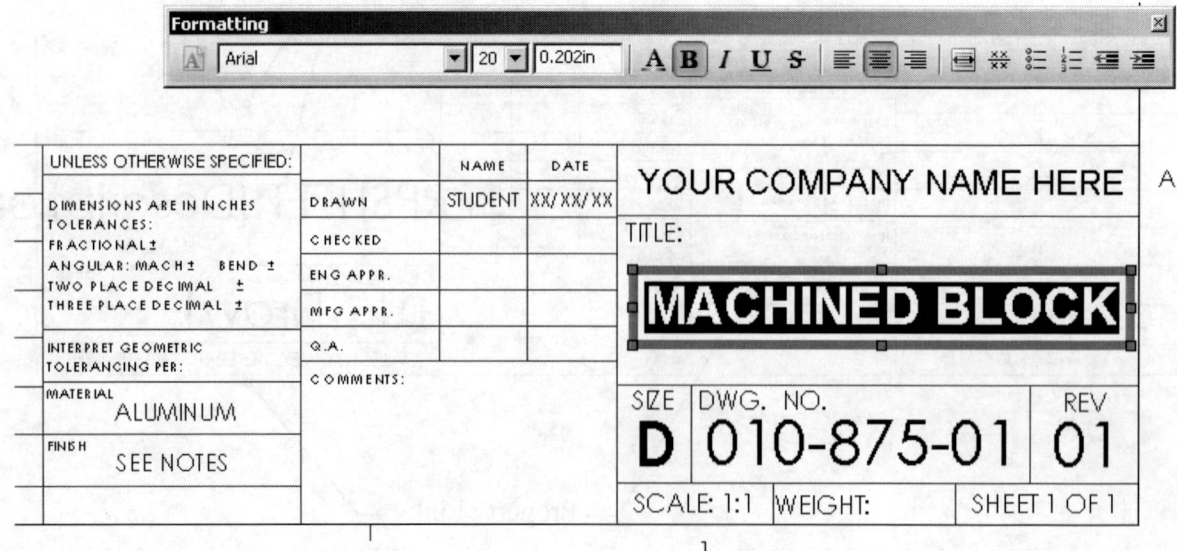

- Click **OK** ✅.

5. Switching back to the drawing Sheet:

- Right click in the drawing and select **Edit Sheet**.

- The Drawing Sheet "layer" is brought back up on top.

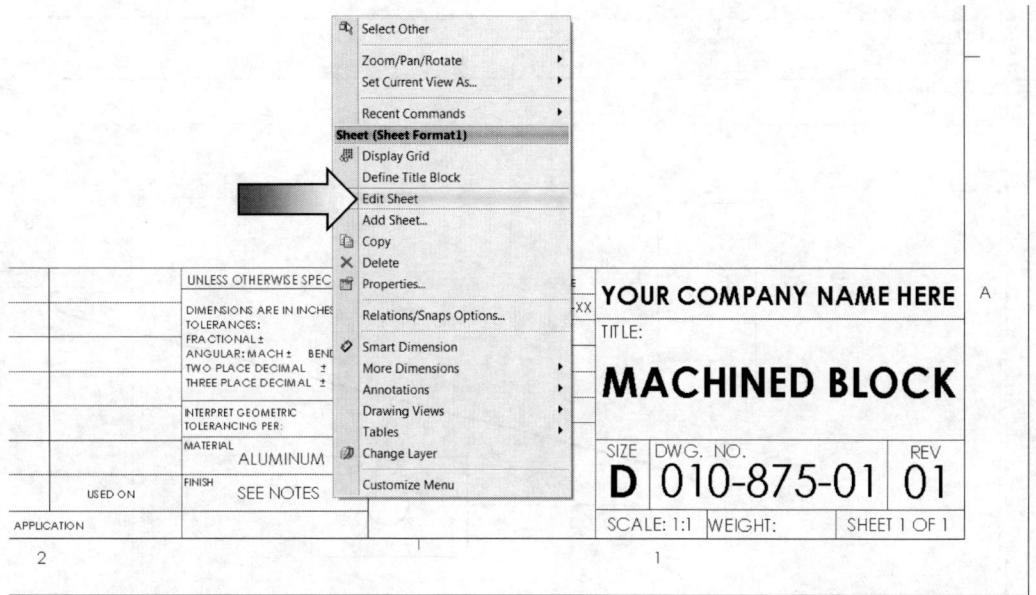

6. Using the View-Palette:

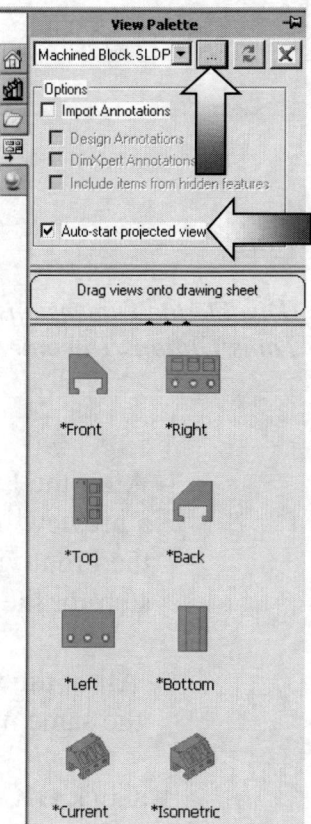

- The **View Palette** is located on the right side of the screen in the Task Pane area, click on its icon to access it.

Note: *If the drawing views are not visible in the View Palette window, click the Browse button [...] and open the part Machined block.*

- The standard drawing views like the Front, Right, Top, Back, Left, Bottom, Current, Isometric, and Sheet Metal Flat-Pattern views are contained within the View Palette window.

- These drawing views can be dragged into the drawing sheet to create the drawing views.

- The **Auto Start Projected View** checkbox should be selected by default.

7. Using the View Palette:

- Click/Hold/Drag the Front view from the View-Palette (arrow) and drop it on the drawing sheet, approximately as shown. Make sure the Auto-Start projected view checkbox is enabled (arrow).

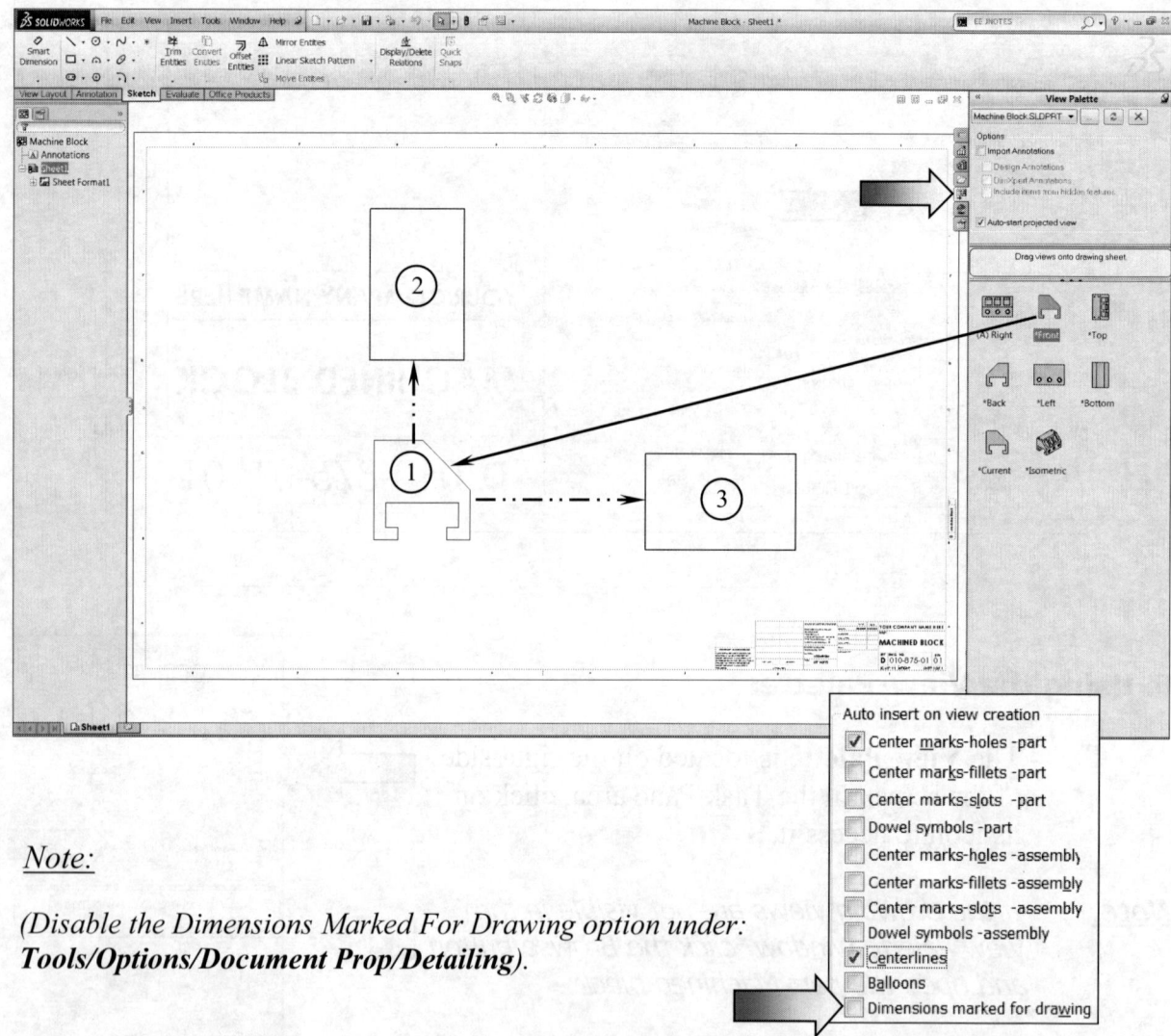

Note:

(Disable the Dimensions Marked For Drawing option under:
Tools/Options/Document Prop/Detailing)*.*

- After the Front view is placed (position 1), move the mouse cursor upward, a preview image of the Top view appears, click in an approximate spot above the Front view to place the Top view (position number 2); repeat the same step for the Right view (position 3).

- All of the views from the View-Palette can be added to the drawing by using the same method.

- Click **OK** ✅ when you are finished with the first three views.

8. Adding an Isometric view:

Standard 3 View
Model View
Projected View
Auxiliary View
Section View
Detail View
Broken-out Section
View Layout
Annotate
Sketch
Evaluate
Office Products

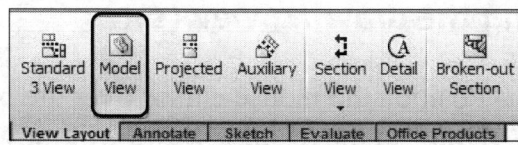

- Switch to the **View Layout** tab.

- Click Model View or select **Insert / Drawing View / Model View**.

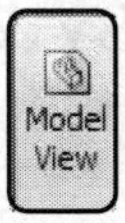

- Click the NEXT arrow .

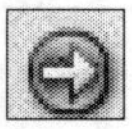

- Select **Isometric** (Arrow) from the Model View properties tree and place it approximately as shown.

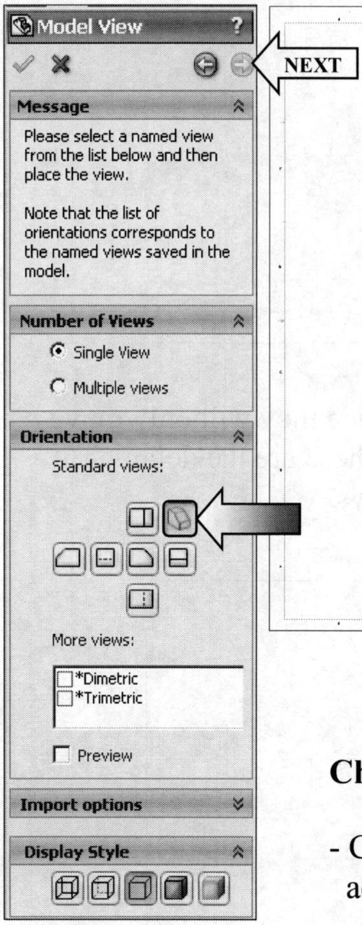
Model View
NEXT
Message
Please select a named view from the list below and then place the view.
Note that the list of orientations corresponds to the named views saved in the model.
Number of Views
Single View
Multiple views
Orientation
Standard views:
More views:
*Dimetric
*Trimetric
Preview
Import options
Display Style

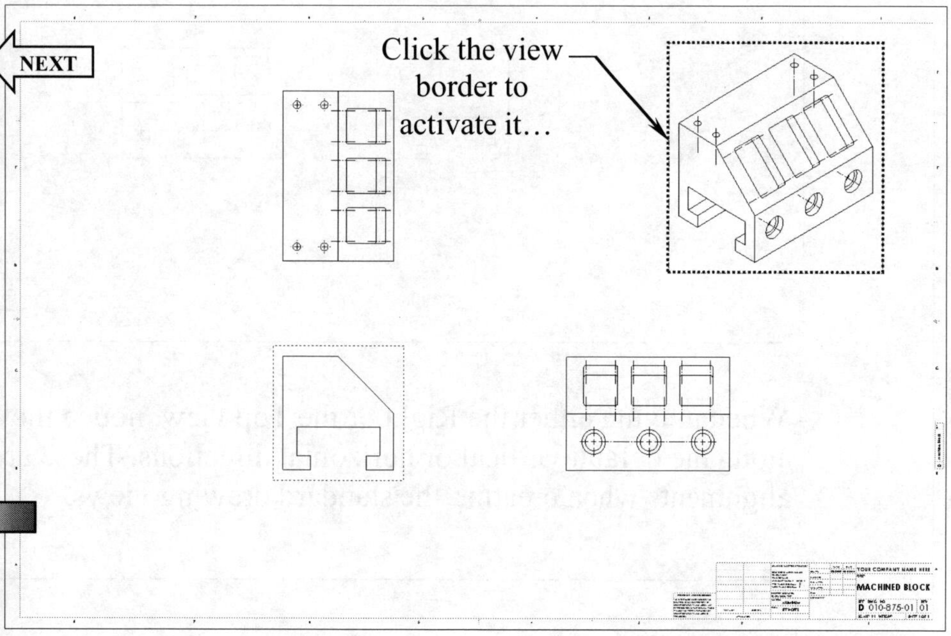
Click the view border to activate it…
MACHINED BLOCK

Changing the view scale:

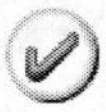

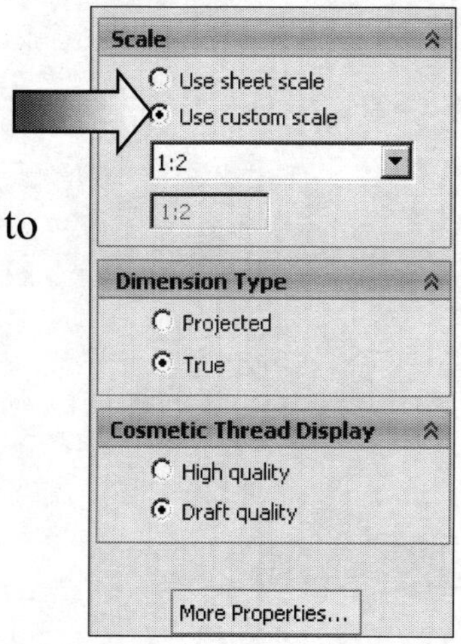
Scale
Use sheet scale
Use custom scale
1:2
1:2
Dimension Type
Projected
True
Cosmetic Thread Display
High quality
Draft quality
More Properties...

- Click the border of the isometric view to activate.

- From the FeatureManager tree select: **Use Custom Scale** option and set the scale to **1:2**.

- Click **OK** .

9. Moving the drawing view(s):

- Position the mouse cursor over the border of the Front view and "Click/Hold/ Drag" to move, all 3 views will move at the same time. By default, the Top and the Right views are automatically aligned with the Front view.

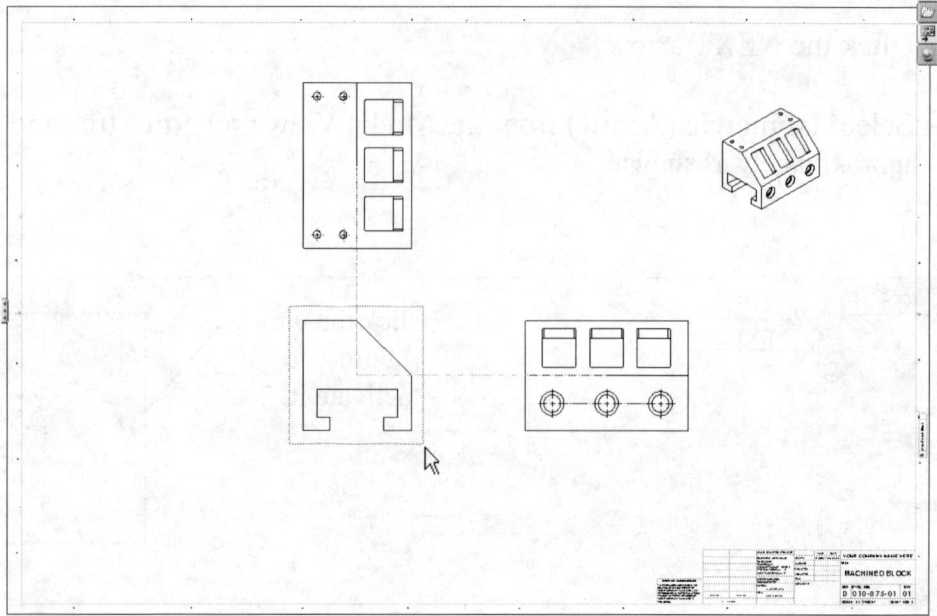

- When moving either the Right or the Top view, notice they will only move along the default vertical or horizontal directions. These are the default alignments when creating the standard drawing views.

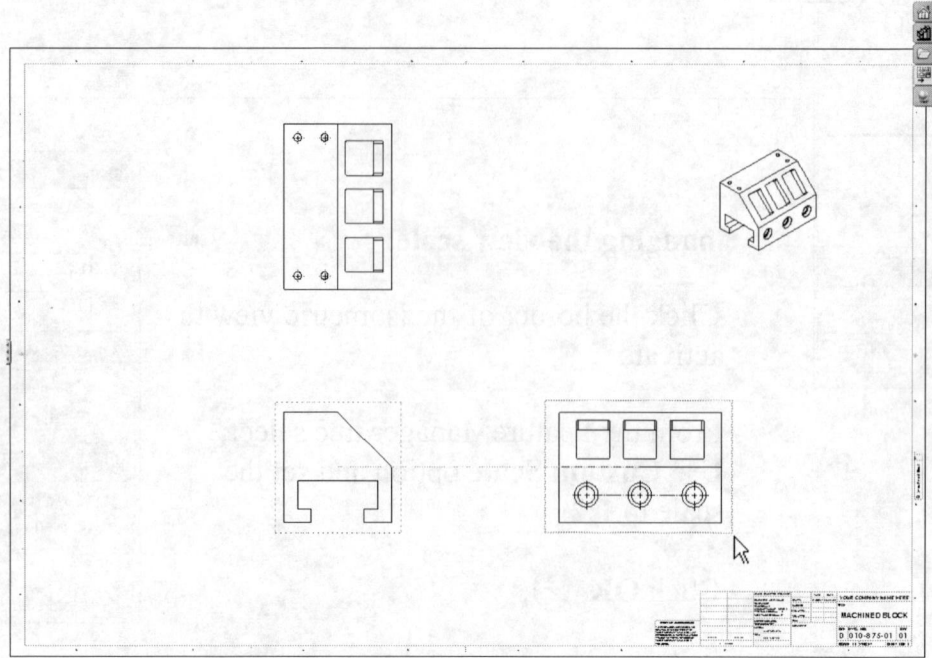

10. Breaking the alignments between the views:

- Right click inside the Top view or on its dotted border and select: **Alignment / Break-Alignment***.

- The Top view is no longer locked to the default direction, it can be moved freely.

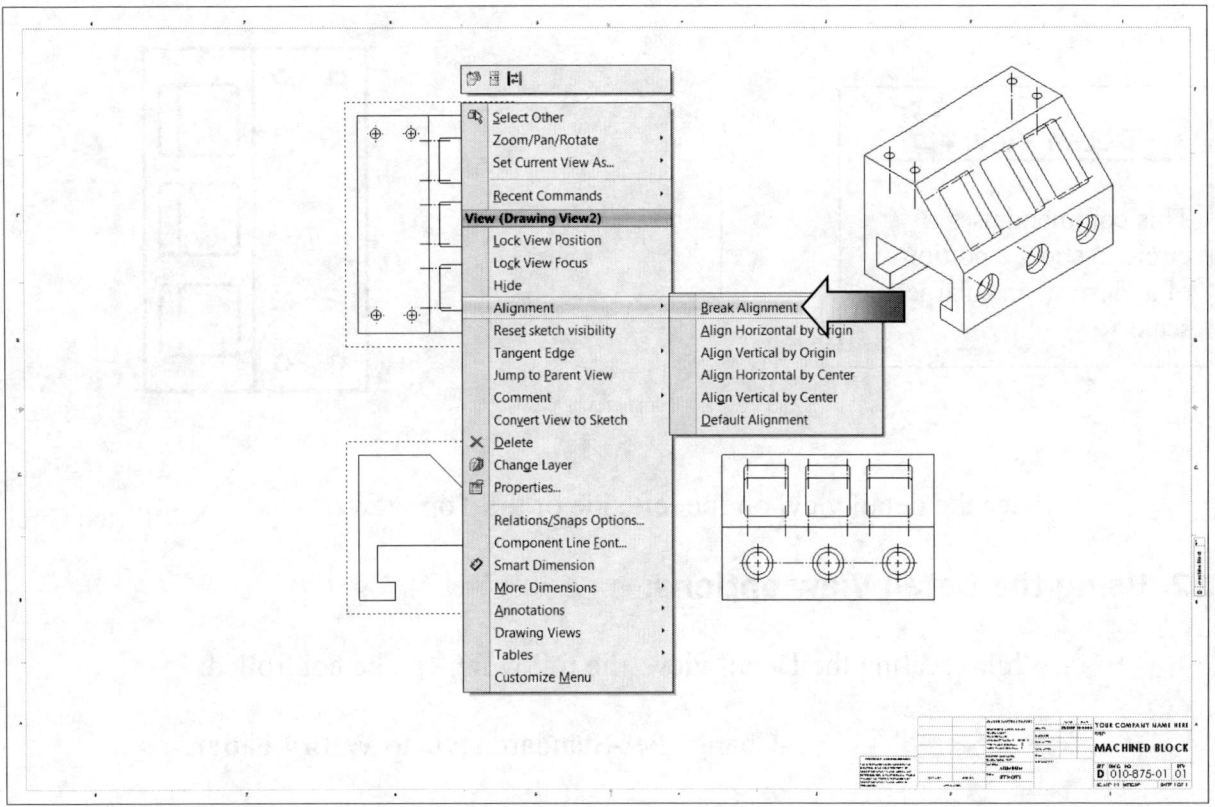

- Dependent views like Projected Views, Auxiliary Views, Section views, etc. will be aligned automatically with the views from where they were created. Their alignments can be broken or also reverted back to their default alignments.

- Independent views can also be aligned with other drawing views by using the same alignment options as shown above.

* To re-align a drawing view:

- Right click on the view's border and select **Alignment / Default-Alignment**.

11. Creating a Detail View:

- Click 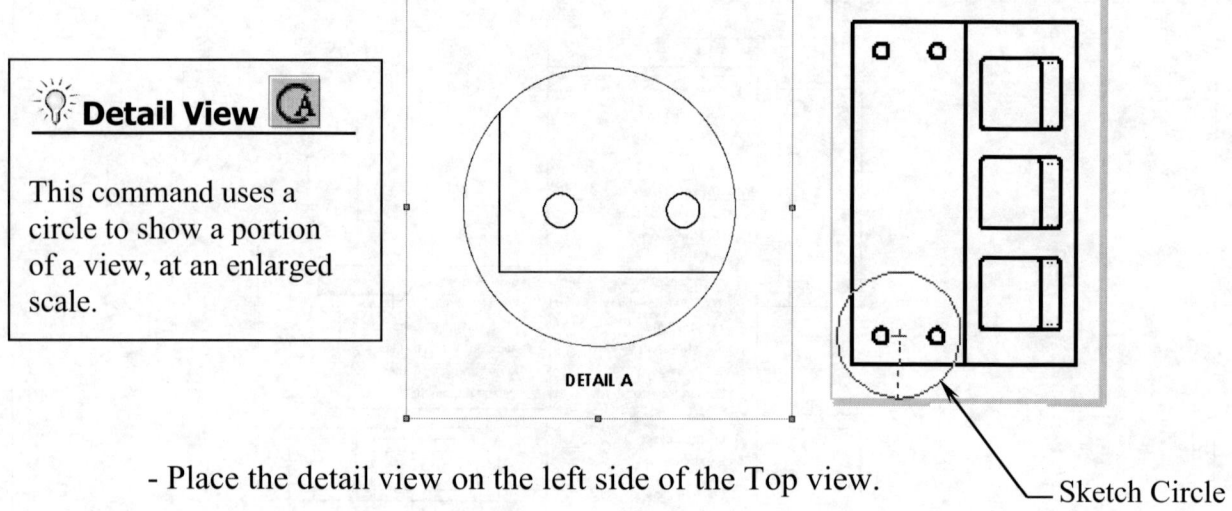 or select **Insert / Drawing View / Detail**.

- Sketch a circle approximately as shown on the Top drawing view.

- The system creates a Detail view automatically at the default 2 to1 scale.

> ☀ **Detail View** Ⓐ
>
> This command uses a circle to show a portion of a view, at an enlarged scale.

DETAIL A

Sketch Circle

- Place the detail view on the left side of the Top view.

12. Using the Detail View options:

- While creating the Detail view, the following can be controlled:

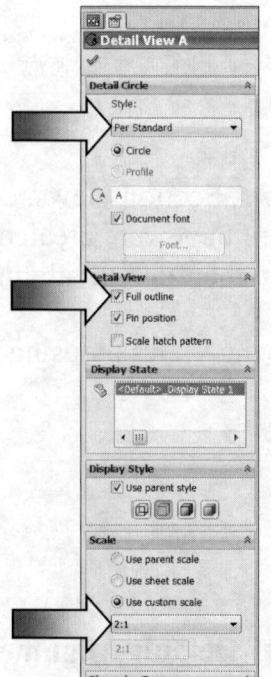

- Change Per-Standard style to **With Leader**.

- Enable **Full Outline**.

- Use Custom scale of **2:1**.

- Click **OK** ✔.

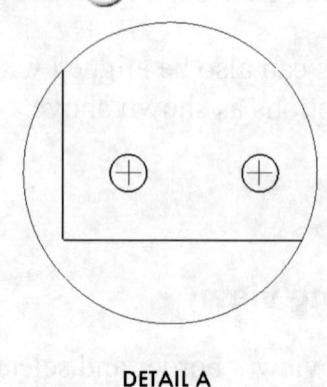

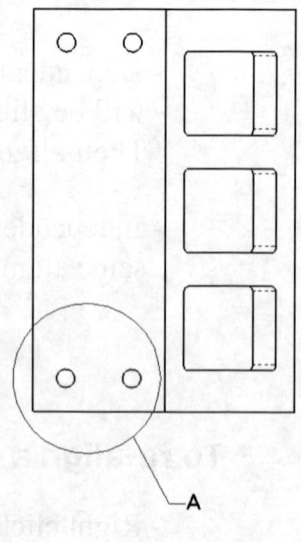

DETAIL A
SCALE 2 : 1

-A

13. Creating a Projected View:

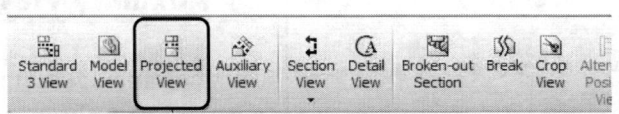

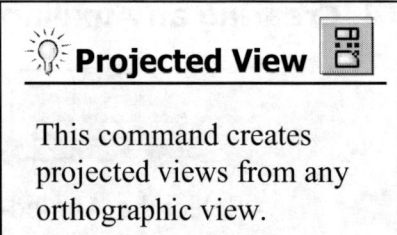

Projected View

This command creates projected views from any orthographic view.

- Click on the Front view's border to activate.

- Click 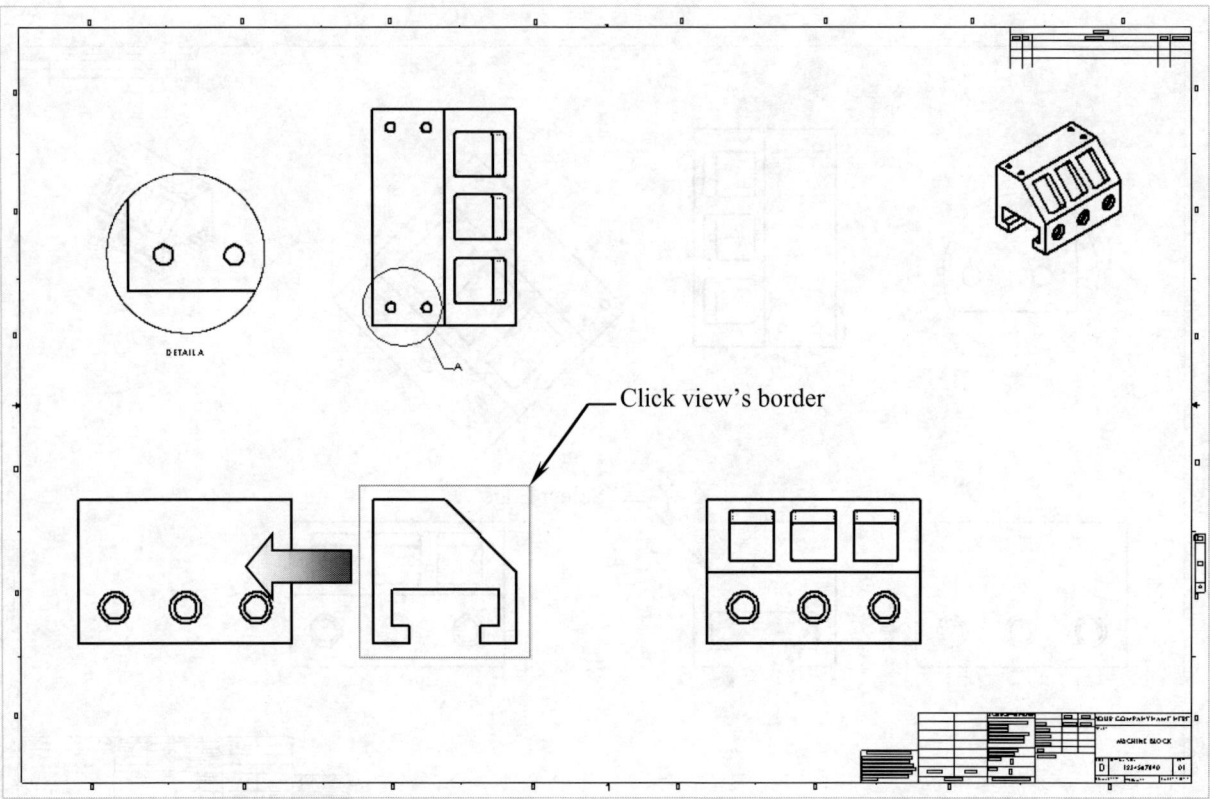 or select **Insert / Drawing View / Projected**.

- The preview of a projected left side view is attached to the mouse cursor, place it on the left side of the Front view.

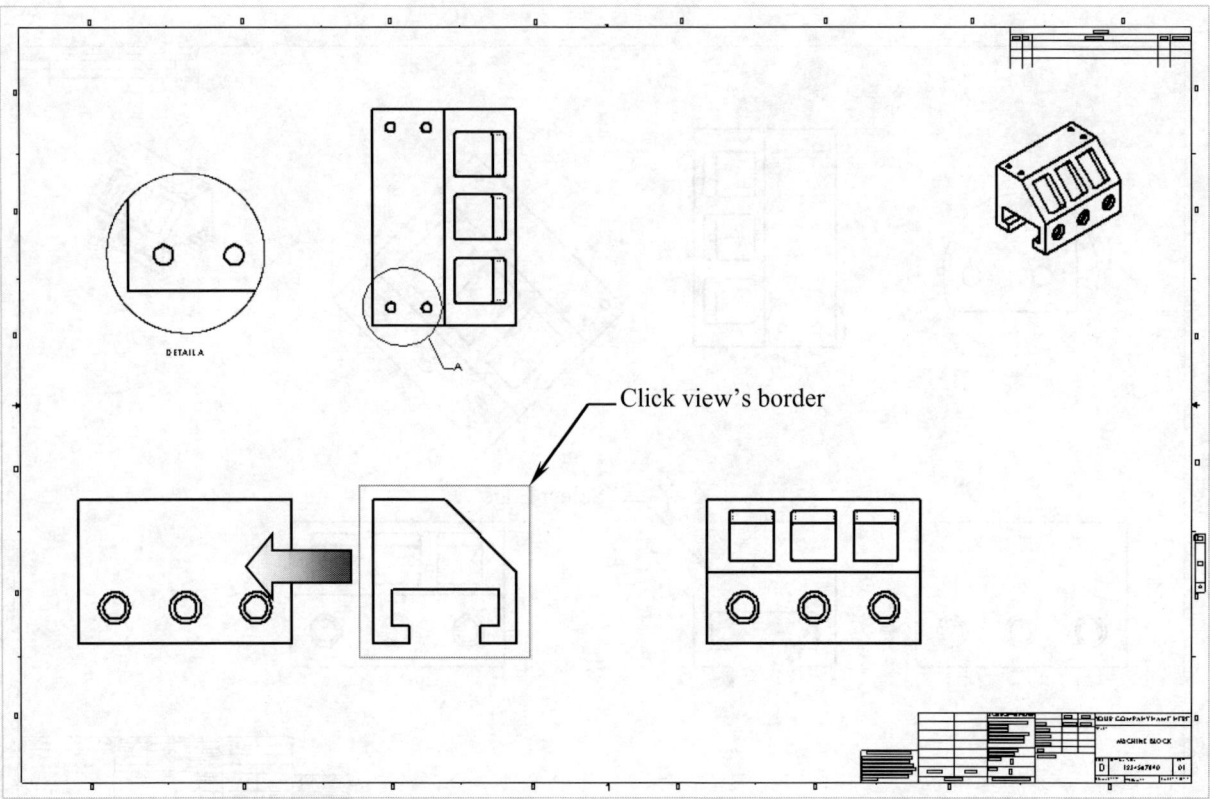

Click view's border

- Notice this view is also aligned automatically to the horizontal axis of the Front view. It can only be moved from left to right.

- For the purpose of this lesson, we will keep all of the default alignments the way SolidWorks creates them. (To break these default alignments at any time, simply right click on their dotted borders and pick Break-Alignment).

- This left side view can also be dragged and dropped from the View Palette.

14. Creating an Auxiliary View:

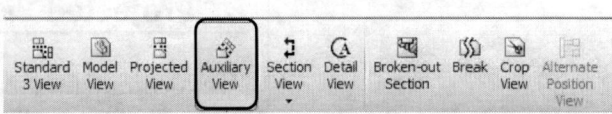

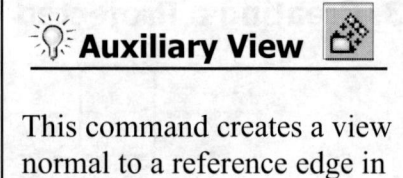

Auxiliary View

This command creates a view normal to a reference edge in an existing view.

- Select the Angled-Edge as indicated.

- Click 🎇 or select **Insert / Drawing View / Auxiliary**.

- The system creates an Auxiliary view and attaches it onto your cursor.

- Place the Auxiliary view approximately as shown.

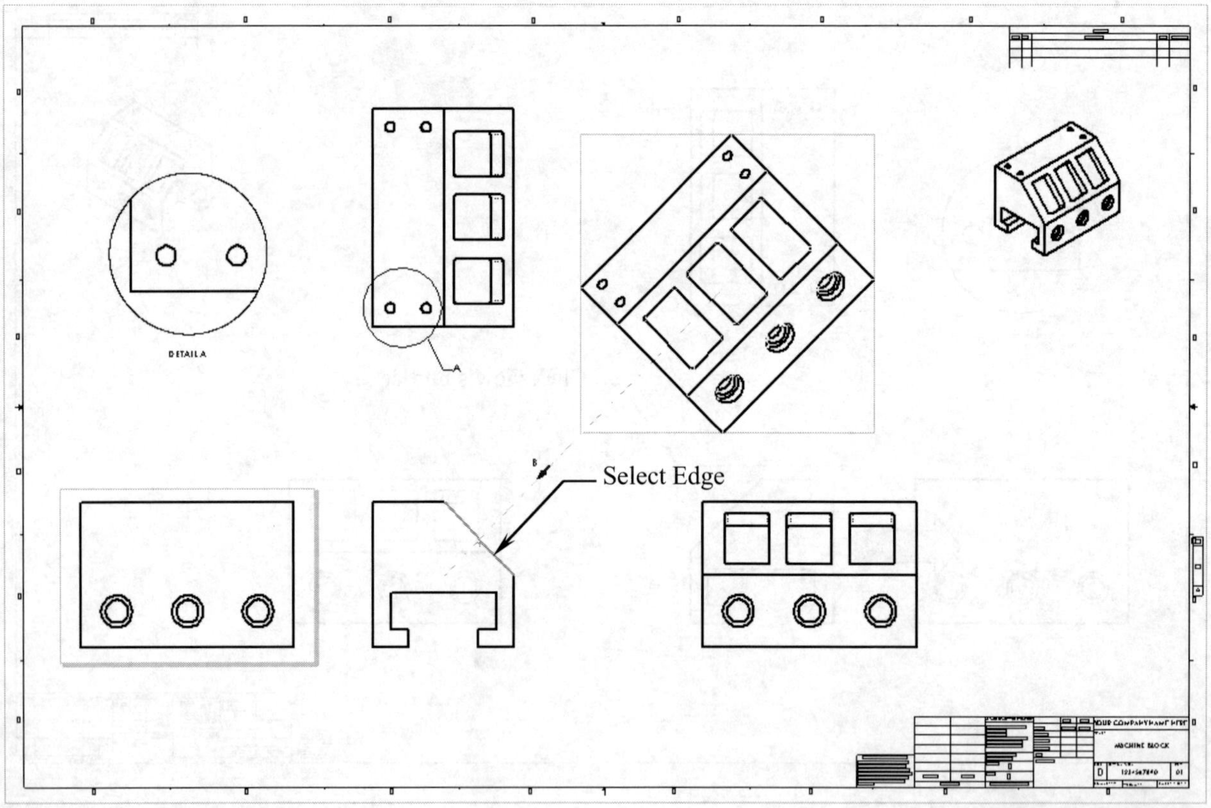

DETAIL A

Select Edge

- The Auxiliary view is also aligned to the edge from which it was originally projected.

- The projection arrow can be toggled on and off from the Properties tree (arrow).

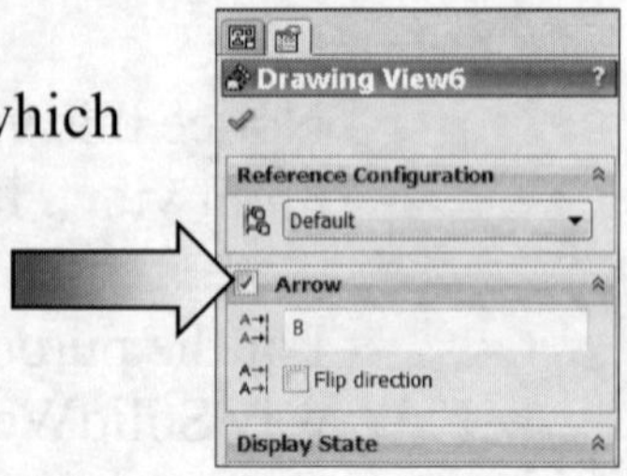

- Use the Break-Alignment option if needed to rearrange the drawing views to different locations.

15. Creating a Section View:

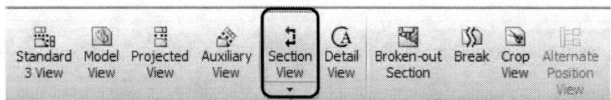

- Click or select **Insert / Drawing View / Section**.

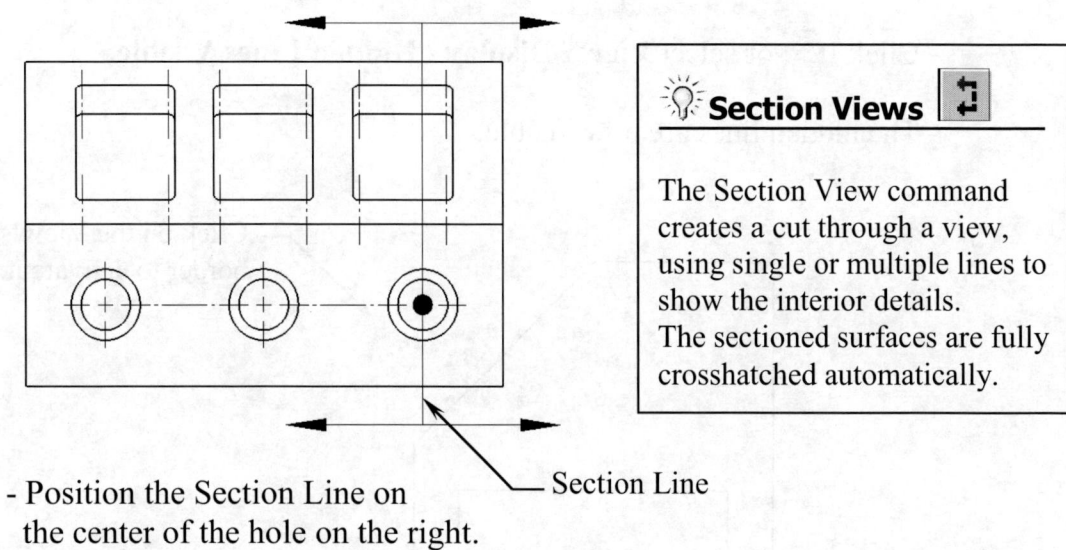

> ☼ **Section Views** 🔁
>
> The Section View command creates a cut through a view, using single or multiple lines to show the interior details.
> The sectioned surfaces are fully crosshatched automatically.

Section Line

- Position the Section Line on the center of the hole on the right.

- The preview of a section view appears, move the mouse cursor to the right-side and click **OK** (the check button) to place it.

- The Section view is aligned horizontally with the view from which it was created and the cross-hatches are added automatically.

- To change the direction of the cut:

* Double Click on the section line and click Rebuild – OR –
* Enable Flip Direction checkbox in the FeatureManager tree (arrow).

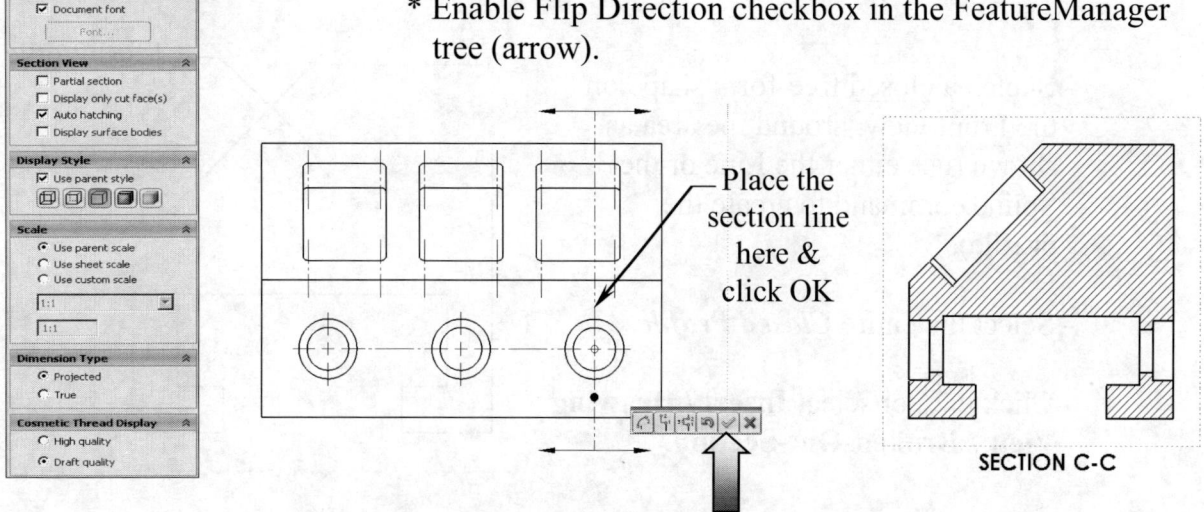

Place the section line here & click OK

SECTION C-C

16. Showing the hidden lines in a drawing view:

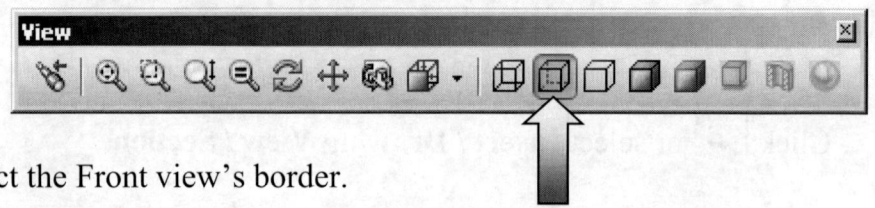

- Select the Front view's border.

- Click 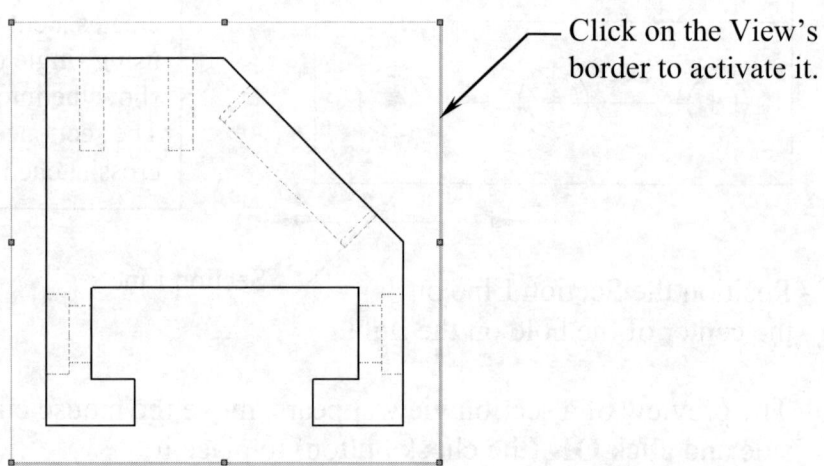 or select **View / Display / Hidden Lines Visible**.

- The hidden lines are now visible.

Click on the View's
border to activate it.

17. Creating a Broken-Out-Section:

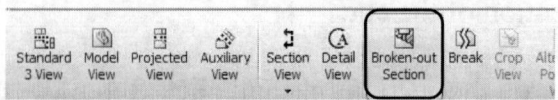

> ⌇ **Broken Out Section View**
>
> Creates a partial cut, using a closed profile, at a specified depth to display the inner details of a drawing view.

- Sketch a <u>closed</u> free-form shape on the Front view, around the area as shown (use either the Line or the Spline command to create the profile).

- Select the entire ***Closed Profile.***

- Click 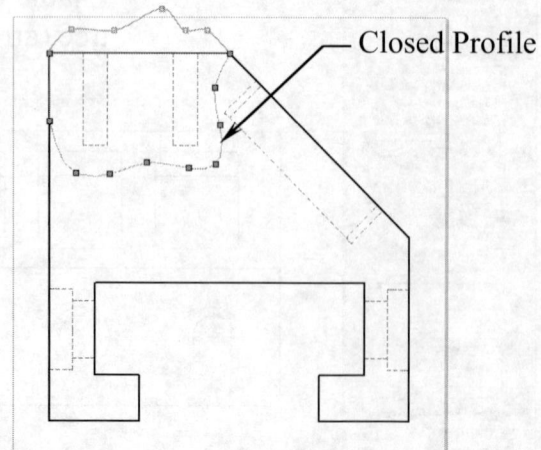 or select **Insert / Drawing View / Broken-Out-Section**.

Closed Profile

- Enable the **Preview** check box in the Properties tree

- Enter **.500** in. for Depth

- Click **OK** .

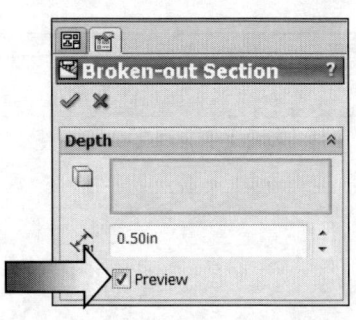

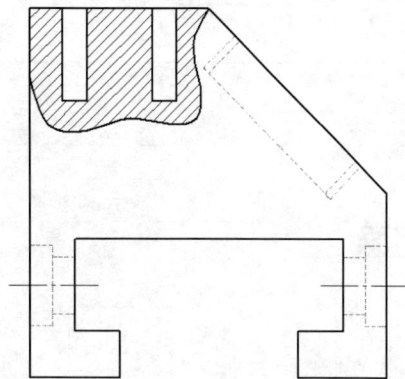

18. Adding a Cutaway view: (Previously created as a Configuration in the model).

- Click or select **Insert / Drawing View / Model**.

- Click on one of the view borders, the Model View Properties tree appears.

- Select **Isometric** (arrow) under Orientation window; use **Custom Scale** of **1:2**.

- Place the new Isometric view below the other isometric view.

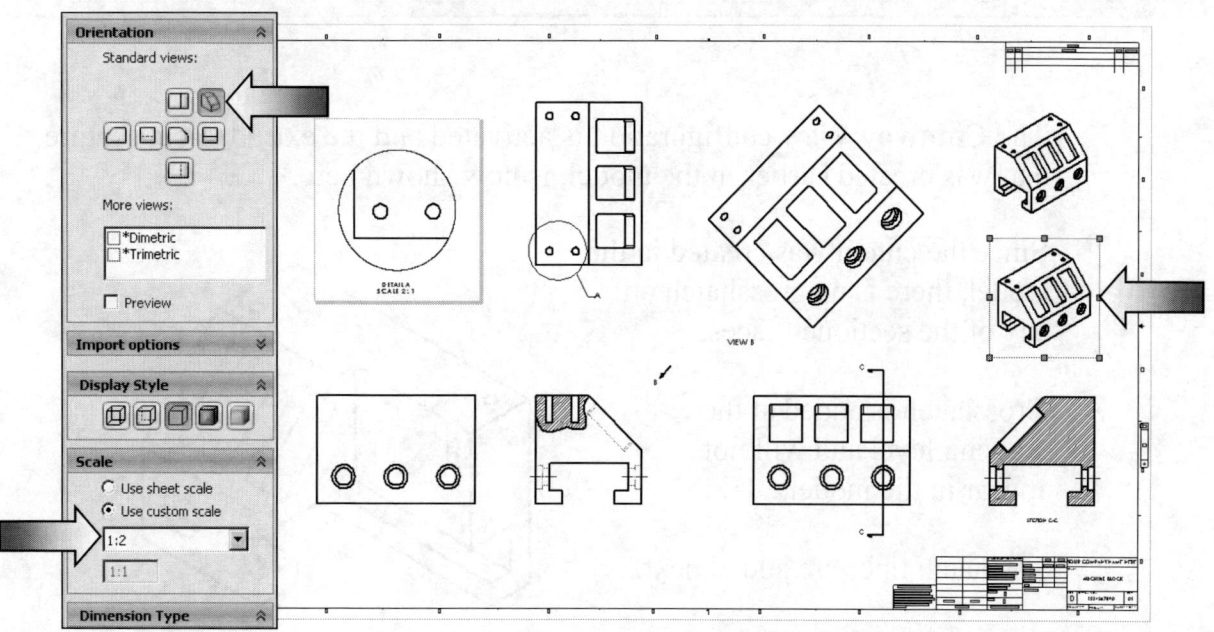

19. Changing Configurations: (From Default to Cutaway View).

- Click the Isometric view's border.

- On the Properties tree, select the **Cutaway View** configuration from the list.

- Click **OK** | OK | .

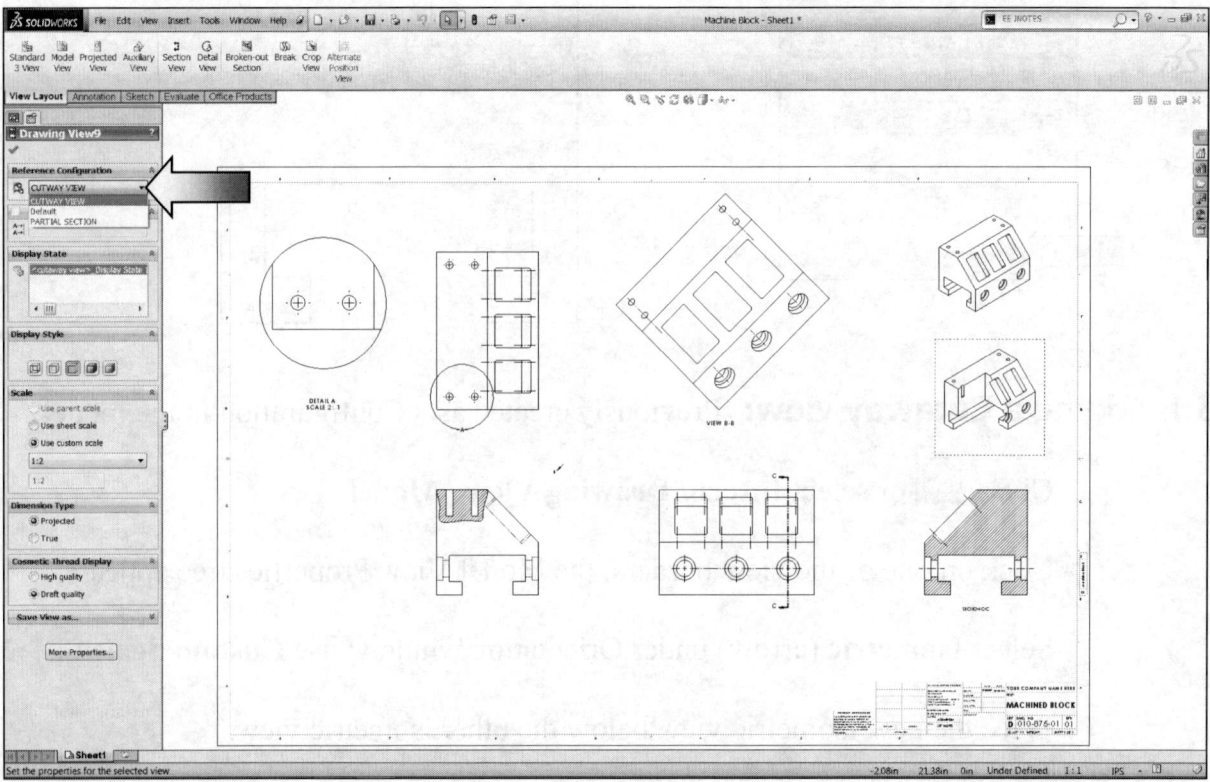

- The **Cutaway View** configuration is activated and the extruded-cut feature that was created earlier in the model, is now shown here.

- Since the cutout was created in the model, there is no crosshatch on any of the sectioned faces.

- Crosshatch is added at the drawing level and will not appear in the model.

- The hatch lines are added next...

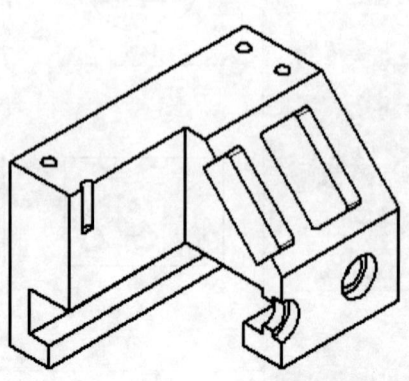

20. Adding crosshatch to the sectioned surfaces:

- Crosshatch is added automatically when section views are made in the drawing, since the cut was created in the model, we will have to add the hatch manually.

- Hold down the CONTROL key and select the 3 faces as indicated.

- Click 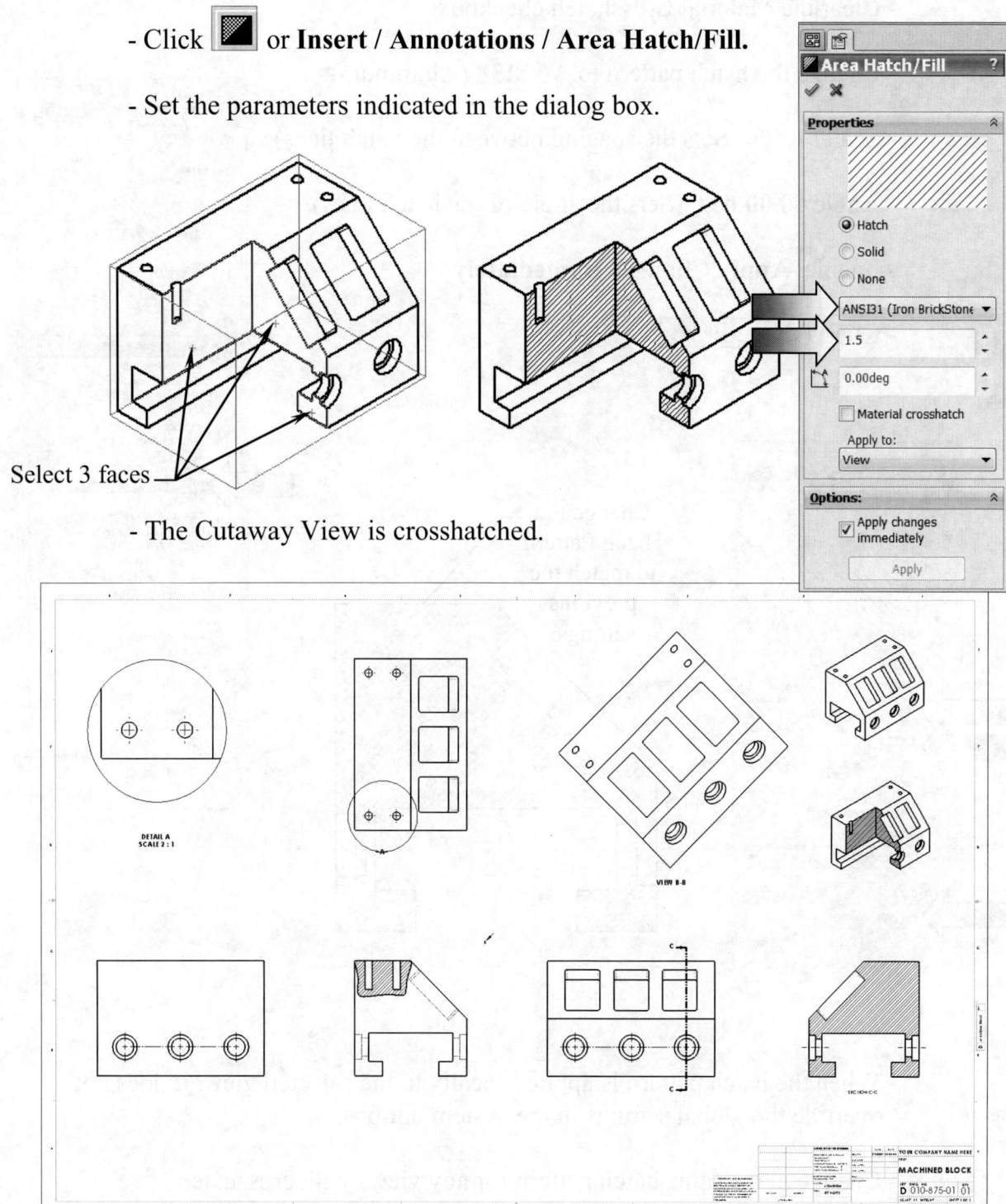 or **Insert / Annotations / Area Hatch/Fill.**

- Set the parameters indicated in the dialog box.

Select 3 faces

- The Cutaway View is crosshatched.

21. Modifying the crosshatch properties:

- Zoom in 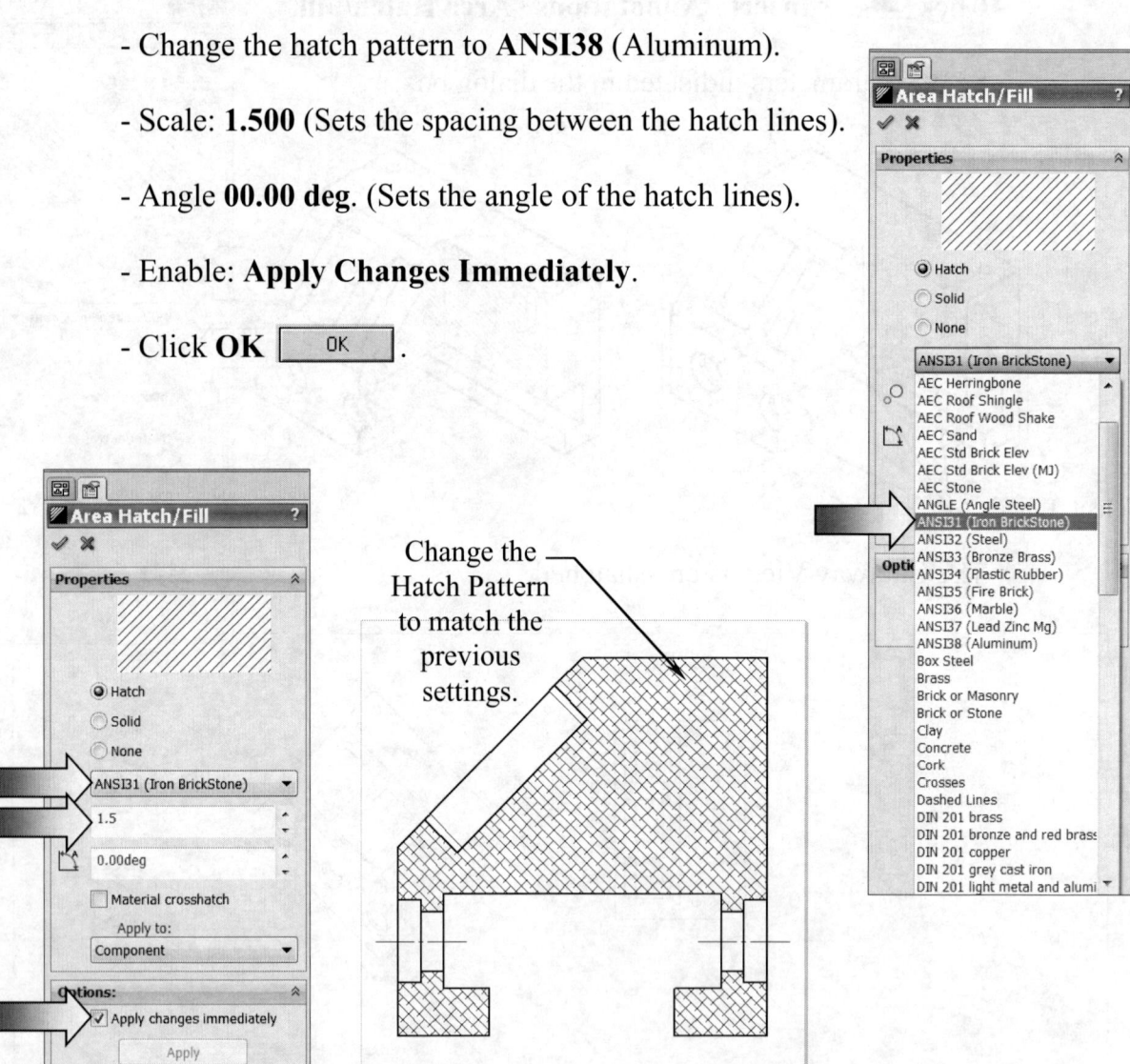 on the **Section C-C**.

- Click inside the hatch area, the **Area Hatch / Fill** properties tree appears.

- Clear the Material Crosshatch checkbox.

- Change the hatch pattern to **ANSI38** (Aluminum).

- Scale: **1.500** (Sets the spacing between the hatch lines).

- Angle **00.00 deg**. (Sets the angle of the hatch lines).

- Enable: **Apply Changes Immediately**.

- Click **OK** OK .

Change the Hatch Pattern to match the previous settings.

SECTION C-C

- When the hatch pattern is applied locally to the selected view, it does not override the global settings in the system options.

- Change to the same hatch pattern for any views with crosshatch.

22. Saving your work:

- Select **File / Save As /**

- Enter **Machine Block-Drawing Views** for file name and click **Save**.

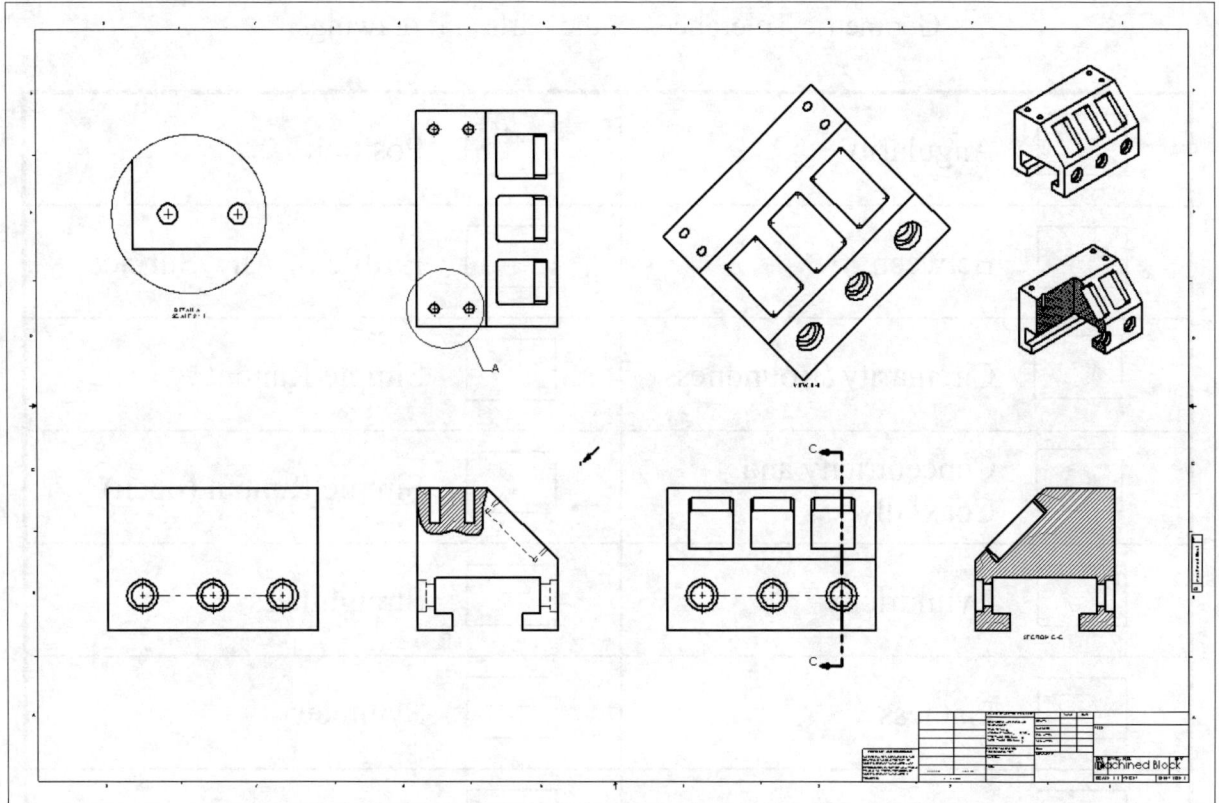

- The drawing views can also be changed from Wireframe to Shaded ⬚⬚ .

- The color of the drawing views is driven by the part's color. What you see here in the drawing is how it is going to look when printed (in color).

- Modifying the part's color will update the color of the drawing views automatically.

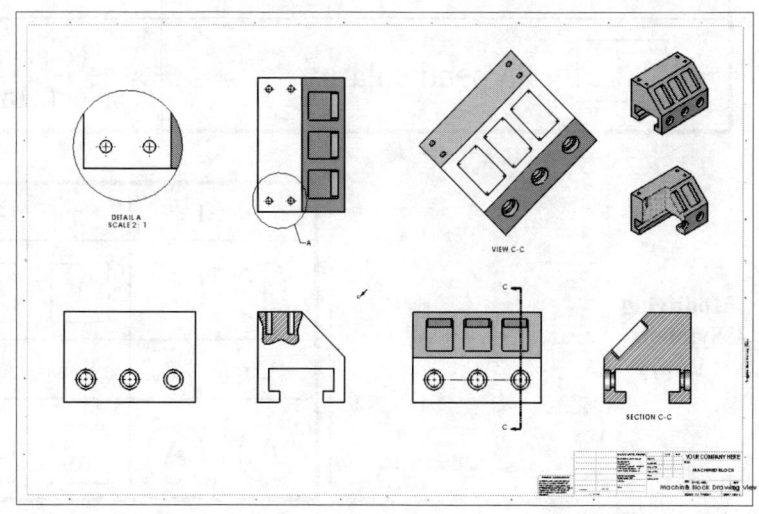

Geometric Tolerance & Flag Notes

Geometric Tolerance Symbols **GCS** are used in a Feature Control Frame to add Geometric Tolerances to the parts and drawings.

Symbol	Name	Symbol	Name
∠	Angularity	⊕	Position
↔	Between	⌓	Profile of Any Surface
○	Circularity (Roundness)	↗	Simple Runout
◎	Concentricity and Coaxially	↗	Simple Runout (open)
⌭	Cylindricity	—	Straightness
▱	Flatness	≡	Symmetry
⌒	Profile of Any Line	↗↗	Total Runout
//	Parallelism	↗↗	Total Runout (open)
⊥	Perpendicularity	To access the symbol libraries, select: **Insert / Annotations / Note**	

Modifying Symbols Library

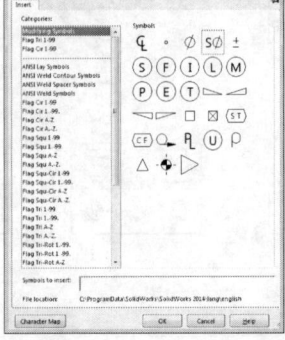

Circle 1-99	Square 1-99	Square/Circle 1-99	Triangle 1-99
(1.) (1)	1. 1	(1.) (1)	△1. △1
Circle A-Z	Square A-Z	Square/Circle A-Z	Triangle A-Z
(A.) (A)	A. A	(A.) (A)	△A. △A

Modifying & Hole Symbols

Modifying Symbols `MC`

Symbol	Name	Symbol	Name
℄	Centerline	ⓉT	Tangent Plane
▫	Degree	◺	Slope (Up)
⌀	Diameter	◿	Slope (Down)
S⌀	Spherical Diameter	◹	Slope (Inverted Up)
±	Plus/Minus	◸	Slope (Inverted Down)
Ⓢ	Regardless of Feature Size	□	Square
Ⓕ	Free State	⊠	Square (BS)
Ⓛ	Least Material Condition	⟨ST⟩	Statistical
Ⓜ	Maximum Material Condition	⌒	Flattened Length
Ⓟ	Projected Tolerance Zone	ꓝL	Parting Line
Ⓔ	Encompassing	SolidWorks supports **ASME-ANSI Y14.5** Geometric & True Position Tolerancing

⌴ Counterbore (Spot face)   ⌵ Countersunk   ▽ Depth/Deep   ⌀ Diameter

ASME (American Society for Mechanical Engineering)
ANSI Y14.5M (American National Standards Institute)

SYMBOLS DESCRIPTION

ANGULARITY:
The condition of a surface or line, which is at a specified angle (other than 90°) from the datum plane or axis.

BASIC DIMENSION: 1.00
A dimension specified on a drawing as BASIC is a theoretical value used to describe the exact size, shape, or location of a feature. It is used as a basis from which permissible variations are established by tolerance on other dimensions or in notes. A basic dimension can be identified by the abbreviation BSC or more readily by boxing in the dimension.

CIRCULARITY (ROUNDNESS):
A tolerance zone bounded by two concentric circles within which each circular element of the surface must lie.

CONCENTRICITY:
The condition in which the axis of all cross-sectional elements of a feature's surface of revolution are common.

CYLINDRICITY:
The condition of a surface of revolution in which all points of the surface are equidistant from a common axis or for a perfect cylinder.

DATUM:
A point, line, plane, cylinder, etc., assumed to be exact for purposes of computation from which the location or geometric relationship of other features of a part may be established. A datum identification symbol contains a letter (except I, C, and Q) placed inside a rectangular box.

DATUM TARGET:
The datum target symbol is a circle divided into four quadrants. The letter placed in the upper left quadrant identifies its associated datum feature. The number placed in the lower right quadrant identifies the target; the dashed leader line indicates the target on far side.

FLATNESS:
The condition of a surface having all elements in one plane. A flatness tolerance specifies a tolerance zone confined by two parallel planes within which the surface must lie.

MAXIMUM MATERIAL CONDITION: Ⓜ

The condition of a part feature when it contains the maximum amount of material.

LEAST MATERIAL CONDITION: Ⓛ

The condition of a part feature when it contains the least amount of material. The term is opposite from maximum material condition.

PARALLELISM: //

The condition of a surface or axis which is equidistant at all points from a datum plane or axis.

PERPENDICULARITY: ⊥

The condition of a surface, line, or axis, which is at a right angle (90°) from a datum plane or datum axis.

PROFILE OF ANY LINE: ⌒

The condition limiting the amount of profile variation along a line element of a feature.

PROFILE OF ANY SURFACE: ⌓

Similar to profile of any line, but this condition relates to the entire surface.

PROJECTED TOLERANCE ZONE: Ⓟ

A zone applied to a hole in which a pin, stud, screw, etc. is to be inserted. It controls the perpendicularity of any hole, which controls the fastener's position; this will allow the adjoining parts to be assembled.

REGARDLESS OF FEATURE SIZE: Ⓢ

A condition in which the tolerance of form or condition must be met, regardless of where the feature is within its size tolerance.

RUNOUT: ↗

The maximum permissible surface variation during one complete revolution of the part about the datum axis. This is usually detected with a dial indicator.

STRAIGHTNESS: —

The condition in which a feature of a part must be a straight line.

SYMMETRY: ═

A condition wherein a part or feature has the same contour and sides of a central plane.

TRUE POSITION: ⊕

This term denotes the theoretically exact position of a feature.

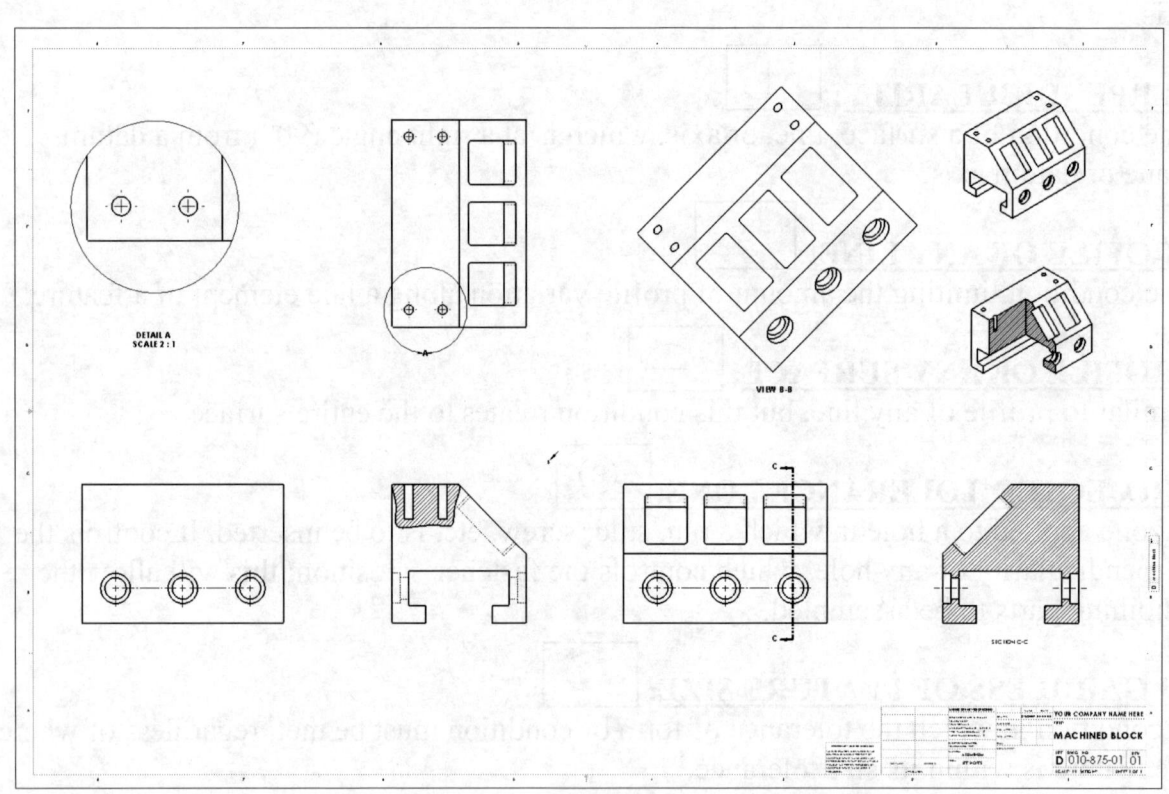

DETAIL A
SCALE 2 : 1

VIEW B-B

SECTION C-C

YOUR COMPANY NAME HERE
MACHINED BLOCK
D 010-875-01 01

CHAPTER 17

Detailing

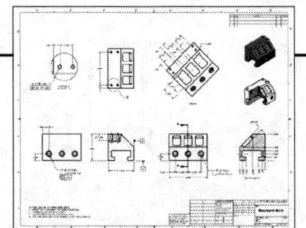

Detailing a drawing
Machined Block Details

- After the drawing views are all laid out, they will be detailed with dimensions, tolerances, datums, surface finishes, notes, etc.

- To fully maintain the associations between the model dimensions and the drawing dimensions, the Model Items options should be used. If a dimension is changed in either mode (from the solid model or in the drawing) they will both be updated automatically.

- When a dimension appears in gray color it means that the dimension is being added in the drawing and it does not exist in the model. This dimension is called a Reference dimension.

- SolidWorks uses different colors for different types of dimensions such as:
    * Black dimensions = Sketch dimensions (driving).
    * Gray dimensions = Reference dimensions (driven).
    * Blue dimensions = Feature dimensions (driving)
    * Magenta dimensions = Dimensions linked to Design Tables (driving).

- For certain types of holes, the Hole-Callout option should be used to accurately call out the hole type, depth, diameter, etc...

- The Geometric Tolerance option helps control the accuracy and the precision of the features. Both Tolerance and Precision options can be easily created and controlled from the FeatureManager tree.

- This chapter discusses most of the tools used in detailing an engineering drawing, including importing dimensions from the model, and adding the GD&T to the drawing (Geometric Dimensions and Tolerancing).

Machined Block
Detailing

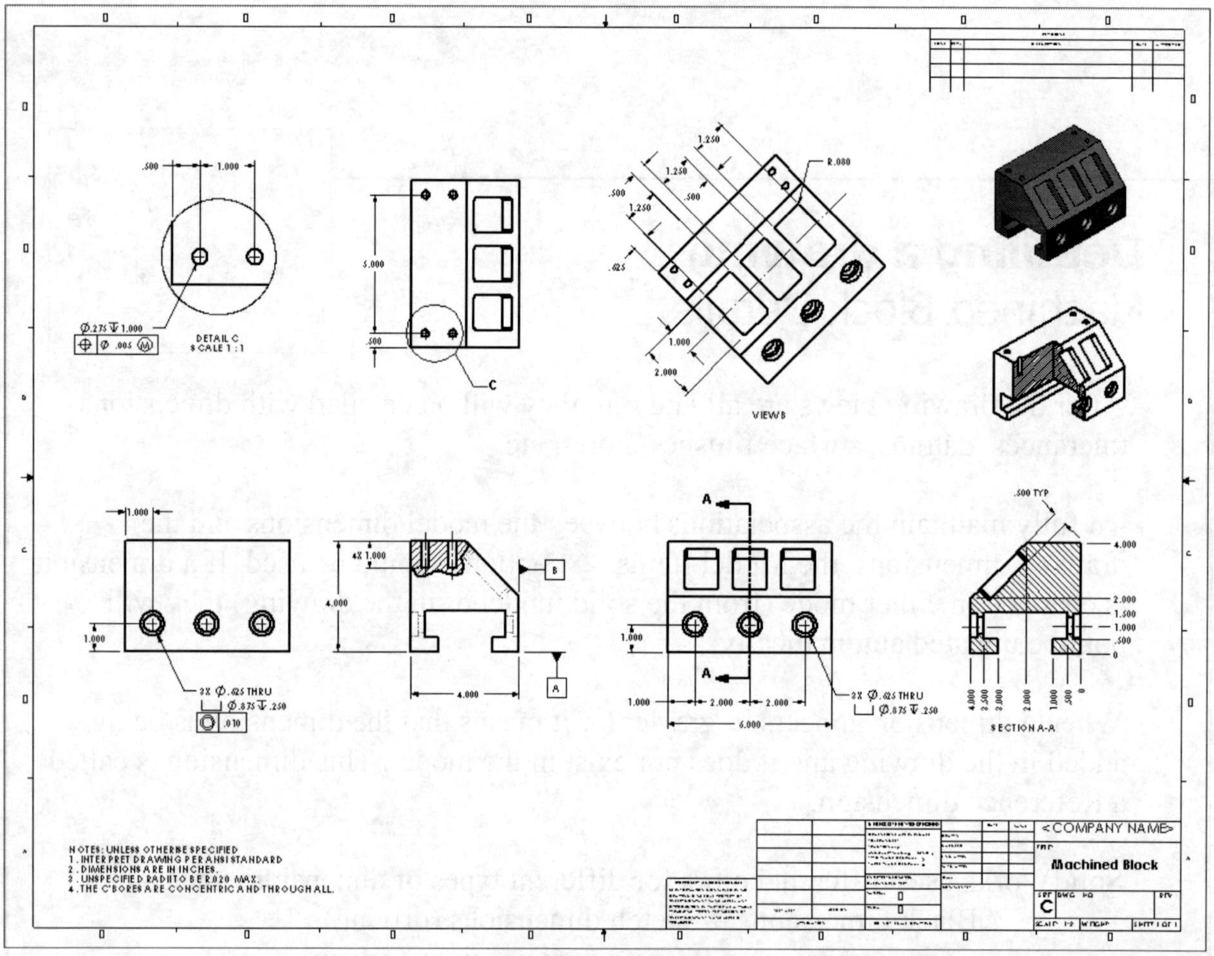

Dimensioning Standards: **ANSI**

Units: **INCHES** – 3 Decimals

Third Angle Projection

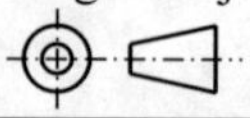

Tools Needed:

 Model Dimensions

 Geometric Tolerance

 Datum Feature Symbol

 Surface Finish

 Hole Callout

 Note

1. Opening the previous file:

- Click **File / Open** and open the previous drawing document **Machined Block**.

2. Inserting dimensions from the model:

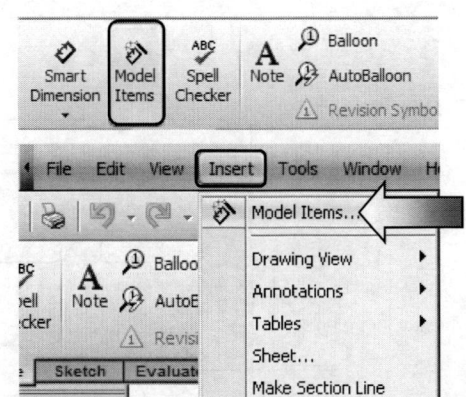

- Dimensions previously created in the model can be inserted into the drawing.

- Click the **Right** drawing view's border.

- Click 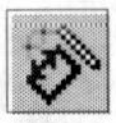 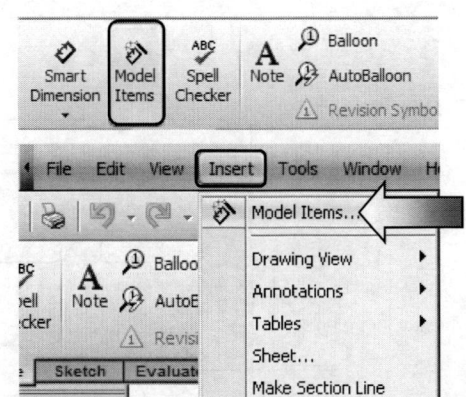 or select **Insert / Model Items**.

- For Source/Destination: **Entire Model**.

- Under Dimensions: Enable **Eliminate Duplicates**.

- Under Options: Select **Use Dimension Placement in Sketch**.

- Click **OK** ✓.

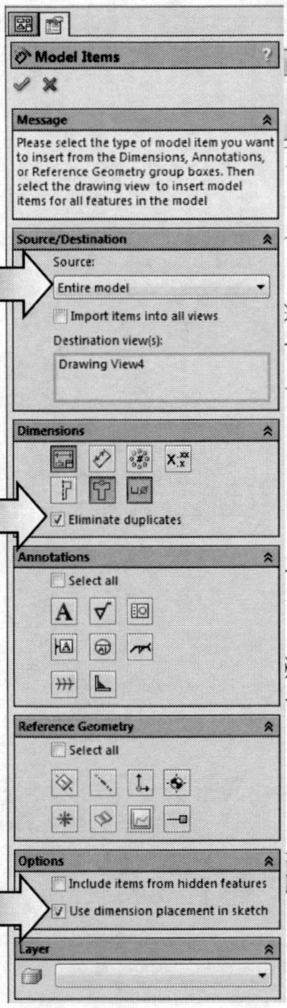

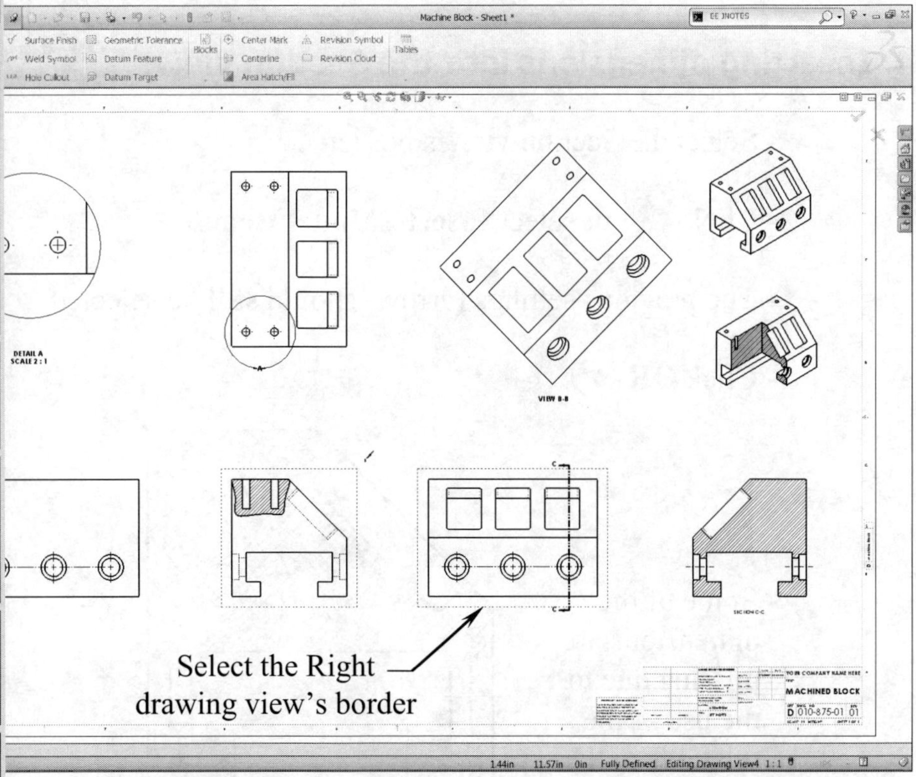

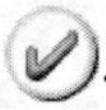

Select the Right
drawing view's border

- The dimensions that were created earlier from the model into the selected drawing view.

3. Re-arranging the new dimensions: Zoom in 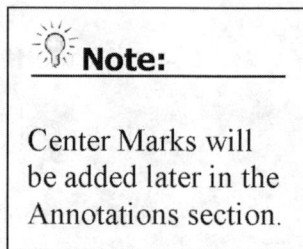 on the Right drawing view.

- Keep only the hole location dimensions and delete the others. The hole types and sizes will be added later. Also add any missing dimensions manually.

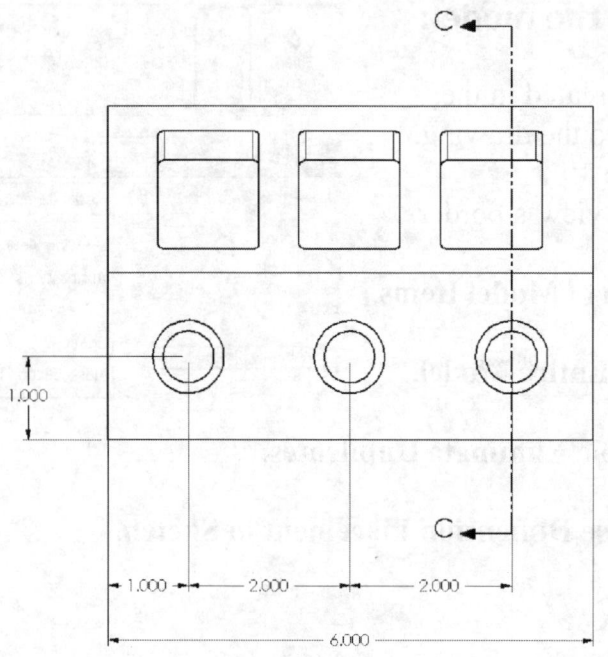

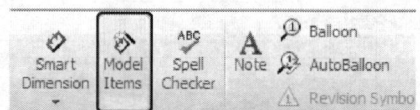

4. Inserting dimensions into the Section view:

- Select the Section view's border.

- Click 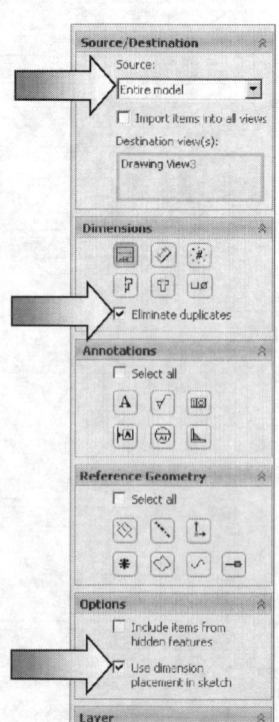 or select **Insert / Model Items**.

- The previous settings (arrow) should still be selected.

- Click **OK** ✓

- Some of the dimensions are missing due to the use of the relations in the model.

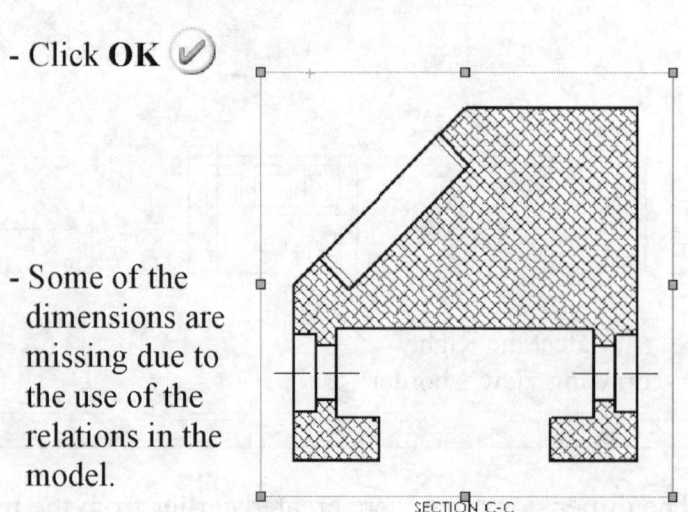

SECTION C-C

- The dimensions from the model are imported into the Section view.

- Use the Smart Dimension tool 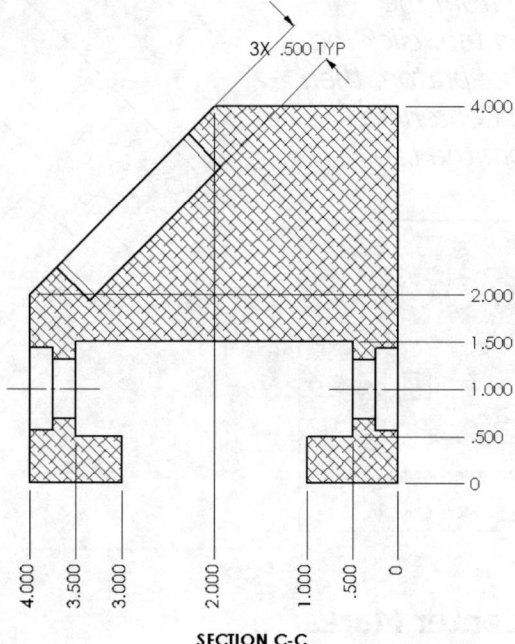 to add any missing dimensions.

- These dimensions are attached to the drawing view and will move with the view.

- If any of these dimensions are changed, both the model and the drawing views will also change accordingly.

SECTION C-C

5. Repeating step 4: Insert the model's dimensions into the Top view.

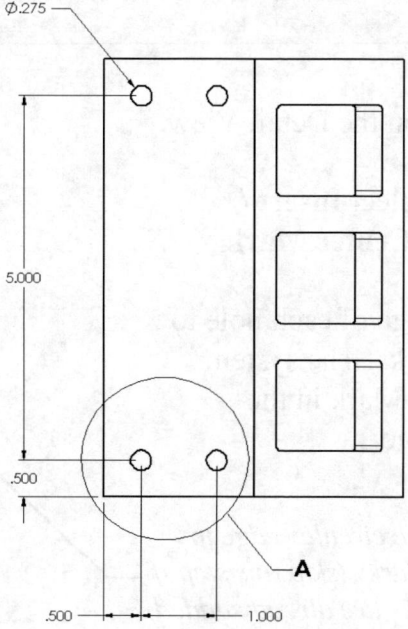

6. Adding dimensions to the Auxiliary view:

- Add any missing dimensions to the drawing view using the Smart Dimension command.

NOTE: To add the Centerline symbol, select the Note command from the Annotation tab, click the Add Symbol button, then select the Centerline option from the list.

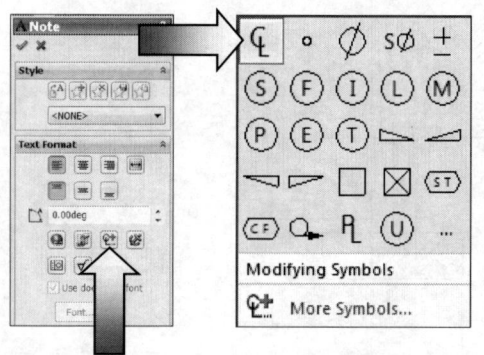

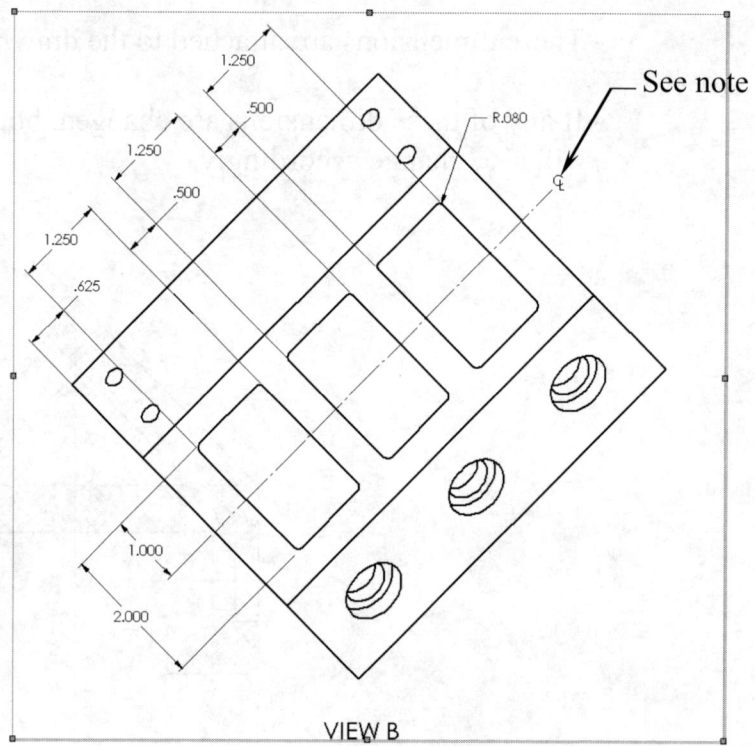

See note

VIEW B

7. Adding the Center Marks:

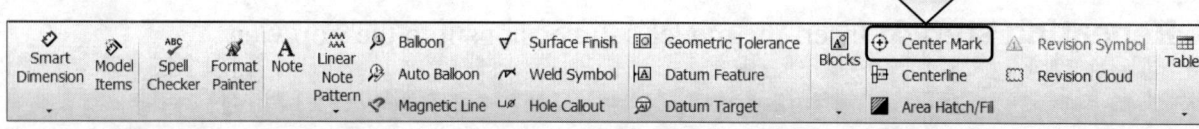

- Zoom in on the Detail View.

- Click or select **Insert / Annotations / Center Mark**.

- Click on the edge of each hole to add Center Marks. The system places a Center Mark in the center of the hole.

Click on the circular edge to add Center Marks (skip this step if the center marks are already added).

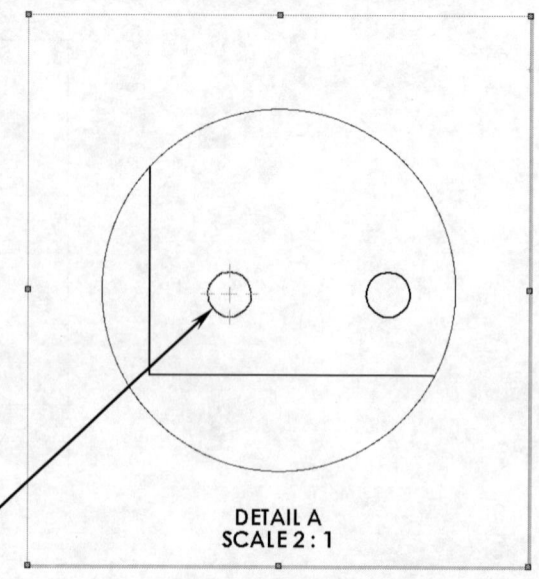

DETAIL A
SCALE 2 : 1

8. Adding center marks to the other holes:

- Click 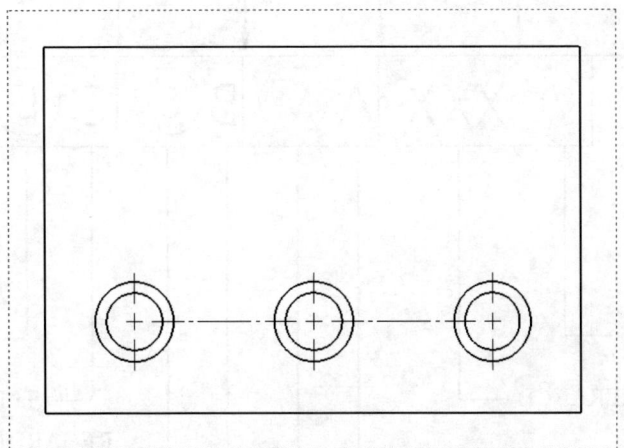 or select **Insert / Annotations / Center Mark**.

- Add a center mark to other holes by clicking on their circular edges.

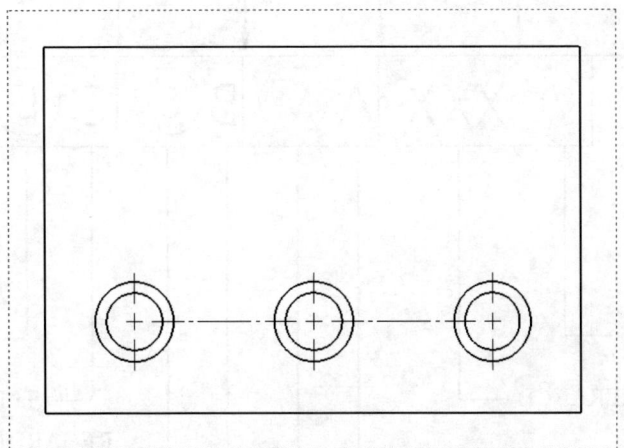

9. Adding the Datum Feature Symbols:

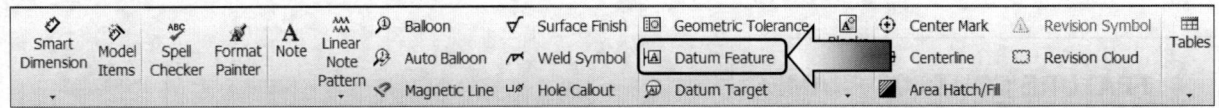

- Click ⊞A or select **Insert / Annotations / Datum Feature Symbol**.

- Select edge 1 and place **Datum A** as shown.

- Select edge 2 and place **Datum B** as shown.

Datum Feature

A symbolic language used on engineering drawings for explicitly describing nominal geometry and its allowable variation.

1982 Datum symbol

1994 Datum symbol

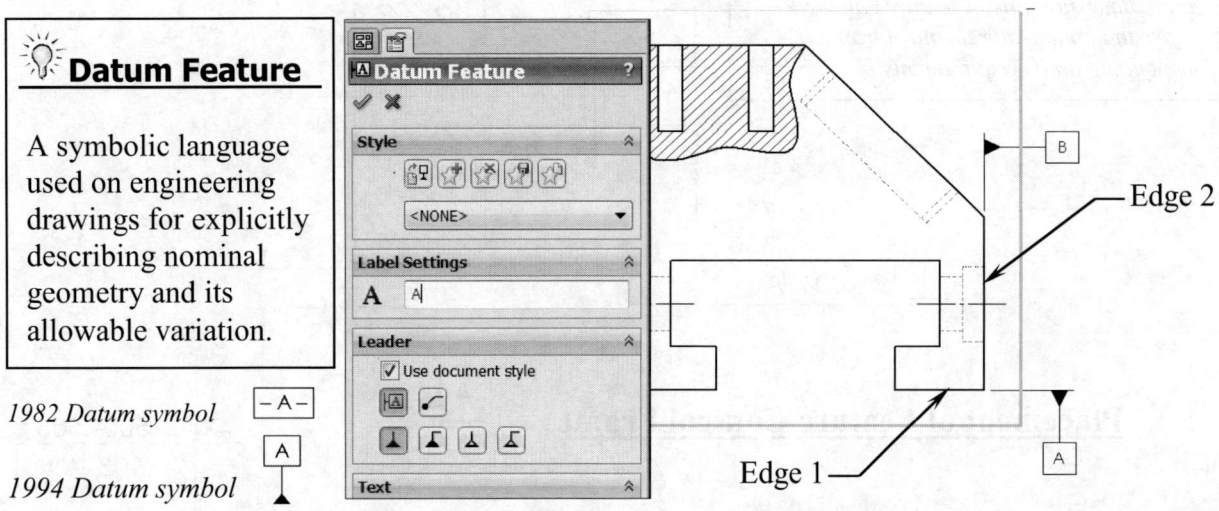

Datum Reference & Geometric Tolerance Examples

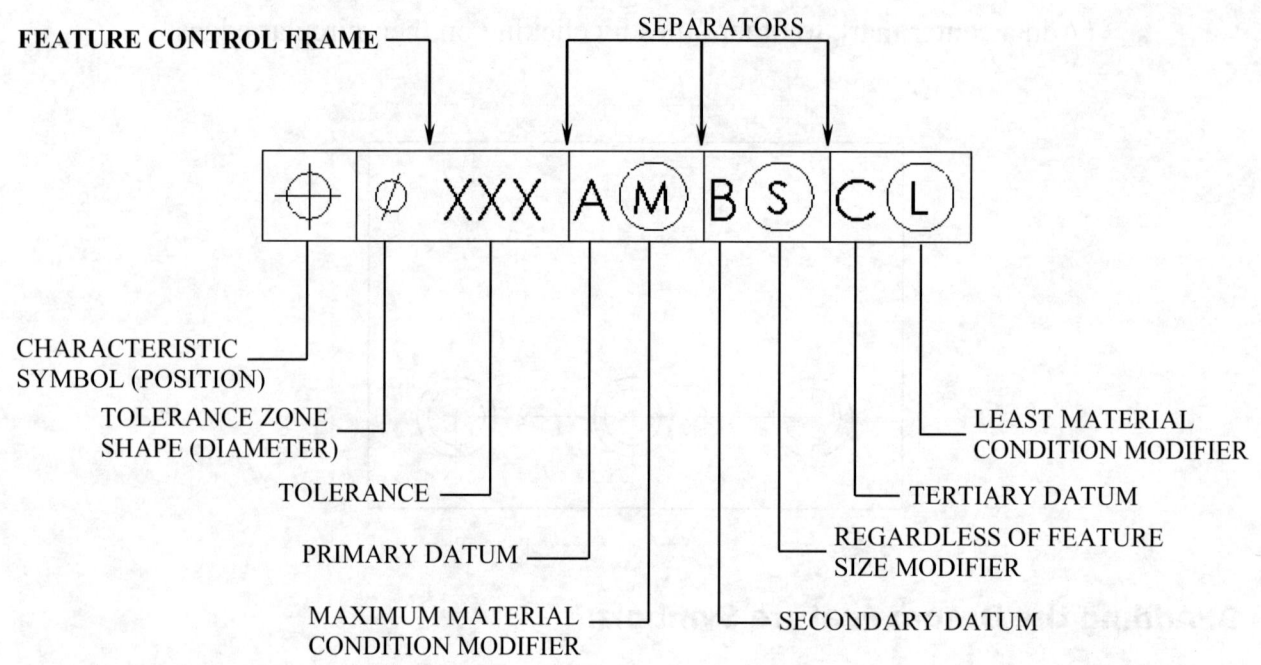

💡 FEATURE CONTROL FRAMES

A feature control frame symbolizes the tolerance requirements for a feature of a part. It can be added to a drawing note for a feature tolerance, or can be specified by running a leader line from the feature control frame directly to the feature. The box may be attached to an extension line from the feature or it can be placed on a dimension line. A feature can have more than one feature control frame, depending on its requirements.

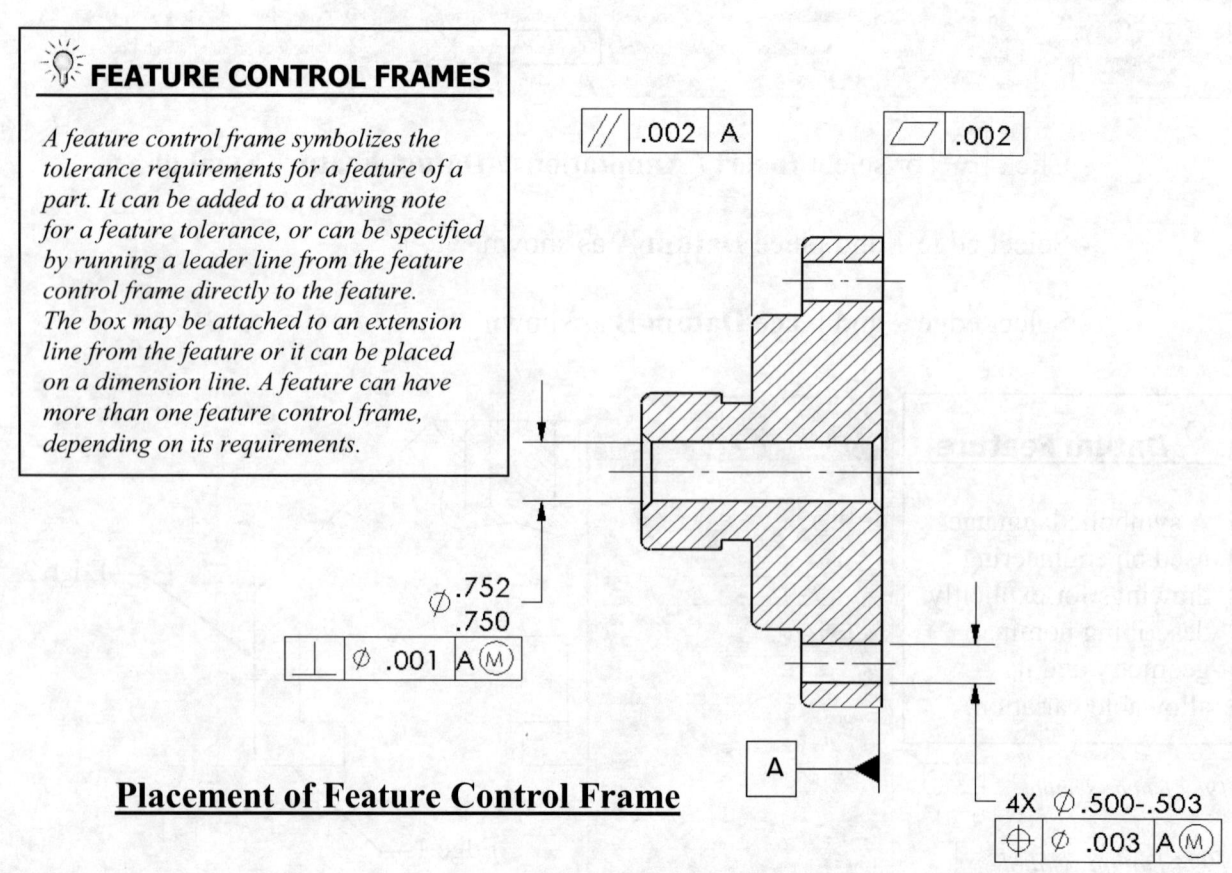

Placement of Feature Control Frame

10. Adding hole specifications using the Hole-Callout:

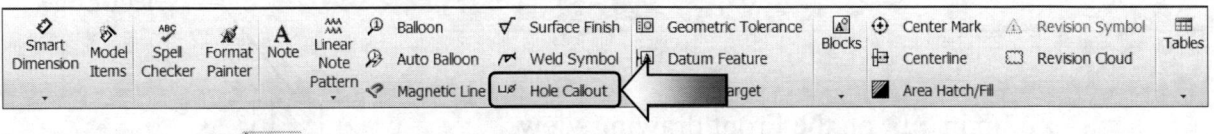

- Click or select **Insert / Annotations / Hole Callout**.

- Select the edge of the C'bore and place the callout below the hole.

- The system creates a callout that includes the diameter and the depth of the hole and the C'bore.

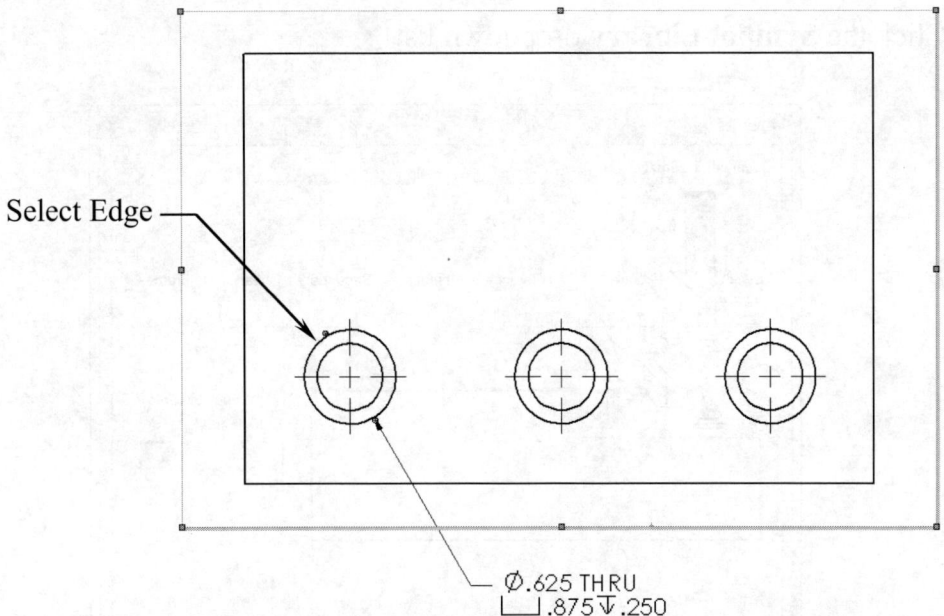

Select Edge

⌀.625 THRU
⊔.875 ▽.250

11. Adding Geometric Tolerances:

- Geometric dimensioning and tolerancing (GD&T) is used to define the nominal (theoretically perfect) geometry of parts and assemblies to define the allowable variation in form and possibly size of individual features and to define the allowable variation between features. Dimensioning and tolerancing and geometric dimensioning and tolerancing specifications are used as follows:

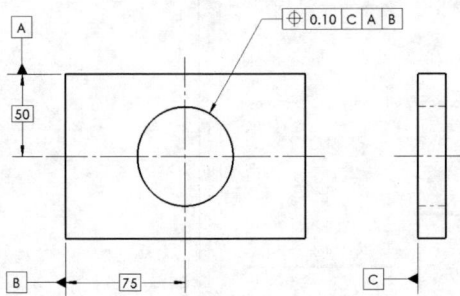

* Dimensioning specifications define the nominal, as-modeled or as-intended geometry. One example is a basic dimension.

* Tolerancing specifications define the allowable variation for the form and possibly the size of individual features and the allowable variation in orientation and location between features. Two examples are linear dimensions and feature control frames using a datum reference.

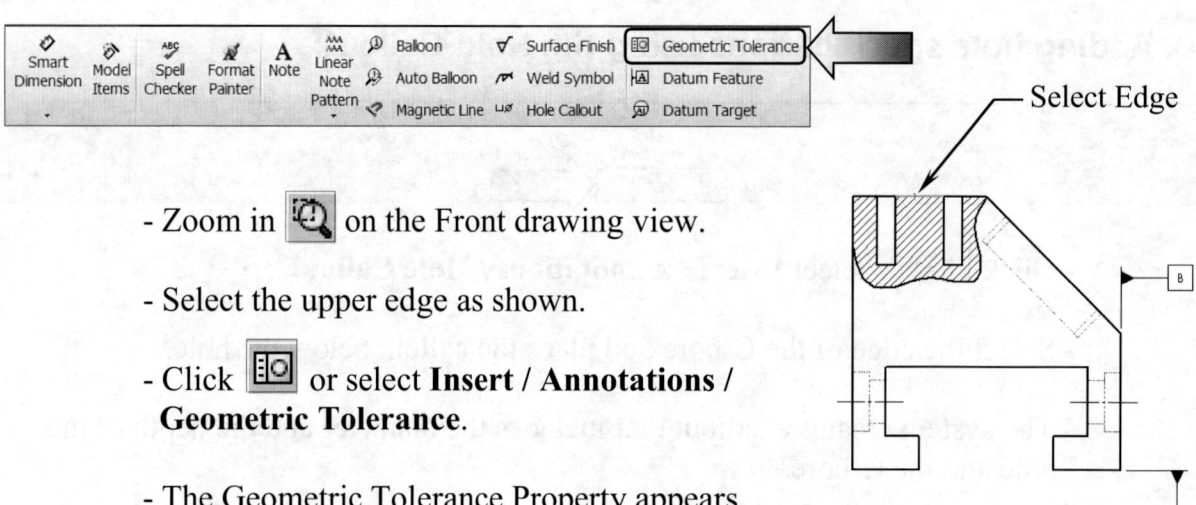

Select Edge

- Zoom in 🔍 on the Front drawing view.

- Select the upper edge as shown.

- Click 📷 or select **Insert / Annotations / Geometric Tolerance**.

- The Geometric Tolerance Property appears.

- Click the **Symbol Library** dropdown list ▾ .

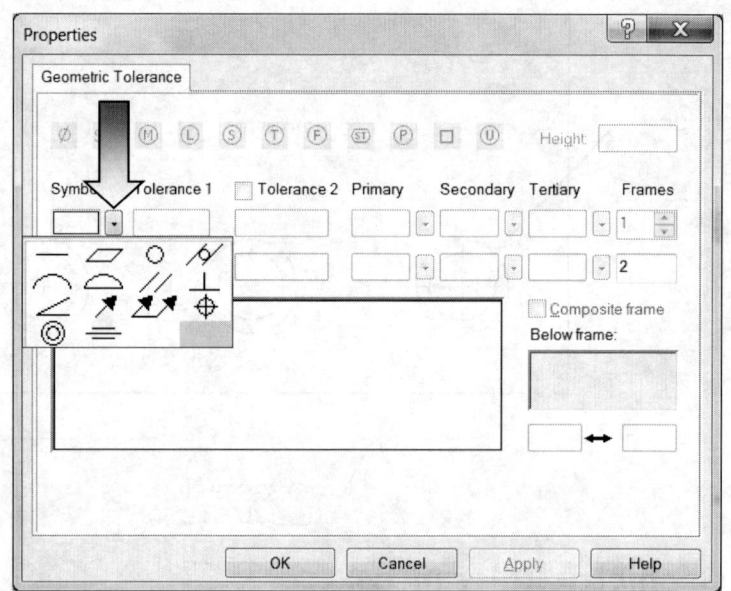

- Select **Parallelism** ⫽ from the **Symbol** library list.

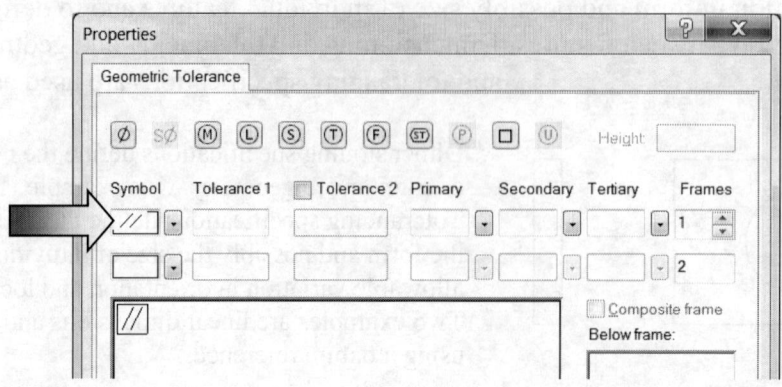

- Enter **.010** under Tolerance 1.

- Enter **A** under Primary reference datum (arrow).

- Click **OK** [OK] .

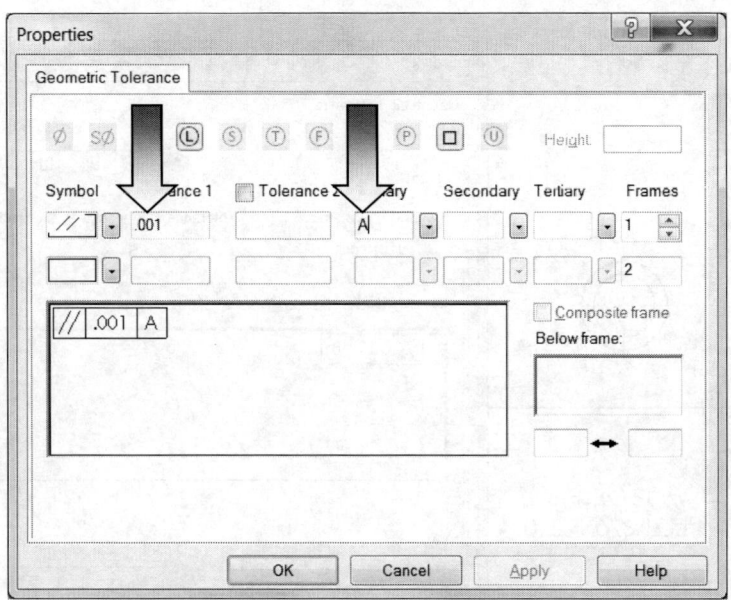

12. Align the Geometric Tolerance:

- Drag the Control Frame towards the left side until it snaps to the horizontal alignment with the upper edge, then release the mouse button.

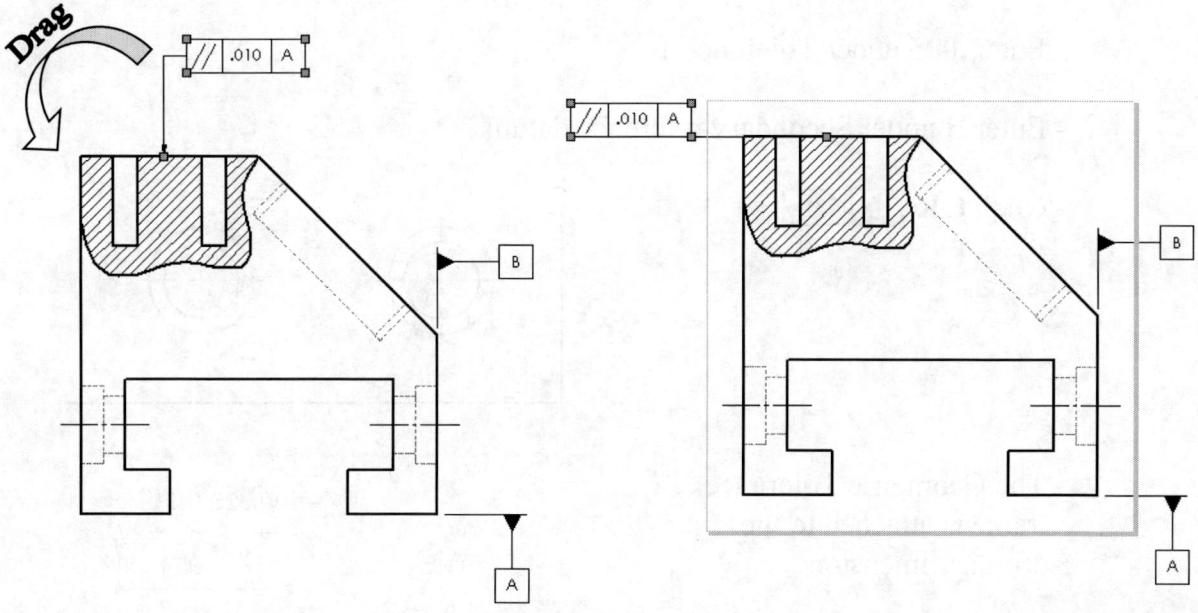

13. Attaching the Geometric Tolerance to the Driving dimension:

- Select the C'bore dimension. By pre-selecting a dimension, the geometric-tolerance will automatically be attached to this dimension.

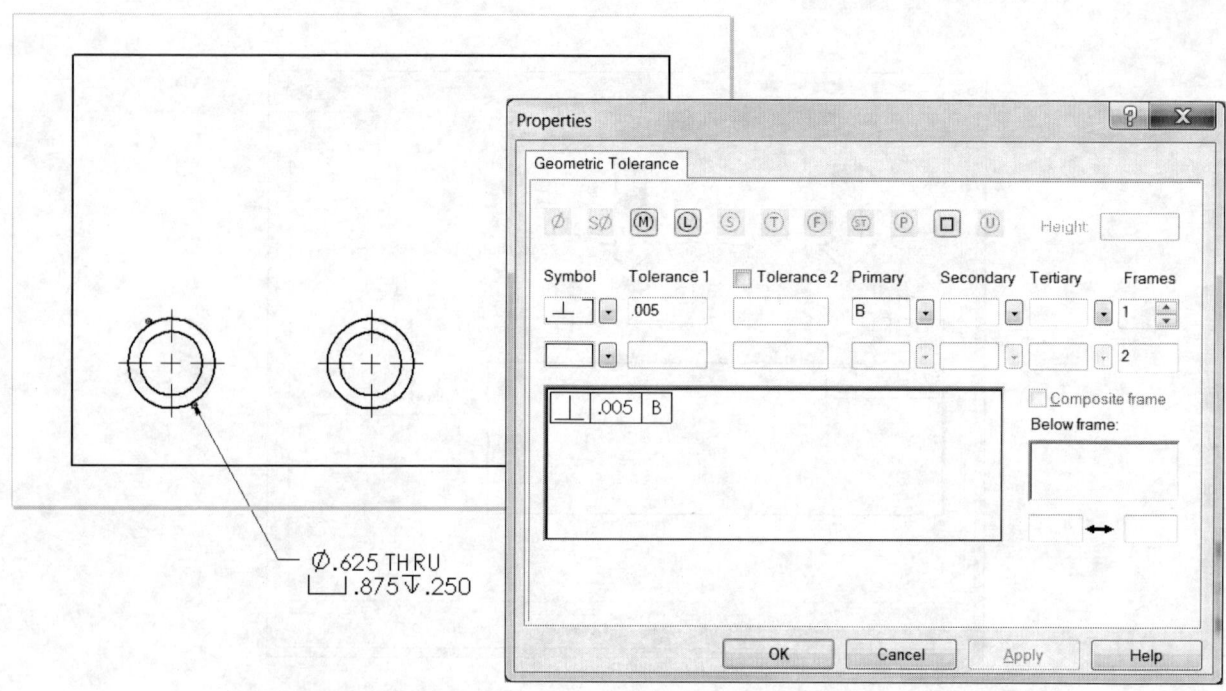

- Click 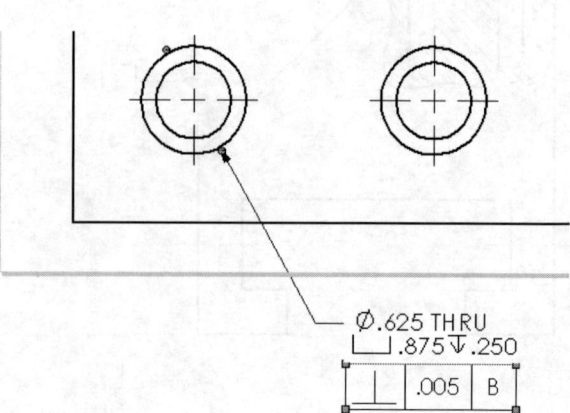 or select **Insert / Annotation / Geometric Tolerance**.

- Click the **Symbol Library** dropdown list ▾.

- Select **Perpendicularity** ⟂ from the Symbol library list.

- Enter **.005** under Tolerance 1.

- Enter **B** under Secondary reference datum.

- Click **OK** ⟦ OK ⟧ .

- The Geometric Tolerance frame is attached to the driving dimension.

14. Adding Tolerance/Precision to dimensions:

- Select the dimension **.500** (circled).

- The dimension properties tree pops up, select **Bilateral** under the Tolerance/
Precision section.

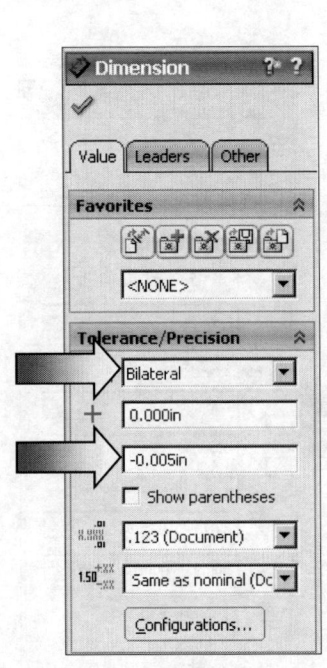

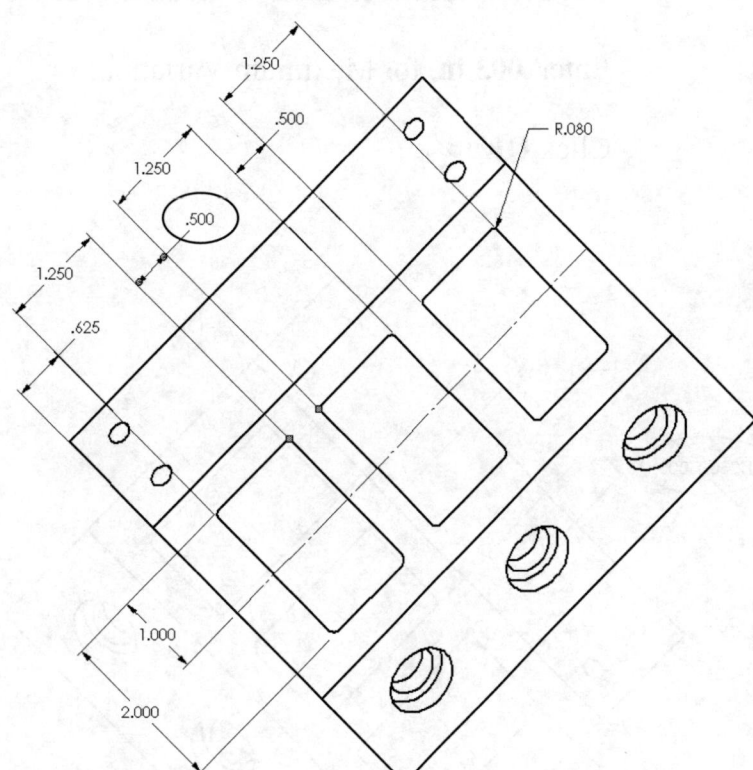

VIEW B

- Enter **.000 in**. for Max variation.

- Enter **.005 in**. for Min variation.

- Click **OK** ✓.

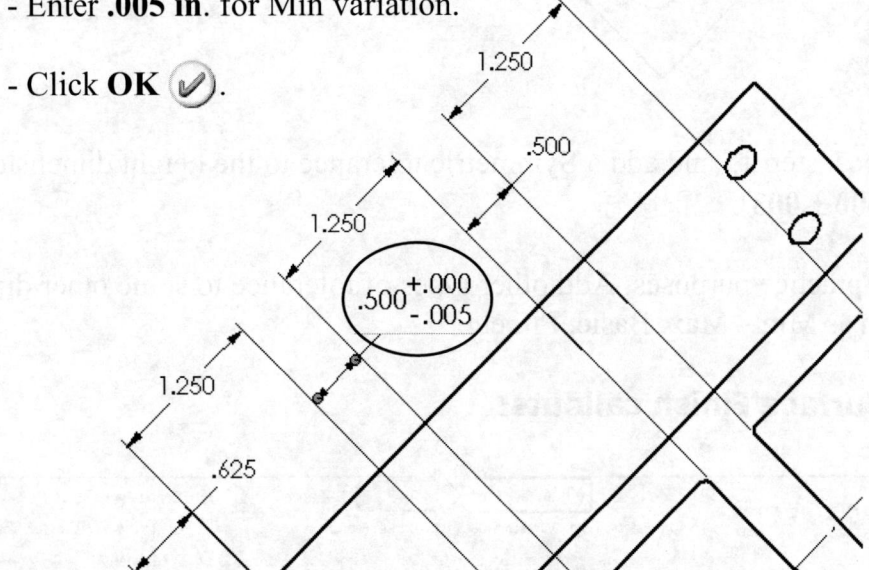

15. Adding Symmetric tolerance to a dimension:

- Select the width dimension **1.250** (circled) and the dimension properties tree appears 🔲 🔲 .

- Choose **Symmetric** under Tolerance/Precision list (arrow).

- Enter **.003 in**. for Maximum Variation.

- Click **OK** ✅ .

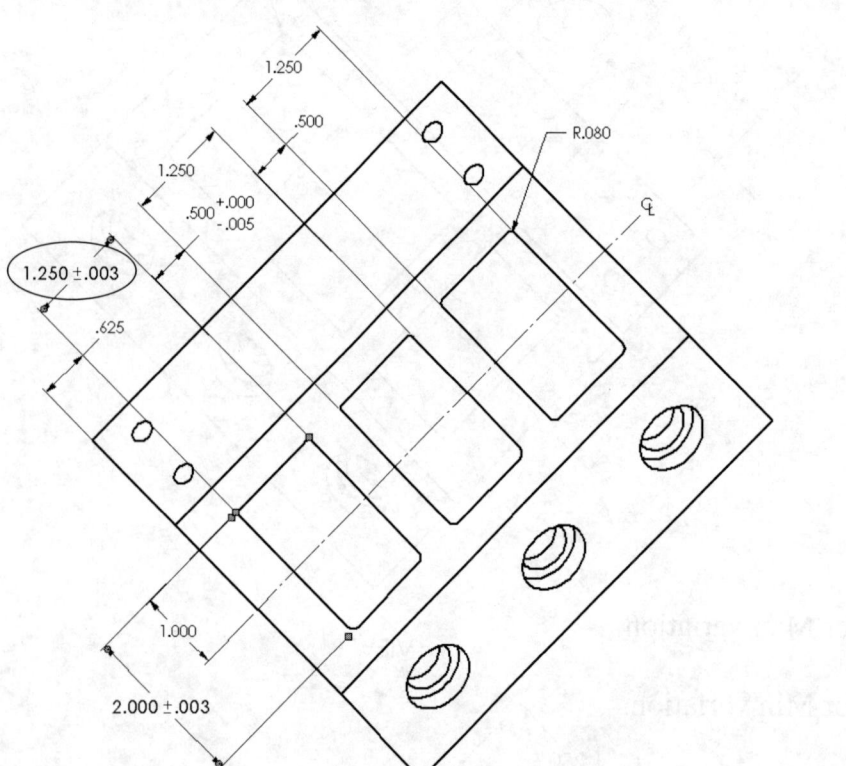

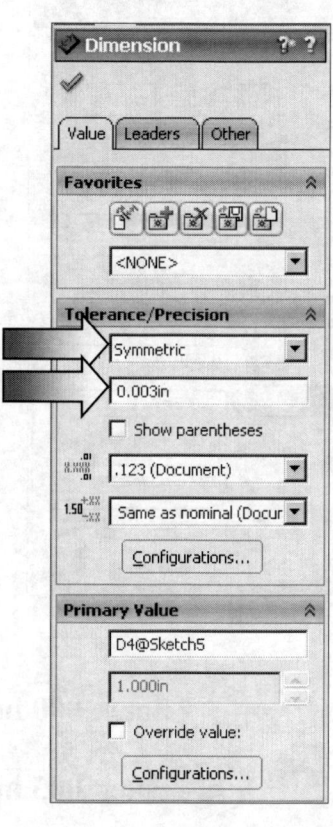

- Repeat step 15 and add a Symmetric tolerance to the height dimension: (**2.000 ±.003**).

- For practice purposes: Add other types of tolerance to some other dimensions such as Min – Max, Basic, Fit, etc..

16. Adding Surface Finish callouts:

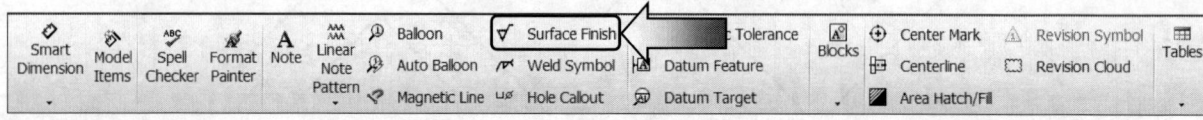

- Surface finish is an industrial process that alters the surface of a manufactured item to achieve a certain property. Finishing processes such as machining, grinding, or buffing, may be applied to improve appearance and other surface flaws, and control the surface friction.

- Zoom in on the Section C-C.

- Select the edge as indicated.

- Click or select **Insert / Annotations / Surface Finish**.

- Choose **Machining-Required** under Symbol.

- Under **Maximum Roughness**, enter: **125**

- Under Leader, select: **Bent leader.**

- Click **OK**.

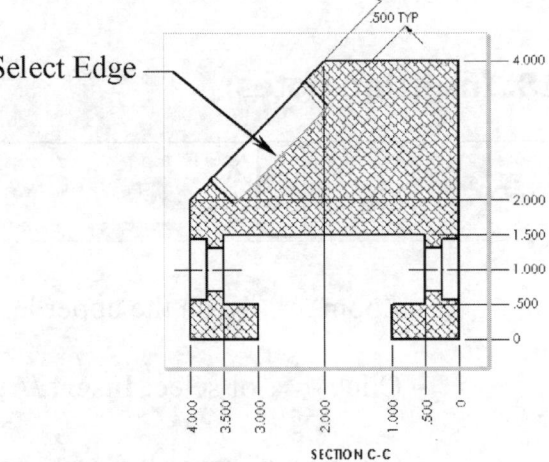

SECTION C-C

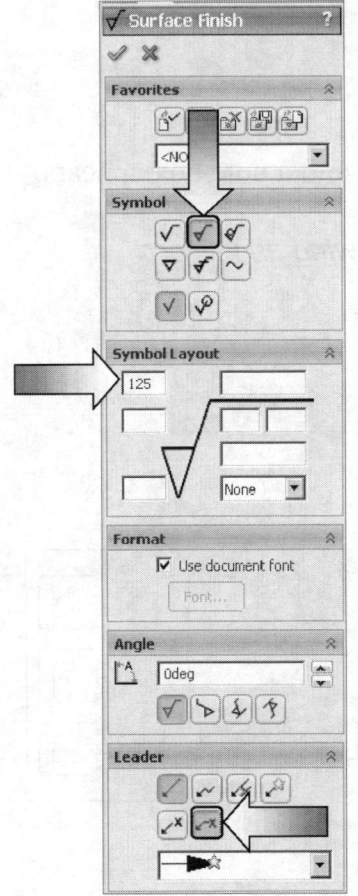

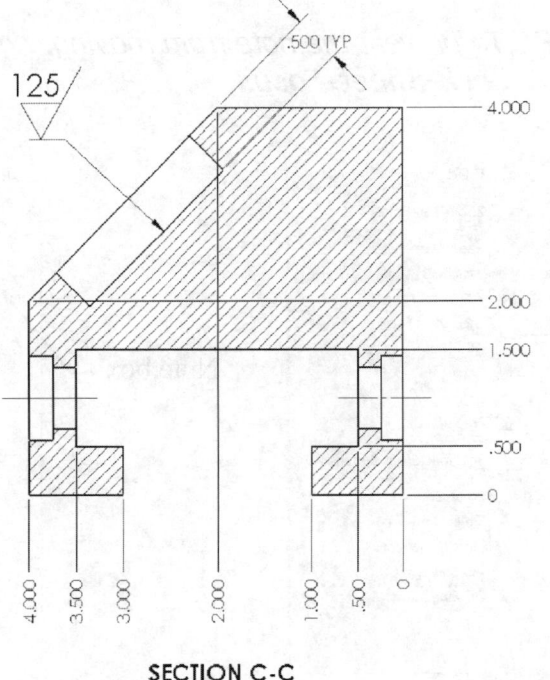

SECTION C-C

17. Adding non-parametric callouts:

- Click 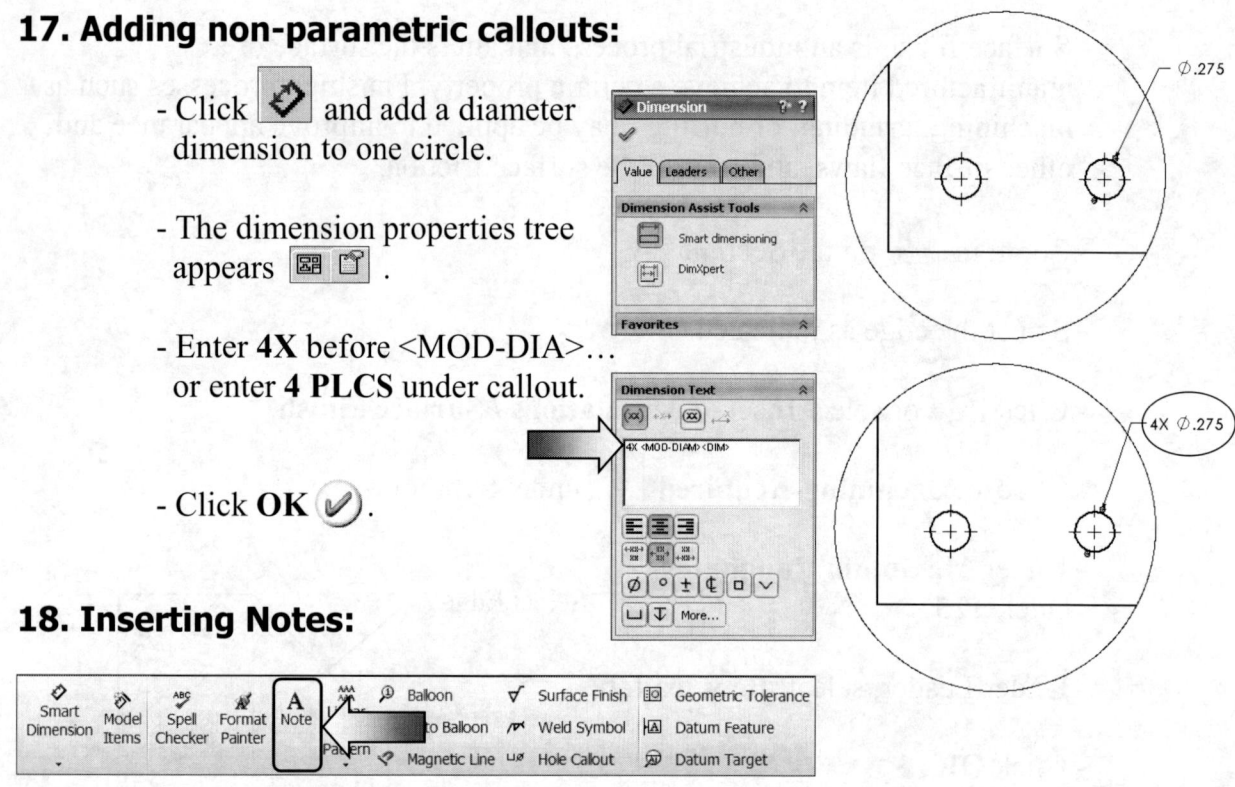 and add a diameter dimension to one circle.

- The dimension properties tree appears ⊞ ⌐ .

- Enter **4X** before <MOD-DIA>… or enter **4 PLCS** under callout.

- Click **OK** ✓.

18. Inserting Notes:

- Zoom in 🔍 on the upper left side of the drawing.

- Click **A** or select **Insert /Annotations / Note**.

- Click on an upper left area, approximately as shown, and a note box appears.

NOTE: _To prevent the note from moving, right click in the drawing and select: Lock-Sheet-Focus._

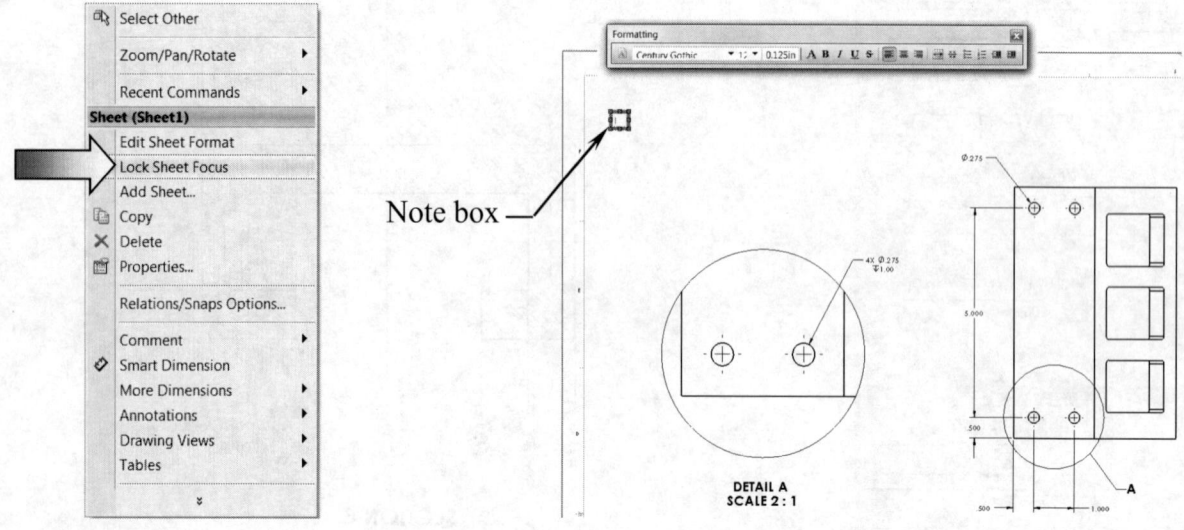

Note box

DETAIL A
SCALE 2 : 1

- Enter the notes below:

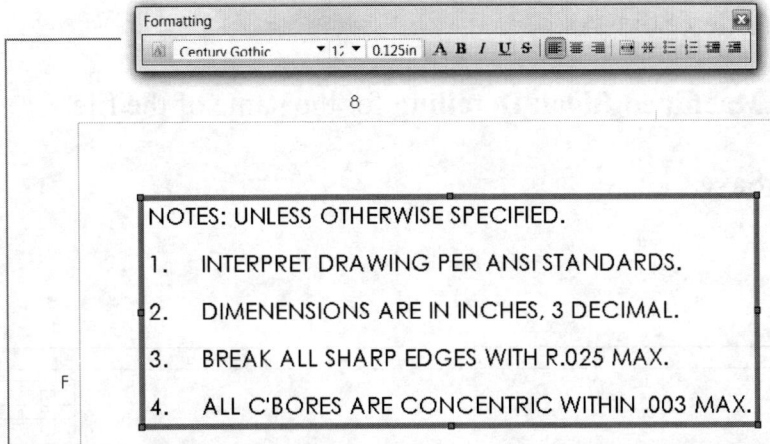

- Click **OK** ✓ when you are finished typing.

19. Changing document's font:

- Double click anywhere inside the note area to activate.

- Highlight the entire note and select the following:

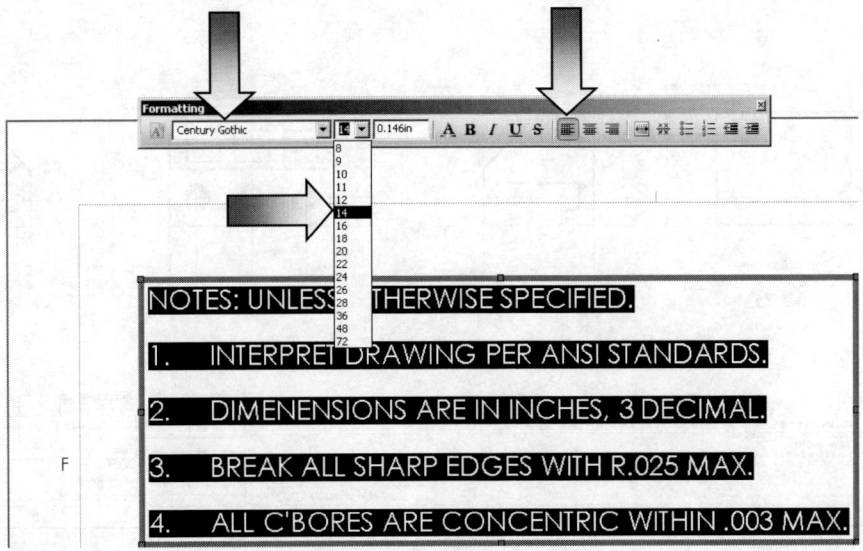

- Font: **Century Gothic**.

- Point size: **14**.

- Alignment: **Left**.

- Click **OK** ✓.

20. Saving your work:

- Select **File / Save As**.

- Enter **Machined Block Detailing** for the name of the file.

- Click **Save**.

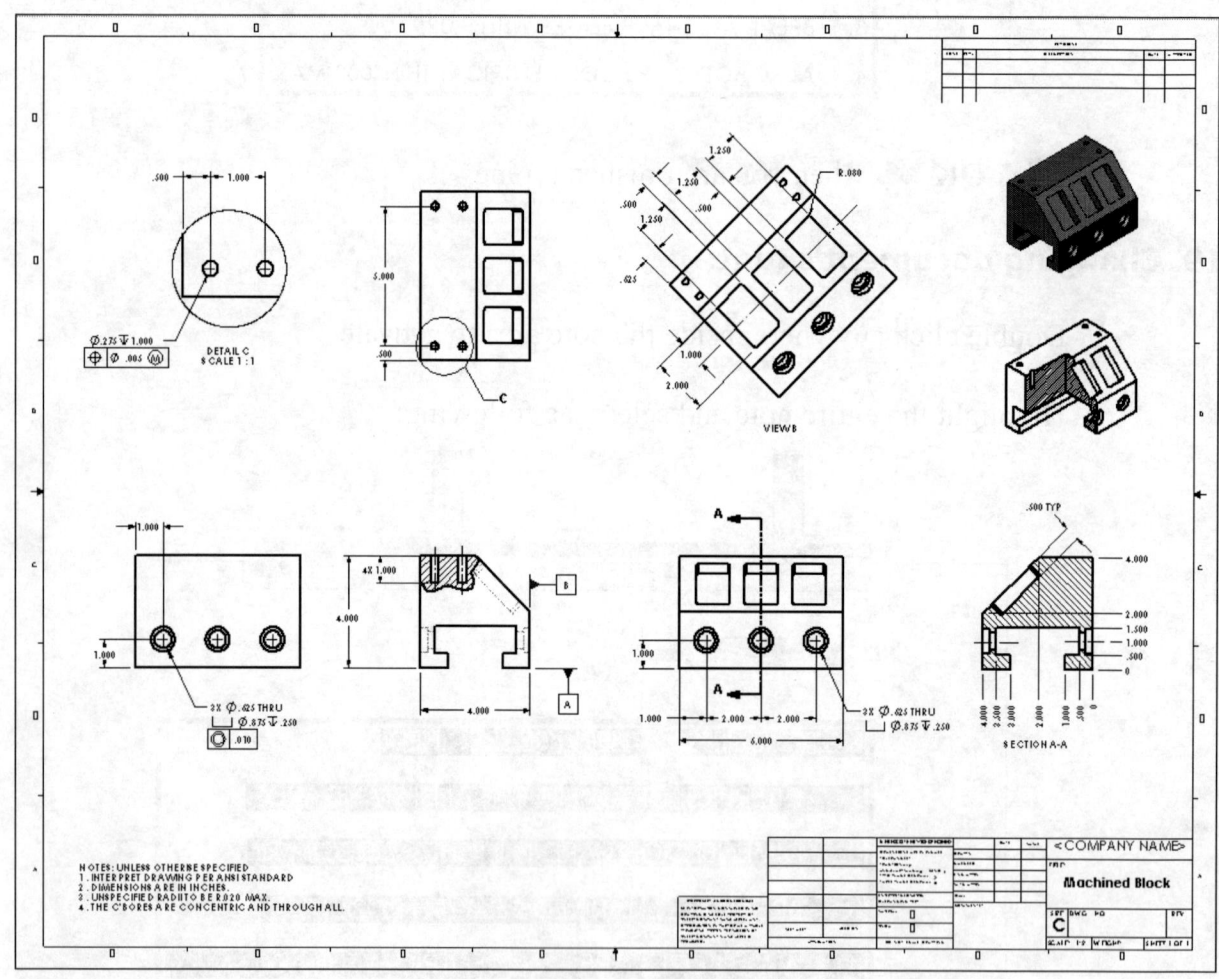

Questions for Review

Drawing & Detailing

1. Existing text in the title block can be edited when the Sheet-Format is active.
   a. True
   b. False

2. The standard drawing views can be created using the following method:
   a. Use Insert / Drawing views menu
   b. Use the Model-View command
   c. Drag and drop from an open window
   d. All of the above

3. View alignments can be broken or re-aligned.
   a. True
   b. False

4. The Detail-View scale cannot be changed or controlled locally.
   a. True
   b. False

5. The Projected view command projects and creates the Top, Bottom, Left, and Right views from another view.
   a. True
   b. False

6. To create an Auxiliary view, an edge has to be selected, not a face or a surface.
   a. True
   b. False

7. Only a single line can be used to create a Section view. The System doesn't support a multi-line section option.
   a. True
   b. False

8. Hidden lines in a drawing view can be turned ON / OFF locally and globally.
   a. True
   b. False

9. Configurations created in the model cannot be shown in the drawings.
   a. True
   b. False

1. TRUE
2. D
3. TRUE
4. FALSE
5. TRUE
6. TRUE
7. FALSE
8. TRUE
9. FALSE

Exercise: Detailing I

1. <u>Create</u> the **part** <u>and</u> the **drawing** as shown.

2. The Counter-Bore dimensions are measured from the Top planar surface.

3. Dimensions are in inches, 3 decimal places.

4. The part is symmetrical about the Top reference plane.

> (To create the "Back-Isometric-View" from the model: hold the Shift key and push the Up arrow key twice. This rotates the part 180°, and then insert this view to the drawing using the **Current-View** option).

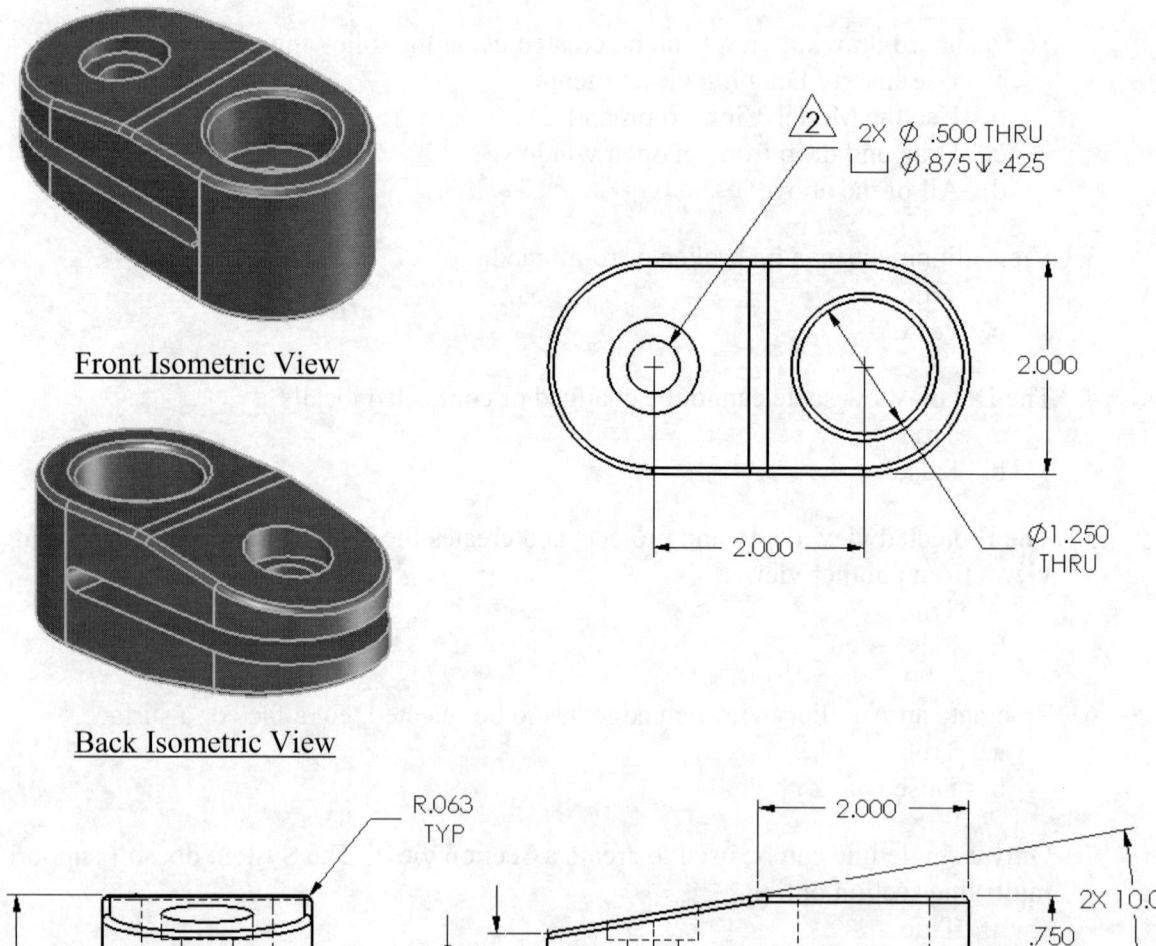

Front Isometric View

Back Isometric View

5. Save your work as: **Clamp Block**.

Exercise: Detailing II

1. <u>Open</u> the part named **Base Mount Block** from the Training Files folder.
2. Create a drawing using the provided details.
3. Create the Virtual-Sharps where needed prior to adding the Ordinate Dimensions.
   (To add the Virtual Sharps: Hold the Control key, select the 2 lines, and click the Sketch-Point command).

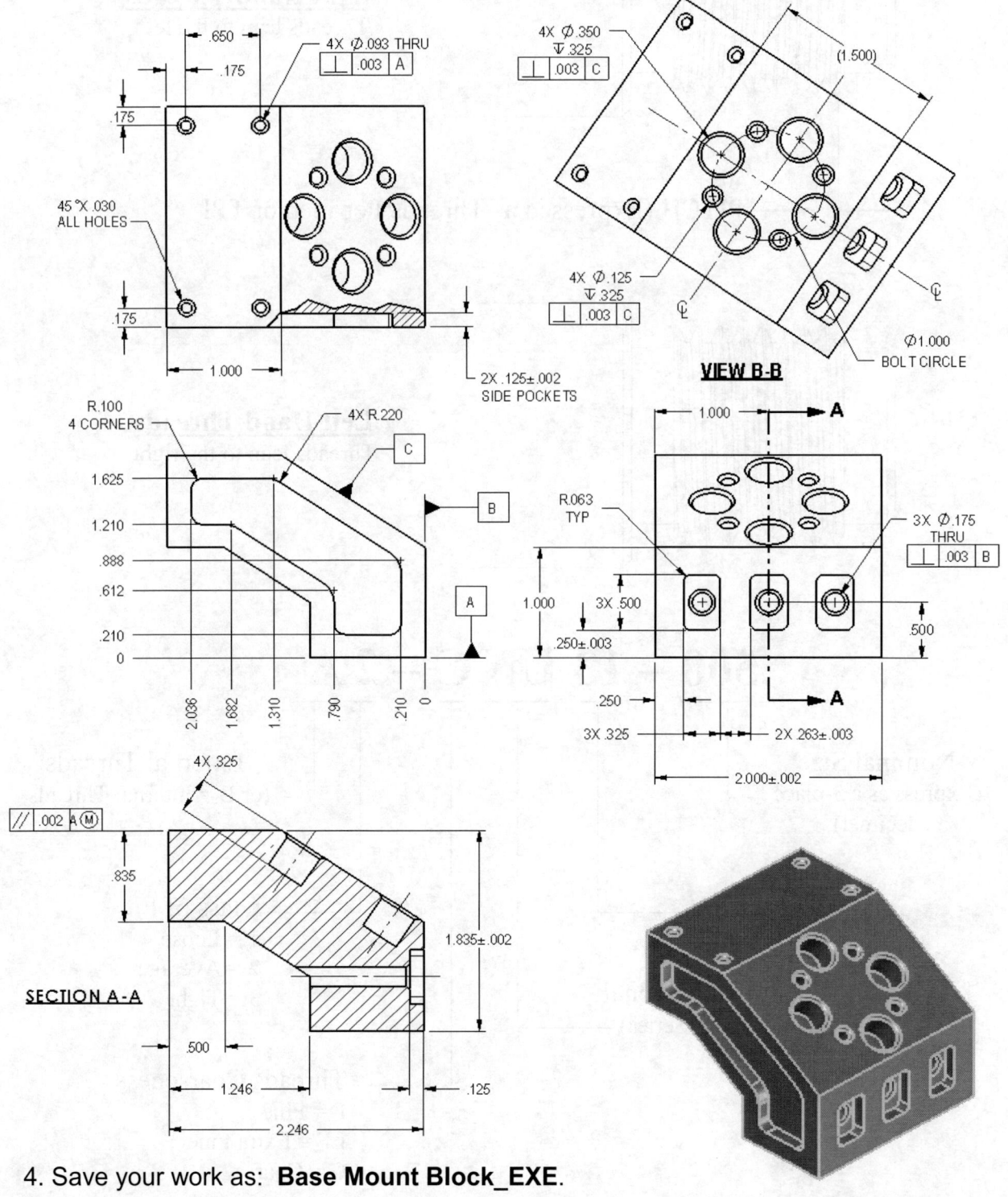

4. Save your work as: **Base Mount Block_EXE.**

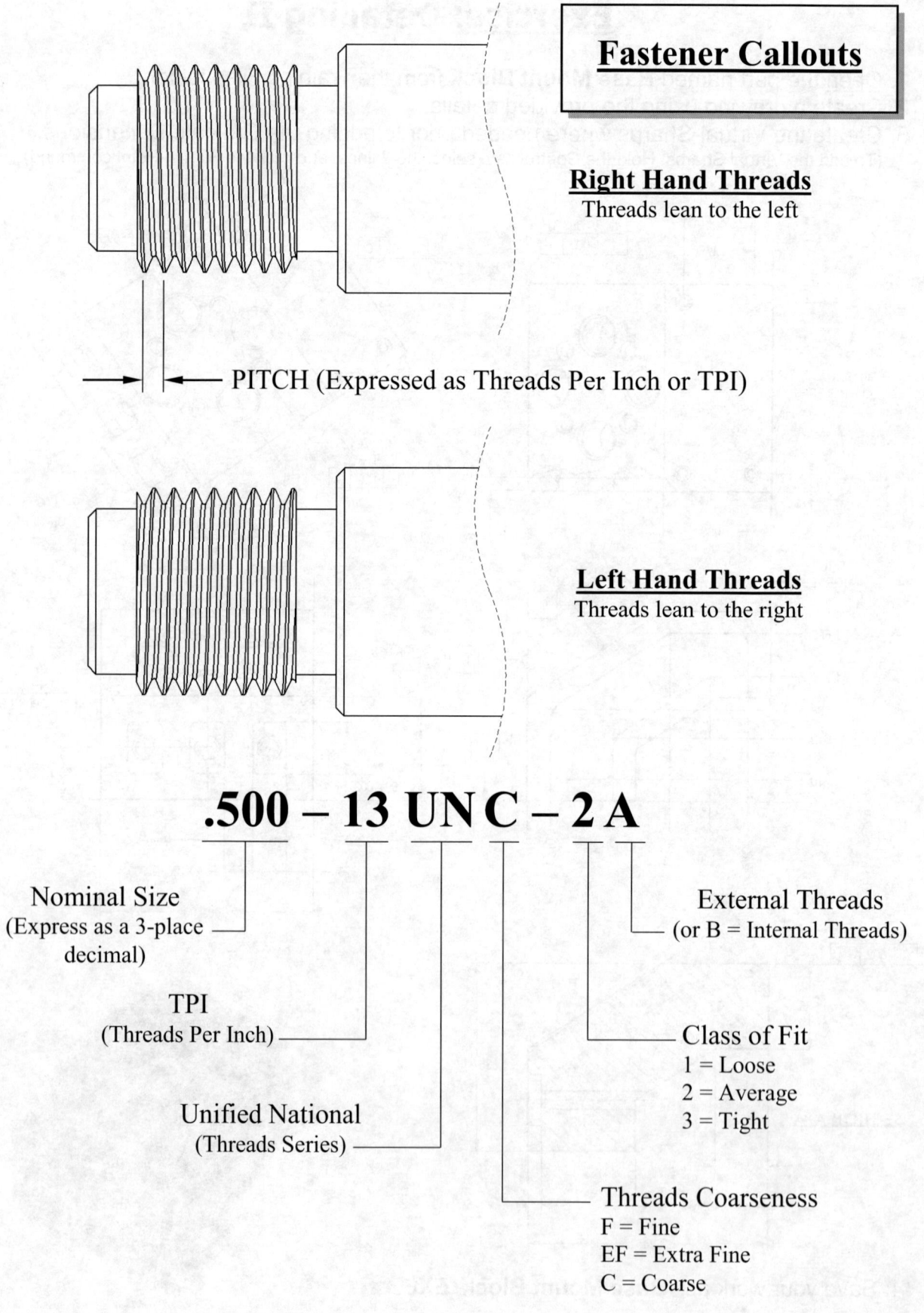

Fastener Callouts

Right Hand Threads
Threads lean to the left

PITCH (Expressed as Threads Per Inch or TPI)

Left Hand Threads
Threads lean to the right

.500 – 13 UN C – 2 A

Nominal Size
(Express as a 3-place decimal)

TPI
(Threads Per Inch)

Unified National
(Threads Series)

External Threads
(or B = Internal Threads)

Class of Fit
1 = Loose
2 = Average
3 = Tight

Threads Coarseness
F = Fine
EF = Extra Fine
C = Coarse

Thread Nomenclature

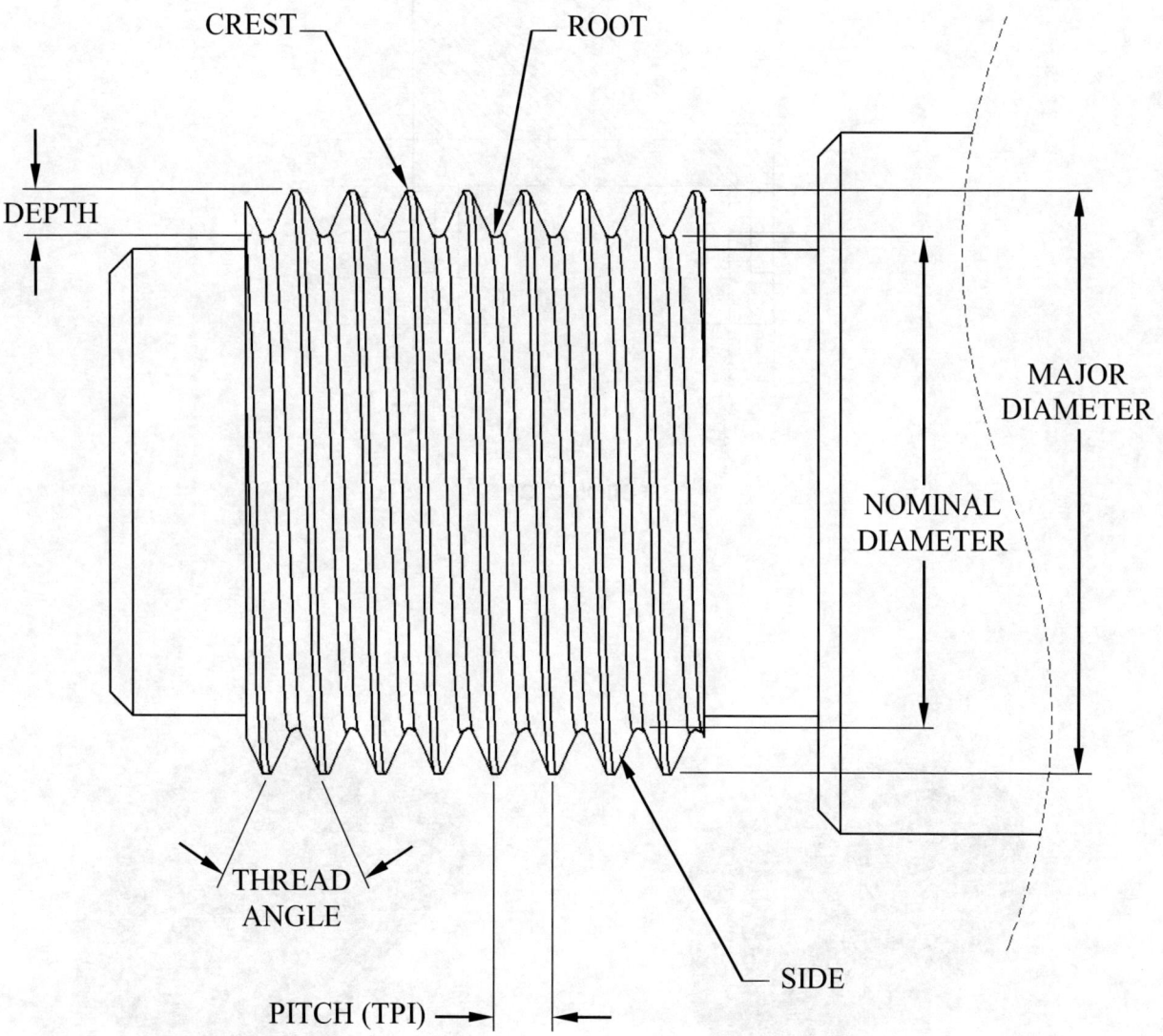

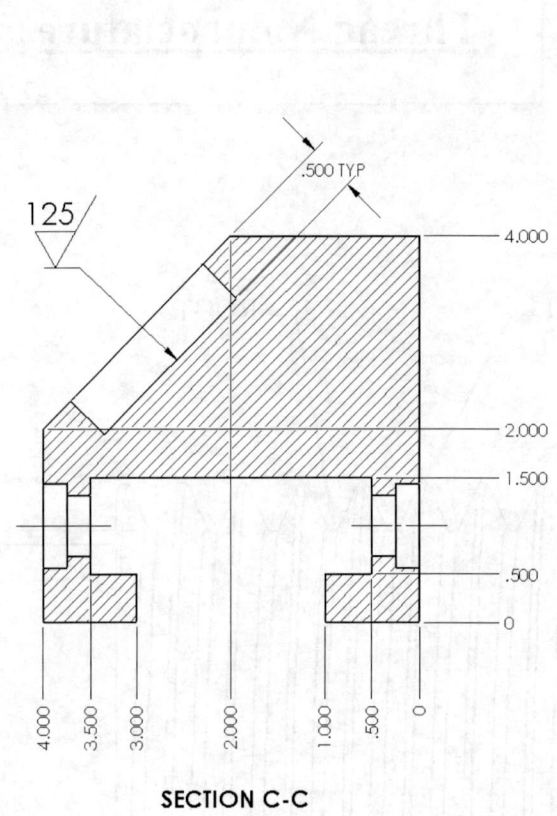

.500 TYP

125

4.000

2.000

1.500

.500

0

4.000
3.500
3.000

2.000

1.000
.500
0

SECTION C-C

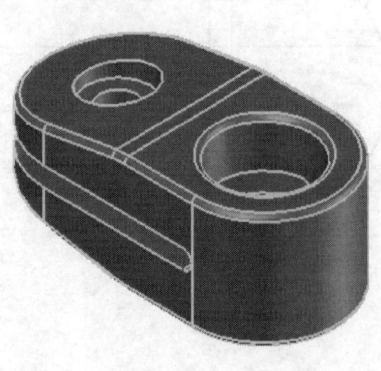

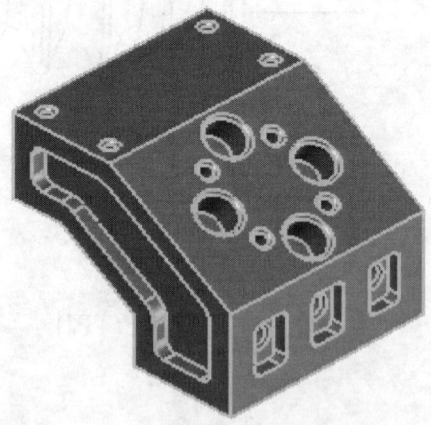

CHAPTER 18

Sheet Metal Drawings

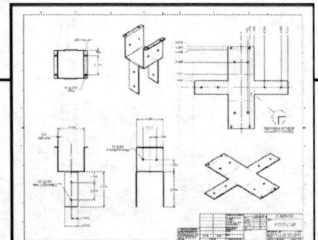

Sheet Metal Drawings
Post Cap

- When a *sheet metal Drawing* is made from a *sheet metal Part*, the SolidWorks software automatically creates a Flat Pattern view for use in conjunction with the Model View command.

- Any drawing views can be toggled to show the flattened stage, along with the bend lines. By accessing the Properties of the view, you can change from Default (Folded) to Flattened.

- By default, the Bend Lines are visible in the Flat Pattern but the Bend-Regions are not. To show the bend-regions, open the sheet metal part and right click the **Flat-Pattern** in the FeatureManager design tree, select **Edit Feature** and clear **Merge Faces**. You may have to rebuild the drawing to see the tangent edges.

- Both of the Folded and Flat Pattern drawing views can be shown on the same drawing sheet if needed. The dimensions and annotations can then be added to define the views.

- Changes done to the Sheet Metal part **will** reflect in the drawing views and the drawing itself can also be changed to update the sheet metal part as well. To prevent this from happening several options are available, refer to the Online Help from within the SolidWorks software for more details.

    - This exercise will guide you through the basics of creating a sheet metal drawing and the use of the Default/Flat-Pattern configurations.

Post Cap
Sheet Metal Drawings

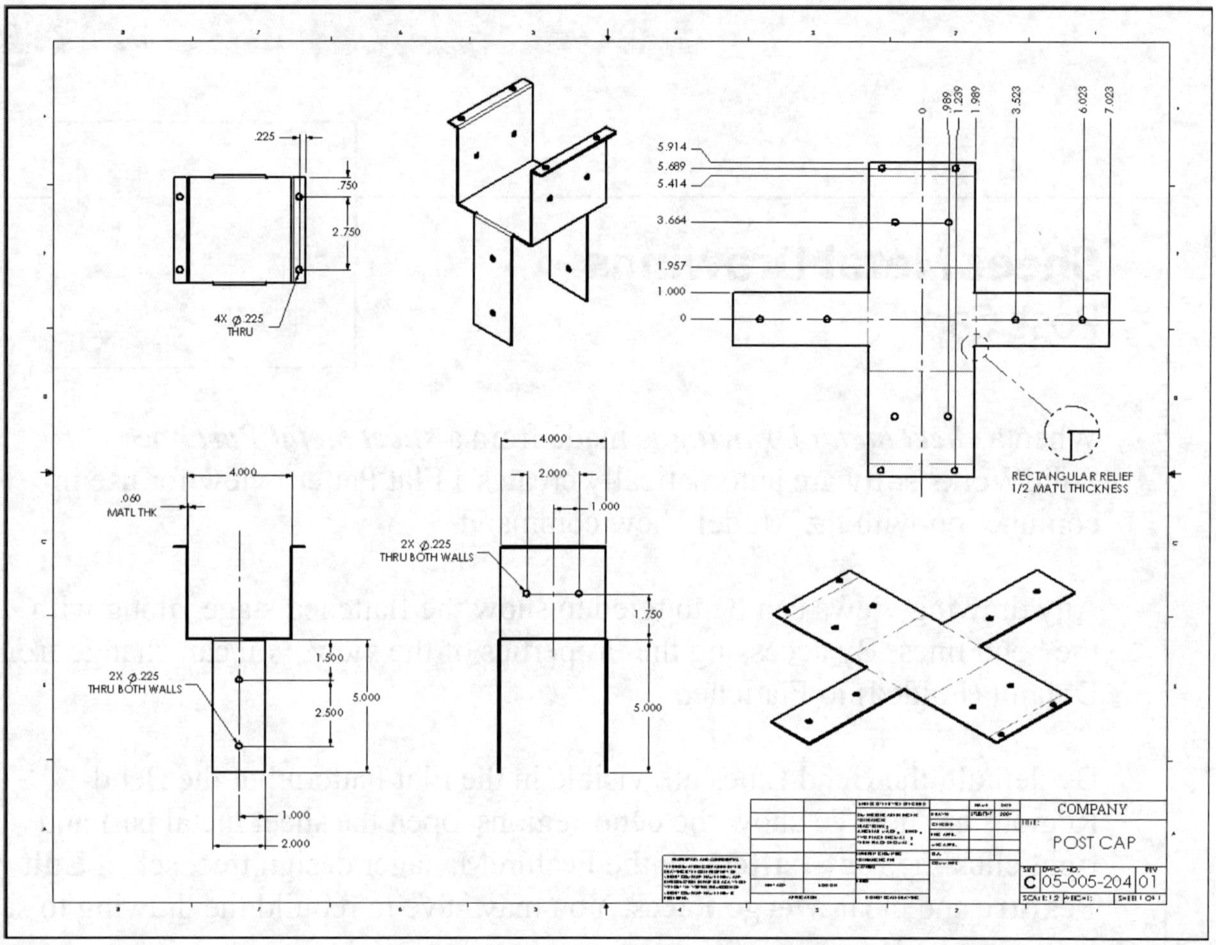

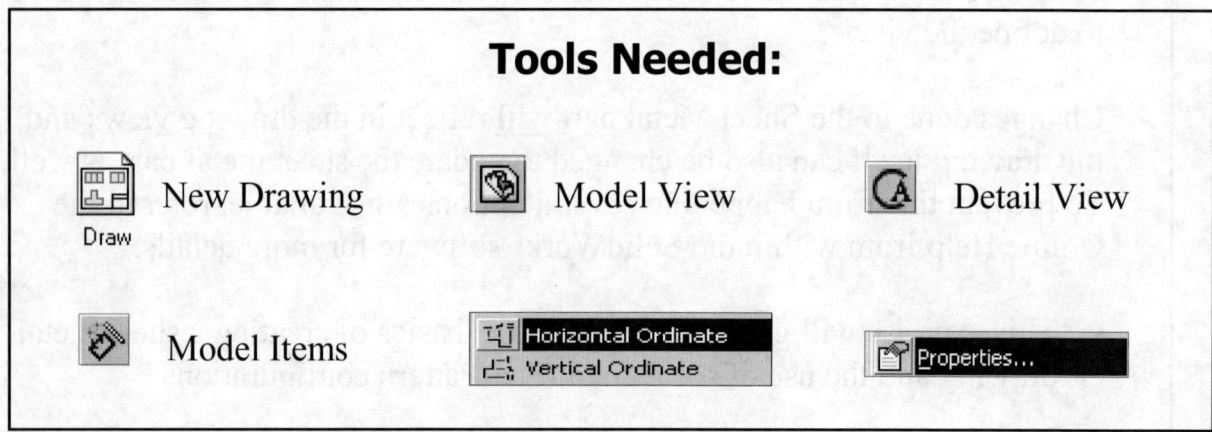

Dimensioning Standards: **ANSI**
Units: **INCHES** – 3 Decimals

Third Angle Projection

Tools Needed:

New Drawing
Draw

Model View

Detail View

Model Items

Horizontal Ordinate
Vertical Ordinate

Properties...

1. Starting a new drawing:

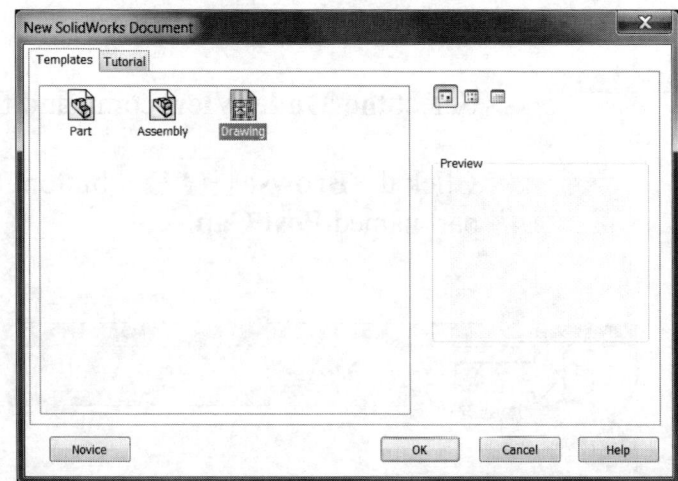

- Select **File / New / Draw** and click **OK**.

- *NOTE: If you have already created and saved a template, you can browse and select the same template for this drawing.*

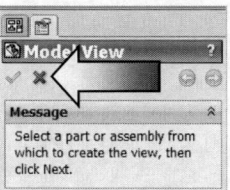

- Click the **Cancel** button (arrow) to exit the insert part mode. The drawing paper size, drawing view scale, and the projection angle must be set first.

- If the Sheet Properties dialog does not appear, right click in the default paper and select Properties.

- Set **Scale** to **1** to **1** and set **Type of Projection** to **Third Angle**.

- Select **C-Lanscape** sheet size.

- Enable **Display Sheet Format** and click **OK** | OK | .

- Go to **Tools / Options** and change the **Units** to **IPS** (Inch / Pound / Second).

(The document units can also be changed at the bottom right corner of the screen.

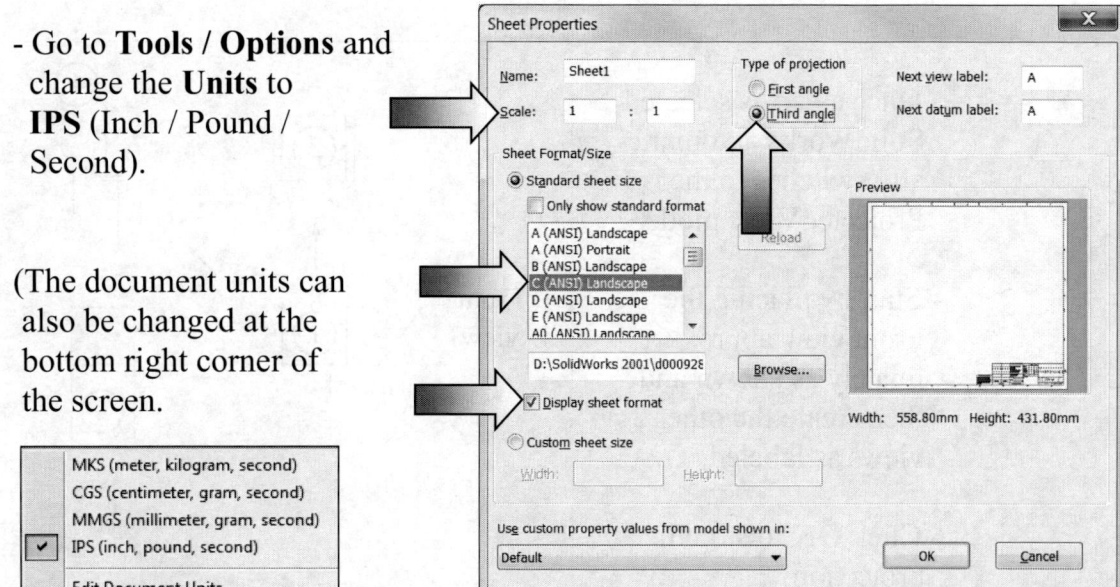

2. Creating the 3 Standard Views:

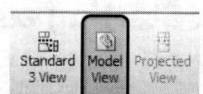

- Select **the Model View** command from the View Layout tab.

- Click the **Browse** Browse... button, from the training files to locate and open the part named **Post Cap**.

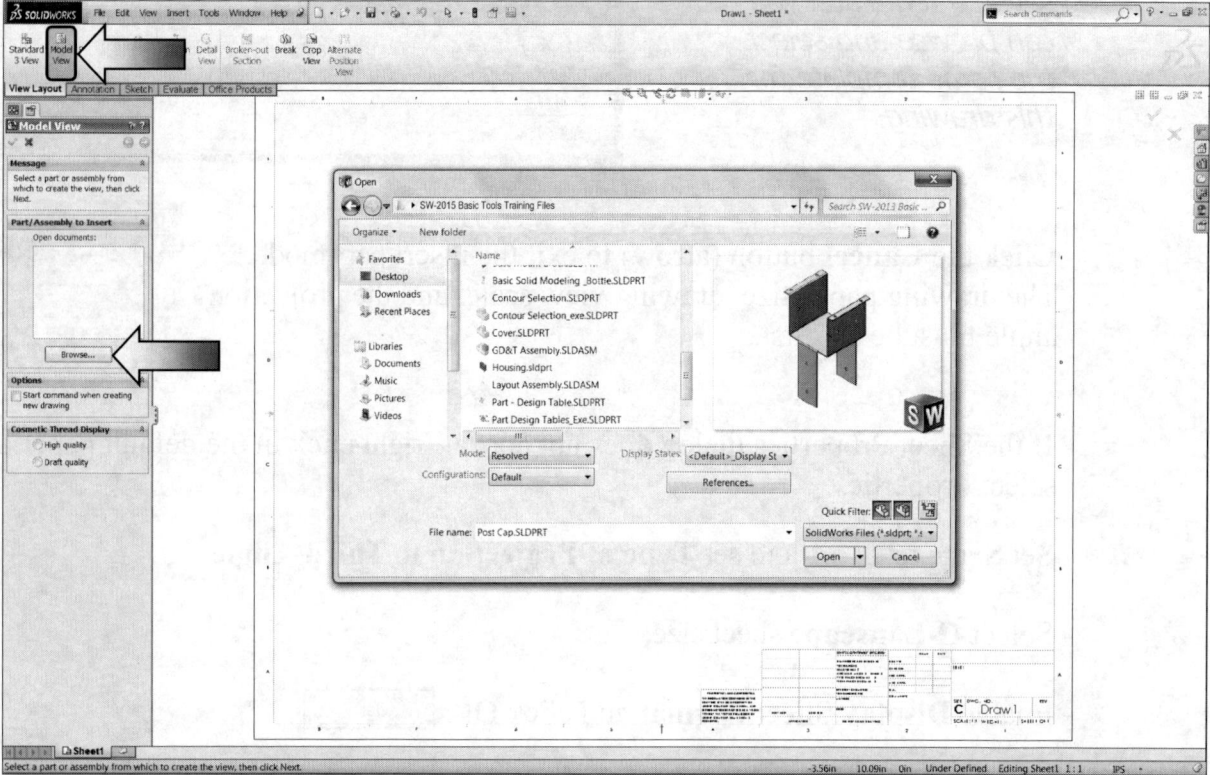

- Once a part is selected SolidWorks automatically switches to the ProjectedView mode.

- Start by placing the Front view approximately as shown and then create the other 3 views as labeled.

- Click **OK** to stop the projection.

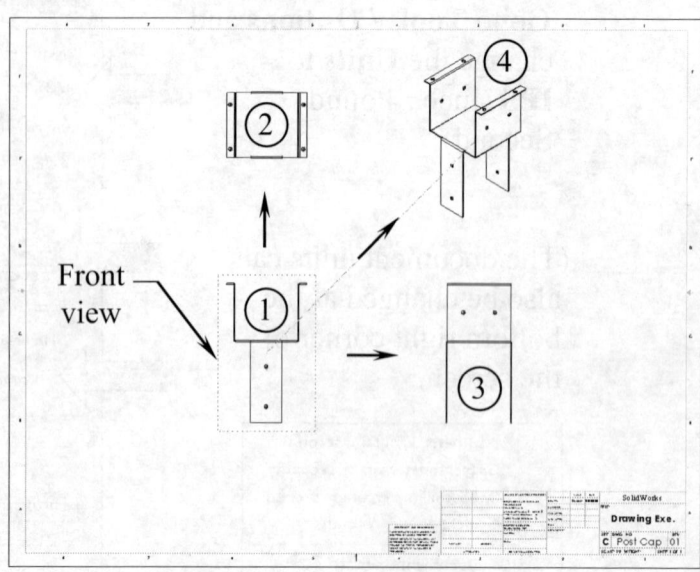

3. Re-arranging the drawing views:

- Re-arrange the drawing views to the approximate positions by dragging on their borders. A flat-pattern view will be placed on the right side of the drawing.

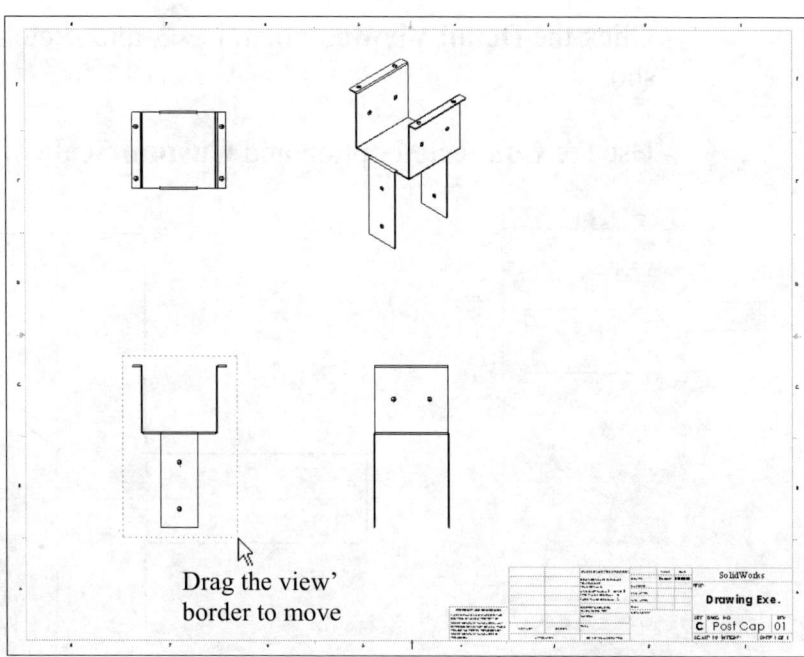

Drag the view' border to move

4. Creating the Flat Pattern drawing view:

- Select the **Model View** command 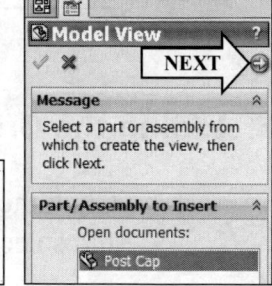, click Next 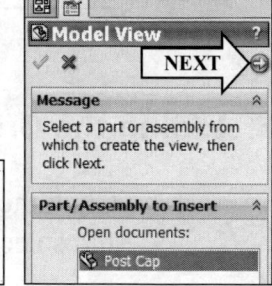, select the **Flat-Pattern** view (Arrow) from the list and place it approximately as shown.

- Bend notes must be turned off <u>prior</u> to creating the Flat Pattern view (**Tools/Option/ Document Properties/Sheet Metal**).

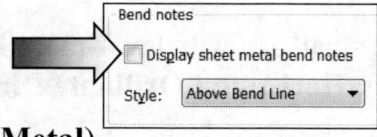

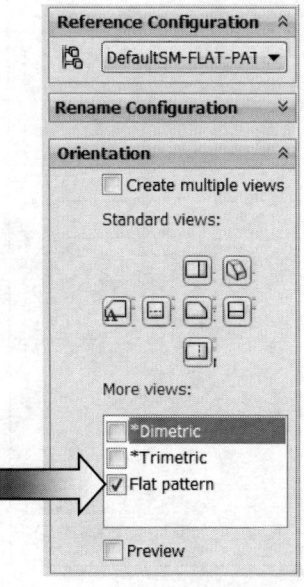

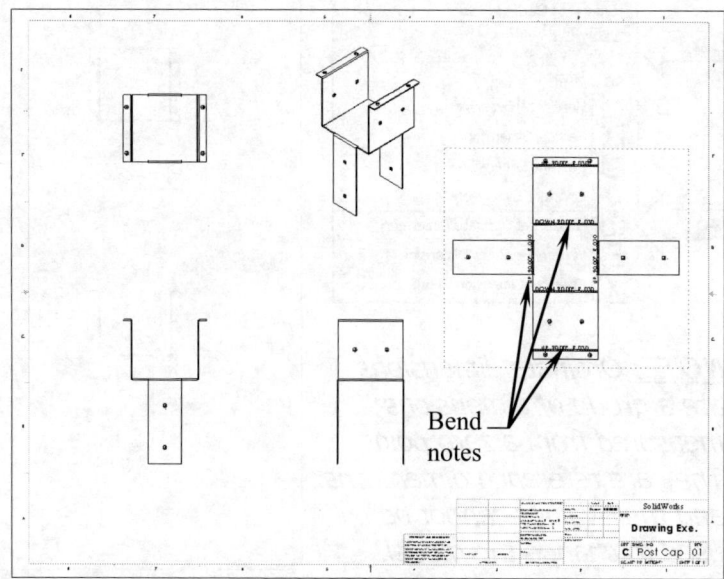

Bend notes

5. Creating a Detail view:

- Click the **Detail View** command 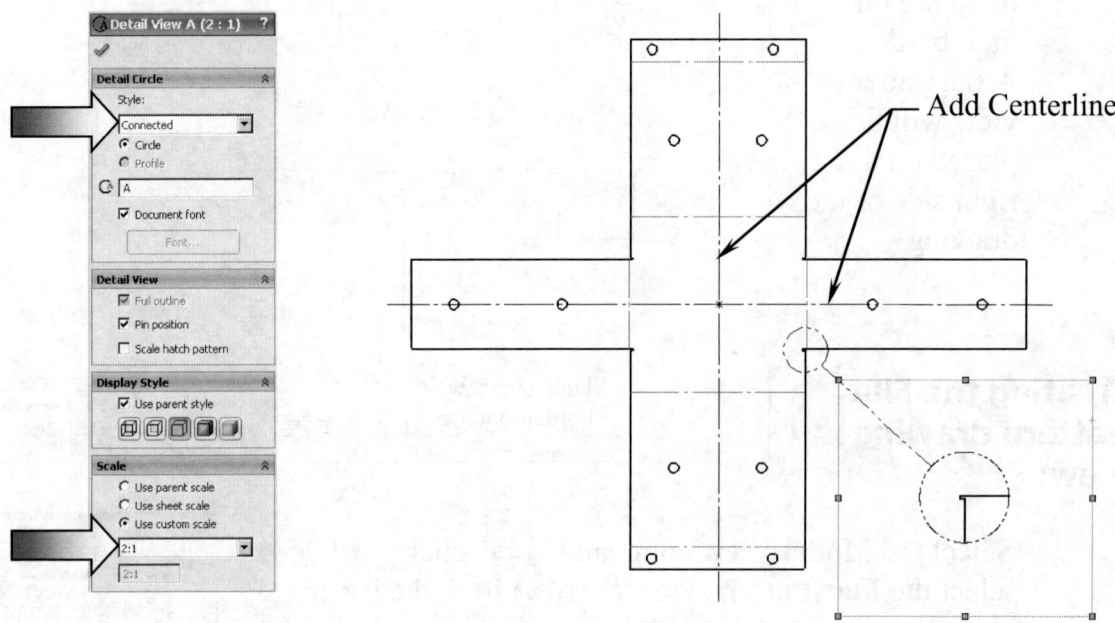 and sketch a Circle approximately as shown.

- Use the **Connected** option and **Custom Scale** of **2:1** (arrows).

Add Centerlines

6. Adding the Ordinate dimensions:

- Click the small arrow below **Smart Dimension** to access its options, and select: **Horizontal Ordinate Dimension** (arrow).

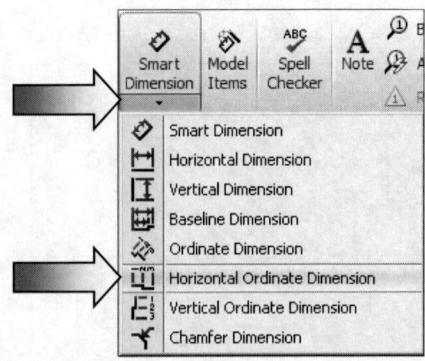

NOTE: _Ordinate dimensions are a group of dimensions measured from a zero point. They are reference dimensions and their values cannot be used to change the model._

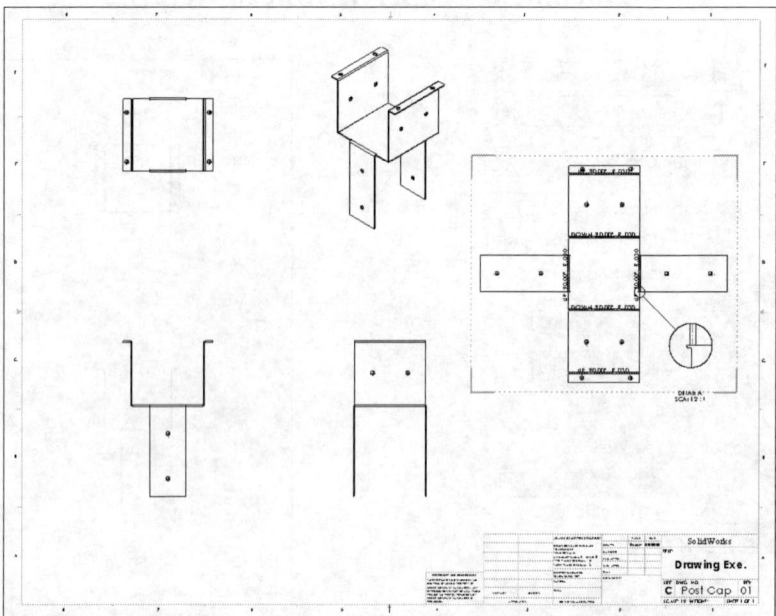

- Starting at the Vertical Centerline, add the Horizontal Ordinate dimensions as shown here.

- Click the drop down arrow under Smart Dimension and select: **Horizontal Ordinate Dimension**

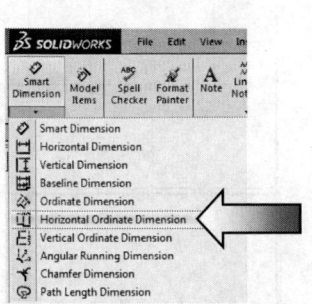

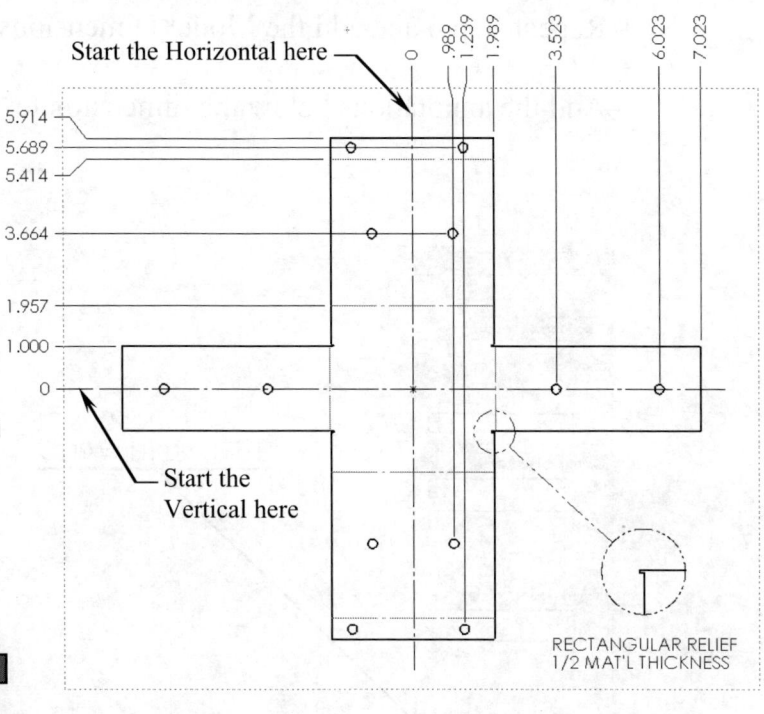

Start the Horizontal here

Start the Vertical here

RECTANGULAR RELIEF
1/2 MAT'L THICKNESS

- Add the Vertical Ordinate dimensions as shown in the drawing view above.

7. Adding the Model dimensions:

- Select the Front view's border to activate it.

- On the **Annotation** tab, click the **Model Items** button, select: **Entire Model** and **Eliminate Duplicates**.

- Click **OK** ⊘.

- Modify the dimensions and add the depth and the thickness callouts as shown.

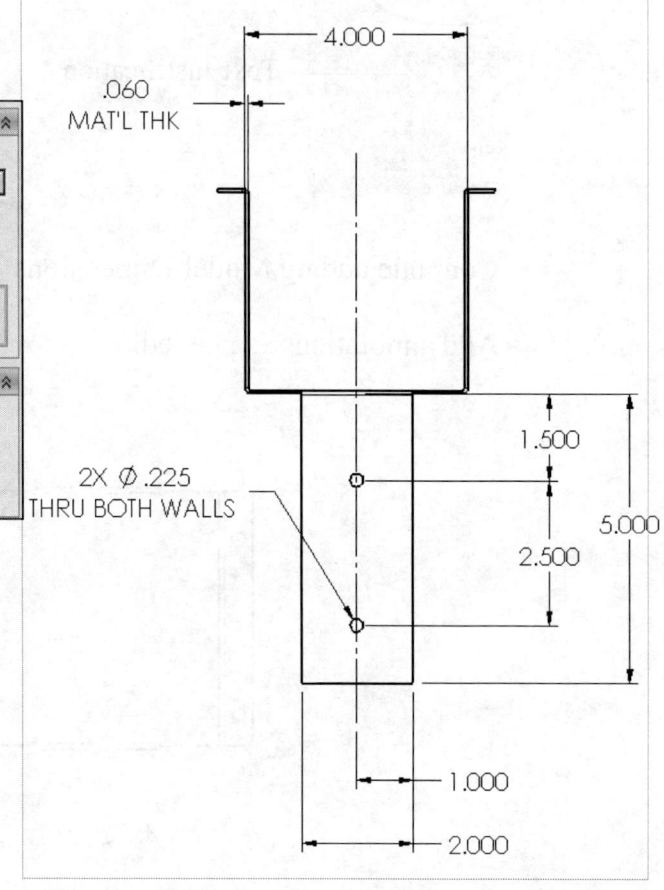

4.000

.060
MAT'L THK

1.500

2X Ø .225
THRU BOTH WALLS

5.000

2.500

1.000

2.000

- Repeat step 6 and add the Model Dimensions 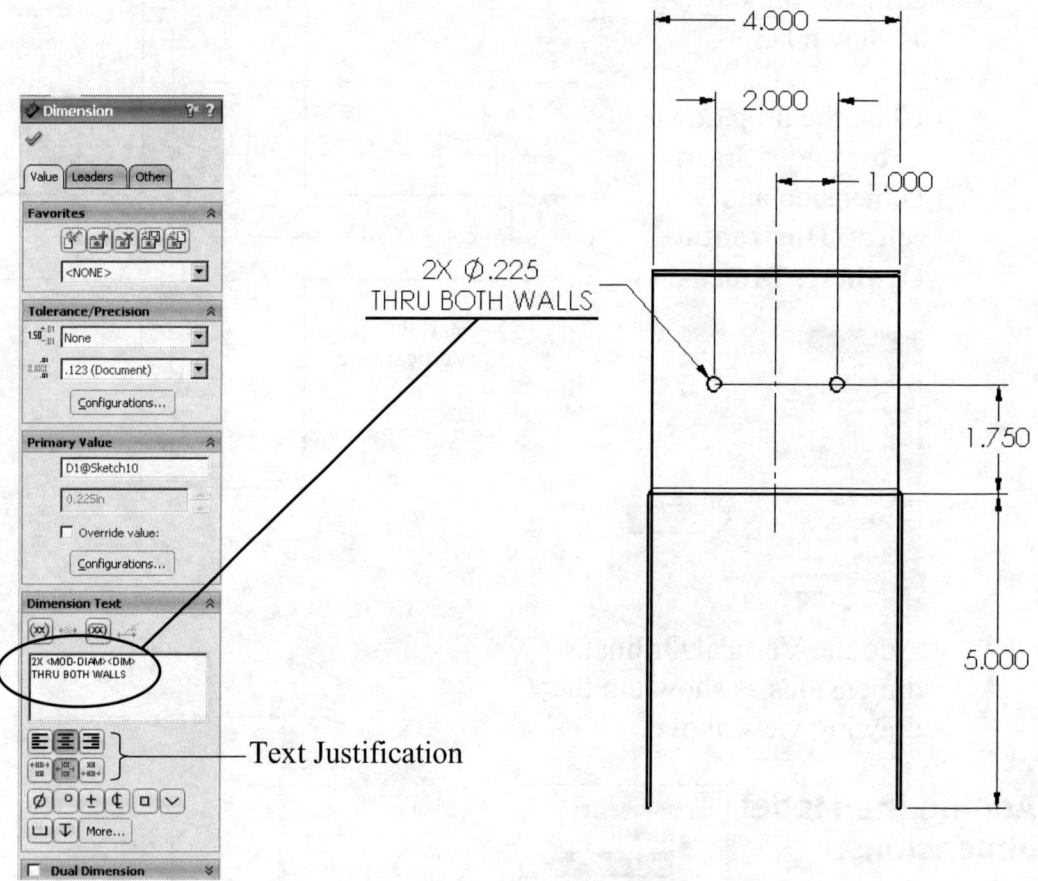 to the Right drawing view.

- Add the annotations below the dimension text (Circled).

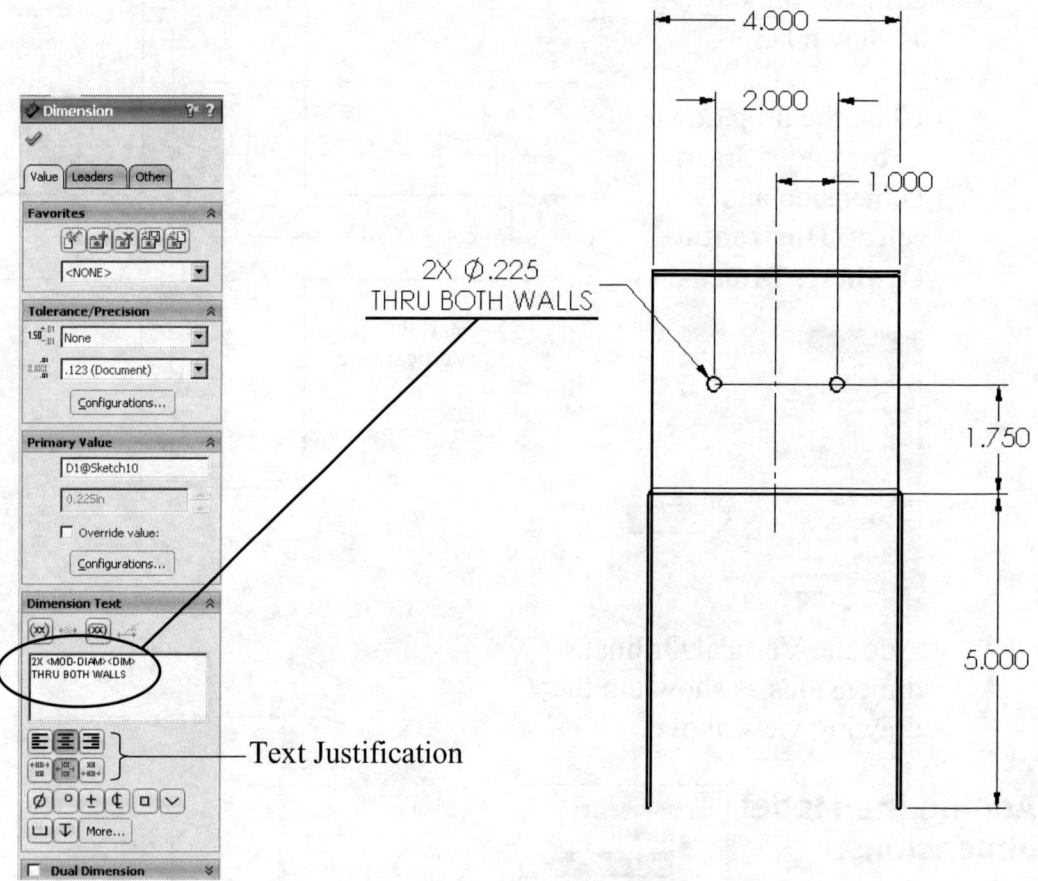

- Continue adding Model Dimensions 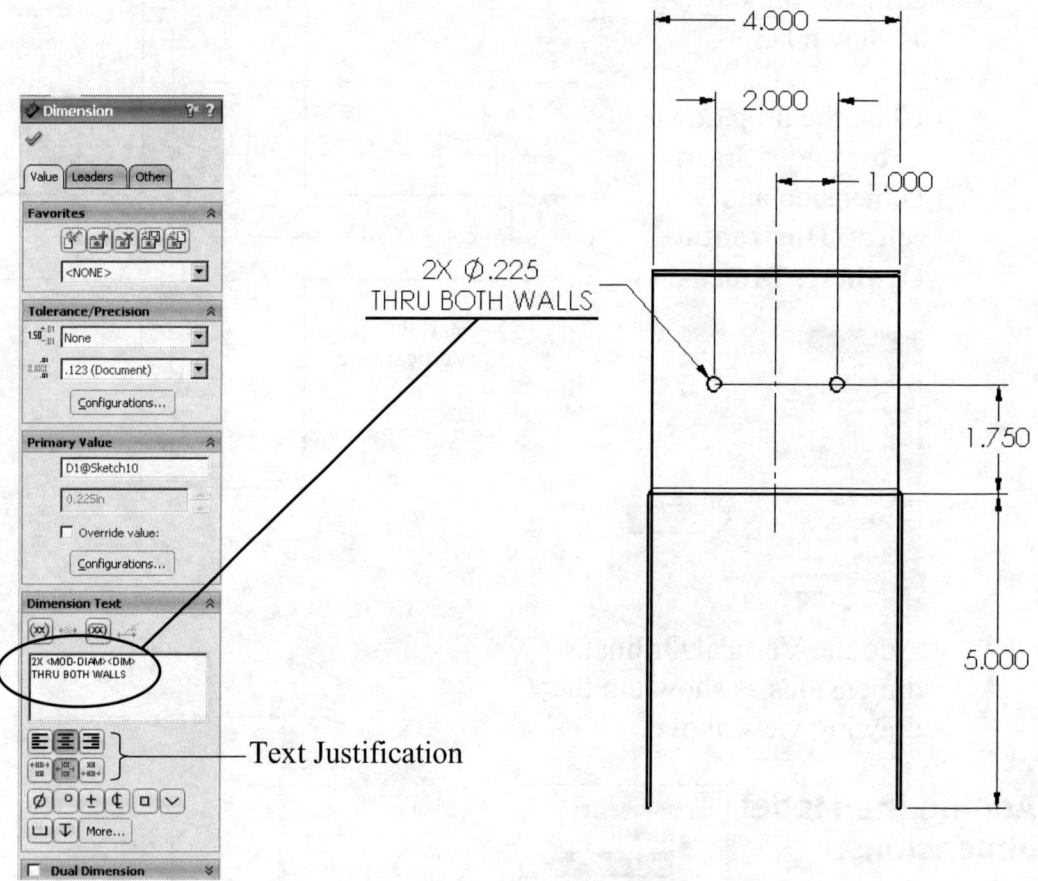 to the Top drawing view.

- Add annotations as needed.

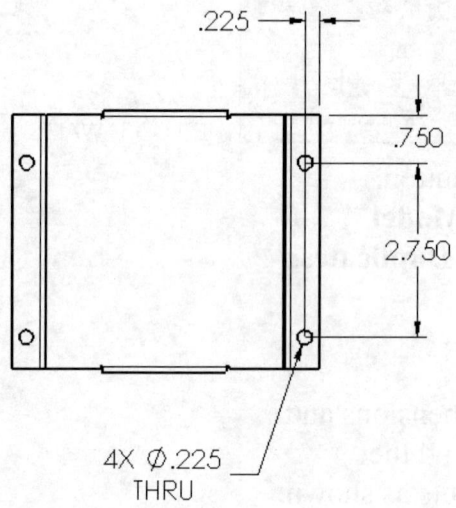

8. Creating the Isometric Flat Pattern view:

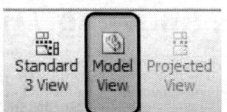

- Click the **Model View** command from the View Layout tab   .

- Click the **Next button** ⊖ , select the Isometric View from the menu and place it below the flat-pattern view.

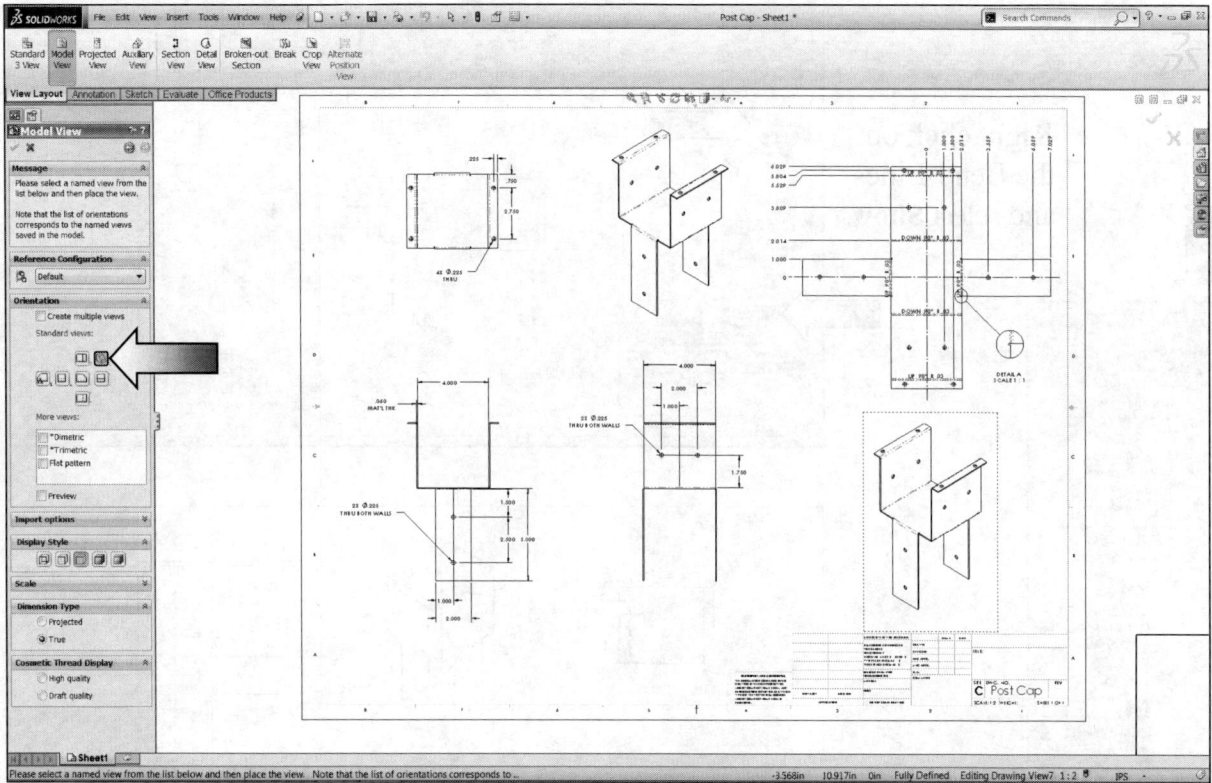

- A drawing view can also be copied and pasted using Ctrl+C and Ctrl+V.

- Under the Reference Configuration section to change the **Default** configuration to **SM-Flat-Pattern** configuration (arrow).

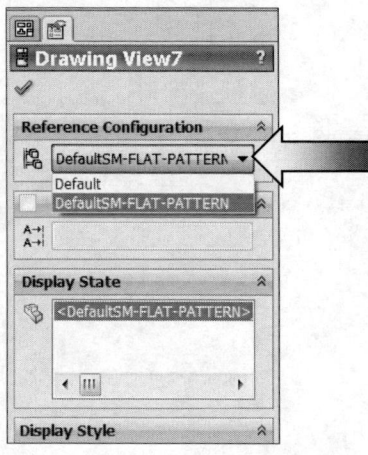

- Click **OK** ___OK___ .

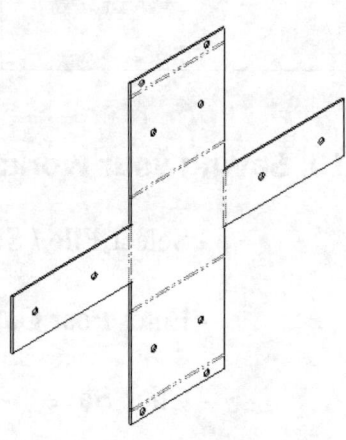

- The flat pattern of the sheet metal part appears. The bend lines and bend regions are also visible in this view.

9. Showing /Hiding the Bend Lines:

- Click the DrawingManager tab (arrow), scroll down the tree and expand the last drawing view in the FeatureManager tree (click the + symbol).

- Expand the Flat Pattern feature.

- Right click on the Bend-Lines and select **Show**.

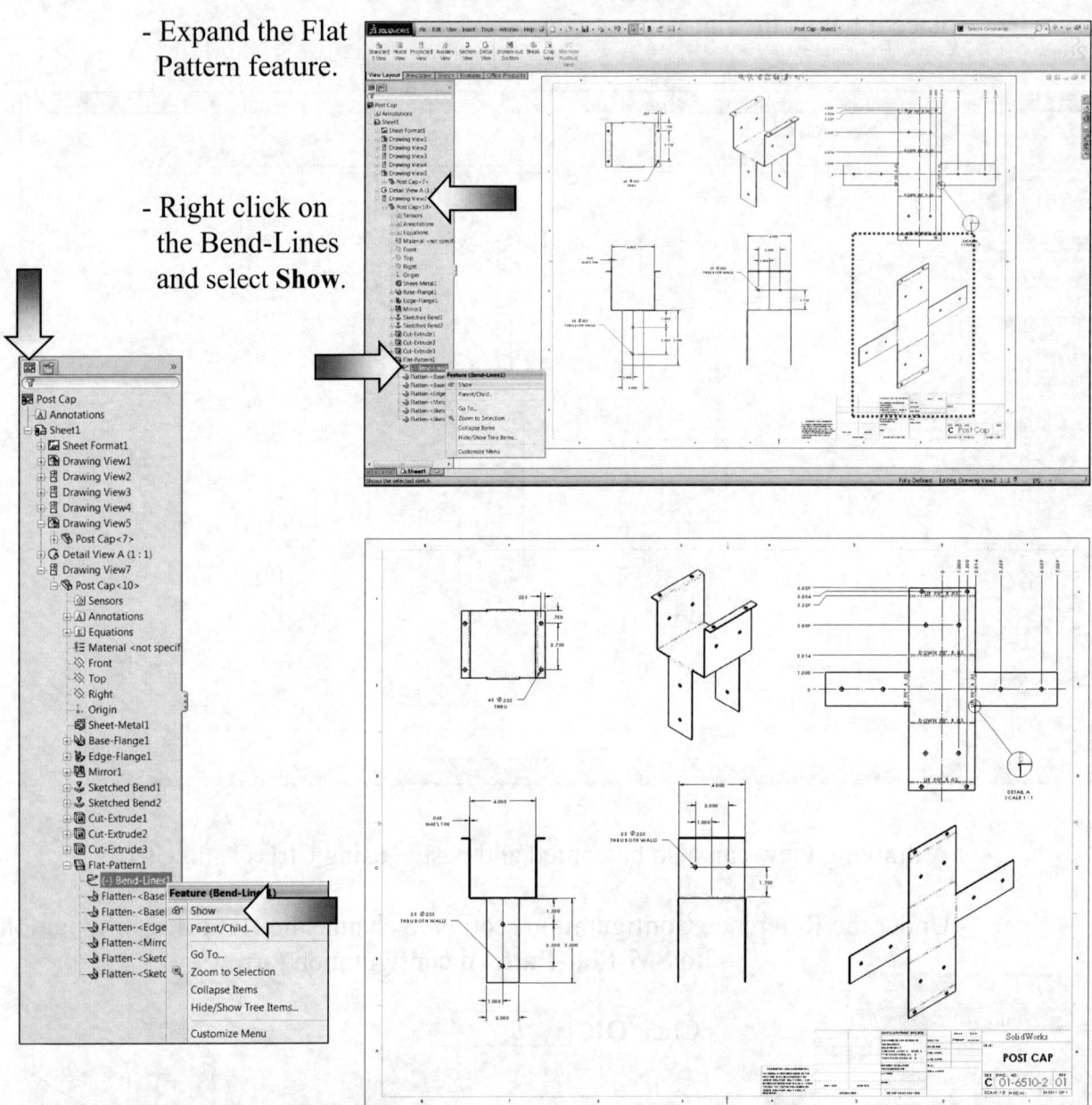

10. Saving your work:

- Select **File / Save As**.

- Enter **Post Cap.slddrw** for the name of the file.

- Click **Save**.

CHAPTER 18 (cont.)

2D to 3D Conversion

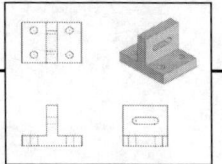

2D to 3D
Converting 2D AutoCAD files to 3D SolidWorks Parts

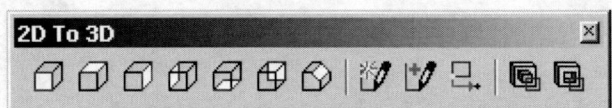

- The 2D to 3D options allow sketches and/or drawings created in SolidWorks or other CAD programs, like AutoCAD, to be converted into 3D solids.

- The sketches can be created in SolidWorks or imported as a DWG or DXF from other CAD sources. In either case, the sketch or the drawing should be a single sketch imported into a part template.

- The drawing can be Cut and Pasted into a sketch in a part template or can be imported into SolidWorks as a sketch in a part template, using the SolidWorks DXF/DWG import options.

- Once the drawing is imported or a sketch is created, follow the four easy steps to convert your sketch into a solid:

   * Edit the sketch.   * Extract the sketches (Front, Top, Right...)
   * Align the sketches.   * Extrude the sketch.

- This chapter and its exercises will guide you through some of the easiest techniques in converting an AutoCAD 2D drawing into a SolidWorks 3D model, as well as using a built-in utility program called DXF/DWG Import by SolidWorks.

2D to 3D Conversions
Converting 2D AutoCAD DWG to 3D SolidWorks Model

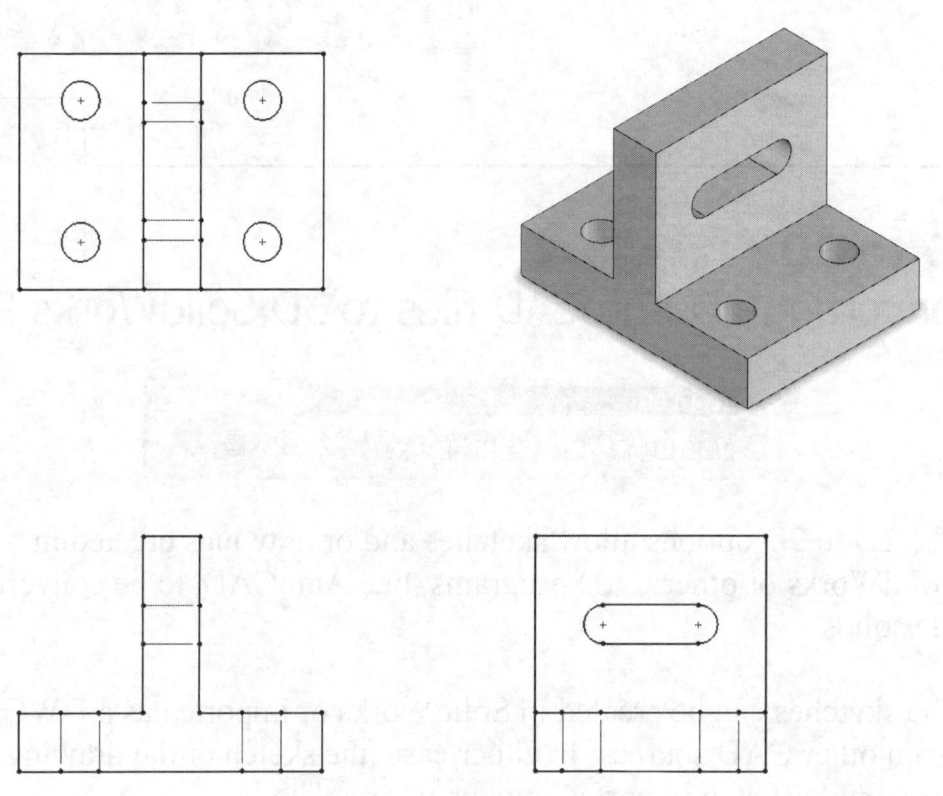

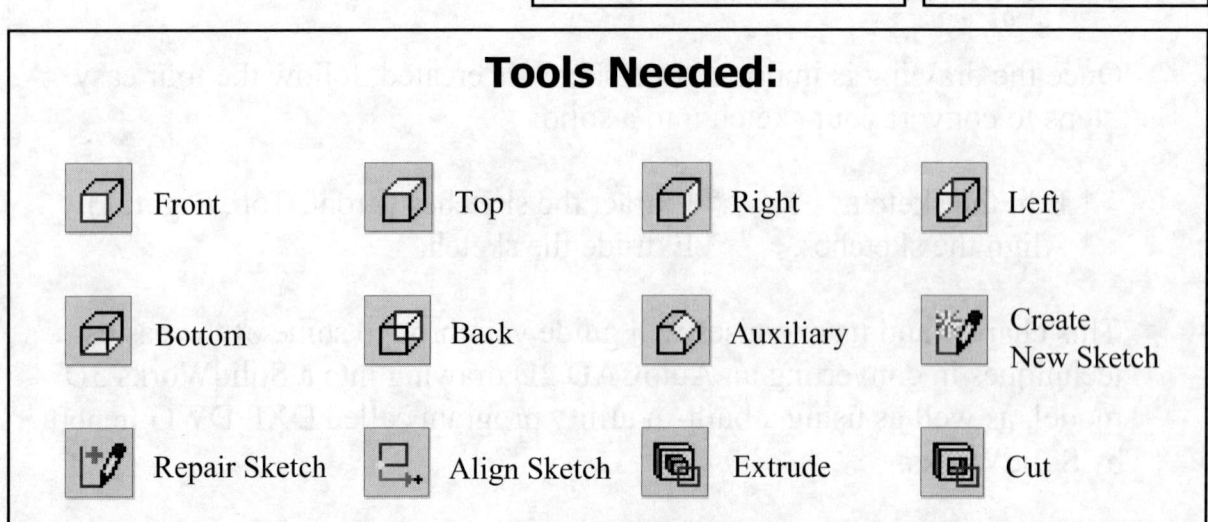

Dimensioning Standards: **ANSI**	Third Angle Projection
Units: **INCHES** – 3 Decimals	

Tools Needed:

Front	Top	Right	Left
Bottom	Back	Auxiliary	Create New Sketch
Repair Sketch	Align Sketch	Extrude	Cut

1. Creating the drawing in AutoCAD®:

- The orthographic views below have already been created in AutoCAD.

- The drawing has also been saved as **2Dto3D.dwg**.

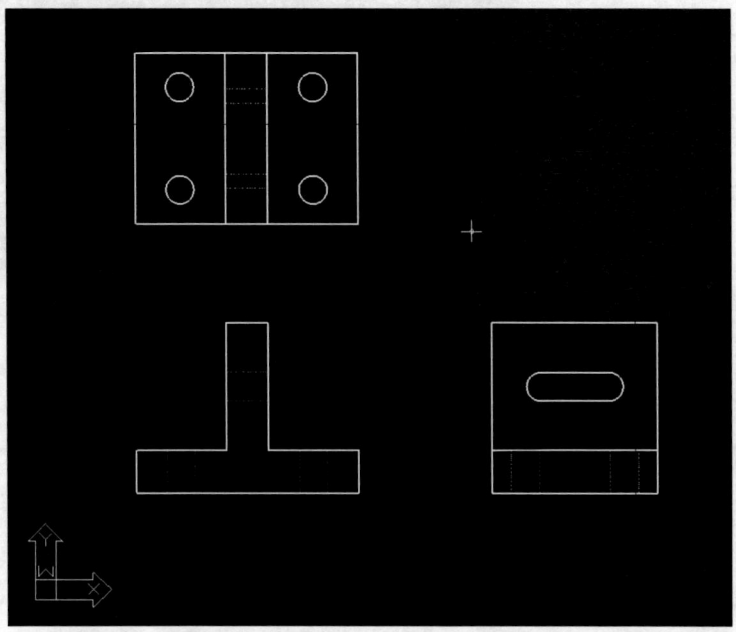

2. Opening the AutoCAD drawing from SolidWorks:

- In SolidWorks, click **File / Open**.

- Change the Files of Type to **Dwg** (*dwg), select the file **2Dto3D** and **open**.

- In the DXF / DWG Import dialog box select: **Import To New Part**.

- Click Next Next >.

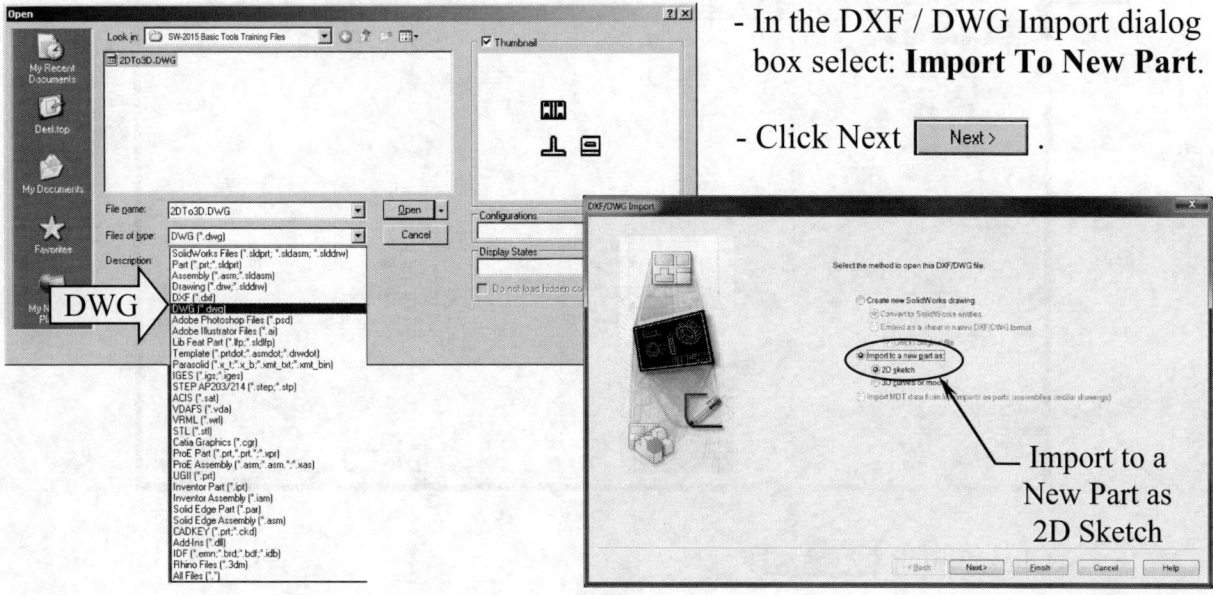

Import to a
New Part as
2D Sketch

- In the Document Settings dialog box, select **All Selected Layers** and **Add-Constraints** checkboxes.

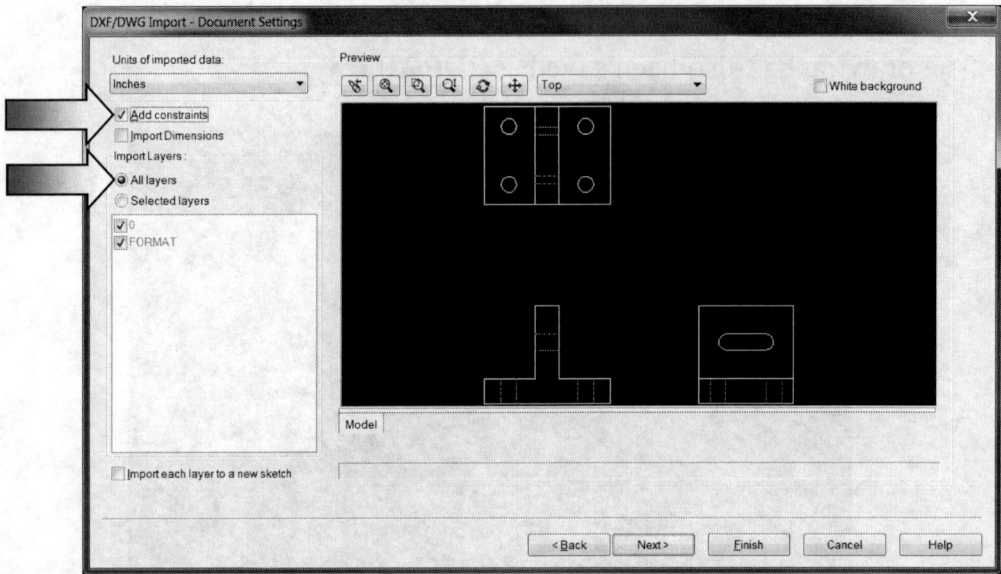

- Click **Next** [Next >] .

- In the Drawing Layer Mapping dialog, select / set the following:

    * Merge points closer than **0.001**

    * White Background: **Enabled**.

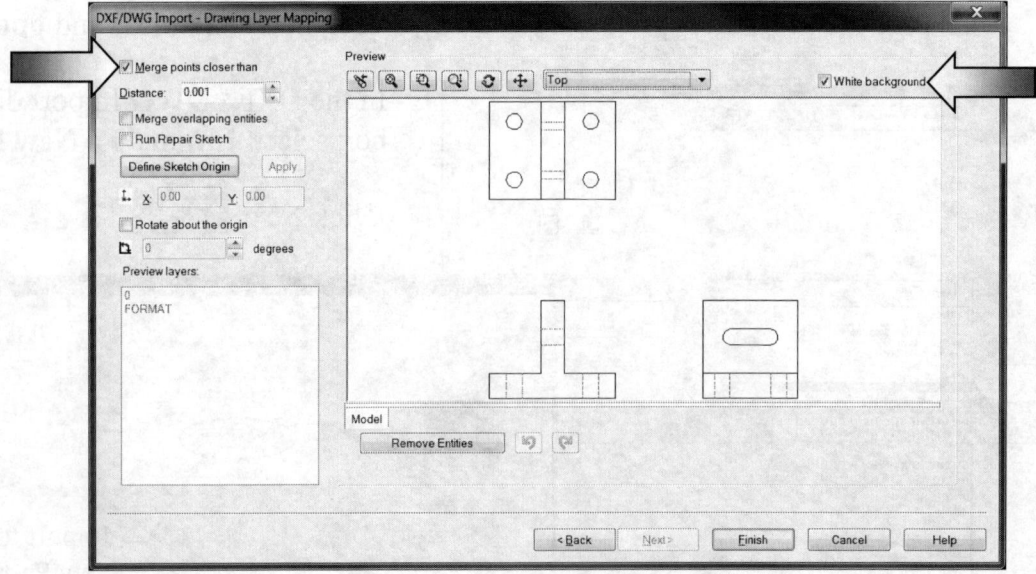

- Click Finish [Finish] .

- The AutoCAD drawing is placed on the SolidWorks' Front plane as a sketch.

- A 2D-To-3D toolbar pops up on the screen. (The 2D-To-3D toolbar can be toggled on/off under View / Toolbars / 2D-To-3D).

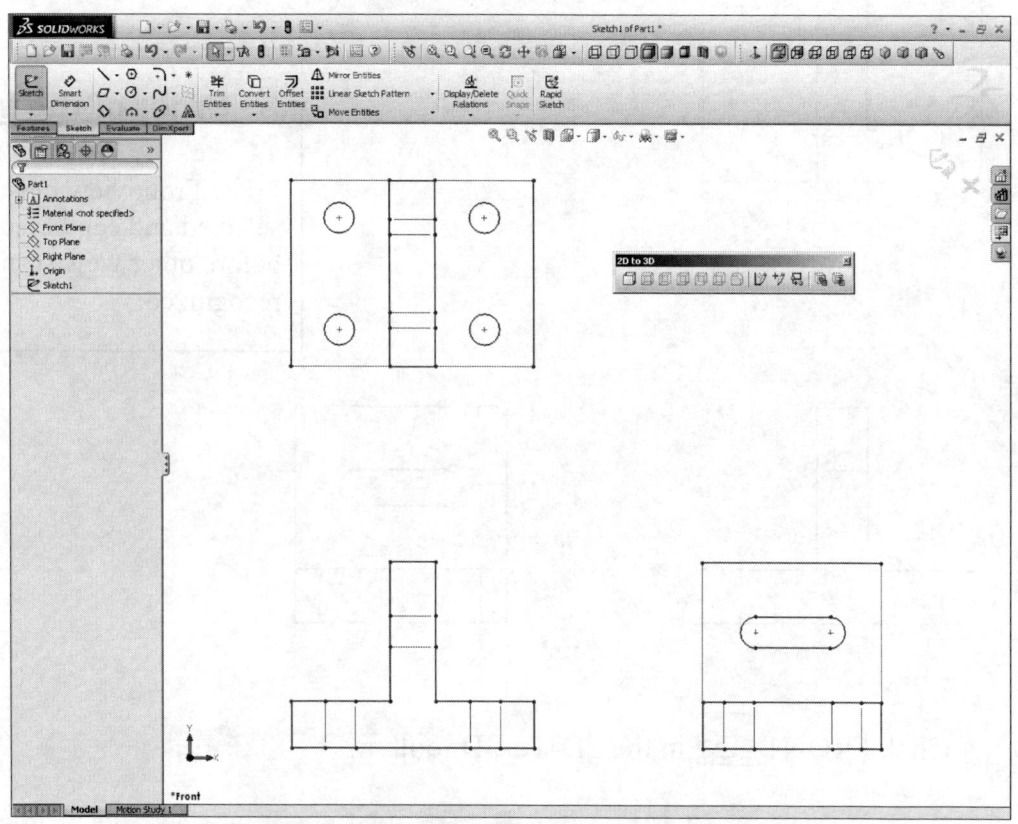

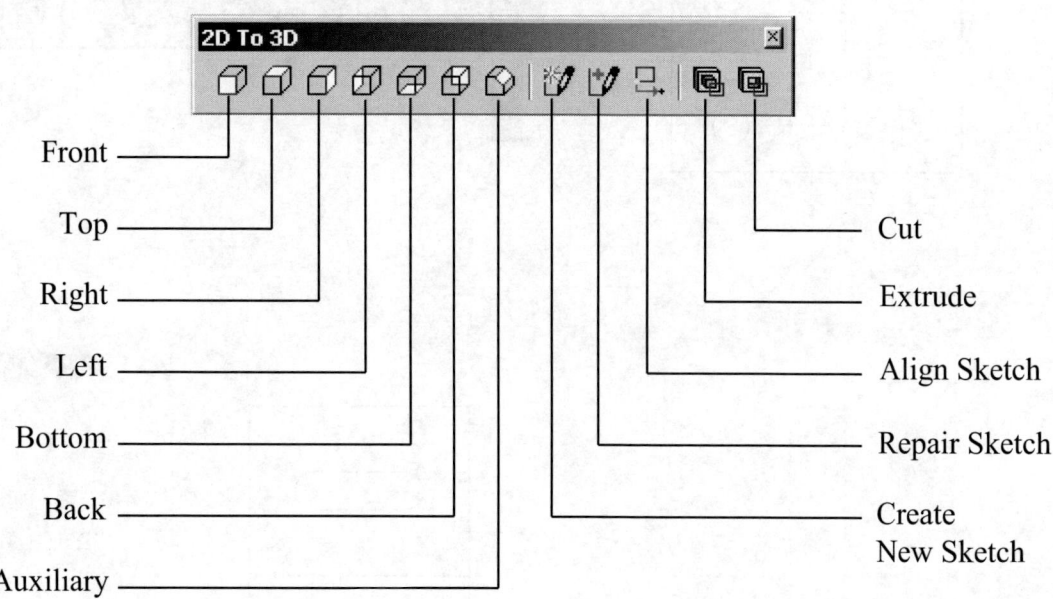

Front —————————— Cut

Top —————————— Extrude

Right —————————— Align Sketch

Left —————————— Repair Sketch

Bottom —————————— Create
New Sketch

Back

Auxiliary

3. Converting the sketches:

- Drag select (click-hold-drag) the Front view.

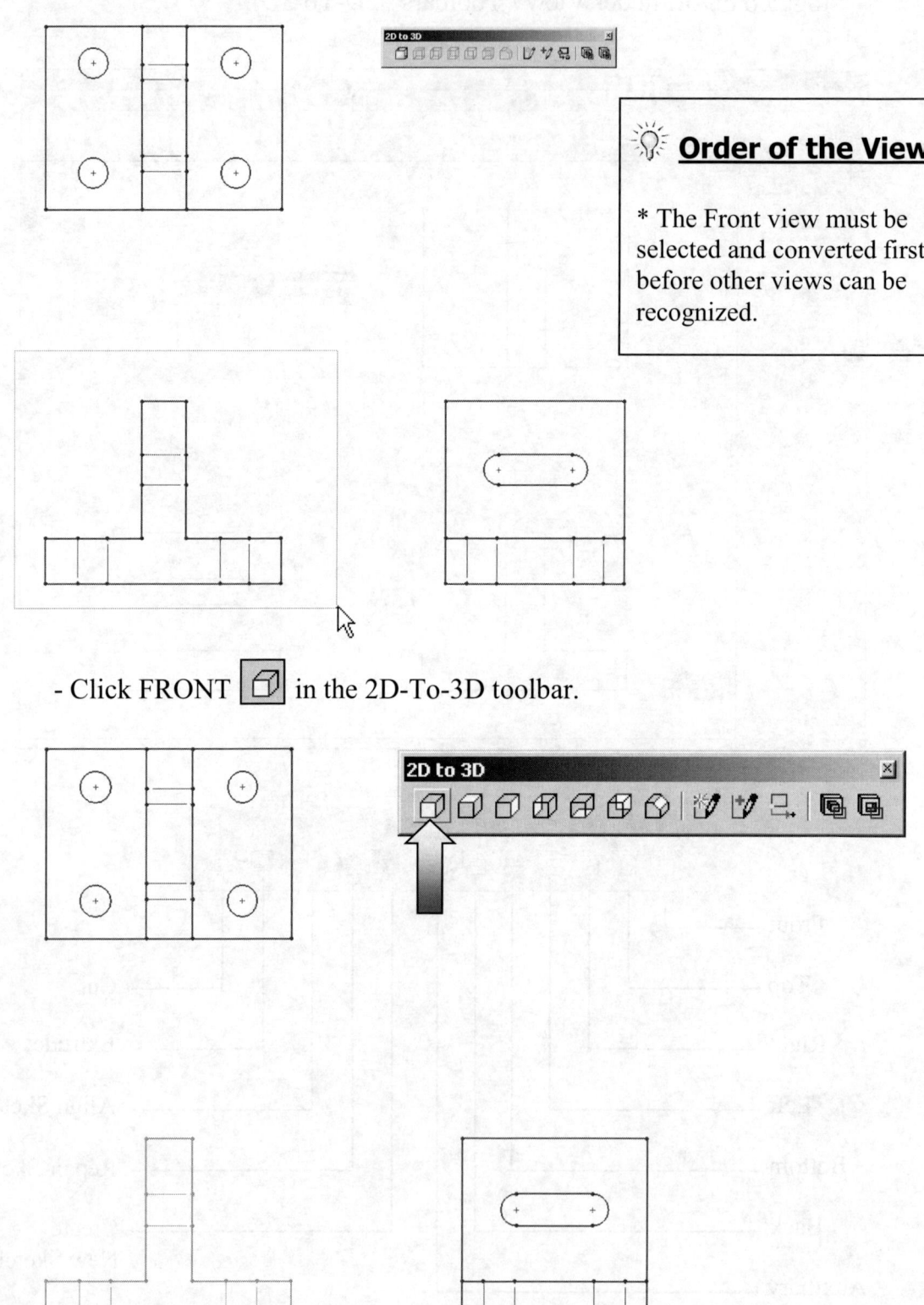

🔆 **Order of the Views**

* The Front view must be selected and converted first before other views can be recognized.

- Click FRONT ⬜ in the 2D-To-3D toolbar.

- The Front view is converted and turned into gray color.

- Drag select (click-hold-drag) the Top view.

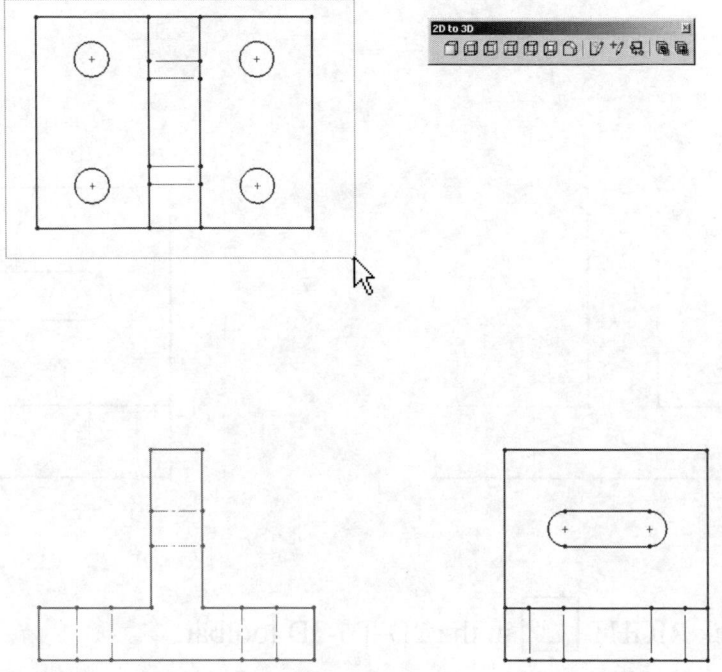

- Click TOP 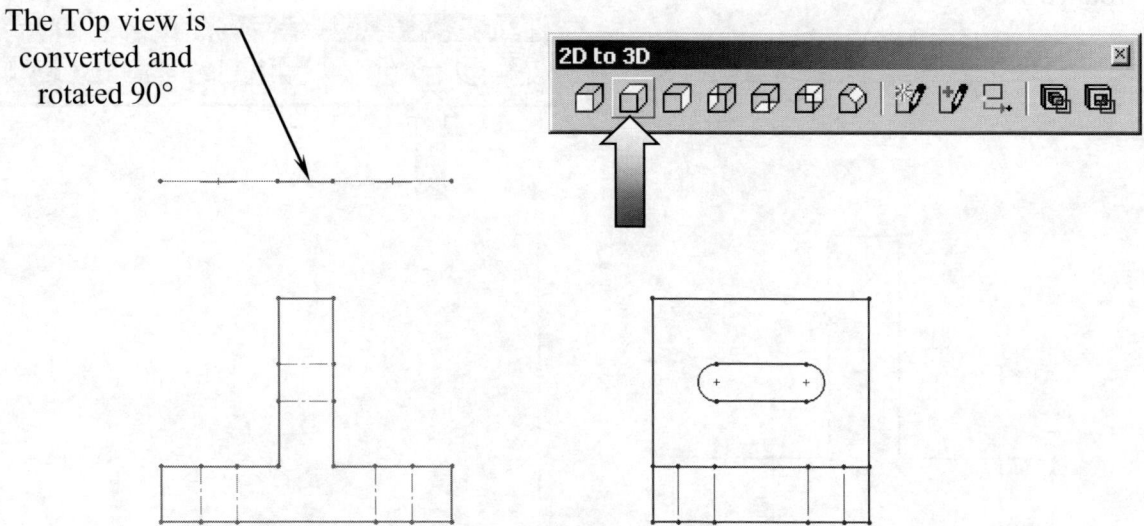 in the 2D-To-3D toolbar.

- The Top view is converted and rotated 90°.

The Top view is converted and rotated 90°

- Drag select (click-hold-drag) the Right view.

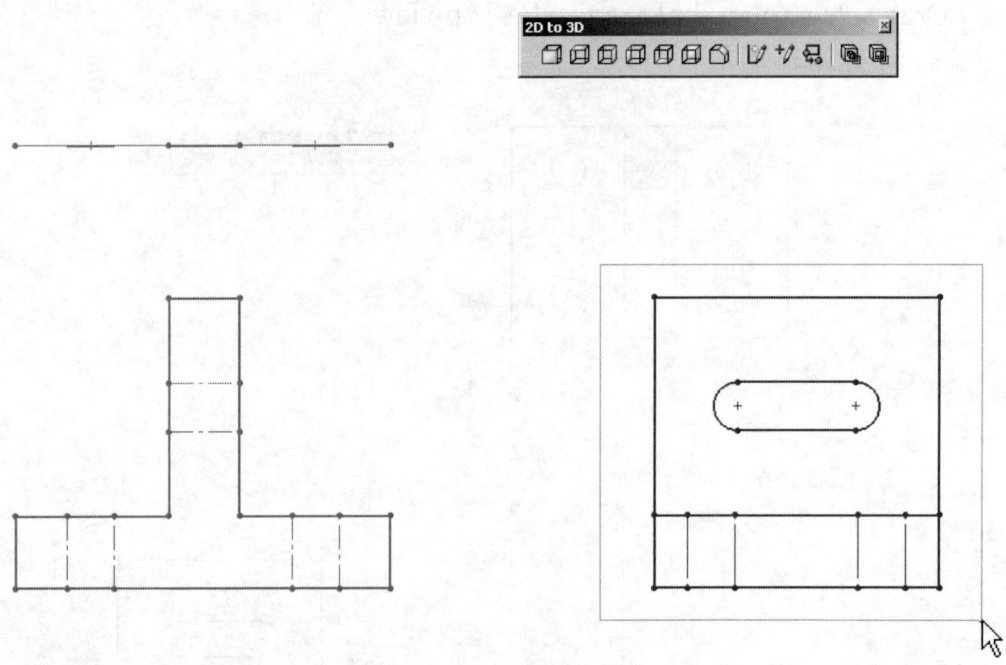

- Click RIGHT ⬛ in the 2D-To-3D toolbar.

- The Right view is converted and rotated 90°.

The Right view is
converted and
rotated 90°

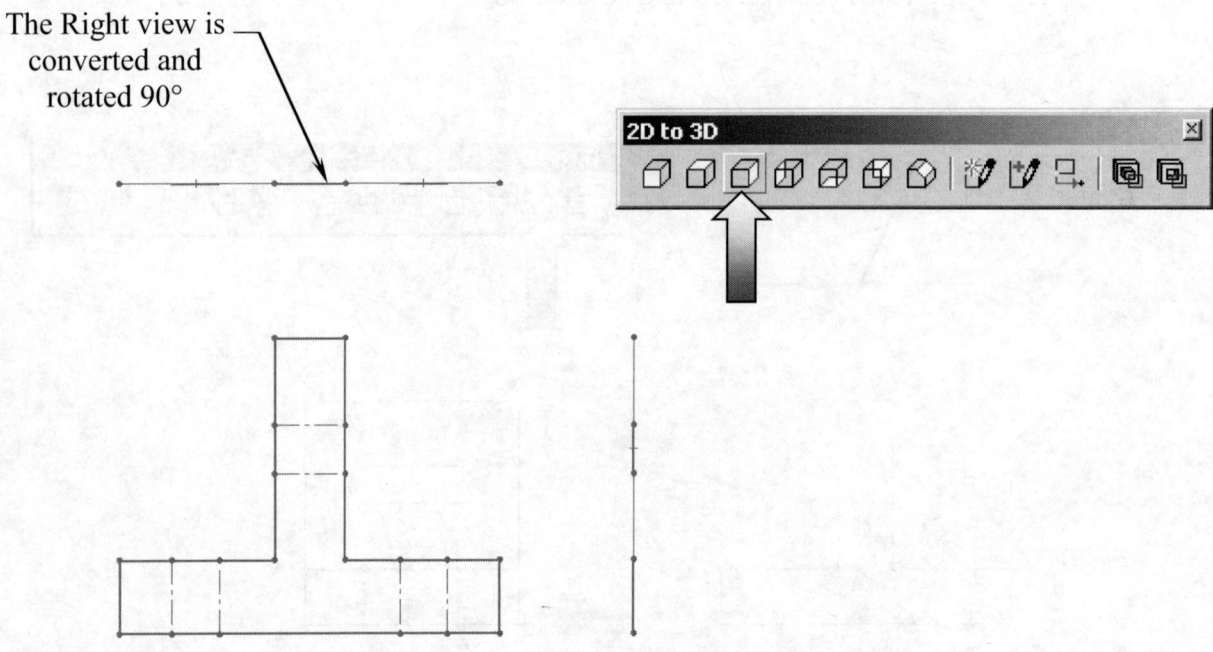

- Change to the Isometric view 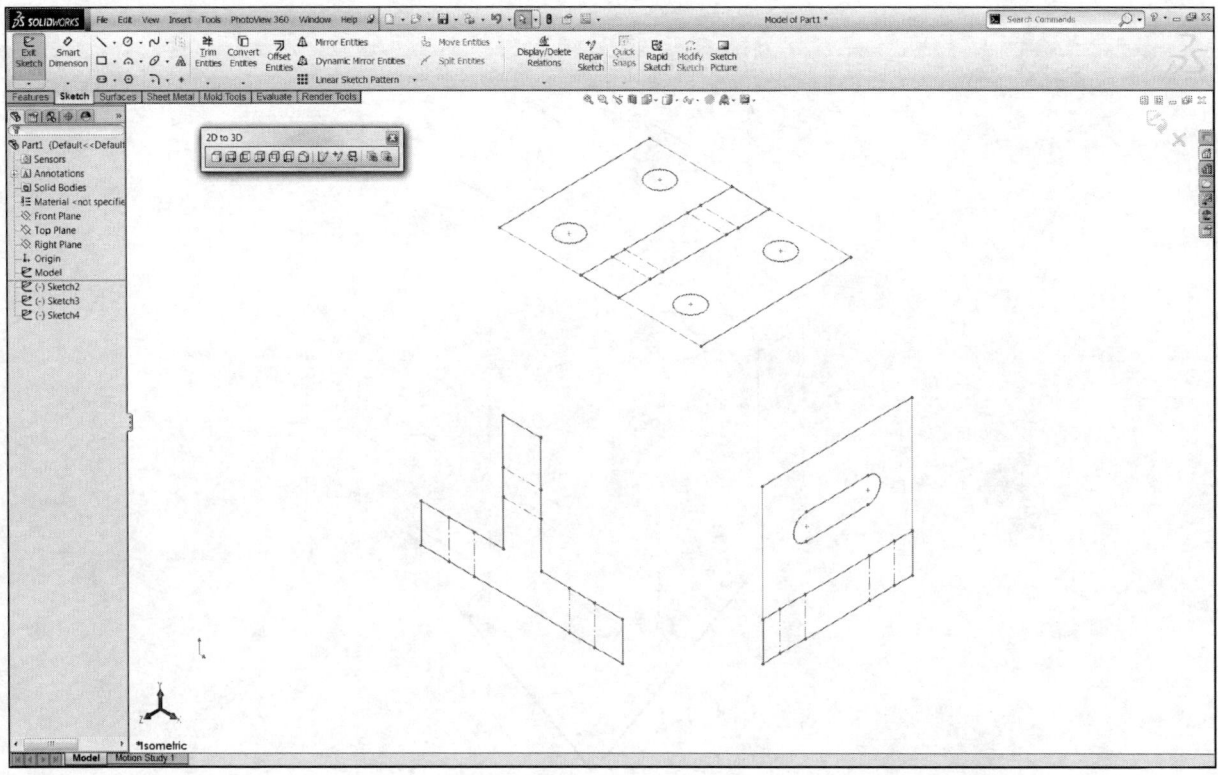 (or press Ctrl + 8), the next step is to align the sketches before making the extrusions.

4. Aligning the three views:

- While holding the CONTROL key, select the **left-edge** of the Top view and the *left-edge* of the Right view as shown.

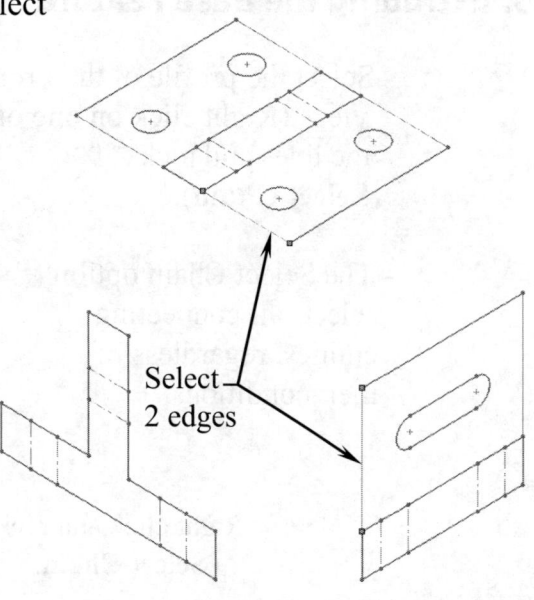

- Click Align Sketch on the 2D-To-3D tool bar.

- The 2 selected views are aligned.

Select 2 edges

- Change to the Right view to verify the result of the alignment.

- Repeating step 4:

- Repeat step number 4 and align the 2 bottom lines between the Front and the Right views.

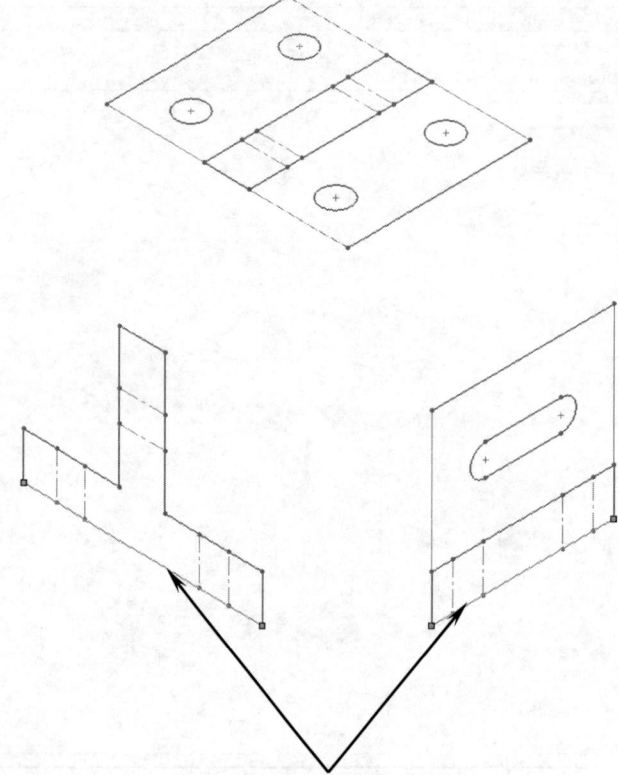

Align the 2 bottom lines.

5. Extruding the Base Feature:

- Select the profile of the Front view. (Right click on one of the lines and pick: **Select Chain**).

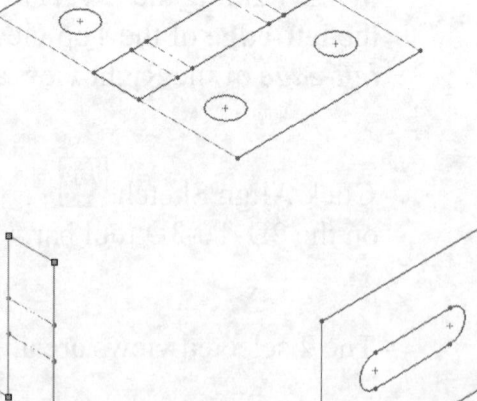

- The Select Chain option selects all connecting entities, regardless of their conditions.

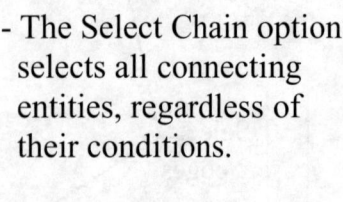

Right click and pick —— **Select Chain**.

- Click Extrude 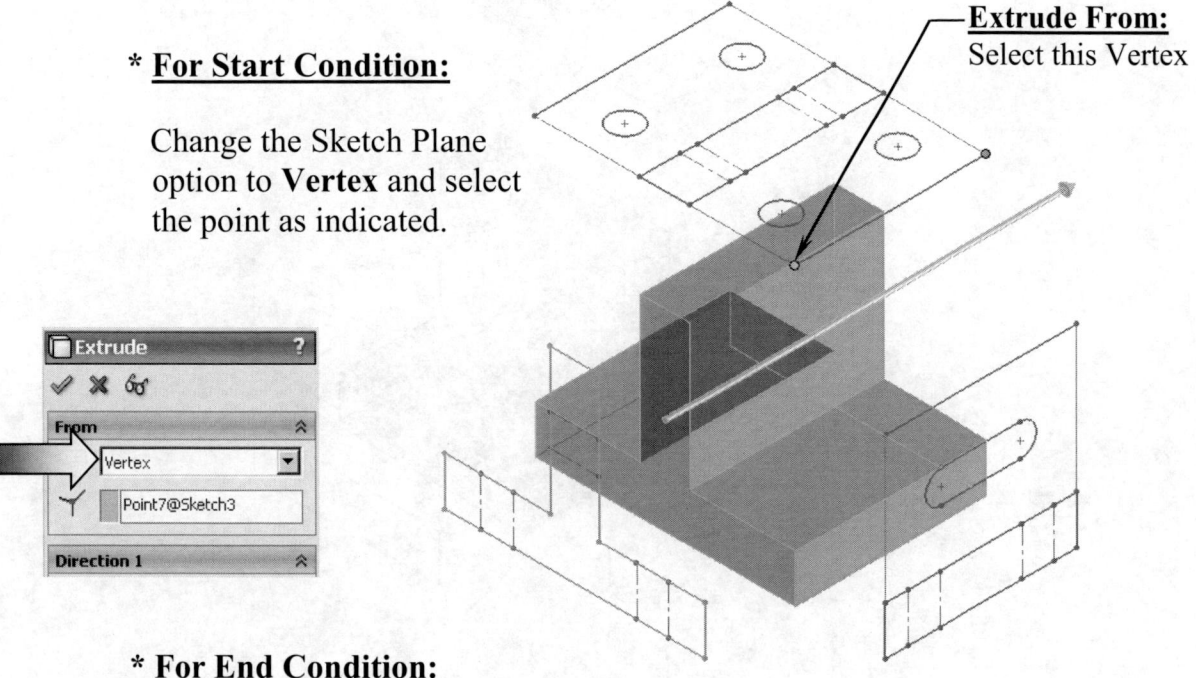 on the 2D-To-3D toolbar or select **Tools / Sketch Tools / 2D-To-3D / Extrude**.

* For Start Condition:

Change the Sketch Plane option to **Vertex** and select the point as indicated.

Extrude From:
Select this Vertex

* For End Condition:

Change the Direction 1 to **Up To Vertex** and select the point as indicated.

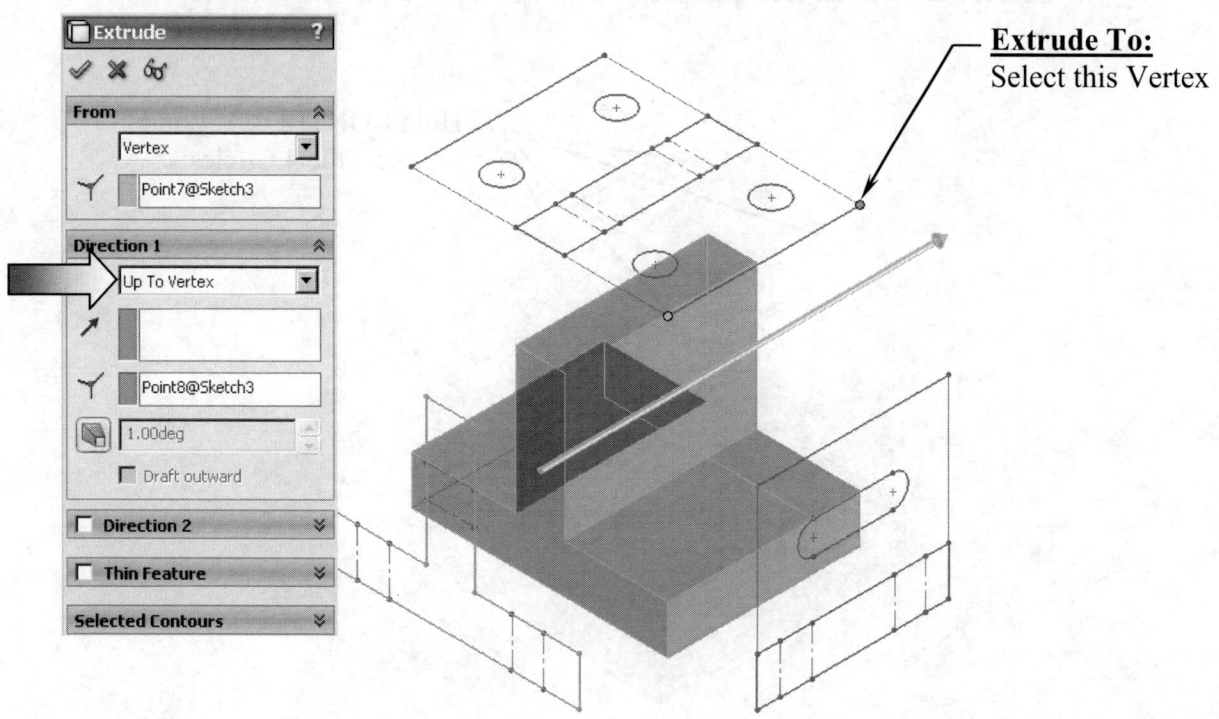

Extrude To:
Select this Vertex

- The solid feature is created from an imported drawing and is centered between the three views.

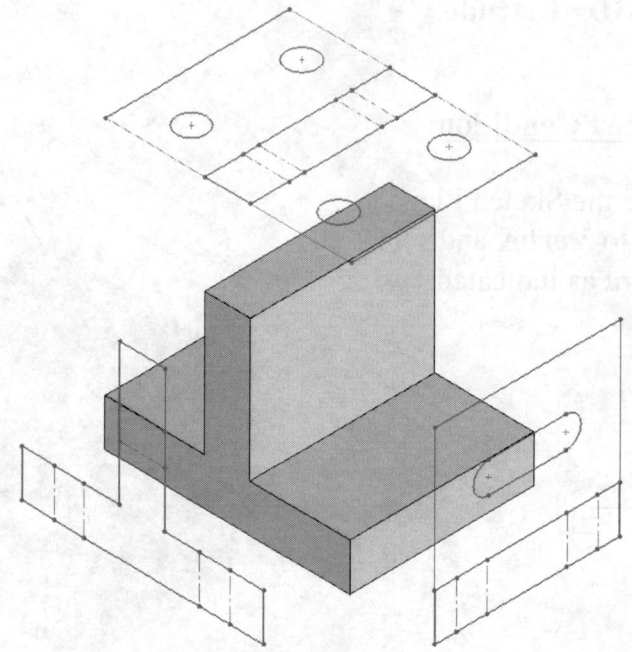

6. Creating the first Cut extrude, the 4 Holes:

- Select the **four circles** and press **Cut** 🔲 on the 2D-To-3D toolbar.

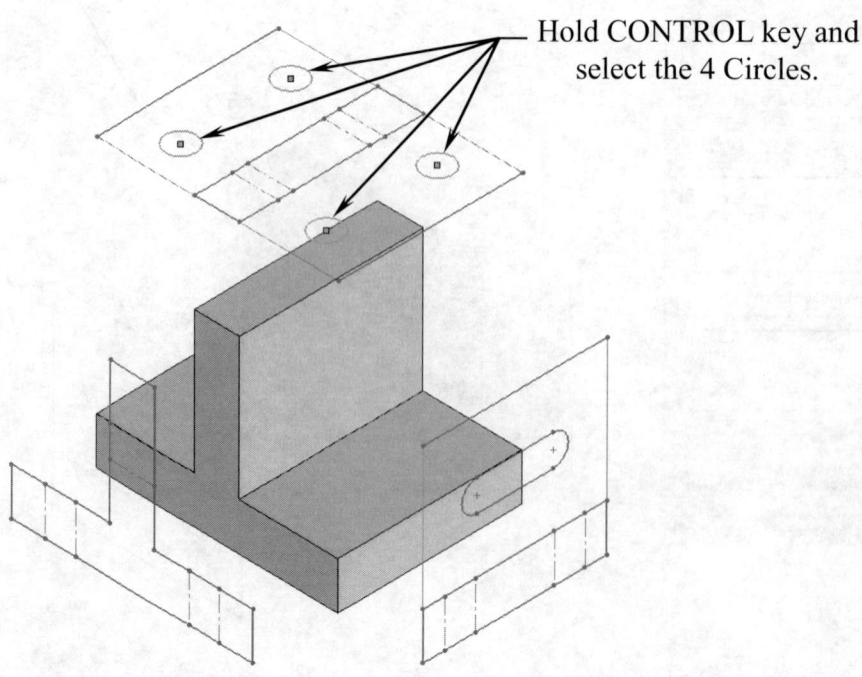

Hold CONTROL key and select the 4 Circles.

- Change the Direction 1 to **Through All**.

- Click **OK** 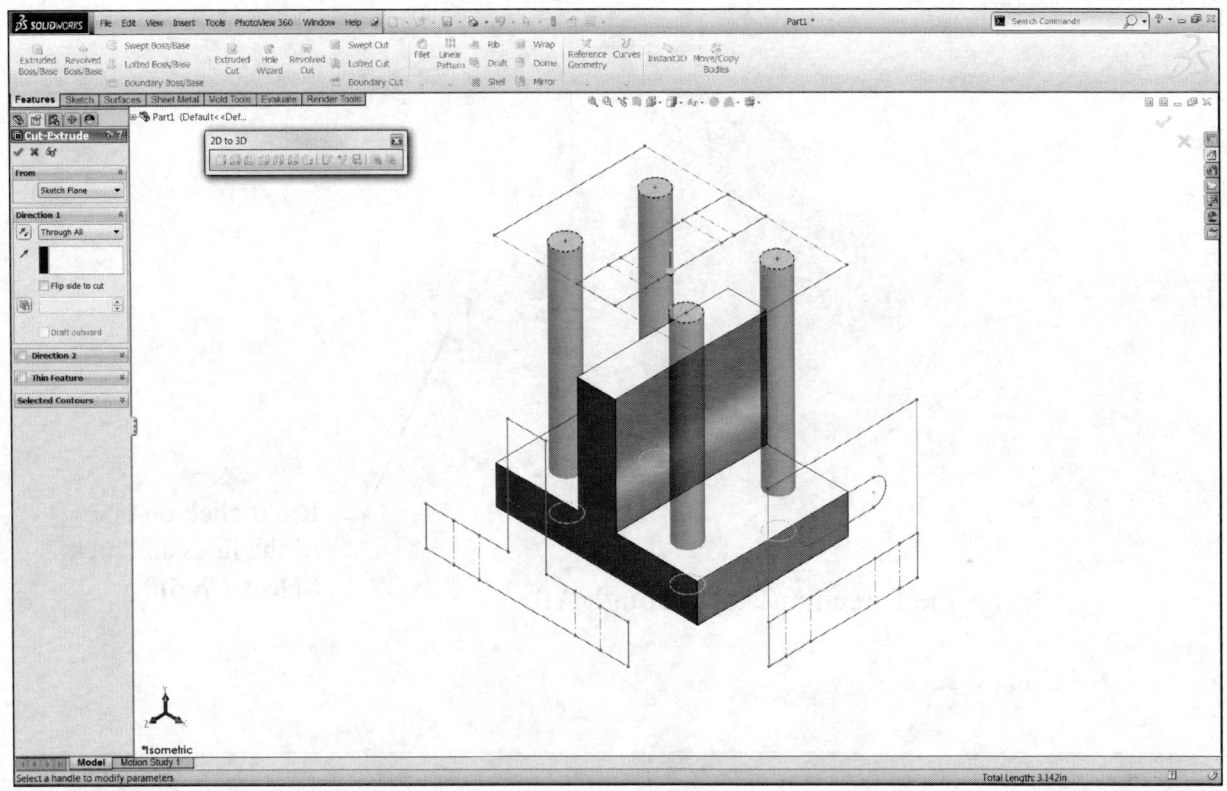.

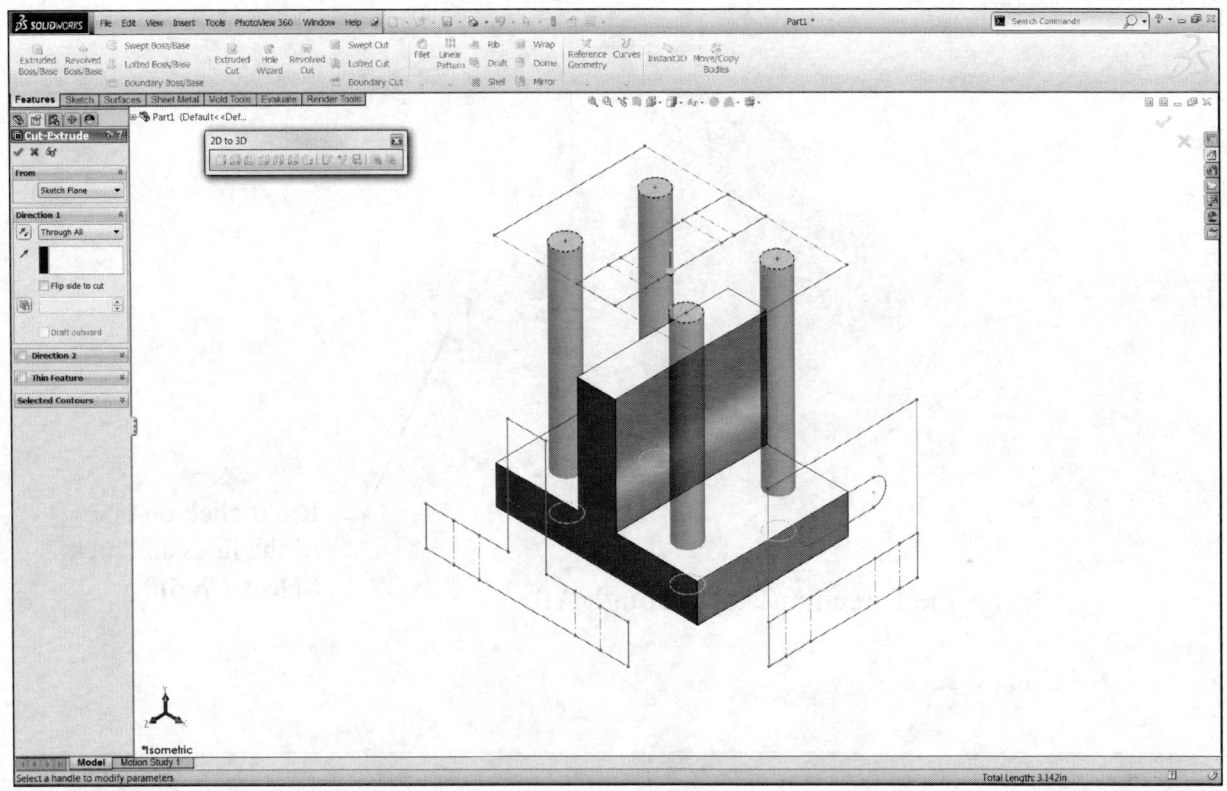

- The Cut feature is created; rotate the part to verify the result.

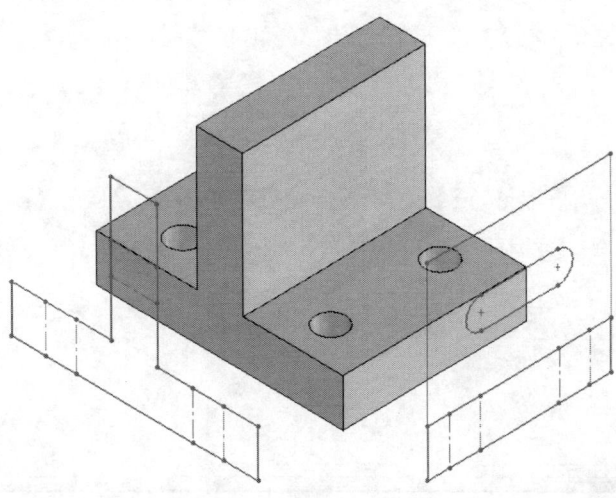

7. Create the second Cut extrude, the Center Slot:

- Right click on one of the lines of the slot and pick **Select-Chain**.

- Press **Convert To Cut** 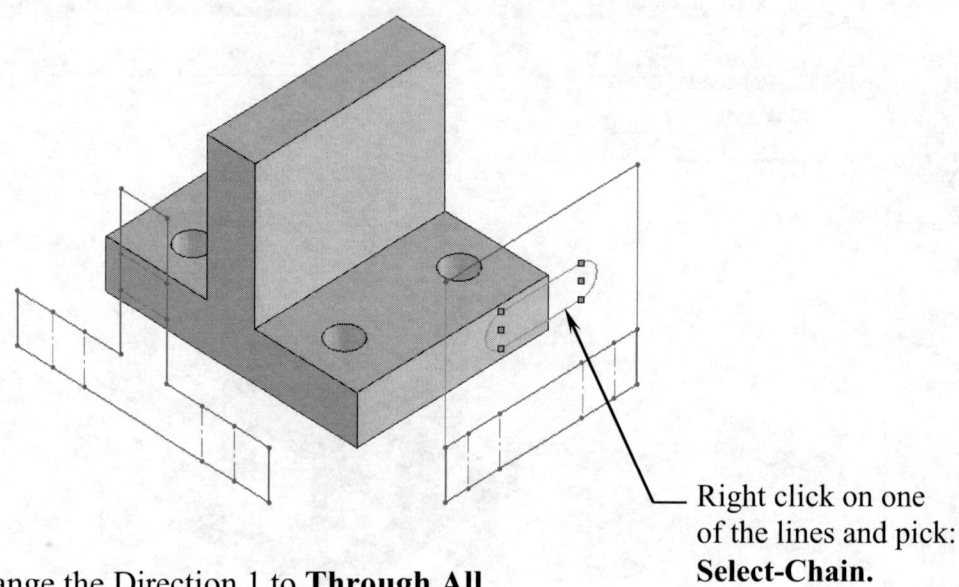 on the 2D-To-3D toolbar.

Right click on one
of the lines and pick:
Select-Chain.

- Change the Direction 1 to **Through All**.

- Click **OK** .

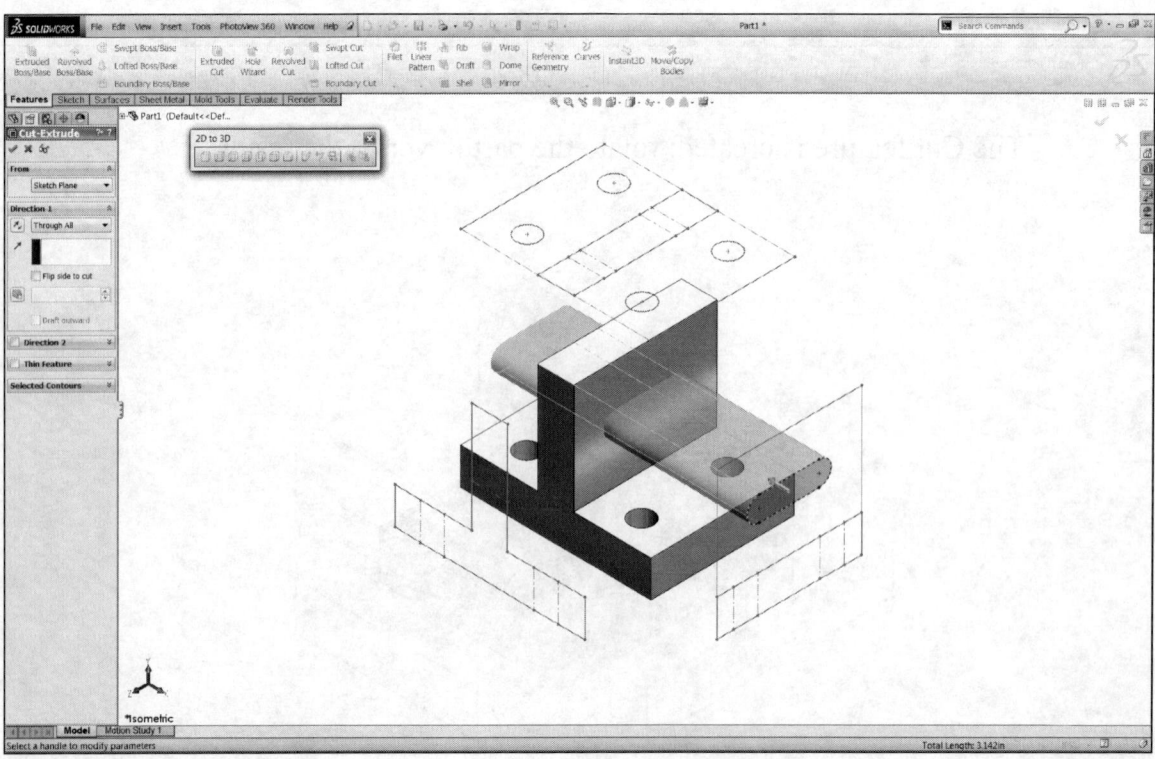

- The Slot feature is created; rotate the model to check out the cut.

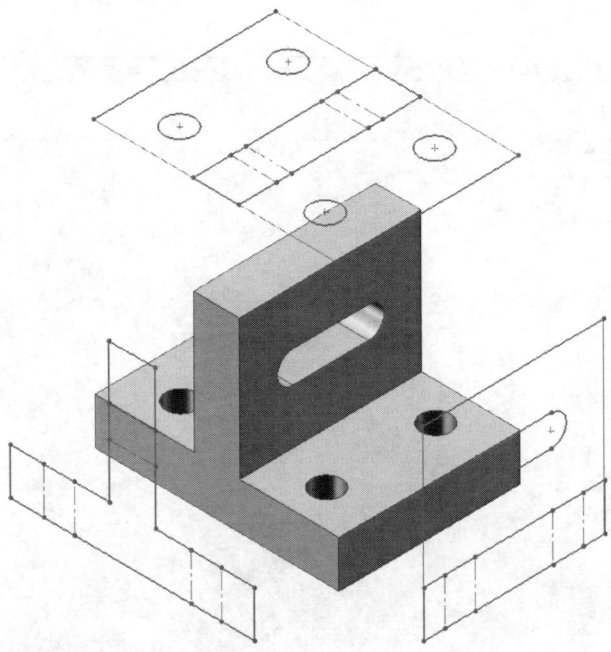

8. Hiding the Front sketch:

- Right click on one of the lines of the Front sketch and select **Hide.**

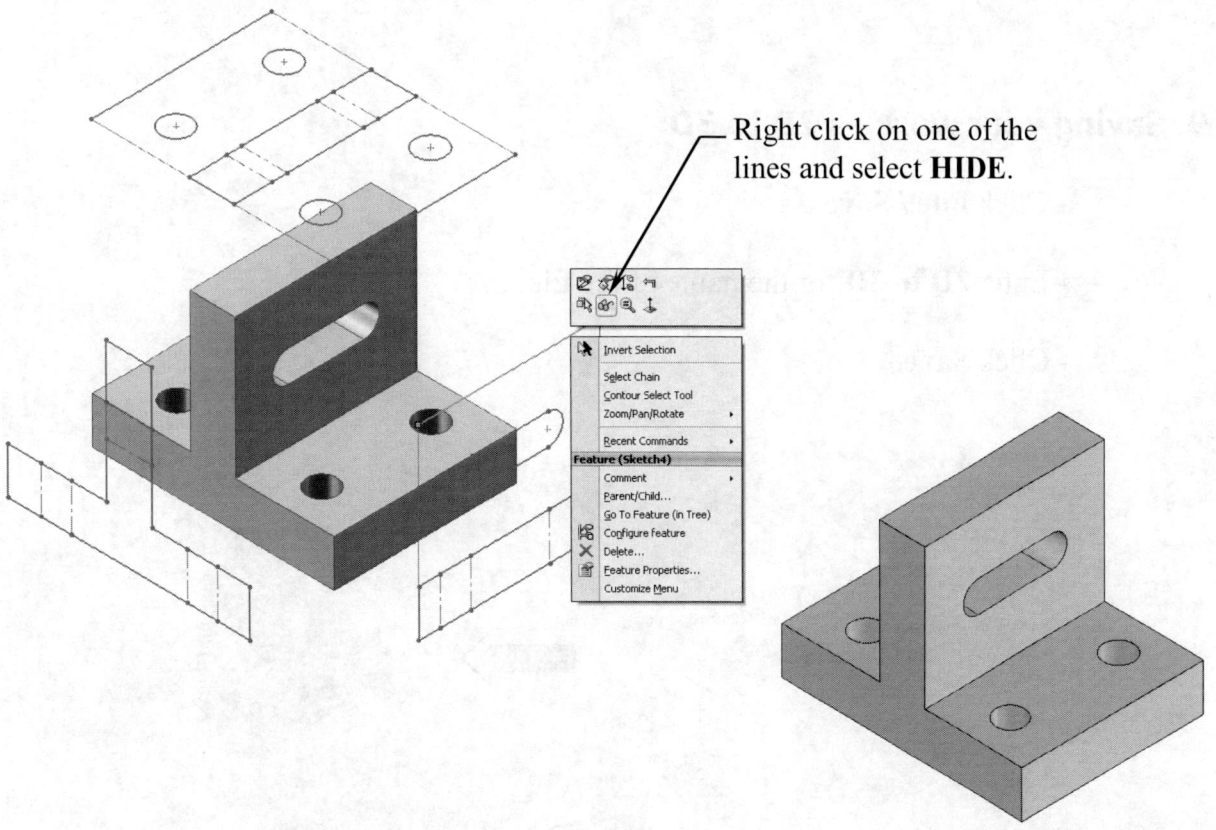

Right click on one of the
lines and select **HIDE.**

- The AutoCAD drawing has been converted into SolidWorks 3D solid model.

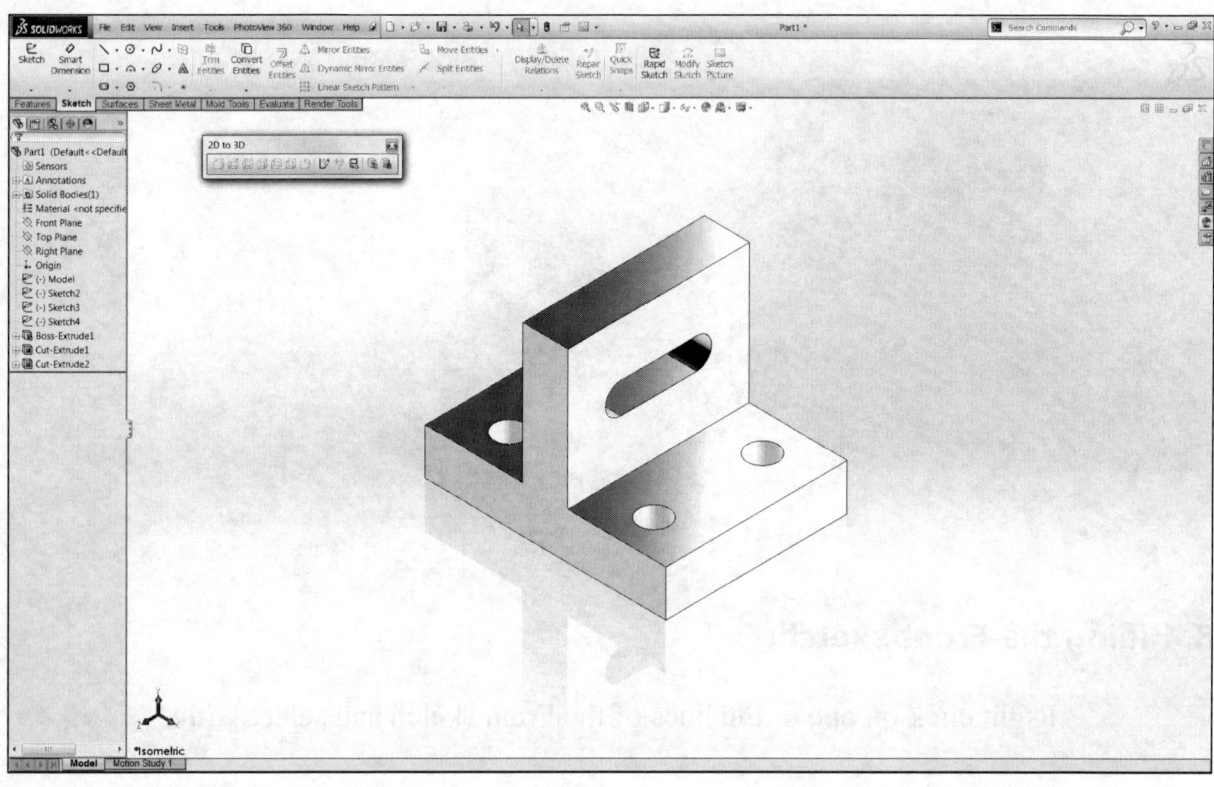

9. Saving your work as 2D to 3D:

- Click **File / Save As**.

- Enter **2D to 3D** for the name of the file.

- Click **Save**.

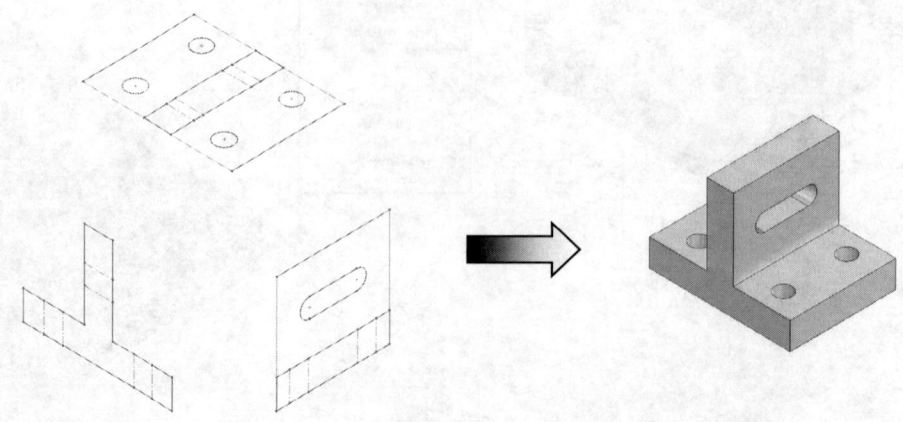

Questions for Review

2D To 3D Conversion

1. The 2D to 3D option allows sketches created in SolidWorks or other CAD software to be converted into 3D solid models.
    a. True
    b. False

2. Both .DXF and .DWG formats are supported for 2D to 3D conversion.
    a. True
    b. False

3. A .DWG document can be inserted into a new SolidWorks drawing or to a new part as a sketch.
    a. True
    b. False

4. The Front view does not have be selected and converted first, no sequence is required.
    a. True
    b. False

5. After the views are converted, they should be aligned with each other.
    a. True
    b. False

6. To select all sketch entities in a view press Control + A.
    a. True
    b. False

7. Before extruding, one view should be selected and a line or a dimension should be used to specify the depth.
    a. True
    b. False

8. A closed sketch profile can be used to make an Extruded-Cut only, not an Extruded-Boss.
    a. True
    b. False

7. True	8. False
5. True	6. False
3. True	4. False
1. True	2. True

Exercise: Modeling & Detailing III

1. Create the **part** and **drawing** as shown.
2. Dimensions are in inches, 3 decimal.
3. All connected edges are tangent.
4. Save the solid model and drawing as: **2D to 3D Part**.

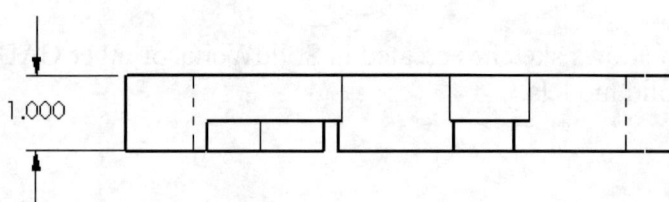

1.000

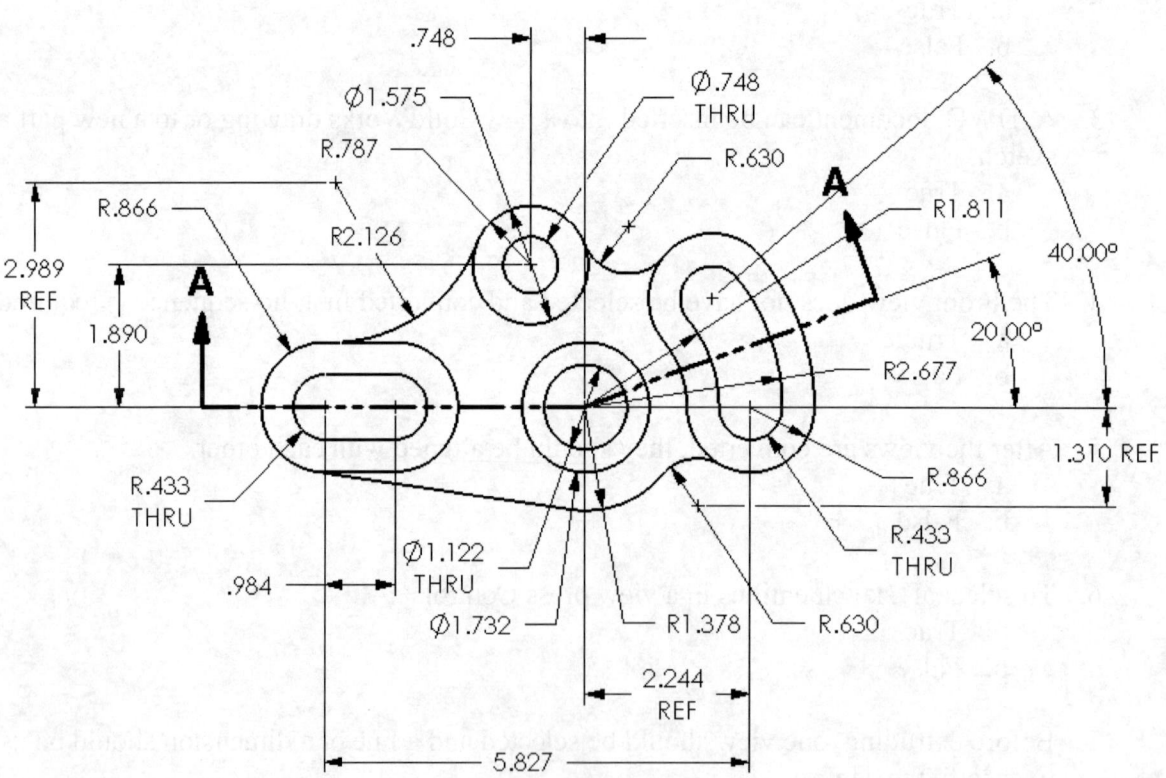

.748

Ø1.575

R.787

R.866

R2.126

2.989
REF

A

1.890

R.433
THRU

.984

Ø1.122
THRU

Ø1.732

R1.378

R.630

Ø.748
THRU

R.630

A

R1.811

40.00°

20.00°

R2.677

1.310 REF

R.866

R.433
THRU

2.244
REF

5.827

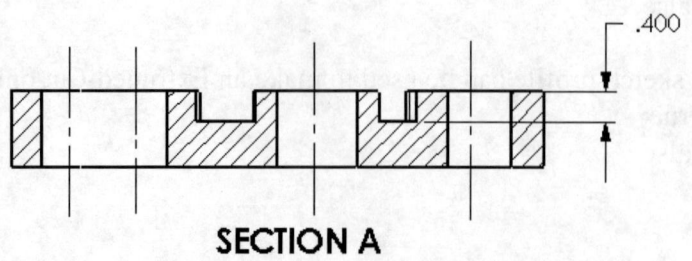

.400

SECTION A

CHAPTER 18 (cont.)

e-Drawings

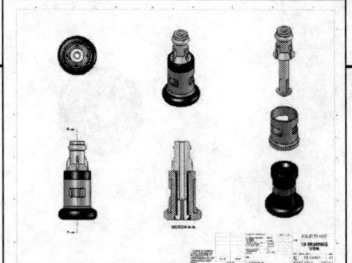

eDrawing & 3D Drawing View

Soft-lock Assembly

eDrawing:

- eDrawing is one of the most convenient tools in SolidWorks to create, share, and view your 2D or 3D designs.

- The eDrawing Professional allows the user to create eDrawing markup files (***.markup**) that have markups, such as text comments and geometric elements.

- With eDrawing 2015 and SolidWorks® 2015, you can create an eDrawing from any CAD model or assembly from programs like AutoCAD®, Creo®, and others.

- The following types of eDrawing files are supported:
  * 3D part files (***.eprt**)
  * 3D assembly files (***.easm**)
  * 2D drawing files (***.edrw**)

3D Drawing View:

- The 3D drawing view mode lets you rotate a drawing view out of its plane so you can see components or edges obscured by other entities. When you rotate a drawing view in 3D drawing view mode, you can save the orientation as a new view orientation.

- 3D drawing view mode is particularly helpful when you want to select an obscured edge for the depth of a broken-out section view. Additionally, while in 3D drawing view mode, you can create a new orientation for another model view. 3D drawing view mode is not available for detail, broken, crop, empty, or detached views.

Soft-Lock Assembly
SolidWorks e-Drawing & 3D Drawing View

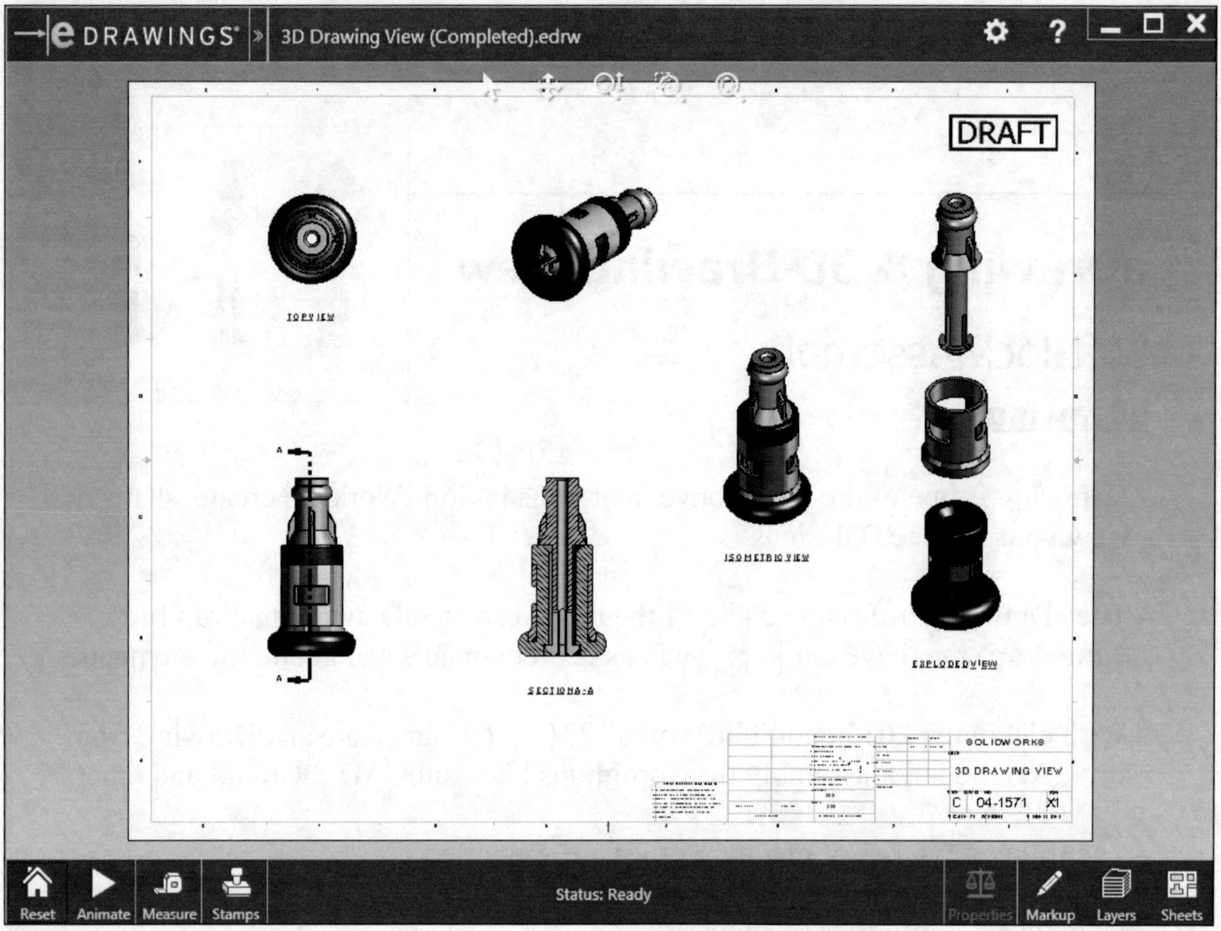

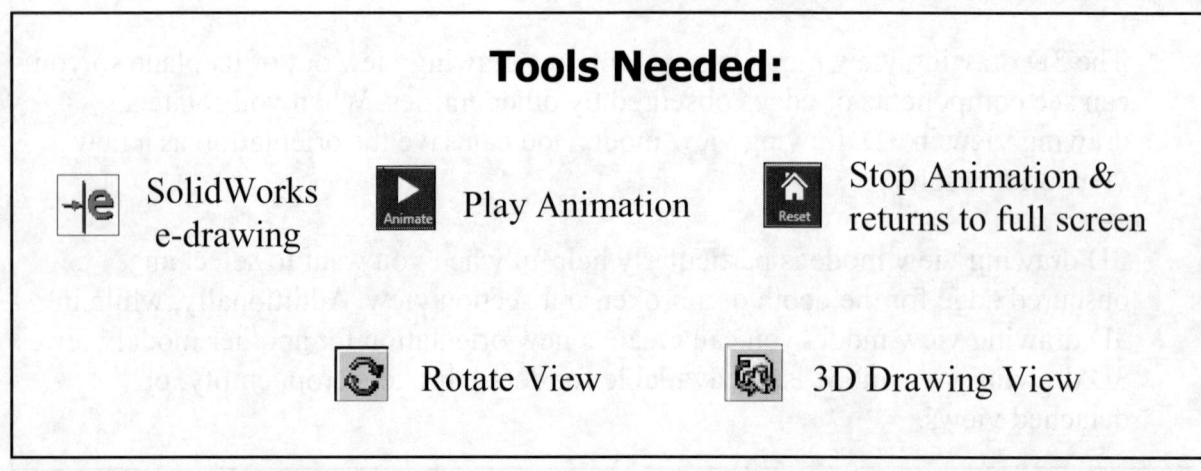

Dimensioning Standards: **ANSI**	Third Angle Projection
Units: **INCHES** – 3 Decimals	⊕ ◁

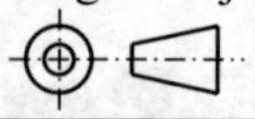

Tools Needed:

⊩e SolidWorks e-drawing	▶ Animate Play Animation	⌂ Reset Stop Animation & returns to full screen
	↻ Rotate View	🔄 3D Drawing View

1. Opening an existing drawing:

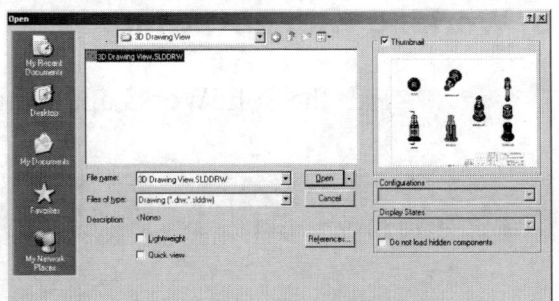

- Click **File / Open**.

- Select **3D Drawing View.slddrw**
  from the Training Files folder and
  open it.

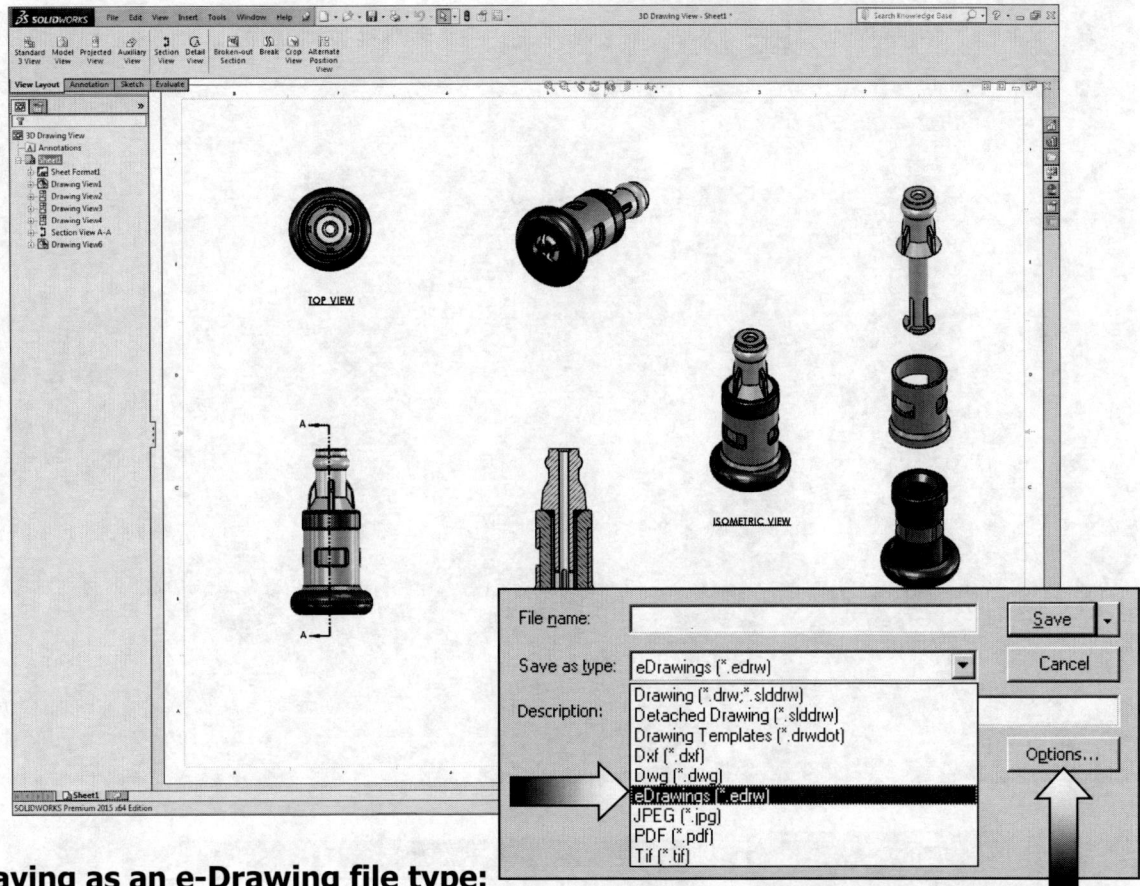

2. Saving as an e-Drawing file type:

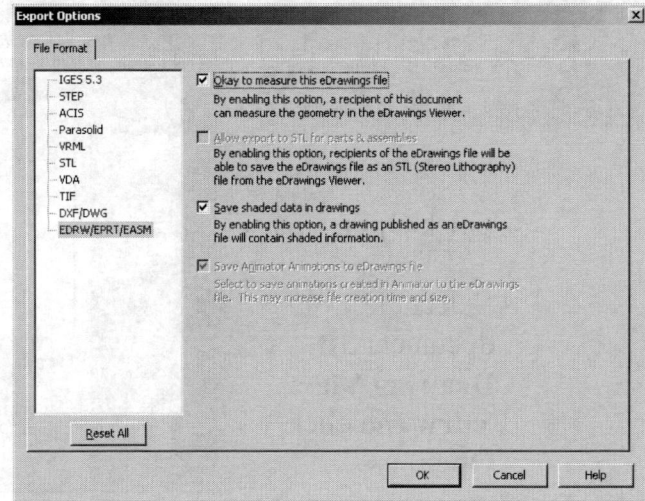

- Select **File / Save As.**

- Change the file format
  to **eDrawing** (*.edrw).

- Enter **3D Drawing View**
  as the file name.

- Click the Options button and
  enable **OK to Measure**.

- Click **Save**.

3. Working with eDrawing:

- Exit the SolidWorks application and launch the **e-Drawing** program .

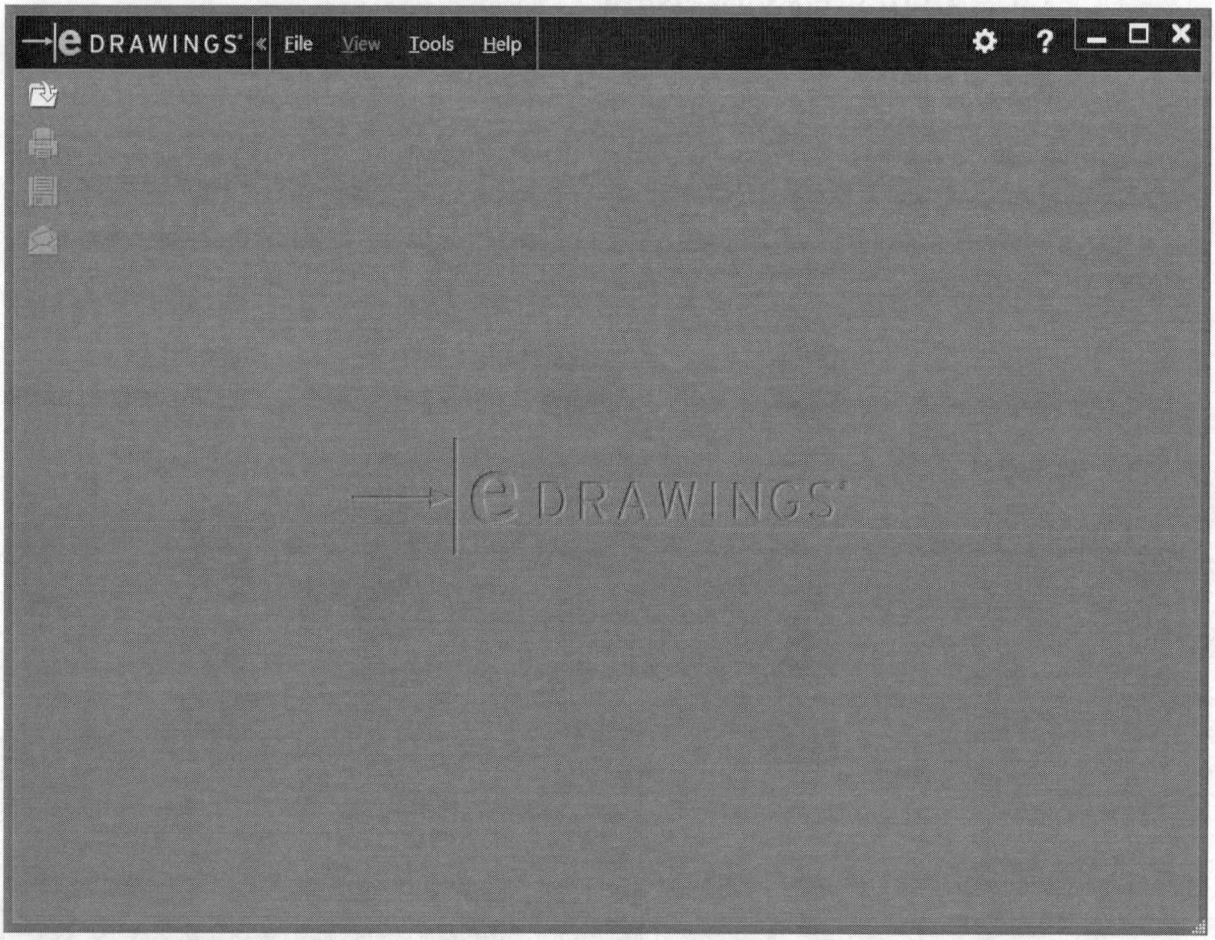

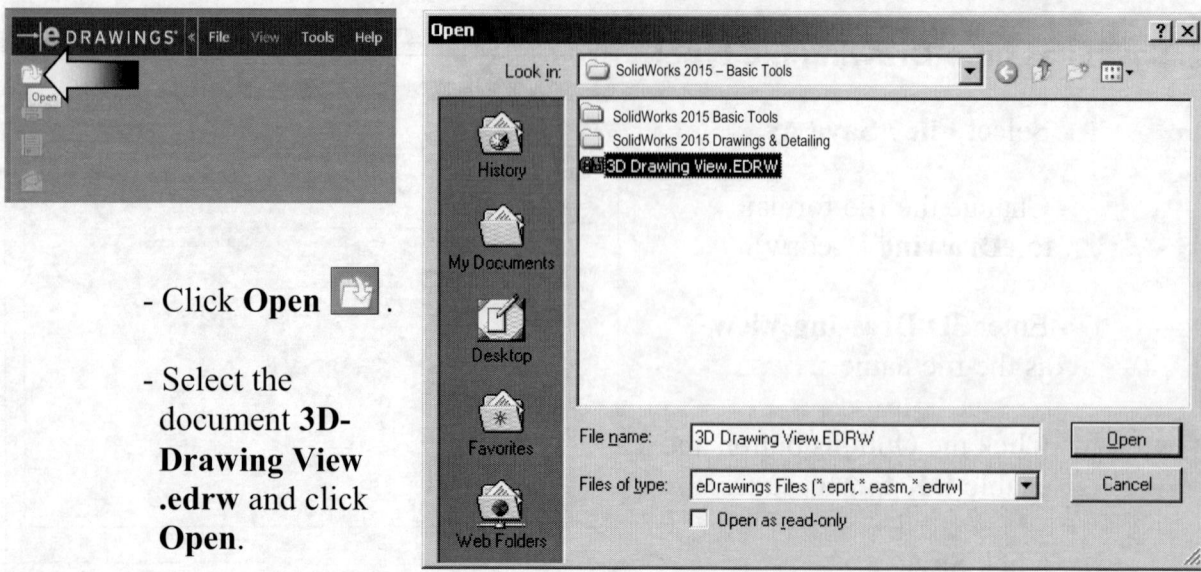

- Click **Open** .

- Select the document **3D-Drawing View .edrw** and click **Open**.

- The previously saved drawing is opened in the new User Interface 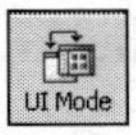 .

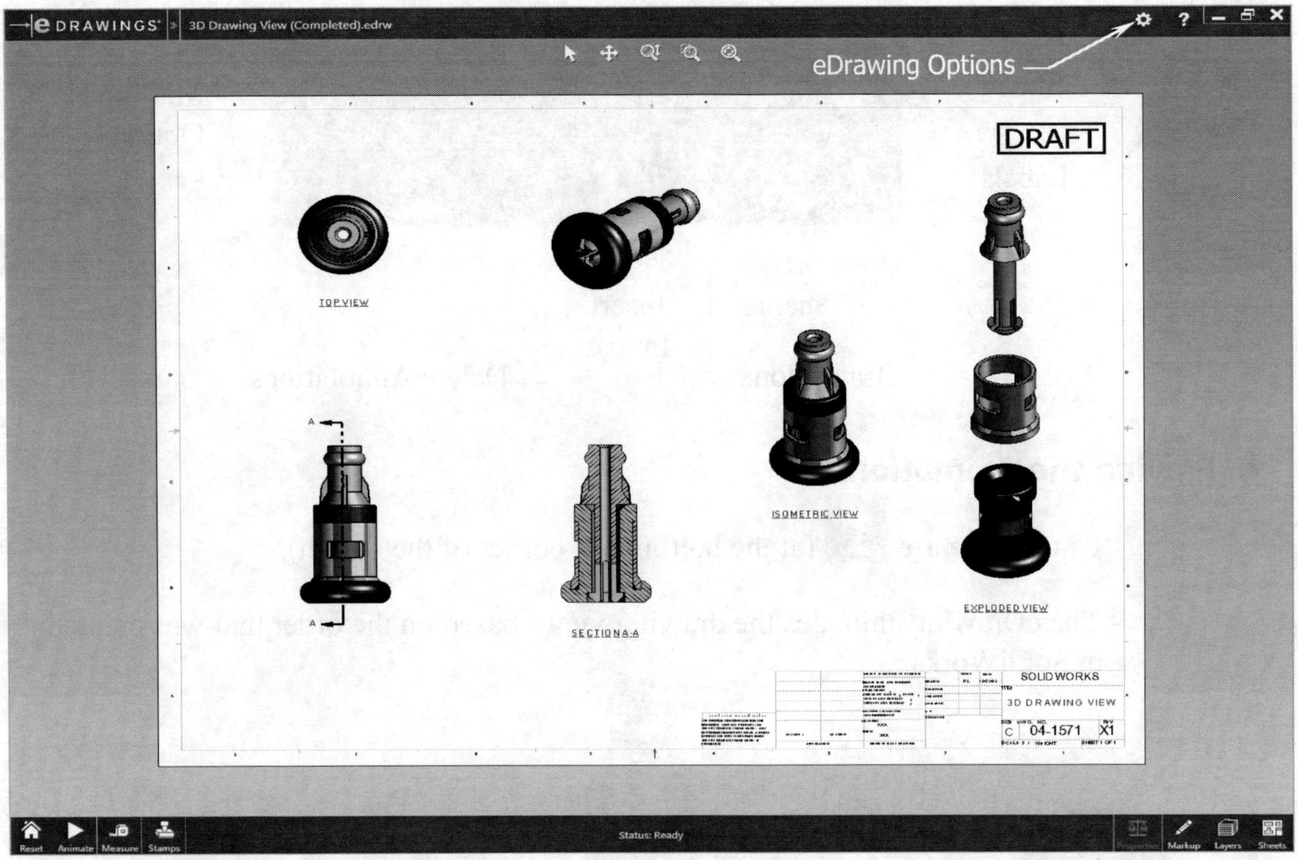

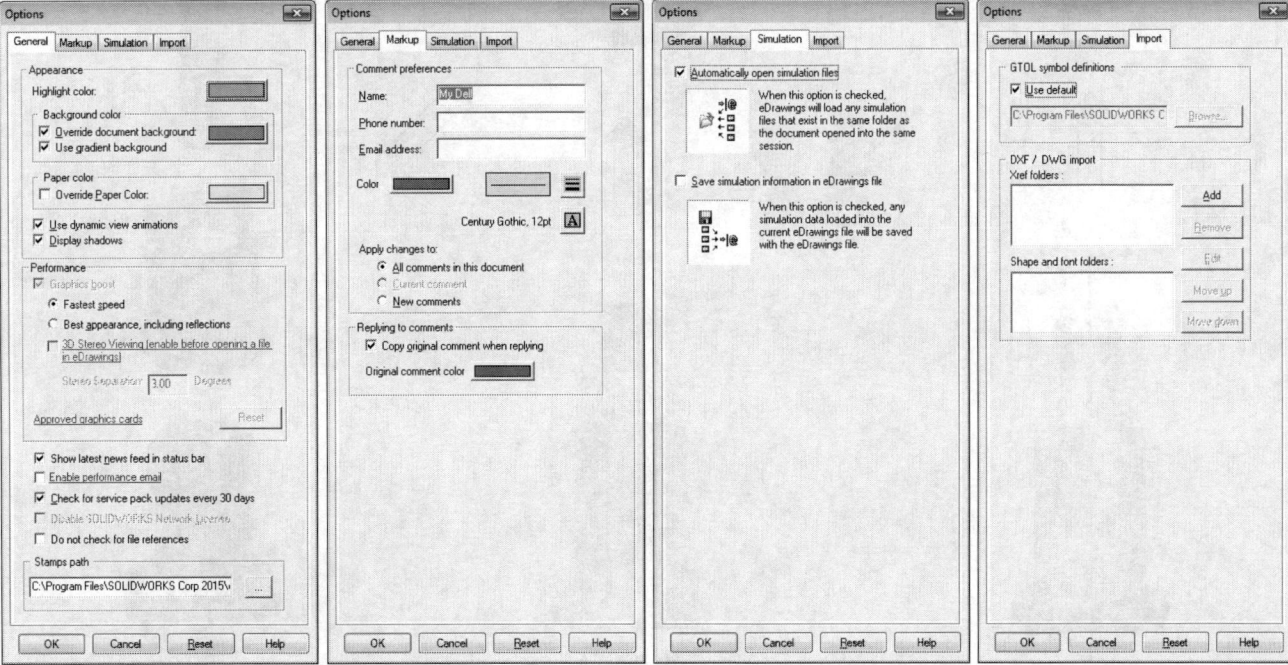

- The eDrawing Options:

- The **Markup** toolbar:

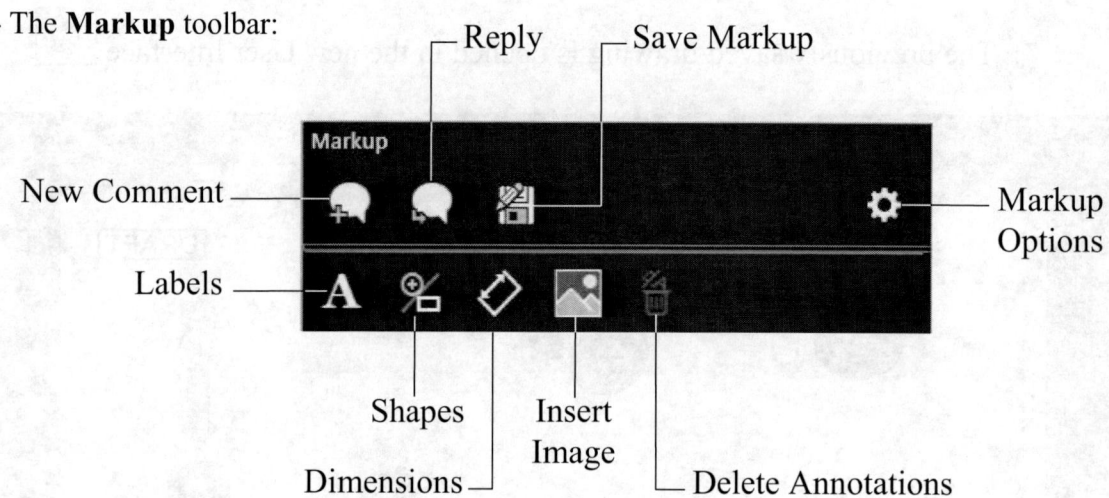

Reply — Save Markup

New Comment —

Markup Options

Labels —

Shapes

Dimensions

Insert Image

Delete Annotations

4. Playing the Animation:

- Click **Animate** (at the bottom left corner of the screen).

- The eDrawing animates the drawing views based on the order that was created in SolidWorks.

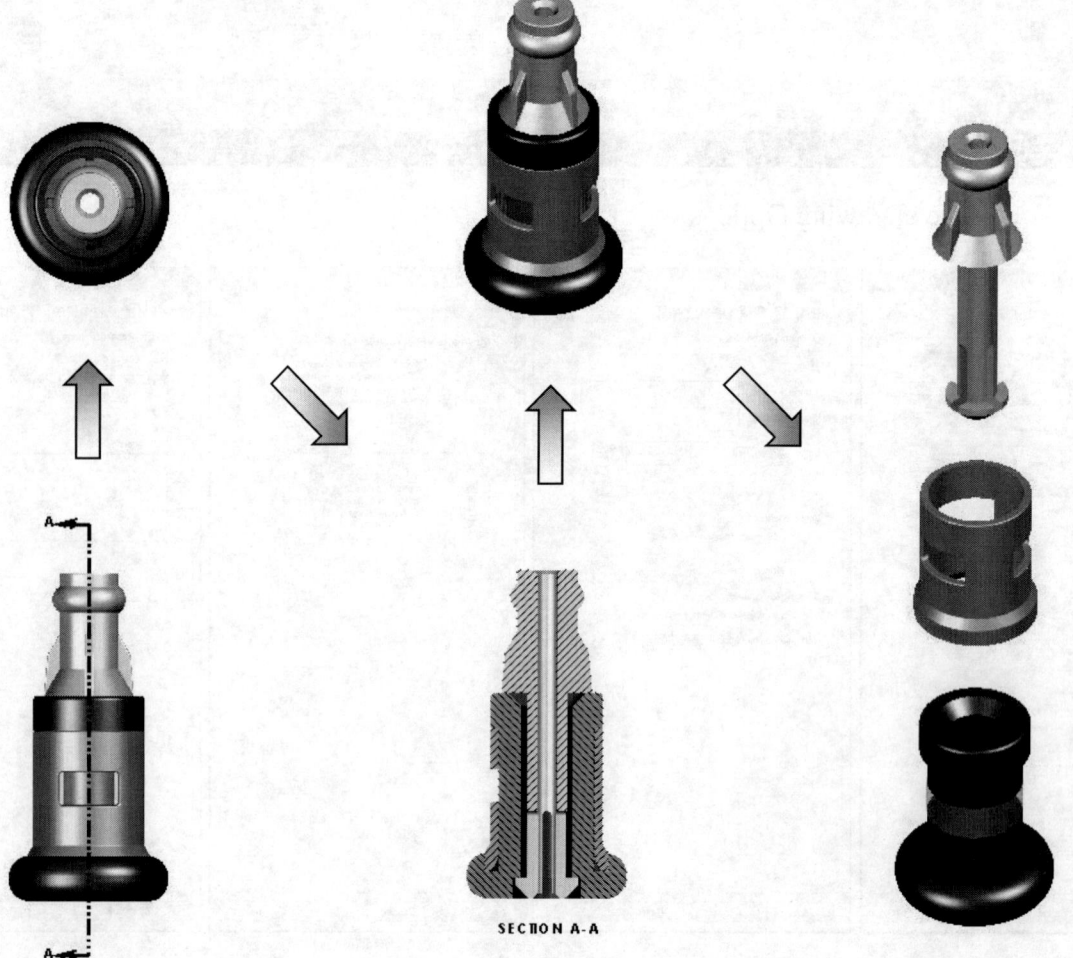

SECTION A-A

- Click **Reset** to stop the animation.

- The Reset command also returns the eDrawing back to its full page mode.

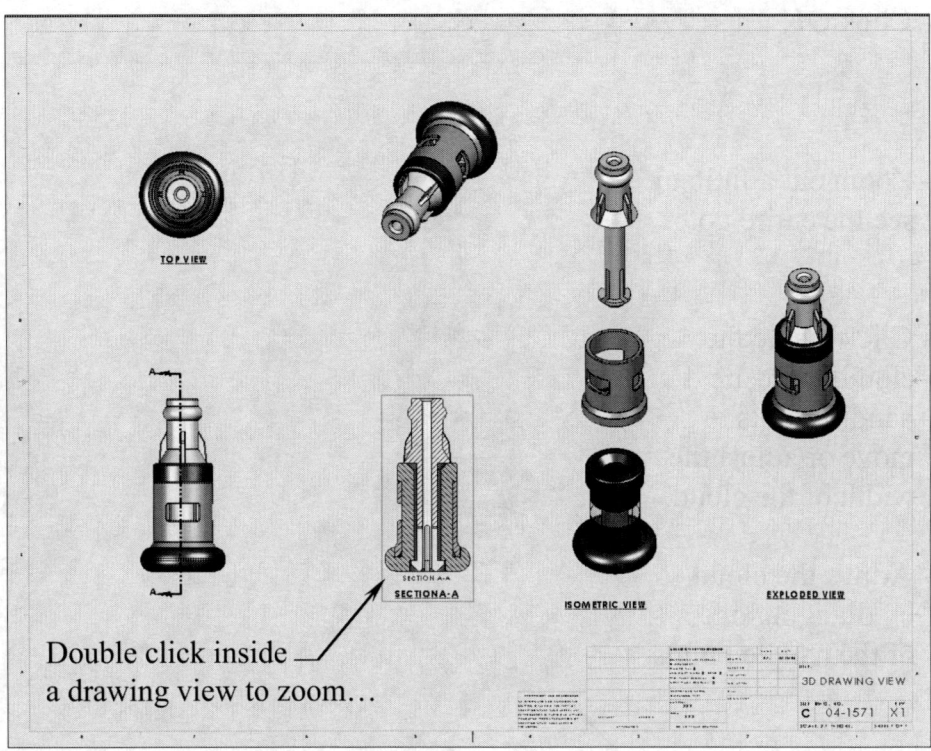

Double click inside
a drawing view to zoom…

- Double click inside the Section view to zoom and fit it to the screen.

5. Adding the markup notes:

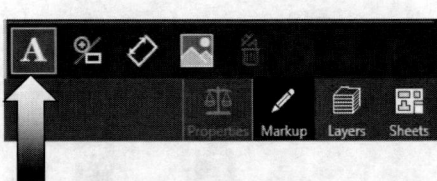

- Click the **Labels** button and select the **Cloud-With Leader** command (2nd arrow).

- Click on the **Edge** of the bottom bore hole and place the blank note on the lower left side.

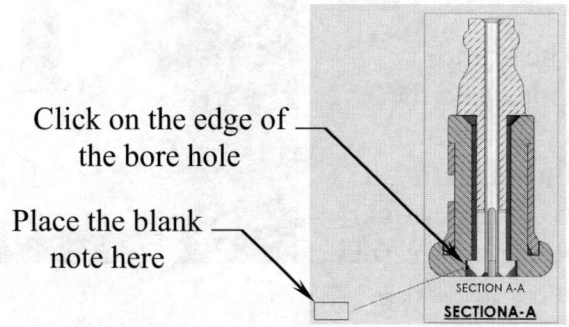

Click on the edge of
the bore hole

Place the blank
note here

- Enter the note:
Increase the Bore Diameter by .015".

- Click **OK**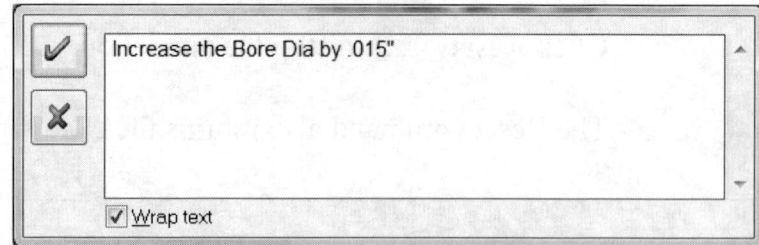

- Zoom out a little to see the entire note.

- Click inside the cloud; there are 4 handle points to move or adjust the width of the cloud.

- Adjust the cloud by dragging one of the handle points.

Drag handle point

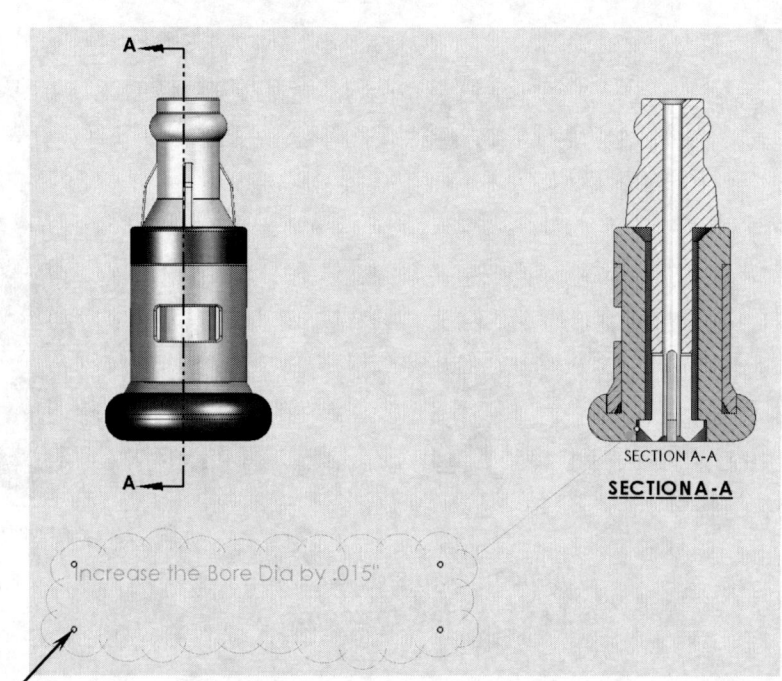

6. Adding a "Stamp":

- Click the **Stamp** button.

- Select the **DRAFT** stamp from the list.

- The stamp appears on the top left corner drawing. Drag it to the upper right corner and resize it.

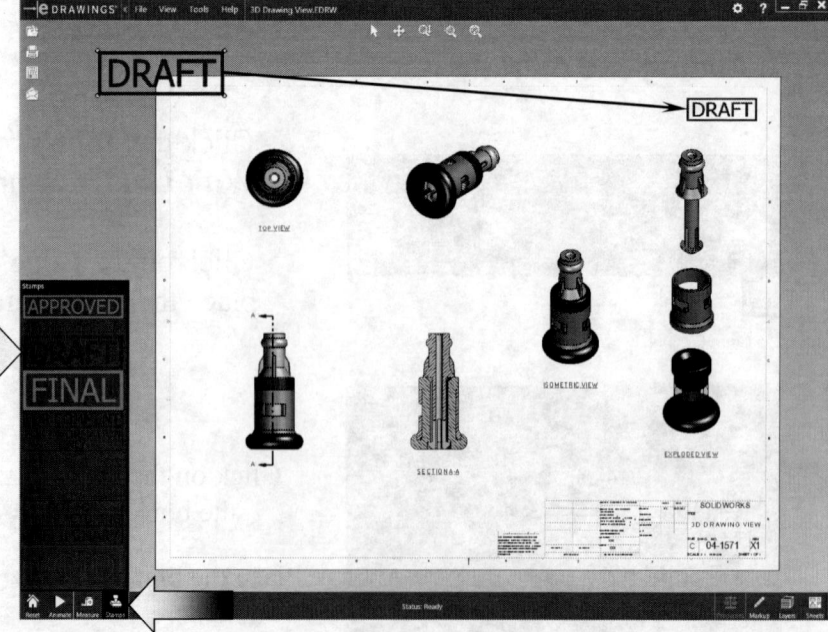

- Click the **Reset** button ![Reset] to return to the full drawing mode.

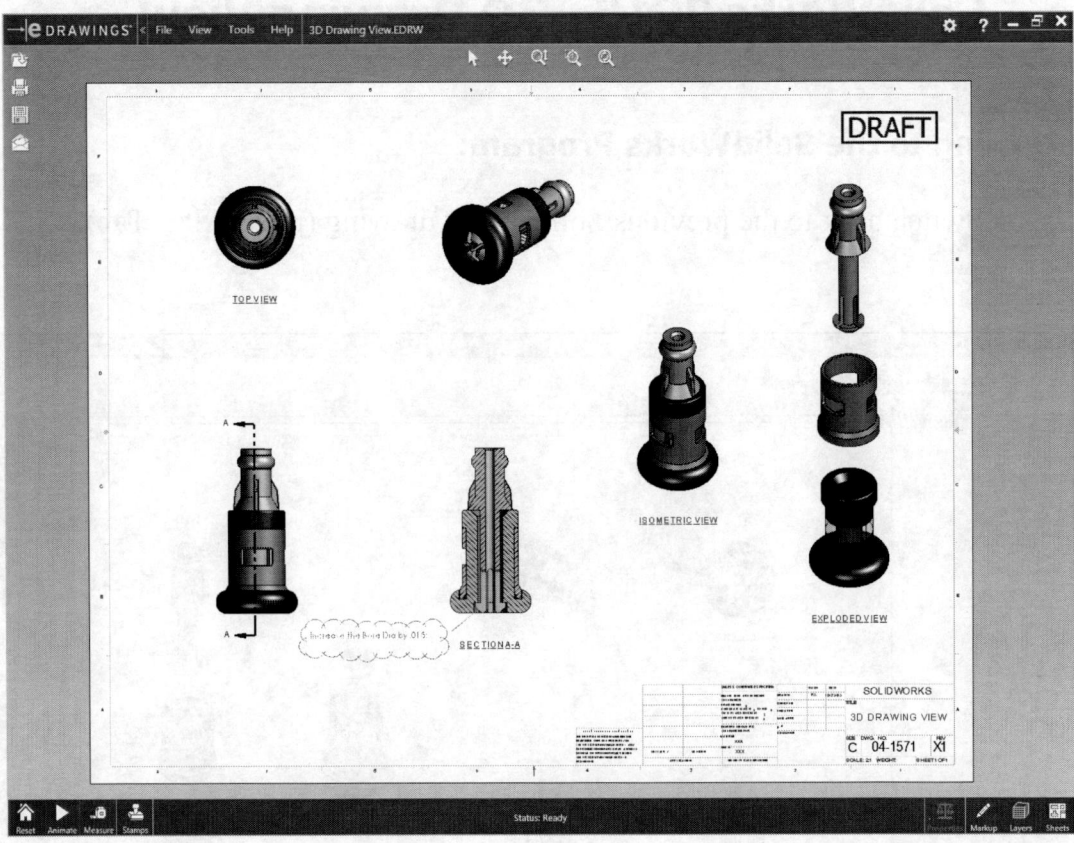

7. Saving as Executable file type:

- Click **File / Save As**.

- Select **eDrawing Executable Files (*.exe)** from the Save As Type menu & click **Save**.

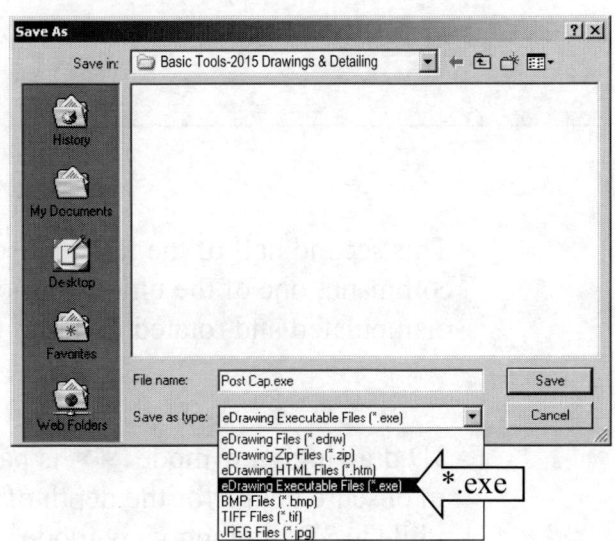

NOTES:

The .exe files are much larger in file size than the standard .edrw.

The .edrw files require eDrawing Viewer or the eDrawing Program itself to view.

Continue...

SolidWorks 2015 - 3D Drawing View

8. Returning to the SolidWorks Program:

- Switch back to the previous SolidWorks drawing (press Alt + Tab).

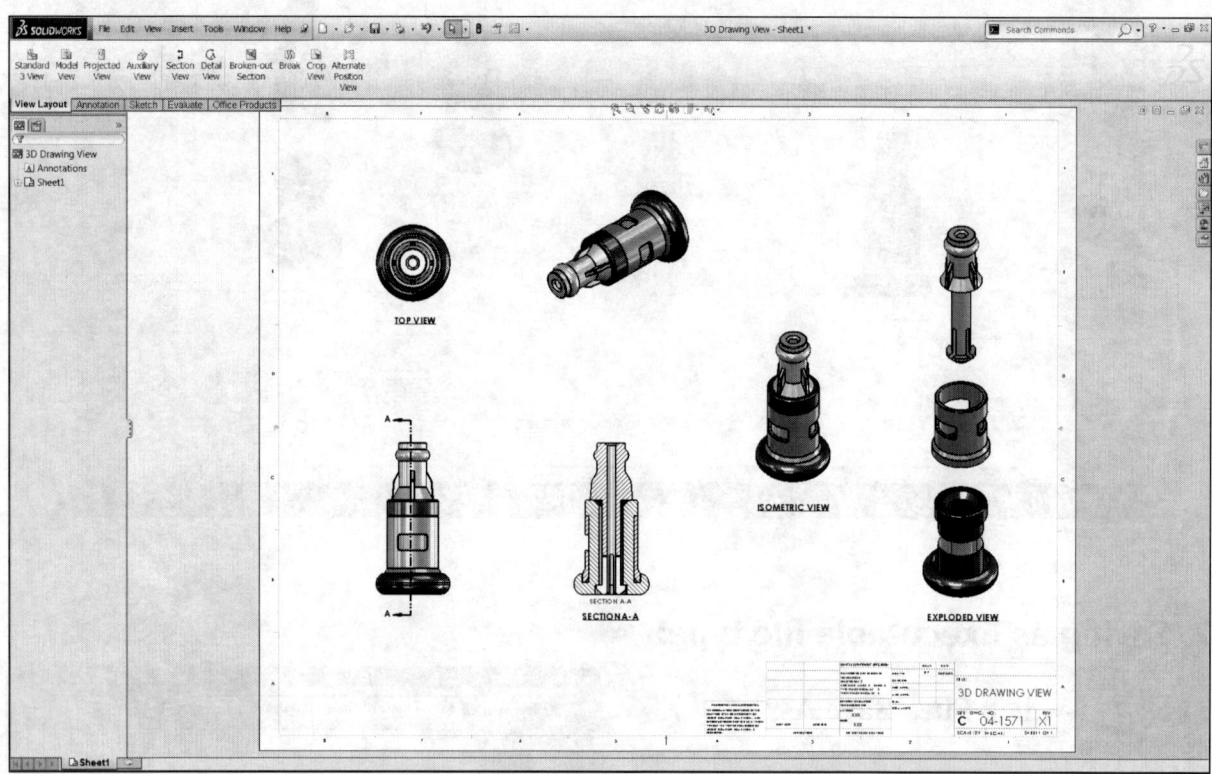

- This second half of the lesson discusses the use of the 3D Drawing View command, one of the unique options that allows a flat drawing view to be manipulated and rotated in 3D to make selections of the hidden entities.

- 3D drawing view mode is particularly helpful when you want to select an obscured edge for the depth of a broken-out section view. Additionally, while in 3D drawing view mode, you can create a new orientation for another model view.

9. Using the 3D Drawing View command: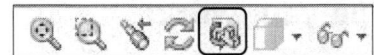

- Create <u>a new Front view</u> and then click the drawing view's border to activate it.

- Click the 3D Drawing View icon ![icon] from the View toolbar (or under the **View / Modify** menus).

- Select the Rotate tool ![icon] and rotate the Front drawing to a different position approximately as shown.

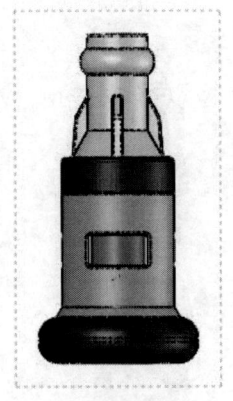

Front Drawing View

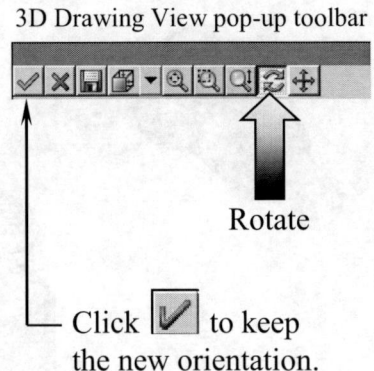

3D Drawing View pop-up toolbar

Rotate

Click ☑ to keep the new orientation.

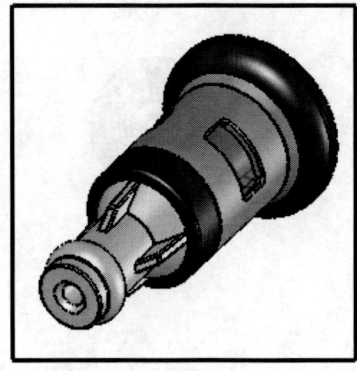

New 3D Drawing View

10. Saving the New-View orientation:

- Click Save ![icon] on the 3D Drawing View pop-up toolbar.

- Enter: **3D Drawing View** in the Named View dialog. This view orientation will be available under **More Views** in the **Model View PropertyManager** the next time you insert a model view.

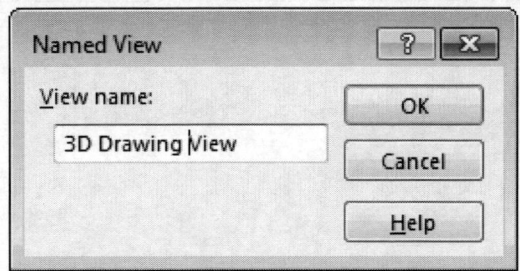

11. Saving your work:

- Click **File / Save As**.

- Enter **3D DrawingView** as file name.

- Click **Save**.

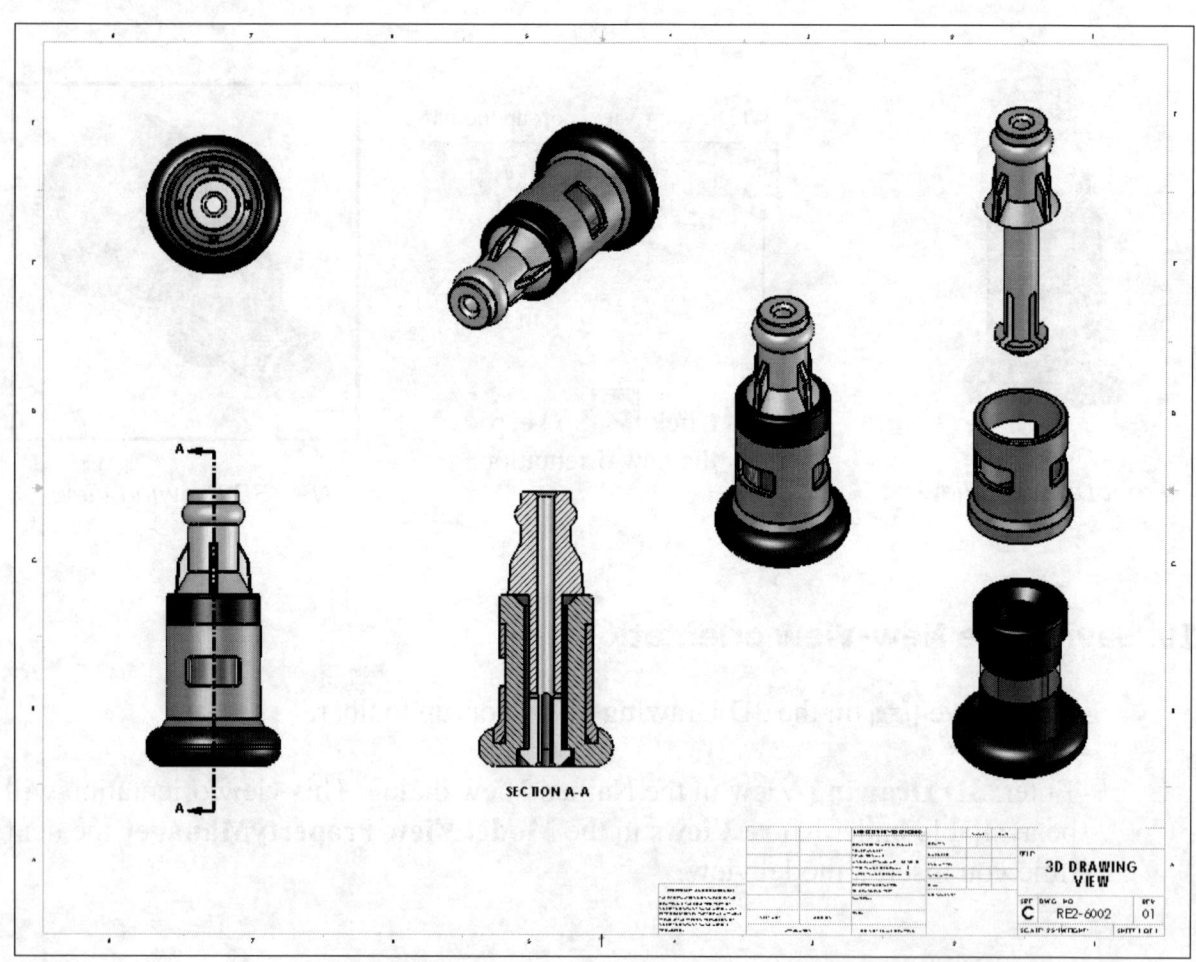

SECTION A-A

3D DRAWING VIEW

CHAPTER 19

Configurations - Part I

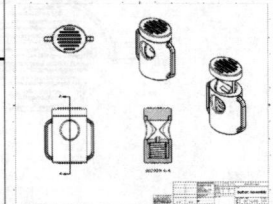

Configurations – Part I
Part, Assembly & Drawing

- Configurations is one of the unique options in SolidWorks which allows the users to create multiple variations of a part or assembly within the same document.

- Configurations provide a convenient way to develop and manage families of parts with different dimensions, components, or other parameters.

- In a **Part document**, configurations allow you to create families of parts with different dimensions, features, and custom properties.

- In an **Assembly document**, configurations allow you to create:

    * Simplified versions of the design by suppressing or hiding the components.

    * Families of assemblies with different configurations of the components, parameters, assembly features, dimensions, or configuration-specific custom properties.

- In a **Drawing document**, you can display different views of different configurations that you created earlier in the part or assembly documents by accessing the properties of the drawing view.

- This chapter will guide you through the basics of creating configurations in the part and assembly levels. Later on, these configurations will be called up in a drawing to display the changes that were captured earlier.

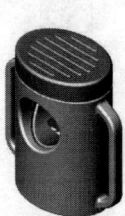
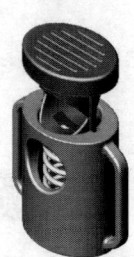
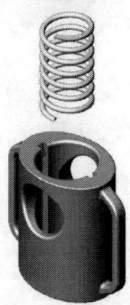

Configurations – Part 1
Part, Assembly & Drawing

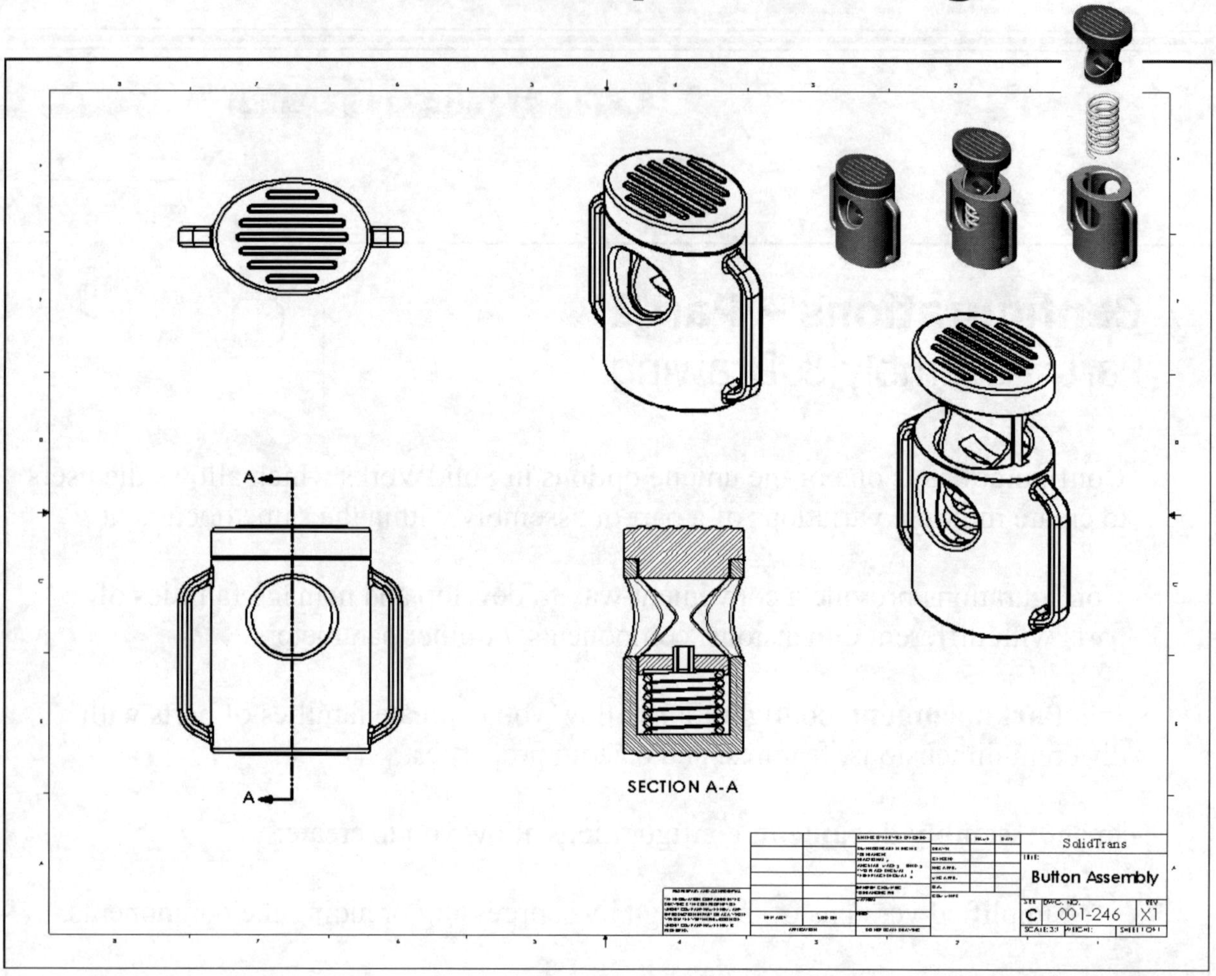

SECTION A-A

			SolidTrans
		TITLE	**Button Assembly**

SIZE: **C** | DWG. NO. 001-246 | REV X1

Dimensioning Standards: **ANSI**	Third Angle Projection
Units: **INCHES** – 3 Decimals	

Tools Needed:

 Part document

Part

 Assembly document

Assembly

 Drawing document

Drawing

Add Configuration

Default
Expanded

1. Opening the existing Assembly Document:

<u>Go to:</u>   Training Files folder
            Button Assembly folder
            Open **Button Assembly.sldasm**

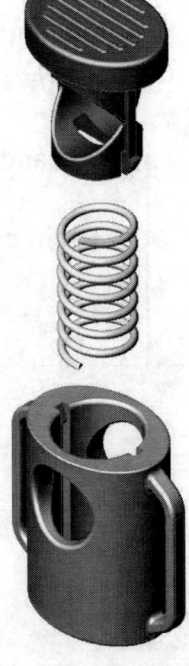

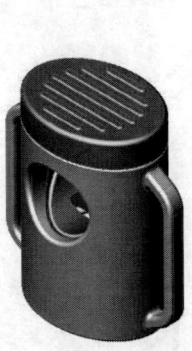

2. Using Configurations in the Part mode:

- From the FeatureManager tree, right click on **Button Spring** and select **Open Part.**

- Change to the **ConfigurationManager** tree.

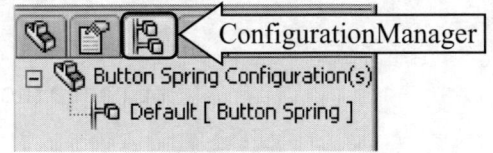

- Right click over the part named Button Spring and select **Add Configuration**.

- Enter **Compressed** under **Configuration Name.**

- Under **Comment**, enter: **Changed Pitch Dim from .915 to .415**

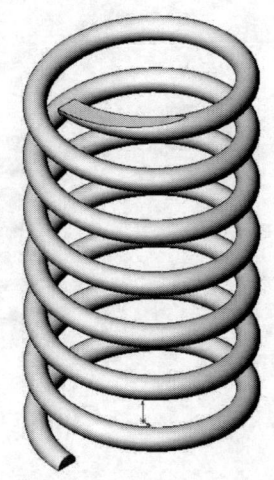

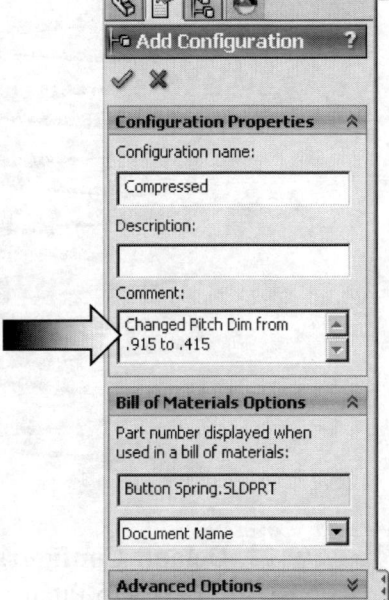

- Click **OK** ✓.

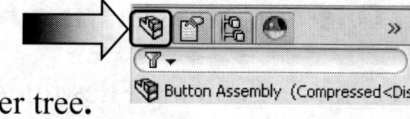

3. Changing the Pitch:

- Switch back to the FeatureManager tree.
(arrow).

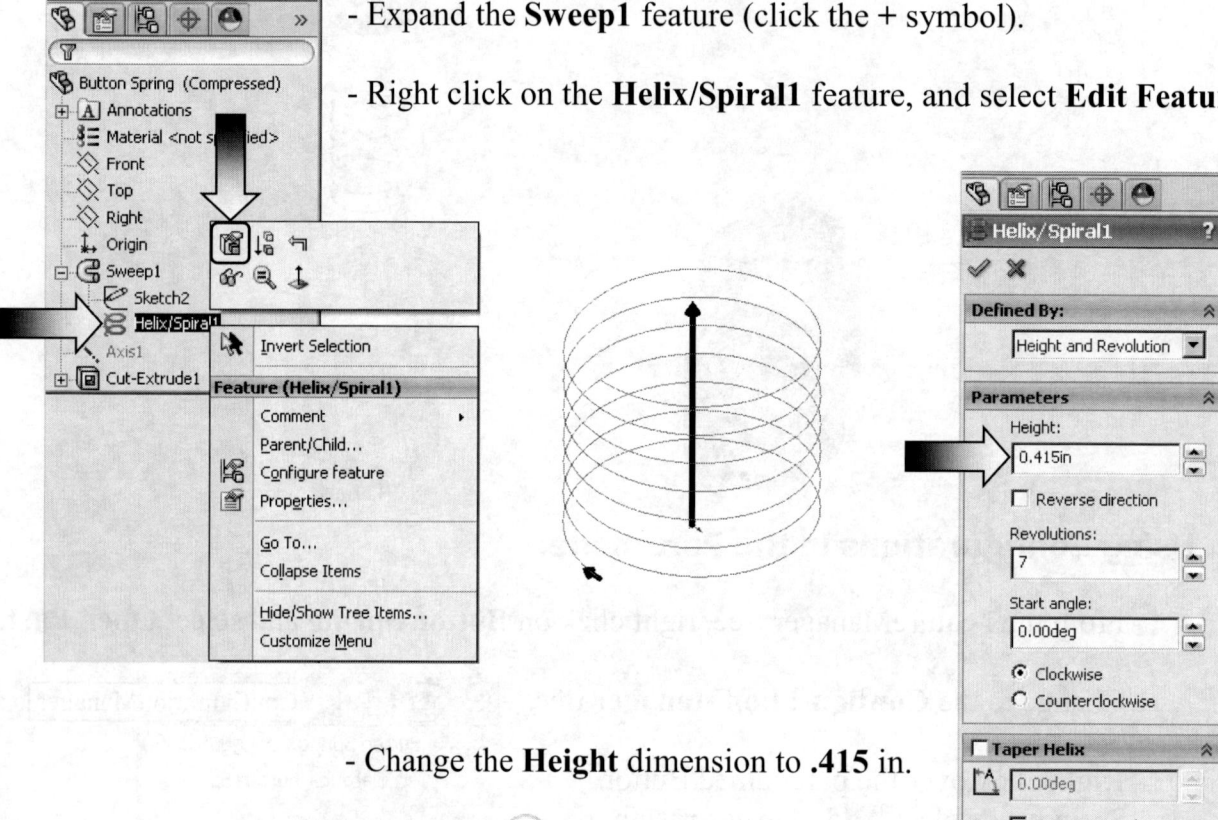

- Expand the **Sweep1** feature (click the + symbol).

- Right click on the **Helix/Spiral1** feature, and select **Edit Feature**.

- Change the **Height** dimension to **.415** in.

- Click **OK** ⊘.

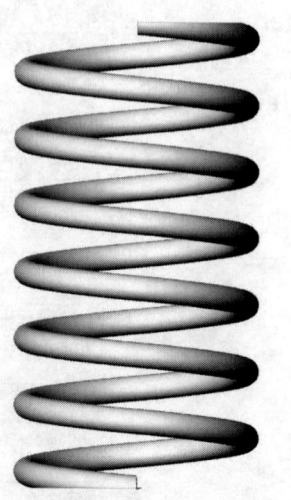

Default Configuration
(.915 Pitch)

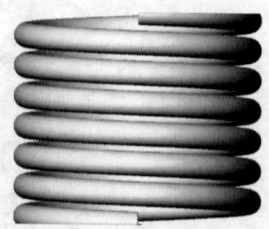

Compressed Configuration
(.415 Pitch)

4. Using Configurations in the Assembly mode:

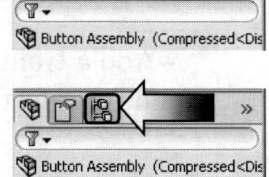

- Switch back to the Assembly document (**Ctrl + Tab**).

- Change to the **ConfigurationManager** tree.

- Right click on the name of the assembly and select: **Add Configuration**.

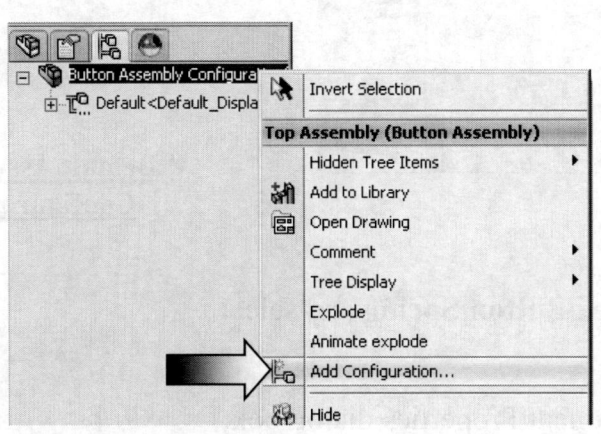

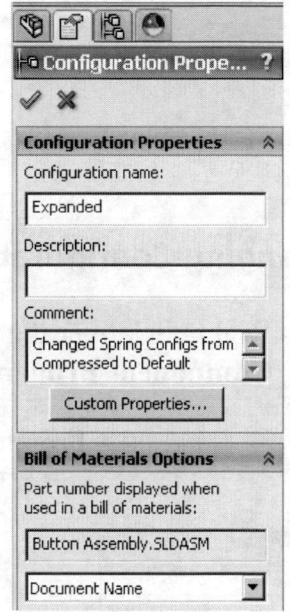

- Enter **Expanded** for Configuration Name.

- Click **OK** ✓ .

5. Changing the Mate conditions:

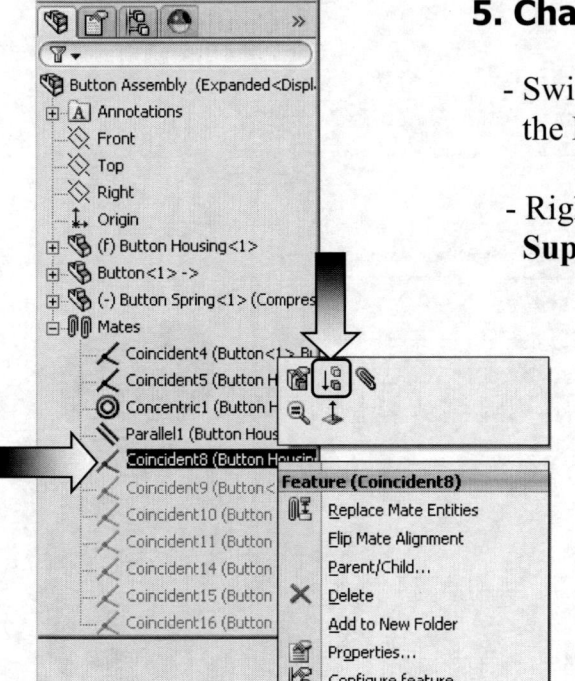

- Switch back to the **FeatureManager** tree and expand the Mates group.

- Right click on the mate Coincident8 and select: **Suppress**.

- By suppressing this mate, the Button (upper part) is no longer locked to the Housing and new Mates can be added to re-position it.

6. Adding new Mates:

- Add a **Coincident** Mate between the 2 faces of the two locking features.

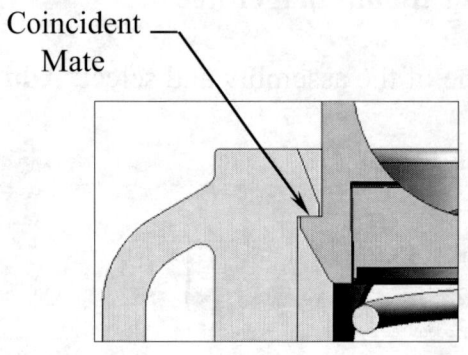

Coincident Mate

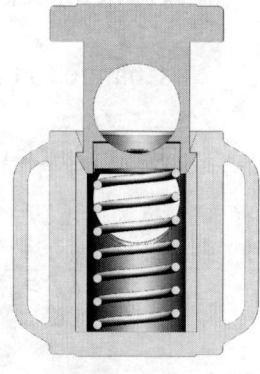

Default Assembly Configuration

7. Changing Configuration:

- Right click over the part named **Button Spring** and select **Component Properties**.

- From the Component Properties dialog box, select the **Default** Configuration.

- Click **OK** ✓.

Compressed Assembly Configuration

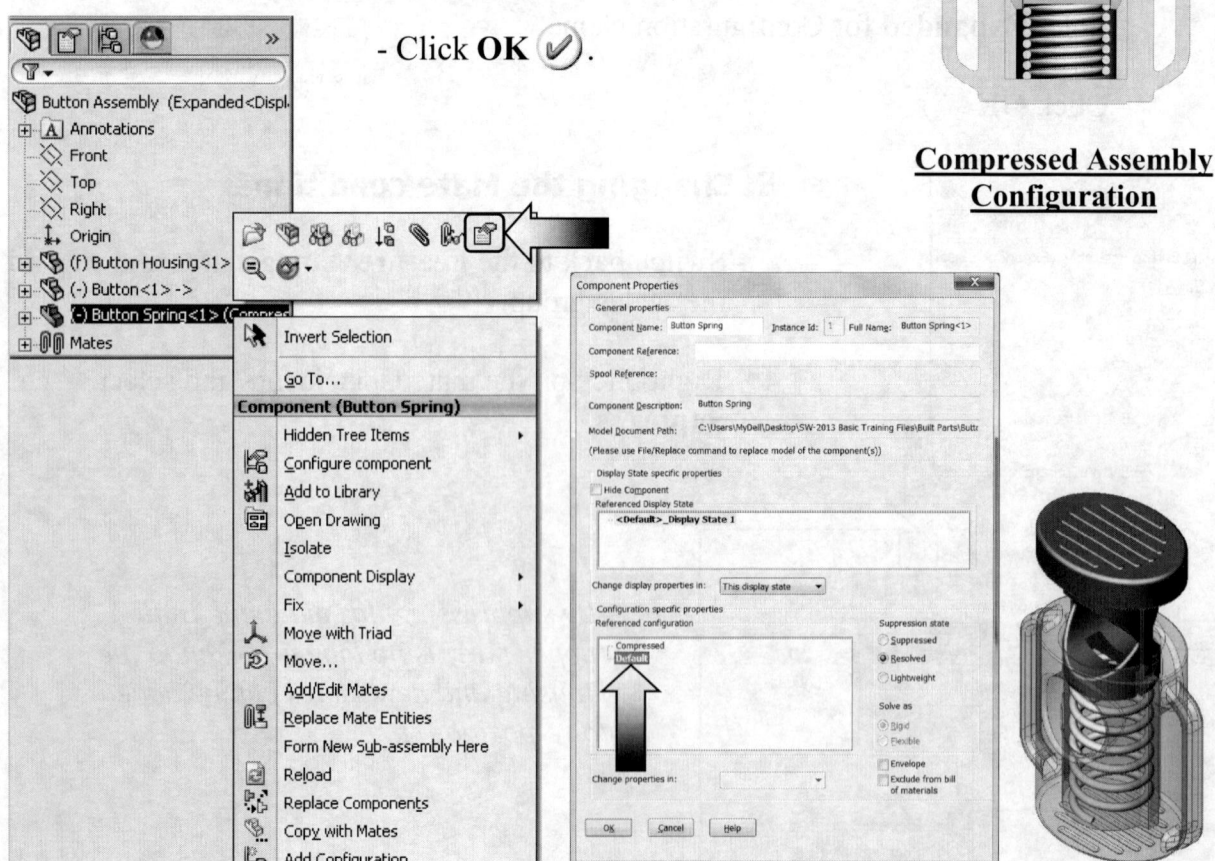

8. Using Configurations in the Drawing:

- Start a New drawing document; Go to **File / New / Draw** (or Drawing).

- Use **C-Landscape** paper size, **Scale: 3:1**

- Create the 4 standard views as shown below (using the **Default** Configuration).

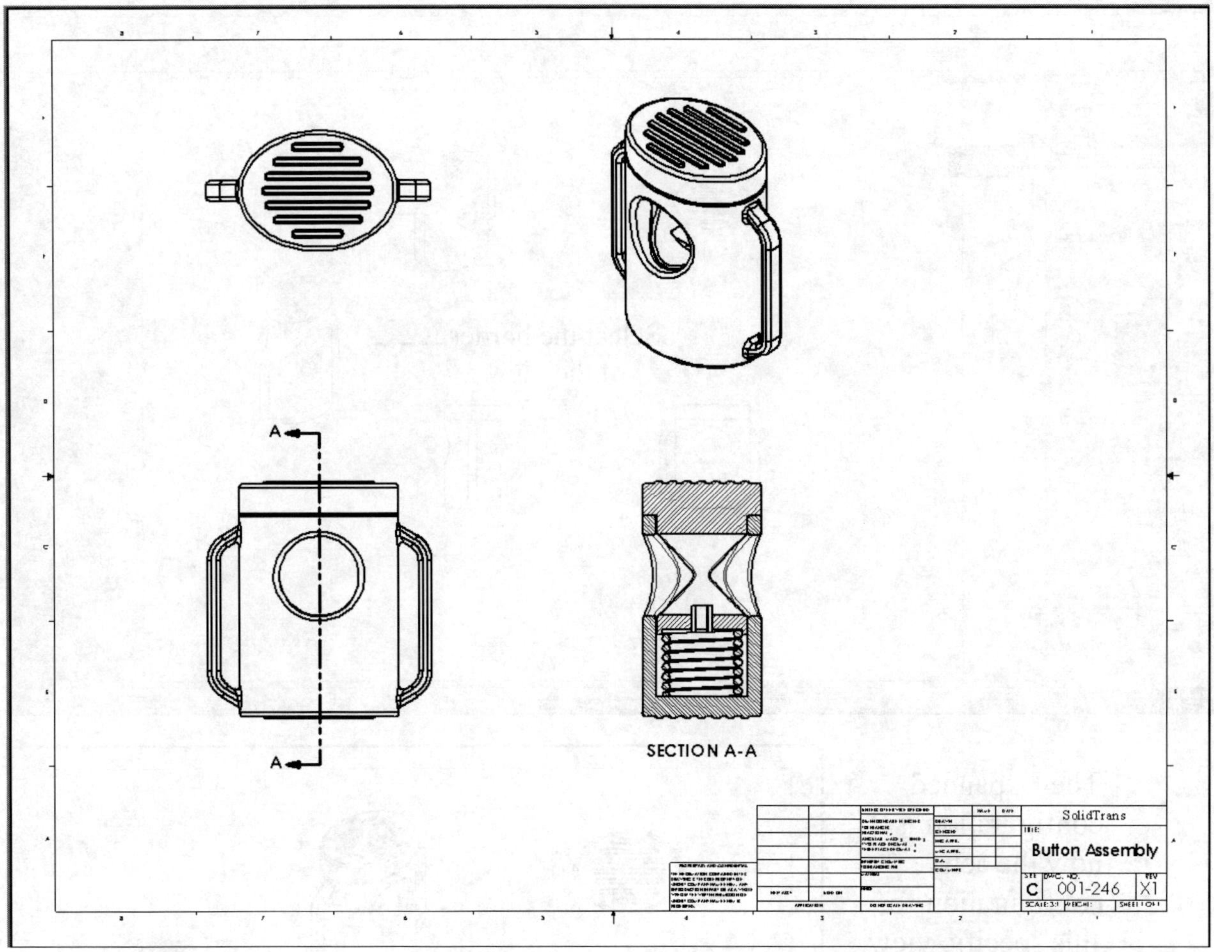
A
A
SECTION A-A
SolidTrans
Button Assembly
C
001-246
X1

9. Creating a 2nd Isometric view:

- Create another Isometric view and place it approximately as shown.

SECTION A-A
Button Assembly

Note: *Copy and Paste also works; first select the Isometric view and press Ctrl+C, then click anywhere in the drawing and press Ctrl+V).*

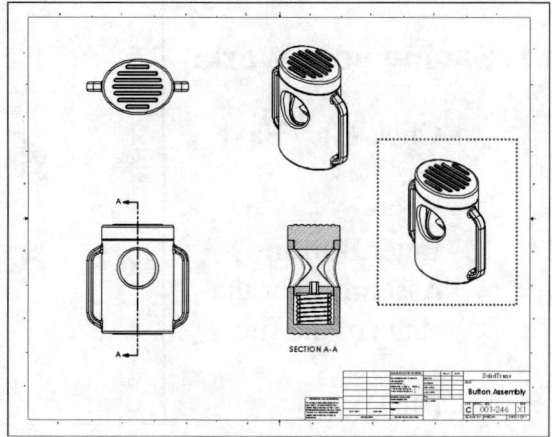

10. Changing the Configuration of a drawing view:

- Click the dotted border of the new isometric view.

- Change from the **Default** configuration to **Expanded** configuration (arrow).

- Click **OK** ✓.

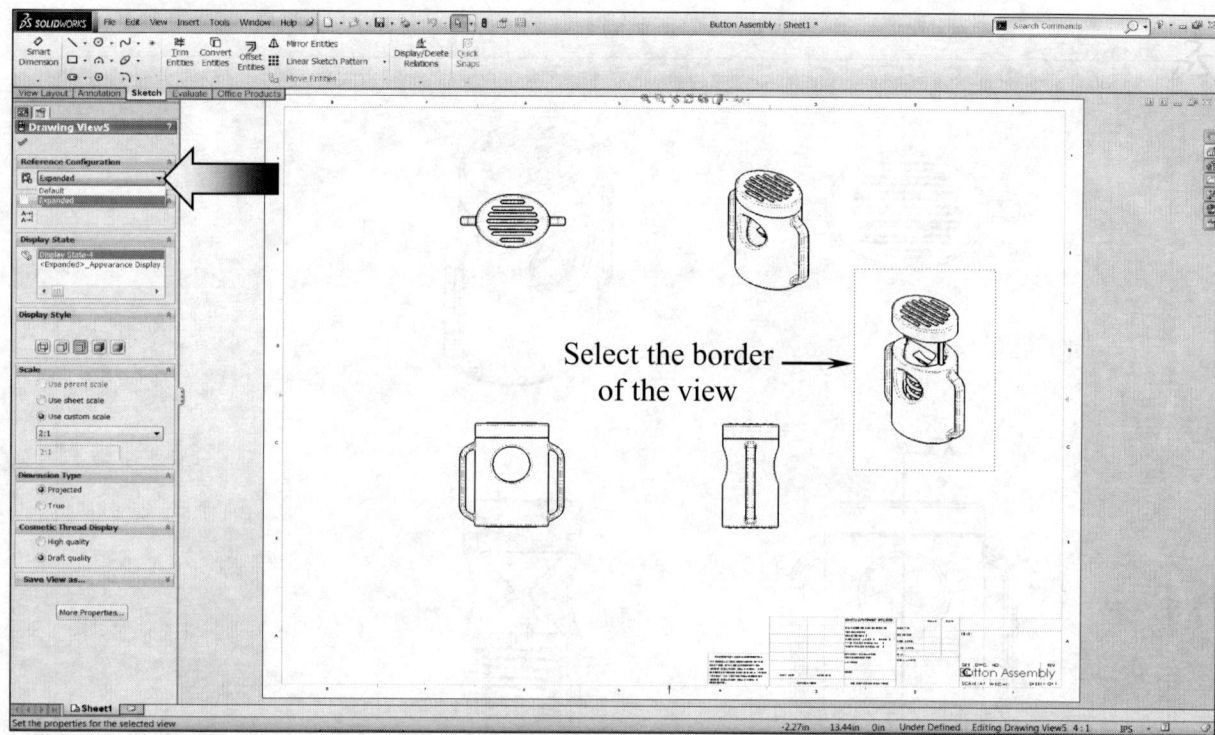

Select the border
of the view

- The Expanded configuration is now the active configuration for this specific view.

11. Saving your work:

- Click **File / Save As**.

- Enter **Button Assembly** for the name of the file.

- Click **Save**.

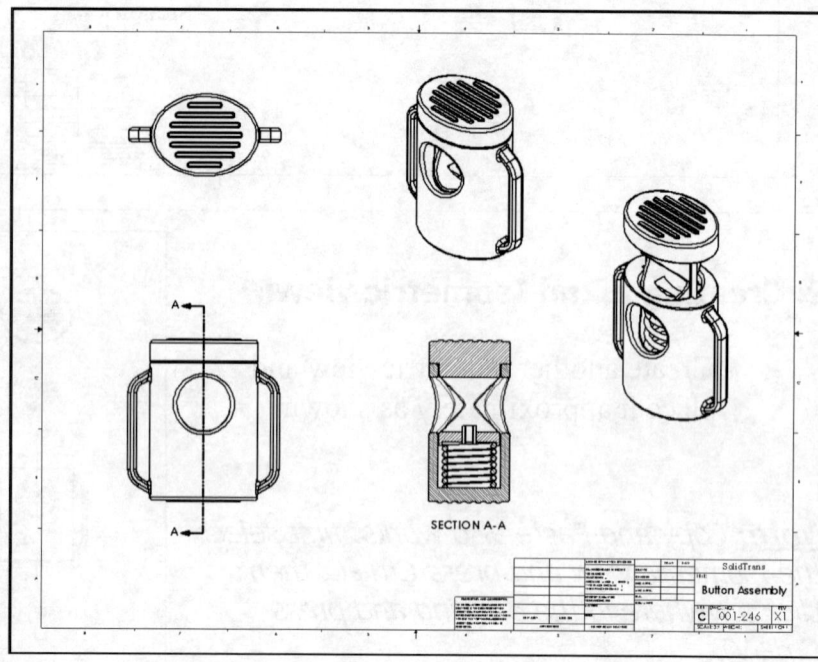

CHAPTER 19 (cont.)

Configurations – Part II

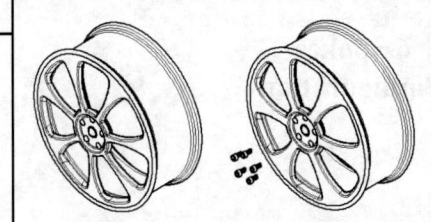

Configurations – Part II
Part / Assembly / Drawing

Configurable Items for Parts:

Part configurations can be used as follows:
* Modify feature dimensions and tolerances.
* Suppress features, equations, and end conditions.
* Assign mass and center of gravity.
* Use different sketch planes, sketch relations, and external sketch relations.
* Set individual face colors.
* Control the configuration of a base part.
* Control the configuration of a split part.
* Control the driving state of sketch dimensions.
* Create derived configurations.
* Define configuration-specific properties.

Configurable Items for Assemblies:

Assembly configurations can be used as follows:
* Change the suppression state (**Suppressed**, **Resolved**) or visibility (**Hide**, **Show**) of components.
* Change the referenced configuration of components.
* Change the dimensions of distance or angle mates, or suppression state of mates.
* Modify the dimensions, tolerances, or other parameters of features that belong to the assembly. This includes assembly feature cuts and holes, component patterns, reference geometry, and sketches that belong to the <u>assembly</u> (not to one of the assembly components).
* Assign mass and center of gravity.
* Suppress features that belong to the assembly.
* Define configuration-specific properties, such as end conditions and sketch relations.
* Create derived configurations.
* Change the suppression state of the Simulation folder in the Feature Manager design tree and its simulation elements (Suppressing the folder also suppresses its elements).

Configurations – Part II
Part, Assembly & Drawing

**6 Spokes
Configuration**

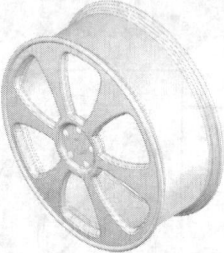

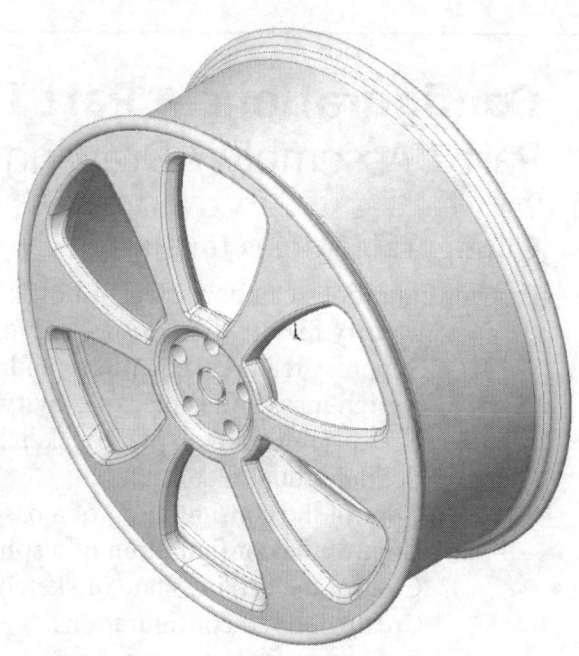

**7 Spokes
Configuration**

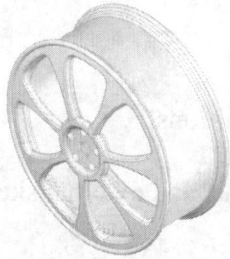

**7 Spokes with Bolts
Configuration**

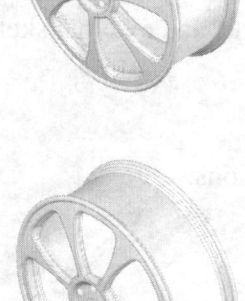

Dimensioning Standards: **ANSI**	Third Angle Projection
Units: **INCHES** – 3 Decimals	

Tools Needed:

 Part document
Part

 Assembly document
Assembly

 Drawing document
Drawing

 Feature Manager

 Configuration Manager

Part Configurations

This section discusses the use of Configurations in the part level, where the driving dimensions of the spokes-pattern will be altered to change the number of spokes in the part.

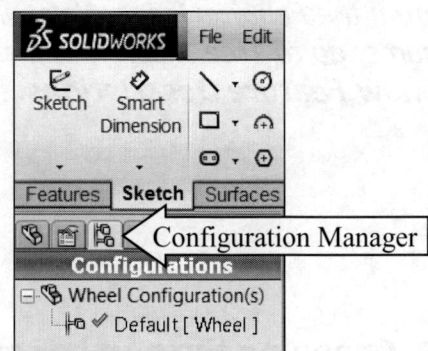

Opening the existing file:

    * Go to the Training Files folder
    * Wheel Assembly folder.
    * **WHEEL.sldprt**

1. Part Configurations:

    - Change to the ConfigurationManager tree:

    - We are going to create a new configuration to capture the change in the Spoke feature.

2. Creating a new configuration:

    - Right click on the name Wheel Configuration and select **Add Configuration**.

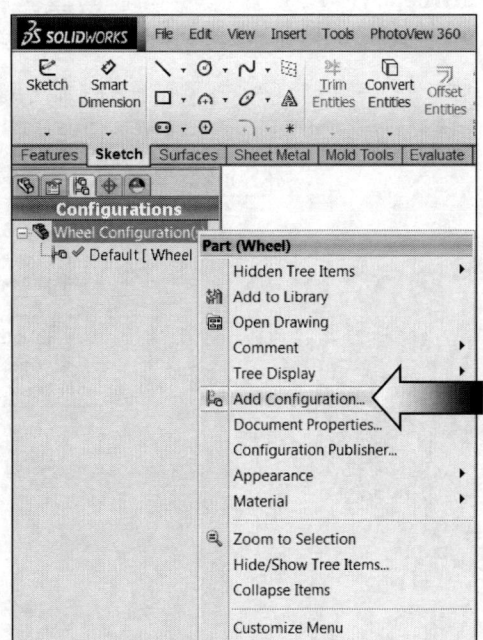

- For Configuration Name, enter:
7 Spokes (arrows).

- Under Description, enter:
Modified the No. of Spokes Pattern.

- Click **OK** 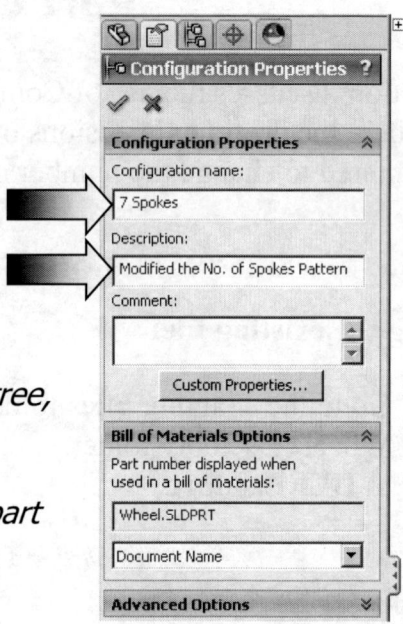.

NOTE:

To display the description in the FeatureManager tree, do the following:

From the FeatureManager tree, right click on the part name, go to Tree-Display, and select:
Show Feature Descriptions.

3. Changing the number of the Spokes:

- Switch back to the FeatureManager tree.

- Right click on the **Spokes Pattern** feature and select **Edit Feature** (Arrow).

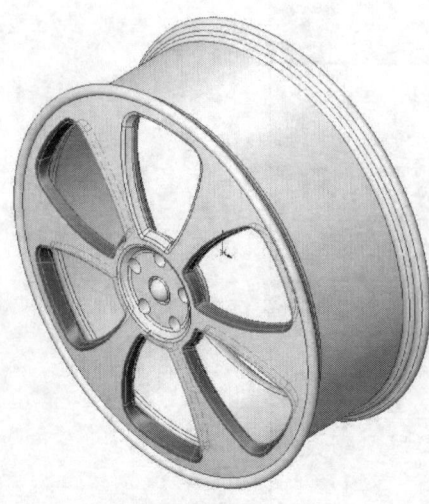

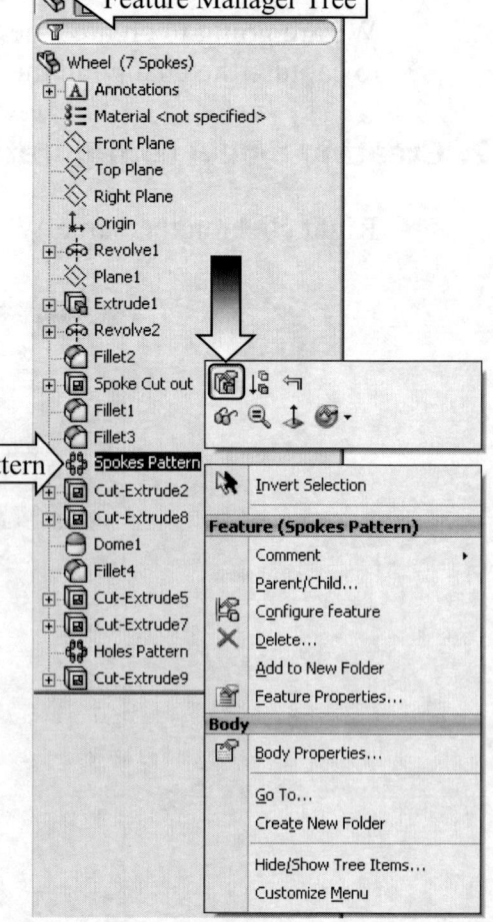

- Change the number of
  instances to **7** (Circled).

- Click **OK** ✅.

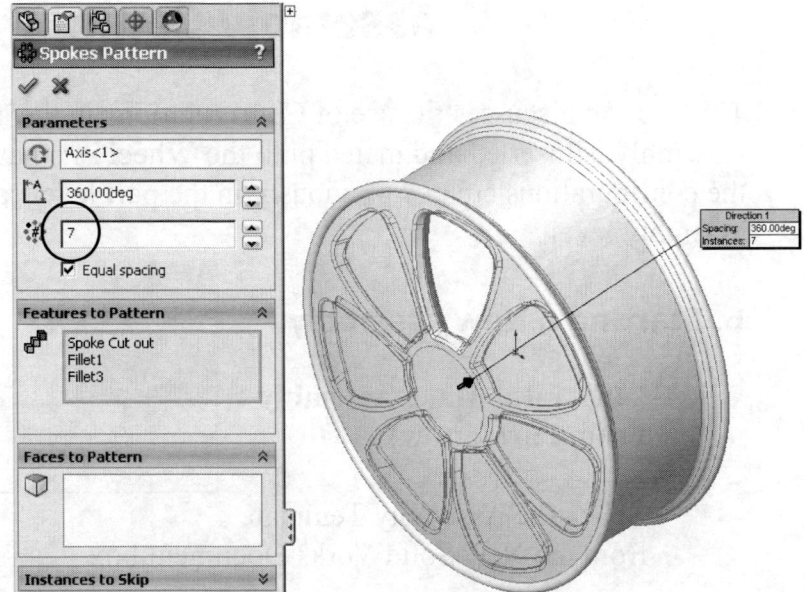

NOTE:

*Equations can be used to
change the number of spokes
and achieve the same result.*

4. Viewing the configurations:

- Change to the ConfigurationManager tree.

- Double click on the **Default** configuration to see the
  6-Spokes design.

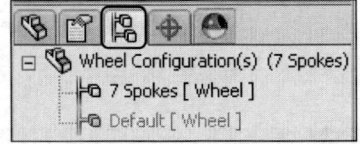

- Double click on the **7 Spokes** configuration to view
  the new changes.

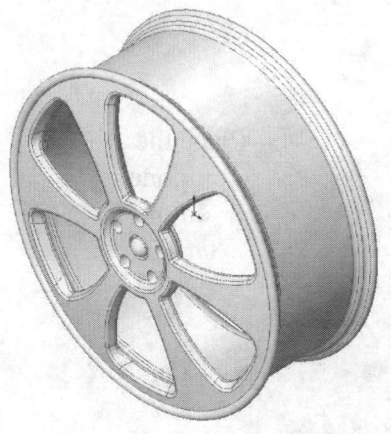

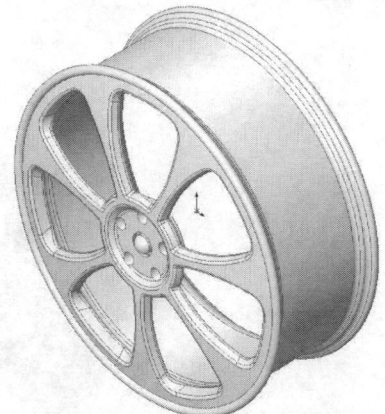

6 Spokes   **7 Spokes**

5. Saving the part:

- Save the part as a copy and name it: **Wheel.sldprt**

Assembly Configurations

This section discusses the use of Configurations in the assembly level, where a Sub-Assembly is inserted and mated onto the Wheel as a new configuration, and any of the configurations created previously in the part level can be selected to use in the assembly level.

6. Starting a New assembly:

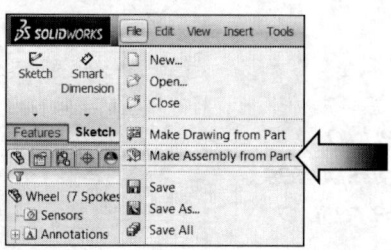

- Click **File / Make Assembly From Part** (arrow).

- Select the Assembly Template from the New SolidWorks Document box.

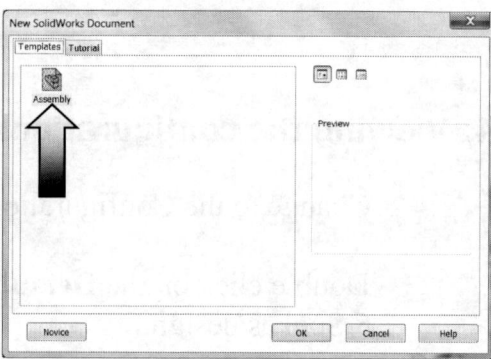

- Click the Origin Point to place the component. (If the Origin is not visible, enable it from the View / Origins menus).

- The 1st part in the assembly document is the Parent Component, it should be fixed on the origin.

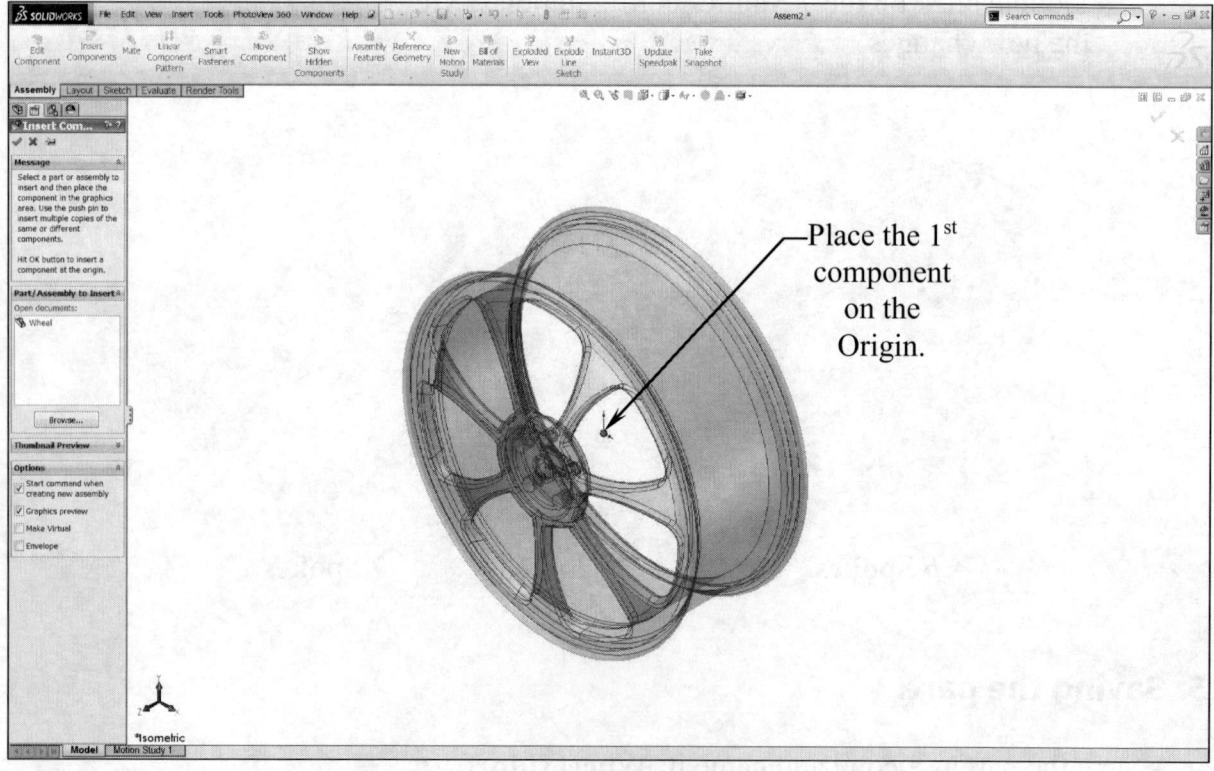

Place the 1st component on the Origin.

7. Assembly Configurations:

- Change to the ConfigurationManager tree.

- Right click on the Assembly's name and select **Add configuration** (Arrow).

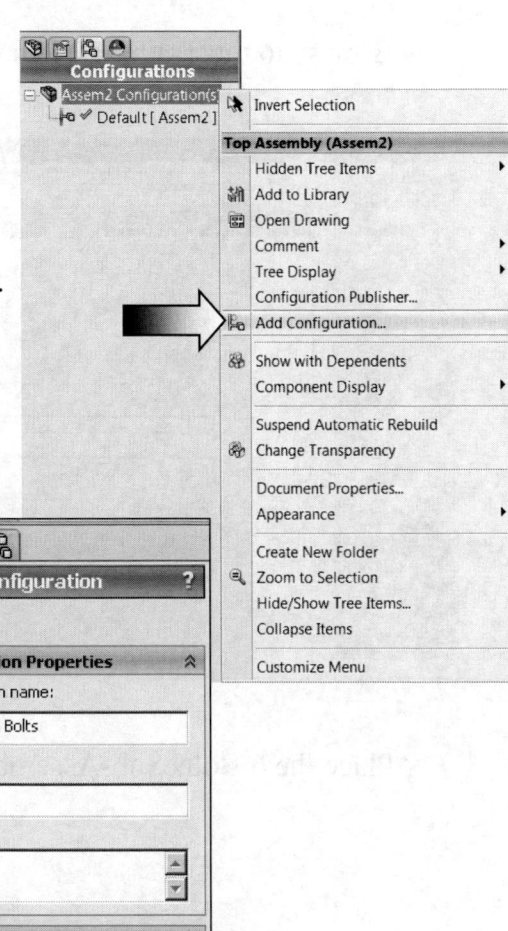

- For Configuration Name, enter: **Wheel With Bolts**.

- Click **OK** 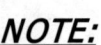.

NOTE:

A set of Bolts, which was saved earlier as an assembly document, is going to be inserted into the Top Level Assembly and becomes a Sub-Assembly.

8. Inserting the Sub-Assembly:

- Click **Insert Components**.

- Click the Browse... button.

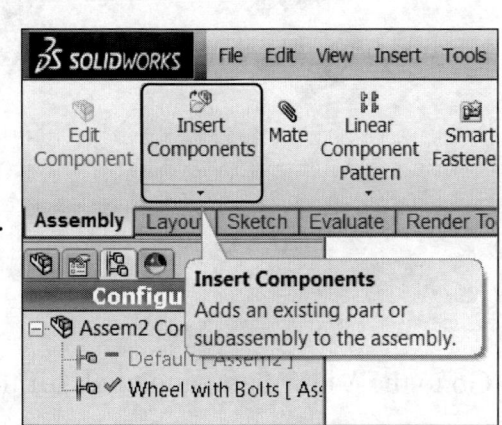

- Browse to the Training Files folder, locate and open the **Bolts Sub-Assembly**.

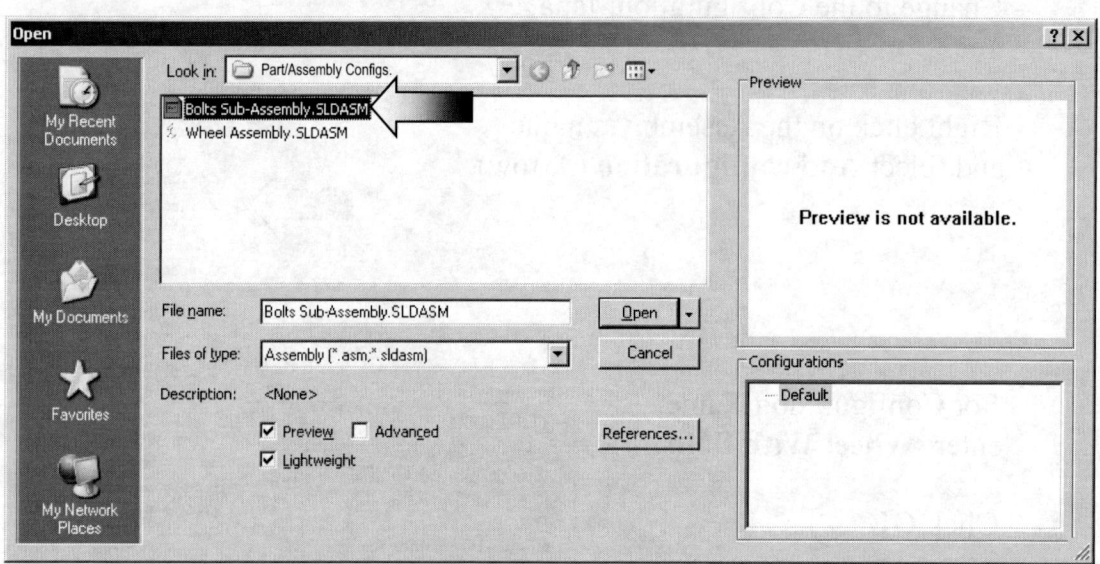

- Place the 6 Bolts Sub-Assembly approximately as shown.

Place the Bolt-Assembly approximately here.

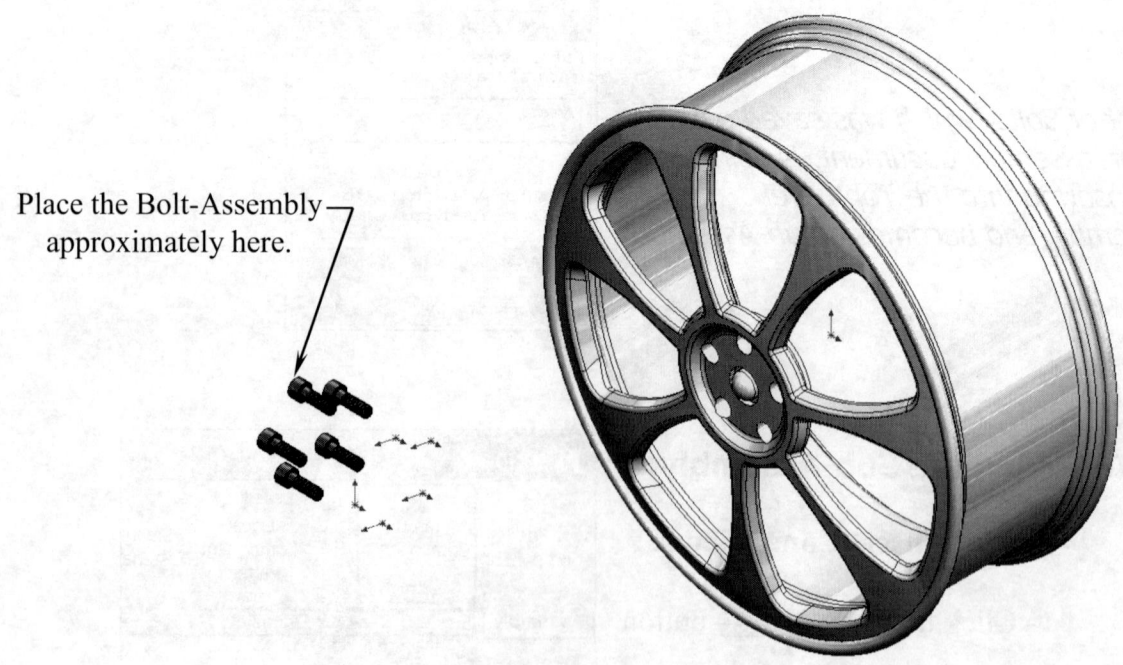

- Go to the View menu and click off the Origins option to hide them.

9. Mating the Sub-Assembly:

- Enable **Temporary Axis** from the **View** menu.

- Click **Mate** 🖉 or select **Insert / Mate**.

- Select the center Axis of one of the Bolts and the mating Holes (pictured).

Select 2 Axis

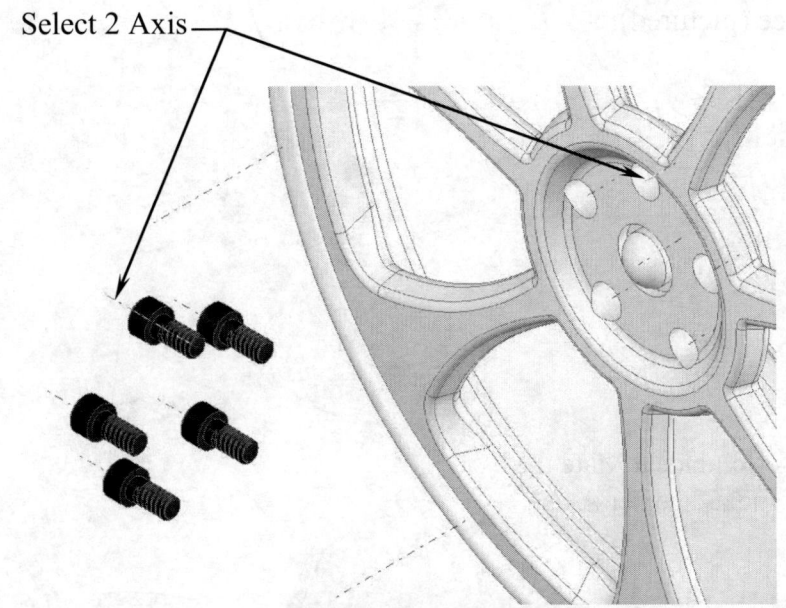

- The system selects the Coincident mate automatically.

- Click either **Align** or **Anti-Align**, to flip the Bolts to the proper direction.

- Click **OK** ✅.

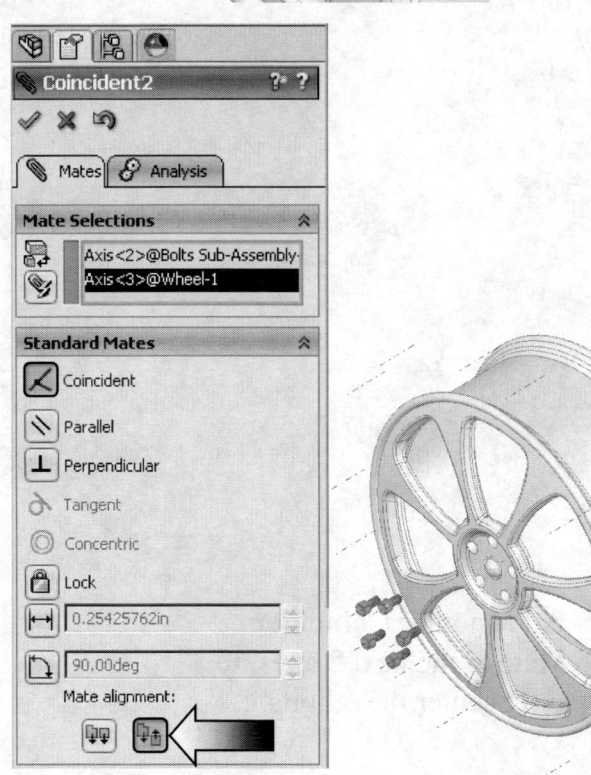

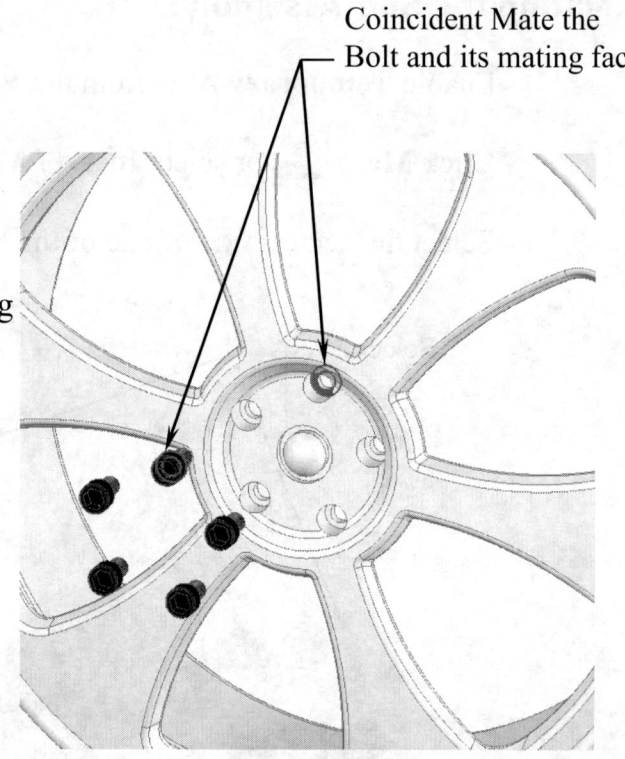

Coincident Mate the
Bolt and its mating face.

- Add a **Coincident** Mate
between the Bottom Face of
one of the Bolts and its mating
surface (pictured).

- Click **OK** ✅.

Coincident Mate the
next 2 center Axis.

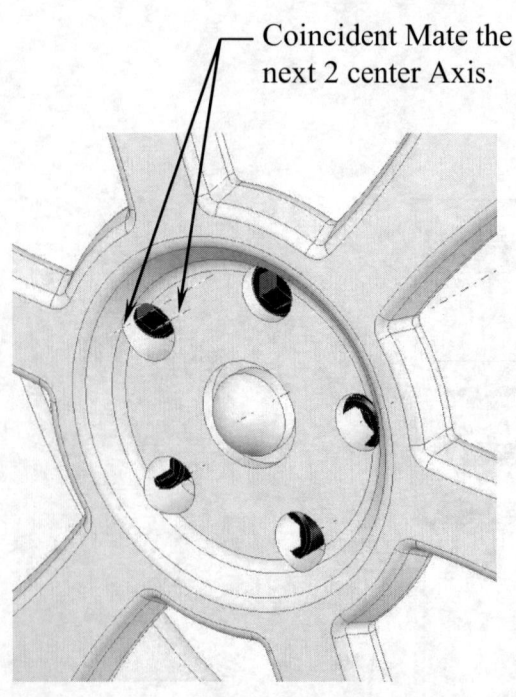

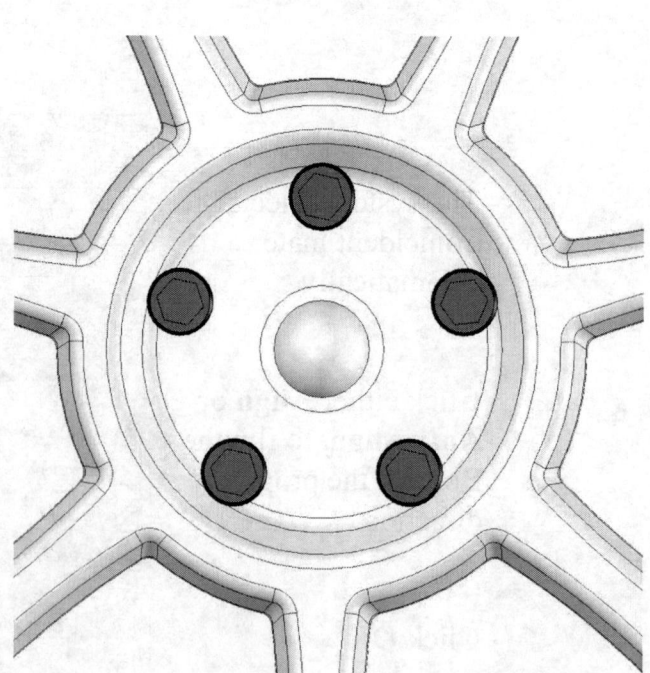

- Add another **Coincident**
Mate to the next 2 axes, to
fully center the 6 bolts.

The Completed Assembly.

10. Viewing the Assembly Configurations:

- Change to the ConfigurationManager tree.

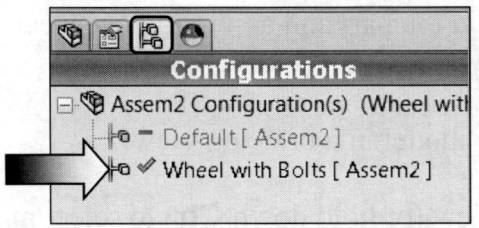

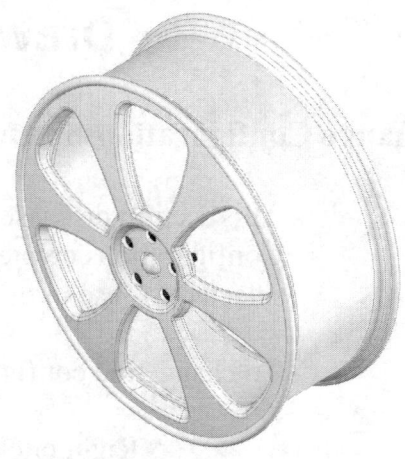

Wheel With Bolts Configuration

- Double click on the **Default** configuration.

- The Bolts Sub-Assembly is **Suppressed**.

- The **7 Spokes** pattern is displayed.

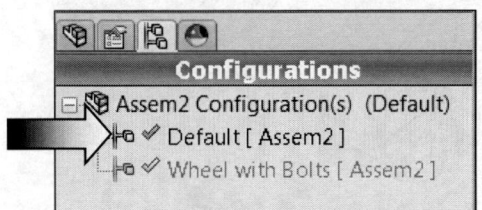

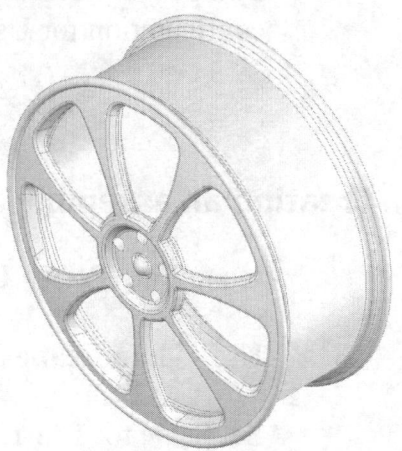

Default Configuration

- Make any necessary changes to the Number of Spokes pattern by accessing the Component's Properties and its Configurations.

  - An assembly exploded view may need to be created for use in the drawing later.

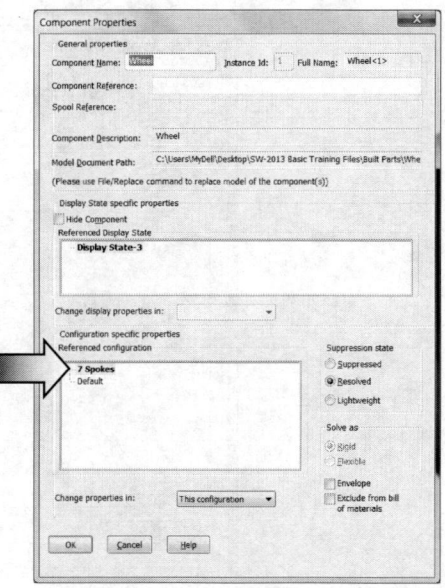

11. Saving your work:

- Save as **Part-Assembly Configurations**.

Drawing Configurations

Change Configurations in Drawing Views

- This section discusses the use of Configurations in the drawing level, where Configurations created previously in the part and assembly levels can be selected for use in the drawing views.

- To change the configuration of the model in a drawing view:

  * Right click a drawing view (or hold down **Ctrl** to select multiple drawing views, then right click) and select **Properties**.

- In the dialog box under **Configuration information**, select a different configuration for **Use- named configuration**.

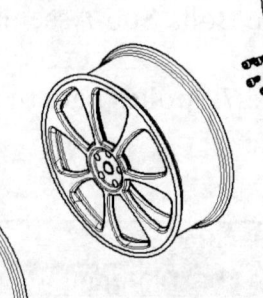

1. Creating an assembly drawing:

- Go to **File / New / Drawing**.

- Use **C-Landscape** paper size.

- Set **Scale** to: **1 to 1**.

- Set the **Projection** to **3rd Angle**.

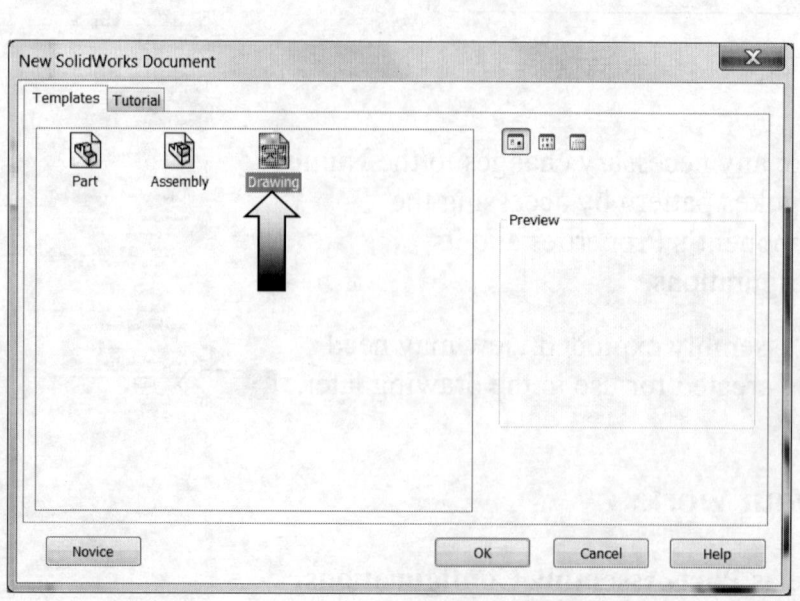

2. Creating the standard drawing views:

- Select **Model View** command 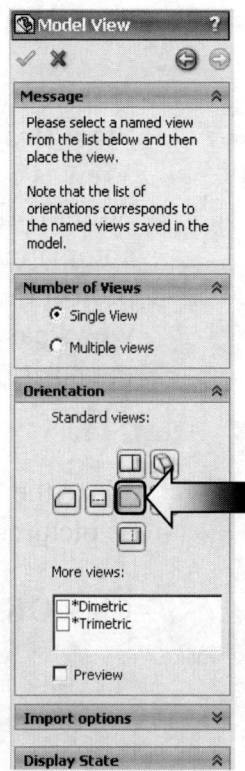.

- Click **Browse** Browse... .

- Select the **Wheel Assembly** and click **Open**.

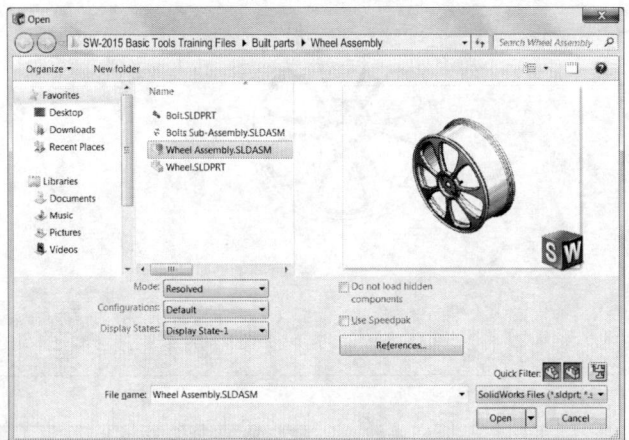

- Select the **FRONT** view from the Standard Views dialog and place it approximately as shown.

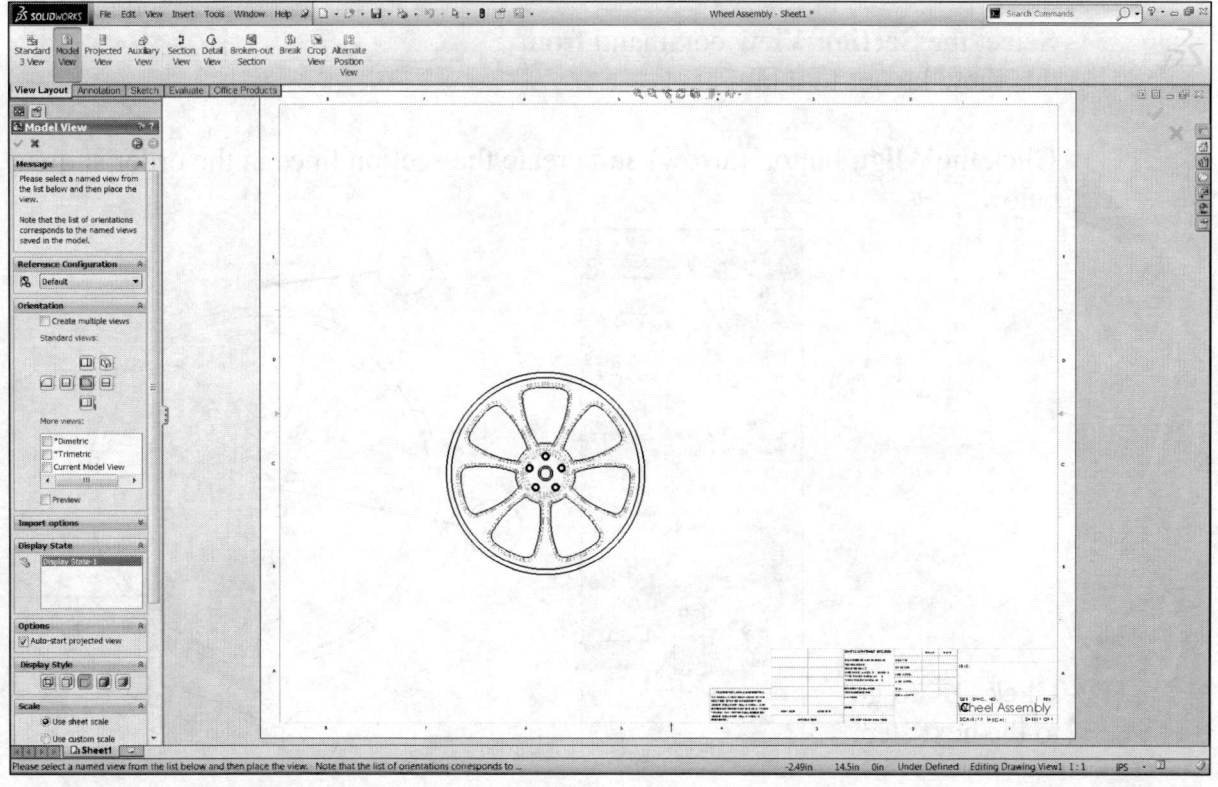

3. Auto-Start the Projected-View:

- If the option **Auto-Start Projected-View** is enabled, SolidWorks will automatically project the next views based on the position of the cursor.

- Place the Top view as pictured.

- Click **OK** ✓.

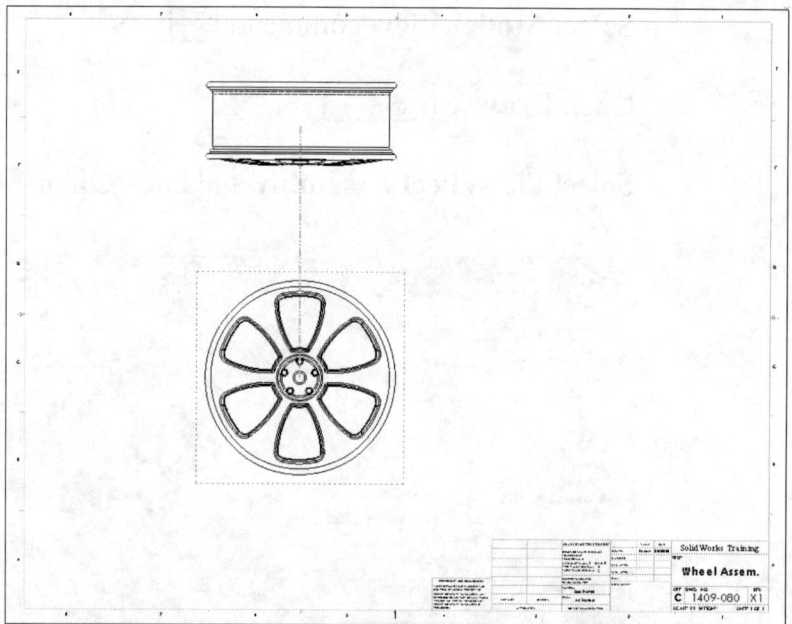

4. Creating the Aligned Section View:

- Select the Front drawing view's border to activate it.

- Select the **Section View** command from the View layout tool tab.

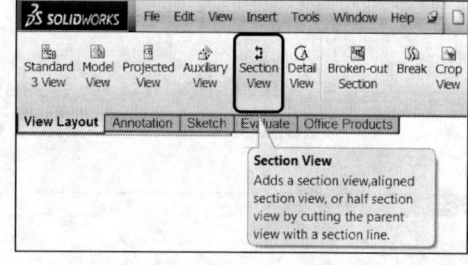

- Click the **Align** button (arrow) and create the section lines in the order shown below.

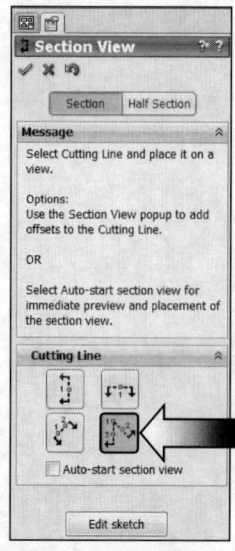

- Click **OK** to go to the next step.

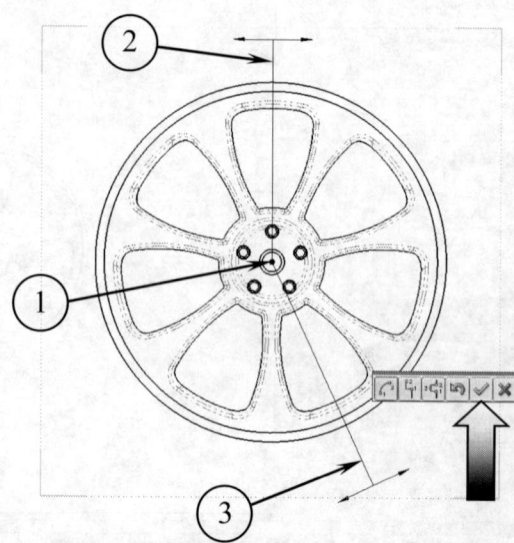

- **Section Scope**: is an option that allows components to be excluded from the section cut. In other words, when sectioning an assembly drawing view, you will have an option to select which component(s) is going to be effected by this section cut. This option is called Section Scope.

- In the Section Scope dialog box, enable **Auto Hatching** and if necessary, click **Flip Direction**.

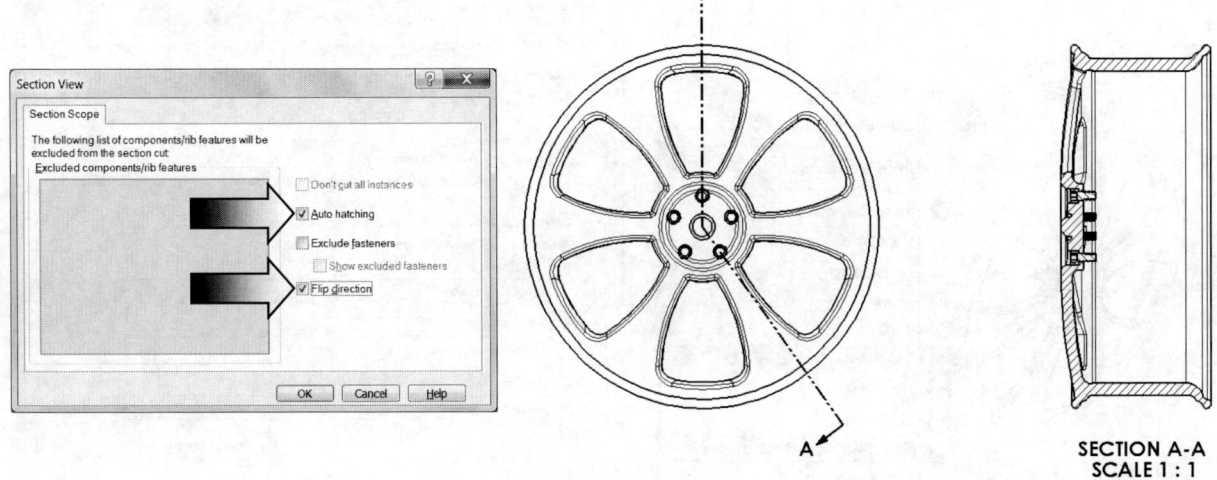

SECTION A-A
SCALE 1 : 1

5. Creating the Isometric view:

- Select the **Model View** command .

- Click **Next** .

- Select **Isometric** view from the Standard Views list.

- Place the Isometric view on the lower right side of the drawing.

- Click **OK** .

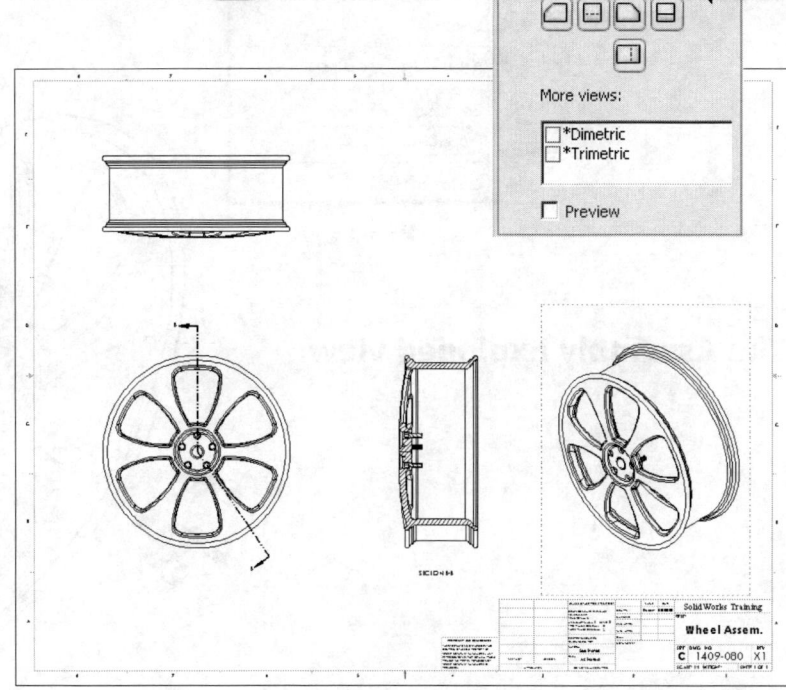

Displaying the Exploded View: (An exploded view must be created from the assembly level prior to showing it in the drawing).

- Right click on the Isometric drawing view's border and select **Properties**.

- Enable the **Show in Exploded State** check box (This option is also available on PropertyManager in the newer releases of SolidWorks).

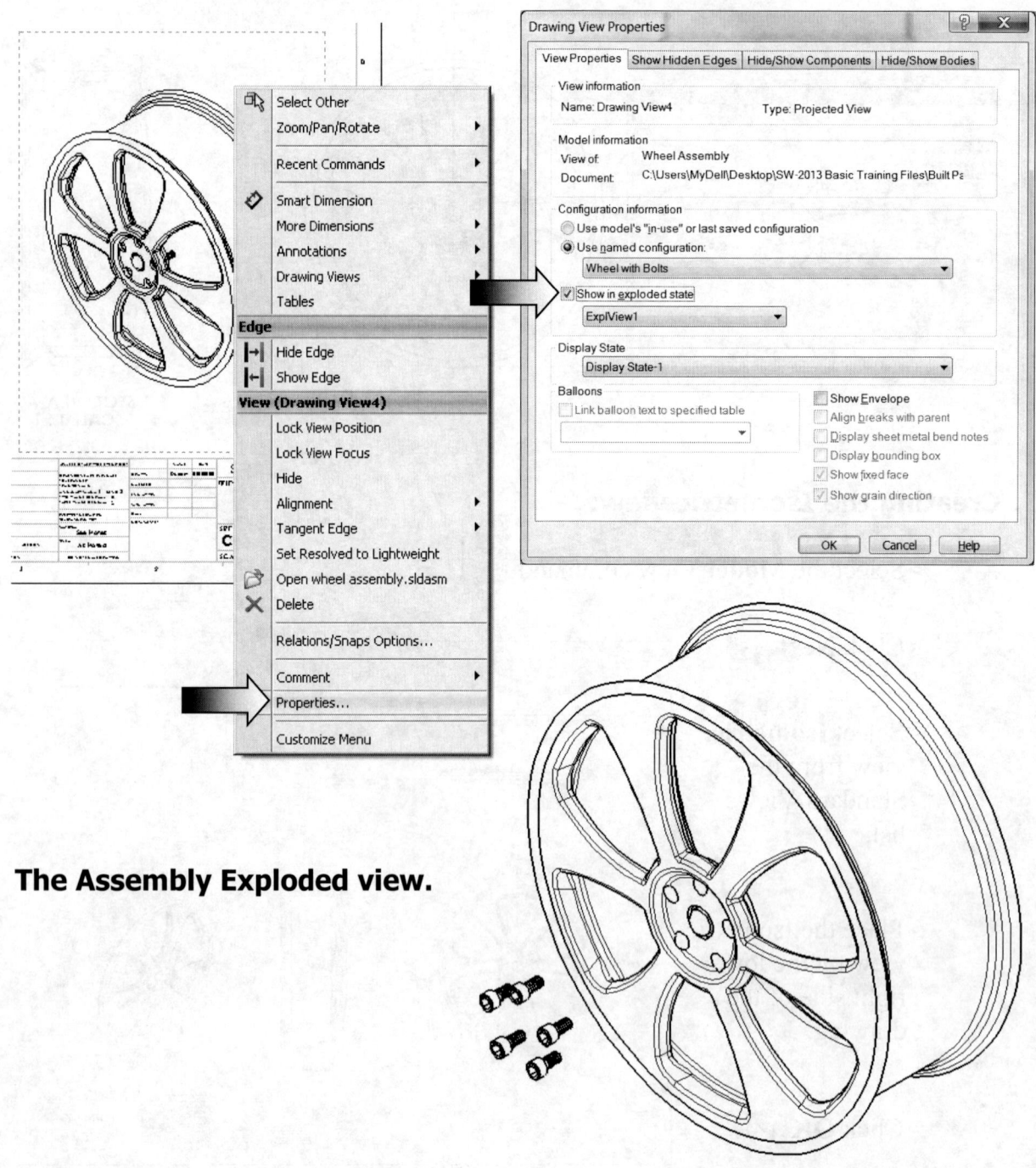

The Assembly Exploded view.

6. Changing Configurations:

- Use the **Model View** command and create 2 more Isometric views.

- Right click on the new Isometric drawing view's border and select **Properties**.

- Select the **Default** configuration.

- Set the 2nd Isometric view to the **6-Spokes** configuration (Switch to the Assembly document to modify the configurations).

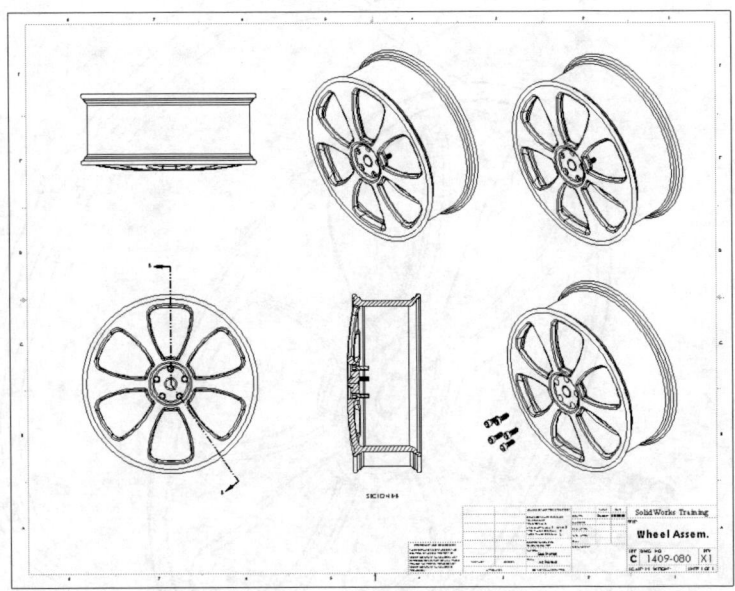

7. Adding Annotations:

- Click Note $\boxed{\mathbf{A}}$ and add the call-outs under each drawing views as shown.

* 6 SPOKES CONFIGURATION.

* 7 SPOKES CONFIGURATION.

* 6 SPOKES WITH BOLTS CONFIGURATION.

8. Saving your work:

- Click **File / Save As**.

- Enter: **Drawing Configurations** for the name of the file.

- Click **Save** and close all documents.

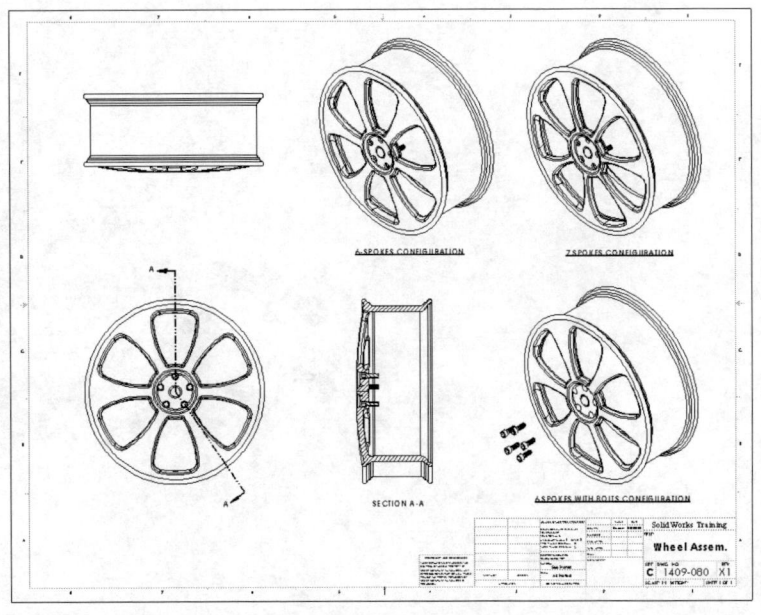

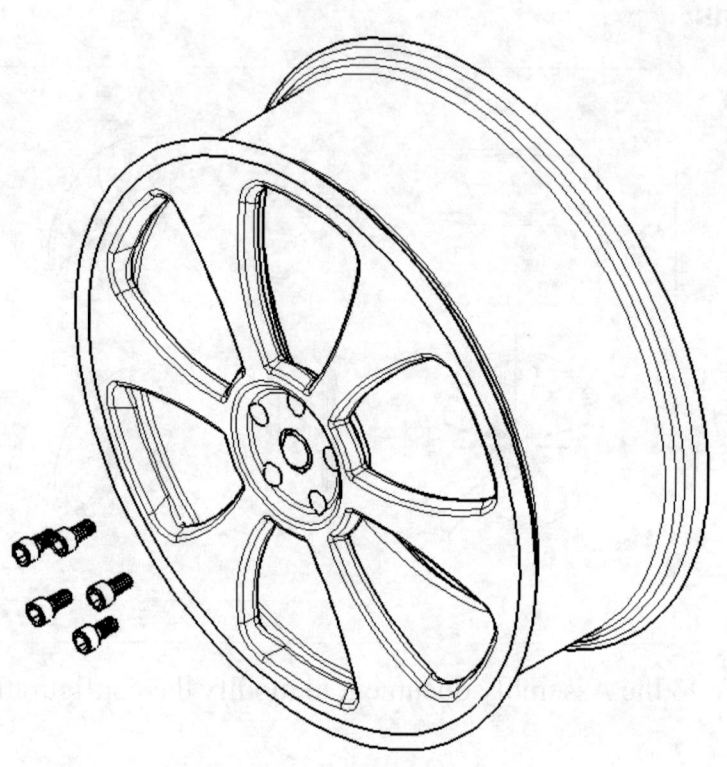

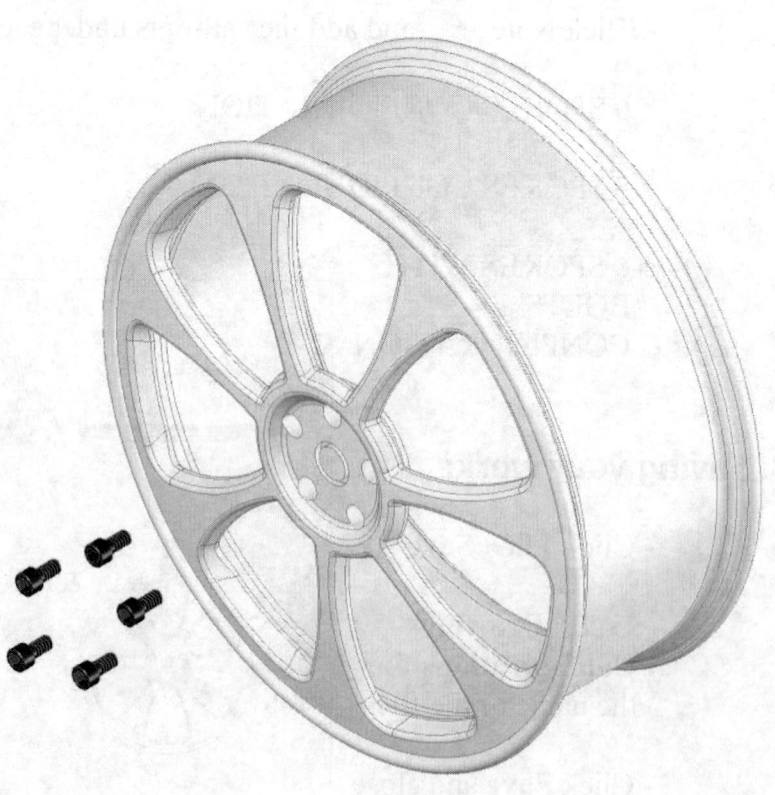

CHAPTER 20

Design Tables

Design Tables in Part, Assembly & Drawing

Design Table Parameters	Description (Legal values)
$PARTNUMBER@_____	- For use in a bill of materials.
$COMMENT@_____	- Any description or text string.
$NEVER_EXPAND_IN_BOM@_____	- Yes/No to expand in B.O.M.
$STATE@_____	- Resolved = R, Suppressed = S
$CONFIGURATION@_____	- Configuration name.
$SHOW@_____	- Has been obsoleted.
$PRP@_____	- Enter any text string.
$USER_NOTES@_____	- Enter any text string.
$COLOR@_____	- Specifying 32-bit RGB color.
$PARENT@_____	- Parent configuration name.
$TOLERANCE@_____	- Enter tolerance keywords.
$SWMASS@_____	- Enter any decimal legal value.
$SWCOG@_____	- Enter any legal x,y,z value.
$DISPLAYSTATE@_____	- Display state name.

In a Design Table, you will need to define the names of the configurations, specify the parameters that you want to control, and assign values for each parameter. This chapter will guide you through the use of design tables in both the part and assembly levels.

Part, Assembly & Drawing
Design Tables

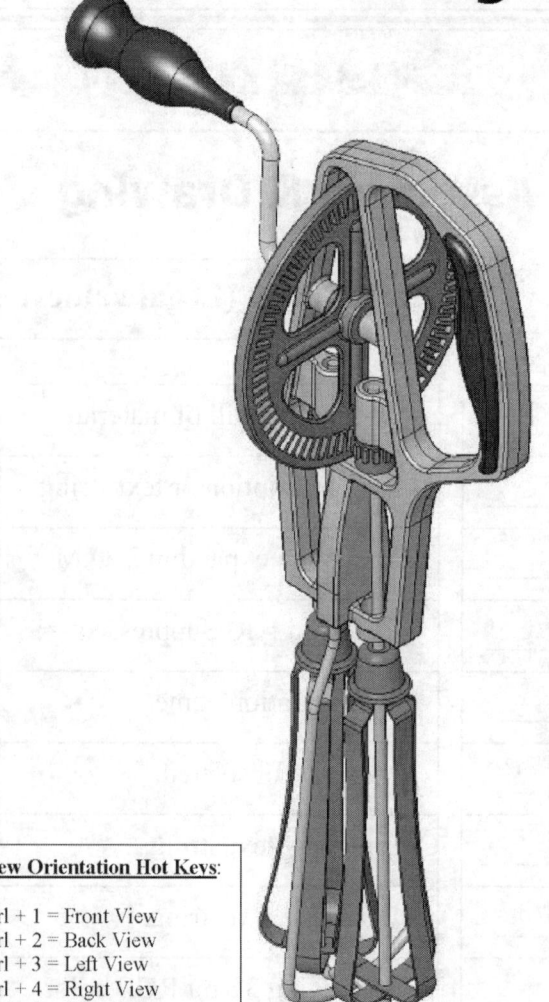

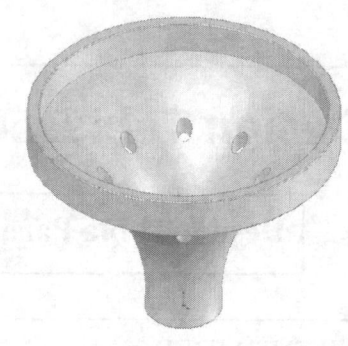

Design Table for: Egg Beater

	A	B	C	D	E	F	G	H	I	J
1	Design Table for: Egg Beater									
2		$state@Egg Beater Handle<1>	$state@Main Gear<1>	$state@Support Rod<1>	$state@Right Spinner<1>	$state@Left Spinner<1>	$state@Right Spinner<2>	$state@Left Spinner<2>	$configuration@Crank Handle<1>	
3	Default	R	R	R	R	R	R	R	Default	
4	Config1	R	S	S	S	S	S	S	Oval Handle	
5	Config2	R	R	S	S	S	S	S	Default	
6	Config3	R	R	R	S	S	S	S	Oval Handle	
7	Config4	R	R	R	R	S	S	S	Default	
8	Config5	R	R	R	R	R	S	S	Oval Handle	
9	Config6	R	R	R	R	R	R	R	Default	
10										

Sheet1

Dimensioning Standards: **ANSI**
Units: **INCHES** – 3 Decimals

Third Angle Projection

Tools Needed:

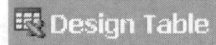 Design Tables / Microsoft Excel

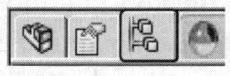 ConfigurationManager

Part - Design Tables

1. Copying the document:

- <u>Go to:</u> The Training Files folder, Design Tables folder **Part Design Table.sldprt**

- **OPEN** a copy of the part document named: **Part Design Table.sldprt**

- This exercise discusses the use of Changing Feature Dimensions and Feature Suppression-States in a Design Table.

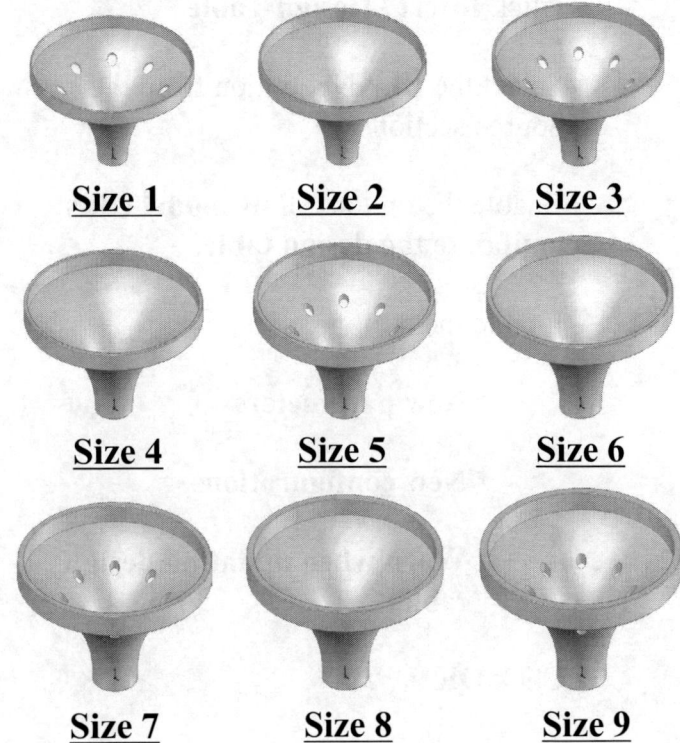

Size 1   Size 2   Size 3

Size 4   Size 5   Size 6

Size 7   Size 8   Size 9

- The names of the dimensions will be used as the column Headers in the design table.

- Go to the **View** menu and enable the option: **Dimension Names** (arrow).

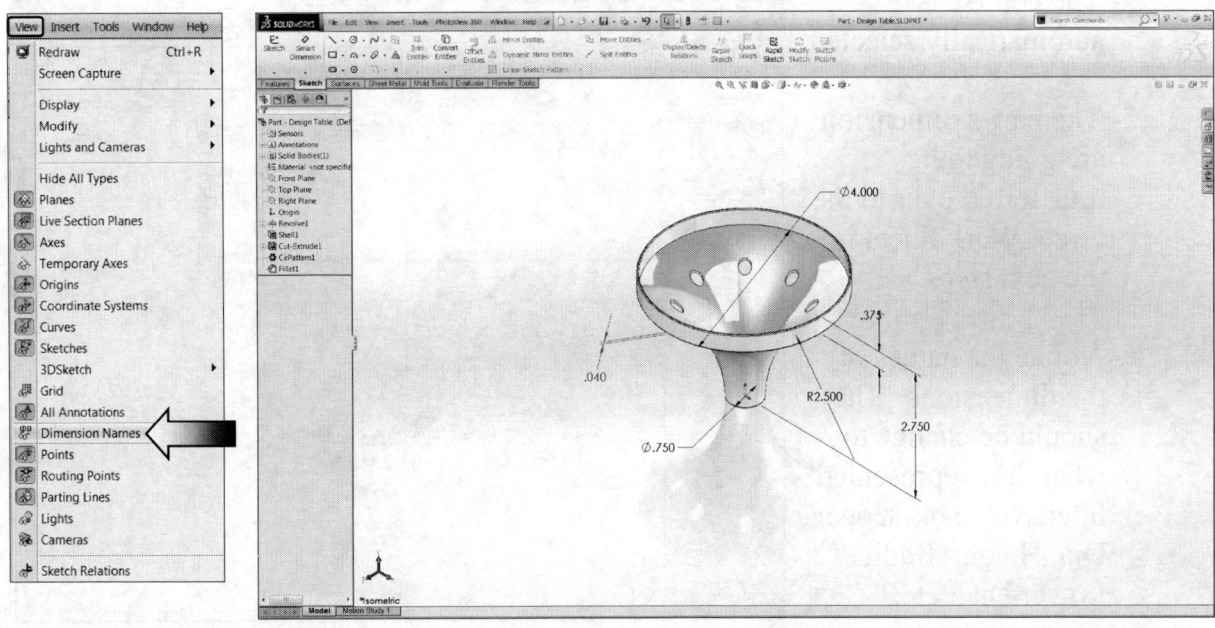

2. Creating a New Design Table:

- Click **Insert / Design Table**.

- Select the **BLANK** option from the Source section.

- Enable the option **Allow model edits to update the design table**.

- Enable the options:

    * **New parameters**

    * **New configurations**

    * **Warn when updating design table**

- Click **OK** ✓.

- Click **OK** in the Add Rows and Columns Dialog box.

- The Microsoft Excel Work Sheet opens up.

- The cell A1 is filled in with the part's name.

- The cell B2 is automatically selected.

- The part's dimensions are going to be transferred over to the Excel Work Sheet in the next steps.

- Notice the names of the dimensions? They should be change to what they represented like: Wall Thk, Upper Dia, Height, Radius, Lower Dia., etc.

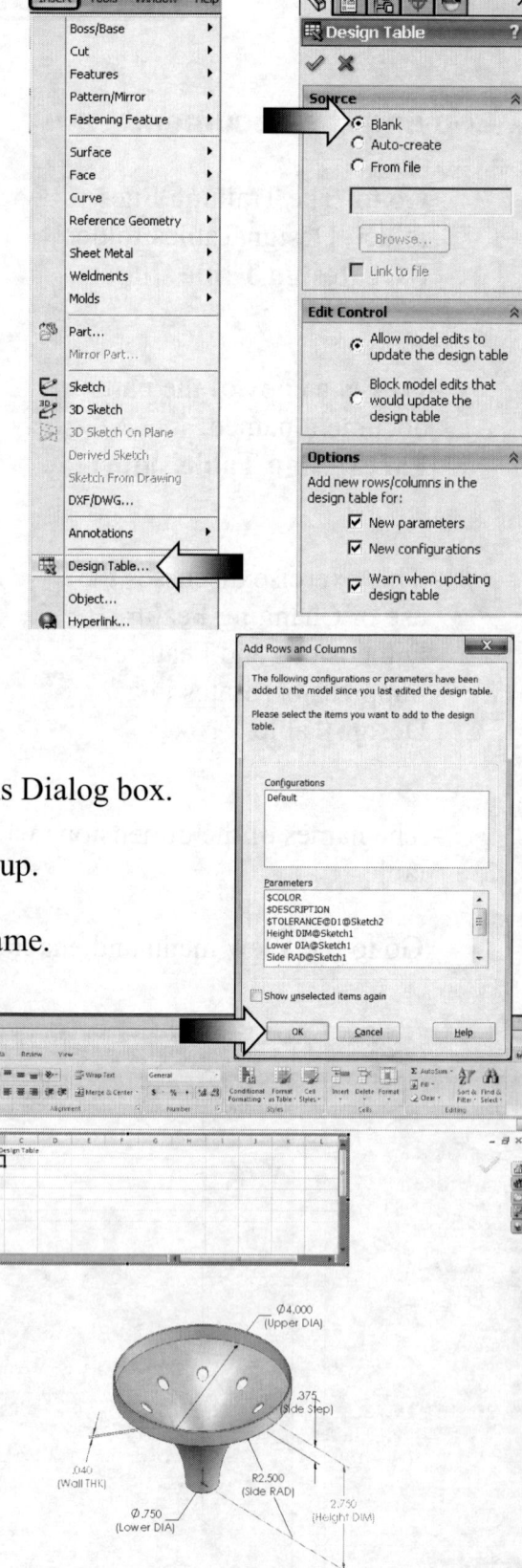

3. Transferring the Dimensions to the Design Table:

- Make sure the cell B2 is selected.

- Double click on the Height Dim **2.750**

- The dimension is transferred over to cell B2.

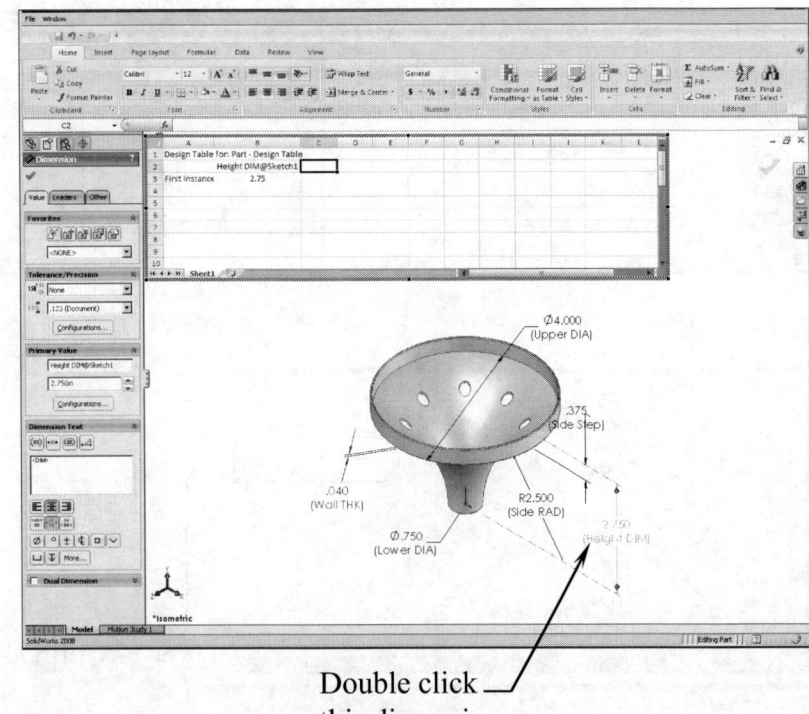

Double click this dimension

- Repeat the same step and transfer the other dimensions in the order as shown.

- Add configs. names: Size1 thru Size9.

	Height DIM@Sketch1	Upper DIA@Sketch1	Lower DIA@Sketch1	Side RAD@Sketch1	Side Step@Sketch1	Wall THK@Shell1
Size1	2.75	4	0.75	2.5	0.375	0.04
Size2						
Size3						
Size4						
Size5						
Size6						
Size7						
Size8						
Size9						

Design Table for: Part - Design Table

4. Using Excel's Addition Formula:

- Select the cell B4, type the equal sign (=), click the number **2.75** in cell B3, and then enter **+.125**

- Copy the formula to the cells below:

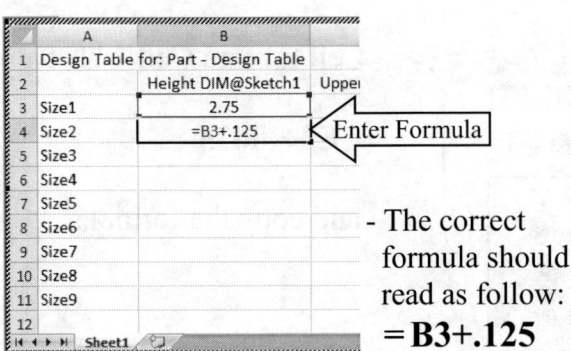

Enter Formula

- The correct formula should read as follow:
= **B3+.125**

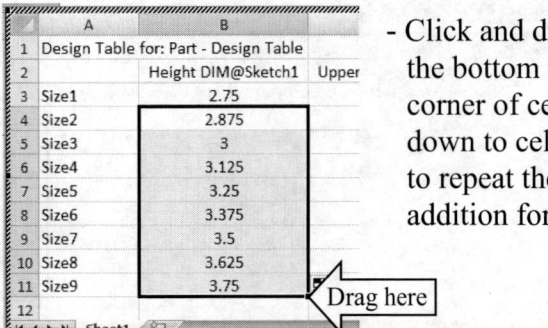

- Click and drag on the bottom right corner of cell B4, down to cell B11 to repeat the addition formula.

Drag here

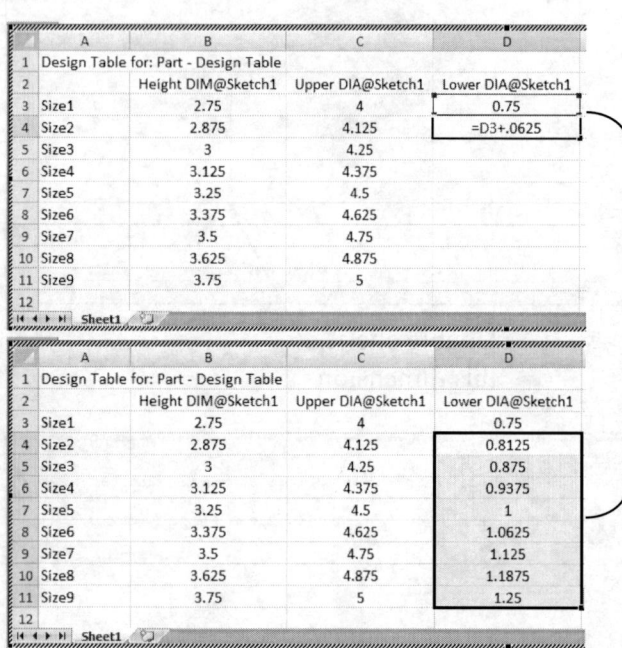

- In cell C4 type:

$$= C3+.125$$

and copy the formula thru cell C11.

	A	B	C	D
1	Design Table for: Part - Design Table			
2		Height DIM@Sketch1	Upper DIA@Sketch1	Lower DIA@Sketch1
3	Size1	2.75	4	0.75
4	Size2	2.875	4.125	=D3+.0625
5	Size3	3	4.25	
6	Size4	3.125	4.375	
7	Size5	3.25	4.5	
8	Size6	3.375	4.625	
9	Size7	3.5	4.75	
10	Size8	3.625	4.875	
11	Size9	3.75	5	

- Cell D4 thru Cell C11, type:

$$= D3+.0625$$

and copy the formula.

	A	B	C	D
1	Design Table for: Part - Design Table			
2		Height DIM@Sketch1	Upper DIA@Sketch1	Lower DIA@Sketch1
3	Size1	2.75	4	0.75
4	Size2	2.875	4.125	0.8125
5	Size3	3	4.25	0.875
6	Size4	3.125	4.375	0.9375
7	Size5	3.25	4.5	1
8	Size6	3.375	4.625	1.0625
9	Size7	3.5	4.75	1.125
10	Size8	3.625	4.875	1.1875
11	Size9	3.75	5	1.25

	A	B	C	D	E
1	Design Table for: Part - Design Table				
2		Height DIM@Sketch1	Upper DIA@Sketch1	Lower DIA@Sketch1	Side RAD@Sketch1
3	Size1	2.75	4	0.75	2.5
4	Size2	2.875	4.125	0.8125	=E3+.0625
5	Size3	3	4.25	0.875	
6	Size4	3.125	4.375	0.9375	
7	Size5	3.25	4.5	1	
8	Size6	3.375	4.625	1.0625	
9	Size7	3.5	4.75	1.125	
10	Size8	3.625	4.875	1.1875	
11	Size9	3.75	5	1.25	

- Cell E4 thru Cell E11, type:

$$= E3+.0625$$

and copy the formula.

	A	B	C	D	E
1	Design Table for: Part - Design Table				
2		Height DIM@Sketch1	Upper DIA@Sketch1	Lower DIA@Sketch1	Side RAD@Sketch1
3	Size1	2.75	4	0.75	2.5
4	Size2	2.875	4.125	0.8125	2.5625
5	Size3	3	4.25	0.875	2.625
6	Size4	3.125	4.375	0.9375	2.6875
7	Size5	3.25	4.5	1	2.75
8	Size6	3.375	4.625	1.0625	2.8125
9	Size7	3.5	4.75	1.125	2.875
10	Size8	3.625	4.875	1.1875	2.9375
11	Size9	3.75	5	1.25	3

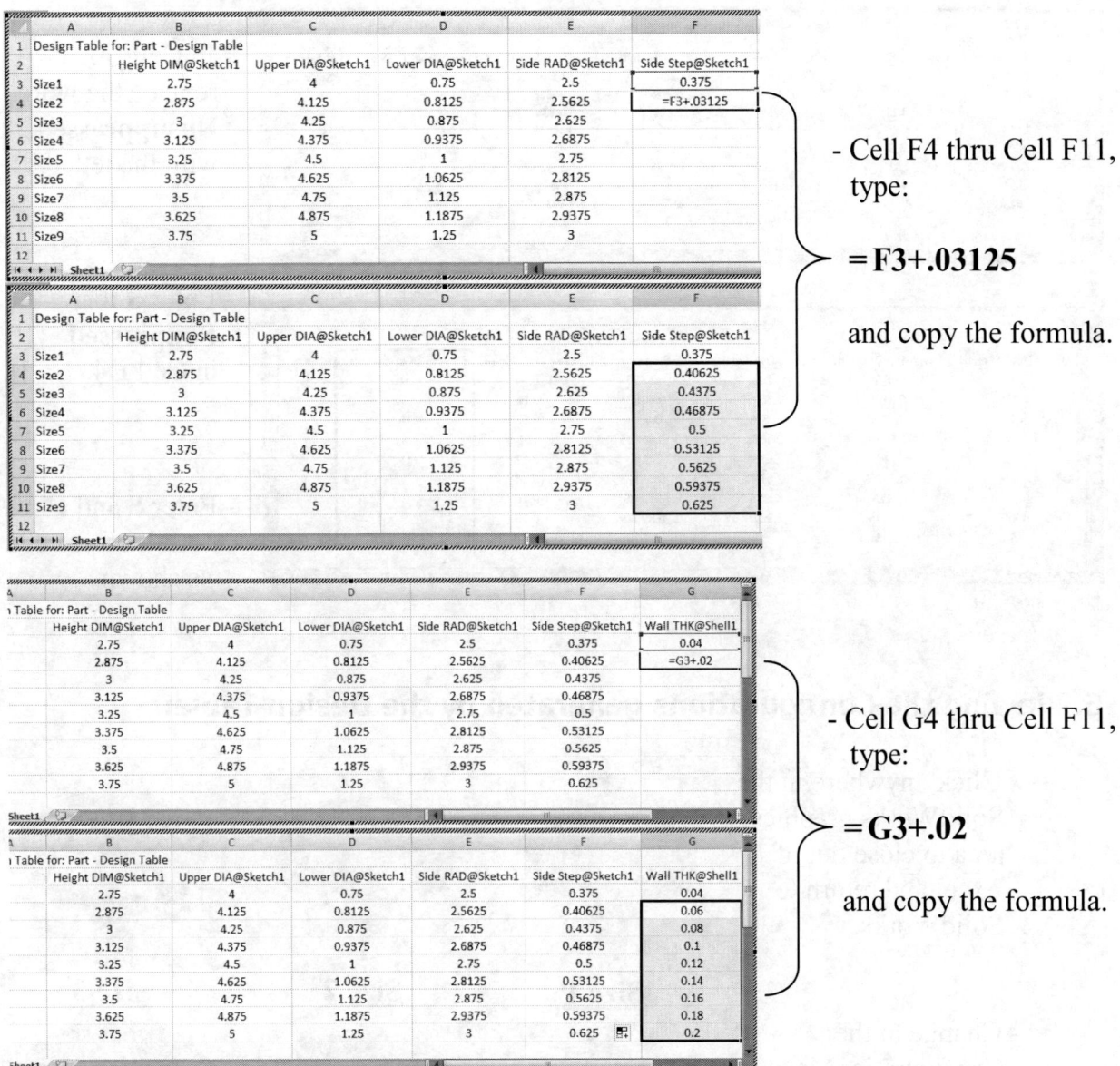

	A	B	C	D	E	F
1	Design Table for: Part - Design Table					
2		Height DIM@Sketch1	Upper DIA@Sketch1	Lower DIA@Sketch1	Side RAD@Sketch1	Side Step@Sketch1
3	Size1	2.75	4	0.75	2.5	0.375
4	Size2	2.875	4.125	0.8125	2.5625	=F3+.03125
5	Size3	3	4.25	0.875	2.625	
6	Size4	3.125	4.375	0.9375	2.6875	
7	Size5	3.25	4.5	1	2.75	
8	Size6	3.375	4.625	1.0625	2.8125	
9	Size7	3.5	4.75	1.125	2.875	
10	Size8	3.625	4.875	1.1875	2.9375	
11	Size9	3.75	5	1.25	3	
12						

Sheet1

- Cell F4 thru Cell F11, type:

=F3+.03125

and copy the formula.

	A	B	C	D	E	F
1	Design Table for: Part - Design Table					
2		Height DIM@Sketch1	Upper DIA@Sketch1	Lower DIA@Sketch1	Side RAD@Sketch1	Side Step@Sketch1
3	Size1	2.75	4	0.75	2.5	0.375
4	Size2	2.875	4.125	0.8125	2.5625	0.40625
5	Size3	3	4.25	0.875	2.625	0.4375
6	Size4	3.125	4.375	0.9375	2.6875	0.46875
7	Size5	3.25	4.5	1	2.75	0.5
8	Size6	3.375	4.625	1.0625	2.8125	0.53125
9	Size7	3.5	4.75	1.125	2.875	0.5625
10	Size8	3.625	4.875	1.1875	2.9375	0.59375
11	Size9	3.75	5	1.25	3	0.625
12						

Sheet1

B	C	D	E	F	G
Table for: Part - Design Table					
Height DIM@Sketch1	Upper DIA@Sketch1	Lower DIA@Sketch1	Side RAD@Sketch1	Side Step@Sketch1	Wall THK@Shell1
2.75	4	0.75	2.5	0.375	0.04
2.875	4.125	0.8125	2.5625	0.40625	=G3+.02
3	4.25	0.875	2.625	0.4375	
3.125	4.375	0.9375	2.6875	0.46875	
3.25	4.5	1	2.75	0.5	
3.375	4.625	1.0625	2.8125	0.53125	
3.5	4.75	1.125	2.875	0.5625	
3.625	4.875	1.1875	2.9375	0.59375	
3.75	5	1.25	3	0.625	

Sheet1

- Cell G4 thru Cell F11, type:

=G3+.02

and copy the formula.

B	C	D	E	F	G
Table for: Part - Design Table					
Height DIM@Sketch1	Upper DIA@Sketch1	Lower DIA@Sketch1	Side RAD@Sketch1	Side Step@Sketch1	Wall THK@Shell1
2.75	4	0.75	2.5	0.375	0.04
2.875	4.125	0.8125	2.5625	0.40625	0.06
3	4.25	0.875	2.625	0.4375	0.08
3.125	4.375	0.9375	2.6875	0.46875	0.1
3.25	4.5	1	2.75	0.5	0.12
3.375	4.625	1.0625	2.8125	0.53125	0.14
3.5	4.75	1.125	2.875	0.5625	0.16
3.625	4.875	1.1875	2.9375	0.59375	0.18
3.75	5	1.25	3	0.625	0.2

Sheet1

5. Controlling the Suppression-States of the holes:

- Select the cell **H2** and double click on the **CutExtrude1** to transfer to cell H2.

C	D	E	F	G	H
Table					
Upper DIA@Sketch1	Lower DIA@Sketch1	Side RAD@Sketch1	Side Step@Sketch1	Wall THK@Shell1	
4	0.75	2.5	0.375	0.04	
4.125	0.8125	2.5625	0.40625	0.06	
4.25	0.875	2.625	0.4375	0.08	
4.375	0.9375	2.6875	0.46875	0.1	
4.5	1	2.75	0.5	0.12	
4.625	1.0625	2.8125	0.53125	0.14	
4.75	1.125	2.875	0.5625	0.16	
4.875	1.1875	2.9375	0.59375	0.18	
5	1.25	3	0.625	0.2	

Select Cell H2

- Part - Design Table (Default)
- Annotations
- Material <not specified>
- Front Plane
- Top Plane
- Right Plane
- Origin
- Revolve1
- Shell1
- Cut-Extrude1 ← Double click
- CirPattern1
- Fillet1

	Height DIM@Sketch1	Upper DIA@Sketch1	Lower DIA@Sketch1	Side RAD@Sketch1	Side Step@Sketch1	Wall THK@Shell1	$STATE@Cut-Extrude1
1	for: Part - Design Table						
3	2.75	4	0.75	2.5	0.375	0.04	UNSUPPRESSED
4	2.875	4.125	0.8125	2.5625	0.40625	0.06	
5	3	4.25	0.875	2.625	0.4375	0.08	
6	3.125	4.375	0.9375	2.6875	0.46875	0.1	
7	3.25	4.5	1	2.75	0.5	0.12	
8	3.375	4.625	1.0625	2.8125	0.53125	0.14	
9	3.5	4.75	1.125	2.875	0.5625	0.16	
10	3.625	4.875	1.1875	2.9375	0.59375	0.18	
11	3.75	5	1.25	3	0.625	0.2	

Sheet1

- In Cell H3, replace the word **Unsuppressed** with the letter **U**.

	Upper DIA@Sketch1	Lower DIA@Sketch1	Side RAD@Sketch1	Side Step@Sketch1	Wall THK@Shell1	$STATE@Cut-Extrude1
3	4	0.75	2.5	0.375	0.04	U
4	4.125	0.8125	2.5625	0.40625	0.06	S
5	4.25	0.875	2.625	0.4375	0.08	U
6	4.375	0.9375	2.6875	0.46875	0.1	S
7	4.5	1	2.75	0.5	0.12	U
8	4.625	1.0625	2.8125	0.53125	0.14	S
9	4.75	1.125	2.875	0.5625	0.16	U
10	4.875	1.1875	2.9375	0.59375	0.18	S
11	5	1.25	3	0.625	0.2	U

Sheet1

- Enter **S** for: **Suppressed** in Cell H4.

- Enter **S** and **U** for all other cells as shown.

6. Viewing the Configurations generated by the Design Table:

- Click anywhere in the SolidWorks graphics area to close out of Excel and return to SolidWorks.

- Change to the ConfigurationManager tree.

- Double click on Size2 and then other sizes to see the parts that were created by the Design Table.

- Save your work as: **Part - Design Table**.

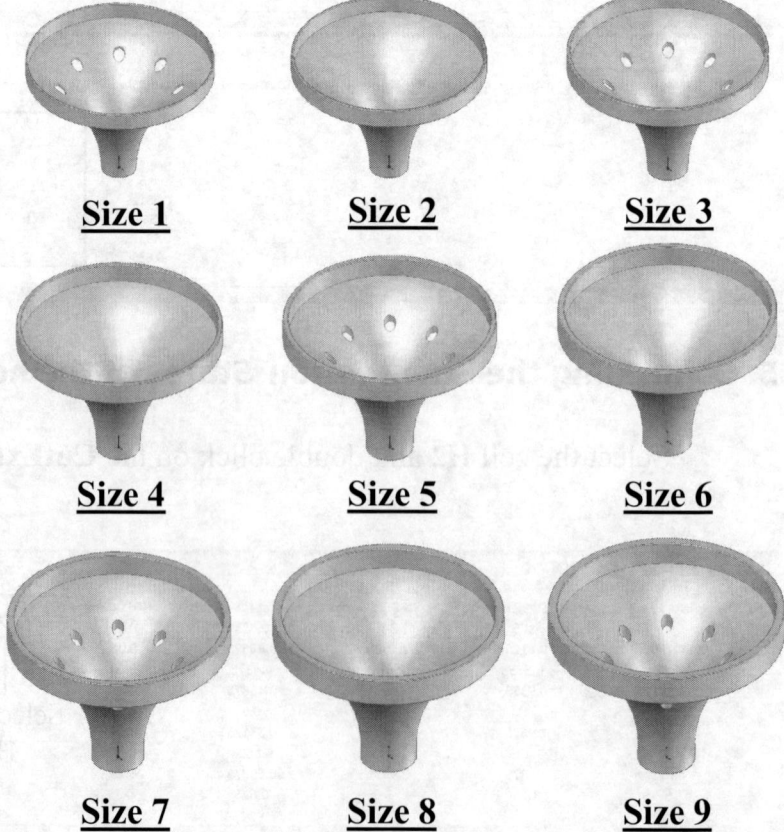

Size 1   Size 2   Size 3

Size 4   Size 5   Size 6

Size 7   Size 8   Size 9

Assembly - Design Tables

1. Copying the Egg Beater Assembly:

- <u>Go to:</u> The Training Files folder
      Design Tables folder
      Egg Beater Assembly Folder.

- Copy the Egg-Beater-Assembly folder to
  your computer.

- **Open** the **Egg Beater Assembly.sldasm**

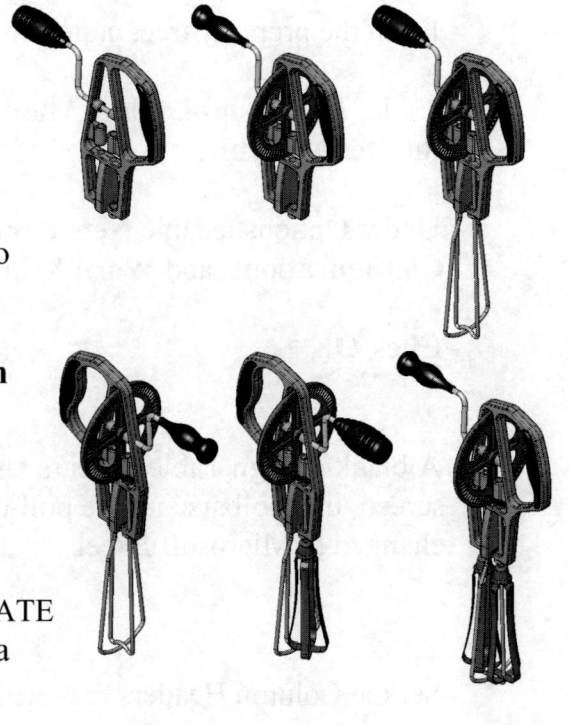

- This exercise discusses the use of the STATE
  and CONFIGURATION parameters in a
  Design Table.

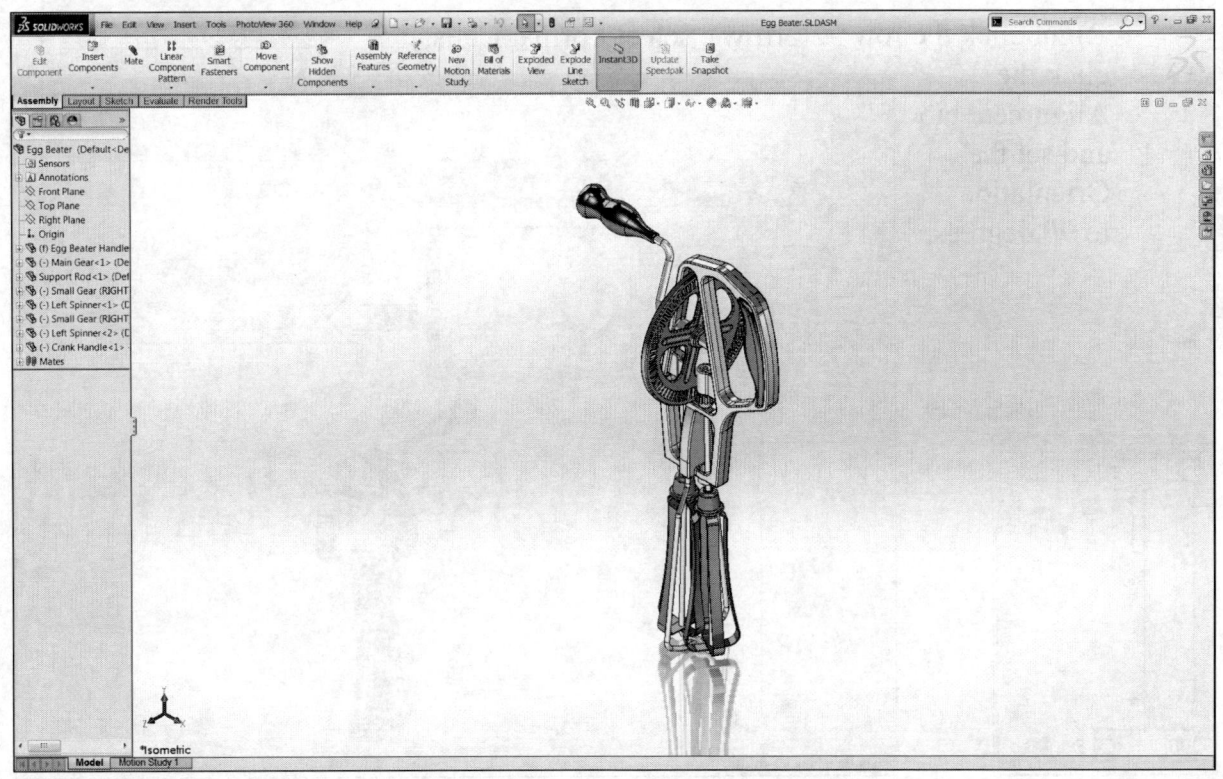

2. Creating a new Assembly Design Table:

- Select **Insert / New Design Table**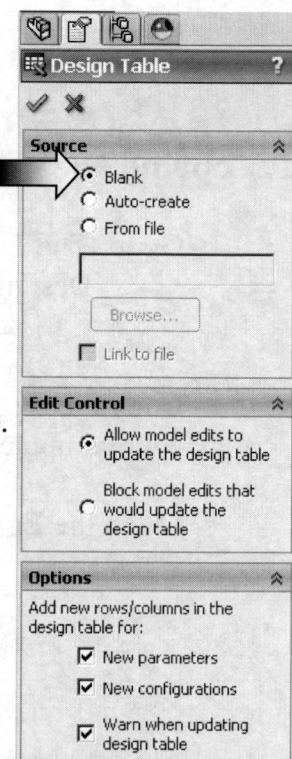

- From the property tree, under Source, select **Blank**.

- Under Edit Control, select **Allow Model Edits to Update the Design Table**.

- Under Options, enable **New Parameters**, **New Configurations**, and **Warn When Updating Design Table**.

- Click **OK** ✓ .

- A blank Design Table appears and overlays the SolidWorks screen, the toolbars and the pull-down menus are now changed to Microsoft Excel.

- Set the Column Headers to Vertical Alignment.

- Right click the row #2(arrow), select Format Cells, click the Alignment tab and set the Orientation to 90 degrees.

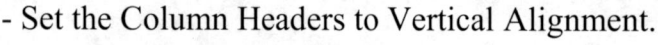

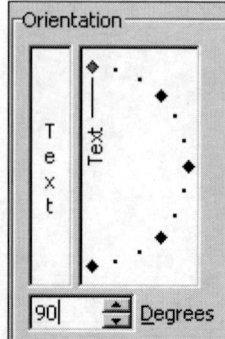

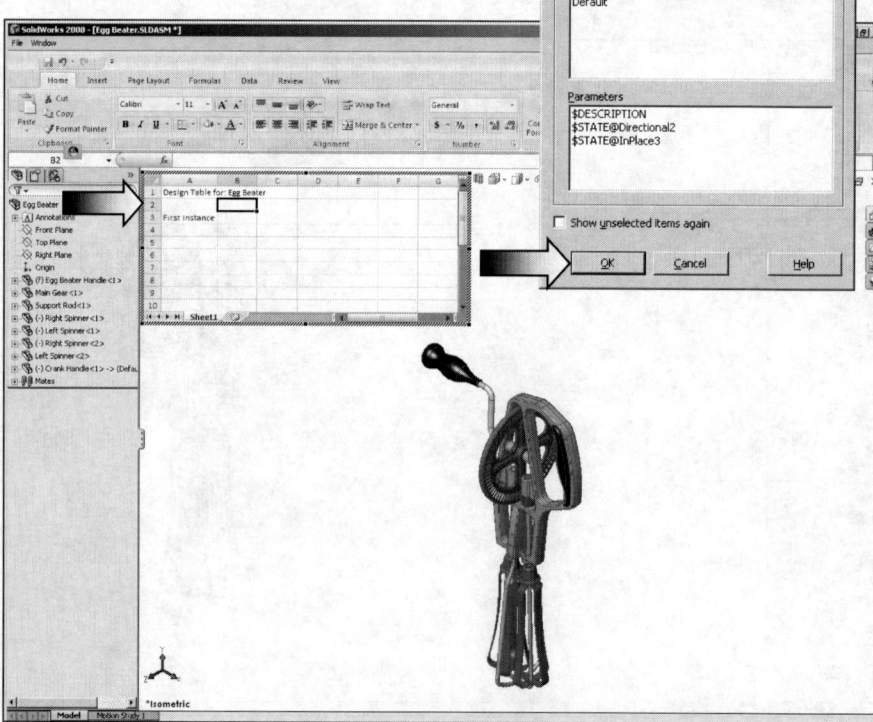

NOTE:

To create a design table, you must define the names of the configurations that you want to create, specify the parameters that you want to control, and assign values for each parameter.

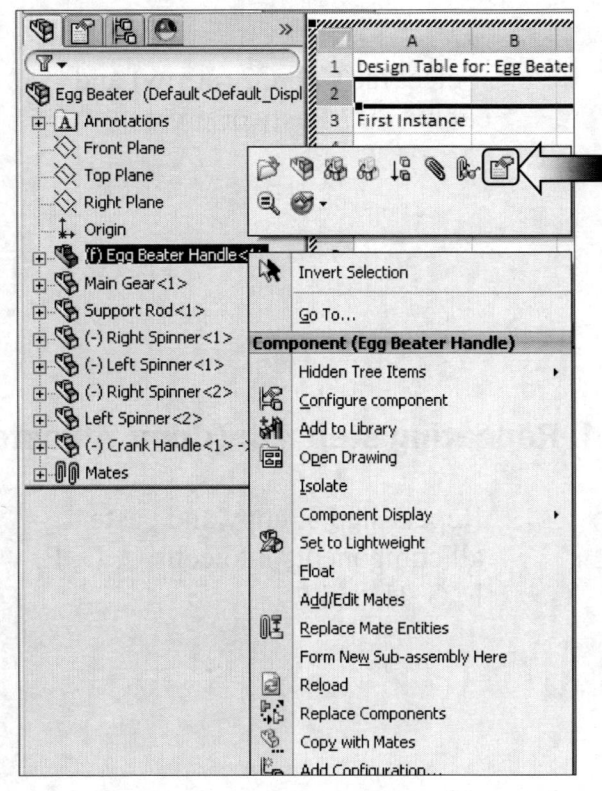

3. Defining the column headers:

- We are going to copy the name of of each component and paste it to the Design Table. They will be used as the Column Headers.

- Right click on the part named Egg Beater Handle and select: **Component Properties** (Arrow).

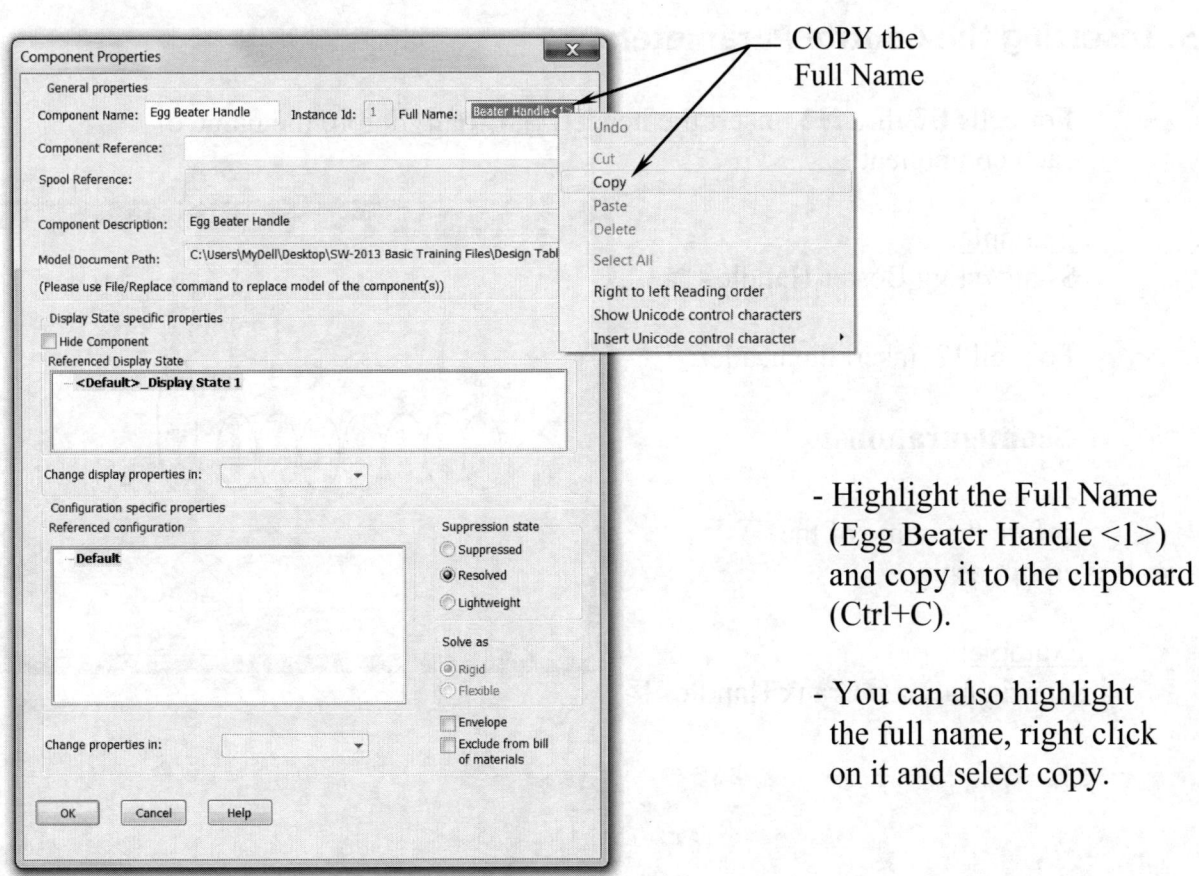

COPY the
Full Name

- Highlight the Full Name (Egg Beater Handle <1>) and copy it to the clipboard (Ctrl+C).

- You can also highlight the full name, right click on it and select copy.

- Select the Cell C2 (arrow) and
  click **Edit / Paste** or press
  Ctrl+V.

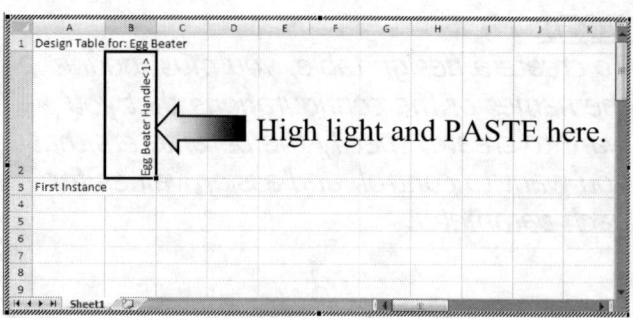

High light and PASTE here.

4. Repeating step #3: (Copy & Paste all components)

- Repeat step 3, copy and paste
  all components into cells C, D, E,
  F, G, H, and I.

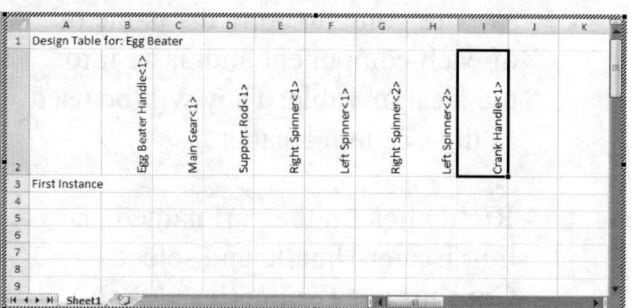

5. Inserting the Control Parameters:

- For cells **B2** thru **H2**, insert the header: **$state@** before the name of
  each component.

Example:
$state@Egg Beater Handle<1>

- For cell **I2**, insert the header:

$configuration@

before the name of the
component.

Example:
$configuration@Crank Handle<1>

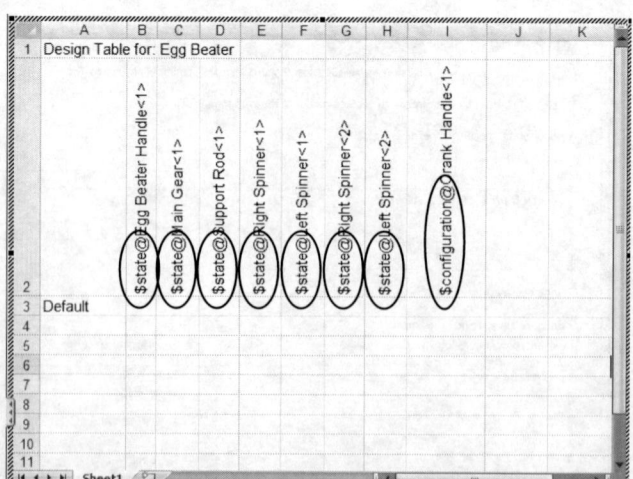

6. Adding the configuration names:

- The actual part numbers can be used here for the name of each configuration.

- Starting at **Cell A4**, (below Default), enter **Config1** thru **Config5** as shown.

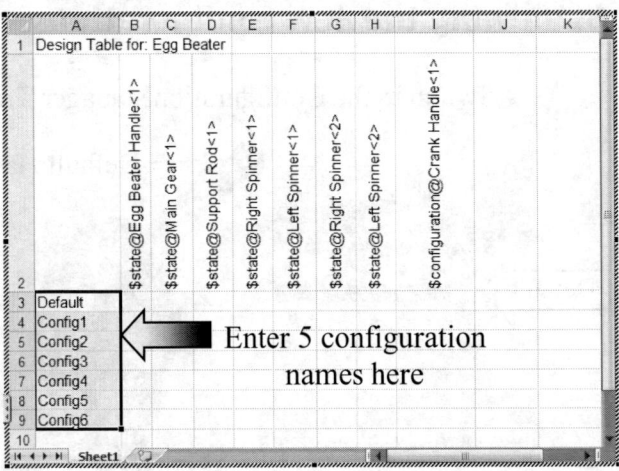

Enter 5 configuration names here

7. Assigning the control values:

- To prevent mistakes, type the letter R and letter S in each cell.

- Enter the values R (Resolved) and S (Suppressed) into their appropriate cells, from column B through column H.

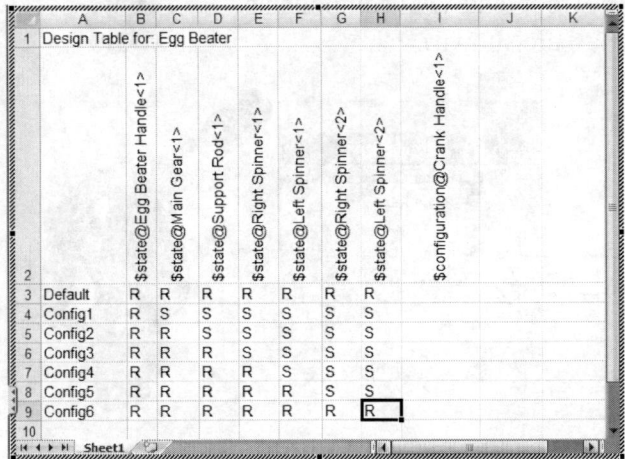

- For Column I, we will enter the names of the configurations instead.

- Select the cell **I3** and enter: **Default**.

- Select the cell **I4** and enter **Oval Handle**.

- Repeat the same step for all 6 configs.

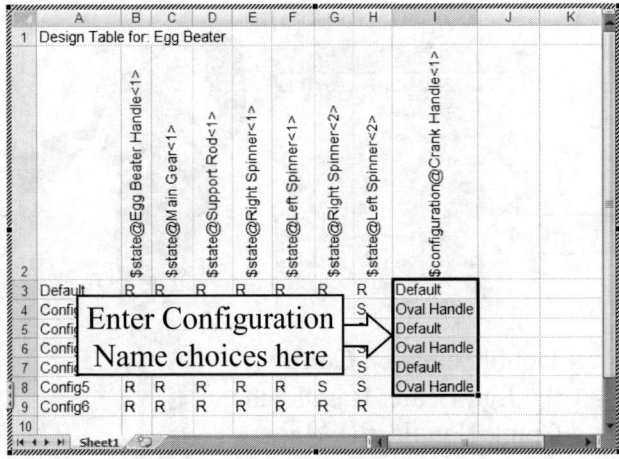

Enter Configuration Name choices here

8. Viewing the new configurations:

- Switch to the ConfigurationManager Tree.

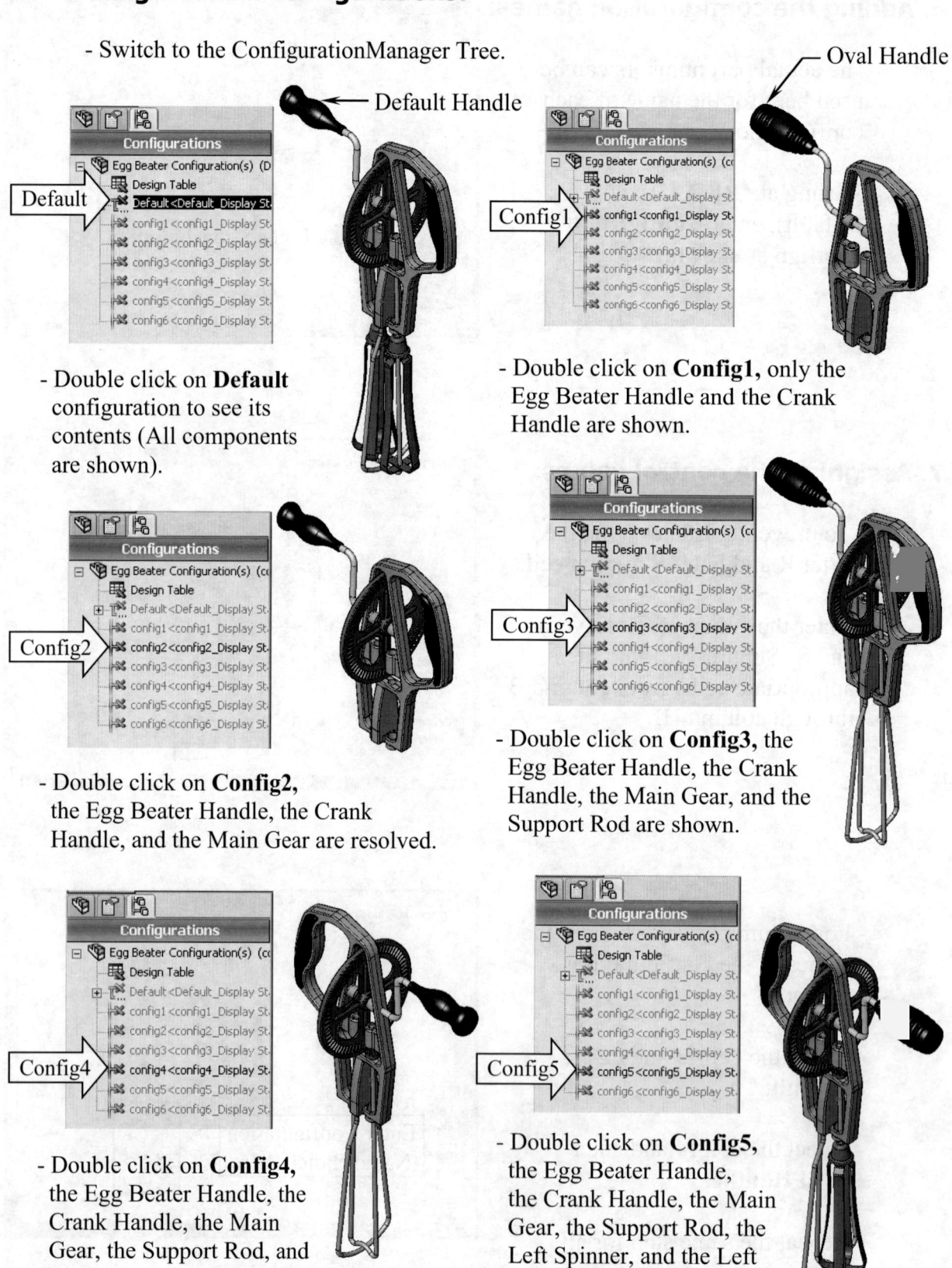

- Double click on **Default** configuration to see its contents (All components are shown).

- Double click on **Config1,** only the Egg Beater Handle and the Crank Handle are shown.

- Double click on **Config2,** the Egg Beater Handle, the Crank Handle, and the Main Gear are resolved.

- Double click on **Config3,** the Egg Beater Handle, the Crank Handle, the Main Gear, and the Support Rod are shown.

- Double click on **Config4,** the Egg Beater Handle, the Crank Handle, the Main Gear, the Support Rod, and the Left Spinner are resolved.

- Double click on **Config5,** the Egg Beater Handle, the Crank Handle, the Main Gear, the Support Rod, the Left Spinner, and the Left Mixer are resolved.

Exercise: Part Design Tables

1. Open the existing document named: **Part Design Tables_EXE** from the Training folder.
2. Create a design table with 3 different sizes using the dimensions provided in the table.
3. Customize the table by merging the cells, adding colors, and borders.
4. Use the instructions on the following pages, if needed.

	Lower Boss Thickness@Sketch	Upper Boss Thickness@Sketch	Center Hole@Sketch1	Upper Boss Dia@Sketch1	Lower Boss Dia@Sketch1	D1@Revolve1	Bolt Cicle@Sketch2	Hole on Flange@Sketch2	D3@CirPattern1	D1@CirPattern1
						Design Table for: Part Design Tables_Exe				
Size 1	0.25	0.25	0.5	1	2	360	1.5	0.25	360	4
Size 2	0.375	0.375	0.625	1.25	2.25	360	1.75	0.275	360	4
Size 3	0.5	0.5	0.75	1.5	2.5	360	2	0.3	360	4

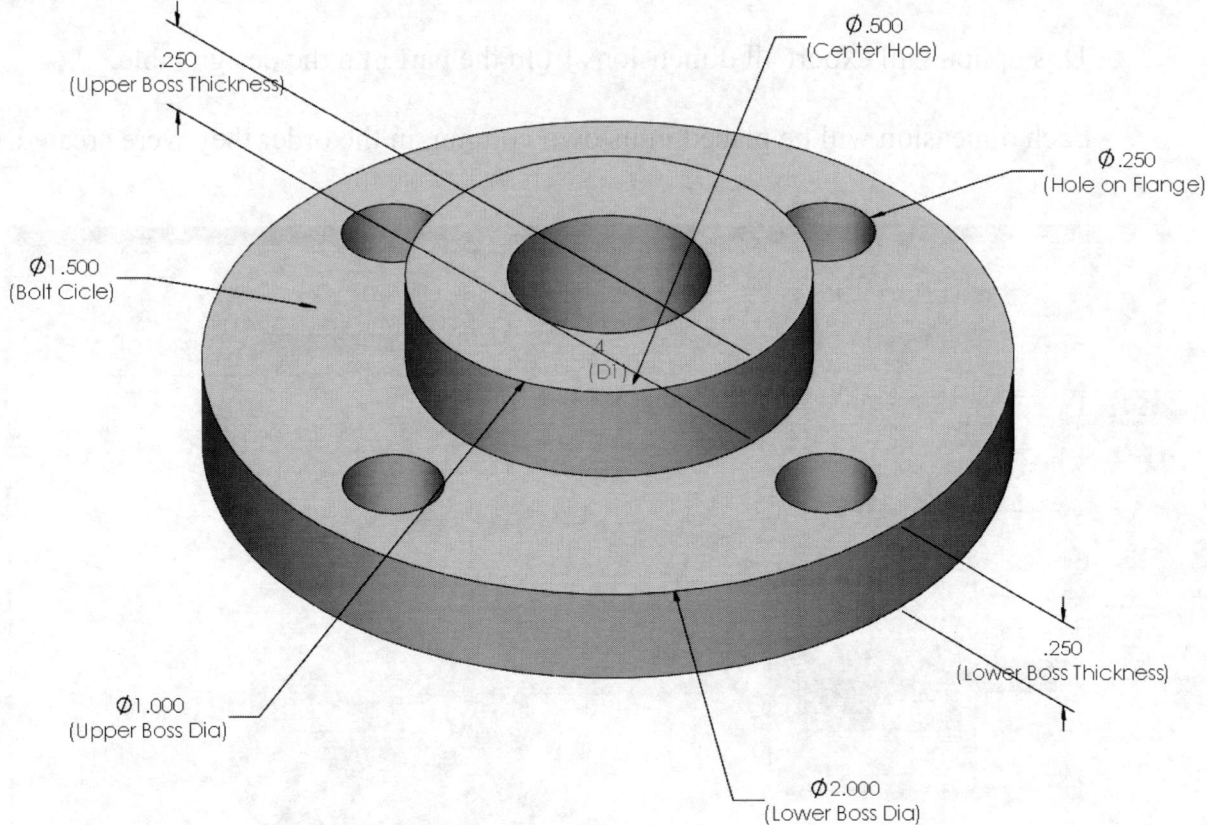

1. Opening the Master part file:

   - From the training files, open the part named: **Part Design Tables_Exe**.
   The dimensions in this part have been renamed for use in this exercise.

2. Inserting a design table:

- From the **Insert** menu click **Tables / Design-Table**.

- Click the **Auto Create** button (default).

- Leave all other options at their default settings.

- Click **OK**.

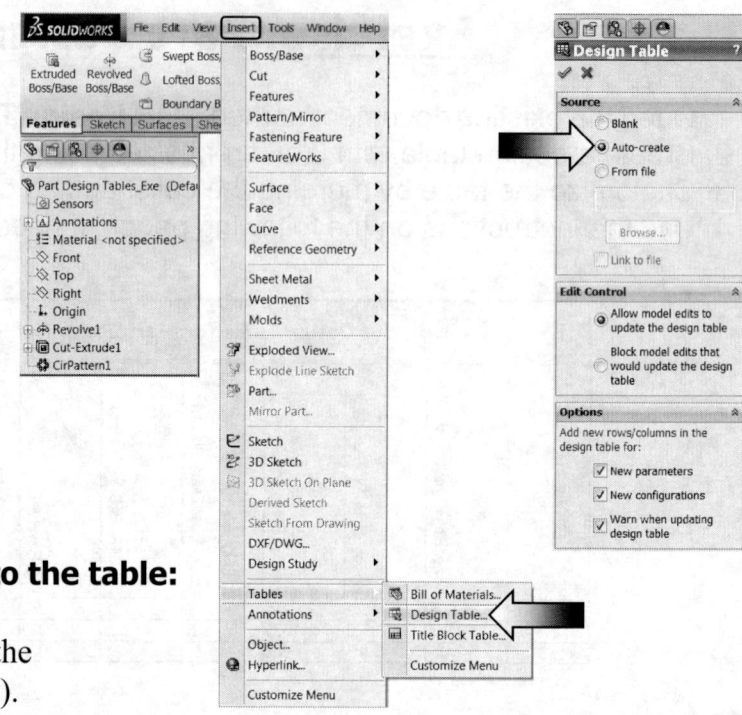

3. Adding model dimensions to the table:

- **Select all dimensions** in the Dimensions dialog (arrow).

- This option will export all dimensions from the part into the design table.

- Each dimension will be placed in its own column, in the order they were created.

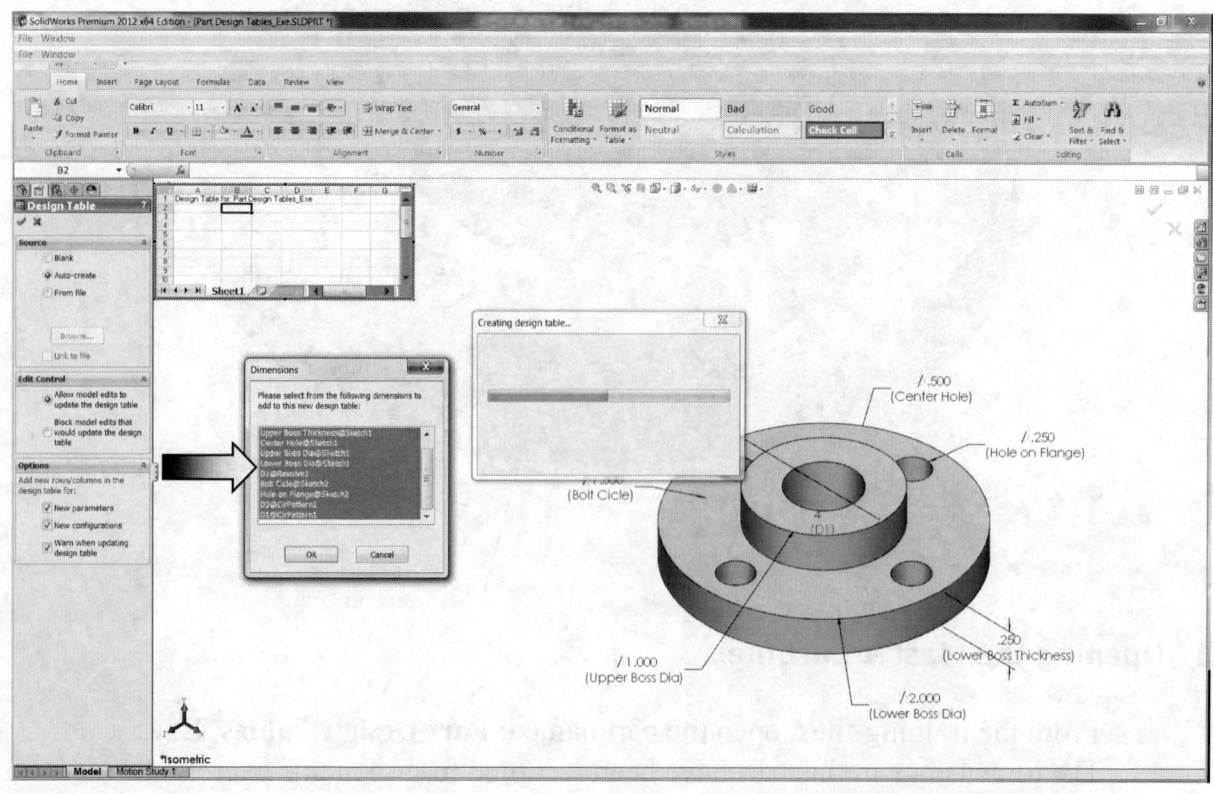

4. Changing the Configuration names:

- For clarity, change the name Default to **Size 1**.

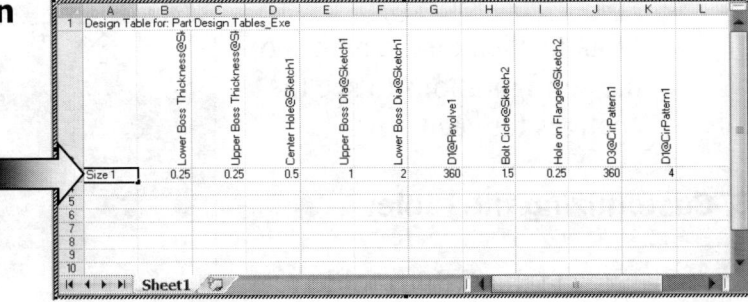

- Create the next 2 configurations by adding the names **Size 2** and **Size 3**, on cell A4 and A5.

- Enter the **new dimensions** for the next 2 sizes.

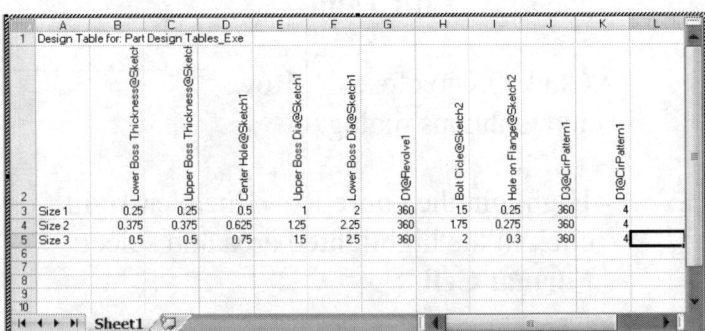

5. Viewing the new configurations:

- Click in the background anywhere. SolidWorks report dialog appears showing 3 new configurations have been generated by the design table.

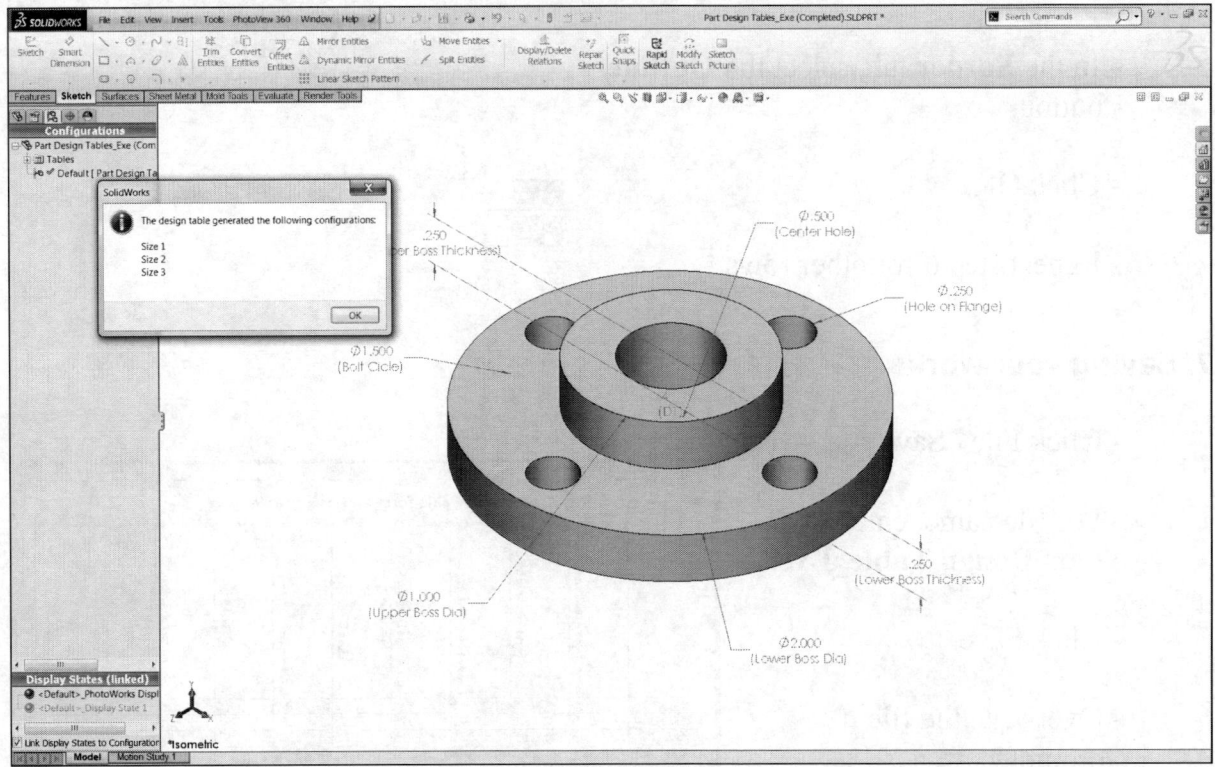

- Double click on the names of the configurations to see the changes for each size.

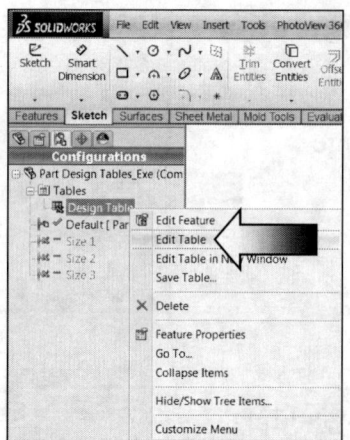
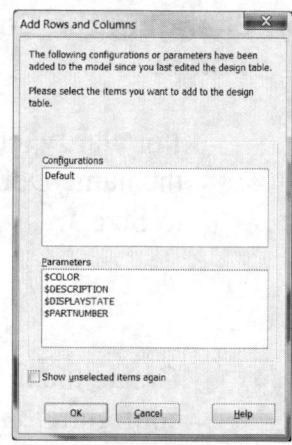

6. Customizing the table:

- Expand the **Tables** folder, right click on Design Tables and select **Edit Table**.

- Click OK to close the Rows and Columns dialog.

- Highlight the entire Row1 header, right click in the highlighted area and select: **Format Cell**.

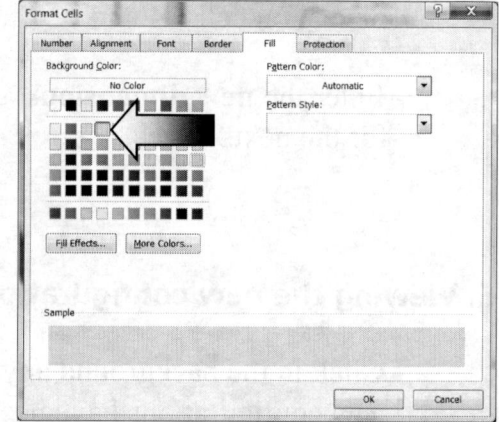

- Click the **Fill** tab and select a color for Row1.

- Change to the **Alignment** tab and enable the **Wrap Text** and **Merge Cells** check-boxes.

- In the **Border** tab, select the **Outline** button.

- Click OK.

- Repeat step 6 for other rows.

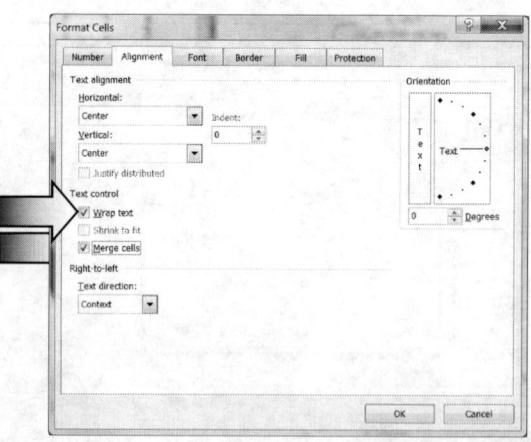

7. Saving your work:

- Click File / Save As.

- For file name, enter: **Part Design Table_Exe**.

- Click Save.

- Overwrite the file if prompted.

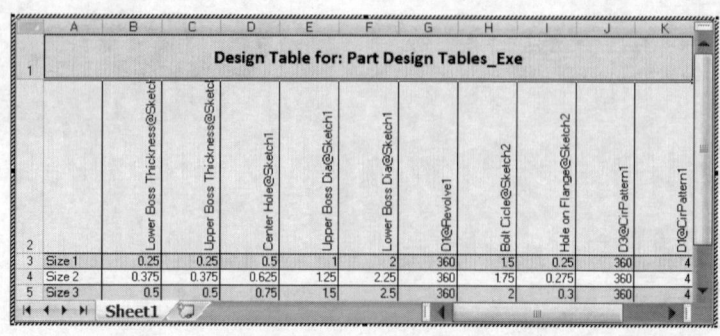

Level 2 Final Exam (1of2)

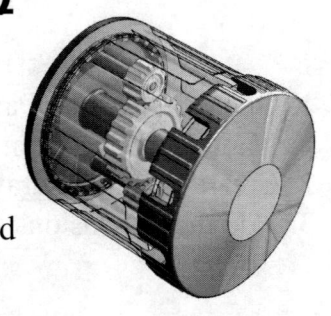

1. Open the existing assembly document named:
   Assembly Motions from the Level 2 Final Exam folder.
2. Create an <u>assembly drawing</u> as shown.
3. Modify the Bill of Materials to match the information provided in the BOM.

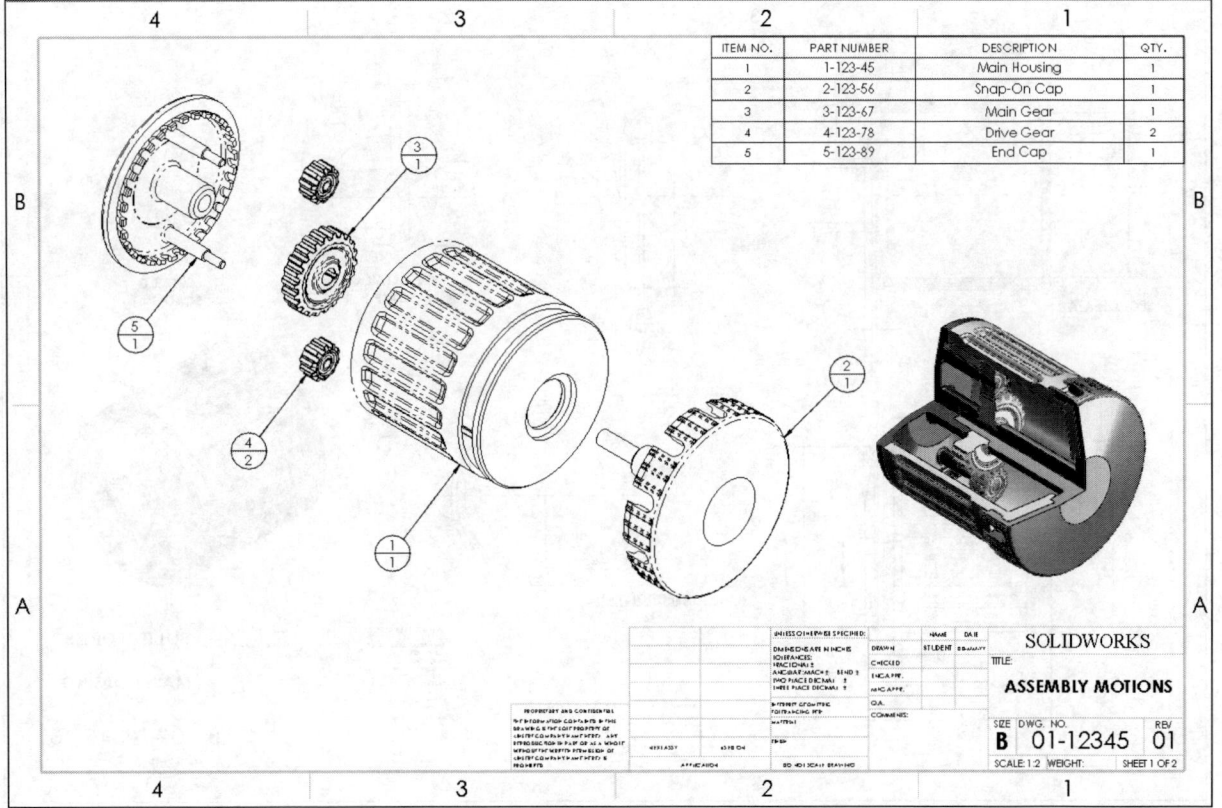

		ITEM NO.	PART NUMBER	DESCRIPTION	QTY.
2		1	1-123-45	Main Housing	1
3		2	2-123-56	Snap-On Cap	1
4		3	3-123-67	Main Gear	1
5		4	4-123-78	Drive Gear	2
6		5	5-123-89	End Cap	1

4. Modify the Balloons to include the Quantity.
5. Fill out the title block with the information shown.
6. Save your drawing as: **L2 Final Assembly Drawing**.

Level 2 Final Exam (2of2)

1. Open the existing Part document named:
   Main Housing from the Level 2 Final Exam folder.
2. Create a <u>detailed drawing</u> shown below.
3. Add the dimensions as shown in each drawing view.

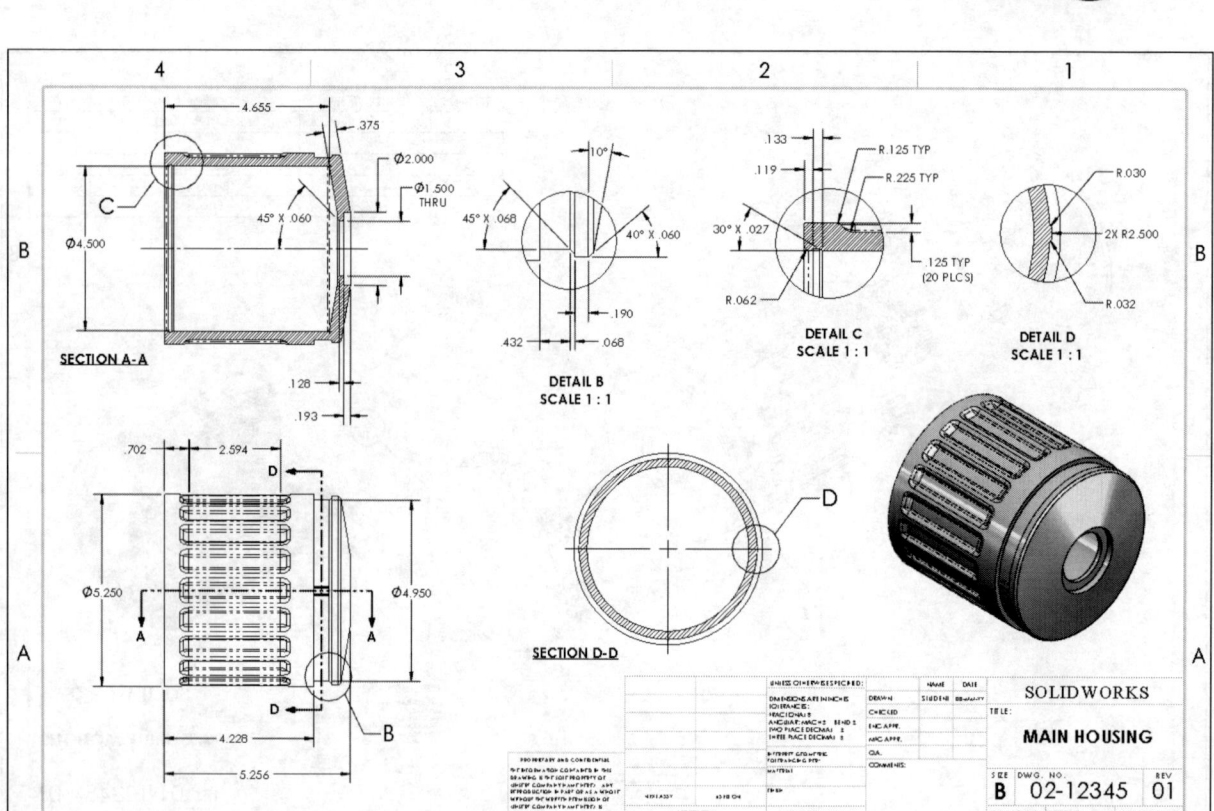

4. Add any missing dimensions as reference dimensions.
5. Fill out the title block with the information shown.
6. Save your drawing as:
   L2 Final Detailed Drawing.

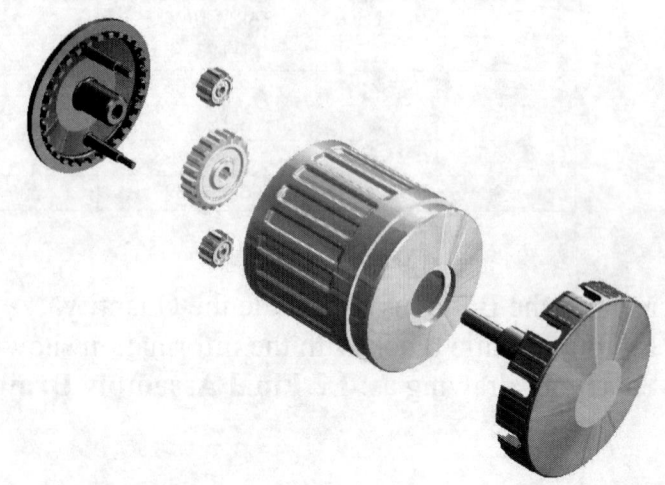

TABLE OF U.S. MEASURES

LENGTH

12 inches	=	1 foot
36 inches	=	1 yard (or 3 feet)
5280 feet	=	1 mile (or 1760 yards)

AREA

144 square inches (in)	=	1 square foot (ft)
9 ft	=	1 square yard (yd)
43,560 ft	=	1 acre (A)
640 A	=	1 square mile (mi)

VOLUME

1728 cubic inches (in³)	=	1 cubic foot (ft)
27 ft	=	1 cubic yard (yd)

LIQUID CAPACITY

8 fluid ounces (fl oz)	=	1 cup (c)
2 c	=	1 pint (pt)
2 pt	=	1 quart (qt)
4 pt	=	1 gallon (gal)

WEIGHT

16 ounces (oz)	=	1 pound (lb)
2000 lb	=	1 ton (t)

TEMPERATURE Degrees Fahrenheit (°F)

32° F	=	freezing point of water
98.6° F	=	normal body temperature
212° F	=	boiling point of water

TABLE OF METRIC MEASURES

LENGTH

10 millimeters (mm)	=	1 centimeter (cm)
10 cm	=	1 decimeter (dm)
100 cm	=	1 meter (m)
1000 m	=	1 kilometer (km)

AREA

100 square millimeters (mm)	=	1 square centimeter (cm)
10,000 cm	=	1 square meter (m)
10,000 m	=	1 hectare (ha)
1,000,000 m	=	1 square kilometer (km)

VOLUME

1000 cubic millimeters (ml)	=	1 cubic centimeter (cm)
1 cm	=	1 milliliter (mL)
1,000 m	=	1 Liter (L)
1,000,000 cm	=	1 cubic meter (m)

LIQUID CAPACITY

10 deciliters (dL)	=	1 liter (L) - or 1000 mL
1000 L	=	1 kiloliter (kL)

MASS

1000 milligrams (mg)	=	1 gram (g)
1000 g	=	1 kilogram (kg)
1000 kg	=	1 metric ton (t)

TEMPERATURE Degrees Celsius (°C)

0° C	=	freezing point of water
37° C	=	normal body temperature
100° C	=	boiling point of water

CHAPTER 21

Using the Intersect Feature

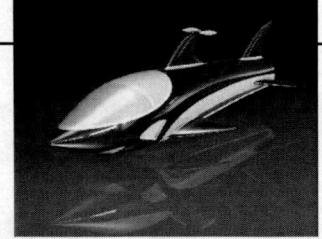

Using the Intersect Feature
Water Warrior Submarine

The Intersect command creates new geometry by intersecting the existing solids, surfaces, or planes.

For example, a solid can be used to add open surface geometry, remove material, or create geometry from an enclosed volume. With the Intersect tool solid bodies can also be merged, or cap some surfaces to define closed volumes.

Surface, Body, or
Plane to Intersect

Regions to Exclude
from Solution

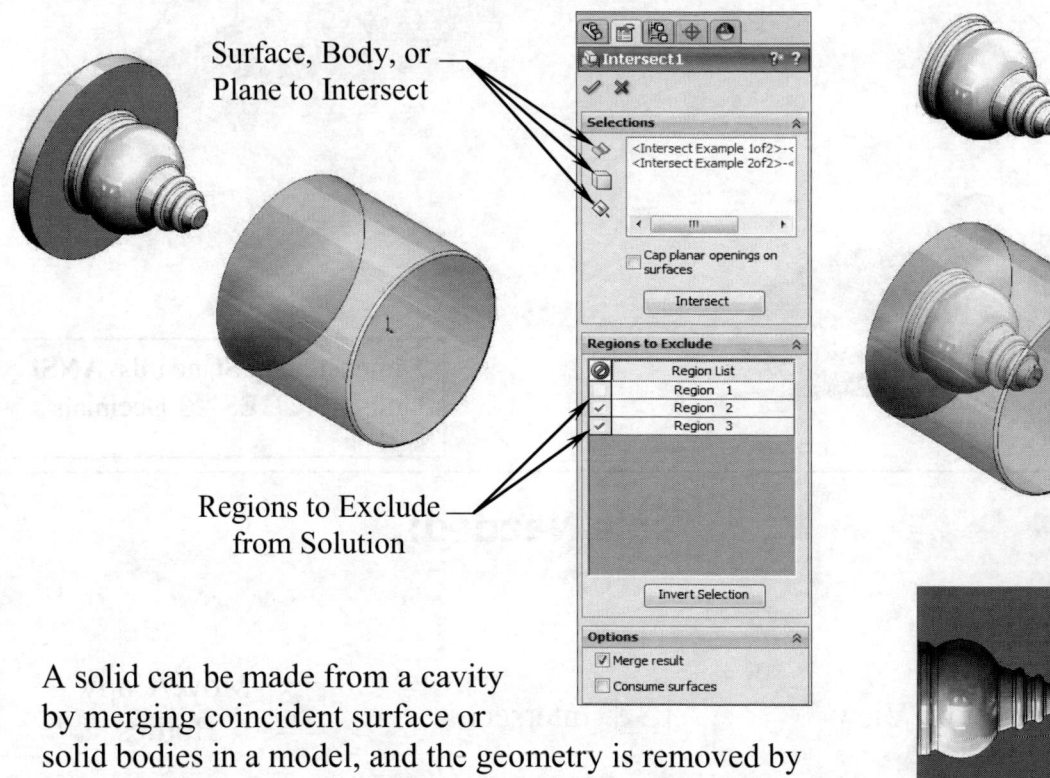

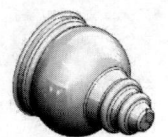

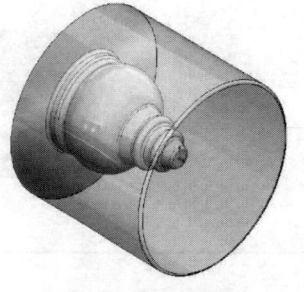

A solid can be made from a cavity
by merging coincident surface or
solid bodies in a model, and the geometry is removed by
defining the bodies that enclose the cavity.

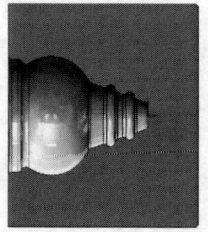

Water Warrior Submarine
Using the Intersect Feature

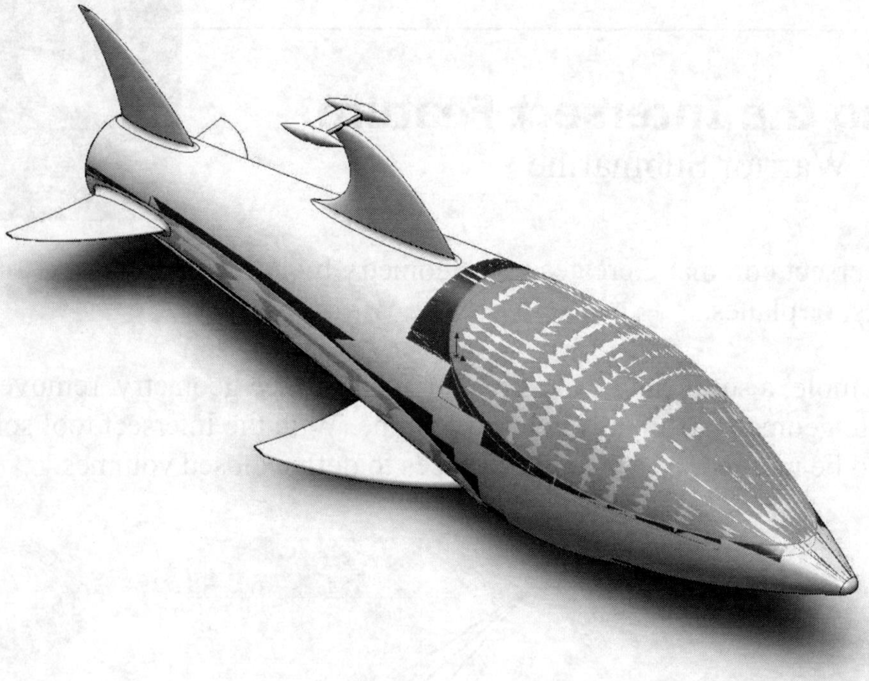

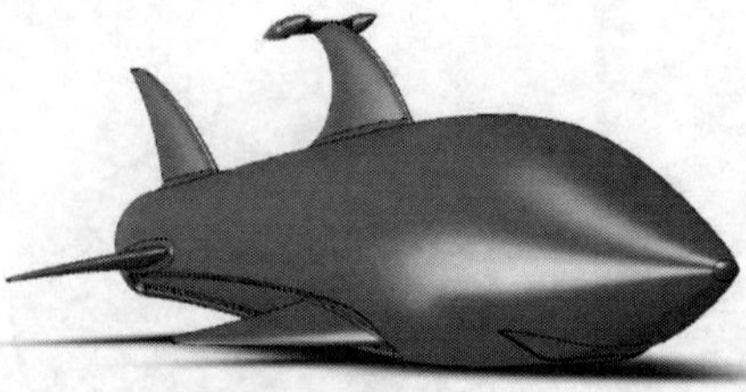

Dimensioning Standards: **ANSI**
Units: **INCHES** – 3 Decimals

Tools Needed:

 Section View

 Intersect

Move/Copy
Bodies

1. Opening the 1st part of the document:

- Click **File / Open**.

- Browse to the Training Files folder, locate and open the document named:
  Water Warrior Submarine Body.

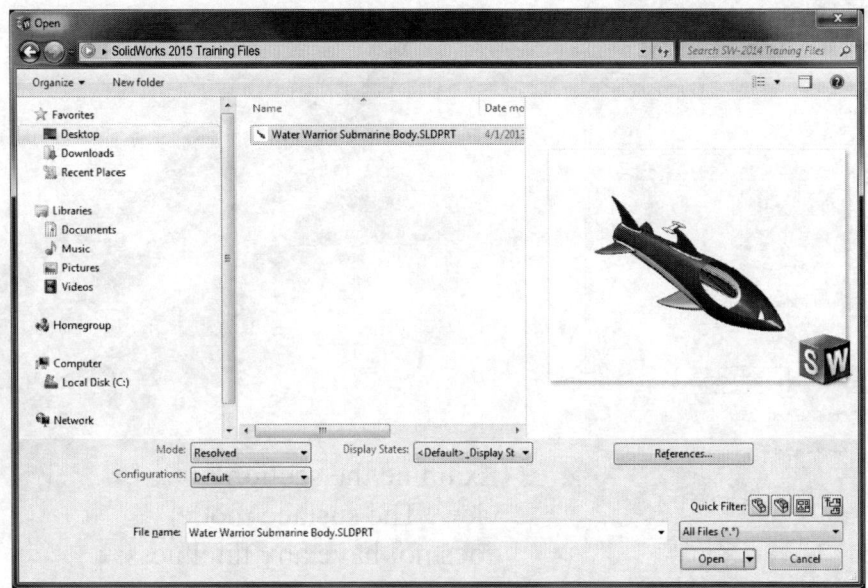

- This model is a surface-model, it does not have any thickness to it.

- A second surface model will get inserted into this same document, located over the cockpit area, as pictured below.

- After placed into position, the two surface bodies will be used to create a solid enclose volume with the intersect tool.

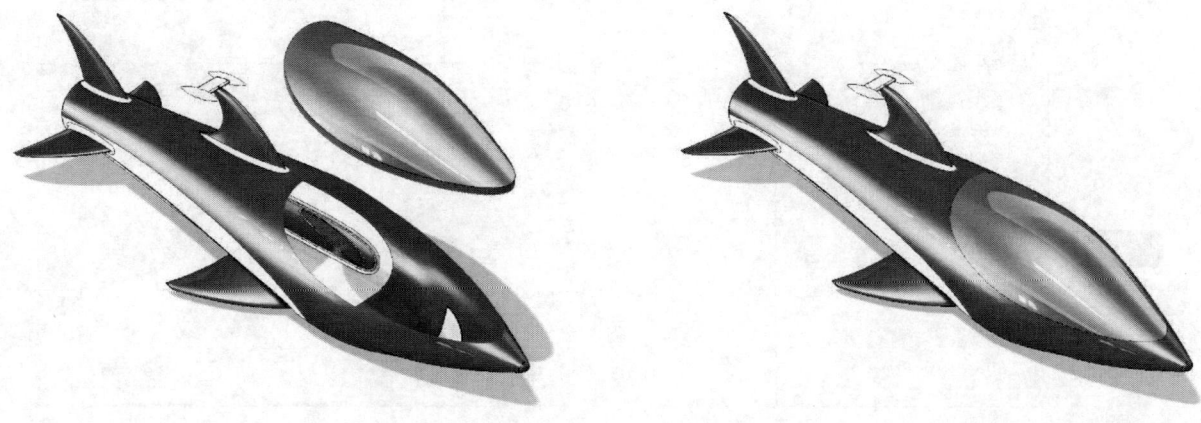

2. Viewing the inside details:

- Click the **Section View** command from the View Heads-Up toolbar.

- Use the **Front** reference plane and create a section at **0.00"** distance (Default).

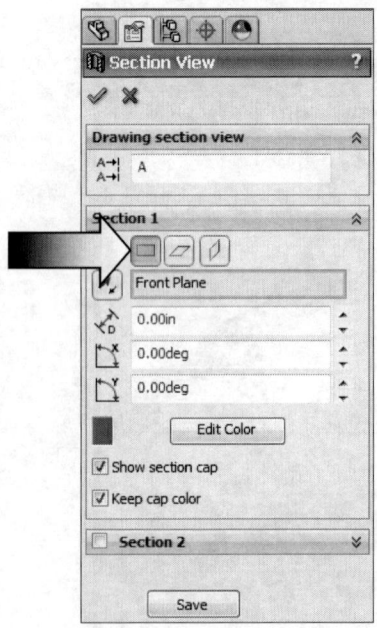

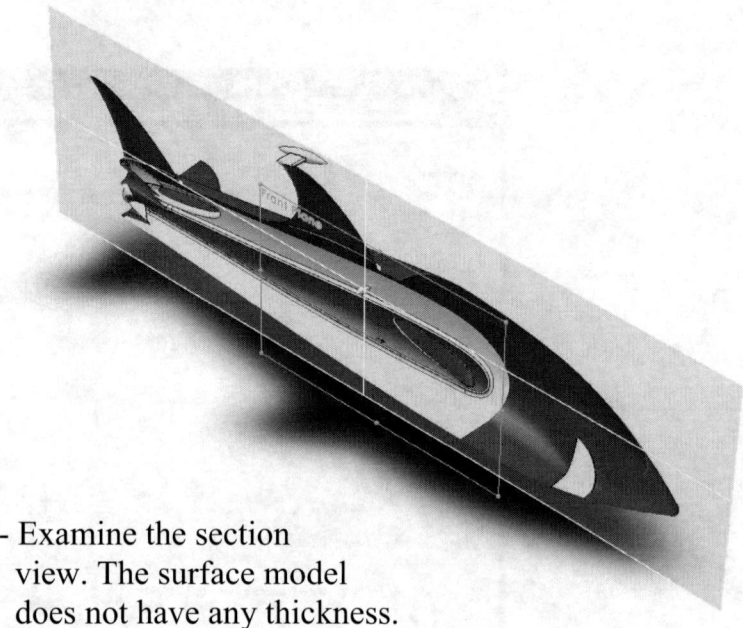

- Examine the section view. The surface model does not have any thickness.

- **Exit** out of the Section View command.

3. Inserting the 2nd surface body:

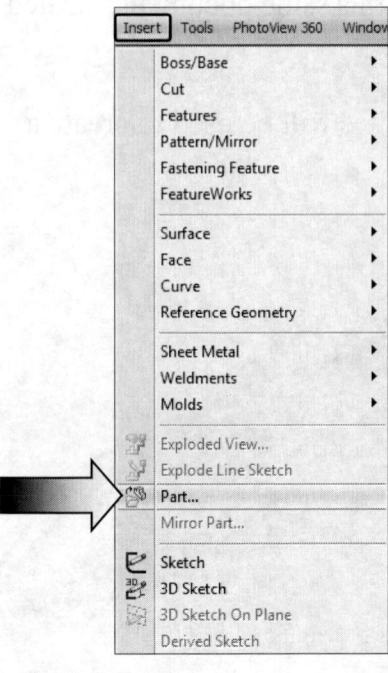

- Select **Insert / Part** (arrow).

- Browse to the Training Files folder, locate and open the document named: **Water Warrior Submarine Cockpit**.

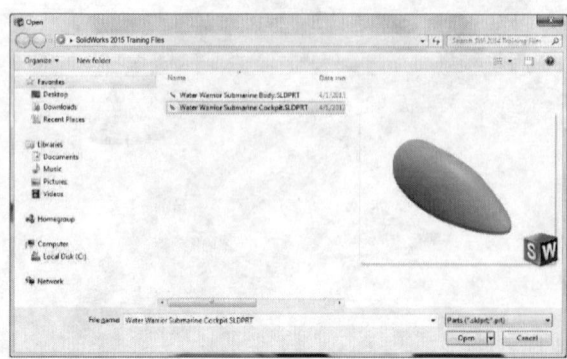

- In the **Insert Part** dialog, enable the Solid Bodies and the Surface Bodies checkboxes, clear all others (arrow).

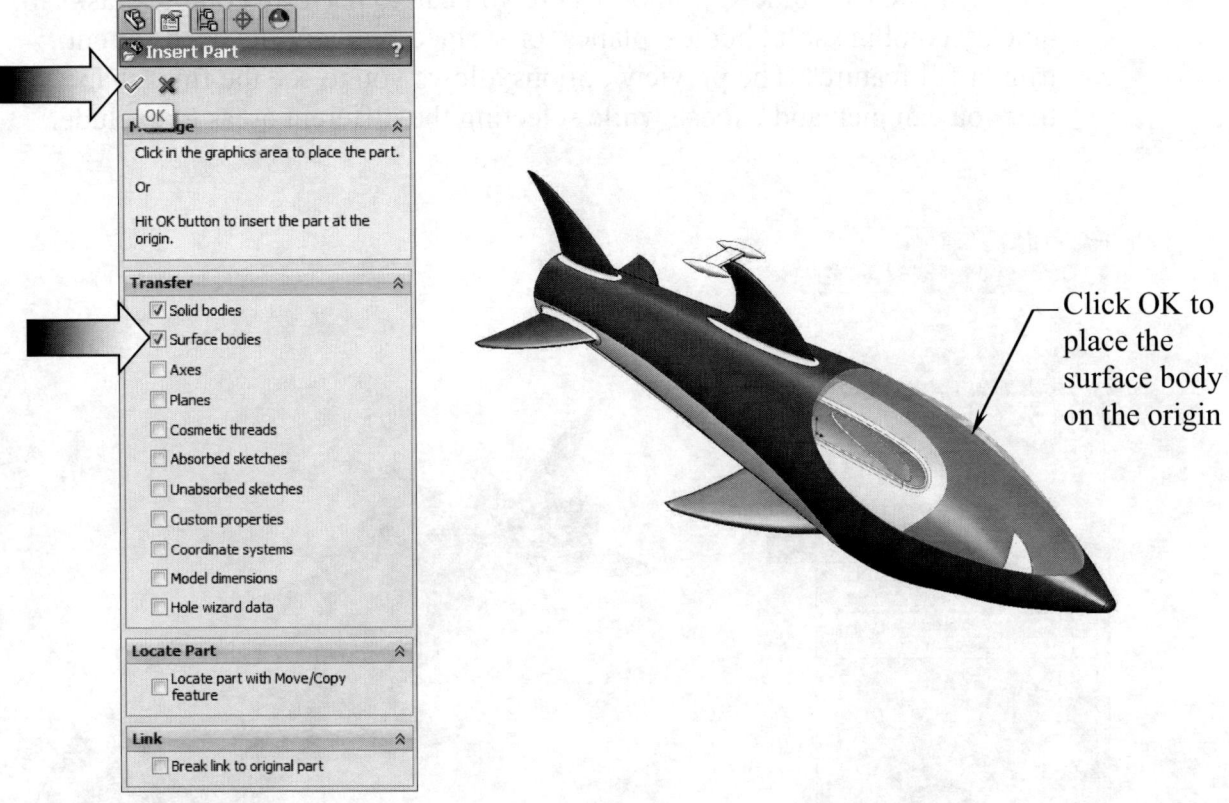

Click OK to place the surface body on the origin

- Click **OK** to place the surface body on the origin (arrow).

4. Creating a section view:

- Click the **Section View** command from the View Heads-Up toolbar once again.

- Use the **Front** reference plane and create a section at **0.00"** distance (Default), similar to the last one.

- Zoom in and examine the section view. Both surface bodies have no thickness to them at this point, but they will become a single solid body after the intersect feature is performed.

5. Creating an Intersect feature:

- The Intersect command is similar to the options Combine-Add, Combine-Subtract, and Combine-Common where you can to perform complex tasks to quickly combine solid bodies, planes, or surfaces without the need for cut, trim or fill features. The preview options allows you to see the final shape that you can pick and choose while selecting the different areas to exclude.

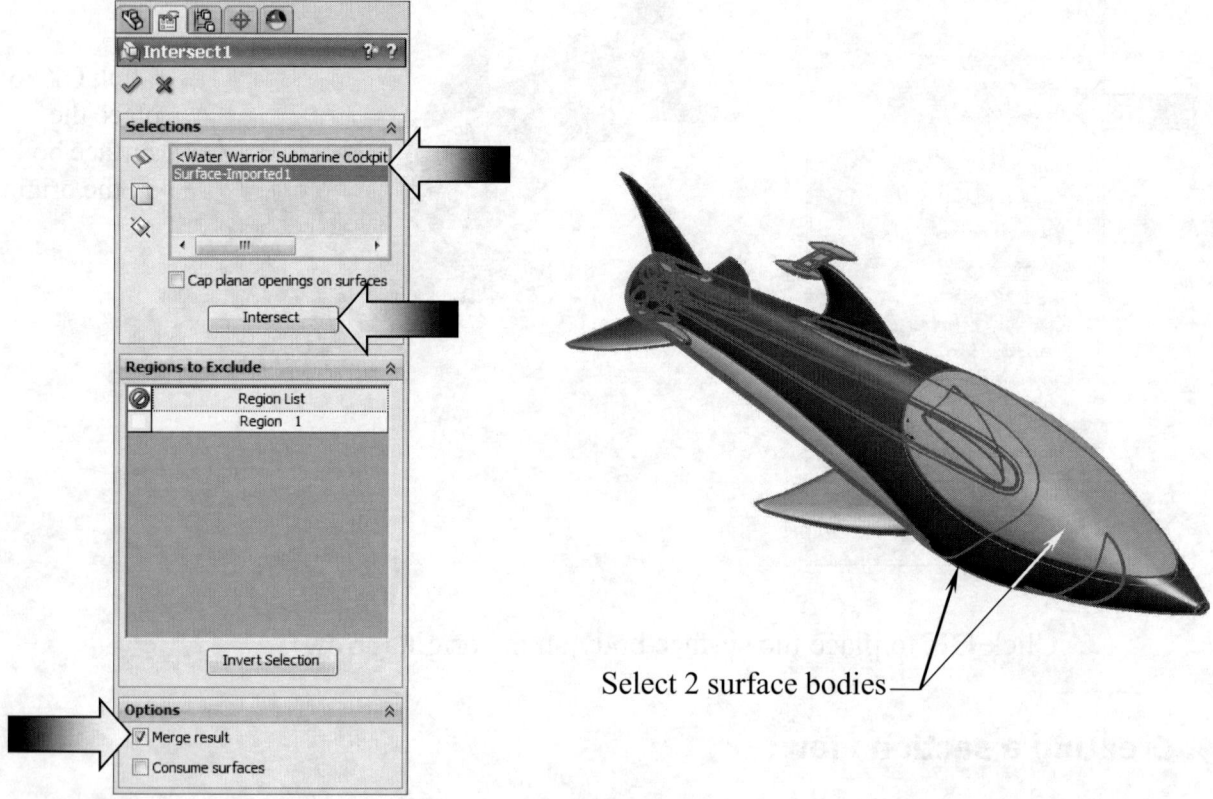

Select 2 surface bodies

- Select **Insert / Features / Intersect**.

- Select the **2 surface bodies** either from the Feature tree or directly from the graphics area (arrow).

- Click the **Intersect** button (arrow). Do not select anything inside the Regions to Exclude section.

- Enable the **Merge Result** checkbox

- Click **OK**.

- The resulting solid body.

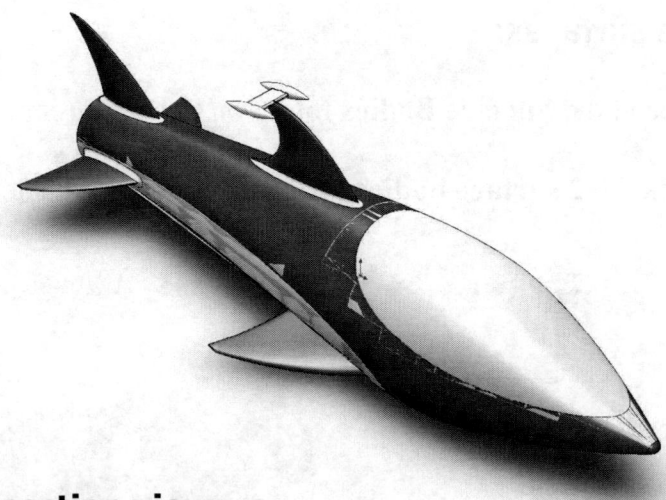

6. Creating another section view:

- Click the **Section View** command once again.

- Use the same settings as the last one and create a section through the center of the model.

- The Intersect operation has converted the 2 surface bodies into a single solid.

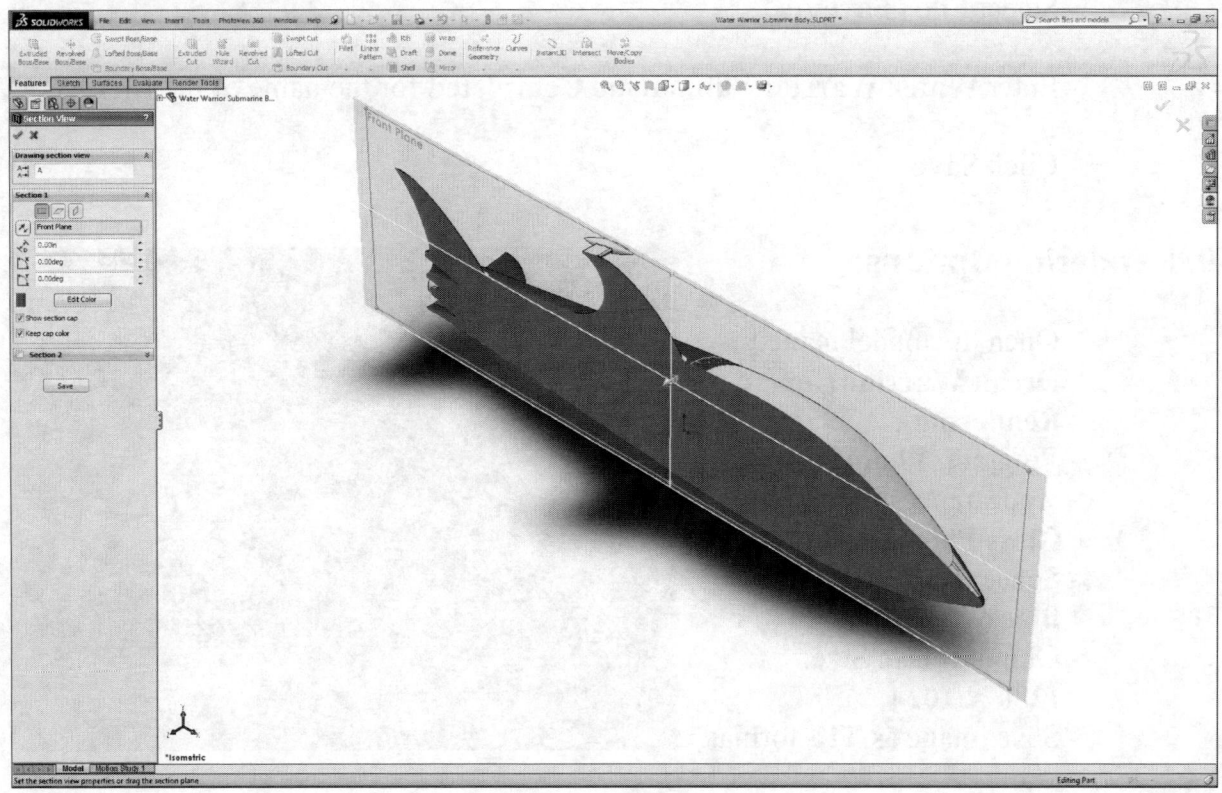

- **Exit** the Section View command.

7. Hiding the surfaces:

- Expand the **Surface Bodies** folder on the Feature tree.

- Click the **2 surface bodies** inside this folder and select **Hide** (arrow).

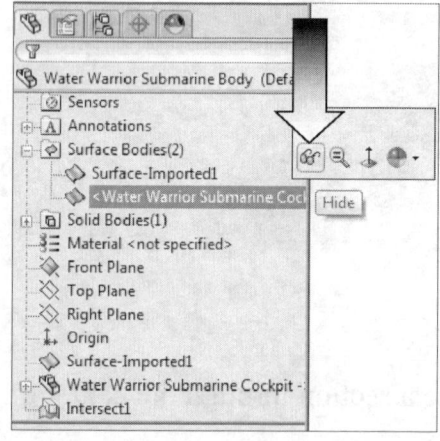

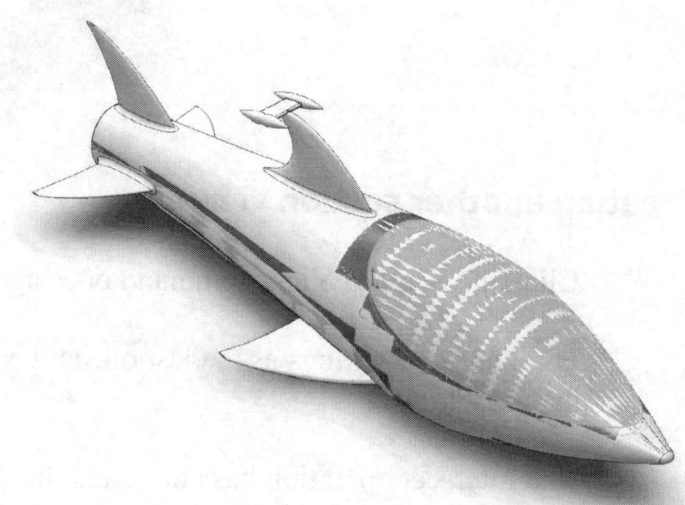

8. Saving your work

- Select **File / Save As**.

- Enter **Water Warrior Submarine Completed** for the name of the file.

- Click **Save**.

9. Rendering Options:

- Open the model named:
  Ocean Warrior (for Rendering).
- Program: **PhotoView 360**
- Appearance: **Black High Gloss Plastic**
- Scene: **Reflective Floor Black**.
- Output Image Size:
  1280 X 1024
- Save image as **TIF** format.

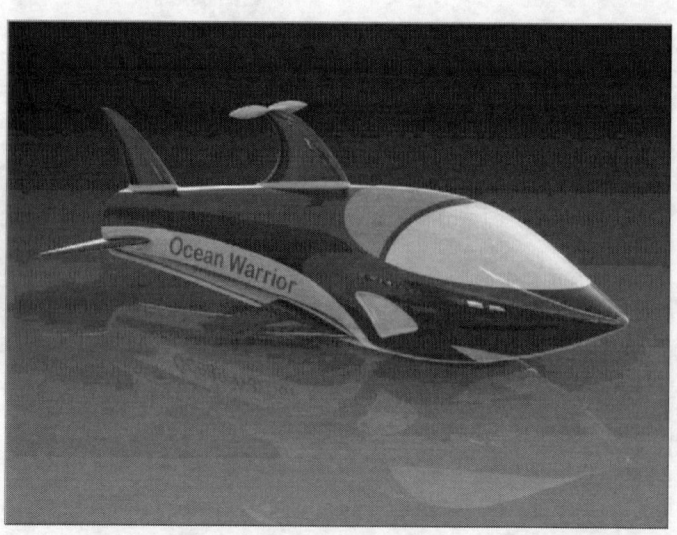

Exercise: Using the Intersect Feature

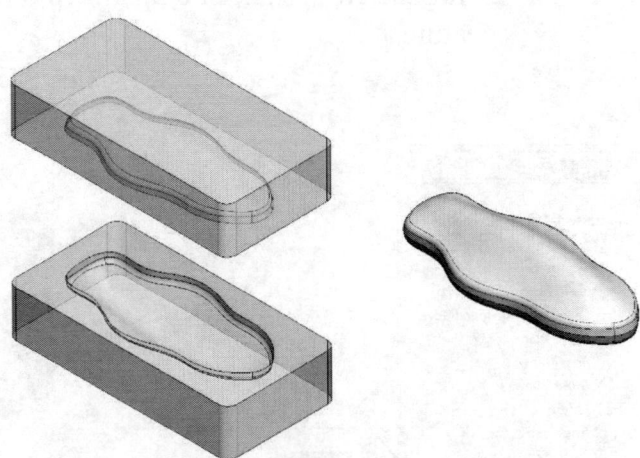

Similar to the options in the Combine command, the Intersect command enables you to perform complex tasks to quickly combine solid bodies, planes, or surfaces without the need for cut, trim or fill features. The preview options allow you to see the final shape that you can pick and choose while selecting the different areas to exclude.

This exercise discusses another use of the Intersect command where 2 cavity models are used to create a solid model as pictured.

1. Opening a SolidWorks document:

    - Click **File / Open**.

    - Browse to the Training Files folder, locate and open the document named:
    Intersect_Cavity.

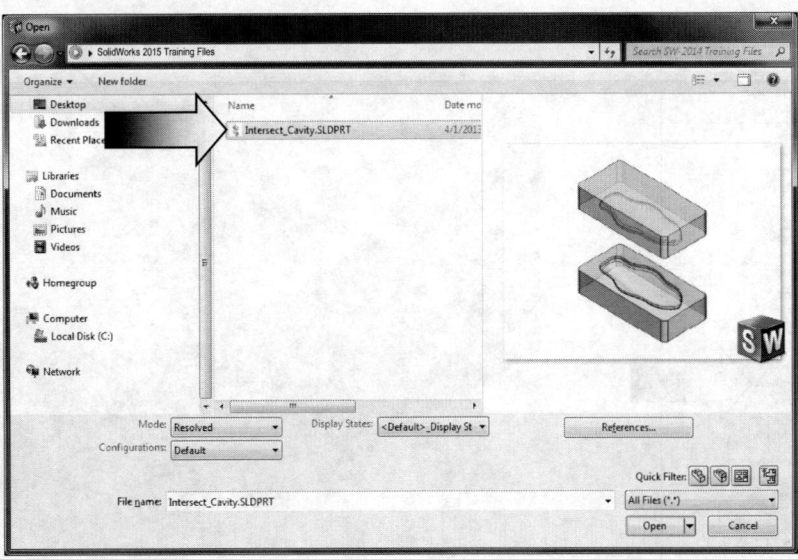

    - This document has 2 solid bodies and their feature histories are omitted to help focus on the Intersect feature.

2. Rolling back:

- Drag the Roll-back line up 1 step to temporarily suppress the Body-Move feature.

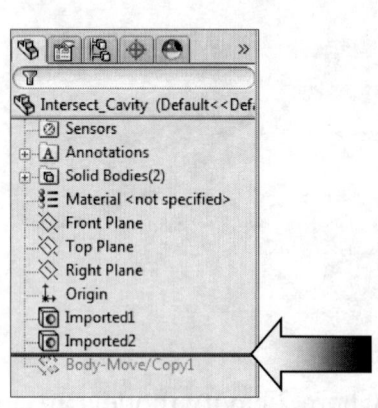

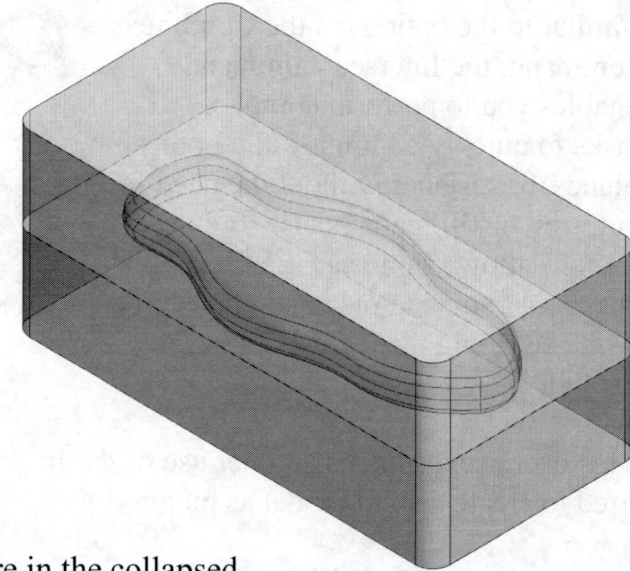

- Make sure the 2 solid bodies are in the collapsed position before moving to the next step.

3. Creating an Intersect feature:

- Select **Insert / Features / Intersect** (arrow).

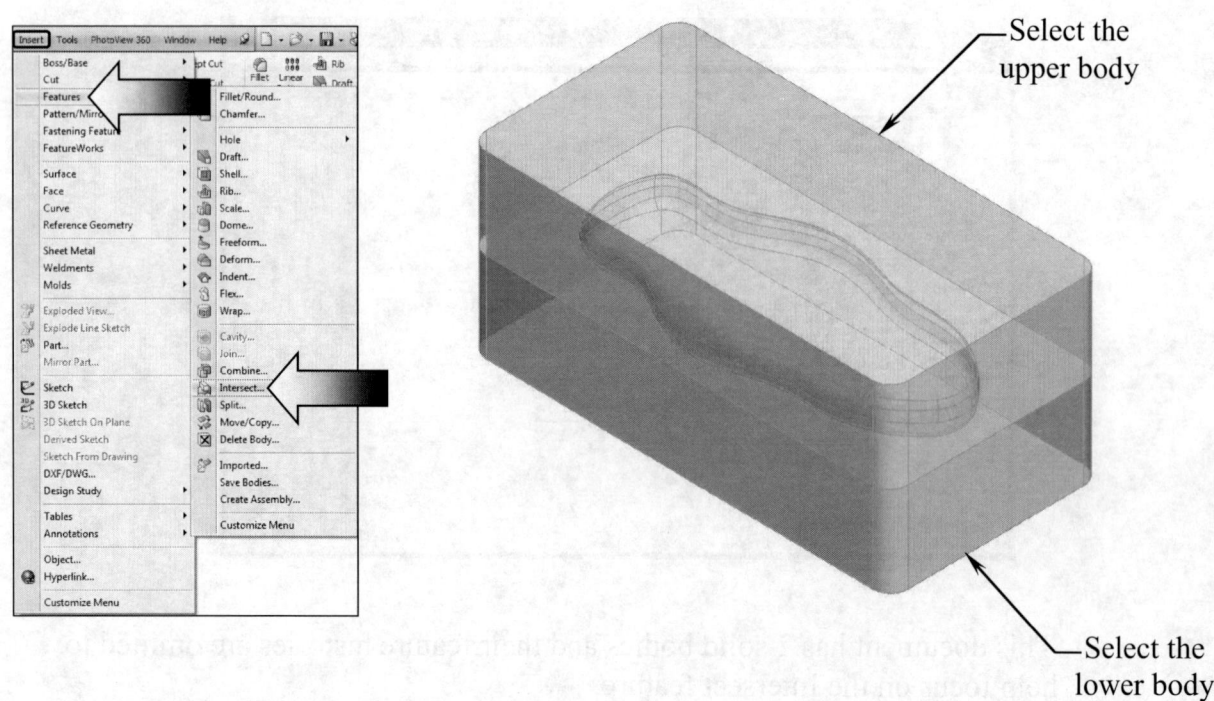

Select the upper body

Select the lower body

- Select the 2 solid bodies as noted.
- Click the **Intersect** button (arrow) after selecting the 2 solid bodies.

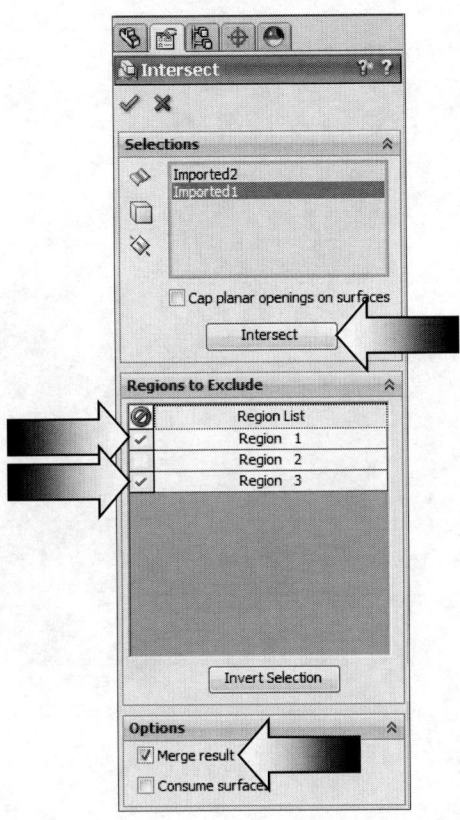

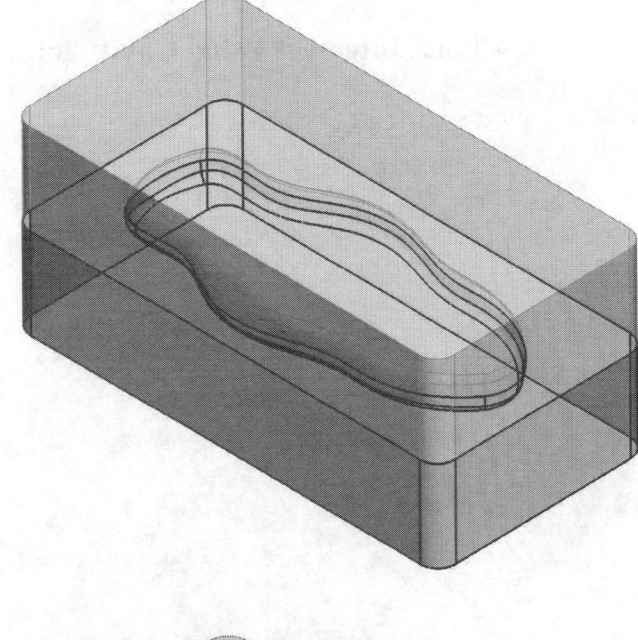

- Explore the options in the
  Regions to Exclude section
  by checking the checkboxes
  for each of the solid body.

- The Preview shows the different
  results when the checkboxes are
  enabled or disabled.

- Select the **Region1** and the **Region3** checkboxes
  to exclude the 2 solid bodies from this operation.

- Enable the **Merge Result** checkbox.

- Click **OK** to complete the Intersect
  operation.

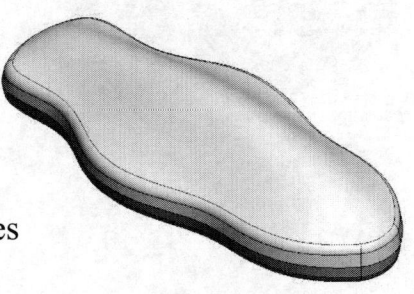

- A solid model is created from the cavities
  of the 2 solid bodies.

4. Saving your work:

- Select **File / Save As**.

- Enter **Intersect Using Cavity** for the name of the file.

- Click **Save**.

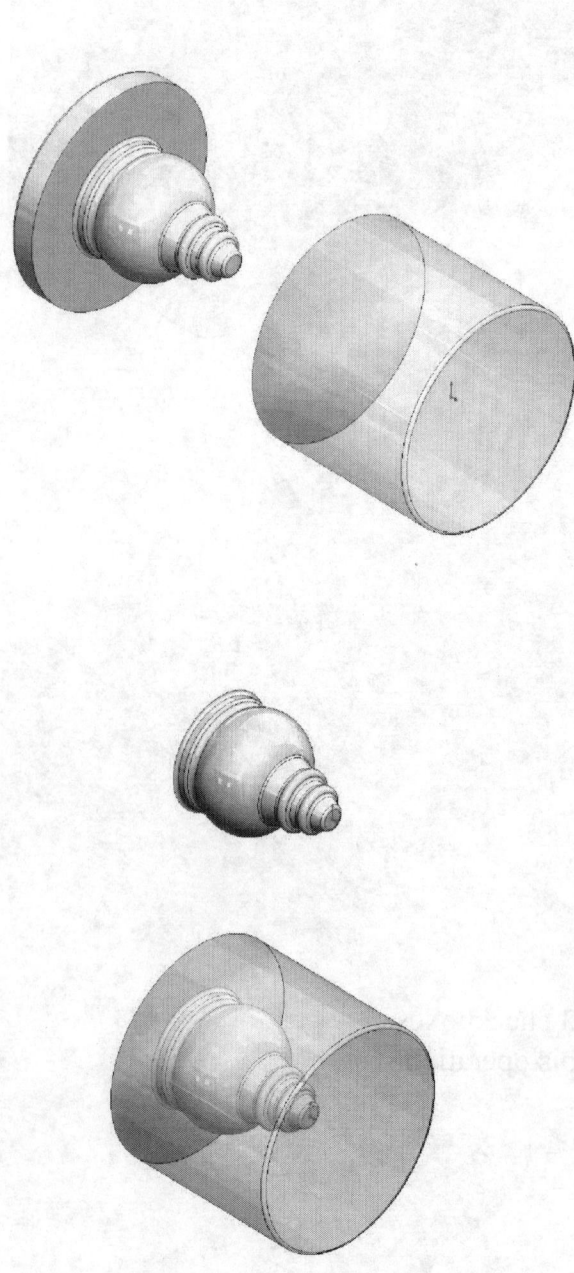

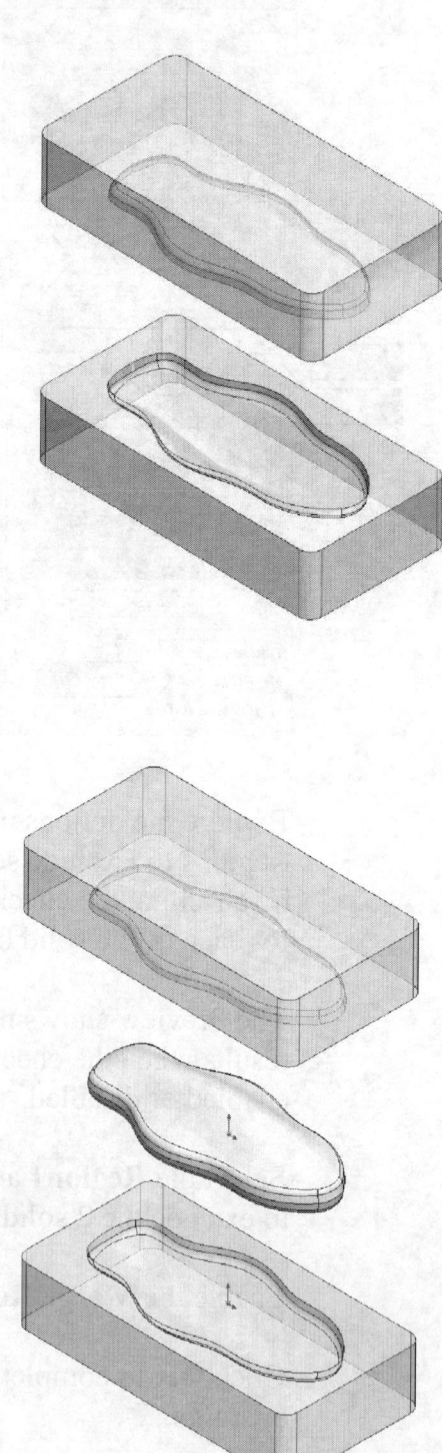

CHAPTER 21

Repairing Part Errors

Understanding and Repairing Part Errors

When an error occurs, SolidWorks will try and solve it based on the settings below:

To pre-set the rebuild action:

A. Click **Options** [icon] (Standard toolbar) or **Tools**, **Options**.

B. Select **Stop**, **Continue**, or **Prompt** for **When rebuild error occurs**, then click **OK**. With **Stop** or **Prompt**, the rebuild action stops for each error so you can fix feature failures one at a time.

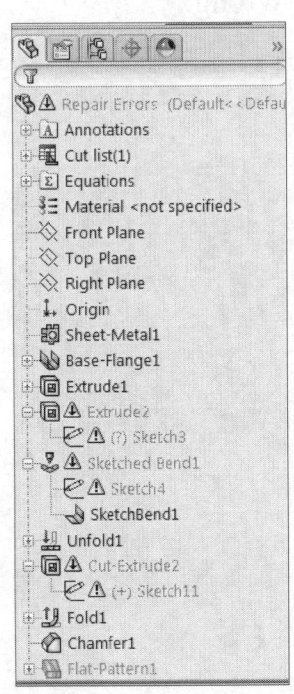

Indicates an error with the model. This icon appears on the document name at the top of the FeatureManager design tree, and on the feature that contains the error. The text of the part or feature is in red.

Indicates an error with a feature. This icon appears on the feature name in the FeatureManager design tree. The text of the feature is in red.

Indicates a warning underneath the node indicated. This icon appears on the document name at the top of the Feature-Manager design tree and on the parent feature in the FeatureManager design tree whose child feature issued the error. The text of the feature is in Olive Green.

Indicates a warning with a **feature** or **sketch**. This icon appears on the specific feature in the FeatureManager design tree that issued the warning. The text of the feature or sketch is in Olive Green.

1. Opening a part document:

- Insert the Training File folder, browse to the Repair Errors folder, and open the part named: **Repair Errors**.

- When opening a document that contains errors, the What's Wrong dialog box will appear and display where the errors are located and suggest some solutions in solving them.

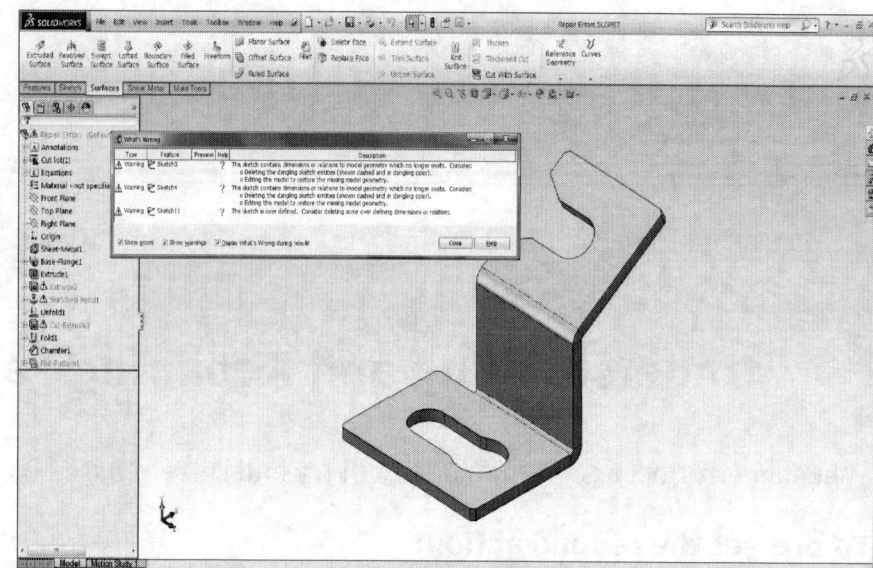

- **Expand** each feature on the FeatureManager tree and hover the pointer over the **Sketch3**.

- An explanation about the error or the warning is displayed in the tooltip. This is the same as right clicking on the error and selecting What's Wrong.

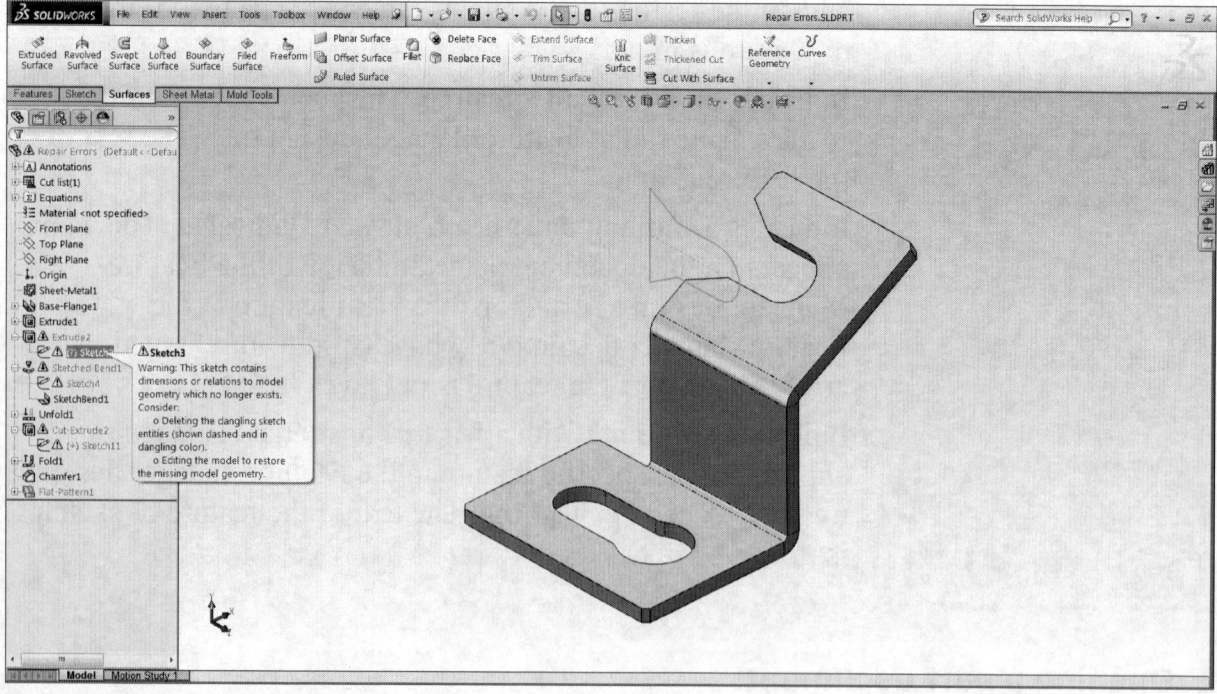

- Another way to see the explanation about the error is to right click on the error and select: What's Wrong.

- The What's Wrong dialog box pops up displaying the same explanation about the selected error. Enable the **Show Warnings** checkbox (arrow) to see the warnings after each rebuild.

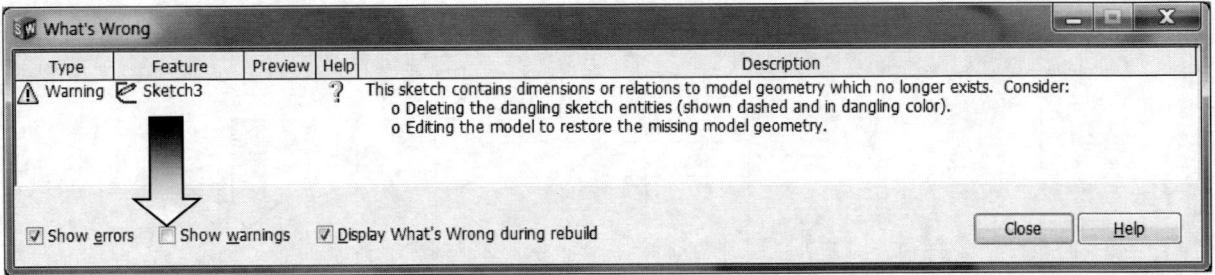

- From the Sketch toolbar click the **Display / Delete-Relations** button.

- The relations or dimensions that contain errors will appear in different colors, Olive Green in this case.

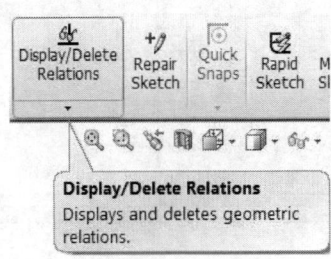

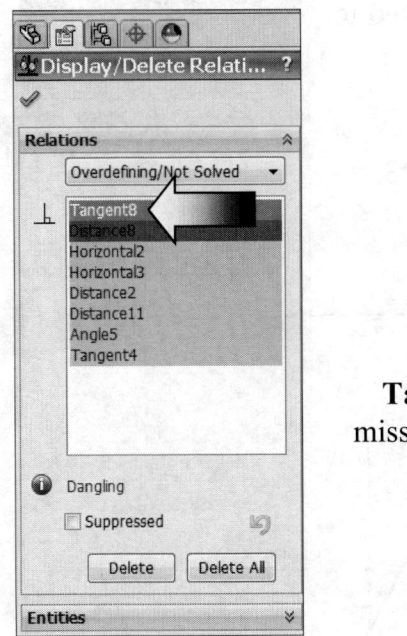

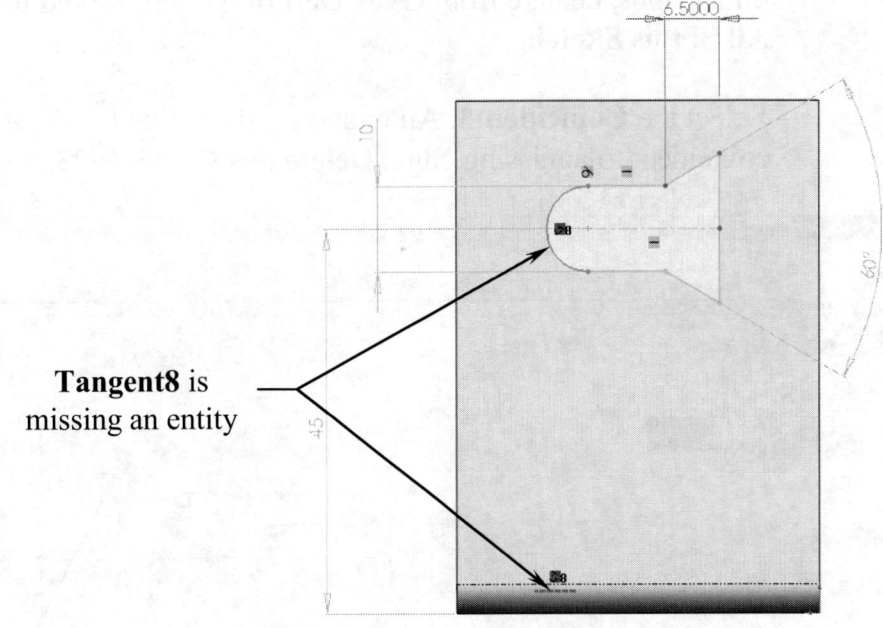

Tangent8 is missing an entity

- **Select** the relation **Tangent8** from the relation dialog box. An arc and the missing entity are highlighted. The missing entity appears in **Red** along with an **Olive Green** tangent symbol above.

- **Delete** the **Tangent8** relation.

- A message on the bottom right of the screen appears, indicating that: **The sketch can now find a valid solution**.

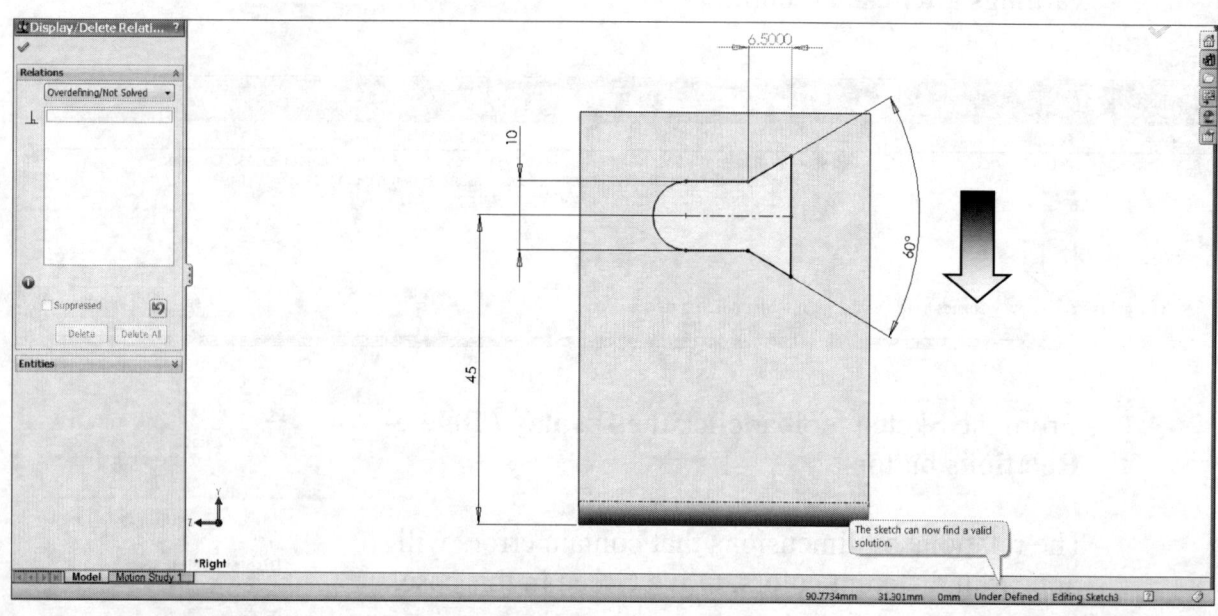

- To see the status for the rest of the relations and dimensions, change from **Over Defining / Not Solved** to **All in this Sketch**.

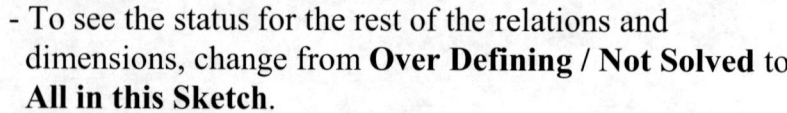

- Select the **Coincident3**. An endpoint of the line is coincident to a missing edge. **Delete** this Coincident3.

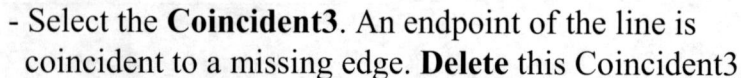

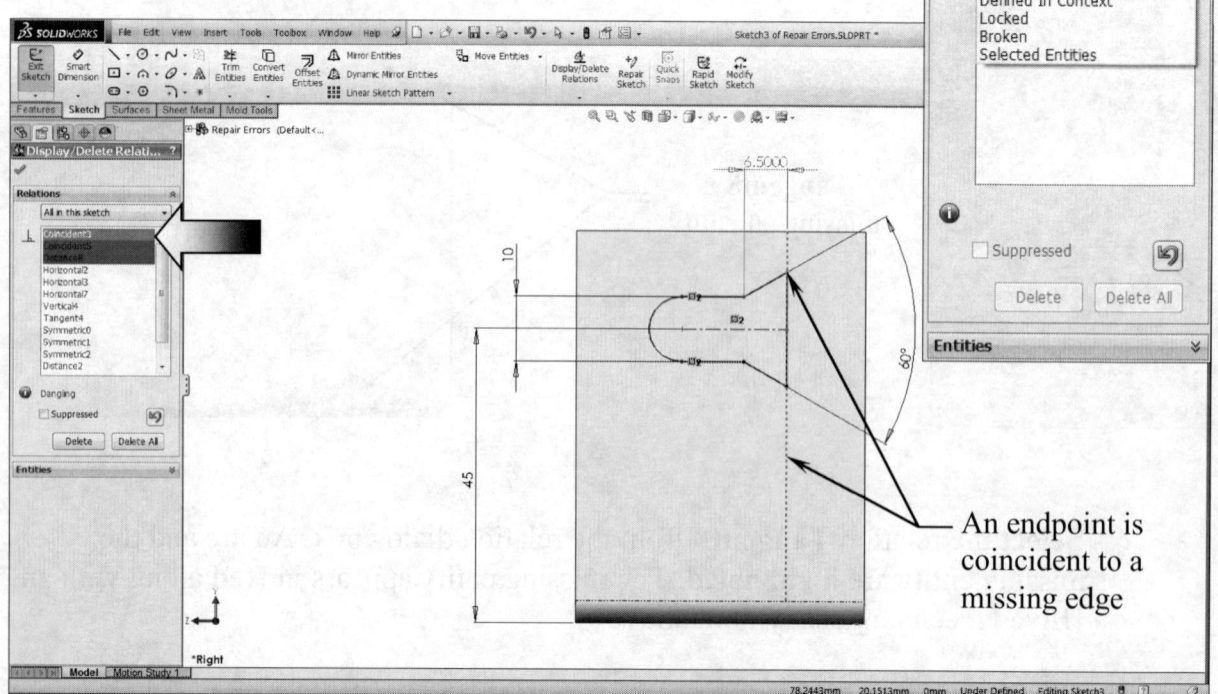

An endpoint is coincident to a missing edge

- **Delete** also the **Coincident5**. It's missing the same edge as the previous relation.

- The dimension **6.500** is dangling. It was also measured to a missing entity, **delete it**.

- **Add** 3 new dimensions as indicated to fully define this sketch. **Exit** the sketch when completed.

Delete this
Dangling dimension

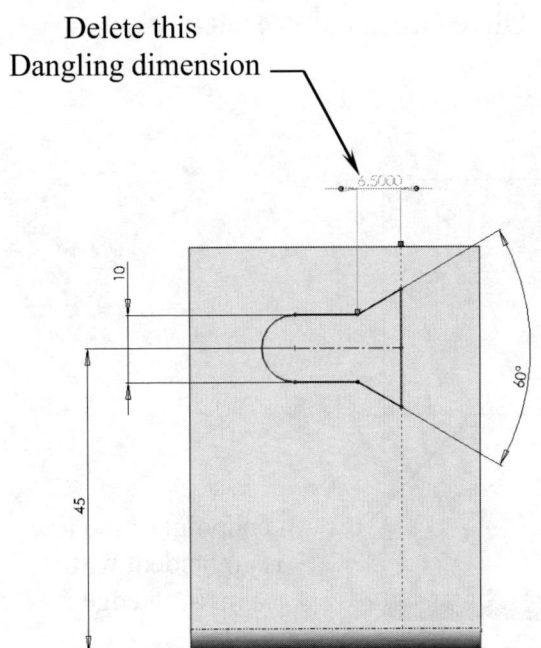

Add 3 new
dimensions

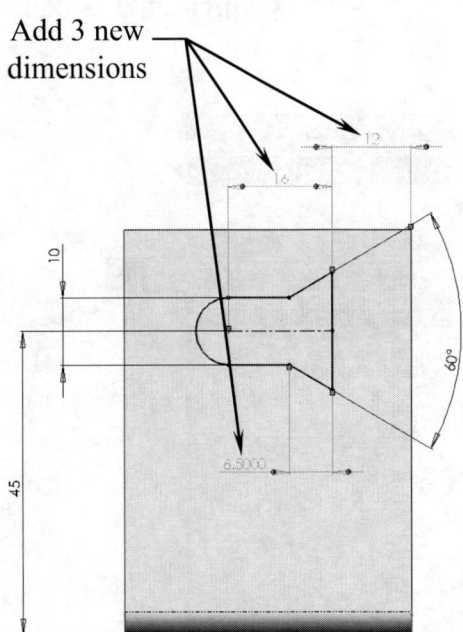

- After exiting the sketch, SolidWorks continues to report other errors still remaining in the part. The **Sketch4** and **Sketch11** still need to be repaired.

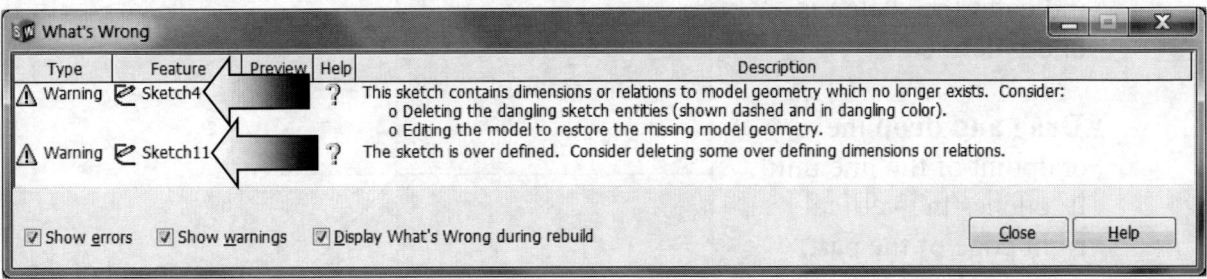

- **Close** the What's Wrong dialog box.

2. Repairing the 2nd error:

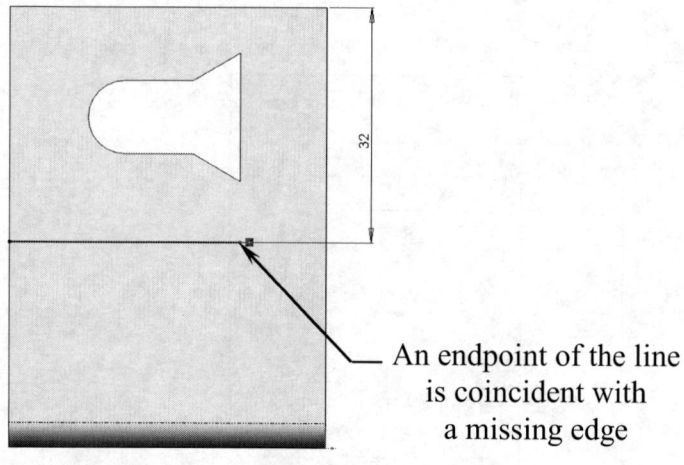

- Right click the **Sketch4** (under the Sketched Bend1 feature) and select **Edit Sketch**.

- Click the **Display / Delete Relations** button once again.

- Change the display relations option to **Dangling** (arrow).

- The **Coincident1** is dangled and has the Olive Green color. **Delete it**.

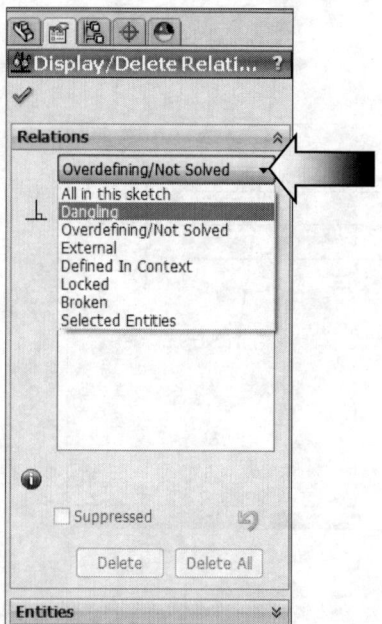

An endpoint of the line is coincident with a missing edge

- The endpoint of the line turns to Blue color. This indicates the sketch is under defined.

- **Drag and drop** the endpoint of the line until it touches the vertical right edge of the part. A coincident relation should be created automatically.

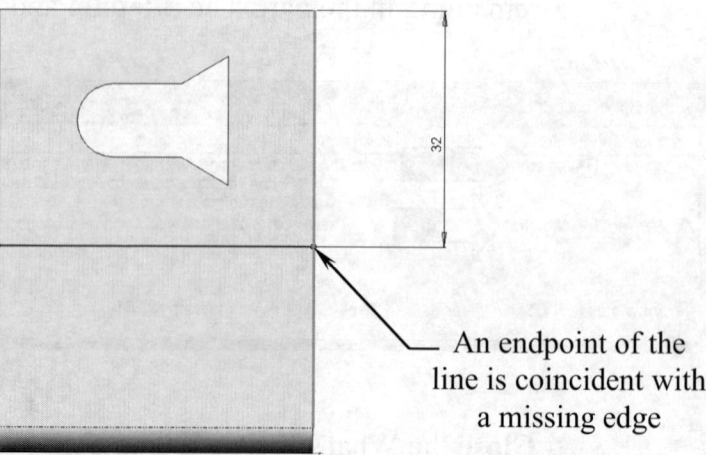

An endpoint of the line is coincident with a missing edge

- **Exit** the sketch or press **Control + Q**.

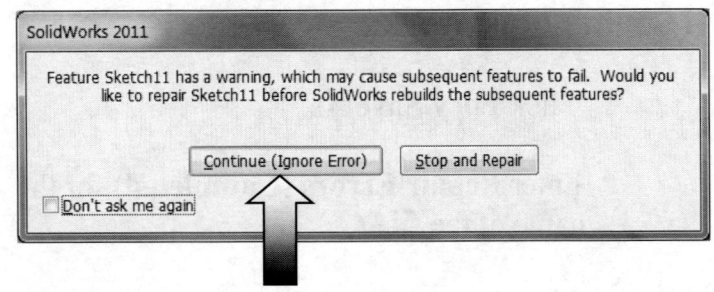

- SolidWorks continues to report the last error in the model. Click the **Continue (Ignore Error)** button to continue.

3. Repairing the 3rd error:

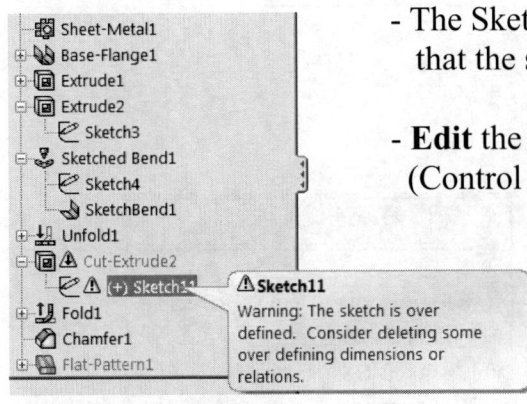

- The Sketch11 has a plus sign next to its name, this indicates that the sketch is Over Defined.

- **Edit** the **Sketch11**. Change to the Top orientation (Control + 5).

- Click the **Display / Delete Relations** button.

- Set the display relations option to: **Over Defining / Not Solved**.

- Select the **Collinear1** from the list. This relation shows a **Magenta** color next to its Collinear symbol.

- Delete the **Collinear1** from the list.

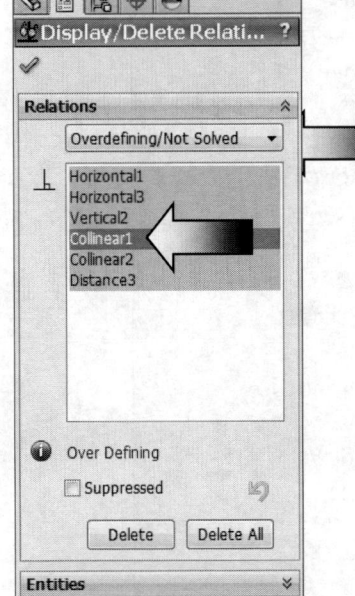

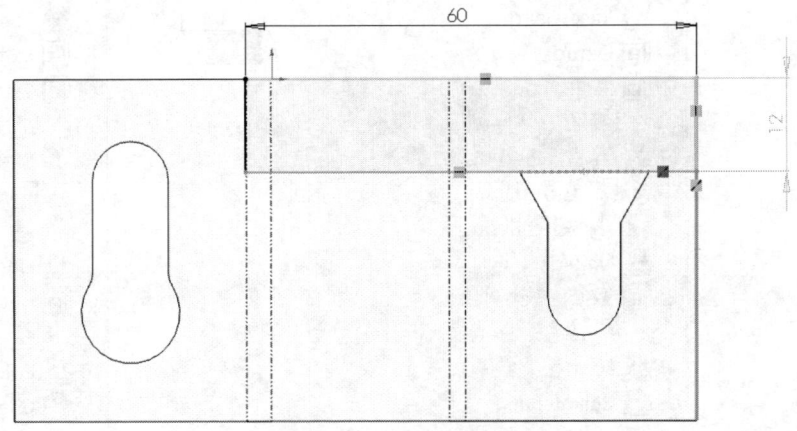

- This last step should bring the sketch back to its Fully Defined status.

- **Exit** the sketch or press **Control + Q**.

4. Saving your work:

- Click **File / Save As**.

- Enter **Repair Errors (Completed)** for the name of the file.

- Click **Save**.

- All errors have been repaired. The Feature-Manager tree is now free of errors.

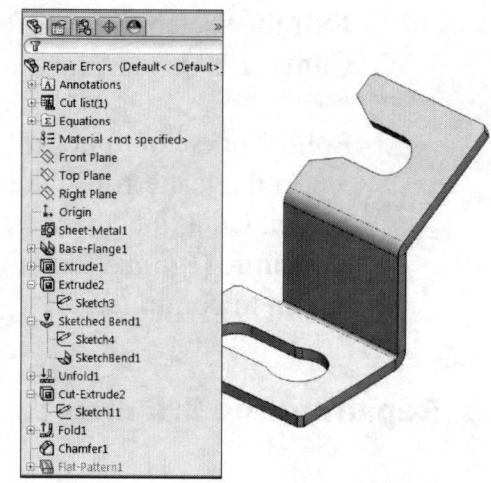

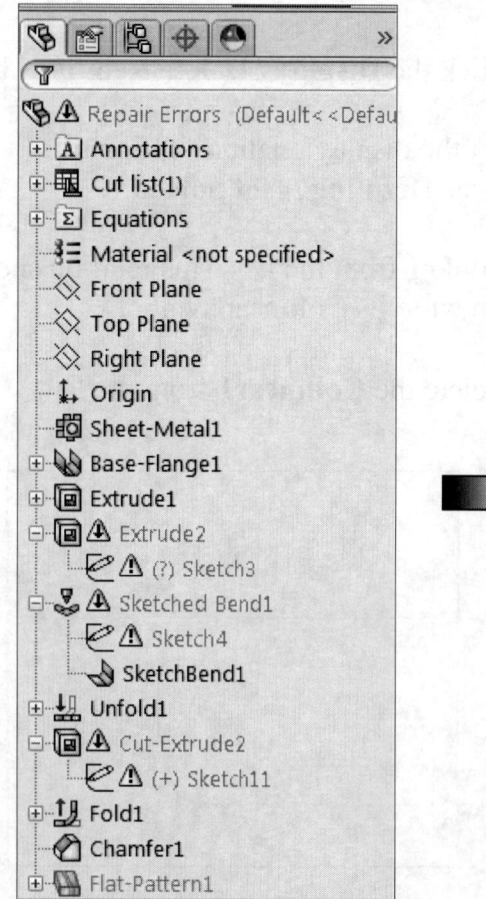

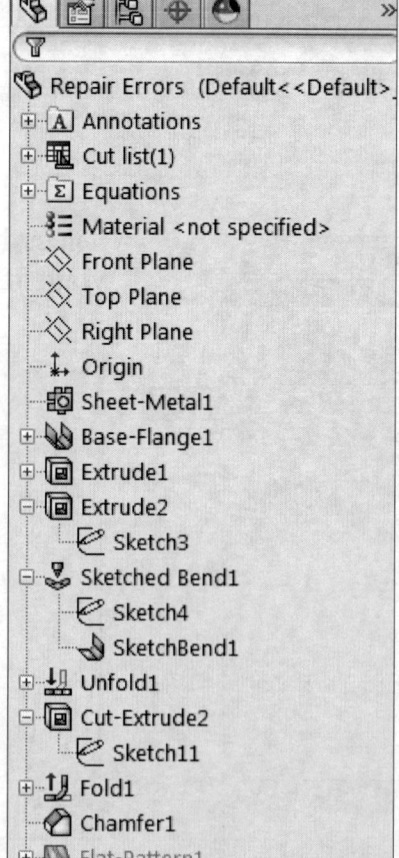

- Close all documents.

SolidWorks 2015

Certified SolidWorks Associate (CSWA)

Certification Practice for the Associate Examination

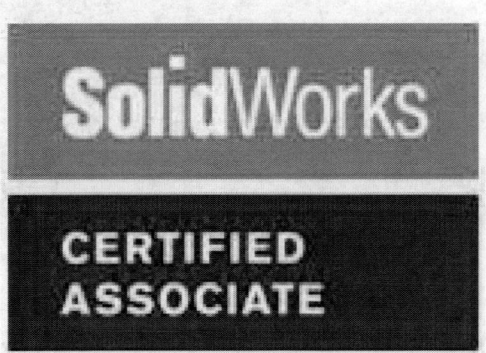

Courtesy of Paul Tran, Sr. Certified SolidWorks Instructor

CSWA – Certified SolidWorks Associate

As a Certified SolidWorks Associate (CSWA), you will stand out from the crowd in today's competitive job market.

The CSWA certification is proof of your SolidWorks expertise with cutting-edge skills that businesses seek out and reward.

Exam Length: 3 hours

Minimum Passing grade: 70%

Re-test Policy: There is a minimum 30 day waiting period between every attempt of the CSWA exam. Also, a CSWA exam credit must be purchased for each exam attempt.

All candidates receive electronic certificates and a personal listing on the CSWA directory when they pass *(Courtesy of SolidWorks Corporation)*.

- CSWA Sample Certificate -

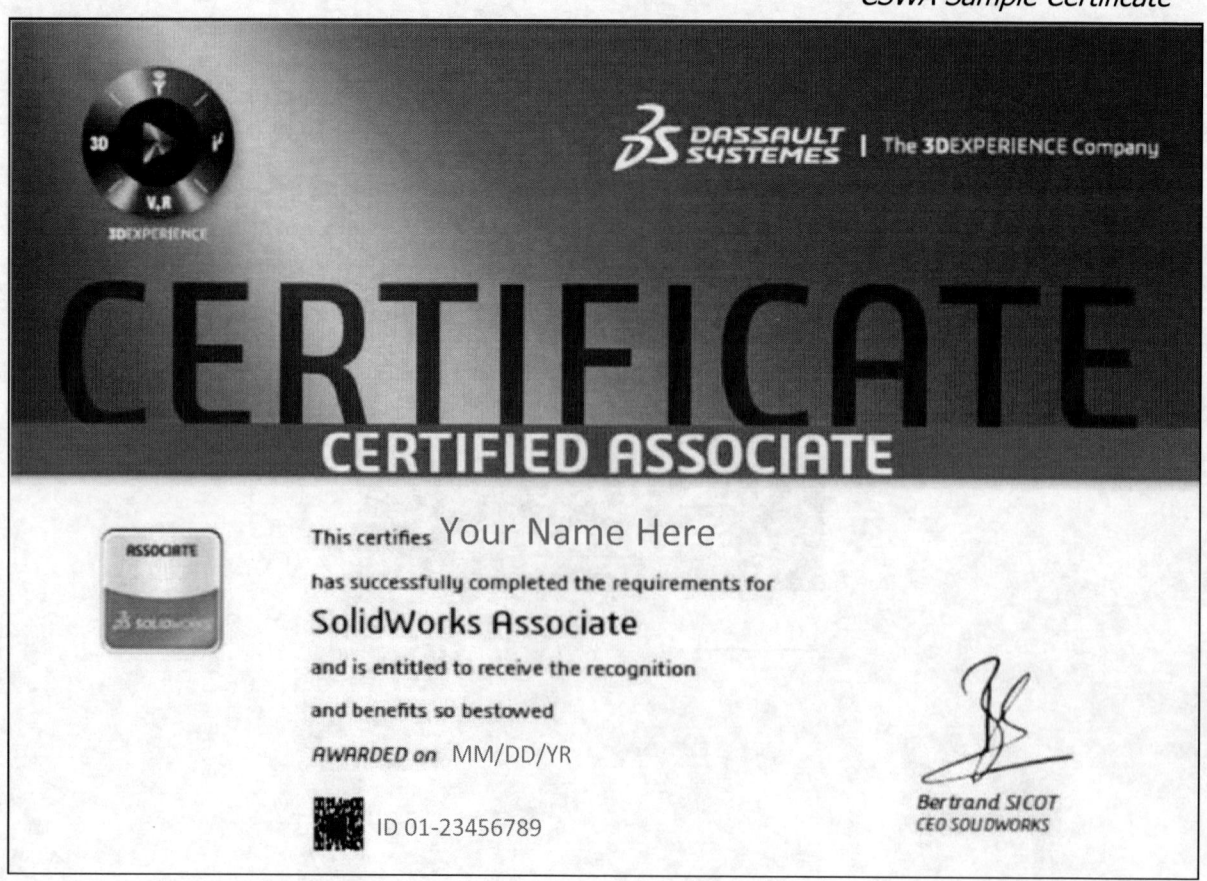

Certified-SolidWorks-Associate program (CSWA)
Certification Practice for the Associate-Examination

> Drawings, Parts & Assemblies

Complete all challenges within 180 minutes

(The following examples are intended to assist you in familiarizing yourself with the structure of the exams and the method in which the questions are asked).

Drafting competencies

Question 1:

Which command was used to create the drawing View B below? (Circle one)

A. Section View

B. Projected

C. Crop View

D. Detail

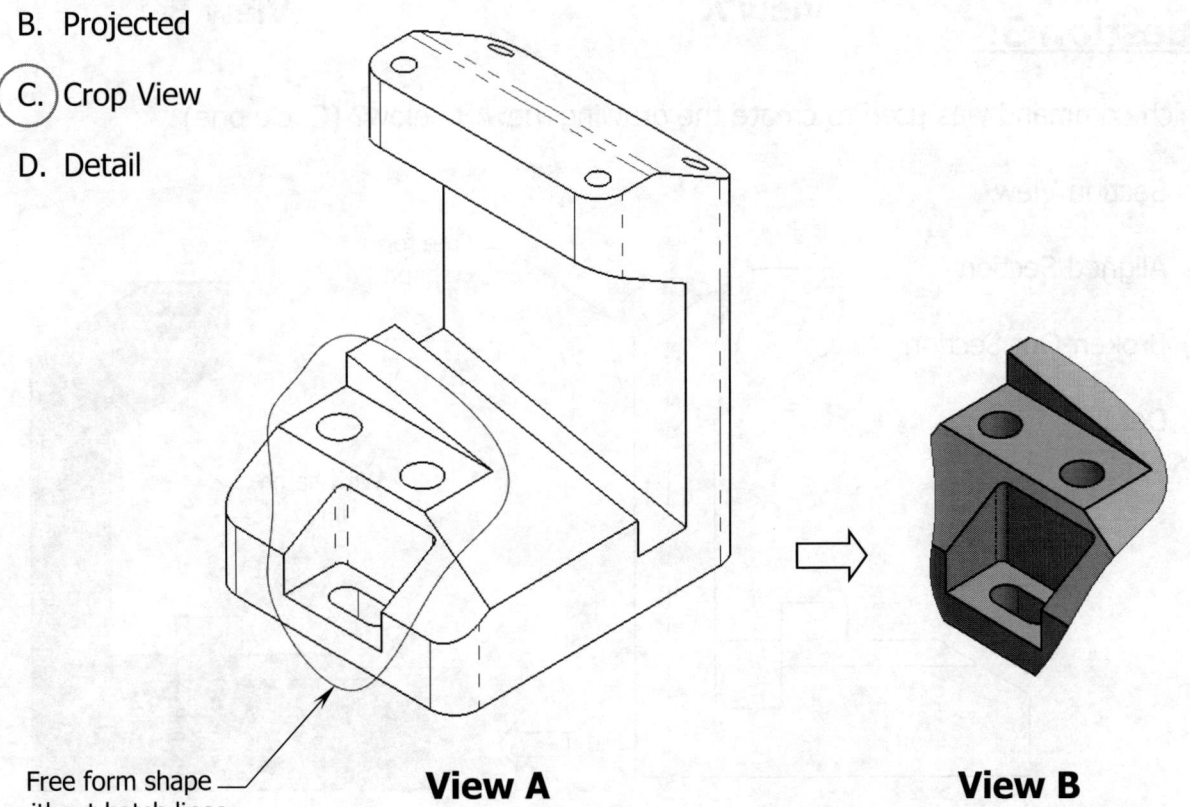

Free form shape without hatch lines

View A

View B

Question 2:

Which command was used to create the drawing View B below? (Circle one)

A. Section View

B. Crop View

C. Projected

D. Detail

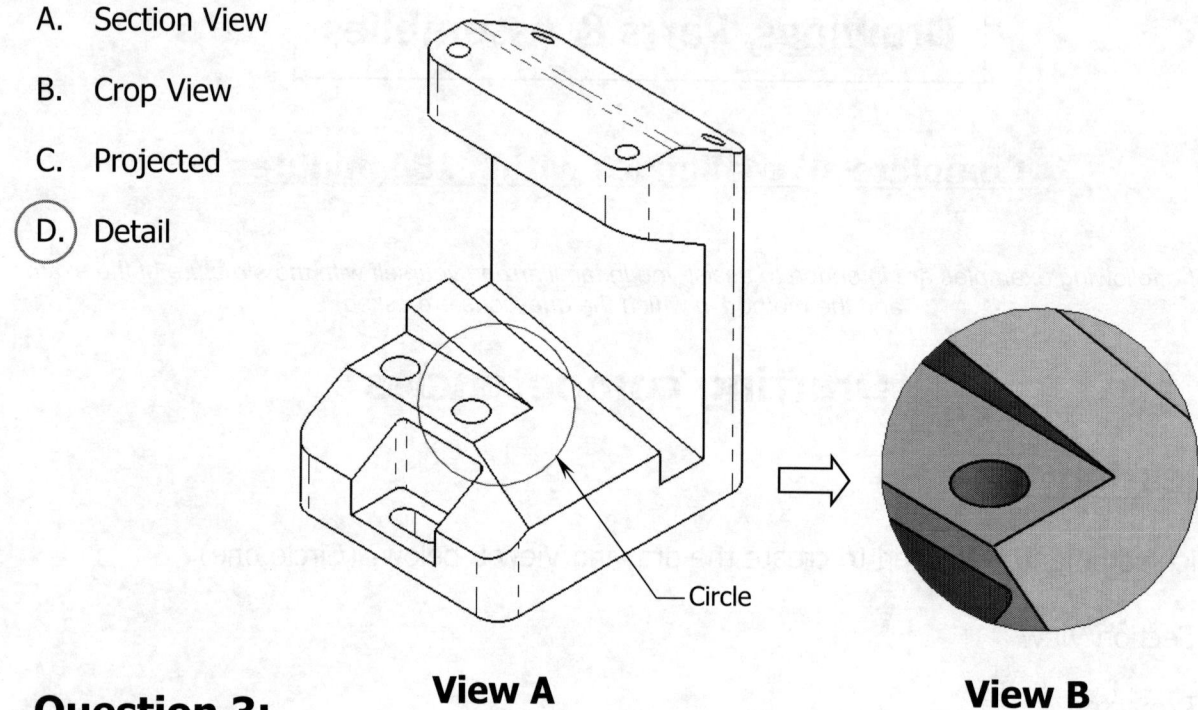

View A

Circle

View B

Question 3:

Which command was used to create the drawing View B below? (Circle one)

A. Section View

B. Aligned Section

C. Broken-Out Section

D. Detail

Free form shape

With hatch lines

View A

View B

Question 4:

Which command was used to create the drawing View B below? (Circle one)

A. Alternate Position View

B. Multiple Positions

C. Exploded View

D. Copy & Paste

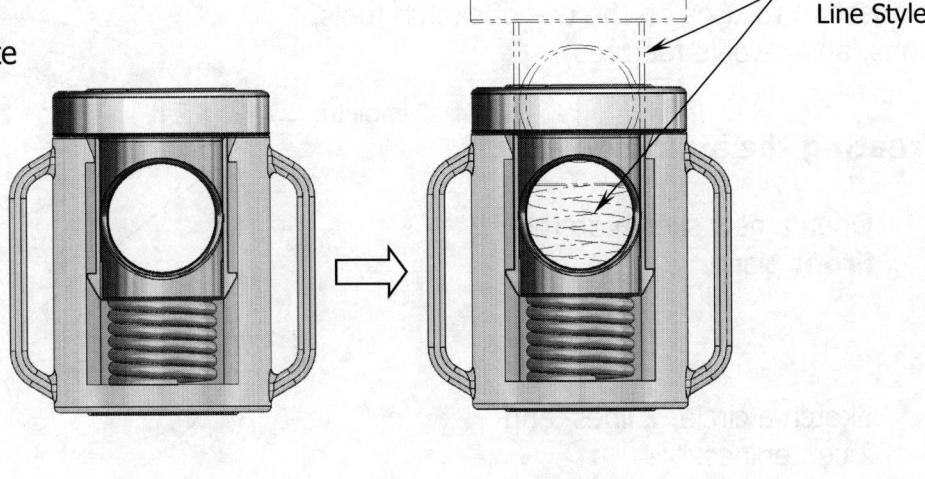

Phantom
Line Style

View A   **View B**

Question 5:

Which command was used to create the
drawing View B below? (Circle one)

A. Aligned Section View

B. Horizontal Break

C. Vertical Break

D. Broken Out Section

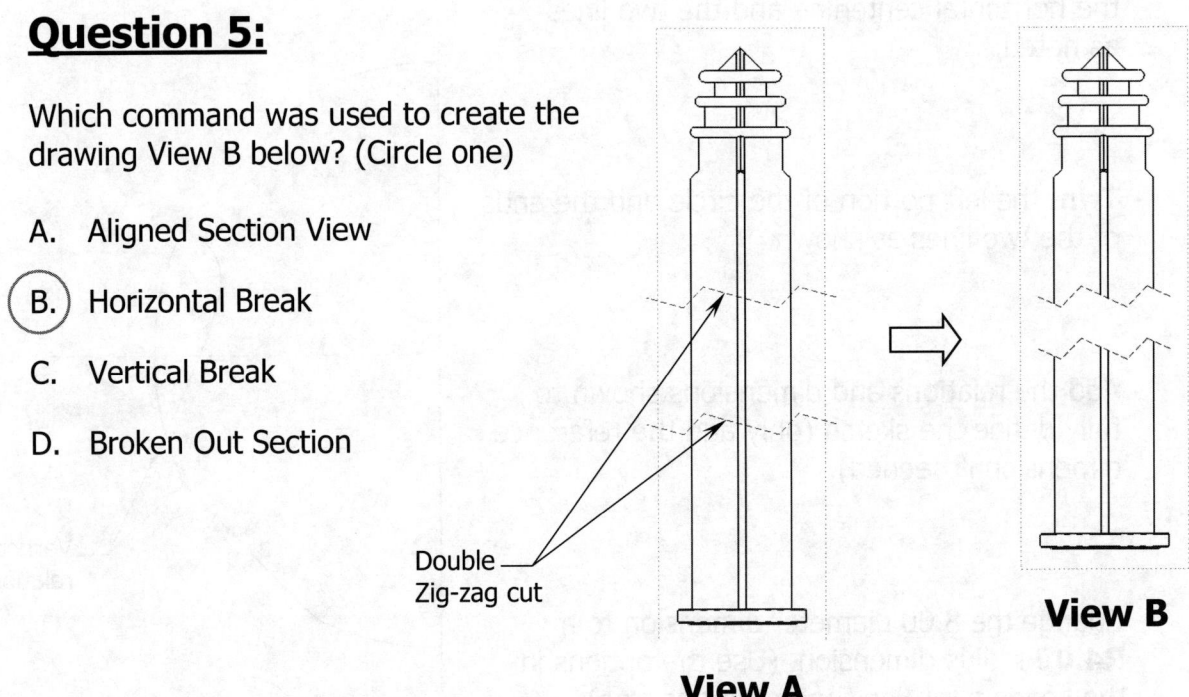

Double
Zig-zag cut

View A   **View B**

Question 6: Basic Part Modeling (1 of 4)

- Create this part in SolidWorks.
- Origin: **Arbitrary**
- Material: **1060 Alloy Steel**

- Unit: **Inches, 3 decimals**
- Drafting Standards: **ANSI**
- Density: **0.098 lb/in^3**

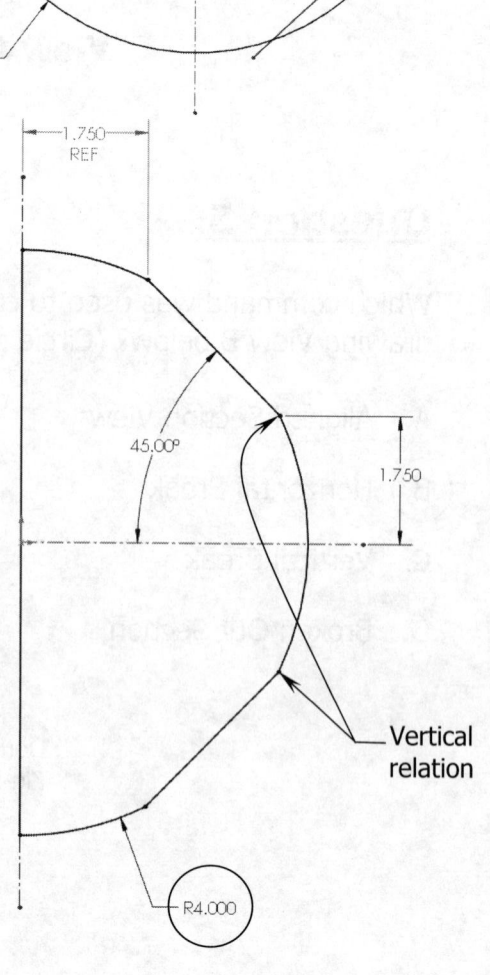

(This question focuses on the use of sketch tools, relations, and revolve features).

1. Creating the main body:

- Open a new sketch on the **Front** plane.

- Sketch a circle, 2 lines, and 2 centerlines.

- Add a **Symmetric** relation between the horizontal centerline and the two lines as noted.

- **Trim** the left portion of the circle and the ends of the two lines as shown.

- Add the relations and dimensions shown to fully define the sketch (only add the reference dimension if needed).

- Change the 8.00 diameter dimension to a **R4.00** radius dimension. (Use the options in the Leaders tab, on the Properties tree).

2. Extruding the base feature:

- Click **Extruded Boss/Base**.

- Use **Mid-Plane** type.

- Thickness: **16.00 in**.

- Click **OK**.

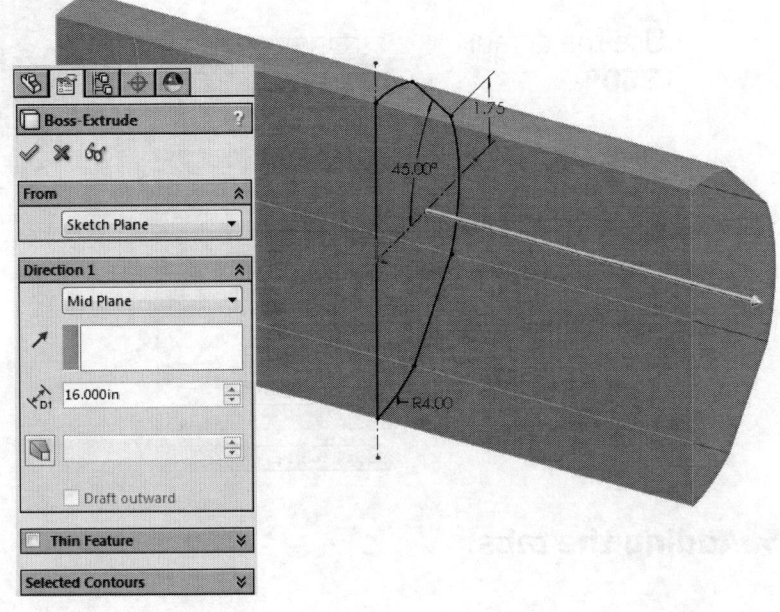

3. Creating the bore hole sketch:

- Open a new sketch on the **front face** as noted.

- Sketch the profile shown below and add dimensions/relations to fully define the sketch.

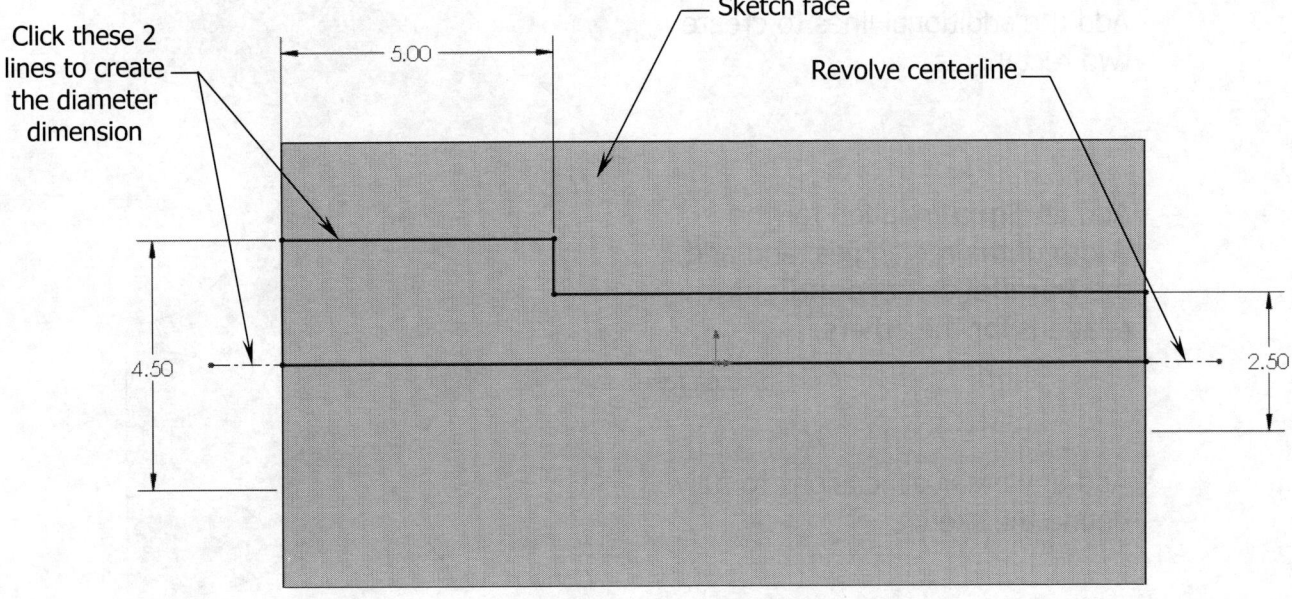

4. Creating a revolved cut:

- Click **Revolved-Cut**.

- Use the default **360°**.

- Click **OK**.

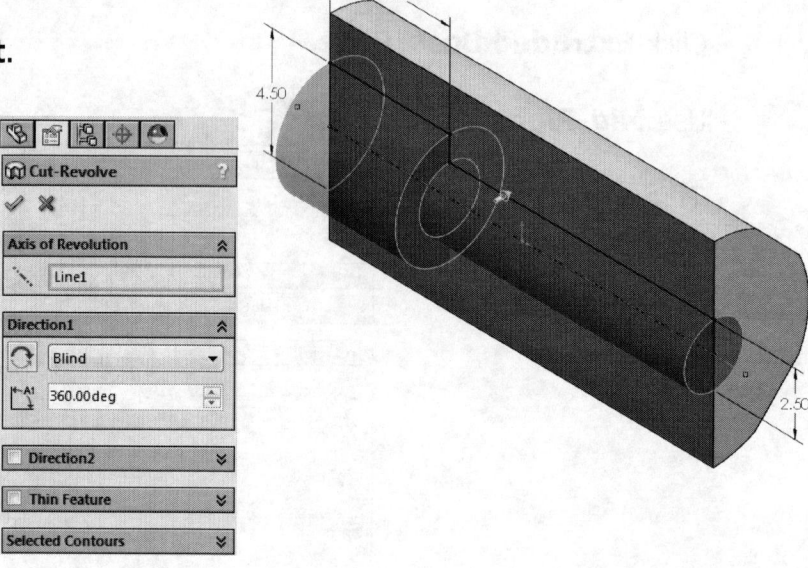

5. Adding the tabs:

- Open a new sketch on the **planar face** of the left end.

- Select the two angled edges and click **Convert Entities**.

- Add the additional lines to create two rectangles.

- Add an **Equal** relation for the Width of the rectangles, and add the **Parallel** or **Perpendicular** relations for the others.

- Add any other dimensions to fully define the sketch.

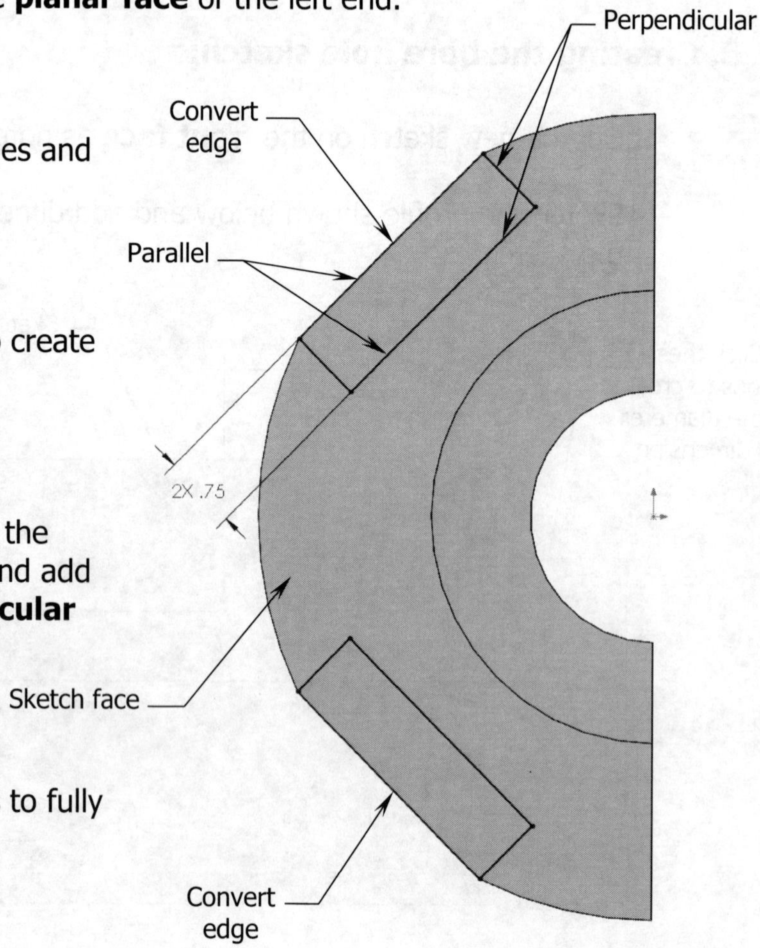

Perpendicular

Convert edge

Parallel

2X .75

Sketch face

Convert edge

6. Extruding the tabs:

- Click **Extruded Boss/Base**.

- Use the default **Blind** type.

- Enter **1.00 in**. for depth.

- Click **OK**.

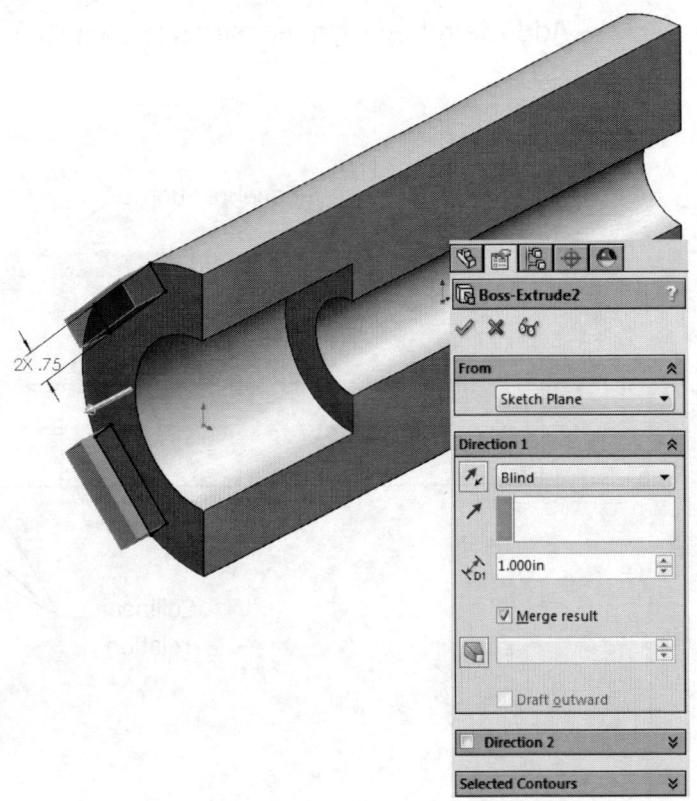

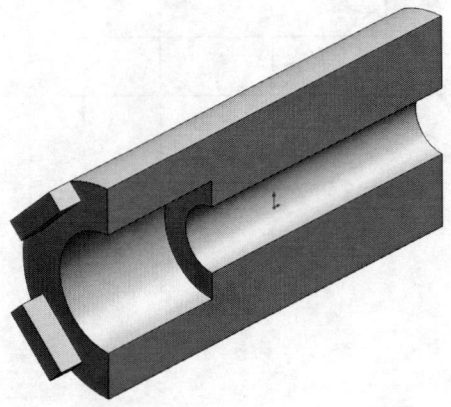

7. Creating the cut features:

- Open a new sketch on the **Top** plane.

- Sketch 2 rectangles and make the lines on the bottom **Collinear** with the edge of the model (see next page).

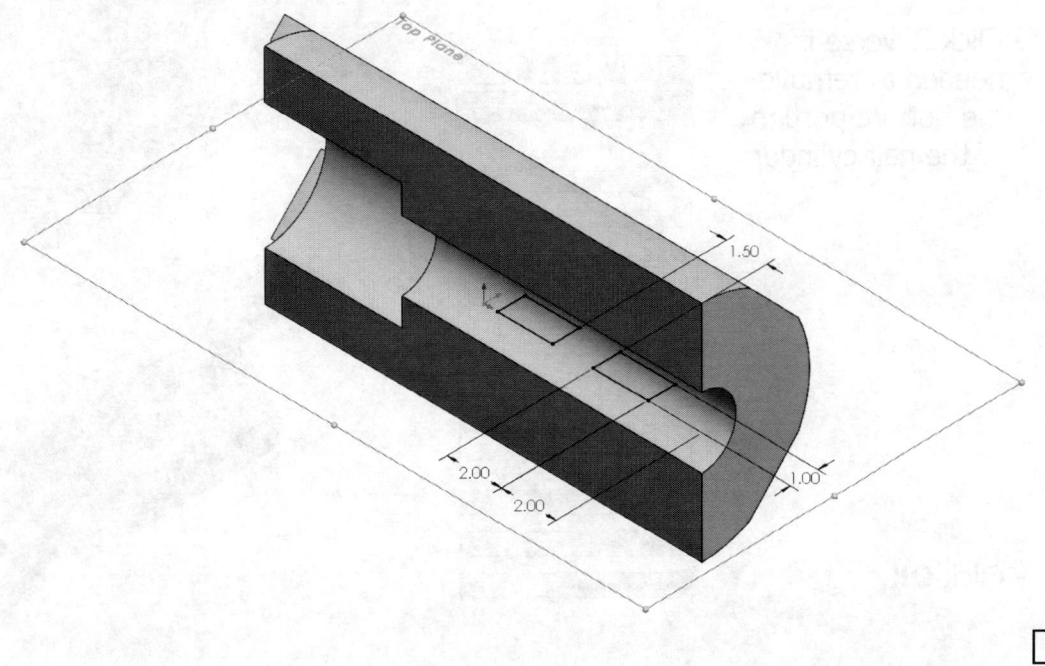

Next ▷

- Add the relations/dimensions shown to fully define the sketch.

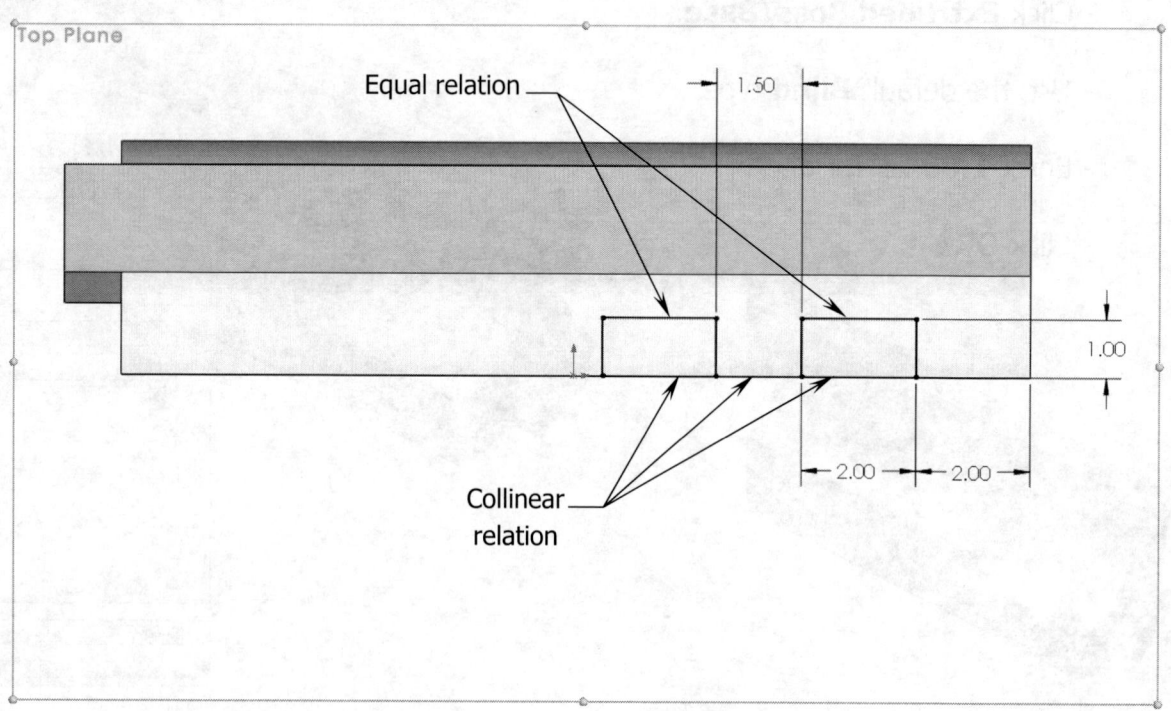

Top Plane

Equal relation

1.50

1.00

Collinear relation

2.00   2.00

8. Extruding the cuts:

- Click **Extruded-Cut**.

- Use the **Through All** type.

- Click Reverse if needed to remove the bottom portion of the half cylinder.

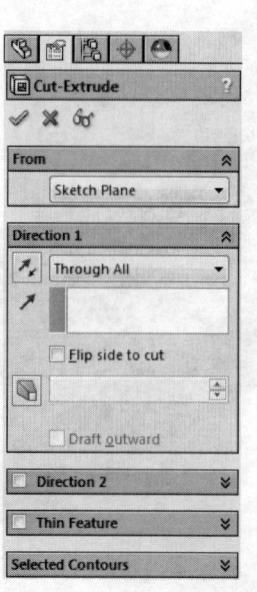

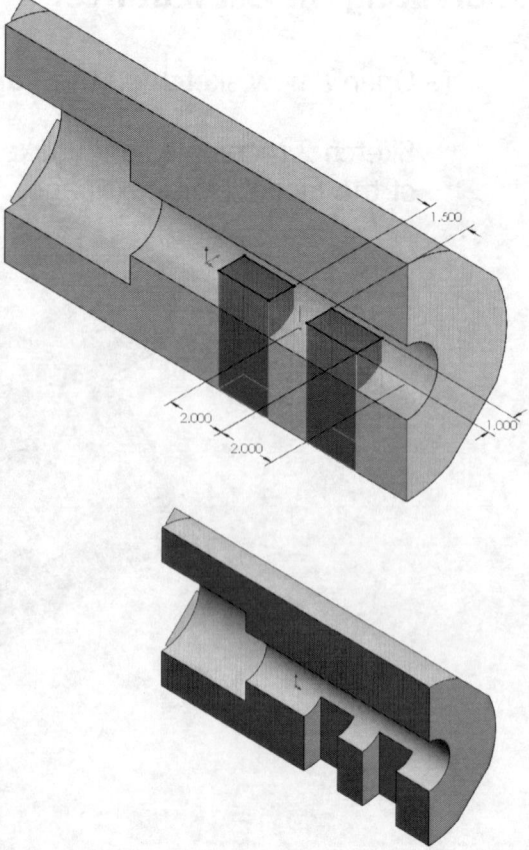

- Click **OK**.

9. Adding another cut feature:

- Open a new sketch on the **planar face** as noted.

- Sketch the profile and add the dimensions below to fully define the sketch.

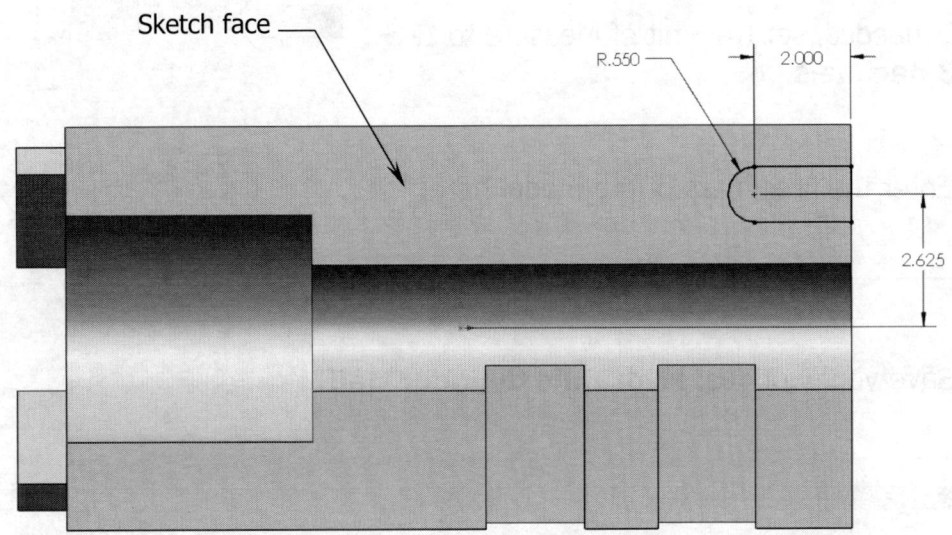

Sketch face

R.550   2.000

2.625

10. Extruding a cut:

- Click **Extruded-Cut**.

- Use the default **Blind** type.

- Enter **.750 in**. for depth.

- Click **OK**.

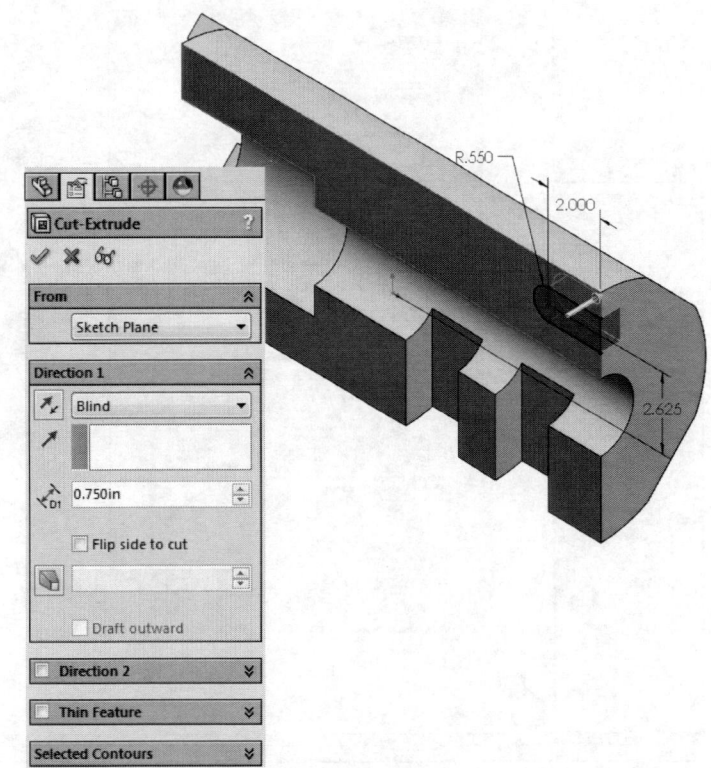

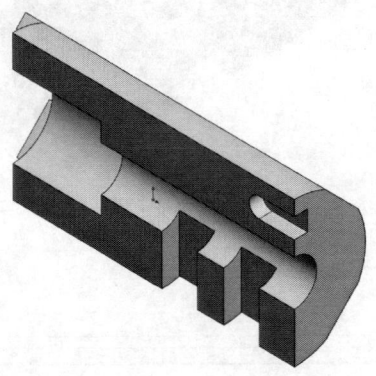

11. Calculating the Mass:

- Be sure to set the material to **1060 Alloy**.

- Switch to the **Evaluate** tab.

- Click **Mass Properties**.

- If needed, set the Unit of Measure to **IPS**, **3 decimals**.

- Enter the final mass of the model here:

_____ lbs.

- Save your work as: **Hydraulic Cylinder Half.**

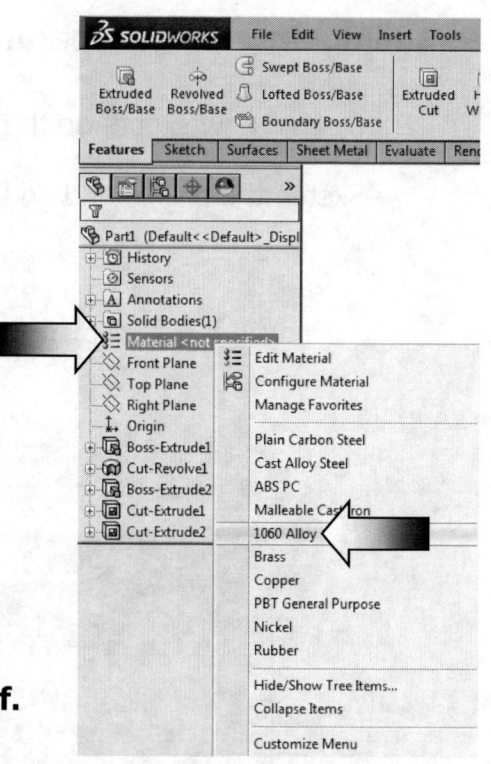

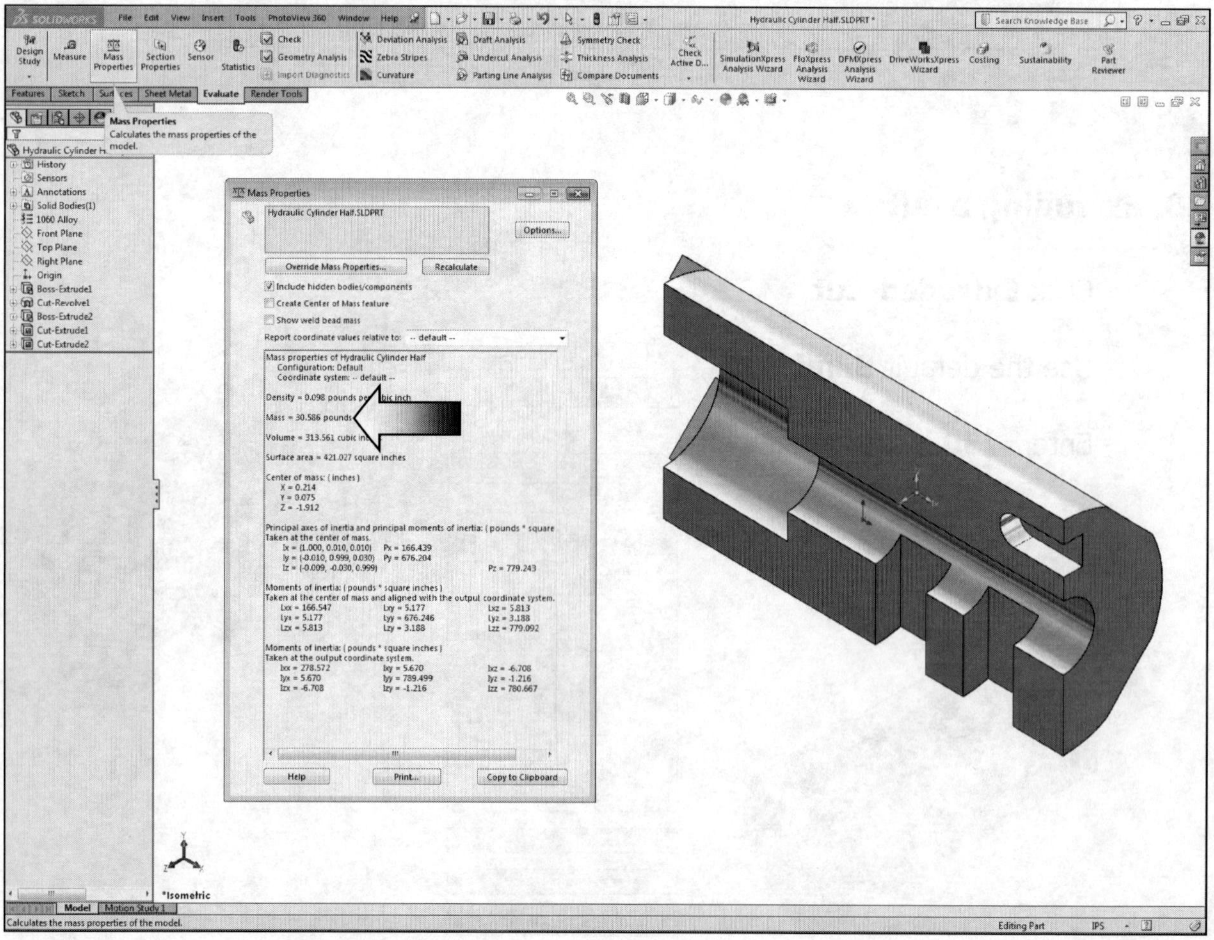

Question 7: Basic Part Modeling (2 of 4)

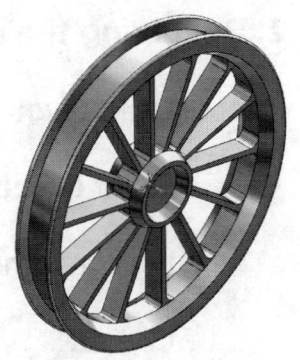

- Create this part in SolidWorks.
- Origin: **Arbitrary**
- Material: **1060 Alloy**

- Unit: **Inches**, **3 decimals**
- Drafting Standards: **ANSI**
- Density: **0.098 lb/in^3**

(This question focuses on the use of sketch tools, relations, and circular pattern feature).

1. Creating the main body:

- Open a new sketch on the **Front** plane.

- Sketch the profile using the Mirror function to ensure all entities are symmetrical about the vertical centerline.

- Add the dimensions and relations needed to fully define the sketch.

*Note: Hold the **Shift** key when adding the 1.00" dimension.

- Add a horizontal centerline and use it as the revolve line in the next step.

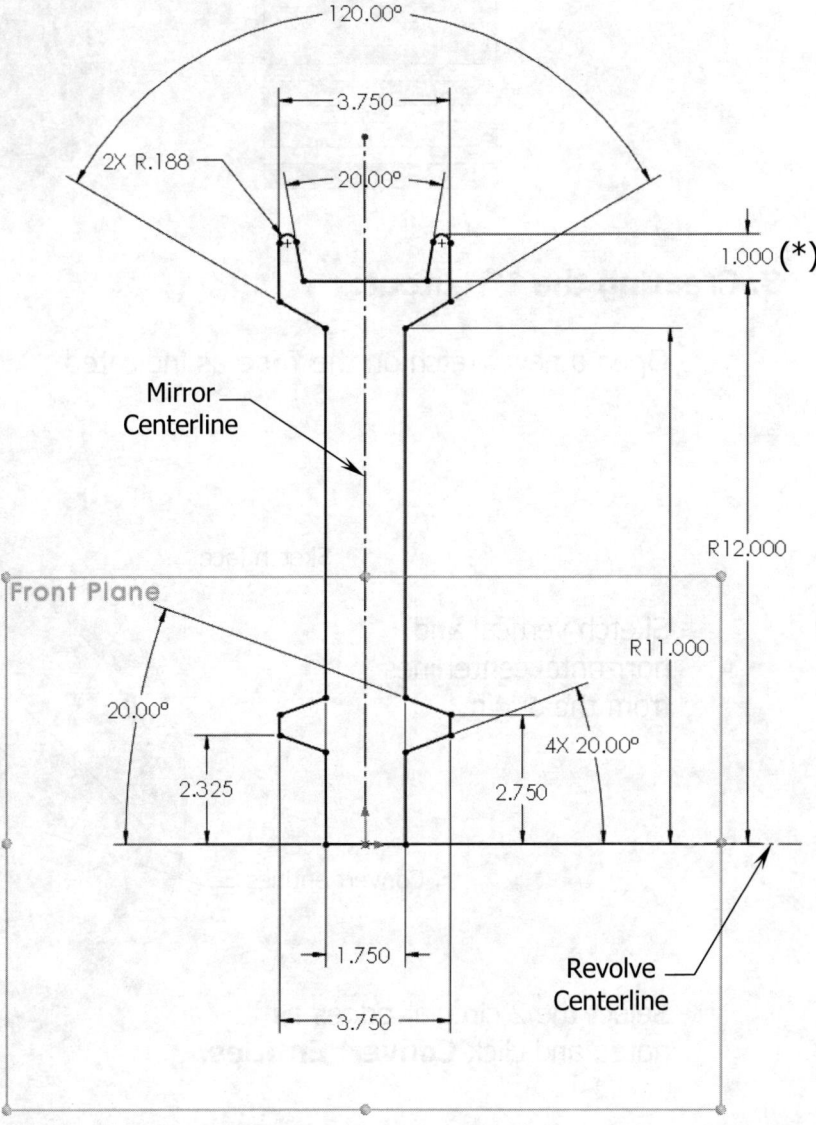

2. Revolving the main body:

- Click **Revolved Boss/Base**.

- Select the **horizontal centerline** as the Axis of Revolution.

- Use the **Blind** type and the default **360°**.

- Click **OK**.

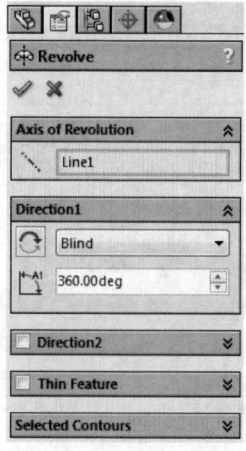

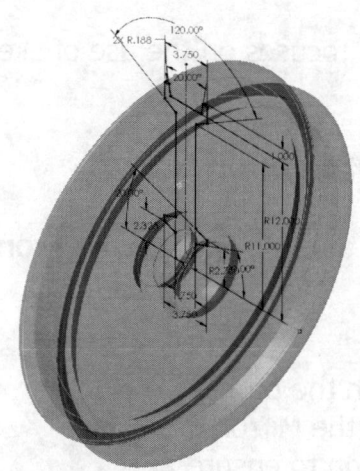

3. Creating the 1st cutout:

- Open a new sketch on the **face** as indicated.

- Sketch vertical and horizontal centerlines from the origin.

- Select the 2 circular edges as noted and click **Convert Entities**.

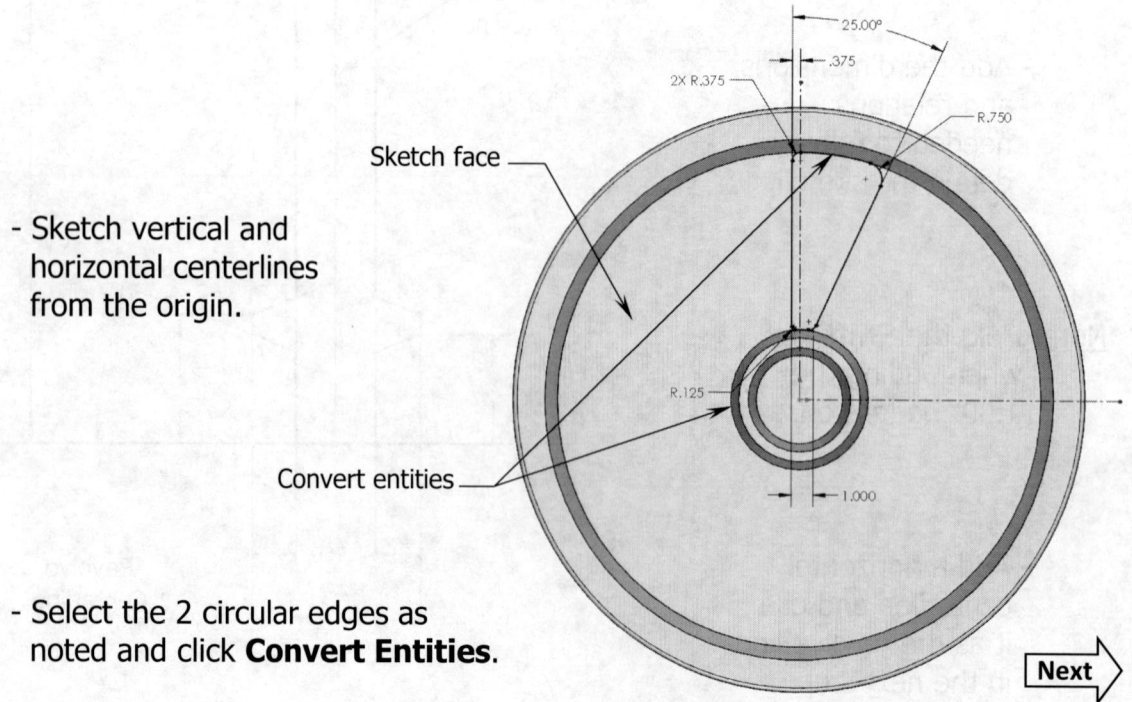

Sketch face

Convert entities

Next

- **Trim** the sketch entities to create one continuous closed contour.

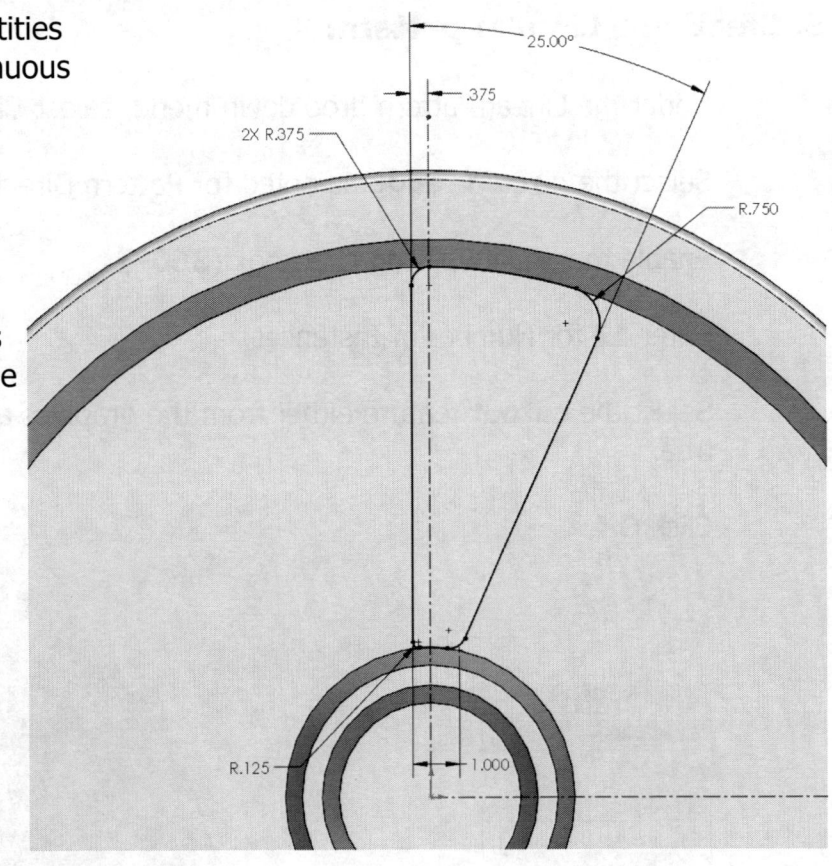

- Add the dimensions shown to fully define the sketch before adding the sketch fillets.

- **Note:**
  There are three different fillet sizes in this sketch.

4. Extruding a cut:

- Click **Extruded-Cut**.

- Use the **Through All** type.

- Click **OK**.

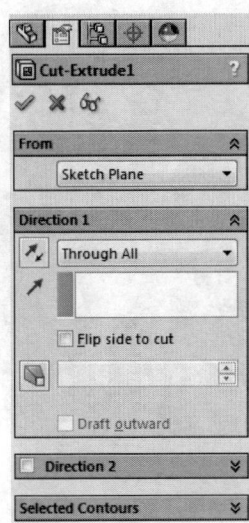

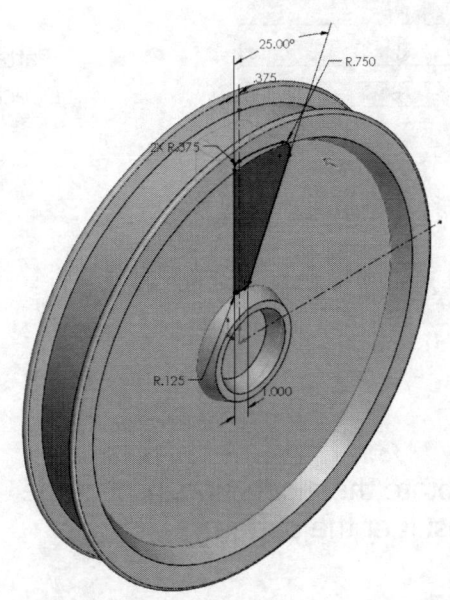

5. Creating a Circular pattern:

- Under the Linear Pattern drop down menu, select **Circular Pattern**.

- Select the **circular edge** as noted for Pattern Direction.

- Enable the Equal Spacing checkbox (**360°**).

- Enter **12** for Number of Instances.

- Select the **cutout** feature either from the graphics area or from the feature tree.

- Click **OK**.

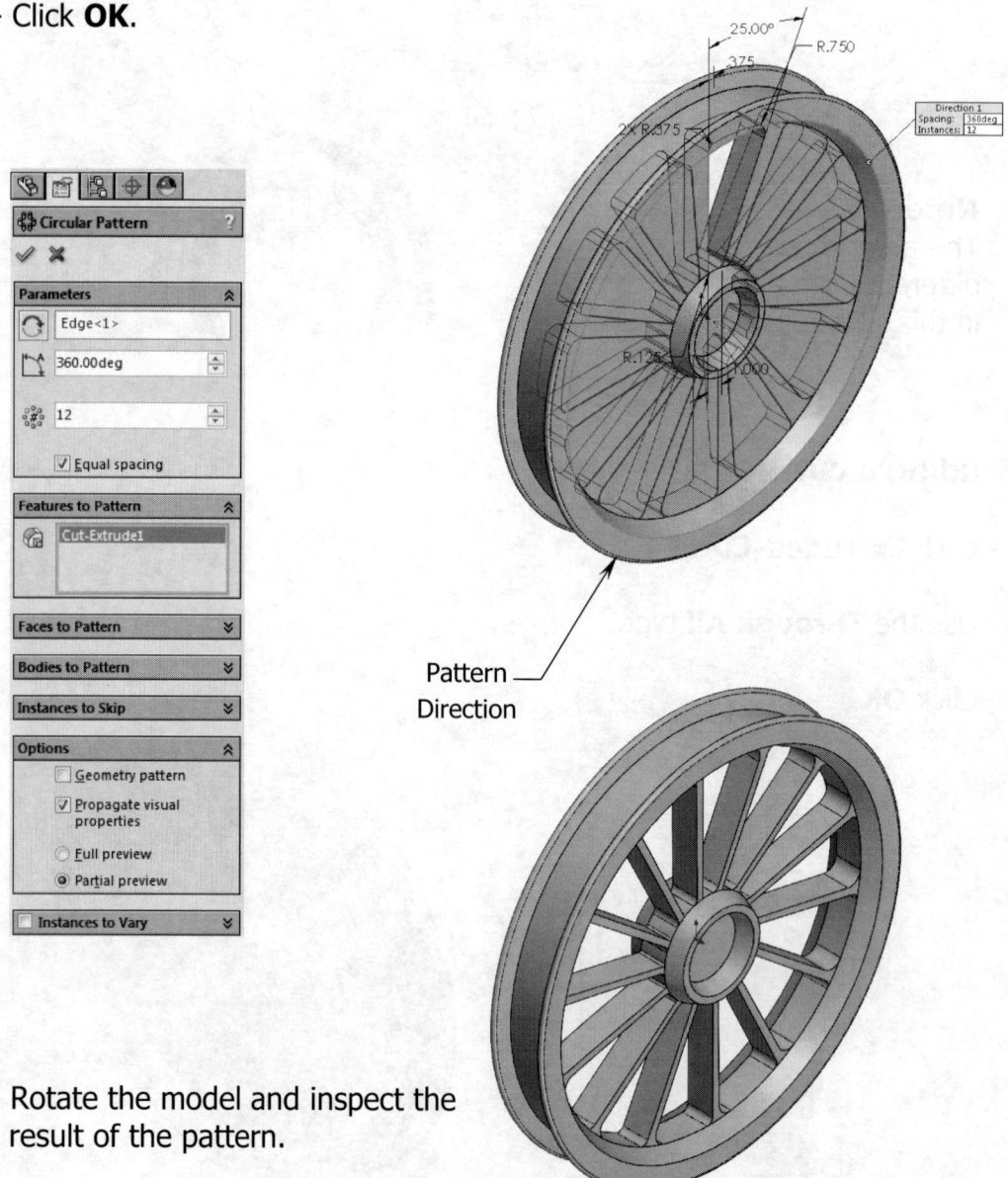

Pattern Direction

- Rotate the model and inspect the result of the pattern.

6. Calculating the Mass:

- Be sure to set the material to **1060 Alloy**.

- Switch to the **Evaluate** tab.

- Click **Mass Properties**.

- If needed, set the Unit of Measure to **IPS**, **3 decimals**.

- Enter the final mass of the model here:

_____ lbs.

- Save your work as: **CSWA_Wheel**.

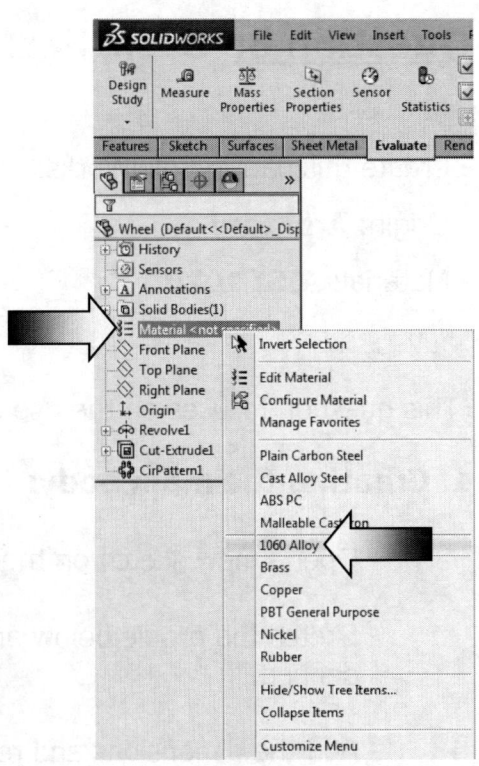

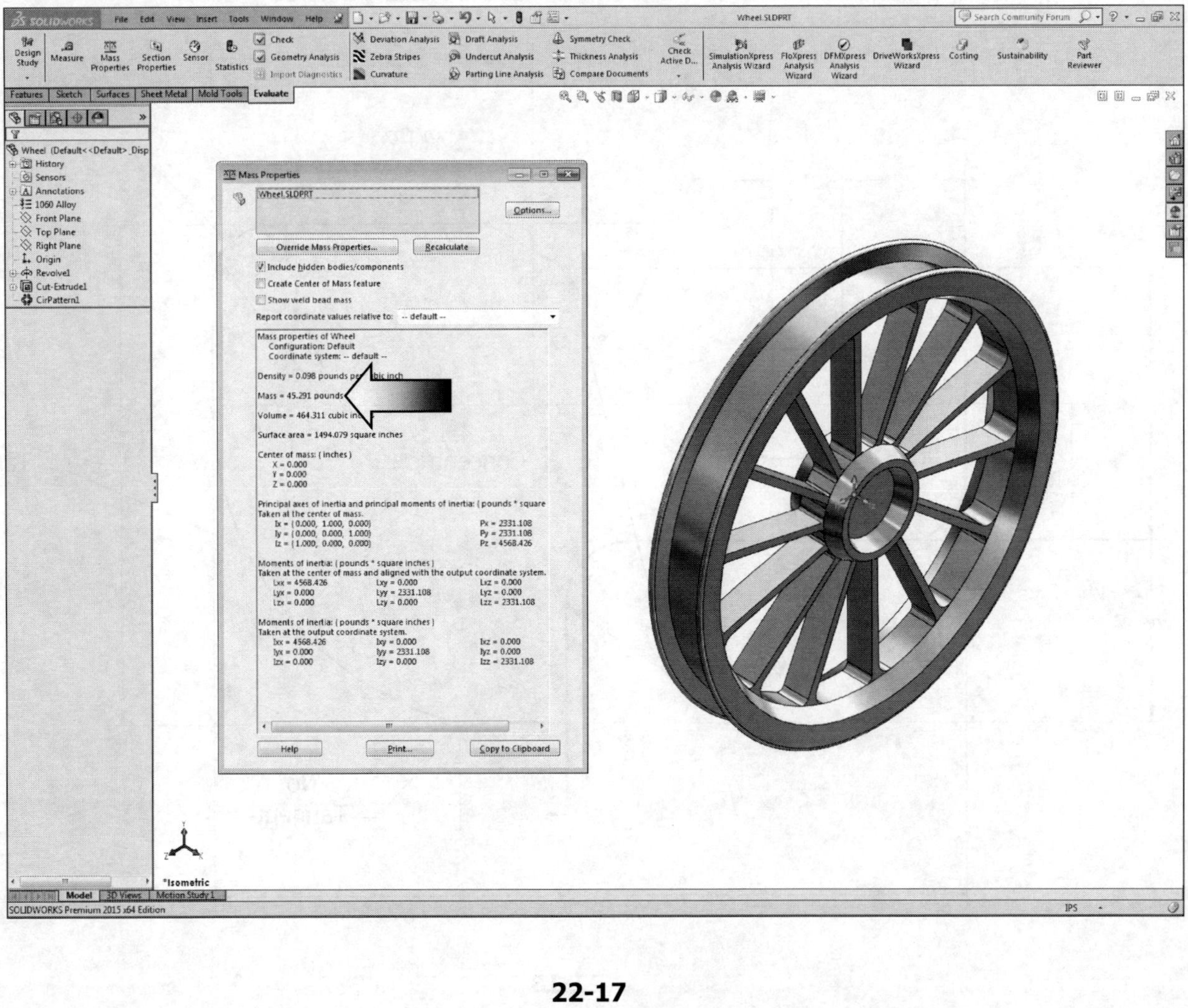

<u>Question 8:</u> Basic Part Modeling (3 of 4)

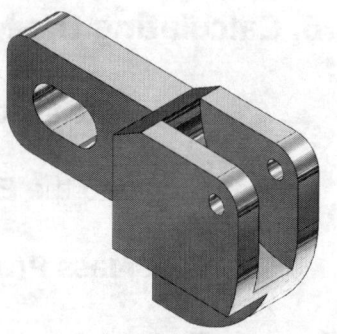

- Create this part in SolidWorks.   - Unit: **Inches**, **3 decimals**

- Origin: **Arbitrary**   - Drafting Standards: **ANSI**

- Material: **AISI 1020**   - Density: **0.285 lb/in^3**

(This question focuses on the use of sketch tools, relations, and extrude features).

1. Creating the main body:

- Open a new sketch on the **Front** plane.

- Sketch the profile below and only add the corner fillets after the sketch is fully defined.

- Add the dimensions and relations as indicated. Do not add the reference dimension (1.417), use it to check or measure the geometry only.

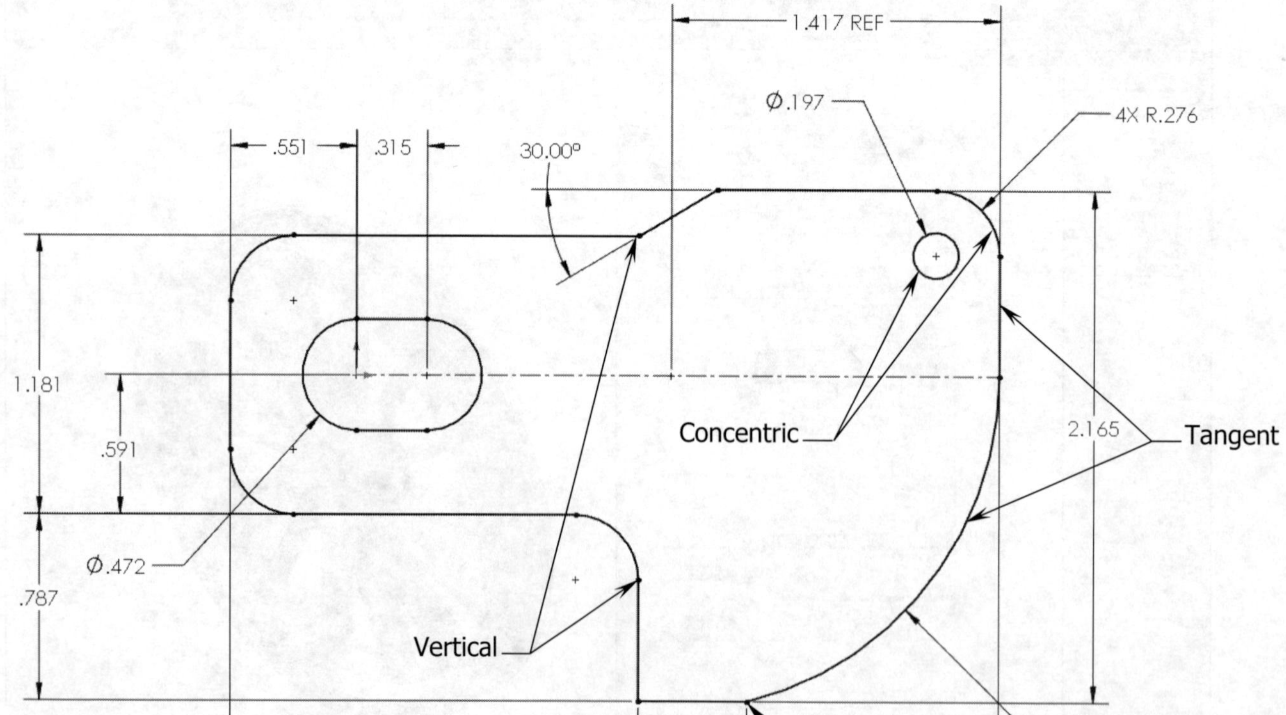

1.417 REF

Ø.197

4X R.276

.551   .315   30.00°

1.181

.591

Ø.472

.787

Concentric

2.165

Tangent

Vertical

.472

No Tangent

R1.417

3.346

2. Extruding the base:

- Click **Extruded Boss/Base**.

- Select the **Mid Plane** type.

- Enter **1.00 in**. for depth.

- Click **OK**.

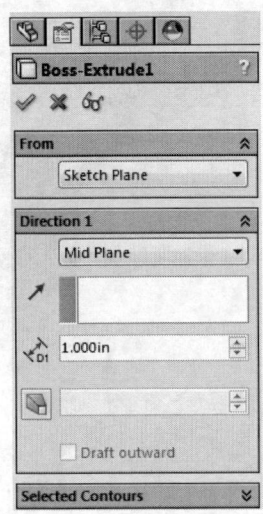

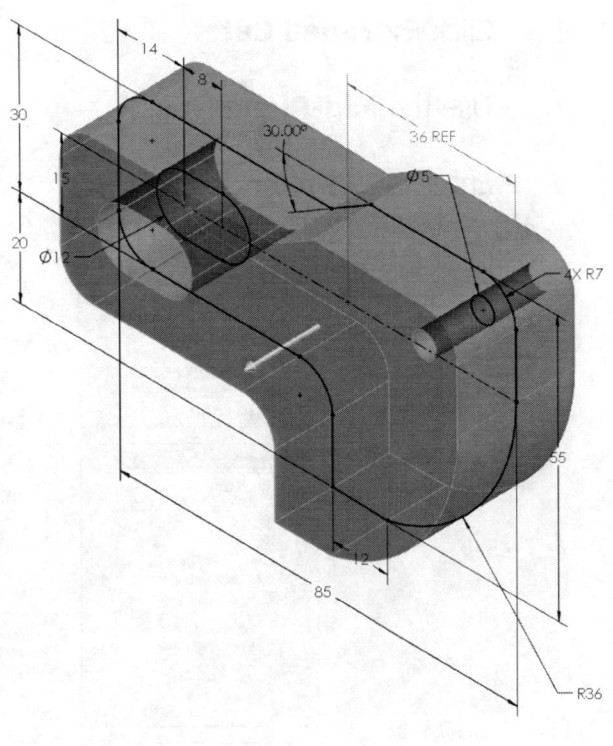

3. Creating the center cutout:

- Open a new sketch
on the **Front** plane.

- Sketch a
circle on the
upper right
corner of
the model.

- Add the dimensions
to fully define the
sketch, as shown.

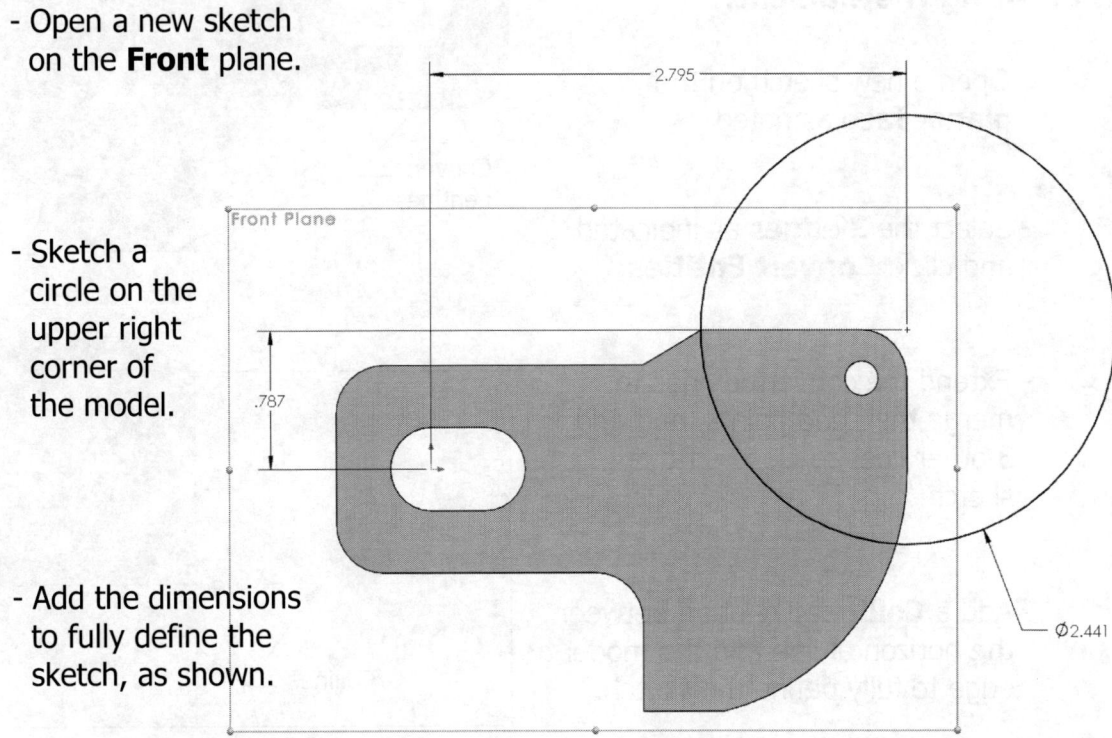

4. Extruding a cut:

- Click **Extruded Cut**.

- Use the **Mid-Plane** type.

- Enter **.475 in**. for depth.

- Click **OK**.

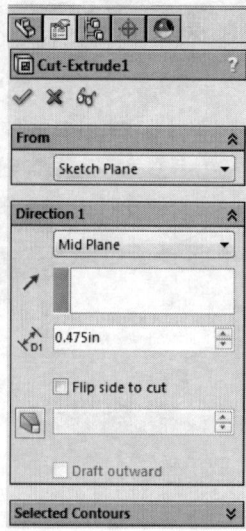

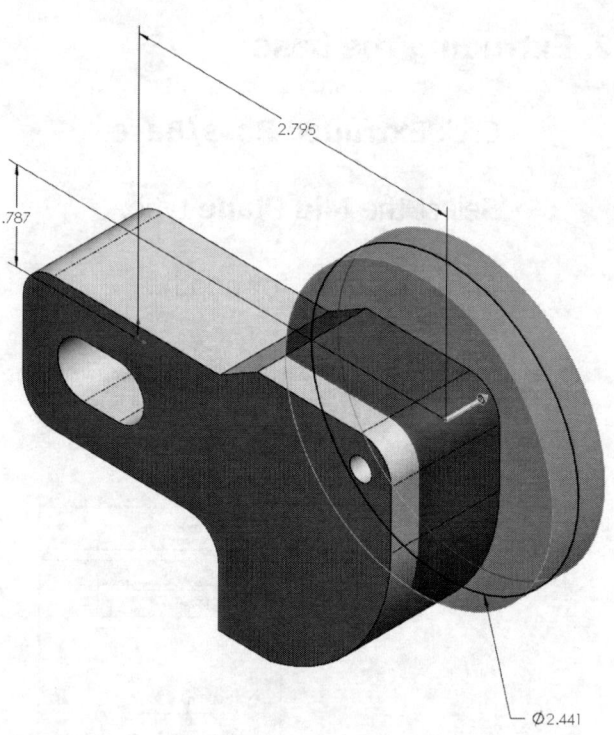

5. Creating the side cut:

- Open a new sketch on the **planar face** as noted.

- Select the **3 edges** as indicated and click: **Convert Entities**.

- Extend the converted lines to merge their end points, and add 3 other lines to close off the sketch.

- Add a **Collinear** relation between the horizontal line and the model edge to fully define the sketch.

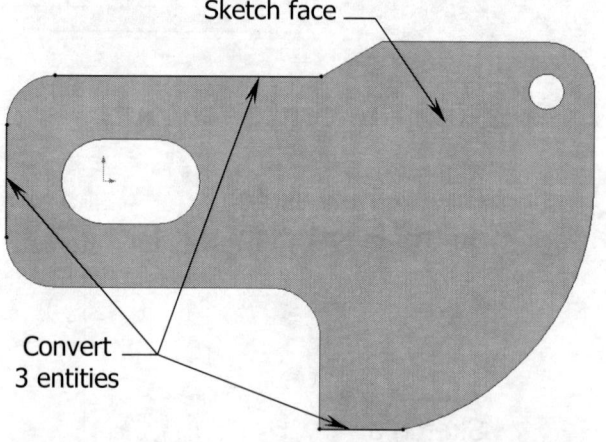

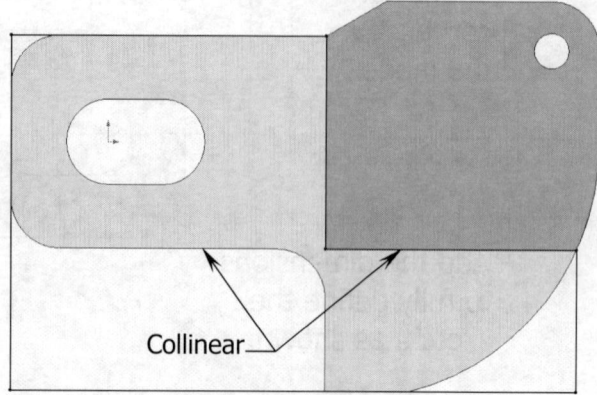

6. Extruding a cut:

- Click **Extruded Cut**.

- Use the default **Blind** type.

- Enter **.492 in**. for depth.

- Click **OK**.

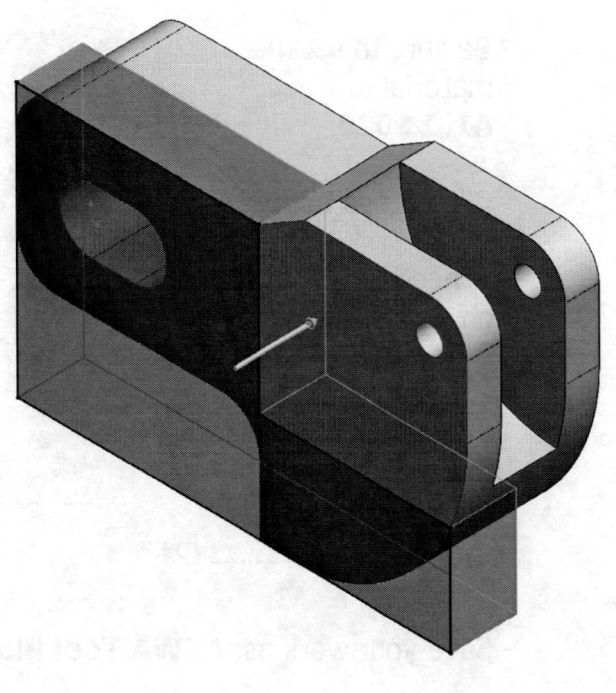

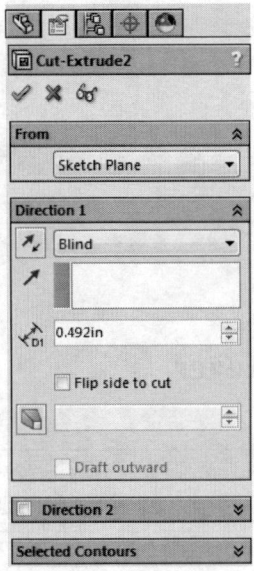

- Rotate the model to verify the result of the cut.

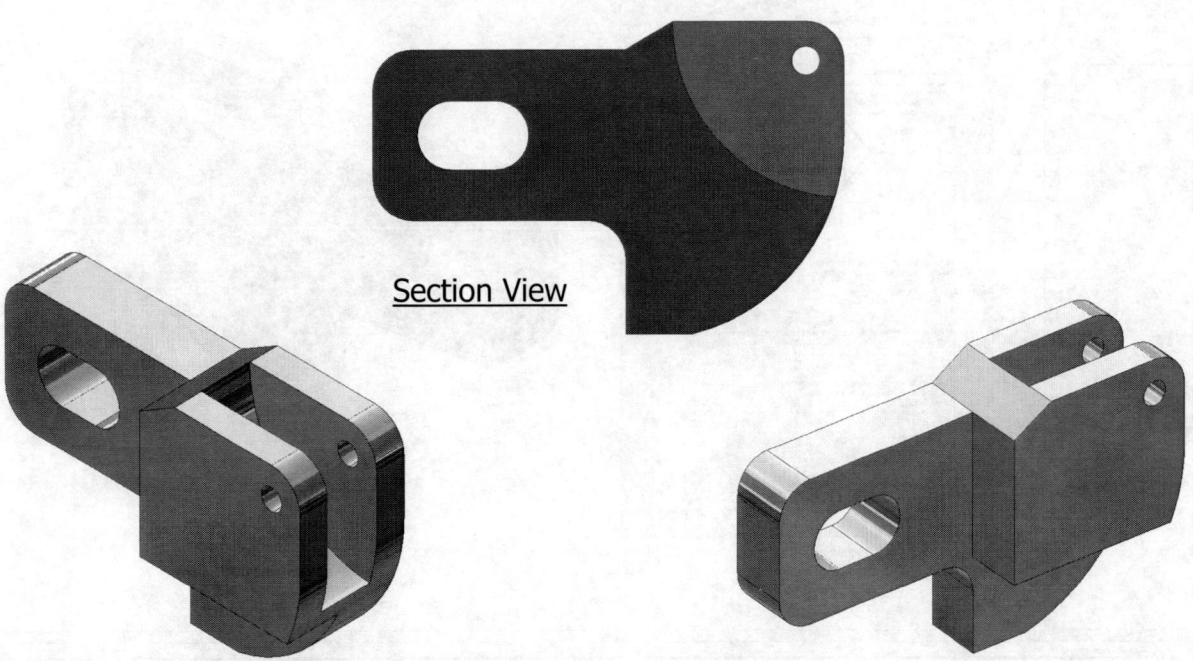

Section View

7. Calculating the Mass:

- Be sure to set the material to: **AISI 1020**.

- Click **Mass Properties**.

- If needed, set the Unit of Measure to **IPS**, **3 decimals**.

- Enter the final mass of the model here:

_____ lbs.

- Save your work as: **CSWA Tool Block Lever.**

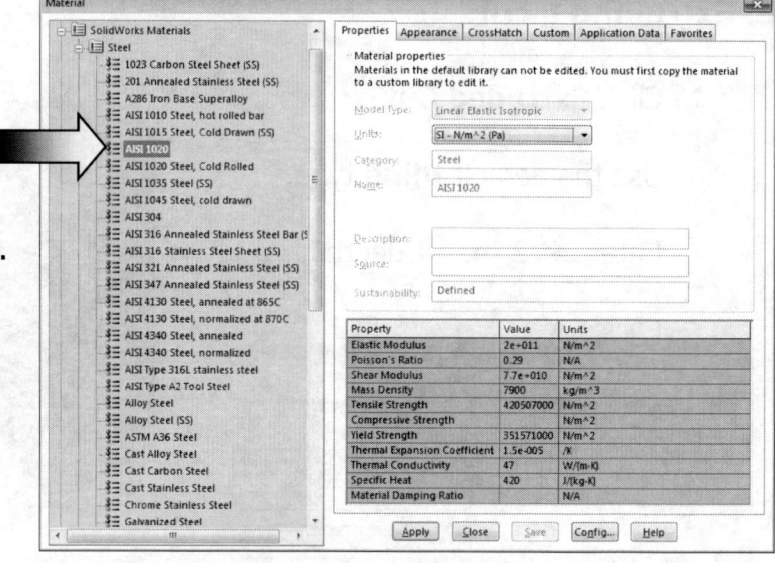

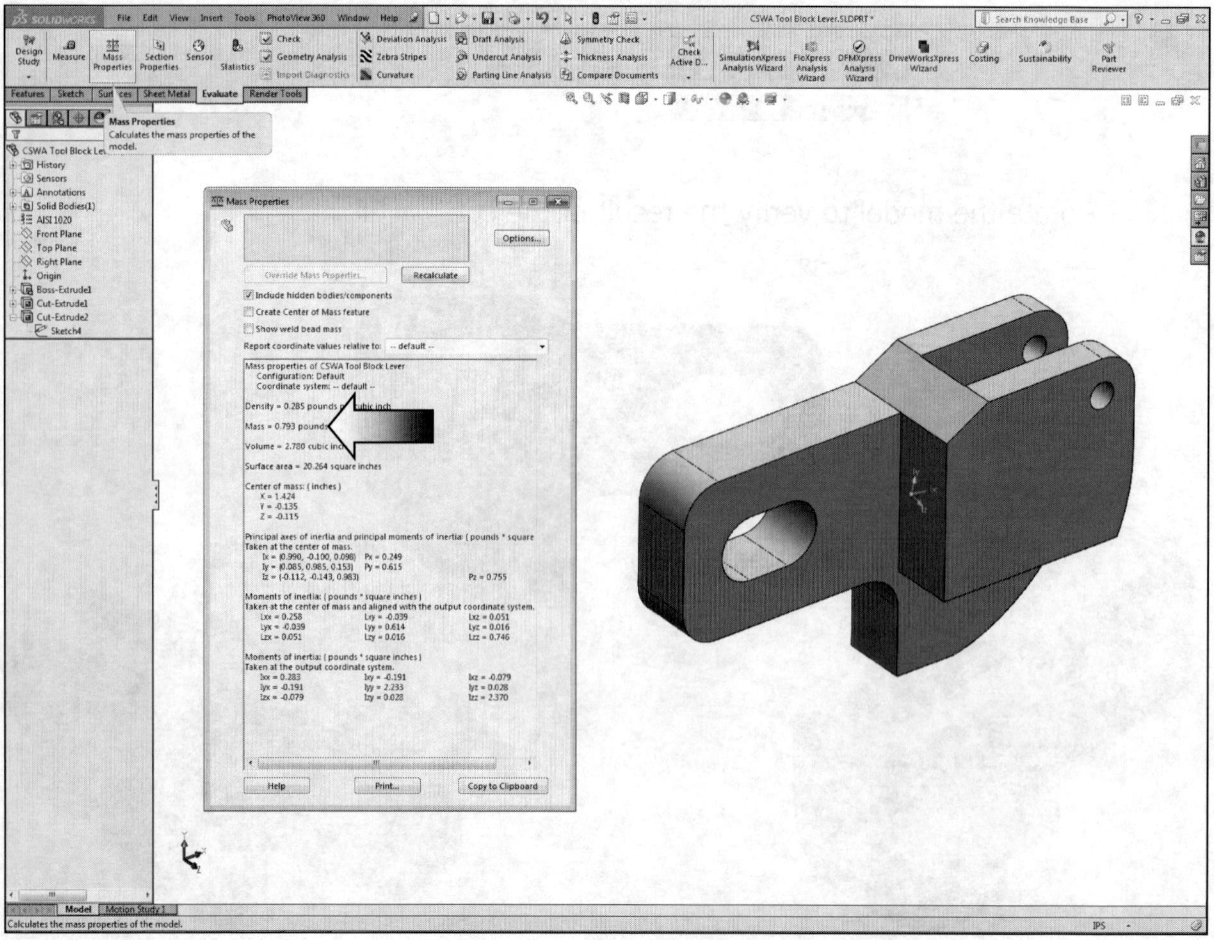

Question 9: Basic Part Modeling (4 of 4)

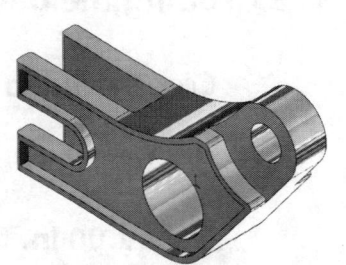

- Create this part in SolidWorks.
- Origin: **Arbitrary**
- Material: **AISI 1020**

- Unit: **Inches, 3 decimals**
- Drafting Standards: **ANSI**
- Density: **0.285 lb/in^3**

(This question focuses on the use of sketch tools, relations, and extrude features).

1. Creating the main body:

- Open a new sketch on the **Front** plane.

- Sketch the profile below and keep the origin in the center of the large hole.

- Add the dimensions/relations as shown to fully define the sketch.

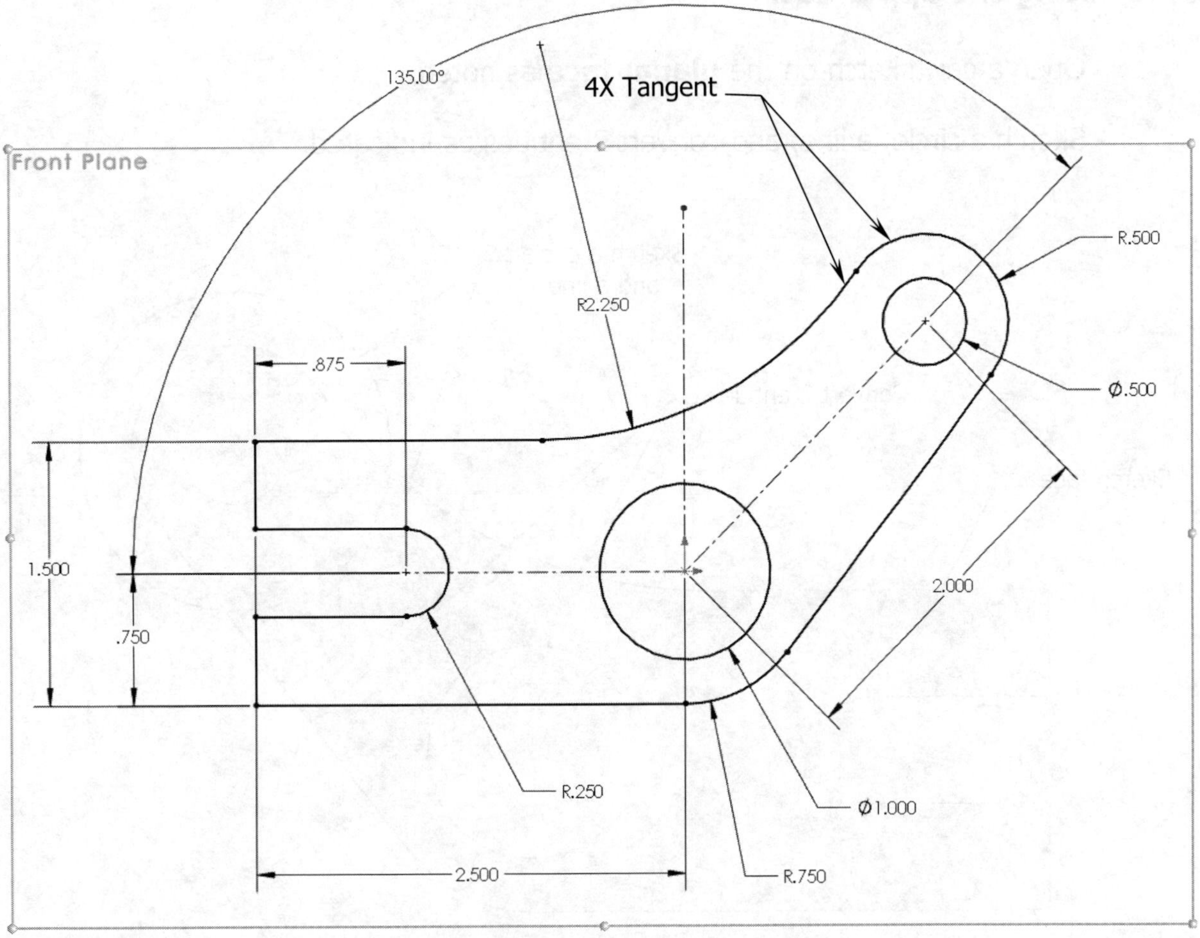

135.00°

4X Tangent

Front Plane

R.500

R2.250

Ø.500

.875

2.000

1.500

.750

R.250

Ø1.000

2.500

R.750

2. Extruding the base:

- Click **Extruded Boss/Base**.

- Use the **Mid-Plane** type.

- Enter **1.00 in**. for depth.

- Click **OK**.

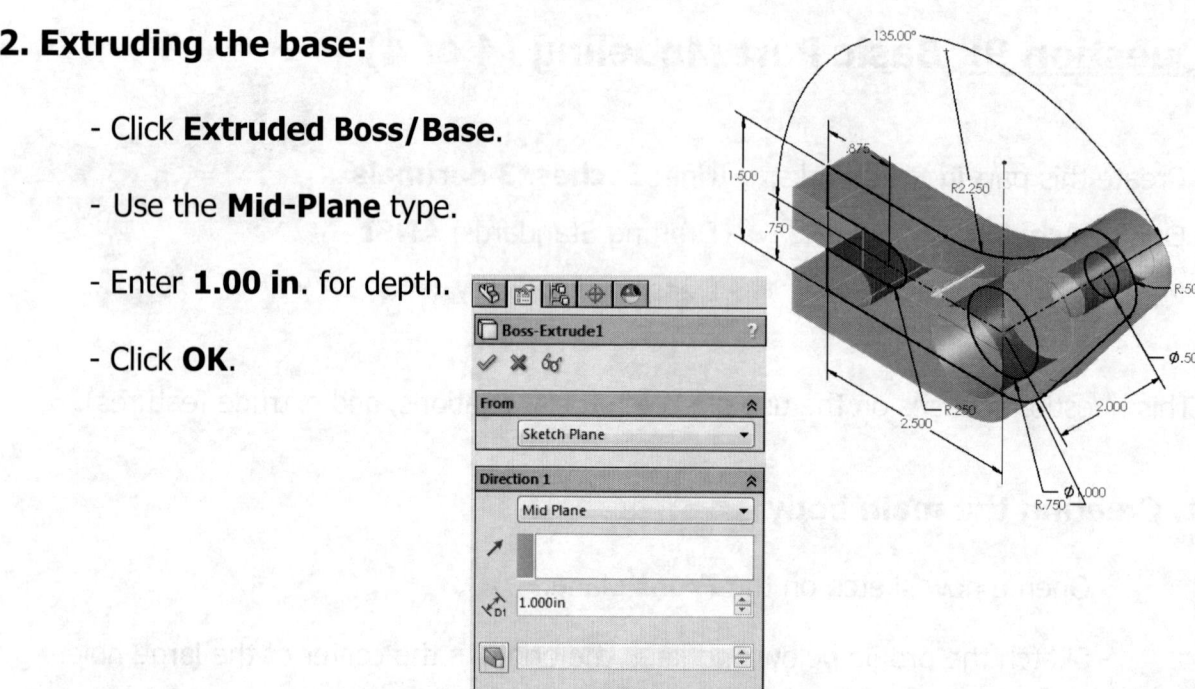

3. Creating the upper cut:

- Open a new sketch on the **planar face** as noted.

- Sketch a circle, a line, and convert 2 entities as indicated.

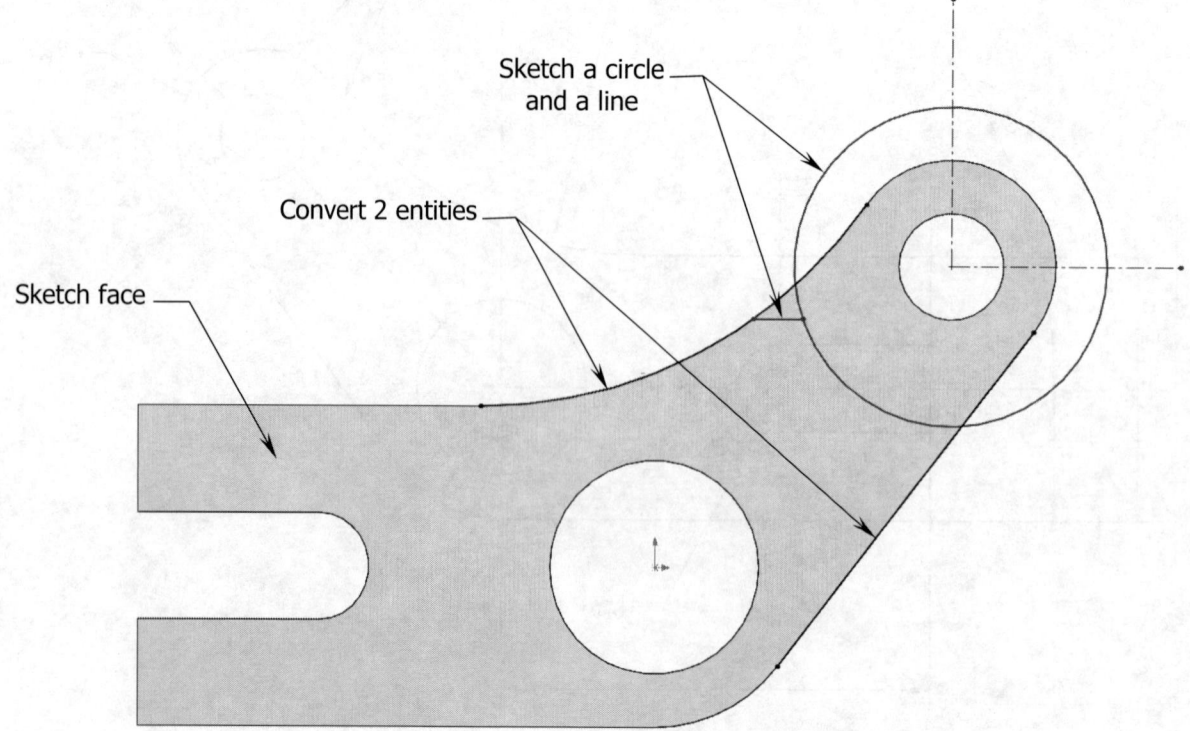

Sketch a circle and a line

Convert 2 entities

Sketch face

- The center of the circle is coincident with the center of the existing hole.

- Trim the entities and add the dimensions shown to fully define the sketch.

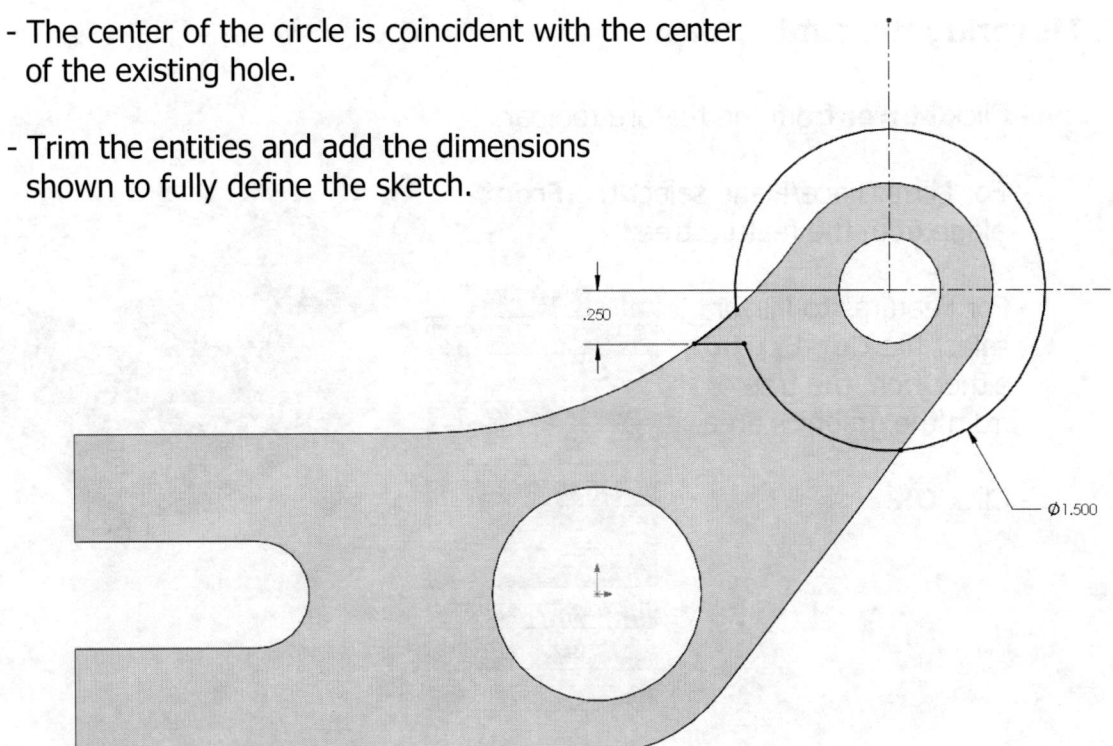

4. Extruding a blind cut:

- Click **Extruded Cut**.

- Use the default **Blind** type.

- Enter **.250 in**. for depth.

- Click **OK**.

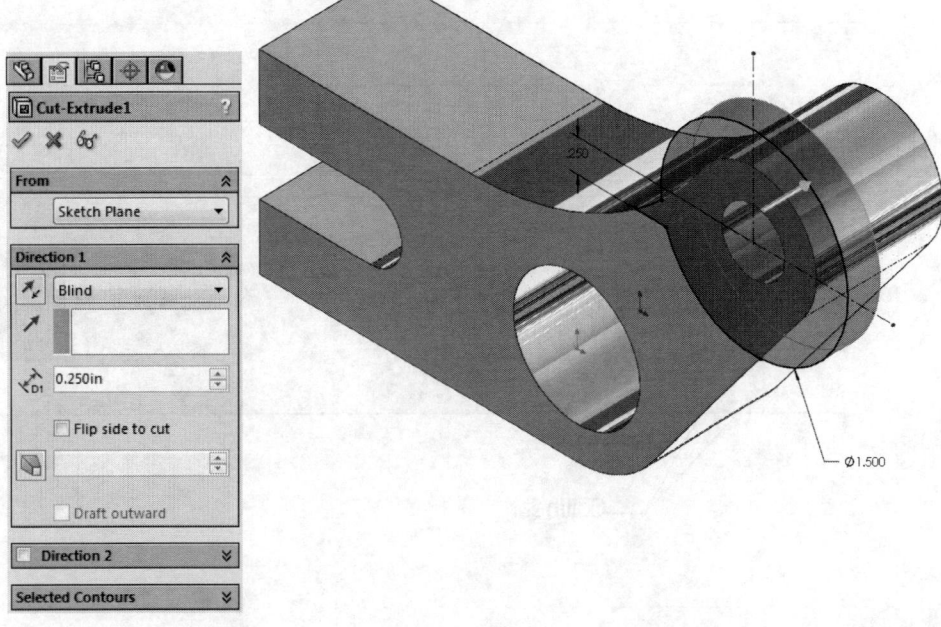

5. Mirroring the cut feature:

- Click **Mirror** from the feature toolbar.

- For Mirror Face/Plane select the **Front** plane from the feature tree.

- For Features to Mirror select the **Cut-Extrude** either from the tree or from the graphics area.

- Click **OK**.

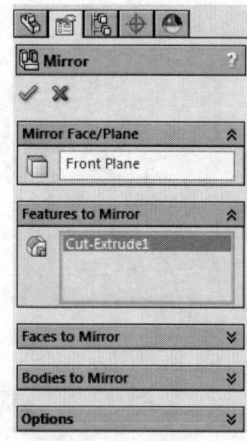

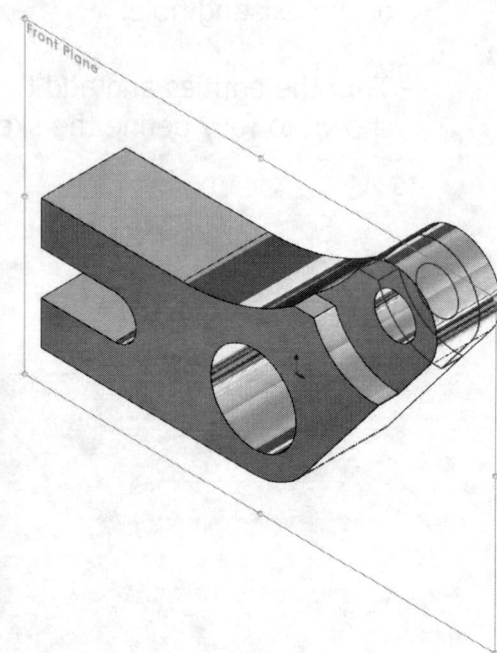

6. Creating the center cut:

- Open a new sketch on the **Top** plane.

- Sketch a rectangle approximately as shown.

- Add the dimensions/relations needed to fully define the sketch.

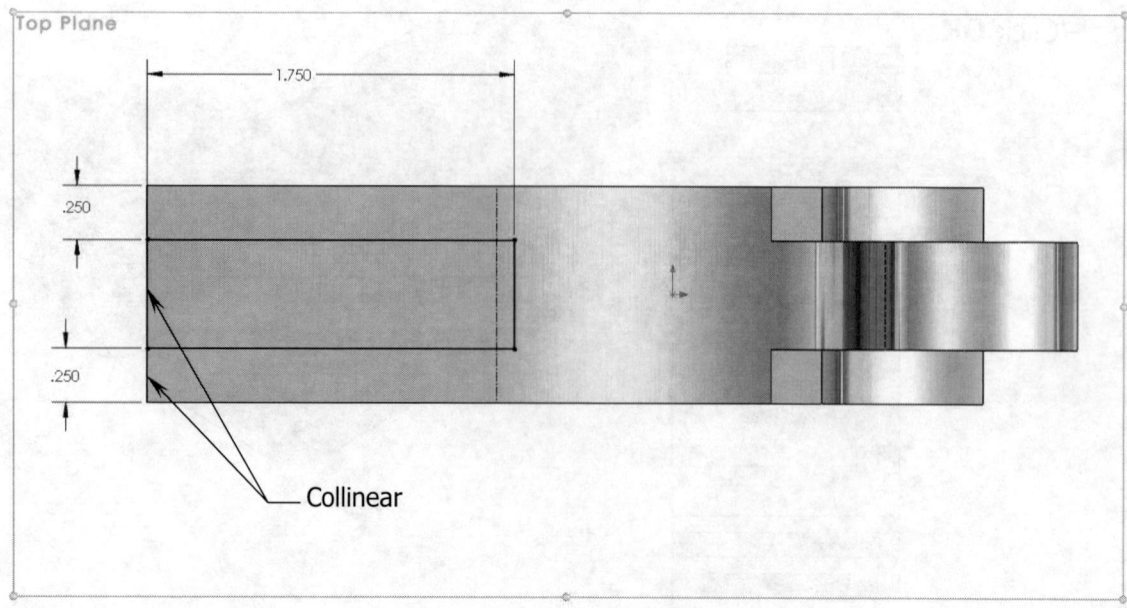

7. Extruding a through cut:

- Click **Extruded Cut**.

- Use the **Through All-Both** type.

- The 2nd direction is selected automatically.

- Click **OK**.

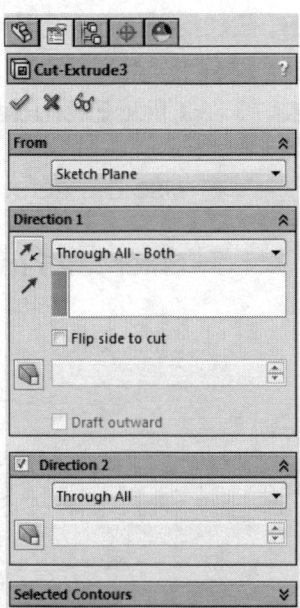

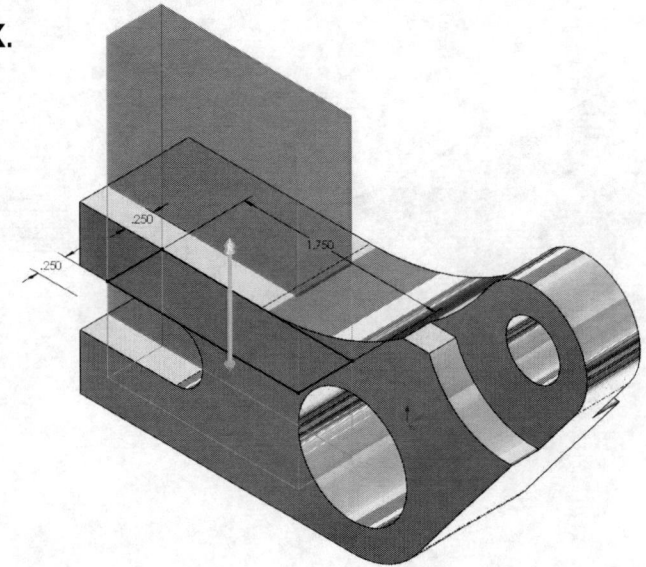

8. Creating a recess feature:

- Open a new sketch on the **planar face** as noted.

- While the selected face is still highlighted click **Offset Entities**.

- Enter **.080 in**. for offset distance and click the Reverse checkbox if needed to place the offset entities on the **inside**.

- Close the Offset Entities command.

Sketch face

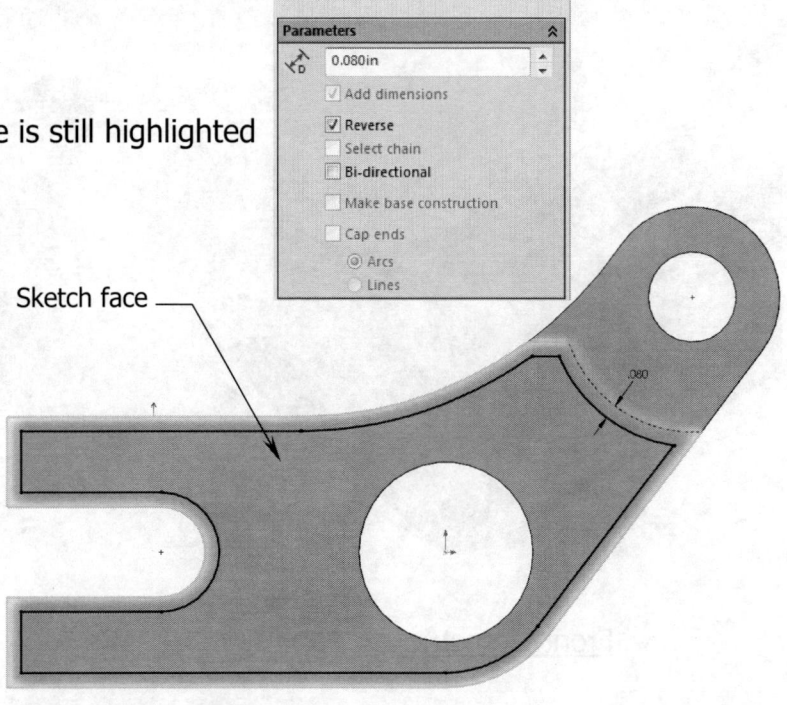

9. Extruding a blind cut:

- Click **Extruded Cut**.

- Use the default **Blind** type.

- Enter **.125 in**. for depth.

- Click **OK**.

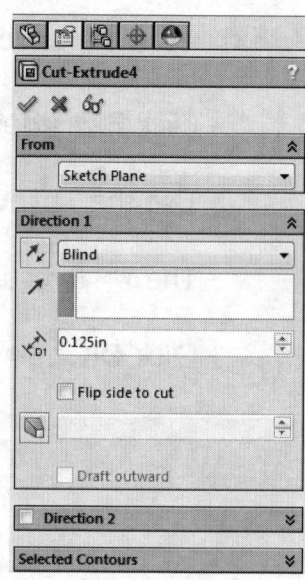

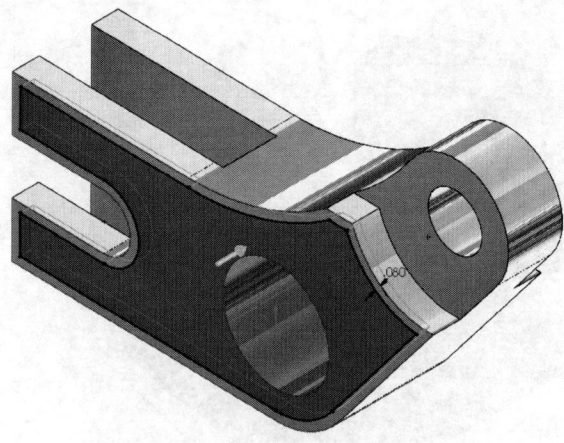

- Rotate the model to verify the result of the cut feature.

Note: The recess feature is only added to one side. Do not mirror it.

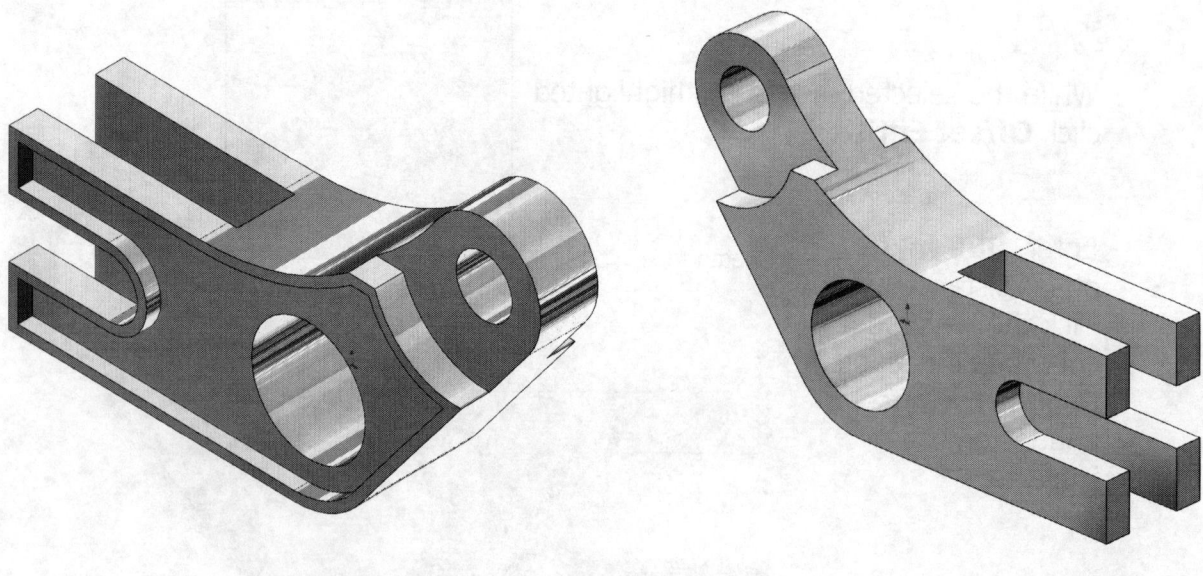

Front Isometric   Rear Isometric

10. Calculating the Mass:

- Be sure to set the material to: **AISI 1020**.

- Click **Mass Properties**.

- If needed, set the Unit of Measure to **IPS**, **4 decimals**.

- Enter the final mass of the model here:

_____ lbs.

- Save your work as: **CSWA Bracket**.

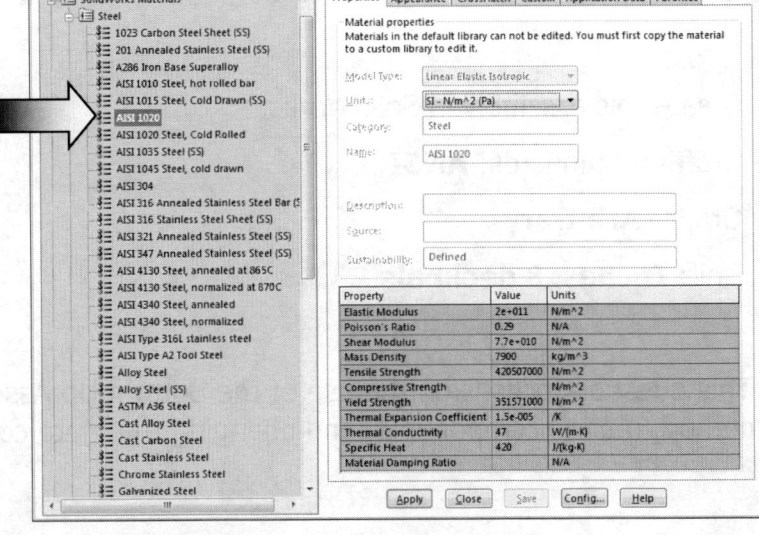

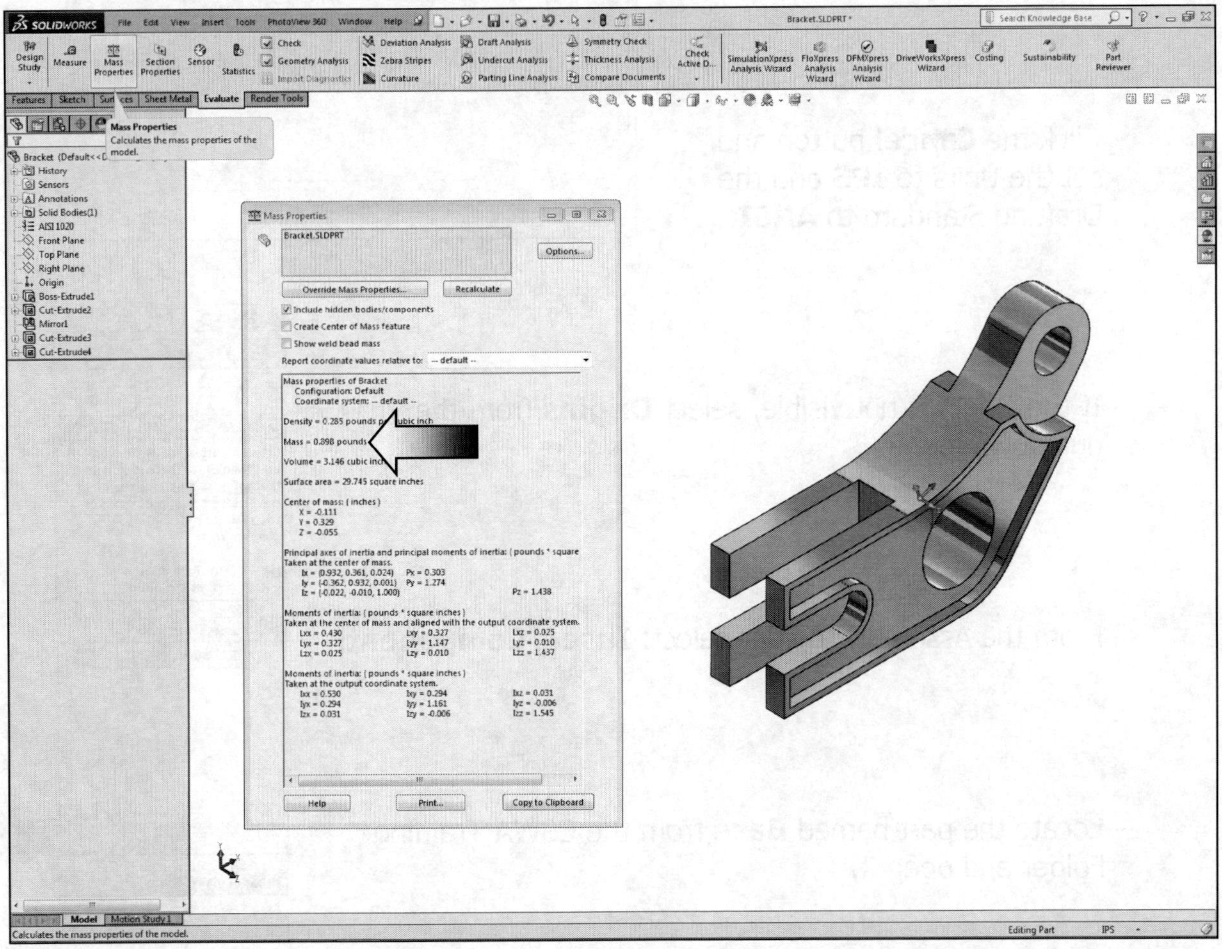

Question 10: Bottom Up Assembly (1 of 2)

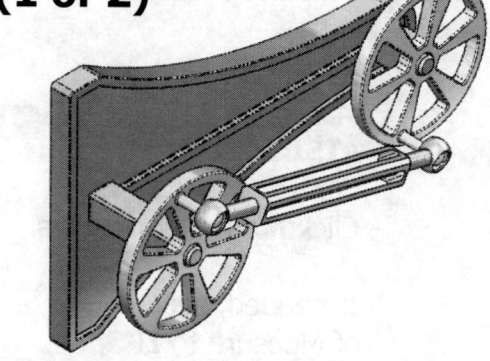

- Create this assembly in SolidWorks.

- Drafting Standards: **ANSI**

- Origin: **Arbitrary**

- Unit: **Inches, 3 decimals**.

(This question focuses on the use of the Bottom Up Assembly method, mating components, and changing the mate conditions).

1. Creating a new assembly:

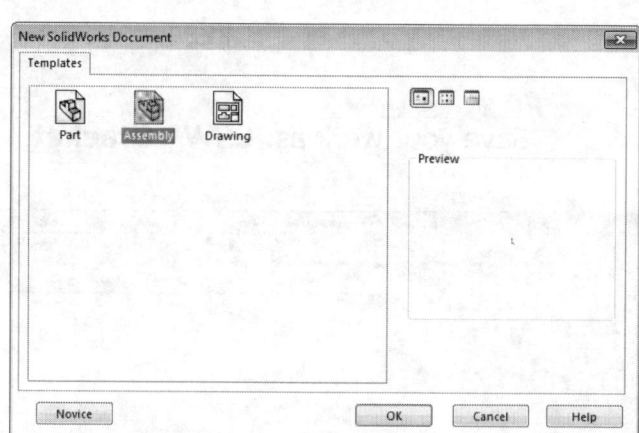

- Select: **File, New, Assembly**.

- Click the **Cancel** button and set the Units to **IPS** and the Drafting Standard to **ANSI**.

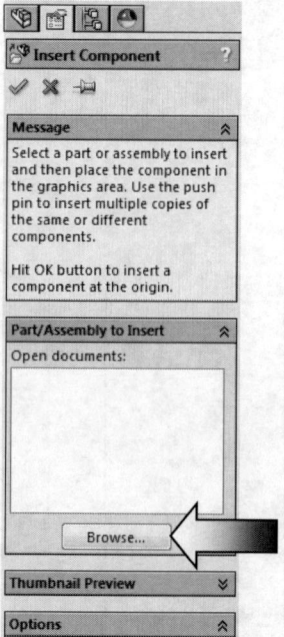

- If the Origin is not visible, select **Origins** from the View pull down menu.

- From the Assembly toolbar select: **Insert Component**.

- Locate the part named **Base** from the CSWA Training Folder and open it.

- Place the 1st component on the assembly's origin.

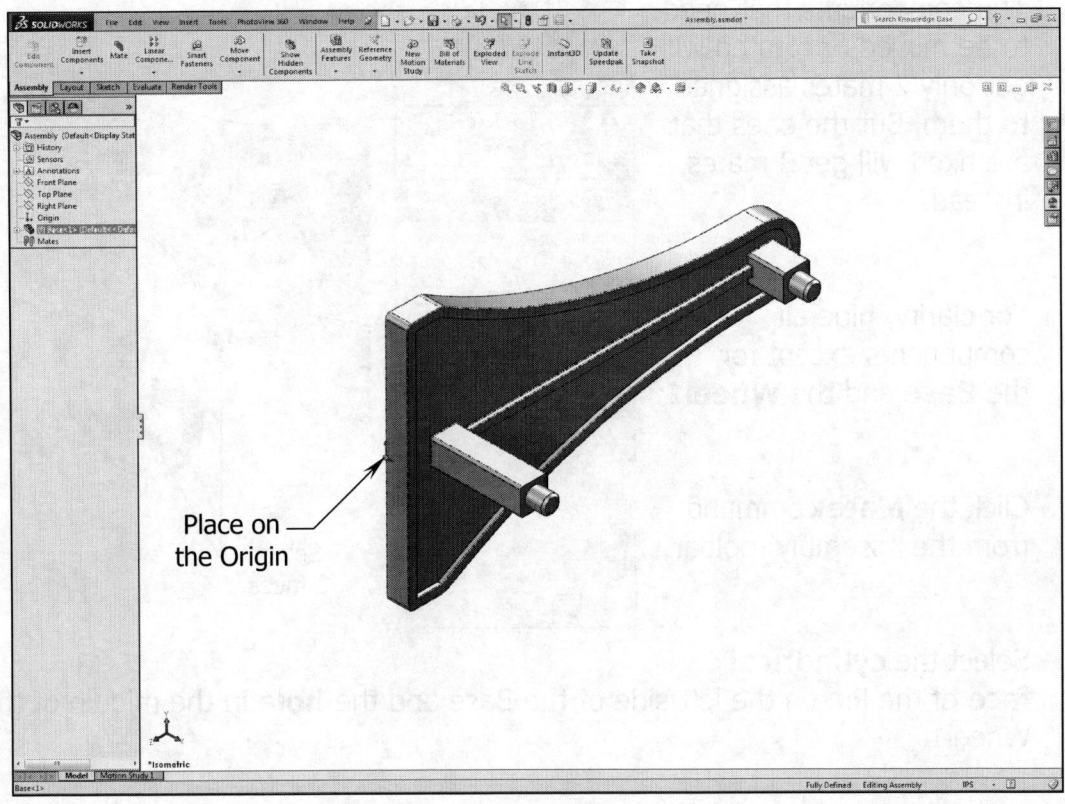

Place on
the Origin

2. Inserting other components:

- Insert the rest of the components into the assembly as labeled.

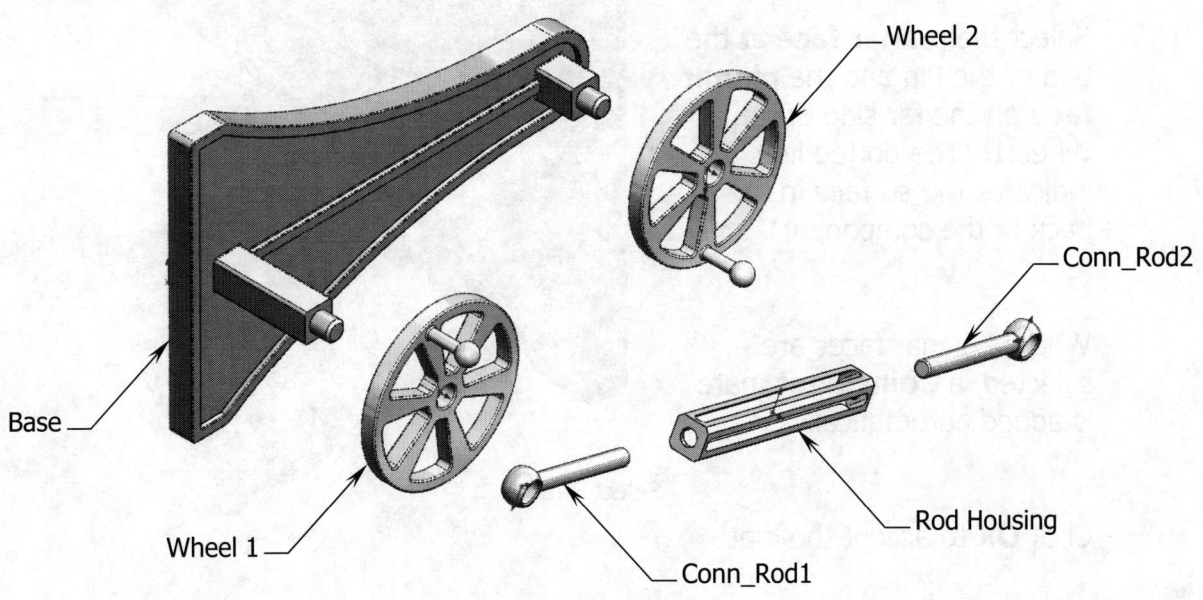

Wheel 2

Conn_Rod2

Base

Rod Housing

Wheel 1

Conn_Rod1

3. Mating the components:

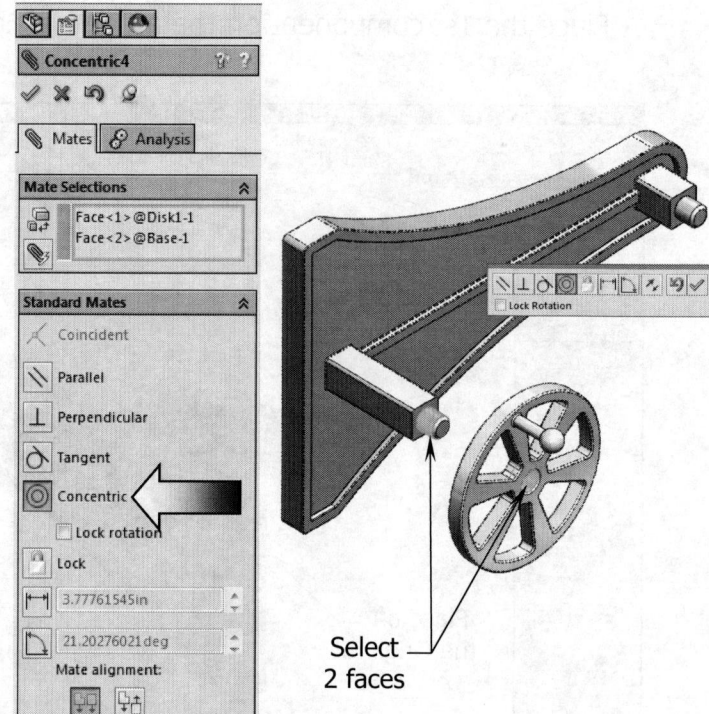

- The components that need to be moved or rotated will get only 2 mates assigned to them. But the ones that are fixed will get 3 mates instead.

- For clarity, hide all components except for the **Base** and the **Wheel1**.

- Click the **Mate** command from the Assembly toolbar.

- Select the **cylindrical face** of the Pin on the left side of the Base and the **hole** in the middle of the Wheel1.

- A **Concentric** mate is selected automatically.

- Click **OK** to accept the mate.

- Select the **planar face** at the end of the Pin and the **planar face** on the far side of the Wheel1. (The dotted line indicates the surface in the back of the component).

- When 2 planar faces are selected, a **Coincident** mate is added automatically.

- Click **OK** to accept the mate.

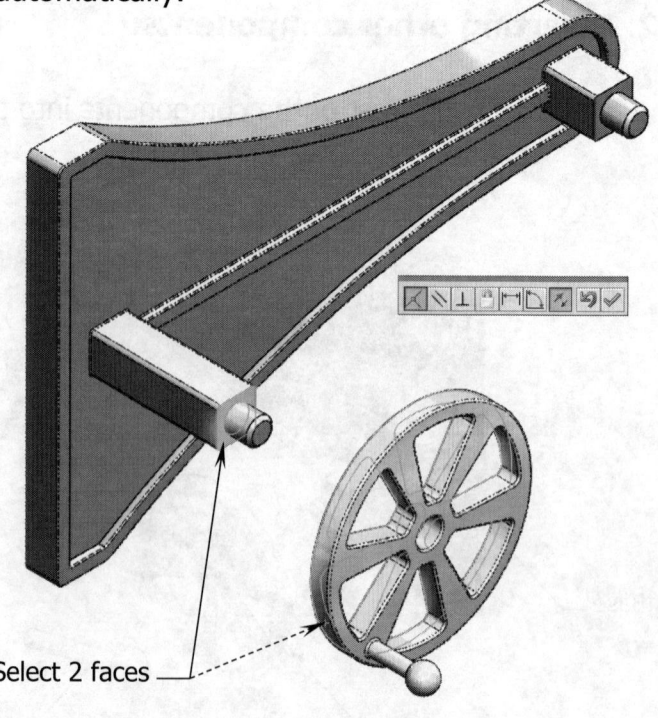

4. Mating the Wheel2 to the Base:

- Show the component **Wheel2**.

- Click the **Mate** command if it is no longer active.

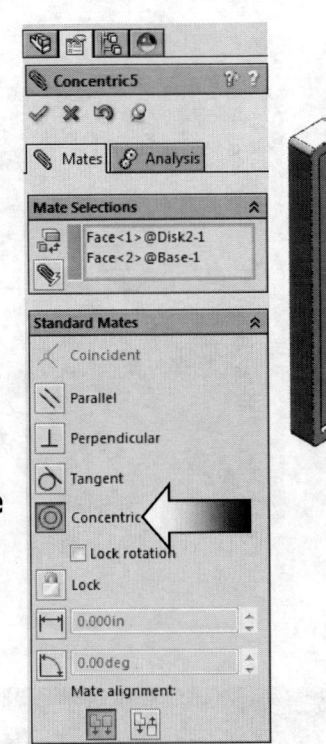

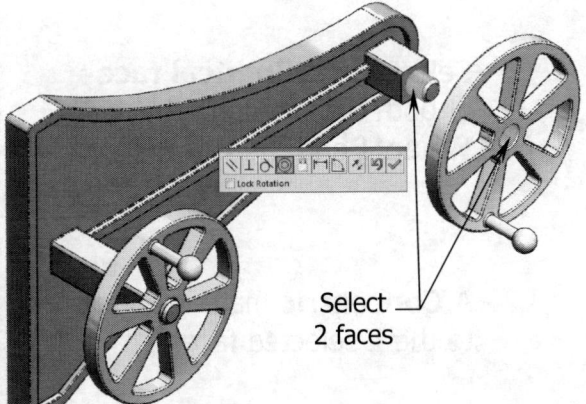

Select 2 faces

- Add a **Concentric** mate between the **cylindrical face** of the 2ⁿᵈ Pin and the **hole** in the middle of the Wheel2.

- Click **OK**.

Select 2 faces

- Next, select the **planar face** at the end of the Pin and the **planar face** on the far side of the Wheel1.

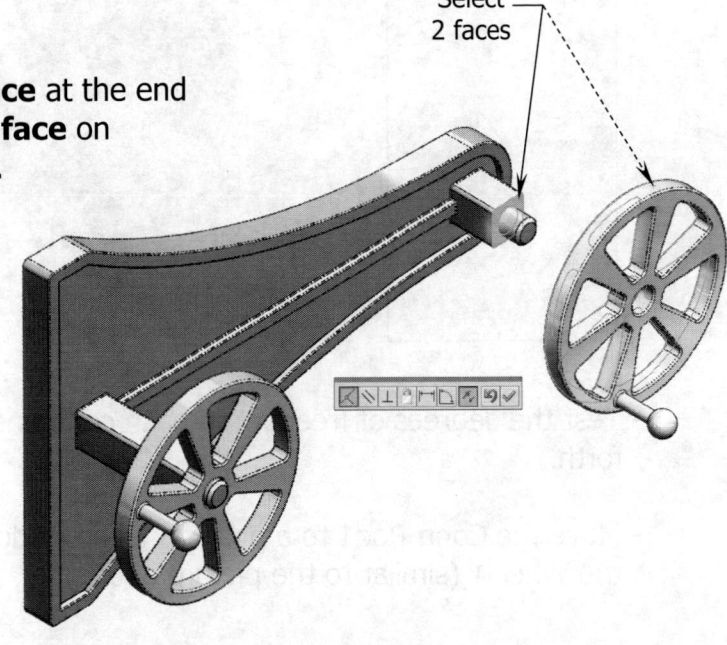

- A **Coincident** mate is added automatically.

- Click **OK**.

5. Mating the Conn-Rod1 to the Wheel1:

- Show the component **Conn-Rod1**.

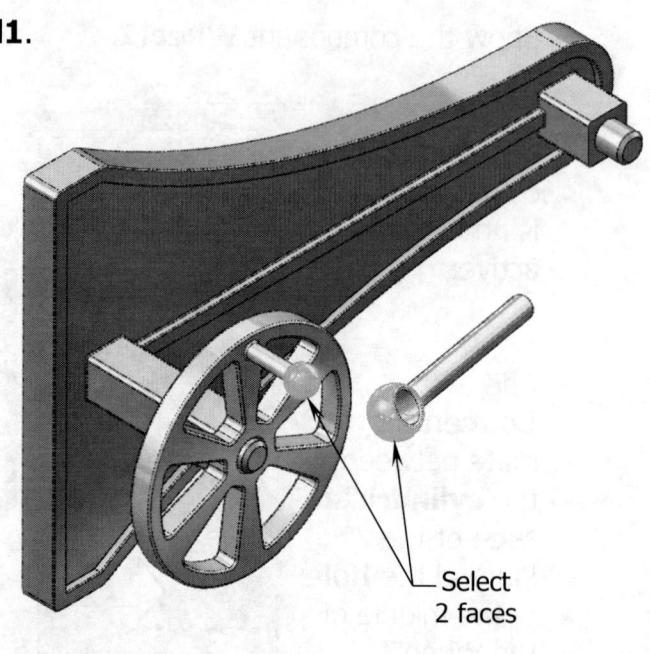

- Select the **cylindrical faces** of both components, the **Wheel1** and the **Conn-Rod1**.

- A **Concentric** mate is added to the 2 selected faces.

Select 2 faces

- Click **OK**.

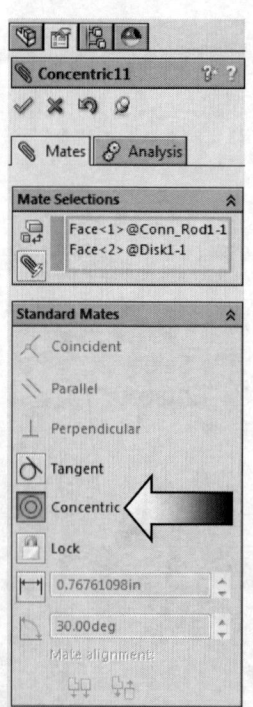

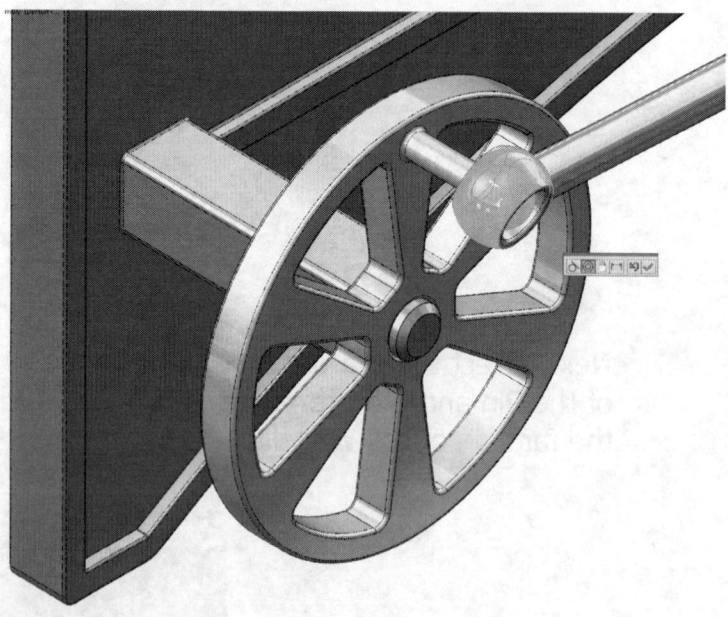

- Test the degrees of freedom of each component by dragging them back and forth.

- Move the Conn-Rod1 to a position where it does not interfere with the knob in the Wheel1 (similar to the picture above).

6. Mating the Conn_Rod2 to the Wheel2:

- Show the component **Conn_Rod2**.

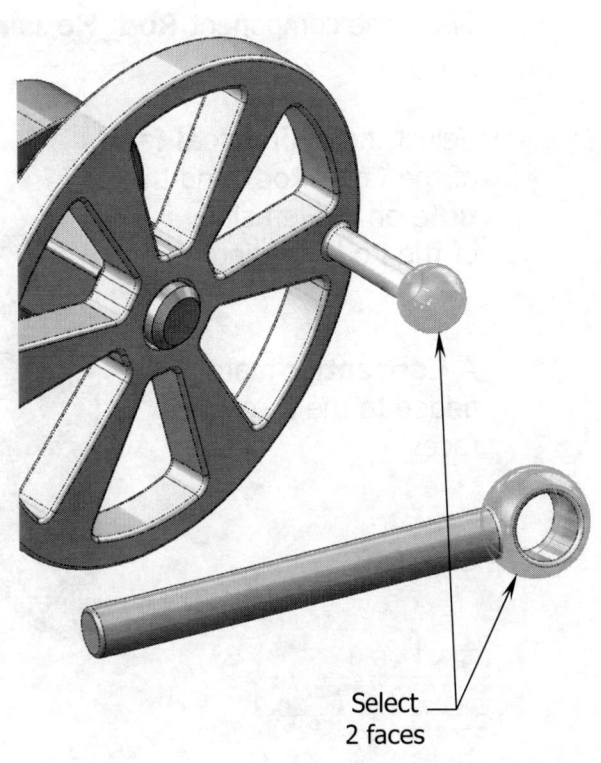

- Select the **cylindrical faces** of both components, the **Conn-Rod2** and the **Wheel2** as pictured.

- Another **Concentric** mate is added to the 2 selected faces.

- Click **OK**.

Select 2 faces

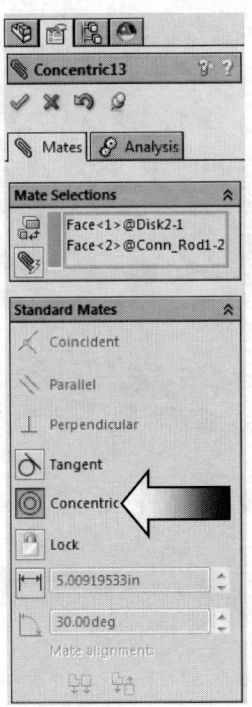

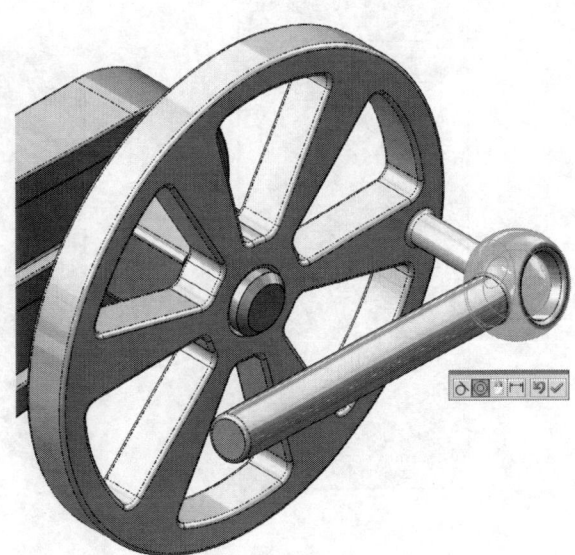

- Drag the Conn_Rod2 back and forth to test it.

- Move the Conn_Rod2 to the position similar to the one pictured above.

7. Mating the Rod_Housing to the Conn_Rods:

- Show the component **Rod_Housing**.

- Select the **cylindrical face** of the Conn-Rod1 and the **hole** on the left side of the Rod_Housing.

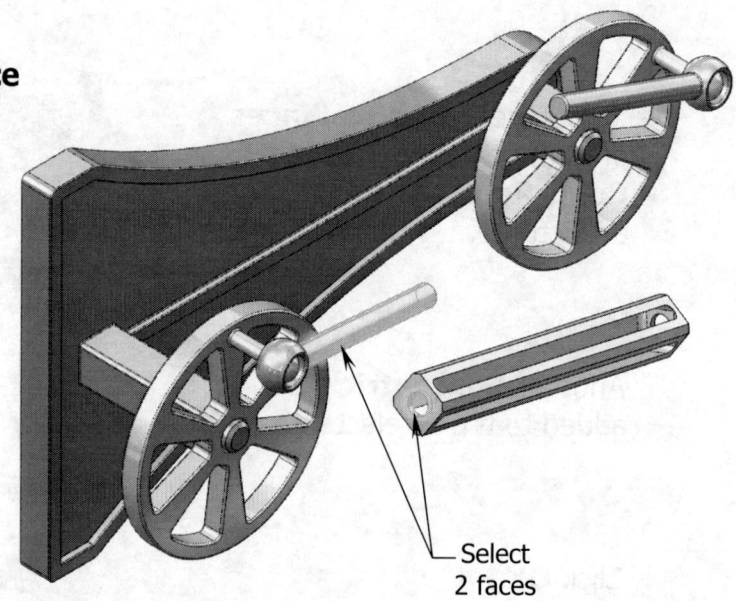

- A **Concentric** mate is added to the 2 selected faces.

- Click **OK**.

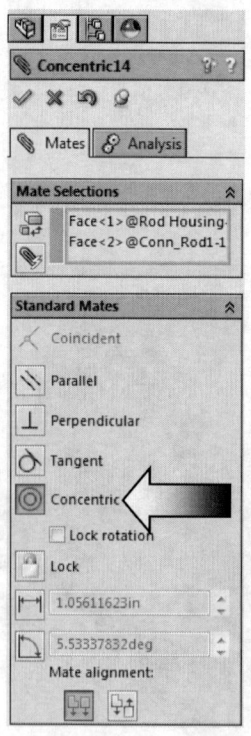

Select 2 faces

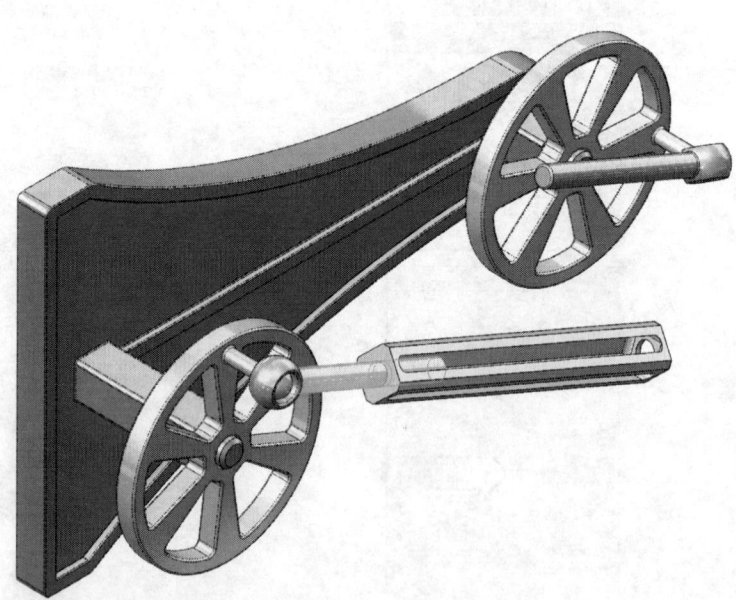

- Test the Rod_Housing by dragging it back and forth. It should be constrained to move only along the longitudinal axis of the Conn-Rod.

- Move the Rod_Housing to a position similar to the one pictured above.

- Zoom in to the right side of the assembly. We will assemble the Conn_Rod2 to its housing.

- Click the **Mate** command if it is no longer selected.

- Select the **cylindrical face** of the Conn-Rod1 and the **hole** on the right side of the Rod_Housing.

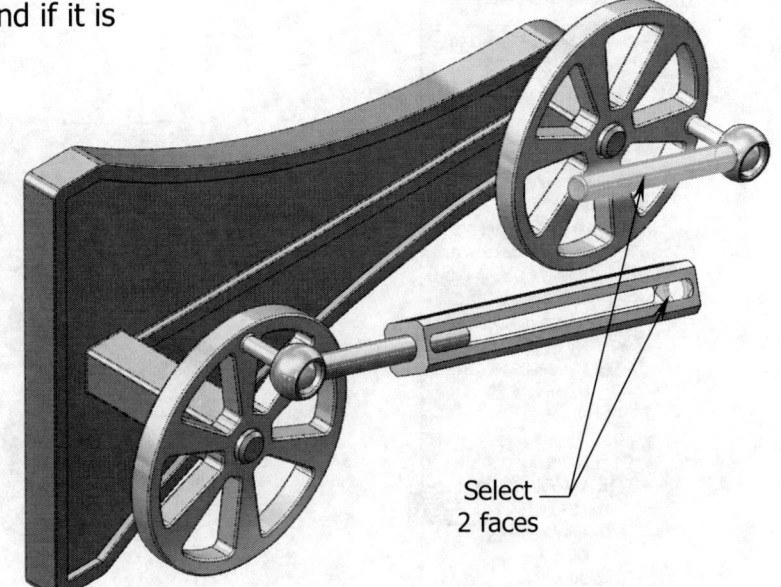

Select 2 faces

- Another **Concentric** mate is added to the 2 selected faces.

- Click **OK**.

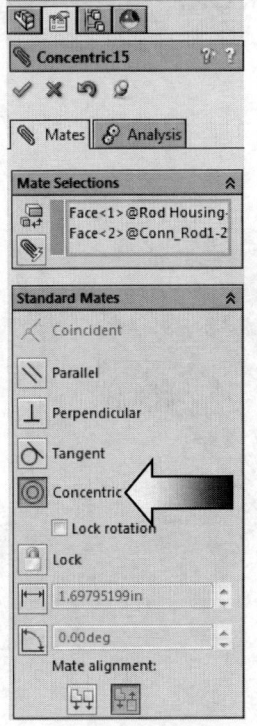

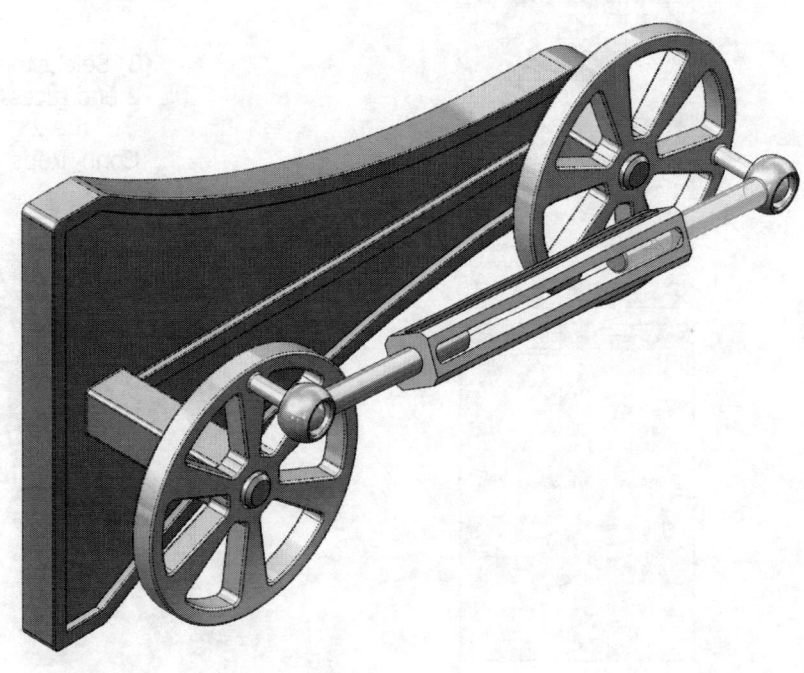

8. Adding a Symmetric mate:

- Using the Feature tree, expand the Rod-Housing and select its **Front** Plane (A).

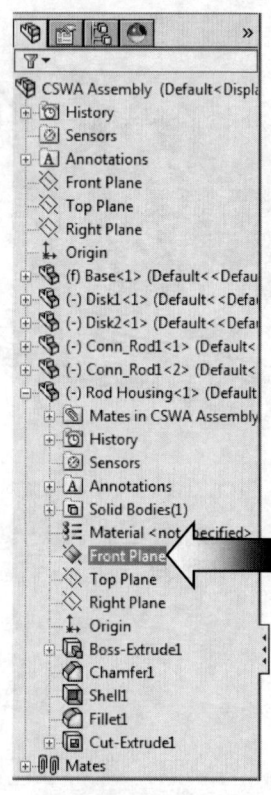

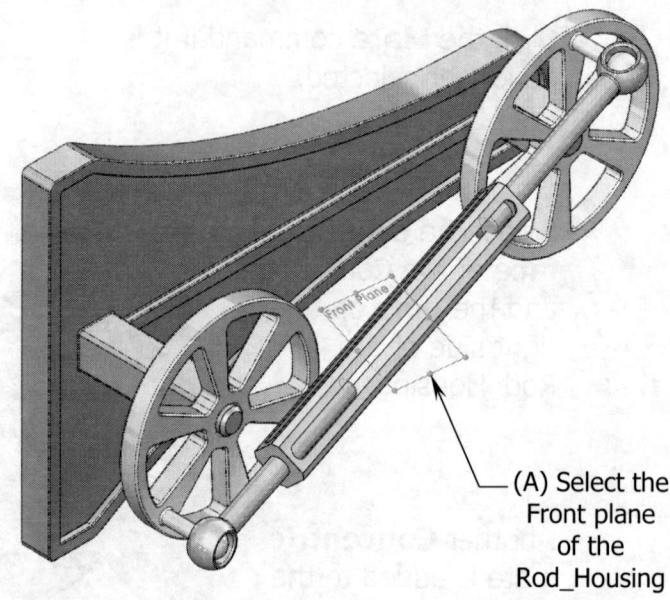

(A) Select the
Front plane
of the
Rod_Housing

- Change to the **Advanced Mates** section and select the **Symmetric** button (B).

- The 2 ends are spaced evenly. Click **OK**.

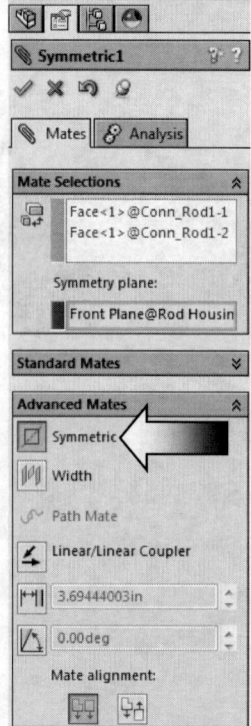

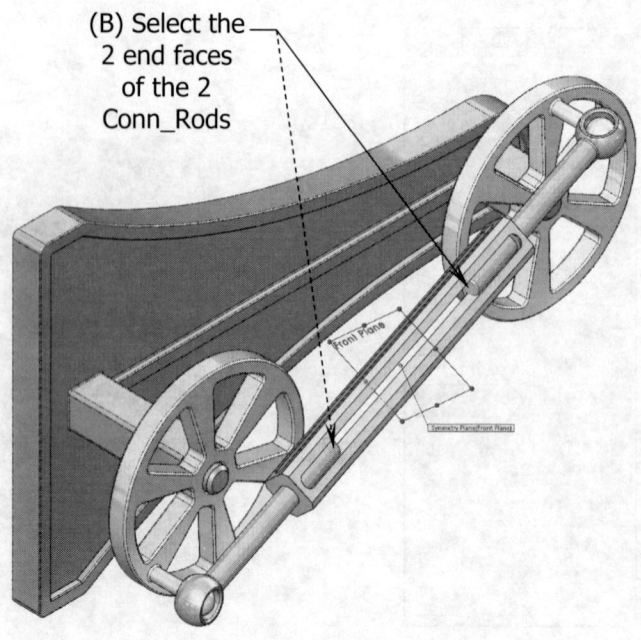

(B) Select the
2 end faces
of the 2
Conn_Rods

9. Testing the assembly motions:

- <u>Exit</u> out of the Mate mode.

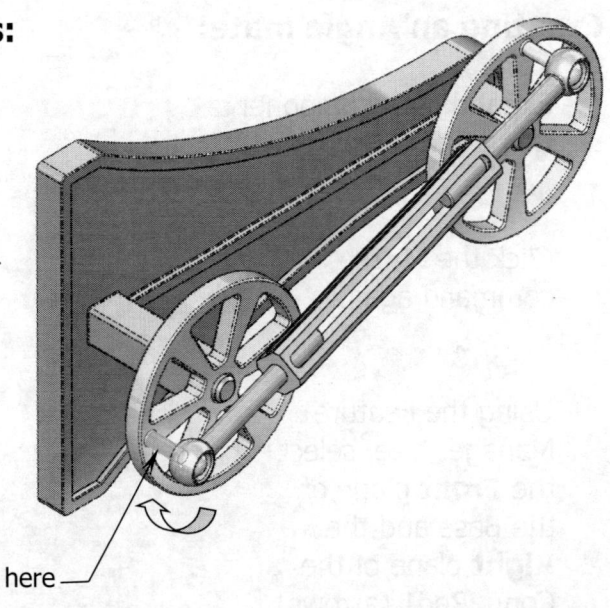

- Drag the handle on the Wheel1 as indicated.

- When the Wheel1 is turned it moves the Conn-Rod1 with it and at the same time, the Rod_Housing and the Conn_Rod2 are also moved along.

Drag here

- Without a **Limit** mate the 2 Conn-Rods will collide with each other, but since Limit mate is not part of the question, we are going to use an alternate method to test the motion of this assembly.

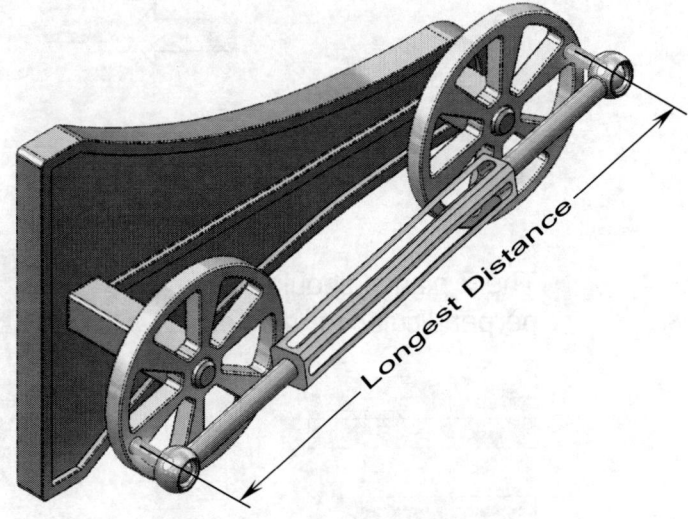

Longest Distance

- Drag the handles on both wheels to fully extend them to their longest distance (approximately as shown).

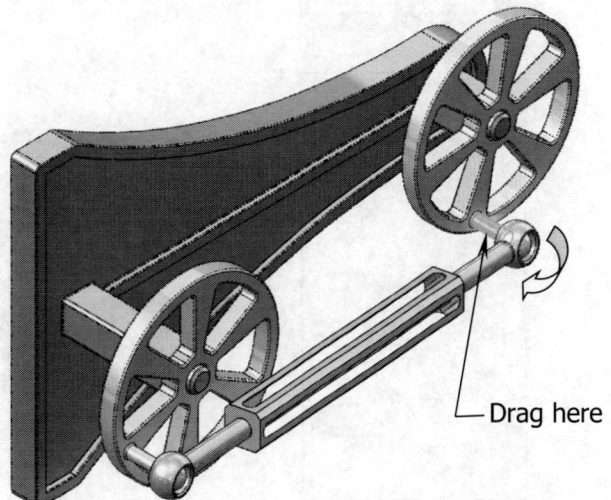

- Drag the handle on the Wheel2 in either direction. The Wheel2 should move both Con_Rods and the Rod_Housing with it but without any collisions.

Drag here

10. Creating an Angle mate:

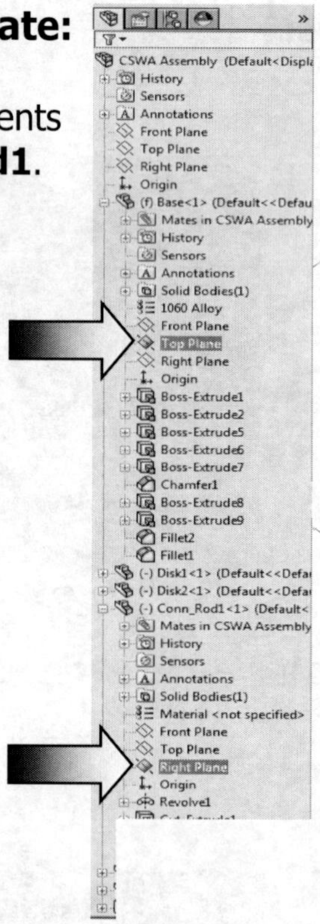

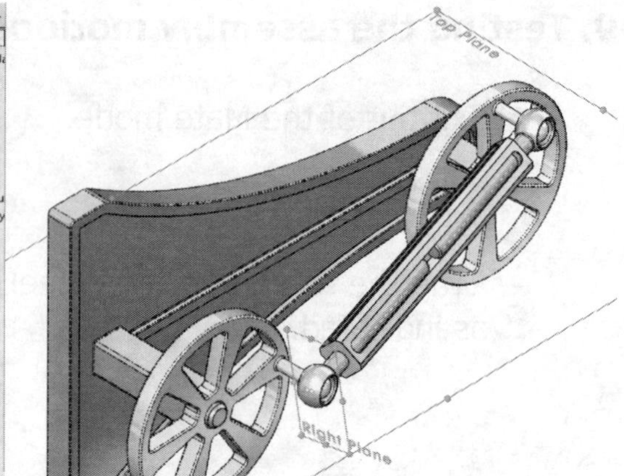

- Expand both components **Base** and **Conn_Rod1**.

- Click the **Mate** command again.

- Using the Feature Manager tree, select the **Front** plane of the Base and the **Right** plane of the Conn_Rod1 (arrows).

- Select the **Angle** button and enter **90°**. Click **OK**.

- The 2 planes should be perpendicular to each other.

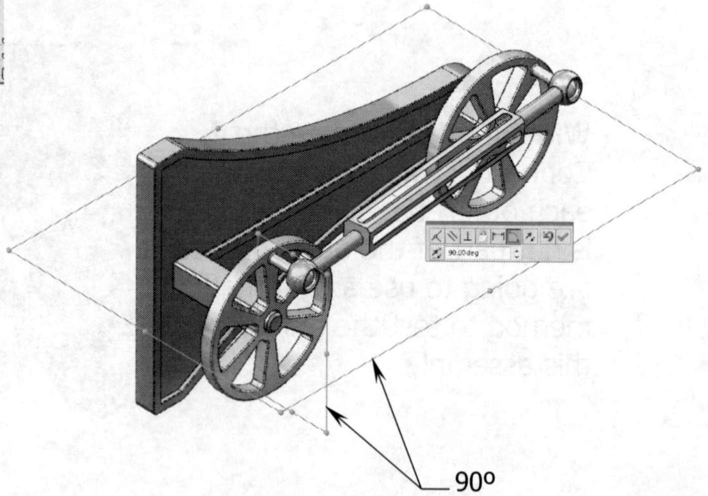

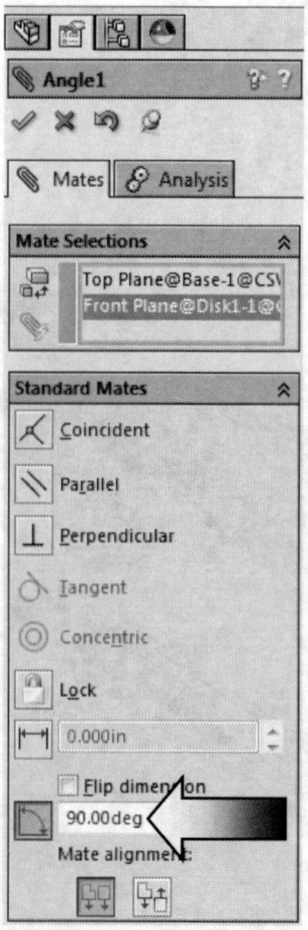

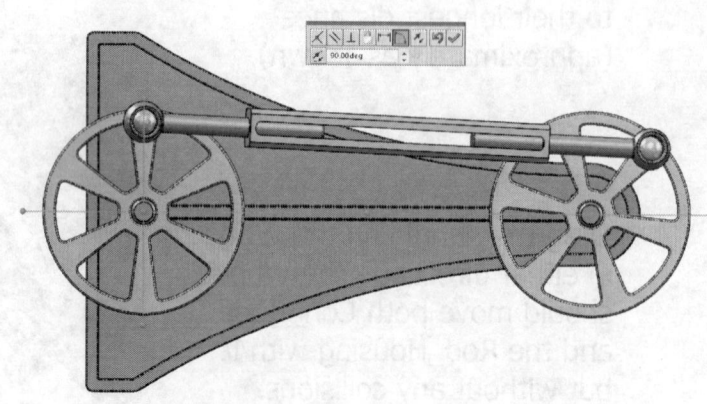

90°

Angle1

Mates | **Analysis**

Mate Selections

Top Plane@Base-1@CSV
Front Plane@Disk1-1@

Standard Mates

- Coincident
- Parallel
- Perpendicular
- Tangent
- Concentric
- Lock

0.000in

☐ Flip dimension

90.00deg

Mate alignment

11. Measuring the distance:

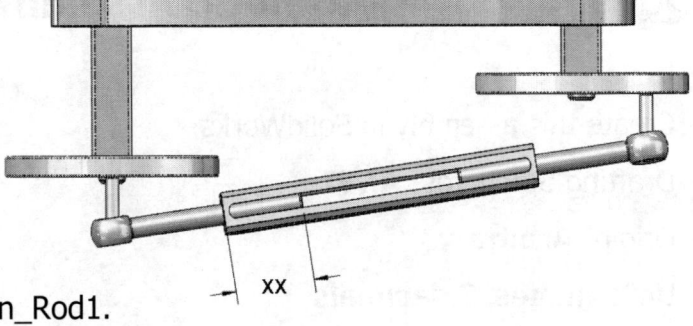

- Switch to the **Evaluate** tab.

- Select the **Measure** command and measure the distance between the **left end** of the Rod_Housing and the **end face** of the Conn_Rod1.

- Enter the distance (in inches) here: _____

12. Changing the mate Angle:

- Expand the **Mates Group** at the bottom of the Feature tree (arrow).

- <u>Edit</u> the **Angle mate** and change the angle to **180°.** Click **OK**.

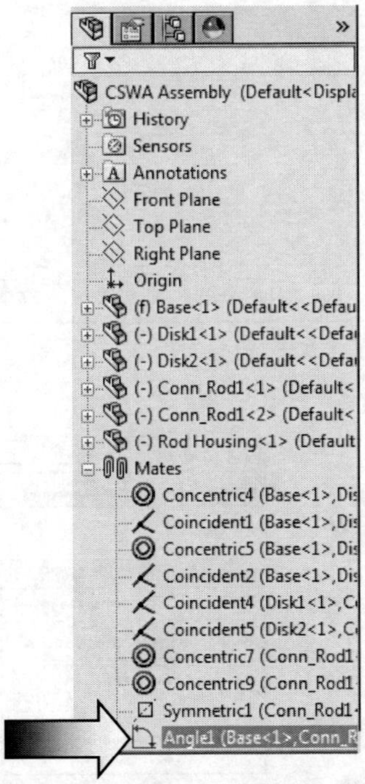

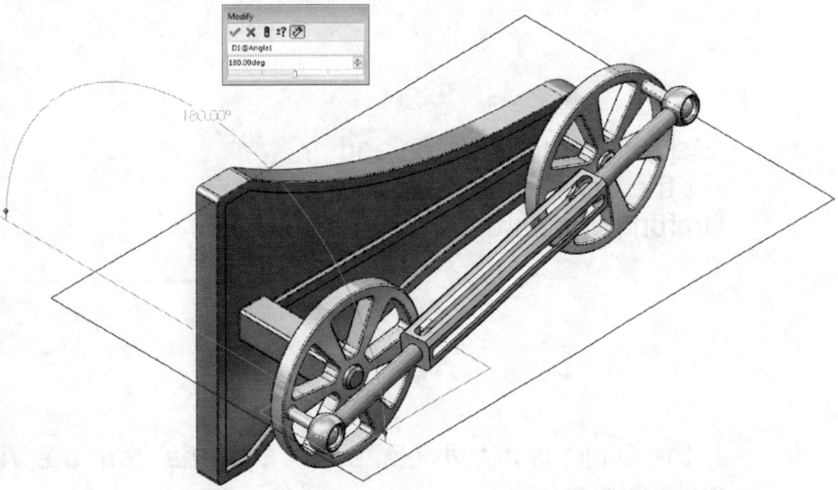

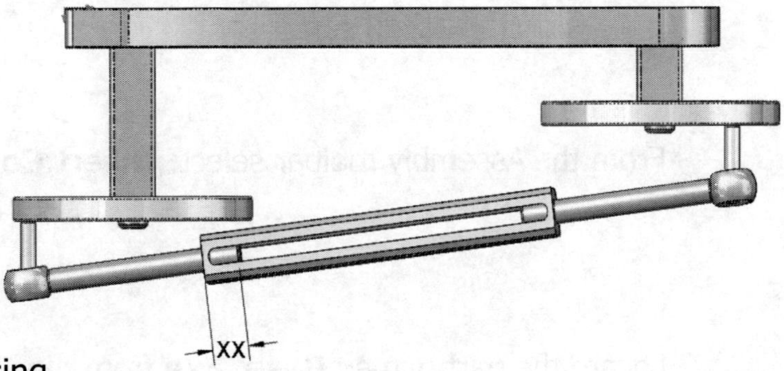

13. Measuring the distance:

- Measure the final distance between the **left end** of the Rod_ Housing and the **end face** of the Conn_Rod1.

- Enter the distance (in inches) here: _____

Question 11: Bottom Up Assembly (2 of 2)

- Create this assembly in SolidWorks.

- Drafting Standards: **ANSI**

- Origin: **Arbitrary**

- Unit: **Inches**, **3 decimals**

(This question focuses on the use of Bottom Up Assembly method, mating components, and changing the mate conditions).

1. Creating a new assembly:

- Select: **File, New, Assembly**.

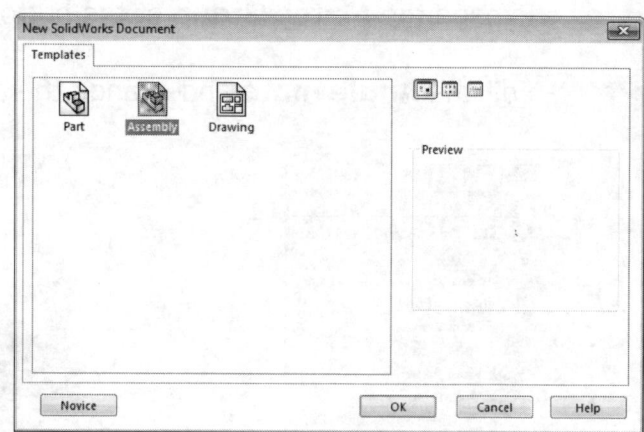

- Click the **Cancel** button and set the Units to **IPS** and the Drafting Standard to **ANSI**.

- If the Origin is not visible, select **Origins** from the View pull down menu.

- From the Assembly toolbar select: **Insert Component**.

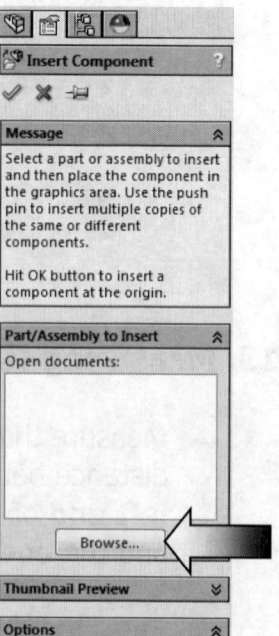

- Locate the part named **Base_Exe** from the CSWA Training Folder and open it.

- Place the 1st component on the assembly's origin.

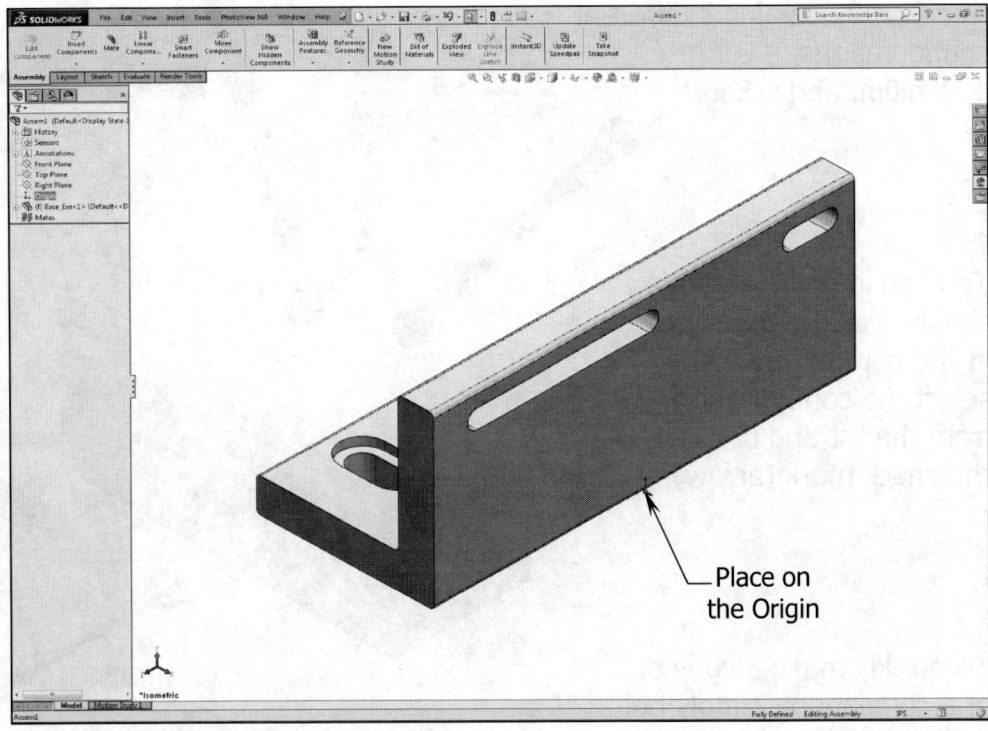

Place on the Origin

2. Inserting other components:

- Insert the rest of the components into the assembly as labeled.

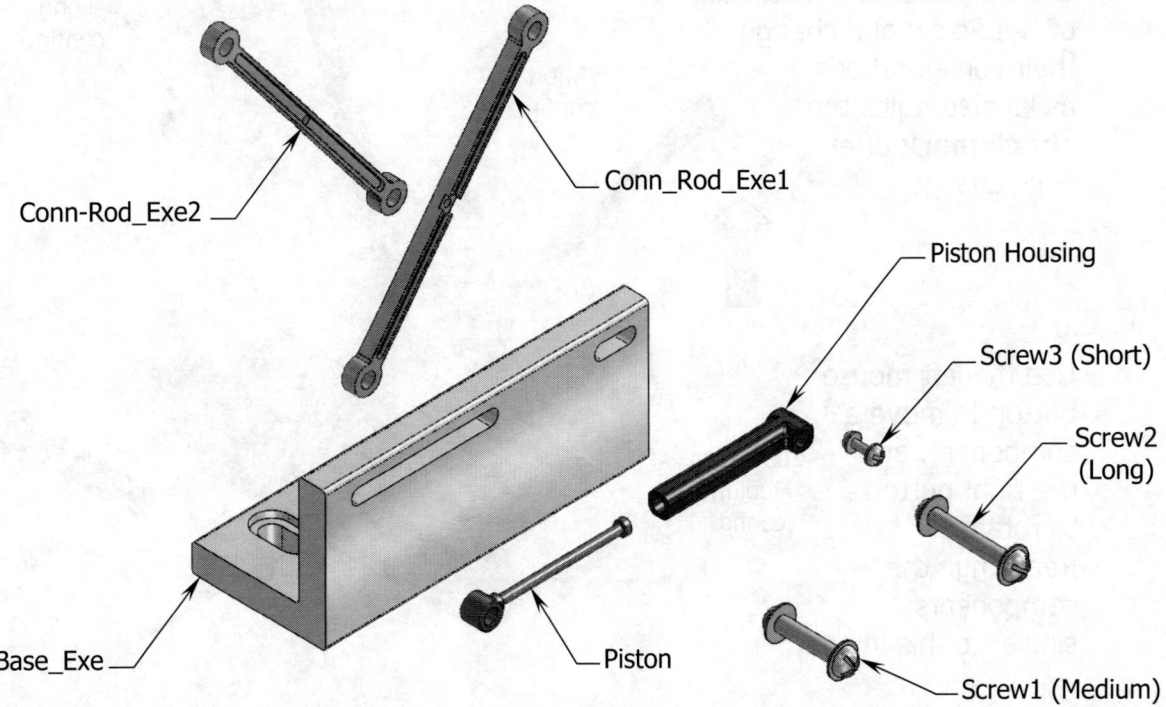

Conn-Rod_Exe2

Conn_Rod_Exe1

Piston Housing

Screw3 (Short)

Screw2 (Long)

Base_Exe

Piston

Screw1 (Medium)

3. Changing configurations:

- The Screw contains 3 different configurations, a Long, a Medium, and a Short.

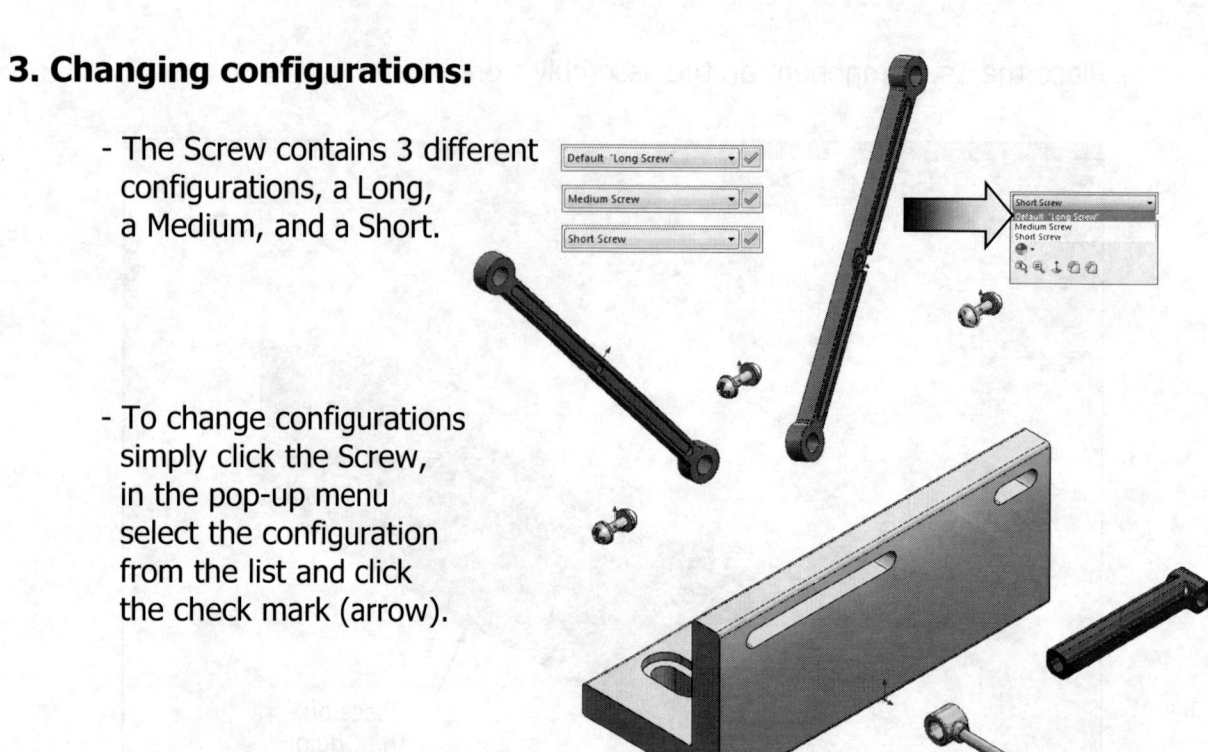

- To change configurations simply click the Screw, in the pop-up menu select the configuration from the list and click the check mark (arrow).

- To quickly make a copy of of a component, simply hold the Control key and drag it a side.

- Create a total of 3 instances of the Screw and change their configurations as labeled. Click the **check mark** after each change

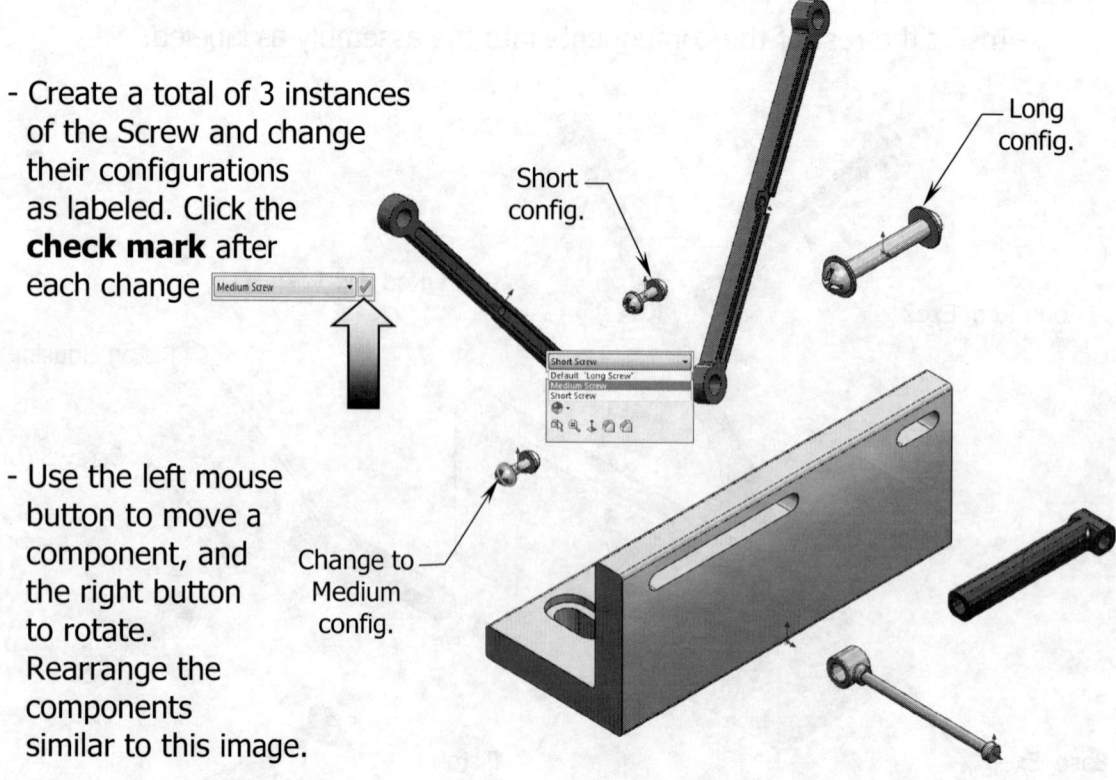

- Use the left mouse button to move a component, and the right button to rotate. Rearrange the components similar to this image.

4. Mating the Piston Housing:

- Click the **Mate** command again to reactivate it.

- Select the **face of the slot** of the Base_Exe and the **hole** in the Piston Housing.

- A **Concentric** mate is selected automatically for the selection.

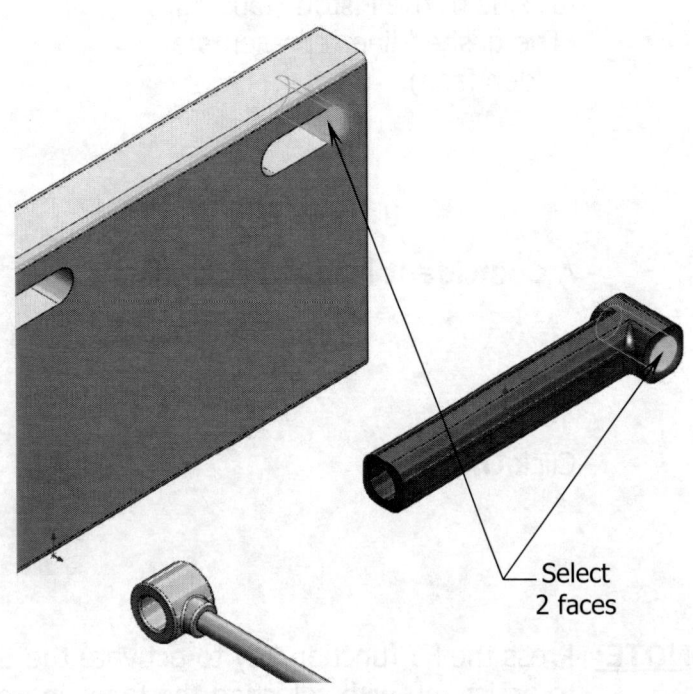

Select 2 faces

- Click **OK** to accept the mate.

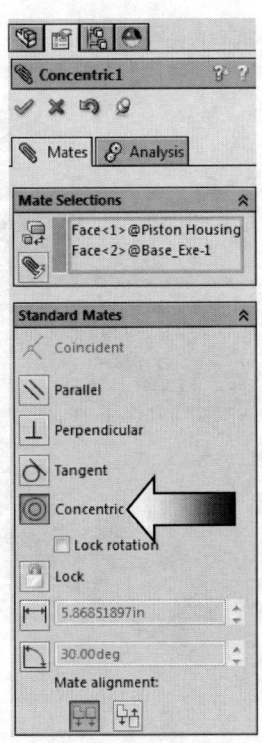

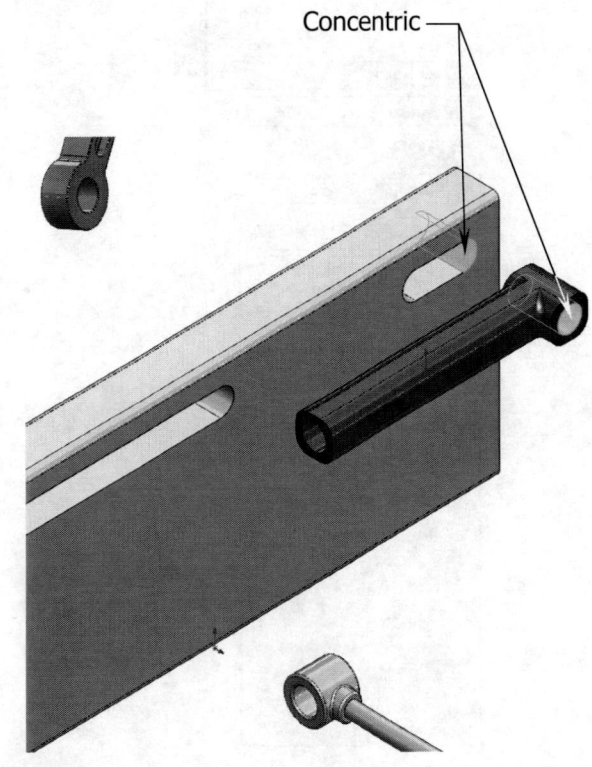

Concentric

- Select the **planar face** in the back of the Base_Exe and the **planar face** on the far side of the Piston Housing. (The dashed line represents a hidden face).

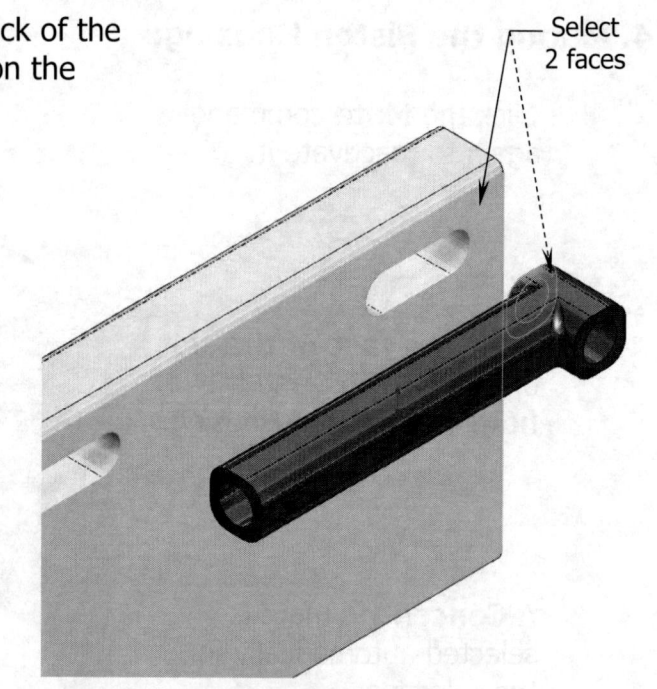

Select 2 faces

- A **Coincident** mate is selected.

- Click **OK**.

NOTE: Press the F5 function key to activate the Selection-Filters and use the Filter-Faces to assist you with selecting the faces more precisely and easily.

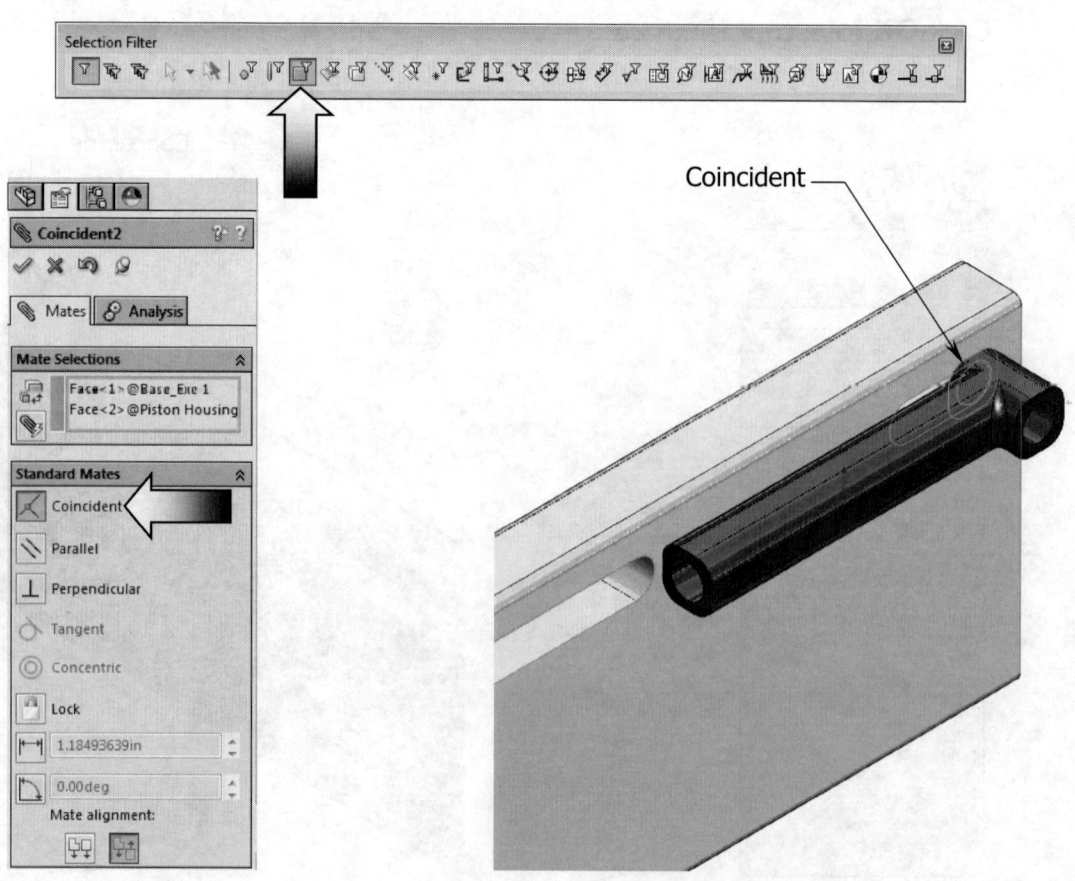

Coincident

5. Mating the Conn-Rod_Exe1:

- Move the Conn-Rod_Exe1 closer to the Base_Exe as pictured, it will be mated to the Piston Housing.

- Click the **Mate** command if it is no longer active.

- Select the **hole** in the Conn-Rod_Exe1 and the **hole** in the Piston Housing.

- A **Concentric** mate is selected.

- Click **OK**.

Select 2 faces

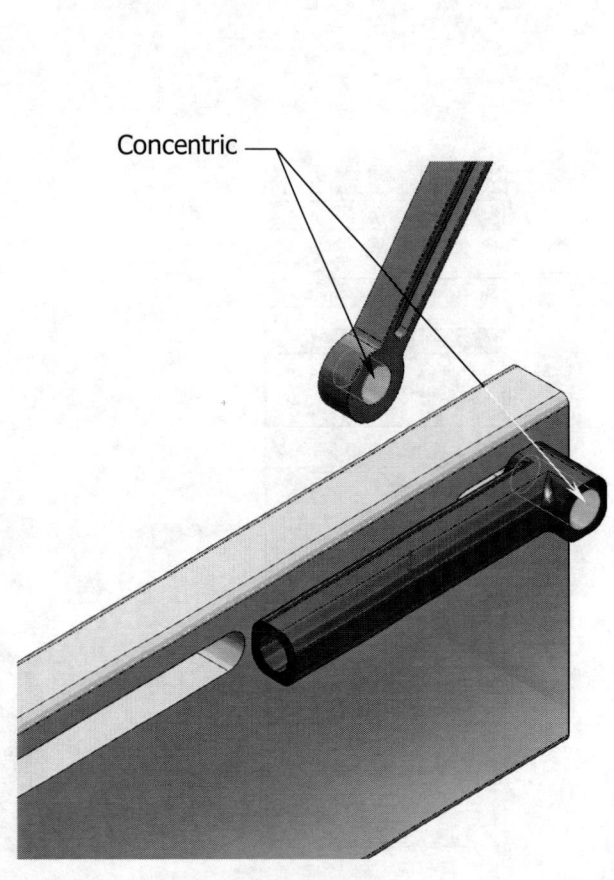

Concentric

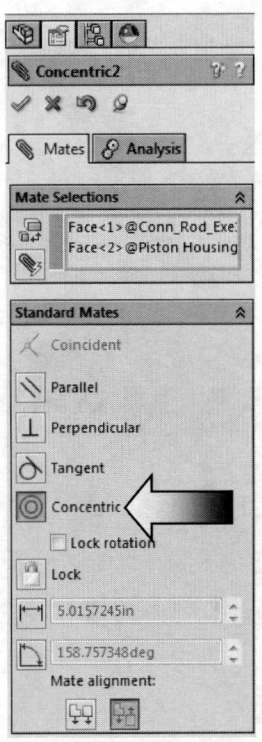

- Select the **planar face** in the front of the Conn-Rod_exe1 and the **planar face** on the far side of the Piston Housing.

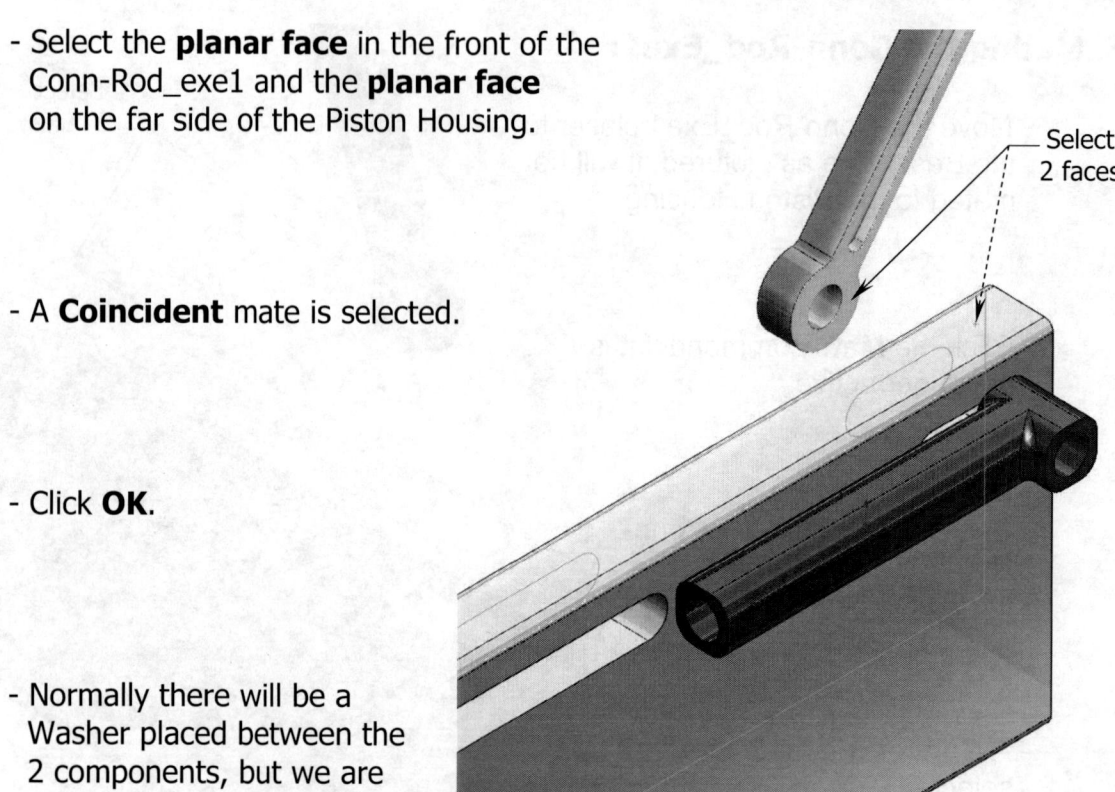

Select 2 faces

- A **Coincident** mate is selected.

- Click **OK**.

- Normally there will be a Washer placed between the 2 components, but we are going to omit it because this assembly does not need one.

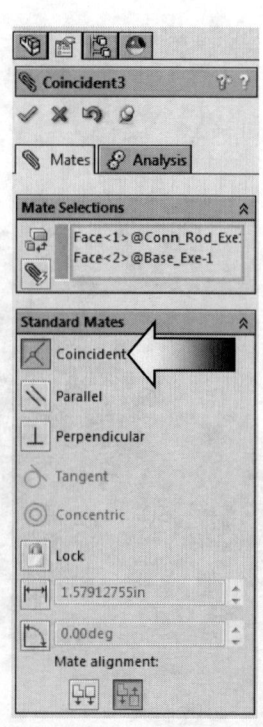

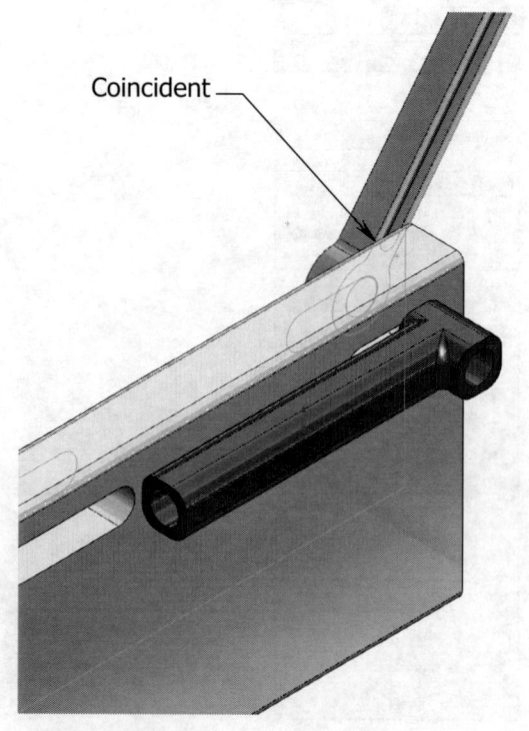

Coincident

6. Mating the Long Screw:

- Move the Long screw closer as pictured, it will be mated to the Conn-Rod_Exe1.

- Ensure that the mate command is still active.

- Select the **cylindrical face** of the Long Screw and the **hole** in the Piston Housing.

- A **Concentric** mate is selected automatically.

- Click **OK**.

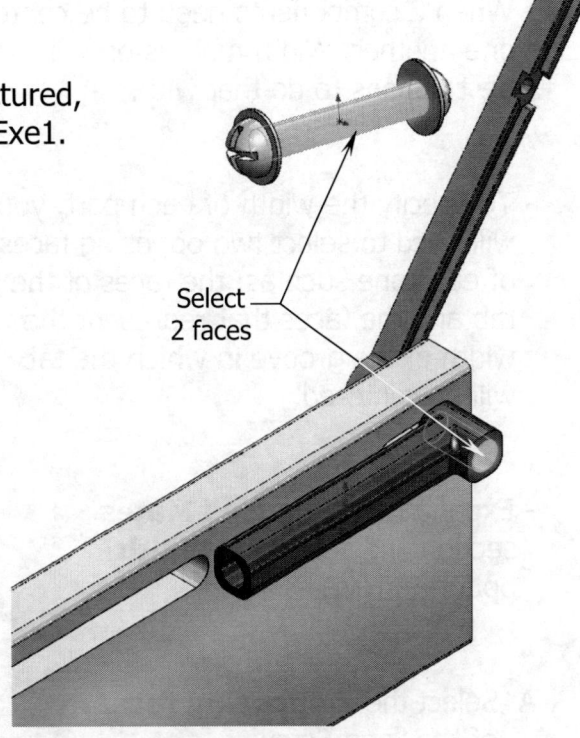

Select 2 faces

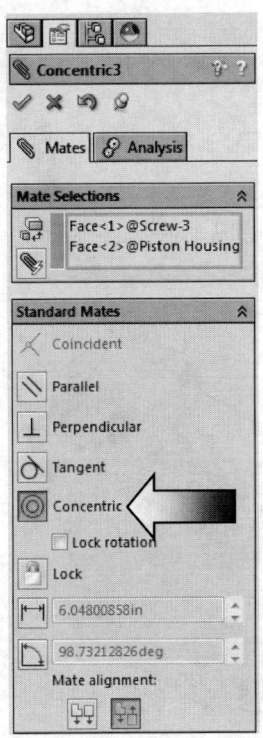

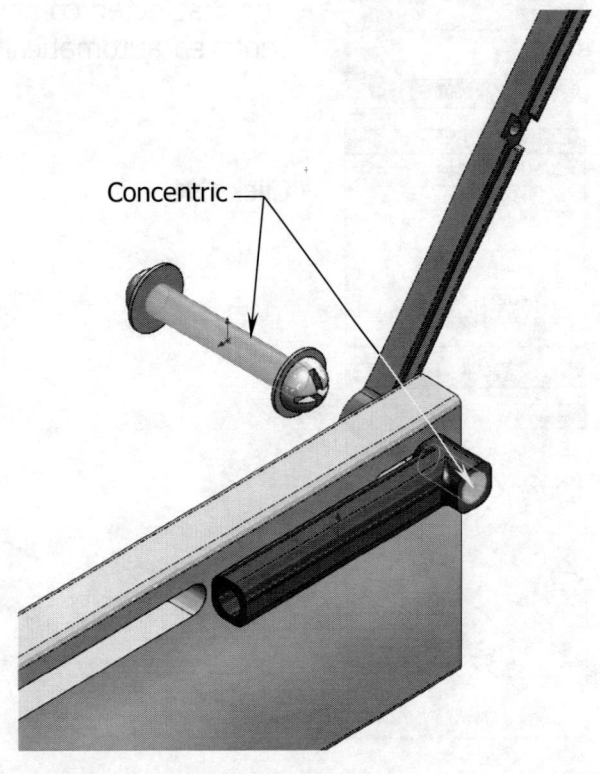

Concentric

- When 2 components need to be centered with one another, Width mate is one of the best options to do that with.

A. Select 2 opposing faces for Width

- To specify the width of each part, you will need to select two opposing faces of each one such as: the faces of the tab and the faces that represent the width of the groove in which the tab will be centered.

B. Select 2 opposing faces for Tab

- Expand the **Advanced Mates** section and select the **Width** option (arrow).

A. Select the **2 opposing faces** of the Long Screw.

B. Select the **2 opposing faces** of the Piston Housing and the Conn-Rod_exe1.

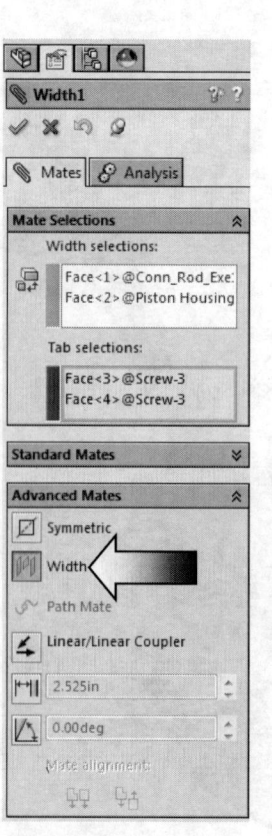

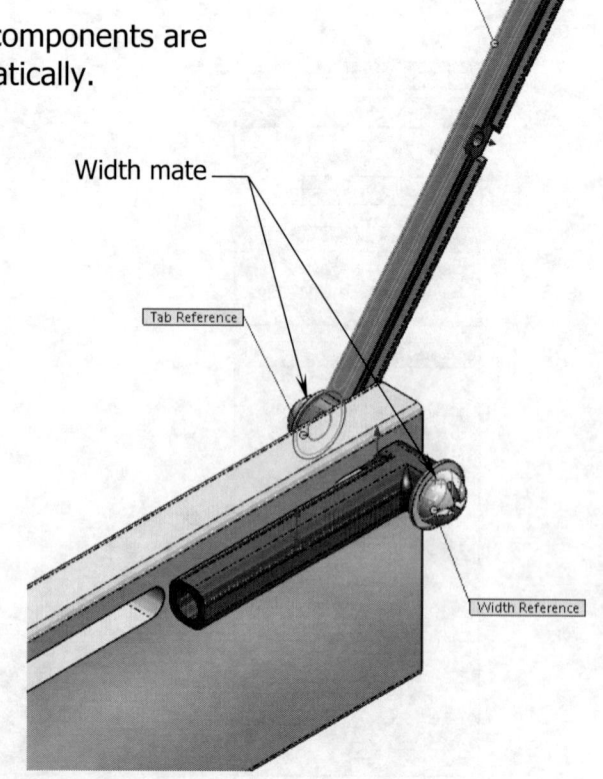

- The 2 selected components are centered automatically.

- Click **OK**.

Width Reference

Width mate

Tab Reference

Width Reference

7. Mating the Piston to its Housing:

- Move the Piston closer to the Piston Housing as pictured.

- Select the **cylindrical face** of the Piston and the **hole** in the Piston Housing as indicated.

- A **Concentric** mate is selected but the alignment is incorrect.

Select 2 faces

- Locate the **Align/Anti Align** buttons (arrow) at the bottom of the Standard Mates section.

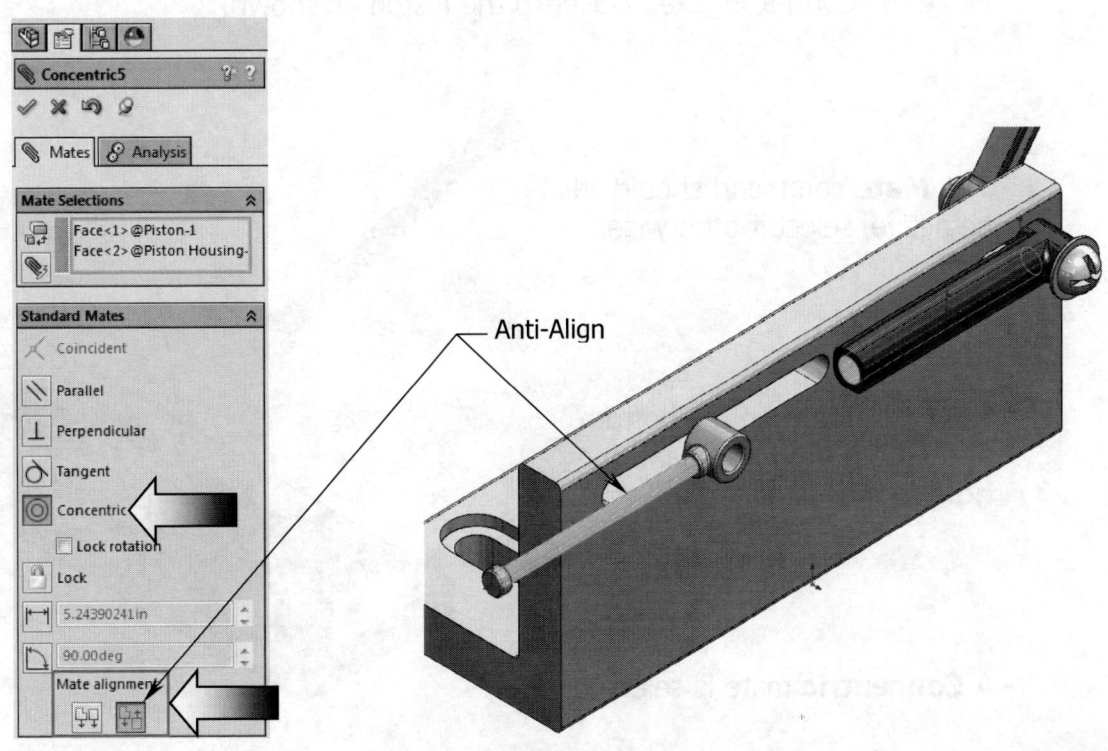

Anti-Align

- Toggle the **Align/Anti Align** buttons (arrow) to flip the Piston to the correct orientation.

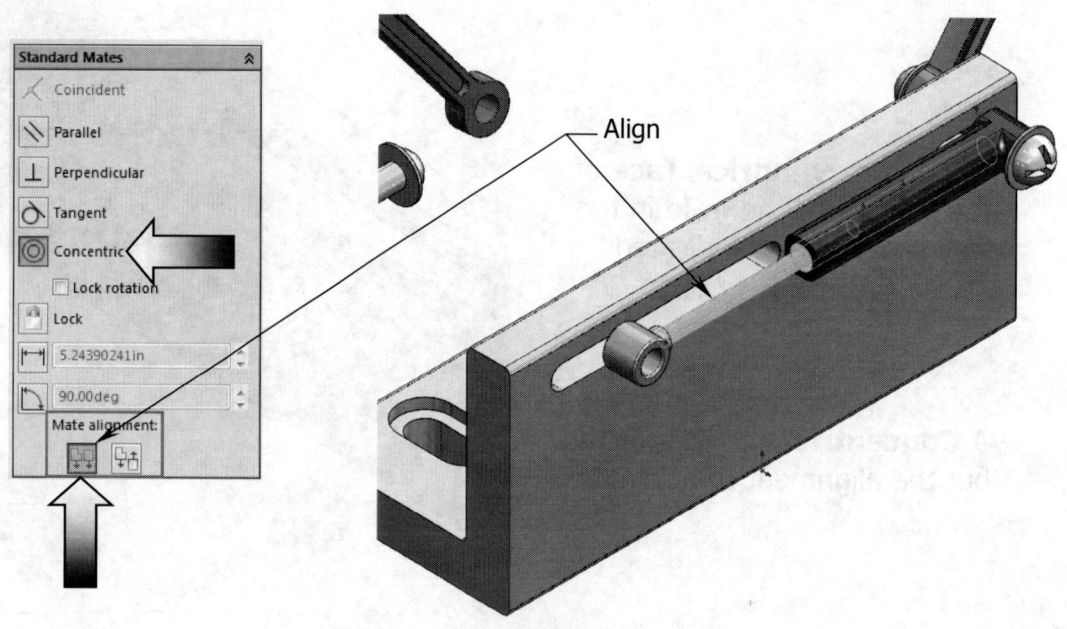

8. Mating the Conn_Rod_Exe2 to the Piston:

- Move the Conn-Rod_Exe2 closer to the Piston as shown.

- The **Mate** command should still be active, select it otherwise.

- Select the **hole** on the bottom of the Conn-Rod_exe2 and the **hole** in the Piston.

- A **Concentric** mate is selected.

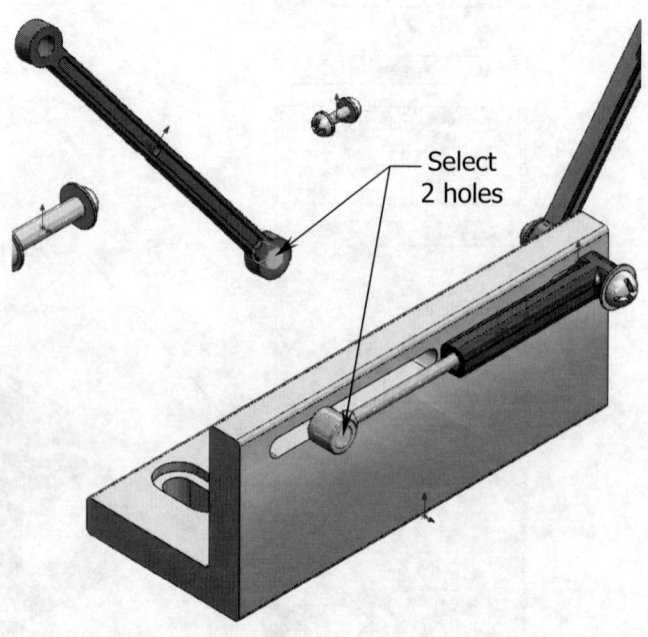

- Click **OK** to accept the concentric mate.

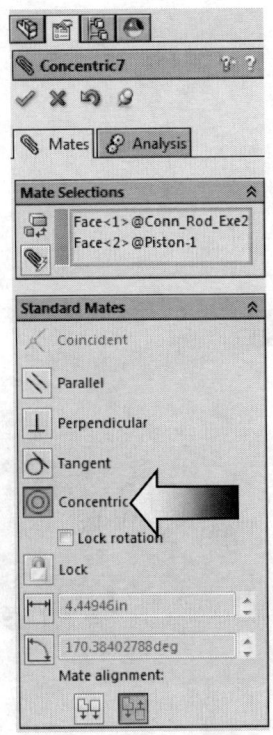

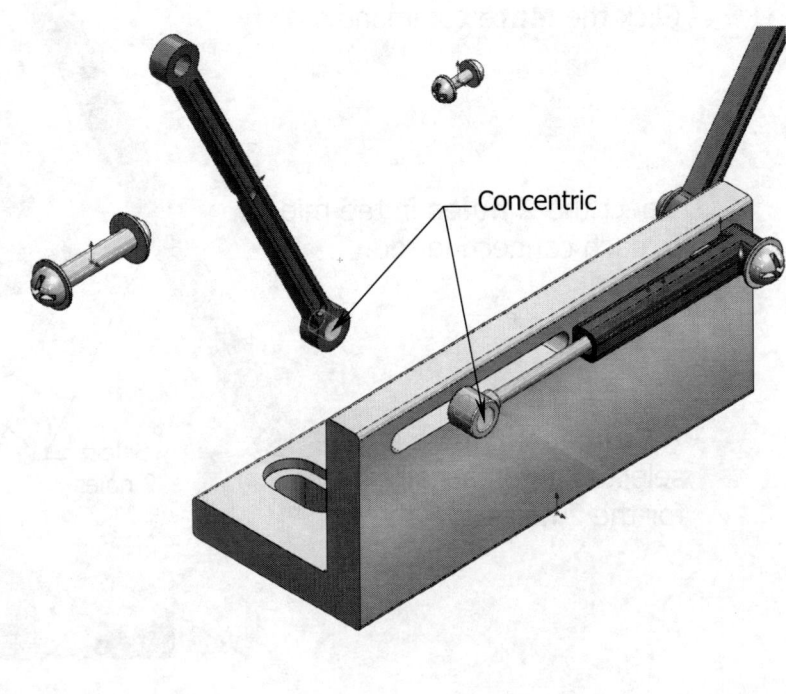

Concentric

9. Rearranging the components:

- Drag the top of the Conn_Rod_Exe2 to the right, and drag the top of the Conn_Rod_Exe1 to the left.

- From the right view orientation the 2 Conn-Rods should look similar to the one pictured below.

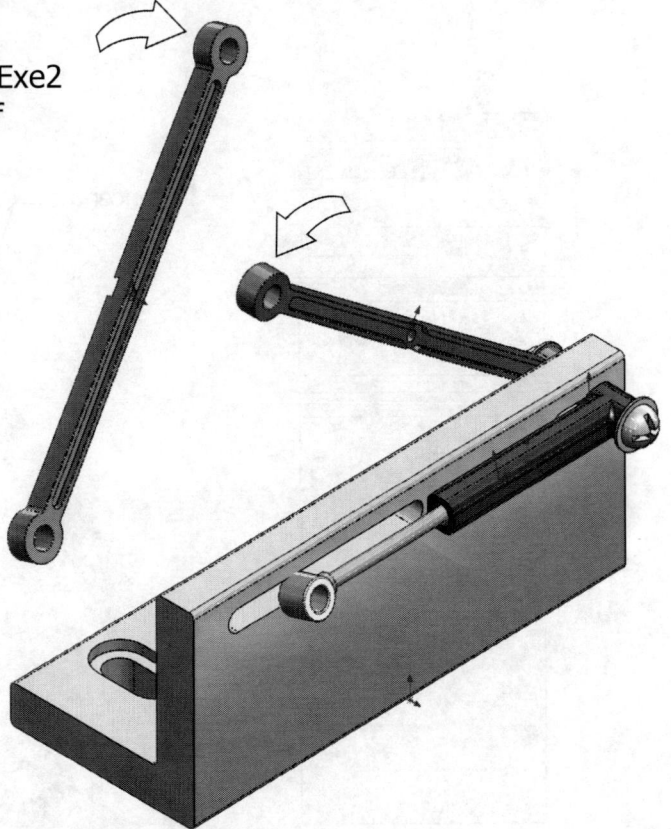

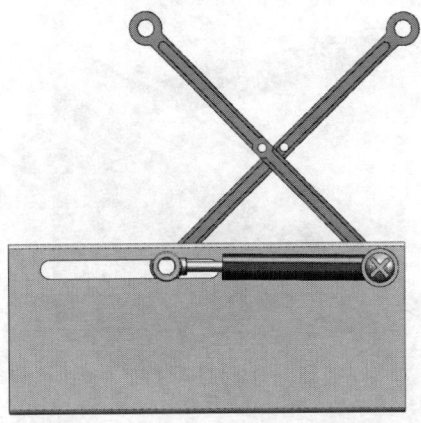

10. Mating the two Connecting Rods:

- Click the **Mate** command.

- Select the **2 holes** in the middle of each connecting rod.

- A **Concentric** mate is selected automatically for the 2 holes.

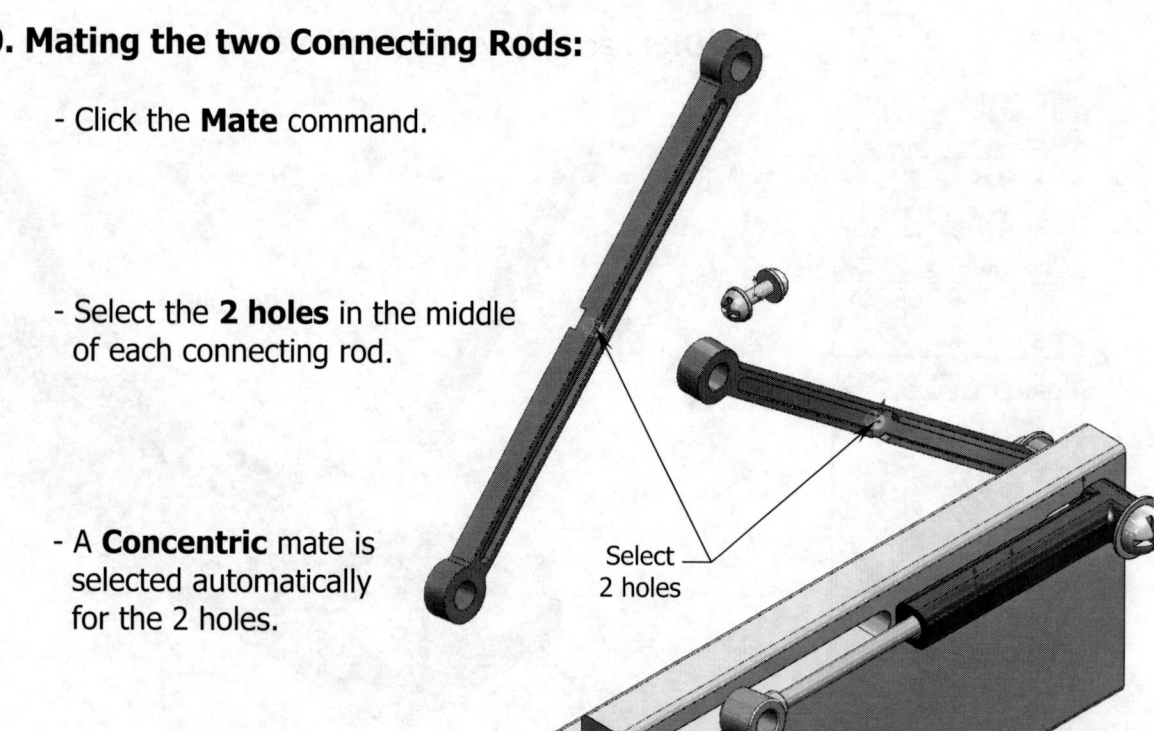

Select
2 holes

- Click **OK**.

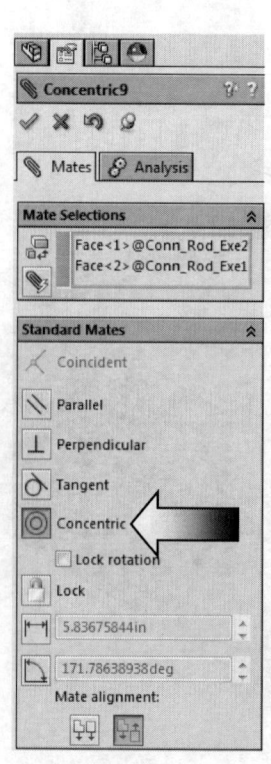

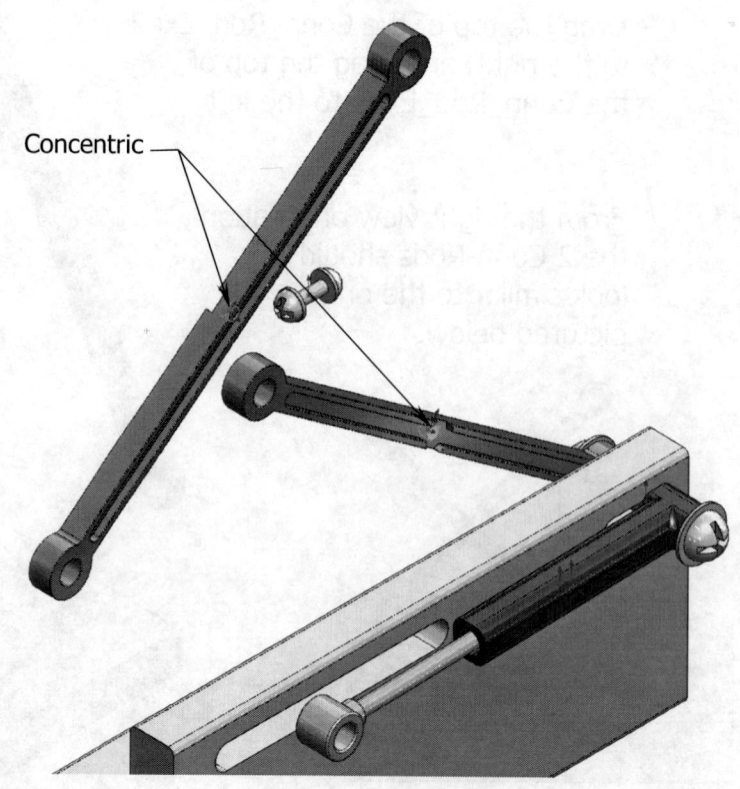

Concentric

- For the coincident mate, select **the face in the front** of the Conn_Rod_Exe2 and **the face on the far side** of the Conn_Rod_Exe1.

- The dashed line represents the hidden face on the rear of the component.

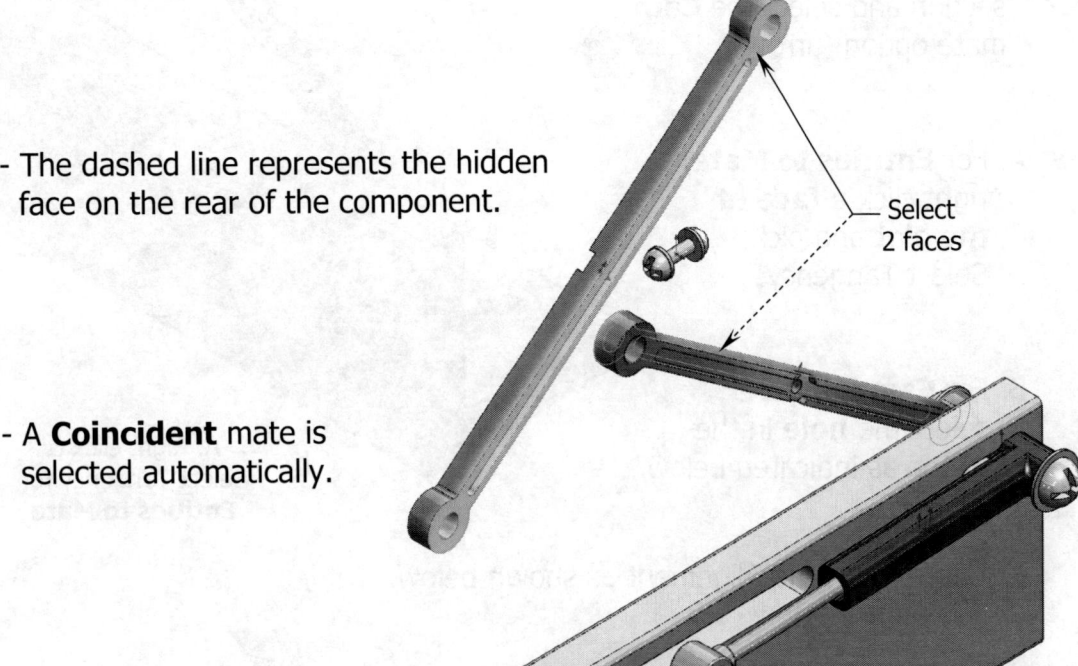

Select 2 faces

- A **Coincident** mate is selected automatically.

- Click **OK**.

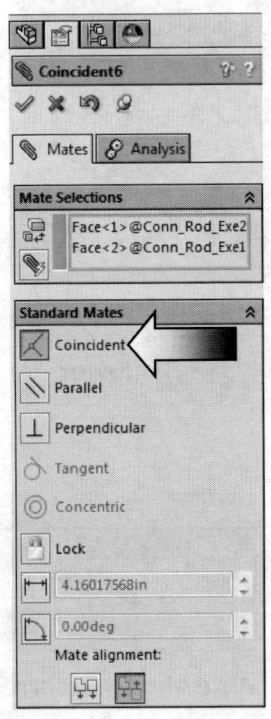

- The front face of the Conn_Rod2 moves forward and touches the back face of the Conn-Rod1.

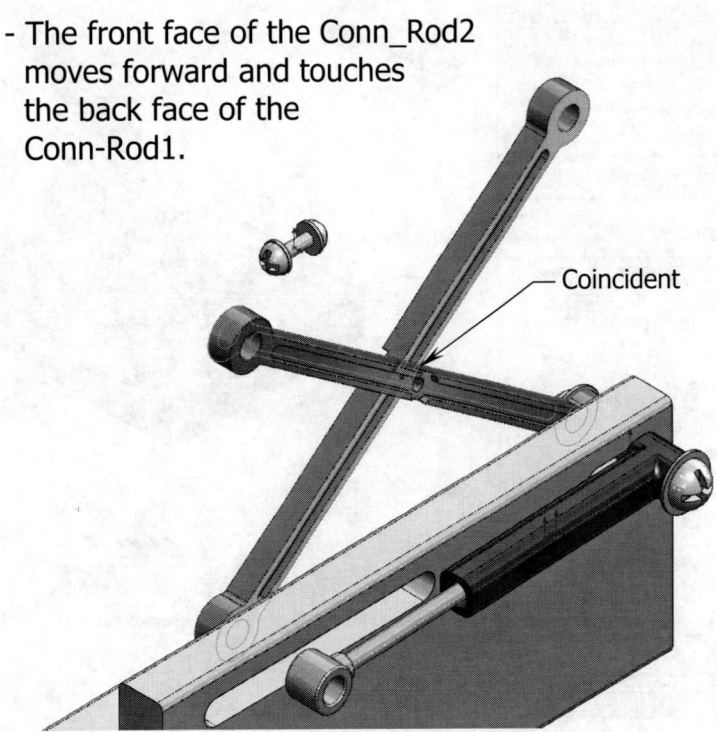

Coincident

11. Adding a Cam mate: (Note: The Slot mate option is only available in SW-2014 or newer).

- Expand the **Mechanical Mates** section and select the **Cam** mate option (arrow).

A. For **Entities to Mate**, right click **a face of the slot** and pick: Select Tangency.

B. For **Cam Follower**, select the **hole** in the Piston as indicated below.

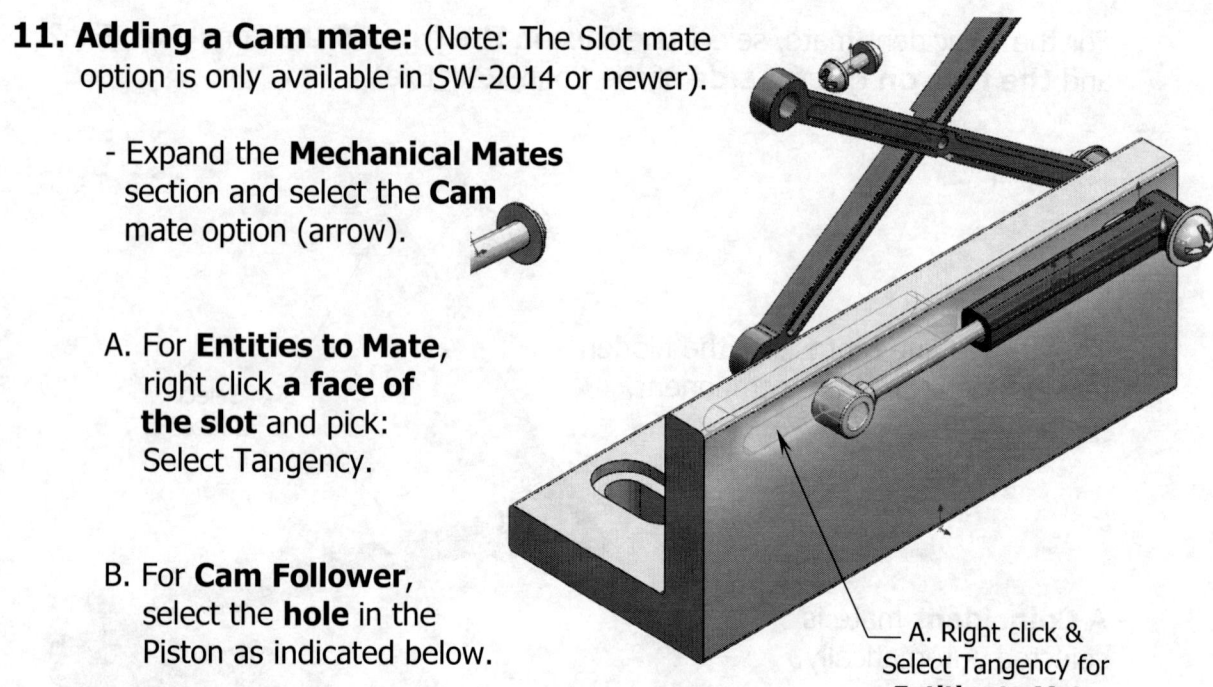

A. Right click & Select Tangency for **Entities to Mate**

- Double check the Alignment as shown below.

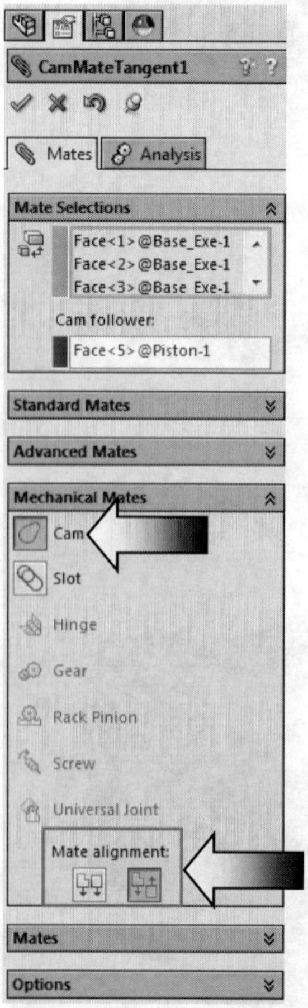

Mate Selections
Face<1>@Base_Exe-1
Face<2>@Base_Exe-1
Face<3>@Base_Exe-1

Cam follower:
Face<5>@Piston-1

Standard Mates
Advanced Mates
Mechanical Mates
- Cam
- Slot
- Hinge
- Gear
- Rack Pinion
- Screw
- Universal Joint

Mate alignment:

Mates
Options

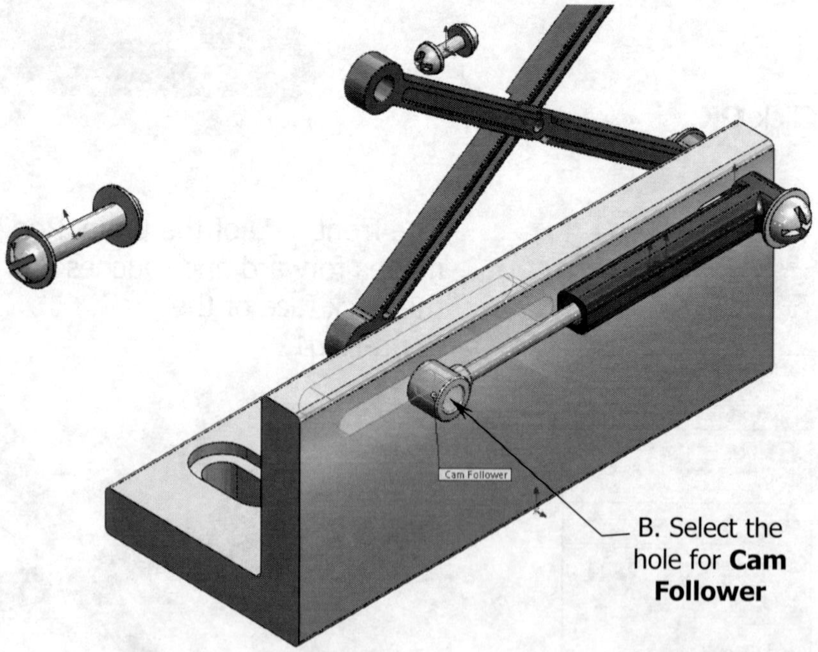

B. Select the hole for **Cam Follower**

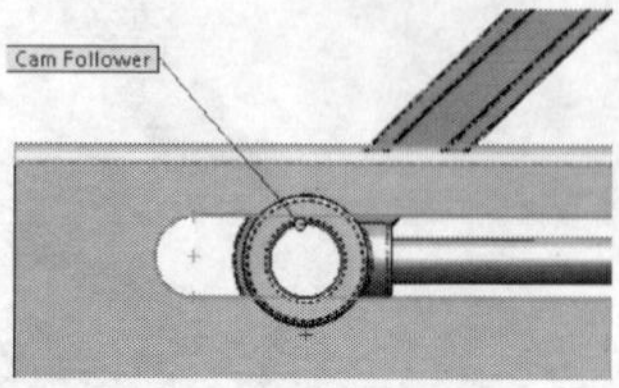

Align - Correct

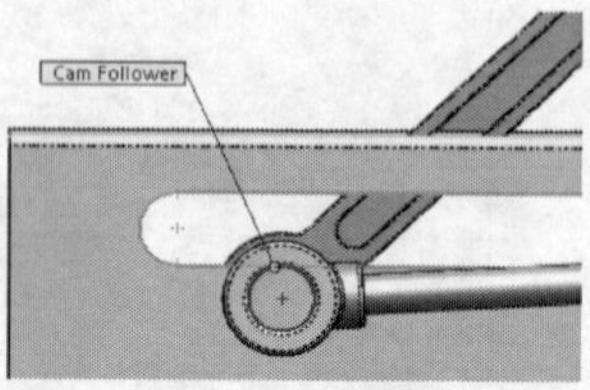

Anti-Align - Incorrect

12. Mating the Medium Screw:

- The **Mate** command should still be active.

- Select the **body** of the Medium Screw and the **hole** in the Piston as indicated.

- A **Concentric** mate is selected.

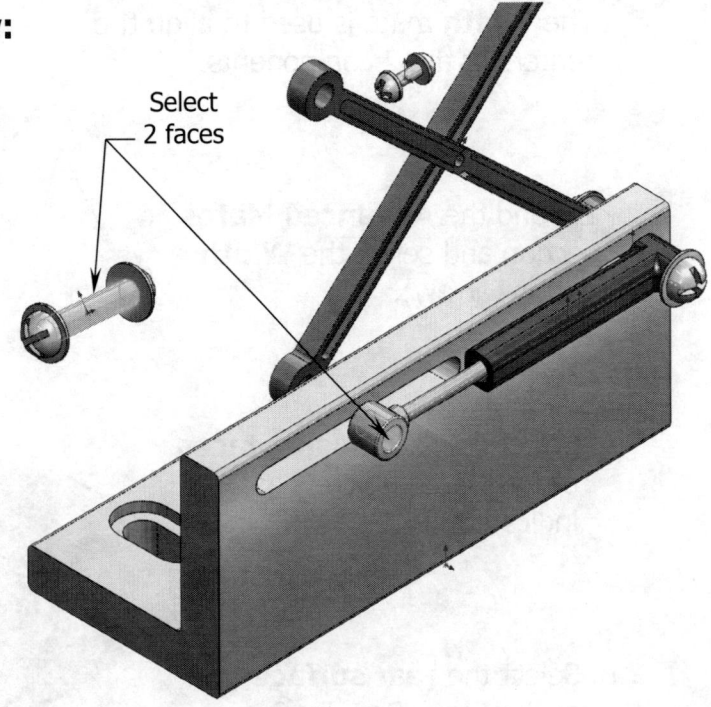

Select 2 faces

- Click **OK**.

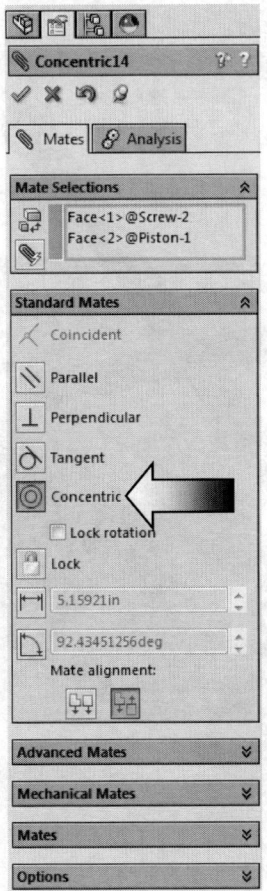

- The cylindrical body of the Medium Screw is rotated and constrained to the center axis of the hole.

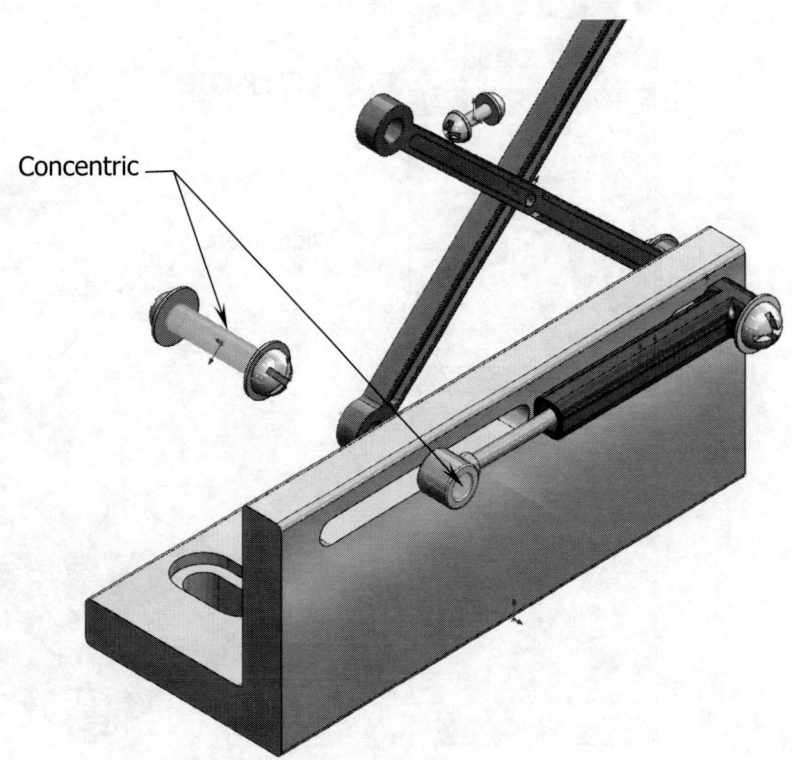

Concentric

- The **Width** mate is used to align the centers of the 2 components.

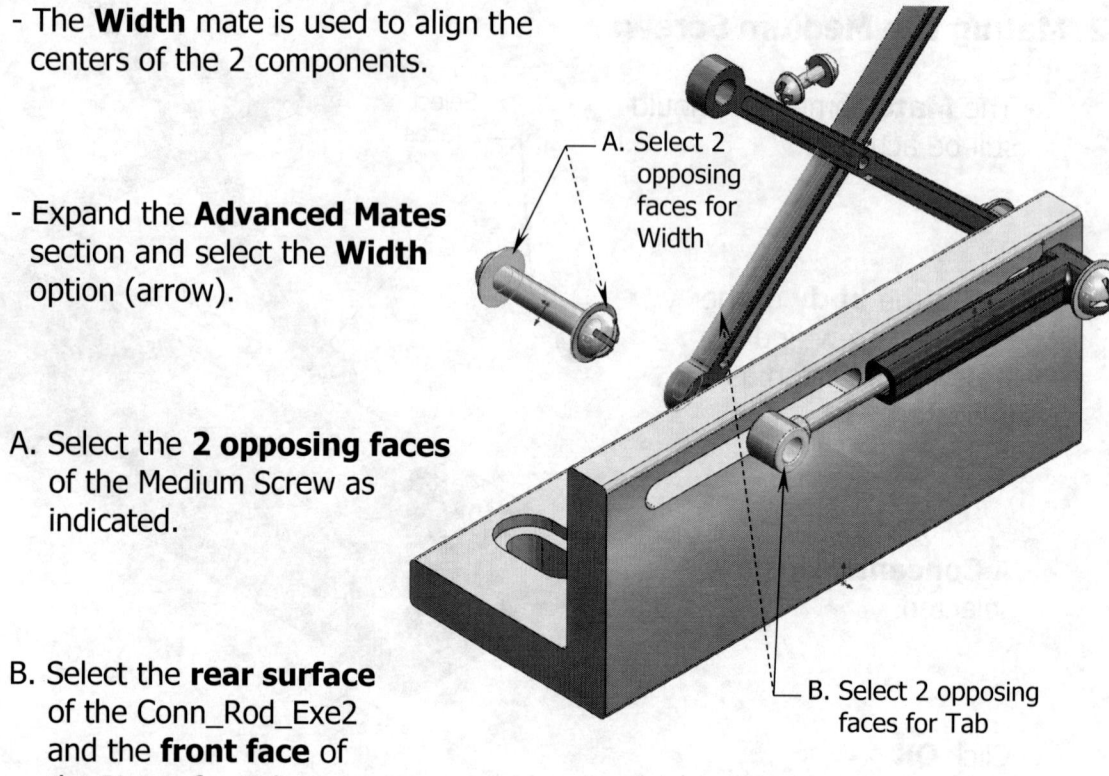

A. Select 2 opposing faces for Width

- Expand the **Advanced Mates** section and select the **Width** option (arrow).

A. Select the **2 opposing faces** of the Medium Screw as indicated.

B. Select the **rear surface** of the Conn_Rod_Exe2 and the **front face** of the Piston for Tab.

B. Select 2 opposing faces for Tab

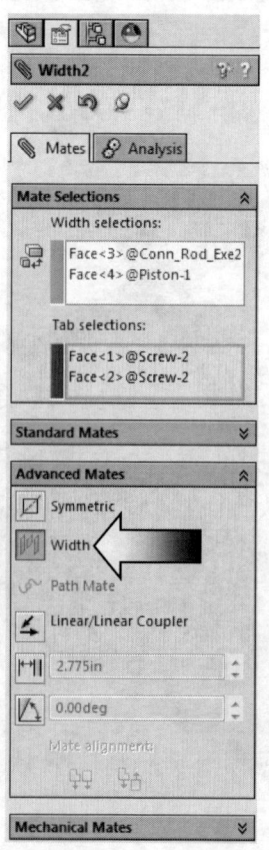

- The 2 selected components are centered automatically.

- Click **OK**.

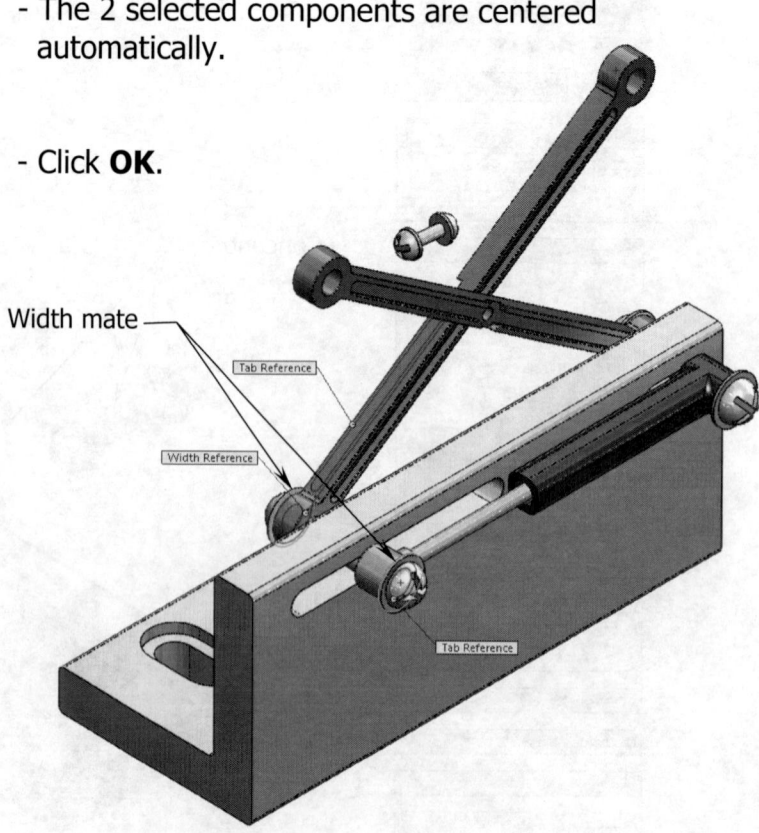

Width mate

13. Mating the Small Screw:

- Click the **Mate** command if it is no longer active.

- Select the **cylindrical face** of the Small Screw and the **hole** in the Conn-Rod_Exe1.

- A **Concentric** mate is selected.

- Click **OK** to accept the mate.

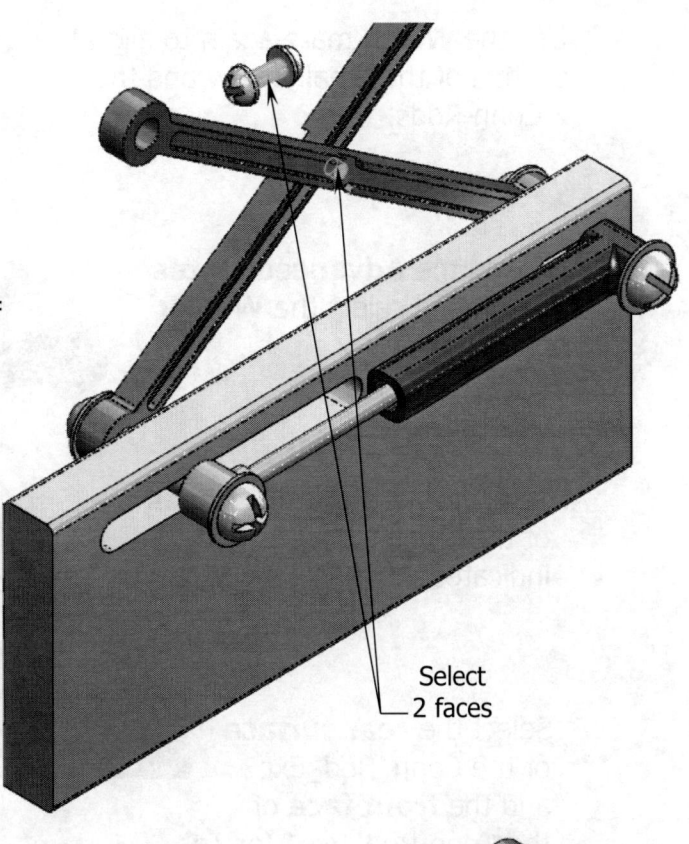

Select
2 faces

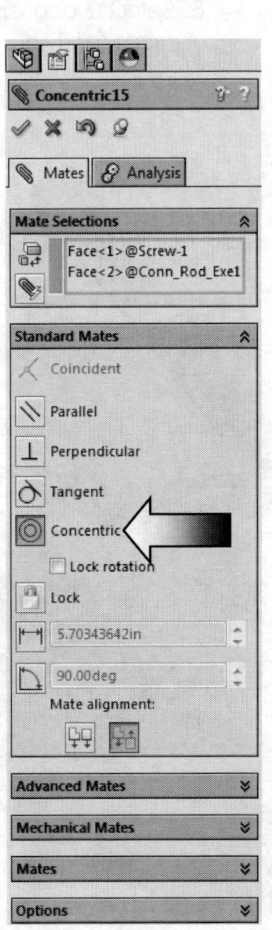

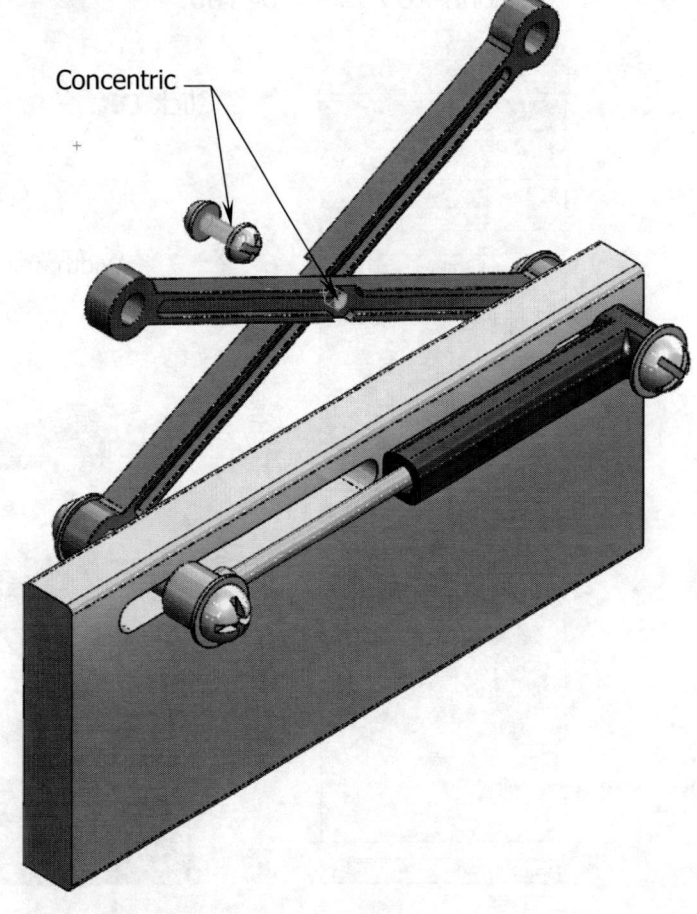

Concentric

- Use the **Width** mate again to align the centers of the Small Screw and the 2 Conn-Rods.

- Expand the **Advanced Mates** section and select the **Width** option (arrow).

A. Select the **2 opposing faces** of the Small Screw as indicated.

B. Select the **rear surface** of the Conn_Rod_Exe2 and the **front face** of the Conn-Rod_Exe1 for Tab.

- Click **OK**.

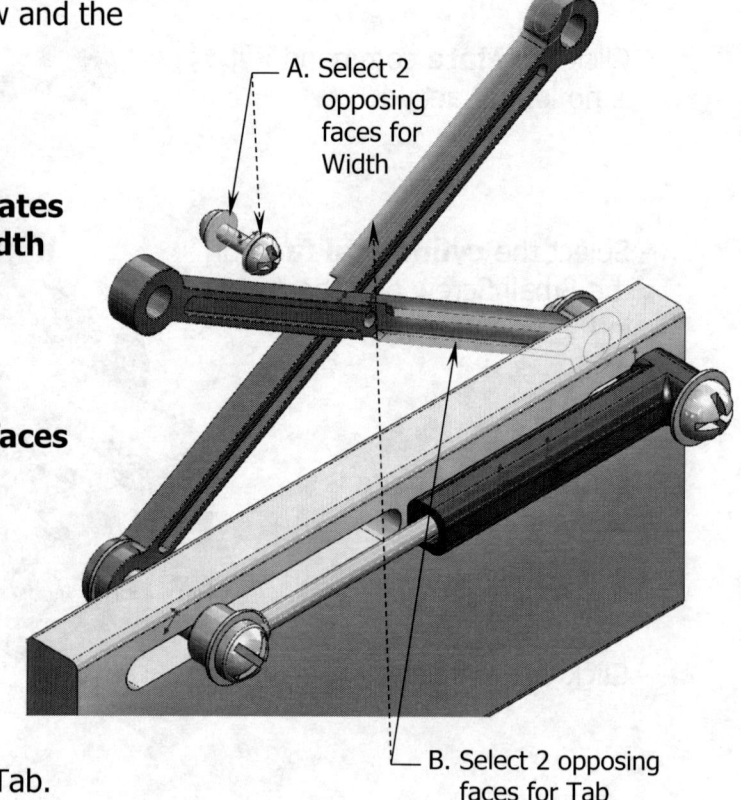

A. Select 2 opposing faces for Width

B. Select 2 opposing faces for Tab

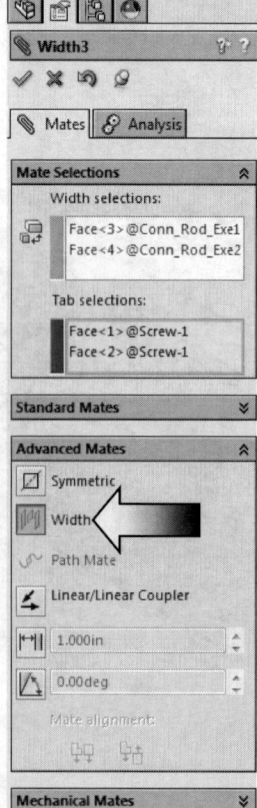

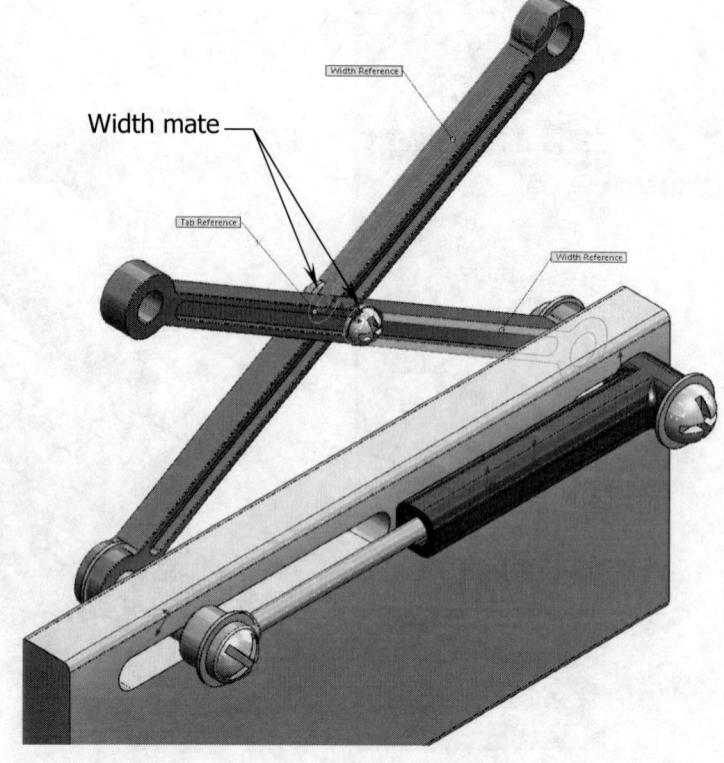

Width mate

14. Mating an Angle Mate:

- After all components have been assembled, a reference location needs to be established so that the center of mass can be measured from it.

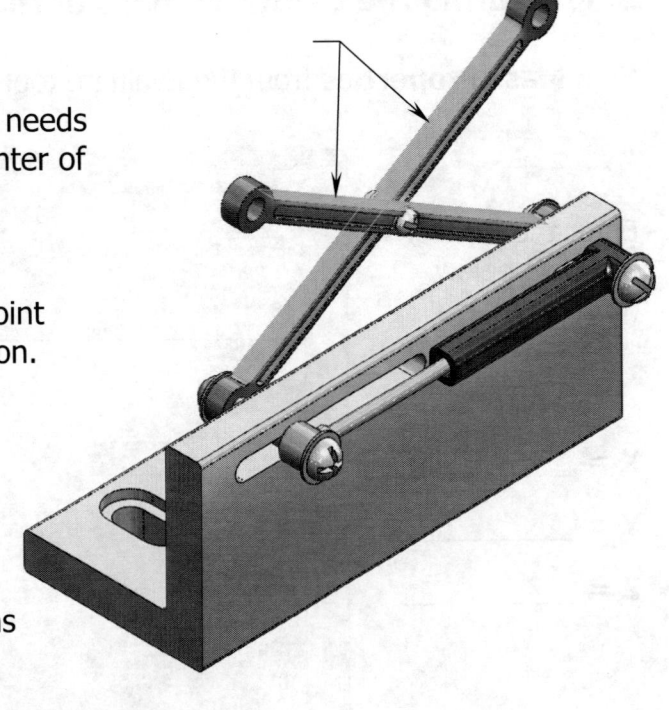

- An Angle mate is used at this point to establish the reference location.

- Click the **Mate** command if it is not active.

- Select the **2 faces** of the 2 arms as indicated.

- Click the **Angle** button (arrow) and enter **60°**.

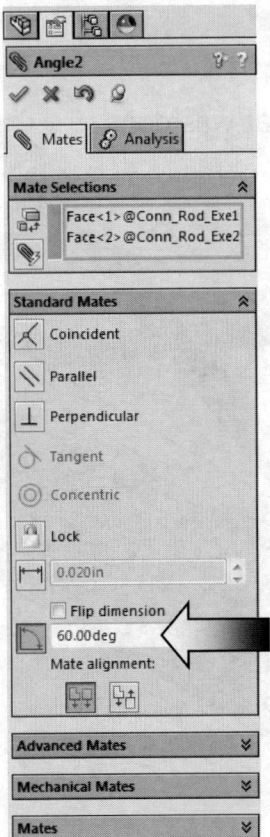

- The 2 arms move to the position similar to the image below. Click **OK**.

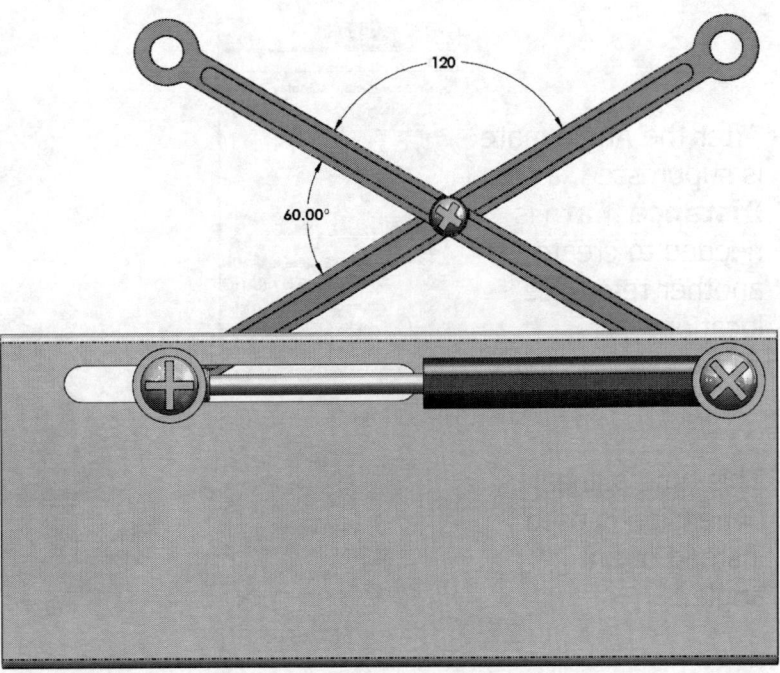

15. Measuring the Center of Mass of the assembly:

- Click **Mass Properties** from the Evaluate tool tab.

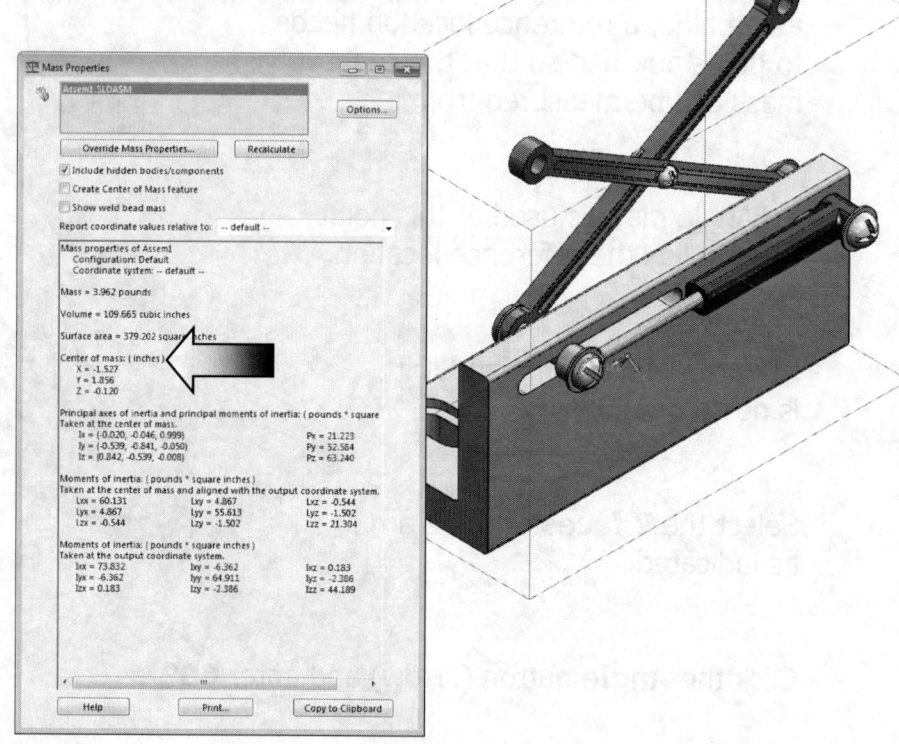

- Enter the **Center of Mass** below (in Inches)

X = _____

Y = _____

Z = _____

16. Suppressing a mate:

- Expand the **Mates Group** and suppress the Angle mate that was done in step number 14.

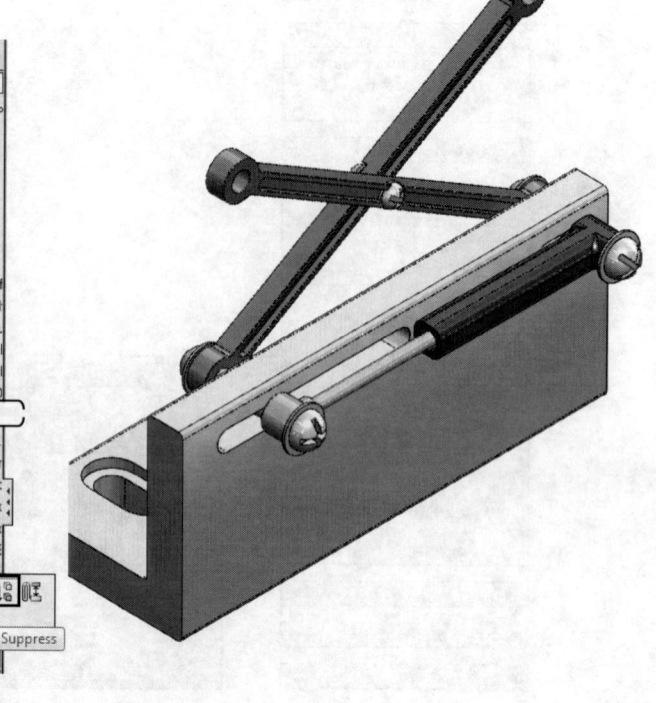

- After the Angle mate is suppressed, a **Distance Mate** is needed to create another reference location.

- This time a linear dimension is used instead of an angle.

17. Creating a Section View:

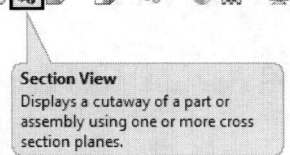

- Click the **Section View** command from the View (Heads Up tool bar).

Section View
Displays a cutaway of a part or assembly using one or more cross section planes.

- Select the **Right Plane** as cutting Plane and enter **.400"** for **Offset Distance**.

- Click the Reverse button if needed to remove the front portion of the assembly

- Click **OK** to close out of the section command.

18. Measuring the distance:

- The Section View allows us to see the inside of the Piston Housing. We will need to create a distance Mate between the end of the Piston and the inside face of the Piston Housing.

- Switch back to the Evaluate tab and click the **Measure** command.

- Measure the distance between the 2 faces as indicated.

- Push **Esc** to exit the measure tool.

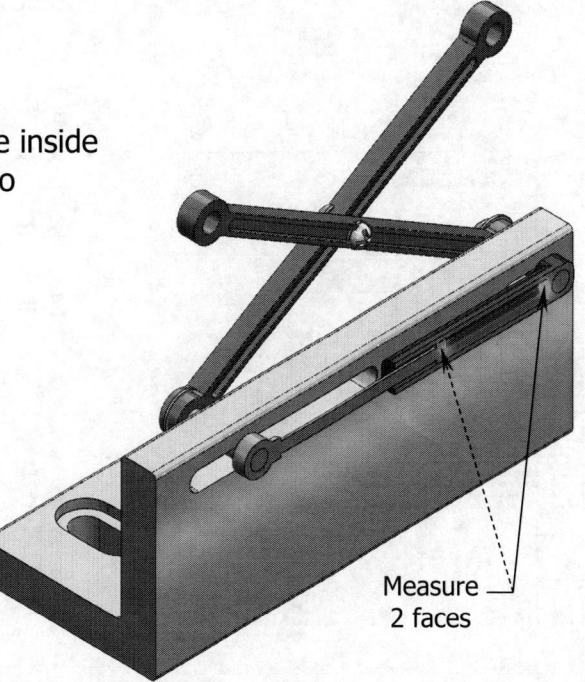

Measure
2 faces

19. Creating a Distance Mate:

- Click the **Mate** command.

- Select the **2 faces** that were used in the last step.

- Click the **Distance** button (arrow) and enter **1.00"**.

- The 2 Arms move to a new position (which equivalents to about 84.66deg).

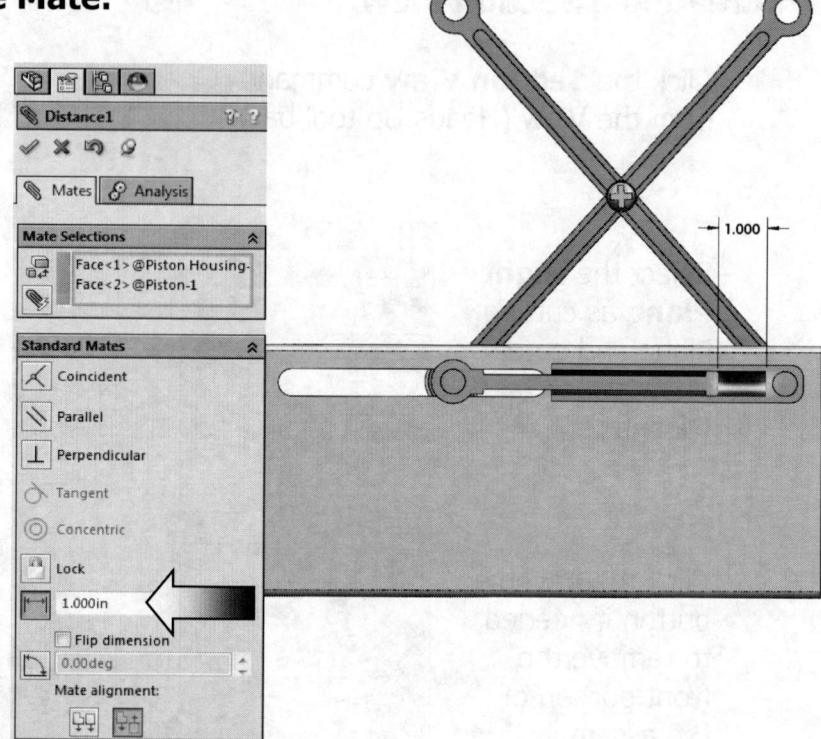

20. Measuring the Center of Mass of the assembly:

- Click **Mass Properties** from the Evaluate tool tab.

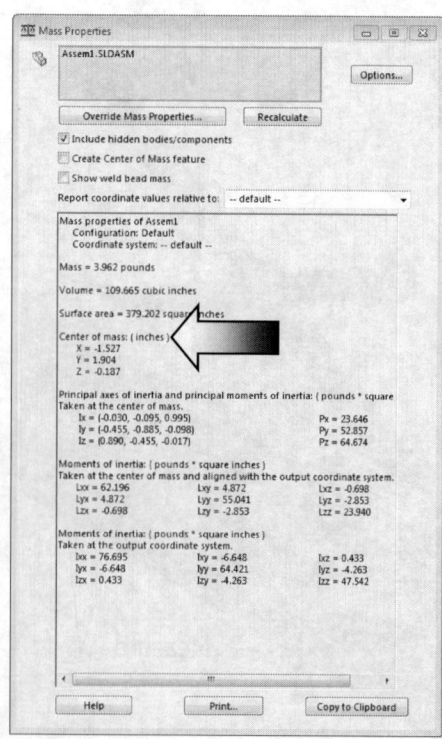

- Enter the Center of Mass below: (in Inches)

X = _____

Y = _____

Z = _____

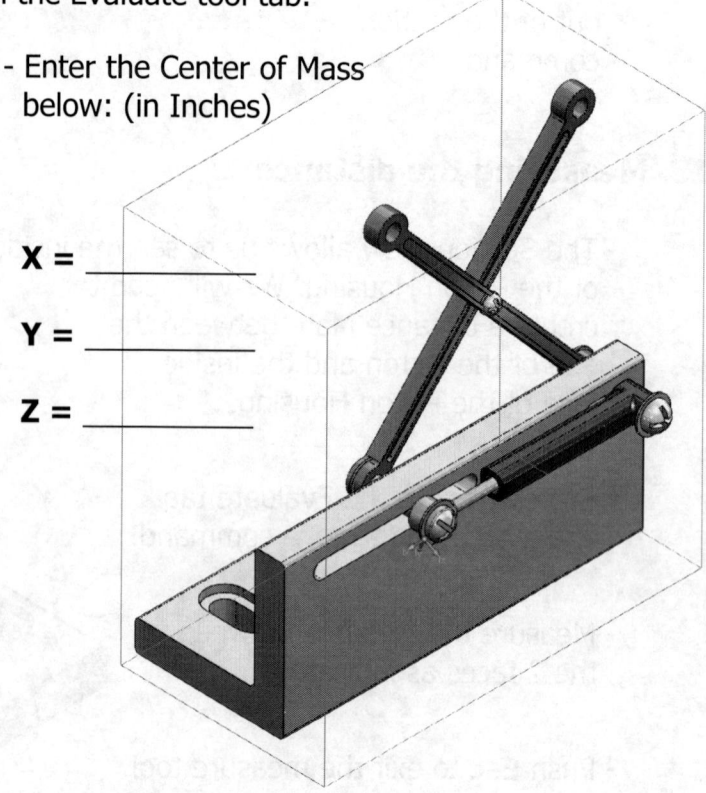

- Practice this material two or three times and time yourself to see if you could complete all challenges within a three hour time frame.

- When you are ready to take the CSWA exam, go to the web link below and purchase the exam using a credit card:
  www.solidworks.com/cswa

- The test costs $99 for a student or customer without a maintenance subscription, but the exam is free of charge for customers who have purchased the maintenance subscription. For more information, go to the quick link within the same webpage above and select: *Certification offers for subscription service customers.*

- As of the writing of this text, there are total of **65822** certified **Certified SolidWorks Associate (CSWA)** users world-wide. Go to the link below and enter your state to find out how many CSWA are in your state:
  https://solidworks.virtualtester.com/#userdir_button

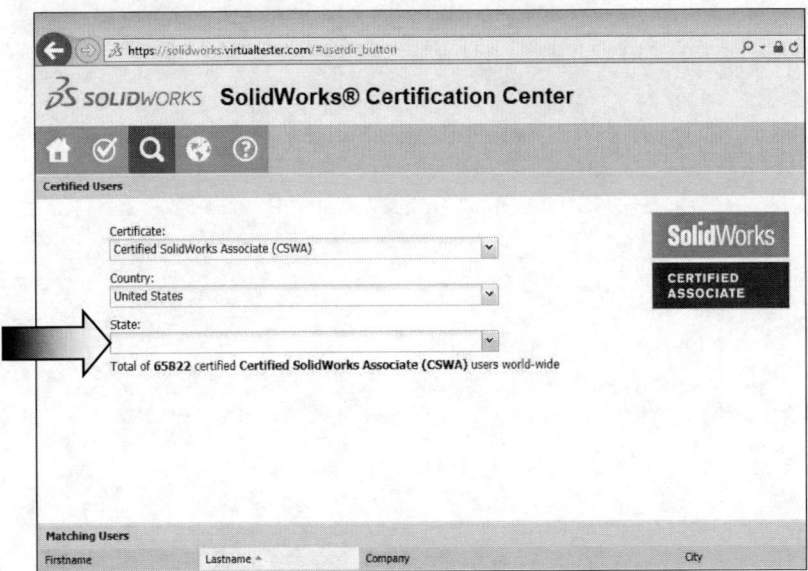

- Exam Length: 3 hours

- Minimum Passing grade: 70%

- Re-test Policy: There is a minimum 30 day waiting period between every attempt of the CSWA exam. Also, a CSWA exam credit must be purchased for each exam attempt.

- All candidates receive electronic certificates and personal listing on the CSWA directory when they pass. You can also update or change your log in information afterward.

- Dual monitors are recommended but not required. You could save up to 10-15 minutes if you do not have to switch back and forth between the exam and the SolidWorks application.

Glossary

Alloys:

An Alloy is a mixture of two or more metals (and sometimes a non-metal). The mixture is made by heating and melting the substances together.

Example of alloys are Bronze (Copper and Tin), Brass (Copper and Zinc), and Steel (Iron and Carbon).

Gravity and Mass:

Gravity is the force that pulls everything on earth toward the ground and makes things feel heavy. Gravity makes all falling bodies accelerate at a constant 32ft. per second (9.8 m/s). In the earth's atmosphere, air resistance slows acceleration. Only on airless Moon would a feather and a metal block fall to the ground together.

The mass of an object is the amount of material it contains.

A body with greater mass has more inertia; it needs a greater force to accelerate.

Weight depends on the force of gravity, but mass does not.

When an object spins around another (for example: a satellite orbiting the earth) it is pushed outward. Two forces are at work here: Centrifugal (pushing outward) and Centripetal (pulling inward). If you whirl a ball around you on a string, you pull it inward (Centripetal force). The ball seems to pull outward (Centrifugal force) and if released will fly off in a straight line.

Heat:

Heat is a form of energy and can move from one substance to another in one of three ways: by Convection, by Radiation, and by Conduction.

- Convection takes place only in liquids like water (for example: water in a kettle) and gases (for example: air warmed by a heat source such as a fire or radiator). When liquid or gas is heated, it expands and become less dense. Warm air above the radiator rises and cool air moves in to take its place, creating a convection current.
- Radiation is movement of heat through the air. Heat forms a match, sets molecules of air moving, and rays of heat spread out around the heat source.
- Conduction occurs in solids such as metals. The handle of a metal spoon left in boiling liquid warms up as molecules at the heated end move faster and collide with their neighbors, setting them moving. The heat travels through the metal, which is a good conductor of heat.

Inertia:

A body with a large mass is harder to start and also to stop. A heavy truck traveling at 50mph needs more power brakes to stop its motion than a smaller car traveling at the same speed. Inertia is the tendency of an object either to stay still or to move steadily in a straight line, unless another force (such as a brick wall stopping the vehicle) makes it behave differently.

Joules:

The Joules is the SI unit of work or energy.
One Joule of work is done when a force of one Newton moves through a distance of one meter.
The Joule is named after the English scientist James Joule (1818-1889).

Materials:

- Stainless steel is an alloy of steel with chromium or nickel.

- Steel is made by the basic oxygen process. The raw material is about three parts melted iron and one part scrap steel. Blowing oxygen into the melted iron raises the temperature and gets rid of impurities.

- All plastics are chemical compounds called polymers.

- Glass is made by mixing and heating sand, limestone, and soda ash. When these ingredients melt they turn into glass, which is hardened when it cools. Glass is in fact not a solid but a "supercooled" liquid, it can be shaped by blowing, pressing, drawing, casting into molds, rolling, and floating across molten tin, to make large sheets.

- Ceramic objects, such as pottery and porcelain, electrical insulators, bricks, and roof tiles are all made from clay. The clay is shaped or molded when wet and soft, and heated in a kiln until it hardens.

Machine Tools:

Are powered tools used for shaping metal or other materials, by drilling holes, chiseling, grinding, pressing or cutting. Often the material (the work piece) is moved while the tool stays still (lathe), or vice versa, the work piece stays while the tool moves (mill).
Most common machine tools are: Mill, Lathe, Saw, Broach, Punch press, Grind, Bore and Stamp break.

CNC

Computer Numerical Control is the automation of machine tools that are operated by precisely programmed commands encoded on a storage medium, as opposed to controlled manually via hand wheels or levers, or mechanically automated via cams alone. Most CNC today is computer numerical control in which computers play an integral part of the control.

3D Printing
All methods work by working in layers, adding material, etc. different to other techniques, which are subtractive. Supports needed because almost all methods could support multi material printing, but it is currently only available in certain top tier machines.

A method of turning digital shape into physical objects. Due to its nature, it allows us to accurately control the shape of the product. The drawback is size restraints and materials often not durable.

While FDM doesn't seem like the best method for instrument manufacturing, it is one of the cheapest and most universally available methods.

EDM
Electric Discharge Machining.

SLA
Stereo Lithography.

SLM
Selective Laser Melting.

FDM
Fused Deposition Modeling.

SLS
Selective Laser Sintering.

J-P
Jetted Photopolymer (or Polyjet)

Newton's Law:
1. Every object remains stopped or goes on moving at a steady rate in a straight line unless acted upon by another force. This is the inertia principle.
2. The amount of force needed to make an object change its speed depends on the mass of the object and the amount of the acceleration or deceleration required.
3. To every action there is an equal and opposite reaction. When a body is pushed one way by a force, another force pushes back with equal strength.

Polymers:
A polymer is made of one or more large molecules formed from thousands of smaller molecules. Rubber and Wood are natural polymers. Plastics are synthetic (artificially made) polymers.

Speed and Velocity:
- Speed is the rate at which a moving object changes position (how far it moves in a fixed time).
- Velocity is speed in a particular direction.
- If either speed or direction is changed, velocity also changed.

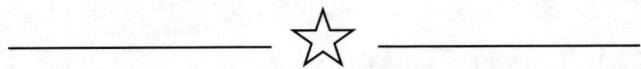

Absorbed
A feature, sketch, or annotation that is contained in another item (usually a feature) in the FeatureManager design tree. Examples are the profile sketch and profile path in a base-sweep, or a cosmetic thread annotation in a hole.

Align

Tools that assist in lining up annotations and dimensions (left, right, top, bottom, and so on). For aligning parts in an assembly.

Alternate position view

A drawing view in which one or more views are superimposed in phantom lines on the original view. Alternate position views are often used to show range of motion of an assembly.

Anchor point

The end of a leader that attaches to the note, block, or other annotation. Sheet formats contain anchor points for a bill of materials, a hole table, a revision table, and a weldment cut list.

Annotation

A text note or a symbol that adds specific design intent to a part, assembly, or drawing. Specific types of annotations include note, hole callout, surface finish symbol, datum feature symbol, datum target, geometric tolerance symbol, weld symbol, balloon, and stacked balloon. Annotations that apply only to drawings include center mark, annotation centerline, area hatch, and block.

Appearance callouts

Callouts that display the colors and textures of the face, feature, body, and part under the entity selected and are a shortcut to editing colors and textures.

Area hatch

A crosshatch pattern or fill applied to a selected face or to a closed sketch in a drawing.

Assembly

A document in which parts, features, and other assemblies (sub-assemblies) are mated together. The parts and sub-assemblies exist in documents separate from the assembly. For example, in an assembly, a piston can be mated to other parts, such as a connecting rod or cylinder. This new assembly can then be used as a sub-assembly in an assembly of an engine. The extension for a SolidWorks assembly file name is .SLDASM.

Attachment point

The end of a leader that attaches to the model (to an edge, vertex, or face, for example) or to a drawing sheet.

Axis

A straight line that can be used to create model geometry, features, or patterns. An axis can be made in a number of different ways, including using the intersection of two planes.

Balloon

Labels parts in an assembly, typically including item numbers and quantity. In drawings, the item numbers are related to rows in a bill of materials.

Base
The first solid feature of a part.

Baseline dimensions
Sets of dimensions measured from the same edge or vertex in a drawing.

Bend
A feature in a sheet metal part. A bend generated from a filleted corner, cylindrical face, or conical face is a round bend; a bend generated from sketched straight lines is a sharp bends.

Bill of materials
A table inserted into a drawing to keep a record of the parts used in an assembly.

Block
A user-defined annotation that you can use in parts, assemblies, and drawings. A block can contain text, sketch entities (except points), and area hatch, and it can be saved in a file for later use as, for example, a custom callout or a company logo.

Bottom-up assembly
An assembly modeling technique where you create parts and then insert them into an assembly.

Broken-out section
A drawing view that exposes inner details of a drawing view by removing material from a closed profile, usually a spline.

Cavity
The mold half that holds the cavity feature of the design part.

Center mark
A cross that marks the center of a circle or arc.

Centerline
A centerline marks, in phantom font, an axis of symmetry in a sketch or drawing.

Chamfer
Bevels a selected edge or vertex. You can apply chamfers to both sketches and features.

Child
A dependent feature related to a previously-built feature. For example, a chamfer on the edge of a hole is a child of the parent hole.

Click-release
As you sketch, if you click and then release the pointer, you are in click-release mode. Move the pointer and click again to define the next point in the sketch sequence.

Click-drag
As you sketch, if you click and drag the pointer, you are in click-drag mode. When you release the pointer, the sketch entity is complete.

Closed profile
Also called a closed contour, it is a sketch or sketch entity with no exposed endpoints; for example, a circle or polygon.

Collapse
The opposite of explode. The collapse action returns an exploded assembly's parts to their normal positions.

Collision Detection
An assembly function that detects collisions between components when components move or rotate. A collision occurs when an entity on one component coincides with any entity on another component.

Component
Any part or sub-assembly within an assembly

Configuration
A variation of a part or assembly within a single document. Variations can include different dimensions, features, and properties. For example, a single part such as a bolt can contain different configurations that vary the diameter and length.

ConfigurationManager
Located on the left side of the SolidWorks window, it is a means to create, select, and view the configurations of parts and assemblies.

Constraint
The relations between sketch entities, or between sketch entities and planes, axes, edges, or vertices.

Construction geometry
The characteristic of a sketch entity, that the entity is used in creating other geometry but is not itself used in creating features.

Coordinate system
A system of planes used to assign Cartesian coordinates to features, parts, and assemblies. Part and assembly documents contain default coordinate systems; other coordinate systems can be defined with reference geometry. Coordinate systems can be used with measurement tools and for exporting documents to other file formats.

Cosmetic thread
An annotation that represents threads.

Crosshatch
A pattern (or fill) applied to drawing views such as section views and broken-out sections.

Curvature
Curvature is equal to the inverse of the radius of the curve. The curvature can be displayed in different colors according to the local radius (usually of a surface).

Cut
A feature that removes material from a part by such actions as extrude, revolve, loft, sweep, thicken, cavity, and so on.

Dangling
A dimension, relation, or drawing section view that is unresolved. For example, if a piece of geometry is dimensioned, and that geometry is later deleted, the dimension becomes dangling.

Degrees of freedom
Geometry that is not defined by dimensions or relations is free to move. In 2D sketches, there are three degrees of freedom: movement along the X and Y axes, and rotation about the Z axis (the axis normal to the sketch plane). In 3D sketches and in assemblies, there are six degrees of freedom: movement along the X, Y, and Z axes, and rotation about the X, Y, and Z axes.

Derived part
A derived part is a new base, mirror, or component part created directly from an existing part and linked to the original part such that changes to the original part are reflected in the derived part.

Derived sketch
A copy of a sketch, in either the same part or the same assembly that is connected to the original sketch. Changes in the original sketch are reflected in the derived sketch.

Design Library
Located in the Task Pane, the Design Library provides a central location for reusable elements such as parts, assemblies, and so on.

Design table
An Excel spreadsheet that is used to create multiple configurations in a part or assembly document.

Detached drawing
A drawing format that allows opening and working in a drawing without loading the corresponding models into memory. The models are loaded on an as-needed basis.

Detail view
A portion of a larger view, usually at a larger scale than the original view.

Dimension line
A linear dimension line references the dimension text to extension lines indicating the entity being measured. An angular dimension line references the dimension text directly to the measured object.

DimXpertManager
Located on the left side of the SolidWorks window, it is a means to manage dimensions and tolerances created using DimXpert for parts according to the requirements of the ASME Y.14.41-2003 standard.

DisplayManager
The DisplayManager lists the appearances, decals, lights, scene, and cameras applied to the current model. From the DisplayManager, you can view applied content, and add, edit, or delete items. When PhotoView 360 is added in, the DisplayManager also provides access to PhotoView options.

Document
A file containing a part, assembly, or drawing.

Draft
The degree of taper or angle of a face, usually applied to molds or castings.

Drawing
A 2D representation of a 3D part or assembly. The extension for a SolidWorks drawing file name is .SLDDRW.

Drawing sheet
A page in a drawing document.

Driven dimension
Measurements of the model, but they do not drive the model and their values cannot be changed.

Driving dimension
Also referred to as a model dimension, it sets the value for a sketch entity. It can also control distance, thickness, and feature parameters.

Edge
A single outside boundary of a feature.

Edge flange
A sheet metal feature that combines a bend and a tab in a single operation.

Equation
Creates a mathematical relation between sketch dimensions, using dimension names as variables, or between feature parameters, such as the depth of an extruded feature or the instance count in a pattern.

Exploded view
Shows an assembly with its components separated from one another, usually to show how to assemble the mechanism.

Export
Save a SolidWorks document in another format for use in other CAD/CAM, rapid prototyping, web, or graphics software applications.

Extension line
The line extending from the model indicating the point from which a dimension is measured.

Extrude
A feature that linearly projects a sketch to either add material to a part (in a base or boss) or remove material from a part (in a cut or hole).

Face
A selectable area (planar or otherwise) of a model or surface with boundaries that help define the shape of the model or surface. For example, a rectangular solid has six faces.

Fasteners
A SolidWorks Toolbox library that adds fasteners automatically to holes in an assembly.

Feature
An individual shape that, combined with other features, makes up a part or assembly. Some features, such as bosses and cuts, originate as sketches. Other features, such as shells and fillets, modify a feature's geometry. However, not all features have associated geometry. Features are always listed in the FeatureManager design tree.

FeatureManager design tree
Located on the left side of the SolidWorks window, it provides an outline view of the active part, assembly, or drawing.

Fill
A solid area hatch or crosshatch. Fill also applies to patches on surfaces.

Fillet
An internal rounding of a corner or edge in a sketch, or an edge on a surface or solid.

Forming tool
Dies that bend, stretch, or otherwise form sheet metal to create such form features as louvers, lances, flanges, and ribs.

Fully defined
A sketch where all lines and curves in the sketch, and their positions, are described by dimensions or relations, or both, and cannot be moved. Fully defined sketch entities are shown in black.

Geometric tolerance

A set of standard symbols that specify the geometric characteristics and dimensional requirements of a feature.

Graphics area

The area in the SolidWorks window where the part, assembly, or drawing appears.

Guide curve

A 2D or 3D curve used to guide a sweep or loft.

Handle

An arrow, square, or circle that you can drag to adjust the size or position of an entity (a feature, dimension, or sketch entity, for example).

Helix

A curve defined by pitch, revolutions, and height. A helix can be used, for example, as a path for a swept feature cutting threads in a bolt.

Hem

A sheet metal feature that folds back at the edge of a part. A hem can be open, closed, double, or tear-drop.

HLR

(Hidden lines removed) A view mode in which all edges of the model that are not visible from the current view angle are removed from the display.

HLV

(Hidden lines visible) A view mode in which all edges of the model that are not visible from the current view angle are shown gray or dashed.

Import

Open files from other CAD software applications into a SolidWorks document.

In-context feature

A feature with an external reference to the geometry of another component; the in-context feature changes automatically if the geometry of the referenced model or feature changes.

Inference

The system automatically creates (infers) relations between dragged entities (sketched entities, annotations, and components) and other entities and geometry. This is useful when positioning entities relative to one another.

Instance

An item in a pattern or a component in an assembly that occurs more than once. Blocks are inserted into drawings as instances of block definitions.

Interference detection
A tool that displays any interference between selected components in an assembly.

Jog
A sheet metal feature that adds material to a part by creating two bends from a sketched line.

Knit
A tool that combines two or more faces or surfaces into one. The edges of the surfaces must be adjacent and not overlapping, but they cannot ever be planar. There is no difference in the appearance of the face or the surface after knitting.

Layout sketch
A sketch that contains important sketch entities, dimensions, and relations. You reference the entities in the layout sketch when creating new sketches, building new geometry, or positioning components in an assembly. This allows for easier updating of your model because changes you make to the layout sketch propagate to the entire model.

Leader
A solid line from an annotation (note, dimension, and so on) to the referenced feature.

Library feature
A frequently used feature, or combination of features, that is created once and then saved for future use.

Lightweight
A part in an assembly or a drawing has only a subset of its model data loaded into memory. The remaining model data is loaded on an as-needed basis. This improves performance of large and complex assemblies.

Line
A straight sketch entity with two endpoints. A line can be created by projecting an external entity such as an edge, plane, axis, or sketch curve into the sketch.

Loft
A base, boss, cut, or surface feature created by transitions between profiles.

Lofted bend
A sheet metal feature that produces a roll form or a transitional shape from two open profile sketches. Lofted bends often create funnels and chutes.

Mass properties
A tool that evaluates the characteristics of a part or an assembly such as volume, surface area, centroid, and so on.

Mate
A geometric relationship, such as coincident, perpendicular, tangent, and so on, between parts in an assembly.

Mate reference
Specifies one or more entities of a component to use for automatic mating. When you drag a component with a mate reference into an assembly, the software tries to find other combinations of the same mate reference name and mate type.

Mates folder
A collection of mates that are solved together. The order in which the mates appear within the Mates folder does not matter.

Mirror
(a) A mirror feature is a copy of a selected feature, mirrored about a plane or planar face.
(b) A mirror sketch entity is a copy of a selected sketch entity that is mirrored about a centerline.

Miter flange
A sheet metal feature that joins multiple edge flanges together and miters the corner.

Model
3D solid geometry in a part or assembly document. If a part or assembly document contains multiple configurations, each configuration is a separate model.

Model dimension
A dimension specified in a sketch or a feature in a part or assembly document that defines some entity in a 3D model.

Model item
A characteristic or dimension of feature geometry that can be used in detailing drawings.

Model view
A drawing view of a part or assembly.

Mold
A set of manufacturing tooling used to shape molten plastic or other material into a designed part. You design the mold using a sequence of integrated tools that result in cavity and core blocks that are derived parts of the part to be molded.

Motion Study
Motion Studies are graphical simulations of motion and visual properties with assembly models. Analogous to a configuration, they do not actually change the original assembly model or its properties. They display the model as it changes based on simulation elements you add.

Multibody part
A part with separate solid bodies within the same part document. Unlike the components in an assembly, multibody parts are not dynamic.

Native format
DXF and DWG files remain in their original format (are not converted into SolidWorks format) when viewed in SolidWorks drawing sheets (view only).

Open profile
Also called an open contour, it is a sketch or sketch entity with endpoints exposed. For example, a U-shaped profile is open.

Ordinate dimensions
A chain of dimensions measured from a zero ordinate in a drawing or sketch.

Origin
The model origin appears as three gray arrows and represents the (0,0,0) coordinate of the model. When a sketch is active, a sketch origin appears in red and represents the (0,0,0) coordinate of the sketch. Dimensions and relations can be added to the model origin, but not to a sketch origin.

Out-of-context feature
A feature with an external reference to the geometry of another component that is not open.

Over defined
A sketch is over defined when dimensions or relations are either in conflict or redundant.

Parameter
A value used to define a sketch or feature (often a dimension).

Parent
An existing feature upon which other features depend. For example, in a block with a hole, the block is the parent to the child hole feature.

Part
A single 3D object made up of features. A part can become a component in an assembly, and it can be represented in 2D in a drawing. Examples of parts are bolt, pin, plate, and so on. The extension for a SolidWorks part file name is .SLDPRT.

Path
A sketch, edge, or curve used in creating a sweep or loft.

Pattern
A pattern repeats selected sketch entities, features, or components in an array, which can be linear, circular, or sketch-driven. If the seed entity is changed, the other instances in the pattern are updated.

Physical Dynamics

An assembly tool that displays the motion of assembly components in a realistic way. When you drag a component, the component applies a force to other components it touches. Components move only within their degrees of freedom.

Pierce relation

Makes a sketch point coincident to the location at which an axis, edge, line, or spline pierces the sketch plane.

Planar

Entities that can lie on one plane. For example, a circle is planar, but a helix is not.

Plane

Flat construction geometry. Planes can be used for a 2D sketch, section view of a model, a neutral plane in a draft feature, and others.

Point

A singular location in a sketch, or a projection into a sketch at a single location of an external entity (origin, vertex, axis, or point in an external sketch).

Predefined view

A drawing view in which the view position, orientation, and so on can be specified before a model is inserted. You can save drawing documents with predefined views as templates.

Profile

A sketch entity used to create a feature (such as a loft) or a drawing view (such as a detail view). A profile can be open (such as a U shape or open spline) or closed (such as a circle or closed spline).

Projected dimension

If you dimension entities in an isometric view, projected dimensions are the flat dimensions in 2D.

Projected view

A drawing view projected orthogonally from an existing view.

PropertyManager

Located on the left side of the SolidWorks window, it is used for dynamic editing of sketch entities and most features.

RealView graphics

A hardware (graphics card) support of advanced shading in real time; the rendering applies to the model and is retained as you move or rotate a part.

Rebuild

Tool that updates (or regenerates) the document with any changes made since the last time the model was rebuilt. Rebuild is typically used after changing a model dimension.

Reference dimension

A dimension in a drawing that shows the measurement of an item, but cannot drive the model and its value cannot be modified. When model dimensions change, reference dimensions update.

Reference geometry

Includes planes, axes, coordinate systems, and 3D curves. Reference geometry is used to assist in creating features such lofts, sweeps, drafts, chamfers, and patterns.

Relation

A geometric constraint between sketch entities or between a sketch entity and a plane, axis, edge, or vertex. Relations can be added automatically or manually.

Relative view

A relative (or relative to model) drawing view is created relative to planar surfaces in a part or assembly.

Reload

Refreshes shared documents. For example, if you open a part file for read-only access while another user makes changes to the same part, you can reload the new version, including the changes.

Reorder

Reordering (changing the order of) items is possible in the FeatureManager design tree. In parts, you can change the order in which features are solved. In assemblies, you can control the order in which components appear in a bill of materials.

Replace

Substitutes one or more open instances of a component in an assembly with a different component.

Resolved

A state of an assembly component (in an assembly or drawing document) in which it is fully loaded in memory. All the component's model data is available, so its entities can be selected, referenced, edited, and used in mates, and so on.

Revolve

A feature that creates a base or boss, a revolved cut, or revolved surface by revolving one or more sketched profiles around a centerline.

Rip

A sheet metal feature that removes material at an edge to allow a bend.

Rollback
Suppresses all items below the rollback bar.

Section
Another term for profile in sweeps.

Section line
A line or centerline sketched in a drawing view to create a section view.

Section scope
Specifies the components to be left uncut when you create an assembly drawing section view.

Section view
A section view (or section cut) is (1) a part or assembly view cut by a plane, or (2) a drawing view created by cutting another drawing view with a section line.

Seed
A sketch or an entity (a feature, face, or body) that is the basis for a pattern. If you edit the seed, the other entities in the pattern are updated.

Shaded
Displays a model as a colored solid.

Shared values
Also called linked values, these are named variables that you assign to set the value of two or more dimensions to be equal.

Sheet format
Includes page size and orientation, standard text, borders, title blocks, and so on. Sheet formats can be customized and saved for future use. Each sheet of a drawing document can have a different format.

Shell
A feature that hollows out a part, leaving open the selected faces and thin walls on the remaining faces. A hollow part is created when no faces are selected to be open.

Sketch
A collection of lines and other 2D objects on a plane or face that forms the basis for a feature such as a base or a boss. A 3D sketch is non-planar and can be used to guide a sweep or loft, for example.

Smart Fasteners
Automatically adds fasteners (bolts and screws) to an assembly using the SolidWorks Toolbox library of fasteners.

SmartMates
An assembly mating relation that is created automatically.

Solid sweep
A cut sweep created by moving a tool body along a path to cut out 3D material from a model.

Spiral
A flat or 2D helix, defined by a circle, pitch, and number of revolutions.

Spline
A sketched 2D or 3D curve defined by a set of control points.

Split line
Projects a sketched curve onto a selected model face, dividing the face into multiple faces so that each can be selected individually. A split line can be used to create draft features, to create face blend fillets, and to radiate surfaces to cut molds.

Stacked balloon
A set of balloons with only one leader. The balloons can be stacked vertically (up or down) or horizontally (left or right).

Standard 3 views
The three orthographic views (front, right, and top) that are often the basis of a drawing.

StereoLithography
The process of creating rapid prototype parts using a faceted mesh representation in STL files.

Sub-assembly
An assembly document that is part of a larger assembly. For example, the steering mechanism of a car is a sub-assembly of the car.

Suppress
Removes an entity from the display and from any calculations in which it is involved. You can suppress features, assembly components, and so on. Suppressing an entity does not delete the entity; you can unsuppress the entity to restore it.

Surface
A zero-thickness planar or 3D entity with edge boundaries. Surfaces are often used to create solid features. Reference surfaces can be used to modify solid features.

Sweep
Creates a base, boss, cut, or surface feature by moving a profile (section) along a path. For cut-sweeps, you can create solid sweeps by moving a tool body along a path.

Tangent arc
An arc that is tangent to another entity, such as a line.

Tangent edge
The transition edge between rounded or filleted faces in hidden lines visible or hidden lines removed modes in drawings.

Task Pane
Located on the right-side of the SolidWorks window, the Task Pane contains SolidWorks Resources, the Design Library, and the File Explorer.

Template
A document (part, assembly, or drawing) that forms the basis of a new document. It can include user-defined parameters, annotations, predefined views, geometry, and so on.

Temporary axis
An axis created implicitly for every conical or cylindrical face in a model.

Thin feature
An extruded or revolved feature with constant wall thickness. Sheet metal parts are typically created from thin features.

TolAnalyst
A tolerance analysis application that determines the effects that dimensions and tolerances have on parts and assemblies.

Top-down design
An assembly modeling technique where you create parts in the context of an assembly by referencing the geometry of other components. Changes to the referenced components propagate to the parts that you create in context.

Triad
Three axes with arrows defining the X, Y, and Z directions. A reference triad appears in part and assembly documents to assist in orienting the viewing of models. Triads also assist when moving or rotating components in assemblies.

Under defined
A sketch is under defined when there are not enough dimensions and relations to prevent entities from moving or changing size.

Vertex
A point at which two or more lines or edges intersect. Vertices can be selected for sketching, dimensioning, and many other operations.

Viewports
Windows that display views of models. You can specify one, two, or four viewports. Viewports with orthogonal views can be linked, which links orientation and rotation.

Virtual sharp

A sketch point at the intersection of two entities after the intersection itself has been removed by a feature such as a fillet or chamfer. Dimensions and relations to the virtual sharp are retained even though the actual intersection no longer exists.

Weldment

A multibody part with structural members.

Weldment cut list

A table that tabulates the bodies in a weldment along with descriptions and lengths.

Wireframe

A view mode in which all edges of the part or assembly are displayed.

Zebra stripes

Simulate the reflection of long strips of light on a very shiny surface. They allow you to see small changes in a surface that may be hard to see with a standard display.

Zoom

To simulate movement toward or away from a part or an assembly.

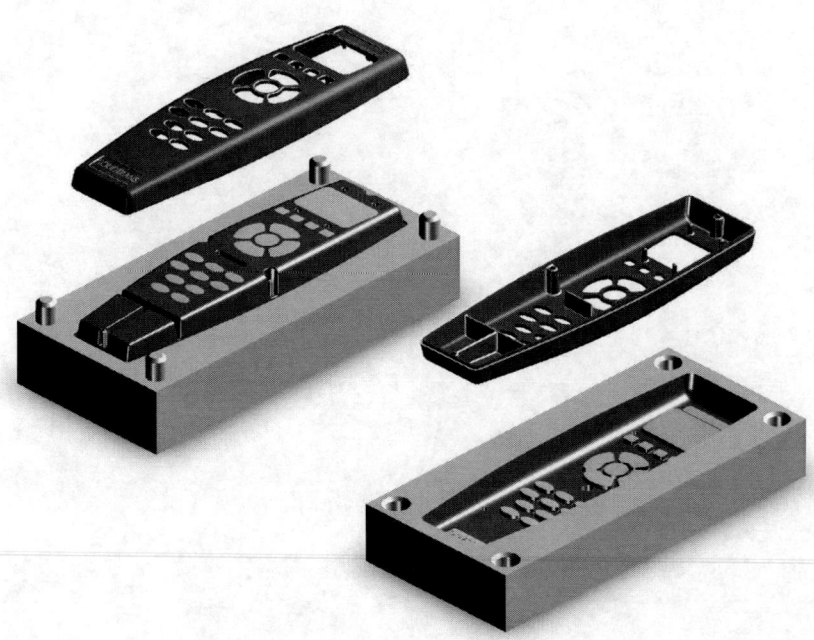

Index

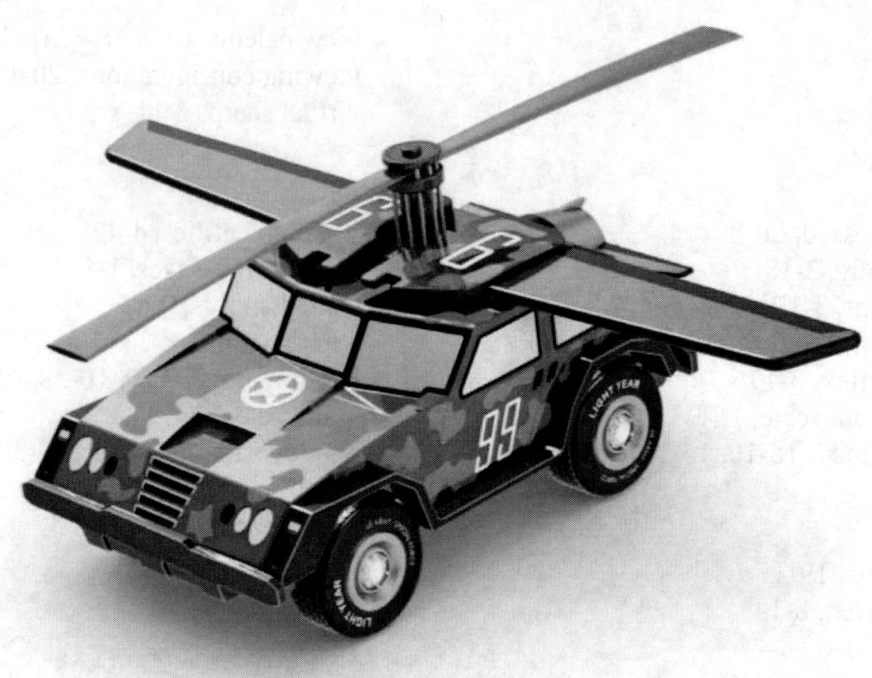

SolidWorks® Quick-Guide

Quick Reference Guide To SolidWorks® Command Icons & Toolbars

The STANDARD Toolbar

- Creates a new document.
- Opens an existing document.
- Saves an active document.
- Make Drawing from Part/Assembly
- Make Assembly from Part/Assembly
- Prints the active document.
- Displays full pages as they are printed.
- Cuts the selection & puts it on the clipboard.
- Copies the selection & puts it on the clipboard.
- Inserts the clipboard contents.
- Deletes the selection.
- Reverses the last action.
- Redo the last action that was undone.
- Rebuilds the part / assembly / drawing.
- Saves all documents.
- Changes the color of the current selection(s).
- Edits material.
- Closes an existing document
- Shows or hides the Selection Filter toolbar.
- Shows or hides the Web toolbar.
- Displays Help topics for SolidWorks.
- Displays full pages as they will be printed.

The STANDARD Toolbar (Cont.)

- Loads or unloads the 3D instant website add-in
- Select tool.
- Reloads the current document from disk.
- Places an online order for a rapid prototype part.
- Checks read-only files for write access.
- Show/Edit the properties of the current selection.
- Changes options settings for SolidWorks.
- Tiles windows vertically, as non-overlapping.
- Tiles windows horizontally, as non-overlapping.
- Opens another window for the active document.

The SKETCH TOOLS Toolbar

- Sketches a rectangle from the center.
- Sketches a centerpoint arc slot.
- Sketches a 3-point arc slot.
- Sketches a straight slot.
- Sketches a centerpoint straight slot.
- Stretches sketch entities and annotations.
- Inserts an Equation Driven Curve.
- Sketches a 3-point arc.
- Inserts a picture into the sketch background.
- Creates sketched ellipses.

The SKETCH TOOLS Toolbar

Selects items for commands to act on.

Sets up Grid parameters.

Creates a sketch on a selected plane or face.

Creates a 3D sketch.

Scales/Translates/Rotates the current sketch.

Moves or copies sketch entities and annotations.

Scales sketch entities and annotations.

Sketches an angle rectangle from the center.

Sketches a parallelogram.

Sketches a line.

Creates a center point arc: center, start, end.

Creates an arc tangent to a line.

Sketches splines on a surface or face.

Sketches a circle.

Sketches a circle by its perimeter.

Sketches a partial ellipse.

Makes a path of sketch entities.

Mirrors entities dynamically about a

Insert a plane into the 3D sketch.

Rotates sketch entities and

Copies sketch entities and

Sketches on a plane in a 3D sketch.

Moves sketch entities without solving dimensions or relations.

The SKETCH TOOLS Toolbar (Cont.)

 Partial ellipses.

 Adds a Parabola.

 Creates sketched splines.

 Sketches a polygon.

 Sketches a rectangle.

 Sketches a parallelogram.

 Creates points.

 Creates sketched centerlines.

 Adds text to sketch.

 Converts selected model edges or sketch entities to sketch segments.

 Creates a sketch along the intersection of multiple bodies.

 Converts face curves on the selected face into 3D sketch entities.

 Mirrors selected segments about a centerline.

 Fillets the corner of two lines.

 Creates a chamfer between two sketch entities.

 Creates a sketch curve by offsetting model edges or sketch entities at a specified distance.

Fits a spline to selected entities.

Trims a sketch segment.

Extends a sketch segment.

Splits a sketch segment.

Construction Geometry.

 Creates linear steps and repeat of sketch entities.

 Creates circular steps and repeat of sketch entities.

Quick Reference Guide To SolidWorks® Command Icons & Toolbars

The SHEET METAL

Inserts a FlattenBends & a ProcessBends feature, A sheet metal feature will be added.

Shows flat pattern for this sheet metal part.

Shows part without inserting any bends.

Inserts a rip feature to a sheet metal part.

Inserts a Sheet Metal Base Flange or a Tab feature.

Inserts a Sheet Metal Miter Flange feature.

Folds selected bends.

Unfolds selected bends.

Inserts bends using a sketch line.

Inserts a flange by pulling an edge.

Inserts a sheet metal corner feature.

Inserts a Hem feature by selecting edges.

Breaks a corner by filleting/chamfering it.

Inserts a Jog feature using a sketch line.

Inserts a lofted bend feature using 2 sketches.

Creates inverse dent on a sheet metal part.

Trims out material from a corner, in a sheet metal

Inserts a fillet weld bead.

Converts a solid/surface into a sheet metal part.

Adds a Cross Break feature into a selected face.

The SURFACES Toolbar

Deletes a face or a set of faces.

Creates mid surfaces between offset face pairs.

Patches surface holes and external edges.

The SURFACES Toolbar (cont.)

Creates an extruded surface.

Creates a revolved surface.

Creates a swept surface.

Creates a lofted surface.

Creates an offset surface.

Radiates a surface originating from a curve, parallel to a plane.

Knits surfaces together.

Creates a planar surface from a sketch or A set of edges.

Creates a surface by importing data from a file.

Extends a surface.

Trims a surface.

Generating MidSurface(s).

Surface Flatten.

Replaces Face with Surface.

Patches surface holes and external edges by extending the surfaces.

Creates parting surfaces between core & cavity surfaces.

Inserts ruled surfaces from edges.

The WELDMENTS Toolbar

Creates a weldment feature.

Creates a structure member feature.

Adds a gusset feature between 2 planar adjoining faces.

Creates an end cap feature.

Adds a fillet weld bead feature.

Trims or extends structure members.

The DIMENSIONS/RELATIONS Toolbar

Inserts dimension between two lines.

Creates a horizontal dimension between selected entities.

Creates a vertical dimension between selected entities.

Creates a reference dimension between selected entities.

Creates a set of ordinate dimensions.

Creates a set of Horizontal ordinate dimensions.

Creates a set of Vertical ordinate dimensions.

Creates a chamfer dimension.

Adds a geometric relation.

Automatically Adds Dimensions to the current sketch.

Displays and deletes geometric relations.

Fully defines a sketch.

Scans a sketch for elements of equal length or radius.

Automatically recognize tolerance features.

Creates linked, unlinked, or collection pattern feature.

Paints faces of toleranced features in different colors.

Adds DimXpert location dimension.

Adds DimXpert datum.

Copies existing tolerance scheme to current configuration.

Adds DimXpert size dimension.

Adds DimXpert geometric tolerance.

Deletes all tolerance data base.

Adds new TolAnalyst.

Did you know??

* Ctrl+Q will force a rebuild on all features of a part.
* Ctrl+B will rebuild the feature being worked on and its dependants.

The STANDARD VIEWS

Front view.

Back view.

Left view.

Right view.

Top view.

Bottom view.

Isometric view.

Trimetric view.

Dimetric view.

Normal to view.

Links all views in the viewport together.

Displays viewport with front & right views

Displays a 4 view viewport with 1st or 3rd Angle of projection.

Displays viewport with front & top

Displays viewport with a single

The Block Toolbar

 Makes a new block.

 Edits the selected block.

 Inserts a new block to a sketch or drawing.

 Adds/Removes sketch entities to/from blocks.

 Updates parent sketches effected by this block.

 Saves the block to a file.

 Explodes the selected block.

 Inserts a belt.

The FEATURES Toolbar

Creates a boss feature by extruding a sketched profile.

Creates a revolved feature based on profile and angle parameter.

Creates a cut feature by extruding a sketched profile.

Creates a cut feature by revolving a sketched profile.

Creates a sweep feature by sweeping a profile along a path curve.

Creates a cut by sweeping a closed profile along an open or closed path.

Creates a cut by removing material between two or more profiles

Creates a cut by thickening one or more adjacent surfaces.

Adds a deformed surface by push or pull on

Creates a lofted feature between two or more profiles.

Creates a solid feature by thickening one or more adjacent surfaces.

Creates a filled feature.

Chamfers an edge or a chain of tangent edges.

Inserts a rib feature.

Scales model by a specified factor.

Creates a shell feature.

Applies draft to a selected surface.

Creates a cylindrical hole.

Inserts a hole with a pre-defined cross section.

Puts a dome surface on a face.

Puts a shape feature on a face.

Applies global deformation to solid or surface bodies.

Wraps closed sketch contour(s) onto a face.

Moves / Sizes features.

Suppresses the selected feature or component.

Un-suppresses the selected feature or component.

Flexes solid and surface bodies

Creates a linear pattern using the selected feature(s).

Creates a circular pattern using the selected feature(s).

Mirrors a feature about a plane.

Creates a Curve Driven Pattern.

Creates a Sketch Driven pattern.

Creates a Table Driven Pattern.

Inserts a split Feature.

Combines two or more solid bodies.

Joins bodies from one or more parts into a single part in the context of an assembly.

Deletes a solid or a surface.

Inserts solid(s) or surface(s) into an existing open document.

Inserts a part from file into the active part document.

Moves/Copies solid and surface bodies or moves graphics bodies.

Merges short edges on faces

Pushes solid / surface model by another solid / surface model

Moves face(s) of a solid

Area fills faces or bodies into one or more contours.

Inserts holes into a series of parts.

Returns suppressed items with dependents to the model.

Cuts a solid model with a surface.

Adds material between profiles in two directions to create a solid feature.

Cuts a solid model by removing material between profiles in two directions.

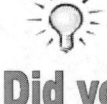

Did you know??

* Right-mouse drag a component in an assembly rotates it.
* Left-mouse drag a component in an assembly moves it.

Extracts core(s) from existing tooling split

 Constructs a surface patch

 Moves face(s) of a solid

 Finds & creates mold shut-off surfaces

 Inserts cavity into a base part.

 Scales a model by a specified factor.

 Applies draft to a selected surface.

 Inserts a split line feature.

 Creates an offset surface.

 Creates parting lines to separate core & cavity surfaces

 Creates a planar surface from a sketch or A set of edges.

 Knits surfaces together.

 Analyzes draft angles of faces, based on a mold pull direction.

 Inserts ruled surfaces from edges.

 Creates parting surfaces between core & cavity surfaces

 Creates multiple bodies from a single body.

 Inserts a tooling split feature.

 Identifies faces that form undercuts.

 Creates parting surfaces between the core & cavity.

 Inserts surface body folders for mold operation.

 Turns selection filters on and off.

 Clears all filters.

 Selects all filters.

 Inverts current selection.

 Allows selection of edges only.

 Allows selection of faces only.

 Adds filter for Surface Bodies.

 Adds filter for Solid Bodies.

 Adds filter for Axes.

 Adds filter for Planes.

 Adds filter for Sketch Points.

 Adds filter for Sketch Segments.

 Adds filter for Midpoints.

 Adds filter for Center Marks.

 Adds filter for Centerline.

 Adds filter for Dimensions and Hole Callouts.

 Adds filter for Surface Finish Symbols.

 Adds filter for Geometric Tolerances.

 Adds filter for Notes / Balloons.

 Adds filter for Weld Symbols.

 Adds filter for Datum Targets.

 Adds filter for Cosmetic Threads.

 Adds filter for blocks.

 Adds filter for Dowel pin symbols.

 Adds filter for connection points.

 Allows selection filter for vertices only.

 Allows selection of weld symbols only.

 Allows selection of blocks only.

 Adds filter for routing points.

The **FLYOUT** Toolbar

 2D to 3D.

 Align.

 Annotation.

 Assemblies.

 Curves.

 Dimensions / Relation.

 Drawings.

 Features.

 Fonts.

 Line Formats.

 Macros.

 Molds.

 Reference Geometry.

 Quick snap filters.

 Selection Filters.

 Sheet Metal.

 Simulation.

 Sketch.

 SolidWorks Office.

 Splines.

 Standard.

 Standard Views.

 Surfaces.

 Tools.

 View.

 Web.

 Weldments.

 Block commands.

 Explode sketch commands.

 Table commands.

 Fastening feature commands.

 Creates a rounded internal or external fillet.

 Linear Patterns Features, Faces and Bodies.

 Creates various corner treatments.

 Displays Deletes geometric relations.

 Creates dimensions for one or more entities.

 Adds an existing part or assembly.

 Linear Patterns components in assembly.

 Moves components in assembly.

 Adds section view with a section line.

 Creates various assembly features.

 Toggles various view settings.

The **SCREEN CAPTURE** Toolbar

 Copies the current graphics window to the clipboard.

 Records the current graphics window to an AVI file.

 Stops recording the current graphics window to an AVI file.

The **Explode Line Sketch** Toolbar

 Adds a route line that connect entities.

 Adds a jog to the route lines.

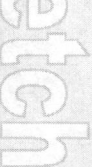

The LINE FORMAT Toolbar

Changes layer properties.

Changes line color.

Changes line thickness.

Changes line style.

Hides a visible edge.

Shows a hidden edge.

Changes line display mode.

The 2D-To-3D Toolbar

Makes a Front sketch from the selected entities.

Makes a Top sketch from the selected entities.

Makes a Right sketch from the selected entities.

Makes a Left sketch from the selected entities.

Makes a Bottom sketch from the selected entities.

Makes a Back sketch from the selected entities.

Makes an Auxiliary sketch from the selected entities.

Creates a new sketch from the selected entities.

Repairs the selected sketch.

Aligns a sketch to the selected point.

Creates an extrusion from the selected sketch segments, starting at the selected sketch point.

Creates a cut from the selected sketch segments, optionally starting at the selected sketch point.

The ALIGN Toolbar

Aligns the left side of the selected annotations with the leftmost annotation.

Aligns the right side of the selected annotations with the rightmost annotation.

Aligns the top side of the selected annotations with the topmost annotation.

Aligns the bottom side of the selected annotations with the lowermost annotation.

Evenly spaces the selected annotations horizontally.

Evenly spaces the selected annotations vertically.

Centrally aligns the selected annotations horizontally.

Centrally aligns the selected annotations vertically.

Compacts the selected annotations horizontally.

Compacts the selected annotations vertically.

Aligns the center of the selected annotations between

Creates a group from the selected items

Deletes the grouping between these items

Aligns & groups selected dimensions along a line or an arc

Aligns & groups dimensions at a uniform distanc

The SIMULATION Toolbar

Stops Record or Playback.

Records Simulation.

Replays Simulation.

Resets Components.

Adds Linear Motor.

Adds Rotary Motor.

Adds Spring.

Adds Gravity.

The MACRO Toolbar

Runs a Macro.

Stops Macro recorder.

Records (or pauses recording of) actions to create a Macro.

Launches the Macro Editor and begins editing a new macro.

Opens a Macro file for editing.

Creates a custom macro.

The TABLE Toolbar

 Adds a hole table of selected holes from a specified origin datum.

 Adds a Bill of Materials.

 Adds a revision table.

 Displays a Design table in a drawing.

 Adds a weldments cuts list table.

 Adds a Excel based of Bill of Materials

 Adds a general table to a drawing sheet.

The REFERENCE GEOMETRY

 Adds a reference plane

 Creates an axis.

 Creates a coordinate system.

 Adds a reference point

 Specifies entities to use as references using SmartMates.

The SPLINE TOOLS Toolbar

 Adds a point to a spline.

 Displays points where the concavity of selected spline changes.

 Displays minimum radius of selected spline.

 Displays curvature combs of selected spline.

 Reduces numbers of points in a selected spline.

 Adds a tangency control.

 Adds a curvature control.

 Adds a spline based on selected sketch entities & edges.

 Displays all handles of selected splines.

 Displays the spline control polygon.

The ANNOTATIONS Toolbar

 Inserts a note.

 Inserts a surface finish symbol.

 Inserts a new geometric tolerancing symbol.

 Attaches a balloon to the selected edge or face.

 Adds balloons for all components in selected view.

 Inserts a stacked balloon.

 Attaches a datum feature symbol to a selected edge / detail.

 Inserts a weld symbol on the selected edge / face / vertex.

 Inserts a datum target symbol and / or point attached to a selected edge / line.

 Selects and inserts block.

 Inserts annotations & reference geometry from the part / assembly into the selected.

 Adds center marks to circles on model.

 Inserts a Centerline.

 Inserts a hole callout.

 Adds a cosmetic thread to the selected cylindrical feature.

 Inserts a Multi-Jog leader.

 Selects a circular edge or and arc for Dowel pin symbol insertion.

 Toggles the visibility of annotations & dimensions.

 Inserts latest version symbol.

 Adds a cross hatch patterns or solid fill.

 Adds a weld symbol on a selected entity.

 Adds a weld bead caterpillar on an edge.

The "Feathers"

 Lightweight component.

Out-of-Date component.

Hidden Lightweight component.

 Hidden, Out-of-Date and Lightweight.

The DRAWINGS Toolbar

Updates the selected view to the model's current stage.

Creates a detail view.

Creates a section view.

Inserts an aligned section using the selected line or section line.

Unfolds a new view from an existing view.

Generates a standard 3-view drawing (1st or 3rd angle).

Inserts an auxiliary view of an inclined surface.

Adds an Orthogonal or Named view based on an existing part or assembly.

Adds a Relative view by two orthogonal faces or planes.

Adds a Predefined orthogonal projected or Named view with a model.

Adds an empty view.

Adds vertical break lines to selected view.

Crops a view.

Creates a Broken-out section.

Inserts an Alternate Position view.

The QUICK SNAP Toolbar

Snap to points.

Snap to center points.

Snap to midpoints.

Snap to quadrant points.

Snap to intersection of 2 curves.

Snap to nearest curve.

Snap tangent to curve.

Snap perpendicular to curve.

Snap parallel to line.

Snap horizontally / vertically.

Snap horizontally / vertically to points.

Snap to discrete line lengths.

Snap to grid points.

Snap to angle.

The LAYOUT Toolbar

Creates the assembly layout sketch.

Sketches a line.

Sketches a rectangle.

Sketches a circle.

Sketches a 3 point arc.

Rounds a corner.

Trims or extends a sketch.

Adds sketch entities by offsetting faces, Edges curves.

Mirrors selected entities about a centerline.

Adds a relation.

Creates a dimension.

Displays / Deletes geometric relations.

Makes a new block.

Edits the selected block.

Inserts a new block to the sketch or drawing.

Adds / Removes sketch entities to / from a block.

Saves the block to a file.

Explodes the selected block.

Creates a new part from a layout sketch block.

Positions 2 components relative to one another.

Moves a component within the degrees of freedom defined by its mates.

The CURVES Toolbar

Projects sketch onto selected surface.

Inserts a split line feature.

Creates a composite curve from selected edges, curves and sketches.

Creates a curve through free points.

Creates a 3D curve through reference points.

Helical curve defined by a base sketch and shape parameters.

The VIEW Toolbar

Displays a view in the selected orientation.

Reverts to previous view.

Zooms out to see entire model.

Zooms in by dragging a bounding box.

Zooms in or out by dragging up or down.

Zooms to fit all selected entities.

Dynamic view rotation.

Scrolls view by dragging.

Displays image in wireframe mode.

Displays hidden edges in gray.

Displays image with hidden lines removed.

Controls the visibility of planes.

Controls the visibility of axis.

Controls the visibility of parting lines.

Controls the visibility of temporary axis.

Controls the visibility of origins.

Controls the visibility of coordinate systems.

Controls the visibility of reference curves.

Controls the visibility of sketches.

Controls the visibility of 3D sketch planes.

Controls the visibility of 3D sketch

Controls the visibility of all annotations.

Controls the visibility of reference points.

Controls the visibility of routing points.

Controls the visibility of lights.

Controls the visibility of cameras.

Controls the visibility of sketch relations.

Redraws the current window.

Rolls the model view.

Turns the orientation of the model view.

Dynamically manipulate the model view in 3D to make selection.

Changes the display style for the active view.

Displays a shade view of the model with its edges.

Displays a shade view of the model.

Toggles between draft quality & high quality HLV.

Cycles through or applies a specific scene.

Views the models through one of the model's cameras.

Displays a part or assembly w/different colors according to the local radius of curvature.

Displays zebra stripes.

Displays a model with hardware accelerated shades.

Edits the real view appearance of entities in the model.

Applies a texture to entities in a model.

Changes the visibility of items in the graphics area.

Controls visibility of the sketch grid.

The TOOLS Toolbar

 Calculates the distance between selected items.

 Adds or edits equation.

 Calculates the mass properties of the model.

 Checks the model for geometry errors.

 Inserts or edits a Design Table.

 Evaluates section properties for faces and sketches that lie in parallel planes.

 Reports Statistics for this Part/Assembly.

 Deviation Analysis.

 Runs the SimulationXpress analysis wizard Powered by SolidWorks Simulation.

 Checks the spelling.

 Import diagnostics.

 Runs the DFMXpress analysis wizard.

 Runs the DriveWorkXpress wizard.

 Runs the SolidWorksFloXpress analysis wizard.

The ASSEMBLY Toolbar

 Creates a new part & inserts it into the assembly.

 Adds an existing part or sub-assembly to the assembly.

 Creates a new assembly & inserts it into the assembly.

 Turns on/off large assembly mode for this document.

 Hides / shows model(s) associated with the selected model(s).

 Toggles the transparency of components.

 Changes the selected components to suppressed or resolved.

 Toggles between editing part and assembly.

 Inserts a belt.

 Inserts a new part into an assembly.

 Smart Fasteners.

 Positions two components relative to one.

 External references will not be created.

 Moves a component.

 Rotates an un-mated component around its center point.

 Replaces selected components.

 Replaces mate entities of mates of the selected components on the selected Mategroup.

 Creates a New Exploded view.

 Creates or edits explode line sketch.

 Interference detection.

 Changes assembly transparency.

 Shows or Hides the Simulation toolbar.

 Patterns components in one or two linear directions.

 Patterns components around an axis.

 Toggles the transparency of components Between 0 and 75 percent.

 Toggles between editing a Part and Assembly.

 Adds fasteners to the assembly using Toolbox.

 Displays statistics and check the health of The current assembly.

 Patterns components relative to an existing Pattern in a part.

 Shows hidden components.

 Toggles large assembly mode for this document

 Checks assembly hole alignments.

 Mirrors subassemblies and parts.

To add or remove an icon to or from the toolbar, first select:

Tools/Customize/Commands

Next select a **Category**, click a button to see its description and then drag / drop the command icon into any toolbar.

Rotate the model

* Horizontally or Vertically:	Arrow keys
* Horizontally or Vertically 90°:	Shift + Arrow keys
* Clockwise or Counterclockwise:	Alt + left or right Arrow
* Pan the model:	Ctrl + Arrow keys
* Zoom in:	Z (shift + Z or capital Z)
* Zoom out:	z (lower case z)
* Zoom to fit:	F
* Previous view:	Ctrl+Shift+Z

View Orientation

* View Orientation Menu:	Space bar
* Front:	Ctrl+1
* Back:	Ctrl+2
* Left:	Ctrl+3
* Right:	Ctrl+4
* Top:	Ctrl+5
* Bottom:	Ctrl+6
* Isometric:	Ctrl+7

Selection Filter & Misc.

* Filter Edges:	e
* Filter Vertices:	v
* Filter Faces:	x
* Toggle Selection filter toolbar:	F5
* Toggle Selection Filter toolbar (on/off):	F6
* New SolidWorks document:	F1
* Open Document:	Ctrl+O
* Open from Web folder:	Ctrl+W
* Save:	Ctrl+S
* Print:	Ctrl+P
* Magnifying Glass Zoom	g
* Switch between the SolidWorks documents	Ctrl + Tab

Double click the **SW-2015 Sample Settings** to install the sample keyboard shortcuts and use the **Sample Part Template** (included) to try out the hot keys (below).

Function Keys

F1	SW-Help
F2	2D Sketch
F3	3D Sketch
F4	Modify Sketch
F5	Selection Filters
F6	Move (2D Sketch)
F7	Rotate (2D Sketch)
F8	Measure
F9	Extrude
F10	Revolve
F11	Sweep
F12	Loft

Sketch

C	Circle
P	Polygon
E	Ellipse
O	Offset Entities
R	Corner Rectangle
Alt + C	Convert Entities
M	Mirror
Alt + M	Dynamic Mirror
Alt + F	Sketch Fillet
T	Trim
Alt + X	Extend
D	Smart Dimension
Alt + R	Add Relation
Alt + P	Plane
Control + F	Fully Define Sketch

SW-Quick-Guide, Part of SolidWorks Basic Tools and Advanced Techniques

SolidWorks® Quick-Guide by Paul Tran – Sr. Certified SolidWorks Instructor
© Issue 11 / Jan-2015 - Printed in The United State of America – All Rights Reserved